BLUMGART'S
Surgery *of the* Liver, Biliary Tract and Pancreas

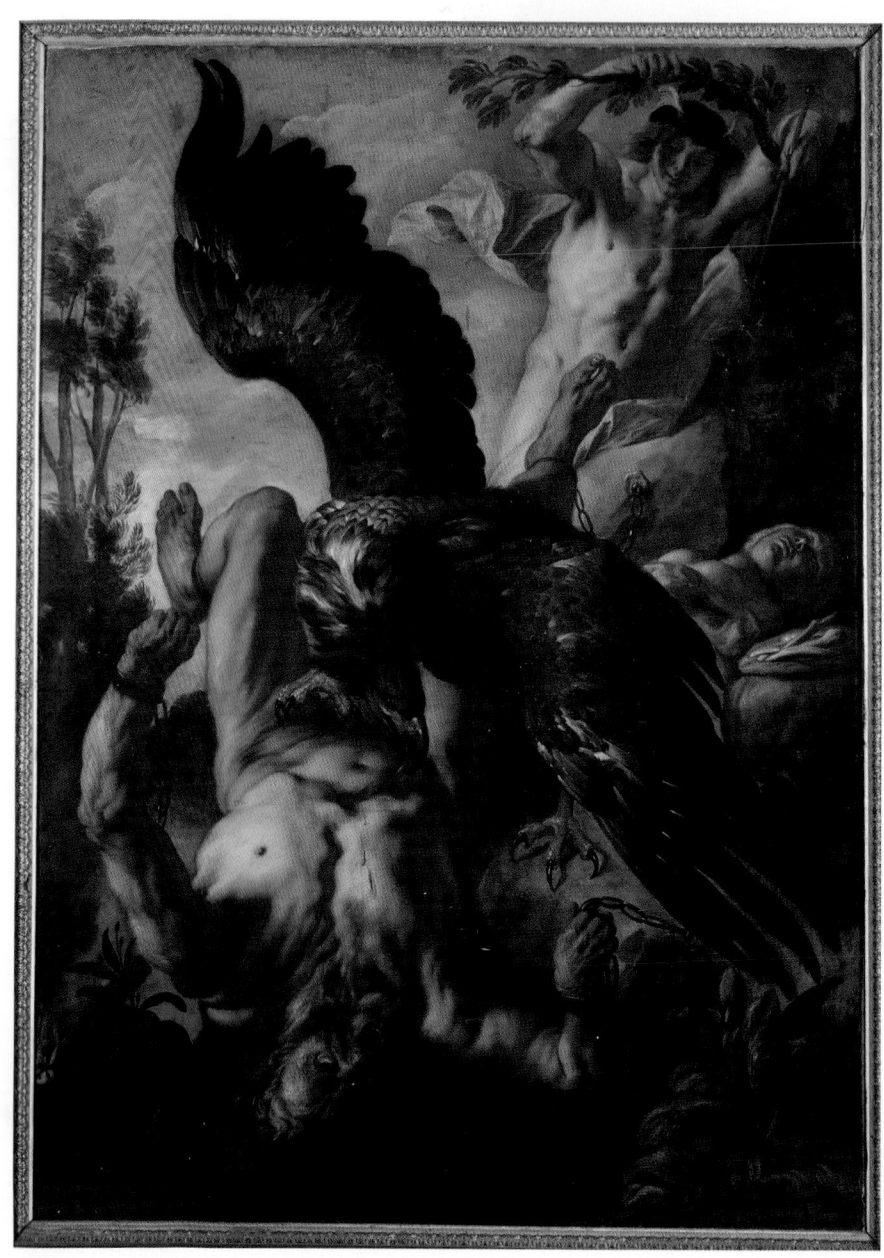

Prometheus, chained to the rocky Mount Caucasus, has his liver eaten by the eagle of Zeus.
Prometheus by Jacob Jordaens, 1640.
Walraff-Richartz Museum & Foundation Corboud, Cologne, Germany.
Photo: Rheinisches Bildarchiv Cologne, rba_c007696

BLUMGART'S
Surgery *of the* Liver, Biliary Tract and Pancreas

7th EDITION | VOLUME 2

EDITOR-IN-CHIEF

William R. Jarnagin, MD, FACS

ASSOCIATE EDITORS

Peter J. Allen, MD
William C. Chapman, MD, FACS
Michael I. D'Angelica, MD, FACS
Ronald P. DeMatteo, MD, FACS
Richard Kinh Gian Do, MD, PhD
Jean-Nicolas Vauthey, MD, FACS

EDITOR EMERITUS

Leslie H. Blumgart, BDS, MD, DSc(Hon),
  FACS, FRCS(Eng, Edin), FRCPS(Glas)

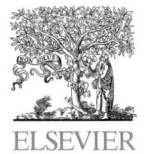

ELSEVIER

Elsevier
1600 John F. Kennedy Blvd.
Ste 1800
Philadelphia, PA 19103-2899

Executive Content Strategist: Jessica McCool
Content Development Specialist: Casey Potter
Senior Content Development Manager: Laura Schmidt
Publishing services Manager: Deepthi Unni
Project Manager: Aparna Venkatachalam
Design Direction: Maggie Reid

Printed in India
Last digit is the print number: 9   8   7   6   5   4   3   2

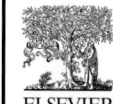 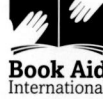

This book is dedicated to Dr. Leslie H. Blumgart. Known as the "Professor," a term of respect and admiration, he is truly a giant in the field, one of the pioneering surgeons who helped establish and develop HPB surgery as a specialty in its own right. He served as a mentor and role model for a generation of surgeons, who strive to maintain the high standards that he established. For all that he has done for us and for the field of HPB surgery, we will be forever grateful.

EDITORS

EDITOR-IN-CHIEF

William R. Jarnagin, MD, FACS
Chief, Hepatopancreatobiliary Surgery
Benno C. Schmidt Professor of Surgical Oncology
Memorial Sloan Kettering Cancer Center;
Professor of Surgery
Weill Medical College of Cornell University
New York, New York

ASSOCIATE EDITORS

Peter J. Allen, MD
Professor of Surgery
Department of Surgery
Memorial Sloan Kettering Cancer Center
New York, New York

William C. Chapman, MD, FACS
Professor
Chief, Division of General Surgery
Chief, Abdominal Transplantation Section
Washington University School of Medicine
St. Louis, Missouri

Michael I. D'Angelica, MD, FACS
Attending Surgeon
Hepatopancreatobiliary Surgery
Enid A. Haupt Chair in Surgery
Memorial Sloan Kettering Cancer Center;
Associate Professor
Department of Surgery
Weill Medical College of Cornell University
New York, New York

Ronald P. DeMatteo, MD, FACS
Vice Chair, Department of Surgery
Chief, Division of General Surgical Oncology
Leslie H. Blumgart Chair in Surgery
Memorial Sloan Kettering Cancer Center
New York, New York

Richard Kinh Gian Do, MD, PhD
Associate Professor of Radiology
Weill Medical College of Cornell University;
Assistant Attending Physician
Department of Radiology
Memorial Sloan Kettering Cancer Center
New York, New York

Jean-Nicolas Vauthey, MD, FACS
Professor of Surgical Oncology
Chief, Hepato-Pancreato-Biliary Section
Bessie McGoldrick Professor in Clinical Cancer Research
Department of Surgical Oncology
University of Texas MD Anderson Cancer Center
Houston, Texas

EDITOR EMERITUS

Leslie H. Blumgart, BDS, MD, DSc(Hon), FACS, FRCS(Eng, Edin), FRCPS(Glas)
Member
Professor of Surgery and Attending Surgeon
Memorial Sloan Kettering Cancer Center;
Professor of Surgery
Weill Medical College of Cornell University
New York, New York

Ghassan K. Abou-Alfa, MD, MBA
Attending Physician
Medicine
Memorial Sloan Kettering Cancer Center
Professor
Medicine
Weill Medical College at Cornell University
New York, New York

Jad Abou-Khalil, MDCM MSc FRCSC
Assistant Professor of Surgery
Hepato-Biliary and Pancreatic Surgery
The Ottawa Hospital,
Clinician Investigator
Clinical Epidemiology
The Ottawa Hospital Research Institute,
Ottawa, Ontario, Canada

Alexandra W. Acher, MD
Department of General Surgery, Division of Surgical
    Oncology
University of Wisconsin,
Madison, Wisconsin

Rene Adam, MD, PhD
Professor of Surgery
Department of Hepato-Biliary Surgery
Paul Brousse Hospital,
Paris Saclay University,
Director of University Research Unit
"Chronotherapy, Cancers and Transplantation"
Paris-Saclay University,
Villejuif, French Guiana

Pietro Addeo, MD PhD
Attending Surgeon
Hepato-Pancreato-Biliary Surgery and Liver Transplantation
University of Strasbourg,
Strasbourg, France

Anil Kumar Agarwal, MS, MCh, FRCS, FACS
Director Professor & Head
GI Surgery & Liver Transplant
GB Pant Institute of Postgraduate Medical Education &
    Research & MAM College, Delhi University,
New Delhi, India

Davit L. Aghayan, MD, PhD
Postdoctoral Researcher
The Intervention Center
Oslo University Hospital,
Oslo, Norway
Visiting Professor
Department of Surgery N1
Yerevan State Medical University after M. Heratsi,
Yerevan, Armenia

Ola Ahmed, MD
Department of Abdominal Organ Transplantation
Washington University School of Medicine,
St Louis, Missouri

Matthew J. Aizpuru, MD
Resident Physician
Surgery
Mayo Clinic,
Rochester, Minnesota

Marc-Antoine Allard, MD, PhD
Centre Hépatobiliaire
Hôpital Paul Brousse,
Villejuif, France

Peter J. Allen, MD
Professor of Surgery
Chief of Surgical Oncology
Surgery
Duke University, School of Medicine
Durham, North Carolina

Thomas A. Aloia, MD, MHCM
Professor of Surgery
Surgical Oncology
UT MD Anderson Cancer Center,
Houston, Texas

Fernando A. Alvarez, MD
Chief
Division of HPB Surgery, Department of Surgery
Clínica Universitaria Reina Fabiola,
Córdoba, Argentina

Neda Amini, MD
Surgical resident
Surgery
Sinai hospital of Baltimore,
Baltimore, Maryland

Jesper B. Andersen, PhD
Associate Professor and group leader
University of Copenhagen,
Department of Health and Medical Sciences
Biotech Research and Innovation Centre,
Copenhagen, Denmark

Christopher D. Anderson, MD
James D. Hardy Chair
Department of Surgery
University of Mississippi Medical Center,
Jackson, Mississippi

Roi Anteby, MD MPH
Postdoctoral Research Fellow
Surgery
Massachusetts General Hospital,
Boston, Massachusetts
Resident
General Surgery
The Chaim Sheba Medical Center,
Tel Hashomer, Ramat Gan, Israel

Vittoria Arslan-Carlon, MD, FASA
Chief, Anesthesiology Service
Anesthesiology and CCM
Memorial Sloan Kettering Cancer Center,
New York, New York

Beatrice Aussilhou, MD
Department of HPB Surgery and Liver Transplantation
Hôpital Beaujon
Clichy, France

Joseph Awad, MD
Professor
Medicine-Gastroenterology and Hepatology
Vanderbilt University
Chief
Transplant Service
VA Tennessee Valley,
Nashville, Tennessee

Michele L. Babicky, MD
Hepatobiliary & Surgical Oncology
Center for Advanced Surgery
The Oregon Clinic,
Medical Director, Hepatobiliary & Pancreatic Cancer Program Program
Providence Portland Medical Center,
Portland, Oregon

Philippe Bachellier, MD, PhD
Professor and Chairman
Hepato-Pancreato-Biliary Surgery and Liver transplant,
Pôle des Pathologies Digestives, Hépatiques et de la
Transplantation Hôpital de Hautepierre-Hôpitaux
Universitaires de Strasbourg
University of Strasbourg,
Strasbourg, France

Vinod P. Balachandran, MD
Assistant Attending
Department of Surgery
Assistant Member
Immuno-Oncology Service, Human Oncology and Pathogenesis Program
Memorial Sloan Kettering Cancer Center
Member
Parker Institute for Cancer Immunotherapy
David M. Rubenstein Center for Pancreatic Cancer Research
Memorial Sloan Kettering Cancer Center,
New York, New York

Fiyinfolu Balogun, MD, PhD
Assistant Attending Physician
Gastrointestinal Oncology, Medicine
Memorial Sloan Kettering Cancer Center,
New York, New York

Andrew S. Barbas, MD
Surgery
Duke University,
Durham, North Carolina

Jeffrey Stewart Barkun, MD, MSc, FRSC (C)
Professor of Surgery, McGill University
Surgery
Hepatobiliary & Transplant Surgery
Surgery
McGill University Health Centre,
Montreal, Quebec, Canada

Claudio Bassi, FRCS, FACS, FEBS
Surgery
Pancreas Institute University of Verona,
Verona, Italy

Olca Basturk, MD
Associate Professor
Pathology
Memorial Sloan Kettering Cancer Center,
New York, New York

Maria del Pilar Bayona Molano, MD, DR-IR
Associate Professor
Interventional Radiology
UT Southwestern Medical Center,
Dallas, Texas

Rachel E. Beard, MD, FACS
Assistant Professor
Surgery
Rhode Island Hospital and Alpert Medical School of Brown University,
Providence, Rhode Island

Jacques Belghiti, MD
Emerite Professor
HPB Surgery & Liver Transplantation
Hospital Beaujon,
Clichy, France

Sean A. Bennett, MD, MSc, FRCSC
Assistant Professor
Surgery
Queen's University,
Kingston, Ontario, Canada

William Bernal, MD, FRCP, FFICM
Professor
Liver Intensive Therapy Unit
Institute of Liver Studies, Kings College Hospital,
London, England

Anton J. Bilchik, MD, PhD
Professor of Surgery, Chief of Medicine
Surgical Oncology
Saint John's Cancer Institute,
Santa Monica, California

Franz Edward Boas, MD, PhD
Associate professor
Interventional radiology
City of Hope Cancer Center,
Duarte, California

Morgan Bonds, MD
Assistant Professor of Surgery
Surgical Oncology
University of Oklahoma,
Norman, Oklahoma

Brooke C. Bredbeck, MD
House Officer
Surgery
University of Michigan,
Ann Arbor, Michigan

Lynn Brody, MD
Clinical Member
Radiology
Memorial Sloan Kettering Cancer Center,
New York, New York

Karen T. Brown, MD, FSIR
Professor
Department of Radiology
University of Utah Health Science Center,
Interventional Radiologist
Department of Radiology
University of Utah,
Salt Lake City, Utah

Jordi Bruix, MD, PhD
Senior Consultant
Bclc. Liver Unit
Hospital Clinic
Barcelona, Spain

Elizabeth M. Brunt, MD
Emeritus Professor (retired)
Pathology and Immunology
Washington University School of Medicine
St Louis, Missouri

Markus Büchler, Professor of Surgery, MD
Professor
Department of General,
Visceral and Transplantation Surgery
University of Heidelberg,
Heidelberg, Germany

Mark P. Callery, MD
William V. McDermott Professor of Surgery
Surgery
Harvard Medical School,
Chief, Division of General Surgery
Beth Israel Deaconess Medical Center,
Boston, Massachusetts

Juan C. Camacho, MD
Assistant Attending Radiologist
Interventional Radiology
Memorial Sloan Kettering Cancer Center,
New York, New York

Andre Campbell, MD
Professor of Surgery
UCSF, Department of Surgery
Zuckerberg San Francisco General Hospital and Trauma
    Center
San Francisco, California

Danielle H. Carpenter, MD
Associate Professor
Department of Pathology
Saint Louis University School of Medicine,
St Louis, Missouri

C. Ross Carter, MD, FRCS
West of Scotland Pancreatic Unit
Glasgow Royal Infirmary,
Glasgow, Scotland

Chung Yip Chan, MBBS, MMed(Surg), FRCS(Edin), MD
Department of Hepatopancreatobiliary and Transplant
    Surgery
Singapore General Hospital,
Singapore

See Ching Chan, MS, MD, PhD, FRCS
Honorary Clinical Professor
Surgery
University of Hong Kong,
Hong Kong, China

Rohit Chandwani, MD, PhD
Assistant Professor
Surgery/Cell & Developmental Biology
Weill Cornell Medicine,
New York, New York

William C. Chapman Sr., MD
Professor of Surgery
Surgery
Washington University in St Louis,
St Louis, Missouri

Harvey S. Chen, MD
General Surgeon
Department of Surgery
UCLA Medical Center,
Los Angeles, California

Daniel Cherqui, MD
Professor
HPB Surgery and Liver Transplantation
Paul Brousse Hospital - Paris Saclay University,
Villejuif, France

TT Cheung, MBBS, MS, MD, FRCS, FACS, FCSHK, FHKAM
Clinical Associate Professor
Chief of Division of Hepatobiliary and Pancreatic Surgery
The University of Hong Kong,
Hong Kong, China

Adrian Kah Heng Chiow, MBBS(Melb), FRCS(Ed), FAMS
Hepatopancreatobiliary Unit, Department of Surgery
Changi General Hospital,
Singapore

Clifford S. Cho, MD
C. Gardner Child Professor
Department of Surgery
University of Michigan Medical School,
Ann Arbor, Michigan

Yun Shin Chun, MD, FACS
Associate Professor
Surgical Oncology
The University of Texas MD Anderson Cancer Center,
Houston, Texas

Bryan M. Clary, MD, MBA
Professor and Chair
Department of Surgery
University of California at San Diego,
San Diego, California

Jordan M. Cloyd, MD
Surgical Oncologist
Surgery
The Ohio State University,
Columbus, Ohio

Maria V. Coats, PhD FRCS
Consultant HPB Surgeon
West of Scotland Pancreatic Unit
Glasgow Royal Infirmary,
Glasgow, United Kingdom

Joshua T. Cohen, MD
Resident
Department of General Surgery
Brown University,
Providence, Rhode Island

Kevin Christopher Conlon, MB, MCh, FRCSI, FRCSEd, FRCSGlas, FACS, MBA, MA, FTCD
Professor and Academic Head
Department of Surgery
Trinity College Dublin, Tallaght, Dublin 24
Consultant HPB Surgeon
Department of HPB Surgery
St Vincents University Hospital,
Consultant Surgeon
Tallaght University Hospital,
Dublin, Ireland

Louise C. Connell, MB Bch BAO, BSc, MRCPI
Medical Oncologist
Medicine, Gastrointestinal Oncology
Memorial Sloan Kettering Cancer Center,
New York, New York

Carlos Uriel Corvera, MD
Professor, Chief of Liver,
Biliary and Pancreatic Surgery
Surgery
UCSF, School of Medicine
Attending Surgeon
Surgery
VA Medical Center,
San Francisco, California

Anne M. Covey, MD
Attending Interventional Radiologist
Diagnostic Radiology
Memorial Sloan-Kettering Cancer Center,
Professor of Radiology
Diagnostic Radiology
Weill Medical College of Cornell University,
New York, New York

Christopher H. Crane, MD
Chief, Gastrointestinal Section
Radiation Oncology
Memorial Sloan Kettering Cancer Center,
New York, New York

John M. Creasy, MD
Fellow, Complex General Surgical Oncology
Department of Surgery
Duke University Medical Center,
Durham, North Carolina

Jeffrey S. Crippin, MD
Marilyn Bornefeld Chair in Gastrointestinal Research and Treatment
Internal Medicine
Washington University School of Medicine,
St Louis, Missouri

Nick Crispe
Professor
Pathology
Adjunct Professor
Immunology
University of Washington
Seattle, Washington

Michael I. D'Angelica, MD, FACS
Enid Haupt Chair in Surgery
Surgery
Memorial Sloan Kettering Cancer Center
Professor of Surgery
Surgery
Weil Cornell School of Medicine
New York, New York

Leonardo Gomes Da Fonseca, MD
Clinical Oncology
Instituto do Cancer do Estado de Sao Paulo,
University of Sao Paulo,
Sao Paulo, Brazil

Hany Dabbous
Professor
Tropical Medicine
Ain Shams University,
Cairo, Egypt

Christopher Danford
Gastroenterologist
Gastroenterology
Intermountain Medical Group,
Salt Lake City, Utah

Michael Darcy, MD
Professor, Interventional Radiology
Radiology
Washington University in St Louis,
St Louis, Missouri

Mark Davenport, ChM, FRCS (Eng), FRCS (Paeds)
Professor
Paediatric Surgery
Kings College Hospital,
London, United Kingdom

Yakira David, MBBS
Fellow
Gastroenterology
Icahn School of Medicine at Mount Sinai,
New York, New York

Ryan William Day, MD
Clinical Fellow
Division of Transplant Surgery
University of California, San Francisco,
San Francisco, California

Jeroen de Jonge, MD, PhD
Assistant Professor
Hepatobiliary and Transplant Surgery. Erasmus MC
Transplant Institute
Erasmus MC Rotterdam,
Rotterdam, Netherlands

Eduardo de Santibanes, MD, PhD
Professor
Surgery
University of Buenos Aires.,
Buenos Aires, Argentina

Martin de Santibañes, MD, PhD
Associate Professor of Surgery
Hepato-Biliary-Pancreatic unit and liver transplantation unit
Hospital Italiano,
Buenos Aires, Argentina

Roeland F. de Wilde, MD, PhD
Surgeon
HPB- & Transplant Surgery
Erasmus MC University Medical Center,
Rotterdam, Netherlands

Jean Robert Delpero,
Emeritus Professor
Department of Surgery
Institut Paoli Calmettes,
Marseille, France

Ronald P. DeMatteo, MD, FACS
The John Rhea Barton Professor and Chair
Department of Surgery
The University of Pennsylvania Health System,
Philadelphia, Pennsylvania

Danielle K. DePeralta, MD
Assistant Professor
Surgical Oncology
Northwell Health,
New York, New York

Niraj M. Desai, MD
Assistant Professor
Department of Surgery
Johns Hopkins University School of Medicine
Baltimore, Maryland

Shannan M. Dickinson, MBBS, FRANZCR
Assistant Attending
Department of Radiology
Memorial Sloan Kettering Cancer Center,
New York, New York

Euan J. Dickson, MBChB, MD, FRCS
Consultant Surgeon
West of Scotland Pancreatic Unit
Glasgow Royal Infirmary
Glasgow, United Kingdom

Christopher John DiMaio, MD
Director of Interventional Endoscopy,
Professor of Medicine
Division of Gastroenterology
Icahn School of Medicine at Mount Sinai
New York, New York

Richard Kinh Gian Do, MD, PhD
Associate Attending
Radiology
Memorial Sloan Kettering Cancer Center,
New York, New York
Associate Professor
Radiology
Weill Medical College of Cornell University,
New York, New York

Safi Dokmak, MD, PhD
HPB Surgery & Liver Transplantation
Hopital Beaujon,
Clichy, Hauts de seine, France

Majella Doyle, MD, MBA
Professor of Surgery
Department of Surgery
Washington University,
St Louis, Missouri

Jeffrey A. Drebin, MD, PhD
Chair
Department of Surgery
Memorial Sloan Kettering Cancer Center,
New York, New York
Professor
Department of Surgery
Weill Cornell Medical College,
New York, New York

Michael R. Driedger, MD
Surgical Oncology Specialist
Division of Hepatobiliary and Pancreatic Surgery
Mayo Clinic,
Rochester, Minnesota
General Surgery
Hepato-Pancreato-Biliary Surgery
Atrium Health,
Charlotte, North Carolina

Vikas Dudeja, MBBS, FACS
Associate Professor
Surgery
University of Alabama at Birmingham,
Birmingham, Alabama

Mark Dunphy, DO
Assistant Attending Physician
Radiology
Memorial Sloan Kettering Cancer Center,
New York, New York

Truman M. Earl, MD, MSCI
Professor of Surgery,
Chief Division of Transplant and Hepatobiliary Surgery
Department of Surgery,
Division of Transplant and Hepatobiliary Surgery
University of Mississippi Medical Center,
Jackson, Mississippi

Tomoki Ebata, MD, PhD
Professor and Chairman
Division of Surgical Oncology, Department of Surgery
Nagoya University Graduate School of Medicine,
Nagoya, Japan

Brett Logan Ecker, MD
Clinical Fellow
Department of Surgery
Memorial Sloan Kettering Cancer Center,
New York, New York

Bjorn Edwin, MD, PhD
Professor
The Intervention Centre
Oslo University Hospital,
Oslo, Norway
Professor
Department of HPB Surgery
Oslo University Hospital,
Oslo, Norway
Professor
Institute of Clinical Medicine
University of Oslo,
Oslo, Norway

Aslam Ejaz, MD, MPH
Assistant Professor
Department of Surgery
The Ohio State University,
Columbus, Ohio

Imane El Dika, MD
Assistant Attending
Department of Medicine
Memorial Sloan Kettering Cancer Center
New York, New York

Itaru Endo, MD, PhD
Professor
Department of Gastroenterological Surgery
Yokohama City University Graduate School of Medicine,
Yokohama, Japan

C. Kristian Enestvedt, MD, FACS
Associate Professor
Department of Surgery; Division of Abdominal Organ
Transplantation/Hepatobiliary Surgery; School of Medicine
Oregon Health & Science University,
Portland, Oregon

R. Eliot Fagley, MD
Section Head for Critical Care Medicine and Chief of Staff
Anesthesiology and Pain Medicine
Virginia Mason Medical Center
Seattle, Washington

Sheung Tat Fan, MD, PhD., D.Sc.
Emeritus Professor of Surgery
Department of Surgery
The University of Hong Kong
Hong Kong, China
Director
Liver Surgery and Transplant Centre
Hong Kong Sanatorium & Hospital,
Hong Kong, China

Olivier Farges, MD, PhD
Department of hepato-biliary and pancreatic surgery
Department of Surgery
Hôpital Beaujon, AP-HP, University Paris 7,
Clichy, France

Michael Steven Farrell, MD, MS
Acute Care Surgeon
Trauma
Lehigh Valley Health Network,
Allentown, Pennsylvania

Benjamin David Ferguson, MD, PhD
Assistant Professor
Department of Surgery
University of New Mexico
Albuquerque, New Mexico

Joana Ferrer-Fàbrega, MD, PhD
Associate Professor. Consultant
HepatoBilioPancreatic Surgery and Liver & Pancreatic
Transplantation Unit. ICMDiM.
Hospital Clínic. University of Barcelona,
Barcelona, Spain

Cristina R. Ferrone, MD
Professor of Surgery
Surgery
Massachusetts General Hospital,
Boston, Massachusetts

Ryan Fields, MD, FACS
Chief, Surgical Oncology; Professor of Surgery
Surgery
Barnes-Jewish Hospital & The Alvin J. Siteman
Comprehensive Cancer Center at Washington University
School of Medicine,
Kim & Tim Eberlein Distinguished Professor
Surgical Oncology
Washington University School of Medicine,
Co-Leader
Solid Tumor Therapeutics Program
Alvin J. Siteman Comprehensive Cancer Center
St Louis, Missouri

Mary Fischer, MD
Anesthesiology and Critical Care
Memorial Sloan Kettering Cancer Center,
New York, New York
Associate Professor
Anestesiology
New York Columbia Weill Medical College,
New York, New York

Yuman Fong, MD
Sangiacomo Chair and Chairman
Department of Surgery
City of Hope National Medical Center,
Duarte, California

Philippa Francis-West, PhD
Professor
Craniofacial
King's College London,
London, United Kingdom

Åsmund Avdem Fretland, MD, PhD
Attending Surgeon
The Intervention Centre
Oslo University Hospital
Attending Surgeon
Department of Hepato-Pancreato-Biliary Surgery
Oslo University Hospital
Oslo, Norway

Jonathan A. Fridell, MD
Chief, Abdominal Transplant Surgery
Surgery
Indiana University School of Medicine,
Indianapolis, Indiana

Scott L. Friedman, MD
Fishberg Professor of Medicine
Division of Liver Diseases
Icahn School of Medicine at Mount Sinai
Dean for Therapeutic Discovery
Icahn School of Medicine at Mount Sinai
New York, New York

Eva Galka, MD, FACS
Associate Professor of Surgery
Department of Surgery, Division of Hepatobiliary, Pancreatic,
& Gastrointestinal Surgery
University of Rochester,
Rochester, New York

David A. Geller, MD, FACS
Richard L. Simmons Professor of Surgery, Chief,
Division of Hepatobiliary and Pancreatic Surgery
Surgery
University of Pittsburgh,
Pittsburgh, Pennsylvania

Scott R. Gerst, MD
Attending Radiologist
Radiology
Memorial Sloan Kettering Cancer Center,
Director
Diagnostic Radiology, David H Koch Ctr for Cancer Care
Diagnostic Radiology
Memorial Sloan Kettering Cancer Center
New York, New York

Justin Theodore Gerstle, MD
Chief, Pediatric Surgery Service
Surgery
Memorial Sloan Kettering Cancer Center
New York, New York
Associate Professor
Surgery
Weill Cornell Medical College, Cornell University
New York, New York

Sepideh Gholami, MD
Assistant Professor
Surgery
University of California, Davis
Sacramento, California

Richard Gilroy, MBBS, FRACP
Medical Director of Hepatology and Liver Transplantation
Internal Medicine
Intermountain Medical Center
Murray, Utah

Brian K.P. Goh, MBBS, MMed, MSc, FRCSEd
Senior Consultant
Hepatopancreatobiliary and Transplant Surgery
Singapore General Hospital
Singapore
Clinical Professor
Duke-National University of Singapore Medical School
Singapore

Gregory J. Gores, MD
Executive Dean for Research, Professor of Medicine
Division of Gastroenterology and Hepatology
Mayo Clinic,
Rochester, Minnesota

John A. Goss, MD
Surgery
Baylor College of Medicine,
Houston, Texas

Brittany Dalia Greene, MD
Resident
Division of General Surgery, Department of Surgery
University of Toronto
Toronto, Ontario, Canada

Bas Groot Koerkamp, MD, MSc, PhD
Associate Professor of Surgery
Surgery,
Division of Hepatopancreatobiliary Surgery and Abdominal
    Transplantation
Erasmus MC,
Rotterdam, Netherlands

Thilo Hackert, MD, MBA
Professor
Department of Surgery
University of Heidelberg
Heidelberg, Germany

Kate Anne Harrington, MB BCh BAO, FFR RCSI
Radiology
Memorial Sloan Kettering Cancer Center
New York, New York

Ewen M. Harrison, MB ChB, PhD, FRCS
Professor of Surgery and Data Science
Centre for Medical Informatics, Usher Institute
University of Edinburgh
Edinburgh, United Kingdom
Consultant HPB Surgeon
Clinical Surgery
Royal Infirmary of Edinburgh
Edinburgh, United Kingdom

Kiyoshi Hasegawa, MD, PhD
Professor
Hepato-Biliary-Pancreatic Surgery Division
Department of Surgery
Graduate School of Medicine, University of Tokyo
Tokyo, Japan

Haley Hauser, BA
Research Project Associate
Gastrointestinal Oncology Service, Department of Medicine
Memorial Sloan Kettering Cancer Center
New York, New York

Julie K. Heimbach, MD
Professor of Surgery
transplantation surgery
Mayo Clinic
Rochester, Minnesota

Alan W. Hemming, MD, MSc
Professor of Surgery
Surgery
University of Iowa
Iowa City, Iowa

Jonathan Hernandez, MD
Principal Investigator
Surgical Oncology
National Institute of Health
Bethesda, Maryland

Yuki Homma, MD, PhD
Department of Gastgroenterological Surgery
Yokohama City University
Yokohama, Japan

Christine A. Iacobuzio-Donahue, MD, PhD
Attending Pathologist
Pathology
Memorial Sloan Kettering Cancer Center
Affiliate Member
Human Oncology and Pathogenesis Program
Memorial Sloan Kettering Cancer Center
Director
David M. Rubenstein Center for Pancreatic Cancer Research
Memorial Sloan Kettering Cancer Center
New York, New York

Rami Imam, MD
Anatomic Pathologist
NYU Langone Hospitals
New York, New York

Oscar Cesar IMVENTARZA Sr., MD
Chief Liver Transplantation
Surgery & Transplantation
Hospital Garrahan,
Buenos Aires, Argentina
Chief Liver Transplantation
Surgery & Transplantation
Hospital Argerich
Buenos Aires, Argentina

Matthew Kalahasty Iyer, MD, PhD
Fellow
Department of Surgery
Duke University Hospital
Durham, North Carolina

William R. Jarnagin, MD, FACS
Chief, Hepatopancreatobiliary Service
Leslie H. Blumgart Chair in Surgical Oncology
Memorial Sloan-Kettering Cancer Center
New York, New York
Professor of Surgery
Weill Medical College of Cornell University
New York, New York

Shiva Jayaraman, MD, MESc, FRCSC, FACS
Associate Professor of Surgery
Surgery
University of Toronto
HPB and General Surgeon
Surgery
St. Joseph's Health Centre, Unity Health Toronto
Scientist
Li Ka Shing Knowledge Institute
Unity Health Toronto
Toronto, Ontario, Canada

Maria Jepperson
Radiologist
Radiology
Intermountain McKay-Dee Hospital
Murray, Utah

Michelle R. Ju, MD
Resident
Surgery
University of Texas Southwestern Medical Center
Dallas, Texas

Sean J. Judge, MD
Resident
Department of Surgery
University of California
Sacramento, California

Christoph Kahlert, MD
Universitätsklinikum Carl Gustav Carus Dresden
Klinik und Poliklinik für Viszeral-, Thorax- und Gefäßchirurgie
Universitätsklinkum Dresden
Dresden, Germany

Patryk Kambakamba, MD
Hepatobiliary Group
St. Vincent's University Hospital
Dublin, Ireland
MD
Department of Surgery
Cantonal Hospital of Winterthur
Winterthur, Switzerland

Ivan Kangrga, MD, PhD
Professor and Vice Chair for Health System Liaison
Department of Anesthesiology
Washington University in St. Louis, School of Medicine
St Louis, Missouri

S. Cheenu Kappadath, PhD
Professor
Department of Imaging Physics
UT MD Anderson Cancer Center
Houston, Texas

Paul J. Karanicolas, MD, PhD, FRCSC, FACS
Associate Professor
Surgery
University of Toronto
Toronto, Ontario, Canada

Seth S. Katz, MD,PhD
Assistant Clinical Member
Radiology
Memorial Sloan Kettering Cancer Center
New York, New York

Yoshikuni Kawaguchi, MD, MPH, PhD
Associate Professor/Lecturer
Hepato-Biliary-Pancreatic Surgery Division
Department of Surgery
The University of Tokyo
Tokyo, Japan

Kaitlyn J. Kelly, MD
Assistant Professor of Surgery
Division of Surgical Oncology
University of California San Diego
San Diego, California

Nancy E. Kemeny, MD
Professor of Medicine
Weill Medical College of Cornell University;
Attending Physician
Solid Tumor—GI Division
Memorial Sloan-Kettering Cancer Center
New York, New York

Adeel Khan, MD, MPH
Associate Professor of Surgery
Division of Abdominal Transplant, Department of Surgery
Washington University in St Louis
St Louis, Missouri

Tahsin M. Khan, MD
Surgical Oncology Research Fellow
Surgical Oncology Program
National Cancer Institute, National Institutes of Health,
Bethesda, Maryland

Heung Bae Kim, MD
Professor of Surgery
Department of Surgery
Harvard Medical School
Boston, Massachusetts
Director, Pediatric Transplant Center; Weitzman Family
Chair in Surgical Innovation
Boston Children's Hospital
Boston, Massachusetts

Woon Cho Kim, MD, MPH
Clinical Fellow
Surgery
University of California San Francisco
San Francisco, California

T. Peter Kingham, MD
Assistant Professor
Surgery
Memorial Sloan Kettering Cancer Center
New York, New York

Joseph Kingsbery, MD
Gastroenterologist
Medicine
Bay Ridge Gastroenterology
Brooklyn, New York
Clinical Instructor
Medicine
NYU Grossman School of Medicine
New York, New York
Clinical Instructor
Medicine
NYP Weill Cornell
Brooklyn, New York

Allan D. Kirk, MD, PhD
Professor and Chairman
Department of Surgery
Duke University
Durham, North Carolina

Russell C. Kirks Jr., MD
Hepatobiliary and Pancreatic Surgeon
St Joseph's/Candler
Savannah, Georgia

David Klimstra, MD
Chairman
Department of Pathology
Memorial Sloan-Kettering Cancer Center
New York, New York
Professor
Department of Pathology and Laboratory Medicine
Weill Medical College of Cornell University
New York, New York

Stuart Knechtle, MD, FACS
William R. Kenan, Jr. Professor of Surgery
Surgery
Duke University School of Medicine
Durham, North Carolina
Executive Director
Duke Transplant Center
Duke University School of Medicine
Durham, North Carolina

Jonathan B. Koea, MHB(Hons), MD
Professor
Department of Surgery
North Shore Hospital
Auckland, New Zealand
Professor
Department of Surgery
University of Auckland
Auckland, New Zealand

Norihiro Kokudo, MD, PhD
Professor
Surgery
National Center for Global Health and Medicine, 1-21-1
Toyama, Shinjuku-ku
Tokyo, Japan

Kevin M. Korenblat, MD
Professor of Medicine
Department of Internal Medicine
Washington University School of Medicine,
St Louis, Missouri
Medical Director, Liver Transplant
Barnes-Jewish Hospital
St Louis, Missouri

Lucy Zumwinkle Kornblith, MD
Assistant Professor of Surgery
Department of Surgery, Division of Trauma and Surgical
Critical Care
University of California San Francisco
San Francisco, California

Geoffrey Wayne Krampitz, MD, PhD
Assistant Professor
Surgery
Thomas Jefferson University
Philadelphia, Pennsylvania

Simone Krebs, MD
Assistant Attending
Department of Radiology
Molecular Imaging and Therapy Service
Memorial Sloan Kettering Cancer Center
New York, New York
Assistant Professor
Department of Radiology
Weill Cornell Medicine
New York, New York

Takafumi Kumamoto
Department of Gastroenterological Surgery
Graduate School of Medicine Yokohama City University
Yokohama, Japan

Choon Hyuck David Kwon, MD, PhD
Director of Laparoscopic Liver Surgery
General Surgery
Cleveland Clinic
Cleveland, Ohio
Professor of Surgery
General Surgery
Lerner College of Medicine of Case Western University,
Cleveland, Ohio
Section Head of HPB Surgery
General Surgery
Cleveland Clinic
Cleveland, Ohio

Kelly J. Lafaro, MD, MPH
Assistant Professor
Department of Surgery
Johns Hopkins University
Baltimore, Maryland

Hauke Lang, MA, MD, FACS
Professor
General, Visceral and Transplantation Surgery,
Unimedizin Mainz
Mainz, Germany

Michael J. LaQuaglia, MD
Clinical Fellow
Pediatric Surgery
Memorial Sloan Kettering Cancer Center
New York, New York

Michael P. LaQuaglia, MD
Joseph H. Burchenal Professor
Department of Surgery and Pediatrics
Memorial Sloan Kettering Cancer Center
New York, New York
Professor of Surgery
Department of Surgery
Weill Cornell Medical School
New York, New York

Nicholas F. LaRusso, MD
Charles H. Weinman Professor of Medicine
Molecular Biology and Biochemistry Internal Medicine
Mayo Clinic
Rochester, Minnesota

Rachel M. Lee, MD, MSPH
Resident Physician
Department of Surgery
Emory University
Atlanta, Georgia

**Ser Yee Lee, MBBS, MMed(Surgery), MSc, FAMS,
    FRCSEd, FACS**
Senior Consultant
Department of Hepatopancreatobiliary and Transplant
    Surgery
Singapore General Hospital
Singapore
Associate Professor
Duke - National University of Singapore (NUS) Graduate
Medical School
Singapore
Senior Consultant
Surgical Associates
Mount Elizabeth Medical Centre
Singapore

Riccardo Lencioni, MD
Professor
Department of Radiology
University of Pisa School of Medicine
Pisa, Italy
Director
Cancer Imaging Program
Pisa University Hospital
Pisa, Italy

Javier C. Lendoire, MD,PhD
Vice-Chairman
Liver & Transplant Unit
Hospital Dr Cosme Argerich
Buenos Aires, Argentina
Chairman
Liver Transplant Division
Instituto de Trasplantes y Alta Complejidad (ITAC)
Buenos Aires, Argentina

Galina Levin, MD
Associate Attending
Radiology
Memorial Sloan Kettering Cancer Center
New York, New York

Kewei Li, MD, PhD
Department of Pediatric Surgery
West China Hospital of Sichuan University
Chengdu, China

Michael E. Lidsky, MD
Assistant Professor
Surgery
Duke University
Durham, North Carolina

Jessica Lindemann, MD, PhD
General Surgery Resident
Department of Surgery
Washington University School of Medicine
St Louis, Missouri

David Linehan, MD
Professor, Chair
Surgery
University of Rochester
Rochester, New York

Roberto Carlos Lopez-Solis, MD, FACS
Associate Professor
General Surgery
West Virginia University School of Medicine
Morgantown, West Virginia

Patrick Daniel Lorimer, MD
General Surgeon
Surgical Oncology
Arizona Advanced Surgery, LLC
Scottsdale, Arizona

Ka Wing Ma
Orthopaedic surgeon
The University of Hong Kong
Pokfulam, Hong Kong

Shishir K. Maithel, MD, FACS
Professor of Surgery
Division of Surgical Oncology, Department of Surgery
Emory University, Winship Cancer Institute
Atlanta, Georgia

Giuseppe Malleo, MD, PhD
Associate Professor of surgery
Department of Surgery, Dentistry, Pediatrics and Gynecology
Unit of Pancreatic Surgery,
University of Verona Hospital Trust
Verona, Italy

Giovanni Marchegiani, MD, PhD
Dr Giovanni Marchegiani
Department of Surgery
Verona University Policlinico Borga Roma
Verona, Italy

James F. Markmann, MD, PhD
Chief, Division of Transplant Surgery
Surgery
Massachusetts General Hospital
Boston, Massachusetts
Claude E. Welch Professor of Surgery
Harvard Medical School
Boston, Massachusetts

J. Wallis Marsh, MD, MBA
Professor and Chairman
Surgery
West Virginia University School of Medicine
Morgantown, West Virginia

Robert CG Martin II, MD, PhD
Professor of Surgery
Sam and Loita Weakley Endowed Chair of Surgical Oncology
Surgery, Division of Surgical Oncology
University of Louisville
Louisville, Kentucky

Marco Massani, MD
Chief
Department of Surgery, Division of First General Surgery,
Hepato-Pancreato-Biliary Regional Referral Centre
Azienda ULSS 2 Marca Trevigiana, Ospedale Ca' Foncello,
Treviso, Italy

Ryusei Matsuyama, MD, PhD
Associate Professor
Gastroenterological Surgery
Yokohama City University School of Medicine
Yokohama, Japan

Aaron W.P. Maxwell, MD
Director of Interventional Oncology
Assistant Professor of Diagnostic Imaging
Department of Diagnostic Imaging
The Warren Alpert Medical School of Brown University,
Providence, Rhode Island

Oscar M. Mazza, MD
Professor of Surgery
Chief of Hepato-Biliary- Pancreatic Unit
Hospital Italiano
Buenos Aires, Argentina

Ian D. McGilvray, MD, PhD
Professor of Surgery
Surgery
University of Toronto
Toronto, Ontario, Canada
Head
Hepatopancreatic Biliary Surgical Oncology
University Health Network
Toronto, Ontario, Canada
Director
Toronto Video Atlas of Surgery
University Health Network
Toronto, Ontario, Canada

Caitlin A. McIntyre, MD
Fellow in Surgical Oncology
Department of Surgery
Memorial Sloan-Kettering Cancer Center
New York, New York

Sophia K. McKinley, MD, EdM
Resident physician
Surgery
Massachusetts General Hospital
Boston, Massachusetts

Josc Melendez
Vice President and Chief Medical Officer
HCA Healthcare
St. Mark's Hospital
Salt Lake City, Utah

Emmanuel Melloul, MD
Lausanne University Hospital
Visceral Surgery
Lausanne University Hospital
Lausanne, Switzerland

Robin B. Mendelsohn, MD
Associate Attending
Medicine, Gastroenterology, Hepatology and Nutrition
    Service
Memorial Sloan Kettering Cancer Center
New York, New York

Takashi Mizuno, MD., PhD.
Associate Professor
Division of Surgical Oncology, Department of Surgery
Nagoya University Graduate School of Medicine
Nagoya, Japan

Hunter Burroughs Moore, MD, PhD
Assistant Professor
Surgery-Transplant
University of Colorado
Denver, Colorado

Cristina Mosconi, MD
Department of Radiology
IRCCS Azienda Ospedaliero-Universitaria di Bologna,
Bologna, Italy

Santosh Nagaraju
Transplant Surgeon
Charleston Area Medical Center Health System
Charleston, West Virginia

Masato Nagino, MD, PhD
Professor and Chairman
Division of Surgical Oncology, Department of Surgery
Nagoya University Graduate School of Medicine
Nagoya, Japan

David M. Nagorney, MD, FACS
Professor of Surgery
Department of Surgery
Mayo Clinic
Rochester, Minnesota

Satish Nagula, MD
Associate Professor
Division of Gastroenterology, Department of Medicine
Icahn School of Medicine at Mount Sinai
New York, New York

Amit Nair, MD, FRCS
Assistant Professor
Division of Transplantation/Hepatobiliary Surgery
University of Rochester Medical Center
Rochester, New York

Navine Nasser-Ghodsi, MD
Fellow
Gastroenterology & Hepatology
Mayo CLinic
Rochester, Minnesota

Nadia Naz, MD, FAAP
Clinical Assistant Professor
Division of Gastroenterology, Hepatology, Pancreatology, and
    Nutrition
University of Iowa Health Care
Iowa city, Iowa

John P. Neoptolemos, BA, MB, BChir, MA (Cambridge), MD, FRCS, FMedSci.
Professor of Surgery
Department of General, Visceral and Transplantation Surgery
University of Heidelberg,
Heidelberg, Baden-Württemberg

James Neuberger, DM, FRCP
Hon Consultant Physician
Liver Unit
Queen Elizabeth Hospital
Birmingham, United Kingdom

Nicole M. Nevarez, MD
Surgical Resident
Department of Surgery
University of Texas Southwestern
Dallas, Texas

Timothy E. Newhook, MD
Assistant Professor
Surgical Oncology
The University of Texas MD Anderson Cancer Center,
Houston, Texas

Takehiro Noda, MD, PhD
Associate Professor
Department of Gastroenterological Surgery
Osaka University
Suita, Japan

Scott L. Nyberg, MD, PhD
Professor
Surgery
Consultant in Transplantation Surgery
Department of Transplantation Surgery
Mayo Clinic,
Rochester, Minnesota

Elisabeth O'Dwyer, MB BCh BAO
Molecular Imaging and Therapeutics Service
Memorial Sloan Kettering Cancer Center
New York, New York

Colm J. O'Rourke, BA(Hons.), PhD
Assistant Professor
BRIC, Department of Health & Medical Sciences
University of Copenhagen
Copenhagen, Denmark

Bruno C. Odisio, MD
Associate Professor
Interventional Radiology
The University of Texas MD Anderson Cancer Center,
Houston, Texas

RYOSUKE okamura, MD, PhD
Assistant Professor
Department of Surgery
Kyoto University Hospital
Kyoto, Japan

Karl Jürgen Oldhafer, Prof. Dr.
Department of Surgery
Asklepios Hospital Barmbek
Hamburg, Germany

Kim M. Olthoff, MD
Donald Guthrie Professor of Surgery
Division of Transplant Surgery, Department of Surgery
University of Pennsylvania
Associate Director
Penn Transplant Institute
Philadelphia, Pennsylvania

Franklin Olumba, MD
Research Fellow
Surgery
Washington University in St Louis School of Medicine
St Louis, Missouri

Susan Orloff, MD, FACS, FAASLD
Professor of Surgery and Chief, Division of Abdominal
Organ Transplantation/Hepatobiliary Surgery
Department of Surgery
Adjunct Professor
Department of Microbiology & Immunology
Oregon Health & Science University
Portland, Oregon

Christine E. Orr, MD, FRCPC
Assistant Professor
Department of Pathology and Molecular Medicine
Queen's University
Kingston, Ontario, Canada

Eileen M. O'Reilly, MD
Section Head, HPB/Neuroendocrine; Co-Director
Medical David M Rubenstein Center for Pancreas
Cancer Research
Medicine
Memorial Sloan Kettering Cancer Center
Professor of Medicine
Medicine
Weill Medical College of Cornell University
New York, New York

Chandrasekhar Padmanabhan, MD
Assistant Professor
Surgery
Vanderbilt Univeristy Medical Center
Nashville, Tennessee

Alessandro Paniccia, MD
Assistant Professor of Surgery
Department of Surgery
University of Pittsburgh
Pittsburgh, Pennsylvania

Theodore N. Pappas, MD
Professor
Surgery
Duke University
Durham, North Carolina

Valérie Paradis, MD, PhD
Professor
Pathology
Beaujon hospital,
Clichy, France

Rowan W. Parks, MD, FRCSI, FRCSEd
Professor
Clinical Surgery
University of Edinburgh
Edinburgh, United Kingdom

Timothy M. Pawlik, MD, MPH, MTS, PhD
Professor and Chair
Department of Surgery
The Ohio State University
Columbus, Ohio
The Urban Meyer III and Shelley Meyer Chair for Cancer
    Research
Wexner Medical Center at The Ohio State University
Columbus, Ohio

Cassandra D. Pierce-Raglione, MD
Director Emeritus
Surgical Oncology
Providence Portland Medical Center
Portland, Oregon

Venu G. Pillarisetty, MD
Professor
Surgery
University of Washington
Seattle, Washington

James Francis Pingpank Jr., MD
Associate Professor of Surgery
Department of Surgery
University of Pittsburgh
Surgical oncologist
UPMC Hillman Cancer Center
Pittsburgh, Pennsylvania

Henry A. Pitt, MD
Distinguished Professor of Surgery
Surgery
Rutgers RWJ Medical School
Chief of Oncologic Quality
Rutgers Cancer Institute of New Jersey
New Brunswick, New Jersey

Patricio M. Polanco, MD
Associate Professor
Surgery
University of Texas Southwestern Medical Center
Dallas, Texas

James J. Pomposelli, MD, PhD
Surgical Director of Liver Transplantation
Professor of Surgery
Department of Surgery
University of Colorado, Anschutz Medical Campus
Aurora, Colorado

John A. Powelson, MD
Associate Professor
Department of Surgery
Indiana University Medical School
Indianapolis, Indiana

Naveen Premnath, MD
Hematology and Oncology
University of Texas southwestern
Dallas, Texas

Motaz Qadan, MD, PhD
Associate Professor of Surgery; Gapontsev Family
Endowed Chair in Surgical Oncology
Surgery
Massachusetts General Hospital
Boston, Massachusetts

Nitya Raj, MD
Assistant Attending Physician
Department of Medicine,
Division of Gastrointestinal Medical Oncology
Memorial Sloan Kettering Cancer Center
New York, New York

Srinevas Reddy, MD
Faculty
Surgical Oncology
Ascension Columbia St. Mary's Hospital
Milwaukee, Wisconsin

Diane Reidy-Lagunes, MD, MS
Associate Attending
Medicine
MSKCC
Associate Professor of Clinical Medicine
Weill Cornell Medical College
New York, New York

Marsha Reyngold, MD, PhD
Assistant Attending
Department of Radiation Oncology
Memorial Sloan-Kettering Cancer Center
New York, New York

Teresa C. Rice, MD
Assistant Professor
Department of Surgery, Division of Transplant Surgery
Medical University of South Carolina
Charleston, South Carolina

Robert W. Rickert, Bachelor of Arts
Medical Student
Department of Surgical Oncology
University of Louisville
Louisville, Kentucky

John Paul Roberts, MD
Professor
Surgery
University of California San Francisco
San Francisco, California

Piera Marie Cote Robson, PhD, NP
Clinical Nurse Specialist
Departments of Nursing and Radiology
Memorial Sloan Kettering Cancer Center
New York, New York

Flavio G. Rocha, MD
Associate Professor of Surgery
Division of Surgical Oncology
Hedinger Chair and Division Head
Surgery, Division of Surgical Oncology
OHSU School of Medicine
Portland, Oregon

Garrett R. Roll, MD, FACS
Associate Professor
Department of Surgery, Division of Transplant
University of California San Francisco
San Francisco, California

Vineet Syan Rolston, MD
Assistant Professor
Gastroenterology
Memorial Sloan Kettering Cancer Center
New York, New York

Maxime Ronot, MD PhD
Professional
Radiology
Beaujon University Hospital
Clichy, France

Alexander S. Rosemurgy II, MD
Director of Hepatopancreaticobiliary Surgery
Surgery
Advent Health Tampa
Tampa, Florida

Charles B. Rosen, MD
Professor
Department of Surgery
Mayo Clinic
Rochester, Minnesota

Chady Salloum,
Doctor
Service de chirurgie hepatobiliopancreatique et transplantation
Hopital Paul Brousse Centre hepatobiliaire
Villejuif, France

Roberto Salvia, MD, PhD
Chief Executive of the Verona Pancreas Institute
Department of Surgery
Pancreas Institute
Verona, Italy

Hrishikesh Samant, MD FACG
Transplant Hepatologist
Hepatology
Ochsner Transplant Institute
New Orleans, Louisiana
Associate Professor
Gastroenterology and Hepatology
Lousiana State University Health
Shreveport, Louisiana
Director Hepatology
Gastroenterology and Hepatology
Ochsner-LSU
Shreveport, Louisiana

Kazunari Sasaki, MD
Clinical Associate Professor
General Surgery
Stanford University
Stanford, California

Mark A. Schattner, MD
Chief Attending
Department of Medicine
Division of Gastroenterology, Hepatology, and Nutrition,
Memorial Sloan Kettering Cancer Center
New York, New York

Gabriel T. Schnickel, MD, MPH
Professor of Surgery
Division of Transplant and Hepatobiliary Surgery, Department
    of Surgery
UC San Diego
San Diego, California

Richard D. Schulick, MD, MBA, FACS
Professor and Chair
Department of Surgery
Director
University of Colorado Cancer Center
University of Colorado School of Medicine
Aurora, Colorado

Max E. Seaton, MD
Surgical Oncology Fellow
Department of Surgery
Jackson Memorial Hospital / University of Miami
Miami, Florida

Yongwoo David Seo, MD
Resident Physician
General Surgery
University of Washington
Seattle, Washington

Jigesh A. Shah, D.O.
Assistant Professor
Surgery
UT Southwestern Medical Center
Dallas, Texas

Kevin N. Shah, MD
Assistant Professor
Surgery
Duke University Medical Center
Durham, North Carolina

Wong Hoi She, MBBS, FRCS, FCSHK, FHKAM
Consultant
Surgery
Queen Mary Hospital, The University of Hong Kong
Hong Kong, China

Junichi Shindoh, MD, PhD
Surgeon-in-chief
Hepatobiliary-pancreatic Surgery Division
Toranomon Hospital
Tokyo, Japan

Chaya Shwaartz, MD
Assistant Professor of Surgery
Abdominal Transplant & HPB Surgical Oncology
Department of General Surgery
University Health Network
Toronto, Ontario, Canada

Jason K. Sicklick, MD, FACS
Professor
Departments of Surgery and Pharmacology
Division of Surgical Oncology
University of California San Diego Cancer Center
University of California San Diego School of Medicine
UC San Diego Health
San Diego, California

Robert H. Siegelbaum, MD
Associate Attending Radiologist
Department of Radiology
Memorial Sloan Kettering Cancer Center
New York, New York

Martin Derrick Smith, MBBCh, FCS(SA), FEBS FRCS(Edin)
Professor
Surgery
University of the Witwatersrand, Johannesburg
Johannesburg, Gauteng

Kevin C. Soares, MD
Assistant Attending
Department of Surgery
Memorial Sloan Kettering Cancer Center
New York, New York
Assistant Professor
Department of Surgery
Weill-Cornell Medical College
New York, New York

Constantinos T. Sofocleous, MD, PhD, FSIR, FCIRSE
Interventional Oncologist/Radiologist
Department of Radiology
Memorial Sloan-Kettering Cancer Center
Professor Interventional Radiology
Weill-Cornell Medical College
New York, New York

Stephen B. Solomon, MD
Chief, Interventional Radiology Service
Director, Center for Image-Guided Intervention
Memorial Sloan-Kettering Cancer Center
New York, New York

Sanket Srinivasa, MBChB, PhD, FRACS
Consultant Surgeon
Waitematā District Health Board
North Shore Hospital
Auckland, New Zealand

Patrick Starlinger, MD, PhD
Associate Professor
Surgery
Mayo Clinic
Rochester, Minnesota

Tommaso Stecca, MD
Department of Surgery
Division of First General Surgery,
Hepato-Pancreato-Biliary Regional Referral Centre
Azienda ULSS 2 Marca Trevigiana, Ospedale Ca' Foncello,
Treviso, Italy

John A. Steinharter, MS
Hepatopancreatobiliary Service
Memorial Sloan Kettering Cancer Center
New York, New York
Medical Student
Robert Larner, MD College of Medicine UVM,
Burlington, Vermont

Camille Stewart, MD
Surgical Oncology Fellow
Surgery
City of Hope National Medical Center
Duarte, California

Lygia Stewart, MD
Professor of Surgery
Department of Surgery
University of California San Francisco and SF VAMC,
San Francisco, California
Chief General Surgery
Department of Surgery
San Francisco VA Medical Center
San Francisco, California

Janis Stoll, MD
Associate Professor of Pediatrics
Gastroenterology, Hepatology and Nutrition
Washington University School of Medicine
St Louis, Missouri

Iswanto Sucandy, MD FACS
Director
Hepatobiliary Surgery
Advent Health Tampa
Tampa, Florida
Associate Professor
Surgery
University of Central Florida
Florida

Paul V. Suhocki, MD
Associate Professor
Department of Radiology
Duke University Medical Center
Durham, North Carolina

James H. Tabibian, MD, PhD, FACP
Associate Professor
Vatche and Tamar Manoukian Division of Digestive Diseases
David Geffen School of Medicine at UCLA
Los Angeles, California
Director of Endoscopy
Department of Medicine, Division of Gastroenterology
Olive View-UCLA Medical Center
Sylmar, California

Nobuyuki Takemura, MD, PhD
Hepato-Biliary Pancreatic Surgery Division
Department of Surgery
National Center for Global Health and Medicine (NCGM),
Tokyo, Japan

Laura H. Tang, MD, PhD
Attending Pathologist
Pathology and Laboratory Medicine
Memorial Sloan-Kettering Cancer Center
New York, New York
Professor of Pathology
Department of Pathology and Laboratory Medicine
Weill Cornell Medical College
New York, New York

Cornelius A. Thiels, DO, MBA
Assistant Professor
Department of Surgery
Mayo Clinic
Rochester, Minnesota

Taner Timucin, MD, PhD
Associate Professor
Surgery & Immunology
Mayo Clinic
Chair
Division of Transplantation Surgery
Mayo Clinic
Rochester, Minnesota

Samer Tohme, MD
Assistant Professor of Surgery
Surgery
University of Pittsburgh
Pittsburgh, Pennsylvania

Guido Torzilli, MD, PhD, FESA, FACS, FAFC(Hon), FCBCD(Hon), FCHB(Hon)
Director
Division of Hepatobiliary and General surgery
Humanitas Research Hospital - IRCCS
Rozzano, Milano
Professor & Chairman
Director
General Surgery Residency Program
Humanitas University
Rozzano, Milano, Italy

Hop S. Tran Cao, MD, FACS
Associate Professor
Department of Surgical Oncology
The University of Texas MD Anderson Cancer Center
Houston, Texas

Simon Hing Yin Tsang, MB ChB, FCSHK, FHKAM
Honorary Clinical Associate Professor
Department of Surgery
The University of Hong Kong
Hong Kong, China
Consultant Surgeon
Department of Surgery
Queen Mary Hospital
Hong Kong, China

Simon Turcotte, MD, MSc
Associate Professor of Surgery
Hepatopancreatobiliary Surgery
Full Scientist
Cancer Axis
Centre de Recherche du Centre Hospitalier de l'Université de
   Montréal
Montréal, Quebec, Canada

Thomas van Gulik, MD, PhD
Professor
Department of Surgery
Amsterdam University Medical Centers, University of
   Amsterdam
Amsterdam, Netherlands

Andrea Vannucci, MD
Associate Professor of Anesthesiology
Department of Anesthesia and Critical Care
University of Chicago - Pritzker School of Medicine
Chicago, Illinois

Jean-Nicolas Vauthey, MD
Professor of Surgery
Surgical Oncology
MD Anderson Cancer Center
Houston, Texas
Fort Worth Living Legend Chair for Cancer Research
Chief of Hepatopancreatobiliary Surgery Section
Dallas Texas

Jack R. Wands, MD
Director
Gastroenterology/Liver Research Center
Rhode Island Hospital
Providence, Rhode Island

Julia Wattacheril, MD, MPH
Associate Professor of Medicine
Medicine
Columbia University College of Physicians and Surgeons,
New York, New York

Sharon Marie Weber, MD
Tim and MaryAnn McKenzie Chair of Surgical Oncology
Surgery
University of Wisconsin
Director for Surgical Oncology
UW Carbone Cancer Center
University of Wisconsin
Chair
Surgical Oncology
University of Wisconsin
Fellowship Director
Surgical Oncology
University of Wisconsin
Madison, Wisconsin

Alice C. Wei, MD MSc FRCSC FACS
Associate Attending Surgeon
Surgery
Memorial Sloan Kettering Cancer Center
New York, New York
Associate Professor
Surgery
Weill Medical College of Cornell University
New York, New York

Matthew Weiss, MD, MBA
Deputy Physician-in-Chief, Director of Surgical Oncology
Department of Surgery
Northwell Health Cancer Institute
Lake Success, New York

Jürgen Weitz, Professor, MD, MSc
Chair
Department of Gastrointestinal, Thoracic and Vascular
   Surgery
University Hospital Carl Gustav Carus,
Technische Universität Dresden
Managing Director
National Center for Tumor Diseases (NCT/UCC)
Dresden, Germany

Andrew David Wisneski, MD
Resident & Research Fellow
Surgery
University of California San Francisco
San Francisco, California

Christopher L. Wolfgang, MD, PhD
Chief, Surgical Oncology; Professor of Surgery,
Pathology and Oncology
Department of Surgery
The Johns Hopkins Hospital
Baltimore, Maryland

Dennis Yang, MD
Advanced Endoscopy Fellow
Gastroenterology
Advent Health
Director
Center for Interventional Endoscopy
Advent Health
Orlando, Florida
Professor
Medicine
Loma Linda University Health
Loma Linda, California

Hooman Yarmohammadi, MD
Associate Attending of Radiology
Radiology
Memorial Sloan-Kettering Cancer Center
New York, New York

Charles J. Yeo, MD, FACS
Samuel D. Gross Professor & Chair
Department of Surgery
Sidney Kimmel Medical College at Thomas Jefferson
   University
Philadelphia, Pennsylvania

**Theresa Pluth Yeo, PhD, MPH, AOCNP, ACNP-BC,
   FAANP**
Co-Director Jefferson Pancreas Tumor Registry
Department of Surgery
Professor
Jefferson College of Nursing
Acute Care Nurse Practitioner
Advanced Oncology Nurse Practitioner
Surgery
Thomas Jefferson University Hospital
Philadelphia, Pennsylvania

Adam Yopp, MD
Associate Professor
Surgery
UT Southwestern Medical Center
Dallas, Texas

Herbert Zeh, MD
Professor and Chair of Surgery
Surgery
UT Southwestern Medical Center
Dallas, Texas

Fangyu Zhou, MD
Postdoctoral Research Associate
Surgery
Washington University School of Medicine
St Louis, Missouri

Gazi B. Zibari, MD
Academic Chairman Dept of Surgery Program Director
Surgery Residency
Transplant
Willis Knighton Health System
Director, John C. McDonald Regional Transplant Center
Transplant
Willis Knighton Health System
Director, WK Advanced Surgery Center
Willis-Knighton Health System
Shreveport, Louisiana

George Zogopoulos, MD, PhD, FRCS(C), FACS
Associate Professor
Surgery and Oncology
McGill University
Attending Surgeon
Hepato-Pancreato-Biliary and Abdominal Organ Transplant
   Surgery
McGill University Health Centre
Montreal, Quebec, Canada

The seventh edition of *Blumgart's Surgery of the Liver, Biliary Tract, and Pancreas* was forged largely during the global COVID-19 pandemic, one of the most significant and devastating healthcare crises of the past century. As such, this has been among the most challenging editions to complete but is ultimately faithful to its long history and Dr. Leslie Blumgart's vision of embracing change to keep the book relevant to its readers. The COVID pandemic has profoundly impacted and disrupted all our lives, both professionally and personally, in ways none of us could ever have imagined. The completion of the seventh edition under such difficult circumstances thus represents a notable achievement and, on behalf of the section editors, I extend my sincere thanks to everyone who contributed.

The seventh edition once again relies heavily on associate editors to comprehensively cover the extraordinary advances over the past 5 years. As world-renowned experts in the field, the associate editors bring great insight to the book based on extensive personal experience. Dr. Jean-Nicolas Vauthey of the University of Texas MD Anderson Cancer Center once again joins Dr. William Chapman of Washington University in St. Louis in taking primary oversight of sections dealing largely with hepatic resection and transplantation, reflecting the substantial contributions they have made in these areas. Drs. Ronald DeMatteo, Michael D'Angelica, and Peter Allen bring their expertise to bear in the sections on basic science/physiology, biliary tract, and pancreatic disease, respectively. Dr. Richard Kinh Gian Do's substantive improvements in the sections on liver, biliary, and pancreatic imaging include moving from modality-based to disease-based descriptions. Dr. T. Peter Kingham joins the editorship for this edition, taking charge of an expanded section on the technical aspects of liver, biliary, and pancreatic resection, including transplantation and minimally invasive approaches.

The current edition reflects advances in the molecular biology of benign and malignant HPB diseases, as well as significant improvements in imaging, therapeutics, and overall disease management. Indeed, since the last edition, great advances have been made in many areas, most notably in our understanding of the molecular underpinnings of malignant disease and the related explosion of treatment options, imaging technology, and minimally invasive/robotic surgery, and these are prominently featured in their respective sections.

As previously described, the organization of the book has been modified in that the sections on radiology are no longer separated by modality but rather by organ and disease type to provide a more rational view of imaging assessment. In addition, the technical aspects of HPB resectional surgery is now focused in a separate section. Furthermore, several new chapters have been added, while others have been expanded.

The general format has been maintained by covering all surgical aspects of the management of HPB disorders, whereas the radiologic, endoscopic, and other nonsurgical approaches are presented in detail and highlighted when they represent the preferred therapy. As with past editions, contributors were chosen largely based on their expertise and were asked to discuss specific topics based not only on the published literature but also on their own views and personal experience. Toward that end, overlap between chapters and discussion of controversy was encouraged to allow for conflicting points of view.

The initial section remains dedicated to general topics of HPB anatomy, physiology, and pathophysiology and thereby provides a solid foundation on which the remainder of the book is constructed. Chapter 2, "Surgical and Radiologic Anatomy of the Liver, Biliary Tract, and Pancreas," remains the cornerstone of this section; one of the most important chapters in the entire book, it provides the basis for understanding much of the material presented in subsequent chapters on physiology, molecular biology and immunology, imaging, and perioperative management.

In summary, the seventh edition attempts to include all aspects of the anatomy, pathology, diagnosis, and surgical and nonsurgical treatments related to HPB disorders, and all of the changes that have occurred since the last edition. We hope the work is of value to a wide range of readers, from seasoned HPB practitioners to surgical trainees and physicians in related disciplines. We have expanded our list of contributors to ensure the broadest and most contemporary viewpoints possible.

I would like to again express sincere thanks to the co-editors who have collaborated with me in this project, as well as all the contributors who generously gave their time to make this seventh edition possible. We hope that the readers find this text to be a valuable resource for many years to come.

W.R. Jarnagin, MD
New York, New York, 2022

ACKNOWLEDGMENTS

The Editors are indebted to our colleagues in surgery and other disciplines for their enthusiastic support and insightful contributions. We thank them for updating their areas of expertise, detailing recent advances, and highlighting areas of controversy and differing opinion – without them, this project would never have been possible. Special thanks to our respective staffs in New York, St. Louis, Houston, Durham (NC), and Philadelphia who have assisted in the preparation of this work. Finally, special thanks and appreciation are due to Erin Patterson, who provided much needed editorial support, and to Dee Simpson, Casey Potter, and all of the staff of our esteemed publisher, Elsevier, for their great support throughout the project.

CONTENTS

PART 7

Hepatic Disease

SECTION I. Inflammatory, Infective, and Congenital

A. Hepatitis

CHAPTER 68

Chronic hepatitis: Epidemiology, clinical features, and management

Christopher D. Anderson and Jeffrey S. Crippin

Surgery in the patient with chronic hepatitis can create multiple dilemmas in the preoperative, perioperative, and postoperative phases. Preoperatively, assessment of the stability of the patient's liver disease can be crucial in decisions regarding a surgical procedure (see Chapter 4). Intraoperatively, both technical and anesthesiology considerations will potentially affect the outcome (see Chapters 26 and 101). Postoperative care involves strategies to prevent or treat acute hepatic decompensation, bleeding, and infections. This chapter will cover the chronic hepatitides and address the issues facing the hepatologist and hepatobiliary surgeon.

CHRONIC HEPATITIS

Hepatitis, in general, means "liver inflammation." Most associate the term with a viral infection; however, a number of different processes and agents can lead to an inflamed liver. Other than viral infections, other relatively common causes of hepatitis include alcohol, hepatotoxins (including medicines), autoimmune disorders, and fat (see Chapters 69 and 74). The other important definition, for purposes of this discussion, is "chronic" versus "acute" hepatitis. Chronic hepatitis implies the presence of hepatic inflammation for a period longer than 6 months. Routinely, this is based on the presence of elevated transaminases, that is, aspartate aminotransferase (AST) and alanine aminotransferase (ALT). Although liver inflammation can certainly occur in the absence of elevated transaminases, establishing the diagnosis of chronic hepatitis is dependent on elevations of the AST and ALT for at least 6 months. Thus the finding of elevated transaminases during an evaluation of a potential patient for surgery should lead to a careful assessment, as it pertains to the clinical issues at hand. However, the presence of a single set of elevated transaminases does not necessarily imply an acute or chronic process. For example, a patient with transaminases in the range of 1000 to 1500 IU/L, in the face of a common bile duct gallstone causing obstruction, is distinctly different from a patient with acute cholecystitis seen with a history of elevated transaminases in the range of three to four times the upper limit of normal and an ultrasound showing fatty infiltration of the liver. Thus the clinical setting and history for any particular patient is of crucial importance when evaluating

a patient for hepatobiliary surgery. A basic working knowledge of each of the chronic hepatitides will facilitate evaluation of the patient facing surgery.

Chronic Hepatitis C

Epidemiology

Hepatitis C virus (HCV) is an RNA virus and a member of the family Flaviviridae. This disease affects approximately 1.6% of the American population, with estimates at three to four million infected.[1] Most commonly, the disease is transmitted by blood-to-blood contact. Before the availability of the hepatitis C antibody test in the early 1990s, posttransfusion hepatitis C was a common means of transmission. However, the availability of reliable assays has led to a marked decrease in the incidence of posttransfusion hepatitis C.[2] Currently, the risk of posttransfusion hepatitis C is approximately 1 in 2 million transfusions. The much more common risk factor for contracting hepatitis C is intravenous drug use. Other needle-stick exposures, such as tattoos and occupational exposure, account for a much lower percentage of cases. Sexual transmission is likewise a low risk, particularly among monogamous partners. However, the prevalence of hepatitis C is much higher at sexually transmitted disease clinics, affecting nearly 10% of nonintravenous drug-using patients seen at such clinics,[3] presumably related to sexual promiscuity and traumatic sex, with increased risk of blood-borne exposure. Vertical transmission occurs in 4% to 6% of children of hepatitis C viremic mothers, with the incidence increasing to 10% to 11% of children of mothers with human immunodeficiency virus (HIV)/HCV co-infection.[4] Inhalation of cocaine has been raised as a potential risk factor, based on the transmission via blood on straws used to snort the inhaled agent.[5] This risk factor has been questioned, with the issue that inhaled cocaine may be associated with other high-risk behavior that is, in fact, the mode of transmission.

Presentation

Patients with chronic hepatitis C are frequently asymptomatic, although many have nonspecific symptoms, usually related to fatigue, myalgias, arthralgias, and/or right upper quadrant discomfort. Most patients are only diagnosed when they seek medical care for other reasons or have the symptoms just mentioned and are found to have mild elevations of the transaminases. However, as many as 30% of patients will have normal transaminases at any one time, as the transaminases may wax and wane with time.[6] Thus a history of any of the risk factors outlined earlier should lead to serologic testing to rule out hepatitis C. Due to the absence of risks factors in some patients, the Centers for Disease Control and Prevention (CDC) recommended one time screening with a hepatitis C antibody in those born from 1945 to 1965.[7]

Diagnosis

The standard screening study for hepatitis C is an enzyme-linked immunosorbent assay (ELISA) for antibody to hepatitis C. This is the standard test used by blood banks around the country and has a sensitivity and specificity in high-risk populations ranging from 98% to 100%.[8] If a patient has a known risk factor and elevated transaminases, a positive hepatitis C antibody study by ELISA is consistent with the diagnosis of hepatitis C. The presence of hepatitis viremia is confirmed with a reverse transcriptase polymerase chain reaction (PCR). Unfortunately, the PCR may take days to a week to get results, depending on the frequency of testing at the local laboratory. Patients can have a positive antibody study without viremia, if the acute infection spontaneously resolved, an event that occurs 15% to 40% of the time.[9] Antibody positivity frequently persists indefinitely, but does not imply infection if viremia is absent, based on an undetectable viral load by PCR. Patients will have one of six genotypes, which are variants in the hepatitis C genome that mainly reflect responsiveness to antiviral therapy.[10] A genotype need not be checked if only screening a patient before surgery. However, if antiviral therapy is considered, a genotype will provide important information regarding the chance of a virologic response and the length of therapy. Genotype 1 is the most common genotype in the United States, accounting for 70% of cases. Genotype 2 accounts for 15% of cases and genotype 3 for another 10% of cases.[10] Genotype 4 is occasionally seen in the United States, although it is more commonly seen in the Middle East and northern and central Africa. Genotypes 5 and 6 are seen in the United States, although rarely, with a higher prevalence in South Africa and Southeast Asia, respectively.

Natural History

The course of hepatitis C is quite variable and can be influenced by a number of factors. Progression of the disease is routinely measured by decades. One commonly quoted figure is that 20% of those with the disease for at least 20 years will have cirrhosis (see Chapter 74). It is important to keep in mind that this implies that 80% of those with the disease for 20 years do not have cirrhosis. Another important consideration in determining the extent of the disease at the time of surgical evaluation is knowledge of when the disease was contracted. For example, if the patient knows they received a blood transfusion at the time of a motor vehicle accident 35 years ago, they have probably had the disease for 35 years. Likewise, a patient with an extensive history of intravenous drug use as a young adult has likely had the disease for several decades, if currently in the sixth or seventh decade of life. The disease takes an accelerated course in patients with excessive alcohol use,[11] contraction of the disease at a later age, and co-infection with HIV or the hepatitis B virus.[12,13]

Treatment

Hepatitis C treatment was previously centered around the use of pegylated interferon (PEG IFN) and ribavirin. This treatment was poorly tolerated, associated with a 45% to 50% response rate for genotype 1 patients, and lasted for 24 to 48 weeks. The addition of a protease inhibitor markedly improved response rates; however, significant side effects were seen, often leading to dose reduction, treatment cessation, or hospitalization.

In the fall of 2014, two new regimens were added to the available treatments. Sofosbuvir was combined with ledipasvir, an NS5a inhibitor, in a single-pill regimen for patients with genotype 1. Following 12 weeks of therapy, sustained virological response (SVR) rates of 95% were seen with 12 weeks of therapy. Patients with cirrhosis required 24 weeks of therapy, although with similar rates of response.[14] Currently, five different oral agents are commonly used: sofosbuvir/ledipasvir (genotypes 1 and 4), elbasvir/grazoprevir (genotypes 1 and 4), sofosbuvir/velpatasvir (all genotypes), glecaprevir/pibrentasvir (all genotypes), and sofosbuvir/velpatasvir/voxilaprevir (all genotypes with previous non-response to agents listed). Treatment routinely lasts from 8 to 12 weeks, depending on the agent, with response rates in the range of 95% and higher. Side effects tend to be mild, with rare need to discontinue treatment.

Drug–drug interactions can either increase or decrease drug levels; thus, careful attention to the list of other medications is crucial to safely treating chronic hepatitis C.[14,15]

If undetectable viremia is achieved during therapy, a viral load is routinely checked 3 months following the end of therapy. An undetectable viral load at that point is consistent with an SVR or "cure." Long-term studies have shown this response is durable, with undetectable viral loads persisting indefinitely,[16] unless the patient is reinfected due to reexposure through intravenous drug use or high-risk sexual contact. Patients who do not respond to antiviral therapy may benefit from a treatment trial with a different agent.

Surgery in the Patient With Hepatitis C

In the noncirrhotic patient with hepatitis C undergoing hepatopancreatobiliary surgery, no special precaution need be taken. The risk of decompensation postoperatively is solely associated with the presence of advanced fibrosis and is not associated with the presence of the HCV itself (see Chapters 74 and 101) If a patient happens to be on antiviral therapy at the time of surgery, the best action is to ask a hepatologist to assess the situation. In most cases, antiviral therapy need not be stopped in the face of surgery. Antiviral therapy can be stopped if more pressing issues are at hand. Stopping antiviral therapy for a period of weeks may necessitate restarting treatment.

Hepatitis B
Epidemiology

Hepatitis B virus is a DNA virus representing the number one cause of chronic viral hepatitis worldwide, with more than 2 billion people infected at some point and more than 350 million infected chronically.[17] More than 45% of the world's population lives in endemic areas, particularly in Asia and sub-Saharan Africa.[18] More than 8% of the population in these areas is positive for hepatitis B surface antigen (HBsAg). The prevalence is much lower on the North American continent, affecting less than 2% of the population overall. In the United States, approximately 73,000 new cases occur each year, with approximately 1.25 million patients infected chronically.[19] However, due to the mobility of the world's population, the possibility of acute or chronic hepatitis B must be considered in patients who have come to the United States from endemic areas, for professional, educational, and/or personal reasons. Changes in patterns of immigration will likely increase the prevalence of the disease by as much as a factor of two.

Transmission

In the United States, the most common means of transmission is via permucosal or percutaneous exposure to blood or body fluids.[20] Thus sexual transmission and parenteral exposure via needle sticks account for the majority of cases. Vertical transmission is relatively rare in this country, due to the identification of HBsAg-positive mothers and the administration of hepatitis B immunoglobulin and the hepatitis B vaccine at the time of birth. Failure to administer these agents frequently leads to chronic infection in the neonate, due to the inability of an immature immune system to eradicate hepatitis B viremia.[21]

Presentation

Acute hepatitis B has a wide range of presentations, ranging from a subclinical disease to acute liver failure. The disease tends to be associated with more severe symptoms as the age of the patient increases. Malaise, arthralgias, anorexia, jaundice, and anorexia may be present. Chronic hepatitis B routinely is often not associated with symptoms, although vague, nonspecific symptoms may be present. Differentiating fatigue, arthralgias, and myalgias from other systemic diseases may be difficult.

Diagnosis

The presence of acute or chronic hepatitis B requires the presence of the HBsAg. If this test is negative, the patient does not have hepatitis B. On occasion, a patient with acute hepatitis B may be seen without HBsAg and without hepatitis B surface antibody (HBsAb), because the virus is being eradicated. This is referred to as the "core window." During this phase, only the immunoglobulin M hepatitis B core antibody (IgM HBcAb) is present, thus its presence on acute hepatitis panels available through commercial laboratories. Chronic hepatitis B is only diagnosed when HBsAg is present more than 6 months following the onset of the acute infection. If HBsAg is positive, the evaluation includes assessment for the presence of the hepatitis B e antigen (HBeAg), hepatitis B e antibody (HBeAb), and hepatitis B viremia with a hepatitis B virus DNA level by PCR. Along with the transaminases, these tests guide decisions regarding the need for antiviral therapy. Imaging studies are only required if there is a suspicion of advanced fibrosis, based on the presence of complications of end-stage liver disease, hypoalbuminemia, a prolonged prothrombin time, and/or thrombocytopenia. Sonography is a reasonable first step, although other cross-sectional imaging studies may be indicated, depending on the sonographic findings. Similar to hepatitis C, there are different hepatitis B genotypes. Eight different hepatitis B genotypes exist, with genotypes A and C most common in the United States. Routine checks of the genotype are unnecessary with regard to screening; however, the genotype can be useful in predicting the response to antiviral therapy.

Natural History

Acute hepatitis B in the adult resolves spontaneously in 90% of cases. The other 10% of cases with persistent HBsAg require careful assessment and follow-up. Within the last decade, the natural history of chronic hepatitis B has been rewritten. Previously, patients either were "chronic carriers" or had "chronic hepatitis B." Chronic hepatitis B now is defined more as a spectrum of disease states that slowly evolve from one to another. Patients contracting hepatitis B in the perinatal period frequently maintain high levels of hepatitis B viremia with normal transaminases.[22] This may persist for decades. This "immune tolerant" phase is characterized by the absence of or, at most, minimal liver injury. Current guidelines recommend observation with regular follow-up of liver biochemistries and hepatitis B serologies and a viral load. Spontaneous HBeAg to HBeAb seroconversion occurs at a rate of 8% to 12% of patients per year.[23] An exacerbation of hepatitis B may accompany seroconversion, with marked elevations of the transaminases. Many of these patients (67%–80%) enter the "inactive carrier state," with absent or low-level viral replication, normal transaminases, and minimal histologic damage.[23] However, 10% to 30% of HBeAb-positive patients continue to have elevated transaminases, viral replication, and histologic damage.[24] As many as 20% of HBeAb-positive patients may revert back to HBeAg positive, with elevated viral loads and transaminases.[24]

Treatment

Patients with acute hepatitis B are treated supportively. There is no indication for antiviral therapy, because 90% of cases resolve spontaneously, and two studies have shown no benefit to the use of antiviral therapy in accelerating resolution.[25,26] Cases of chronic hepatitis B must be carefully assessed to determine the appropriate treatment for the appropriate patient. Guidelines have been published by several professional societies. The key themes throughout all the published guidelines include (1) if the transaminases are normal, observe, even if there is a detectable viral load; (2) consider treatment if the transaminases are elevated or if there is significant histologic damage; and (3) consider treatment in all cirrhotics with chronic hepatitis B. Medical management is centered around the use of nucleoside/nucleotide analogues. The nucleoside/nucleotide analogues are relatively nontoxic and easy to take, although years of treatment may be necessary before seroconversion occurs. Entecavir and tenofovir are potent suppressants of hepatitis B viral replication.[27] Lamivudine, the mainstay of therapy over a decade ago, is not considered first-line therapy due to high levels of drug resistance. PEG IFN offers a defined treatment length of 48 weeks; however, weekly subcutaneous injections and significant side effects make it a rare choice among many clinicians. The nucleoside/nucleotide analogues lead to eradication of viral replication in approximately 80% of cases, with HBeAg seroconversion in as many as 22% of patients, whereas PEG IFN leads to HBeAg seroconversion in as many as 34% of cases.[27]

Surgery in the Patient With Chronic Hepatitis B

No special precautions are necessary in the patient with chronic hepatitis B, unless the patient has cirrhosis (see Chapter 74). Otherwise, surgery can proceed as scheduled. If the patient is on antiviral therapy, discontinuation of the antiviral agent can lead to replicative rebound, resulting in an acute hepatitis and, potentially, liver failure. Thus antiviral agents should not be stopped suddenly until the case can be discussed with a hepatologist. Any HBsAg-positive patient not on an antiviral agent should be considered for prophylactic antiviral therapy if immunosuppressive therapy or chemotherapy is started.[27] Flares of hepatitis following immunosuppressive therapy or chemotherapy, even to the point of hepatic decompensation and death, have been reported in patients without previous evidence of viral replication.[28]

Nonalcoholic Steatohepatitis

Epidemiology

Nonalcoholic steatohepatitis (NASH) (see Chapter 69) is slowly becoming the most common liver disease seen worldwide. Nonalcoholic fatty liver disease (NAFLD) has a prevalence of 3% to 23% of the North American population.[29,30] The prevalence of fatty liver disease has paralleled the increase in body weight seen globally. Nearly 75% of those with obesity or type 2 diabetes mellitus have NAFLD,[30] and approximately 20% of obese patients have NASH.[31] The increase in body mass seen in the United States during the last 25 years suggests the prevalence will rise before it falls.

Presentation

Patients are usually without symptoms. During routine physical examinations and health screens, abnormal transaminases are a frequent presenting problem. Right upper abdominal quadrant fullness or pain, in the absence of other causes, is a common complaint. Patients routinely have multiple features of the metabolic syndrome, including hyperlipidemia, hyperglycemia/diabetes mellitus, and hypertension. All of these issues appear to be related to the development of insulin resistance.[32]

Diagnosis

The definitive diagnosis of NAFLD is made histologically. This does not imply a biopsy is obtained in all cases, however. The finding of elevated transaminases in an obese patient suggests the diagnosis; however, other causes of chronic liver disease must be ruled out. Alcoholic steatohepatitis is the first consideration, although this may be limited by the honesty of the patient and whether family members are aware of alcohol ingestion. If heavy alcohol use is unlikely, viral hepatitis serologies, autoimmune serologies, iron studies, and a ceruloplasmin level should be checked. If these studies are negative/normal, the next step is imaging of the liver, either sonographically or with cross-sectional imaging. Fatty infiltration of the liver is only detected if greater than 30% of the parenchyma is infiltrated with fat.[33] If fat is detected, a liver biopsy is not required. Many hepatologists proceed with a liver biopsy if there is a question of another liver disease, for instance, borderline autoimmune serologies or mildly elevated iron studies, or if there is some question of the presence of moderate to severe fibrosis. The biopsy can be used to rule out other liver diseases and as a means of staging the amount of fibrotic tissue. The latter is seen as "incentive" to patients for a dedicated weight-loss program. Biopsies from patients with NASH show fat and inflammation, although distinguishing the findings from alcoholic steatohepatitis may be difficult.

Natural History

Hepatic steatosis occurs with minimal or no inflammatory changes histologically. NASH is associated with necroinflammatory changes. Steatosis with or without inflammation may progress to fibrosis and cirrhosis; however, the risk of fibrosis progression is lower in patients with steatosis alone.[34] Natural history studies are relatively few in number, due to small numbers and limited long-term follow-up. However, NASH progresses to cirrhosis in 15% to 20% of cases.[35] Progression is obviously shorter in patients seen with advanced fibrosis, although 30% of patients will have progression of fibrosis over 5 years[36] (see Chapter 74).

Treatment

Despite multiple trials of medical treatments, the mainstay of therapy for NASH remains weight loss.[37] Decreased dietary intake, ideally complemented by an exercise program, will lead to weight loss, a decrease in hepatic fat, and lower transaminases. Weight loss in the amount of 10% to 15% of the current body weight over the course of a year is a reasonable and attainable goal for most patients. However, bariatric surgery, and its frequently accelerated weight loss, is not harmful and has been associated with histologic improvement.[38]

Medical therapy for NASH has been the source of multiple drug trials. The thiazolidinediones have been associated with improvement of transaminases and a decrease in histologic fat.[39] However, weight gain is a potential side effect, thus use of this class of medications solely to improve NASH is not standard of practice. If a patient is diabetic and has NASH, use of pioglitazone or rosiglitazone may be considered. Vitamin E has been associated with improved liver tests and decreased hepatic histologic inflammation[40]; however, its effect on disease progression is unclear. Obeticholic acid has been studied with evidence of improved fibrosis.[41] However, weight loss and exercise remain the foundation of NASH treatment.

Surgery in the Patient With Nonalcoholic Steatohepatitis

Routinely, no special precautions need be taken for the operative candidate with NASH in the absence of cirrhosis. However, large hepatic resections in patients with fatty livers have been associated with decompensated liver disease postoperatively[42,43] (see Chapters 98 and 101). Thus careful assessment of the patient considered for hepatic resection must take all of these factors into account. A liver biopsy may provide the necessary information regarding baseline hepatic histology, the extent of fatty infiltration and fibrosis, and the presence of other conditions that may lead to postoperative decompensation.

Autoimmune Hepatitis

Epidemiology

Autoimmune hepatitis is a chronic, usually progressive, liver disease with an incidence among Northern Europeans of 1.9 per 100,000 population[44] and 1 per 200,000 in the United States[45] Although often characterized as a disease of middle-aged women, all ages may be affected, including the very young and the elderly. Women are affected more often than men. Patients frequently have a coexisting autoimmune disease; thus, a history of thyroid disease, rheumatoid arthritis, or psoriasis, among others, should at least raise the possibility of the diagnosis in a patient seen with elevated liver biochemistries.[46]

Presentation

Patients present in several ways, ranging from relatively asymptomatic elevations of the transaminases to cirrhosis to acute liver failure, the latter two preceded by relatively nonspecific symptoms of fatigue and malaise of varying duration. As many as 40% of patients are seen with systemic complaints and an acute illness, with fever, arthralgias, myalgias, and skin rash possible. This can progress to acute liver failure with hepatic encephalopathy within 8 weeks of the onset of symptoms, potentially leading to death or need for a liver transplant (see Chapter 77) Autoimmune hepatitis historically accounts for 5% to 6% of liver transplants done in the United States.

Diagnosis

No single test or finding leads to the diagnosis of autoimmune hepatitis. Other causes of acute and chronic liver disease must be ruled out. Thus viral serologies, iron studies (hereditary hemochromatosis), serum ceruloplasmin (Wilson disease), $\alpha 1$-antitrypsin level and phenotype, drug-induced hepatotoxicity, alcoholic liver disease, and NASH must be ruled out, based on historic, serologic, radiologic, and histologic data. Autoimmune serologies are helpful, particularly when present at a titer of greater than 1:80. Antinuclear antibodies and anti–smooth muscle antibodies are frequently present; however, their absence does not rule out the disease. The anti–liver/kidney microsomal antibody is much less common (<5% of cases) in the United States. Other autoimmune serologies occur even less commonly and are not routinely checked in clinical practice.

Histologic features are the foundation of the diagnosis; however, serologic and clinical findings may lead to the diagnosis, even in the absence of classic histologic findings. Characteristic histologic findings include interface hepatitis, previously known as "piecemeal necrosis," and a portal plasma cellular infiltrate. However, other liver diseases, such as Wilson disease, chronic hepatitis C, and drug-induced hepatotoxicity can have similar histologic features. Thus the issues outlined earlier regarding careful assessment and evaluation for other acute and chronic liver diseases cannot be forgotten. Histologic features of other autoimmune liver diseases, such as primary biliary cirrhosis, may suggest the presence of an overlap syndrome, featuring serologic and histologic features of both diseases.

Natural History

Untreated, autoimmune hepatitis is often a progressive disease, with death occurring in 40% of untreated patients. In those surviving the initial illness, another 40% progress to cirrhosis, with the potential manifestations of end-stage liver disease, including ascites, portal hypertension, and hepatic encephalopathy. Not unexpectedly, severe histologic damage on the initial liver biopsy is a poor prognostic factor. Although transaminase elevations do not always correlate with the amount of liver damage or prognosis in other liver diseases, persistent transaminase elevations greater than 10 times the upper limit of normal are associated with higher rates of early mortality. Patients with milder laboratory and histologic findings have a less severe course; however, cirrhosis still develops in approximately 50% of patients over a period of 15 years.[47] Thus early diagnosis and treatment is crucial to prolonging long-term survival.

Treatment

Indications for treatment must be individualized, although clearly more severe cases should be started on therapy immediately. Patients with histologic features and transaminases greater than 10 times the upper limit of normal should be treated. Lower-level transaminase elevations in combination with bridging necrosis and/or lobular necrosis should also be treated. The potential risks and benefits of treatment should be considered in patients without the findings just mentioned; however, due to the progressive nature of the disease, most experienced hepatologists routinely treat patients with transaminase elevations and even mild histologic changes.

Immunosuppressive therapy is the key to controlling this progressive disease. Although treatment protocols vary by center and clinician, corticosteroid-based treatment is most common. Oral prednisone, at a dose of 30 to 60 mg daily, is usually started in most cases, even in patients with coexistent diseases that potentially could be affected, for instance, diabetes mellitus. Due to the adverse effects associated with long-term high-dose corticosteroid therapy, the dose is tapered over varying amounts of time, ranging from weeks to months. Due to the potential for disease flares as the corticosteroid dose is tapered, most start azathioprine, at a dose of 50 mg daily, along with corticosteroids, or within 2 to 3 months of the initiation of treatment.[47] Azathioprine is usually not effective for 4 to 8 weeks after initiation, thus, many clinicians start it with prednisone, rather than delaying. Ninety percent of adults show marked improvement in laboratory studies and symptoms within 2 weeks of starting therapy; however, disease remission is uncommon in less than 12 months. Thus azathioprine is continued after prednisone is tapered off. As the prednisone is tapered, any elevation in transaminases can be addressed with an increase in dose, but the long-term side effects associated with corticosteroids make this a less than ideal choice. Thus increased doses of azathioprine, incrementally increased to a maximum dose of 2 mg/kg/day, are routinely used if the disease flares during the steroid taper.

Depending on the severity of the histologic damage seen initially, most clinicians continue the azathioprine at least for a period of 1 to 2 years. Even with normal transaminases, a significant number of patients will have ongoing interface hepatitis on immunosuppressive therapy. Thus any attempt to stop immunosuppressive therapy should be preceded by a liver biopsy to assess the histologic response to therapy. As a rule, more severe initial changes will take longer to correct and will lag biochemical improvement. Many clinicians see autoimmune hepatitis as a "chronic" disease that will inevitably flare off therapy; clearly, however, some patients go into remission and can remain off therapy without histologic progression. Patients tapered off therapy should be followed with liver biochemistries at least twice a year, because relapses may occur without symptoms. Reinstitution of immunosuppressive therapy leads to improvement in most patients within 2 years and should lead to indefinite immunosuppressive therapy with azathioprine and, in some cases, prednisone, based on liver biochemistries.[47]

The complications of long-term corticosteroid therapy are well known and need not be outlined. However, the short- and long-term consequences associated with azathioprine are less well known and worth listing. Bone marrow suppression, with anemia, leukopenia, and thrombocytopenia, is the most common laboratory abnormality. Symptomatically, nausea, vomiting, and abdominal pain may lead to cessation of therapy due to intolerance. Acute pancreatitis is rare, as is hepatoxicity, usually marked by sinusoidal obstructive syndrome or cholestasis, both of which usually respond to drug cessation. Long-term, malignancy can occur, usually in the form of lymphoma or leukemia.[48] However, one series of patients with autoimmune hepatitis followed during 20 years showed no incidence of malignancy.[49] Allopurinol should never be used in patients on azathioprine. Allopurinol inhibits xanthine oxidase, an enzyme necessary for the breakdown of azathioprine. If this enzyme is inhibited, the half-life of azathioprine is prolonged and can be toxic, with profound bone marrow suppression. Other agents have been used for the treatment of autoimmune hepatitis, although the experience is predominantly anecdotal. Mycophenolate mofetil, another lymphocyte inhibitor used in solid-organ transplant recipients, can be substituted for azathioprine in cases of intolerable side effects, with comparable efficacy, based on a relatively limited experience.

Surgery in the Patient With Autoimmune Hepatitis

No special precautions need be taken in patients with autoimmune hepatitis requiring surgery. Patients with acute autoimmune hepatitis with signs of acute liver failure or cirrhosis clearly are at risk; however, indications for surgery in this setting would likely be only of an emergent nature (see Chapter 75). All the risks and benefits of surgery must be carefully considered. In the patient with well-controlled autoimmune hepatitis on maintenance immunosuppression, the risk of liver decompensation and/or a disease flare is small, as long as patients are maintained on their medications. Stress doses of corticosteroids should be considered if a patient is on corticosteroids or has recently been tapered off. If a patient is on azathioprine monotherapy preoperatively, the dose should be restarted as soon as possible postoperatively. A prolonged absence of gut motility should lead to discussion with a hepatologist regarding the need for intravenous steroids to keep the disease in remission. Routinely, a few days off immunosuppressive therapy will not lead to a disease flare; thus, the potential risks and benefits associated with corticosteroids need to be carefully considered. Patients with advanced cirrhosis routinely are not surgical candidates, except in cases of emergent and/or life-threatening events requiring surgical intervention. Finally, the degree immunosuppression associated with corticosteroids and azathioprine has not routinely affected wound healing or postoperative recover.

SUMMARY: APPROACH TO SURGERY IN PATIENTS WITH LIVER DISEASE

Partly due to the epidemic of obesity and NAFLD, increasing numbers of patients with chronic liver disease are undergoing nonhepatic and nontransplant operations. Liver disease, especially significant fibrosis or cirrhosis, represents a significant risk factor for perioperative morbidity and mortality (see Chapters 75 and 101). Any clinically evident signs of liver dysfunction should raise concern, particularly for intraabdominal operations. Although there is no absolute consensus on risk quantification, it is clear the perioperative risk in patients with liver disease increases with the severity of liver dysfunction.[50] Perioperative risk in these patients can be quantified using the Childs-Turcotte-Pugh (CTP) score and/or the Model for End-Stage Liver Disease (MELD)[50–52] (see Chapter 4). The MELD score can discriminate risks to a finer degree than the CTP score and has evolved as the best predictor of 30- and 90-day operative mortality.[50] Furthermore, the perioperative mortality risk greatly increases in patients with MELD scores greater than 10 to 15.[50,53–56] There is also utility in MELD-based variants in making more refined predictions regarding surgical risk.[53,56]

Ultimately, the indication for surgery, that is, elective or emergent, along with the patient's estimated operative risk from liver disease, must be considered as the operative plan is developed. These factors should clearly influence the informed consent for the patient and family. When possible, patients should be referred to a specialty liver care center where preoperative optimization should be carried out via a multidisciplinary team approach.

References are available at expertconsult.com.

CHAPTER 69

Hepatic steatosis, steatohepatitis, and chemotherapy-related liver injury

Samer Tohme, Srinevas K. Reddy, and David A. Geller

Fatty liver disease (FLD), comprising hepatic steatosis or steato-hepatitis with or without associated fibrosis, and hepatic sinusoidal injury (SI) are emerging challenges at the forefront of hepatobiliary surgery. Because of the high prevalence of metabolic syndrome elements (hypertension, diabetes mellitus, obesity, and dyslipidemia), many patients considered for hepatic resection for benign or malignant indications will have nonalcoholic fatty liver disease (NAFLD). In parallel with the metabolic syndrome epidemic, NAFLD is the most common chronic liver disease in the Western hemisphere. It is estimated that by 2050, NAFLD will be both the most common cause of hepatocellular carcinoma (HCC) and indication for liver transplantation in the United States. Because of potential survival benefits from perioperative chemotherapy for initially resectable and "conversion" chemotherapy for initially unresectable colorectal cancer liver metastases (CRCLM), FLD, and SI in the background liver will be more commonly encountered during hepatic resection. Understanding the effects of background liver injury on postoperative outcomes is crucial to efforts aimed at improving the safety of liver resection (see Chapters 74 and 89).

HISTOPATHOLOGY OF FATTY LIVER DISEASE AND SINUSOIDAL INJURY

Fatty Liver Disease

NAFLD comprises nonalcoholic fatty liver (NAFL), also known as "simple steatosis," and nonalcoholic steatohepatitis (NASH) (see Chapter 74). Grossly, a fatty liver is characterized by hepatomegaly, yellow appearance, and rounded edges (Fig. 69.1A). Hepatic steatosis is defined as abnormal macrovesicular or microvesicular triglyceride accumulation in at least 5% of hepatocytes diagnosed histologically or by radiologic imaging.[1–4] NAFL was traditionally thought of as a benign condition with a low likelihood of progression to NASH and associated fibrosis.[3,5,6] However, several studies dispute whether NAFL and NASH represent a spectrum of FLD (i.e., progression from steatosis to steatohepatitis) or distinct diseases.[7–10] Moreover, although progression is more rapid in NASH, patients with NAFL (including those with inflammatory components insufficient for a NASH diagnosis) can also experience fibrosis progression.[4,9,11]

NASH encompasses a pattern of injury characterized by hepatic steatosis, lobular inflammation, and hepatocyte ballooning with or without associated fibrosis (Fig. 69.2A). In adults, the initial injury usually occurs in the perivenular (zone 3) portion of the hepatic acinus, which is the least oxygenated and most prone to free radical–mediated injury. This is in contrast to other chronic liver diseases in which marked portal inflammation is observed early in the disease course. However, with worsening disease, the injury may progress to all zones. Ballooning injury, a requirement for the diagnosis of NASH, is

a condition in which hepatocytes become enlarged and the cytoplasm becomes irregularly clumped with clear, nonvesiculated areas with or without residual fat droplets.[1–4,12–14] Borderline steatohepatitis includes some but not all of these features.[12] The most common standardized method for evaluating NASH is a validated histologic scoring system developed by the Pathology Committee of the NASH Clinical Research Network. This NAFLD activity score (NAS) includes potentially reversible features of steatohepatitis, including steatosis (score 0–3), lobular inflammation (0–3), and hepatocyte ballooning (0–2). A total NAS of 5 or greater correlated with the diagnosis of steatohepatitis.[4,15] Importantly, NASH diagnosis should be made based on a recognized pattern of liver injury and not simply by a numerical score. Recent studies demonstrate that using a particular NAS threshold missed 40% to 45% of patients with steatohepatitis as diagnosed by experienced hepatobiliary pathologists and that NAS thresholds were not correlated with liver-related mortality.[16–18]

Early liver fibrosis and cirrhosis is commonly associated with NASH (see Chapters 7 and 74). Early characteristic patterns of fibrosis that are due to NASH include delicate collagen strands that may isolate one or more hepatocytes (see Fig. 69.2B) and perisinusoidal "chicken-wire" fibrosis. In more advanced stages, periportal fibrosis may occur with possible progression to bridging fibrosis.[12] Of patients with NASH, 25% to 30% have advanced fibrosis on diagnosis, 10% to 15% of which have cirrhosis. Moreover, fibrosis progression has been noted on serial biopsies in 25% to 37% of cases with older age and greater body mass index (BMI) at diagnosis risk factors for this fibrosis progression.[6,19–21] Importantly, many of the histologic features of NASH disappear when advanced fibrosis or cirrhosis develops, a finding known as "burned out" NASH.[4,17,21–23] Given the similarities in the profile of metabolic syndrome elements observed in several studies between patients with NAFLD and cryptogenic cirrhosis, it is widely thought that as many as 50% to 70% of traditionally diagnosed cryptogenic cirrhosis can be ultimately traced back to NASH.[3,6,21,24–28]

Importantly, FLD has many causes that may synergistically augment background liver injury. Potential risk factors include alcohol use, elements of the metabolic syndrome, hereditary disorders, and drug-induced injury, particularly from chemotherapeutics. There are few reliable, consistent histologic criteria that differentiate between causes of FLD.[29,30] For inclusion in clinical trials and cohort studies, the consumption threshold used to define the nonalcoholic nature of FLD is arbitrarily set at fewer than 21 and 14 drinks per week for men and women, respectively.[2] Yet because patients often experience multiple insults, FLD should be considered one histopathologic injury with multiple nonexclusive causes that may synergistically augment liver injury.[30]

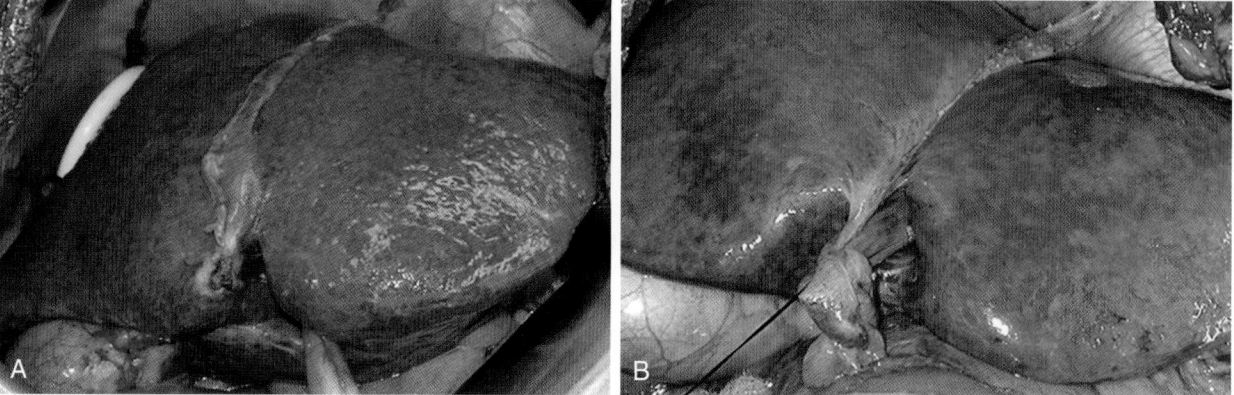

FIGURE 69.1 **A,** Intraoperative gross photograph of a fatty liver. Note the hepatomegaly, yellow appearance, and rounded edges. **B,** Intraoperative photograph of a liver with sinusoidal obstructive syndrome. Note the patchy blue mottled appearance. (Courtesy Michael Choti, MD.)

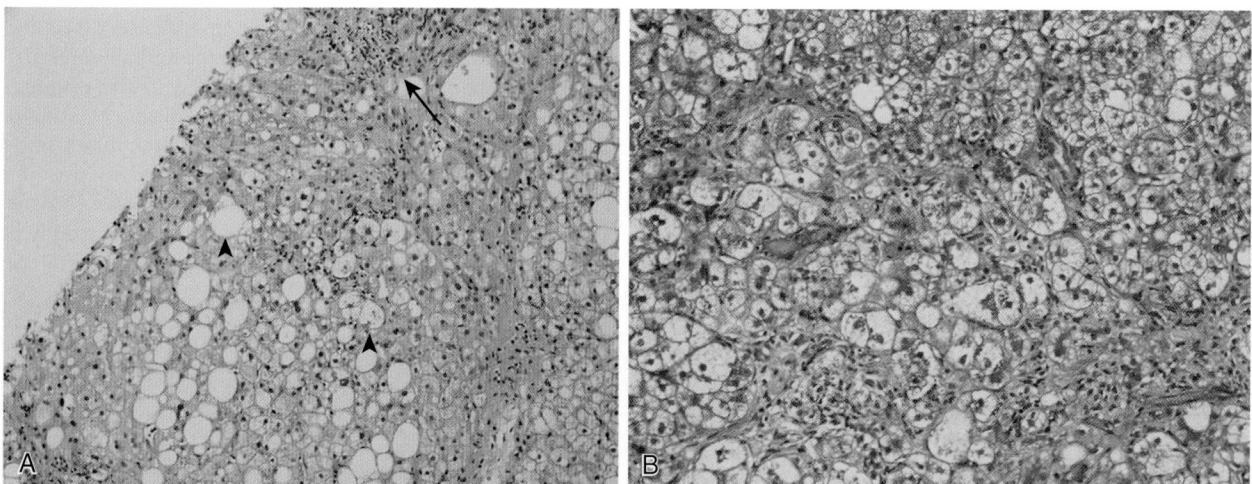

FIGURE 69.2 **A,** Steatohepatitis with moderate steatosis, lobular inflammation *(arrow),* and hepatocyte ballooning degeneration *(arrowheads)* observed. Stained with hematoxylin and eosin, magnification ×200. **B,** Steatohepatitis with hepatocyte ballooning degeneration (throughout specimen) and trichome staining showing pericellular fibrosis. Stained with Masson trichrome, magnification ×200. (Courtesy Schuyler O. Sanderson, MD.)

Sinusoidal Injury

Hepatic SI from chemotherapeutics has a recognized histologic pattern originally observed in bone marrow transplant recipients (see Chapters 7 and 74) Grossly, a liver affected by severe SI has a mottled blue appearance (see Fig. 69.1B). Injury to the sinusoidal endothelial cells leads to subintimal thickening, extravasation of erythrocytes into the subendothelial space, and hepatocyte plate disruption[31-33] (Fig. 69.3A). This congestion blocks venous outflow resulting in sinusoidal dilatation and deposition of extracellular collagen leading to perisinusoidal fibrosis. At later stages, this injury can obliterate central venules, leading to sinusoidal obstructive syndrome[31] (see Fig. 69.3B). Thus perisinusoidal fibrosis, sinusoidal capillarization, hepatocyte atrophy and plate disruption, centrilobular necrosis, and nodular regenerative hyperplasia can all be observed after initial SI.[34] Nodular regenerative hyperplasia is characterized by the diffuse transformation of normal hepatic parenchyma into small, regenerative nodules that compress surrounding parenchyma and can cause portal hypertension.[33] SI and associated lesions are categorized as mild (centrilobular involvement limited to one third of the lobular area); moderate

(centrilobular involvement extending to two thirds of the lobular area); and severe (complete lobular involvement or centrilobular involvement extending to adjacent lobules with bridging congestion).[33]

EPIDEMIOLOGY OF FATTY LIVER DISEASE

The prevalence of NAFLD is increasing worldwide at approximately the same rate as obesity.[4,35] In parallel with the metabolic syndrome epidemic, NAFLD is the most common chronic liver disease in the developed world. The global prevalence of NAFLD in the general population has been estimated to be 25%, whereas the global prevalence of NASH has been estimated to range from 3% to 5%.[36] As age increases so does the prevalence of NAFLD and NAFLD-related fibrosis. This could be driven by a higher prevalence of metabolic conditions in older individuals. Regarding sex, studies from Asia found that even after adjusting for age and the presence of type 2 diabetes, along with other diseases, the prevalence of NAFLD was 4.2% higher in women.[37,38] In contrast, a number of studies from the United States and Europe have reported a higher prevalence of

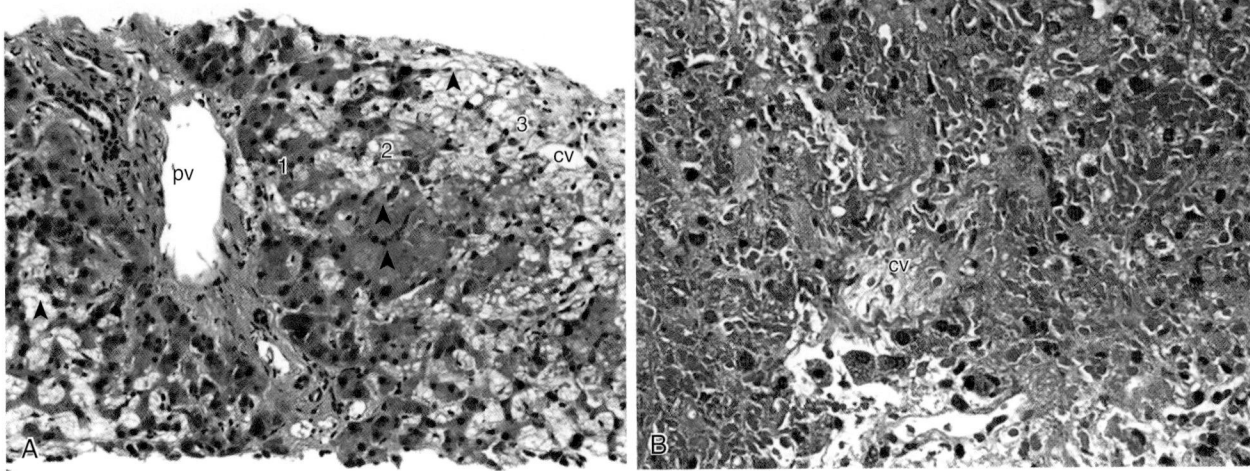

FIGURE 69.3 A, Sinusoidal obstructive syndrome affecting all zones of the liver *(numbered),* with extensive loss of hepatocytes in zone 3. Note the extensive sinusoidal congestion and dilatation *(arrowhead).* **B,** Severe sinusoidal obstructive syndrome with central vein *(cv)* obliteration and no viable hepatocytes. Stained with hematoxylin and eosin, magnification ×200. *pv,* Portal vein. (Courtesy Schuyler O. Sanderson, MD.)

NAFLD in men.[39,40] The risk of NAFLD also differs with race and ethnicity. The highest prevalence of NAFLD is observed in Hispanics, followed by non-Hispanic white individuals, and the lowest prevalence is observed in African Americans (10%).[36] Despite a higher prevalence in the obese, NAFLD does occur in 7% to 15% of lean patients and is associated with Hispanic ethnicity, diabetes mellitus, and hypertension.[41,42] The prevalence of lean NAFLD in the United States was reported to be 7%, whereas the prevalence of lean NAFLD in rural areas of some Asian countries can be up to 30%.[36] Importantly, NASH can be found concurrently with other chronic liver diseases in 5% to 18% of cases.[43–46] Superimposed NASH may act synergistically with hepatitis C virus (HCV) or hepatitis B virus (HBV) to promote advanced fibrosis and worse outcomes.[46–48]

As a result of its emerging prevalence, NAFLD and NASH are rapidly becoming a major indication for liver transplantation in the United States.[36] Between 2004 and 2013, new wait list registrants with NASH increased by 170%—more than any other disease cause. An analysis of the Scientific Registry of Transplant Recipients from 2012 to 2016 found that NASH was the fastest increasing indication for liver transplantation among those listed, positioning NASH to become the most common indication for liver transplantation in the United States in the near future.[49] NASH is also the most rapidly growing indication for liver transplantation in patients with HCC in the United States, with an increase of 4-fold from 2002 to 2012.[50]

DIAGNOSIS

Liver biopsy provides a direct measure of liver fibrosis; however, it is an invasive procedure that carries risks. In addition, current histopathologic fibrosis staging systems provide only a semiquantitative measure of fibrosis, which may not be sensitive to subtle changes in fibrosis over time (see Chapter 74). The optimal method for evaluating liver fibrosis should be accurate, reproducible, and dynamic in how it responds to the change in fibrosis levels over time. In lieu of histopathologic assessment, the gold standard for diagnosis of FLD and SI, noninvasive assessments, have variable accuracy. Noninvasive tests, including blood-based biomarkers and imaging techniques, such as elastography, are generally preferred by patients and physicians in routine clinical practice. Routine liver enzyme tests are insensitive, because 80% of patients with NAFLD will have normal aminotransferase levels.[4,51] More complex biomarker blood tests, such as Enhanced Liver Fibrosis (ELF) Score, Hepascore, and Fibrospect II, incorporate some of the direct markers of fibrogenesis and fibrinolysis are generally more accurate than "simple" biomarkers in predicting advanced fibrosis and cirrhosis.[52] Ultrasound characteristics of fatty liver include hepatomegaly, diffuse increase in echogenicity of liver parenchyma resulting from intracellular accumulation of fat and vascular blunting.[5,53] However, conventional ultrasound can miss up to 22% of cases of steatosis.[54] Key limitations of ultrasound are interobserver and intraobserver variability[53] and the inability to distinguish between simple steatosis and NASH.[4] On computed tomography (CT) scan, hepatic steatosis has low attenuation and appears darker than the spleen (see Chapter 14). This is based on the fact that attenuation of fat is much lower than that of soft tissue (Fig. 69.4). Similar to ultrasound, CT is excellent at diagnosing moderate to severe steatosis (>30%) but less effective with milder steatosis.[53] With intravenous contrast, CT has a sensitivity of 50% to 86% and specificity of 75% to 87% for detecting hepatic steatosis greater than 30%.[5,55,56] Currently, the best validated methods for noninvasive imaging are transient elastography using ultrasound (such as FibroScan) and magnetic resonance elastography (MRE)[52] (Fig. 61.5) (see Chapters 14 and 74). MRE appears more accurate than sonographic elastography and is not significantly affected by obesity but is costly, time-consuming to perform, and not widely available.[52] Emerging technologies including three-dimensional MRE and genetic prediction models may improve on the accuracy of currently available noninvasive tests to predict fibrosis and NAFLD.

NONALCOHOLIC STEATOHEPATITIS AND HEPATOCELLULAR CARCINOMA

Concomitant increases in the incidence of HCC and prevalence of NAFLD suggests that a substantial proportion of HCC arises

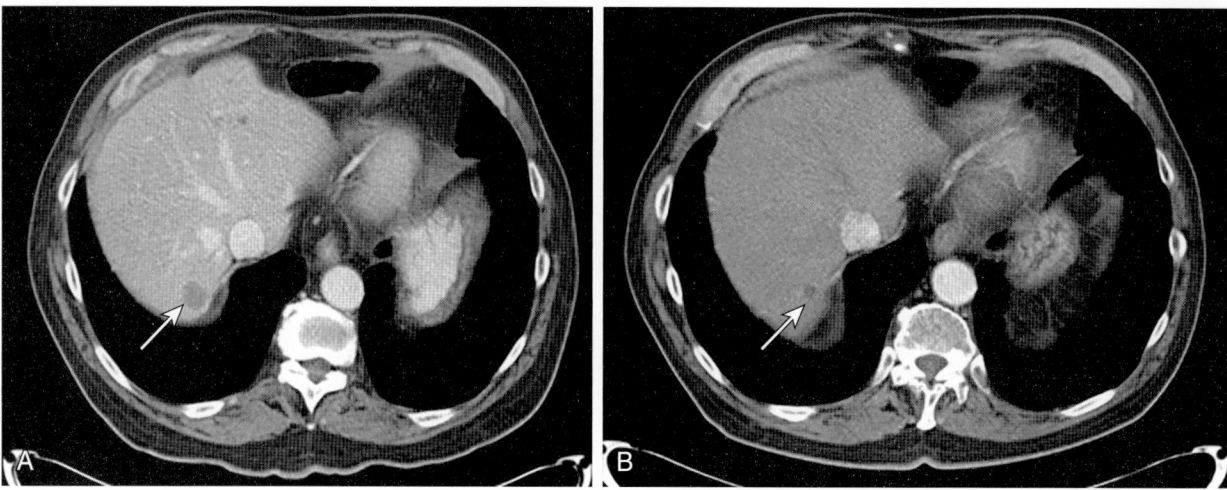

FIGURE 69.4   Effects of eight cycles of preoperative FOLFIRI (folinic acid [leucovorin], 5-fluorouracil [5-FU], and irinotecan [Campto]) for colorectal cancer liver metastases. Note the shrinkage in liver metastases *(arrow)* in prechemotherapy computed tomography (CT) scan **(A)** relative to postchemotherapy image **(B)**. Also note the relative increased density of the background liver (from steatohepatitis) on the postchemotherapy CT scan due to chemotherapy-induced liver injury.

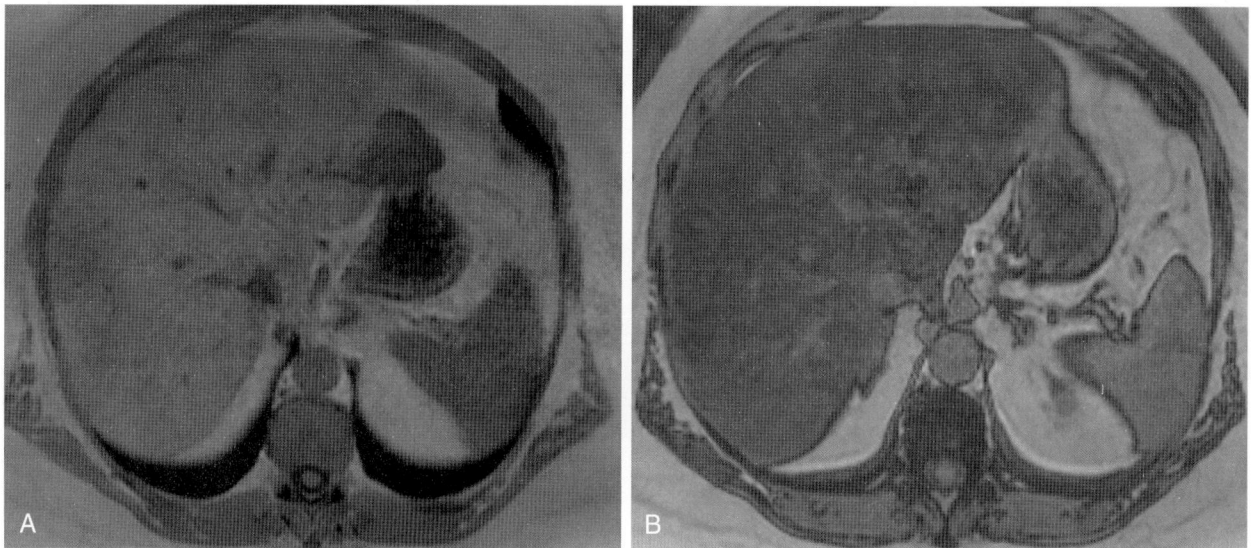

FIGURE 69.5   Magnetic resonance imaging displaying a fatty liver.   Note the signal drop-out when comparing the in-phase **(A)** with opposed-phase **(B)** images.

as the result of hepatocellular injury from NASH (see Chapters 7, 74, 87, and 89). In the United States, HCC is the fastest rising cause of cancer-related deaths in both sexes.[57] HCC incidence rates have increased in each successive cohort born between 1900 and 1959.[58] Comparative prospective cohort studies demonstrate that the incidence of HCC in the setting of NASH-cirrhosis is lower compared with that in HCV- or HBV-related cirrhosis.[4,7,59–61] Despite the lower odds ratio, the overall greater prevalence of NAFLD means that FLD contributes more toward HCC on a population level.[62] In a study of HCC in patients 68 years and older identified from the SEER-Medicare databases, the population-attributable fraction of diabetes and obesity was 36.6%, greater than that of alcohol (23.5%), HCV (22.4%), and HBV (6.3%).[63] Assuming that only 10% of the approximately 90 million people in the United States with NAFLD have NASH, that only 25% of these will develop

cirrhosis, and that only 25% of these patients will develop HCC, more than 500,000 subjects in the United States are at risk for HCC as a result of NAFLD alone.[24] Between 15% and 50% of HCC arises in the setting of cryptogenic cirrhosis.[21] Given similar associations between obesity and diabetes mellitus with NASH-cirrhosis and cryptogenic cirrhosis, NASH likely accounts for the majority of HCC arising in cryptogenic cirrhosis.[21,64] Risk factors for HCC in the setting of NASH include advanced age, advanced fibrosis, diabetes mellitus, obesity, and the rs738409 single nucleotide polymorphism of palatin-like phospholipase domain-containing 3 (PNPLA3), which encodes for adiponutrin, a triacylglycerol lipase that mediates triglyceride lipolysis in hepatocytes.[20,65–68] Visceral fat accumulation and older age have also been shown to be risk factors for cancer recurrence after RFA of HCC among NASH patients who were previously treatment naïve.[69]

Caution must be exercised when examining series that ascribe HCC arising in patients with the metabolic syndrome and without histologic examination of the background liver as resulting from NASH. Deleterious effects of metabolic syndrome elements itself (rather than associated liver injury) may lead to HCC.[62,70–72] Diabetes and obesity have been shown to promote HCC in the setting of chronic liver diseases other than NAFLD, such as hepatitis viral infections and alcoholic liver disease.[8,70,73,74] Background steatosis also affects survival after HCC treatment because of other background liver diseases. Among 188 patients who underwent resection of early-stage HCC because of HBV (75%) or HCV (23%), background hepatic steatosis and steatohepatitis were associated with poorer overall survival after resection among all patients and among patients with and without cirrhosis.[75]

HCC in the setting of NASH has distinctive features when compared with other chronic liver diseases (see Chapters 68, 74, 87, and 89). NASH patients with HCC are more often female, are older at HCC diagnosis, have higher BMI, and more often have components of the metabolic syndrome compared with counterparts with HCV infection or alcoholic liver disease.[7,20,60,76,77] We compared outcomes of 52 patients who underwent liver resection or transplantation for HCC in the setting of histologic documented NASH with 162 counterparts with HCV and/or alcoholic liver disease.[76] As found in other studies, 29% of patients with NASH-HCC did not have bridging fibrosis or cirrhosis, suggesting that NASH itself may be carcinogenic independent of cirrhosis.[21,76,78] As a result, patients with surgically treatable HCC in the setting of NASH had lower Model for End-Stage Liver Disease

(MELD) scores and better synthetic function at HCC diagnosis compared with counterparts with HCV and/or alcoholic liver disease. As in other studies, we found that no difference in recurrence-free survival between NASH-HCC and HCV/ethyl alcohol (ETOH)-HCC patients (median 60 vs. 56 months). In contrast, overall survival was longer among NASH patients (median not reached vs. 52 months, $P = .009$). Given similarities in tumor stage and clinicopathologic characteristics, most patients had early-stage HCC and well-compensated disease at HCC diagnosis, and the most common cause of death was liver failure, this difference in overall survival was likely due to the more severe background liver disease among patients with HCV-ETOH. Similar studies are summarized in Table 69.1.

HCC in livers with background steatohepatitis have a characteristic appearance labeled "steatohepatitic hepatocellular carcinoma (SH-HCC)." These tumors have features resembling nonneoplastic steatohepatitis, including large-droplet steatosis, ballooning of malignant hepatocytes, pericellular fibrosis, and intratumoral inflammatory cell infiltration (Fig. 69.6).[85,86] The largest liver resection series of SH-HCC comprises 51 patients, nearly half of which occurred in the setting of HCV.[86] In comparison to conventional HCC, background steatosis and steatohepatitis was more commonly observed in SH-HCC compared with conventional HCC (53% vs. 9%, $P < .0001$). Steatohepatitic features did not affect overall or disease-free survival after liver resection. Other studies have also noted the higher prevalence of metabolic syndrome elements and background NAFLD between SH-HCC and conventional HCC.[87,88]

TABLE 69.1   Studies Comparing Hepatocellular Carcinoma in Background Nonalcoholic Steatohepatitis Versus Other Chronic Liver Diseases

REFERENCE	PATIENTS	THERAPY	DFS	OS	COMMENTS
Sadler (2018)[79]	60 NASH vs. 869 non-NASH	Transplant	5-yr 89% vs. 66% ($P = .08$)	5-yr 80% vs. 78% ($P = .1$)	No difference in tumor recurrence (13% vs. 14%), greater proportion of extrahepatic recurrence in NASH. NASH protective for recurrence in tumors outside Milan (HR 0.21).
Lewin (2017)[80]	271 NASH vs. 3462 non-NASH	Transplant			NASH has lower likelihood of high-risk explant features.
Weinman (2015)[81]	45 NASH vs. 1074 non-NASH	Transplant, resection, regional, systemic, supportive		Median survival 11.3 vs. 15.5 ($P = .3$)	Only a small number of NASH-HCC received resection or transplant
Hernandez-Alejandro (2012)[82]	102 NASH vs. 283 HCV	Transplant	5-yr 80% vs. 70%	—	Vascular invasion and poor differentiation more common in NASH-HCC.
Reddy (2012)[76]	52 NASH vs. 162 HCV ± ETOH	Resection and transplant	Median 60 vs. 56 mo	Median not reached vs. 52 mo	NASH patients older; more often female and had the metabolic syndrome. Overall survival difference statistically significant.
Tokushige (2010)[83]	34 NASH vs. 56 HCV	Resection, ablation, TACE	Median 34.8 vs. 34.8 mo	—	Tumor size and fibrosis stage risk factors for recurrence among NASH patients.
Wakai (2011)[84]	17 NAFLD vs. 61 HBV vs. 147 HCV	Resection	5-yr 66% vs. 39% vs. 25%	5-yr 59% vs. 63% vs. 57%	NAFLD patients older, higher BMI, and larger tumors. Recurrence-free survival difference statistically significant.

BMI, Body mass index; *ETOH,* ethyl alcohol; *HBV,* hepatitis B virus; *HCC,* hepatocellular cancer; *HCV,* hepatitis C virus; *HR,* hazard ratio; *NAFLD,* nonalcoholic fatty liver disease; *NASH,* nonalcoholic steatohepatitis; *TACE,* transarterial chemoembolization.

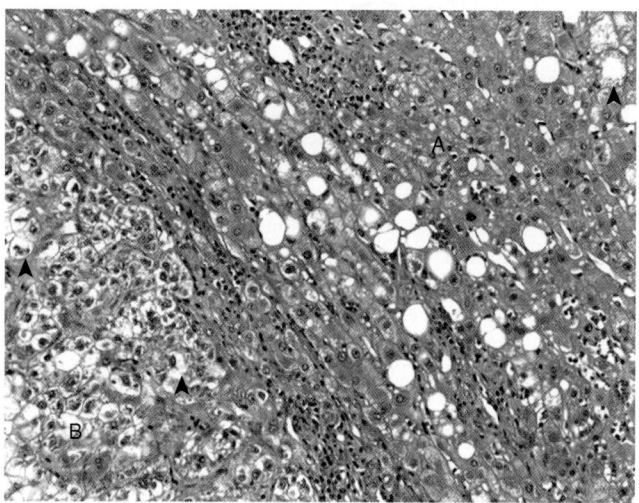

FIGURE 69.6 **Steatohepatitic-hepatocellular carcinoma (HCC) in the setting of nonalcoholic steatohepatitis.** Note the steatosis and hepatocyte ballooning degeneration *(arrowheads)* in the background liver *(A)* and HCC *(B).* Stained with hematoxylin and eosin, magnification ×200. (Courtesy Schuyler O. Sanderson, MD.)

CHEMOTHERAPY-MEDIATED HEPATOTOXICITY

As perioperative chemotherapy is part of the treatment for CRLM, consideration of chemotherapy-associated liver injury is important (see Chapters 90 and 98). Types of liver injury are specific to regimen of chemotherapy. 5-Fluorouracil has long been recognized in causing "simple" hepatic steatosis in 30% to 47% of treated patients.[31,32] Steatosis and steatohepatitis have been associated with diabetes, obesity (as measured by BMI), and irinotecan therapy in many studies,[89–91] a relationship confirmed by animal models.[92] Other studies have noted only a relationship with irinotecan and steatohepatitis, but not steatosis.[93,94] A two-phase mechanism by which irinotecan may cause steatohepatitis has been proposed in which components of the metabolic syndrome (especially insulin resistance) leads to excess fatty-acid deposition in hepatocytes resulting in increased production of reactive oxidation species. These steatotic hepatocytes are more susceptible to another insult (e.g., chemotherapy treatment) acting as a "second hit" leading to further mitochondrial damage and generation of more reactive oxidation species–mediated hepatocyte damage.[31,32] Studies showing that both metabolic factors and irinotecan therapy contribute to steatohepatitis or that suggest a synergistic relationship between obesity and irinotecan in promoting steatohepatitis support this hypothesis.[89,93] Finally, some reports note no association between any chemotherapy agent and steatohepatitis—citing only a relationship with obesity.[95–97] Grossly, fatty livers with steatohepatitis exhibit a yellow appearance with rounded edges (see Fig. 69.6A). Reasons for this lack of association include discrepancies in histopathologic assessment, the overall relatively high prevalence of NAFLD attenuating the influence of chemotherapy on FLD, and differences in interval between last dose of chemotherapy and hepatic resection and durations of preoperative treatment.[94]

Oxaliplatin treatment before liver resection for CRCLM is associated with hepatic SI. Up to 74% of patients treated with oxaliplatin will have some degree of SI with moderate to severe injury in 54% of patients.[33] Sinusoidal obstruction, centrilobular perisinusoidal and venular fibrosis, and nodular regenerative hyperplasia have been reported with oxaliplatin therapy.[33,94,96,97] The appearance of these livers is a striking patchy "blue" mottling. These more severe manifestations of SI are associated with prolonged therapy, particularly with more than six cycles of treatment.[98–102] However, SI has been observed with less than six cycles of oxaliplatin.[34] Through mechanisms not yet defined, concomitant bevacizumab reduces both the frequency and severity of SI.[33,94,99,103,104]

SAFETY OF LIVER RESECTION WITH FATTY LIVER DISEASE AND SINUSOIDAL INJURY

Many risk factors predisposing to background liver injury are associated with poor outcomes after liver resection (see Chapters 101 and 102). The presence of the metabolic syndrome and individual elements are associated within superficial surgical-site infections, sepsis, acute renal failure, and cardiopulmonary morbidity and mortality after liver resection.[105–107] NASH has been shown to be an independent risk factor for subclinical atherosclerosis,[108] atherosclerosis progression,[109] and overall cardiovascular morbidity.[110] Thus the presence of NASH may increase the likelihood of cardiopulmonary morbidity after liver resection.[71] Prospective randomized controlled trials have shown an increase in postoperative morbidity—particularly bile leaks—after liver resection with preoperative chemotherapy. In the EORTC 40983 Intergroup trial, patients treated with six cycles of FOLFOX before liver resection had an increased proportion of postoperative complications (25% vs. 16%, P = .04), particularly bile leaks (8% vs. 4%,).[111] A phase II trial of FOLFIRI + bevacizumab for initially resectable CRCLM reported a bile leak proportion of 32.4%.[112] Although many scoring systems have been developed to noninvasively measure NASH-associated fibrosis[55,113,114] that predict long-term mortality and cirrhosis development,[115–117] the use of these scoring systems for the safety of liver resection has not been evaluated.

Several series have analyzed the impact of underlying liver injury on postoperative outcomes after partial hepatectomy (Table 69.2). A meta-analysis shows that both mild (relative risk [RR], 1.53 [1.27–1.85]; P < .001) and moderate-severe (RR, 2.01 [1.66–2.44]; P < .001) steatosis is associated with increased complications after major liver resection (more than three segments), but only moderate-severe steatosis was associated with increased postoperative mortality (RR, 2.79 [1.19–2.79]; P = .02).[118] Among patients with the metabolic syndrome, resection of HCC in the setting of a NAS of 2 or greater was independently associated with severe cardiorespiratory and liver-specific complications.[119]

Other studies have noted that elements associated with liver injury such as chemotherapy treatment[120] or components of the metabolic syndrome are associated with poor outcomes after liver resection. However, these studies are unable to determine if the poor outcomes are due to the result of histologic injury to the underlying liver or from other side effects of these elements that predispose to liver injury. To address this issue, we performed a cohort-matched comparison of noncirrhotic patients with hepatic steatosis greater than 33% or steatohepatitis with respective matched controls with no underlying liver disease.[121] Controls were selected not only for demographics, comorbid conditions, and extent of hepatic resection, but also for possible causes of FLD. Thus our study uniquely accounts for the morbidity derived from these factors separate from underlying liver

TABLE 69.2 Studies Evaluating Outcomes After Liver Resection With Background Steatosis, Steatohepatitis, or Sinusoidal Injury

REFERENCE	PATIENTS	MORBIDITY	MORTALITY	COMMENTS
Reissfelder (2014)[91]	None-light inflammation (n = 87) Mild-severe inflammation (n = 37)	54% vs. 23% P = .04	—	—
Aloia (2006)[98]	HCN/RNH (n = 22) No HCN/RNH (n = 70)	—	—	HCN/RNH associated with need for blood transfusion.
Wolf (2013)[89]	Steatosis (n = 134) No steatosis (n = 250)	38% vs. 35% P = NS	0% vs. 1.2% P = NS	No injury was associated with liver-related, infectious, or major morbidity.
	Steatohepatitis (n = 16) No steatohepatitis (n = 368)	63% vs. 35% P = NS	0% vs. 0.8% P = NS	
	SI (n = 39) No SI (n = 344)	46% vs. 35% P = NS	0% vs. 0.9% P = NS	
Gomez (2007)[123]	Steatosis (n = 194) No steatosis (n = 192)	49.5% vs. 22.4% P < .001	2.6% vs. 1.0% P = NS	
McCormack (2007)[124]	Steatosis (n = 58) No steatosis (n = 58)	50% vs. 25% P = .007	8.5% vs. 1.7% P = 0.21	Matched cohort study. Major resections only. Increased blood loss and frequency of blood transfusions with hepatic steatosis.
Vauthey (2006)[93]	Steatohepatitis (n = 34) No steatohepatitis (n = 372)	—	14.7% vs. 1.6% P = 0.001	Irinotecan was associated with steatohepatitis.
Makoweic (2011)[95]	Steatosis (n = 37) No steatosis (n = 65)	60% vs. 42% P = NS	NS	No histologic injury was associated with liver-related morbidity.
	Moderate-severe steatohepatitis (n = 23) None-mild steatohepatitis (n = 79)	61% vs. 44% P = NS	NS	
	Moderate-severe SI (n = 40) None-mild SI (n = 62)	50% vs. 47% P = NS	NS	
Nakano (2008)[125]	SI (n = 20) No SI (n = 16)	40.0% vs. 6.3% P = .026	NS	Major resections only. No influence of steatosis on post-operative outcomes.
Ramos (2016)[126]	Steatosis (421) No steatosis (513)	32% vs. 31% NS	3.2% vs. 3.5% NS	Resection for colorectal liver metastases, steatosis had a better 5 yr-survival on univariate.
D'Assignies (2016)[127]	Steatosis (n = 25) No steatosis (n = 100)	48% vs. 28% P = .04	NS	Steatosis defined by MRI liver fat fraction >5%, longer hospital stays, more pulmonary complications and more severe postoperative complications.
Reddy (2012)[76]	Steatosis (n = 72) No steatosis (n = 72)	34.7% vs. 44.4% P = NS	4.2% vs. 1.4% P = NS	Matched cohort study. Steatohepatitis associated with liver-related morbidity.
	Steatohepatitis (n = 102) No steatohepatitis (n = 102)	56.9% vs. 37.3% P = .008	3.9% vs. 1.0% P = NS	

HCN, Hemorrhagic centrilobular necrosis; *RNH,* regenerative nodular hyperplasia; *MRI,* magnetic resonance imaging; *NS,* not significant; *SI,* sinusoidal injury.

injury and assesses the impact of this injury on postoperative outcomes on patients with a variety of benign and malignant diagnoses, unlike most other studies, which exclusively examine patients with CRCLM (see Table 69.2). We observed that patients with steatohepatitis had higher overall (56.9% vs. 37.3%, P = .008) and hepatic-related (28.4% vs. 15.7%, P = .043) morbidity after liver resection compared with matched controls. In contrast, there was no difference in any postoperative outcome between patients with hepatic steatosis and matched controls. The deleterious effects of steatohepatitis were maintained on multivariable analysis in the entire study population for overall (RR, 2.32 [1.27–4.24]; P = .007) and hepatic-related (RR, 2.72 [1.20–6.17]; P = .016) morbidity. Importantly, the cause of background liver injury was not associated with hepatic-related postoperative outcomes, indicating that hepatic-related morbidity in patients with steatohepatitis is the result of liver injury and not from other side effects derived from factors that predispose to this injury. Our results also

stress the importance of discerning between steatosis and steatohepatitis and may explain the inconsistency regarding the impact of severity of steatosis on postoperative outcomes observed in other studies.[71,122]

Knowledge of background hepatic injury will alter preoperative management aimed at improving the safety of liver resection. Patients with suspected NAFLD should be subjected to extensive cardiopulmonary evaluation to avoid corresponding postoperative morbidity. A key factor in determining postoperative outcome after resection is the volume of liver remnant as this is a surrogate for liver function. With normal liver, a 20% liver remnant is sufficient. However, at least 30% is required for liver subject to steatohepatitis or SI and 40% more required with a cirrhotic liver.[128] Recognition of these liver injuries may alter treatment strategies aimed at increasing anticipated liver remnant volume before liver resection with preoperative portal vein embolization or employment of combination resection and ablation as a parenchymal-sparing strategy.[128–131]

SECTION I. Inflammatory, Infective, and Congenital

B. Liver Infection and Infestation

CHAPTER 70

Pyogenic liver abscess

Martin de Santibañes, Oscar Mazza, and Eduardo de Santibañes

OVERVIEW

Pyogenic liver abscess (PLA) may be solitary or multiple collections of pus within the liver, the result of bacterial infection. PLA causes significant morbidity, mortality, and increased consumption of healthcare resources. PLA represents the most common visceral abscess, with an incidence of 5 to 20 in 100,000 hospitalizations in the Western population.[1] In 1938 Ochsner et al.[2] reported the first series of patients with hepatic abscesses in the modern surgical era treated by surgical drainage. This study included 47 patients and reported an overall survival of 67%. The advent of antibiotic therapy marked the basis of the contemporary treatment of liver abscesses, becoming a major part of the therapy, combined with surgical drainage. The first landmark report in minimally invasive treatment of liver abscess was that of McFadzean et al. in 1953.[3] They presented a group of 14 patients who underwent percutaneous drainage for PLAs with no deaths within the group. Although potentially effective for dealing with the acute problem, such approaches are associated with the disadvantage of overlooking the underlying abdominal pathology because of the lack of surgical exploration.

The development of clinical ultrasound (US) in the 1960s and the introduction of computed tomography (CT) in the 1970s represent the two major advances in the diagnosis and treatment of PLAs. Surgical exploration as a diagnostic tool was replaced by abdominal imaging, thus allowing minimally invasive techniques to become the first choice of treatment. Currently, percutaneous needle aspiration (PNA) and percutaneous catheter drainage (PCD) have become standard methods for both single and multiple PLAs (see Chapter 31). Surgical debridement, done either in an open or a laparoscopic fashion, has a limited therapeutic role for patients in whom nonoperative treatment fails or in those requiring surgical treatment for the underlying cause of the abscess. In addition, surgical exploration may be indicated as the initial procedure when coexistence of peritonitis is suspected as result of abscess rupture into the peritoneal cavity.

ETIOLOGY

During the 19th century, PLAs were well known as a complication of acute appendicitis. Since then, etiology and presentation have dramatically changed. Inflammatory abdominal diseases are no longer the most common underlying conditions for PLAs, being replaced in later decades by a higher incidence of biliary causes, including malignancies, immunocompromised status, and advanced age.[4] In 1996 Huang et al. (1996)[1] presented a review that spanned more than 40 years in the treatment of PLAs. They analyzed and compared patterns of clinical presentation in 80 patients treated between 1952 and 1972 with a second group of 153 patients treated from 1973 to 1993. The authors concluded that the increased incidence of biliary malignancies as a cause of PLAs was due to a more aggressive approach in the treatment of this pathology, which includes more frequent instrumentation of the biliary tree (see Chapters 30, 31, 51, and 52). Hilar cholangiocarcinoma was the most frequent single condition found during the second period reviewed, with the use of biliary stents and broad-spectrum antibiotics leading to the emergence of mixed bacterial and fungal infections (see Chapters 51 and 52). Biliary malignancy was an important risk factor for hospital mortality.[5]

Elucidating the underlying condition that caused a liver abscess is as important therapeutically as the correct treatment of a PLA. In a simplified schema, infection may get to the liver by five different avenues: (1) portal vein, (2) hepatic artery, (3) biliary tree, (4) adjacent organ infection, and (5) direct trauma to the liver. The term *cryptogenic PLA* applies when no underlying pathology is identified (Box 70.1).

Portal pyemia is often a consequence of intraabdominal infection, such as acute appendicitis or diverticulitis. The incidence of this mechanism as a cause of PLA has markedly decreased in the past years. However, portal vein patency must be evaluated with Doppler US or dynamic CT scan in patients with PLAs (see Chapter 14). Gastrointestinal (GI) malignancies, such as colorectal adenocarcinoma or even gastric carcinoma, may also lead to a disruption of the mucosal barrier, leading to pyemia and liver abscess in the absence of liver metastasis.[6] This phenomenon should be particularly considered in the evaluation of patients with a cryptogenic PLA.[7] Adequate investigation of etiology after PLA treatment may lead to a diagnosis of an underlying disease previously unknown for the patient.[8]

Hematogenous spread of infection through the hepatic artery may also cause PLA. Frequent examples are bacterial endocarditis and intravenous drug abuse, but certain immunosuppressive conditions may also be associated with this mechanism. Liver cirrhosis is often associated with immunodeficiency, and the incidence of liver abscesses in cirrhotic patients compared with the general population is increased (see Chapters 10 and 74).[9] Loss of hepatic filter function, impaired immunity, and frequent

---

BOX 70.1   Classification of PLA According to the Underlying Mechanism of Dissemination

Hepatobiliary
Cholelithiasis
  Benign strictures
  Acute cholangitis
  Periampullary tumors
  Gallbladder cancer

Portal
Diverticulitis
  Anorectal suppuration
  Pelvic suppuration
  Postoperative sepsis
  Intestinal perforation
  Pancreatic abscess
  Appendicitis
  Chronic inflammatory bowel disease
  Colonic cancer
  Gastric cancer

Arterial
Endocarditis
  Vascular sepsis
  Ear, throat, nose, or dental infection

Traumatic
Open or closed abdominal trauma
  Chemoembolization
  Percutaneous ethanol injection or radiofrequency ablation

Adjacent Abdominal Pathology
Acute cholecystitis
  Gastroduodenal perforation
  Colonic perforation
  Cryptogenic

PLA, Pyogenic liver abscess.

---

abdominal infections may also be responsible factors. Immunosuppressive drug use, alcoholism, chronic pancreatitis, pyelonephritis, and acquired immunodeficiency syndrome are also associated with PLA.[1]

Adult liver transplant recipients differ from the general population with respect to the type of PLA they contract, the reasons for which are many: reconstructed biliary anatomy, recurrent hospitalizations, poor clinical condition, and immunosuppression. A recent study showed that patients with post–liver transplant PLA were more likely to have lower body mass index ($P = .006$), to have renal failure ($P = .031$), and to have undergone retransplantation ($P = .002$). A history of hepatic artery thrombosis ($P = .010$), the presence of Roux en-Y hepatojejunostomy ($P < 0.001$), and longer organ ischemia time ($P = .009$) were independent predictors for the development of post–liver transplant PLA.[10]

The incidence of diabetes mellitus varies among different series, but its presence is associated with a 10-fold increased risk for PLA compared with that of the general population. Diabetes mellitus was the most common comorbidity in a report of PLA from Taiwan and was present in 41 (16%) of 253 patients with PLA.[11] Type 2 diabetes mellitus was significantly associated with increased hazard of PLA (hazard ratio [HR], 2.88; 95% confidence interval, 2.73–3.04). Age and gender may significantly modify the relationship between type 2 diabetes mellitus and PLA, with a higher HR noted in male patients and those less than 45 years old.[12]

Biliary pathology has become the most identifiable cause of PLA in recent decades.[13] In this group of patients, infection may have different etiologies. Bile duct strictures, common bile duct stones, and hepatolithiasis are benign conditions that are associated with PLA (see Chapters 33, 34, 37, 39, and 41–44). Benign diseases are more commonly reported in Asia[5]; in Western countries, however, biliary malignancy is a more prevalent condition. Instrumentation of bile duct obstruction by endoscopic stenting or percutaneous drainage is a frequent cause of cholangitis and PLA. Malignancy is a predictor of higher recurrence and mortality rates. The mortality rate of PLA caused by underlying malignant disease is almost twice as high as that of nonmalignant disease.[14] In addition, a population-based study demonstrated that the incidence of GI cancer is increased more than 4-fold among patients with PLA compared with control participants. Patients with PLA had a higher incidence of colorectal cancer, followed by cancers of the biliary tract, pancreas, and small intestine.[15] The authors suggest further evaluation of these patients to allow early diagnosis of these malignancies.

Direct liver contamination by adjacent organ infection may produce a PLA, with acute cholecystitis the most common example (see Chapter 34). However, gastric and duodenal perforation directly into the liver may also give rise to a PLA. Perforation secondary to foreign bodies, mainly from fish bones, have been also reported. In addition, liver parenchyma may become infected after direct damage. Intrahepatic biloma, hematoma, and necrotic parenchyma are favorable conditions for development of a PLA. This is a well-known consequence of blunt or penetrating liver trauma and liver resections.

In recent decades, local treatments for liver tumors have become a widespread alternative for many patients. These local techniques include ethanol injection, transarterial chemoembolization, selective internal radiation therapy, and radiofrequency ablation (RFA) (see Chapters 94 and 96), which induce tumor necrosis either by chemical or thermal tissue destruction. In all these patients, PLA is a potentially life-threatening complication that may occur up to 5 months after a successful procedure. Transarterial liver embolization may be helpful in patients with hepatocellular carcinoma or liver metastases of GI sarcomas and neuroendocrine tumors. The incidence of liver abscess after this procedure is low. Ong et al. (2004)[16] reported PLAs in 0.26% of 3878 embolizations; the mortality rate in these patients was 33%. Patients with bilioenteric anastomosis are at particular risk for this complication. The odds ratio (OR) for developing PLA in this population was 894 in a series from Philadelphia.[17] Subjacent pathology is not a predisposing factor for this complication,[18] but RFA of liver tumors may also cause a PLA. In a multicenter study from Italy, Livraghi et al. (2003)[19] reported 2320 patients with 3554 lesions, with a 0.3% incidence of PLA. This incidence was slightly higher (1.7%) in another group of patients with hepatocellular carcinoma treated by RFA.[20] De Baere et al. (2003)[21] reported a 100% incidence of liver abscess in patients with prior bilioenteric anastomosis who underwent RFA. A further prospective analysis showed an incidence of PLA of 50% in patients with biliary diversions, but the risk was not increased if this diversion was performed synchronously with the ablation procedure.[22]

In some patients with a PLA, no underlying cause is identified; they are considered to have a cryptogenic PLA. These cases account for as many as 67% in some published data.[11] Patients with cryptogenic PLA are at a 7-fold increased risk of having colorectal cancer. A screening colonoscopy may be considered in the population with cryptogenic PLA, especially if

TABLE 70.1 Demographics, Origin, and Mortality Rates of PLAs in Eastern and Western Series

REFERENCE, COUNTRY, YEAR	NO. PATIENTS	AGE (YEARS)	DIABETES (%)	BILIARY (%)	CRYPTOGENIC (%)	SOLITARY (%)	RIGHT LOBE (%)	MORTALITY (%)
Mangukiya, India, 2012[24]	400	35	—	15.5	56	50	83	—
Chen et al., Taiwan, 2008[11]	253	56.4	41.9	29.6	67.2	67.6	71.5	9.1
Lok et al., Hong Kong, 2008[5]	111	62.6	18.9	22.5	53	80.2	67.6	11.7
Eroles Vega et al., Spain, 2008[25]	68	63	6	37	35	56	19	—
Seeto & Rockey, United States, 1996[26]	142	51	15	37	40	61	58	10
Czerwonko et al., Argentina, 2018[10]	142	60	—	47.9	23.2	45.8	63.4	7.7
Alvarez et al., Spain, 2001[13]	133	16-92 (range)	12	18.5	25.5	73	71.5	14

PLAs, Pyogenic liver abscesses.

positive for *Klebsiella pneumoniae.*[23] Etiology and presentation are summarized in Table 70.1.[24–26]

INCIDENCE

PLA is a rare disease, and actual incidence rates are poorly described in the literature. However, recent investigations demonstrated a marked increase of PLA incidence in the general population in the last few years. Huang et al. (1996)[1] showed that PLA accounted for 13 per 100,000 hospital admissions in 1973, which increased to as many as 20 per 100,000 only 20 years later. In a recent study from a teaching hospital in the United Kingdom, PLA had an incidence of 18.5 per 100,000 hospital admissions, with an estimated crude incidence of 2.3 cases per 100,000 general population.[8]

Two recent studies demonstrated this tendency in both Eastern and Western countries. In 2008 Tsai et al. published an analysis of PLA in the Taiwanese population from 1996 through 2004. The incidence of PLA rose from 11.15 to 17.59 cases per 100,000 inhabitants over the period of study, with more than 30,000 cases occurring in this period. Of these patients, 62% were male; the age of highest incidence in men was 80 to 84 years, and for women it was 85 to 89 years. Factors associated with PLA were diabetes, malignancy, renal disease, and pneumonia. The incidence of liver abscess is high among end-stage renal disease dialysis patients. In addition to the well-known risk factors of liver abscess, two other important risk factors, peritoneal dialysis and polycystic kidney disease, were found to predict liver abscess in end-stage renal disease dialysis patients.[27] Mortality rates, however, decreased from 12.33% in 1996 to 9.72% in 2004.

The second, a national series from Denmark,[28] analyzed 1448 cases in a 25-year period; 54% were male. The incidence of PLA in Danish men was 6 per million in 1977 and 18 per million in 2002. In women, the incidence rose from 8 per million to 12 per million in the same period. Mortality rates in 1977 were 40% and 50% for men and women, respectively, and decreased to a global rate of 10% in 2002.

CLINICAL PRESENTATION

Liver abscesses may have a broad array of symptoms and physical findings, which may vary according to the patient's underlying condition. Cryptogenic lesions are often found after several days of nonspecific symptoms. The most frequent clinical features include fever of more than 38°C and chills. Other symptoms that may be present are general malaise and anorexia. Patients may also have abdominal pain, nausea and vomiting, diarrhea, and weight loss. Although more often found with abscesses of biliary origin, jaundice may be an indicator of systemic sepsis response, and septic shock may be a dramatic form of the presentation. There are no significant differences in clinical presentation between single and multiple lesions, although single PLAs are more frequent in the right lobe of the liver. These symptoms may be present from several days up to several weeks before hospital admission.[26,29] In another group of patients, PLA is a consequence of an underlying pathologic process that may lead to a faster diagnosis. Benign or malignant biliary disease, intraabdominal infections, and abdominal surgery are frequent causes of abscesses, and imaging studies should be systematically carried out to exclude the presence of a PLA in a septic patient. Another study compared the clinical presentations among different causative pathogens, including *K. pneumoniae,* and there were no significant differences among the causative pathogens.[30]

Finally, some patients may be seen with systemic complications as a result of metastatic septic lesions that originate from a PLA. Although rare, cases of endophthalmitis; meningitis; cellulitis; lung abscess; prostate, kidney, and joint infections; pulmonary emboli; and even cardiac tamponade due to pericardiac effusion have been reported in the literature.[31,32] Infection by *K. pneumoniae* genotype K1 and immunosuppression resulting from diabetes mellitus and alcohol intake may be predisposing factors for these complications.[33,34]

The risk factors associated with PLA mortality include gender, jaundice, rupture of liver abscess, and multiple organ failure. Multiple organ failure, initial low blood pressure, and initial respiratory distress are poor prognostic factors that result from higher disease severity contributing to higher mortality.[35]

DIAGNOSIS

The most common laboratory findings are nonspecific alterations as a result of infection. In a large series from Hong Kong, low albumin levels were found in 92.8% of patients seen with PLAs.[5] Leukocytosis (74.8%), increased alkaline phosphatase (72.1%), and elevated alanine aminotransferase levels (ALT; 58.6%) were frequent laboratory abnormalities also present

TABLE 70.2 Laboratory Data of 72 Patients With PLA on the First Day of Intensive Care

VARIABLE	SURVIVORS (n = 52)	NONSURVIVORS (n = 20)	P VALUE
WBC count (10³/mm³)	16.5 ± 18	16.4 ± 14	.99
Hemoglobin (g/dL)	11.3 ± 2	10.4 ± 3	.17
Platelet (10³/mm³)	202 ± 175	196 ± 133	.89
ALK-p (IU/L)	182 ± 134	168 ± 105	.75
AST (IU/L)	127 ± 176	562 ± 1571	.28
ALT (IU/L)	105 ± 144	234 ± 468	.09
Total bilirubin (mg/dL)	2.5 ± 2	2.6 ± 2	.89
C-reactive protein (mg/dL)	25.8 ± 10	23.8 ± 9	.61
BUN (mg/dL)	32 ± 22	38 ± 19	.29
Creatinine (mg/dL)	1.9 ± 2	2.9 ± 2	.02
Albumin (g/dL)	2.2 ± 0.6	1.9 ± 0.5	.11
Prothrombin time(s)	16 ± 5	21 ± 5	.01

Data are expressed as mean ± standard deviation.

ALK-p, Alkaline phosphatase; *ALT*, alanine aminotransferase; *AST*, aspartate aminotransferase; *BUN*, blood urea nitrogen; *PLA*, pyogenic liver abscess; *WBC*, white blood cell.

From Chen SC et al. Comparison of pyogenic liver abscesses of biliary and cryptogenic origin: An eight-year analysis in a university hospital. *Swiss Med Wkly*. 2005;135:344–351.

in these patients. Jaundice may be seen in as many as 50% of patients, and alkaline phosphatase, γ-glutamyl transferase, erythrocyte sedimentation rate, and glutamic-oxaloacetic transaminase levels are usually elevated.[35] Alvarez et al. (2001)[13] analyzed laboratory data obtained from patients younger than and older than 60 years. The only significant difference between these two groups was that older patients tended to present with higher blood urea nitrogen and serum creatinine levels. Hemoglobin level, serum C-reactive protein, blood urea nitrogen, creatinine levels, prothrombin time, and total bilirubin levels must be part of systematic laboratory tests in patients with PLA.

Some findings at presentation may be prognostic and associated with increased mortality rate. Chen et al. (2008)[36] presented a review of 72 patients admitted to the intensive care unit. Low levels of serum albumin, increased serum creatinine, and prolonged prothrombin time were significant risk factors for death. These authors' findings are shown in Table 70.2.

The clinical investigations used to evaluate liver abscesses have changed in recent decades. Plain radiographs may be part of the routine evaluation, but these play a minor role in PLA diagnosis. Indirect findings in chest and abdominal radiographs may include atelectasis, an elevated right hemidiaphragm, pleural effusion, enlargement of the liver shadow, and, exceptionally, an air-fluid level in gas-forming bacterial infections.

US imaging is usually the first diagnostic approach in these patients (see Chapter 14). Although US examination may not detect small lesions and those located on the dome, it has several advantages. It is fast, inexpensive, and provides information about biliary tract and gallbladder pathology, the most prevalent conditions that predispose to PLA. The images obtained by this procedure vary according to different stages of evolution of the disease. Anechoic images are infrequent, with most lesions being hypoechoic; most abscesses present with a smooth wall, which thickens with chronicity. Some abscesses have inhomogeneous content, and if pus becomes thick, the lesion may be confused

with liver parenchyma. Gas within an abscess is hyperechoic and casts shadows. Doppler scan should be routinely performed; this may help in differentiating solid tumors, show vessels surrounding the abscess, and, most important, evaluate portal vein patency.

CT has a sensitivity of more than 97% in detecting PLA and is considered the most important imaging modality (see Chapter 14). Examination should be routinely performed with intravenous contrast enhancement. During the arterial phase, parenchyma surrounding the abscess may show segmental enhancement as a result of altered portal microcirculation in the infected tissue. The typical CT image description of PLA is that of a target-like sign that appears as a single or multiloculated mass with a central hypodense region and peripheral contrast enhancement during the portal phase of examination.

CT scan offers the advantage of detecting other intraabdominal pathology that may be the cause of the abscess, such as acute diverticulitis or appendicitis. It may also provide information about portal vein patency and may demonstrate local complications that may include pleural effusion, vascular complications, and spontaneous rupture into the peritoneal cavity, retroperitoneum, and even the pericardium.[37] Finally, CT scan is generally necessary to guide percutaneous drainage of the abscess (Fig. 70.1).

Magnetic resonance imaging (MRI) is an alternative to CT for the diagnosis of PLA. In MRI sequences, PLA appears much the same as other fluid-containing lesions: hypointense in T1-weighted and hyperintense in T2-weighted images (see Chapter 19). After contrast administration, most PLAs show a hyperintense enhancement rim, which may persist in later phases.[38] Infected tumors or metastases may show the same pattern, and differentiation by MRI may be difficult, although diffusion techniques may play a role in distinguishing between benign and neoplasic lesions. MRI is not widely accepted as a first-line diagnostic approach for several reasons: examinations take more time, patient cooperation is needed, and MRI cannot be used as guidance for percutaneous treatment. Nevertheless, it has the advantage of providing data regarding the biliary tract in patients with underlying biliary pathology, findings that could change the therapeutic approach (Fig. 70.2).

Nuclear medicine has a limited role in PLA diagnosis, but in case of doubt, it may be helpful for detecting intraabdominal abscesses. This may be important, for example, in a patient with polycystic liver disease and suspected infection of a single lesion. Indium-111 leukocyte scintigraphy readily detects most hepatic abscess. Gallium-67 may also be used, but it is normally taken up by the liver, making interpretation of the results more difficult. In both cases, prior technetium-99m sulfur colloid scan provides more diagnostic accuracy.[39]

Conflicting results have been reported regarding PLA characteristics according to different origins.[40] Single lesions tend to be cryptogenic, whereas multiple abscesses are more likely to have a biliary origin.[13,41] Regardless of etiology, patients are most commonly seen initially with a single lesion.[42] In both single and multiple forms, abscesses are more frequently located in the right hepatic lobe, followed by a left and bilateral distribution.[11,26]

A PLA less than 2 cm in diameter is described as a *microabscess*. Multiple microabscesses may present as widely scattered lesions or with a cluster pattern that tends to aggregate focally.[43] The diffuse miliary pattern of pyogenic microabscesses is usually staphylococcal in origin, the result of hematogenous spread of an endovascular infection. The cluster pattern is often associated with coliform and enteric organisms and may occur in cholangitic abscesses secondary to biliary obstruction. It is

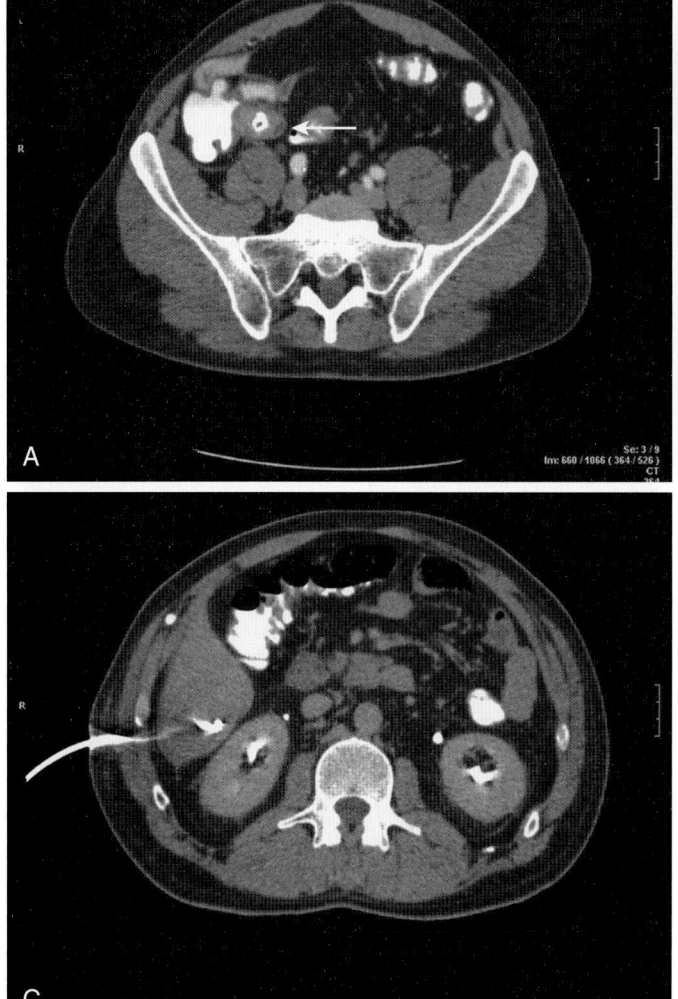

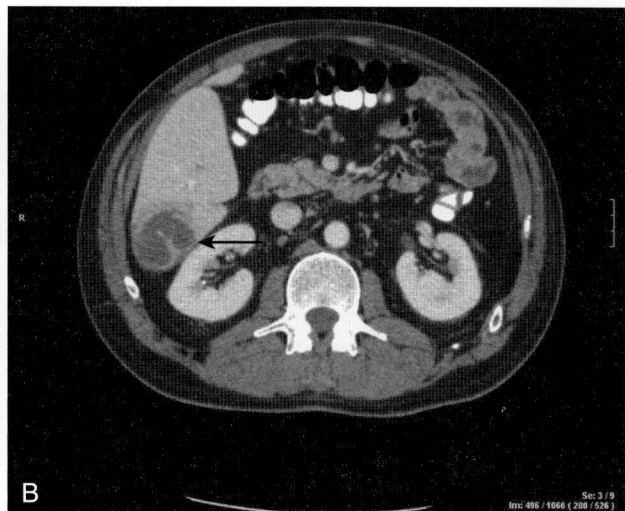

FIGURE 70.1 **A 50-year-old patient seen with fever, leukocytosis, and nonspecific abdominal pain**. **A,** Computed tomography scan showed an inflammatory process in the terminal ileum *(arrow)*. **B,** A single pyogenic liver abscess in the portal phase is located in the posterior segment of the right hepatic lobe *(arrow)*. **C,** Percutaneous drainage was placed at examination.

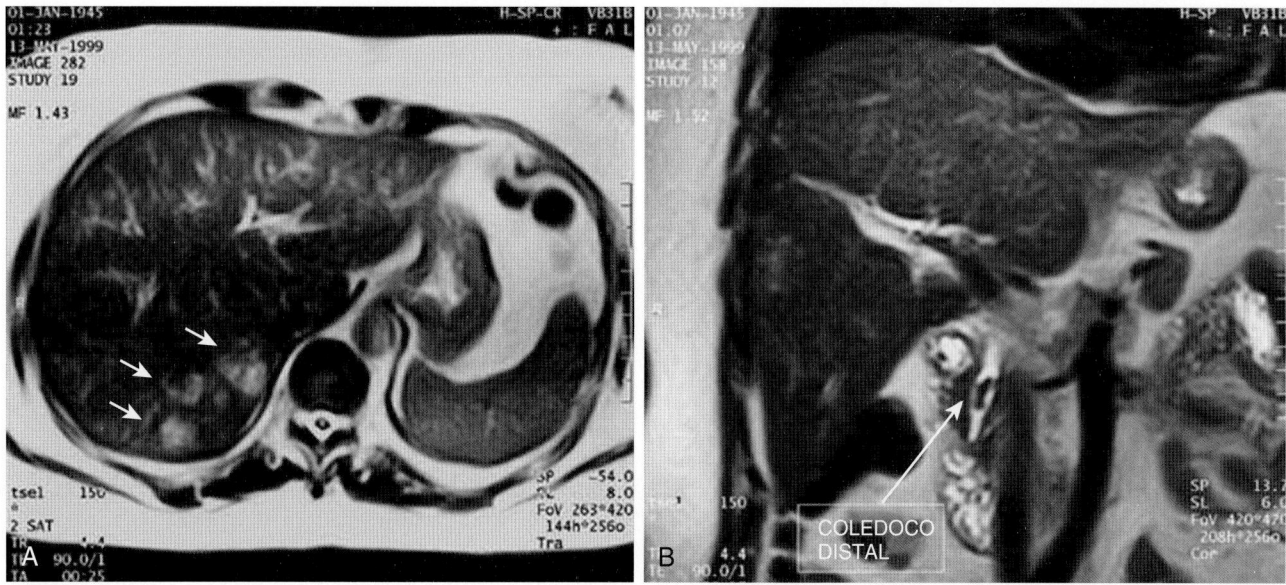

FIGURE 70.2 **A,** Magnetic resonance (MR) image of the liver showing three small pyogenic liver abscesses (PLAs) in the right posterior segment of the liver *(arrows)*. **B,** MR cholangiopancreatography demonstrates a stone in the distal common bile duct originating in the PLAs *(arrow)*.

probable that the clustering of pyogenic microabscesses is an early stage of an evolving pyogenic abscess cavity, and the tendency of coliform microabscesses to coalesce into a larger abscess with intercommunicating cavities explains the success of single-catheter drainage of multiseptate PLAs.

MICROBIOLOGY

Although PLAs may originate from a broad spectrum of microorganisms, the underlying etiology and geographic location of PLAs are often related to specific pathogens. Identification of pathogens may be achieved by direct puncture of the abscess or by blood cultures. The positive abscess culture rates are higher than those of blood culture samples, and only as many as 50% of patients with PLA have both cultures positive.[40] Moreover, negative abscess cultures may be found in 20% of patients.[5] Poor culture technique may be the reason in some cases, but negative cultures can also be caused by the use of broad-spectrum antibiotics before cultures are obtained. Patients with cryptogenic PLAs are more likely to have negative cultures from the blood, whereas patients with PLAs secondary to biliary tract disorders are more likely to have positive cultures from blood and aspirated pus.[26]

In Asian populations, *K. pneumoniae* is the most frequent pathogen associated with cryptogenic PLAs. The incidence of infection with *K. pneumoniae* appears to have markedly increased in this population, ranging from 50% to 88% of all cases occurring in Taiwan in the last few decades to become an endemic disease. *K. pneumoniae* serotype K1 has been observed worldwide and is the most prevalent type among all 77 serotypes.[44] Diabetes mellitus is suggested to be an important risk factor, but the pathogenesis is still unclear. No mutations or clonal spread strains have been found. Environmental or host factors may be responsible for the different incidence rates in Asia compared with Western series.[45] Although PLAs secondary to *K. pneumoniae* infections are associated with an increased risk of septic metastases, overall mortality, even in populations of patients with diabetes, is decreased in this group of patients.[46,47] *K. pneumoniae* K2 is the most frequently isolated serotype after K1, but this serotype has been much less studied.[48]

Gas-forming PLAs are uncommon and often associated with compromised immunity in patients with diabetes, and they present higher mortality rates than non–gas-forming PLAs. *Escherichia coli*, *Enterobacteriaceae*, and *K. pneumoniae* are well-known gas-forming microorganisms. The mechanisms of gas formation involves mixed acid fermentation of glucose, increased production of gas, impaired transportation of gas, and equilibrium between the gas in local tissues and that in abscesses.[49]

E. coli is the most common pathogen in Western countries, in both monomicrobial and polymicrobial isolates, followed by *Streptococcus milleri*. Anaerobes may also be cultured from PLAs, and *Bacteroides* spp. are the most common isolated organisms.[8,41]

An abscess secondary to biliary tract disease or originating from a GI source is more likely to be polymicrobial with aerobic gram-negative organisms and anaerobes. PLAs that result from hematogenous spread, on the other hand, are more likely to be monomicrobial, and staphylococci and streptococci are the most frequent bacteria isolated in these patients. A summarized spectrum of possible pathogens is listed in Box 70.2. The isolation of multidrug-resistant bacteria can be found in up to 11% of patients, and could be explained by the presence of patients with chronic disease and history of prolonged hospitalizations.[10,11]

BOX 70.2 Selected Causative Microorganisms of PLAs

Gram-Negative Aerobes
Escherichia coli
Klebsiella pneumoniae
Pseudomonas aeruginosa
Proteus spp.
Enterobacter cloacae
Citrobacter freundii

Gram-Positive Aerobes
Streptococcus milleri
Staphylococcus aureus
Enterococcus spp.

Gram-Negative Anaerobes
Bacteroides spp.
Fusobacterium spp.

Gram-Positive Anaerobes
Clostridium spp.
Peptostreptococcus spp.

PLAs, Pyogenic liver abscesses.

TREATMENT

The basis for treatment of PLAs relies on complete drainage of pus and infected debris, initiation of adequate antibiotic therapy, and resolution of the underlying cause (see Chapter 31). Modern imaging techniques allow accurate diagnosis, localization, and assessment of dimensions and actual number of lesions (see Chapter 14). US is usually performed as the initial diagnostic approach, and CT scan should be routinely performed, either in cryptogenic suspected lesions or in secondary abscesses. The aim of CT examination is to achieve a complete evaluation of the abdominal cavity to assess any underlying condition that may need further or concomitant treatment. If a biliary origin is suspected, magnetic resonance cholangiopancreatography may be useful to assess the hepatic abscess and completely evaluate the biliary tree. Abdominal imaging has replaced surgical exploration as a diagnostic tool, making possible the high success rates of the percutaneous approach.

During the past several years, treatment of PLAs has shifted toward minimally invasive percutaneous treatment. Nevertheless, treatment options include a wide spectrum that ranges from antibiotic therapy alone to major operative interventions that could include liver debridement and/or resection. Adequate antibiotic selection is critical in the treatment of PLAs. Blood samples should be obtained before starting antibiotics, if possible, but not at the expense of treatment delay in an unstable patient. Broad-spectrum parenteral therapy must begin as soon as possible. Fine-needle aspiration (FNA) or percutaneous drainage may increase the risk of bacteremia, even in stable conditions, so close monitoring of the patient during and after the procedure is always indicated.

The choice of the antimicrobial agent depends on the epidemiology, the patient's background, and the underlying disease, if present, and should be adjusted according to geographic differences and local antimicrobial treatment policies. Empiric treatment of a cryptogenic abscess should be directed to cover the most commonly found organisms: gram-negative bacilli, anaerobes, and microaerophilic streptococci. A classic regimen of ampicillin, an aminoglycoside, and metronidazole may be a first therapeutic approach. Other options include combinations of third-generation cephalosporins or quinolones with metronidazole.

Patients who come to medical attention with secondary PLAs should be treated according to epidemiology and risk factors. Abscess secondary to acute cholangitis after biliary instrumentation and postoperative abscess after abdominal surgery should be treated as nosocomial infections, with a distinct epidemiology and flora compared with cryptogenic lesions. Antibiotic selection should be based primarily on the patient's clinical history and local resistance patterns. Imipenem-cilastatin, vancomycin, and piperacillin-tazobactam therapies should be considered in these cases. A sample culture, whenever possible, is mandatory, and when information regarding the organism and antibiotic sensitivity becomes available, modifications can be instituted.

PLAs must be treated with a prolonged course of antibiotics. Initially, antibiotics should be administrated parenterally. This therapy must be maintained until stabilization of the patient's condition is achieved and for at least 2 weeks thereafter. Criteria for clinical stability include subjective and objective evidence of improvement in the inflammatory response produced by the infection. The patient should be afebrile, with a white cell count trend toward normal and adequate oral intake and GI absorption. The patient may then be switched to oral antibiotic therapy, perhaps even continued on an outpatient basis for at least 2 more weeks. This sequential modality has proven effective in the treatment of PLAs compared with continuous intravenous administration, reducing both the cost of therapy and the length of hospital stay.[50]

Drainage of all lesions may not be possible in patients with multiple small abscesses. In such cases, percutaneous puncture of any of the abscess may be indicated for isolation of the causative bacteria for a rational antibiotic therapy (Fig. 70.3). If a biliary origin of these lesions is suspected, biliary decompression is mandatory, either by endoscopic, percutaneous, or surgical means (see Chapters 29, 30, and 42). The mortality rates reported in patients with multiple liver abscesses are high, ranging from 22% to 44%. However, Giorgio et al. (2006)[51] reported 0% mortality in 39 patients treated with an aggressive approach consisting of PNA of all visible lesions under sonographic guidance and antibiotic therapy.

Drainage of pus is usually necessary for an effective resolution and to shorten the duration of antibiotic therapy, especially in lesions greater than 5 cm in diameter. Drainage can be achieved by nonsurgical methods, such as PCD or PNA. Either open drainage or laparoscopic drainage approaches can be used surgically. Surgical drainage is used only in patients who do not respond to such treatment and currently may be possible laparoscopically.

Percutaneous Treatment

During the last 2 decades, results in patients seen with PLAs have improved as a result of improvements in radiologic diagnosis and percutaneous treatment alternatives. Percutaneous drainage is a safe and effective treatment for almost all PLAs[52] (see Chapter 31). This procedure can be performed under sonographic or CT guidance. The US examination provides real-time guidance of the needle, and it is fast and reliable (Fig. 70.4). Fluoroscopy control and operating theaters under aseptic conditions are recommended. The freehand technique allows dynamic changes in the needle pattern and does not have the limitations of attached needle guides. CT guidance is recommended for multiple abscess drainage, when multiple catheters may be placed, or in cases of hazardous anatomic locations. Local anesthesia and minimal sedation is used for most of these procedures.[51]

After aspiration of a PLA to obtain samples for culture and to confirm the diagnosis, the treatment options are complete aspiration of pus (PNA) or catheter drain insertion (PCD). Controversy persists regarding the optimal procedure, particularly for small abscesses. The first randomized trial conducted by Rajak et al. in 1998[53] showed 100% resolution of PLAs in the PCD group with a 60% success rate in the FNA group. Although FNA patients were given only a second chance of aspiration before placement of a PCD, the thick, viscous nature of the pus was considered a major cause of failure in this group. In a subsequent randomized study conducted by Yu et al. in 2004[54] using intermittent needle aspiration, no significant differences were found between PCD and FNA, suggesting that FNA may be as effective as catheter drainage. However, a tendency toward a shorter hospitalization and lower mortality rate was found in the FNA group. Finally, a third trial randomly assigned 60 patients to FNA or PCD.[55] The authors succeeded in all 30 patients undergoing one or two PCDs. In the FNA group, a 33% failure rate was reported after three aspiration procedures. None of the patients with multiloculated lesions was effectively treated by FNA. The authors recommended PCD as first-line treatment option but considered FNA a valid alternative in simple abscesses smaller than 50 mm in diameter. Several nonrandomized studies report experiences with both therapeutic approaches with good results. The clinical experience of the treating physicians is important in the evaluation of each patient. FNA could be considered as an alternative to routine PCD in patients with small uniloculated lesions, no viscous content, and no communication with the biliary tree.

Regarding the effectiveness of treatment, a current meta-analysis showed a higher rate of success, clinical improvement, and days to achieve a 50% reduction in abscess cavity size in the PCD group compared with the PNA group. This may be a convincing argument in support of the PCD method. No

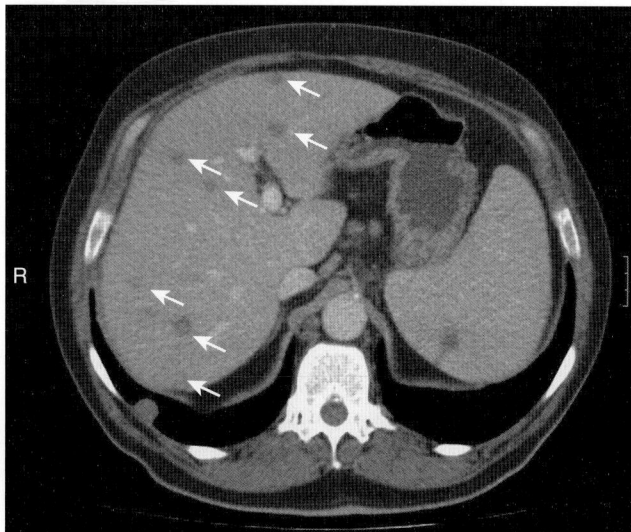

FIGURE 70.3 Multiple microabscesses *(arrows)* in a patient after left colectomy as a result of colon carcinoma. He received intravenous antibiotic therapy for 6 weeks and recovered.

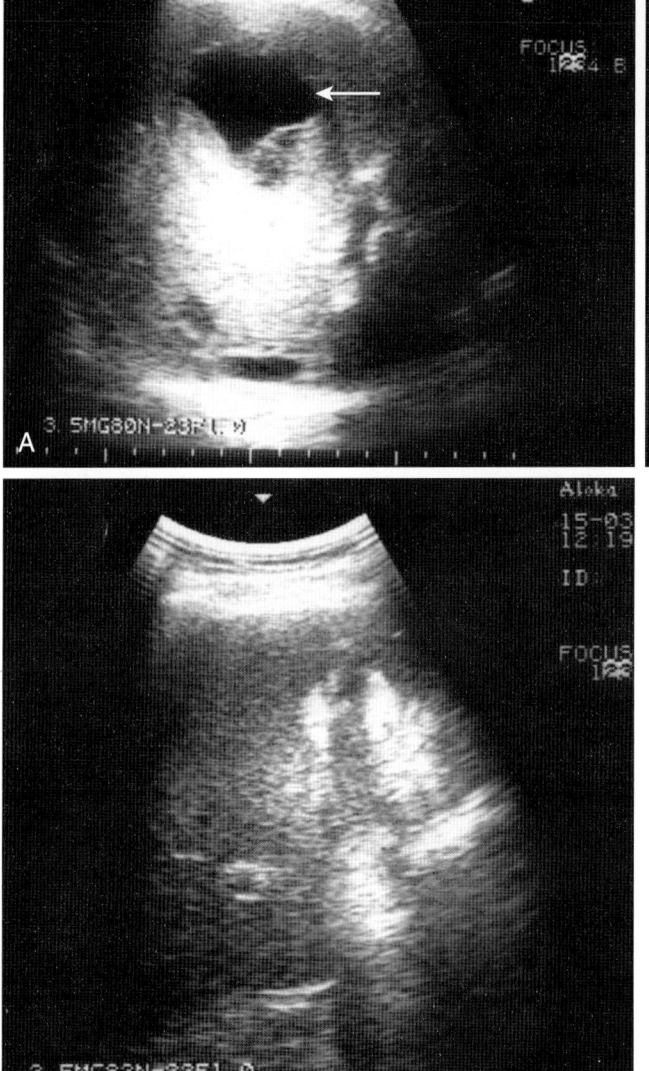

FIGURE 70.4   **A,** Ultrasound-guided drainage of a postoperative pyogenic liver abscess *(arrow)*. **B,** Real-time control showing catheter placement. **C,** After drainage control, showing complete collapse of the cavity.

significant differences were found in duration of hospitalization or procedure-related complication.[56]

Placement of a PCD may cause bacteremia in spite of antibiotic administration. The most important preventive measure is to avoid excessive manipulation of infected pus. Overdistention of the abscess with contrast agents during the procedure and saline injections to wash the cavity are associated with an increased risk of bacteremia and are therefore not recommended.[57] Flushing the catheter may be useful for maintaining its patency, especially in cases of viscous pus. Furthermore, in such cases, larger catheters may be needed to drain the cavity efficiently. In some cases, after apparent successful drainage, imaging may show incomplete evacuation of the abscess cavity, and repositioning of the catheter, or even placement of additional catheters, may be necessary. An intercostal approach may cause pneumothorax, pleural effusion, or contamination of the pleural space, and a chest tube should be placed without removal of the abscess drain.

Failure of PCD may occur in as many as 10% of patients, and the chronicity of a PLA may result in a thick, fibrous rind that will not collapse. In other cases, a cluster of abscesses may be misinterpreted as a multiloculated PLA on imaging, and the absence of communication with the main cavity results in incomplete drainage. Persistent drainage of bile through the catheter after several days or weeks is commonly seen when the abscess communicates with the biliary tree (Fig. 70.5). Endoscopic retrograde cholangiopancreatography with endoscopic sphincterotomy and transpapillary stent may help resolve this problem. Sugiyama and Atomi (2002)[58] found that in all cases of biliary communication, complete cure of abscesses after PCD required additional treatment to relieve the obstruction.

Surgical Treatment

Surgical treatment of PLAs as a first therapeutic approach is not usually indicated. Percutaneous procedures have been increasingly performed, leaving surgical drainage to salvage cases

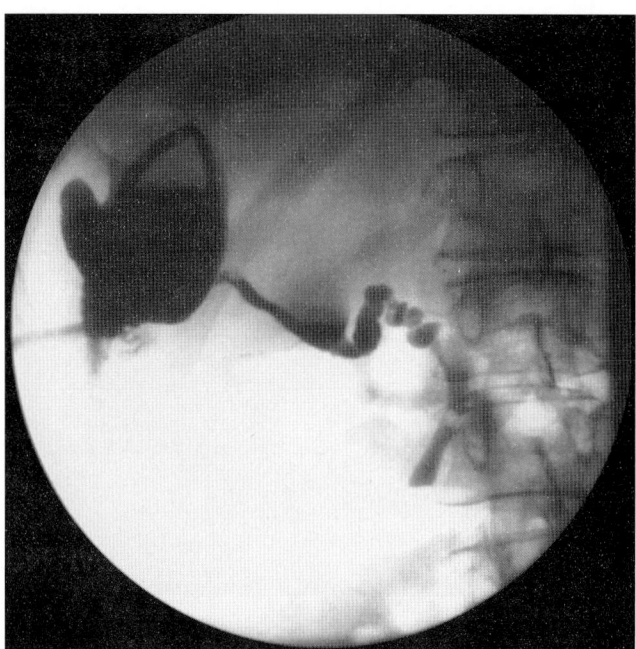

FIGURE 70.5 Percutaneous fistulogram showing a pyogenic liver abscess in communication with the gallbladder and the presence of a common bile duct stone.

in which percutaneous treatment fails.[59] However, surgical treatment of PLAs may be indicated in certain specific clinical situations.

Primary surgical therapy is indicated in patients with intraperitoneal rupture, in which complete exploration and lavage of the abdomen are indicated. Laparoscopic approach combined with intraoperative US examination appears to be a minimally invasive therapeutic option for this rare condition.[60] In some other patients, surgery may be indicated for the treatment of complications of the percutaneous drainage, such as bleeding or intraperitoneal leakage of pus.

Patients with an underlying pathology that needs surgical resolution can undergo treatment for the liver abscess during the same operation, as in cases of acute cholecystitis presenting with an adjacent abscess. It must be emphasized, however, that percutaneous drainage is indicated if surgery must be delayed for further stabilization of a critically ill patient.

Large, multiloculated abscesses containing thick pus are more prone to not respond to percutaneous treatment. In these patients, complete evacuation and removal of necrotic tissue and debris may be more easily achieved surgically.[61] Percutaneous drainage may, on the other hand, delay effective treatment, which would increase the number of treatment failures, secondary procedures, and length of hospital stay.[59] Failure to institute appropriate surgical treatment in a timely fashion could be harmful in critically ill patients who require urgent resolution of the septic illness[62] and in whom salvage surgery may be associated with a mortality rate of 46%.[63] However, a multidisciplinary team of surgeons and interventional radiologists is mandatory for treating patients in these complex situations. Laparoscopic drainage may play an important role in diminishing wound-related complications. With a laparoscopic approach, intraoperative US plays an important role to assess location and extension of the lesion[64]; however, it should be emphasized that an open approach should be used

if there is any question regarding the adequacy of drainage being achievable laparoscopically. No prospective studies compare open versus laparoscopic approach in the treatment of PLAs. Wang et al. (2004)[65] presented a retrospective comparison of 5 patients treated with open drainage versus 18 patients who underwent laparoscopic approach. Although mortality rate in the series was 0%, the laparoscopic group had shorter operating times and earlier oral intake in the postoperative period, with less intraoperative blood loss and shorter hospitalization. Given the bias associated with patient selection, these results cannot be taken as evidence of the superiority of the laparoscopic approach but only as evidence that laparoscopic treatment is feasible in selected patients.

In all cases, when operating on a patient with a PLA, localization of the abscess should be assisted by means of intraoperative US for a complete examination of the liver to exclude associated lesions (see Chapter 24). In superficial lesions, the pus can be evacuated with needle aspiration to avoid peritoneal contamination, and the abscess cavity can then be opened to break up loculations and remove any debris from the cavity wall. Closed suction drainage should be considered in most cases. In lesions located deep within the liver parenchyma, an extended hepatotomy to reach the lesion may be necessary, but this maneuver may increase the risk of postoperative bile leak; for these cases, the placement of intrahepatic catheter drainage under US guidance may be an effective alternative.

Liver resection for the treatment of PLAs is rare because almost all PLAs can be cured by either percutaneous or operative drainage, but in some cases, PLAs with different physical and etiologic characteristics may need a different surgical approach. Liver atrophy and multiple abscesses may be the consequences of chronic obstruction of a segmental bile duct branch as a result of hepatolithiasis or intrahepatic strictures (see Chapters 39, 41, 42, and 44). Resection of the affected liver segments is the recommended treatment for these patients. Although more frequent in the left lobe, this condition may also be present in the right lobe of the liver. This aggressive approach is also indicated for multiple pyogenic abscesses with severe destruction of surrounding liver parenchyma.[29] In an impressive series, Strong et al. (2003)[66] reported 49 patients who underwent liver resections for PLAs during a 15-year period. Indications for surgery were failure of medical treatment or underlying hepatobiliary pathology. Two deaths (4%) occurred after intraperitoneal rupture of the PLA.

Treatment Summary

Parenteral antibiotic therapy should be started as soon as possible in patients with PLAs. In stable patients, blood specimen samples for culture before therapy can be useful, but delaying therapy is not advisable. A combination of ampicillin, aminoglycoside, and metronidazole or a third-generation cephalosporin plus metronidazole are both effective schemes for therapy. In multiple small lesions, FNA under CT or US guidance is advised to obtain samples for culture. Solitary nonloculated cysts smaller than 50 mm can be treated by puncture and aspiration alone, but biliary tree communication must be excluded in these cases; otherwise, a PCD must be placed.

Imaging and clinical response are good indicators of treatment success. On occasion, a residual cavity may persist despite drainage. In this situation, if the patient remains asymptomatic and the lesion imaging is stable, no further procedure may be needed.[67] After clinical stabilization, antibiotics may be switched to oral administration. A complete course of 4 weeks of antibiotics is recommended, although some authors suggest 2 weeks of treatment.[68]

Surgical debridement is indicated for the failure of nonoperative approaches for suspected intraperitoneal rupture of the abscess or in patients who need surgery to address underlying pathology. Laparoscopic drainage may be attempted in these cases. Finally, liver resection may be indicated in patients with hepatolithiasis, complex bile strictures, or liver atrophy.

OUTCOME AND PROGNOSIS

After successful treatment, recurrence of a PLA is rare; however, it is important to differentiate PLA recurrence from relapse as a result of incomplete treatment. Some patients with underlying risk factors may be at risk for recurrence. Cheng et al. (2008)[69] reported 601 patients with PLAs with a median follow-up of 72 months. Recurrence rates were low in the cryptogenic (2%) and diabetes (4.4%) groups compared with those whose disease was of a biliary origin (23.8%). Except for patients with biliary pathology, recurrences tended to be caused by the same organisms that generated the first PLA. However, the authors found no difference in recurrence rates comparing *E. coli* and *K. pneumoniae* organisms as causative agents. In another study, 14% of the patients who survived the first episode exhibited recurrence in the first year of follow-up. All the recurrences were ipsilateral to the lesions of the first event. Multidrug-resistant bacteria isolation and a history of cholangitis were also found as independent risk factors for recurrence in the first year.[10]

PLA is a potentially life-threatening disease. Since the first report by Oschner et al. in 1938,[2] improvement in antibiotic therapy, new imaging techniques, and minimally invasive procedures have significantly decreased mortality. In series published in the last 2 decades, mortality rates ranged between 6% and 20%.[70] Abscesses caused by *K. pneumoniae* have a higher risk of metastatic infection; however, mortality rates in these patients are lower compared with those whose PLA is caused by other organisms, even if compared with *E. coli* infections.[47] Diabetes is a well-known risk factor for PLA, but mortality rates in patients with diabetes are not increased compared with the general population in both Eastern and Western series.[13,46] Liver cirrhosis is a strong risk factor for PLA and is associated with poor prognosis and high short-term mortality rates.[9] In general, the prognosis of patients with malignancy is poor, but in the absence of comorbidities, age is not associated with worse prognosis.[13]

Systemic response to septic injury is a major determinant of outcome. This may be indicated by the presence of septic shock, clinical jaundice, coagulopathy, leukocytosis, and hypoalbuminemia. Findings of an Acute Physiologic, Age, and Chronic Health Evaluation (APACHE II) score of 15 or higher at admission, multidrug-resistant isolates, gas-forming abscesses, anaerobic infections, and a blood urea nitrogen level of 7.86 mmol/L or greater have been identified as high mortality–associated risk factors.[11] In a recent series, 11 of 142 patients died during hospitalization (7.8%). Cause of death was multiorgan failure due to severe sepsis in all but one patient, who suffered a massive pulmonary embolism. Mortality was associated with serum bilirubin >5 mg/dL and bilateral involvement in multivariate analysis.[10]

References are available at expertconsult.com.

CHAPTER 71

Amebiasis and other parasitic infections

Hrishikesh Samant, Hany Dabbous, and Gazi B. Zibari

AMEBIC LIVER ABSCESS

History

The earliest report of amebiasis is probably the Sanskrit document *Brigu-samhita*, written about 3000 BCE, referring to bloody mucoid diarrhea.[1] Assyrian and Babylonian texts refer to blood in the feces, suggesting the presence of amebiasis in the Tigris-Euphrates basin before the sixth century BCE, and it is possible that hepatic and perianal abscesses described in both *Epidemics* and *Aphorisms* in the *Corpus Hippocratorum* refer to amebiasis.[2,3] After the death of Hippocrates in 356 BCE, Alexander the Great became king of Macedonia. In Alexander's eastern campaign, he reached an area where amebiasis was endemic, and he died on the return trip at the age of 33 years, probably of an amebic liver abscess (ALA).[4]

In 1818, Ballingall[5] described a surgical technique to drain liver abscesses. In 1828, James Annesley gave detailed descriptions of "hepatic dysentery."[6] The connection between amebic dysentery and liver abscesses was described by the English physician William Budd,[7] but Charles Morehead, professor of Medicine and first principal of Grant Medical College, Bombay, India, was the first to report a case of hepatic abscess, in 1848.[8]

Entamoeba histolytica was discovered by Friedrich Lösch in 1873 in Russia.[9] Lösch recognized amebae in the colon and terminal ileum accompanying acute dysentery.[8] He gave descriptions of amebae, including structure, size, motility, intracytoplasmic elements, and drawings. Lösch named the amebae after his patient; *Amoeba coli* was proved later on sequencing of the genome, and a calreticulin-like protein and Golgi apparatus were detected in the amebae.[10,11]

Stephanos Kartulis, a Greek physician, found amebae in intestinal ulcers in patients from Egypt in 1885 and noted that he never found amebae from nondysenteric cases.[12] In 1890, Osler reported a young physician who died of ALA after an attack of dysentery. The report by William Thomas Councilman and Henri Lafleur, working at Johns Hopkins in 1891, represents a definitive statement about the pathologic processes of amebiasis, amebic dysentery, and ALA at the end of the nineteenth century.[13] Schaudinn did differentiate between harmless *Entamoeba coli* and pathogenic *E. histolytica*.[8] In 1901, Harris produced ALAs by intrarectal infection of puppies with *E. histolytica* cultivated *E. histolytica* in vitro, introducing the term *amebiasis*. In 1952, Hoare reported that *E. histolytica* had three phases.[14,15] Species of amebae found in human host—*Entamoeba gingivalis*, *Entamoeba coli*, *Iodamoeba bütschlii*, and *Entamoeba hartmanni*—were discovered between 1849 and 1919.[8]

A plant alkaloid, concessine, was found to kill *E. histolytica*.[1] The first effective treatment came from Brazil in the form of ipecac; emetine was isolated from ipecac in the nineteenth century. Leonard Rogers, professor of pathology at Medical College Hospital in Calcutta, India, reported successful treatment of both intestinal and hepatic amebiasis by injectable salts of emetine.[16] The 1930s witnessed the introduction of two important hydroxyquinolines introduced by Anderson and Koch in 1931 and by a number of others.[17] Although largely replaced by imidazoles in the 1980s, hydroxyquinolines remain useful today. In 1966, Powell et al. demonstrated the effectiveness of metronidazole as an amebicidal agent in both intestinal and extraintestinal amebiasis.[18]

Epidemiology

Amebiasis occurs worldwide but predominantly seen in developing countries. Old textbooks often reported one tenth of the world population infected with *E. histolytica*, with 100,000 deaths per year due to invasive amebiasis.[19] These estimates could be confounded as it dates before the separation of *E. histolytica* from the morphologically identical, nonpathogenic *Entamoeba dispar* and *Entamoeba moshkovskii*.[20–22] *E. dispar* infection is ten times more common than infection with *E. histolytica*.[23] Molecular techniques allow construction of more reliable map of endemic regions of *E. histolytica* amebiasis around the world, such as on the Asian subcontinent (India, Bangladesh), Africa, Asian Pacific (Thailand, Japan), and South and Central America (Mexico, Colombia).[24,25] Infection is common in these countries given poor sanitation and low socioeconomic status. Amebiasis, caused by *E. histolytica*, is second most common cause of parasite infection-related mortality worldwide and estimated to account for 40,000 to 74,000 deaths annually. More recent data show that amebiasis caused about 55,000 deaths in 2010, down from 68,000 in 1990 worldwide.[26,27]

The exact burden of amebiasis in developing countries is difficult to quantify because of variations in study designs, sample sizes, and sensitivity of diagnostic tests used. Reported seroprevalence of *E. histolytica* in some rural communities of Mexico is as high as 42%.[28] The annual incidence of amebic dysentery in children in Bangladesh is reported as 11%.[29] In the large Global Enteric Multi-Center Study (GEMS) from various countries, *E. histolytica* has the highest hazard ratio for death in the second year of life.[30] The annual incidence of ALA averaged 21 cases per 100,000 inhabitants in Hue City, Vietnam.[31] Recent data from 115 cases of liver abscesses from tertiary care center in India showed 88% positivity for *E. Histolytica* with nested multiplex PCR test.[32]

Infection is becoming more common in developed countries because of increased migration and travel from endemic countries. Although the incidence of amebiasis is low in United states, at least five deaths per year were reported as amebiasis related.[33] In the United States and Europe, patients infected with the human immunodeficiency virus (HIV) have increased risk of amebiasis.[34] Recent reports from other industrialized countries such as Japan, for example, have shown high rates of invasive amebiasis in HIV-infected persons.[35]

Organism

E. histolytica is a protozoan with two forms: trophozoite and cyst. Cysts constitute the infective form through fecal-oral transmission by food, water, or direct person-to-person contact. Cysts survive the acid of the stomach and travel through the small intestine, and within the terminal ileum or colon, trophozoites emerge to complete the life cycle.[36] Cysts can survive for 45 minutes in feces lodged under fingernails and for 1 month in soil at 10°C. They remain infective in fresh water, seawater, and sewage but are destroyed by drying, iodine, and heat. They are not killed by chlorination used to purify drinking water.[37] The genus *Entamoeba* includes the pathogenic species *E. histolytica* and nonpathogenic *E. hartmanni*, *E. coli*, *Entamoeba polecki* (in swine), and *E. moshkovskii* (from sewage).[36] There are four species of human intestinal amebae with identical morphologic characteristics: *E. histolytica*, *E. dispar*, *E. moshkovskii*, and *Entamoeba bangladeshi*.[38] The study of zymodemes, patterns of the electrophoretic mobility of isoenzymes, genetic differences using RNA and DNA probes, and the use of polymerase chain reaction (PCR) amplification became more reliable in their identification.[39] Encoding genes for transcription factors have been cloned for *E. histolytica*.[40]

Host Factors

The major reservoir for *Entamoeba* spp. is the human being. Breastfed neonates have a low incidence as a result of the presence of immunoglobin A (IgA) and low iron content in breast milk.[41] A diet rich in iron and carbohydrates predisposes to invasive amebiasis and *HLA-DR3* gene expression is an independent risk factor for ALA.[42]

Although immunosuppression is considered an important risk factor for invasive amebiasis in Asian Pacific countries, others mention there is no particular susceptibility for developing invasive forms of amebiasis in immunosuppressed individuals.[43–45] Nevertheless, some HIV infections have been detected during admission of patients with ALA. On the other hand, the natural history of the disease seems to be the same in immunocompetent patients.[46]

Pathogenesis

The disease course is determined by three virulence factors: lectin (a surface protein), amebapores (small peptides), and cysteine proteases. The virulence of different strains of E histolytica is variable.[47] Trophozoite adhesion to the colonic wall is mediated by lectin, which results in persistent infection, and caspase 3 activation, which is a crucial step in cell necrosis and abscess formation.[48] Amebapores are inserted by the trophozoite into the host cell, where they puncture the lipid bilayer and form a portal of entry into the host. Amebapores result in colloid osmotic lysis of the cell.[49] Cysteine proteases contribute to degradation of the extracellular matrix proteins and disruption of cell monolayers.[50] Other amebic molecules such as lipophosphopeptidoglycan, peroxiredoxin, arginase, and lysine, and glutamic acid-rich proteins are also implicated in the pathogenesis of amoebiasis.[51]

It is anticipated that antiamebic antibodies protective against invasive infection would block lectin binding and neutralize amebapore and cysteine proteases. It has been suggested that the proteophosphoglycans (PPGs) in the amebic glycocalyx may participate in *E. histolytica* pathogenicity because the closely related, nonpathogenic *E. dispar* lacks a significant glycocalyx surface layer.[52] Furthermore, antibodies that bind to

PPGs neutralize liver abscess formation.[53] PPGs are anchored into the parasite cell membrane by a glycosylphosphatidylinositol (GPI) moiety. Synthesis of the GPI anchor requires a cascade of enzymes, including mannosyltransferase 1 (PIG-M1), whose blockage reduces GPI synthesis and PPGs in trophozoites.[54] In addition, experimental evidence suggests that liver cell necrosis is increased when neutrophils are present along with *E. histolytica*.[55]

Normal blood flow in the portal vein is about 1.4 L/min, pressure is 12 to 15 mm Hg, and erythrocyte velocity is 8 to 18 cm/sec. In comparison, sinusoidal blood flow is extremely low (3.4–0.16 mL/min), as is red blood cell velocity 0.1 mm/sec[56] (see Chapter 5). Forces exerted on a parasite that adheres to the endothelium are thus much lower in the sinusoids and may partly explain why the parasite crosses the endothelium within these structures. Lack of tight junctions in liver sinusoidal endothelial cells can facilitate crossing by the parasite, creating a larger breach when reaching the hepatic parenchyma.[57]

Publication of the *E. histolytica* genome facilitated transcriptome studies of the parasite.[58] Microarrays have been used to compare virulent and avirulent trophozoites (those unable to form liver abscesses) from the same strain.[59] Overexpression of peroxiredoxin and rubrerythrin genes in virulent parasites is of interest for ALA development because inflammatory cell recruitment and subsequent inflammation are features of liver infection by *E. histolytica*.[60]

Molecular Genetics

Molecular genetics has contributed to better understanding of amebiasis pathogenesis. The Institutes for Genomic Research have recognized that *E. histolytica* has a small, highly repetitive genome rich in adenosine-thymidine and densely packed sequences, but it lacks introns.[61] Although some regions of the genome encode highly conserved proteins, other areas exhibit high degrees of polymorphism.[62] Sequencing of the *E. histolytica* genome has revealed at least 44 genes.[63] The purification of trophozoites from different organs of the same patients revealed that their tropism was linked to different genotypes.[64]

Host Defense

It has not been definitively established which mechanism is responsible for invasion or recurrence. The first line of defense is the innate immunity that recognizes pathogen-associated molecular patterns (PAMPs) that trigger an inflammatory response. Natural killer T cells activated by *E. histolytica* are important in the control of ALA.[65] Interferon-γ (IFN-γ) initiates inflammation through macrophage production of tumor necrosis factor (TNF) and nitrous oxide (NO) synthesis by polymorphonuclear cells and macrophages. In vitro, the effects of IFN-γ can be bypassed by the recognition of PPGs of *E. histolytica* by Toll-like receptors (TLRs) 2 and 4, which results in direct production of TNF and interleukin (IL)-12 and IL-8.[66] This shows the importance of early recognition of PPGs and inflammatory cell recruitment during ALA onset.[67]

Complement cannot prevent invasion because it is absent from gut mucosal secretions, and amebic cysteine proteases degrade C3a and C5a.[68,69] Neutrophils fail in initial host defense.[70] The second line of adaptive immune response constituted by activated lymphocytes and macrophages is the important effector mechanism against *E. histolytica*.[71] *E. histolytica* infection elicits mucosal IgA and serum IgG response to lectin protein shown to be protective against infection in addition to epitope-specific antibodies that inhibit adherence to target cells.[72,73] The galactose/*N*-acetyl-d-galactosamine–binding (Gal/GalNAc) lectin isolates from three distinct areas of the world—Bangladesh, Republic of Georgia, and Mexico—retains remarkable sequence conservation, and is recognized as a potential vaccine target.[74,75] Serum IgG response to the lectin protein does not provide protection against infection.[76]

Pathology

The development of ALAs is a serious complication of infection by *E. histolytica* and is the most common extraintestinal form of invasive amoebiasis. Trophozoites that successfully penetrate the colonic mucosal barrier cause invasive disease, enter the portal system, and travel to the liver. Amebic colitis and ALA rarely occur simultaneously, and the colonic lesions are usually silent; direct extension to the liver and lymphatic spread do not occur. The cecum is the most common site of amebic colitis, and the right lobe of the liver is more commonly affected because of drainage of the right portal branch from the right side of the colon. The condition usually starts as diffuse amebic hepatitis; liver cells undergo liquefactive necrosis, starting in the center and spreading peripherally to produce a cavity full of blood (Fig. 71.1) and liquefied liver tissue resembling anchovy

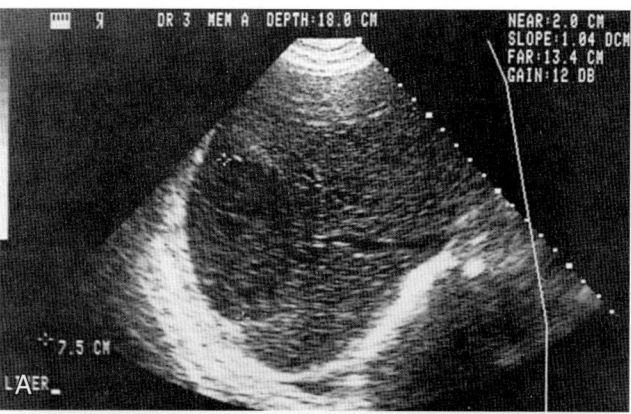

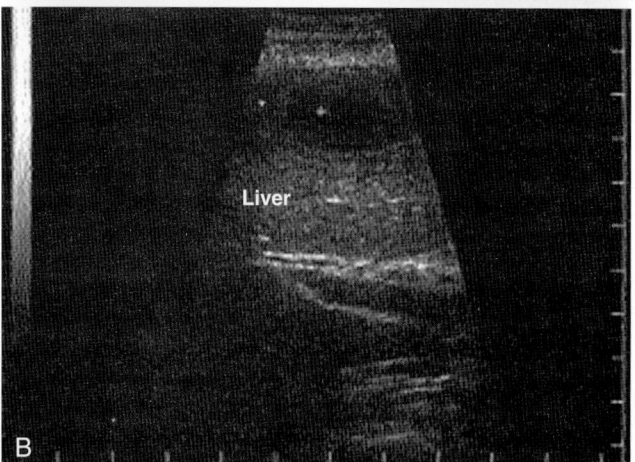

FIGURE 71.1 A, Ultrasound showing a typical liver abscess in a 36-year-old man. The abscess is peripherally located and 7.5 cm in diameter, with a poor rim, internal echoes, and distal sonic enhancement. **B,** Ultrasound showing a typical liver abscess in the left lobe. (**A,** Courtesy Professor M.S. Khuroo, Sher-I-Kashmir Institute of Medical Sciences, Srinagar, India. **B,** Courtesy Professor A.K. El Dory, Ain Shams University, Cairo.) (See Chapter 14.)

sauce; it has no odor and is sterile. The fluid itself is free from any amebae, which may be found at the expanding edge of the abscess cavity with little inflammation. Amebae are known to lyse neutrophils, and the release of neutrophilic mediators may promote hepatocyte death and extension of the abscess. Secondary bacterial infection may occur spontaneously, altering the color, odor, and consistency of the pus. Lack of fibrotic response by the surrounding tissue with centrifugal extension results in extension of the abscess to the Glisson capsule, which is resistant to the amebae. Typically, ALAs are solitary, large, and located in the right liver. Left lobe abscesses are less common, but because of the smaller volume of the left liver, abscesses in this location are more prone to rupture the capsule.[41] Vascular and biliary structures may traverse the abscess cavity; because of the intrahepatic covering of the Glisson capsule, such structures are resistant to the process of liquefactive necrosis. However, these structures can be mistaken for septa within the abscess cavity and fracturing of these strands can lead to hemorrhage or biliary leak, or it can create a communication between the vascular and biliary channels and result in hemobilia and jaundice.[77] The abscess wall is typically ill defined with a minimal host response of fibrous tissue, but long-standing abscesses may develop a fibrous wall and may even calcify.[78] In treated cases, complete resolution is the rule, but it may take 6 months to 2 years or longer than the usual time for pyogenic abscesses to resolve.[41,79]

Clinical Presentation

Most *E. histolytica* infections are asymptomatic or present as mild, "noninvasive" disease. Asymptomatic carriers, or *cyst passers,* may excrete cysts for a short period, but the majority of these patients clear the infection within 12 months. Patients with confirmed *E. histolytica* infection, even if they are asymptomatic, should be treated to eliminate the organism and prevent further transmission.[80] The time between penetration of colonic mucosa and damage to hepatic parenchyma is unknown. Active diarrhea usually occurs in less than 30% of patients at any time before presentation despite intestinal infection by *E. histolytica.* Symptomatic amebic colitis presents as diarrhea with blood and mucus in stools and the presence of hematophagous trophozoites (trophozoites with ingested red blood cells) in stools or tissues.[81] However, in most cases of ALAs, standard stool microscopy results are negative, but in research studies, cultures of stool were positive for *E. histolytica* in more than 75% of patients with ALA.[82] Although *E. dispar* is considered to be nonpathogenic, there have been reports of ALA and diarrhea.[83,84] Similarly, nonpathogenic *E. moshkovskii* has been associated with diarrhea.[85] The pathogenicity of *E. bangladeshi* needs further investigation.[86]

The peak incidence of ALA is between 20 and 60 years of age; thus it is predominantly a disease of young men. ALA is 10 times more common in adults than in children and is 3 to 10 times more common in males.[86,87] Children (especially neonates), pregnant women, and women in the postpartum period have an increased risk of severe disease and death. Treatment with steroids, malignancy, malnutrition, alcoholism, men having sex with men, advanced age, and malnutrition could be considered risk factors for severe disease.[88]

Concomitant hepatic abscess is found in only one third of patients with amebic colitis. The duration of symptoms is usually 10 days. In nonendemic regions, such as Western Europe and the United States, patients usually report travel to an endemic area in the previous 2 to 5 months (median, 3 months), although a prolonged latency may occur.[86,89] Patients with ALA start reporting nonspecific symptoms such as anorexia, nausea, vomiting, and acute colitic illness. Abdominal pain and fever are the cardinal symptoms of the disease, seen in 90% of patients or more. Other signs and symptoms vary according to the site and the size of the abscess. The chief symptom is typically the abrupt onset of right upper quadrant pain radiating to the right shoulder and scapular area. The pain increases with coughing, deep breathing, and walking. If the abscess is in the left liver, the pain may be epigastric, precordial, or retrosternal and may radiate to the left shoulder. Abscesses located on the inferior aspect of the liver may manifest in a manner similar to peritonitis resulting from any upper abdominal cause. On occasion, the presentation is insidious, lasting 2 or more weeks; in such patients, significant weight loss may occur.[41] One report has suggested that ALAs can be silent and asymptomatic.[90]

Abdominal examination usually reveals a tender, soft hepatomegaly accompanied by overlying muscle guarding and intercostal tenderness. Jaundice is often seen, although it was previously reported to be a prominent feature in only 5% to 8% of patients[84]; biliary communication of ALA had been reported in up to 27%.[91,92] Because the right posterior-superior surface of the liver is the most common site of ALA, it is always accompanied by right basal lung signs as a result of pleural effusion, empyema, or lung abscess.[93] On the other hand, left liver abscess may be complicated by pericardial friction, and abscesses in this location can extend into the pericardium, a sign associated with a very high mortality rate.[94] Hepatic failure, ascites, and splenomegaly may occur in 15% of patients who have multiple abscesses. Hepatic encephalopathy in patients with ALA may result from a combination of right hepatic vein occlusion, pylephlebitis, and occlusion of several portal vein radicles.[95] Clinically, the usual differential diagnosis includes acute cholecystitis, hepatitis resulting from viral or other causes, and pyogenic liver abscess. With atypical presentation, hepatocellular carcinoma, a hepatic hydatid cyst, or a simple cyst may be considered.[41] Approximately three quarters of patients with an ALA have leukocytosis. Eosinophilia is rare, but mild anemia may occur in half of patients and is multifactorial. Hyperbilirubinemia is present in only a small proportion of cases.

In chronic liver abscess, the alkaline phosphatase level tends to be elevated, and the AST level tends to be within normal limits. Chest radiography typically shows elevation of the right dome of the diaphragm with an anterior bulge on the lateral view, atelectasis of the right lung, and pleural effusion. Amebic lung abscess with concurrent lung cancer, but without either a liver abscess or amebic colitis, although extremely uncommon, has been recently reported.[96,97]

Diagnosis

Diagnostic tests for intestinal amebiasis and also used as community screening procedure include (1) microscopic examination of unfixed fecal samples, (2) the Ritchie method of fecal concentration, (3) staining of alcohol-fixed stools, (4) Robinson in vitro culture, (5) stool antigens, (6) serology (indirect hemoagglutination test [IHAT], enzyme-linked immunosorbent assay [ELISA], and immunofluorescence test), (7) isoenzyme electrophoresis of stool for zymodeme identification, and (8) PCR.

Stool microscopy is still by far the most commonly used method for diagnosis of intestinal amebiasis around the world.

It can distinguish the *E. histolytica* cyst (four nuclei, centrally located endosome, and round chromatoidal body) from cysts of other nonpathogenic protozoa but not from cysts of commensals *E. dispar* and *E. moshkovski*. Direct microscopic examination is less sensitive than Robinson culture and zymodeme identification, the gold standards.[98]

Stool antigen tests can overcome some of the limitations of microscopy but be reported with variable sensitivity and specificity in low-endemic regions.[99] Benefits of stool antigen tests are rapid, differentiating of pathogenic strains and diagnosis of early infection in endemic areas where serology is less useful.[100]

DNA-based PCR is rapid and sensitive to detect cysts in the stool (<5) and in fluids aspirated from ALA.[39] In 2007, Helmy used nested PCR and restriction enzyme digestion (RED) to distinguish *E. histolytica* from *E. dispar*.[101] Currently, a number of PCR assays, such as conventional PCR, nested PCR, real-time PCR (RT-PCR), multiplex PCR, and loop-mediated isothermal amplification assay, are commercially available.[100] These PCR tests are extremely sensitive and considered the gold standard for diagnosis but still largely underused because of cost and requirement for technical expertise.[102]

Serologic tests are very useful when *E. histolytica* is present in extraintestinal sites. Amebic serology is highly sensitive and specific in the differentiation between pyogenic and amebic hepatic abscess. Currently, ELISA for detection of the galactose-inhibitable adherence protein in serum and feces and IHAT appear to be the most reliable tests, with sensitivity and specificity greater than 95%, with a reversal rate of 82% after 1 week of treatment with metronidazole.[103,104] Serology detects antibodies specific for *E. histolytica* in approximately 70% with active intestinal infection and 10% who are asymptomatic cyst passers.[23] Serologic results becomes positive after 2 weeks of initial infection. Antibody titers peak by the second and third months, decrease to lower levels by 9 months, and revert to negative by 12 months. Because antibodies persists over years, positive serologic findings may not necessary means active infection.[105]

Imaging

Ultrasonography (US) for diagnosis of ALA has an accuracy of 90% (see Chapter 14). It will show an abscess located in contact with the liver capsule (see Fig. 71.1) as round or oval, with well-defined margins; they are hypoechoic and clearly defined from normal liver parenchyma with distal enhancement (Figs. 71.2–71.4).[106] In 80% of patients, the abscess is single in the right lobe and in 10% in the left lobe; 6% in the caudate lobe are single, and the remaining are multiple abscesses.[107] In early stages, amebic abscess appears as a subtle area of decreased echogenicity, and US diagnosis is not pathognomonic; complicated cysts, hematomas, metastases, and amebic abscesses may mimic each other.[108] Only 40% of patients have typical US features of ALA. The mean resolution time for ALA is 7 months, and complete resolution may take up to 2 years. On occasion, percutaneous diagnostic aspiration may be needed to differentiate amebic from pyogenic liver abscess.[109] Although pyogenic liver abscesses tend to resolve earlier (within 2–4 months), ALAs acquire a more echogenic and fibrous wall in 8 to 16 weeks and begin to resemble, but must be differentiated from an encapsulated tumor. With time, resolution may be complete, or the result may be a residual cystic cavity that resembles a simple cyst of the liver.[110]

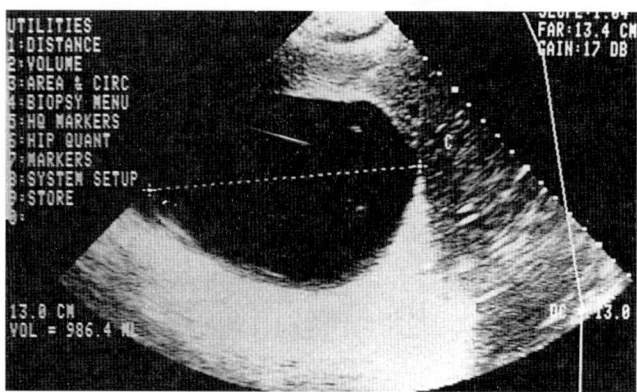

FIGURE 71.2 Ultrasound showing an abscess with more liquid contents in a 25-year-old man. The distal sonic enhancement has resulted in a "white out" of structures distal to the abscess cavity. (Courtesy Professor M.S. Khuroo, Sher-I-Kashmir Institute of Medical Sciences, Srinagar, India.)

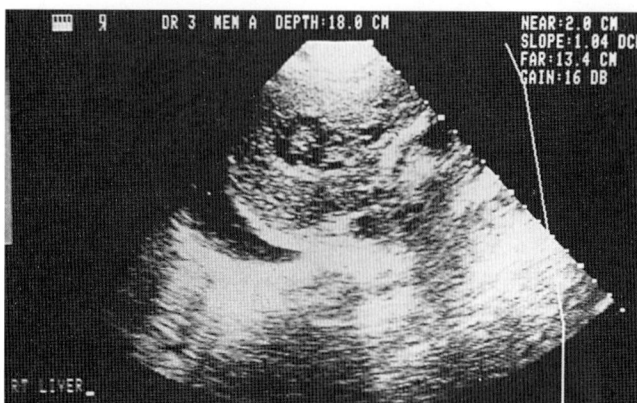

FIGURE 71.4 Ultrasound showing a typical metastatic "target" deposit in a 45-year-old woman. The central location, smaller size, and poor distal enhancement differentiate it from an amebic abscess. The presence of ascites is visible. (Courtesy Professor M.S. Khuroo, Sher-I-Kashmir Institute of Medical Sciences, Srinagar, India.) (See Chapter 14.)

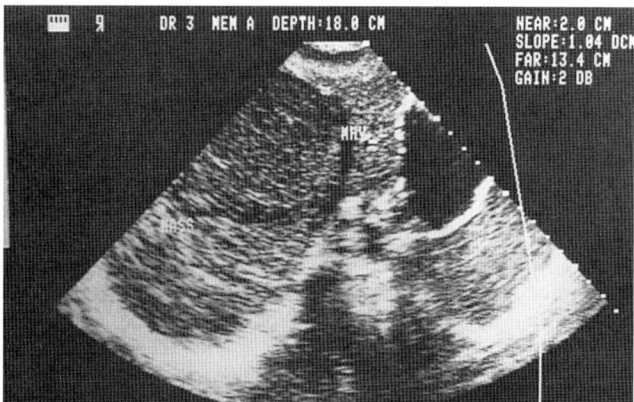

FIGURE 71.3 Ultrasound from a 50-year-old woman with a right liver mass initially mistaken for amebic liver abscess but proven on further investigation to be a tumor. There is a mixed-echo pattern with hyperechoic and medium-level echoes, no clear margin, and no distal sonic enhancement typical of an amebic abscess. *MHV*, Middle Hepatic vein. (Courtesy Professor M.S. Khuroo, Sher-I-Kashmir Institute of Medical Sciences, Srinagar, India.)

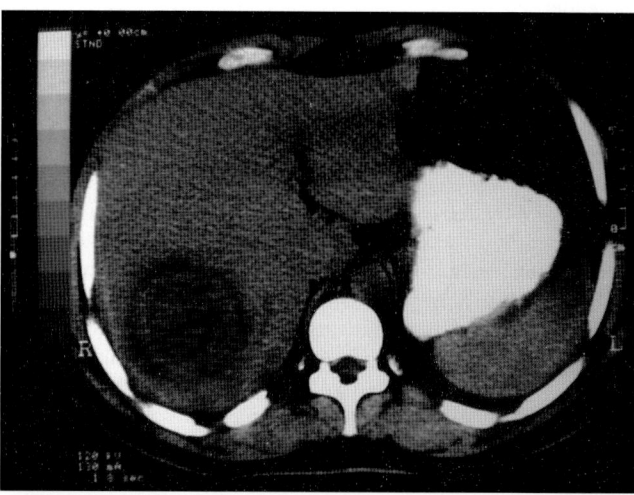

FIGURE 71.5 Computed tomographic image showing a typical liver abscess with an enhancing wall and peripheral zone of edema. (Courtesy Professor A.K. El Dory, Ain Shams University, Cairo.) (See Chapter 14.)

Computed tomography (CT) does not add to the diagnostic accuracy of US in acute stages, except in evaluation of imminent rupture of an abscess or for detection of small lesions (see Chapter 14). ALAs usually appear on CT with contrast as rounded, well-defined lesions with complex fluid.[111] The most characteristic finding is an enhancing wall with a peripheral zone of edema around the abscess (Fig. 71.5). The abscess cavity may show multiple septa (more with pyogenic abscesses), fluid and debris levels, air bubbles, or hemorrhage. CT may detect extension of ALAs to other organs.[111]

Magnetic resonance imaging (MRI) (see Chapter 14) is not superior to CT in the diagnosis of ALA, but it may be useful in differentiating it from a hepatic neoplasm. ALAs appear as heterogeneous cavities that are hypointense on T1-weighted images and hyperintense on T2-weighted images. The abscess margin may show incomplete hyperintense rings with perilesional edema on T2-weighted images. After treatment, the abscess cavity becomes homogeneous, and complete concentric rings appear as a result of periabscess fibrosis and hemosiderin deposits.[112]

Liver scan with gallium citrate and technetium-labeled sulfur colloid radionuclide show ALAs as "cold" spots, whereas pyogenic lesions are seen as "hot" spots.[113] This method is largely limited in diagnosis because of the availability of better imaging modalities.

Role of Aspiration

US- or CT-guided aspiration (Fig. 71.6) is often justified on the basis that the diagnosis would be "more certain," or that the abscess can be "aspirated to dryness" at the time of therapeutic aspiration. PCR may detect *E. histolytica* DNA in ALA pus as well as in the saliva of patients.[114,115] No randomized controlled trial has shown that aspiration is beneficial in survival, length of hospitalization, or time to become afebrile compared with treatment with antiamebic drugs alone, and aspiration may only confuse the diagnosis by revealing atypical pus or

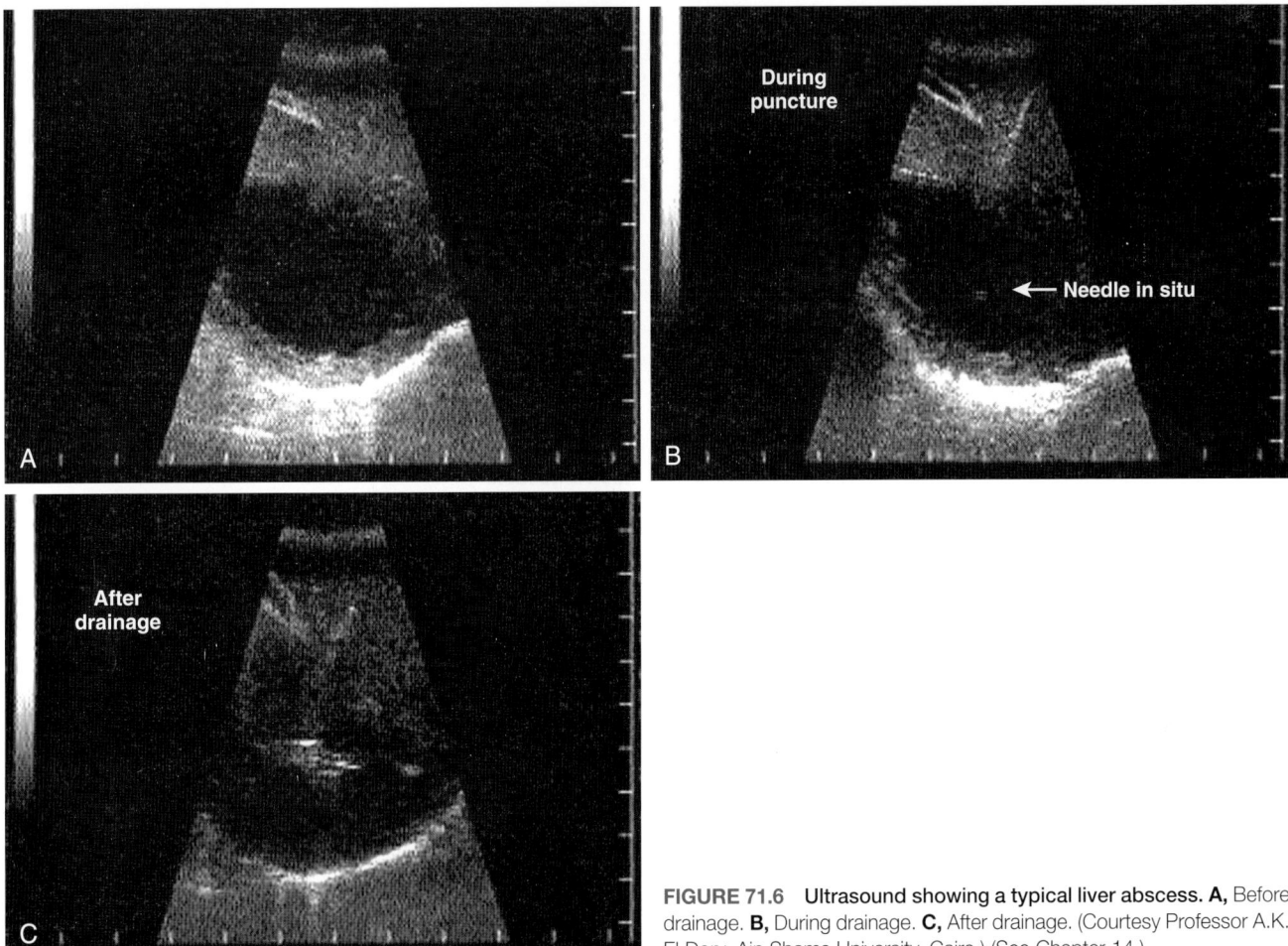

FIGURE 71.6   Ultrasound showing a typical liver abscess. **A,** Before drainage. **B,** During drainage. **C,** After drainage. (Courtesy Professor A.K. El Dory, Ain Shams University, Cairo.) (See Chapter 14.)

blood.[80,116–118] Clinical improvement invariably occurs with antiamebic therapy alone in uncomplicated cases. When the differential diagnosis in a given case includes operable neoplasm or hydatid disease, aspiration is risky and may be contraindicated.[75]

Therapeutic aspiration should be reserved for the following situations:

1. Serology is inconclusive and differential diagnosis is pyogenic liver abscess.
2. A therapeutic trial with antiamebic drugs is deemed inappropriate, as in pregnancy.
3. The liver abscess is secondarily infected (15% of cases) (see Chapter 72).[119]
4. Rupture is imminent in an extremely large abscess (>10 cm), especially if pericardial rupture from a left lobe abscess appears likely.[116]

The following factors predict the need for aspiration: (1) age 55 years or older, (2) an abscess 5 cm or more in diameter, and (3) failure of medical therapy after 7 days.[120] In endemic areas, because of late presentation and existence of multiple abscesses, up to 50% of patients may require aspiration.[121] A single aspiration may be sufficient for diagnostic purposes, but it is inaccurate to recommend it because the characteristic "anchovy paste" characteristic of amebic abscess may not be found; when performed as part of therapy, it will likely be inadequate. Percutaneous catheter drainage is better than percutaneous needle aspiration for management of large liver abscesses (>10 cm) in terms of duration to attain clinical relief and duration for which parenteral antibiotics are needed.[122]

Complications

The most common complications of ALA arise from rupture of the abscess into surrounding organs or anatomic spaces. Communication occurs into the peritoneum, viscera, and large vessels on one side of the diaphragm and the pleura, bronchi, lungs, and pericardium on the other.[123]

Peritoneal and Visceral Involvement

Peritonitis with amebiasis is due to rupture of an ALA in 78% of patients and perforated or necrotizing amebic colitis in the other 22%.[124,125] Spontaneous rupture of ALA may occur in 2.7% to 17% of cases.[126,127] Adherence of the liver abscess to the diaphragm, abdominal wall, omentum, or bowel tends to confine contamination and lead to rupture into hollow viscera, such as the stomach or colon.[128] Rare complications of amebic colitis include appendicitis, perianal cutaneous amebiasis, and rectovaginal fistulae.[129,130]

A hepatogastric, hepatoduodenal, or hepatocolonic fistula and acute hepatic failure may occur from ruptured ALA. Free rupture into the peritoneal cavity is uncommon and usually occurs only in a nutritionally depleted patient.[131] Bloody diarrhea may occur in colonic rupture, and hematemesis may occur in cases of hepatogastric fistula. US and CT often show a perihepatic fluid collection in cases of ALA that are reactive or with actual leaks from the abscess cavity.[111] Management of abscesses that extended into the peritoneal cavity with aggressive surgical approaches were associated with increased mortality rates and have now been replaced by increasingly successful attempts at percutaneous drainage of the liver abscess and the extravasated pus.[124,126,127,132]

Absolute indications for laparotomy include a doubtful diagnosis; concomitant hollow viscus perforation with fistulization, resulting in life-threatening hemorrhage or sepsis; and failure of conservative management. At laparotomy, the liver abscess, which usually appears as a tan-colored bulge on the surface, must be handled gently. Septa running across the cavity are usually blood vessels and bile ducts traversing the abscess cavity. Hemorrhage can be difficult to control, and postoperative bile leaks may result. Endoscopic stenting or nasobiliary drainage may be required in cases of biliary communication.[133] Irrigation of the abscess cavity with saline is usually sufficient and may be followed by the installation for 3 to 5 minutes of a solution of 65 mg of emetine hydrochloride in 100 mL of normal saline. Tube drains are inserted and retained as necessary. Hollow viscus perforations must be dealt with on an individual basis, with exteriorization, proximal diversion, or serosal patch closure.[73] Postoperative intravenous metronidazole is combined with broad-spectrum antibiotics, and dehydroemetine is added if no cardiac contraindication exists. The mortality rate of viscus perforation ranges from 12% to 50%.[127]

Thoracic and Pleuropulmonary Involvement

Pulmonary complications occur in 7% to 20% of patients with ALA.[80] A sympathetic right-sided effusion is the most common pulmonary complication and usually does not require treatment itself. Other thoracic complications include rupture of the abscess into the pleural cavity or into the bronchial tree. This condition manifests as dyspnea and dry cough with right basal crepitations and collapse of the right lung in addition to the abdominal signs. A pleural rub may also be found. Sudden onset of coughing with expectoration of copious quantities of chocolate-colored sputum occurs if the abscess ruptures into bronchi.[134,135] There are several routes of pulmonary infection, including direct hematogenous and inhalational amebiasis.[136] Thoracocentesis is the main line of treatment. In case of aspiration and intercostal tube drainage, care is taken to go high on the right lateral side of the chest near the axilla. Ineffective early drainage of the amebic empyema is usually complicated by secondary infection that requires aggressive surgical procedures, such as pulmonary decortication, because the fibrous tissue can be dense enough to complicate thoracoscopic surgical techniques.[73]

Lung abscess rarely occurs, and it is walled off from the pleural and peritoneal cavities; surgical intervention is not required because postural drainage, bronchodilators, and antiamebic drugs may suffice. Metronidazole is effective, but emetine produces a rapid response and may be required in cases of metronidazole resistance.[137]

Vascular and Pericardial Involvement

Some cases of vascular complications have been reported, such as Budd-Chiari syndrome and right atrial and inferior vena cava thrombosis, complicating multiple large ALAs.[138-140] Surgical removal of the thrombus may be required.

Abscess rupture into pericardium is rare but serious, occurring in 1.3% to 2% of patients, with mortality rates from 30% to 60%.[136] Abscesses of the left lobe of the liver or those more centrally located are more prone to pericardial complications that range from asymptomatic pericardial effusion to cardiac tamponade.[141] Although left lobe abscesses resolve equally well with antiamebic drugs, as do right-sided abscesses, the detection of pericardial thickening or pericardial effusion may constitute an indication for aspiration of a left-sided ALA.[111,142] In cardiac tamponade, pericardiocentesis must be performed, along with drainage of the liver abscess followed by antiamebic drugs, namely metronidazole. Dehydroemetine is used with caution because of its cardiotoxicity.[73]

Chemotherapy

Metronidazole

Metronidazole is the drug of choice for invasive colitis and ALA. The oral dose of metronidazole is 500 to 750 mg three times daily for 7 to 10 days in adults and 35 to 50 mg/kg in three divided doses for 10 days in children, with a cure rate of more than 90%.[143]

Hepatopulmonary amebiasis was found to respond equally to doses of 400 and 800 mg three times daily given over 5 days.[135] The intravenous route is also highly effective at a recommended dose of 500 mg every 6 hours. Metronidazole reaches high concentrations in the liver and intestine and crosses the placenta and the blood–brain barrier. Its use is contraindicated in the first trimester of pregnancy and must be used cautiously in the second and third trimesters; breastfeeding should be discontinued during its use. The response of patients with ALA to metronidazole is profound, with improvement in symptoms within 72 to 96 hours. However, a luminal agent such as paromomycin (30 mg/kg three times daily for 5–7 days), iodoquinol (650 mg orally three times daily for 20 days), or diloxanide furoate (500 mg orally three times daily for 10 days) should also be used to eradicate intestinal colonization.[80]

Over 5 days, an 85% cure rate is achieved, which may increase to 95% after 10 days.[134] From 5% to 15% of patients with ALA may be resistant to metronidazole,[142] but this may not be a major clinical problem[143]; most reports of "drug resistance" reflect delayed resolution of either clinical symptoms or US findings and not a true resistance documented by drug failure. Experimental resistance may be related to inducing superoxide dismutase in vitro.[86] Alternative to medical therapy, percutaneous aspiration, or surgical intervention usually must be considered in patients who do not respond.[142] In countries where they are available, tinidazole, ornidazole, and nitazoxanide are alternative agents for the treatment of ALA; these drugs are administered for only a few days.[144-146] One study of a single 2-g dose of either tinidazole or ornidazole gave a success rate of 94% in both treatment arms.[144] Other studies have shown a success rate of almost 100% for patients treated with tinidazole for 2 to 3 days.[145-147] Secnidazole has a longer half-life, and a single daily dose of 2 g for 5 days is effective.[148] Satranidazole showed lower incidence of side effects and better tolerance than metronidazole in a randomized, single-blind trial of 49 patients with ALA.[149]

Other Medications

Emetine hydrochloride is effective against trophozoites and reaches amebicidal concentrations in tissues rather than intestine.

Emetine is administered by intramuscular or deep subcutaneous injection in a dose of 1 mg/kg/day (maximum, 60 mg/day) for 10 days. The patient must be placed on complete bed rest. Tissue levels persist for 40 to 60 days, and re-administration should be avoided for 6 weeks. Side effects include myositis at the injection site, hypotension, tachycardia, chest pain, dyspnea, and abnormalities on electrocardiogram, including T-wave inversion and prolonged Q-T interval. The drug is contraindicated in renal, cardiac, and muscular disease and is used cautiously in children and elderly patients.[73] Emetine or dehydroemetine is valuable in treatment of hepatopulmonary amebiasis.[134,137,142]

Chloroquine phosphate is antimalarial and is effective in patients with resistance to emetine and pulmonary amebiasis but has no luminal amebicidal activity.[134] Chloroquine is administered orally in a dose of 1 g (600 mg base) per day for 2 days, followed by 500 mg (300 mg base) per day for 2 to 3 weeks. It is contraindicated in patients with retinopathy, but it has been used in pregnant patients.[134] Diloxanide is ineffective in invasive amebiasis and is used for treatment of asymptomatic carriers. Nitazoxanide has shown efficacy in amebic dysentery. The recommended dose is 500 mg three times daily for 10 days. No serious side effects are reported.[150] Further studies are warranted in hepatic amebiasis. Trifluoromethionine is a lead compound, but a single subcutaneous or oral dose prevented the formation of ALA in a rodent model.[151]

Therapeutic Strategy

Oral metronidazole is administered as a single drug, with concomitant correction of hypoprothrombinemia, hypoproteinemia, and anemia. If dramatic improvement occurs in 48 to 72 hours, only a complete course of metronidazole treatment is required. A luminal agent, such as diloxanide furoate (500 mg three times daily for 10 days) or paromomycin (30 mg/kg/day in three doses for 10 days), must be administered after metronidazole therapy for eradication of intestinal infection as part of a complete treatment regimen.[80]

In patients who do not respond satisfactorily, emetine or dehydroemetine is added. Evidence of pulmonary, peritoneal, or pericardial extension is an indication for aspiration of the liver abscess with an intercostal tube or catheter drainage. Percutaneous catheter drainage is usually recommended for abscesses larger than 10 cm in diameter and for left lobe liver abscess, failure of medical treatment for 7 days, and failure to differentiate the abscess from a pyogenic abscess.[122] The following are predictive of the need for aspiration: (1) age older than 55 years, (2) abscess greater than 10 cm in diameter, and (3) failure of medical therapy after 7 days.[120] Late presentation with the existence of multiple abscesses may require aspiration, but prompt medical care decreases the need. Laparotomy is usually reserved for patients with suspected peritonitis, fistulization, or secondary infection with sepsis after failure of above measures.[121]

A review of literature reported a mortality rate for patients with ALA of 4%.[84] In patients treated with amebicidal drugs alone, the mortality rate was less than 1%.[80] Independent risk factors for death include serum bilirubin greater than 3.5 mg/dL; encephalopathy; hypoalbuminemia, defined as less than 2 mg/dL; and multiple abscess cavities or total abscess volume greater than 500 mL.[152,153] Rupture into the peritoneal cavity and the pericardium is responsible for most deaths. Patients treated with early and aggressive surgery as advocated by some authors did not show a remarkable improvement in mortality rate, although in the series by Balasegaram, the hospital stay was probably reduced.[126,132] Ruptured ALA occurs in 2% to 17% of patients, with reported mortality rate of 6% to 50%. These patients usually constitute a major risk for surgery and anesthesia.

Prevention

In addition to regular sanitary measures that include proper washing of vegetables and fruits as well as drinking only bottled water in endemic areas, modern biologic techniques have helped characterize amebic antigens that show great promise in the development of a vaccine. No prophylactic vaccine is currently available for amebiasis, but efforts to better define antigenic candidates and wider use of animal models are encouraging.[154–156] A codon-optimized DNA vaccine has been tested in a murine model and was found to be useful in stimulating type 1 cellular immune response and serum antibodies.[157] Gal-lectin based vaccinations have conferred some protection in various animal models.[158] Other examples, a serine-rich *E. histolytica* protein has been expressed in avirulent vaccine strains of *Salmonella*.[159] A synthetic, enhanced, intranasal lectin-based amebiasis subunit has been extensively studied as attractive candidates for vaccine development.[160] In addition, galactosamine-inhibitable lectin shows promise in animal studies.[66]

Cell-mediated immunity may be sufficient for vaccine protection from intestinal amebiasis with significant IFN-γ, IL-2, IL-12, IL-10, and IL-17 production with recombinant vaccines.[161] Gram-negative bacteria expressing *E. histolytica* antigens may constitute a suitable oral vaccine carrier against invasive ameobiasis.[65] Thus various amebic proteins associated with virulence have been studied as potential vaccine targets and development of both parental and oral vaccine for human is in progress.

LIVER FLUKE DISEASE

Fasciola hepatica, Clonorchis sinensis, and opisthorchiasis are the major liver flukes (see Chapter 45). They are unsegmented leaf-shaped trematodes. Although they have common features with respect to structure and life cycle, with accidental infection of humans, there are some epidemiologic differences. The Western Hemisphere is free of the disease, but clinical manifestations may occur in natives of these areas several years after emigration to other countries. The first report of *C. sinensis* infection was described in a Chinese carpenter residing in Calcutta, India.[162]

Fascioliasis

Zoonotic disease is caused by *F. hepatica* (temperate) and *Fasciola gigantica* (tropical), the causative agents of fascioliasis in cattle and sheep (see Chapter 45). Human infections with *F. hepatica* are found in areas where sheep and cattle are raised and where humans consume raw watercress, including Europe, the Middle East, and Asia.[73] Infections with *F. gigantica* have been reported in Asia, Africa, and Hawaii. Prevalence is high in Bolivia (65%–92%), Ecuador (24%–53%), Egypt (2%–17%), and Peru (10%). In hyperendemic areas of Bolivia, 68% of children are infected; 11% of Ethiopians who emigrated to Israel are also infected.[73] An estimated 2.4 million people are infected with liver flukes worldwide.[163] The incidence in humans is estimated to be only 1%, and most patients are encountered as sporadic cases or in small community outbreaks.[164]

A distinct syndrome of fascioliasis, termed *halzoun* in Lebanon and *marrera* in Sudan, can result from consuming raw liver of an infected sheep, goat, or cow. The living fluke adheres to the posterior pharyngeal wall, causing severe pharyngitis and laryngeal edema. Similarly, disease can follow consumption of sashimi of bovine liver served in "yakitori" bars in Japan if the liver is contaminated with juvenile worms.

Morphology and Life Cycle

F. hepatica is a flat, leaflike, hermaphrodite trematode 15 to 30 mm long, 10 mm thick, and 3 mm wide that inhabits the bile ducts and gallbladder of the host. When the eggs in mammalian stool are deposited in tepid water (22°–26°C), miracidia appear, develop, and hatch in 9 to 14 days. These miracidia then invade many species of freshwater snails, in which they multiply as sporozoites and redia for 4 to 7 weeks. They leave as free-swimming cercaria that subsequently attach to watercress, water lettuce, mint, parsley, or khat. Free-swimming cercaria may remain suspended in the water and encyst over a few hours. When humans consume contaminated plants or water, larvae excyst in the duodenum, migrate through the bowel wall and peritoneal cavity, and penetrate the Glisson capsule, actions that initiate the acute larval, hepatic, and invasive stages of human infection, in which the parasites eat their way down to the bile ducts. Larvae sometimes also travel to ectopic body sites. This stage may last 3 to 4 months, during which the larvae mature and migrate through liver into large hepatic and common bile ducts. Mature flukes consume hepatocytes and duct epithelium and reside for years in the hepatic and common bile ducts and occasionally in the gallbladder; this is the chronic adult biliary stage of infection. Adult fluke worms produce eggs about 4 months (range, 3–18 months) after infection; these eggs traverse the sphincter of Oddi and intestine and then continue the cycle of infection. Acute and chronic stages can overlap, particularly in a high-level infection. The life cycle takes about 5 months, 3 months of which are required for the journey through the human host. The adult worms that develop in the bile ducts at the end of this period have a life span of 3 to 4 years. The parasite may invade other organs during migration, such as the urinary tract, and cause hematuria. Ectopic fascioliasis may affect the peritoneum, muscles, brain, and subcutaneous tissues.[165]

Pathology

Early during infection, hepatic lesions may be white or gray nodules on the liver capsule, subcapsular tracts, and, rarely, a localized hepatic mass. Later, the worm enters the biliary system. *F. hepatica* is a relatively large parasite. In the intrahepatic ducts, the worms move to and fro, and the spinous nature of the integument causes extensive destruction of the biliary epithelium; in this way, the presence of the parasite stimulates fibrosis in the bile duct wall (Fig. 71.7). Serious infection may be associated with hepatic and biliary fibrosis, hepatic necrosis, abscess formation, cholangiohepatitis, impaired nutrition, and death. A liver biopsy may reveal a nonspecific round cell infiltration of portal tracts, and cholangiocarcinoma may occur in association with fascioliasis.[73]

Clinical Features

Eating watercress and drinking contaminated water in an endemic area are the likely routes of infection. Clinical symptoms and signs, together with radiologic findings, are the mainstay of diagnosis. The acute phase usually lasts 4 months and is caused by the migration of the immature fluke through the hepatic parenchyma, leading to hemobilia. Patients usually develop

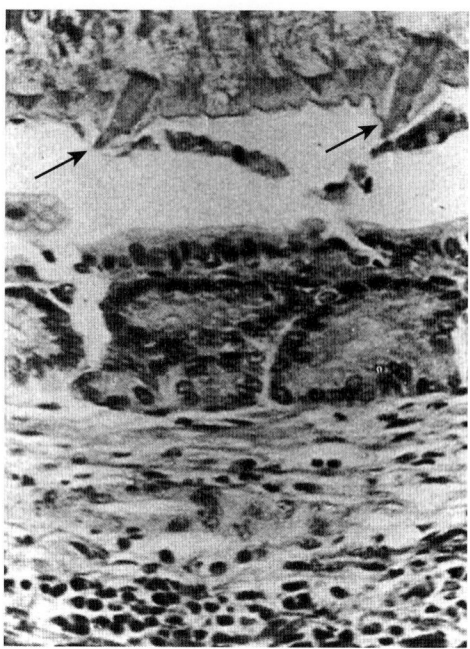

FIGURE 71.7 Spines of *Fasciola hepatica (arrows)* damaging the biliary epithelium (original magnification, ×500). (Courtesy Professor M.S. Khuroo, Sher-I-Kashmir Institute of Medical Sciences, Srinagar, India.) (See Chapter 45.)

right upper quadrant pain, hepatomegaly, fever, vomiting, diarrhea, anemia, hypergammaglobulinemia (especially IgG and IgE), and allergic reactions.[166]

On US examination of the intrahepatic and extrahepatic bile ducts, no motile echogenic images are seen.[167] The findings in the liver parenchyma are nonspecific, although suspected nodules or cavitary lesions might warrant further imaging. The characteristic sonographic features such as heterogeneity of the liver with multiple poorly defined hypoechoic-isoechoic lesions, and multiple echogenic nonshadowing particles in the gallbladder or common bile ducts may be seen. Nonetheless, the differential diagnosis of fascioliasis versus other hepatic lesions may still be difficult.[168] CT is the most useful method for diagnosis; it can show peripherally located hypodense lesions, usually on the right lobe, with peripheral enhancement on contrast scans, arranged in a track-like fashion with no coalescence into a larger abscess cavity, such as is seen in pyogenic abscesses. MRI usually adds nothing and cannot show the track-like appearance of the lesions.[169] After infection of the biliary tract or gallbladder, an asymptomatic clinical phase starts during which the flukes mature into adult form. This is followed by the chronic phase, caused by the adult fluke within the biliary system, during which the symptoms persist more than 4 months, are more discrete, and reflect intermittent biliary obstruction and inflammation. The main symptoms include recurrent episodes of biliary colic, cholangitis, and cholecystitis accompanied by constitutional upset, jaundice, anemia, hypoproteinemia, and edema. The liver may be tender and enlarged with splenomegaly. Motile echogenic images with biliary mud can be seen in the gallbladder and bile ducts on US during this phase (Fig. 71.8). Real-time sonography may show the worm moving inside the gallbladder. Biliary duct dilation is common, and MRI cholangiography may show signal loss in the large bile ducts consistent

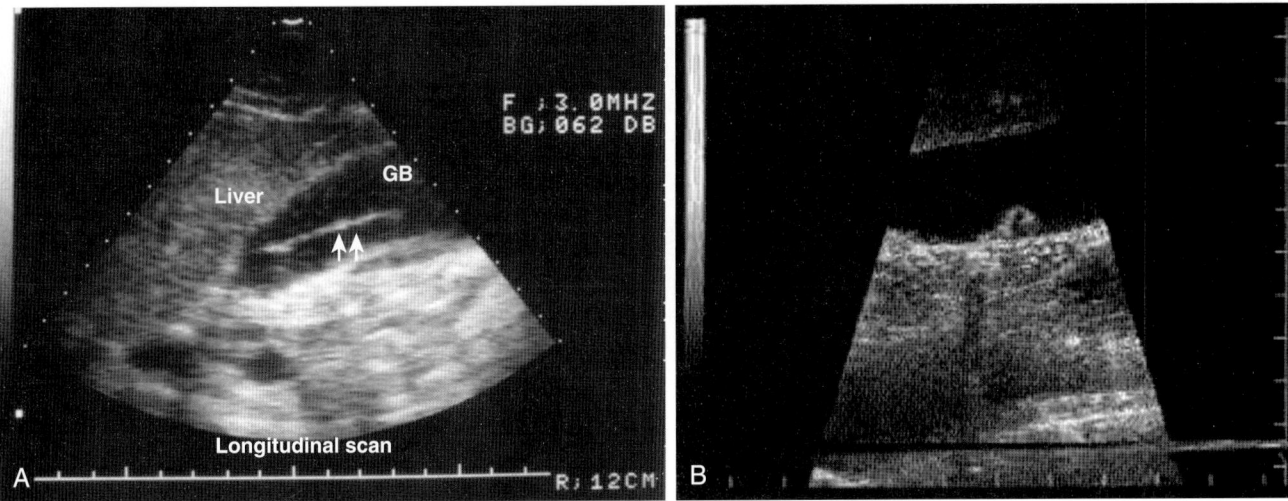

FIGURE 71.8 Ultrasound of *Fasciola hepatica* moving inside the gallbladder *(GB)* as an echogenic mass *(arrows)*. **A,** Longitudinal view. **B,** Transverse view. (Courtesy Professor A.K. El Dory, Ain Shams University, Cairo.) (See Chapter 45.)

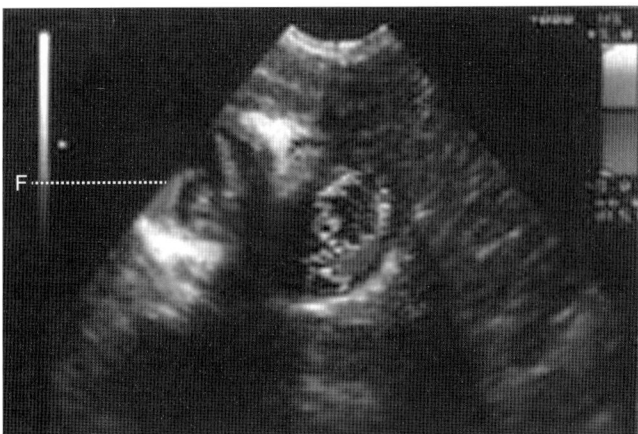

FIGURE 71.9 Endoscopic ultrasound of *Fasciola hepatica* inside the common bile duct as an echogenic mass in a transverse view. *F,* Indicates *Fasciola* worm. (Courtesy Professor A.K. El Dory, Ain Shams University, Cairo.) (See Chapter 45.)

with flukes or edema.[170] Diagnosis of fascioliasis by endoscopic ultrasound (Fig. 71.9) has also been reported.[171,172] Liver biopsy is not indicated for diagnosis and usually reveals necrotic debris, track-like destruction of parenchyma, polymorphonuclear infiltration with abundant eosinophils, Charcot-Leyden crystals, granulomas with or without eggs, fibrosis, and bile duct proliferation.[173] Eosinophilia may be 50% or more of the total white blood cell count and is seen regardless of the clinical stage of infection; it also may be seen in asymptomatic contacts of the patient, who have latent infection.[167,174] It has been reported that eosinophilia could be absent in chronic cases in endemic areas, and anemia is usually present.[175,176] Liver function tests show features of cholestasis. Hemoglobinuria is often present because the flukes can penetrate and lodge in the kidneys during migration through the peritoneal cavity. Adult flukes and eggs are absent from the feces and bile during the acute phase, and even in the chronic phase, so stool examination may not be diagnostic. Repeated stool analysis is required because of intermittent secretion of ova. Serologic modalities include complement fixation test, indirect fluorescent antibody test, IHAT, and counterimmunoelectrophoresis may be used with neither low specificity nor sensitivity.[175]

A specific serologic test to detect IgG antibodies to a crude *Fasciola* worm antigen preparation has been found to be positive in 97% to 100% of patients.[177] A variety of different antigens, such as Fas2, CL1, SAP2, and FhSAP2, have been used. Fas2 is a major cysteine proteinase antigen of *F. hepatica* (E/S protein of the adult parasite). Fas2-ELISA detects the IgG antibodies against the antigen Fas2. The Arc II detects a mosaic of antigens, including the Fas2. Fas2-ELISA is more specific than Western blot and Arc II.[178] The largest human diagnostic study was carried out in Peru, where the Fas2-ELISA (cathepsin L1–based antibody) was validated, including 634 infected children from endemic areas. The sensitivity was 92.4% and specificity was 83.6%, with a negative predictive value of 97.2%.[179] RT-PCR on stool is emerging as a new diagnostic test with higher sensitivity, but is not yet commercially available.[180]

The findings on imaging have already been described, and a differential diagnosis from necrotic hepatic neoplasms and liver abscesses must be made (see Chapters 14 and 66).[170] At laparoscopy or laparotomy, the characteristic features of hard, grayish white nodules on the liver surface with subcapsular channels may be seen in 55% to 75% of patients. Portal lymph nodes are often enlarged, and the common bile duct may be dilated. The diagnosis of fascioliasis should be considered in patients with a history of ingestion of raw watercress or other aquatic plants or those who have recently traveled to an endemic area and develop prostration, cholangitis, hepatosplenomegaly, anemia, and eosinophilia. The acute parenchymal phase is usually difficult to diagnose except by serologic tests for *Fasciola*. *Pseudofascioliasis* refers to the presence of eggs in the stool, which results not from an actual infection but from recent ingestion of infected liver containing eggs. This can be avoided by eating a liver-free diet several days before stool examination.[73]

Consequences of Chronicity of Infection in Fascioliasis

Recent studies have shown a strong association between fascioliasis and liver fibrosis (see Chapter 7). It seems that hepatic fibrosis may evolve in some susceptible hosts, depending on the time and burden of infection. Liver cirrhosis has been reported in infected children and adults, especially those with high-density infections (see Chapter 74).[181,182] New data on the pathogenesis of hepatic involvement associated with *F. hepatica* infection have implicated cathepsin L1 and its collagenolytic function, associated with tissue invasion with proteolytic activity, leading to collagen type I expression and ultimately hepatic fibrosis (Marcos 2002, unpublished observation).[183] On the contrary, chronic infection may also cause a persistent immunosuppressed status, suggesting that the infected host may be susceptible during chronic infection to other T helper cell type 2 (Th2)-associated pathogens.[184]

Treatment

Emetine and chloroquine may be successful in the short term, but recurrence is the rule because these drugs have no effect on the parasite. Fasciolae are also usually refractory to praziquantel. The drug of choice for both phases of *Fasciola* infection is triclabendazole, 10 mg/kg orally, repeated after 12 hours, and it can be used even in the presence of biliary obstruction.[175,185] Cure rates of 90% have been reported, with no significant drug-related side effects. The most frequent adverse event is biliary colic caused by the passage of dead or dying parasites passing through the bile ducts. Bithionol is an alternative, available as 200-mg tablets at a daily dose of 30 mg/kg/day, to a total therapeutic dose of 150 mg/kg. The drug is administered on alternate days in three divided doses after meals. Nausea, abdominal pain, diarrhea, and photosensitivity are the most common side effects. Clinical improvement is gradual and occurs over 2 to 3 weeks.[73] Family members need screening with serologic studies and treatment even if asymptomatic to avoid future complications

Surgical treatment may be indicated for diagnosis or for cholangitis (see Chapter 43). On occasion, a live worm may be found in the gallbladder or the bile duct, or the worm may find its way out through the T-tube placed at surgery.[186] Endoscopic retrograde cholangiopancreatography (ERCP) may be used to relieve obstruction with removal of the worm. Rarely, percutaneous transhepatic cholangiography (PTC) may be an alternative with failed ERCP (Fig. 71.10; see Chapter 29).

Prevention

Infection can be prevented by avoiding ingestion of raw freshwater plants in endemic areas. Proteomics and genomics have led to identification of molecules, including cathepsin L, glutathione-S-transferase, leucine aminopeptidase, and fatty acid–binding proteins.[187] The feasibility of inducing protective responses by vaccine has been proven only in laboratory and large animals studies; human data are lacking.

Biliary Clonorchiasis

See Chapter 45.

Epidemiology

C. sinensisis is endemic in northeast China, southern Korea, Japan, Taiwan, northern Vietnam, and the far eastern part of Russia.[188–190] In general, the infection is acquired by eating raw or uncooked cyprinoid fish products in rural areas (see Chapter 45).

Morphology and Life Cycle

C. sinensis is 10 to 25 mm long, 3 to 5 mm wide, pink, and transparent when alive but hard, friable, and black when

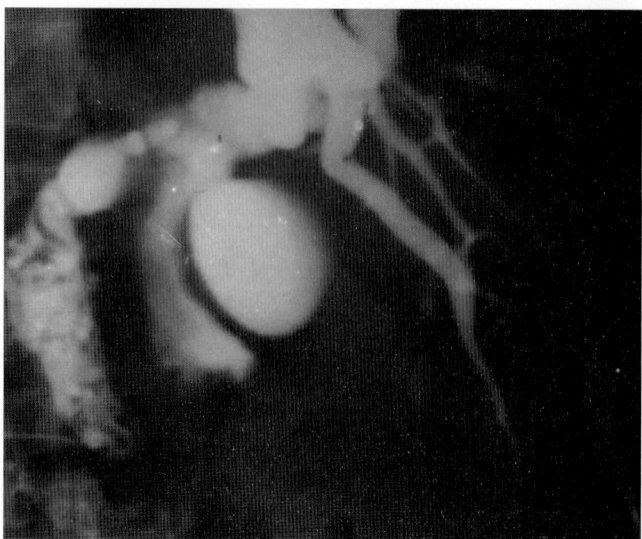

FIGURE 71.10 Percutaneous transhepatic cholangiography of *Fasciola hepatica* inside the common bile duct. (Courtesy Professor A.K. El Dory, Ain Shams University, Cairo.) (See Chapter 45.)

dead.[191] Adult worms inhabit the intrahepatic ducts and may migrate down the common bile duct but tend to die in the gallbladder. In heavy infection, they may be found in the pancreatic duct. Cysts from infected fish are digested by gastric juice; larvae then migrate from the duodenum into the common bile duct upward until they lodge in a duct that is too small for further passage. Eggs laid in bile ducts reach the intestine to be excreted in feces, and the life cycle continues in fresh water in the snail and grass plant or black carp, the intermediate hosts. The cercarial forms that emerge from the snail in fresh water attach to and penetrate the fish, with encysted metacercariae developing in the muscles; humans acquire the infection by ingesting the fish.[73]

Pathology

Irritation by the worm causes the biliary epithelium to undergo hyperplasia, which may progress to metaplasia and adenomatous hyperplasia. In the initial stages, periductal inflammation is mild, and dilation of the small- and medium-sized ducts in the periphery of the liver may occur.[191,192] Metaplastic changes occur early in biliary epithelium, transforming normal cells into mucin-producing cells, which results in highly mucinous bile. This results in stagnation of bile with repeated cholangiohepatitis that eventually kills the worms. This may lead to ductal fibrosis and stricturing with formation of calcium bilirubinate calculi and sepsis resulting from infection by *Escherichia coli* and anaerobic streptococci.[192–194] Progression to biliary cirrhosis is unusual, but there is an increased incidence of cholangiocarcinoma in patients infected with *C. sinensis* (see Chapters 50 and 51).[191,192,195] The etiology of cholangiocarcinoma is multifactorial. Carcinogens in infected individuals may be prone to malignant changes when hyperplasia of bile duct cells occurs.[195]

Relationship to Recurrent Pyogenic Cholangitis

Of patients with recurrent pyogenic cholangitis, 50% are infected with *C. sinensis*.[194,196,197] It is prudent to investigate patients with cholangitis or cholangiocarcinoma who reside in endemic areas for evidence of *Clonorchis* infection because screening for latent infection may be appropriate in relatives and close contacts of patients who test positive for *Clonorchis*.[73] See Chapter 44 for more information.

Clinical Features

The clinical features are independent of the severity of infestation. In an endemic area, 86% of 1091 patients screened by stool examination were found to have clonorchiasis. Only one patient had intrahepatic stones, and the 8% incidence of gallbladder stones was related more to ethnicity than to infection with *C. sinensis*.[198] The classic signs associated with clonorchiasis are those of recurrent pyogenic cholangitis.[1100,200] When clonorchiasis is acalculous, it is usually asymptomatic. Early symptoms include general malaise, abdominal discomfort, and diarrhea. Screening investigations may show eosinophilia with fluctuating jaundice or elevated liver enzymes.[192] Clonorchiasis occurs equally in males and females, with peak incidence in the second and third decades of life.[193] Another study showed that men are more commonly affected.[192] Anemia and hypoproteinemia are common. Jaundice varies in intensity, and progression to cirrhosis results in splenomegaly. Evidence of pancreatitis also may be found. Plain radiographs of the abdomen may reveal gas in the biliary tree, but stones are rarely visualized. US and CT detect ductal dilation and calculi; however, contrast imaging of the biliary tract is essential to delineate the distribution of stones and strictures and to plan operative therapy. The common bile duct and hepatic ducts are usually dilated, but definite stenosis is seen in only 5%. Cholangiocarcinoma may be intrahepatic, hilar, or extrahepatic.[193,201]

Diagnosis

The diagnosis of clonorchiasis with cholangitis depends on high index of suspicion. Elevated eosinophil counts warrant a search for the parasite, and fecal examination for eggs has been used for diagnosis of clonorchiasis.[202] The gold standard detection method for clonorchiasis is formalin ethyl-acetate concentration technique (FECT).[203] Detection of specific antibodies and circulating antigen by Dot-ELISA has been described.[204–206] Monoclonal antibody–based ELISA (Mab-ELISA) is most sensitive and specific tests and these coproantigen tests are increasingly used as diagnostic tools.[207] These serologic assays do not distinguish active from past infection. Concurrent clonorchiasis may be diagnosed by stool examination and serologic ELISA test in cases of fascioliasis.[208] Other methods for diagnosis include intradermal test with diluted antigens of *C. sinensis*, radiologic studies of the liver, and bile examination for eggs, metacercariae, and cercariae.[192,209] Of these, the intradermal test is the easiest to perform, but it has low specificity.[209] Paramyosin (CsPmy) is a myofibrillar parasitic protein whose gene has been identified. Induction of host IgG suggests that paramyosin may be a diagnostic antigen or a vaccine for clonorchiasis.[210] RT-PCR appears to be a powerful tool for both the detection and quantification of *C. sinensis* infections and is now commercially available.[211] Diagnostic methods such as detection of extracted parasite DNA in stool samples by loop-mediated isothermal amplification (LAMP) have been developed.[212]

Treatment

Praziquantel (Biltricide) is the drug of choice. The dosage schedule is usually 25 mg/kg three times daily at 5-hour intervals in 1 day (total dose, 75 mg/kg) for 1 or 2 days, with a cure rate of 83% to 85%.[213] Praziquantel side effects include headache, dizziness, insomnia, nausea, and vomiting. Albendazole also has shown good efficacy in treatment of *Clonorchis* infection.[214] Antibiotics may be needed for associated pyogenic cholangitis, and interventional procedures are required in cases complicated by calculus formation. Endoscopic and minimally invasive techniques have the advantage of reduced morbidity over open surgery.[215] Patients referred to surgery are complicated cases in whom multiple endoscopic (ERCP) or percutaneous (PTC) procedures have failed.

Prevention

Education to reduce consumption of undercooked fish, strict hygiene measures, and mass drug administration are a few approaches to prevention.

Biliary Opisthorchiasis

Opisthorchiasis is caused by *Opisthorchis viverrini* and *Opisthorchis felineus*, the latter of which is endemic in the southeast Asia, Soviet Union, Kazakhstan, and Ukraine[216] (see Chapter 45). The infection is acquired by eating raw or uncooked cyprinoid fish products in rural areas or dishes such as *koi-pla*.[217]

These small flukes migrate to the liver through the duodenum by the ampulla of Vater into the bile ducts, where they matu3re into adult worms in less than a month. The adult flukes reside in medium-sized and small intrahepatic bile ducts and occasionally in extrahepatic bile ducts, the gallbladder, and pancreatic duct, where they can live for many years; in the liver, they can live for decades.[175] See Chapter 45 for more information on opisthorchiasis.

Clinical Features

Because *Opisthorchis* flukes do not penetrate the liver parenchyma, their disease manifestations are caused by the obstruction of the biliary tract, where they can cause prominent inflammation. Flukes can occasionally gain access to the pancreatic tract, where they can cause obstruction and pancreatitis.

OPISTHORCHIS VIVERRINI. In acute infection, only 5% to 10% of heavily infected patients have symptoms, such as right upper quadrant pain, flatulence, fatigue, and a hot sensation over the abdomen. In the chronic phase, mild hepatomegaly occurs. Jaundice and splenomegaly are rare, but intrahepatic duct stones and recurrent cholangitis are common (see Chapters 39 and 43). Whenever jaundice and ascending cholangitis are detected, fluke-related cholangiocarcinoma should be suspected (see Chapters 50 and 51).

OPISTHORCHIS FELINEUS. In acute infection, symptoms occur 2 to 4 weeks after eating raw fish and include fever, nausea, vomiting, abdominal pain, malaise, arthralgia, lymphadenopathy, and skin rash.[218] Eosinophilia is common during the initial 2 to 6 weeks of infection, with raised liver enzyme levels. In chronic infection, eosinophilia is milder. Patients may come to medical attention with suppurative cholangitis and liver abscess because of biliary obstruction.

CONSEQUENCES OF CHRONICITY OF INFECTION IN OPISTHORCHIASIS. The higher the intensity and the higher the anti–*O. viverrini* antibody titers, the higher the risk for cholangiocarcinoma.[219] The International Agency for Research on Cancer recognizes this parasite as a category I carcinogen. The lesions that predispose to malignant changes in *O. viverrini* are dilation of subcapsular medium and large bile ducts with prominent fibrotic wall, periductal inflammatory cell infiltration, goblet cell metaplasia, epithelial and adenomatous hyperplasia, and periductal fibrosis. The pathogenesis of *O. viverrine*–mediated hepatobiliary changes may be due to mechanical irritation or its metabolic products.[220,221] Several *N*-nitrosol compounds and their precursors occur at low levels in fermented food, such as preserved mud fish paste *(pla ra)*, a condiment that is a ubiquitous component of the cuisine of northeastern Thailand and Laos.[222] Few patients with infection show certain cytokine gene polymorphisms resulting in aberrant cytokine production with an increased risk of fibrosis and cholangiocarcinoma.[223]

Diagnosis of Opisthorchiasis

Opisthorchiasis is diagnosed by detection of eggs in feces. In light infections—those with fewer than 10 adult worms in the biliary tract—a PCR assay detecting the DNA of the adult parasite in stools may be helpful.[224] Amongst newer diagnostic tests, urine antigen detection is an emerging method for diagnosis of opisthorchiasis.[203] Because antigen tests become negative after 1 month after treatment, it can differentiate recent infection from past infection. However, its important limitation is cross-reactivity with other helminths (intestinal flukes).[225] There are PCR-based methods for detecting Opisthorchis eggs in stool, but they are still not available commercially.[211]

Treatment of Opisthorchiasis

Praziquantel is the drug of choice for *O. viverrini* and *O. felineus* treatment. For *O. viverrini*, a single dose (40–50 mg/kg) of praziquantel treatment is indicated, with a cure rate between 91% and 97%.[213] Tribendimidine has shown good in treatment of opisthorchiasis.[226]

Biliary Ascariasis

See Chapter 45.

Epidemiology

Ascaris lumbricoides is a roundworm that commonly infects more than a quarter of the population in Asia, Africa, and Central America as well as those who have emigrated to the United States from these areas.[227] Clinical symptoms occur in individuals who have a heavy worm burden.[228] When confined to the intestine, *Ascaris* infestation is usually asymptomatic, although ascariasis is an important cause of biliary disease in areas of the world where the rate of *Ascaris* infection is high. Tropical and subtropical regions with poor socioeconomic conditions and fecal contamination of the soil around dwellings and farms are main sources of infection.[229,230] Infection becomes symptomatic when the worms enter the biliary tract.[229,231] Kamiya et al.[232] reported that more than 11% of patients with gallbladder or biliary tract complications had *Ascaris* worms in their biliary tract. The incidence of gallstones in developing and developed countries is similar, and it is unnecessary to consider ascariasis as an etiologic factor in all patients diagnosed with gallstone disease who hail from an endemic area.[198,229]

The adult worm in humans inhabits the small intestine, mainly the jejunum, where the fertilized female lays eggs. These ova are excreted in host feces and can survive environmental conditions. In warm moist soil, the ova undergo maturation and are able to infect humans if the egg is swallowed. Mature ova hatch in the duodenum, releasing larvae that penetrate the mucosa of the proximal intestine to enter the portal venous blood, in which they are carried through the liver and via the right side of the heart to the pulmonary capillary bed. Here, larvae develop further, penetrating alveoli traveling up the trachea, entering the esophagus, and returning to the intestine. In the jejunum, they mature to adults, reach 20 to 30 cm in length, and have a life span of 1 to 2 years.[73]

Pathology

The adult *Ascaris* reaches the duodenum either because of increased worm burden in the jejunum or as a consequence of increased intestinal motility.[233] The ability of *A. lumbricoides* to enter the common bile duct, especially with heavy duodenal infection, is well known. Usually only one or two worms enter the biliary system, but massive infection may occur. The worm head moves first through the ampulla of Vater to the common bile duct, cystic duct, and intrahepatic ducts; because the length of the extrahepatic tree is only 4 to 10 cm, part of the worm may remain in the duodenum.[234] In 2002, Kamiya et al.[232] reported that 95% of the worms found in the biliary tract were located in the hepatocholedochus, whereas only 3% were found in the gallbladder and even more rarely in the intrahepatic ducts. Migration into the biliary tract has been reported to be frequent after cholecystectomy, sphincterotomy, sphincteroplasty, choledochostomy, or biliary enteric anastomosis, presumably from increased space in the bile duct after gallbladder removal and increased release of cholecystokinin and secretin, which relaxes the sphincter of Oddi.[235] Biliary migration is commonly seen in women, especially pregnant women; this is due to high levels of progesterone, which also relaxes the sphincter of Oddi.[236] Children are at lower risk for biliary migration because of the small diameter of their ductal systems.[237]

The worm tends to move out of the biliary tract within 24 to 36 hours of inducing biliary or pancreatic symptoms, and the detection of live ascarids in the duodenal lumen is considered strong evidence of biliary ascariasis. The impacted worm causes spasm of the sphincter of Oddi, resulting in partial biliary obstruction and colicky pain, and cholangitis can occur after mechanical obstruction (see Chapter 43). Suppurative cholangitis may extend to intrahepatic ducts and cause multiple cholangiolitic liver abscesses. Acalculous cholecystitis, empyema of the gallbladder, and, less commonly, necrosis and perforation of the bile duct may occur.[238] Dead worms cannot leave the bile duct; rather they disintegrate, providing a nidus for stones and provoking a chronic inflammatory response that leads to ductal strictures. Calculi associated with ascariasis are of the calcium bilirubinate type, with the exception that ascarid ova or debris usually can be identified in the calculus.[231,239] *Escherichia coli*, the pathogen usually identified with calcium bilirubinate stones, is frequently encountered in suppurative cholangitis.[239] Another factor that may facilitate stone formation is the albuminoid membrane that covers most of the eggs and is not found in any other parasite. Worms reaching the intrahepatic ducts may become impacted or invade the liver parenchyma to form nests of worms.[240] Unable to extricate themselves, the worms die. The resultant cholangiolitic abscess may enlarge and present on the surface or rupture into the peritoneal cavity. Extension of the abscess through the diaphragm can cause bronchopleural fistula and lung abscess, a well-known and potentially fatal complication.[238,241] The presence of dead worms in the bile duct also induces an intense eosinophilic inflammation that precipitates a fibromatous reaction. Eventually, the dead worms are surrounded by calcification, and the ongoing inflammation results in biliary stricture formation.[242] Based on the aforementioned pathologic features, biliary ascariasis has been classified as *uncomplicated* and *complicated*.[73]

Clinical Features

Biliary ascariasis in the pediatric age group is most commonly seen in children aged 2 to 8 years. In endemic areas, adults are frequently affected, and mean age at presentation is 35 years. For unknown reasons, women are three times more likely to be affected than men; in children, a similar sex difference has not been noted. The mean duration of symptoms varies from 4 to 6 years, and 40% of patients may give a history of biliary surgery. In one large series, 80% of patients had undergone either cholecystectomy or endoscopic sphincterotomy.[243] Microscopic examination of stool and bile samples in these patients gives a positivity rate for *A. lumbricoides* of nearly 100%.[244] Vomiting of worms is common, as well as a history of passing worms in the stool.[230,241]

The most common presentation is usually with sudden severe upper abdominal colic with tenderness and guarding localized to the right upper quadrant or epigastrium. If present, fever is usually low grade, and jaundice, marked toxemia, and hepatomegaly are usually absent. Worms are rarely seen in the gallbladder, and the US finding of distention, wall edema, and intraluminal sludge completely resolves, usually within 2 weeks. Endoscopic examination is difficult to perform and unnecessary in the acute phase, but, if done, it may show duodenal or ampullary worms. ERCP has been commonly used for both diagnosis and removal of worms from the biliary tract (Fig. 71.11) and is particularly valuable when used with real-time US, with a sensitivity of 100%.[245]

ACUTE SUPPURATIVE CHOLANGITIS. Worms in the bile duct may block the cystic duct, leading to acute acalculous cholecystitis or empyema of the gallbladder (see Chapter 34). Worms may also occlude the accessory cystic duct.[246] Biliary stasis as a result of spasm of the sphincter of Oddi, coupled with intestinal contents carried by the worm into biliary tract, lead to pyogenic cholangitis.[242] This appears with right hypochondrial pain, fever, jaundice, tender hepatomegaly, and leukocytosis. Apathy, hypotension, metabolic acidosis, and electrolyte disturbances signify a grave prognosis. US may show worms in the biliary tree, and endoscopy may visualize pus, a tubular filling defect not suggestive of a tumor or stone on cholangiography, or a worm emerging from the ampulla (Fig. 71.12). See Chapter 43 for more information on cholangitis. Rarely worms can be aspirated from biliary tree during percutaneous cholangiography (Fig 71.13)

HEPATIC ASCARIASIS. No clinical features distinguish hepatic ascariasis from suppurative cholangitis. The diagnosis is usually made by US, and aspirated pus might yield the ova of *A. lumbricoides*. The right lobe is more commonly affected, and rupture into the peritoneal cavity is a recognized complication.[242]

ACUTE PANCREATITIS. The character of the pain with acute pancreatitis varies, but an increase in serum amylase confirms diagnosis. Although encountered half as often as the purely biliary presentation, the condition was seen in only 31 of 500 patients in the series by Khuroo et al.[244] and Lloyd.[230] Severe pancreatitis with progression to hemorrhagic pancreatitis or pancreatic fluid collections occurred in only one tenth of these cases. Sandouk et al.[243] reviewed 300 patients with pancreatic ascariasis in Syria and showed that US, along with clinical findings, was the mainstay of diagnosis, similar to another review of 14 patients.[247] See Chapters 54 and 55 for more information on pancreatitis.[243,248]

Late Complications

Late complications include intraductal calculi and biliary strictures.

Diagnosis

LABORATORY STUDIES. Stool analysis is usually the investigation of choice in the search for ascarid ova or remnants of dead worms, and results may approach 100%.[244] Stool concentration

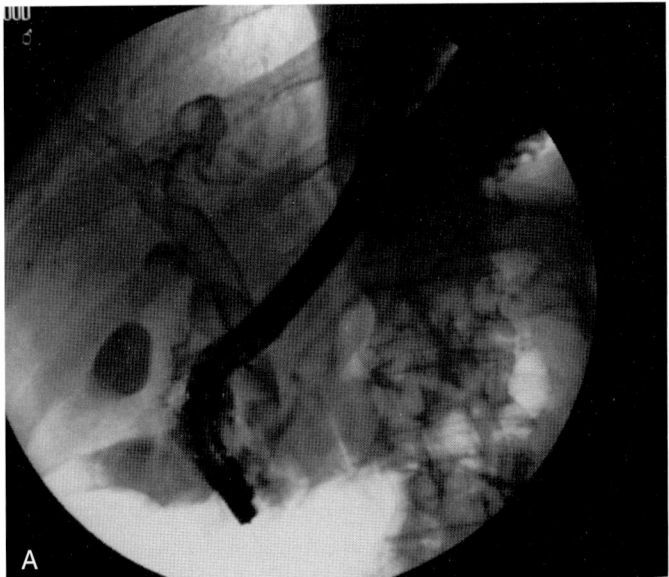
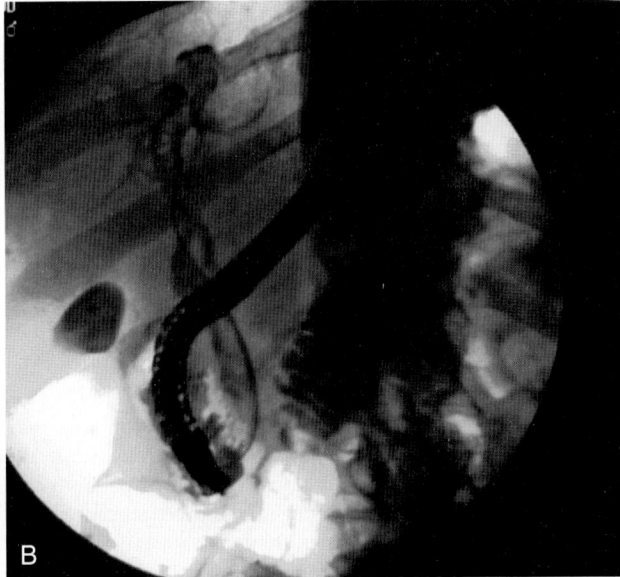

FIGURE 71.11 **Endoscopic retrograde cholangiography of biliary ascariasis. A,** Inside the common bile duct. **B,** Trial of removal using Dormia basket. (Courtesy Professor A.K. El Dory, Ain Shams University, Cairo.) (See Chapter 45.)

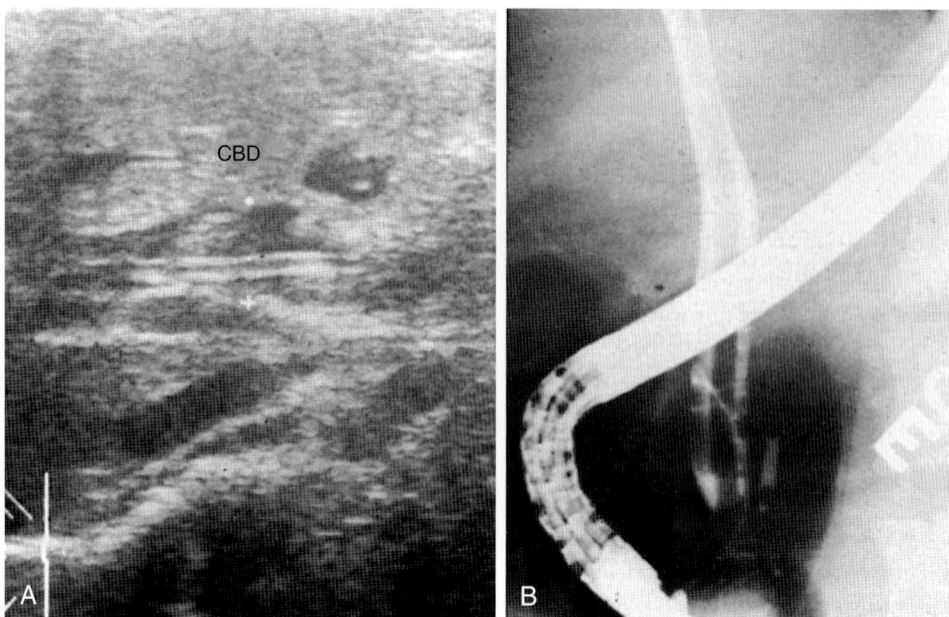

FIGURE 71.12 **A,** Ultrasound of a 30-year-old woman with biliary colic of 7 days' duration, showing the dilated common bile duct *(CBD)* with an echogenic tubular structure in the lumen and no distal shadowing. **B,** Endoscopic retrograde cholangiopancreatography in the same patient reveals the worm in the CBD and across the papilla. (Courtesy Professor M.S. Khuroo, Sher-I-Kashmir Institute of Medical Sciences, Srinagar, India.) (See Chapter 45.)

methods for detection of *Ascaris* eggs include Kato-Katz and FLOTAC techniques.[249] PCR has better sensitivity and specificity compared with microscopy but is not available for commercial use.[250] Serologic tests detecting IgG antibodies to *A. lumbricoides* are mainly use for epidemiologic research. These antibodies do not have any protective role. Leukocytosis greater than 12,000/mm³ usually denotes suppurative biliary and hepatic complications. The eosinophil count is seldom elevated more than 5%. Hyperbilirubinemia occurs in hepatopancreatobiliary ascariasis.[240] Elevation of alkaline phosphatase and transaminases may occur when cholangitis supervenes, and pancreatitis is suggested if serum amylase is greatly elevated. Normal liver enzymes and amylase levels have been reported in a case of recurrent *Ascaris*-related pancreatitis as a result of worm migration.[251] Specific serologic tests are available that can be used to monitor successful treatment but are not commonly used in clinical practice.[252]

DIAGNOSTIC IMAGING. Abdominal radiographs may confirm the presence of intestinal worms in 90% of children (see Chapters 14 and 16). On occasion, air is seen in the biliary tree or in hepatic or subphrenic abscesses.[240] US is the imaging modality of choice because it shows dilated bile ducts containing linear or round areas of increased echogenicity representing worms.[253,254] Other findings were gallbladder distention with sludge inside, an edematous wall, and a mildly dilated biliary tree.[252] This may mimic gallbladder cancer.[255] Real-time scanning may reveal the diagnostic movement of active worms within the biliary system. Multiple bile duct worms have a spaghetti-like appearance, with alternating echogenic and echolucent strips; if densely packed in the bile duct, they may appear as a hyperechoic pseudotumor.[242] On transverse scanning, the biliary worm produces a bulls-eye appearance.[256] Other characteristic appearances include single or multiple long, linear echogenic

strips within the bile duct without acoustic shadowing.[257] US is useful for identifying intrahepatic worms and abscesses and for monitoring the response of lesions to therapy. Ascarid liver abscesses characteristically contain echogenic worm debris; CT does not offer significant advantage over real-time US, and it is less sensitive.[245] A thin line of dye is occasionally seen within the corpus of a worm that has swallowed dye, and the worm is easily visualized on an unenhanced scan within the biliary tree.[258]

Endoscopy may reveal a worm in the duodenum, and occasionally a worm may be seen impacted in or protruding from the ampulla of Vater. ERCP has been done safely, even in the acute setting, and it shows worms in the extrahepatic and intrahepatic biliary tree, including liver abscesses and cases of recurrent pancreatitis.[241,250] Biliary strictures can be studied, and endoscopic extraction of worms and biliary decompression may succeed in aborting an attack of severe cholangitis.[244] Magnetic resonance cholangiopancreatography (MRCP) is a useful modality in pancreaticobiliary ascariasis. The worms are described as linear, hyperintense tubular structures with a central hypointense area.[259] Endoscopic US has been shown to document biliary ascariasis.[260] Percutaneous transhepatic cholangiography has been used in cases of failed ERCP to visualize and relieve obstruction in the abnormal biliary tree containing worms.[240] Adult worms or debris may be identified in the aspirated bile.

Management

The management strategy for ascariasis includes conservative measures, endoscopic extraction, or surgical intervention. Without appropriate nonoperative management, worms spontaneously return to the duodenum in 98% of children and 94% of adults.[230,238,244] Parenteral antispasmodic drugs and analgesics to relax the sphincter of Oddi and relieve biliary colic, nasogastric

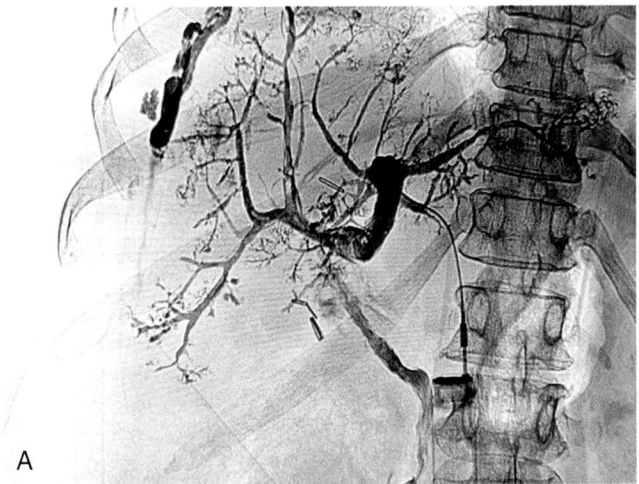

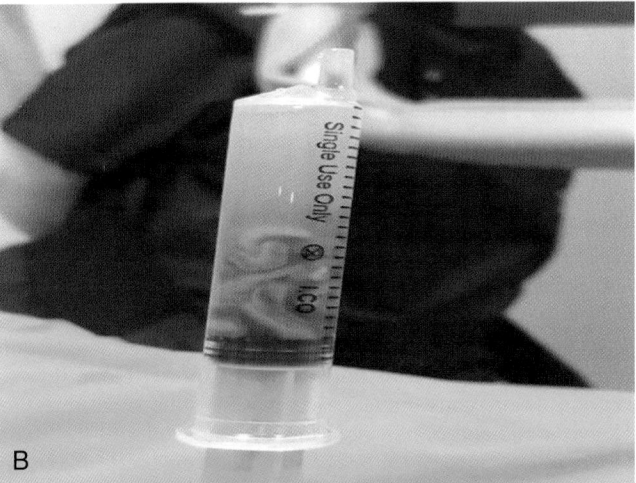

FIGURE 71.13 A, Percutaneous cholangiogram showing dilated left hepatic duct. **B,** Biliary ascaris aspirated from percutaneous drain (Courtesy Karim Abdeltawab, professor of interventional radiology, Ain Shams University) (See Chapter 45.)

decompression, and intravenous fluids are recommended in the acute stage. Successful elimination of an adult *Ascaris* worm from the gallbladder 7 days after killing it with albendazole has been documented[261]; however, oral anthelmintic drugs may not be helpful in the treatment of biliary ascariasis because of poor enterohepatic circulation.[233] Administration of piperazine citrate through the nasobiliary catheter has been shown to be effective.[262] However, some investigators think this approach should not be used because it has been reported to cause paralysis or death of the worm in the bile duct, and this dead worm may act as a nidus for future stone formation.[242] Albendazole (400 mg/day for 1 day) or mebendazole (100 mg twice daily for 3 days) and pyrantel pamoate (single dose of 11 mg/kg to a maximum of 1 g) are the preferred agents, and cure can be achieved in nearly 100% of cases. The safety of these drugs in pregnant women and children younger than 2 years is not established; in this situation, piperazine is safe in a single dose of 75 mg/kg (maximum, 3.5 g) on 2 consecutive days. Other agents that have shown some efficacy in treatment of ascariasis include ivermectin, nitazoxanide, and levamisole. Stool examination is required to confirm eradication of the infection, and follow-up US is needed to look for intraductal worms. ERCP is recommended if symptoms or US

abnormalities persist beyond 2 weeks with suspected pancreaticobiliary ascariasis. Anthelminthic medications help to reduce morbidity associated with infection but does not prevent reinfection because agents are active against adult worms but not against larvae.[263] To prevent reinfection in endemic areas, anthelmintic therapy must be repeated every 2 months in patients who are cured.[244]

The problem of reinfection of the bile ducts after operative or endoscopic removal of worms has led to important modifications in the interventional approach previously advocated.[230,238] Preoperative eradication of intestinal worms ideally should be done before endoscopic or surgical manipulation of the common bile duct. Severe persistent pain unresponsive to anthelmintics is an indication for ERCP and endoscopic removal of intrabiliary worms. In an endemic area, multiple reinvasions of the bile ducts by worms are seen in patients who have undergone endoscopic sphincterotomy.[244]

It would seem to be of paramount importance to preserve the sphincter of Oddi.[242,244,264] Failure of response to conservative management with increasing jaundice may indicate coexisting stones in the common bile duct.[244,263] When skilled endoscopic intervention has failed or is unavailable, a PTC procedure or surgery is recommended, a situation more likely to occur in children than in adults.[265] Laparoscopic common bile duct exploration, with removal of the worm and a cholecystectomy, was reported by Astudillo et al.[266]

Conservative management includes treatment of pain with analgesics, treatment of pyogenic cholangitis with antibiotics, and oral administration of anthelmintic drugs. This management strategy is applied for a few days, and its success is judged by symptomatic improvement. The symptoms usually resolve with this approach within 3 days in 60% to 80% of patients.

Worm extraction with biliary drainage may be lifesaving in patients with severe cholangitis, and it is successful in all patients from the papillary opening and in more than 90% of patients from the bile ducts.[242] Biliary cannulation in these patients is easier to achieve because the passage of worms across the sphincter makes it patulous.[244] Worms can be extracted across the papillary opening by using grasping forceps or a Dormia basket; polypectomy snares should be avoided because the snare may cut the worm, leaving a remnant that may lead to stone formation. If the worms are unable to come out or are dead, they can be pulled out using a Dormia basket or a biliary occlusion balloon.[267] Total clearance of bile ducts may require multiple endoscopic sessions. Endoscopic papillary balloon dilation has been described in nonendemic areas to remove the worm and associated calculi.[247] When the worm cannot be reached by conventional ERCP, Sandouk et al.[268] have suggested using the whirlpool jet technique. Early ERCP should be performed when pancreaticobiliary ascariasis is suspected in cases of repeated pancreatitis after cholecystectomy and sphincterotomy, even with normal liver enzymes, because of worm migration.[250]

Surgical intervention is required when the *Ascaris* organisms enter the intrahepatic ducts, leading to the formation of stones, strictures, and abscesses and when gallbladder ascariasis is present (see Chapters 39, 42, and 43).[242] Laparoscopic extraction of live worms from the bile duct also has been reported in the literature.[269] Overall, 20% of patients with biliary ascariasis need surgery.[270] An initial operative cholangiogram helps define the extent of the infection (see Chapter 23). Worms are removed through a longitudinal choledochotomy because compression of the liver often propels intrahepatic worms toward the common bile duct. Choledochoscopy is also valuable, especially if worms, debris, or stones are impacted in the intrahepatic ducts.

The evacuated biliary tree is irrigated with saline and closed over a large-bore T-tube. Intraoperative cholangiography through the T-tube is done to identify residual worms. The liver may contain granulomatous nodules or abscesses, and worms under the liver capsule can be extracted by incision and drainage of the abscess. Removal of all worms from the intestine by enterostomy is an important part of the operation to prevent biliary reinfestation, a serious complication that may require reoperation.

Postoperatively, a broad-spectrum antibiotic is prescribed. Worms identified in the bile duct at this point should be managed conservatively because the worm may spontaneously return to the intestine. Irrigation of the T-tube with saline may help, but anthelmintics should not be administered through the T-tube; this would kill the worm in the common bile duct and prevent spontaneous evacuation. Endoscopic extraction may be successful if the worm is impacted around the T-tube or can be removed by applying suction to a T-tube and gently withdrawing it with the worm. If these measures fail, reoperation is necessary with preoperative oral anthelmintics.[73]

Full recovery is the rule, with a mortality rate of 1% or less. Worm reinvasion after successful initial management is always symptomatic and may occur in 30% of those treated.[244] A careful search for biliary lithiasis in the intrahepatic and extrahepatic bile ducts and management of sepsis and biliary strictures should result in a good prognosis. MRCP and ERCP should always be considered in cases of repeated pancreatitis. Recurrent pyogenic cholangitis, liver abscesses, and granuloma necessitate surgery.

Prevention

In endemic areas, school screening may be effective in the detection and early treatment of asymptomatic carriers. Health education, good sanitation, and early medical therapy of intestinal ascariasis are the best ways to prevent reinfection.

BLOOD FLUKES

Schistosomiasis

Schistosomiasis is sometimes referred to as *bilharziasis* after Theodor Bilharz, who first identified the parasite in 1852. Schistosomiasis is caused by infection with blood flukes known as *schistosomes*. It can be associated with serious morbidity and mortality and may cause anemia, chronic pain, diarrhea, exercise intolerance, malnutrition, bladder cancer, portal hypertension, and central nervous system complications.[271] Chronic complications usually occur in individuals who live in endemic areas and have recurrent exposure. However, schistosomiasis can also cause complications in people with even brief exposures, such as travelers.[272] Three major species and two less common species produce infection in humans. Of the major species, *Schistosoma mansion* is common in tropical and subtropical areas of sub-Saharan Africa, the Middle East, South America, and the Caribbean. *Schistosoma japonicum*, prevalent in Asia, can provoke intestinal and hepatic complications. *Schistosoma haematobium* is common in North Africa, sub-Saharan Africa, the Middle East, Turkey, and India and predominantly

leads to renal and bladder sequelae, although on occasion it results in liver disease. The minor species include *Schistosoma mekongi* and *Schistosoma intercalatum*, both of which can also induce intestinal and liver disease. More than 200 million people worldwide are estimated to have schistosomiasis, a disease responsible for more than 200,000 deaths annually.[273]

Life Cycle

The life cycle of schistosomiasis is complex and requires both intermediate and definitive hosts. The adult worms are approximately 1 to 2 cm in length with a cylindrical body, two terminal suckers, a blind digestive tract, and reproductive organs.[274] The male schistosome forms a groove, where the female resides. Females produce hundreds to thousands of eggs per day. After contact with water, the ovum releases miracidium, which seeks an intermediate host in the snail. After 4 to 6 weeks, the miracida multiply asexually into sporocysts and later into cercariae. The cercariae leave the snail and seek a definitive host, where they develop into adult worms. As the definitive host, humans acquire schistosomiasis by contact with fresh water. Cercariae penetrate the intact skin of humans and become schistosomulae, which migrate from the skin into blood and lymph vessels and are carried to the heart and lungs. They then migrate through pulmonary capillaries into the left side of the heart and then into the arterial circulation, where they are carried to the mesenteric arteries, splanchnic arteries, and portal veins; they subsequently reach the liver, where they mature into adults over a period of 1 to 4 weeks.

Different species have a propensity to affect different organs. The adult worms migrate against portal blood flow to varying destinations: mesenteric venules of the small intestine (*S. japonicum* and *S. mekongi*), mesenteric venules of the colon (*S. mansoni* and *S. intercalatum*), and the vesical venous plexus (*S. haematobium*). Adults remain in these blood vessels for life, residing in permanent copulation and adhering to the wall of the blood vessels. Worms survive for 5 to 7 years but can persist up to 30 years.[275] Female worm begins to produce eggs, which travel hematogenously to other sites or traverse from vascular space through host tissues to the lumina of intestine or urinary bladder. The eggs are then variably excreted in the feces (*S. mansoni, S. japonicum, S. haematobium, S. intercalatum,* and *S. mekongi*) or the urine (*S. haematobium*).

Pathogenesis

Unless adult worms migrate to an unusual location, such as the spinal cord or brain, little damage occurs to the host, whereas cellular infiltrate is consistently found around the eggs.[276] Eggs released into the bloodstream can invade local tissues, release toxins and enzymes, and provoke a Th2-mediated immune response. Inflammation and granuloma formation occur around deposited eggs and lead to fibrosis of affected tissues.[277] *S. mansoni, S. japonicum, S, mekongi,* and *S. intercalatum* eggs tend to either penetrate the bowel adjacent to the mesenteric vessels or travel by the portal venous system to the liver. In the bowel, granulomatous inflammation around the invading eggs can result in intestinal schistosomiasis characterized by ulceration and scarring.[278]

In the liver, eggs lodge in presinusoidal radicles of the portal vein, where they elicit a granulomatous fibrosing reaction that blocks venous blood flow. Portal hypertension results, with compensatory portosystemic blood flow and late progressive liver damage (see Chapter 74) Symmers pipestem fibrosis is pathognomonic. It is distinct from cirrhosis because there is no hepatocyte dysfunction; instead, the portal hypertension results from fibrosis within blood vessels. Eggs of *S. haematobium* usually affect the urinary tract; however, this parasite may be associated with hepatic damage.

The interaction between the parasite and host immune response is complex. Immunity to infection with any schistosome species is both innate and acquired. It is the host's immune response to invading eggs that is the major cause of clinical disease. A host-mediated type 2 Th2 fibrogranulomatous inflammatory response occurs, which may result in activation of hepatic stellate cells, the mediators of fibrosis.[279]

The age-intensity curve in endemic areas characteristically shows a rise in intensity of infection during the first 2 decades of life, followed by a decline in adults, with possible acquired immunity to adult worms. The behavioral factors (e.g., walking barefoot and swimming) may play a role in the incidence of infections in children compared with adults.

Clinical Picture

Most patients are asymptomatic, and symptoms depend on the stage of disease. The different species of *Schistosoma* cause varying clinical complications. Acute symptoms may present as swimmer's itch or Katayama fever. Symptoms are also more likely to occur in travelers and other nonimmune hosts. Lymphadenopathy, eosinophilia, and hepatosplenomegaly may be prominent findings. The diagnosis of Katayama fever relies on appropriate epidemiology and consistent clinical findings.[273]

Symptoms of chronic infection often begin insidiously and are progressive without treatment. Intestinal schistosomiasis may cause chronic or intermittent abdominal pain and diarrhea with iron-deficiency anemia secondary to ulceration and polyps. Acute appendicitis also has been described in one case report.[280] Hepatic schistosomiasis can lead to hepatomegaly and severe splenomegaly in children and adolescents. Chronic hepatic schistosomiasis develops years later in young and middle-aged adults, with a long duration of intense infection, splenomegaly, and portal hypertension (see Chapter 76). However, hepatocellular function remains normal. Leading causes of morbidity and mortality include the formation of ascites and esophageal bleeding from varices. Urinary schistosomiasis may be asymptomatic or may cause hematuria, and symptoms related to anemia may be present. Squamous cell carcinoma of the bladder and nephritic syndrome may occur.[281]

Schistosomiasis can sometimes be associated with serious neurologic complications. Pulmonary manifestations can also be seen in people with hepatosplenic disease as a result of heavy infections with *S. mansoni*, *S. japonicum*, or *S. haematobium* infection. Presinusoidal portal hypertension fosters the development of portosystemic collateral vessels that allow *Schistosoma* eggs to embolize into the pulmonary circulation, leading to granulomatous pulmonary endarteritis. Pulmonary hypertension and cor pulmonale gradually ensue with dyspnea as the principal symptom. As disease evolves, the heart enlarges and pulmonary arteries dilate to aneurysmal proportions, representing end-stage, irreversible alterations.[282] Recurrent urinary tract infections or bacteremia as a result of *Salmonella* infection are classic complications of schistosomiasis.[283] It has been postulated that infection with *S. haematobium* may increase the risk of HIV infection.[284] Persons with hepatitis B or C viruses have more severe disease.

Diagnosis

Complete blood count may show anemia, leukopenia, or thrombocytopenia as a result of hypersplenism with hypercellular marrow, portal hypertension, or varices. The liver profile is usually normal except in cases of coinfection. Eggs in the stool or urine are often used as a test, and rectal snips as well as circulating antigen are specific and sensitive to detect active infection and assess treatment. Serology usually detects previous exposure, and abdominal US shows splenomegaly and periportal fibrosis.[273] These laboratory tests have poor sensitivity when infection is early and there is need for more sensitive tests in strategies to eliminate of schistosomiasis in endemic regions. There is some progress in use of genomic tests targeting schistosome DNA sequences, which can help species-specific diagnosis even in the absence of excreted eggs.[285] PCR assays for stool, urine, and serum have been developed with better sensitivity in early infection for diagnosis of schistosomiasis.[286] However, the tests have remained as research tool due to cost.

Treatment

Praziquantel is the drug of choice for treatment of schistosomiasis. *S. haematobium*, *S. mansoni*, and *S. intercalatum* can be treated with 40 mg/kg in one or two doses, whereas the dosage for *S. japonicum* and *S. mekongi* is 60 mg/kg in two or three doses at least 3 hours apart. No serious side effects are reported, and treatment is efficacious in about 85% to 90%.[280] In addition to anthelmintic therapy, patients with severe portal hypertension and esophageal varices may also benefit from treatment with propranolol and/or sclerotherapy band ligation or shunt procedures (see Chapters 80, 81, 82, 83, 84, 85).[282]

Despite its demonstrated efficacy in decreasing recurrent variceal hemorrhage, enthusiasm for surgery has declined over the last 2 decades, due in part to the more easily administered techniques of endoscopic therapy or intervention. Orthotopic liver transplant is the only treatment that corrects the portal hypertension and also corrects the liver failure when it occurs. (see Chapter 105)

Acknowledgment

The authors acknowledge the contributions of Hanny Dubbous, P.G. Thomas, and N. Garg to this chapter.

References are available at expertconsult.com.

CHAPTER 72

Hydatid disease of the liver

Javier C. Lendoire, Emmanuel Melloul, and Oscar Cesar Imventarza

INTRODUCTION

Hydatid disease, or cystic echinococcosis (CE), is a worldwide parasitic zoonosis, caused by the larval stages of the metacestode *Echinococcus granulosus*.[1] Three more species of Echinococcus of public health concern have been recognized: *Echinococcus multilocularis*, causing alveolar echinococcosis, which will be discussed in the next section of this chapter; and *Echinococcus vogeli* and *Echinococcus oligarthus*, both causing polycystic echinococcosis.[2] Hydatid disease is the most prevalent and accounts for more than 95% of the estimated 2 to 3 million cases of echinococcosis in the world.[3] The definitive hosts of this parasite are usually members of the canid family, such as dogs, which develop the adult worm in the gut following ingestion of the larvae, present in the tissues of the intermediate hosts, usually sheep.[4] When infected, humans develop visceral hydatid cysts, which are fluid-filled structures limited by a parasite-derived membrane that contain a germinal epithelium.[2] Hydatid cysts usually affect the liver (50%–70%), followed by the lungs (20%–30%) and less frequently the spleen, kidney, heart, bones, central nervous system, and other organs.[5] Cysts can remain asymptomatic for years, but as they increase in size symptoms and complications can arise.[6] Up to a third of affected patients can develop complications such as secondary infection of the cyst cavity, biliary fistula, and rupture into the peritoneal and pleural cavity.[7] Therefore it is important to strictly abide by treatment guidelines to decrease the rate of possible complications. The modern treatment of liver hydatid cyst (LHC) varies from surgical intervention to percutaneous drainage or medical therapy.[8] Surgery remains the only definitive treatment for large, active, symptomatic, or complicated hydatid cysts.[9] Surgical management has evolved from open surgery to an increase in the application of the laparoscopic approach.[10] Percutaneous techniques can be a good alternative to surgery in selected patients with uncomplicated cysts or high-risk medical status performance.[11] Medical therapy is used for inoperable cases, for disseminated systemic disease, or as a complementary therapeutic option in percutaneous or surgical approaches to prevent postoperative recurrence.[12]

This zoonosis represents a major public and economic health problem due to the health costs generated for patient care; those affected by the disease may require prolonged hospitalizations with loss of quality of life, working days, and uprooting as they must move to urban centers for definitive care. Also, significant economic losses happen due to seized viscera or reduced production of wool or meat in infected animals. Prevention is the most effective and efficient way to control hydatid disease, and the development of health education and promotion activities in the community is essential.[3]

ECHINOCOCCUS GRANULOSUS

Echinococcus granulosus (EG), from a taxonomic perspective, is currently considered a multispecies complex referred to as EG sensu lato (s.l.). The species identified in this complex are EG sensu stricto (genotypes G1/G2/G3), Echinococcus equinus (genotype G4), Echinococcus ortleppi (genotype G5), Echinococcus canadensis (genotypes G6/G7/G8/G9/G10), and Echinococcus felidis (lion strain). Genotype 1 (G1) is the most widely distributed species at the global level and accounts for approximately 80% of human cases of hydatid disease.[13] Genotypes G2, G5, G6, G7, G8, and G9 have also been documented to infect humans.[14]

The adult worm of EG, 3 to 6 mm long, consists of scolex (head) bearing a rostellum with a double row of numerous hooks, four prominent suckers, a short neck region, and the strobilae (body) with three proglottids—usually one immature, one mature, and one gravid.[3] The last is the largest and bears the mature eggs.[5] On maturity each gravid proglottid can contain an average of 587 fertile eggs, which are eliminated with the dog's feces. A complete life cycle of the EG requires two hosts, a carnivore and a herbivore, and takes 32 to 80 days (Fig. 72.1). The adult tapeworm lives in the intestine of the dog, which is the most common definitive host.[2] Gravid proglottids release microscopic ovoid eggs (30–40 µm) that are passed in the feces and are immediately infectious. Echinococcus eggs contain a hexacanth embryo (oncosphere or first larval stage) surrounded by a thick keratinized wall and are extremely resistant, enabling them to withstand a wide range of environmental temperatures for many months. After ingestion by a suitable intermediate host (sheep, goat, swine, cattle, horse, camel), eggs hatch in the small intestine and release six-hooked oncospheres that penetrate the intestinal wall and migrate through the circulatory system into various organs, especially the liver and lungs. In these organs, the oncosphere develops into a thick-walled hydatid cyst that enlarges gradually, producing protoscolices and daughter cysts that fill the cyst interior. The definitive host becomes infected by ingesting the cyst-containing organs of the infected intermediate host. After ingestion, the protoscolices evaginate, attach to the intestinal mucosa, and develop into adult stages. Humans are aberrant intermediate hosts; they become infected by ingesting eggs either from direct contact with a contaminated dog or by ingesting contaminated water, food, or soil. Oncospheres are released in the intestine, and hydatid cysts develop in a variety of organs.[15] These cysts grow at a rate of 1 to 5 cm/year and may remain undetected for years, so they can reach very large sizes before becoming clinically evident. If cysts rupture, the liberated protoscolices may create secondary cysts in other sites within the body (secondary echinococcosis).[16]

Hydatid cysts are usually unilocular and can range anywhere from 1 to 20 cm in diameter. Cystic growth is expansive by concentric enlargement. They tend to affect the right lobe more frequently than the left lobe due to the nature of the portal blood flow.[1] There are three layers in a hydatid cyst: pericyst, ectocyst, and endocyst (Fig. 72.2). The pericyst or adventitial layer is the outermost layer, which is entirely made up of host

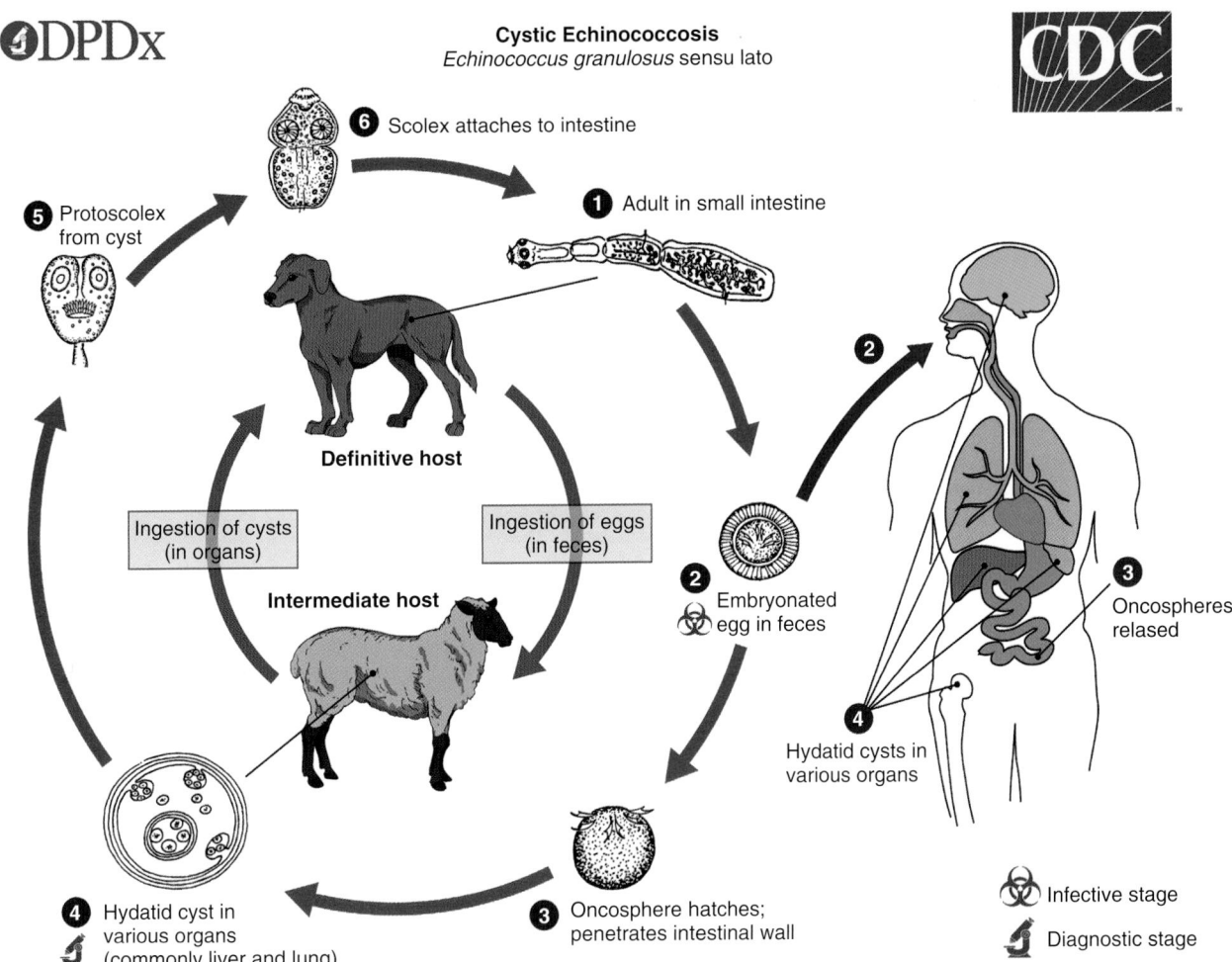

FIGURE 72.1 **Process of life cycle of cystic echinococcosis.** The adult *Echinococcus granulosus* (1) resides in the small intestine of the definitive host. Gravid proglottids release eggs (2) that are passed in the feces. After ingestion by a suitable intermediate host, eggs hatch in the small intestine and release six-hooked oncospheres (3) that penetrate the intestinal wall and migrate through the circulatory system into various organs. In these organs, the oncosphere develops into a thick-walled hydatid cyst (4) that enlarges gradually, producing protoscolices and daughter cysts that fill the cyst interior. The definitive host becomes infected by ingesting the cyst-containing organs of the infected intermediate host. After ingestion, the protoscolices (5) evaginate, attach to the intestinal mucosa (6), and develop into adult stages (1) in 32 to 80 days. Humans are aberrant intermediate hosts and become infected by ingesting eggs (2). Oncospheres are released in the intestine (3), and hydatid cysts develop in a variety of organs (4).

tissues in response to the expanding parasite. The host cellular inflammatory reaction is initiated in the early stages of postoncospheral development, and the initial intensity of this reaction varies between hosts and governs the fate of the developing metacestode. If too intense it will cause the degeneration and eventual death of the parasite, whereas in suitable intermediate hosts the initial reaction resolves, leaving a fibrous capsule.[17] With time, the adventitial layer may calcify, either partially or totally.[18] The ectocyst is the middle acellular layer, which is the elastic, laminated membrane resembling egg white that protects the cyst.[5] It provides a physiochemical barrier with apparent multifunctionality, allows passage of nutrients, and is easily separable from the adventitia. Finally, the endocyst or the germinal epithelium is the innermost layer, which is the only living component, being responsible for the formation of the other layers as well as the hydatid fluid and brood capsules (see Fig. 72.2). Undifferentiated cells in the germinal layer produce invaginations into the cyst cavity, forming the brood capsules.[19] It surrounds a cavity filled with hydatid fluid. Hydatid fluid is clear and contains electrolytes and proteins. Cyst fluid is clear or pale yellow, has a neutral pH, and contains sodium chloride, proteins, glucose, ions, lipids, and polysaccharides. The fluid is antigenic and may also contain protoscolices and hooklets. When vesicles rupture within the cyst, protoscolices pass into the cyst fluid and form a white sediment known as hydatid sand.[19] Daughter cysts have a structure similar to the mother cysts, including a laminated and germinative membrane, cyst fluid, brood capsules, and protoscolices. The only difference is the absence of an adventitial layer.[17]

EPIDEMIOLOGY

EG sensu lato has a worldwide geographic distribution with endemic foci present on every inhabited continent (Fig. 72.3).[20] Some areas, such as Central Asia, present a high prevalence of both EG and Echinococcus multilocularis.[21] In regions where CE is endemic, incidence rates in humans can exceed 50 per 100,000 person-years. The global burden of hydatid disease is estimated at 1 million at any one time.[22] The greatest prevalence of hydatid disease in human and animal hosts is found in

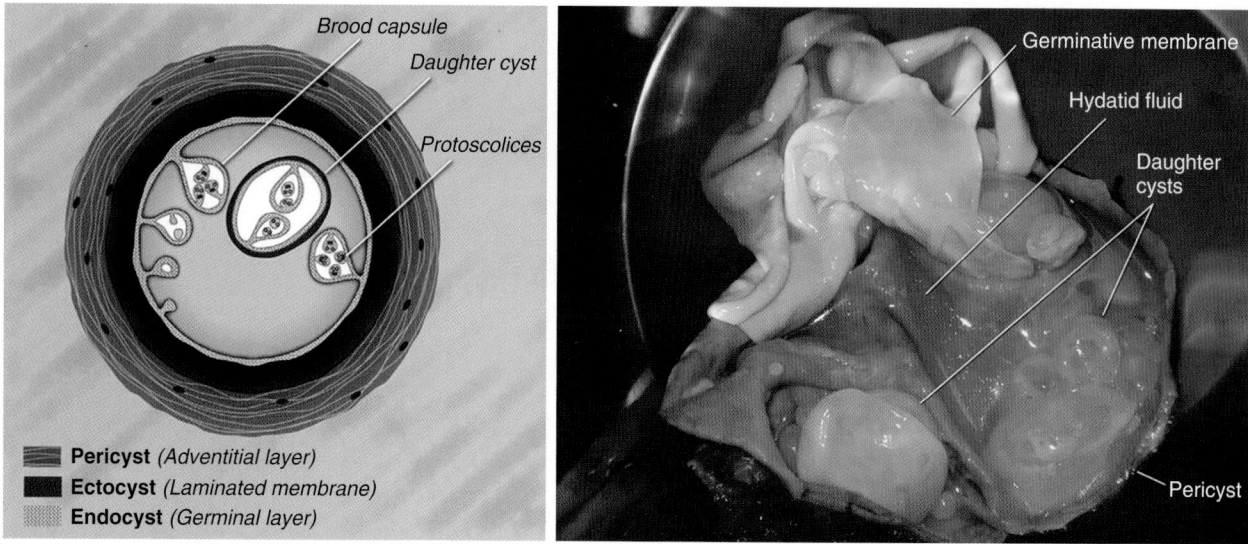

FIGURE 72.2 Schematic representation and explant specimen after surgery of a viable uncomplicated liver hydatid cyst. There are three layers: pericyst, ectocyst, and endocyst. The endocyst or germinal epithelium is the only living component of the cyst that generates hydatid fluid and brood capsules and is responsible for the formation of the other layers. (Scheme modified from Thompson RCA. Biology and Systematics of Echinococcus. In: Thompson RCA, Deplazes P, Limbery AJ, eds. *Advances in Parasitology. Echinococcus and Echinococcosis Part A.* Vol. 95. Academic Press is an imprint of Elsevier; 2017:91, Fig. 7.)

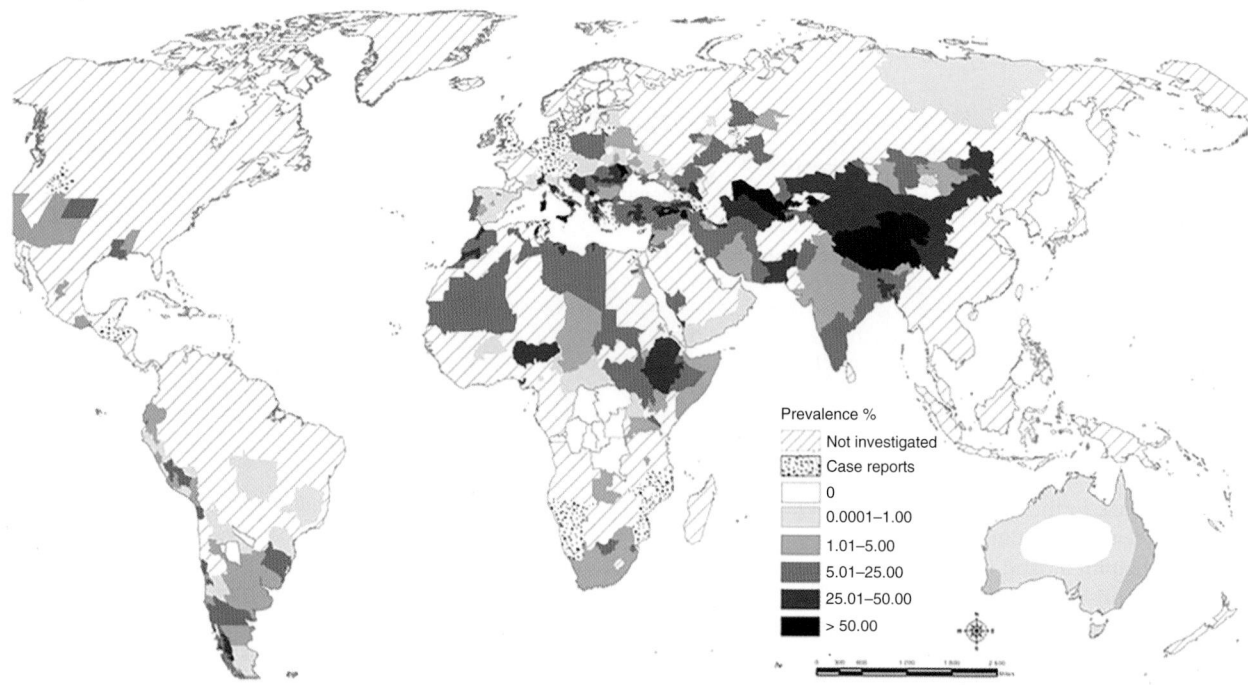

FIGURE 72.3 Map with the global distribution of Echinococcus spp. causing cystic echinococcosis (CE) mainly from domestic intermediate hosts (not included are the cervid genotypes of Echinococcus canadensis and Echinococcus equinus). In addition, in areas where data of domestic intermediate hosts are missing, case reports of CE in wild intermediate hosts are given as dotted areas. (From Deplazes P, Rinaldix L, Alvarez Rojas CA, et al. Global distribution of alveolar and cystic echinococcosis. *Adv Parasitol.* 2017;95:315–493.)

countries of the temperate zones, including several parts of Eurasia (the Mediterranean regions, southern and central parts of Russia, central Asia, China), Australia, some parts of the Americas (especially South America), and north and east Africa.[23] The distinct genetic types of EG, based on morphology, host specificity, and molecular characteristics, include two sheep strains (G1 and G2), two bovid strains (G3 and G5), a horse strain (G4), a camelid strain (G6), a pig strain (G7), and a cervid strain (G8). A ninth genotype (G9) has been described in swine in Poland and a tenth strain (G10) in reindeer in Eurasia.[14] The most frequent strain associated with human hydatid disease appears to be the common sheep strain (G1).[1] This strain appears to be widely distributed in all continents (Fig. 72.4).[14] Highest rates of infection are recorded in communities involved in extensive sheep farming, and epidemiologic studies suggest that this genetic variant is the principal

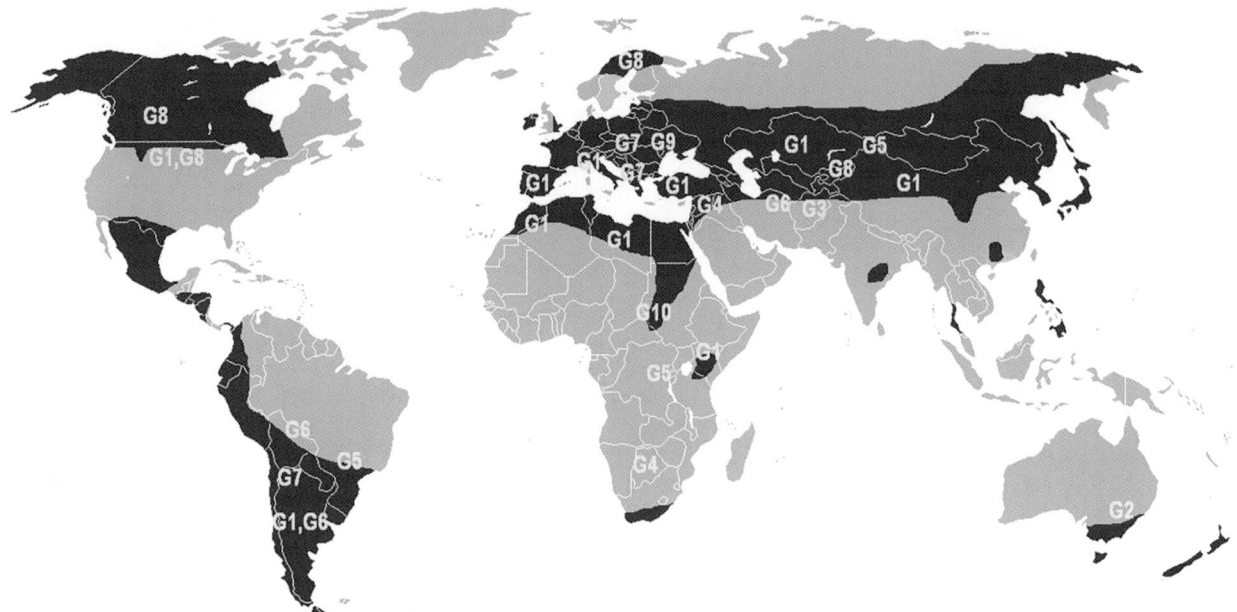

FIGURE 72.4   Map showing the worldwide distribution of the zoonotic strains of Echinococcus granulosus and geographic endemicity.

strain infecting humans.[3] In Europe, EG is present in most countries. Annual incidence rates of 4 to 8 per 10^5 population have been reported in the Mediterranean regions.[14,24] Fourteen countries reported 412 confirmed cases of CE in 2017. This was an 11% decrease compared with 2016, when 465 confirmed cases were reported. Bulgaria accounted for 53% of the cases in 2017 and Germany for 18%. The majority (35%) of CE cases were observed in the age group 25 to 44 years, followed by the age group 45 to 64 years (25%). Increasing country-specific trends were observed in Austria, Germany, Lithuania, and Poland, and decreasing trends in Slovakia and Spain.[25] Hydatid disease is a serious health problem in Turkey with 5.7 per 10^5 population and a high prevalence in regions of the Anatolian peninsula.[26] In central Asia and western China at least 270 million people (58% of the total population) are at risk for hydatid disease.[27] The infection rate of females in China has been assessed to be considerable higher than that of males because of their role in the home activities, including feeding dogs, collecting yak dung for fuel, and milking livestock. This nomadic or seminomadic pastoral lifestyle is one of the most important risk factors for hydatid disease in China.[14] In Australia, where EG established viable reservoirs in native wallabies and kangaroos, the highest rates recorded have been in rural northeast and southeast New South Wales with 23.5 per 10^5 population.[9] In South America, the disease is endemic or hyperendemic in Argentina, Uruguay, Chile, Southern Brazil, and mountain regions of Perú and Bolivia.[13] In a 5-year period, 29,556 cases of CE were reported to official authorities in the five countries belonging to the Sub-Regional Initiative for the control of EG (Argentina, Brazil, Chile, Peru, and Uruguay), with an incidence rate range between 0.012 and 13 per 100,000 inhabitants according to the country.[28] Argentina shows three high-incidence areas: the Patagonia region, in the south of the country (where the provinces of Neuquén and Chubut show the highest national rates), the Northwest region (including the provinces of Catamarca, Santiago del Estero, and Salta), and

the province of Entre Ríos in the East. Neuquén is one of the provinces with higher hydatid disease endemicity in Argentina, despite the fact that provincial sanitary authorities have carried out a control program of EG since 1970; the mean annual incidence of human EG in Neuquén is 8.9 per 10^5 inhabitants.[29] In selected areas of other South American countries, hydatid disease has been recorded as 6 to 20 per 10^5, such as in the south of Chile.[14] The global burden of hydatid disease has been calculated to be of approximately 1 to 3 million disability-adjusted life years (DALYs) annually. In addition, the economic burden of this disease to the global livestock industry has been estimated at over $3 billion per annum. Despite the substantial socioeconomic impact, echinococcosis remains a neglected zoonosis in certain countries.[22] A study performed in Salamanca Province, Spain, demonstrated a diminished incidence of hydatid disease in recent years, although active transmission remains in pediatric and young patients.[30] Continuous education and training for the relevant health professionals is still needed because hydatid disease is endemic in many countries.[20]

COMPLICATIONS

The natural history of hydatid cyst can be divided into two phases. In the first phase of cyst growth, rupture can occur when the pressure of the hydatid liquid becomes greater than the resistance of the hydatid wall (pericyst). The second phase is of ageing and progressive involution as a consequence of the overproduction of scolices and daughter cysts. During this phase the hydatid cyst will be full of scolices and membranes that replace the hydatid liquid, and calcifications occur in the pericyst.[13] Hydatid cyst in the liver may cause symptoms resulting from compression, distortion of neighboring structures or viscera, infection, and erosion into the bile duct, the pleural space, or the peritoneal cavity.[7] Less frequently the cyst may communicate with the digestive tract and the bronchial tree.[7] Complications are usually observed in one third of patients with hydatid disease of the liver (HDL).

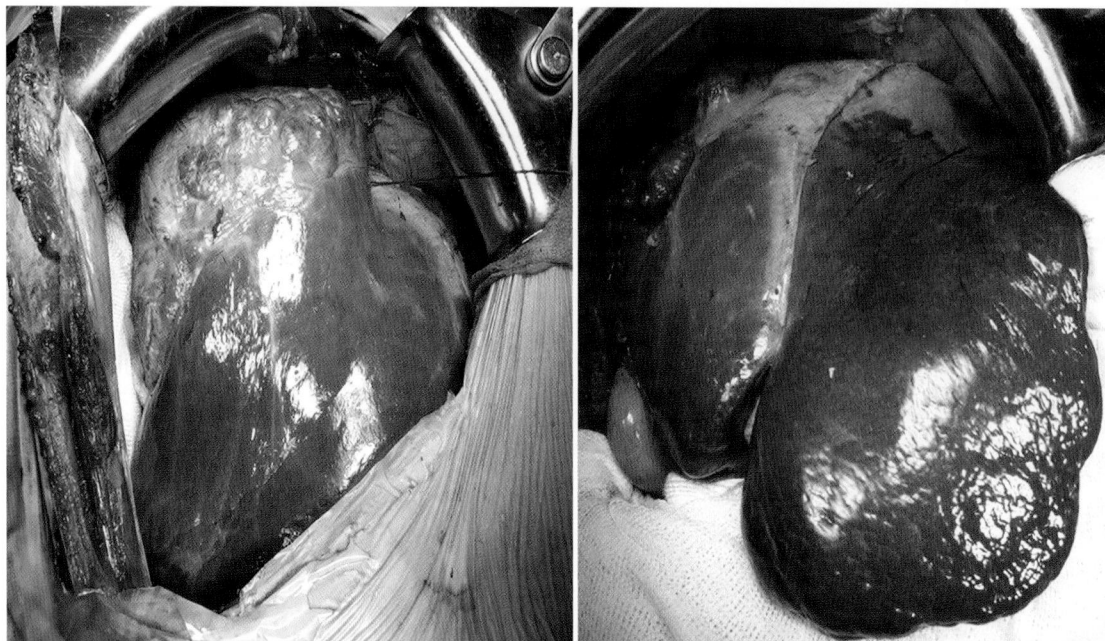

FIGURE 72.5   Clinical photograph of a patient operated on for a hydatid cyst located in the right lobe. **A,** The presence of an atrophied right hemiliver due to cyst compression. **B,** The enlargement of the left lobe (more pronounced in segments II and III) due to compensatory regeneration.

Compressive Effects

Liver hydatid cyst (LHC) growth may lead to significant mass effect to adjacent structures, including biliary tree, portal vein, hepatic veins, right diaphragm, stomach, and kidney.[7] Enlargement of the cyst tends to occur toward the surface of the liver and is commonly seen in the presence of atrophied lobes or segments containing hydatid cysts with enlargement of the residual hepatic parenchyma due to compensatory regeneration[31] (Fig. 72.5). Depending on the location, large cysts can cause compression of the bile ducts and obstructive jaundice[32] (Fig. 72.6). Compression and displacement of hepatic veins and inferior vena cava (IVC) may lead to secondary Budd-Chiari syndrome (see Chapter 86). Clinical manifestations include abdominal pain, jaundice, and swelling of the lower limbs.[7] Ascites and venous thrombosis may also develop in these patients. Portal vein obstruction is a rare complication, more commonly reported in hydatid cysts located around the hilum; it is generated by a decreased portal vein inflow and thrombosis with cavernous transformation and is commonly associated with presinusoidal portal hypertension.[33]

Infection

Secondary bacterial infection occurs in approximately 10% of hydatid cysts but is usually latent and subacute. Hydatid cysts may become infected after an episode of bacteremia or due to the communication with the bile duct and is clinically translated by pain in the right hypochondrium, hepatomegaly, and fever.[34]

Cyst Rupture

Intrabiliary Rupture

Cistobiliary communication is the most common complication of HDL and one of the most serious, occurring in up to 42% of patients in some series.[34] Two theories have been postulated about its pathogenesis: the first asserts that the compression of

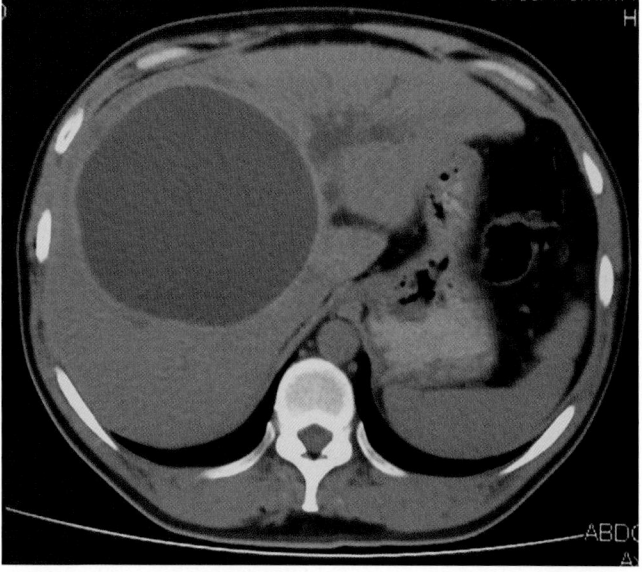

FIGURE 72.6   Diagnostic computed tomography scan of a central liver hydatid cyst with compression of the bile duct. Note the dilatation of the biliary duct at the level of the left lateral sector of the liver.

the LHC on the wall of the bile duct causes progressive necrosis and finally a communication between the cysts and the biliary tree; the second hypothesis states that after the trapping of small biliary radicals in the pericystic wall, high intracystic pressure (35 cm H_2O) causes atrophy first and then subsequently the rupture of biliary radicals.[35,36] It has been reported that up to 90% of the liver hydatid cysts have some kind of communication during their evolution.[37] Clinical manifestations depend mainly on the size of the biliocystic communication. Minor communications (<5 mm) lead to cystic fluid drainage, whereas

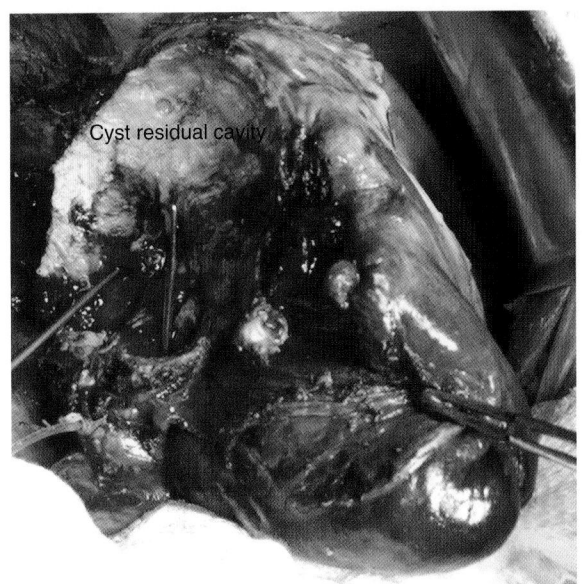

Cyst residual cavity

FIGURE 72.7 Surgical photograph of a right liver hydatid cyst treated with a partial pericystectomy. Note the major biliary communication demonstrated by the passage of the surgical explorer into the residual cyst cavity.

major ruptures (3%–17%) allow the passage of the cyst contents (hydatid membrane and daughter cysts) into the bile duct.[35] The classic triad of biliary rupture in cystic hydatid disease (biliary colic, jaundice, and urticaria), eventually associated with fever (in case of cholangitis), is more frequent in patients with major communications[37] (Fig. 72.7). In cases of intrabiliary rupture smaller than 5 mm, it is exceptional to find hydatid material in the bile duct. In some patients, jaundice can be temporarily relieved following biliary communication due to reduction of intracystic pressure.[36] Migration of daughter cysts through the biliocystic communication can lead to a secondary obstruction at the level of the duodenal papilla.[38] Minor leaks of the cyst can produce flushing and urticaria, and major rupture can lead to potentially fatal anaphylactic reaction.[5]

Communication between the cysts and the biliary tree occurs more frequently in those cysts located in the center of the liver, near the hilum, most commonly in the right hemiliver[36] (see Fig. 72.7). From 114 cases of cystobiliary ruptures reported in three studies, 65% were located in the right hemiliver, 21% in the left hemiliver, and 14% presented a bilateral distribution.[36,39,40] Because cystobiliary rupture is a major risk factor for morbidity, preoperative and intraoperative identification of predictive factors is a relevant issue.[35,41] Size of the cyst has always been reported as an important predictor for the presence of cystobiliary communications. A cutoff value in size from 7.5 cm to 14.5 cm was demonstrated in different studies, but the most commonly reported was 10 cm.[36,37,40,41] Other predictors described are a fibrotic or calcified pericystic wall, the number of cysts, cyst Gharbi type IV, and preoperative laboratory findings such as leukocytosis, eosinophilia, hyperbilirubinemia, and elevated alkaline phosphatase (ALP) and gamma glutamyl transpeptidase (GGT).[36,37,39,40,41]

Peritoneal Rupture

Intraperitoneal rupture of a hydatid cyst may result from trauma or spontaneously when the intracystic pressure increases more than 50 cm H_2O.[42] It is the third most common complication

(1%–16%) after intrabiliary rupture and allergic reactions.[42] The main risk factors predisposing to peritoneal rupture include young age, cyst diameter greater than 10 cm, and superficial cyst location. Young age is a risk factor because of the greater frequency of traumatic events in this population.[42] Clinical signs and symptoms of intraperitoneal cyst ruptures may vary widely among patients. The most frequent symptoms are mild or severe abdominal pain, nausea, vomiting, and some allergic reactions that span a wide range.[43] Antigenic fluid released into the peritoneal cavity and absorbed into the circulation is the cause of the acute allergic manifestations.[42] If the content of the rupture is purulent or associated with the biliary tract, it may cause peritoneal irritation, and acute abdominal pain may occur.[44,45] Approximately 16.7% to 25% of patients with hydatid cyst rupture develop minor allergic reactions, such as urticaria and macular eruption, and 1% to 12.5% of patients develop more severe allergic reactions such as peripheral edema, syncope, or anaphylaxis.[46] If the rupture is insidious, the release of brood capsules, scolices, and even daughter cysts from a ruptured hydatid cyst into the peritoneal cavity leads to multiple cysts in the peritoneal cavity. This phenomenon is called *secondary echinococcosis*.[47]

Intrathoracic Rupture

LHC located at the dome of the liver can grow and erode through the diaphragm to involve the thoracic cavity.[48] Intrathoracic rupture is a serious complication that can damage the pleura, pulmonary parenchyma, and bronchi. Its frequency appears to decline from 16% to 2.5% of the reported cases.[49] Intrathoracic evolution of a hydatid cyst depends on several factors: the intimate contact of the hepatic dome with the diaphragm; the thoracoabdominal pressure gradient, which tends to aspirate the contents of the liver cyst toward the thoracic cavity; the erosion of the diaphragm by ischemia-necrosis caused by eventual inflammation and superinfection of the cyst; and the corrosion of all tissues in contact with the bile[49] (Fig. 72.8). The cyst, after having passed through the diaphragm, can be fistulized in the bronchi, generally of the lower and/or middle lobe. Initially, a hydatid pneumonia is generated that is followed by an intraparenchymal cavity where bronchi will eventually become fistulized constituting a biliobronchial fistula, the ultimate stage of this severe complication.[50] The clinical presentation is predominantly pulmonary (cough, expectoration, and dyspnea) with abdominal symptoms being less frequent.[51] Hemoptysis, hydatid vomica, and bilioptysis are clinical manifestations of the biliobronchial fistulization.[50] Bilioptysis, a pathognomonic sign, is clinically evident in 28.6% to 40.6% of the cases.[49]

Cutaneous Fistulization and Other Complications

Spontaneous cyst-cutaneous fistula is an extremely rare complication of LHC, usually occurring silently, in elderly people.[52] Spontaneous cyst rupture in the gastrointestinal tract also is infrequent, in only 0.5%; patients can present with hydatidemesis (hydatid cysts and membranes in the vomitus) and/or hydatidenteria (passage of hydatid membranes in the stools).[53]

Exceptionally, a subacute chronic fistula may be created between the cyst and the IVC, with transit of daughter cyst or membranes into the bloodstream and then to the right atrium, causing a pulmonary embolism. The most severe complication of the cysto-venous communication is acute exsanguinating hemorrhage or anaphylactic shock, which may have a high mortality. The fact that the intracystic pressure is higher than the central venous pressure may facilitate the passage of material into the IVC.[54]

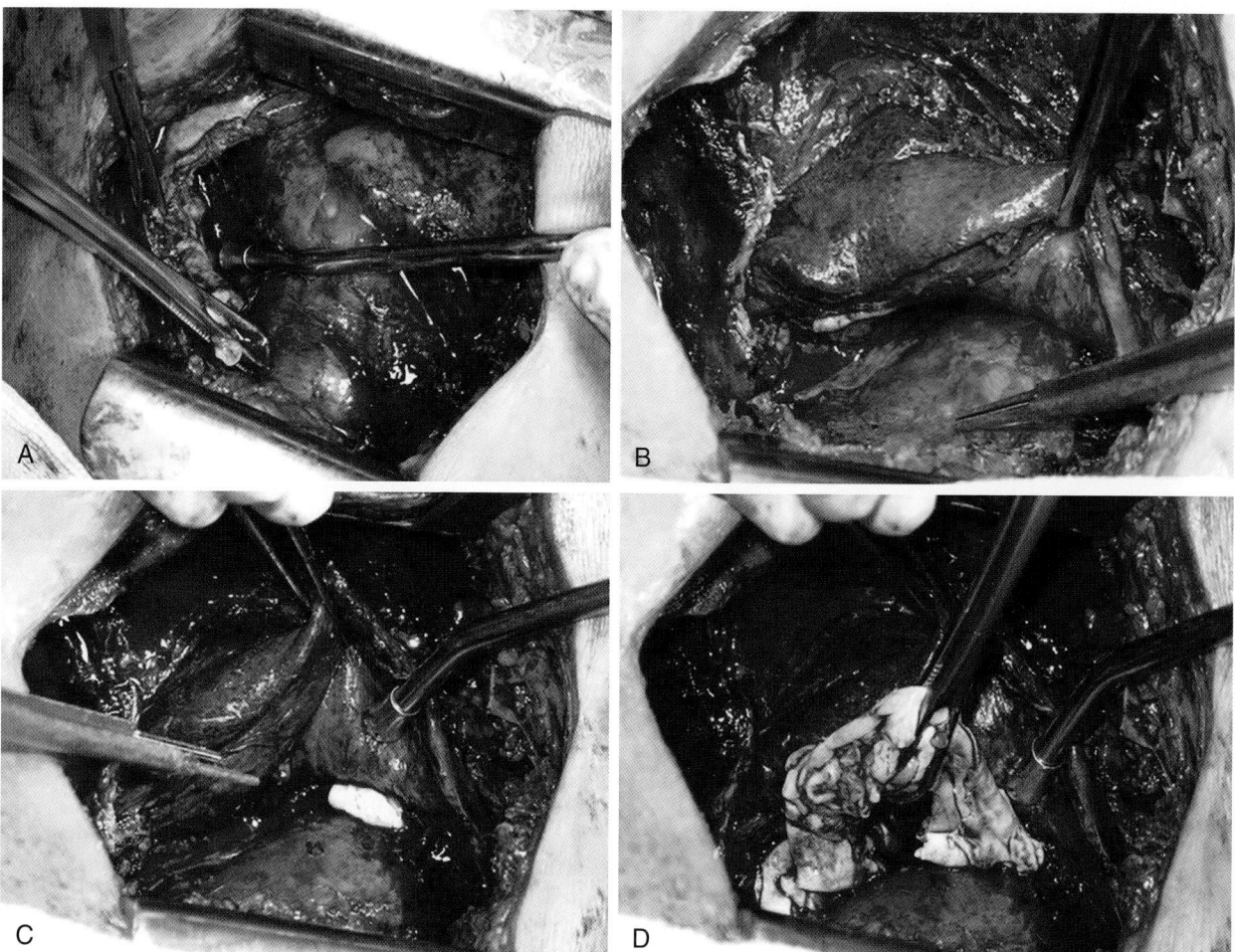

FIGURE 72.8 Operative views after a thoracotomy for an intrathoracic rupture of a right liver hydatid. The cysts located at the dome of the liver eroded through the diaphragm (a) to involve the thoracic cavity. Release of the inflammatory pulmonary adhesions with the diaphragm (b). Conservative treatment of the pulmonary cyst—note the removal of the germinative membrane with a Foerster clamp (c, d).

DIAGNOSIS

Humans are usually asymptomatic for an infection with EG for a long time. The growth of the cyst in the liver is variable, ranging from 1 to 5 mm in diameter per year. Most primary infections consist of a single cyst, but up to 20% to 40% of infected people have multiple cysts. The symptoms depend not only on the size and number of cysts, but also on the mass effect within the organ and on neighboring structures.[15] HDL diagnosis is based on a combination of clinical findings, imaging techniques, and serology, usually in conjunction with a history of exposure or immigration from an endemic area. Proof of the presence of protoscolices may be given by microscopic examination of the fluid and histology. False-positive reactions may occur in persons with other tapeworm infections, cancer, or chronic immune disorders. Whether the patient has detectable antibodies depends on the physical location, integrity, and viability of the cyst. Patients with senescent, calcified, or dead cysts usually are seronegative.[2]

The introduction of ultrasound for the diagnosis of human abdominal echinococcosis in the early 1970s was of special relevance for mass screening of populations. Mass screening has proven a reliable and relatively cheap method for demonstrating the true extent of human hydatid disease.[55] Ultrasound

examination is the basis of hydatid cyst diagnosis in abdominal locations, at both the individual and population level. In 1995, the World Health Organization–Informal Working Group on Echinococcosis (WHO-IWGE) developed a standardized classification that could be applied in all settings to replace the plethora of previous classifications and allow a natural grouping of six cyst types into three relevant groups (active, transition, inactive).[56] An expert consensus on the clinical management of patients with CE established that the diagnosis may be defined according to three situations:[57]

- *Possible case:* Any patient with a clinical or epidemiologic history, and imaging findings or serology positive for CE.
- *Probable case:* Any patient with the combination of clinical history, epidemiologic history, imaging findings, and serology positive for CE on two tests.
- *Confirmed case:* The above, plus either (1) demonstration of protoscolices or their components, using direct microscopy or molecular biology, in the cyst contents aspirated by percutaneous puncture or at surgery, or (2) changes in ultrasound appearance.

In most cases, the diagnosis is incidental, when ultrasonography or a computed tomography (CT) scan is indicated for investigation of other pathology or in patients with abdominal pain or anomalies of liver blood tests. The most common symptom, when it occurs, is right upper quadrant or epigastric pain, and the most common findings on examination are an enlarged liver and a palpable mass. Pressure effects are initially vague and may include nonspecific pain, cough, low-grade fever, and the sensation of abdominal fullness. As the mass grows, the symptoms become more specific because the mass impinges on or obstructs specific organs.[58]

Laboratory Tests

Laboratory tests are rarely abnormal in patients with uncomplicated hydatid cysts. Serum alkaline phosphatase levels are raised in one third of the patients. In patients with rupture of the cyst in the biliary tree, marked and transient elevation of cholestatic enzyme levels occurs, often in association with hyperamylasemia and eosinophilia. CE is one of the few parasitic infections in which the basis for laboratory diagnosis is primarily serology.[57] Different immunologic methods have been used for this differential and specific diagnosis.[116]

Echinococcus spp. can survive in humans for a long time through active regulation of the host immune response by the secretion of proteins at the interface of parasite and host tissues. Profiling hydatid cyst fluid protein composition and excretory/secretory products provides valuable information on parasite survival strategies and the molecular mechanisms of parasite-host interaction. In addition, analysis of the protein profiles can help in identifying potential molecular markers for developing diagnostic and follow-up tools. Proteomic analysis of the composition of cyst/vesicular fluids has identified hundreds of proteins from both Echinococcus spp. and the host that may help differentiate subpopulations of patients in the future.[59] Characterization of ES proteins from EG adult worms and protoscoleces also shows promise for identification of potential diagnostic markers.[60-63]

Serologic Tests

In humans, infection with EG induces an antibody response, most commonly IgG (predominantly IgG1 and IgG4), followed by IgM, IgA, and IgE. In 30% to 40% of the patients no antibodies are detectable, even with circulating antigens, indicating the presence of different mechanisms for the inhibition of host immune response.[1] Serologic tests in hydatid disease are used for the differential diagnosis of a cystic liver mass, for epidemiologic surveillance, and for post-treatment follow-up. Serology for diagnosis of hydatid disease dates from the early use of the complement-fixation (CF) test in the first decade of this century (Ghedini, 1906), the hemagglutination test, the bentonite-flocculation test, the latex-agglutination test, and the Cassoni intradermal skin test. Other techniques, such as hemagglutination and flocculation, appear to be more sensitive than the CF test. At present, serologic tests usually are based on the reaction and precipitation of the test antigen and the circulating antibodies in the host. The sensitivity and specificity of the tests depend on the quality of antigens. Antibody detection remains the method of choice.[64] EG antigen B and antigen 5 (Ag5) are the most specific antigens used for immunologic diagnosis.[65]

Immunoelectrophoresis (IEP) diagnostic values range from 91% to 95% in hydatid disease. IEP is not suitable for epidemiologic surveillance; rather, it is used for post-treatment follow-up.

Enzyme-linked immunosorbent assay (ELISA) for Echinococcus IgG is the quantitative determination of IgG antibodies (total and subclasses) against EG in human serum.[66] For detection of antibodies against EG infection, crude or purified antigens are used, and, by purification of the antigens, specificity of the test increases significantly. The reported sensitivity of this test varies from 88.23% to 100%.[67]

Blotting. Western immunoblotting, which provides fractionation of the parasite antigens, results in higher sensitivity and specificity. Sensitivity of 72% to 97% and specificity of 96% to 100% have been reported for this test in diagnosis of hydatid disease.[65]

DNA detection. Recently developed DNA-based methods, such as quantitative and/or nested polymerase chain reaction (PCR) assays, are highly sensitive, reasonably specific, and able to distinguish Echinococcus species from each other and from other cestodes; they can discriminate the various genotypes of EG, including following clinical biopsy of a suspected case, and identify infected mammalian host species.[68]

To compare serologic results between various studies, one needs to have a good knowledge of the nature and composition of antigens as well as geographic area of the studied cohort (endemic versus nonendemic area), strain of EG in circulation, and clinical data of patients.[65]

Imaging (see Chapter 14)
Radiology

Plain radiographs of the abdomen and chest may reveal a thin rim of calcification delineating a cyst, or an elevated hemidiaphragm, poorly moving right diaphragm, and hepatomegaly. These signs are nonspecific. Calcification is seen at radiography in 20% to 30% of hydatid cysts and usually manifests with a curvilinear or ring-like pattern representing calcification of the pericyst.[18]

Ultrasound

Ultrasound is the screening method of choice and primary diagnostic technique, with a diagnostic accuracy of 90%. Advantages of ultrasound diagnosis include the possibility for wide geographic coverage reaching populations with difficult access to health care, the early diagnosis at primary health care facilities, and the appropriate clinical management and timely treatment with local follow-up. Findings usually seen in solitary cysts are an anechoic univesicular cyst with well-defined borders and enhancement of back-wall echoes in a manner similar to simple or congenital cysts.[69] The cyst wall usually has a hypoechoic layer, flanked by an echogenic line on either side. Features that suggest hydatid etiology include dependent debris (hydatid sand) moving free with change in position; presence of wall calcification or localized thickening in the wall corresponding to early daughter cysts; separation of membranes (ultrasonic water lily sign) due to collapse of germinal layer seen as an undulating linear collection of echoes; and daughter cysts, probably the most characteristic sign with cysts within a cyst, producing a cartwheel or honeycomb cyst. When the matrix composed of detached membranes, broken daughter cysts, scolices, and hydatid sand fills the cyst, the cyst can appear as a solid mass.[1] Multiple cysts with normal intervening parenchyma present a differential diagnosis with necrotic secondaries, polycystic liver disease, abscess, chronic hematoma, and biliary cysts. Complications may be evident such as echogenic cysts in infection or signs of biliary obstruction (dilated bile ducts with images corresponding to hyperechoic vesicles or hydatid membranes within the biliary tract) usually implying a biliary communication.[16]

TABLE 72.1 Comparison of Gharbi's and World Health Organization–Informal Working Group on Echinococcosis (WHO-IWGE) Ultrasound Classification

CLASSIFICATION			
GHARBI	WHO-IWGE	DESCRIPTION	ACTIVITY
I	CE1	Unilocular, echo-free cyst, often double walled. "Snowflake effect" apparent on shifting the patient's position due to free-floating protoscolices	Active
III	CE2	Multivesicular, multiseptated cysts. Cyst septations produce "wheel-like" structures. Daughter cysts visible as "rosette-like or honeycomb-like" structures	Active
II	CE3A	Cyst with partial or total detachment of the laminated layer with floating undulating hyperechoic membranes showing the dual wall and "water lily" sign	Transitional
III	CE3B	Daughter cysts in solid matrix	Transitional
IV	CE4	Heterogeneous cyst with appearance of a "ball of wool"; no daughter cysts	Inactive
V	CE5	Solid matrix with calcified wall; degree of calcification varies from partial to complete	Inactive

CE, Cystic echinococcosis.

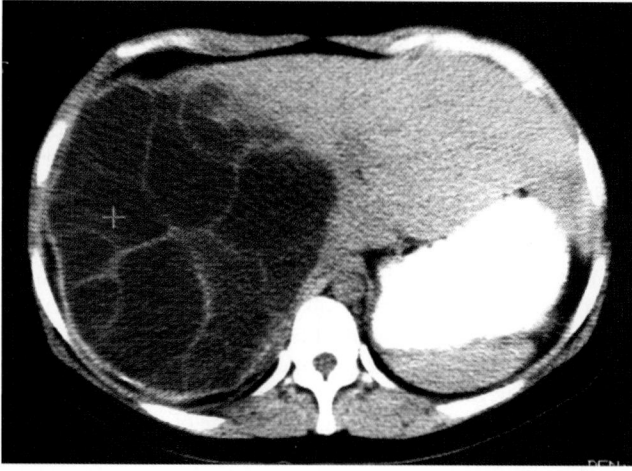

FIGURE 72.9 Diagnostic computed tomography of a liver hydatid cyst type CE2 involving the right lobe plus segment IV. Note the compression of the IVC and hypertrophy of segments II/III of the left lobe. *IVC,* Inferior vena cava

The classification system developed by Gharbi et al in 1981[70] was revised by the WHO-IWGE and is currently the screening method of choice (Table 72.1). The WHO-IWGE classification allows grouping of cysts into active, transitional, and inactive, which is relevant for treatment planning and follow-up.[64,71] The relevance of ultrasound extends to its application in endemic areas as focused assessment of specific conditions with ultrasound can be taught to nonspecialists in short courses, such as the focused assessment with ultrasound for echinococcosis (FASE) training course implemented in Argentina since 2000.[72] Investment in equipment and FASE-like training courses should be part of public health policies for hydatid disease.[73,74]

Contrast-enhanced ultrasound may be used to distinguish hydatid cyst from neoplasm; the absence of contrast enhanced in the LHC due to fluid-filled avascular cysts may be demonstrated. Perifocal inflammatory reactions, as nodular zones of peripheral ring enhancement, are seen.[75] Intraoperative ultrasonography is an important investigation tool during surgery for hydatid cyst of the liver. Ultrasound also has a crucial role in the guidance for percutaneous treatments.[64,76,77]

Computed Tomography

Computed tomography (CT) is not as operator dependent as ultrasound, and it gives the surgeon an accurate roadmap of the sites of the cysts in the liver. Multidetector row CT has the highest sensitivity of imaging of the cyst (94%–100%).[78] It is the best mode to detect the number, size, and location of the cysts (Fig. 72.9). It may provide clues to the presence of complications such as infection and intrabiliary ruptures. CT scanning has the advantages of inspecting any organ, detecting smaller cysts when located outside the liver, locating cysts precisely, and sometimes differentiating parasitic from nonparasitic cysts. Measurement of cyst density appears to be an additional tool to differentiate parasitic from nonparasitic cysts and for follow-up studies during chemotherapy.[69] Together with ultrasound, CT can determine the degree of calcification of a cyst, which, according to a recent study, is not conclusive of disease regression and may occur in all cyst stages[18] (Figs. 72.10 and 72.11).

Magnetic Resonance Imaging

Magnetic resonance imaging (MRI) is superior to CT in demonstrating the internal composition of cysts, the cyst wall defects, potential biliary involvement, and neural involvement.[69] On T2-weighted MRI, hydatid liver cysts present frequently a low signal intensity rim, represented by the pericyst, rich in collagen.[69] Daughter cysts, if present, are seen as cystic structures attached to the germinal layer that are hypointense relative to the intracystic fluid on T1-weighed images.[69] After the intravenous injection of gadolinium contrast agent the pericyst may show slight enhancement. MRI is the best diagnostic method to demonstrate the floating membranes or incipient detachment of the membranes. Secondary to damage or degeneration of the hydatid cyst, the membranes collapse and MRI shows the typical "snake sign."[1] Diffusion-weighed MRI is particularly useful in differentiating hydatid from simple liver cysts and the different hydatid cyst types.[79] MRI may have some advantages over CT scanning in the evaluation of postsurgical residual lesions, recurrences, and selected extrahepatic infections.[32] It is also superior in identifying changes of the intrahepatic and extrahepatic venous system (obstruction, thrombosis, invasion) and in identifying cystobiliary fistulas[80] (Fig. 72.12). Previous studies demonstrated that MRI reproduces the ultrasound-defined features of cystic echinococcosis (CE) better than CT. If ultrasonography cannot be performed owing to cyst location or patient-specific reasons, MRI with heavily T2-weighted series is preferable to CT.[81] Magnetic resonance cholangiopancreatography (MRCP) is useful to study potential involvement of the biliary tree as cystobiliary communications or biliary dilatations secondary to compression of cysts.[69]

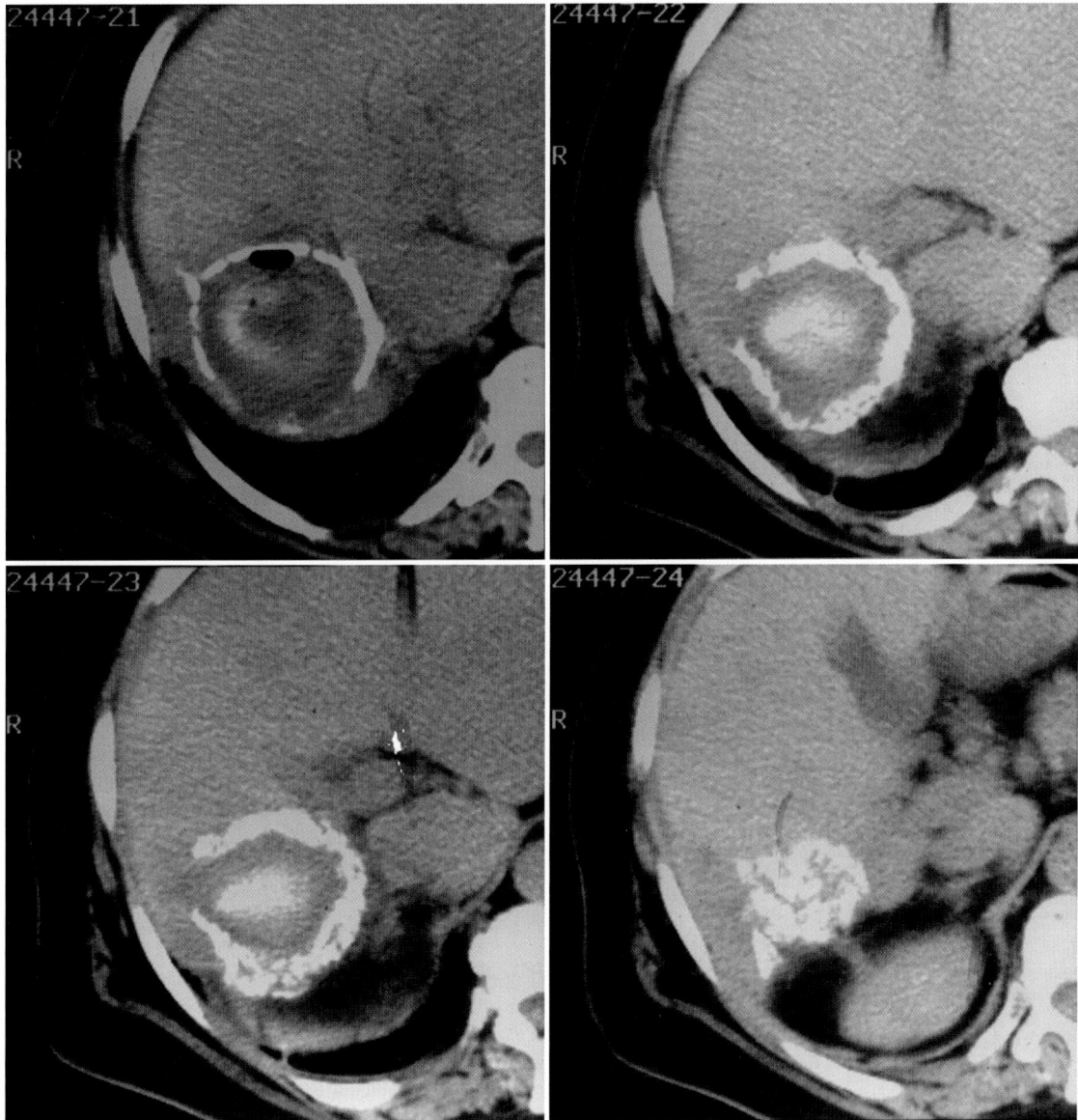

FIGURE 72.10 Diagnostic computed tomography sequence of a CE5 calcified liver hydatid cyst. Note that the calcification is extensive, nearly complete, with thick calcified walls (CALC3).[18]

Endoscopic Retrograde Cholangiopancreatography

Suspected minor cystobiliary communications should be investigated by noninvasive methods such as MRCP, ultrasound, and CT (see Chapter 14). Endoscopic retrograde cholangio-pancreatography (ERCP) remains an important tool in cases where a major rupture into the biliary tree has occurred, allowing both the diagnosis of a major biliary communication and clearance of the common bile duct before surgery or intervention by the means of sphincterotomy.[37] Therapeutic ERCP is indicated for early (persistent biliary fistula and obstructive jaundice) and late (sclerosing cholangitis, sphincter of Oddi stenosis) postoperative biliary events, of which biliary fistulas are the most common. If biliary strictures accompany biliary fistula, sphincterotomy needs to be supplemented with biliary stenting. Nasobiliary drainage is an option in cases with biliary sepsis, particularly when the bile ducts are filled with hydatid elements[38] (see Chapters 45 and 71).

Multimodality Imaging Approach for Complications of Liver Hydatid Cysts

Complications of liver hydatid disease occur in about one third of patients and may potentially be life threatening if not promptly diagnosed. Adequate knowledge of diagnostic imaging clues of complications of liver echinococcosis is crucial to guide the clinical, radiologic, and therapeutic management.[7]

INTRABILIARY RUPTURE. Communicating rupture of LHC within the biliary tree is usually seen on ultrasound as echogenic LHC with a hypoechoic or snowstorm pattern; in case of perforation, rounded or linear hyperechoic structures without posterior shadowing can be detected within the common bile duct. Hydatid material into the biliary tract is evident as high attenuation/intensity content in the common bile duct on CT and T1-weighted MRI and as hypointense filling defect on T2-weighted MRI or MRCP. MRI may show the direct fistulous

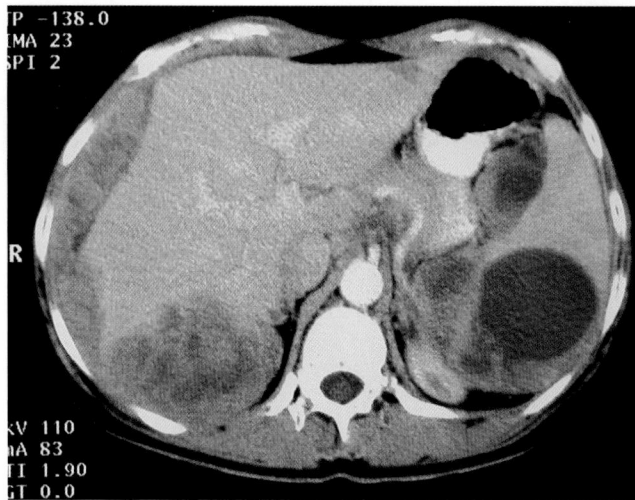

FIGURE 72.11 Diagnostic computed tomography of a CE4 solid heterogeneous liver hydatid cyst. Note that the omentum is surrounding the right liver surface and a simultaneous splenic hydatic cyst is present.

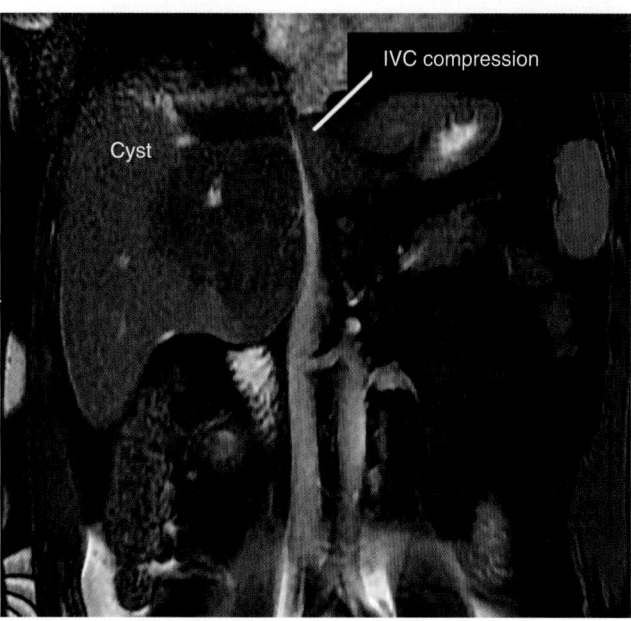

FIGURE 72.12 Diagnostic magnetic resonance imaging of a right liver hydatid cyst that produce compression and displacement of the inferior vena cava (IVC) behind the hepatic veins or the right atrial cavity, type 1 of the classification shown in Table 72.2.[54]

TABLE 72.2	Classification of Liver Hydatid Cysts According to the Localization and Type of Contact With the IVC[54]
Type I	Cysts located in segment VIII, I and IVA in contact with the IVC behind the hepatic veins or the right atrial cavity
Type II	Large cysts localized in segment VI and/or II/III/IV with lateral contact with the IVC
Type III	Large centrally located cysts with encasement of the IVC and massive IVC involvement

IVC, Inferior vena cava.

postoperative biliary fistula, and therefore MRI should be preferred over ERCP for the diagnosis.[38]

RUPTURE OF HEPATIC HYDATID CYSTS INTO ADJACENT VISCERA. CT and MRI characteristically demonstrate daughter cysts within the peritoneal cavity (see Chapter 14). Pelvic hydatid cysts may mimic adnexal cystic masses, and the identification of peripheral calcifications, floating membranes, or daughter cysts in hydatid cysts is crucial for differential diagnosis.[46] In patients with communicating rupture of LHC with the thoracic structures, chest x-ray and CT may show pleural effusion, elevation of the diaphragm, lung consolidation, or laminated atelectasis at the lung bases.[50]

SUPERINFECTION OF HEPATIC HYDATID CYSTS. Ultrasound and CT may demonstrate multiple confluent intrahepatic lesions with poorly defined margins, associated with the presence of air and air-fluid level. However, these findings may also be present in uninfected ruptured cyst. Contrast-enhanced CT and MRI may demonstrate an enhancing rim lesion in case of liver abscess and hypervascular areas in the contiguous liver parenchyma, which may reflect inflammatory changes occurring in case of superinfection. The combination of these imaging findings with history of LHC, pain, fever, and leukocytosis should prompt the diagnosis of LHC suppuration.[82]

VASCULAR COMPLICATIONS. LHC growth may lead to significant mass effect on adjacent vascular structures, including portal and suprahepatic veins (see Fig. 72.9). Ultrasound, CT, and MRI usually show LHC located in the hepatic dome, extrinsic compression of hepatic veins or IVC, and ascites. According to the preoperative imaging studies, hydatid cysts in contact with the IVC are classified as shown in Table 72.2.[54]

In summary, ultrasound or CT imaging outcomes allow a confident diagnosis of LHC, and no further test is usually needed (see Chapter 14). If reliable ultrasound or CT imaging diagnosis is not possible, MRI and further serologic tests can be performed to reach the final diagnosis. Regarding complications, ultrasound should be performed as the first imaging technique, but it is usually not sufficient for the assessment of complications of LHC. Depending on availability and patient compliance, CT and MRI may be performed alone or in sequence for a more comprehensive diagnostic assessment of complications of LHC.

TREATMENT

General Considerations

Although most patients with hydatid disease are asymptomatic or paucisymptomatic, treatment should be generally implemented

track between the LHC and biliary tree as well as the leakage of hepatobiliary contrast agent from the biliary tract into the LHC when using hepatobiliary-specific contrast agent (see Chapter 14). Indirect signs of communicating rupture on CT and MRI include the presence of intracystic fat—due to the lipid content of the bile—or air content and air-fluid levels.[79,80] ERCP has a high sensitivity (86% to 100%) in the diagnosis of intrabiliary rupture as it directly demonstrates linear wavy filling defects of laminated hydatid membrane into the common bile duct, the duodenum, or protruding from the ampulla of Vater, and may show the communication with the introduction of a catheter from biliary ducts directly into the hepatic hydatid cyst. However, ERCP may promote the formation of to prevent complications, such as infection, rupture of the cyst to adjacent structures, or anaphylaxis. Currently four major treatment options are available: surgery, interventional approaches, medical therapy, and follow-up with no specific treatment ("wait and see").[8,83] No consensus has been established on the optimal treatment for HDL due to a lack of longitudinal controlled studies or randomized clinical trials.[84] Decisions should be made according to status performance of the patient, characteristics of the cysts, physician and team expertise, medical resources available, and adherence of patients to long-term monitoring.[2] The main goals of treatment are to ensure complete elimination of the parasite (including the destruction or resection of the germinal layer) and the prevention of recurrent disease with a low rate of morbidity and mortality.

Surgical Treatment

Common Principles and Indications

Surgery remains the gold standard treatment and is the most common approach for treating HDL, although removal of the parasitic mass is not always 100% effective. The main principles of hydatid surgery are as follows: (1) remove all infective components contained in the cyst; (2) avoid spillage of cyst contents into the abdomen; (3) address the residual cavity; and (4) search for and manage any communication with the biliary tract or adjacent structures.

Surgery is the treatment of choice in complicated cysts, large CE2 and CE3b cysts with multiple daughter cysts, and superficial cysts that may rupture spontaneously or because of trauma. The surgical procedures indicated in uncomplicated HDL should be individualized and evaluated against other options. Contraindications to surgery are diffuse hepatic cysts, cysts that are difficult to access, dead cysts, inactive cysts that can be partially or totally calcified (CE4, CE5), very small cysts, and cysts in patients who are not suitable for surgery due to their general condition.[12]

Surgical Approach

Surgical approaches to LHC can be divided into conservative surgery, when the pericyst is not resected but the germinal and ectocyst (laminated membrane) are resected; and radical surgery, when the pericyst is included in the resection.

CONSERVATIVE SURGERY. Conservative surgery is a safe and technically simple procedure that requires short operative time and can be employed regardless of where the cyst is located. The conservative approach is primarily supported by general surgeons from endemic areas who emphasize the need for a safe and reliable first-line treatment.[85-87] After a complete exploration of the peritoneal cavity, the area around the cysts is covered and isolated with packs that can be immersed in a scolicidal agent. Surrounding tissues should be protected from spread of parasites during the cyst evacuation. Then the cyst is punctured and/or incised at its most accessible part (Fig. 72.13). All contents are aspirated and the germinative membrane is removed with forceps. The cavity is flushed with a scolicidal agent, and the pericyst is cleaned and removed from daughter cysts. It is important to inspect the inner surface of the residual cavity, peeling the laminated membrane to reduce thickness of the pericyst and remove daughter cysts hidden in the pericyst layer (exogenous daughter cysts).[12] Then the cyst is deroofed by partial resection of the projecting part of the pericyst. Residual cavity is examined for biliary fistulas and treated by omentoplasty and/or drainage. The omentum has a natural absorptive capacity that decreases the risk of infection and minimizes fistula formation.[88] Capitonnage, an obliterative procedure that sutures the cystic wall, is another option still used in endemic regions for treatment of the residual cavity[85] (Fig. 72.14). Management of biliary fistulas is described later in this chapter. The conservative techniques offer the advantage of a straightforward approach that can be performed in low-complexity centers. Disadvantages are the risk for chemical cholangitis due to the scolicidal agents, especially if there is a biliary fistula, and anaphylactic reactions due to spillage of cystic contents.[6]

RADICAL SURGERY. This approach involves resection of the pericystic membrane and the parasitic contents with or without liver resection. The first technique, commonly referred to as pericystectomy (also known in the literature as cystopericystectomy, capsulectomy, radical cystectomy, and subadventitial

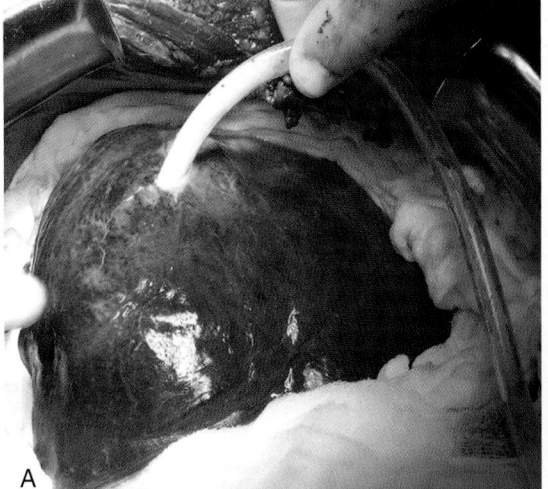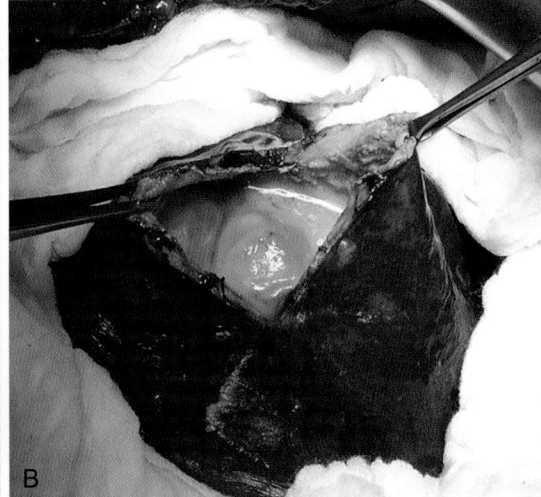

FIGURE 72.13 Operative view of the first surgical steps in the conservative approach. Note that area around the cysts is covered and isolated with packs that can be immersed in a scolicidal agent. Surrounding tissues should be protected from the spread of parasites during the cyst evacuation (a). Then the cyst is punctured and/or incised at its most accessible part (b).

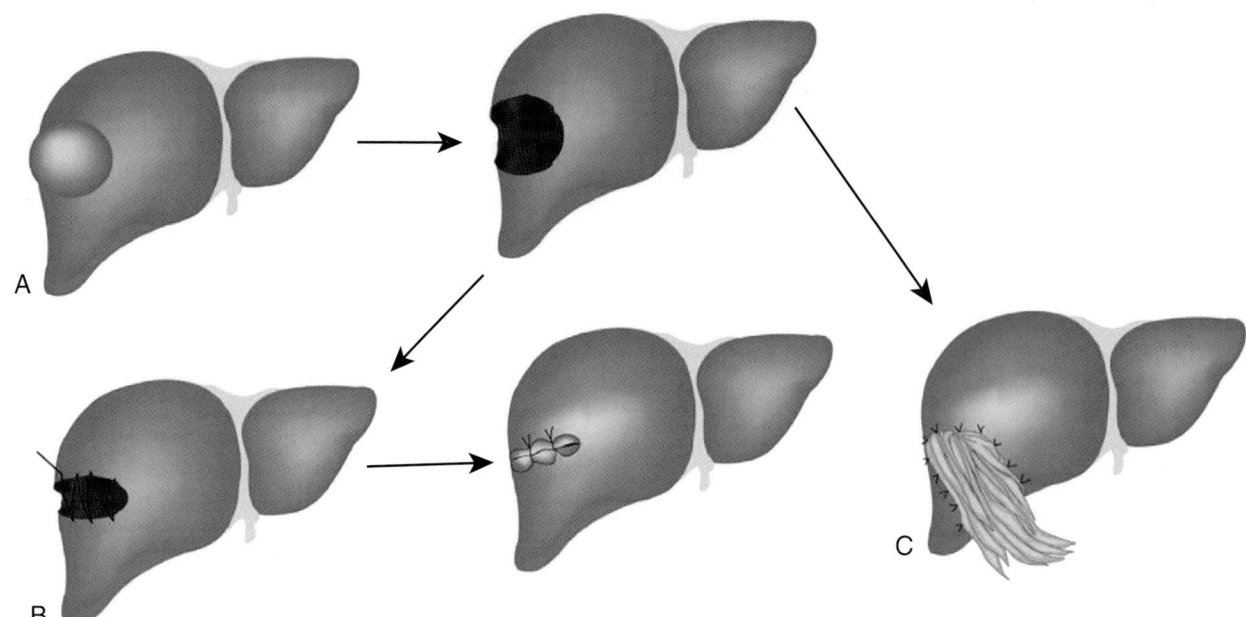

FIGURE 72.14 Flowchart with the schematic representation of the surgical options for the management of the residual cavity in conservative surgery for hydatid liver cysts. Following evacuation and partial resection of the cyst the cavity can be address with capitonnage **(B)** or omentoplasty **(C).** (From Duek F, Lendoire JC. What approach is best for hepatic hydatid cyst? B) Surgical. In: Chu Q, Vollmer C, Zibari G, Orloff S, Williams M, Gimenez M. *Hepato-pancreato-biliary and transplant surgery, practical management and dilemmas.* Beaux Books, 2018:188–200.)

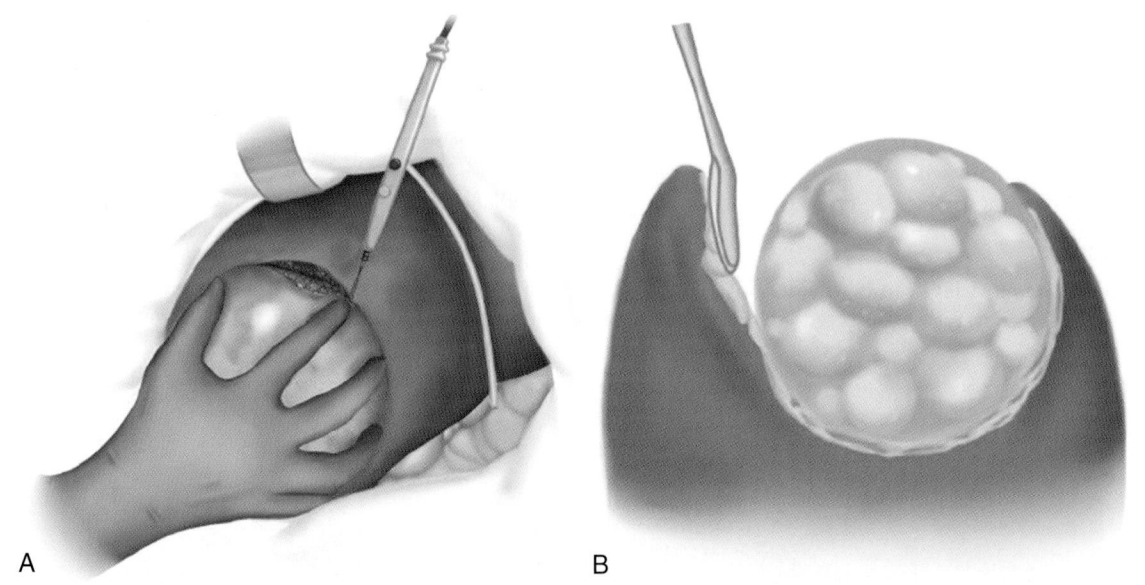

FIGURE 72.15 Schematic representation of the radical technique of close pericystectomy. (From Duek F, Lendoire JC. What approach is best for hepatic hydatid cyst? B) Surgical. In: Chu Q, Vollmer C, Zibari G, Orloff S, Williams M, Gimenez M. *Hepato-pancreato-biliary and transplant surgery, practical management and dilemmas.* Beaux Books, 2018:188–200.)

cystectomy), follows the periadventitial plane created by the cyst as possible, but without injuring vascular or biliary structures[27,89,90] (Fig. 72.15). Ideally, a total pericystectomy should be attempted, although a subtotal pericystectomy may be required to avoid injuring major vascular structures such as suprahepatic veins commonly displaced and involved by the cyst. Thus radical surgical techniques can also be divided into

"closed techniques," which do not violate the cyst wall, and "open techniques," which include a partial or total cyst excision after opening and sterilizing the cyst[91] (Figs. 72.15 and 72.16). As an example, a peripherally located small LHC can be address with a "closed total pericystectomy," whereas a big centrally located cyst can be treated with an "open subtotal pericystectomy." A subtotal radical pericystectomy requires at least

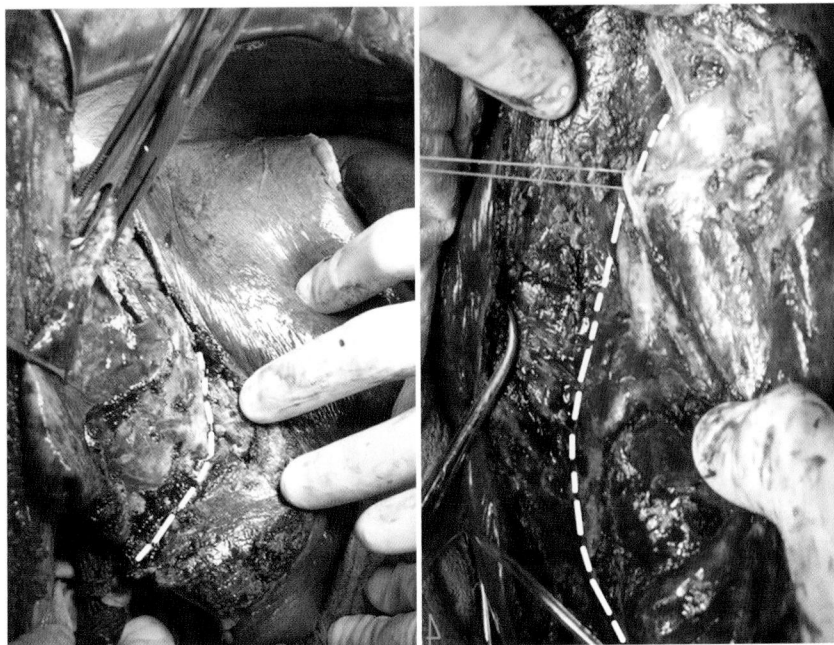

FIGURE 72.16 Operative views of the radical technique open pericystectomy. Note that the plane of transection follows the periadventitial plane created by the cyst without injuring vascular or biliary structures.

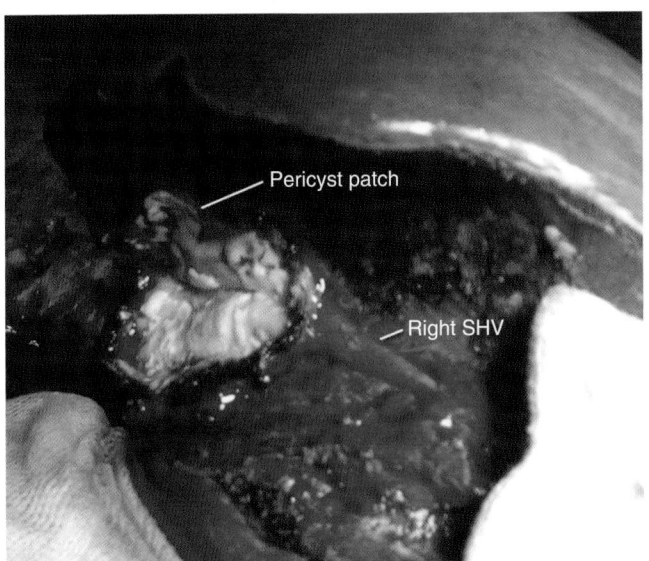

FIGURE 72.17 Operative views of a partial pericystectomy in a patient with a hydatid cyst in contact with the IVC type 1. Note the pericyst patch left over the confluence of the RHV with the IVC. *IVC,* Inferior vena cava; *RHV,* right suprahepatic vein.

80% removal of the cystic wall. Advantages of the pericystectomy include the preservation of normal liver parenchyma and the complete resection of the parasite and the pericyst, resulting in a resilient residual cavity that is easy to obliterate and allows for adequate treatment of eventual biliary communications. During the pericystectomy, a fragment of pericyst can be left in place to avoid dangerous dissection in contact with vascular or biliary structures[12] (Fig. 72.17).

The second radical technique described for the treatment of hydatid cysts is liver resection. Anatomic or nonanatomic liver resections are radical techniques that may be necessary in selected cases, but one should always weigh the risks and benefits of such radical procedures, keeping in mind that LHC is a benign disease. Liver resection is usually performed in multiple unilobar cysts, large cysts occupying almost the entire lobe, complicated cysts, those near large vascular or biliary structures, and peripherally located cysts, usually in the left lateral segment, for pedunculated lesions.[92] Parenchymal-sparing techniques should be pursued if possible. In selected cases, major hepatectomy is required, more frequently in recurrent hydatid cysts after suboptimal treatment or in cysts with severe involvement of the right or left bile duct at the hilar plate without the possibility of reconstruction.[93,94]

HYDATID CYST IN CONTACT WITH INFERIOR VENA CAVA. This localization of hydatid cyst represents a challenge for hepato-pancreato-biliary surgeons. Usually asymptomatic, when the involvement of the IVC does cause symptoms, they are very severe an may have two specific causes: IVC thrombosis due to cystic compression, which may evolve into cavernomatosis, and Budd-Chiari syndrome, depending on the location of the thrombus.[16] Although the literature is scarce, the most widely accepted approach is conservative surgery. The decision must be based on the location of the cyst, length, circumferential contact with IVC, symptoms, whether the cyst is recurrent, and the technical training of the surgeon. According to Ramia et al.,[54] classification of hydatid cyst with IVC contact, in types I and III a conservative surgery is indicated more frequently due to the complexity and morbidity of performing radical procedures (see Fig. 72.17). Type II cysts, with longer side IVC contact, are those cysts that most frequently allow performance of total cystectomy, but this is not always feasible.

SCOLICIDE SUBSTANCES. The intraoperative dissemination of protoscolex-rich hydatid fluid during surgery or percutaneous procedures for LHC is a cause of recurrence.[95] Injection of a protoscolecide into hydatid cysts to reduce the risk of spillage of viable protoscoleces and possible recurrence is an integral part of the surgical technique employed by many surgeons around the world.[96] Also, the scolicidal agent can be used to protect surrounding organs during the surgical procedure.[48] A broad spectrum of protoscolicidal agents, from warm water to the highly toxic formalin, have been tested over the past 50 years, but the feasibility, safety, and efficacy of many of these compounds have generally not been determined. Serious complications have limited the use of some of these; formalin and betadine should never be used under any circumstances.[97] However, the majority, albeit less harmful than these two compounds, resulted in serious biliary, gas embolism, renal, and toxic complications that limited their use; toxicity to bile duct mucosa explains why communication between the CE and the bile ducts must be carefully checked before the use of any protoscolicidal agent.[37] There have been considerable efforts made to discover additional potential protoscolecides, including plant extracts and the use of physical methods in vitro, but details of their clinical application are lacking.[97] WHO-IWGE recommended 20% hypertonic saline as the preferred protoscolecide in surgery and 20% hypertonic saline or 95% alcohol in percutaneous procedures, but rigorous, high-quality comparative studies on these protoscolecidal agents are still awaited.[96]

LAPAROSCOPIC TECHNIQUE. Laparoscopic management of LHC has been a controversial topic because of the concern of spillage and anaphylaxis. Since the first laparoscopic procedure was performed in 1992, this technique has been confirmed to be feasible and safe, avoiding a laparotomy.[10,78] Early reports of laparoscopic treatments of hydatid cysts were confined to simple conservative procedures, but the refinements in the laparoscopic techniques have allowed for conditions that traditionally would have done by the open technique to be done laparoscopically (i.e., total or subtotal pericystectomy, liver resection).[98–100] The ideal cases for a laparoscopic cystectomy are uncomplicated cysts with location in the anterior segments, preferably in the liver periphery away from major vessels and ducts. Deep parenchymal cysts or those close to the main vasculature structures are usually not amenable to a radical laparoscopic approach. In general, an open approach or in selected cases a conservative laparoscopic surgery will be the most appropriate technique in these cyst locations. One advantage of laparoscopy in conservative surgery is that the laparoscope can enter the cyst cavity and allow detailed inspection. Because of its 3-fold larger image, it better shows bile duct leakage within the cysts.[101]

Based on the learning curve, an expansion of the application of laparoscopic radical techniques to more complex hydatid cysts had been shown.[99] Laparoscopic pericystectomy combines the advantages of a radical surgical procedure and those of minimally invasive surgery (Fig. 72.18). However, one should be mindful that radical surgery should be performed in high-volume centers that have a great deal of expertise in hepato-pancreato-biliary surgeries and laparoscopy. Compared with the open approach, the laparoscopic approach has shown in small series advantages such as less blood loss, shorter hospital stays, better cosmetic effect, faster recovery time, and lower wound infection rates.[100,102] However, there are no randomized controlled trials comparing both approaches; most of the published studies are noncomparative; and the only

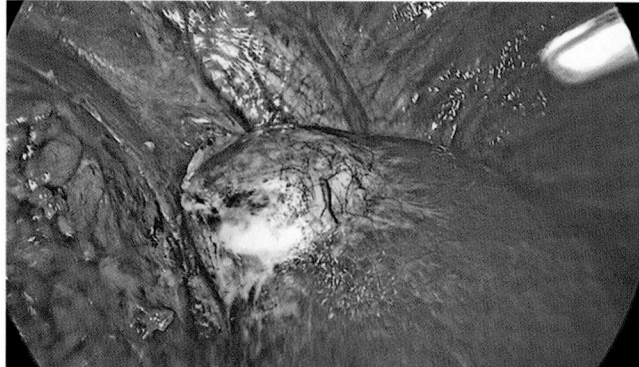
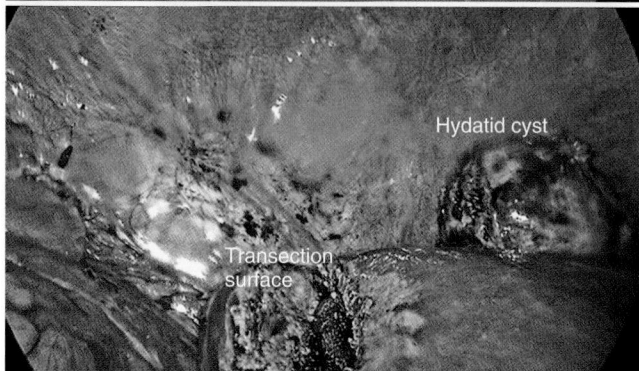

FIGURE 72.18 Surgical photographs of a laparoscopic close pericystectomy for a liver hydatid cyst located on segments 7/8. Note the parenchyma transection surface with a hemostatic agent and the cyst pervious to bag extraction. (Courtesy Mariano Massa, MD.)

meta-analysis demonstrated no significant trends in morbidity, mortality, recurrence, and cure rate.[102] Recently, Magistri et al.[103] published the largest experience with the robotic approach for radical procedures in hydatid cysts. In 15 patients treated by liver resection (67%) and pericystectomy (33%) the authors demonstrated the safety and effectiveness of this approach, also in difficult segments of the liver, with short recovery and no site recurrence.[103]

Results of Surgical Treatment

An analysis of the results of surgical treatment in patients with hydatid liver disease, published in the last 7 years, is presented in Table 72.3.

MORBIDITY AND MORTALITY. Overall postoperative morbidity ranges between 9% and 42%. Surgical complications including biliary fistula, intraabdominal abscess, wound infection, and hemorrhage are major problems in the postoperative period, but are usually associated with complicated hydatid cysts. Although conservative surgical procedures are still the preferred technique for many surgeons, several studies have demonstrated fewer complications after radical approaches.[89,108,105] An evidence-based study by Manterola et al.[110] with 11,403 patients demonstrated that a conservative approach was a significative risk factor for developing postoperative complications. Other predictive factors for morbidity are age, previous surgery for hydatid cyst, cyst size greater than 10 cm, multiple cysts, centrohepatic cyst location, and the presence of cystobiliary communications.[110,111] Generally, postoperative mortality ranges from 0% to 3.2%.[108,112] The value of the surgical technique was

TABLE 72.3 Analysis of the Results of Surgical Treatment According to the Surgical Technique in Series With >100 Patients Treated for Liver Hydatid Cysts and Published in the Last 7 Years

REFERENCE, YEAR	NUMBER OF PATIENTS	CS (%)	RS (%)	LAP (%)	MORBIDITY (%)	MORTALITY (%)	RECURRENCE (%)
Mehrabi Bahar,[85] 2014	155	100	—	—	9.68	0	0
Manterola,[104] 2014	126	0	100	—	10.3	0	0.8
El Malki,[86] 2014	493	83	17	—	17.5 CS 16.5 RS 19	0.4 CS 0.5 RS 0	3.6 CS 5.8 RS 3
Tuxun,[98] 2014	914	89	11	95	15	0.22	1.1
Yucel,[87] 2015	425	85.5	12.3	1.7	2.6	0	4.5
He,[105] 2015	1267	62.5	37	—	28 CS 35 RS 17	1.7 CS 1.7 RS 0	4.6 CS 6.7 RS 1.2
Georgiou,[89] 2015	232	67	33	—	28 CS 29.3 RS 11.7	1.7 CS 2.7 RS 0	8.6 CS 12 RS 0
Benkabbou,[106] 2015	820	78	22	—	18.7 (*)	0.6	—
Ran,[107] 2015	112 (**)	77	23	—	28 CS 15 RS 19	0	2.6 CS 3.4 RS 0
Pang,[108] 2017	4127	55.1	44.9	—	31 CS 41 RS 18	3.2 CS 3.2 RS 3.4	7.7 CS 12 RS 2
Jaén-Torrejimeno,[109] 2019	238	44,5	55.5	—	42 CS (****)	0.4	7.2 No dif.
Julien,[91] 2020	116	16	84	0.8	9 (***)	1	2

CS, Conservative surgery; *Lap,* Laparoscopic approach; *RS,* radical surgery.

Notes: (*) intraabdominal complications; (**) pediatric patients; (***) Clavien III, IV, V; (****) risk factor for morbidity.

reinforced in a recent study that demonstrated that closed surgical resection techniques are associated with lower rate of severe complications and mortality (Dindo-Clavien III-IV-V) in comparison with the open surgical procedures.[91]

RECURRENCE. Recurrence of hydatid cyst is defined as the appearance of new and growing hydatid cysts after therapy. It includes reappearance and growth at the site of a previously treated hydatid cyst (local recurrence) or the development at a new distant site (i.e., peritoneal cavity) due to spillage.[113] After surgery, all patients treated for a primary LHC should undergo abdominal ultrasound surveillance. It is usually recommended at the first month after discharge, every 6 months during the first 4 years, and then annually thereafter, to detect recurrences.[96] In the case of highly suspected HDL recurrence on an ultrasound, abdominal CT scan should be performed. Recurrence is characterized by the appearance of a new cyst, undetected by radiologic exploration before the surgery or by the surgeon during the procedure, whether in the first liver location of the hydatid cyst or in another liver segment. Recurrence rates of LHC range from 0% to 8.6% (see Table 72.3). Despite advances in surgical techniques, recurrence remains one of the major problems in the management of hydatid disease. It can be seen in intervals from 3 months to 20 years after the first operation.[113] Some authors report a significant rate of recurrence after conservative surgery.[86,89,105,112,114] They report that recurrences with conservative surgery are due to the possibility of leaving material on the outer surface of the pericyst (exogenous vesiculation) or peritoneal soiling during the cyst's emptying.

However, surgeon skill and experience can be a critical determining factor independent of the technique used.[113] Treatment options for local recurrences are similar to those for the primary disease.

Treatment of Complicated Hydatid Cysts

Rupture in the Biliary Tracts

The management strategy of a cistobiliary communication depends on when it is diagnosed. Preoperatively diagnosed frank fistula presenting with obstructive jaundice and/or cholangitis can be effectively managed by ERCP, which is both diagnostic and therapeutic[38] (see Chapters 20 and 30). Preoperative therapeutic ERCP has a reported success rate of 80% to 100% and can be used when hydatid membranes and/or daughter cysts that generate biliary obstruction are demonstrated by cholangiography. Endoscopic sphincterotomy, extraction by balloon or basket catheter, nasobiliary drainage, and biliary stenting are some of the therapeutic methods that can be performed by ERCP.[38] Routine preoperative ERCP was recommended by some authors to assess the presence of cistobiliary fistulas in order to reduce postoperative bile leaks after surgery; however, there is no consensus supporting such a recommendation.[115] Overall success rate of endoscopic management can range from 70% to 86%, but not all centers in endemic regions have this procedure available.[35]

Intraoperatively diagnosed cistobiliary communications can be managed by several surgical techniques such as simple suturing, suturing with biliary decompression, or transfistular

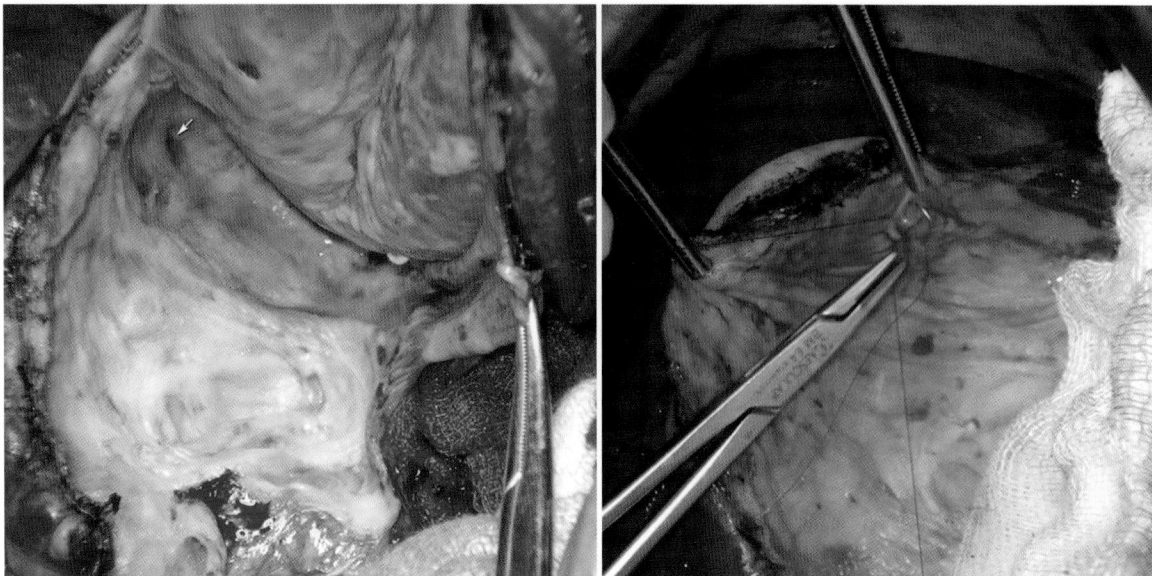

FIGURE 72.19 Surgical photographs of a minor cistobiliary fistula (<5 mm) after partial pericystectomy *(arrow)* and surgical treatment by suturing.

biliary drainage. The indication depends on the characteristics of the fistula (size, location), proximity to the vessels, involvement of hilar confluence, and surgeon experience.[37] If the fistula is less than 5 mm, it can be treated by suturing it on the healthy tissue after removal of the capsule of the cyst along with drainage (Fig. 72.19). However, the main disadvantage of this technique is the risk of prolonged biliary leakage and subphrenic abscess formation. Suture with biliary decompression can be established by means of a transcystic tube (through the cystic duct after cholecystectomy) or a T-tube through choledochotomy.[36,116] (see Chapter 37). Transfistular internal drainage is performed by a transhepatic-cystic choledochostomy, offers a low rate of postoperative biliary fistula, and can be an option also in patients with impaired general conditions and/or uncontrolled sepsis.[106] Some authors proposed a more radical approach (pericystectomy, hepatectomy) in the presence of large cistobiliary communications (>5 mm) when upstream atrophy of the liver parenchyma is present and in cysts located in the hilar plate[34] (Fig. 72.20). In selected patients with large perihilar cystobiliary communications with no upstream liver parenchyma atrophy, a conservative procedure with a Roux-en-Y hepaticojejunostomy had also been proposed.[34,42] Postoperative mortality in patients with biliary rupture ranges from 1.25% to 7% and is caused mainly by sepsis and liver failure. Postoperative morbidity is between 16.7% and 55%, higher than observed in patients operated on for LHC without intrabiliary rupture. The complications reported are biliary fistula (5%–27%), wound infection, pulmonary complications, bilioma, bleeding, and abscess formation.[35]

Rupture in the Peritoneum

Intraperitoneal hydatid cyst rupture is a life-threatening complication because it causes serious hemodynamic instability and allergic reactions. Medical treatment should be initiated as soon as possible at the emergency unit after confirming the diagnosis.[46] According to a recent review with a total of 194 cases of peritoneal rupture in 13 studies, there is no consensus about the best surgical treatment option.[46] Each case should be evaluated separately according to the general principles of

hydatid cyst surgery.[42] The peritoneal cavity should be washed with scolicidal solutions. Perforated cyst cavities should be carefully evaluated. Remaining cyst contents should be evacuated, and the free edges of the cystic cavity should be widely excised. Surgical treatment of the primary cyst should be the aim if the patient condition allows, more frequently by a conservative technique.[43] Antihelmintic treatment should be administered as soon as possible for patients diagnosed with intraperitoneal rupture to prevent disease recurrence due to overlooked cyst contents during surgery.[44]

Rupture in the Thorax

The objective of the treatment of hydatid cysts ruptured in the thorax is to dry up the biliobronchial fistula, treat its etiology, and correct the associated thoracoabdominal lesions.[49] The first stage of preparation for the intervention must include respiratory physiotherapy, well-adapted antibiotic therapy, blood transfusion in the event of anemia, and caloric and electrolyte equilibration.[50] Several approaches have been proposed: thoracotomy alone, thoraco-phrenolaparotomy, and laparotomy alone or associated with thoracotomy. Some authors have proposed a preoperative endoscopic sphincterotomy for fistula drainage.[50] The surgical treatment of a biliobronchial fistula generally has five objectives: (1) treatment of endothoracic lesions; (2) treatment of liver hydatid cysts after hepatodiaphragmatic disconnection; (3) investigation and treatment of biliary fistulas; (4) repair of the diaphragm; and (5) adequate drainage of the pleural and hepatic cavity (the cystic cavity and/or the interhepatodiaphragmatic space)[51] (see Fig. 72.8). Frequently, an excision of pulmonary parenchyma as a segmental or lobar resection is required.[51] Postoperative complications (16%) are common, most frequently pleuropulmonary suppurations. Prognosis is severe, with mortality ranging from 8.9% to 39%.[49]

Percutaneous Treatment

Since the late 1980s a number of techniques for percutaneous treatment of LHC have been developed, in which, after percutaneous aspiration of the cyst under ultrasonography or CT guidance, a scolicidal agent is injected into the cyst cavity with

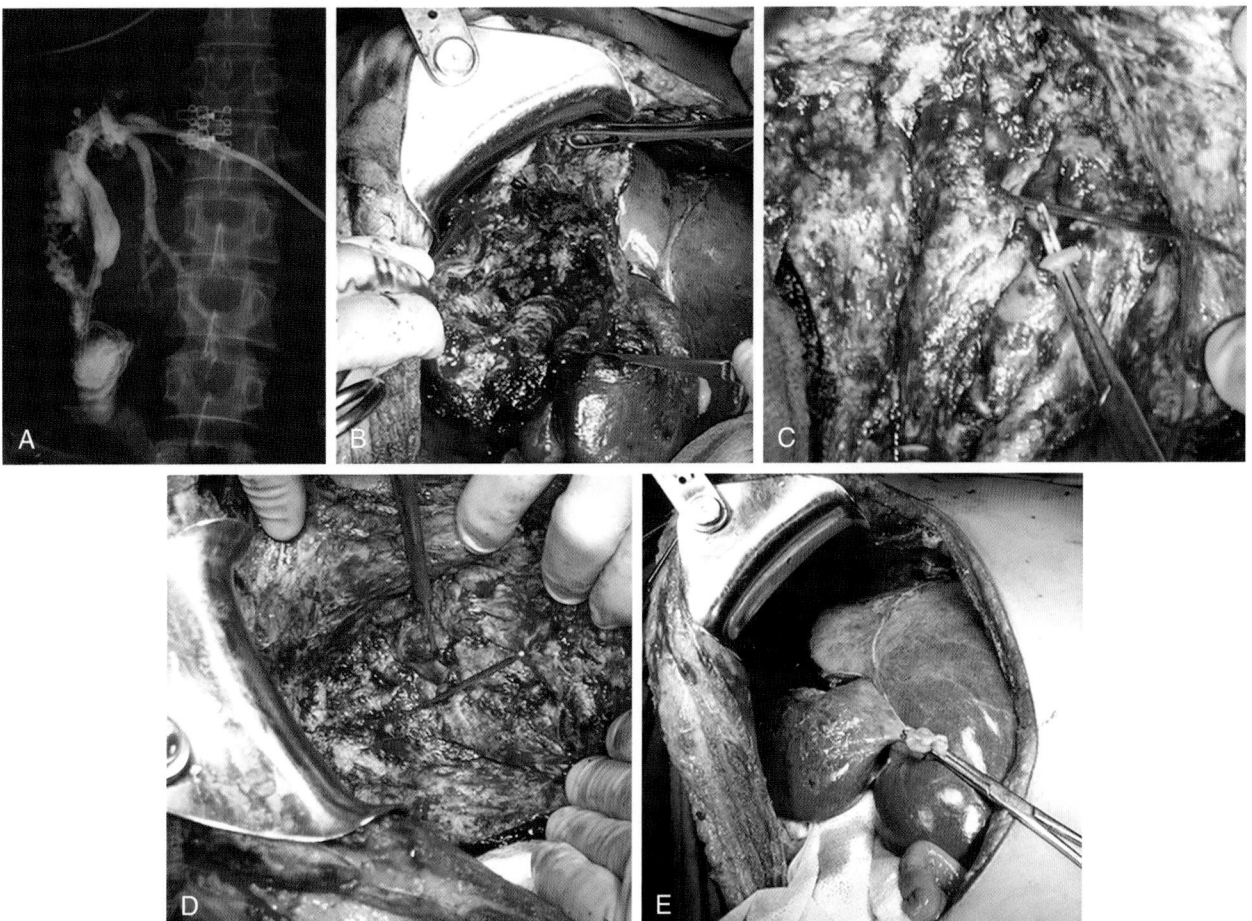

FIGURE 72.20   Diagnostic intraoperative cholangiography (a) and operative views of a major cistobiliary fistula (<5 mm) due to biliary rupture of a right liver hydatid cyst (b). Note the right bile duct opened in the cyst cavity (surgical explorator) (c). The blue plastic stent from the left duct can be seen (d). Treatment by a right hepatectomy was performed (e).

or without reaspiration of the cyst contents.[117] The first one described was the puncture, aspiration, injection, and reaspiration (PAIR) technique.[118] The procedure consists of puncturing the cyst by a Seldinger technique, aspiration of 20% of the cyst volume, and cystography injecting 10% of the estimated volume of contrast medium. If no contrast extravasation outside the cyst is detected, as much of the cyst fluid as possible is aspirated and scolicidal agents as 30% hypertonic saline are injected to an estimated one-third of the cyst volume, waiting then for 10 to 15 minutes. After this period, all fluid in the cyst is reaspirated. The aim of the PAIR technique is the destruction of the germinal layer.[119] Modifications of the PAIR procedure, without reaspiration of the cyst contents and with repetition of the procedure at an interval of 3 to 7 days, have also been developed.[117]

Other percutaneous procedures are those aiming at the evacuation of the entire endocyst, also known as catheterization techniques (PAIDS and MoCaT) or percutaneous evacuation of cyst content (PEVAC). These techniques are usually indicated in cysts larger than 6 cm. The PAIDS procedure is a standard catheterization; following puncture and aspiration of the cyst contents and injection of the scolicidal agent, a small-caliber catheter (6–8 French) is placed in the cavity under fluoroscopic guidance. All the fluid in the cyst cavity is reaspirated

through the catheter. The catheter is kept in place until the fluid drainage is less than 10 mL/day, at which time a cystogram is obtained under fluoroscopy to exclude the possibility of a cistobiliary communication. Then 95% ethanol at an amount of 30% to 50% of the estimated cyst volume is injected into the cyst cavity to sclerose the cyst wall. After 15 minutes, all fluid is reaspirated and the catheter removed. If the daily drainage is more than 10 mL, the catheter is left in place until the amount has dropped and the sclerosing procedure is repeated before removal. In the MoCaT and PEVAC, both modified catheterization techniques, the major advantage is that it removes the cyst contents as well as cystic and solid (degenerated membranes and pieces of daughter vesicles) components of the cyst through a 14- or 16-French catheter.[120]

The main indications for percutaneous treatment are active LHC; a stage approach based on the WHO-IWGE is recommended.[96,121]

- WHO types CE1 and CE3a can be treated either by PAIR or PAIDS. The PAIR technique is used for cysts smaller than 5 to 6 cm in diameter.[120,122] Advantages of the catheter technique are the easy management in case of obstruction over a needle procedure and the easy control of the fistula in case of the presence of an undetected cystobiliary communication.[122] Some studies have demonstrated a lower complication rate and shorter hospital stay.[117] A meta-analysis published in 2017 compared PAIR versus laparoscopic surgery in 57 studies with a total of 2832 patients (PAIR group $n = 1650$ and laparoscopic group $n = 1182$). A statistically significant advantage of the PAIR procedure on cure rate, postoperative complications, and mortality was demonstrated, but recurrence was lower in the laparoscopic group.[102] Further studies comparing different treatment methods are still pending.[120]

• WHO types CE2 and CE3b. Percutaneous treatment of CE2 and CE3b cysts has been a challenge since the 1990s. PAIR and the standard catheterization technique PAIDS demonstrated high recurrence rates (32%–61.5%) in these cyst types.[123] The MoCaT technique resulted in lower recurrence rate (3.8%) although it had a higher complication rate, such as cistobiliary fistula and abscess.[124] Prospective studies are needed to compare modified catheterization techniques with surgery, which at the present time is the most standard procedure in CE2 and CE3b cysts.[123]

Medical Treatment

Medical treatment in hydatid disease is used for reducing cysts, decreasing infectivity, and avoiding relapses. Drugs are also useful in disseminated or inoperable CE as the sole modality of treatment.[125] Systemic antiinfective treatment of hydatid disease relies on continuous administration of two benzimidazole carbamates, albendazole (ABZ) and mebendazole (MBZ), which are drugs clinically efficient to interrupt the larval growth of EG. Mebendazole was the first benzimidazole used that proved effective for the treatment of echinococcosis.[126] Because of its increased bioavailability and easier administration to patients, ABZ has become the antiinfective treatment of choice for echinococcosis, at an average dosage of 10 to 15 mg/kg/day.[127] Fatty meals increase the bioavailability of the benzimidazoles.[128] After oral ingestion ABZ is rapidly metabolized (first-pass metabolism in the liver) into the active form albendazole sulphoxide, which inhibits tubulin polymerization in the parasite microtubules and inactivates cell division.[127] Although ABZ sulphoxide has been shown to penetrate both the hepatic and the nonhepatic hydatid cysts, the prognostic value of plasma cyst concentrations has not been determined yet.[127,129] Intracystic concentrations of ABZ have been demonstrated to be satisfactory despite interpatient variability, and higher values have been found in small or calcified cysts.[129] Therefore current recommendations for medical treatment alone are for cyst types CE1 and CE3 ≤5 cm.[48] Currently, MBZ is only an alternative drug for those patients who have experienced complications with ABZ.[126] Praziquantel (40–50 mg/kg/day), an isoquinolone derivative used against HDL, has shown efficacy in combination with benzimidazoles.[128] Praziquantel is probably an ideal agent for prophylaxis in the preoperative and postoperative setting to prevent implantation of protoscoleces and subsequent recurrence.[96] Combined treatment increases the levels of ABZ sulphoxide in serum and cystic fluid.[126,128] It is unlikely to be as effective as ABZ in treating the whole cyst, as it is less active against the germinal layer of the hydatid cyst.[125]

Antiinfective treatment alone is reserved for small or medium-sized isolated cysts or, alternatively, multiple and inoperable cysts in the liver and/or in multiple organs. Recent cysts and/or those with thin walls are more accessible to drugs.[130] Medical treatments can result in significant regression in 30% to 50% and cure in about 30%.[130] A combination of interventional

techniques plus ABZ is recommended and is used routinely with PAIR and other percutaneous techniques.[119] It is less widely used with surgery, although it was demonstrated that preoperative and postoperative use of ABZ decreases the viability of cysts at the time of surgery and significantly reduces the chances of cyst recurrence.[131,132] In a review of 72 publications with more than 10,008 patients treated for CE, 7% stated that ABZ was not given and 20% did not report any use of prophylaxis.[121] A recent meta-analysis by Velasco-Tirado et al.[125] that analyzed 33 studies (11 randomized controlled trials) established that treatment outcomes are better when surgery or PAIR is combined with benzimidazole drugs given before and/or after the operation. ABZ chemotherapy was found to be the primary pharmacologic treatment to be considered, and the combined treatment with ABZ plus praziquantel resulted in higher scolicidal and anticyst activity and was more likely to result in cure or improvement relative to ABZ alone.[125]

Criteria for curtailing antiinfective treatment are clearly missing. Based on pharmacologic evidence and the relatively low and slow efficacy of ABZ to kill protoscoleces, a reasonable indication would be to administer ABZ from 1 week before to 2 to 3 months after the interventional procedure (surgery or PAIR) whenever the cyst has been opened.[96,133] Side effects of albendazole therapy include mild abdominal pain, nausea, vomiting, pruritis, dizziness, alopecia, rash, and headaches. Occasionally, leukopenia, eosinophilia, icterus, and mild elevation in transaminase levels are seen. Thus all patients should have monitoring of leukocyte counts and liver function tests. Contraindication to chemotherapy include pregnancy, chronic hepatic diseases, and bone marrow depression.[128]

Watch-and-Wait Approach

In 2010 Frider, a hepatologist from Argentina who dedicated his life to the study of hydatid disease, published an interesting review about the dilemma of whether "to treat or not to treat" asymptomatic carriers.[130] Follow-up of these patients and demonstration by ultrasound of the evolution of cysts over time, their spontaneous disappearance, and the absence or slow growth through long-term longitudinal studies were critical to propose noninterventional studies in selected patients. The "watch-and-wait" strategy is recommended for degenerating CE4 cysts and all CE5 type cysts. According to a recent study the presence of detachment of the laminated membrane of the cyst and pericyst degenerative changes such as thickening or calcification of any grade justifiably exempts asymptomatic univesicular liver hydatid cysts from any treatment.[134] In another recent study, 98% of 53 patients with CE4–CE5 cysts observed for at least 2 years remained stable, without complications, strengthening the conviction that the watch-and-wait approach is a safe and useful method for the clinical management of inactive asymptomatic LHD. This avoids overtreatment of these patients, with attendant and unjustified risks and costs.[135] The watch-and-wait approach may also be suitable for other cyst types (e.g., small CE1 cysts). However, prospective studies are needed.

Follow-up, Prevention, and Control

A close follow-up of patients with hydatid disease should also be undertaken for at least 5 years because of the high rates of relapse after surgery and the uncertainty of complete cure after drug treatment and/or percutaneous procedures.[96] Initially patients should be seen every 6 months for the first 2 years, and then once a year depending on the appropriate clinical setting.[5] Regular tests of blood counts and serum transaminases are necessary to assess the safety of management within the first 6 months after initiation of antiinfective treatment, because hepatic toxicity and leukopenia are the most severe adverse effects and may prevent ABZ use in some patients. ABZ sulphoxide measurements are extremely useful to assess the patient's observance and to adjust drug dosages.[96]

The WHO has listed echinococcosis as one of the 17 neglected diseases targeted for control or elimination by 2050. Current prevention and control of hydatid disease relies on the provision of safe animal slaughtering conditions (offal destruction and preventing dogs from feeding on infected organs of ungulates) and on dosing dogs with praziquantel.[5] Vaccination of sheep with the EG95 vaccine has been promoted as a complementary intervention to eliminate EG transmission, and there have been trials of this approach in China and South America. For most countries where hydatid disease is endemic, however, the logistics and costs of vaccinating sufficient numbers of animals may preclude widespread application of the vaccine.[96]

ECHINOCOCCUS MULTILOCULARIS

Alveolar echinococcosis (AE) is caused by ingestion of eggs of Echinococcus multilocularis, found in the excrement of foxes.[136] It is endemic in the Northern Hemisphere, including North America and several Asian and European countries, such as France, Germany, Switzerland, and Austria.[137] The ingested eggs develop into an alveolar structure composed of small vesicles that grow slowly and are able to reach a diameter of 15 to 20 cm.[136,138] Each vesicle has the same wall structure as Echinococal cyst (EC).[136] Compared with encapsulated growth of EC, AE presents an infiltrative neoplastic growth with potential metastasis to adjacent and distant organs such as lungs, spleen, bone, and brain.[139] Serology tests (ELISA, Western blot) have a high diagnostic sensitivity of 90% to 100%, with a specificity of 95% to 100%.[57] Western blot allows one to distinguish between Echinococcus granulosus– and Echinococcus multilocularis–infected patients in 76% of cases.[140] However, serologies do not allow one to distinguish active from inactive forms of both echinococcoses. AE usually has an asymptomatic phase between 5 and 15 years before the development of symptoms, which are related to mass effect such as abdominal pain, weight loss, or fatigue.[141]

Imaging Findings

Ultrasound may show a mass with irregular limits and scattered calcification, surrounded by a hyperechogenic ring and a hypoechogenic center with multivesicular appearance.[138] Central necrosis may give the appearance of a cystic-like structure.[142] On unenhanced CT, AE lesions appear as tumor-like masses with irregular borders, with heterogeneous internal structures and multiple calcifications (Fig. 72.21). No significant intralesional enhancement is seen on contrast-enhanced CT, whereas mild enhancement can be seen in the peripheral tissue on delayed phase.[143] On MRI, AE is visible in the form of small round cysts with a weak enhanced solid component.[144] The lesion can be large and irregular, which is clearly shown on T2-weighted imaging. T1-weighted images reveal more clearly the hepatic extension than CT, especially to hepatic veins, vena cava, and perihepatic spaces.[144]

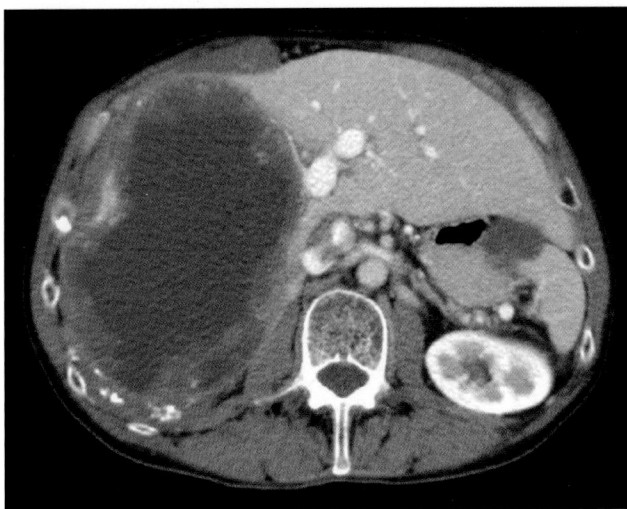

FIGURE 72.21 Computed tomography image of alveolar echinococcosis. The lesion appears as a tumor-like mass with irregular borders, heterogeneous internal structures, and multiple distributed calcified foci (white arrows).

Fluorodeoxyglucose positron emission tomography (FDG-PET) is useful for the detection of metabolic activity in AE.[145] It is therefore used for the assessment of lesion metabolism and the continuation or withdrawal of antiparasitic treatment. However, sophisticated equipment and high cost widely limit FDG-PET use for routine evaluation.[145]

Management

AE typically grows along the biliary tract and therefore may infiltrate the liver diffusely beyond the primary mass.[146] The surgical management of AE is similar to that of a hepatic malignancy.[136] Radical resection is the only curative procedure, even though it is often difficult to achieve because of echinococcal dissemination (Fig. 72.22).[137] It should be followed by a 2-year period of antihelminthic therapy (e.g., benzimidazole) and patients should be monitored for at least 10 years, because of the risk of recurrence.[137,147] Curative surgery is performed by open or laparoscopic surgery depending on the experience of the surgical team. Palliative resections are typically not indicated, because endoscopic treatments of biliary complications and long-term benzimidazole therapy represent efficient alternatives to surgery.[148] Liver transplantation is indicated in advanced cases with liver failure and inability to achieve a radical resection.[149] The absence of extrahepatic localizations is mandatory for such cases.[57] Of note, liver transplantation as an alternative to palliative surgery has not been shown superior compared with long-term conservative therapy. In a recent review by Salm et al.,[148] the authors observed that strategies changed from a relatively high rate of reductive to more curative surgeries in recent years. Most authors showed no benefit of reductive surgeries compared with medical treatment alone, and some reported worse survival due to a higher rate of progression and complications. Based on that, the WHO recommends to avoid reductive surgery for AE and to perform curative resections whenever possible.[57] According to the different series, the average rate of curative resections is 63% (range, 21%–87%).[148]

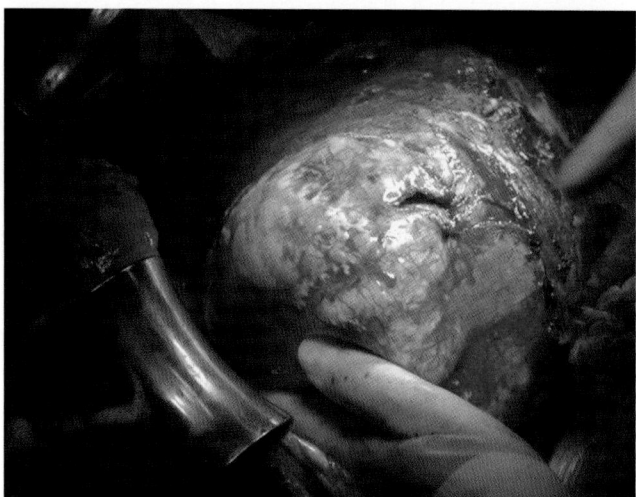

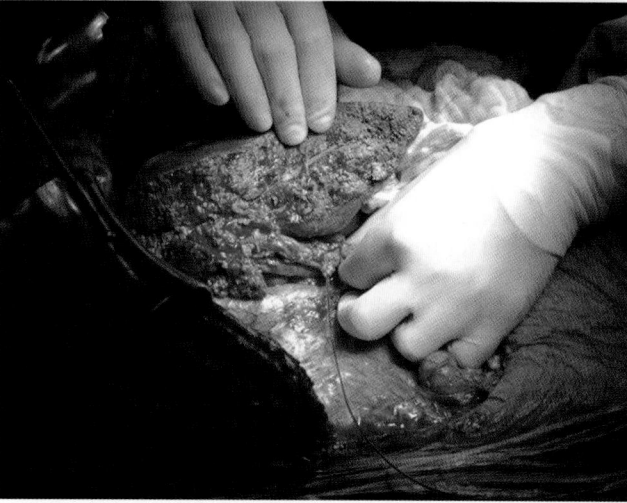

FIGURE 72.22 Radical resection of alveolar echinococcosis. **A,** Intra-operative view of large tumor located in the right liver. **B,** View after right hepatectomy. A transcystic catheter was placed in the bile ducts to perform a leak test using methylene blue cholangiography.

Some studies recommend combining liver resection with adjacent organs such as diaphragm, adrenal gland, lung, pancreas, or stomach.[150] However, it is unclear if such extensive surgery is indicated in AE. A recent case series suggested ex vivo liver resection with autotransplantation as a therapeutic alternative for patients with advanced AE.[151] However, a 30-day mortality of 7% with an overall mortality of 12% (>90 days) was excessively high, with a median follow-up of 22 months only. Therefore any indication for such extensive surgery is questionable and should be balanced with the satisfying results of conservative lifelong medical treatment with benzimidazoles.

Laparoscopic liver resection for oncologic disease is feasible and safe; however, little is known on its use for AE. Preliminary results are promising and are in line with results observed for oncologic disease in experienced hands.

The role of surgical margins has been studied and seems to be significantly correlated with local recurrence and overall survival. Experts recommend a 20 mm margin-free resection to avoid local recurrence.[57] However, data are scarce to support this recommendation. The reported safety margin range from 1 to 20 mm. Nevertheless, a safe distance of at least 1 mm combined with adjuvant benzimidazole therapy for at least 2 years results in long-term disease-free survival.[150] Future studies on AE should incorporate the extent of the disease, as it is an important cofounding factor.

To summarize, although complete liver resection combined with benzimidazole therapy is the only curative treatment of AE, lifelong benzimidazole therapy alone also significantly improved survival so far. Treatment should be tailored to patient condition and performed ideally in high-volume centers due to the specificity and rarity of the disease. Liver transplantation and extensive surgery should be reserved for exceptional cases, because good results are obtained with benzimidazole therapy alone. When the surgical option is used, achieving R0 resection should be the ultimate goal.

The references for this chapter can be found online by accessing the accompanying Expert Consult website.

SECTION I. Inflammatory, Infective, and Congenital

C. Nonparasitic Liver Cysts

CHAPTER 73

Simple cysts and polycystic liver disease: Clinical and radiographic features and surgical and nonsurgical management

Béatrice Aussilhou and Olivier Farges

The entity common to simple cysts and polycystic liver disease (PCLD) is a malformation, lined by a nonatypical biliary-type epithelium that does not communicate with the biliary tree. This differentiates these diseases from hydatid cysts (see Chapter 72), cystic hepatobiliary neoplasms (see Chapter 88B), and cystic dilation of the intrahepatic bile ducts (see Chapter 46).

Simple cysts and PCLD do not simply differ in term of number of cysts; as will be seen, simple cysts are frequently multiple, whereas the extent of disease in PCLD is highly variable. PCLD is currently a well-described genetic disease that comes in two forms: with and without adult dominant polycystic kidney disease (ADPKD).

Symptoms, when present, are associated either with an increase in the size of single cysts or, for PCLD, in the increase in the size of the whole liver. Apart from acute complications, the most frequent of which is intracystic bleeding, these symptoms have frequently evolved progressively for a prolonged period of time (years). It may therefore be difficult for clinicians to differentiate those related to the cyst(s) or to the associated conditions. It may even occasionally take some time to understand the true severity of cyst-related symptoms that some patients have unconsciously become used to.

Most patients with simple cysts or PCLD are asymptomatic and require no treatment. When indicated, the aim of treatment in patients with single cysts is to either destroy the epithelial lining of the cyst with sclerotherapy or create a communication between the cyst lumen and the peritoneal cavity by fenestration. In patients with PCLD, treatment aims at reducing the volume of the hepatomegaly and promoting the regeneration of noncystic liver (hepatectomy) or at replacing the entire liver (transplantation). For patients with PCLD, the treatment is a major procedure, and medical alternatives are still under development. Although only a limited number of surgical teams perform major partial hepatectomy because of the rarity of the indications and complexity of the procedure, a number of new medical treatments besides somatostatin analogues are at the experimental phase.

SIMPLE CYSTS OF THE LIVER

Simple cysts of the liver are cystic formations containing serous fluid that do not communicate with the intrahepatic biliary tree. Numerous terms have been used to designate this lesion, including biliary cyst, nonparasitic cyst of the liver, benign hepatic cyst, congenital hepatic cyst, unilocular cyst of the liver, and solitary cyst of the liver. The last designation is inappropriate because, as mentioned later, simple cysts are often multiple. Simple cysts occur frequently in the general population. Most simple cysts are less than 3 cm in diameter, are easily identified by ultrasound (US), and are asymptomatic. Symptoms, when present, occur in larger cysts and are usually associated with intracystic bleeding that changes the morphologic appearance of the cyst. Most often, a hemorrhagic cyst can be falsely taken for another cystic tumor.

It is in this circumstance that differential diagnosis with other cysts, most notably cystadenomas or hydatid disease, may prove difficult.

Pathology and Pathogenesis

Macroscopically, a simple cyst of the liver has a spherical or ovoid shape. The diameter ranges from a few millimeters to 20 cm or more. The cyst does not communicate with the intrahepatic bile ducts. Small cysts are surrounded by normal hepatic tissue. Large cysts produce atrophy of the adjacent hepatic tissue; a huge cyst may result in complete atrophy of a hepatic lobe, with compensatory hypertrophy of the other lobe. Atrophy respects the large bile ducts and blood vessels, which appear to be abundant in the atrophic tissue in contact with the cyst. Large bile ducts and blood vessels persisting after atrophy may protrude and form folds over the inner surface of the cyst. There is no septation; the cysts are unilocular. The cystic fluid is usually clear; however, intracystic bleeding is relatively common, and the fluid may be brownish when this is the case. Even when a simple cyst is apparently unique, imaging studies disclose the presence of one or more small additional cysts in most

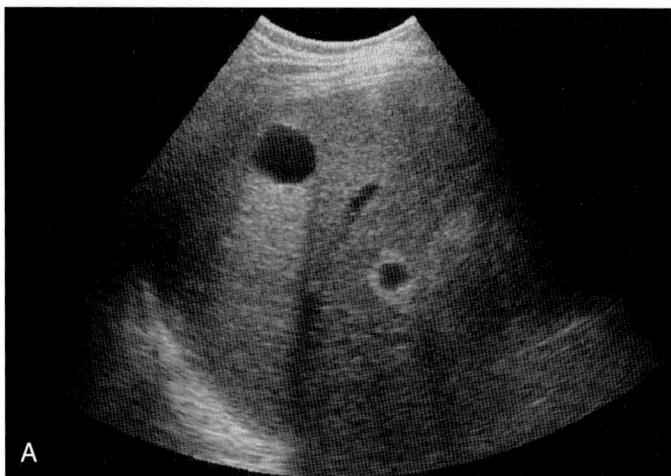 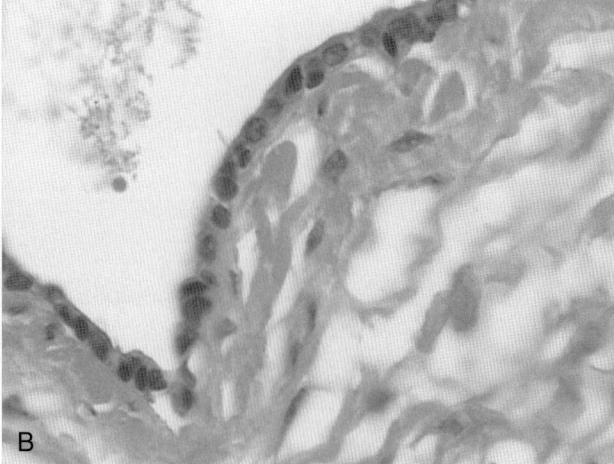

FIGURE 73.1 Ultrasound of a simple cyst of the liver **(A)** and microscopic view of its epithelial lining **(B).** (See Chapter 14.)

patients. In a few cases, simple cysts are multiple, resembling the liver cysts of PCLD, criteria for distinguishing both conditions are given later.

Microscopically, the cysts appear to be bordered by a single layer of cuboidal or columnar epithelial cells, resembling biliary epithelial cells (Fig. 73.1). The cells are uniform, without any atypia. Stroma is absent in small cysts and reduced to a thin layer of connective tissue in large cysts. Simple cysts of the liver are regarded as a congenital malformation. An aberrant bile duct would have lost communication with the biliary tree and would dilate progressively. Liver cyst epithelial cells retain differentiated secretory function; they secrete fluid and generate a positive luminal pressure that may be greater than 30 cm H_2O, which accounts for most symptoms. The composition of the fluid, which contains water and mineral electrolytes without bile acids and bilirubin, is close to that of the normal secretion of the epithelium of the bile ducts. It is not toxic for the peritoneum, which is the rationale for cyst fenestration.

Prevalence and Etiology

Simple cysts have long been considered rare. By 1971, only 350 cases had been reported,[1,2] and early estimates from autopsy studies were less than 1%.[3] The development of imaging techniques revealed, however, that simple cysts are much more frequent. Prevalence in US studies is 3% to 5%,[4,5] was 18% in a more recent spiral computed tomography (CT) study of an adult population,[6] and 24% when using non–contrast-enhanced magnetic resonance imaging (MRI).[7] These discrepancies are explained by the usual small size of most cysts, which are discovered only with accurate imaging techniques. An association between simple hepatic cysts and simple renal cysts has been documented[6] but is unexplained.

The incidence of simple cysts is age and gender related. Simple cysts are uncommon before age 40 years, and their incidence increases sharply thereafter. Simple cysts also are larger in adults older than 50 years than in younger individuals[3] The female-to-male ratio is 1.5:1 for all simple cysts shown at necropsy or imaging. In symptomatic or complicated simple cysts, however, it is 9:1.[2] Huge cysts affect women older than 50 years almost exclusively. Based on these observations, the diagnosis of simple cysts should be retained with caution when a large

and/or symptomatic cystic mass is observed in a male patient or in a young woman.

Manifestations and Diagnosis

In most cases, simple cysts—all small cysts but also most large cysts—are asymptomatic and fortuitously shown by US or CT (see Chapter 14). Only some large cysts produce abdominal pain or discomfort. Because of the high prevalence of simple cysts in adults, the fortuitous coincidence of this lesion and another hepatic or extrahepatic disease is common. The causal relationship between abdominal pain or discomfort and a simple cyst of the liver must be admitted with caution and accepted only if the cyst is large and the other possible causes of the symptoms have been excluded. At clinical examination, only large cysts can be palpated as spherical tumors. In most cases, the fluid content of the tumor can be suspected. In some cases, the cyst is so tense that it may be taken for a solid tumor. The condition of individuals with simple cysts of the liver is good. Liver function tests are normal; abnormal liver function tests in a patient with simple cyst of the liver are not related to the cyst and are caused by another liver disease, except when the cysts compress bile ducts. The cyst fluid contains high concentrations of cancer antigen (CA) 19-9 and carcinoembryonic antigen (CEA) but low concentrations of tumor-associated glycoprotein-72.[8] This may translate to slightly increased serum concentrations of these tumor markers, most notably CA19-9.[9]

US is the best procedure for recognizing simple cysts (see Chapter 14). A simple cyst is a circular or oval, totally anechoic lesion, with sharp, smooth borders and strong posterior wall echoes, indicating a well-defined tissue-fluid interface.[10] There is accentuation of the echoes beyond the cyst compared with echoes at a similar depth transmitted through normal adjacent liver tissue (see Fig. 73.1). Accentuation of the echoes beyond the cyst, so-called *acoustic posterior enhancement*, which indicates that the lesion is fluid-filled, is observed only when the deep tissue transmits US and is not seen when a total reflector, such as gas or bone, lies behind the cyst or when the cyst is very posterior. There is neither wall nor septation, but a false image of septation may be seen when two cysts are adjacent. In some patients, intracystic echoes or material can be detected following intracystic bleeding (see later).

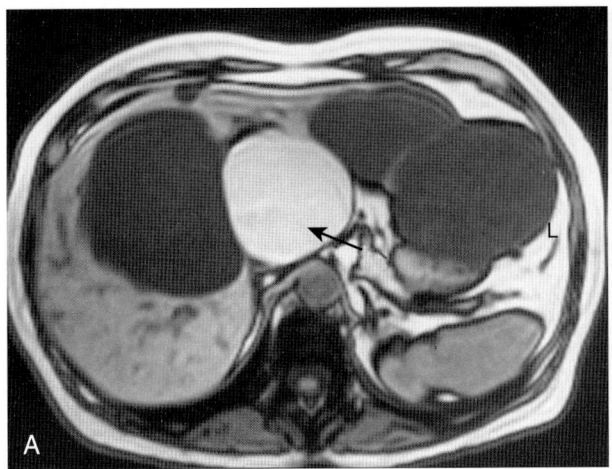 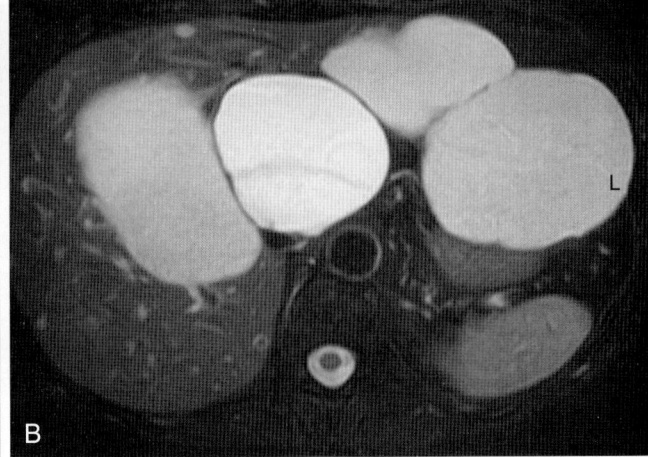

FIGURE 73.2   **Magnetic resonance imaging of a patient with multiple cysts.** All cysts are hyperintense on T2-weighted images **(B)**, whereas on T1-weighted images **(A)**, cysts are hypointense except for one cyst, which is hyperintense as a result of intracystic bleeding *(arrow)*. (See Chapter 14.)

The other imaging procedures have less utility in diagnosis compared with US and are generally not required. CT confirms the presence of one or several round or oval, water-dense lesions, without septations or intracystic formations; dynamic CT shows that they are avascular (see Chapter 18). In small cysts, recognition of water density may be difficult (the average density of the cyst being obscured by the density of the adjacent liver tissue), and an apparent increase in density may be observed after intravenous (IV) injection of contrast medium. However, CT is not a good imaging method to explore cysts. On MRI, the cyst is homogeneous, very hypointense on T1-weighted images, and very hyperintense (as the gallbladder content) on T2-weighted images (Fig. 73.2). Contrast US shows no enhancement of the cyst wall.[11]

If the patient is living or has been living in an area where hydatid disease is endemic, or if there is any doubt about a possible hydatid cyst, serologic tests for this parasitic infection (although its accuracy is fairly low) as well as MRI should be performed (see Chapters 19 and 74).

Course and Complications

In most cases, simple cysts are asymptomatic and remain silent; repeated US studies usually show no appreciable changes during years, and surveillance is not required. In some patients, the cysts grow slowly. In a few patients, the size of the cysts increases rapidly; such a course, which may be associated with severe pain and discomfort, is observed almost exclusively in women older than 50 years.

Complications are uncommon. Intracystic bleeding is the most frequent.[2,12] It is presumed to result from the erosion of an artery adjacent to the cyst. The clinical manifestations consist of sudden, severe pain and increase in the size of the cyst. The pain resolves in a few days. In a few cases, pain is mild or absent. There is no evidence of anemia, and the biologic liver tests show only a moderate elevation of γ-glutamyltransferase.

On US, echoic material, corresponding to clots, is present within the cyst (Fig. 73.3); usually this echoic material is mobile, sliding in the inferior part of the cyst (see Chapter 14). Hemorrhagic cysts also become hyperintense on T1-weighted MRI, whereas uncomplicated cysts are hypointense (see Fig. 73.2; see also Chapter 14). After gadolinium injection, there is frequently

an enhancement of the periphery of the cyst when hemorrhage is recent, which corresponds to compressed liver parenchyma (Fig. 73.4). Communication with the bile duct lumen, presumably also by an erosive mechanism, may develop. Bacterial infection is, in contrast, exceptional.[13] It seems to be more frequent in the presence of renal insufficiency, dialysis, and, above all, in polycystic liver. In that case, a positron emission tomography (PET)–CT can be useful to localize the infected cyst among other cysts. In general, a giant infected cyst can be diagnosed with CT scan. In case of infected giant cyst, medical treatment is insufficient, and prolonged drainage or a surgical approach is necessary.

Spontaneous rupture into the peritoneal cavity (Fig. 73.5)[14,15] or, more rarely, the pleural cavity or the duodenum[16] is exceptionally rare. In contrast to hydatid cysts, peritoneal perforation of simple cysts is self-limited. Severe hemoperitoneum has been described only in patients receiving anticoagulation[17,18] with very few exceptions.[19]

There are also anecdotal case reports of traumatic rupture of simple cysts mimicking an acute surgical abdomen.[20]

Because simple cysts are tense, they may compress the bile ducts or the inferior vena cava (IVC; Fig. 73.6), and although anecdotal, pulmonary embolism after clot formation has been reported.[21] Acute Budd-Chiari syndrome (see Chapter 86) has also been reported.[22] As will be discussed later in this chapter, with these conditions, compression of biliary branches or hepatic veins is a potential source of intraoperative or postoperative complications.

Differential Diagnosis

Hydatid cysts, liver abscesses, and cystadenomas and cystadenocarcinomas are the main differential diagnosis (especially when simple cysts have become atypical). They are addressed in Chapters 72, 70, and 88B, respectively.

Embryonal sarcomas are mostly observed in children between the ages of 2 and 15 years and are exceptional in adults. The tumor is usually large and poorly differentiated with abundant myxoid or necrotic content. Although the tumor may appear as cystic on CT and MRI, because of the very high water content of the myxoid stroma, US shows that it is, in fact, solid. Late-phase imaging after contrast injection during CT and

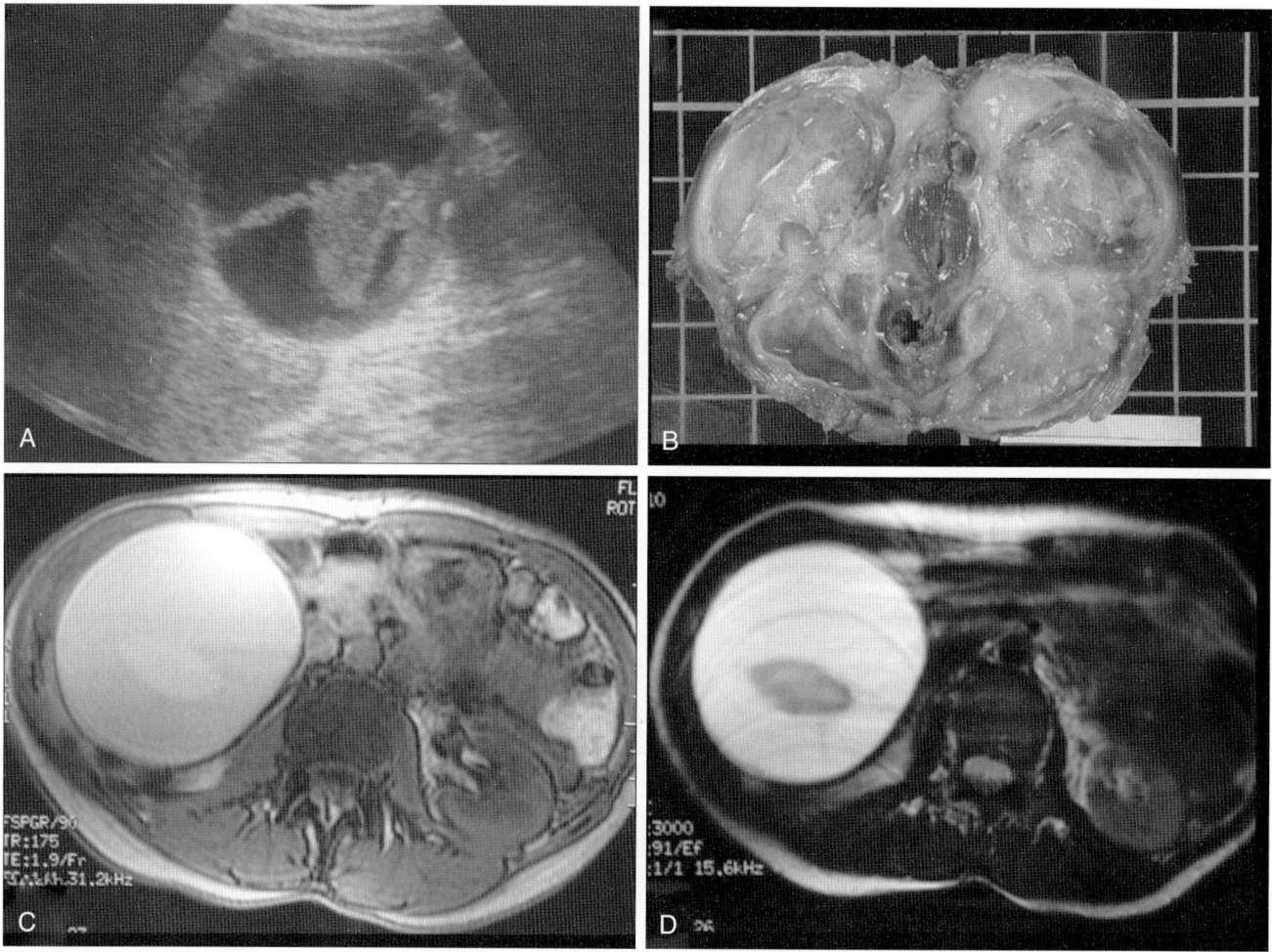

FIGURE 73.3 **Hemorrhagic simple cyst of the liver. A,** Ultrasound view. **B,** Macroscopic view of the resected specimen. **C** and **D,** Magnetic resonance imaging views. (See Chapter 14.)

MRI shows late enhancement, which is incompatible with a cystic tumor.

Other primary tumors, including hepatocellular carcinoma and cholangiocarcinoma, may occasionally be cystic. The cystic appearance corresponds to necrosis that may be either spontaneous (in particular for rapidly growing tumors) or treatment induced. However, with few exceptions, these tumors remain mostly solid. Giant hemangiomas may occasionally present as partly cystic. This corresponds to noncirculating areas. Hemangiomas are hypointense on T1-weighted images and hyperintense on T2-weighted images (as any cystic lesion), but the kinetics of contrast enhancement is typical (see Chapter 19).

Intrahepatic pseudocysts in the context of acute pancreatitis or pancreatic ducts rupture are exceptional, with less than 20 reported cases[23] (see Chapter 55). They may be located in the left side of the liver (along the lesser omentum) or the right side of the liver (along the right portal vein). They have a subcapsular location, a hemorrhagic or necrotic content, and a fibrous wall that enhances at the late phase of the injection. Magnetic resonance cholangiopancreatography (MRCP) is useful to (occasionally) document rupture of the pancreatic duct (see Chapter 17). Liver hematomas are rarely spontaneous and usually appear in the context of trauma or liver surgery. They have also been described in association with hepatocellular

carcinoma, liver adenoma or, very rarely, metastases. When occurring at the end of a pregnancy, HELLP (hemolysis, elevated liver enzymes, low platelet count) syndrome should be suspected. Clinical symptoms are usually obvious with pain and sometimes hypotension. When the clots are fresh, these hematomas are spontaneously echogenic on US, hyperdense on CT scan, hyperintense on T1-weighted, and hypointense on T2-weighted MRI sequences. At a later phase, clots liquefy, and the content appears cystic.

Bilomas are cystic lesions containing bile as a result of spontaneous, traumatic, or iatrogenic bile duct rupture. These may be surrounded by a fibrous capsule. Biliary anomalies (dilation, stenosis, or a combination of these) are frequent.

Ciliated Hepatic Foregut Cysts

Ciliated hepatic cysts have been described in all areas where the foregut extends during the embryonic period, including the sublingual area, esophagus, stomach, ileum, pancreas, and gallbladder. They also may be present within the liver. Although extremely rare, ciliated hepatic cysts warrant special consideration.

When located within the liver, ciliated cysts are located within the liver parenchyma and have a characteristic four-layer border that consists of a pseudostratified ciliated columnar

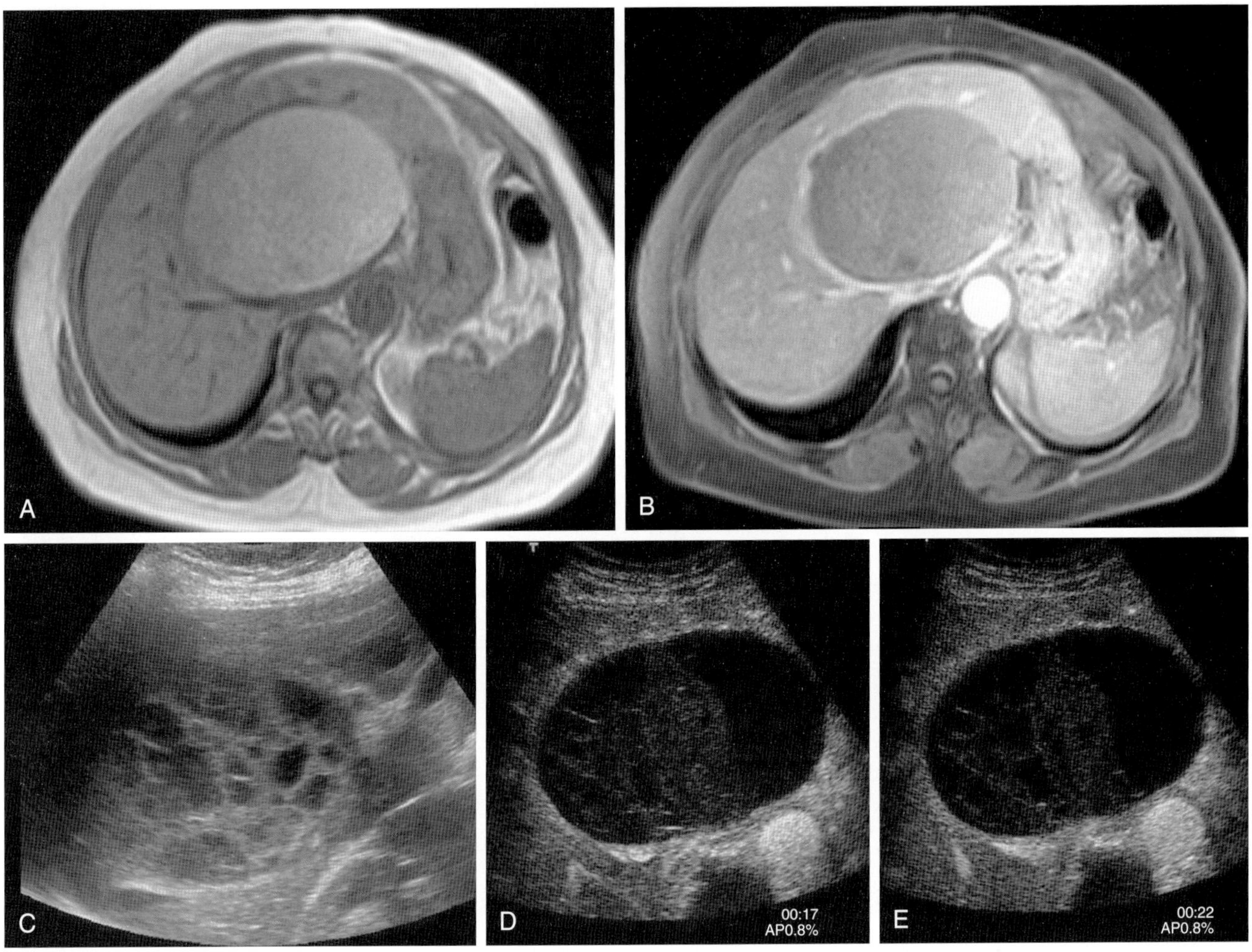

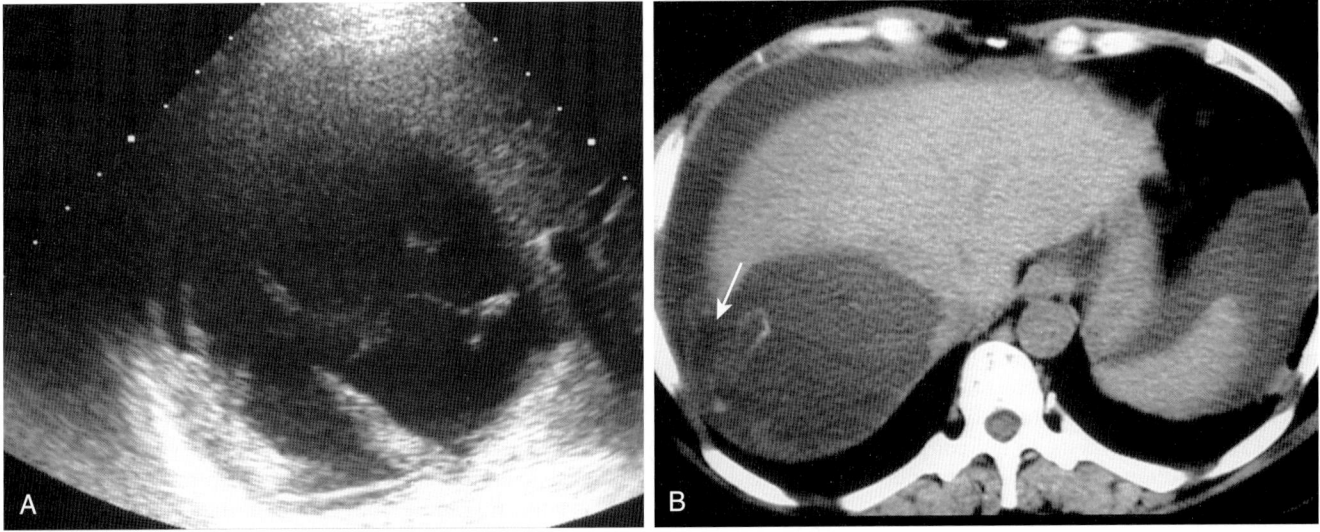

FIGURE 73.4   Example of a hemorrhagic simple cyst. The cyst is hyperintense on T1-weighted images **(A),** and there is peripheral enhancement after injection of gadolinium **(B)** because of compression of the adjacent liver. On ultrasound, the cystic lesion as echogenic and anechogenic portions **(C),** but the echogenic portions do not enhance during contrast ultrasound **(D and E).**

FIGURE 73.5   Spontaneous rupture of a simple cyst. Ultrasound **(A)** and computed tomography scan **(B).** The cystic lesion is heterogeneous and ill-limited. A communication is visible with the peritoneal cavity *(arrow)* where ascites is visible.

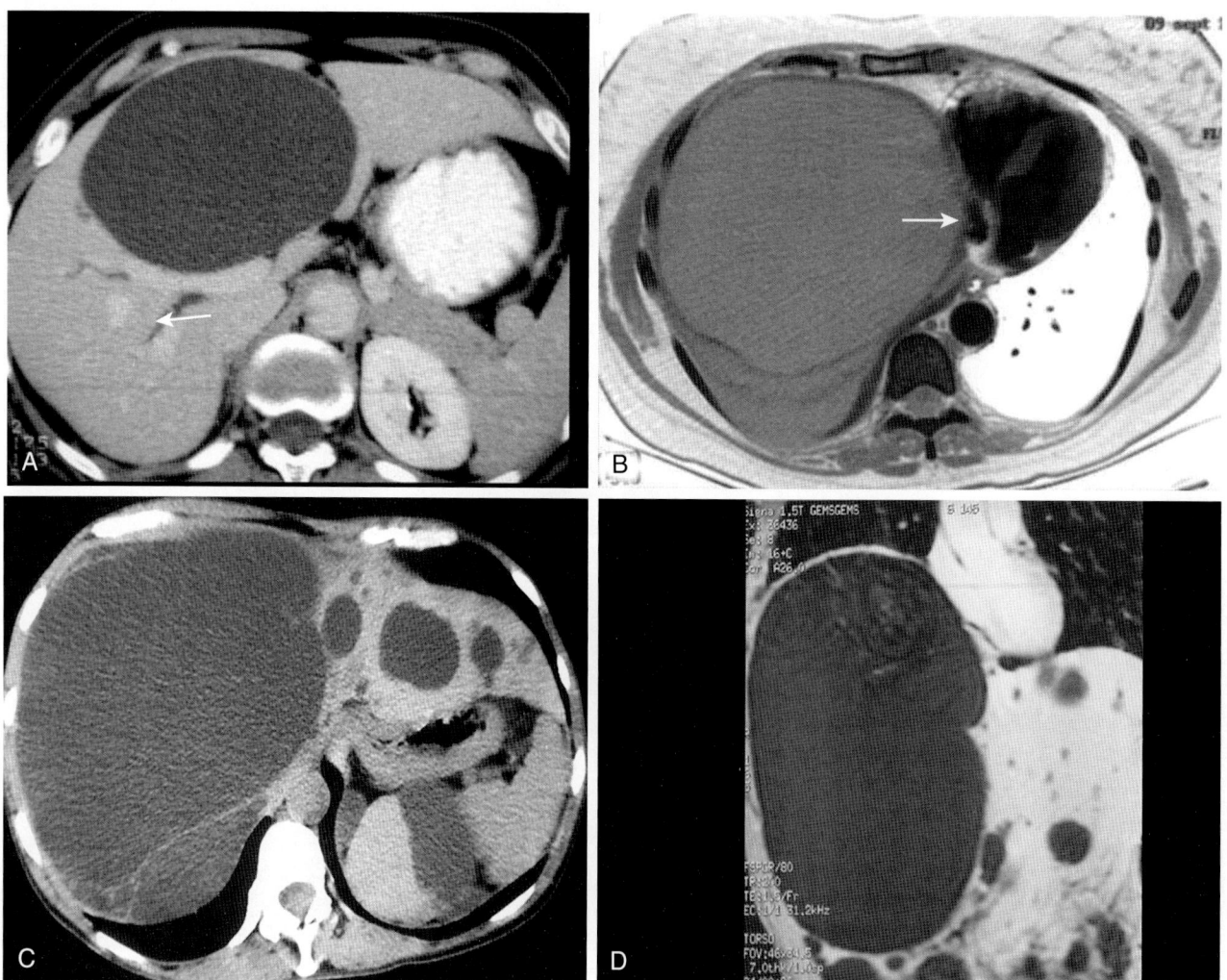

FIGURE 73.6 Compression by hepatic cysts of the biliary confluence **(A)** with enlarged bile ducts upstream *(arrow)*, the inferior vena cava **(B)** with a small clot in the caval lumen *(arrow)*, the stomach indirectly by a large cyst of the right liver rotating the left lateral section **(C)**, the diaphragm, and the right atrium **(D)**.

epithelium covering a subepithelial connective tissue, smooth muscle bundles, and an outer fibrous capsule. The lining epithelium may secrete fluid of different composition (from nearly water to viscous or mucous), which explains why its echogenicity may be variable and why calcifications may be present, although exceptionally. The second characteristic of these cysts is that they are subcapsular, usually located on the anterior surface of the liver close to the insertion of the falciform ligament. Two-thirds are localized in the left lobe of the liver in segment IV, but right lobe cysts also have been described.[24,25] The final characteristic of these cysts is that they are classically unilocular and usually less than 4 cm in diameter. Typically, these cysts do not communicate with the biliary system, although this has been reported, particularly in children.

Ciliated hepatic cysts, although known since 1857, are rare, with approximately 100 cases reported in the literature, most in the past 20 years.[26] There is no gender predominance, and the age of the patients ranges from newborn with prenatal diagnosis[27] to 82 years (mean age, 48 years).

Most ciliated hepatic foregut cysts are asymptomatic (two-thirds of reported patients) and discovered incidentally during abdominal imaging studies or surgical explorations. Abdominal symptoms are rare, probably because of their small size. When present, the most frequent symptom is epigastric or right upper quadrant abdominal pain that can be observed even with small cysts because of their subcapsular location.

The three characteristics on imaging are their predominant location in segment IV, their small size (4 cm ± 2 cm), and their subcapsular location. Most (>90%) are unilocular. Two-thirds of the cysts are hypoechoic on US, are hypodense on CT, and do not enhance after injection of contrast material (Fig. 73.7). They are anechoic as formal biliary cysts in less than 5%.[28] Some ciliated cysts also may have an atypical solid tumor appearance on CT and a noncystic appearance on US (hyperechoic), probably as a result of mucinous material, calcium, and cholesterol crystals within the cyst. On MRI, the lesion is highly hyperintense on T2-weighted images but highly variable on T1 sequences, being hyperintense in 52%, isointense in 24%, and hypointense in 14%. When atypical on imaging, the

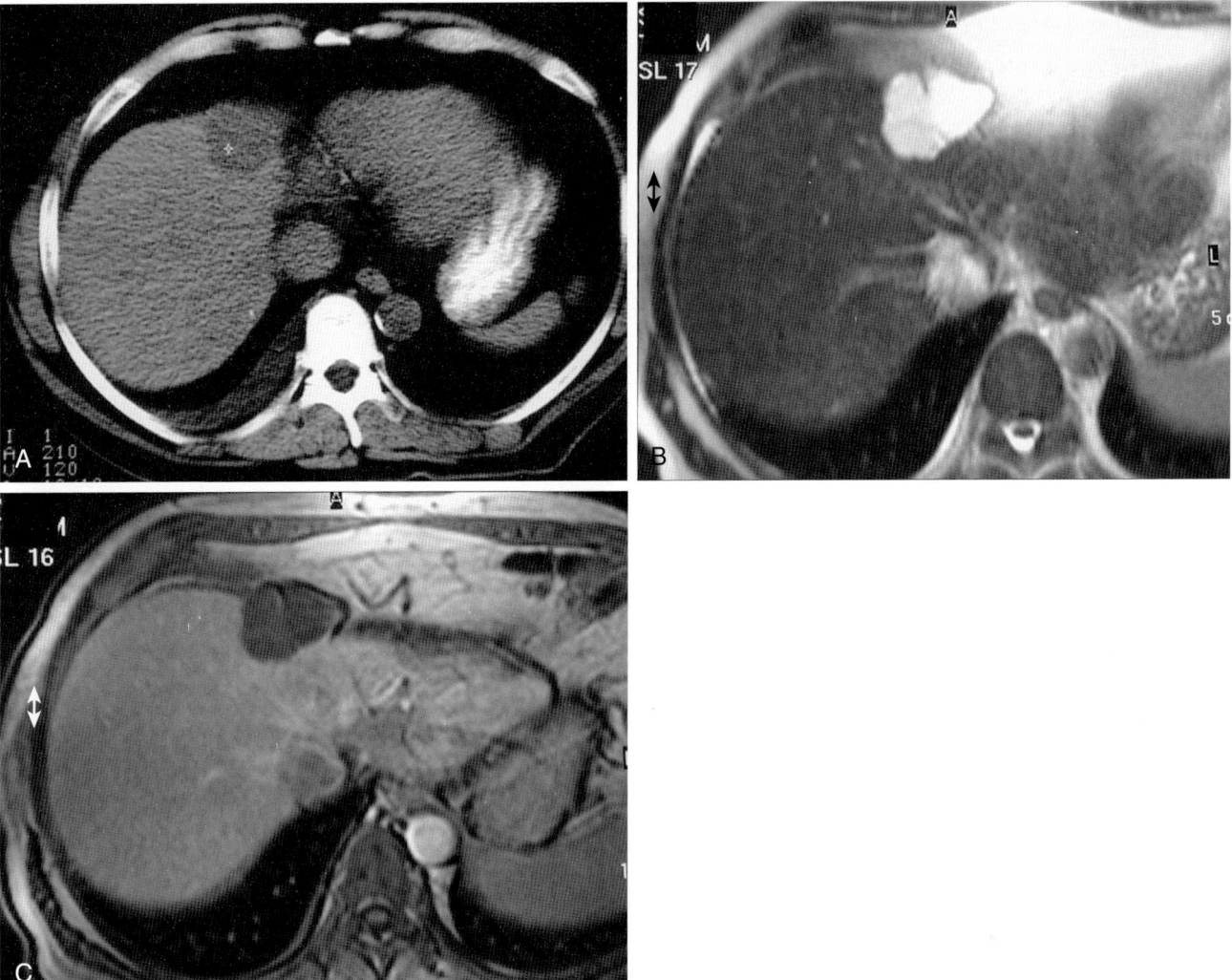

FIGURE 73.7   Ciliated hepatic foregut cyst. Computed tomography (CT) scan and magnetic resonance imaging. On CT scan without injection, the tumor is hypodense, subcapsular and is located in the upper part of segment IV **(A)**. It is hyperintense on T2-sequences **(B)** and hypointense on T1 sequences after injection of gadolinium **(C)**.

differential diagnosis includes cystadenoma or cystadenocarcinoma (see Chapter 88B) and may be difficult, especially because CA19-9 may be expressed by the epithelium of the ciliated cysts, and its serum level may be slightly elevated.[29] Fine-needle aspiration cytology may be helpful by showing ciliated pseudostratified tall columnar epithelial cells suspended in a mucous background. The presence of these cells is virtually diagnostic of this condition, and the positive predictive value of aspiration is 76%.[26]

Ciliated hepatic foregut cysts are usually thought to follow a benign course. Compression of adjacent structures is extremely rare, with a single case report of portal compression resulting in portal hypertension[30] and another in jaundice.[31] Malignant transformation into squamous cell carcinoma has been reported in four patients in recent years,[31–34] whereas one other patient had extensive squamous metaplasia,[35] yielding a risk of malignancy of less than 5%. Because this transformation has occurred in patients with cysts larger than 7 cm, most authors agree that excision is indicated when the cyst is larger than 4 to 5 cm, enlarges, shows abnormalities in its wall, or is symptomatic, although other authors have broader indications.

Management

Asymptomatic liver cysts, even when large, need no treatment and do not require surveillance. A small percentage of patients have symptoms related to an increase in the size of cysts, which is often correlated with an intracystic hemorrhage or a cystic infection. Caution must be exercised when considering whether a simple cyst is symptomatic when it is smaller than 8 cm or when it does not protrude outside of the liver surface without a compression of a close organ. If this is not the case, or if symptoms are vague, US-guided aspiration of the cyst may be attempted as a therapeutic test. If this does not result in improvement of symptoms, further treatment is not required. When aspiration is effective at relieving symptoms, the cyst is symptomatic. Improvement, however, is transient, because the cyst inevitably recurs after simple aspiration,[36] and more effective and durable treatment should be considered.

It is unclear whether treatment is indicated in patients who are asymptomatic but have evidence on imaging of compression of the bile ducts, the vena cava, or of portal or hepatic veins by the cysts. When a patient is completely asymptomatic and

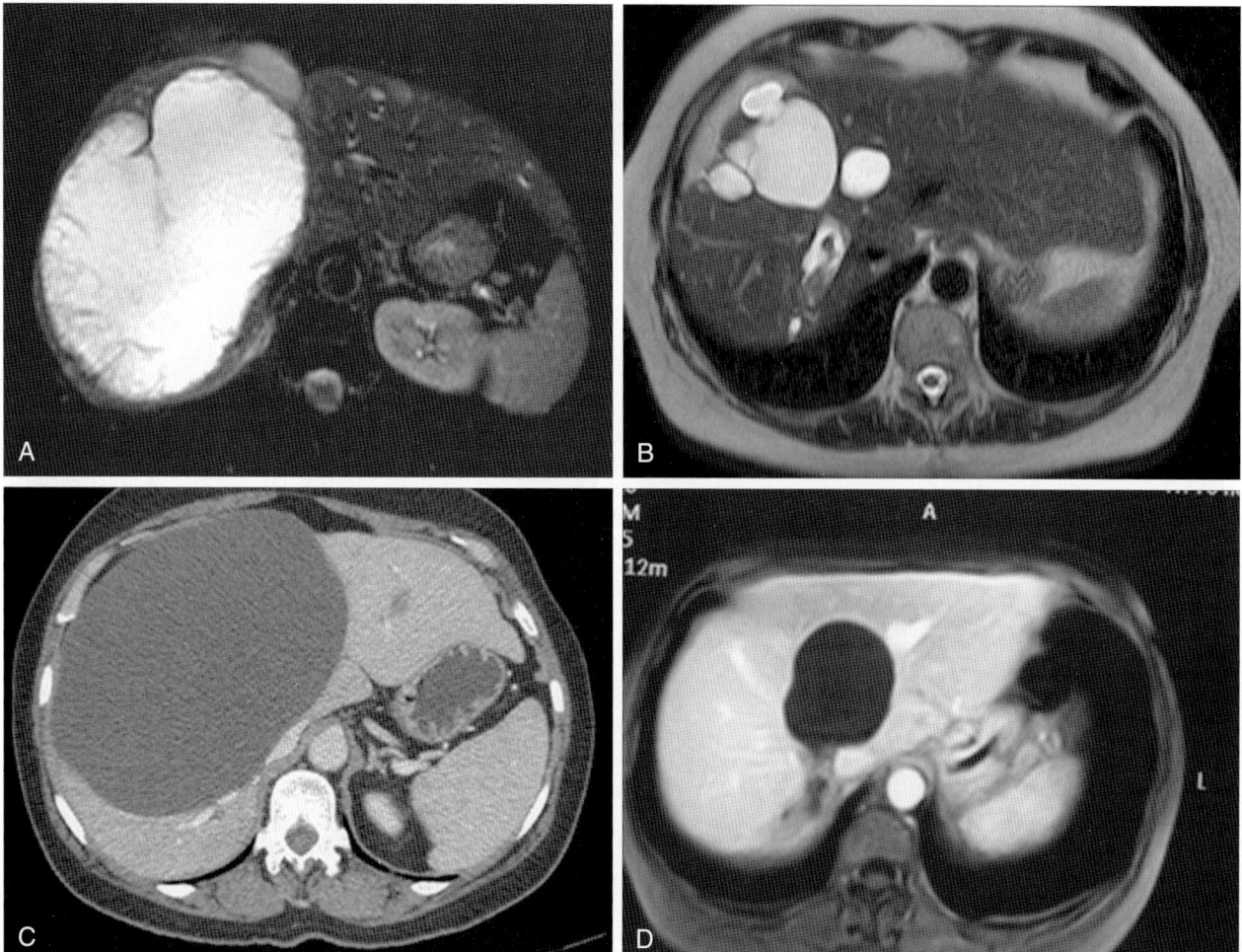

FIGURE 73.8 Biliary cysts before (**A** and **C**) and after (**B** and **D**) alcohol sclerotherapy. In the first patient (**A** and **B**), vascular pedicles were compressed, and marked atrophy persisted despite reduction in the size of the cyst. In the second patient (**C** and **D**), hepatic vein compression persisted despite size reduction.

there is no vascular or parenchymal consequence of the compression of the vena cava or the hepatic vein, no treatment is required. Treatment can be considered when there is a compression of the hepatic vein and vascular abnormalities in the noncystic liver parenchyma, or if there is ascites, reflecting a "suffering" noncystic liver parenchyma, even if the patient is asymptomatic. However, if these anomalies are unilateral (i.e., at least one hemiliver has normal biliary drainage and normal inflow and outflow), our opinion is that treatment is not required because the stenosis is not always reversible (Fig. 73.8).

Treatment of symptomatic cysts relies on the destruction of the epithelial lining (sclerotherapy) or on the creation of a communication between the cyst and the peritoneal cavity (unroofing, also known as fenestration). Sclerotherapy is performed under US guidance, whereas unroofing is currently mostly performed by laparoscopy. Hence symptomatic patients today are most likely to undergo a minimally invasive procedure. This should not lead to an extension of the indications because complications, occasionally severe ones, may occur. It is also important to warn patients early on that these treatments aim at transforming a large, symptomatic cyst into a small, asymptomatic one, and that they should not worry if some anomalies persist on imaging after the procedure.

Sclerotherapy

Method

Sclerotherapy aims to destroy the epithelium lining the inner surface of the wall to stop intracystic fluid secretion. Under US guidance, the cyst is located and punctured, and a small drainage catheter is introduced using the Seldinger technique. Injection of water-soluble contrast media ensures that no communication with the bile duct exists and that no leak into the peritoneal cavity is present, both of which are contraindications to continuing with the procedure.[37]

The most frequently used sclerosing agent is 95% ethanol, as for renal cysts. Minocycline hydrochloride, otherwise used for pleurodesis or, more recently, ethanolamine oleate,[38,39] and hypertonic saline and bleomycin[40] have been proposed as alternatives. Radiofrequency ablation (RFA) has also been performed, although reports are only anecdotal.

The amount of ethanol injected should be limited because alcohol sclerotherapy is associated with an increase in blood alcohol concentration, peaking 3 to 4 hours after treatment.[41] Because massive ethanol intoxication leading to coma has been reported after injection of 240 mL in a 3500 mL cyst,[42] the volume of alcohol should not exceed 100 to 120 mL. To

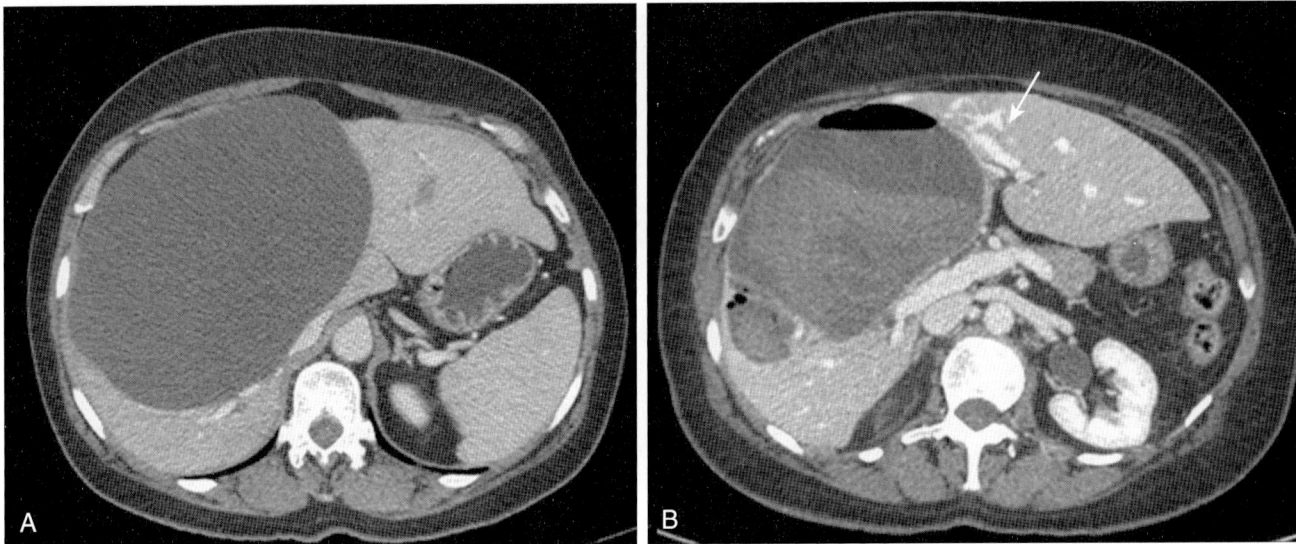

FIGURE 73.9   Biliary cyst before **(A)** and after **(B)** sclerotherapy by ethanol. Sclerotherapy was complicated by hemorrhage (dense content). Note the presence of hepatic vein collateral circulation adjacent to the cyst that could have been inadvertently injured during sclerotherapy *(arrow)*.

ensure that the sclerosant comes in contact with the entire surface, the patient is rolled in different positions. Alcohol is then aspirated and the catheter removed. The procedure is performed with the patient under light general anesthesia because it is painful.

Several protocols have been designed that differ in the duration of alcohol retention in the cyst (from 10 to 240 minutes) and in the number of sessions (single or multiple).[37,41,43,44] Comparative studies are lacking, but a single study showed that 120- and 240-minute retention times yield comparable results.[41] More recently, Larssen et al. suggested that a single procedure of sclerotherapy with a short period of exposure of ethanol (during 20 minutes maximum) can be sufficient to relieve symptoms in the long term (median of 56 months), with no sign of recurrence.[45] Long-acting somatostatin analogues administered 2 weeks before and 2 weeks after sclerotherapy did not improve cyst reduction or clinical response in a randomized controlled trial (RCT).[46]

Prolonged catheter drainage with negative pressure of the cyst without sclerotherapy has been shown to be as effective as alcohol injection in a single RCT.[47] This result mainly shows that an important aspect of percutaneous treatments in general is to achieve collapse of the cystic cavity.

Limitations

Although the alcohol injected should not exceed a certain amount, the size of the cyst in itself is not a limitation. Provided the cyst collapses after aspiration, the sclerosant will come into contact with the epithelial lining. It is also possible to repeat the procedure if required.

An absolute contraindication, which should be formally and completely excluded by a fistulography before the injection, is the presence of a communication between the cyst and the biliary tract. Simple cysts do not normally have such a communication, but fistulization may occur, presumably by erosion.

Recent intracystic bleeding with fresh blood in the cyst is also a contraindication for most physicians; in such cases, sclerotherapy should be delayed by 3 months.[48]

Complications

Although the injection is painful (which is why the procedure is performed under general anesthesia), pain resolves rapidly, and most patients are discharged the next day. Transient neuropsychic disorders secondary to diffusion of alcohol through the cyst wall have been reported. Intracystic bleeding or cystic infection is rare but potentially severe (Fig. 73.9). It should be realized that vessels are compressed at the periphery of enlarged cysts because of the high intracystic pressure and are therefore not visible; however, bleeding may occur once the cysts have emptied if a vessel has been inadvertently punctured.

Inflammatory changes are frequent after sclerotherapy and may interfere with imaging follow-up. They may also increase the difficulty of subsequent fenestration if sclerotherapy has been ineffective.

Long-Term Outcome

An initial systematic literature review published in 2001 identified 112 patients treated by alcohol sclerotherapy and 17 treated with minocycline hydrochloride instillation.[49] In most patients, a complete or partial regression of the cyst was seen, but follow-up was short overall. Although the technique has developed, the reported experience since then has been limited. A recent systematic review on 16 studies involving 526 patients showed a 90% to 100% volume reduction in studies with a follow-up of 12 months or more and disappearance of symptoms in 79% to 100% of patients in series published over the past 20 years.[50] Hemorrhagic cysts with hemorrhagic aspirate can be associated with a lower reduction of the volume of the cyst at 1 month, which can be a risk factor of incomplete clinical response.[51]

An early morphologic assessment, usually by US, is frequently performed. However, patients should be warned that this is likely to show the persistence of the cyst, although at a smaller size; this is not predictive of symptomatic recurrence. Moreover, the cyst volume reduction is not the best reflection of the success of the aspiration sclerotherapy procedure; instead, the assessment of the symptoms is the best predictive factor of the success of this treatment.[52] In practice, several

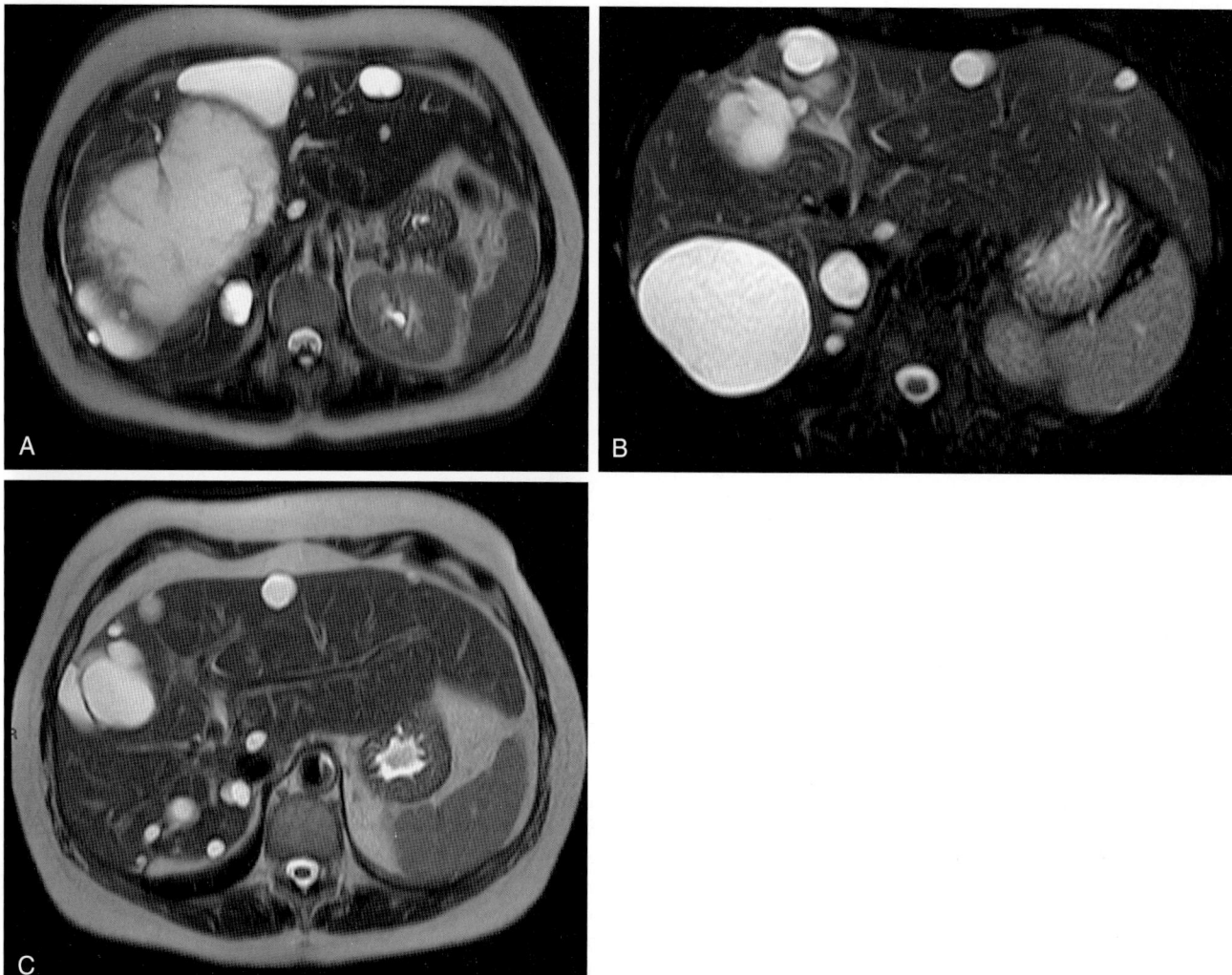

FIGURE 73.10 **Magnetic resonance imaging follow-up of a cyst after sclerotherapy with ethanol.** **A,** Before therapy. **B,** Six months later, the cyst has decreased. **C,** Eighteen months later, the cyst has disappeared.

months—perhaps up to a year—may be required to achieve optimal efficacy after alcohol sclerotherapy (Fig. 73.10).

Fenestration

Method

The surgical treatment of choice for a single, large, symptomatic cyst is fenestration that consists of an excision of the roof of the cyst to establish a large communication between the cyst and the peritoneal cavity. Fluid continues to be produced by the epithelial lining, but it is reabsorbed by the peritoneum, and the cyst cavity collapses. This treatment is extremely simple because symptomatic cysts are virtually always large and have a protrusion of part of their wall outside the liver. Only the protruding part of the cyst wall should be excised; there is no need to enter the liver parenchyma, which is the main cause of intraoperative and postoperative bleeding or biliary leaks, nor is there a need to remove the cyst completely.

The procedure has initially been described as laparotomy but is currently most often performed as laparoscopy, which offers the advantage of being less invasive and ensuring a quicker recovery.[53,54] It was also established that laparoscopic fenestration improves long-term quality of life (QOL).[55] In a systematic review and meta-analysis of 62 studies including 1314 patients who had laparoscopic fenestration of symptomatic cysts, the postoperative morbidity, major morbidity rates, and major mortality rates were 10.8%, 3.3%, and 1.0% respectively; symptomatic long-term relief was observed in 90.2% of the patients.[56]

No prospective series compared the results of laparoscopic and open fenestration but recent meta-analysis and a subsequent retrospective analysis showed no difference in terms of recurrence rate or improvement of QOL between laparoscopic or open fenestration.[57,58]

A pneumoperitoneum is established, the cyst is punctured and incised with either scissors or electrocautery, and the cyst wall is widely excised. If transection is performed along a thin part of adjacent parenchyma to ensure a wider opening (i.e., if the protruding part of the cyst is small), endovascular staplers may occasionally be used to secure vasculobiliary structures that are compressed at the periphery of the cyst wall. The internal lining of the cyst is examined, and if a biliary communication is suspected, intraoperative cholangiography should be performed. Some investigators have advocated treating the remnant cyst epithelium by argon laser beam coagulation or

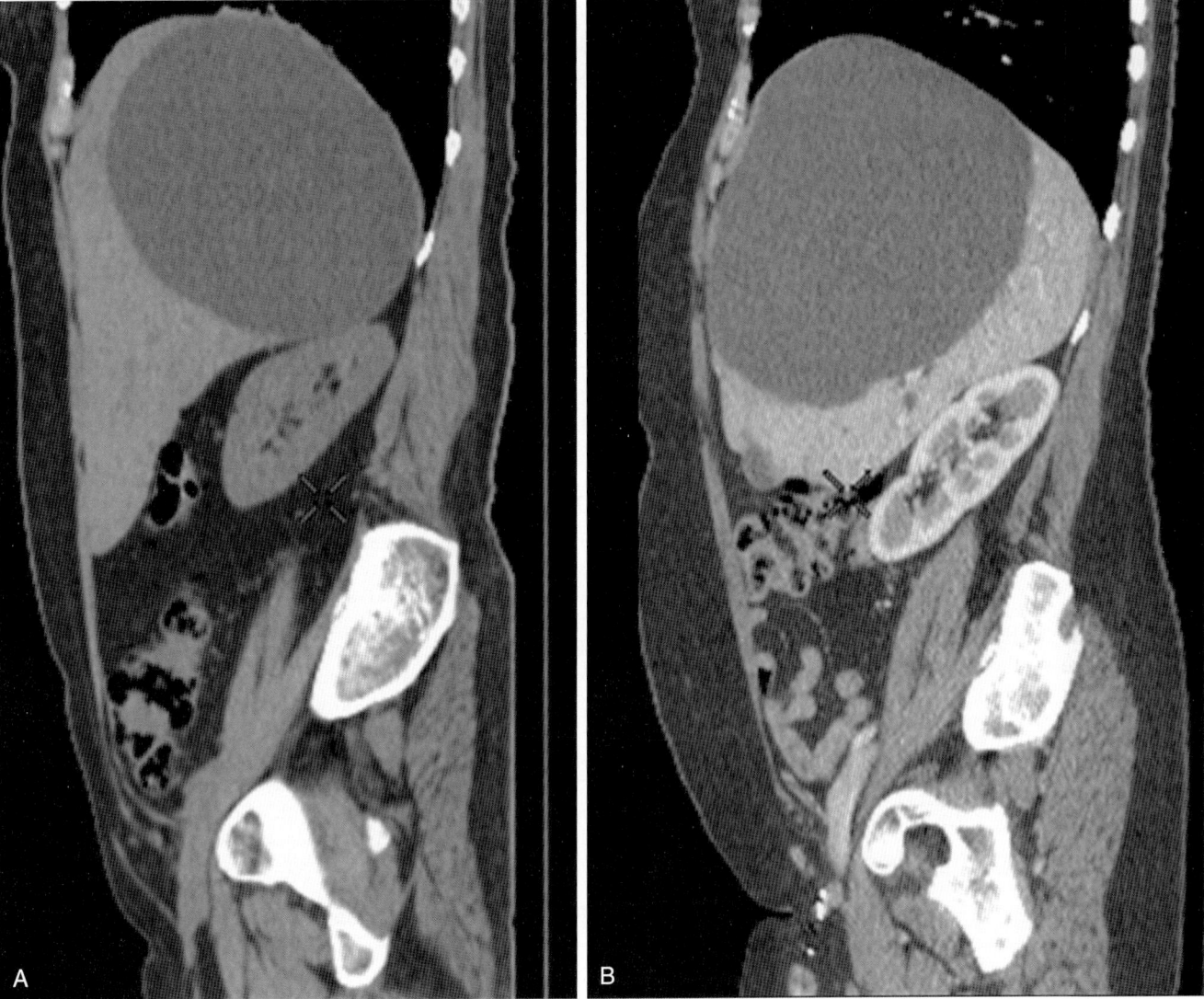

FIGURE 73.11   Two examples of large cysts located in the right liver *(transverse view)*. A cyst with a predominantly posterior development **(A)** may be more difficult to fenestrate by laparoscopy than an anterior cyst **(B),** and sclerotherapy may be more successful.

electrocoagulation to destroy the epithelium. In any case, the excised portion of the cyst is sent for pathologic analysis. Suction drainage is optional.

Limitations

Cysts protruding into segments VII or VIII are not formal contraindications to laparoscopic fenestration, but the procedure is unlikely to be very successful in such a case because limited access will prevent wide unroofing. In addition, the margins of the opening may adhere to the diaphragm, and the risk of postoperative cyst recurrence is increased as a result of contained secretion. There is also a risk of intraoperative injury to the diaphragm (Fig. 73.11). Open fenestration is a wise alternative in this circumstance.

Complications

The most severe intraoperative complication is bleeding, and transfusion has occasionally been required.[59] This occurs when the liver parenchyma, not the cyst wall, is opened and when the cyst compresses vascular structures, in particular the suprahepatic

veins. Conversion, the most frequent indication for which is bleeding, is required in less than 5% of patients.

Postoperative complications are rare, and patients are usually discharged after 1 to 3 days. No deaths have been reported, and morbidity ranges between 0% and 15%.[59,60] The most severe complications include biliary leak and hemorrhage, which result from reexpansion of biliary and vascular structures that were compressed at the interface between the cyst wall and the parenchyma and that were inadequately secured. If the periphery of the opened cyst is thick, it should be closed with running sutures; an alternative is to use an endovascular stapler on these portions of the cyst wall because it allows wide fenestration while maintaining hemostasis. Ascites is very rare after fenestration of simple cysts, unlike PCLD (see later).

Long-Term Outcome

Long-term efficacy of fenestration for simple cysts is still somewhat unclear. Reported experience is limited, follow-up is usually short, and results are not always stratified according to the number of cysts (i.e., simple cysts vs. PCLD). Furthermore, cyst recurrence, symptomatic recurrence, and the need for additional treatment are not always distinguished. It is usually assumed that although cysts may recur in one-third to one-half of patients, symptomatic recurrence occurs in less than 5%[61-63]; however, higher figures of symptomatic recurrence (15%–20%) have been reported.[56,60,64-67] Persistent symptoms may be related to technical failure or reflect inaccurate selection, with some patients undergoing surgery for non–cyst-related symptoms.

A more precise comparison of preoperative and postoperative symptoms has recently been published.[59] Abdominal pain was improved in 91% of patients and disappeared in 68%. Other symptoms, including impaired gastrointestinal transport, early satiety, nausea, vomiting, and acid reflux, disappeared in 53% of the patients. Overall, within 1 year of surgery, 32% of the patients experienced or had persistent subjective symptoms in this series, but this rate decreased to 7% and 2% after 3 and 5 years, respectively. During follow-up, 9% required reoperation.

Sclerotherapy Versus Fenestration

Although both techniques have been used for years, no randomized or prospective comparative analysis has been done. As a rule, the severity of symptoms that leads to treatment has not been standardized, and recurrence is poorly defined. It would seem that both methods are almost as effective.[49,65,68] Our policy is to systematically attempt sclerotherapy first, whatever the size of the cyst; fenestration is indicated in cases of recurrence, but location of the protruding part of the cyst may influence this choice, or when the patient wants to be relieved of the pain immediately (see Fig. 73.11).

POLYCYSTIC LIVER DISEASE

Polycystic liver disease, or more precisely, diseases, is a genetic disorder responsible for the progressive development of multiple cysts in the liver. This entity was initially considered to exclusively develop in the context of ADPKD.[69] However, identification of families with PCLD but no ADPKD[70,71] proved that PCLD may also occur alone. These two forms of PCLD (with or without ADPKD) are linked to distinct gene mutations. Both, however, have an autosomal dominant transmission and almost identical clinical courses. Of note, one-third of patients with isolated PCLD may have a few kidney cysts (usually one or two)[72] as does the general population of adult patients.[6] Distinction between the two forms of PCLD is addressed later.

Genetics

PCLD Associated With ADPKD

PCLD associated with ADPKD is linked to mutations in either the *PKD1* or *PKD2* gene. *PKD1*[73] is located on the short arm of chromosome 16 and encodes polycystin-1; its mutation accounts for 85% of mutations in ADPKD patients. Most of the remainder is related to a mutation in *PKD2*[74], which is located on chromosome 4 and encodes polycystin-2. *PKD1* mutation is associated with more renal cysts, larger cysts, more prevalent hypertension, and faster progression to the end stage of renal disease than *PKD2* mutation. GANAB mutation has also more recently been shown to cause ADPKD (as well as autosomal-dominant PCLD [ADPCLD]).[75]

Isolated PCLD (Without ADPKD)

Isolated PCLD without ADPKD is associated with heterozygous mutation in either the protein kinase C substrate 80K-H (*PRKCSH*), *SEC63*, *LRP5* or, very rarely, *GANAB* genes. These genes affect the endoplasmic reticulum and function in the early secretory route of the cell. *PRKCSH* is located on the short arm of chromosome 19, which encodes the protein hepatocystin.[76] Hepatocystin functions as the β-subunit of α-glucosidase 2 and is involved in the protein folding processes and quality control of newly synthesized glycoproteins.[77] *SEC63* is located on the long arm of chromosome 6 and encodes the SEC63 protein, which is involved in protein transport across the endoplasmic reticulum membrane.[78] However, these mutations only explain 25% to 40% of cases,[79] which suggests that there are other gene mutations involved. Recent studies suggest that these may include ALG8 and SEC61B[80] as well as ALG9.[81]

The Two-Hit Theory

PCLDs have an autosomal dominant phenotype but are considered to be a recessive disease at the molecular level because they require a second somatic mutation. According to this theory, there is a germline mutation in either *PKD1* or *PKD2*. However, cell proliferation and cyst formation occurs in individual cells that have, in addition, received a second loss-of-function somatic mutation in the other gene copy.[82] This second hit explains that affected cells are few and that cysts develop from place to place and may also account for the extreme heterogeneity of the disease. This theory has been designed for PCLD associated with ADPKD and also confirmed for isolated PCLD.[83] The molecular mechanism of cyst formation has been the subject of reviews.[84]

Pathology and Pathogenesis

Liver cysts in PCLD are macroscopically and microscopically similar to simple cysts of the liver, and their number and distribution are highly variable. They are lined by a single-layered epithelium that has phenotypic and functional characteristics of biliary epithelium.[85] It retains, in particular, secretory capacity and responsiveness to secretin.[86] The cysts result from abnormal remodeling of the ductal plate and mainly arise from dilation of biliary microhamartomas, also known as *von Meyenburg complexes*, which have lost their communication with the biliary tree.[87] Some cysts also arise from peribiliary glands surrounding large intrahepatic bile ducts (Fig. 73.12).[88]

The mechanism of cyst expansion is still not fully explained but shares most mechanisms involved in the development of renal cysts. It results from a combination of proliferation of epithelial cells, remodeling of the extracellular matrix required for the cyst to invade the surrounding liver parenchyma,[89] and neovascularization resulting in increased density of the vascular bed surrounding the cysts.[90,91]

Microvilli and long cilia normally present on cholangiocytes (just as in the kidney tubules) are thought to play a dominant role. They are mechanosensory organelles that may be bended by bile flow but can also be reactive to hormones, morphogens, or growth factor stimuli, or even function as sensors of cell injury. They modulate intracellular concentrations of intracellular levels of cyclic adenosine monophosphate (cAMP) and calcium ions (Ca^{2+}), which are mediators of proliferation and secretory activity of cholangiocytes. In PCLD,

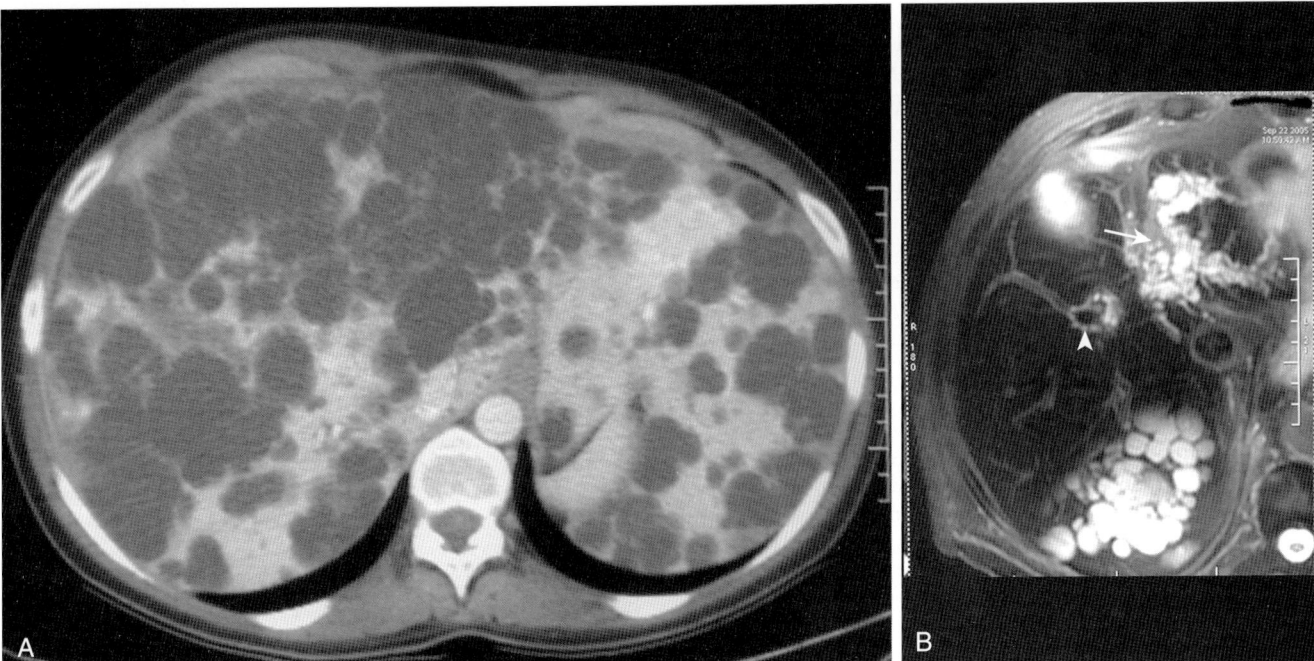

FIGURE 73.12   Polycystic liver disease. Cysts arise peripherally **(A)** or from peribiliary glands **(B)**. Note that they are prominent around the left bile duct *(arrow)* but can also be seen around the right portal pedicle *(arrowhead)*.

these cilia progressively disappear from the luminal surface of the epithelium while cysts enlarge.[92] Their absence could impair Ca^{2+}-dependent counterregulation of cAMP, which is a key determinant of cholangiocyte proliferation. It is unclear whether the disappearance of these cilia is a primary event or results from increased pressure. Of note, however, is that polycystin-1 and polycystin-2 are localized to the cilia, and their absence as a result of a *PKD1* or a *PKD2* mutation could result in ciliary dysfunction. In patients with isolated PCLD, it has been postulated that polycystins could be the target of aberrant maturation of newly synthesized glycoprotein caused by *PRKCSH* or *SEC63* mutations.

Two other targets of cell cycle have been identified. One is the mammalian target of rapamycin (mTOR)-mediated signaling cascade,[93] which explains the interest from the industry for mTOR inhibitors. The other is through micro-RNAs, which are small noncoding RNAs that inhibit target messenger RNA transcripts via sequence-specific base paring. Micro–RNA-15a, in particular, is downregulated in cyst epithelium, resulting in an overexpression of Cdc25A, which activates the cyclin-dependent kinase progression of cell cycle.[94]

Fluid secretion by the cyst-lining epithelium may also contribute to cyst expansion. Ciliary dysfunction could also play a role because it has also been shown to result in maintenance of an immature phenotype by biliary epithelial cells, with postnatal expression of developmental proteins. A variety of cytokines and growth factors present at increased concentration in the cysts have been implicated in cyst growth by autocrine/paracrine signaling.[91,92,95] Angiogenic factors, in particular, could play a role by promoting vascularization of the cyst but also by directly stimulating cholangiocytes. Furthermore, the epithelium stains positive for insulin growth factor-1 (IGF-1) and its receptor, as well as for estrogen receptors,[92] and is particularly sensitive to such signaling.

All of these observations and hypotheses account for the rationale of using vasopressin antagonists or somatostatin analogues (known to inhibit cAMP), sirolimus (inhibitor of mTOR signaling), or vascular endothelial growth factor (VEGF) inhibitors in the treatment of PCLD (see later). The presence of estrogen receptors also provides a rationale for the influence of the estrogen status of the patients on the clinical course of their disease. In particular, women with ADPKD are more likely to develop hepatic cysts than men,[96] nulliparous women are less likely to develop hepatic cysts than multiparous women,[97] and oral contraceptives or postmenopausal hormonal substitutive therapy increases the number and size of the liver cysts.[98]

Epidemiology

PCLD Associated With ADPKD

ADPKD occurs in approximately 1 in every 800 live births and is characterized by progressive development and enlargement of fluid-filled cysts, leading ultimately to renal failure in 50% of affected individuals. PCLD is the most frequent extrarenal-associated condition, but liver cysts develop later than renal cysts. Their prevalence increases with age and was recently evaluated by MRI in a young adult population with relatively preserved kidney function to be 58% in patients aged 15 to 24 years, 85% in those aged 25 to 34 years, and 94% in those aged 35 to 46 years.[99] Overall prevalence is the same in men and women, but as for simple cysts, women have a more severe liver disease than men, and multiparity as well as use of oral contraceptive drugs or estrogen replacement therapy (ERT) also tends to worsen the condition.[98–101] Prevalence of liver cysts is also correlated with kidney volume and renal cyst volume.[99]

Isolated PCLD

Isolated PCLD has been considered rare, with an estimated incidence of less than 0.01%. Compared with PCLD associated with ADPKD, the overall incidence of isolated PCLD is, in fact, only slightly lower.[102] However, in clinical series dealing with symptomatic patients, it is two to five times less frequent,[103,104] which may reflect the milder course of isolated PCLD. As for PCLD associated with ADPKD, cysts increase with age, and although the disease is transmitted equally in men and women, 85% of symptomatic patients are women (van Keimpema et al., 2010).

Manifestations and Diagnosis

Symptoms

In most patients, the liver cysts are small and sparse and remain clinically silent. Even with massive organ enlargement, significant hepatic complications remain fairly uncommon, although patients (or others) may have noted a protuberant abdomen. A few patients (up to 20%) develop symptoms that may include abdominal pain or discomfort, early satiety, shortness of breath, and leg edema. These result from compression of the stomach, diaphragm, and IVC either by single large cysts (see Fig. 73.6) but much more frequently because of the enlargement of the whole liver (Fig. 73.13C). Because symptoms have progressively evolved during a prolonged period of time, patients occasionally tend to have become used to these discomforts and to either be unaware of them or to minimize them. In that respect, the development of a specific assessment scale may prove useful.[105] At clinical examination, the liver may reach an enormous size, and its inferior border is frequently palpated in the iliac fossa. The cysts may be so tense that they can be confused with solid tumors.

Previous history of self-resolving acute abdominal pain is not unusual and may be the result of spontaneous bleeding within one or more cysts. However, these episodes may remain clinically silent. While the disease progresses, denutrition may develop and may be associated with ascites and/or pleural effusion (Fig. 73.14). Body weight is an inaccurate marker because muscular loss correlates with the progressive increase in the weight of the liver, which may reach more than 10 kg. One should instead focus on the thickness of the muscles of the abdominal wall or the psoas muscle on imaging studies.

Typically, patients referred to surgeons are women between 35 and 50 years; their liver cysts have been diagnosed 10 years previously, and symptoms have become incapacitating for 6 to 18 months. Clinical manifestations (as well as complications and management) are the same whether PCLD is isolated or associated with ADPKD.[103,106]

Biology

The only abnormality may be an increase in γ-glutamyl transferase or alkaline phosphatase, but this is infrequent. Although liver cysts may diffusely involve the liver, the hepatic parenchymal volume is preserved,[107] and there is therefore no sign of liver failure. When present, a superimposed cause of chronic liver disease is likely. This lack of influence on liver function explains that polycystic livers from even brain-dead donors have been used in the context of emergency liver transplantation.[108]

Imaging

US shows multiple, fluid-filled, round or oval cysts with sharp margins in the liver (and the kidneys when associated with

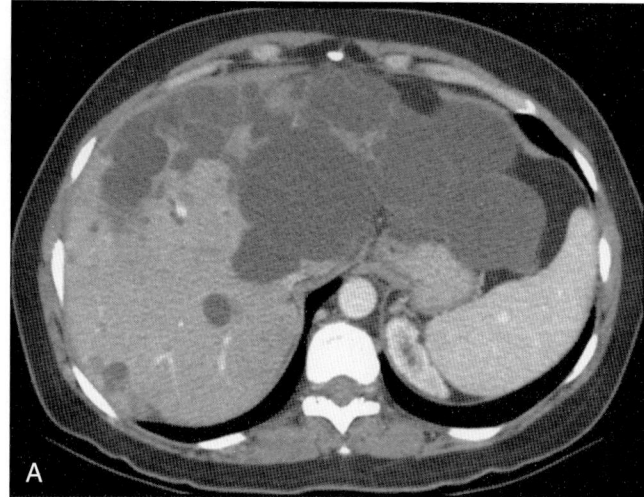

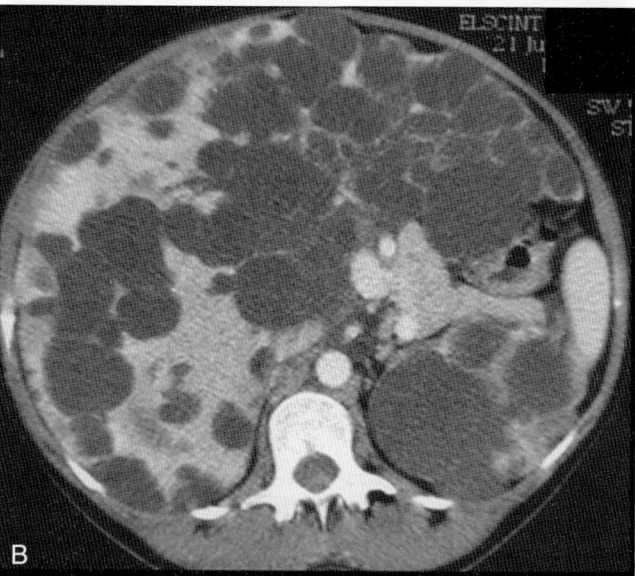

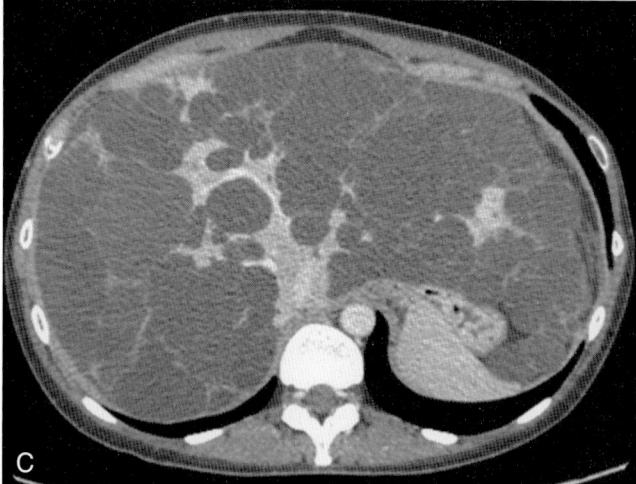

FIGURE 73.13 Representative examples of the heterogeneity of polycystic liver disease. A, Limited extension: There are several large cysts, but large areas of noncystic liver remain. **B,** Intermediate form: Intermediate size cysts are scattered throughout the liver, but some areas of noncystic liver remain. **C,** Severe form: Almost all the liver is replaced by cysts, whereas there is likely vascular injury within the few remnant noncystic areas.

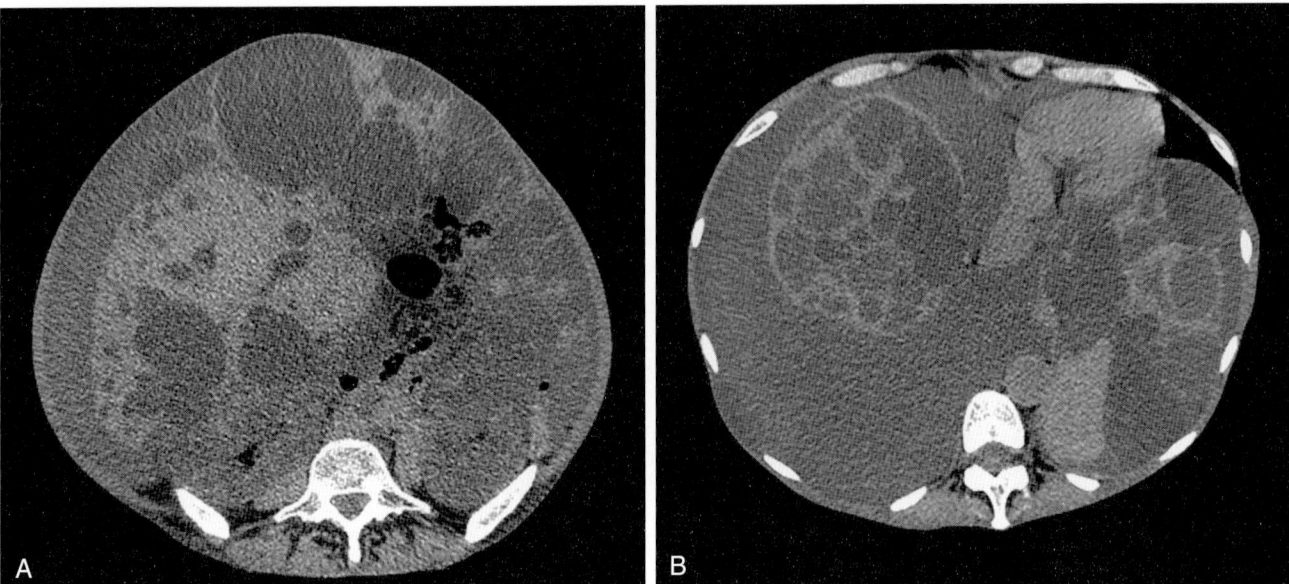

FIGURE 73.14   Two examples of polycystic liver disease associated with malnutrition (note that muscles of the abdominal wall are very thin), ascites **(A)** and pleural effusion **(B)**.

ADPKD; see Chapter 14). Coalescent cysts may give a false image of septation. On CT, the cysts have fluid attenuation values of −5 to +20 Houndsfield units and have distinct margins with the parenchyma. Calcification of the cysts has been reported but is rare.[109,110] Considering the high prevalence of associated ADPKD, injection of contrast agents should be used with extreme caution. The cysts do not show contrast enhancement, and it may be extremely difficult to identify the vascular structures (as well as biliary structures or even normal landmarks of the liver). Similar to simple cysts, uncomplicated cysts of PCLD are very hyperintense on T2-weighted MRI and very hypointense on T1-weighted MRI (see Chapter 14). Cysts complicated by hemorrhage become hyperintense on T1 MRI (see Fig. 73.2). PCLD may be associated with peribiliary cysts that may be difficult to identify but can be suspected when tubular structures run parallel to portal branches, mimicking a biliary dilation (see Fig. 73.12).[111]

In the perspective of treatment, attention should be paid to the following:

- The severity of cystic involvement (see Fig. 73.13). In a small subset of patients, symptoms are not related to the size of the whole liver but to one or two large cysts. These patients should be identified because their management is the same as those with simple cysts but targeted to the large cysts.
- The distribution of the cysts, which is frequently uneven, with some areas relatively spared (in particular segment V or VI), which is the rationale for liver resection.
- Peribiliary cysts or cysts located around the biliary confluence as well as those located in the vicinity of the termination of the hepatic veins. Right hepatic vein compression is frequent and results in an easily identifiable collateral circulation between the right and middle hepatic vein (Fig. 73.15), which can be a source of intraoperative bleeding.

Natural History

In patients with ADPKD, the number and size of the liver cysts are greater in women than in men, increase with patient age, and correlate with the size of the kidney[99] and the severity of kidney dysfunction. Pregnancy, multiparity, and use of female steroid hormones further increase the risk of severe hepatic cystic disease.[98] The natural course is highly variable from one individual to another or within the same family members, but the progression is fairly linear for a given patient. Hence age at the time of diagnosis, first symptoms, incapacitating symptoms, and kidney involvement are useful markers to predict the future need for transplantation. Although the lifespan of patients with ADPKD has lengthened with dialysis and transplantation, liver-related symptoms have become more frequent.

In patients with isolated PCLD, the liver involvement also correlates with female gender and number of pregnancies[106] (Van Keimpema et al., 2010). Apart from kidney symptoms that are absent, the course is the same as that of PCLD associated with ADPKD.[103]

Complications

Within Cysts

Bacterial infection is the most severe complication and, although very rare, can be severe enough to threaten a patient's life.[112,113] Symptoms may include fever, chills, and right upper quadrant pain or less typical symptoms. Cyst infection has mainly been observed in patients with ADPKD under dialysis or in those with immunosuppressive drugs after renal transplantation.[114] It is exceptional, if it exists at all, in patients with isolated PCLD[103,106] (van Keimpema et al., 2010). Differentiating infection within kidney or liver cysts is difficult. The infected cysts can be recognized by US and CT (see Chapters 15 and 18), which show echoic material (corresponding to pus) within the cysts.[113] Thickened irregular cyst wall, hyperdense content, and fluid-fluid or air-fluid levels may also be seen. PET with ^{18}F-fluorodeoxyglucose–labeled leucocytes or ^{111}In-labeled leukocyte scintigraphy may be used to document and localize infection.[115,116] Treatment of infected cysts should

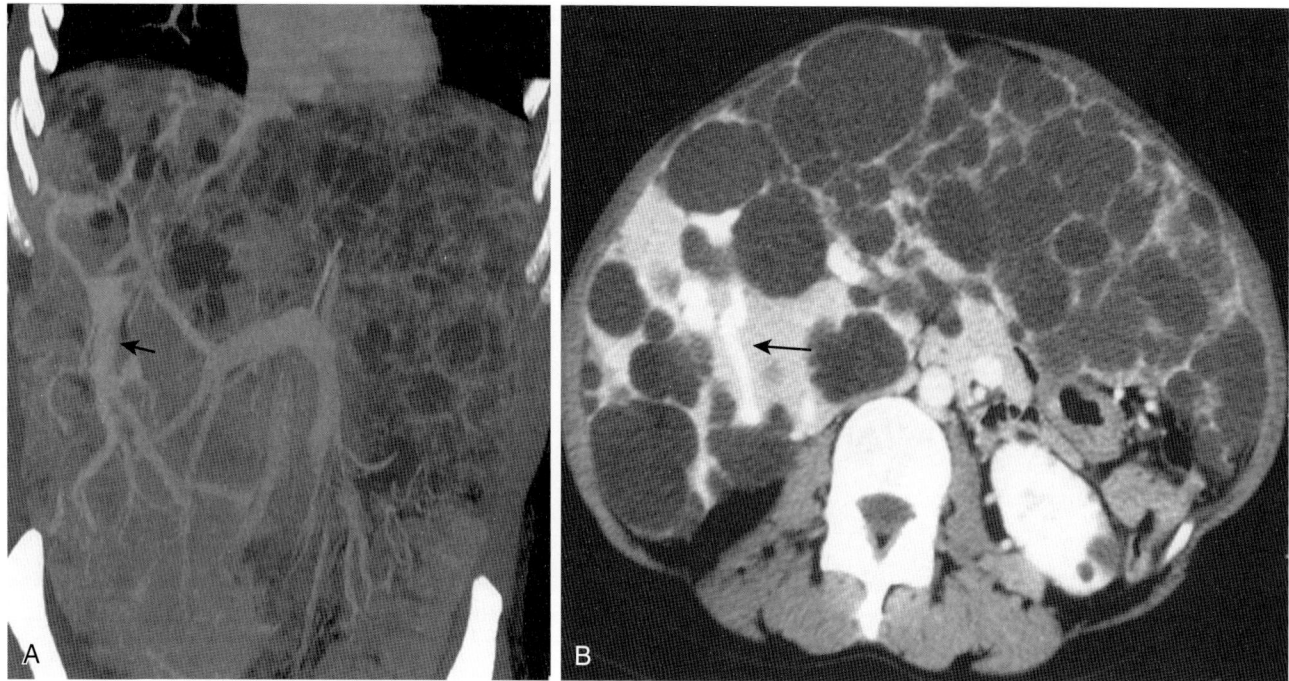

FIGURE 73.15   Polycystic liver disease resulting in compression of hepatic veins. A collateral circulation between the right and middle hepatic vein is visible *(arrow)*. **A,** longitudinal view; **B,** transversal view.

include aspiration/drainage in addition to antibiotics, provided the infected cyst has been identified.[113]

A recent retrospective study has recently suggested that in patients with repetitive cyst infections, decontamination of the digestive tract may reduce recurrence of cyst infections.[117]

Intracystic bleeding is, in contrast, very frequent and may occasionally be mistaken for cyst infection.

Although it has been claimed that malignant transformation could occur, it is still unclear if the hepatic cysts predisposes to the development of cholangiocarcinoma; we believe that it does not.

From Cyst Compression

Cholestasis secondary to compression of the bifurcation by large cysts[118,119] or peribiliary cysts may occur. Jaundice is, in contrast, rare and may result from progressive or acute enlargement of cysts (the latter in case of intracystic bleeding). A mild dilation of the common bile duct is also not unusual.[120]

Portal hypertension with ascites, or even variceal bleeding, as a result of portal or hepatic vein compression has been described.[121–124] Severe forms may also occur in the few patients with ADPKD who have associated congenital hepatic fibrosis or in patients with autosomal recessive PKD in whom, however, liver cysts are rare.

Compression of adjacent organs by the enlarged liver is responsible for most symptoms (see earlier), but less common is the compression of the right atrium that may result in hypotensive episodes[125] or the IVC.

The parenchymal impact of hepatic (or portal) vein compression is frequent. In our experience with liver resection or transplantation, they are present in more than 75% of patients and include centrilobular fibrosis, sinusoidal congestion, peliosis, and nodular regenerative hyperplasia (Fig. 73.16).

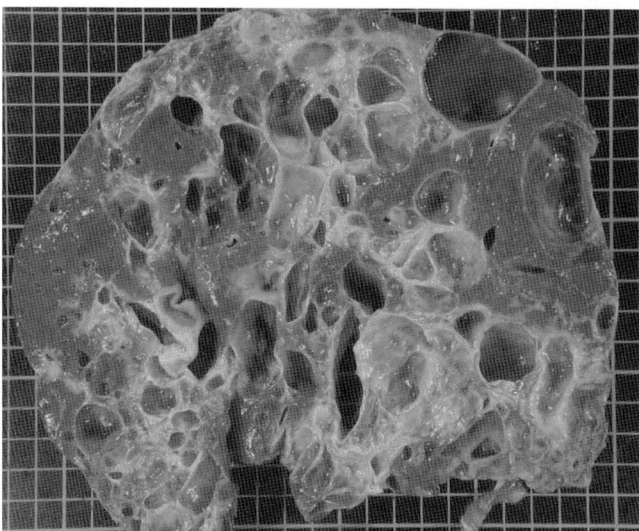

FIGURE 73.16   Macroscopic view of a resected specimen of polycystic liver disease. Because of compression by cysts or inflow/outflow obstruction, microscopic injuries are frequent.

From Associated Conditions

ADPKD is well known for other extrarenal manifestations than the liver. These include, most notably, intracranial aneurysms but also dolichoectasias, thoracic aortic and cervicocephalic artery dissections, and coronary artery aneurysms. These vascular diseases have directly been linked to *PKD1* or *PKD2* mutations in experimental models.[126]

The incidence of cerebral aneurysms is 8%, three to four times higher than in the general population.[127] It has been linked to a mutation in the 5′ region of *PKD1* (rather than the 3′ region), and the main risk factor is therefore a family history of intracerebral aneurysms or subarachnoid hemorrhage (SAH).[128] In this context, the incidence is 16%. Most of these aneurysms are small (<6 mm in diameter) and do not seem to be at increased risk of growth or rupture compared with the general population.[129] Widespread screening is not indicated and should be restricted to individuals with a family history of aneurysm or SAH, previous aneurysm rupture, preparation for major elective surgery, high-risk occupations (such as airline pilots), and patient anxiety despite adequate information.[127] The ideal method is MRI.

Mitral valve prolapse and pericardial effusion are also frequent, found in 25% and 35% of patients with ADPKD, respectively. They are generally well tolerated and do not require therapeutic intervention.[130,131]

Cerebral aneurysms and mitral valve abnormalities have been reported with the same or a slightly lower incidence in patients with isolated PCLD.[103,106]

Staging

Several systems have been proposed to grade the severity of PCLD, and the rationale behind their design is different.

Gigot's classification relies on CT imaging and was designed to identify the indications and limits of fenestration in the treatment of PCLD.[132] The classifications are type I, limited number (<10) of large cysts (>10 cm); type II, diffuse involvement of liver parenchyma by multiple medium-sized cysts, with remaining large areas of noncystic liver parenchyma on preoperative CT; and type III, massive, diffuse involvement of liver parenchyma by small- and medium-sized liver cysts and only a few areas of normal liver parenchyma between cysts. The drawback of this classification is that because the distribution of cysts is uneven, some patients may seem to have either one or the other type, depending on the CT slice.

Qian's classification has been used in the context of familial screening and relies on cyst number and the presence of symptomatic hepatomegaly[106]: grade 0, 0 cysts; grade 1, 1 to 10 cysts; grade 2, 11 to 20 cysts; grade 3, more than 20 cysts; and grade 4, more than 20 cysts and symptomatic hepatomegaly. It has, however, no contribution to the selection of treatments.

Schnelldorfer's classification aims at differentiating patients who could benefit from resection or transplantation. It is apparently more complex but in fact more reliable.[104] It takes into account the presence of symptoms (absent, mild, or severe), the number and size of the cysts, the presence of relative normal areas of liver parenchyma (≥2 sectors, ≥1 sector, or <1 sector), and whether there is an isosectoral portal or hepatic vein occlusion of the preserved sector.

DIFFERENTIATION AMONG SIMPLE CYSTS, ISOLATED PCLD, AND PCLD ASSOCIATED WITH ADPKD

The distinction between isolated PCLD and PCLD associated with ADPKD relies on the number of kidney cysts and a familial history. In adults with a positive family history, the diagnosis of ADPKD is established by radiologic evidence of at least two unilateral or bilateral cysts in persons younger than 30 years, at least two cysts in each kidney in persons 30 to 59 years, and at least four cysts in each kidney in persons 60 years or older.[133] Of note, one-third of patients with isolated PCLD may have a few kidney cysts (usually one or two) (van Keimpema et al., 2010), as does the general population of adult patients,[6] and in the absence of a family history, the diagnosis of ADPKD is retained if more than five kidney cysts in either one or both kidneys are visible on CT.

Unlike ADPKD, there are no clinical guidelines as to what distinguishes PCLD from simple cysts (that are frequently multiple). Surgical series have in the past used a threshold of 5 or 6 cysts, whereas for others, involvement of greater than 50% of the parenchyma was required. These differences should be taken into account when analyzing the results of these series. More recently, in the case of family screenings, it has been proposed that sporadic cases of PCLD are defined by the presence of more than 15 to 20 cysts, whereas when there is a positive familial history, the presence of 4 cysts is sufficient.[103,106]

For neither form of PCLD is genetic testing required or useful in clinical practice, in particular because not all mutations have been identified yet.

Differential Diagnosis for Multiple Cysts

Biliary hamartomas, also known as von Meyenburg complexes, also correspond to an anomalous arrangement of the ductal plate (see Chapter 90A). They are well known by pathologists and surgeons because they are a frequent finding during liver surgery. They may be observed within an otherwise normal liver (6% of the population) but may also be associated with Caroli disease, congenital hepatic fibrosis, and PCLD, in which they are particularly prevalent (virtually constant). Identification of this entity is important because they may be mistaken for liver metastases. As such, these biliary hamartomas are asymptomatic and discovered incidentally. They range in size from 2 to 10 mm and may appear on US as hypoechogenic, hyperechogenic, or heterogeneous, depending on their size, associated biliary dilation, and fibrous stroma.[134] They are hypodense on CT and do not enhance. They are very hypointense on T1-weighted images, very hyperintense on T2-weighted images, and are best seen on MRCP sequences (Fig. 73.17; see Chapter 19).

Caroli disease is addressed in Chapter 46.

Peribiliary cysts arise from cystic enlargement of peribiliary glands located in and around the walls of extrahepatic and large intrahepatic bile ducts. These cysts may have a diameter as large as 2 cm. They are mainly observed in the context of a severe chronic liver disease, including cirrhosis with portal hypertension or PCLD and after liver transplantation. They are usually asymptomatic, but obstructive jaundice has been reported. Imaging features, when known, are easily recognized. On US, the cysts are located along the main bile ducts or within portal tracts beside portal veins. On MRCP, they may mimic an enlarged bile duct, but smaller biliary branches upstream are not dilated. Increase in size and diameter is possible but rare.[135]

Cystic Metastases

They are solid tumors, and their cystic form is rare. The cystic component may be partial or total. Cystic metastases frequently arise from neuroendocrine, sarcomas, melanomas, or, occasionally, bronchial or breast primaries. They can also result from ovarian or pancreatic cystadenocarcinomas. Finally, although very rare, metastases from anal carcinoma are frequently cystic. If the primary tumor is unknown, the presence of peripheral hypervascularization and multiplicity of the lesions should raise the suspicion of this diagnosis. MRI diffusion sequences may also be helpful.

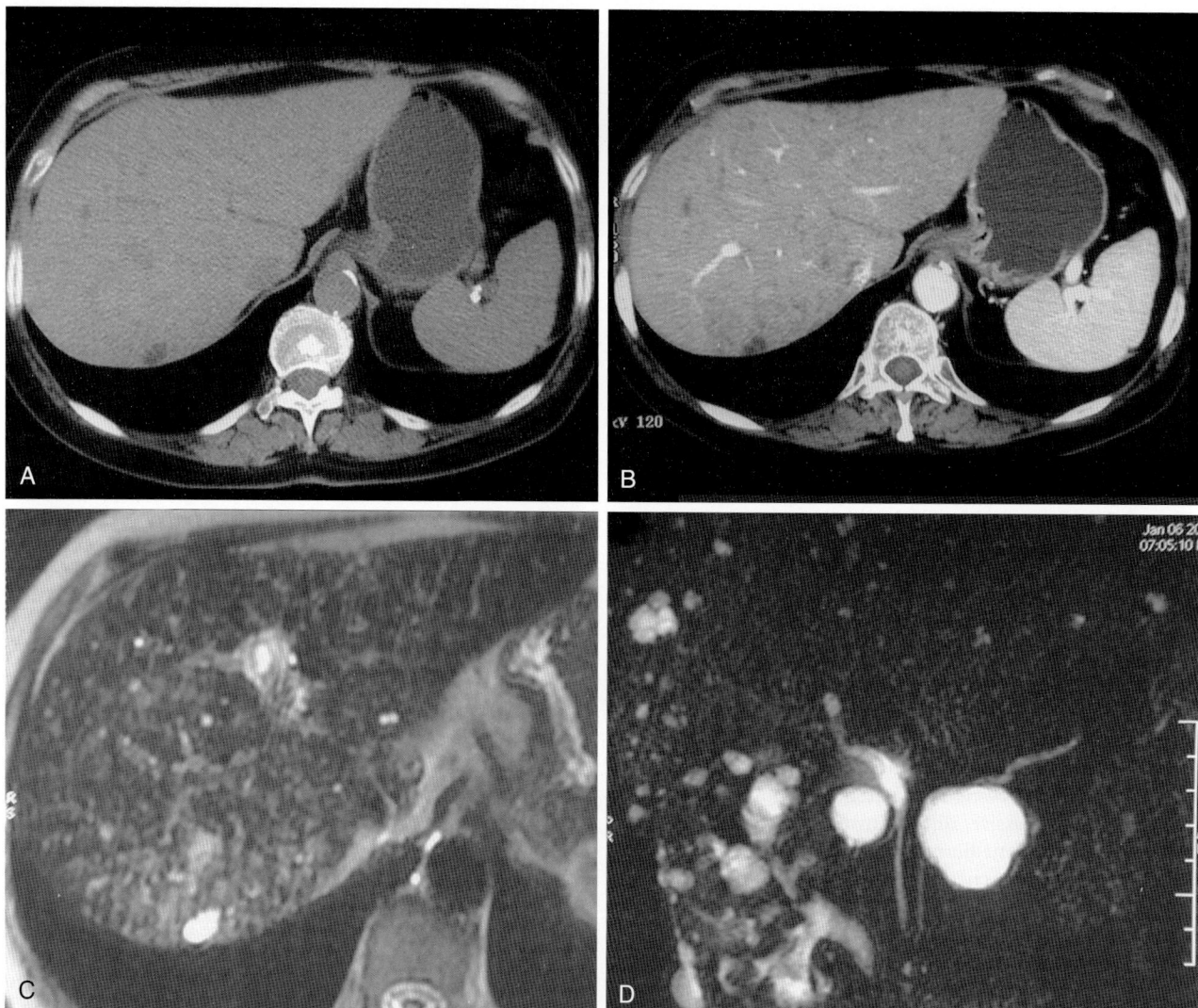

FIGURE 73.17. **Biliary hamartoma.** On computed tomography (CT) scan, hypodense lesions are visible **(A)** that do not enhance after injection **(B)** but become more visible. They are better seen on T2-weighted image **(C)** and on magnetic resonance cholangiopancreatography sequence **(D)**. (See Chapter 14.)

Management

Symptoms in PCLD are associated mainly with the volume of the entire liver rather than with the volume of a specific cyst. Although palliation with percutaneous alcohol sclerotherapy or laparoscopic fenestration has been reported, neither proves effective in the long term in the most frequent forms of PCLD.[136] The aim of treatment is instead to decompress and reduce the size of the entire liver or to remove as many cysts as possible. In highly symptomatic patients, these objectives can be achieved by open fenestration, liver resection, or liver transplantation. Patients should be carefully informed of the limitations and risks of these procedures. Medical alternatives have been recently introduced, although larger studies are required to confirm their clinical impact.

Nonsurgical Treatments

Medical Treatment

Currently, medical treatments available to reduce symptoms related to hepatomegaly and slow down the evolution of renal

insufficiency are somatostatin analogs. There are other potential treatments that can slow down the production of fluid by the cholangiocytes underlying the cysts, including the signaling pathways.[137] For example, there is interest in the inhibition of cholangiocyte autophagy.[138] However, most of these new treatments are still at the animal or development stage and the only approved and effective treatment remains somatostatin analogues.

SOMATOSTATIN ANALOGUES. Cyclic adenosine monophosphate is a potent mediator of cholangiocyte proliferation and secretion of fluid into cysts. Somatostatin receptors are expressed on cholangiocytes; when triggered, this activates a signaling cascade that suppresses cAMP. Somatostatin blunts hepatic cyst expansion by blocking secretin-induced cAMP generation.[139] It also suppresses the expression of IGF-1, VEGF, and other cystogenic growth factors and downstream signaling from their receptors.[140] A recent review of the literature has confirmed the efficacy on hepatic cysts' growth of somatostatin analogues.[141]

Two precursor RCTs have for the first time demonstrated that 6 or 12 months of treatment with lanreotide, a long-acting somatostatin analogue, was associated with a significant reduction of liver volume in patients with PCLD, with or without ADPKD, compared with placebo-treated controls.[142,143] This was especially the case in patients with larger livers; however, this decrease in volume was limited overall, on average 3% to 5%[144,145]; severity of abdominal symptoms was not improved,[143] although some features of QOL scores were. Furthermore, treatment beyond 6 to 12 months provided little, if any, further reduction in total liver volume, and once treatment was stopped, liver volume rebounded toward baseline.[146] Pooled data from RCTs suggest that this treatment should be targeted toward younger women.[147]

In a recent RCT on 175 patients with ADPKD followed for 120 weeks, a group of 93 patients who were treated by lanreotide was compared with a control group of 82 patients who received standard care including blood pressure control, sodium-restricted diet, and hypertensive agents without lanreotide. The treatment with lanreotide for 120 weeks reduced the growth of liver significantly (decreasing by 1.99% in the lanreotide group versus increasing by 3.92% in the control group). Growth was still reduced at 4 months after the last injection of lanreotide.[148]

AVOIDANCE OF ESTROGEN REPLACEMENT THERAPY. Avoidance of ERT would seem logical as a medical treatment for PCLD because hepatic cystic disease may worsen under the influence of hormones of pregnancy or exogenous female steroid hormones.[149] However, proof that avoidance is effective is lacking, and the benefits and drawbacks should be discussed on an individual basis.

MAMMALIAN TARGET OF RAPAMYCIN INHIBITORS. mTOR also regulates secretion and proliferation of biliary and cystic epithelium. Follow-up of transplant recipients with ADPKD whose immunosuppression contained sirolimus has shown that both the native kidney[93] and liver volume[150] decreased compared with those of patients who received the more classic calcineurin inhibitor immunosuppression. The clinical impact of this size reduction was not assessed. Trials have been launched in ADPKD patients to halt the progression of kidney disease with no significant effect on the progression of renal cysts.[151–153] An RCT has failed to demonstrate a benefit of everolimus when added to octreotide.[154] There is therefore currently not enough evidence to support the use of mTOR in PCLD patients.

ARTERIAL EMBOLIZATION. Transcatheter embolization, also known as *renal contraction therapy*, has been advocated in Japan since the mid-1990s for patients with ADPKD,[155] and it has been applied to PCLD since the early 2000s.[156] The rationale is that kidney cysts are supplied by well-developed arteries and that hepatic cysts in ADPKD patients are mostly supplied from hepatic arteries but not from portal veins. Embolization may use microcoils or polyvinyl alcohol particles, ranging in size from 150 to 250 μm, and targets hepatic artery branches supplying the hepatic segments mainly replaced by the cysts[156,157]. Considering the extent of the disease and the number of small-branch arteries to occlude, the procedure is demanding. Initial experience reported a reduction in intrahepatic cyst volume (from 6.667 ± 2.978 cm^3 to 4.625 ± 2.299 cm^3), whereas the volume of hepatic parenchyma increased.[156] These authors'

updated experience showed a 5% reduction in liver volume at 6 months and 9% at 12 months.[158] Improvement of symptoms was observed in most patients but required several months to be optimal. No major complications were reported except for classic but occasionally severe postembolization syndrome.[156–159] Because targeted segments are those that also have an occluded portal flow, it is possible that the procedure acts as a hepatectomy, favoring regeneration of noncystic parenchyma.

Series of arterial embolization predominantly come from Japan; experience with this technique appears very limited elsewhere, and prospective RCTs are lacking.

Cyst-Targeted Treatments

As a rule, percutaneous sclerotherapy and laparoscopic fenestration are futile in highly symptomatic patients with massive, diffuse involvement of the liver. However, some patients may have one to five large cysts coexisting with a varying number of very small cysts. In these patients, symptoms are related only to the large cysts, which should be treated individually, as if they are a single cyst.[48] The small cysts, which are often located deep in the liver, should not be treated.

PERCUTANEOUS SCLEROTHERAPY. Percutaneous sclerotherapy is usually considered ineffective in patients with PCLD because symptoms are related to the multiplicity of the cysts, which cannot all be targeted. Furthermore, the rigid architecture of the parenchyma, as well as the presence of smaller adjacent cysts, prevents cyst collapse. Symptomatic recurrence requiring additional treatment occurs in most patients[65]; however, a small subset of patients have one or a few strategically located large cysts (>6 cm) that may account for at least part of the symptoms and can be managed as simple cysts. The technique and results do not differ from those for simple cysts. Cyst resolution is gradual and may only be optimum within 1 year of therapy.

Fenestration
Technique and Indication

Initially described by Lin and colleagues,[160] the aim of fenestration is to unroof as many cysts as possible, starting with superficial cysts and proceeding stepwise to the deeper cysts. Open fenestration was historically the standard therapy, but a laparoscopic approach has also been used recently; with few exceptions, this does not allow sufficient and safe access to the deeper cysts and, as a rule, a laparoscopic approach is contraindicated.[62,161] The exceptions are patients with a limited number of large and superficial cysts that can be individually treated as single cysts (Fig. 73.18).

In a recent meta-analysis and systematic review,[124] the authors compared the results of laparoscopic fenestration for simple cysts and for PCLD: patients with PCLD were more likely to have symptomatic recurrence and reintervention (33.7% vs. 9.6% and 26.4% vs. 7.1%, respectively). Complications were also more frequent in PCLD patients (29.3% vs. 10.8%). So we think that fenestration should be reserved for simple cysts and is not the best approach for PCLD.

Complications

The main intraoperative hazard is inadvertent injury of vascular structures that are compressed at the periphery of the cysts. What looks like a simple membrane between two cysts may, in

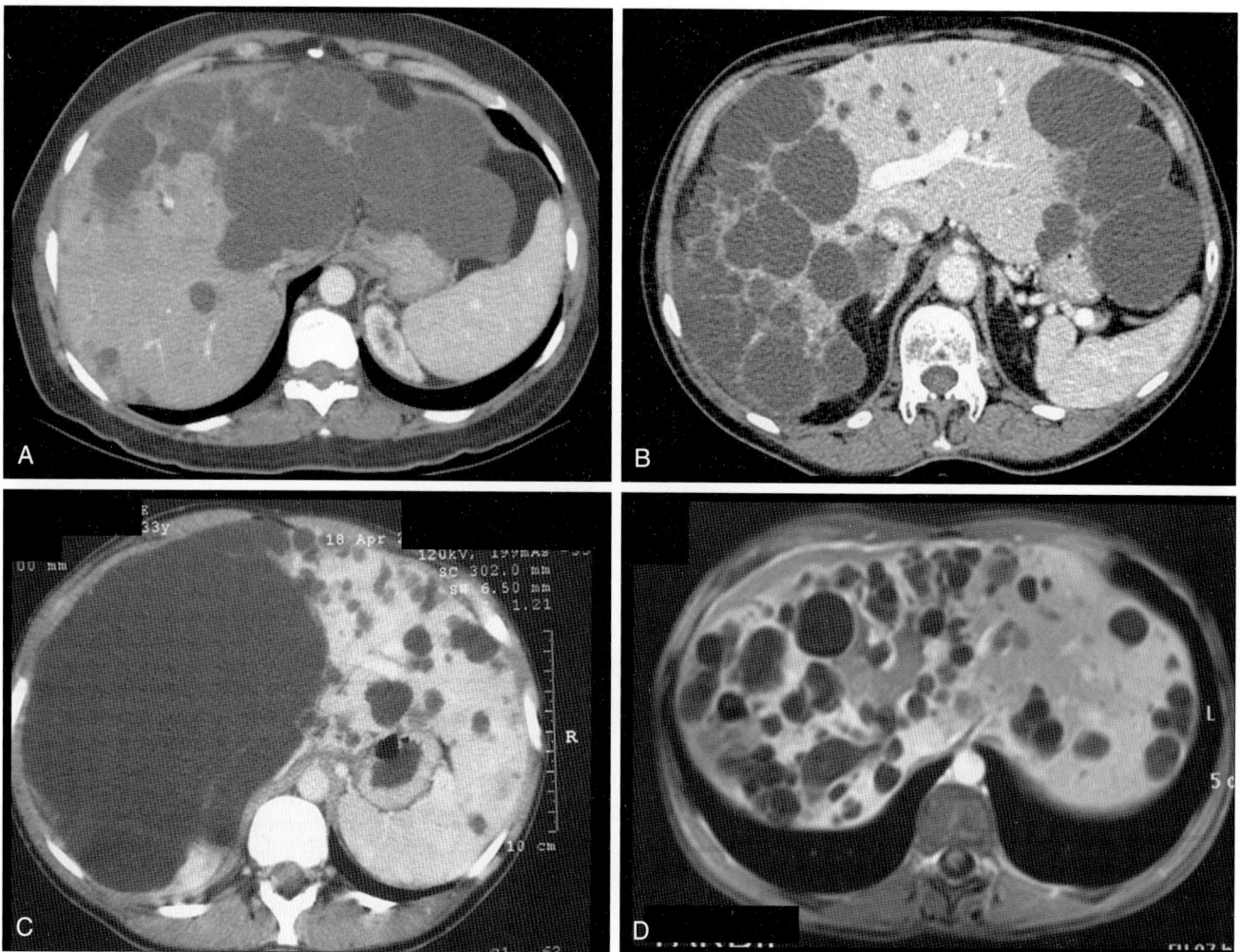

FIGURE 73.18   **Examples of patients with polycystic liver disease but with limited cyst involvement, in whom laparoscopic fenestration of the cysts could be considered. A,** Cysts are mainly located in the left lateral section. **B,** Fenestration of the cysts in the left lateral section is likely to be effective, whereas fenestration of those in the right liver is not because the cysts are small and deeply located. **C** and **D,** The same patient before and after fenestration of a large cyst in the right liver. Note that the large cysts collapse, small cysts remain, and the obstruction of the termination of the hepatic vein persists, which can account for some persisting symptoms of congestion.

fact, be a large hepatic vein; therefore it may be wise to puncture it with a fine needle before widely opening it. Hemorrhage from hepatic vein injury can be massive in patients with PCLD because the termination of the hepatic vein is frequently compressed by cysts, resulting in outflow obstruction. Biliary injury may also occur when cysts located around the biliary confluence are approached. As for hepatic veins, the biliary confluence may be compressed between adjacent cysts, thus becoming unrecognizable. Most complications occur when deeper, localized cysts are treated.

Fenestration for PCLD is associated with a higher incidence of postoperative biliary leak compared with fenestration for simple cysts. This occurs particularly when cysts are left untreated around the biliary confluence (Fig. 73.19). Performing intraoperative cholangiography to ensure that biliary drainage of both hemilivers is normal at the end of the procedure is advisable.

Postoperative ascites is also a frequent complication. It may result in delayed wound healing or in ascites superinfection. The mechanism is probably multifactorial and includes persistent secretion by the epithelial lining, relative outflow obstruction

when cysts around the termination of the hepatic veins are not unroofed, or impaired kidney function.

Mortality, although at low rates, has been reported, and morbidity averages 31% (Table 73.1).

Outcome

The incidence of symptomatic recurrence overall is 35% (see Table 73.1). Results are largely influenced by morphologic aspects of the disease.

Treatment of Intracystic Complications

In the case of intracystic bleeding, only symptomatic treatment of pain is required. Patients who are treated by anticoagulation should be hospitalized and monitored, because it is in this setting that severe complications have been described. If pain persists after 3 months, sclerotherapy of the hemorrhagic cyst may be considered.

In the case of cyst infection, the prolonged use of antibiotics may not be completely useful. Often, a prolonged drainage of the infected cyst is required and, in case of failure, surgical

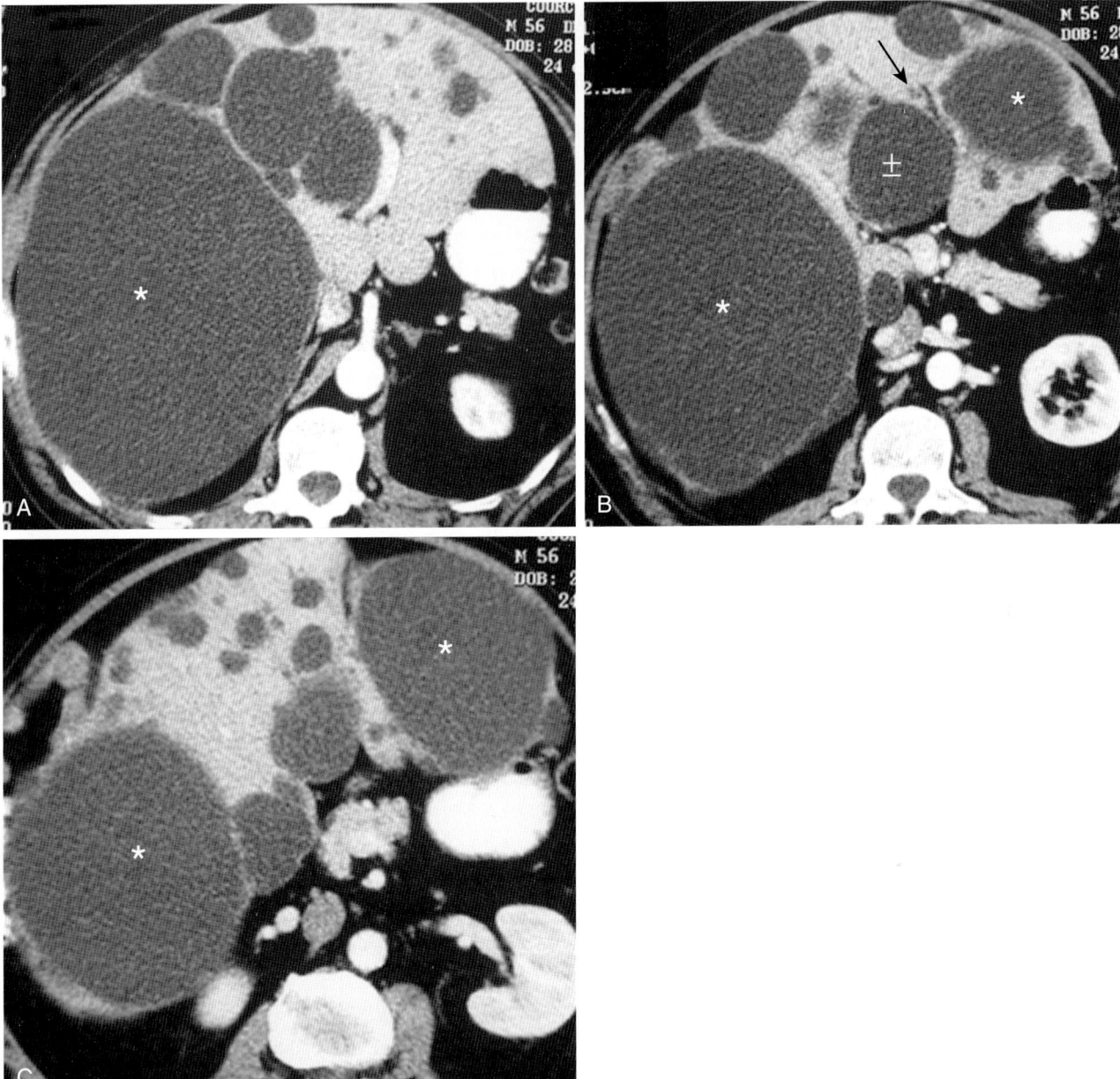

FIGURE 73.19   A–C, preoperative imaging in a patient who underwent laparoscopic fenestration of multiple cysts, resulting in a postoperative biliary leak. The two fenestrated cysts are marked by an asterisk. Note the small enlarged bile duct *(arrow)* upstream of a cyst close to the biliary confluence (±). The patient was reoperated by open surgery to close the leak and unroof the central cyst (±).

treatment consisting of fenestration of the cyst by laparoscopy or laparotomy.

Hepatectomy

Partial liver resection has been proposed, in combination with fenestration of the remnant liver, to reduce liver volume and increase regeneration of the noncystic liver[174] (see Chapter 101). This is made possible by the frequently asymmetric distribution of the cysts, with some areas being relatively spared (Fig. 73.20). Regeneration is associated with expansion of these areas, whereas the volume of the remaining small cysts remains unchanged or progresses very slowly. Although this technique is highly successful in some patients, it is technically demanding, associated with a high morbidity rate, and its indications are

becoming more selective and restrictive. This technique is efficient only if the quantity of resected liver is sufficient and exceeds three segments. In our experience, a left lateral sectionectomy is associated with a high rate of symptomatic recurrence.

Technique

The site and extent of resection are dictated by the location of the cysts, and surgery aims at removing as much cystic liver as possible. Care should be taken, however, to leave a sufficient amount of functional remnant liver (see Chapters 101 and 102). In particular, evidence of congestion related to outflow obstruction should be ruled out. This can be done on imaging by carefully analyzing the termination of the hepatic veins after reconstruction

TABLE 73.1 Treatment of PCLD by Fenestration in Clinical Series

REFERENCE, YEAR	NO. PATIENTS (OPEN/LAPAROSCOPIC)	DEATHS (n)	MORBIDITY (n)	RECURRENT SYMPTOMS (n)	FOLLOW-UP
Van Erpecum et al., 1987[162]	9 (9/0)	1	0	1	<12 mo
Turnage et al., 1988[163]	5 (5/0)	1	1	2	10 mo
Sanchez et al., 1991[164]	7 (7/0)	0	NA	4	18 mo
Farges & Bismuth, 1995[165]	13 (13/0)	0	9	3	84 mo
Morino et al., 1994[62]	9 (9/0)	0	4	4	NA
Kabbej et al., 1996[161]	13 (0/13)	0	6	10	26 mo
Gigot et al., 1997[132]	10 (8/2)	0	6	2	71 mo
Koperna et al., 1997[166]	39 (34/5)	0	NA	7	75 mo
Martin et al., 1998[167]	13 (6/7)	0	4	7	37 mo
Marks et al., 1998[168]	7 (0/7)	0	4	0	NA
Katkhouda et al., 1999[169]	8 (0/8)	0	3	1	NA
Hansman et al., 2001[61]	2 (2/0)	0	0	2	NA
Fiamingo et al., 2003[170]	6 (0/6)	0	3	1	34 mo
Robinson et al., 2005[136]	11 (0/11)	0	2	6	41 mo
Konstadoulakis et al., 2005[171]	9 (0/9)	1	0	2	26 mo
Barahona-Garrido et al., 2008[172]	16 (12/4)	0	4	3	68 mo
Erdogan et al., 2007[65]	4 (2/2)	0	2	3	15 mo
Van Keimpema, et al., 2008[173]	12 (0/12)	0	3	1	18 mo
Gall et al., 2009[60]	24 (11/13)	0	8	17	77 mo
Loehe et al., 2010[59]	22 (6/16)	0	5	—	76 mo
Schnelldorfer et al., 2009[104]	10 (8/2)	0	0	—	96 mo
Kamphues et al., 2011[55]	31 (0/31)	0	0	13	49 mo
Bernts et al., 2019[56]	146 (0/146)	0	43	48	30 mo
TOTAL	426	3	107 (25%)	137 (32%)	

NA, Not available; *PCLD*, polycystic liver disease.

and looking for a collateral circulation between hepatic veins, usually running close to the liver surface. A biopsy may also be useful, although the interpretation of results is not standardized.

The liver resection is most often a left hepatectomy or a right hepatectomy. In case of left-sided resections, an associated segment I resection may be considered if this segment is also involved with cysts. The main hazard is injury of the hepatic vein or of the biliary confluence, a danger compounded by the fact that the usual landmarks are displaced by the cysts and are hardly recognizable. Intraoperative US is of little help because vascular and biliary structures are compressed, and the presence of cysts interferes with visualization. Extensive fenestration of the larger cysts is performed first to decompress the liver, gain access to its dome, and mobilize the right or left triangular ligaments. Transection is performed either in the noncystic parenchyma or proceeding stepwise between the cystic cavities. When approaching the biliary confluence, the surgeon should always bear in mind that glissonian pedicles are compressed between the cysts and that no cyst wall should be cut before the surgeon is sure that this is not the case. An intraoperative cholangiography may prove useful. The same holds true for the hepatic veins close to their termination.

After hepatectomy, the remnant liver is widely fenestrated (see Fig. 73.20). Intraoperative cholangiography may be advisable to ensure that no bile duct injury has occurred and that bile drains freely (i.e., that a deeply situated cyst does not compress the remnant right or left duct). Considering the high rate of biliary leak, a leakage test should also be performed; it is also

wise to place running sutures along the transected cyst walls. After right-sided resections, care should be taken to secure the remnant liver in a stable position, resulting in adequate venous outflow. A suction drain is frequently left in the abdomen.

Morbidity and Mortality

Hepatectomy for PCLD, although a benign disease, is a demanding procedure with a definite risk of mortality and high morbidity rates, even when performed by highly experienced hepatopancreatobiliary surgeons. The main intraoperative risk is bleeding, and perioperative transfusions are required in 50% to 80% of patients. Injury to the main bile ducts within the liver remnant occurs in 5%.[104,175]

Mortality rates in the literature average 4% (Table 73.2) and have been related to abdominal sepsis, acute Budd-Chiari syndrome, and complications related to treatment of complications. Intracranial hemorrhage from ruptured aneurysms has also been described.

Morbidity rates average 64% (see Table 73.2), but some consider that it is virtually constant. The most frequent complications are ascites and pleural effusion, and the mechanism is likely the same as for fenestration: persistent fluid secretion by the remnant epithelial lining and relative outflow obstruction. However, increased portal pressure and lymphatic leakage associated with liver resection increase this risk. Furthermore, patients undergoing liver resection, rather than fenestration, tend to have more severe PCLD with malnutrition. Although ascites resolves in most patients within 1 month, some have

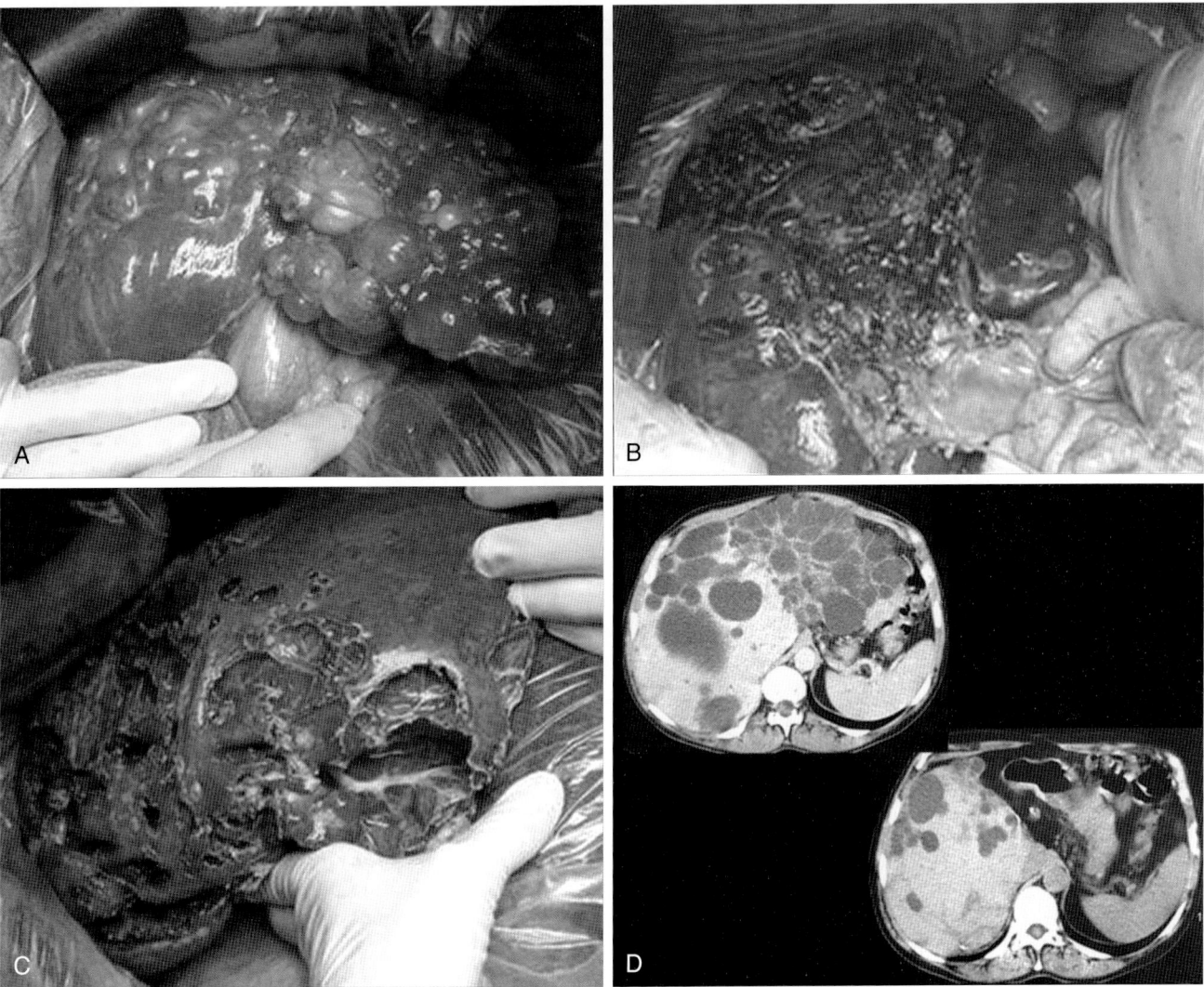

FIGURE 73.20   Principle of liver resection for polycystic liver disease. A, The liver is massively enlarged, but some areas of noncystic liver remain. **B,** An extended left hepatectomy is performed. **C,** The remaining right liver is widely fenestrated. **D,** Preoperative and postoperative computed tomographic scan shows an expansion of the noncystic liver.

required stenting of the IVC or hepatic veins to resolve outflow obstruction.[104,185] The next most frequent complications are hemorrhage and biliary leak; approximately 10% of patients require reoperation for management of these. In contrast, liver failure is infrequent unless a major vascular structure has been inadvertently injured. Hepatectomy is usually not performed in patients with severe kidney failure. In those with moderate impairment, although a slight transient deterioration of kidney function may be observed, most patients have recovered their preoperative creatinine levels by the time of discharge. Prolonged fever with no obvious cause is observed in 10% of patients (see Chapter 28).

Preoperative risk factors for complications include kidney dysfunction, ascites, denutrition, and parenchymal changes with venous collaterality because of hepatic vein outflow obstruction.[104,186,187] The vascular compressions cause venous congestion in the remnant liver to be preserved and can contraindicate the partial resection. In the presence of these symptoms, liver transplantation may be required (see Chapters 26–28).

Long-Term Outcome

Results are highly variable among series and among patients. This reflects the diversity of the clinical and morphologic situations and the extent of resection. The average reduction in hepatic volume achieved ranges between 50% and 75%,[104,175] which results in considerable objective and subjective improvement in greater than 75% of the patients (Fig. 73.21). In a retrospective study[188] of 186 patients, postoperative liver volume was reduced by an average of 61% with an important complications rate of 21% and a mortality rate of 2.7%; however, they showed a sustained response in the improvement of the symptoms. A recent study of 18 patients who underwent fenestration and partial hepatectomy showed improvement of the symptoms 6 months after surgery and QOL with a significant decreased volume of the liver (50%).[117] In this study, the follow-up was too short but the results in term of symptoms were in favor of the partial resection.

Our updated experience (unpublished yet) of 74 partial hepatectomies confirms that partial hepatectomy is safe and efficient mainly in Gigot II PCLD and provided the resected volume

TABLE 73.2 Treatment of PCLD by Combined Resection and Fenestration

REFERENCE, YEAR	NO. PATIENTS	MORTALITY	MORBIDITY	RECURRENT SYMPTOMS	FOLLOW-UP
Turnage et al., 1988[163]	3	2 (67%)	2 (67%)	33%	10 mo
Vauthey et al., 1991[176]	5	0	5 (100%)	0	14 mo
Newman et al., 1990[a,177]	9	1	5	1	17 mo
Henne-Bruns et al., 1993[178]	8	0	3 (38%)	50%	15 mo
Madariaga et al., 1993[179]	2	0	NA	0	>96 mo
Que et al., 1995[a,174]	31	1 (3%)	15 (48%)	3%	28 mo
Soravia et al., 1995[180]	10	1 (10%)	2 (20%)	33%	68 mo
Koperna et al., 1997[166]	5	0	NA	0	—
Martin et al., 1998[167]	9	0	6	0	NA
Vons et al., 1998[181]	12	1 (8%)	10 (83%)	2	34 mo
Hansman et al., 2001[61]	2	0	0	0	NA
Yang et al., 2004[182]	7	0	7 (100 %)	0%	20 mo
Li et al., 2008[183]	21	0	16 (76%)	14%	61 mo
Schnelldorfer et al., 2009[*,104]	124	4 (3%)	78 (63%)	—	96 mo
Aussilhou et al., 2010[175]	45	2 (4%)	32 (71%)	30%	41 mo
Bernts et al., 2020[184]	18	0	2 (11%)	5.5%	6 mo
TOTAL	253	10 (4%)	161 (64%)		

[a]Studies held at the same institution.
NA, Not available; *PCLD*, polycystic liver disease.

exceeds 50% of the total liver volume. The improvement in QOL is sustained until at least 5 years after resection.[175]

Symptoms may recur because of the enlargement of some cysts that were left untreated, and such patients may benefit from targeted treatments, sclerotherapy in particular. In addition, other recurrences are related to the progressive reexpansion of the entire liver. It has recently been estimated that after 4 years of follow-up, the liver was on average 11% larger than the initial remnant volume after resection.[104] However, half of the patients have stable volumes, a difference that may also reflect the variable natural history of the disease.

There is very preliminary evidence that laparoscopic partial liver resection is an option with resected volume of parenchyma and efficacy on symptoms equivalent to those achieved by laparotomy.[189]

Transplantation

Because PCLD is a genetic disease, liver transplantation is the only curative treatment (see Chapters 105 and 125). As for any benign disease, there is some reluctance to perform this high-risk procedure for this indication, considering that liver function is preserved (see Chapter 111). Nevertheless, some patients with massive liver involvement have incapacitating symptoms that may be life threatening (ascites, denutrition); in this situation, and when liver resection is considered too high risk with little anticipated efficacy, liver transplantation is the only option (Fig. 73.22). QOL is excellent after transplantation despite the need for long-term immunosuppression.

In countries where graft allocation is patient oriented, based on the Model for End-Stage Liver Disease criteria, exceptions have been implemented because patients with PCLD who do not have liver failure would otherwise have no chance to undergo transplantation.[190]

Technique

Most transplantations have been performed with livers from brain-dead donors, although living donors have also been used.[191] The technique is the same as that for other indications, but, as for hepatectomy, extensive fenestration is required first to gain access to the liver. The IVC can be preserved, which is important in the context of living donation, but transient clamping may be necessary to achieve this. A transient portocaval shunt is required in most instances because PCLD does not induce portal hypertension with spontaneous portosystemic shunts. Liver transplantation for PCLD is more demanding than for other indications because the hepatic pedicle is stretched and because of compressive adhesions of the cysts and the IVC. Total liver exclusion may be required during removal of segment I (see Chapters 109, 121, and 125).

To avoid massive hemorrhagic procedure during total hepatectomy, an exposure left lateral sectionectomy may be helpful because it facilitates total hepatectomy with vena cava preservation.

In patients with ADPKD, simultaneous kidney transplantation is most often indicated in case of renal insufficiency[66] except if renal insufficiency is slight and stable, in which case single-liver transplantation appears safe, provided renal-sparing immunosuppression is used. Secondary kidney transplantation may be required in half of the patients, with the drawback of a lack of immune protection against rejection, unlike what is observed when the liver and kidney are transplanted from the same donor.[192–194] However, it seems better to perform combined transplantation to avoid two surgical interventions and to emphasize preemptive kidney transplantation.[195]

Perioperative Risk

Liver transplant for PCLD is particularly demanding in patients who have undergone previous procedures, in particular open surgery. Virtually all patients require an intraoperative transfusion. The reported mortality rate is 14% overall (Table 73.3) and is higher than for other elective indications.[196] It is mainly related to sepsis. As for other indications of transplantation, perioperative mortality and morbidity, in particular from sepsis, are increased in patients with the most severe forms of the disease (see Chapter 120). Such severe forms are usually associated with malnutrition.[193,197] A previous

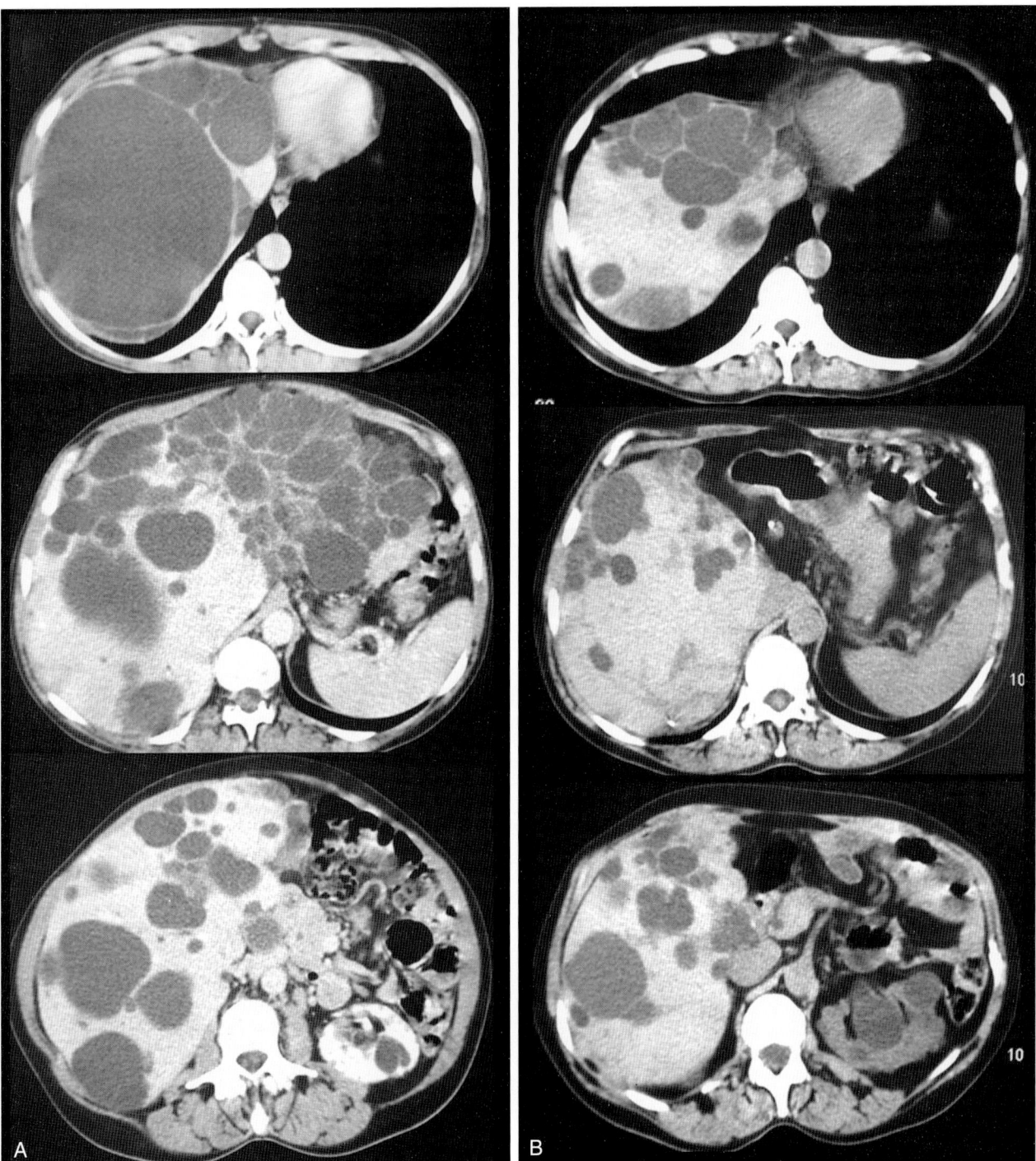

FIGURE 73.21 **Computed tomographic scan in a patient who had undergone left hepatectomy and fenestration of the right liver for polycystic liver disease. A,** Preoperative view. **B,** View 24 months after surgery.

history of fenestration or resection increases the postoperative mortality and morbidity.[198] Therefore, when transplantation will likely be indicated at some stage of the disease, fenestration and resection should be considered with caution.

Long-Term Outcome

The 5-year survival rate in the registries is 80% to 84%, higher than for most other indications. Survival rates at 5 years as high as 92.3% have been reported,[209] although most recent figures remain at 85%.[210]

QOL is excellent.[206] The short-term prognosis is the same as for liver transplantation for other indications.[211] Short- and long-term results are the same for liver transplantation and for combined transplantation of liver and kidney.

CONCLUSION

Treatment is only indicated when symptoms related to cysts are present. Single large cysts can be equally treated by sclerotherapy or laparoscopic fenestration. In patients with symptoms

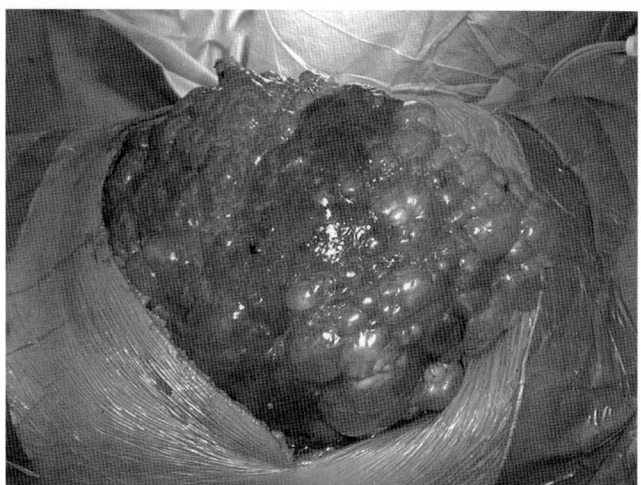

FIGURE 73.22 Intraoperative view of a patient undergoing liver transplantation for polycystic liver disease. Note that the liver is massively enlarged, and there is hardly any spared area of noncystic liver.

TABLE 73.3 Liver Transplantation With or Without Kidney Transplantation for Highly Symptomatic PCLD in the Literature and Reported Deaths

REFERENCE, YEAR	NO. PATIENTS	LT	LT + KT	DEATHS
Starzl et al., 1990[199]	4	2	2	1
Uddin et al., 1995[200]	3	3	0	1
Klupp et al., 1996[201]	10	5	5	1
Washburn et al., 1996[202]	5	4	1	1
Lang et al., 1997[197]	17	9	8	5
Swenson et al., 1998[203]	9	6	3	1
Jeyarajah et al., 1998[192]	6	3	3	2
Pirenne et al., 2001[193]	16	15	1	2
Becker et al., 2003[204]	17	0	17	3
Gustafsson et al., 2003[205]	7	4	3	0
Kirchner et al., 2006[206]	36	21	15	5
Ueno et al., 2006[194]	14	9	5	1
Krohn et al., 2008[207]	14	11	3	1
Taner et al., 2009[196]	13	6	7	3
Schnelldorfer et al., 2009[104]	7	4	3	2
Aussilhou et al., 2010[175]	27	4	23	4
Le Roy et al., 2019[208]	15	4	11	0
TOTAL	220	11	110	33 (15%)

KT, Kidney transplantation; *LT,* liver transplantation; *PCLD,* polycystic liver disease.

related to a limited number of large cysts, fenestration is the treatment of choice (Fig. 73.23). In PCLD patients whose symptoms cannot be linked to one or a few large cysts, treatment may range from observation to transplantation, depending on the severity of symptoms and whether areas of noncystic parenchyma can be preserved. Liver resection and, to some extent, fenestration should be avoided if liver transplantation is anticipated, considering the likelihood of cyst progression and the added complexity of the liver transplant procedure, if prior cyst fenestration or resection has been performed.

References are available at expertconsult.com.

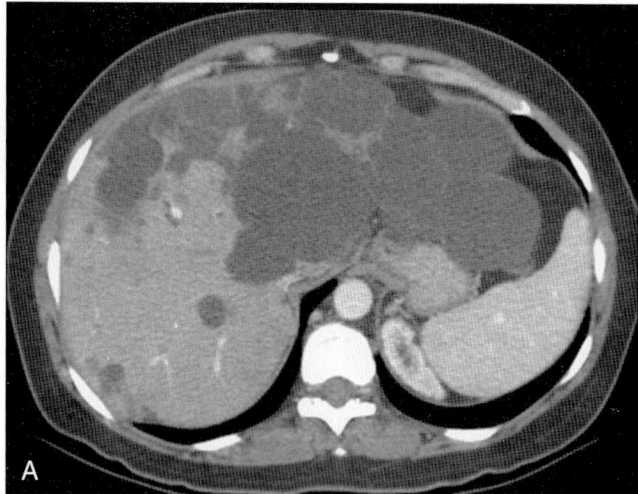

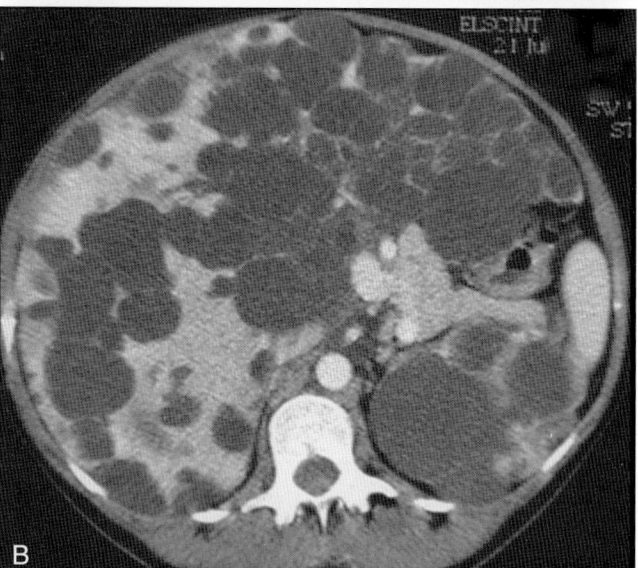

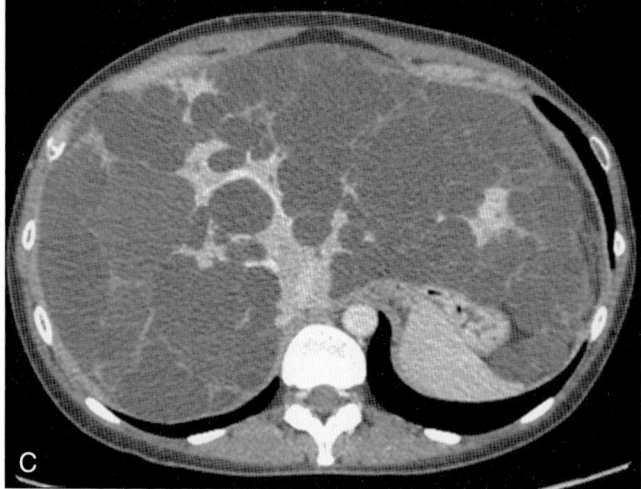

FIGURE 73.23 Treatment according to severity of polycystic liver disease. A, A mild form can be treated by laparoscopic fenestration or hepatectomy. **B,** A moderate form in which fenestration is unlikely to be effective; left hepatectomy can be considered because the future remnant liver is large and has normal inflow and outflow. **C,** A severe form requiring liver transplantation.

SECTION I. Inflammatory, Infective, and Congenital

D. Hepatic Cirrhosis, Portal Hypertension, and Hepatic Failure

CHAPTER 74

Cirrhosis and portal hypertension: Pathologic aspects

Elizabeth M. Brunt and Danielle H. Carpenter

OVERVIEW

Cirrhosis, the final stage of untreated chronic liver disease (see Chapter 7), is primarily attributable to alcohol abuse, viral hepatitis C (see Chapter 68), and, increasingly, nonalcoholic steatohepatitis (NASH; see Chapter 69) in the United States (US).[1] The true prevalence of cirrhosis is unknown because in early, developing stages, the condition may be asymptomatic. Nevertheless, cirrhosis is the 11th most common cause of death in adults in the US and accounts for up to 41,743 deaths per year in adults.[2]

In autopsy series, cirrhosis is documented in 5% to 10% of cases, but autopsy subjects may not be representative of the general population.[3] Currently, clinicians[4] and pathologists alike[5] consider cirrhosis as a *process* with many stages, rather than a single entity; in this conceptual framework, only the final end stage requires transplant as definitive treatment, whereas the preceding stages can be managed with more aggressive preventative medical therapies.[6]

The cirrhotic liver functions markedly less efficiently than normal liver, but it is the aberration of the portal blood flow with resultant portal hypertension that causes the most significant complications of cirrhosis.[6] In addition, cirrhosis itself is a major predisposing condition to hepatocellular carcinoma (HCC; see Chapter 89) and is increasingly recognized as a predisposing condition for intrahepatic cholangiocarcinoma (iCCA; see Chapter 50) and other primary liver carcinomas of mixed hepatocellular-biliary phenotypes. This predisposition to malignancy is likely because of the inflammatory microenvironment, as well as the recognized plasticity of cell types within the liver.[7] However, the cirrhotic liver is considered to be resistant to metastases from extrahepatic tumors.

Interestingly, portal hypertension may occur in the absence of significant matrix deposition and the structural alterations of cirrhosis, a condition referred to as *noncirrhotic portal hypertension* (see Chapter 74). The underlying conditions associated with noncirrhotic portal hypertension may be idiopathic but are broadly subdivided into *prehepatic, intrahepatic,* or *posthepatic* in terms of clinical presentation and for management considerations. This chapter focuses on the histopathologic features of cirrhosis and noncirrhotic portal hypertension.

PATHOGENESIS AND REVERSIBILITY OF CIRRHOSIS

The transformation of normal hepatic architecture through fibrosis (aberrant matrix deposition) to cirrhosis results from progressive deposition of mixed connective tissue in regions of "extinct" parenchyma, angiogenesis, and vascular remodeling, regardless of the underlying etiology. Fibrogenesis is a dynamic, complex, and highly regulated process, triggered by liver parenchymal injury and mediated by the interplay of cellular necrosis and apoptosis on one hand (see Chapter 7) and inflammatory cascades that include immune cells (see Chapter 10), cytokines, and chemokines (see Chapter 11) on the other hand, which result in activation of specific matrix-producing cells.[8,9] These cells are resident hepatic stellate cells and portal myofibroblasts. During fibrogenesis, prevention of matrix degradation by metalloproteinases is orchestrated by the release of potent tissue metalloproteinase inhibitors; apoptosis of fibrogenic hepatic stellate cells is also inhibited (Figs. 74.1 and 74.2). Scar formation is the consequence of an imbalance favoring collagen synthesis and deposition versus degradation and resorption (see Chapter 7). In addition, basement membrane components and connective tissue formed by activated hepatic stellate cells along the hepatic plates results in "capillarization" of the sinusoids, a process that virtually excludes the exchange of molecules (such as albumin and clotting proteins) between hepatocytes and sinusoidal blood. Sinusoidal endothelial fenestrations are closed in capillarization.

Established cirrhosis, traditionally considered an irreversible process, has been shown otherwise from accumulating evidence by pathologists[10] from treatment trials with pretreatment and posttreatment biopsies for viral hepatitis B (HBV), C (HCV), and hereditary hemochromatosis. A study by Poynard and colleagues (2002)[11] that analyzed 3010 patients with chronic HCV in four major clinical trials found reversal of cirrhosis reported in 75 (49%) of 153 patients with baseline cirrhosis. Although Pol et al. (2004)[12] showed reversal of cirrhosis in 7.8% of 64 immunocompetent patients with HCV-related cirrhosis at 4.6-year mean interval, resolution of cirrhosis was shown in 2 patients upon examination of the liver explants at transplantation. Similarly in HBV, Sun and colleagues (2017)[13]

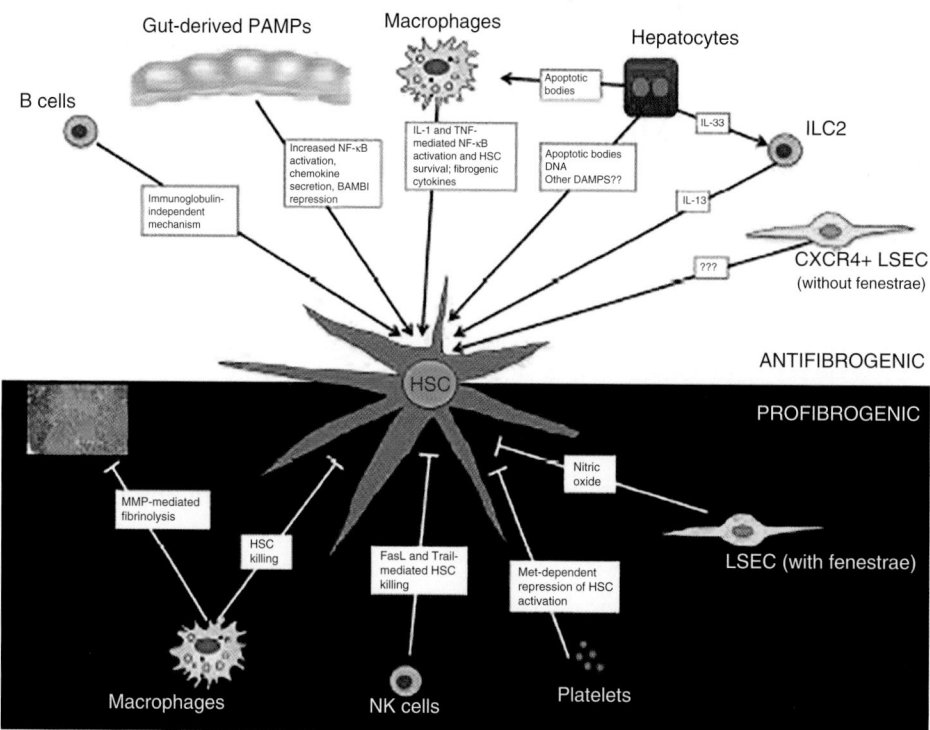

FIGURE 74.1 **Fibrogenesis.** This figure highlights the cell-cell interactions of matrix production and resolution. (From Seki E, Schwabe RF. Hepatic inflammation and fibrosis: Functional links and key pathways. *Hepatology.* 2015;61:1066–1079; see Chapter 7.)

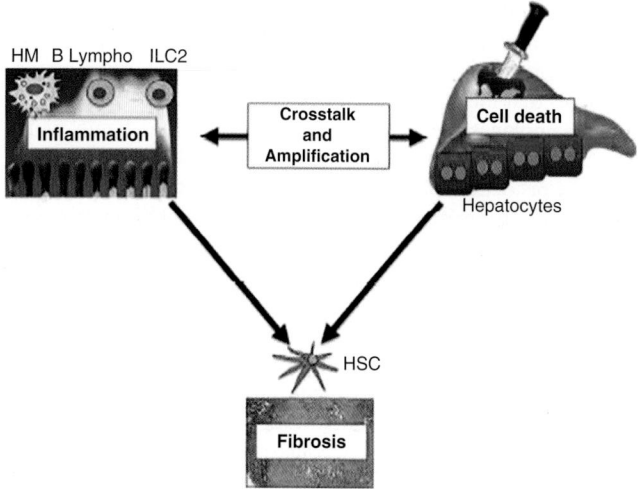

FIGURE 74.2 Links of cell death, various forms of inflammatory responses, and fibrosis are shown in this figure. *B lympho,* B lymphocyte; *HM,* hepatic macrophage; *HSC,* hepatic stellate cell; *ILC2,* type 2 innate lymphoid cell. (From Seki E, Schwabe RF. Hepatic inflammation and fibrosis: Functional links and key pathways. *Hepatology.* 2015;61: 1066–1079; see Chapters 7 and 10.)

recently proposed a novel classification scheme, the "Beijing Classification" to systematically categorize fibrosis progression and regression based on a cohort of 71 HBV-treated subjects in whom cirrhotic regression was noted from 72% (pretreatment) to 52% in post-treatment biopsies. Falize et al. (2006)[14] analyzed 36 hereditary hemochromatosis patients and demonstrated that regression of fibrosis was seen in 69% of those with bridging fibrosis and in 35% of patients with cirrhosis after

venesection therapy. Regression of cirrhosis has also been reported in patients with other diseases, including alcoholic liver disease (ALD), autoimmune hepatitis (AIH), and primary biliary cholangitis.[15-17] One mechanism proposed for repopulation of hepatic parenchyma is via "stem/progenitor" cells derived from the distalmost biliary tree. Recent studies using routine and immunostains have characterized the progression of "liver buds" as they mature into hepatocytes.[18]

The proposed mechanisms for breakdown and remodeling of liver fibrosis include loss of activated stellate cells via apoptosis, decreased expression of matrix metalloproteinase inhibitors, and increased production and activity of metalloproteinases or collagenases[9] (see Chapter 7). Currently, the extent to which cirrhosis is truly reversible is the subject of debate, and an important question not often addressed is the extent to which actual parenchymal and vascular architecture can be restored even if scar tissue is resorbed.[19] Considerations include sampling differences or interpretation errors in the studies showing reversibility; these questions rely on comparisons with prior biopsies for convincing answers. Regardless, these discussions have important clinical implications. Finally, Lee and Friedman (2014)[20] have introduced an ongoing discussion that even with viral cure in HCV, a minority of subjects actually do continue with progressive disease (fibrosis) and HCC (see Chapter 89).

ROLE OF LIVER BIOPSY IN ADVANCED LIVER DISEASE

Investigation of patients with chronic liver disease, and cirrhosis and portal hypertension involves multiple disciplines and clinical tools, including pathology, radiology, clinical chemistry, virology, serologic testing, and, more recently, molecular testing.

Liver biopsy evaluation is diminishing while more serum markers and imaging tests gain traction in clinical practice[6]; however, in cases with unknown clinical diagnoses, liver biopsy can still be considered a primary diagnostic tool, despite the drawback of invasiveness[21,22] (see Chapter 23). In fact, liver biopsy can serve several important purposes, such as establishing or confirming the clinical concern of cirrhosis or alternative explanation for portal hypertension; assessing the possible underlying causes of disease; distinguishing dysplastic nodules from HCC; and providing tissue for chemical, biochemical, molecular, or ultrastructural studies.[23]

To obtain representative liver tissue for most types of analysis in nonfocal disease processes, needle biopsy, rather than wedge biopsy, has proved to be the most useful technique. This procedure can be done percutaneously with or without ultrasound guidance, via the transjugular route when pressure measurements are needed, or during surgical procedures (see Chapters 22 and 87). A cutting needle or the Menghini aspiration needle may be used. If cirrhosis is suspected, a cutting needle is the preferred method of biopsy because the result is less likely to be fragmented, as often occurs with an aspiration needle. A continuous piece of tissue of "adequate" size (both length and diameter) is important in avoiding sampling error. Traditionally, it has been recommended that an adequate biopsy specimen should be no smaller than 20 gauge and at least 1.5 cm in length, or it should contain at least five portal tracts.[22] For accurate and reliable grading and staging of chronic viral hepatitis, however, studies have shown that a biopsy specimen of at least 2 cm that contains at least 11 complete portal tracts is needed.[24]

Usually performed during open surgery or laparoscopy, wedge biopsy is discouraged for evaluation of diffuse parenchymal liver diseases, such as cirrhosis, because this technique samples primarily the subcapsular liver parenchyma, which may contain misleading fibrous septa that extend from the capsule deep into the underlying parenchyma and can be easily confused or overinterpreted as fibrosis (Fig. 74.3). A wedge biopsy is most suitable for evaluation of visible focal lesions present on or immediately below the capsule. Even during open surgery, a needle biopsy to sample deep liver parenchyma is preferable for evaluation of diffuse disease.[24]

Prompt fixation of the liver biopsy specimen in buffered formalin is vital to high-quality histology. Many special stains and analyses, such as iron or copper quantitation, and molecular and genomic analyses can be performed on formalin-fixed, paraffin-embedded (FFPE) tissue. If an unusual metabolic disorder is suspected and electron microscopic examination is expected, prebiopsy discussion with the pathologist is useful so that additional fresh tissue can be fixed in glutaraldehyde. For final interpretation of any liver tissue, sufficient clinical information is necessary.

The safety of liver biopsy depends on operator experience as well as the underlying condition of the liver, as noted in a large study.[25] The most serious complications are rare and include bleeding (0.6%–0.7%), and death (0.2%).[25] Extrahepatic or intrahepatic tumor seeding from biopsy and/or ablation of tumor is a dreaded but rare complication.[26]

MORPHOLOGIC FINDINGS IN CIRRHOSIS

Grossly, the liver with established cirrhosis exhibits a nodular appearance that diffusely involves the entire liver (Fig. 74.4). The cirrhotic liver is firm and may be enlarged or shrunken. The parenchyma may be tan, yellow (when fatty), or dark green when there is bile stasis. The nodules' sizes may be a clue to the underlying disease: "micronodular" cirrhosis, in which nodules are <3 mm is prototypic of ALD. Mixed micromacronodular cirrhosis is the most common. Large, bulging nodules that are notably discolored from background are worrisome for malignancy, particularly HCC.

Microscopically, the liver parenchyma is divided by interconnecting, variable-sized fibrous septa that contain profiles of lymphatic and vascular lumina, as well as epithelial-lined ductular structures and diverse inflammatory cell types; the septa divide the parenchyma into the nodules that typically no longer retain an identifiable terminal hepatic venule. However, identifiable portal tracts may be found within the septa. Some "hints" of the preceding liver disease may be retained in or near the portal tracts: lymphoid aggregates in HCV or HBV, granulomatous cholangitis in primary biliary cholangitis (PBC), complete absence or replacement of ducts by scar in primary sclerosing cholangitis (PSC). The normal portal-central relationship is

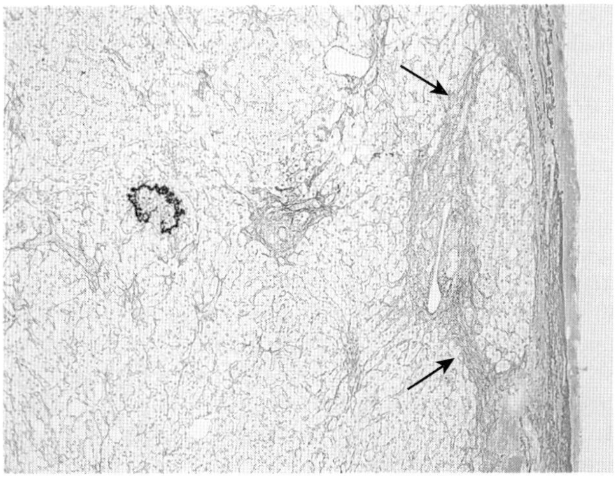

FIGURE 74.3 Wedge biopsy showing overestimation of fibrosis just beneath the liver capsule (Gomori reticulin stain). *Arrows* indicate fibrous septa extending into the hepatic parenchyma.

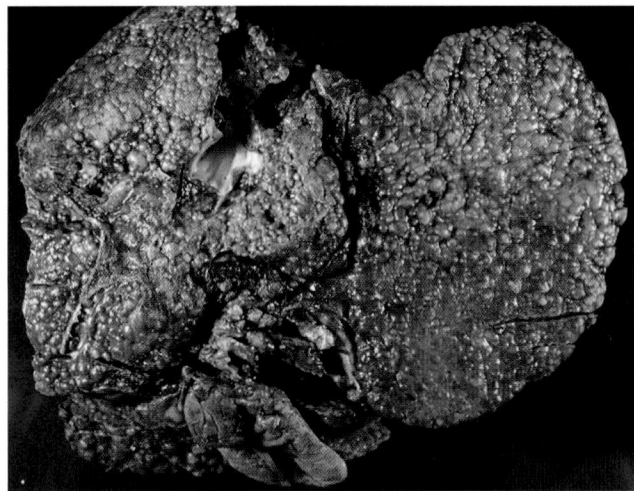

FIGURE 74.4 Gross appearance of cirrhotic liver showing diffuse involvement of the entire liver by regenerative nodules and fibrous scar.

lost; the exception to this remodeling is biliary cirrhosis, in which the terminal hepatic venule may retain its central location. The hepatocytes within the nodules may appear morphologically normal, may be undergoing active injury from the disease process, or may show evidence of regeneration. The latter may be characterized by thickened cell plates with as many as two cells across; anisonucleosis; large-cell change with maintenance of nuclear/cytoplasmic (N/C) ratio; or small, crowded cells with increased N/C ratios. The reticulin stain is useful to show cord thickening.

Along the edges of septa, there are recognizable biliary structures admixed with connective tissue and inflammation. This process of epithelial-mesenchymal-inflammatory interaction at the interface with damaged hepatocytes is referred to as *the ductular reaction*, a prototypic response that occurs in all forms of chronic liver disease, albeit with differing appearance depending on the exact disease process.[27] The epithelial component within this rim is progressively attenuated and ultimately lost concurrently with neoplastic progression of the intranodular hepatocytes from cirrhosis to dysplastic nodule to encapsulated HCC.[28] This can be appreciated by immunohistochemical staining with antibodies to biliary keratins 7 or 19.

Biliary cirrhosis is caused by disorders such as PBC, PSC or secondary sclerosing cholangitis, and biliary atresia. This type of cirrhosis exhibits unique morphologic features appreciated microscopically and characterized by a highly irregular "jigsaw puzzle" or "geographic" nodular pattern (Fig. 74.5). As noted, the terminal hepatic venule may be retained, and loss or effacement of native bile ducts by either lymphoid aggregates or scar tissue may be evident. Ductular reaction (proliferation) may be more pronounced than in other types of cirrhosis. A characteristic clue to biliary cirrhosis is the constellation of findings in periseptal hepatocytes referred to as *cholate stasis (chronic cholestasis)*. These findings include periseptal hepatocyte swelling/ballooning, Mallory-Denk bodies (Mallory's hyaline), and granules of copper deposition. In addition, foam cell aggregates may be seen in the sinusoids of the nodules. Some investigators have attributed abundant large-cell change to chronic cholestasis. Another subtle histologic clue to biliary cirrhosis is the presence of nodular regenerative hyperplasia within the regenerative nodules.

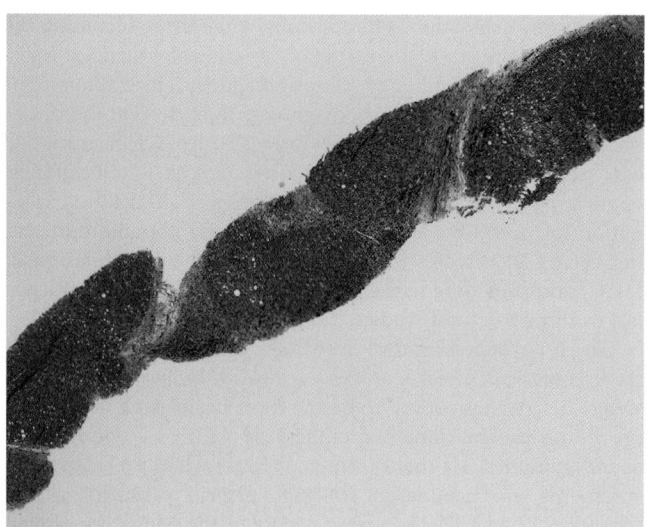

FIGURE 74.6 Cirrhosis visible on a needle biopsy specimen (Masson trichrome stain).

Recognition of cirrhosis can be straightforward when an adequate biopsy specimen is examined, even on hematoxylin and eosin–stained sections. It may be helpful to use Masson trichrome or another connective tissue stain to highlight the dense perisinusoidal fibrosis of alcoholic hepatitis, nonalcoholic steatohepatitis and cirrhosis. Connective tissue stains are particularly helpful to discern if the broken edges of fragmented needle biopsy specimens are because of a tissue plane, or artefact, as a thin layer of collagen adheres to the curved edge of a cirrhotic nodule (Fig. 74.6).

Another significant clue to cirrhosis is the numerous vascular channels within septa that traverse or course across the core biopsy.

On the other hand, cirrhosis may be difficult to diagnose on needle biopsy specimens; for instance, when a macronodule is sampled or is "incomplete" (incomplete septal cirrhosis), it may create challenges, but morphologic clues exist. In the last case, although the complete spectrum of morphologic features of cirrhosis are not exhibited, the vascular relationships are markedly altered, and ectatic, eccentrically located portal veins parallel to abnormally thin septa may be noted. In addition, some septa may be seen to extend into the parenchyma and end blindly. This type of "incomplete septal cirrhosis" is common in HBV-related liver disease.

Additional stains considered routine by liver pathologists in evaluation of liver biopsies include the iron stain and periodic acid–Schiff stain after diastase digestion (PAS-d). The former is useful in detecting and relaying semiquantification of hepatocellular iron, detecting reticuloendothelial iron, and highlighting intracanalicular bile plugs. PAS-d is useful in detecting the variable-sized periportal eosinophilic "globules" that accumulate in the endoplasmic reticulum when a Z allele is present in subjects with either MZ or ZZ α_1-antitrypsin deficiency. PAS-d also is quite helpful in noting bile duct basement membranes, perisinusoidal basement membranes, and PAS-d–laden Kupffer cells and portal and septal macrophages characteristic of recent necroinflammatory activity.

Not all larger nodules detected in cirrhotic livers are malignant. A macroregenerative nodule or large regenerative nodule usually measures 0.5 to 1.5 cm and is rarely 5 cm or more in

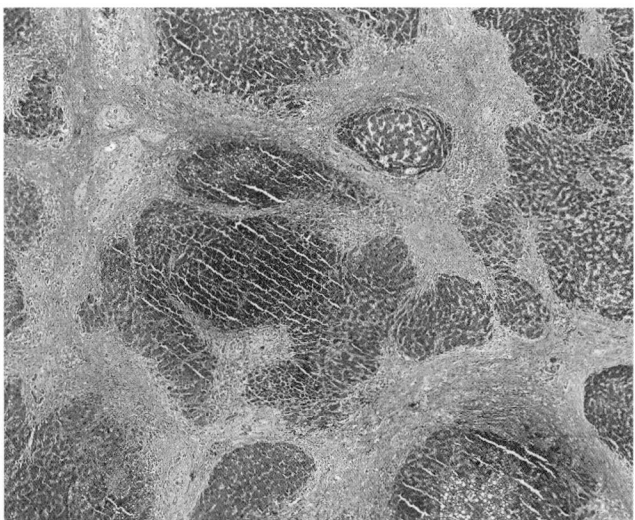

FIGURE 74.5 Biliary cirrhosis exhibiting a "jigsaw puzzle" pattern (Masson trichrome stain).

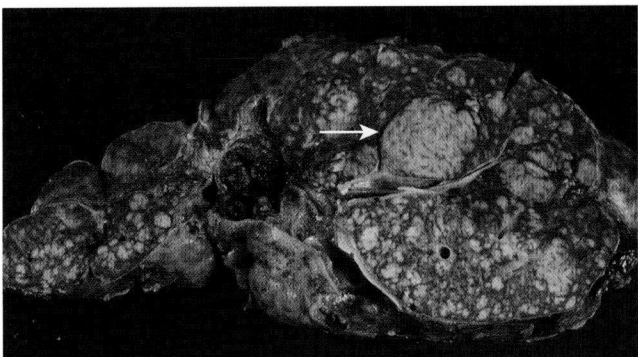

FIGURE 74.7 Gross photomicrograph of hepatocellular carcinoma *(arrow)* in a cirrhotic liver. The tumor stands out from the background cirrhosis.

diameter.[29] It is seen more commonly in macronodular cirrhosis and may be distinct from surrounding cirrhotic nodules on gross examination. Histologically, a macroregenerative nodule may contain portal structures or short fibrovascular septa. The hepatocytes within the nodule are similar to the hepatocytes in smaller cirrhotic nodules but almost always exhibit hyperplastic change, evidenced by thickened plates. The clonal nature of the macroregenerative nodule has been shown, and its malignant potential is low but unquestioned.[30]

A dysplastic nodule is a premalignant lesion that usually measures more than 0.5 cm.[29] Evolution to HCC within months or a few years has been well documented.[31] A high-grade dysplastic nodule exhibits more clear-cut architectural or cytologic atypia, such as bulging or map-like clonal growth; pseudoglandular formation; unpaired arteries; and small-cell change characterized by increased cell density, high N/C cell ratio, and nuclear hyperchromasia. These morphologic changes are insufficient, however, for the diagnosis of HCC because a dysplastic nodule does not invade the surrounding stroma or blood vessels, and it maintains cell plates no more than three cells wide.[32]

Distinguishing a high-grade dysplastic nodule from well-differentiated HCC can be extremely difficult or impossible from a needle biopsy specimen, although it may be less ambiguous when an explant is examined (Fig. 74.7; see Chapter 89).[33] Identification of ductular reaction at the periphery aids in positive identification of cirrhosis or dysplastic nodule.[28,34] Clinical management of patients with cirrhosis and dysplasia in biopsy specimens is challenging.

Assessment of Underlying Etiology in Cirrhosis

Cirrhosis is best classified by its underlying etiology if possible (Box 74.1), which can be determined by clinical history and laboratory investigation in many but not all cases. Morphologic examination may help establish the diagnosis or guide the clinical investigation. In the following discussion, the morphologic features characteristic of many chronic liver diseases that commonly cause cirrhosis are discussed. At end-stage liver disease, however, the histopathologic findings may no longer be evident, even to experienced hepatopathologists. Many cases of "cryptogenic" cirrhosis represent burned-out processes, for which no identifying clinical or morphologic features remain. These cases are frequently because of ALD, AIH, and nonalcoholic steatohepatitis (NASH). The possible contribution of underlying genetic abnormalities and as yet unnamed viral agents is not known but deserves exploration.

BOX 74.1 Causes of Cirrhosis

Chronic Hepatitis
Chronic hepatitis B
Chronic hepatitis delta
Chronic hepatitis C
Autoimmune hepatitis

Fatty Liver Diseases
Alcoholic liver disease
Nonalcoholic steatohepatitis

Chronic Biliary Diseases
Primary biliary cholangitis
Primary sclerosing cholangitis
Extrahepatic biliary atresia
Other causes of biliary obstruction

Genetic Diseases
Hereditary haemochromatosis
Wilson disease
α_1-Antitrypsin deficiency
Other rare genetic diseases

Vascular Diseases
Venous outflow obstruction (Budd–Chiari syndrome)
Sinusoidal obstruction syndrome
"Cardiac cirrhosis"

Drugs
Other Rare Causes

From Burt AD, Ferrell LD, Hübscher SG. *MacSween's Pathology of the Liver*, 7th ed. Elsevier: 2018.

Alcoholic Liver Disease

Excessive alcohol consumption is arguably the leading cause of liver disease in the Western world, which encompasses a clinicopathologic spectrum that includes fatty liver, alcoholic hepatitis, and alcoholic cirrhosis. Alcoholic cirrhosis, or Laënnec cirrhosis, is classically micronodular and may retain some of the features of alcoholic hepatitis. The liver is firm, and may appear pale or yellow, enlarged, greasy, or shrunken on gross examination. Histologically, in the initial stages, lesions predominate in the perivenular region (zone 3) of the acinus and include various combinations of steatosis (fat), hepatocyte ballooning, Mallory-Denk bodies, and satellitosis. Steatosis may be predominantly macrovesicular, defined by the presence of large fat droplets in the cytoplasm of hepatocytes displacing the nuclei. Microvesicular steatosis can also be seen, often in clusters of hepatocytes that also contain megamitochondria, and is characterized by fine fat droplets surrounding the centrally-retained nuclei. Alcoholic *hepatitis* is characterized by an inflammatory infiltrate rich in neutrophils, most frequently distributed in the lobules adjacent to hepatocytes containing Mallory-Denk bodies (i.e., satellitosis), and dense, perisinusoidal fibrosis (Fig. 74.8). Lymphocytes and histiocytes also may be present in portal tracts,[35] sometimes in the form of lipogranulomas. In the portal and periportal regions, ductular reaction with numerous neutrophils may occur. Cholangiolitis, cholangiolar (ductular) cholestasis, and canalicular bile plugs are worrisome lesions for concomitant pancreatitis and/or sepsis. A scoring system for 90-day prognosis has been validated, based on relevant histologic features.[36]

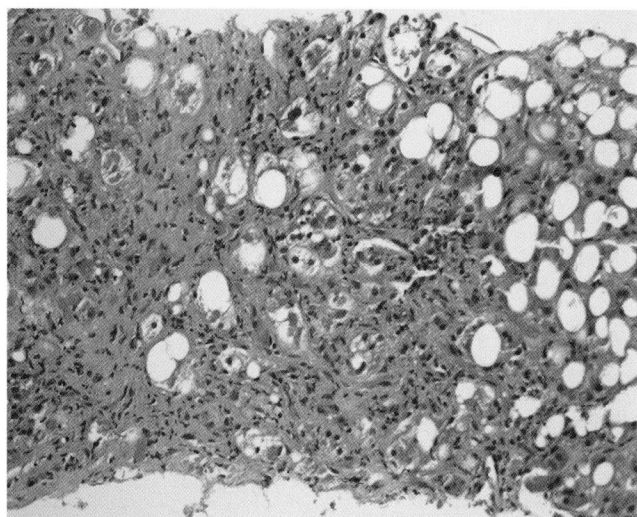

FIGURE 74.8 Alcoholic hepatitis characterized by macrovesicular steatosis, hepatocyte ballooning, lobular neutrophilic infiltration, and presence of Mallory-Denk bodies.

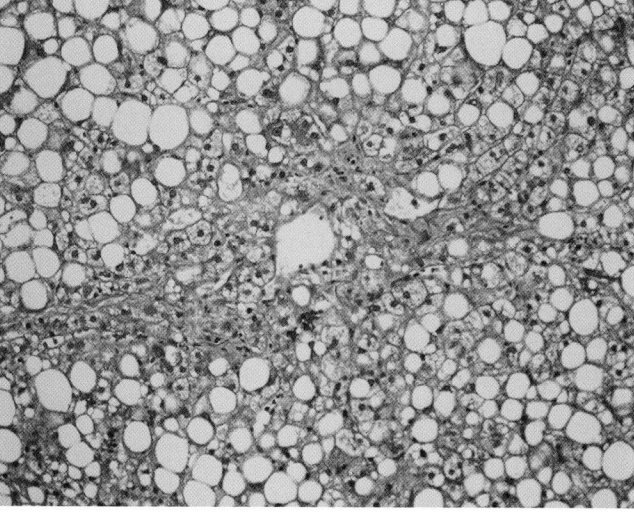

FIGURE 74.9 Zone 3 "chicken wire" perisinusoidal fibrosis; this feature can be seen in nonalcoholic and alcoholic steatohepatitis (Masson trichrome stain).

The patterns of fibrosis in alcoholic hepatitis are characteristic. Fibrosis usually involves the terminal hepatic venules, leading to the thickening of the wall; luminal occlusion may be seen with necrosis of adjacent hepatocytes and Mallory-Denk bodies within remaining hepatocytes, a lesion referred to as *central hyaline necrosis.* Subendothelial fibrosis is a venoocclusive lesion of alcoholism that may be noted even in end-stage cirrhotic livers. Fibrosis may extend into the lobules in perisinusoidal spaces as delicate or dense strands, giving rise to a distinctive "chicken wire" pericellular (perisinusoidal) distribution. Trichrome stain is particularly useful in detecting this unique form of fibrosis. With time, the liver may be replaced by micronodular cirrhosis; often, the septa of ALD are quite broad as manifestations of the microvascular obliteration.[37] As alcoholic cirrhosis progresses, the aforementioned morphologic features may become less obvious. The liver may shrink and be nearly replaced by fibrosis, and the cirrhosis may evolve into a macronodular or mixed nodular architecture with characteristic broad septa. Steatosis, ballooning, and Mallory-Denk bodies may not be discernible, especially in patients who have stopped consuming alcohol for several months or longer.

Nonalcoholic Fatty Liver Disease

NAFLD, the umbrella term for fatty liver that includes steatosis (NAFL), steatohepatitis (NASH), and cirrhosis, is the most common cause of liver test elevation in the world and closely follows ALD for liver transplantation in the US.[38] (see Chapter 69). Prevalence studies estimate that approximately 30% of the US population is affected by fatty liver; of these individuals, 15% to 20% are at risk for progression to cirrhosis.[39] Projections are for 100 million US citizens to be affected by NAFLD by 2030.[38] These increasing risks include not only cirrhosis and HCC but also the larger associated metabolic processes, obesity, type 2 diabetes, and associations with cardiovascular diseases.

Histopathologic differences and similarities of NASH and ALD are reviewed elsewhere.[37] Pertinent to this chapter are the following. Most, but not all, of the histopathologic features described in alcoholic hepatitis can be found in NASH; lesions of injury can be seen in cirrhosis of both ALD and NAFLD.

These mainly include steatosis, which is predominantly macrovesicular (large droplet or mixed large and small droplets); hepatocyte ballooning; lobular inflammation, which is usually mild and includes neutrophils; small lipogranulomas; and varying amounts of perisinusoidal fibrosis (Fig. 74.9). The presence of marked portal inflammation, particularly when accompanied by lymphoid aggregates or abundant plasma cells, should raise the suspicion of concurrent disease, such as chronic viral hepatitis or AIH,[40] and extensive portal chronic inflammation in the absence of an overlapping disease has been shown to correlate with advanced NASH and more severe clinical metabolic features.[41] In addition, Mallory-Denk bodies may or may not be seen in NASH; if present, they may be poorly formed. In contrast to ALD, in which Mallory-Denk bodies may be present in apoptotic hepatocytes, in NASH they are restricted to ballooned hepatocytes. Recently, an immunohistochemical stain to detect loss of K8/18 in ballooning, as well as presence of clumped K8/18 in Mallory-Denk bodies, has been introduced.[42] If numerous Mallory-Denk bodies are present in the background of steatohepatitis, an alcoholic origin is more likely.[37] Likewise, marked cholestasis is highly unlikely in precirrhotic NASH but can occur in ALD. The broad septa of ALD are rare in NAFLD as well.

Fibrosis in NASH begins in the pericentral perisinusoidal spaces; with time, portal and periportal fibrosis develop, and eventually bridging fibrosis and cirrhosis may occur. This typically does not obliterate the terminal hepatic venules, another feature dissimilar to alcoholic hepatitis. A grading and staging system has been proposed for NASH primarily based on the extent and severity of the constellation of steatosis, ballooning change, the grade of lobular and portal inflammation, and the stage of fibrosis and remodeling.[43] Similar to the widespread use of grading and staging in other forms of chronic liver disease, this proposal was made in recognition of the unique features of steatohepatitis to facilitate further reproducible evaluation for clinical and laboratory investigation. A revision of this system by the National Institute of Diabetes and Digestive and Kidney Diseases–sponsored NASH Clinical Research Network is used widely in clinical trials.[44]

As NASH fibrosis progresses, it is recognized that most of the described histologic features may no longer be present. However, it is incorrect to assume that all cases of "cryptogenic cirrhosis" are NASH cirrhosis because ALD and AIH may also result in cirrhosis without characteristic features of the underlying disease process. Only a prior liver biopsy showing evidence of NASH can be accepted as evidence, and the diagnosis then is no longer "cryptogenic" but is NASH-cirrhosis.

True "cryptogenic cirrhosis" deserves its own diagnostic category and clinical evaluation for other possible entities.

Chronic Hepatitis C

Before the new interferon (IFN)-sparing curative therapies for HCV, cirrhosis developed in a high proportion of patients infected with HCV, especially patients with a long duration of infection, concurrent alcohol consumption, coinfection with HBV or human immunodeficiency virus (HIV), nonresponse to antiviral therapy, and men (see Chapter 68). Interestingly, even after virologic cure, a small number of individuals from large clinical trials (7%–13%) continue to have fibrosis progression or even cirrhosis.[20] HCV-related cirrhosis is virtually always macronodular or mixed macronodular and micronodular. The fibrovascular septa vary in width and usually are infiltrated by mononuclear cells, predominantly lymphocytes, but also include plasma cells and eosinophils. Lymphoid aggregates, often with well-formed germinal centers, are characteristic, although not pathognomonic (Fig. 74.10). A mild degree of bile duct damage (the Poulsen lesion) also may be seen in some cases, and interface hepatitis may also be present. The lobular inflammation is typically spotty and mild, with or without acidophilic bodies. Subendothelial inflammation in portal veins, identical to endotheliitis, also may occur in HCV infection. No reliable antibody for immunohistochemical detection of HCV proteins has been found.

Chronic Hepatitis B

Chronic hepatitis secondary to HBV infection is another common cause of cirrhosis[45,46] (see Chapter 68). Compared with hepatitis caused by HCV, HBV hepatitis may exhibit more severe portal and lobular necroinflammation, particularly when

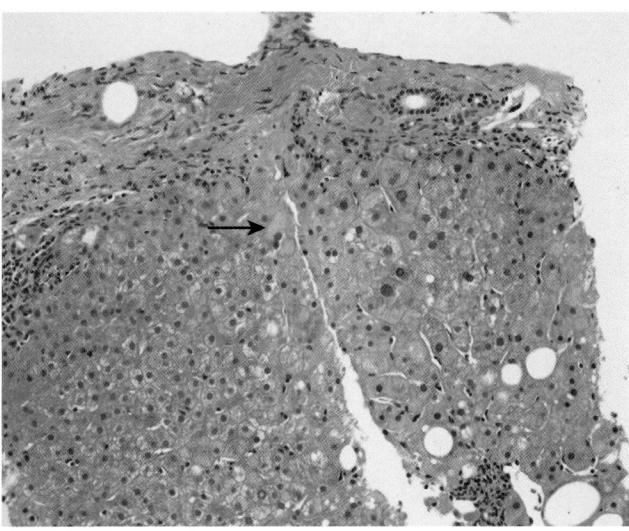

FIGURE 74.11 Ground-glass hepatocytes *(arrow)* in chronic hepatitis B virus.

there is an acute exacerbation. Confluent or multiacinar bridging necrosis with collapse of the lobular framework may be seen. A relatively specific finding in chronic HBV hepatitis is the presence of "ground-glass" inclusions within hepatocytes, which are uniform, pale, or eosinophilic cytoplasmic alterations resulting from enriched smooth endoplasmic reticulum filled with hepatitis B surface antigen (Fig. 74.11). However, changes resembling ground-glass inclusions have been observed in a variety of conditions.[47] A definitive diagnosis can be established by histochemical stains (orcein, Victoria blue) or with immunohistochemical detection of hepatitis B surface antigen in the cytoplasm (as inclusions or diffusely) or along the membranous surface and hepatitis B core antigen in the nucleus.

Coinfection or superinfection with hepatitis D virus (HDV) in HBV patients usually causes more severe liver damage and accelerates the development of cirrhosis.[48] Immunohistochemical detection of HDV intranuclear antigen is helpful in establishing the diagnosis.

Autoimmune Hepatitis

The diagnosis of AIH relies on a constellation of clinical, laboratory, and histopathologic findings; clinically, AIH may include cirrhosis either as an end result or at presentation. Histopathologic examination of liver tissue serves important roles in confirming clinical concern and excluding diseases secondary to other etiologies.[49] Classic AIH exhibits a dense portal, septal, and lobular mononuclear cell infiltrate, with marked periportal or periseptal interface hepatitis enriched in plasma cells. The presence of numerous plasma cells in portal inflammation and within lobular foci of necrosis and the formation of hepatitic "rosettes" are characteristic (Fig. 74.12). In severe cases, confluent or bridging necrosis may be seen, sometimes accompanied by pseudoacinar formation. Predominantly centrilobular necrosis with relatively mild portal inflammation also has been described in AIH.[50] Fibrosis may rapidly progress in untreated patients. At the cirrhotic stage, the liver parenchyma is divided by broad, fibrous bands into variable-sized nodules, similar to those caused by alcoholic or chronic viral hepatitis; plasma cells and rosettes may become less prominent. Burned-out AIH may be a cause of so-called "cryptogenic" cirrhosis.

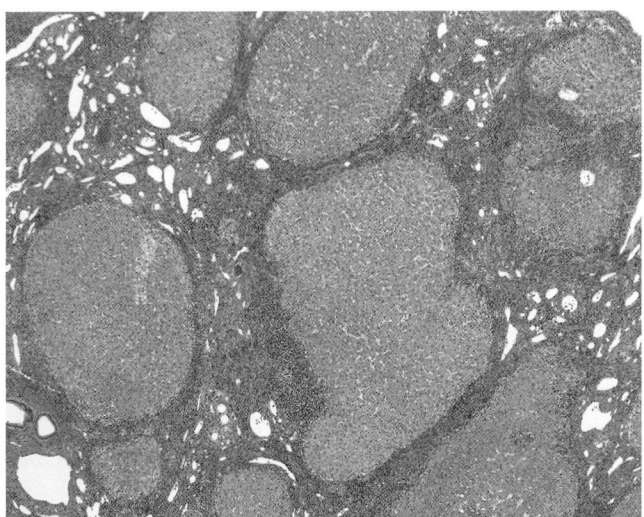

FIGURE 74.10 Hepatitis C virus cirrhosis with characteristic septal lymphoid aggregates.

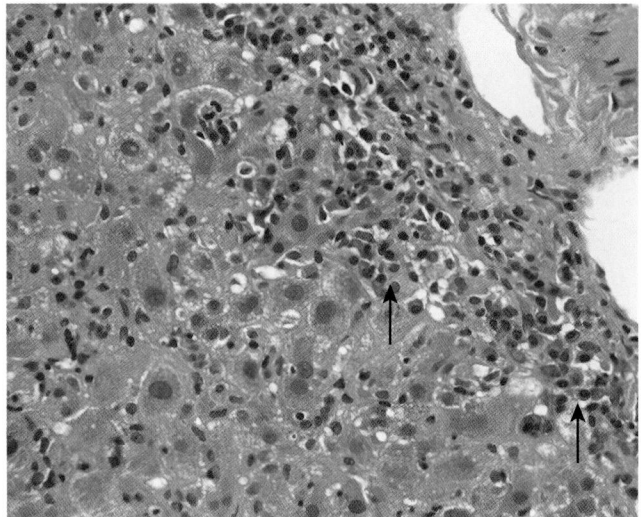

FIGURE 74.12 Autoimmune hepatitis may be characterized by hepatitic "rosettes" and numerous plasma cells *(arrows)* in the portal tracts and lobules.

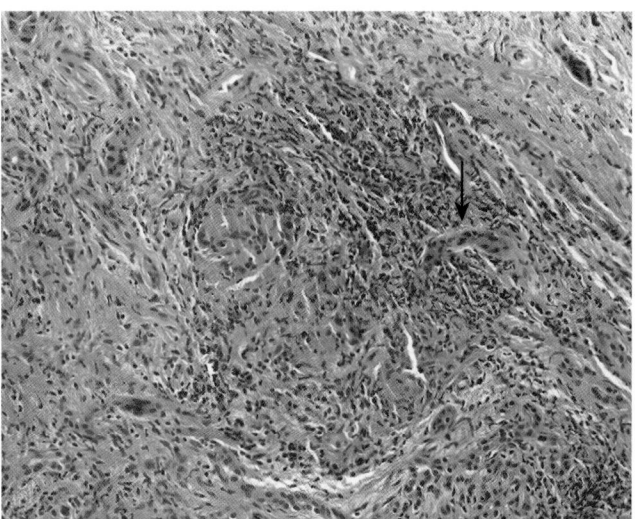

FIGURE 74.13 Florid duct lesion with granulomatous portal inflammation and damaged bile duct *(arrow)* in early-stage primary biliary cholangitis.

Primary Biliary Cholangitis

PBC is an autoimmune disorder predominantly of women during or after childbearing years that leads to progressive destruction of intrahepatic bile ducts.[51] The pathogenesis is multifactorial and remains poorly understood. Lesions of the early stages of mixed chronic portal inflammation with lymphocytes, plasma cells, eosinophils, and the pathognomonic "florid duct lesion," characterized by lymphocytic or granulomatous bile duct infiltration (Fig. 74.13) can remain even in late-stage disease. Ductular reaction, interface hepatitis, and periportal changes collectively referred to as "cholate stasis" with foamy changes of hepatocytes and copper deposition are more common in advanced stages. In the setting of positive serum antimitochondrial antibody (AMA), the florid duct lesion is essentially diagnostic. The affected ducts may rupture, or the duct epithelium may exhibit degenerative change. With progression,

ductopenia becomes evident, and features of chronic cholestasis are dominant throughout the parenchyma. True cirrhotic remodeling is seen only at the late stage of PBC; it is commonly inhomogeneously distributed (the "jigsaw" pattern of biliary cirrhosis) and may be micronodular. A periseptal rim of pallor is noted because of cholate stasis. Florid duct lesions and granulomas may continue to exist where native bile ducts have not been completely destroyed. Canalicular bile stasis (cholestasis) with bile plugs may be seen in the late stage; this finding is regarded as hepatic decompensation.

Features of AIH may occur with or may precede those of PBC; when these occur simultaneously, it is referred to as overlap syndrome or autoimmune cholangitis, regardless of serum autoantibodies. The dominant histopathologic process (hepatitis vs. biliary) determines treatment.[52] Residual lesions may or may not be seen in advanced stages (i.e., cirrhosis).

HCC is now known to occur with the same frequency in PBC as in cirrhotic HCV[53]; non-response to ursodeoxycholic acid (URSO) is the primary risk factor for HCC, independent of disease stage and gender.[54]

Primary Sclerosing Cholangitis

PSC, an idiopathic inflammatory and fibrosing process, segmentally affects both the extrahepatic and intrahepatic biliary tree, resulting in biliary strictures and ultimately, biliary cirrhosis[55,56] (see Chapter 41). PSC is strongly associated with inflammatory bowel disease, particularly ulcerative colitis, and with the development of cholangiocarcinoma (see Chapters 50 and 51), as well as colorectal carcinoma, gallbladder carcinoma (see Chapter 49) and HCC (see Chapter 89). This still enigmatic disease more commonly affects young men. The definitive diagnosis of PSC rests on characteristic imaging findings; liver biopsy is too selective in this inhomogeneous process. Characteristic histopathologic features include concentric, "onion-skin" periductal fibrosis; however, this merely indicates chronic biliary obstruction of any cause and thus is not pathognomonic. The involved duct epithelium exhibits atrophic and degenerative changes; a characteristic fibro-obliterative scar eventually replaces the bile duct (Fig. 74.14). Thus PSC is one of the disease processes

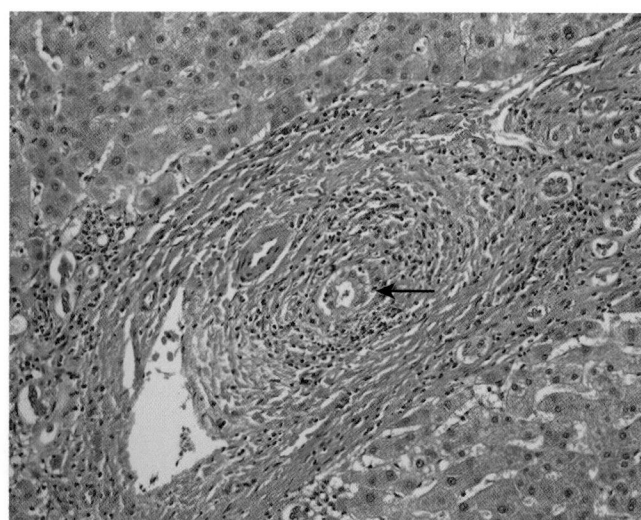

FIGURE 74.14 Characteristic concentric onion-skin periductal fibrosis in primary sclerosing cholangitis. The residual duct epithelial cells show atrophic and degenerative changes *(arrow)*.

among the differential for ductopenia and features of chronic cholestasis; others include various medications and viral infections, graft versus host disease, sarcoidosis, PBC, and idiopathic ductopenia.[57]

Cholangiocarcinoma, a dreaded and challenging complication for screening in PSC, has an incidence of 400- to 1500-fold increased lifetime risk greater than the general population and occurs within the first year of diagnosis of PSC in up to 50%.[58] Careful evaluation of explant livers for occult cholangiocarcinoma with thorough sampling of all hilar tissue is recommended. Although cirrhosis may occur, CCA is not reported in small-duct PSC (see Chapters 50 and 51).

Hereditary Hemochromatosis

Hereditary hemochromatosis (HH) is an autosomal recessive disorder that results in iron overload in several organs. Cirrhosis is a recognized complication, if untreated. HH is because of abnormal genetic control and expression by the liver of the master iron regulator hepcidin. There are several genetic mutations that result in metabolic iron overload, but the best known is associated with homozygous C282Y mutations of the *HFE* gene.[58,59] Iron deposition initially occurs in zone 1 (periportal) hepatocytes, with a decreasing gradient toward the centrilobular area. The iron granules are concentrated along the border of the canaliculi; this is best shown by modified Perls' Prussian blue stain (Fig. 74.15). With progression, untreated HH results in iron deposition throughout the entire lobule, and iron granules are seen not only in hepatocytes but also in Kupffer cells, biliary epithelial cells, and portal macrophages. Kupffer cell clusters, or siderotic nodules, are common, and usually little to no significant portal and/or lobular inflammation is evident. This pattern of iron deposition is not restricted to HH because any form of ineffective erythropoiesis may also result in it; thus the diagnosis rests with genetic testing.

Fibrosis in HH is portal based. When cirrhosis develops, it is typically micronodular with portal to portal bridging and retention of the terminal hepatic venules. Hepatocytes in cirrhotic nodules remain iron loaded, typically exhibiting a periseptal distribution pattern. The presence of iron-free nodules or foci are concerning for dysplasia or HCC because neither retain

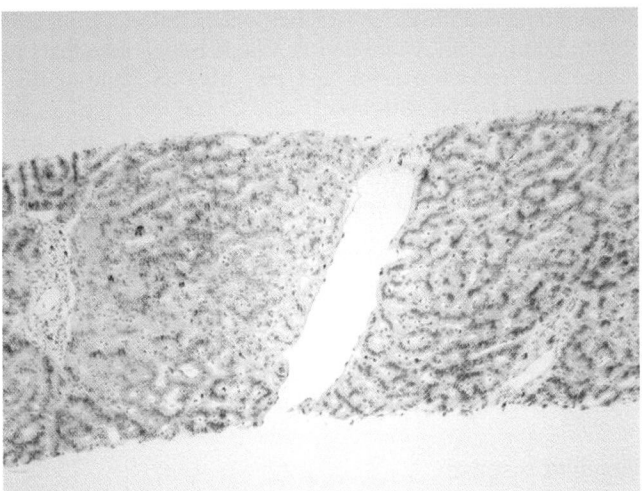

FIGURE 74.15 Massive hepatocellular iron deposition in case of hereditary hemochromatosis (C282Y homozygous) illustrates the pericanalicular location in the hepatocytes with a periportal to centrolobular gradient (Perls' Prussian blue stain).

iron even in iron-loaded livers. The risk of HCC is markedly increased in C282Y homozygous HH and is most often seen in the setting of cirrhosis.[60]

Secondary iron overload in the liver is a common finding in a variety of nonbiliary conditions, including hepatic necrosis and cirrhosis.[60] Stainable iron may be detected in cirrhosis from chronic HCV and HBV, alcoholic steatohepatitis and NASH, and cirrhosis unrelated to homozygous HH. Iron deposition in these conditions is usually mild and rarely exceeds 2+ when a semiquantitative histologic score of 1 to 4 is used. Iron granules may be found in hepatocytes, Kupffer cells, and endothelial cells of the sinusoids or large vessels. If a higher score is appreciated in hepatocytes (e.g., 3+ or 4+, which is more commonly associated with C282Y homozygous HH), age-adjusted chemical quantitation of iron concentration, the hepatic iron index, or genetic testing for *HFE* mutations should be performed. Patients with chronic viral hepatitis or steatohepatitis who also have an increased liver iron content have a higher chance of harboring at least one C282Y *HFE* mutation. It has been suggested that these patients are less likely to respond to venesection therapy and are also more prone to fibrosis and cirrhosis.[61]

Wilson Disease

Wilson disease is an autosomal recessive inherited metabolic disorder of copper metabolism. Any young to middle-aged patient with otherwise unexplained cirrhosis, chronic liver disease, or fulminant liver failure (with hemolytic anemia) clinically should be investigated for Wilson disease,[62] particularly when neuropsychiatric symptoms are involved. Morphologic features in the liver vary as widely as the potential clinical presentations and may show overlapping features of acute injury overlaid on previously unsuspected chronic liver disease (cirrhosis). At the precirrhotic stage, lymphocytic portal inflammation with interface hepatitis that mimics chronic viral hepatitis or AIH may be evident. Hepatocytes may show variable degrees of steatosis, necrosis, anisocytosis, and anisonucleosis. In later stages, atypical lipofuscin, canalicular cholestasis, and hepatocellular and Kupffer cell iron accumulation may be noted. Periportal hepatocytes may contain glycogenated nuclei and Mallory-Denk bodies, and cirrhosis is usually micronodular. Because of the spectrum of clinical and histologic features of Wilson disease, the differential diagnoses are broad and include chronic hepatitis (viral, AIH, drug-induced), steatohepatitis, PBC or PSC, iron overload and non-Wilson copper toxicosis.

Copper and copper-binding protein accumulation may be shown on tissue sections by histochemical techniques, such as rhodanine, rubeanic acid, orcein, or Victoria blue stains (Fig. 74.16) and are most likely present in cirrhosis. In early stages, copper is cytoplasmic and not readily detectable; in later stages, copper is predominantly lysosomal and more readily detectable. Thus a negative copper stain does not exclude Wilson disease. It is also important to recall that copper deposition also may occur in chronic cholestatic liver diseases, such as PBC or PSC, usually in zone 1, or in periseptal hepatocytes in cirrhosis. Copper quantitation by biochemical assay in hepatic tissue is the diagnostic test for Wilson disease, which can be performed reliably on FFPE tissue. A value of greater than 250 µg/g dry hepatic tissue has been used as a cutoff value.

Currently, plasma-based genetic testing has not yet become practical for clinical diagnosis because of the number of genetic mutations in *ATP7B* copper transport gene that may result in this disease.

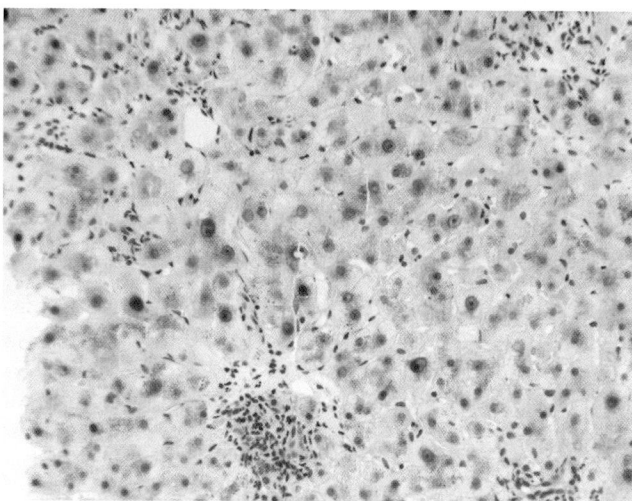

FIGURE 74.16 Abundant copper deposition (red granules) in an end-stage case of Wilson disease (rhodanine stain).

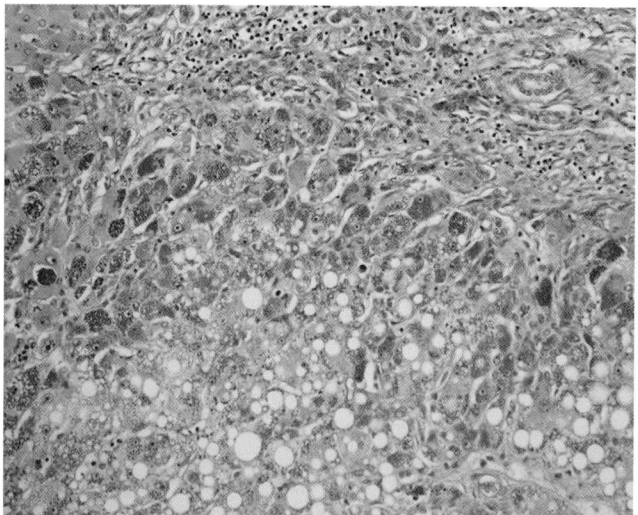

FIGURE 76.17 Varying sizes and shapes of diastase-resistant hyaline globules in periseptal hepatocytes in α_1-antitrypsin deficiency (periodic acid–Schiff stain after diastase digestion).

α_1-Antitrypsin Deficiency

Liver injury in α_1-antitrypsin deficiency results from retention of mutant α_1-antitrypsin protein translated from at least one Z allele, leading to an intracellular injury cascade culminating in liver cell death.[63] The histopathologic hallmark of the disease is the presence of eosinophilic globules of varying sizes that contain the misfolded mutant α_1-antitrypsin accumulated in the endoplasmic reticulum of zone 1 hepatocytes, in patients older than infants. These globules are best shown by PAS-d stain (Fig. 74.17), but immunohistochemical stain is confirmatory. The globules can be seen in homozygous (PiZZ) and heterozygous (PiMZ) patients, which may be determined by serum protein electrophoresis or genomic DNA analysis. Liver disease and cirrhosis are commonly thought only to develop in homozygous patients, although retrospective studies have shown a 3-fold to 5-fold overrepresentation of heterozygous patients in groups with chronic liver disease,[65] suggesting heterozygous MZ status may predispose patients to liver injury by other disease. When

chronic hepatitis is seen in α_1-antitrypsin deficiency, other causes, such as HCV or alcohol, should be excluded.[66] Cirrhosis developing from α_1-antitrypsin deficiency can be micronodular, macronodular, biliary, or mixed in pattern. Dysplasia and HCC may occur in cirrhotic livers.

Cryptogenic Cirrhosis

In approximately 10% to 15% of patients with cirrhosis, no clinically or pathologically identifiable cause of cirrhosis is identified. However, accumulating evidence suggests that a large proportion of cryptogenic cirrhosis may represent burned-out NAFLD. This suggestion is based on reported biopsy series of diagnosed NASH, followed by subsequent cirrhosis with complete loss of the features of active steatohepatitis. In addition, several authors have shown that many of these patients have type 2 diabetes, obesity, or both, compared with patients with cirrhosis of other etiologies.[65-68] Development of posttransplant NAFLD also is frequent in this group of patients,[68] but whether this represents actual recurrence of NASH or de novo NASH remains an area of discussion.[69]

An autoimmune etiology also has been proposed based on clinical and histopathologic findings,[70,71] but autoantibodies may no longer be detectable in these cases.[72] PSC and alcoholic cirrhosis may present as otherwise cryptogenic cirrhosis, and a case report documented prior biopsy-proven Budd-Chiari syndrome presenting as cryptogenic cirrhosis 34 years later.[73] Mutations in cellular keratins[74] or canalicular transporter proteins[75] may also result in cryptogenic cirrhosis. Finally, the possibility of an as yet unknown viral infection or metabolic condition cannot necessarily be excluded by histopathology alone in cryptogenic cirrhosis. Evaluation of patients with unexplained cirrhosis should include careful review of all prior liver biopsy specimens, especially those from several years prior.

NONCIRRHOTIC PORTAL HYPERTENSION

An increase in the pressure of the portal venous system can be seen in a heterogeneous group of prehepatic, intrahepatic, and posthepatic conditions in the absence of cirrhosis (Box 74.2; see Chapters 76 and 79). The etiopathogenetic mechanisms leading to portal hypertension in these conditions, the clinical presentation, and the prognoses vary widely.[78] Portal hypertension in Budd-Chiari syndrome (see Chapter 86) is secondary to posthepatic vein obstruction and may have an acute or subacute clinical course with liver failure. Portal hypertension associated with infiltrative amyloid or hematologic disorders, such as leukemia, mastocytosis, and Gaucher disease, is believed to occur primarily at the intrahepatic sinusoidal level. Precirrhotic alcoholic hepatitis also may cause portal hypertension because of hepatocyte swelling, sinusoidal fibrosis, and central sclerosis, which may be more insidious clinically. Liver biopsy functions to confirm the absence of cirrhosis and helps establish or suggest an alternative diagnosis.[21] The histopathologic features of several selected entities associated with noncirrhotic portal hypertension are discussed briefly.

Vascular Disease
Venous Outflow Obstruction

Obstruction of hepatic venous outflow (posthepatic obstruction) increases sinusoidal pressure and results in subsequent portal hypertension. Etiologic possibilities include congestive heart

BOX 74.2   Causes of Noncirrhotic Portal Hypertension

Prehepatic
Extrahepatic portal vein obstruction or compression
Portal or splenic vein thrombosis
Arterioportal shunt or fistula
Massive splenomegaly

Intrahepatic
Nodular regenerative hyperplasia
Alcoholic hepatitis
Drugs and toxins
Granulomatous disease (sarcoidosis, schistosomiasis)
Amyloidosis
Venoocclusive disease
Congenital hepatic fibrosis
Hereditary hemorrhagic telangiectasia
Idiopathic noncirrhotic portal hypertension (INCPH)/Portosinusoidal
  vascular disease (PSVD)

Posthepatic
Budd-Chiari syndrome
Congestive heart failure
Inferior vena cava (IVC) obstruction
Constrictive pericarditis
Tricuspid valve disease

Da BL, Koh C, Heller T. Noncirrhotic portal hypertension. *Curr Opin Gastroenterol.* 2018;34(3):
140–145; Rajekar H, Vasishta RK, Chawla YK, Dhiman RK. Noncirrhotic portal hypertension. *J Clin
Exp Hepatol.* 2011;1(2):94–108.

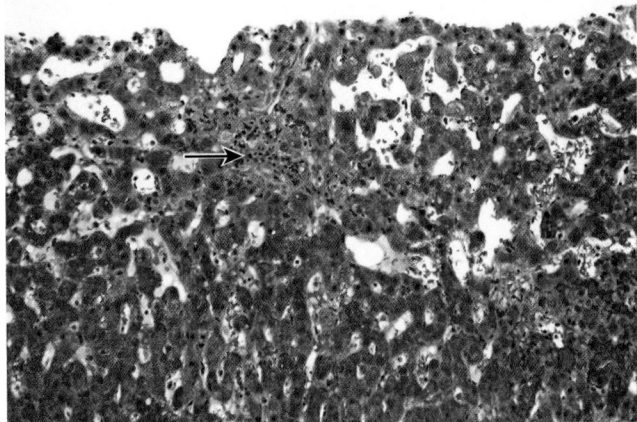

FIGURE 74.18 This connective tissue stain highlights the lesions of venoocclusive disease (sinusoidal obstruction syndrome). The remnants of the wall of the terminal hepatic venule are seen *(arrow);* necrosis and dropout of the perivenular, zone 3 hepatocytes are demonstrated (Masson trichrome stain).

failure (CHF), narrowing or occlusion of large hepatic veins (Budd-Chiari syndrome; see Chapter 86), or obliteration of the terminal or sublobular hepatic veins. The mechanistically unique lesion known as "sinusoidal obstruction syndrome" (or venoocclusive disease) that occurs in bone marrow transplant recipients is not included in this category, however. Liver injury caused by CHF is characterized by zone 3 sinusoidal dilation (also known as congestion) and, when severe or acute, leads to extravasation of red blood cells into the space of Disse, displacing hepatocytes from the hepatic cords. Hepatocellular necrosis is uncommon unless accompanied by systemic hypotension and hypoperfusion. The portal tracts are typically unremarkable and devoid of significant inflammatory cell infiltration. In long-standing cases, zone 3 hepatocytes exhibit atrophic change and are often no larger than a small nucleus, with markedly attenuated cell plates. Lipofuscin pigment and sinusoidal lining-cell iron may accrue. Perivenular fibrosis and bridging fibrosis may replace the withered cords. Rarely septal formation, reverse lobulation, and cardiac cirrhosis occur in refractory cases.

Budd-Chiari syndrome results from obstruction at any level of the hepatic venous system between the liver and the inferior vena cava (IVC) or the right heart atrium. It may result from a variety of thrombotic and nonthrombotic causes, among which hypercoagulable states secondary to myeloproliferative disorders are the most common.[79] The histopathologic features of Budd-Chiari syndrome are similar to those of CHF, but acute onset also may give rise to a hemorrhagic appearance within zone 3, with extravasation of red blood cells into the space of Disse replacing hepatocytes within the cords, and significant hepatocyte loss. If unrelieved, Budd-Chiari syndrome results in cord atrophy, replacement by fibrosis, and eventual cirrhosis. Interestingly, a ductular reaction has been reported in as many as 47% of cases [80]; this finding, along with elevated alkaline phosphatase, can result in a mistaken impression of a cholestatic process.

In contrast to Budd-Chiari syndrome, venoocclusive disease, now known as sinusoidal obstruction syndrome (SOS),[81] rarely results in cirrhosis and has variable clinical manifestations that range from elevation of liver function tests to portal hypertension, life-threatening ascites, and liver failure. The process affects the distal sinusoids, the intrahepatic portion of the hepatic venous system, and the terminal hepatic and sublobular veins. It has been stressed that the injury is to the sinusoidal lining cells and surrounding hepatocytes. SOS is most common after bone marrow or hematopoietic stem cell transplantation, is more likely to occur in persons infected with HCV, and is associated with conditioning chemotherapeutic agents (see Chapters 69 and 98) and hepatic radiation.[82-84]

Oxaliplatin-based chemotherapy is increasingly recognized as a cause of marked damage to the sinusoids, with the subsequent risks of nodular regenerative hyperplasia, perisinusoidal and outflow vein fibrosis, and potentially liver failure[85] (see Chapters 69 and 98). Patients usually are seen within 30 days after chemotherapy; however, late-onset venoocclusive disease has been reported[86] (Fig. 74.18). Bridging fibrosis, cirrhosis, or nodular regenerative hyperplasia may ensue in recovery.

Portosinusoidal Vascular Disease (Idiopathic Noncirrhotic Portal Hypertension)

Broadly speaking, idiopathic noncirrhotic portal hypertension (INCPH) includes any number of disorders causing portal hypertension in the absence of cirrhosis, portal vein thrombosis, or other known cause. Heterogenous but common histologic features amongst these cases have led to a variety of terms, including *hepatoportal sclerosis, incomplete septal cirrhosis,* and *obliterative portal venopathy,* and are believed to represent the effects of longstanding portal venous insufficiency. Portal vein stenosis, herniated portal vein branches, hypervascularized portal tracts, and abnormal periportal (shunt) vessels may all be seen in INCPH to varying degrees and depending on distribution (Fig. 74.19).[87,88] These portal-based histologic findings, in addition to nodular regenerative hyperplasia (NRH; see later), have been increasingly

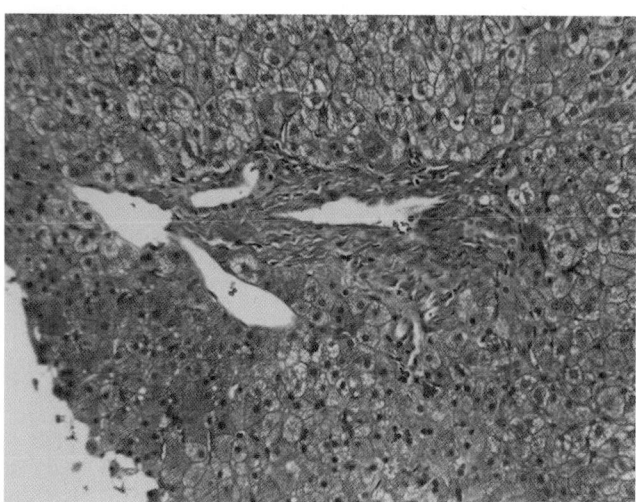

FIGURE 74.19 Portal changes in portosinusoidal vascular disease (PSVD)/idiopathic noncirrhotic portal hypertension (INCPH) include herniated portal vein branches and portal fibrosis, pictured here, among others (Masson trichrome stain).

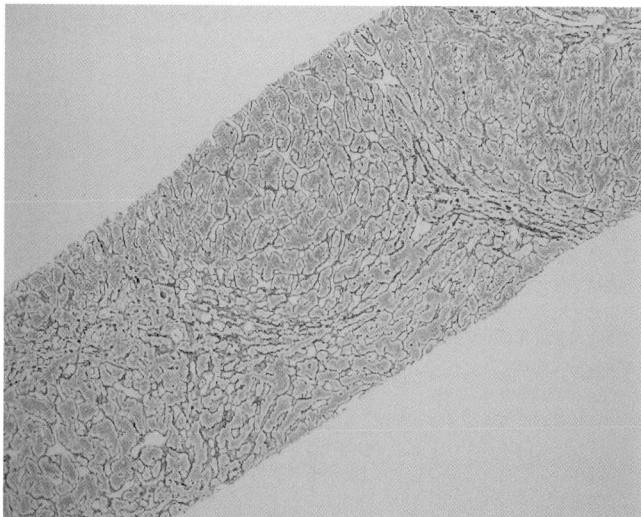

FIGURE 74.20 Reticulin stain highlights nodularity of the parenchyma in nodular regenerative hyperplasia; no scar tissue (fibrous septum) is present (Sweet's reticulin).

recognized in patients before development of portal hypertension, prompting proposal of a more encompassing term: portosinusoidal vascular disease (PSVD).[77,78,89]

Although the etiology is obscure, there is a common association of PSVD/INCPH with immunologic disorders; immunologic disturbance is thus thought to be involved in pathogenesis. Bacterial infection leading to repeated stimulation also has been proposed as a candidate mechanism, but this remains speculative. In addition, some authors[90,91] suggest that prothrombotic disorders and thromboembolism play a role in etiopathogenesis. A recent review suggests it is a combination of recurrent infections and thrombotic disorders that results in the condition.[76]

The vascular pathologic changes in PSVD/INCPH may or may not be related to the initiating factors.[91] Histologic findings are heterogeneous and often subtle and may be missed on a needle biopsy specimen. Nevertheless, biopsy is essential to rule out cirrhosis or clearly identifiable causes of portal hypertension, such as schistosomiasis or amyloid. Macroscopically, the liver may have a reduced mass, and the surface may be irregularly undulant or finely wrinkled, because of subcapsular parenchymal atrophy.[92] The cut surface may show portal and perivascular fibrosis, dilation and wall thickening of the veins, and unusual distribution and approximation of the portal and outflow vascular structures. Microscopically, the most specific signs of PSVD include (1) NRH (see later); (2) obliterative portal venopathy in which portal veins are thickened, stenotic, or replaced by fibrosis; and/or (3) incomplete septal fibrosis seen as incomplete, blind-ended septa partially surrounding rudimentary nodules. Other portal tract vascular abnormalities (multiple arteries or periportal vascular channels), nonzonal sinusoidal dilatation, and architectural irregularities (distortion of the regularly distributed portal tracts and central veins) are also suggestive of PSVD, especially with clinical signs of portal hypertension.[88,89]

Nodular Regenerative Hyperplasia

In addition to an important pattern in PSVD/INCPH, NRH is associated with a wide range of conditions, mainly including hematologic disorders, connective tissue diseases, and medications.

Portal hypertension has been reported in approximately half of patients with NRH.[93] The pathogenesis is unclear but may involve intrahepatic portal venous thrombosis, leading to a microcirculatory disturbance in the liver that causes localized ischemia with atrophy and compensatory hepatocyte hyperplasia. The liver may be normal sized or enlarged when associated with a hematologic disease. On cut surface, the liver is diffusely nodular in appearance, with nodules ranging from 0.1 to 1 cm in diameter. Microscopically, the nodular appearance is best appreciated with reticulin stain (Fig. 74.20), which highlights regenerative nodules with atrophic hepatocytes at the edges; little to no fibrosis is present. Some nodules may result in compression of the outflow vein to give the appearance of the "new moon." Nodular regenerative hyperplasia differs from cirrhosis in that fibrosis, if present, is minimal, and the portal tract distribution is usually unaltered. These characteristic features may be shown more easily on a wedge biopsy specimen and may be difficult to appreciate on a needle biopsy specimen.

Schistosomiasis

In endemic areas, infestation by *Schistosoma japonicum* or *S. mansoni* is a frequent cause of portal hypertension.[94] The mechanism involves ova deposition in the portal venules, which incites a granulomatous inflammatory response and extensive, so-called *clay pipe stem fibrosis*, leading to hemodynamic disturbance. Definitive diagnosis can be made by showing the presence of schistosomal ova (see Chapters 45 and 71).

Congenital Hepatic Fibrosis

Congenital hepatic fibrosis is a developmental disorder that results in portal hypertension in children, and rarely in adults, but not in cirrhosis (see Chapters 1 and 76). It is included in the spectrum of conditions referred to as fibropolycystic liver disease (see Chapter 73). The liver is usually enlarged and firm. Microscopically, the portal tracts are expanded by mature fibrous tissue and may show portal-to-portal bridging fibrous bands that do not have the characteristic features of inflammation in septa described earlier. An increased number of aberrant duct profiles are distributed at the periphery of the fibrous

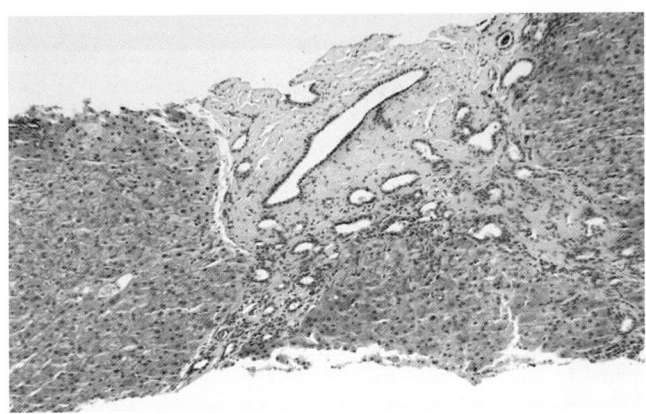

FIGURE 74.21   Congenital hepatic fibrosis. The duct plate abnormality is manifested by remnant ductal profiles along the limiting plate; some of the duct structures contain inspissated bile.

bands and portal tracts; no necrosis and no parenchymal remodeling are noted (Fig. 74.21). Inspissated bile may be noted in these ductal lumina, and portal vein branches may be hypoplastic or absent, but the hepatic artery branches may be hypertrophic and numerous,[95] suggesting arteriovenous anastomosis.

Drugs and Toxins

Chronic liver injury attributable to drugs or toxins may cause extensive fibrosis and, rarely, cirrhosis, leading to portal hypertension. Drug-induced cirrhosis accounts for less than 1% of cases in transplant databases. Well-known examples include methotrexate, chronic hypervitaminosis A, amiodarone, and valproic acid. Certain herbals have also been associated with cirrhosis, including Bush tea (pyrrolizidine alkaloids) and comfrey.[96] Toxins include long-term arsenic (in vineyard workers) and vinyl chloride exposures. A comprehensive and updated review of cases and known mechanisms of action can be found at http://livertox.nlm.nih.gov (see Chapters 69 and 98).

CONCLUSION

Long-standing portal hypertension causes serious extrahepatic complications. Common presentations include esophageal varices with variceal bleeding, portal hypertensive gastropathy, congestive splenomegaly with hypersplenism, and ascites with spontaneous bacterial peritonitis. Portal hypertension also contributes to the development of hepatic encephalopathy and hepatorenal syndrome. In general, portal hypertension secondary to a noncirrhotic etiology has a better prognosis than portal hypertension caused by liver cirrhosis because of maintained synthetic function in the former. Pathologic recognition of the characteristic morphologic features of many commonly encountered disorders underlying cirrhosis and noncirrhotic portal hypertension can aid in clinical management of patients with portal hypertension with and without cirrhosis.

References are available at expertconsult.com.

CHAPTER 75

Nonhepatic surgery in the cirrhotic patient

Truman M. Earl, Franklin Olumba, and William C. Chapman

OVERVIEW

Chronic liver disease and cirrhosis were the eleventh leading cause of death in the United States and resulted in more than 44,358 deaths in 2019.[1] Chronic viral infection (see Chapter 68) and alcohol abuse account for the majority of the disease burden globally, but the incidence of obesity-associated nonalcoholic fatty liver disease (see Chapter 69) accounts for an ever-increasing proportion of cases, especially in Western societies.[1] Clinicians continue to gain knowledge and skills to care for patients with cirrhosis in the end stages of their disease, and this has led to a significant increase in the number of patients with comorbid liver disease and cirrhosis encountered in both general and specialty surgical practice.

Cirrhosis can have dramatic effects on multiple organ systems, making surgery on the cirrhotic patient a complex and difficult undertaking (see Chapters 74 and 77). A population-based study demonstrated that people with cirrhosis, in particular those with portal hypertension, have significantly worse outcomes after elective operations than those without cirrhosis.[2] The mere act of opening the abdominal wall in a cirrhotic patient with portal hypertension causes collateral blood vessels to dilate and may lead to systemic hypotension and hepatic decompensation secondary to ischemia.[3,4] Numerous other physiologic alterations in the cirrhotic patient also require added attention perioperatively to their volume status, dosing of many common anesthetics and analgesics, and management of any coagulopathies.[5]

Extrahepatic surgery in the cirrhotic patient may be a formidable undertaking. Increased risk has led some to advise avoidance of surgery unless absolutely necessary.[6,7] However, cirrhotic patients are more likely to undergo emergency surgery than patients without cirrhosis despite worse outcomes in the emergency setting.[8–11] These patients have a 4-fold to 10-fold higher postoperative mortality rate following emergency procedures and a major complication rate 5-fold to 7-fold higher than for elective procedures.[12] For this reason, necessary extrahepatic surgeries undertaken in the elective setting are likely to be safer for the cirrhotic patient. The objective of this chapter is to provide practical knowledge on how to evaluate these patients before surgery, as well as current information on some of the most commonly performed procedures in this unique population.

EVALUATION AND STRATIFICATION OF LIVER DISEASE (SEE CHAPTER 4)

The decision regarding whether a cirrhotic patient is medically fit to undergo an operation can be difficult to make. Many factors must be considered, but the most important are the magnitude (emergent vs. elective) and type of proposed operation (major abdominal vs. orthopedic vs. high-risk cardiac), the nonhepatic comorbidities of the patient, and the severity of the liver disease. Numerous factors have been correlated with poor outcome in patients with cirrhosis—including low albumin levels, blood transfusion requirements, abnormal coagulation, and ascites—and various scoring systems to gauge these have evolved. The first developed scoring system was the Child-Turcotte-Pugh (CTP) system, which incorporates several objective and subjective variables to stratify severity of liver disease. Two older studies of operative mortality in cirrhotic patients produced nearly identical results with CTP scores of A, B, or C showing operative mortality rates of 10%, 30%, and 80%, respectively.[13,14] A retrospective review of 64 cirrhotic patients undergoing various intraabdominal and thoracic surgeries from 1999 to 2005 suggested a 1-year operative mortality rate in patients with CTP A, B, or C of 9%, 29%, and 70%, respectively. They compared the strengths of three scoring systems, further discussed below, and concluded that CTP was slightly better at estimating 30-day morbidity in this patient population.[15]

The Model for End-Stage Liver Disease (MELD) score was developed to predict death after transjugular intrahepatic portosystemic shunt (TIPS) (see Chapter 85) to stratify the risk of progression to liver failure and the need for liver transplantation. What followed was establishment of the MELD score to predict morbidity and death after nonshunt abdominal surgery.[8,16,17] As with CTP, MELD correlates with risk of postoperative death (Figs. 75.1 and 75.2). Several reports have found that MELD is superior to CTP in predicting postoperative morbidity and mortality.[17,18] More recently, integrated MELD (iMELD), which incorporates both serum sodium and age into risk calculation, has been found to be superior to both CTP and standard MELD in mortality prediction for cirrhotic patients undergoing emergency surgery.[19] Interestingly, the survival rates from the more recent series indicate a fairly dramatic improvement in survival compared with older series (Fig. 75.3).

In addition to factors considered in MELD and CTP scoring, other factors have been identified for risk stratification and prediction in cirrhotic patients undergoing major operations (see Chapter 26). These include elevated creatinine level, chronic obstructive pulmonary disease (COPD), male gender, and an American Society of Anesthesiologists (ASA) class of IV or V.[20] Teh et al.[21] developed the Mayo model and demonstrated ASA classification as a useful marker to further stratify the comorbid illness in cirrhotic patients preoperatively. This case-control study of cirrhotic patients who underwent major nontransplant operations identified MELD score, ASA class, and age as predictors of perioperative death. An ASA class of IV was equivalent to the addition of 5.5 MELD points in added risk, and age greater than 70 years was equivalent to three additional MELD points. A single point increase in MELD score was associated with a 15% increase in perioperative death in the first year. Emergency surgery predicted in-hospital death, although patients undergoing emergency operations had a higher median MELD score. ASA class V was the strongest predictor of 7-day mortality, and MELD score was the most

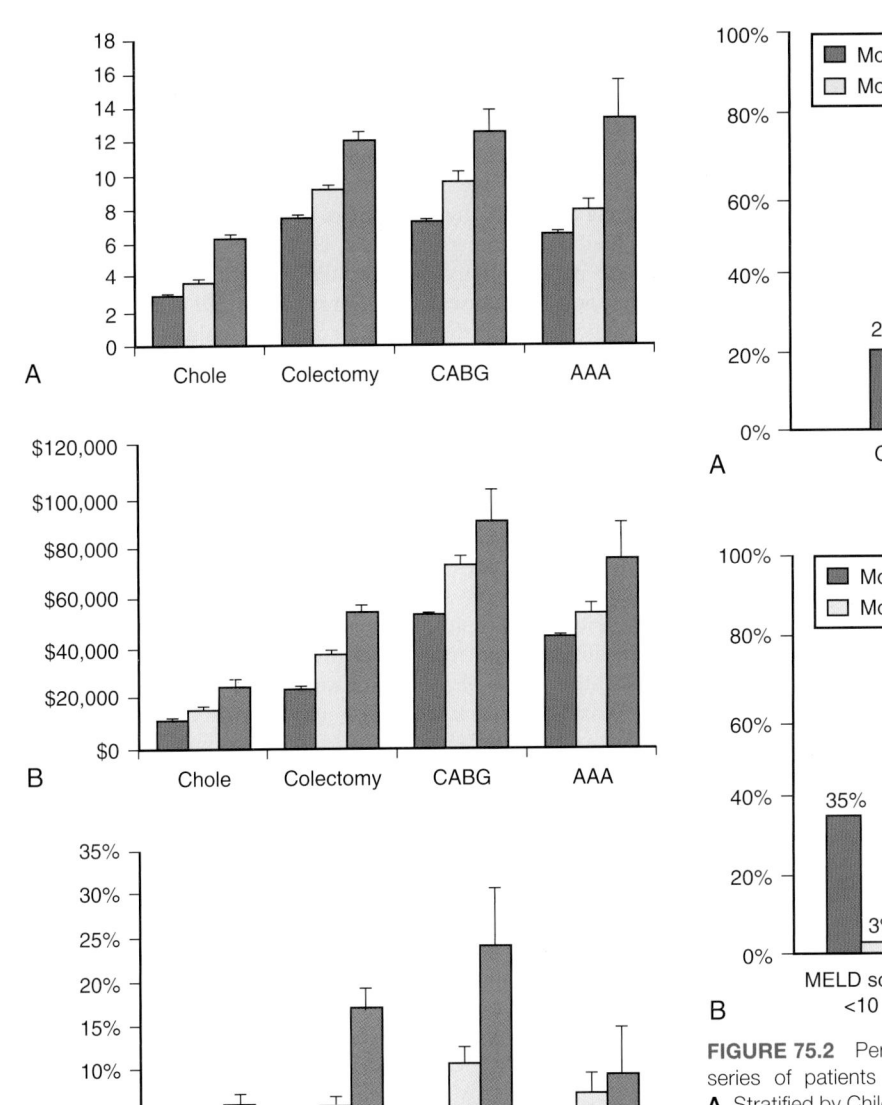

FIGURE 75.1 Outcomes for patients who underwent four index operations (cholecystectomy [Chole], colectomy, coronary artery bypass grafting [CABG], and abdominal aortic aneurysm [AAA]). **A,** Length of stay. **B,** Total charges. **C,** Mortality rate. Normal, light gray; cirrhosis, medium gray; cirrhosis complicated by portal hypertension, dark gray. (Modified from Csikesz NG, Nguyen LN, Tseng JF. Nationwide volume and mortality after elective surgery in cirrhotic patients. *J Am Coll Surg.* 2009;208:96–103.)

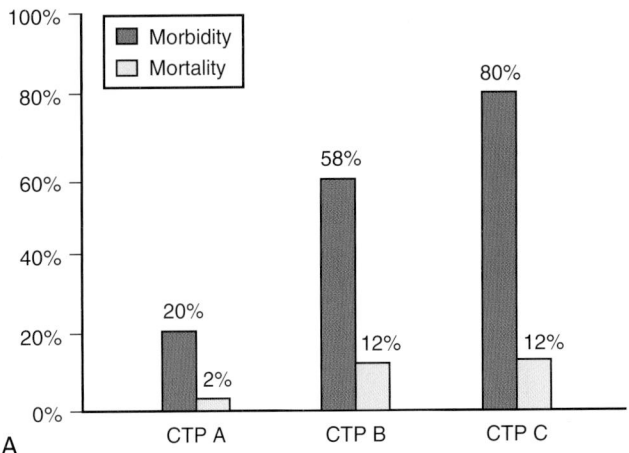
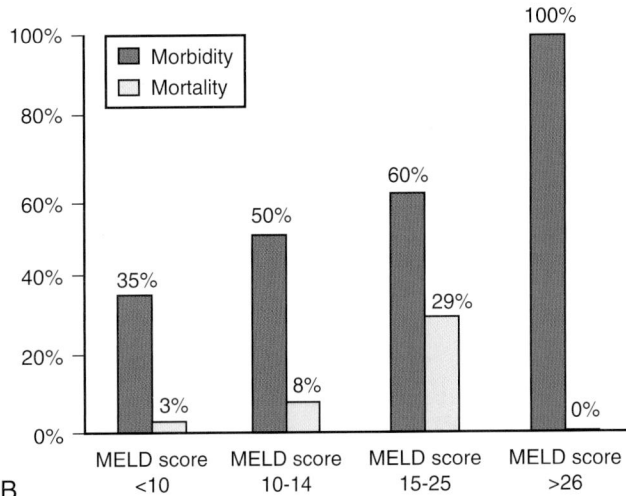

FIGURE 75.2 Perioperative morbidity and mortality rates in a recent series of patients who underwent nonhepatic abdominal surgery. **A,** Stratified by Child-Turcotte-Pugh (CTP) class. **B,** Stratified by Model for End-Stage Liver Disease (MELD) score. (Modified from Telem DA, Schiano T, Goldstone R, et al. Factors that predict outcome of abdominal operations in patients with advanced cirrhosis. *Clin Gastroenterol Hepatol.* 2010;8:451–457.)

robust predictor beyond 7 days. The median survival of patients in this series was 4.8 years for a MELD score of 0 to 7, 3.4 years for a score of 8 to 11, 1.6 years for 12 to 15, 64 days for 16 to 20, 23 days for 21 to 25, and 14 days for 26 or greater. Newer models have been developed in recent years that aim to incorporate more granular data than the Mayo model. Sato et al.[22] created the ADOPT-LC score incorporating patient age, CTP, Charlson comorbidity index, and duration of anesthesia in surgery into a risk model for in-hospital mortality of cirrhotic patients undergoing elective major surgical procedures in Japan. They found the aforementioned factors to be most predictive of in-hospital mortality and, when incorporated into a

model, produced a better Area Under Curve than CTP score alone (0.881 vs. 0.803; $P = 0.01$). One of the latest models, the VOCAL-Penn model, used data on 4712 surgical procedures (among abdominal wall reconstruction, vascular, cardiac, chest, orthopedic, and abdominal surgeries) in 3785 cirrhotic patients to develop a model more predictive of postoperative mortality than the Mayo risk score, MELD, MELD-Na, or CTP at 30 and 90 days.[23] The VOCAL-Penn model included many of the same predictors as the Mayo model but also featured emergency indication and a surgery-specific category. The investigators were able to achieve a C-statistic for prediction of postoperative mortality significantly higher than all other model scores at 30 and 90 days in both their derivation and validation cohorts. However, this and other models developed in recent years have yet to be externally validated, and CTP and MELD-Na remain the commonly used models for morbidity and mortality prediction specifically in cirrhotic patients undergoing surgical procedures.

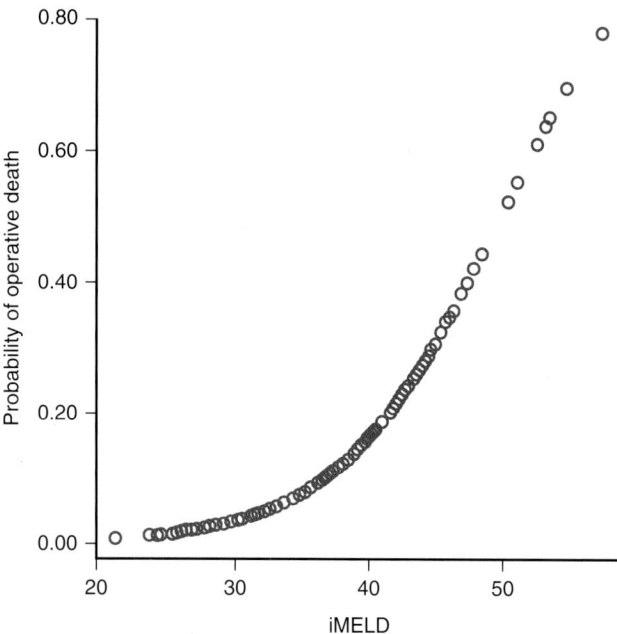

FIGURE 75.3 Relationship between the predicted probability of operative death and Integrated Model for End-Stage Liver Disease (iMELD) in 190 patients with cirrhosis who underwent operation. (Modified from Costa BP. Value of MELD and MELD-based indices in surgical risk evaluation of cirrhotic patients: Retrospective analysis of 190 cases. *World J Surg.* 2009;33:1711.)

PERIOPERATIVE MANAGEMENT AND OPTIMIZATION

The perioperative management of patients with cirrhosis involves aggressive attempts to control the various manifestations of their underlying disease. Much of this is covered at length in other chapters (see Chapters 26 and 77). Nonetheless, a few considerations are worth mentioning here.

In patients with liver cirrhosis the protein-energy malnutrition can range from 20% to 60% depending on clinical stage of chronic liver disease, placing them at an increased risk for developing a variety of postoperative complications, such as wound dehiscence, infections, reaccumulation of ascites, and death.[24,25] Nutritional status should be evaluated preoperatively; when found to be deficient, efforts should be undertaken to improve it (see Chapter 26).

Classically, cirrhotic patients were thought to be in a hypocoagulable state due to impaired hepatic synthesis of clotting factors, decreased vitamin K stores, thrombocytopenia and abnormal laboratory tests of coagulation such as prothrombin time (PT), international normalized ratio (INR), and activated partial thromboplastin time. The literature now supports a hypothesis of "rebalanced hemostasis" due to concomitant decreases in both procoagulant and anticoagulant proteins.[26] Thrombocytopenia is compensated by increases in von Willebrand factor and factor VIII levels. These alterations are not detected on standard laboratory measures of coagulation parameters. Moreover, when spontaneous bleeding does occur, it is usually of hemodynamic origin due to the presence of portal hypertension.[27] In the operating room, careful tissue handling and the maintenance of a low central venous pressure are other factors that can help to minimize blood loss.[28] Direct measurements of clot formation,

propagation, and fibrinolysis, such as thromboelastography, have proven useful in limiting blood product utilization during liver transplantation and may be helpful in reducing bleeding in other situations.[29-31] If significant bleeding arises, administration of cryoprecipitate, diamino-8-D-arginine vasopressin, antifibrinolytics, or recombinant factor VIIa may be necessary to reverse coagulopathy and control hemorrhage.[32]

In the perioperative period, altered mental status in a cirrhotic patient should be thoroughly evaluated. Only after all other potential causes have been ruled out can hepatic encephalopathy be reliably diagnosed. Lactulose should be administered and titrated for three soft bowel movements a day. Rifaximin has been shown to effectively reverse hepatic encephalopathy, and concomitant administration with lactulose was found to be more effective than lactulose alone in a randomized trial of encephalopathic patients.[33] Postoperatively, the administration of narcotics and other sedating medications should be kept to a minimum. There is no role for prophylactic lactulose therapy for asymptomatic cirrhotic patients undergoing surgery[32] (see Chapter 77).

Perioperative fluid management in cirrhotic patients can be very difficult. Patients with cirrhosis should be adequately resuscitated to avoid hypotension and hepatic ischemia, but fluids should also be given judiciously to minimize bleeding attributable to portal hypertension and the accumulation of ascites postoperatively. One center that performs a large volume of surgery on patients with end-stage liver disease limits the infusion of crystalloid solutions in the perioperative period.[34] Instead, all patients with advanced liver disease are placed on a postoperative sodium-poor albumin drip until they can resume oral intake. Albumin infusion has been shown to have a number of beneficial effects in cirrhotic patients beyond simple volume expansion and increase in plasma oncotic pressure.[35] It reduces mortality in patients with spontaneous bacterial peritonitis; improves outcome following large-volume paracentesis; and, in combination with vasoconstrictors, is useful in the management of hepatorenal syndrome. These effects of exogenous albumin are due to volume expansion, immunomodulation, and endothelial stabilization through increase in the effective albumin concentration.[35]

Ascites increases the risk of postoperative renal failure, infections, and wound dehiscence. Even if ascites is drained at the time of surgery, it rapidly reaccumulates in the postoperative period. Medical therapy, which includes salt restriction and diuretics, is typically considered the first line of treatment. TIPS, however, may be considered a first-line treatment for refractory ascites and may be placed before elective surgery to help control ascites throughout the entire perioperative period.[36-38] Moreover, TIPS may also reduce the risk of significant perioperative bleeding. In one of the largest series on the use of TIPS in patients undergoing major extrahepatic surgery, 25 cirrhotic patients with a mean MELD score of 15 ± 7.6 underwent TIPS at a median of 20 days before major abdominal and cardiothoracic operations. Blood transfusions were relatively minimal in the series, with a median of 3 units for abdominal operations (range, 0–21) and 4 units for cardiothoracic operations (range, 0–20). With a median follow-up of 33 months, actuarial 1-year patient survival was 74%, and the three postoperative deaths in the series occurred in patients with MELD scores higher than 24, all of whom underwent emergent surgery.[39] Studies that compare outcomes after surgery with preoperative TIPS placement versus those with no

TIPS, however, are lacking. Also, the optimal time interval between TIPS placement and elective surgery is unclear, but it is common for a period of several weeks to be required to see a clinical improvement in ascitic volume after TIPS; therefore shunts should probably be placed several weeks before planned operations (see Chapter 85.

SPECIFIC PROCEDURES

Cholecystectomy

The incidence of gallstones in patients with cirrhosis is twice that of the general population as a result of increased intravascular hemolysis and decreased gallbladder motility and emptying[40–42] (see Chapter 33). In the 1980s, rates of major morbidity and mortality in patients with cirrhosis undergoing cholecystectomy were as high as 35% and 25%, respectively.[13,43–45] Postoperative death occurred secondary to blood loss, sepsis, and liver failure. Almost invariably, these procedures were performed as open laparotomy. At that time, the presence of cirrhosis was considered a contraindication for the laparoscopic approach, based on the assumption that it would lead to increased rates bleeding and liver failure.[46] However, numerous studies have demonstrated favorable morbidity and minimal to no mortality in patients with early cirrhosis (CTP class A and B) undergoing laparoscopic cholecystectomy.[47–54] A meta-analysis comparing laparoscopic cholecystectomy in cirrhotic and noncirrhotic patients demonstrated significantly higher rates of morbidity (21% vs. 8%, respectively; $P < .001$), intraoperative bleeding (26% vs. 3%; $P < .001$), and open conversion (7% vs. 4%; $P < .05$), but no difference was reported in terms of wound infection and mortality rates between the two.[53] A more recent VA Surgical Quality Improvement Program analysis confirmed similar results with 18.7% morbidity and 3.8% mortality rates.[55] MELD score was a significant predictor of both complications and 90-day mortality with odds ratio (OR) 1.1 (confidence interval [CI] 1.02–1.20; $P = .016$) and OR 1.21 (CI 1.08–1.35; $P = .01$), respectively. Current data still support the use of CTP class for assessment of mortality risk in patients with liver cirrhosis undergoing laparoscopic cholecystectomy.

Laparoscopic cholecystectomy offers improved visualization for meticulous dissection and avoids the need for a large subcostal or upper midline incision (see Chapter 36). It is associated with less operative blood loss, shorter operative time, and decreased length of hospital stay versus the open procedure in cirrhotic patients.[56] Furthermore, a retrospective study from the National Inpatient Sample (NIS) demonstrated increased in-hospital morbidity and mortality in cirrhotic patients undergoing open cholecystectomy compared with laparoscopic cholecystectomy.[57] Meta-analysis comparing laparoscopic and open approaches in cirrhotics found that laparoscopic cholecystectomy appeared to be associated with shorter operative time, reduced complication rates, and reduced length of hospital stay.[55,58]

Some specific technical considerations must be considered when performing laparoscopic cholecystectomy in a cirrhotic patient. In placing the umbilical port, particular care must be taken to avoid venous collaterals and the umbilical vein. One approach may be to place one of the other ports first, such as the subxiphoid port, in order to then place the umbilical port under direct visualization. Transillumination of the abdominal wall helps the surgeon to avoid these and other venous collaterals during trocar placement or by use of preoperative computed

tomography if one was performed.[59] Furthermore, the subxiphoid port should be placed off midline to avoid the falciform ligament and the recanalized umbilical vein. Careful traction on the gallbladder helps to avoid avulsion and undue bleeding as it is dissected off the liver. Instruments such as the Harmonic Scalpel (Ethicon, Somerville, NJ) or LigaSure (Covidien, Mansfield, MA) may also be used to help control bleeding during the dissection.[60–63] A subtotal or supracystic cholecystectomy, leaving part of the gallbladder wall attached to the liver bed and ligating the cystic duct from within the gallbladder with a purse-string suture, is an option in patients with large pericholecystic venous collaterals,[64] as is the case generally for the "difficult gallbladder" (see Chapters 34 and 36). In a 2015 systematic review and meta-analysis of subtotal cholecystectomy for "difficult gallbladders" (which included cholelithiasis and cholecystitis in CTP class A and B cirrhotics) it was found that subtotal cholecystectomy had a similar morbidity rate compared with total cholecystectomy done for simple cases (also see Chapter 34).[65] Trocars should also be removed under direct visualization to ensure adequate abdominal wall hemostasis at the end of the procedure. Finally, if anatomy is unclear or any doubt exists as to the safety of continuing laparoscopically, the procedure should be converted to open. In patients with advanced cirrhosis (CTP class C), cholecystectomy in general is associated with very poor outcomes.[66] Despite the lack of controlled trials, the literature supports the use of alternatives to cholecystectomy, such as a percutaneous cholecystostomy, in this high-risk group.[50,66,67] An alternative option is an endoscopically placed cystic duct stent, although the expertise for this is not widely available and there is a lack of studies demonstrating convincing superiority to percutaneous approach in this high-risk group.[68–70]

Both CTP and MELD are useful predictors of postoperative morbidity and mortality and few data support one scoring system over the other (see Chapter 4). CTP A and B patients can be operated on with acceptable outcomes. The exact cutoff value for MELD varies among studies.[18,67] In CTP classes A and B patients and, in general, in patients with MELD score less than 15, laparoscopic cholecystectomy can be considered but should likely be performed at centers experienced in managing cirrhosis. In patients with class C cirrhosis, surgery should be deferred until liver disease is better compensated, and alternate interventions, such as percutaneous cholecystostomy or endoscopic stenting, should be employed either as definitive therapy or as a bridge to cholecystectomy under better circumstances.

Herniorrhaphy

Umbilical hernias occur in up to 20% of patients with cirrhosis. The pathogenesis of umbilical hernias in the setting of cirrhosis is multifactorial; ascites causes increased intraabdominal pressure, poor nutritional status leads to decreased abdominal muscle mass and fascial strength, and umbilical vein dilation results in enlargement of the preexisting supraumbilical fascial opening.[71] In addition to the risks of bowel incarceration and strangulation that affect all patients with umbilical hernias, additional unique risks accompany having an umbilical hernia and cirrhosis. Skin ulceration over the hernia may be associated with the leakage of ascites, sac rupture, bacterial peritonitis, and even evisceration, with very high attendant rates of morbidity and mortality. Although rare, spontaneous umbilical rupture and ascites leak known as "Flood syndrome" is associated with up to a 60% perioperative mortality rate and has been shown to correlate independently with an adverse outcome after emergent repair.[34,72]

Historically, mortality rates for umbilical hernia repair (UHR) in patients with cirrhosis were prohibitively high, and the prevailing opinion among surgeons was that uncomplicated hernias should be left untreated.[73,74] UHR was only undertaken when complications, such as incarceration, strangulation, skin breakdown, impending rupture, or overt rupture, necessitated immediate intervention. In the present era, however, outcomes appear to be significantly improved for elective and even complicated UHR in patients with end-stage liver disease. Most series published in the literature since the early 1980s have reported few to no perioperative deaths and relatively low morbidity, although most of them have been relatively small retrospective studies.[75-78]

Marsman et al.[79] looked at outcomes of elective UHR versus conservative management in patients with umbilical hernias, cirrhosis, and ascites. Seventeen patients with a median MELD score of 23 (range, 18–26) underwent elective UHR, and another 13 patients, also with a median MELD score of 23 (range, 18–27), were observed. In the elective UHR group, 3 patients (18%) had local wound complications, but there were no instances of hepatic decompensation or perioperative death. In contrast, in the group that was observed, 10 patients (77%) developed complications, including nine cases of incarceration and one spontaneous rupture with evisceration; these led to emergency UHR in six patients, and there were two perioperative deaths (15%). Several other studies have found increased complications of patients treated emergently and advocate for elective repair of suitable patients not expecting imminent liver transplantation.[11,80]

A retrospective review of the Veterans' Affairs National Surgical Quality Improvement Program (VA NSQIP) database analyzed the results of UHR in 127 cirrhotic and 1294 noncirrhotic patients.[10] It determined that UHR performed electively in patients with cirrhosis was associated with an outcome similar to that in patients without cirrhosis. When UHR was performed emergently, however, patients with cirrhosis had significantly worse outcomes than those without. One drawback of this study was that the authors were not able to classify the degree of hepatic impairment among the patients with cirrhosis.

In patients with ascites, UHR has been combined with peritoneovenous (PV) shunting, closed-system suction drainage, or temporary peritoneal dialysis catheters to help manage ascites as the repairs heal.[76,81-84] A review of published studies compared UHR with concomitant interventions to control ascites versus repair alone and determined that uncontrolled ascites was associated with a relative risk ratio of 8.51 (95% CI, 2.69–26.9) for hernia recurrence.[85] Although PV shunting cannot be recommended in the current era because of the associated complications and high incidence of shunt occlusion, TIPS has been used more recently to successfully reduce refractory ascites in the period surrounding UHR.[34,86] Although the therapeutic benefit of TIPS for refractory ascites is well documented, no studies exist regarding its efficacy to reduce complications of elective umbilical hernia repair. It is, however, an important consideration in the management of ascites in patients under consideration for hernia repair.

Whether nonabsorbable mesh should be used for the repair in cirrhotic patients is another issue of debate. Traditionally, the use of foreign material has been avoided in the repair of complicated hernias. However, some evidence suggests that nonabsorbable mesh may be used successfully, even when ascites is present.[77,87] A study published in 2010 prospectively randomized 80 CTP class A and B patients with cirrhosis and an umbilical hernia to either primary tissue repair with sutures or mesh repair with polypropylene onlay.[84] Surgical site infection occurred at a higher rate in the mesh group (16%) versus suture repair (9%), but the difference was not significant. Furthermore, all infections were successfully managed conservatively and did not require mesh removal. At a minimum of 6 months of follow-up, hernias recurred in 14% of patients in the suture repair group and in only 3% of patients in the mesh repair group ($P < .05$). Current data support the use of mesh for umbilical hernia repair in cirrhotic patients, even those with ascites, and may reduce risk of recurrence. In those patients with well-compensated disease, elective repair may be advocated due to high risk of complications following emergent repair.[80]

The results of inguinal hernia repair in this patient population are similar to those for umbilical herniorrhaphy.[88-90] Outcomes after elective repair do not vary between cirrhotic and noncirrhotic patients, although outcomes after emergent repair of an incarcerated or strangulated inguinal hernia are significantly worse in patients with cirrhosis.[91] It appears that cirrhotic patients may safely undergo inguinal hernia repair with mesh; local wound complications, if they do arise, are usually easily treated.[89,90] Moreover, quality of life improves after elective inguinal hernia repair in symptomatic patients with cirrhosis.[88] In short, it is reasonable, and the data would suggest even advisable, to repair hernias electively in patients with cirrhosis. However, as with any elective operation, patients should be well compensated and ascites controlled.

Colectomy

Compared with cholecystectomy and herniorrhaphy, considerably less data are available on colon resection in patients with chronic liver disease and cirrhosis. Available data suggest that colectomy is particularly high risk for those with cirrhosis and portal hypertension with mortality rates around 20% to 25%.[92-94] Emergent colectomy is associated with an even higher mortality rate: up to 36% in patients with cirrhosis who have portal hypertension and 21% in those with portal hypertension who did not have cirrhosis.[94]

In a large, population-based study, Nguyen et al.[94] found that patients with cirrhosis and cirrhosis with portal hypertension had significantly higher in-hospital mortality than patients with no cirrhosis (14% and 29% vs. 5%, respectively, $P < .0001$). Extraintestinal complications, such as pulmonary and wound complications, are increased in patients with cirrhosis and portal hypertension.[95] In another retrospective, single-center study that included 41 cirrhotic patients undergoing colorectal surgery (CTP class A, 40%; class B, 49%; class C, 12%), the presence of preoperative ascites was significantly linked to postoperative morbidity.[93] As with other abdominal procedures, MELD has been shown to be an independent predictor of postoperative mortality following colorectal surgery.[96]

When feasible, the laparoscopic approach for colectomy may be advantageous in this patient population. A recent retrospective review of NSQIP data looked at laparoscopic versus open partial colectomy for colon cancer in patients with ascites.[97] The authors found that laparoscopic colectomy was associated with decreased complications (adjusted OR 0.7 95% CI 0.4–1.0, $P = 0.046$) and shorter hospital stay (9 days vs. 15 days, adjusted $\beta = -4.2$, 95% CI -7.7 to -0.7, $P = 0.018$). The cohort undergoing laparoscopic colectomy notably had fewer preexisting comorbidities and smoked less, although they were similar in ASA classification and functional status. Nonetheless, laparoscopic colectomy is feasible in well-selected cirrhotic patients and may offer benefit over traditional open resection in terms of complication burden.

Bariatric Surgery

Because of the high incidence of nonalcoholic fatty liver disease (NAFLD) and its association with the metabolic syndrome, chronic liver disease is not infrequent among patients being considered for bariatric procedures. The finding of overt cirrhosis is estimated to occur in 1.4% of patients undergoing these operations.[98] Of 2119 patients undergoing laparoscopic roux-en-Y gastric bypass, 30 were found to be cirrhotic with all patients classified as CTP class A. Nine patients experienced complications and the average length of stay was 4 days. Mosko et al.[99] analyzed patients undergoing bariatric procedures in the Nationwide Inpatient Sample (NIS) from 1998 to 2007 and found higher mortality rates among cirrhotics. After adjusting for covariates, the adjusted odds ratio of mortality for compensated and decompensated cirrhosis compared with noncirrhotic patients was 2.17 (95% CI, 1.03–4.55) and 21.2 (95% CI, 5.39–82.9), respectively.

Despite the increased risk, several reports document the reversal of even advanced liver disease after surgical weight loss.[100–102] Improvements in fibrosis, necroinflammatory changes, and steatosis have been documented after surgical weight loss (see Chapter 7). Therefore it appears that bariatric surgery may be reasonable in patients with early fibrosis and possibly in those with well-compensated cirrhosis. As outlined earlier, the risk inherent to the procedure, severity of liver disease, and comorbid conditions must be considered individually along with the potential benefit of surgical weight loss.

The choice of weight loss procedure in those deemed candidates is also unclear.[103,104] The optimal procedure regarding weight loss remains under intense debate in the bariatric surgical community and is beyond the scope of this chapter. However, the suggestion has been made that sleeve gastrectomy may be the procedure of choice in patients with cirrhosis because of minimal bleeding complications, protection from malabsorption associated with other bariatric procedures, preservation of endoscopic access to the biliary tree, and potential improvement in transplant candidacy.[105,106] No studies evaluating the use of adjustable gastric bands in cirrhotic patients are available.

Cardiac Procedures

Cardiovascular risk factors occur at greater rates among those with cirrhosis than among the general population.[107] Because of these and other factors, cardiac surgery is becoming increasingly more frequent in patients with end-stage liver disease, in particular those awaiting liver transplantation.[108] Cardiac surgery, however, is extremely risky in patients with cirrhosis. Mortality rates are as high as 50% to 80% in patients with advanced liver disease undergoing cardiac surgery with cardiopulmonary bypass (CPB) because of high rates of infection, gastrointestinal complications, and bleeding.[109–111]

Outcomes for cirrhotic patients undergoing cardiac surgery have variably been associated with serum bilirubin and platelet count.[112–115] More consistently, however, outcomes have been linked to the preoperative CTP or MELD score. CTP class B and C and/or a MELD score greater than 13 to 15 have been shown to correlate with a significantly increased risk for postoperative complications and death in cirrhotic patients undergoing cardiac procedures, in particular those involving CPB.[108,113,114,116,117] One systematic review including 939 patients undergoing cardiac surgeries found mean in-hospital mortality rates of 8.92%, 31.38%, and 47.62% and late mortality rates (death after hospital discharge) of 20.58%, 43.58%, and 56.48% for CTP classes A, B, and C, respectively.[118]

CPB induces the production of inflammatory cytokines and other vasoactive substances and leads to further derangements in hemodynamics, coagulation, and immune function. Advanced cirrhosis (CTP class B and C) is considered a contraindication for CPB.[113,114,116] A few reports, however, have described successful on-pump valve procedures in patients with advanced liver disease.[119–121] By preoperative optimization of hepatic status, aggressive administration of platelets and fresh frozen plasma throughout the perioperative period, and dilutional ultrafiltration (DUF) during CPB, these investigators were able to curtail the negative effects of CPB in patients with decompensated disease. DUF in particular helps to minimize hemodilution and remove inflammatory mediators produced during CPB.[120]

Another option that has shown modest success in patients with moderate to severe cirrhosis in need of coronary artery bypass (CAB) is off-pump (OPCAB) surgery.[116,122,123] OPCAB may reduce bleeding and transfusion requirements. In analysis of the NIS databases, Gopaldas et al.[124] found that cirrhosis was independently associated with increased mortality, morbidity, length of stay, and hospital charge. However, in patients undergoing OPCAB the presence of cirrhosis did not affect mortality or morbidity unless there was severe liver dysfunction. Those undergoing on-pump CAB had increased mortality and morbidity regardless of severity of liver disease.

Thoracic Procedures

The literature on thoracic surgery in patients with cirrhosis primarily describes thoracoscopic procedures for the treatment of hepatic hydrothorax, a complication that occurs in approximately 4% to 12% of cirrhotic patients.[125,126] It is a symptomatic transudative pleural effusion that is believed to arise secondary to tiny defects in the diaphragm that allow ascites to flow from the high-pressure peritoneal cavity into the low-pressure pleural space.[127,128] Hepatic hydrothorax may result in significant respiratory compromise, and initial treatments include sodium restriction, diuretics, frequent thoracenteses, and TIPS (see Chapter 85). When these fail, or patients are not candidates for TIPS, indwelling tunneled pleural catheters, video-assisted thoracoscopic surgery (VATS) with closure of obvious diaphragmatic defects, and mechanical or chemical pleurodesis are options that may allow prolonged symptomatic relief.[129–133] Problems with indwelling catheters include infection risk, occlusions, and pain around the catheter site.[134] Potential complications of pleurodesis include empyema and persistent leakage of high volumes of ascites from the chest tube site. Nonetheless, the procedure is relatively well tolerated and is associated with success rates of up to 80%, even in patients with advanced cirrhosis.[135] However, no guidelines yet exist for the optimal procedure in cases of refractory hepatic hydrothorax, and many of these patients are already candidates for orthotopic liver transplantation.

Cirrhosis is present in approximately 4% to 7% of patients undergoing esophagectomy in some series.[136–138] Actual rates of cirrhosis in patients with esophageal neoplasms are likely higher than reported, because alcohol plays an important role in the pathogenesis of both diseases. Stage for stage, many more cirrhotics than noncirrhotics would be deemed unsuitable for surgery. Unlike gastric resection, esophagectomy in cirrhotic patients is actually associated with relatively few deaths as a result of postoperative liver failure, in theory because of the radical gastroesophageal devascularization and postoperative anorexia, which may lead to a significant reduction in alcohol consumption.[137] Nonetheless, esophagectomy in cirrhotic patients is associated with much higher rates of surgical morbidity and mortality compared with noncirrhotics, in the range of 31% to 87% and 17% to 26%, respectively.[136-138] Perioperative bleeding, ascitic effusions, pneumonia, and sepsis are the most common complications and cause the majority of postoperative deaths. Significant preoperative coagulopathy, hyperbilirubinemia (>3 mg/dL), weight loss (>10%–15% of body weight), and CTP classes B and C are associated with the highest rates of postoperative death and may be considered contraindications for surgery. For patients surviving the immediate postoperative period, however, overall survival appears to be similar to that of noncirrhotic patients undergoing the same procedures.[137,139]

Trauma

Cirrhotic patients represent approximately 1% to 1.5% of the trauma population and an even greater proportion of those sustaining blunt trauma.[140,141] In these patients, falls are the most common cause of injury (43%), followed by assault.[140,142] Complications occur in up to 10% of patients and primarily include acute respiratory distress syndrome, trauma-associated coagulopathy, pneumonia, and sepsis.[140,143] In-hospital mortality rates are high, in the range of 22% to 33%. The CTP classification appears to be associated with a stepwise increase in the risk of death: 8.0% in class A, 32.3% in class B, and 45.5% in class C.[144]

Cirrhotic trauma patients are significantly more likely than those without cirrhosis to undergo laparotomy, and splenectomy is one of the most common operations performed.[140,143] This is not surprising given the prevalence of portal hypertension and splenomegaly among these patients. Among cirrhotic patients,

nonoperative management of splenic injury fails in up to 92% of patients and cirrhosis is an independent risk factor for splenectomy in blunt trauma patients.[145-147] Multivariate analyses from several studies have demonstrated that after laparotomy, 40% to 55% of cirrhotic patients ultimately die in the hospital, versus only 15% to 24% of those who avoid laparotomy.[140,143,144,148]

Obviously, management of these patients is highly complex. The American College of Surgeons recommends that trauma patients with a history of cirrhosis be transferred to a trauma center, if they are not at one already,[149] and should be very carefully resuscitated and monitored in an intensive care setting. Bleeding complications are common, and coagulopathy and hypothermia should be aggressively corrected. Because these patients are almost routinely malnourished, nutritional support should be started early, arguably with branched chain amino acid supplementation.[150,151] It is imperative to promptly diagnose injuries in these patients, although interventions should be undertaken judiciously.

SUMMARY

In general, nonhepatic elective surgery may be safely performed in patients with well-compensated cirrhosis. There is certainly almost always an increase in morbidity and mortality when compared with patients without chronic liver disease; however, often these are not prohibitive. The severity of liver failure as judged by the CTP or MELD scoring systems appears to be the most important factor in determining postoperative outcomes. CTP class A or B cirrhotic patients and those with a MELD score less than 15 are often suitable operative candidates, depending on the magnitude and necessity of the procedure. Emergency operations carry greater risk, as does comorbid illness and age. Postoperative complications such as liver decompensation, infection, renal failure, and ascites should be anticipated. Perhaps most important, operations on cirrhotic patients should be performed only after medical optimization of liver disease and only by centers experienced in managing end-stage liver disease.

The references for this chapter can be found online by accessing the accompanying Expert Consult website.

CHAPTER 76

Portal hypertension in children

Nadia Naz and Janis M. Stoll

Normal pressure in the portal venous system ranges from 5 to 10 mm Hg. Portal hypertension is defined as portal venous pressure exceeding 10 mm Hg. Hepatic venous pressure gradient (HVPG) is a surrogate marker of portal hypertension. Normal HVPG is between 1 and 4 mm Hg. Portal hypertension develops when HVPG is more than 5 mm Hg. HVPG greater than 10 mm Hg is the prediction of the development of varices in adults.[1] Data are limited in children but suggest that there may be similar pressure thresholds for the development of complications in the pediatric population.[2]

PATHOPHYSIOLOGY OF PORTAL HYPERTENSION (SEE CHAPTERS 5 AND 74)

The portal system is a low-pressure venous system that carries partially oxygenated blood to the liver, whereas the liver receives highly oxygenated blood through hepatic arteries. Both systems combine within the sinusoidal spaces. Portal hypertension occurs when there is either increased portal resistance or increased portal blood flow. Varices are abnormal venous communications between the portal and systemic circulation that develop to decrease the pressure in the portal venous system.

Etiology (see Chapter 74)

In broad terms, portal hypertension is divided into two categories, cirrhotic secondary to chronic liver disease and noncirrhotic, for example, due to portal venous occlusion, congenital hepatic fibrosis (CHF), nodular regenerative hyperplasia (NRH), nonalcoholic fatty liver disease (NAFLD), sinusoidal obstruction syndrome (SOS), rare metabolic diseases (Gaucher and Zellweger syndromes), schistosomiasis, and hepatoportal sclerosis. On the other hand, pediatric portal hypertension can be categorized into three main types, prehepatic, hepatic, and posthepatic, as described in Box 76.1. Overall, the most common cause of portal hypertension in children is as a result of intrahepatic, sinusoidal causes from a variety of liver diseases predominantly from biliary atresia. Extrahepatic portal vein obstruction (EHPVO) is the most common cause of noncirrhotic portal hypertension in children. Causes of EHPVO are summarized in Box 76.2.

Clinical Presentation (see Chapter 79)

Gastrointestinal Bleeding

Gastrointestinal hemorrhage from variceal bleeding is the most frequent presentation (in about two-thirds of cases) of portal hypertension in children (see Chapters 80–83). Varices are abnormal venous communications between the portal and systemic circulation that develop to decrease the pressure in the portal venous system (see Chapter 5). [8]When the portal vein is congested, collateral blood vessels develop at the junction of the high-pressure portal vein and low-pressure systemic vein forming varices, mainly in the esophagus and stomach but also around the umbilicus and rectum. Gastroesophageal varices are more prone to bleeding because of their location and exposure to acid and food. In children with short bowel syndrome, stomal varices are a site for low resistance and a common source of hemorrhage. Gastrointestinal bleeding can present with hematemesis or melena. Gastrointestinal bleeding from ruptured varices often follows upper respiratory tract infection, fever, or nonsteroidal antiinflammatory drug (NSAID) ingestion. It can also occur in the setting of prolonged gastroesophageal reflux as a result of erosions over the varices. In adults HVPG of 12 mm Hg appears to predict the risk of bleeding from esophageal varices.[1] There is limited data; however, mortality associated with first variceal bleed in children has been reported close to 1%.[3–7] This may be because biliary atresia and extrahepatic portal vein thrombosis are two common causes of portal hypertension in children, and portal hypertension develops during the early course of these disease processes when the liver is very well compensated.

The classification of esophageal varices is based on endoscopic findings. There are some interobserver variations regarding the grading of esophageal varices. The most accepted classification is as follows[8]:

Grade 0   No esophageal varices

Grade 1   Small and nontortuous esophageal varices

Grade 2   Tortuous varices but limited to less than one-third of the distal esophageal radius

Grade 3   Large and tortuous esophageal varices occupying greater than one-third of the distal esophagus radius

According to the Japanese Research Society for Portal Hypertension, grading of esophageal varices can also be described as follows[9]:

Grade 1: Flattened by insufflation.

Grade 2 and 3: Not flattened by insufflation. Confluency differentiates grade 2 from 3, with grade 3 confluent around the circumference of the esophagus.

Splenomegaly

Splenomegaly is the second most common finding in children with portal hypertension. Hypersplenism manifests as left upper quadrant discomfort or pain; incidental finding on physical exam; and less commonly by thrombocytopenia, leukopenia, petechia, or ecchymosis. Splenic size does not appear to correlate with portal hypertension.[10,11] It rarely requires surgical intervention in cases of symptomatic anemia or severe physical discomfort.[12]

BOX 76.1   Causes of Portal Hypertension in Children

Prehepatic
Portal vein thrombosis
Superior mesenteric vein thrombosis
Splenic vein thrombosis
Congenital stenosis of the portal vein

Hepatic
Presinusoidal
Idiopathic portal hypertension
Primary sclerosing cholangitis
Primary biliary cirrhosis
Sinusoidal
Biliary atresia
Autoimmune hepatitis
Wilson disease
Hepatitis B and C
α_1 Antitrypsin deficiency
Glycogen storage disease type IV
Toxins (vitamin A toxicity)
Cystic fibrosis
Congenital hepatic fibrosis
Caroli disease
Choledochal cyst
Familial cholestasis
Gaucher disease
Steatohepatitis
Peliosis hepatis
Schistosomiasis

Post Sinusoidal/Post Hepatic
Budd-Chiari syndrome
Hepatic vein occlusion
Congestive right-sided heart failure
Inferior vena cava obstruction

BOX 76.2   Causes of Extrahepatic Portal Vein Obstruction

Idiopathic
Prothrombotic state
   Portal vein injury
   Umbilical vein catheterization
   Abdominal surgery
   Trauma
   Liver transplantation
Local inflammatory conditions
   Intraabdominal abscess
   Abdominal sepsis
   Inflammatory bowel disease
   Pancreatitis
   Omphalitis
   Severe dehydration

Ascites

Ascites is one of the major complications of portal hypertension. It likely develops because of sodium and fluid retention as a result of increased portal pressure. Ascites might be a presenting sign in 7% to 21% of children with portal hypertension.[13] Paracentesis in children is safe but only reserved for cases when ascites is refractory for treatment and causing respiratory compromise or concern for peritonitis to perform cell count and culture. Treatment includes salt restriction and diuretic therapy. The diuretic of choice is spironolactone, but combination treatment with furosemide might be necessary for patients who do not respond to spironolactone alone. Albumin infusion may be needed to increase intravascular osmotic pressure followed by diuretic dosing.

Hepatopulmonary Syndrome

Hepatopulmonary syndrome (HPS) is characterized by abnormal blood oxygenation as a result of intrapulmonary vascular dilation in advanced liver disease. There are two forms of HPS, type I and type II. In type I the vessels enlarge such that the red blood cells traveling through the center of the vessel do not have significant contact time with the oxygen-rich alveoli. In type II HPS the diffusion perfusion mismatch is presumed to be caused by arteriovenous communications completely bypassing alveoli. The most common symptom is exertional dyspnea, but others include fatigue, palpitations, syncope, and chest pain.

Other clinical presentations of portal hypertension include hepatic encephalopathy, growth failure, coagulopathy, biliopathy, and increased intestinal permeability.

Diagnosis of Portal Hypertension (see Chapter 79)

HVPG is a surrogate marker to measure portal venous pressure. It is measured by introducing a catheter, which is wedged into the hepatic vein via the femoral or transjugular approach. This pressure is known as wedge hepatic venous pressure (WHVP). The catheter is then retracted into a free-flowing hepatic vein, and this pressure is known as free hepatic venous pressure (FHVP). The difference between WHVP and FHVP is known as HVPG. HVPG measurements are feasible in the pediatric population, but given the invasive nature of the procedure HVPG should only be performed by clinicians with complete understanding of the specific elements required for accurate measurements. In children with chronic liver disease who require a liver biopsy for clinical indication or children with heart disease who require cardiac catheterization, HVPG measurements can be performed at the same time. Normal HVPG ranges from 1 to 4 mm Hg. Portal hypertension develops when HVPG exceeds more than 5 mm Hg. The cause of portal hypertension can be roughly suggested by the HVPG. In presinusoidal obstruction HVPG is normal; however, WHVP is elevated. In portal hypertension secondary to cirrhosis, usually, both HVPG and WHVP are increased.

Management of Portal Hypertension in Children

There has been continuous advancement in understanding and optimizing the management of portal hypertension in adults. There are limited numbers of randomized trials and prospective data in children regarding the management of pediatric liver diseases, and most recommendations are extrapolated from adult studies, expert opinions, and pediatric case series. As portal hypertension can result from intrahepatic or extrahepatic causes, management is tailored based on the etiology and functionality of the liver (see Chapter 79).

Prediction of Varices

In recent years, there has been advancement in developing scores to stratify children for variceal screening. In 2017 Witters and colleagues[14] introduced King's variceal prediction score (K-VaPS), which was adapted from the adult equivalent of utilizing spleen size and serum albumin and was validated prospectively in a cohort of 124 children. It showed a receiver operating characteristic (ROC) of 0.818 in the detection of a grade greater than or equal to 2 varices secondary to chronic liver disease. Another scoring system known as the Clinical Prediction Rule[15] was developed using platelet count, spleen size, and serum albumin. It showed an ROC of 0.80 and was developed by analyzing 108 children. It predicts esophageal varices secondary to both chronic liver disease or portal vein thrombosis. The Varices Prediction Rule[16] (with an ROC of 0.75) was specifically developed for infants with biliary atresia to predict significant varices utilizing platelet count and serum albumin at 6 months post-Kasai portoenterostomy.

Preprimary Prophylaxis

The aim of preprimary prophylaxis is the early treatment of portal hypertension to prevent or delay the development of esophageal varices. In the animal model, propranolol therapy resulted in a significant reduction in the development of portal hypertension, portal-systemic shunting, and portal venous inflow.[17,18] Only a few studies were performed on humans. A randomized control trial was performed in 231 cirrhotic patients using the nonselective β-blocker (NSBB) timolol. This study showed that NSBBs did not prevent the formation of varices and were even associated with an increased number of adverse events requiring discontinuation of treatment.[19] Currently there is no indication to use β-blockers to prevent the formation of varices.[20]

Primary Prophylaxis

Primary prophylaxis of variceal bleeding in adults with cirrhosis is widely accepted[21] (see Chapters 74, 79, and 80). Existing uncertainties in children of the risk and benefits related to the use of NSBBs appeared to be low mortality associated with the first bleed from varices. A recent concern includes neurodevelopmental consequences of repeated general anesthesia in young children that would be required for primary endoscopic prophylaxis,[22,23] causing difficulty in creating a clear consensus on primary prophylaxis in children.[24] Given the invasive nature of the endoscopic procedure and the need for repeated use of general anesthesia, there has been interest in the development of noninvasive predictors of varices to identify high-risk patients, as described in the earlier section "Prediction of Varices"; however, these tests are not sufficiently accurate. Surveillance endoscopy for prophylactic therapy with endoscopic variceal ligation (EVL) may be justifiable in specific clinical circumstances, such as when the clinician feels the risk of mortality from the first variceal hemorrhage is greater than that for children in general (e.g., when a child is not in reasonable proximity to medical care that can provide life-saving treatments for variceal hemorrhage). As a result of the unfavorable adverse effect profile of endoscopic sclerotherapy (EST), it is not indicated for primary prophylaxis.

Therapy of Bleeding Esophageal Varices

Acute bleeding from esophageal varices is an emergency that requires immediate medical attention. Blood volume and fluid resuscitation to achieve hemodynamic stability is the most important step (see Chapters 80 and 81). The goal of resuscitation is to preserve tissue perfusion. Central venous oxygen saturation and venous lactate can be useful to assess adequate tissue perfusion. Vital signs, particularly tachycardia and hypotension, can

be helpful to assess the amount of blood loss. Patients on a prophylactic β-blocker may not have compensatory tachycardia and may develop significant hypotension without an increase in heart rate. Fluid resuscitation in the form of crystalloids followed by red blood cell transfusion is critical. Red blood cell transfusion should be provided conservatively to maintain a hemoglobin level usually between 7 and 8 g/dL,[25] but it also should be individualized depending on the presence of other underlying factors including lung disease, cyanotic congenital heart disease, age, hemodynamic status, or ongoing bleeding. Recommendations regarding the management of coagulopathy from hepatic dysfunction and thrombocytopenia are not conclusive. Prothrombin time (PT)/international normalized ratio (INR) is not a reliable indicator of coagulopathy or bleeding in patients with cirrhosis, and evidence in support to correct PT/INR is lacking. In the setting of acute hemorrhage plasma and clotting, factor support is recommended in general; however, in the setting of acute variceal hemorrhage, the goal should not be to normalize the clotting abnormality but to prevent the risk of fluid overload and its consequences (brain edema, pulmonary edema, or rebleeding from varices). Vitamin K deficiency should be corrected if present. In the case of profound thrombocytopenia (<20,000) administration of platelets should be considered. In adults the use of recombinant factor VIIa is not effective[26] and is not recommended in children for acute variceal hemorrhage. Data are lacking on the prevalence of bacterial infections in children with variceal hemorrhage. A high index of suspicion should be maintained and timely institution of intravenous antibiotic therapy should be considered given the high risk of potentially fatal infection.

Endoscopy

Once the patient is stabilized, endoscopy is recommended in any patient who presents with upper gastrointestinal bleeding and whose esophageal varices are the cause of bleeding, ideally within 24 hours (see Chapter 81). There are two therapeutic options, EVL and EST. EVL is the recommended form of therapy for acute esophageal variceal bleeding because it is easier, safer, and has significantly lower overall complications and mortality.[27,28] In infants and children in whom ligation is technically difficult EST is the recommended form of endoscopic therapy. For sclerotherapy a variety of agents have been used (sclerosants, ethanolamine/tetradecyl sulfate) and these are injected either intravariceally or paravariceally until bleeding stops. In the setting of emergency sclerotherapy, there is a significant risk of bacteremia and antibiotics should be considered when suspected.

Pharmacologic therapy with vasoactive drugs (vasopressin, octreotide, somatostatin, etc.) should be started as soon as possible before endoscopy is performed and can be continued up to 5 days (see Chapters 80 and 81). Vasopressin efficacy is believed to be caused by direct vasoconstrictor activity on splanchnic arterioles and precapillary sphincters, with secondary reduction in portal venous blood flow and pressure. Vasopressors are long-acting and have been widely used; they are given as a bolus followed by continuous infusion. Somatostatin and its synthetic homologous octreotide are also shown to decrease splanchnic blood flow. Their effect on acute hemorrhage appears to be similar with fewer side effects. IV H_2 receptor blockers and proton pump inhibitors should also be considered to decrease the risk of bleeding from erosions or ulcerations.

Balloon Tamponade

Balloon tamponade is rarely indicated in cases of massive bleeding when the primary measures described previously failed to control the bleeding. This procedure is mainly used as a bridge until definitive treatment (endoscopic or portosystemic shunting surgery, etc.) can be instituted (for a maximum of 24 hours due to risk of pressure ulceration) and facilitated by trained staff and physicians in intensive care unit settings (see Chapter 81).

Treatment Failure

Rebleeding within 5 days can be managed by a second endoscopy. Persistent bleeding resistant to pharmacotherapy and endoscopy is managed by a transjugular intrahepatic portosystemic shunt (TIPS). Failure of TIPS or lack of expertise in TIPS in small children necessitates consideration of portosystemic shunting (see Chapters 83–85).

Secondary Prophylaxis

EVL is the preferred therapy for secondary prophylaxis in children with chronic liver disease.[29] Every 2 to 4 weeks following ligation therapy until complete ablation then every 6 to 12 months to treat if varices recur. There is insufficient data on the use of NSBB as monotherapy or an adjunct to therapy with EVL. EST is recommended in infants or small children in whom EVL is not possible. If EVL or EST cannot be performed, an NSBB may be considered but data on its efficacy, safety, and the appropriate dose are lacking, and there is a risk of masking tachycardia caused by hypovolemia during a major bleeding episode. If an NSBB is used, response to therapy by measuring HVPG is desirable (see Chapter 80).

Surgical Management

Transjugular Intrahepatic Portosystemic Shunt (see Chapter 85)

Surgical therapy in the form of shunts is usually the last option in cases of acute, persistent, and uncontrollable bleeding. TIPS is considered in children with severe portal hypertension secondary to chronic liver disease when they are nonresponsive to endoscopic therapy and NSBBs. It appears to decrease portal pressure acutely. Risks associated with shunts include shunt occlusion and the risk of hepatic encephalopathy.

Management of Gastric Varices

In children, studies are limited to the case reported or series when considering a recommendation for the management of gastric varices. Endoscopic therapy with tissue adhesive (e.g., N-butyl-cyanoacrylate or N-butyl-2-cyanoacrylate plus methacyloxysulfolane) may be considered for acute bleeding from isolated gastric varices and type 2 gastroesophageal varices. Data are lacking on safety and efficacy of balloon-occluded retrograde transvenous obliteration used for isolated gastric fundal varices. TIPS and/or portosystemic shunt therapy may be considered as an alternative approach to treating bleeding gastric varices.[29]

Extrahepatic Portal Vein Obstruction

EHPVO is defined as the obstruction of the extrahepatic portion of the portal vein with or without the involvement of an intrahepatic portal vein. It is a chronic process with the development of cavernous transformation and may include occlusion of other veins including splenic, superior mesenteric, and coronary veins. Causes are heterogeneous and listed in Box 76.2. EHPVO is a noncirrhotic, nonmalignant form of portal hypertension. About 70% of children with EHPVO present with upper gastrointestinal hemorrhage.[30] A major concern of EHPVO arises from its complications including variceal bleeding, hypersplenism, and portosystemic shunting. Restoration of blood flow through a portal vein by meso-Rex bypass (MRB) to prevent complications is the main mode of therapy (see Chapter 84).

Diagnosis

Diagnosis of portal vein obstruction is made by color Doppler ultrasonography (CDUSG) or cross-sectional imaging including magnetic resonance portovenogram (MRP). These images show evidence of portal vein occlusion, the presence of intraluminal material, or the presence of portal vein cavernosa. Both modalities may complement each other in preoperative assessment of EHPVO; however, MRP is found to have higher sensitivity compared with CDUSG[30] (see Chapter 14).

Management

Meso-Rex Bypass

According to Baveno VI Pediatric Satellite Symposium, MRB is the preferable preprimary and primary approach in children with EHPVO.[24] MRP is a bypass between a superior mesenteric vein and rex recessus (a remnant of ductus venosus). To consider MRB the following criteria should be met: the absence of underlying liver disease with normal HVPG, the absence of a prothrombotic state, body weight greater than 8 kg, favorable anatomy (retrograde internal jugular venogram); patent superior mesenteric, splenic, and bilateral internal jugular veins; absence of significant cardiovascular abnormalities; and pulmonary hypertension (see Chapters 83 and 84).

SUMMARY

There is a diverse range of therapeutic options for the management of pediatric patients presenting with complications of portal hypertension. A careful assessment of the pediatric patient with portal hypertension is of utmost importance to determine how best to manage the potential complications with pharmacologic, endoscopic, or surgical procedures. A multidisciplinary team approach to these complex patients is often necessary to best determine the course of action in a patient who may require liver transplantation in the future.

The references for this chapter can be found online by accessing the accompanying Expert Consult website.

CHAPTER 77

Management of liver failure

William Bernal

Acute liver failure (ALF), a term that is equivalent to the now archaic "fulminant hepatic failure," evolves after a catastrophic insult to the liver and results in the development of the dual characteristics of coagulopathy and encephalopathy within a matter of days or weeks of the liver injury.[1] The absence of a previous diagnosis of liver disease is another requirement, with the exception of severe reactivations of hepatitis B. Patients with acute presentations of Wilson disease are also included within the definition of ALF despite having established cirrhosis at presentation. ALF should not be confused with the more recent concept of acute-on-chronic liver failure (ACLF), which occurs in patients with cirrhosis and is often precipitated by infection or gastrointestinal hemorrhage. The principles of management are similar in some respects (e.g., encephalopathy, coagulopathy) but very different in others (e.g., cerebral edema is almost exclusively observed in ALF). This chapter will be based mainly on ALF unless specified otherwise (see Chapter 74).

Acute liver failure is best considered as an umbrella term for a heterogenous condition that incorporates a range of clinical syndromes. The dominant factors that give rise to this heterogeneity include the underlying etiology, the age of the patient, and the duration of time during which the disease evolves. Natural history studies indicate that survival rates without liver transplantation range from 10% to 90%, with the best outcomes seen in patients with rapidly evolving pregnancy-related syndromes, severe acetaminophen hepatotoxicity, and hepatitis A. Survival rates are worse in older patients and, possibly, in very young children. The rate of progression of the disease is used to subclassify patients into groups with differing clinical problems and outcomes. There is a lack of universal agreement on terminology, but the main options in use are the terms *hyperacute* (encephalopathy within 7 days of the onset of jaundice), *acute* (encephalopathy within 8–28 days of the onset of jaundice), and *subacute liver failure* (encephalopathy more than 28 days of the onset of jaundice), which will be used in this chapter.

ETIOLOGY OF ACUTE LIVER FAILURE

ALF remains a rare condition in the West, with probably fewer than 5 cases per million population per year. Viruses and drugs account for the majority of cases, but there is a significant variation in the patterns seen worldwide (Table 77.1).[1] In the West, there has been a trend toward more cases associated with acetaminophen and fewer from an identifiable viral infection. A number of patients have no definable cause, which is a condition referred to as *acute liver failure of indeterminate etiology* in this chapter, but also known as *seronegative hepatitis* and previously as *non–A to E hepatitis*. Most of the drug-induced cases are rare idiosyncratic reactions, but some, such as acetaminophen, are at least in part dose-related toxic events (see Chapters 68 and 69).

Viral (see Chapter 68)

ALF is a very uncommon complication of hepatitis A infection, occurring in 0.1% to 0.3% of hospitalized cases and in 0.4% of all cases seen in the United States. The incidence of ALF following hepatitis B was 1% to 4% of hospitalized patients. In early studies, hepatitis D coinfection or superinfection was thought to increase the risk because it was found in 30% to 40% of patients with ALF due to hepatitis B, compared with 5% to 20% of less severe cases. Vaccination and antiviral therapy have altered the observed pattern of hepatitis B–related ALF, which is now often seen in patients with previously subclinical, non-cirrhotic hepatitis B infection with a "reactivation" phenomenon following therapeutic immunosuppression, often after chemotherapy for malignancy.[2] The risk of ALF after exposure to hepatitis C appears to be very low, but it has been described. Hepatitis E is common in parts of Asia and Africa, and the risk of ALF ranges from 0.6% to 2.8% to greater than 20% in pregnant women, and is particularly high during the third trimester. Hepatitis E is also encountered in Europe and the United States and may account for some cases that would previously have been described as indeterminate hepatitis.

Indeterminate hepatitis is a common cause of ALF in some parts of the Western world. Most cases are sporadic, and unidentified toxins or autoimmune processes may be the underlying mechanisms. Very detailed case scrutiny will identify a known etiology in some cases, but in others the cause remains obscure.[3] Middle-aged females are most frequently affected, and the risk for ALF has been calculated at 2.3% to 4.7% of hospitalized cases.

Drugs

Acetaminophen (paracetamol) overdose and liver injury from the resultant hepatotoxicity is the most common cause of ALF in the United Kingdom and the United States. In the United Kingdom, it is usually taken with suicidal or parasuicidal intent, but in the United States, up to half of cases apparently follow therapeutic use.[4] This is either because of unintentional overdosing or accelerated metabolism in people with liver enzyme induction as a consequence of antiepileptic therapy or regular alcohol usage. Legislation limiting the quantities of acetaminophen that can be purchased in the United Kingdom has been credited with reducing hospitalizations for ALF by about 50% by limiting the size of overdose.

The risk of developing ALF secondary to an idiosyncratic reaction ranges from 0.001% for nonsteroidal antiinflammatory drugs to 1% for the isoniazid/rifampicin combination. The diagnosis is made on the basis of a temporal relationship between exposure to the drug and the development of ALF. The more common offending drugs are listed in Box 77.1. Most cases develop during the patient's first exposure to the drug but some, such as halothane, occurred in sensitized individuals on the second or subsequent exposure. Nontherapeutic drugs also

TABLE 77.1 Geographic Variation in the Etiology of Acute Liver Failure

	UNITED KINGDOM (%)	UNITED STATES (%)	JAPAN (%)	INDIA (%)
Acetaminophen	57	46	0	0
Drug reactions	11	11	7	4
Indeterminate	17	6	38	41
Hepatitis A or B	7	12	41	18
Hepatitis E	1	—	0	28
Other causes	7	25	14	9

BOX 77.1 Examples of Drugs Causing of Acute Liver Failure

MECHANISM OF LIVER INJURY

Dose-Related	Idiosyncratic	
Acetaminophen	Allopurinol	Monoamine oxidase inhibitors
Anabolic steroids[a]	Amiodarone	**Nonsteroidal anti-inflammatory drugs**
HAART drugs	**Carbamazepine**	Phenytoin
Sulfonamides	Disulfiram	Propylthiouracil
Sodium valproate[a]	**Ecstasy**[a]	Pyrazinamide
	Flutamide	**Rifampicin**
	Gold	Statins[a]
	Halothane	Sulfonamides
	HAART drugs	Terbinafine
	Isoniazid	Tetracycline
	Ketoconazole	Tricyclic antidepressants
	Methyldopa	

[a]Both dose-related and idiosyncratic mechanisms illustrated.
HAART, Highly active antiretroviral therapy.
Note: Drugs more commonly implicated are shown in bold.

cause ALF, for instance, Ecstasy (methylenedioxymethamphetamine), which has been associated with a number of clinical syndromes ranging from rapidly progressive hyper-ALF associated with malignant hyperpyrexia to subacute liver failure.

Other Etiologies

ALF associated with pregnancy is rare, complicating approximately 1:100,000 pregnancies, and tends to occur during the third trimester.[5] Three discrete entities have been described but considerable overlap is frequently observed. Acute fatty liver of pregnancy usually occurs in primigravidae carrying a male fetus and is characterized by severe microvesicular steatosis. The HELLP syndrome is defined as the combination of hemolysis, elevated liver enzymes, and low platelet count. ALF complicating preeclampsia or eclampsia typically exhibits very high serum aminotransferase levels and abnormal tissue perfusion patterns on computed tomography scanning, which reflect the microvascular infarction characteristic of this condition.

Wilson disease may present as ALF, usually during the second decade of life. It is characterized clinically by a Coombs-negative hemolytic anemia and demonstrable Kayser-Fleischer rings in the majority of cases. The serum ceruloplasmin levels are usually, but not invariably, low, and the serum and urinary copper levels are increased. Poisoning with *Amanita phalloides* (mushrooms) is most commonly seen in Central Europe, South Africa, and the

west coast of the United States. Severe diarrhea, often with vomiting, is a typical feature and commences 5 or more hours after ingestion of the mushrooms, and liver failure develops 4 to 5 days later. Autoimmune chronic hepatitis may present as ALF but is usually beyond rescue with corticosteroid or other immunosuppressive therapy. Budd-Chiari syndrome may present with ALF, and the diagnosis is suggested by hepatomegaly and confirmed by the demonstration of hepatic vein thrombosis. Ischemic hepatitis resulting from hypoperfusion due to systemic shock or cardiac failure is increasingly recognized as a cause of ALF, especially in older patients. Malignancy infiltration, especially with lymphoma, may masquerade as ALF and is typically associated with hepatomegaly and again seen in older patients.

DIAGNOSIS

The cardinal features of ALF are encephalopathy and coagulopathy. The diagnosis of encephalopathy is usually obvious on clinical evaluation and ranges from drowsiness to advanced coma. However, in subacute liver failure, clinical evidence of encephalopathy can remain subtle until the disease is advanced, and psychometric testing may be useful to establish the diagnosis and facilitate timely intervention with liver transplantation. The diagnosis of encephalopathy is supported by elevated arterial ammonia levels. Hypoglycemia should be excluded as an alternative explanation for impaired mental function.

Once a clinical diagnosis of ALF has been established, the next step is to determine the etiology. This may be obvious from the patient's history when acetaminophen or mushroom ingestion is responsible for the liver injury. In other cases, a systematic approach is required. The appropriate investigations required in all patients are outlined in Table 77.2, whereas those that are relevant in specific circumstances are listed in Table 77.3. Imaging of the liver serves to assess the size and shape of the liver, which is usually small, and screen for portal hypertension. The detection of portal hypertension does not always indicate chronic liver disease because ascites and/or splenomegaly may be seen in subacute liver failure, as well as the acute presentation of Wilson disease.

Histologic assessment of liver tissue may sometimes aid the diagnosis of the cause of ALF (see Chapter 68, 69, and 74). Confluent necrosis is the most common histologic finding, and this may be zonal or panlobular. Necrosis that is zonal and coagulative or eosinophilic is more likely to be secondary to a toxic insult or ischemia. The features of necrosis and parenchymal collapse may be interspersed with evidence of regeneration, either occurring in a diffuse pattern of small areas throughout the liver or in randomly occurring larger nodules that give the "map-like" pattern that has been described in this condition. The latter pattern is most commonly seen in patients with subacute liver failure.

TABLE 77.2 Core Investigation of Etiology of Acute Liver Failure

ETIOLOGY	INVESTIGATION
Hepatitis A (HAV)	IgM anti-HAV
Hepatitis B ± D (HBV, HDV)	IgM anticore, HBV DNA (HBsAg may be negative)
Hepatitis E (HEV)	IgM anti-HEV
Acetaminophen	Drug levels in blood

HBsAg, Hepatitis B surface antigen; *IgM,* immunoglobulin M.

TABLE 77.3 Extended Investigation of Etiology of Acute Liver Failure

ETIOLOGY	INVESTIGATION
Idiosyncratic drug reactions	Eosinophil count, histology
Autoimmune	Autoantibodies, immunoglobulins
Pregnancy-related syndromes	
Fatty liver	Ultrasound, uric acid, histology
HELLP syndrome	Platelet count
Toxemia	Serum aminotransferases
Wilson disease	Urinary copper, ceruloplasmin, hemolysis screen, slit-lamp examination
Budd-Chiari syndrome	Ultrasound or venography
Malignancy	Imaging, histology, bone marrow
Ischemic hepatitis	Aminotransferases, echocardiography
Other viral Infections	IgM and nucleic acids for CMV, EBV, HSV, VZV, Parvovirus.

CMV, Cytomegalovirus; *EBV,* Epstein-Barr virus; *HELLP,* hemolysis, elevated liver enzymes, and low platelet count; *HSV,* herpes simplex virus; *VZV,* varicella zoster virus.

BOX 77.2 Findings Suggestive of Acute Alcoholic Hepatitis

Hepatomegaly
Marked elevation of γ-glutamyl transferase
High white cell count not responding to antibiotics
Elevated immunoglobulin A level
Appearance of fatty infiltration on ultrasound

Histologic features may suggest specific diagnoses, including sodium valproate toxicity, malignant infiltration, Wilson disease, pregnancy-related syndromes, and Budd-Chiari syndrome. Sodium valproate toxicity is characterized by microvesicular steatosis. Screening for malignant infiltration as the cause of ALF is one of the stronger indications for performing a liver biopsy, especially when the liver is enlarged. Patients with Wilson disease presenting as ALF usually have established cirrhosis, commonly associated with interface hepatitis resembling autoimmune disease, hepatocyte ballooning, and steatosis (see Chapter 74). Liver histology may be useful in making a precise diagnosis within the spectrum of pregnancy-related liver diseases. The histologic features of Budd-Chiari syndrome (see Chapter 86) are extreme sinusoidal dilation, congestion, and coagulative necrosis.

Liver biopsy may also be of assistance in differentiating ALF from established cirrhosis and from acute alcoholic hepatitis, whether or not it is associated with cirrhosis. The former scenario can usually be distinguished on clinical grounds, but acute alcoholic hepatitis can present with clinical features very similar to subacute liver failure. A history of high alcohol consumption may not be available, but the diagnosis of acute alcoholic hepatitis is suggested by the investigational findings outlined in Box 77.2.

PROGNOSIS

In ALF, the grade of encephalopathy correlates strongly with outcome, and this is true for both the grade of encephalopathy at the time of presentation to a specialist unit and the maximum grade attained. The prognosis worsens further when complications such as cerebral edema, renal failure, and cardiovascular instability co-exist. However, other patients with ALF have a very poor prognosis despite the absence of cerebral edema and renal failure. This is especially true of patients with subacute liver failure who, in addition, often do not manifest severely abnormal coagulation parameters but have negligible capacity for native liver regeneration.

The use of transplantation intensified the need for early indicators of prognosis so that those in need of this intervention could be identified in advance of the full clinical consequences of liver failure. The King's College and Clichy criteria were early examples of prognostic models, but at least 20 different approaches to the evaluation of likely outcome have now been described.[6] Some of these, such as Model for End-Stage Liver Disease, are applicable to most etiologies, although it remains true that acetaminophen-related liver injury behaves very differently from most other causes of ALF. Other models are specific to single underlying etiologies. Some models are composites of clinical and laboratory information, and some are modified by patient age (see Chapters 105 and 107).

Assessment of the volume of viable hepatocytes by histologic examination is considered by some to be of prognostic value, but the potential for sampling error is considerable. The critical mass that suggests a good prognosis has been calculated as 25% to 0%. A small liver on clinical or radiologic assessment, or, more particularly, a liver that is found to be shrinking rapidly, is another indicator of poor prognosis that is especially useful in subacute liver failure.[7]

MANAGEMENT

Overall Strategy

In ALF, the overall strategy is a combination of intensive medical care (see Chapter 26) and liver transplantation in selected patients (see Chapters 105 and 107). The use of liver support devices is restricted to clinical trials (see Chapter 78), but therapeutic plasma exchange may have a role for some patients.[8] Management starts with identification of etiology and an initial assessment of prognosis that is then progressively updated. Appropriate patients should be referred to specialist centers, where a decision on the need for immediate liver transplantation is made. Supportive care is provided to prevent the development of complications and maintain metabolic and cardiorespiratory stability to optimize conditions for native liver regeneration. Patients are then monitored for those complications that may develop, and these are treated as they emerge to the point of recovery, death, or transplantation.[9]

Patients with ACLF also require, and benefit from, intensive monitoring. This is especially appropriate when the deterioration has been triggered by a specific reversible complication and in patients who are active or appropriate candidates for liver transplantation. Ascites and bleeding varices are frequently important components of the clinical problem, and the management of these is discussed separately in Chapters 79 to 85.

General Measures

There are a number of drugs with well-defined roles in specific etiologies of ALF. *N*-acetylcysteine is established as an effective antidote to acetaminophen hepatotoxicity when given within

16 to 24 hours of the overdose, based on blood levels of the drug. However, clinical benefit was also suggested with later administration associated with reduced mortality and the incidence of cerebral edema. A trial of n-acetylcysteine in non-acetaminophen etiologies of ALF with early disease also suggested clinical benefit in this group.[10] Penicillin, and possibly silymarin, should be added at the earliest opportunity to the standard supportive measures in patients with *A. phalloides* toxicity. Patients with Wilson disease or autoimmune hepatitis presenting with ALF rarely respond to penicillamine or immunosuppressive therapy, respectively.[11] Some cases with severe acute alcoholic hepatitis benefits from corticosteroid therapy but not from pentoxifylline.

MANAGEMENT OF SPECIFIC COMPLICATIONS (SEE ALSO CHAPTER 26)

Encephalopathy

Encephalopathy is invariably present in ALF and is often present in ACLF. Patients with grades 1 and 2 encephalopathy exhibit degrees of drowsiness or mild disorientation, but they can be easily roused and respond appropriately to verbal stimuli. Patients with chronic liver disease will often have a hepatic flap and fetor hepaticus, in contradistinction to patients with ALF and an equivalent degree of encephalopathy. In ALF, progression to grade 3 encephalopathy is diagnosed when the patient becomes very confused and, at best, obeys simple commands. Grade 4 encephalopathy signifies deep coma, with the patients responsive only to painful stimuli. Patients reaching grades 3 and 4 are intubated and placed on supported ventilation at this stage of disease evolution.[9]

Encephalopathy with ACLF is also managed with airway protection for advanced grades, and with standard therapeutic measures of rehydration, electrolyte correction, and lactulose and phosphate enemas, usually with good effect. There is no place for protein restriction, but treatment of triggering events is of key importance (Box 77.3). In contrast, these "standard" therapeutic agents of lactulose and enemas are not utilized in ALF, with the exception of patients with subacute liver failure who may benefit from some of the measures used in chronic liver disease. However, these approaches are ineffective in the treatment of the more rapidly progressive encephalopathy characteristic of the hyperacute and acute syndromes. In this setting ammonia is recognized as the neurotoxin of primary importance and the prompt control of hyperammonemia forms an important clinical goal. Arterial concentrations above 150 μmol/L, particularly if sustained, are associated with a significantly increased risk of cerebral edema and intracranial hypertension, and measures are instituted to rapidly control and lower these elevations.[9] This may include the use of hemofiltration through

standard continuous renal replacement therapy, and very short-term deferment of nutritional support for protein restriction. Ammonia-lowering medications including L-*o*rnithine L-*a*spartate (LOLA) appear ineffective, although trials of alternative agents are ongoing.

Cerebral edema was a common complication of severe encephalopathy in ALF, especially hyperacute and ALF but less so in subacute liver failure. It was a major cause of death and frequently disqualified patients from liver transplantation. In many centers it is now seen in only a small minority of cases, likely reflecting the effectiveness of neuroprotective measures employed in those patients assessed to be at high risk of the complication. These include control of blood ammonia concentration, high level sedation, temperature control and avoidance of fever and hypercapnia, metabolic stability, and maintenance of serum sodium levels in the 145 to 150 mmol/L range.[9] When present, the clinical features of cerebral edema include systemic hypertension, "decerebrate" posturing, hyperventilation, abnormal pupillary reflexes, and ultimately, impairment of brain-stem reflexes and functions. Cerebral edema has only been described in a small number of cases in patients with cirrhosis.

Intracranial pressure (ICP) monitoring is acknowledged to be reasonably safe but is now mainly reserved for patients with other clinical or radiologic evidence of intracranial hypertension and those at high risk who are undergoing liver transplantation. Treatment of surges in ICP that may compromise brain-stem function and lead to death is focused on the use of osmotherapy with intravenous bolus therapy with either hypertonic saline or mannitol. Acute, but not chronic, hyperventilation may be of benefit in reducing critical surges in intracranial hypertension and employed as an emergency temporizing intervention in parallel with use of other medication.

In the later stages of the neurologic complications, where elevations in ICP become refractory to standard therapies, treatment is focused on preserving cerebral perfusion and other second-line therapies may be employed. These may include thiopentone, indomethacin employed as a cerebral vasoconstrictor, or the utilization of induced moderate hypothermia. At this stage of the complication, spontaneous recovery is unlikely without liver transplantation, and hepatectomy is sometimes useful to secure transient improvement while awaiting a graft.

Infection

Infection is a prominent complication in all varieties of liver failure. In ALF, it is one of the most common causes of death and has an integral role in the evolving cycle of hemodynamic instability and multisystem failure. It also frequently disqualifies potential candidates from emergency liver transplantation. Infection may be difficult to detect with confidence, because there is a poor correlation between the presence of infection and the classic indicators of fever and elevation of white cell counts. Bacterial infection may occur in as many as 80% of cases, and fungal infection in 30%. Systemic fungal infection is notoriously difficult to diagnose in the setting of ALF, and a high index of suspicion is required, especially in high-risk patients. Risk factors for both bacterial and fungal sepsis include severity of liver injury, co-existing renal failure, cholestasis, and need for liver transplantation. Surveillance cultures are required on a regular basis, and fungal biomarker tests utilized to guide antifungal therapies, particularly if transplantation is considered a likely option.

BOX 77.3 Common Precipitants of Acute Hepatic Encephalopathy

Infection
Constipation
Dehydration or over diuresis
Gastrointestinal bleed
Large protein dietary intake
Narcotic drugs
Benzodiazepines

Early clinical trials of prophylactic antibiotics demonstrated that systemic use reduced the incidence of culture-positive bacterial infection by half, but this strategy was associated with the emergence of highly resistant organisms in as many as 10% of cases, without improvement in mortality. However, a low threshold for the use of prophylactic systemic antibiotics is recommended, particularly when liver injury is severe, extrahepatic organ failure including encephalopathy is evolving or established, systemic inflammatory response syndrome (SIRS) is present, or when there has been an unexplained deterioration in condition.[9] Precise regimens used are determined by local antibiotic policy.

Infection is a key precipitant of acute on chronic liver failure and must be actively sought out and excluded at the very earliest stages of deterioration. Again, many infections may not have typical signs and symptoms of sepsis; rather, they manifest as worsening of features of hepatic decompensation or renal function, and in many no organism is identified. When present, infections are often nosocomial in origin and may have extended antimicrobial resistance patterns. In patients with chronic liver disease who develop sepsis, early delivery of effective antibiotics is key, as there is a close relation between survival and delayed and/or inappropriate antibiotic treatment. Spontaneous bacterial peritonitis is a particularly important infection to consider in this setting, and the diagnosis can only be excluded with confidence if the white cell count in ascites is less than $250/mm^3$.

Hemodynamic Instability

The hemodynamic changes in liver failure are similar to those observed in the SIRS. Circulating volume is frequently depleted because of low oral intake and vomiting and/or diarrhea. In parallel, the early hemodynamic profile reflects a hyperdynamic circulation with increased cardiac output and reduced systemic peripheral vascular resistance. Profound vasodilation may cause further relative hypovolemia, and invasive monitoring is used to determine appropriate fluid regimens and adequate intravascular volumes. Progressive disease leads to circulatory failure, either as a result of a falling cardiac output or an inability to maintain an adequate mean arterial pressure. This is a common mode of death in liver failure.

Circulatory failure is initially managed with volume resuscitation utilizing appropriate combinations of colloid, crystalline fluids, and blood products. Hypotension occurring despite adequate intravascular volumes is treated with vasopressor agents, using norepinephrine as the primary vasopressor and adjunctive use of vasopressin or terlipressin by infusion.[9] Use of inotropic agents to augment cardiac output may be required but mandates invasive hemodynamic monitoring to assess both requirement and response, recognizing that in some cases a low cardiac output may be a primary or contributory cause of liver hypoperfusion or congestion, and a driver of liver injury. Some patients with both ALF and acute on chronic liver failure who develop resistance to inotropes may have relative adrenal insufficiency, which responds to administration of hydrocortisone.

Renal Failure

However defined, renal dysfunction and failure is common in patients with liver failure. In ALF between 40% and 80% of patients are classified as having acute kidney injury (AKI), which is associated with increasing age, an acetaminophen etiology, and the development of infection. It may have a multifactorial etiology and in at least some patients with acetaminophen overdose is an early consequence of direct drug toxicity. Early renal dysfunction is also seen in Wilson disease and pregnancy-related syndromes. Urea synthesis is impaired in ALF, and serum creatinine levels are preferred for the purposes of monitoring renal function.

AKI is also a frequent complication of chronic liver disease, occurring in up to 50% of hospitalized patients, and is a strong predictor of poor survival in both the short and longer term. Here the broad heading of AKI encompasses subtypes, conventionally considered as resulting from hepatorenal syndrome (HRS-AKI) and non-HRS-AKI, with the former resulting from the classical functional pathophysiologic mechanisms associated with portal hypertension, splanchnic vasodilation, and renal vasoconstriction. Non-HRS-AKI may result from a multitude of other insults ranging from pre-renal insults such as from hypovolemia and renal insults from sepsis or drug-induced tubular injury, and both may be superimposed on underlying intrinsic renal disease. In practice there is probably overlap between HRS-AKI and non-HRS-AKI, particularly in ACLF and multiorgan failure (MOF) where "pure" HRS-AKI probably represents the minority of cases.

Optimization of intravascular filling is essential in patients with deteriorating renal function. Terlipressin in combination with albumin infusions is widely used in Europe in the management of AKI in chronic liver disease, and there is evidence to suggest this strategy improves renal function and survival rates. The metabolic complexity of combined liver and renal failure in the setting of ALF suggests early intervention with renal replacement therapy is prudent, preempting standard indications. Continuous hemofiltration systems are associated with less hemodynamic instability and run a lower risk of aggravating latent or established cerebral edema than intermittent hemodialysis and are associated with improved survival.[12] The role for renal support therapy is less well defined in ACLF. Its use is most clear-cut when the magnitude of liver failure is of limited severity, where there is an option for "rescue" liver transplantation, or when there are other indications of improving organ failure.

Metabolic Abnormalities

Hypoglycemia is common in ALF and can induce reversible impairment of consciousness before the onset of classic encephalopathy. Other signs and symptoms of hypoglycemia are often masked, and regular blood glucose monitoring is required. Metabolic acidosis is present in 30% of patients in whom ALF develops after an acetaminophen overdose and is associated with a particularly high mortality. This acidosis precedes the onset of encephalopathy and is independent of renal function. In contrast, a metabolic acidosis is found in 5% of patients with other etiologies of ALF, occurring later in the disease process and also associated with a poor outcome. Blood lactate is frequently elevated in this setting and probably reflects the combination of increased production from peripheral dysoxia and impaired clearance from compromised liver function. Elevated blood lactate frequently improves with restoration of circulating volume with intravenous fluids. Persistent elevation is a marker of illness severity and poor prognosis.

In most etiologies of ALF, alkalosis is the dominant acid-base abnormality, and it may be associated with hypokalemia. Hyponatremia may reflect sodium depletion in patients with vomiting or may be dilutional due to inappropriate fluid resuscitation. A risk factor for the development of cerebral edema, its correction is an important early target for metabolic stabilization. Hypophosphatemia is most frequently encountered in acetaminophen-induced ALF when renal function is preserved and may be profound.

Hyponatremia is the dominant abnormality seen in ACLF. This does not reflect sodium depletion because total body sodium levels are almost always above normal in these patients. The hyponatremia may be diuretic induced in patients with ascites, and withdrawal of diuretic therapy is advised if the serum sodium is less than 130 mEq/L. Refractory hyponatremia is conventionally managed by fluid restrictions of 800 to 1500 mL/day, depending on severity. Hemofiltration may be used to correct hyponatremia in severe cases or when the serum sodium is less than 120 mEq/L immediately before liver transplantation to reduce the risk of central pontine myelinolysis associated the rapid increase in serum sodium levels that inevitably occurs in the intraoperative and perioperative periods.

Coagulopathy

As the liver is responsible for the synthesis of most of the coagulation factors (except factor VIII, which is produced by endothelial cells) and some of the inhibitors of coagulation and fibrinolysis, coagulopathy is a near universal feature of liver failure. In ALF, circulating levels of fibrinogen; prothrombin; and factors V, VII, IX, and X are reduced, and serial measurements of prothrombin time are widely used as an indicator of the severity of liver damage. However, the functional consequences are complex as most patients seem to have a state of "rebalanced hemostasis" resulting from the parallel loss of procoagulant and anticoagulant factors and there is no great increased risk of bleeding; some patients may be hypercoagulable. Spontaneous bleeding is seen in fewer than 15% of cases, and the risk of bleeding with less invasive procedures such as central venous catheter placement and even transjugular liver biopsy is relatively small.[13] Correction of coagulopathy complicates prognostic evaluation and should be reserved for active bleeding and more invasive procedures such as surgery or insertion of ICP monitoring devices, although thrombocytopenia is common and may be corrected. The role of pharmacologic venous thromboembolism prophylaxis is yet to be defined.

The severity of the abnormality of standard laboratory measures of coagulation is usually less marked in ACLF, and thrombocytopenia in this setting is usually due to hypersplenism. However, the functional hemostatic phenotype is complex with a state of rebalanced but unstable hemostasis common.

Patients with decompensated disease may tend toward a prothrombotic state, whereas those with associated MOF may trend toward hypocoagulability with impaired fibrinolysis.[14] Bleeding in critically ill patients with chronic liver disease mostly results from portal hypertension and spontaneous hemorrhage is uncommon.[15] There is thus a limited role for prophylactic use of blood products; procedure-related bleeding is also very uncommon, and its risk is principally determined by the nature of the procedure and operator experience. Fresh frozen plasma use in patients who are not bleeding is best avoided. Administration may have minimal effects on functional measures of hemostasis, but its expansion of circulating volume may increase portal pressure and portal hypertensive bleeding risk.[16,17]

Nutrition (see Chapter 26)

Although most patients with ALF are well nourished at the onset of the illness, it is important to institute nutritional support as soon as possible. Most patients are catabolic with high rates of energy expenditure from systemic inflammation and liver regeneration. As with other critical illness, early nutritional support through the enteral route and using standard feed formulation is preferred. As discussed earlier, in those with very severe hepatic impairment and considered at high risk of cerebral edema, transient protein restriction may be considered.[18] When protein is reintroduced serial monitoring of blood ammonia concentration is required.

Nutritional support in ACLF is equally as important but subject to more constraints. Unlike ALF, these patients are frequently undernourished before the onset of the episode of ACLF and the presence of undernutrition is an unequivocal marker of poor prognosis. Enteral nutrition should be started early, once hemodynamically stabilized. Insertion of a nasogastric tube for enteral feeding in patients with esophageal varices is associated with a low risk of bleeding and is not contraindicated but is usually deferred until 24 to 48 hours after bleeding is controlled. Nutritional support goals are for the provision of 20 to 30 kcal/kg ideal body weight per day, increasing over the course of illness from acute to recovery phases, and with protein/amino acid of 1.2 to 1.5 g/ kg ideal body weight per day.[18,19] There are no current recommendations for routine use of specific enteral feed formulas, or for the use of protein restriction.

The references for this chapter can be found online by accessing the accompanying Expert Consult website.

CHAPTER 78

Support of the failing liver

Harvey S. Chen, Matthew Aizpuru, Kewei Li, and Scott L. Nyberg

FAILING LIVER

A failing liver is a serious condition that warrants a multimodal approach (see Chapter 77). The best treatment for a failing liver in the setting of acute liver failure (ALF; no history of liver disease) or acute-on-chronic liver failure (ACLF; history of chronic liver disease or cirrhosis) is liver transplantation (see Chapter 105).[1] Supportive therapy, however, in ALF, ACLF, and posthepatectomy liver failure (PHLF) may be used to determine whether liver function will return to baseline or to bridge the patient until an organ becomes available (see Chapter 77).

The incidence of ALF in the United States is more than 2500 persons per year, but the number is much higher for patients with ACLF (>200,000).[2] The outcome of ALF varies by etiology. Those with favorable prognoses are acetaminophen overdose, hepatitis A, and ischemia, with approximately 60% spontaneous survival.[3] Etiologies with poor prognoses are drug-induced ALF, hepatitis B, and idiopathic cases, with approximately 25% spontaneous survival (see Chapter 77).

The aim of support therapy in the setting of liver failure is to return the patient to the compensated state. Several promising approaches to supportive therapy have been and continue to be evaluated, including cell transplantation and the application of extracorporeal liver support. These approaches are most promising in the setting of ALF and PHLF because of the possibility of complete recovery without imposing adverse sequelae, such as lifelong immunosuppression with liver transplantation. A failing liver may not regenerate or recover completely; therefore buying time to bridge to liver transplantation can be lifesaving. The interest in liver-assist devices is great because of high mortality rates, increasing wait lists, an expansion of indications for transplantation, and major liver resections.

This chapter emphasizes novel and promising techniques, such as extracorporeal liver support, cell transplantation, and tissue engineering. A historic summary of the different attempts to support the failing liver is also reviewed. Extracorporeal liver support is divided into *biologic* and *nonbiologic* systems.

NONBIOLOGIC LIVER SUPPORT

Historic Blood Purification Options

Throughout the 1960s and 1970s, it was believed that small (molecular weight cut-off <5 kDa) dialyzable molecules caused coma in ALF.[4,5] As a result, numerous attempts were made to treat ALF patients with hemodialysis[6] and charcoal hemofiltration[7] for removal of these small toxins. Although case reports[8] and controlled studies[7] of both therapies have shown reversal of hepatic encephalopathy and improved survival, neither therapy has been proven successful in prospective randomized trials of either ALF or ACLF.

Plasma Exchange and Hemodiafiltration

Plasma exchange was a natural outgrowth of the less effective blood-exchange transfusion technique. The goals of plasma exchange in ALF are to reduce the level of circulating toxins and to replace deficient essential factors, such as clotting factors produced by the liver. Plasma exchange is achieved by apheresis, with removal of the patient's jaundiced plasma and replacement with normal plasma. The results of early clinical trials were discouraging; encephalopathy often improved temporarily, but patient survival was not affected. Therapeutic gains, such as reduction in serum bilirubin and partial recovery from coma, were short lived and seen predominantly in patients with drug-induced ALF.[9-11] In addition, a significant complication rate was reported with plasma exchange, including chemical toxicity, viral infections, and death from lung and brain complications.[12]

Clemmesen and colleagues[13] investigated the effect of repeated, high-volume (15% of body weight) plasma exchange in 23 patients: 14 patients with ALF and 9 with ACLF (Table 78.1). The etiologies of ALF were acetaminophen in 8, hepatitis in 3, and nonhepatitis (A, B, C) in 3. Of the patients with acetaminophen intoxication, 25% died, and 21% were bridged to transplantation.

A recent multicenter, prospective, randomized control trial in Europe[15] recruited 182 ALF patients and randomized them to high volume-plasma exchange (HVP) versus standard medical treatment (SMT) groups. Overall survival between HVP and SMT groups was 59% versus 48%. A significant survival benefit was seen in a subgroup of patients who did not receive a liver transplant. This study further demonstrated significantly reduced proinflammatory cytokines (tumor necrosis factor [TNF]-α, interleukin [IL]-6, IL-4, IL-10, and transforming growth factor [TGF]-β) in the HVP group, which may represent a decreased systemic inflammatory response and explain the favorable outcome in these patients.

Despite its limitations and unproven efficacy, plasma exchange continues to be a frequently used method of liver support in patients with ALF. It is used for the correction of coagulopathy and for nonspecific removal of accumulated toxins.

Albumin Dialysis

The Molecular Adsorbent Recycling System (MARS) and Prometheus liver dialysis systems are two extracorporeal therapies that facilitate removal of nonpolar toxins by albumin in patients with ALF and ACLF.

MARS

MARS (Gambro-Baxter, Deerfield, IL) was developed in the early 1990s.[33] Briefly, MARS is a two-circuit system composed of a blood circuit and a secondary albumin circuit; these are

TABLE 78.1   Overview of Important Nonbiologic and Biologic Extracorporeal Liver Support Device Trials

NONBIOLOGIC DEVICES	TYPE OF TRIAL	AUTHOR	YEAR	NO. OF PATIENTS	INDICATION	SURVIVAL % DEVICE + SMT	SMT
Charcoal hemoperfusion	RCT	O'Grady et al.[7]	1988	62	ALF	34% (10/29)	39% (13/33)
BioLogic-DT	CT	Ellis et al.[14]	1999	10	ALF	0% (0/5)	0% (0/5)
Plasma exchange	Uncontrolled	Clemmesen et al.[13]	1999	23	ALF, ACLF	53%* (8/15)	
Plasma Exchange	RCT	Larsen et al.[15]	2016	182	ALF	59%[a] (54/92)	48%[a] (43/90)
Plasma Exchange		Zhou et al.[16]	2017		ALF		
MARS	RCT	Heemann et al.[17]	2002	23	ACLF	92% (11/12)	55% (6/11)
MARS	RCT	Saliba et al. FULMAR trial[18]	2013	102	ALF	85%[a] (45/53)	76%[a] (37/49)
MARS	RCT	Banares et al. RELIEF trial[19]	2013	180	ACLF	61% (58/95)	59% (55/94)
Prometheus	Uncontrolled	Rifai et al.[20]	2003	11	ACLF, HRS	27% (8/11)	
Prometheus	Uncontrolled	Grodzicki et al.[21]	2009	52	ALF, PHLF	54%[a] (28/52)	
Prometheus	RCT	Kribben et al. HELIOS Trial[22]	2012	145	ACLF	66% (51/77)	63% (43/68)

BIOLOGIC DEVICES	TYPE OF TRIAL	AUTHOR	YEAR	NO. OF PATIENTS	INDICATION	SURVIVAL % BAL + SMT	SMT
ELAD	CT	Ellis et al.[23]	1996	240	ALF, PNF	78%[a] (7/9)	33% (1/3)
ELAD	RCT	Thompson et al.[24]	2018	203	ALF (alcoholic hepatitis)	51% (49/96)	50% (53/107)
HepatAssist	RCT	Demetriou et al.[25]	2004	171	ALF, PNF	71%[a] (60/85)	62%[a] (53/86)
Latvian Trial	CT	Margulis et al.[26]	1989	126	ALF, ACLF, Sepsis	67% (37/59)	40% (27/67)
TECA-Hybrid Artificial Liver Support System	Uncontrolled Phase 1	Xue Y et al.[27]	2001	6	ALF, ACLF, PHLF	33% (2/6)	
BLSS	Uncontrolled Phase 1	Mazariegos et al.[28]	2001	4	ALF, ACLF	25%[a] (1/4)	
AMC-BAL	Uncontrolled Phase 1	van de Kerkhove et al.[29]	2002	12	ALF	100%[a] (12/12)	
RFB	Uncontrolled Phase 1	Morsiani et al.[30]	2002	7	ALF, PNF	86%[a] (1/7)	
MELS	Uncontrolled Phase 1	Sauer et al.[31]	2003	8	ALF, ACLF	100%[a] (8/8)	
Hybrid-BAL	Uncontrolled Phase 1	Ding et al.[32]	2003	12	ALF	75% (3/12)	

[a]Survivors include patients bridged to liver transplantation.

ACLF, Acute-on-chronic liver failure; *ALF*, acute liver failure; *AMC-BAL*, Amsterdam Medical Center Bioartificial Liver; *BLSS*, Bioartificial Liver Support System; *CT*, controlled trial; *ELAD*, extracorporeal liver-assist device; *HRS*, hepatorenal syndrome; *MARS*, Molecular Adsorbent Recycling System; *MELS*, modular extracorporeal liver support; *Phase I*, safety assessment trial; *PHLF*, post-hepatectomy liver failure; *PNF*, primary nonfunction; *RCT*, randomized controlled trial; *RFB*, Radial-Flow Bioreactor; *SMT*, standard medical therapy; *TECA*, Hong Kong TECA LTD Co.

separated by a high-flux dialyzer membrane with a pore size and nominal molecular weight cut-off (MWCO) of approximately 60 kDa. The pore size of this membrane makes it impermeable to albumin (67 kDa) but permeable to smaller water and nonpolar waste substances. On the opposing side of this membrane is an albumin circuit that consists of supraphysiologic levels (>10%) of human albumin dialysate. Waste removal occurs by diffusion via the concentration gradient between the patient's blood and the albumin dialysate in the secondary circuit. The high concentration of albumin is believed to facilitate removal of nonpolar molecules known to bind to albumin. Detoxification of these nonpolar waste molecules occurs when the albumin passes over adsorbent columns, including an anion exchange resin column and an activated charcoal column.[34] The secondary circuit also includes a conventional low-flux dialysis for detoxification of water-soluble molecules.

One of the earlier MARS trials was an uncontrolled trial of 13 patients who had not responded to SMT of ACLF.[35] The etiologies of cirrhosis were hepatitis C in 1 patient and alcohol abuse in the rest; the precipitating events were unknown in 10 cases. This early, uncontrolled study showed an overall survival of 69% (9/13). A larger randomized controlled trial (RCT) of the MARS system plus SMT (*n* = 39) versus SMT alone (*n* = 31) in the treatment of hepatic encephalopathy in advanced cirrhosis was reported by Hassanein and colleagues.[36] This trial demonstrated that the use of MARS therapy was associated with an earlier and more frequent improvement of grades 3 and 4 hepatic encephalopathy compared with SMT alone. This 5-day trial did not assess the role of MARS therapy on survival of cirrhotic patients.

The RELIEF trial evaluated survival of ACLF patients treated with MARS at 19 European centers.[19] This prospective

RCT of MARS treatment included 102 patients randomized to MARS therapy ($n = 95$) or SMT alone ($n = 94$). The trial showed that MARS therapy had an acceptable safety profile; there were, however, no significant differences in survival between the groups (61% vs. 59%). Possible explanations for the nonsignificant results of the RELIEF trial included no use of extra albumin and insufficient treatment dosage.

In contrast to ACLF, the FULMAR trial evaluated survival of ALF patients treated with MARS.[18] This prospective RCT of MARS treatment included 102 patients randomized to MARS therapy ($n = 53$) or SMT alone ($n = 49$). The study showed overall high survival rates: Survival at 6 months was greater after MARS treatment (85% vs. 76%); however, this difference did not reach a statistically significant level ($P = .28$). A limitation of this study was its short interval from randomization to liver transplantation (approximately 16 hours). This short interval prohibited definitive evaluation of efficacy of the MARS device. Moreover, this study reflects the high efficacy of liver transplantation, with 1-year survival rates approaching and often exceeding 90%.

Along with hepatic encephalopathy, MARS has been shown to improve other secondary complications of ALF, including renal dysfunction, pulmonary dysfunction, jaundice, and systemic inflammation associated with lowering of both systemic vascular resistance and mean arterial pressure (MAP).[37] One prospective RCT of MARS showed significant improvement in survival in patients with hepatorenal syndrome.[38] MARS therapy has been associated with prolonged relief of intractable pruritus in patients with cholestatic liver disease.[39] In addition, Novelli and colleagues[40] showed that MARS therapy was associated with an improvement in Model for End-Stage Liver Disease (MELD) scores at 1 and 3 months after treatment.

There are very few trials comparing plasma exchange and albumin dialysis devices. The most recent study[16] compared plasma exchange alone versus double plasma molecular adsorption system with plasma exchange in 67 patients with toxic hepatic failure. They found no difference in mortality, but improvement in hepatic encephalopathy with the addition of albumin dialysis.

Prometheus

Prometheus (Fresenius Medical Care, Waltham, MA) is another form of albumin dialysis. Prometheus functions by detoxifying fractionated plasma as it passes through two adsorption columns. Prometheus and MARS differ in the MWCO of their blood-separation membranes. MARS uses a 50- to 60-kDa MWCO membrane that prevents passage of albumin from the blood, whereas Prometheus uses a larger porosity membrane with 250-kDa MWCO that allows the passage of albumin. Therefore greater potential removal of albumin-bound toxins from the patient's blood is possible with the Prometheus system.[20] There have, however, been concerns of lowering the patient's albumin levels using Prometheus[41] and concerns of losing clotting factors, presumably because of reduction in protein C and protein S concentrations after the fractionation and adsorption process.[42]

The HELIOS trial was an RCT to assess survival of ACLF patients treated with fractionated plasma separation (FPSA).[22] Patients with ACLF were randomly allocated to groups treated with FPSA plus SMT ($n = 77$) or SMT alone ($n = 68$). Primary endpoints were survival probabilities at days 28 and 90, irrespective of liver transplantation. The study showed no significant differences in either 28- or 90-day survival. There was, however, improved survival in a subgroup analysis of patients with hepatorenal syndrome and in patients with a MELD score greater than 30.

BIOLOGIC LIVER SUPPORT

Standard medical therapy alone has been associated with less than 50% recovery from ALF (see Chapter 77); therefore an effective liver support device to reduce the need for liver transplantation and increase the possibility of spontaneous recovery is needed. Many investigators believe that liver support at this level of complexity requires the use of a biologic component that includes a mammalian liver tissue preparation. Accordingly, investigators have used various biologic configurations to support a failing liver consisting of whole livers, hepatocyte transplantation, primary hepatocytes, and hepatocyte-based cell lines. However, factors such as device complexity, shortage, uncertain availability of high-quality liver tissues, and immunologic barriers have prevented the widespread use of bioartificial liver (BAL) support systems.

Ex Vivo Liver Perfusion

In 1965 Eiseman and colleagues[43] reported the use of xenogeneic (porcine) liver hemoperfusion to treat eight comatose patients. None of these patients survived, but transient clinical improvement, such as awakening from the comatose state, was reported. Later, in 1967, Burnell and colleagues[44] reported the use of human-human cross-circulation in the treatment of three patients with fulminant hepatic failure. Moreover, livers from a variety of species (e.g., porcine, dog, bovine) have been used.[43,45,46] Evident after the treatments were symptoms of hyperacute rejection, such as gastrointestinal bleeding, hemolysis, and thrombocytopenia, and less specific symptoms, such as fever and nausea, that would subside after each session. Hemoperfusion of human organs not suitable for transplantation were also reported, including two of three patients bridged to transplantation in 1993.[47]

Hepatocyte Transplantation

Transplantation of hepatocytes is promising for patients with inherited liver disorders, such as tyrosinemia[48] and hyperbilirubinemia Crigler-Najjar syndrome,[49] which eventually lead to liver failure. The possibility of treating liver insufficiencies with hepatocyte transplantation has been investigated over the years. The infusion of purified glucocerebridase in patients with enzyme disorders, such as Gaucher disease, has been attempted.[50] Allogeneic hepatocyte transplantation to animals with enzyme deficiencies is a promising option. Studies in the mid-1970s showed conjugation of bilirubin in Gunn rats with deficiency in the enzyme uridine diphosphate glucuronyltransferase after alloinfusion of functional hepatocytes in the portal vein (PV) alone[51] and both the PV and intramuscularly.[52] Later, a group at University of Minnesota transplanted hepatocytes both intraportally and intraperitoneally in rats to support the recovery of ALF induced by dimethylnitrosamine.[53]

Experimental models of liver failure and genetic defects of liver metabolism indicate that transplanted hepatocytes can assume the full range of functions of intact whole livers.[54] Intraportal infusions of hepatocytes in humans succeeded the intraportal infusion of purified enzymes. A limiting factor of enzyme therapy has been the short-term efficacy. The indications for hepatocyte transplantation have in humans been ALF,[55] as a bridge to liver

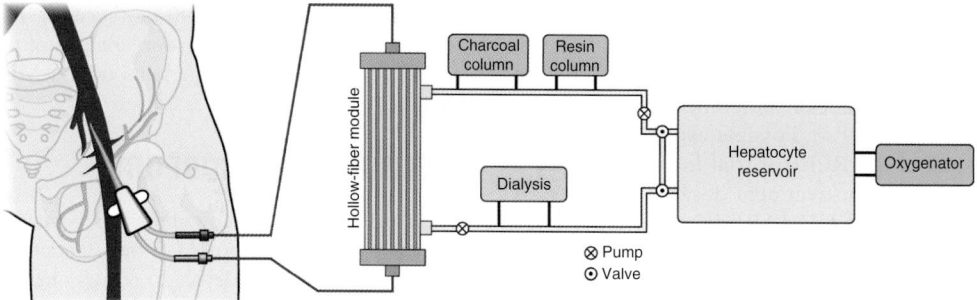

FIGURE 78.1 **A schematic overview of a generic bioartificial liver (BAL).** The BAL consists of two extracorporeal circuits: a blood circuit and an albumin circuit in direct contact with the biologic component, liver cells. A semipermeable membrane consisting of a hollow-fiber module in this example separates the two compartments. The molecular weight cut-off of the semipermeable membrane may range from 65 kDa to 0.2 mµ. The albumin circuit consists of supraphysiologic levels of albumin (>10%). The patient's blood is detoxified by removal of waste molecules across the membrane into the albumin solution. The waste molecules are eliminated from the albumin solution when it is perfused through the charcoal and resin columns or exposed to hepatocytes within the hepatocyte reservoir. Depending on the hydration status and kidney function of the patient, water can be removed from the albumin solution as ultrafiltrate from a high-flux dialysis module. This cycle is repeated continuously during extracorporeal BAL therapy.

transplantation,[56] as treatment for ornithine transcarbamylase deficiency,[57] and allogeneic hepatocyte transplantation in humans for Crigler-Najjar syndrome type 1.[49] These disorders have partially been corrected by hepatocyte transplantation, and these attempts have shown a proof of principle for cell transplantation therapy.[58,59]

Extracorporeal Hepatocyte Systems

Because of the scarcity of donor livers, it is valid to search for artificial means of liver replacement and/or support. The development of a BAL is a formidable task that must take into account the vast functions of the liver; this organ is not like the kidneys or lungs, which in a supportive context have one or two functions that must be replaced. To achieve these effects, a BAL should be able to lower blood levels of substances toxic to the brain, liver, and other organs, and it should provide whole-liver functions that are impaired or lost. The concept of BAL support was developed by Sorrentino in 1956,[60] who demonstrated more than 50 years ago that fresh liver tissue homogenate converts urea from ammonium chloride and metabolizes ketone bodies, barbiturates, and salicylic acid. It was not until the mid-1970s, however, that Wolf and colleagues[61] placed hepatoma cells in the extra-fiber space of the hollow-fiber cartridge and showed that an extracorporeal device was capable of performing liver-specific functions, such as conjugating bilirubin. The first clinically applied BAL support was by Matsumura and colleagues[62] in California, where a 45-year-old patient experienced hepatic failure because of an inoperable bile duct carcinoma. The device contained isolated rabbit hepatocytes separated from the patient's blood by a dialysis membrane. Figure 78.1 depicts a schematic overview of a modern generic BAL.

Clinical Trials of Bioartificial Liver Devices

Nine BAL devices have been evaluated in clinical trials (see Table 78.1). Only HepatAssist and Extracorporeal Liver-Assist Device (ELAD) systems have been evaluated in RCTs to date. The other BAL systems have only undergone phase I trials and will not be emphasized. These systems differ in perfusion rate, cell source, cell mass, and duration of treatment (continuous vs. intermittent).

HepatAssist System

The first BAL device to be evaluated in a multicenter prospective RCT was the HepatAssist System (Circe Biomedical, Lexington, MA).[25] The HepatAssist System used a hollow-fiber–based configuration with a membrane pore size of approximately 0.15 µm to separate the patient's plasma from 7 billion primary porcine hepatocytes (approximately 75 g) in the device. This was the first biologically based liver-assist device to be evaluated in a US Food and Drug Administration (FDA)–approved pivotal trial. This trial enrolled a total of 171 patients (86 controls and 85 BAL treated, including 147 ALF patients). The overall 30-day survival was 71% for the BAL group and 62% for the control group that received SMT. A trend was seen toward a better survival in the BAL group, although this difference did not reach statistical significance. Significant improved survival was found in a subgroup of patients with known etiology of ALF treated with BAL. Side effects of ALF included thrombocytopenia, renal failure, and increased intracranial pressure. The incidence of these side effects was higher in controls, but again the difference did not reach statistical significance. The authors concluded that the HepatAssist System, and its use of xenogeneic pig hepatocytes, was safe with regard to zoonosis; all patients tested negative for porcine endogenous retrovirus after treatment.

Extracorporeal Liver-Assist Device

The ELAD (Vital Therapies, San Diego, CA) was inoculated with a human hepatoblastoma cell line (C3A) loaded in a hollow-fiber cartridge. Ellis and colleagues[23] evaluated the ELAD in an RCT of patients with ALF. Two groups of patients were studied: those judged to be potentially recoverable (group 1, 17 patients) and patients who already fulfilled criteria for transplantation (group 2, 7 patients). Patients were randomly allocated to ELAD treatment or control (SMT alone). The etiologies of ALF were acetaminophen overdose in 17 cases, non-A non-B fulminant viral hepatitis in 5 cases, and hepatotoxicity from antituberculous chemotherapy in 2 cases. Of those who received ELAD treatment, 7 (78%) of 9 survived compared with 6 (75%) of 8 in the control group (group 1). Only 1 (33%) of 3 patients from group 2 who received BAL treatment survived compared with 1 (25%) of 4 in the control group.

In 2007, 54 patients with ACLF were studied in an RCT of ELAD at two different centers in China.[63] The endpoint was 30-day survival. A significant difference was reached between the control group, with 47% (9/19) survival, and the ELAD-treated group, with 86% (30/35) survival.

A third generation of ELAD was soon developed and underwent a multicenter RCT to study ALF patients with severe alcoholic hepatitis.[24] This study showed no significant overall survival between ELAD and SMT group (51% vs. 50%). Subgroup analysis demonstrated higher mortality in the ELAD group in patients with MELD scores of at least 28 (68.9% vs. 55.3%, P = .15). Specifically, patients with Cr greater than 1.5 mg/dL and international normalized ratio (INR) greater than 2.5 have higher mortality. Patients with age younger than 46.9 and MELD scores of less than 28 did show survival benefit.

Extracorporeal Liver Support and Study End Points

Should survival be the most important endpoint to assess liver support? The ideal clinical endpoint is transplant-free survival, thus assessing the impact of a therapy on avoiding liver transplantation and its short-term and long-term morbidities. There are, however, other important endpoints, such as improvement in symptoms (i.e., pruritus, encephalopathy, jaundice, coagulopathy, renal dysfunction, pulmonary function, systemic hemodynamics).

There are conflicting results revealed by meta-analyses performed in an attempt to address whether or not extracorporeal liver support therapy improve survival in patients with either ACLF or ALF. The earliest systematic reviews performed by the Cochrane group[64,65] suggested that nonbiologic support systems reduce mortality in ACLF compared with SMT. A meta-analysis by Khuroo and colleagues,[66] however, failed to show a significant survival benefit with MARS treatment (nonbiologic) compared with SMT alone. A more current review from 2019 included the most studies to date and separated ALF from ACLF.[67] This analysis concluded that liver support therapy reduced hepatic encephalopathy in patients with liver failure, and it may provide more survival benefit for patients with ACLF than ALF.

The results to date do not justify use of nonbiologic liver support devices for all patients with liver failure. However, use of the nonbiologic therapy in select groups of patients, such as drug overdose or severe hepatic encephalopathy, may be justifiable.

POSTHEPATECTOMY LIVER FAILURE

The application of liver support devices in PHLF is an emerging indication.[68] The need for liver support is based on increased rates of severe postoperative mortality and overall liver-related morbidity with major hepatectomies[69] (see Chapters 101 and 102). Major hepatectomy is associated with reduced synthetic, detoxification, and immune responses with potentially life-threatening complications, such as hepatic encephalopathy, increased susceptibility to infections and sepsis, renal failure, coagulopathy, and hemodynamic instability (see Chapters 101 and 102).[70-72] Thus the term *major hepatectomy*, defined as resection of three or more segments, is based on the association of greater morbidity and mortality.[73,74] The indications for major hepatectomies have expanded during the last 20 years, and also high-risk patients with steatosis, fibrosis, and chemotherapy-induced liver injury are included.[71] Treatment options of PHLF include intensive medical care focused on treating the

complications until the remnant liver recovers. These patients often require prolonged stays in intensive care units (ICUs) and endure protracted recovery.[75] Liver support devices may be considered and, as a last resort, (rescue) liver transplantation.

There are reports of the use of MARS for the treatment of PHLF.[76,77] These two reports were uncontrolled evaluations of nonbiologic liver support systems. Grodzicki and colleagues[21] reported use of Prometheus for PHLF. There is only one study that reported the use of a biologic support system for PHLF.[27]

These preliminary results are promising. RCTs are warranted in evaluating liver support devices in PHLF. Future studies should address when to initiate liver support therapy and the duration of therapy.

FUTURE DIRECTIONS

BAL devices that have reached clinical trials have been inoculated with hepatocytes from either primary or transformed sources. The trials performed so far have shown safety and proof of concept; however, efficacy data to convincingly demonstrate support of a patient with a failing liver are still missing. Limitations of the first-generation BAL systems have included excess device complexity,[78] insufficient dose of hepatocytes to support a failing liver,[26] and loss or absence of differentiated function.[79] To address these limitations, a number of research efforts are underway. Various novel configurations have been undertaken to improve hepatocyte viability and functional activity in the quest to improve device efficacy. For example, promising reports have shown that combining different cell types of the liver in coculture with hepatocytes more closely mimics the liver environment in vivo.[80-82] As another example, Nyberg and colleagues[83] have developed a novel method of forming hepatic spheroids through gentle oscillation in a rocked bioreactor. Compared with traditional monolayer systems, spheroids show superior function in albumin production, phase I and phase II metabolism, and ureagenesis. In addition, suspension culture of hepatocyte spheroids is capable of supporting 250 to 500 g of primary hepatocytes. This cell mass is a significant increase versus first-generation devices. A calculated dose exceeding 150 g of viable hepatocytes is needed in a BAL to effectively detoxify ammonia, assuming a clinical production rate of 400 μmol/hr of ammonia.[84] This device has already undergone rigorous large animal model studies and showed significant survival benefit in pigs with drug-induced ALF[85] and PHLF.[86]

Improved detoxification through enhanced mass transfer is another important aspect of future BAL designs. Optimal mass transfer is achieved with a semipermeable membrane of porosity that provides efficient waste removal and an effective immunologic barrier to protect nonautologous cells in the BAL. A study showed improved mass transfer of toxins with a 400-kDa cut-off membrane compared with a 70-kDa membrane.[84] However, porosity greater than 400 kDa, which includes apheresis membranes, may allow large fluxes of plasma proteins and immune-mediated damage of nonautologous hepatocytes in the BAL.[87,88]

An abundant source of metabolically active hepatocytes is essential to any successful BAL system. Porcine hepatocytes have been used, but immunologic concerns and theoretical risks of zoonosis have limited their acceptance.[89,90] Meanwhile, immortalized human hepatocytes fail to express a full battery of hepatocyte functions (i.e., ammonia detoxification, phase I and phase II metabolic activities) and carry theoretical risks of malignant spread to an immunocompromised transplant recipient.[91] These risks of porcine and transformed human cells have led researchers to explore alternative options for production of human stem-cell derived hepatocyte-like cells in vitro.[92] In vivo differentiation and expansion of hepatocyte-like cells has also been pursued because solely in vitro efforts have been of limited success.

One promising system for expansion of human hepatocytes in vivo uses u-plasminogen activator–transgenic severe combined immunodeficiency (u-PA/SCID) mice.[93-95] These transgenic mice express u-PA under the transcriptional control of a hepatotoxic albumin promoter.[94] Taking advantage of their immunodeficient state, human hepatocytes can be successfully transplanted into these mice without rejection. While the recipient murine hepatocytes die, healthy, unaffected human hepatocytes expand unopposed within the mouse liver, yielding chimeric human/mouse livers.[96] This system has led to engraftment levels exceeding 50%. Critics of the SCID-mouse system point to difficulties in animal husbandry, maintenance of mutant phenotype, renal disease in the transgenic mice, and a narrow window for human hepatocyte transfer.[95]

In response to concerns over the SCID-mouse system, an alternative approach has been used to expand human hepatocytes with other transgenic mice. Using immunodeficient $Rag2^{-/-}/Il2rg^{-/-}$ mice, researchers sought to generate an essential hepatocyte deficit and a selective pressure for the stable engraftment of human hepatocytes.[97] Fumarylacetoacetate hydrolase (FAH) is an essential enzyme in tyrosine catabolism. Mice deficient for FAH develop tyrosinemia and liver disease in the absence of the protective drug 2-(2-nitro-4-trifluoromethylbenzoyl)-1,3-cyclohexanedione, better known as NTBC.[98] $FAH^{--}/RAG2^{-/-}Il2rg^{-/-}$ triple-knockout mice were shown to be a successful model of stable engraftment and proliferation of human hepatocytes for the treatment of FAH deficiency.[99] Animals in this system are easily bred, devoid of renal disease, and transplantable at a range of ages.

Novel systems for in vivo[94,97] and in vitro expansion of human hepatocytes are still early in development.[100,101] Critical to any system used to expand human hepatocytes is the ability to produce a large quantity of stable, healthy cells with normal hepatocyte phenotypes. In this regard, in vivo systems appear to be more advanced than in vitro systems; however, in vivo systems are currently limited by the number of hepatocytes that can be expanded from a mouse—approximately 5 g.[102] To overcome the size limitations of the mouse model, a FAH-deficient pig was cloned.[103] Furthermore, transcriptor activator–like effector nuclease (TALEN) technology has been applied to generate combined SCID and inactivated RAG2 minipigs. These animals were subsequently injected with induced pluripotent stem cells, resulting in mature teratomas with all three germ layers.[104] Reprogramming strategies may be more successful if the approach is less aggressive by omitting the step of embryonic dedifferentiation before maturation.[105] When transplanted with human hepatocytes, the pig has the potential to repopulate with human hepatocytes on a large scale, providing a practical source of hepatocytes for cell-based BAL devices.

Interesting and promising approaches to hepatocyte production have been made with stem cells.[106,107] Embryonic stem cells are pluripotent, meaning they have the potential to differentiate into most cell types and therefore could be a source of human hepatocytes. This would also increase the possibility of obtaining unlimited numbers of human hepatocytes and thus further the development of cell-based therapies for liver diseases. The potential uses for stem cells are numerous.[108,109] Drawbacks to stem cell–produced hepatocytes are the limited number of approved human cell lines; the lack of recognition of how to control the development of immature stem cells to mature, phenotypic, liver-specific cell types; and the possibility of teratoma formation.[110] However, cocultivation with endothelial cells and mesenchymal stroma cells can potentially overcome these drawbacks by enhancing differentiation and bud structure formation.[111]

Tissue engineering provides an exciting new frontier to support of the failing liver. Similar to cardiac studies with decellularized hearts, current efforts are aimed at decellularization of whole livers from donor animals (rodent or porcine) to create a scaffold on which to regenerate a suitable donor organ.[112] The decellularization process completely eliminates donor cells while preserving the extracellular matrix and vasculature-reducing potential immune complications.[113] Early work in rodents demonstrates that a decellularized implanted rat liver can support in vitro recellularization with maintenance of cell viability and function.[114] More recently, Shaheen and colleagues have examined the use of decellularized porcine livers revascularized with human umbilical vein endothelial cells and transplanted into pigs.[115] They found that these bioengineered livers can remained perfused up to 15 days without anticoagulation and that human endothelial cells colonize the sinusoids of the liver and express endothelial markers similar to normal liver tissue. Significant research efforts have been dedicated to regeneration as a solution to the lack of high-quality and readily available organs for transplantation in support of the failing liver.

The references for this chapter can be found online by accessing the accompanying Expert Consult website.

CHAPTER 79

Management of ascites in cirrhosis and portal hypertension

Kevin M. Korenblat

A BRIEF HISTORY OF ASCITES AND PORTAL HYPERTENSION

Ascites is the pathologic accumulation of fluid in the peritoneal cavity. It is both the most frequent and prominent clinical sign of liver disease. Notwithstanding the near reflexive association of ascites with liver disease, the formation of ascites is caused by a variety of conditions that range from benign to sinister.

Descriptions of ascites exist in human history from as distant as 1600 years Before the Common Era. Hindu medical treatises, the Ebers Papyrus of Ancient Egypt, and Mesoamerican figurines with a protuberant abdomen and everted umbilicus[1] testify to the experience of many cultures with ascites. Hippocrates, though lacking any knowledge of hepatic physiology, presciently observed "when the liver is full of fluid and this overflows into the peritoneal cavity, so that the belly becomes full of water, death follows."[2] Even the term *ascites*—derived from the Greek *askos*, a bag made of leather or sheepskin used to contain liquids—reflects its ancient origins.[3]

CLINICAL FINDINGS

Common physical examination findings of ascites include diastasis of abdominal muscles, umbilical herniation, and bulging flanks. In the supine position, fluid pools in the flanks where percussion may be dull compared with more tympanic areas of the central abdomen. The examination findings are easily elicited with large-volume ascites. The findings are less obvious in those with smaller ascites volumes, obesity, and concomitant organomegaly.

Ultrasound is the best imaging modality for the detection of ascites; it is inexpensive, avoids ionizing radiation, is performed as point-of-care testing, and has the added benefit of capturing the liver architecture and portal vein patency (see Chapter 13).

Ascites is graded by its volume. Grade 1 ascites is mild and detectable only by radiographic imaging. Grades 2 and 3 reflect moderate and severe ascites, respectively. In the latter, there is obvious abdominal distention, which is frequently associated with the discomfort of a protuberant abdomen, particularly in previously asthenic individuals.

PORTAL HYPERTENSION AND MECHANISMS OF ASCITES FORMATION

Ascites is the most common complication of portal hypertension arising from cirrhosis and the annual incidence is 5% to 10%.[4] Ascites development is associated with a median survival of 2 years[5,6] and, absent an earlier development of other signs or symptoms, heralds the change from a compensated to a decompensated state.

Portal hypertension can arise from cirrhotic and noncirrhotic disease, though as a manifestation of portal hypertension, ascites is more common in disorders that increase hepatic sinusoidal pressure from either sinusoidal hypertension or postsinusoidal processes (heart failure, venous outflow obstruction such as Budd-Chiari syndrome; see Chapter 86). By comparison, ascites is less frequent in presinusoidal portal hypertension (e.g., extrahepatic portal vein thrombosis).

The splanchnic circulation consists of all the vasculature arising from the celiac, superior mesenteric, and inferior mesenteric arteries (see Chapters 2 and 5). Splanchnic arterioles are partially constricted under basal conditions and are responsive to a myriad of endothelial-derived substances, circulating vasoactive agents, and neurotransmitters.[7]

The majority of the blood flow into the liver arises from the venous drainage of the splanchnic organs and conveyed into the liver by the portal circulation. Under normal conditions, portal blood (and hepatic arterial blood) enter the sinusoids at the portal tract and transverse the sinusoids to reach the hepatic vein. Sinusoids are separated from cords of hepatocytes by liver sinusoidal endothelial cells (LSECs), whose properties of being both fenestrated and lacking a basement membrane allow oxygen, cells, and plasma components to diffuse into the space of Disse wherein reside the hepatic stellate cells (HSCs) (see Chapter 7).

HSCs are the principal collagen-producing cells of the liver and elaborate extracellular matrix in response to liver injury rendering the fenestrations of the LSECs ineffective (see Chapter 7). These architectural changes in the hepatic microcirculation result in the *static* contribution to portal hypertension. Based on studies in animal models, these static changes account for 80% of the increase in resistance to portal flow. The remaining 20% of the resistance reflects *dynamic* forces influenced by HSCs that acquire a contractile, pericyte-like function.[8] Molecular signaling to the HSCs through increased sensitivity to endothelin; ligand of the CXC chemokine receptor 4; dysfunctional nitric oxide–mediated signaling between LSECs and HSCs; and microvascular thrombosis have all been studied as mechanisms to explain LSEC response.[9]

In the splanchnic circulation, different but equally important changes occur that contribute to portal hypertension. The most determinative change is splanchnic arterial vasodilation. In experimental models of cirrhosis, vasodilation is mediated by nitric oxide (NO)–dependent and NO-independent processes.[10] An incomplete list of NO-independent processes includes vasodilatory natriuretic peptides, endocannabanoids, impaired sympathetic nervous system signaling, and overactivity of the enzyme heme oxygenase. Vasodilation in the splanchnic circulation decreases the effective arterial circulation, and increases in cardiac output compensate for the change.

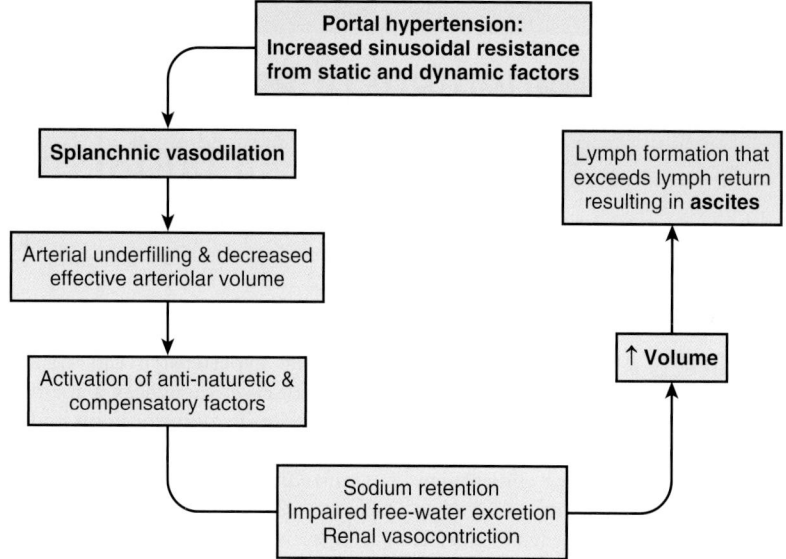

FIGURE 79.1 Flowchart of the pathophysiologic processes that link the development of portal hypertension in cirrhosis to the ascites development.

To date, none of the signaling pathways that result in either dynamic HSC effects or splanchnic vasodilation has translated into therapies to counteract portal hypertension. In comparison, there are emerging therapies that may reduce or reverse hepatic fibrosis.[11]

With the progression of portal hypertension, additional compensatory mechanisms marshal to maintain the arterial circulation in the face of even greater increases in splanchnic vasodilation. These mechanisms include activation of the renin-angiotensin-aldosterone system and sympathetic nervous system stimulation of renal sodium retention. Nonosmotic release of arginine vasopressin (antidiuretic hormone [ADH]) is an additional compensatory mechanism to increase the effective arterial volume, even at the expense of tonicity; this is often the mechanism for hyponatremia in decompensated cirrhosis.

The cumulative effects of increased hydrostatic pressure in the hepatic microcirculation, increased splanchnic volume, and hyperdynamic circulation (increased flow) lead to hepatic lymph formation in excess of its removal (Fig. 79.1). The excess fluid weeps into the peritoneal cavity and is recognized as ascites.

EVALUATION OF ASCITES

Cirrhotic ascites is translucent but commonly takes on a yellow or amber color. The fluid typically has a low leukocyte (less than 100 µL/mm³) and red blood cell content. The protein content is typically less than 2.5 mg/dL, and the protein content varies inversely with the severity of the portal hypertension. High protein content (ascites fluid protein greater than 2.5 mg/dL) is commonly seen in ascites arising from venous outflow obstruction from heart failure.[12]

Measurement of the serum albumin ascites gradient (SAAG) is both a highly accurate and clinically facile technique for assessing the origins of ascites. The SAAG is calculated by subtracting the concentration of albumin in the ascites from that in the plasma. With an approximately 97% accuracy, a difference (called the *gradient*) greater than 1.1 g/dL indicates the presence of portal or sinusoidal hypertension.[13]

Opacification of the ascites fluid can arise from a number of disparate processes. Bloody ascites (hematocrit >0.5%) can be seen in traumatic paracentesis, spontaneous rupture of hepatocellular cancer, or hemorrhagic pancreatitis. Chylous ascites is milky in appearance from increased concentration of chylomicron-rich triglycerides (ascites triglyceride >100 mg/dL).[14,15] It arises from disruption of lymphatic flow, most commonly lymphagiectasia or lymphoma, but it can also occur with disseminated mycobacterial infections,[16] cancers[17] (Kaposi sarcoma, carcinoid tumors), abdominal trauma, or surgical disruption of the cisterna chyli. Cirrhotic ascites can also take on a chylous appearance owing to rupture of abdominal lymphatics from portal hypertension. In these cases, known as pseudo-chylous ascites, the triglyceride concentration is generally less than the threshold value of ascites triglyceride found in cases not arising from portal hypertension.

Both malignancy and tuberculosis peritonitis can result in ascites, and in both circumstances, the SAAG is less than 1.1 g/dL. Confusion may arise when liver disease coexists, as in the case of tuberculosis and alcohol-related liver disease. The diagnosis of malignant ascites is established by the finding of cancer cells within the peritoneal cavity. This can be diagnosed by cytology in combination with immunohistologic staining.[18]

The peritoneum is a common site of involvement in tuberculosis, and in the United States the peritoneum is the sixth most common extrapulmonary site. Peritoneal cell counts typically vary between 500 and 1500 cells/mm³ with a lymphocyte predominance in 68%, although the absence of a lymphocyte predominance does not exclude tuberculosis, particularly in patients with renal failure in whom the cells are mostly neutrophils. Mycobacterial culture of the fluid has a diagnostic sensitivity of 34% and requires several weeks of incubation.[19] Measurement of adenosine deaminase activity in the peritoneal fluid has been proposed as another diagnostic test with high sensitivity and specificity,[20] although the positive predictive value has been reported to be low in the setting of concomitant cirrhosis. Of all the diagnostic strategies, laparoscopy with peritoneal biopsy affords the highest sensitivity and specificity and permits exclusion of other granulomatous and nongranulomatous processes that can produce low-SAAG ascites. The ascites concentration of lactate dehydrogenase (LDH) tends to be higher than that of serum LDH in malignant ascites and less than half that of serum in tuberculous ascites.

MANAGEMENT OF ASCITES

The primary goal of ascites management is to reduce ascites volume. This can be achieved by strategies that increase renal sodium excretion, mechanically remove the ascites, or reduce portal hypertension. It is only with reduction of portal hypertension that the fundamental physiologic mechanism responsible for ascites is addressed. Choosing the most appropriate therapy must consider the volume of ascites, the severity of the underlying liver disease, and the presence of renal dysfunction or electrolyte disorders.

Dietary Sodium Restriction

Renal sodium retention is a compensatory response to decreases in effective arteriolar volume, and dietary sodium restriction is one strategy that can tip the balance in favor of net sodium loss. First studied over 60 years ago,[21] dietary salt restriction has been shown to decrease the rate of ascites accumulation and increase urine volume. The median sodium consumption among adults in the United States is 3232 mg per day.[22] Patients with mild degrees of cirrhotic portal hypertension have a baseline rate of sodium excretion of at least 40 mEq/day.[23] Consequently, those with ascites are commonly advised to restrict dietary salt intake to less than 1.5 to 2 grams per day (54 to 68 mEq/day),[24] the lower values considered adequate for daily needs. Although seemingly a simple intervention, success with dietary salt restriction is difficult. Most sodium consumed is added in commercial food processing, and the patient's actual consumption may be unapparent unless food labeling is scrutinized.

Medical Management

Most patients at some point require diuretics (Table 79.1). Between 500 and 750 mL per day of ascites can be mobilized

TABLE 79.1 Diuretics and Dosages Used in the Management of Ascites

MEDICATION	STARTING DOSE	MAXIMAL DOSE
Aldosterone Antagonists		
Spironolactone	50–100 mg daily	400 mg daily
Amiloride[a]	5 mg daily	10 mg daily
Eplerenone[a]	50 mg daily	100 mg daily
Loop Diuretics		
Furosemide	20–40 mg daily	160 mg daily
Arginine Vasopressin Receptor Antagonists		
Tolvaptan[b]	15 mg daily	

Initial and maximal dosages of diuretics used in the treatment of cirrhotic ascites. The combination of an aldosterone antagonist and loop diuretics is more effective than either class of diuretic alone.

[a]Amiloride and eplerenone are most commonly used as a substitute for spironolactone when spironolactone use results in gynecomastia.

[b]Use tolvaptan only with extreme caution in cirrhotic ascites and preferably under the guidance of a physician with experience with its use.

without intravascular depletion, and greater amounts of ascites fluid losses may be tolerable in the presence of edema, which tends to act as a buffer. The avoidance of rapid fluid loss is critical because precipitous and excessive intravascular volume contraction can give rise to kidney injury.

Aldosterone Antagonists

The aldosterone antagonists, spironolactone, amiloride, and eplerenone, can be used as monotherapy or in combination with loop diuretics. These agents prevent sodium reabsorption in the distal tubule and cortical collecting duct. Although aldosterone antagonists are weak natriuretics, they are effective in cirrhotic ascites.

Urine sodium excretion and plasma aldosterone concentration are inversely related in cirrhosis, and a greater sensitivity to the dose-response curve is observed in those with ascites. One explanation for the effectiveness of this group of diuretics is that they target the functional hyperaldosteronism common in cirrhosis that would otherwise promote sodium reabsorption in the cortical collecting duct of the sodium filtered in the loop of Henle. In addition, unlike other diuretics that require access to the tubular lumen, spironolactone enters the principal cell of the collecting duct from the plasma compartment and thereby circumvents decreases in renal blood flow and hypoalbuminemia commonly encountered in patients with cirrhosis that might otherwise reduce diuretic activity.

Spironolactone is commonly started at 50 to 100 mg daily. The dose can be doubled every 3 days to a maximum of 400 mg per day. Its long half-life makes daily dosing permissible even at maximal dosages. Both hyperkalemia and hyponatremia may occur and require dose reduction or drug discontinuation. A recognized side effect of spironolactone in men is tender gynecomastia. This occurs because of greater exposure to estradiol by increases in peripheral conversion of testosterone to estradiol and greater bioavailability of estradiol displaced from sex hormone–binding globulin. When this occurs, amiloride (5 to 10 mg per day) or eplerenone (50 to 100 mg per day) can be substituted.[25]

Loop Diuretics

Though loop diuretics are often unsuccessful as monotherapy for ascites, the combination of a loop diuretic and an aldosterone antagonist is the most commonly prescribed combination for moderate to severe ascites. The most commonly used loop diuretic is furosemide, beginning at doses of 20 to 40 mg daily. The dose is doubled in a coordination with increases in spironolactone and, like spironolactone, a 4-fold increase in dose (160 mg daily) is considered a maximal dose. An added benefit of loop diuretics is that they counteract the hyperkalemia associated with aldosterone antagonists, and they may also benefit those who develop edema with ascites.

Although the parenteral administration of loop diuretics is a common therapy for edema in heart and renal failure, this should be avoided in the management of ascites because it may precipitate acute kidney injury. Successful use of diuretics requires diligent monitoring for electrolyte disorders and azotemia. Advanced cirrhosis is often associated with a catabolic state and lean muscle mass loss. Consequently, seemingly modest increases in serum creatinine may reflect significant impairment of glomerular filtration rate.

The development of azotemia should prompt dose reduction or cessation of diuretics. Renal dysfunction may also be a sign or a complication of liver disease, including spontaneous bacterial peritonitis or gastrointestinal (GI) bleeding from portal hypertension. In these and similar situations of acute decompensation, diuretics should be discontinued until the condition improves or resolves.

Arginine Vasopressin Receptor Antagonists

The nonosmotic release of ADH is a compensatory mechanism for the decrease in effective arterial volume that occurs with splanchnic vasodilation with cirrhosis. ADH exerts its effects through the arginine vasopressin receptor-2 (AVPR2); the receptor is predominantly expressed in the distal convoluted tubule and collecting ducts of the kidney. Satavaptan is a selective AVPR2 receptor antagonist that has been tested in clinical studies of both the syndrome of inappropriate ADH release and hyponatremia occurring with cirrhosis.[26] These medications should be used with great caution. The hyponatremia that develops in cirrhosis can be managed by other means, including diuretic withdrawal, albumin infusions, or hypertonic saline; and concerns have been raised about the safety of long-term use of an oral formulation (tolvaptan) in the setting of chronic liver disease.[27]

Refractory Ascites

Refractory ascites is ascites that persists despite dietary sodium restriction and high-dose diuretics (spironolactone 400 mg per day; furosemide 160 mg per day). *Diuretic-intolerant* ascites describes diuretic failure because of intolerant side effects (e.g., kidney injury, hyponatremia, hypotension) that prevent the attainment of a dose sufficient to effect ascites control. The clinical significance of refractory ascites should not be underestimated; the survival curves of individuals with refractory ascites approximates those with type II hepatorenal syndrome, also called hepatorenal syndrome–nonacute kidney injury (HRS-NAKI).[28-30]

Before labeling a patient with refractory ascites, it is important to exclude excessive sodium intake or other medications that may influence diuretic response. In particular, nonsteroidal antiinflammatory agents, including aspirin, may decrease diuretic response and contribute to kidney injury.

Treatment options for refractory ascites include therapeutic paracentesis, transjugular intrahepatic portosystemic shunt (TIPS; see Chapter 85), various peritoneal shunting procedures, and liver transplantation.

Paracentesis

Large-volume paracentesis, also known as therapeutic paracentesis, was the most effective treatment in practice before the development of modern diuretics, after which the practice fell out of favor until it was reintroduced in 1987 as safe and effective.[31]

A number of large-bore needles (15 gauge or smaller) of various configurations and features have been introduced for paracentesis. The procedure can be done with or without ultrasound guidance. Commonly chosen sites for needle placement are over the right or left lower quadrant; fluid is removed by gravity, peristaltic pumps, or vacuum suction. No single technique is superior to the other.

Potential immediate adverse events from paracentesis include hematoma and peritoneal hemorrhage. Leakage of ascites can be reduced by introducing the needle in a "Z-track" fashion. Modest leaks are best controlled by covering the site with

an ostomy appliance, but larger leaks may require the site of leakage to be sutured. No compelling data are available to suggest that repeated large-volume paracentesis predisposes to bacterial peritonitis. There is also no evidence to suggest that the typical patient with large-volume cirrhotic ascites is at risk for an abdominal compartment syndrome; thus paracentesis should not be expected to improve kidney function simply by decreased peritoneal ascites volume.

There are two central debates in paracentesis. The first centers on the maximal volume of fluid that can be removed at one time, and the second is whether circulatory volume expanders are required. Because ascites is extravascular fluid, paracentesis can be safely done until fluid withdrawal is complete. Immediately after paracentesis, cardiac stroke volume and output increase, and the renin-angiotensin-aldosterone (RAA) axis is suppressed. At greater than 12 hours after paracentesis a rebound increase in the RAA and increased arterial vasodilation occur. These changes are reflected in a reduction in systemic vascular resistance and form the basis of the postparacentesis circulatory dysfunction,[32] a condition associated with renal dysfunction, a higher incidence of hyponatremia, and decreased survival rate.

The administration of volume expanders at the time of paracentesis is principally done to ameliorate these changes and applies to both adults and children.[33] Studies comparing albumin to other agents (saline, colloidal starches) have shown it to be more effective in preventing circulatory dysfunction in paracentesis when the volume removed is greater than 5 L. In practice, 12.5 g of 25% albumin can be infused for every 2 L of ascites removed. The timing of administration has not been rigorously studied, but because of the long circulatory half-life of albumin, its administration after completion of paracentesis is likely to be sufficient. The benefits of albumin notwithstanding, no compelling data are available to suggest that albumin administered with paracentesis improves patient survival.

The intermittent, chronic administration of albumin independent of its use with paracentesis has, however, emerged as a strategy for the management of decompensated cirrhosis. In some but not all trials, the chronic administration of albumin was associated with decreased rates of paracentesis and refractory ascites.[34] These studies reflect a growing appreciation for potential antiinflammatory properties of albumin, and the potential role of damaged (oxidized) albumin as its own proinflammatory signal.[35]

Transjugular Intrahepatic Portosystemic Shunt (TIPS)

TIPS (see Chapter 85) was first introduced experimentally in 1969, and the first performance of TIPS with a metallic stent in a human was in 1988.[36] The purpose of the TIPS is to create a pathway to bypass sinusoidal hypertension and thereby relieve portal hypertension. In multiple, randomized clinical trials, TIPS placement in those with refractory ascites has been associated with substantially greater sustained relief of ascites compared with paracentesis.[37-40]

The early clinical experience with TIPS used bare metal stents, which were prone to occlusion. In the early 2000s, stents partially covered with expanded polytetrafluoroethylene (ePTFE) became more widely used and, eventually, preferred for their favorable rates of patency. The clinical trials with ePTFE stents also demonstrated a transplant-free survival benefit not seen in earlier studies.[41]

The magnitude of portal decompression necessary to effect ascites resolution is not known. The most common indirect measure of portal hypertension is the hepatic venous pressure gradient (HVPG). The HVPG is measured by hepatic vein catherization with a balloon-tipped, pressure-transducing catheter, and the HVPG necessary for control of ascites is unknown.

A critical component to the success of TIPS is proper patient selection. TIPS is contraindicated in those with pulmonary hypertension and heart failure with reduced ejection fraction. Situations in which TIPS placement is not technically possible include extensive (and unrecanalizable) portal vein thrombosis, or infiltrative hepatocellular cancer.

The periprocedural TIPS mortality risk is low, between 1.7% and 3%. Unlike procedure-related mortality, for which no risk predictions are available, several systems have been offered to predict the short-term (typically within 90 days of TIPS) survival. Scoring systems include serum bilirubin alone, the Acute Physiology and Chronic Health Evaluation II (APACHE II), Child-Turcotte-Pugh (CTP) class, and the Model for End-Stage Liver Disease (MELD) (see Chapter 4). The simplest of these is serum bilirubin as a predictor of 30-day mortality, with a 40% increased risk of death for each 1 mg/dL increase above 3 mg/dL.[42,43] Although the contemporary version of MELD (incorporating serum sodium) is most commonly used for liver transplant organ allocation in the United States, it was originally developed to predict the 3-month mortality after TIPS.[44] Decreased survival after TIPS has been reported with MELD scores of 15 and greater. In patients with high MELD scores, the risks and benefits of TIPS should be carefully considered, as should the patient's candidacy for liver transplantation as an alternative to TIPS or to rescue following clinical deterioration post-TIPS.

The other major risk of TIPS is post-TIPS encephalopathy. This risk is estimated to be 20% to 37%.[45] In most cases, the encephalopathy is manageable with standard medication. Rarely, the confusion refractory to treatment requires narrowing the diameter or complete TIPS occlusion. In some studies, the risk of hepatic encephalopathy in similar between those randomized to TIPS and those randomized to repeated session of large-volume paracentesis.[41,46]

Peritoneovenous Shunt

Peritoneovenous shunting (PVS) was introduced by Leveen in 1974 for the management of refractory ascites.[47] The shunt is a plastic cannula subcutaneously tunneled with one end in the peritoneal cavity and the other in the central venous circulation. One-way flow is established by a pressure-sensitive valve positioned between the two ends. These shunts go by a variety of names, including Leveen, Minnesota, and Denver shunts, which reflect proprietary differences in technical details. The placement of shunts results in increases in plasma volume, glomerular filtration rate, and urine sodium excretion. All these effects reflect favorable physiologic changes to decrease ascites formation; however, PVS use is very uncommon in contemporary current practice. One reason for its lack of use is that 40% of shunts stop working within 1 year of placement. Another reason for their unpopularity is the adverse events reported with their use, which include pulmonary edema, disseminated intravascular coagulation, and peritonitis.

A more contemporary version of peritoneal shunting is a proprietary automated, low-flow shunt that is placed between the peritoneum and urinary bladder, permitting ascites removal through micturition.[48] The placement of peritoneal drains that can be intermittently accessed for fluid removal is generally not done because of the risk of infection and precipitating electrolyte and kidney dysfunction, though their feasibility continues to be studied and occasionally used for palliation.[49]

Liver Transplant

Liver transplantation is effective in both relieving ascites and improving survival (see Chapter 105), and in all patients with refractory cirrhotic ascites, consideration should be given to liver transplantation as a treatment option. Although cases of persistent ascites have been reported after liver transplantation, these cases are uncommon and generally arise for reasons different than those before transplant.[50]

COMPLICATIONS

Hepatic Hydrothorax

Hepatic hydrothorax is the pleural effusion in those with end-stage liver disease and portal hypertension that occur in the absence of other conditions expected to cause the effusion.[51] It has been proposed that intraabdominal pressure from ascites leads to herniation of the peritoneum through gaps in the diaphragm that eventually rupture in the pleural cavity resulting in egress of ascites from the peritoneal cavity into the negative pressure space of the pleural cavity. These areas of communications have been shown by following the transdiaphragmatic passage of tracers (air, dyes, and radiolabeled substances) and by direct thoracoscopic visualization of the defects. Hydrothorax is uncommon; the reported incidence is 5% to 12%, which is remarkably similar to the incidence of hydrothorax with continuous ambulatory peritoneal dialysis. The effusions are mostly right sided but can be left sided or bilateral and present in patients with minimal or no abdominal ascites.

Respiratory symptoms encountered with a hydrothorax include dyspnea, fatigue, and nonproductive cough. The relationship between hypoxemia and hydrothorax is more complex. Hypoxemia requires ventilation-perfusion mismatching, and the mere presence of a hydrothorax alone, even one large enough to opacify a hemithorax, does not always result in resting hypoxemia. When deoxygenation is documented, the possibility of an underlying acute or chronic parenchymal lung disease or the hepatopulmonary syndrome should be considered as a cause of hypoxemia before attributing it to the hydrothorax.

Hepatic hydrothorax should be suspected in any patient with cirrhosis and portal hypertension with a pleural effusion. Diagnostic thoracentesis should be performed as a starting point in the evaluation. The hepatic hydrothorax is transudative by traditional criteria. Tracking the migration of technetium-99m–labeled albumin or sulfur colloid has been proposed and used to establish the diagnosis of hydrothorax, although in practice such tests are rarely used. Rather, the diagnosis is reasonable in the setting of a rapidly recurring transudative effusion in a patient with cirrhosis in whom other diseases that predispose to transudative effusion have been excluded. If doubt persists, measurement of the hepatic venous pressure gradient can help support the diagnosis and exclude right-sided heart failure.

Therapeutic thoracentesis is safe and can provide immediate relief from dyspnea. By comparison, tube thoracostomy, also known as chest tube placement, should be avoided. Prominent complications associated with chest tube placement for hydrothorax include infection and acute renal failure, the latter likely reflecting large volume losses.

The principles of management of a hydrothorax are similar to those of ascites. Dietary salt restriction followed by diuretics is the first line of treatment. Even if these treatments are modestly successful, they may still be inadequate to relieve symptoms given the small capacitance of the pleural space. In these situations, TIPS should be considered early in the care. Although the data supporting a role for TIPS in hepatic hydrothorax are less established than those for ascites, in one study a favorable clinical response was achieved in 79% and 75% at 1 and 6 months, respectively.[52] Not surprisingly, liver transplantation is also an effective treatment of hydrothorax.

Surgical repair of the diaphragmatic defects has been described in small series of patients. Obvious limitations to the procedure are the operative morbidity and mortality in patients with end-stage liver disease. Management of hydrothorax is particularly challenging in individuals in whom TIPS is contraindicated and in those in whom hydrothorax is refractory to TIPS. One therapy used for refractory hydrothorax is tunneled pleural catheters originally employed for malignant effusions.[53] The risk of infection is theoretically reduced because the catheters are tunneled and it is a closed system. Further, because they are designed for periodic use, the rate of fluid loss can be controlled.

Spontaneous Bacterial Peritonitis

Spontaneous bacterial infection of the cirrhotic ascites in the absence of suppurative infection or bowel perforation. This condition, termed *spontaneous bacterial peritonitis* (SBP), has emerged as one of the most common and feared complications of cirrhotic ascites. The prevalence and consequences of SBP are substantial: between 10% and 27% of patient with cirrhosis who have ascites will have SBP at the time of hospitalization.[54] SBP is both a potentially lethal complication and a marker of decreased survival. Twenty years ago, studies of patients presenting with their first episode of SBP reported a mortality rate of 47%. Those who survived the immediate infection still faced a high risk of dying, and in a majority of these late deaths, renal failure played a significant role.

The forces that promote infection of the ascites remain incompletely understood. The most common organisms to cause SBP are enteric gram-negative aerobic bacteria, and studies of cirrhosis in animal models show increased bacterial translocation. There are also recent trends to more gram-positive bacteria[55] and quinolone-resistant bacteria, the latter by virtue of the increased use of quinolone antibiotics.

The cirrhotic host may also be uniquely susceptible to infection as a combined effect of decreased reticuloendothelial and leukocyte function and diminished opsonic activity of ascites fluid. The opsonic activity correlates with ascites protein levels, and patients with ascites protein less than 10 g/L have a greater probability of developing peritonitis than with higher ascites protein levels.

Symptoms of SBP are varied and protean. Obvious symptoms include fever and abdominal pain, bur more subtle symptoms are those of decompensation of liver disease, including acute kidney injury, hepatic encephalopathy, and jaundice. GI bleeding as a manifestation of SBP illustrates the interrelatedness of these functions in cirrhosis. GI bleeding can both promote bacterial translocation, and therefore increase the risk of SBP, and bacterial infection can result in further mesenteric vasodilation, which increases the risk of portal hypertensive bleeding. Prophylactic antibiotics given at the time of variceal bleeding, for instance, decreases the risk of rebleeding.[56] Most important, patients with SBP can be asymptomatic.

Paracentesis to exclude SBP should be performed in all subjects with new-onset ascites and in those with a change in clinical condition. The diagnosis of SBP rests on the demonstration of an abnormally high neutrophil count in the ascites fluid or culture of an organism from the fluid. The combination of two positive findings is properly termed *spontaneous bacterial peritonitis*. By comparison, *culture-negative neutrascites* (CNNA) is the appropriate term when neutrascites is present but no organisms are recovered with culture. These terms notwithstanding, the natural history of SBP and CNNA are indistinguishable and should be treated identically. *Bacterascites* is the term applied to a positive ascites culture in the absence of neutrascites. Limited data on this subset of patients suggest that the infection may be transient.

The conventional threshold to diagnose SBP is a neutrophil count greater than 250 polymorphonuclear (PMN) cells per microliter (Fig. 79.2). This threshold is associated with the highest sensitivity to detect infection and has been a reliable biomarker over many years of study. Ascites PMN counts require adjustment when the ascites is bloody or the paracentesis traumatic. Inoculating ascites directly into blood culture media at the bedside increases the likelihood for recovery of organisms.

Particularly high neutrophil counts or the recovery of multiple microbiologic organisms should raise concern for secondary peritonitis that would reflect either a suppurative abdominal infection or bowel perforation. Measurement of ascites fluid protein, LDH, and glucose can help distinguish between spontaneous and secondary peritonitis. Secondary peritonitis should be strongly suspected when any two of the three conditions are met: glucose levels are less than 50 mg/dL; ascites protein concentration is greater than 1 g/dL; and the ascites LDH is greater than the upper limits of the reference range of serum LDH.

Antimicrobial therapy should be started either empirically if there is a clinical suspicion for SBP or promptly after the diagnosis. The initial treatment should be parenteral and cover the most frequent organisms. In common practice, the antibiotics of choice are third-generation cephalosporins, particularly cefotaxime or ceftriaxone. Other antibiotic choices may be influenced by local microbial resistance patterns, medication allergies, or a prior pattern of infection. Five days of therapy are as efficacious as 10 days of therapy. Antifungal therapy is generally not required as first-line therapy; however, it may have a role in those after abdominal surgery who develop SBP while receiving antibacterial therapy, patients with persistent neutrascites despite adequate antibacterial therapy, or patients with secondary peritonitis.

The administration of intravenous albumin has emerged as a critical adjunct to antibiotics for the treatment of SBP. The major benefit of albumin is the prevention of acute kidney injury, which occurs in as many as 30% of those with SBP despite effective antibiotic therapy. In a foundational trial comparing a control group that received antibiotics alone to a group that received albumin and antibiotics, the rates of renal impairment were reduced from 33% to 10%, and the hospital mortality rate was reduced from 29% to 10%, respectively.[57] The dose of albumin used was 1.5 g/kg body weight at diagnosis and 1 g/kg body weight on day 3. Patients with preexisting kidney disease and

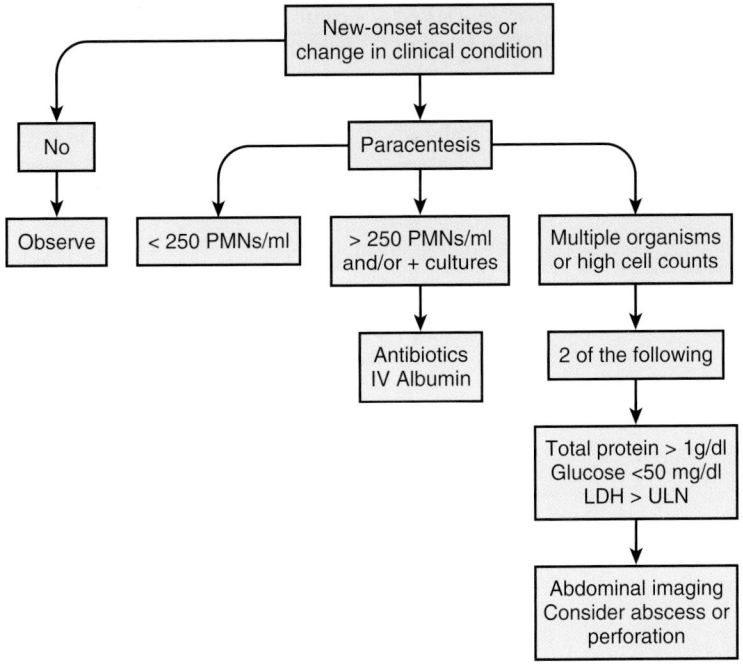

FIGURE 79.2 Flowchart for the evaluation of ascites for spontaneous bacterial ascites.

TABLE 79.2   Historical and Newly Proposed Classification System for the Hepatorenal Syndrome and Associated Criteria

HISTORICAL CLASSIFICATION	PROPOSED CLASSIFICATION		CRITERIA
HRS type 1	HRS-AKI		Absolute increase in sCR ≥0.3 mg/dL within 48 hours and/or Urinary output ≤0.5 mL/kg body weight ≥6 hours or Percent increase in sCr ≥50% using the last available value of outpatient sCr within 3 months as the baseline value
HRS type 2	HRS-NAKI		eGFR <60 mL/min per 1.73 m² for <3 months in the absence of other causes
		HRS-AKD	Percent increase in sCr <50% using the last available value of outpatient sCr within 3 months as the baseline value
		HRS-CKD	eGFR <60 mL/min per 1.73 m² for ≥3 months in the absence of other causes

AKD, Subacute kidney disease; *AKI,* acute kidney injury; *CKD,* chronic kidney disease; *eGFR,* estimated glomerular filtration rate; *HRS,* hepatorenal syndrome; *NAKI,* nonacute kidney injury; *sCR,* serum creatinine.

Modified from Angeli P, Garcia-Tsao G, Nadim MK, Parikh CR. News in pathophysiology, definition and classification of hepatorenal syndrome: A step beyond the International Club of Ascites (ICA) consensus document. *J Hepatol.* 2019;71(4):811–822.

serum bilirubin concentrations greater than 4 mg/dL appeared to derive the greatest benefit based on subgroup analysis.

Antibiotic prophylaxis has also been proposed for those with prior episodes of SBP or in those with ascites protein content less than 10 g/L. Clinical studies have shown strategies that use primary and secondary prophylaxis to reduce episodes of SBP and short-term mortality risk[58,59]; however, many studies lack a robust methodology and concerns persist that long-term antibiotic therapy will result in the selection for antibiotic-resistant organisms.

Acute Kidney Injury

Acute kidney injury (AKI) does not arise as a direct consequence of ascites; however, the same pathophysiologic process that results in ascites can lead to kidney dysfunction (see Chapter 77). To compensate for the decrease in effective arteriolar volume central

to portal hypertension, compensatory mechanism to preserve renal perfusion can result in intense intrarenal arterial vasoconstriction and, at the extreme, kidney injury. Precipitants of kidney injury in cirrhosis are typically those that result in worsening systemic vasodilation (infection) or decreased effective arteriolar volume (hypovolemia, GI hemorrhage).

This process, historically called the hepatorenal syndrome (HRS), is divided into two forms: HRS type 1 and HRS type 2. HRS type 1 is a rapidly progressive form resulting in oliguric renal failure within 2 weeks. HRS type 2 is a slowly progressive form of renal dysfunction with a natural history similar to that seen with refractory ascites. Both types occur in subjects with advanced liver disease, large-volume ascites, and hyperbilirubinemia.[60]

A proposed revised nomenclature uses the terms HRS-AKI in place of HRS type 1 and HRS-NAKI (non-AKI) for HRS type 2.[61] HRS-NAKI is further subdivided into that occurring in the context of subacute kidney disease (HRS-AKD) or chronic kidney disease (HRS-CKD). The revision also aligns with Kidney Disease Improving Global Outcomes (KDIGO) classification system (Table 79.2).

Treatment of AKI involves volume expansion, typically in the form of albumin infusion alone or in combination of vasoconstrictors. Current vasoconstrictors in use include the combination of midodrine and octreotide[62] or terlipressin.[63,64] Terlipressin is a synthetic peptide with vasocontrictive activity on the vasopressin (V1) receptor on vascular and extravascular muscle cells. Renal replacement therapy can be performed as a temporizing measure but is seldom sustainable because of the development of profound vasoplegia. Liver transplantation is the most effective treatment for these types of kidney injury.

CHAPTER 80

Medical management of bleeding varices: Primary and secondary prophylaxis for variceal bleeding

Richard Gilroy, Christopher Danford, and Maria Jepperson

INTRODUCTION

The presence of portal hypertension is a prerequisite for the development of, and bleeding from, varices. Portal hypertension is defined by a portal venous pressure exceeding the inferior vena cava pressure by more than 5 mm Hg (see Chapters 74, 76, and 79). Measuring the free hepatic vein pressure and subtracting this from the wedged hepatic vein pressure, commonly known as the hepatic venous pressure gradient (HVPG), is the most common approach for establishing an increased gradient. A normal HVPG is between 3 and 5 mm Hg. An HVPG greater than 10 mm Hg is designated "clinically significant portal hypertension" (CSPH) With a gradient greater than 10 mm Hg. CSPH is a harbinger for the development of varices and gradients greater than 10 correlate with bleeding risk. Varices may occur anywhere in the portal venous circulation with esophageal varices the most common and the most likely to bleed. The likelihood of esophageal varices being present runs parallel to the severity of liver disease, as measured by Child-Turcotte-Pugh (CTP) classification; 43% of CTP class A and 75% of CTP class C have esophageal varices (see Chapters 4, 5, and 79).

Although varices generally develop in the presence of cirrhosis, varices may also develop in the absence of intrinsic liver disease. This most often occurs when obstruction to the portal vein, splenic vein, or another large mesenteric vein occurs generally from thrombosis, most often secondary to phlebitis following an infection (see Chapter 74). Table 80.1 details the causes of portal hypertension. In those with liver disease, the likelihood of variceal bleeding increases as liver function declines. In addition, the presence of other complications of cirrhosis, like spontaneous bacterial peritonitis (SBP), hepatocellular carcinoma, and portal vein thrombosis (PVT) independently increase the risk for bleeding form varices.

When bleeding occurs, the event contributes morbidity to an often already compromised state. Bleeding events in patients with end-stage liver disease are common causes of acute-on-chronic liver failure (ACLF), and each bleeding event contributes independently to mortality. The risk for mortality associated with a bleed is greatest in those bleeding with higher Model for End-Stage Liver Disease (MELD) scores, and historically the likelihood for mortality approached 30% to 50%[1] (see Chapter 4). Current data fortunately illustrate the 6-week mortality following a portal hypertensive bleed to be substantially less than this.[1–4] Changes to several aspects of clinical care and near universal adoption of standardized evidence-based approaches to acute event management and to secondary prophylaxis has likely led to reductions in mortality.[5–24] The current 6-week mortality risk following a variceal bleed is now approximately 15%.[2–4]

In studies designed specifically to assess whether timing of endoscopy impacts outcome with acute bleeding events, early endoscopy, defined as occurring in less than 6 hours, has not shown diminished mortality, although early endoscopy may diminish cost.[25] Endoscopy in most instances should be undertaken within 24 hours of hospitalization and following the establishment of hemodynamic stability (see Chapter 81). There are some instances during which early endoscopy (i.e., within 6 hours) may benefit particular subgroups at high risk for early mortality and in which certain therapeutic options may be limited. Examples of such patient groups include those with a MELD score greater than 18, those with a CTP score greater than 12, those with unfavorable anatomy for interventional radiology, and those with significant premorbid encephalopathy.[26,27] Endoscopic management of acute bleeding from esophageal varices is accomplished with band ligation, and Following the initial endoscopy, timely follow-up endoscopy at 2 weeks is important along with repeat endoscopy preferably every 2 weeks until the varices are completely ablated. Best illustrating the role and success of this and other available medical therapies in the primary and secondary prophylaxis against variceal bleeding are diminishing mortality rates in patients with cirrhosis and the decline in liver transplant waiting list mortality despite rising MELD scores in those listed for transplantation.[2,28–30] These findings also underscore the utility of an early diagnosis of esophageal varices through aggressive screening strategies, careful surveillance for small varices, and the role of prophylactic therapies with nonselective β-blockade and/or band ligation in the management of varices (see Chapter 81).

NATURAL HISTORY OF VARICES

The diagnosis of esophageal varices should be considered in any patient with cirrhosis[31–33] (see Chapters 5 and 74). The likelihood of discovering varices in any patient correlates with the severity of the underlying liver disease. The prevalence of esophageal varices among patients with compensated cirrhosis is about 30% to 40%, whereas it approaches 85% among patients with decompensated cirrhosis.[34] In patients with compensated cirrhosis without varices, esophageal varices develop at a rate of 7% to 8% per year and progress from small to large varices at a rate of 10% to 12% per year. The propensity for developing varices increases with the development of clinical decompensation. The incidence of bleeding in those with varices is approximately 10% to 15% per year in patients with high-risk varices. Factors independently associated with variceal bleeding, beyond liver disease severity, include the size of the varices, coloring on the varices, a history of previous bleeding, HVPG, ACLF, PVT, liver stiffness measured by transient

TABLE 80.1 Locations and Pathologies Leading to Portal Hypertensions

LOCATION	PATHOLOGY
Prehepatic	Portal vein thrombosis Mesenteric or splenic vein thrombosis Congenital stenosis of the portal vein Extrinsic portal vein compression Arteriovenous fistula of the mesenteric circulation Splenomegaly
Intrahepatic-presinusoidal	Schistosomiasis Hepatoportal sclerosis Primary biliary cirrhosis Sarcoidosis Sclerosing cholangitis Congenital hepatic fibrosis Hepatic arterioportal fistula Intrahepatic portal vein obstruction (e.g., tumor or cyst associated)
Intrahepatic-sinusoidal	Cirrhosis Nodular regenerative hyperplasia Steatohepatitis Acute hepatitis Toxin (e.g., arsenic, vinyl chloride)
Intrahepatic-Post-sinusoidal	Budd-Chiari syndrome Sinusoidal obstruction syndrome/veno-occlusive disease (SOS/VOD)
Extrahepatic	Restrictive cardiomyopathy Constrictive pericarditis Congenital heart disease Pulmonary hypertension

elastography, and active alcohol use.[35,36] Bleeding from varices is rare if the HPVG is less than 12 mm Hg.[35,36] Albeit uncommonly measured endoscopically, the degree of pressure within the varix and the wall tension of the varix correlate with the probability for bleeding.[37] Figure 80.1 illustrates the evolution of portal hypertension complication.

Management of the Acute Hemorrhage (see Chapter 81)

When bleeding occurs, resuscitation is immediately initiated with care to avoid over-resuscitation. Excessive resuscitation increases plasma volume and thereby portal pressure, which may contribute to ongoing bleeding risk.[35,38] However, adequate and timely resuscitation are critical to diminish the likelihood of developing an acute kidney injury. For transfusion, in those with cirrhosis, a hemoglobin threshold of 7 g/dL is suggested. With active bleeding, in particular when hemodynamic instability is present, immediate cross-matching is imperative and earlier initiation of transfusion will often occur. However, a restrictive transfusion strategy should be employed with a hematocrit or hemoglobin target of 21% to 24% or 7 to 8 g/dL, respectively. These targets, in high-quality studies, are associated with increased survival and lower HVPGs when compared with liberal transfusion strategies.[9,38–40] Patients with portal hypertension have preexisting hypotension and in resuscitating those with bleeding a target systolic blood pressure between 90 and 100 mm Hg and target heart rate less than 100 beats/min are recommended. Because of the use of nonselective β-blockers (NSBBs) in some, tachycardia is not always present in these patients. Accordingly, targets for resuscitation during an active bleed include restoration of the hematocrit to 24%, maintaining fibrinogen levels greater than or equal to 120 mg/dL, where possible increase platelet counts to 50,000, administer intravenous antibiotics and vasoactive medication (octreotide or terlipressin) during the resuscitation, and undertake endeavors to optimize renal function.[41] Interestingly, across the majority of studies examining variceal bleeding, the use of therapeutic anticoagulation before a bleeding event was not identified as an independent risk factor variceal hemorrhage, although no study has been performed to examine bleeding risk in those on anticoagulation in contrast to peptic ulcer bleeding. Anticoagulation is less commonly used in those with cirrhosis.

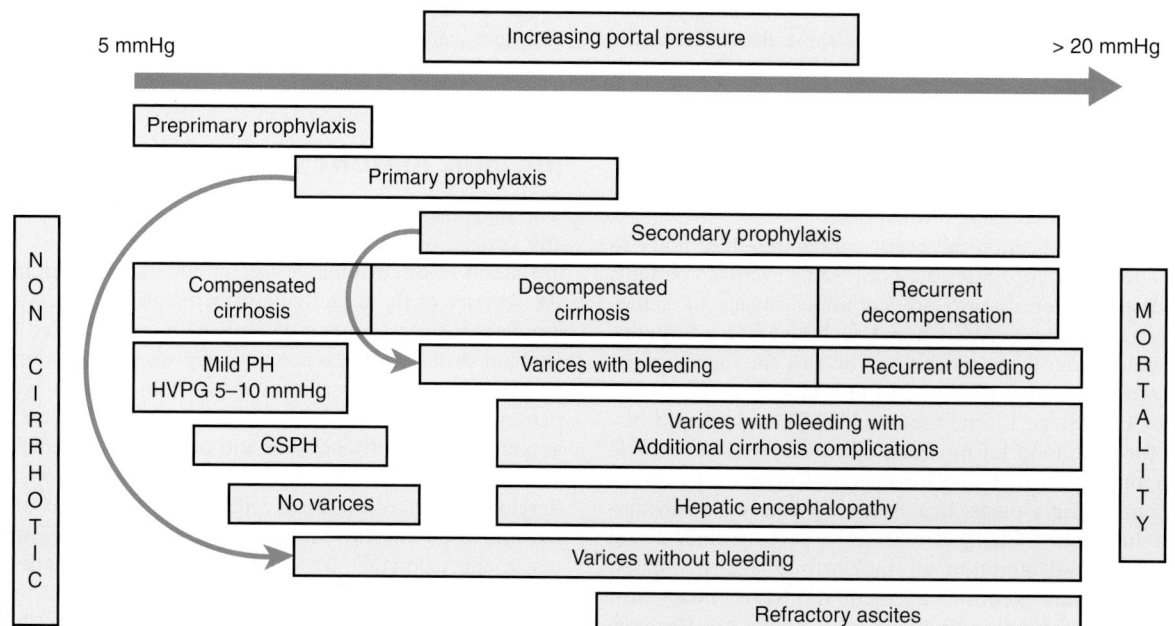

FIGURE 80.1 Evolution of portal hypertension complication. *CSPH,* Clinically significant portal hypertension; *HVPG,* hepatic venous pressure gradient.

Sites and the Propensity to Variceal Bleeding

Although variceal bleeding is most common in cirrhotic patients, it is important to remember other etiologies, such as peptic ulcer disease, are also common causes of acute upper gastrointestinal bleed.[42] When variceal in origin, the most common source is esophageal varices (70%) and the most common location is just above the gastroesophageal junction.[42] Signs of the site of bleeding include a clot overlying a varix, a white plug also known as a fibrin plug on the varix, or active extravasation of blood from the side of a varix during endoscopy. It is not uncommon, however, to fail to identify the specific site of bleeding at the time endoscopy. In instances where an acute gastrointestinal bleed occurs, in the presence of varices and in the absence of an alternative site to explain blood loss, band ligation starting at the gastrointestinal junction should occur when varices are present. It is also important to note that when bleeding occurs as an initial event, and in the absence of other complications of cirrhosis, the 5-year mortality is relatively low at 20%. In contrast, when bleeding occurs in the presence of other complications of cirrhosis, the transplant-free survival falls to less than 20% at 5 years.[43]

Gastric varices are present in 20% of patients with cirrhosis. They bleed less commonly than esophageal varices, and a greater likelihood for these being present occurs with aberrancies to the portal circulation (for example, splenic vein thrombosis). Gastric varices account for 5% to 10% of all variceal hemorrhages and bleeding from these is associated with significantly greater mortality than esophageal varices. In contrast, rectal varices are far more common than gastric varices and are present in 44% of patients with cirrhosis and in 59% with a history of esophageal varices (59%); however, they only account for less than 5% of all portal hypertensive bleeds.[44]

Ectopic varices are an uncommon cause of variceal bleeding and account for up to 5% of all bleeding events.[45] Ectopic varices that are associated with bleeding are most often located in a stoma or surgical anastomosis and then, in decreasing order, the duodenum, jejunum/ileum, rectum, and colon.[45,46] Ectopic varices are more common when extrahepatic thrombosis within the portal circulation occurs.[45–47] Portal biliopathy, an uncommon clinic complication of portal hypertension, occurs most commonly when cirrhosis exists in the presence of an extrahepatic PVT and these rarely bleed in the absence of a surgical intervention such as an endoscopic retrograde cholangiopancreatography (ERCP).[48–52] Finally, another rare site of ectopic bleeding associated with portal hypertension includes vessels in the peritoneal cavity or those associated with a recanalized umbilical vein.[51,52] Bleeding from these sites is very rare and generally associated with trauma or iatrogenic injury. The presence of varices in these locations should be considered when planning a procedure, such as a paracentesis; however, the presence of varices will rarely preclude a procedure.

Stages of Portal Hypertension

Cirrhosis, which is often the consequence of a chronic and progressive liver disease, is the most common cause of portal hypertension (see Chapter 74). After developing cirrhosis, patients move through stages of portal hypertension. Table 80.2 outlines the stages of portal hypertension and details the clinical objectives for each stage. For all chronic liver diseases, the primary objective is to arrest and, where possible, reverse the process that caused cirrhosis. Examples of this include eradication or suppression of viral hepatitis in those with hepatitis C or hepatitis B (see Chapter 68), abstinence from alcohol in those with alcoholic liver disease, and weight loss in those with nonalcoholic steatohepatitis (see Chapter 69). When portal hypertension is present (HVPG >5 mm Hg), patients are initially compensated, meaning cirrhosis in the absence of any decompensating event (ascites, encephalopathy, variceal hemorrhage) and without CSPH (HVPG 5–10 mm Hg) or with CSPH (HPVG >10 mm Hg). The final phase is decompensated cirrhosis, and commonly this population has an HPVG greater than 12 mm Hg. In each phase of portal hypertension associated with cirrhosis the therapeutic objectives and approaches differ.

Compensated Cirrhosis Without Clinically Significant Portal Hypertensions

In those with compensated cirrhosis without CSPH the goal of therapy is largely confined to management of the underlying cause of cirrhosis. In compensated cirrhosis without CSPH, and in contrast with those with cirrhosis and CSPH, patients have a normal cardiac index as opposed to an increased cardiac index, which is seen in decompensated disease.[53] Accordingly, those with compensated cirrhosis without CSPH (HPVG <10) obtain no benefit from medical treatments for portal hypertension as the treatments are designed to diminish the cardiac output; in patients with cirrhosis without CSPH the cardiac output is normal.[53]

Compensated Cirrhosis With Clinically Significant Portal Hypertension

Identifying those with CSPH commences with the clinical examination. CSPH is present in all patients with signs of

TABLE 80.2	Stages of Portal Hypertension in Cirrhosis, Clinical Manifestations, and Goals of Therapy Disease					
DISEASE STAGE	**COMPENSATED CIRRHOSIS**			**DECOMPENSATED CIRRHOSIS**		
HVPG	<10 mm Hg	≥10 mm Hg (CSPH)		≥12 mm Hg		
Varices	Absent	Absent	Present	Present		
Complications of portal hypertension	Absent	Absent	Absent	Acute variceal bleed	Prior variceal bleed without complications	Prior variceal bleed with complications
Goals of therapy	Prevent CSPH	Prevent decompensation	Prevent decompensation	Control bleed	Prevent further bleeds and decompensation	Prevent further decompensation and mortality

CSPH, Clinically significant portal hypertension; *HVPG,* hepatic venous pressure gradient.
Adapted from Chandra R, Kapoor D, Tharakan A, Chaudhary A, Sarin SK. Portal biliopathy. *J Gastroenterol Hepatol.* 2001;16(10):1086–1092.

decompensation (ascites, hepatic encephalopathy) and in those clinical signs of portal hypertension (splenomegaly, caput medusae). In these patients variceal screening is always indicated. In those with cirrhosis and without signs of decompensation or portal hypertension, a liver stiffness measurement less than 20 kPa by transient elastography and platelet count greater than 150,000/mm³ defines a group unlikely to have CSPH and patients not requiring screening endoscopy.[32,33] However, all patients with CSPH (HPVG >10 mm Hg), and in all with a liver stiffness >20 kPa and platelet count less than 150,000/mm, screening endoscopy should be offered.

The gold standard for screening for esophageal varices is upper gastrointestinal endoscopy. Albeit other tests may provide similar information, like capsule endoscopy or endoscopic ultrasound (EUS), which both have a limited role, although EUS has some very specific therapeutic roles in the management of gastric and ectopic varices.[54,55] In all patients with evidence of CSPH, an ultrasound of the liver with Doppler of the portal vein is indicated. Whenever possible, a triple-phase contrast cross-sectional imaging study of the abdomen should be considered to evaluate patients with portal hypertension and, in all patients with PVT, a contrast imaging study is required to define the portal venous anatomy. Contrast imaging studies better exclude pathologies that might lead to thrombosis, like hepatocellular carcinoma. The contrast imaging studies also provide a road map for potential intervention in instances where interventional radiology may be considered to manage refractory bleeding or portal vein recanalization.

In those with cirrhosis with CSPH and without varices, timolol, an NSBB, was examined in a multicenter study by the Portal Hypertension Collaborative Group. This placebo-controlled study failed to demonstrate a statistical difference in the development of varices between groups, although it did show a greater number of serious adverse reactions in the treatment arm when compared with the placebo.[56] Accordingly, NSBBs should not be given to patients with cirrhosis and without varices.[56,57]

Compensated Cirrhosis With Clinically Significant Portal Hypertension and Small Varices

Patients with small varices without high-risk features in general should not be treated with medical therapies. A meta-analysis of six studies demonstrated nothing to support the use of NSBBs in cirrhotic patients with small varices.[53] The same meta-analysis highlights that there was significant heterogeneity in the study design of those studies that entered into the meta-analysis and that the studies often lacked adequate follow-up data.[53] In a subgroup analysis, NSBBs were recommended for patients with small varices possessing stigmata reflecting a risk for bleeding, like red wales; however, these stigmata are rare in those with small varices.[53] The North Italian Endoscopic Club (NIEC) index, first published in 1988 and later revised, is a detailed scoring system used to better define the risk for variceal bleeding. The list contains clinical, laboratory, and endoscopic features that, when used collectively, assist in predicting the risk for variceal bleeding.[57,58] This validated score is useful for identifying individuals in whom primary prophylaxis provides the greatest benefit (Table 80.3).[59]

Primary and Secondary Prophylaxis

Primary prophylaxis aims to prevent a disease or injury before it ever occurs. Secondary prophylaxis is an intervention that diminishes the likelihood of the event recurring. With both primary and secondary prophylaxis for variceal bleeding, the primary end point of variceal bleeding must be balanced against the side effects of the intervention to prevent it. Another important secondary end point in prophylaxis, when applying or not applying a treatment or intervention it is the overall mortality associated with the action compared with no action or any existing standard of care.

Primary Prophylaxis and Esophageal Varices

Primary prophylaxis with either NSBB, carvedilol, or variceal band ligation (VBL) is recommended for patients at increased risk for variceal bleeding, including those with medium or large varices or those with small varices with red wale signs (Table 80.4). NSBBs work by reducing portal pressure via blockade of β_1- and β_2-adrenergic receptors. The activity of NSBB decreases cardiac output and increases splanchnic vasoconstriction. Carvedilol possesses β-blocker and anti–α_1-adrenergic activity, which lowers both intrahepatic and portosystemic vascular resistance. Compared with placebo, NSBBs and VBL both reduce the risk of a first bleed from varices in randomized controlled trials (RCTs) and meta-analyses.[60,61] Carvedilol is equivalent to, or more effective than, VBL in preventing a first variceal bleed.[11,62] The decision to use NSBBs, VBL, and carvedilol remains largely left to patient and physician preference, relative or absolute contraindications, and any history of previous adverse events associated with the therapy. Although meta-analyses have suggested decreased bleeding risk with VBL compared with NSBBs,[61,63,64] NSBBs have been shown to improve overall mortality compared with placebo, which has not been demonstrated with VBL.[61] Up to 15% of patients will have contraindication to NSBBs, whereas another 15% will experience dose-limiting side effects such as fatigue and dizziness, requiring dose reduction or discontinuation.[65] Importantly, the efficacy of NSBBs requires judicious assessment for adequacy of dosing, and assessment for adverse events, to ensure efficacy. Unfortunately, this is something that is less likely achieved outside of clinical studies[59] (Fig. 80.2).

Among NSBB trials that repeated endoscopy after NSBB initiation, no change was noted in variceal size and repeat endoscopy to evaluate efficacy of NSBB therapy is not recommended.[34] NSBBs are titrated to a heart rate of 55 to 60 beats/min, whereas carvedilol has no heart rate goal and is generally started at 3.125 mg twice daily or 6.25 mg once daily and, if tolerated, is titrated up to 6.25 mg twice daily. VBL is recommended every 2 to 4 weeks until varices are eradicated followed by surveillance endoscopy at 6 months following eradication and then every 6 to 12 months thereafter as ongoing surveillance. After successful placement of a transhepatic portosystemic shunt (TIPS), surveillance endoscopy is not indicated, except in instances of TIPS dysfunction or occlusion.

Other medications have been trialed for the primary prevention of variceal bleeding. These alternate medical therapies have either insufficient data or lack of effect to support their use. Isosorbide mononitrate, although it may lower portal pressure, has not been found to be effective in reducing bleeding risk or mortality compared with placebo.[61] Angiotensin II receptor blockers (ARBs) may reduce portal pressure; however, they have shown variable results in reducing bleeding in the absence of concurrent NSBB.[60] ARBs have not been studied specifically in primary prophylaxis of variceal bleeding and cannot be recommended in 2021.[66,67] Similarly, statins are not

TABLE 80.3 North Italian Endoscopy Club Index

Estimated 1-year percentage probability of bleeding by variceal size and presence of red wale sign by Child-Pugh class

| | CTP A | | | CTP B | | | CTP C | | |
	SMALL	MEDIUM	LARGE	SMALL	MEDIUM	LARGE	SMALL	MEDIUM	LARGE
Red Wale Signs									
Absent	6	10	15	10	16	26	20	30	42
Mild	8	12	19	15	23	33	28	38	54
Moderate	12	16	24	20	30	42	36	48	64
Severe	16	23	34	28	40	52	44	60	76

Pocket chart for calculation of NIEC index[a]

		POINTS
CTP Class		
A		6.5
B		13
C	f	19.5
Varix Size		
Small		8.7
Medium		13
Large		17.4
Red Wale		
Absent		3.2
Mild		6.4
Moderate		9.6
Severe		12.8

[a]Calculated by adding the above three variables

Cumulative percentages of patients bleeding among 321 patients with cirrhosis and varices classified according to NIEC index

| RISK CLASS | NIEC INDEX | NUMBER WHO BLED/TOTAL | RATE OF BLEEDING (%) | | |
			6 MONTH	1 YEAR	2 YEAR
1	<20.0	6/63	0	1.6	6.8
2	20.0-25.0	12/76	5.4	11	16
3	25.1-30.0	14/63	8	14.8	25.5
4	30.1=35.0	18/56	13.1	23.3	27.8
5	35.1-40.0	24/48	21.8	37.8	58.8
6	>40.0	7/11	58.5	68.9	68.9

CTP, Child-Turcotte-Pugh; *NIEC,* North Italian Endoscopy Club Index.
Adapted from de Franchis R, Eisen GM, Laine L, et al. Esophageal capsule endoscopy for screening and surveillance of esophageal varices in patients with portal hypertension. *Hepatology.* 2008;47(5):1593–1603.

effective at reducing HVPG when added to an NSBB and are not recommended for primary prophylaxis.[68] Statins use importantly, is assuming an increasing role in other areas of cirrhosis management.[58]

Combination therapy of VBL plus propranolol was not more effective than VBL alone in preventing first variceal bleed or death. The combination of NSBB and VBL was associated with an increase in adverse events.[69] Similarly, combination VBL plus NSBB versus NSBB alone has not been shown to lessen the risk of a first bleed and combination therapy was associated with increased adverse events.[70] In 2021 the Cochrane Collaborative performed a network analysis of 66 RCTs examining primary prevention for variceal bleeding and concluded that low-certainty evidence supported that β-blockers, VBL, or β-blockers plus nitrates decrease mortality compared with no intervention in people with high-risk esophageal varices and concurrent cirrhosis,

whereas VBL was associated with a greater frequency of severe adverse events when compared with the other interventions.[71]

Surgical shunts were initially attempted in the 1960s for primary prophylaxis of variceal bleeding (see Chapter 83). The shunts were effective in reducing bleeding in those patients who underwent surgical shunting, although a substantial risk for complications and mortality accompanied shunt surgery compared with no intervention, and the patients' CTP scores correlated with the risk for mortality benefit.[72] By extension, TIPS is also not recommended for primary prophylaxis and its perioperative role will be discussed later. The relative and absolute contraindications to a TIPS are detailed in Table 80.4. When a TIPS is placed in the presence of a relative contraindication actions should be taken to mitigate the impact of relative contraindication, for instance, treatment with antibiotics before placement of a TIPS in those with a history of cholangitis.

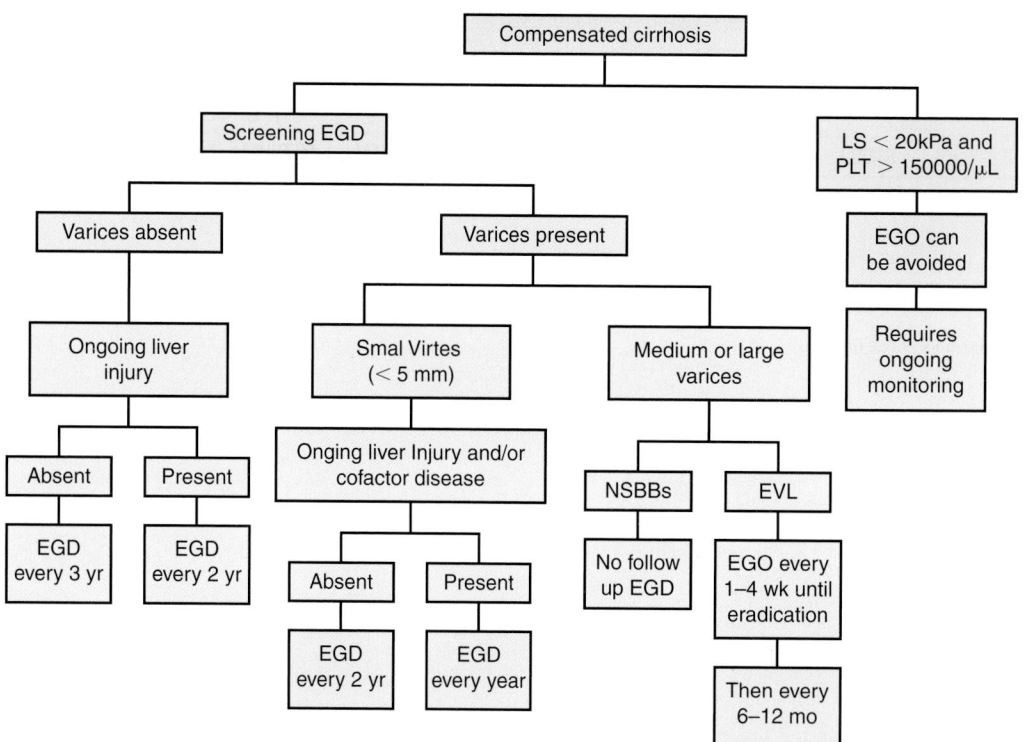

FIGURE 80.2   **Algorithm for variceal screening.** *EGD,* Esophagogastroduodenoscopy; *EGO EVL, LS, NSBB,* nonselective β-blocker; *PLT,.*

TABLE 80.4   Relative and Absolute Contraindications to Transhepatic Portosystemic Shunt Placement

Relative

1.   Hepatic encephalopathy
2.   MELD score >15
3.   Coagulopathy or severe thrombocytopenia
4.   Pulmonary hypertension (mean pulmonary arterial pressure >30 and <45 mm Hg)
5.   Portal vein thrombosis
6.   Hepatocellular carcinoma
7.   History of cholangitis
8.   Multiple hepatic cysts

Absolute

1.   Refractory hepatic encephalopathy
2.   Severe heart failure
3.   Severe pulmonary hypertension
4.   Severe tricuspid regurgitation
5.   Bacteremia/sepsis
6.   Active cholangitis
7.   Unrelieved biliary obstruction

MELD, Model for End-Stage Liver Disease.

Although trials are more limited in patients with noncirrhotic portal hypertension, both NSBBs and VBL appear to be equally effective in primary prophylaxis of variceal bleeding in this setting.[73]

Primary Prophylaxis Gastric Varices

Only one trial has evaluated primary prophylaxis of gastric variceal bleeding. This study included patients with gastroesophageal varices type 2 with eradicated esophageal varices or large isolated gastric varices type 1. Patients were randomized to cyanoacrylate injection ($n = 30$), β-blocker ($n = 29$), or no treatment ($n = 30$).[74] Patients who underwent cyanoacrylate injection were less likely to bleed (10%) compared with both NSBB (38%) and no treatment (53%). However, survival was similar between NSBB and cyanoacrylate injection, and given the potential benefits of β-blockers outside of bleeding prophylaxis in cirrhosis, and the limited access to expertise and training in cyanoacrylate injection, one cannot recommend one therapy over the alternative (Table 80.5).

TABLE 80.5   Management of Varices

LOCATION	PRIMARY PROPHYLAXIS	SECONDARY PROPHYLAXIS
Esophageal: Low-risk (small varices without stigmata)	None	N/A
High-risk (large varices or small varices with stigmata)	NSBB/carvedilol or VBL	NSBB/carvedilol + VBL
Gastric (fundal)	Cyanoacrylate or NSBB	TIPS BRTO ± TIPS Cyanoacrylate[a]
Ectopic	None (rectal), unknown for other locations	TIPS ± embolization BRTO ± TIPS VBL Cyanoacrylate[a] Surgical[a]

[a]Choice of therapy for secondary prophylaxis in gastric and ectopic varices should be individualized based on anatomy, degree of portal hypertension, encephalopathy risk, and center expertise.
BRTO, Balloon-occluded retrograde transvenous obliteration; *NSBB,* nonselective β-blocker; *TIPS,* transjugular intrahepatic portosystemic shunt; *VBL,* variceal band ligation.

Similar to esophageal varices, TIPS is not recommended as a primary prophylaxis irrespective of size of the gastric or esophageal varices or the NIEC score. This recommendation is based on the higher mortality rate in those undergoing TIPS compared with no NSBB or carvedilol and the propensity for a TIPS to result in hepatic encephalopathy. Balloon-occluded retrograde transvenous obliteration (BRTO) of gastric varices has also not been studied for primary prophylaxis and similarly cannot be recommended for this reason (see Chapter 85).

Secondary Prophylaxis Esophageal Varices

In patients who have recovered from an initial or subsequent esophageal variceal bleed, combination therapy with NSBB and VBL is recommended over monotherapy (see Table 80.5). This position is supported by a meta-analysis showing reduced re-bleeding risk in those receiving combination therapy compared with VBL alone.[75] There is no significant difference associated with substituting carvedilol for a NSBB in secondary prophylaxis.[76,77] One study did suggest a potential mortality benefit for NSBB and ISMN compared with NSBB and VBL,[78] although this was never substantiated in subsequent studies.[75]

Patients who underwent TIPS during an acute episode of bleeding (or following the bleeding event) do not require further treatment of varices or follow-up endoscopies to survey or eradicate varices, provided the TIPS remains patent and without dysfunction. Evidence to support dysfunction includes the persistence of ascites after TIPS placement, gastrointestinal bleeding following placement of the TIPS, or dysfunction as measured by Doppler velocities on ultrasound. Velocities in the shunt should range between 90 and 190 cm/s and a peak velocity above or below this range indicates probable dysfunction associated with stenosis of the TIPS[79] (Fig. 80.3; see Chapter 85).

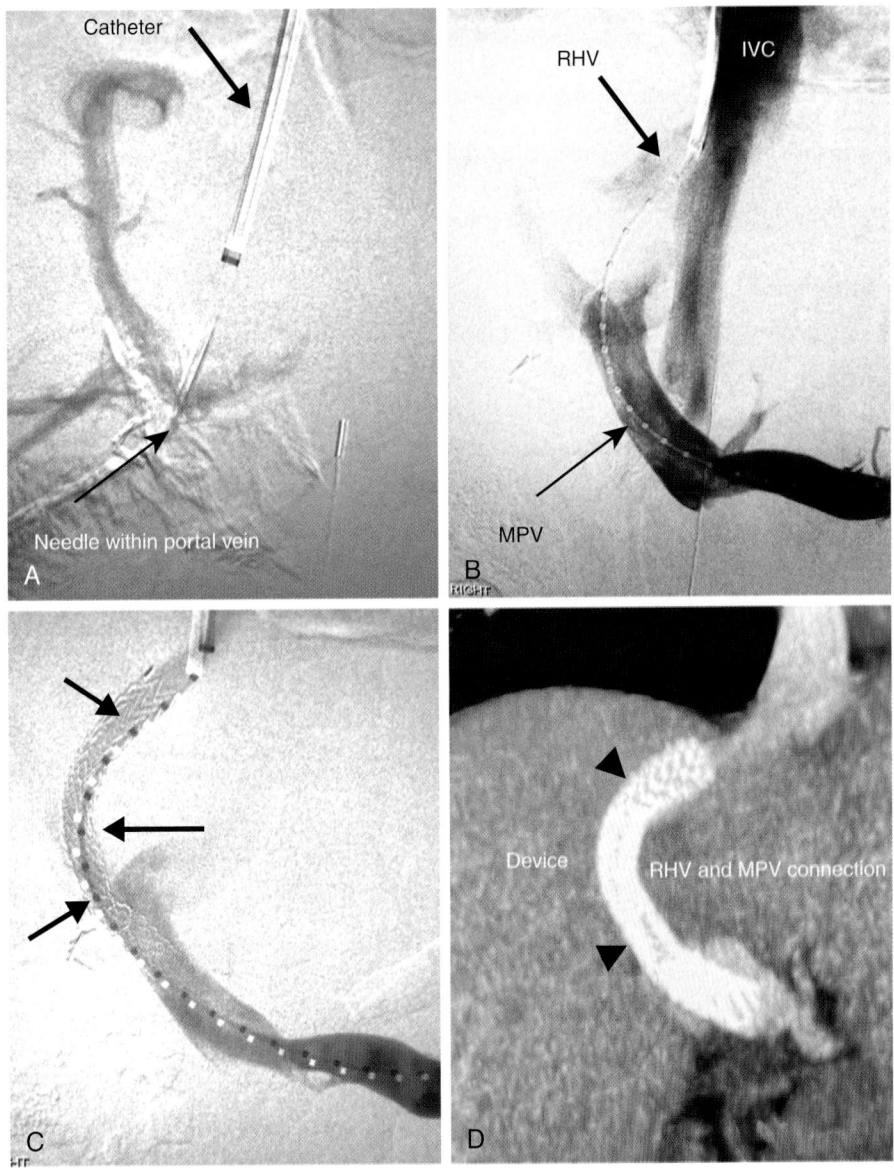

FIGURE 80.3 Transhepatic portosystemic shunt placement. A, Introduction of needle though catheter within the right hepatic vein to opacify the portal vein. **B,** Catheter and wire connecting inferior vena cava *(IVC)* with the portal vein from the right hepatic vein. **C,** Deployment of the stent over the wire to connect the hepatic and portal veins. **D,** Deployed stent decompressing the portal venous system through the stent. *MPV,* main portal vein; *RHV,* right hepatic vein.

In those patients who rebleed following initiation of secondary prophylaxis (NSBB plus VBL), TIPS is recommended to salvage the situation, provided no contraindications exist. TIPS can also be considered as secondary prophylaxis in those with successful initial control of variceal bleeding in instances where the risk for rebleeding is high (CTP class C and B patients with active bleeding at the time of endoscopy), although again provided that contraindications to a TIPS are absent. Of 359 patients, in one multicenter study, admitted with a variceal bleed it was noted that only 63 patients were randomized to answer this question. In this subset of patients, an early TIPS was associated with lower risk of rebleeding and diminished mortality. This multicenter study did exclude patients with a CTP score less than 7 or greater than 13.[80] A subsequent meta-analysis confirmed a survival benefit in CTP class B or C with active bleeding who undergo early TIPS.[81] Although one study did include CTP class B without active bleeding and indicated a survival benefit to TIPS in this population, this remains controversial[18] (see Chapter 85).

In a trial comparing simvastatin in addition to standard of care (NSBB + VBL) to NSBB and VBL alone, simvastatin was found to reduce mortality in CTP class A and B patients, although there was no change in rebleeding risk.[82] In that mortality benefit was not the primary outcome for this study, and in the absence of confirmation of these results in subsequent studies, the use of statins in variceal bleeding cannot yet be recommended.

Secondary Prophylaxis Gastric Varices

The optimal treatment for secondary prophylaxis of bleeding in gastric (primarily fundal) varices is not well defined and largely depends on center expertise. One study compared cyanoacrylate injection with propranolol and found cyanoacrylate injection to be superior to NSBB in both rebleeding and mortality.[83] In a subsequent study the addition of NSBB to cyanoacrylate injection did not provide any additional benefit to cyanoacrylate alone.[84]

TIPS has been compared with cyanoacrylate injection and TIPS was found to be more effective in preventing rebleeding from gastric varices (11% vs. 38%). However, there was no difference in mortality between the two groups and encephalopathy was significantly higher in the TIPS group.[85] Cyanoacrylate has the ability to embolize and it is relatively strongly contraindicated in patients with hepatopulmonary syndrome or in those with intracardiac shunting. Training and expertise in the appropriate use of this agent is also limited and this accordingly limits the ability to recommend its use outside of specific centers.

BRTO, in randomized studies, has not been compared directly with TIPS, cyanoacrylate injection, or medications in preventing rebleeding from gastric varices, although it has been shown to be effective.[86] In the acute setting, BRTO may be more effective than TIPS in acutely controlling bleeding, rebleeding, and mortality while diminishing the likelihood of encephalopathy, although these data are nonrandomized and retrospective.[87] However, in a 2020 systematic review and meta-analysis of 7 studies comprising 676 patients the authors concluded that although the technical success, hemostasis rates, and complication rates associated with TIPS and BRTO were similar, BRTO was associated with lower rates of rebleeding, postprocedure hepatic encephalopathy, and mortality at 1 year.[64] BRTO is also more likely to be effective than TIPS for diminishing the risk of rebleeding in those with left-sided portal hypertension, and comparative studies of BRTO with surgical shunts or splenectomy to manage left-sided portal hypertension are not available. Although BRTO is associated with lower rates of encephalopathy, it does have the potential to worsen portal hypertension and to increase the size and bleeding risk associated with esophageal varices.[86] For this reason, BRTO may be used in tandem with TIPS in those where HVPG exceeds 12 mm Hg on completion of the BRTO procedure. In instances where PVT is present in the setting of bleeding from gastric varices, a BRTO may be contraindicated in the absence of the recanalization of the portal vein and placement of a TIPS as in this setting a BRTO could lead to extensive mesenteric congestion and venous infarction (Fig. 80.4; see Chapter 85).

In summary, the selection of therapy for the prevention of rebleeding in gastric varices is complicated and must consider local expertise, encephalopathy risk, and the degree of portal hypertension (see Table 80.4). In choosing among the options that include cyanoacrylate injection, TIPS, and BRTO, data are insufficient to direct a recommendation to one therapy over another and the choice and technical approaches associated with the choice of therapy must be individualized to the patient's circumstances.

Rectal Varices

Bleeding from rectal varices is rare, and there are no prospective trials evaluating the efficacy of different interventions for managing acute bleeding or secondary prophylaxis. One retrospective analysis did examine sclerotherapy versus band ligation for primary or secondary prophylaxis in 34 patients. This study found a nonsignificant lowering of recurrent bleeding (defined as either bleeding or return of varices with red wale signs) in the sclerotherapy arm (33%) compared with band ligation (55%), although recurrence was high in both groups.[88] Cyanoacrylate injection has been reported to be effective in case reports but has not been compared with other interventions.[89]

TIPS, with or without concomitant embolization of the vein feeding the rectal varices, appears to be more effective than endoscopic therapy in reducing the risk for recurrent bleeding, as seen in a small retrospective study. In this study that included 12 patients with active bleeding rectal varices, bleeding recurred in only one patient (8.3%) following the intervention. The number of patients who underwent concomitant embolization of rectal varices was not reported in this study, although 5 of 27 in the total cohort underwent embolization.[90] BRTO has also been shown to be effective in managing rectal varices, although the published experience is confined to case reports and small series.[91] The surgical management of rectal varices, when employed, consists of circumferential stapling of rectal varices using the same device used in hemorrhoidectomy. The largest series is limited to a case series of nine patients who failed endoscopic and medical therapy and the treatment was universally effective[92] (see Table 80.5 and Chapter 85).

Ectopic Varices

Similar to rectal varices, there are no guidelines or large-scale studies comparing therapies to guide treatment of ectopic varices. The management of ectopic varices largely depends on the portal venous anatomy and the hospital's clinical expertise and skills. Ligation, cyanoacrylate injection, sclerotherapy, TIPS with or without embolization, and BRTO have all been reported to be effective in individual case reports. The largest

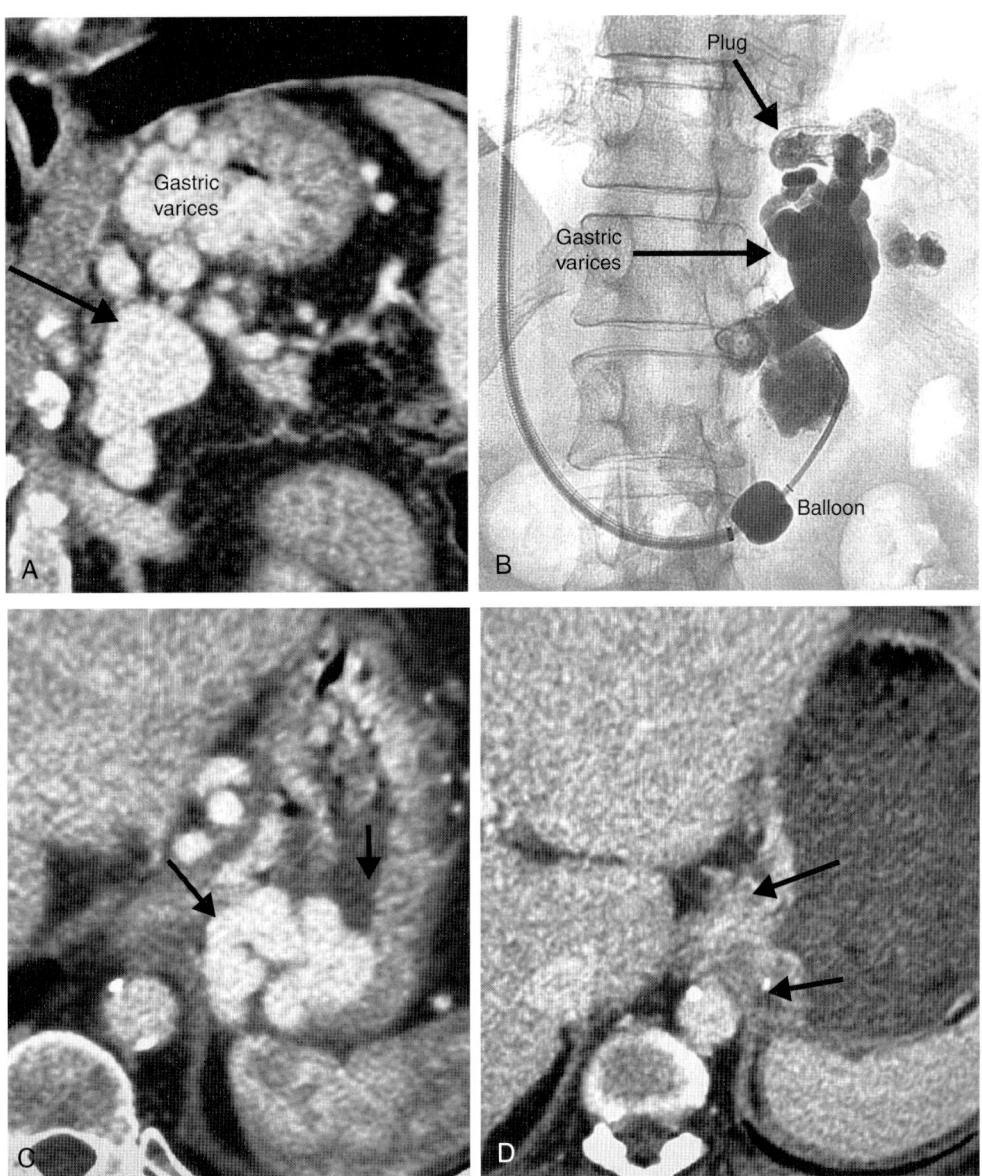

FIGURE 80.4   Balloon-occluded retrograde transvenous obliteration (BRTO). A, Computed tomographic image of gastric varices with *arrow* marking spontaneous shunt connecting the left renal vein to the gastric varices. **B,** Catheter entering through the inferior vena cava then through the spontaneous shunt to occlude shunt and gastric varices. **C,** Cross-sectional image of gastric varices before occlusion. **D,** Cross-sectional image 6 months after the procedure of the ablated gastric varices.

retrospective studies have examined TIPS with or without embolization in 60 patients (29 stomal varices, 16 duodenal, 15 other). Rebleeding occurred in 14 (23%), although this was due to shunt dysfunction in 2 and in these patients resolved with shunt revision.[90,93] Embolization alone to ectopic varices is not recommended because of high rebleeding rates[94] (see Table 80.4; Fig. 80.5).

Portal Vein Thrombosis and Portal Vein Recanalization

PVT occurs in 20% of patients with cirrhosis and is more common in those with hepatocellular carcinoma than in those without (see Chapters 74 and 89). In cirrhosis, PVT is uncommonly associated with a specific procoagulant disorder, whereas in noncirrhotic patients, procoagulant disorders are more common and a history of prior surgery, intraabdominal infections, abdominal trauma, or umbilical vein cannulation as a child is

more likely. PVT, if present at the time of liver transplantation, is associated with increased blood loss, morbidity, and mortality during and following liver transplantation and diminished posttransplant portal vein patency. In a meta-analysis of 8 studies containing 353 cirrhotic subjects, the use of anticoagulation was associated with increased portal vein recanalization and reduced progression of thrombosis when compared with patients who do not receive anticoagulants. Importantly, these benefits were realized with no excess of major and minor bleeding events and lower incidence of variceal bleeding.[95] When mechanical recanalization to the portal vein is necessary, a transhepatic approach with thrombectomy and often with a concurrent TIPS to assist with portal venous flow is employed.[96] The latter also appears to significantly improve patency and flow in the portal circulation following the procedure. In some instances, a trans-splenic approach without a TIPS may be

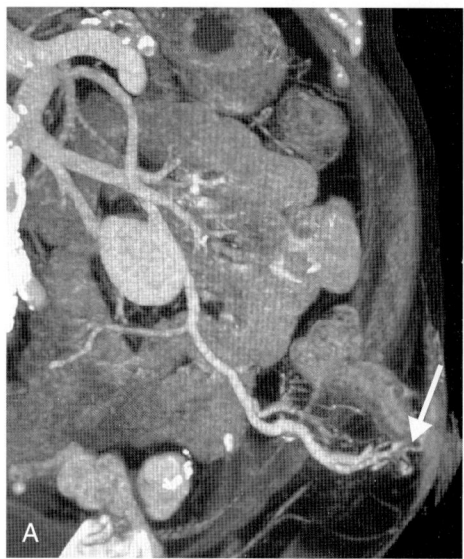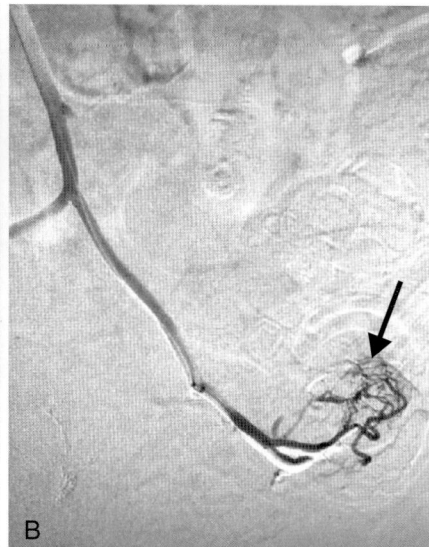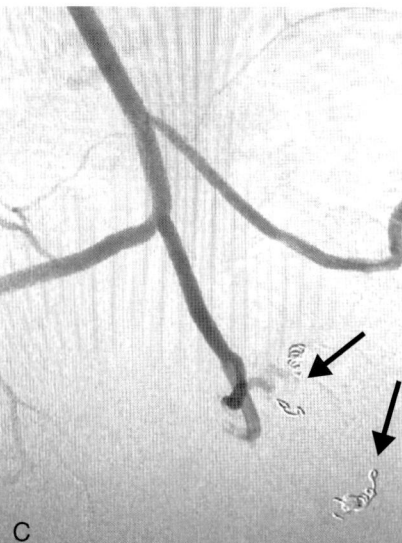

FIGURE 80.5 Ectopic varices. A, Computed tomography illustrating mesenteric vein associated with peristomal (ectopic) varices. **B,** Catheter with the vessel illustrating opacification of the peristomal veins. **C,** Coil occlusion of the veins and tributaries backfilled with glue.

considered as an alternative way to reestablishing portal venous flow, thereby diminishing portal venous pressure.[97] Illustrated in Figures 80.5 to 80.8 are the outcomes of portal vein recanalization without a TIPS in a patient with bleeding duodenal varices with concurrent portal biliopathy (see Fig. 80.6B) and portal, mesenteric, and splenic vein occlusion with refractory anemia from gastrointestinal blood loss where portal and mesenteric vein recanalization was performed pretransplant with placement of a concurrent TIPS.

Portal Hypertensive Gastropathy

Portal hypertensive gastropathy (PHG) can be a source of blood loss and may lead to anemia in those with cirrhosis with or without varices. PHG is more common in those with varices and more commonly a source of blood loss as a patient's clinical status declines. Data are lacking to support NSBB for primary prophylaxis in PHG; however, data are present to support NS-BBs, carvedilol, and TIPS in secondary prophylaxis in PHG.[33,98]

Special Populations

Pregnancy

Variceal bleeding is the leading cause of maternal mortality in pregnant patients with portal hypertension.[99] Risk of bleeding is highest in the second and third trimester; therefore screening endoscopy is recommended in the second trimester. In patients with preexisting varices, there is a 25% to 35% risk of variceal bleeding during pregnancy with mortality rates as high as 50% in patients with cirrhosis and between 2% and 6% in patients with noncirrhotic portal hypertension.[100,101] Expert opinion is that patients found to have medium or large varices or small varices with high-risk stigmata should undergo prophylactic band ligation and those without high-risk varices should be started on an NSBB as the benefit is felt to outweigh potential risk.[102,103]

Perioperative Management for Those With Clinically Significant Portal Hypertension

No prospective randomized studies examining whether interventions improve clinical outcomes for patients with CSPH

undergoing surgery exist. Without prospective randomized studies of TIPS or medical management versus no intervention before abdominal surgery in those with CSPH it is difficult to provide recommendations (see Chapters 75 and 85). In those retrospective studies that are available, the populations undergoing TIPS before abdominal surgeries were largely confined to patients with MELD scores less than 10 and with average CTP scores around 6.[59,104–107] In these studies control arms were not available and a lack of comparative data between the studies prevents the pooling of data. Accordingly, it is not possible to provide an evidence-based recommendation regarding prophylactic preoperative TIPS placement for cirrhotic patients undergoing abdominal surgery. Until such a time that evidence is available the decision to do a preoperative TIPS needs careful consideration and individualization of the therapy to the patient's situation and careful reflection and tracking of outcomes under a formalized clinical review process following these procedures. Ultimately, it is imperative to design prospective, multicenter, and potentially randomized studies of preoperative TIPS in populations in which perceived benefit exists, for instance, those with esophageal, abdominal, or pelvic malignancies in which surgery has curative intent.

Multidisciplinary Care

Optimal management, for patients with complications of chronic liver disease, requires a coordinated multidisciplinary structure.[108,109] Within this, open lines of communication between specialties must be present and prospective monitoring of the outcomes of interventions must be in place. Accordingly, multidisciplinary meetings and case conferences, with shared decision making, are central to the delivery of care. This is particularly important when coordinating sequential procedures on different days in the same patient. Prospective clinical follow-up and the monitoring of outcomes is also essential, and all systems are best served when the processes are associated with a robust quality assessment and performance improvement (QAPI) platform.[110,111]

It is not uncommon in the management of patients with end-stage liver disease that one procedure or investigation is later followed by a second procedure or investigation. On occasion,

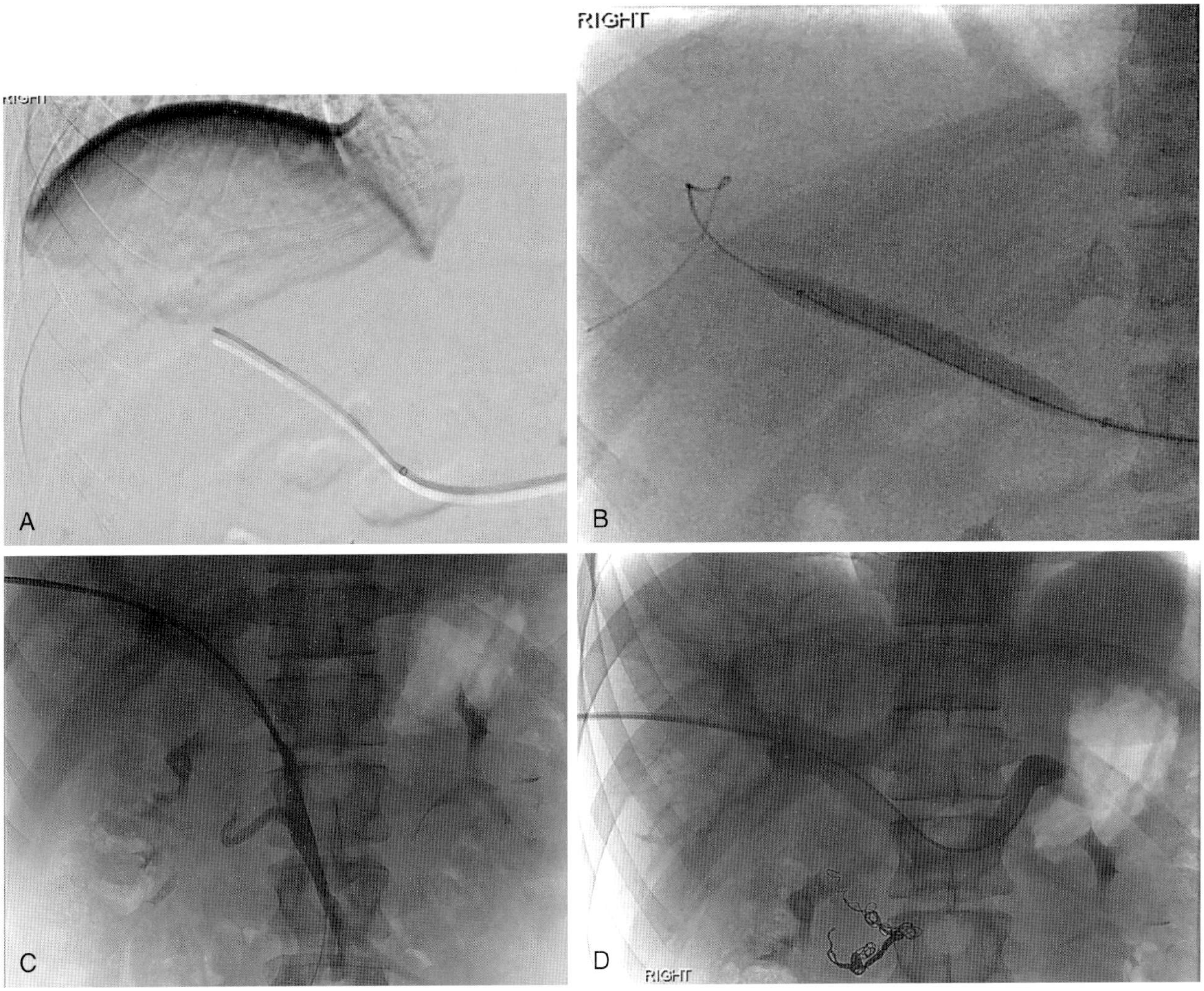

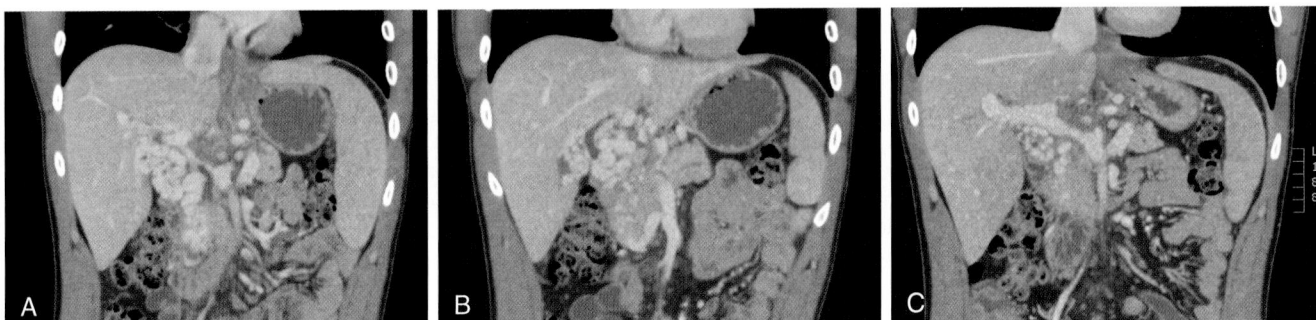

FIGURE 80.6   Recanalization of an extrahepatic portal and mesenteric vein thrombosis. A, Trans-splenic approach to intrahepatic portal vein. **B,** Balloon dilation of portal vein remnant. **C,** Transhepatic approach to superior mesenteric vein obstruction. **D,** Outcome of portal vein recanalization.

FIGURE 80.7   Extrahepatic portal vein thrombosis and outcome with recanalization. A, Extrahepatic portal vein thrombosis. **B,** Portal biliopathy and duodenal varices. **C,** Recanalize portal vein with decompression of the biliary tree and duodenal varices.

procedures to manage portal hypertension require revision, or the procedure that is to be performed occurs in a different department or location and by a provider not intimately connected to the decision. Multidisciplinary meeting minutes address potential deficiencies created and ensure that the best care is always provided. In addition, and although one procedure may address a particular problem, the procedure itself might create another, with a notable and common example of the development or worsening of hepatic encephalopathy following TIPS placement for either bleeding esophageal varices. An established multidisciplinary structure, within which the roles and responsibilities for each member are defined, allows for facilitated care delivery and improved outcomes and diminished costs to the patient and the system.[109]

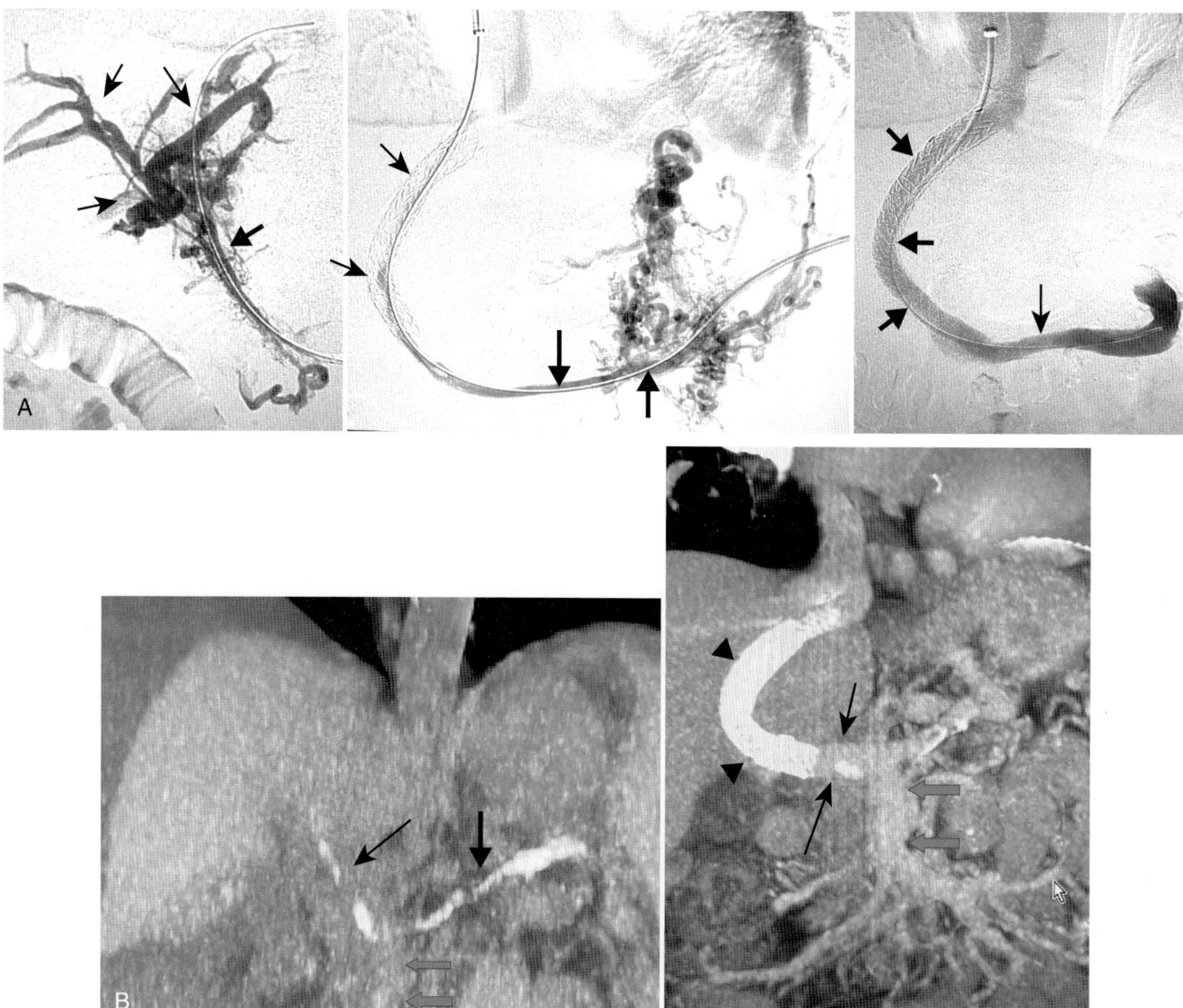

FIGURE 80.8 **A,** Portal vein recanalization and transjugular intrahepatic portosystemic shunt placement. **B,** Portal vein recanalization for refractory gastrointestinal bleeding and diuretic resistant ascites.

CONCLUSION

Evidence supports primary and secondary prophylaxis in patients with esophageal varices, particularly in those with stigmata of risk for bleeding. Several novel therapeutic options to manage varices exist and require additional randomized multicenter studies to define the benefits to these and their specific role in the management of portal hypertension. When appropriately selected, primary and secondary prophylaxis diminishes both morbidity and mortality in those in whom the intervention is applied.

The references for this chapter can be found online by accessing the accompanying Expert Consult website.

CHAPTER 81

Portal hypertensive bleeding: Acute management

Joseph Awad and Julia Wattacheril

OVERVIEW

The most important aspect of care in patients with suspected variceal or other portal hypertensive hemorrhage is adequate resuscitation and stabilization while directed diagnostic maneuvers and therapies are being coordinated (see Chapters 26 and 80). Although this chapter focuses on acute esophageal variceal bleeding, many of the principles and therapies may apply to other sources of portal hypertensive bleeding. Acute variceal hemorrhage is associated with a 15% to 20% mortality rate at six weeks.[1,2] Although evidence supports the use of endoscopy for diagnosis and treatment, insufficient resuscitation in an inappropriate environment can lead to significant periprocedural complications, while excessive resuscitation can promote bleeding. Appropriate pharmacotherapy is effective in controlling variceal hemorrhage in some patients and can be started immediately in any hospital, regardless of endoscopic staff availability.

The morbidity of patients who are seen with acute variceal hemorrhage is strongly influenced by their reason for recent decompensation (see Chapter 77). In most instances, early resuscitative measures, followed by pharmacotherapy and endoscopy, allow improvement in hepatic synthetic function and provide time to address more definitively the overall management of the patient and any recurrent bleeding (see Chapter 80). In patients with life-threatening exsanguination or who are refractory to pharmacotherapy and endoscopic intervention, balloon tamponade is a useful maneuver until the patient is stable enough for endoscopy or transjugular intrahepatic portosystemic shunting (TIPS). TIPS and other interventional radiologic procedures are being recommended earlier in the course of disease and are generally used for short-term and midterm stabilization (see Chapter 85) as a bridge to a more definitive therapy like transplantation. Shunt operations (see Chapters 83 and 84) have traditionally been reserved for individuals for whom transplantation or radiologic interventions are not an option but who have a reasonable chance of operative survival.

EMERGENCY MANAGEMENT

Before any diagnostic maneuvers can be performed (e.g., endoscopy), support of the circulating blood volume with adequate resuscitation is imperative. This is best achieved in an intensive care unit (ICU), although resuscitation should begin wherever the patient presents for medical attention (see Chapter 26). Additionally, in patients with significant bleeding or decreased consciousness, endotracheal intubation should be expedited. Isotonic crystalloid is the first replacement fluid of choice, but typed and cross-matched blood products are often needed for patients with variceal hemorrhage. Evidence supports the use of colloids versus crystalloid and packed red blood cells, with the end points of optimal hemodynamics and oxygen transport.[3] Maintenance of hemoglobin values of approximately 7 to 9 g/dL are recommended; higher blood volumes are associated with increased portal pressures, higher rebleeding rates, and higher mortality rates.[4] Other measures of the adequacy of resuscitation include systolic blood pressures of 90 to 100 mm Hg, central venous pressures of 9 to 16 mm Hg, and adequate urine output. When the adjusted prothrombin time (PT) is prolonged by more than three to four seconds, fresh frozen plasma is likewise recommended but may not be as beneficial as expected from the improvement in PT. Fibrinogen supplementation has been helpful in liver transplantation and may have a role.[5] Similarly, if significant thrombocytopenia contributes to coagulopathy, platelet transfusion should commence. Recombinant factor VIIa has not been shown to benefit patients with cirrhosis with gastrointestinal (GI) hemorrhage versus standard therapy.[6]

Complications from variceal bleeding contribute to overall morbidity and mortality related to chronic liver disease. Preventing these complications can therefore have a significant impact on the short-term mortality rate associated with variceal bleeding. Antibiotic prophylaxis has been shown to decrease variceal rebleeding and bacterial infection.[7,8] Systematic reviews have shown decreased mortality rates with antibiotic prophylaxis in the setting of cirrhotic GI bleeding.[9] Based on a number of positive studies the choice of antibiotic should be dictated by patient tolerance, local antibiotic availability, and susceptibility issues and should broadly cover gram-negative rods and oral gram-positive organisms.

Controlling Acute Hemorrhage: Pharmacologic Agents (see Chapter 80)

Coupling pharmacologic measures and endoscopy with the initiation of preventative measures provides the most sustainable results when attempting to control acute GI hemorrhage in patients with advanced liver disease. The specific drugs are widely available, generally safe, and can be initiated as soon as variceal hemorrhage is suspected. Drugs such as somatostatin or its analogues octreotide and vapreotide work by constricting arterial and thus venous splanchnic blood flow, thereby reducing portal hypertension acutely. In randomized controlled trials comparing these vasoactive agents with other ones, including vasopressin and terlipressin, no significant differences in bleeding control were reported, although vasopressin and more recently terlipressin were associated with more adverse events.[2,10,11] Currently, an initial bolus dose of octreotide 50 μg intravenously, followed by 50 μg/hr, is recommended. Duration usually extends from 72 hours to five days, and recurrent bleeding should be treated with an additional bolus dose. Only octreotide and vasopressin are currently available in the United States.

Controlling Acute Esophageal Variceal Hemorrhage: Endoscopic Therapy

The two main endoscopic therapeutic choices are endoscopic variceal ligation (EVL) and sclerotherapy. The former is preferred, given its superior control of bleeding and reported decreases in rebleeding rates, mortality rates, and esophageal complications. Both techniques require a skilled endoscopist; however, when both groups were treated with somatostatin concomitantly, failure rates of EVL were estimated at 10% compared with 24% of sclerotherapy patients. Failure to control acute bleeding is also significantly more frequent in the sclerotherapy group[2] (see Chapter 80).

After adequate sedation and diagnostic endoscopy, EVL should commence. The decision regarding whether to start with a standard 2.8-mm gastroscope versus a therapeutic endoscope is practitioner dependent, given the improved potential for clot removal by irrigation with the latter. Once a variceal source has been identified, the endoscope should be removed, and a multibanding kit should be applied with a standard gastroscope. Bands should be applied to any vessels actively spurting blood or displaying stigmata of recent hemorrhage, such as red wale marks, white nipples, and/or adherent blood clots. Other vessels should then be ligated, starting as close as possible to the esophagogastric junction. The varix is drawn into the ligator by applying suction, and a band is then applied as shown in Figure 81.1.

When considering sclerotherapy, two techniques of sclerosant injection are generally in use, and the choice of which to use is somewhat institutionally and regionally influenced. Sclerosants can be injected into the varix itself (intravariceally) or adjacent to it (paravariceally); both techniques appear to be effective. Often a paravariceal injection results inadvertently from an intravariceal injection attempt, given the technical challenges in an acutely bleeding patient. Sodium morrhuate and sodium tetradecyl sulfate are the two sclerosants most commonly used

in the United States, and each varix should be injected with 1 to 2 mL of sclerosant just above the esophagogastric junction and 5 cm proximal. Some endoscopists find sclerotherapy effective when active bleeding impairs visualization for EVL. On occasion, application of sclerotherapy sufficiently impedes bleeding enough to allow band ligation. Adverse events include fever, retrosternal pain, dysphagia, esophageal ulceration and delayed bleeding, injection-induced bleeding, esophageal perforation and stricture, mediastinitis, pleural effusion, acute respiratory distress syndrome, and infection.

Tamponade Techniques

A correctly placed balloon tube can temporarily control acute variceal bleeding. The balloon tube is primarily used when patients have continued, active bleeding despite attempted control by emergency endoscopic therapy. A balloon tube may also be inserted when massive variceal bleeding obscures visibility during emergency endoscopy; both are relatively uncommon circumstances. Balloon tube tamponade has also proved to be lifesaving during the transfer of patients to a tertiary care center, to control a subsequent major bleed while awaiting emergency endoscopy, or while preparing for alternative therapy when endoscopic therapy fails (e.g., a further major, acute variceal bleed after two emergency endoscopic treatments during a single hospital admission).

The balloon tube should be inserted by a practitioner familiar with the technique (details to follow). The tube should be left in place for as short a time as needed for resuscitation, endoscopic treatment, or radiologic intervention. Bleeding that continues after tube insertion warrants additional assessment regarding correct placement and potential for repeat endoscopy. In these cases, a bleeding lesion below the balloon in the distal stomach or duodenum that was missed at the first diagnostic endoscopy is usually the culprit.[12]

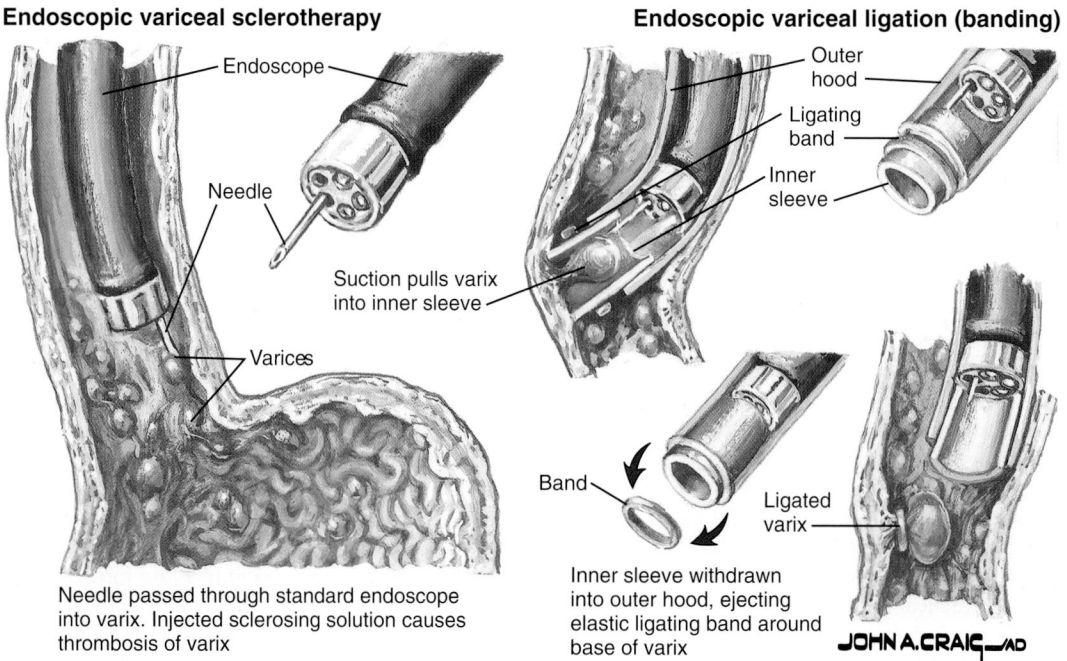

Endoscopic variceal sclerotherapy

- Endoscope
- Needle
- Suction pulls varix into inner sleeve
- Varices

Needle passed through standard endoscope into varix. Injected sclerosing solution causes thrombosis of varix

Endoscopic variceal ligation (banding)

- Outer hood
- Ligating band
- Inner sleeve
- Band
- Ligated varix

Inner sleeve withdrawn into outer hood, ejecting elastic ligating band around base of varix

JOHN A. CRAIG—AD

FIGURE 81.1 Variceal bleeding ligation techniques. (Netter illustration from www.netterimages.com. Copyright Elsevier, Inc. All rights reserved.)

TECHNIQUE. After confirming a complete air seal, the deflated lubricated tube is passed via the mouth through a bite guard placed between the teeth. The tube is inserted as far as possible. To confirm the balloon's position in the stomach, the epigastrium is auscultated while instilling air via the aspirating lumen of the gastric tube with a 50-mL syringe. Thereafter, the gastric balloon is cautiously inflated via its lumen to 100 mL in 50-mL increments. Inflation should be easy. If the tube is curled in the esophagus, resistance is felt and the inflation must be stopped immediately; otherwise, the esophagus may be damaged. If the gastric balloon has been easily inflated, it is pulled up until it is seated firmly against the esophagogastric junction. Then the position of the tube is confirmed radiographically before another 150 to 200 mL of air is added to the balloon.

Tension on the tube is often maintained by taping it to the face mask of an American football helmet. Alternatively, a split tennis ball strapped to the tube at the mouth guard can be used to protect the patient's lips from the pressure of the tennis ball. Adequate tension on the gastric balloon should be checked regularly at the mouth. Inflation of the esophageal balloon is not usually necessary, because traction on the gastric balloon is generally sufficient to compress gastric veins that feed esophageal varices. If esophageal balloon inflation is required, a three-way stopcock and a blood pressure manometer are used to inflate the esophageal balloon to 40 mm Hg before clamping the tube. This pressure needs to be checked regularly, and the balloon should be deflated hourly to prevent esophageal necrosis. The fourth lumen, which opens in the esophagus, is placed on constant suction; the gastric lumen is used for suction and to administer medication such as lactulose.

Patients with a balloon tube in place are monitored carefully in an ICU. When the balloon tube has been inserted and fixed and bleeding has been arrested, resuscitation is continued, clotting abnormalities are corrected, and the patient is made as fit as possible for the necessary subsequent management. Ideally, the balloon tube should be removed within 24 hours.[13]

Gastric Varices

Approximately 20% of patients with cirrhosis have gastric varices, either in isolation or associated with esophageal varices. Bleeding from gastric varices carries greater risk and is associated with increased mortality rates.[14] In these cases, endoscopic variceal obturation (EVO) with *N*-butyl-cyanoacrylate (BCA) has been demonstrated as superior to EVL in controlling initial hemorrhage, as well as controlling rebleeding.[15,16] In the United States, where BCA is approved for cerebral arteriovenous malformations but not for gastric varices, 2-octyl-cyanoacrylate has been used instead (approved for wound closures); adverse events have been noted and include thromboembolic events and bacteremia (prophylactic antibiotics are recommended). Its use requires specialized endoscopic training. In situations where this is not available, primary placement of TIPS is preferred[17] (see Chapter 85). TIPS is also effective in controlling acute hemorrhage from gastric varices. Decreased recurrent bleeding has been demonstrated in patients undergoing TIPS versus EVO[18] but carries a higher rate of encephalopathy. More recently, additional transvenous means to embolize gastric varices, including balloon-occluded retrograde transvenous obliteration through the left renal vein, have been developed.[19] One advantage of this approach is the avoidance of shunting of blood away from the liver, reducing the risk of hepatic encephalopathy and liver failure after the procedure. However, ascites can increase.

Ectopic Varices

Ectopic varices are those in an atypical location (nonesophageal or nongastric). Bleeding from ectopic varices accounts for approximately 1% to 5% of variceal bleeding.[20] Most ectopic varices arise from global portal hypertension, but they may be related to regional thrombosis. They commonly occur at prior surgery sites, where the healing process promotes venous connections between a high-pressure portal system and the lower-pressure systemic circulation. Common sites include the duodenum, anorectal region, umbilicus, and ostomies. Patients typically bleed into the lumen of the GI tract, but peritoneal and retroperitoneal bleeding can occasionally occur. Given their relatively rare occurrence, treatment recommendations have been made based on case reports, case series, and small reviews, but not randomized controlled trials.

Imaging and endoscopy techniques have allowed approximation of the prevalence of ectopic varices. Anorectal varices have been reported in 10% to 40% of patients with cirrhosis; duodenal varices have been reported in 40% of patients with portal hypertension as seen during angiography. Fortunately, bleeding from these lesions is quite rare.

Peristomal/stoma varices are seen in patients with ostomies who have, or later develop, portal hypertension such that alternatives to creating an ostomy should be considered in these patients. Although more common in those with significant intrahepatic portal hypertension, they are particularly insidious and can bleed at a hepatic venous pressure gradient of less than 12 mm Hg. Peristomal varices are most common on the skin near the stoma rather than deep within the stoma. Thus it is important to remove the skin covering around the stoma and apply direct pressure or local treatment to the bleeding vessel.

Initial management remains the same as in esophageal variceal bleeding, namely, to provide adequate clinical assessment and resuscitative measures, hemodynamic support, and antibiotic prophylaxis. Vasoactive drugs are reasonable to use, and endoscopy should proceed with goals similar to those for therapy of variceal bleeding.

Band ligation of ectopic varices has been limited to a few reports and mainly involves varices in the rectum and duodenum. Banding can be performed when the diameter of the varix does not exceed the endoscope diameter. More studies have evaluated the role of sclerotherapy in ectopic varices, but the results were less than optimal. Colorectal varices respond less often to sclerotherapy, possibly as a result of the dilution of sclerosant to an ineffective concentration in these larger varices.

Embolization with coils, gel foam, collagen, autologous blood clot, or thrombin has been effective in interventional radiology as an adjunct to band ligation or TIPS. Occlusion of the supplying vein decreases blood supply to the varix itself. Steel coils, placed via interventional techniques, are most effective in achieving total focal occlusion. Success rates for bleeding cessation are reported to be greater than 90%; however, the underlying portal hypertension is not treated.

Surgical treatment, including direct focal devascularization, is effective and usually performed in the presence of portal vein occlusion or advanced cirrhosis. Some of the direct approaches used are oversewing of varices via duodenotomy, duodenal dearterialization and stapling, circumferentially stapled anoplasty, and double-selective shunting. Nonselective portosystemic shunts (see Chapters 85 and 86) are much more invasive and are therefore less commonly used.[20]

Portal Gastropathy and Gastric Antral Vascular Ectasia

Portal gastropathy is rarely a cause of rapid life-threatening bleeding, but it can be severe enough to require daily transfusion. This situation is most common in the presence of gastric antral vascular ectasia (GAVE), a condition well described by its name. GAVE can occur without portal hypertension but is especially difficult to manage in the presence of portal hypertension. The antrum often has a red, longitudinally striped appearance that gives this condition its alternative name, *watermelon stomach*. In the absence of portal hypertension, this cause of chronic blood loss and iron deficiency anemia can be treated with argon plasma coagulation (APC) or antrectomy. However, APC in the setting of portal hypertension is much less effective and can even cause a worsening of bleeding. Unfortunately, TIPS shunting has also been of little benefit, and antrectomy is usually too risky to be considered.

Recently, banding of antral mucosa has been described as a treatment for this condition. As many as 12 bands can be placed per session, with approximately three sessions required to complete the treatment course. Banded mucosa is sloughed and replaced by mucosa without ectatic blood vessels. Wider experience with this modality will help determine the place of banding in this difficult to manage condition.[21]

RECURRENT BLEEDING

GI hemorrhage in patients with cirrhosis either recurs or cannot be controlled in approximately 2% to 13% of cases despite coordinated efforts with directed therapy. In these cases, shunt therapy is indicated. In Child-Turcotte-Pugh class A (compensated) cirrhotic patients, surgical shunts (see Chapters 83 and 84) have proven efficacious. However, in most acute and later recurrences, TIPS is the preferred mechanism of portal decompression (see Chapter 84). In addition to serving as a bridge to liver transplantation in patients not responding to pharmacologic and endoscopic therapy, TIPS is sometimes thought to be advantageous because of the lower portal pressures during transplantation; however, once the portal vein is clamped the advantage is lost. A TIPS functions as a nonselective shunt, and the development of encephalopathy or worsening of existing encephalopathy should be considered before implantation. Stenosis or occlusion may develop in as many as 50% of patients within one year with bare metal stents; however, results are improved when stents covered with polytetrafluoroethylene are used. Both types of stents can be restored with angiographic interventions.

In patients for whom shunts are not available (anatomic limitations, portal vein thrombosis), other therapies may have to be considered. In recurrent gastric variceal hemorrhage, BCA had lower rates of rebleeding (15% vs. 55%) and mortality (3% vs. 25%) during a median of 26 months, according to a randomized trial.[22] In Europe, self-expandable covered metal stents to control refractory variceal bleeding without fluoroscopic guidance have been investigated and may be a viable alternative to balloon tamponade. These stents are not available in the United States.[23]

In the era of TIPS, an extensive gastric and lower esophageal devascularization together with transection of the lower esophagus is rarely required (see Chapter 82). The extensive abdominothoracic Sugiura procedure developed in Japan has been replaced by a transabdominal procedure in most institutions.[13]

No Therapy: Observation Only

Patients with end-stage liver disease who are not candidates for transplantation and who are seen with major esophageal variceal bleeding complicated by multiorgan failure perhaps should not be subjected to the most invasive procedures described. Withholding treatment in these circumstances, in which the chances of meaningful survival is remote at best, is a difficult clinical and ethical decision but one that must be considered, discussed, and accepted in the appropriate clinical scenario.

References are available at expertconsult.com.

CHAPTER 82

Portal hypertensive bleeding: Operative devascularization

Anil Kumar Agarwal

TREATMENT OF ESOPHAGOGASTRIC VARICES

This chapter addresses the role of devascularization procedures in the management of portal hypertensive bleeding. The management of variceal bleeding is based on the underlying cause, liver function, presentation, and the patient's clinical condition. Several nonsurgical therapeutic options are available to manage an acute bleeding episode and prevent subsequent episodes (see Chapters 80, 81, and 84). The roles of other treatment modalities, including pharmacotherapy (see Chapter 80), endoscopic therapy (see Chapter 81), transjugular intrahepatic portosystemic shunt (TIPS) (see Chapter 85), and portosystemic shunts (see Chapters 84 and 85), are discussed in other chapters in this book.

Bleeding from esophageal and gastric varices is the most life-threatening acute manifestation of portal hypertension and is a cause of significant morbidity and mortality.[1,2] Variceal bleeding is commonly from esophageal varices, and although primary hemorrhage from gastric varices is uncommon, it is more difficult to control and has higher morbidity and mortality.[3,4] The mortality from an acute episode of bleeding depends on the patient's liver function status and clinical status. With the advent of pharmacologic agents, endoscopic procedures, including sclerotherapy, variceal band ligation, and glue injection, and radiologic procedures, such as TIPS and balloon-occluded retrograde transvenous obliteration (see Chapter 30), improved control of variceal bleed has been possible.[1,5,6] In the last decade, with standardized approaches using these nonsurgical options in patients with acute variceal hemorrhage, the mortality rate, which was reported as high as 30% to 40%, has come down to 14% to 15%.[7,8]

Of patients with variceal bleeding, 10% to 15% do not respond to nonoperative methods and require surgical intervention.[9] Surgical options include shunt and nonshunt procedures. The role of shunts is discussed in Chapters 84 and 85. In patients with chronic liver disease and significant functional compromise, nonselective shunts have an unacceptably high incidence of encephalopathy and hepatic decompensation.[10,11] In advanced stages of liver failure, liver transplantation will be a definitive treatment (see Chapter 105), with other modalities bridging the interim waiting period. Devascularization procedures are directed toward varices in the esophagus and the stomach. Compared with TIPS and surgical shunts, the devascularization procedures maintain portal perfusion and hepatocyte function, thereby resulting in a much lower incidence of postoperative hepatic dysfunction and encephalopathy. Besides, the applications of shunting operations are limited in patients with extensive thrombosis of the mesenteric venous system, in both cirrhotic and noncirrhotic settings. In addition, nonshunting operations do not alter vascular anatomy and do not complicate future liver transplant surgery, although they can cause significant upper abdominal adhesions, which may be associated with increased bleeding at the time of transplantation.

Devascularization procedures are now performed less frequently; however, when most nonsurgical measures fail in an emergent scenario, and when radiologic therapies are not feasible, their role still exists in the surgical armamentarium available to salvage critical situations of variceal bleeding.[12] In elective situations in patients without cirrhosis with no shuntable vein and difficult-to-obliterate varices, devascularization is the best and, at times, the only option available.

Indications

Devascularization procedures aim to control bleeding from varices in the esophagogastric region. They do not control bleeding from ectopic varices, nor do they treat the underlying disease. However, splenectomy, which is part of most described devascularization procedures, can effectively treat hypersplenism and improve liver function in some patients because of the favorable changes in splanchnic hemodynamics.[13] Devascularization procedures can be used for primary prophylaxis of variceal bleeding, to control acute bleeding, or to prevent recurrent bleeding from esophagogastric varices.

The indications for devascularization procedures can be discussed in two scenarios: (1) patients with underlying chronic liver disease and (2) patients with a healthy liver, as in extrahepatic portal vein obstruction (EHPVO) and noncirrhotic portal fibrosis (NCPF).

In the current era, transplantation of the liver being a well-established modality (see Chapter 105), there are only a few indications for devascularization for the treatment of esophagogastric varices in patients with chronic liver disease. The recent American Association for the Study of Liver Diseases practice guidelines does not include devascularization procedures in their recommended practice guidelines in the acute or prophylactic setting.[14] This may perhaps be due to the fact that the majority of patients of portal hypertension in the United States have a cirrhotic cause, and the options of nonsurgical modalities, as well as liver transplantation, are more easily available. However, in other parts of the world where the facilities are not as well developed, devascularization procedures still have a significant role to play, especially in the emergency management of esophagogastric variceal bleeding.[15]

Devascularization, therefore, has a role as an emergency procedure when other nonsurgical methods have failed or are not a feasible option to control acute variceal bleeding or recurrent bleeding. It has been demonstrated that rebleeding after two sessions of emergency variceal sclerotherapy is unlikely to respond to further endoscopic therapy, and devascularization may be used in noncirrhotic patients and in cirrhotic patients when other modalities such as TIPS (see Chapter 85) are not feasible or not available.[15,16] Additionally, in patients who are not candidates for transplantation and have high-grade varices with symptomatic hypersplenism, devascularization is performed for primary prophylaxis of bleeding and treatment of hypersplenism. Devascularization is contraindicated in severely compromised liver dysfunction, as in Child-Pugh C patients, except perhaps as a "last ditch" effort. Occasionally, when TIPS is unavailable, this procedure has been used as a bridge to liver transplantation because, unlike a portocaval shunt, it does not alter the vascular anatomy and complicate future transplantation surgery.[17]

In a noncirrhotic cause, for example, EHPVO and NCPF, shunt surgery is usually the preferred option (see Chapters 83 and 84) However, devascularization is indicated in patients with noncirrhotic portal hypertension with unfavorable vascular anatomy, such as the absence of a shuntable vein in patients with extensive mesenteric venous thrombosis or an inadequate vein size to permit a shunt, which often may be detected intraoperatively.[18–20] In noncirrhotic patients with acute variceal bleeding, devascularization is indicated when other modalities have failed to control acute bleeding and the patient is unstable to undergo a shunt procedure, even when the shunt is technically feasible. In one series, 16 of 114 patients (14%) with EHPVO underwent devascularization.[18] The procedure has been reported to give good results in children with massive splenomegaly with hypersplenism secondary to EHPVO.[21,22] Goyal et al.[23] suggested that esophagogastric devascularization is an operation that can be performed even in hospitals where facilities and expertise for shunt procedures and interventional procedures like TIPS are not available.

The devascularization procedure may be indicated in some other situations, such as portal biliopathy in the absence of a shuntable vein[24] and chronic pancreatitis with portal hypertension.[25]

In this chapter, splenectomy alone has not been separately considered because, in noncirrhotic patients needing splenectomy for symptomatic hypersplenism, a shunt is commonly added if there is a shuntable vein.[26] In noncirrhotic patients with an unshuntable vein and patients with chronic liver disease, splenectomy is combined with esophagogastric devascularization. In addition, isolated splenectomy as a means of secondary prophylaxis for variceal bleeding has a 30% to 50% failure rate and hence is not advocated,[27,28] except in the instance of left-sided portal hypertension (i.e., isolated splenic vein thrombosis).

SURGICAL ANATOMY, PATHOPHYSIOLOGY OF VARICES, AND EFFECTS OF DEVASCULARIZATION
Anatomy and Pathophysiology

To understand the basis of devascularization, the underlying anatomy that results in esophagogastric varices must be understood (see Chapter 2). When portal hypertension develops, there is a diversion of portal venous blood away from the liver to join the low-pressure systemic circulation by collateral pathways—natural portosystemic shunts (see Chapters 74 and 80). The esophagogastric region is the main site of natural portosystemic shunting. The coronary and other gastric veins are connected to tributaries of the superior vena cava by collateral channels in the submucosa of the esophagus, and in the periesophageal area (adventitial plexus). The drainage is

mainly into the submucosal and subepithelial veins of the esophagus by the gastroesophageal junction. The increased blood flow and resistance in the muscularis layer of the esophagus contribute to the increase in venous pressure, resulting in the formation of dilated and tortuous varices. A three-dimensional observation reveals the intrinsic and extrinsic veins in the esophageal wall.[29] The intrinsic veins (intramural vessels), including the submucosal, subepithelial, and the intraepithelial veins, are strongly implicated in the development of varices. Periesophageal veins comprise the extrinsic vein system and branch veins (extramural vessels) from the periesophageal collaterals enter the esophageal wall and feed the varices.

In portal hypertension, the increased venous pressure can produce varices throughout the length of the esophagus and down into the upper stomach; however, the bleeding from esophageal varices usually occurs in the lowest 5 cm of the esophagus. In the stomach, although varices are seen more often on the lesser curve, it is the less common fundal varices that are more dangerous and likely to lead to exsanguinating hemorrhage.[30] Therefore a technique targeting extramural and intramural vessels in this vulnerable area would help in controlling or preventing bleeding from esophageal varices.

Devascularization being a variceal-directed ablative surgery, aims at the obliteration of varices or disconnection of the esophagogastric veins from the hypertensive portal tributaries. The goal of the esophagogastric devascularization is to disconnect the esophagus and stomach from this collateral system while maintaining a portosystemic shunt in place by the adventitial plexus surrounding the esophagus.[31] Most of the described devascularization procedures have two major components:

1. Devascularization of the esophagogastric region to reduce bleeding from the esophagogastric varices.
2. Splenectomy, which decreases portal flow and thereby pressure, facilitates esophagogastric devascularization, and also effectively deals with hypersplenism, if present.

The devascularization of the esophagogastric region is achieved by interruption of the extramural and the intramural vessels feeding gastroesophageal varices with the maintenance of hepatic portal perfusion. Based on the targeted vessels the surgical procedures can be conceptually classified as:

1. Devascularization procedures (Hassab type) that targets extramural vessels feeding gastroesophageal varices
2. Devascularization procedures (Sugiura type) that focus on extramural and intramural vessels feeding gastroesophageal varices and preserving the longitudinal esophageal vessels, thereby maintaining the spontaneous portoazygos flow in the region

Evolution of Devascularization Procedures

The evolution of devascularization procedures can be divided into three stages. In the early 1950s and 1960s, surgery was directed toward ligation/transection of varices and esophageal transection. Boerema and Crile, in 1950, reported ligation of esophageal varices with unsatisfactory results. Walker, in 1964, reported transthoracic esophageal transection. Along similar lines, gastroesophageal resection,[32–38] upper gastric transection[39–41] and transabdominal esophageal transection[42,43] were also reported in the period, with unsatisfactory outcomes.

In the late 1960s and early 1970s, Hassab and Sugiura developed the two successful procedures named after them that describe systematic devascularization of the esophagogastric region together with splenectomy. Hassab, in 1967,[44] described an esophagogastric devascularization completely performed through the abdominal route in portal hypertension, secondary to schistosomiasis. In 1973, Japanese surgeons Sugiura and Futagawa[45] described a transthoracic esophageal devascularization combined with esophageal transection and an abdominal approach for splenectomy and upper stomach devascularization with vagotomy and pyloroplasty. Hassab[44] and Sugiura and Futagawa[45] reported good results and laid the foundation for the currently practiced devascularization procedures. Both Hassab and Sugiura procedures were subsequently modified, and currently the modified versions of these two procedures is commonly used.[46–53] During the last decade, devascularization procedures are frequently performed using a minimally invasive approach.[54–56] Of the two devascularization procedures, conceptually, the Sugiura-type procedures result in more thorough devascularization by interrupting extramural perforating veins and intramural portosystemic shunt feeding the varices.[52,53] In addition, it is the most physiologic procedure because the periesophageal spontaneous portocaval shunt is preserved to preclude a postoperative rise in portal pressure. However, despite suboptimal devascularization, Hassab-type procedures are commonly used, especially in the minimally invasive approach, perhaps because of technical simplicity and the option of effectively managing post-devascularization residual varices using an endoscopic approach.[55–57]

HASSAB AND MODIFIED HASSAB DEVASCULARIZATION PROCEDURE

Hassab developed a devascularization procedure in 1957 and reported a cumulative experience of 355 cases in 1967. Even though in this series the procedure of gastroesophageal devascularization with splenectomy was applied in cases of portal hypertension secondary to bilharzial (schistosomiasis) infestation, the procedure is recommended for other causes as well.

The Hassab devascularization procedure is performed through an abdominal incision. The options for incision include midline, extended left subcostal, or L-shaped, depending on the size of the spleen. The left lobe of the liver is freed from its attachments. Splenic artery ligation followed by splenectomy is performed. Splenectomy and ligation of short gastric veins is followed by ligation of the vessels ascending through the hiatus and the diaphragm. The gastrohepatic ligament is incised. A major part of the gastrohepatic ligament containing the left gastric vessel is divided between ligatures. The peritoneum over the intraabdominal part of the esophagus is reflected, and the abdominal esophagus is circumferentially dissected and looped with umbilical tape. This is followed by the devascularization of 3 to 4 inches (7–10 cm) of the lower esophagus and proximal stomach along with vagotomy and pyloroplasty (Fig. 82.1). The abdomen is closed after the placement of a drain in the region.

An important aspect of the Hassab procedure is the absence of esophageal transection. Hassab[44] suggested that portoazygous disconnection without esophageal transection was sufficient and reported that varices disappeared completely or improved in 91% of patients. However, Nakamura et al.,[58] based on endoscopic ultrasonography findings, reported that the Hassab type gastroesophageal decongestion and splenectomy is effective for the extramural connections but not for the intramural connections resulting in recurrent esophageal varices. Later Hassab[59] suggested that combined sclerotherapy or endoscopic ligation

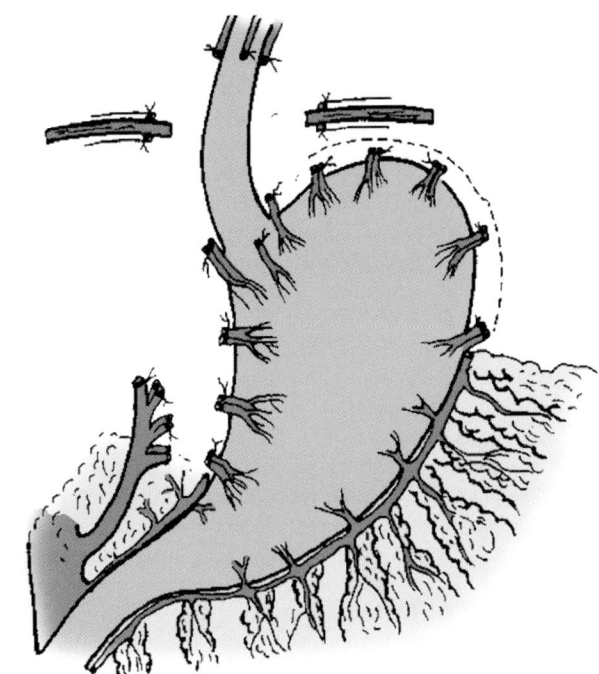

FIGURE 82.1 Diagrammatic representation of the Hassab procedure. (From Hassab MA. Gastroesophageal decongestion and splenectomy in the treatment of esophageal varices in bilharzial cirrhosis: further studies with a report on 355 operations. *Surgery.* 1967;61:170–176.)

could reduce rebleeding if there were missed obliterated esophageal perforators or if devascularization at operation was incomplete. Another critical aspect of the Hassab procedure is that the main trunk of the left gastric vessels was not preserved and the division of the left gastric vein could disrupt the spontaneous portacaval shunt between left gastric and paraesophageal veins. Disruption of the spontaneous shunt at the gastroesophageal area increases portal pressure and promotes the formation of a new collateral pathway leading to recurrence of esophageal varices and exacerbation of portal hypertension gastropathy.[60] Therefore selective devascularization of only the branch veins that enter the wall of the esophagus and stomach was proposed as a modification of the Hassab procedure.[60,61] A meta-analysis of seven randomized controlled trials (RCTs) and seven nonrandomized observational clinical studies compared perioperative outcomes and postoperative complications between selective and nonselective (division of left gastric vessels) gastroesophageal devascularization.[62] The patients who underwent selective gastroesophageal devascularization had less portal hypertensive gastropathy, rebleeding, and postoperative mortality. However, selective gastroesophageal devascularization may not be feasible in all patients. If the paraesophageal veins directly enter the esophageal wall, or if it is difficult to identify the paraesophageal vein because of the extensive varicose vessels, the left gastric vein needs to be ligated to block abnormal blood flow to the esophagogastric varices.

SUGIURA AND FUTAGAWA DEVASCULARIZATION PROCEDURE

Sugiura and Futagawa devised this devascularization procedure in 1967 and published their initial experience of 84 patients in 1973 and, subsequently, a larger experience of 671 patients in

1984. The procedure consists of a transthoracic and an abdominal procedure performed through two separate incisions. The thoracic procedure involves extensive paraesophageal devascularization up to the inferior pulmonary vein and esophageal transection. The inferior pulmonary vein is the landmark for the upper extent of devascularization because the drainage from varices to bronchial and azygous veins begins at that level. The abdominal procedure includes splenectomy, devascularization of the abdominal esophagus and upper half of the stomach with selective vagotomy, and pyloroplasty.

Contrary to general belief, Sugiura and Futagawa performed the two parts of the operation as a single stage in 55 of the 84 patients. In 29 poor-risk patients, the two parts of the operation, that is, thoracic and abdominal, were done in two stages 4 to 6 weeks apart, with transthoracic being the first stage in 21 patients and transabdominal in 8 patients.

The Sugiura and Futagawa procedure resembles the Hassab procedure in terms of performing splenectomy and devascularization directed to the paraesophagogastric area. However, in contrast to the Hassab procedure, only the transverse branches to the esophagus are ligated, preserving the paraesophageal longitudinal channels and left gastric vessels. In addition, esophageal transection is added to disrupt intramural portosystemic connections and prevent revascularization of the esophageal varices from the intramural vessels. Thus the Sugiura procedure divides extramural perforating veins and intramural portosystemic shunt feeding the varices while preserving periesophageal portocaval shunt. Splenectomy and preservation of portacaval shunt between left gastric and paraesophageal veins reduces portal pressure but not to the extent of a total shunt procedure, thus lessening the risk of hepatic decompensation.

Sugiura-Futagawa Operation: Thoracic Procedure

In the thoracic component of the operation, a left lateral thoracotomy is performed in the sixth intercostal space and the mediastinal pleura is incised. Care is taken to preserve the dilated collateral veins running parallel to the esophagus, and only the shunts (vascular channels) from these to the esophagus are completely ligated and divided. The lower part of the esophagus is surrounded by a plexus of adventitial veins that run parallel to the esophageal wall and communicate with the submucosal variceal channels by perforating veins (Fig. 82.2). These perforating veins must be completely and systematically ligated and divided to devascularize the esophagus. Approximately 30 to 50 of these shunting (perforating) veins along the 12 to 18 cm of the thoracic esophagus are meticulously ligated and divided from the upper edge of the inferior pulmonary vein to the diaphragm. The hiatus is now devascularized, and the lower esophagus is transected at the level of the diaphragm. The posterior muscular layer was left intact in the original description, and approximately 70 to 90 interrupted sutures are placed to occlude the divided varices. Because of the high risk of an esophageal anastomotic leak, esophageal transection is not done in the patients who had recently received endoscopic sclerotherapy or variceal band ligation. After closing the thoracotomy over a drain, a laparotomy is performed.

Sugiura-Futagawa Operation: Abdominal Procedure

Laparotomy is performed through an upper midline incision with left lateral extension. The first step is to perform a splenectomy, followed by devascularization of the greater curvature and abdominal part of the esophagus. The posterior vagus

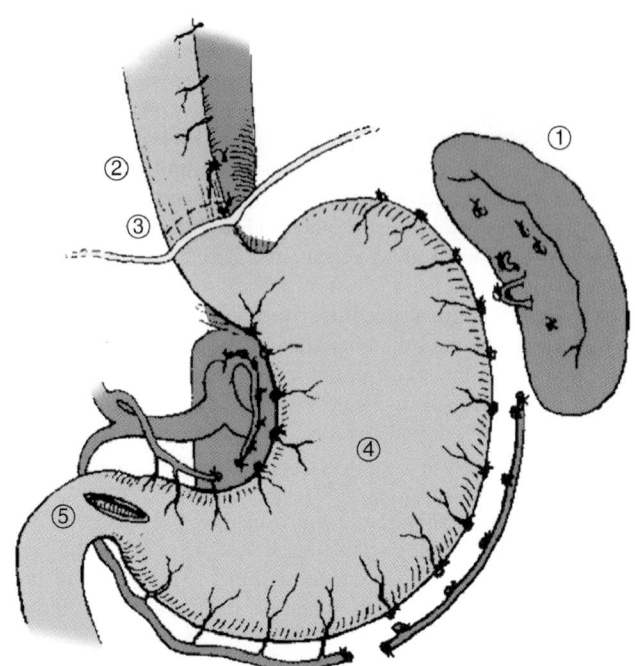

FIGURE 82.2 Sugiura procedure includes *1,* splenectomy; *2,* devascularization of 8 to 10 cm of the esophagus; *3,* transection and end-to-end anastomosis of the lower esophagus 4 to 5 cm above the gastroesophageal junction; *4,* devascularization of the lesser and greater curvatures of the stomach; and *5,* pyloroplasty. (From Selzner M, et al. Current indication of a modified Sugiura procedure in the management of variceal bleeding. *J Am Coll Surg.* 2001;193:166–173.)

nerve is divided at this step because of its proximity. Lesser curvature devascularization follows, and the cardioesophageal branches of left gastric vessels (but not the main left gastric) are ligated and divided. The length of devascularization is approximately 6 to 7 cm along the lesser curvature. The esophagus and cardia are completely mobilized and freed from the adjacent structures. Devascularization is facilitated by the division of the anterior vagus nerve, and for this reason a pyloroplasty is performed. A drain is placed in the splenic fossa.

In 1984 Sugiura and Futagawa reported the outcomes of 671 patients who underwent their devascularization procedure. The 203 (30%) patients had prophylactic, 363 (54%) patients had elective, and 105 (16%) patients had an emergency procedure. The cause of portal hypertension was cirrhosis in 495 patients, EHPVO in 39 patients, and other causes in the remaining 137 patients. Overall operative mortality was 4.9%, with 13.3% mortality in the emergency setting and 3% in the elective setting. In patients with cirrhosis, Child-Pugh status–based mortality was 0% for 244 Child-Pugh class A patients, 2% for 251 class B patients, and 16% for 176 class C patients. There were no operative deaths among Child-Pugh class A and B patients who underwent a prophylactic devascularization procedure. The overall survival rate was 46% for class C patients compared with 86% and 81% for class A and B patients, respectively. Late deaths were due to hepatic failure and hepatocellular carcinoma and not to variceal bleeding. The 10-year actuarial survival rate in patients with cirrhosis was 55% in emergency cases, 72% in prophylactic cases, and 72% in elective cases. The corresponding survival rates in patients without cirrhosis were 90% in emergency cases, 96% in prophylactic cases, and 95% in elective cases. The incidence of recurrent variceal bleeding was only 1.5%, and 5.2% developed recurrent varices. There was no postoperative variceal bleeding in prophylactic cases.

MODIFIED SUGIURA-FUTAGAWA DEVASCULARIZATION PROCEDURE

The original Sugiura-Futagawa procedure produced excellent results in Japan; however, the results could not be duplicated in the West, and the procedure was thought to be time-consuming and technically too complex. This procedure was modified by several surgeons using an exclusive abdominal approach and stapled transection of the esophagus, achieving results similar to those with the combined thoracic and abdominal approach.[46,48,63] The standard modifications include completing the entire procedure by the abdominal approach and esophageal transection using staplers. Antireflux surgery was added in some series. In 1974, Van Kemmel was the first to use a circular stapling device for performing esophageal transection. Peracchia et al.,[63] in 1980, modified the technique by adding antireflux cardioplasty. Ginsberg et al.[46] in 1982 modified the original operation by performing proximal gastric vagotomy (preserving main vagal trunk and thereby avoiding pyloroplasty) and using a circular end-to-end anastomosis stapler through a left thoracoabdominal incision for esophageal transection. A loose fundal wrap was also performed.

All the modifications suggested and practiced have at the core splenectomy, gastroesophageal devascularization, and esophageal transection to interrupt extramural and intramural vessels, with variations being the use of an exclusive abdominal approach, the technique of esophageal transection, vagal preservation, and antireflux surgery.*

Author's Approach

The modified Sugiura procedure used at our institute includes splenectomy with esophagogastric devascularization done using a transabdominal approach. Because highly selective vagotomy is performed, a drainage procedure is not added. In addition, fundoplication is not performed. The extent of devascularization on the esophagus includes 7 to 10 cm of distal esophagus, preserving longitudinal periesophageal veins (Fig. 82.3A); on the stomach, up to the incisura along the lesser curve of stomach, preserving the left gastric vein, and two thirds along the greater curvature of stomach, preserving the gastroepiploic arcade (see Fig. 82.3B). Esophageal transaction is performed by using an end-to-end anastomosis stapler (Fig. 82.4). Alternatively, stapling of the anterior and posterior walls can be achieved by using a thoracoabdominal stapler (without a cutter) introduced by enterotomy on either side. Previous sclerotherapy induces periesophageal fibrosis, which poses a threat of injuring the esophageal wall during devascularization. When the esophagus is inflamed because of multiple sessions of sclerotherapy, especially in the acute setting, the stapling is done just below the gastroesophageal junction.[70] Occasionally, fundic resection is performed for bleeding from large fundic varices.[71,72] Sometimes, early gastrotomy is done to oversew gastric varices in acutely bleeding gastric varices. When the Sengstaken-Blakemore tube is used for temporary control of bleeding, we first perform the

*References 19, 46, 50, 51, 53, 47, 64 to 69.

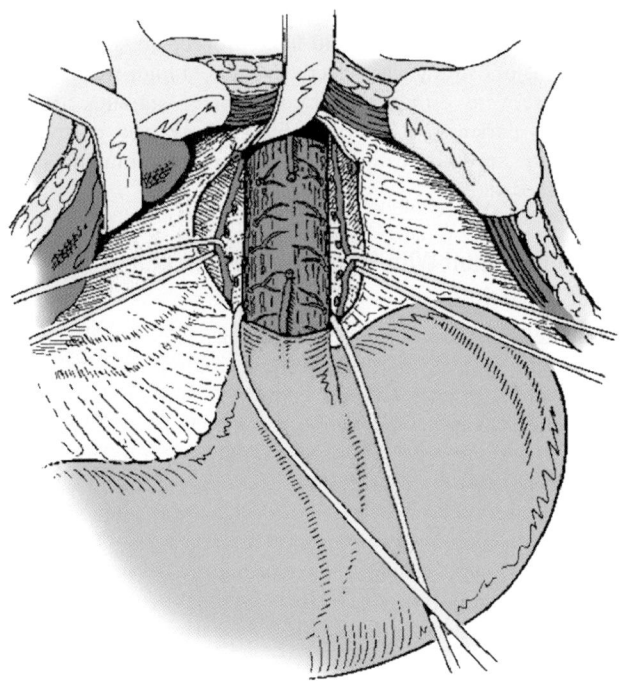

FIGURE 82.3 Modified Sugiura procedure performed at our center. **A,** Devascularization of 7 to 10 cm of distal esophagus and **(B)** on the stomach up to the incisura along the lesser curve of the stomach, preserving the left gastric vein, two thirds along the greater curvature of stomach (60%–70% of stomach), preserving right gastric arcade.

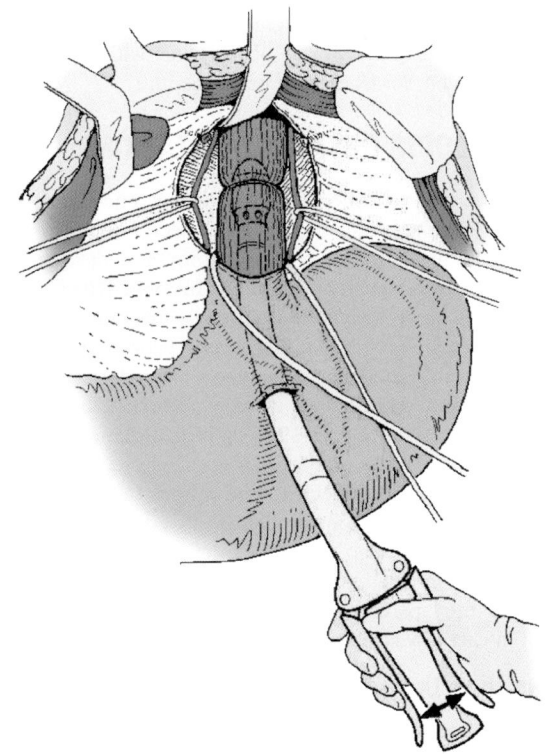

FIGURE 82.4 Esophageal transection by a mechanical stapler. The head of the circular stapler has been closed, and the esophageal anastomosis has been completed.

esophagogastric devascularization and splenic artery ligation without deflating the tube and later proceed to splenectomy. Feeding jejunostomy was selectively used in high-risk patients who underwent esophageal transection or stapling. In this group of patients, a Gastrografin swallow was performed around the seventh postoperative day before commencement of oral feeds.

Combined Shunt With Devascularization and Other Procedures

Combined procedures consisting of splenectomy, splenorenal shunt, and esophagogastric devascularization have been described in series from Chinese centers.[73–78] In a meta-analysis of these data, the hemodynamic parameters showed a significant decrease of portal vein pressure, portal vein diameter, and free portal pressure in the combined group compared with the devascularization group. The authors claim that combined procedures integrate the advantages of shunt surgery with those of devascularization, including maintaining the normal anatomic structure of the portal vein.[78] However, we think that it defeats the very reason for performing a devascularization procedure instead of shunting because devascularization is often performed in patients in whom a shunt is either not feasible or considered to be unsafe. The results of this combined procedure have not been compared with shunt alone. At best, it could imply that patients chosen for a shunt procedure may benefit from the addition of limited devascularization.

A more radical approach, in the form of partial or total esophagogastrectomy with the jejunal or colonic conduit for bypass has been suggested by some authors.[32,34,38,79] However, such extensive complex surgical procedures require multiple anastomoses and therefore are not popular in these often-unstable patients. These are useful only as a last resort in patients with extrahepatic portal obstruction with unshuntable veins and a failed devascularization procedure.

LAPAROSCOPIC DEVASCULARIZATION

Although the laparoscopic approach has become the standard practice for various indications for splenectomy, the reported experience with laparoscopic splenectomy and devascularization in portal hypertension is limited. In 1994 Kitano et al.[80] first described laparoscopic-assisted devascularization in seven patients with cirrhosis with bleeding esophageal varices. Manzano-Trovamala et al.[81] in 1996 performed the totally laparoscopic devascularization. Hashizume et al.[82] performed the Hassab procedure laparoscopically in 1998. Several authors have subsequently performed a devascularization procedure by a minimally invasive approach with several modifications, with excellent results.[83–92] Devascularization through a single port has also been described.[93–95] Jiang et al.[94] in 2009 compared open and laparoscopic splenectomy with azygoportal devascularization and concluded that the laparoscopic procedure was a safe and effective method in carefully selected patients.

Laparoscopic Devascularization: Procedure

The patient lies supine and is strapped to the table to allow for changes in position. The camera port is a 10-mm port at the umbilicus. The other ports used are 12 mm at the left midclavicular line and two 5-mm ports at the epigastrium and left anterior axillary line (Fig. 82.5). The patient is placed in the reverse Trendelenburg position, and the splenic hilum is exposed by dividing the splenogastric, gastrocolic, and splenocolic ligaments. The splenic artery is ligated at the superior border of the pancreas if feasible. The remaining attachments (splenophrenic and splenorenal) are divided so that the spleen now has only the hilar attachments left. Splenic vessels are divided with a laparoscopic vascular stapler. The greater curvature devascularization is performed using an ultrasonic dissector or LigaSure (Covidien/Medtronic, Minneapolis, MN). The posterior gastric vein, the main branch of the gastric coronary vein, and the left gastric artery are identified and divided with clips or stapler. The lesser curvature is devascularized in a similar manner. The esophagus is pulled inferiorly, and the lower 6 to 10 cm of the esophagus is devascularized. The spleen is placed in a retrieval bag, morcellated, and extracted from the 12-mm trocar. Kawanaka et al.[57] reported the safety and efficacy of customized laparoscopic devascularization for gastric varices based on computed tomography (CT) vascular anatomy. In patients with posterior and short gastric vein as the afferent feeding veins of the gastric varices, laparoscopic splenectomy with left gastroesophageal devascularization was performed. A total laparoscopic devascularization, including left gastric vessels, was performed in patients with the left gastric vein as the feeding vein. The feasibility of vagus nerve preserving laparoscopic devascularization has been recently reported.[97,98] However, thermal damage to the vagus nerve can still happen in a proportion of patients because of the use of energy devices.

RESULTS AND OUTCOME

Operative Mortality

The postoperative mortality of devascularization procedures has been variably reported in different series based on the case-mix, that is, cirrhotic or noncirrhotic, and whether it was an emergency or an elective procedure. On one end of the spectrum, there are patients with normal liver function (NCPF or EHPVO) being operated in an elective setting, in which the mortality is low,[18,19,23] whereas the mortality for patients with chronic liver disease with decompensation being operated in an emergency setting tends to be high.[66,99,100]

The overall operative mortality rate of the Hassab procedure in Egypt[44] was reported as 12.4%, and 8.5% for the Sugiura procedure and its modifications in Japan.[48,101] When the devascularization operation is used as an emergency procedure, the operative mortality increases significantly to 38.4% in the Hassab[44] and 20.6% in the Sugiura procedure.[48] Sugiura and Futagawa[99] reported an overall operative mortality of 4.9%, with 13.3% in emergency and 3% in elective cases (Table 82.1). In patients with cirrhosis, the Child-Pugh status–based mortality was 0% for 244 Child-Pugh class A patients, 2% for 251 class B patients, and 16% for 176 class C patients. In the Western series, the operative mortality of the operation performed as an emergency procedure for variceal bleeding varied between 22% and 100%.[100] Better results in the Japanese series were attributed to the fact that most patients with cirrhosis in Japanese series were nonalcoholic. Although alcohol-related chronic liver disease has been considered by some authors to be at higher risk for postoperative complications because of other coexisting diseases and malnutrition, others found no significant difference in the outcomes of patients with alcoholic versus nonalcoholic cirrhosis.[45,98,100]

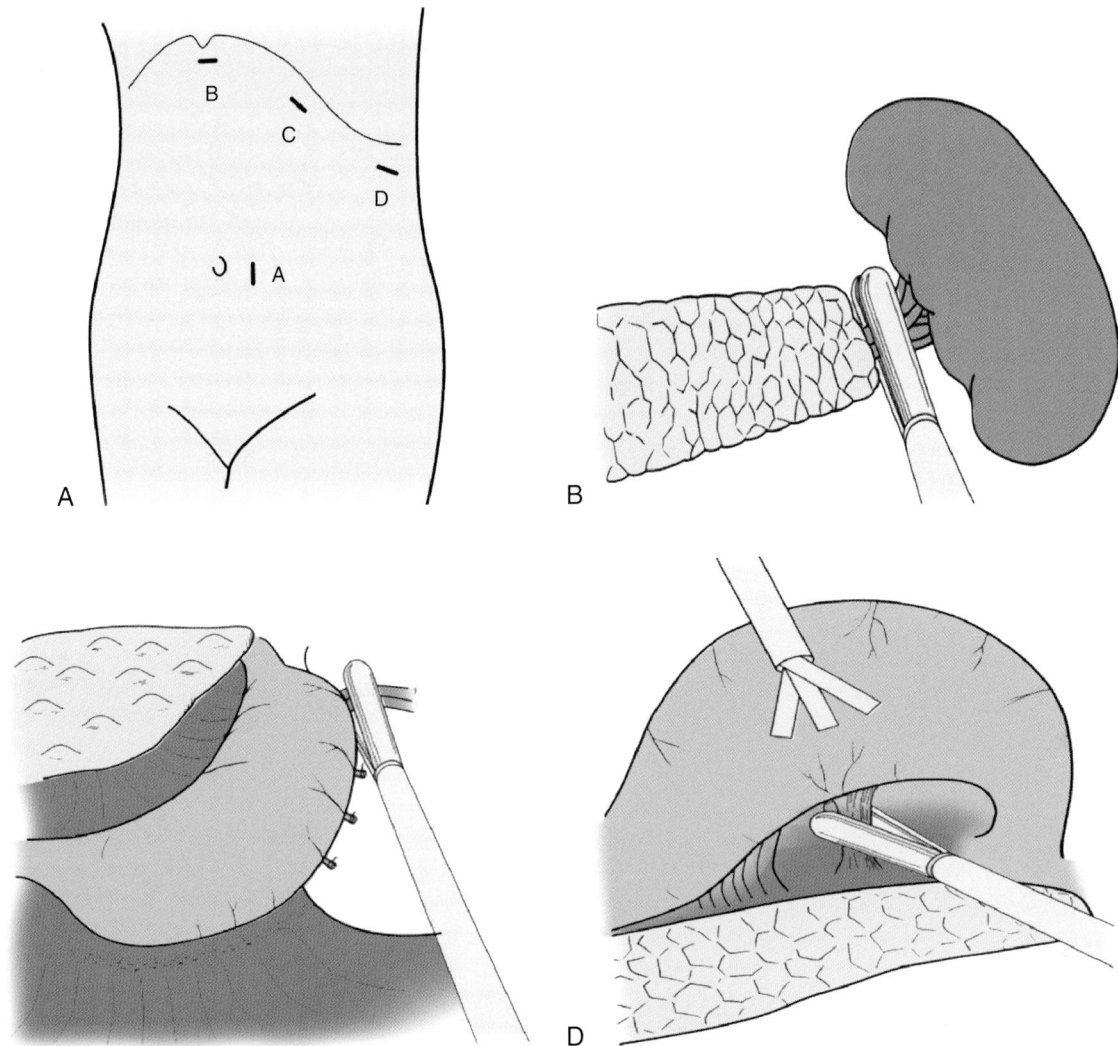

FIGURE 82.5   Port sites. A, Close to the umbilicus, where a laparoscope is inserted (**B–D**); in the left upper abdomen along the subcostal line is where 12-mm trocars are inserted. **B,** The splenectomy is completed, and the splenic artery and vein are cut. **C,** Devascularization along the fundic area is done after dissecting the posterior wall of the stomach. **D,** Devascularization along the lesser curvature, including the left gastric artery and vein, is done while the greater curvature of the stomach is lifted up. (From Hashizume M, et al. Laparoscopic gastric devascularization and splenectomy for sclerotherapy-resistant esophagogastric varices with hypersplenism. *J Am Coll Surg.* 1998;187:263–270.)

In patients with cirrhosis, the major cause of mortality is hepatic decompensation and not variceal bleeding. However, in patients with a noncirrhotic cause, variceal bleeding rather than liver failure is the common cause of death following acute variceal bleeding. In an analysis of 3588 operated patients from 59 Japanese centers, Inokuchi[48] reported that postoperative variceal bleeding accounted for only 8.7% of the deaths, whereas 45% of deaths were attributed to liver failure. The high rate of mortality is reported in patients with Child-Pugh C cirrhosis who undergo surgery for acute variceal bleeding that was not controlled by other means, as a "last-ditch effort."[112] Qazi et al[97] reported mortality in Child-Pugh A, B, and C as 12% to 14%, 30% to 50%, and 80%, respectively, for the modified Sugiura procedure.

Operative Morbidity

The outcomes, including morbidity and mortality, in various devascularization operations, are summarized in Tables 82.1

and 82.2. The morbidity is related to the underlying liver dysfunction and the surgical technique used. The risk of esophageal leak and stenosis is attendant with esophageal transection and gastric outlet obstruction when a vagotomy is done without pyloroplasty.

Complications are limited in patients with noncirrhotic cause (EHPVO, NCPF) or bilharzial cause compared with patients with chronic liver disease. The rate of esophageal leakage and stenosis with the Sugiura and modified Sugiura procedures incorporating esophageal transection are 5% to 14% and 2% to 28%, respectively. Some authors have suggested that avoiding esophageal transection can avoid these complications while maintaining comparable rebleed rates.[65,114] However, others have argued that esophageal transection is a very important component of the procedure to reduce variceal recurrence and will result in a significantly higher failure rate if esophageal transection is not performed.[53,101] We routinely perform esophageal transection and avoid this only in cases of a friable

TABLE 82.1 Outcomes of Devascularization in Various Series

AUTHOR, YEAR	N	REBLEEDING RATE (%)	CHRONIC ENCEPHALOPATHY (%)	ESOPHAGEAL LEAK (%)	ESOPHAGEAL STRICTURE (%)	PORTAL VEIN THROMBOSIS (%)	OPERATIVE MORTALITY (%)	SURVIVAL RATE (%)
Hassab and Modified Hassab Procedure								
Hassab, 1967[44]	355	2.3	0.3	—	—	1.4	12.4	—
Lu et al., 1990[101]	73	11.3	0	—	—	—	—	5-yr survival: 85.5% 10-yr survival: 75.8% 15-yr: survival: 70.4%
Abu-Elmagd et al., 1993[102]	108	17	4.2	—	—	—	4.2	5-yr survival: 73%
Makdissi et al., 2010[103]	97	14.6	0	—	—	—	6.2	—
Liu et al., 2013[104]	562	9.7	3.2	—	—	5.5	4.6	Late mortality of 15.1% (various causes)
Yang L et al., 2013[77]	207	5.8 (14.9% late rebleed in survivors)	1.5%	—	—	7.9	2.9	3-yr survival: 95.5%
Zhang et al., 2019[53]	91	30.8	16.9	—	—	4.2	4.4	5-yr survival: 71.4%
Ma et al., 2020[15]	151	17.2	NA	—	—	16.6	NA	5-yr survival: 77.9%
Sugiura Procedure								
Sugiura and Futagawa, 1984[997]	671	1.5	0	6	2	0.74	5	10 yr actuarial survival Noncirrhotic (Em/Prop/Elect): 90%/96%/95% Cirrhosis (Em/Prop/Elect): 55%/72%/72%
Dagenais et al., 1994[105]	21	26	0	14	37	—	10	—
Mariette et al., 1994[67]	39	24	0	—	28	—	0	—
Modified Sugiura Procedure								
Peracchia et al., 1980[63]	15	0	0	—	26.7	—	6.7	—
Ginsberg et al., 1982[46]	20	0	0	0	20	—	20	—
Umeyama et al., 1983[50]	101	15.7	—	—	—	—	11.8	5-yr survival IPH: 72% Cirrhosis: 55%
Inokuchi, 1985[48]	3136	7	5	7	13	—	9	5-yr survival: 69.7%
Orozco et al., 1992[104]	100	8	3	6	—	—	22	69 (at 10 yr)
Idezuki et al., 1991[107]	532	20%	NA	NA	NA	NA	5	10-yr survival EHPVO: 90.6% IPH: 76.7% Cirrhosis: 32%
Mathur et al., 1997[66]	65	6.3	—	6	8.5	—	27.6	72 (at 33 mo)
Mercado et al., 2002[108]	87	11	0	1.2	2.6	—	1.2	—
Ma et al., 2004[109]	160	3.8	2.5	0	0	—	0	97.5
Qazi et al., 2006[97]	142	6.9	0	5.6	4.6	6.3	12.7	CTP A: 44 CTP B: 22.5 CTP C: 0 (at 15 yr)
Zhang et al., 2019[53]	81	19	11.1	0	4.8	3.2	3.7	5-yr survival rate 75.3%

CTP, Child-Turcotte-Pugh score; EHPVO, extrahepatic portal venous obstruction; Elect, elective; Em, emergency; ET, emergency thoracotomy; IPH, idiopathic portal hypertension; Prop, prophylactic. NA, Not available.

TABLE 82.2	Operative Mortality Rates of Devascularization Procedures for Esophagogastric Varices							
	NO. PATIENTS				**OPERATIVE MORTALITY RATE (%)**			
PROCEDURE	**TOTAL**	**ELECTIVE**	**EMERGENCY**	**CTP C***	**TOTAL**	**ELECTIVE**	**EMERGENCY**	**REFERENCES**
Hassab	355	316	39	—	12.4	9.2	38.4	Hassab, 1967[44]
Laparoscopic Hassab	250	—	—	7	2	—	—	Zheng et al., 2018[55]
Sugiura	671	566	105	176	4.9	3.4	13.3	Sugiura and Futagawa, 1984[99]
Modified Sugiura	854	754	100	—	7.1	4	31	Inokuchi, 1985[48]
	20	16	4	4	20	0	100	Ginsberg et al., 1982[46]
	22	22	—	—	5	5	—	Orozco et al., 1998[111]
	81	81	0	11	3.7	3.7	—	Zhang et al., 2019[53]

*Number of Child-Turcotte-Pugh (CTP) class C patients included.

esophagus or one that has undergone recent multiple sessions of sclerotherapy. The staple line can be protected with a fundal wrap in selected cases.

The incidence of postoperative ascites has ranged widely, from 3% to 33%, based on the severity of cirrhosis, the extent of splanchnic venous thrombosis, and preoperative presence of ascites. In series reporting a high rate of postoperative ascites, it usually resolves within a few months.[100] Devascularization procedures do not usually result in deterioration of liver function, and encephalopathy is generally not exacerbated. Although patients with Child-Pugh C are likely to have poor outcomes with high morbidity regardless of the type of non-transplant treatment modality, devascularization cannot be considered to be contraindicated because it is the only salvage option that remains when other modalities have either failed or are not available[99] (see Chapter 77). Improvement in liver function observed in some patients after devascularization might be due to the changes of splanchnic hemodynamics, namely, decreased portal pressure and flow combined with the increased flow in the hepatic artery.[13]

Portal vein thrombosis may be linked to thrombocythemia or to a decrease in portal blood flow after splenectomy[115–118] and affects 5.6% to 6.6% patients. The actual rate may be higher because reported rates usually include only symptomatic cases. Preoperative high portal vein flow and wider diameters of the portal vein and splenic vein are important risk factors for portal vein thrombosis after devascularization. Unexplained fever and abdominal pain by the end of the first postoperative week should be assessed by ultrasound Doppler and contrast CT. Acute portal vein thrombosis should be treated with anticoagulation for a period of 3 to 6 months with careful monitoring. A recent meta-analysis[119] reported that prophylactic low-molecular-weight heparin (LMWH) might decrease the incidence of portal vein thrombosis after splenectomy without increasing the risk of bleeding. However, the two RCTs included in the meta-analysis did not show benefit with LMWH. Hence, the role of routine prophylactic LMWH after devascularization needs further evaluation.

Efficacy: Control of Variceal Hemorrhage

The best way to evaluate a devascularization procedure would be determining its efficacy in controlling acute bleeding and prevention of rebleeding. Its impact on variceal grade reduction will indicate long-term efficacy. Immediate control of bleeding is achieved in 95% to 100% of patients.* Although the initial devascularization procedures, such as esophageal transection

alone or splenectomy alone, do not yield satisfactory results, the Hassab procedure, the Sugiura procedure, and its modifications resulted in good control of variceal bleeding, with a resultant decrease in recurrence of bleeding and improved survival. The Hassab and Sugiura procedures report rebleeding rates of 6.2% to 8.3% and 1.5% to 16%, respectively.[27,106,121–124]

Unlike the Sugiura procedure, which targets extramural and intramural vessels, the Hassab operation devascularizes only the extramural vessels. Some studies comparing the modified Hassab and Sugiura procedures reported a trend toward better control of recurrent variceal bleeding after the modified Sugiura procedure with comparable operating time and morbidity.[53,125] In addition, the modified Sugiura procedure was reported to be more effective than the Hassab procedure for the treatment of rebleeding after endoscopic variceal ligation.[52] However, other studies comparing devascularization procedures with or without esophageal transection have shown comparable rebleeding rates.[65,114] In the absence of high-level evidence, a Sugiura type of devascularization with interruption of intramural and extramural vessels feeding varices is preferred whenever feasible. In high-risk patients, esophageal transection could be omitted, but the principle of maintaining a periesophageal spontaneous portocaval shunt should be followed for better postoperative outcomes.

Survival Outcome

Survival figures have been variably quoted in different series depending on the type of patients included in the series—with and without liver dysfunction. Although in the setting of cirrhosis, the survival rate is determined by the underlying liver disease, in patients with a normal liver, as in NCPF or EHPVO, a control of rebleeding procedure will translate into overall improved survival of these patients.

The 5-year survival rate with the Hassab operation ranges from 73% to 85%, seemingly better than that of other devascularization procedures. However, these results may be attributed to the preserved liver function in schistosomal portal hypertension. The 5-year survival rate of the Sugiura and modified Sugiura operations is approximately 70% and dramatically decreases to approximately 30% in the emergency setting. In the setting of cirrhosis, the major factor determining survival is the status of liver disease. Qazi et al.[97] published outcomes on 142 consecutive patients in whom nonoperative management with endoscopic sclerotherapy failed, requiring

*References 9, 44, 48, 66, 99, 104, 120.

TABLE 82.3 Outcomes in Laparoscopic Devascularization Series

AUTHOR, YEAR	N	POSTOPERATIVE MORBIDITY, n (%)	MORTALITY (%)	REBLEED RATE, (%)	ENCEPHALOPATHY (%)	FOLLOW-UP (mo)
Hashizume et al., 1998[82]	10	0	0	0	NA	8–20
Yamamoto et al., 2006[89]	7	0	1	0	NA	NA
Hong et al., 2007[136]	23	5 (21.7)	0	0	NA	NA
Wang et al., 2008[87]	25	8 (32)	0	0	0	3–60
Jiang et al., 2009[94]	28	5 (17.9)	0	0	0	1–34
Zheng et al., 2012[116]	24	4 (16.7)	0	0	NA	3–36
Luo et al., 2011[137]	30	3 (10)	0	NA	NA	NA
Wang et al., 2012[138]	20	2 (10)	0	0	0	18
Ando et al., 2012[139]	6	4 (66.7)	0	NA	NA	NA
Cheng et al., 2014[84]	188	78 (41.5)	0	3.7	1.1	2–65
Chen et al., 2018[54]	55	17 (30.9)	0	0	3.6	NA
Zheng et al., 2018[55]	250	33 (13.2)	2	3.6	1.6	4–75
Luo et al., 2020[56]	30	10 (33.3)	0	0	6	12

NA, Not available.

devascularization in the emergency setting. In this study, 15-year survival rates were recorded based on the Child-Pugh classification at the time of procedure. These authors found a 44% survival rate in patients with Child-Pugh A, 22.5% in patients with Child-Pugh B, and 0% in patients with Child-Pugh C. In most series, the 5-year overall survival rate has ranged from 58% to 93%.[99] Even though the rate of rebleeding is lower with the devascularization procedures compared with endoscopic treatment and TIPS,[126,127] devascularization is not a competing modality. It is usually the last resort in cirrhotic patients when other modalities have failed or are not feasible. Improvement in liver function observed in some patients after devascularization might be due to the splenectomy-related changes of splanchnic hemodynamics, namely, decreased portal pressure and flow.[13]

Long-term outcomes of devascularization are much better in noncirrhotic portal hypertension. Mathur et al.[66] reported a 5-year survival of 88% in a series of 68 patients (44 EHPVO, 22 NCPF) who underwent devascularization with an operative mortality of 4%, rebleeding rate of 11% (5% variceal), and an esophageal stricture rate of 15%. A Mexican series reported similar results in 38 patients with EHPVO undergoing the one-stage or two-stage Sugiura procedure.[69] Goyal et al.[23] reported a rebleeding rate of 10% and a 95% overall survival among 22 patients with NCPF undergoing esophagogastric devascularization at a mean follow-up of 4 years.

Devasularization Versus Shunt

In comparison with surgical shunts, devascularization was found to have superior survival and less incidence of encephalopathy rate in RCTs[128,129] (see Chapters 83 and 84). Rebleeding was less with shunt surgery in another RCT.[130] In subsequent Egyptian series, devascularization was found to be better than shunt procedures in patients with high-grade chronic hepatitis[104] and nonalcohol-related chronic liver disease.[131] The selective shunt was preferred over devascularization in schistosomal patients in the presence of a shuntable vein.

Zong et al.[130] performed a meta-analysis of the available studies up to December 2013 to evaluate the effectiveness of devascularization and shunt procedures in terms of recurrent postoperative bleeding, postoperative hepatic encephalopathy,

ascites, operative mortality, and long-term survival rates. The study included 1716 patients, of which 770 underwent devascularization, and in 946 a shunt was performed. Although there was no significant difference in the mortality rate and overall survival, the recurrent bleeding rate was significantly higher in the devascularization group than the shunt group, the rate of encephalopathy was lower in the devascularization group, and ascites control was better in the shunt group.

Laparoscopic Devascularization

Laparoscopic devascularization with splenectomy (see Fig. 82.5) is a technically challenging procedure because of the coagulopathy related to poor liver function and potential bleeding after an injury to collaterals or the splenic capsule. The advent of hemostatic tools, such as clips, monopolar or bipolar coagulation, ultrasonic coagulation, LigaSure vessel sealing system, and vascular stapler, have permitted laparoscopy in devascularization procedures.[80,83,85-92,130] The hand-assisted laparoscopic procedure can be resorted to in difficult situations. Published laparoscopic series are summarized in Table 82.3. Laparoscopic procedures appear to be associated with longer operative time but less blood loss and transfusion, shorter postoperative hospital stay, and lower complication rates compared with open procedures (Table 82.4).[54,56,86,131] Several individual and systematic reviews have established laparoscopic devascularization as a safe and effective modality.[82,85,96,131-133]

Two meta-analyses[82,140] comparing laparoscopic esophagogastric devascularization with open devascularization reported that intraoperative blood loss, postoperative complications, and hospital stay were lower in the laparoscopic group. However, operation time was longer in the laparoscopic group. The results of these meta-analyses suggest that laparoscopic devascularization is a safe, minimally invasive alternative for patients with liver cirrhosis and portal hypertension. In the last decade, a significant proportion of devascularization procedures are done using a minimally invasive approach. However, the level of evidence supporting laparoscopic devascularization is not high, because the majority of the studies included in the meta-analysis are nonrandomized comparative studies. Thus there is a need for well-designed RCTs to prove the benefit of minimally invasive devascularization procedures conclusively.

TABLE 82.4 Comparison of Laparoscopic and Open Devascularization Series

AUTHOR, YEAR	PROCEDURE	NUMBER	OPERATIVE TIME (min)	BLOOD LOSS (ml)	TRANSFUSION (%)	HOSPITAL STAY (DAYS)	COMPLICATIONS (%)
Jiang et al., 2009[94]	Lap	26	235 ± 36	200 ± 30	23.1	6.5 ± 2.3	15.4
	Open	26	178 ± 47	420 ± 50	38.5	11.7 ± 4.5	42.3
Luo et al., 2011[137]	Lap	30	232 ± 75	550 ± 350	13.3	6.5 ± 2.5	10
	Open	35	230 ± 98	1850 ± 177	NA	12.5 ± 3.0	11.4
Ando et al., 2012[136]	Lap	6	341 ± 94	531 ± 390	0	19.8 ± 8.7	16.7
	Open	33	222 ± 52	778 ± 555	NA	35.6 ± 16.9	24.2
Zheng et al., 2012[116]	Lap	24	210 ± 61	90 ± 44	NA	NA	16.7
	Open	30	190 ± 31	350 ± 157			33.3
Chen et al., 2018[54]	Lap	55	230 ± 24	244 ± 25	NA	9.5 ± 1.9	17
	Open	72	203 ± 30	336 ± 40		14.2 ± 2.4	37
Zheng et al., 2018[55]	Lap	250	223 ± 18	208 ± 19	31	8	13.2
	Open	203	188 ± 12	298 ± 26	36	12	15.3
Luo et al., 2020[56]	Lap	30	119 ± 18	142 ± 33	23.3	8.1 ± 1.3	33.3
	Open	38	219 ± 31	285 ± 77	47.4	11.3 ± 1.3	57.9

Conclusion

Although no single surgical treatment is recognized as an ideal approach for all cases of portal hypertension with variceal bleeding, the choice of surgical treatment for these patients must weigh the risks of recurrent bleeding and decompensation, taking into account the patient's hemodynamics, the underlying cause and severity of liver dysfunction, transplant candidacy, availability of a shuntable vein, local expertise, and alternative treatment strategies available. A devascularization procedure is a very effective tool that must be available in the armamentarium of the surgeon to deal with the difficult problem of variceal bleeding when all other options have failed or are unavailable.

References are available at expertconsult.com.

CHAPTER 83

Portal hypertensive bleeding: The role of portosystemic shunting

Stuart J. Knechtle, Jigesh A. Shah, and Paul Suhocki

OVERVIEW

Esophageal varices develop in patients with portal hypertension, most commonly secondary to hepatic cirrhosis (see Chapters 74, 76, and 80). They occur most frequently in the distal esophagus, although they may be accompanied by gastric varices. Rupture of varices is associated with massive upper gastrointestinal (GI) bleeding with an attendant high mortality rate. Therapy aimed at the prevention and treatment of bleeding varices has included pharmacologic, endoscopic, radiologic, and surgical strategies (see Chapters 80–85). All of these therapies have evolved technically and increasing clinical experience has resulted in a more accurate definition of the role of each treatment modality. This chapter discusses the appropriate role of surgical shunts for the management of bleeding esophageal varices. However, an understanding of the role of surgical therapy also requires an understanding of the context in which it is applied. The natural history of bleeding esophageal varices is discussed first, followed by a description of the roles of alternative therapies. In current medical practice, it is most appropriate to apply surgical shunts within the context of medical (see Chapter 80) and endoscopic management (see Chapter 81), transjugular intrahepatic portosystemic shunts (TIPS; see Chapter 85), and liver transplantation (see Chapter 105). Clearly, liver transplantation has evolved as the definitive therapy for portal hypertension associated with liver disease and appropriately far surpasses shunt surgery by sheer volume in current clinical practice. Many patients are treated sequentially with more than one modality, and algorithms are presented to help establish the appropriate clinical context for surgical shunt therapy.

NATURAL HISTORY OF ESOPHAGEAL VARICES

Esophageal varices may produce massive upper GI bleeding that is difficult to control. Not all varices bleed, and not all patients with cirrhosis or portal hypertension will develop esophageal varices. Clinical studies have sometimes included control groups without medical intervention, and analysis of these trials has helped define the natural history of esophageal varices. In a series of 819 patients, 46% with biopsy or clinical evidence of cirrhosis and no history of bleeding had esophageal varices by endoscopy.[1]

Over time, varices may appear, disappear, or change in size depending on alterations in patient physiology. A study of 84 patients with cirrhosis without previous bleeding who were monitored by serial endoscopy over 2 years showed that 31% of patients without varices progressed to large varices over 2 years, whereas in 70% of patients with small varices, the varices enlarged after 2 years.[2,3] Dagradi studied the influence of alcohol on varices in patients with cirrhosis and found that variceal length increased in 65% of patients with cirrhosis who continued to consume alcohol, but it decreased in 80% of patients with cirrhosis who abstained from alcohol. Baker and colleagues[4] reported that varices regress in 25%, disappear in 32%, and progress in 21% of patients with cirrhosis whose varices are monitored by endoscopy (see Chapter 80).

Most bleeding episodes in long-term studies occur during the first 1 to 2 years after identification of varices.[4–7] Average mortality rates after bleeding from esophageal varices are 23% at 1 year, 34% at 2 years, and 58% at 3 years (see Chapters 80 and 81). Approximately one-third of deaths in patients with known esophageal varices are attributable to upper GI bleeding; a larger proportion die as a result of liver failure. The mortality rate directly attributable to variceal hemorrhage is 10% to 17% for cirrhotic patients.[4,7,8] In patients with varices, upper GI bleeding is attributable to variceal hemorrhage in roughly two-thirds of patients.[9] Clinical parameters associated with increased risk of hemorrhage and death from esophageal varices include large varices, those with cherry-red spots,[3] concurrent gastric varices,[10] Child-Turcotte-Pugh (CTP) classification, continued alcohol use,[3] and infection.[11] Death correlates closely with CTP classification[12] and with Modified End-Stage Liver (MELD) score[13,14] (see Chapter 4).

Rebleeding and mortality rates markedly increase after varices bleed. Studies have reported rebleeding rates to be 30% within 6 weeks of an initial variceal hemorrhage[15,16] and 60% to 75% within 1 year.[4,16] Esophageal varices are the cause of bleeding in approximately 16% of hospital admissions for upper GI bleeding.[17] Mortality rates from all causes within 1 year of initial hemorrhage have been estimated at 40% to 66%.[15,16,18,19] The risk of dying increases while the interval between initial and second hemorrhage decreases.[9] If patients survive for more than 12 weeks after a variceal hemorrhage, the risk of rebleeding or dying returns to that of patients who have never bled.[9] With regard to children, the risk of mortality has not been well characterized after a first bleed in the setting of portal hypertension, but the first bleed appears to be only rarely fatal and the associated morbidity is not well characterized.[20]

PHARMACOLOGIC MANAGEMENT OF PORTAL HYPERTENSION

Prophylaxis

β-Blocker therapy has been studied to test its efficacy in preventing primary variceal hemorrhage in patients with known varices (see Chapter 80). Nadolol is an essential *nonselective β-blocker*, blocking both β1 and β2 receptors. Patients given nadolol were compared with untreated control individuals. Nadolol reduced the incidence of bleeding from 35% ± 3% to 12% ± 3%, and the incidence of fatal bleeds was reduced from 18% ± 3% to 10% ± 2%. There was no difference in the overall mortality rate.[21] This study has been used to support the use of prophylactic β-blockade to prevent initial variceal hemorrhage. More recently, carvedilol, a nonselective β-blocker with additional α$_1$-blocking effect, appears to be better at reducing the hepatic venous wedge pressure gradient when compared with nonselective agents such as nadolol, and has gained interest as primary prophylaxis against variceal bleeding.[22]

Nitrates are vasodilators whose action is mediated by nitric oxide on vascular smooth muscle. Nitroglycerin decreases portal pressure in patients with cirrhosis when high doses are used.[23] In animal studies, nitroglycerin lowered portal pressure 13% and systemic blood pressure decreased 25%. This drug lowers portal pressure less than systemic pressure. Nitrates in combination with β-blockade may offer prophylaxis against an initial variceal bleed.

Clinical randomized controlled trials (RCTs) comparing nonselective β-blockers (propranolol or nadolol) with no therapy in cirrhotic patients showed that drug treatment effectively reduced the risk of a first variceal hemorrhage.[21] The combination of isosorbide mononitrate and β-blockade further reduces portal pressure and has been shown in three studies to effectively reduce the risk of a first variceal bleed compared with β-blockade alone.[24–26] These investigations have noted, however, the difficult problem of compliance, particularly in patients with alcoholism. In addition, fatigue may be a side effect of therapy with β-blockade, and even more seriously, if patients do bleed, their ability to compensate for blood loss by tachycardia is compromised.

Acute Variceal Hemorrhage (see Chapter 81)

The posterior pituitary hormone vasopressin causes splanchnic arteriolar vasoconstriction, reducing portal blood pressure by approximately 15% when given intraarterially or intravenously.[27,28] Intravenous use is preferred for safety and convenience, and the optimal dose of the drug is 0.3 to 0.4 U/min intravenously. As a result of simultaneous vasoconstrictive effects on the cardiac, mesenteric, and cerebral circulations, the complications increase when doses of 0.5 to 0.7 U/min are administered. It is not necessary to taper the dose; the infusion can be stopped when the therapeutic end point is reached. In a controlled study comparing vasopressin with no therapy, approximately half of the patients on vasopressin stopped bleeding, but this result did not differ from control subjects.[27,29]

Nitroglycerin is often administered concurrently with vasopressin to reduce the systemic vasoconstrictive effects of vasopressin, and it may further reduce portal pressure. Nitroglycerin infusion begins at 40 μg/min and is titrated to a mean arterial blood pressure of 65 to 75 mm Hg.[30]

Octreotide reduces bleeding[31] and enhances the results of sclerotherapy.[32] Somatostatin and octreotide are endogenous peptides that act by reducing splanchnic, hepatic, and azygos blood flow.[33] Their principal advantage versus vasopressin is that they do not cause vasoconstriction of the myocardial and cerebral circulations. Somatostatin and octreotide should be administered continuously at 250 μg/hr and increased to 500 μg/hr if bleeding continues. Preliminary studies demonstrated that octreotide helped arrest acute variceal bleeding in six of six patients.[34,35] RCTs comparing somatostatin or octreotide with vasopressin versus no infusion have shown equivocal

results, which suggests that vasopressin and somatostatin have similar efficacy.[36–38] Neither vasopressin, somatostatin, nor terlipressin has been approved by the US Food and Drug Administration for treatment of variceal bleeding, although these agents are commonly used for this purpose. A prospective RCT showed equivalence of terlipressin, somatostatin, or octreotide, followed by endoscopic treatment of acute variceal bleeding.[39]

Prevention of Rebleeding After Initial Control

Propranolol was shown by Lebrec and colleagues[40,41] to reduce rebleeding significantly after acute variceal hemorrhage (see Chapter 80). This effect may be mediated by a decrease in cardiac output (β$_1$-blockade), increased splanchnic arteriolar resistance (β$_2$-blockade), and consequent decrease in portal blood flow[42] and collateral blood flow via the azygos venous system.[43] β-Blockade is not widely used in the United States to prevent rebleeding after an episode of variceal hemorrhage because endoscopic ligation is preferred, and β-blockade after acute bleeding has not been shown to reduce mortality.[44] Meta-analysis comparing β-blockade with endoscopic therapy demonstrated a nonstatistically significant decrease in pooled relative risk for bleeding in the sclerotherapy group and no difference in mortality between the two groups.[31] An RCT showed, however, that isosorbide mononitrate (80 mg/day) in combination with nadolol (80 mg/day) was more effective than sclerotherapy in reducing rebleeding,[25] and complications were less frequent in the group treated with drugs (16% vs. 37%). A Taiwan study reported that following endoscopic variceal ligation (EVL) to control acute variceal bleeding, proton pump inhibitor infusion was similar to combination with vasoconstrictor infusion in terms of initial hemostasis, very early rebleeding rate, and associated with fewer adverse events.[45] In summary, multimodal pharmacologic therapy plays a principal role in the United States in the prevention of rebleeding.[46]

ENDOSCOPIC THERAPY OF VARICEAL HEMORRHAGE

Prophylaxis

The use of prophylactic sclerotherapy to prevent a first hemorrhage was studied in three meta-analyses[44,47,48] (see Chapters 80 and 81). One study concluded that paravariceal injection with polidocanol decreased mortality rates.[47] The other two reports found that prophylactic sclerotherapy did not reduce bleeding or mortality rate and concluded that sclerotherapy was not indicated in this setting.[31,44,48] The largest trial of prophylactic sclerotherapy was the Veterans Affairs (VA) cooperative trial. This trial included 281 patients but was prematurely closed because of excess mortality rate in the sclerotherapy group.[49] Sclerotherapy prevented variceal hemorrhage but substituted bleeding from sclerotherapy-induced ulceration. This study effectively ended the use of prophylactic sclerotherapy in the United States.

Acute Variceal Hemorrhage

When it became apparent that the once predominant therapy for variceal hemorrhage (emergency surgical shunts) was not improving survival but substituting death from liver failure for death from bleeding, endoscopic variceal injection was evaluated as a less invasive therapy (see Chapter 81). In 1980 a prospective randomized trial with 107 patients from King's

College Hospital showed control of bleeding by sclerotherapy in 57% of 51 treated patients compared with 25% of 56 patients treated medically.[50] Two years later, a follow-up study showed improved patient survival with sclerotherapy compared with controls who received blood transfusions, vasopressin, and a Sengstaken-Blakemore tube when necessary.

When interpreting this and subsequent trials, it is important to understand that the King's College trial had more nonalcoholic patients than alcoholic patients (60 vs. 47) and had patients with relatively mild liver failure (74 were CTP class A or B; 33 were class C). The more patients in any study of variceal hemorrhage who are alcoholic or who have CTP class C liver disease, the more difficult it is to show a survival advantage of therapy. Death from bleeding in such patients tends to be replaced by death from liver failure[51] (see Chapter 77). The VA cooperative study showed no reduction of long-term survival when acute hemorrhage was treated with sclerotherapy.[52]

EVL was developed as an endoscopic alternative to sclerotherapy, potentially lowering the risk of ulceration and perforation of the esophagus.(see Chapters 80 and 81). Seven prospective RCTs compared EVL with endoscopic sclerotherapy.[53–57] In all studies, EVL and sclerotherapy were equally effective in controlling active bleeding. Complications were significantly lower with EVL in all studies. No esophageal strictures were seen in patients treated with EVL compared with 5% to 33% of patients treated with sclerotherapy. The development of the multiband ligating device, which allows banding without repeated reinsertions of the endoscope, made this modality of endoscopic control of varices much more attractive such that it has become the endoscopic therapy of choice.[58]

Prevention of Rebleeding

Although EVL effectively stops acute variceal bleeding, rebleeding remains a problem, and intermediate (2- to 5-year) survival is not improved in many trials. A confounding variable confusing interpretation of the results in many of these trials is continued alcoholism. Alcohol abstinence for 6 months, CTP class, and aspartate aminotransferase level all were independent predictors of survival in the VA trial.[52] When EVL was compared with sclerotherapy, rebleeding rates were significantly decreased with EVL in three studies,[53,56,59] and mortality rates were significantly lower in three studies.[56,57] As a result, EVL has emerged as the principal therapy in preventing rebleeding (see Chapters 80 and 81).

Following an episode of variceal bleeding, prophylactic antibiotics decreases the risk of rebleeding and is superior to use of antibiotics in response to signs and symptoms of infection. Ceftriaxone 1 g intravenously every day for up to 7 days or norfloxacin 400 mg orally daily for up to 7 days is recommended.[60]

Transjugular Intrahepatic Portosystemic Shunt (see Chapter 85)

The development and clinical use of TIPS for the treatment of portal hypertension first occurred in the 1990s, and its use for the treatment of variceal hemorrhage and portal hypertension has since expanded.[61,62] Currently, TIPS has proven to be the treatment of choice for patients with portal hypertension who are at high risk of variceal bleeding and is detailed elsewhere (see Chapter 87).[63] Advances in radiology have facilitated the placement of TIPS in more complex and high-risk patients and

will be described herein. Fluoroscopy had been used by itself for many years to create a TIPS following its introduction in 1989.[64] Transabdominal ultrasound was later added to help guide the needle from hepatic vein to portal vein (PV). These two modalities together are useful for constructing a TIPS within the confines of the liver capsule but do not allow for safe shunt creation outside of the liver capsule. Newer imaging and instrumentation have since made the extrahepatic splanchnic and systemic veins usable targets for creating shunts outside of the liver. They have also reduced the operative time and radiation dose of the procedure, making it safer for pregnant women, pediatric patients, and the operator. With this the technical success rate has been reported at 98%, with a 30-day mortality rate of less than 3%.[65] Furthermore, in patients with CTP class C cirrhosis, the placement of a TIPS has been shown to reduce the rate of rebleeding from 60% to 70% to 40% to 50% and decrease the risk of mortality from 40% to 20% to 35%.[65]

One new tool now used for TIPS is the intracardiac echocardiography (ICE) catheter (Irvine Biomedical, Irvine, California). This intravascular ultrasound catheter is positioned inside of a vein or artery to give the operator a sagittal view of structures lying far beyond the vessel wall. For the Budd-Chiari patient with no suitable hepatic veins for a TIPS, the ICE catheter is positioned in the intrahepatic inferior vena cava (IVC). It allows the operator to steer the transjugular or transfemoral curved needle through the wall of the IVC, through liver tissue, and into the intrahepatic PV under direct ultrasound visualization for creating a direct intrahepatic portacaval shunt (DIPS).[66]

The ICE catheter also facilitates mesocaval shunt creation for the patient with extrahepatic occlusion of the main PV (see Chapter 84). The superior mesenteric vein (SMV) or the confluence of the SMV and the splenic vein is visualized through the wall of the IVC. The radiologist can advance the needle through the wall of the IVC to the SMV or the confluence under direct ultrasound guidance in preparation for a mesocaval shunt.[67]

In creating extrahepatic portal systemic shunts, it is necessary to see important organs that may lie within the planned path of the proposed shunt. These organs are often obscured from view by gas or bony structures when using ultrasound. To circumvent these technical limitations, many angiographic suites are now equipped with cone beam computed tomography (CT), which uses fluoroscopy data to generate cross-sectional imaging. Although it does not provide the spatial resolution and image quality of a conventional CT scanner, cone beam CT supplies images that are adequate for planning a safe needle trajectory from one vein to another. This ensures that a percutaneous splenorenal shunt does not pass through the pancreatic tail, kidney, duodenum, or colon.

The stiff needle used for radiologic shunts may not be able to pass through the often circuitous venous routes necessary for creating a deep extrahepatic shunt. The PowerWire (Baylis Medical, Burlington, MA) is a useful tool in this setting. Radiofrequency energy is used to heat the tip of the wire for effortless passage of the wire through tissues. In creating a side-to-side splenorenal shunt (Figs. 83.1–83.3), the heated PowerWire tip burns through the walls of the splenic vein and the renal vein and any intervening tissue (see Fig. 83.3). The wire then maintains access from the splenic vein to the renal vein while the shunt is dilated and the stent is placed (Figs. 83.4 and 83.5).

Chronic occlusion of the main PV or splenic vein is often seen in cirrhotic patients due to low portal blood flows. A TIPS

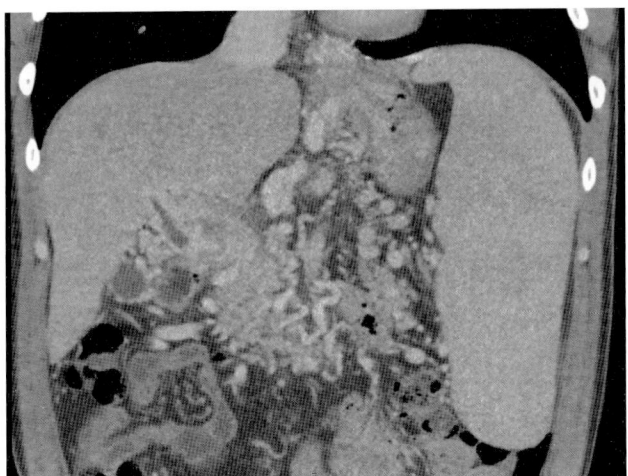

FIGURE 83.1 Computed tomographic (CT) coronal imaging of the abdomen demonstrating extensive chronic cavernous transformation and collateralization from portal hypertension and portal vein thrombosis (see Chapters 13 and 14). (Courtesy P. Suhocki, Duke University Medical Center, Durham, NC.)

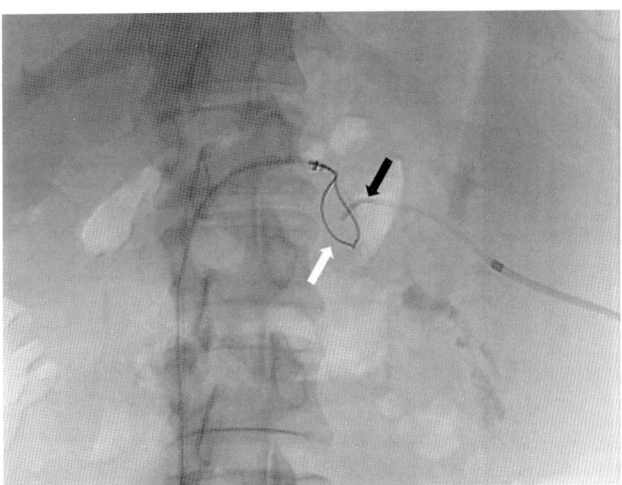

FIGURE 83.3 Fluoroscopic image of a sheath and snare in the left femoral vein (*white arrow*) via the left femoral vein.   Direct access to the splenic vein *(black arrow)* will facilitate later central access. (Courtesy P. Suhocki, Duke University Medical Center, Durham, NC.)

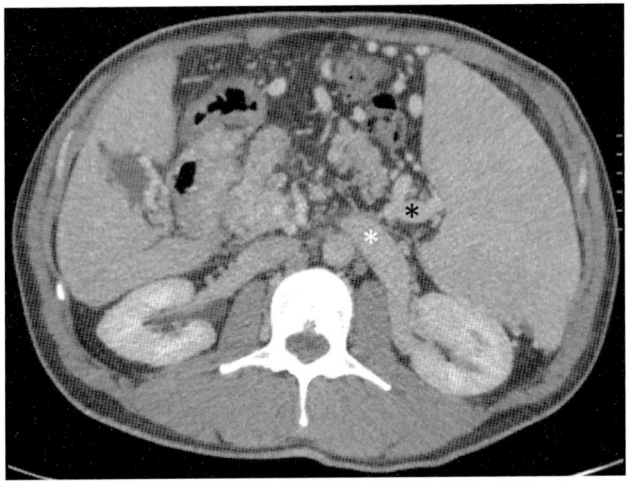

FIGURE 83.2 Computed tomographic (CT) axial imaging demonstrating patent renal vein *(white asterisk)* and patent proximal splenic vein *(black asterisk)* for subsequent splenorenal shunt (see Chapters 13 and 14). (Courtesy P. Suhocki, Duke University Medical Center, Durham, NC.)

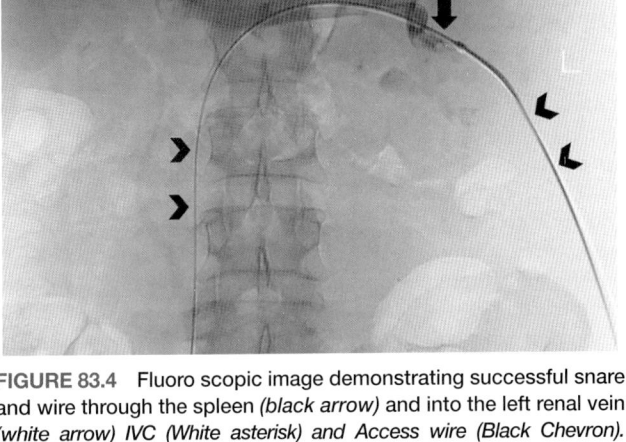

FIGURE 83.4 Fluoro scopic image demonstrating successful snare and wire through the spleen *(black arrow)* and into the left renal vein *(white arrow)* IVC *(White asterisk)* and Access wire *(Black Chevron)*. Subsequent contrast administration demonstrates communication of the splenorenal shunt with inferior vena cava (IVC) drainage. (Courtesy P. Suhocki, Duke University Medical Center, Durham, NC.)

by itself will not lower venous pressures throughout the portal circulation in this setting. Patency of these veins must first be reestablished by performing catheter-directed thrombolysis and thrombectomy. Balloon angioplasty of the veins with or without stenting is often required. A TIPS placed at the same time will maintain rapid blood flow in the vein to ensure continued patency. This is often performed in preparation for orthotopic liver transplantation obviating the need for placing a venous conduit at the time of surgery.[68]

Creation of a TIPS shunt is not necessary for the noncirrhotic patient with sinistral portal hypertension in whom splenic vein thrombolysis and thrombectomy can reestablish blood flow from the left upper quadrant toward a normal liver. If such attempts at venous recanalization fail and the splenic vein stump and renal vein anatomy are favorable, a percutaneous splenorenal shunt

can be considered.[69] If anatomy is unfavorable, the spleen can be embolized with particulate material to significantly reduce splenic volume and lower the risk of variceal bleeding.[70] In the noncirrhotic patient with widely patent PVs, the presence of an arterioportal fistula must always be considered as the cause of portal hypertension. Albeit rare, this congenital or posttraumatic entity can easily be treated with coil or plug embolization of the feeding artery.[71] Endoscopic creation of an intrahepatic portal systemic shunt has been described in a study of five swine[72] and all animals survived 2 weeks before necropsy, which showed no bleeding related to the shunts.

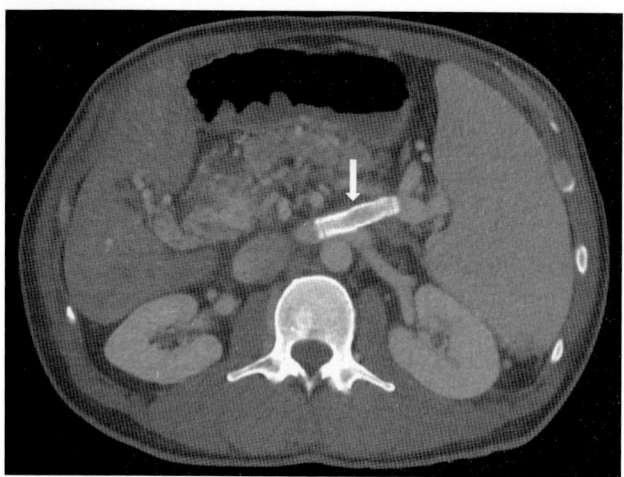

FIGURE 83.5 Computed tomographic (CT) axial imaging demonstrates a stent placement in a completed percutaneous distal splenorenal shunt. (Courtesy P. Suhocki, Duke University Medical Center, Durham, NC.)

Modern day stents used for TIPS are polytetrafluoroethylene (PTFE) covered primarily because of less associated need for intervention, less shunt dysfunction, and better outcomes.[119] Primary patency (patency without radiologic intervention to revise the TIPS) has been reported to be between 56% and 75% after 6 years.[73] Primary assisted patency (patency after revision) has been reported to be 77% to 96% after 6 years with median survival of 42.8 months.[73] If post-TIPS ultrasound reveals narrowing or thrombosis of the shunt, patency can be restored by repeat balloon dilation and stenting or by thrombectomy. Color Doppler ultrasound of TIPS is routinely performed at 1- and 6-month intervals to evaluate luminal narrowing or increased flow velocity, suggesting impending thrombosis of the TIPS. The rate of TIPS restenosis or occlusion is higher than the rate of recurrent symptoms because, in some patients, occlusion does not produce symptoms. Intra-stent stenosis, previous splenectomy, and shortening of the hepatic veins as a result of stenting are all factors leading to TIPS occlusion.[74]

Although the ability of TIPS to prevent an initial variceal hemorrhage has not been studied, patients awaiting liver transplantation who have intractable ascites are often treated with TIPS as a means of bridging to liver transplantation. Despite not being a true study of prophylaxis, these patients seem to be at low risk of bleeding given their lower portal pressure. Additionally, TIPS is effective in controlling acute variceal hemorrhage when medical management or EVL or both are ineffective (see Chapter 85). When used as primary therapy for acute variceal bleeding, TIPS may reduce treatment failure and mortality rate in high-risk patients. Most commonly TIPS has been used to prevent recurrent variceal hemorrhage.

SURGICAL SHUNTS FOR BLEEDING ESOPHAGEAL VARICES

Prophylactic Surgery

Early trials of prophylaxis for variceal bleeding compared portacaval shunts with medical therapy. Although bleeding was effectively prevented, survival was not significantly enhanced with surgery because of a marked increase in deaths from accelerated hepatic failure[75] (see Chapter 77). Because only one-third of patients with varices eventually bleed, surgery cannot be justified as prophylaxis and is not recommended in this setting (see Chapter 84).

In a prospective, controlled study to evaluate prophylactic surgery in 112 patients with portal hypertension and esophageal varices, Inokuchi and colleagues[76] found the bleeding rates were 19.2% in the medical group and 0% in the surgical group. No difference was reported in the survival rate between the two groups at 2-year follow-up, and prophylactic surgery led to a prevention of esophageal bleeding without any increase in the mortality rates. This is the only study to support a role for prophylactic surgery, but it should be noted that the majority of these patients had posthepatic cirrhosis with reasonably well-preserved liver function.

Acute Variceal Hemorrhage

At most American centers, pharmacologic and endoscopic therapy are first used to treat bleeding esophageal varices (see Chapter 81). Patients who do not respond to EVL are referred for consideration for TIPS or a surgical shunt. Although emergency surgical shunts prevent bleeding more effectively than sclerotherapy, overall mortality rate is equivalent.[31,77]

Although nonoperative therapies are useful for initial management of bleeding esophageal varices, if these measures fail to control bleeding, emergency surgery should be promptly considered.[78] Emergency surgical shunts normalize portal pressure immediately and effectively control variceal hemorrhage, but emergency surgery has been associated with a mortality rate of 20% to 55%.[31,77]

The high risk of dying after placement of an emergency shunt is presumably related to the frequent decompensation of liver function and associated comorbidity at the time of an acute bleed. Outcomes correlate with CTP classification and MELD score (see Chapter 4) rather than with the type of shunt performed. Liver failure and encephalopathy often ensue and are the proximate causes of death associated with emergency surgery in most series.

In choosing which surgical shunt to use for emergency control of bleeding, the portacaval shunt (see Chapter 84) is an acceptable choice because it effectively decompresses the portal venous system and can usually be rapidly constructed. An end-to-side portacaval shunt is adequate, although patients with ascites should have a side-to-side portacaval shunt to relieve their ascites as well. A series by Orloff and colleagues[79] showed the usefulness of the portacaval shunt in the emergency setting. Other functional side-to-side shunts, such as the mesocaval shunt and proximal splenorenal shunt (see Chapter 84), also effectively decompress the PV and relieve esophageal variceal bleeding, and they should be effective for relief of ascites. In contrast to portacaval shunts, these shunts do not require dissection in the porta hepatis and do not complicate future liver transplantation. In appropriately selected patients, a DSRS also may be used in the emergency setting to relieve variceal hemorrhage in patients with a large, patent splenic vein and absent or medically controlled ascites.[80]

Prevention of Rebleeding After Initial Control

In view of the disadvantages of emergency shunts, the more attractive role of surgical shunts is in the elective setting to prevent recurrent variceal hemorrhage. Because the natural history of variceal hemorrhage places patients who have bled once at high risk for rebleeding, definitive therapy ought to be considered after control of the acute hemorrhage (see Chapters 80 and 81). In an appropriately selected patient, surgical shunts substantially reduce the risk of recurrent bleeding, maintain stable liver function, and obviate the need for repeated endoscopic procedures. In the current era, TIPS placement may have equal or superior outcomes compared with surgery and is certainly less invasive.[81] The role of TIPS versus a surgical shunt for prevention of rebleeding was clarified by a randomized clinical trial comparing the two treatments in patients who did not respond to medical therapy.[82] No difference was found in rebleeding rates (5.5% for distal splenorenal shunt [DSRS] vs. 10.5% for TIPS; P value not significant), encephalopathy, or survival. TIPS patients required more interventions, although the study used noncovered stents. TIPS was slightly more cost-effective than DSRS at 1 year,[83] and the study concluded that the two treatments were of equal efficacy in preventing recurrent variceal hemorrhage.

Shunts are characterized depending on whether they completely divert (nonselective), partially divert (partially selective), or compartmentalize (selective) the portal venous circulation. Relative to nonselective shunts, the goal of partial and selective shunts is to preserve hepatic portal perfusion and minimize the risk of progressive liver failure and encephalopathy while preventing variceal bleeding.

General Aspects of Nonselective Shunts (see Chapter 84)

The end-to-side portacaval shunt was the first experimental shunt performed in dogs.[84] This shunt is the prototype of the nonselective shunt and has been compared in RCTs with conventional medical management for the treatment of portal hypertension and its complications.[85]

When the end-to-side portacaval shunt was compared with the side-to-side shunt in a controlled trial, no significant clinical differences were noted between these two shunts.[86] The interposition mesocaval shunt, also a nonselective shunt, was studied in a randomized trial comparing it with the direct side-to-side portacaval shunt, and no clinical or hemodynamic differences were evident.[87] The same series documented a high graft thrombosis rate after the mesocaval shunt. Nevertheless, the mesocaval shunt avoids dissection in the porta hepatis, which is an advantage for future liver transplant candidates. An additional option is a central or proximal splenorenal shunt with splenectomy. In the current era, indications for a nonselective shunt include an emergency shunt for variceal hemorrhage, an elective shunt in the presence of significant ascites, and treatment of Budd-Chiari syndrome. In some patients not suited for a selective shunt, a nonselective shunt might serve as a long-term bridge to hepatic transplantation when bleeding is not controlled endoscopically or by TIPS.

Budd-Chiari syndrome (see Chapter 86) with ascites, abdominal pain, and portal hypertension is an indication for a side-to-side portacaval shunt, although again TIPS is a preferable option if technically feasible.[88] A side-to-side shunt is necessary because the PV serves as the major efferent conduit in this syndrome. If the disease is fulminant, or if cirrhosis has developed secondary to long-standing hepatic venous occlusion, liver transplantation is a preferable option. If liver transplantation is not anticipated and if TIPS or DIPS is not available, a side-to-side portacaval shunt may be the appropriate

procedure. Often the caudate lobe enlarges after occlusion of the major hepatic veins because the caudate lobe communicates directly with the vena cava and may become the major route of venous outflow from the liver. Massive hypertrophy of the caudate lobe may prevent a side-to-side portacaval shunt from being technically possible because of caudal expansion of the caudate lobe that is interposed between the PV and the IVC and prevents their side-to-side anastomosis. In this setting a mesocaval shunt may be technically more feasible.

When Budd-Chiari syndrome involves occlusion of the hepatic portion of the IVC, the infrahepatic vena cava develops collaterals to the azygos venous system. These collaterals permit the portal circulation to be decompressed into the IVC via a mesocaval shunt, and a mesoatrial shunt is generally not required in such patients. Although a mesoatrial shunt circumvents an occluded IVC, it is a long shunt with a poor patency rate and has been associated with poor outcomes. Successful management of Budd-Chiari syndrome requires accurate diagnosis and treatment of the underlying hypercoagulable state. TIPS can also be used in patients with Budd-Chiari syndrome as a less invasive treatment option compared with surgical shunting. Long-term anticoagulation is usually necessary to prevent shunt thrombosis in both surgically treated and TIPS-treated patients.

General Aspects of Distal Splenorenal Shunt

Warren and colleagues[89] introduced the selective DSRS (see Chapter 84) with the goal of preserving hepatopetal blood flow in the PV while decompressing esophageal varices. The distal splenic vein is anastomosed to the left renal vein, and collateral vessels are ligated, such as the coronary and gastroepiploic veins connecting the superior mesenteric and gastrosplenic components of the splanchnic venous circulation (Fig. 83.6). This procedure compartmentalizes the portal venous circulation into a high-pressure superior mesenteric venous system to perfuse the liver and a decompressed gastrosplenic venous system to avoid variceal bleeding.[90]

In patients with advanced ascites, the DSRS is contraindicated because lymphatics are transected during the dissection of the left renal vein and the liver continues to have elevated sinusoidal pressures. In such patients, the DSRS may worsen ascites rather than relieve it. Warren's claim that the operation effectively accomplishes its goal of preserving hepatic function better than nonselective shunts remains controversial. Controlled trials have shown decreased portosystemic encephalopathy after the DSRS. Henderson and colleagues[91] showed that portal flow is maintained in most patients with nonalcoholic cirrhosis and noncirrhotic portal hypertension, but portal flow rapidly collateralizes to the shunt in patients with alcoholic cirrhosis, particularly if alcohol consumption continues. Failure to ligate the coronary vein results in early loss of hepatopetal portal flow.

Despite surgical interruption of collaterals that connect the superior mesenteric venous system to the gastrosplenic system, collaterals gradually develop through a pancreatic network termed the pancreatic siphon. Surgical splenopancreatic disconnection improves selectivity of the DSRS, especially in alcoholic cirrhotic patients; however, the complete dissection and ligation of multiple splenopancreatic venous tributaries, to disconnect the splenic vein from what is often a very fibrotic pancreas, is technically demanding and frequently bloody, and the clinical benefits of this extension of the procedure have not been clearly shown.

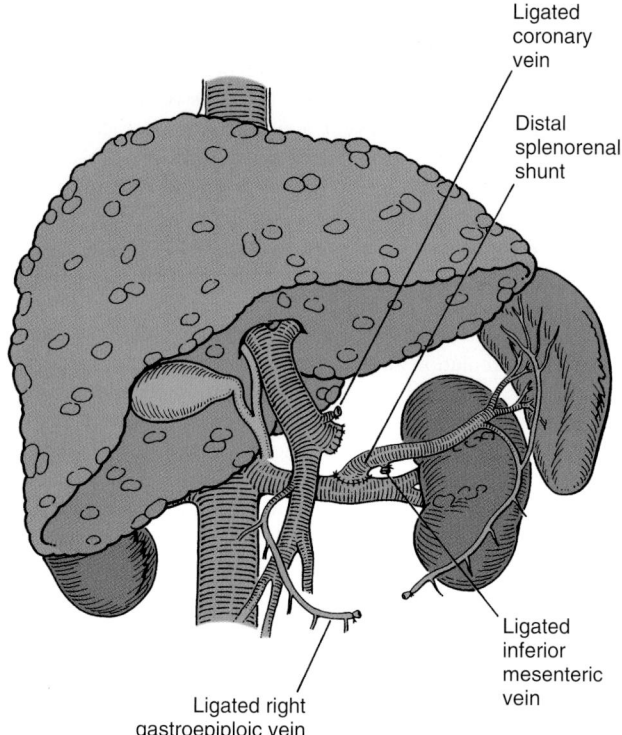

FIGURE 83.6 Distal splenorenal shunt requires ligation of the coronary vein. Drainage of the splenic vein is into the left renal vein. The right gastroepiploic vein also is ligated and divided (see Chapter 84). (From Knechtle SJ, ed. *Portal Hypertension: A Multidisciplinary Approach to Current Clinical Management.* Futura, 1998:175–202.)

Visceral or CT angiography should be done in any patient considered for a surgical shunt and especially before a DSRS, which requires a patent splenic vein, preferably at least 7 mm in diameter. Patients who have undergone splenectomy and those who have a thrombosed splenic vein are not candidates for this shunt procedure.

Six of seven controlled trials comparing the DSRS with non-selective shunts have evaluated alcoholic cirrhotic patients and were summarized by Jin and Rikkers.[92] None of these trials showed a survival advantage of either procedure. Four of seven trials showed less encephalopathy after a selective shunt, whereas the other trials showed no difference in encephalopathy rates. Rebleeding rates did not differ between the two shunt groups, although one trial noted a higher rate of rebleeding after DSRS.

When the DSRS was compared with repeated endoscopic therapy, rebleeding was less frequent with selective shunts, but hepatic portal perfusion was better maintained by sclerotherapy. Encephalopathy rates were similar in both groups.[93,94] These two studies suggested that sclerotherapy effectively controls initial bleeding, but patients who do not respond to sclerotherapy should promptly undergo surgery. Another indication for surgery, rather than endoscopic therapy, is poor access to advanced medical care. Such patients benefit from an initial selective shunt, rather than long-term endoscopic therapy, because the latter requires multiple visits to a medical center.

Partial Shunt

The partial shunt proposed by Sarfeh and colleagues[95] is a means of decompressing varices while preserving hepatic portal perfusion (see Chapter 84). An 8-mm or 10-mm PTFE graft is interposed between the PV and IVC. A prospective randomized trial of partial (8-mm diameter) and nonselective (16-mm diameter) interposition portacaval shunts showed a lower frequency of encephalopathy after the partial shunt, but similar survival was reported after both types of shunts.[96] The largest series of partial shunts was reported by Rosemurgy and colleagues[97] and included 170 patients older than 18 years. Small-diameter H-graft shunts were performed in patients who did not respond to endoscopic variceal ablative therapy (56% alcoholic, 44% nonalcoholic); 38% were CTP class A or B and 62% were CTP class C. Variceal bleeding after shunt placement was very uncommon (2%). Actual survival was superior to that predicted by MELD scores but did parallel the degree of hepatic reserve. Small-diameter H-graft shunting was encouraged in those patients who were neither eligible nor suitable for liver transplantation.[97]

TYPES OF SHUNTS: TECHNICAL ASPECTS (SEE CHAPTER 84)

Portacaval Shunt

Nonselective portacaval shunts can be performed by using a side-to-side method, an end-to-side method, or with an interposition graft to create a functional side-to-side shunt (see Chapter 84). Side-to-side shunts have the advantage of relieving ascites by reducing intrahepatic sinusoidal pressure in addition to decreasing the portal venous pressure gradient. They also are effective in decompressing varices and preventing recurrent variceal bleeding. The current recommended indication for a portacaval shunt would be for a patient with significant ascites and bleeding varices unresponsive to nonsurgical treatment who would not be a future candidate for liver transplantation. Patients who may eventually receive a liver transplant ideally should not be treated with such a shunt; rather, they should have a shunt in which the dissection is performed outside the porta hepatis. Portacaval shunts involving dissection in the hilum of the liver inevitably result in postoperative scarring in the hilum and make subsequent liver transplantation more difficult, with the added potential morbidity and mortality. Nevertheless, liver transplantation in patients with previous portacaval shunts can be done safely. If liver transplantation is not anticipated as a future option, a portacaval shunt is technically more straightforward than a DSRS and is a shorter operation in an unstable, actively bleeding patient.

A side-to-side portacaval shunt is performed through a transverse upper abdominal incision. The common bile duct is encircled and retracted to the patient's left. If a replaced right hepatic artery arises from the superior mesenteric artery, this also needs to be encircled and retracted to the left, which makes the exposure of the PV more difficult. The PV is dissected and encircled with a vessel loop, and the IVC is dissected and encircled with a vessel loop between the lower edge of the liver and the right renal vein. Partially occluding vascular clamps are placed on the IVC and PV, and the two are approximated. A venotomy is made longitudinally in each vein approximately 2 cm in length and stay sutures of 6-0 polypropylene are placed at the corners. These stay sutures are tied down, and the anastomosis is performed with a running technique. Vascular clamps are removed, and the wound is checked for hemostasis. The completed anastomosis is shown in Figure 83.7.

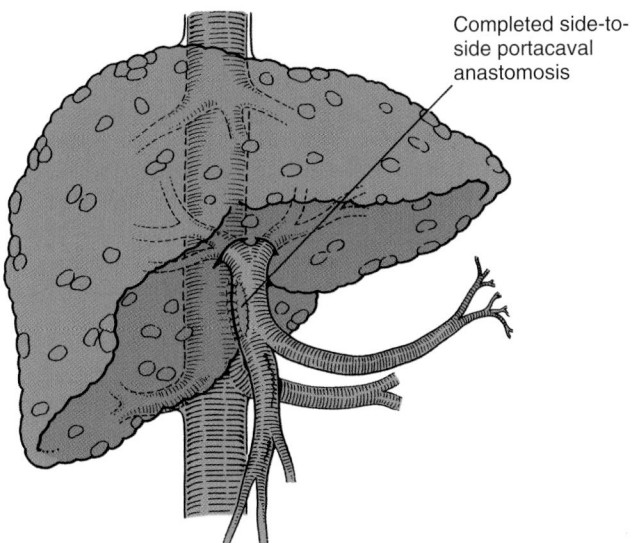

Completed side-to-side portacaval anastomosis

FIGURE 83.7 The completed anastomosis of a side-to-side portocaval shunt normalizes portal pressures and results in hepatofugal blood flow through the shunt (see Chapter 84). (From Knechtle SJ, ed. *Portal Hypertension: A Multidisciplinary Approach to Current Clinical Management.* Futura, 1998:175–202.)

Mesocaval Shunt (see Chapter 84)

A mesocaval shunt may be indicated as a long-term bridge to liver transplantation or as definitive therapy in patients whose bleeding is not controlled by endoscopic methods or who have not responded to TIPS placement (see Chapter 85). Although a PTFE or Dacron graft is commonly used as a conduit between the SMV and IVC, we have used an internal jugular vein autograft for this purpose. The better long-term patency rate for a vein graft favors the use of autologous vein over prosthetic material; however, a synthetic graft is more commonly used and avoids the surgical morbidity of jugular vein procurement. Mesocaval shunts are not difficult technically and have the advantage of keeping the area of dissection away from the porta hepatis, which is an advantage if liver transplantation is a future consideration. Its disadvantage is the long course around the duodenum and relatively poor long-term patency.

The mesocaval shunt is performed through a transverse upper abdominal incision. By elevating the transverse colon, the middle colic vein can be identified as it courses toward its junction with the SMV. The SMV is anterior and to the right of the superior mesenteric artery. After dividing overlying peritoneum and fat, there is generally a segment approximately 2 cm or 3 cm in length that is free of other venous tributaries. This segment of the SMV is dissected free and encircled, and the IVC can be dissected through the right colon mesentery; it is optimal to dissect a segment of IVC that is caudal to the duodenum so that the duodenum does not interfere with shunt placement. Next, the IVC is encircled with a vessel loop. The mesocaval shunt should take as straight a path as possible from the SMV to the vena cava rather than coursing around the duodenum, which may compress the graft.

Jugular Vein Conduit

When using a jugular vein conduit, the left neck is generally preferred because the left jugular vein is often slightly longer

than the right jugular vein (Fig. 83.8). An incision similar to a carotid endarterectomy incision is made along the anterior border of the sternocleidomastoid muscle. The platysma muscle is divided, and the jugular vein is identified. Branches are doubly ligated and divided, and the jugular vein is dissected free from the clavicle to the mastoid. It is ligated with silk ties proximally and distally, and the graft segment is excised and placed in sterile saline until it is used. Next, the neck wound is closed, and the proximal end of the jugular vein graft is anastomosed end to side to the SMV with running 6-0 polypropylene (see Fig. 83.8). The distal end of the graft is anastomosed end to side to the IVC also with running 6-0 polypropylene. Partial occlusion clamps are placed on the SMV and IVC during construction of the anastomoses; after completion, the clamps are removed and shunt flow is assessed with an electromagnetic or ultrasonic flowmeter. Flow should be 1 to 2 L/min, and significantly lower flow rates should prompt inspection of the graft for technical problems.

Meso-Rex Shunt (see Chapters 76 and 84)

Patients who experience extrahepatic PV occlusion as the cause of portal hypertension and variceal hemorrhage may *not* have cirrhosis or advanced fibrosis of the liver. If they have a patent intrahepatic left PV and a patent SMV or suitable other collateral vein, they may be candidates for a meso-Rex shunt that places a venous conduit from the SMV to left PV. This shunt may use the autologous left internal jugular vein as a conduit. The significant advantage of the meso-Rex shunt is that it restores portal blood flow to the liver and relieves portal hypertension, an ideal combination that may preserve liver integrity

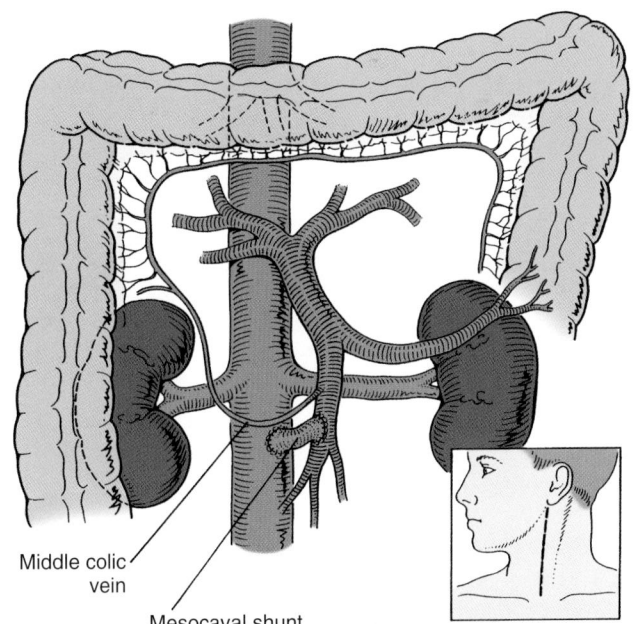

Middle colic vein

Mesocaval shunt

FIGURE 83.8 The left jugular vein provides an ideal autologous endothelialized vein graft for a mesocaval shunt and is approached through the incision shown *(inset)*. The vein can be excised from the clavicle to the angle of the mandible. The proximal end of the vein should be anastomosed to the superior mesenteric vein (SMV) (see Chapter 84). The completed mesocaval shunt uses an 8- to 10-cm graft to decompress the SMV into the vena cava. (From Knechtle SJ, ed. *Portal Hypertension: A Multidisciplinary Approach to Current Clinical Management.* Futura, 1998:175–202.)

and function long term. This shunt is more commonly used in children, although selected adults may benefit as well.

The meso-Rex shunt benefits from preoperative planning and imaging, although surgical exploration provides move definitive evaluation of the SMV and left PV as inflow/outflow, respectively. The surgical dissection follows the round ligament to the left PV, which if patent allows restoration of portal inflow to the liver via the graft. A suitable conduit, generally the left jugular vein, reconstructs flow from the SMV to the liver (Fig. 83.9). Although the cumulative experience with the meso-Rex shunt is modest, the outcomes have been encouraging with respect to long-term results.[98] A recent consensus conference advocated for more common application of this shunt in children with extrahepatic PV occlusion, allowing preservation of liver function with its associated benefits.[20]

Distal Splenorenal Shunt (see Chapter 84)

A DSRS is performed through a transverse upper abdominal incision. The gastrocolic omentum is taken down such that the right gastroepiploic vein is divided, but the short gastric veins are left intact. The splenic flexure of the colon is mobilized and retracted caudally. The inferior border of the pancreas is retracted anteriorly and cranially to expose the posterior aspect of the pancreas and the splenic vein, which is dissected free from the pancreas, and all tributaries are ligated and divided. The coronary vein may be one of its branches, or it may enter the PV.

The splenic vein dissection is generally the most challenging aspect of the procedure and may be particularly difficult in patients with pancreatic fibrosis from chronic pancreatitis. The splenic vein is dissected medially to its confluence with the SMV and laterally to a point that allows the vein to be brought down to the renal vein without kinking or tension. If splenopancreatic dissection is a goal of the procedure, the dissection continues all the way to the spleen such that all pancreatic tributaries are ligated and divided (Fig. 83.10).

The left renal vein is dissected next, and adjacent lymphatics are ligated to avoid the complication of chylous ascites. The left adrenal vein is ligated and divided to assist in mobilization of the left renal vein. The gonadal vein and descending lumbrical veins are left intact to give additional venous outflow to the shunt. If a circumaortic left renal vein is present with a small anterior branch, decompression may be compromised. In this case, anastomosis directly to the IVC should be considered (i.e., a distal splenocaval shunt).[99] A vessel loop is placed around the left renal vein, and an adequate length of splenic vein should be dissected such that when it is divided at the PV, it can reach the left renal vein easily without tension.

Identification and ligation of the coronary vein is an essential component of the operation. It is preferable to ligate the coronary vein at its junction with the portal or splenic vein. The coronary vein also can be ligated at the superior border of the pancreas, just before it extends along the lesser

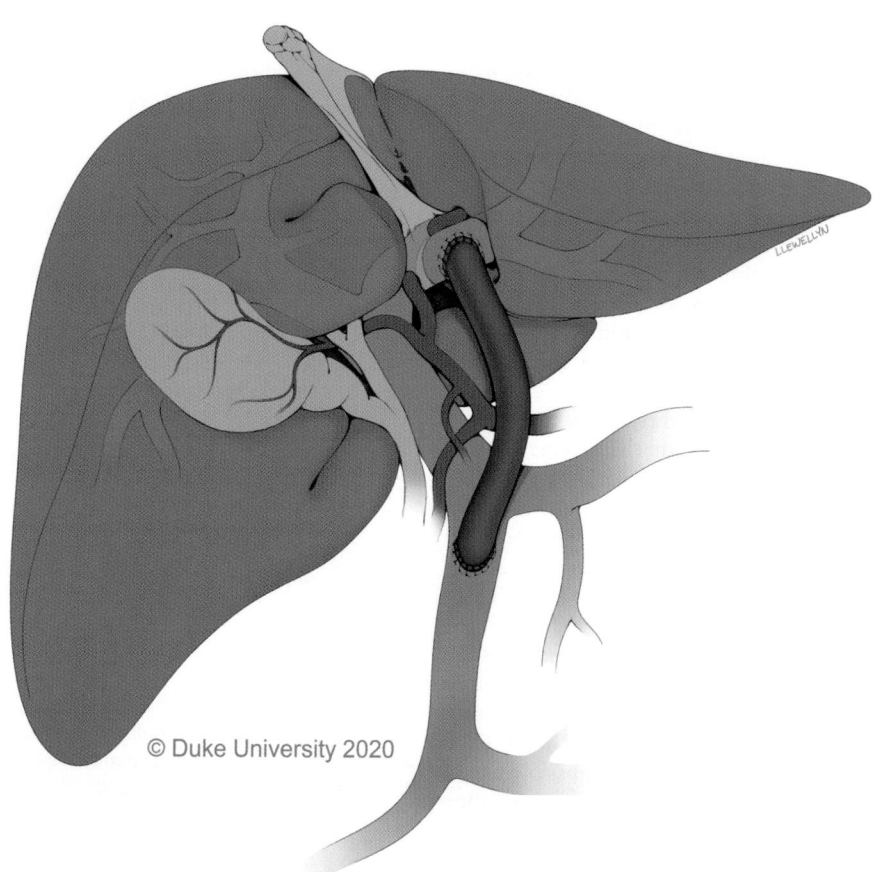

© Duke University 2020

FIGURE 83.9 Creation of the meso-Rex shunt by dissection of the round ligament to the left portal vein, allowing restoration of portal inflow to the liver via the graft via the superior mesenteric vein (SMV) (see Chapters 76 and 84).

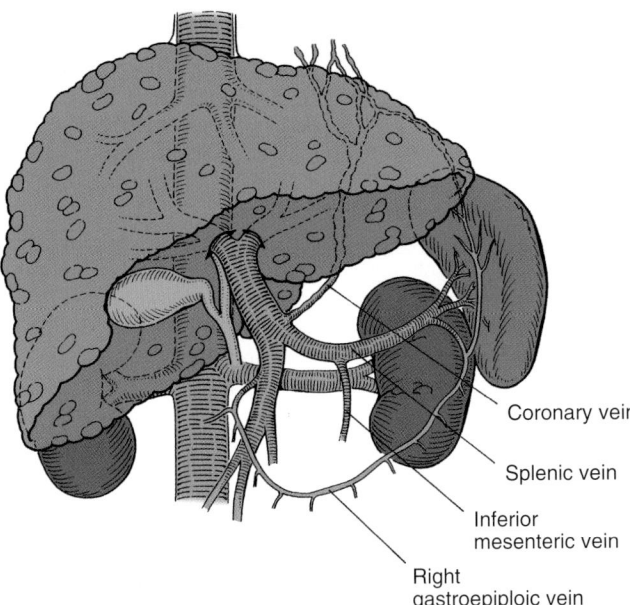

FIGURE 83.10   **The relevant anatomy exposed for a distal spleno-renal shunt.** The short gastric veins are left intact. The coronary vein and right gastroepiploic veins are ligated (see Chapter 84). (From Knechtle SJ, ed. *Portal Hypertension: A Multidisciplinary Approach to Current Clinical Management.* Futura, 1998:175–202.)

curvature of the stomach. The coronary vein is generally large and attenuated and must be ligated if the shunt is to be selective. Blood flow through the completed shunt (see Fig. 83.6) can be measured with a flowmeter and is generally 300 to 1000 mL/min.

Minimally Invasive Approaches to Creation of Portosystemic Shunts

With the advent of TIPS methodology by interventional radiologists, portosystemic shunts have been created with minimally invasive techniques and ever-improving long-term patency. For instance, the RCT comparing DSRS and TIPS[120] showed no superiority of DSRS over TIPS. Many clinicians would recommend TIPS as a long-term solution for selected patients and reserve surgical shunts for situations in which TIPS is not feasible. Furthermore, several reports of a DSRS being placed either through the retroperitoneum[69] or via the left renal vein into the splenic vein (personal communication from Suhocki et al.) have shown the possibility of creating a selective shunt by minimally invasive techniques (see Fig. 83.5). As intravascular stent techniques, design, and placement continue to improve, these alternatives may increasingly provide attractive alternatives to the ever-rarer application of surgical shunts.

Devascularization Procedures for Bleeding Esophageal Varices (see Chapter 82)

Surgical devascularization procedures were developed with the intent of disconnecting varices from the hypertensive portal venous system, decreasing the risk of variceal hemorrhage. In contrast to most shunts, these procedures avoid encephalopathy by preserving hepatic portal perfusion. The gold standard of devascularization procedures has become the Sugiura procedure, which consists of thoracic esophageal transection and devascularization, followed weeks later by laparotomy to control

bleeding from esophageal varices.[100] The Sugiura procedure differs from other devascularization procedures in that extensive esophageal and gastric devascularization are performed in a manner that preserves the venous collaterals connecting the coronary vein to the azygos system, which discourages varices from reforming. The initial report by Sugiura and Futagawa[100] included 276 patients and described an operative mortality rate of 4.3% and recurrence of varices in 2.3% after follow-up of 1 to 10 years. Actuarial 1-year survival was 83%. Survival according to CTP classification was 95% for class A, 87% for class B, and 57% for class C. Survival was better after an elective procedure than after an emergency operation.

The outstanding results achieved in the Japanese series have not been duplicated elsewhere. Many surgeons outside Japan have used modifications of the Sugiura procedure to control bleeding esophageal varices, particularly in patients with extensive mesenteric venous thrombosis or in those with a previous failed surgical shunt. Orozco and colleagues[101] reported a 10-year experience with the elective Sugiura procedure using a one-stage transabdominal approach. Mortality rate correlated with CTP class. The Toronto experience with the modified Sugiura procedure was reported by Dagenais and colleagues in 1994[102] and included a 22% operative mortality rate when the procedure was used in the emergency setting; the 5-year survival rates were 100% for CTP class A, 43% for class B, and 25% for class C patients. In a series of 32 patients undergoing transabdominal esophagogastric devascularization for variceal bleeding, 11 of the 12 patients without liver disease survived more than 10 years. The other 20 patients with cirrhosis had a 5-year survival rate of 51%.[103] This experience suggests that esophagogastric devascularization is an effective alternative to shunt surgery, particularly in patients whose underlying condition is diffuse splanchnic venous thrombosis in the absence of liver disease. The only prospective, randomized clinical trial comparing the Sugiura procedure with selective or total shunts was performed in patients with bilharzial cirrhosis (caused by the ova of *Bilharzia* and occurring commonly in Egypt) and bleeding varices.[104] This trial concluded that patients treated with devascularization were more likely to survive longer without encephalopathy compared with patients treated with a shunt.[104,105]

Patients with portal venous anatomy unsuitable for surgical shunts, those who have had shunt failures, and those who do not respond to medical management may be considered for devascularization procedures. Patients who progress to CTP class C liver failure should be considered for liver transplantation. Devascularization procedures should be reserved for those rare patients with bleeding varices refractory to medical management and who also are ineligible for TIPS, a surgical shunt, or liver transplantation.

Liver Transplantation for Bleeding Esophageal Varices

Definitive therapy for patients with advanced liver failure (CTP class B or C) is liver transplantation (see Chapter 105). Variceal hemorrhage is the most common clinical manifestation of portal hypertension to prompt liver transplant evaluation. The acute management of variceal hemorrhage in liver transplant candidates begins with endoscopic diagnosis and EVL where feasible, in combination with pharmacologic therapy, TIPS, or both for failures of endoscopic management. In view of the strong correlation between CTP class and long-term outcome, seen with virtually every form of therapy for bleeding varices, compelling evidence suggests that liver transplantation should be the treatment of choice for such patients with advanced liver disease. In the current era, each of the treatments discussed so far, including surgical shunts, should be used in a complementary fashion, and some patients require sequential application of the various modalities. Naturally, liver transplantation is the ultimate solution to cirrhosis and end-stage liver failure when these are the underlying cause of portal hypertension and variceal hemorrhage.

Because of the disparity between the number of patients awaiting liver transplantation and the supply of donor livers, transplantation is generally accompanied by an unpredictable waiting period that varies depending on the supply of donor livers. Average waiting times for liver transplantation in the United States vary depending on blood type and United Network for Organ Sharing (UNOS) regions.[106] Operative morbidity and mortality associated with liver transplantation correlate with the preoperative condition of the recipient. For this reason, it is advisable to use alternative measures to arrest variceal hemorrhage and to optimize the medical condition of the patient before proceeding to liver transplantation. Liver transplant programs in the United States preclude active alcoholics from liver transplantation and generally require at least a 6-month period of abstinence. This therapy generally is unavailable to active alcoholics with variceal hemorrhage, and such patients may need to be considered for temporizing alternative therapies. Because of immediate normalization of portal pressure, liver transplantation is effective therapy for bleeding esophageal varices resulting from underlying portal hypertension.[107]

A portacaval shunt or surgical shunt involving dissection in the porta hepatis makes subsequent liver transplantation more difficult technically. If liver transplantation is anticipated after a surgical shunt, a shunt should be performed outside the porta hepatis whenever possible. Distal splenorenal and mesocaval shunts are the preferred shunts for such patients.[108,109] A surgical shunt may be an attractive means of controlling variceal hemorrhage in a patient who may not need liver transplantation for several years. Most patients eligible for liver transplantation with CTP class C cirrhosis require transplantation in the short term and are managed more appropriately with TIPS as a bridge to liver transplantation. TIPS may significantly improve the CTP class and may reduce morbidity for patients awaiting liver transplantation.[110]

Meso-Rex Shunt for Portal Vein Occlusion After Liver Transplantation

Especially in children, extrahepatic PV thrombosis may occur long after liver transplantation, generally seen many months or years after surgery (see Chapter 76). Often it manifests as portal hypertension, with GI bleeding from the Roux-en-Y, worsening splenomegaly, or even encephalopathy.[111,112] This problem, limiting PV blood flow to the liver and creating portal hypertension, can be addressed with an SMV to left PV shunt graft, termed the *meso-Rex shunt* because it is placed in the rex recessus space by following the round ligament to the left PV (see Fig. 83.9). An autologous vein is used to create such a shunt, which relieves portal hypertension and restores physiologic blood flow to the liver.[113] Young children seldom experience life-threatening variceal bleeds and the vast majority can be managed medically in combination with planned surgical shunts or liver transplantation.

Extrahepatic Portal Vein Thrombosis

Extrahepatic PV thrombosis is a relatively uncommon cause of portal hypertension and variceal bleeding (see Chapter 74). Management of this entity is distinctly different from that of patients with cirrhosis because these patients usually have a normal liver, and survival is not limited by progression of the underlying liver disease. The etiology of PV thrombosis includes direct causes, such as neonatal peritonitis, trauma, and tumors of the porta hepatis, and congenital abnormalities of the PV, and indirect causes such as neonatal systemic sepsis, dehydration, and hypercoagulable states. PV thrombosis results in presinusoidal portal hypertension and the development of hepatopetal collaterals, which often maintain excellent portal perfusion.

Experience in the treatment of variceal bleeding as a result of PV thrombosis indicates three possible treatment options. Expectant medical management of each acute bleeding episode is tempting because the bleeding is generally well tolerated when the liver is normal. This approach may be appropriate in infants because bleeding tends to be self-limited, and half of these patients outgrow their variceal bleeding without therapy. Endoscopic variceal ablation and surgery should certainly be considered in the adult population, in whom the mortality rate for variceal hemorrhage approaches 20% over time with recurrent bleeding.[89] It must be remembered that the same normal liver that allows patients to tolerate conservative management of bleeding also makes them excellent candidates for more aggressive treatment. Typically, the acute episode of variceal bleeding can be managed by resuscitation, vasopressin or octreotide infusion, and then endoscopic variceal ablation.[114]

If bleeding becomes recurrent, evaluation of the portal, mesenteric, and splenic veins is performed with CT angiography to include venous phases and/or magnetic resonance angiography (see Chapters 13). If the spleen is in situ and the splenic vein is patent, the patient is an excellent candidate for the DSRS, although central splenorenal shunts and mesocaval shunts can also be used if the SMV is also open. If the splenic vein is also occluded or if the spleen is absent, further endoscopic variceal ablation should be attempted. If this fails, exploration is performed. In rare cases, a shuntable vein can be found, such as the coronary vein (a coronary caval shunt). Most often, if the spleen has not already been removed at a previous operation, usually for thrombocytopenia, a gastric devascularization with splenectomy is required. Recurrent variceal hemorrhage after devascularization can occur in 20% to 30% of patients, which requires further endoscopic variceal ablation but rarely esophagogastrectomy.[115]

Present Role of Surgical Shunts

A shunt may serve as a long-term bridge to liver transplantation in patients who are deemed to be acceptable candidates for liver transplantation. Clearly, the vast majority of patients with underlying liver disease and portal hypertension are currently treated with liver transplantation if they are acceptable candidates. Consistent with the previously mentioned observations, surgical shunts generally are reserved for patients with good hepatic reserve and variceal bleeding. Excellent results are achieved in this setting.[116]

An algorithm summarizing current decision making in the management of variceal hemorrhage is shown in Figure 83.11. Patients are divided into those potentially eligible for a liver

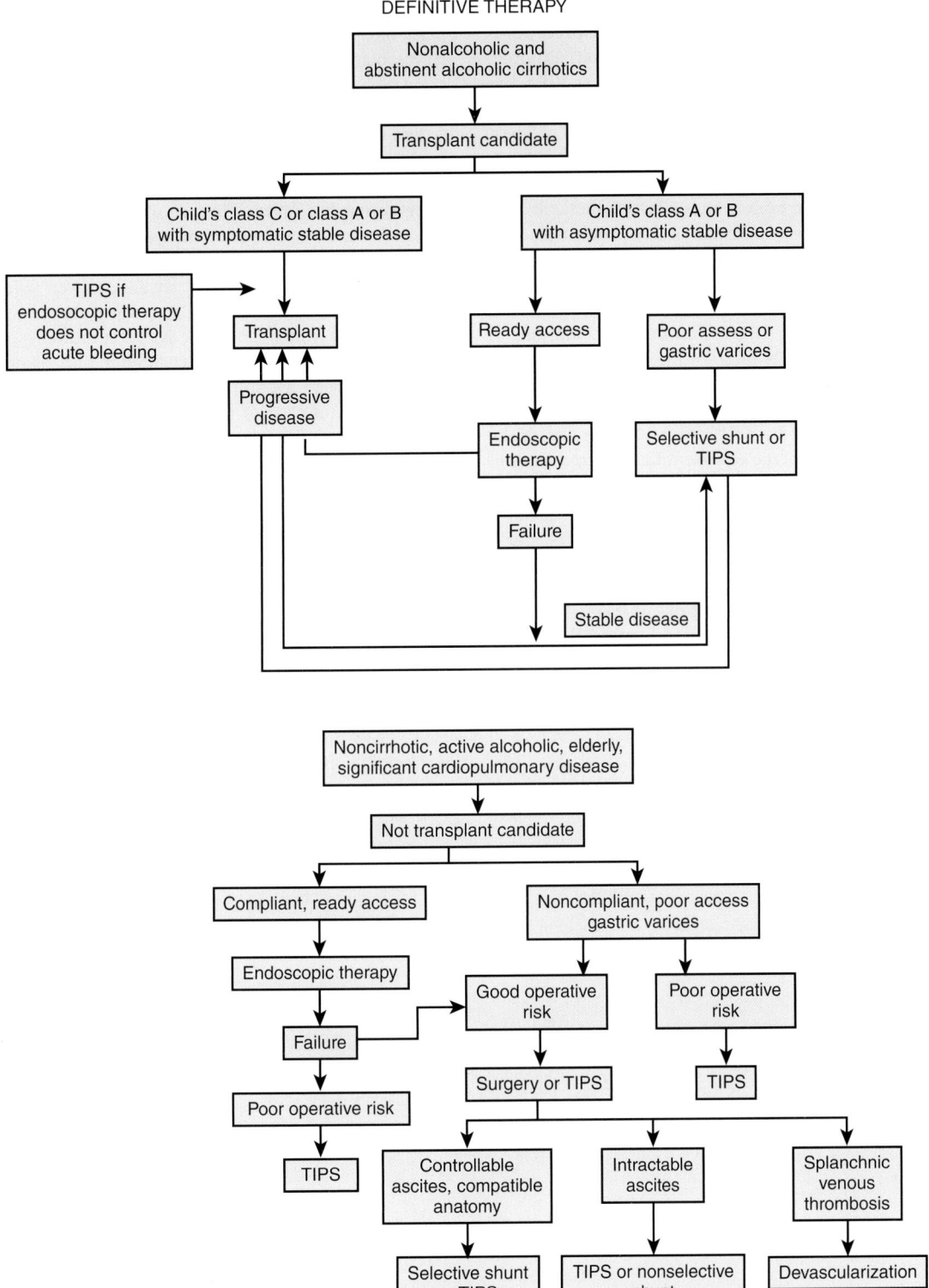

FIGURE 83.11 Algorithm for definitive therapy of variceal hemorrhage. *TIPS,* Transjugular intrahepatic portosystemic shunt. (From Rikkers LF. Portal hypertension. In: Levine BA, et al., eds. *Current Practice of Surgery.* Vol 3. Churchill Livingstone; 1995.)

transplant versus ineligible patients. The sequential use of various modalities is illustrated. The current use of procedures performed for variceal hemorrhage suggests that although banding continues to be used frequently, the use of TIPS has dramatically increased, as has liver transplantation. Nonselective shunts are rarely used today, and selective shunts are performed in a highly select group of patients.

During the past 25 years, liver transplantation and TIPS (see Chapters 85 and 105) have evolved into effective therapies and have substantially affected management of this problem and indirectly changed the risk status (CTP class or MELD) of patients undergoing shunts. Analysis of this group of patients shows that, in recent years, the CTP class has progressively improved, and the need for emergency surgery has declined. The use of nonselective shunts declined because of the development of effective alternatives, such as EVL and TIPS, and because advanced liver failure with ascites was managed by liver transplantation, sometimes preceded by TIPS. Consequently, less risky patients were selected to undergo elective shunts for treatment of variceal bleeding. The incidence of postoperative encephalopathy decreased, and long-term (10-year) survival improved, especially because shunt patients could be salvaged if they experienced liver failure postoperatively.[117]

Another role for portosystemic surgical shunts is in children with variceal hemorrhage after endoscopic therapy. Excellent results have been achieved in children with meso-Rex, distal splenorenal, and mesocaval shunts to prevent bleeding[118] (see Chapter 76).

SUMMARY

The clinical management of bleeding esophageal varices has changed radically during the last 25 years. Recent changes include the improved patency of TIPS, the technical ability to place alternative portosystemic shunts by minimally invasive intravascular techniques, and improved outcomes in liver transplantation. The excellent efficacy of EVL and its lower complication rate favor its increased use. Similarly, the minimally invasive nature of the TIPS procedure and its successful implementation by interventional radiologists has reduced further the need for surgical shunts. TIPS is being increasingly used when endoscopic intervention has failed. The use of expanded PTFE (ePTFE)-covered stents, rather than bare stents, allows better patency rates over time for TIPS. Liver transplantation is routinely recommended for patients with advanced liver failure. Surgical shunts are used more selectively, and with better results than in an earlier era when they were more commonly performed. A multidisciplinary approach to evaluation and treatment of variceal hemorrhage has improved the outcomes of these patients. Selective use of each of the therapies, alone or in combination with other modalities, results in improved outcomes.

We consider the current role of surgical shunts to be (1) less frequent than in the previous era; (2) of benefit in the emergency setting in adults only when other modalities, including medical therapy, endoscopic control, or TIPS, have failed; (3) occasionally useful in the elective setting as a long-term bridge to liver transplantation; (4) useful in the elective setting as definitive therapy for patients with noncirrhotic portal hypertension or CTP class A cirrhosis if TIPS or intravascular DSRS (as shown) are not feasible; and (5) a beneficial treatment for Budd-Chiari syndrome when TIPS is not technically feasible. We prefer the selective DSRS in patients without ascites because of its lower risk of portosystemic encephalopathy and its potential for preserving portal blood flow.

References are available at expertconsult.com.

CHAPTER 84

Techniques of portasystemic shunting: Selective and nonselective shunts

Alexander S. Rosemurgy and Iswanto Sucandy

INTRODUCTION

Surgical shunts for portal hypertension and variceal bleeding are rarely undertaken today, making this chapter either irrelevant or more important than ever. I believe the latter. The decline in surgical shunting is generally a consequence of the perceived outcomes with transjugular intrahepatic portosystemic shunt (TIPS) and the concept of TIPS as a bridge to transplantation (see Chapter 85). The results with TIPS have been shown in several trials to be inferior to and never better than surgical portal decompression, and its role in bridging to transplantation seems too often an illusion because the bridge is seldom "crossed."[1–6] Accelerating the decline in surgical shunting is the loss of shunting in the armamentarium of most surgeons. No longer is surgical shunting "fair game" on the written or oral exams for board certification. No longer are patients with upper gastrointestinal (GI) hemorrhage routinely cared for on surgical services. Rarely are surgeons consulted regarding patients with bleeding varices or gastropathy. Generally, the decision to apply portal decompression for bleeding varices is now made without the involvement of surgeons, but rather using intensivists, hepatologists, interventional radiologists, and gastroenterologists.

To wit, the UK guidelines on the management of variceal hemorrhage in cirrhotic patients state that TIPS be used for patients who rebleed despite combined variceal banding/ligation and noncardioselective β-blocker therapy (or when monotherapy with variceal banding/ligation or noncardioselective β-blocker therapy is used because of intolerance or contraindications to combination therapy) and in selected patients because of patient choice.[7] Where TIPS is not feasible in Child A or B patients, these guidelines suggest that "shunt surgery" can be used where local expertise and resources allow. How can patients knowledgably choose? "Shunt surgery" is excessively broad, reflecting nonsurgeons' view of and understanding of surgery. Furthermore, patients of Child class C consume fewer resources after operative portal decompression than after TIPS.[8]

The American College of Gastroenterology (ACG) & American Association for the Study of Liver Diseases (AASLD) Joint Clinical Guidelines state that TIPS is indicated in patients in whom hemorrhage from esophageal varices cannot be controlled or in whom bleeding recurs despite combined pharmacologic and endoscopic therapy[9] and should be considered in patients in whom hemorrhage from fundal varices cannot be controlled or in whom bleeding recurs despite combined pharmacologic and endoscopic therapy. Herein, to the detriment of the guidelines, there is no mention of operative shunting.

Others also state the role of operative shunting with silence, denoting their perception of its role. So stated, combined treatment with vasoactive drugs, prophylactic antibiotics, and endoscopic techniques is the recommended standard of care for patients with acute variceal bleeding.[10] To others, surgical shunts are considered only when all other treatment modalities fail.[11]

There is also a belief that the disorder of cirrhosis and bleeding varices or portal gastropathy has changed based on the decreasing number of patients undergoing portal decompression for bleeding varices or portal gastropathy.[12] Whether this decrease is because patients are identified earlier in the course of their disorder, gastroenterologists are better at caring for these patients so that portal decompression is unnecessary, or the care of these patients is so decentralized that their numbers go unrecognized and unreported is unknown (see Chapters 74 and 81).

With that preamble, this chapter brings together a summary of the shunt procedures that were the backbone for the control of variceal bleeding for half a century ending early in the 21st century. Even as these surgical shunts evolved with improving outcomes, other therapies—pharmacologic (e.g., beta blockade), endoscopic (e.g., variceal banding/sclerotherapy), and radiologic (e.g., TIPS)—were evolving, generally for the benefit of patients (see Chapters 80, 81, and 85). It is unfortunate that the role of surgical shunting has diminished to the extent it has because its application is now unreasonably infrequent.

PREOPERATIVE ASSESSMENT

Patient assessment before any shunt procedure is similar and is based on:
1. Underlying liver disease and its severity
2. Abdominal venous anatomy and patency
3. Overall performance status

Clinical and lab assessment with determination of Child class and Model for End-Stage Liver Disease (MELD) score are the best tools for assessment of the severity of liver disease (see Chapter 4). Stated better, outcome after shunting is related to hepatic reserve, which is not measured well with conventional "liver function tests," which, in fact, are not "tests" of liver function at all. Child class, 60 years since its description, is probably the best predictor of outcome after shunting.[13] Vascular imaging is performed with color-flow Doppler ultrasound, computed tomography (CT) venography, or magnetic resonance imaging (MRI) venography (see Chapter 14). If venous anatomy is not apparent after these studies, something is wrong. Occlusion versus patency versus recanalization must be resolved and may sometimes require angiography/portal venography.

Overall status is assessed by American Society of Anesthesiologists (ASA) score or Eastern Cooperative Oncology Group (ECOG) score for general performance activities. Detail is beyond the scope of this chapter, but centers managing patients with portal hypertension should have standard approaches to general assessment of these patients.

Options for patients include:

1. Endoscopic variceal sclerotherapy (EVS) or banding (EVB): For patients amenable to definitive control of esophageal varices. Bleeding gastric varices/gastropathy requires one of the following options (see Chapters 80 and 81).
2. Devascularization operations: Indicated to separate the portal circulation from the gastroesophageal variceal complex. Ascites, among many issues, seem to plague these patients postoperatively (see Chapter 82).
3. TIPS: Not our preferred choice because of high failure rates within the first year (about 50%) and excessive diversion of nutrient hepatic blood flow with dramatic diminution of effective hepatic blood flow and resultant progressive hepatic dysfunction[1,14] (see Chapter 85).
4. Operative shunting: Our choice when option #1 is not indicated or possible (see Chapter 83).

PORTACAVAL SHUNTS

Portacaval shunts decompress the portal system by direct means and are referred to as "central shunts" or "nonselective shunts"; the terms are used interchangeably. They were the only successful therapy in the first three-quarters of the 20th century because of limitations of endoscopy and interventional radiology. There are three variations for portacaval shunts:

1. End-to-side
2. Side-to-side (small diameter or large diameter)
3. Interposition, which may be either large or small in diameter

The exposure and set up of the portal vein (PV) and inferior vena cava (IVC) is similar for all these options, but the anastomoses are different. This section will describe and illustrate the techniques (see Chapter 83).

Access

Patients are positioned for a portacaval shunt in a 30-degree left lateral decubitus position with rolled sheets under the patient's right side. A transverse incision is used to divide the right rectus abdominis muscle and a (short) portion of the obliques and transversus abdominis muscles. Self-retaining retractors are placed over the (padded) gallbladder and hepatic flexure to expose the hepatoduodenal ligament.

Exposure and Dissection

A limited Kocher maneuver is undertaken, using electrocautery generously, from the foramen of Winslow dividing tissue caudally to expose the anterior surface of the IVC. The peritoneal covering to the IVC contains small collateral vessels that can be controlled with cautery, and dissection of the fibroareolar tissue encasing the IVC is carried out (using a conventional plastic sucker with a Russian forceps holding the IVC) caudally to the level of the renal veins (Fig. 84.1); ultimately 100% of the IVC is freed of overlying tissue, unless an interposition shunt is used. Once mobilization is complete, a vessel loop or umbilical tape is placed around the vena cava, which should elevate the IVC toward the PV without difficulty. For an interposition shunt, mobilization of the IVC only needs to involve dissection of the ventral 50% of the IVC.

The hepatoduodenal ligament is then incised posteriorly and laterally with electrocautery, and the PV is identified. The

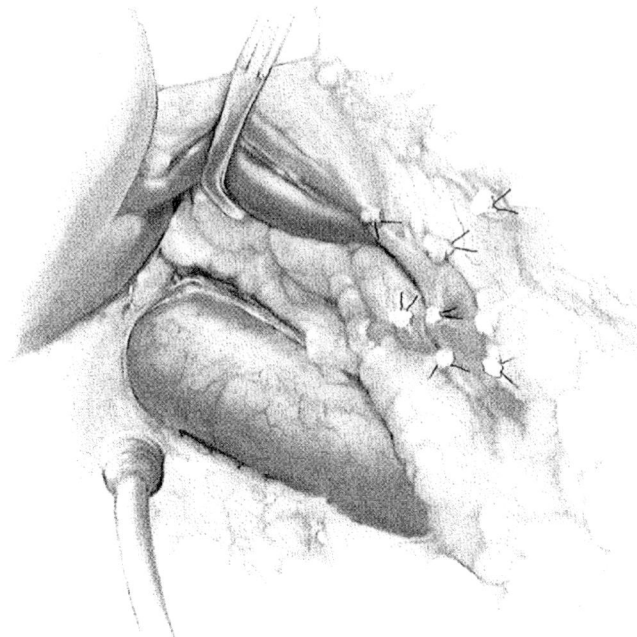

FIGURE 84.1 Kocherization and preparation of the vena cava. (From Rosemurgy AS, Korkolis DP. 8-mm interposition portacaval shunt. In Clavian P, Sarr M, Fong Y, eds. *Atlas of Upper Gastrointestinal and Hepato-Pancreato-Biliary Surgery*. Springer; 2007:675–685.)

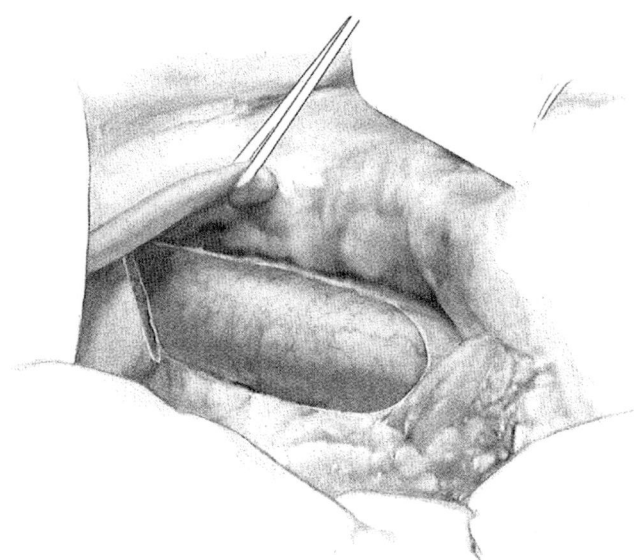

FIGURE 84.2 Exposure of portal vein. (From Rosemurgy AS, Korkolis DP. 8-mm interposition portacaval shunt. In Clavian P, Sarr M, Fong Y, eds. *Atlas of Upper Gastrointestinal and Hepato-Pancreato-Biliary Surgery*. Springer; 2007:675–685.)

common bile duct and replaced/accessory right hepatic artery (if present) are retracted ventrally and medially with a vein retractor held from the left side of the operating table. Whatever shunt is used, it is important to identify and preserve an accessory or replaced artery to avoid deficiencies in liver blood flow after shunting. The dissection is carried out along the long axis of the PV in a cranial to caudal fashion, gently lifting the fibroareolar tissue away from the vein, which should be grasped with a Russian forceps (Fig. 84.2). Dissection should be circumferential with a vessel loop placed around the PV; the vessel loop is used to retract the vein laterally as it is mobilized to its bifurcation distally (i.e., towards the liver) and to the pancreas proximally.

Adequate mobilization of both IVC and PV is judged by raising the IVC ventrally and retracting the PV posterolateral with their respective vessel loops. Usually, a portion of the caudate lobe requires resection to allow the two vessels to be brought into appropriate propinquity without tension. The caudal tip of the caudate lobe can be grasped with a ringed forceps, retracted caudally, and removed with electrocautery. If bleeding is notable, pressure should be placed on the caudate edge and applied, using a retractor if need be. The bleeding generally stops with this; electrocautery reapplication may be necessary.

The Anastomoses

Regardless of the shunt approach undertaken, pressures in the portal system (i.e., the PV) and IVC before and after shunting must be measured, with the patient momentarily off the ventilator. After shunting, the portal pressure should be assayed proximal to portacaval anastomosis.

End-to-side portacaval shunt anastomoses are begun by dividing the PV at its bifurcation and turning the PV posteriorly for anastomosis to the IVC. A longitudinal strip of IVC is excised to give a "window" that ensures adequate outflow for the shunt. The anastomosis is completed with either interrupted or continuous sutures (my choice but do not "purse string" the anastomosis).

This shunt fell out of favor and use beginning in the 1960s, in general, because it only decompressed the portal system and splanchnic circulation, including varices, but did not decompress the high-pressure cirrhotic liver sinusoids. As such, it did not alleviate ascites. Furthermore, this shunt diverted all portal blood flow from the liver and, thereby, greatly reduced effective hepatic blood flow and was, thereby, associated with progressive liver failure.

A side-to-side portacaval shunt is a vein-to-vein side-to-side anastomosis. A Satinsky clamp is securely (i.e., closed all the way so the vein wall does not slip out) placed on the ventral aspect of the IVC, and two right-angled vascular clamps are ultimately placed approximately 5 cm apart on the PV. A 2.5-cm longitudinal strip of IVC is excised to give a "window" that ensures adequate outflow for the shunt. A 2.5-cm opening is made along the posterolateral aspect of the PV to line up the veins for anastomosis (Fig. 84.3A). Beginning in the middle of the left or back wall of the anastomosis, a 5-0 double-armed polypropylene suture is used in a running manner to the cephalad and caudal extents (see Fig. 84.3B). The sutures are tied at each corner of the anastomoses (at the cephalad and caudad extents). The right side or front wall is completed with two 5-0 polypropylene sutures, beginning at each corner; these are tied to the free ends of the posterior layer, and the right side is run from each end toward the midportion of the anastomosis (see Fig. 84.3C). Before tying the sutures together, the vascular clamps are partially released, beginning with the IVC, to release thrombus that may have formed. Upon completion of the anastomosis, the clamps are sequentially released, beginning with the IVC (i.e., the outflow), followed by the distal PV clamp and finally the proximal PV vein clamp. Pressure measurement in the PV and IVC should show a minimal (i.e., 0–4 mm Hg) gradient across the anastomosis.

Small-diameter prosthetic interposition H-graft portacaval shunt involves placement of a prosthetic graft between the PV and the IVC. Exposure for this anastomosis differs from a side-to-side anastomosis in that the IVC does not need to be circumferentially mobilized to allow tension-free approximation of the PV and IVC; the IVC is only mobilized enough to safely side clamp it for placement of the graft (i.e., about 50% of the

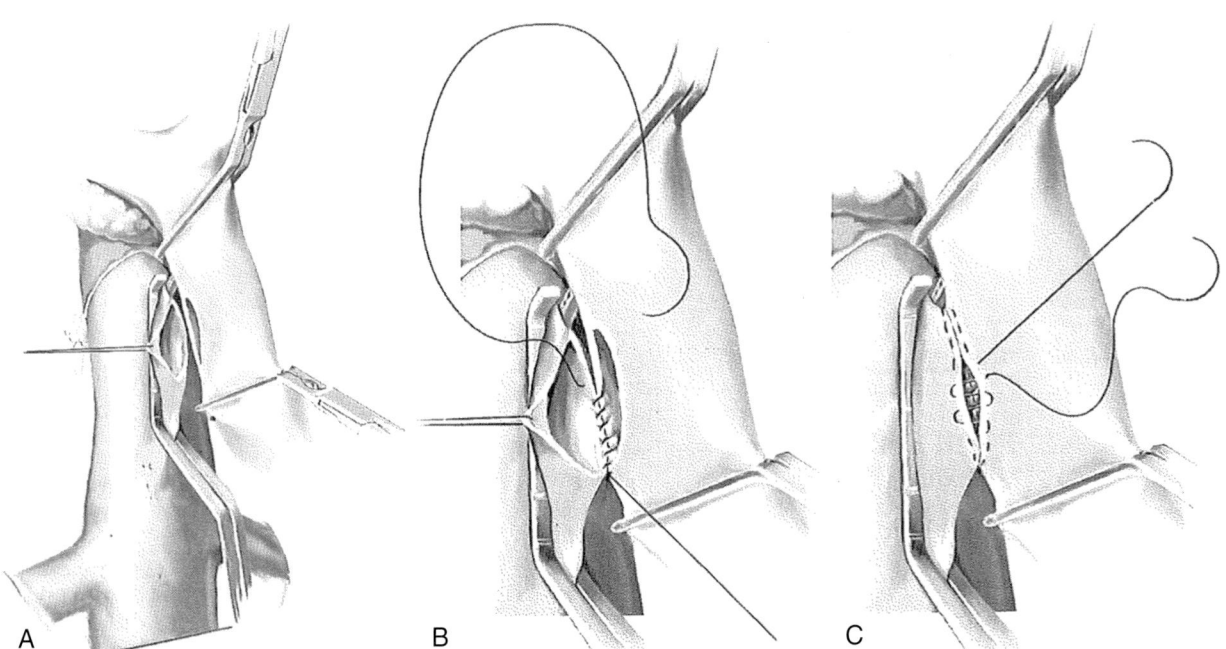

FIGURE 84.3 Three steps in a side-to-side portocaval anastomosis. A, Initial set-up for portocaval shunt. **B,** Posterior wall of anastomosis. **C,** Completion of anastomosis. (From Orloff M, Orloff S. Portacaval shunts: Side-to-side and end-to-side. In Clavian P, Sarr M, Fong Y, eds. *Atlas of Upper Gastrointestinal and Hepato-Pancreato-Biliary Surgery.* Springer; 2007:687–702.)

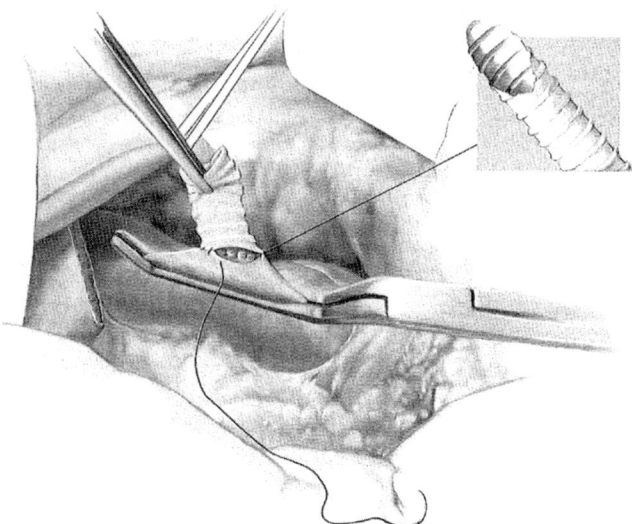

FIGURE 84.4 Graft-caval anastomosis. (From Rosemurgy AS, Korkolis DP. 8-mm interposition portacaval shunt. In Clavian P, Sarr M, Fong Y, eds. *Atlas of Upper Gastrointestinal and Hepato-Pancreato-Biliary Surgery.* Springer; 2007:675–685.)

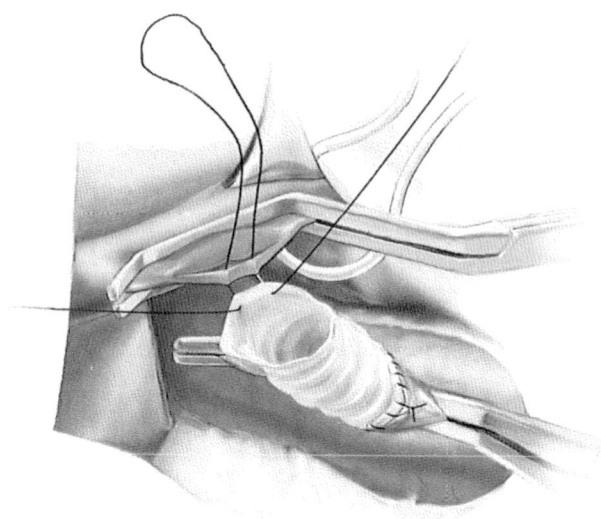

FIGURE 84.5 Portal vein–graft anastomosis. (From Rosemurgy AS, Korkolis DP. 8-mm interposition portacaval shunt. In Clavian P, Sarr M, Fong Y, eds. *Atlas of Upper Gastrointestinal and Hepato-Pancreato-Biliary Surgery.* Springer; 2007:675–685.)

IVC should be freed of overlying tissue). The graft used for the prosthetic small-diameter interposition portacaval shunt is an 8 to 10 mm (PVs larger than 1.5cm require a 10-mm graft) externally ring-reinforced polytetrafluoroethylene (PTFE) graft and is fashioned to measure 3.0 cm from toe-to-toe and 1.5 cm from heel-to-heel, with the ends beveled at 90 degrees to each other. Because the PV is naturally oriented approximately 60 degrees to the IVC, the bevels of each end of the graft are at about 90 degrees to each other (Fig. 84.4). Once the graft is cut to size, it is placed in a syringe full of heparinized saline. With a finger over the tip of the syringe, suction is placed on the syringe. Dislodged air bubbles will emanate from the graft, and vigorous tapping on the side of the syringe will facilitate their dispersal. By removing air from the graft, heparin will completely permeate the prosthesis and facilitate Doppler ultrasound evaluation postoperatively and promote graft patency.

A Satinsky clamp is placed on the anterior wall of the IVC and fully closed to prevent the wall of the IVC slipping from the clamp. A portion of the IVC wall is then excised that should measure approximately 4 mm long and 2 mm wide; this promotes graft outflow. The anastomosis of the graft to the IVC is sewn with running 5-0 polypropylene suture, beginning at the cephalad end of the anastomosis and progressing along the back, or left, or medial wall (see Fig. 84.4). The anastomosis is begun by placing a horizontal mattress suture at the cephalad heel of the anastomosis. The suture is run inside-out on the vein and outside-in on the graft until beyond the toe of the graft. At this point, the other limb of the 5-0 polypropylene is used to complete the lateral (or right) wall of the anastomosis (see Fig. 84.4). The IVC-graft anastomosis is assessed (for leak) by occluding the graft with a right-angle clamp and releasing the Satinsky clamp. When the clamp is replaced on the IVC, the graft is irrigated with heparinized saline to remove blood and clot.

The PV graft anastomosis is made on the posterolateral wall of the PV. The PV is grasped and retracted laterally, and a right-angled side-biting vascular clamp is placed on it (Fig. 84.5). The PV need not be completely occluded to perform the anastomosis, but it usually is. A venotomy is made with an 11-blade

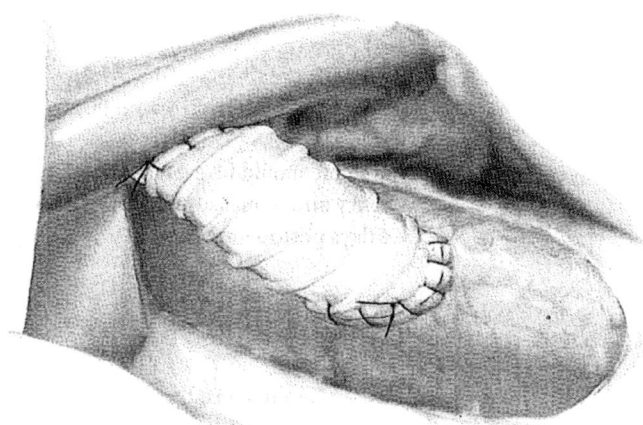

FIGURE 84.6 The completed small-diameter prosthetic H-graft portacaval shunt. (From Rosemurgy AS, Korkolis DP. 8-mm interposition portacaval shunt. In Clavian P, Sarr M, Fong Y, eds. *Atlas of Upper Gastrointestinal and Hepato-Pancreato-Biliary Surgery.* Springer; 2007:675–685.)

scalpel, extended with Potts scissors, and a retraction suture (5-0 polypropylene) placed on the midportion of the ventral wall of the PV to facilitate exposure (not shown in Fig. 84.5). The anastomosis begins at the midposterior wall using a double-armed 5-0 polypropylene suture, with an initial horizontal mattress (inside-out on the vein and outside-in on the graft) followed by running the sutures to the corners (see Fig. 84.5). Once the back row is complete, the suture is drawn tight with a nerve hook; the back wall will not be seen again so make sure the back wall is tight. The front wall is then sewn with each free end of the double-armed suture, converging upon the midportion. Before closure, the PV clamp is partially released to blow clot and debris, and with the clamp reapplied, vigorous irrigation of the graft and PV with heparinized saline is carried out. The sutures are tied and the clamp on the IVC is removed before removing the clamp on the PV. A palpable thrill should be present in the IVC cephalad to the anastomosis (Fig. 84.6).

A metallic clip is placed on the IVC cephalad and caudad to the cava-graft anastomosis to allow interventional radiologists to identify and cannulate the anastomosis.

Pressures in the PV and IVC are again measured. A gradient of less than 10 mm Hg, a decrease in PV pressure of more than 10 mm Hg, an increase in IVC pressure, and a thrill in the IVC cephalad to the shunt assures graft function and patency. A gradient of 4 to 6 mm Hg is ideal; this is partial portal decompression (to a normal PV-IVC gradient).

MESOCAVAL SHUNTS

In the 1970s, mesocaval shunts were undertaken with interposition autologous, homologous, heterologous, and synthetic grafts. The prosthetic mesocaval shunt was popularized by Drapanas who emphasized operating away from the liver hilum (see Chapter 83).

These shunts directly decompress the portal system (they are central, nonselective shunts). Mesocaval shunts belong to the general category of side-to-side portosystemic shunts and, as such, decompress both the high-pressure splanchnic circulation and high-pressure hepatic sinusoids of the cirrhotic liver (if the PV is patent). The degree of decompression, and with this the percent loss of portal flow to the liver, is dependent on the diameter and length of the shunt. The length of a mesocaval shunt is much longer than an interposition portacaval shunt, which increases the risk of thrombosis in the graft. Also, the smaller the diameter of the graft, the higher the likelihood of graft thrombosis.

Their primary indication for these shunts now is portal hypertension with an obstructed (e.g., clotted) PV.

Access

A transverse supraumbilical incision is used. When the peritoneum is opened, ascites is removed, and the abdomen is explored; a self-retaining retractor is placed to provide maximal exposure. Exposure of the superior mesenteric vein (SMV) and IVC occurs in the infracolic compartment of the abdomen, so the transverse mesocolon is retracted cephalad and the small intestine is retracted caudad and to the left to expose the root of the mesentery.

Exposure and Dissection

A transverse incision is made through the peritoneum, just below the middle colic vein, to locate and initiate dissection of the SMV (Fig. 84.7). The superior mesenteric artery usually is located ventral and to the left of the SMV; however, these relationships are inconstant and Doppler ultrasound may help identify the vascular structures. Once identified, the SMV is mobilized and skeletonized from the caudal border of the pancreas to the confluence of the ileocolic and jejunal veins, which form the SMV. Small branches are doubly ligated and divided, and large branches are controlled with vessel loops. The SMV is dissected bluntly on the anterior surface, and sharp dissection is limited until the vein and all tributaries are identified. Usually, a large tributary vein enters the right posterior lateral border of the SMV between the ileocolic and middle colic veins. Care is required; the inferior mesenteric vein enters the left side of the SMV rather than the splenic vein in about 50% of patients. During dissection of the SMV, multiple lymphatic channels and lymph nodes are encountered and should be ligated before division to prevent uncontrolled lymph flow after the procedure,

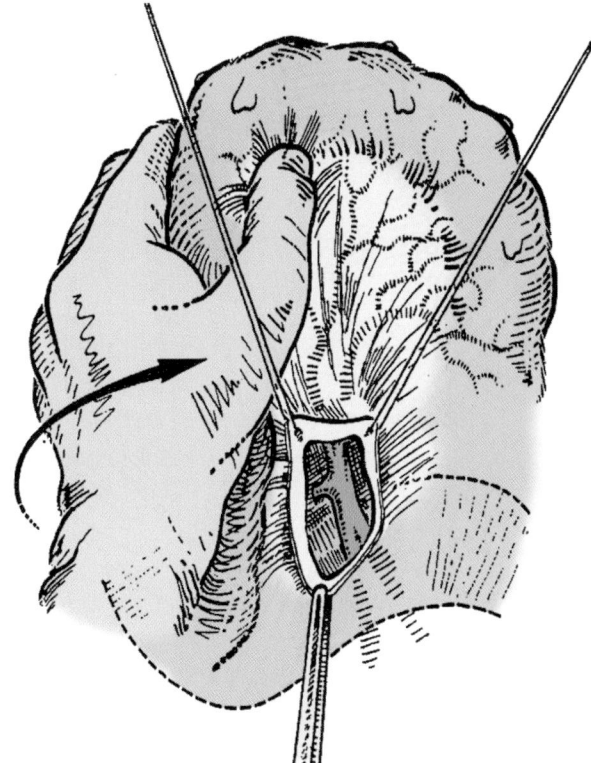

FIGURE 84.7 Exposure of the superior mesenteric vein.

which would contribute to postoperative ascites. Ideally, a 6- to 7-cm length of large-diameter SMV should be exposed circumferentially and mobilized to accommodate the graft. If the SMV is quite short, the ileocolic vein and/or middle colic vein may be sacrificed (Fig. 84.8).

The IVC is identified by a direct approach through the right colonic mesentery. The distal second portion and third portion of the duodenum are mobilized with a limited Kocher maneuver, again ligating and dividing the large lymphatic channels in the retroperitoneum. A 6- to 7-cm length of IVC is dissected along the anterior and lateral borders, freeing about 50% of its diameter. It is not necessary to mobilize the cava circumferentially but only enough to allow placement of a large side-biting Satinsky clamp for partial occlusion (Fig. 84.9; see also Fig. 84.8). After mobilization of the SMV and IVC, soft tissue between these structures can be divided to allow the graft to take an optimal (i.e., shortest) route.

Anastomosis

The IVC graft anastomosis is performed first. A large side-biting Satinsky clamp is placed on the cava and an ellipse of anterior IVC wall is excised to promote graft outflow. Using angled Pott scissors, the venotomy is enlarged to the same diameter, usually 8 to 12 mm, as the chosen externally ringed polytetrafluoroethylene (PTFE; preferred) or internal jugular vein graft (see Fig. 84.9). If the opening is too large, the graft does not assume a circular shape at the anastomosis.

The cava-graft anastomosis is deep in the most dependent area of the wound, and good exposure is difficult, yet essential. The duodenum is retracted superiorly (see Fig. 84.9), and the rest of the viscera are retracted inferiorly and to the left. Two corner sutures are placed using 5-0 polypropylene suture at

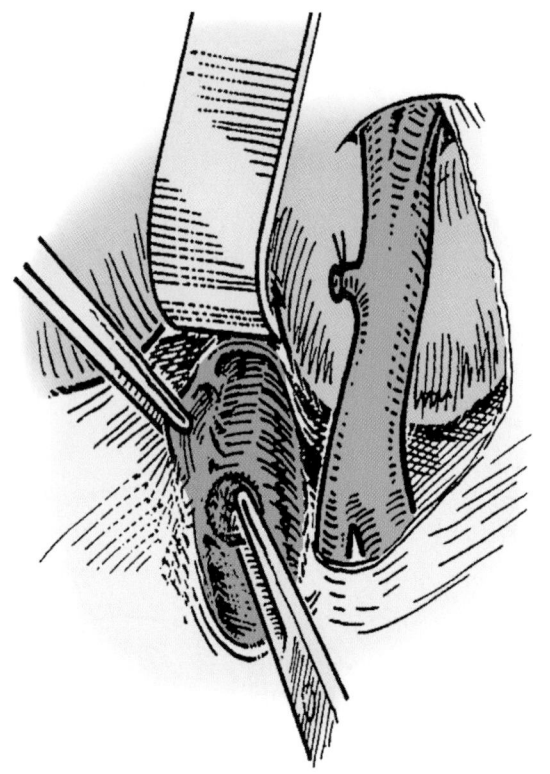

FIGURE 84.8   Dissection of the anterior and lateral aspect of the inferior vena cava and its relationship to the superior mesenteric vein.

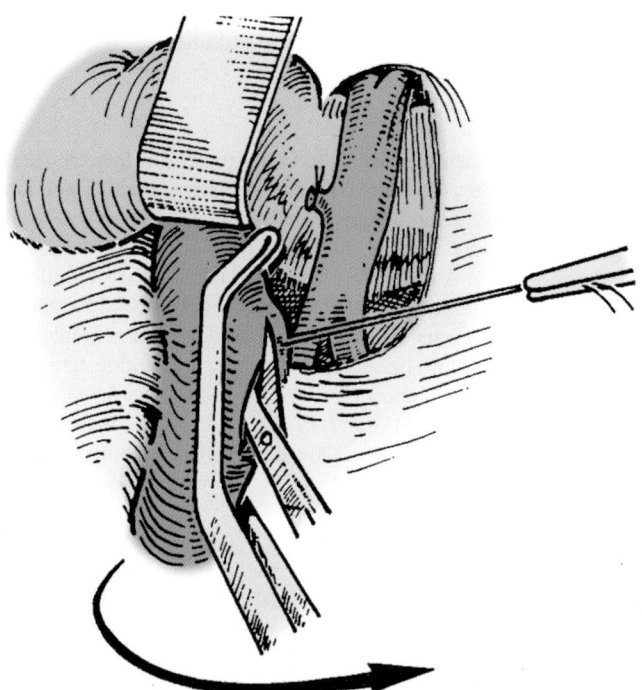

FIGURE 84.9   Inferior vena cava venotomy.

each end of the venotomy, and these are tied to position the graft over the venotomy. A stay suture also is placed midway along the medial cava venotomy lip for gentle traction to distract it away from the lateral suture line. The Satinsky clamp is rotated to the patient's left, and the right side of the anastomosis is completed

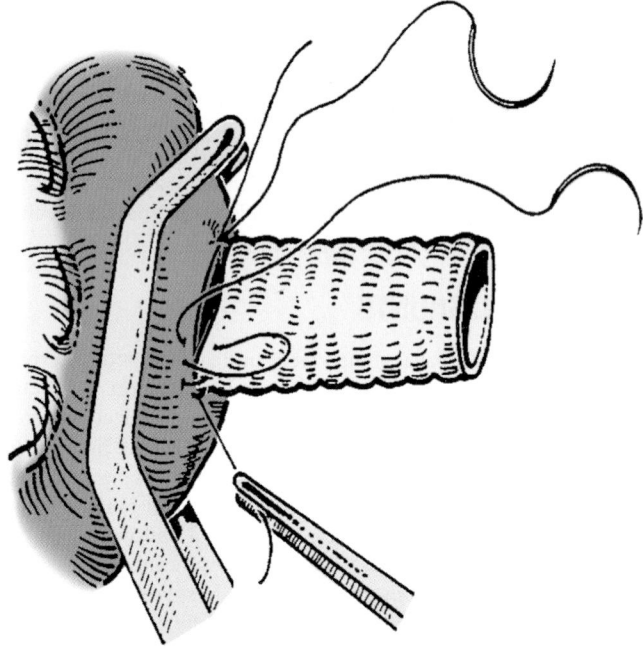

FIGURE 84.10   The inferior vena cava and graft are rotated medially, and the right lateral suture line is performed first.

first. It is sewn from inferior (i.e., caudad) as a continuous suture outside-in on the graft and inside-out on the vein to the superior (i.e., cephalad) corner stitch (Fig. 84.10). The Satinsky clamp is now rotated to the patient's right, and a suture is run cephalad-to-caudad to complete the left side of the anastomosis. Hemostasis at this anastomosis is checked by placing a right angle on the prosthesis, and the Satinsky clamp is released. Any leaks are repaired, the Satinsky clamp is reapplied to the IVC any remaining blood is suctioned from the graft lumen and the lumen is irrigated with heparinized saline.

The length of the graft is crucial; it must be determined before doing the SMV-graft anastomosis (Fig. 84.11). The graft assumes a C configuration (and is often called a "C shunt") as it passes caudad around the lower border of the third portion of the duodenum, then ventral to the third portion of the duodenum and uncinate process, before it is finally is anastomosed obliquely to the anterior-lateral (i.e., ventral and a bit on the left side of the SMV) surface of the SMV. If the graft is too short, undue tension is placed on the suture line, and the SMV is retracted and distorted. If the graft is too long, it becomes redundantly bowed and distorted when the clamps are removed. It also is helpful to mark the graft to maintain proper orientation. When the appropriate length is determined, the graft is cut obliquely to correspond to its angle to the SMV (Fig. 84.11). Two vascular clamps are applied proximally and distally on the SMV, and the vein is partially rotated to allow the anastomosis to be performed on the anterior-left lateral aspect of the vein. A small ellipse is excised from the SMV, and the venotomy is extended proximally and distally using angled Potts scissors to match the length of the obliquely cut graft. Sutures are placed at cephalad and caudad ends of the venotomy and graft using 5-0 polypropylene suture to approximate the vein and graft (see Fig. 84.11). The right suture line (i.e., the back wall) is completed first in a continuous fashion from within the graft and vein, from cephalad to caudad corners

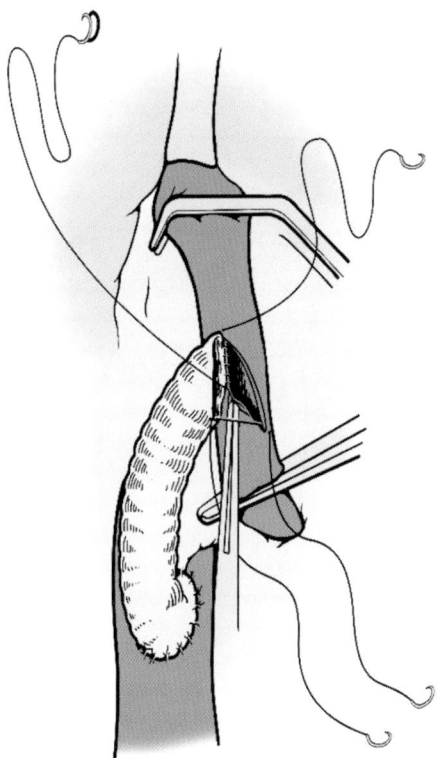

FIGURE 84.11 After occlusion with vascular clamps, the superior mesenteric vein (SMV) venotomy is performed at the anterior-lateral aspect of the SMV, and the SMV-graft anastomosis is started. (Illustration courtesy Dominic Doyle, Medical Arts Group, Vanderbilt University.)

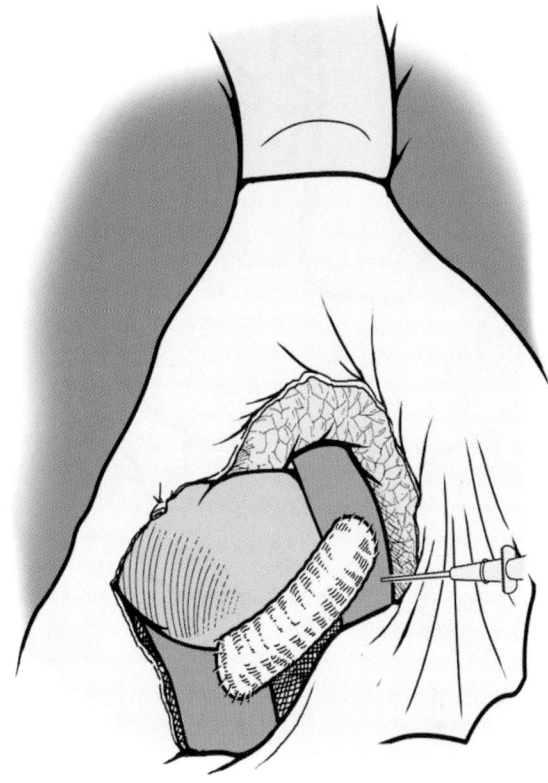

FIGURE 84.12 After completion of the interposition mesocaval shunt, the portal system pressures are measured. (Illustration courtesy Dominic Doyle, Medical Arts Group, Vanderbilt University.)

(see Fig. 84.11). The left suture line is then sewn by rotating the vein to the patient's right for better exposure, again running from cephalad to caudad.

The Satinsky clamp on the IVC is removed first, and anastomotic leaks are repaired. The clamps are removed from the SMV, and flow is allowed through the shunt; gentle pressure may be applied to the anastomoses for hemostasis. Pressures in the SMV and IVC are again measured and the gradient between them should be 0 to 6 mm Hg, depending on the graft diameter and length. A physiologic gradient of 4 to 6 mm Hg is ideal. The completed mesocaval interposition shunt is shown in Figure 84.12.

DISTAL SPLENORENAL SHUNT

The distal splenorenal shunt (DSRS) came on the shunt scene in the 1970s when Warren and Zeppa introduced the concept of selective (i.e., noncentral) gastroesophageal variceal decompression. This shunt compartmentalizes the abdomen, with the shunt decompressing the esophageal and gastric varices through the spleen to the left renal vein, while portal hypertension and portal flow to the liver is (hopefully) maintained (to varying degrees) in the SMV and PV axis. This shunt became widely used for four decades and was extensively studied in randomized trials against total shunts, endoscopic therapy, and TIPS (see Chapter 83).

Access

The patient is positioned on the table with the left arm at the side and the left side slightly elevated. Hyperextending the operating table to open the angle between the left lower ribs and iliac crest aids in exposure and access to the tail of the pancreas.

The preferred incision is a long left subcostal incision, extended across the right rectus muscle. A fixed retractor system is placed to facilitate and maintain exposure.

Exposure and Dissection

Access to the splenic and left renal veins is through the lesser sac to expose the pancreas and retroperitoneum (Fig. 84.13). The gastroepiploic arcade is interrupted from the pylorus to the first short gastric vessels; the left gastroepiploic vein is divided. Exposure is greatly enhanced by taking down the splenic flexure of the colon (the lienocolic ligament is very vascular), which gives access to the inferior margin of the pancreas from the mesenteric vessels to the splenic hilum. The pancreas is then fully mobilized, using electrocautery, along its inferior border over its entire length so that it is turned completely on its cephalad side. The inferior mesenteric vein is the first venous landmark identified and should be traced up to its entry into the SMV or splenic vein and then divided to aid further exposure.

The SMV and splenic vein junction is identified, initially on its dorsal surface, as a safe plane for initial dissection. The splenic vein is then isolated along its inferior and posterior aspect with dissection occurring directly on the vessel (Fig. 84.14). With the posterior plane free, attention turns to the ventral and more difficult plane of dissection on the splenic vein. Tributaries rarely enter the ventral surface of the PV; this plane between the neck of the pancreas and the PV should be opened first, lifting the pancreas ventrally, then the pancreas should be cautiously

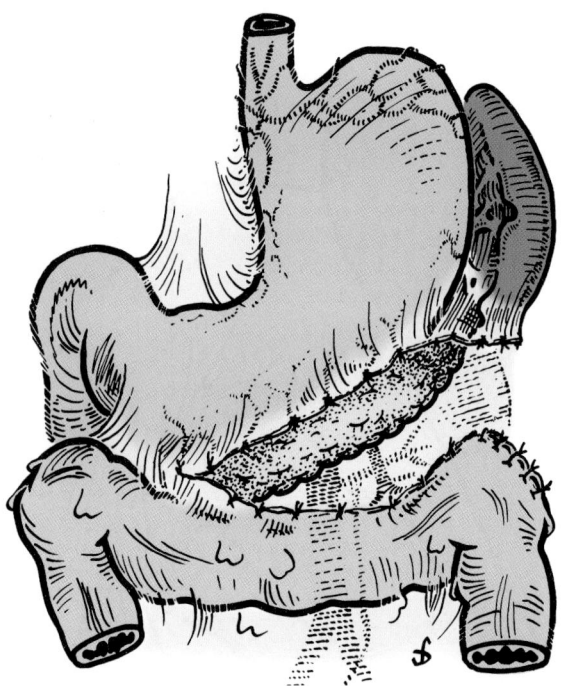

FIGURE 84.13 The pancreas is mobilized from the superior mesenteric vein to the spleen by dividing the posterior parietal peritoneum along its inferior margin.

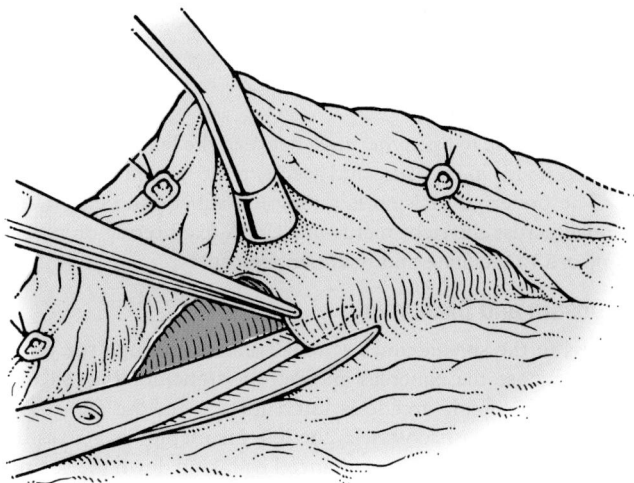

FIGURE 84.14 The splenic vein is dissected initially along its inferior and posterior edge. This dissection must be directly on the vein.

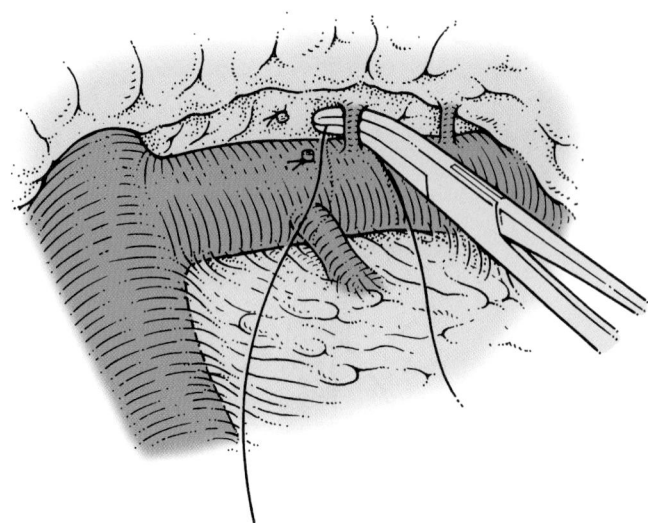

FIGURE 84.15 Isolation of tributaries from the pancreas into the splenic vein requires their dissection at right angles to the splenic vein. These vessels have thin walls and require gentle dissection.

separated and dissected from the anterior and superior surfaces of the splenic vein. The key is to dissect the pancreas off the splenic vein rather than the vein from the pancreas. This requires a delicate touch and is best achieved by spreading the tissues gently in the line of the tributaries and at right angles to the splenic vein. This isolates the tributaries, and when identified, a fine right-angle clamp is passed around them, with a 3-0 tie on the vein side and a clip on the pancreatic side (Fig. 84.15). As much of the splenic vein as possible should be dissected in this manner before dividing the splenic vein at the superior mesenteric vein junction. It is ideal to carry this dissection out into the splenic hilum to achieve a pancreatic-splenic disconnect; this minimizes chances of recollateralization between the portal and systemic systems.

The left renal vein is isolated and mobilized from the retroperitoneum before dividing the splenic vein at the superior mesenteric junction. Preoperative vascular imaging should have shown the anatomy and defined any abnormality: a circumaortic left renal vein is found in 16% of the population, and in 4%, the left renal vein is totally retroaortic; the latter may preclude construction of a distal splenorenal shunt. In circumaortic anatomy, the anterior branch is usually larger and is adequate for outflow for a distal splenorenal shunt. The retroperitoneum is opened just to the left of the superior mesenteric artery and ventral to the aorta; these landmarks are identified by palpation. The divided tissue ventral to the left renal vein should be ligated because there are many lymphatics in it, and ligation minimizes the risk of postoperative chylous ascites. Initial dissection should be minimal to identify the left renal vein, which should be mobilized over an adequate length to allow it to be brought up into a side-biting vascular clamp. The left adrenal vein should be divided, whereas the gonadal vessel is left intact, because it can serve as an outflow tract. The vein should be mobilized over approximately 3 cm, and as a guide, the anastomosis usually is made just ventral to the adrenal vein orifice.

Division of the splenic vein at the SMV junction lines up the splenic and left renal veins for anastomosis. A lateral venorrhaphy is undertaken along the SMV and the splenic vein is controlled with a bull dog or similar vascular clamp. At this point the surgeon must judge whether enough splenic vein has been dissected free of the pancreas to allow it to come down to the left renal vein without kinking or tension. In the event that more dissection of the splenic vein is needed, this can now be performed more easily because the vein can be manipulated downward, as shown in Figure 84.16. The disadvantage of this manoeuvre is that the pressure in the splenic vein has increased with ligation, which leads to greater risk of tearing of the small tributaries or the splenic vein.

Anastomosis

This is performed without tension, and usually the splenic vein needs to be trimmed so that when the clamps are removed, the vein is not redundant and lies without kinking. This alignment

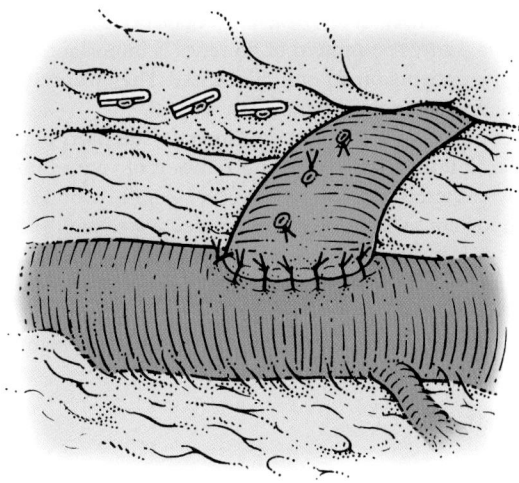

FIGURE 84.18 The anterior row of the anastomosis is completed with interrupted sutures.

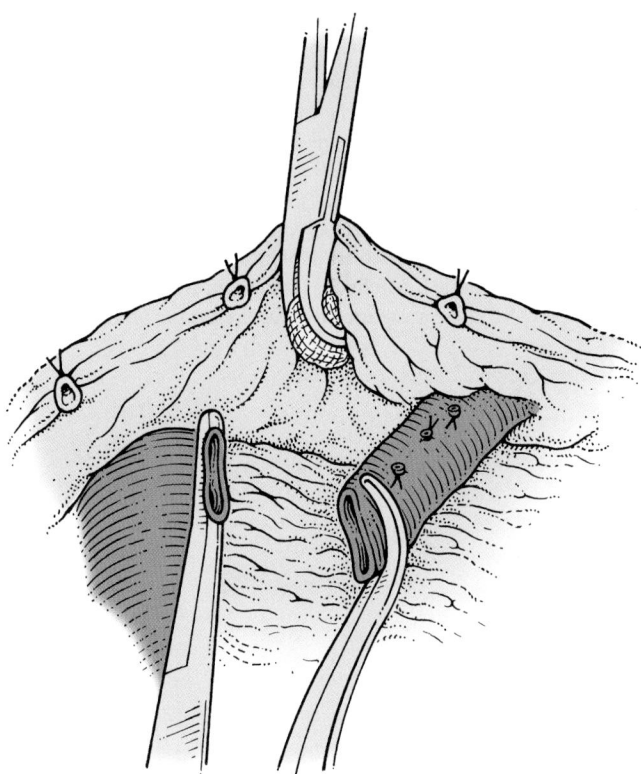

FIGURE 84.16 Division of the splenic vein allows the angle between the pancreas and vein to be opened. This improves exposure for dissection of small tributaries to the splenic vein at the cost of increased pressure in the vein.

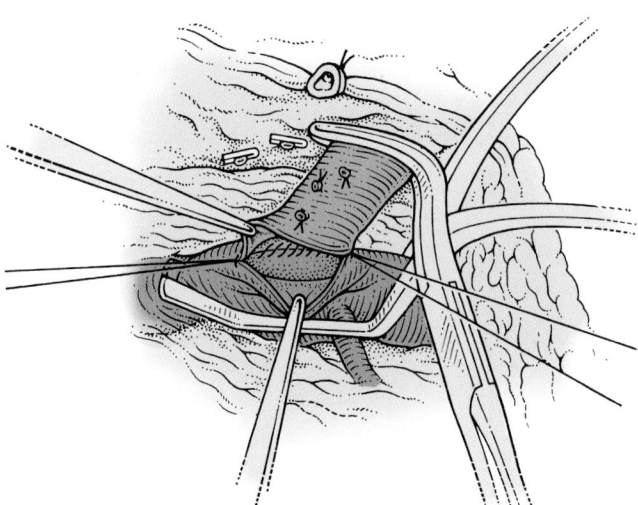

FIGURE 84.17 The posterior anastomosis is made with a running suture. The clamps must be held for a tension-free anastomosis.

can be difficult to judge, particularly if the two veins are overlying each other. The position of the clamps and trimming of the splenic vein are shown in Figure 84.17. The left renal vein is opened over sufficient length without removing an ellipse. The posterior row of the anastomosis is completed with a running suture, with stay sutures placed at both corners, and the suture is run outside-in inside-out; the ventral row is usually interrupted

to avoid risk of a "purse-string" effect. The completed anastomosis is shown in Figure 84.18.

Portal Azygos Disconnection

The final step is interrupting the main paths by which the high-pressure PV attempts to reconnect to the now low-pressure splenic vein. These paths are by:
1. Transpancreatic collaterals
2. Collaterals along the mesocolon to the inferior ramus of the splenic vein
3. The left and right gastric venous systems

The pancreatic siphon of large collaterals flowing through the pancreas can be prevented by dissecting the splenic vein completely out of the pancreas and into the splenic hilum as previously noted. The collaterals that develop in the mesocolon have a final common pathway in the splenocolic ligament to the lower pole of the spleen and do not develop if the splenic flexure is taken down as described earlier. The transgastric collaterals are minimized by ligating the left and right gastric veins.

Abdominal closure should be in two layers of the transverse incision with a running nonabsorbable suture. No drains are placed.

COMMON THEMES IN PERIOPERATIVE AND POSTOPERATIVE MANAGEMENT

The majority of patients having any of the surgical shunts described herein have underlying cirrhosis as the cause of their portal hypertension. This dictates the need for careful team management with some important differences from the typical surgical patient. The risks lie in decompensation of their liver disease with jaundice, ascites, encephalopathy, and increased susceptibility to infection. General points to minimize these risks are:
- Careful preoperative selection and preparation. Optimize nutritional and fluid balance status preoperatively.
- An intraoperative liver biopsy should be done on all these patients as an assessment of the activity and stage of the underlying liver disease.
- Fluid management, both intraoperatively and postoperatively, aims at minimizing sodium retention, which will aggravate ascites. These patients are better "run dry" in contrast to the normal surgical patient. However, it is easier to treat

ascites than liver failure. Ensure organ perfusion and avoid oliguria. Early resumption of diuretics is important.

- Get the patients on an oral diet ASAP. They will do a better job maintaining their fluids than we will.
- Infection prevention measures include standard perioperative antibiotic prophylaxis, and removal of central lines and Foley catheters as soon as possible. Careful wound closure is important as leaking ascites creates a very high risk of infection. If it occurs, run a nylon suture along the incision.
- Shunt patency should be assessed in all patients at 5 to 7 days. This can be done with ultrasound in most patients, but direct shunt catheterization—with measure of portosystemic pressure gradient—is advocated by some.

OUTCOMES

Cirrhosis and portal hypertension are formidable foes. Portosystemic shunting, in its many varieties, has unfairly and irresponsibly been excluded from healthcare's armamentarium against portal hypertension. TIPS is not the answer because of its high one-year failure rate,[1] diversion of excessive portal blood flow resulting in progressive hepatic dysfunction,[14] and illusionary relationship with transplantation.[6]

We wish to thank J. Michael Henderson, MD and C. Wright Pinson, MD for their assistance in prior iterations of this chapter.

References are available at expertconsult.com.

CHAPTER 85

Transjugular portosystemic shunting (TIPS): Indications and technique

Pilar Bayona Molano and Michael Darcy

INTRODUCTION

Besides the well-established role of transjugular intrahepatic portosystemic shunt (TIPS) in the treatment of portal hypertension, additional indications in noncirrhotic, presurgical, and oncologic patients, as well as portal vein thrombosis, have evolved over the past several years. In presurgical patients, TIPS has been used before major interventions such as colectomy in efforts to reduce the risk of intraoperative bleeding. In anticipation of liver or multivisceral transplant TIPS has become a tool to reestablish physiologic portal venous flow, especially in cases of portal vein thrombosis, to avoid organ hypoperfusion and improve outcomes.[1] Portal vein recanalization–TIPS (PVR-TIPS) may achieve recanalization in patients even with complete portal vein thrombosis. Bureau et al.[2] demonstrated in a randomized controlled trial that polytetrafluoroethylene (PTFE)–coated TIPS led to an increase in transplant-free survival in patients with cirrhosis and recurrent ascites, widening the possibilities to not only bridge patients but use TIPS as definitive therapy. Berry et al.[3] reported from an analysis of the UNOS (United Network for Organ Procurement) database the benefit of TIPS to reduce the mortality rate in the waiting list.

Currently, with the advance of locoregional therapies to bridge or downstage liver tumors, it is not uncommon to face the need of treating patients with TIPS requiring other therapies such as transarterial chemoembolization (TACE), yttrium-90, or ablation. This makes it necessary to have extensive multidisciplinary evaluation for correct selection and to prevent complications that could affect the quality of life and expectancy. The concomitant use of TIPS and intraarterial chemoembolization has been reported as safe and effective in patients with hepatocellular carcinoma (HCC) undergoing liver transplantation.[4] Technically, TIPS is still a challenging intervention, requiring, along with the conventional approach, the development of technologic tools to aid portal venous access and decompression, including intravascular ultrasound (IVUS) guidance, cone beam computed tomography (CT), and new control expandable stents.

INDICATIONS

In 2009 the American Association for the Study of Liver Diseases (AASLD) published practice guidelines that include the primary and secondary roles of TIPS for portal hypertension[5] (see Chapters 74, 77, and 78). Since then, multiple updates have been written, including the use of PTFE-covered stents to improve patency, the use of TIPS for Budd-Chiari syndrome (see Chapter 86), and specific algorithms as a second-line therapy for the management of ascites.[6,7] The European Association for the Study of the Liver (EASL) produced clinical guidelines for the management of patients with decompensated cirrhosis, using evidence from PubMed and Cochrane database searches before March 2018 and guided by a panel of experts.[8] The value of TIPS versus a surgical shunt in the prevention of variceal rebleeding in patients who have failed medical therapy, as well as the cost analysis, has been clarified by the publication of a controlled trial comparing TIPS versus distal splenorenal shunt (DSRS). It was concluded that TIPS was slightly more cost effective than DSRS at year 5, but these two approaches were of equal efficacy in the prevention of variceal rebleeding.[9,10] Current indications from multiple clinical trials are listed in Box 85.1.

Authors have identified predictor scales, including the Model for End-stage Liver Disease (MELD), Child-Turcotte-Pugh (CTP), Apache II, and more recently the Garcia-Pagan score, this last one to predict the survival of patients with Budd-Chiari syndrome undergoing TIPS (see Chapter 4). Despite multiple attempts to develop new predictive models, MELD and CTP are still the best predictors of post-TIPS survival. In 2010 a randomized trial described that early preemptive TIPS, performed within 72 hours of an acute episode of variceal bleeding, demonstrated an increased survival benefit for patients who were Child-Pugh class C and with no increase in the risk of hepatic encephalopathy.[11]

Acute Variceal Hemorrhage (see Chapters 80 and 81)

Increased portal pressure is a determining factor for both variceal rupture and the severity of the bleeding episode. The common hemodynamic end point after decompressing the portal vein is a portosystemic gradient of 12 mm Hg. Clinical success is indicated by cessation of demonstrable gastrointestinal bleeding, transfusion requirements, pharmacologic support, or balloon tamponade, and by return of hemodynamic stability with or without performance of adjunctive variceal embolization when indicated.[12] The main downfall to TIPS has been the development of new hepatic encephalopathy or exacerbation of existing encephalopathy, occurring in 20% to 31% of cases[13] (see Chapter 79). It is for this reason that TIPS has been recommended only after failure of medical management and not as front-line therapy for variceal bleeding. The concept of early TIPS within 72 hours from the initial bleeding episode (ideally ≤24 hours) was described for patients at high risk of first-line treatment failure (i.e., Child-Pugh class B with active bleeding at index endoscopy or in Child-Pugh class C score lower than 14 points). Early TIPS demonstrates an important advantage in terms of absolute risk reductions of mortality in high-risk patients with MELD ≥19 or Child-Pugh C cirrhosis.[14,15] Multiple studies and one meta-analysis have all shown significantly improved survival with stent graft TIPS compared with medical/endoscopic therapy.[16,17]

BOX 85.1   Transjugular Intrahepatic Portosystemic Shunt (TIPS): Current Indications

Uncontrollable esophageal or gastric variceal hemorrhage
Current or prior variceal hemorrhage that is not amenable to initial or continued endoscopic therapy
Prophylaxis against recurrent variceal bleed in high-risk patients (5 days from initial bleeding)
Recurrent bleeding from ectopic varices or stomas, for which nonselective beta-blockers and/or endoscopic treatment fails
Portal hypertensive gastropathy or enteropathy (transfusion dependent and not responding to medical therapy)
Refractory ascites
Hepatic hydrothorax
Portal vein thrombosis
Budd-Chiari syndrome
Hepatorenal syndrome
Decompression of portosystemic collaterals before abdominal surgical procedures
Portal hypertension associated with malignancies (palliation)
Hepatopulmonary syndrome* in study

*In the hepatopulmonary syndrome, the role of TIPS is still unclear, and it is hypothesized that it can be as a result of lessening of intrapulmonary vascular dilations (IPVDs).[13] However, it has been shown to improve hypoxemia in some patients and can be safely performed for the treatment of other complications of portal hypertension in the presence of hepatopulmonary syndrome and reasonably used as a bridge toward liver transplant.[13]

Isolated Gastric Varices and Portal Gastropathy

The risk of bleeding for gastric varices has been reported at about 10% to 16% per year.[18] Sarin classification is the most used to classify gastric varices and is based on the endoscopic and anatomic characteristics.[19] The approach for cardiofundal varices Gastroesophageal varices type 1 in Sarin's classification (GOV 1), considered an anatomic continuation of the esophageal varices, has been described with a relative consensus that they be treated like the esophageal varices with medical and endoscopic therapy as a first-line and TIPS as a second-line treatment. Isolated gastric varices often appear as a result of portomesenteric vein thrombosis and are associated with spontaneous portosystemic shunts. Some reports suggest that the use of cyanoacrylate may be the elective treatment for gastric varices followed by repeated sessions of glue injection along with nonselective beta-blockers as secondary prophylaxis.[20] A randomized trial[21] showed that rebleeding was significantly less frequent in the TIPS group compared with variceal obliteration with endoscopic cyanoacrylate injection (see Chapters 80 and 81).

Portal hypertensive gastropathy (PHG) might be clinically important because it is sometimes responsible for insidious blood loss (chronic iron deficiency anemia) and in exceptional cases even overt acute bleeding. In patients with medically refractory PHG and compensated cirrhosis, TIPS has been shown to improve the endoscopic appearance and decrease the transfusion requirement. In one of the largest studies (40 patients with PHG) endoscopic improvement was detected between 6 weeks and 3 months after TIPS placement.[22]

Ectopic Varices

Ectopic varices are defined as large pressurized portosystemic venous collaterals occurring anywhere in the abdomen except in the gastroesophageal region and account for up to 5% of all variceal bleeding.[23] These collaterals occur where the portal venous system is in juxtaposition to the systemic venous system. After development of intrahepatic portal hypertension, these shunts act to divert flow from the increased intrahepatic vascular

resistance. The varices can be related with prior abdominal surgeries in ostomies, or can appear in unusual locations such as ovaries and bladder. They have also been associated, in the absence of portal hypertension, with congenital anomalous portosystemic anastomoses, abnormal vessel structures, arteriovenous fistulae, or thromboses. TIPS decompression provides primary intervention or salvage modality in cases of bleeding; however, although ectopic varices decompress through different pathways, the rebleeding rate is higher. Therefore the combination with embolization has been reported to be superior to TIPS alone.[24]

Ascites

Early investigators recognized that TIPS led to a reduction or resolution of ascites in many patients (see Chapter 79). Several studies have tried to determine positive predictors of post-TIPS ascites resolution. MELD score, aspartate transaminase levels, hepatic-portal venous gradient, creatinine levels, glomerular filtration rate, and platelet count have been found to predict a good response to TIPS.[25,26] In general, 54% to 79% of patients show significant ascites resolution after TIPS.[44–46] A recent randomized trial found covered stents for TIPS to increase the proportion of patients with cirrhosis and recurrent ascites who survive transplantation-free for 1 year, compared with patients given repeated large-volume paracenteses and albumin. These findings support TIPS as the first-line intervention in such patients.[27]

Hepatic Hydrothorax

TIPS is reserved for patients with hepatic hydrothorax who are refractory to medical management (see Chapter 79). Liver transplantation, if indicated, constitutes the best long-term treatment option for patients with refractory hepatic hydrothorax[28] (see Chapter 105). TIPS has been considered as definitive treatment or bridge to transplantation in patients with refractory hepatic hydrothorax.[29] Patients requiring multiple thoracenteses or chest tubes can benefit from TIPS, with a beneficial response reported in 74% to 79% of patients undergoing the procedure.[30,31] Of those who respond, about two thirds have complete resolution of the hydrothorax, and the remainder experience partial resolution of the effusion but are symptomatically improved, with either decreased or resolved dyspnea. In our experience,[32] the patients who showed no clinical response to TIPS were all critically ill with elements of multiorgan failure, and 30-day mortality was 83%. Thus TIPS is unlikely to be helpful as a last-ditch effort to improve pulmonary function in severely ill patients on mechanical ventilation.

Portal Vein Thrombosis

TIPS in portal vein thrombosis (PVT) is considered in select cases of obstructive PVT with worsening symptomatic portal hypertension but only in select institutions where expertise in performing this procedure optimally is available.[33] Excellent rates of improvement and recanalization of PVT with TIPS have been reported; however, anticoagulation is also associated with similar results.[34,35] In addition, portal vein recanalization (PVR) and TIPS creation (PVR-TIPS) has been performed in patients with PVT to improve their candidacy for transplantation by providing a patent portal vein at the time of transplantation and treat portal hypertension symptoms, decreasing the mortality on the liver transplant waiting list[36,37] (Fig. 85.1). The goal is to permit a physiologic portal vein reconstruction, which has demonstrated similar survival to that of patients without PVT.[38,39] Although this can often still be accomplished from a

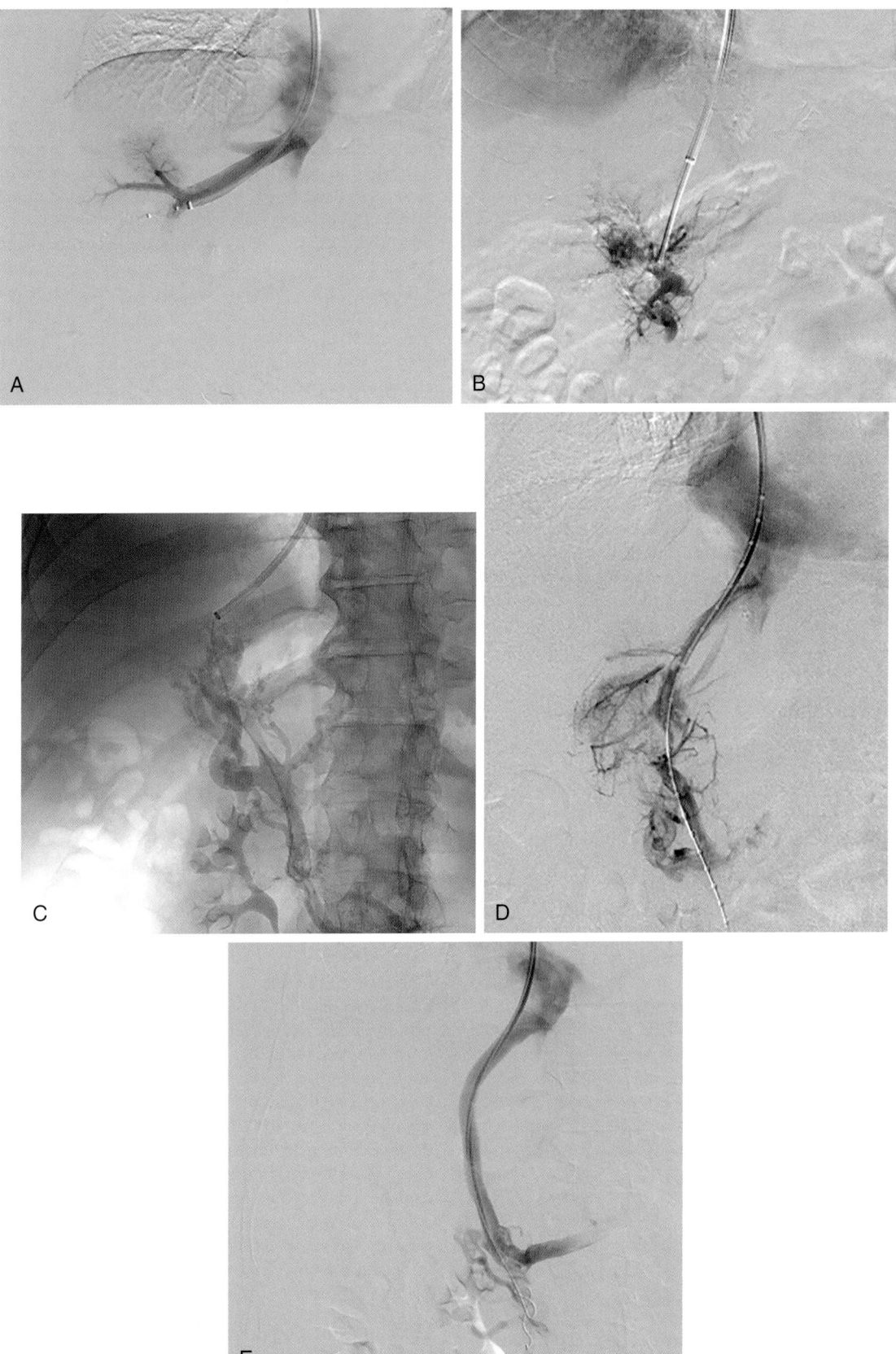

FIGURE 85.1   Patient with cavernous transformation of the portal vein requiring transjugular intrahepatic portosystemic shunt (TIPS) for portal hypertension. **A,** Initial venogram with the catheter in the right hepatic vein. **B,** A Colapinto needle (Cook Medical) used to target the portal vein collaterals. It is inserted through an introducer extending from the right internal jugular vein across the right atrium and hepatic vein. **C,** Venogram with the catheter at the SMV (Superiotr Mesenteric Vein) demonstrating cavernous transformation of the portal vein without visualization of a main residual vessel. **D** and **E,** The shunt tract was measured using a marker catheter. The stent was deployed from the collateral vein draining the portomesenteric vein confluence into the hepatic vein confluence. Final TIPSogram demonstrated widely patent stent and no further filling of portal venous collaterals.

transjugular route, use of a percutaneous transhepatic or transsplenic access is sometimes needed to initially recanalize the portal vein (Fig. 85.2). Thornburg et al.[40] reported 60 successful cases of transsplenic PVR-TIPS with no cases of recurrent PVT following transplantation and 5-year overall survival rate of 82%. In the acute PVT setting, TIPS constitutes a mechanical tool to reestablish the venous outflow when the intrahepatic portal venous branches are thrombosed and provides an access route to perform thrombectomy and portomesenteric venous lysis. The technical success rate for establishing a shunt and maintaining patency of the portal system is generally 70% to 100%,[41,42] with the technical failures a result of the inability to traverse the portal occlusion. However, in patients in whom the occlusion has progressed to cavernous transformation, the technical success rate in some studies has been as low as 35%.[43,44] Recently, the use of transsplenic approach has become more common for PVR-TIPS even in the setting of cavernous transformation.

If a large enough extrahepatic collateral vessel is present it can be used as a valid "landing zone" for the portal side of the TIPS. Malignant portal vein thrombosis due to hepatocellular carcinoma has been sometimes felt to be a contraindication for TIPS. However, several studies have shown that TIPS can still be done in this setting with very high technical success rates, low complications, and good relief of both variceal bleeding and intractable ascites.[45,46] In patients with a reasonable life expectancy TIPS can be considered for palliation of portal hypertensive symptoms despite malignant thrombosis.

Budd-Chiari Syndrome

TIPS is an alternative treatment in Budd-Chiari syndrome (BCS) after failed medical therapy and other endovascular therapies such as angioplasty and stent insertion on the hepatic veins or inferior vena cava (IVC) (see Chapter 86). In patients without a remaining hepatic vein stump or complete occlusion, a direct portosystemic shunt (DIPS) is an option, with a puncture from the intrahepatic IVC into the liver parenchyma to target the portal vein via the caudate lobe. If a remnant of the hepatic vein (HV) is available, the needle passing across the liver parenchyma can start from the HV stump, if it can be engaged. If the HV stump cannot be engaged, passes can be made directly from the IVC itself. The needle pass should start from the retrohepatic segment of the IVC to avoid the chance of hemorrhage. Garcia-Pagan et al.[7] reported long-term outcomes for patients with severe BCS treated with TIPS even in high-risk patients, suggesting that TIPS may improve survival. They also identified a small subgroup of BCS patients with poor prognosis despite TIPS who could possibly benefit from early OLT.[7]

Preoperative Decompression

For patients with severe portal hypertension that requires colonic resection, the operative mortality can be high (see Chapter 75). Portal hypertension poses a risk in terms of dilated collateral veins, increased risk of operative bleeding, and the possibility of portal hypertension–related ascites, causing infectious complications or incisional ascites leakage postoperatively. Recent reports showed good results using TIPS for portal decompression to allow safe laparoscopic colonic resection.[47] One unresolved question concerns how much time to allow between the TIPS and the operation to ensure optimal decompression of the dilated collateral veins. Although waiting a few weeks after portal decompression seems prudent, one group reported safely operating 2 days after TIPS.[48]

TIPS Pretransplant

Multiple studies have reported the effect of TIPS on liver transplant outcomes. Guerrini et al.[49] reported that patients with TIPS had a lesser risk of mortality 1 year after LT compared with those without TIPS. Other studies showed no difference in terms of graft outcomes with TIPS pretransplant.[50,51] In a cohort study, 1081 patients undergoing liver transplant were analyzed, 130 with TIPS before transplant. The results demonstrated a more severe underlying liver disease in patients with TIPS compared with those without TIPS, as characterized by greater MELD scores, greater serum bilirubin levels, and lesser platelet counts. In addition, the presence of hepatocellular carcinoma or hepatitis C virus, which negatively affects graft survival, was observed less frequently in patients with TIPS. The authors suggest that pretransplant TIPS placement increases graft portal flow but does not compromise surgical outcomes after liver transplantation[49] (see Chapters 105 and 106).

Hepatorenal Syndrome

TIPS improves several hemodynamic variables and therefore its role in improving hepatorenal syndrome has been described, but the effect on the survival of patients with poor liver function is limited (see Chapters 74, 77, and 79). Furthermore, plasma renin activity, aldosterone, and noradrenaline concentrations improve gradually after TIPS insertion, suggesting a positive effect on systemic underfilling, an important factor in hepatorenal syndrome.[52] Malinchoc et al.[53] reported a negative correlation between the creatinine concentrations before TIPS, with an elevated creatinine concentration being a negative predictive factor for survival after TIPS. However, multiple studies, including a meta-analysis by Salerno et al.,[54] failed to demonstrate that correlation. Studies have reported that TIPS improves posttransplant graft and patient survival significantly, possibly due to an improved pretransplant renal function and portal blood supply of the graft.[55]

Hepatopulmonary Syndrome

The role of TIPS in this pathology is unclear. Its safety was questioned because hypoxemia may increase the risk of complications during the procedure, but also because it might increase intrapulmonary vascular dilations (IPVDs) and worsen oxygenation, exacerbating the hyperdynamic circulatory state; however, no complications were reported.[56] A systematic review evaluated a total of 12 patients with hepatopulmonary syndrome; 10 patients underwent TIPS and 9 (75%) had improvement of oxygenation but by unclear mechanisms. A possible explanation for this finding was that portal decompression could decrease the production of local and systemic vasodilators such as nitric oxide and carbon monoxide, which can be implicated in the development of IPVDs[57] (see Chapters 76, 79, and 105).

TIPS and Oncologic Patients

TIPS has been considered in certain reports as a palliative tool for refractory ascites due to metastatic disease[58] (see Chapters 90, 91, and 92). Luo et al.[59] studied a large cohort of patients with cirrhosis and HCC who underwent TIPS for recurrent variceal bleeding and/or ascites. Of a total of 217 patients, 97.69% of the TIPS procedures were completed successfully,

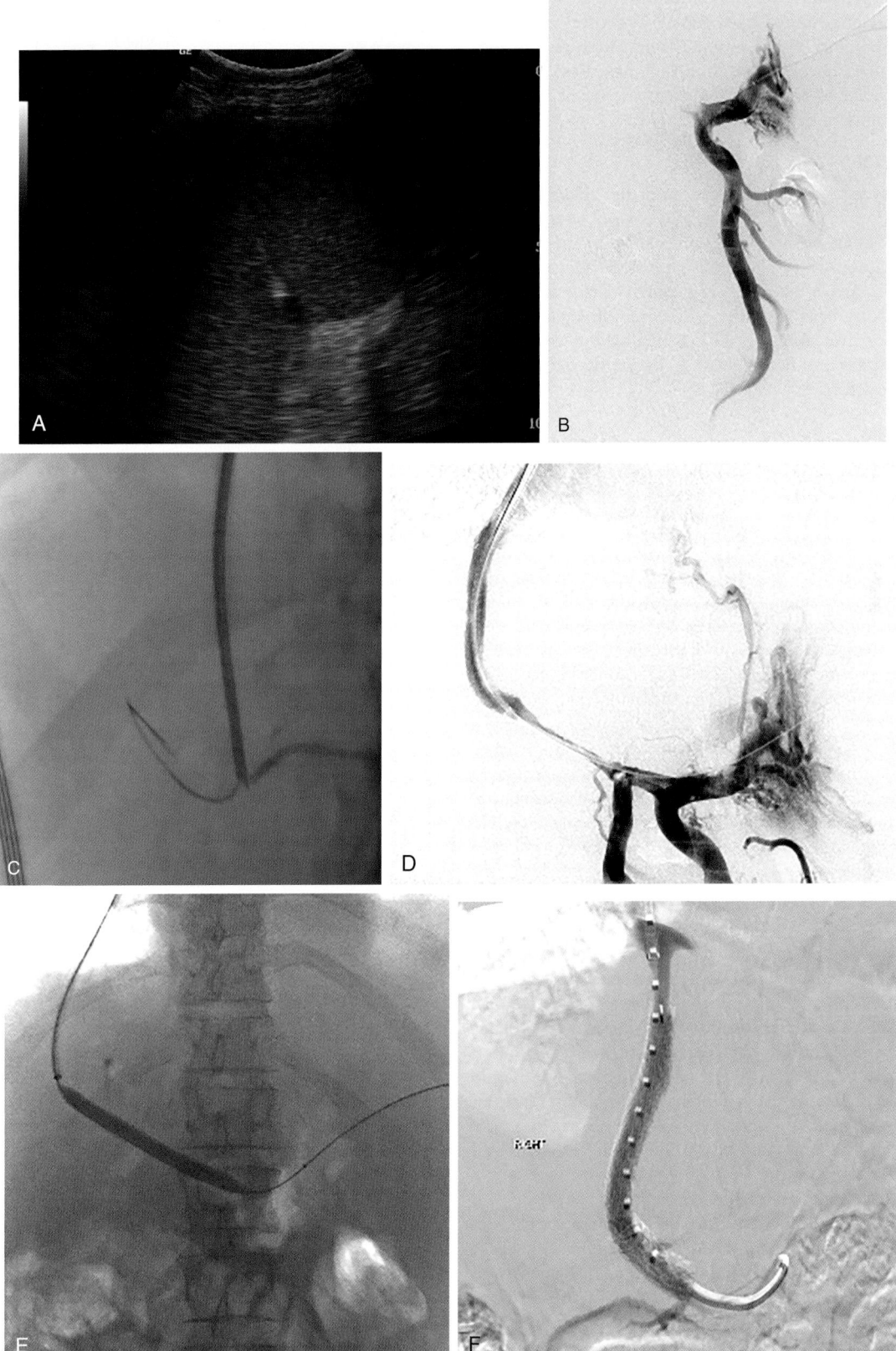

FIGURE 85.2 Transsplenic recanalization of the portal vein: patient with portal vein thrombosis requiring transjugular intrahepatic portosystemic shunt (TIPS) for intractable ascites. **A,** Transsplenic access and catheterization of the splenic vein using ultrasonographic guidance. **B,** Contrast injection in the splenic vein through a catheter demonstrated occlusion of the main portal vein and opacification of the inferior mesenteric vein (IMV) with retrograde flow. **C,** A wire was manipulated across the remnant main portal vein and is used as a target to create the shunt. A Colapinto needle (Cook Medical) is advanced from the hepatic vein through the liver into the main portal vein remnant. **D** and **E,** A wire was inserted throughout the tract and the tract was dilated. **F,** A final TIPSogram demonstrated widely patent shunt without visualization of retrograde flow or varices.

with no serious procedure-related complications, such as tumor rupture or bleeding, either from tumor puncture or directly from venous puncture in the tumor tissue. These results suggested that, if there is strict selection of suitable cases combined with the experience of skilled TIPS placement, severe complications will continue to be rare.[59]

Polycystic Liver

A polycystic liver presents additional anatomic challenges (see Chapter 73). Preprocedure CT scans can be used to analyze the distribution of cysts and their position relative to the right hepatic and portal veins. The planned tract may be adjusted based on this analysis. It has been reported that IVUS enabled safe creation of an intrahepatic portosystemic shunt in a patient with severe Polycystic liver disease (PCLD), highlighting the benefits of direct visualization of needle passage for portosystemic shunt creation in this setting.[60]

CLINICAL ASSESSMENT AND RISK EVALUATION FOR PATIENTS UNDERGOING TIPS PROCEDURE

The safety of TIPS interventions is grounded in proper selection of patients, performance of the procedure, and post-TIPS surveillance. Patients who receive TIPS are at risk for encephalopathy, renal dysfunction, cardiac dysfunction (high cardiac output), liver failure, respiratory complications (portopulmonary hypertension), infections, coagulopathy, and electrolyte disturbances (hyponatremia), among others. For these reasons a patient's cardiovascular status and hepatic, hematologic, nutritional, and renal functions should be carefully evaluated. Ideally, clinical assessment will include complete history, physical examination, and laboratory studies with complete blood count, serum liver enzymes, coagulation parameters, echocardiography, and triple-phase CT and/or liver vascular ultrasound if contrast injection is not appropriate. The contraindications should be identified in the initial assessment and according to the risk they are classified as absolute or relative.[61] Box 85.2 shows a list of the absolute and relative contraindications for TIPS procedure.

Patient Selection Criteria

Laboratory tests are performed to look for coagulopathy, liver or renal failure, and systemic infection, as well as to establish MELD or Child-Pugh classification (see Chapter 4). To improve the patient's clinical state, hematocrit and coagulation deficit (fresh frozen plasma if international normalized ratio [INR] is >1.8, platelet infusion if count is <50,000 × 10^9/L, or according to the center's standards) should be corrected. The acutely bleeding patient must be hemodynamically stabilized during the procedure.[62]

Cardiologic evaluation should demonstrate or rule out preexisting cardiac dysfunction. Patients with cirrhosis can develop hyperdynamic circulation due to persistent splanchnic vasodilation. Cardiac output will increase after TIPS insertion as portomesenteric venous flow is bypassed to the systemic circulation, and this can aggravate any preexisting heart failure. In patients with any cardiac history, transthoracic echocardiography is beneficial to evaluate for possible heart failure and tricuspid valve regurgitation that will require optimization before TIPS is considered. In addition, the left ventricular function and pulmonary pressure are important parameters that can contraindicate the procedure due to the expected increase in right heart and pulmonary pressures with increased preload after shunting.[61] Prospective studies have identified aortic

---

BOX 85.2 Absolute and Relative Contraindications for Patients Undergoing TIPS Procedure

Absolute Tips Contraindications
Congestive heart failure (particularly right-sided heart failure)
Severe tricuspid regurgitation
Severe pulmonary hypertension (mean pulmonary pressure greater than 45 mm Hg)
Uncontrolled infection or biliary obstruction

Relative Tips Contraindications
Obstruction of all hepatic veins
Complete portal vein thrombosis
Hepatocellular carcinoma (especially if centrally located)
Severe coagulopathy (INR greater than 5)
Thrombocytopenia (platelet count less than 20,000/cm^3)
Moderate pulmonary hypertension
Recurrent or persistent severe spontaneous hepatic encephalopathy
Advanced liver failure (bilirubin greater than 5 mg/dL or Model for End-stage Liver Disease [MELD] score greater than 17)
Cardiac dysfunction (ejection fraction less than 60%), cardiac diastolic dysfunction
Advanced age (>69 years old)
Extensive polycystic liver disease

INR, International normalized ratio; *TIPS,* transjugular intrahepatic portosystemic shunt.

---

stenosis as a risk factor of cardiac decompensation within 1 year after TIPS. Diastolic dysfunction estimated using the E/A ratio (early maximal ventricular filling/late filling velocity) is a promising predictor of death in patients with cirrhosis who are treated with TIPS. In normal subjects the E/A ratio is greater than 1, otherwise the diastolic ventricular function is considered impaired.[63] Other reports demonstrated that diastolic dysfunction, indicated by reduced E/A ratio, is prevalent in advanced cirrhosis and is associated with reduced ascites clearance and increased mortality after TIPS, possibly related to worsening of hemodynamic dysfunction in the post-TIPS period.[64] Additionally, brain natriuretic peptide (BNP) greater than 40 pg/mL was associated with development of cardiac failure.[65] Reduced functional residual capacity due to ascites and hepatic hydrothorax impairs respiratory function.

Pulmonary function test (spirometry) can identify respiratory dysfunction, and chest radiograph may reveal presence and extension of fluid collection inside the thorax. When respiratory function is compromised, drainage of these fluid collections may be required. This is normally performed on the day before the TIPS procedure and should involve the use of albumin for volume replacement (8 g per 2.5 liters drained) to avoid postparacentesis circulatory dysfunction and renal impairment.[61] Baseline renal impairment may be attenuated by correction of hyponatremia, volume expansion with human albumin solution, and the use of acetylcysteine for 48 hours, although there is a lack of trial evidence to support this.[61] Active spontaneous bacterial peritonitis (SBP) is a potential risk for contamination of the stent graft being implanted. The prevalence of SBP in hospitalized cirrhotic patients ranges between 10% and 30%. The diagnosis is established with an ascites polymorphonuclear (PMN) count greater than 250/mm.[66] Thus if the indication for TIPS is not an emergency, the procedure is usually postponed until the SBP has cleared.

Prognostic capabilities for prediction of mortality at 30 days and 90 days demonstrated with the receiver operating characteristic curves after TIPS placement were better for MELD and MELD-Na when compared with bilirubin, Child-Pugh, Emory, prognostic index (PI), acute physiology and chronic health evaluation (APACHE 2), and Bonn TIPS early mortality (BOTEM).[67] Rubin et al.[68] found that the pre-TIPS APACHE II score was the single determinant most strongly associated with decreased survival in the month after a TIPS procedure. Patients undergoing an emergency TIPS procedure who have a Child-Pugh score of 12 or higher along with an APACHE II score of 18 or higher (or patients with a PI of 18 or higher) are expected to have a very high risk of early death after the procedure[69] (see Chapter 4). Garcia-Pagan et al.[70] described a score predicting the probability of mortality or requiring a liver transplant after TIPS in patients with Budd-Chiari syndrome based on age, bilirubin, and INR. Patients with a score greater than 7 have a high probability of mortality or requiring liver transplantation after TIPS placement in Budd-Chiari syndrome patients.[70]

Diagnostic Imaging

Preprocedural cross-sectional imaging is crucial to evaluate vascular patency and anatomic variants of the portal and hepatic vein circulation, as well as the liver arterial supply. Liver vascular ultrasound can be used pre-TIPS but can have limitations depending on the body habitus.[71] The presence of portal vein thrombosis, patency of the splenic and mesenteric veins, and evidence of cavernous transformation may technically challenge the access into the portal vein and can help to determine if additional percutaneous transsplenic or transhepatic access is necessary. Evaluation of patency and potential flow limiting stenosis of the hepatic artery, celiac artery, or superior mesenteric artery, as well as the presence of a replaced or accessory hepatic artery, is crucial to anticipate any potential liver hypoperfusion after TIPS. Biliary abnormalities can precipitate infection or fistulae and need to be identified and treated before proceeding with TIPS. The presence and location of liver lesions and tumor vascular invasion can preclude TIPS feasibility and need to be evaluated (see Chapters 2, 14, and 15).

Anesthesia Evaluation

TIPS is painful and typically requires general anesthesia. Hemodynamic changes, fluid shifts, hemorrhage, transfusion of blood products, and use of vasoactive pressor during TIPS procedure can be difficult to manage by the interventionist. Performing TIPS procedures under general anesthesia allows a dedicated anesthesiologist to manage these complex and frequently critically ill patients, freeing the interventionist to concentrate on the technical aspects of the procedure.[94] If moderate sedation is used, anticipation of the most painful portions of the procedure may allow for deeper sedation during these segments[71] (see Chapters 26 and 106).

Antibiotic Prophylaxis

During the intervention, inadvertent puncture of the biliary ducts or contamination with skin or enteric flora can result in systemic infection or "endotipsitis" (i.e., infection of the stent). The incidence of endotipsitis has been reported in the literature up to 1% to 2%,[72] and the diagnosis is frequently made by exclusion of other sources. Long-term antibiotics including coverage for gram-negative organisms and fungi may be necessary. For coverage of biliary and enteric flora, much wider spectrum coverage is necessary.[71]

TIPS TECHNIQUE

Modifications to the initial described technique have been evolving in order to reduce complications. Those changes include the insertion of a control expandable PTFE-covered stent graft, a multistep dilation of the shunt, and intravascular ultrasonography guidance.

Catheterization of the Hepatic Vein

The procedure is started by accessing the jugular vein. If both internal jugular veins are occluded, collateral veins or external jugular veins can sometimes be used for access. Next, a hepatic vein (HV) is catheterized as the starting point for creating the transhepatic tract; typically, the right HV is usually chosen because of its larger size.

Mapping the Portal Vein

Multiple mapping methods to access the portal vein have been developed, including the use of CO_2 wedged hepatic venography, IVUS guidance, a delayed venous angiographic phase, or fusion of preexisting CT or magnetic resonance imaging (MRI) using a special software added to real-time fluoroscopy. A recanalized umbilical vein can be percutaneously punctured and a catheter can be advanced into the portal vein to take a venogram and target it. Other invasive methods are used and are more important when portal vein thrombosis is present. Those methods include transhepatic puncture of the portal vein or transsplenic puncture of the splenic vein, in which case a catheter is advanced into the Superior Mesenteric Vein (SMV) confluence and main portal vein if it is still present. Some of these methods imply a higher risk of bleeding.

Carbon dioxide (CO_2) venogram is obtained using nonballoon or balloon end hole catheters with a wedged location in the proximal hepatic vein to diffuse the gas across the hepatic sinusoids into the portal vein. The major reported complication of this technique is potential hepatic capsular rupture, which has been more frequently associated with very peripherally positioned end hole catheters.[73,74] While the balloon catheter is in place, it is recommended to measure free and wedged HV pressures to determine the Hepatic Venous Pressure Gradient (HVPG) or sinusoidal gradient and confirm the presence of portal hypertension before creating the TIPS. Monescillo et al.[75] have demonstrated that stratifying patients into low-risk (HVPG <20 mm Hg) and high-risk (>20 mm Hg) categories predicts the risk of recurrent bleeding and the chance of medical treatment failure. However, these pressures can be misleading; PVT may artifactually lower the wedged pressure because it is a presinusoidal obstruction. Also, some patients who have gigantic varices or spontaneous portosystemic venous shunts decompressing the portal vein may have normal portal pressures even when measured directly in the portal vein. The decision to proceed with a TIPS is often is based on other clinical and endoscopic evidence of portal hypertension, not on the HVPG measurement alone.

The use of IVUS with a 90-degree side-fire intracardiac echocardiography (ICE) catheter has been implemented to provide real-time ultrasound guidance to target specific segments of the portal vein. In a retrospective study of 109 patients comparing safety and effectiveness of IVUS-guided portal vein access with fluoroscopic TIPS technique, IVUS guidance demonstrated shorter portal vein access times, decreased needle pass–related capsular perforations, and reduced radiation dose.[76] A second study with 68 patients reported that IVUS facilitated successful TIPS creation in patients with challenging anatomy and reduced important procedure metrics, including radiation exposure, contrast agent volume, and overall procedure duration, compared with fluoroscopically guided TIPS creation.[77] Technically, two separate venous accesses are obtained, the second to insert and manipulate the 5- to 10-MHz IVUS probe.

The critical aspects that IVUS affects are to select the most appropriate hepatic vein based on proximity to the portal vein and visualization of the needle tip under real-time IVUS guidance as it is advanced in small increments toward the desired portal vein branch. The needle trajectory is adjusted as needed based on the anatomy and angulation of the targeted portal vein. IVUS guidance may benefit patients with compromised renal function by decreasing the volume of contrast used throughout the procedure. It may also reduce the risk of acute renal failure or nephrotoxicity, which is reported in up to 4% of cases.[78]

If the patient has a large umbilical vein collateral on the anterior abdominal wall, this can be punctured and used as a pathway to feed a catheter into the portal system. Through this catheter, contrast can be injected to delineate the portal anatomy, plus the catheter can be positioned to act as a real-time target for the transhepatic needle passes.

Additional approaches include percutaneous transhepatic puncture of the portal vein and percutaneous access of the splenic vein. In both scenarios, a direct portal venography using a catheter is obtained to establish a target. Recently, three-dimensional path planning software programs for use in modern angiographic units have been implemented that permit use of a preexisting CT or MRI to create a portal vein map and fuse it with cone beam CT using it as guidance in real-time fluoroscopy (Fig. 85.3).

TIPS Access and Shunt Insertion

Typically, the preferred target is the intrahepatic portal vein, because extrahepatic access increases the risk of intraabdominal hemorrhage. Routinely, the right portal vein from the right hepatic vein is the first choice for interventionists considering it to be associated with high success rate.[79] Studies have reported that TIPS created through the left portal vein were associated with a significantly lower rate of encephalopathy than right portal vein TIPS.[80,81]

A variation on TIPS is the direct intrahepatic portosystemic shunt (DIPS) procedure (Fig. 85.4). With this technique, a direct puncture is made from the intrahepatic IVC segment into the portal vein with or without IVUS guidance. The reported primary patency of DIPS at a mean of 256 days follow-up was 100%.[82]

Initial venography is performed to verify the correct portal vein access, to identify the point of entry into the portal system, and to make sure that a hepatic arterial branch was not inadvertently entered. Pressures should next be measured via the portal vein catheter and in the right atrium. This is necessary to establish the baseline pressures and portosystemic gradient, not only to confirm portal hypertension but to provide a baseline value against which the TIPS results will be compared. As mentioned before, a normal portal pressure needs to be evaluated in the clinical context and will not preclude the insertion, especially when portosystemic shunts are identified.

The tract is measured from the entry point in the portal vein back to the HV-IVC junction. It has been shown that patency is lower if the stent does not extend all the way to this point,[83] because stenosis can form above a TIPS even in short segments of uncovered HV (Fig. 85.5).

Regarding TIPS before liver transplant, multiple anatomic details should be considered. TIPS can complicate liver transplant operations by having the stent extend extrahepatically into the outflow of hepatic vein, the inferior vena cava, the main portal vein, or mesenteric vein (see Chapters 109 and 125). The exact incidence of adding difficulty to transplantation surgery is unknown but is thought to be relatively uncommon.[84] Few reports have described the impact of TIPS extending in the right atrium or main portal vein requiring surgical strategies such as direct anastomosis onto the TIPS–portal vein complex or latero-lateral cavo-caval anastomosis with running suture included the stent and the wall of the vein.[85,86]

The current standard of care is to use a stent graft and most used is the Viatorr device (W. L. Gore Inc., Flagstaff, AZ), which was specifically designed for TIPS. It has a 2-cm long, bare stent component that sits in the portal vein and a stent-graft segment

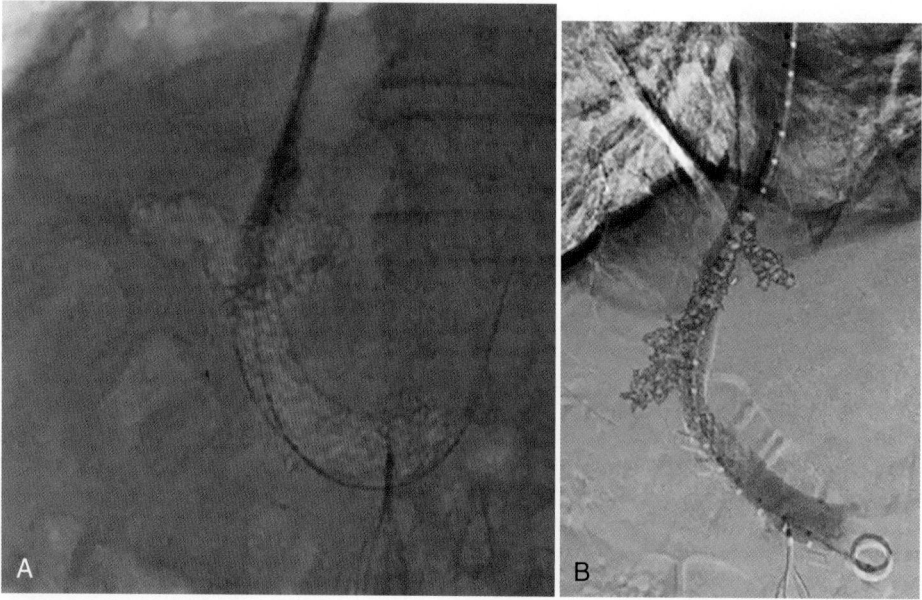

FIGURE 85.3 Three-dimensional (3D) mapping used during transjugular intrahepatic portosystemic shunt (TIPS) for accessing the portal vein. It is obtained as a result of fusion based on axial computed tomography image overlapped with a cone beam evaluation. A 3D map of the portal vein is available in real time during fluoroscopy and can be used as a target. **A,** In this case a wire was placed in the portal vein and the tract was dilated using an angioplasty balloon before inserting the stent. **B,** A TIPSogram is done through a marker pigtail that helps to measure and confirm the appropriate length and location of the shunt. A fused 3D map of the hepatic veins was used to identify the anatomic location of the distal end of the stent.

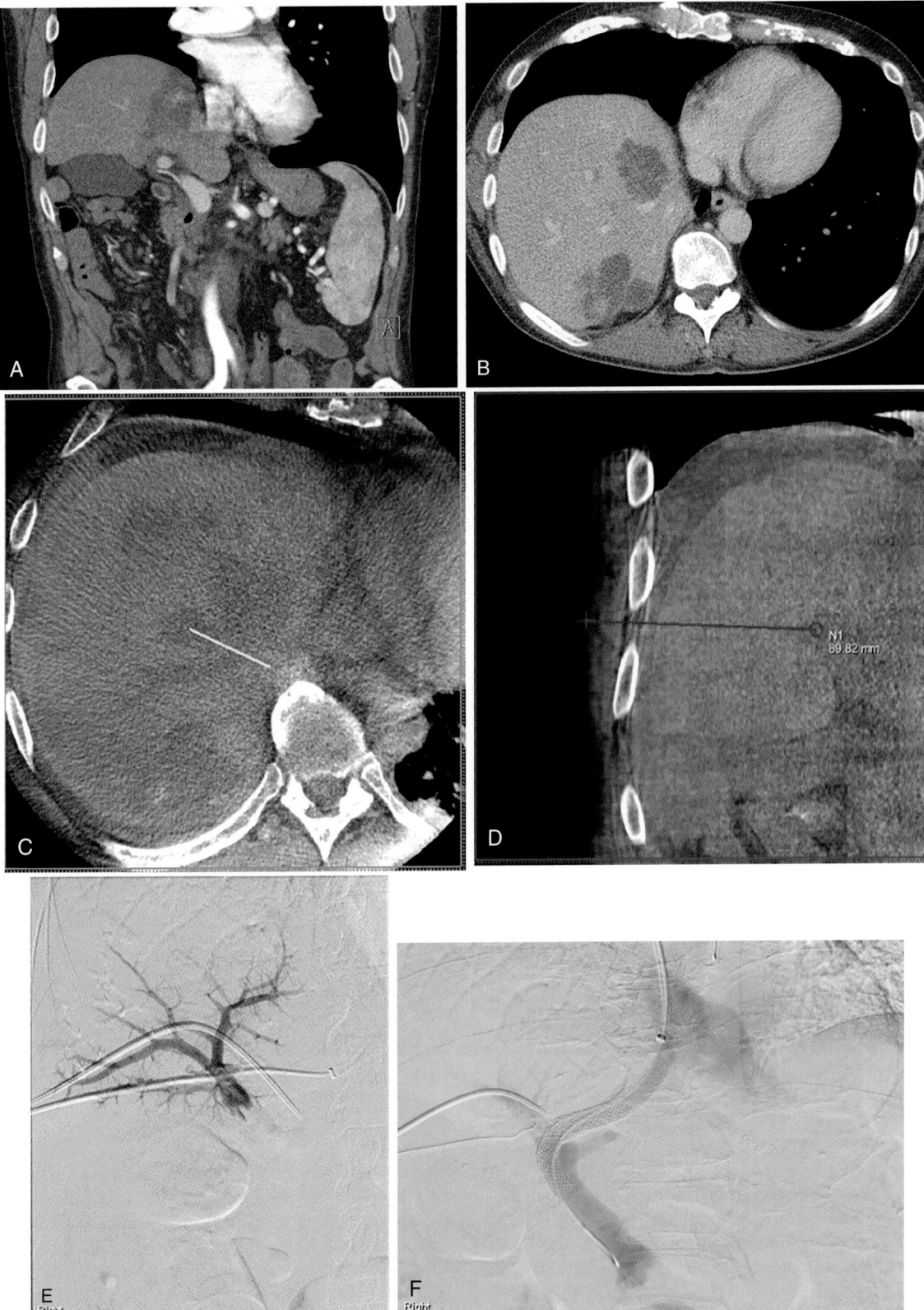

FIGURE 85.4   Direct portosystemic shunt (DIPS) in a patient with liver metastases. **A** and **B,** Computed tomography (CT) of abdomen with contrast, coronal and axial views, demonstrating multiple liver metastases involving the confluence of the hepatic veins. **C** and **D,** Cone beam CT (Dyna Ct) demonstrating the transparenchymal and percutaneous planning of DIPS using three-dimensional I-Guide software (Siemens). The demarked tracts preclude the puncture of the liver lesions. **E,** Direct percutaneous portogram and parallel percutaneous access across the portal vein into the inferior vena cava with portogram using the coaxial system of a vascular introducer. **F,** DIPSogram with injection in the main portal vein demonstrated widely patent shunt.   *Continued*

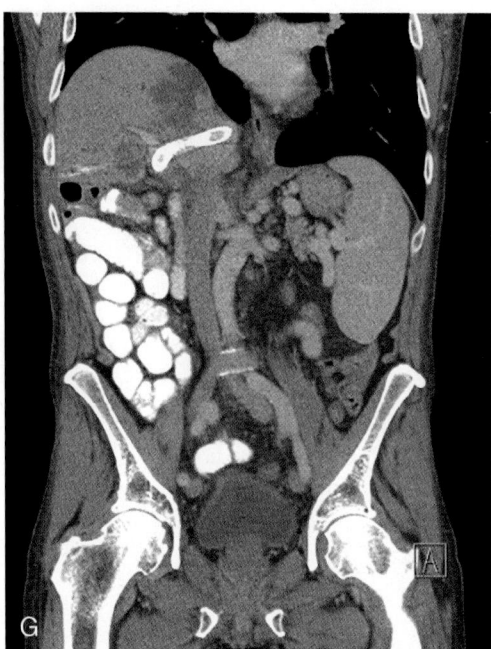

FIGURE 85.4, cont'd   G, Post-DIPS contrast CT of the abdomen showed the stent around the lesions without crossing them.

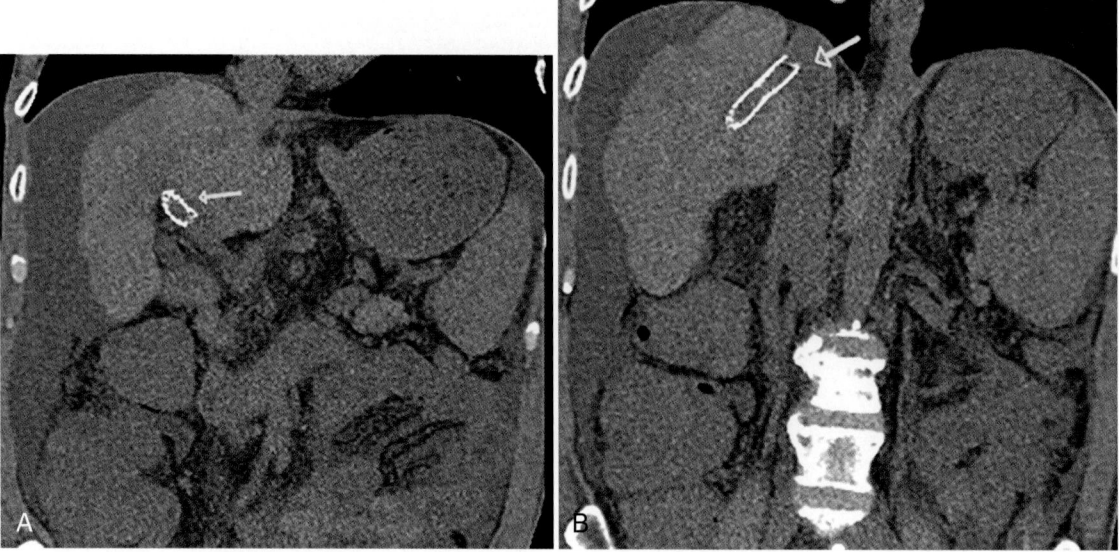

FIGURE 85.5   Post-TIPS noncontrast computed tomography of the abdomen demonstrating the appropriate location of the stent into the proximal portal vein at the confluence of the intrahepatic branches in **A** and 1 to 5 mm in the hepatic vein–inferior vena cava junction on **B** *(yellow arrows).*

length varying from 4 to 8 cm covering the parenchymal tract. Studies to date have shown significantly improved patency compared with stent grafts created with bare metal stents. For example, a randomized trial between Viatorr and bare-stent TIPS reported 2-year primary patency rates of 76% and 36%, respectively.[87] Besides the patency of TIPS, crucial factors to consider are the final stent diameter and portosystemic gradient (PSG). Complications related to portosystemic shunting, such as Hepatic Encephalopathy (HE), accelerated liver failure, hepatic insufficiency, and congestive heart failure, have been associated with overshunting and final shunt diameter. One concern that arose when stent grafts were first used was an increased potential for encephalopathy; however, encephalopathy rates have actually been lower with stent grafts than with bare metallic stents.[88,89]

Some authors have reported success with preemptive underdilation of the PTFE-covered Viatorr stents in patients with a high risk for post-TIPS encephalopathy, such as by dilating the 10-mm stent with an 8-mm balloon or varying balloon dilation within the stent to create an hourglass shape.[90] The multistep dilation strategy, with modulation of the TIPS diameter, deploying the stent at a diameter smaller than the nominal one as a first approach, has been recommended in the most recent consensus on TIPS management to prevent complications.[91] Aside from this concept, a newly available Viatorr TIPS endoprosthesis with controlled expansion (Viatorr CX) offers the operator the option to dilate the TIPS between 8 and 10 mm. MELD scores have also significantly improved in the Viatorr CX patients compared with noncontrolled TIPS expandable groups.[78,92]

BOX 85.3   Complications Related to TIPS Procedure

Transient arrhythmia or sustained supraventricular or ventricular tachycardia
Capsular puncture or perforation
Injuries of the kidney, bowel, gallbladder, or pancreas
Extrahepatic puncture of the main portal vein
Inadvertent puncture of the hepatic artery
Arterioportal fistulae
Intrahepatic biliary duct puncture
Biliary fistulae, hemobilia, cholangitis, sepsis, and stent infection
TIPS stent migration
Undesired migration of embolization material
Rupture of varices during embolization
Hepatic encephalopathy
Liver failure and hepatic insufficiency
Segmental liver infarctions
Acute kidney injury (higher-impact patients with emergent TIPS for acute bleeding)
Severe allergy to iodinated contrast medium
Increased radiation dose

TIPS, Transjugular intrahepatic portosystemic shunt.

After stent-graft deployment, repeat portal venogram is performed, and pressure measurements are taken to confirm proper placement of the device, assess for complications related to stent placement, and ensure that the portal system has been adequately decompressed. The venogram should show good flow through the shunt and no further flow in varices or collateral pathways. Pressure measurements should show a successful reduction in the portosystemic gradient. Typically, the target is to get the portosystemic gradient below 12 mm Hg, the commonly accepted threshold below which variceal bleeding is unlikely. However, resolution of ascites may require a slightly lower PSG, down around 8 mm Hg. If the PSG is too high, careful venography and a pull-back pressure measurement are necessary to ensure that the tract is fully stented and that there are no kinks or thrombi that might be limiting flow through the shunt. In some patients, the gastroesophageal varices may still fill on the post-TIPS venography despite adequate lowering of the PSG. These pathways may be so large that the resistance to flow through them is the same as or less than the resistance to flow through the TIPS; therefore embolization of these vessels may be needed to eliminate flow through them and redirect flow through the shunt.

COMPLICATIONS

The reported risk related to TIPS for minor complications is 4%, and for major complications it is 3%[71,93] (Box 85.3). Advancing wires across the heart can precipitate transient arrhythmia. Occasionally, a sustained supraventricular or ventricular tachycardia requires urgent treatment. These patients also often exhibit electrolyte imbalances aggravating the risk of arrhythmia.

Inadvertent puncture of the hepatic artery occurs with an incidence of approximately 6%.[94] In general, transjugular hepatic arterial puncture carries low clinical significance because the rate of symptomatic arterial injuries is less than 2%.[95] Puncture of the hepatic artery can precipitate severe complications, including hemorrhage, pseudoaneurysm formation, vascular dissection or occlusion, and arterioportal fistula, which may result in worsening of preexisting portal hypertension. Segmental liver infarctions can be secondary to portal or hepatic vein thrombosis

but are also related to hepatic arterial injury. Clinical outcomes varied significantly, from transient problems to acute liver failure with high mortality rates, and depending on the severity the patients may require liver transplantation.[96]

Also, unrecognized selection of the inferior accessory right hepatic vein can increase the risk of accidental capsular puncture as well as injuries of the kidney, bowel, gallbladder, or pancreas. The reported rate of gallbladder puncture is under 10%, and that of right kidney is 1.5%.[97] If the hemodynamic status changes due to capsular puncture, the initial treatment is to tamponade with the balloon and embolize the vessel using coils. Extrahepatic puncture of the main portal vein can be associated with massive hemoperitoneum, which can lead to death.[98,99]

Intrahepatic biliary duct puncture can occur in up to 5% of cases.[97] A fistulous communication between biliary and vascular system may result in hemobilia, cholangitis, sepsis, and stent infection.

Stent migration during deployment has also been described, but the risk is low at 1%.[97] More common is the stent graft assuming an unexpected straighter shape after deployment or after removal of the guidewire, which can result in retraction of the cranial end from the hepatic venocaval junction requiring additional stenting. Malposition or migration of a TIPS stent into the suprahepatic vena cava, right atrium, or main portal vein potentially complicates native hepatectomy and graft implantation.[49,100]

Undesired migration of embolization material is a risk when varices or competitive portosystemic shunts are either sclerosed or embolized after TIPS. Also, overinjection of liquid embolic material can lead to rupture of varices.

TIPS Reduction

Multiple techniques have been implemented to reduce the size of TIPS for patients with refractory encephalopathy. In patients with decompensated liver failure, the benefit of the reduction has been controversial, with some studies reporting no benefit.[101] The goal is to reduce the shunt diameter or completely occlude the stent to improve hepatopetal portal flow into the liver, increasing the ammonia metabolism and therefore decreasing the bloodstream levels. The decision of shunt reduction versus occlusion should be evaluated in the setting of possible complications of portal hypertension after the occlusion such as gastroesophageal variceal hemorrhage, mesenteric thrombosis, and intestinal ischemia.

Transjugular Shunt Dysfunction

TIPS dysfunction with recurrence or persistence of portal hypertension symptoms may represent either TIPS dysfunction or, more uncommonly, the need for placement of a second, parallel TIPS (more common when ascites or hepatohydrothorax is a symptom). In the first instance, Doppler ultrasound should be performed to evaluate for velocities of the main portal vein and shunt.[102] If the velocities measure ≤50 cm/sec or greater than 250 cm/sec, there may be a high degree of stenosis. In these cases, patients must undergo a TIPSogram with angioplasty or restenting if the MELD score permits that. In 2006 Helmy et al.[103] described 40 patients who received parallel TIPS with the TIPS insufficiency. After a mean follow-up period of 11.6 months, both the parallel shunts and the index shunt in the nonparallel shunt group behaved in a similar way regarding the cumulative primary shunt patency rates.[103]

The references for this chapter can be found online by accessing the accompanying Expert Consult website.

CHAPTER 86

Budd-Chiari syndrome and veno-occlusive disease

C. Kristian Enestvedt and Susan L. Orloff

Among the etiologies of portal hypertension, those caused by postsinusoidal obstruction are seen infrequently by most clinicians. Nonetheless, these disease processes represent complex clinical challenges and require a thorough knowledge of the available diagnostic and treatment modalities. Included in this group are Budd-Chiari syndrome and veno-occlusive disease. The latter condition is also referred to as *sinusoidal obstruction syndrome* and is most often seen after myeloablation with chemotherapy or radiation therapy before hematopoietic stem cell transplant.

BUDD-CHIARI SYNDROME

Budd-Chiari syndrome (BCS) is a group of disorders caused by occlusion of the major hepatic veins, the inferior vena cava (IVC), or both at or near the level of the hepatic vein ostia. Although a brief discussion of this clinical phenomenon first appeared in a book by Budd[1] in 1845, Lambron in 1842 is said to have reported the first case. In 1899 Chiari collected 10 cases and reported three personal cases and presented the first thorough clinicopathologic description of the syndrome, including the hypothesis that the underlying mechanism was endophlebitis of the hepatic veins. The weight of evidence, however, favors the current opinion that the primary process is usually thrombotic rather than inflammatory. Since publication of the initial description, more than 8000 cases of BCS have been described in the medical literature. In recent years the incidence has increased substantially, most likely as a result of increased awareness of BCS, improvements in diagnostic methods, and widespread use of thrombogenic agents, such as oral contraceptives.[2,3] Nevertheless, BCS remains a relatively uncommon condition. Contemporary reports place the incidence of BCS between 0.2 and 2 per 1 million population, but these numbers are not well established and show substantial regional and geographic variation.[4]

Obstruction of hepatic venous outflow produces intense congestion of the liver and the clinical manifestations of ascites, hepatomegaly, and abdominal pain. Depending on the rapidity and extent of obstruction of hepatic venous outflow, the course of BCS may be rapid or chronic, progressing to death in weeks or leading to death from liver failure or bleeding esophageal varices after an illness of months or occasionally years. In Western countries, a rapid course is common, and the outcome is often fatal in reported cases. With prompt diagnosis and improved therapeutics, however, this condition can be managed as a chronic condition or cured entirely. Effective surgical therapy developed at highly specialized centers enables durable decompression of the obstructed hepatic vascular bed. As a result, the previously dismal outlook for patients with BCS has improved considerably. The advent of less invasive measures, notably the introduction and wide adoption of transjugular intrahepatic portosystemic shunt (TIPS) and hepatic vein stent, has further reduced the morbidity related to BC (see Chapter 85).

For patients in whom these measures fail, liver transplantation remains a viable option, with excellent results despite recurrent disease in some reports (see Chapter 105). Many centers have adopted a stepwise approach to treatment, converting this once uniformly fatal process to a well-controlled, manageable condition.

Predisposing Conditions

Specific conditions are known to predispose to the development of BCS (Box 86.1). During the past 60 years, a marked change has been observed in the frequency with which a known cause or predisposing condition has been identified in patients with BCS. In the classic collective review of 164 cases of BCS reported by Parker in 1959,[5] a predisposing condition or etiology could not be identified in 70% of the patients. In recent years, the incidence of idiopathic cases of BCS has plummeted to less than 30%,[6-11] an improvement attributed to two factors: (1) a greater awareness of BCS and (2) improved diagnostic tools to identify the anatomic lesions and to diagnose thrombogenic hematologic disorders. In fact, many experts agree that there may be multiple predisposing risk factors for the development of this syndrome.

Regional variation in etiology between the East and West in the predisposing conditions and in the anatomic pattern of BCS has been recognized for some time (Table 86.1). The classic description of BCS falls under the primary designation and is directly attributable to thrombosis at the hepatic veins. Membranous obstruction of the vena cava (MOVC) is rare in the West, but it is a frequent cause of BCS in Eastern countries such as Japan, China, and India, as well as South Africa. In the West, thrombosis of the major hepatic veins alone is substantially more common than thrombosis or occlusion of the IVC, whereas in India, China, and Japan, IVC occlusion is much more common than hepatic vein occlusion alone. In North America, the acute or subacute forms of BCS predominate, and chronic BCS is observed less frequently, whereas in the East, the reverse is observed. In the West, BCS is seldom found during pregnancy or the postpartum period, whereas in India, pregnancy is a major predisposing condition for BCS. The same difference is seen in the incidence of infections, such as hepatic amebiasis (see Chapters 45 and 71), which are rare in the West but are reported frequently in series of BCS from India. The use of oral contraceptives (OCs) has been frequently associated with BCS in the United States, where OC use is widespread. Finally, an important distinction in etiology regarding the prevalence of myeloproliferative disorders (MPDs) highlights additional geographic differences. A recent study from China observed that MPDs were uncommon in the BCS cohort examined, whereas this is a frequent finding in Western studies.[12,13]

Hematologic Disorders

Hematologic diseases that cause vascular thrombosis are the most common conditions that predispose to BCS in North

---

BOX 86.1   Conditions Predisposing to Budd-Chiari Syndrome (BCS)

Primary BCS
Hematologic disorders
  Polycythemia vera
  Paroxysmal nocturnal hemoglobinuria
  Essential thrombocythemia
  Primary erythrocytosis
  Myelofibrosis
  Acute leukemias and lymphomas
  Hemolytic anemias
  Protein C deficiency
  Protein S deficiency
  Antithrombin III deficiency
  Lupus anticoagulant (antiphospholipid syndrome)
  Factor V Leiden mutation
  JAK2 V617F mutation
  Prothrombin (factor II) mutation
  Antiphospholipid syndrome
  Hyperhomocysteinemia
Oral contraceptives
Pregnancy and postpartum
Connective tissue disorders
  Behçet's syndrome
  Sjögren's syndrome
  Mixed connective tissue disease
  Sarcoidosis
  Rheumatoid arthritis
  α_1-Antitrypsin deficiency
  Idiopathic hypereosinophilia syndrome
  Systemic lupus erythematosus
Membranous obstruction of inferior vena cava

Secondary BCS
Malignant neoplasms
  Hepatocellular carcinoma
  Renal cell carcinoma
  Adrenal carcinoma
  Leiomyosarcoma of inferior vena cava
  Others (carcinomas of lung, pancreas, and stomach; melanoma;
    reticulum cell sarcoma; adrenal sarcoma; tumor of right atrium)
Infections
  Amebic liver abscess
  Aspergillosis
  Hydatid disease
  Schistosomiasis
  Syphilitic gumma
  Filariasis
Trauma
Iatrogenic
  Malposition/occlusion of transjugular intrahepatic portosystemic shunt
  Caval filter dysfunction

TABLE 86.1   Differences Between West and East in Predisposing Conditions and Anatomic Patterns of Budd-Chiari Syndrome (BCS)

FEATURE	WEST	EAST
Membranous obstruction of the IVC	Rare	Frequent
Hepatic vein occlusion predominates	+	−
IVC occlusion predominates	−	+
Acute or subacute BCS predominates	+	−
Chronic BCS predominates	−	+
Pregnancy/postpartum	Uncommon	Frequent
Infection	Rare	Common
Oral contraceptives	Frequent	Uncommon
Myeloproliferative disease	Common	Rare

IVC, Inferior vena cava.

---

the series of 77 cases reported by Orloff et al.,[15] 31% had polycythemia vera, and its association with BCS was noted to diverge from the classic description of BCS in several ways. First, it was found more often in young adults, rather than in middle-aged and elderly patients. Second, polycythemia vera has been shown to be responsive to treatment with hydroxyurea, which should be started as soon as the disease is discovered and continued for life. Other treatments for polycythemia vera include serial phlebotomy, anagrelide, interferon alfa-2b, and ruxolitinib, recently approved by the US Food and Drug Administration (FDA). Whatever treatment regimen is used, the disease runs a benign course if treated early.

Paroxysmal nocturnal hemoglobinuria (PNH) is another hematologic disorder associated with BCS.[16–19] It was responsible for 6.7% of the cases in the collected series of Mitchell et al.[8] and 12% of the cases in the series of Valla et al..[19] In all the hematologic disorders associated with hepatic vein thrombosis, but particularly in PNH, thrombosis of other splanchnic vessels and even extraabdominal vessels has been observed.[20] When diagnosed early, PNH should be treated with eculizumab to prevent long-term sequelae.

While hematologic diagnosis has become progressively more sophisticated, many other thrombogenic conditions have been identified in BCS, including other myeloproliferative states (e.g., essential thrombocythemia, primary erythrocytosis, myelofibrosis) and thrombophilic states, such as protein C deficiency, protein S deficiency, antithrombin III deficiency, and antiphospholipid syndrome with lupus anticoagulant or anticardiolipin antibodies or both.[7,11,21–30] Patients with the factor V Leiden mutation, which leads to activated protein C resistance, have a 5-fold to 10-fold increase in the risk of thrombosis if they are heterozygotic and a 50-fold to 100-fold increase if they are homozygotic.[23,31,32] More recent evidence indicates that multiple prothrombotic factors acting concurrently are involved in a substantial percentage of patients with BCS.[32,33] Rarely, hematologic malignancies, such as acute leukemia and lymphoma, have been associated with BCS.

In 2005 identification of the underlying cause of BCS was enhanced by the discovery of a very reliable and noninvasive marker for chronic MPDs. The marker is the gain-of-function mutation V617F of the *JAK2* gene.[34–41] By combining identification of this marker with results of bone marrow histology and clonality assay, more than 50% of BCS cases have been found to be caused by an underlying chronic MPD.[42]

America and Western Europe. Of disorders with thrombotic tendencies, myeloproliferative diseases (MPDs) are most often associated with BCS. A review of reported cases indicates myelodysplasia as an underlying etiology in approximately half of affected patients.[14] A recent meta-analysis of BCS studies implicates MPD in 40.9% of 1062 reported cases of BCS.[13] Historically, *polycythemia vera* has been the most frequently occurring of the MPDs in BCS patients, constituting 8.5% of the cases of BCS in the collected series of Parker[5] and 10.4% of the cases in the collected series of Mitchell et al..[8] However, in contemporary series the prevalence is considerably higher. In

It cannot be overemphasized that every patient found to have BCS should undergo a thorough hematologic evaluation. The assessment is an expansion of the workup proposed by Mahmoud and Elias[43] and others[4,44] (Box 86.2). With these studies, it should be possible to diagnose all the known predisposing thrombogenic hematologic disorders associated with BCS. If this evaluation is uniformly performed, the incidence of idiopathic BCS will likely continue to decline.

Oral Contraceptives

An increased incidence of thromboembolic phenomena involving various blood vessels and organs in women taking OCs has been well established. The first case of BCS associated with OC use was reported by Ecker and McKittrick,[45] 5 years after these drugs became available commercially. Since then, more than 200 cases of BCS in patients taking OCs have been described,[2,3,32,46,47] and the increasing overall incidence of BCS in recent years has been attributed partly to the widespread use of these agents. In the collective review reported by Mitchell et al.,[8] use of OCs was believed to be responsible for 9.4% of BCS cases from 1960 to 1980. Valla et al.[3] reported a relative risk of 2.37 for hepatic vein thrombosis among OC users, similar to that of cerebrovascular accident (stroke), myocardial infarction, and venous thromboembolism. Recent literature, however, has questioned the strength of the association between OCs and venous thrombotic disease. It has been proposed that OCs are not a primary cause of BCS but contribute to thrombosis only if there is an underlying hematologic disorder.[3] In addition to causing BCS, OCs have been linked to other liver disorders, including veno-occlusive disease, portal vein thrombosis, cholestasis, hepatocellular adenoma, and possibly hepatocellular carcinoma and angiosarcoma.[47,48]

Pregnancy and Postpartum

Budd-Chiari syndrome has been observed in women during pregnancy and, more often, during the postpartum period. The first case of BCS reported by Chiari[49] occurred in a woman who developed the disorder after childbirth. In the collective review by Mitchell et al.,[8] 9.9% of BCS cases occurred during pregnancy or postpartum, and in a series of 105 patients with BCS observed from 1963 through 1978, Khuroo and Datta[50] reported 16 patients (15.2%) with BCS after pregnancy; 8 patients died, and 7 were lost to follow-up after discharge. The hypercoagulable state that is known to occur during pregnancy is presumed to be responsible for the association with BCS, although only 1 of 77 cases of BCS occurred peripartum in a recently reported large series.[15] As with OCs, it is increasingly clear that many patients in whom BCS develops in association with pregnancy may also have an underlying thrombophilia, either inherited or acquired.[51]

Malignant Neoplasms

Occlusion of the suprahepatic IVC by invasive tumors has been the cause of BCS in numerous case reports. This etiology represents prototypical secondary BCS. The most common cancers associated with BCS are hepatocellular carcinoma (see Chapter 89), renal cell carcinoma, adrenal carcinoma, and leiomyosarcoma of the IVC. An example of a cholangiocarcinoma occluding the intrahepatic portion of the IVC is shown in Fig. 86.1A. Other malignancies that have been infrequently associated with BCS include carcinomas of the lung, pancreas, and stomach; melanoma; reticulum cell sarcoma; adrenal sarcoma; and sarcoma of the right atrium.

Infections

Infections involving the liver were believed to be responsible for 3% of BCS cases reviewed by Parker,[5] 9.9% of the cases reported by Mitchell et al.,[8] and none of the cases in sizable series reported in more recent years. The most common infections associated with BCS are those caused by parasites, particularly amebic liver abscesses, hydatid disease, and schistosomiasis (see Chapters 73 and 74). Syphilitic gumma of the liver accounted for 1.8% of BCS cases in Parker's review but has not been reported as a cause of BCS in recent years. Aspergillosis involving the hepatic veins and IVC has been a rare cause of BCS. In India, Victor et al.[52] provided evidence that filariasis can cause BCS. These cases represent rare entities that are infrequently reported in BCS literature, but may be more prevalent than reported in developing countries where health reporting is limited.

Trauma

Abdominal trauma may in particular circumstances predispose patients to the development of BCS (see Chapter 113). Trauma was responsible for 1.2% of BCS cases reported by Parker[5] and 2.4% of the cases reviewed by Mitchell et al..[8] Blunt and penetrating trauma have been implicated occasionally in BCS patients, in whom severe liver injury leads to deep laceration at the level of the hepatic veins. Endothelial injury at this location can lead to thrombosis, scar, and ultimately the development of BCS.

Connective Tissue Disorders

Occasional cases of BCS have been reported in association with various connective tissue and autoimmune diseases, most of which are known to have thrombotic tendencies, including Behçet's disease, Sjögren's syndrome, mixed connective tissue disease, sarcoidosis, and rheumatoid arthritis. Numerous cases of BCS in patients with Behçet's disease have been described.[53,54] A recent large series examining vascular complications in 5970 patients with Behçet's disease reported BCS in

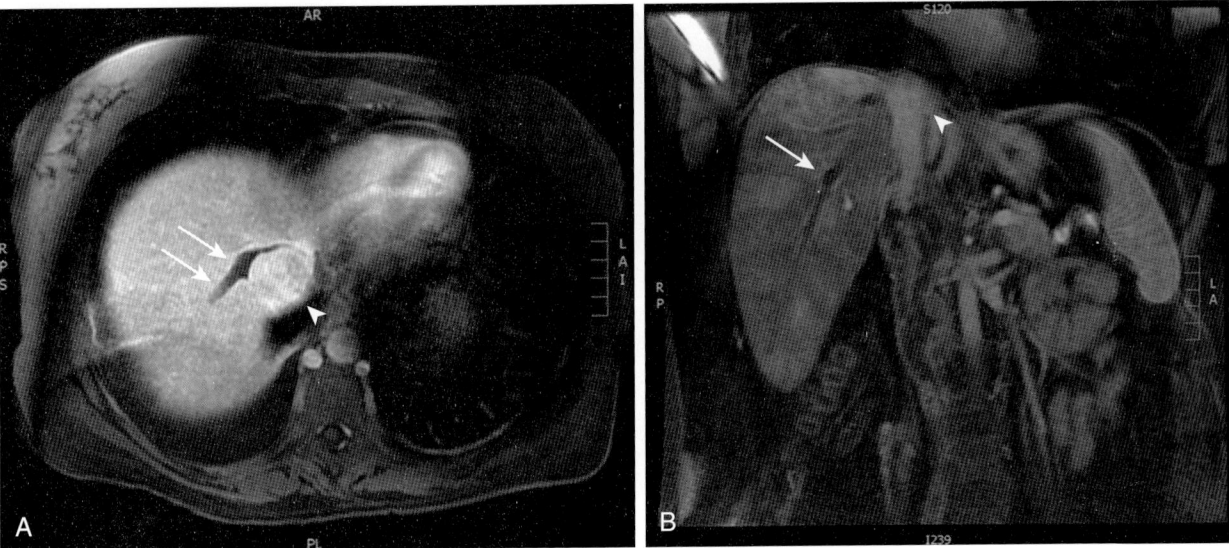

FIGURE 86.1   Axial **(A)** and coronal **(B)** magnetic resonance images demonstrate leiomyosarcoma *(white arrows)* of the intrahepatic inferior vena cava *(white arrowhead)* with nonopacification of the obstructed right hepatic vein (see Chapters 14 and 15).

2.4% of the 882 affected patients.[55] Median time from diagnosis to development of BCS was 2.3 years.

Membranous Obstruction of the Vena Cava (MOVC)

More than 600 cases of BCS resulting from MOVC have been reported from Japan,[56–61] China[62–64] and other parts of Asia, India,[50] and South Africa.[65] In the United States and Europe, MOVC is rare. A congenital cause of this condition has been proposed, but evidence strongly suggests it represents the end result of acquired thrombosis.[58,66,67]

MOVC usually runs a chronic course during many years, and extensive hepatic fibrosis or cirrhosis and portal hypertension will have developed in most patients by the time they come to medical attention. An increased incidence of hepatocellular carcinoma has been observed in association with MOVC.[58,65] The therapeutic implications of this condition and other forms of IVC occlusion are distinctly different from those of occlusion confined to the major hepatic veins.

Miscellaneous Rare Conditions

Other conditions that have been rarely associated with BCS include inflammatory bowel disease, hepatic torsion after partial resection of the liver, live-donor liver transplantation of the left lateral section, lipoid nephrosis, and protein-losing enteropathy. The latter two conditions are associated with a prothrombotic condition that may predispose patients to BCS.

Pathology

The liver receives approximately one-fourth of the cardiac output through its dual afferent blood supply: the portal vein and hepatic artery. After perfusing the sinusoids, the blood is returned to the heart through the hepatic veins and IVC. Obstruction to the egress of blood from the liver at any point along the outflow route results in numerous serious hemodynamic and morphologic alterations. There is a marked increase in intrahepatic pressure, which is reflected by a similar increase in portal pressure (see Chapters 5 and 74). The increased intrahepatic pressure causes extravasation of plasma from the liver sinusoids and lymphatics with formation of ascites (see Chapter 79).

Obstruction to the egress of blood from the liver also results in dilation of the sinusoids and intense centrilobular congestion of the hepatic parenchyma, which is greatest around the terminal hepatic venules (central veins) (Fig. 86.2). Ischemia, pressure necrosis, and atrophy of the parenchymal cells in the center of the liver lobule are apparent. With persistence of the obstruction, the necrotic parenchyma is replaced by fibrous tissue and regenerating nodules of liver tissue. The end result is cirrhosis of the type associated with chronic congestive heart failure, often referred to as *congestive hepatopathy*. The rapidity with which cirrhosis develops is related to the severity of outflow obstruction, but it is not unusual for cirrhosis to occur within months.[5] This pathophysiology is similar to that seen after liver transplantation in the patient with anastomotic venous outflow obstruction, with similar clinical manifestations.

The reversibility of liver damage in BCS is a direct function of the extent and duration of hepatic venous outflow obstruction. Early in the course of the disease, relief of the obstruction can be expected to result in reversal of the parenchymal and hemodynamic abnormalities. Late in the course, the damage to the hepatic parenchyma becomes irreversible; thus the timing of therapy has profound implications for the prognosis.

Three major hepatic veins—the right, left, and middle—conduct blood into the IVC from the bulk of the hepatic parenchyma. The left and middle hepatic veins usually form a common trunk just before joining the IVC, and several small hepatic veins, often termed *short hepatic veins*, enter directly into the retrohepatic IVC and drain the caudate lobe and small central regions of the right and left lobes of the liver (see Chapter 2). Initially, occlusion is limited to one or two of the major veins. During variable intervals, all three of the major hepatic veins become occluded. The small hepatic veins that join the retrohepatic IVC, particularly the veins draining the caudate lobe, often are spared. These veins ultimately form the basis for intrahepatic shunts because they are the only site for adequate parenchymal drainage.

In most patients with BCS, occlusion of the hepatic veins is caused by thrombosis.[5] The thrombus undergoes organization and ultimately is converted to fibrous tissue that permanently

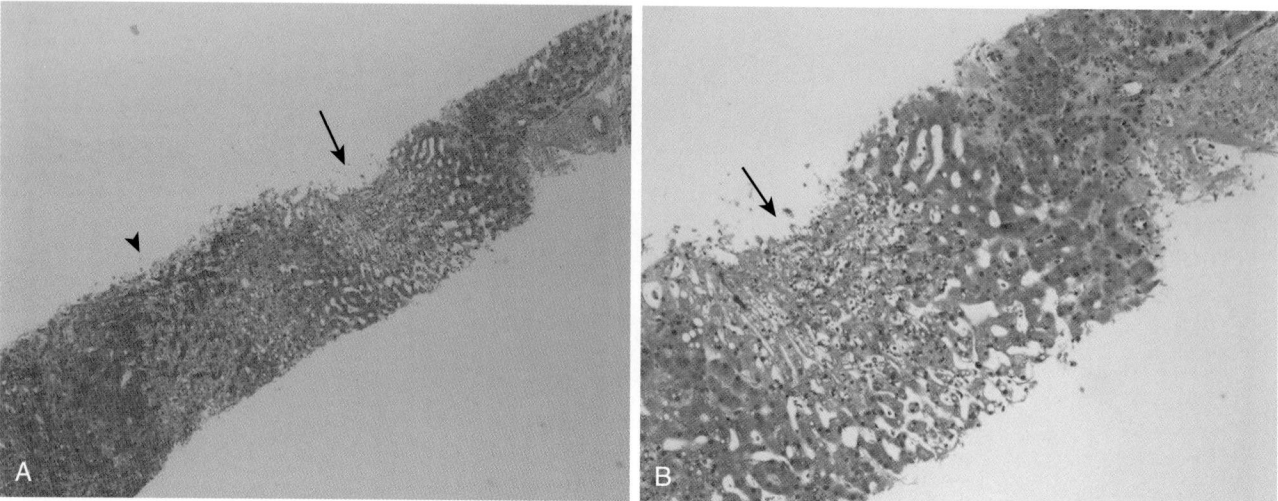

FIGURE 86.2 Liver biopsy demonstrating typical characteristics of venous outflow obstruction under low **(A)** and high **(B)** power. Note the marked sinusoidal congestion *(black arrowhead)* and hepatocyte atrophy *(black arrow)* (see Chapter 74).

occludes the veins. Although recanalization of the occluded veins sometimes occurs, it rarely results in effective new outflow channels. Indeed, chronic congestion of the liver leads to some degree of irreversible parenchymal injury. Retrograde propagation of the thrombus into smaller hepatic veins is typically found. Prograde propagation of the thrombus from the hepatic veins into the IVC, with partial or complete occlusion of the IVC, sometimes occurs and greatly changes the therapeutic approach and prognosis. With the use of imaging studies (e.g., angiography) and portosystemic pressure measurements, it is important to determine whether the IVC has become involved in the occlusive process.

In membranous obstruction of the IVC, the "membrane" varies from very thin to several centimeters thick and usually contains fibrous tissue, smooth muscle, and elastic tissue. The location and extent of the membrane vary considerably, and in some cases a long segment of IVC has been replaced by fibrous tissue. Occlusion of one or more of the major hepatic veins often has been associated with membranous obstruction of the IVC. MOVC has been reported to be the most common cause of BCS in Japan,[56,57,59–61,67] India,[50] and China,[62–64,68] and in the Bantu population of South Africa.[65] Although some experienced authors have proposed a congenital cause,[56,57,59,60,65] a strong argument has been made that suggests MOVC is the end result of thrombosis of the IVC, often occurring early in life.[58] Most of the cases have run a chronic course before discovery, and when first seen by a physician, patients have extensive hepatic fibrosis or cirrhosis with portal hypertension and all its manifestations. The therapeutic considerations in patients with MOVC differ from those in patients with BCS caused by obstruction of the hepatic veins.

Clinical Manifestations

The clinical manifestations and course of BCS are determined by the extent of occlusion of the hepatic venous outflow system and the rapidity with which the venous occlusion becomes complete. Patients can have an acute or subacute course (typical for patients in Western countries), with rapid progression of liver disease and its consequences during a few weeks to a few months. In some patients, however, BCS develops insidiously, with clinical manifestations appearing gradually during months

or years. Patients with MOVC observed in Japan, China, India, and South Africa often come to the physician for the first time with manifestations of well-established cirrhosis after tolerating symptoms for many years. The chronic form of BCS, regardless of etiology, is characterized by portal hypertension and its clinical sequelae.

In 77 patients reported by Orloff et al.,[15] 12 were referred with advanced cirrhosis, and the remaining 65 patients were referred at a mean 14 weeks after onset of BCS (range, 4–78 weeks). Of the 65 patients, 59 (91%) were referred at less than 18 weeks after onset of symptoms, relatively early in the course of BCS. However, in another contemporary single-center experience, most patients presented with advanced disease at diagnosis, with 92% exhibiting ascites and 55% with cirrhosis.[69] In the collected series of Mitchell et al.,[8] which excluded patients with MOVC, two-thirds had symptoms for less than 3 months and 83% had symptoms for 6 months or less at diagnosis. In his collected series of 133 patients, Parker[5] observed that 57% had symptoms for 3 months or less, and 71% had been symptomatic for 6 months or less.

Symptoms

Patients with BCS can present with most of the myriad symptoms associated with acute or chronic liver failure (see Chapter 77). The initial symptom in the majority of patients is abdominal distention secondary to ascites, which increases progressively over a few weeks (see Chapter 79). Abdominal distention caused by ascites occurs at some time in almost every patient with BCS. Most patients report abdominal pain that is dull, nagging, and chronic. The spectrum of pain is localized to the right hypochondrium, diffuse in the upper abdomen, or diffuse throughout the abdomen. The underlying pathophysiology is likely distention of the liver capsule from intense hepatic congestion or rapid accumulation of ascites. Many patients with acute BCS report striking and progressive weakness as a manifestation of their severe illness, with abrupt onset. Additionally, these patients are often malnourished, may exhibit severe anorexia, and can exhibit mild jaundice.

CHRONIC LIVER DISEASE. Patients with the chronic forms of BCS, such as MOVC, often have the usual symptoms of cirrhosis and portal hypertension, including upper gastrointestinal bleeding secondary to ruptured esophagogastric varices (see Chapters 80 and 81), hepatic encephalopathy, hepatorenal syndrome (see Chapter 77), and edema of the lower extremities (see Chapter 81). Peripheral edema is particularly prominent in patients with MOVC, and some experience varicose veins of the legs.[5,65]

Physical Examination Findings

Massive ascites on physical examination is one of the most common presenting signs at the time of BCS diagnosis. The reported incidence of ascites ranges from 83% to 100% in the larger reported series.[5,8,15,69] Hepatomegaly resulting from severe congestion of the liver occurs in most patients. Over time, this may dissipate to a degree, and in the chronic forms of BCS, hepatomegaly may not be as striking because the liver becomes cirrhotic and contracts. Substantial muscle wasting as a result of loss of lean body mass during a relatively short time is observed in many patients. Signs of portal hypertension are often exhibited, including distention of abdominal veins and palpable splenomegaly. Edema of the lower extremities or lower trunk may indicate involvement of the IVC in the occlusive process, although it is a common finding in patients with liver failure of various etiologies, including BCS. Also, patients with chronic BCS may have the usual manifestations of chronic liver disease: spider angiomata, palmar erythema, asterixis, breast hypertrophy, testicular atrophy, fetor hepaticus, and jaundice.

Diagnostic Studies

Ultrasonography

Real-time and Doppler duplex ultrasonography (US) of the liver has been shown to be of diagnostic value in BCS.[70–80] Findings include (1) absence of normal hepatic veins draining into the IVC with flat or reversed flow, (2) an abnormal intrahepatic network of comma-shaped venous structures, (3) thrombus in the IVC and flat or reversed flow in patients with IVC thrombosis, and (4) enlargement of the caudate lobe. Ascites has been shown regularly. US with Doppler may be used as an initial screening tool, with confirmation by computed tomography (CT), magnetic resonance imaging (MRI), or venography for a definitive diagnosis. Furthermore, US can be used as an appropriate guide to treatment and for surveillance after TIPS placement. Appropriate direction and flow velocity are key requirements for verification of TIPS patency (Fig. 86.3) (see Chapter 14).

Computed Tomography

Contrast-enhanced CT of the liver has considerable diagnostic value in BCS.[70,81–86] CT findings can be quite specific depending on the time course of BCS. In the early, acute period, CT demonstrates a liver with smooth contour (absent cirrhosis), lack of contrast enhancement in hepatic veins at both venous and delayed phases, compression of the intrahepatic IVC, and frequently the presence of ascites (Fig. 86.4A and B). In the subacute period, patchy enhancement is a harbinger of deranged blood flow through the liver (see Fig. 86.4C). Often, hepatomegaly is observed, with caudate hypertrophy and central enhancement (see Fig. 86.4D and E). Collateral vessel development is frequently seen with intrahepatic shunting. In the chronic phase, the liver can appear nodular and cirrhotic. Regenerative nodules often form, with arterial enhancement persisting through the venous phases, in contrast to hepatocellular carcinoma, which typically demonstrates washout in the venous phase. In the chronic stages, IVC occlusion may be observed (see Chapter 14).

Magnetic Resonance Imaging

Magnetic resonance imaging (MRI) is capable of showing patency or obstruction of the hepatic veins and is particularly effective in visualizing the entire length of the IVC. Imaging features are similar to those seen with CT scan. MRI has been useful in differentiating the acute form of BCS from the subacute and chronic forms.[81,83,84,87] MRI is an especially effective modality for patients with renal dysfunction, provided there is a relatively preserved glomerular filtration rate (>40). New contrast agents for MRI can even be used in the setting of chronic or acute kidney disease[19]. Furthermore, MRI is useful in differentiating regenerative nodules from hepatocellular carcinoma based on T2-weighted signal characteristics (Fig. 86.5A).[73] Similar to CT, MRI is efficacious at demonstrating intrahepatic collaterals and shunting (see Fig. 86.5B and C) (see Chapter 14).

Hepatic Venography and Pressure Measurements

Angiographic examination of the IVC and hepatic veins with pressure measurements is the diagnostic study of greatest value in BCS, particularly if interventional radiology or surgical therapy is contemplated. Venography remains the gold standard for diagnosis of BCS. This study may occasionally be combined with hepatic and superior mesenteric arteriography and indirect portography (see Chapters 4, 5, and 21). In BCS confined to the hepatic veins, the IVC is patent, and IVC pressure is relatively normal for

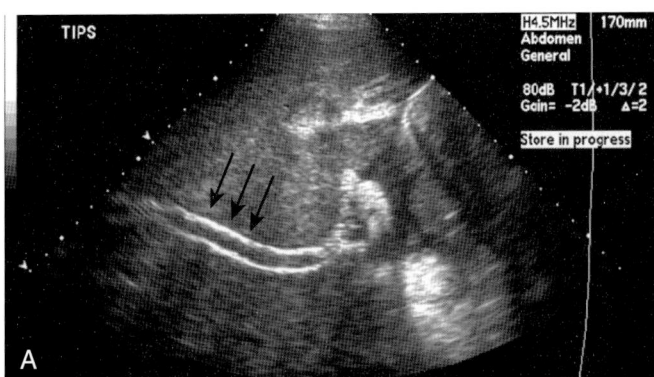
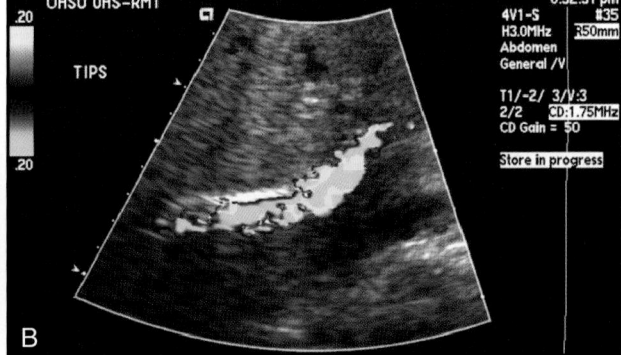

FIGURE 86.3 B-mode **(A)** and color Doppler **(B)** ultrasound images showing patent transjugular intrahepatic portosystemic shunt *(arrows)* with appropriate flow direction and velocity.

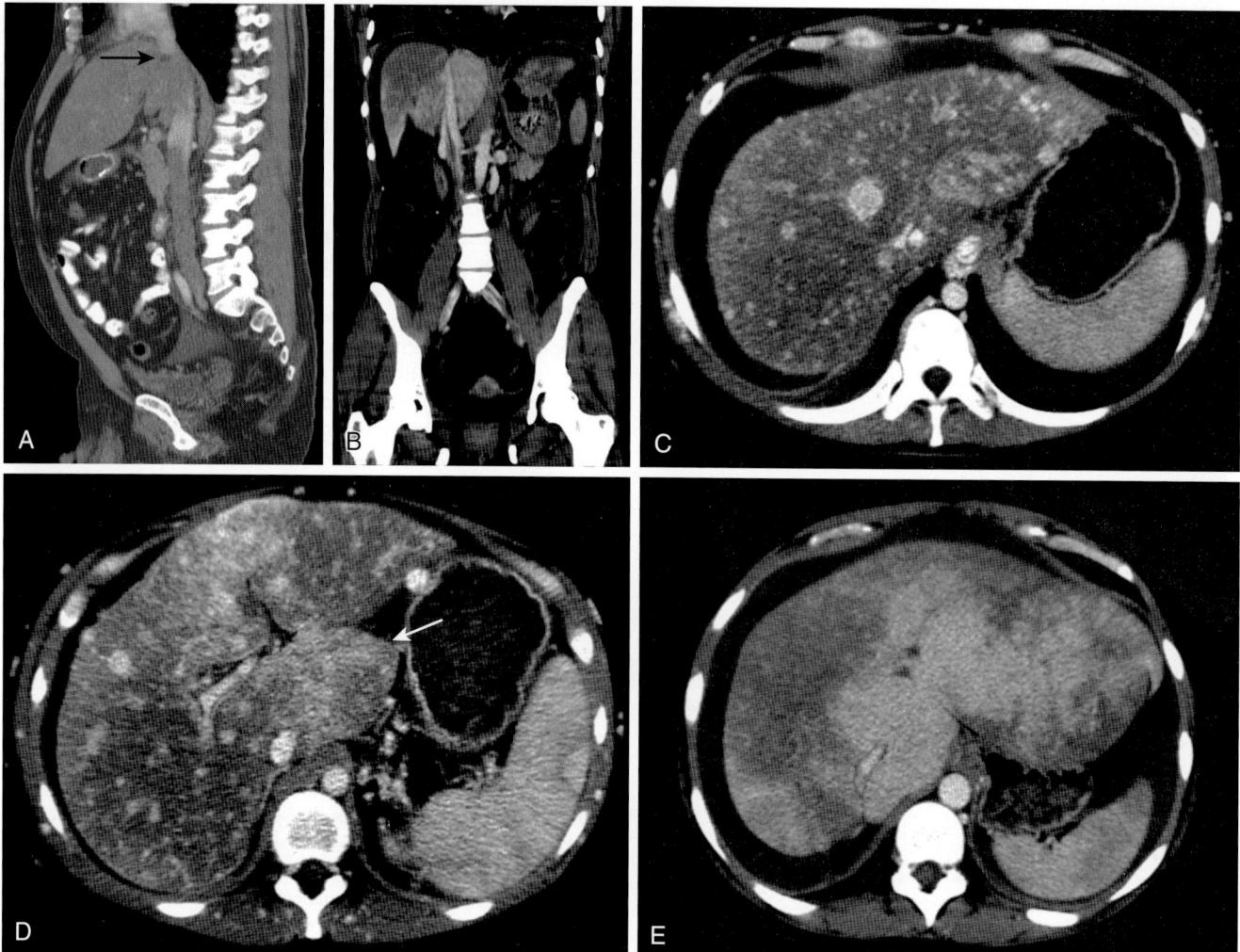

FIGURE 86.4 Early in the acute setting, Budd-Chiari syndrome is demonstrated on sagittal **(A)** and coronal **(B)** computed tomographic images, with subtle thrombosis in the hepatic veins with nonopacification *(black arrow)* and a smooth liver contour. With time, prominent intrahepatic vessels can be seen **(C)**, ascites develops, significant caudate hypertrophy occurs **(D,** *white arrow***)**, and heterogeneous enhancement is seen with central hyperenhancement and peripheral hypoenhancement **(E)** (see Chapter 14).

patients with ascites. A patent IVC is a prerequisite for portacaval shunt (PCS) and is a crucial finding (see Chapters 83 and 84). In some patients, the IVC is moderately compressed in its retrohepatic course by the enlarged liver and, in particular, by a hypertrophied caudate lobe (Fig. 86.6A). This finding usually is not clinically significant unless severe compression precludes surgical shunting. In some cases, an IVC stent can be placed percutaneously by the interventional radiology team, to expand the compressed IVC and allow appropriate portal decompression by the surgical shunt.[88–91]

The most important angiographic finding is the demonstration by hepatic venography of occlusion or marked narrowing of the major hepatic veins. In some cases, patent hepatic vein orifices cannot be identified, which is indirect evidence that all the major hepatic veins are occluded. Usually, however, it is possible to enter at least one major hepatic vein and show the presence of a thrombus or narrowing and distortion of the vein (see Fig. 86.6B). Injection of dye in the wedged hepatic venous position often shows a characteristic spider-web pattern of small hepatic venous collaterals connecting to portal or systemic veins (see Fig. 86.6C). Wedged hepatic vein pressure (WHVP) usually

is greatly elevated, which reflects the obstruction to hepatic venous outflow. In patients with hepatic vein occlusion alone, IVC pressure is substantially lower than WHVP.

Most often in contemporary management, venography is a platform for interventional radiology procedures. These include TIPS placement, catheter-directed thrombolysis, mechanical thrombectomy and balloon angioplasty, and recanalization of an occluded hepatic vein or vena cava with stent placement (Fig. 86.7). An additional advantage of hepatic venography is facilitating transjugular liver biopsy. Use of hepatic venography offers an essential guide and road map for surgical therapy in BCS.[81,83]

Liver Biopsy

Percutaneous or transjugular needle liver biopsy yields histologic findings characteristic of BCS early in the disease course; along with hepatic angiography, it provides conclusive diagnostic information.[92] The diagnostic features are quite spectacular and include intense centrilobular congestion combined with centrilobular loss of parenchyma and necrosis (see Fig 86.2). Mild to moderate fibrosis of the liver parenchyma is found in

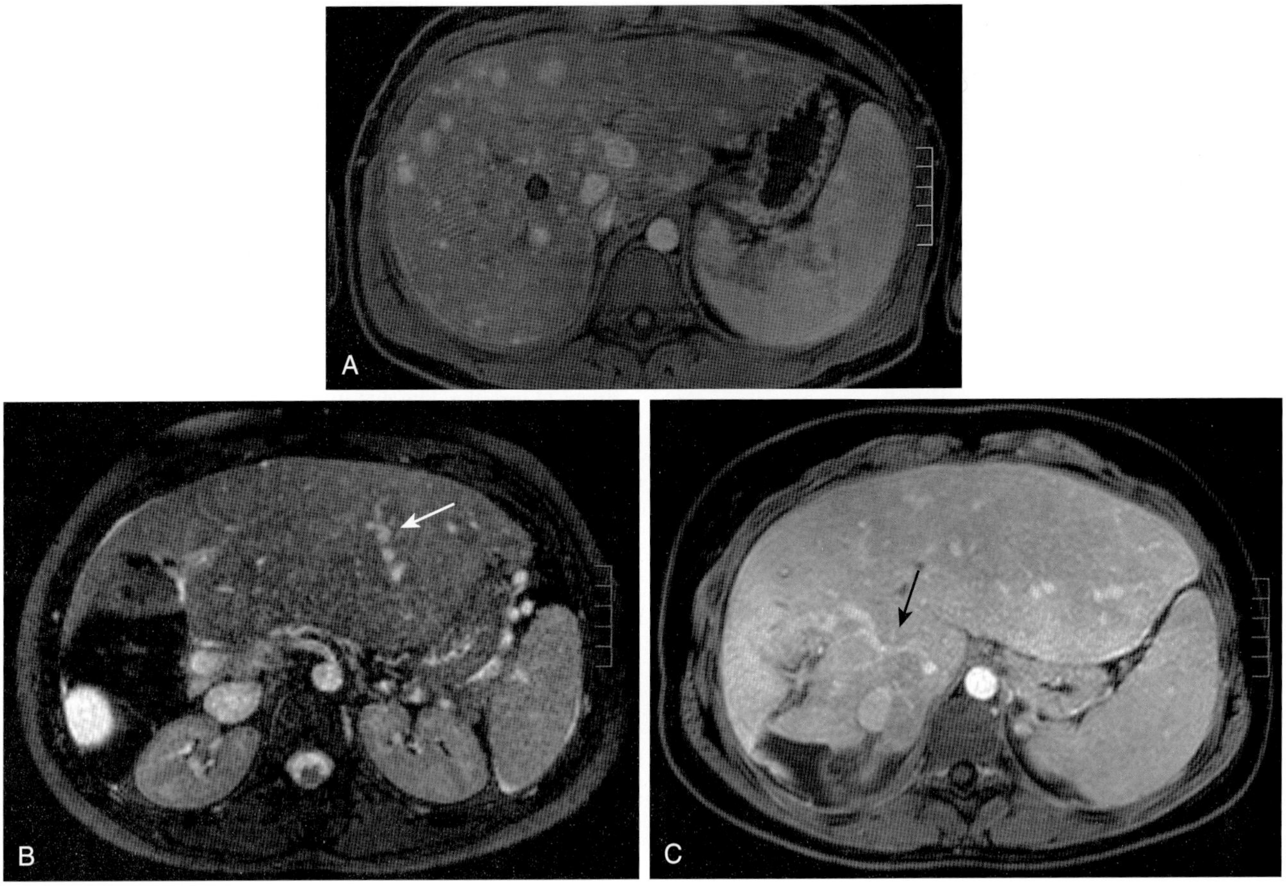

FIGURE 86.5 Further sequelae seen on axial magnetic resonance images include development of diffuse nodular disease (**A**); growth of large intrahepatic, often comma-shaped collaterals (**B,** *white arrow*); and intrahepatic shunts (**C,** *black arrow*) between the portal system and the caudate lobe (see Chapter 14).

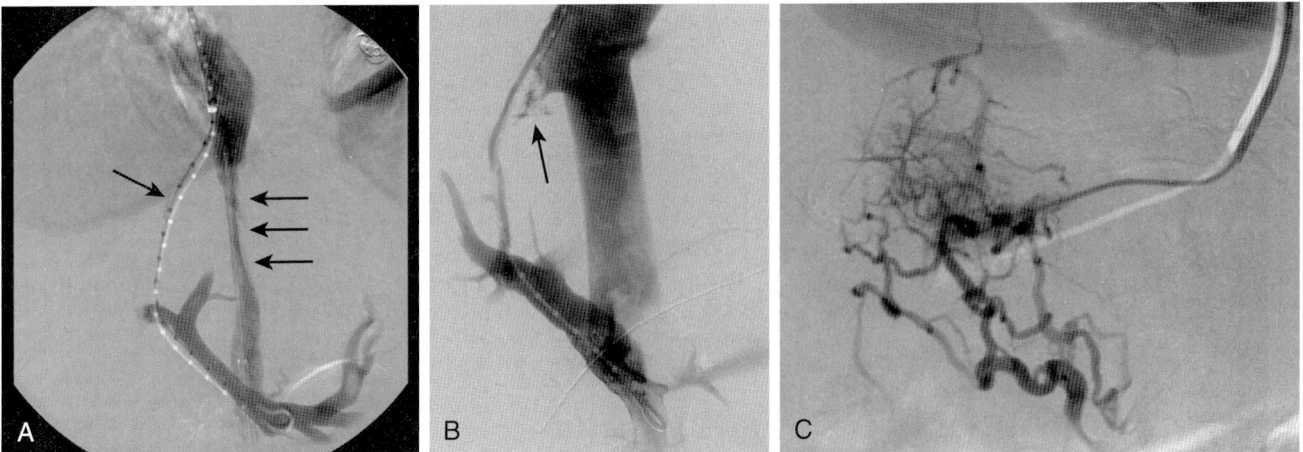

FIGURE 86.6 Venogram of the inferior vena cava demonstrates compression of the intrahepatic portion of the cava (**A,** *black arrows*) during placement of a transjugular intrahepatic portosystemic shunt *(single black arrow)*. Most often, one of the occluded veins can be cannulated, often showing thrombus (**B,** *black arrow*). Further injection after accessing the hepatic vein may demonstrate the classic "spider web" pattern of small, intrahepatic venous collaterals (**C**).

early and subacute disease, but in chronic or rapidly progressive disease, cirrhosis similar to congestive hepatopathy of cardiac origin develops. In fact, cirrhosis has been observed within months of the onset of symptoms. Only two other conditions, the latter of which is referenced above, constrictive pericarditis and congestive heart failure, produce a histologic picture similar to that seen in the acute stage of BCS. Both of these cardiac

disorders can be eliminated easily from consideration by appropriate cardiac functional studies.

Abnormal Liver Function Tests

Liver chemistries, synthetic, and biliary excretory functional tests are usually abnormal in BCS, although the type of abnormality varies and is nondiagnostic. Many patients have transaminase

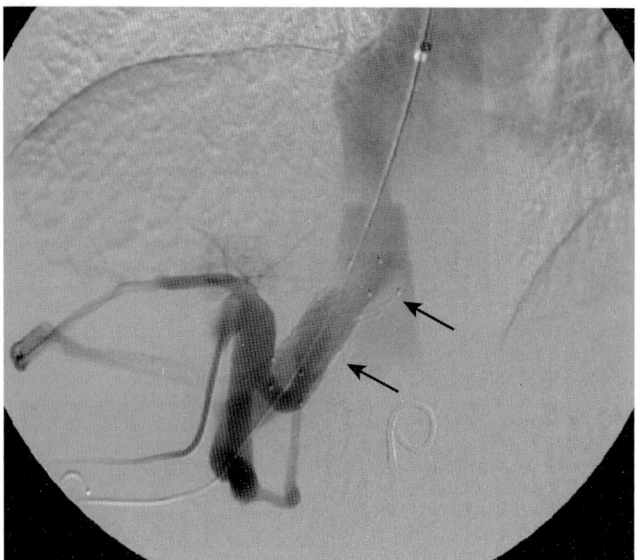

FIGURE 86.7 Venogram showing stent placement *(black arrows)* in a recanalized right hepatic vein.

elevations 3 to 10 times normal limits, indicating varying degrees of ongoing liver injury. Synthetic and excretory liver dysfunction may be seen with abnormal international normalized ratio (INR) and bilirubin levels. These biochemical abnormalities are not specific to BCS but indicate significant hepatic dysfunction and are an important part of the diagnostic workup.

Nonsurgical Therapy

The objectives of nonoperative therapy of BCS are to (1) remove the cause of the venous thrombosis, (2) relieve the high pressure and congestion within the liver, (3) prevent extension of the venous thrombosis, and (4) reverse the massive ascites. These objectives are quite challenging to accomplish.

Medical therapy alone to treat BCS has seen limited success. Most reports indicate failure of medical therapy and the need for additional interventions. However, systemic anticoagulation is a mainstay of therapy for patients with a history of BCS, whether they were treated with interventional radiologic measures, surgical shunting, or transplantation. Contemporary management prescribes heparin for treatment of the acute-onset BCS while definitive management planning is underway. Long-term therapy with anticoagulation is essential to prevent recurrence. Most often, this is accomplished with warfarin, for a goal of INR in the 2 to 3 range. However, newer anticoagulation medications are gaining favor that do not require laboratory monitoring. A direct oral anticoagulant medication such as apixaban or rivaroxaban, for example, is indicated for a wide array of uses and may be considered in BCS.

In BCS caused by hematologic disorders, such as polycythemia vera and PNH, some dramatic responses to intravenous (IV) heparin therapy have been reported, although relapses have been common.[16,18,20] Long-term anticoagulation with oral warfarin has been recommended to follow the initial IV use of heparin during the acute phase of BCS, although initiation or enhancement of bleeding is a potential complication of anticoagulant therapy, particularly in patients in whom cirrhosis and esophageal varices develop.

Thrombolytic therapy with urokinase or streptokinase has been used in many patients in an attempt to dissolve the thrombi and restore hepatic venous outflow.[7–10,14,93–104] The experience with thrombolytic therapy has been recorded in anecdotal reports with relatively short follow-up. Approximately one-third of patients were believed to have had a clinical response to treatment for periods of 2 months to 1 year. Half of the patients died as a result of BCS during the brief periods of observation. In the small-number experience of Powell-Jackson et al.,[100] all four patients who received thrombolytic treatment in the acute phase of BCS died without evidence of a response. However, thrombolytic therapy combined with angioplasty has produced more durable results in select contemporary reports. In a recent series from China, 12 of 13 patients had patent hepatic veins without recurrent thrombosis after a mean follow-up of 24 months. The one initial treatment failure was salvaged by repeat angioplasty.[105]

In current Western practice, tissue plasminogen activator (tPA) is the direct thrombolytic agent of choice. Administration is best accomplished with catheter-directed methods, although systemic delivery has been described for other indications. Careful monitoring is required for systemic delivery in particular because of a high risk of bleeding. Single case reports have described successful thrombus resolution with systemic thrombolysis alone.[106] In addition to tPA administration, percutaneous mechanical thrombectomy has been reported as a successful method of clot extraction in BCS.[107,108]

Anticoagulant therapy has been used widely in BCS to prevent propagation of the thrombi.[4,8,10,14,16,18,20,46,50,100,102,104,109,110] Most reports of the effectiveness of this form of treatment have been anecdotal and lack long-term follow-up. There is no evidence that the use of either heparin or warfarin (Coumadin) brings about dissolution of established thrombosis. As previously mentioned, many of the patients who are seen with BCS have a concomitant prothrombotic state, and most need to be placed indefinitely on anticoagulant therapy after intervention to prevent recurrent thrombosis. This is true for patients irrespective of therapeutic intervention. Newer oral anticoagulants, such as the factor Xa inhibitors (rivaroxaban, apixaban, and edoxaban) and the direct thrombin inhibitors (e.g., dabigatran), although not initially approved for BCS, will likely see application in the BCS population in the near future.

Control of ascites is feasible in some patients with BCS by use of the usual diuretic regimens, although ascites is resistant to therapy in many patients (see Chapter 79). Therapeutic measures include stringent sodium restriction, administration of diuretic drugs, and repeated IV infusion of albumin, particularly as a replacement of ascitic fluid after paracentesis if required for symptom control. Renal function should be monitored closely during diuretic therapy to avoid precipitating the hepatorenal syndrome, which may complicate cases of chronic BCS. There is no evidence that control of ascites alone influences long-term outcome.

Interventional Radiologic Therapy
Percutaneous Transluminal Angioplasty

Use of percutaneous transluminal angioplasty has been reported in more than 300 patients with BCS[111–124] (see Chapters 21 and 85). Most of the patients had chronic liver disease of long duration, and many had obstruction of the IVC of the membranous or segmental type. The obstructed vein was dilated with one or more balloon catheters. In all cases, the portosystemic pressure gradient that existed before balloon dilation was substantially reduced or eliminated at the time of dilation. Stenosis often

TABLE 86.2 Intraoperative Pressure Measurements* in 65 Patients With Budd-Chiari Syndrome Who Underwent Surgical Portal Decompression

	PRESHUNT PRESSURES					POSTSHUNT PRESSURES				
GROUP	PV	IVC	PV-IVC GRADIENT	RA	PV-RA GRADIENT	PV	IVC	PV-IVC GRADIENT	RA	PV-RA GRADIENT
Hepatic Vein Occlusion Alone SSPCS (n = 39)										
Mean	376	132	244	—	—	166	161	5	—	—
Range	265 to 438	74 to 250	134 to 338	—	—	116 to 292	118 to 284	−12 to 40	—	—
IVC and Hepatic Vein Occlusion Mesoatrial Shunt (n = 8)										
Mean	320	305	9	101	211	244	—	—	147	78
Range	274 to 368	256 to 348	−8 to 46	90 to 112	162 to 256	196 to 248	—	—	124 to 162	52 to 94
IVC and Hepatic Occlusion Combined PCS and CAS (n = 18)										
Mean	308	296	12	112	196	170	164	6	148	22
Range	266 to 348	264 to 320	−8 to 34	95 to 125	140 to 240	158 to 184	160 to 178	−6 to 10	136 to 162	8 to 42

*In millimeters (mm) of saline.

CAS, Cavoatrial shunt; *IVC*, inferior vena cava; *PCS*, portacaval shunt; *PV*, portal vein; *RA*, right atrium; *SSPCS*, side-to-side portacaval shunt.

From Orloff MJ, Isenberg JI, Wheeler HO, Daily PO, Girard B. Budd-Chiari syndrome revisited: 38 years' experience with surgical portal decompression. *J Gastrointest Surg.* 2012;16(2):286–300.

recurred, however, and required repeated balloon dilation. Most of the patients have not had long-term follow-up, so it is difficult to evaluate the ultimate effectiveness of percutaneous transluminal angioplasty. Of the few patients who have been observed for several years, the long-term success rate is less than 50%,[114,117,118,123] although Wu et al.[120] reported restenosis in only 1 of 41 patients during follow-up of 32 (±12) months. A recent randomized controlled trial confirmed the high rates of restenosis with angioplasty alone, but showed striking success for angioplasty combined with stenting.[125]

The use of expandable metallic stents has been added to the interventional radiologic armamentarium in an attempt to maintain prolonged patency of the IVC.[112,113,116,121,126] Patients treated by transluminal angioplasty should have careful follow-up that includes venography and portosystemic pressure measurements every 3 to 6 months to detect recurrent stenosis of the IVC in the initial postprocedural period. Serial follow-up with Doppler US thereafter is recommended at a minimum. For patients not considered surgical or transplant candidates, in particular those who do not yet have end-stage cirrhosis and portal hypertension, angioplasty with stenting may be the best option. Several recent series exemplify the technical and clinical value of angioplasty with stenting. Cheng et al.[127] performed recanalization angioplasty on 162 patients with BCS reporting on a multi-institutional experience in China. While the lesions were somewhat heterogeneous with varying degrees of hepatic vein (HV) occlusion, technical success was achieved in 106 of 109 patients with IVC-only lesions and 51 of 53 patients who had involvement of the HVs. The techniques employed were also fairly heterogeneous and included angioplasty alone, angioplasty with stenting, and both interventions in combination with thrombolytic therapy. The latter was used for an average of 5 days' duration. The change in portosystemic pressures demonstrated across the lesions were statistically significant and showed nearly immediate pressure normalization after recanalization. Overall success was 96.6% (157/162) with 5 technical failures. The median follow up was 15 months, and at 2 years symptom-free survival was 82% with initial treatment and 92% when reintervention groups were considered. The authors describe important technical pearls, for instance, that the approach to the RHV is optimal for success via a transjugular approach, and frequently they employed access via both the femoral and jugular veins. In the rare instance where recanalization of the HVs fails, attempts to access the large accessory veins via direct puncture from the cava may relieve portal hypertension.

To better assess the relative benefit of angioplasty with stenting versus angioplasty alone, Wang et al.[125] performed a randomized controlled trial of two BCS cohorts. A total of 88 patients were divided into angioplasty alone (45) or angioplasty plus routine stenting (43) groups. Restenosis was significantly more frequent in the angioplasty-only group (18 patients vs. 1 patient, $P < .01$), as was symptom recurrence (18 vs. 5, $P < .01$) as shown in Table 86.2. Recurrence of portal hypertension complications was seen in 29% versus 9% ($P = .03$). Restenosis, overall survival, and symptom-free recurrence are shown in Fig. 86.8, with the accompanying hazard ratios per event. On multivariable analysis, the predictors of restenosis included angioplasty only, which was also the only predictor of symptom recurrence. In summary, the authors concluded that angioplasty plus routine stenting conferred an absolute risk reduction for restenosis of 35.6%. As treatment for this condition moves further toward an IR-first approach, stenting with angioplasty should be considered standard practice unless technically unfeasible.

Transjugular Intrahepatic Portosystemic Shunt

Transjugular intrahepatic portosystemic shunt (TIPS; see Chapter 85) is a side-to-side portacaval shunt (SSPCS) inserted percutaneously under radiographic visualization and control. As such, TIPS is based on the same rationale for relieving hepatic venous outflow obstruction and intrahepatic portal hypertension as the surgical SSPCS. The attractiveness of TIPS is that it can be done without a major surgical abdominal operation in patients who have liver disease and thus are often

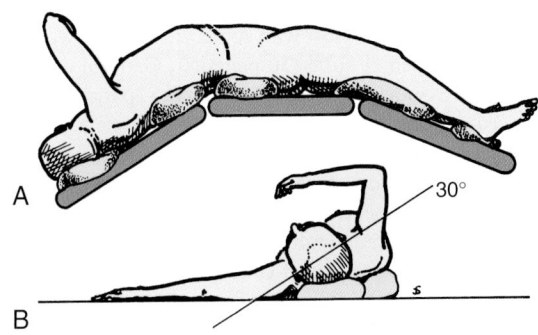

FIGURE 86.8 Position of patient for side-to-side portacaval shunt.

quite ill. Its major disadvantage is a substantial incidence of occlusion of the TIPS that may require repeated revision and hospitalization and often involves recurrence of symptoms. In some patients who have complete occlusion of the hepatic veins or complete occlusion of the IVC, an additional disadvantage is technical inability to insert the TIPS. Insertion of the TIPS by direct puncture of the retrohepatic IVC, which sometimes is the only way that the shunt can be created, may be associated with a substantial incidence of complications.[128]

Between 1995 and 2004, there were many reports of TIPS treatment of BCS, each involving a few patients.[129–138] The largest and longest reported experience with TIPS in BCS during that period was that of Rössle et al.[128] at the University Hospital of Freiburg, Germany, who described their experience with 35 patients—11 acute, 13 subacute, and 11 chronic—who were followed for a mean of 37 (± 29) months. Shunt failure occurred in seven patients (20%): two were technical failures, two required liver transplantation (LT) (one died), and three died after TIPS. Excluding the two patients who required LT but including the two who could not have TIPS for technical reasons, the 5-year survival rate was 74%. TIPS occlusion requiring revision occurred in 19 (58%) of 33 patients. One patient required 10 revisions during a follow-up period of 53 months.

Results reported by others were not as good as those of the Freiburg group. Mancuso et al.[133] described a series of 15 patients, with five deaths and one technical failure, a 40% negative outcome. Cejna et al.[130] reported a series of eight patients; two (25%) died 2 weeks after TIPS, one developed TIPS occlusion requiring LT, and three others required two to seven revisions for TIPS stenosis. Only two (25%) of eight of the initial series of patients had revision-free TIPS patency. Perello et al.[139] reported a series of 13 patients with three shunt failures (23%). The failures included one death, one TIPS thrombosis that necessitated a surgical shunt, and one patient who required LT. Of the remaining 10 patients, 7 (70%) experienced TIPS occlusion. In 5 of these, TIPS dysfunction had not been corrected. These initial, underpowered series describing the early experience for TIPS in BCS were not encouraging.

Since 2004 use of TIPS in BCS has increased substantially, mainly in Europe, in part as a result of the availability of polytetrafluoroethylene (PTFE)–covered stents. Most of the reports have involved retrospective reviews of small numbers of cases followed for short periods. In 2006 Rössle et al.[140] reported results of TIPS with PTFE-covered stents in 112 patients, 17 of whom had BCS. Of these, 12 patients were lost to follow-up, and 16 experienced TIPS failure. The 1-year TIPS failure rate was 10%, 22 patients died, and three underwent LT. The mortality rate without and with the patients lost to follow-up was 20% and 30%, respectively. The authors concluded that the TIPS procedure was improved by the PTFE-covered stent. More recent reports of TIPS treatment for BCS include an experience totaling more than 120 patients, most with similar results (Attwell et al.[141] [17 patients]; Eapen et al.[142] [30 patients]; Gandini et al.[143] [13 patients]; Hernandez-Guerra et al.[144] [25 patients]; Murad et al.[145] [16 patients]; Plessier et al.[146] [20 patients]).

In a multicenter review conducted by Garcia-Pagán et al.,[147] 124 BCS patients treated with TIPS in six European centers were analyzed retrospectively for 1993 to 2006. It is noteworthy that 147 of 221 patients with BCS were eligible for TIPS, but 14 were excluded for technical contraindications, and attempts at TIPS failed in an additional 9 patients. Thus, in a population of patients with BCS, only 60% actually underwent TIPS. Twenty-two patients had complications associated with the

TIPS procedure, and two died as a result. Sixty-one (41%) of the 124 patients had TIPS dysfunction during follow-up that required restenting in 35, angioplasty in 20, and thrombolysis in 6 patients. Portosystemic encephalopathy developed in 21% of patients within 1 year. During follow-up, 16 patients died (13%), and 8 required LT (6.5%). Actuarial LT-free survival at 1, 5, and 10 years was 88%, 78%, and 69%, respectively.

During the past 2 decades, results for interventional radiologic treatment alone in BCS have improved steadily. Primary patency has dramatically improved with the advent of covered stents and is better than 75% in larger series, with secondary patency of 99% at a mean follow-up of 82 months.[148] In one single-center experience, long-term follow-up included 72% survival at 10 years. The largest reported systematic review looked at 2255 patients treated with percutaneous techniques.[149] This meta-analysis included 29 studies in patients who underwent recanalization or TIPS. The restenosis rate at 1 year in the TIPS group was 12% (95% confidence interval [CI], 8%–16%). Survival at 1 and 5 years in the TIPS group was 87.3% and 72.1%, respectively. Overall survival for any interventional strategy was 92% at 1 year and 76% at 5 years.

Surgical Therapy

Side-to-Side Portacaval Shunt

With the advent and increasing adoption of interventional radiologic techniques for treatment of BCS, surgical techniques are becoming something of a lost art. These procedures are crucial options for some patients, however, and require the skill and experience typically seen only in specialized centers. Historically, definitive management of BCS centered ultimately on the use of various surgical shunt procedures (see Chapters 83 and 84). Treatment by direct SSPCS or its hemodynamic equivalents—the portacaval interposition graft, mesocaval interposition graft, or splenorenal shunt—of BCS caused by occlusion of the hepatic veins has been reported in almost 400 patients.[62,64,99,100,110,150–179] Of these, SSPCS proved to be the most widely applied and durable. This technique is indicated only in patients with BCS who have a patent IVC and an IVC pressure that is substantially lower than WHVP or portal pressure. *Obstruction or occlusion of the IVC is a contraindication to PCS.* It is not unusual for patients with BCS caused by hepatic vein occlusion to have an elevated pressure in the IVC as a result of caval compression by an enlarged, congested liver, massive ascites, or both. The absolute level of IVC pressure is not crucial to the effectiveness of SSPCS, as long as the portal pressure is substantially higher than caval pressure, and the IVC is shown to be patent. In the event that caval compression persists after SSPCS, an IR-placed caval stent can be used to expand the retrohepatic caval compression, and this approach will afford complete resolution of ascites and peripheral edema.

Figs. 86.8 to 86.17 describe the technique for SSPCS.

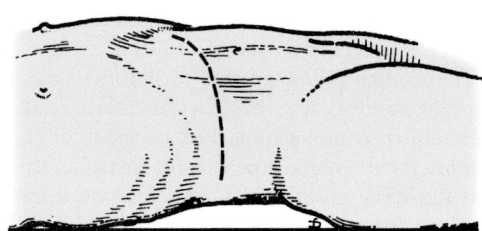

FIGURE 86.9 Long, right subcostal incision used for side-to-side portacaval shunt.

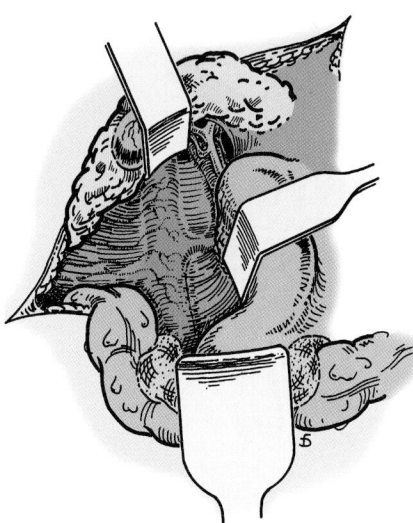

FIGURE 86.10   Exposure of the operative field for side-to-side portacaval shunt.

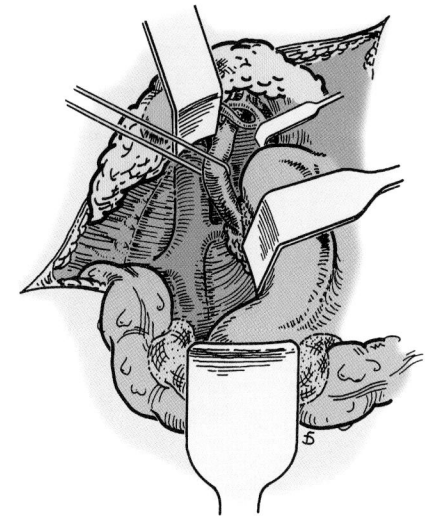

FIGURE 86.13   Mobilization of a long length of portal vein, including the segment behind the pancreas, in preparation for side-to-side portacaval anastomosis (see Chapter 84).

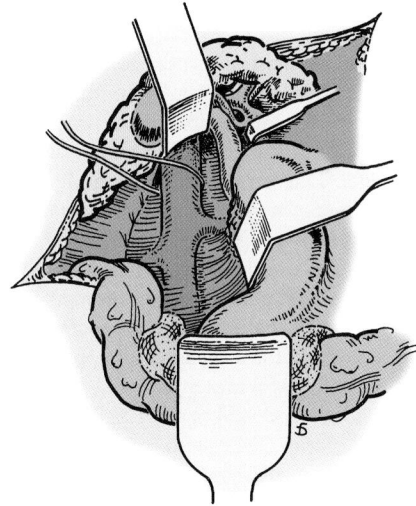

FIGURE 86.11   Circumferential isolation of the inferior vena cava between renal veins and liver in preparation for side-to-side portacaval anastomosis (see Chapter 84).

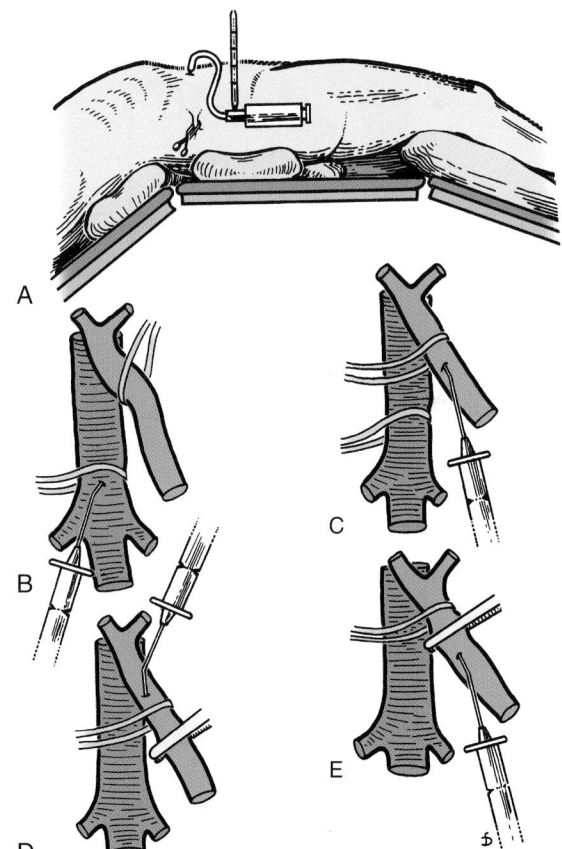

FIGURE 86.14   Measurement of pressures in the inferior vena cava (IVC) and portal vein (PV) with a saline (spinal) manometer by direct needle puncture before performance of portacaval anastomosis. All portal pressures are corrected by subtracting the IVC pressure from the portal pressure. Pressures in the IVC and PV are measured again after completion of the shunt. **A,** For all pressure measurements, the bottom of the manometer is positioned at the level of the IVC, which is marked on the skin surface of the body with a towel clip. **B,** IVC pressure. **C,** Free portal pressure. **D,** Hepatic occluded portal pressure, obtained on the hepatic side of a clamp occluding the portal vein. **E,** Splanchnic occluded portal pressure, obtained on the intestinal side of a clamp occluding the portal vein.

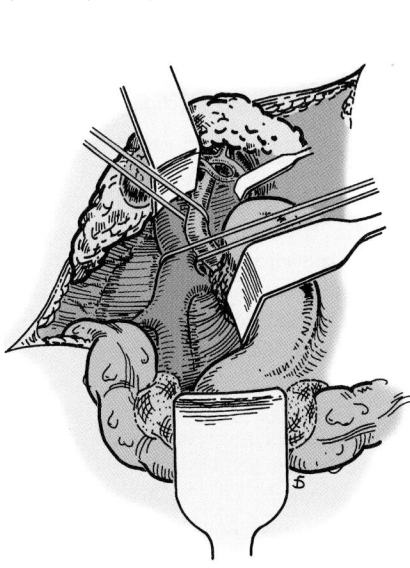

FIGURE 86.12   Exposure of portal vein in preparation for side-to-side portacaval anastomosis (see Chapter 84).

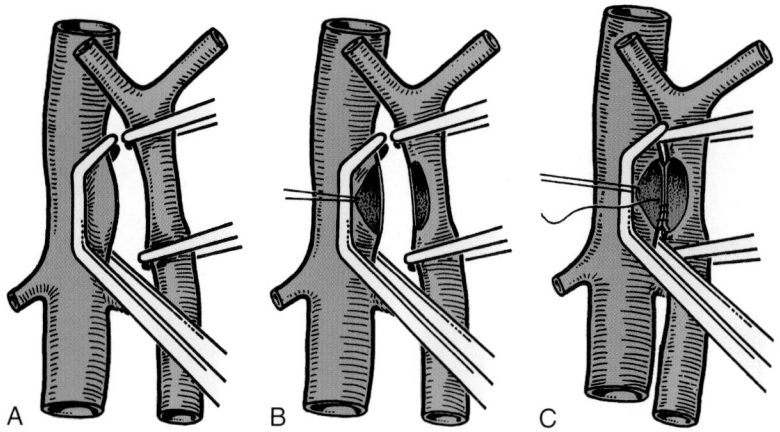

FIGURE 86.15 Side-to-side portacaval anastomosis. **A,** Placement of clamps on the inferior vena cava (IVC) and portal vein (PV). **B,** Strips of IVC and PV 2.5 cm in length have been excised. **C,** Placement of a posterior row of continuous 5-0 vascular suture from inside the lumina of IVC and PV (see Chapter 84).

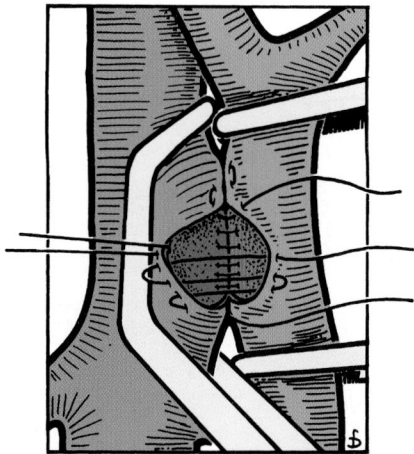

FIGURE 86.16 Side-to-side portacaval anastomosis. Placement of anterior row of two continuous everting sutures of 5-0 vascular material (see Chapter 84).

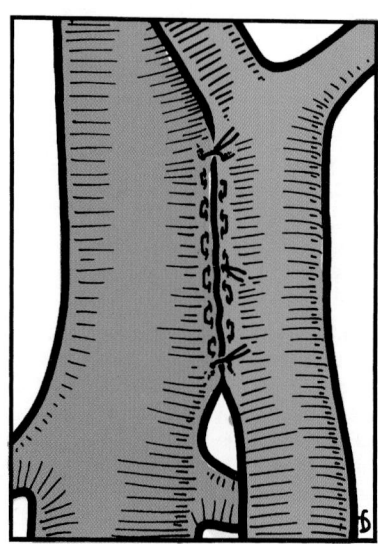

FIGURE 86.17 Completed side-to-side portacaval anastomosis (see Chapter 84).

Mesoatrial Shunt

When BCS is caused by thrombosis of the IVC and the hepatic veins, SSPCS and equivalent decompressive procedures are ineffective, because the high pressure in the infrahepatic IVC does not permit adequate decompression of the portal system and liver. Under such circumstances, a mesoatrial shunt has been advocated. Synthetic Dacron or Gore-Tex grafts ranging from 14 to 20 mm in diameter have been used in most cases and have been connected end-to-side to the superior mesenteric vein (SMV) in the abdomen and the right atrium (RA) in the thorax.

In the mesoatrial shunt, a midline laparotomy combined with a median sternotomy is the standard approach. The SMV is isolated circumferentially for a distance of approximately 3 cm in the root of the small bowel mesentery, and the pericardium is opened to expose the lateral wall of the RA. The graft is anastomosed to the side of the SMV with continuous 5-0 vascular suture, tunneled through the root of the transverse mesocolon and greater omentum, then passed anterior to the stomach and left lobe of the liver into the mediastinum through an opening made in the anterior diaphragm. Alternatively, the graft can be tunneled behind the right lobe and through a fenestration in the diaphragm. The prosthesis is anastomosed to the side of the RA with a monofilament vascular suture (see Chapter 84).

Combined SSPCS and Cavoatrial Shunt

The combined procedure is performed through a long, right subcostal incision for the PCS and a median sternotomy for the cavoatrial shunt (CAS) (Figs. 86.18 and 86.19). After completion of the SSPCS, a 20-mm-diameter, ring-reinforced Gore-Tex graft is anastomosed to the side of the IVC at the level of the PCS. The graft is channeled anterior to the liver through an opening made in the right leaf of the diaphragm and is anastomosed to the side of the RA.

Surgical Outcomes

Success rates of portal decompression in BCS have ranged from 85% to 97% after direct SSPCS[150,153,161,167,172,173,180] and 67% after splenorenal shunt.[62,150,167,168] Mesocaval or portacaval interposition grafts with autologous internal jugular vein have been reported in approximately 50 patients with BCS, most of them in France, with a success rate of 89%.[153,159,167,172,173,178] Mesocaval

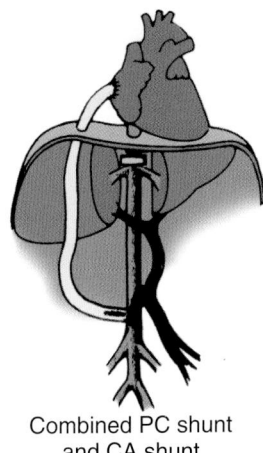

Combined PC shunt
and CA shunt

FIGURE 86.18 Combined side-to-side portacaval (PC) shunt and cavoatrial (CA) shunt using a 20-mm ring-reinforced Gore-Tex graft. The operation was done in 18 patients with Budd-Chiari syndrome secondary to inferior vena cava occlusion. (From Orloff MJ, Daily PO, Girard B. Treatment of Budd-Chiari syndrome due to inferior vena cava occlusion by combined portal and vena caval decompression. *Am J Surg.* 1992;163:137–143.)

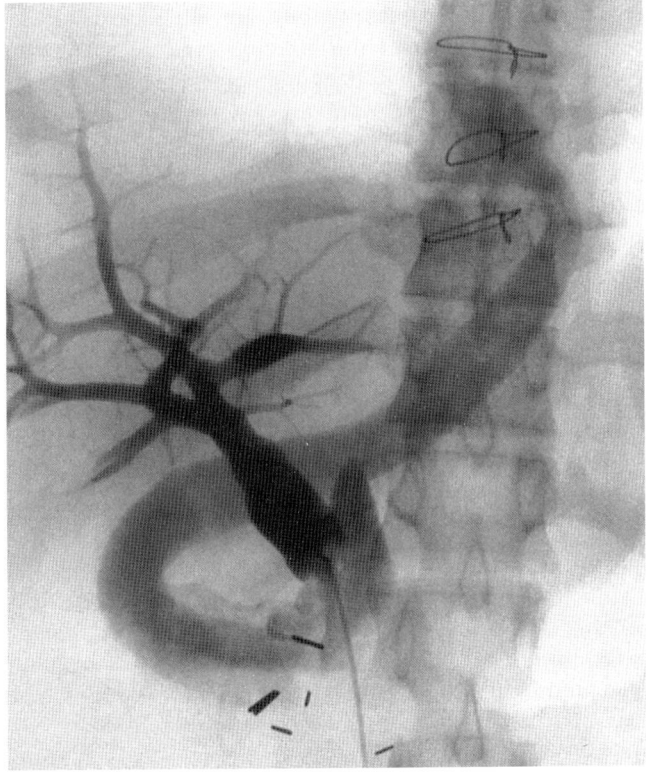

FIGURE 86.19 Shunt catheterization and venogram showing patency of the portacaval shunt (PCS) and cavoatrial shunt (CAS) 1 year after performance of combined PCS and CAS in a patient with Budd-Chiari syndrome secondary to inferior vena cava occlusion. Serial angiographic studies showed patency and excellent function of the PCS and CAS in all patients. (From Orloff MJ, Daily PO, Girard B. Treatment of Budd-Chiari syndrome due to inferior vena cava occlusion by combined portal and vena caval decompression. *Am J Surg.* 1992;163:137–143.)

or portacaval interposition grafts using synthetic materials, such as Dacron or PTFE (Gore-Tex), have been successful in approximately 52% of 39 patients with BCS, which is the lowest success rate of the various in-continuity portal decompressive procedures.[62,150,161,162,165,167,168,173] Although all three shunts are hemodynamically similar, synthetic interposition portacaval or mesocaval grafts and the splenorenal shunt are probably inferior to direct SSPCS in the treatment of BCS. Occlusion of the shunt is a serious complication that may result in death; the splenorenal shunt and the synthetic interposition grafts have a substantial incidence of thrombosis, not only in BCS, but also in other diseases that cause portal hypertension.[161,181–184]

The largest single-center experience of surgical treatment for BCS, which included SSPCS, mesoatrial shunt, and combined SSPCS with CAS, was reported by Orloff et al.[15] in 2012. Table 86.3 summarizes long-term results, with follow-up of 5 to 38 (mean, 15) years. In total, 38 patients (97%) recovered from the SSPCS procedure and were long-term survivors, with an overall survival rate of 95%. All the survivors have remained free of ascites without requiring diuretic therapy.

Liver biopsies and angiographic or US studies were performed periodically for 37 years after surgical shunt therapy in the 38 survivors (see Table 86.3). Cirrhosis persisted in three patients who had established cirrhosis at the shunt operation, including one patient with Beh√ßet's disease. In 97% of the survivors, no evidence of hepatic congestion or necrosis was found in the follow-up biopsy specimens.[15] Mild to moderate fibrosis was found in 42% of the patients; 50% had normal liver biopsy specimens (Fig. 86.20). Angiography or US showed patency of the PCS and IVC, and pressure measurements showed a widely patent anastomosis with a gradient that ranged from 0 to 44 mm saline and averaged 4 mm across the shunt. Two patients with polycythemia vera developed thrombosis of the PCS 1 week and 3 months postoperatively. Both patients underwent reoperation with thrombectomy and reconstructed portacaval anastomosis with an H-graft of autologous internal jugular vein and required lifelong anticoagulation with warfarin. One patient has remained well for 28 years since revision of the shunt. Unfortunately, the other patient developed recurrent shunt thrombosis and required LT.

For mesoatrial shunt recipients, five (63%) of the eight patients subsequently developed thrombosis of the graft and died of liver failure. Three of the deaths occurred during the first postoperative year, one occurred in the second year, and one occurred in the fifth year. All five patients developed recurrence of ascites, and three developed portosystemic encephalopathy while their hepatic function deteriorated. The three long-term survivors of the mesoatrial shunt (38%) have been followed up for 20+ years with patent shunts and no clinical signs of BCS. Accordingly, mesoatrial shunt suffers from a fairly high thrombosis rate, and future therapy in these patients may likely require a combination of interventional, medical, and surgical techniques.

In the results for the combined shunt, all 18 patients survived the operation and are alive 5 to 25 years postoperatively (see Table 86.3). Mean follow-up is 12 years. All patients are free of ascites, and none requires diuretics; hepatomegaly and splenomegaly are gone; and liver function tests results are normal in all survivors, with no instance of portosystemic encephalopathy.

TABLE 86.3   Long-Term Results of Portal Decompression Operations in 65 Patients With Budd-Chiari Syndrome

	HEPATIC VEIN OCCLUSION ALONE	IVC AND HEPATIC VEIN OCCLUSION	
	SSPCS	MESOATRIAL SHUNT	COMBINED SSPCS AND CAS
No. patients	39	8	18
Onset to Operation (Weeks)			
≤17 (%)	92	88	100
Mean	16	12	15
Range	4 to 78	7 to 19	10 to 18
Follow-up (Years)			
Mean	15	17	14
Range	5 to 38	20 to 24	5 to 25
Ascites (%)	0	63	0
Need for diuretics (%)	0	63	0
Abnormal liver function tests (%)	8	63	0
Portosystemic encephalopathy (%)	0	38	0
Employed or housekeeping (%)	95	25	94
Survival (%)			
30-day	97	100	100
Current	95	38	100

CAS, Cavoatrial shunt; *IVC,* inferior vena cava; *SSPCS,* side-to-side portacaval shunt.

From Orloff MJ, Isenberg JI, Wheeler HO, Daily PO, Girard B. Budd-Chiari syndrome revisited: 38 years' experience with surgical portal decompression. *J Gastrointest Surg.* 2012;16(2):286–300.

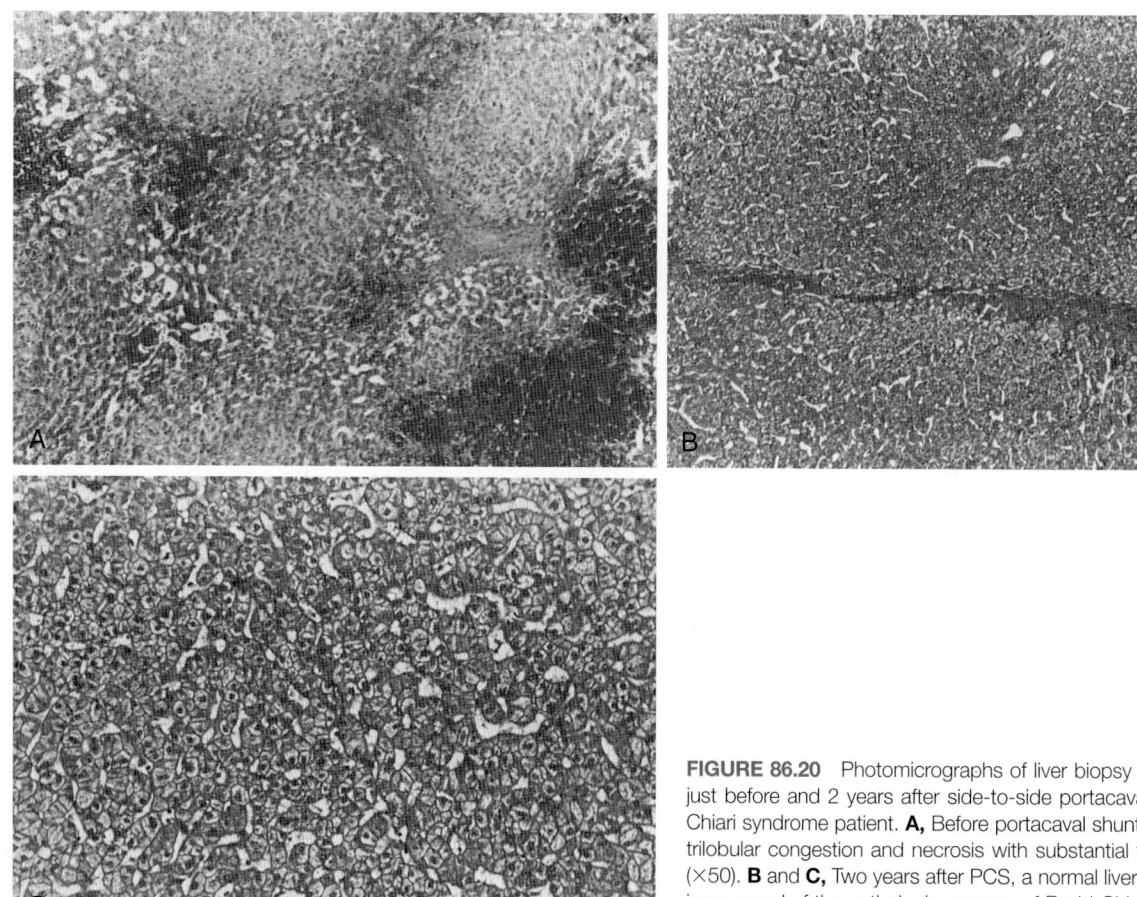

FIGURE 86.20 Photomicrographs of liver biopsy specimens obtained just before and 2 years after side-to-side portacaval shunt from Budd-Chiari syndrome patient. **A,** Before portacaval shunt (PCS), intense centrilobular congestion and necrosis with substantial fibrosis can be seen (×50). **B** and **C,** Two years after PCS, a normal liver architecture, a striking reversal of the pathologic process of Budd-Chiari syndrome, can be seen (**B,** ×80; **C,** ×160.)

Other series of mesoatrial shunting that involve five or more patients have been reported, although follow-up generally has been relatively short. Stringer et al.[185] of London reported excellent results in five patients, but follow-up of 9 to 16 months was too short to warrant conclusions. Wang et al.[63,68] of Beijing reported survival of 61% and 50% at 5 and 10 years, respectively, in 70 patients, but their reports contain insufficient details to determine how many of these patients had patent and functioning grafts, how well the patients were followed, or the exact nature of the BCS being treated. Emre et al.[186] reported 85% survival in 13 patients during follow-up of 1 to 76 months, with one known thrombosed shunt. Behera et al.[187] of Chandigarh, India, described 100% graft patency during 6 to 71 months of follow-up of 10 patients, with survival of 90%. Khanna et al.[188] reported a 62% survival rate in 13 patients during follow-up of 2 months to 7.5 years.

The combined surgical experience for BCS emphasizes the importance of performing SSPCS, mesoatrial shunt, or combined SSPCS and CAS early in the disease course. Hepatic venous outflow obstruction produces widespread destruction of the hepatic parenchyma by pressure necrosis and ischemia, and the liver damage becomes irreversible in a surprisingly short time; some patients developed cirrhosis within 3 or 4 months of the onset of symptoms. Thus the relief of ascites is much less important than decompressing the liver, and referral for surgical intervention should be made early in the course of BCS to salvage the liver and avoid LT.

Membranous Obstruction of Vena Cava: Surgical Options

Patients with MOVC described in the literature largely have had a chronic disorder that has progressed to cirrhosis and portal hypertension by the time they came to medical attention. The lesion causing IVC obstruction has varied from a thin membrane located in the suprahepatic IVC to an extensive area of stenosis involving the retrohepatic IVC.

When the area of IVC obstruction is short and is located at or above the level of the hepatic vein orifices, two treatment options are available: percutaneous transluminal angioplasty and transcardiac membranotomy. Early reported experience with percutaneous transluminal angioplasty in MOVC was limited to short follow-up with high rates of recurrent IVC thrombosis or stenosis.[56,114,118,119,123,124,189–191] Long-term IVC patency has been achieved in more recent reports, however, indicating that many of these patients can be treated with interventional techniques particularly when stenting is used.[192]

For circumstances in which percutaneous approaches are unavailable or inappropriate, transcardiac membranotomy has been the most frequently used treatment of MOVC when the membrane is thin. The technique involves fracture of the membrane by the finger or a dilator inserted through the right atrial appendage (Fig. 86.21). More than 125 cases have been described, with a successful outcome in 70% to 90% during follow-up that ranged from 2 months to 7 years but generally was brief.[56,57,60,61,62,64,65,190,193–196]

When more than a thin membrane causes obstruction of the IVC, and particularly when a long area of stenosis involves the retrohepatic IVC, the treatment options are different and consist mainly of direct excision and repair of the involved area of IVC (endovenotomy) or a cavoatrial bypass graft. A direct attack on the lesion generally has involved excising the obstructing tissue in the lumen of the IVC and repairing the vein with a synthetic or pericardial patch graft. Twelve such attempts have

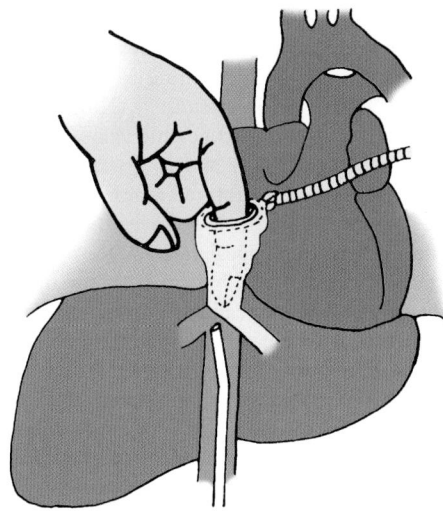

FIGURE 86.21 Technique of transcardiac membranotomy. (From Iwahashi K. Surgical correction of the inferior vena cava obstruction with Budd-Chiari syndrome. *Arch Jpn Chir.* 1981;50:559–570.)

been described in the literature, with success in five patients and failure in seven, four of whom died.[56,57,190] Koja et al.[197] (Kuniyoshi et al.,[198]) reported direct removal of the IVC obstruction under partial cardiopulmonary bypass in 32 patients with impressive results, although the reported follow-up was short. The alternative approach is an IR-guided angioplasty with stent. This approach is gaining form and will likely replace most surgical treatments.

Use of a cavoatrial bypass graft has been reported in 11 patients who had a long segment of IVC stenosis. The procedure succeeded during short periods of follow-up in three patients and failed in eight, four of whom died.[56,61,199–201] When the IVC obstruction involves or extends below the orifices of the hepatic veins, cavoatrial bypass does not decompress the liver. Under such circumstances, consideration should be given to adding SSPCS to the cavoatrial bypass. The combined procedure of IVC and portal decompression has not been reported in MOVC.

Surgical Removal of Venous Obstruction

Senning[202,203] reported a direct method of removing obstruction of the IVC and hepatic veins in patients with chronic BCS. The operation is performed with cardiopulmonary bypass and involves opening the suprahepatic IVC and RA, removing any vena caval thrombus, resecting the dorsocranial part of the liver containing the confluence of the occluded major hepatic veins, and reconstructing the hepatic outflow tract by suturing the RA to the liver capsule. Since his initial description, Senning[204] and others[205] have reported the results of the operation in 17 patients, 2 of whom (12%) died within 2 weeks of operation and 4 of whom died later. Actuarial 1-year and 3-year survival rates were 76% and 57%, respectively; LT was required for two patients, and three developed recurrent thrombosis. During follow-up of 7 months to 11 years, 10 (67%) of the 15 early survivors had prolonged relief of BCS.

Kawashima et al.[206] reported success of the Senning operation in five of seven patients during follow-up of 2 months to 5 years, and Nakao et al.[207] described success in two patients followed for 1 to 2 months. In a modification of the operation,

Koja et al.[197] (Kuniyoshi et al.,[198]) described direct removal of the IVC obstruction under partial cardiopulmonary bypass in 32 patients with chronic BCS resulting from IVC obstruction of 1 to 42 years' duration. Koja et al.[197] (Kuniyoshi et al.,[198]) reopened the IVC and occluded hepatic veins under direct vision without resecting the liver and reconstructed the hepatic outflow tract with a patch graft of autologous pericardium. Many of the patients had cirrhosis or severe fibrosis of the liver, and 29 of the 32 had esophageal varices. No operative deaths were reported. During 1.5 to 17 years of follow-up, there were four late deaths, and hepatocellular carcinoma developed in seven patients. Survival rates at 5 and 10 years were 93.6% and 81%, respectively. In a follow-up to their 1998 report, in 2009 Kuniyoshi et al. reported their results from 1979 to 2008 in 53 patients.[208] Overall mortality was 32%, and total obstruction or severe stenosis of the reconstructed IVC developed in 14% of survivors. Based on the accumulated experience, it does not appear that radical open-end venectomy is the first-choice procedure for IVC occlusion and should only be used for patients with no other viable options.

Liver Transplantation

Indications

Liver transplantation is a radical, drastic treatment for BCS, but it is effective when a patient's life is at stake and other therapeutic options have been exhausted or are not technically feasible (see Chapter 105). LT is not in competition with TIPS, stenting, SSPCS, or any other type of treatment but rather can be very useful in far advanced, decompensated liver disease, when liver dysfunction has progressed beyond salvage with other portal decompression procedures.

It is imperative that the indications for the use of LT in BCS be established and clearly understood. Indications include the following:
1. Cirrhosis with progressive liver failure that has reached the point of permitting a reasonable prediction that the patient will die within 1 year—the most common indication for LT and the same used widely in other liver diseases[209,210]
2. Failure of a portosystemic shunt or TIPS, usually because of thrombosis, with persistence or recurrence of symptoms and signs of BCS
3. BCS with unshuntable portal hypertension secondary to thrombosis of the PV, splenic vein, and much of the SMV—a rare indication that applies only if patent blood vessels are available to vascularize the liver allograft
4. Acute fulminant hepatic failure

Outcomes

To date, the English literature contains reports of more than 1000 patients with BCS who have undergone LT; Table 86.4 summarizes these reports. The largest number of case reports have come from reviews of 248 patients registered in the European Liver Transplantation Registry and 510 patients registered in the United Network for Organ Sharing (UNOS) Liver Standard Transplant Analysis and Research files. All the reports were based on retrospective reviews of medical records (see Chapter 105).

As shown in Table 86.4, the indications for LT varied greatly, and it cannot be said that LT was done in patients who had 1 year or less to live because of cirrhosis with progressive liver failure. In several series the indications were not clearly stated.[211–214] Ulrich et al.[215] reported 12% of the 39 patients

TABLE 86.4 Indications for Liver Transplantation in 15 Retrospective Series of Budd-Chiari Syndrome (BCS) Reported in the Literature

REFERENCE	NO. PATIENTS	INDICATIONS FOR OLT
Srinivasan et al., 2002[220]	19	Failed shunt, 5
		Acute liver failure, 6
		Chronic liver failure, 8
Melear et al., 2002[212]	17	Not stated
Hemming et al., 1996[161]	10	Failed shunt, 3
		Advanced cirrhosis, 4
		IVC obstruction, 2
Ringe et al., 1995[213]	43	Unclear, 39
		Failed shunt, 4
Knoop et al., 1994a, 1994b[221,222]	8	Child class C, 5
		Child class B, 3
Galati et al., 1993[223]	32	Failed shunt, 2
		Cirrhosis—?
		Hepatic necrosis–?
Shaked et al., 1992[224]	14	Failed shunt, 2
		Advanced cirrhosis, 4
		Poor synthetic function, 8
Halff et al., 1990[216]; Iwatsuki et al., 1991[225]	32	Failed shunt, 5
		Intractable ascites, 17
		Recurrent variceal bleeding, 14
		Encephalopathy, 15
Sakai & Wall, 1994[226]	11	Chronic BCS, 5
		Acute fulminant BCS, 3
		Failed shunt, 3
Jamieson et al., 1991[211]	26	Failed shunt, 2
		Unclear, 24
Ulrich et al., 2008[215]	42	Cirrhosis, 11
		Portal vein occlusion, 10
		Hepatic necrosis, 12
		Severe acute liver failure, 8
		Hepatocellular carcinoma, 3
		Hepatic artery occlusion, 2
Cruz et al., 2005[227]	11	Failed TIPS, 5
		Failed PSS, 1
		Intractable ascites, 1
		Portal-systemic encephalopathy, 3
Plessier et al., 2006[146]	11	Failed therapy with anticoagulation and TIPS, 11
Mentha et al., 2006[217] European Liver Transplantation Registry, 1988–1999	248	Fulminant hepatic failure, 47
		Renal failure, 40
		Portal vein thrombosis, 47
		Failed PSS, 49
		Failed TIPS, 11
		Failed percutaneous angioplasty, 18
Segev et al., 2007[214] (UNOS Registry, 1987-2006)	510	Not reported

IVC, Inferior vena cava; *OLT,* orthotopic liver transplantation; *PSS,* portosystemic shunt; *TIPS,* transjugular intrahepatic portosystemic shunting; *UNOS,* United Network for Organ Sharing.

were Child-Turcotte-Pugh (CTP) class A, and 57% were class B, obviously not in liver failure. The report of Halff et al.[216] stated, "The decrease in synthetic function was not as severe as in many other causes of end-stage liver disease." Every series had some patients who underwent LT because of a failed portosystemic shunt. In the registry review of Mentha et al.,[217] 49 of the 248 patients had failure of a portosystemic shunt.[218,219]

Table 86.5 shows the survival statistics in the reported series.[220–227] All the studies suffer from short follow-up of many patients, sometimes less than 1 year. A substantial variation in patient selection was apparent from one series to the next, particularly with regard to severity of liver disease, so comparisons are difficult. The early mortality in series that had 10 or more patients ranged from 5% to 36% and averaged 15%. The 5-year survival rate, when reported, ranged from 45% to 95% and averaged 71%. Segev et al.,[214] in their UNOS registry review, reported that since introduction in 2002 of the Model for End-Stage Liver Disease (MELD) scoring system for organ allocation by disease severity, 3-year patient survival has increased from 72.6% to 84.9%, and 3-year graft survival has increased from 64.5% to 80.6%.

Most of the series did not report the results of pathologic examination of the explanted liver in the patient with BCS. The reports of Ringe et al.[213] on 43 patients, Halff et al.[216] on 32 patients, Sakai and Wall[226,228] on 11 patients, and Srinivasan et al.[220] on 19 patients described the findings in the host liver, however, and confirmed the clinical impression that many patients underwent LT without having decompensated liver disease. Only 17 of the 43 patients of Ringe et al.[213] had cirrhosis; the others had congestion alone (14 patients) and fibrosis alone, lesions that are found in the early stages of BCS. Similarly, in the report of Halff et al.,[216] none of the 32 patients had cirrhosis, and Sakai and Wall[228] reported that 3 of 11 of their patients had central congestion and necrosis but no fibrosis or cirrhosis.

An important concern about LT in BCS is recurrence of BCS in the transplanted liver.[227,229,230] Table 86.6 shows the incidence of recurrent BCS in the liver allograft. Some investigators reported no recurrence of BCS, whereas others[216,221,222,227] reported substantial recurrence rates of 13% to 27% despite treatment with anticoagulants. Most series have shown a substantial incidence of posttransplant thrombosis in other splanchnic blood vessels, particularly in the PV (range, 9%–40%), often

---

TABLE 86.5 Survival After Liver Transplantation for Budd-Chiari Syndrome Reported in the Literature

REFERENCE	NO. PATIENTS	FOLLOW-UP (mo)	EARLY MORTALITY (%)	SURVIVAL ≥1 YEAR (%)
Srinivasan et al., 2002[220]	19	1 to 119	5	1 to 119 mo (84)
				1 yr (95)
				5 yr (95)
				10 yr (78)
Melear et al., 2002[212]	17	1 to 158	6	1 to 158 mo (88)
				1, 5, and 10 yr: NR
Hemming et al., 1996[161]	10	?	10	1 yr (82)
				5 yr (67)
Ringe et al., 1995[213]	43	2 to 137	30	1 yr (69)
				5 yr (69)
Knoop et al., 1994a, 1994b[221,222]	8	4 to 59	13	1 yr (88), >1 yr: NR
Galati et al., 1993[223]	9	2 to 60	0	2 to 60 mo (100)
Shaked et al., 1992[224]	14	2 to 60	14	1 yr (86)
				3 yr (76)
Halff et al., 1990[216]	32	12 to 132	25	1 yr (69)
Iwatsuki et al., 1991[225]				5 yr (45)
Sakai & Wall, 1994[226]	11	12 to 72	36	1 to 6 yr (64)
Jamieson et al., 1991[211]	26	12 to 60	31	1 yr (69)
				5 yr (50)
Ulrich et al., 2008[215]	42	1 to 203 (median 96)	7	1 yr (92)
				5 yr (89)
				10 yr (83.5)
Cruz et al., 2005[227]	11	1 to 132	18	1 yr (81)
				5 yr (65)
				10 yr (65)
Plessier et al., 2006[146]	11	17 to 56	9	1 yr (91)
				3 yr (91)
Mentha et al., 2006[217]	248	Long-term via registry (mean, 48)	13	1 yr (76)
				5 yr (71)
				10 yr (68)
Segev et al., 2007[214]	510	Long-term via registry	15	1 yr (82)
				3 yr (76)

NR, Not reported.

TABLE 86.6 Reported Rates of Recurrence of Budd-Chiari Syndrome and Other Thrombosis After Liver Transplantation for Budd-Chiari Syndrome

REFERENCE	NO. PATIENTS	RECURRENCE NO.	RECURRENCE %	OTHER THROMBOSIS NO.	OTHER THROMBOSIS %
Srinivasan et al., 2002[220]	19	2	11	2	11
Melear et al., 2002[212]	17	0	0	3	18
Ringe et al., 1995[213]	43	0	0	10	23
Hemming et al., 1996[161]	10	0	0	1	14
Knoop et al., 1994a, 1994b[221,222]	8	1	13	1	13
Shaked et al., 1992[224]	14	0	0	NR	NR
Halff et al., 1990[216]	23	3/18	17	4	22
Sakai & Wall, 1994[226]	11	0	0	1	9
Jamieson et al., 1991[211]	26	2	8	5	19
Ulrich et al., 2008[215]	42	3	7	5	12
Cruz et al., 2005[227]	11	3	27	3	27
Plessier et al., 2006[146]	11	1	9	4	36
Mentha et al., 2006[217]	248	5	2	35	14
Segev et al., 2007[214]	510	7	8	36	40

NR, Not reported.

with disastrous consequences. The frequent development of thrombosis makes it mandatory that patients receive early and lifelong anticoagulation therapy after LT. At the same time, it should be recognized that one of the potential benefits of LT in certain thrombogenic disorders, such as antithrombin III deficiency and protein C deficiency, is correction of the underlying defect by transplantation of a liver from a normal donor.

It has been suggested that LT is preferable to SSPCS in the treatment of BCS because if SSPCS fails, the risk of performing subsequent LT is increased. It has been proposed that mesocaval shunt is preferable to SSPCS because it is advantageous to avoid dissection of the hepatic hilum should subsequent LT be required.[153,231] In 11 more recent studies, previous portosystemic shunt, regardless of type, had no influence on the outcome of LT.[232–239] AbouJaoude et al.[232] emphasized that thrombosis of a portosystemic shunt may seriously compromise performance of LT. Long-term shunt patency should therefore be the main factor that determines the type of shunt selected for the potential LT candidate, which applies even more to patients with BCS. Direct PCS has had a thrombosis rate of 0.5% or less compared with occlusion rates of 24% to 53% reported for mesocaval interposition shunts using synthetic grafts.[15,161,240–243] Mesocaval interposition shunts using autologous internal jugular vein grafts, which have been used widely

in France, have shown patency rates comparable to direct SS PCS.[153,159,178]

Orthotopic liver transplantation is the appropriate treatment in the late stages of BCS, when the liver disease is no longer reversible, and when stabilization of progressive hepatic decompensation is impossible. Most patients who are candidates for LT should be in CTP class C.

In considering treatment of BCS by LT, it is important to take into account the downside of such therapy: (1) the vast shortage of donor livers to treat the many patients who need LT; (2) long wait times where disease progression can lead to drop-off; (3) the unpredictable availability of donor organs; (4) the need for and consequences of lifelong immunosuppression; and (5) the high cost of LT, which may or may not be cost-effective depending on the alternative therapies pursued and the potential repeat interventions required (see Chapter 105).

VENO-OCCLUSIVE DISEASE

In 1954 Bras et al.[244] coined the term *veno-occlusive disease* (VOD) to describe a common liver disease in Jamaican children caused by the ingestion of "bush teas" made from plants of the *Crotolaria* and *Senecio* genera, which contain the well-known hepatotoxic pyrrolizidine alkaloids. VOD of the liver, more recently called sinusoidal obstruction syndrome (SOS), may mimic BCS clinically, because both conditions involve hepatic venous outflow obstruction. However, VOD involves the sinusoids and the central and sublobular hepatic veins within the liver rather than the hepatic veins.[245–247] The underlying process in VOD is subendothelial sclerosis of the hepatic veins and sinusoids secondary to endothelial injury caused by toxic agents, such as pyrrolizidine alkaloids, antineoplastic drugs, radiation, or stem cell transplant. More than 20 drugs have been implicated, most notably busulfan, 6-mercaptopurine, azathioprine, and cyclophosphamide. Thrombosis of the small hepatic veins may occur after damage to the venous intima. Electron microscopic studies of liver biopsy specimens obtained from children with VOD caused by pyrrolizidine poisoning showed marked endothelial damage in the sinusoids and subterminal and terminal hepatic veins in all zones of the liver, with extravasation of erythrocytes into the space of Disse and narrowing of the lumen where the sinusoid entered the central vein.[248]

Similar to BCS, hemorrhagic necrosis of the liver parenchyma around the centrilobular veins occurs early in the course of VOD. Extensive occlusion of the small hepatic veins ultimately leads to diffuse fibrosis and cirrhosis. Patients with VOD caused by chronic pyrrolizidine poisoning often have well-established cirrhosis when first seen by a physician. VOD that develops as a complication of therapy for another condition—such as occurs during cancer chemotherapy, radiation therapy, or bone marrow transplantation (BMT)—usually is detected early in the course of disease.

Symptoms and Signs

Veno-occlusive disease has been observed in individuals of all ages, including infants and adults in their sixth decade; however, VOD caused by pyrrolizidine alkaloids has been seen most frequently in infants and children. The clinical manifestations depend on the disease stage at which the patient seeks medical treatment.[248–252] The acute stage is often preceded for 1 or 2 weeks by a febrile illness with upper respiratory symptoms, vomiting and diarrhea, or both. The patient then experiences abrupt onset of abdominal pain, weakness, anorexia, fever, and abdominal distention secondary to ascites.[245,253,254] Jaundice is the rule, and splenomegaly with thrombocytopenia is common. Some patients experience edema of the lower extremities and occasionally of the hands and face, and physical examination in the acute phase invariably shows hepatomegaly and ascites. Many patients have splenomegaly; some have distention of the superficial veins of the abdominal wall, and some have peripheral edema and a pleural effusion. Those patients who develop VOD after bone marrow transplantation usually experience the clinical features within 3 weeks after transplantation. Many patients have died during the acute stage from liver failure, bleeding esophageal varices, or intercurrent infection.

Patients other than BMT recipients may be initially seen in the chronic stage of VOD with the usual clinical manifestations of cirrhosis of the liver: ascites, hepatomegaly, splenomegaly, wasting, abdominal venous distention, spider angiomata, palmar erythema, asterixis, and peripheral edema. Bleeding from esophageal varices is a major cause of death in the chronic stage, and cirrhosis of the liver has been observed 3 months after acute onset of VOD.[250]

Diagnostic Studies

The diagnosis of VOD is strongly suspected when, in the proper setting, such as following BMT, ascites, jaundice, hepatomegaly, and right upper quadrant abdominal pain develop in patients.[253] The most important diagnostic study in VOD is needle liver biopsy, which shows the specific abnormality of extensive occlusion of the small hepatic veins within the liver.[248,250,252,255] In the acute stage of VOD, an additional biopsy finding is centrilobular hemorrhagic necrosis of the hepatic parenchyma. In the chronic stage of VOD, the biopsy specimen shows diffuse fibrosis or cirrhosis of the liver (see Chapter 74).

Angiographic studies are not as helpful in VOD as they are in BCS. The major hepatic veins and IVC are normal on venography, but WHVP is invariably elevated, a finding that supports the diagnosis of VOD. Findings on hepatic arteriography and indirect portography are similar to the findings in BCS. Because of the significant risk of bleeding after BMT, it is safest in such patients to perform liver biopsy by the percutaneous transjugular route. WHVP can be measured at the same time. Imaging studies, including Doppler US, CT, and MRI, are important adjuncts to exclude BCS.

Liver function test results are invariably abnormal in VOD and do not differ from the results seen in BCS; these abnormalities reflect serious hepatic dysfunction but are not specific for VOD. After BMT, elevated plasma levels of plasminogen activator inhibitor 1 (PAI-1) have been reported to be a useful marker in distinguishing VOD from several other causes of posttransplant hepatic dysfunction, such as graft-versus-host disease, drug-induced hepatotoxicity, sepsis, and viral hepatitis.[256] PAI-1 has been implicated in the pathology of VOD.

Treatment

Substantial experience has been reported with treatment of patients with VOD caused by pyrrolizidine alkaloids.[249,250,252,257] If such patients are seen during the acute stage of VOD, the initial treatment consists of withdrawal of the causative agent and measures to support the damaged liver. Approximately one-fourth of patients recover from the acute phase with supportive medical therapy, approximately one-fifth die of liver failure or bleeding esophageal varices, and the remainder experience a chronic condition that waxes and wanes while cirrhosis of the liver evolves. SSPCS is indicated during the acute phase in patients who bleed from esophageal varices and in patients who, within 4 to 8 weeks of onset, show no signs of recovery, such as disappearance of ascites, improvement in liver function, and improvement in the characteristic lesions seen on percutaneous needle biopsy of the liver. Serial liver biopsy specimens are helpful in assessing the course of the disease.

During the past decade there has been a marked increase in the use of BMT and a corresponding increase in the frequency of VOD. This increase has given rise to numerous trials of various interventions aimed at preventing and treating VOD. In mild forms of VOD, spontaneous recovery is reported in 70% to 85% of patients.[253] However, severe forms do not resolve without treatment.[258]

Agents studied in prophylaxis of VOD include defibrotide, ursodeoxycholic acid (UDCA), tPA, antithrombin III (ATIII), prostaglandin E_1 (PGE$_1$), and anticoagulation with low-dose heparin.[253,259] Of these, the most promising is defibrotide. In five retrospectively controlled studies of VOD prophylaxis, the incidence and severity of VOD were reduced by defibrotide.[260-264] In five of the trials, UDCA showed a significant benefit, with reductions in both incidence of VOD and mortality.[265-270]

Pharmacologic options for the treatment of established VOD include defibrotide, tPA, ATIII, and methylprednisolone. Of these, defibrotide has been subject to the most extensive investigation. In six studies of defibrotide treatment of patients with established VOD, all or most at high risk with multiorgan failure, 36% to 76% had complete remission of VOD.[271-276] Encouraging responses to defibrotide have been found in children as well as following liver transplantation.[273,277]

Use of tPA in treatment of VOD has been evaluated in several series totaling 130 patients.[253,278] The response rate has approached 30% in the largest series[279]; however, no response was seen in patients with renal, respiratory, or multiorgan failure. Moreover, severe bleeding developed in 24%. Thus administration of profibrinolytics and anticoagulants should be avoided in these patients, but conversely, these agents have benefit early in the course of VOD.

Several studies of ATIII in treatment of VOD have been reported. In a retrospective review of the largest series (48 patients), Peres et al.[280] observed that ATIII failed to reduce the incidence of VOD but seemed to be beneficial in mild to moderate VOD and especially in severe VOD. These results were similar to those of Haussmann et al.[281] in pediatric patients.

A single study investigated methylprednisolone treatment of VOD, with results suggesting a therapeutic benefit.[282] However, prospective comparative studies are needed to warrant use of this agent.

Transjugular intrahepatic portosystemic shunting has been used in a small number of patients with VOD. Senzolo et al.[253] summarized the results of TIPS in 27 patients with generally severe VOD, 24 of them following BMT. All but three of the BMT patients died. Available data suggest that although portal hypertension and ascites improve after TIPS, long-term efficacy and overall survival remain poor.[283-289]

Because of the high mortality rate of severe VOD after BMT, LT warrants consideration (see Chapter 105). Experience with LT in severe VOD is limited, with case reports in the literature on 12 patients,[290-296] with 5 of the 12 long-term survivors. The problems associated with use of LT, not unique to VOD, include predicting which patients will not survive despite other forms of treatment; the timing of the LT operation, before multiorgan failure is so severe that survival is not possible; and obtaining a suitable liver graft. One-fourth of patients with VOD experience the severe form of the disease. The causes of death in severe VOD are hepatic failure, renal failure secondary to hepatorenal syndrome, respiratory failure from pulmonary VOD or infection, gastrointestinal bleeding, sepsis, and congestive heart failure. In the Seattle study of a cohort of 355 patients, the mortality rate of severe VOD was 98%.[297]

Side-to-side portacaval shunt has been used effectively in severe VOD after BMT, but the experience has been limited because of a general reluctance to subject these very ill patients to a major operation despite their almost certain death without effective nonsurgical treatment.[298] Experience is similarly small with the use of TIPS in severe VOD secondary to BMT, and its role remains to be defined.

SUMMARY

Budd-Chiari Syndrome

Although no etiologic or predisposing condition can be identified in some cases of BCS, in recent years an underlying disorder has been found in more than 70% of patients. The most common conditions that predispose to BCS are hematologic disorders with thrombotic tendencies, such as polycythemia vera and paroxysmal nocturnal hemoglobinuria. Evidence indicates that multiple prothrombotic hematologic factors acting concurrently are involved in many patients with BCS. In the Western experience, hematologic factors play a primary role, whereas in the East, membranous obstruction of the vena cava is common.

The pathologic lesion of BCS is thrombosis of the major hepatic veins or the inferior vena cava (IVC) or both, which results in hepatic venous outflow obstruction; intrahepatic and portal hypertension; dilation of the liver sinusoids; intense centrilobular congestion of the hepatic parenchyma; and ischemia, pressure necrosis, and atrophy of the parenchymal cells in the center of the liver lobule. Early in the course of BCS these lesions are reversible, if the obstruction is relieved. Persistence of the high pressure and congestion within the liver results in irreversible damage, hepatic fibrosis, and progression to cirrhosis, often within months. The two paramount dangers in BCS are development of irreversible liver damage and extension of thrombosis from the hepatic veins into the IVC. The most striking difference between the East and West in the pathology of BCS is the site of the venous occlusion causing hepatic outflow obstruction: in the East, it is usually in the IVC; in the West, it is most often in the major hepatic veins.

The diagnosis of BCS in the initial weeks and months is based on finding the typical symptoms and signs combined with abnormal results of several diagnostic studies (US, CT, MRI, or angiographic examination of IVC and hepatic veins). Liver biopsy reveals the typical lesions of obstruction to hepatic venous outflow: intense centrilobular congestion and centrilobular loss of parenchyma and necrosis. Liver function tests invariably show significant hepatic dysfunction. In surgical patients with BCS confined to the hepatic veins, the clinical manifestations and results of diagnostic studies are confirmed by the findings of marked ascites; an enlarged, congested liver; splenomegaly; extensive portosystemic collateral veins; IVC pressure that is substantially lower than portal vein (PV)

pressure; portal hypertension; and a markedly elevated hepatic occluded portal pressure, which sometimes is higher than the free portal pressure.

Treatment of BCS has evolved; initial experience predominantly led to surgical intervention, but percutaneous techniques have supplanted surgical shunt procedures as a more popular upfront treatment strategy, with surgical therapy reserved for those patients who are not able to undergo interventional radiologic procedures, or those who do not respond to this strategy, or other medical approaches. Nonsurgical therapy of BCS includes medical treatment with thrombolytic agents, anticoagulants, and diuretics and interventional radiologic therapy consisting of transluminal angioplasty, venous stenting, and TIPS. Additional techniques include infusion of thrombolytic agents, such as streptokinase, urokinase, or tPA, or recanalization with mechanical thrombectomy. Anticoagulant therapy to prevent propagation of the thrombi has produced a limited, short-term response when used alone but is an essential component of long-term management in any patient with an underlying prothrombotic state.

Radiologic therapy consisting of percutaneous transluminal angioplasty with and without the use of metallic stents has had some short-term success in patients with chronic BCS resulting from stenosis of the IVC. The TIPS procedure is used with increasing frequency for all forms of BCS. The advantage of TIPS is that it does not require a major operation; disadvantages are a high rate of TIPS stenosis and occlusion requiring repeated revision, frequent recurrence of symptoms, and numerous radiologic procedures and hospitalizations. The incidence of TIPS occlusion has decreased greatly with the introduction of PTFE-covered stents.

Side-to-side portacaval shunt has proved to be the most effective therapy of BCS caused by thrombosis of the hepatic veins; it converts the valveless PV into an outflow tract, decompressing the obstructed hepatic vascular bed. Splenorenal shunt, interposition mesocaval shunt, and portacaval shunt using synthetic grafts are hemodynamically similar to SSPCS but are inferior operations in BCS because of a high incidence of thrombosis and occlusion. Interposition shunt using an autogenous internal jugular vein H-graft has produced results similar to those of direct SSPCS. Important technical features of SSPCS are proper positioning of the patient; use of a long, right subcostal incision; and extensive mobilization of the IVC and PV so that the two vessels can be brought together. SSPCS is contraindicated when BCS is caused by thrombosis or occlusion of the IVC. In these patients, a mesoatrial shunt has been used with some short-term success, although incidence of thrombosis of the bypass graft is high. The combined cavoatrial shunt/SSPCS has replaced the mesoatrial shunt as the preferred treatment for BCS caused by IVC occlusion.

Liver transplantation is indicated in patients with chronic BCS who have cirrhosis with progressive hepatic failure and in patients who have had an unsuccessful portosystemic shunt. In approximately 1043 patients with advanced liver disease secondary to BCS, LT has resulted in a mean actuarial 5-year survival rate of 71%. BCS recurred in 13% to 27% of the liver grafts, and thrombosis of other blood vessels, particularly the PV, occurred in 9% to 40% of patients. LT and SSPCS are not competing forms of treatment; LT is appropriate therapy in late stages of BCS, when the liver disease no longer can be reversed by SSPCS.

The most effective treatment strategy for BCS involves a multidisciplinary approach that includes hepatologists, hematologists, interventional and diagnostic radiologists, and transplant surgeons. Initial measures most frequently use the less invasive percutaneous approaches. Although surgical therapy with portacaval shunt is losing popularity globally, it should remain a crucial tool in the management of BCS patients. Careful integration of all treatment options in a stepwise method, with inclusion of the patient in the clinical decision making, will produce successful and durable outcomes.

Veno-occlusive Disease

Also called *sinusoidal obstruction syndrome*, VOD is a group of disorders in which hepatic venous outflow obstruction is caused by subendothelial sclerosis of the sublobular hepatic veins, terminal hepatic venules, and sinusoids within the liver. VOD is caused by antineoplastic drugs, ingestion of plants containing pyrrolizidine alkaloids, and irradiation of the liver. In the Western Hemisphere the most frequent cause is bone marrow transplantation (BMT). Extensive occlusion of the small hepatic veins results in centrilobular hemorrhagic necrosis of the liver parenchyma, which progresses to diffuse fibrosis and cirrhosis. Although it can occur at any age, VOD caused by pyrrolizidine alkaloids has been observed most often in children; after a prodromal febrile illness, acute-onset abdominal distention from ascites ensues, along with abdominal pain, hepatosplenomegaly, weakness, and sometimes jaundice and peripheral edema.

The most important symptoms and signs of VOD after BMT are ascites, jaundice, and abdominal pain. Some patients recover from the acute stage of VOD, but approximately one-fifth of patients with pyrrolizidine poisoning die; cirrhosis develops rapidly in the remainder, with all its clinical manifestations. Mortality from severe VOD after BMT has been reported at 98%. The most important diagnostic study in VOD is percutaneous needle liver biopsy, which shows the specific abnormality of extensive occlusion of the small hepatic veins within the liver and centrilobular hemorrhagic necrosis.

Substantial experience with treatment of VOD involves patients who ingested pyrrolizidine alkaloids. In the acute stage, supportive medical therapy is used. SSPCS is indicated during the acute stage if bleeding esophageal varices develop, or if the clinical and liver biopsy signs of hepatic venous outflow obstruction do not subside after 4 to 8 weeks. In the chronic phase of VOD, with the usual manifestations of cirrhosis, SSPCS is recommended even before variceal hemorrhage has occurred.

Mortality in patients with chronic VOD is high, and the major cause of death is bleeding esophageal varices (see Chapter 81). Medical therapy of the many patients who have developed VOD after BMT has included defibrotide, tPA, ursodeoxycholic acid, antithrombin III, prostaglandin E_1, anticoagulation with low-dose heparin, and high-dose corticosteroids. None of these agents has been uniformly effective, but the most promising agent in prophylaxis and treatment of VOD is defibrotide, reported to produce a complete response rate of 36% and a 100-day survival rate of 35% in severe VOD. In addition, SSPCS, TIPS, and LT have been used in a few patients with severe VOD. These procedures have had some success and deserve further evaluation, particularly because one-fourth of patients with VOD experience the severe form, and again, BMT-associated mortality in severe VOD is reportedly 98%.

The references for this chapter can be found online by accessing the accompanying Expert Consult website.

SECTION II. Neoplastic

A. General

CHAPTER 87

Tumors of the liver: Pathologic aspects

Valérie Paradis

Liver tumors encompass a large spectrum of benign and malignant neoplasms, both primary and metastatic. In addition, a variety of nonneoplastic tumor-like masses deserve attention because they can simulate neoplasms. Despite the major advances in imaging procedures, the definitive diagnosis of a liver tumor continues to be based primarily on accurate examination and interpretation of histologic material. The roles of the pathologist are to establish the histologic type of the tumor, estimate its potential behavior, guide for the choice of the most relevant therapy, and assess any pertinent prognostic indicators.

According to their histogenesis, primary intrahepatic tumors are classified into three main categories: hepatocellular, biliary, and mesenchymal tumors, although there are additional rare entities. Liver tumor classification has recently been refined, especially in regard to their molecular characteristics; this chapter will present the main pathologic aspects of intrahepatic liver tumors according to the 5th edition of the World Health Organization (WHO) classification.[1]

HEPATOCELLULAR TUMORS

Hepatocellular Carcinoma

See Chapter 89.

Clinical and Epidemiologic Background

Hepatocellular carcinoma (HCC) accounts for 75% to 85% of primary malignant liver tumors in adults, ranking as the sixth most common cancer and the fourth leading cause of cancer-related death worldwide.[2,3]

One of the striking characteristics of HCC is the marked geographic variation in its frequency, which is mainly related to geographic distribution of chronic liver disease–related risk factors (see Chapters 68 and 74). East Asia and sub-Saharan Africa have a very high incidence, whereas Italy, Spain, and Latin American countries are at intermediate risk. A relatively low but increasing incidence is found in Western Europe, the United States, Canada, and Scandinavia.[4-6] The major known risk factors for HCC are hepatitis viruses (chronic hepatitis B [HBV] and hepatitis C [HCV]), toxic agents (alcohol and aflatoxins), metabolic diseases (metabolic syndrome, α-1 antitrypsin deficiency and Wilson disease), hereditary hemochromatosis, and immune-related diseases (primary biliary cirrhosis and autoimmune hepatitis). Given that the burden of chronic liver diseases is expected to rise, it is expected that the incidence of HCC will also increase in the future, especially with the pandemic obesity and metabolic syndrome.[7-10] In addition, despite very effective treatment for viral hepatitis, the risk of developing cancer persists in HCV infection after viral eradication and remains significant in hepatitis B[11-13] (see Chapters 68 and 74).

HCC is primarily a disease of older men, and its incidence generally increases with age. In Western Europe and the United States, most patients with HCC are between 50 and 75 years of age. It occurs more frequently in men than women with a male-to-female ratio ranging from 2:1 to 9:1, although the reason is not clear.[14] Serum α-fetoprotein (AFP) is elevated in most symptomatic tumors, but small cancers are associated with lesser or even normal levels. Thus serum AFP is not a reliable diagnostic test for HCC screening patients with cirrhosis.[15]

The association between cirrhosis and HCC is well established. Indeed, 60% to 90% of HCC arises in cirrhotic livers. Conversely, approximately 1% to 3% of patients with cirrhosis will develop HCC annually. It is admitted that HCC usually occurs after a mean delay of 10 years after the constitution of liver cirrhosis. This observation is highly consistent with a multistep process that implies progressive malignant transformation of preneoplastic lesions such as macroregenerative and dysplastic cirrhotic nodules. This progression parallels the growing accumulation of genetic and epigenetic abnormalities into liver cells from regenerative to malignant nodules. Nevertheless, it has been widely recognized that in patients with metabolic syndrome, HCC may develop in absence of advanced liver fibrosis in up to 45% of cases, suggesting the involvement of specific mechanisms probably related to the pathogenesis of the underlying disease rather than fibrosis alone.[16-20]

Pathologic processes of HCC are peculiar for several aspects. Indeed, its morphologic patterns are varied beyond the classic classification based on growth pattern and tumor differentiation (see Chapter 74). Furthermore, molecular pathogenesis of HCC is complex, involving different molecular pathways that may reflect different etiologic factors and various underlying liver disease conditions, and it may help in identification of new therapeutic targets.[21-23] Accordingly, a pathomolecular classification of HCC describing the main histologic subtypes related to molecular alterations has been proposed.[24]

Gross Pathology

HCC can adopt a wide range of gross configurations. Several macroscopic classifications have been proposed, but their clinical relevance has not yet been proven.

Tumor size ranges from less than 1 cm (occult HCC) to over 30 cm in diameter. At time of diagnosis, the mean size of HCC arising on cirrhotic liver is usually inferior to those occurring in nonfibrotic liver. HCC tumors less than 2 cm are recognised as "small" or "early HCC".[25] Small HCCs have been subdivided into vaguely nodular and well-circumscribed HCC, two patterns with differences in prognosis, with the vaguely nodular form having a better prognosis than the well-circumscribed one.[25,26] Although the diagnosis of large HCC relies mainly on imaging modalities, biopsy is often requested for the diagnosis of these small nodular lesions.

At gross examination, overt HCC may display a nodular, infiltrative, or diffuse macroscopic pattern.[27] The nodular (expanding) pattern is the most common type. It is typically seen in association with cirrhosis. This group of HCCs is characterized by a sharp demarcation between the tumor mass and the compressed and partly atrophic surrounding parenchyma (Fig. 87.1). The nodule may be single or multiple across the liver when developed as a complication of cirrhosis. When nodules are multiple, small nodules, less than 1 cm in diameter and adjacent to the main tumor nodule (usually within 2 cm), they are considered satellite nodules (Fig. 87.2). In cases of multiple HCCs, nodules may represent either multifocal independent tumors or intrahepatic metastasis. Such distinction is quite impossible based on pathologic study alone but could be addressed with surrogate molecular analysis.[28,29] On cut section, nodular HCC is circumscribed totally or partly by a fibrous capsule.[30] Capsule formation is considered to begin at a tumor diameter of at least 10 mm or greater because no distinct capsule was noted in lesions less than 10 mm.[31] The prognostic significance of

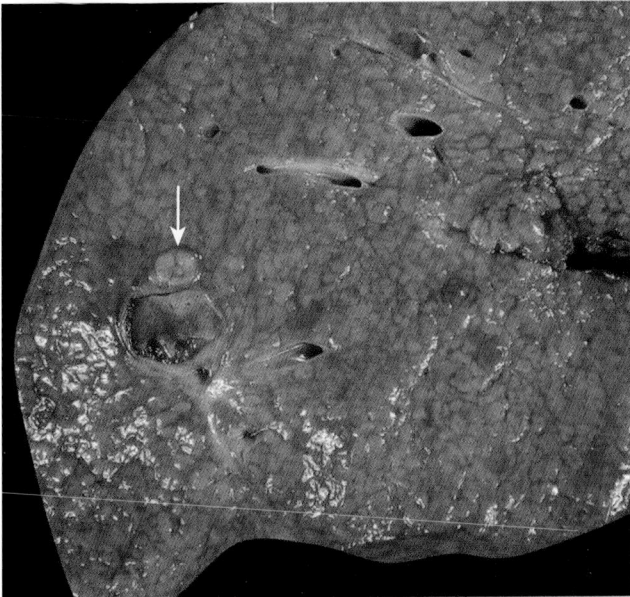

FIGURE 87.2 Hepatocellular carcinoma. The tumor is massively necrotic with minute satellite nodules in the close vicinity (arrow).

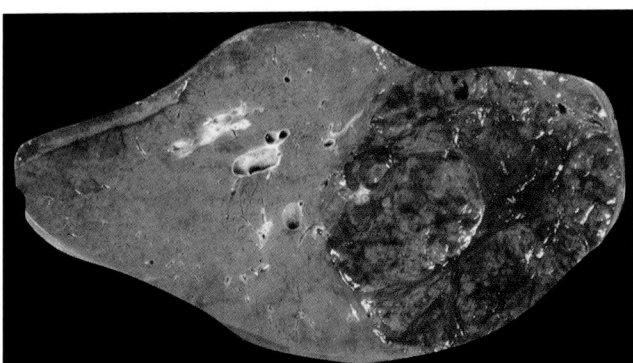

FIGURE 87.3 Hepatocellular carcinoma. The tumor forms soft masses with cholestatic foci and area of hemorrhage and necrosis.

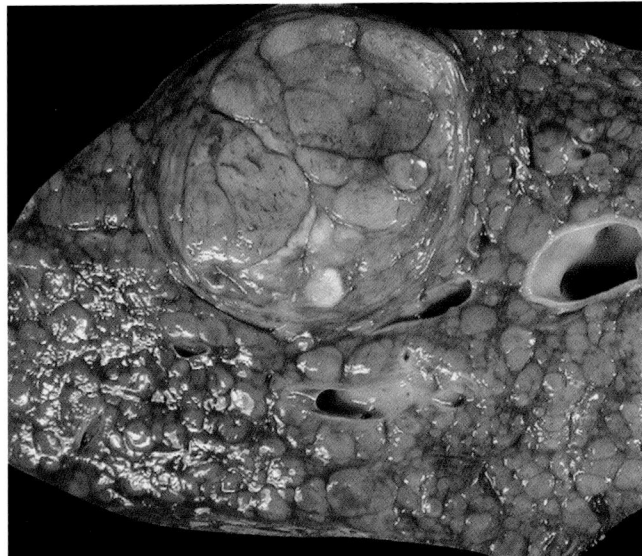

FIGURE 87.1 Hepatocellular carcinoma developed on liver cirrhosis. Hepatocellular carcinoma developed in a cirrhotic liver with an expanding growth pattern. The tumor is sharply demarcated from the surrounding parenchyma and limited by a fibrous capsule. Note the distorted hepatic vessels forming curved structures at the periphery of the tumor, suggesting an expanding growing pattern.

capsule formation has not yet been definitively settled. HCCs typically form soft masses that vary in color from gray, light brown, or yellow-green, depending on their content of fat or bile, often punctuated by foci of hemorrhage or necrosis when the tumor reaches a significant volume (Fig. 87.3).

The infiltrative (massive) pattern is usually characterized by a large single mass that occupies a substantial portion of the liver. The lesion is poorly circumscribed with ill-defined, invasive borders (Fig. 87.4).[32] On cut section, the tumor extends into and distorts the adjacent nontumor tissue, interdigitating with surrounding parenchyma. Vessels are incorporated into and not displaced by the tumor mass so that tortuous vessels around the tumor are not so obvious.[33]

The diffuse (or cirrhotomimetic) pattern is the least common and represents a widespread infiltration by numerous small nodules that virtually replace the entire liver. In this pattern, the tumor consists of several unconnected small tumors of roughly similar size. Multicentric origin or intrahepatic spread after portal vein invasion have been discussed as pathogenic mechanisms (Fig. 87.5).[34]

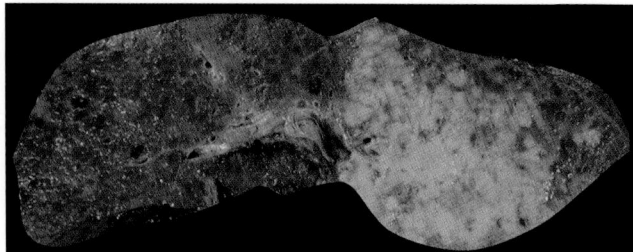

FIGURE 87.4 Hepatocellular carcinoma with an infiltrative growth pattern.   The tumor is poorly circumscribed and extends into the surrounding cirrhotic parenchyma. No rim of compressed tissue or capsule is visible.

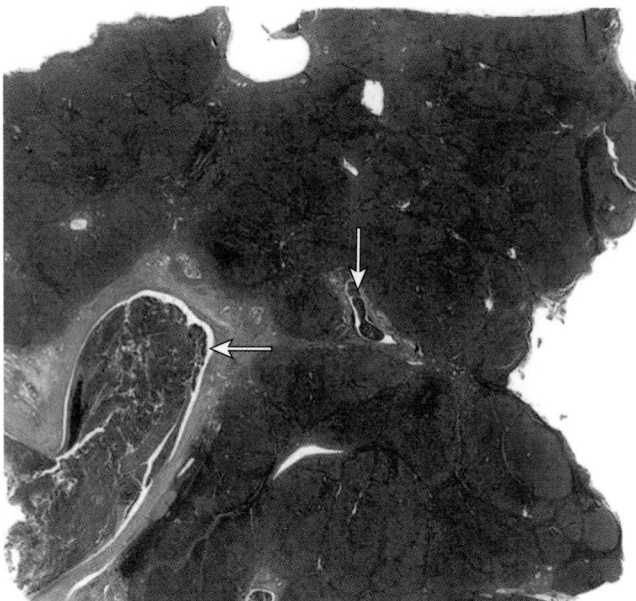

FIGURE 87.6 Hepatocellular carcinoma with vascular invasion.   Invasion of a dilated large portal vein and a small vein *(arrows)* by a tumoral thrombus in a cirrhotic liver close to a hepatocellular carcinoma.

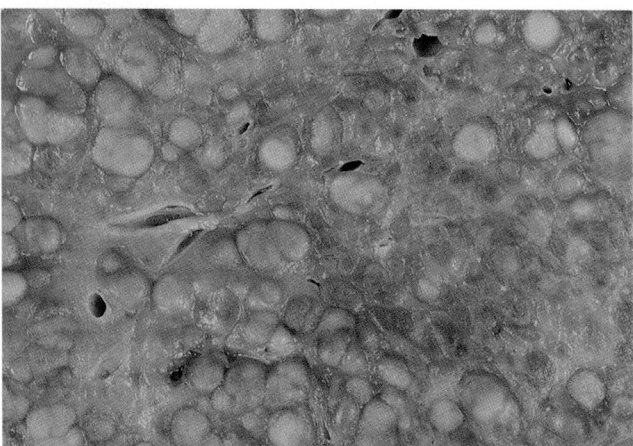

FIGURE 87.5 Hepatocellular carcinoma with a diffuse pattern of growth.   The liver is quite totally replaced by numerous small tumoral round nodules.

Pedunculated HCC is noted in rare instances, presumably reflecting an origin from an accessory hepatic lobe.[35] The identification of the pedunculated form of HCC is significant because even in the case of large tumors, limited resection may give excellent results.

This gross classification has limitations because categorization of a tumor within one single growth pattern may be difficult. Expanding HCC may show areas of infiltrative pattern. Finally, along with the diffuse pattern, which is associated with a dismal prognosis, differentiation between expanding and infiltrative patterns does not appear to be a prognostic indicator.

In advanced HCC, invasion of large veins is common even at gross examination (see Chapter 14). The portal vein is more often involved than hepatic veins, inferior vena cava, or right atrium (Fig. 87.6). Portal vein invasion may be associated with thrombosis. Vascular invasion should be determined with care at the initial gross examination (macrovascular invasion). In some instances, intravascular tumor plugs in the close periphery of a large tumor may be difficult to distinguish from satellite tumor nodules. Invasion of large bile ducts producing biliary obstruction and hemobilia might be occasionally found.

Histopathology

Histopathologic evaluation is no more systematic before treatment because dynamic imaging has high diagnostic accuracy

for tumors larger than 2 cm. When imaging remains inconclusive, ultrasound (US)-guided biopsy is indicated, especially in nodules smaller than 2 cm in diameter, a situation in which biomarkers have low predictive values and hyperarterialization may be incomplete or absent. For nodules smaller than 1 cm, biopsy is generally not recommended because of its limited performance. These diagnostic criteria have been endorsed by most international liver diseases associations.[15,36] Nevertheless, and despite the major advances in radiologic procedures, the definitive diagnosis continues to be often primarily based on accurate examination and interpretation of histologic material for any small or atypical nodule. Moreover, a more active biopsy strategy is increasingly proposed, aiming to adapt therapeutic strategies.

Histopathologically, the diagnosis of HCC is based on the resemblance between tumor cells and normal hepatocytes.[37] Therefore the microscopic evaluation entails the assessement of cytologic characteristics of tumoral cells and evaluation of their architectural pattern.[38,39] Tumoral cells may present varying degrees of hepatocellular differentiation within a single tumor. Nuclei are usually basophilic, often irregular with prominent nucleoli and a high nuclear-to-cytoplasmic ratio. In well-differentiated HCC, the tumor cells may closely resemble normal hepatocytes with a polygonal shape, distinct cell membranes, and eosinophilic granular cytoplasm (Fig. 87.7). Bile canaliculi often can be seen by light microscopy or demonstrated by immunostaining. When dilated, they might contain bile pigment, a characteristic feature of hepatocellular differentiation. Accumulation of glycogen or fat in tumor cells may produce a clear cell appearance (Fig. 87.8). Mallory-Denk bodies, hyaline globules, or eosinophilic ground-glass–like cytoplasmic inclusions can be observed.[40]

As the tumor evolves to poorly differentiated phenotype, cell-to-cell heterogeneity, bizarre nuclei, or giant tumoral cells

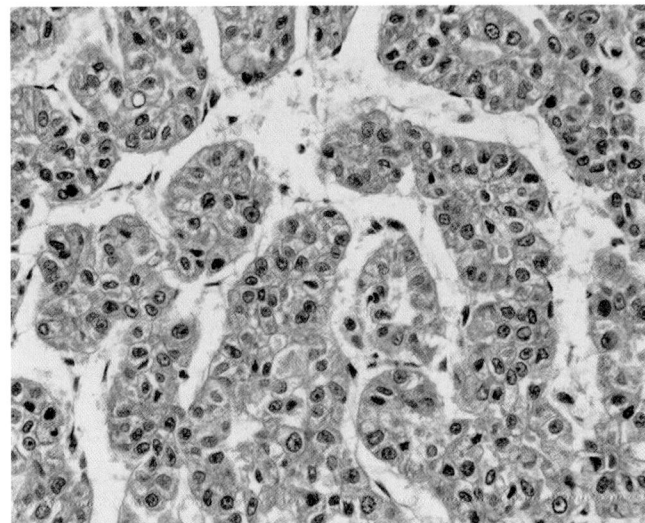

FIGURE 87.7   Well-differentiated hepatocellular carcinoma. Tumor cells are organized in enlarged trabecula (>6 cell plates) and more or less resemble normal hepatocytes with a polygonal shape, distinct cell membranes, and clear cytoplasm with a high nuclear-to-cytoplasmic ratio.

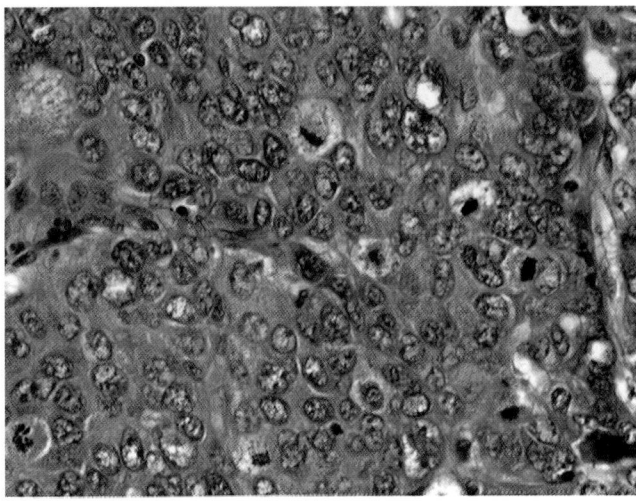

FIGURE 87.9   Poorly differentiated hepatocellular carcinoma. The tumor is highly cellular with tumoral cells organized in large trabeculae with bizarre nuclei, mitosis, and apoptotic bodies.

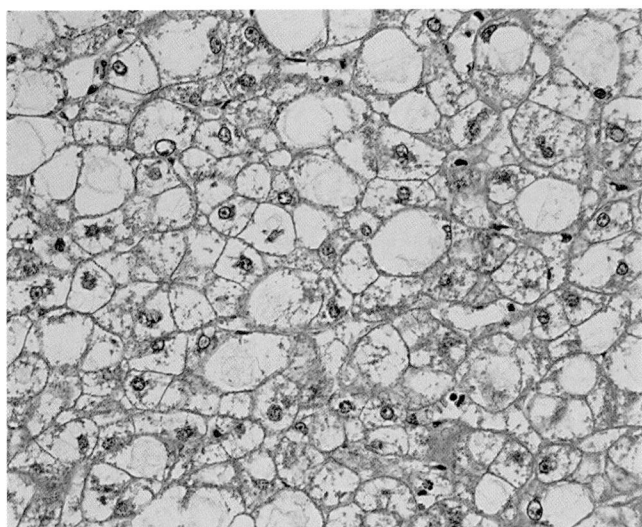

FIGURE 87.8   Hepatocellular carcinoma with clear cell pattern. Malignant tumor cells of various sizes are enlarged with a clear cytoplasm.

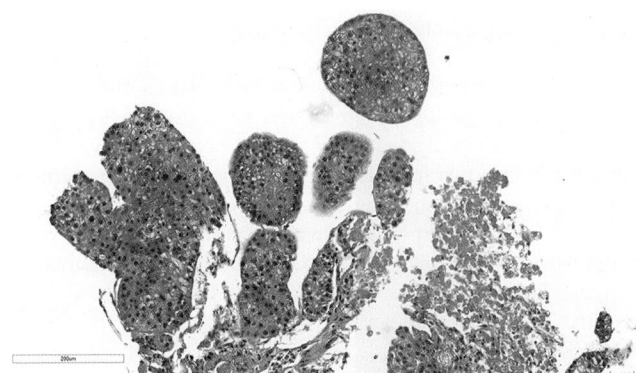

FIGURE 87.10   Hepatocellular carcinoma with a macrotrabecular pattern. Biopsy specimen showing tumor trabeculae are composed of more than six cell plates, outlined by endothelial cells.

may appear. Mitosis and apoptotic bodies can be observed (Fig. 87.9). Different degrees of cellular differentiation are usually present within a single large tumor, although small HCCs tend to be more homogeneous.

Growth Patterns

The arrangement of the cells contributes to the variety of microscopic appearances. On this basis, three main growth patterns that may co-exist within a nodule are described. The main architectural patterns of growth of HCC are as follows:

1. Trabecular growth, in which tumoral hepatocytes are arranged in plates varying in thickness from 2 to over 20 cells. Macrotrabecular pattern is commonly used for trabecular proliferations being at least 7 cells thick (Fig. 87.10). This feature resumes the normal trabecular arrangement of liver plates. Neoplastic cells are organized along simplified sinusoids lined by flat endothelial cells, with few or no Kupffer cells. Compared with normal liver plates, the reticulin framework is commonly sparse or absent.

2. A compact or solid pattern occurs when the trabeculae are closely aligned, and the sinusoids become compressed and unapparent. It may co-exist with a macrotrabecular pattern and shows a worse prognosis.[24]

3. The acinar or pseudoglandular pattern results from either gland-like dilatation of the canaliculi between tumor cells (lumens can contain bile) or central degeneration of trabeculae (lumen containing mainly degenerative products with fibrin) (Fig. 87.11). Like the trabecular pattern of growth, stroma is typically sparse. The lack of a desmoplastic stroma reaction is a helpful diagnostic clue when other glandular malignant epithelial neoplasms, especially cholangiocarcinomas, are discussed. On occasion, large vascular lakes resembling peliosis can develop within the pseudoglandular formations.

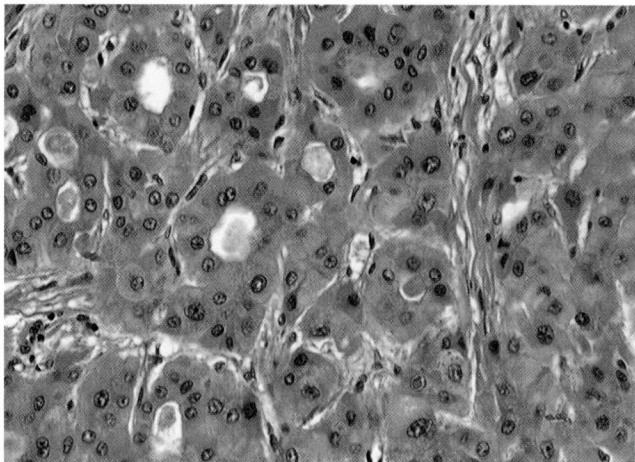

FIGURE 87.11 Hepatocellular carcinoma with pseudoglandular pattern. Hepatocytes display gland-like organization around dilated canaliculi between tumor cells with or without bilirubinostasis.

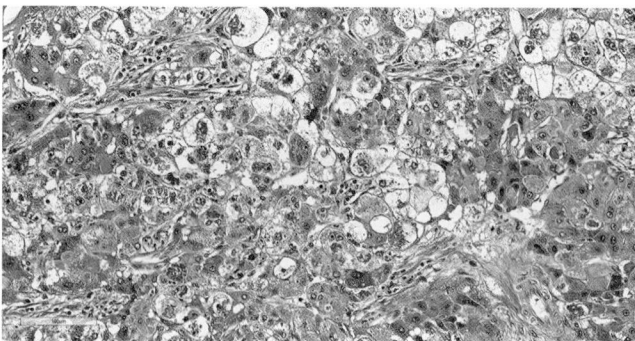

FIGURE 87.12 Steatohepatitic subtype of hepatocellular carcinoma. Tumor is predominantly composed of large, ballooned cells with Mallory-Denk bodies, some inflammation and pericellular fibrosis.

Hepatocellular Carcinoma Subtypes

HCCs can be further classified into subtypes that represent distinct clinicopathologic entities. High-throughput molecular studies have provided several molecular classifications of HCC, identifying different subclasses, mostly linked to clinical context (including etiologic factors) and prognosis (including tumor recurrence and survival).[21,22,41–47] Schematically, HCCs are divided into two main groups, one associated with chromosomal stability and showing a better prognosis, and the other associated with chromosomal instability and showing a worse prognosis. Based on the G1 to G6 classification, a pathomolecular classification has been proposed based on pathologic features specifically associated with the molecular patterns[24] (see Chapter 9B).

STEATOHEPATITIC SUBTYPE. Initially described HCV infection in transplanted patients and then in patients with alcoholic or metabolic clinical context, the steatohepatitic subtype (SH-HCC) is characterized by morphologic hallmarks recapitulating the nonalcoholic steatohepatitis (NASH) picture, including steatosis, ballooning malignant hepatocytes, Mallory-Denk bodies within tumor cells, inflammatory infiltrates, and pericellular fibrosis[40] (Fig. 87.12). To note, there is no consensual definition of SH-HCC, which may be referred to as HCC showing an SH pattern in more than 5% to more than 50% of tumor area according to the series. In addition, the number of elementary features (steatosis, ballooned cells, Mallory-Denk bodies, inflammation, and fibrosis) required for the diagnosis may vary.[48–50]

Macroscopically, SH-HCC is nodular, well-limited, and more yellowish (because of steatosis) compared with other subtypes (Fig. 87.13).[48] In one study, SH-HCC tended to be smaller and better differentiated independently of the presence of cirrhosis in the background liver.[50] These HCCs were assigned to the G4 transcriptomic subgroup characterized by a lack of Wnt/β-catenin pathway activation and low GS expression.[24,51] Although no significant changes in the gene involved in lipid metabolism were observed, activation of the interleukin-6 (IL-6)/AKT/STAT pathway was frequent in this subgroup, which is consistent with the involvement of this pathway in the transition from nonalcohol fatty liver (NAFL) to NASH.[24]

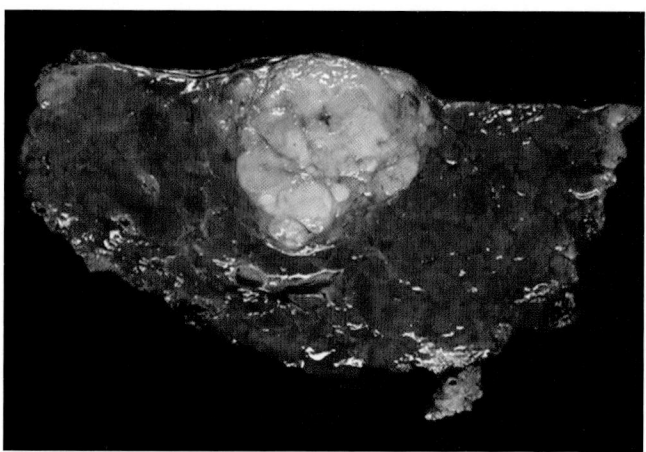

FIGURE 87.13 Steatohepatitic subtype of hepatocellular carcinoma. Macroscopic view showing a 3-cm nonencapsulated yellowish tumoral nodule.

Immunophenotypically, in addition to the common markers of HCC (glypican-3, heat shock protein-70 [HSP-70] and glutamine synthetase [GS]) ballooned tumor hepatocytes are negative for cytokeratin (CK) 8/18, except for the Mallory-Denk bodies, which are also labeled by ubiquitin.[40,48,49] Additionally, SH-HCCs are diffusely stained with sonic hedgehog ligand, and a minority of them express progenitor markers, including SALL4, EpCAM, and CK19.[51]

Whether SH-HCC may present a better or worse prognosis compared with conventional HCC remains difficult to conclude, because available data are derived from resected or transplanted patients. Nevertheless, nearly all failed to show any statistical difference in terms of overall survival or disease-free survival.[48,50] Such clinical behavior is supported by the less aggressive histologic phenotype with a lack of satellite nodules and microvascular invasion that SH-HCC seems to display.[24]

CLEAR CELL HCC. Clear cell HCC, defined by the predominant (>80%) proliferation of clear cell morphology from glycogen accumulation, accounts for aproximately 5% of overall HCC.[52] The clear cell variant has been associated with a better prognosis, but the survival advantage, if present, is minor and has not been confirmed.[53] Clear cell HCC may be associated with hypoglycemia and hypercholesterolemia, and sudden death from severe hypoglycemia has been reported.[54,55] This subtype is not clearly associated with specific molecular features thus far.

MACROTRABECULAR-MASSIVE HCC.

This subtype, observed in 10% to 20% of HCCs, is defined by a predominant (>50% of total tumoral area) macrotrabecular (>6 cells thick) architectural proliferation (see Fig. 87.10).[24] It is more frequently observed in the context of HBV infection, associated with high AFP serum levels, and exhibits features of worse prognosis, including vascular invasion and satellite nodules.[22,24,56] Macrotrabecular-massive HCC clustered with the G3 transcriptomic subgroup is linked to cell cycle activation and chromosomal instability. *TP53* mutations and/or *FGF19* amplifications are common hallmarks.

CTNNB1-MUTATED HCC.

HCCs with mutations in *CTNNB1* (which encodes β-catenin, a molecule of the Wnt signaling pathway playing a role in liver physiology and zonation) are generally well-differentiated hepatocellular neoplasms characterized by trabecular and pseudoglandular architectural patterns, intratumoral cholestasis, and lack of immune infiltrates (see Fig. 87.11). These tumors cluster with the G5 and G6 transcriptomic subgroups, display expression of genes involved in hepatocellular differentiation, and function as well in bile uptake.[57,58]

SCIRRHOUS HCC.

Scirrhous HCC is a rare (~5% of HCCs) but distinctive variant characterized by abundant, dense fibrous stroma and compressed, sometimes elongated, malignant hepatocytes (Fig. 87.14). The tumor tends to occur in an older age group, affect men and women equally, and might be associated with hypercalcemia.[59] Although generally smaller in size, they exhibit granular eosinophilic cytoplasm, vesicular nuclei, and conspicuous nucleoli. Bile pigment can sometimes be discerned. Scirrhous HCC is characterized by the expression of progenitor markers, including CK19 and CD133 and also demonstrates activation of transforming growth factor-beta (TGF-β) pathway/epithelial-to-mesenchymal transition.[24,60]

LYMPHOCYTE-RICH HCC.

The lymphocyte-rich HCC subtype is very rare (<1%) and refers to HCC showing massive infiltration of lymphocytes, mimicking lymphoepithelioma tumors, which can be observed in various organs, including the nasopharynx. Nevertheless, although such tumors may be associated with EBV, EBV appears not be involved in the development of lymphocytic-rich HCC.[61] Compared with other subtypes, lymphocytic-rich HCC is characterized by a better prognosis.

OTHER SUBTYPES OF HCC.

Besides the main HCC subtypes, several others have been reported based on specific morphologic

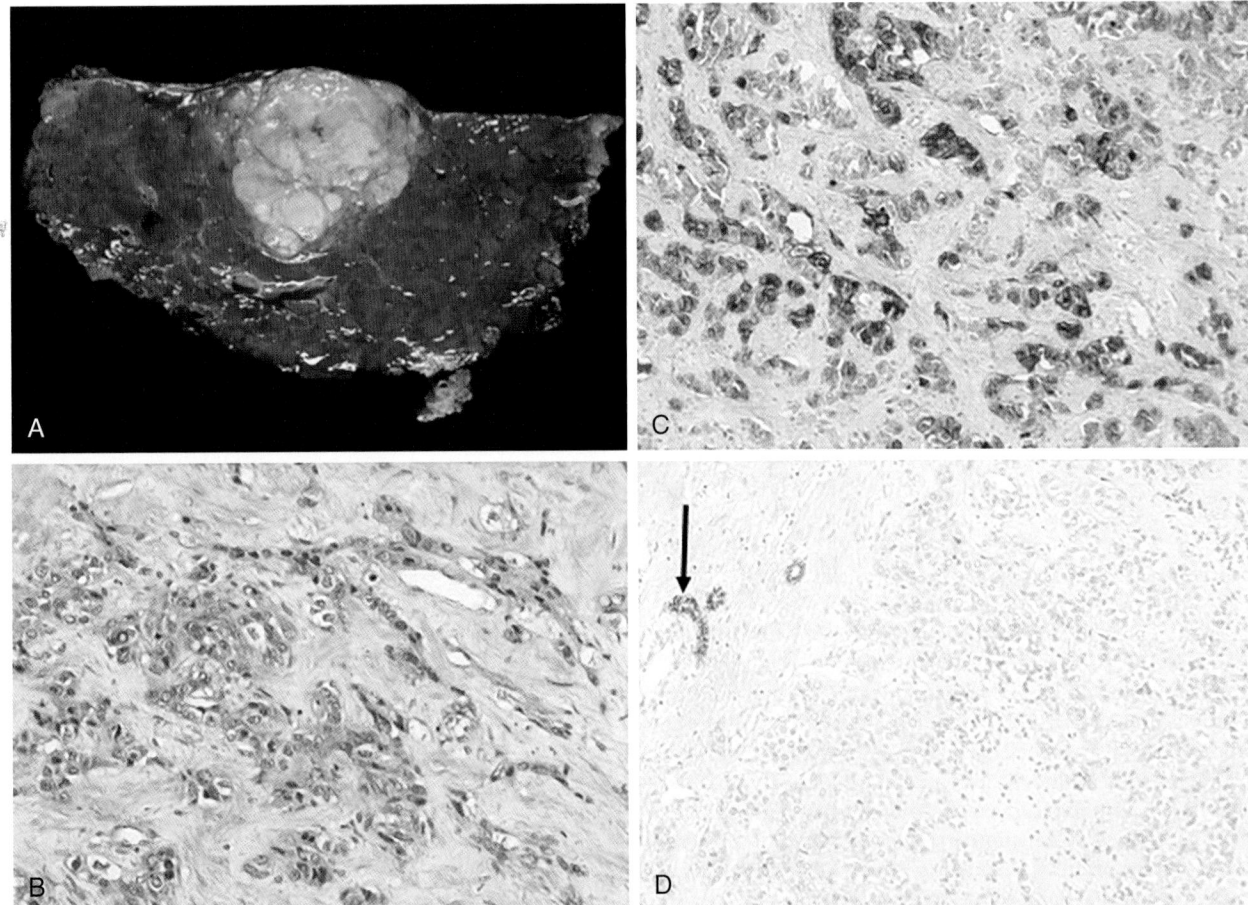

FIGURE 87.14   Scirrhous hepatocellular carcinoma. A, Macroscopic view showing a poorly limited nodule within a noncirrhotic liver. **B,** Histologically, presence of an abundant, dense fibrous stroma with compressed, sometimes elongated, malignant hepatocytes. **C,** Tumor cells are positive for glypican-3 and **(D)** negative for CK7 (CK7-positive entrapped bile ducts *arrow*).

and/or molecular features. Among them, sarcomatoid HCC is characterized by a sarcomatous-appearing component of spindle-shaped or giant tumor cells.[62] The elongated spindle cells are arranged in bundles, occasionally with interlacing or storiform patterns. The giant cells are multinucleated, markedly pleomorphic, and cytologically anaplastic, and osteoclast-like giant cells are described in some instances.[63] These tumors have been referred to as carcinosarcomas. The sarcomatoid component varies in its extent, and histologic transitions with the carcinomatous elements are often noted. The spindle-shaped cells are typically immunoreactive for keratin and AFP.[64] Sarcomatoid changes have been described with resistance to targeted therapies.[65]

The chromophobe variant is composed of tumoral cells with a pale chromophobe cytoplasm showing in some places striking nuclear atypias.[66] Whereas no specific clinical correlations have been reported, this chromophobe HCC is associated with the alternative lenghtening of telomere phenotype, a telomerase-independent mechanism identified in other malignancies.[66]

A small subset of HCC is characterized by the production of granulocyte colony-stimulating factor, resulting in intratumoral infiltration of neutrophils.

Using microarray technology, several studies have shown that a subset of adult HCC display phenotypical traits of progenitor cells. These tumors retain stem cells markers and express CK19, a marker of biliary lineage. Interestingly, worse survival was demonstrated for this subgroup.[67–69] This phenotype is associated with *TP53* mutations and particular subclasses of HCC (G1–G3).[24,60,67]

HCC IN NONCIRRHOTIC LIVER. This group encompasses several entities. HCC might develop during the evolution of a chronic fibrosing liver disease, at the stage of incomplete cirrhosis (septal fibrosis). This is especially common in the context of chronic HBV infection and more often reported in patients with nonalcoholic fatty liver disease (NAFLD) given the rising prevalence of metabolic syndrome worldwide.[9,16,18,70–72] Because of the possible reversibility of cirrhosis, it is not known whether HCCs in incomplete cirrhosis develop during an ongoing fibrogenesis or along the reversion of cirrhosis. Finally, HCC may also arise from the malignant transformation of preexisting hepatocellular adenoma (see later) (see Chapter 88A).

Among HCCs developed in a normal background liver, the fibrolamellar variant was first delineated as a distinct entity in 1980.[73] In a population-based study, fibrolamellar HCC constituted 0.85% of all cases of primary liver cancer and 13.4% of all cases in patients younger than 40 years.[74] Clinically, it occurs in young people with equal sex ratio, and no association with chronic liver disease, cirrhosis, or any other known predisposing risk factors.[75] Characteristic genetic abnormalities have been suggested.[76,77] In addition, overexpression of neuroendocrine genes, including prohormone convertase 1, neurotensin, delta/notch-like epidermal growth factor–related receptor and calcitonin, has been reported in fibrolamellar HCC.[78] These data are consistent with description of neurosecretory granules in tumoral cells by electron microscopy and may support the potential efficiency of chemotherapeutic and targeted therapies.[78] More importantly, a chimeric transcript resulting from an approximately 400-kilobase deletion on chromosome 19 was specifically identified in a set of fibrolamellar HCCs. The fusion transcript encodes a chimeric protein coupling a segment of the HSP (DNAJB1) with the catalytic domain of protein kinase A.[79] Later, messenger RNA (mRNA) and long intergenic non-coding RNA (lncRNA) signatures, highlighting the key role for protein kinase A signaling, were specifically reported in this subtype.[80]

On gross examination, fibrolamellar HCC is firm, mostly well-defined but unencapsulated single nodule that ranges from 5 cm to over 20 cm.[81] On cut section, the tumor is gray to brown with scalloped borders and a solid consistency (Fig. 87.15). Prominent fibrous septa subdivide the mass and may connect with a central zone of scarring (Fig. 87.16). Such features may be confusing with focal nodular hyperplasia. In addition, there are several reports in the literature of fibrolamellar HCC spatially associated with focal nodular hyperplasia, although filiation between these two lesions have never been convincingly demonstrated.[82] Calcifications may be observed.

The distinctive histologic features are fibrous stroma and large eosinophilic tumor cells (Fig. 87.17).[83] The stroma comprises

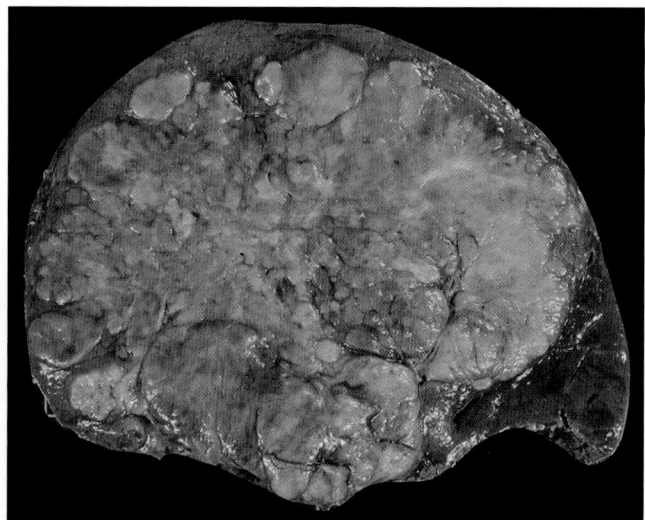

FIGURE 87.15 Fibrolamellar hepatocellular carcinoma. Large lobulated tumor, well-delineated from normal surrounding liver.

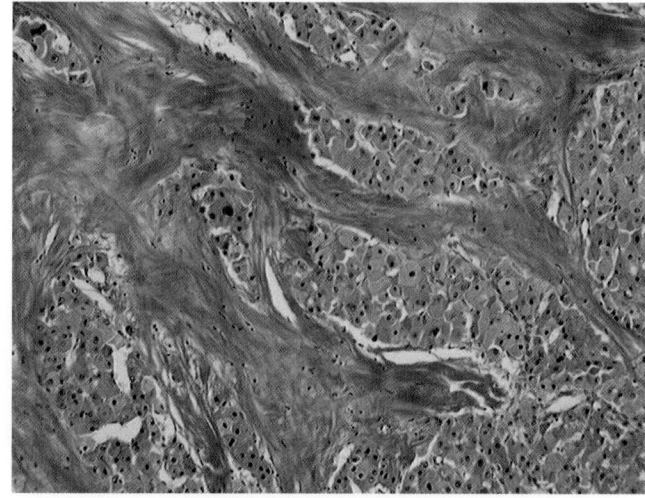

FIGURE 87.16 Fibrolamellar hepatocellular carcinoma. The tumor is composed of large eosinophilic tumor cells organized in cords between dense acellular fibrous bands.

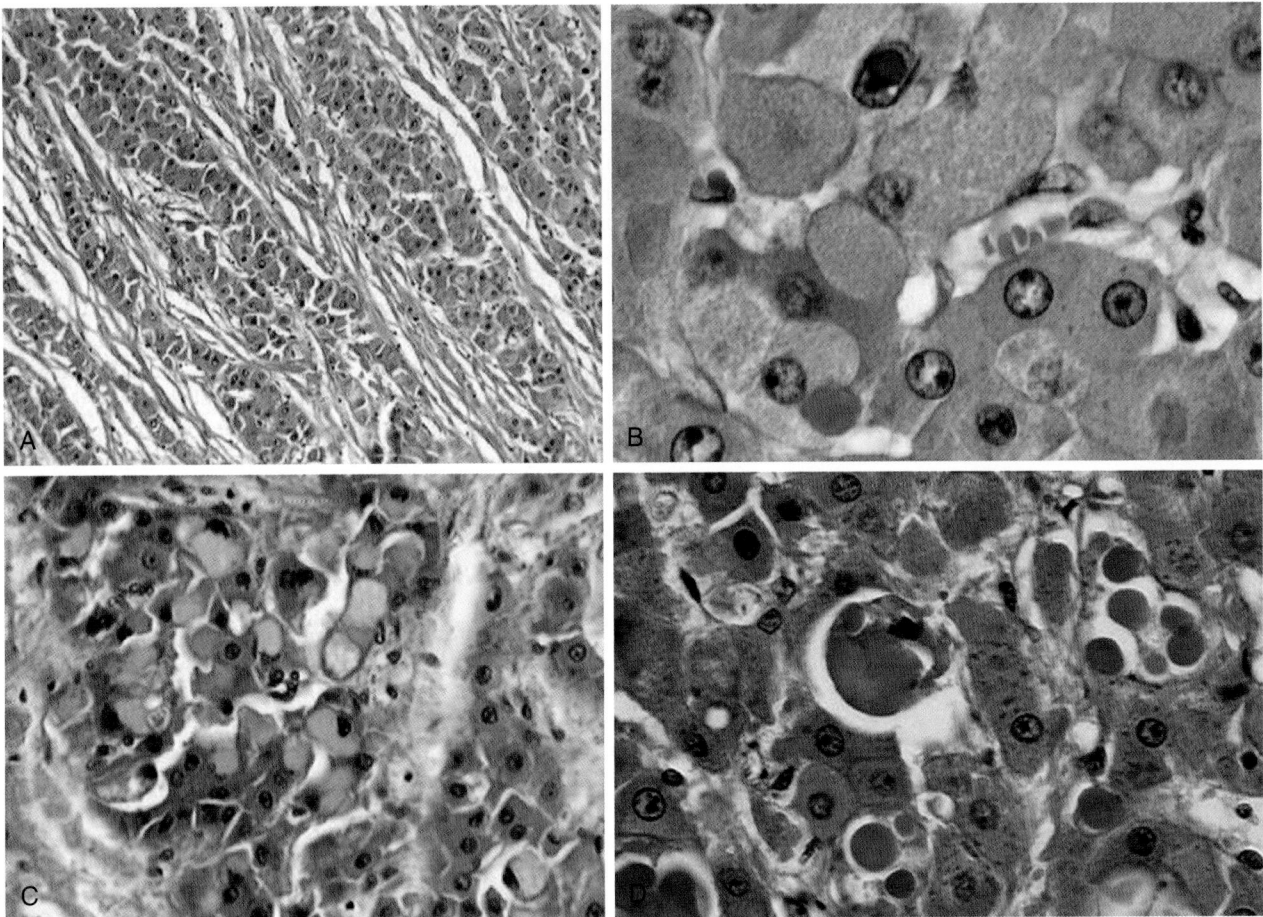

FIGURE 87.17   Fibrolamellar hepatocellular carcinoma.   A, Tumoral cells organized in trabeculae along fibrous septa. **B,** High magnification showing large eosinophilic tumoral cells with intracytoplasmic ground-glass pale bodies. **C,** Intracytoplasmic pale bodies. **D,** Intracytoplasmic eosinophilic globules of various size.

dense fibrous bands of varying thickness that are organized around nests, cords, and sheets of neoplastic cells.[84] The tumor cells are usually larger than normal hepatocytes and display abundant, granular, and deeply eosinophilic cytoplasm with prominent nucleoli. Bile pigment is common and fat or glycogen accumulation sometimes seen. Most fibrolamellar HCCs are histologically of low grade, mitoses are usually sparse, and nuclear pleomorphism or multinucleation is infrequent. Cytoplasmic inclusions of various types are common, including ground-glass pale bodies, eosinophilic cytoplasmic globules of variable periodic acid–Schiff (PAS) positivity, and, rarely, Mallory bodies (see Fig. 87.17). Fibrolamellar HCCs express CK7 abundantly and, in some cells, biliary-type CK19.[85] Interestingly, tumor cells from fibrolamellar HCC also display CD68 positivity with a granular or stippled cytoplasmic staining.[86]

Fibrolamellar HCC tends to be slow-growing and frequently surgically resectable with a better prognosis than other types.[87] Successfully resected patients have a good chance of long-term survival despite extrahepatic recurrences. Transcriptomic data identified two distinct clinical subgroups of fibrolamellar HCC showing different evolutive course.[78] Noteworthy, conventional HCC may display, at varied extent, morphologic features of the fibrolamellar type. Despite the presence of this fibrolamellar component, these so-called mixed-fibrolamellar HCCs (FLC/HCCs) keep clinicopathologic characteristics of conventional tumors, mostly observed in older patients with preferentially liver recurrences.[88] An extensive molecular study recently demonstrated that such mixed FLC/HCCs define a subgroup associated with *BAP1* (gene encoding BRCA1-associated protein-1) inactivation related to mutations or translocations.[89] None of them carried the *DNAJB1-PRKACA* fusion as observed in the fibrolamellar subtype. Compared with conventional HCC, FLC/HCCs are more often observed in women in absence of chronic liver disease but display a poorer prognosis.[89]

Histologic Grading

Grading of HCC relies on the Edmondson and Steiner system, which subdivided HCC into four grades, I to IV, on the basis of histologic and cytologic resemblance to normal liver.[90] This grading has been shown to correlate with the DNA content and cellular proliferation indices of the tumor.[91] Grade I is the well-differentiated one, in which hepatocytic-like cells are arranged in thin trabeculae. Small HCCs tend to be grade I, although they are often not uniform in their differentiation. Grade II HCCs are composed of larger tumor cells with abnormal nuclei. Glandular structures may be present. In grade IV, neoplastic cells are much less differentiated with hyperchromatic nuclei and loss of trabecular pattern. In fact, most HCCs present as grade II or III.[92] Therefore, and as for other carcinomas, there is a general tendency to summarize the grading to a three-scale system with well-, moderately- and poorly differentiated HCC. Tumor grade is used to predict patient survival and disease-free survival after resection and liver transplantation as well, with the worst grade tending to drive prognosis.[93–95] Importantly, grading obtained from the needle biopsy correlates well with the grading performed in the respective resection specimen.[96]

Hepatocellular Carcinoma Staging

Several staging systems have been proposed for HCC.[97,98] The main prognostic factors are related to tumor stage (number and size of nodules, presence of vascular invasion, extrahepatic spread), liver function (defined by Child-Pugh class, bilirubin, albumin, portal hypertension), and general health status. Tumor-node-metastasis (TNM) staging takes into account the size of the nodule, presence of vascular invasion, and number of nodules. The cause has not been identified as an independent prognostic factor.

Size is a major prognostic factor. Small or minute carcinomas have a better prognosis, although with larger cancers, the tumor size does not directly correlate with outcome. The presence of satellite nodules around the main tumor has been recognized as a prognostic factor in several studies. Improved survival has been associated with tumors that are encapsulated or fail to invade surrounding hepatic parenchyma.[99–101]

Macroscopic and microscopic vascular invasion are among the relevant histoprognostic criteria and should be mentioned. Vascular invasion is a known predictor of recurrence and survival, directly associated with histologic differentiation, degree, and size of the main nodule.[102,103] Characteristically, the prevalence of microscopic vascular invasion increases with tumor size, with up to 60% to 90% in nodules above 5 cm in size.[104]

A major influence on clinical status of the patient is the presence or absence of cirrhosis, which thus becomes a leading indicator for survival (see Chapter 74). Therefore simultaneous biopsy of nontumoral liver is of major importance and should be systematically performed to contribute to therapeutic decisions and assist the pathologist in identification of very-well-differentiated HCC.

Premalignant Hepatocellular Lesions and Small Hepatocellular Carcinoma

From experimental hepatic carcinogenesis and epidemiologic studies, it appears that liver carcinogenesis follows a multistep process. Although a few HCCs arise in normal liver, the vast majority of them develop from the stepwise pathway of normal liver → fibrosis → cirrhosis → HCC. Therefore cirrhosis is recognized as a precancerous condition.

There is consensus to support that HCC results from cumulative genetic and epigenetic events that may differ according to the cause of the chronic background liver disease. Although recurrent gene abnormalities have been reported in fully developed HCC, there is a paucity of knowledge regarding the early molecular events associated with HCC[105–107] (see Chapter 9B).

Several studies using different approaches have looked for early molecular abnormalities in regular cirrhosis. Molecular markers have been evaluated in macronodules and none of the oncogenes or tumor suppressor genes involved in advanced HCC have been repeatedly found altered in the precancerous lesions. By contrast, proliferation markers, neoangiogenesis, telomerase expression, allelic losses, and clonality have been studied with more consistent results. Interestingly, using clonal analysis these studies convincingly demonstrated that among

cirrhotic micronodules that appear similar on light microscope, some are already monoclonal (neoplastic) and other polyclonal (regenerative).[29,108] Telomerase, an enzyme that allows unrestricted cell proliferation and is specifically expressed in cancer, can be detected in some but not all of these clonal micronodules without any remarkable histopathologic features.[109] More recently, *TERT* promoter mutations have been reported as the most frequent mutations in liver carcinogenesis, with an increasing rate from dysplastic nodules (<20%) to HCC (~60%).

Morphologically, several terms have been used in the past to define the intermediate lesions such as adenomatous hyperplasia and atypical adenomatous hyperplasia, but in 1995 the International Working Party proposed a unified nomenclature that has gained wide acceptance and is still currently used.[110] This classification was recently reviewed and completed by an international group that added to the panel definitions of the early and small HCC.[25]

MACROREGENERATIVE NODULE. Macroregenerative nodules (MRNs) are tumor-like hepatocellular masses that can arise in the setting of cirrhosis. These lesions have increasingly been detected resulting from both improved radiographic imaging techniques and more widespread screening of cirrhotic patients. Most MRNs are large, discrete nodules ranging from 1 to 3 cm in diameter. There is no minimum size threshold for definition because MRNs have to be appreciated according to the size of background cirrhotic nodules (2-fold to 3-fold larger than cirrhotic nodules).[111,112] Macronodules are often well-limited and surrounded by condensed connective tissue (Fig. 87.18). MRNs are common; they have been found after careful inspection in about 10% of cirrhotic livers at autopsy or at time of transplantation. Histologically, most MRNs are indistinguishable from the usual parenchymal nodules seen in cirrhosis. Normal-appearing hepatocytes are arrayed in plates of one or two cells thickness limited by a regular sinusoid lining and bounded by typical fibrous septa containing blood vessels, bile ductules, and varying degrees of inflammatory infiltration.

DYSPLASTIC NODULE. Dysplastic nodules (DNs) are sizable lesions arising in cirrhosis that differ from the surrounding liver

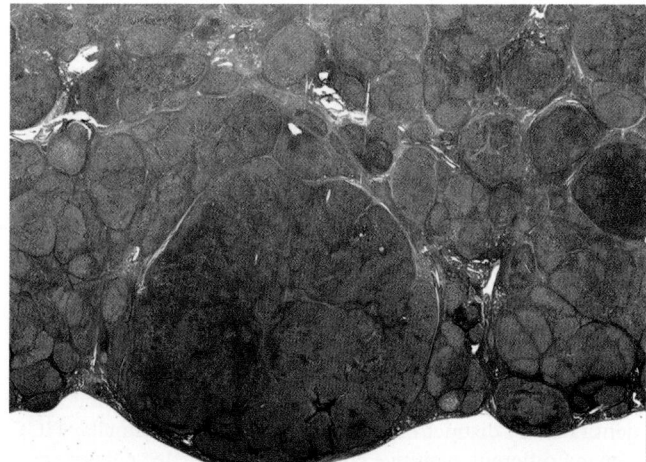

FIGURE 87.18 Low magnification of a benign regenerative macronodule in a cirrhotic liver. Macronodule is well demarcated from surrounding liver. Fibrous septa and portal tracts are still present within macronodule.

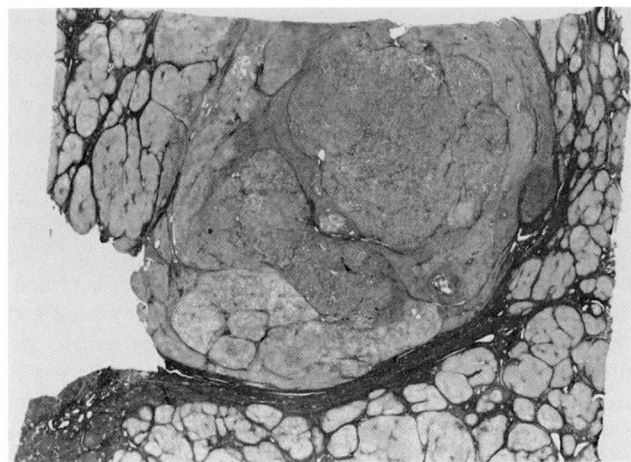

FIGURE 87.19 A macronodule with a nodule-in-nodule pattern of growth. An expansile proliferative basophilic zone is located within a macronodule.

parenchyma in size, color, texture, and degree of bulging of the cut surface. Based on microscopic features, DNs are further subdivided into low grade (LG-DN) and high grade (HG-DN), the latter being closer to HCC in the spectrum of

hepatocarcinogenesis.[25,110,113] Briefly, LG-DNs display features suggestive of a clonal cell population but lack architectural atypia whereas HG-DNs show cytologic and architectural atypias but insufficient for a diagnosis of malignancy (Fig. 87.19). Although dynamic imaging may help differentiate DNs from small HCCs, liver biopsy remains the gold standard.[114]

The premalignant nature of DN is supported by different clues, including the common association with HCC in resected and explanted end-stage cirrhotic livers, with the presence of hepatocellular cytoarchitectural abnormalities featuring a lesion on the way to HCC[115–117]; the morphologic evidence of neoangiogenesis under the form of unpaired arteries supporting the abnormally ongoing vascular supply[118,119]; and the detection of both genetic and epigenetic changes greater than those in the surrounding tissues but less frequent and consistent than in HCC; and their natural history showing an increased risk for malignant transformation compared with control cirrhotic nodules.[120,121] Among the various cytologic alterations that characterized DNs are enlarged, crowded, or irregular nuclei with patent nucleoli, increased nuclear-to-cytoplasmic ratio (Fig. 87.20A–B). Atypical architectural findings involve expansile proliferative zones sometimes located within an MRN (nodule-in-nodule formations), increased number of unpaired arteries, focal loss of associated reticulin framework, and foci of abnormal structural patterns, including

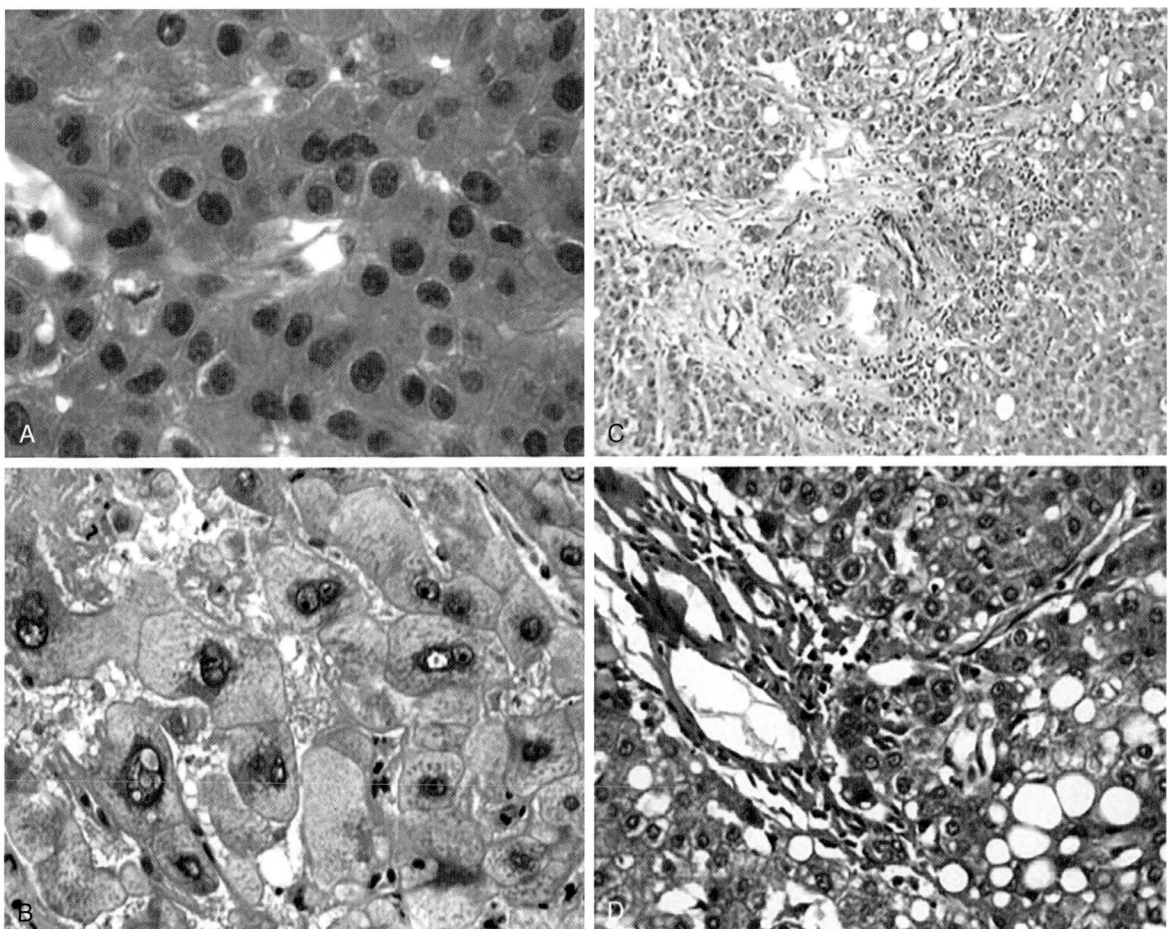

FIGURE 87.20 Histologic features discriminating hepatocellular nodules less than 2 cm in cirrhotic liver. A, Small liver cell changes: foci of small liver cells with increased nuclear/cytoplasmic ratio. **B,** Large liver cell changes: cluster of abnormal large liver cells with dystrophic nuclei. **C,** Isolated arteries within the nodules. **D,** Stromal invasion: liver cells.

irregular thickening of the hepatic plates (see Fig. 87.20C).[110] Stromal invasion, defined as the presence of tumor cells invading into the portal tracts or fibrous septa, is, according to Eastern pathologists, the most relevant feature in discerning HG-DN from small HCCs (see Fig. 87.20D).[25] The degree and extent of these features vary greatly among cases, thus forming a histologic continuum that stretches between ordinary macroregenerative nodules and obvious HCC.[122] Immunohistochemical markers such as glypican 3, HSP-70, GS, and arginase-1 have been recently evaluated. Alone or in combination, they have good accuracy to discriminate HCC from precancerous lesion in surgical specimens but also in liver biopsy.[123–126]

DNs must be differentiated from dysplastic foci, which are defined as microscopic changes incidentally recognized in cirrhotic tissue. According to histopathologic criteria, dysplastic foci are split into large or small liver cell changes (see Fig. 87.20A–B). Although large liver cell change (previously large liver cell dysplasia) consists of abnormal but nonneoplastic hepatocytes that are a predictor of HCC development, small liver cell change is composed of neoplastic cells that are direct precursors of HCC.[127,128]

SMALL HCC. A small liver cancer is currently defined as HCC with a maximum diameter of less than 2 cm.[34] Small HCCs have been further divided into two different entities: early HCC (eHCC) and small progressed HCC (small pHCC). Macroscopically, eHCC shows a vaguely nodular pattern, nonencapsulated, with indistinct margins. Histologically, eHCCs are well-differentiated without vascular invasion. In contrast, small pHCCs show distinct margins, commonly delimited by a fibrous capsule.[25] Microscopically, small pHCCs are well to moderately differentiated with obvious stromal invasion and diffuse sinusoidal capillarization. They have already acquired an ability to invade the vessels and metastasize (Fig. 87.21).[129–131] On the liver biopsy sample, the difference between these two different entities cannot be recognized because it requires the notion of gross features that are not recognizable in small fragments. The differential diagnosis between eHCC and HG-DN may be challenging on a biopsy specimen and then requires additional immunophenotypic markers, including glypican 3, HSP-70, and GS, as indicated previously.

NATURAL HISTORY OF PREMALIGNANT LESIONS AND DIAGNOSTIC CHALLENGE. Few prospective studies have been conducted in large series of histologically proven nonneoplastic nodules detected by

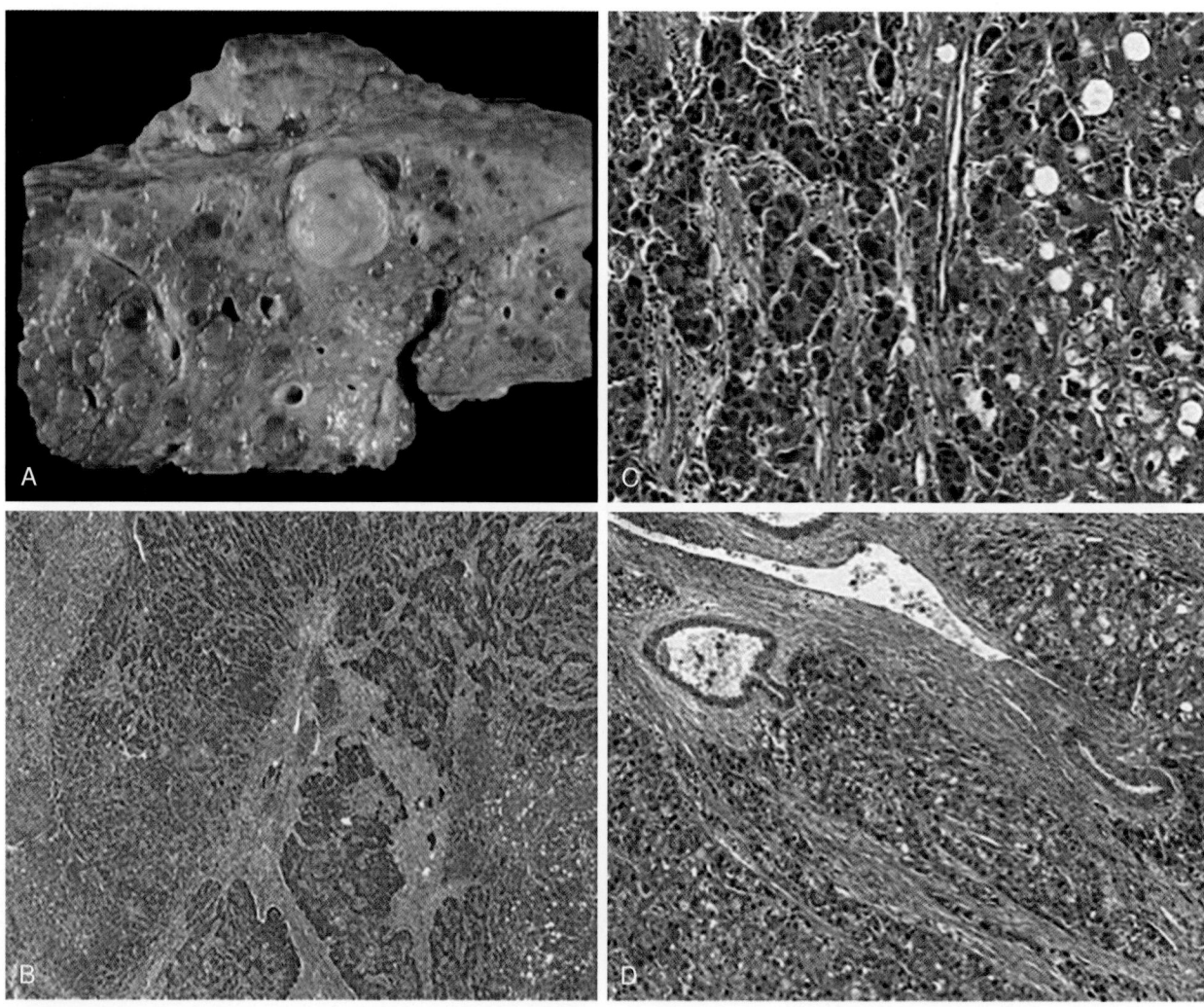

FIGURE 87.21 Small progressed hepatocellular carcinoma (HCC).   A, Macroscopic view showing a small less than 2 cm HCC with distinct margins. **(B–C)** Histologically, the hepatocellular proliferation is heterogeneous with well-differentiated and moderately differentiated areas. **D,** Presence of portal vein invasion.

US during surveillance programs in cirrhosis. Taken together, they have shown that only a minority of macroregenerative or dysplastic nodules (LG-DNs) became malignant, those transforming are mostly in the group of HG-DNs. Furthermore, 40% to 60% stabilized and a few definitely disappeared during follow-up.[132–134] Most of these nodules are 1 to 2 cm, so they seldom display a diagnostic pattern at imaging. Therefore histologic assessment is needed at baseline, and it is worth repeating when sampling is not adequate. Whether HCC regularly develops from DN along the sequence low grade → high grade → early and small pHCC is still unclear. This hypothesis is supported by the feature called nodule-in-nodule, which has been reported mainly in the Eastern literature.[135,136] However, HCC has also been found to originate from outside DNs during the surveillance of cirrhotic patients, supporting that HCC can also develop de novo by skipping the gradual transition of the sequence.[133]

Hepatoblastoma

Hepatoblastoma is the most common primary liver tumor of childhood, accounting for 45% of the malignant hepatocellular neoplasms of infants and young children.[137] Almost all cases of hepatoblastoma occur during the first 3 years of life (median age of 18 months), although rare cases have been described in older children.[138] Serum AFP is markedly elevated in 90% of cases. Although most cases are sporadic, they also can be associated with congenital or genetic disorders, including Beckwith-Wiedemann syndrome, Wilms tumor, familial adenomatous polyposis, glycogen storage disease, and various congenital anomalies.[139,140]

The large majority of hepatoblastomas show genetic alterations of the WNT/β-catenin signaling pathway.[141,142] Gene expression profiling has identified two different classes of hepatoblastoma, one displaying greater genetic instability (gains of chromosomes 8q and 2p), overexpression of progenitor cell markers, and MYC signaling upregulation, which is associated with a more aggressive clinicopathologic phenotype.[143]

Hepatoblastomas are typically solitary masses, mostly located in the right lobe, well-circumscribed, and occasionally encapsulated, with size ranging from 5 to 20 cm in diameter.[137] The cut surface of hepatoblastoma has a bulging, lobulated contour and a variable tan to light brown to gray-white appearance with occasional foci of hemorrhage, cystic degeneration, necrosis, or calcification (Fig. 87.22).[138]

Histologically, hepatoblastoma is composed predominantly of immature liver cells resembling either fetal or embryonic hepatocytes. They are classified by the International Pediatric Liver Tumors Consensus Classification as either epithelial or mixed epithelial and mesenchymal.[144]

The fetal pattern is made of thin trabeculae or nests of hepatocytes smaller than normal with a uniform monotonous appearance, an abundant polygonal cytoplasm, and round regular nuclei with inconspicuous nucleoli. Nuclear pleomorphism is minimal and mitoses are few. Foci of extramedullary hematopoiesis are a common finding (Fig. 87.23). The embryonal pattern is made of solid nests or glandular structures with pseudorosettes. Cells are less mature, small, dark, and poorly defined, with enlarged nuclei and coarse chromatin (Fig. 87.24). Scattered mitoses are regularly noted, with foci of necrosis occasionally seen. Fetal and embryonal patterns often co-exist, and transitions between the two are frequently present. In addition to the two major patterns, other types are described. The small cell undifferentiated pattern consists of

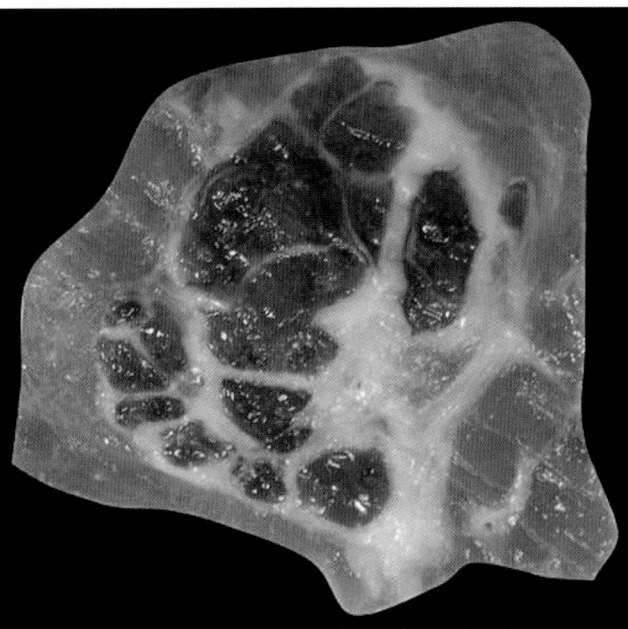

FIGURE 87.22 Hepatoblastoma. Well-limited tumor with lobulation, hemorrhagic foci, and areas of cystic degeneration. (Courtesy Dr. M. Fabre.)

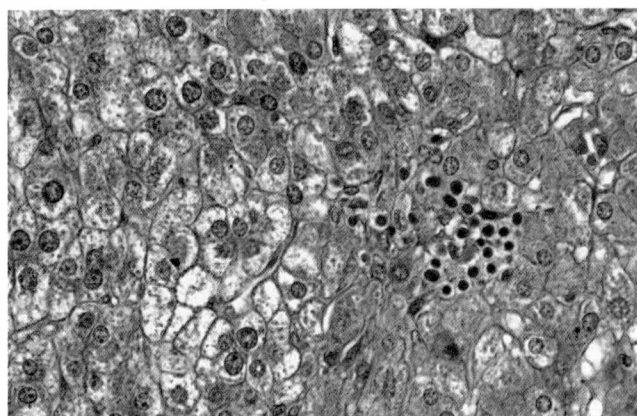

FIGURE 87.23 Fetal type of hepatoblastoma. Tumoral hepatocytes are smaller than normal, with an abundant polygonal cytoplasm and round regular nuclei organized in thin irregular plates with a dark foci of extramedullary hematopoiesis. (Courtesy Dr. M. Fabre.)

small uniform cells similar to those of neuroblastoma with scanty cytoplasm, hyperchromatic nuclei, and frequent mitoses.[145] Other patterns include the macrotrabecular and the cholangioblastic.

The mixed hepatoblastomas combine the epithelial component with mesenchymal-derived tissues of various differentiations. Usually this consists of osteoid-like material, sometimes focally calcified, or primitive spindle cells occurring in fasciculated or loose myxoid arrangements. Rarely, trabecular bone formation or cartilaginous or rhabdomyoblastic differentiation is identified.

Immunohistochemistry, useful for identifying residual tumor tissue after chemotherapy, includes markers of the WNT/β-catenin signaling pathway (/β-catenin nuclear positivity in tumoral cells), AFP, and glypican-3.

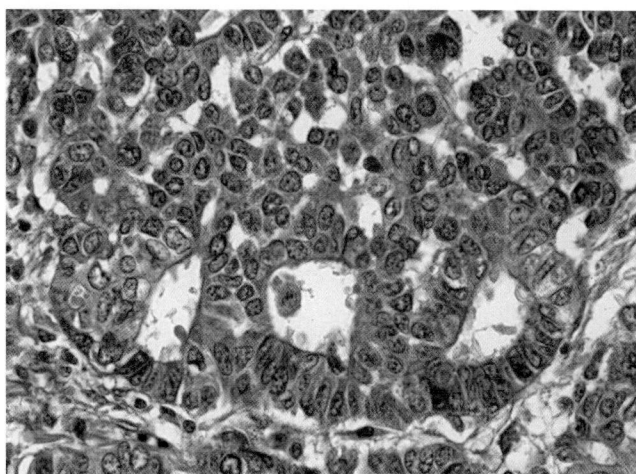

FIGURE 87.24 Embryonal type hepatoblastoma. Tumoral cells are less mature, made of small, dark, angular cells with compact cytoplasm and poorly defined outlines. (Courtesy Dr. M. Fabre.)

Hepatoblastoma is an aggressive neoplasm that invades locally and spreads to regional lymph nodes, lungs, adrenal glands, brain, and bone marrow. Main prognostic parameters include tumor extension, presence of metastasis at the diagnosis, and serum AFP level.[146,147] Once stage is taken into account, the various histologic subtypes become less important prognostic indicators.[148] Nonetheless, tumors of pure fetal-type histologic findings with low mitotic activity tend to have the best prognosis.[149]

Benign Liver Cell Tumors

Benign hepatocellular lesions encompass two main entities, focal nodular hyperplasias (FNHs) and hepatocellular adenomas (HCAs), that strongly differ in term of pathogenesis, clinical presentation, and behavior (see Chapter 88A). Both groups are mainly observed in young women, usually in the context of oral contraception and develop in an otherwise normal liver. Whereas HCA is a neoplastic clonal and proliferative lesion, there is now consensus on the polyclonal, nonneoplastic, and reactive origin of FNH.[150–152]

FOCAL NODULAR HYPERPLASIA. FNHs are 10 times more frequently observed than HCAs. This is the second most common benign liver process, after hemangioma. It is predominantly diagnosed in women of 30 to 50 years of age as a solitary nodule in two thirds of cases. Most FNHs are diagnosed incidentally, but some are revealed by clinical symptoms or biologic alterations such as pain, liver mass, or increased γ-glutamyl-transferase. However, complications such as rupture or bleeding are exceptional, and thus far no evidence of malignant transformation has been reported. The diagnosis of FNH is strongly suggested by imaging techniques so that histopathologic examination is required for diagnosis in a minority of cases[153,154] (see Chapter 14) When performed, the diagnosis of FNH on fine needle biopsy specimens might be occasionally difficult because the fibrous septa and thick abnormal arteries, the hallmarks of FNH, are usually missing.[155,156]

On gross examination, FNH usually appears as a solitary rounded mass, discrete pale to beige and well delineated from background normal liver but without defined fibrous capsule

(Fig. 87.25A). On cut surface, FNHs display a variegated and partly nodular organization with frequently (but not always) a central stellate scar with radiating fibrous cords that are also visualized at imaging.[157,158]

The typical histopathologic features of classic FNH include fibrous septa containing large dystrophic arteries with a peripheral ductular reaction and absence of interlobular bile ducts (see Fig. 87.25B–C). Hepatocytes are usually normal, arranged in normal or mildy thickened plates without cytologic atypia lined by a well-preserved sinusoidal framework. Steatosis or cholestatic degeneration with Mallory bodies may be seen. FNH has been classified into classic FNH and nonclassic forms.[158] In nonclassic forms of FNH, the diagnosis may remain difficult because some of the distinguishing pathologic features may be inapparent. The latter consist of hepatocyte nuclear factor (HNF) without central scar, mixed hyperplastic and adenomatous form, HNF with steatosis, steatohepatitis, and a form with atypia of large cell type.[158,159] There is now strong evidence, based on clonal features and the angiopoietin gene expression profile, that the previously so-called telangiectatic variant of FNH in fact may belong to the group of HCAs (see later).[159] Immunohistochemistry may provide interesting information. Immunostaining with GS showing broad, anastomosing areas of positive hepatocytes adjacent to hepatic veins, described as a map-like pattern, is highly consistent with the diagnosis of FNH and suggests a focal maintenance of lobular organization (see Fig. 87.25D).[160] A further study showed that the phenotype of endothelial cells lining the vascular channels in FNH differ from those in the remaining liver, associated with a downregulation of angiotensin-converting enzyme-1/CD143.[161]

FNH and FNH-like nodules are now well known to develop in the context of vascular liver diseases, including Budd-Chiari syndrome[162,163] (see Chapter 86), portosystemic shunts (see Chapter 84), portal vein thrombosis, portal vein agenesis, and other circulatory disorders of the liver, such as hereditary telangiectasia, and cirrhosis, supporting the concept of a vascular trigger in the pathogenesis of FNH.[164–166] Evidence supports that FNH is a hyperplastic reaction resulting from an arterial malformation related to an increased arterial blood flow.[157]

Similar to HCA, FNH has been observed in association with the use of oral contraceptives, although the relationship remains controversial. FNH may occur together with HCA. FNH has been found to be associated with a variety of nonhepatic tumors and tumor-like conditions, including hemangioma of the liver, hepatoblastoma, and several other tumors (e.g., in siblings with glioblastoma).[167,168] The significance of these associations is unclear but suggest that the pathogenesis of FNH is probably heterogeneous.

Hepatocellular Adenomas

HCA is a rare, benign liver cell neoplasm strongly associated with oral contraceptive (OC) use and androgen steroid therapy.[167,168] Its estimated incidence is 0.1 per year per 100,000 in non-OC users, and reaches 3 to 4 per 100,000 in long-term OC users. HCA size may decrease in size after OC cessation or after menopause. HCA can also occur spontaneously or in association with underlying metabolic diseases, including type 1 glycogen storage disease, iron overload related to β-thalassemia, and diabetes mellitus. Therefore HCAs represent a heterogeneous group of tumors, in which histopathologic features may vary according to the etiologic background.

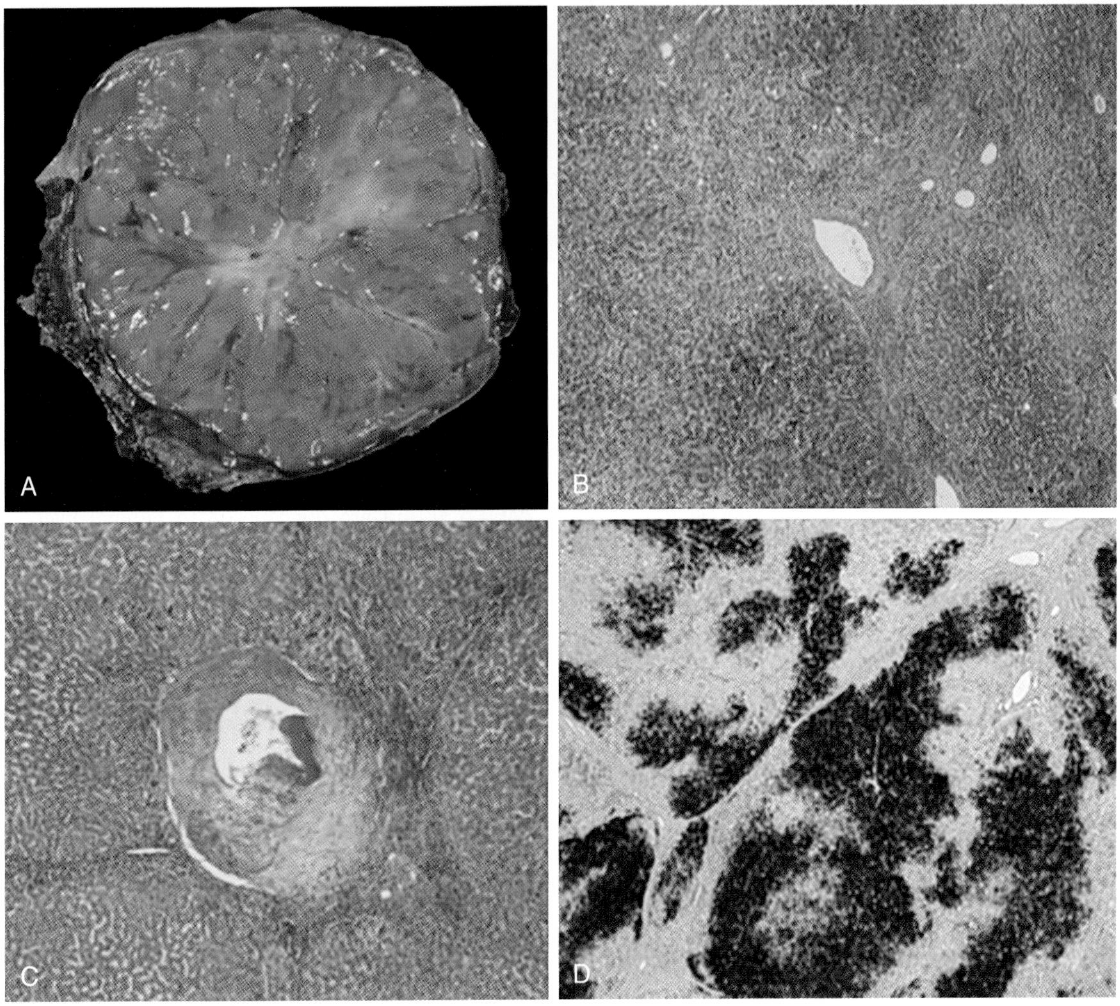

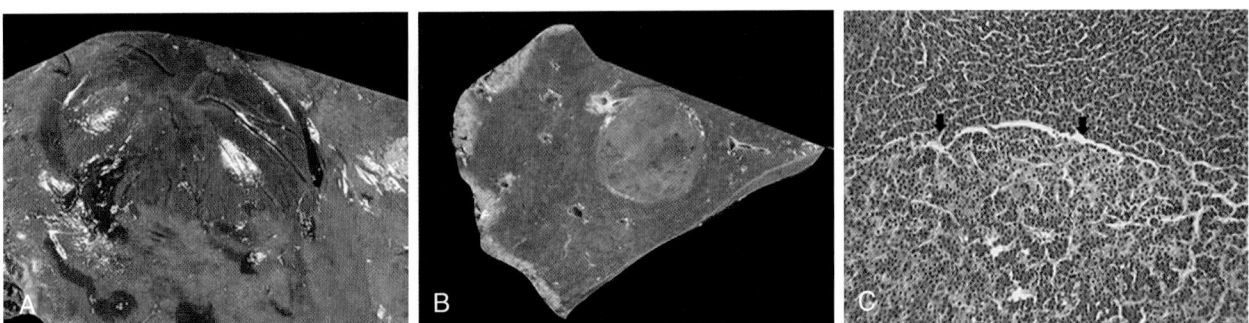

FIGURE 87.25 Focal nodular hyperplasia. A, Macroscopic view showing a well-limited nodular lesion with central stellate scar and radiating fibrous cords. **B,** Histologically, fibrous septa delineating hepatocellular nodules. **C,** Central scar containing large dystrophic artery with thick irregular wall. **D,** "Map-like pattern" of glutamine synthetase immunoexpression.

FIGURE 87.26 Hepatocellular adenoma. A, External view of a superficial tumor bulging under the capsule with large subcapsular and dilated vessel. **B,** On cut section, soft, well-delineated tumor with little or no fibrous capsule and small heterogeneous foci of hemorrhage. **C,** Histologically, proliferation of benign hepatocytes of normal size with a normal nuclear/cytoplasmic ratio pushing the normal liver parenchyma (arrows).

HCAs are usually solitary, sometimes pedunculated, with size ranging from a few mileometers to 30 cm. Large subcapsular vessels are commonly observed for large superficial tumors (Fig. 87.26A). On cut sections, the tumor is soft, white to brown, well-delineated, with little or no fibrous capsule (see Fig. 87.26B). Heterogeneous areas of necrosis and/or hemorrhage may be observed, preferentially in tumors of large size.

Histologically, HCA consists of a proliferation of benign hepatocytes of normal size or slightly enlarged with a normal nuclear-to-cytoplasmic ratio (see Fig. 87.26C). Hepatocytes are arranged in a trabecular pattern without any residual portal tracts. Mitoses are unusual. Small, thin, and unpaired vessels without other portal tract elements, including connective tissue, bile ducts, or ductular reaction, are usually found throughout the tumor. The cytoplasm of hepatocytes may be normal, clear glycogen-rich, or fatty. Cellular atypias can be impressive, especially in patients who have taken steroids for many years. In that context, differential diagnosis with HCC may be difficult. Vascular changes including sinusoidal dilatation, peliosis, infarcts, and hemorrhage are frequent. These changes may leave edematous or fibrotic regions, often with hemosiderin-laden macrophages.

Compared with patients with FNH, patients with HCA are more likely to present with symptoms such as abdominal pain, spontaneous bleeding, and hemorrhage, with an increased risk according to the size for tumors larger than 5 cm in diameter.[169] The risk for malignant transformation of HCA ranges between 4% and 10%, with a higher rate in males, in large HCA, and also varies with HCA subtype.[16,169,170] In addition, recent evidence suggests that metabolic syndrome may favor development of HCC in a preexisting HCA.[16] Increased incidence of metabolic syndrome may partly explain the rising incidence of malignant transformation of HCA, especially in the male population.[171]

Multiple HCAs and so-called adenomatosis are not uncommon (Fig. 87.27). Classically, liver adenomatosis is defined when at least 10 nodules are present.[172,173] Patients with multiple HCAs are predominantly females, but the use of OCs appears to be less prevalent.[174] Patients with glycogen storage disease type I are also at risk of developing multiple HCAs.[175] Nevertheless, these tumors share the same clinical and imaging characteristics independently of their number.[169,176] In addition, recent studies indicate that the risk for complications, including bleeding and malignant transformation, is similar to that in patients with solitary HCA and is not influenced by the number of tumors.[160,169] The three main morphologic patterns of liver adenomatosis have been described: the steatotic form, the peliotic/telangiectatic form, and the mixed form.[176] Of note, the proportion of steatotic HCAs is higher and presence of microadenomatous foci in the nontumoral liver is more often observed in patients with liver adenomatosis.[169]

MOLECULAR CLASSIFICATION OF HEPATOCELLULAR ADENOMAS. Molecular comprehensive studies have gained further insights in the knowledge of HCA demonstrating some degree of molecular and histologic heterogeneity among HCAs.[152] This approach also allowed the identification of genetic alterations associated with the malignant transformation of HCA.[177]

To date, HCAs are subdivided into four main subtypes according to phenotypical and molecular features, the HNF1α-mutated steatotic (H-HCA), the inflammatory (I-HCA), the

β-catenin–mutated HCA (β-HCA), and, more recently described, the sonic hedgehog HCA (sh-HCA).[159,178–180] Importantly, surrogate immunophenotypic markers linked to the genetic abnormalities may be used for the classification of the main groups of HCA.[151] Finally, a minor group of HCAs remains unclassified because they do not display any specific morphologic or genotypic features. Figure 87.28 illustrates the three main HCA subtypes (see Chapter 9B).

The first group of HCAs (H-HCA) displays biallelic mutations of the *TCF1* gene inactivating the hepatocyte nuclear factor 1α (HNF1α) transcription factor. This homogeneous group is phenotypically characterized by marked steatosis, absence of cytologic abnormalities, or inflammatory infiltrates (see Fig. 87.27). Whereas both HNF1α mutations are somatic in most cases, patients with inherited mutation in one allele of HNF1α and an additional somatic mutation may develop HCA in the context of maturity-onset diabetes of the young type 3 (MODY3) and are predisposed to familial liver adenomatosis.[180,181] Immunophenotypically, H-HCAs are characterized by the absence of liver fatty-acid binding protein in tumor cells compared with a cytoplasmic staining in normal hepatocytes.

The second group of HCAs (I-HCA) comprises well-delineated, unencapsulated tumors with areas of vascular changes without any fibrous scar (Fig. 87.29).[159,182,183] Histologically, the hepatocellular proliferation contains small clusters of arteries embedded in collagen often associated with an inflammatory infiltrate (lymphocytes and macrophages) and occasionally ductular proliferation. In addition, foci of sinusoidal dilation and peliotic changes are usually present. Mild or significant steatosis also may be observed within tumoral cells. Although commonly observed in women using OCs, I-HCAs are often reported in patients with increased body mass index (BMI) associated with inflammatory syndrome (increased C-reactive protein [CRP fibrinogen serum levels]).[184] Although, this HCA subtype displays distinct genetic mutations, the cardinal feature is the activation of the JAK/STAT pathway, resulting in the inflammatory phenotype of HCA and explain activation of the acute inflammatory phase observed in tumoral hepatocytes.[185] The most frequent mutations (~60%) are observed in the *IL6ST* gene that encodes the signaling coreceptor gp130,[185,186] followed by mutations of *STAT3* and *GNAS*, accounting for 5% each.[152] Immunophenotypically, tumor cells express acute-phase inflammatory proteins, including serum amyloid A and CRP. GS may be focally expressed by tumoral hepatocytes, mostly around veins.

The third group of HCAs (β-HCA) includes subtypes showing activation of the WNT signaling pathway, which results from mutations or deletion of CTNNB1 (encoding β-catenin). This group is composed of three subtypes according to the degree of WNT signaling pathway activation that are closely related to the genetic alterations and then associated with a varied potential of malignant progression.[187] Accordingly, large deletions and most hotspot mutations of exon 3 lead to high levels of β-catenin activation and exon 3 S45 and exon 7/8 mutations lead to moderate and low activation of the pathway, respectively. The subtype with exon 3 abnormalities is mostly encountered in male patients and frequently shows significant cell atypias, pseudoglandular formations, and pigment accumulation (bile, lipofuschins). Among the three subtypes, the one with exon 3 abnormalities (except S45) displays the highest risk for malignant transformation into HCC.[178,186] Immunophenotypically, activation of WNT signaling pathway may be identified by β-catenin and/or GS expression, the latter marker being more

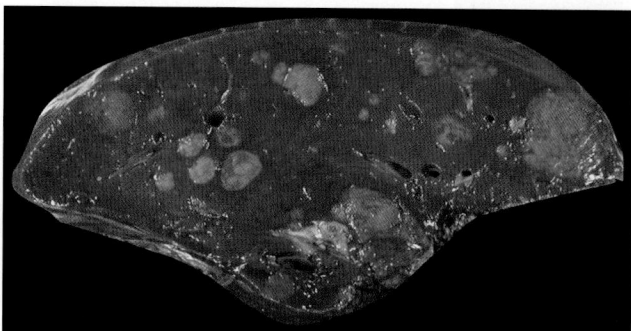

FIGURE 87.27 Liver adenomatosis. Macroscopic view showing multiple hepatocellular adenomas of various sizes are dispersed throughout the liver.

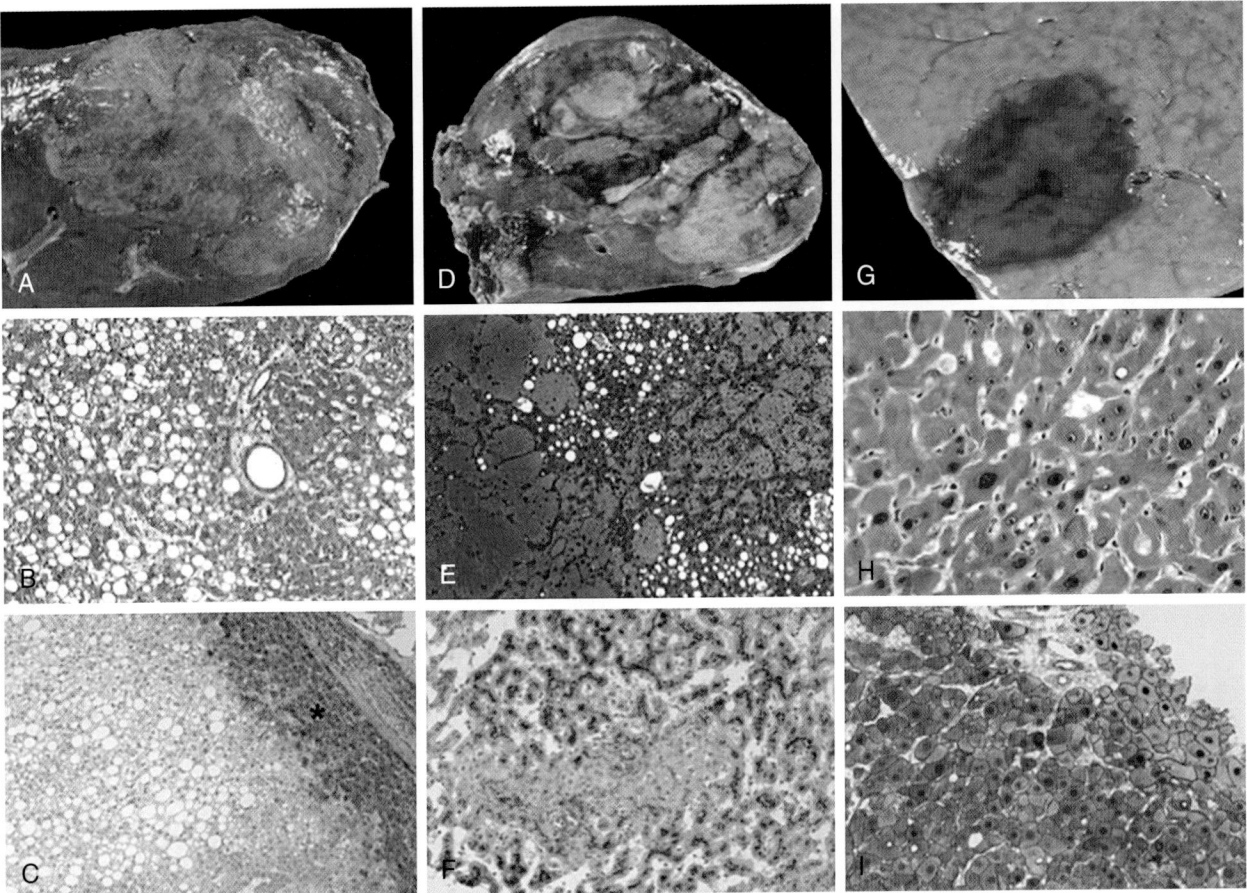

FIGURE 87.28   Pathomolecular subtypes of hepatocellular adenomas.   A–C, Steatotic hepatocellular adenoma (HCA). **A,** Cut section showing a well-limited soft yellow tumor. **B,** Histologically, most tumor hepatocytes are steatotic. **C,** Tumor cells are negative for liver fatty acid binding protein (compared with adjacent nontumoral liver (*)). **D–F,** Inflammatory HCA. **D,** Cut section showing a large nodule unencapsulated with congestive areas. **E,** Histologically, hepatocellular proliferation with extensive dilated and congestive sinusoids. **F,** The tumoral cells are positive for serum amyloid A. **G–I,** β-Catenin–activating HCA. **G,** Cut section showing well-limited cholestatic nodule. **H,** Significant cellular atypias are observed in some tumoral hepatocytes with increased nuclear-to-cytoplasmic ratio. **I,** β-Catenin immunostaining is observed in some tumoral cells.

sensitive. In HCA associated with exon 3 abnormalities (except S45), nuclear β-catenin staining is observed in some tumoral cells (usually focal) and a diffuse, homogeneous, and strong GS staining is present. In HCA with exon 3 S45 mutation, very few to no β-catenin–positive nuclei may be observed and GS shows a heterogeneous GS (starry-sky) pattern with a diffuse reinforcement at the peripheral border. In HCA with exon 7/8 mutations, a faint GS immunostaining may be present in some cases, mostly in a perivascular location, sometimes associated with an incomplete reinforcement at the border.[186] Importantly, some I-HCAs may also exhibit WNT signaling pathway activation regardless of the nature of the genetic abnormalities.

A fourth group of HCA (sh-HCA) has been identified, characterized by the activation of the sonic hedgehog pathway related to deletions of *INHBE*, leading to the fusion of *INHBE* and *GLI1*.[180] This group, accounting for around 4% of HCA, is associated histologic and symptomatic bleeding (see Fig. 87.29). As sh-HCAs are more often observed in patients with increased BMI, some degree of steatosis may be observed in nontumoral liver. Immunophenotypically, increased GLI1 and prostaglandin D synthase is observed in tumoral cells.[180] A distinct group of HCAs at high risk of bleeding has been highlighted using a global proteomic approach. They are characterized by an upregulation

of the arginine synthesis pathway and display overexpression of argininosuccinate synthase 1 in tumor cells.[188]

Finally, a small group of HCAs without any characteristic morphologic features or the genetic abnormalities previously described still remains.

In surgical series of HCA, steatotic and inflammatory subtypes appear to be equally distributed, accounting for 85% of overall HCA and β-catenin–mutated HCA are reported in 10%. Importantly, around 10% of HCA are mixed, inflammatory HCA with β-catenin–activating mutations.

Borderline Atypical Hepatocellular Adenomas

In some cases, the differential diagnosis of HCA and well-differentiated HCC may be difficult because these borderline/atypical hepatocellular neoplasms do not meet all morphologic criteria unequivocal for a diagnosis of HCC.[189–191] Such terminology also has been proposed for HCAs arising in an atypical context such as male sex or female sex outside the common age ranking (younger than 15 or older than 50 years of age). In practice, most of these lesions share the pathologic and molecular characteristics of β-HCA, which are recognized to display the highest risk for malignant transformation into HCC. The malignant progression from HCA to HCC follows a molecular

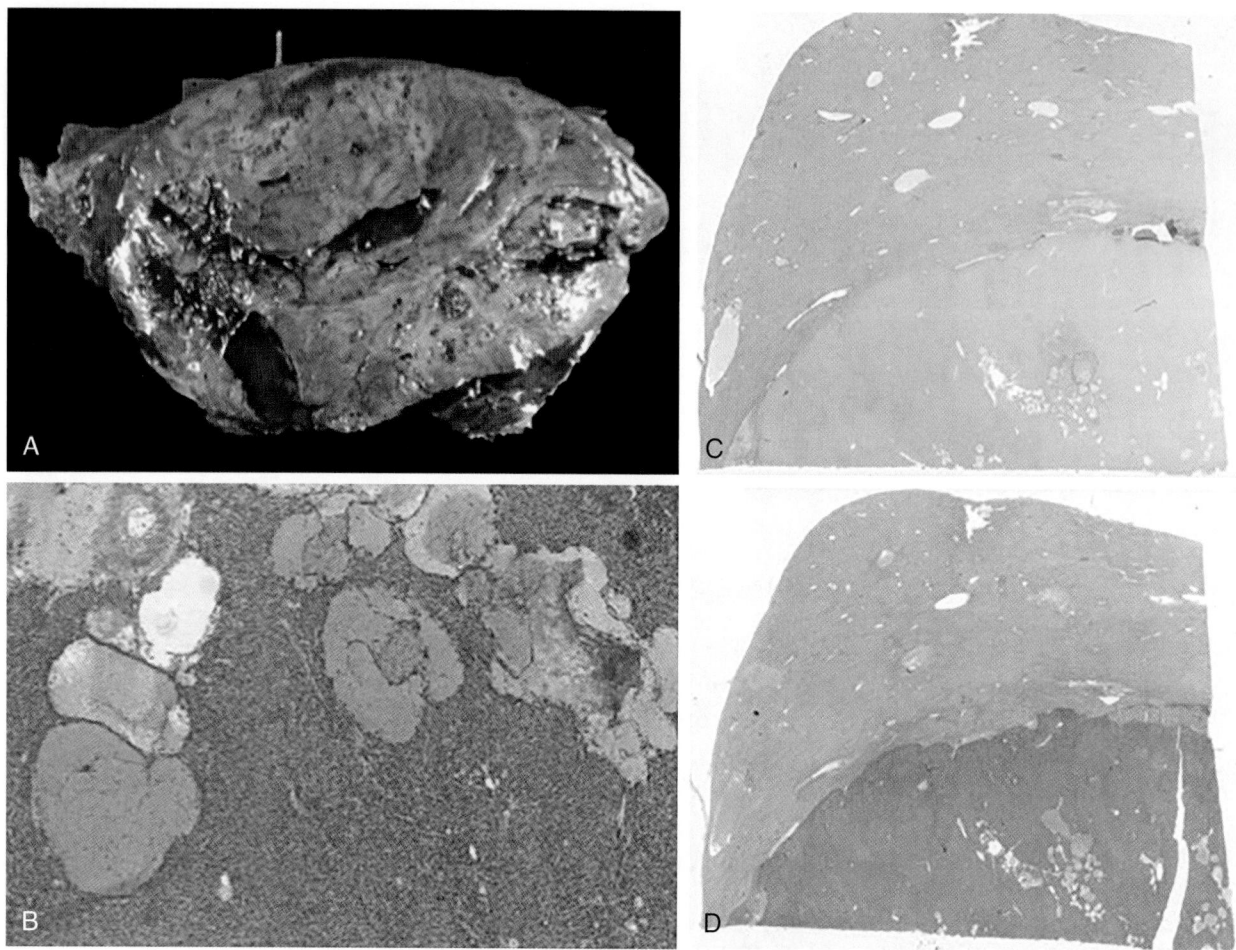

FIGURE 87.29   Hepatocellular adenoma with activation of the sonic hedgehog pathway.   A, Cut section showing a large soft nodule with extensive hemorrhagic areas. **B,** Histologically, the hepatocellular proliferation is unremarkable except for the presence hemorrhagic spaces. **C,** The tumoral hepatocytes are negative for serum amyloid A. **D,** Tumor cells express Prostaglandin D synthase compared with the absence in adjacent nontumoral liver.

stepwise process with β-catenin mutations as first hit and *TERT* promoter mutations as second hit.

BILIARY CELL TUMORS

Cholangiocarcinoma

See Chapters 50 and 51.

Epidemiology and Clinical Background

Cholangiocarcinomas (CCs) are malignancies with biliary differentiation that develop along the biliary tree.[192] It is the second most frequent primary malignant tumor of the liver (5%–15% of liver primary malignancies).[193,194] CC is mainly observed in adults with a peak incidence between 60 and 70 years and a male-to-female ratio of 1.5.[195] These tumors are classified according to their anatomic location into intrahepatic (IH-CC) and extrahepatic (EH-CC).[194] CCs developed within the intrahepatic bile ducts are referred as peripheral CCs and those arising in the bifurcation of the common bile duct as hilar CCs (or Klatskin tumor) and those in the extrahepatic bile ducts as extrahepatic CCs.[196] Hilar tumors are the most common, accounting for 60% to 70% of CCs, whereas peripheral tumors and tumors located in the extrahepatic bile duct represent 5% to 10% and 20% to 30% of CCs, respectively.[193,197]

The prevalence of CC shows a wide geographic distribution largely because of variations in regional environmental risk factors, with the highest incidence observed in Asian countries where parasitic infections (*Opisthorchis viverrini* and *Clonorchis sinensis*) are endemic[198–200] (see Chapter 45). Importantly, the incidence of CC is rising in most countries, including nonendemic areas. This increase is specifically observed for IH-CCs (including hilar tumors), whereas the incidence of EH-CC is stable or even decreased.[4,197,201]

Although several risk factors for CC are well-established, most occur in patients without evident predisposing factors.[202] Primary sclerosing cholangitis (PSC), associated with ulcerative colitis, is one of the most recognized risk factors (see Chapter 41). Indeed, patients with PSC display a 1.5% cumulative annual risk of developing CC per year and 10% to 20% will eventually develop CC.[203] Fibropolycystic liver diseases, including choledocal cyst, Caroli syndrome (see Chapter 46), and congenital hepatic fibrosis, are also common risk factors,[204] and infections with parasitic liver flukes, such as *O. viverrini* and *C. sinensis*, contribute to the high incidence of CC in Asia[200,205] (see Chapter 45). Hepatolithiasis (see Chapters 39 and 44), cholelithiasis, cholangitis (see Chapter 43), chronic pancreatitis, and use of Thorotrast are also risk factors.[202,206,207] More recently, associations of CC with obesity, diabetes, human immunodeficiency virus infection, HCV infection, and alcoholic liver disease have been reported in large population databases.[194] Recent advances in identification of specific pathways and gene abnormalities involved in CC development have been reported underlying potential drug targets[105,208–210] (see Chapters 9B and 9E).

Clinical symptoms at time of diagnosis depend on the anatomic location, the growth types of CCs, and TNM stage.[193] Although IH-CCs are usually discovered at a late stage (see Chapter 50), hilar and EH-CC usually present earlier with cholestasis (see Chapter 51). The prognosis of CC is dismal, partly related to its propensity to invade directly adjacent liver parenchyma and spread along the portal pedicles. Presence of perineural and vascular invasion is frequent in the hilar tumors. In the intraductal growth type, tumor often spreads intraluminally along the ducts. Intrahepatic metastases develop in nearly all advanced cases. The incidence of metastases to regional lymph nodes is higher than in HCC. Blood-borne spread occurs later, particularly to the lungs.[197,211,212] Small duct CCs with cholangiocarcinoma differentiation shows better overall survival.[213] In cirrhotic patients, prognosis of IH-CC is similar to that of HCC, whereas it is worse in noncirrhotic patients.[214]

Pathology

Most CCs develop in a noncirrhotic liver. The Liver Cancer Study Group proposed a classification of CCs based on their growth pattern with three main types: mass-forming, periductal infiltrating, and intraductal growing.[215] These patterns are associated with different clinical evolution, the intraductal growing and the periductal infiltrating showing the best and worse prognosis, respectively (65% survival at 5 years compared with <5%).[211,212,216]

The mass-forming type is defined by a single nodular lesion developed in the liver parenchyma. The tumor is usually well-delineated, not encapsulated, and gray to white, with a firm and solid consistency (Fig. 87.30A). In the case of large tumors, adjacent satellite tumoral nodules are commonly observed. The periductal infiltrating type spreads along the portal tracts with stricture of the involved ducts, potentially leading to obstructive dilatation and cholangitis of the peripheral bile ducts (see Fig. 87.30B). The intraductal growing type is a polypoid or papillary tumor developed within dilated bile-duct lumen (see Fig. 87.30C). This type represents malignant progression of biliary papillomatosis or intraductal papillary neoplasm of the bile duct (see later). These three patterns may overlap in the same tumor. Although most CCs occur in a background of normal liver, recent reports suggest that cirrhosis, independently to its origin, increases 10 times the risk for patients to develop CC (see Fig. 87.30D).[217]

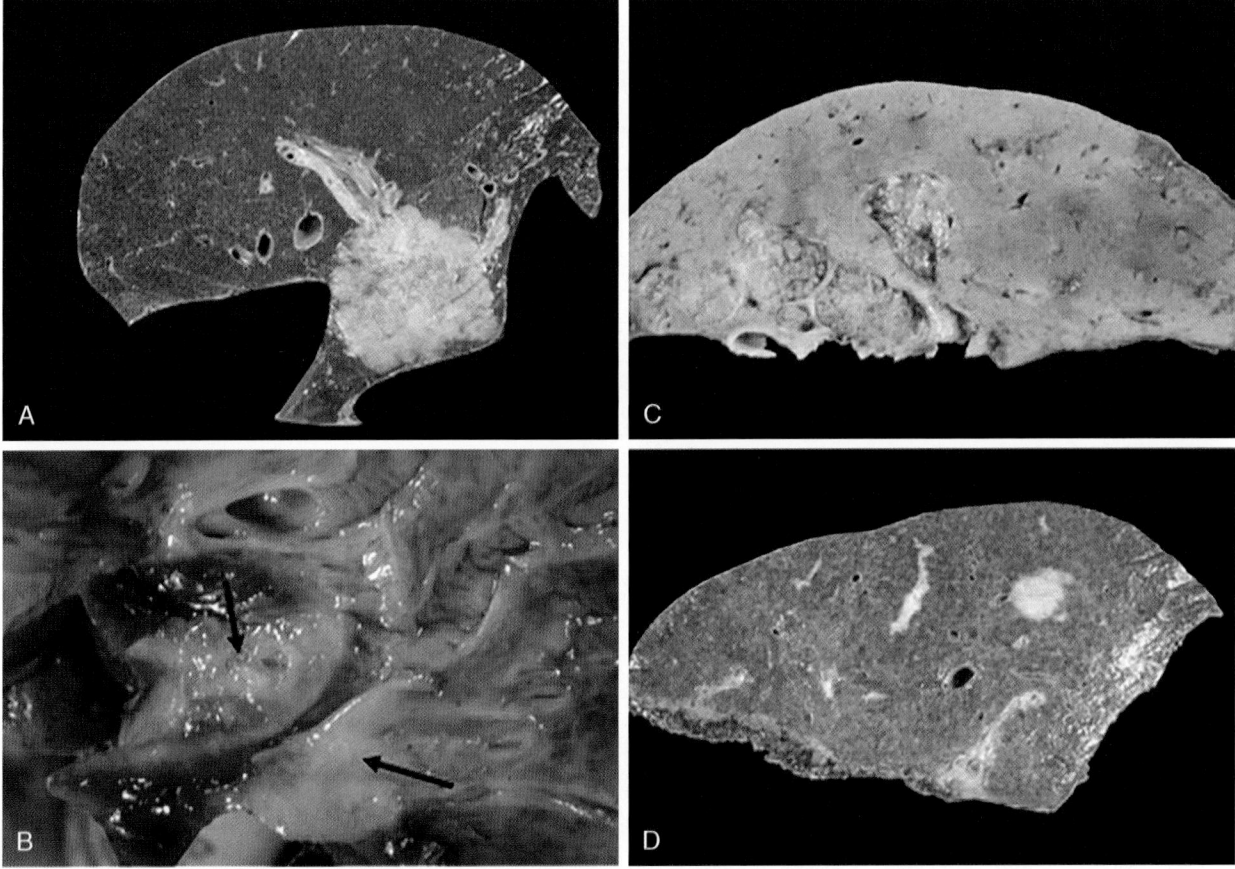

FIGURE 87.30 Growth patterns of cholangiocarcinoma. A, Mass-forming type: well-limited unencapsulated tumor gray to white with fibrous aspect developed in a normal but cholestatic liver. **B,** Periductal infiltrating type: infiltrating tumor *(black arrows)* developed along the hilum, leading to narrowing bile duct and obstructive dilatation of peripheral intrahepatic bile ducts. **C,** Intraductal growing type: endoluminal papillary proliferation growing into the bile ducts in a normal liver. **D,** Cholangiocarcinoma arising in cirrhotic liver: small and solitary well-limited unencapsulated white tumor developed on a cirrhotic liver.

The mass-forming CC is the most common form, accounting for approximately two thirds of cases, followed by mixed mass-forming and periductal infiltrating observed in 25% of cases. The pure peri-infiltrating type and the intraductal growth pattern are rare.[218] CCs arising in the intrahepatic small bile ducts or ductules usually present as the mass-forming type, whereas CCs arising in the intrahepatic large bile ducts (hilar CC) present as any of the three types.[219]

Most CCs are adenocarcinomas with a prominent fibrous stroma. CCs can be graded into well-differentiated, moderately differentiated, or poorly differentiated adenocarcinomas according to their morphology. Most CCs are well-differentiated tumors with a glandular or tubular pattern of growth, although micropapillary, acinar, or cord-like patterns also occur. The tumoral cells, resembling their normal counterpart, are small or medium-sized, cuboidal or columnar, with small nuclei and nucleoli (Fig. 87.31A). Cytoplasm is usually pale, slightly eosinophilic, and sometimes more abundant and clear. Mucus secretion may be highlighted by Alcian blue staining, although the amount is usually small. Less differentiated tumors may show cribriform formations and/or a cord-like pattern, and poorly differentiated cancers are characterized by marked cellular pleomorphism. Hilar and EH-CC are more often well-differentiated compared with peripheral CCs.[220] Presence of dense hyaline fibrous stroma is a key feature of CC (see Fig. 87.31A). Usually, the center of the tumor is densely sclerotic and hypocellular and there may be focal calcifications, whereas the periphery of the tumors is more cellular. CCs frequently infiltrate portal tracts, invading portal vessels (Fig. 87.32C). Perineural invasion is a frequent finding in hilar CCs (see Fig. 87.32D).[220] Because CCs originate from biliary epithelial cells, tumoral cells display immunostaining with anti–CK7 and CK19, carcinoembryonic antigen, and epithelial membrane antigen (see Fig. 87.31B). The keratin profile is particularly useful for the differentiation of IH-CC from metastatic carcinoma derived from colorectal origin: CK7 is constantly expressed in CC, whereas CK20 is constantly expressed in metastatic colon carcinoma.[221]

Intrahepatic CCs have been recently divided into two main subtypes: small duct and large duct.[222] Small duct CCs preferentially develop in the hepatic parenchyma (see Fig. 87.31C). Large duct IH-CCs arise in the large intrahepatic bile ducts near the hilum and resemble perihilar and EH-CCs (see Fig. 87.31D). The main characteristics of both subtypes are detailed in Table 87.1.

Several histologic variants have been reported, including adenosquamous and squamous carcinoma, mucinous carcinoma, signet-ring cell carcinoma, clear cell carcinoma, mucoepidermoid

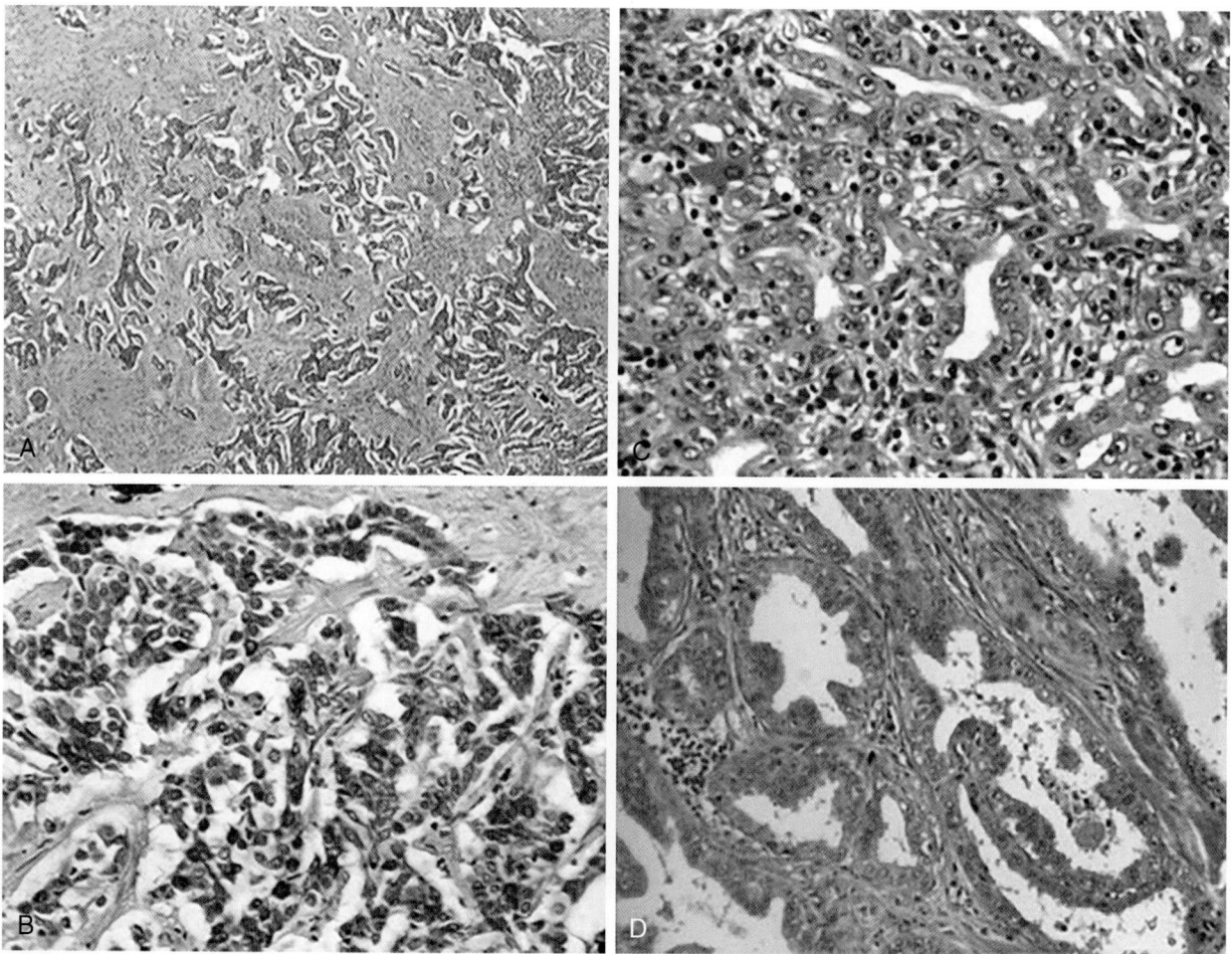

FIGURE 87.31 **Histologic features of cholangiocarcinoma.** **A,** Low magnification showing a well-differentiated adenocarcinoma characterized by a prominent fibrous stroma. **B,** Tumor proliferation expresses cytokeratin 7. **C,** Small duct type of cholangiocarcinoma with a glandular pattern composed of small cuboidal eosinophilic cytoplasm. **D,** Large duct type of cholangiocarcinoma with larger glandular structures.

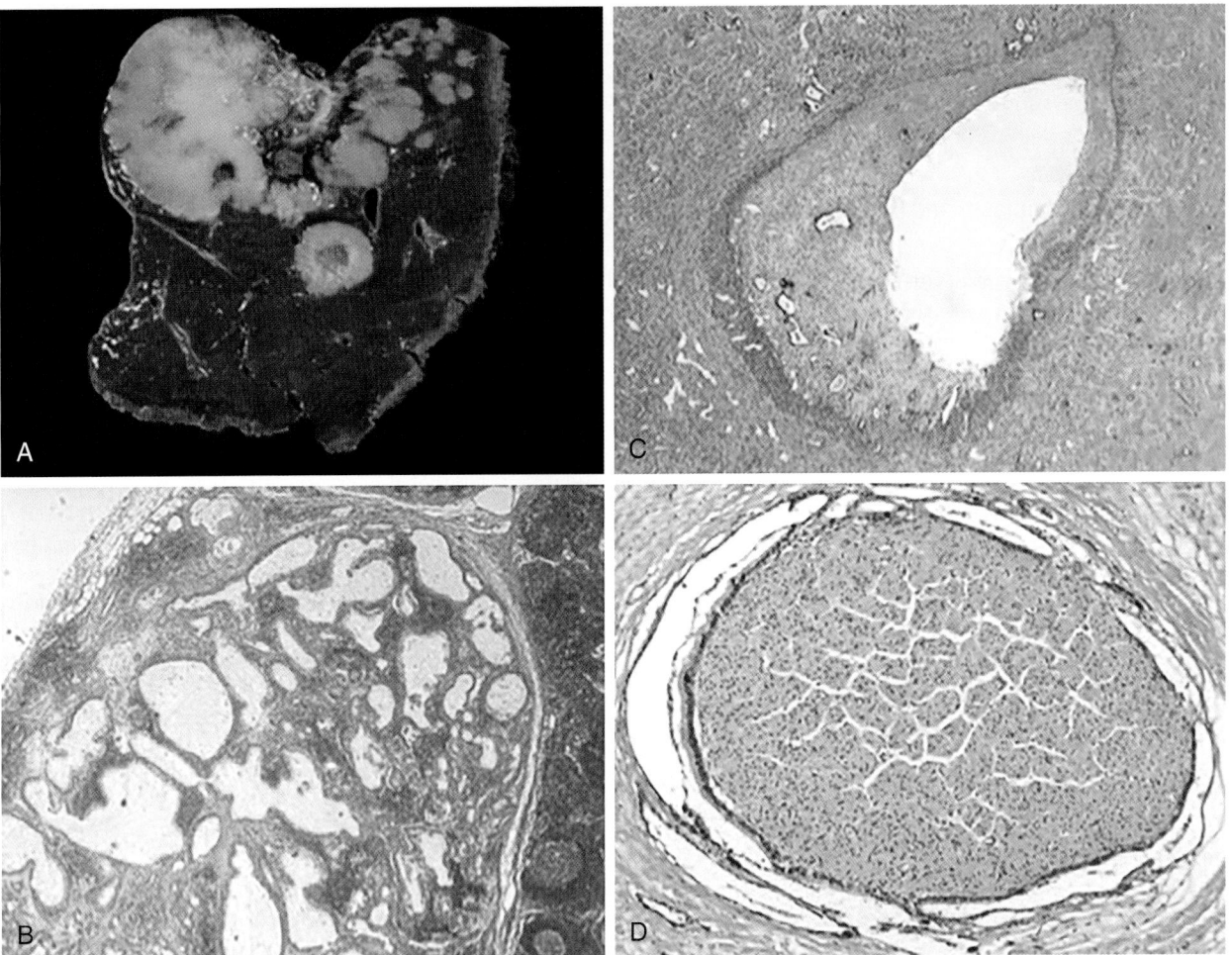

FIGURE 87.32 Histoprognostic factors of cholangiocarcinoma. A, Gross macroscopy showing a mass-forming type of cholangio-carcinoma with satellite nodules around. **B,** Presence of a lymph-node metastasis (residual lymph node on the right). **C,** Vascular section invaded by carcinomatous glands. **D,** Perineural invasion with tumoral cells lining the nerve structure.

TABLE 87.1	Subtypes of Intrahepatic Cholangiocarcinomas	
	SMALL DUCT TYPE	LARGE DUCT TYPE
Location	Peripheral liver parenchyma	Perihilum
Macroscopic growth pattern	Mass forming	Periductal infiltrating, ± mass forming
Risk factors	Cirrhosis	Primary sclerosing cholangitis, hepatolithiasis, liver fluke infection
Preneoplastic lesions	Unknown	Biliary intraepithelial neoplasm, intraductal papillary neoplasm
Histology	Ductal and tubular patterns, fibrous stroma Small to medium-sized cells No mucin production	Tubular pattern Desmoplastic reaction Columnar cells Mucin secretion common
Perineural/ lymphatic invasion	Rare	Frequent

carcinoma, lymphoepithelioma-like carcinoma, and sarcomatous CC. In addition, cholangiolocarcinoma (previously included in combined hepatocellular-cholangiocarcinomas), and CC with ductal plate malformation pattern are subtypes of small duct IH-CC (Fig. 87.33).

The diagnosis of IH-CC may be challenging, with the main diagnostic issue concerning the differential diagnosis between CC and metastatic carcinomas. In that setting, fine needle aspiration, and especially cytologic smears, have been shown as performant in core biopsy with a specificity of 100%, a sensitivity of 84%, and no false-positive cases of CC.[223–225] In contrast, biopsy is much more limited in cases of extrahepatic strictures. Additional approaches, including evaluation of ploidy, fluorescence *in situ* hybridization (FISH), and other biomarkers have been shown to increase sensitivity (up to 34%) and specificity (up to 98%).[224,226–228]

Molecular Pathology

A large set of molecular alterations have been described in CC, including mutations in *KRAS, TP53, IDH1/2, ARID1A, BAP1, BRAF,* and *EGR* (see Chapter 9E). In addition, other alterations involving oncogenetic pathways, mutations *(MET, PIK3CA),* and gene fusions *(FGFR2)* have been reported.[229–231]

In parallel, integrative analysis of expression and genetic alterations described two main biologic classes of IH-CC, including an inflammation class characterized by activation of inflammatory signaling pathways and a proliferative class characterized by oncogenic signaling pathways, the latter being associated with a worse prognosis.[230]

Intraductal Papillary Neoplasm and Biliary Intraepithelial Neoplasia

Intraductal papillary neoplasm of the liver and bile ducts (IPNB), previously recognized as biliary papilloma/papillomatosis, is the macroscopic premalignant lesion that may transform into large duct IH-CC.[232] It is a rare condition characterized by the multicentric proliferation of columnar epithelium within the large bile ducts, although it can diffuse anywhere in the large intrahepatic or extrahepatic bile ducts. IPNB is a disease of middle age or older adults, and men are affected about twice as often as women. Grossly, the neoplasm forms a polypoid mass, mostly characterized by papillary proliferation, inside the bile duct lumen (Fig. 87.34A). Skipped areas may be present.[233] The surface epithelial cells covering these papillae are pancreatobiliary, gastric, or intestinal type cells (see Fig. 87.34B). Although often cytologically benign, the cells can display greater degrees of nuclear atypia; in situ or invasive carcinoma is occasionally noted. This invasive tumor may be a conventional tubular type of adenocarcinoma, or in 10% to 15% of cases a mucinous (colloid) adenocarcinoma.[233–235] Oncocytic variants of biliary papillomatosis have been reported, with clinical features similar to those of their nononcocytic counterparts. The invasive tumors associated with these oncocytic papillary lesions is also oncocytic, because of the presence of abundant cytoplasmic mitochondria.[236] IPND development follows a multistep process of carcinogenesis associated with accumulation of gene mutations involving in oncogenic pathways (*KRAS* mutation, *TP53* mutation, loss of p16).

Biliary intraepithelial neoplasia (BIN) is a microscopic noninvasive precursor lesion of large duct IH-CC.[237] BIN is defined by a flat or micropapillary dysplastic lesion with multilayered nuclei.[238] The abnormal cells have an increased nuclear-to-cytoplasmic ratio, partial loss of nuclear polarity, and nuclear hyperchromasia. They are divided into low-grade (regrouping former BIN-1 and -2), and high-grade (former BIN-3) according to the severity of cytoarchitectural atypias (Fig. 87.35).[239] Chronic biliary inflammation may induce neoplastic changes of biliary epithelium.[240] BIN cases display *KRAS* mutations in the early stages and then *TP53* mutations arise.[241–243]

Combined Hepatocholangiocarcinoma

Combined hepatocholangiocarcinoma (cHCC-CC) is a rare but increasingly recognized neoplasm in the liver, accounting for approximately 5% of primary liver malignancies.[244–246] It shares unequivocal features of both HCC and CC as defined by the WHO classification.[247] Depending on various investigations, patients with combined HCC-CC share similar clinical and pathologic features with patients with HCC or CC.[246,248–251]

Although a unified histopathologic criteria for combined HCC-CC is still not available, it is generally accepted that a firm diagnosis of combined HCC-CC requires evidence of HCC

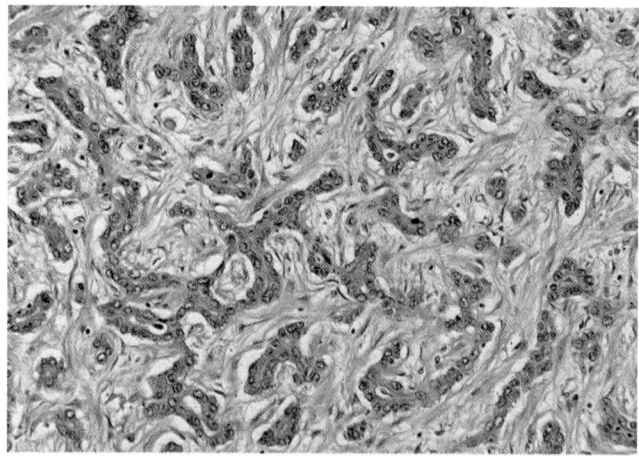

FIGURE 87.33 Cholangiolocarcinoma. Small monotonous tubular formations resembling ductular proliferation within dense fibrous stroma.

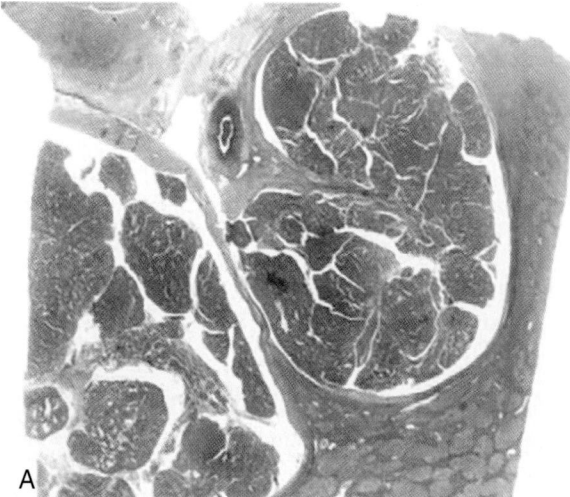
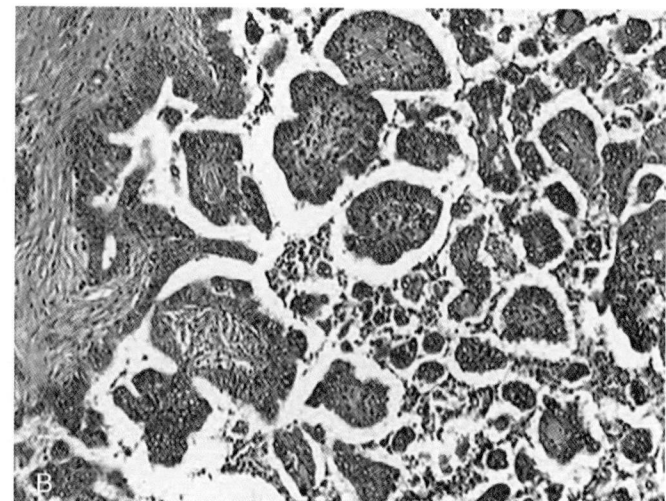

FIGURE 87.34 Biliary papillomatosis. A, Low magnification showing bile duct lumen covered by papillary excrescences. **B,** Tumoral papillae with fibrous stalk covered by proliferation of cuboidal cells.

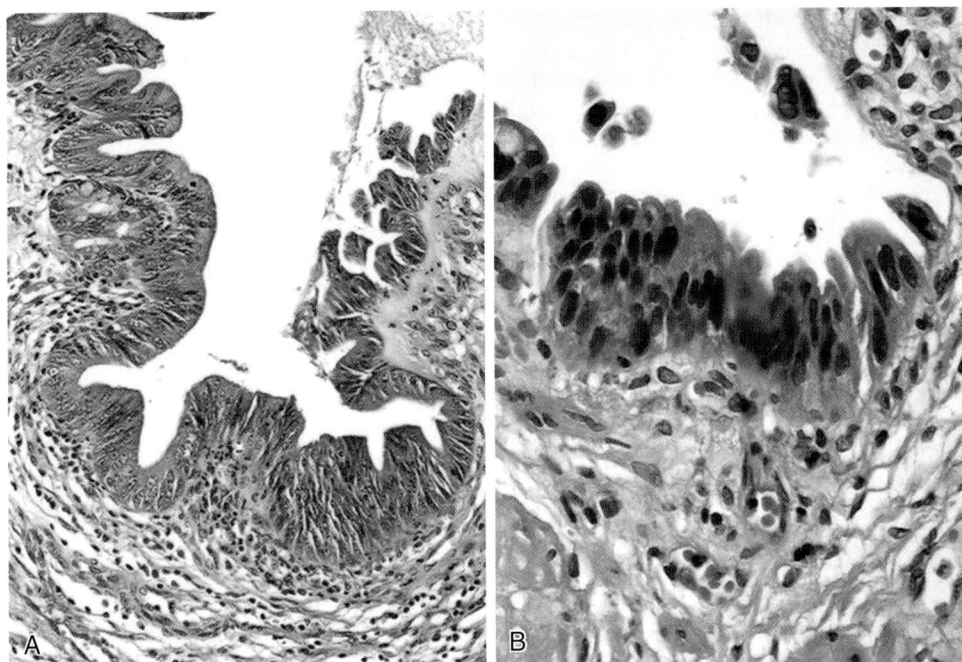

FIGURE 87.35 Biliary intraepithelial neoplasia (BIN). A, Low-grade BIN (former BIN-2) characterized by micropapillary projections lined by multilayered cells with cell atypias. **B,** High-grade BIN (former BIN-3) with atypical cells showing increased nuclear-to-cytoplasmic ratio, loss of nuclear polarity, and nuclear hyperchromasia.

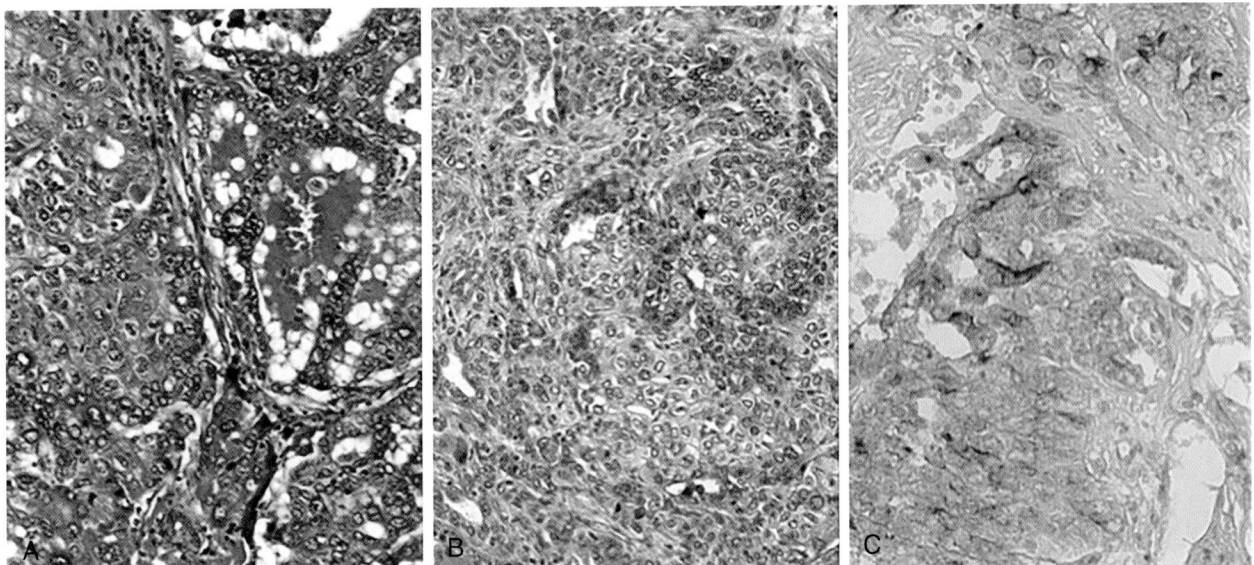

FIGURE 87.36 Hepatocholangiocarcinoma. A, Association of a hepatocellular differentiation *(right part)* with trabecular and solid growth pattern and cholangiocarcinoma differentiation *(left part)* with glandular structures lined by biliary-type epithelium. **B,** Transitional aspect with intermediate tumoral cells. **C,** CD133 immunostaining in the transition area.

differentiation such as trabecular growth pattern, bile production, bile canaliculi, and clear evidence of CC, such as true glandular structures formed by biliary-type epithelium, mucin production, or prominent desmoplastic stoma (Fig. 87.36A).[246,252,253] Transition aspect, composed of small uniform cells with scant cytoplasm, may be seen (see Fig. 87.36B). There are no minimum cutoff amounts of the different components required for the diagnosis of cHCC-CC. When the tumor is entirely composed of a transition pattern, a diagnosis of intermediate cell

carcinoma is proposed.[254–256] Separate HCC and CC coincidentally found in the same liver is generally considered a collision tumor and is excluded by the WHO classification of combined HCC-CC. This has been further supported by the genetic findings that two independent neoplastic clones develop at close proximity, and hence no histologic transitions exist.[257]

The cell of origin of combined HCC-CC has been a matter of debate. The fact that the HCC and CC elements intermingle with each other in a transitional area in most combined

HCC-CC strongly supports that both components of the cancer derive from the hepatic progenitor cells. Several molecular investigations support this hypothesis because single clonal tumor with homogeneous genetic background in both HCC and CC components of combined HCC-CC was demonstrated, suggesting that histologic diversity of HCC-CCC is a phenotypic expression of divergent differentiation potential of a single clone.[257–259] Stem cell features may be highlighted by immunohistochemistry studies based on positivity with CK19, CD56, EpCAM, cKit, and CD133 (see Fig. 87.36C).

Mucinous Cystic Neoplasm

Mucinous cystic neoplasms (MCNs) were previously reported separately as biliary cystadenoma and cystadenocarcinoma (see Chapter 88B). They correspond to cyst-forming epithelial neoplasms showing no communication with the bile duct associated with ovarian-type subepithelial stroma. They are divided into MCN with low/intermediate grade dysplasia or high-grade dysplasia. In some cases, invasive carcinoma may occur.

MCN is an uncommon cystic neoplasm that accounts for less than 5% of all intrahepatic biliary cysts.[260] The histogenesis of MCN remains uncertain, although an origin from embryonic foregut rests has been advanced.[261] Almost all of these tumors occur in middle-aged women, with a peak incidence in the fifth decade.[262] They are characteristically large multiloculated cysts (2.5–28 cm) without communication with the intrahepatic biliary system (Fig. 87.37A). The tumor is solitary and spherical and contains white to yellow to brown mucinous or gelatinous material. Individual locules vary in size, and the internal surface is typically smooth with occasional trabeculations or papillations.[260] If solid areas are present, concern should be raised for an invasive component.[262,263]

Histologically, the cysts are lined by a simple columnar to cuboidal epithelium with mucin-filled cytoplasm. On occasion, the epithelium can be pseudostratified or focally ulcerated, and goblet cells or squamous cells are sometimes seen. Nuclear atypias and mitoses are rare, but their presence should raise the possibility of complicating cystadenocarcinoma. Underneath is an ovarian type of hypercellular stroma, which is absent in cases arising in men.[262] Typically, this stroma is densely cellular and composed of closely packed spindle cells reminiscent of ovarian stroma (see Fig. 87.37B). This stroma stains with antibodies to estrogen and progesterone receptor, and growth can occur during hormone replacement therapy and pregnancy.[264] The vast majority of MCNs are low/intermediate-grade dysplasia. In MCNs with high-grade dysplasia, the presence of invasive carcinoma must be carefully screened. It mostly occurs in large tumors as tubulopapillary or tubular adenocarcinomas.[265] *KRAS* mutations are observed in around 20% of MCNs, mostly in those with high-grade dysplasia.[265]

Prognosis of MCN is excellent in the absence of invasive carcinoma and if complete resection is achieved.[266] In cases of an invasive component, the prognosis seems to be better than that for classic intrahepatic cholangiocarcinoma.

Other Benign Cystic and Bile Duct Lesions

See Chapters 48, 73, and 88.

Ciliated Hepatic Foregut Cysts

Ciliated hepatic foregut cyst is a rare lesion, generally solitary and unilocular.[267] This lesion is of small size (<3 cm), lined by a characteristic ciliated pseudostratified columnar epithelium with mucous cells and an underlying fibrous wall containing abundant smooth muscle.[268] Occasional cases of squamous carcinoma arising in a ciliated hepatic foregut cyst has been reported.[268] Because these features are similar to those seen in bronchial and esophageal cysts, an analogous origin from the embryonic foregut is suggested.[269]

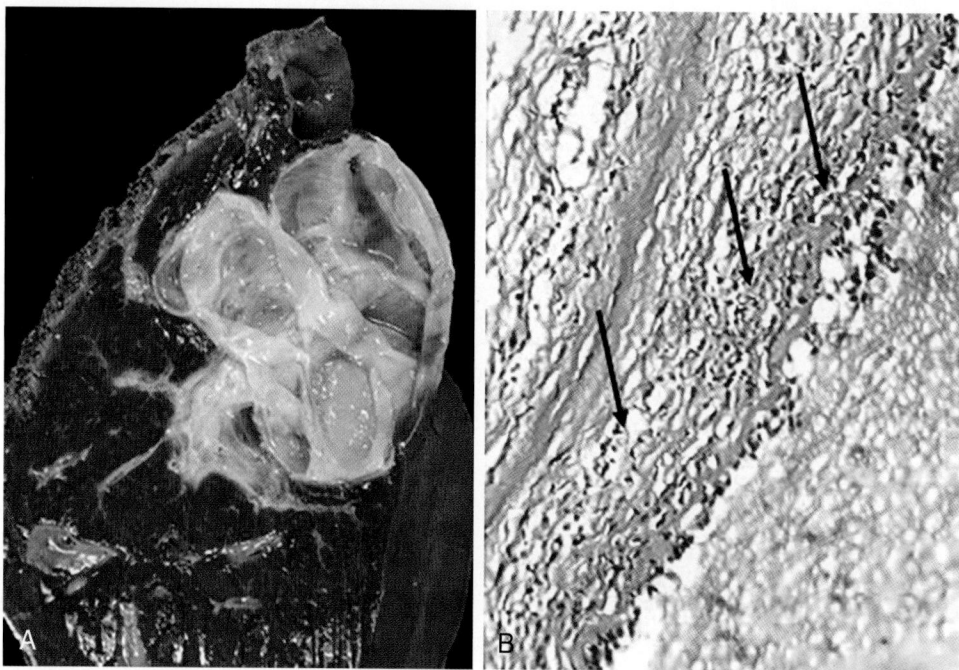

FIGURE 87.37 **Mucinous cystadenoma neoplasm.** **A,** Macroscopic view showing a multiloculated cyst with smooth and white internal surface. **B,** Histologically, the cyst is lined by epithelial cells covering a densely cellular stroma *(arrows).*

Bile Duct Adenoma

Bile duct adenoma is an incidental finding often discovered at surgery because most of them develop superficially under the Glisson's capsule.[270,271] It is an inconsequential lesion that may be mistaken for bile duct hamartoma or metastatic carcinoma.[272] Almost all bile duct adenomas are less than 1 cm in diameter, although cases up to 4 cm have been recorded. The lesion typically appears as a discrete white nodule, usually solitary and subcapsular in location with a firm consistency and unencapsulated margin. Histologically, bile duct adenoma is made of a compact proliferation of small ductules with small or inapparent lumens lined by cuboidal epithelium with slightly basophilic cytoplasm and bland, regular nuclei. Mitoses, cytologic atypia, and nuclear pleomorphism are absent. Ductular structures are surrounded by a fibrotic hyalinized stroma that can distort duct structures. Portal tracts are often entrapped within the tumor, and scattered inflammatory cells are sometimes seen. Malignant transformation has not been clearly documented.

MESENCHYMAL TUMORS

Benign Mesenchymal Tumors

See Chapter 88A.

Hemangioma

Hemangioma is the most common primary tumor of the liver, with a prevalence in autopsy surveys ranging from 0.4% up to 20%.[273] The lesion is discovered at all ages and in both sexes, although they are more frequent in older age groups and, in most series, favor women.[274]

The vast majority of hemangiomas are clinically silent and discovered incidentally during radiologic examination, surgery, or autopsy. However, larger tumors can occasionally become clinically evident with abdominal discomfort, hepatomegaly, or a palpable abdominal mass.[275] Rare reports describe spontaneous rupture with hemoperitoneum or a bleeding diathesis with hypofibrinogenemia or platelet sequestration and consequent thrombocytopenia (Kasabach-Merritt syndrome).[276] Hemangiomas can be correctly identified in most instances by radiographic imaging. Needle biopsy is not necessary and is, in fact, contraindicated because of the risk of severe hemorrhage.

Most hemangiomas are solitary lesions less than 4 cm in diameter (Fig. 87.38). Multiple tumors are seen in up to 25% of cases, and hemangiomas up to 30 cm have been recorded. The tumors can occur anywhere in the liver but are frequently located immediately beneath the hepatic capsule. The cut surface demonstrates a soft, dark-red, spongy mass with blood-filled cavities and occasional foci of thrombosis, scarring, or calcification. Most are well-demarcated from the surrounding liver. Histologically, hemangiomas are composed of dilated vascular spaces lined by flattened endothelial cells and supported by connective tissue septa. The septa consist of poorly cellular fibrous bands with varying degrees of myxoid change and scarring. Thick-walled blood vessels and scattered bile ducts are sometimes found in larger septa. The vascular spaces are frequently the sites of thrombi in various stages of organization. Hemangiomas may also demonstrate involutional changes with extensive hyalinization, obliteration of the vascular channels, and sometimes calcification.

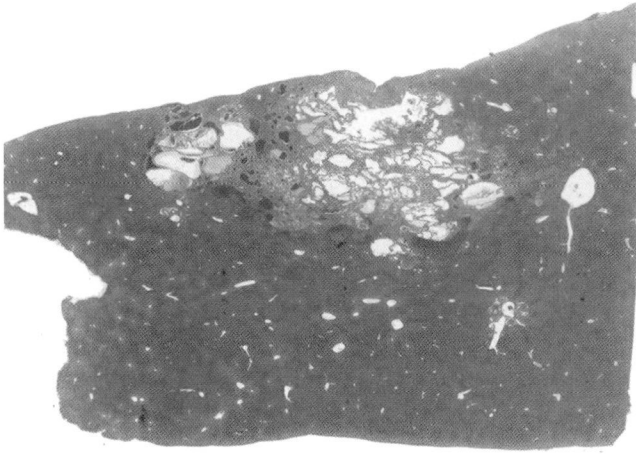

FIGURE 87.38 Hemangioma. At low magnification, the lesion is made of vascular cavities, some filled with blood, well-demarcated from the surrounding liver.

Hepatic Small Vessel Neoplasm

This entity, recently described, is considered a benign/low-grade vascular tumor, mostly observed in adults (mean age 54 years).[277] These tumors are relatively small (2 cm in diameter), poorly defined, and have infiltrative borders. Histologically, they correspond to proliferation of small, thin-walled vessels lined by flattened to plump endothelial cells. The main differential diagnosis is hepatic angiosarcoma. Whereas the Ki-67 proliferation index is low in hepatic small vessel neoplasm, it is usually higher than 10% in angiosarcoma. Interestingly, activating hot-spot *GNAQ* mutations are observed in two thirds of this entity.[277]

Hepatic Infantile Hemangioma

Hepatic infantile hemangioma (previously referred to as infantile hemangioendothelioma) is a benign pediatric vascular proliferation of the liver. Although uncommon, it is nonetheless the predominant hepatic neoplasm of the first year of life and only a few cases have been reported in adults. Most cases manifest clinically with hepatomegaly, diffuse abdominal enlargement, or a palpable abdominal mass. The prognosis is generally good because the tumors undergo usually spontaneous involution and can completely regress.[278] However, a potentially life-threatening feature is not uncommon because of arteriovenous shunting through the tumor that may result in cardiac failure with a reported mortality rate of about 25%.[279] Typically, infantile hemangioendothelioma appears as sharply defined but nonencapsulated masses, ranging from 1 to 15 cm in diameter. On cut section, the lesion is well delineated with a gray-tan to pink color and firm or spongy appearance. Central hemorrhage, necrosis, fibrosis, or calcification can be noted in larger lesions.

Histologically, the tumor is characterized by a proliferation of small, irregular vascular channels that are lined by a single layer of plump endothelial cells. These channels display small, often compressed lumens and contain varying quantities of red blood cells. The endothelial cells are uniform with almost no mitoses. The fibrous stroma is composed of scattered fibroblasts and collagen fibers. Small bile ducts are scattered through the mass. The tumor generally grows by expanding into adjacent liver, although hepatic plates can sometimes be entrapped along its advancing edge. The lining endothelial cells express CD31, CD34, and GLUT1.[280]

Some infantile hemangiomas may demonstrate atypical histologic features with atypical crowded and multilayered endothelial cells showing hyperchromatic nuclei and occasional mitoses. This atypical pattern has been referred to as type 2, as contrasted with the more common type 1 pattern. Most of the type 2 tumors pursue a benign course, but some exhibit more aggressive behavior with extensive local growth and in some instances, metastases. Consequently they have been considered by some investigators to be a low-grade childhood form of angiosarcoma.[281]

Mesenchymal Hamartoma

Mesenchymal hamartoma is a benign tumor arising in children younger than 2 years of age, although sporadic examples are described in adolescents and adults.[282] It is thought to arise from a developmental abnormality in the formation of ductal plates during late embryogenesis and related to disordered mesenchymal-epithelial transformation. Although some cases are discovered incidentally, most are clinically evident because of their large size causing progressive abdominal distention or a palpable abdominal mass.

The tumor appears grossly as a solitary, expanding mass ranging from 3 to 30 cm in diameter. Typically the tumor is well demarcated from the adjacent liver, although an infiltrative border or satellite lesions is not so rare.[283] On cut surface, the lesion is composed of multiple small cysts. These cysts are filled with clear or mucoid fluid, lined by a smooth surface and surrounded by a myxoid tissue with fibrous bands.[284]

Histologically, mesenchymal hamartoma is characterized by the association of loose connective tissue and epithelial bile ducts in varying proportions, arranged in lobulated islands. The mesenchymal component consists of elongated bland cells within an edematous myxoid stroma containing varying amounts of collagen. Focally, this stroma undergoes cystic degeneration, yielding a lymphangiomatous appearance and giving rise to the grossly visible cysts. In addition, numerous thick-walled veins, foci of extramedullary hematopoiesis, and scattered bile ducts can be observed. The ducts often exhibit branching or cystically dilated lumen. Bile duct cells can be atrophic or hyperplastic. Small clusters of unremarkable hepatocytes lacking a lobular arrangement are interspersed within the tumor.[283] Mesenchymal hamartoma is characterized by a benign course in the majority of cases when entirely resected.[285]

Angiomyolipoma

Angiomyolipoma (AML), belonging to the group of perivascular epithelioid cell tumors (PEComas), is a rare mesenchymal tumor occurring at a median age of about 45 years, predominantly in women, with a ratio of 5:1.[286] Ten percent of cases occur in the setting of tuberous sclerosis, usually associated with co-existing renal AML.[287] Size ranges widely from 1 cm to over 20 cm. Tumor is usually single, but multiple tumors in the liver and multiorgan involvement have been described.[288,289] There has been only one report of malignant degeneration in a liver AML.[290]

Most AMLs are well circumscribed but not encapsulated (Fig. 87.39A). AMLs have three key components, thickened-wall blood vessels, adipocytes, and epithelioid cells. Epithelioid cells, commonly the dominant component, are often ultimately associated with the blood vessel walls (see Fig. 87.39B). Some tumors contain a spindle cell component. Extramedullary hematopoiesis is frequently observed.[291] The mitotic index is usually low. AMLs are positive for smooth muscle actin (desmin, SMA) and melanocytic markers (HMB45, melan A).[292]

The histogenesis of AML is unclear. Recent studies suggest that AML is a clonal proliferation that favors a neoplastic process.[293] Strong arguments suggest that the three cell types are derived from a single precursor cell present in the perivascular space, the perivascular epithelioid cells.[291,294]

Lipoma

Lipomatous tumors are rarely found in the liver. Most occur in adults as asymptomatic lesions, incidentally detected by radiographic imaging. Typically, the tumors are solitary masses ranging from 1 to 20 cm. Microscopically, they are composed of mature adipose tissue, either pure or accompanied by a vascular, hematopoietic, or myeloid component. Depending on the constituents, the tumor is designated as pure lipoma, angiolipoma, or myelolipoma.[295,296]

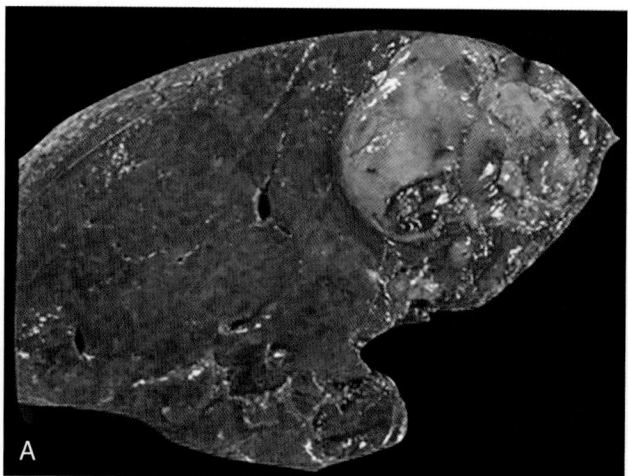
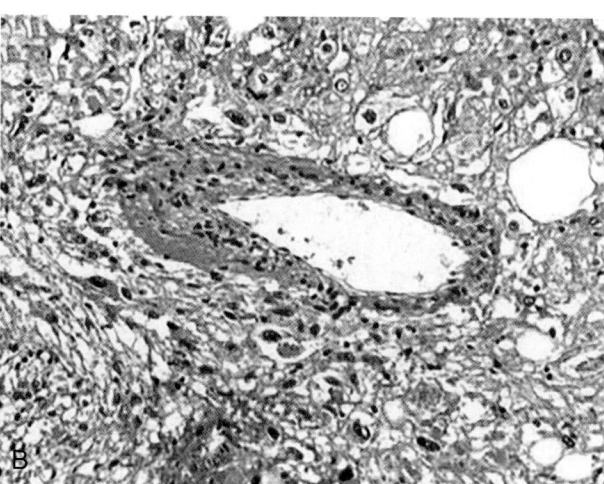

FIGURE 87.39 Angiomyolipoma. A, Macroscopic view showing a well-circumscribed soft white nodular lesion with foci of hemorrhage. **B,** Histologically, the lesion is composed of myoid cells with fat droplets and thick-walled vessels.

Inflammatory Myofibroblastic Tumor

Inflammatory myofibroblastic tumor (IMT) is a fibroblastic/myofibroblastic neoplasm of intermediate biologic behavior, rarely described in the liver. Histologically, IMT is made of fascicles of uniform spindle cells arranged in a myxoid or collagenous stroma with a prominent inflammatory infiltrate.[297] Mitotic activity is low. Tumor cells are positive for SMA, less frequently for desmin, and may express keratin markers. Importantly, around two thirds of IMTs display rearrangements of the *ALK* locus, leading to overexpression of ALK by immunohistochemistry.[298,299]

Solitary Fibrous Tumor

Solitary fibrous tumor (SFT) is a fibroblastic tumor of the adult that can be associated with hypoglycemia. Histologically, SFT is composed of bland ovoid to spindle cells arranged in poorly defined fascicles associated with prominent, thin-walled, dilated, and branching blood vessels. The tumor cells are positive for CD34 and STAT6 (related to gene fusions involving *STAT6*).[300,301] Most SFTs show a benign behavior.

Malignant Mesenchymal Tumors

Epithelioid Hemangioendothelioma

Epithelioid hemangioendothelioma (EHE) is a low-grade malignant tumor of endothelial origin that can occur in several sites, including the liver. At time of diagnosis, most patients are in their fourth or fifth decades of life, with about 60% of the patients being women.[302] Unlike with hepatic angiosarcoma, no strong etiologic associations or predisposing factors have been identified, although a relationship with long-term OC use has been suggested.[303]

EHE tends to be an indolent and slowly growing tumor, but the natural history can vary considerably.[304] Most patients have a prolonged survival, whereas others suffer rapid deterioration with early death from hepatic failure or extensive tumor spread.[303,305] Metastases commonly involve the lung, spleen, abdominal lymph nodes, omentum, and peritoneum. Even with metastatic disease, some patients can survive for many years, although the distinction between metastatic spread and multicentric disease is sometimes difficult.[306] The best treatment strategy in EHE remains poorly defined even if data suggest that liver transplantation might be proposed even in patients with extrahepatic metastasis.[307-309] In addition to tumor burden, extrahepatic metastasis, resectability, age, and absence of comorbidity, the pattern of progression (stability versus slow progression versus rapid progression) also should be assessed before therapeutic decision and especially liver transplantation.

In approximately 80% of cases the tumor is multifocal with involvement of both lobes by tumor nodules of various sizes. These nodules are white to tan, with a firm consistency, sometimes located beneath the capsule leading to a capsular retraction at imaging (Fig. 87.40A).[310,311] The background liver is generally normal.[302]

Histologically, the tumor comprises small groups of tumor cells surrounded by a distinctive and often abundant stroma of varying myxoid or sclerotic character. The neoplastic cells display abundant eosinophilic cytoplasm and large vesicular and

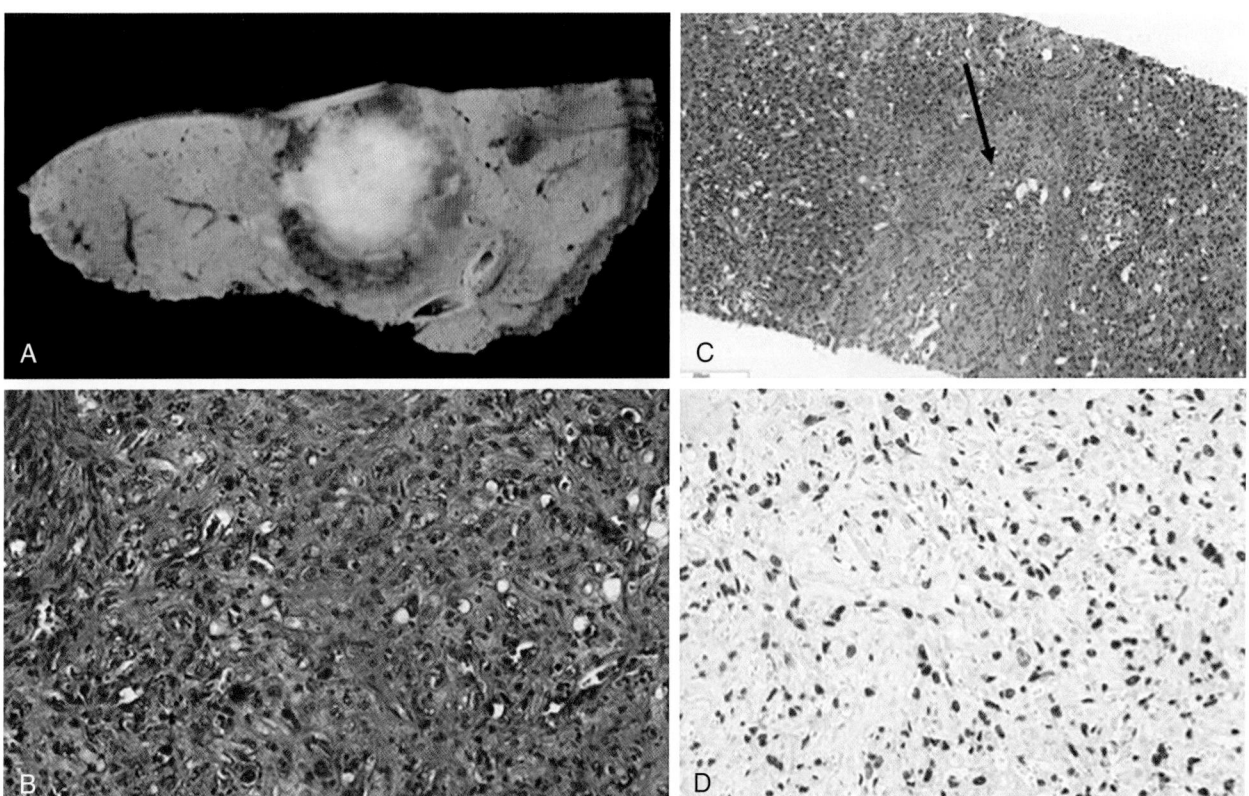

FIGURE 87.40   Epithelioid hemangioendothelioma. A, Macroscopic view showing a white, firm nodule with hyperhaemic margin. **B,** Histologically, the tumor is composed of groups of epithelioid tumor cells with mild atypias and cytoplasmic vacuoles in some of them. **C,** Tumor cells invade the hepatic vein *(arrow).* **D,** Tumors cells are positive for erg, a vascular marker, by immunohistochemistry.

hyperchromatic nuclei with variable nucleoli. These cells show their endothelial origin by displaying one or more intracytoplasmic vacuoles that represent intracellular vascular lumina (see Fig. 87.40B). In addition, they can form small capillary-like lumina, which sometimes contain red blood cells.[311] Toward its center the tumor ultimately becomes densely sclerotic, often with focal calcification, and the tumor cells can be difficult to discern. At the actively proliferating margin of the tumor, the neoplastic cells infiltrate the sinusoids, resulting in ductular transformation, atrophy, and eventual obliteration of the adjacent hepatic plates. The underlying lobular architecture is frequently preserved. The tumor also invades the central veins, portal veins branches, and larger blood vessels (see Fig. 87.40C). This intravascular growth appears as intraluminal papillary clusters or tuft-like projections.[274] Tumor cells are positive for endothelial markers (factor VIII–related antigen, CD34, CD31, and erg) at immunohistochemistry examination (see Fig. 87.40D).[312] Based on a reciprocal translocation t (1;3)(p36;q25), a consistent *WWTR1-CAMTA1* fusion gene has been found in around 90% of HEE.[313] Additional gene fusions have been identified, including *YAP1-TFE3* fusion in HEE without *CAMTA1-WWTR1* fusion.[314] Detection of *CAMTA1-WWTR1* fusion by FISH, RT polymerase chain reaction, or nuclear CAMTA1 expression on immunohistochemistry studies are useful to confirm the diagnosis of HEE because it has not been identified in other human tumors, especially liver angiosarcoma.[314,315]

Angiosarcoma

Although exceptional, hepatic angiosarcoma is the most common primary sarcoma of the liver.[316–318] Association with exposure to Thorotrast, vinyl chloride monomer, or inorganic arsenical compounds have been identified in 25% to 40% of angiosarcomas.[316–323] With control of exposure to vinyl chloride in workers in the 1970s, the incidence of hepatic angiosarcoma declined. The peak incidence is in the sixth and seventh decades of life, and approximately 75% of the patients are men. Rare cases are reported in children, most in association with infantile hemangioendothelioma.

Patients with angiosarcoma usually have symptoms at presentation, including abdominal pain, fatigue, weight loss, hepatosplenomegaly, ascites, jaundice, and anemia. Rupture of angiosarcoma with intraperitoneal hemorrhage may be observed in about 25% of patients.[325] The prognosis of patients with angiosarcoma is very poor.[324,325] Most patients deteriorate rapidly and die within 6 months of diagnosis, usually from hepatic failure, extensive tumor burden, or tumor rupture. Distant metastases, most commonly to the lungs, regional lymph nodes, spleen, or bone marrow, are noted in over half the patients.[322]

On gross examination, angiosarcomas typically appear as multiple gray or hemorrhagic masses scattered throughout both liver lobes (Fig. 87.41A). The size varies greatly between 0.1 and 5 cm, and tumors have a spongy consistency with irregular, ill-defined borders. Less often the tumor is represented by a large solitary mass, typically over 15 cm in diameter.

The histologic appearance is characterized by a proliferation of malignant endothelial cells with pale ill-defined cytoplasm and enlarged, pleomorphic, and hyperchromatic nuclei (see Fig. 87.41B). The cells usually assume an elongated orientation, but they can also appear rounded or polygonal with conspicuous cytoplasm and prominent nucleoli. Mitoses, although in variable number, are often numerous and bizarre. In some cases, the cells show evidence of phagocytic behavior.[274,326] The tumor infiltrates preexisting vascular structures and eventually destroys the hepatic parenchyma. With early involvement, the malignant cells line the sinusoids and separate the hepatic plates. With progression, the hepatocytes are ultimately replaced by fibrosis while the sinusoids dilate, producing irregular pelioid-like vascular spaces of varying size. These spaces are lined by multilayered tumor cells, sometimes in a papillary arrangement, and contain blood and necrotic debris. Extramedullary hematopoiesis is often present.[329] The tumor also invades central veins or portal vein branches. This can lead to luminal occlusion with subsequent hemorrhage, necrosis, and infarction.

In angiosarcomas associated with Thorotrast, vinyl chloride, and arsenic exposure, an initial precursor stage that precedes the development of overt tumor has been recognized with hypertrophy and hyperplasia of endothelial cells together with reactive hepatocyte alterations.[328] Similarly to EHE, angiosarcomas express endothelial markers such as CD31 and CD34 on immunohistochemistry study.[329] *KRAS* mutations have been described in sporadic cases as well as *TP53* mutations in vinyl chloride–related angiosarcoma.[330–332]

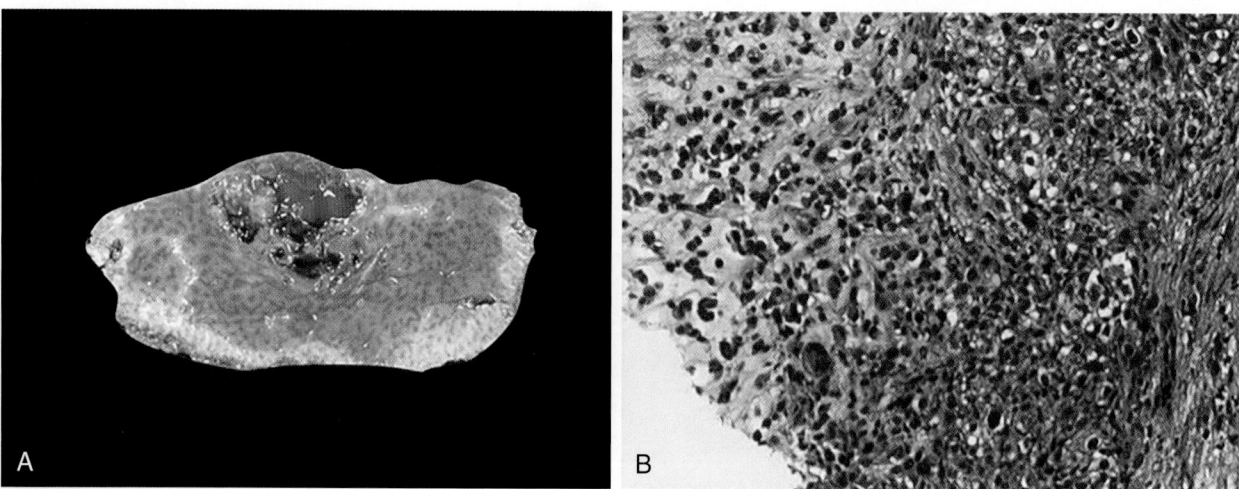

FIGURE 87.41 **Angiosarcoma.** **A,** Macroscopic view showing an hemorrhagic mass, ill-limited from surrounding liver. **B,** Histologically, the proliferation is made of malignant endothelial cells with ill-defined cytoplasm and enlarged, pleomorphic, and hyperchromatic nuclei.

Surgical resection seems the best therapeutic option offering a median survival between 17 and 19 months,[325,333] at least better than liver transplantation.[334,335]

Embryonal Sarcoma

Embryonal sarcoma of the liver is a highly malignant childhood neoplasm.[336] It is the third most common hepatic mesenchymal malignancy in the pediatric population, after hepatoblastoma and HCC. The peak incidence is between 5 and 15 years, with an age range that extends from newborn infants to almost 30 years of age.[283,336,337] The prognosis of embryonal sarcoma is very poor. Death often occurs because of massive local tumor growth with direct extension into contiguous structures and even through the diaphragm.

On gross examination, the tumors are large, well-demarcated masses, usually 10 to 30 cm in diameter, with a soft gelatinous consistency.[338] Most of the tumors occupy the right lobe of the liver. The cut surface is variegated with areas of solid gray-white tumor interrupted by foci of cystic degeneration, hemorrhage, and necrosis.[336]

Histologically, the tumors are composed of malignant spindle-shaped cells separated by myxoid stroma.[339] The neoplastic cells are grouped into closely packed sheets or fascicles or scattered loosely in the stroma. They vary greatly in size and have pleomorphic, hyperchromatic nuclei, inconspicuous nucleoli, and poorly defined borders. Mitoses are often numerous and bizarre, and multinucleated tumor giant cells can be seen. A characteristic finding is the presence of PAS-positive and diastase-resistant eosinophilic globules within tumor cells and in the extracellular stroma.[340] The myxoid stroma, which dominates the less cellular portions of the tumor, harbors numerous thin-walled veins and often contain foci of extramedullary hematopoiesis. Areas of hemorrhage and necrosis are frequent, and bands of dense hyalinized collagen are occasionally noted. The periphery of the tumor typically entraps bile ducts that are cystically dilated and lined by a cuboidal epithelium that often displays hyperplastic or atypical features. The tumor lacks histologic evidence of cellular differentiation, and its histogenesis remains uncertain.[341] Embryonal sarcoma should represent a primitive mesenchymal neoplasm capable of divergent differentiation.[342] Although behavior may be aggressive, a favorable outcome is observed in cases of surgically resected tumors.

Other Sarcomas

Most primary hepatic sarcomas occur in adults between 40 and 60 years of age who present with signs and symptoms indicative of a hepatic mass. These primary hepatic sarcomas should be distinguished from metastatic involvement by sarcomas of other organs and from sarcomatoid HCC.[64] The overall prognosis is poor, with most patients dying within a year of diagnosis.

Hepatic sarcomas histologically resemble their soft tissue counterparts. Among the types reported are fibrosarcoma, follicular dendritic cell sarcoma, desmoplastic nested single cell tumor, malignant fibrous histiocytoma, hemangiopericytoma, osteosarcoma, malignant schwannoma, and dedifferentiated liposarcoma. Leiomyosarcomas are described arising within the hepatic parenchyma, from the ligamentum teres, and from the hepatic vein, where they have been associated with the Budd-Chiari syndrome.[343,344]

Kaposi sarcoma is seen primarily in the setting of acquired immunodeficiency syndrome (AIDS). Histologically, the tumor is characterized by multifocal nodules composed of proliferated spindle cells with slit-like spaces that contain extravasated erythrocytes. These lesions are predominantly centered on portal tracts, but they also spread into and destroy the parenchyma.[274]

Hepatobiliary rhabdomyosarcoma is a rare neoplasm that usually arises from the common bile duct.[345] Most patients are young children, with exceptional cases reported in adults.[137,346] Histologically the tumor resembles botryoid-type embryonal rhabdomyosarcomas occurring elsewhere in the body. Soft polypoid masses protrude into the ductal lumen and are covered by intact, ulcerated, or inflamed biliary epithelium. The tumor is composed of small hyperchromatic cells with variable eosinophilic cytoplasm and rare cross-striations. Beneath the biliary epithelium, the cells are densely packed and form a so-called cambium layer, whereas deeper in the tumor, they are separated by a loose myxoid stroma. The diagnosis is secured by immunohistochemical demonstration of desmin, muscle-specific actin, myoglobin expression, or the ultrastructural finding of the characteristic myofilaments.

MISCELLANEOUS TUMORS

Inflammatory Pseudotumor

Inflammatory pseudotumors of the liver are nonneoplastic masses of unknown cause (see Chapter 48). They occur at any age and clinically manifest with abdominal pain together with various systemic manifestations, including low-grade fever, weight loss, leukocytosis, anemia, and inflammatory syndrome.[347] Although the cause is unknown, a yet-unidentified infectious or immunoglobulin G4 (IgG4) autoimmune-related process has been suggested.[348,349]

The masses are often solitary and range between 2 and 25 cm in diameter. They have a variable histologic appearance consisting of proliferated fibroblasts and myofibroblasts, lymphocytes (sometimes with lymphoid follicles), plasma cells, eosinophils, and neutrophils. Fibrosis or granulation tissue–like zones can be conspicuous, particularly in the central portions of the mass. Multinucleated or foamy macrophages, phlebitis, and granulomas are sometimes noted. Inflammatory pseudotumor may regress.

Others

Several examples of malignant rhabdoid tumor of the liver have been recognized. These tumors are highly aggressive neoplasms with a distinctive histologic appearance.[350] Rare cases of primary hepatic germ cell tumors of several types, including teratomas, yolk sac tumors, and choriocarcinoma, have been described. The combination of yolk sac tumor and hepatoblastoma has been described.[351] These tumors exhibit malignant behavior, although occasional long-term survival has been obtained with cancer chemotherapy.

Squamous carcinoma of the liver is uncommon, with most cases developing within simple hepatic cysts, various forms of fibropolycystic liver disease, or teratomas.[352]

Adrenal rest tumor and pancreatic heterotopia have been described and might be misleading.[353]

HEMATOPOIETIC NEOPLASMS

Primary Hepatic Lymphoma

Liver may represent the sole site of involvement by malignant lymphoma, but these primary hepatic lymphomas are uncommon, although hepatitis C infection may be a risk factor.[354,355]

On gross examination, most cases are characterized by a single large mass or, less often, multiple discrete nodules. Rarely the liver is diffusely infiltrated without a well-defined mass lesion. The tumors are predominantly classified as non-Hodgkin lymphomas of the diffuse large cell type, with occasional examples of small noncleaved or cleaved varieties such as the mucosa-associated lymphoid tissue (MALT).[356,357] Most of the tumors are phenotypically of B-cell lineage, although occasional T-cell lymphomas are also described. The neoplastic lymphocytes expand the portal tracts and invade into adjacent parenchyma to form large infiltrative nodules. The lobules are otherwise little affected, although occasional cases, particularly with T-cell lymphomas, demonstrate sinusoidal infiltration.[358]

Secondary Involvement

All varieties of lymphomas, leukemias, and hematopoietic proliferations can secondarily affect the liver, usually as a manifestation of disseminated disease and often in conjunction with splenic involvement.

As a general rule, the low-grade non-Hodgkin lymphomas tend to produce multiple portal-based infiltrates, whereas the intermediate- and high-grade types give rise to large irregular tumor masses. Sinusoidal involvement is uncommon except with peripheral T-cell lymphomas.[358–360]

Hepatic involvement in Hodgkin disease can manifest as large irregular masses or as small, diffusely distributed nodules. The characteristic infiltrate, which predominantly affects portal tracts, consists of a polymorphous collection of Reed-Sternberg cells or variants together with small lymphocytes, large mononuclear cells, plasma cells, eosinophils, and neutrophils in varying numbers.[361]

Leukemias of both acute and chronic types tend to permeate the sinusoids with malignant cells, with involvement of the portal tracts additionally noted with the lymphoid varieties. Hepatic involvement is especially common and conspicuous in hairy cell leukemia.[362]

Langerhans cell histiocytosis involves the liver in about 40% of cases.[363] The most important clinical manifestations include jaundice and portal hypertension resulting in part from infiltration of large bile ducts to produce a sclerosing cholangitis–like picture.

The liver is commonly involved in generalized mastocytosis. Mast cells accumulate principally in the portal tracts and are accompanied by varying degrees of periportal fibrosis and, on occasion, cirrhosis.

METASTASIS

Metastases are by far the most common form of hepatic malignancy, accounting for over 95% of the total. In autopsy series, liver metastases are noted in about 40% of patients with malignant tumors, the sites of origin including virtually every organ in the body.[364] The more frequent primary sites include carcinomas of the colon, pancreas, lung, and breast in adults, and neuroblastoma, Wilms tumor, and rhabdomyosarcoma in pediatric patients.[365] Although the origin of the tumor is often known when metastases are biopsied, carcinomas of the pancreas, stomach, and lung are particularly notorious for being occult primary neoplasms. Evaluation of mitotic index in liver metastasis of neuroendocrine tumor is important for prognosis and treatment but hampered by a certain degree of heterogeneity within the tumor.[366]

Grossly, metastatic tumors in the liver are almost always multiple, but they can appear as solitary nodules, confluent masses, or small diffusely infiltrative lesions that can mimic cirrhosis (Fig. 87.42).[367] The size range varies considerably. Typically these tumors are gray-to-yellow nodules, sometimes complicated by central necrosis, umbilication, or cystic change, and they can occur anywhere within the parenchymal mass.[365] Some metastases may display prominent fibrous changes.

In general, metastatic tumors maintain the histologic features seen in their primary location. A desmoplastic stroma is common with metastatic adenocarcinomas, especially those from the pancreas or breast, and the overall picture cannot be distinguished from cholangiocarcinoma. Some metastatic tumors tend to infiltrate the sinusoids, and tumors such as small cell carcinoma and melanoma can grow within the hepatic plates and replace the liver cells.

The references for this chapter can be found online by accessing the accompanying Expert Consult website.

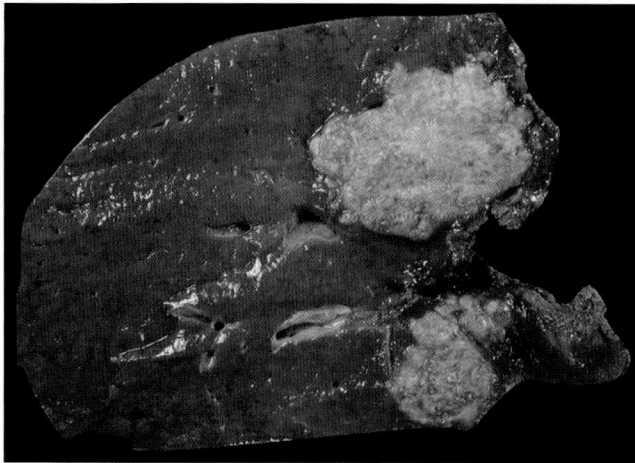

FIGURE 87.42   Liver metastasis. Confluent and infiltrative masses of varying size made of pale nodules with central necrosis.

SECTION II. Neoplastic

B. Benign and Premalignant Tumors

CHAPTER 88A

Benign liver lesions

Safi Dokmak and Maxime Ronot

The widespread use of medical imaging (see Chapter 14), such as hepatic ultrasonography (US), computed tomography (CT) scan, and magnetic resonance imaging (MRI), has led to the increased detection of asymptomatic tumors. In the absence of underlying chronic liver disease, the vast majority of these lesions correspond to benign liver tumors, including cystic and solid lesions. Cystic tumors will be discussed in Chapter 88B. Clonal analysis shows that these benign lesions contain a broad spectrum of regenerative and true neoplastic processes (Table 88A.1; see Chapter 87). Based on the cell of origin, the most frequent solid benign tumors may be classified into two groups according to their epithelial or mesenchymal origins. Epithelial lesions include hepatocellular focal nodular hyperplasia (FNH) and hepatocellular adenoma (HCA), and cholangiocellular tumors (bile duct adenoma). Mesenchymal tumors originating from blood vessels include hemangioma; those originating from adipose tissue include angiomyolipoma; and those originating from muscle tissue include leiomyoma. Apart from HCA and angiomyolipoma, which could be associated with serious complications requiring surgery, the vast majority of solid benign liver lesions remain asymptomatic, are not subject to malignant transformation, do not increase in volume, and therefore do not require any treatment or follow-up.[1,2] In this setting, the understanding of clinical, biologic, radiologic, and pathologic characteristics of each tumor is important to achieve both accurate diagnosis and appropriate management. Advances in imaging studies now allow precise noninvasive diagnosis in the majority of cases, which reduces the place of percutaneous biopsy to limit patients and restricts the place of resection for final diagnosis only to exceptional cases. The most frequent benign liver cell lesions include hemangioma, FNH, and HCA. Because radiologic imaging is of critical importance in diagnosis and management, there is considerable emphasis on the role of radiologic study (see Chapter 14).

CAVERNOUS HEMANGIOMA

Hepatic hemangiomas are probably the most common of all solid liver tumors, accounting for up to 70% of all benign liver lesions.[3] These tumors occur at all ages. However, because of the difference of histologic structure between adult and infantile forms and because of various clinical presentations, they must be regarded as separate entities.[4] Only hemangioma of the liver in adults will be considered in this chapter (see Chapter 87).

Pathogenesis and Pathology

The prevalence of hemangioma in the general population ranges from 3% to 20%[3,5,6] with a large predominance in women, with a 5:1 female/male ratio.[7-9] In adults, hemangiomas are usually found in patients at a mean age of 50 years, equally in the left and right lobes of the liver. The vast majority of hemangiomas are less than 5 cm in diameter and are rarely pediculated. Hemangiomas measuring 10 cm or more are referred to as "giant hemangiomas" and can present with fibrosis, thrombosis, and calcifications. The pathogenesis of hemangioma remains largely unknown. Some of these tumors have estrogen receptors and accelerated growth has been observed with high estrogen states, such as those associated with puberty, pregnancy, oral contraceptive (OC) use, and androgen treatment (see Chapter 87). These findings suggest that hormonal effect may be one of the pathogenic mechanisms,[9,1] especially in giant hemangiomas, supporting that US monitoring in pregnant women with giant hemangiomas should be advocated.[11] Macroscopic examination demonstrates well-delineated, red-blue, flat lesions that may partially collapse on sectioning. Similar to imaging findings, some degrees of fibrosis, calcification, and thrombosis may be observed, most commonly on the largest lesions. Microscopically, hemangiomas are made of cavernous vascular spaces lined by flattened endothelium underlying fibrous septa of various widths (see Chapter 87). Small hemangiomas may become entirely fibrous, appearing as "a solitary fibrous nodule."

Clinical and Biologic Data

The vast majority of hemangiomas are asymptomatic and found incidentally during US examination or CT examination (see Chapter 14) of the abdomen for unrelated reasons.[9] Although the majority of hemangiomas remain stable in size,[12,13] tumor enlargement greater than 5% may be observed in up to 45% of the lesions. A strong correlation has been demonstrated between initial mean linear dimension and tumor growth, and large lesions show significantly higher growth over time.[12] The prevalence and growth of hemangiomas is very related to the age, with a low prevalence in the 20- to 29-year-old group and higher growth rate in the 30- to 39-year-old group.[14]

Hepatic hemangiomas are usually asymptomatic but pain and discomfort are the most frequent symptoms. It is not always easy to attribute pain to hemangiomas, especially for

TABLE 88A.1   Overview of Benign Liver Lesions

LESION	TYPE	COMMENTS
Epithelial Lesions		
Hepatocytes	Hepatocellular adenoma	Very rare Several subtypes Associated with oral contraceptives, obesity, and genetic factors. High rate of complications Bleeding and malignant transformation
	Focal nodular hyperplasia	Rare Female predominance No risk of complication
	Nodular regenerative hyperplasia	Very rare Associated with systemic diseases and drugs Portal hypertension
	Focal fatty change	Common Associated with diabetes, obesity, hepatitis C virus, malnutrition, and anomalies of venous drainage No risk of complication
Biliary Cells	Bile duct adenoma	Rare No risk of complication
	Biliary hamartoma (Von Meyenburg complex)	Very rare Development anomaly No risk of complication
Nonepithelial Lesions		
Mesenchymal	Hemangioma	Common Female predominance Very low risk of complication
	Angiomyolipoma	Rare Associated with tuberous sclerosis Malignant transformation if > 5 cm
	Lipoma, leiomyoma, lymphogioma	Exceptional No risk of complication
	Hepatic small vessel neoplasm	Recently described new entity No complication
Heterotopia	Spleen, adrenal, pancreatic, or gastric	Exceptional Very low risk of complication
Others	Peliosis hepatis	Exceptional Associated with androgens, oral contraceptives, drugs, malignancies, tuberculosis, systemic diseases Very low risk of complication by liver rupture
	Inflammatory pseudotumor	Very rare Associated with general syndromes No risk of complication
	Solitary fibrotic tumor	Sequela of a previous infection/liver tumor No complication

small ones, because pain related to an uncomplicated hemangioma can be because of associated disorders such as gallbladder disease, hepatic cysts, gastroduodenal ulcers, or a hiatal hernia.[15,16] Large hemangiomas can be asymptomatic or may manifest as an abdominal mass[17] and exceptionally as fever.[18] Compared with those located the right liver, large lesions located in the left lobe of the liver may cause pressure effects on the stomach with resulting symptom.[19] Exceptionally large hemangiomas may cause compression of bile ducts resulting in jaundice,[20,21] of the vena cava with lower limb edema,[22] of the hepatic veins, and of the portal vein. Liver biologic tests, including alkaline phosphatase and γ-glutamyl transferase, are normal. Normal laboratory tests associated with a large hepatic tumor with mild symptoms could be of help in the diagnosis of hemangioma.

Complications are mostly observed in large hemangiomas and can be divided into (1) alterations of internal architecture, such as with inflammation; (2) coagulation abnormalities; and (3) compression of adjacent structures. Inflammatory processes complicating giant hemangiomas are rarely observed, but their prevalence is probably underestimated. In this situation, first described by Bornman and colleagues,[13,23] inflammation may occur as a consequence of the thrombosis of a part of the hemangioma. Signs and symptoms of this process include low-grade fever, weight loss, abdominal pain, accelerated erythrocyte sedimentation rate, anemia, thrombocytosis, and increased fibrinogen level, which contrast with otherwise normal white blood cell count and liver function tests. The imaging features are those of a giant hemangioma, but inner thrombosis can be depicted. Clinical and laboratory abnormalities disappear after surgical excision of the hemangioma.[23–25]

Kasabach-Merritt syndrome is an exceptional complication of hepatic hemangioma in adults[26] (see Chapter 87). This coagulopathy, which consists of intravascular coagulation, clotting, and fibrinolysis within the hemangioma, may progress to secondary increased systemic fibrinolysis and thrombocytopenia.[27,28] The syndrome is reversible after removal of the hemangioma.

Intratumoral hemorrhage or rupture is rare. It can occur spontaneously or secondary to anticoagulation therapy or blunt trauma.[29] Spontaneous rupture of a hemangioma is exceptional, reported mainly as case reports, with less than 100 indisputable cases reported to date.[29-31] The mean size of hemangiomas with spontaneous rupture is 11 cm (1–37 cm), and the reported mortality has decreased over the past 20 years. Meanwhile, nonspontaneous rupture occurs more frequently in patients aged younger than 40 years.[29] This rare complication may occur in association with Kasabach-Merritt syndrome and is associated with a short-term mortality rate of 35%.[31] Taking into account the high prevalence of these tumors, however, the extremely low incidence of this complication should not interfere with therapeutic management or with specific advice given to patients who are often worried by the presence of a vascular liver tumor.[32] Preventive surgery is not advocated because mortality has been reported after liver resection for benign diseases.[33,34]

Imaging

On US, the classic sonographic appearance of hemangioma is that of a homogenous hyperechoic mass with sharp margins, measuring less than 3 cm in diameter and associated with acoustic enhancement (Fig. 88A.1; see Chapter 14). No vascular pattern is usually identified on color Doppler. Other investigations are required when US does not show typical patterns. Contrast-enhanced US reveals peripheral globular enhancement on arterial and portal venous phases and an isoechoic pattern on late phase in most atypical hemangiomas.[35]

Criteria for the diagnosis of hemangioma on CT scan include (1) low attenuation on noncontrast CT, (2) peripheral and globular enhancement of the lesion followed by a central enhancement on contrast CT, and (3) contrast enhancement of the lesion on delayed phases[36] (see Chapter 14). Among these criteria, the presence of peripheral puddles at the arterial phase has a sensitivity of 67%, a specificity of 99%, and a positive predictive value of 86% for the diagnosis of hemangioma.[37] On MRI, hemangioma appear hypointense on T1-weighted sequences and strongly hyperintense on heavily T2-weighted sequences (Fig. 88A.2). Dynamic multiphasic T1-weighted sequences after extracellular gadolinium chelate administration show findings similar to that on contrast-enhanced CT phases (Fig. 88A.3).[38] After injection of hepatobiliary MR contrast agents such as gadoxetic acid, hemangiomas are hypointense or have incomplete enhancement compared with the background liver during the transitional because of rapid and conspicuous uptake of contrast by hepatocytes, especially in the noncirrhotic liver. Complete

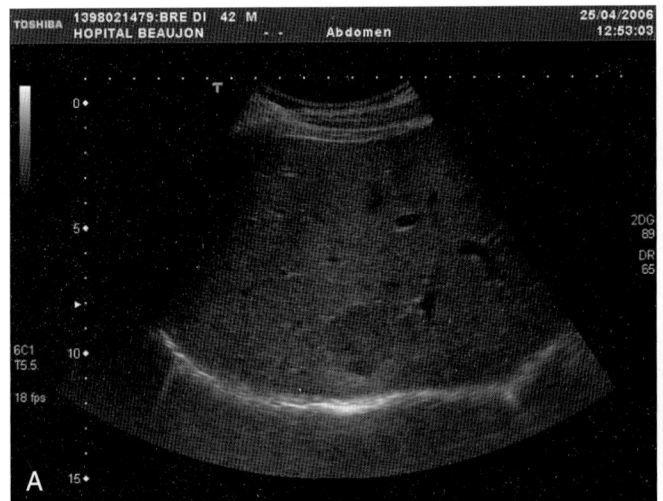

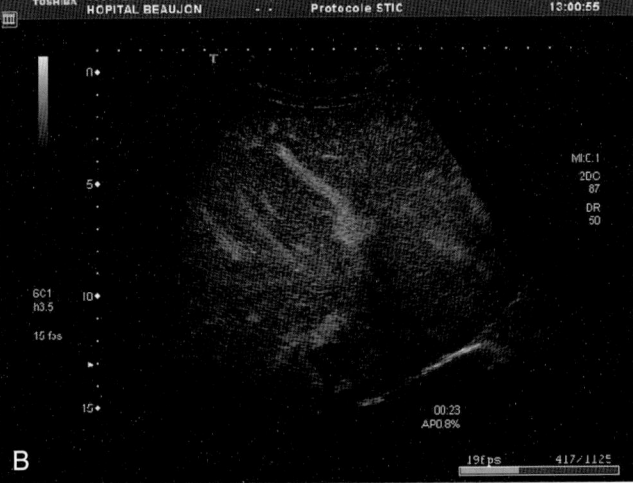

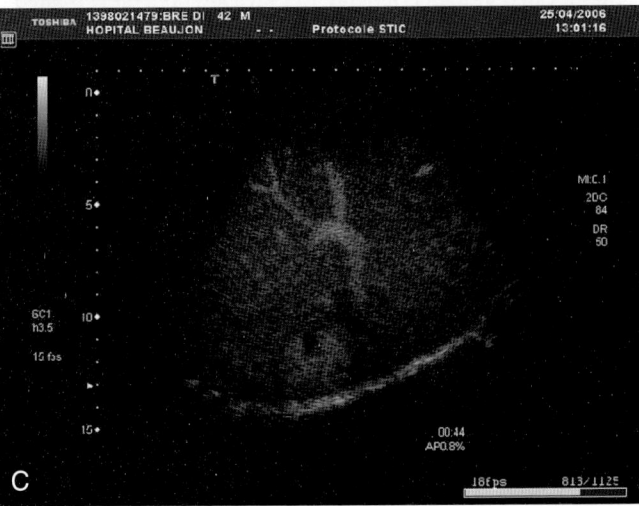

FIGURE 88A.1   Hemangioma. Ultrasound (**A**) shows a hypoechoic liver lesion with posterior acoustic enhancement. Contrast-enhanced ultrasound (**B** and **C**) demonstrates peripheral puddling, followed by complete and delayed enhancement (see Chapter 14).

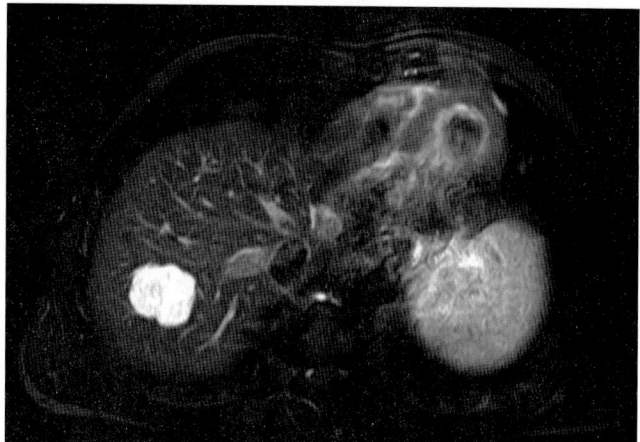

FIGURE 88A.2 Hemangioma T2-weighted magnetic resonance imaging shows typical bright signal (see Chapter 14).

hypointensity on hepatobiliary phase images, known as the "pseudo washout sign," is therefore usually observed in hemangiomas, especially in rapidly enhancing or small ones.[39]

The two most common imaging atypias are found in giant hemangiomas and in rapidly filling hemangiomas. Giant hemangiomas, which are defined as exceeding 6 to 12 cm in diameter, are often heterogeneous with marked central areas corresponding to thrombosis, extensive hyalinization, and fibrosis.[40,41] However, the typical features are present. Rapidly filling hemangiomas occur significantly more frequently in small lesions (42% of hemangiomas < 2 cm in diameter).[42] CT and MRI show an immediate homogeneous enhancement at the arterial phase. Their diagnosis is based on strong hyperintensity on T2-weighted images, the parallelism enhancement with arterial structures, and the persistent enhancement on delayed-phase imaging. The other atypical hemangiomas are very uncommon and include very slow–filling hemangiomas, calcified hemangiomas, hyalinized hemangiomas, cystic hemangiomas, pedunculated hemangiomas, hemangiomas with fluid-fluid levels that contain fluid of different attenuations on CT and intensities on MRI corresponding to the sedimentation level, and hemangiomas with capsular retraction. In these rare lesions, US, CT, and MRI are less reliable, and second-line imaging such as contrast-enhanced ultrasound (CEUS) may be helpful.

Hemangiomas associated with inflammatory response syndrome are usually because of acute thrombosis of a part or all the hemangioma and can be diagnosed by showing spontaneous hyperattenuation on unenhanced CT scans. Hemangiomas developing in an abnormal liver are also difficult to diagnose. In fatty livers, these lesions usually appear isoechoic or hypoechoic with US and hyperattenuating with unenhanced CT.[43] MRI with T2-weighted sequences showing strong hyperintensity, and fat-suppressed sequences and opposed T1-weighted sequences, are crucial for diagnosis in this setting. With progressive cirrhosis, hemangiomas, which are filled with blood, are prone to be compressed by the cirrhotic architecture[44] and are therefore likely to decrease in size and become more fibrotic, which may make them more difficult to diagnose by imaging.[45] In this clinical setting, US cannot confidently make the diagnosis of hemangiomas because half of the hyperechoic lesions are hepatocellular carcinomas (HCCs).[46] Nevertheless, the typical appearance is often depicted on cross-sectional imaging.[47]

Altogether, imaging, and especially MRI, is able to diagnose liver hemangiomas in almost all cases, and liver biopsy should be restricted only to exceptional cases. In these situations, biopsy of hemangiomas may be performed without significant risk of hemorrhage[48,49] and allows an overall accuracy of 96%.[48]

Management

Whatever the size, there is no treatment for asymptomatic hemangioma. When the diagnosis is established, it is not necessary to adopt therapeutic or specific lifestyle measures. The patient should be reassured about the rare occurrence of growth and the extremely low risk of complications. Therefore there is no argument for interrupting OCs, avoiding pregnancy, or giving specific advice to interrupt sporting activities. Apart from very specific situations, a follow-up is not justified. Although in specialized centers liver resection mortality for benign lesion is almost nil, there is a risk of intraoperative bleeding and postoperative biliary fistula, which should be considered unacceptable considering the benign nature of these lesions.

Indications for treatment include severe symptoms and complications[50–52] (see Chapter 101). Inability to exclude malignancy should be an exceptional indication for resection. Before considering surgery or any other treatment, other causes of pain should be excluded. Surgical resection remains the definitive treatment, but the last decade showed the widespread use of nonsurgical options like transarterial embolization and ablation. Patients should be managed in specialized units where all surgical and nonsurgical options are available. To our knowledge, radiotherapy[53] and hepatic artery ligation, which were described many years ago for the treatment of liver hemangiomas, are no longer practiced.

Surgical resection is the treatment of choice.[16,17,33] It can be done by an open or minimally invasive approach and consists of resection or enucleation of the hemangioma (see Chapter 101). The widespread use of laparoscopy should not modify the rare indications for surgery for this benign disease, but when surgery is indicated, the laparoscopic approach is an excellent option because there is no liver disease and large margins are not needed. The minimal approach is suitable for peripheral lesions and those located in anterolateral segments of the liver.[54–56] Minimally invasive right hepatectomy can be done if the transection plane is free of intrahepatic collateral circulation. The choice between enucleation and resection requires consideration of the size and anatomic location of the lesion. Hemangiomas located in the peripheral liver area are preferably treated by enucleation, whereas tumors deeply located are more safely resected with a formal anatomic liver resection.[57–59] Comparative studies between resection and enucleation showed similar results and the risk of bleeding was not necessarily related to the size but to the location of lesions and to adjacent vascular structures.[60–62] During surgery, early arterial ligation may be considered to allow manual decompression of large hemangioma and to facilitate their manipulation and enucleation.[53] Several studies have shown that resection of benign diseases, including symptomatic hemangiomas, relieves symptoms and improves quality of life in the vast majority of selected patients, especially when a laparoscopic approach is preferred.[17,63,64] In the absence of improvement, surgical complications should be ruled out, and the cause of symptoms initially attributed to hemangioma should be reconsidered.

Finally, many comparative studies have shown that resection for liver hemangiomas may carry a higher relative risk for severe

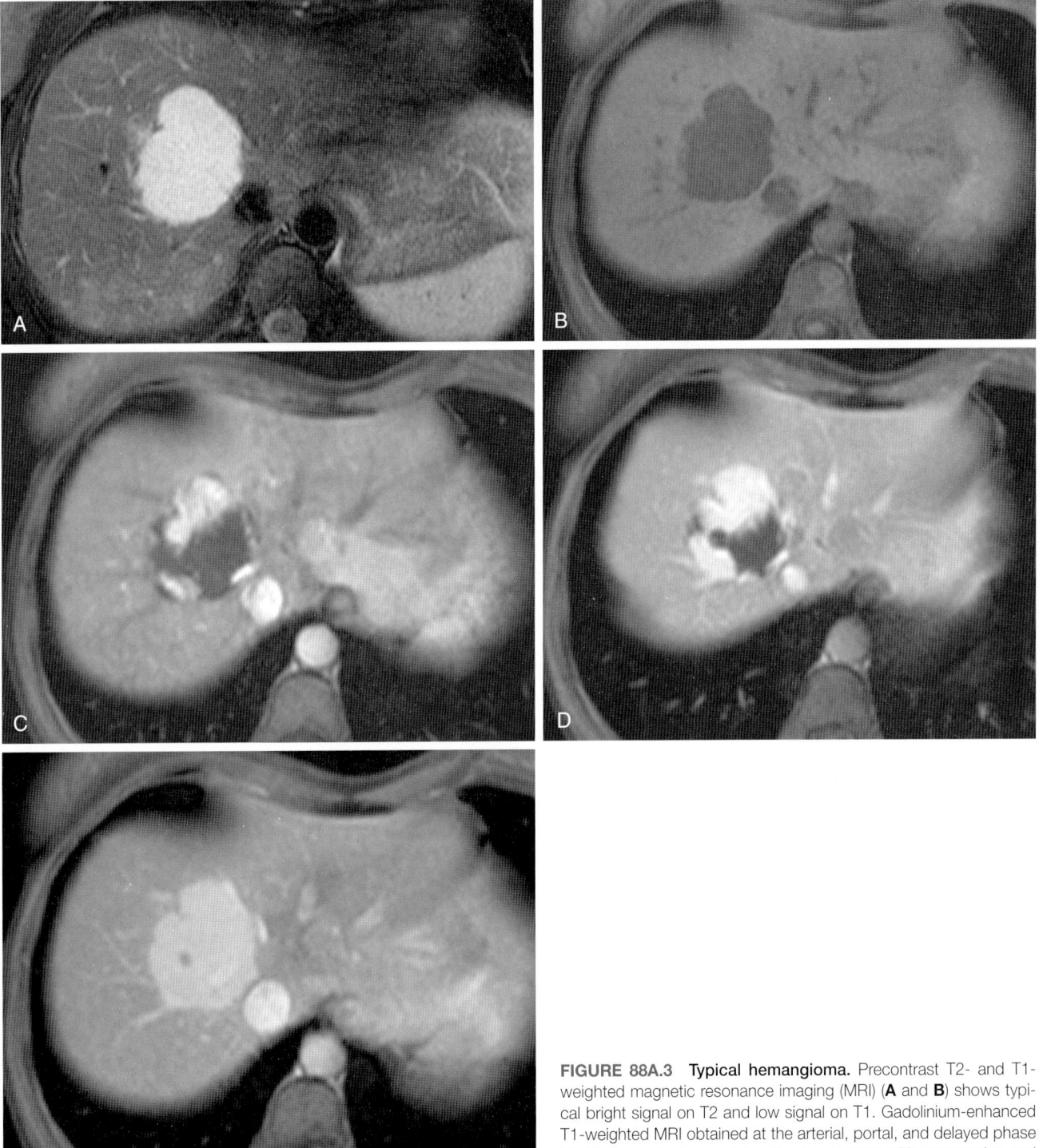

FIGURE 88A.3 Typical hemangioma. Precontrast T2- and T1-weighted magnetic resonance imaging (MRI) (**A** and **B**) shows typical bright signal on T2 and low signal on T1. Gadolinium-enhanced T1-weighted MRI obtained at the arterial, portal, and delayed phase (**C–E**) shows typical peripheral enhancement with progressive and complete filling over time (see Chapter 14).

complications[65,64] compared with simple observation. In a large population (n = 492) with long-term follow-up (11 ± 6.4 years), life-threatening complication occurred in 7% of operated patients and in 2% of nonoperated ones.[65] All these studies state that observation is preferred and that surgery should be reserved for patients with severe symptoms and should be done in specialized units.[65–67]

Transarterial embolization or chemoembolization have been proposed for the treatment of liver hemangiomas,[68–72]

but indications and results remain unclear. A review article reporting on 1284 patients reported a high success rate (90%), but results are difficult to interpret. Indeed, the primary outcome was the size reduction and not symptom relief, and indications for treatment were not well-detailed in more than two-thirds of cases. When provided, the main indications for treatment were severe symptoms in only one-third of cases. Severe complications occurred in 3% of patients, and the majority (90%) of patients showed only partial relief of symptoms.[73] Radiofrequency ablation (RFA) has been re- ported as an alternative treatment for liver hemangiomas be- tween 5 to 10 cm in diameter.[74–76] These procedures can be performed percutaneously or under laparoscopic control for subcapsular lesions to avoid injury to adjacent structures.[75–78] A high success rate has been reported,[75,78] but morbidity was reported to be frequent[78] and severe when the procedure was performed on hemangiomas greater than 10 cm,[79] especially because of acute renal failure secondary to massive intravas- cular hemolysis.[80] Using the same principles, percutaneous and laparoscopic microwave ablations were recently described for the treatment of hepatic hemangiomas.[81–83] Although the results of nonsurgical options are encouraged, they cannot be recommended in routine practice. These procedures should be evaluated in patients with severe symptoms and compared with the classical surgical treatment.

Liver transplantation has also been successfully used in ex- ceptional situations to treat symptomatic patients with techni- cally unresectable and complicated giant hemangiomas or hemangiomatosis with cardiopulmonary complications[84–88] (see Chapter 105). These patients typically have extremely large hemangiomas with hepatomegaly and complications such as severe portal hypertension.[89] About 25 cases have been re- ported in the literature, and the main indications for liver trans- plantation were respiratory distress, massive hemorrhage, Kasa- bach-Merritt syndrome, and failure of previous treatment.[90] The long-term results are excellent.

FOCAL NODULAR HYPERPLASIA

Pathogenesis and Pathology

FNH is a benign, tumor-like condition predominantly diag- nosed in women 30 to 50 years of age. Most FNHs and their surrounding liver parenchyma express estrogen but not proges- terone receptors.[91] Yet, most cohort and clinical studies found no influence of OCs[92,93] and pregnancy[10,94,95] on tumor growth (see Chapter 87).

FNH is considered a hyperplastic reaction resulting from arterial malformation.[96] This hypothesis, which suggests that increased arterial flow hyperperfuses the local liver paren- chyma, leading to secondary hepatocellular hyperplasia, has been reinforced by molecular analyses showing that FNH involves polyclonal regenerative processes.[97–99] Molecular pro- files of FNHs show deregulation of genes involved in vascular remodeling, such as for angiopoietins, with a characteristic increase in the angiopoietin 1 (responsible for vessel forma- tion)/angiopoietin 2 (which acts as an antagonist of angio- poietin 1) ratio, which strongly supports the theory of a vascular hyperplastic reaction resulting from arterial malfor- mation.[100] In addition, upregulation of extracellular matrix genes associated with activation of the transforming growth factor-β signaling pathway and overexpression of Wnt/ β-catenin target genes (such as *GLUL*, which encodes gluta- mine synthetase) has been reported.[99] Indeed, FNHs display a typical map-like pattern of glutamine synthetase expression on immunohistochemistry, in which positivity is predominantly observed in hepatocytes at the periphery of the nodules.[101] The heterogeneous distribution of glutamine synthase is caused by β-catenin activation without β-catenin–activating mutations, in accordance with polyclonal origin, and could be the result of abnormal arterial blood flow.[99]

The fact that FNH accounts for a regenerative process in- duced in a specific vascular territory could explain the absence of changes in size in the vast majority of cases. This also likely explains the occurrence of these lesions in patients with vascu- lar disorders of the liver, including Budd-Chiari syndrome,[102] hereditary hemorrhagic telangiectasia,[103] congenital absence of portal flow/portosystemic shunt,[104–106] portal thrombosis with subsequent hepatic arterialization,[107] or in the population who received chemotherapy for pediatric cancers,[108] stem cell trans- plantation, or hepatic metastases.[109] Such regenerative focal processes are also described in cirrhotic tissue with the so- called FNH-like macronodules.

Histologically, FNHs display a typical pathologic pattern. Grossly, FNH is a well-circumscribed, unencapsulated, and usually solitary mass, and it is characterized by a central fibrous scar that radiates into the liver parenchyma (Fig. 88A.4). His- tologically, FNH is composed of benign-appearing hepatocytes arranged in nodules that are partially delineated by fibrous septa originating from the central scar, and the main diagnostic feature is the presence of large and dystrophic arteries in the fibrous septa (see Chapter 87).

Besides this classic form of FNH, several variant lesions are described with increased frequency and commonly classified as "nontypical FNH" by radiologists. This group is somehow het- erogeneous, including FNH without central fibrous scar and FNH containing fat.[110] However, in this group of atypical FNH, molecular analyses showed that lesions displaying telan- giectatic changes, so-called "telangiectatic form of FNH," were, in fact, clonal processes and should be regarded as a variant form of liver cell adenoma rather than FNH.[111,112]

Clinical and Biologic Data

FNH represents the second most frequent solid benign lesion, with an estimated prevalence of approximately 1%.[113] These lesions occur predominantly in women with a female/male ratio of 9:1. In female patients, FNHs are often discovered between 30 and 40 years of age, whereas men with FNH are usually older.[110] Most FNHs are asymptomatic and are discovered in- cidentally during liver US examination. Although FNH is mainly a solitary lesion, multiple FNHs can be observed in 20% of the cases and can be associated with hemangiomas or with HCAs.[114–116] In a few patients with a large tumor, FNH can be discovered by abdominal pain or discomfort. Large le- sions located in the left lobe of the liver may cause pressure effects on adjacent structures, with resulting symptoms. The lesion may be felt when pedunculated and may be responsible for acute episodes of pain because of the torsion of the pedicle. Large FNHs that develop below the Glisson capsule can be responsible for pain,[117] but in most cases, pain related to FNH is probably because of associated disorders.

Complications of FNH, such as rupture or bleeding, have been initially reported. They actually occur in so-called *telangi- ectatic FNH*, which should now be classified as hepatocellular adenoma. No malignant transformation of FNH has been clearly established. A reduction in size after menopause can be observed, but in the vast majority of cases, FNH remains stable in size, even after interruption of OCs or pregnancy.[93] However, some case reports showing regression of FNH after discontinu- ation of OCs have been recently described.[118–121]

Hepatic biologic tests are normal in almost 80% of cases.[122] A mild elevation of γ-glutamyl transferase and alkaline phos- phatases may sometimes be observed in patients with a large

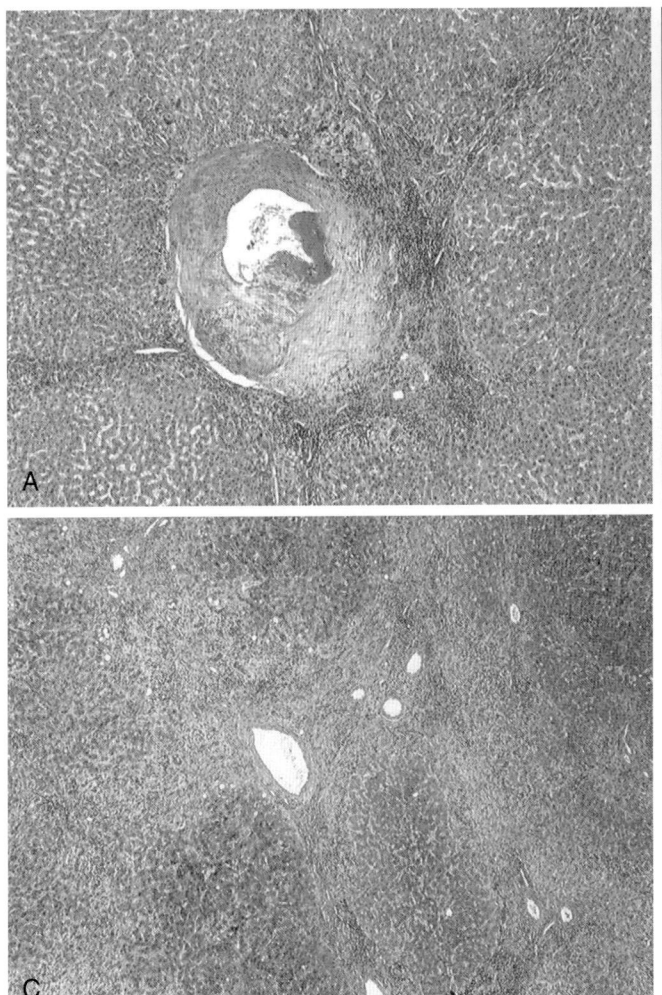

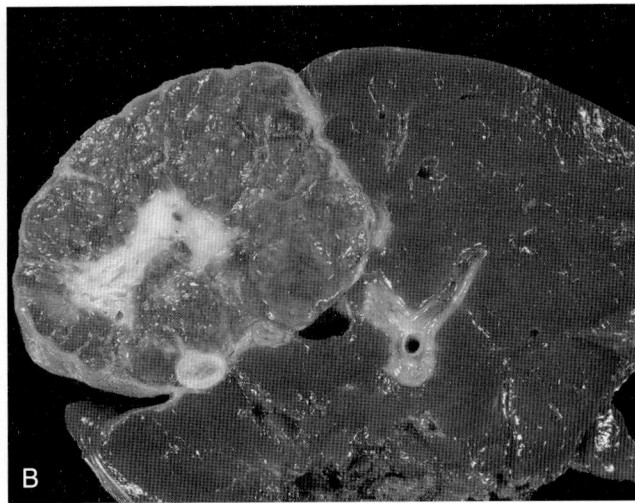

FIGURE 88A.4 A macroscopic view of focal nodular hyperplasia (FNH), which is well circumscribed and displays a central fibrous scar that radiates and delineates liver parenchyma nodules.

FNH that causes extrinsic compression of intrahepatic biliary ducts or hepatic veins.[122,123] The presence of a slight elevation of serum aminotransferase levels could be because of the presence of associated steatosis in the underlying liver parenchyma.

Imaging

Regardless of the imaging modality, FNHs are associated with several findings (Fig. 88A.5; see Chapter 14): lack of capsule, often with lobulated contours; lesion homogeneity, except the central scar; US echogenicity; CT attenuation; MRI signal intensity similar to or slightly different from that of the adjacent liver on precontrast US, CT, or MRI[117,124]; and strong and homogeneous enhancement on arterial-phase CEUS, CT, or MRI, with a central vascular supply becoming similar to the adjacent nontumorous liver on portal and delayed phases.[45,104] The central scar is best seen on MRI, being hypointense won precontrast T1-weighted images, strongly hyperintense on T2-weighted images, and hyperintense on delayed phase because of the accumulation of extracellular contrast material in the fibrous tissue.[125,126] Most FNHs are isointense or hyperintense in the hepatobiliary phase, unlike HCAs, HCCs, and nonhepatocellular tumors.[127,128] Because none of these individual imaging features is completely specific to FNH, diagnosis is based on a combination of features. Diagnosis of FNH is certain when all findings are met and very likely when four of the findings are seen. MRI has the highest sensitivity (70%) and a specificity of almost 100% for the differentiation of FNH from other benign lesions.[129] However, the diagnostic performance of CEUS is higher than MRI for small FNHs (<3 cm).[130]

FNHs can have an unusual appearance if fat is present (mimicking HCAs), or if there is an atypical scar or calcifications. However, when all typical features are present, these findings should not modify the diagnosis.[131] In patients with atypical MRI results, liver biopsy is indicated. In the setting of an atypical MRI result, abnormal arteries, fibrous bands, ductular reaction, and cholestasis are probably the most discriminating diagnostic features of FNHs.[132] More recently, the use of surrogate immunohistochemical markers has been shown to help diagnosis. For example, glutamine synthetase expression increases positive diagnosis from 53.3% to 93.3%.[133]

Management

Whatever the size and the number of lesions, there is no treatment for asymptomatic FNH when the diagnosis is firmly established. In addition, the occurrence of this lesion in men should not modify the indication of conservative treatment.[134–136] FNH has no risk of malignant transformation, and there is no risk of complications. The patient should be reassured about the absence of complications and the natural

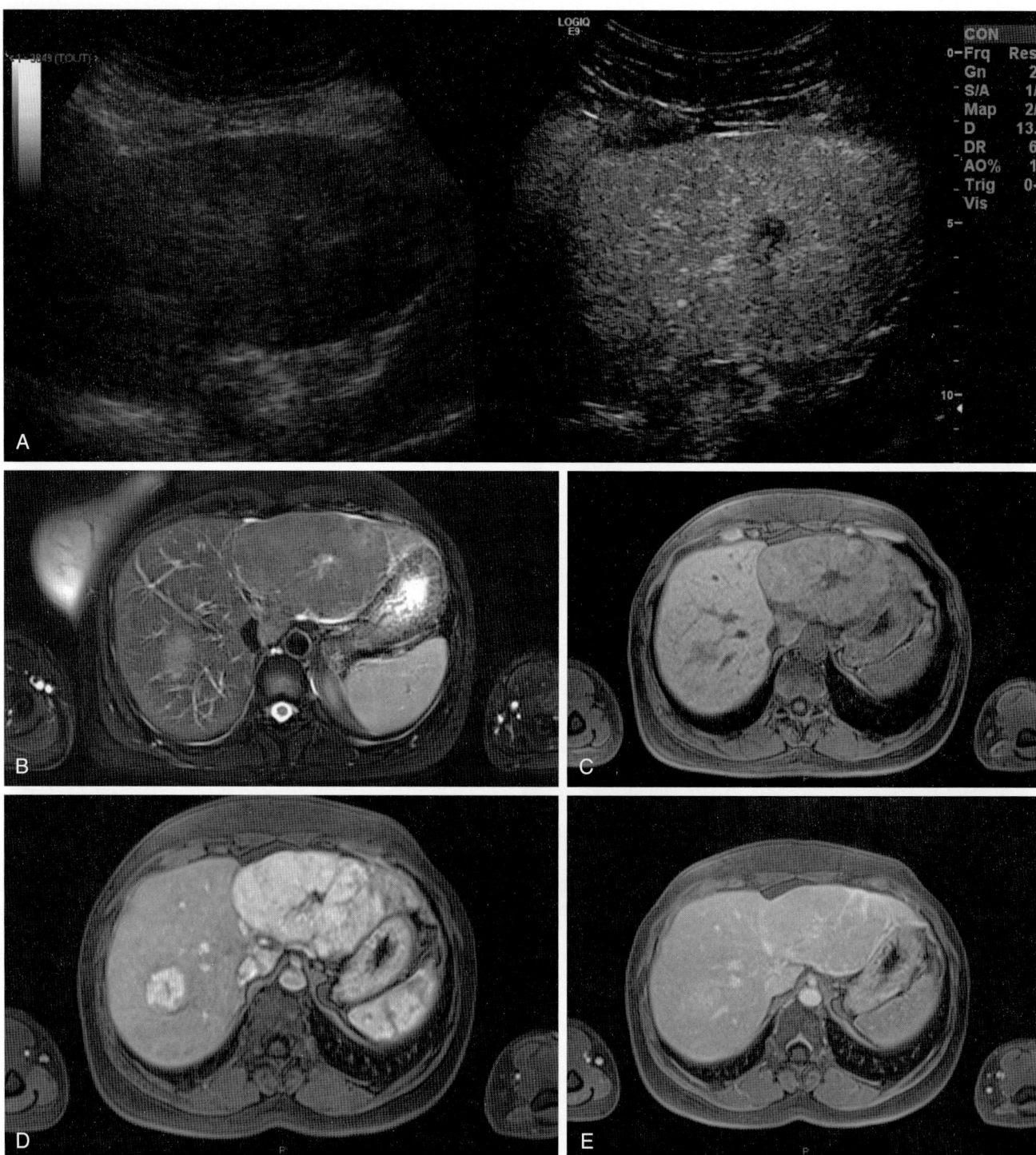

FIGURE 88A.5 **Typical focal nodular hyperplasia (FNH).** Contrast-enhanced ultrasound (**A**) demonstrates strong and homogeneous enhancement apart from the central scar that remains hypoechoic. Precontrast T2- and T1-weighted magnetic resonance imaging shows two FNHs that are isointense on T2 (**B**) and hypointense on T1 (**C**). Gadolinium-enhanced T1-weighted magnetic resonance imaging obtained at the arterial and delayed phase (**D** and **E**) shows strong and homogeneous enhancement of the lesion with progressive fading. The central scar is hyperintense on T2 and enhances on delayed imaging. Note that the central scar is more evident in the large FNH (see Chapter 14).

history of this lesion, which remains stable, could decrease, and may even disappear after the fifth decade. Therefore there is no argument for interrupting OCs or avoiding pregnancy.[52] In a study including 20 pregnant women with FNH of a mean size of 58.5 mm (± 22.7 mm), the follow-up showed partial regression (50%), stability (35%), and slight increase (15%)

with no complication.[94] Likewise, when diagnosis is established, follow-up is not justified.

Surgical resection is restricted to symptomatic patients (see Chapter 101). Symptomatic patients with confirmed FNH should be thoroughly investigated to exclude other etiologies before attributing symptoms to the liver lesion. In some series,

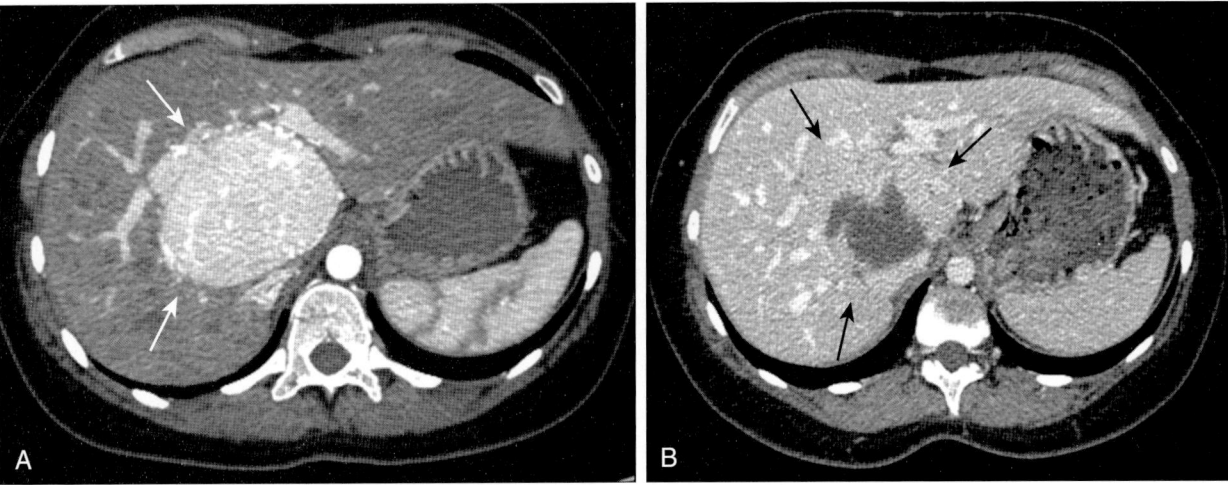

FIGURE 88A.6   Focal nodular hyperplasia before and after arterial embolization. Abdominal computed tomography scan with contrast medium injection on arterial and portal phases. **A,** Homogeneous centrohepatic focal nodular hyperplasia shows an immediate and intense enhancement during arterial phase *(white arrows).* **B,** Postembolization aspect of the lesion. Note size decrease and complete devascularization of the center of the lesion appearing as a homogeneous unenhanced central area *(black arrows).*

the main indication for surgery was an uncertain diagnosis.[137,138] Nowadays, such an indication should be exceptional and only validated after thorough concentration with very experienced radiologists, possibly after liver biopsy. The development of laparoscopy should not extend the indication of resection. Resection, which should be performed in specialist hepatobiliary units, is clearly indicated in patients with large symptomatic FNH located in the left liver and in those with a pedunculated lesion. Given the frequent existence of large vessels surrounding the lesion, liver resection with a surgical margin is preferred over enucleation and surgical difficulty should not be underestimated, even for peripheral lesions. Limited liver resection is advocated with low morbidity.[139] In some symptomatic patients with large FNH located in the right liver or in segment I, and necessitating difficult or risky resection, transarterial embolization has been advocated as a first step to confirm the implication of the lesion in symptoms.[140,126] Data show that this is an attractive treatment that may both decrease the size of the lesion and relieve symptoms[141–143] (Fig. 88A.6). It is currently the most successful and most often proposed treatment after surgery.[144] However, even though arterial embolization might be efficient, there is currently no rationale to support its routine use. No series of percutaneous ablation for the treatment of symptomatic FNH were described in the literature.

HEPATOCELLULAR ADENOMA

Introduction

HCA is a group of rare, benign liver neoplasms with a strong predominance in young women (female/male ratio, 9:1) taking OCs. Obesity and genetic alterations have emerged as more frequent risk factors. Although its prevalence in the general population is less than 0.05%, it has long been of interest given its potential complications, which include hemorrhage and malignant transformation into HCC.[2] This interest has increased in the last decade because of major progress in understanding risk factors, as well as the clinical, radiologic, and histologic aspects of this disease. HCA is no longer considered

a single entity of surgical indication whatever the size but is now divided into three radiologic (inflammatory, HNF1A, and classic) and at least five histologic (HNF1A, inflammatory, β catenin, sonic hedgehog, and unclassified) subtypes with different risks of complications[145] (see Chapter 87).

Risk Factors for Hepatocellular Adenoma

Before the introduction of OCs, HCAs were rarely reported in the medical literature. These tumors became widely recognized in the 1970s after numerous case reports from the United States and other countries of liver tumors in women who used OCs.[146] It has been reported that the hormonal background had a role in the pathogenesis of HCA. Estrogens have consistently been reported as a predominant factor, significantly and independently correlating with the development of HCA.[147] In women taking OCs, the positive correlation with HCA incidence is dose dependent.[148,149] Consequently, spontaneous regression of HCAs after withdrawal of estrogens has been reported.[150–152] However, no satisfactory causal explanation for the association of OC use and the occurrence of HCAs currently exists because regression after withdrawal of OC occurs inconsistently and the widespread use of low-content estrogen has not eliminated the risk of developing HCA, which suggests that other factors, mainly genetic and environmental, might also contribute to the pathogenesis of this disease. The development of HCA could be the consequence of the promotion of *HNF1α* gene mutations after estrogen exposure[2] or germline heterozygous CYP1B1 mutations leading to decreased activity of an enzyme involved in estrogen metabolism.[153] The influence of obesity on the development of HCA has also been suggested because the prevalence of HCA is higher in obese patients.[154] Many studies demonstrate that HCA is currently more frequently observed in obese patients and in those with metabolic syndrome and steatohepatitis[155–160] (see Chapter 69), with overweight and obese patients representing between 38% and 73% of patients with HCA.[159,160] There is a shift away from modern OC and toward obesity and metabolic syndrome being the dominant and emerging risk factors for HCA.[161] Androgen also contributes to the pathogenesis of

HCA, with tumors having been reported in patients who have Fanconi's anemia treated with androgen, in athletes who have taken steroids, and in patients with high levels of endogenous androgens.[162–166] HCA may also occur in association with certain metabolic diseases such as type 1 glycogen storage disease (GSD),[167–169] high triglyceride concentrations,[169] and iron overload related to beta-thalassemia or hemochromatosis.[170] Familial cases have been reported in patients with maturity-onset diabetes type 3 (MODY 3)[171,172] and the McCune–Albright syndrome.[2] HCA can also occur in patients with hepatic vascular abnormalities such as portosystemic shunts with portal deprivation,[173–175] with Budd-Chiari syndrome and other vascular diseases,[176] and, rarely, in cirrhosis.[177,178] Other rare causes include polycystic ovary syndrome related or not to sodium valproate leading to hyperandrogenemia,[179–181] patients with Turner syndrome receiving growth hormone therapy,[182] patients with Hurler syndrome with severe immune deficiencies,[183] and adults with history of childhood cancer (leukemia) and treated by hematopoietic stem cell transplants with irradiation or estrogen therapy.[184] HCA is rare in men (10%), and androgen use, metabolic syndrome and steatohepatitis, type 1 GSD, and portosystemic shunts with portal deprivation should be systematically considered.

Clinical Presentation

The mean age at presentation is 37 (16–62) and the mean size is 8.4 cm (±4.2; range: 1–22).[154] HCA is usually asymptomatic and discovered incidentally during nonrelated imaging studies for nonspecific abdominal pain or abnormal hepatic function tests. The most common symptom is abdominal pain[154,185] observed with large or pedunculated HCA. Acute pain can be related to bleeding. HCA may rarely present with fever, anemia, or pruritus. Half of patients have multiple tumors (>2 HCAs).[154] Mild cholestasis or cytolysis can be observed in patients with large HCAs or in patients with underlying steatosis.[154] Alpha-fetoprotein (AFP) serum level should be systematically performed, but it is usually normal even in HCA with malignant transformation. Inflammatory markers (C-reactive protein [CRP], fibrinogen, and platelets) may be increased with inflammatory HCA.[186] The diagnosis of HCA is based on imaging studies, including contrast-enhanced CT scan and MRI.[187,188] Tumor subtyping is done with MRI[189,190] and by liver biopsy if needed.

Histology

HCA is a heterogeneous disease that includes several tumor subtypes associated with various risks of complications.[191] Large subcapsular vessels are commonly found on macroscopic examination. On cut sections, the tumor is well-delineated, sometimes encapsulated, and of fleshy appearance, ranging in color from white to brown (Fig. 88A.7; see Chapter 87). HCA frequently displays heterogeneous areas of necrosis and/or hemorrhage. Histologically HCA consists of a proliferation of benign hepatocytes arranged in a trabecular pattern. However, the normal liver architecture is absent. Hepatocytes may have intracellular fat or increased glycogen. Five main subtypes of HCA have been identified based on mutations in specific oncogenes and tumor suppressor genes: *HNF1α* inactivated HCAs (HNF1A); inflammatory HCAs (IHCA); β-catenin–mutated HCAs (b-HCA); sonic hedgehog HCA; and unclassified subtypes. The main histologic hallmarks of the different subtypes (see the chapter on the pathologic aspects of liver tumors) can be briefly summarized as follows:

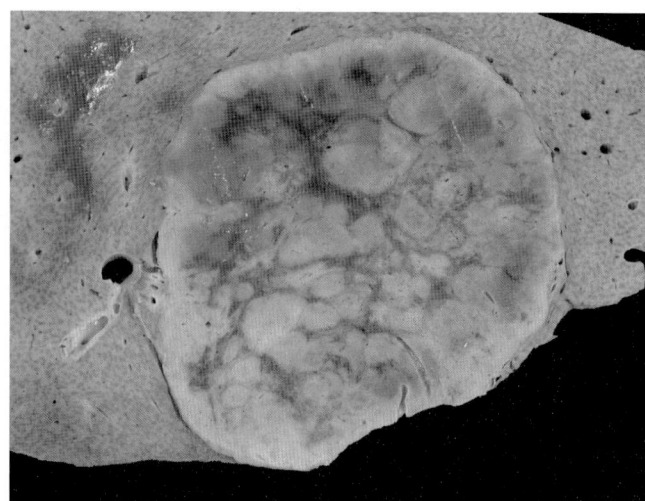

FIGURE 88A.7   Macroscopic aspect of hepatocellular adenoma. The lesion is well delineated, unencapsulated, and tan to yellow with some vascular changes (see Chapter 87).

HNF1A

This subtype is characterized by bi-allelic inactivating mutations of HNF1A (hepatocyte nuclear factor 1α). HNF1A is a key transcription factor that controls several metabolic pathways in the hepatocyte, including estrogen metabolism and fatty acid synthesis deregulation with liver fatty acid binding protein (LFABP), down-expression leading to fatty acid accumulation, and steatosis in the tumor hepatocyte. The HNF1A mutation was identified in young patients with a familial context of MODY 3[192] and was later described in some familial cases of adenomatosis and MODY 3.[193] However, adenomatosis is infrequent in MODY 3, thus other genetic or environmental factors are probably involved in the development of HCA.[194,195] The HNF1A subtype is associated with intermediate levels of estrogen exposure.[194] On histology, HNF1A is characterized by prominent steatosis associated with an absence of LFABP expression in tumor hepatocytes compared with the normal high expression in nontumor hepatocytes.[196,197]

Mutated β Catenin

This subtype involves mutations of CTNNB1 (protein coding gene) coding for β catenin, leading to impaired β-catenin phosphorylation that induces the translocation of β catenin in the nucleus and expression of Wnt/β-catenin genes such as GLUL (coding for glutamine synthase) and LGR5. These mutations are associated with a higher risk of malignant transformation (see Chapter 89). These mutations are also observed in colorectal cancer and medulloblastoma. It has recently been shown that mutations on exon 3, but not 7 or 8, are associated with the risk of malignant transformation.[194] These tumors are more commonly related to androgen than estrogen intake (both endogenous and exogenous androgen exposure) and are more frequently observed in men; most HCAs that develop from anabolic steroids are β-catenin mutated.[152,194] However, women who develop β-catenin HCA have been less exposed to estrogen.[194] Morphologically, this subtype is characterized by cellular atypia.[191] Tumor hepatocytes demonstrate strong and homogenous glutamine synthetase positivity (β-catenin target gene) and nuclear expression of β catenin in some tumor hepatocytes, with high specificity and low sensitivity.[191] This variability and heterogeneity may challenge the diagnostic process based on biopsy; molecular analysis is required for an accurate histologic diagnosis. For exon 7/8 mutations, glutamine synthetase expression is heterogeneous and less marked, with no β-catenin nuclear staining.[198]

Inflammatory Hepatocellular Adenoma

This is the most frequent subtype, resulting from the activation of the IL-6/JAK/STAT pathway in tumor hepatocytes with overexpression of acute phase inflammatory proteins such as CRP and serum amyloid A (SAA). It is an inflammatory syndrome, so anemia and fever may be observed, and is considered to be a paraneoplastic syndrome induced by uncontrolled production of cytokines.[186] Inflammatory HCA can also involve the β-catenin mutation. Therefore alterations of the Wnt/β-catenin pathway should be searched for in the presence of inflammatory HCA. This subgroup is mainly observed in obese patients with extensive exposure to OCs.[194] Morphologically, these tumors are characterized by the presence of small arteries, inflammatory matrix, and sinusoidal dilatation.[199] Tumor hepatocytes exhibit cytoplasmic expression of SAA and CRP on immunohistochemistry induced by STAT3 activation.[196,200] They can also contain steatosis and can present with a mutated β catenin.[196]

Sonic Hedgehog Hepatocellular Adenoma

The sonic hedgehog mutation (5% of HCA cases) was recently isolated from the subgroup of unclassified HCA. This mutation results in uncontrolled activation of the sonic hedgehog pathway because of the overexpression of GLI1.[194] It seems that it is associated with a higher risk of clinical and histologic bleeding. It is mainly observed in obese patients with extensive exposure to OCs.[194]

Unclassified

No genetic alterations can be identified in less than 10% of HCAs.

Considering that mutated β catenin can be on exon 3 or exons 7 or 8 and that inflammatory HCA can be mixed (inflammatory and mutated β catenin), theoretically eight subgroups of HCA can be defined.[194]

Diagnostic Pathway

Imaging findings widely vary according to the subtype of HCA (see Chapter 14). HNF1A HCAs appear homogeneous on MRI and have a variable signal on T2-weighted sequences; they are usually slightly hyperintense on non–fat-suppressed sequences and isointense or hypointense on T2-weighted fat-suppressed sequences. A diffuse and homogeneous signal dropout on chemical shift T1-weighted sequences is the most striking finding[189,190] (Fig. 88A.8). The sensitivity of MRI ranges from 87% to 91%, and the specificity ranges from 89% to 100%.[189,190]

On MRI (Fig. 88A.9), IHCA shows a strong hyperintense signal on T2-weighted images that might be either diffuse or appear as a rim-like band in the periphery of the lesion, defining the atoll sign.[201] On T1-weighted sequences, lesion signal intensity varies from isointense to hyperintense. When hyperintensity is present, it persists on fat-suppressed sequences and opposed-phase sequences. The sensitivity and specificity of MRI ranges from 85% to 88% and 88% to 100%, respectively, when a markedly hyperintense signal on T2-weighted images and persistent enhancement on delayed phase is present.[189,190]

The two other subtypes, b-HCA and unclassified HCA, are less characteristic on imaging and have similar findings to other hepatocellular tumors (mainly arterial enhancement and portal or delayed washout). b-HCA and unclassified subtypes might have heterogeneous content, but no feature can differentiate them from HCC. Because the accuracy of MRI for diagnosing and subtyping HCAs is good, the usefulness of biopsy results for decision making is limited, which reduces its diagnostic place.[202] CEUS is useful for differentiating HCA from FNH, but its value for HCA subtyping is limited.[189,203]

As previously stated, liver-specific contrast agents are useful for the differential diagnosis of HCA and FNH because most FNH are isointense or hyperintense on hepatobiliary phase, whereas most HCAs are hypointense compared with the liver parenchyma.[204] Nevertheless, several authors have reported cases of partially or completely hyperintense HCA on HBP images.[205,206] Importantly, Reizne et al. showed that isointensity or hyperintensity of HCAs on HBP does not necessarily correspond to an increased hepatospecific contrast-agent uptake. In IHCA, tumor hyperintensity on precontrast images and the underlying steatosis likely explain such isointensity or hyperintensity, which do show reduced HBP contrast-agent uptake. On the other hand, marked contrast uptake can be observed, especially in BHCA.[207] Because of these limitations in imaging diagnosis, we recommend percutaneous biopsy to differentiate atypical FNH from HCAs and to identify b-HCA in patients with tumors 5 cm or more that are not considered for resection.[145,154]

Multiple Adenoma and Adenomatosis

Adenomatosis (>10 HCAs) was initially described by Flejou et al. as being more frequent in men with a higher rate of complications[208] and being associated with liver steatosis.[209] Adenomatosis has been observed in obese patients and is associated with microadenomas and the HNFA1 subtype, but the risk of complications is not increased compared with patients with single or multiple HCAs (2–10).[154] In fact, multiple HCAs (>2 HCAs) are more frequently observed but the risk of complications or bleeding is not increased.[154,210–212,185] Thus management should be based on the size and not the number of tumors,[154] limiting the indications for liver transplantation.

Risk Factors for Complications

Bleeding

Bleeding is the most frequent complication of HCA and may be clinical (acute pain and large zones of bleeding on imaging) or subclinical, with small areas of bleeding in HCA discovered on imaging or histology. Although the prevalence of subclinical bleeding is high (30%–60%),[154] the clinical impact of this complication is unknown. Clinical bleeding is the most important complication and is observed in 20% to 25% of cases in surgical series.[154,172,213] This may be overestimated because data on prevalence are mainly based on surgical series, which mainly treat complicated HCAs. In most cases, bleeding HCAs are discovered when the episode of bleeding occurs, and it is less frequent to diagnose bleeding in an observed HCA.[214] The clinical presentation is that of an acute right upper quadrant and lower chest pain that can mimic pulmonary embolism in some patients. Hemodynamic stability must be rapidly obtained after careful resuscitation. Bleeding may be intratumoral alone with or without parenchymal extension, and in 10% of

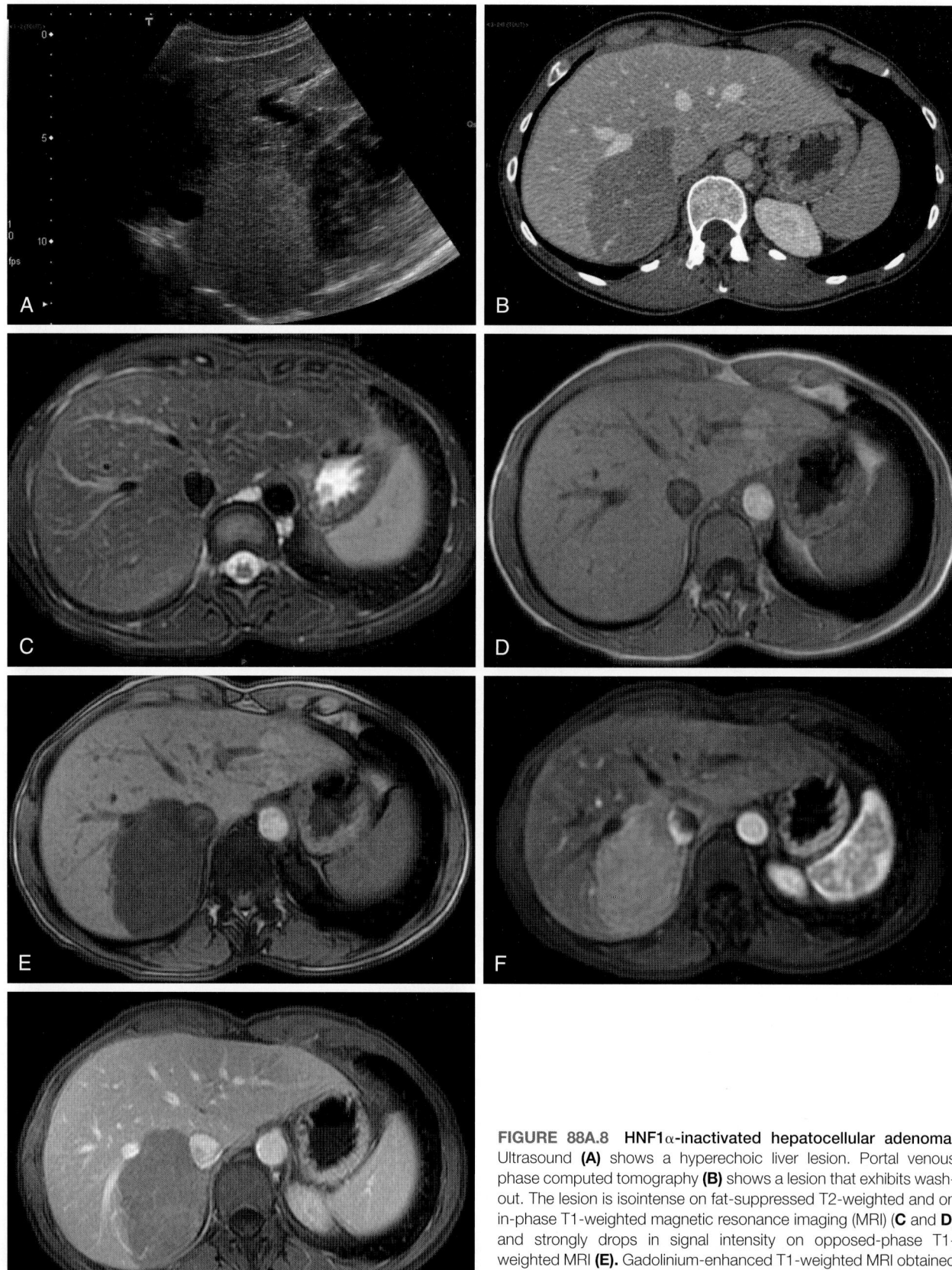

FIGURE 88A.8   HNF1α-inactivated hepatocellular adenoma. Ultrasound **(A)** shows a hyperechoic liver lesion. Portal venous phase computed tomography **(B)** shows a lesion that exhibits washout. The lesion is isointense on fat-suppressed T2-weighted and on in-phase T1-weighted magnetic resonance imaging (MRI) **(C** and **D)** and strongly drops in signal intensity on opposed-phase T1-weighted MRI **(E).** Gadolinium-enhanced T1-weighted MRI obtained at the arterial and delayed phase **(F** and **G)** shows strong lesion enhancement on arterial phase and washout on delayed phase (see Chapter 14).

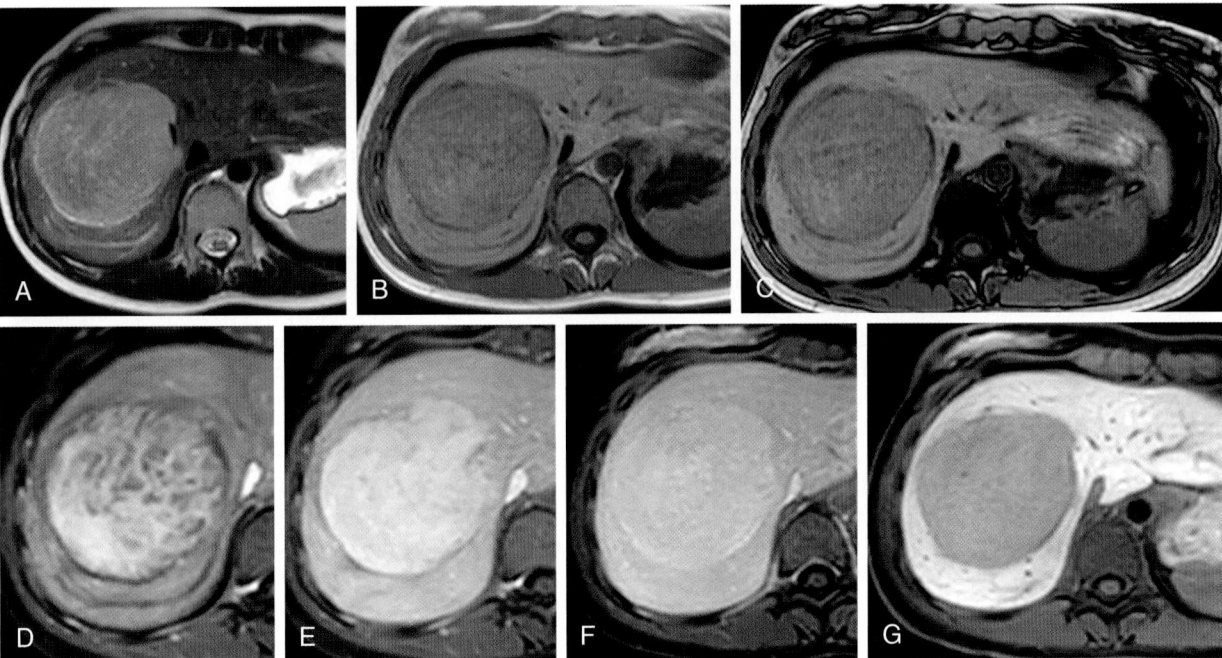

FIGURE 88A.9   Inflammatory hepatocellular adenomas of the right liver in a 23 year-old obese female patient. On hepatospecific magnetic resonance (MR) contrast-enhanced magnetic resonance imaging (MRI), the lesion is hyperintense on fat-suppressed T2-weighted and on in-phase T1-weighted images **(A, B)** with no signal dropout on opposed-phase T1-weighted images **(B)** because of absence of fat. On dynamic phases **(D–F)** the lesion shows marked lesion enhancement on arterial phase **(D)** and persistent enhancement on portal venous **(E)** and delayed phase **(F)**. On hepatobiliary phase **(G)**, the lesion is homogeneously hypointense (see Chapter 14).

cases, it is associated with hemoperitoneum.[154] The main risk factor of bleeding is the presence of sonic hedgehog HCA, IHCA, and tumor size, with a 5% risk in HCA less than 5 cm and 25% in HCA greater than 5 cm.[154,194,210,213–215] Other risk factors are exophytic lesions or lesions located in the left lateral segments and with peripheral arteries visualized on imaging,[215] as well as hormone use within the last 6 months.[210] HNFA1 HCAs have a very low risk of bleeding (<10%).[154]

Malignancy

Malignant transformation is the second most common complication of HCA (see Chapter 89). There is no specific clinical or radiologic presentation and in most cases the diagnosis is made on the specimen after resection. The AFP level is usually normal, and malignant transformation is suggested in cases of rapid growth of tumors. In clinical practice, it may be very difficult to differentiate between malignant HCA and well-differentiated HCC that develops on a normal liver in young women with or without elevated AFP levels. On histology, the presence of both adenomatous tissue and HCC foci is highly suggestive of the diagnosis of preexisting HCA.[216,217] The risk of malignancy might be overestimated as a consequence of the preferential inclusion of resected lesions in the reported series, and some well-differentiated HCCs might have been inappropriately classified as transformed HCAs. The most important risk factors for malignancy are male sex and tumor size. The risk of malignant transformation in men and women is greater than 50% and less than 5%, respectively.[154,216,218,219] Malignant transformation is mainly observed in HCAs greater than 5 cm and has been found in large HCAs (>8 cm)[210,220,221] but is rare in HCAs that are less than 5 cm.[154] Certain retrospective studies have shown an increased risk

of malignancy in b-HCA[154,185] with mutations on exon 3 but not on 7 and 8.[198] The risk of malignant transformation is moderate with IHCA and very low with HNFA1 HCA.[154] HCC within HCA are typically well-differentiated, with a normal serum α-fetoprotein level. They are devoid of vascular invasion or satellite nodules, are usually diagnosed post-hoc on the resected HCA specimen, and are associated with a favorable prognosis after local resection.[154]

Management

A better understanding of the disease and the risk factors for complications has shifted the treatment from resection of all HCAs to a much more conservative approach in which the place of surgery is decreasing. When a diagnosis is made, underlying risk factors should be managed in all cases, including mainly OC withdrawal[222,223] and weight loss.[52] A period of 6 months is usually needed to observe an effect on tumor size, but it was demonstrated recently that this period can be prolonged to 12 months, especially on large HCAs, to obtain a significant reduction in size.[224] Encouraging results were recently reported with weight loss alone in obese patients.[225] If the tumor does not regress to a size without risk (<5 cm), several treatment options may be discussed, including surgical resection, transarterial embolization, percutaneous ablation, and, more rarely, liver transplantation

Uncomplicated Hepatocellular Adenoma

The decision to perform invasive treatment is based on a patient's sex, the size of the largest tumor, and HCA subtype.[2,154] In men, HCA should be resected whatever the size because of the high risk of malignancy (>50%; see Chapter 103B). In men with GSD, however, the risk of malignancy is low,[168,226,227] close to that observed in HNFA1, and resection can be less aggressive and limited only to large HCAs. In women, only large HCAs (>5 cm) should be resected and HCAs less than 5 cm can be observed, except in b-HCA cases.

The New Classification and the Role of Liver Biopsy

Although the new classification has significantly increased the understanding of the disease, its influence on patient management is limited because of the absence of validation. In most cases, HCA diagnosis and subtyping can be obtained from MRI.[190,228] Therefore the usefulness of biopsy for decision making is reduced.[202] The main indication of preoperative biopsy is to diagnose b-HCA and mixed HCA (IHCA and b-HCA) but in most cases, biopsy is not required because results would not change the therapeutic approach. In men, the only indication is to confirm HNFA1 subtype in patients with multiple HCAs to avoid large resection or liver transplantation. In women, HCAs greater than 5 cm should be resected irrespective of subtype. Molecular subtyping should be considered in the following situations: (1) to diagnose b-HCA in HCAs less than 5 cm (this is still a matter of debate given the very low risk of complication of these small lesions); (2) If observation of large HNFA1 (5–8 cm) is suggested (in this setting, histologic confirmation of HNF1A subtype may allow for conservative management with regular follow-up regardless of the size, given the extremely low risk of complication); and (3) To tailor the surgical strategy or in case of prospective evaluation of its role. Finally, current invasive tests are insufficiently sensitive to diagnose b-HCA, which is made indirectly by measuring glutamine synthetase on immunohistochemistry with heterogeneity of expression in the nucleus and the cytoplasm.[2,229,230] Thus management strategy should remain based on sex and tumor size, with liver biopsy performed to refine the management and surgical strategy.

Bleeding Hepatocellular Adenoma

Hemodynamic stability must be obtained in the presence of hemodynamic instability and patients should be managed in an intensive care unit (ICU).[214,231] Emergency surgical resection should no longer be performed because this procedure requires a large incision, extended liver resection (resection of HCA and hematoma), and transfusion and is associated with a high morbidity, a long hospital stay,[154] and mortality.[232] In case of urgent surgery, packing is preferred to liver resection to decrease morbidity and mortality[233] (see Chapter 113). Modern management includes stabilization with or without transfusion, transarterial embolization, and delayed surgical resection.[233-236] Transarterial embolization is indicated within the first 2 to 3 days after the complication occurs and is best performed using catheterization of the artery feeding the territory of the lesion (Fig 88A.10; see Chapters 21, 94A, and 115). Within the first week after the procedure, the patient might complain of persistent pain, have episodes of fever, and present with right pleural effusion. Elevated aminotransferase levels generally return to normal 1 week after the procedure. The patient can then be discharged after cessation of OC and advocated weight loss. Delayed resection is performed 3 to 6 months after embolization once the parenchymal hematoma has disappeared and consists, in the majority of cases, of laparoscopic minor liver

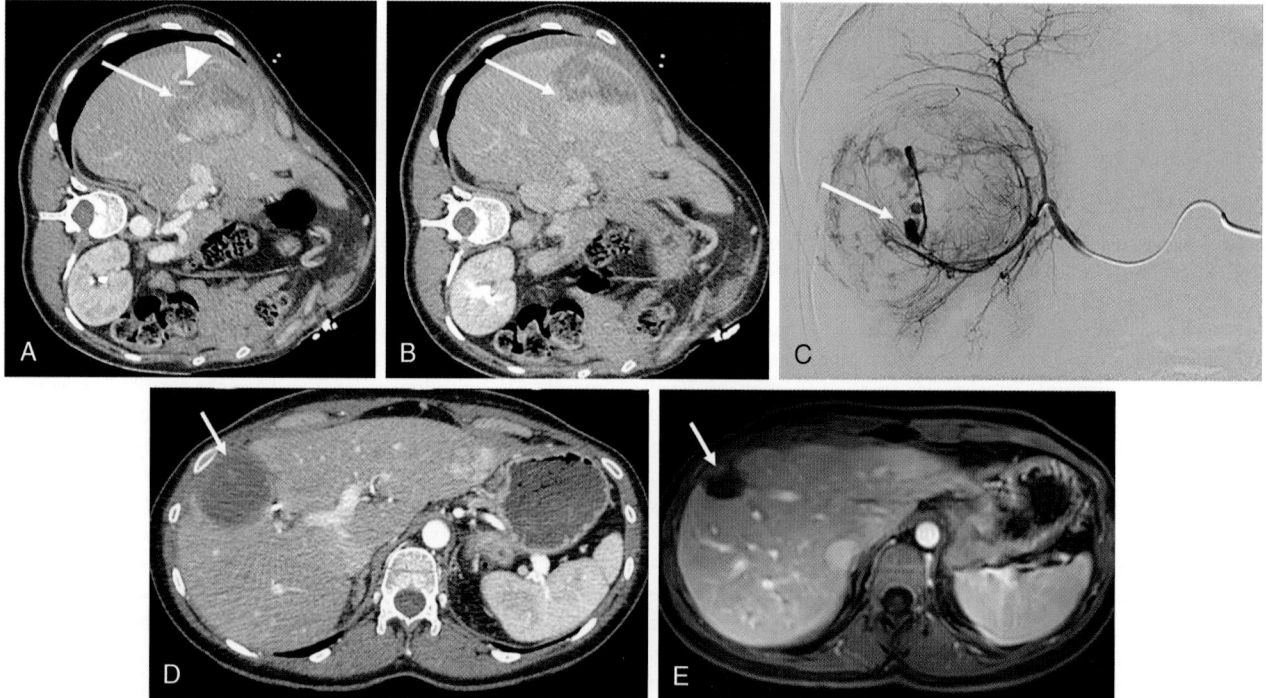

FIGURE 88A.10 Bleeding hepatocellular adenoma successfully treated with transarterial embolization in a 29-year-old pregnant female patient. The patient experienced abdominal pain. Contrast-enhanced computed tomography (CT) (**A** and **B**) shows a heterogeneous focal lesion in the right liver *(arrow)* with active bleeding on arterial phase *(arrowhead in* **A**). Digital subtracted angiography (**C**) shows the tumor blush and the active bleeding *(arrow)* that was treated with coils. Contrast-enhanced CT performed 3 months after the embolization shows a round nonenhancing lesion, corresponding to the completely necrotic adenoma *(arrow in* **D**). Contrast-enhanced magnetic resonance imaging (MRI) performed 5 years after the treatment shows that the lesion progressively decreased in size, with no tumor recurrence (**E**) (see Chapter 94).

resection with lower morbidity and shorter hospital stay.[214,215] In about one-third of cases, complete necrosis can be observed without any residual tumor tissue and a conservative nonoperative approach can be proposed (see Fig. 88A.10). This high rate of necrosis observed mainly after embolization has led us to discuss transarterial embolization for any bleeding HCA to increase the complete necrosis rate.[214] Observation can also be discussed if bleeding HCAs have shrunk to less than 5 cm because recurrent bleeding in the same HCA is rare, and the risk of malignancy is very low.[214] Although there are no data in the literature, biopsy of the viable tissue can be discussed just before the embolization to reach the diagnosis of ruptured HCA because the radiologic diagnosis can be challenging at admission because of bleeding and necrosis. In this situation, however, the diagnosis of HCA can be established based on clinical data because HCA remains the most frequent cause of liver bleeding in a young female.

Indications for Embolization in Bleeding Hepatocellular Adenoma

The efficacy of transarterial embolization on tumor regression in bleeding HCAs has led some authors to consider using this vascular procedure in nonbleeding HCAs (see Chapter 94A). However, its role in nonbleeding HCA is a subject of debate. Many retrospective studies have shown a significant decrease in the size of nonbleeding HCA after embolization.[237–239] For some authors, this treatment is mainly effective in patients with multiple and small HCA (<3 cm)[220] and in those with adenomatosis.[240] In a recent large multicenter study evaluating the effect of embolization in nonbleeding HCA ($n = 36$), severe complications were reported in less than 10%, but this treatment was efficient because the median size decreased from 70 mm to 45 mm ($P < .001$).[241] This treatment should be applied with caution because severe necrosis on the normal liver can be observed.

Malignancy Associated with Hepatocellular Adenoma

If a malignant HCA is suspected preoperatively (rapid growth, slight elevation of AFP, satellites nodules), anatomic liver resection is recommended, as for HCC, especially in patients with a normal liver, making major liver resection safe. If the diagnosis is made postoperatively, there is no need for additional surgery if the resection is performed with free surgical margins because the risk of satellite nodules or vascular invasion is rare.[154,210] On the other hand, if resection is not satisfactory or is incomplete, we suggest a second intervention for complete resection.

Surgical Resection

When possible, the laparoscopic approach should be the standard procedure because HCA is a benign disease occurring in young women, with long-term parietal benefits of the approach. The advantages of the laparoscopic approach for morbidity and hospital stay compared with open surgery were recently reported in a large study.[242] Resection with margins of a few millimeters is sufficient but care should be taken in some patients because it can be difficult to differentiate between adenomatous tissue and the normal liver parenchyma.

Percutaneous Ablation

Ablation by radiofrequency and more rarely by microwave[243] has already been described with good results[244–249] and a low recurrence rate[246,247] (see Chapter 96). However, in most of those studies ablation was performed on small HCAs of less than 5 cm for which treatment is not needed. However, ablation can be an interesting option for the treatment of limited-size HCAs (4–5 cm) during pregnancy,[250] recurrence after resection,[246] difficult intraoperative locations or the need for major liver resection,[248] and for small b-HCAs.

Indications for Liver Transplantation (See Chapter 105)

One of the major advantages of the clinical, genotypic, and phenotypic classification of HCA is to limit the indications for liver transplantation, which are rare.[145,211] In women with multiple HCA, only HCA greater than 5 cm should be resected, and remnant HCA less than 5 cm remains stable in most cases. In the European Liver Transplant Registry, only 49 liver transplantations were performed between 1986 and 2013 for liver adenomatosis.[251] It should be noted that with the routine and frequent use of modern imaging for abdominal complaints, massive adenomatosis with large HCAs involving both liver lobes[252] has become rare. The main indications for liver transplantation are symptomatic uncontrolled GSD with multiple HCA,[253] recurrent HCA many years after resection of transformed HCA, and patients in whom liver resection is risky because of vascular anomalies[254] (HCA and portocaval shunt) or because of the presence of underlying liver disease such as Budd-Chiari syndrome or other chronic liver diseases.

Pregnancy

Pregnancy has been contraindicated in patients with HCA because of the risk of growth with subsequent rupture or bleeding. This complication, which can lead to maternal and fetal mortality, is rare and was reported mainly in case reports,[255–257] but the natural history of HCA from diagnosis to treatment has completely changed in the past 15 years and HCA is no longer considered to be a contraindication to pregnancy. We followed 15 pregnancies in 11 women including 9 with residual HCA. HCA did not recur in any of the women without residual HCA (6 pregnancies) and two of those with residual HCA ($n = 9$) experienced moderate progression without complications.[154] In another study, 17 pregnancies were followed in 12 women with HCAs of less than 5 cm. Progression occurred in 4 cases, requiring a cesarean in 2 (>34 weeks) and preventive percutaneous ablation.[258] In a recent multicentric study, prospective evaluation of growth of HCAs of less than 5 cm was assessed in pregnant women with regular follow-up by ultrasound. Forty-eight women were followed during 51 pregnancies. Growth (>20%) was observed in 13 (25%) with a median increase of 14 mm (interquartile range [IQR] 8–19) and one HCA increase to greater than 70 mm that was treated at 26 weeks of pregnancy by embolization. Other pregnancies proceeded without complications.[259] According to literature data and when the diagnosis is made before pregnancy, HCA greater than 5 cm should be treated and HCA less than 5 cm can be regularly followed by US every 2 to 3 months. In this situation, there is a place for ablation and embolization mainly for HCA between 3 to 5 cm. If the diagnosis of HCA greater than 5 cm is made during pregnancy, a discussion and collaboration is needed between gynecologist, surgeon, hepatologist, and interventional radiologist. The decision of abortion or not depends on the risk of complications and the week of gestation, but pregnancy is often allowed with very close observation in a specialized unit where complications can be managed. OC use is not absolutely contraindicated and low-estrogen content OC or progesterone-based OC can be used if there are gynecologic indications for this treatment.

Follow-Up

The nonoperative management of lesions that were classically considered high risk probably justifies the approach of close monitoring until sufficient evidence of the outcomes of less stringent follow-up has been obtained. The growth of residual HCA after resection was studied in two recent large series. The first series studied the long-term evolution of HCA in 118 patients. After a median follow-up of 5 years, MRI showed stability or regression in 78%, including 71% after resection of multiple HCA and 90% after resection of solitary HCA. Risk factors for progression were multiple tumors and HNFA1 inactivated subtype.[260] In another multicenter study including 134 patients, the median number of residual HCAs was three. Follow-up showed regression (25%), stability (62%), and growth of at least one lesion (11%); 3 patients (2%) developed new lesions, and 4 patients underwent re-intervention, including one male. No risk factors were found for growth.[261] This favorable evolution of HCA suggests that after diagnosis or management, a yearly CT scan or MRI and even US is sufficient at first, then every 2 years in case of stability. Follow-up may be discontinued after menopause because changes are rare after this age. In a recent study, radiologic follow-up in 48 women with HCA in the post-menopausal period showed undetectable lesions (44%), stability (33%), or significant regression (19%).[262] In all cases, it is very rare to observe complications of residual HCA or newly developed HCA.

OTHER LESIONS

Fatty Lesions of the Liver

Angiomyolipoma (see Chapter 87)

Hepatic angiomyolipomas are rare mesenchymal tumors formed from smooth muscle cells, adipose tissue, and proliferating blood vessels, which belong to the group of tumors with a perivascular epithelioid cell differentiation, referred to as *perivascular epithelial cell tumors* (PEComas).[263] This group also includes angiomyolipomas of other sites, lymphangioleiomyomatosis, clear-cell myomelanocytic tumors, and clear-cell "sugar" tumors. All PEComas share morphologic and immunophenotypic features, such as epithelioid or occasionally spindled cells associated with blood vessel walls, and immunostaining of both melanocytic (HMB-45 and/or Melan-A) and smooth muscle (actin and/or desmin) markers.[264,265] Hepatic angiomyolipomas are mostly sporadic but can be linked to tuberous sclerosis, and in this situation, the kidney involvement is more frequent and constantly present when the liver involvement is present.[263,266]

These tumors are more frequent in women (ratio 3:1) aged 30 to 50 years (median age, 44 years),[267-269] are often greater than 5 cm in diameter,[270] and might increase in size.[269,271] Discovery of hepatic angiomyolipomas is incidental during routine imaging in approximately 40% of cases because patients are usually asymptomatic and have normal liver test results, or the discovery may be the consequence of symptoms related to the size of the tumor, or of nonspecific symptoms such as weight loss.[270] The tumor can occur as a solitary mass or as multiple lesions when associated with tuberous sclerosis.[272-274] In about 10% of cases, hepatic angiomyolipomas have aggressive behavior

like a malignant tumor, including local recurrence after resection[274-276,268,269] and distant metastases.[277-279,271] In surgically treated patients, the estimated risk of mortality is less than 1%.[269]

The appearance of angiomyolipoma on imaging is inconsistent because of the varying content of the three components (smooth muscle cells, adipose tissue, and proliferating blood vessels) and the rarity of the lesion, and the frequent resemblance to HCA and carcinoma when the amount of fat is small leads to routine consideration of percutaneous biopsy. On contrast-enhanced imaging (CEUS, CT, or MRI; Fig. 88A.11), angiomyolipomas typically appear markedly enhanced on the arterial phase without washout on the portal or delayed phases.[280] When present, macroaneurisms (large central vessels) within the lesions are highly characteristic (see Chapter 14).

Liver biopsy is mandatory for most patients with angiomyolipomas, and histologic diagnosis is based on the identification of the different components. Histologic diagnosis might be challenging in patients with lesions that have prominent proliferation of epithelioid cells and a scarcity of adipose tissue. The accuracy of diagnosis is aided by staining for melanocytic markers such as HMB-45, which stains the epithelioid component.[281]

When a diagnosis for angiomyolipoma is established, careful observation with serial imaging follow-up is recommended in asymptomatic patients who have lesions less than 5 cm in diameter.[282] For lesions greater than 5 cm, a more aggressive approach should be undertaken. As a matter of fact, these lesions have the highest risk of malignant transformation, especially when major epithelioid content is present. Liver resection remains the treatment of choice for hepatic angiomyolipoma greater than 5 cm in diameter[268,69,271,275] (Fig. 88A.12; see Chapter 101). Because the lesion can have aggressive behavior, oncologic liver resection is advocated and recurrence was described even after R0 resection.[275] Nonsurgical treatment by transarterial embolization[269,275] and RFA[268] have been described, but it is too early to clearly identify their indications and benefits (see Chapters 94 and 96). Few cases of liver transplantation were reported, the main indications being nonresectability,[283,284] multiple lesions with tuberous sclerosis,[285] and misdiagnosis for HCC.[279]

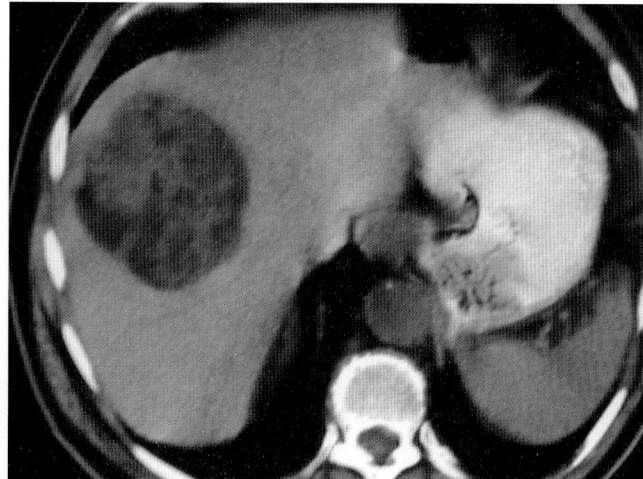

FIGURE 88A.11   Typical angiomyolipoma. Precontrast computed tomography shows a heterogeneous lesion that contains fat (see Chapter 14).

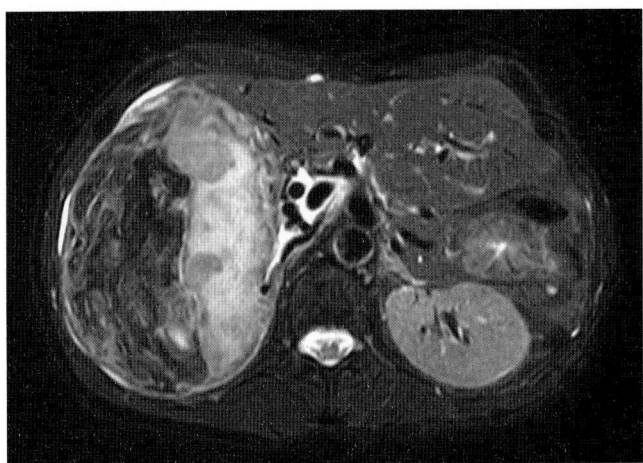

FIGURE 88A.12 Large hepatic angiomyolipoma requiring resection for the risk of malignant components. Lesion heterogeneity is well demonstrated on magnetic resonance imaging (see Chapter 14).

Lipoma (see Chapter 87)

Hepatic lipoma is a very rare liver tumor that can mimic angiomyolipoma (see Chapter 89) with nearly no publication on the subject in the last decade. They are homogeneous and circumscribed, show fat attenuation on CT, and do not enhance after intravenous injection of contrast material. On MRI imaging, lipomas are hyperintense on T1-weighted images and moderately hyperintense on T2-weighted images. The key finding is the drop in signal intensity on fat-suppressed MR sequences.[286] Contrary to fatty hepatocellular tumors that contain fat, lipomas do not drop in signal intensity on opposed-phase T1-weighted MR images. Microscopic analysis shows well-differentiated adipose tissue without any significant changes. Contrary to other benign liver tumors, lipomas have been more associated to liver steatosis.[287] There is no need for resection of lipoma.[288,289]

Biliary Hamartoma (see Chapter 87)

These lesions are also known as the Von Meyenburg complex and usually present as multiple and small (<5 mm) nodules scattered throughout the liver. Their prevalence in adults is approximately 5% in autopsy series, and they are particularly frequent in patients with congenital hepatic fibrosis or polycystic liver disease.[290] Biliary hamartomas include abnormal development of small intrahepatic bile ducts and are composed of bile ductules, inflammatory cells, and fibrosis (see Table 88A.1).[291] Contrary to bile duct adenomas, no *BRAF* V600E mutations have yet been identified in biliary hamartomas.[292] The main practical problem raised by this tumor is for the pathologist because its possible discovery during surgery for carcinoma of another abdominal organ leads the surgeon to perform a biopsy for frozen section diagnosis.[293] The pathologist who is unaware of this rare entity may be puzzled and tempted to call the lesion metastatic carcinoma. Otherwise, hamartomas are easily recognized on heavily T2-weighted MR images and appear as multiple small lesions that are strongly hyperintense. The "starry sky" appearance on MRI is very suggestive of the diagnosis.[294,295] The diagnosis is often mistaken for Caroli disease, but these lesions do not communicate with bile ducts.[296] These lesions are benign and can be associated with increased

carbohydrate antigen (CA19-9).[297] Biliary hamartomas are almost always asymptomatic and complications are very rare. These include portal hypertension,[298] cholangitis,[299,300] and malignant degeneration.[301]

Bile Duct Adenoma (see Chapter 87)

Bile duct adenoma (BDA), also called *benign cholangioma*, is a benign and asymptomatic lesion that is typically discovered incidentally in imaging studies, during surgery, or at autopsy.[302] BDAs are usually small in size (<5 mm), well circumscribed, and subcapsular (see Chapter 89). These lesions include the proliferation of noncystic biliary structures within a dense fibrous stroma.[303] The overlapping histologic features with biliary hamartomas have led some authors to sometimes consider BDAs a variant of biliary hamartomas; however, the recent identification of *BRAF* V600E mutations in more than half of cases of BDAs support a different pathogenesis process. This finding has also led some authors to support an "adenoma to carcinoma" sequence in the occurrence of *BRAF*-mutated intrahepatic cholangiocarcinoma[292,304] (see Chapter 9E). On imaging, most lesions are hypoechoic to liver parenchyma on US, hypodense with unenhanced CT hypointense relative to liver on T1-weighted images, hyperintense on T2-weighted images, and hyperintense on diffusion-weighted imaging (DWI). Arterial-phase hyperenhancement is often depicted; without washout, the persistence of hyperenhancement on venous and delayed phases is probably related to the fibrous stroma, which is a characteristic component of this lesion. Clinically significant differential diagnosis of BDA includes HCC, metastatic disease, and cholangiocarcinoma. The presence of persistent enhancement on portal venous or delayed-phase images argue against HCC and metastatic disease. Imaging features of BDA may overlap with cholangiocarcinoma; however, the lack of additional biliary ductal abnormalities (e.g., biliary dilation or strictures) may help in differentiating the two entities.[305] Historically, BDAs were considered indolent. Hence resection was not justified, and the only clinical significance of these lesions was in the possible confusion with metastatic carcinoma during surgery.[306] Whether the identification of oncogenic mutations should lead to changing the current nonaggressive policy regarding these lesions remains to be assessed.

Inflammatory Pseudotumors (see Chapters 48 and 87)

Inflammatory pseudotumors of the liver (IPLs), also known as inflammatory myofibroblastic tumors, are rare benign lesions affecting 0.2% to 0.7% of patients referred to hepatobiliary units.[307–309] Commonly found in the lung, recent data suggest the liver to be the first affected organ followed by the lung and the gastrointestinal tract.[310] Inflammatory pseudotumors are considered to be a result of an exaggerated inflammatory response, often associated with various inflammatory diseases.[311] It has been hypothesized that IPLs originate from a dendritic cell origin.[312] The etiology of IPL is not well understood but might be caused by underlying microbial infection, obliteration of portal vessels, or immunoglobulin G4 (IgG4)-related sclerosing cholangitis.[313] IPLs are slightly more common in men and in non-European populations, occur at an average age of 50 to 65 years,[314,308] and are mainly located in the right liver.[315] Underlying chronic liver disease or cirrhosis can be present,[315] and many cases were reported with Epstein-Barr virus (EBV).[316]

IPLs are symptomatic in 80% to 90% of patients. Common presenting symptoms include fever, abdominal pain, weight loss, and fatigue.[312,308] In some cases of perihilar IPL, jaundice and cholangitis might be the revealing symptoms and mimic hilar cholangiocarcinoma.[317,318] There are no recommendations for distinguishing these two diagnoses. In a clinical setting, when a patient presents with hilar stenosis, several diagnoses should be considered. The most frequent situation corresponds to tumoral stenosis, and other diagnoses include autoimmune cholangiopathy, primary sclerosing cholangitis, IPL, and several other rare diseases. In the absence of typical clinical features rendering the diagnosis of malignancy unlikely, patients often undergo resection (when possible), and a diagnosis is made on the operative specimen. Abnormal blood liver test results are seen in less than 20% of patients with IPL, with mild elevations of γ-glutamyl transferase and alkaline phosphatases. Hematologic test results are usually normal but reveal an inflammatory syndrome in one-third of patients.

On imaging, there are three different patterns. First, lesions can be ill-defined, large (median, 4–5 cm in diameter), heterogeneous, and hyperenhanced on arterial phase. On MRI, the lesion is often hypointense on T1-weighted sequences and isointense or hyperintense on T2-weighted sequences.[308,319] Second, the IPL may be encapsulated, often discovered fortuitously, appearing as a solitary necrotic nodule of the liver.[320] Third, IPL may appear as an ill-defined lesion with periportal infiltration, dilated bile ducts, and enlargement of hepatic lymph nodes on CT and MRI[319] (Fig. 88A.13).

Histologic examination shows that IPLs are mainly composed of spindle cells and polymorph inflammatory cells. Anomalies of portal vein branches with thrombophlebitis in close contact with the lesion are commonly described. Periportal inflammation of the parenchymal cells is associated with destruction of bile ducts and intrahepatic extension of inflammatory disease.

Diagnosis of IPL remains challenging, and therapeutic management is based on accurate diagnosis in only 50% of patients.[309,312] Most common initial diagnoses after laboratory and imaging investigations include malignant lesions (such as cholangiocarcinoma) and liver abscess in 50% and 20% of patients, respectively.[312,308] Low diagnostic accuracy emphasizes the need for liver biopsy, which should be repeated until other diagnoses have been ruled out. Histologic analysis of biopsy material results in surgery being avoided in 75% of patients with IPL.[312,321] Indeed, IPLs are benign lesions with no malignant potential, and thus undertaking surgical treatment can be risky and dangerous, such as in IPL mimicking hilar cholangiocarcinoma, which requires major liver resection. When the diagnosis is certain, conservative options, including simple surveillance, steroids, and antibiotics, might be attempted with complete regression rates of greater than 90%.[312,322,323,308,321] The rationale for using steroids would be the autoimmune etiology resembling IgG4-related sclerosing cholangitis, which often responds well to steroids. Several physicians use antibiotics because of the possible infectious etiology of IPL. Even though the benefit of

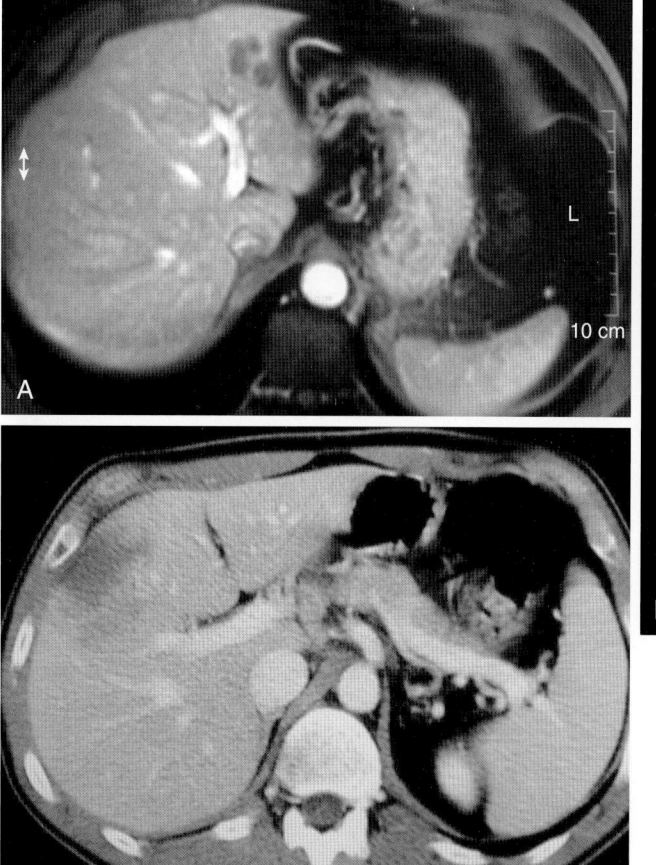

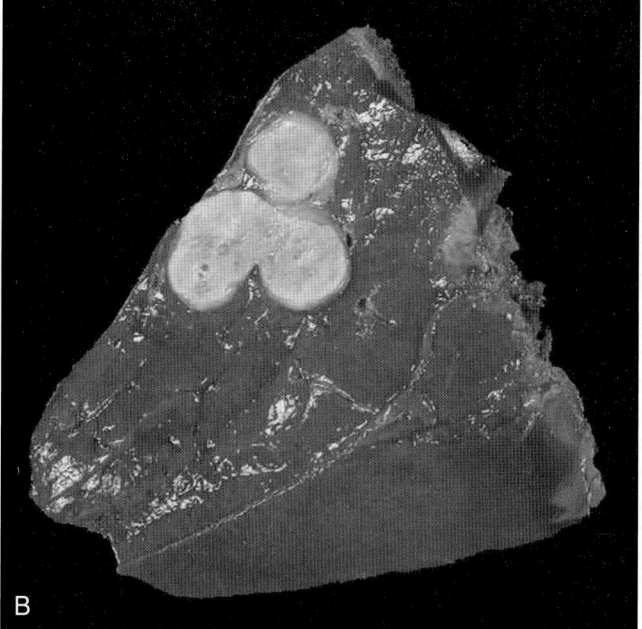

FIGURE 88A.13 Inflammatory pseudotumor of the liver. **A,** Solid and necrotic appearance on postgadolinium T1-weighted magnetic resonance imaging sequence. **B,** Macroscopic analysis shows a subcapsular, well-limited, trefoil-shaped, white lesion corresponding to necrosis. A thin fibrous capsule is observed at the border of the lesion. **C,** Aggressive pattern mimicking cholangiocarcinoma on computed tomography (see Chapter 14).

one medical option over another has not been clearly established, there might be a role for steroids in the control of symptoms such as fever and jaundice, when present.[312]

Rare Tumor or Pseudotumor (see Chapters 48 and 87)

Solitary Fibrotic Tumor

Also known as solitary necrotic tumor, solitary fibrotic tumor is an uncommon liver tumor (see Chapter 89). Slightly more frequent in men, with a mean age at presentation of 60 years, most patients are asymptomatic.[324] Solitary fibrotic tumors are usually unique, well limited, and small (<2 cm).[273] Histologically, a central necrotic core is surrounded by a hyalinized fibrotic capsule containing collagen and elastin fibers with inflammatory cellular infiltration. Calcifications may also be observed. The etiology of this lesion is still uncertain, but possible causes include sclerosing hemangioma, trauma, and infections, especially a parasitic infection such as a hydatid cyst or tuberculosis.[324–326] On imaging, diagnosis might be challenging because the lesion can mimic liver malignancy, especially metastases.[327,328] Progressive enhancement can be very intense on delayed phase and is related to abundant collagen.[329] Most lesions show hypoattenuation of precontrast CT, hypointensity on T1-weighted imaging, and variable signal on T2-weighted images depending on the content. Absence of enhancement on all dynamic phases after contrast administration may help discriminate these lesions from metastatic liver tumors and intrahepatic cholangiocarcinoma.[330] Noticeably, a pronounced peripheral enhancement on delayed- or very delayed-phase images is highly suggestive of the diagnosis.[331]

Solid fibrotic tumors are assumed to be benign, and absence of symptoms would favor a nonoperative management. However, association with extrahepatic malignancy like colorectal cancer may be observed and suggest the possible theory of necrosis of small foci of metastases.[332,324] Therefore given the frequent absence of reliable preoperative diagnosis on imaging and unspecific results of tumor biopsy, resection seems to be justified.[333]

Lymphangioma

Lymphangiomas are benign neoplasms that are regarded as malformations arising from sequestrations of lymphatic tissue that fail to communicate with the normal lymphatic system during embryogenesis.[334] Lymphangiomas are more frequently found in the neonatal period and childhood and less frequently during adulthood.[335,336] The occurrence of solitary lymphangioma in the liver is extremely rare, and only a few cases have been reported to date.[337] In adults, these lesions are generally small (<4 cm) and asymptomatic, but some cases of giant lesions have been reported.[338–342] On imaging, this lesion shows a solid and cystic component and may contain small peripheral calcification. Hence differential diagnoses include other cystic neoplasms such as bile duct cyst (see Chapter 46), biliary cystadenoma (see Chapter 88B), or hepatic hydatidosis (see Chapter 72).[343] Histologically, it is a benign lesion composed of vascular lymphatic spaces lined by regular cells. Immunohistochemistry using D2-40, LYVE-1, and Prox-1 markers is helpful to discriminate lymphatic from vascular endothelium and may be of value in establishing a diagnosis of lymphangioma.[337] Given their extremely low incidence, no practical management can be recommended, even though resection of symptomatic giant lesions may be advocated.

Leiomyoma

Hepatic leiomyomas are very rare benign liver tumors developed from the smooth muscles of the vessels or bile ducts[344,345] and about 30 cases were reported in the literature.[346] These lesions mostly occur in women,[347] and an association has been observed with immunodeficiency status, such as human immunodeficiency virus (HIV) and EBV infections, as well as organ transplantation.[348–350] In this latter situation, lesions are often discovered during follow-up and at a smaller size than in patients without immunosuppressive disorders.[351,352] On imaging, the lesions are hypoechoic on US and hypoattenuating on CT scan with variable enhancement after injection of contrast material. On MRI, leiomyomas are hypointense on T1-weighted sequences and strongly hyperintense on T2-weighted sequences.[353] Histologic features include spindle cell proliferation without nuclear atypia, hemorrhage, or necrosis. Immunoreactivity with mesenchymal markers shows positivity of the cell proliferation with vimentin and smooth muscle actin. Because of the nonspecific radiologic findings, liver resection is usually recommended.

Heterotopic Tissue

The presence of heterotopic tissue within the liver has been described, and diagnosis is usually established after surgical excision.

The most frequent is liver splenosis, which corresponds to autotransplantation of splenic tissue occurring after traumatic splenic rupture or, less frequently, after surgical rupture during splenectomy.[354,355] Case reports are frequent in the literature. Splenosis is asymptomatic, most often located in the left liver, with a mean size of about 4 cm, and multiple lesions can be observed.[356] The presence of associated peritoneal nodules is suggestive of the diagnosis of splenosis.[357] On imaging, the lesion exhibits features of a hyper-enhanced tumor with washout on the delayed phase. These radiologic features make the differential diagnosis with another hyper-enhanced liver tumor very difficult and can be misinterpreted on standard preoperative evaluation as HCC or metastatic disease.[358–363] Diagnosis can be suspected using scintigraphy of technetium-99m–labeled heat-denatured red blood (see Chapter 18) and established with liver biopsy.[355,364,365]

Hepatic endometriosis is a rare lesion and less than 40 cases were reported in the literature. It occurs in two-third of cases in women of childbearing period, with a mean age of 39 years, but may also occur after menopause.[366,367] Women most often are nulliparous and in about 30% to 40% of cases, no history of pelvic endometriosis is found.[367] The exact pathogenesis of hepatic endometriosis is poorly understood and seems to be multifactorial, involving retrograde menstruation, lymphatic dissemination, iatrogenic cell dissemination, and coelomic metaplasia.[366,368,369] These lesions are generally larger than 5 cm, can be of cystic appearance,[368,370,371] and are often discovered during workup for abdominal symptoms,[369] which are not related to menstruation in the vast majority of cases.[366,369] These lesions are usually developed within the liver but subcapsular and hepatic pedicle locations were described.[372,373] Preoperative diagnosis is extremely challenging given the absence of any specific clinical or radiologic features and often requires resection.[369]

Other heterotopic tissues mainly include adrenal, pancreatic, and gastric tissues located around the bile ducts.[374–377]

Hepatic Pseudolesions

The development of more and more sophisticated imaging modalities has led to the identification of several intrahepatic abnormalities, especially after injection of contrast material. Although these "pseudolesions" are not true liver lesions, they can mimic liver tumors.

Perfusion Disorders

These abnormalities are the consequence of the hyperarterialization of a liver segment because of decreased or absent portal vein flow (see Chapter 5). Perfusion disorders are seen on CT and MRI after injection of contrast material, predominate on arterial or portal phase, and disappear or attenuate on delayed phase (see Chapter 14). These perfusion disorders result from portal obstruction, compression, or an arterioportal shunt.[378] In general, they have typical straight borders corresponding to segmental or subsegmental locations. Diagnosis can be more difficult in patients with small peripheral or central "pseudonodular" shaped lesions, such as in cirrhosis because of arterioportal shunts. In case of hepatic vein obstruction, these abnormalities are not systematized (mosaic form) because of the rapid development of interhepatic veins shunts.[379]

Parenchymal Compression

Parenchymal compression, when localized, can give the aspect of a pseudolesion because of impaired enhancement in the compressed territory in the portal phase but without hyperarterialization on the arterial phase. In this case, the pseudolesion has no vascular topography and can be exacerbated by deep inspiration because of compression by ribs and diaphragm.[379]

Confluent Fibrosis

Confluent fibrosis can also mimic a tumor. This feature is mainly observed in chronic liver disease, corresponds to parenchymal extinction, and is located in segments IV and VIII with capsular retraction.[379]

Postradiation Pseudolesion

Pseudolesion of liver parenchyma can be observed after radiation. Previous history of radiation therapy and straight borders without anatomic distribution are highly suggestive. Because of associated fibrosis, atrophy of the involved segment can be observed with compensatory hypertrophy.[379]

Peliosis

Peliosis is a rare condition characterized by multiple, small, blood-filled pools in liver parenchyma of various sizes, varying from 1 mm to several centimeters without lobular systematization. This lesion, which results from focal rupture of sinusoidal walls, is mostly observed in adult patients after systemic chemotherapy for colorectal liver metastases using oxaliplatin.[380] It can also be associated with androgenic-anabolic steroids,[381,382] OCs,[148,383] HIV infection,[384] corticotherapy for systemic lupus erythematous[385,386] or idiopathic thrombocytopenic purpura,[387] hepatitis viral B and C,[388,389] kidney transplant recipients,[390,391] or severe tuberculosis and malignancies such as Hodgkin lymphoma.[392] Imaging findings often mimic

true tumors because they are well-delineated, strongly hyperintense on T2-weighted MRI, and enhance on arterial-phase CT or MRI (see Chapter 14). The persistent contrast uptake within the lesion is because of the blood-pooled condition.[393] Histologically, this lesion can lead to extensive fibrosis resulting from parenchymal destruction and collapse.[394] In general, peliosis is asymptomatic, but severe complications such as spontaneous liver rupture with subsequent bleeding[395–399] after percutaneous liver biopsy[400] or hepatopulmonary syndrome have been reported.[401] Exceptionally portal hypertension and liver failure were reported.[391,402] The treatment includes withdrawal of the possible causative agents, which can lead to regression of the disease.

Focal Fatty Changes

Hepatic steatosis is generally a diffuse process. However, heterogeneous focal fat distribution, presented as spared liver areas (without steatosis) or areas that are fattier than the rest of liver parenchyma, can also be present.[403] Although the pathogenesis is not well understood, regional hypoxia of hepatic tissue is thought to play a role.[404] The majority of patients have underlying conditions such as diabetes, obesity, hepatitis C, nonalcoholic steatohepatitis (NASH; see Chapter 69), and malnutrition. Lesions are often discovered incidentally on imaging studies. Focal steatosis is mainly localized in segment IV.[379] An anomalous venous drainage was suspected some years ago when using CT arterial portography, which often showed lack of enhancement of the posterior part of segment IV, leading to the assumption that venous supply to this territory did not come directly from the portal vein, but perhaps from the gastric vein or duodenopancreatic venous arcade.[405–407] Later, the "venous theory" was completed by the "insulin theory."[408] Insulin, which stimulates the conversion of glucose to fatty acids has a variable concentration in the portal vein tributaries. This explains why aberrant right gastric veins (with low insulin concentration) that drain directly into the segment IV result in focal fatty sparing in a patient with liver steatosis. Conversely, aberrant duodenopancreatic arcades (with high insulin concentration) that drain directly into the segment IV result in focal fatty steatosis.[409] In patients with a steatotic liver, focal fatty sparing may be seen around the gallbladder fossa in segments IV and V. Interestingly, these pseudolesions are seen much more often in patients with an intact gallbladder than in patients with previous cholecystectomy (78% vs. 33%).[410] Focal fatty sparing around the gallbladder is also very likely to be related to venous drainage because there are almost always small cystic veins (with low insulin concentration) that drain directly into the liver and are subsequently interrupted by cholecystectomy.

Another aspect is the nodular aspect, which can mimic liver metastasis.[411,412] In rare instances, liver steatosis appears as multiple lesions distributed throughout the liver parenchyma mimicking liver tumors and especially liver metastases. The lesions are hyperechoic and homogeneous with US, hypoattenuating in all CT phases, with enhancement theoretically parallel to that of the liver. Their signal intensity drops on opposed-phase T1-weighted MR images confirming that the lesions contain fat (see Chapter 14). The findings suggestive of pseudotumoral nodular steatosis are the multiplicity of lesions, their small size (<2 cm) liver, and the inconsistent but very pathognomonic presence of a fattier border in the periphery of the lesions.[408,413]

REGENERATIVE PROCESSES

Nodular Regenerative Hyperplasia

Nodular regenerative hyperplasia (NRH) is a relatively rare, benign, diffuse, micronodular transformation of the liver that has been referred to by many names in the literature, including nodular transformation, noncirrhotic nodulation, and partial nodular transformation. NRH is a distinct disease entity characterized by diffuse involvement of the liver with nodules composed of hyperplastic hepatocytes, and it should not be confused with the regenerative nodules of cirrhosis or FNH[414] (see Chapter 87). The pathogenesis of NRH is not well known. One of the proposed theories hypothesizes that a primary vascular process leads to obliteration of portal vein, which, in turn, induces ischemia, atrophy of hepatocytes in the central zone, and the proliferation of hepatocytes.[415] The other theory proposes that a preneoplastic process leads to NRH because of the reported high prevalence of hepatocyte dysplasia (20%–42%) and HCC formed in livers of patients with NRH.[416,417] The prevalence of NRH is reported to be about 2%.[7]

This entity was classically associated with a wide spectrum of systemic diseases and drugs, including myeloproliferative and lymphoproliferative disorders, chronic vascular disorders, rheumatologic and collagen vascular diseases (rheumatoid arthritis, Felty's syndrome, polyarteritis nodosa, amyloidosis, and primary biliary cirrhosis),[418–420] primary hypogammaglobulinemia,[421] common variable immunodeficiency,[422] monoclonal antibody for breast cancer,[423,424] solid-organ transplantation,[425,426] HIV infection,[427–429] hereditary hemorrhagic telangiectasia,[430] hepatoportal sclerosis, congenital absence of the portal vein,[431] portal venopathy,[432] and malignant disease.[433] This disease is also associated with the use of drugs, such as steroids,[434] azathioprine for inflammatory bowel disease,[435–438] and chemotherapeutic agents. Currently, this lesion is considered the most severe induced histologic liver lesion in patients treated with oxaliplatin-based chemotherapy for colorectal liver metastases, with an incidence reaching up to 24%,[380,439–442] and it can be associated with high postoperative morbidity in case of major liver resection.

Clinically, NRH is usually asymptomatic with preserved liver function[443,419] and low risk of liver insufficiency leading to liver transplantation.[444,429] However, portal hypertension may be observed in 30% of patients, with subsequent esophageal varices, splenomegaly, and ascites[443,416,419] (see Chapter 74). Fatal bleeding from varices has also been observed occasionally.[419] The risk of transformation into HCC or cholangiocarcinoma is rare.[417,445–447] Biologically, more than two-thirds of patients show abnormal liver tests. In patients undergoing chemotherapy for colorectal liver metastases, an aspartate aminotransferase–to–platelet ratio index (APRI score) greater than 0.36 and platelet count less than $100.10^3/mm^3$ are predictive of the presence of NRH.[448,441] Imaging findings are not specific, and histologic examination is often warranted. On imaging, three presentations are possible. First, liver imaging is unremarkable. Second, imaging shows signs of noncirrhotic portal hypertension without any liver nodules. Third, NRH appears as multiple liver nodules with or without portal hypertension. In most cases, imaging shows normal hepatic parenchyma. When nodules are seen, they have a variable enhancement, and they are hyperintense on T1-weighted images and isointense or hypointense to normal liver on T2-weighted images.[449–451]

Contrary to FNH, the central scar is lacking. Differences between these two lesions is mainly based on the presence of multiple, small nodules, signs of portal hypertension, and clinical context. Accurate diagnosis should be confirmed with histologic examination before treatment. In highly suspicious cases, percutaneous needle biopsy can establish the diagnosis.[440] In doubtful cases with a negative percutaneous biopsy, open biopsy is indicated to obtain an adequate sample of hepatic tissue because percutaneous needle biopsies may give falsely normal results.[7]

Management depends on the clinical symptoms. In asymptomatic patients, no treatment is recommended. The effect of the withdrawal or specific treatment of the possible causative disease or agents on the course of this entity is not well known. For patients receiving oxaliplatin-based chemotherapy, associated use of bevacizumab seems to limit the development of NRH[380,441] and regression can be observed several months after withdrawal of chemotherapy.[452] In patients with complications of portal hypertension, appropriate management includes drug therapy, endoscopic therapy, transjugular intrahepatic shunt, portocaval shunt,[7] or splenic artery ligation[453] if necessary. Because of the high postoperative morbidity in case of anticipated major liver resection in a patient receiving oxaliplatin-based chemotherapy,[441] biologic evaluation using both the APRI score and platelet count should be routinely performed, and preoperative liver biopsy may be proposed. If NRH is diagnosed, major liver resection should be avoided or prepared by portal vein embolization or splenic artery ligation.[453]

Focal Nodular Hyperplasia-Like Lesions

FNH-like lesions are lesions that histopathologically resemble FNH but are seen in patients with liver disease or liver vessels abnormalities. The most common causes of liver diseases responsible of FNH-like lesions development are Budd-Chiari syndrome,[102] hereditary hemorrhagic telangiectasia,[103] congenital hepatic fibrosis,[454–456] surgery for congenital heart diseases (Fontan surgery) with associated liver disease,[457] portosinusoidal vascular disease,[458] and cirrhosis.[459] All these diseases induce severe liver flow alterations with decreased portal vein blood flow and marked increased hepatic artery blood flow.[107,104] FNH-like lesions may be a hepatic response to increased arterial inflow. Similarly, FNH-like lesions have been reported in patients with cavernous transformation of the portal vein[107]; imaging findings of the FNH-like lesions are similar to the FNHs arising on normal liver, and they may contain a central scar. Because the liver signal is abnormal in Budd-Chiari syndrome, the FNH-like lesions are mostly hyperintense on T1-weighted and hypointense on T2-weighted images. However, they still enhance strongly at the arterial phase. Contrary to FNHs, they may become more numerous and grow or disappear over time. Washout on portal venous or delayed phase is observed in up to one-third of tumors, limiting the value of these features for the differentiation with HCC.[460] Other features, including signal on precontrast T1 and T2 images, AFP serum level, and appearance on liver-specific enhanced hepatobiliary phase images are therefore useful for the diagnosis.[461]

Hepatic Small Vessel Neoplasm

This rare liver vascular neoplasm composed of small vessels with an infiltrative border was recently described in 17 patients.[462] These tumors were not typical of liver hemangiomas and angiosarcoma was suspected related to the infiltrative aspect. It occurs mainly in men with a mean age of 54 years (24–83) and an average size of 2.1 cm (0.2–5.5 cm). The final diagnosis is made on histology with immunohistochemical staining and the Ki-67 proliferative index is most helpful to exclude malignancy. The most frequent presentation was incidental, no complication was encountered, and no recurrence was reported after complete resection[462] (see Chapter 87).

Acknowledgments: The authors would like to thank Pr Jacques Belghiti, Pr Valérie Vilgrain, Pr Valérie Paradis and Dr François Cauchy, who participated and contributed to drafting and writing the previous editions of this chapter.

The references for this chapter can be found online by accessing the accompanying Expert Consult website.

Cystic hepatobiliary neoplasia

Olivier Farges and Valérie Paradis

OVERVIEW

The vast majority of nonparasitic cystic lesions of the liver are simple cysts. They are unilocular, do not communicate with the biliary tree, have a serous content, and although the epithelium does divide to account for volume expansion, they are not considered tumors and have no malignant potential. Furthermore, they do not tend to recur after partial resection. These lesions are described in detail in Chapter 73. Although primary or secondary solid hepatic malignancies may become cystic as a result of tumor necrosis, it is extremely rare for them to be totally cystic. However, this has been described in case reports for embryonic liver sarcoma, malignant fibrous histiocytoma, or metastases from a variety of primaries, most including neuroendocrine tumors or even colorectal primary tumors.[1-4]

Primarily cystic hepatobiliary neoplasms that constitute another group of cystic tumors are extremely rare. These tumors are of biliary origin and include both benign (with malignant potential) and malignant tumors that have initially been given the names of *cystadenoma* and *cystadenocarcinoma*[5]; however, increasing evidence, in particular from Asian authors, suggests that biliary cystic neoplasia include a wider group of entities that resemble those described in the pancreas as being either mucinous cystic neoplasms (MCNs) or intraductal papillary mucinous neoplasms (IPMNs).[6,7] The main difference relates to the presence or absence of an ovarian stroma (OS) and whether a luminal communication exists between the tumor and the bile ducts (see Chapter 89).

Given this confusion and based on the evolution of the classification of pancreatic mucinous cysts, the latest World Health Organization (WHO) *Classification of Tumours of the Digestive System,* published in 2010, proposed that the disease entity previously designated as "biliary cystadenoma/adenocarcinoma" should instead be classified as either MCN when an OS is present or IPMN of the bile duct (IPMN-B) when the tumor communicates with the biliary tree.[8] However, some cystic neoplasms of the liver with mucinous epithelium may lack both OS and bile duct communication or at least a communication is not always demonstrated.[9] The ratio of MCN to IPMN-B seems to vary between geographic areas, being greater than 1 in the West and less than 1 in Asia[10] (see Chapter 89).

Detailed characteristics of these tumors are not always described in the literature, and the WHO-2010 classification is not widely applied even today,[11,12] casting some confusion on previous descriptions and reports of cystadenoma. Although the same confusion has been observed for cystic tumors of the pancreas, the clinical and pathologic differentiations of these two tumors are accepted worldwide now that a consensus on the definition of *pancreatic* MCNs has been reached.[13,14] A second problem in analyzing the literature is that because of the rarity of the tumor, the number of large series remains very limited, and most references are case reports.

DEFINITION

The initial definitions of cystadenoma by Edmondson in 1958[15] and by Wheeler and Edmondson in 1985[16] were strict and included three distinctive features: the lesion should be (1) multilocular (composed of multiloculated cysts), (2) lined by a columnar epithelium, and (3) accompanied by a densely cellular ovarian-like stroma (see Chapter 87).

This definition was revisited in 1994 by Devaney and colleagues after retrospective analysis of a larger series of 70 patients. Although most fulfilled the criteria set out by Edmondson and Wheeler, that definition was considered too restrictive because the presence of an OS was inconsistently observed. Furthermore, not all cystadenoma-like lesions they saw were multilocular, and the epithelium lining was not exclusively of the columnar type; it was associated in one-third with a cuboidal epithelium. This led the authors to suggest that lesions diagnosed as cystadenoma (or cystadenocarcinoma) should include cystic tumors both with and without OS as well as those having a unilocular gross appearance. More precisely, only 14% of the tumors they observed lacked OS, and only a single patient had a unilocular tumor, which actually was a cystadenocarcinoma.

Although this landmark study showed that cystadenoma-like lesions encompass different entities (those with OS were exclusively observed in women and those without were observed in both sexes, with potentially different courses, which will be discussed later) this revision might have introduced some confusion because a detailed pathologic description of tumors subsequently reported as being cystadenoma (cystadenocarcinoma) has not always been provided, and some occasionally resemble atypical benign cysts or cystic forms of intrahepatic cholangiocarcinoma (ICC), rather than genuine cystadenoma (or cystadenocarcinoma), on the imaging or pathologic pictures illustrating these series and case reports.

It has been suggested that by differentiating biliary cystic tumors based on their stroma and communication between the tumor and the bile duct, two groups of biliary tumors could be identified that are the counterparts of pancreatic cystic neoplasms. The first group, MCN, has OS, typically does not communicate with the bile duct, and is the biliary counterpart of pancreatic mucinous cystadenoma. The second group lacks OS, communicates with the biliary ducts, and is referred to as IPMN-B, similar to the IPMN of the pancreas (IPMN-P; see Chapter 60). Although most cases of IPMN-B present as tubular or fusiform dilation of the involved bile duct, some may present as cystic dilations. The latter is known as cyst-forming IPMN-B and resembles cyst-forming branch-duct IPMN-P.

MUCINOUS CYSTIC NEOPLASMS OF THE LIVER (HEPATOBILIARY CYSTADENOMA WITH OVARIAN STROMA)

The most classic primary cystic tumors of the liver are hepatobiliary cystadenoma. Being of biliary origin, these tumors may occur anywhere along the biliary tree, including the common hepatic duct, cystic duct, or gallbladder, but the most frequent location, found in 83% to 94% of the patients, is the liver.[11,17,18] These tumors are well known because of their inherent risk of malignant transformation, common to all adenomatous lesions. The risk of malignant transformation of hepatobiliary MCN of the liver (MCN-L), however, remains somewhat ill-defined.

Incidence

Cystadenomas are exceedingly rare. No accurate incidence estimates are available, but the two largest series included 52 and 54 patients,[10,18] and most studies have involved fewer than 10 patients; in the early 2000s, it was estimated that fewer than 200 patients had been reported.[19] It is frequently quoted that intrahepatic cystadenomas constitute less than 5% of cystic lesions of the liver based on an old report,[20] but this figure is likely overestimated; it has since become obvious that the prevalence of simple cysts of the liver in the adult population is higher than previously thought.

Pathology (see Chapter 87)

Cystadenomas are almost always solitary, and they may range in size from less than 1 to 40 cm; they are generally large, with a mean diameter of 15 cm,[17] which suggests that they are probably slow growing. Cystadenomas have been reported to develop equally in the right and left liver or to involve both lobes (approximately 33% each)[18,21]; however, a striking feature in our experience, as well as in recent series, is the very high proportion of tumors occurring in the left paramedian section (segment IV) or the left liver.[11,22-24] Pictures of cystadenoma provided in the literature also show tumors in this location almost exclusively; an example is shown in Figure 88B.1.

Cystadenomas are grossly lobulated and multiloculated and usually contain clear to mucinous fluid.[17] Hemorrhagic fluid

may be present,[23] but this is very rare and should raise the suspicion of malignancy.[17] A bilious content is similarly very unusual[17] because lack of communication with the biliary tree is a distinctive feature; however, fistulization of cystadenoma in the biliary tree has been reported,[25,26] the same as for pancreatic mucinous cystadenoma, which may explain the bilious content.

The internal lining is generally smooth but may contain microscopic or, more rarely, macroscopic polypoid lesions projecting into the lumen (Fig. 88B.2). This internal lining has three distinct layers: (1) an epithelial layer, (2) a mesenchymal stroma, and (3) an outer layer of collagen connective tissue that separates it from the adjacent parenchyma (Fig. 88B.3).

The epithelial lining, as for pancreatic cystadenoma, consists of glandular, nonciliated cells arranged in a single flat row with occasional papillary or polypoid projections, pseudostratifications, and crypt-like invaginations. In two-thirds of the patients, the epithelium is columnar, but in one-third, it consists of a combination of columnar and cuboidal epithelium. The epithelial lining may show denuded areas with chronic inflammation and hemorrhage. The columnar cells contain histologically benign-appearing, basally located nuclei and intracellular mucin. However, mucinous epithelium may be lacking in up to 20% of the cases,[11] which may represent the initial phase of the tumor with the appearance of mucinous epithelium representing the next phase in tumorigenic progression.[27]

The lining epithelium occasionally shows papillary infoldings, and mild epithelial atypia with a slight increase in the size of the basally located nuclei has been reported to be at least focally present in most patients. More severe dysplasia, consisting of a multilayer appearance of hyperchromatic cells with loss of polarity, appears much less frequently. Foci of intestinal metaplasia are also rare, seen in the form of numerous goblet cells. Atypia and metaplasia are suggestive of a high risk of malignant transformation.[18]

Phenotype has been further characterized in a limited number of patients. The epithelium shows strong and diffuse cytoplasmic staining with antibodies against carcinoembryonic antigen (CEA) and cancer antigen (CA) 19-9, whereas CA-125 staining is focal or absent.[28,29] It also stains positive for cytokeratin-7 (CK-7), CK-19, CK-8, and CK-18,[30] which supports

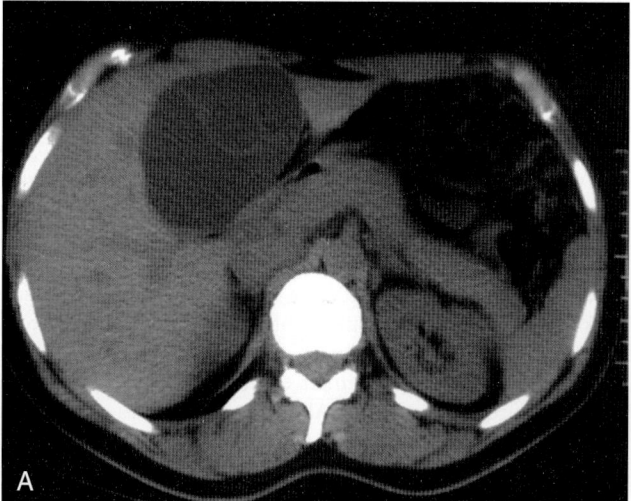
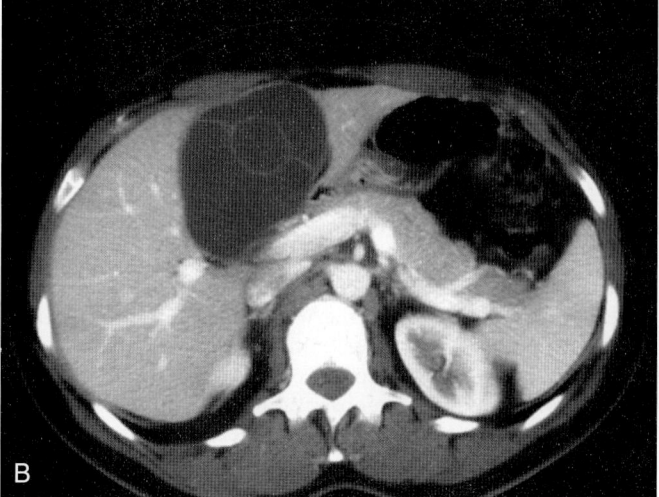

FIGURE 88B.1 Cystadenoma with ovarian-like stroma. The cyst has a thin wall and septa that enhance after injection of contrast agent **(B)**, versus **(A)** without injection. Note that the tumor is in segment IV, which occurs frequently (see Chapter 14).

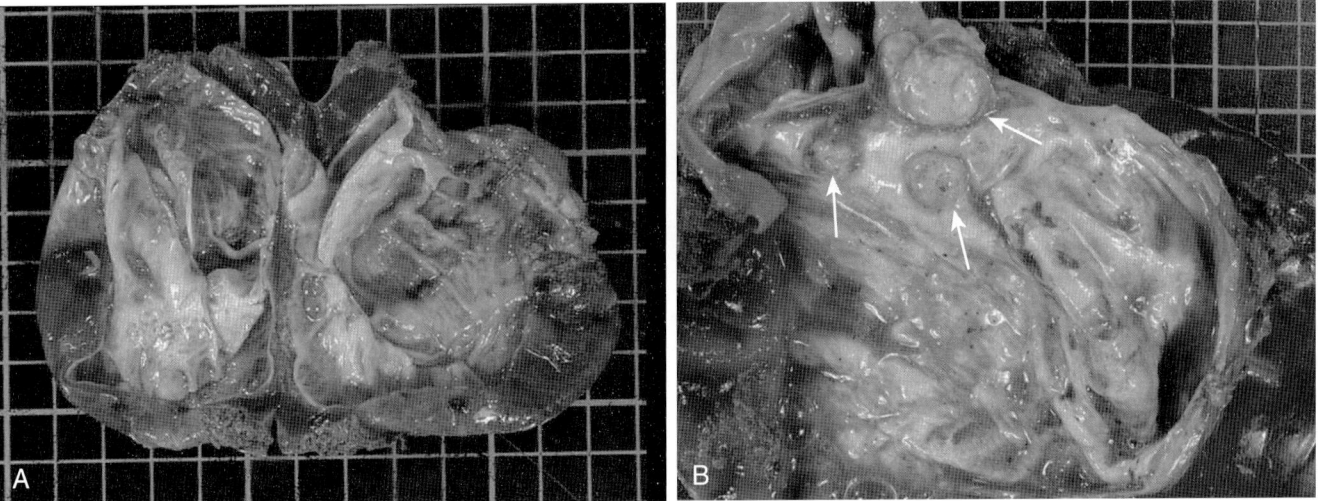

FIGURE 88B.2   Cystadenoma with ovarian-like stroma. The internal lining is smooth but may contain microscopic **(A)** or macroscopic **(B)** polypoid lesions *(arrows; see Chapter 87).*

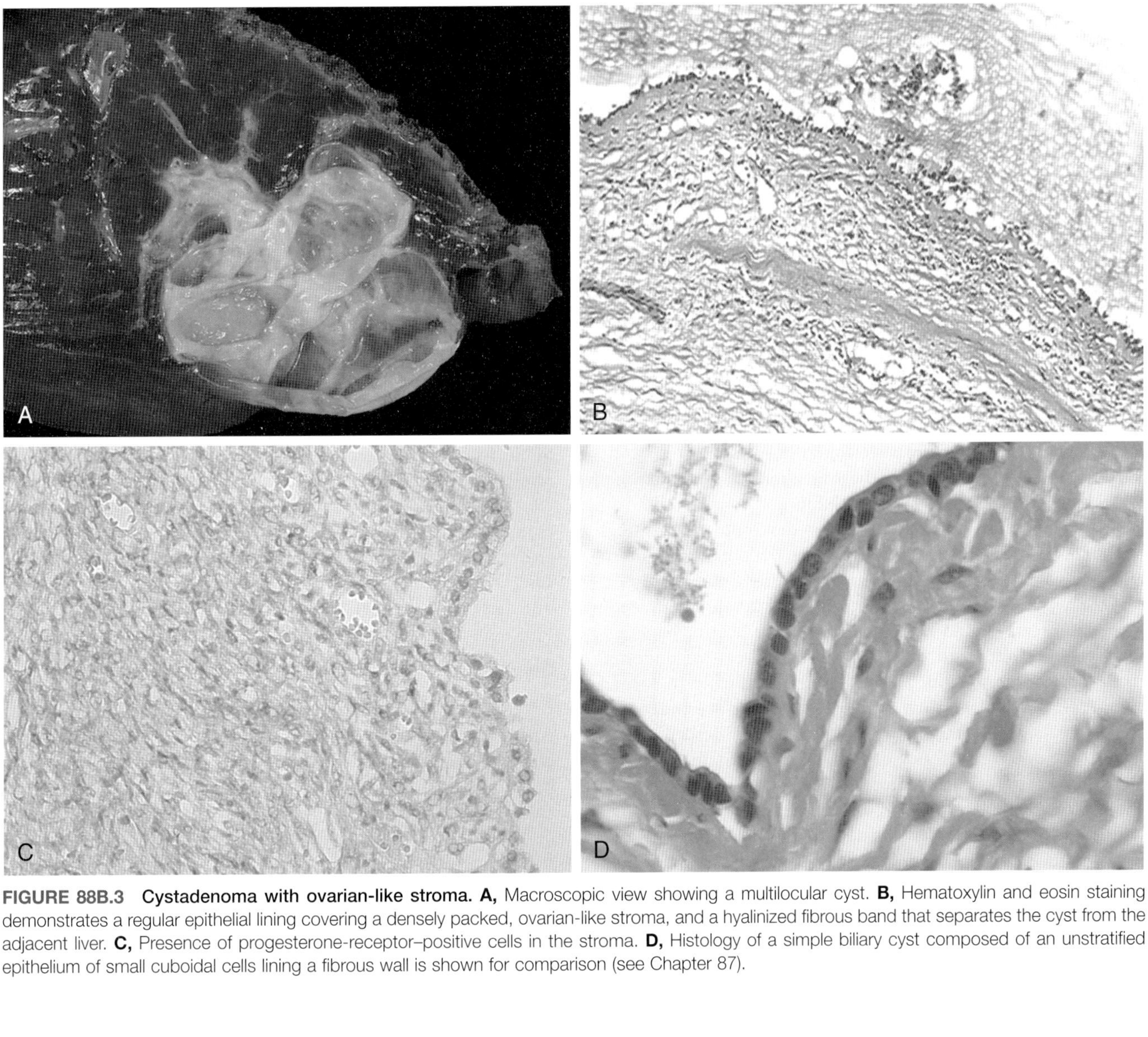

FIGURE 88B.3   Cystadenoma with ovarian-like stroma. A, Macroscopic view showing a multilocular cyst. **B,** Hematoxylin and eosin staining demonstrates a regular epithelial lining covering a densely packed, ovarian-like stroma, and a hyalinized fibrous band that separates the cyst from the adjacent liver. **C,** Presence of progesterone-receptor–positive cells in the stroma. **D,** Histology of a simple biliary cyst composed of an unstratified epithelium of small cuboidal cells lining a fibrous wall is shown for comparison (see Chapter 87).

a biliary origin, and it is negative for inhibin-α,[30,31] vimentin,[31] and estrogen or progesterone receptors,[32] and CD56 is only expressed focally.[33]

The *stroma* consists of a compact arrangement of bland, spindle-shaped cells with round to oval nuclei. This appearance is reminiscent of OS, hence the name given to these tumors. However, it has also been found to resemble the primitive mesenchymal elements associated with the developing biliary system in the fetus. This stroma may be abundant or diffuse in approximately half of the patients but at the other extreme may only be focal in 10% of the patients[11] and mitotic activity is not prominent. It expresses estrogen and progesterone receptors, as does the stroma of pancreatic cystadenoma[32,34]; inhibin-α, a gonadal protein that has a more limited expression in the sex cord–stromal tissue, is also expressed in both hepatic and pancreatic mucinous cystadenoma[35,36] and in sex cord–stromal tumors. They are immunoreactive with α–smooth muscle actin, vimentin, but also desmin. There is no immune reaction with CEA, CA19-9, or CA-125.[18,28]

A *densely hyalinized pseudocapsule* surrounds the tumor and separates it from the adjacent liver tissue, which explains how these tumors can be enucleated.

Despite the similarities between hepatic and pancreatic mucinous cystadenomas, few studies have compared the phenotypes of both lesions. One reported denser and more abundant stroma, more intense estrogen or progesterone receptors, and more inhibin-α in hepatic than in pancreatic cystadenomas, but the significance of this is unclear.[35]

Risk Factors and Origin

There are no clearly identified risk factors apart from sex because cystadenomas with OS are exclusively observed (or at least in more than 90% as for pancreatic cystadenoma) in women. However, a history of previous oral contraceptive use does not appear to be a distinctive feature.[18] Several hypotheses have been raised based on some pathologic features of the tumor, most notably the presence of an ovarian-like stroma or the occasional presence of eosinophilic or endocrine cells. It is still unclear whether cystadenomas are of congenital origin or are acquired neoplastic lesions.

The resemblance is striking among cystadenomas with OS located in the liver, pancreas, retroperitoneum, and ovary.[37–39] The particular OS common to these locations contains estrogen and progesterone receptors and inhibin-α.[35] These similarities suggest a common pathway of tumor development, although simultaneous occurrences of hepatic cystadenoma with pancreatic[40] or ovarian cystadenoma[41] are exceedingly rare.

One hypothesis is that during embryonic development, ectopic ovarian cells would have migrated to the liver or pancreas, released hormones and growth factors, and caused endodermally derived epithelium to proliferate and finally to form a tumor.[42] The right and left primordial gonads are indeed located directly under the diaphragm before their descent, at the level of the dorsocranial side of the liver and the tail of the pancreas, respectively. Furthermore, the cells covering the gonads show an activated morphology in contrast to the peritoneal epithelium elsewhere,[43] which suggests that they have the ability to detach from the gonadal surface, cross the peritoneal cleft, and attach to the peritoneal surface of nearby organs. This hypothesis would explain the predominance of cystadenoma in the body or tail of the pancreas, rather than in the head, as well as the apparent predominance of liver cystadenoma in

segment IV. Splenogonadal fusion has also been documented,[44] and demonstration of endocrine cells in about 50% of cystadenomas is a distinctive feature[44] compatible with the hypothesis of these tumors developing from peribiliary glands.

The OS resembles the primitive embryonic mesenchyma of embryonic gallbladder and large bile ducts that contribute to the connective tissue surrounding the bile ducts,[29] and it has therefore also been suggested that these tumors could derive from ectopic embryonal tissue destined to form the gallbladder[29] or from ectopic embryonic rests of primitive foregut sequestered within the liver.[16]

Presentation

Intrahepatic biliary cystadenoma with an OS is exclusively observed in women, with few exceptions. Age at diagnosis is highly variable, between 1 year[45] and 70 years, but it peaks in the fourth or early fifth decade. In most patients, the tumor is discovered during the workup of epigastric or right upper quadrant pain or vague abdominal complaints that include abdominal discomfort or swelling. Palpation of an abdominal mass that moves freely with respiration is also a classic circumstance of diagnosis. Because the tumor may grow to a considerable size, a gradual increase in abdominal girth and/or compression of the stomach or duodenum may also occur; however, because of the slow progression of the neoplasm, the onset of symptoms tends to be insidious and to have evolved for a prolonged period of time before treatment.[21,46] This may explain why large tumors are over-represented in most reports of cystadenomas. With the increasingly liberal use of imaging to investigate even the most minor symptoms, cystadenomas are often discovered incidentally, and it is possible that a significant proportion are not identified or are mistaken for simple cysts[46] (see Chapter 73).

More acute episodes of pain have been reported in up to 35% of the patients, and most of these are related to biliary obstruction.[21,47] This is biologically witnessed by concomitant cytolysis or cholestasis. Jaundice or itching[48] may also be present, whereas cholangitis is rare. Typically, such episodes are transient, and any jaundice tends to resolve spontaneously, which is compatible with the migration of mucous material or tumor embolus from the cyst into the bile duct (Fig. 88B.4). Such tumor protrusion in the bile duct lumen has been reported even for small cystadenomas less than 4 cm in diameter.[46] An alternative mechanism of obstruction is simple compression of the biliary confluence by the cystadenoma. Other causes of acute presentation have included tumor rupture,[49] superinfection, bleeding,[50] and caval compression,[51] but these are rare.

Diagnosis
Differential Diagnosis

Apart from the other cystic tumors addressed in this chapter, most notably cystadenocarcinoma, the main differential diagnosis of cystadenoma is simple cysts that have become atypical on imaging studies as a result of intracystic bleeding[52] or previous sclerotherapy[53] (see Chapter 73). The risk of mistaking a cystadenoma for a benign cyst is that this lesion may be treated by simple unroofing, which is an inappropriate treatment associated with a high risk of recurrence (see "Management" later); to mistake a simple or atypical cyst for a cystadenoma is to perform an occasionally risky and

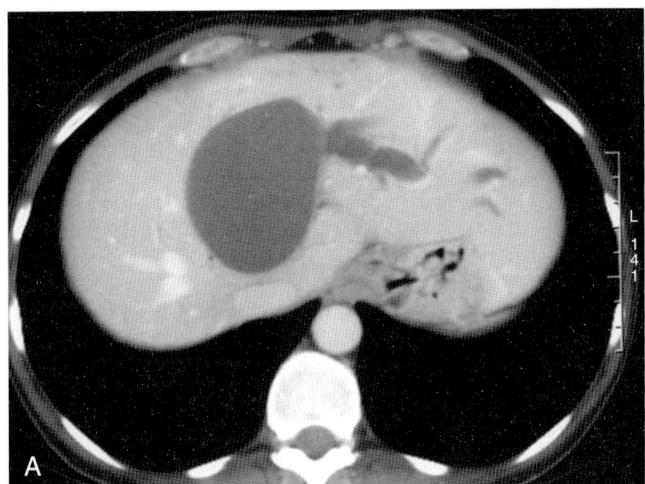 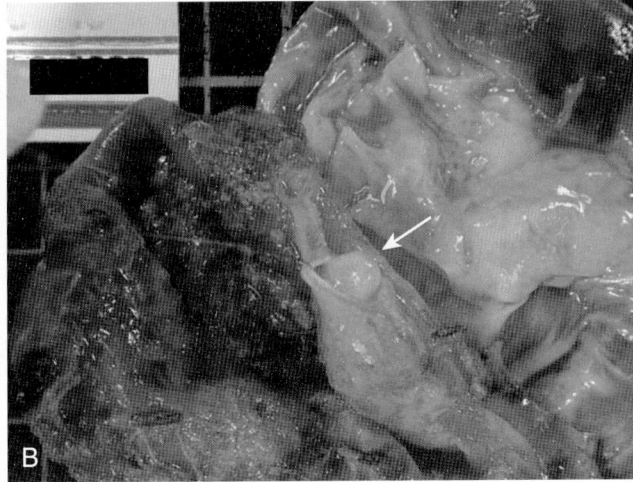

FIGURE 88B.4   Cystadenoma with ovarian-like stroma with tumor protrusion in the bile duct. **A,** Note the presence of dilated bile ducts upstream of the cyst located in segment IV. **B,** Tumor *(arrow)* protruding into the left bile duct on the resected specimen (see Chapters 14, 87).

unwarranted resection because simple cysts do not require complete resection. Considering the very high incidence of simple cysts, the latter is probably much more common, and it has been shown that a cystadenoma-like lesion is almost as likely to be a simple cyst as to be a cystadenoma.[24,54-56] Clinical history is totally unreliable in the diagnosis of hemorrhagic cysts because intracystic hemorrhage can occur in the absence of any symptoms,[52] and the diagnosis mainly relies on imaging (see Chapter 14).

Alternative differential diagnoses include nonsuppurative granulomatous infection of a simple cyst,[57] hepatic abscess[58] (see Chapter 70), echinococcal cysts[59] (see Chapter 72), mesenchymal hamartoma[60] (see Chapter 88A), ciliated hepatic foregut cysts (see Chapter 88A), intrahepatic lymphangioma (see Chapter 88A), cystic hemangioma (see Chapter 88A), cystic forms of hepatocellular carcinoma (see Chapter 89), ICC (see Chapter 50), mucin-producing metastases from thyroid or colon carcinoma, and cystic metastases of the ovary, of melanoma, and of kidney and neuroendocrine tumors.[61] They have also been occasionally confused with pancreatic cysts.[28]

Imaging (see Chapter 14)

The characteristic ultrasonographic (US) finding for biliary cystadenoma is an anechoic mass with echogenic internal septations (Fig. 88B.5). Papillary projections into the cystic space may also be seen. On computed tomography (CT) scans, the lesions appear as multiloculated hypodense masses with a well-defined wall. The content demonstrates fluid attenuation because of the presence of mucin, blood, or bile. Fine septal calcifications may occasionally be seen, and both the wall and the septations enhance after administration of contrast material (see Fig. 88B.1).

With magnetic resonance imaging (MRI), cystadenoma is typically seen as a fluid-containing multilocular cyst with homogeneous high signal intensity on T2-weighted images and homogeneous low or isosignal intensity on T1-weighted images.[23] These signals may vary depending on the content of the cystic fluid. Mucinous fluid will appear with an isosignal, serous fluid with a hyposignal, and hemorrhagic fluid with a hyperintense signal that can only be seen in the lower part of a fluid-fluid level. Thin internal septal structures separate fluid-filled spaces. These, along with the wall of the lesion, are contrast enhanced (Fig. 88B.6).

Contrast US is a reliable exploration that shows a typical honeycomb enhancement pattern of the cyst wall and septa.[62-64] An intracystic structure of complicated simple cysts corresponds to clots and is not enhanced.[65] Although the periphery of simple cyst may show enhancement, this corresponds to compressed adjacent liver, and this should be differentiated from enhancement of the cyst wall of cystadenoma (see Fig. 88B.5).

As for other cystic lesions, CT scan is less reliable and accurate than US or MRI (see Chapter 14). Cystadenoma in particular may wrongly appear unilocular on CT scan, whereas US[66] and MRI[23,67] will visualize the internal septa. Two additional features besides multilocularity may help in the differential diagnosis of simple cysts: They are frequently multiple,[68] whereas cystadenomas are single lesions, and although biliary dilation has been considered uncommon, a mild enlargement upstream of the tumor is probably more frequent than previously thought; using higher resolution imaging, enlargement was observed in one- to two-thirds of the patients in a recent series.[24,69] Along the same line, an increase in serum alkaline phosphatase levels has recently been shown to be a feature distinctive from simple cysts.[24]

Cytology and Tumor Markers

CYTOLOGY. Aspiration cytology is either nonspecific or shows chronic inflammatory exudates with large numbers of neutrophils, lymphocytes, and macrophages. A few groups of nonatypical bland cuboidal-to-columnar epithelial cells, occasionally arranged in papillary clusters, may be seen.[28]

TUMOR MARKERS. Unlike for the pancreas, measurement of tumor markers in hepatobiliary cystic lesions has been infrequently performed, and results are confusing. Early case reports have pointed to a link between cystadenoma and CA19-9 by showing its expression by epithelial lining and by revealing increased intracystic and serum concentrations.[70,71] However, CA19-9 is also expressed by normal biliary epithelial cells, and very high levels have occasionally been measured in the bile of patients with various nontumoral conditions.[55,72,73]

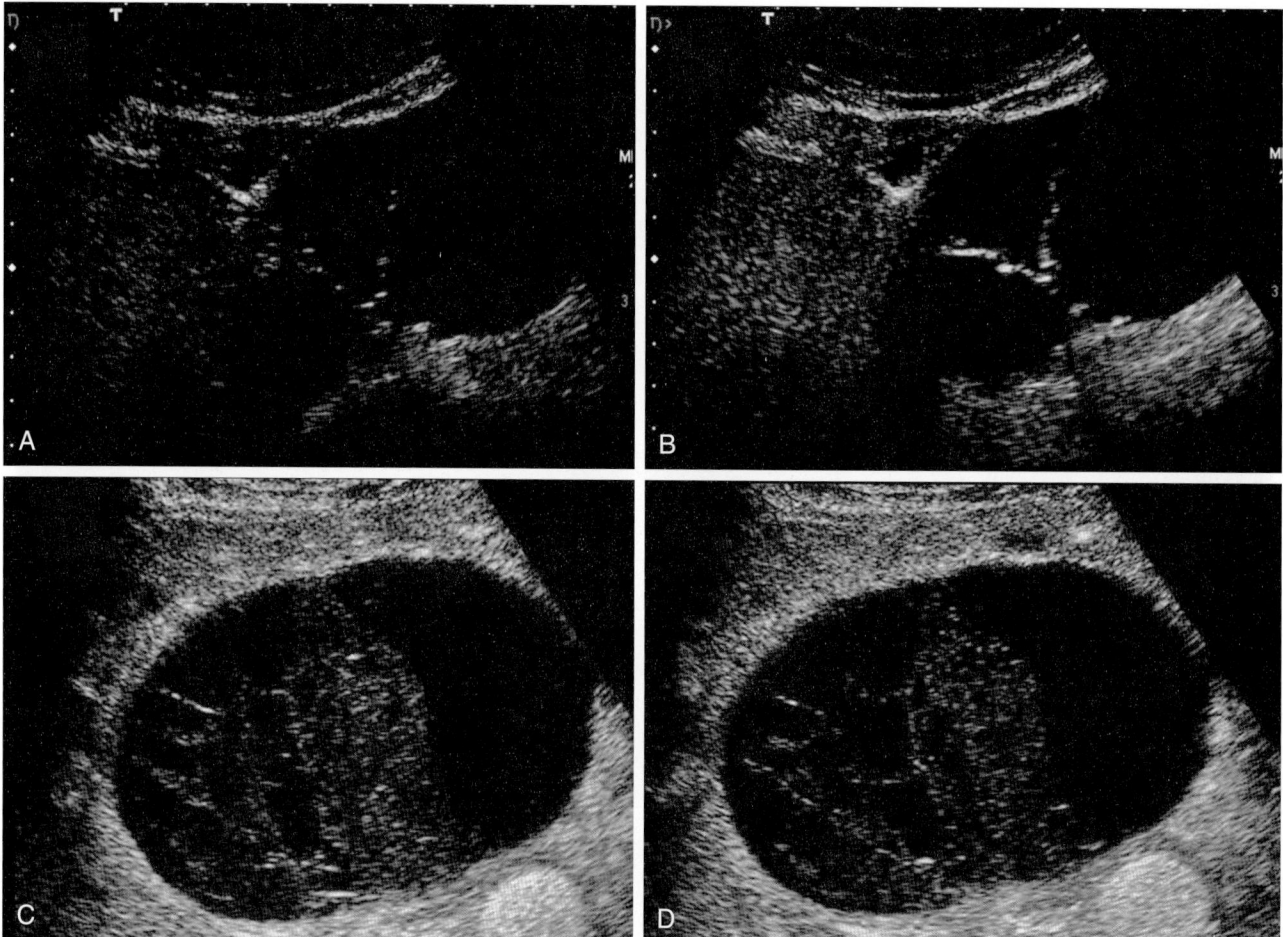

FIGURE 88B.5 Ultrasound (US) and contrast US of a cystadenoma with ovarian-like stroma **(A** and **B)** and of a hemorrhagic simple cyst **(C** and **D)**. Normal US **(A** and **C)** and contrast US **(B** and **D)** are shown. The septa are enhanced in the cystadenoma, but in hemorrhagic cysts, the intracystic material corresponds to clots and does not enhance (see Chapter 14).

It is also expressed by the epithelium lining simple cysts of the liver[74] and in the cystic fluid of simple cysts.[74–76] An increased serum concentration of CA19-9 in these patients has even been reported and can occasionally be very high, probably as a result of communication of the cyst with the circulation. Four studies have shown that cyst concentration[24,75,77] and serum concentration of CA19-9[74,75] are comparable in patients with cystadenoma and simple cysts. As will be discussed later, CA19-9 is also inaccurate in differentiating cystadenoma from cystadenocarcinoma.[72]

It has also been suggested that a CEA concentration greater than 600 ng/mL in the supernatant of cystic liver lesions could accurately differentiate cystadenoma or cystadenocarcinoma from benign, nonmucinous cysts.[77] The epithelial lining of cystadenoma indeed stains positive for CEA[28]; however, this has not been confirmed in subsequent studies, in which concentrations in cystadenoma and simple cysts were comparable.[24,55,75,77] In contrast, intracystic concentration of tumor-associated glycoprotein-72 is increased in cystadenoma and low in simple cysts, and this proved reliable to differentiate both lesions.[76]

Complications

Cystadenoma with an OS is considered a precancerous lesion, as will be detailed later. Malignancy arises in most cases from the epithelium lining (cystadenocarcinoma), but sarcomatous

transformation of the OS has also been reported.[21] No specific feature has been clearly linked to a higher risk of malignancy, apart from the presence of epithelial atypia (dysplasia) or intestinal metaplasia. The odds ratio for their association with malignancy in landmark series has been calculated to be 8 (95% confidence interval [CI], 2.4–27.0) and 2.4 (95% CI, 1.2–3.5), respectively.[18] The rate of transformation has ranged between 2% and 30% but, as previously mentioned, most series lacked a stringent requirement of OS for the diagnosis. When this definition is applied, two studies found a concordant rate of approximately 5%.[10,11] Of note and as for the OS, the carcinomatous transformation may be very focal, underlying the need for extensive sampling of the entire specimen for accurate diagnosis and staging.

Series comparing resected biliary and pancreatic MCN have yielded conflicting results in terms of prevalence of dysplasia, with one reporting a slightly lower prevalence of low-/intermediate-grade dysplasia for pancreatic MCN than for liver MCN[10] and another a lower prevalence of high-grade dysplasia or carcinoma in situ for biliary MCN than for pancreatic MCN.[11]

Although cystadenoma with an OS by definition does not communicate with the biliary tree, fistulization in the bile duct may occur. Ensuing symptoms are usually related to the migration of the mucinous cystic content. The incidence of this complication is unknown because it is only documented by

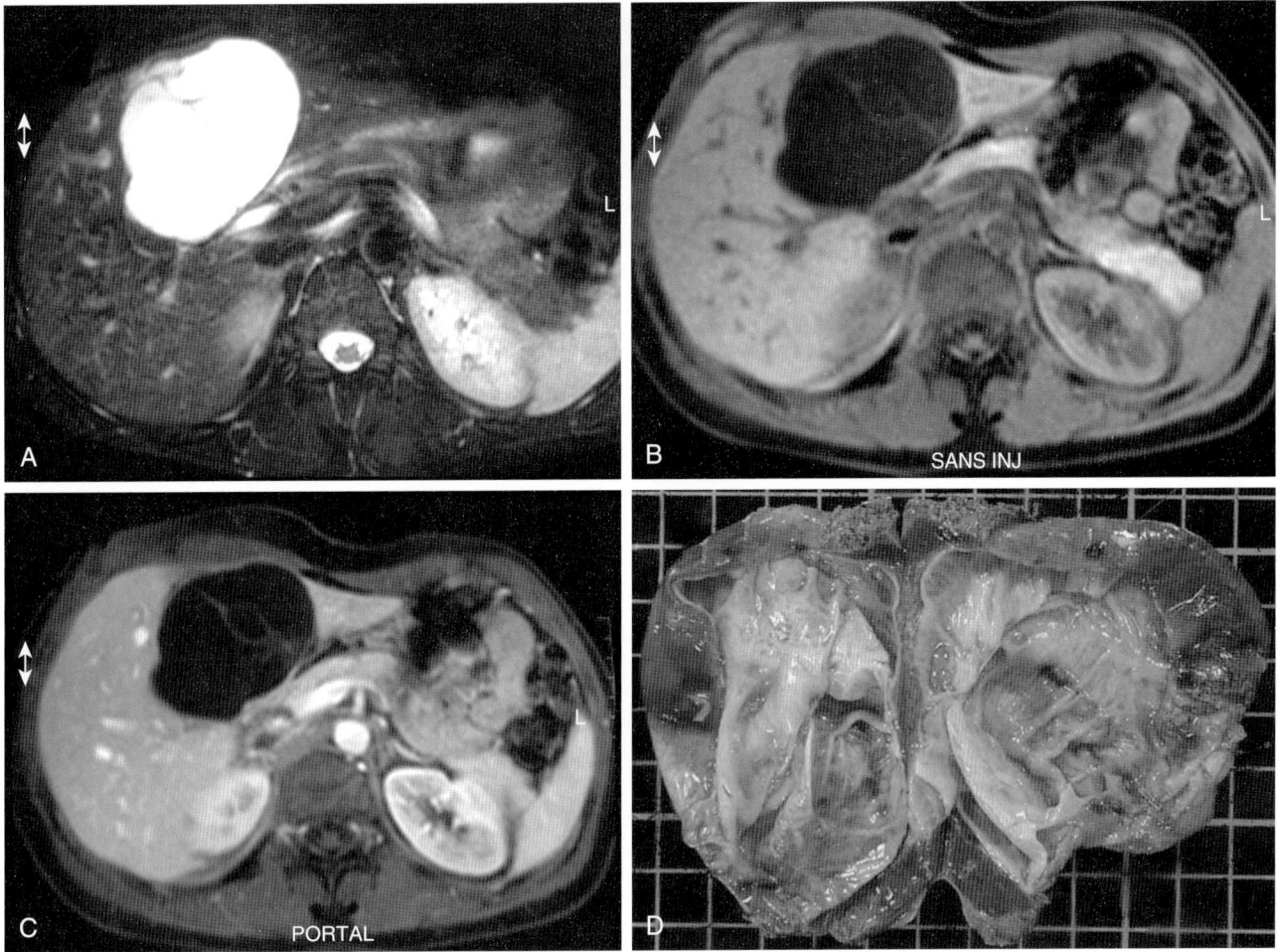

FIGURE 88B.6   Magnetic resonance imaging of a cystadenoma with ovarian-like stroma **(A–C)** and macroscopic view **(D)**. Specimen is the same as in Figure 88B.1. **A,** The tumor is hyperintense on T2-weighted images. **B,** Septa are visible on T1-weighted images. **C,** Tumors enhance after injection of gadolinium (see Chapter 14).

endoscopic retrograde cholangiopancreatography (ERCP) and intraoperative cholangiography (IOC), which are not routinely performed. Other complications have included rupture in the peritoneal cavity, superinfection, bleeding, and caval compression, as previously mentioned.

Management

Cystadenomas require complete excision to prevent recurrence of symptoms and malignant transformation (see Chapter 101). Evidence that partial excision, aspiration, and external or internal drainage are ineffective is that recurrence has been noted very early on[16,18,20,50] and that 40% to 50% of the patients culled by tertiary referral centers had undergone such previous treatments before referral.[22,45,78–80] Updated evidence is shown in Table 88B.1 and in a recent systematic review that reported an 82% recurrence rate after fenestration or marsupialization.[12] Recurrence occurs at a mean of 21 months but may be delayed up to 4 years,[80,81] and recurrences up to 15 years after an initial operation have even been suggested.[11] This may explain why recurrence after incomplete resection has not been systematically observed because most studies only have short-term follow-up.[50,82,83] Development of a cystadenocarcinoma after partial resection of a cystadenoma has also been documented.[21,84–86]

Fenestration of the cystadenoma with fulguration of the internal cystic lining has been attempted with occasionally adequate long-term success,[45] but experience is too limited to recommend this strategy. Although not documented, it is likely that some small cystadenomas mistaken for simple cysts have also been successfully treated with percutaneous ethanol injection. Ethanol is indeed effective in the management of simple cysts, hydatid disease, and hepatocellular carcinoma; however, this cannot be currently recommended, especially because most cystadenomas are large and ethanol injection induces morphologic changes that prevent accurate follow-up of the cyst wall. In any case, the clinician should not entirely rely on intraoperative frozen-section biopsies to differentiate simple cysts and cystadenoma because these can be falsely negative even when repeated.[83,80]

Surgery can consist of partial hepatectomy or enucleation as there is a dissection plane between the cystadenoma and the adjacent parenchyma (see Chapter 101). Care should be taken when the cyst lies in segment IV so as not to injure the biliary bifurcation. IOC should be performed to document a potential biliary communication and exclude the presence of mucus or tumor material in the bile duct. Treatment of extrahepatic cystadenoma should include bile duct resection and bilioenteric reconstruction rather than simple enucleation from the bile duct wall. As for other tumors, laparoscopic resection can be an

TABLE 88B.1		Outcome After Fenestration of Cystadenoma			
REFERENCE	**SIZE (cm)**	**OS**	**FENESTRATION**	**RECURRENCE**	**FOLLOW-UP (mo)**
Akwari et al., 1990[21]	NA	+	Open	Yes, clinical	2
	8	+	Open	Yes, clinical	0.5
	11	+	Open	Yes, clinical	36
Gadzijev et al., 1996[87]	NA	+	Open	Yes, clinical	24
Regev et al., 2001[88]	NA	+	Laparoscopic	Yes, clinical	NA
	NA	+	Laparoscopic	Yes, clinical	NA
	NA	+	Laparoscopic	Yes, clinical	NA
Dixon et al., 2001[89]	NA	+	Open	Yes, imaging	NA
Tan et al., 2002[90]	NA	+	Laparoscopic	Yes, clinical	20
Koffron et al., 2004[91]	NA	+	Laparoscopic	No	NA
Erdogan et al., 2006[43]	NA	+	Open	Yes, clinical	72
Teoh et al., 2006[56]	17	+	Laparoscopic	Yes, imaging	3
	17	+	Laparoscopic	Yes, imaging	3
	18	+	Open	No	6
Delis et al., 2008[78]	NA	+	Laparoscopic	Yes, clinical	NA
	NA	+	Laparoscopic	Yes, clinical	NA
Korobkin et al., 1989[66]	NA	NA	Open	Yes, clinical	60
	NA	NA	Open	Yes, clinical	360
Zacherl et al., 2000[92]	NA	NA	Laparoscopic	Yes, imaging	3
Vogt et al., 2005[80]	NA	NA	Laparoscopic	Yes, clinical	13
	NA	NA	Laparoscopic	Yes, clinical	120
	NA	NA	Laparoscopic	Yes, imaging	6
	NA	NA	Laparoscopic	Yes, clinical	3
	NA	NA	Laparoscopic	Yes	8
	NA	NA	Open	Yes	4
	NA	NA	Open	Yes	3
Thomas et al., 2005[45]	NA	NA	Unstated	Yes	NA
	NA	NA	Unstated	Yes	NA
	NA	NA	Unstated	Yes	NA
	NA	NA	Unstated	Yes	NA
	NA	NA	Unstated	Yes	NA
	16	NA	Laparoscopic + fulguration	No	12
	16	NA	Laparoscopic + fulguration	No	72
Barabino et al., 2004[82]	16	−	Laparoscopic	No	24
Fiamingo et al., 2004[93]	10	−	Laparoscopic	No	24
Veroux et al., 2005[94]	12	−	Laparoscopic	No	14
Manouras et al., 2008[83]	16	−	Laparoscopic	No	6
Lee et al., 2015[95]	NA		Unstated	No	Lost for follow-up
	NA		Unstated	No	Lost for follow-up
	NA		Unstated	No	Lost for follow-up
	NA		Unstated	Yes	(a)
	NA		Unstated	Yes	(a)
	NA		Unstated	Yes	(a)
	NA		Unstated	Yes	(a)
	NA		Unstated	Yes	(a)

−, Absent; +, present; follow-up, time to recurrence or duration of follow-up; *NA,* not available; *open,* open surgery; *OS,* ovarian stroma.
(a), median disease free survival for these 5 patients was 4 months.

option for trained surgeons.[91,94,96] A single case of recurrence after complete resection has been reported.[16]

HEPATOBILIARY CYSTADENOMA WITHOUT OVARIAN STROMA

Although the latest version of the WHO classification considers that the presence of an OS is a prerequisite for the diagnosis of MCN, some cystadenomas have been reported that do not have OS, even recently.[9] Before considering this diagnosis, several samples of the specimen should be analyzed; as in some patients, the OS may be only focally present.[11,18] It is unclear, however, whether cystadenoma without an OS is a discrete entity or whether it is, in fact, an IPMN-B (see later) in which the communication with the biliary tree could not be demonstrated. Although cystadenoma with and without an OS have very similar clinical and morphologic features, a distinctive characteristic is that the former only develops in women, whereas the latter may develop in both sexes.

Incidence

The largest surgical series of cystadenoma, with or without an OS, published over the past 15 years have, as a rule, included a higher number of tumors with OS than without in a ratio of 5:1 to 10:1 (Table 88B.2)[17,18,43,88]; however, others have reported equal numbers,[31,80] lower numbers,[97] and in one study, virtually all lesions described as "cystadenoma" lacked OS.[91] This discordance is puzzling but probably speaks to the lack of strict pathologic definition of this entity. It is likely that a number of tumors previously diagnosed as cystadenoma without an OS were, in fact, simple cysts of the liver that had a multilocular appearance as a result of intracystic bleeding or because several cysts were juxtaposed. They might also have included cystic forms of IPMN-B, which is addressed separately in this chapter.

Pathology

Cystadenomas without OS are typically multilocular and have a mucinous content (Fig. 88B.7). The epithelium is phenotypically similar to the classic cystadenoma (see earlier). Devaney and colleagues (1994)[18] did not observe areas of atypia or dysplasia in this variant, but others have.[31] These tumors also tend to more frequently communicate with the biliary tree than cystadenoma with an OS. In particular, a higher proportion of patients are seen with bilious fluid within their cyst[17]; however, data are scarce, and ERCP and IOC have not been routinely performed. When a communication is documented, the tumor should be currently considered an IPMN-B (see Chapter 87).

The phenotype of the epithelium lining cystadenoma without an OS has been very inconsistently characterized but has been reported to stain positive for CK-7, CK-8, CK-18, CK-19, mucin 1 (MUC1), MUC5, and MUC6 but not for CEA, CA19-9, or MUC3.[105,107] This phenotype is close to that of large bile ducts (see Chapter 89).

PRESENTATION AND DIAGNOSIS

Unlike those with OS, cystadenomas without OS have been described in both sexes, and the female/male ratio is actually close to 1 based on the rare available data.[17,18,31] Otherwise, age (peaking between 40 and 60 years), symptoms, and size of the cyst are comparable.[17] Imaging studies have up to now been

TABLE 88B.2 Cystadenomas and Cystadenocarcinomas With and Without an Ovarian Stroma

REFERENCE	OS	CYSTADENOMA (NO. PATIENTS)	CYSTADENOCARCINOMA (NO. PATIENTS)
Ishak et al., 1977[20]	+	8	6
Wheeler & Edmondson, 1985[16]	+	13	4
Akwari et al., 1990[21]	+	44	9
Devaney et al., 1994[18]	+	44	6
	−	8	12
Buetow et al., 1995[17]	+	22	4
	−	5	3
Tsiftsis et al., 1997[98]	NA	2	1
Shimada et al., 1998[55]	NA	1	1
Owono et al., 2001[31]	+	2	0
	−	2	3
Hansman et al., 2001[79]	NA	7	1
Regev et al., 2001[88]	+	8	0
	−	0	1
Ammori et al., 2002[99]	NA	6	2
Hai et al., 2003[100]	+	0	1
	−	3	2
Koffron et al., 2004[91]	+	6	1
	−	27	0
Vogt et al., 2005[80]	+	10	1
	−	8	3
Thomas et al., 2005[45]	+	18	1
Oh et al., 2006[101]	+	5	2
	−	2	4
Daniels et al., 2006[22]	+	12	0
Lewin et al., 2006[23]	+	4	0
	−	2	1
Lim et al., 2007[69]	+	14	3
Koea, 2008[102]	NA	3	2
Pojchamarnwiputh et al., 2008[103]	NA	5	7
Lee et al., 2009[104]	NA	6	4
Seo et al., 2010[24]	NA	13	7
Choi et al., 2010[75]	NA	17	0
Erdogan et al., 2010[47]	+	12	1
	−	1	1
Zen et al., 2014[10]	+	71	67
Total	+	293	106 (26%)
	−	58	30 (34%)
	NA	58	24 (29%)

Percentage refers to the proportion of cystadenocarcinoma among cystadenomatous tumors.
−, Absent; +, present; NA, not available; OS, ovarian stroma.

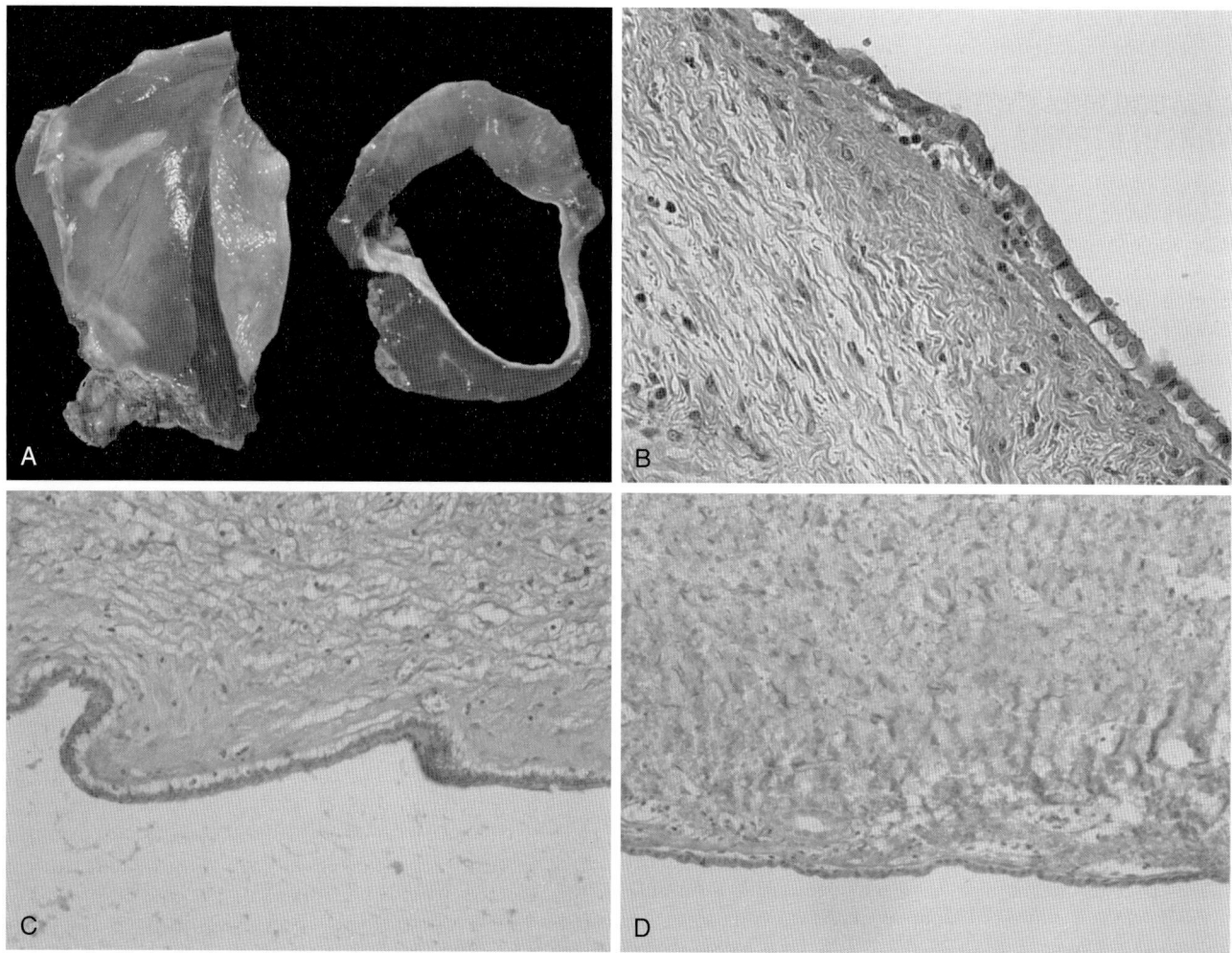

FIGURE 88B.7 Cystic mucinous tumor without ovarian-like stroma. **A,** Macroscopic view showing a unilocular cyst. **B,** Hematoxylin and eosin staining demonstrates cyst lining by an unstratified epithelium of regular cuboidal cells lying on a fibrous wall without ovarian-like stroma. **C,** Mucin production is observed in epithelial lining cells. **D,** No progesterone receptor immunostaining was observed in the fibrous wall (see Chapter 87).

unable to differentiate between cystadenoma with and without an OS.[17,23,31] In the cystic fluid, CA19-9 appears always increased, and CEA levels are also increased in most patients.[91,93]

Natural History and Management

Very little data are available on the natural history of cystadenoma without an OS. Case reports suggest that it may undergo morphologic changes with a progressive increase in diameter, mural thickening, development of papillary nodules, and subsequent malignant transformation.[107,108] These changes have been observed over a prolonged period of time (10 years). Whether cystadenoma with and without an OS has the same malignant potential is unclear. It is accepted, however, that both require complete resection. IOC should be performed to document a potential biliary communication. If present, the diagnosis of IPMN-B should be considered and ruled out by frozen-section analysis.

CYSTADENOCARCINOMA

Definition and Incidence

Cystadenocarcinomas are very rare primary cystic tumors that do not primarily communicate with the biliary tree; they are lined by a tubulopapillary malignant epithelium (Fig. 88B.8; see Chapter 87). Single case reports exist in which malignancy was an adenosquamous carcinoma,[18] or it developed in the stroma.[21] Cystadenocarcinoma was first described in 1943 by Willis, but by 2000, only 100 had been reported in the literature,[109,110] and they were considered to account for only 0.4% of hepatic malignancies.[111] Most have been found in the liver, with only anecdotal reports of locations in the extrahepatic bile duct and the gallbladder in particular.[112] As for cystadenomas, these are usually stratified in two groups depending on the presence or absence of an OS[20,70]; however, some pathologists are reluctant to consider the diagnosis of cystadenocarcinoma when the OS is lacking because these may correspond to cystic variants of mass-forming ICC or to malignant IPMN-B.[6,7] The distinction is not purely academic because these tumors have distinct modes of spread and prognoses that could influence management. This should be taken into account when analyzing the literature, and even when reading this section.

Epidemiology and Presentation

Overall female/male ratio is 2:1, but cystadenocarcinomas with OS are exclusively observed in women, whereas those without OS are twice as frequent in men.[109] Although the age

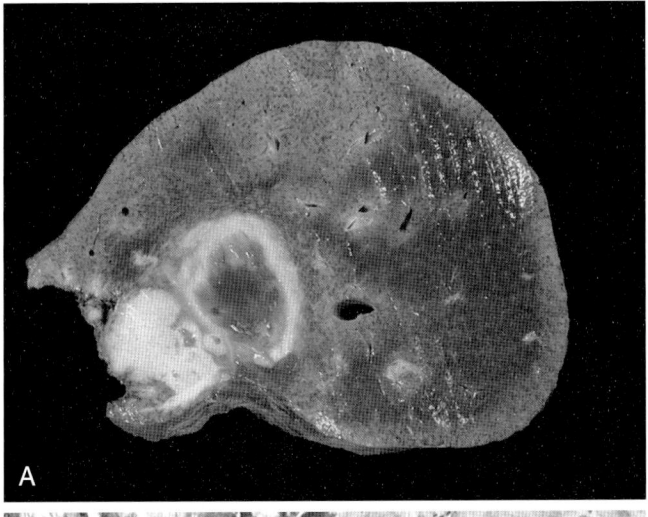
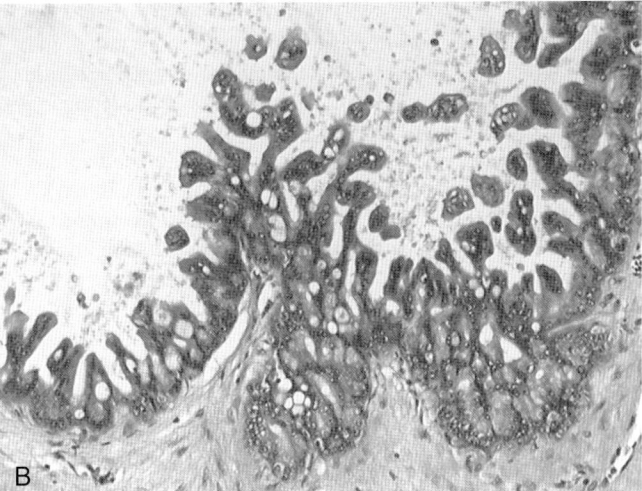
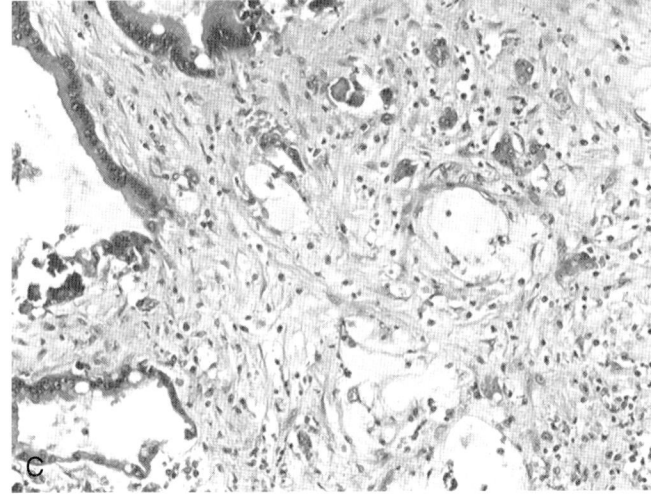

FIGURE 88B.8 **Cystadenocarcinoma. A,** Macroscopic view showing a complex lesion with cystic and solid parts. **B,** Hematoxylin and eosin (H&E) staining demonstrates infiltrative isolated carcinomatous cells or those forming variably sized glands. **C,** H&E staining of the cystic part of the tumor characterized by epithelial papillary proliferations of high-grade dysplasia (see Chapter 87).

range is wide—from 18 to 88 years—it peaks in the late 50s and 60s,[24,110,113] approximately 15 to 20 years later than cystadenomas. This difference is especially obvious for lesions with OS.[16–18,21]

Although usually nonspecific, symptoms are virtually always present and are initially rather indolent.[113] They are common to cystadenoma and include abdominal swelling, discomfort, pain, or palpation of an abdominal mass. Biliary obstruction with jaundice is reported in 20% of the patients, related to biliary compression or migration of mucus or tumor material. Acute symptoms may otherwise occur as a result of intracystic hemorrhage or tumor rupture. As a rule, diagnosis is delayed, and the mean time interval between first symptoms and treatment is 29 months[110]; one case was reported of a cystadenocarcinoma being discovered 1 year after bone metastasis.[114]

Origin and the Cystadenoma-Cystadenocarcinoma Sequence

Cystadenocarcinoma has no identified risk factors, and its origin is unknown but is usually assumed to represent the malignant counterpart of cystadenoma. The proliferating epithelial cells indeed resemble those observed in cystadenoma; both express a biliary-type phenotype, and typical areas of cystadenoma (benign columnar epithelium) coexist with malignant papillary epithelium in most patients (up to 90%).[110] Longitudinal morphologic studies of single patients whose cystic lesions were followed for more than a decade have also shown the progressive development of typical cystadenocarcinoma.[107,115] As a whole, cystadenocarcinomas also tend to be larger and to be discovered 5 to 10 years later than cystadenoma.[110] The transition from one to the other is thought to occur through dysplasia or metaplasia that may be observed within cystadenoma (see "Pathology" earlier). This applies to both intrahepatic[20,107] and extrahepatic cystadenoma[116,117] and to cystadenomas both with and without OS.[118]

The risk of malignant transformation of cystadenoma into cystadenocarcinoma is unknown because the tumor is rare and limited data are available. A rough estimate can be made by comparing the relative proportion of "cystadenoma" and cystadenocarcinoma in published series (see Table 88B.2). Among resected patients, 15% of tumors with OS were malignant. Although biased, this estimate is consistent with that reported for choledochal cysts, which are also premalignant lesions. In contrast, the proportion of cystadenocarcinoma is apparently much higher among tumors without OS or an undefined stroma (see Table 88B.2). The reason for this discrepancy is unclear, which does not necessarily imply that cystadenomas without OS are at greater risk of malignant transformation. These could also include ICC mistaken for cystadenocarcinoma (see Chapter 50) or malignant IPMN-B (papillary cholangiocarcinoma; see "Cystic Variants of Intraductal Papillary Mucinous Neoplasm of the Bile Duct" later in this chapter).

The time necessary for a cystadenoma, with or without OS, to undergo malignant change and subsequently become invasive in the cyst wall, the adjacent parenchyma, or neighboring organs is unknown. Case reports have shown that a lesion may remain morphologically unchanged for years, but that once mural nodules appear, these may progress within a few months.[107] The propensity of, and time necessary for, the malignant epithelial proliferation to become invasive is also unknown. It has been reported that in approximately one-third[18] to one-half[110,119] of the patients who had undergone surgery, the tumor was confined to the cyst, which may explain the very high survival rates reported after complete resection. However, parenchymal extension appearing as satellite nodules or perineural and lymphatic invasion for tumors located close to a glissonian pedicle does exist, and distant metastases are present at the time of diagnosis in 20% of the patients.[110]

Diagnosis

Cystadenocarcinoma could theoretically be mistaken for metastases from cystadenocarcinoma of the ovary or pancreas, but these are usually multiple, whereas cystadenocarcinomas are, as a rule, single lesions. The main difficulty lies in how best to differentiate them from cystadenoma on the one side and from cystic variants of mass-forming ICC or malignant IPMN-B on the other side. It could be argued that these distinctions are of little practical importance because all require resection; however, the extent of resection may differ.

Gross Morphology and Imaging

Cystadenocarcinoma shares most of the morphologic and radiologic features of cystadenoma (see Chapter 87). The lesions are solitary[24] and usually large, with an average diameter of 12 cm but growing up to 40 cm[110]; they can also be small,

and cystadenocarcinoma of less than 5 cm have been reported, including one being 2 cm.[23,67,110] Therefore a small tumor is not evidence that a lesion is benign. Macroscopically, they more frequently have a hemorrhagic or bilious content,[17] and hemorrhage or nodularity within the cyst wall is evident.[17,23,24]

On imaging, cystadenocarcinomas are also more frequently associated with larger septa; intrahepatic cysts debris; bile duct dilation[12,24]; enhancement of mural nodules on CT scan, MRI, or contrast US[12,66,103,120]; and coarse calcifications along the wall or septa[12,17,66] (Fig. 88B.9; see Chapter 14). However, all of these features can also be observed in nonmalignant cystadenoma,[75,108] and differentiating both tumors on macroscopy or imaging alone has up to now proven very difficult.[17,100] Case reports exist of fluorodeoxyglucose positron-emission tomography/CT positivity,[121] but the accuracy of this exploration has not been evaluated.

Biology

An increase in serum tumor markers CEA and CA19-9 is very rare and, when present, is usually mild.[100,110] This has also been described, in particular for CA19-9, in cystadenoma both with and without an OS,[71,100,122,123] and serum levels greater than 50,000 μ/mL have been reported.[124] Accordingly, serum tumor markers CEA and CA19-9 are not helpful in differentiating cystadenocarcinoma from cystadenoma,[125] although a recent systematic review found a slightly higher proportion of cystadenocarcinoma patients with serum tumor markers above the normal upper range.[12]

Cyst Content

Cystic fluid analysis does not provide discriminant information. The content is usually hemorrhagic, bilious, or mixed. Although in earlier case reports, fine-needle aspiration cytology was found to be useful,[127,128] more recent studies have shown that malignant or even atypical cells are very infrequently retrieved.[24,100]

Although inconsistently measured, CA19-9 and CEA concentrations are usually increased in the cystic fluid; this increase, however, is comparable to that observed in cystadenomas, and CA19-9 is present at very high concentrations in most

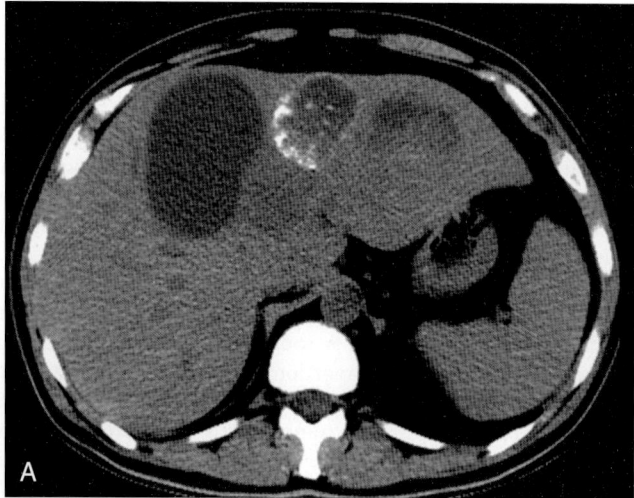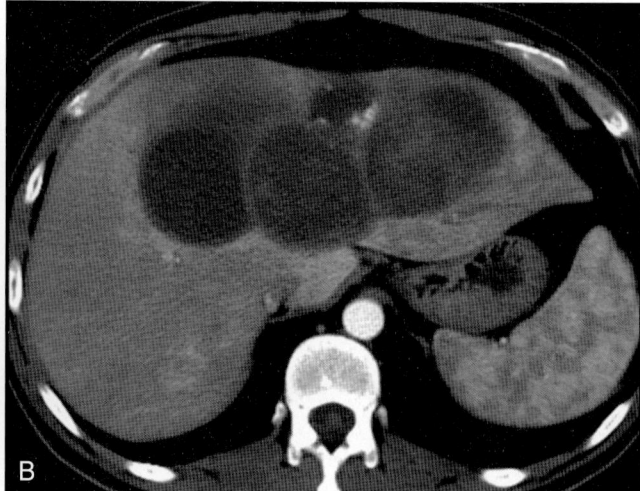

FIGURE 88B.9 **Computed tomographic appearance of a cystadenocarcinoma. A,** Gross calcifications are present along the cyst wall. **B,** Heterogeneous tissue material enhances within the cyst lumen after injection of contrast agent (see Chapter 14).

patients,[24,100] although it has been reported to be normal in a patient whose cystadenocarcinoma did not stain positive for this tumor marker.[72] Although some patients may have CEA levels higher than those observed in cystadenoma or simple cysts, most have normal or mildly elevated concentrations that are therefore not discriminant.[24] This is consistent with the observation that the epithelium of both cystadenoma and cystadenocarcinoma stain positive for CEA.[128]

Cyst sampling should, in any case, be performed with caution because cystadenocarcinomas, and biliary tumors in general, have a high propensity for peritoneal seeding that has been observed after this procedure.[119,129] Pleural effusion, presumed to be related to aspiration cytology, has also been reported.[100]

Treatment

Surgery should consist of complete resection (see Chapter 1010), and IOC should be considered because some of these tumors may communicate with the biliary tree (see Chapter 24). Because tumor extension cannot be reliably assessed on preoperative imaging, it is advisable to perform a formal resection with a wide margin rather than an enucleation. Resection of the biliary confluence followed by a hepaticojejunostomy may be required if the tumor lies close to the biliary confluence. Every effort should be made not to open the cyst because peritoneal carcinomatosis has been observed after accidental cyst rupture despite negative cytology for tumor cells in cystic fluid.[130] Partial resection of cystadenocarcinoma with an OS is associated with a dismal prognosis.

After complete resection, the prognosis appears better overall than that of patients with hepatocellular carcinoma (see Chapter 89) or cholangiocarcinoma (see Chapter 50). After complete resection, 5-year survival can be as high as 65% to 70%.[46,80,110,113,125] Cystadenocarcinomas associated with OS tend to have a more favorable course than those not associated with OS[18,131] with less frequent parenchymal, vascular, and lymphatic invasion.[100] It is unclear, however, whether this relates directly to the presence of an OS; to sex (cystadenocarcinomas with an OS are exclusively observed in women), as shown for other malignancies; or to tumor invasiveness.

CYSTIC VARIANTS OF INTRADUCTAL PAPILLARY MUCINOUS NEOPLASM OF THE BILE DUCT

IPMN-B is a relatively new, distinct pathology characterized by intraluminal papillary proliferation in the bile ducts that produce mucin.[132] They almost exclusively occur in the intrahepatic bile ducts or the left or right bile ducts, do not have an OS, and probably correspond to entities previously described using the terms *biliary papilloma, mucin-producing ICC, intraductal mucosal-spreading mucin-producing peripheral cholangiocarcinoma, intraductal growth–type peripheral cholangiocarcinoma,* and *intraductal variant of peripheral cholangiocarcinoma.*[133] These tumors have striking clinical, histologic, and phenotypic similarities with IPMN-P,[6,134–136] and both may occasionally coexist in the same patient[137,138] (see Chapters 59 and 60). IPMN-B may also develop in the extrahepatic bile ducts, including the biliary confluence, in which case it shows more difference with IPMN-P and a higher prevalence of invasive carcinoma.[139]

IPMN-B may macroscopically be divided into two types. The *ductectatic type* evidences diffusely dilated bile ducts, and the *cystic type* appears as a large cystic mass.[140] A parallel has therefore been drawn between branch duct cystic IPMN-P and cystic variants of IPMN-B that are thought to develop from small bile ducts. Because these variants of IPMN-B have both cystic (mucin) and solid (papillary projection) compartments, they may resemble cystadenoma or cystadenocarcinoma[69,141,142] and might have been mistaken for them in the past. The reason why an IPMN-B exhibits cystic tumor formation rather than localized segmental dilation is unclear. One hypothesis is that if the IPMN arises in a large bile duct, this bile duct will further increase in size as a result of increased pressure, and the mucus will prevent drainage. The other hypothesis is that these cystic IPMN arise from peribiliary glands located within the wall of or scattered in the surrounding connective tissue of the large bile ducts[143,144] (see Chapter 87).

Definition and Etiology

IPMN-B, including its cystic variants, has mainly been described in the East, initially in patients with hepatolithiasis (see Chapter 39) or *Clonorchiasis* infection (see Chapter 45).[145] It develops in the bile duct lumen and is characterized by innumerable frond-like papillary infoldings, which consist of columnar epithelial cells surrounding slender fibrovascular stalks supported by connective tissue from the lamina propria. Further stratification is based on the presence and severity of atypia of the biliary epithelia: *Type 1* is low-grade dysplasia, *type 2* is high-grade dysplasia, *type 3* is in situ and microinvasive adenocarcinoma, and *type 4* is invasive adenocarcinoma (see Chapter 87). Types 3 and 4 are associated with papillary tumor tissue and mucobilia in the large, dilated ducts containing stones, whereas this is frequently absent in type 1 lesions, and intraductal spreading is virtually constant. This description was somewhat confusing because these tumors had been observed in a specific context of chronic biliary inflammation; however, it has subsequently been described in the absence of such conditions,[6,146,147] although etiology remains unknown. IPMN-B are much more prevalent in the East than in the West, and the ratio of IPMN-B to MCN is 6:1 in Asia and 1:3 or 1:6 in the West.[10]

Pathology (see Chapter 87)

Cystic IPMN-B morphologically is multilocular and frequently contains mucinous fluid (Fig. 88B.10). It may also occasionally be hemorrhagic.[6] Papillary mural nodules within an otherwise smooth or finely granular wall are virtually constant except in totally benign lesions.[148] In situ or invasive adenocarcinomas are particularly prevalent in IPMN-B and are present overall in up to 60% to 70% of the patients, and even higher rates have been found in the cystic variant.[148,149] This may either be a mucinous carcinoma, associated with profuse mucous secretion; a tubular adenocarcinoma, invading the bile duct wall with abundant fibrous stroma at the base of the papillary lesions and commonly associated with vascular, lymphatic, and perineural invasion; or a combination of these.[6,7]

As for IPMN-P, the lining epithelia of IPMN-B has been classified into a *pancreatobiliary type, intestinal type, gastric type,* and *oncocytic type,*[7] although these subtypes may occasionally coexist. More simply, it can be categorized as a *columnar type,* which resembles the intestinal type of IPMN-P, and a *cuboidal type,* which resembles the pancreatobiliary type or oncocytic variant of IPMN-P.[147] In one study, both were observed in the cystic form of IPMN-B, whereas only the columnar type was observed in the ductectatic form (see Chapter 87).

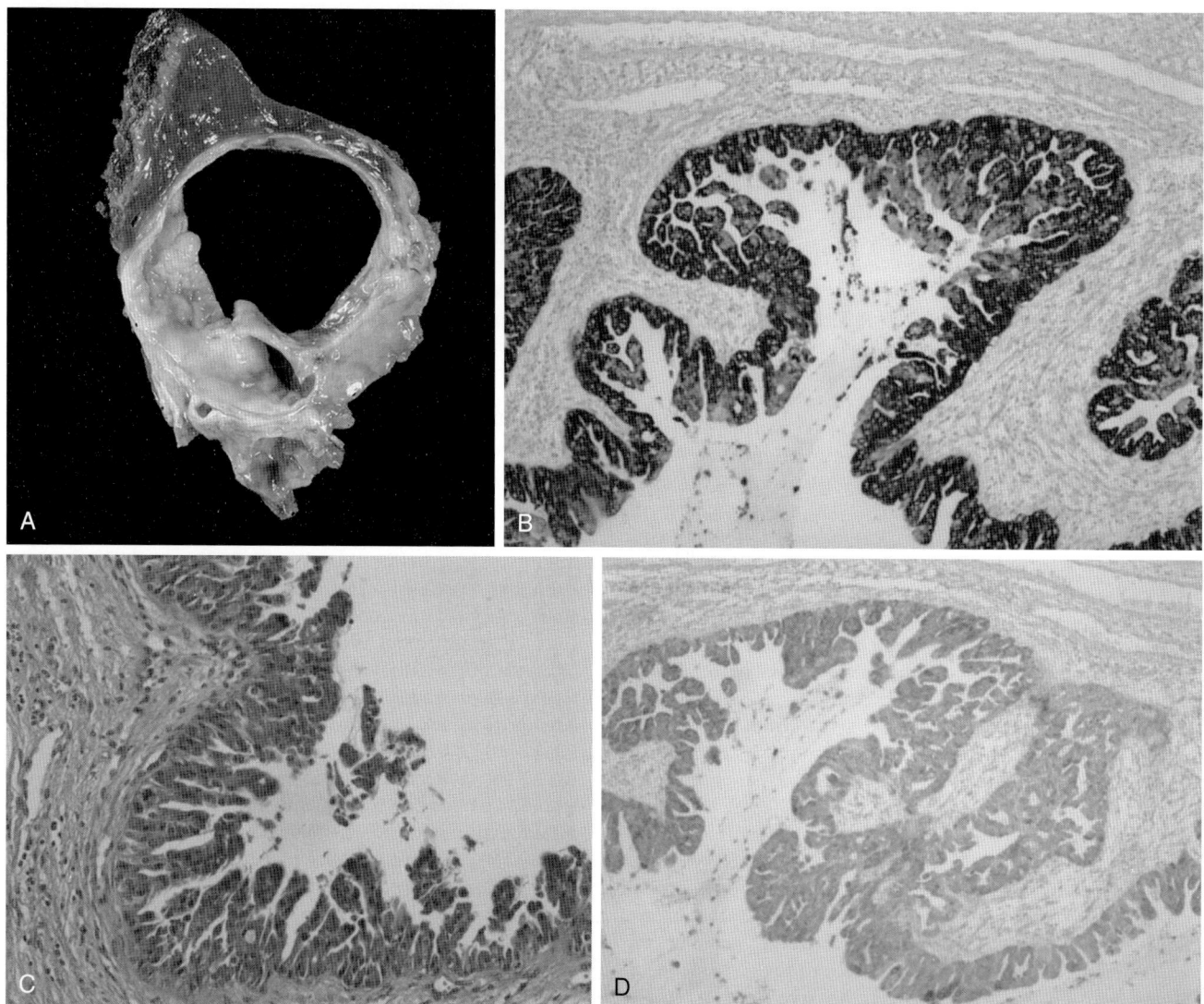

FIGURE 88B.10 Intraductal papillary mucinous neoplasia of the bile ducts. **A,** Macroscopic view showing a multilocular cyst characterized by papillary mural nodules within a smooth wall. **B,** The lining epithelium is composed of papillary projections made of several layers of atypical cells. No features of mural invasion are present. **C,** Epithelial proliferation is strongly positive for mucin 5 (MUC5). **D,** Cell proliferation displays slight mucin 1 (MUC1) staining (see Chapter 87).

A parallel has been established between the cell type and the incidence of malignant changes. Cuboidal pancreatobiliary oncocytic-type epithelium is more frequently—actually, almost always—associated with the presence of carcinoma than the columnar type, but this is more frequently a superficial (in situ) tumor than an invasive one.[6,147]

The epithelium stains positive for CK-7 (biliary phenotype) and occasionally and inconsistently for CK-20 (intestinal phenotype). CA19-9 is observed diffusely, and CEA is restricted to areas of high-grade dysplasia and sometimes carcinoma.[6,7]

Although MUC5AC is expressed in virtually all patients (gastric phenotype), MUC2 (intestinal phenotype) is more frequent in the columnar type, and MUC6 is more often seen in the cuboidal type.[6,7,147] MUC1 is, in contrast, not expressed except in some invasive areas of tubular cholangiocarcinomas, in which MUC2 expression may disappear.[6,7,147]

More recently, a collaborating consensus study by Japanese and Korean pathologists[139] introduced a new classification of IPNM-B: (1) type 1 is defined as a neoplasm showing well-organized and relatively uniform papillary growth with thin fibrovascular stalks. In addition to the fine papillary architecture, tubular or slightly complex architectural components rarely coexist. Gross mucin is common. In many cases, the tumor is composed of high-grade lesions, but rarely low/moderate-grade lesions may coexist. This type is predominant in intrahepatic IPMN-B; (2) type 2 is defined as showing complex papillary growth with thick papillae or irregular branching. Tubular, cribriform, and solid components may also be observed. This type is predominant in extrahepatic distal IPMN-B. These two types are associated with distinct pathologic and molecular phenotypes as well as prognosis.[150] Type 1 IPMN-B has a noninvasive phenotype, intestinal and oncocytic subtypes, overt mucin production, and a 5-year survival of 91%. Type 2 IPNM-B is associated with an invasive phenotype, the pancreatobiliary subtype, and worse prognosis compared with the type 1 with a 5-year survival of 59%.

Diagnosis

Cystic variants of IPMN-B develop almost equally in both sexes and peak in the sixth decade, which is 10 to 20 years more than for cystadenoma with an OS.[6,147] Many patients are asymptomatic, with their tumor discovered during a general health examination, but epigastralgia, jaundice, and cholangitis may occur. Cystic variants cannot be differentiated from cystadenoma or cystadenocarcinoma by their diameter, which may range between 2 and 17 cm,[69,151] nor can they be discerned by thickness of septa or presence of calcifications[69]; however, cystic variants are more frequently associated with prominent or large (>1 cm) mural nodules and bile duct dilation distal to the tumor. The latter is because of the issue of mucus from the cyst in the bile ducts. Communication with the biliary lumen is indeed a key feature,[105] but CT and MRI are insufficient to show the luminal communication,[69,143,151] probably because it is too narrow. Preoperative ERCP or IOC is more reliable; in contrast, macroscopic examination of the specimen is inaccurate.[6]

Complications

The two main complications of cystic variants of IPMN-B relate to the migration of mucus or tumor material in the bile ducts and to malignant transformation. Mucobilia may result in transient symptoms of biliary obstruction, and biliary obstruction by mucus has occasionally resulted in bile duct rupture.[152] Malignant transformation is particularly frequent, although the stage of malignancy is less advanced than for other biliary tumors.[7] Because most of these tumors show malignant changes at the time of diagnosis, they are likely slow growing. High-grade dysplasia and invasive carcinoma seem more prevalent in IPMN-B than in IPMN-P.[10]

Management and Prognosis

Cystic IPMN-B requires resection, and an IOC should be performed to document the biliary communication and rule out the presence of mucus in the bile duct (see Chapters 24 and 101). Because IPMN-B may spread superficially along the lumen of the bile ducts or be present in adjacent ducts, simple enucleation of the cyst may be insufficient. Formal hepatectomy should be performed, occasionally with extrahepatic bile duct resection and lymph node sampling. Even in patients with associated carcinoma, the prognosis is better than after resection of intrahepatic or hilar cholangiocarcinoma.[6,7,147,148] Five-year survival is 61% and may be as high as 80% for those patients with the cuboidal cell type. Survival after resection of malignant IPMN-B is adversely impacted by the presence of the columnar cell type[147] and MUC1 expression.[147,153]

CONCLUSION

Cystic tumors of the liver are rare and include different entities that should be stratified with regard to content (mucinous or nonmucinous), tumor stroma (presence or absence of an OS), and relation to the bile ducts (communicating with the lumen or not). Cystic tumors with an OS (cystadenoma) occur in women, do not typically communicate with the bile duct, and, in most cases, are adenomas, although no reliable criterion differentiates them from cystadenocarcinoma. Malignant transformation may occur in up to 5%, although higher figures have been reported in the past. IPMN-B lesions may have a cystic appearance, occur in both sexes, and communicate with the biliary lumen, although this may be difficult to document; they may spread beyond the cystic mass in the adjacent bile ducts and frequently harbor severe dysplasia or malignancy, which may be either invasive or superficial. These lesions share several features and are currently considered to be the counterparts of the same lesions occurring in the pancreas; in any event, they require complete resection. Cystadenoma without an OS is an ill-defined entity that is no longer accepted by pathologists worldwide because they may include some IPMN-B or atypical cysts.

References are available at expertconsult.com.

SECTION II. Neoplastic

C. Malignant Tumors

CHAPTER 89

Hepatocellular carcinoma

Leonardo Gomes da Fonseca, Joana Ferrer-Fàbrega, and Jordi Bruix

OVERVIEW

Hepatocellular carcinoma (HCC) is the most common primary liver tumor and results in approximately 800,000 deaths globally per year. Worldwide, liver tumors represent the fourth leading cause of cancer death and the sixth most common neoplasia.[1] Its incidence presents marked geographic differences, therein Asia and sub-Saharan Africa constitute high-risk areas with yearly incidence exceeding 20 cases per 100,000 population.[2] Incidence rates and mortality are increasing in many parts of the world including North America, Latin America, and Central Europe, whereas it appears to be decreasing in Japan.[3–6] The prevalence is 3-fold higher in males compared with females and the peak incidence is around the sixth and seventh decade of life.[7]

HCC usually develops in the setting of chronic liver disease, particularly in patients with cirrhosis (see Chapter 74). The main background etiologies are chronic viral hepatitis B (HBV) and C (HCV) infections, alcoholic liver disease, and metabolic dysfunction-associated fatty liver disease (MAFLD)[8] (see Chapters 68, 69, and 74). The burden of risk factors, as well as the geographic distribution, are being reshaped by the implementation of universal HBV vaccination, the widespread use of direct-acting antiviral (DAA) drugs against HCV, and the growing occurrence of MAFLD-associated comorbidities (obesity, diabetes, dyslipidemia, and others) that frequently overlap with excessive alcohol consumption.[9]

Because HCC is a major global health problem, preventive and therapeutic strategies are areas of increasing interest among clinical researchers. Nevertheless, the 5-year survival rate is between 5% and 15%,[10,11] which reflects the challenging management of these patients.

This chapter provides an overview of the epidemiology, diagnosis, and therapeutic approaches to HCC.

EPIDEMIOLOGY, RISK FACTORS, AND PREVENTION

Cirrhosis is the major determinant of HCC and can be caused by viral infections (HBV and HCV), MAFLD, alcohol intake alpha-1 antitrypsin deficiency, and hereditary hemochromatosis, among others (see Chapter 74). One-third of cirrhosis patients will develop HCC throughout their lifetime, with an annual risk of 1% to 8%, depending on the etiology. The risk is

greater the more relevant the signs are and the more severe the liver disease is.[12]

The geographic distribution of HCC varies widely according to ethnic groups and regions, with a clear association with exposure to hepatitis viruses and environmental pathogens. The majority of cases (80%) occur in sub-Saharan Africa and West Asia, where there is a high prevalence of HBV infection and exposure to aflatoxin B1, a mycotoxin produced by *Aspergillus* species that induces a specific p53 mutation that offers proliferation advantages. In addition to cirrhosis, the risk of developing HCC among patients with chronic HBV is related to high viral load, active viral replication, genotype C, and the presence of liver dysfunction. HBV-related HCC can develop even in the absence of cirrhosis in 20% to 30% of the cases, and inactive HBV carriers are also at increased risk because of HBV gene integration into the host genome.[13,14] A significant impact on reducing HCC-related deaths through HBV vaccination has been reported in endemic areas, such as Taiwan.[15]

In Japan and Western countries (especially Europe and the United States), the main risk factor is chronic HCV infection. HCC in patients with HCV occurs almost exclusively in the setting of advanced stage liver disease or cirrhosis. There is increasing evidence that HCV treatment decreases, but does not eliminate, the risk of HCC.[16] The rate of HCV-related HCC is expected to decrease or stabilize in the coming years[17] because of the effectiveness of DAAs in inducing a sustained virologic response in higher rates compared with the ancient interferon-based regimens. A meta-analysis has shown that sustained virologic response is associated with a reduced risk of developing HCC.[18] On the other hand, it has been hypothesized that the use of DAAs in patients previously treated for HCC may be related to early recurrences with aggressive biological behaviour, which raises concern on the wide applicability of DAA in patients with past HCC.[19] This is still a highly controversial issue with major heterogeneity between different studies preventing a robust conclusion.

A noticeable transition in risk factors has been observed in Western countries. There is growing evidence that MAFLD is an increasingly frequent liver condition in patients who develop HCC, often associated with other comorbidities such as obesity, hypertension, and diabetes,[8] but clearly overlapping with alcohol consumption (see Chapter 69). It is likely that MAFLD causes HCC via cirrhosis, but the precise pathogenesis has not yet been elucidated because some cases are reported to happen in the absence of cirrhosis.[8] A national United States registry on liver transplantations between 2002 and 2016 showed that HCV and alcohol intake etiologies remained stable, HBV decreased, and there was a relevant increase in the so-called "non-alcoholic steatohepatitis" that nowadays has been grouped under the new name of MAFLD.[8,17,20] This trend projects an ascending burden of MAFLD-related HCC in the coming years and the need to implement strategies to prevent and reduce risk factors associated with metabolic syndrome. However, in patients with MAFLD the main cause of death is because of cardiovascular events, thus stressing the need for a multiorgan approach beyond individual specialities to manage these patients.[21]

Protective factors include HBV vaccination and antiviral treatment for both HBV and HCV[9,22] (see Chapter 68). Proper controls in healthcare settings prevent HCV dissemination through blood transmission. Alcohol intake should be the target of health campaigns in the community and aflatoxin contamination of food can be prevented by avoiding grain storage in humid conditions. Also, the epidemic of obesity must be controlled by health education. Secondary prevention in patients with chronic liver disease requires the prior recognition of affected individuals, but no proof of the cost-effectiveness of population screening for liver disease has been offered. Finally, observational studies support that statins,[23] aspirin,[24] and coffee consumption[25] reduce the risk of HCC, but additional evidence is needed to clarify if any alimentary or pharmacologic measure impacts in reducing the risk of HCC.

MOLECULAR PROFILE

Hepatocarcinogenesis is a complex process in which several molecular landmarks and signaling pathways are involved (see Chapter 9B). Genomic analyses are predominantly restricted to early-stage resected HCC samples, which inadvertently depicts early genetic and epigenetic events that might not reflect intermediate and advanced stages. Nevertheless, there has been accumulating knowledge of some of the molecular hits behind the initiation and progression of HCC.

The most frequent alterations described are related to telomerase maintenance (telomerase reverse transcriptase [TERT] promoter), CTNNB1/Wnt-Beta-catenin pathway activation, p53 mutations, and MAP kinase signaling. Moreover, some targetable pathways are explored in translational research, such as the activation of c-MET, fibroblast growth factor receptor (FGFR), vascular endothelial growth factor receptor (VEGFR), and transforming growth factor beta (TGF-β), among others.[26,27] (Targeted therapies will be discussed elsewhere in this chapter.)

A first molecular-based classification divided HCC into two classes: the proliferative class, which is tagged by activation of RAS pathway, FGF amplification, HBV infection, and poor prognosis, and the nonproliferative class, which is characterized by Wnt-Beta-catenin alterations and HCV infection.[28]

In another approach based on whole-genome sequencing, three HCC integrated clusters were identified. Cluster 1 has low mutation frequency of CTNNB1, low expression of TERT, and was associated with early stage and Asian origin. Clusters 2 and 3 have higher prevalence of TERT promoter and CTNNB1 mutations, whereas cluster 3 also presents with high p53 mutations occurrence.[29]

Limitations of HCC molecular profiling rely on the need to distinguish "driver" events (those that are fundamental for neoplastic transformation and therefore with potential therapeutic applicability) from "passenger" events. Besides, genetic variations are heterogeneous through time, between tumor sites in the same individual, or even within a single tumor site. In spite of the advances in molecular characterization of HCC, these findings have not yet translated into substantial changes in the clinical setting.

SCREENING STRATEGIES

The purpose of screening is to reduce mortality through early detection at a stage amenable to be treated with curative modalities. Several uncontrolled studies suggest that screening for HCC results in a higher proportion of early diagnoses, higher cure rates, and better prognosis.[30,31] A Chinese study of more than 18,000 participants randomized patients with chronic HBV infection to perform screening with ultrasound and serum alpha-fetoprotein (AFP) every 6 months. HCC mortality was significantly reduced in the screening group (83.2 vs. 131.5 per 100,000 person).[32] This trial, however, had low adherence among the participants and was carried out in a population with a particular risk factor (HBV). Even though the data have not been reproduced globally and it seems unfeasible for ethical reasons, the use of screening in patients with cirrhosis is widely established in clinical practice.

The selection of individuals to screening is determined by the risk of developing HCC, life expectancy, and local health structure conditions that allow for proper treatment. Cost-effectiveness studies suggest that screening should be applied when the risk of HCC is at least 1.5% per year, regardless of the etiology of liver disease.[31] This includes all patients with cirrhosis who are potential candidates to receive anti-tumor treatment, in addition to some subgroups without cirrhosis with chronic HBV infection and high-risk according to recently proposed scores, such as PAGE-B[33] or Toronto- THRI.[34] Cirrhotic patients with sustained virologic response after treatment for HCV must remain under screening because this condition does not eliminate the risk of HCC.[18]

On the other hand, it is not clear whether noncirrhotic patients with HCV (e.g., with bridging fibrosis) should be screened. Still, for nonviral etiologies such as MAFLD, it is not defined which subgroups benefit from screening. This is because of the heterogeneous incidence of HCC within these scenarios and the fact that the HCC can arise even in the absence of cirrhosis.

Ultrasonography is the screening study of choice because it balances cost and availability (see Chapter 14). Sensitivities of 60% to 80% and specificity greater than 90% are reported for screening liver tumors[35] using ultrasonography. The use of serum AFP measurement is commonly applied. However, this marker has low sensitivity because, in general, it is not increased in small tumors and may be altered because of the underlying liver disease, as well as in patients with cholangiocarcinoma (CC). Cirrhosis is also a risk factor for CC and hence a primary hepatic mass associated to increased AFP may correspond to either HCC or CC. Other biomarkers are being analyzed for their role in early detection such as des-y-carboxyprothrombin, AFP-lectin, and glypcan-3.

The recommended screening interval is semiannual. This recommendation is based on estimates of tumor growth rate and illustrated by a prospective study that showed better performance of 6-month than 12 month interval in detecting early lesions, and the 3-month interval increased the detection of small nodules without impacting survival.[36] The role of other imaging methods, such as computed tomography (CT) and magnetic resonance imaging (MRI) as screening for HCC is not yet established.

The European Association for the Study of the Liver (EASL)[9] and the American Association for Study of Liver Disease (AASLD)[22] recommend abdominal ultrasonography every 6 months. Because of the suboptimal accuracy of the AFP serum level, the determination of this marker is optional.

CLINICAL PRESENTATION

There is a range of clinical presentations for patients with HCC, from asymptomatic (as in cases diagnosed in screening programs) to severe symptoms. Symptoms may occur because of the underlying cirrhosis (ascites, jaundice, abdominal collateral circulation, upper digestive hemorrhage, hepatic encephalopathy) or because of tumor growth and spread (abdominal pain, weight loss, palpable abdominal mass, dyspnea, and bone pain).

A sudden worsening of liver function in a patient with otherwise stable chronic liver disease should be investigated for the possibility of HCC. Ascites and variceal bleeding may develop because of portal or hepatic vein invasion. Paraneoplastic syndromes such as diarrhea, hypoglycemia, erythrocytosis, and hypercalcemia may also be present and are generally associated with poor prognosis.[37]

DIAGNOSIS

For patients with cirrhosis, the diagnosis can be made using dynamic contrast-enhanced imaging techniques based on the neovascularization process that occurs during the hepatocarcinogenesis. Malignant lesions develop blood supply from the hepatic artery, unlike the nontumor liver parenchyma whose supply is predominantly from the portal system. For this reason, HCC nodules show contrast uptake in the arterial phase and "wash-out" in the venous and late phases (Fig. 89.1). This pattern has a sensitivity of around 80% and a specificity of

at least 90% in liver nodules larger than 2 cm in the context of cirrhosis[38] (see Chapter 14).

On detection of an abnormal finding in ultrasonography, further evaluation must be performed. Nodules measuring less than 1 cm in a cirrhotic liver may not correspond to a malignant focus in greater than 60% of cases, so close follow-up in 3 to 4 months is recommended. In a cirrhotic liver, nodules larger than 1 cm can be diagnosed as HCC if the vascular profile on imaging techniques is typical.[9,22] In these cases, a single dynamic imaging technique can establish the diagnosis (e.g., CT or MRI; see Chapter 14). If the characteristic dynamic profile is not recognized, fine-needle biopsy is recommended. It must be stressed that biopsy is not 100% sensitive; hence a negative result does not exclude HCC. Other tumor markers, such as protein induced by vitamin K absence (PIVK), AFP fractions, and glypican-3, have been proposed to be used alone or in combination with AFP, but their usefulness in routine clinical practice has not been established.[39] Immunohistochemical markers, such as Hsp-70, glypcan-3, and glutamine synthetase, can increase the specificity of the histologic diagnosis, but do not replace expert pathology analysis.[40] In the context of a noncirrhotic liver, the diagnosis must be made by histology.

The American College of Radiology has proposed a system for estimating the likelihood of malignancy. This system is called the Liver Imaging Reporting and Data System (LI-RADS) and classifies lesions into 5 categories, from definitely benign (1) to definitely malignant (5), with the objective of providing guidance for subsequent management.[41] LI-RADS may be useful for homogenous reporting but seems to aggregate little changes to what is already the current practice based on the well-established radiologic criteria. Prospective studies to define the role of LI-RADS in the clinical realm are awaited[42] (see Chapter 14).

STAGING AND PROGNOSTIC EVALUATION

Considering that the majority of patients with HCC have associated liver disease, prognostic evaluation should assess not only the extent of tumor involvement but also the severity of liver function impairment. In addition, performance status

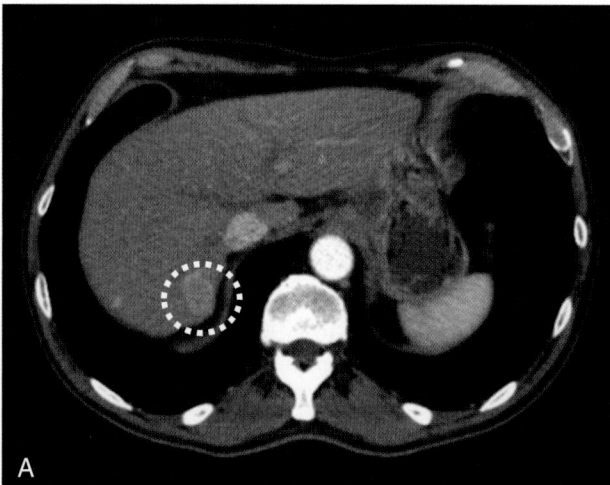 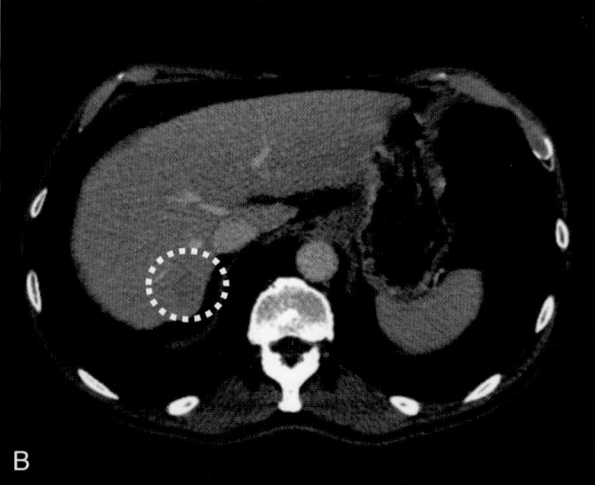

FIGURE 89.1 Computed tomography (CT) scan depicts a 3.5-cm nodule in segment VII, hypervascular in arterial phase **(A)** and faint hypovascular in portal phase **(B)**. (See Chapter 14.)

TABLE 89.1	Prognostic Systems to Predict Outcome in Hepatocellular Carcinoma Patients				
PROGNOSTIC SYSTEM (YEAR)	**NO.**	**TUMOR STAGE**	**LIVER FUNCTION**	**HEALTH STATUS**	**STAGES**
Okuda (1985)	850	Tumor involvement > 50%	Bilirubin, albumin, ascites		I, II, III
CLIP (1998)	435	Tumor morphology, AFP, portal vein invasion	Child-Pugh		0–6
GRETCH (1999)	761	Portal vein invasion and AFP	Bilirubin, alkaline phosphatase	Karnofsky	A–C
AJCC TNM (2002)		Number of nodules, tumor size, portal vein invasion, metastases			I, II, III, IV
CUPI (2002)	926	TNM and AFP	Bilirubin, ascites, alkaline phosphatase	Symptoms	Score 0–12 3 risk groups
JIS (2003)	722	TNM by LCSGJ	Child-Pugh		0–5
SLiDe (2004)	177	TNM by LCSGJ	Liver damage by LCSGJ, PIVKA		0–3
Tokyo (2005)	403	Number of nodules and tumor size	Albumin, bilirubin		0–8
Taipei Integrated (2010)	2030	Total tumor volume and AFP	Child-Pugh		0–6
BCLC (1999)		Number of nodules, tumor size, portal vein invasion metastases	Child-Pugh, portal hypertension	PS	0, A-D
Yau (2014)	3856	Number of nodules, tumor size, portal vein invasion	Child-Pugh	PS	9 stages I–Vb

AFP, α-Fetoprotein; *AJCC*, American Joint Commission on Cancer; *BCLC*, Barcelona Clinic Liver Cancer; *CLIP*, Cancer of the Liver Italian Program; *CUPI*, Chinese University Prognostic Index; *JIS*, Japan Integrated Scoring; *LCSGJ*, Liver Cancer Study Group of Japan; *PIVKA*, protein induced by vitamin K absence or antagonist; *PS*, performance status; *SLiDe*, (S, stage; Li, liver damage; De, des-gamma-carboxy prothrombin score); *TNM*, tumor-node-metastasis classification from the AJCC/UICC; *UICC*, Union Internationale Contre Cancer [International Union against Cancer].

and cancer-related symptoms are key determinants of survival. A number of systems and algorithms have been proposed to predict prognosis for HCC, such as the Cancer of the Liver Italian Program (CLIP) score, the Tumor-Node-Metastasis (TNM), the Hong Kong Liver Cancer staging system, the albumin-bilirubin (ALBI) score, and the Okuda system[43-47] (Table 89.1).

The Barcelona Clinic Liver Cancer (BCLC) strategy has been widely validated in assessing prognosis because it incorporates all relevant dimensions to predict prognosis: tumor burden, liver function, and cancer related symptoms (Fig. 89.2). Its original version was in 1999 and over the years it has incorporated updated concepts in the management of HCC.[48,49] The BCLC classification includes five stages (0, A, B, C, and D) according to prognostic variables related to liver function (preserved or end-stage liver disease), status performance according to the Eastern Cooperative Oncology Group (ECOG) scale, and tumor burden. Because it links staging, prognosis prediction, clinical decision-making and treatment indication, the BCLC classification has become a widely accepted clinical tool for treatment decision making.[9,22] Also, it has been shown that the BCLC staging system outperforms other prognosis systems[50] (see Chapter 4).

The very early (BCLC 0) and early (BCLC A) stages correspond to patients with a single tumor of up to 2 cm and single lesions irrespective of size or up to 3 nodules of up to 3 cm, respectively, in the absence of vascular invasion and cancer symptoms and with preserved liver function. These patients should be considered for local treatments with a curative intention such as surgical resection, liver transplantation, or percutaneous ablation. Their 5-year survival ranges from 50% to 70%.[51,52] Intermediate stage (BCLC B) includes those patients who have multifocal tumors with preserved liver function. These cases should be considered for transarterial chemoembolization (TACE), which may achieve a 50% survival rate at 3 years.[53] Tumors should be able to be selectively approached

to prevent damage to the nontumoral liver and liver disease should be compensated (no clinically relevant ascites in need of treatment). Tumors that present with diffuse, infiltrative or extensive bilobar involvement should be considered for systemic therapies.

The advanced stage (BCLC C) includes patients with preserved liver function and with one or more of the following characteristics: extrahepatic dissemination, vascular invasion, or nonsevere impairment of functionality (ECOG 1–2). These patients benefit from systemic treatment with the aim to increase survival and improve quality of life. Sequences of systemic agents provide an extended overall survival (OS) of around 2 years.[54]

Finally, terminal stage (BCLC D) is characterized by liver dysfunction or severe functional impairment (ECOG 3–4). This group has a dismal prognosis and should receive best supportive care to minimize symptoms.

TREATMENT APPROACHES

Appropriate treatment selection is complex and patients with HCC should ideally be managed in reference centers with multidisciplinary teams including hepatologists, surgeons, radiologists, pathologists, radiation oncologists, and clinical oncologists. The level of evidence for many modalities is limited to cohort studies and retrospective series, whereas there are randomized studies performed in the setting of intermediate and advanced stages. Thus major research is needed in several scenarios.

Treatment alternatives include local (resection, transplantation, and ablation), intra-arterial (TACE and transarterial radioembolization [TARE]) and systemic therapies (tyrosine kinase inhibitors, monoclonal antibodies, and immunotherapy). Guidelines and algorithms are useful for conceptualization and standardization, but the approach should be personalized according to each individual context.

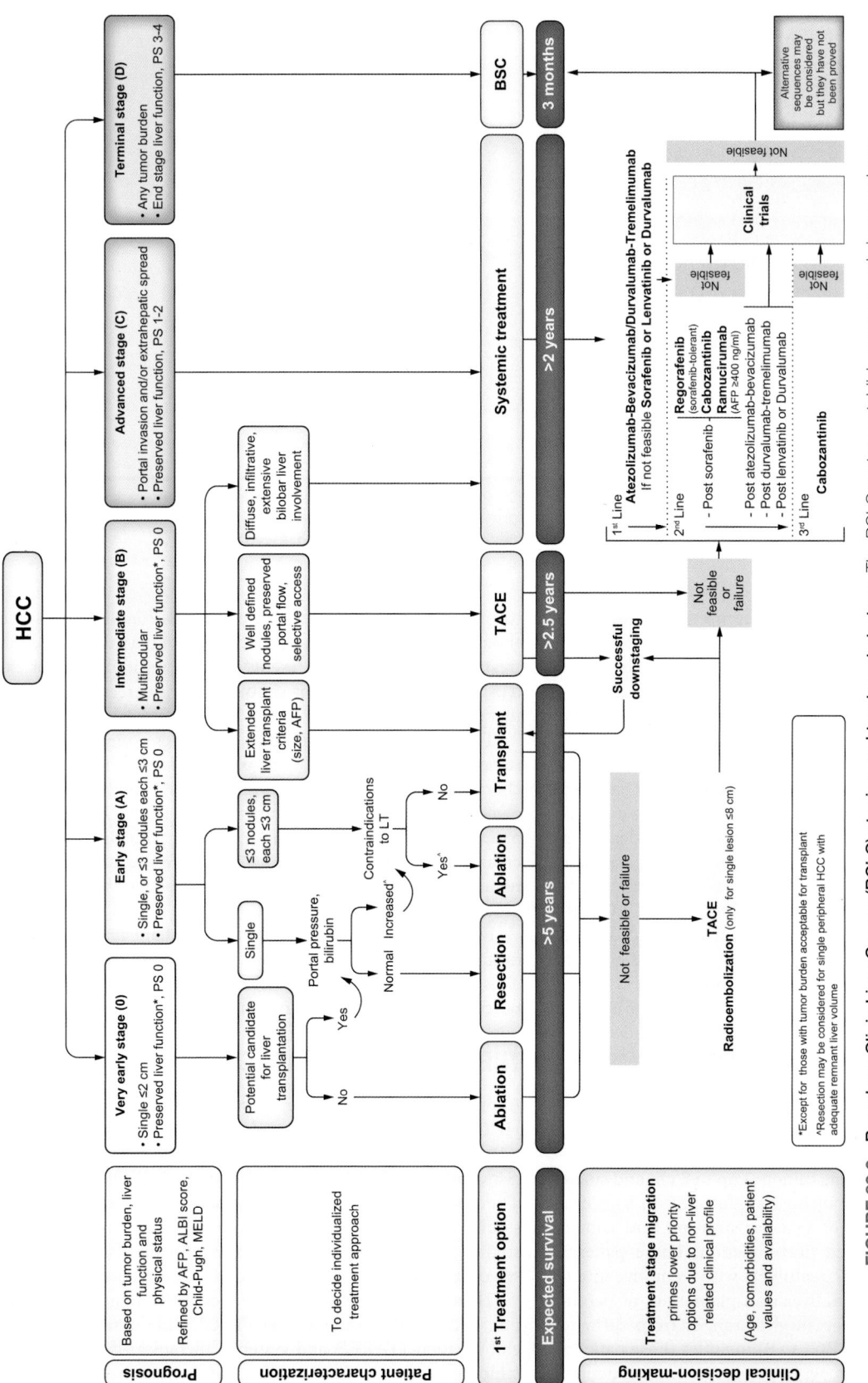

FIGURE 89.2 Barcelona Clinic Liver Cancer (BCLC) staging and treatment strategy. The BCLC system establishes a prognosis in accordance with the 5 stages that are linked to first-line treatment recommendation. The expected outcome is expressed as median survival of each tumour stage according to the available scientific evidence. Individualised clinical decision-making, according to the available data on November 15, 2021, is defined by teams responsible for integrating all available data with the individual patient's medical profile. Note that liver function should be evaluated beyond the conventional Child-Pugh staging. *AFP*, alpha-fetoprotein; *ALBI*, albumin-bilirubin; *BCLC*, Barcelona Clinic Liver Cancer; *BSC*, best supportive care; *ECOG-PS*, Eastern Cooperative Oncology Group-performance status; *LT*, liver transplantation; *MELD*, model of end-stage liver disease; *TACE*, transarterial chemoembolisation. From: Reig M, Forner A, Rimola J, Ferrer-Fàbrega J, Burrel M, Garcia-Criado A, Kelley RK, Galle PR, Mazzaferro V, Salem R, Sangro B, Singal AG, Vogel A, Fuster J, Ayuso C, Bruix J. BCLC strategy for prognosis prediction and treatment recommendation: The 2022 update. J Hepatol. 2022 Mar;76(3):681-693. doi: 10.1016/j.jhep.2021.11.018. Epub 2021 Nov 19. PMID: 34801630; PMCID: PMC8866082.

Surgery

Liver resection is the treatment of choice for localized HCC in the absence of cirrhosis (see Chapters 101, 102, and 118). Patients with compensated cirrhosis should be thoroughly evaluated for the risk of decompensation. In cases with severe liver dysfunction, however, surgery is formally contraindicated (see Chapter 120).

Assessment of liver function is crucial to achieving favorable outcomes (see Chapter 4). Postoperative mortality is significant reduced in those patients with normal bilirubin and absence of clinically significant portal hypertension.[52] Thrombocytopenia, esophageal varices, ascites, and splenomegaly are indirect markers of portal hypertension. Nevertheless, hepatic vein catheterization is the most accurate tool to measure portal pressure, and hepatic pressure gradient less than 10 mm Hg is the best cutoff value.[55] Alternatively, clinically significant portal hypertension may be established by elastography, avoiding the need for hepatic vein catheterization.[56] In selected patients, 5-year survival rate reaches 70% to 80% with surgical resection. Patients with portal hypertension are at high risk for liver decompensation and death after surgery, with survival rates at 5 years of 50%.[52,55,57]

Optimal results with resection are demonstrated in single lesions, although in some groups, selected cases with two or three nodules may be considered for resection after careful evaluation. The tumor size is not a limiting factor, but the risk of recurrence is higher the larger the tumor is. Vascular invasion denotes an elevated risk of systemic recurrence and therefore should be ideally managed with systemic therapy. Even so, some groups advocate that patients with segmental vascular invasion may benefit from resection.[58]

Despite advances in diagnostic capacity, underestimation of tumour extension continues to be a possibility. It is therefore essential to have an intraoperative ultrasound to detect potential unrecognised nodules between 0.5 and 1 cm and optimize the surgical resection efficacy, while at the same time being instrumental to perform anatomical resections (Fig. 89.3). Advances in laparoscopic-robotic surgery allow a less invasive surgical treatment and provide comparable results in terms of

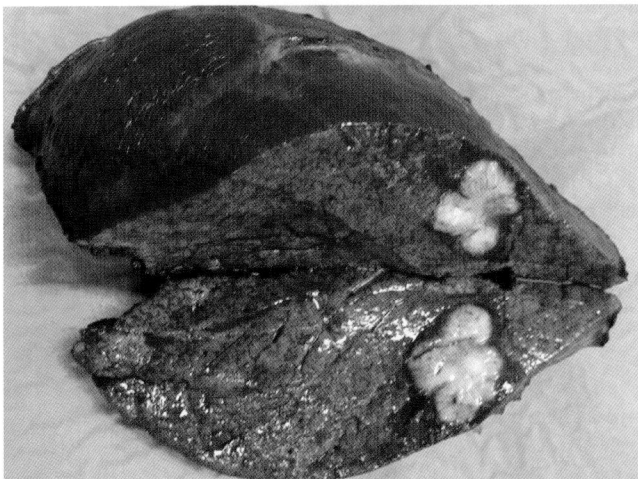

FIGURE 89.3 Surgical specimen of a segmental hepatic resection. Segment-oriented resections maximize the elimination of tumor satellites, although this goal may be hampered by tumor size and growth pattern. (See Chapters 101 and 102.)

survival with lower perioperative morbidity and shorter hospital stays.[59,60]

Three international consensus conferences were held in 2008 in Louisville in the United States,[61] in 2014 in Morioka, Japan,[62] and in 2017 in Southampton, UK,[63] which provided up-to-date summaries of the status and perspective of laparoscopic liver resection. No differences in operative time, blood loss, intraoperative complications, hospital stay, and morbidity were found in laparoscopic liver resection for cirrhotic compared with noncirrhotic patients. In fact, a laparoscopic approach appears to reduce the incidence of postoperative ascites, liver failure, and morbidity with no difference in overall or disease-free survival at 2 years. The minimally invasive approach could play a role in the context of "expanding indications" beyond the "ideal candidate"[64,65] (see Chapters 127D and 127E).

Disease recurrence after resection might be predicted by pathologic findings such as poor differentiation degree, presence of satellites/multifocality, and the existence of microvascular invasion. Because of the high risk of recurrence, at the BCLC, we have proposed enlistment for transplantation in those patients with resected HCC who have pathology-registered pejorative histologic markers ("ab initio indication").[66]

There is no proof of benefit of any adjuvant therapy to prevent recurrence and thus no approach should be recommended.

Liver Transplantation

Liver transplantation has the advantage of approaching both the tumor and the underlying liver disease and is recommended as the first-line option for HCC within Milan criteria[9,22] (see Chapters 105 and 108).

The Milan criteria (1 nodule ≤ 5 cm or even 3 nodules ≤ 3 cm, in the absence of portal invasion or extrahepatic disease[67]) are widely used, although there are increasing data suggesting the potential benefit of liver transplantation in cases with larger tumor burden (e.g., using the University of California San Francisco [UCSF] expanded criteria).[68] Within Milan criteria, the 5-year survival rate is 60% to 80%, with a recurrence rate of less than 15%.[67] The level of AFP can also be used, once levels greater than 1000 ng/mL are associated with high risk of recurrence.[69,70]

Bridging therapies, such as TACE or ablation (see Chapters 94 and 96), are often needed for patients on the waiting list to reduce the risk of tumor progression, especially when the time on the list is longer than 6 months. Likewise, downstaging using locoregional therapies can be used to increase eligibility for liver transplantation, but the key in such instance is what criteria should be used for staging and potential downstaging. Results with downstaging are variable, mainly because of differences in eligibility criteria. Although successful downstaging can tend to be lower in more liberal criteria, rates of downstaging achievement can reach up to 90% when more strict criteria are applied.[71]

Living donor liver transplantation offers the possibility to avoid waiting lists for a deceased organ, which can be an important benefit in HCC patients because it reduces the dropout rate and time to transplant.[72] In addition to reducing the risk of dropout, living donor transplantation has the potential to provide access to liver transplantation for patients who otherwise would not be eligible for a deceased-donor liver according to Milan criteria. On the other hand, it is important to mention that living-donor transplantation must be restricted to centers of excellence to minimize donor risk and optimize recipient outcome (see Chapters 109 and 121).

Percutaneous Ablation (see Chapter 96)

Percutaneous treatment is proposed for patients with liver-only disease who are not candidates for surgery or transplantation.[73] Radiofrequency and microwave ablation are the main techniques, but ethanol injection can be used in particular situations, such as tumor in a subcapsular location or in the vicinity of the gallbladder, blood vessels, or heart. The best results with ablation are achieved in solitary tumors smaller than 2 cm,[74] where these techniques may achieve complete necrosis and recurrence rates comparable to resection. However, tumors between 2 to 3 cm or up to three nodules may also be treated percutaneously.[75–77] It has been suggested that resection was not superior to ablation in tumors of up to 3 cm, but there is a need for further comparative trials to validate these findings.[77,78]

External radiotherapy and stereotactic body radiation therapy have been explored in some settings (e.g., segmental portal vein invasion) with encouraging results but still lacks robust evidence on safety and efficacy[79,80] (see Chapter 95).

Intra-arterial Therapy

Patients with liver-only HCC without vascular invasion who are not amenable to resection, transplantation, or ablation should be considered for intra-arterial therapies[9,22] (see Chapter 94). These therapies aim to induce tumor necrosis, exploiting the predominant arterial blood supply of HCC. This allows for the selective infusion of embolizing particles coupled or not with cytotoxic agents or for the intraarterial infusion of radioactive isotopes.

Intra-arterial drug-eluting beads that slowly release chemotherapy or conventional chemoembolization using emulsion of cytotoxic agents with lipiodol followed by spongostan injection seem to have similar efficacy, but the former is suggested to have less toxicity and better tolerance.[81] Both techniques are preferred over bland embolization, although there is no firm evidence to support or refute the superiority of one over another.[82,83]

Randomized trials and metanalysis confirmed that TACE improves survival in cases not suitable for curative treatment.[84,85] Current expected median survival in patients selected according to evidence-based recommendations is around 30 months and may even exceed 40 months.[53]

Absolute contraindications to TACE include decompensated cirrhosis or severely reduced portal vein flow (tumoral or nontumoral portal vein thrombosis). It is crucial to assess liver function before and after every procedure to prevent liver function deterioration.[86] In the absence of objective response to TACE or untreatable progression, systemic therapy should be considered as part of stage migration strategy.[87]

TARE uses the injection of 90-Ytrium-labeled spheres without the need for macroembolization. There are no robust randomized studies comparing TARE with TACE; however, data suggest comparable tumor control rates.[88] In patients with BCLC C stage, TARE was not superior to sorafenib,[89,90] and it also failed to enhance the benefit of sorafenib in combination.[91] More studies are needed to place TARE into the treatment algorithms and define subgroups that benefit from this therapy.

Systemic Treatment

Systemic therapies are recommended for patients with preserved liver function who present with extrahepatic spread, have macrovascular invasion, or are ineligible for liver-directed modalities because of refractoriness or contraindication (see Chapter 99).

Until 2007, limited therapies existed for advanced stage disease. Previous studies with conventional chemotherapy (e.g., doxorubicin and platinum combinations) have resulted in significant toxicities and modest efficacy.[92,93] Nevertheless, there has been a resurgence of enthusiasm with the increasing knowledge on molecular mechanisms, intracellular signaling pathways, and angiogenesis. Subsequently, molecularly targeted agents such as sorafenib and regorafenib proved survival superiority over supportive care and pioneered the era of systemic treatment in HCC.[94]

Sorafenib, a tyrosine kinase inhibitor with antiangiogenic and antiproliferative activity, was the first drug to demonstrate increased OS in patients with advanced HCC. A survival benefit was shown both in Western and in Asian population.[95,96] Regorafenib has shown a significant increase in survival in patients with advanced HCC who had progressed on sorafenib.[97] An exploratory analysis showed that the sequence sorafenib-regorafenib provided a median survival of 26 months, which reflects a significant advance in the treatment of advanced HCC.[54]

Novel agents have shown improved outcomes in prospective randomized studies. Lenvatinib, another tyrosine kinase inhibitor, proved to be noninferior to sorafenib in the first line and was approved as an alternative to sorafenib.[98] After progression to sorafenib, regorafenib, cabozantinib (both as second- or third-line), and ramucirumab (in patients with AFP of at least 400 ng/mL) can be used based on positive results of phase III trials.[97,99,100]

The liver is a complex immunologic organ because of its physiologic immunotolerance, the abundance of immunosuppressive molecules (such as PD-1 and PDL-1), and the fact that HCC develops mostly under chronic inflammation conditions.[101] Immunity-modulating therapies are being studied in many active clinical trials. Preliminary results with immunotherapy based on anti-PD1 antibodies (nivolumab and pembrolizumab) showed encouraging response rates[102,103] but have not compared favorably with sorafenib (in the first line)[104] or placebo (in the second line)[105] (see Chapter 10).

Combinations of targeted therapies and immunotherapy are gaining prominence in the treatment of HCC. The combination of atezolizumab (anti-PDL1 antibody) and bevacizumab (anti-VEGF antibody) has shown to improve survival in a phase 3 trial in first-line versus sorafenib, which included HCC patients with very well preserved liver function.[106] Similarly, the combination of durvalumab (an anti-PDL1 antibody) plus a single dose of tremelimumab (an anti-CTLA-4 antibody) improved survival over sorafenib and durvalumab was non-inferior to sorafenib according to randomized phase III trial.[107] Other combinations with encouraging results are nivolumab plus ipilimumab,[108] and lenvatinib plus pembrolizumab.[109]

Considering the increasing alternatives, the standard of care in advanced HCC is based on the selection of candidates (based on performance status, liver function, degree of portal hypertension, and comorbidities), definition of the most suitable sequence of drugs, and expected incidence and severity of adverse events.[110] Interestingly, some adverse events such as dermatology reaction under sorafenib or regorafenib are associated with better outcomes.[111] Thus these should be seen positively and not as unnecessary treatment interruptions.

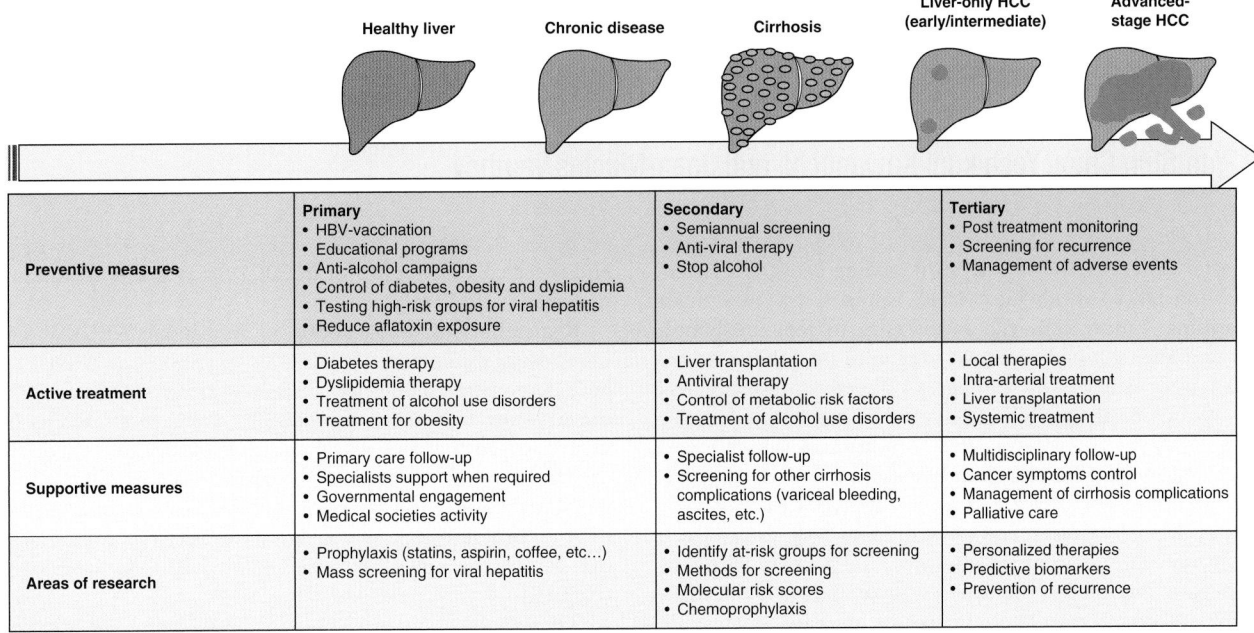

	Healthy liver → Chronic disease → Cirrhosis → Liver-only HCC (early/intermediate) → Advanced-stage HCC		
	Primary	**Secondary**	**Tertiary**
Preventive measures	• HBV-vaccination • Educational programs • Anti-alcohol campaigns • Control of diabetes, obesity and dyslipidemia • Testing high-risk groups for viral hepatitis • Reduce aflatoxin exposure	• Semiannual screening • Anti-viral therapy • Stop alcohol	• Post treatment monitoring • Screening for recurrence • Management of adverse events
Active treatment	• Diabetes therapy • Dyslipidemia therapy • Treatment of alcohol use disorders • Treatment for obesity	• Liver transplantation • Antiviral therapy • Control of metabolic risk factors • Treatment of alcohol use disorders	• Local therapies • Intra-arterial treatment • Liver transplantation • Systemic treatment
Supportive measures	• Primary care follow-up • Specialists support when required • Governmental engagement • Medical societies activity	• Specialist follow-up • Screening for other cirrhosis complications (variceal bleeding, ascites, etc.)	• Multidisciplinary follow-up • Cancer symptoms control • Management of cirrhosis complications • Palliative care
Areas of research	• Prophylaxis (statins, aspirin, coffee, etc…) • Mass screening for viral hepatitis	• Identify at-risk groups for screening • Methods for screening • Molecular risk scores • Chemoprophylaxis	• Personalized therapies • Predictive biomarkers • Prevention of recurrence

FIGURE 89.4   Interventions in the natural history of hepatocellular carcinoma *(HCC)* development in progressive liver diseases and strategies targeting each specific clinical context.

FUTURE PROSPECTS

Prevention of HCC in patients with chronic liver disease is essential, and advances have been achieved with antiviral treatment and HBV vaccination. A trend toward increasing rates of MAFLD-related HCC underscores the need to broaden the preventive focus to causes of metabolic syndrome, such as obesity, diabetes, and dyslipidemia.

Novel biomarkers and imaging tools may allow detection of dysplastic nodules before their malignant transformation or early-stage disease suitable for curative treatment. Early diagnosis implies better outcomes, but even after local treatment, the probability of recurrence is a matter of concern. Adjuvant treatments, such as immune-oncology agents, are promising strategies to be tested in this setting. Close follow-up is warranted because some of the local recurrences are still suitable for curative treatment.

However, a significant proportion of patients are still diagnosed with advanced stage, and many recurrences occur outside the liver. Systemic treatment is, probably, the most evolving field in HCC, moving from a context in which there were no effective drugs in the early 2000s to a situation with several options (Fig. 89.4). Active translational research should help to develop predictive biomarkers, opening the doors to the much-expected personalized medicine and precision oncology, already in place in many neoplasms, but not in the field of primary liver cancer.

The references for this chapter can be found online by accessing the accompanying Expert Consult website.

CHAPTER 90

Hepatic metastasis from colorectal cancer

Yun Shin Chun, Yoshikuni Kawaguchi, and Jean-Nicolas Vauthey

Colorectal cancer (CRC) is the third leading cause of cancer-related mortality worldwide.[1] CRC spreads via two main mechanisms: cancer cells can metastasize to regional lymph nodes and then through central lymphatics into the systemic circulation, or cancer cells can spread directly to the liver via portal venous drainage.[2] The likelihood of presenting with or developing metastases is associated with primary tumor T and N stage and the presence of lymphovascular invasion. Approximately 15% to 25% of patients with CRC present with synchronous liver metastases, and an additional 20% to 30% will develop metachronous liver metastases.[3] In patients with isolated hepatic metastases, the extent of liver disease is the main determinant of survival. The outcome of untreated metastatic CRC is well-documented in older literature.[4] The median survival of untreated CRC with synchronous liver metastases is only 5 to 10 months.

Liver resection is the mainstay of treatment for colorectal liver metastases (CLM) and represents the only potentially curative treatment option. Surgical resection of CLM is associated with a 5-year overall survival (OS) rate of 58%.[5] However, only 10% to 20% of patients present with resectable disease. For patients eligible for liver resection, disease recurrence rates of up to 66% are reported.[6] This chapter will review initial assessment of patients with CLM and strategies to increase resectability and reduce recurrence rates. In addition, innovations in perioperative management, emerging data on biomarkers, and controversies will be discussed.

PRINCIPLES OF MEDICAL TREATMENT OF METASTATIC COLORECTAL CANCER

Advances in systemic therapy for metastatic CRC have resulted in significant improvements in patient survival (Fig. 90.1; see Chapters 97 and 98). Historically, median survival of patients receiving palliative treatment with 5-fluorouracil (5-FU) alone was limited to 6 to 12 months. First-line combination therapy regimens with oxaliplatin or irinotecan have led to median survival rates of 30 months.[7] Targeted therapies in combination with first-line cytotoxic agents have led to further improvements in response rates and survival.

Cytotoxic Agents (see Chapter 98)

Since the 1950s, 5-FU has been the cornerstone of treatment for metastatic CRC. Leucovorin (LV), also known as folinic acid, enhances the activity of 5-FU by stabilizing binding of 5-FU to its target, thymidylate synthase. Irinotecan, a topoisomerase inhibitor, was approved by the United States Food and Drug Administration (FDA) in 2000 for first-line treatment of metastatic CRC, based on two randomized controlled trials (RCTs) showing improved response and OS rates with the addition of irinotecan to 5-FU/LV.[8,9] Oxaliplatin is a platinum derivative that exerts synergistic cytotoxicity with 5-FU

and received FDA approval in 2004 for first-line treatment of metastatic CRC.[10,11]

Regimens with a backbone of infusional 5-FU/LV, combined with oxaliplatin (FOLFOX) or irinotecan (FOLFIRI), have demonstrated objective response rates greater than 50% in the first-line treatment of metastatic CRC. Four RCTs have demonstrated that FOLFOX and FOLFIRI have similar clinical efficacy, and the choice of regimen can be tailored to the individual patient and toxicity profiles.[12] Capecitabine is an oral fluoropyrimidine that is converted to 5-FU in tumor tissues that can be combined with oxaliplatin (XELOX) or irinotecan (XELIRI).

The combination of 5-FU, LV, oxaliplatin, and irinotecan (FOLFOXIRI) for unresectable metastatic CRC was compared with FOLFIRI in a phase III RCT by the Gruppo Oncologico Nord Ovest.[13] FOLFOXIRI was associated with significantly higher response rates, progression-free survival (PFS), and OS. However, toxicity was greater in the FOLFOXIRI arm, with statistically significant greater incidence of grade 2 to 3 neuropathy and grade 3 to 4 neutropenia.

Biologic Therapies

Biologic agents in combination with first-line chemotherapy have shown promising results. Bevacizumab, a monoclonal antibody against vascular endothelial growth factor, is associated with improved survival when added to irinotecan or oxaliplatin-based regimens in the first-line metastatic setting.[14,15] Cetuximab is a monoclonal antibody directed against epidermal growth factor receptor (EGFR). Mutations in *KRAS*, which lies downstream in the EGFR signaling pathway, are associated with resistance to cetuximab. For *KRAS* wild-type tumors, the addition of cetuximab to FOLFIRI or FOLFOX is associated with improved response rates and PFS.[16,17] Panitumumab is another monoclonal antibody directed against EGFR, which has similar efficacy and toxicity as cetuximab.[18]

Metastatic CRC patients with *BRAF* V600E mutations have particularly poor outcomes, with median OS of only 4 to 6 months after failure of initial treatment. In CRC, monotherapy with *BRAF* inhibitors is ineffective because of pathway reactivation through EGFR signaling. The recently published BEACON trial showed improved OS and response rates with triplet therapy of encorafenib, binimetinib, and cetuximab, over the control group of cetuximab and irinotecan.[19] Combination therapy with encorafenib, a *BRAF* inhibitor, anti-EGFR therapy (cetuximab), and binimetinib, a selective inhibitor of mitogen-activated protein kinase (MAPK) kinase, overcomes the limitations of *BRAF* inhibition alone.

Perioperative Chemotherapy for Resectable Disease

After potentially curative resection of CLM, two-thirds of patients suffer disease recurrence, and half of these recurrences occur in the liver.[6] In efforts to improve relapse rates, perioperative chemotherapy was compared with surgery alone in the

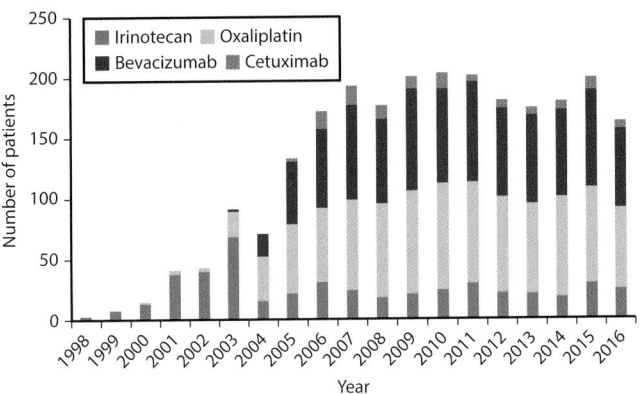

FIGURE 90.1 Number of patients treated with cytotoxic and biologic agents before resection of colorectal liver metastases at The University of Texas MD Anderson Cancer Center.

European Organisation for Research and Treatment of Cancer (EORTC) intergroup trial 40983 (EPOC).[20] Patients with resectable CLM, up to 4 in number, were randomized to perioperative FOLFOX or hepatectomy alone. Among 342 eligible patients, median PFS was 20.9 months in the perioperative chemotherapy arm, compared with 12.5 months in the surgery alone arm ($P = .035$). OS rates were similar between the two arms. More recently, the New EPOC study showed a detrimental effect on survival with the addition of cetuximab to perioperative chemotherapy for patients with *KRAS* exon 2 wild-type, resectable CLM.[21]

In the adjuvant setting, an RCT of adjuvant 5-FU/LV versus surgery alone showed improved 5-year disease-free survival (DFS) with adjuvant treatment (33.5% vs. 26.7%, $P = .028$) but no statistically significant benefit in OS.[22] This trial was suspended because of slow accrual and enrolled 173 patients from 47 hospitals in a 10-year time period. In a subsequent randomized study, FOLFIRI compared with 5-FU/LV after CLM resection had no significant impact on DFS or OS.[23] These results are congruent with the lack of efficacy of FOLFIRI for adjuvant treatment of stage III CRC.[24,25]

Conversion Therapy for Borderline Resectable Disease

A study published in 2004 of over 1000 CLM patients showed that 12.5% of patients with initially unresectable CLM achieved sufficient downsizing with systemic therapy to undergo hepatic resection. Among these patients with initially unresectable disease, 5-year OS after hepatectomy was 33%.[26] Most of the patients in this study received oxaliplatin-based chemotherapy. FOLFOXIRI has been shown in RCTs to improve resectability rates over FOLFOX or FOLFIRI.[13,27] However, hepatotoxicity with FOLFOXIRI can be significant, as described later in this chapter.

Biologic agents have also been shown to increase resectability rates. In a recent RCT of 241 patients with unresectable, *RAS*-mutated CLM, the addition of bevacizumab to FOLFOX increased objective response rates and conversion to resectability, with 22.3% of patients undergoing R0 resection after FOLFOX plus bevacizumab, compared with 5.8% of patients after FOLFOX alone ($P < .01$).[28] Similarly, cetuximab added to FOLFOX or FOLFIRI for *RAS* wild-type CLM increased resectability rates in retrospective and prospective studies.[29,30]

Hepatic Arterial Infusion Chemotherapy (see Chapter 97)

The rationale for infusion of chemotherapy directly into the hepatic artery is the liver's dual blood supply, with metastases perfused predominantly via the hepatic artery, in contrast to portal blood supply to normal liver. Thus hepatic arterial infusion (HAI) delivers chemotherapy preferentially to tumor over normal liver parenchyma. Floxuridine (FUDR), a metabolite of 5-FU, has been extensively studied for HAI because of its high first-pass extraction in the liver, thereby minimizing systemic exposure.

In 1999 an RCT of adjuvant 5-FU plus HAI-FUDR compared with 5-FU alone after CLM resection demonstrated significantly higher 2-year OS in the HAI-FUDR group (86% vs. 72%, $P = .03$).[31] Two-year hepatic recurrence-free survival (RFS) was also significantly higher with HAI-FUDR (90% vs. 60%, $P < .001$). More recently, a phase II single-arm study of HAI-FUDR plus systemic therapy for 64 patients with initially unresectable CLM reported response and conversion to resectability rates of 73% and 52%, respectively.[32]

Disadvantages of HAI chemotherapy include biliary toxicity, which can be mitigated with the concurrent infusion of dexamethasone and avoidance of systemic administration of bevacizumab. Hepatic toxicity with HAI oxaliplatin reportedly occurs more frequently than with systemic oxaliplatin.[33] In addition, multidisciplinary expertise in surgery, nuclear medicine, interventional radiology, and gastroenterology is required for placement and management of HAI pumps.

Chemotherapy-Associated Hepatotoxicity

A study published in 2006 from The University of Texas MD Anderson Cancer Center (MDACC) demonstrated associations between oxaliplatin and sinusoidal injury and between irinotecan and steatohepatitis (Fig. 90.2).[34] Oxaliplatin-related sinusoidal injury can progress to nodular regenerative hyperplasia and clinically significant portal hypertension. Splenomegaly and thrombocytopenia are surrogates for oxaliplatin-induced sinusoidal injury.[35] In the MDACC study, steatohepatitis, but not sinusoidal injury, was associated with higher mortality after CLM resection (14.7% vs. 1.6%, $P = .001$; see Chapter 98).

FOLFOXIRI is associated with high response rates but correspondingly high rates of liver toxicity. In a pooled analysis of 37 patients who underwent R0 hepatectomy after FOLFOXIRI for initially unresectable disease, sinusoidal dilation and steatosis were identified in 100% and 76% of resected specimens, respectively.[36]

Strategies to mitigate the negative effects of chemotherapy-associated hepatotoxicity include limiting preoperative chemotherapy to up to six cycles, sufficient time interval between chemotherapy and liver resection, and the use of bevacizumab with oxaliplatin to protect from sinusoidal injury. In the EPOC trial, patients who received six cycles of preoperative FOLFOX had higher rates of reversible postoperative complications than those who underwent surgery alone (25% vs. 16%, $P = .0401$).[20] In a study from Memorial Sloan-Kettering Cancer Center (MSKCC), maximum radiologic response in CLM was observed after 2 to 4 months of chemotherapy; if continued beyond 4 months, there was little gain in therapeutic benefit.[37] Twelve or more cycles of preoperative chemotherapy are associated with significantly higher rates of severe sinusoidal injury, postoperative major morbidity, and mortality.[38]

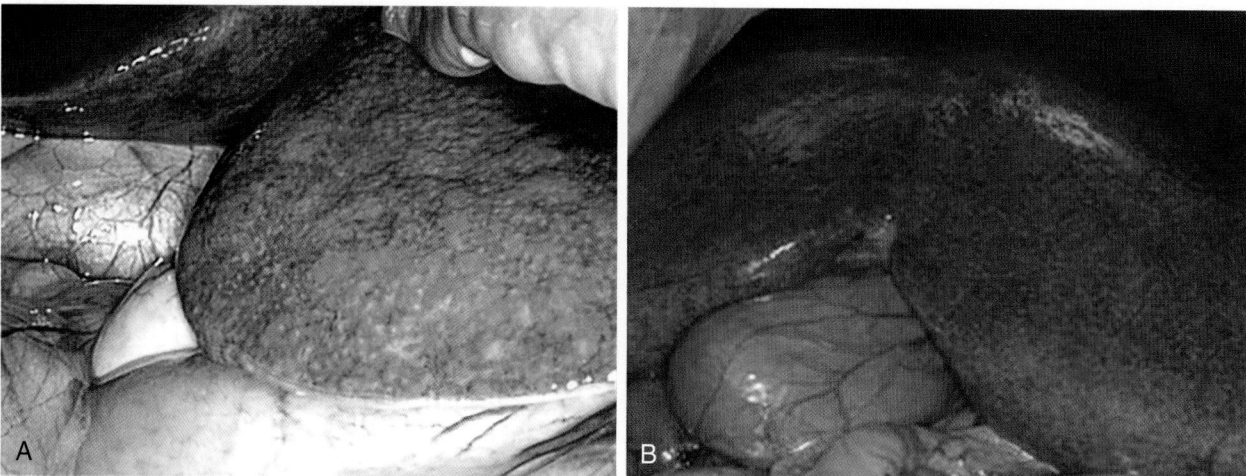

FIGURE 90.2   Intraoperative photos of oxaliplatin-induced "blue" liver from sinusoidal injury **(A)** and irinotecan-induced "yellow" liver from steato-hepatitis **(B).**

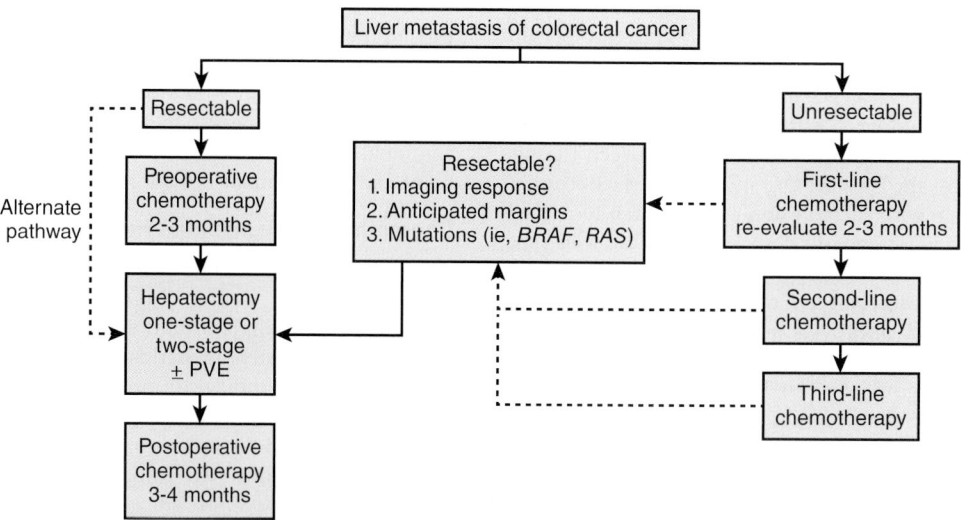

FIGURE 90.3   Treatment algorithm for patients presenting with resectable and initially unresectable colorectal liver metastases. *PVE,* Portal vein embolization. (From Chun YS, Vauthey JN. Local therapy for colorectal liver metastases: Establishing today's level of evidence and defining tomorrow's roadmap. *J Natl Cancer Inst.* 2017;109[9].)

A longer interval between chemotherapy and CLM resection is associated with lower morbidity but should be balanced with the risk of disease progression during the treatment-free interval. The risk of postoperative complications is reportedly twice as high among patients with interval between chemotherapy and CLM resection of up to 4 weeks, compared with 5 to 8 weeks.[39] Thus an interval of 5 weeks is recommended between chemotherapy and surgery. Despite its antiangiogenic effects, bevacizumab can also be administered 5 weeks before hepatectomy without an increase in postoperative complications.[40]

Treatment Sequencing

For patients with resectable and initially unresectable CLM, treatment sequencing integrates short courses of chemotherapy, evaluation of response, tumor genetics, and one- or two-stage hepatectomy (TSH) with portal vein embolization (PVE) when indicated (Fig. 90.3). The choice of first-line therapy with FOLFOX or FOLFIRI depends on toxicity profiles, particularly

hepatic sinusoidal injury and peripheral neuropathy with oxaliplatin and steatohepatitis and gastrointestinal toxicity with irinotecan. Patients with baseline splenomegaly are at risk for severe sinusoidal injury with oxaliplatin, whereas patients with hepatic steatosis, obesity, and diabetes are at risk for developing steatohepatitis with irinotecan. Given the improved pathologic response with bevacizumab and its protective effect on oxaliplatin-associated sinusoidal injury, FOLFOX plus bevacizumab is a commonly used first-line regimen.[41,42]

PREOPERATIVE EVALUATION OF PATIENTS WITH COLORECTAL LIVER METASTASES

Criteria for Resectability

Preoperative evaluation of patients with CLM begins with assessment of their physical fitness to undergo hepatectomy, including chronic comorbidities, acute infectious or thrombotic processes, underlying liver impairment, and performance status. In particular, given the cardiovascular demands of low central venous pressure anesthesia and possible portal pedicle clamping, any history of cardiac or pulmonary disease must be investigated because these patients are at significant risk for intraoperative and postoperative complications (see Chapters 25, 26, and 28). Age alone does not constitute a contraindication in the absence of other medical factors.[43]

Evaluation of oncologic resectability involves complete radiologic staging, biomarkers and other prognostic factors, response to systemic therapy, and endoscopic evaluation if the primary tumor is intact. The goals of this assessment are to determine that the primary tumor site is either completely treated or amenable to simultaneous or future resection and to quantify the number and location of extrahepatic disease (EHD).

Technical resectability of intrahepatic disease is defined as the ability to achieve a margin-negative resection while preserving adequate biliary drainage and vascular inflow and outflow, and sparing at least two contiguous hepatic segments with future liver remnant (FLR) volume of more than 20% with normal liver, more than 30% after extensive chemotherapy, and more than 40% with cirrhosis.[44]

Preoperative Imaging (see Chapter 15)

High-quality, contrast-enhanced cross-sectional imaging is essential to identify liver metastases and their relationship to major vessels and bile ducts and to evaluate the quality of nontumoral liver and anticipated FLR volume. The quality of baseline imaging is critically important before systemic therapy, which can lead to disappearing metastases and induce changes in the liver parenchyma that reduce the sensitivity of radiologic exams.

Computed Tomography

Contrast-enhanced computed tomography (CT) of the chest, abdomen, and pelvis is the primary imaging modality for staging patients with metastatic CRC because of its wide availability, fast scanning speed, and low cost. CT scans image with high resolution the lungs, solid intra-abdominal organs, lymph nodes, and soft tissues. High-quality multidetector CT entails a quadruple-phase protocol through the liver that includes precontrast, arterial, portal venous, and delayed phases. Slice thickness should not exceed 5 mm. The portal venous phase is the most important for identifying CLM because they are not typically well-vascularized. Arterial phase images are useful to distinguish metastatic disease from benign vascular lesions, such as hemangiomas, and to identify arterial anatomy. Coronal and sagittal reconstructions are performed to further delineate anatomy. Three-dimensional reconstructions can be rendered to calculate FLR volumes.[45]

Magnetic Resonance Imaging

Magnetic resonance imaging (MRI) is technically more demanding with slower image sequencing than CT. Consequently, MRI requires more engaged patient cooperation to tolerate multiple breath-holds and sequences. The sensitivity of MRI versus CT in detection of CLM depends on imaging techniques and protocols, use of hepatobiliary contrast agents with MRI, and underlying liver disease, particularly steatosis.[46,47]

Positron Emission Tomography (see Chapter 18)

In the United States, the use of positron emission tomography (PET)-CT for staging and diagnosis of CRC was approved by

Medicare in 2001.[48] A limitation of PET is lack of adequate specificity, with false-positive results in the setting of inflammation. Additional limitations include poor sensitivity for lesions less than 1 cm, a significant drop in sensitivity during administration of systemic therapy, and a low degree of anatomic detail.

Single institution retrospective studies have suggested that PET-CT has improved detection over CT alone to detect hepatic and extrahepatic metastases.[49] However, in an RCT of patients with metachronous, resectable CLM, PET-CT compared with CT alone did not affect surgical planning or long-term patient outcomes.[50] PET scans may be useful to rule out EHD in patients with high-risk, borderline-resectable disease.

Treatment Sequencing With Synchronous Metastases

For patients presenting with synchronous disease, the decision to perform staged or simultaneous resection of the primary tumor and liver metastases depends on the extent of disease, symptoms, and magnitude of anticipated surgery. After confirmation that the patient does not require palliative primary tumor resection or bowel diversion, most patients are advised to initiate short-course systemic therapy. The second decision point is to determine the surgical treatment sequence: simultaneous resection or staged primary-first or reverse liver-first.

Benefits of simultaneous resection include resection of all disease under one general anesthesia and lower cost.[51] Low-risk colorectal and hepatic resections can be combined with low morbidity rates, but high-risk colorectal plus major hepatectomy is associated with mortality and major morbidity rates of 5% and 55%, respectively.[52] Therefore most patients requiring complex liver and colorectal procedures should undergo staged resection.

The traditional staged approach entails primary tumor resection, followed by systemic therapy and hepatectomy. Potential benefits of the traditional staged approach include definitive treatment of the primary tumor and selection of patients with favorable biology for hepatectomy who do not have significant disease progression after primary resection and systemic therapy.[51] A potential drawback of the traditional approach is delayed treatment of metastatic disease, particularly if the patient suffers a complication after colorectal surgery.

The liver-first, reverse approach was initially proposed in 2006 with the intent of treating liver metastases early because prognosis in most patients is determined by their metastatic disease.[53] In a liver-first sequence, patients whose primary tumors are asymptomatic receive systemic therapy first, followed by hepatectomy and subsequently primary tumor resection. The risk of primary tumor-related complications with the reverse approach is low.[54] Bleeding from the primary tumor can be managed with transfusion and chemotherapy and does not pose a contraindication to the reverse approach. However, patients whose primary tumors cannot be traversed with a pediatric colonoscope or have perforation are not candidates for the reverse approach, and instead should undergo resection of the primary tumor in a staged or synchronous fashion.

A recent multicenter trial from France randomized 85 patients with resectable, synchronous CLM to simultaneous or traditional delayed liver resection.[55] The primary outcome of 60-day major morbidity rate was similar in both groups (49% simultaneous and 46% delayed resection). After 2 years, a trend toward improved OS and DFS was observed in the simultaneous

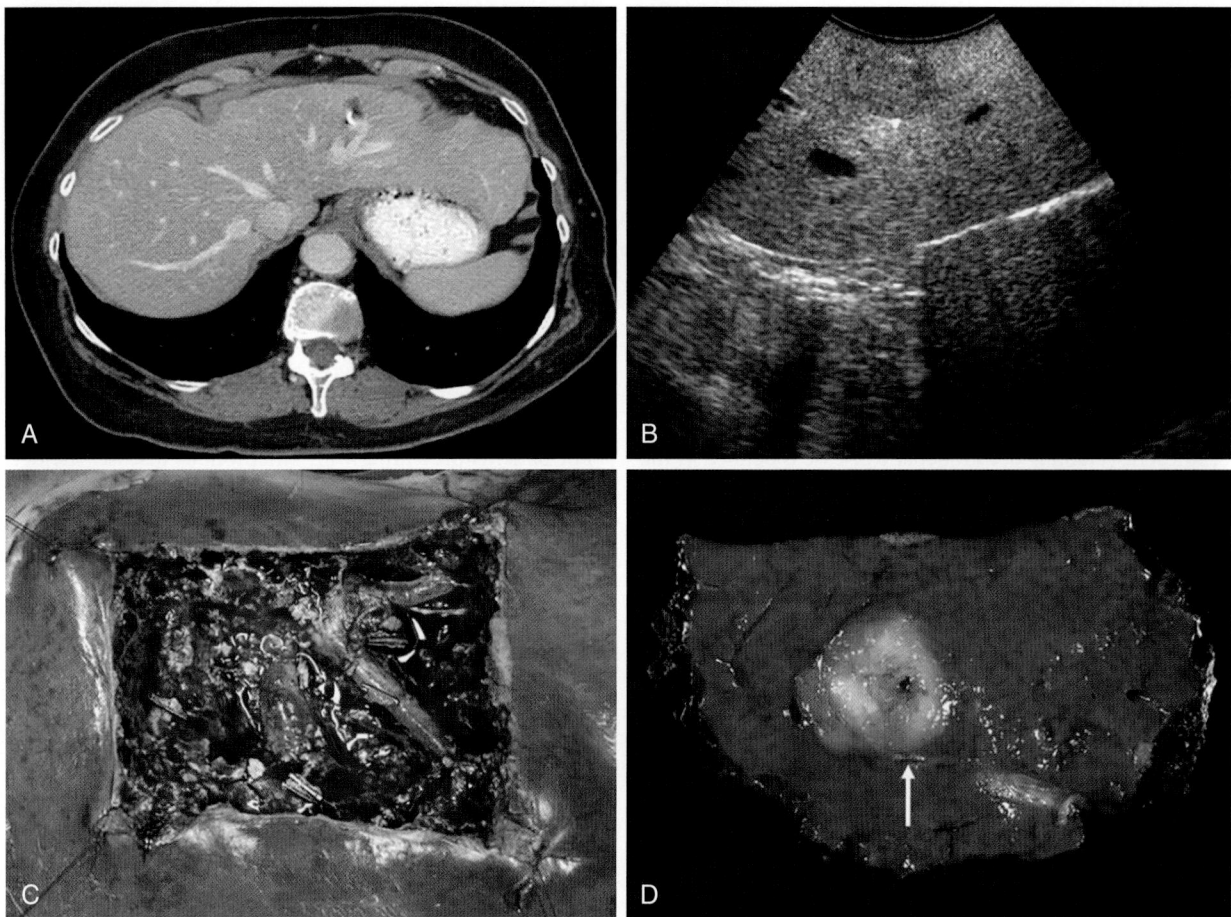

FIGURE 90.4   **A,** Computed tomography scan of small segment II liver metastasis marked with fiducial. **B,** Intraoperative ultrasound shows hyperechoic coil. **C,** Intraoperative photo after targeted, parenchymal-sparing resection. **D,** Pathologic examination demonstrates fiducial at posterior margin of metastasis *(white arrow)*. (From Zalinski S, Abdalla EK, Mahvash A, Vauthey JN. A marking technique for intraoperative localization of small liver metastases before systemic chemotherapy. Ann Surg Oncol. 2009;16[5]:1208–1211.)

resection group (*P* = .05). In the delayed resection group, 8 patients did not undergo hepatectomy, mainly because of disease progression. Limitations of the trial include the long study duration of 10 years, trend toward patients with more favorable characteristics in the simultaneous resection group, and variability in timing of hepatectomy in the delayed resection group, ranging from 8 to 49 weeks.

Preoperative Fiducial Placement for Disappearing Liver Metastases

The rate of radiologically disappearing liver metastases (DLMs) after chemotherapy ranges from 5% to 24%, depending on the size of CLM.[56] In addition, chemotherapy-associated changes to the nontumoral liver parenchyma can obscure visualization of metastases by intraoperative ultrasound (IOUS; see Chapters 24 and 103). Despite radiologic disappearance, complete pathologic response is observed in a minority of DLM. Therefore the goal of CLM resection is to remove all metastases visualized before chemotherapy.

For metastases at risk of disappearing with chemotherapy, percutaneous placement of a fiducial marker before chemotherapy enables intraoperative localization and targeted parenchymal-sparing resection (Fig. 90.4).[57] Fiducial marker placement is not necessary if the lesion at risk of disappearing is located within the field of planned resection or is subcapsular and likely to be identified by visualization or palpation.

PERIOPERATIVE MANAGEMENT

Perioperative principles for resection of CLM are similar to other hepatic resections, including anesthesia, enhanced recovery, venous thromboembolism prophylaxis, and strategies to reduce bile leak (see Chapters 25–27). For open hepatectomy, choice of incision includes subcostal or midline, with J or L extensions across the abdomen to enhance exposure. For resections of the left liver and anterior segments, midline incision is often sufficient. For access to the retrohepatic vena cava, particularly in obese patients, a reverse L incision provides optimal exposure and maximizes safety.[58]

Role of Laparoscopic Staging

Before the development of sophisticated abdominal imaging, laparoscopy played a role in staging patients with metastatic CRC, particularly those with poor prognostic factors.[59] Given the fidelity of current imaging, there are relatively few indications for diagnostic laparoscopy. Because a negative laparoscopy lengthens anesthetic time and increases operating costs, the technique is now reserved for patients deemed to be at high risk for unresectable disease.

Intraoperative Staging and the Role of Ultrasound

The abdomen should be explored for evidence of extrahepatic metastases. IOUS is essential to delineate intrahepatic anatomy, particularly hepatic vein tributaries and portal vein branches, and can be performed before liver mobilization (see Chapters 24 and 103). For parenchymal-sparing resections, IOUS is indispensable for marking the intended line of transection, particularly for lesions located deep in the liver parenchyma. After scoring the liver capsule along these planes, a properly positioned US probe perpendicular to the capsular mark will confirm an adequate margin from the transection line to the tumor (Fig. 90.5). As transection progresses, ultrasound is repeated to maintain relationships among the transection plane, major vascular structures, and the tumor.[60]

Although not widely available, the use of contrast-enhanced IOUS has been reported from several groups outside the United States.[61] In a series of 60 patients from the UK with metastatic CRC, the accuracy of preoperative MRI/CT, standard IOUS, and contrast-enhanced IOUS was 74%, 79%, and 96%, respectively.[62]

Transection Techniques

Selection and use of the increasing number of devices and techniques for liver transection are discussed elsewhere (see

Chapters 101 and 118). For liver metastasectomy, these are generally divided between instruments that crush and divide the liver (staplers and vessel-sealing devices) and dissection instruments. Given the frequent need to complete parenchymal-sparing and extended hepatectomies along nonanatomic planes, most surgeons prefer the parenchymal transection techniques that entail a dissection with visualization of the intrahepatic structures. Instruments such as the Cavitron ultrasonic surgical aspirator allow for curvilinear transection planes, individual control of small intrahepatic structures, and minimal damage to the remnant liver.[63]

After major hepatectomy, interrogation of the security of bile duct closure on the transection surface has been shown to reduce the risk of clinically significant bile leak and nonbilious collections (deep organ space infection).[64,65] Likewise, these tests obviate the need for prophylactic transperitoneal drains. Topical coagulant agents have not been shown to reduce postoperative bleeding or bile leak.[66]

Minimally Invasive Surgery

Two recent RCTs have compared minimally invasive and open liver resection for resectable CLM. Both the OSLO-COMET and LapOpHuva trials were single-center studies that excluded major hepatectomy.[67,68] In both trials, postoperative complication rates and hospital length of stay were lower in the minimally invasive arm. Careful patient selection and surgeon experience are critical for achieving optimal outcomes with minimally invasive resection of CLM (see Chapter 127).

Perioperative Morbidity and Mortality

Postoperatively, meticulous management of metabolic derangements and monitoring of liver function and coagulation factor abnormalities are required (see Chapter 26). Most patients undergoing CLM resection do not have liver cirrhosis but may have chemotherapy-related hepatic injury. After CLM resection, morbidity and mortality rates reflect the extent of hepatectomy, surgeon and hospital volume, and underlying patient comorbidities.[69] Classification systems based on the complexity and difficulty of hepatic resection have been developed that correlate with postoperative morbidity rates.[70]

Contemporary series report that up to one-third of patients will experience a complication (Table 90.1; see Chapter 28). The incidence of cardiovascular and thrombotic complications is about 5%, most commonly arrhythmia.[71,72] Pulmonary complications, reported in 7.5% of patients, are related to the large upper abdominal incisions, postsurgical sympathetic pleural effusions, and failure to mobilize patients early. Liver insufficiency and liver failure remain the most dangerous liver-related complications and occur in 3% to 8% of patients after major hepatectomy.[73,74] Other hepatobiliary complications include bile leak in 4% of patients and perihepatic abscess in 2% to

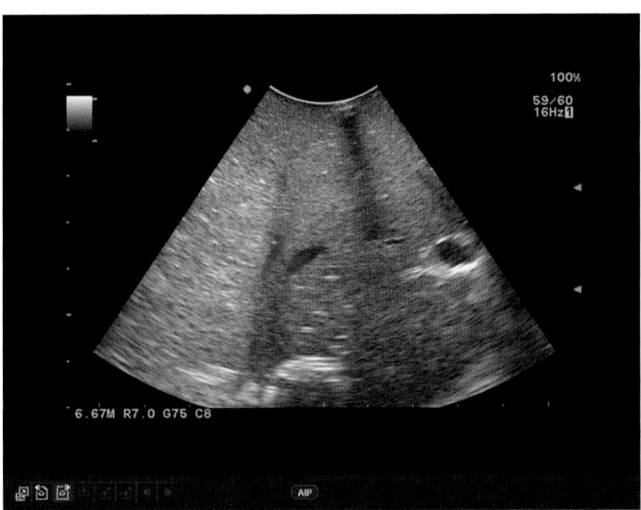

FIGURE 90.5 Ultrasonographic parenchymal transection/margin assessment. With the probe aligned perpendicular to a cautery-scored capsular mark, the image demonstrates the distance from the large tumor *(hyperechoic white area)* and hepatic veins *(central anechoic structures)* to the proposed transection line *(linear hypoechoic shadow)*.

TABLE 90.1 Morbidity and Mortality Rates After Resection of Colorectal Liver Metastases				
STUDY	NO. OF PATIENTS	MORBIDITY	MAJOR MORBIDITY	MORTALITY
Tamandl, 2015[72]	746	37%	17.3%	0.5%
Lordan, 2017[78]	479	32.8%	6.5%	2.3%
Wiseman, 2019[79]	2832	33%	–	0.7%
Elfrink, 2020[80]	4639		6.2%	1.4%
Olthof, 2020[81]	3846	10.5%	–	1.9%

10%.[75,76] Significant hemorrhage is rare (1%–3%) but can be an important cause of early perioperative mortality. To assess and compare postoperative complications accurately, morbidity, mortality, and readmissions should be recorded and reported for 90 days after surgery.[77]

Mortality associated with an elective liver resection for CLM has decreased significantly because of advances in the understanding of liver anatomy, surgical techniques, diagnostic and interventional radiology, and anesthesia. In the past decade, major series of CLM resection report mortality rates of less than 3% (see Table 90.1). These rates are notable because they have declined despite the use of more complex and radical procedures. The majority of posthepatectomy deaths occur from perioperative hemorrhage or liver failure.

STRATEGIES TO INCREASE RESECTABILITY (SEE CHAPTER 102)

In addition to the systemic therapy discussed earlier in this chapter, other strategies to increase resectability of CLM include TSH, completion ablation, PVE (see Chapter 102C), and nonanatomic parenchymal-sparing resection (see Chapter 102A).

Two-Stage Hepatectomy

TSH entails a sequential strategy for bilateral CLM that cannot be resected in a single procedure (Fig. 90.6). In the first stage, metastases in the FLR are resected, typically with partial hepatectomy. If indicated, PVE is performed between the two stages to ensure adequate FLR volume. Systemic therapy is not routinely administered between the two stages but is indicated for patients with significant tumor progression. TSH carries a risk of dropout between the first and second stages in 11% of patients, most from disease progression.[82] A minority of patients have insufficient hypertrophy of the FLR after PVE that precludes the second-stage hepatectomy. Despite the presence of multiple, bilateral metastases, patients who complete TSH have 5-year OS rates of up to 51%, partly because of the test of time between the two stages to select patients with favorable tumor biology.[83] Additionally, liver venous deprivation (combined hepatic vein embolization and PVE) has been recently reported as a safe approach leading to a superior degree of hypertrophy and kinetic growth rate compared with PVE alone, and it should be considered as a new approach before major hepatectomy in patients with a very small FLR.[84,85]

Completion Ablation

Techniques, indications, and results of liver ablation have evolved over time (see Chapter 96). For CLM, a phase II RCT assigned patients with unresectable, liver-only metastases to chemotherapy plus local ablation or chemotherapy alone (CLOCC).[86] Patients in the ablation arm had significantly higher 5-year OS (43.1% vs. 30.3%, P = .01). For resectable CLM, ablation is associated with higher local recurrence rate of 37%, compared with 11% and 4% after hepatectomy, with or without a positive margin, respectively.[87,88]

For patients with otherwise unresectable disease, completion ablation is a strategy to safely resect all but one to two small metastases and preserve liver parenchyma.[89] After hepatectomy, the remaining one to two metastases are treated with percutaneous ablation under CT guidance. Contrast-enhanced CT during ablation is critical to evaluate the extent of tumor and intraprocedural ablation zone. Completion ablation is associated with lower rates of postoperative complications and local tumor progression than intraoperative ablation.[90]

PROGNOSTIC AND PREDICTIVE FACTORS

Patient outcomes after CLM resection are heterogeneous, with subsets of patients succumbing early to disease recurrence. Thus accurate risk stratification is needed to optimize patient selection for surgery. Although prior studies have demonstrated adverse outcomes associated with greater number and size of CLM, synchronous disease, and EHD, more recent studies demonstrate that long-term survival can be achieved despite the presence of negative prognostic factors.

Number and Size of Liver Metastases

Historically, patients with at least four CLM and/or tumor diameter greater than 5 cm were not considered for hepatic resection because of poor outcomes.[91] However, because of safer surgery, effective systemic therapies, and improved understanding of tumor biology, number and size of CLM are no longer contraindications to surgery.

Extrahepatic Disease

Previously, the presence of nonpulmonary EHD was considered a contraindication to CLM resection.[92] More recently, studies have shown that in highly selected patients, resection of CLM and EHD can result in long-term survival. However, 84% to 90% of patients suffer disease recurrence after a median of 8 months.[93,94] The prognosis of patients undergoing resection

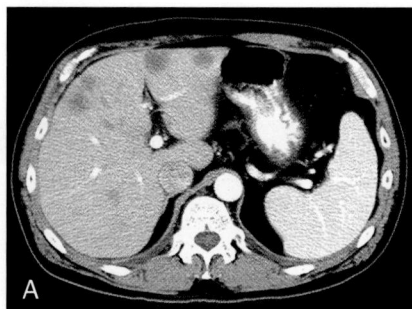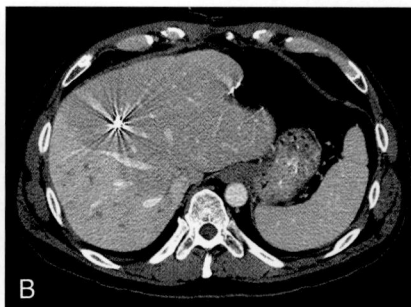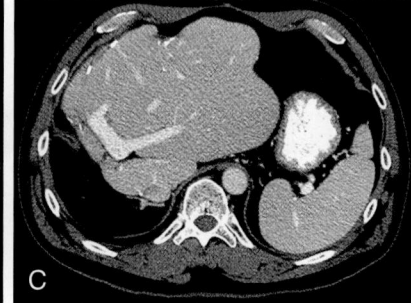

FIGURE 90.6   A, Computed tomography scans showing multiple, bilateral liver metastases treated with systemic therapy. **B,** After first-stage partial left hepatectomy and portal vein embolization. **C,** After second-stage extended right hepatectomy.

of CLM and EHD partly depends on the site of EHD. Lung metastases are associated with the best outcomes, with 5-year OS of 32% to 50%.[95] Portal lymph nodes or limited peritoneal disease reportedly has intermediate 5-year OS rates after resection of 24% to 42%, although patient populations in published series are heterogeneous with small sample sizes.[93,94] Retroperitoneal lymph nodes and multiple anatomic sites of EHD have particularly poor 5-year OS rates of 7% to 14%. A recent study from MDACC and the University Hospital of Lyon highlights the importance of molecular factors in selecting patients for resection of CLM and EHD.[96] Among 109 patients undergoing resection of CLM and various extrahepatic sites of disease, including the lungs, peritoneum, or portal lymph nodes, 28% of patients had co-mutation of *RAS/TP53*, which was an independent predictor of OS (5-year OS 25% vs. 50%, with and without *RAS/TP53* co-mutation, P = .02; Figure 90.7).

Predictive Models and Clinical Risk Scores

Several scoring systems and predictive models have been developed to estimate prognosis and guide selection of patients for CLM resection (Table 90.2). The most recognized and widely used scoring system is the clinical risk score from MSKCC published in 1999, which assigns one point to each of the following factors: (1) node-positive primary, (2) disease-free interval of less than 12 months between resection of primary and presentation of CLM, (3) carcinoembryonic antigen (CEA) greater than 200 ng/mL, (4) more than one liver metastasis, and (5) CLM size greater than 5 cm.[97]

New scoring systems have been developed that integrate the systemic inflammatory response using the neutrophil-to-lymphocyte ratio and molecular factors.[102] In a study of 608 patients undergoing CLM resection, a scoring system composed of three factors (*RAS* mutation, CLM size > 5 cm, and node-positive primary) accurately stratified OS and RFS.[103]

Primary Tumor Location

The location of the primary tumor in the right (cecum to hepatic flexure) versus left colon (splenic flexure to rectum) is emerging as a significant prognostic and predictive factor in localized and metastatic CRC. Right-sided tumors are associated with worse

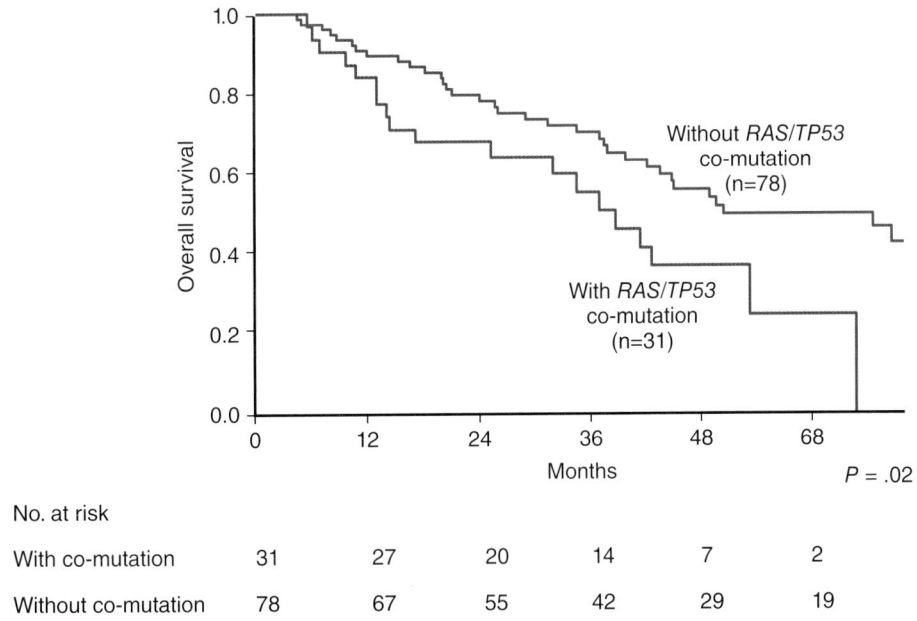

FIGURE 90.7 Overall survival after resection of colorectal liver metastases and extrahepatic disease by co-mutation of RAS-TP53. (From Lillemoe HA, Passot G, Kawaguchi Y, et al. RAS/TP53 co-mutation is associated with worse survival after concurrent resection of colorectal liver metastases and extrahepatic disease. *Ann Surg.* 2020. Online ahead of print.)

TABLE 90.2	Prognostic Factors Included in Traditional Scoring Systems for Patients Undergoing Resection of Colorectal Liver Metastases							
STUDY	NO. OF PATIENTS	PRIMARY TUMOR	DFI	TUMOR SIZE, cm	TUMOR NUMBER	CEA, ng/mL	RESECTION MARGIN	OVERALL SURVIVAL: LOW VS. HIGH-RISK
Nordlinger, 1996[a,98]	1568	Serosal invasion, node positive	< 24 mo	≥ 5	> 3	> 30	< 1 cm	2-yr: 79% vs. 43%
Fong, 1999[93]	1001	Node positive	< 12 mo	> 5	> 1	> 200	–	5-yr: 60% vs. 14%
Iwatsuki, 1999[b,99]	243	–	≤ 30 mo	> 8	≥ 3	–	–	5-yr: 48.3% vs. 0%
Zakaria, 2007[c,100]	662	Node positive	< 30 mo	> 8	> 1	–	–	5-yr: 55% vs. 20%
Rees, 2008[d,101]	929	Poorly differentiated, node positive	–	≥ 5	> 3	> 60	Positive	5-yr: 64% vs. 2%

Scoring systems include [a]age > 60 years, [b]bilateral metastases, [c]hepatoduodenal lymph node metastasis and blood transfusion, and [d]extrahepatic disease.
CEA, Carcinoembryonic antigen; *DFI,* disease-free interval; *mo,* months; *yr,* years.

survival after CLM resection and higher prevalence of *BRAF* mutations.[104,105] Primary tumor location also predicts response to anti-EGFR therapy. In clinical trials of *RAS* wild-type metastatic CRC, anti-EGFR therapy was not beneficial for patients with right-sided primary tumors.[106] In contrast, primary tumor location did not affect the efficacy of bevacizumab.[107]

Response to Preoperative Systemic Therapy

Pathologic response to systemic therapy is an important surrogate marker of tumor biology and an independent predictor of survival after CLM resection (Fig. 90.8).[108] Pathologic response can be stratified by the percent of viable tumor cells,

with at least 50% viable tumor cells classified as minor response; 1% to 49% viable tumor cells, major response; and 0% viable tumor cells, complete response. In a study from MDACC of 305 patients undergoing CLM resection, 5-year OS rates were 75%, 56%, and 33% with complete, major, and minor pathologic response, respectively ($P < .05$). Among preoperative systemic therapy regimens, 5-FU plus oxaliplatin and bevacizumab was an independent predictor of pathologic response.

Response to systemic therapy is conventionally assessed radiologically using the Response Evaluation Criteria in Solid Tumors (RECIST), which is based on reduction in tumor size. For patients receiving chemotherapy with bevacizumab, morphologic changes in liver metastases seen on CT correlate better than RECIST with pathologic response and survival.[109] An optimal morphologic response is defined as homogeneous attenuation of metastases, sharp tumor-liver interface, and absence of peripheral enhancement (Fig. 90.9).

MOLECULAR DETERMINANTS OF OUTCOME

Advances in next-generation sequencing have led to the identification of distinct molecular subtypes of CRC that determine patient outcomes and response to therapy. In the 1990s, DNA mismatch repair deficiency leading to microsatellite instability-high (MSI-H) tumors was identified as an important factor in colon carcinogenesis. However, MSI-H tumors affect less than 2% of patients undergoing CLM resection. In contrast, somatic gene mutations, particularly *RAS* and *BRAF*, have emerged as important predictive and prognostic biologic factors in CLM (Fig. 90.10).

RAS

Three *RAS* genes encode proteins KRas, NRas, and HRas, which are members of the family of small GTPases in the MAPK signaling cascade (Fig. 90.11). The MAPK pathway transmits extracellular signals to the nucleus and regulates cellular proliferation, differentiation, and apoptosis. *RAS* mutations lead to constitutive activation of the Ras protein, resulting in resistance to therapies that target EGFR, which lies upstream of Ras in the MAPK pathway.

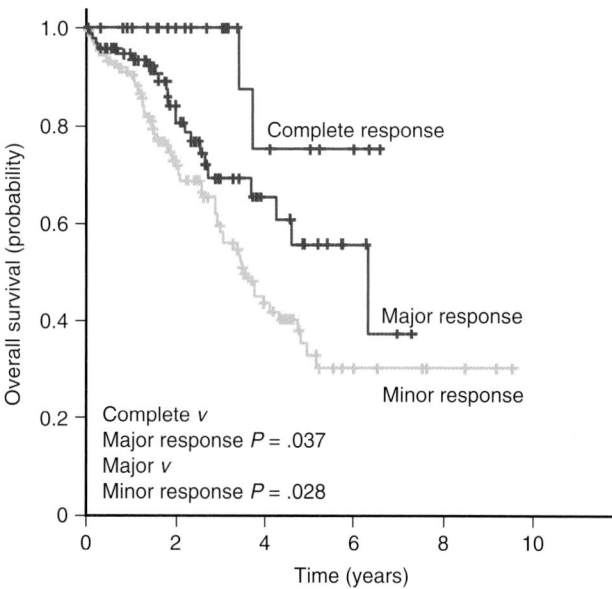

FIGURE 90.8 Overall survival after resection of colorectal liver metastases, stratified by degree of pathologic response to preoperative systemic therapy. (From Blazer DG, 3rd, Kishi Y, Maru DM, et al. Pathologic response to preoperative chemotherapy: A new outcome end point after resection of hepatic colorectal metastases. *J Clin Oncol.* 2008;26[33]: 5344–5351.)

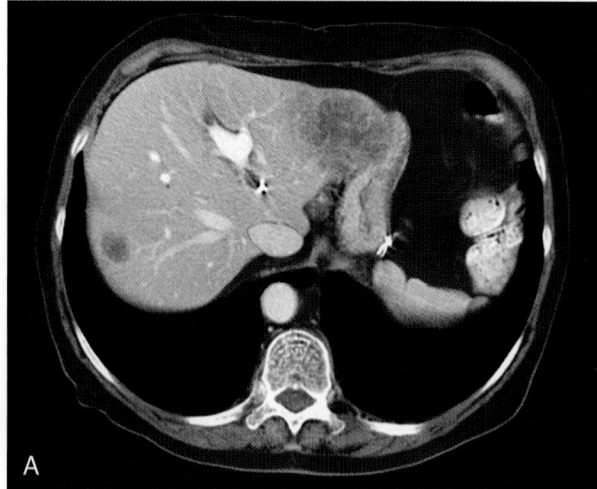
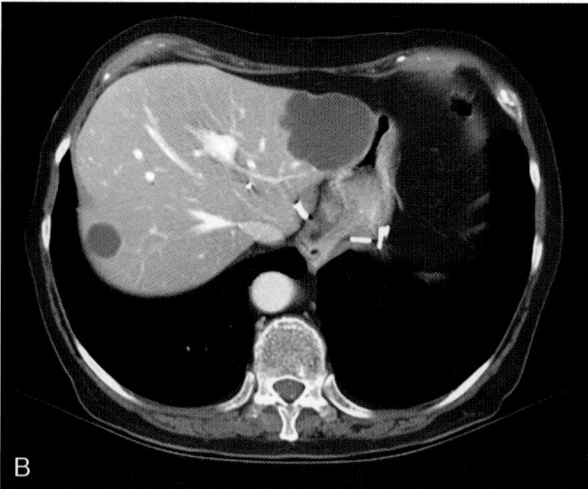

FIGURE 90.9 **A,** Baseline computed tomography of colorectal liver metastases. **B,** Optimal morphologic response after FOLFOX and bevacizumab. (From Chun YS, Vauthey JN, Boonsirikamchai P, et al. Association of computed tomography morphologic criteria with pathologic response and survival in patients treated with bevacizumab for colorectal liver metastases. *JAMA.* 2009;302[21]:2338–2344.)

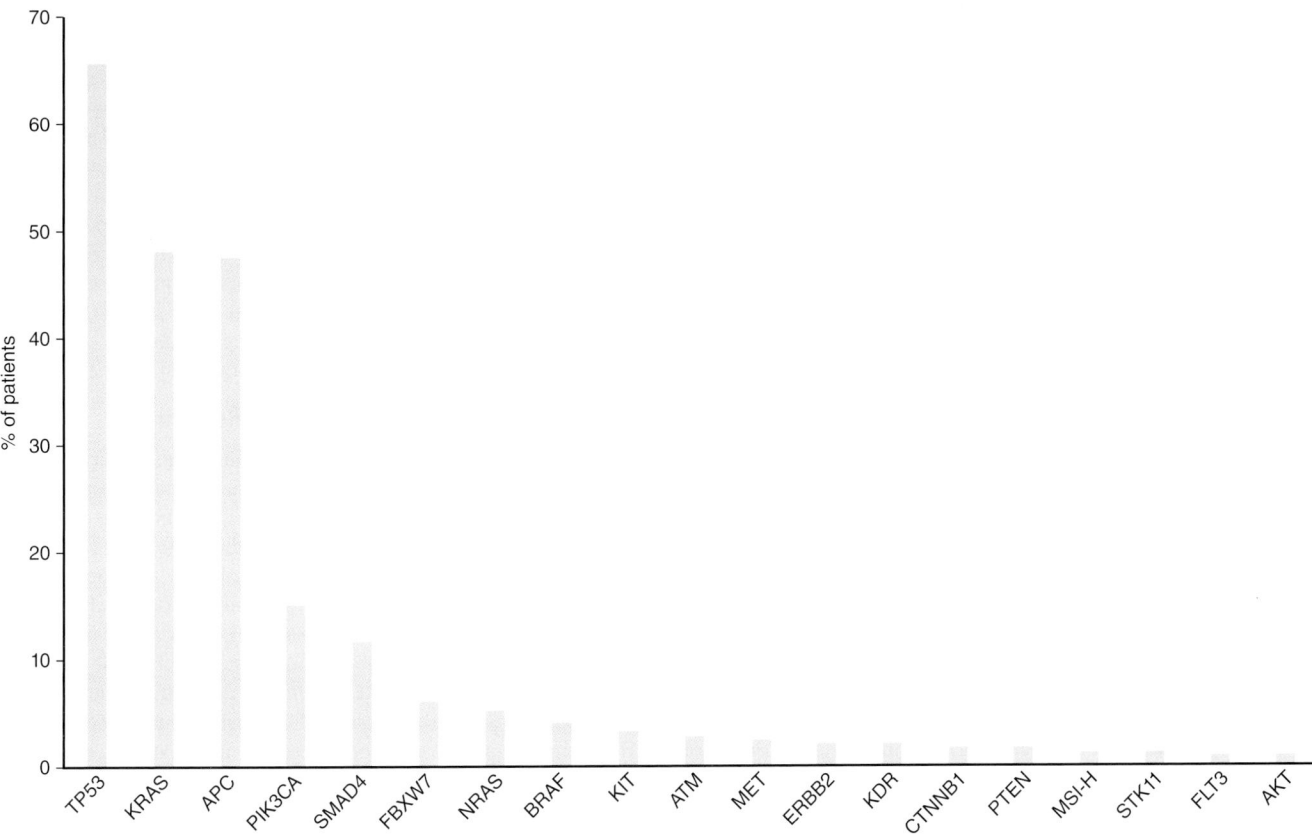

FIGURE 90.10 Frequency of somatic gene mutations among patients undergoing resection of colorectal liver metastases. (From Chun YS, Passot G, Yamashita S, et al. Deleterious Effect of RAS and evolutionary high-risk TP53 double mutation in colorectal liver metastases. *Ann Surg.* 2019;269[5]:917–923.)

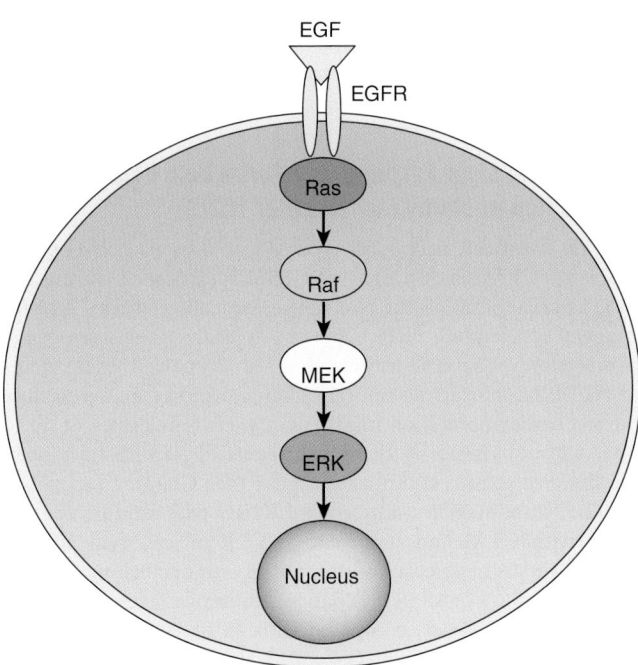

FIGURE 90.11 Interactions between epidermal growth factor receptor *(EGFR)*, Ras, and Raf in mitogen-activated protein kinase *(MAPK)* signaling cascade.

A study published in 2013 of 193 patients undergoing CLM resection who did not receive anti-EGFR therapy demonstrated significantly lower 3-year OS of 52.2% with a *RAS* mutation, compared with 81% *RAS* wild type (P = .002).[110] In addition, *RAS* mutation predicted recurrence in the lungs (3-year lung RFS rate, 34.6% vs. 59.3%, P < .001). A meta-analysis of 1181 patients undergoing CLM resection confirmed worse OS with *KRAS* mutations.[111]

BRAF

BRAF is a member of the rapidly accelerated fibrosarcoma (Raf) family of cytosolic protein kinases that transduces signals downstream of Ras, leading to activation of the MAPK signaling cascade (see Fig. 90.11). *BRAF* mutations, identified in 8% to 12% of all patients with metastatic CRC, are associated with aggressive disease and poor survival.[112,113] Patients with *BRAF* mutations are less likely to have liver-limited metastatic disease compared with *BRAF* wild-type patients. In a multicenter study of 1497 patients undergoing CLM resection, 35 patients (2%) had *BRAF* mutations.[114] Median OS and RFS rates were significantly shorter with a *BRAF* mutation (OS, 40 vs. 81 months; RFS, 10 vs. 22 months; both P < .001).

The most common *BRAF* mutation is V600E, leading to an amino acid change from valine (V) to glutamic acid (E) at codon 600. Up to a quarter of *BRAF* mutations in CRC encode non-V600 mutations.[112] Recently, *BRAF* mutations have been categorized into three classes based on kinase activity and signaling mechanisms.[115] Class I mutants are V600 mutations, which result in 500-fold to 700-fold increased kinase activity and greater activation of the MAPK pathway than *RAS* mutations. Class II mutants, which include mutations in codons 464, 469, 597, and 601, have kinase activity that is less than V600 mutants. Class III mutants, which include mutations in codons 594 and 596, have low or no kinase activity but increase MAPK signaling via enhanced binding to the Ras protein. A large, pooled analysis of metastatic CRC patients demonstrated that non-V600E *BRAF* mutations are associated with excellent prognosis, with median OS rate of 60.7 months, compared with 11.4 and 43.0 months with V600E mutation and *BRAF* wild-type, respectively ($P < .001$).[116] However, this improved prognosis with non-V600E mutations has not been shown in series of CLM resection, likely because of the small numbers of patients.

SMAD4

SMAD4 is a tumor suppressor gene central to transforming growth factor-β signaling that is associated with chemoresistance and poor prognosis in stages I to IV CRC.[117] *SMAD4* mutations are identified in 13% of patients with both resectable and unresectable CLM and associated with worse 3-year OS after CLM resection (62% vs. 82%, $P < .001$).[118]

Co-Occurring Genomic Alterations

Somatic gene mutations occurring concurrently as double or triple mutations are increasingly recognized as stronger determinants of tumor biology than a single gene mutation. *TP53*, the most frequently mutated gene in CLM, does not affect prognosis when considered in isolation.[119] However, double mutation in both *TP53* and *RAS* is associated with significantly worse 5-year OS after CLM resection of 20.6%, compared with 60.0% without double mutation ($P < .001$). Poor outcomes have also been observed among patients with double mutation in *BRAF* and *TP53*.[120]

Further supporting the importance of co-occurring genomic alterations, a recent study from MDACC showed that triple mutation in *RAS*, *TP53*, and *SMAD4* is associated with significantly worse survival than single or double mutation of these genes.[121]

RECURRENCE AFTER RESECTION OF COLORECTAL LIVER METASTASES

Although the cure rate for liver metastasectomy is considered to be about 20%, most patients undergoing CLM resection die from recurrent disease.[122] These patients likely harbored occult disease at the time of surgery that ultimately progressed. Recurrences occur in the liver in 60% of patients and exclusively in the liver in up to 40%.[123]

Postoperative Follow-Up

Most recurrences develop within the first 2 years of CLM resection. Surveillance strategies after CLM resection have been poorly studied, and no consensus exists regarding the extent and frequency of follow-up.[124] Early detection of recurrent disease provides an opportunity for potentially curative repeat hepatectomy, ablation of small liver metastases, and treatment of extrahepatic recurrence, particularly recurrent colorectal disease and limited pulmonary metastases. A typical follow-up regimen is physical examination, serum CEA level, and CT of the chest, abdomen, and pelvis every 3 to 4 months for the first 2 years

and every 6 months for the next 2 to 3 years, and an annual visit 5 years after resection. Subsequently, long-term survivors can be monitored with annual CEA levels.

A recent study of over 1000 patients showed that the risk of recurrence peaks approximately 1 year after CLM resection, declines from 1 to 4 years, and remains stable after 4 years (Fig. 90.12A).[125] Risk factors for recurrence at time of resection are primary lymph node metastasis, multiple liver metastases, CLM diameter greater than 5 cm, and *RAS* mutation. In patients who remain disease-free at 2 years, *RAS* mutation remains the sole risk factor for recurrence. These data suggest that surveillance algorithms can be tailored to patients' risk of relapse and time elapsed since CLM resection (see Fig. 90.12B).

Re-Resection for Recurrence after Resection

For patients with recurrent CLM who have a good performance status and adequate hepatic reserve, repeat hepatectomy may be considered. In carefully selected patients, repeat hepatectomy is associated with survival rates similar to those after the first hepatectomy.[126] Factors associated with adverse outcomes after re-resection include recurrence less than 6 months after initial resection, *RAS* mutation, and positive margins at the first or repeat resection.[126–128] From a technical standpoint, the presence of adhesions and the altered anatomy of the liver, particularly the position of the vasculature and biliary system, make these operations challenging. Contemporary series of repeat liver resections report an operative mortality rate of 0% and a perioperative complication rate that is similar to initial resections.[128,129] These favorable outcomes reflect careful patient selection.

AREAS OF CONTROVERSY AND FUTURE DIRECTIONS

Efforts to increase resectability and improve survival for patients with CLM include associated liver partition and portal vein ligation for staged hepatectomy (ALPPS; see Chapter 102D), R1 margin resection, and liver transplantation (see Chapter 105). These innovations hold promise for selected patients, but rigorously tested data with long-term follow-up are needed before acceptance as standard of care.

Associating Liver Partition and Portal Vein Ligation for Staged Hepatectomy (see Chapter 102D)

ALPPS has been proposed as an alternative to conventional TSH for CLM. A concern with TSH is drop-out during the time interval between the two stages, typically 8 weeks. ALPPS triggers accelerated FLR hypertrophy and enables two-stage completion within a short period of 1 to 2 weeks. Initial studies of ALPPS reported alarmingly high morbidity and mortality rates. Furthermore, high intrahepatic recurrence rates of up to 60% were observed.[130] Technical details of ALPPS have been modified to reduce complication rates (see Chapter 123).

The Scandinavian multicenter LIGRO trial randomized patients with CLM and standardized FLR of less than 30% to ALPPS versus hepatectomy after portal vein occlusion.[131] In the ALPPS arm, 44 of 48 (92%) patients underwent resection of all grossly visible disease, compared with 28 of 49 (57%) patients after portal vein occlusion ($P < .001$). Rates of major morbidity, 90-day mortality, and R0 resection were not significantly different between the two arms. The LIGRO trial investigators named the non-ALPPS arm as conventional TSH. However, 55% of

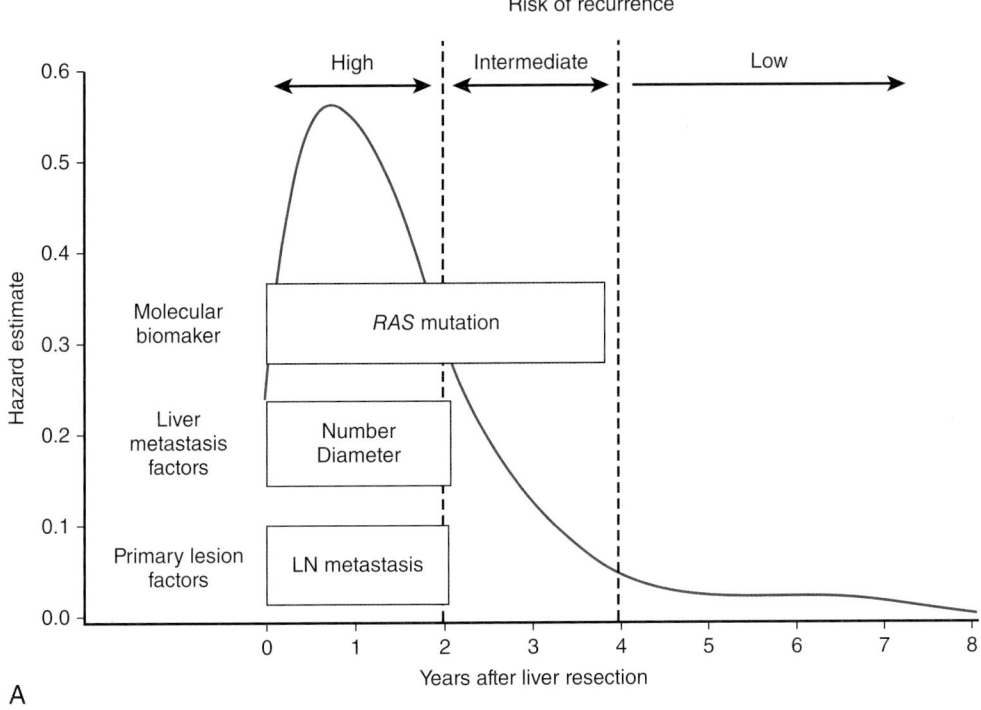

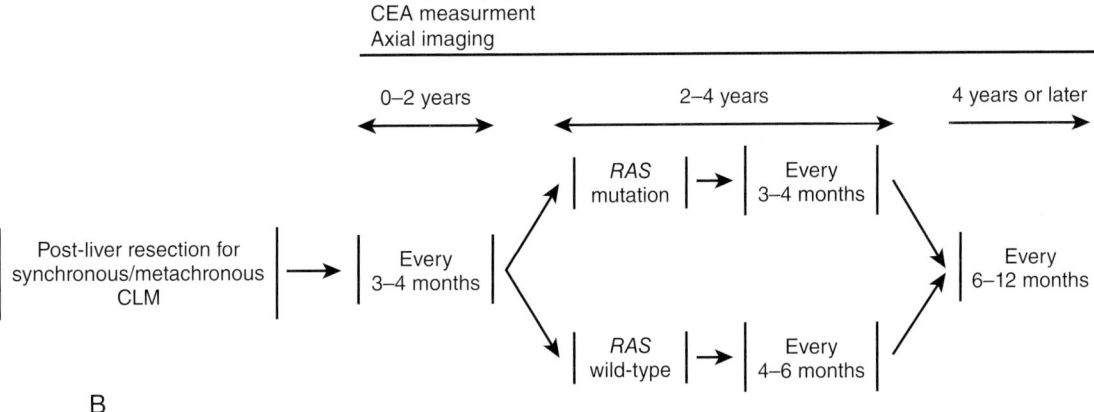

FIGURE 90.12   Changes in risk of recurrence and prognostic factors over time **(A)** and proposed surveillance algorithm stratified by *RAS* mutation and time elapsed since resection of colorectal liver metastases **(B)**. *CLM*, Colorectal liver metastases; *LN*, lymph node. (From Kawaguchi Y, Kopetz S, Lillemoe HA, et al. A new surveillance algorithm after resection of colorectal liver metastases based on changes in recurrence risk and RAS mutation status. *J Natl Compr Canc Netw.* 2020;18[11]:1500–1508.)

the patients in the purported TSH arm underwent one-stage hepatectomy, including patients who underwent ablation of metastases in the FLR. In the non-ALPPS arm, the primary reason for non-completion of resection was insufficient FLR hypertrophy, which occurred in more patients after portal vein ligation than PVE. In contrast, most published series of TSH with PVE report disease progression, not insufficient hypertrophy, as the primary reason for drop-out.[82,132]

Resection Margin

The prognostic impact of residual microscopic disease at the resection margin (R1 resection) and width of negative margin is controversial. Historically, a resection margin of 1 cm was recommended, based on studies published in the 1980s showing better survival with resection margins of at least 1 cm.[91,133] A more recent multi-institutional study of over 500 patients undergoing CLM resection demonstrated that the width of negative margin, from 1 mm to 1 cm or greater, did not affect recurrence or survival rates.[88] Blurring the lines further on the importance of resection margins, a 2008 study of 436 patients undergoing CLM resection demonstrated similar OS rates after R0 and R1 resection.[134] In this study, R1 resection was associated with higher rate of overall intrahepatic recurrence, but not with marginal recurrence.

Most studies define R1 resection as tumor-free margin of less than 1 mm. Patients with resection margins between 0.1 and 0.9 mm are reported to have survival that is worse than patients with resection margin of at least 1 mm but better than those with tumor cells at the margin.[135] Multiple studies demonstrate that the prognostic impact of a positive margin is contingent upon other factors such as response to systemic therapy, suggesting that a microscopically positive margin is a surrogate marker of aggressive tumor biology, rather than a predictor of worse survival due to marginal recurrence.[136,137] Based on current data, the goal of CLM resection is a microscopically negative margin.

Liver Transplantation (see Chapter 105)

Historically, 5-year OS after liver transplantation for CLM was dismal, only 18%, and was largely abandoned.[138] Interest in liver transplantation for CLM has been resurrected by a prospective protocol from Oslo University Hospital, the SECA study.[139] Norway is fortunate to have a surplus of liver grafts and short time on the waiting list for a deceased donor liver of less than 1 month. Inclusion criteria for the SECA protocol included unresectable CLM; no EHD by PET, CT, bone scan, and staging laparotomy; R0 resection of the primary tumor, Eastern Cooperative Oncology Group (ECOG) performance status of 0 or 1, and a minimum 6 weeks of chemotherapy. Post-transplant immunosuppression included sirolimus, an mTOR (mammalian target of rapamycin) inhibitor with antineoplastic effects. The initial report included 21 patients enrolled over a prolonged period of more than 4 years. After median follow-up after transplant of 27 months, estimated 5-year OS of 60% was reported; however, 6 patients (29%) died of disseminated cancer after median of 26 months, including a patient who died 6 months after transplantation. Twenty patients (95%) suffered disease recurrence, most often in the lungs.

In SECA-II, more stringent inclusion criteria were applied to a study population of 15 patients, including at least 10% response to chemotherapy and greater than 1-year interval between dates of CRC diagnosis and listing for liver transplant.[140] After median follow-up of 36 months, 5-year OS of 83% was reported, but DFS was significantly lower, 35% at 3 years. Currently, prospective trials investigating liver transplantation for CLM are ongoing in Canada and Europe. However, in many countries, the feasibility of liver transplantation for CLM is limited by the critical organ shortage.

CONCLUSION

For medically fit patients with metastatic CRC to the liver, hepatic resection is the standard of care and is associated with 5-year OS rates approaching 60%. In the hands of expert surgeons, hepatic metastasectomy can be performed with low morbidity and mortality. Advances in systemic therapy, diagnostic and interventional radiology, and perioperative management have expanded the number of patients eligible for resection. Increasingly refined surgical approaches combined with molecular analysis-driven prognostication and treatment will continue to improve the cure rate in patients with a disease that was believed to be terminal just a few decades ago.

The references for this chapter can be found online by accessing the accompanying Expert Consult website.

CHAPTER 91

Hepatic metastasis from neuroendocrine cancers

M. D. Smith and J. W. Devar

OVERVIEW

The liver is the most common site of metastasis for all neuro-endocrine neoplasms and second only to regional lymph nodes as the dominant site of metastases from all gastrointestinal (GI) tract malignancies. In patients with neuroendocrine liver metastases (NELMs) the cause of death is from local progression in the liver resulting in liver failure. The progress made and the accumulated experience documenting the survival potential of hepatic resection for selected patients with colorectal metastases has driven the investigation of this approach for other malignancies metastatic to the liver; there are fundamental biological differences in neuroendocrine tumors (NETs), and evidence for a similar approach in NELMs has not yet been proven. As yet, no randomized prospective data (or level 1 evidence) has evaluated liver-directed therapies (resection, transplantation, ablation, intra-arterial therapy) for patients with NELM. Consensus guidelines have been developed,[1–8] however, because of a paucity of level 1 data, recommendations have weak evidentiary support and appropriate patient selection for the various therapies continues to be debated. Clinical decisions therefore are based on experience, and guidelines are based on a lower level of evidence. Published data also originate in high-volume centers of excellence, and the generalizability is not proven. The role of the multidisciplinary team (MDT) is essential in individualizing patient care.

The recent advances in imaging have been valuable in both the morphologic and functional characterization of the disease. Contrast-enhanced ultrasound (US), contrast-enhanced dynamic computed tomography (CT), and magnetic resonance imaging (MRI) with diffusion-weighted imaging and liver-specific contrast have improved the diagnosis and characterization of NELM (see Chapter 15). Isotope scanning with positron emission tomography (PET)/CT has progressed significantly and become the standard against which other modalities will be compared (see Chapter 18).

Despite the absence of level 1 data, accumulated clinical experience suggests that cytoreduction through liver-directed therapies is beneficial for symptom control and survival. Furthermore, cytoreduction has been demonstrated to be safe (see Chapter 101).

Liver-directed therapy of NELM is appealing because GI NET has a route of metastatic dispersal similar to colorectal metastases, through the portal venous system; moreover, the natural history of NETs is typically prolonged compared with other GI tract malignancies and, in fact, with other solid tumors. Initial experience with hepatic resection for metastatic NET suggested that patients might benefit in terms of survival and symptom relief from clinical endocrinopathies when antihormonal and antineoplastic therapies were ineffective.[9] In addition to the prolonged natural history of NET and the clinically significant endocrinopathies, several other observations have supported further assessment of liver-directed

therapies: (1) the prolonged presence of intrahepatic disease before evidence of extrahepatic progression, (2) the impression that the severity of clinical endocrinopathy correlates with the intrahepatic volume of metastatic disease, (3) the resectability of the primary and regional NET despite metastatic disease, and (4) the presence of normal, nonmetastatic liver. Finally, it is important to note that much of the experience quoted in this chapter has not incorporated the newer classifications, including grade and differentiation, into the analysis of the data. This is common in the studies evaluating the use of systemic therapies, including targeted therapies, peptide receptor radionuclide therapy (PRRT), and somatostatin analogues (SSAs) (see Chapter 65). The use of the classification system facilitates the understanding of the different first-, second-, or third-line therapies in the development of treatment algorithms. This chapter details the clinical data supporting liver-directed therapy for NELM and presents the current outcomes for resection, transplantation, and intraarterial, ablative, and systemic therapies for NELM.

CLASSIFICATION OF GASTROENTEROPANCREATIC NEUROENDOCRINE TUMORS

Most NELMs are of GI or pancreatic origin, so-called gastroenteropancreatic (GEP) tumors[10] (see Chapter 65).

The GEP NETs have been divided into two broad types: *functional* and *nonfunctional,* either of which may or may not be associated with hormone production that causes a clinical endocrinopathy. Regardless of origin, NETs are similar histopathologically. Many histologic and morphologic features are shared by both benign and malignant tumors. Importantly, only the confirmed presence of metastases confers an unequivocal diagnosis of malignancy.

Clinical behavior for NETs has ranged from an indolent to an aggressive clinical course with rapid cancer progression and death. For GEP NETs, two classification schemes have been used.[11,12] Broadly, these classifications stratify patients with malignant GEP NETs into *low-grade* (well-differentiated) or *high-grade* (poorly differentiated) NETs (World Health Organization [WHO] classification). In 2017 the WHO revised the classification system, which emphasizes the proliferation index and the tumor differentiation. In general, only patients with liver metastases from well-differentiated (low-grade) NETs, rather than poorly differentiated (high-grade) NETs, are approached surgically. Limited evidence is emerging suggesting that there may be a role for surgery in poorly differentiated NELMs.[13]

The tumor-node-metastases (TNM) staging has been described, which correlated with survival.[14–18] Another classification system is based on the number and extent (or pattern) of hepatic metastases identified on radiologic imaging: a single metastasis (type I) of any size or location, an isolated metastatic bulk accompanied by smaller lesions (type II), and disseminated

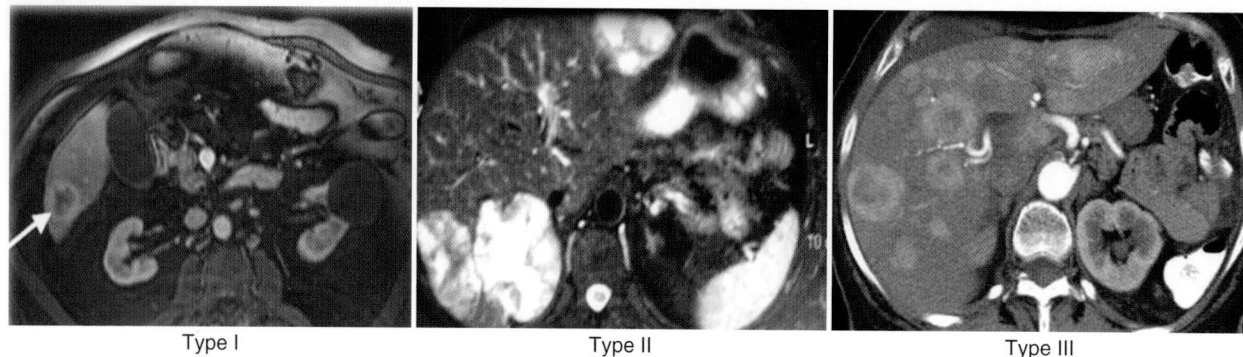

Type I   Type II   Type III

FIGURE 91.1   Classification of types of neuroendocrine liver metastases by distribution in the liver.

metastatic spread through both liver lobes (type III) (Fig. 91.1). The three groups reportedly differ significantly in regard to tumor-related characteristics and help determine a therapeutic approach that correlates with long-term survival.[19] The published guidelines by the North American Neuroendocrine Tumors Society highlight the importance of a uniform approach to pathology reporting. This is especially relevant regarding differentiation and grade of individual tumors, which have a major impact on prognostication and choice of therapy.[20]

GI NETs produce a variety of proteins and peptide hormones.[21,22] Almost all NETs are positive for neuroendocrine markers chromogranin A and neuron-specific enolase. The serum levels correlate poorly with prognosis[23]; however, they are useful for clinical follow-up.[24,25] Pancreatic NETs (pNETs) produce a wide variety of one or more peptides: gastrin, insulin, glucagon, and vasoactive intestinal polypeptide, among others.[26,27] Nonfunctional pNET implies the production of an inactive peptide or subclinical hormone or no peptide production.

Small Intestinal Carcinoids

Small intestinal carcinoids represent the most common GI carcinoid tumor and metastasize to the liver not infrequently.

It is important to recognize carcinoid heart disease in patients with GI carcinoids undergoing evaluation for resection. Approximately 20% of patients with carcinoid syndrome will have clinically evident carcinoid heart disease, and an even larger proportion will have occult heart disease detectable by echocardiography.[28] The confirmation of carcinoid heart disease requires a thorough cardiac evaluation.[29] The major consequence of carcinoid heart disease is the presence of right heart failure and the elevated systemic venous pressures that can cause a pulsatile liver (implying hepatic vein pressures >25 mm Hg), which precludes hepatic resection. The presence of clinically significant carcinoid heart disease dictates medical treatment, and occasionally valve replacement, before resection of the primary small intestinal carcinoid and the NELMs.[30] Survival after surgical repair of carcinoid heart disease is improved compared with medical treatment, even without surgical treatment of hepatic metastases.[31] Some patients may be candidates for hepatic resection after repair of carcinoid heart disease, depending on objective decreases in systemic venous hypertension and the degree of functional cardiac improvement.[32,33] Conversely, hepatic resection has been associated with decreased cardiac progression of the carcinoid heart disease and improved prognosis.[34]

Any patient with carcinoid syndrome requires preoperative and intraoperative SSA therapy to prevent a *carcinoid crisis*,[35] a clinical syndrome of life-threatening intraoperative hypotension or hypertension and severe flushing with or without concurrent bronchospasm or arrhythmias. To date, the frequency and factors predictive of this perianesthetic complication remain unknown. Prevention is essential, and appropriate treatment should be prescribed in all patients undergoing intervention for metastatic carcinoid tumors.[36] Short-acting analogues are preferred, even if the patient has received the long-acting analogue within 30 days. Management should consist of subcutaneous short-acting SSA therapy immediately preoperatively, followed by intravenous infusion of the SSA throughout the operation and continued administration in the early postoperative period. Additional intraoperative increases in SSA infusion rates are appropriate for unexplained intraoperative hemodynamic instability.

The 5-year survival for localized small intestinal carcinoid ranges from 78% to 93% and in metastatic disease decreases to 19% to 38%.[37]

Pancreatic Neuroendocrine Tumors

An aggressive operative approach is generally warranted for pNETs (see Chapter 65).[38,39] Resection remains the treatment of choice for patients with localized NET of the pancreas and for selected patients with hepatic metastases.[40] Resection of the primary NET and the regional lymph nodes is generally possible despite their often large size. The extent and type of pancreatectomy is dictated by the site of the primary NET; pancreatoduodenectomy is used for NETs of the head of the pancreas (see Chapters 117A and 127C) and distal pancreatectomy/splenectomy for NETs of the body and tail of the pancreas (see Chapters 117B and 127B). Alternatively, enucleation may be used selectively for small (<1–2 cm) superficial NETs. For patients with NETs invading adjacent structures or the GI tract, en-bloc resection is recommended. Laparoscopic pancreatectomy currently is applicable for resection of many pNETs.[41,42] Concurrent laparoscopic resection of the primary pNET and hepatic metastases may be feasible selectively. Concurrent resection of primary pNET and hepatic metastases can be performed safely, although staged resections may be preferable, particularly in patients with involvement of the head of the pancreas,[43] to avoid the development of hepatic abscesses. Overall actuarial 5-year survival rates for pNETs range from 45% to 63%, with a median survival of about 4 years.[6]

Epidemiology of Neuroendocrine Tumors

NETs are more common in woman than in men and are associated with a high socioeconomic status. Localized disease has the best prognosis, with 5-year survivals ranging between 78% and 93%. In metastatic NETs the 5-year survival is poor, at 19% to 38%, although survival has increased in the last two decades.[37,44,45] This improvement in survival is likely due to refinement in surgical techniques and newer novel targeted agents that have been introduced into the management of these tumors. NETs metastatic to the liver have the worst prognosis. Poorly differentiated NETs and rapidly progressive NELMs (>25% volume increase on two consecutive CT scans within 3 months) negatively affected survival.[46] Until now, no series of liver resections has reported the proliferation index, the differentiation and the degree of liver involvement, which makes it difficult to ascertain the overall survival in each category within the WHO 2017 classification.

The Surveillance, Epidemiology, and End Results (SEER) database showed that 27% of NETs at presentation were associated with distant metastases.[37] This is in contrast with European databases, which show that distant metastases are present in 44% to 73% of patients presenting to specialized centers. Metastases are generally found in the liver and lymph nodes and in less than 15% of patients, metastases are found in the bones. However, bony metastases are generally grossly underestimated because of the lack of adequate imaging.

Overall the metastatic potential of NETs is lower than that of adenocarcinomas. Similar to that of carcinoid tumors, the 5-year survival of patients with pNETs ranges from 30% to 40%, with a median survival of approximately 40 months.[47] Up to 75% of patients who present with midgut or hindgut tumors are likely to have liver metastases, in particular, the nonfunctioning group and those with a pancreatic primary tumors (likely to be high grade) have the highest rate of liver involvement.[48] In a series of 35 patients with hepatic metastases, 60% of which were metastatic gastrinomas, the 5-year survival was approximately 70%. With more than 75% tumor replacement the 5-year survival was only 24%, whereas 5-year survival approached 80% for less than 50% tumor replacement.[49]

RADIOLOGIC ASSESSMENT OF NEUROENDOCRINE LIVER METASTASIS

The radiologic assessment of NELMs is essential in diagnosis planning and management. There is an increasing need to individualize patient care and make clinical decisions based on guidelines; therefore the information from the radiologic assessment is important for the MDT evaluation (see Chapters 15 and 18). It is important to establish the site, number, and extent of lesions, as well as the relationship to the vasculature and biliary structures. As with any liver resection, the future liver remnant must be determined (see Chapter 102). Imaging is important in determining the pattern of liver disease because this affects treatment decisions and also may have prognostic value.[19] Three patterns of liver disease are described (also mentioned under the classification section, see Fig. 91.1). The simple, or type I, pattern refers to a single liver metastasis of any size and location, the complex, type II, pattern refers to a bulk of disease in one liver lobe with smaller lesions in the other lobe, and the diffuse, or type III, pattern describes disseminated multifocal spread through both liver lobes. Type III represents the majority (70%–80%) of patients who are also not candidates

for curative hepatectomy. There are two broad groups of investigations: anatomic and functional imaging. US and contrast-enhanced CT (CECT) are predominantly anatomic, and MRI can combine both. Radioisotope scanning is functional imaging, but the addition of high-quality PET/CT can provide some anatomic detail.

Ultrasound

The appearance of NELM on US is variable and ranges from a hypoechoic to hyperechoic lesion, although a mixed type is more common (see Chapter 15). A central cystic appearance also may be present. Even though the hypervascular nature of these lesions can be demonstrated on color Doppler, this is best demonstrated with contrast-enhanced US (CEUS). CEUS can also identify lesions not usually seen on US; however, it is currently not available for routine use.

Contrast-Enhanced Computed Tomography Scanning

CECT has been the routine cross-sectional imaging modality of choice for NELMs, but this is changing (see Chapter 15). Not only will CECT identify more lesions than CEUS but it is also very useful in elucidating the vascular anatomy. Because of the hypervascular nature of the NELM, multiphase contrast CT is indeed essential.

Magnetic Resonance Imaging

MRI is rapidly becoming the imaging modality of choice for NELMs because it combines morphologic identification with some functional modalities (see Chapter 15). Using hepatic arterial-phase and fat-suppression T2-weighted images, more lesions are identified than with CECT, particularly lesions smaller than 5 mm. Diffusion-weighted MRI (DWI) and liver-specific contrast use the biologic nature of NETs and the physics of DWI combined with apparent diffusion coefficient mapping to enhance the ability of this imaging modality to identify more lesions in the liver.

Radioisotope Scanning

The technology of radioisotope scanning in imaging NELMs has evolved over a relatively short period (see Chapter 18). Using the presence of somatostatin receptors (SSTRs) on the tumor cell surface, especially SSTR subtype 2, octreotide radio-labeled scanning, or the octreoscan, was introduced to identify and functionally characterize NETs. Unfortunately the early technology suffered from poor image quality and spatial resolution. Nonetheless, over the past two decades numerous chelator-conjugated SSAs were developed, specifically DOTA-conjugate peptides such as DOTA-TATE, DOTANOC, and DOTATOC (Fig. 91.2) These short amino acid–chelator conjugates demonstrated a greater affinity for the SSTR compared with that of an octreoscan. DOTA agents can be labeled with gallium-68 (^{68}Ga), a generator-eluted positron emitter that enables PET imaging and thus provides improved image quality and spatial resolution. ^{68}Ga-DOTA–conjugated somatostatin binds SSTR-expressing tumors and can identify lesions with a resolution of less than 5 mm. These ^{68}Ga-conjugated radiopharmaceuticals have become the reference standard imaging modality for NELM with a sensitivity of 82% to 100% and a specificity of 67% to 100% in low-grade NETs. In addition, it may identify extrahepatic disease (sensitivity and specificity 85%–96% and 67%–90%, respectively) especially subcentimeter bone metastasis in low-grade NETs.[50,51]

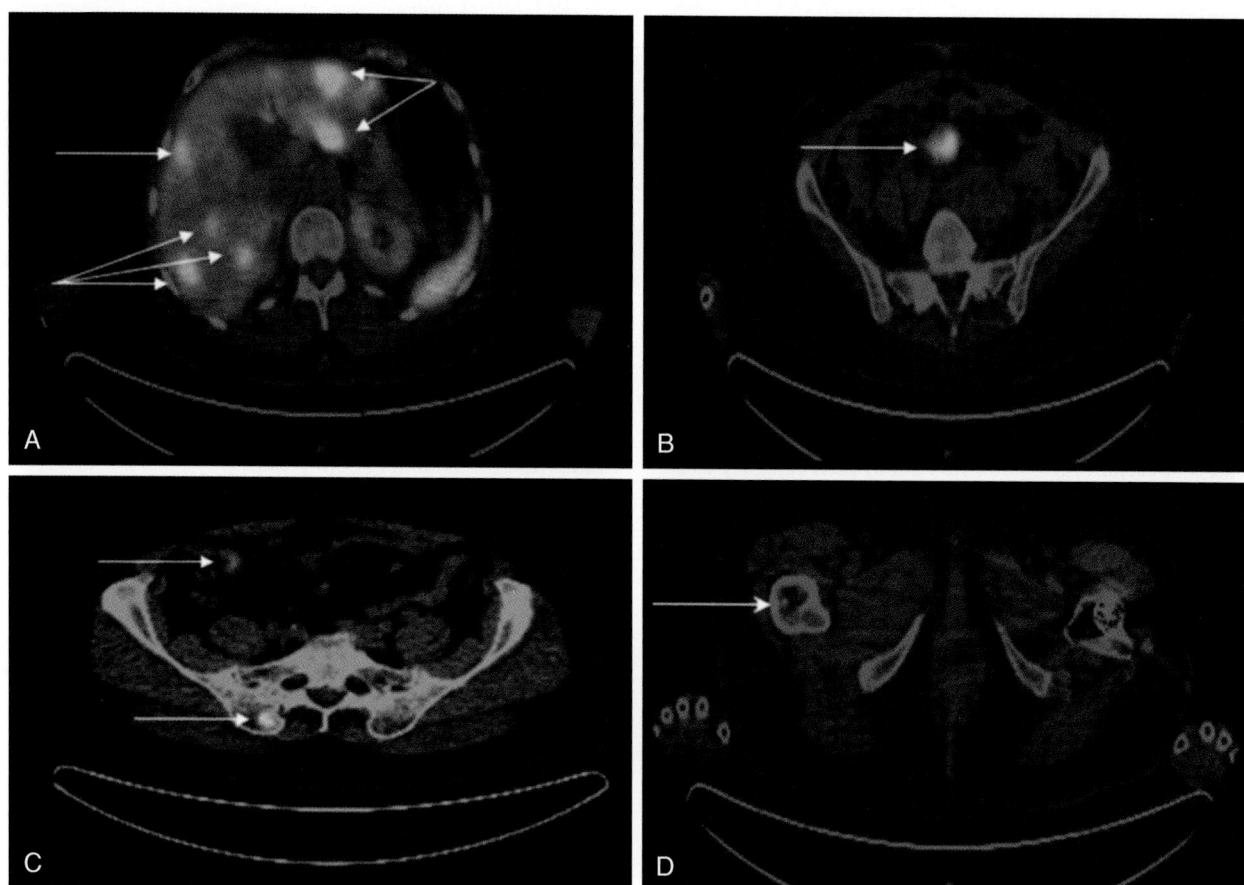

FIGURE 91.2 Imaging findings with ⁶⁸Ga-DOTA-TATE positron-emission tomography/computed tomography in a patient with bilobar liver metastases (**A,** *arrows*) from a neuroendocrine neoplasm of the distal ileum (**C,** *arrow*). Also depicted are mesenteric lymph node metastases (**B,** *arrow*), a pelvic bone metastasis (**C,** *bottom arrow*), and a small metastatic deposit in the right femur (**D,** *arrow*) (see Chapter 18).

This modality has been shown to alter the treatment decisions in up to 60% of patients by escalating or deescalating treatment options.[50,51] In a recent systematic review and meta-analysis that reported on a total of 1561 patients, change in management occurred in 44% (range, 16%–71%) of NELM patients after SSTR PET/CT. In a subgroup who had an initial indium-111 octreoscan, after the addition of an SSTR PET/CT, the information led to a change in management in 39% (16%–71%), demonstrating the superiority of the PET/CT.[52]

There is some suggestion that the use of dual imaging with both ⁶⁸GA-DOTA and 2-[¹⁸F]fluoro-2-deoxy-D-glucose (FDG)–PET/CT may have the benefit of identifying high-grade lesions with Ki67 greater than 10%, the latter of which may have a reduced expression of SSTRs and therefore better identification by FDG, which will, in turn, predict worse prognosis. ¹⁸F-FDG-PET provides complementary diagnostic information and is of value for NET patients with negative SSTRs findings or a high proliferation index.[53] ⁶⁸Ga-somatostatin receptor PET/CT should therefore be used in grade 1/2 NETs. 2-[¹⁸F]fluoro-2-deoxy-D-glucose (FDG)-PET/CT can be used to assess resectability of hepatic metastases in grade 2 NETs, and potentially in combination with ⁶⁸Ga-somatostatin receptor PET/CT.[7]

There remains debate about the timing of SSTR scintigraphy in relation to the administration of SSA therapy. However, no recommendation is possible based on the current evidence.

The choice of imaging modality has significant ramifications for treatment decisions in some NELM patients. Having enough imaging data may influence the correct choice of treatment or even the extent of treatment. The combination of morphologic and functional imaging is crucial in decision making. Given the current value of peptide receptor radioisotope therapy in treatment, as defined by the Netter 1 trial,[54] such functional imaging becomes even more essential when planning therapy.

LIVER-DIRECTED THERAPY

Hepatic Resection for Neuroendocrine Metastases

The current mainstay of treatment for NELM of GI origin is resection (see Chapters 101, 102, and 118). There is no level 1 evidence showing improved survival after resection of NELM. Furthermore, the appropriate selection of patients for resection and the definition of resectability remain debatable. Patients with G1/G2 NELM with type I (single metastasis, limited to one lobe) metastasis and selected patients with type II NELMs (isolated metastatic bulk accompanied by smaller lesions in the contralateral lobe) may be candidates for liver resection with curative intent. Those who have extrahepatic disease also may be candidates provided that the extrahepatic disease can be completely resected. Only up to 20% of patients are eligible for this approach.[7] A small proportion of patients may be rendered resectable with advanced surgical procedures that focus on ensuring adequate future liver remnant function. These may include two-step resections with right or left portal vein embolization or the associated liver partition and portal vein ligation (ALPPS) procedure (see Chapter102D).

Although hepatic resection for malignancy is used most often with curative intent, recurrence (or persistence) after resection of NELM is almost universal.[55,56] The tumor biology of NETs is typically indolent, shifting the treatment paradigm to long-term management and symptom palliation rather than cure, using combinations of liver-directed therapy (resection, transplantation, ablation, intraarterial therapy).

Traditionally, resection of NELMs has been recommended if the primary tumor and regional disease were resectable or resected and a minimum of 90% of the volume of hepatic metastases were resectable or ablatable.[48] In the early 1990s, debulking hepatic resection could be performed safely, and overall survival approached 75% at 4 years.[57] Survival did not differ significantly between complete (R0) or incomplete (R1 to R2) resections, and mean duration of symptomatic response was nearly 2 years. In a landmark study in 2003, Sarmiento et al.[55] showed that symptoms resolved in 98% of patients. Median time to recurrence of symptoms was 45 months, but 40% of patients were asymptomatic at 5 years. Overall survival was 61% and 35% at 5 and 10 years, respectively, and perioperative mortality rate was 1.2%. Recurrence, however, was 84% at 5 years and 94% at 10 years.

A review of the current literature on hepatic resection for NELMs is summarized in Table 91.1 The cumulative findings support the efficacy of hepatic resection for NELM. Overall 5-year survival has ranged from 41% to 82%. Operative mortality has been low, at approximately 1%. Resolution of endocrine symptoms has exceeded 90% in most series, although duration of response was not frequently reported. Despite the margin status (R0, R1 vs. R2), overall survival has not differed significantly in most series, although a recent international multicenter analysis did demonstrate a significantly decreased survival for R2 resections in patients with endocrinopathies.[58] Although the accumulated clinical experience supports cytoreduction of NELM to control symptoms and prolong survival,

evidence by clinical trials to determine the optimal liver-directed therapies is lacking; for example, comparison between R0/R1 resection versus R2 resection versus intraarterial therapy have been lacking and further studies have been recommended.[3]

An additional consideration is the pattern of metastatic disease and the extent of resection required. An R0 or R1 hepatic resection of NELM is challenging for patients presenting with bilobar synchronous hepatic metastases (type II) (Fig. 91.3). Approaches used for metastatic colorectal cancer to the liver have been used for NELM. Preoperative portal vein embolization with staged hepatic resection has been used successfully. Conventional two-stage hepatectomy, including either portal vein ligation or embolization, has been proposed for patients with large tumor burden.[59] In this latter study on two-stage hepatectomy, 23 patients were included and only 19 proceeded to the second step. Of the 19 patients, 14 (74%) had an R0 resection. The morbidity of the first step was 17% and after the second step was 21%. The 2-, 5- and 8-year disease-free survival (DFS) and overall survival rates were 85%, 50% and 26% and 94%, 94%, and 79%, respectively.

The evidence for the use of ALPPS for staged hepatectomy is scant, and data from the International ALLPS registry included only 21 patients with NELM between 2010 and 2017 (see Chapter 102D). R0 resection was achieved in 19 patients at stage 2.[60] Median follow-up was 28 months (range, 19–48 months) and the median DFS was 17.3 months, 1-year DFS was 73.2% and 2-year DFS was 41.8%. Median overall survival could not be established because of the short-term follow-up. The morbidity after the first stage was 29% and 52% after the second stage. It was reported that the Clavien-Dindo classification 3b morbidity was 9%, with a mortality rate of 5% at 90 days.

Although the overall survival at 2 years did not differ in the two previously mentioned studies,[59,60] the 2-year DFS was significantly better with the two-stage hepatectomy at 85% versus 41.8% with ALLPS. It is important to note that these are retrospective studies with small numbers and currently no conclusions can be made.

High-grade NETs are generally excluded from resection because of the aggressive biologic processes of these tumors, and they are typically treated with systemic therapy. However

TABLE 91.1 Selected Hepatic Resection Study Results Stratified on the Basis of Margin Status

AUTHOR AND YEAR	TOTAL PATIENT NUMBER	N	R0/R1 OS	PFS	N	R2 OS	PFS
Sarmiento et al. 2003	170		76%	—	95	—	9%
Mazzaferro et al. 2007	36	36	85%	—	—	—	—
Kianmanesh et al. 2008	41(23)*		79%				
Scigliano et al. 2009	41	37	R0: 88% R1: 82%		4	50%	0%
Frilling et al. 2009	119	23	100%	96%	—	—	—
Saxena et al. 2011	74	48	98 months		26	27 months	Median: 24 months
Maxwell et al. 2016	228	—	—	—	108	Median: 10.5 years 5 year: 76%	Median: 2.2 years
Fairweather et al. 2017	649	58	5 year: 90% 10 year: 70%	NR	—	—	—

N, Number of patients undergoing hepatectomy; NR, not recorded; OS, overall survival; PFS, progression-free survival.
*Figures representing the first and second step of the two-step hepatectomy.

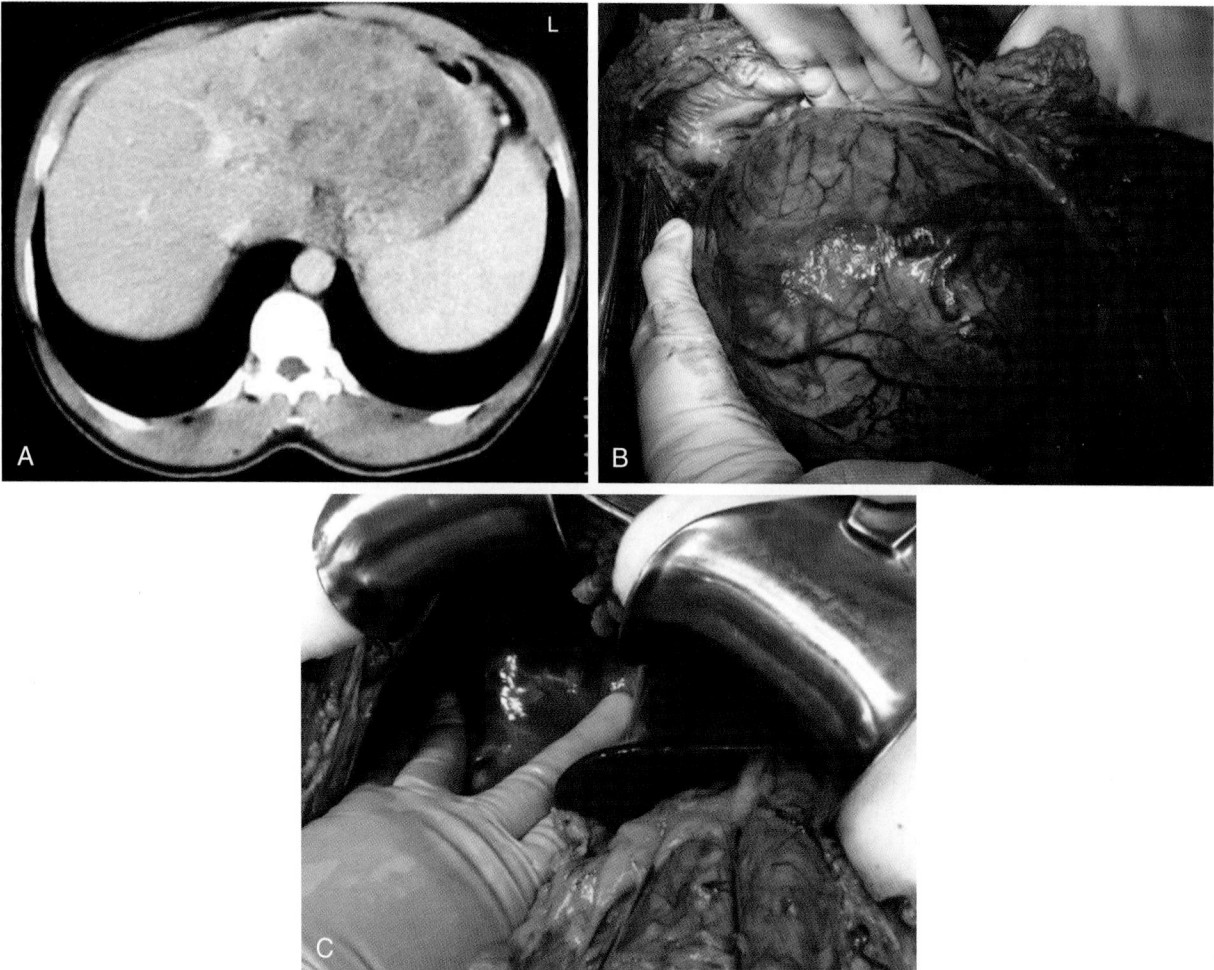

FIGURE 91.3 **Male patient who presented with a nonfunctional pancreas neuroendocrine tumor. A,** Preoperative computed tomography scan (see Chapter 15). **B,** Operative specimen. **C,** Intraoperative picture of multiple neuroendocrine liver metastases in right lobe.

limited data are emerging for poorly differentiated NETs (grade 3b), suggesting there may be a role for resection. Classically these patients undergo systemic chemotherapy, with a median overall survival of 11 months. In a case series of 32 patients with neuroendocrine carcinomas undergoing resection with or without ablation, 75% of patients had poorly differentiated tumors. Overall survival at 3 and 5 years was 47% and 43%. However, median recurrence of disease was noted at 8.4 months. There was a trend to better progression-free survival (PFS) and overall survival with Ki67 between 21% and 54%.[13] Further robust data are required to adopt a resection strategy for these high-grade NETs (WHO 3b).

Single-stage extended hepatic resection combined with ablation also has been reported.[61] However, the enthusiasm for extended resections must be tempered by the realization that the overall frequency of recurrence or progression after hepatic resection is approximately 60% to 80% at 5 years and nearly 100% by 10 years, and the removal of large volumes of normal liver with extended resections may limit future therapeutic options.

Data looking at the site of recurrence after resection was reported in the multi-institutional analysis of 322 patients with NELMs. In the 209 (64.9%) who developed recurrence after resection, the site of recurrence was noted in 169 patients, with liver-only recurrence in 65.7%, extrahepatic recurrence only in 11.2%, and both intrahepatic and extrahepatic recurrence in 23.1%. The most common modality used to treat hepatic recurrence was repeat resection in 36% of patients and intraarterial therapy in 21.4%. The 10-year overall survival was 60.3% and 52%, respectively.[62]

Intrahepatic progression of NELMs after resection, regardless of the perceived completeness of resection, requires subsequent liver-directed therapy. Similar to the initial resection, the extent and distribution of hepatic recurrence dictates the choice of therapy.

Metastatic NETs that preclude ablation or resection is treated by bland embolization, chemoembolization, or radioembolization. Systemic chemotherapy in the absence of extrahepatic disease is limited to patients who have reached the limits of liver-directed therapy. A schema for management of neuroendocrine metastases to the liver is outlined in Figure 91.4.

Debulking Resection

In the surgical treatment of liver metastasis from other cancers the eligibility criteria have been well described. The intention is to completely resect all liver disease. With respect to the future liver remnant, in general, disease is limited to one portion of the liver allowing resection by nonanatomic resections, lobectomies,

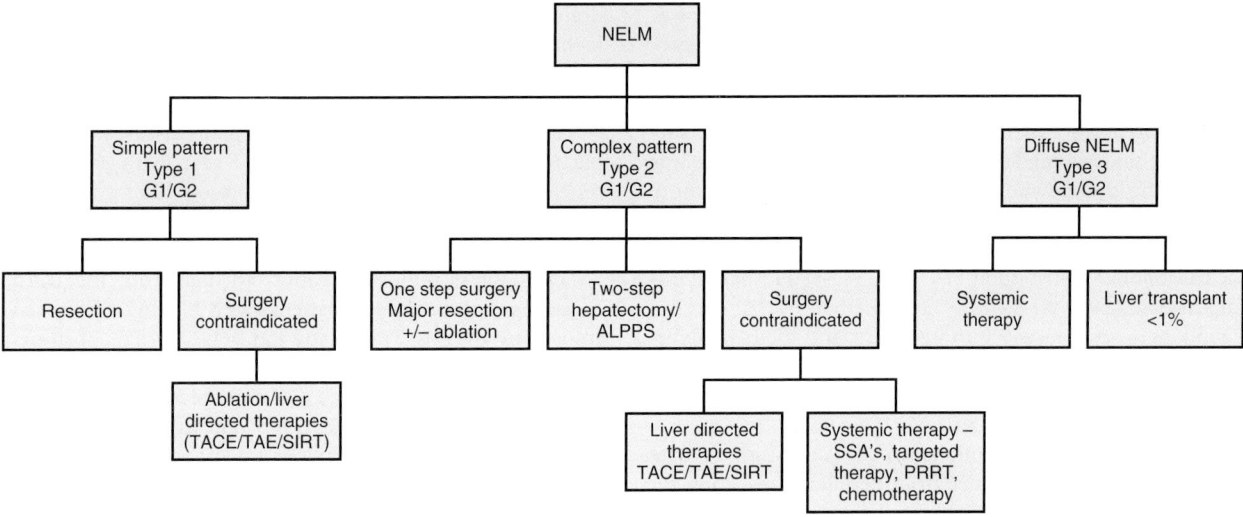

FIGURE 91.4   Algorithm for the treatment of neuroendocrine liver metastases.

and trisegmentectomies. Positive margins are associated with recurrence and poor outcomes. The same expectation is not necessarily true for NELMs. Only 20% of NELMs are eligible for curative resections.[63]

In studies reporting the outcome from liver resection for hepatic metastases from NETs, PFS for R0, R1, and R2 resections are not large despite a decrease in overall survival.[58,64] The main outcome difference based on the margin status is disease control. In addition, the morbidity and mortality rates are very good, with approximately 20% morbidity and less than 3% mortality. These data support the earlier study by McEntee's group in 1990 that reported good outcomes for patients who have functional NET with NELM.[65] Debulking in that era was introduced to treat the hormone symptoms. In 2003 the landmark paper by Sarmiento et al.[55] demonstrated that the benefit from debulking was both for reduction in hormonal-related symptoms and an improvement in overall survival; thus this procedure was also of benefit in patients with symptomatic nonfunctional NELM. In addition the outcome for the various primary sites, especially pancreas versus midgut, were similar. Moreover, the authors supported the requirement for a greater than 90% reduction in tumor burden.

The options for treatment have progressed since then, including the introduction of SSA therapy into routine management of patients with both functional and nonfunctional tumors. Improvement in surgical techniques and the addition of other liver-directed therapies, such as the combination of resection with ablation therapies, have been introduced, but a good level of evidence from comparative studies is still lacking.

A number of studies reporting on outcomes for liver resection in general have included patients whose procedures may be classified as cytoreduction surgery. The use of the term *cytoreduction* is confusing because most patients undergoing liver resection with curative intent recur between 5 and 10 years postoperatively. Therefore most curative surgeries could be considered palliative or cytoreductive. When considering resections without a curative intent and not surgery undertaken with the intention of complete resection, the term *debulking* is appropriate. It is the outcomes in this group of patients that are considered in this section.

The current indications for debulking include hormonal symptoms not responsive to medical therapies or symptoms because of the local effects of the large size of the tumor not responding to other therapies.

A number of studies have also shown that the presence of extrahepatic disease did not influence the decision to perform debulking surgery[66]; however, it would have an impact on the decision to perform curative surgery when a worse outcome can be expected.[58] In 2014 Graff-Baker et al.[67] strongly recommended that even if extrahepatic disease is discovered at operation with a debulking intent, surgery should not be aborted. The vast majority of patients with metastatic NETs die of liver failure and not from the extrahepatic disease, and studies have shown no difference in survival between patients with and those without extrahepatic disease.[63]

The traditional requirement for a greater than 90% debulking was recently challenged.[67,68] In a study including patients with extrahepatic disease, Graff-Baker's group reviewed their retrospective data dividing patients into three groups: 70% to 90%, 90% to 99% and 100% resections. They reported a disease progression of 27.3%, 27.3%, and 31.6%, respectively. The overall disease-specific survival at 5 years was 90%. The only factor that influenced prognosis was patients younger than 50 years. Their data support a reevaluation of the cutoff volume for debulking surgery. Thus the duration of response should be proportional to the extent of the debulking or cytoreduction of the NELM and the growth rate of the residual tumor.[69] Reduction of more than 90% of the volume of hepatic metastases can result in significantly different residual cancer volumes based on variations of the metastatic volume. Both time to recurrence of symptoms and survival are related to residual metastatic cancer volume. The maximal clinical impact of cytoreduction may not be realized by more than 90% cytoreduction of NELM, but by the minimization of residual metastatic cancer volume that is not the resected volume but rather the residual tumor volume. In attempting to minimize the residual tumor volume, theoretically, resection (or transplantation) offers the possibility of a more "complete" cytoreduction without affecting other treatment options. The sequential combination of resection with other liver-directed therapies may be indicated to truly minimize the residual tumor volume.

In 91.5% of cases, patients will show significant improvement in their symptoms after cytoreduction. In patients presenting with an endocrinopathy, 89.8% had symptomatic improvement.

When comparing patients who underwent debulking surgery to those undergoing surgery with a curative intent, it was found that the group who had debulking surgery had more symptoms (75% vs. 63%), had higher grade tumors (35% vs. 13%), were likely to be synchronous at presentation (70% vs. 59%), had bilobar distribution (76% vs. 53%), and had extrahepatic disease (19% vs. 8%).[67,70] The median overall survival for debulking resections is 7.0 to 9.6 years, and the 5-year survival is 61% to 88%.[61,67,68,70] The 5-year disease-specific survival is 90%, with median overall survival similar between functional and nonfunctional NELM.[67]

Osborne's group in 2006 published the only study to date that has compared the outcomes from debulking resection for metastatic NETs to other liver-directed therapy, in particular, embolization. Although the results can be difficult to interpret, the results for symptom relief were better for debulking surgery (69% vs. 59%) and the symptom-free interval was also longer for debulking surgery (56 months vs. 37 months). Moreover, the mean survival benefit was greater in debulking surgery (32 ± 18.9 months vs. 24 ± 15.8 months). The authors concluded that debulking surgery should be pursued whenever possible, even if complete resection may not be achievable.[71]

In patients who respond to chemotherapy, additional cytoreduction is a valid and direct method of providing relief from symptoms. Very few of the systemic therapies will result in a measurable response according to Response Evaluation Criteria in Solid Tumors (RECIST) and thus will not single-handedly increase the proportion of patients who can have complete resections.

The ultimate choice of which liver-directed therapy to use is individualized; however, it is significantly influenced by the extent and pattern of metastatic disease in the liver. Focusing on minimizing any residual disease, the definition of resectable liver disease is more restrictive. Patients with limited unilobar or bilobar disease can be considered for resection, with or without adjunctive measures such as ablation, again assuming all identifiable disease can be addressed in this manner. However, those patients with a diffuse metastatic burden are unlikely to benefit from surgical resection with gross disease remaining and are likely more appropriate for consideration of either transplantation or catheter-based therapies.

Hepatic Transplantation for Neuroendocrine Metastases

Resection for liver metastases with intent to cure is realistic in only approximately 20% of patients presenting with liver metastases (see Chapters 105 and 108B). In light of the fact that the 80% will have either complex type II or diffuse type III patterns of metastases (as described earlier), other strategies are required to achieve a possible cure. What makes liver transplant attractive is the fact that up to 50% of metastases may be missed on current imaging modalities,[72] and thus an incomplete R0 resection may have implications for overall survival. In the initial phases of orthotopic liver transplantation (OLT), outcomes were poor and strategies at determining criteria for OLT were debated. Currently criteria for transplantation are still not well defined. Mazzaferro et al.[73] and other groups have suggested that transplant be limited to patients with low-grade tumors, the primary tumor should be drained by the portal venous system and resected, and liver involvement should be limited to less than 50%. Disease progression should be stable for 6 months and limited to a younger age group (50–60 years).

It is essential to exclude extrahepatic disease with imaging, particularly ^{68}Ga-octreotate PET/CT scan, with a specific focus on excluding nodal and bony metastases.[74] Before transplantation a staging laparotomy or laparoscopy may be considered to rule out peritoneal deposits.[75]

The largest published cohort to date from the European registry reported on 213 patients with NELM who received a transplant over a 27-year period. The 90-day postoperative mortality was 10%, the 5-year survival was 52%, and nearly 60% had disease recurrence.[76] A more recent systematic review found a 5-year survival of 70.7%.[77] The difference in long-term outcomes is most likely explained by patient selection and differences in data reporting.

Factors associated with poor long-term survival include synchronous resection of the primary tumor at liver transplant, presence of hepatomegaly because of tumor bulk, poorly differentiated tumors, margin-positive resection, and lymph node–positive disease. Other factors include a Ki67 index greater than 10%.[4,6,76,78]

The European NeuroEndocrine Tumor Society (ENETS) consensus guideline suggests that the inclusion criteria for liver transplantation for NELM include a well-differentiated G1/G2 tumor, Ki67 index less than 10%, stable disease for 6 months, age younger than 55 years, and primary tumor removed at least 6 months before the procedure.[4,6] The authors of these guidelines indicate that using these criteria, less than 1% of NELMs would be suitable for transplantation. There is a suggestion in the literature that tumors arising from the GI tract have a better outcome than pNETs after transplantation.[76,79]

The Organ Procurement and Transplant Network has proposed recommendations for selecting patients in the United States. Their age limit is 60 years, and they have specific guidelines for imaging, time interval, type of diagnostics, and radiographic characteristics.

Single-center series reporting on hepatic transplantation for NELM are small, and follow-up has been limited. Overall survival has ranged from 50% to 100% at 1 year and 36% to 89% at 5 years, but DFS has been infrequent. Overall 5-year survival is similar to that for transplantation for hepatocellular carcinoma (HCC) but remains less than transplantation for nonmalignant indications. In the European registry, 17% of the patients died from early or late complications of transplantation without evidence of persistent or recurrent disease. Symptomatic relief from clinical endocrinopathies has been uniformly complete, but duration of symptom relief after OLT has not been clearly documented. Rates of recurrence are generally similar to those after resection, with criteria of patient selection for OLT likely accounting for this finding.

Although the survival data have improved, caution in selection of NELM patients for hepatic transplantation is still advised and the benefit of OLT for NELM should be balanced between the shortage of organs and the potential clinical benefit. At this stage, standardization of patient selection criteria, immunosuppressive regimens, and an MDT are needed. Because of a lack of level 1 evidence, the recommendations to endorse OLT for extensive NELM warrants ongoing deliberation and requires robust data to guide practice.

Ablation

The initial evidence supporting ablation for NELM was based on the data from other liver malignancies (see Chapter 96A). There is no good evidence for its use, but there is significant support for its inclusion in treatment strategies.[4–6,8] A number of techniques, including cryotherapy and percutaneous ethanol injection, are no longer in common clinical practice (see Chapter 96D). Their role and outcomes are of historical value only. The current technologies include radiofrequency ablation (RFA) (see Chapter 96B) and microwave ablation (MWA) (see Chapter 96C). RFA is the best described, but there are some important benefits for MWA that will be discussed in this chapter. Ablative techniques are most effective in patients with a low tumor volume (lesions between 1 and 5 cm) and best indicated for a limited number of metastases (fewer than 5 or 6 lesions).[48]

Radiofrequency Ablation of NELM

Currently, RFA is the most widely used ablative technique for hepatic tumors because of its versatility, ease of use, and relatively low risk of complications[80–83] (see Chapter 96B). However, its utility for NELM will be limited by the disease extent in most patients. It is well tolerated with a 10% morbidity and a mortality rate of 0.7%.[84] Complications include bleeding, wound infections, pneumonias, urinary tract infections, and liver abscess formation. Mean hospital stay for RFA is 1.1 days.

The application of RFA for NELM arose after its efficacy was established in the treatment of HCC and metastatic colorectal cancer. Reports of RFA specifically for NELM have been limited. RFA has been used both on its own and as an adjunct to resection. Objective tumor destruction has been well documented and has been shown to be effective in local tumor control. Local tumor control was achieved in 82% to 98% of metastases, although duration of follow-up was short.[56,80,85,86] Local recurrence has ranged from 3% to 22% of metastases.[7,87] Local liver recurrence was observed in 7.9%, but new tumors are reported in up to 63% at a medium of 30 months.[88] Improved survival with RFA for NELM has been demonstrated for selected patients (84% at 3 years and 53% at 5 years).[7,89,90] In addition, a median survival time of 3.9 years from the time of first ablation and a medium DFS of 1.3 years has been shown.[88,91] Successful ablation typically occurred in the treatment of metastases smaller than 3 cm[86,92,93]; only 50% of tumors greater than 5 cm were ablated completely, even with repeated ablation.[94]

Duration of follow-up is insufficient to determine actual durability of local control, given the protracted natural history of NETs. Progression of hepatic metastases occurs in about 30% of patients within 2 years.[87] Specific factors of the hepatic metastases, such as site, degree of necrosis or fibrosis, and hormonal markers, have not yet been correlated to RFA response.

RFA effectively relieves clinical endocrinopathies related to NELM. Some degree of symptom relief has been reported in nearly 90% of patients after ablation, and duration of relief from symptoms usually is 10 months or longer.[87,88,95] A systematic review demonstrated a 92% symptom improvement after RFA lasting a median of 14 to 27 months.[84] Recurrence of symptoms was common, occurring in 63% to 87% and 5-year survival rates of 57% to 80%. It is important to note that 48% of these patients had concomitant liver resections. These findings are similar to those reported after hepatic resection of NELM.[49,55]

In the setting of extrahepatic disease, isolated hepatic ablation will have a limited effect on symptoms[95]; however, clinical efficacy will depend on the volume, site of extrahepatic tumor, and the specific hormone expression.

Serum and urine NET markers are generally proportional to tumor volume. The response of such markers to RFA has been variable. In a study of 34 patients treated with intraoperative RFA, only 65% had a decrease in serum tumor markers. Persistence of elevated tumor markers after RFA likely reflects patient selection, completeness of ablation, and occult or overt NELM. A favorable response in reduction of serum tumor markers after ablation may predict the durability of symptomatic response and may be associated with improved survival and decreased incidence of disease progression.[87]

Microwave Ablation

MWA therapy is a local treatment by which tumors are destroyed by coagulation from the passage of microwaves into tissue (see Chapter 96C). MWA emerged as a reliable technique under a variety of clinical situations. Two main zones are described after ablative therapy: central and transitional. No viable cells were demonstrated in 93% of lesions after treatment, even up to 6 cm in diameter.[96] Although data comparing RFA with MWA are awaited, the results reported in observational studies indicate that MWA may have a role when larger ablation zones are required.[97] The benefit of MWA in the zone close to vessels and bile ducts has been described. In addition, there is some suggestion that the zone of ablation may be larger with microwave. There is no study with a direct comparison of these two technologies.

Ethanol Ablation of Hepatic Neuroendocrine Metastases

Ethanol ablation has been used in patients with NELM to the liver[81,98,99] (see Chapter 96D). Several studies have documented a complete intrahepatic response in patients with NELM with percutaneous ethanol injection.[100] Percutaneous ethanol injection has been used primarily in patients in whom thermal ablation of metastases are associated with risk of damage to adjacent to structures. Selective ethanol ablation can be performed on metastases adjacent to vital structures, such as the hepatic flexure of the colon; those adjacent to large vessels vulnerable to the heat-sink effect; and those adjacent to central bile ducts, where subsequent biliary stricture may occur. Moreover, metastases of very small size can be ablated successfully with ethanol, with limited effects to adjacent liver.

Cryoablation of Hepatic Neuroendocrine Metastases

Intraoperative cryoablation is effective in the treatment of primary and secondary tumors of the liver[101–106] (see Chapter 96D). Based on a collective review of 1990s literature, local recurrence develops in approximately 30% of cryoablated tumors.[103] Comparatively, cryoablation has been associated with greater local recurrence (14% vs. 2%) and a greater frequency of complications (41% vs. 3%) than RFA for patients with both primary and secondary hepatic tumors.[82,107]

Cryoablation for NELM is limited to ablation performed intraoperatively.[103,108–110] Most often, cryoablation was performed as an adjunct to resection of the primary tumor and hepatic metastases and local control of NELM occurred in 95% of treated metastases.[103,107,110] Some degree of relief of symptoms has been shown in all patients, regardless of the percentage of tumor volume ablated.[103,108,110] Moreover, adjuvant therapy with a long-acting SSA after ablation can prolong symptom-free survival.[107]

Guidelines for Ablation

General guidelines for the ablation of hepatic metastases are analogous to the treatment of hepatocellular carcinoma and colorectal metastases. Given the prolonged survival and clinical endocrinopathies associated with NELMs, broader application of ablation as a component of multimodal treatment is recommended. Indeed, because reports have shown that cytoreduction of NETs can consistently improve both patient symptoms and survival, the corollary of aggressive ablation of progressive NELMs should provide similar patient benefit.

Three clinical scenarios exist for ablation of NELM: (1) as an adjunct to concurrent surgical resection of hepatic metastases, (2) as treatment of limited hepatic metastases in patients unfit for operation, and (3) as the primary hepatic therapy when clinical expertise or intraoperative circumstances preclude safe resection. Palliation of symptoms is an important aim for all patients with functional neuroendocrine symptoms.

RFA complements intraoperative resection of NELMs. Given the extensive hepatic tumor burden typically encountered, ablation affords selective treatment of metastases located deep in the liver or in sites not amenable to resection after partial hepatectomy. Adjunctive RFA optimizes debulking of hepatic metastases, reduces the extent of resection, and increases the number of patients who may benefit from cytoreductive surgery.

Resection is precluded in many patients with NELM because of the extent of tumor burden, comorbid disease, or prior hepatic resection. In such patients, percutaneous ablation allows less invasive tumor debulking and may have some advantage over chemotherapy alone, as some have suggested in colorectal liver metastases.[111] Generally speaking, if the metastasis is visible with imaging, it can usually be treated with percutaneous ablation.

Several case series have compared the outcomes of hepatic resection versus other liver-directed therapies. A single-center series showed better overall survival for 58 hepatic resections versus other ablative strategies. They reported a 5-year survival for resection 90%, RFA 84%, chemoembolization 55%, systemic therapy 58%, and observation alone 38%.[112]

In a recent meta-analysis of studies investigating intervention for liver metastases rising from GEP NETs, four studies reported outcomes on any surgery versus chemotherapy.[113] The meta-analysis demonstrated a statistically significant 5-year overall survival in favor of any surgery when compared with chemotherapy (odds ratio [OR], 0.05; 95% confidence interval [CI], 0.01–0.21; $P < .0001$). This may infer that ablation, as part of a debulking strategy, is better than chemotherapy (Fig. 91.5).

In patients with one or two very small hepatic metastases, surgical resection might be considered overly aggressive given the effectiveness of percutaneous RFA in treating such tumors (Fig. 91.6). Percutaneous treatment is typically performed on an outpatient basis and obviates the longer hospitalization after resection. Moreover, given the invariable recurrence of metastases after surgical resection,[55] percutaneous ablation is well suited for the patient who has undergone prior liver surgery. Although repeat resection is possible in a limited number of patients,[114] ablation can be easily performed on multiple occasions based on occurrence of new metastases.

RFA of neuroendocrine hepatic metastases allows a relatively noninvasive mechanism to treat symptoms, similar to the role of hepatic resection. Ablation may not be indicated for treating local pressure symptoms but can be used to manage

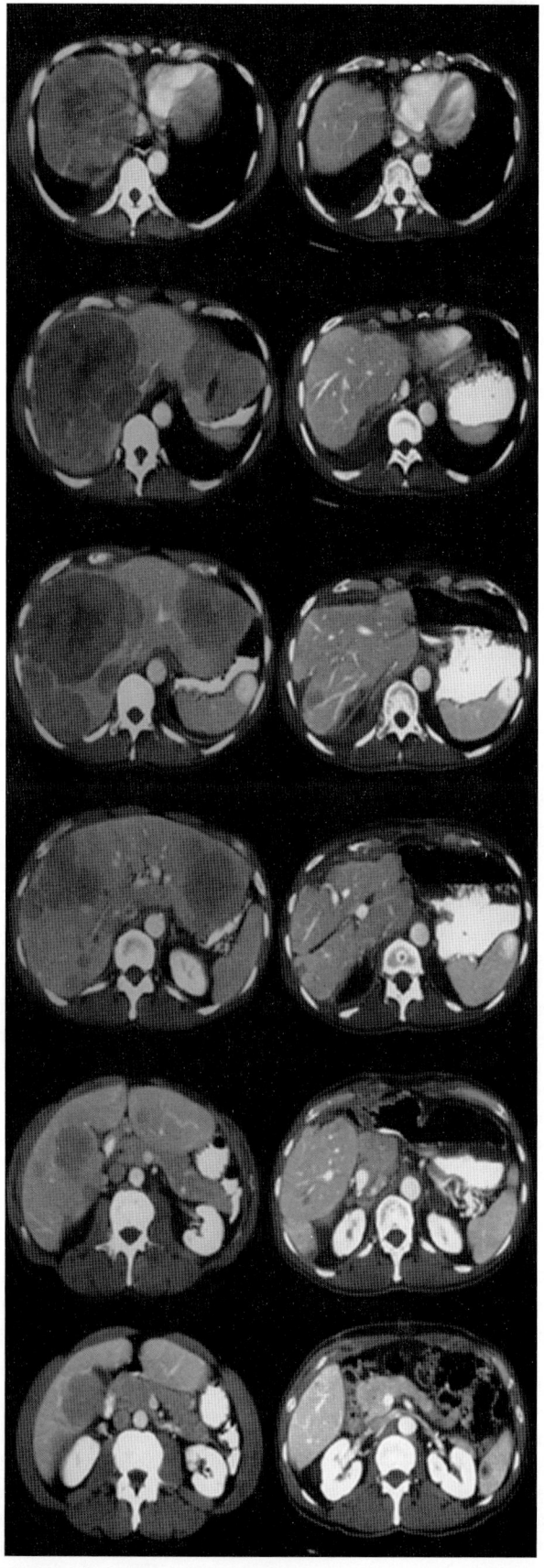

FIGURE 91.5 Computed tomography images in a patient with metastatic carcinoid tumor before *(left)* and 18 months after *(right)* cytoreductive hepatic resection. Intrahepatic recurrences were ablated by percutaneous radiofrequency ablation (see Chapters 15 and 96B).

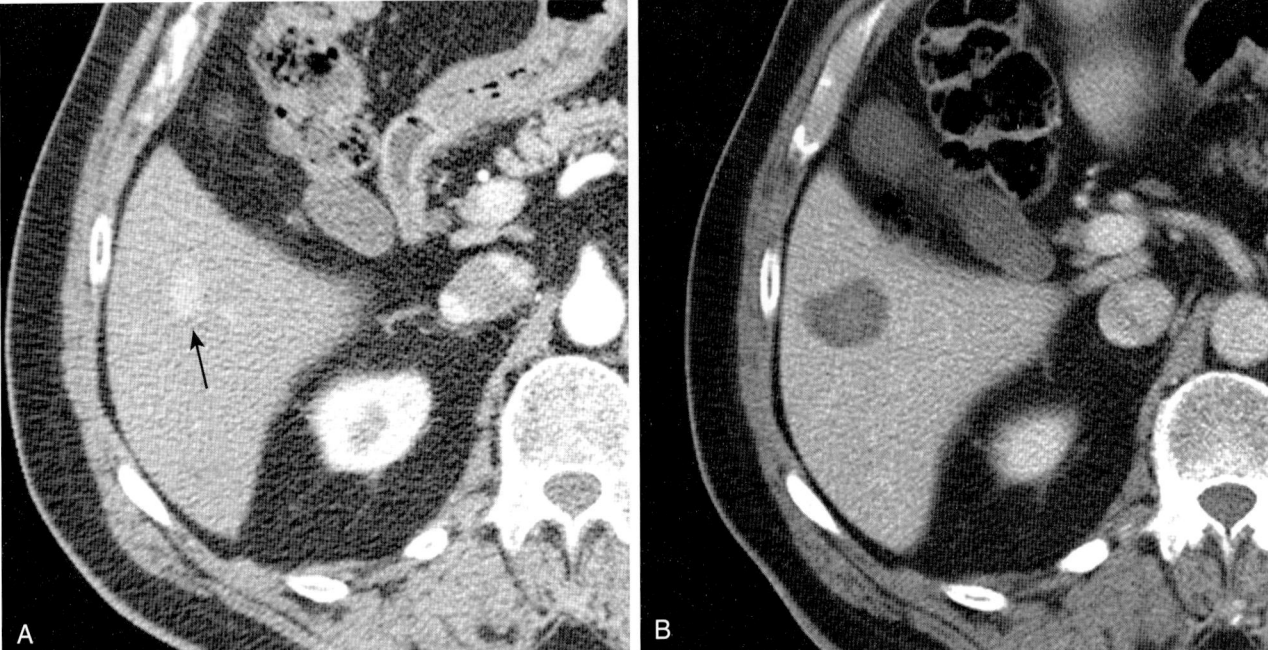

FIGURE 91.6 Percutaneous radiofrequency ablation (RFA) of metastatic carcinoid in a nonsurgical patient. **A,** Computed tomography (CT) with intravenous contrast shows a subtle, hyperenhancing, solitary 2.3-cm metastasis in the right lobe of the liver *(arrow)*. Given limited disease and surgical risk in this 115-kg patient, the metastasis was treated with radiofrequency ablation. **B,** CT image obtained 3 months after ablation shows no recurrent tumor (see Chapters 15 and 96B).

endocrinopathies. There is some evidence that RFA can result in an overall survival benefit, but the impact on other symptoms is not clear. The focus of such ablative treatment is usually 2-fold, both debulking of the patient's hepatic tumor and secondary symptom management.

Embolization

Neuroendocrine metastases are intensely hypervascular. Hepatic arterial embolization (HAE) results in ischemia of the metastases and variable tumor necrosis, which can alleviate symptoms or endocrinopathies[115] (see Chapter 94). Hepatic arterial embolization, or in combination with intraarterial chemotherapy (HACE) has been used for relief of symptoms. Repeated embolization is possible depending on the interventional vascular technique used, selective or nonselective. Hepatic arterial embolization with or without HACE has been used for relief of symptoms. Most studies have used a combination of doxorubicin or streptozocin.

Objective complete or partial tumor responses to embolization alone range from 30% to 70% with similar symptom relief response rates of 73% to 100%, tumor marker response rates of 57% to 91%, and response on imaging of 33% to 50%.[35,116,117] Intermittent or temporary dearterialization with the use of an implantable hepatic artery drug-eluting beads provides similar symptomatic relief for 6 to 12 months.[118] Duration of response has ranged from 15 to 30 months. The 5-year survival for HACE and HAE is 50% to 83% and 40% to 67%, respectively, but no benefit to overall survival has yet been demonstrated[4,6,117] (see Chapter 94A). To date, there are no randomized trials comparing embolization with and without chemotherapy, indicating a significant difference in outcomes or response and observational data have shown no statistical difference between the two

groups.[119,120] A combination of chemoembolization with hepatic artery chemoinfusion for patients with unresectable hepatic disease has achieved better than 3-year survival for the majority of patients.[121] Patients with hormonally functional disease may have a statically significant improved survival compared with nonfunctional NETs: median survival of 38.6 versus 27.7 months.[122]

Mortality rates of 0 to 3.3% have been reported. Complications are generally tolerable. The most notable complication is postembolization syndrome, consisting of nausea, right upper quadrant abdominal pain, fever, and elevation of serum transaminases, usually lasting for 3 to 7 days. Parenteral analgesia, intravenous hydration, and antipyretics are often necessary. Antibiotic prophylaxis is recommended for embolization. Other complications include gallbladder necrosis, hepatic abscess formation, and renal failure. Patients with large (>5–10 cm) metastases and those with more than 50% to 70% hepatic replacement are at greater risk of complications. Sequential lobar embolization may reduce the severity of postembolization syndrome and may lower the risk of complications. Although drug-eluting beads may have high response rates, reported serious complications such as bilomas and hepatic abscess formation resulted in a phase II trial being prematurely discontinued because of the serious adverse events.[123,124]

Contraindications to embolization procedures include occlusion of portal venous inflow and previous pancreaticoduodenectomy, mainly as a result of an increased occurrence of hepatic abscess. Large hepatopulmonary shunts can be occluded but are considered a relative contraindication. Patients planned for liver transplantation may experience vascular alterations making transplant more challenging; these are a relative contraindication. Patients with severe comorbidities should not undergo embolization.[4,6]

Radioembolization with yttrium-90 (^{90}Y) has been used in the setting of NELM (see Chapter 94B). Limited data have suggested that the toxicity may be less than with HACE or HAE. Radiologic response has been demonstrated in 22% to 70% of patients, and 3-year survival is 40% to 50%.[125-133] The survival rates after radioembolization were reported according to grade in a recent systematic review and were 71, 56, and 28 months for grades I, II, and III, respectively.[127] In addition in functioning NETs, 69% had improvement in symptoms. This treatment also may be effective in patients who have irresectable NELM and who had unsuccessful HAE or HACE. Although theoretically radioembolization can be used more often because of the greater patency of lobar arteries to the liver compared with bland embolization, cost efficacy, durability, and functional liver status after repeat radioembolization have not been demonstrated. This approach remains investigational.

Surgery versus Embolization

Two publications have compared surgery to intraarterial therapies (IATs). The first was a systematic review and meta-analysis. It showed a significant overall survival benefit in favor of surgery (OR, 0.18; 95% CI, 0.05–0.61; P = .006).[113] Similar results were reported in a large multicenter study. Further analysis in this group showed that IATs were effective in retarding tumor progression and palliating symptoms. At a median follow-up of 25.8 months, response by RECIST criteria was partial, stable, or progressive in 6.3%, 40.6%, and 33.3%, respectively. Median and 5-year survival for surgery versus IAT was 123 months and 74%, and 34 months and 30%, respectively.[122] The survival benefit from surgery included patients with symptoms and more than 25% hepatic tumor involvement, but there was no difference in patients with asymptomatic disease and more than 25% hepatic involvement. These authors therefore recommend that in asymptomatic patients with more than 25%, IAT should be considered and surgery alone reserved for asymptomatic patients with low-volume disease or symptomatic patients with high-volume disease.

SYSTEMIC TREATMENT OF NEUROENDOCRINE LIVER METASTSES

Systemic therapy is mainly reserved for advanced locoregional or metastatic disease that is unresectable. In general there are accepted guidelines that have been suggested and treatment is based on the proliferation index and the differentiation. According to the WHO classification,[4] in general, chemotherapy is reserved for WHO grade 3b NETs and intermediate to well-differentiated NETs that are rapidly progressive (see Chapter 65). This section discusses treatment related to the nonresectable NELMs or patients whose disease has recurred after liver-directed therapy. Systemic therapy has two broad intentions. The first is to address the functional symptoms to improve quality of life, and the second is the antineoplastic effect aimed at improving overall survival. The most common functional NETs are from the midgut and produce carcinoid syndrome. Carcinoid syndrome occurs in 2 to 8.4 new cases per 100,000 persons per year.[5,134] SSAs are the preferred first-line treatment option in functional GEP-NETs.

Systemic Therapy for Carcinoid Syndrome

Carcinoid syndrome is mediated by multiple hormones, predominantly serotonin, and is expressed as flushing (94%), diarrhea (78%), carcinoid heart disease (20%–53%), and/or abdominal pain (51%). The role of SSAs in the treatment of the diarrhea and flushing was first described in 1978.[135] The effect of SSAs is mediated through type 2 and type 5 SSTRs, inhibiting the cellular release of the hormone. SSAs have been associated with a biochemical response in 70% of patients, and symptomatic relief is experienced in 60% to 90%.[35] In the latter study, objective reduction in tumor size of greater than 50% of the largest diameter, occurred in less than 10% of patients. Stabilization of NETs has been observed in 36% to 70% for a median duration of 12 months. As expected, symptomatic response has been correlated with improved quality of life, although response to SSA therapy varies by primary site of the NET and its SSTR expression. As noted previously, short-acting SSA therapy is used to prevent or treat the carcinoid crisis periprocedurally for any intervention, including resection, transplantation, ablation, or embolization. In general, SSA treatment is well tolerated. Steatorrhea, diarrhea, abdominal discomfort, and biliary sludge or gallstones can develop but rarely preclude continued use.[136] Over a decade ago the long-acting analogues of somatostatin, such as lanreotide and long-acting octreotide, became available and still remain the mainstay for long-term symptomatic treatment.[137] Despite the effectiveness of SSAs, tachyphylaxis does occur after prolonged use. Serotonin-3 receptor antagonists (ondansetron) and antidiarrheal therapy in combination with SSAs may be useful once tachyphylaxis occurs.

Pasireotide, a more recently developed SSA with affinity for multiple SSTRs, was thought to potentially have a better clinical impact on carcinoid syndrome. In a randomized phase III study of pasireotide long-acting release (LAR) versus high-dose octreotide, LAR failed to show superiority.[138]

For patients who had refractory symptoms despite maximal doses of SSAs, the addition of interferon-alpha (IFN-α) was suggested for symptom control.[139] However, the side effect profile of IFN-α is significant and poorly tolerated, and with newer drugs available there is a limited role for this combination

More recently telotristat etiprate, a novel inhibitor of tryptophan hydroxylase, the rate-limiting enzyme in the biosynthesis of serotonin has been investigated. The multicenter randomized, double-blind, placebo-controlled phase III trial TELESTAR reported a reduction of 40% of bowel movements per day, thus improving quality of life. Importantly, stool form improved in 20% and flushing in 27%.[140]

Antineoplastic Therapy
Somatostatin Analogues

SSAs may inhibit the cell cycle and increase apoptosis. The indirect effects include immune modulation, antiangiogenesis, and growth factor inhibition. The antiproliferative effect was initially evaluated in the PROMID study.[141] A total of 85 patients with well-differentiated, metastatic midgut NETs were randomized into the placebo or octreotide LAR groups. A difference, in favor of LAR, of 8.3 months in tumor progression was observed. However, there was no difference in overall survival between these two groups (see Chapter 65).

Similarly, a phase III study, CLARINET, revealed a PFS for lanreotide versus placebo. This was the first study to show improved disease-free progression with SSAs in pNETs.[142]

Interferon-Alpha

IFN-α has antineoplastic, proapoptotic, cytotoxic/cytostatic, and immune modulatory effect in NETs. It has been considered as a second-line option in progressive NETs on SSAs therapy. Tumor response rates of 10% have been reported. Despite a pegylated formulation the several side effects are still present and not well tolerated. With the introduction of newer novel therapeutic options with higher efficacy and lower side effects, there seems to be limited application of IFN-α.[143]

Newer Drugs and Targeted Therapy

mTOR Inhibitors

The mechanistic target of rapamycin (mTOR) pathway plays an important role in the regulation of proliferation in NETs. The phase III RADIANT 3 trial showed that for well-differentiated low- or intermediate-grade pNETs there was a PFS benefit of 11 months with everolimus against 4.6 months with placebo, which was statistically significant, and an overall survival benefit of 6.3 months, which was not statistically significant.[144] The RADIANT 4 trial confirmed that this improved PFS also applied to midgut and lung NETs.[145] However, there was no overall survival benefit in the RADIANT 4 trail. Everolimus has been deemed safe but does have serious grade 3 and 4 drug-related adverse events (diarrhea, infections, anemia, fatigue, and hyperglycemia), which may limit its tolerability and, consequently, patient compliance (see Chapter 65).

Tyrosine Kinase Inhibitors

Sunitinib is a multitargeted tyrosine kinase inhibitor that inhibits multiple angiogenic factors, including the vascular endothelial growth factor receptor 1-3, stem cell factor, and the platelet-derived growth factor receptors.[146] The Sunitinib (SUN 1111) phase III trial, involving pNETs, reported PFS of 11.4 months compared with placebo of 5.5 months.[147] The study was prematurely discontinued because of higher rates of adverse events and deaths in the placebo group. As with everolimus, there was no benefit to overall survival. Several adverse events were noted with Sunitinib, including hypertension, diarrhea, nausea, vomiting, skin toxicity, asthenia, and fatigue, but fewer grade 3 or 4 toxicities are observed when compared with those with chemotherapeutic agents (see Chapter 65).

Peptide Receptor Radionucleotide Therapy

PRRT combined with an SSA allows targeted delivery of radionuclides to tumor cells expressing high levels of SSTR (see Chapters 18 and 65). The radiolabeled SSAs combine yttrium or lutetium (^{90}Y or ^{177}Lu), with a carrier molecule, generally octreotide, and a chelator, usually DOTA.[148] The ^{177}Lu radionuclide is characterized by the emission of beta-rays, which have an immediate tissue penetration. Treatment response is directly related to the expression of SSTRs in the tumor. The Netter-1 trial randomized 229 patients with well-differentiated metastatic midgut NETs that were progressive on SSAs. The trial was randomized to receive a ^{177}Lu DOTA-TATE or double dose of octreotide (60 mg/28 days). Median PFS was not reached in the ^{177}Lu DOTA-TATE arm versus 8.4 months in the double-dose octreotide arm. This study reported a 79% reduction in the risk

of progression or death and an overall response rate of 18% in the PRRT group compared with 3% in the control arm.[54] PRRT is generally well tolerated, and adverse events include nausea, fatigue, and abdominal pain and are related to the amino acid infusion for renal protection. Long-term side effects include renal failure, acute leukemia, or myelodysplastic syndrome in 1% to 2% of cases.[149]

SYSTEMIC CHEMOTHERAPY

Systemic chemotherapy is generally reserved for patients with advanced or progressive disease, particularly where other treatments have failed[150,151] (see Chapter 65). Patients with pNETs are more responsive to chemotherapy than those with carcinoid tumors.[151] Streptozocin-based combinations with 5-fluorouracil (5-FU) and doxorubicin have resulted in objective responses in 45% to 69%[152,153]; however, a later study reported disappointing results using a 5-FU and streptozocin combination.[154] Median duration of response for high-grade NETs is about 8 to 9 months. Carcinoid tumors are less sensitive to cytotoxic agents because of the preponderance of low-grade malignant (well-differentiated) histology and low proliferation index.[155] Dacarbazine, 5-FU, and epirubicin combination therapy has achieved an objective tumor response in approximately 30% of patients with carcinoid tumors, and the median duration of response for carcinoid tumors is about 6 months.[35,155] Some success has been achieved with hepatic artery infusional cisplatin in metastatic pNET.[156] The combination of temozolomide and capecitabine is gaining popularity, but data for the use of temozolomide are limited. It may be considered if streptozocin/5-FU is unavailable. Reported objective response rates from small prospective and retrospective studies range between 15% and 70% and particularly with locally advanced and metastatic pNETs.[157] Data supporting the combination of temozolomide and capecitabine can be found in this retrospective review of seven patients with pNETs who had disease progression after long-acting octreotide, chemotherapy, and other liver-directed therapies.[158] The total response rate was 43%, and clinical benefit was 71%. The median duration of response was 8 months. Grade 3 toxicity included thrombocytopenia and fatigue. More data are required in prospective trials with larger numbers to confirm the findings discussed here.

For advanced poorly differentiated NETs, that is WHO grade 3b, a combination of cisplatin and etoposide is the standard of care. Second-line therapy includes FOLFOX and FOLFIRI.[4] Because there are so many treatment options for patients with GEP-NETs, it is vital that an algorithm be followed in these patients with metastatic disease. There is evidence that the median survival of patients is greater than three times higher in high-volume centers and that data are consistent across centers of excellence.[159] It is therefore vital that these patients with NELMs are treated at high-volume centers and in the setting of a well-established MDT.

The references for this chapter can be found online by accessing the accompanying Expert Consult website.

CHAPTER 92

Hepatic metastasis from noncolorectal nonneuroendocrine tumors

Christoph Kahlert, Ronald P. DeMatteo, and Jürgen Weitz

OVERVIEW

Only 10% of malignant liver tumors are primary liver or bile duct cancers. The vast majority of cancerous hepatic lesions are metastatic lesions originating from extrahepatic primary tumors (see Chapters 90 and 91). The only potentially curative approach for most malignant liver tumors is surgical resection. This procedure can be performed safely with an acceptable risk of perioperative mortality and morbidity[1] (see Chapters 101 and 102).

Recent studies provide evidence that a complex multimodality therapy has improved the clinical outcome of patients with colorectal liver metastases over the last 2 decades. In 2020, patients who underwent a partial hepatectomy for colorectal liver metastases had a median life expectancy of 6.6 years (6.0–8.3 years), and approximately two thirds of the patients are still alive after 5 years if they are treated in high-volume centers.[2] For patients with neuroendocrine liver metastases, surgical resection is associated with 5-year survival rates of approximately 75% and a median overall survival of 125 months.[3,4] In contrast, the role of hepatectomy in patients with liver metastases from noncolorectal, nonneuroendocrine (NCNN) tumors is not well defined, but the number of reports on this topic are increasing.

SERIES SUMMARIZING MULTIPLE PRIMARY TUMOR TYPES

In the past 2 decades, an increasing number of studies reporting the outcome of resection of NCNN metastases have been published. However, despite the fact that partial hepatectomy can be considered as a relatively safe surgical procedure in 2020,[1,2,5] most current reports regarding hepatectomy for metastases of NCNN tumors still combine multiple primary tumor types to obtain a sufficient number of patients to analyze.[6-10] A major objection to liver resection in patients with NCNN is the argument that many NCNN liver metastases originate from extraabdominal primary tumors, which often spread simultaneously to other organs. In this case, a resection of the liver metastases would not be warranted because the extrahepatic disease burden defines the outcome in patients with a multifocal metastatic disease.[7] For selected patients, however, partial hepatectomy for NCNN is associated with long-term survival.

To date, one of the largest cohort of patients with NCNN has been described by Sano et al.[10] In their study, data regarding 1639 hepatectomies performed between 2001 and 2010 for 1539 patients with NCNN were collected from 124 institutions. Most frequently, patients underwent hepatectomy because of noncolorectal liver metastases originating from gastric carcinomas, gastrointestinal stromal tumors (GISTs), biliary carcinomas, ovarian cancer, and pancreatic cancer. The authors of this study report that a R0/1 hepatectomy was achieved in 90% of patients and the in-hospital mortality rate reached 1.5%. Overall survival and disease-free survival (DFS) rates of 1465 patients included in survival analysis were 41% and 21%, respectively, at 5 years, and 28% and 15%, respectively, at 10 years. Among the five most frequent tumor types, patients with a hepatic metastasized GIST ($n = 204$) had the best prognosis and experienced a 5-year and 10-year survival of 72% and 40%, respectively, with a median survival of 100 months. In patients with liver metastases from breast cancer ($n = 74$) the median survival was 62 months, in patients with liver metastases from ovarian cancer ($n = 107$) the median survival reached 65 months. The lowest survival rate was observed in patients with liver metastases derived from pancreatic carcinoma ($n = 77$) and biliary carcinoma ($n = 150$), accounting for a 5-year survival of 31% and 17%, respectively.[10]

Overall, these recent data confirm the results of previous large studies with comparable results such as the report by Adam et al.[6] This study reports the outcome of 1452 patients who had undergone liver resection for liver metastases from noncolorectal tumors in 41 centers. With a mean follow-up of 31 months (range, 0–258 months), the 5-year and 10-year survival rates were 36% and 23%, respectively, and the median overall survival equaled 35 months. The largest subset in this series represented patients with liver metastases from breast cancer ($n = 460$). These patients experienced a 5-year and 10-year survival of 41% and 22%, respectively, with a median survival of 45 months. The second largest subgroups were patients with liver metastases from different types of primary gastrointestinal (GI) cancer. In this cohort, the 5-year survival reached 31% and the median survival was 26 months. The third largest group in this study consisted of patients with liver metastases originating from urologic primary tumors. In this very heterogeneous subgroup, Adam et al.[6] observed the most favorable outcome for patients with adrenal metastases (5-year survival, 66%), followed by testicular metastases (5-year survival, 51%) and renal metastases (5-year survival, 38%).

Andreou et al.[7] performed hepatic resection in 51 patients with liver metastases from a noncolorectal primary. This cohort consisted of 26 patients with a primary tumor from the adrenal gland, 11 patients with thyroid cancer as primary site, 9 patients with a primary testicular germ cell tumor, and 5 patients with a primary ovarian granulosa cell cancer. Ninety-day postoperative morbidity and mortality were 27% and 2%, respectively. After a median follow-up of 20 months, the 5-year overall and recurrence-free survival rates were 58% and 37%, respectively. Noteworthy in this small cohort, they identified only the presence of more than one site of extrahepatic tumor disease as an independent prognostic marker in their multivariate analyses

TABLE 92.1	Primary Tumor Type of Patients Undergoing Liver Resection for Metastatic Noncolorectal, Nonneuroendocrine Tumors
PRIMARY TUMOR	**NO. (%)**
Breast	29 (20)
Melanoma	17 (12)
Reproductive tract	39 (28)
Testicular	20 (14)
Gynecologic	19 (14)
Ovarian	12
Endometrial	4
Cervical	2
Fallopian tube	1
Adrenocortical	15 (11)
Renal	11 (8)
Gastrointestinal	12 (9)
Stomach	3
Duodenal	1
Pancreatic	5
Ampullary	2
Anal	1
Other	13 (9)
Lung	4
Salivary gland	3
Nasopharyngeal	2
Glottal	1
Tonsil	1
Thyroid	1
Sweat gland	1
Unknown	5 (3)

From Weitz J, Blumgart LH, Fong Y, et al. Partial hepatectomy for metastases from noncolorectal, nonneuroendocrine carcinoma. *Ann Surg.* 2005;241(2):269–276. http://journals.lww.com/00000658-200502000-00012.)

(P = .016). In contrast, survival was not affected by the primary tumor type. Based on these observations, the authors concluded that mostly the extrahepatic burden defines the prognosis for patients with NCNN.

The Memorial Sloan Kettering Cancer Center (MSKCC) experience regarding hepatic resection for metastases from NCNN carcinoma was analyzed by Weitz et al.[9] The objectives of this study were to define perioperative and long-term outcome and to define prognostic factors for survival in 141 patients who underwent resection for liver metastases from NCNN carcinoma during the period April 1981 through April 2002. Table 92.1 depicts the primary tumor types. The median operative time was 238 minutes (interquartile range [IQR], 180–321 minutes), and the median blood loss was 600 mL (IQR, 250–1420 mL). The median length of hospital stay was 9 days (IQR, 7–12 days). Of 141 patients, 46 (33%) experienced postoperative complications, but the 30-day mortality rate was 0%. The median follow-up was 26 months, with a median follow-up of 35 months. The 3-year relapse-free survival rate was 30% (median, 17 months), and the 3-year cancer-specific survival rate was 57% (median, 42 months). Primary tumor type and length of disease-free interval from the primary tumor were significant independent prognostic factors for relapse-free and cancer-specific survival (Figs. 92.1–92.3; Table 92.2).[11]

Margin status was significant for cancer-specific survival and showed a strong trend in relapse-free survival. Patients with a primary reproductive tract tumor who underwent R0 resection had the best outcome, with a 3-year cancer-specific survival of 78%. In the group of patients with primary non–reproductive tract tumors, survival after R0 resection was influenced largely by the length of the disease-free interval. Patients with a disease-free interval of 24 months or less achieved a 3-year survival of 36%, but only 5% were free of relapse after 3 years. Patients with a non–reproductive tract primary and a disease-free interval of more than 24 months had a 3-year cancer-specific survival of 72% and a 3-year relapse-free survival of 30%, with 14 5-year survivors in this group.

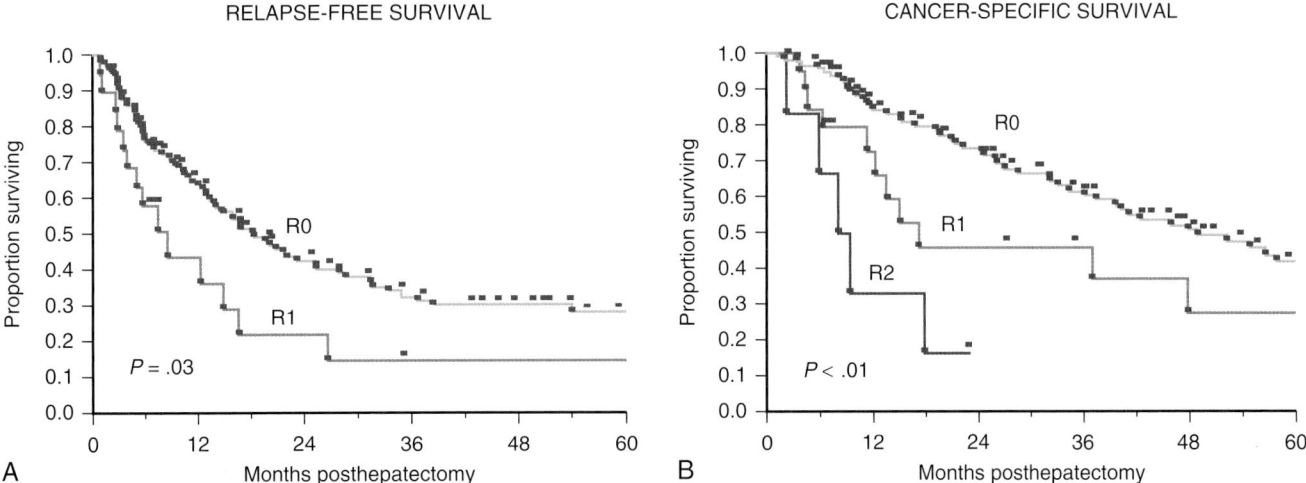

FIGURE 92.1   Survival after resection of hepatic metastases stratified according to margin status (R0, n = 116; R1, n = 19; R2, n = 6). **A,** Relapse-free survival (patients with R2 resection were excluded for relapse-free survival). **B,** Cancer-specific survival. (From Weitz J, Blumgart LH, Fong Y, et al. Partial hepatectomy for metastases from noncolorectal, nonneuroendocrine carcinoma. *Ann Surg.* 2005;241[2]:269–276. http://journals.lww.com/00000658-200502000-00012.)

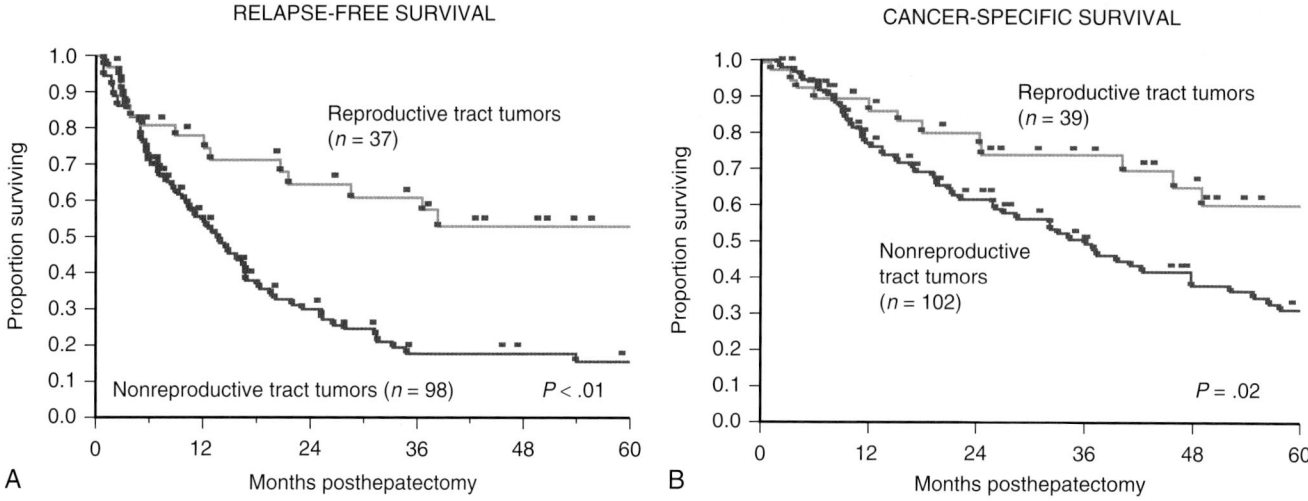

FIGURE 92.2   Survival after resection of hepatic metastases stratified according to primary tumor type (reproductive tract versus nonreproductive tract tumors; patients with R2 resection were excluded for relapse-free survival). **A,** Relapse-free survival. **B,** Cancer-specific survival. (From Weitz J, Blumgart LH, Fong Y, et al. Partial hepatectomy for metastases from noncolorectal, nonneuroendocrine carcinoma. *Ann Surg.* 2005;241[2]:269–276. http://journals.lww.com/00000658-200502000-00012.)

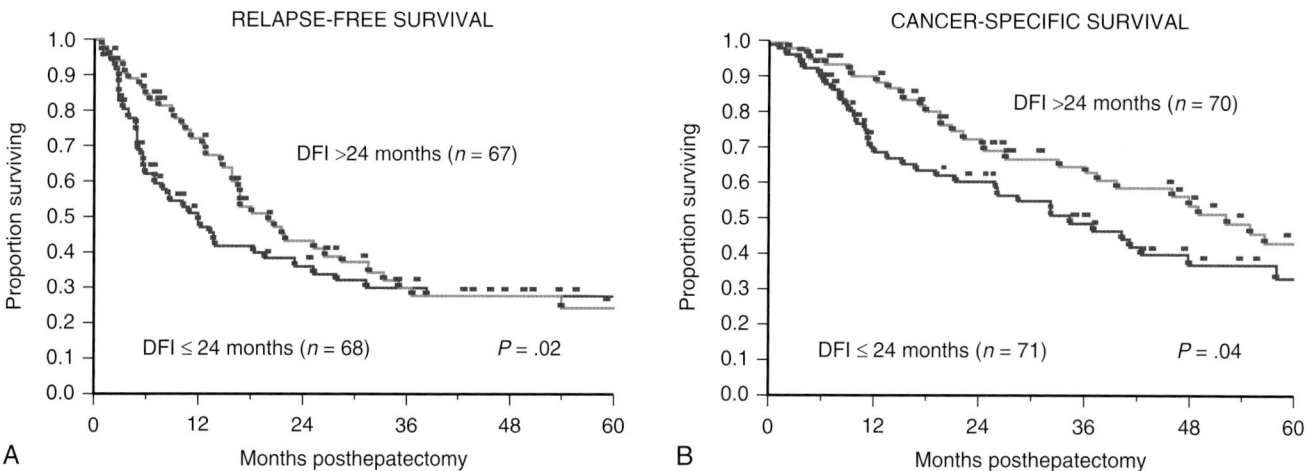

FIGURE 92.3   Survival after resection of hepatic metastases stratified according to disease-free interval *(DFI)*; patients with R2 resection were excluded for relapse-free survival. **A,** Relapse-free survival. **B,** Cancer-specific survival. (From Weitz J, Blumgart LH, Fong Y, et al. Partial hepatectomy for metastases from noncolorectal, nonneuroendocrine carcinoma. *Ann Surg.* 2005;241[2]:269–276. http://journals.lww.com/00000658-200502000-00012.)

Martel et al.[12] performed a hepatectomy in 52 patients with liver metastases from a noncolorectal, noncarcinoid, and non-sarcoma primary tumor. Ninety-day mortality was 0%. The overall 5-year survival rate was 58%, with the following results for various primary tumors: adrenal carcinoma 100% (*n* = 3), breast cancer 85% (*n* = 11), ocular melanoma 66% (*n* = 5), other melanomas 83% (*n* = 6), gastroesophageal cancer 50% (*n* = 7), and renal cell cancer 0% (*n* = 4). The authors pointed out that the overall survival in this highly selected group of patients was similar to results they obtained in 185 patients who underwent liver resection for metastases of colorectal cancer (CRC) during the same period.

In a systematic review, Fitzgerald et al.[8] summarized the benefits of liver resection for NCNN liver metastases. This report includes 3596 patients from 73 studies that were published after 1990. The largest subset of patients had undergone liver resection because of breast cancer metastases (*n* = 1013). The

next two largest populations were patients with liver metastases originating from melanoma (*n* = 643) and from gastric cancer (*n* = 481). In this systematic review, Fitzgerald et al.[8] showed that the longest expected survival is observed for patients with liver metastases derived from genitourinary primaries (median, 63 months; range, 5.4–142 months), followed by patients with breast cancer (median, 44.4 months; range, 8–74 months), patients with GI cancer (median, 22.3 months; range, 5–58 months), and 23.7 months for other tumor types (range, 10–72 months). From their point of view, there is a benefit to resection for patients with NCNN liver metastases. However, the degree of survival advantage is predicated by primary tumor site.[8]

In conclusion, those studies show that the safety of hepatectomy for patients with NCNN metastases has increased substantially for the past 2 decades. More importantly, however, there is an increasing number of patients who show very good results for long-term survival after resection of liver metastases from

TABLE 92.2 Multivariate Analysis of Prognostic Factors of Patients Undergoing Liver Resection for Metastatic Noncolorectal, Nonneuroendocrine Carcinoma

FACTOR	RELAPSE-FREE SURVIVAL[a]		CANCER-SPECIFIC SURVIVAL	
	HAZARD RATIO (95% CI)	P VALUE	HAZARD RATIO (95% CI)	P VALUE
Disease-Free Interval				
≤24 mo	1.4 (1.1-1.8)	.02	1.4 (1.0-1.8)	.03
>24 mo	Reference		Reference	
Primary Tumor				
Adrenocortical	0.9 (0.5-1.6)	<.01	0.7 (0.4-1.3)	.02
Breast	0.9 (0.6-1.5)		1.0 (0.6-1.7)	
Gastrointestinal	0.6 (0.3-1.1)		0.8 (0.3-1.5)	
Reproductive tract	0.4 (0.2-0.6)		0.4 (0.2-0.7)	
Melanoma	1.0 (0.5-1.9)		1.5 (0.7-2.7)	
Renal	1.1 (0.5-2.2)		0.7 (0.3-1.3)	
Other	1.6 (0.8-2.9)		1.7 (0.3-1.3)	
Unknown	Reference		Reference	
Margin Status				
R0	Reference	.08	Reference	<.01
R1	1.8 (0.9-3.2)		2.1 (1.1-4.1)	
R2	ND[a]		2.7 (0.8-7.9)	

[a]Relapse-free survival patients with incomplete macroscopic resection (n = 6) were not included in the analysis.

CI, Confidence interval; ND, not determined.

Data from Weitz J, Blumgart LH, Fong Y, et al. Partial hepatectomy for metastases from noncolorectal, nonneuroendocrine carcinoma. Ann Surg. 2005;241(2):269–276. http://journals.lww.com/00000658-200502000-00012.

NCNN origin. Crucial for this successful surgical treatment of NCNN metastases is the preoperative evaluation and selection of patients based on clinical factors and tumor biology.[13]

Therefore laparoscopy might be a reasonable staging tool for patients with NCNN liver metastases (see Chapter 24). D'Angelica and coworkers[14] examined 30 patients with potentially resectable NCNN tumors based on preoperative imaging. Of these patients, 9 had unresectable disease, 6 of whom were identified by laparoscopy. If possible, laparoscopic liver resection also should be the method of choice for curative resection of NCNN metastases. Triantafyllidis et al.[15] evaluated the perioperative and long‚Äëterm outcomes of laparoscopic liver resections for noncolorectal liver metastases in 56 patients. Major postoperative morbidity was reported to reach 3.6%, and the perioperative mortality was zero. Overall survival rates at 3 and 5 years were 71.4% and 52.9%, respectively, and 8 of 56 (14.3%) patients with NCNN metastases underwent repeat laparoscopic liver resection for recurrent metastatic tumors.

However, the retrospective nature of these studies and the consequent bias related to patient selection represent major limitations. Nevertheless, the general theme is one of potential benefit of hepatic resection in selected patients with limited disease, specific primary tumor types, and a longer disease-free interval.

SERIES FOCUSED ON ONE PRIMARY TUMOR TYPE

Sarcoma

One of the first surgical series of patients with sarcoma metastatic to the liver was composed of 56 patients who underwent liver resection.[16] These patients were selected from 331 patients with liver metastases from sarcomas who had been admitted to MSKCC during the years 1982 through 2000. GISTs (Fig. 92.4) and leiomyosarcomas were the most common histologic findings; no perioperative deaths were reported in patients undergoing complete resection of the tumor, and the 5-year overall survival rate was 30%, with a median of 39 months in

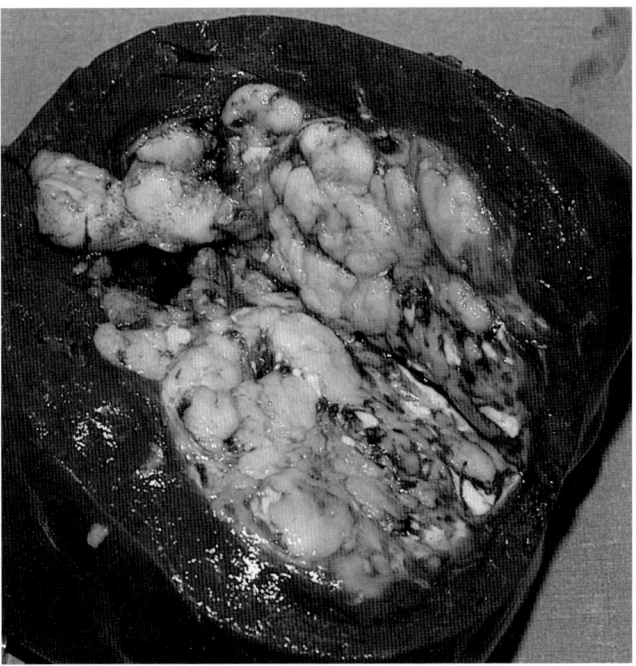

FIGURE 92.4 Right hepatectomy for a liver metastasis from gastrointestinal stromal tumor (see Chapter 118A.)

completely resected patients. Patients who did not undergo complete resection had a 5-year survival of only 4% (Fig. 92.5). A disease-free interval of less than 24 months was a significant adverse prognostic parameter for survival on univariate and multivariate analysis (Fig. 92.6).

In a report from Pawlik et al.,[17] 66 patients undergoing liver resection and/or ablation were included; the 5-year disease-free and overall survival rates were 16.4% and 27.1%, respectively. Patients in whom radiofrequency ablation (RFA) was part of the treatment and patients who did not receive chemotherapy, mostly imatinib mesylate for metastatic GISTs, showed a significantly reduced survival.

The treatment strategy for patients with liver metastases from GISTs has changed since the development of the targeted

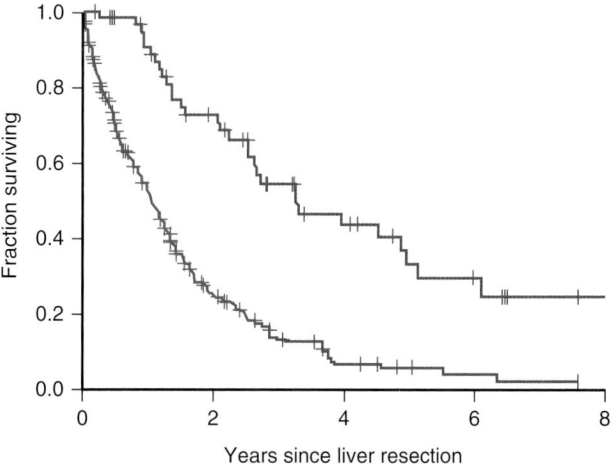

FIGURE 92.5 Disease-specific survival of patients with liver metastases from sarcoma who underwent complete resection (*upper line*, n = 56) versus other treatment (*lower line*, n = 275; P = .0001). (From DeMatteo RP, Shah A, Fong Y, et al. Results of hepatic resection for sarcoma metastatic to liver. *Ann Surg.* 2001;234[4]:540–548. https://pubmed.ncbi.nlm.nih.gov/11573047.)

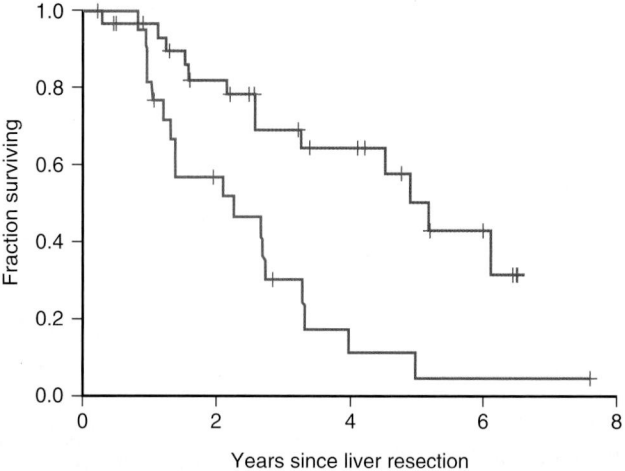

FIGURE 92.6 Disease-specific survival of patients after complete resection of liver metastases from sarcoma with a disease-free interval of more than 2 years (*upper line*, n = 32) versus less than 2 years (*lower line*, n = 24; P = .002). (From DeMatteo RP, Shah A, Fong Y, et al. Results of hepatic resection for sarcoma metastatic to liver. *Ann Surg.* 2001;234[4]:540–548. https://pubmed.ncbi.nlm.nih.gov/11573047.)

agent imatinib mesylate, which achieves dramatic tumor response rates[18,19] such that imatinib is now the first-line treatment. Resection is considered for patients when they reach the maximal response to imatinib if all gross tumors can be removed and for those who have immediate or limited acquired resistance to the drug.[20] In a randomized trial, Xia et al.[21] demonstrated that surgical resection of liver metastases in combination with imatinib results in a significantly longer survival rate than treatment with imatinib alone. However, although patients responding to a preoperative tyrosine kinase inhibitor therapy benefit from surgical resection, there seems to be no advantage from a surgical intervention for nonresponders.[22] For patients with non-GIST sarcoma liver metastases, innovative advances in perioperative therapy have significantly improved the prognosis for long-term survival. Goumard et al. reported a 5-year overall survival rate of 49%, independent of histologic subtype and primary tumor location in a cohort of 126 patients undergoing resection of non-GIST sarcoma liver metastases. ([6]). Among the 65 patients (52%) who received preoperative chemotherapy, radiologic response according to the Choi criteria specifically was associated with improved overall survival ([6]). Based on their data, the authors suggested that in particular the radiologic response to preoperative chemotherapy can be a significant indicator and decision aid for the selection of patients with non-GIST sarcoma liver metastases that are scheduled for hepatectomy ([6]).

Breast Cancer

Breast cancer is the second most common malignant tumor of women in the Western world. In fact, 42,690 breast cancer–related deaths are estimated in the United States in 2020 ([7]). Only in a minor subset (4%–18%) of patients with breast cancer are liver metastases the only sign of disseminated disease (Fig. 92.7).[23–25] Although it has not been formally proven that liver resection prolongs survival for selected patients with liver metastases of breast cancer, 5-year survival was 48% to 61% in more recently published series.[26–28] Patients with liver metastases from breast cancer receiving chemotherapy only rarely, if ever, survive 5 years.[29] In a case-matched control study, Mariani et al.[30] reported that selected patients with liver metastases and no additional extrahepatic disease have a 3-year survival of 80.7% when undergoing surgical intervention. In contrast, matched-control patients without surgical treatment exhibited only a 3-year survival of 51%. Even with aggressive systemic chemotherapy, the median survival for patients with metastatic breast cancer is less than 2 years.[29] Resection for liver metastases in this setting may prolong survival for a subset of highly selected patients and may significantly extend median overall survival.[26]

In contrast to the study by Mariani et al.,[30] Sadot et al.[31] reported a case-control study comparing 69 patients submitted to resection with or without ablation to a matched group of patients treated medically and showed no survival difference between the two groups (50 vs.45 months, P = .5). Of note, there was no difference in outcome between patients treated with resection or ablation in this series.

Table 92.3 summarizes the published studies of liver resection for metastatic breast cancer.[32–34] Meaningful comparisons between these studies cannot be made because they are heterogeneous studies reporting small patient numbers with different inclusion criteria and treatment strategies. Valid criteria for selecting patients who might benefit from hepatic resection for

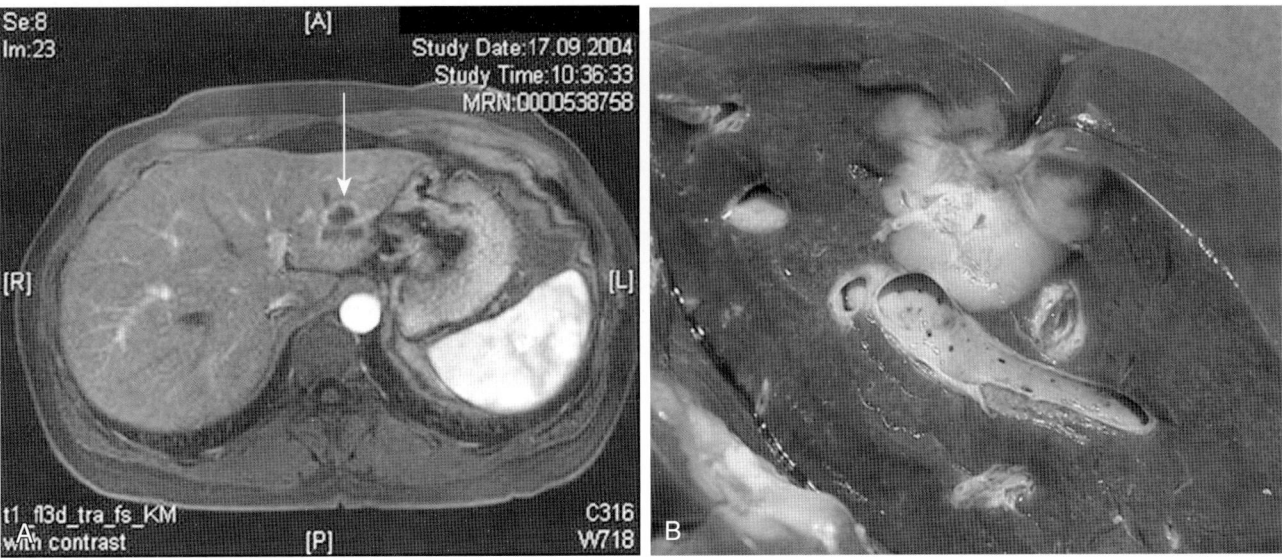

FIGURE 92.7   Liver metastasis of breast cancer. A, Computed tomography scan shows the lesion *(arrow)* to have early peripheral contrast enhancement. **B,** The patient underwent resection of segments II and III; a gross photograph of the sectioned specimen is shown.

TABLE 92.3   Results of Liver Resection for Metastatic Breast Cancer[a]

REFERENCE	NO. PATIENTS	MEDIAN SURVIVAL (MO)[b]	ADVERSE PROGNOSTIC FACTORS	COMMENTS
Sadot et al., 2016[31]	69	50	Node involvement of primary tumor Multiple liver metastases	No extrahepatic disease; case control comparison to medically treated patients; resection and ablation patients combined
Bacalbasa et al., 2014[26]	52	32	Estrogen/progesterone receptor status Node involvement of primary tumor Multiple liver metastases	Inclusion criteria: no extrahepatic disease
Hoffmann et al., 2010[27]	41	34	Positive resection margin Disease-free interval <12 mo	Median overall survival, 58 months
Caralt et al., 2008[32]	12	36	Disease-free interval <24 mo	Seven patients experienced hepatic recurrence
Vlastos et al., 2004[28]	31	63	None	Inclusion criteria: no extrahepatic disease
Elias et al., 2003[24]	54	34	Negative receptor status (odds ratio, 3.5)	Inclusion criteria: no extrahepatic disease, no disease progression on chemotherapy
Pocard et al., 2000[33]	49	42	Short disease-free interval; node-positive primary	Inclusion criteria: good performance status, objective response on chemotherapy, 1-3 liver metastases
Selzner et al., 2000[35]	17	27	Short disease-free interval	6041 patients with breast cancer treated during study interval
Yoshimoto et al., 2000[34]	25	34	None	67% of patients experienced recurrence in the liver

[a]Only series including more than 10 patients are presented.
[b]Overall survival.

metastases of breast cancer cannot be defined at this time. A common recommendation is that patients with extrahepatic disease should not undergo liver resection, even though some studies did not find a worse prognosis for such patients. Some authors also suggest that patients should first undergo systemic chemotherapy and that only patients who do not progress should undergo liver resection.[6] Further negative predictive risk factors advising against a surgical approach are positive lymph node status of the initial breast cancer, occurrence of liver metastases within 1 year after resection of the primary tumor,[30,35] and extensive hepatic lesions requiring a major resection.[6] Moreover, tumor biologic processes have an impact on the prognosis of patients with liver metastases from breast cancer; two studies demonstrated that a positive hormone (estrogen/progesterone) receptor status is associated with increased survival.[26,30] However, formal randomized trials confirming these strategies are still lacking. In a 2009 report regarding RFA, median survival for included patients was 30 months, but the follow-up time was only 19 months and the local tumor progression rate was 25%.[36]

Melanoma

Melanoma was estimated to account for approximately 7% of new cancer cases in men and for 5% of new cancer cases in women in the United States in 2020.[7] Most cases (90%) involved melanoma of cutaneous origin, whereas a small subset was derived from the uvea (5 %) or from other body sites.[37] Depending on the site of the primary melanoma, there is a different pattern of metastatic spread: Cutaneous melanomas disseminate to the liver in 15% to 20% of patients with this metastatic disease. Furthermore, they are often associated with simultaneous extrahepatic disease.[38] In contrast, in 40% of patients with liver metastases from uveal melanoma, the liver is the only organ of the secondary disease without any additional extrahepatic disease.[39] Therefore the number of liver metastases resected from uveal melanoma is nearly equivalent to that of cutaneous melanoma.

Cutaneous Melanoma

Cutaneous melanoma recurs after potentially curative resection in approximately one third of patients, with almost every organ being at risk.[40] Hepatic metastases are diagnosed in approximately 10% to 20% of patients with stage IV melanoma, even though it is well documented that most patients have liver metastases on postmortem examination.[41] In the era before the introduction of targeted therapy in melanoma by BRAF and/or MEK inhibitors, as well as checkpoint inhibitors, most patients were considered to have unresectable melanoma as a result of extrahepatic disease or disseminated hepatic metastases. This point was shown by a study from the John Wayne Cancer Institute and the Sydney Melanoma Unit.[41] During the years 1971 through 1999, a total of 26,204 patients with melanoma were seen in these institutions and 1750 patients (6.7%) had liver metastases. Only 34 patients underwent surgical exploration for attempted liver resection, and hepatectomy was performed in 24 patients. Of these 24 patients, 12 had synchronous extrahepatic disease and 18 could be rendered disease free surgically. The 10 patients who underwent exploration only had a median survival of 4 months; the overall survival of all patients with liver metastases treated nonoperatively was 6 months. Overall survival in the patients who underwent complete resection was 28 months, with a median DFS of 12 months. One patient achieved 10-year survival, and the 5-year overall survival was 29%. Complete gross resection and histologically negative margins were associated with an improved DFS, and complete gross resection showed a trend for improved overall survival ($P = .06$).

From this experience, one might conclude that extrahepatic disease per se is not a contraindication for resection, provided that all disease is resectable. Patient selection is crucial, which is well documented in this study. Only 1.4% of all patients with liver metastases underwent hepatic resection, and these patients had a median disease-free interval of 58 months before presenting with hepatic metastases. Several other small series in the literature mostly comprise fewer than 10 patients undergoing liver resection for metastatic melanoma, with median survival times of 10 to 51 months.[41,42] Repeat hepatic resection might be beneficial for some patients who can be rendered disease free surgically.[43]

However, for the last decade there has been a paradigm shift in the treatment of metastatic melanoma by the innovative introduction of a targeted therapy using BRAF or MEK (MAPK/

ERK) inhibitors or immune checkpoint inhibitors. Current studies have shown that the median survival in selected patients with metastatic melanoma disease and a BRAF V600 mutation can be extended to more than 21 months.[44] Moreover, the combination therapy with dabrafenib and trametinib resulted in an objective rate of tumor response of 64%.[44] This effective systemic therapy also has a powerful impact on patients undergoing resection in metastasized melanoma.[45] Recent studies have shown that patients undergoing hepatectomy for liver metastases of melanoma can experience a 1- and 2-year survival of 51% and 38%, respectively, in the new era of systemic treatment.[46]

These data are encouraging in that targeted therapy might render more patients eligible for a curative surgical approach when they are seen with liver metastases.

Uveal Melanoma

Uveal melanoma is a distinct entity that seems to have different tumor biologic processes, and it commonly spreads to the liver. Approximately 50% to 80% of patients with uveal melanoma in whom distant metastases develop have liver involvement. Mariani et al.[47] investigated the management of liver metastases from uveal melanoma in 798 patients; 255 patients of this cohort received surgical treatment. The median overall survival after hepatic surgery was 14 months compared with 8 months in those who had no surgery. When they performed a survival analysis based on the resection status, they observed a median overall survival of 27 months after R0 resection, 17 months after R1 resection, and 11 months after R2 resection. In a multivariate survival analysis, they identified three further prognostic classifiers: time to liver metastases (>24 months), number of liver metastases resected (≤4 lesions), and absence of miliary disease. Hsueh et al.[48] reported on 112 patients with metastatic uveal melanoma, and 78 patients had liver metastases. A total of 24 patients underwent surgical resection for metastatic disease, 5 with liver metastases. A multivariate analysis showed resection, but not site of metastasis, to be a significant predictor of survival. The median survival for patients undergoing resection was 38 months in this series, with a 5-year survival of 39%. In a report from Pawlik et al.[17] 16 patients with liver metastases from ocular melanoma underwent resection; the median time to recurrence was 8.8 months. Compared with patients undergoing liver resection for metastatic cutaneous melanoma, more patients experienced recurrent disease in the liver (53% versus 17%); however, the 5-year survival was significantly better for metastatic ocular melanoma (21% versus 0%; $P = .015$). Despite these data, most patients with liver metastases from uveal melanoma are not candidates for a complete resection.

For optimal selection of patients who might be eligible for liver resection in case of uveal melanoma, a diligent staging is mandatory. In this context, magnetic resonance imaging (MRI) might be superior to fluorodeoxyglucose positron-emission tomography (FDG-PET), as recently reported in a preliminary study.[49]

Gastric and Pancreatic Cancer

Multimodality approaches have significantly improved the prognosis for patients with metastatic gastric cancer. Several retrospective studies have suggested that surgery for liver metastases arising from gastric adenocarcinoma is reasonable in very carefully selected patients, provided that complete resection seems feasible after careful preoperative staging[50] (Table 92.4[51–55]). Cheon et al.[50] reported on 58 patients with liver-only metastases

TABLE 92.4 Results of Liver Resection for Metastatic Gastric Cancer[a]

REFERENCE	NO. PATIENTS	MEDIAN SURVIVAL[b]	ADVERSE PROGNOSTIC FACTORS	COMMENTS
Schildberg et al., 2012[52]	31	5-year survival, 13%	Synchronous liver metastases R1 and R2 resection	
Takemura et al., 2012[53]	64	34 months	Serosal invasion of the primary tumor, large hepatic tumor (>5 cm),	32 patients received synchronous gastrectomy and hepatectomy; 32 patients underwent metachronous hepatectomy
Garancini et al., 2012[54]	21	11 months, 5-year survival rate 19%	Positive resection margin; >1 liver metastasis; no fibrous pseudocapsule	Three 5-year survivors; 68% of patients developed liver recurrence of metastasis
Ambiru et al., 2001[55]	40	2-year survival, 27%	Synchronous metastases	Six 5-year survivors; 72% of patients developed liver recurrence
Fujii et al., 2001[56]	12	16.3 months	Disease-free interval <12 months; metastases >5 cm	—

[a]Only series including more than10 patients are presented.
[b]Ovserall survival.

from gastric cancer who underwent gastric resection regardless of hepatic surgery. The overall 1-year, 3-year, and 5-year survival rates of those 41 of 58 patients who underwent hepatic resection with curative intent were 75.3%, 31.7%, and 20.8%, respectively, and three patients survived longer than 7 years. Similar encouraging results have been reported in a multi-institutional cohort including 513 patients subjected to hepatectomy for liver metastases originating from gastric cancer with a 5- and 10-year overall survival of 32% and 25%, respectively.[10] Recently, a pilot study established a clinical model to identify a patient population with limited metastatic gastric cancer, which could potentially benefit from surgical intervention after induction chemotherapy.[56] Those data have provided the rationale to launch a prospective, multicenter, randomized, investigator-initiated phase III trial (RENAISSANCE trial) to compare the effect of chemotherapy alone versus chemotherapy, followed by surgical resection on survival and quality of life in patients with limited-metastatic gastric cancer, including patients with a maximum of five metastatic hepatic lesions that are potentially resectable.[56] Similarly designed studies are needed in the future to answer the question of whether patients with liver metastases from gastric cancer actually benefit from a metastasectomy and may even be treated with a curative intent.

For patients with pancreatic ductal adenocarcinoma, only a handful of long-term survivors have been reported after the resection of liver metastases[57] (see Chapter 62). In a report from Shrikhande et al.,[58] 11 patients underwent combined pancreatic and liver resection for metastatic pancreatic cancer, with a median survival of 11.4 months. A recent review on this topic summarized 103 patients who underwent liver resection for metastatic pancreatic cancer; median survival ranged from 5.8 to 11.3 months.[59] Consequently, surgery remains highly controversial. Nevertheless, in the new era of multiagent chemotherapy, highly selected patient groups with oligometastatic pancreatic carcinoma might still benefit from a resection. A systematic review of surgical resection of liver-only synchronous metastases from pancreatic cancer has reported a median survival of 34 to 56 months in those patients with preoperative chemotherapy and good response.[60] However, until sufficient data are available from prospective randomized studies that have recently been initiated,[61] the resection of liver metastases originating from pancreatic ductal adenocarcinoma should remain a case-by-case decision.

For other primary malignant tumors of the pancreas that show a less aggressive tumor biology, such as solid pseudopapillary tumor of the pancreas, resection of liver metastases might be justified.[62]

Renal Carcinoma

Liver metastases develop in approximately 10% to 20% of patients with renal tumors,[63] and they have a dismal prognosis. Less than 10% survive beyond 1 year, and only approximately 2% to 4% experience hepatic disease that is amenable to complete resection. In one series, 88 patients with liver metastases from primary renal tumors were identified; 68 patients underwent metastasectomy of the liver, whereas the remaining 20 patients, who declined surgical treatment, served as a control cohort.[64] The overall survival rate at 5 years after metastasectomy was 62.2%, with a median survival of 142 months. In the comparative group, the 5-year overall survival rate was significantly lower (29.3%), with a median of 27 months ($P = .003$). Patients with a high tumor grade, positive lymph node status at initial diagnosis, synchronous liver metastases, and patients with a reduced physical performance status according to the Eastern Cooperative Oncology Group (ECOG) score showed a worse prognosis. In another report on 31 patients, 5-year overall survival was 39% for the whole patient group and 50% for patients with negative margins.[65] Conclusively, in patients with hepatic metastases from renal tumors who are candidates for a complete resection, surgical exploration may be justified with a curative intent. However, this remains a rare exception and it is estimated that surgical treatment of hepatic metastases is performed in only approximately 1% of patients with liver metastases.[63] Therefore other therapies should be considered, such as hepatic artery embolization and targeted molecular therapy, such as sunitinib.

Reproductive Tract Tumors

Effective chemotherapeutic regimens are available for most reproductive tumors. Resection is only one component of a multimodal approach to the treatment of liver metastases from these tumors. The development of liver metastases is a well-defined adverse prognostic factor for patients with germ cell tumors.[66] Rivoire et al.[67] attempted to define guidelines for the resection of liver metastases from germ cell tumors; these authors examined 37 patients who had undergone liver resection for metastatic germ cell tumors. All patients had received cisplatin-based chemotherapy before surgery. Median survival was 54 months, with an overall 5-year survival rate of 62%. The authors defined three prognostic factors associated with a worse outcome: (1) pure embryonal carcinoma in the primary tumor, (2) liver metastasis greater than 3 cm, and (3) presence of viable residual disease after chemotherapy. Because no patient with liver tumors less than 1 cm had viable disease, the authors recommended a nonsurgical approach for these patients. Men with liver tumors greater than 3 cm in diameter represent a high-risk group that may not benefit from partial hepatectomy, but resection was recommended for the other subgroups.

Hahn et al.[68] presented data regarding 57 patients undergoing liver resection for metastatic testicular cancer after systemic chemotherapy. In 48 patients, concomitant cytoreductive procedures for extrahepatic disease were performed. The overall 2-year survival rate was 97.1%. Pathologic analysis of resected specimens showed either a benign lesion or only necrotic tumor in 58% of specimens. Of 5 patients with active disease and persistently elevated serum markers, 3 died during follow-up, underlining the importance of response to chemotherapy as a predictor of outcome.

Epithelial ovarian cancer is the fifth leading cause of tumor-related death in women in Western countries and is the leading cause of gynecologic cancer death after breast cancer.[7] Less frequent histologic types of ovarian cancer encompass sarcoma, germ cell, and stromal tumors.[69]

Patients with metastatic ovarian or fallopian tube carcinoma usually do not present with isolated liver metastases because the disease is generally diffuse within the abdomen and pelvis. Cytoreductive surgery that reduces disease to less than 1 cm when combined with chemotherapy is an accepted treatment approach. Unlike most other tumors, ovarian cancer is usually confined to the liver surface, and although extensive involvement can be seen, isolated intraparenchymal hepatic metastases are uncommon (Fig. 92.8). For these diseases, liver resection may be necessary to achieve an optimal cytoreduction.

A median overall survival of 62 months after hepatic resection has been described with this approach in 24 patients, with 18 patients having extrahepatic disease at the time of hepatectomy.[70] In this study, complete resection of all gross disease was possible in 21 patients, whereas in 3 patients, tumor debulking to less than 1 cm was performed. Merideth et al.[71] reported 26 patients who underwent liver resection for metachronous metastases from ovarian carcinoma; cytoreduction was suboptimal (residual tumor = 1 cm) in 5 patients. Median disease-related survival was 26.3 months, and a disease-free interval exceeding 12 months and optimal cytoreduction were associated with improved outcome. In a more recent study, Lim et al.[72] have investigated the clinical significance of hepatic parenchymal metastasis in patients with primary epithelial ovarian cancer. This series consisted of 16 patients with hepatic parenchymal lesions secondary to peritoneal seeding (International Federation of Gynecology and Obstetrics [FIGO] stage IV). As control, Lim et al.[72] included 97 patients with ovarian cancer and peritoneal dissemination but without liver metastases (FIGO stage IIIc). Their study revealed that the 5-year progression-free survival rates and the 5-year overall survival rate for patients with stage IIIc disease versus patients with stage IV disease and hepatic parenchymal metastasis from peritoneal seeding were 25% and 23%

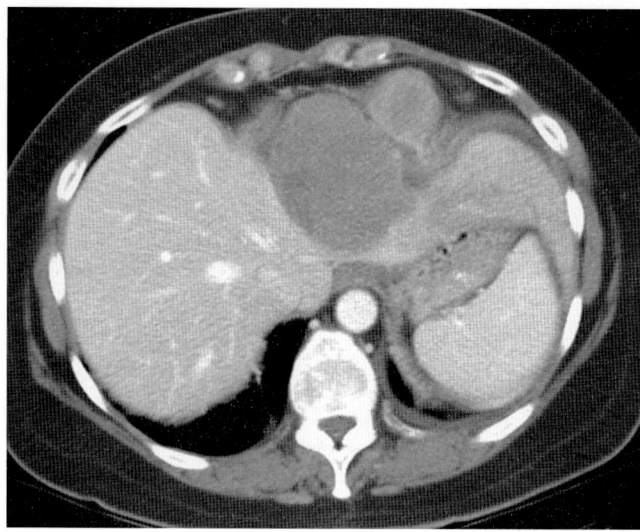

FIGURE 92.8   Axial computed tomographic image of a large ovarian metastasis to the left liver. Note that the tumor extends into the liver from without, with no penetration evident through the liver capsule (see Chapter 15).

($P = .81$) versus 55% and 51% ($P = .57$), respectively. In conclusion, hepatic metastasectomy for ovarian epithelial cancer should be performed only if an optimal cytoreduction of extrahepatic disease can be obtained because there is an inverse correlation between the volume of the residual tumor and the patient overall survival.[73] In this context, patients may benefit from an additional hyperthermic intraperitoneal chemotherapy (HIPEC).[74] However, because this intervention is also associated with a relevant increase in perioperative morbidity and mortality, a diligent patient selection for this multimodal procedure should be performed preoperatively.[74]

Liver resection for metastases from cervical and endometrial cancer has been reported in the literature, with an overall survival of 7 to 50 months.[75,76] Selected patients may benefit from hepatectomy; however, because of the small number of published cases, no general conclusions can be drawn from the available data.

Other Primary Tumors

Resection of liver metastases of lung cancer has been reported, and in selected patients, long-term survival has been achieved. Di Carlo et al.[77] summarized the available data from the literature. Liver resection was performed in 14 patients with liver metastases from lung cancer, and 2 patients lived longer than 5 years.

A report summarized the results of hepatic resection for metastatic squamous cell carcinoma from various primary sites (anus, head/neck, lung, esophagus, and others).[78] The median overall survival was 22 months, with synchronous disease, metastasis size greater than 5 cm, and positive surgical margins being adverse prognostic parameters.

Patients seen with liver metastases from an unknown primary tumor are a challenge to manage because median overall survival is approximately 5 months. Liver resection or ablative therapy might be appropriate for some patients in whom all disease can be destroyed or removed, but a median DFS of only 6.5 months has been reported.[79]

CRITICAL EVALUATION OF LIVER RESECTION FOR METASTATIC NONCOLORECTAL NONNEUROENDOCRINE TUMORS

Before discussing the rationale of liver resection for metastatic NCNN tumors, it is helpful to consider the reasons for the relative success of liver resection for metastatic CRC (see Chapter 90). As a result of the favorable long-term outcome after resection and the improved safety of liver resection, the treatment strategy for patients with liver metastases arising from primary CRCs has changed in the past 2 decades. Mortality, morbidity, and long-term outcome have been improved significantly through patient selection (see Chapters 90 and 101), a refined perioperative management (see Chapter 26), more effective combination chemotherapy or patient-specific targeted therapy (see Chapters 9A, 97, and 98), and the adoption of new surgical procedures such as laparoscopic liver resection[7,80] (see Chapters 127D and 127E). Therefore liver metastases from CRC are no longer viewed as indicators of untreatable, widespread, systemic disease, and cure is still possible with surgery in some patients.

Two different concepts explain the relatively favorable outcome of patients undergoing hepatectomy for liver metastases from CRC. First, the tumor biologic processes of metastatic CRC are likely different from those of other solid tumors; tumor cell dissemination of CRC by the bloodstream may be inefficient and could lead to death of most of the tumor cells shed into the bloodstream before the development of clinically significant metastases. Implantation of circulating colorectal tumor cells in the liver may be particularly effective owing to the expression of particular adhesion molecules.[81-83] The second reason may be the venous drainage of the large intestine by the portal vein to the liver; tumor cells that reach the liver through the portal vein may be effectively entrapped by the liver, preventing systemic spread. If this concept is correct, tumor cells must overcome hepatic filtration to reach the systemic circulation and cause distant metastases.[82]

Both notions are substantiated by clinical and experimental findings. It could be shown that the liver is an effective filter for CRC cells because these cells can be found more frequently in blood samples obtained from the portal vein compared with blood samples from the vena cava.[84,85] Tumor biologic processes are also important, however, because the most relevant prognostic factors after resection of colorectal liver metastases, such as length of disease-free interval and nodal status of primary tumor, are at least in part surrogates for tumor biologic processes.[86]

These concepts are crucial when trying to define the value of surgical resection of noncolorectal liver metastases. Except for GI primaries, the liver is not the primary filter for venous blood from the organs being discussed in this chapter. Liver metastases from non-GI cancers indicate systemic tumor spread; this makes selection of patients with good tumor biologic condition, a crucial factor in offering hepatic resection to patients who may benefit the most. Tumor biologic status depends mainly on the primary tumor type, which is shown by the fact that relapse-free and cancer-specific survival for patients with reproductive tract primary tumors is significantly longer compared with that of patients with non–reproductive tract primary tumors in most studies.

When selecting patients for liver resection, it also is important to select patients with more favorable tumor biologic status within a particular histology condition. Disease-free interval, or the time between the treatment of the primary tumor and the development of liver metastasis, may be a valid surrogate marker in this respect, with a longer disease-free interval being associated with less aggressive tumor biologic status. Most studies support this concept because patients with a longer disease-free interval show a longer relapse-free and cancer-specific survival after hepatectomy.[9]

The biologic behavior of liver metastases also is most likely linked to the behavior of the primary tumor because positive lymph node status or venous invasion of the primary tumor predicts worse outcome after hepatectomy for liver metastases in some studies. Tumor biologic status also appears to determine whether a patient would respond to systemic chemotherapy, which might be an important component when managing these patients, as has been shown for hepatic metastases of reproductive tract primary tumors.

Another important point that should be considered when contemplating hepatic resection for a patient with NCNN metastases is the likelihood of achieving a microscopically complete tumor resection. In most studies, long-term survival can be achieved only if the tumor can be removed completely, which depends on tumor-related factors and surgical expertise at high-volume centers.[87] When summarizing the published data, primary tumor type, length of disease-free interval, and pathologic features of the primary tumor may be valid criteria to assess the potential outcome after a planned hepatic resection for patients with metastatic NCNN tumors. By applying these criteria, long-term survival after potentially curative resection of liver metastases can be achieved.[9,28,52] The use of systemic chemotherapy to assess the biologic behavior of the tumor also should be considered, although randomized trials validating this approach are lacking.

CONCLUSION

Hepatic resection for metastatic NCNN tumors is safe and is associated with a favorable outcome in highly selected patients. Primary tumor type and disease-free interval seem to be valid selection parameters. Because hepatic resection is often the only modality offering a potential cure, it should be considered in some patients with metastases from NCNN tumors.

CHAPTER 93

Hepatic tumors in childhood

Michael J. LaQuaglia, J. Ted Gerstle, and Michael P. LaQuaglia

OVERVIEW

An appreciation of hepatic segmental anatomy (see Chapter 2) has led to major advances in hepatic surgery, especially for tumors. In addition, the well-known but still somewhat mysterious stimulus to hepatic regeneration has allowed larger and more extensive resections. In small infants, 70% to 80% of the liver can be removed safely, greatly increasing the scope for cure. This may be aided by portal vein embolization or ligation (see Chapters 101 and 102) or computer-aided three-dimensional reconstructions that allow "in-silico" tumor resection.[1,2]

Advances have also been made in understanding tumor biology and clinical behavior. This chapter addresses benign and malignant tumors of the liver and biliary tract encountered in infancy, childhood, and adolescence.

HISTORY

From 310 to 280 BCE, Herophilus and Erasistratus first presented a description of hepatic anatomy (see Introduction). In the late 1880s, hepatic resection was attempted, but advances in anesthesia and antisepsis would be required before a successful outcome could be realized. Wendel used avascular anatomic planes in the liver to perform a hepatic resection in 1910,[3] and progress in hepatic surgery has been based on an appreciation of hepatic segmental anatomy as described by Couinaud (see Introduction).[4,5] The distribution of the portal and hepatic veins delimits each hepatic segment, which has a unique portal vein and hepatic artery branch and bile duct. Knowledge of this anatomy allows control of the vascular structures before division of the hepatic parenchyma, making major hepatic resections feasible (see Chapter 2).

Bloodless hepatic dissection is crucial in infants and small children, who may have a total blood volume less than 1 L. In the pediatric literature, Martin and Woodman[6] reported that hepatoblastomas could be treated by hepatic lobectomy, and modern hepatic resection is soundly based on principles of segmental hepatic anatomy.

A second important historic finding was the sensitivity of some tumors, especially hepatoblastoma, to systemic chemotherapy.[7] Chemotherapy caused significant reductions in tumor volume, and previously unresectable hepatoblastomas became resectable.[8,9] Presently, the standard of practice is to administer neoadjuvant systemic chemotherapy to patients with hepatoblastoma, unless the tumor is clearly resectable at diagnosis.

In addition, appreciation of the biology of hepatic epithelial malignancies has increased, especially the differences between hepatoblastoma and hepatocellular carcinoma (HCC) (see Chapter 9C). These differences include the relatively good prognosis of hepatoblastoma compared with HCC in childhood, the importance of complete surgical resection of the primary hepatic tumor, and the association of hepatoblastoma with certain clinical syndromes.[10-15] Finally, the first application of hepatic transplantation to a childhood liver tumor was reported by Heimann et al. in 1987,[16] and a series of pediatric liver tumor patients treated by hepatic transplantation was reported by Tagge et al. in 1992.[17] There is continued interest in use of this modality for unresectable hepatic malignancies in childhood and adolescence[18-20] (see Chapters 105, 108, and 110).

MALIGNANT TUMORS

Primary malignant liver tumors constitute approximately 1.7% of childhood malignancies in Western nations. The overall incidence of primary liver cancer, as published by the Surveillance Epidemiology and End Results (SEER) program, is 16.5 cases per 1 million children in the 0- to 4-year age group, 0.5 cases per 1 million in the 5- to 9-year age group, 0.9 cases per 1 million in the 10- to 14-year age group, and 1.5 cases per 1 million in the 14- to 19-year age group.[21] Liver cancers constitute 0.5% to 2% of all pediatric solid tumors and about 5% of abdominal tumors in childhood.[22] The distribution of the most common malignant hepatic tumors is depicted in Fig. 93.1. Hepatoblastoma is the most common, and its treatment is a success story in pediatric oncology.

Hepatoblastoma

Incidence

Hepatoblastomas are the most common primary hepatic tumors of childhood, constituting 43% to 64% of all hepatic neoplasms in one large series.[22-24] Hepatoblastoma accounts for 91% to 96% of primary hepatic tumors in children younger than 5 years[21,25] but comprises less than 1% of hepatic malignancies when adult age groups are included.[26] The Liver Cancer Study Group of Japan identified 30 hepatoblastomas (0.6%) in a cohort of 4658 patients of all ages diagnosed during a 2-year period.[27]

Each year, hepatoblastoma affects 1 to 2.4 of every 1 million children younger than 15 years,[21,28] and approximately 50 to 70 new cases per year are reported in the United States, with a male/female ratio of 1.7:1.[29] Although hepatoblastoma has been reported sporadically in adults,[30-38] the median age at diagnosis is approximately 18 months, and most cases occur before the age of 3 years.[10] Hepatoblastoma is the most prevalent malignant neoplasm of the fetus and neonate and results in death within 2 years if not treated.[39-43] The incidence of hepatoblastoma from 2007 to 2011 was 4.2 per 1 million children younger than 20 years, and it may be increasing.[21,44] The incidence in the same age group from 1993 to 1997 was 1.2 per 1 million, and this was increased from 0.6 per 1 million from 1973 to 1977.[25] However, this increase may simply be due to improving diagnostic modalities.

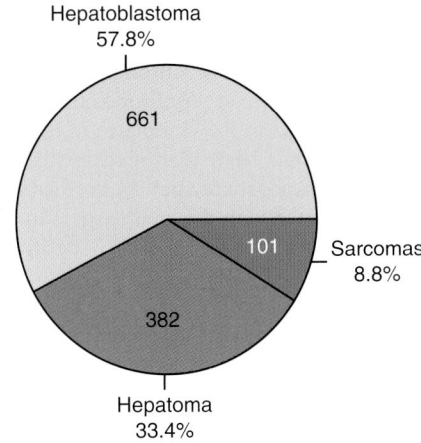

FIGURE 93.1 The frequency distribution of malignant hepatic tumors in childhood as compiled from reported large series. (Modified from Exelby PR et al. Liver tumors in children in the particular reference to hepatoblastoma and hepatocellular carcinoma. *J Pediatr Surg.* 1975;10:329–337; and Weinberg AG, Finegold MJ. Primary hepatic tumors of childhood. *Hum Pathol.* 1983;14:512–537. Used with permission from the American Academy of Pediatrics Surgical Section Survey 1974.)

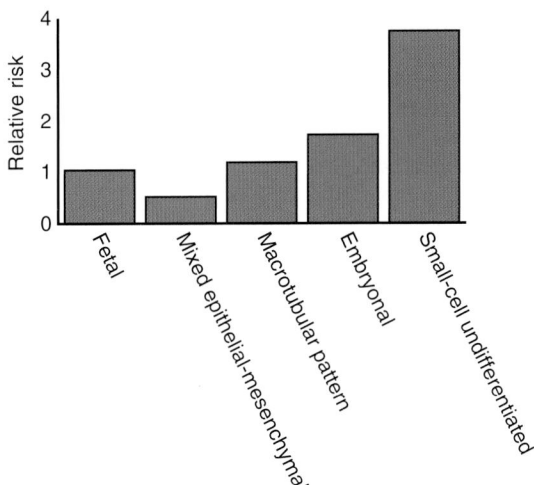

FIGURE 93.2 Graph depicts the risk of death for patients with fetal histology hepatoblastoma adjusted for age, sex, and stage and compared with other histopathologic subtypes.

Hepatoblastoma may occur in siblings.[45–48] It is most strongly associated with familial polyposis,[49,50] Gardner syndrome,[51] and Beckwith-Wiedemann syndrome.[11,14] In familial polyposis, the incidence of hepatoblastoma seems to be increased in first-degree relatives of patients with polyposis. Beckwith-Wiedemann syndrome is associated with Wilms tumor, rhabdomyosarcoma, adrenocortical carcinoma, and hepatoblastoma with a possible association between hepatoblastoma and trisomies 2, 8, 18, and 20.[52,53]

Hepatoblastoma is also associated with low birth weight.[54,55] It is unknown whether the causative agent is developmental abnormalities associated with prematurity or interventions, such as early total parenteral nutrition. These tumors also are reported in patients with congenital anomalies, such as cleft palate, and cardiovascular and renal anomalies, including polycystic kidney and absence of the right adrenal gland.[56] There are also at least two reports of hepatoblastoma occurring in patients with biliary atresia.[57] There are sporadic findings of hepatoblastoma in patients with hepatitis B, but no correlation has been found between the two diseases.[58,59] To date, no evidence associates hepatoblastoma with hepatitis B or C infection or any other chronic viral hepatitis. These patients usually do not have cirrhosis or inborn errors of metabolism.[60,61]

A great advance in developing data-driven models of risk for hepatoblastoma was the institution of the Children's Hepatic Tumors International Collaboration (CHIC).[60,61]

Pathology

Hepatoblastomas are large tumors that can contain fibrous bands, producing a spoked-wheel appearance (see Chapter 87).[62] The five histologic subtypes observed in hepatoblastoma are (1) fetal, (2) embryonal, (3) mixed epithelial, (4) mesenchymal/macrotubular, and (5) anaplastic or small-cell undifferentiated. These subtypes are differentiated based on the findings with light microscopy, but all tumor cells appear smaller than nonneoplastic hepatocytes. Extramedullary hematopoiesis is notably present and may be related to constitutive cytokine production by the tumor cells.[63] The fetal type grows in trabeculae and resembles fetal hepatic cells, whereas embryonic hepatoblastoma cells grow in noncohesive sheets and resemble embryonic cells. Some hepatoblastomas contain mesenchymal tissue along with the epithelial component. Calcification also may appear in these tumors, and one patient was reported with osteosarcomatous elements in the hepatoblastoma and associated pulmonary metastases.[64] The anaplastic or small-cell undifferentiated type consists of small, round blue cells reminiscent of neuroblastoma. This subtype is rare but particularly aggressive, with a strong metastatic potential.[65] The importance of subtyping in hepatoblastoma is due to the association between prognostic risk and subtype, illustrated in Fig. 93.2.[66,67] Some studies have indicated that the fetal histologic subtype has a better prognosis; in contrast, patients with the rare small-cell undifferentiated variant usually do poorly.[65,68]

Basic Biology (see Chapter 9B)

Few cellular models of hepatoblastoma exist, and immortalized cell lines have been difficult to establish. One cell line, isolated from a human hepatoblastoma in 1995, clearly expresses the c-MYC and HRAS1 oncogenes and epidermal growth factor receptor (EGFR).[69] Antibodies that blocked the EGFR inhibited cell growth. Although there has not been a connection established between HRAS and hepatoblastoma, knockdown of c-MYC has led to growth inhibition in hepatoblastoma-derived cell lines HepG2 and Huh6.[70] Another new cell line was established in 2009 from a 5-year-old hepatoblastoma patient and contains an identical genotype to tumor cells, with morphologic, molecular, and immunohistochemical confirmation.[71] Three-dimensional cellular organoid models have also shown promise for maintaining hepatoblastoma lines in culture.[72]

Perhaps the most exciting insight is the association between hepatoblastoma and familial adenomatous polyposis syndrome.[73,74] In one study of 13 hepatoblastomas obtained from nonfamilial adenomatous polyposis patients, 69% had mutations in the adenomatous polyposis coli (APC) gene.[75] In one case of siblings with hepatoblastoma, a shared APC gene mutation was identified.[76] To date, over 100 patients have been described with both hepatoblastoma and familial adenomatous polyposis, with compelling implications regarding screening for both diseases.[77] In addition, the association between hepatoblastoma and β-catenin, an *APC*-regulated protein and transcription cofactor for many proliferation genes, is well studied. In an analysis of 52 hepatoblastoma samples, 48% showed mutations in a region known to regulate activation.[78] Subsequent studies also noted mutations, as well as increased expression of β-catenin in as many as 88% of samples, where it frequently localized to the nucleus.[79-83] When hepatoblastoma samples that contained β-catenin in the nucleus were compared with those that did not, nuclear β-catenin was associated with more aggressive histologic subtypes.[84,85] Moreover, when compounds known to inhibit β-catenin activity were added to hepatoblastoma cell lines in vitro, a reduction in nuclear localization and a dose-dependent inhibition of cell growth were observed.[86] The proliferation-inducing transcriptional coactivator Yes-associated protein (YAP) has also been observed to localize to the nucleus in hepatoblastoma. One study involving 94 tumor samples demonstrated YAP nuclear localization in 85% of cases. Coimmunoprecipitation was then performed between YAP and β-catenin in HepG2 cells, which exhibited an association between the two.[87] This association has been investigated in murine models, where constitutively active YAP and β-catenin led to the development of hepatoblastoma.[88] Similar results were demonstrated when β-catenin was constitutively active with the YAP paralog, transcriptional cofactor with PDZ-binding motif (TAZ).[89] There is evidence that mTOR is a downstream effector of YAP/TAZ/β-catenin activation in hepatoblastoma cells and that mTOR inhibitors have therapeutic potential.[90,91]

Elevated hepatocyte growth factor levels have been demonstrated in the serum of 10 (43%) of 23 patients with hepatoblastoma.[92] Addition of hepatocyte growth factor to hepatoblastoma-derived cell lines has been shown to demonstrate both antiapoptotic and antiproliferative properties, highlighting the need for further study.[93,94]

Small epithelial cells, characteristic of hepatic stem cells, have been observed in human hepatoblastomas of various subtypes.[95] Additionally, various genetic abnormalities have been reported in hepatoblastoma. Chromosome 8q amplification is associated with a worsened prognosis and has been correlated with overexpression of the transcription factor pleomorphic adenoma gene 1 *(PLAG1)*.[96] Telomerase and its regulatory protein expression levels have been correlated with poor outcome in human hepatoblastoma,[97] and tamoxifen may inhibit hepatoblastoma cells by reducing telomerase levels.[98]

Loss of heterozygosity on chromosome 11p15.5, the region associated with Beckwith-Wiedemann syndrome, and on chromosome 1p36 has been described in hepatoblastoma.[99,100] Investigations into both regions suggest that each may contain a tumor suppressor gene, but this has not been proven. Trisomy 20 and trisomy of all or part of chromosome 2 also have been reported.[101] In addition, an abnormality of chromosome 2q may provide a common genetic link between hepatoblastoma and rhabdomyosarcoma.[102] Finally, frequent genetic losses found using comparative genomic hybridization included regions 13q21-q22 (28%) and 9p22-pter (22%), and the most frequent genetic gains were on chromosomes 2q23-q23 (33%) and 1q24-q25 (28%).[103] Differentially expressed microRNA has been shown to be deregulated in hepatoblastoma.[104]

In addition, the well-known thrombocytosis associated with untreated hepatoblastoma is fascinating, as is the presence of extramedullary hematopoiesis. It has been shown that hepatoblastoma cells secrete interleukin (IL)-1β, which causes secretion of IL-6 from surrounding fibroblasts and endothelial cells.[105] Other factors, such as erythropoietin and stem cell factor, have been localized to the cytoplasm of hepatoblastoma cells. Thrombopoietin has been identified in hepatoblastoma tissue and serum from a patient, but its correlation with the thrombocytosis associated with this neoplasm is unclear.[106]

Clinical Findings

The most common presenting sign of hepatoblastoma is an asymptomatic abdominal mass. The child is often in good health, and the tumor usually is discovered incidentally, when an attentive parent, grandparent, or clinician discovers the mass on a routine examination or while bathing the child.[107] Patients with the small-cell undifferentiated variant of hepatoblastoma, who often have distant metastases at diagnosis, are more frequently symptomatic. Accompanying symptoms such as pain, irritability, minor gastrointestinal disturbances, fever, and pallor occur in smaller numbers of patients. Significant weight loss is unusual, although patients may fail to thrive. In most series of hepatoblastomas and HCCs, a few patients present acutely with tumor rupture and intraperitoneal hemorrhage.[108] Rarely, hepatoblastoma manifests with sexual precocity secondary to a β-human chorionic gonadotropin (β-hCG)–secreting tumor,[109] and one patient with a hepatoblastoma was reported presenting with a biliary fistula.[110] Finally, hepatoblastoma may present as a cardiac tumor.[111]

A mild anemia associated with a markedly elevated platelet count is observed in most patients at diagnosis, and the platelet count can range into the millions. As noted previously, the cause is probably secondary to abnormal cytokine release.

Measurement of serum α-fetoprotein (AFP) is well established as an initial tumor marker in the diagnosis of hepatoblastoma and a means of monitoring the therapeutic response.[112] The normal level in most laboratories is less than 20 ng/mL, whereas the AFP level at diagnosis in hepatoblastoma patients can range from normal to significantly elevated (7.7×10^6 ng/mL); it is estimated that the AFP is elevated in 84% to 91% of patients with hepatoblastoma.[67] One study reported a mean AFP level in hepatoblastoma of 3 million ng/mL, whereas the mean in pediatric patients with HCC was approximately 200,000 ng/mL.[113] In infants younger than 1 year, the AFP is normally elevated and is highest at birth (Fig. 93.3).

Some authors suggest that subfractionation more reliably indicates whether the increased AFP is secondary to a hepatoblastoma or HCC (see Chapter 89), an endodermal sinus tumor, or benign liver disease.[114] The half-life of AFP is approximately 6 days, and in one study, 24 (77%) of 31 patients had levels decline postresection by at least 1 log before second-look surgery.[115] Of these patients, 16 (50%) of 32 eventually had AFP levels decline to normal at the end of adjuvant therapy and had no clinical or radiographic evidence of hepatoblastoma at this point. Finally, 15 (94%) of 16 patients who attained a complete response also showed a decline in AFP levels of 2 logs or more before second-look surgery.[112] A large, early decline in AFP levels was an independent predictor of survival in multivariate analysis. It has been suggested that a low initial AFP level, although exceedingly rare, is associated with worse survival.[116] A retrospective analysis of International Society of Pediatric Oncology Liver Group (SIOPEL) groups 1 through 3, which focused on hepatoblastoma patients presenting with

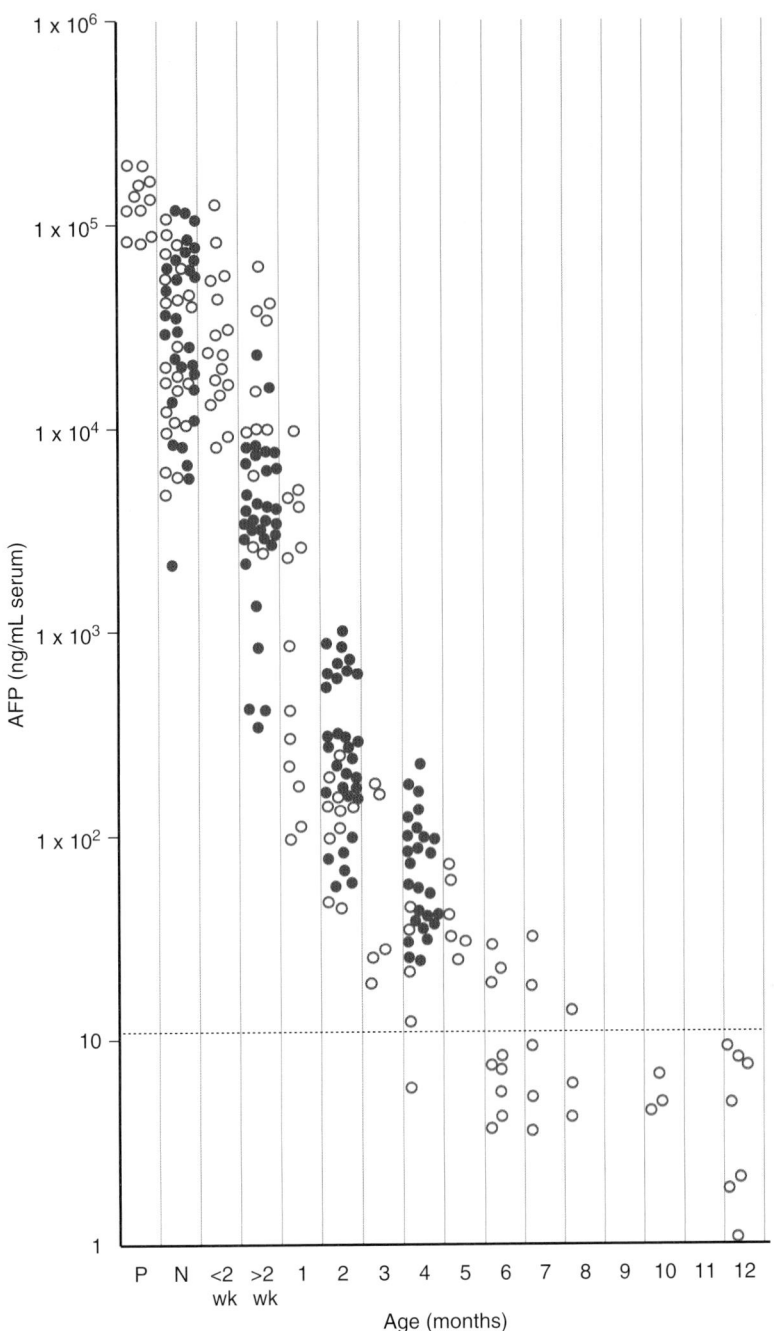

FIGURE 93.3   Graph shows the time decay of α-fetoprotein levels in normal infants during the first year of life. (Used with permission from Wu JT et al. Serum alpha fetoprotein [AFP] levels in normal infants. *Pediatr Res.* 1981;15:50–52.)

AFP levels less than 100 ng/mL (N = 21 patients during a 14-year period), concluded that low initial AFP level was associated with extensive disease at diagnosis, poor response to chemotherapy, and poor outcome.[117] Small-cell undifferentiated hepatoblastomas may also be associated with lower AFP levels.[118] However, the small sample size limits multivariate analysis.

When interpreting the AFP level, it is important to realize that normal levels are very high at birth and decrease during the first 6 months of life. Premature newborns may have AFP levels in the range of 100,000 ng/mL. Term newborns also can have relatively high levels (10^4 to 10^5 ng/mL). By 2 months of age, most infants have levels ranging from 100 to 1000 ng/mL, and

by 6 months, levels should be less than 100 ng/mL. Usually, levels decrease to normal (<20 ng/mL) after 6 to 7 months, but levels may remain elevated for 1 year after birth.[119] AFP may also be elevated in the setting of liver damage, liver regeneration, or the presence of another tumor.

Imaging

The first imaging study is usually an abdominal ultrasound (US) (see Chapter 14). If duplex technique is used, tumor vascularity can be gauged, and the hepatic veins can be assessed.[120] The ultrasonographer also should search for anomalies of the genitourinary system and rule out tumor thrombus in either the

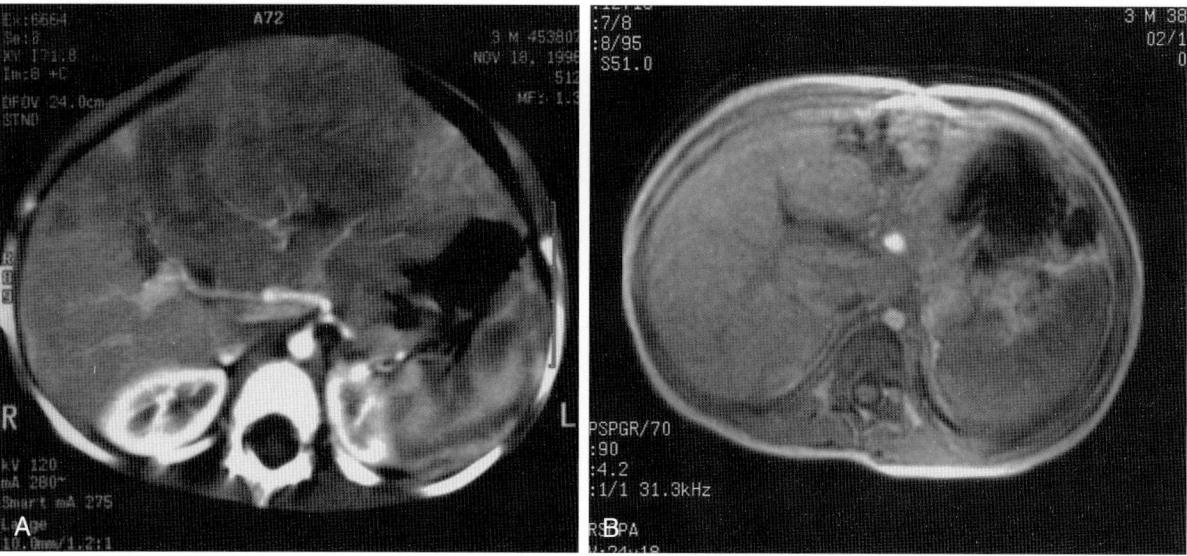

FIGURE 93.4   A, Computed tomographic image of a patient with hepatoblastoma before induction chemotherapy. **B,** Magnetic resonance image of the same patient after four courses of vincristine, cisplatin, and 5-fluorouracil (see Chapter 14).

vena cava or the hepatic veins. Computed tomography (CT) (see Chapter 14) is useful to identify pulmonary metastases, identify diffuse hepatic involvement, and determine resectability. Oral and intravenous contrast material is used (Fig. 93.4A). CT scans can be performed quickly and can be completed in less than 2 minutes in helical scanners; this greatly shortens the required period of sedation for infants or small children, and it has the added advantage of being a quick and reliable screening method for pulmonary metastases. Hepatoblastoma will appear as a well-demarcated tumor without a capsule. CT angiography (CT portography) uses CT with fine cuts and an increased amount of intravenous contrast material to image hepatic tumors and the hepatic venous anatomy. CT portography may provide as much information as magnetic resonance imaging (MRI) (see Chapter 14), which is useful for evaluating hepatic lesions and their relationship to vascular structures. MRI can show the hepatic veins, vena cava, and bile ducts.[121] MRI of a hepatoblastoma patient after neoadjuvant chemotherapy is shown in Fig. 93.4B. Positron-emission tomography has been used to identify hepatoblastoma recurrence and to search for sites of metastatic disease, but it may not be reliable for lesions smaller than 6 to 10 mm[122] (see Chapter 18).

Staging

In the United States, the commonly used staging system is that from the Children's Oncology Group (COG), based on operative findings (Table 93.1). A tumor-node-metastasis (TNM) classification has also been used (Table 93.2).[123] The *PRE-*Treatment *EXT*ent (PRETEXT) system of disease staging has been used extensively by SIOPEL (Fig. 93.5).[124] It relies on radiographic findings before any therapy, including surgery, and does not account for the independent surgeon's judgment at the time of surgery regarding resectability. This staging system is based on Couinaud's system of segmentation of the liver and is thought to predict the degree of tumor infiltration, the extent of surgical resection, and the complexities involved in the resection.[125,126] This system classifies the tumor into one of four categories, depending on which sections of the liver do

TABLE 93.1	Children's Oncology Group Staging for Hepatoblastoma
STAGE I	**COMPLETE RESECTION**
Favorable histology	Purely fetal histology with a low mitotic index
Other histology	All other stage I tumors
Stage II	Gross total resection with microscopic residuals or total resection with preoperative or intraoperative rupture
Stage III	Unresectable tumors as determined by the attending surgeon, partially resected tumors with macroscopic residual involvement, or any tumor with lymph node involvement
Stage IV	Measurable metastatic disease to lungs or other organs

Used with permission from Finegold MJ et al. Liver tumors: Pediatric population. *Liver Transpl.* 2008;14(11):1545–1556, 2008.

not include tumor (Table 93.3).[127] Additional criteria added in 2005 (Table 93.4) further classify these tumors based on local extension, multifocality, rupture, and metastasis.[126,127]

PRETEXT was compared with pathologic findings in 110 patients and was correct in 51%, overstaged in 37%, and understaged in 12%. The authors compared this system with the Children's Cancer Group/Pediatric Oncology Group (CCG/POG) and TNM schemes and claimed a better correlation with risk status. In this study, data from patients who had neoadjuvant chemotherapy were analyzed, whereas a study from the COG analyzed data from patients with a hepatoblastoma at diagnosis and reported that both the COG stage and PRETEXT were useful prognostic indicators. The PRETEXT system has been described as showing improved predictive value for survival compared with other staging classifications.[124] Moreover, this system can be valuable for recognizing patients who are candidates for resection (PRETEXT stages I and II) and those who may benefit from lower dose chemotherapy.[68] It is recommended that all liver tumor patients in future COG studies undergo PRETEXT

TABLE 93.2	Tumor-Node-Metastasis Staging for Hepatic Malignancies

Primary Tumor (T)

TX	Primary tumor cannot be assessed
T0	No evidence of primary tumor
T1	Solitary tumor without vascular invasion
T2	Solitary tumor with vascular invasion or multiple tumors, none >5 cm
T3a	Multiple tumors >5 cm
T3b	Single tumor or multiple tumors of any size involving a major branch of the portal vein or hepatic vein
T4	Tumor(s) with direct invasion of adjacent organs other than the gallbladder or with perforation of visceral peritoneum

Stage Grouping

Stage I	T1	N0	M0
Stage II	T2	N0	M0
Stage IIIA	T3a	N0	M0
Stage IIIB	T3b	N0	M0
Stage IIIC	T4	N0	M0
Stage IVA	Any T	N1	M0
Stage IVB	Any T	Any N	M1

Used with permission from Edge SB et al (eds). *American Joint Committee Cancer Staging Manual,* 7th ed. New York: Springer; 2011, p 242.

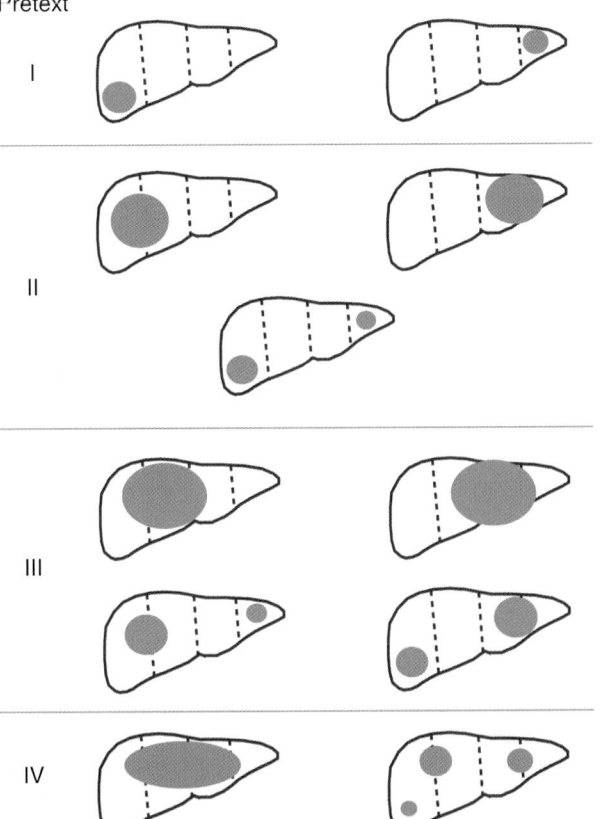

Pretext

I

II

III

IV

FIGURE 93.5 The PRE-Treatment EXTent (PRETEXT) staging system used by the International Society of Pediatric Oncology. The PRETEXT number generally corresponds to the number of liver sections affected by the lesion(s) (see Table 93.3).

TABLE 93.3	PRETEXT Staging System

PRETEXT NUMBER	DEFINITION
I	One section is involved, and three adjoining sections are free
II	One or two sections are involved, but two adjoining sections are free
III	Two or three sections are involved, and no two adjoining sections are free
IV	All four sections are involved

PRETEXT, PRE-Treatment EXTent.

Used with permission from Roebuck DJ et al. PRETEXT: A revised staging system for primary malignant liver tumours of childhood developed by the SIOPEL group. *Pediatr Radiol.* 2005;37:123–132.

TABLE 93.4	PRETEXT Staging: Additional Criteria

C: Caudate lobe involvement	C1: Tumor involving the caudate lobe C0: All other patients All C1 patients are at least PRETEXT II
E: Extrahepatic abdominal disease	E0: No evidence of tumor spread in the abdomen (except M or N) E1: Direct extension of tumor into adjacent organs or diaphragm E2: Peritoneal nodules Add suffix "a" if ascites is present (e.g., E0a)
F: Tumor focality	F0: Patient with solitary tumor F1: Patient with ≥2 discrete tumors
H: Tumor rupture or intraperitoneal hemorrhage	H1: Imaging and clinical findings of intraperitoneal hemorrhage H0: All other patients
M: Distant metastases	M0: No metastases M1: Any metastasis (except E and N) Add suffix or suffixes to indicate location
N: Lymph node metastases	N0: No nodal metastases N1: Abdominal lymph node metastases only N2: Extraabdominal lymph node metastases ± abdominal lymph node metastases
P: Portal vein involvement	P0: No involvement of the portal vein or its left or right branches P1: Involvement of either the left or the right branch of the portal vein P2: Involvement of the main portal vein Add suffix "a" if intravascular tumor is present (e.g., P1a)
V: Involvement of the IVC and/or HVs	V0: No involvement of the HVs or IVC V1: Involvement of 1 HV but not the IVC V2: Involvement of 2 HVs but not the IVC V3: Involvement of all 3 HVs and/or the IVC Add suffix "a" if intravascular tumor is present (e.g., V3a)

HVs, Hepatic veins; *IVC,* inferior vena cava; *PRETEXT,* PRE-Treatment EXTent.

Used with permission from Otte JB: Progress in the surgical treatment of malignant liver tumors in children. *Cancer Treat Rev.* 2010;36:360–371, 2010.

staging. The PRETEXT system was recently updated and clarified to streamline its use in clinical trials.[128]

Treatment

Multiple studies support the effectiveness of systemic chemotherapy combined with complete surgical resection of the primary hepatic tumor.[63,129–131] Survival depends on removal of the primary liver tumor, when imaging suggests that complete resection is feasible.

The first clinical decision is whether to initiate neoadjuvant chemotherapy or proceed with resection. Often, resection is not feasible if tumors are large and involve both hepatic lobes. Preoperative (neoadjuvant) chemotherapy results in tumor shrinkage and makes subsequent resection easier.[9] In one study, the rate of shrinkage was high after initiation of chemotherapy, but it declined after two cycles had been administered (Fig. 93.6).[132] Another study focused exclusively on neoadjuvant therapy in PRETEXT stage III and IV patients and found that the majority of tumors that became resectable required only two cycles of chemotherapy, whereas several more required four cycles.[133] Exquisite clinical judgment and good communication between members of the multidisciplinary team are crucial because approximately 60% of hepatoblastomas are resectable at diagnosis.

To confirm the diagnosis, an initial biopsy is required. For unresectable tumors, the initial surgical procedure should include a diagnostic biopsy and placement of a vascular access device for chemotherapy. A second laparotomy is performed after four cycles of chemotherapy if imaging studies show a good response and the tumor appears resectable.

Complete resection of the primary tumor is necessary for survival and may require extended hepatectomy and/or complex biliary reconstruction (see Chapters 101, 118, and 119). For hepatoblastoma, reports have suggested that gross total resection of the primary lesion may be adequate for cure in chemoresponsive tumors.[134,135] A SIOPEL report demonstrated that, for patients being treated with adjuvant chemotherapy, a microscopically positive resection margin did not affect event-free survival or overall survival.[136]

For resected tumors (stage I) with fetal histology, further therapy is not recommended. All other stage I tumors without pure fetal histology, in addition to stage II patients, should receive four cycles of cisplatin, 5-fluorouracil (5-FU), and vincristine (C5V). Patients with stage III and IV disease should receive four cycles of chemotherapy, followed by resection or transplantation, followed by two more cycles of chemotherapy. C5V is administered, followed by doxorubicin if there is minimal response to C5V. Reports have suggested the use of doxorubicin from the start in this subgroup.[137,138] The combination of cisplatin plus doxorubicin was compared with cisplatin plus 5-FU plus C5V in a combined CCG/POG (intergroup) study.[139] The efficacy was thought to be similar, but more complications resulted with the regimen containing doxorubicin, accounting for equivalent event-free survivals; however, a more detailed review of the analysis suggested that the doxorubicin-containing arm had an improved disease-specific survival. This finding implied that with better management of toxicity, patient outcome might be better with a doxorubicin-containing regimen. In 2009 a trial was published by SIOPEL 3 that randomized 255 "standard-risk" patients (defined as patients with PRETEXT stage I, II, or III and no evidence of extrahepatic disease) into two groups, the first treated with cisplatin alone and the second with cisplatin plus doxorubicin. They reported no difference in achieving resection, or in 3-year event-free or overall survival between these groups, indicating that standard-risk patients may be successfully treated with cisplatin alone.[140] Clinical trials by COG and SIOPEL are planned to evaluate the use of doxorubicin, irinotecan, and other agents, especially in high-risk patients.

In patients with unresectable primary tumors, the use of liver transplantation is increasing (see Chapters 105, 108, and 110). An analysis published in 2005 showed an approximately 80% long-term disease-free survival in those receiving transplantation in large, solitary, or multifocal tumors invading all four sectors of the liver.[141] The United Network for Organ Sharing (UNOS) database consists of more than 200 patients, with a median age of 2.9 years, who underwent orthotopic liver transplantation (OLT) for hepatoblastoma between 1987 and 2006. Approximately half of the patients had a recurrence. Overall survival was 80%, 69%, and 66% at 1, 5, and 10 years, respectively.[142] A 2013 study that queried the UNOS and SEER databases from 1988 to 2010 and 1975 to 2007, respectively, determined that as many as 20% of hepatoblastoma cases are now being referred for OLT, and 5-year survival after transplant is estimated at 73%.[143] In a multicenter review, data on 147 patients with hepatoblastoma were analyzed after liver transplantation. In almost three-quarters of these patients, the original surgery was OLT; the remaining patients either had residual disease after prior resection or had recurrent tumor. The first group of patients had an improved outcome, with 82% overall disease-free survival, compared with 30% in the second group. Smaller, single-center reports have reinforced findings that liver transplantation for hepatoblastoma has the best outcome when done as the primary procedure rather than as a salvage procedure.[144–147]

Transplantation, however, does require the use of immunosuppressive treatment, which comes with its own set of side effects. Moreover, there is in increased chance of thrombosis of the hepatic artery after transplantation in children.[148] The main causes of mortality after transplantation, accounting for 54% of this population, are metastases and recurrence.[142] COG is continuing to investigate the role of liver transplantation in hepatoblastoma. A global database has been instituted to aid in this endeavor (see Chapters 108, 110, and 111).

In one study, the 1-year survival for patients presenting with metastases was no different from that in patients with localized

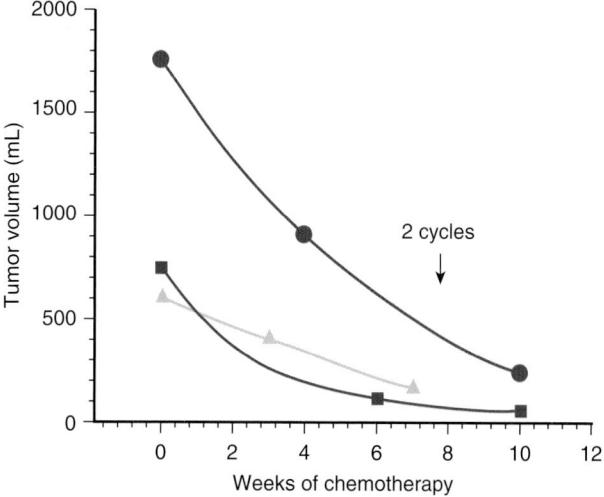

FIGURE 93.6 Tumor volumes of three hepatoblastoma patients are plotted versus time from initiation of chemotherapy. A significant reduction in tumor volume is apparent that is most rapid during the first two cycles of induction chemotherapy. (Used with permission from Medary I et al. Kinetics of primary tumor regression with chemotherapy: Implications for the timing of surgery. *Ann Surg Oncol.* 1996;3:521–525, 1996.)

tumors.[112] In another study by SIOPEL, the 5-year overall and event-free survival for children with hepatoblastoma who presented with pulmonary metastases were 57% and 28%, respectively.[149] This study suggested that 25% to 30% of patients with synchronous pulmonary metastases are curable. It is still necessary to resect the primary liver tumor, and pulmonary metastasectomy should be done only if the primary site is controlled.[135] Many pulmonary metastases resolve with chemotherapy, but thoracotomy and resection are sometimes required for larger or persistent metastatic lesions.[150]

No prospective studies are underway for pulmonary metastasectomy, but one study describes the advantage of pulmonary metastasectomy for diagnosed lesions that remain after neoadjuvant therapy.[151] Some radiation oncologists have treated pulmonary metastases with external-beam radiotherapy in an approach similar to that used for Wilms tumors, but with 18 to 20 Gy administered[152]; however, this may be associated with significant pulmonary toxicity and has not resulted in cure. One case report notes long-term survival in a hepatoblastoma metastatic to the brain, but in general, there is almost no reported cure in patients with spread to sites outside of the lung or local lymph nodes.[153]

Outcome

Following a gross total resection, the 5-year event-free survival is 83%, but this drops to 41% in patients with tumor remaining after surgery.[139] Some patients with microscopic residual tumor are curable with continued chemotherapy and may benefit from external-beam radiotherapy to the primary hepatic site. Resection of many hepatoblastomas may be easier after chemotherapy, and complete resection of the primary hepatic tumor is necessary for survival. In multivariate analysis, factors that have been independent predictors of worse prognosis include a high TNM stage, unresectable tumor, bilobar involvement and multifocality, AFP less than 100 ng/mL or greater than 10^5 ng/mL, distant metastases, embryonal versus fetal histology, and vascular invasion.[154] COG has reported 3-year event-free survival rates of 90%, 50%, and 20% for stages I to II, III, and IV, respectively.[138]

Prognostic Factors

These data have been generated for a large number of patients by the CHIC collaboration.[60,61] Importantly, these prognostic factors are determined at enrollment on study. Negative prognostic factors are PRETEXT IV tumors, distant metastases at diagnosis, unresectable vessel involvement (portal or hepatic vein), extrahepatic tumor extension, multifocal tumor, tumor rupture at presentation, and age at diagnosis of greater than 8 years. Parameters associated with an improved prognosis include PRETEXT I and II tumors, and patients who are from 0 to 2 years of age at diagnosis. An initial AFP of 1000 to 1,000,000 is associated with the best prognosis, whereas an AFP less than 100 has the worst outcome. AFPs that are greater than 1,000,000, or from 100 to 999 have intermediate survival (Figs. 93.7, 93.8, and 93.9).

Future Directions

Advances in the surgical exploitation of the hepatic segmental anatomy (see Chapter 2) and improvements in surgical technique (see Chapters 101, 102, and 118) and perioperative management (see Chapter 26) have allowed more extensive resections so that even very large and bilobar tumors can be

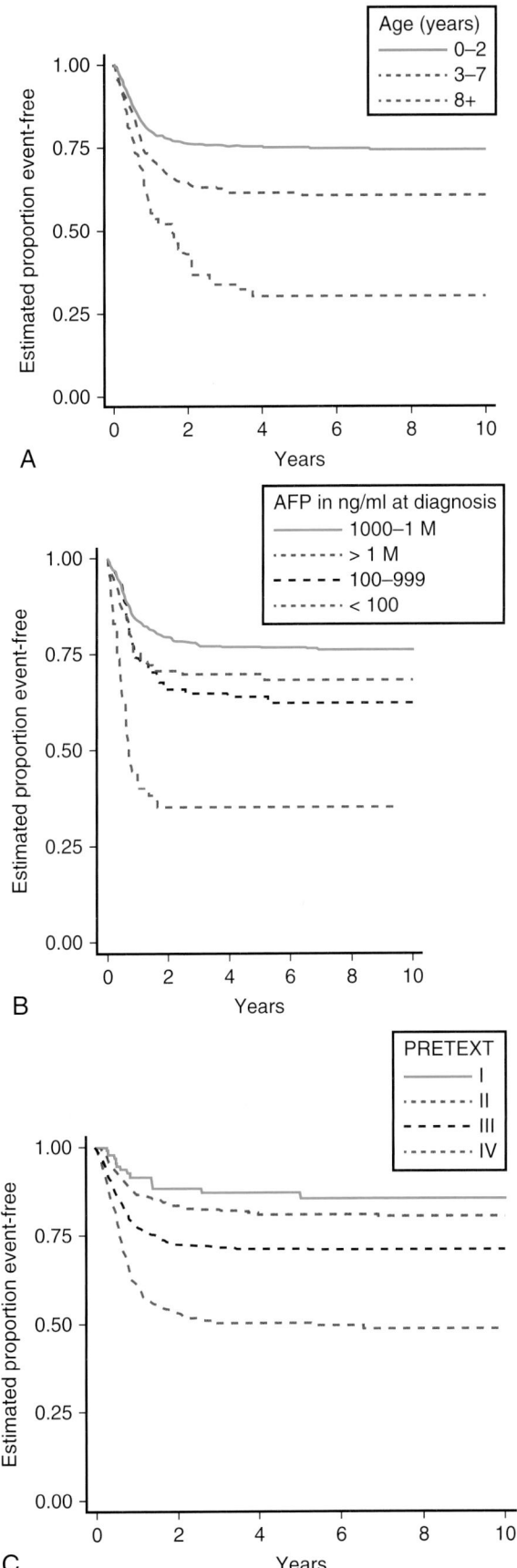

FIGURE 93.7 The impact of **(A)** age at diagnosis, **(B)** alpha-fetoprotein level, and **(C)** PRETEXT stage on event-free survival in patients with hepatoblastoma.

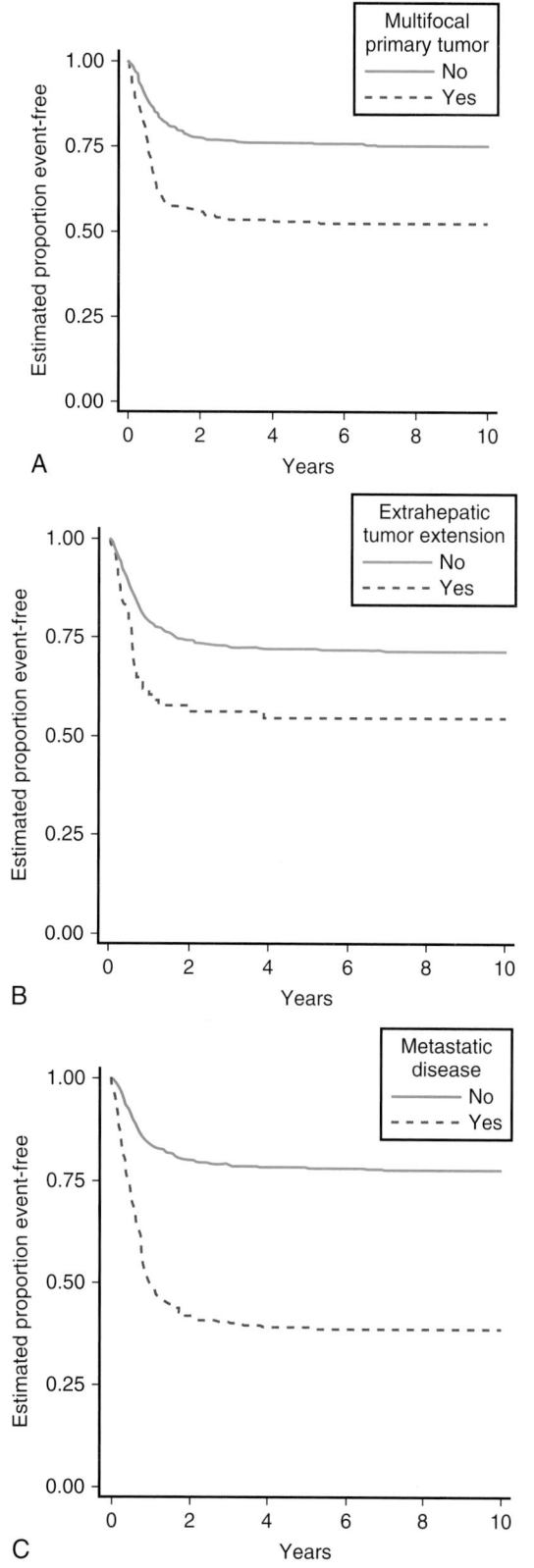

FIGURE 93.8 The impact of **(A)** multifocality, **(B)** extrahepatic extension, and **(C)** presence of distant (pulmonary) metastases on event-free survival in hepatoblastoma.

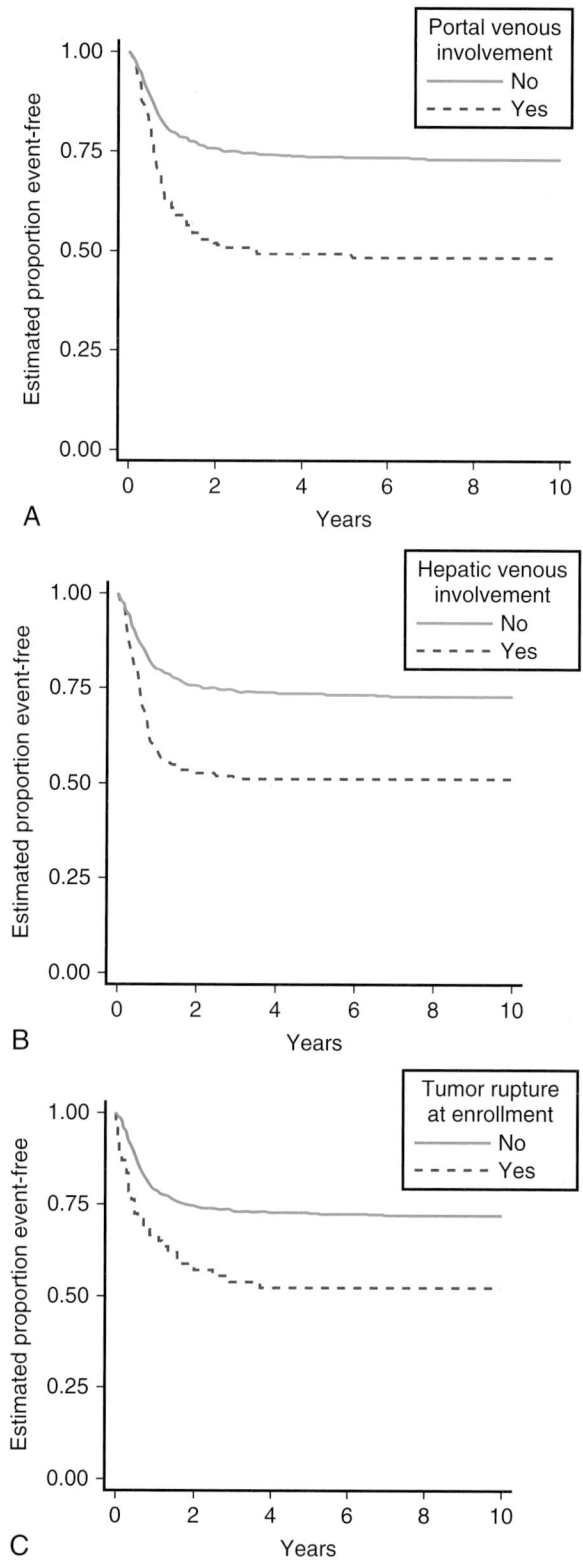

FIGURE 93.9 The impact of **(A)** portal or **(B)** hepatic vein involvement and **(C)** preoperative tumor rupture on event-free survival in hepatoblastoma.

removed successfully. Segmental resection is also feasible and may allow resection of multifocal lesions (see Chapters 102B and 118B).

Various novel treatments are currently under investigation. First, transcatheter selective arterial chemoembolization, which involves the direct injection of chemotherapeutic agents to the tumor, hypothetically decreases systemic toxicity (see Chapter 94). The average decrease in tumor size was 84% in one study,[155] and unresectable hepatoblastomas may become resectable with this intervention.[156] Doxorubicin, cisplatin, and fluorodeoxyuridine have been promising, because these agents have a high hepatic extraction; case reports exist with striking results. For example, Yokomori et al.[157] describe the total regression of a tumor in a 4-month-old infant with fetal hepatoblastoma treated for 1.5 years with 5-FU, vincristine, doxorubicin, and cisplatin. No recurrence was seen after 6 years of follow-up. Risks involved with this technique include infection, thrombosis, or shifting of the catheter. Furthermore, it is challenging to carry out in children, and prospective studies are needed. Other new approaches include treatment with anti-AFP antibodies, IL-2, and viral transfection vectors to attack malignant hepatic cells.[158–161]

Hepatocellular Carcinoma (Hepatoma)

Epidemiology

Hepatocellular carcinoma (HCC) (see Chapter 89) accounts for 22% to 23% of pediatric liver tumors but is rare in infancy.[21,28] Approximately 1.2 cases per 1 million children exist in the United States.[21] The Lung Cancer Study Group of Japan reported no cases in children age 4 years or younger in a series of 2286 patients with histologically reviewed tumors.[27] Historic series without pathology review may report a higher rate of infantile HCC owing to misdiagnosis of some early hepatoblastomas.[10] A 2014 query of the SEER database, with data spanning from 1973 to 2009, reported 218 HCC patients diagnosed before 20 years of age. Of these, 9% were younger than 5 years at diagnosis, and nearly half of that group was in the first year of life. Sixteen percent of tumors were diagnosed in children from 5 to 9 years of age, 27% in children from 10 to 14 years of age, and 48% from 15 to 19 years of age.[162] We have had personal experience of infants with well-documented HCC, and it affects approximately 0.5 children younger than 15 years per 1 million annually. SEER data indicate that HCC accounts for 93% of primary hepatic malignancies in the 15- to 19-year-old age group.[21] The incidence is bimodal, with an early peak that is lower than that of hepatoblastoma. Most of these early cases occur before 5 years of age. A second peak occurs between 13 and 15 years of age. HCC has a male predominance (1.3 to 3.2:1), and in areas endemic for hepatitis B, the male/female ratio may be reversed, at 0.2:1. Approximately 35 to 40 new HCCs are diagnosed per year in the pediatric age group in the United States. Incidence reported for the years 1973 to 1977 versus 1993 to 1997 showed a decrease from 0.45 to 0.29 cases per 1 million.[25]

In contradistinction to HCC in adults, conditions associated with cirrhosis occur in only 30% to 40% of children with HCC; the remaining 60% to 70% of tumors are present without any cirrhosis.[163–168] However, there are certain known risk factors. Hepatitis B and C infection correlates with the incidence of HCC. In Asia, 85% of HCC patients, both adult and pediatric, are hepatitis B surface antigen positive, whereas this is found in only 10% to 25% of patients in the United States (see Chapter 68). The relative risk for the development of HCC is 250:1 for patients with chronic active hepatitis compared with patients without hepatitis surface antigen positivity.[123] Hepatitis C antibodies are found in 20% of patients with HCC. In one report, an infant with a history of neonatal hepatitis developed HCC.[169] A universal vaccination program against hepatitis B has reduced the incidence of HCC in Taiwan. The average annual incidence of HCC in children 6 to 14 years of age declined from 0.70 per 100,000 children in the years 1981 to 1986 to 0.36 in the years 1990 to 1994 ($P < .01$) coincident with widespread administration of the hepatitis B vaccine.[170] The mortality rate also decreased during this period. Antiviral therapy with lamivudine reduced the risk of development of HCC in patients with chronic hepatitis B infection and cirrhosis or fibrosis.[171]

Other conditions associated with the development of HCC include cirrhosis, α_1-antitrypsin deficiency, tyrosinemia, aflatoxin ingestion, hemochromatosis, hepatic venous obstruction, androgen and estrogen exposure, Alagille syndrome (arteriohepatic dysplasia), Thorotrast administration, progressive familial intrahepatic cholestasis, glycogen storage disorders, and congenital portosystemic shunts[172,173] (see Chapter 89). One case of childhood HCC developing in a patient with neurofibromatosis has also been reported.[174]

In one comparative study of pediatric HCC and hepatoblastoma, numerous discriminating features were reported.[175] The mean age at presentation was 18 months for hepatoblastoma versus 10 years for HCC. The initial resectability of HCC was 45% and did not improve with chemotherapy, whereas 91% of hepatoblastomas could be completely resected before or after chemotherapy. Tumor rupture occurred in 36% of hepatoblastomas versus 9% of HCCs. Most important, the survival of patients with HCC was much worse, with an overall 5-year survival of only 24%.[162]

Pathology (see Chapter 87)

HCCs are highly invasive and often multicentric at diagnosis, with frequent hemorrhage and necrosis. Nuclear pleomorphism, nucleolar prominence, and the absence of extramedullary hematopoiesis are observed, and the cells are larger than normal hepatocytes. Low-grade HCCs may look similar to normal hepatocytes, especially if a limited amount of tissue is sampled. Invasiveness, and vascular invasion in particular, is a hallmark of these tumors. Extrahepatic dissemination to portal lymph nodes, lungs, and bones is frequent at diagnosis and strongly affects survival. HCCs naturally progress from capsular invasion to extracapsular extension, then vascular invasion, and finally to intrahepatic metastases.[176] A strong correlation has been found between intrahepatic metastases and portal vein thrombosis; this suggests that efferent tumor vessels anastomose to the portal, rather than hepatic veins, allowing intrahepatic spread and explaining the multicentricity that is a hallmark of HCC.

Biology and Molecular Biology

Most investigations into the basic biology of HCC involve the study of hepatitis B and its relationship to carcinogenesis.[177] In one in vivo model in which rats developed HCC after prolonged feeding with glyceryl trinitrate, *KRAS* point mutations were identified in 8 of 18 animals that developed tumors,[178] and no *TP53* mutations were seen. Another model in mice engineered an inducible mutation in the *YAP* gene, which led to overexpression when the mice were fed doxycycline. These mice began to develop HCC nodules after 8 weeks of YAP overexpression.[179] Cytogenetic data indicate that chromosomal abnormalities are complex, and consistent patterns have historically been difficult to establish (see Chapters 9B and 9C).[180]

Clinical Findings

Children and adolescents with HCC are often seen initially with palpable abdominal masses (40%), but many are asymptomatic at diagnosis.[181] Pain is frequent (38%) and may occur in the absence of an obvious mass. Constitutional disturbances such as anorexia, malaise, nausea and vomiting, and significant weight loss occur with greater frequency. Jaundice is an uncommon feature of either disease, but AFP is elevated in approximately 85% of patients, with most levels greater than 1000 ng/mL.[123] Although elevated, these levels are usually less than those measured in hepatoblastoma patients.

Staging

The PRETEXT staging system listed for hepatoblastoma is also used for HCC in childhood.

Treatment

For more than a quarter century, no significant progress has been made in treatment of the pediatric population with HCC.[165] This tumor remains extremely resistant to current chemotherapy agents, and long-term survival is impossible without complete resection. Because of a high incidence of multifocality within the liver, extrahepatic extension to regional lymph nodes, vascular invasion, and distant metastases, complete resection is often impossible. Infiltration with thrombosis of portal and hepatic venous branches is common, and even the vena cava may be involved. Furthermore, the cirrhosis found in a number of HCC livers may preclude an extensive resection. The first prospective SIOPEL study reported a 36% resectability rate among children with HCC.[182] Even with complete resection, however, the prognosis remains poor secondary to the high rate of recurrence; 5-year survival postresection is reported to be 40%.[162]

Historically, the same chemotherapy protocols used for hepatoblastoma were also applied to HCCs in childhood; however, HCC is rather unresponsive to chemotherapy overall, although cisplatin in particular has shown activity against it (see Chapter 99).[183] The addition of doxorubicin, as well as the VEGF and RAF kinase inhibitor sorafenib, has also shown a modest benefit.[184] The utility of external-beam radiation therapy is unclear; it can aid with temporary control of gross disease, but it has not been shown to reduce the risk of relapse in patients with residual disease after resection. Because of the poor survival of patients with HCC, present thinking is to apply new and innovative approaches to these cancers.

Unresectable HCCs can be palliated with embolization with or without added chemotherapeutic agents or radioisotopes (see Chapter 94).[185] Percutaneous intralesional injection of ethanol also has been of palliative benefit when lesions are small (see Chapter 96D).[186] Radiofrequency ablation (RFA) of these tumors, percutaneously or at laparoscopy/laparotomy, has been associated with tumor resolution and prolonged survival (see Chapter 96B).[187–190] Lin et al.[191] reported that RFA was superior

to ethanol injection in HCCs 4 cm or less in diameter. Moreover, preliminary research using metronomic chemotherapy and adjuvant antiangiogenic treatments is currently under way.[192–195]

Because standard therapies have proven unsuccessful, liver transplantation has been used more widely (see Chapters 105, 108, and 110). The Milan criteria used for adults have been extrapolated to children. They stipulate a single tumor no larger than 5 cm in diameter or as many as three tumors each 3 cm or less in diameter,[194] an absence of macroscopic portal vein invasions, and absence of extrahepatic disease; however, no current data support the efficacy of using the Milan criteria in this population. The UNOS database included information on 41 patients with HCC who received OLT from 1987 to 2006. The overall survival was 86%, 63%, and 58% for 1, 5, and 10 years, respectively. Analogous to hepatoblastoma, mortality was mainly secondary to recurrence, which occurred even more often than it did in hepatoblastoma (86% vs. 54%).[142] A more recent SEER study demonstrated a 5-year survival of 85% after transplant.[172]

Outcome

The overall survival from metastatic or unresectable HCC in childhood approaches zero, and it remains a therapeutic problem (Table 93.5). Occasionally, resection of localized lesions results in long-term survival. The most recent query of the SEER database reports a 5-year overall survival of 45% after successful resection; 42% of patients who underwent surgery were alive after 10 years, and 28% after 20 years.[162] The trend is to separate HCC from hepatoblastoma in clinical studies because of its greatly differing biologic behavior.

Fibrolamellar Variant

Fibrolamellar HCC (FLH) is a histologic variant of the disease first described in 1956. Due to a specific genetic finding, it is becoming clear that FLH is a distinct tumor from HCC that is virally determined or otherwise idiopathic. It is characterized microscopically by bands of collagen that are arranged in a layered, or lamellar, pattern (see Chapters 87 and 89).[196] It is relatively rare, with an age-adjusted incidence of 0.2 per 1 million, and for this reason, large series have been limited. However, a 2012 systematic review published in the *Journal of the American College of Surgeons* synthesized most of the published series, ranging back to 1980 and covering 575 patients.[197] FLH is notable for multiple clinical characteristics that distinguish it from nonfibrolamellar HCC. Typically seen in older children and young adults, the age at diagnosis has been reported as anywhere from 1 to 62 years of age, with an overall median of 21 years. It is exceedingly rare in patients younger than 5 years. Unlike standard HCC, it is equally prevalent in males and females, and only 3% of patients have cirrhotic livers. Furthermore, on multivariate analysis, male gender has been shown to fare better, an observation not seen in standard HCC. At 5 and 10 years, overall survival in males was significantly better than in females, with a hazard ratio of 0.33.[162] FLH has been described as having a lower mitotic index and following a more indolent course compared with standard HCC, and it was once thought to be associated with a better long-term prognosis[198]; however, studies indicate that when stage is controlled for, the survival is similar between standard HCC and its fibrolamellar variant.[199] The tendency of FLH to grow slowly, as a single mass, compared with the early multifocality of standard HCC,

TABLE 93.5   Comparison of Resectability and Survival for Hepatoblastoma and Hepatocellular Carcinoma in Childhood

REFERENCE	HEPATOBLASTOMA		HEPATOCELLULAR CARCINOMA	
	RESECTABILITY (%)	SURVIVAL (%)	RESECTABILITY (%)	SURVIVAL (%)
Exelby et al., 1975	60	35 overall; 60 in complete resection	34	13 overall; 35 in complete resection
Ehrlich et al., 1997	77	87	—	—
Stringer et al., 1995	90	67	—	—
Ni et al., 1991	—	—	9.8	10 at 1 years
Hata, 1990	—	42	—	—
Ortega et al., 1991	48	67	13	21
Douglass et al., 1993	77 (group III)	90% groups I and II; 67% group III	—	—
von Schweinitz et al., 1995a	89	73	—	—
Moore et al., 1997	—	—	33	16.6 at 5 years
Weitman et al., 1997	—	0 progression-free survival at 2 years	—	—
Lee & Ko, 1998	—	47% at 5 years	—	17 at 5 years
Chan et al., 2002	91	—	45	—
Tsai et al., 2004	—	55% at 3 years	—	0 at 3 years

may account for it being diagnosed more often at an early stage. Despite this, 10% of patients may come to medical attention with tumor rupture and a hemoperitoneum.[123]

Biologically, FLH has been noted to coincide with an elevated serum unsaturated vitamin B_{12} binding capacity, as well as elevated neurotensin levels.[197] In contrast to standard HCC, which can have an AFP greater than 100 ng/mL in as many as 85% of patients, AFP is elevated in FLH only 10% of the time.[197,199] One study performed on 15 patients with FLH found a translocation on chromosome 19, leading to a chimeric transcript that merged the activating region of heat-shock protein DNAJB1 with the functional region of protein kinase A, causing it to become hyperactive.[200] Protein kinase A affects many cellular pathways and has been implicated in several other cancers.[201] The translocation was present in 100% of tumor samples, compared with 0% in matched healthy liver controls derived from the same patients, suggesting it plays a role specific to the disease (Fig. 93.10).[200] More recently, four individuals without a DNAJB1-PRKACA fusion but with FLH were identified; three had Carney complex. All had evidence of inhibition of a PRKACA regulatory protein.[202]

Similar to standard HCC, chemotherapy has little efficacy in FLH, and resection offers the only chance of cure (see Chapter 99). FLH is staged using the same PRETEXT criteria as hepatoblastoma and HCC, and like both of these diseases, patients may be offered partial hepatic resection or transplant, depending on the extent of disease. To date, the Milan criteria have typically been applied; however, as with standard HCC, the generalizability of these criteria to the pediatric population is questionable. In contrast to standard HCC, patients with FLH generally have a higher resection rate of 60%, as well as a higher 5-year survival rate of 59% after resection, compared with 40% in standard HCC.[162,197] Even without resection, 20% of FLH patients are reported to be alive after 5 years, compared with 3% of standard HCC patients.

Future Directions

Gene therapy with viral vectors that attack dividing cells is being investigated. Hepatocytes rarely divide unless stimulated by liver resection. Viruses such as herpes attack dividing cells and can be molecularly manipulated to contain cytotoxic genes, and modified herpesvirus can be transfected efficiently into hepatoma cells.[203,204] One group has used an adenovirus vector to deliver murine endostatin to tumors in nude mice injected with HCC cells with a resultant reduction in tumor growth.[205] A number of workers are investigating selective inhibition of the DNAJB1-PRKACA fusion.

Rhabdomyosarcoma of the Extrahepatic Bile Ducts

Incidence

Although embryonal rhabdomyosarcoma of the extrahepatic bile ducts is extremely rare, it is the most frequently seen malignancy in the biliary tree of children.[206] Ten cases were reported in intergroup rhabdomyosarcoma studies I and II, constituting 0.8% of confirmed tumors in those studies.[207] Fewer than 100 cases have been reported since 1975.[208,209]

Pathology

Biliary rhabdomyosarcoma is categorized into five histopathologic subtypes: embryonal, alveolar, botryoid embryonal, spindle cell embryonal, and anaplastic (see Chapter 87). Most tumors are of the embryonal histopathologic subtype, which accounts for 60%. They often show botryoid characteristics similar to other rhabdomyosarcomas that arise in a hollow viscus. Immunohistochemistry and nuclear staining are informative for diagnosis of embryonal rhabdomyosarcoma, as well as desmin and muscle-specific actin.[208,210,211] Distant metastases develop in approximately 40% of patients, but mortality is most often due to the effects of local invasion, including biliary sepsis.[212] Long-term survival is considered to be 60% to 70% and is not dependent on resectability.[194] Rhabdomyosarcoma of the liver and the ampulla of Vater, but not involving the bile ducts, also has been reported but is very rare.[213]

Presentation

These tumors are usually diagnosed from 1 to 9 years of age, with an average age of 3 years, and are seen more frequently in males. The typical presentation includes intermittent jaundice (see Chapter 51) and may include loss of appetite and episodes of cholangitis (Charcot's triad) (see Chapter 43).[194,214]

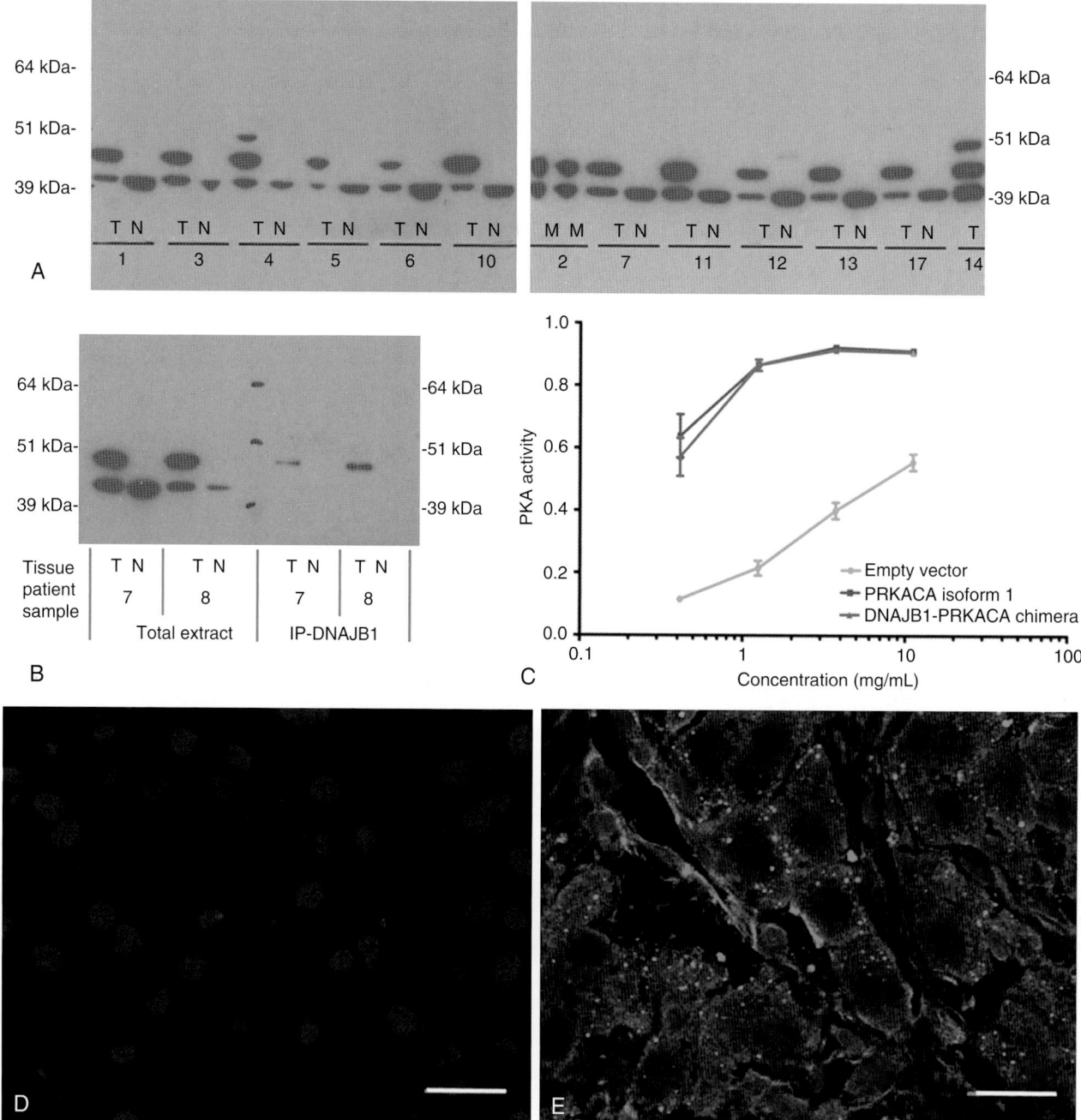

FIGURE 93.10   Tumor-specific expression of a protein consistent with the DNAJB1-PRKACA (heat-shock protein DNAJ–functional domain of protein kinase A [PKA]) chimera. **A,** Immunoblot analysis. Protein extracts of fibrolamellar carcinoma *(T)* and adjacent liver tissue *(N)* were separated by sodium dodecyl sulfate–polyacrylamide gel electrophoresis (SDS-PAGE) and subjected to immunoblot analysis using an antibody to the carboxyl terminus of PRKACA. This analysis revealed the presence of the native PRKACA in all tumors, metastasis and normal samples, and the presence of one additional, apparent higher molecular-weight band in all tumor samples (the predominant chimera). There is a second even higher molecular-weight band (the minority chimera) in the two tumor samples that had demonstrated a second set of RNA reads mapping between exon 2 of DNAJB1 and exon 2 of PRKACA (Patient 4, 14). **B,** Confirmation of chimeric protein. Protein extracts of fibrolamellar carcinoma *(T)* and adjacent liver tissue *(N)* were immunoprecipitated with an antibody to the amino terminus of DNAJB1 and run adjacent to total cell extract on SDS-PAGE. These samples were then subjected to immunoblot analysis using an antibody to the carboxyl terminus of PRKACA. **C,** PKA activity of wild type (WT) PRKACA and chimera are indistinguishable. HEK-293T cells were transfected with an empty control plasmid, a plasmid encoding WT PRKACA, or a plasmid encoding the chimeric DNAJB1-PRKACA. Cell extracts were diluted and assayed for PKA activity. The activity of the WT PRKACA and the chimera PRKACA-DNAJB1 are significantly higher ($P < .001$, two-way analysis of variance) than background kinase activity. Samples were processed in triplicate ± standard error of measurement. **D** and **E,** Immunofluorescence assay. The presence and distribution of PRKACA protein was examined with an antibody against the carboxyl terminus in **(D)** adjacent normal and **(E)** fibrolamellar hepatocellular carcinoma liver tissue from patient 11 and imaged by confocal microscopy. The green areas correspond to PRKACA, and the blue areas correspond to nuclei, which were stained with Hoechst. Scale bar is 20 microns. *IP,* Immunoprecipitation.

Hepatomegaly and a palpable abdominal mass are commonly observed.[212,215] The diagnosis may be confused with hepatitis, with resultant delay in specific therapy, but rhabdomyosarcoma of the bile ducts can also be mistaken for a choledochal cyst (see Chapter 46).[216]

Imaging

Ultrasonography (US) shows a hilar or intrahepatic mass that may be confused with a choledochal cyst (see Chapter 16).[217,218] Although CT or MRI (see Chapter 16) may provide information about extension and metastases,[219] they do not establish the diagnosis. Imaging may be more accurate for extrahepatic ductal involvement.[220] Cholangiography may also be useful, both for mapping disease and anatomic variants. An endoscopic, laparoscopic, or percutaneous transhepatic approach may be taken.[221]

Treatment

Surgical exploration and biopsy are necessary to establish the diagnosis in most cases. Often, a hilar lymph node provides diagnostic material, but carefully sampling the primary tumor may be necessary. A core needle biopsy or aspiration cytology may be adequate for diagnosis, and entry into the bile ducts should be avoided if possible. Intraoperative US (see Chapter 24) is helpful in identifying the course of biliary structures. Initial complete resection before chemotherapy may be difficult or impossible because of the extensive nature of these tumors. Also, microscopic submucosal extension is common, and resection margins are often microscopically positive despite the normal appearance of the intrahepatic bile ducts.

It is probably better to first establish the diagnosis with a biopsy and then begin systemic chemotherapy, which reduces the tumor size and allows a cleaner resection at second-look surgery. During the initial biopsy, hilar and left gastric lymph node sampling is performed to determine whether these nodal echelons require added radiotherapy. In the series reported from the intergroup rhabdomyosarcoma study, 6 of the 10 patients underwent initial resection, but all had microscopic or minimal gross disease left behind.[207] The only 4 survivors were in this group; however, none of the 4 patients in whom resection was not attempted survived. In another report of 3 consecutive cases from a single institution, all patients presented with jaundice, cachexia, and abdominal mass.[206] The tumor arose in the common hepatic duct in 2 children and in the left hepatic duct in the third. The technical difficulty of prechemotherapy resection is illustrated by the fact that intrahepatic extension was noted in all, making complete resection impossible. Two of these patients were alive and disease free at 9 months and 14 years, respectively, whereas the third died as a result of progressive disease at 33 months. All received radiotherapy in addition to multiagent chemotherapy. Jaundice was not a late problem.

The need for aggressive surgical resection of biliary rhabdomyosarcomas was challenged in a report by Spunt et al.[222] They reported 25 patients with this diagnosis from intergroup rhabdomyosarcoma studies I to IV and noted that although only 29% of these patients underwent a gross total resection before or after multiagent chemotherapy, the overall 5-year survival rate was 78%. They concluded that surgery was important for diagnosis and staging but that it was not necessary for long-term survival with present chemotherapeutic agents. They also noted that the use of biliary drains in patients undergoing aggressive surgery was associated with a high rate of serious infections.

The surgical approach is bile duct resection and a Roux-en-Y hepaticojejunostomy (see Chapters 32 and 51). Intraoperative cholangiography is recommended to ensure adequate bile drainage. The 4 of these 10 patients who survived were alive and free of disease from 6 months to more than 6 years from diagnosis. Liver transplant has also been described for unresectable tumor, with 4-year disease-free survival.[223]

Future Directions

Presently, the need for radiation, or even surgical resection, has been questioned. In the future, some of these patients may be treated by chemotherapy alone after establishment of the diagnosis. If a complete radiologic response is documented after neoadjuvant chemotherapy, no further intervention except observation may be needed, although this requires further study. Embryonal rhabdomyosarcoma of the extrahepatic bile ducts is rare, is locally invasive, and requires multidisciplinary treatment. Initial biopsy followed by chemotherapy and resection at a second-look procedure is the standard course.

Embryonal Sarcoma

Incidence

Embryonal sarcoma, also known as malignant mesenchymoma or undifferentiated sarcoma in the older literature, is a rare primary hepatic neoplasm that occurs in older children. In one study, 2 cases were reported out of 1102 (0.2%) primary liver tumors analyzed.[224] Fewer than 200 cases have been reported in the literature.[225] The age at diagnosis ranges from 5 to 16 years.[226,227] Embryonal sarcoma constitutes 14% of malignant liver tumors occurring in children 6 to 10 years of age; however, many of the patients reported recently were older than 10 years.[83,225,228,229]

Pathology

Microscopically, these tumors appear as a pleomorphic or undifferentiated sarcoma, and areas of the liver may be entrapped (see Chapter 87). The cells are spindle or stellate shaped, without prominent nuclei or well-defined cell borders. Mitotic figures are also present within the tumor, and the cytoplasm and extracellular matrix contain eosinophilic granules.[230] Primitive mesenchymal cells with occasional small cysts and ducts lined with benign-appearing epithelium are sometimes present at the periphery.[231] Some reports have suggested that embryonal sarcoma of the liver may represent malignant degeneration of a mesenchymal hamartoma, and the two may be difficult to distinguish on diagnosis.[232–234]

Clinical Presentation

A right upper quadrant abdominal mass and pain are significant presenting symptoms, and fever also may be prominent. Gastrointestinal symptoms and lethargy may also be present.[230] Spontaneous rupture has been reported.[229]

Imaging

Embryonal sarcoma often appears hypodense (dark) on CT and has a bright peripheral fibrous pseudocapsule, as shown in Fig. 93.11. They can be very bulky tumors and sometimes are confused with cystic liver disease.[235,236] These tumors may have

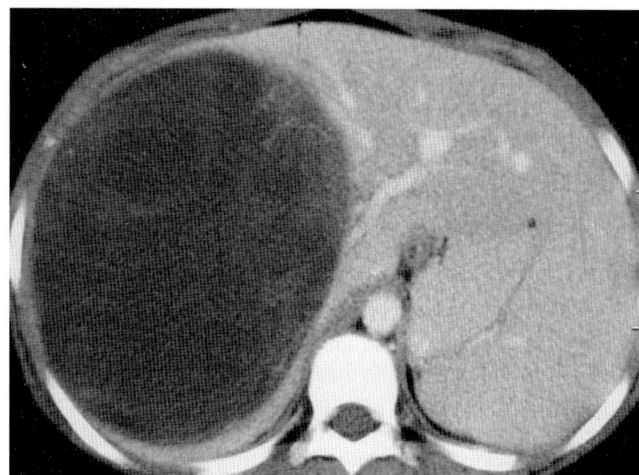

FIGURE 93.11 Computed tomographic image showing the radiologic characteristics of embryonal sarcoma (malignant mesenchymoma) (see Chapter 14).

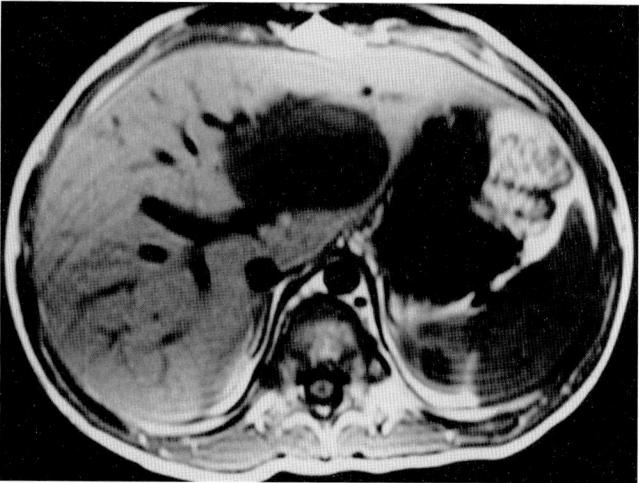

FIGURE 93.12 Leiomyosarcoma of the liver in a patient with acquired immunodeficiency syndrome (computed tomographic scan).

the appearance of a solitary liver cyst in childhood[237] or may mimic a hydatid cyst.[238]

Treatment and Outcome

Embryonal sarcomas of the liver are treated with resection, with or without neoadjuvant chemotherapy, followed by adjuvant chemotherapy.[239] Cisplatin, doxorubicin, cyclophosphamide, dacarbazine, actinomycin, vincristine, and other agents have been used in combination with radiotherapy.[226,227,230] Complete surgical resection should be attempted and usually requires a major hepatectomy for tumor clearance. Orthotopic transplantation has also shown success when clean margins cannot be obtained with a partial hepatectomy. Although past reports have cited a poor prognosis of 20% to 40% disease-free survival, two more recent single-institution series, each with five patients, have reported no recurrence of disease post-treatment, with follow-up ranging from 8 months to 16 years, with a median of 39 months.[225,228] A multi-institutional European study reported disease-free survival of 68% after a median follow-up of 136 months, and a 5-year overall survival of 72%.[240] Survival in this cohort was contingent on the ability to undergo at least an R_1 surgical resection. We have seen long-term survival with a combination of modern multiagent chemotherapy and complete resection.

Leiomyosarcoma

Patients with human immunodeficiency virus (HIV) infection and other immunodeficient patients experience an increasing incidence of smooth muscle tumors (see Chapter 87).[241–243] Although leiomyosarcoma may metastasize to the liver from other sites, primary hepatic leiomyosarcoma has been reported in less than 50 patients. It typically arises from the intrahepatic vascular structures, bile ducts, or ligamentum teres. Patients typically present with nonspecific abdominal pain or gastrointestinal symptoms. Cross-sectional imaging findings may vary. Biopsy will show intersecting bundles of spindle-shaped cells.[243] Adjuvant therapy has not shown significant efficacy; these tumors must be resected for control. They tend to be low grade or have an indeterminate malignant potential. Supportive and antiretroviral therapy is given through the perioperative period. A case of HIV-associated leiomyosarcoma is shown in Fig. 93.12.

Primary Hepatic Rhabdoid Tumor

Incidence

Rhabdoid tumors are very rare, highly malignant, sarcoma-like neoplasms that usually involve the kidney or central nervous system (see Chapter 87).[244] They can be primary in extrarenal sites, including the extremity, paraspinal, cervical soft tissues, and the liver.[245–247] In a literature review of 19 cases of primary hepatic rhabdoid tumor, the median patient age was 16.7 months, and 89% of patients were younger than 2 years. The overall mortality rate was 89%, and the median time to death was 15.3 weeks.[248] A more recent review identified 34 cases reported from 1970 to 2010, of which only 4 patients were alive at the time of publication (88% mortality). The patients who survived had a slightly older median age at diagnosis (12.5 months, compared with 8 months), and 3 of the 4 were female. Multivariate analysis was not possible due to the small sample size.[249]

Pathology

Histopathologic examination shows a high-grade round-cell neoplasm with abundant cytoplasm and containing cells with cytoplasmic filamentous inclusions.[250] The cells are frequently positive for vimentin and cytokeratins, and deletions at chromosome 22q11, often involving the tumor suppressor gene *INI1*, are often seen.[250,251]

Imaging

Rhabdoid tumors have no distinct radiologic features.

Clinical Presentation

The diagnosis may be suspected if widespread metastases, including central nervous system dissemination, are found with a hepatic mass. Cases with spontaneous rupture have been reported.[247,248,252,253]

Treatment

These tumors are highly resistant to treatment. Disease confined to the liver should be resected if possible. Treatment with dose-intense, antisarcoma-type chemotherapy is also warranted.[249]

Outcome

Although an initial period of control is feasible, these tumors are likely to recur and metastasize.

Angiosarcoma

Some authors describe angiosarcoma as the malignant form of hemangioendothelioma in children (see Chapter 87).[254,255] Arsenic exposure has been associated with malignant progression from hemangioendothelioma to hemangiosarcoma[254]; however, no clear association has been reported between angiosarcoma and arsenic, Thorotrast, or vinyl chloride.[256] Angiosarcoma is typically evidenced by a swiftly growing liver. Histologically, hypercellular whorls of spindled sarcoma cells are observed interspersed with bile ducts, blood vessels, and collagen. Intracellular periodic acid–Schiff–positive globules are present in most cases, and focal factor VIII staining may be seen.

Complete resection is required for cure of angiosarcoma, but recurrence rates are high, and the tumor is often not resectable; it is typically present in both lobes of the liver, and consideration should be given to adjuvant chemotherapy. Transplant has historically been rejected due to the rate of recurrence; however, there have been reported cases, with 1 patient still alive after 27 months.[257,258] Early metastasis, most commonly to the lung, is seen frequently.[22,254,259–261] One review stated an average survival of 16 months.[256] In another report of 10 cases of hepatic angiosarcoma in childhood, 6 patients were female and 4 were male.[261] The median age at diagnosis was 3.7 years (range, 1.5–7 years), with a mean follow-up of 10 months, and 6 of 7 patients with follow-up died from disease. A more recent, multi-institutional case series of 8 pediatric patients with hepatic angiosarcoma found evidence of either malignant transformation from, or concomitant development with, infantile hemangioma or hemangioendothelioma in 7 of 8 patients.[262] Two out of eight patients underwent orthotopic liver transplantation as a part of multimodal therapy, and these were the only two patients alive at the time of publication, disease-free at 3.5 years and 5.5 years, respectively.

Malignant Germ Cell Tumors

Primary malignant germ cell tumors of the liver are very rare and may present as teratomas, choriocarcinomas, or yolk sac tumors (see Chapter 87).[263] In childhood, these may respond well to neoadjuvant chemotherapy followed by resection. Usually, a regimen containing cisplatin, ifosfamide, and bleomycin is used. Case reports are exceedingly rare.

Primary Hepatic Non-Hodgkin's Lymphoma

Primary non-Hodgkin's lymphoma of the liver occurs in childhood and may comprise 5% of primary hepatic malignancies in this age group (see Chapter 87).[264] It is primarily a B-cell lymphoma.[265] Burkitt's lymphoma and other types of small-cell, noncleaved lymphoma have been reported.[266,267] One or many lesions may be involved.[268] The primary treatment of lymphoma in childhood is chemotherapy, which usually results in complete resolution of the hepatic mass. Resection is rarely, if ever, indicated but has been described for small tumors.[265]

Hepatic Metastases

The liver is a relatively frequent site of metastatic disease in childhood. Non-Hodgkin's lymphoma, neuroblastoma, rhabdomyosarcoma, rhabdoid tumors, Wilms tumor, desmoplastic small round-cell tumor, adrenal cortical carcinoma, osteogenic sarcomas, and a host of other malignancies may metastasize to the liver. Few data are available to determine the correct surgical approach to these lesions. Criteria for surgical removal of hepatic metastases include control of the primary site, a solitary or limited number of metastases, adequate hepatic reserve, good performance status, and a reasonable expectation of prolonged survival or cure. A helpful finding is some response of the metastatic lesions to adjuvant chemotherapy, and MRI is helpful in the diagnosis and evaluation of hepatic metastases.

We have had experience with 11 patients (age range, 4.3–21 years) who underwent hepatic metastasectomy. The overall survival in this group was 20%, but local hepatic control was greater than 85%. Advantages of hepatic metastasectomy include amelioration of liver function abnormalities, improvement of biliary obstruction, and possibly prolonged survival.[269]

Neuroblastoma

Hepatic metastases from neuroblastoma may be encountered in stage IV neuroblastoma and in newborns and infants with stage IV-S disease. In the latter situation, the liver involvement is a hallmark of the disease.[270] In stage IV-S, hepatic tumors generally resolve, although they may increase alarmingly in size before this happens. The increase in size usually causes pulmonary and vena caval impairment and may require relief by placement of an abdominal silo similar to that used for congenital abdominal wall defects. For stage IV disease, it may be advantageous for patients to undergo hepatic metastasectomy, which may aid in diminution of treatment or prolonged survival.[269] One patient with neuroblastoma and hepatic metastasectomy had disease-free survival with a follow-up time of 59 months.[269] A review of 17 neuroblastoma patients who had liver metastases at diagnosis, and who had survived disease free for at least 5 years, showed that very few of them had long-term liver damage, regardless of the treatment modalities they underwent.[271]

Wilms Tumor

Wilms tumor metastasizes to the liver in approximately 12% of patients,[272] and this usually is associated with unfavorable histology.[273,274] Resection of localized residual disease may be beneficial in well-selected cases. In one report, 15 cases of metastatic Wilms tumor with hepatic metastasectomy were analyzed and showed a 2-year survival of 62% and a 5-year survival of 44%.[275] In one report, 4 patients with Wilms tumors metastatic to the liver underwent hepatic resection with a 2-year survival of 80%, and 2 patients survived 14 and 17 years, respectively.[276] This experience is also noted in other reports of Wilms tumor.[277] However, experience with 3 patients did not show survival greater than 9 months.[269] One large study, which looked at 742 stage IV Wilms tumor patients, found that the presence of liver metastases did not portend a worse prognosis than metastases to other sites. It also concluded that patients did not benefit from hepatic metastasectomy as part of the primary treatment regimen but may benefit from resection of residual metastatic disease after adjuvant chemotherapy and/or radiotherapy.[278]

Osteogenic Sarcoma

Calcified hepatic metastases sometimes may be observed in patients with osteogenic sarcoma.[279] Although pulmonary metastasectomy for this disease is well described,[280–282] the role for hepatic metastasectomy has not been clarified. We reported a case of a child with osteogenic sarcoma with isolated liver metastases resected by a formal right lobectomy. This patient remained without disease for 2 years afterward and then developed recurrence in a limb, which required amputation. Hepatic metastases returned 46 months after this, and the patient died thereafter.[269] In one report of an adult with osteogenic sarcoma metastatic to the liver, the patient underwent radiofrequency thermal ablation, with stabilization of the hepatic lesions, but died 13 months later due to cachexia.[283] Case reports remain exceedingly rare.

Desmoplastic Small Round-Cell Tumor

Hepatic involvement with desmoplastic small round-cell tumor (DSRCT) is frequent and is usually associated with a fatal outcome.[284-286] We published a series of 157 DSRCT patients, of whom 54% had some type of liver lesion. The presence of liver involvement was associated with poorer survival on multivariate analysis, and therefore a scoring system was proposed whereby the presence of hepatic lesions would stratify DSRCT patients into a higher risk group.[287] The pattern of metastases is diffuse, leaving no spared segments that would allow resection, and complete resection is associated with a significant survival advantage in this disease.[288] Future strategies include chemoembolization and arterial infusion therapy. Hepatic radiation to a level of 3000 cGy is ineffective. Reports have shown some promise with radiofrequency ablation, as well as radioactive microspheres.[289,290]

Rhabdomyosarcoma

The liver follows regional lung, lymph nodes, and bone as a site of rhabdomyosarcoma metastases.[291] Resection of liver metastases is usually not feasible because of diffuse hepatic involvement and the presence of metastases in other sites.

Colon Cancer

Colon cancer can occur in childhood.[292] Approximately 50% of these patients have signet ring tumors. The pattern of spread is over peritoneal surfaces, rather than through the portal system, and hepatic metastases usually occur late despite massive peritoneal disease (see Chapter 90).

Malignant Peripheral Nerve Cell Tumor

Malignant peripheral nerve cell tumors are likely to metastasize to the liver in childhood and adolescence. The pattern of metastases is usually miliary, and the tumors do not respond well to chemotherapy.[293]

Adrenocortical Carcinoma

Adrenocortical carcinoma also may metastasize to the liver, although concomitant pulmonary and retroperitoneal metastases are usually also present.[294] Treatment is usually with platinum-based chemotherapy. There is some evidence in adults that hepatic metastasectomy can prolong life by a median of 11.5 months, but recurrence is near.[295] Transcatheter arterial chemoembolization has also shown some promise.[296]

Rhabdoid Tumor

Rhabdoid tumor most commonly originates from the kidney and can metastasize to liver.[250] It also may be primary to the liver, but this is rare. The pattern for hepatic metastases is usually diffuse and is not amenable to surgical resection. Chemotherapy protocols suitable for sarcoma are usually used.[244]

Hepatic Evaluation and Resection
Surgical Anatomy

The schema of hepatic anatomy most useful for the surgeon is based on the work of Couinaud; this is described in other chapters (see Chapter 2). The principles of hepatic resection in small children and infants are the same as those for adults (see Chapters 101 and 102).

Hepatic Regeneration

The liver in a child is able to regenerate quickly, even after massive resection (see Chapter 6) and administration of systemic chemotherapy.[297,298] In most patients, recovery to the normal volume for age is rapid (Fig. 93.13).

EVALUATION OF A CHILD WITH A HEPATIC MASS

Patients presenting with a suspected hepatic mass first undergo a thorough history and physical examination. Blood work

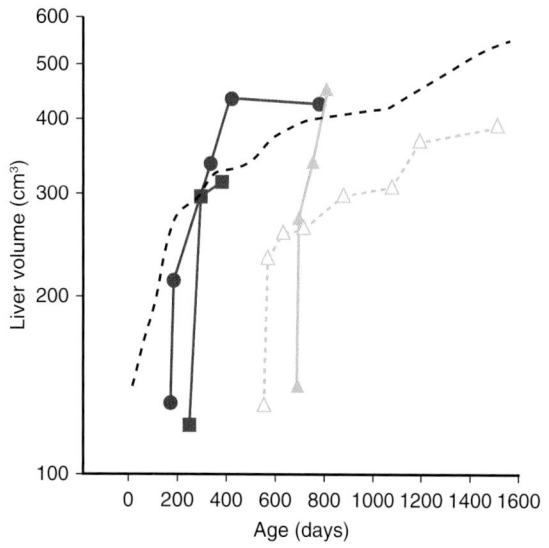
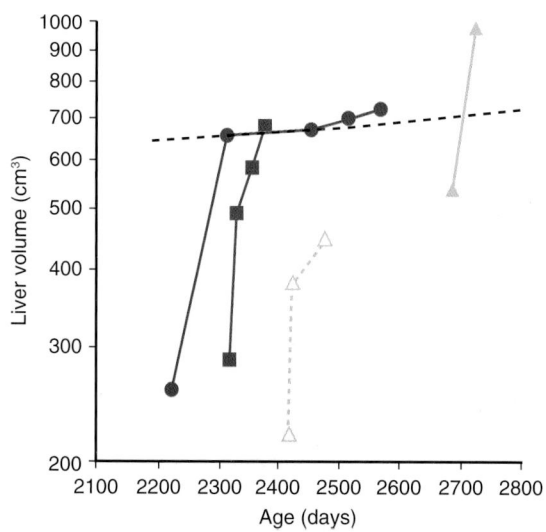

FIGURE 93.13 Graphs show the rapid recovery of hepatic volume to normal levels for age after major resections in childhood. The graphs show regeneration in two different age groups. (Used with permission from Wheatley JM et al. Liver regeneration in children after major hepatectomy for malignancy: Evaluation using a computer-aided technique of volume measurement. *J Surg Res.* 1996;61:183–189, 1996.)

should include a complete blood count, liver function tests, coagulation studies, and tumor markers that should include serum AFP and β-hCG. Doppler US is done to determine whether a mass is cystic or solid, determine the patency of the portal and hepatic veins and vena cava, and identify satellite lesions (see Chapter 14). At present, MRI provides the greatest amount of information concerning the lesion and surrounding veins and bile ducts, and CT portography has been shown to give anatomic information equal to MRI (see Chapter 14). If a malignant tumor is suspected, thoracic CT is done to identify metastases. A tissue diagnosis is mandatory if malignancy is suspected after the workup. Percutaneous needle core or aspiration biopsy is useful for hepatoblastomas but may not be definitive in the case of HCC; open or laparoscopic biopsy is acceptable if necessary. Before exploration, the surgeon must do a thorough diagnostic workup to determine resectability. Often, a team approach with a pediatric surgeon and an experienced hepatobiliary surgeon is helpful.

BENIGN HEPATIC TUMORS (SEE CHAPTERS 87 AND 88)

Benign hepatic tumors accounted for less than 35% of 1250 pediatric liver tumors in one study.[28] Benign tumors of the liver that occur in childhood include hemangiomata or vascular malformations, hepatocytic adenomas, focal nodular hyperplasia, mesenchymal hamartomas, and various types of cysts and cystic disease. The distribution of common benign hepatic tumors of childhood is illustrated in Fig. 93.14.

Hemangiomata and Vascular Malformations

Hemangiomata are lesions characterized by endothelial-lined vascular spaces that vary in size and extent.[299,300] They are sometimes classified as hamartomas and are the most common skin lesions observed in childhood. Hemangioendotheliomas are highly proliferative cellular lesions of variable malignant potential. In contrast, venous malformations and cavernous hemangiomata are distinguished by a lack of cellularity and large vascular spaces. Arteriovenous malformations are the

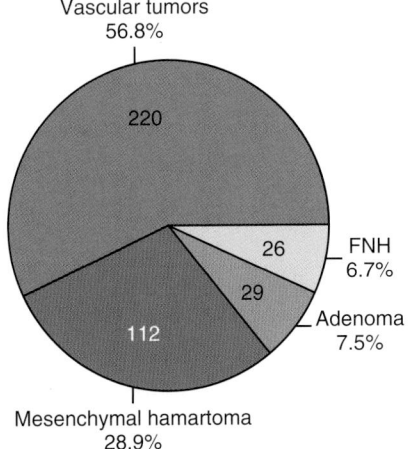

FIGURE 93.14 The frequency distribution of benign hepatic tumors in childhood.[10,22] This graph is based on surgical or pathologic series of patients. With modern imaging techniques, the frequency of asymptomatic vascular tumors discovered incidentally is undoubtedly much higher.[224] *FNH,* Focal nodular hyperplasia.

rarest pathologic subtype and are distinguished by abnormal anastomoses between arteries and veins. Venous malformations, cavernous hemangiomata, and arteriovenous malformations may be associated with significant shunting that results in congestive heart failure.

Incidence

The overall incidence of endothelial-lined vascular tumors of the liver in childhood is probably unknown because many are asymptomatic. Vascular lesions taken together represent 13% to 18% of symptomatic hepatic tumors in childhood.[10,28] Hepatic hemangiomata are more common in girls by 2:1.[301]

Presentation and Diagnosis

An abdominal mass is probably the most frequent sign of a vascular tumor of the liver. Multiple hemispheric, cutaneous hemangiomata may be present and warn the physician of possible visceral lesions. A systolic bruit sometimes can be heard over the enlarged liver. Infants with large, actively perfused vascular lesions may come to medical attention with congestive heart failure. Rarely, jaundice, disseminated intravascular coagulation (DIC), or hemorrhagic shock from intraperitoneal rupture may be present, and rupture can be precipitated by percutaneous needle biopsy.[302]

Imaging studies are usually all that is required to confirm the diagnosis. Tumor extent and tissue characterization are assessed using MRI with standard spin-echo T1-weighted and T2-weighted imaging.[303] Intravenous administration of gadopentetate dimeglumine (gadolinium) can produce greater resolution. Vascular lesions can be seen as intensely white on T2-weighted images, and this study is often accurate enough to be definitive. Contrast-enhanced CT scan will demonstrate a focus with decreased density, with contrast enhancement from the edges toward the middle of the tumor, which will then be homogeneously enhanced.[194] Arteriography is rarely indicated, given the detail and accuracy of modern imaging techniques, and open biopsy can result in massive hemorrhage.

Treatment

Asymptomatic lesions do not require treatment, and many hepatic hemangiomata regress after the first year of life. Patients with congestive heart failure are admitted to the intensive care unit and treated with digitalis and furosemide. Treatments designed to accelerate involution of the hemangioma in these cases have historically included steroids and vincristine. However, more recent evidence has suggested that propranolol, which was incidentally given in the treatment of heart failure, may reduce the tumor size with greater speed and efficacy, and fewer side effects, than previous therapies.[304] This was initially demonstrated in cutaneous hemangiomas but has since been shown to be applicable to hepatic lesions.[305]

If the heart failure remains refractory to these maneuvers, hepatic artery embolization or direct surgical ligation may be necessary.[306,307] Hepatic arterial embolization may be successful in controlling symptoms, but rapid development of collateral vessels can make subsequent resection or embolization difficult. Transfusion of blood and platelets may be required for DIC. Interferon-α (IFN-α) therapy for symptomatic angiomatosis and hemangioendothelioma is being used with success in individual patients.[308]

Patients who are seen in hemorrhagic shock with rupture of a vascular tumor usually require hepatic resection; however, initial hepatic arterial embolization may control bleeding temporarily and may allow stabilization and safer surgery (see Chapters 31 and 115).[309] In some patients, hepatic artery embolization could represent definitive treatment and obviate the need for surgery. Hepatic resection may also be required in some patients in association with congestive heart failure. Blood loss in these complicated procedures may be reduced using hemodilution techniques.[310,311]

Outcome

The overall prognosis for benign hepatic vascular lesions is good. Most patients do not require operative intervention, and most cellular lesions start to regress after the first year of life. Angiosarcomatous degeneration of benign hemangioendotheliomas has been reported in five patients from one institution.[22] Three of the five were treated with radiotherapy to the benign hemangioendotheliomas before the development of angiosarcoma. This and other reports from the literature have correlated radiotherapy of benign vascular tumors with subsequent malignant degeneration, usually to angiosarcoma.[312]

Hemangioendothelioma

The incidence of hemangioendothelioma is 1%, and it is the most prevalent hepatic vascular tumor in pediatric patients younger than 6 months (see Chapter 87).[313] In one report of 16 infants and children with hemangioendothelioma, 15 were seen initially with hepatomegaly, 7 with congestive heart failure, and 4 with associated cutaneous lesions.[314] Kasabach-Merritt syndrome (see Chapter 88A), a platelet-trapping coagulopathy, also has been observed.[315] This phenomenon can produce profound thrombocytopenia, with platelets as low as 6000, and fibrinogen can fall to less than 100 mg/dL. Transfusion of platelets does not reverse the process and may worsen symptoms while the platelets become sequestered in the tumor. However, the transient rise in platelet count may be sufficient for necessary surgical procedures. Otherwise, it is advised to treat patients based on symptoms, as opposed to laboratory values. Severely symptomatic patients may be treated with corticosteroids, IFN-α, vincristine, and other chemotherapeutic agents.[316] These lesions may appear very cellular, but they do not metastasize. If a primary lesion produces symptoms, resection is indicated for relief.

Hemangioblastoma

Hemangioblastoma of the liver usually is associated with von Hippel–Lindau disease.[317] In infancy and childhood, these lesions appear very cellular, but distant metastases are uncommon. Complete resection should be performed and is usually curative. Hemangioblastomas of the central nervous system and retina have been treated with IFN-α2a but without striking resolution, although two retinal lesions showed shrinkage.[318] Radiotherapy and chemotherapy are options for tumors not amenable to surgical resection (see Chapter 87).[319]

Mesenchymal Hamartoma

Mesenchymal hamartomas are usually solitary hepatic masses occurring in infants. They are usually multicystic, and the cysts are lined with flattened biliary epithelium or endothelium. Actively growing mesenchyme is abundant and associated with distended lymphatics. It is postulated that mesenchymal hamartomas arise in areas of focal intrahepatic biliary atresia; this results in distal bile duct obstruction and hepatocellular necrosis.[320] Others have hypothesized that these lesions arise in conjunction with anomalies of vascular development. This explains the occurrence of small hemangiomata observed in close proximity to mesenchymal hamartomas.[321] Cytogenetic analysis has only rarely been performed on these tumors, but a consistent 19q13.4 breakpoint has been identified (see Chapter 87).[322]

Epidemiology

Mesenchymal hamartomas account for 6% of primary liver tumors in childhood, and a male predominance is reported. In one study, 4 of 134 patients with space-occupying liver lesions had mesenchymal hamartomas.[323] Two-thirds of these tumors are diagnosed in infants younger than 1 year, although presentation in the teenage years has been described. In one study of 18 such tumors, the mean age at diagnosis was 16 months.[40]

Presentation and Diagnosis

Most mesenchymal hamartomas are seen as an enlarging abdominal mass or hepatomegaly and are usually not otherwise symptomatic,[321] but they can grow to great size and may cause respiratory distress or evidence of caval obstruction. Mesenchymal hamartomas are typically found within the right lobe of the liver. US, CT, and MRI are the most useful diagnostic studies, although an open biopsy is often necessary to make the diagnosis. Fig. 93.15 shows an MRI of a huge mesenchymal hamartoma. Giant hepatic cysts in fetuses also have been diagnosed on ultrasound.[324]

Treatment

Anatomic resection is effective treatment, especially for large lesions (see Chapters 101, 102, and 118). Because of the mesenchymal component, these lesions have a definite capsule that facilitates enucleation of large, central mesenchymal hamartomas not amenable to lobectomy. Enucleation was done in the case illustrated in Fig. 93.15. Occasionally, it is necessary to marsupialize a large cystic lesion, but only if it is not feasible to remove this lesion completely. This approach may not be successful.[325]

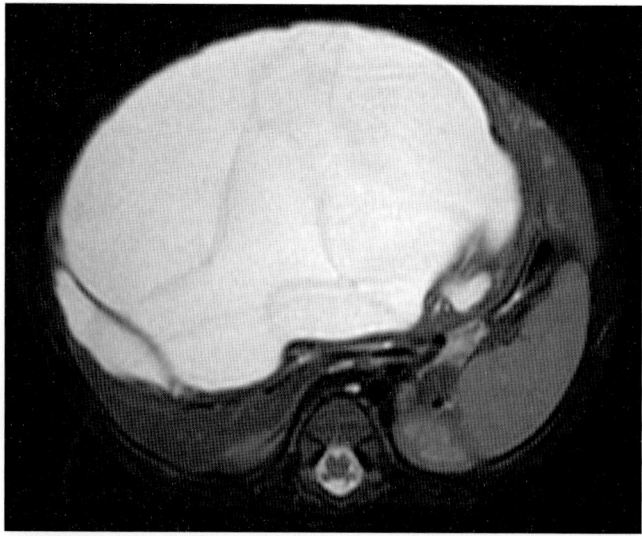

FIGURE 93.15 T2-weighted magnetic resonance image of a massive mesenchymal hamartoma (see Chapter 14).

One report using sequential CT scans documented initial expansion followed by involution of a mesenchymal hamartoma.[326] Because many reports exist describing spontaneous regression, the role of surgery is contested in the asymptomatic patient.[194,327] However, cases in which suspected mesenchymal hamartomas underwent malignant transformation to embryonal sarcomas have also been reported.[194] It has been postulated that in utero decompression of giant hepatic cysts would improve the outcome in these patients.[324]

Outcome

Patients with mesenchymal hamartomas do well with all forms of therapy. In one study of 18 patients, 13 who were available for follow-up were alive and well 1 month to 24 years after treatment (mean, 5 years).[40]

Focal Nodular Hyperplasia and Hepatocellular Adenoma

Focal nodular hyperplasia (FNH) and hepatocellular adenomas are benign hepatocellular proliferations that are more common in adults than in children (see Chapters 87 and 88A). Hepatic adenomas are expected with type I glycogen storage disease after the first decade of life and may be multiple.[328] FNH has also been described in a patient with type I glycogen storage disease.[329] Hepatic adenomas also have grown in patients undergoing androgen therapy for hematologic disorders, after danazol use, and in woman on oral contraceptives.[330] Both tumors have been correlated with a high-estrogen environment.[329] There has been some attention toward FNH developing in children treated for other solid malignancies.[331,332] These authors postulated that a vascular injury secondary to chemotherapy or radiation was the causal factor.

FNH is distinguished from adenoma by the presence of fibrous septa that contain bile ducts and an inflammatory infiltrate. In one report, 5 of 39 unresected hepatic adenomas developed HCC.[333]

Epidemiology

Less than 2% of hepatic tumors in childhood are FNH or hepatocellular adenomas.[22] Both lesions have been described in infants and teenagers. Most patients are younger than 5 years at presentation and predominantly female.[334] An association with contraceptive use has been found in adults, but no defined association between exogenous hormone administration in childhood and adolescence has been reported, although FNH has been reported in an infant antenatally exposed to corticosteroids.[335] In one report of 48 benign liver tumors in childhood, there were 3 cases (6%) of FNH and 2 cases of hepatocellular adenoma (4%).[299]

Presentation and Diagnosis

Patients with hepatocellular adenomas usually come to medical attention with an asymptomatic abdominal mass; they are more likely to be symptomatic and may present with rupture and resultant hemorrhage, causing an acute abdomen. Both FNH and adenoma are well encapsulated on imaging studies. Because FNH is associated with fibrous septa, abdominal US and CT may show a distinctive central "scar." Hepatic adenomas may show encapsulation on imaging studies, but histologic sections may be difficult to distinguish from HCC (see Chapter 14). In childhood, these tumors may attain great size, contributing to symptoms. In one report of six cases in childhood, the average tumor size was 7.5 cm (range, 2.5–10 cm).[336] The tumor was localized to the right lobe in four of the six and was bilobar in

the remaining two. Superparamagnetic oxide–enhanced MRI may discriminate between hepatic adenoma and FNH.[337]

Treatment

It is best to remove adenomas because of the difficulty of differentiating them from low-grade HCCs, uncertainty about future malignant degeneration, and the possibility of rupture and hemorrhage.[338] Resection also results in relief of preoperative symptoms.[339] An anatomic liver resection usually is required, and we have used extended left hepatectomy successfully in children to treat this lesion.[340] Laparoscopic resection of these lesions has also been done,[341,342] and percutaneous RFA has recently become an option for treatment.[343,344] Embolization of unresectable lesions is another alternative, if the masses are large or symptomatic. Unresectable and asymptomatic cases of FNH are observed using serial abdominal US, MRI, and clinical examination. Spontaneous regression has been documented, and patients with symptoms are typically treated with either surgical resection or ablation.[194]

Outcome

Most patients do well after hepatic resection, and in general, anatomic resection provides the best result. In one study of six patients with FNH and two with an adenoma, six were long-term survivors.[336] Three patients with FNH were alive 4 to 17 years after hepatic lobectomy, and two other patients were followed with observation alone and were alive and well 13 and 15 years later. The one death in this group was from leukemia, with an incidental finding of FNH. One of the two patients with an adenoma survived for 10.5 years after lobectomy, whereas the second died as a result of postoperative hemorrhage.

Cysts and Cystic Disease (See Chapters 73 and 90B)

Multiple cases of solitary, congenital, nonparasitic liver cysts in childhood have been reported.[345,346] They are extremely rare but have been increasingly noted as incidental findings on US and CT scans performed for other reasons. Cysts are simple and not multilocular; they often have a bluish appearance at laparotomy, and the wall usually has three layers. The lining is generally cuboidal or columnar, although mucinous or squamous epithelium is reported. The middle layer comprises vascular elements, and the outer layer comprises compressed hepatocytes, collagen, muscle fibers, and bile ducts.[347] The central contents are straw colored and clear and are not under high pressure, as is the case with parasitic cysts. Most of these cysts are located in the right, anteroinferior hepatic lobe (segment V), and occasionally they are pedunculated.

Most solitary cysts are asymptomatic and do not require therapy. Older patients sometimes complain of abdominal pain or sensations of fullness. Rarely, a large cyst ruptures; torsion of a pedunculated cyst has been reported, and 9% of solitary cysts may be associated with extrahepatic biliary obstruction and jaundice secondary to external bile duct compression by the cyst. These cysts do not affect longevity, although malignant degeneration has not been reported. This must be considered when planning therapy. Solitary, asymptomatic cysts do not require therapy. One single-institution study covering 67 cases over 20 years reported symptomatic presentation in only 15%. The mean cyst diameter in the symptomatic group was 13.7 cm, compared with a mean diameter of only 2.1 cm in the asymptomatic group.[348] If the cyst is symptomatic or doubt persists about the diagnosis, simple percutaneous aspiration is usually followed by recurrence, but aspiration followed by injection with ethanol or other compounds (sclerotherapy) may also be an effective treatment.[349] More commonly, operative intervention is required.

Preoperative MRI or Doppler US (see Chapter 14) is necessary to determine proximity to the portal and hepatic veins. Cysts that are neither adherent nor in proximity to these vascular structures are excised. Hepatic lobectomy may be necessary for symptomatic cysts that adhere to major veins, and marsupialization is sometimes a viable alternative. Injection of contrast media into the cyst can rule out a rare communication with the biliary tract. Cysts discovered incidentally at laparotomy should be left alone when less than 5 cm in diameter, but aspiration of cysts that are from 5 to 10 cm in diameter should be performed to confirm the diagnosis. Aspiration is followed by excision of the cyst wall. For large cysts, especially if there has been previous inflammation or the cyst wall is near major venous or biliary branches, an anatomic liver resection is indicated.[350] This resection avoids unnecessary bleeding and risk of postoperative biliary fistula.

Adult-type polycystic disease involving the liver has been reported with right lobar replacement and sparing of the left hepatic lobe;[351] this was effectively treated by right hepatic lobectomy. Embryonal sarcoma of the liver sometimes can be confused with a solitary cyst,[237] and percutaneous needle aspiration and biopsy may be required to establish the diagnosis.

References are available at expertconsult.com.

SECTION II. Neoplastic

D. Treatment: Nonresectional

CHAPTER 94A

Hepatic artery embolization and chemoembolization of liver tumors

Aaron W. P. Maxwell and Constantinos T. Sofocleous

Hepatocellular carcinoma (HCC) is the most common primary liver cancer worldwide (see Chapter 89). Despite the widespread implementation of surveillance programs of high-risk populations, only 20% to 30% of HCC patients are candidates for potentially curative surgical treatment, including hepatic resection (see Chapter 101) and liver transplantation[1] (see Chapters 105 and 108) due to poor liver function, underlying portal hypertension, tumor extent, comorbidities, and other factors. Moreover, even among those patients who ultimately undergo surgical intervention, long-term disease recurrence remains common, with reported rates ranging from 50% to 70% within 5 years.[2] As a result—and in the absence of highly effective systemic therapies—transarterial liver-directed therapies have assumed a central role in the management of patients with malignant liver disease. Transarterial chemoembolization (TACE) has been the most commonly used intervention to achieve liver tumor control and prolong patient survival.[3] TACE should be distinguished from hepatic artery embolization (HAE), wherein embolic material is delivered without a chemotherapeutic agent, and hepatic arterial infusion (HAI) chemotherapy, which involves the administration of one or more intraarterial antineoplastic agents without an associated embolic component.

BASIC PRINCIPLES OF HEPATIC ARTERIAL EMBOLIZATION THERAPY

Blood Supply of Liver Tumors

The liver's unique dual blood supply provides the rationale for arterially directed therapies for liver malignancies (see Chapter 2). Under normal physiologic conditions, the portal vein is estimated to supply approximately 70% to 80% of the normal hepatic blood flow, with the hepatic artery contributing only a minority to parenchymal perfusion. Liver tumors, however, invert this normal arteriovenous ratio and preferentially parasitize hepatic arterial inflow as the dominant source of perfusion, deriving up to 90% to 100% of flow from the hepatic arterial circulation. Directed endovascular occlusion of tumoral arterioles within the liver, therefore, may selectively induce ischemia within the tumor microenvironment while sparing nontumorous liver parenchyma

supplied primarily by the portal vein. Similarly, directed intraarterial chemotherapy infusion leverages this principle to allow for significantly higher concentrations of drug delivery, with an estimated twofold to tenfold increase in the tumor for chemotherapeutic agents such as doxorubicin, cisplatin, mitomycin C, and 5-fluorouracil (5-FU) when compared with conventional systemic intravenous administration methods.[4]

These vascular relationships are not without exception, however, as hepatocarcinogenesis is a complex and multistep process associated with differential arterialization of tumoral blood supply[5] according to the stage of the tumor development (see Chapters 9B and 9C). Whereas encapsulated nodular HCC, for example, commonly demonstrates near-complete supply via the hepatic artery, well-differentiated HCC as well as the extracapsular infiltrating edge of advanced HCC can be supplied all or in part by the portal vein.[6] Similar observations have been made with liver metastases, wherein small lesions—generally less than 200 μm—are supplied almost exclusively by sinusoidal blood while larger lesions undergo progressive arterialization. However, even in an advanced stage, most liver metastases still have a discrete portal blood supply.[7] Accordingly, both early- and late-stage liver metastases may demonstrate a higher propensity toward incomplete response to any hepatic arterial embolization therapy due to differential perfusion from both arterial and portal venous sources.

Transarterial Chemoembolization

The theoretical goal of TACE is to combine the effects of targeted tumor ischemia by embolization with the antineoplastic effects of high-dose intraarterial chemotherapy. To date, there is no consensus on the optimal chemotherapeutic agent or dosing regimen, and the utility of incorporating any chemotherapeutic agent into intraarterial embolization therapy remains fundamentally unproven despite decades of research (see "Hepatic Artery Embolization" later in this chapter). Nevertheless TACE remains widely performed worldwide, and the most commonly used antineoplastic drug is doxorubicin, followed by cisplatin, epirubicin, mitoxantrone, and mitomycin C.[8] Using a traditional (or "conventional") approach to TACE, the chemotherapeutic drug is dissolved in water or a water-soluble contrast agent. The drug is then mixed with ethiodized oil and administered as a water-in-oil-type emulsion (Fig. 94A.1). The pharmacokinetics of the resultant chemotherapy-ethiodized oil emulsions depend substantially on their composition, with greater oil-to-aqueous phase ratios exhibiting superior physical stability and sustained drug release.[9]

When injected into the hepatic artery, ethiodized oil is preferentially accumulated in the tumor via mechanisms that are presently incompletely understood. When intratumoral sinusoids are fully occluded, additional instilled ethiodized oil may flow retrograde into the portal vein via arterioportal communications.[7] This phenomenon allows for transient dual (arterial and portal) embolization of HCC, which may be clinically relevant when attempting to treat extracapsular infiltrative tumors and satellite nodules that are perfused via portal venules (Fig. 94A.2). Once accumulated in tumor vasculature, prolonged retention of ethiodized oil is commonly observed, which may reflect the absence of lymphatics and Kupfer cells within the tumor microenvironment. In contrast, in the normal liver parenchyma, ethiodized oil is nonocclusive and accumulates in the terminal portal venules by way of the peribiliary plexus, passing into the systemic circulation via hepatic sinusoids.[10]

After infusion of the ethiodized oil emulsion during conventional TACE, distal tumor-feeding hepatic arteries and arterioles are embolized. Hepatic artery embolization induces tumoral ischemic necrosis and increases chemotherapeutic drug dwelling time in the tumor by slowing the rate of efflux from the hepatic circulation. Furthermore, ischemic damage by embolization potentiates absorption of chemotherapeutic drugs,

disrupting the function of transmembrane pumps in tumor cells.[11] Proximal arterial occlusion should be avoided as it is associated with the development of collateral pathways of intrahepatic and tumoral perfusion, thereby limiting treatment effects, and may preclude repeat sessions of embolization therapy.

Optimal treatment effects are achieved when the appropriate size of particle embolic is selected. Although distal small particle embolization is known to improve outcomes relative to proximal and large particle treatments, the administration of excessively small particle embolic (especially in tumors with shunts) may be associated with increased risk of toxicity, including hepatic parenchymal infarction, biliary necrosis, and arteriovenous shunting to the lungs or systemic circulation.[12]

Historically, gelatin sponge particles have been the most frequently used agent for embolization during TACE. These particles demonstrate a broad and heterogeneous distribution of sizes—some particles measuring up to 1000 μm and beyond—which generally yield a more proximal embolization. As a pseudo-temporary agent, complete or partial recanalization is known to occur following gelatin sponge embolization over the course of weeks to months. Gelatin sponge has not been associated with significant hepatic parenchymal injury among patients with good hepatic functional reserve,[13] presumably reflective of the larger particle size thereby precluding significant distal small vessel embolization.

Like gelatin sponge, polyvinyl alcohol (PVA) particles are also irregular in shape but have greater size calibration and

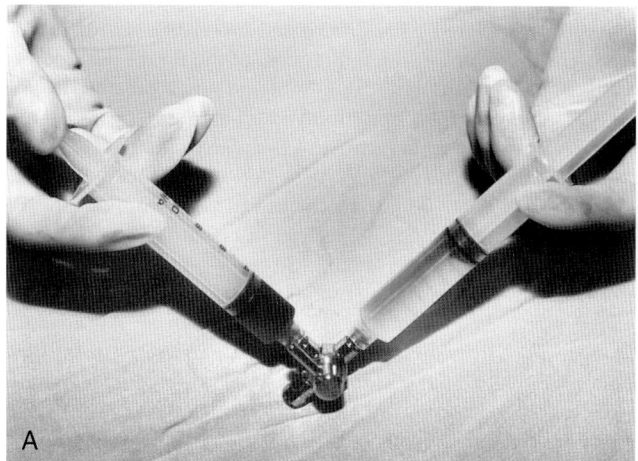
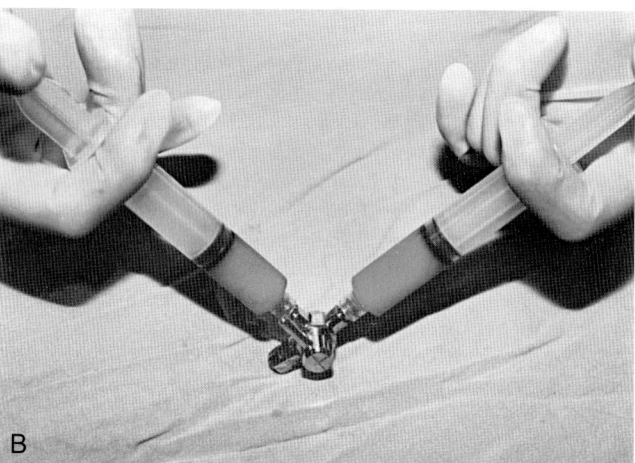

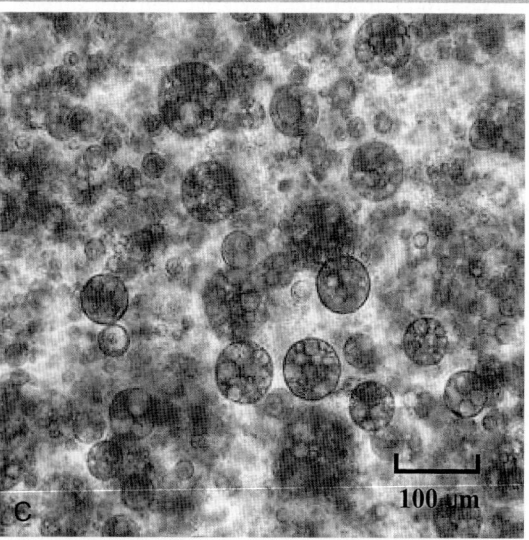

FIGURE 94A.1 Preparation of an emulsion of Lipiodol and doxorubicin hydrochloride. Every 10 mg of doxorubicin hydrochloride was dissolved in 0.5 mL of the water-soluble contrast medium. **A** and **B,** Lipiodol and dissolved doxorubicin hydrochloride were drawn separately into syringes interconnected with a three-way stopcock **(A)** and emulsified by means of vigorous pushing of each syringe alternately **(B). C,** Light photomicrograph shows the formation of oil-in-water–in-oil–type emulsion with variable-sized (10–50 μm) water droplets containing doxorubicin hydrochloride in the oil base.

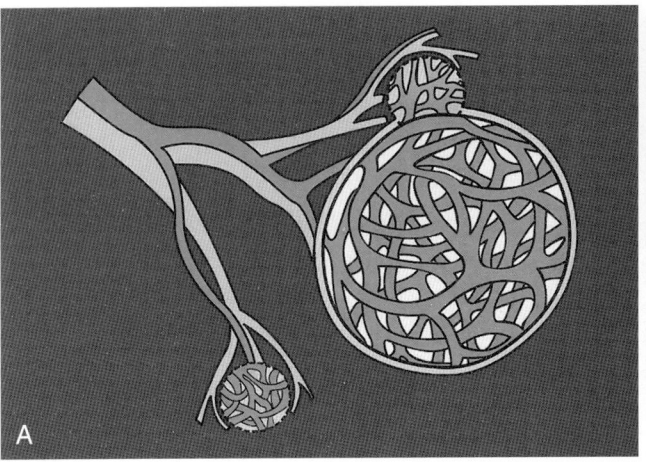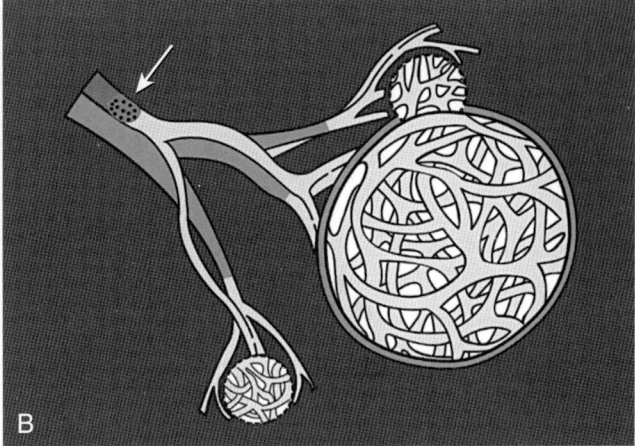

FIGURE 94A.2 The concept of subsegmental or segmental transarterial chemoembolization using Lipiodol. **A,** Exclusive arterial supply for encapsulated nodular hepatocellular carcinoma (HCC) and mixed arterial and portal venous supply for the portion of extracapsular invasion and small HCC without capsule formation. **B,** If a sufficient amount of an emulsion of Lipiodol and chemotherapeutic drug is injected through a tumor-feeding artery, not only the tumor neovasculature is filled with the emulsion but also the peripheral portal veins around the tumor are filled. Subsequent hepatic artery embolization *(arrow)* may result in the effect of combined arterial and portal blockage; tumor fraction with mixed arterial and portal venous supply can be treated effectively by the combined effect of high-dose chemotherapy and ischemia.

are more permanent in nature. PVA induces permanent or semipermanent arterial occlusion and can achieve more distal embolization because of the particles' smaller size (as low as 50–250 μm in diameter). The utilization of calibrated trisacryl gelatin microspheres has more recently come into favor, with the added advantage over other embolic agents of greater precision, in terms of both particle size distribution and particle shape. To date, however, no differences in patient outcomes have been demonstrated following treatment with TACE using different embolic materials, and thus the choice of agent remains largely a reflection of operator preference.

To prevent pulmonary and/or systemic particle embolization during TACE, attention should be paid to the presence or absence of significant arteriovenous and arterioportal shunts. Shunts are associated with larger tumors and may preclude safe administration of TACE therapy.[14] Among patients with significant shunting, large particle embolization is recommended before chemoembolic administration, which may be delayed for up to 1 month to allow for flow redistribution following shunt closure. In cases where particle embolization is not feasible or not effective, the use of sorafenib therapy has been described[15] as an adjunct method for shunt reduction. In rare cases, arterioportal shunt can be sufficiently large resulting in hepatofugal portal flow with ascites and variceal bleeding. In these patients, hepatopetal flow may be restored with shunt embolization, with consequent improved performance status and ascites.[16]

INDICATIONS

The most common indication of TACE is unresectable (and noneligible for ablation) HCC (see Chapter 89). The determination of resectability of HCC should be based on the extent of tumor involvement and underlying liver function. Most patients with HCC have baseline liver cirrhosis (see Chapter 74). Compared with patients without underlying liver disease, cirrhotic patients often require a larger liver remnant after surgery to maintain adequate liver function (see Chapter 102). Accordingly, significantly fewer patients with cirrhosis meet criteria for potentially curative resection when compared with noncirrhotic patients. Patients with poor liver function may not

tolerate extensive arterial embolization because their livers are more dependent on arterial blood supply than normal livers. Moreover, patients with severe cirrhosis are more likely to die of underlying liver disease than of HCC. Thus TACE is typically recommended in patients with reasonably preserved liver function (Child-Pugh class A or B7) and performance status (Eastern Cooperative Oncology Group [ECOG] score 0 or 1).

Several methods have been proposed to provide a clinical classification of HCC, including the French classification, the Cancer of the Liver Italian Program (CLIP), the Chinese University Prognostic index (CUPI), and the Japan Integrated Staging (JIS) staging systems (see Chapter 89). However, these staging systems for predicting prognosis of patients with HCC do not indicate which patients would benefit from TACE. In 2002 the Barcelona Clinic Liver Cancer (BCLC) staging system was developed and subsequently endorsed by both the European Association of the Study of the Liver (EASL) and the American Association of Study of Liver Diseases (AASLD).[17,18] According to the BCLC staging system, TACE is recommended as first-line therapy for intermediate-stage HCC, defined as multinodular disease without macroscopic vascular invasion or extrahepatic spread among patients with favorable performance status. However, less than 15% of the patients with HCC initially present with this stage,[19] and in clinical practice TACE is commonly also employed for patients with early-stage (although larger in size) HCC by BCLC criteria. Recent guidelines for HCC management reported that TACE is the most frequently used first treatment for HCC in Asia and North America.[20]

Spontaneous rupture of HCC is an indication for embolization-based intervention, regardless of underlying liver function (see Chapter 31). Even in patients with advanced liver cirrhosis, nodular HCC showing exophytic growth can be managed safely by selective embolization to prevent tumor rupture without deterioration of liver function.[21]

TACE with or without thermal ablation techniques may play a neoadjuvant role as a downstaging therapy before resection or as a bridge therapy for patients awaiting liver transplantation. Data are conflicting, however, with early reports demonstrating no improvement in overall survival following pretransplant TACE, as well as no change in transplant list dropout rates.[22]

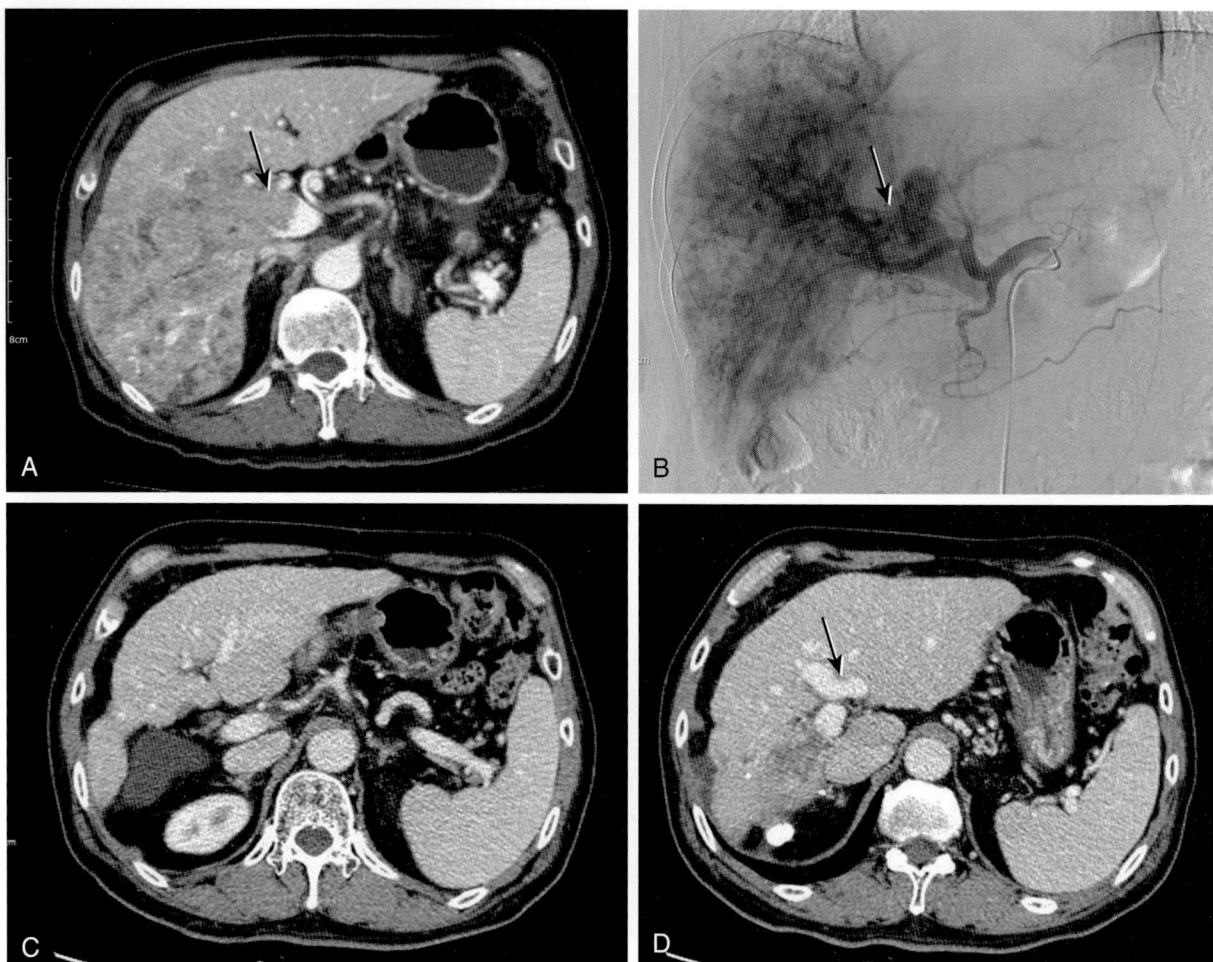

FIGURE 94A.3 Transarterial chemoembolization (TACE) for diffuse hepatocellular carcinoma (HCC) with main portal vein thrombosis in a 70-year-old man. Pre-TACE Child-Pugh score was A6 and serum α-fetoprotein (AFP) level was markedly increased (1298 ng/mL). **A,** Arterial phase computed tomography (CT) scan shows diffuse HCC involving right lobe of the liver extending into the main portal vein *(arrow)*. **B,** Celiac arteriogram shows diffuse hypervascular tumor in right lobe. Note extensive arterioportal shunt through intraportal tumor *(arrow)*. TACE was performed with an emulsion of 6 mL of Lipiodol and 30 mg of doxorubicin hydrochloride, followed by embolization of the right hepatic artery with polyvinyl alcohol (150–250 μm) and gelatin sponge particles. Hepatic artery infusion chemotherapy with cisplain (70 mg) was performed after embolization. **C** and **D,** Two-year follow-up CT after three sessions of TACE shows complete remission of diffuse HCC with recanalization of the main portal vein *(arrow)*. Liver function is still preserved (Child-Pugh score A5), and AFP level is normalized (4.5 ng/mL).

As methodologically sound prospective data are lacking to definitively guide decision making, the use of TACE for these indications remains unproven (see Chapters 101B and 108A).

Beyond primary hepatic malignancy, patients with metastatic liver disease may also benefit from TACE, including patients with neuroendocrine tumors (NETs) (see Chapter 91), gastrointestinal stromal tumors (GISTs), uveal melanoma (see Chapter 92), and other common pathology, including primary breast and lung cancers. The most common indications are rapid progression of liver tumor with stable or absent extrahepatic disease and symptoms related to tumor bulk or hormonal excess, especially among patients with NET. In addition, there has been growing interest in the application of liver-directed therapies such as TACE in the setting of liver-isolated or liver-dominant oligometastatic disease with the goal of generating a prolongation of chemotherapy-free survival.

Generally accepted contraindications to therapy with TACE include patients with decompensated cirrhosis (Child-Pugh B8 or higher) (see Chapter 4) and extensive tumor with massive replacement of both lobes of the liver. Major portal vein invasion has traditionally been considered a contraindication to TACE, but this can be safely and effectively managed by an adjustment of the embolization protocol to reduce the amount of chemoembolic agents and the extent of the embolization, especially in patients with a limited parenchymal tumor and adequate liver function[23,24] (Fig. 94A.3). In addition, active gastrointestinal bleeding, refractory ascites, extrahepatic spread, hepatic encephalopathy, biliary obstruction, documented history of severe allergic reaction to contrast media, and uncorrectable coagulopathy are also considered contraindications to TACE.

PROCEDURE

Before the TACE procedure, comprehensive laboratory testing should be performed, including complete blood cell count, prothrombin time with international normalized ratio, creatinine levels, and liver synthetic function assessment. Baseline tumor markers, where appropriate, should be measured to monitor for changes after treatment. Contrast-enhanced cross-sectional imaging of the liver (multiphase computed tomography [CT] or magnetic resonance imaging [MRI]) should be performed to evaluate the number, size, and segmental location of the tumors,[25] their growth pattern (expansible vs. replacing or infiltrating), and the presence or absence of macroscopic vascular invasion into the hepatic or portal venous systems. In addition, imaging of the chest, abdomen, and pelvis is recommended to document the presence or absence of metastatic disease. Patients are to remain nil per os overnight before the procedure and are kept hydrated with continuous intravenous infusion of crystalloid before, during, and following embolization. Antiemetics and narcotic analgesics are administered intravenously, and patients with documented contrast allergies may receive oral steroids and/or antihistamine therapy before the procedure.

The use of antibiotic prophylaxis before and after embolization has historically been recommended among patients undergoing hepatic embolization therapy, particularly among patients with a biliary enteric anastomosis or prior biliary instrumentation.[26–29] More recent literature suggests that, among patients with an intact sphincter of Oddi, the elimination of postprocedure antibiotics does not adversely affect outcomes among patients with primary and secondary liver tumors receiving embolization-based therapies.[30] This practice is supported in the most recent guidelines on antibiotic prophylaxis published by the Society of Interventional Radiology.[31]

After local administration of anesthetic solution, the Seldinger technique is used to gain access to the common femoral, radial, or other target artery, and initial diagnostic visceral arteriography is performed to determine arterial anatomy of the liver and patency of the portal vein. Anatomic variations of celiac trunk and hepatic arteries are frequently encountered, with common variants including the right hepatic artery arising from the superior mesenteric artery and the left hepatic artery arising from the left gastric artery. For complete angiography, all hepatic arteries should be adequately opacified by selecting an appropriate catheter as well as a corresponding rate and volume of contrast injection. All tumor-feeding arteries should be identified; selective segmental or subsegmental hepatic arteriograms with multiple oblique angles and magnifications are frequently necessary to identify small tumor-feeding arteries. In addition, cone beam computed tomography (CBCT) and CT arteriography have shown particular value in identifying tumoral vascular supply and are robust problem-solving tools for challenging

cases due to the ability to visualize tumor-vessel relationships as a volumetric rendering. Data from a systematic review and meta-analysis of CBCT performed during TACE for HCC demonstrated a sensitivity for tumor detection of 90% relative to 67% with conventional angiography.[32] Similarly, CBCT demonstrated a sensitivity for detection of tumor feeding arteries in 93% of cases compared with 55% using digital subtraction angiography alone.

The treatment protocol should be individualized according to the patient's liver function, extent of tumor, presence or absence of macroscopic vascular invasion, and the patient's baseline functional status. Every effort should be made to preserve nontumorous liver parenchyma from ischemia and cytotoxicity induced by embolization and chemotherapeutic administration, respectively. Selective or superselective administration of chemoembolic has been shown to provide the broadest safety margin, sparing uninvolved liver parenchyma while improving treatment outcomes from TACE, particularly when treating lesions with one or two vascular pedicles that can be targeted selectively.

After an appropriately sized microcatheter is positioned selectively into the tumor-feeding artery in close proximity to the tumor, the ethiodized oil-chemotherapy emulsion is injected. If significant arteriovenous shunting is present, large-particle (300–500 μm) embolization may be used to reduce the risk of passage of the chemoembolic emulsion into the systemic circulation. This can decrease the risks of complications such as oil pulmonary embolism, pneumonitis, paradoxic cerebral ischemia, or systemic toxicity from the distribution of the chemotherapeutic agent.

The amount of oil-chemotherapy emulsion to be injected depends on the size and vascularity of the tumor. The dose of doxorubicin typically ranges from 20 to 75 mg, with a maximum prescribed dose of 150 mg. The generally accepted upper limit of volume for ethiodized oil is 15 mL; however, safe administration of volumes up to or even exceeding 40 mL have been described in patients with large HCC tumor burden.[33] For a small- or medium-sized tumor, sufficient ethiodized oil is injected to saturate the tumor neovasculature and to partially opacify portal venules. The end points for the emulsion administration are stasis in tumor-feeding arteries and/or appearance of ethiodized oil in portal vein branches (Fig. 94A.4).

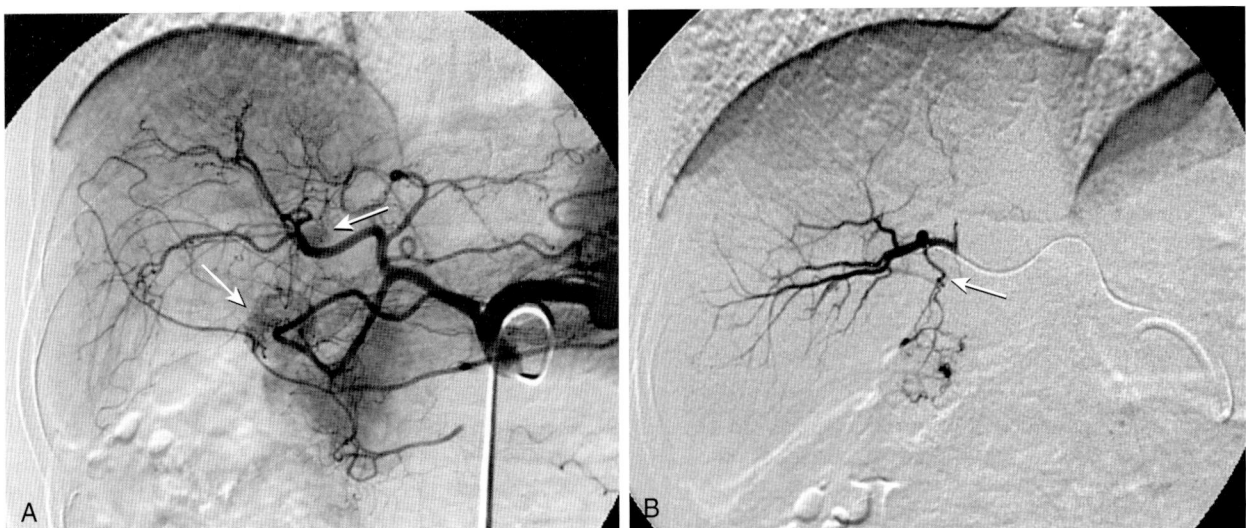

FIGURE 94A.4 Subsegmental transarterial chemoembolization (TACE) in a 43-year-old man with multinodular hepatocellular carcinoma. **A,** Celiac arteriogram shows two hypervascular tumor nodules (arrows) in the liver. **B,** The larger mass is supplied by a feeding artery (arrow) from the right posterior segmental branch.
Continued

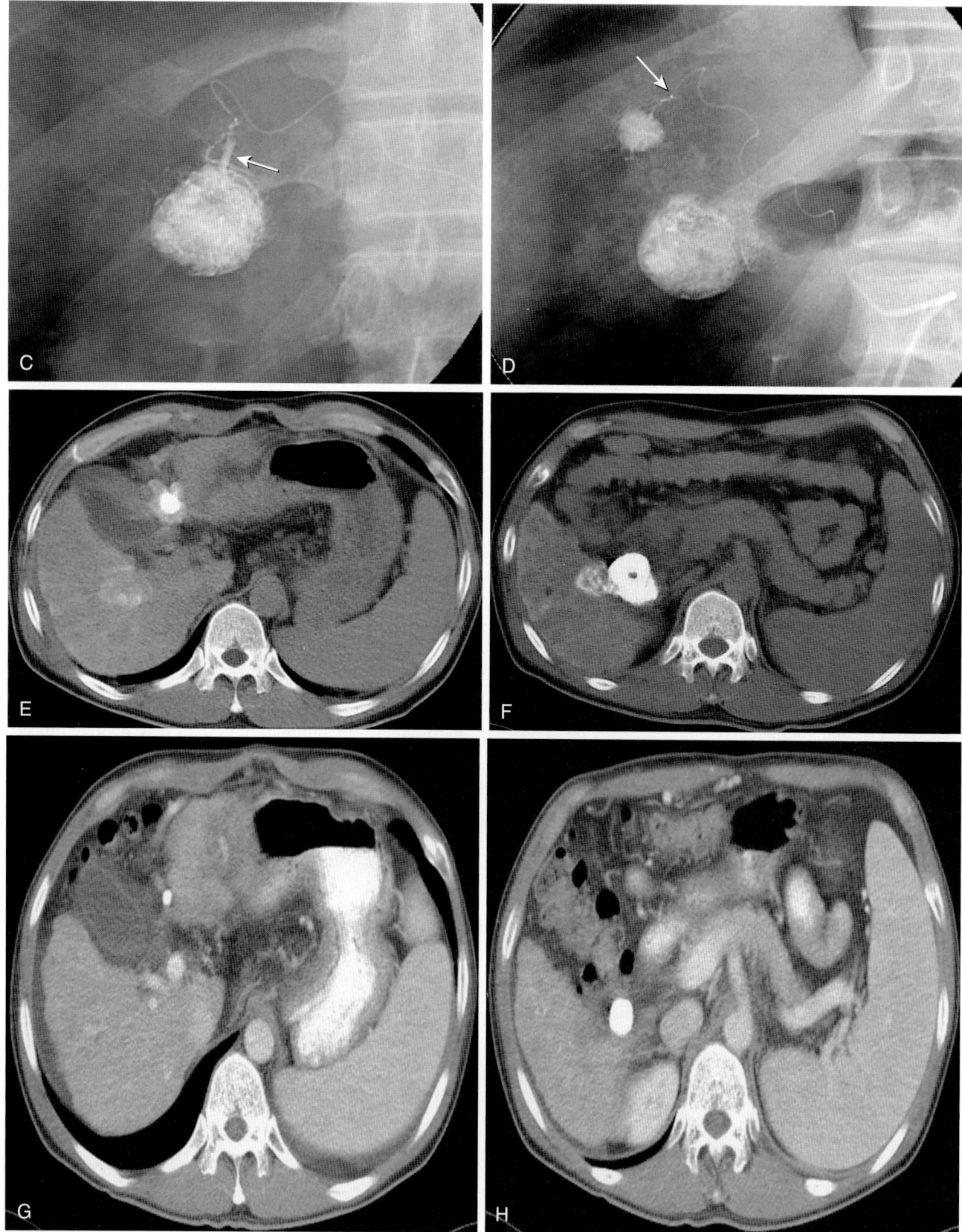

FIGURE 94A.4 cont'd   C, Subsegmental TACE was performed by selective catheterization of the tumor-feeding artery and injection of an emulsion of 5 mL of Lipiodol and 30 mg of doxorubicin hydrochloride. Embolization was not performed because sufficient stagnation of blood flow was achieved after injecting the emulsion. Note the filling with Lipiodol of the peripheral portal branch *(arrow)* accompanying the tumor-feeding artery. **D,** Subsegmental TACE was also performed for the tumor located in hepatic segment IV by selective catheterization of the tumor-feeding artery *(arrow)*. **E** and **F,** Noncontrast computed tomography (CT) reveals compact retention of Lipiodol in the nodules. **G** and **H,** Follow-up CT scan 2 years later shows shrunken tumors without evidence of any viable portion.

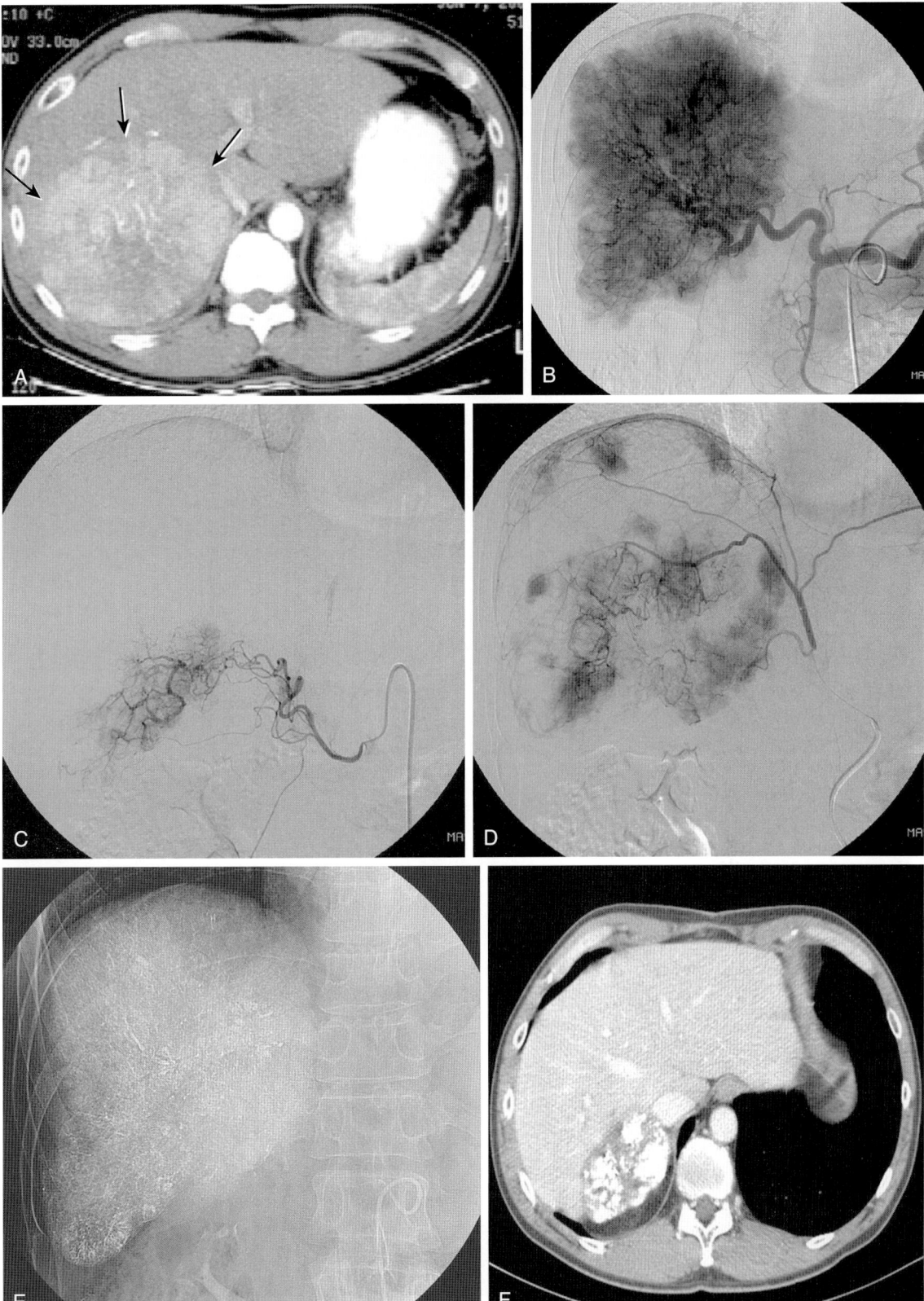

FIGURE 94A.5 A large hepatocellular carcinoma supplied by multiple extrahepatic collaterals in a 43-year-old man. **A,** Arterial phase computed tomography (CT) scan shows a huge hypervascular mass in the right hepatic lobe *(arrows)*. **B,** Celiac arteriogram shows a well-demarcated hypervascular mass with multinodular confluent appearance. **C** and **D,** Selective angiograms of the renal capsular artery **(C)** and the right inferior phrenic artery **(D)** also show multifocal tumor stain. Transarterial chemoembolization was performed with an emulsion of 20 mL of Lipiodol and 100 mg of doxorubicin hydrochloride, followed by embolization with a gelatin sponge at the right hepatic artery and extrahepatic collaterals. **E,** Postembolization plain radiograph shows diffuse uptake of Lipiodol in the tumor. **F,** Follow-up CT scan shows a markedly shrunken primary tumor with a thick capsule, persistent Lipiodol retention, and well-preserved, nontumorous hepatic parenchyma.

After infusion of the emulsion, tumor-feeding hepatic arteries are embolized with the use of gelatin sponge, PVA particles, or other embolic material.

Embolization of extrahepatic collaterals supplying the tumors is crucial to achieve successful outcomes. When a tumor is adjacent to a hepatic bare area or suspensory ligaments, for example, or it invades into an adjacent organ, a selective arteriogram of possible extrahepatic arteries should be obtained. With recent advances in imaging technology, collateral vessels can often be identified by thorough review of preprocedure CT data performed in the arterial phase. Common extrahepatic collaterals include the inferior phrenic artery, omental artery, internal mammary artery, colic branch of superior mesenteric artery, adrenal artery, intercostal artery, renal capsular artery, and gastric arteries[34-40] (Figs. 94A.5 and 94A.6). When the hepatic artery and extrahepatic collaterals supply the tumor, additional TACE or particle embolization of the extrahepatic collaterals should be performed—if deemed safe—in an effort to optimize therapeutic efficacy. These extrahepatic collaterals can also be used as an access route to the tumors in patients with hepatic artery occlusion, an event that can occur in patients who undergo multiple prior TACE or other intraarterial therapies.

Recently, the use of CBCT has assumed a central role in intraprocedural imaging. This technology can provide greater detail regarding relevant vascular anatomy and associated liver

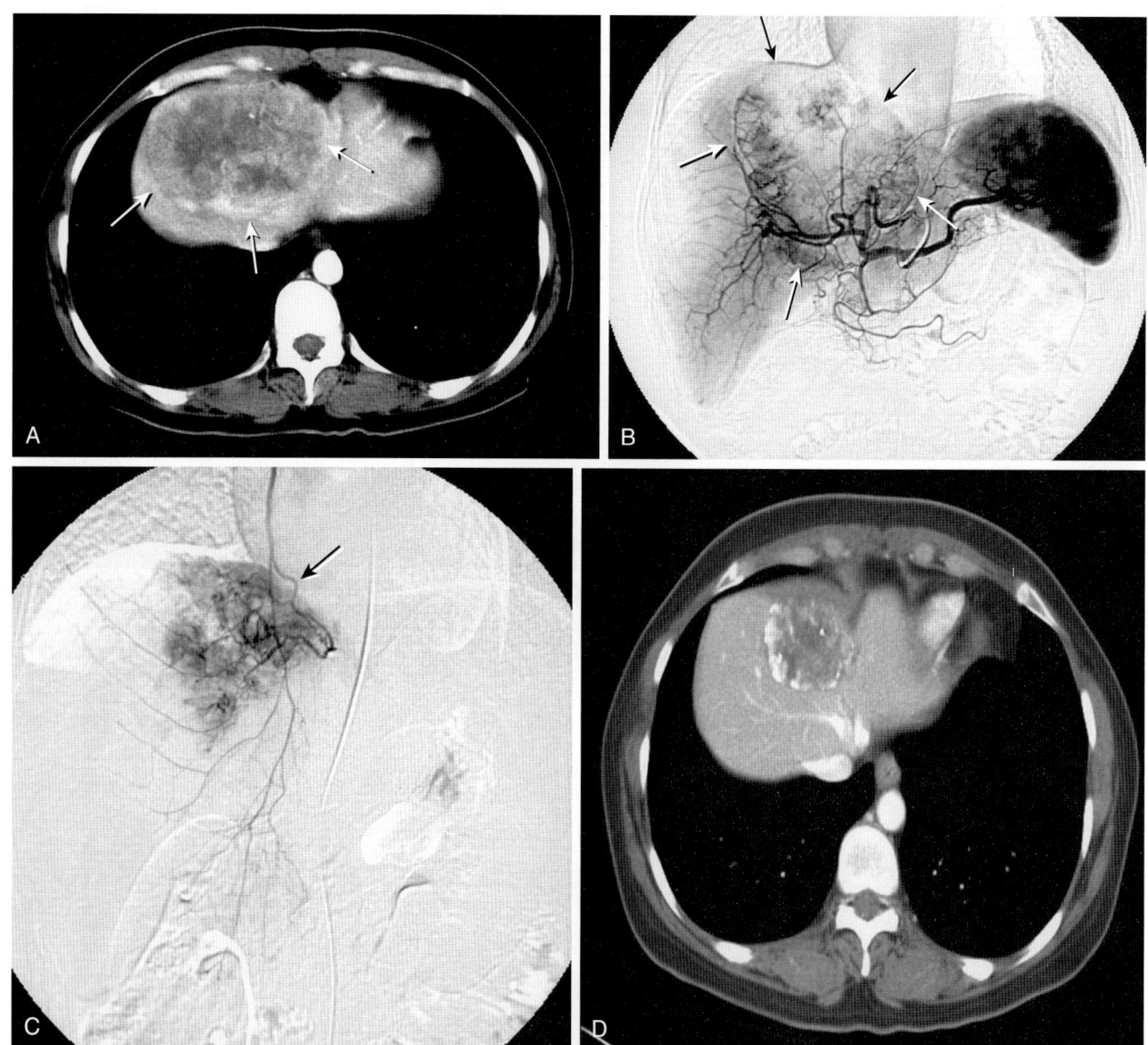

FIGURE 94A.6 Hepatocellular carcinoma supplied by the right internal mammary artery as an extrahepatic collateral at its initial presentation in a 34-year-old woman. **A,** Initial computed tomography (CT) scan shows a large tumor abutting the anterosuperior aspect of the diaphragm *(arrows).* **B,** Celiac arteriogram shows a large hypervascular mass occupying the medial segment of the left hepatic lobe and extending to the adjacent segments *(white arrows).* A defect in tumor stain appears at the superior aspect of the tumor *(black arrows),* suggesting the presence of an extrahepatic collateral supply. **C,** Right internal mammary arteriogram shows tumor stain at the area exactly matched with the defect in tumor stain on the celiac arteriogram. Transarterial chemoembolization was performed with an emulsion of 15 mL of Lipiodol and 50 mg of doxorubicin hydrochloride, followed by gelatin sponge embolization at the right hepatic artery and the diaphragmatic branch of the right internal mammary artery *(arrow).* **D,** Nine-year follow-up CT scans show a markedly shrunken tumor with no evidence of enhancing viable tumor.

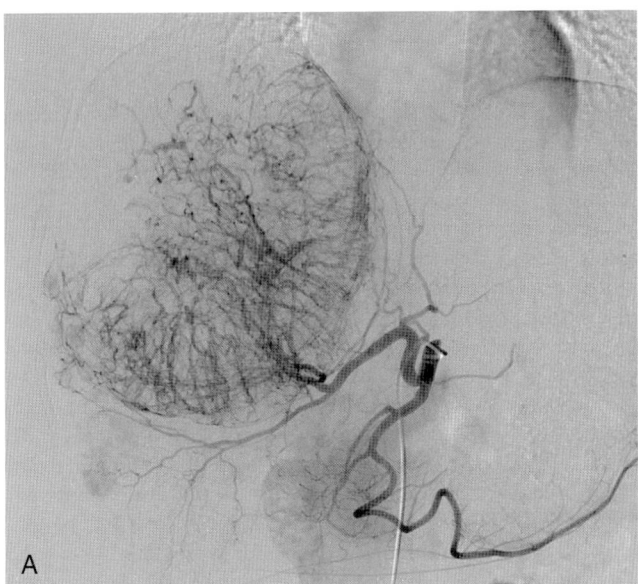 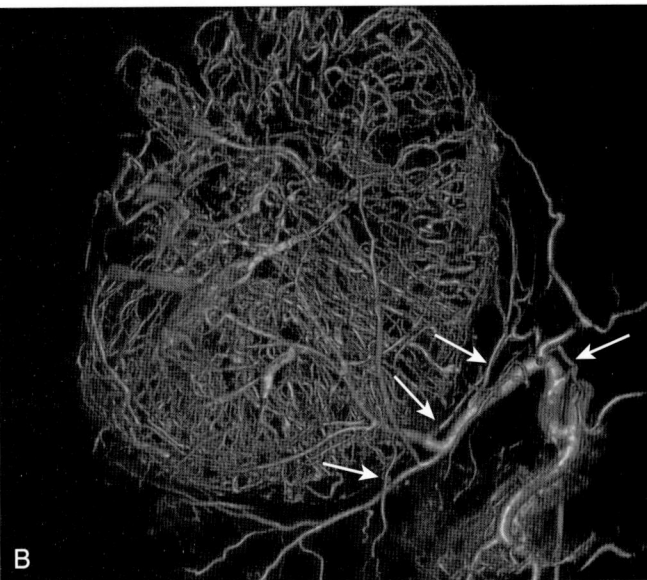

FIGURE 94A.7   Application of cone-beam computed tomography (CT) for transarterial chemoembolization of hepatocellular carcinoma in a 49-year-old man. **A,** Common hepatic arteriography shows a huge hypervascular mass in the right hepatic lobe supplied by multiple feeding vessels. **B,** Three-dimensional volume-rendered image from cone-beam CT clearly demonstrates tumor feeders, including multiple small central feeding vessels *(arrows)*. Real-time interactive anatomic information provided by cone-beam CT helps achieve successful superselective catheterization of tumor feeders and complete chemoembolization.

parenchyma beyond that provided by conventional digital-subtraction angiography (DSA) and fluoroscopy. CBCT allows the operator to recognize tumor-feeding vessels with greater confidence, which may in turn allow for more selective administration of chemoembolic material and thereby decrease the volume of nontumoral liver parenchyma within the treatment zone (Fig. 94A.7). Moreover, CBCT aids in the identification of important extrahepatic arteries, including the supraduodenal and retroduodenal arteries, right gastric artery, phrenic artery, and falciform artery, which may serve as sources of nontarget embolization.[41–43] The relative contribution of individual feeding arteries to tumoral perfusion may also be assessed using CBCT, allowing for more accurate apportionment of chemoembolic material during treatment. Last, as ethiodized oil is intrinsically radiodense, CBCT as well as CT (in hybrid rooms capable of both angiographic and diagnostic helical CT) can be performed following the TACE procedure without injection of additional iodinated contrast media, and the completeness of embolization can be assessed according to the percentage of tumor volume demonstrating retention of the administered oil emulsion. If incomplete coverage of the target lesion(s) is identified, additional angiographic imaging can then be performed before completion of the TACE procedure to identify other sources of hepatic or extrahepatic tumor supply that may require treatment.[44,45]

After the procedure, intravenous hydration is continued, and analgesic and antiemetic medications are supplied on an as-needed basis. Patients can be discharged once they have resumed adequate oral intake and intravenous analgesics are no longer required, which may occur on the day of the procedure or following a short inpatient hospital stay, typically 1 to 2 days in duration. Laboratory studies of liver function and tumor markers (where appropriate) should be repeated 2 to 4 weeks after the procedure. Multiphase contrast-enhanced CT or MRI is recommended every 2 to 3 months after the procedure to

evaluate the efficacy of the treatment and to detect local or distant tumor recurrences. When there is residual/recurrent tumor on follow-up imaging or elevation of tumor markers, patients may return for another session of TACE according to their hepatic functional recovery.

No consensus has been reached on the ideal protocol for repeat TACE, but the additional embolization is generally recommended only when progression of disease is documented radiographically ("on-demand" strategy).[46,47] Among patients without objective response after two treatments, additional TACE procedures should not be performed. Similarly, caution should be exercised in patients who develop clinical or functional deterioration (ECOG performance status greater than 2 or hepatic decompensation) after their initial TACE procedures.[2]

THERAPEUTIC EFFICACY OF CHEMOEMBOLIZATION

Hepatocellular Carcinoma (see Chapter 89)

Numerous studies have shown that TACE induces significant tumor necrosis without negative influence on liver function in selected patients with sufficient hepatic synthetic reserve. The extent of tumor necrosis has been reported to range from 60% to 100%, with higher rates reported among patients treated using selective or superselective chemoembolic administration. In comparison with lobar TACE, selective TACE led to significantly higher rates of mean necrosis (75.1% vs. 52.8%) and complete necrosis (53.8% vs. 29.8%).[48,49] Miyayama et al.[50] treated 123 HCCs smaller than 5 cm using a 2-Fr microcatheter and reported local recurrence rates of 25.6% and 34.7% at 1 year and 3 years, respectively. The rate of local recurrence was significantly lower when a greater degree of portal vein visualization was demonstrated during TACE. However, in large tumors, even though necrosis may appear macroscopically complete, histologic examination often reveals foci of residual viable tumor cells, which may reestablish vascularity and resume growth during the early or late follow-up interval, thereby accounting for the known high rates of recurrence after TACE therapy. Several studies have suggested that tumor characteristics lead to a favorable response after TACE, including small, encapsulated, expansile, hypervascular tumors.[51,52] Pathologically, trabecular-type HCC showed more prominent necrosis than scirrhous, compact, or well-differentiated HCC.[53-55]

The survival benefit associated with TACE has been demonstrated by two randomized controlled trials (RCTs). The first, performed in 2002, demonstrated significantly prolonged overall survival among 40 patients treated with TACE using gelatin sponge and doxorubicin when compared with 35 patients treated with conservative medical therapy alone.[56] This study was pivotal for the establishment of TACE as standard of care therapy of intermediate stage nonresectable HCC. The same study included a third arm—embolization alone using proximally administered gelatin sponge without the administration of intraarterial doxorubin or ethiodized oil—that enrolled 37 patients. Though widely cited as evidence of the superiority of TACE over embolization alone, the trial was ended prematurely following the ninth interim analysis after a survival benefit of TACE was demonstrated relative to the control arm that received medical therapy alone, whereas no survival benefit was demonstrated over those treated with embolization alone. Additionally, two patients within the embolization arm did not receive the embolization procedure but were included based on the intention-to-treat methods of the trial. Accordingly, no conclusions about the relative efficacy of TACE over embolization alone can be drawn from this trial.

A second trial—also published in 2002—compared standard medical therapy alone to TACE performed using gelatin sponge, ethiodized oil, and cisplatin among 80 patients with unresectable HCC evenly randomized between two treatment groups. Survival was significantly prolonged in the TACE group, though the rate of death from liver failure was also significantly increased.

As a result of these investigations, TACE became established as the standard of care for patients who meet the criteria for BCLC intermediate stage HCC. Llovet et al.[56,57] showed that median and 3-year survival rates were 19 to 20 months[57] and 29%,[56] respectively, in BCLC intermediate-stage patients. In 2010 a retrospective study[58] reported that the overall median time-to-progression (TTP) was 7.9 months, and median survivals of patients in stages A, B, and C of the BCLC staging system were 40.0, 17.4, and 6.3 months, respectively. However, TTP is not a validated surrogate for overall survival in hepatocellular carcinoma, and thus the significance of these latter findings is uncertain.

Geographic disparities in the utilization of TACE preclude direct comparison of outcomes in differing populations. The 4966 patients stratified to TACE recommended by the Japanese guidelines showed that 3-year survival of patients with two or three tumors greater than 3 cm or four or more tumors was 55% and 46% in Child-Pugh class A, respectively, and 30% and 22% in class B, respectively.[59] In a study from Japan and Korea, the 2-year survival rate of 99 patients with unresectable HCC was 75.0%. The median TTP was 7.8 months, and the median overall survival period was 3.1 years.[60]

TACE as a neoadjuvant therapy in candidates for hepatic resection is controversial. Several early studies reported a possible survival benefit in patients treated with TACE before resection of HCC when compared with resection alone.[61,62] However, in two subsequent randomized trials,[63,64] preoperative TACE did not improve surgical outcomes, including postoperative recurrence, disease-free survival rates, and overall survival rates. Moreover, the preoperative TACE group had a lower resection rate and longer operative time, thus evaporating enthusiasm for this therapeutic approach.

Liver transplantation (LT) is associated with the best prognosis among patients with early-stage HCC associated with underlying liver cirrhosis (see Chapter 115A). However, because of a steadily increasing waiting time, a substantial proportion of patients are excluded from LT secondary to tumor progression. The cumulative probability of dropout from the waiting list has been reported to range from 7% to 11% at 6 months up to 38% at 12 months following listing for LT.[65] The impact of TACE as a bridge therapy before LT is still uncertain due to absence of controlled studies comparing patients who underwent LT with and without neoadjuvant TACE. The most recent series, including patients treated with TACE before LT, have indicated that the dropout rate due to tumor progression may be lower and ranges between 3.0% and 9.3%, with a mean waiting time on the transplantation list exceeding 6 months.[66-68]

A recurrence rate of less than 15% has been reported in patients within the Milan criteria undergoing LT without preceding neoadjuvant therapies.[69,70] Whether receiving TACE while on the waiting list decreases this rate is still controversial. Two large studies reported low recurrence rates of 7.6% and 10.7% in patients who were treated with TACE before LT.[66,67] However, in a case-control study that included 100 patients who received pretransplant TACE and 100 control patients, pretransplant TACE was not an independent predictor of post-transplantation survival or disease-free survival.[71] More recently, Tsochatzis et al.[72] evaluated 150 consecutive patients and reported significantly lower HCC recurrence after LT in the TACE group (6%) than in the control group (18.1%). No prospective randomized trials have been performed to evaluate the effects of TACE on post-LT recurrence.

TACE has also be employed to downstage patients with advanced HCC and thereby expand selection criteria for LT. However, due to the wide heterogeneity of published techniques—including combination therapies—the true effect of this approach on patient outcomes remains unknown[73-75] (see Chapter 108A). Estimated rates of successful downstaging range from 24% to 71%, and the proportion of patients successfully transplanted ranges from 10% to 67%.[76] The reported survival rates range from 78.8% to 100% and from 54.6% to 93.8% at 3 and 5 years, respectively.[77] Two prospective studies have demonstrated that survival after LT in patients with large tumors successfully downstaged is similar to that of patients who initially met the criteria for LT.[78,79]

Neuroendocrine Tumors (see Chapter 91)

Gastroenteropancreatic neuroendocrine tumors (GEP-NETs) collectively represent the second most common gastrointestinal malignancies after colorectal cancer. The World Health Organization classifies GEP-NETs into grade 1 (G1), grade 2 (G2), and grade 3 (G3) carcinoma, formerly called carcinoid, well-differentiated, and poorly differentiated tumors, respectively.[80] GEP-NETs are metastatic at the time of initial diagnosis in 21%, 30%, and 50% for G1, G2, and G3 tumors, respectively, and may develop in up to 90% of patients over the course of their disease. Tumor grade and metastatic status represent the most important prognostic factors.[81] In general, G1 and G2 tumors are considered potential candidates for locoregional therapies, whereas G3 tumors generally are only candidates for systemic treatment due to rapid progression and widespread metastasis.[82] The development of liver metastasis may induce the systemic release of hormonal agents and invoke symptoms such as rash, hypertension, diarrhea, and electrolyte disorders; these are collectively known as *carcinoid syndrome*. In the later stages of the disease, significant hepatomegaly caused by bulky metastatic tumors may result in progressive pain and dyspnea, and the primary goal of hepatic embolization therapy is to reduce liver tumor burden and palliate symptoms.

TACE is one therapeutic locoregional therapeutic option for patients with liver metastases from GEP-NET. Symptomatic response is obtained in 52% to 86%; the response is even higher when TACE is used as a first-line therapy, with 70% complete symptomatic response and 20% partial response.[83] In a retrospective study by Hur et al.,[84] a median overall survival of 38.6 months was demonstrated (55 months for nonpancreatic NET and 27.6 months for pancreatic NET). In the absence of randomized trials evaluating locoregional therapies, no definitive answers to factors influencing outcomes of treatment can be provided. However, from retrospective series, outcomes are inversely related to the degree of liver replacement by tumor, and after embolization therapy, patients with nonpancreatic NET have significantly prolonged survival compared with patients with pancreatic NET. When employed early in the disease course, TACE is associated with favorable results—including symptom control—and published 5- and 10-year overall survival rates of 83% and 56%, respectively, when used in first-line therapy.[82,83]

High tumor burden—variably quoted as greater than 50% or 75% tumoral involvement—has previously been associated with poor outcomes.[85] In this high-risk population, embolization therapy should be performed in stages, typically as sequential lobar treatments (Fig. 94A.8). For small tumors and for patients with fewer than three tumors, hepatic embolization therapy can be combined with local ablation therapies to maximize tumor necrosis and improve local disease control. Before the introduction of pharmacologic antagonists of tumor metabolites, exacerbation of the symptoms of carcinoid or carcinoid crisis was common after embolization therapy. The increased availability of somatostatin analogs has resulted in a significant reduction of this complication after embolization therapy.

Despite these encouraging reports of success with TACE for treatment of metastatic NET, the potential for long-term

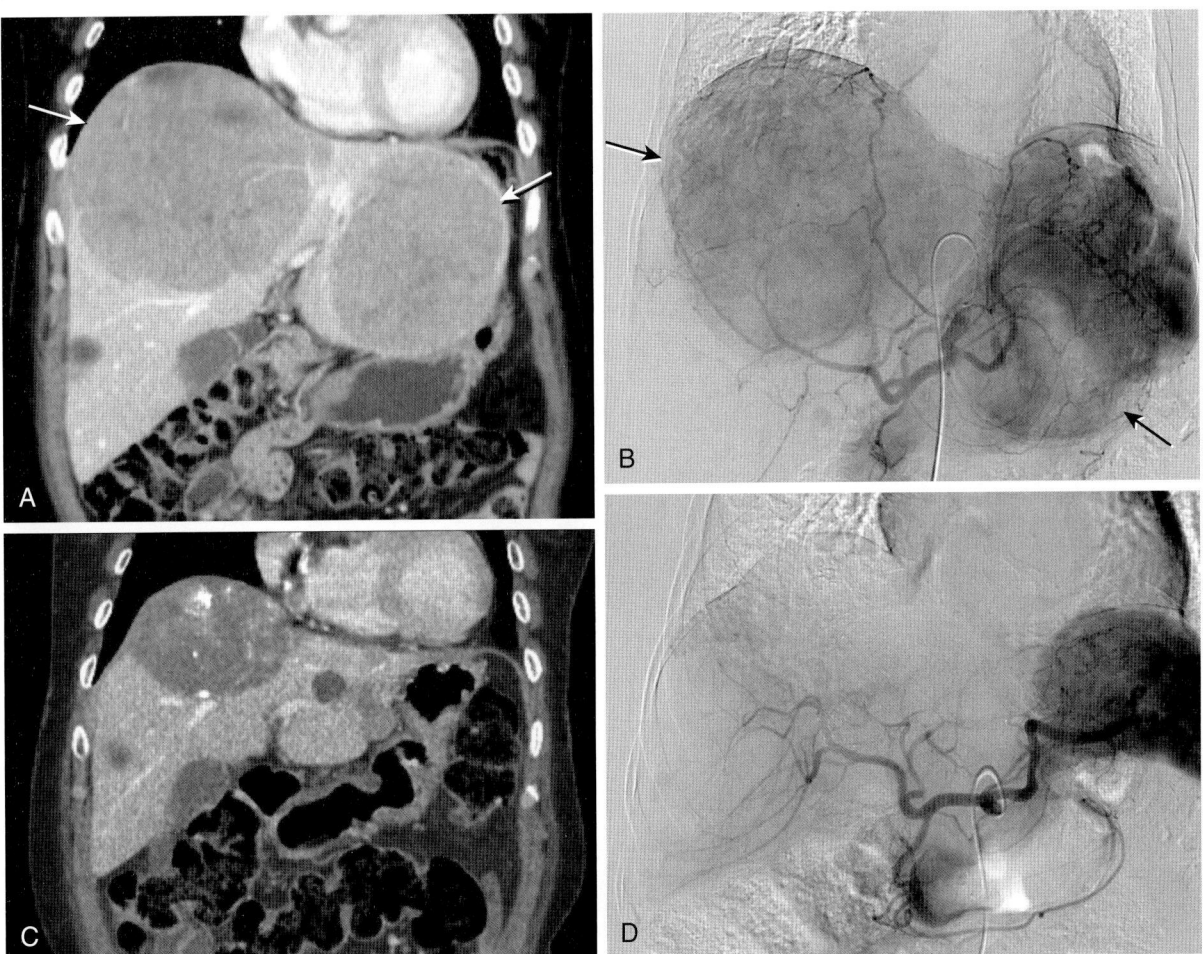

FIGURE 94A.8   Liver metastasis from neuroendocrine tumor with unknown origin in a 74-year-old woman. **A** and **B,** A liver computed tomography (CT) **(A)** and celiac arteriogram **(B)** show multiple hypervascular huge tumors involving more than 50% of the entire liver *(arrows)*. Transarterial chemoembolization (TACE) was performed in staged manner, with only a part of the vascular tumor embolized at each session. **C** and **D,** Thirty-month follow-up CT **(C)** and celiac arteriogram **(D)** after 11 sessions of TACE show markedly improved metastatic lesions.

morbidity remains a concern. Patients with metastatic NET—particularly those with low-grade histology—may experience prolonged survival by undergoing repeated locoregional liver-directed therapies, and hepatic dysfunction can accrue following multiple such interventions. Accordingly, the United States National Comprehensive Cancer Network (NCCN) treatment guidelines currently recommend against the use of TACE using drug-eluting bead (DEB) technology in this patient population due to higher reported rates of toxicity when compared with conventional TACE with ethiodized oil or transarterial embolization alone.

Sarcoma and Gastrointestinal Tumors (see Chapter 92)

A small number of investigations have addressed hepatic embolization therapy for treatment of sarcoma and GISTs. Many gastrointestinal soft tissue neoplasms previously classified as leiomyomas, schwannomas, leiomyoblastomas, or leiomyosarcomas are today classified as GISTs on the basis of molecular and immunohistologic features. The liver is the most common site of metastasis from malignant GISTs. Hepatic resection is the treatment of choice for a single metastasis, but the majority of patients with liver-dominant metastases have unresectable disease. Because this tumor is frequently hypervascular, hepatic embolization therapy has been an effective palliative treatment for unresectable liver metastases (Fig. 94A.9). Because imatinib mesylate (Gleevec), a tyrosine kinase inhibitor (TKI), proved to be highly effective against GISTs, TACE is currently recommended for patients who did not respond to therapy or became resistant to TKI. In a small series, including 26 sessions of TACE in 14 patients with TKI-resistant liver metastasis, the median progression-free survival time was 7.0 months, and the median overall survival was 9.7 months.[86] Cao et al.[87] compared

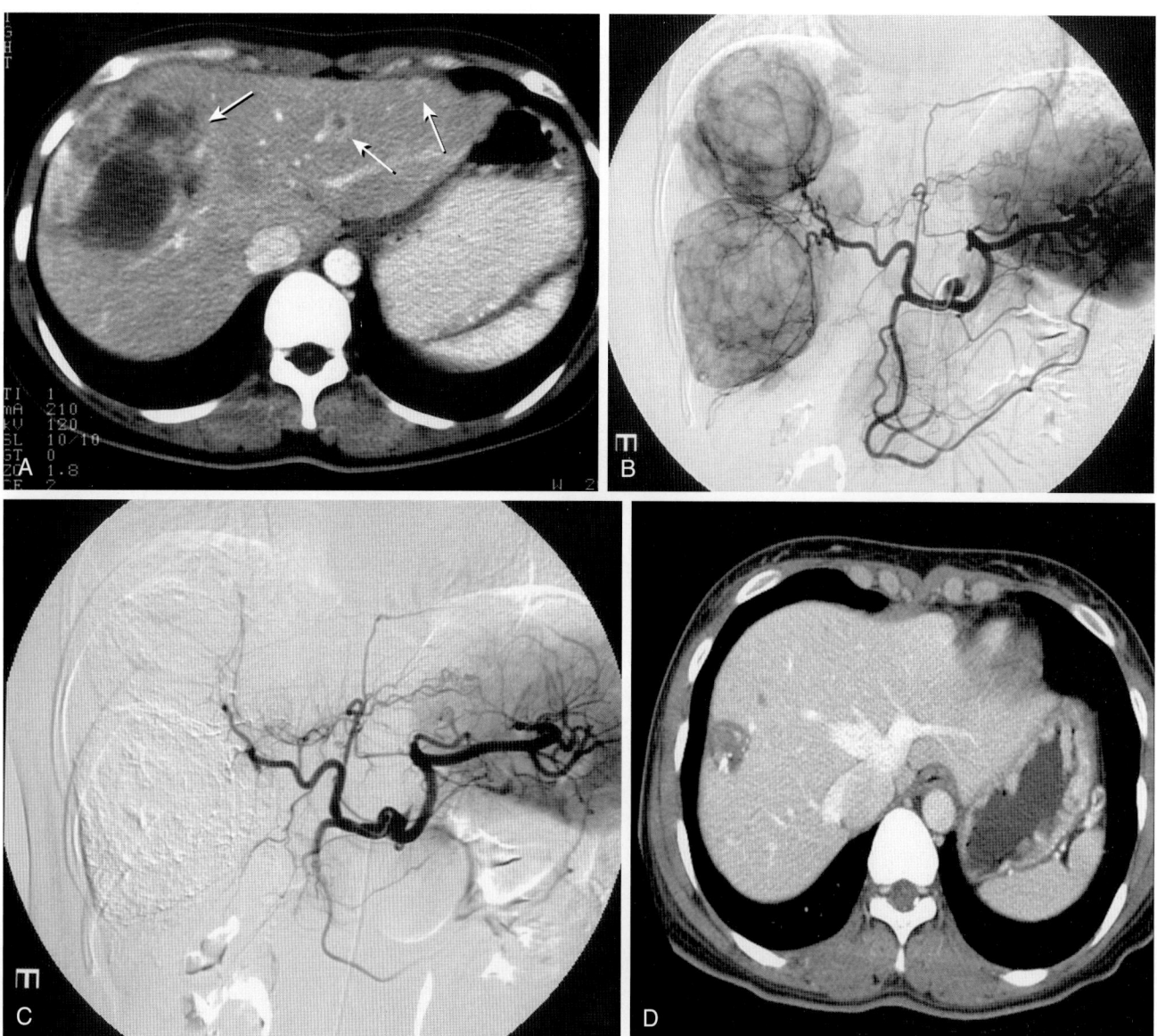

FIGURE 94A.9 Liver metastasis from gastrointestinal stromal tumor of the stomach in a 34-year-old woman. **A,** Computed tomography (CT) scan of the liver shows multiple metastatic tumors in both hepatic lobes *(arrows)*. **B,** Celiac arteriogram shows multiple and variable-sized hypervascular tumors in the liver. **C,** Initial transarterial chemoembolization (TACE) was performed with an emulsion of 10 mL of Lipiodol and 50 mg of doxorubicin hydrochloride, followed by embolization with gelatin sponge particles. Completion arteriogram shows successful devascularization of the tumor. **D,** After three sessions of repeat TACE, 8-year follow-up CT scan shows no evidence of viable tumor in the liver.

TACE versus best supportive care among 60 patients after clinical failure with TKI therapy. The TACE group showed longer median progression-free survival (30.0 weeks vs. 12.9 weeks) and overall survival (68.5 weeks vs. 25.7 weeks) than the control group, with the best prognosis noted among patients without extrahepatic disease at the time of TACE.

Colorectal Metastases (see Chapter 92)

Colon cancer is the second leading cause of cancer-related death in the Western Hemisphere, and liver is the most common site of distant metastasis of colon cancer. Liver metastasis will develop in approximately 50% to 60% of patients with colorectal cancers in their lifetime, and more than half will die of metastatic liver diseases.[88] Hepatic resection is the only potentially curative treatment for liver metastasis from colon cancer, but less than 30% of patients have resectable disease at the time of initial evaluation.[89] Systemic chemotherapy remains the standard of care for patients with irresectable disease, with a median survival of 22 months reported[90] (see Chapters 97 and 98).

Bland hepatic artery embolization and TACE have been used as second-line therapeutic options for hepatic disease progression following systemic chemotherapy. Studies from the early 1990s on 5-FU and melphalan or interferon-α showed promising results in patients with good performance status, no extrahepatic disease, and solitary lesions.[91,92] Subsequently, several TACE series were published in which different treatment regimens were used.[93,94] Vogl et al.[94] published a case series including 463 patients on TACE with starch microspheres and different chemotherapeutic agents (mitomycin C, gemcitabine, irinotecan). They showed 1- and 2-year overall survival rates of 62% and 28%, respectively.

Uveal Melanoma (see Chapter 92)

Uveal melanoma is a rare but highly lethal malignancy with median survival of 2 to 6 months.[95] Liver metastases are found in as many as 40% of patients at the time of initial evaluation, and a sole metastasis is found in more than 80% of patients.[96] Several early case series reported on the use of TACE for local control of metastatic uveal melanoma.[97,98] A retrospective study of 201 patients compared cisplatin-based TACE with systemic chemotherapy and reported a response rate of 36% after TACE compared with less than 1% with systemic therapy.[99] More recent studies performed using varying technical methods and materials have reported median survival rates ranging from 11.5 to 21 months.[100–102] Most recently, Edelhauser et al.[103] performed TACE with fotemustine in 21 patients and achieved improved response rate (43%) and mean survival (28.7 months).

COMPLICATIONS

The overall rate of complications following TACE is approximately 4% and the mortality rate is under 1%.[104,105] Major complications including liver failure or infarction, liver abscess, biliary necrosis, tumor rupture, cholecystitis, and nontarget embolization are uncommon. Important predisposing factors for major complications following conventional lipiodol-based TACE include portal vein occlusion, baseline hepatic dysfunction, biliary obstruction, previous biliary surgery or intervention, large-volume intraarterial administration of ethiodized oil, and nonselective embolization.[26] Recognition of predisposing factors before the procedure, selective embolization with an adequate amount of chemoembolic material, and careful postprocedure patient monitoring are critical to minimize incidence and risks of complications.

Postembolization Syndrome

Postembolization syndrome (PES) occurs in up to 80% of patients and comprises the symptoms of pain, fever, nausea, and vomiting.[104] PES is not considered a complication but rather an expected phase of immediate postprocedure recovery following any hepatic embolization therapy. Though the etiology of the syndrome is not fully understood, it likely reflects a cascade of immunologic phenomena induced by ischemic injury. This generates an abrupt release of tumoral antigens into the systemic circulation, with the resultant proinflammatory cascade provoking the characteristic "flu-like" symptoms experienced by most patients. Similarly, pain reflects local changes from ischemic cell death with additional potential contributing factors, including hepatic capsular distention and nontarget embolization, such as gallbladder ischemia secondary to inadvertent passage of embolic material into the cystic artery.[106] Though patients may experience transient and mild laboratory alterations including leukocytosis or elevated hepatic transaminases, the diagnosis of PES remains fundamentally clinical in nature. PES is self-limiting and requires only supportive management including hydration, antiemetics, analgesics, and antipyretics. PES is the most common reason for hospitalization following TACE and other liver-directed embolization-based therapies.

Liver Failure

The most serious complication of hepatic embolization therapy is liver failure (see Chapter 77). In a retrospective study that included 197 sessions of TACE, acute liver failure developed in 20% of patients, and 3% of these cases were irreversible.[107] Hyperbilirubinemia, prolonged prothrombin time, higher dose of chemotherapeutic drug, and advanced cirrhosis were associated with irreversible failure.[107,108] In general, selective TACE does not affect liver function in patients with Childs class A or B cirrhosis, with most hospitalizations due to liver dysfunction developing in patients with class C disease.

Liver Abscess

Liver abscess is a rare (0.5% to 2%) but potentially fatal complication of hepatic embolotherapies (see Chapter 70). Predisposing factors include portal vein obstruction and treatment of metastatic tumors.[28,109] Prior biliary enteric bypass surgery, sphincter of Oddi dysfunction, and prior biliary intervention are the most important and common predisposing factors leading to abscess development following TACE.[29,109,110] Biliary-concentrated antibiotics such as piperacillin are recommended to prevent liver abscess in these patients[27,111] and should be continued for several days following embolization therapy. Typical clinical manifestations are pain, fever, and leukocytosis, which may present up to 7 to 10 days following embolization therapy. The combination of percutaneous abscess drainage and administration of antibiotics is typically the effective therapy (Fig. 94A.10).

Bile Duct Injury

Both intrahepatic and extrahepatic bile ducts may be damaged by hepatic arterial embolization therapy due to ischemia within the peribiliary capillary plexus. This complication has been

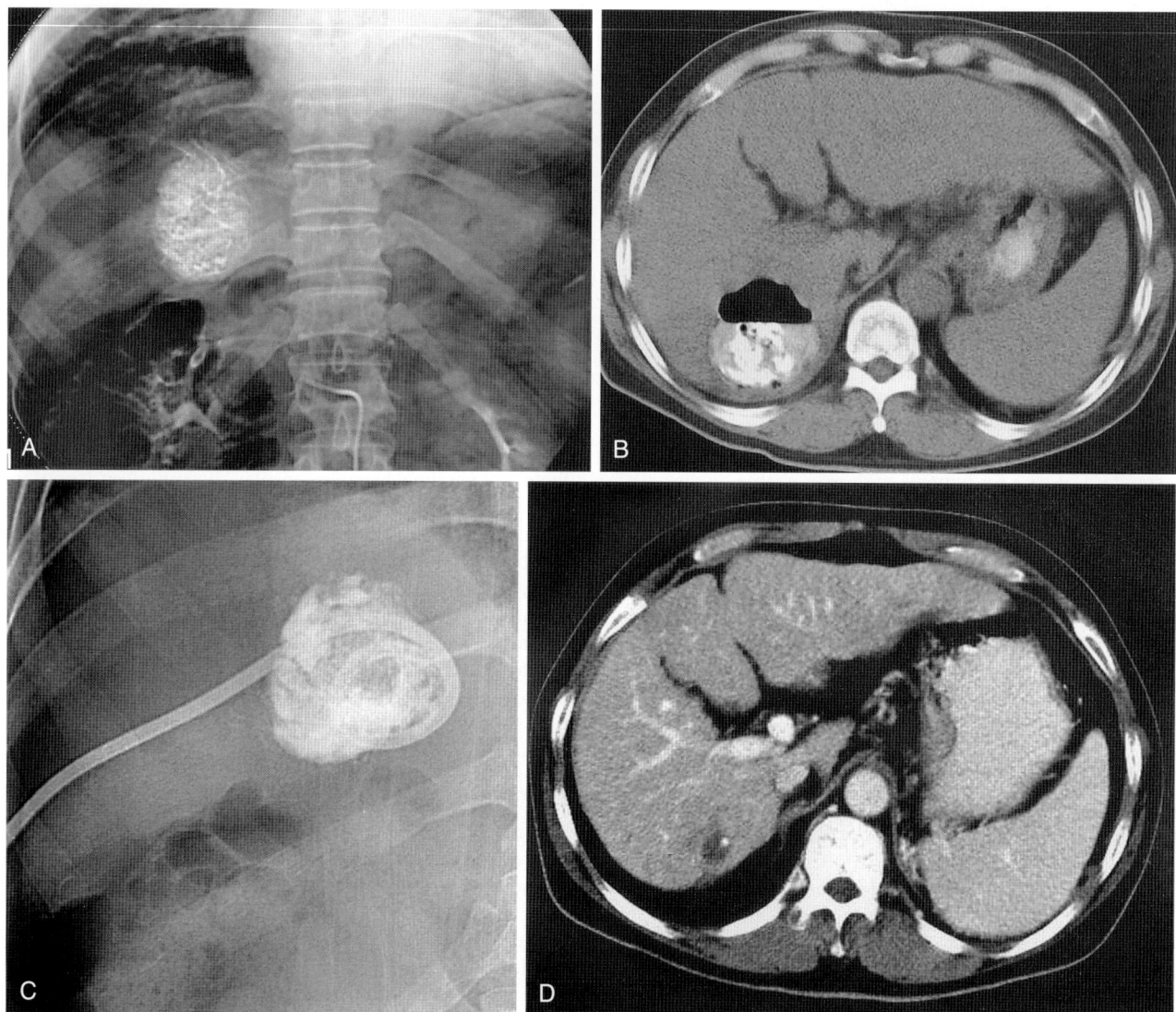

FIGURE 94A.10 Liver abscess formation after transarterial chemoembolization (TACE) and treatment with percutaneous drainage in a 55-year-old man. **A,** Plain radiograph obtained after TACE shows selective Lipiodol accumulation in the tumor. **B,** Noncontrast computed tomography (CT) scan 2 weeks later shows air-fluid level in the tumor. **C,** The abscess cavity is drained with a percutaneous drainage catheter. **D,** Follow-up CT scan 1 month later shows remarkable tumor shrinkage without evidence of viable tumor.

reported in 2% to 12.5% and may manifest as intrahepatic biloma or one or more areas of biliary structure formation[108,112,113] (see Chapter 42). Intrahepatic bile duct injury may cause occlusion of adjacent portal branches, liver parenchymal atrophy, and liver abscess.[114] In 2003 Sakamoto et al.[112] reported that bile duct injury is more frequent following TACE among patients with metastatic tumor, noncirrhotic liver, and in those who underwent selective embolization of distal hepatic arteries. Most patients are asymptomatic, but when signs of cholangitis are present, treatment with antibiotics and percutaneous biliary drainage is often necessary.[115,116]

Extrahepatic Nontargeted Embolization

Nontarget embolization occurs infrequently but may, rarely, be associated with significant toxicity. The gallbladder is the most common organ affected by nontarget embolization.[117] In most cases this is asymptomatic or may manifest with clinical and laboratory features of acute cholecystitis. Rarely, more serious conditions have been reported, including gallbladder perforation,

gangrenous or emphysematous cholecystitis requiring cholecystectomy, or percutaneous cholecystostomy.[118]

Skin complications can develop after TACE or embolization therapy of extrahepatic collateral vessels, especially the internal mammary artery and intercostal artery.[35,119,120] Painful induration and discoloration are often observed, but transmural necrosis requiring skin grafting is exceedingly rare. A characteristic rash can develop within the periumbilical region via nontarget embolization of the falciform artery that may be avoided with pre-embolization coiling—if identified before embolization—or placement of cold packs on the anterior abdominal wall from the xyphoid to the umbilicus to induce local vasoconstriction during embolization therapy.[121]

Gastroduodenal ischemia and ulceration can occur as a result of inadvertent embolization of gastric, gastroduodenal, or pancreaticoduodenal arteries.[122] Rarely, such injuries may progress to perforation and require surgical intervention. Prophylactic coil embolization or temporary balloon occlusion during the embolization procedure can minimize the incidence of this complication.

TACE of the inferior phrenic artery may induce pulmonary toxicity via embolization of small collaterals to the pulmonary arterial and systemic bronchial arterial trees.[37,123] Diaphragmatic paresis resulting in weakness can also develop.[124,125] A potential risk of pulmonary embolism or infarction exists in the presence of an arteriovenous shunt because ethiodized oil emulsion or particles can pass through the shunt. The incidence of pulmonary oil embolization reaches 43% when a large amount of ethiodized oil is used for TACE.[126] Respiratory symptoms of cough, hemoptysis, and dyspnea may develop in 2 to 5 days and are expected to resolve within 10 to 28 days after TACE in most cases, but serious complications such as respiratory arrest may occur. To prevent pulmonary oil embolism, it is recommended to use no more than 15 mL of ethiodized oil, to administer ethiodized oil superselectively, and to carefully look for arteriovenous hepatic shunts on initial arteriograms and during the procedure.[127] Fatal pulmonary embolus has also been reported when embolizing large tumors in the diaphragmatic dome with small particles.[12]

Iatrogenic Vascular Injury

Iatrogenic arterial injury, such as dissection, may occur during hepatic embolization therapy. The two most common sites of dissection are the celiac and proper hepatic artery. Iatrogenic arterial dissection often heals spontaneously but rarely may result in complete obstruction or pseudoaneurysm formation[128] (see Chapter 124). When such injuries occur, they may preclude treatment with TACE or other embolization-based therapies.

Embolization Therapy Combined With Other Treatments

Embolization therapy can be combined with other local treatments to obtain a synergistic effect on tumor necrosis. Combination therapy employing embolization alongside percutaneous ethanol injection (PEI) (see Chapter 96D), thermal ablation (see Chapters 96B and 96C), laser interstitial thermotherapy (LITT) (see Chapter 96C), and radiotherapy (RT) (see Chapter 95) has been studied, and better results were reported with combination treatments than with either of these therapies alone.[129–132]

TACE can be used together with PEI to improve response to therapy. It hypothesizes that PEI effectively ablates much of the central core of the tumor, while TACE targets the periphery, including microscopic areas of disease. In addition, TACE is thought to result in the lysis of intratumoral septa and in the formation of a fibrous wall around the hypervascularized tumors, which enhances the diffusion of ethanol within tumor tissue.[129] Several trials compared PEI-TACE combination therapy with stand-alone treatment.[133–136] In studies with small HCC, the combination therapy improved local recurrence rates and survival rates compared with PEI alone[136] and TACE alone.[135] This synergistic effect of the combination therapy was also demonstrated in larger HCCs.[137] Due to size restrictions with the use of PEI, however, this technique has fallen out of favor at many institutions.

RFA is designed to destroy tumors by heating tissue to lethal temperatures, those exceeding 60°C (see Chapter 98B). It has proved to be an effective treatment of small HCCs, but the tumor volume that can be ablated is limited. Hepatic artery embolization eliminates the heat-sink effect by blood flow; thus it induces a larger ablation area by RFA (Fig. 94A.11). In addition, a larger volume of sublethal hyperthermia around ablation is exposed to synergistic high concentrations of chemotherapeutic

drugs. Many reports have demonstrated this combination to be a useful therapeutic method to control intermediate and large HCCs.[130,138–140] Takaki et al.[141] treated 20 patients with HCCs larger than 5 cm with a TACE-RFA combination and reported a 5-year survival rate of 41%. A randomized trial combining RFA with TACE for treating patients with intermediate (3.1–5 cm) HCC showed a significantly decreased tumor progression rate in the TACE-RFA group compared with the RFA-alone group (6% vs. 39%).[142] A more recent randomized trial of 189 patients with HCC less than 7 cm demonstrated better overall and recurrence-free survival in the combination group.[130] The survival benefit from the TACE-RFA combination has also been reported in meta-analysis studies.[143,144] However, among patients with small HCCs, the enhanced therapeutic efficacy from combination therapy is controversial. A prospective study did not find any benefit in local tumor progression and survival with the combination treatment compared with stand-alone RFA in HCC 3 cm or smaller.[145] Considering the increased cost and patient discomfort of additional TACE, it may be reasonable to restrict this therapy combination to intermediate and large HCCs or small lesions with infiltrative margins.

Several investigators used TACE to downsize a tumor that could be ablated with LITT. Zangos et al.[146] performed repeated TACE (mean, 3.5 sessions per patient) in 48 patients with HCCs 5 to 8 cm in diameter to reach a favorable size for magnetic resonance–guided LITT. Repeated TACE reduced the tumor size in 32 patients (66.7%), and subsequent LITT resulted in a median survival of 36 months after the first treatment. The same combination was used by Vogl et al.,[131] who also showed that TACE can be used as a downsizing tool before LITT in 50.6% of patients with unresectable liver metastasis. Pacella et al.[147] also used LITT to reduce tumor volume and then performed TACE in HCCs up to 9.6 cm in diameter. After this combination treatment, complete response was achieved in 90% of the tumors, with a local recurrence rate of 7% at 3 years.

The combination of TACE and three-dimensional conformal RT has involved three strategies.[148] The most common approach is TACE followed by RT in patients with macroscopic venous invasion, in which RT is used to treat portal vein and inferior vena cava tumor thrombus to enhance the therapeutic effect of TACE. From 40 to 60 Gy during 5 to 6 weeks can be delivered safely to the macrovascular disease.[132,149] In a case-control study of 15 patients, 34.1% who underwent the combination therapy showed complete disappearance of venous tumor thrombi, and 1-year survival rate was improved in the combination group compared with the group that received TACE alone (34.8% vs. 11.4%). A second approach involves RT performed between repeat TACE procedures, with RT used as a planned "consolidation" procedure to target residual viable tumor after TACE.[148] A theoretical benefit of this approach is that the chemotherapeutic drugs retained in the tumor by TACE may have a radiosensitizing effect. In the third approach, repetitive TACE for large HCC is given until optimal response, followed by RT. Tumor shrinkage after TACE allows the use of smaller irradiation fields, which permits higher tumor doses and improves the normal liver tolerance.[132]

Despite the heterogeneity of disease, patients, and treatment techniques, the majority of studies have suggested a benefit of the combination therapy compared with stand-alone therapies in treatment of advanced HCC.[149-152] However, despite these favorable outcomes, patient selection parameters for each combination therapy remain incompletely characterized.

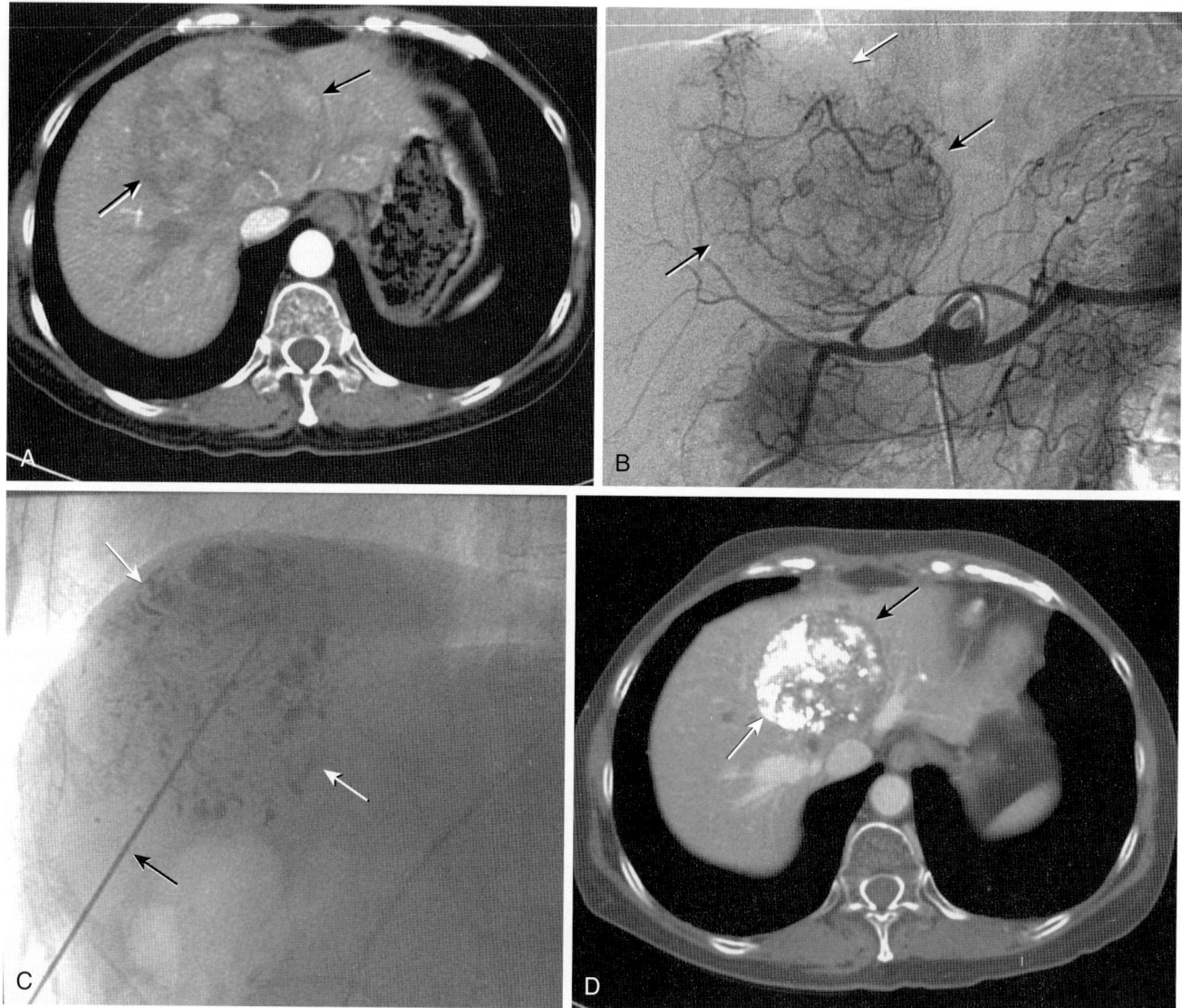

FIGURE 94A.11 Combination therapy using transarterial chemoembolization (TACE) and radiofrequency ablation (RFA) in a 48-year-old woman with large hepatocellular carcinoma (HCC). **A,** Arterial phase computed tomography (CT) shows a heterogeneously enhanced massive HCC *(arrows)*. **B,** Celiac arteriogram shows a hypervascular tumor stain supplied by left hepatic artery *(arrows)*. TACE was performed with an emulsion of 7 mL of Lipiodol and 40 mg of doxorubicin hydrochloride, followed by embolization with gelatin sponge particles. **C,** Immediately after TACE, RFA was performed. Under fluoroscopic guidance, an expandable electrode *(black arrow)* was placed, aiming Lipiodol accumulated in the tumor *(white arrows)*. **D,** Follow-up CT obtained 1 year later shows remarkable tumor shrinkage with no evidence of viable tumor *(arrows)*.

The discovery and use of novel targeted molecular agents have improved long-term outcomes for patients with advanced HCC (see Chapter 99). Sorafenib, an oral multitarget TKI with antiangiogenic and antiproliferative mechanisms, was the first such agent to show clinical benefit. In 2008 sorafenib was demonstrated to prolong median survival and median time to radiologic progression compared with a placebo in an RCT, ushering in a new area of anti-HCC therapeutics and becoming the new standard of care for HCC patients with contraindications to surgical or locoregional therapies.[153]

Because of sorafenib's antiangiogenic properties, it was initially hypothesized that sorafenib administration during and/or after TACE may counteract hypoxia-induced angiogenesis, thereby reducing tumor recurrence and improving long-term patient outcomes. Several noncomparative studies[154–156] and RCTs[157,158] have been performed to evaluate this question.

However, whether the combination together yields any meaningful clinical benefit compared with TACE alone remains unproven. A randomized phase III study comparing sorafenib with placebo following TACE in 458 patients demonstrated no added benefit of sorafenib,[157] and results from the randomized SPACE trial (sorafenib or placebo in combination with TACE for intermediate stage HCC) also failed to demonstrate any significant benefit with regard to tumor progression or overall survival.[158] In addition, results from the IMbrave150 multicenter randomized trial published in 2020 demonstrated that the combination of bevacizumab and atezolizumab was superior to sorafenib with regard to overall survival, progression free survival, and quality of life,[159] calling into question any future applications of sorafenib among patients with unresectable HCC, whether alone or in combination with locoregional therapies.

ALTERNATIVE APPROACHES TO LIVER-DIRECTED INTRAARTERIAL EMBOLIZATION THERAPY

Hepatic Artery Embolization

A long-standing controversy remains regarding the routine administration of antineoplastic drugs during hepatic arterial embolization therapy. Although the concept of delivering high-dose chemotherapy to the tumor is mechanistically sound, no direct evidence exists to support the routine use of TACE over hepatic artery embolization (HAE) alone. In multiple studies, HAE with spherical embolic agents or microspheres has been shown to be as effective as TACE for treatment of both primary and metastatic liver tumors and may be considered at present to be an equivalent treatment option without the added expense and potential local and systemic toxicities of chemotherapy.[160–164]

The microspheres used for HAE and other embolization therapies are composed of an inert elastic polymer with a smooth hydrophilic surface. The spherical shape allows for precise calibration of particle size within a narrow range. They are compressible and have little tendency to clump together, which results in a lower rate of catheter occlusion and better penetration into distal small vessels.[165] Currently, there are several commercially available microspheres, including tris-acyl gelatin microspheres (Embosphere; Merit Medical, South Jordan, UT), spherical PVA (Contour SE [Boston Scientific, Natick, MA], Bead Block [Biocompatibles, Farnham, UK]), and polyphosphazene-coated polymethylmethacrylate microspheres (Embozene; Celonova Bioscience, San Antonio, TX).

The technical details of HAE are similar to those of TACE but with key differences. A thorough clinical evaluation including physical examination, assessment of laboratory values, and review of relevant cross-sectional imaging studies is conducted before each procedure. On the day of embolization, patients are administered a single dose of intravenous antibiotics unless they have a history of biliary enteric anastomosis or incompetent sphincter of Oddi, in which case additional postembolization antibiotics are administered to minimize the risk of infection. Either moderate sedation or general anesthesia may be employed according to operator preference. Arterial access is obtained, after which a 4- or 5-French catheter is used to cannulate the arterial supply to the liver. As the vast majority of HAEs are performed selectively or superselectively, a microcatheter is employed to target segmental or subsegmental hepatic arterial branches for treatment.

With HAE, the primary goal is distal small vessel occlusion usually at the terminal arteriole or capillary level. Because of this, the therapeutic endpoint during the HAE procedure is complete arterial stasis, conventionally defined as five or greater heartbeats without demonstration of antegrade flow within the embolized territory. This endpoint differs from conventional TACE in which reflux of embolic material into portal venules is used to assess the extent of embolization. Additionally, complete arterial stasis may not be desired when TACE is performed, as this has been associated with worse survival outcomes when compared with patients in whom stasis was not achieved during their TACE procedure.[166]

Cone-beam or conventional helical CT performed without the administration of intravenous contrast media immediately following HAE can be used to predict treatment outcomes. When compared with preprocedure imaging, complete coverage of the target lesion(s) by retained high-density contrast material following the embolization procedure has been shown to strongly correlate with the probability of complete response by modified Response Evaluation Criteria In Solid Tumors (RECIST) criteria.[167] Conversely, the presence of one or more deficits in contrast retention within the target lesion(s) portends a poor prognosis and a high likelihood of local recurrence. These findings complement similar findings among patients who have undergone treatment with conventional TACE in which the pattern of lipiodol retention has been shown to correlate with patient outcomes.[168]

Hepatocellular Carcinoma

The most common application of hepatic artery embolization is in the treatment of patients with unresectable hepatocellular carcinoma (see Chapter 89). Techniques have been refined considerably since the first applications of HAE were explored in the 1970s,[169] wherein large gelatin sponge particles or stainless steel coils were administered proximally within one or more tumor-associated arterial branches to induce ischemic cell death, generally before planned surgical resection. Presently, HAE using nondegradable calibrated microspheres is indicated for most patients with one or more hepatocellular carcinoma tumors and a contraindication to resection or liver transplantation who have preserved liver function and favorable performance status. Among appropriately selected patients, HAE is associated with prolonged overall survival and low local and systemic toxicity.

Improved survival with HAE was first demonstrated in a randomized trial by Lin et al.,[170] who compared embolization alone to systemic therapy with the cytotoxic agent 5-fluorouracil. Overall survival in the embolization cohort was 42.2% at 21 months, significantly better than in the chemotherapy cohort. These findings were replicated in subsequent trials, including a randomized trial by Chang et al.[171] comparing HAE to embolization with cisplatin that demonstrated a 24-month overall survival rate of 39.5% among patients in the HAE trial arm.

With greater HAE experience came a better understanding of the role of particle size on treatment effects. In 1997 Sonomura et al.[172] demonstrated greater hepatic necrosis with particle sizes under 500 μm among dogs treated with HAE, and subsequent cohort studies in humans supported this observation. Maluccio et al.[173] performed bland embolization using 45 to 100 μm nonspherical PVA or 40 to 120 μm Embosphere in 322 patients with HCC and reported 1-, 2-, and 3-year overall survival rates of 66%, 46%, and 33%, respectively. In patients without extrahepatic disease or portal vein involvement by tumor, the overall 1-, 2-, and 3-year survival rates increased to 84%, 66%, and 51%, respectively, improved relative to earlier reports using proximal gelatin sponge embolization. Bonomo et al.[174] used 40 μm and/or 100 μm Embozene in 53 HCC patients, and they reported 56% objective response by the RECIST criteria.

More recently, Brown et al.[164] performed a randomized trial comparing HAE using 100- to 300-μm spherical microparticles with doxorubicin TACE using 300- to 500-μm spherical microparticles among 101 patients with unresectable hepatocellular carcinoma. Median progression-free and overall survival with HAE were 6.2 months and 19.6 months, respectively, which were not significantly different between treatment groups (TACE) but were prolonged when compared with a large historic cohort of patients treated with sorafenib chemotherapy as part of the randomized controlled SHARP trial.[153] Adverse events, too, were similar between groups occurring in 38% of HAE patients and 40% of TACE patients. Together, these findings confirmed the superiority of modern HAE techniques over standard-of-care medical therapy while also demonstrating equivalence of HAE with TACE with respect to both treatment outcomes and toxicity among patients with HCC and contraindications to surgical intervention.

As with TACE, HAE may also be used in combination with ablation, allowing for treatment of larger tumors than may be optimally treated with HAE alone. Maluccio et al.[175] compared outcomes among patients with solitary HCC tumors up to 7 cm in size treated with surgical resection or combined HAE and ablation using radiofrequency or ethanol injection. Though the authors reported improved progression-free survival among patients in the surgical cohort, there was no difference in overall survival at 5 years (56% and 58% for HAE/ablation and surgery, respectively). A subsequent analysis of this cohort with a median follow-up interval of greater than 10 years confirmed these findings, with no difference in median overall survival and higher complications among patients who underwent surgical resection.[176]

Neuroendocrine Tumors (see Chapter 91)

Patients with liver-dominant metastatic neuroendocrine tumors—particularly those with low-grade histology—may benefit from hepatic artery embolization, in terms of both overall survival and symptomatic relief. In 1986 Carrasco et al.[177] published the first report of HAE for NET using polyvinyl sponge in 25 patients with symptomatic metastatic carcinoid tumors. Their results demonstrated symptomatic relief in 87% of patients, with 60% of patients alive at a median of 16 months. A subsequent cohort analysis by Erikssen et al.[178] evaluated HAE using gelatin sponge among 12 patients with metastatic pancreatic NET (P-NET) and 29 patients with metastatic nonpancreatic NET (NP-NET). Their results demonstrated a similar objective response rate (52%, NP-NET; 50%, P-NET) and median response duration (12 months, NP-NET; 10 months, P-NET) between the two groups. However, median year overall survival was significantly better among patients with NP-NET (80 months) when compared with P-NET patients (20 months).

As in hepatocellular carcinoma and other malignant disease processes, technologic as well as technical developments have improved outcomes following HAE for NET patients with hepatic metastatic disease. Strosberg et al.[179] reported on outcomes following HAE using polyvinyl alcohol or microspheres among 84 patients with liver metastases from carcinoid or pancreatic NET. The authors found a median overall survival of 36 months and noted few major complications with no therapy-related deaths reported. Zener et al.[180] subsequently evaluated the effects of spherical embolic particle size on outcomes in a cohort of 160 patients with liver metastases from NET. Results demonstrated an improved response rate according to modified RECIST criteria among patients in whom particles less than 100 μm in size were used (64%) when compared with larger particle sizes (42%), though this difference did not translate into improved overall survival. However, tumor histology was noted to strongly predict long-term outcomes after HAE, with a median overall survival of 55 months among patients with well-differentiated or moderately differentiated NET as

compared with 13 months for patients with poorly differentiated or undifferentiated tumors.

The incorporation of cytotoxic chemotherapy into HAE for neuroendocrine tumor has been evaluated in several trials. Pitt et al.[161] retrospectively reviewed outcomes among 100 patients (49 TACE, 51 HAE) with metastatic NET. No differences in morbidity, mortality, or overall survival were observed (median overall survival, TACE: 25.5 months; median overall survival, HAE: 25.7 months). These findings were subsequently replicated in two randomized trials. In 2012 Maire et al.[162] evaluated outcomes in 26 patients (12 TACE, 14 HAE) with metastatic midgut NET and found no statistically significant difference with respect to 2-year progression-free survival (38%, TACE; 44%, HAE) and overall survival (80%, TACE; 100% HAE) between the two treatments. In a separate randomized study by Fiore et al.[160] published in 2014, TACE again failed to demonstrate superiority over HAE, with an overall median progression-free survival of 36 months that did not differ between groups. Together, these and other trials call into question the routine application of TACE among metastatic NET patients. Moreover, Fiore et al.[160] found an improved toxicity profile with HAE and suggested it may be the preferred embolotherapeutic approach for patients with metastatic NET given comparable long-term clinical outcomes and equivalent or possibly favorable morbidity relative to TACE.

A 2014 publication indicated that disease biology and stage may determine outcomes of HAE for NETs.[181] Among 320 consecutive patients analyzed, urgent HAE for refractory symptoms (urgent group, P = .007), greater than 50% liver replacement by tumor (P < .0001), and extrahepatic metastasis (P = .007) were independent predictors for shorter overall survival. Patients with all three risk factors had decreased overall survival versus those with none (median, 8.5 vs. 86 months). Thirty-day mortality was significantly lower in patients treated electively (1%) versus the urgent group (8.5%). Complications were rare in the elective group (3%) whereas they were significantly higher (10.6%) in patients treated urgently for refractory symptomatology. Male sex and urgent HAE for symptoms were independent factors for both higher 30-day mortality rate and complications.

TACE With Drug-Eluting Beads

In an attempt to capitalize on the benefits of calibrated microspheres—reproducible distal small-vessel embolization—while simultaneously employing the theoretical benefits of localized delivery of high-dose, chemotherapy-delivered, drug-eluting beads (DEBs) were designed (Fig. 94A.12). DEBs are composed of a spherical embolic base on which a cytotoxic chemotherapeutic agent has been adsorbed or "loaded." On catheter-directed intratumoral DEB delivery, the drug elutes into the tumor microenvironment, theoretically providing a mechanism for sustained locoregional drug delivery combined with small-vessel ischemia.

Two commercial products are available for use as DEBs: PVA-based microspheres (DC Bead in Europe, LC Bead in the United States; Biocompatibles, Surrey, UK), and superabsorbent polymer (SAP) microspheres (HepaSphere in Europe, QuadraSphere in the United States; Merit Medical, South Jordan, UT). DC/LC Beads consist of nondegradable hydrogel microspheres based on PVA with a smooth surface and a precisely calibrated size that ranges from 100 to 900 μm. They are characterized by a high content of negatively charged 2-acrylamido-2-methylpropanesulfonate (AMPS). The unsaturated AMPS monomer crosslinks the

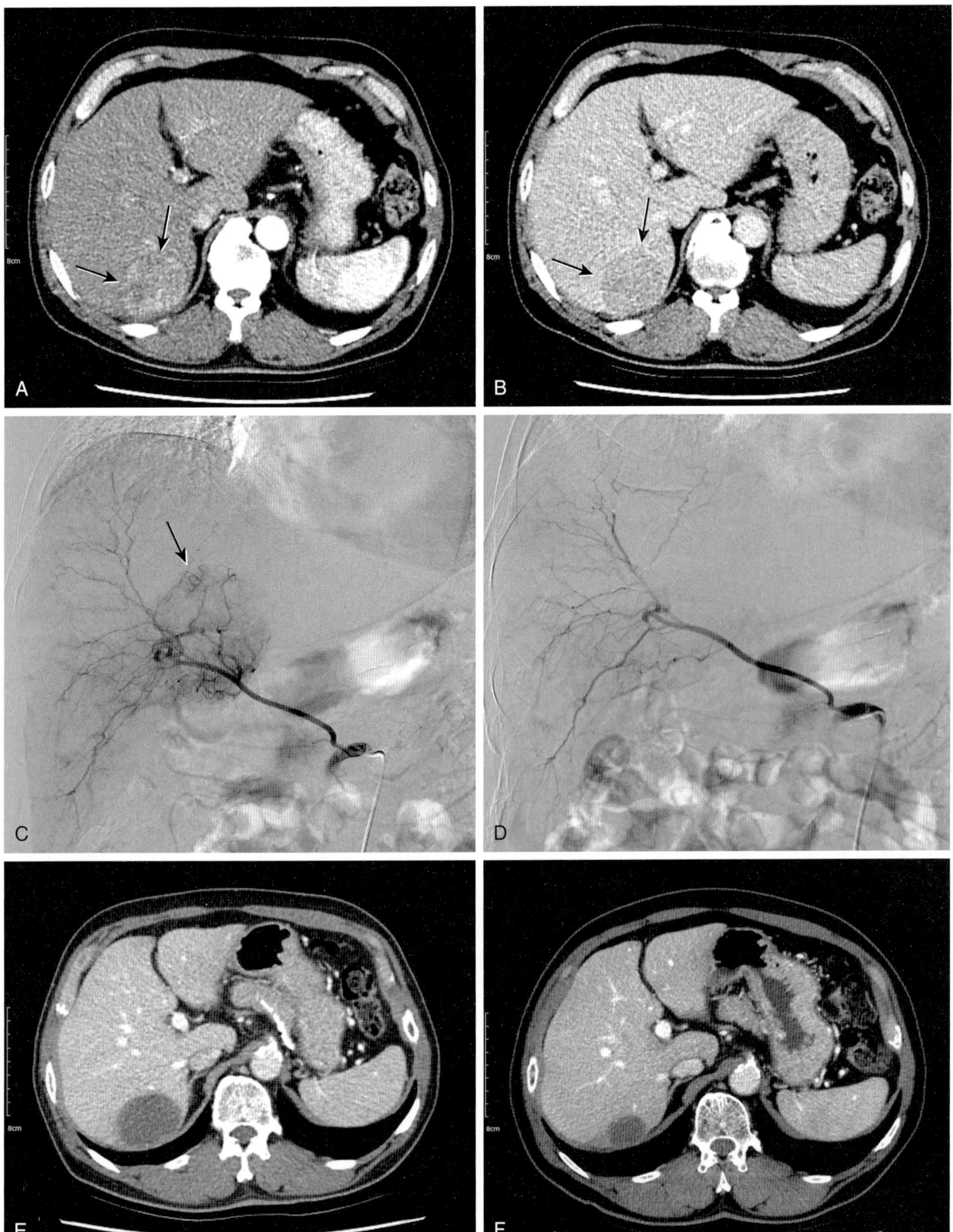

FIGURE 94A.12   Drug-eluting beads–transarterial chemoembolization (DEB-TACE) in a 65-year-old man with high surgical risk due to coronary artery stenosis. **A** and **B,** Arterial **(A)** and portal **(B)** phase computed tomography (CT) scan shows a 5-cm single hepatocellular carcinoma with typical enhancement pattern *(arrows).* **C,** Right hepatic arteriogram shows a hypervascular tumor supplied by multiple tumor-feeding arteries from right posterior hepatic artery *(arrow).* **D,** TACE was performed with 2 vials of DC Beads (100–300 μm) loaded with 100 mg doxorubicin hydrochloride (50 mg per each vial of DC Beads). **E** and **F,** One-month **(E)** and 2-year **(F)** follow-up CT show complete necrosis of the tumor with progressive shrinkage.

PVA backbone, and it allows the load and release of positively charged drugs, such as doxorubicin or irinotecan, by an increased number of negatively charged sulfonate moieties. HepaSpheres or QuadraSpheres are SAP microspheres composed of vinyl alcohol and sodium acrylate copolymer. These particles swell and conform to the vessel lumen. Similar to DC Beads, they can load positively charged drugs.

Despite the theoretical benefits of DEB-TACE over other embolization-based treatment methods, no compelling evidence exists to suggest improved long-term outcomes with DEB-TACE when compared with conventional TACE (cTACE) or HAE. The PRECISION-V RCT failed to demonstrate a statistically significant difference in objective response between the DEB-TACE and cTACE group (51.6 vs. 43.5%).[182] However, DC Beads were associated with improved tolerability, with a significant reduction in serious liver toxicity and a significantly lower rate of doxorubicin-related side effects.[183] In two subsequent RCTs comparing DEB-TACE and TACE, there was no significant difference in time to tumor progression and survival.[184,185] More recently, DEB-TACE was compared with HAE in an RCT evaluating both treatments among 101 patients with unresectable HCC, with results demonstrating no differences with respect to survival, disease progression, response rate, or complications.[164] Together, these data call into question the routine use of DEB-TACE over cTACE or HAE alone, the latter of which is associated with lower costs and lower risk of long-term vascular toxicity compared with either chemotherapy-containing modality.

Early reports of DEB-TACE suggested that postembolization syndrome or systemic adverse effects may occur less frequently.[186,187] However, more recent data have not supported this claim, including a retrospective evaluation of 283 patients treated with DEB-TACE or cTACE, which found significantly greater utilization of analgesics and antiemetics following DEB-TACE within the first 6 to 24 hours of therapy.[188]

Beyond hepatocellular carcinoma, DEB-TACE has also been investigated for the treatment of colorectal liver metastases using irinotecan-loaded microspheres (DEBIRI).[189] In 2011 the use of DEBIRI was evaluated in a multicenter study of 55 patients after progression on systemic chemotherapy.[190] Response rates were 66% at 6 months and 75% at 12 months. Overall survival in this small patient cohort was 19 months, with progression-free survival of 11 months. In 2012 Fiorentini et al.[191] showed a significant survival benefit using DEBIRI (median, 22 months) compared with systemic therapy with irinotecan, FU, and leucovorin (median, 15 months) in a small, multi-institutional phase III RCT. Since the publication of these and other trials showing favorable outcomes with DEBIRI, however, there has been a progressive shift toward the use of yttrium-90 radioembolization for treatment of patients with colorectal liver metastases.

CONCLUSION

Hepatic artery embolization therapy is effective treatment for selected patients with primary and secondary liver tumors that may be employed with either palliative or potentially curative intent in selected patients. TACE—the most commonly utilized arterial embolization therapy for treatment of unresectable HCC worldwide—combines the effects of targeted tumor ischemia by embolization with intraarterial chemotherapy and has been shown in randomized clinical trials to prolong survival when compared with best supportive care. To date, however, neither cTACE nor TACE with DEB-TACE has been shown superior to HAE alone with respect to either survival or disease control, and thus it remains likely that the primary efficacy observed following any of these three interventions relates to the intratumoral ischemia induced by the targeted delivery of embolic material into the tumor microenvironment. Regardless of chosen approach, treatment decisions should be individually tailored according to each patient's condition, with proper patient selection yielding optimal clinical results with low rates of local and systemic toxicity.

References are available at expertconsult.com.

Radioembolization for liver tumors

Cristina Mosconi, S. Cheenu Kappadath, and Bruno C. Odisio

OVERVIEW

Interventional oncology is a rapidly growing branch of interventional radiology that is a vital part of multidisciplinary oncologic care. In the management of patients with liver tumors, the minimally invasive nature of its procedures allows targeted delivery of oncologic treatments, maximizing their local effects while minimizing the systemic exposure to such treatments. In this chapter we discuss the general concepts of transarterial radioembolization with yttrium-90 and its use for the treatment of primary and secondary liver malignancies.

RATIONALE

Biological Effects of Radiation

Radiation is known to damage cellular DNA and ultimately lead to cell death. The energetic electrons that damage cellular DNA may arise from either internal radionuclide decay or from interactions in tissue from external photons/protons. The indirect action is caused by the production of hydroxyl radicals (OH^-) when the secondary electron interacts with a water molecule, which is responsible for two thirds of the x-ray damage to DNA.[1] The main mechanisms of cell death include mitotic death, apoptosis, and the bystander effect.[1]

The basic principle of radiation therapy is to maximize radiation absorbed dose within diseased tissue while sparing dose where disease is absent (see Chapter 95). Among other considerations, external beam radiation dose plans are ultimately limited by radiation to normal tissue at both entry and exit. A benefit to brachytherapy is its ability to emit energy internally, which enables limiting of the normal tissue absorbed doses. Transarterial radioembolization with yttrium-90 is a form of brachytherapy and has often also been referred to as selective internal radiation therapy (SIRT). In conventional radiotherapy, the probability of tumor response is known to be related to the radiation absorbed dose. SIRT has been for many years primarily a palliative treatment, so careful dosimetric treatment planning was not routinely performed and large uncertainties in absorbed dose calculations have been clinically acceptable. However, the potential of SIRT goes well beyond palliation, as demonstrated by recently published correlations between dosimetry and tumor response and survival.[2,3] With recent evidence for tumor and parenchymal dose response thresholds with ^{90}Y radioembolization,[4,5] SIRT has expanded from a whole-liver salvage agent to a precise instrument for definitive, high-dose, conformal radiotherapy.

Transarterial Radiation Delivery

The preferential delivery of SIRT to liver tumors via the transarterial approach is based on two anatomic and pathologic factors: the normal liver parenchyma receives ≥75% of its blood from the portal vein, whereas liver tumors derive 80% to 100% of their blood supply from the hepatic artery[6] (see Chapter 2); and the neovascularization around tumors leads to increased microvascular density in liver lesions compared with normal liver parenchyma. These features mean that when ^{90}Y-microspheres are released into the hepatic artery, they will preferentially accumulate in the periphery of tumors in at least a 3:1 to 20:1 ratio compared with a normal liver.[7]

^{90}Y-microspheres must be deposited in the network of tumor vessels within the tumors.[7] Any particles situated within the afferent tumor vessels, more than 3 mm from the tumor, will not have a direct antitumor effect. For this reason, the particles that are used for SIRT need to be small enough (~20 to 40 mm) to allow optimal penetration and deposition within the tumor plexus, but large enough to prevent the passage of microspheres through the capillary bed into the venous circulation that escapes the liver. The principles and mode of action of SIRT are fundamentally different from transarterial chemoembolization (TACE) (see Chapter 94A); in TACE, the vessels that feed the tumor are filled with chemotherapeutic agents and subsequently embolized with particles to ensure a static, ischemic environment to maximize exposure to those agents and to promote ischemic necrosis. In contrast, optimal perfusion and blood flow are required during SIRT to allow the generation of free radicals by ionization of water molecules near the tumor cell's DNA.

CLINICALLY AVAILABLE ^{90}Y-MICROSPHERES

^{90}Y is a beta particle that decays to ^{90}Zr with a half-life of 64.1 hours. An energetic beta particle with maximum energy of 2.28 MeV is released with every disintegration, which generates bremsstrahlung radiation that subsequently allows confirmation by imaging of treatment delivery and distribution with single-photon emission computed tomography (SPECT)/computed tomography (CT). The mean and maximum tissue penetration depth of the beta particle is 2 to 4 and 11 mm, respectively, with greater than 90% of the ^{90}Y energy distributed within 5 mm of tissue deposition. Uniformly implanted ^{90}Y of activity 1 GBq within 1 kg of tissue leads to a mean radiation absorbed dose of about 50 Gy.

TheraSphere (Boston Scientific BTG, Minneapolis, MN) is a Food and Drug Administration (FDA)–approved microsphere device under humanitarian device exemption for the treatment of unresectable hepatocellular carcinoma. It is made of insoluble, biocompatible glass about 20 to 30 microns in diameters and density of 3.3 g/mL. At time of calibration, the microspheres have specific activity of 2500 Bq/sphere. A 3-GBq vial consists of about 1.2 million spheres. Unit dosages of up to 20 GBq are available and the device has a 12-day shelf life from time of calibration.

SIR-Spheres (Sirtex Medical, Boston, MA) is an FDA-approved microsphere device for the treatment of metastatic CRC. SIR-Spheres consist of insoluble, biocompatible resin about 20 to 60 microns in diameters and density of 1.6 g/mL. At time of calibration, the microspheres have specific activity of 50 Bq/sphere. A 3-GBq vial consists of about 30 to 60 million spheres. Unit dosages are 3 GBq with a shelf life of 24 hours. The activity can be used up to 3 days before expiration providing a range of available activities.

PRETREATMENT PLANNING

Patient Selection

All patients should undergo a multidisciplinary clinical evaluation including professionals from interventional radiology; hepatology; medical, surgical, and radiation oncology; and nuclear medicine. Clinical history, physical examination, and laboratory liver function profiling should be examined carefully. In addition, detailed radiologic imaging is needed, showing unequivocal and measurable evidence of hepatic lesions that cannot be surgically resected or ablated with curative intent, and arterial anatomy conducive for hepatic arteriography.[8] The best candidates for SIRT are patients with unresectable liver-only or liver-dominant tumors.[7]

Dosimetry Methods

TheraSphere

Per the product package insert, the user determines the amount of administered activity based on delivering an average dose assuming uniform particle distribution to total treatment volume. The calculation of the dose requires the volume of the liver to be infused—typically assessed using routine diagnostic CT or magnetic resonance imaging (MRI). The mass in kilograms of the treatment volume is then calculated by multiplying the treatment volume by the tissue density. For a prescribed dose (D) in Gy to the target tissue, the activity (A) in GBq to be administered to the target area of the liver, assuming uniform distribution of microspheres, is calculated as follows: $A = D \times m/50$, where m is the mass of the treatment volume in kilograms.

SIR-Spheres

The model of dosimetry for SIR-Spheres is traditionally based on whole-liver infusion. Per the product package insert, the user establishes the amount of administered activity (A) in GBq based on the body surface area (BSA) of the patient in m^2 that is adjusted by the tumor burden as follows: $A = BSA - 0.2 +$ (Tumor volume [L]/Total liver volume [L]). Ideally, the tumor and total liver volumes will be assessed using routine diagnostic CT or MRI.

Lung Dose

Planar 99mTc-MAA (macroaggregated albumin) scans are used to determine the lung shunt fraction (LSF), which is typically computed from planar scintigrams of lung and liver regions after transarterial administration of the 99mTc-MAA from the planned treatment site. The maximum amount of administered activity is limited to maintain lung mean dose less than 30 Gy per treatment and less than 50 Gy in cumulative treatments. For a given LSF, this maximum amount of administered activity allowed (Amax) is given by the following equation: $Amax = 30 \times m\_lung/(50 \times LSF)$, where m_lung is the mass of the treatment volume in kilograms, usually taken to be 1 kg. Recent studies suggest that planar imaging overestimates lung shunt fraction and that 1 kg does not often represent the true lung mass.[9,10] Consequently, improved methods to calculate LSF and the use of patient-specific lung masses are currently being discussed.

An obvious limitation of these dosimetry methods is that the amount of activity administered is determined with safety in mind, to prevent overdosing to the normal live parenchyma and lungs and to minimize the occurrence of radiation-induced complications, such as radiation pneumonitis and radioembolization-induced liver disease (REILD), respectively. Unlike treatment planning for external beam radiation therapy, the prescribed activities are not determined based on attaining a patient-specific tumor dose threshold. This is thought to result in underdosing in some patients and drive mixed outcomes reported on clinical trials involving radioembolization.[11–13] Furthermore, the patient outcomes following radioembolization will also depend on the actual spatial dose distribution of the activity. The two commonly used dosimetry models that improve on single-compartment package insert dosimetry are the partition model (PM)[14] and voxel dosimetry (VD).[15]

The PM offers improvement over the standard package insert dosimetry by computing doses separately for tumor and normal liver (NL) volumes. Nevertheless, PM can still lead to significant deviations in predicted doses in many cases due to (1) the implicit assumption that microsphere distributions are uniform within each of the tumor and NL compartments, (2) the uncertainty in determining the tumor to NL uptake ratio (TNR) required for PM calculations, and (3) its inability to address multiple tumors with different sizes and/or uptake. VD enables the determination of individual tumor doses and dose distributions rather than aggregating all tumors as a single compartment. This requires quantitative knowledge of the in vivo spatial distribution of the activity concentration in Bq/mL—usually accomplished using Y90 SPECT/CT or Y90 PET/CT. Although the spatial distribution of dose deposition is explicitly accounted for with voxel dosimetry, it demands high-quality input images.

Ultimately, tumor and NL response to radioembolization are dependent on the actual delivered radiation dose distribution. Fundamental differences exist between planning dosimetry using the in vivo distribution of 99mTc-MAA and the actual delivered dose distribution using the in vivo distribution of 90Y-microspheres, which can lead to differences in dose calculation. Such differences can occur from two factors: (1) the inherent image quality differences between MAA-SPECT, 90Y-SPECT, and 90Y-PET (even if the underlying raw signal distribution is identical), and (2) the different in vivo distributions of MAA and 90Y particles that stem from a number of treatment-day–specific parameters such as catheter tip location, flow dynamics, and number of particles. Therefore definitive estimates of tumor and NL doses achieved with radioembolization must be based on posttherapy 90Y-SPECT and 90Y-PET images acquired after Y90 delivery (Fig. 94B.1).

CLINICAL EVIDENCE

Primary Liver Tumors

Hepatocellular Carcinoma (see Chapter 89)

The role of SIRT in hepatocellular carcinoma (HCC) was first explored in the setting of portal vein thrombosis (PVT). In

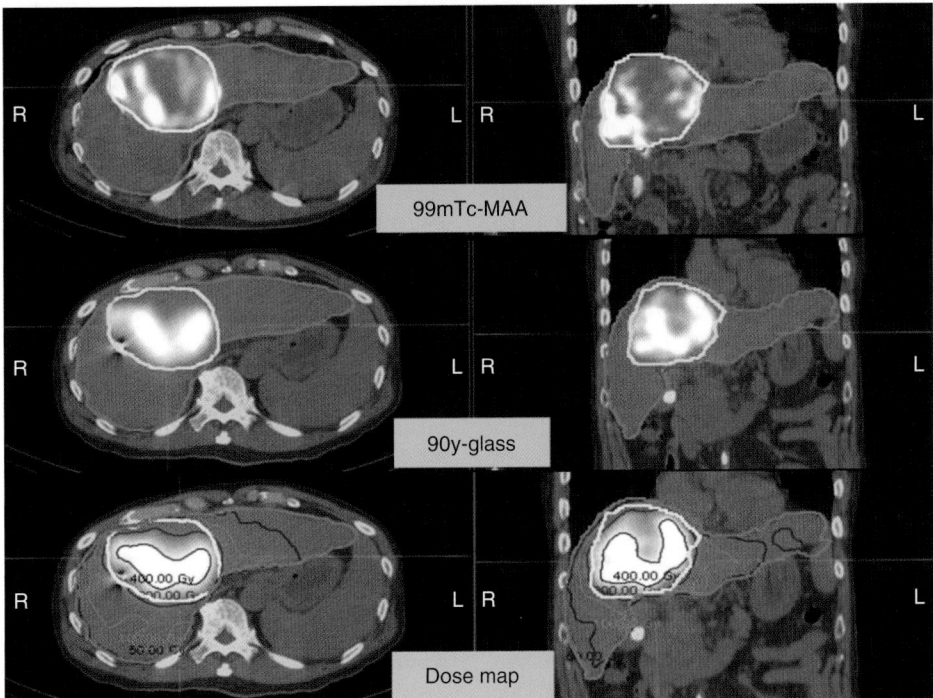

FIGURE 94B.1 Example of the value of imaging and differences in dose estimates based on the model used for dose calculation in a patient with hepatocellular carcinoma (HCC) treated with ^{90}Y-radioembolization (glass microspheres). *Top panel:* ^{99m}Tc-macro-aggregate albumin (MAA) single-photon emission computed tomography (SPECT/CT) images used for planning. *Middle panel:* ^{90}Y-microsphere SPECT/CT images used for treatment delivery verification. *Bottom panel:* Resulting voxel level dose map with isodose lines. The patient has a solitary large HCC *(yellow contour)* with an estimated volume of 449 mL and underwent whole-liver treatment (2036 mL) with 5.51 GBq of activity. The mean dose to whole-liver treatment *(blue contour)* using package insert dosimetry (single-compartment uniform distribution) was estimated to be 118 Gy. The mean dose to the tumor and normal liver compartments based on partition model was estimated to be 306 Gy and 80 Gy, respectively. The actual dose distribution in the tumor and normal liver compartments was heterogeneous as evident by the isodose lines shown on the bottom panel, with large regions of the tumor receiving greater than 400 Gy, and large areas of the normal liver receiving less than 100 Gy.

2004 Salem et al.[16] reported on the safety of SIRT in unresectable HCC patients with PVT. In 2008 a similar two-center phase 2 study investigated the safety of SIRT in 108 unresectable HCC patients with and without PVT of the branch or main portal vein.[17] No cases of radiation-induced gastritis or pneumonitis were reported and there was no increased risk of hepatic failure or encephalopathy in both studies. With the safety profile of SIRT better understood, several studies began to examine long-term treatment outcomes across stages. In the first long-term outcomes analysis for 291 HCC patients treated with SIRT, Salem et al.[18] noted a TTP for the entire patient cohort of 7.9 months varied by Child-Pugh stage (CPS) (see Chapter 4), as did survival outcomes. Even if PVT is not a contraindication for SIRT, prognosis is closely correlated to the PVT extension; in fact, Kulik et al.[17] reported an overall survival (OS) of 4.4 months in patients with main PVT, 9.9 months in patients with branch PVT, and 15.4 months in patients without PVT. Similar results were obtained with the resin microspheres (OS of 9.7, 10.7, and 15.3 months for main PVT, branch PVT, and no PVT, respectively).[19] In 2013 Mazzaferro et al.[20] conducted the first phase 2 study examining the efficacy and long-term outcomes of SIRT. They observed that OS was correlated to CPS and, in particular, with the presence and the extension of PVT, reporting that patients with CPS A and branch PVT had OS similar to that of patients with CPS A without PVT (17 months vs. 18 months). Another European series of 104 patients showed that median OS differed significantly between patients with segmental and lobar/main PVT.[21] More recently, Spreafico et al.[22] proposed a prognostic score for survival, validated by other groups,[23] where the variables independently correlated with OS were bilirubin, extension of PVT, and tumor burden. Likewise, a recent retrospective analysis sought to elucidate baseline patient characteristics and prognostic factors in unresectable HCC patients termed "Super Survivors" (alive greater than 3 years after SIRT). The variables identified were imaging response to SIRT, CPS, PVT, and segmental (versus lobar) SIRT delivery.[24]

In recent years there have been several studies comparing the efficacy of SIRT to TACE (see Chapter 94A) and systemic therapies (see Chapter 99). About SIRT versus TACE, the first paper about this topic was published in 2011, reporting similar survival times (20.5 months vs. 17.4 months, respectively) but longer time-to-progression of SIRT (13.3 months vs. 8.4 months, $P = .046$).[25] Other retrospective studies[26–28] showed similar results, and in 2016 a systematic review and meta-analysis of 5 studies and 553 patients showed no significant survival differences for up to 4 years between the groups.[29] In 2016 the results of the PREMIERE trial, a landmark phase 2 study, discovered a significantly longer median TTP for patients receiving SIRT when compared with TACE (26 months vs. 6.8 months, $P = .0012$), although no differences in survival were noted.[30]

The relative efficacy of SIRT versus sorafenib for advanced HCC patients was evaluated in the SARAH trial,[13] a phase III, randomized, controlled, open-label, multicenter trial that included 459 locally advanced HCC patients or those previously treated with two unsuccessful rounds of TACE. The median OS was not significantly different between the two treatment arms (8.0 vs. 9.9 months for the SIRT and sorafenib groups, respectively). Median PFS was similar between the two groups. Higher rates of treatment-related adverse events were noted in the sorafenib group. Another randomized, phase III, open-label, multicenter trial comparing sorafenib to SIRT in 360 patients with locally advanced HCC with and without vascular invasion (SIRveNIB)[12] reported similar results: median OS was not statistically different between the two groups (8.8 vs. 10.0 months in the SIRT and sorafenib groups, respectively). Both randomized studies were negative and demonstrated no survival benefits for SIRT when compared with sorafenib. However, these results must be interpreted with caution, and there are many questionable points to consider.[31] First of all, failure of rejecting the null hypothesis in a superiority trial should be distinguished from the concept used in a noninferiority trial, in which a noninferiority margin is set a priori and generally larger sample sizes are needed.[32] Consequently, neither the results of SIRveNIB nor the results of SARAH trials could be instrumental to claim for an equivalency between SIRT and sorafenib. A second relevant point is that SIRT is a sophisticated technical procedure that requires high skills, after a considerable learning curve. The expertise in managing such treatment might have been highly heterogeneous in both the SIRveNIB trial (which was conducted at 11 centers, among which only 5 had facilities to perform SIRT) and the SARAH trial (which was conducted at 25 centers). Moreover, considering that SIRT is a form of radiotherapy, dosimetric considerations should be further elucidated; no endpoints regarding tumor-absorbed dose and liver-absorbed dose were planned, whereas a clear tumor dose-response relationship has been demonstrated in several studies.[33] It is important to recognize that these prospective trials, along with SIRFLOX and FOXFIRE discussed later in this chapter, employed rudimentary activity/dose calculation schema that did not differentiate between tumor and normal liver compartments, leading to indeterminant absorbed doses within them.[34] Recent advances in our understanding of SIRT dosimetry demonstrate the benefits of patient-specific dosimetry that results in different treatment strategies for different anatomy, previous treatments, biodistribution, and disease heterogeneity. Recommendation on the clinical and dosimetric considerations for Y90 radioembolization for HCC from an international multidisciplinary working group has been recently published.[35] Finally, SIRT is particularly effective in those patients with PVT limited to primary or secondary order branches of the portal vein; in both studies, subgroup analyses were not designed to target survival differences according to PVT extension.

Intrahepatic Cholangiocarcinoma (see Chapter 50)

Ibrahim et al.[36] conducted a study of 24 patients with histologically proven intrahepatic cholangiocarcinoma (ICC) and reported that median OS was 14.9 months from the time of the first treatment, significantly prolonged in patients with ECOG 0, without PVT and with peripheral tumors. A second and more recent study of the same group[37] confirmed these initial results; survival varied according to the presence of multifocal, infiltrative, or bilobar disease. On a comprehensive review, based on a pooled analysis, Al-Adra et al.[38] found an overall weighted median survival of 15.5 months. However, the authors pointed out the heterogeneity of the study populations included in the pooled OS; in fact, all the studies reported survival since the initiation of SIRT but, in some cases, the patients had undergone systemic chemotherapy before or during the treatment. About this, Edeline et al.[39] and Mosconi et al.[40] showed that SIRT combined with chemotherapy seems to be a promising strategy as first-line treatment for unresectable ICC; Edeline et al.[39] observed median PSF of 10.3 months, longer when chemotherapy was given concomitantly than when chemotherapy was given before SIRT, with respective median of 20.0 versus 8.8 months ($P = .001$) (median OS was not reached). Mosconi et al. showed a median OS of 17.9 months with better significantly median survival in the treatment-naive patients compared with previously treated patients (52 vs. 16 months, $P = .009$).[40,41]

Cucchetti et al.[41] performed a meta-regression study, confirming the following: naive ICC treated with SIRT had a 2-year survival of 50.4% whereas ICC treated after failure/recurrence of a previous treatment had a 2-year survival of 23.6%. They also observed that ICC morphology and location play a relevant role, with a median pooled survival of the infiltrative type of 8.2 months versus 19.3 months of peripheral ICC. Recently a phase 2 clinical trial[42] reported that the combination chemotherapy and SIRT had antitumor activity as first-line treatment of unresectable ICC, and a significant proportion of patients were downstaged to surgical intervention. A recent international multicenter study ($n = 115$) on efficacy and toxicity of radioembolization with 90Y resin microspheres for patients with ICC[43] reported median OS from first diagnosis of 29 months with 1-, 3-, and 5-year OS rates of 85%, 31%, and 8%, respectively. Median OS after treatment was 11 months with 1- and 3-year OS rates of 44% and 4%, respectively.

The most relevant studies published to date on the use of SIRT for primary liver cancer are summarized on Table 94B.1.

Secondary Liver Tumors

Colorectal Liver Metastasis (see Chapter 90)

Liver resection remains the gold-standard local curative therapy for patients with colorectal liver metastasis (CLM) (see Chapter 101). Unfortunately, only 20% of patients with CLM are eligible for resection.[44] Unresectable patients receive systemic therapy with biological agents as neoadjuvant or definitive treatment alone or in combination with some other form of local therapy. In this context, SIRT has been used in clinical practice in combination with first-line systemic therapy as a salvage locoregional therapy and as bridge to surgery. The most relevant prospective studies published to date are summarized on Table 94B.2.[45–48]

SIRT With First-Line Therapy

One of the first studies on the use of SIRT as first-line therapy published by Gray et al.[45] examined its combination with floxuridine hepatic artery infusion (HAI) in a randomized phase III trial. This showed that the addition of a single administration of SIRT to HAI regimen was associated with a statistically significantly longer time to liver progression (15.9 [SIRT + HAI] vs. 9.7 [HAI alone] months, $P = .001$), reduction of carcinoembryonic antigen (CEA) levels, and acceptable safety profile.[45]

TABLE 94B.1   Summary of Results of Selected Published Studies on the Use of SIRT in Patients With Primary Liver Cancers

TUMOR HISTOLOGY STUDY/AUTHOR NAME	STUDY ARMS	STUDY DESIGN	PATIENT POPULATION	SUMMARY OF RESULTS
Hepatocellular Carcinoma				
SARAH Trial[13]	SIRT vs. sorafenib	Phase III, randomized, open-label, multicenter	459 locally advanced HCC patients who failed two rounds of TACE	• No differences in OS (8 vs. 9.9 months) and PFS between two cohorts
SIRveNIB12	SIRT vs. sorafenib	Phase III, randomized, open-label, multicenter	360 locally advanced patients without vascular invasion	• No differences in OS (8.8 vs. 10 months) and PFS between two cohorts
Intrahepatic Cholangiocarcinoma				
Edeline J et al.[42]	Evaluation of SIRT in combination with systemic chemotherapy as first-line treatment	Phase II	41 patients with unresectable ICC who have never received chemotherapy or intraarterial therapy	• Combination chemotherapy and SIRT had antitumor activity as first-line treatment with a median OS of 22 months • Significant proportion of patients (22%) were downstaged to surgical intervention
Mosconi et al.[40]	OS, tumor response, and the safety of radioembolization	Retrospective	23 patients with unresectable ICC	• Longer survival was obtained in treatment-naive patients as compared with patients in whom SIRT was preceded by other treatments, including surgery (52 vs. 16 months, $P = .009$)

ICC, Intrahepatic cholangiocarcinoma; OS, overall survival; PFS, progression-free survival; SIRT, selective internal radiation therapy; TACE, transarterial chemoembolization.

TABLE 94B.2   Summary of Results of Selected Published Studies on the Use of SIRT in Patients With Colorectal Liver Metastasis

STUDY/AUTHOR NAME	STUDY ARMS	STUDY DESIGN	PATIENT POPULATION	SUMMARY OF RESULTS
Gray et al.[45]	Floxuridine HAI alone vs. in combination with single SIRT administration	Phase III, randomized trial	74 patients with bilobar, unresectable CLM	• Improved radiologic response for combined SIRT arm • Improved median time to disease progression in the liver (15.9 [SIRT + HAI] vs. 9.7 [HAI alone] months, $P = .001$)
Van Hazel et al.[46]	5-fluorouracil and leucovorin alone vs. in combination with a single SIRT administration	Phase II, randomized trial	21 patients with untreated advanced CLM (irrespective of extrahepatic disease)	• Improved radiologic response for arm with combined SIRT • Improved median survival for arm with combined SIRT (29.4 vs. 12.8 months, $P = .025$) • Longer time to progression of disease for combined SIRT arm
SIRFLOX Study[11]	First-line mFOLFOX6 ± bevacizumab vs. mFOlFOX6 ± bevacizumab plus with single SIRT administration	Phase III, multicenter, randomized trial	530 patients with treatment-naive liver-only/dominant CLM	• No differences in PFS at any site • Significant improvement PFS in the liver for SIRT combined arm (20.5 vs. 12.6 months, $P = .002$)
Combined analysis of FOXFIRE, SIRFLOX, and FOXFIRE-Global[47]	First-line FOLFOX vs. FOLFOX plus single SIRT administration	Combination of three phase III, multicenter, randomized trials	1103 chemotherapy-naive patients with unresectable CLM	• No improvement in OS • Improvement in liver-specific PFS and best radiologic response for SIRT combined arm • Improvement in OS among patients right-side primary tumors on combined SIRT arm
Hendlisz et al.[48]	Chemorefractory patients treated with 5-FU alone vs. 5-FU plus SIRT	Phase III, multicenter, randomized trial	46 patients with unresectable chemorefractory liver-limited CLM	• Significant improvement on time to liver progression and time to tumor progression on SIRT combined arm • No differences in OS

CLM, Colorectal liver metastasis; HAI, hepatic artery infusion; OS, overall survival; PFS, progression-free survival; SIRT, selective internal radiation therapy.

Subsequently, a phase II randomized study evaluated the use of 5-fluorouracil and leucovorin alone or in combination with a single administration of SIRT.[46] This study demonstrated that the addition of a single administration of SIRT was associated with better median survival (29.4 vs. 12.8 months, $P = .025$), longer time to progression (18.6 vs. 3.6 months, $P < .0005$), and a higher objective response rate.[46]

More recently, with the incorporation of oxaliplatin- and irinotecan-based chemotherapies to colorectal cancer, several studies have evaluated the value of SIRT with such new systemic regimens. Sharma et al.[49] examined on a phase I study the maximum-tolerated oxaliplatin dose as part of FOLFOX regimen to be used in combination with SIRT, defining this as 60 mg/m^2 for the first three cycles. Similarly, van Hazel et al.[50] performed a dose escalation study of irinotecan-naive patients submitted to irinotecan systemic therapy combined with SIRT. A maximum-tolerated dose was not reached. Based on the positive safety profile results of such studies, large-scale studies were conducted to evaluate the efficacy of adding SIRT to the contemporary systemic therapy regimens. The SIRFLOX study, a phase III randomized clinical trial, included 530 patients with treatment-naive liver-only/dominant CLM, and compared standard chemotherapy regimen (mFOLFOX6 ± bevacizumab) alone or in combination with single SIRT administration. Its results showed that its primary endpoint, overall progression-free survival, was not different with the addition of SIRT to the FOLFOX-based first-line chemotherapy. Nevertheless, statistically significantly improvement on median progression-free survival in the liver was noted on the SIRT + systemic arm (20.5 [SIRT + systemic] vs. 12.6 [systemic only] months, $P = .002$).[11] Subsequently, a combined analysis of three multicenter, randomized, phase III trials evaluated overall survival outcomes in 1103 chemotherapy-naive patients with CLM unsuitable for curative resection or ablation who were randomized to FOLFOX alone or in combination with a single SIRT treatment.[47] This analysis also did not show improvement in overall survival with the addition of SIRT to FOLFOX. Despite this negative finding, statistically significantly improvements in liver-specific progression-free survival and best radiologic response were noted among the patients receiving SIRT in combination with FOLFOX.[47] Notably, among a subgroup of 179 patients with right-side primary tumors, OS was improved with the addition of SIRT to the systemic treatment (median, 22.0 [SIRT + systemic] vs. 17.1 months [systemic alone] HR, 0.641; $P = .008$).[51] A potential explanation for the lack of overall survival results reported by these recent studies is the use of the body surface area dosimetry methodology, which might not be the optimal dosimetry methodology. A strong relationship between SIRT dose delivered to the CLM and survival was recently reported on a phase II clinical trial,[52] highlighting the criticality of a more personalized dosimetry approach for patients with CLM undergoing SIRT.

SIRT as Second-Line and Salvage Therapy

SIRT has been used in clinical practice as a second-line monotherapy, with three of the largest retrospective studies showing OS rates ranging from 12 to 14.7 months.[53-55] The role of SIRT as a second-line therapy will be better defined by the EPOCH trial, a multicenter phase III study comparing unresectable CLM patients who failed first-line systemic chemotherapy who received standard of care second-line systemic therapy alone or in combination with SIRT.[56]

The experience with SIRT on patients with chemorefractory disease has been extensively published in the literature. Hendlisz et al.[48] performed a single-center phase III trial in 46 patients with unresectable, chemotherapy-refractory, liver-limited metastatic colorectal cancer comparing 5-FU alone or in combination with SIRT. The study primary endpoint, time to liver progression, was significantly longer on the combination arm (5.5 [SIRT + 5-FU] vs. 2.1 [5-FU only] months, HR = 0.38; 95% CI, 0.20 to 0.72; $P = .003$), and a trend on median OS was observed (10 [SIRT + 5-FU] vs. 7.3 months [5-FU only], HR = 0.92; 95% CI, 0.47 to 1.78; $P = .80$).[48] A prospective phase II multicenter study including 50 patients who failed prior irinotecan- or oxaliplatin-based chemotherapy regimens reported median OS of 12.6 months and both PFS and TTP of 3.7 months.[57] The results of such prospective studies are also reflected on the largest retrospective series, which demonstrated median OS ranging from 9.1 to 11.9 months,[54,55,58,59] and are on a par with the survival rates of modern chemotherapy regimens used in the third-line setting,[60,61] highlighting the potential meaningful survival benefit of SIRT on this patient population.

Yttrium-90 Radioembolization Before Surgical Resection

Limited reports exist in regard to the use of SIRT for borderline resectable patients.[62-64] Justinger et al.[63] reported the use of SIRT in 13 patients with marginally resectable CLM. Twelve patients achieved potentially resectable disease after SIRT. The use of SIRT for radiation lobectomy for providing both local tumor control and future liver remnant hypertrophy was investigated by Vouche et al.[65] in 83 patients with CLM, 8 of whom were treated with a median radiation dose of 107 Gy. The authors concluded that radiation segmentectomy was a safe and effective technique to provide FLR hypertrophy.[65] Further investigations will help in understanding the value and timing of radiation segmentectomy effectiveness in comparison with other liver regenerative techniques.

Breast Cancer Liver Metastasis (see Chapter 92)

SIRT has been advocated for patients with breast cancer metastatic to the liver who have progressed or failed on standard of care polychemotherapy.[66-68] A phase II open-label study of 30 patients who received prior systemic chemotherapy and were submitted to single-session, whole-liver SIRT demonstrated an acceptable toxicity profile with partial response in 61% and stable disease in 35%. Median survival for the responders was 23.6 months versus 5.7 months for nonresponders.[66] On a retrospective single-center analysis of 83 patients, Fendler et al.[68] showed a median OS of 35 weeks. Sequential lobar (instead of whole-liver) SIRT treatment and absence of prior angiosuppressive therapy were associated with lower rate of serious adverse events. Tumor burden greater than 50% and transaminase toxicity grade ≥2 independently predicted short survival.[68] More recently, Deipolyi et al.[69] demonstrated a relationship between imaging response following SIRT and presence of PI3K pathway mutation.

Melanoma Liver Metastasis (see Chapter 92)

Melanomas include cutaneous melanoma, which accounts for greater than 90% of melanoma cases, and ocular (uveal) melanoma, which encompasses 5% of patients, with liver metastases occurring in 15% to 20% of the patients with the cutaneous form and up to 90% of the patients with the ocular form.[70,71]

Recently, remarkable improvements in progression-free and overall survival have been achieved with immunotherapy and molecularly target agents in patients with cutaneous melanoma.[72–74] Unfortunately, such improvements have not been seen for the ocular melanoma subtypes. Moreover, distinct circulating cytokines and clinicopathologic features displayed by patients with melanoma liver metastasis[75] make them less responsive to anti-PD1 and ipilimumab therapy.[76] Therefore treatment methods for specifically improving liver tumor control are needed. Gonsalves et al. performed a phase II trial on the use of SIRT for patients with uveal melanoma who were treatment-naive (group A, $n = 24$ patients) or who had progressed following immunoembolization (group B, $n = 24$ patients). Tumor growth stabilization, a critical variable on patients with uveal melanoma given its aggressive growth pattern, was seen ion 87% and 58.3% of the patients in groups A and B, respectively. Median progression-free and overall survivals for group A were 8.1 and 18.5 months, respectively, and for group B 5.2 months and 19.2 months. No cases of radiation-induced liver disease were recorded.

Neuroendocrine Cancer Liver Metastasis (see Chapter 91)

Neuroendocrine tumors (NETs) are a group of rare hormone-secreting malignancies, with the most common being the carcinoid tumors. Although most often nonfunctional, some NETs produce excessive amounts of hormones associated with debilitating clinical syndromes, such as carcinoid syndrome: vasoactive intestinal tumors (VIPomas), gastrinomas, and somatostatinomas are some examples (see Chapter 65). Metastatic disease to the liver from a primary NET is common. Preprocedure workup includes imaging studies, serum chromogranin A levels, and clinical evaluation with special emphasis on evaluating symptoms related to the carcinoid syndrome. A recent meta-analysis included 424 patients and showed a weighted average disease control rate of 86%, along with a correlation between objective response rate to SIRT with improved median survival.[77] A recent international multicenter study ($n = 244$) on efficacy and toxicity of radioembolization with 90Y resin microspheres[78] demonstrated safety and efficacy of radioembolization in NET patients with a high disease control rate of 91% and alleviation of NET-related symptoms in 79% of symptomatic patients. Currently, treatment guidelines recommend hepatic-directed therapies, including radioembolization, for patients with NET deemed unresectable with low tumor burden who have progressed under octreotide or lanreotide. For patients with clinically significant tumor burden, radioembolization might be offered as an alternative or complementary front-line therapy to octreotide or lanreotide.[79]

POSTTREATMENT MANAGEMENT

Response Assessment

For patients with HCC or ICC, tumor viability-based imaging criteria such as the modified response evaluation criteria in solid tumor (mRECIST) and European Association for the Study of Liver (EASL) are routinely utilized[30,80,81] (see Chapter 13). Such methods utilize arterial tumor enhancement as a surrogate for tumor viability and are considered an accurate predictor of histologic necrosis and are associated with favorable OS following SIRT.[18,82] Typically, changes in arterial enhancement occur up to 2 months following SIRT delivery,[80,81,83] preceding the changes in tumor size, which occurs between 4 and 6 months following SIRT.[80]

For patients with secondary liver cancers, tumor size is used as the main surrogate for tumor response. Therefore it is critical to acknowledge that tumor shrinkage might take several months to occur. Moreover, tumor pseudoprogression following SIRT is not uncommon due to intratumoral edema, hemorrhage, and necrosis. Aiming to address such issues, vRECIST and change in total lesion glycolysis have been utilized.[52,84]

Complications

Postradioembolization Syndrome

The incidence ranges from 20% to 55%[85] and consists of the following clinical symptoms: fatigue, nausea, vomiting, anorexia, fever, abdominal discomfort, and cachexia.

Hepatic Dysfunction

The incidence of radiation-induced liver disease after SIRT administration ranges from 0% to 30%, with most of the reports showing an incidence of 0% to 8% with a lethal outcome of 0% to 5%.[86,87] Radiation-induced liver disease results from the exposure of normal liver parenchyma to high doses of radiation. Clinical correlation is essential; in fact, this may lead to biochemical aberrations with minimal clinical manifestations.

Biliary Sequelae

The incidence of biliary sequelae after SIRT is less than 10%.[85] It results from radiation-induced injury to the biliary structures. The majority of biliary complications are asymptomatic. Radiation cholecystitis requiring surgical intervention is present in less than 1% of cases.[85]

Radiation Pneumonitis

The incidence of radiation pneumonitis is less than 1% if standard dosimetry models are used.[88] Radiation pneumonitis manifests as a restrictive ventilatory dysfunction. On chest CT, it has a bat-wing appearance. Management is medical with steroids. A 99mTc-MAA scan is used for calculating the mean lung doses; values less than 30 Gy per treatment and less than 50q Gy cumulatively are recommended.

Gastrointestinal Complications

With proper percutaneous techniques, the incidence of gastrointestinal (GI) ulceration is well below 5%.[85] The cause of this complication is the ectopic distribution of radioembolic microspheres into the lining of the GI tract. Cases refractory to proton pump inhibitors may require surgical management. Pretreatment angiography is essential for identifying and embolizing the hepaticoenteric collaterals that may supply the GI tract, and 99mTc-MAA scan may help to identify splanchnic flow.[89]

SUMMARY

Transarterial radioembolization with yttrium-90 is a novel, minimally invasive locoregional therapy that has gained acceptance in clinical practice. Its acceptable safety profile, outpatient nature, and growing evidence on efficacy make it an attractive alternative in the management of primary and secondary liver malignancies. Appropriate treatment requires careful patient selection, patient-specific dosimetry, and management from a high-level expertise multidisciplinary/multiprofessional team. The negative results of the most recent trials in respect to the positive impact of this therapy in overall survival outcomes highlight the need for further understanding and application of advanced dosimetry methodologies in order to maximize their oncologic benefit, while preserving patients' nontumorous liver function.

The references for this chapter can be found online by accessing the accompanying Expert Consult website.

CHAPTER 95

External beam radiotherapy for liver tumors

Marsha Reyngold and Christopher H. Crane

HISTORICAL CONTEXT AND WHOLE-LIVER RADIATION THERAPY

The efficacy of radiation therapy (RT) is predicated on the ability to deliver the tumoricidal RT dose while keeping the dose to the surrounding normal tissues the same. The balance between the probability of tumor control and the risk of normal tissue complications is a measure of the therapeutic ratio of the treatment. Irradiation of tumors using external beam RT (EBRT) will expose the surrounding organs to doses that may range up to the prescription dose of the tumor. Unfortunately, doses necessary to achieve tumor control usually overlap with those that can cause complications. In case of liver tumors, doses necessary to control disease are higher than doses that cause dysfunction of the liver parenchyma. Improvements in the therapeutic ratio for liver tumors have been primarily predicated on achieving greater conformality of RT thereby limiting exposure of the liver parenchyma and nearby gastrointestinal (GI) tract to tolerable limits. This is more challenging for larger liver tumors or when there is underlying liver disease.

Early clinical experience that revealed the low tolerance of normal liver parenchyma to RT involved irradiation of the entire liver or large parts of the organ. Radiation-induced liver disease (RILD) was described as a clinical syndrome characterized by hepatomegaly and ascites, often associated with liver function test abnormalities, most consistently with alkaline phosphatase elevation.[1,2] This clinical syndrome was associated with venoocclusive histologic changes characterized by sinusoidal congestion with fibrin deposition in central veins.[2] In the largest series of 40 patients treated with whole-liver doses ranging from 1300 to 5100 cGy, over 40% of patients who received 3800 cGy and above developed RILD, whereas no patient receiving less than 3000 cGy did.[1] Some of the patients with RILD recovered after medical management with diuretics and occasionally steroids; others subsequently died of liver failure. Due to concerns of toxicity arising from large volumes of liver receiving low doses, and despite the fact that a contemporaneous report of 26 hepatocellular carcinoma (HCC) cases treated with RT at Memorial Hospital from 1923 to 1959 with tumor doses ranging from 700 to 4500 cGy (average 2956 cGy) showed regression in 14 cases in patients who received greater than 2000 cGy,[3] the enthusiasm for RT as treatment for liver cancer waned.

The next several decades saw several failed attempts to improve the therapeutic ratio of liver irradiation by varying the fractionation size and/or combining low-dose whole-liver irradiation with cytotoxic or radiopharmaceutical agents.[4,5] Radiation Therapy Oncology Group (RTOG) study 84-05, although conducted for liver metastasis, is notable for reconfirming that dose escalation beyond 30 Gy to the whole liver is associated with high risk of complications.[4] This was a dose escalation study of whole-liver RT delivered in twice-daily fractions of 1.5 Gy based on the assumption that smaller fraction size with the same total dose may potentially lessen the effect on normal tissues and the twice-daily schedule would keep the overall treatment time the same, thus maintaining the treatment efficacy. None of the 122 patients receiving 27 Gy or 30 Gy to the whole liver developed liver injury; 5 of 51 patients receiving 33 Gy did. A subsequent RTOG study conducted in 194 patients with HCC showed that combining low-dose daily whole-liver irradiation to 2100 cGy with chemotherapy or using hyperfractionation to 2400 cGy in twice-daily fractions was associated with response rates of 22% and 18%, respectively.[5] This served as the background for future studies, which hypothesized that smaller liver volumes could tolerate higher RT doses and that higher doses would be more effective.

PARTIAL-LIVER IRRADIATION: THREE-DIMENSIONAL CONFORMAL RADIATION THERAPY (3D-CRT)

Although it was known that normal tissue tolerance depends on the amount of tissue irradiated, it was not until the tools to quantify the relationships became available in the 1980s that partial liver volume dose escalation became feasible.[6,7] The rationale for pursuing partial-liver irradiation was at least in part based on the observation that liver function can be preserved after a significant part of the liver is surgically resected. A clinical protocol carried out at the University of Michigan designed to stay within a given normal tissue complication probability allowed for delivery of focal radiation ranging from 48 to 72.6 Gy in 11 patients with localized HCC and 9 patients with cholangiocarcinoma.[8] These doses were associated with an objective response in 11 of the 11 evaluable patients compared with 1 of 6 patients who received whole-liver irradiation to 36 Gy. Following these initial steps, a series of dose escalation protocols by the same group helped to quantify the relationship between dose, irradiated volume, and RILD, and provided initial data on the dose-response relationship for liver tumors. An important step was development of a model that quantitatively described the probability of normal tissue complication for a given dose and volume irradiated.[9] Using this model with parameters that were revised as more data were accumulated, the investigators gained a better ability to describe the risk of RILD, compare alternate radiation plans, and individualize radiation on the basis of the predicted probability of toxicity. These data also showed that patients with primary liver tumors had a greater risk of RILD than patients with metastatic disease, likely secondary to underlying cirrhosis often associated with the former.

Two consecutive prospective trials conducted between 1996 and 2003 relied on the strategy of maximizing tumor dose using the prospectively validated predictive model of toxicity related to dose and volume of liver treated.[10] In doing so they were able to establish objective volumetric dose parameters or constraints that minimize the risk of RILD and laid the foundation for further study of RT in the treatment of inoperable liver tumors.[11] Between April 1996 and April 2003, 81 patients with primary liver cancers along with 47 patients with colorectal liver metastases were treated with hepatic arterial floxuridine and focal liver RT to 40 to 90 Gy (median, 60.75 Gy) in 1.5-Gy twice-daily fractions with a planned 2-week break. Median survival rates in HCC and cholangiocarcinoma, slightly inferior to colorectal metastatic cancer, were 15.2 and 13.3 months, respectively, with a trend for improved survival with higher doses. Importantly, the total dose was the only significant factor associated with survival. Similar results were noted in a prospective phase II trial from France that included Child-Pugh (CP) A/B cirrhotic patients with small-size HCC (1 nodule ≤5 cm, or 2 nodules ≤3 cm) unsuitable for other curative treatments.[12] Twenty-seven patients were treated with a dosing strategy that conformed to the approach put forth by the University of Michigan, with all except for one patient receiving 66 Gy in 2 Gy/fraction using three-dimensional conformal radiation therapy (3D-CRT). Objective response was 92% with only transient grade 4 liver toxicity noted exclusively in CP B patients. As new technologies emerged, they were investigated in the treatment of primary liver tumors in an effort to achieve even better tumor control.

INTENSITY-MODULATED RADIATION THERAPY AND STEREOTACTIC BODY RADIATION THERAPY

Intensity-modulated radiation therapy (IMRT) is an advanced radiation technology that further improves on the conformality of dose delivery to the target and allows for greater control of doses that spill into normal organs. It involves a computational optimization process that selects RT beam directions and modulates the intensity of each beam to gain the desired target coverage while minimizing the dose to the normal organs based on the tumor target and normal structures outlined by the physician on the simulation computed tomography (CT) or, more recently, magnetic resonance imaging (MRI). IMRT allows for greater control of dose distribution, which makes individual radiation plans more customizable to the patient's individual anatomy. Due to its superior dosimetry, IMRT has significant advantages over 3D-CRT whenever there is a radiosensitive organ such as the stomach or duodenum near the tumor. Stereotactic body radiotherapy (SBRT) usually incorporates IMRT along with image guidance and organ motion management to deliver larger doses per treatment with increased precision.[13] The mechanism of cell killing for these higher doses of RT is predicted to be more multifaceted than that of standard fractionation and may result in a more ablative effect.[14] However, not all the doses delivered with the SBRT technique are high enough to have an ablative effect. Attention should be paid when interpreting the results of SBRT studies whether ablative or nonablative doses are used.

For image guidance, radiopaque fiducial markers can be percutaneously introduced into or at the periphery of the liver tumor to aid with tumor alignment, but soft tissue image guidance is critical to assess the dose delivery to organs in proximity to liver tumors, which move from day to day, such as the stomach and duodenum. The imaging components of radiation treatment delivery systems have evolved from two-dimensional radiographs to three-dimensional CT or MRI that allows for soft tissue visualization. The most significant recent innovation is real-time adaptive planning, which enables changing the radiation dose distribution every day to address changes in internal organ position. This capability is very valuable for left lobe tumors due to the variable relative position of the stomach relative to the liver from day to day.

In the past, respiratory motion and day-to-day organ motion were largely ignored. Larger volumes were treated with lower doses with limited benefit. Motion management techniques were critical innovations that enabled the delivery of ablative doses near radiosensitive organs such as the stomach. Diaphragmatic motion during breathing is associated with significant liver displacement and deformation. The average displacement during quiet breathing in the supine position has been reported by a number of investigators to range between 8 and 25 mm.[15] There are multiple strategies to control or compensate for respiratory motion. The most common and most straightforward technique to control breathing motion is inspiration or expiration breath-hold. Respiratory gating and tracking during treatment are ways to account for breathing motion. Gating allows for the beam to only turn on at the prespecified portion of the breathing cycle, typically end expiration when the diaphragm is still and relaxed. Tracking is an emerging option that allows for the treatment beam to follow the internal motion. Compensating for the range of tumor motion during breathing with or without abdominal compression to minimize diaphragmatic excursion is sufficient for many liver tumors that are not near the stomach, colon, or duodenum. Respiratory gating is available in a number of standard radiation delivery systems. More versatile systems also allow for it to be combined with soft tissue image guidance to address day-to-day organ motion.

Hepatocellular Carcinoma (see Chapter 89)

SBRT was initially developed for intracranial tumors. The first SBRT experience for primary liver tumors was reported as a part of a pilot of extracranial SBRT in 31 patients at the Karolinska Institute using a variety of doses and methodology that evolved over the study period.[16] This study included 8 with HCC and 1 with intrahepatic cholangiocarcinoma (IHCC) treated with 16 to 66 Gy in 1 to 3 fractions, with impressive objective response rates (70%).

Utilizing an individualized dose allocation approach based on the model of toxicity developed by researchers at the University of Michigan, the group at Princess Margaret Hospital was the first to conduct a prospective trial of SBRT in primary liver tumors.[17] The study included 31 patients with unresectable CP A HCC who underwent six-fraction SBRT with a median dose of 36.0 Gy (24.0–54.0 Gy). Median survival of HCC patients was 11.7 months. There was no RILD, but there was a decline in CP classification from A to B in seven patients (17%).

This experience established SBRT as a promising alternative to surgery with several prospective phase I and II trials reported since with durable local control (LC) ranging from 65% to 100% and overall survival (OS) at 1 and 2 years ranging from 55% to 75% and 32% to 84%, respectively (Table 95.1).[18–26] The individual studies differ with regard to fractionation schemes as well as patient characteristics such as tumor size or stage, extent of cirrhosis, proportion of patients with tumor vascular thrombus (TVT), and prior liver-directed therapy.

TABLE 95.1 Select Prospective Phase I/II Studies of SBRT for HCC

STUDY	FRACTIONATION SCHEME	N	MEDIAN SIZE, CM (RANGE)[a]	CP CLASS	TVT	PRIOR LOCAL THERAPY	2Y LC	2Y OS	MEDIAN SURVIVAL, MONTHS	GRADE 3[b] GI/LIVER TOXICITY OR CHANGE IN CP
Mendez Romero et al.[24] (2002-2006)	30-37.5 Gy in 3 25 Gy in 5	8	3.2 (0.5-7.2)	A: 62.5% B: 25%	37.5%	NR	75% (22 mo)	40%	NR	12.5% (12.5% Gr 5 RILD)
Tse et al.[27] (2003-2006)	24-54 Gy in 6	31	[a]173 mL (9-1913)	A: 100%	52%	58%	65% (1Y)	48% (1Y)	11.7	26%
Bujold et al.[28] (2004-2010)	24-54 Gy in 6	102	7.2 (1.4-23.1)	A: 100%	55%	61%	87% (1Y)	34%	17	30% (6.9% Gr 5) 29% and 6% CP class ↓ at 6 and 12 mo
Cardenes et al.[25] (2005-2007)	36-48 Gy in 3 40 Gy in 5	17	4 (2-6)	A: 35% B: 65%	18%	23.5%	100%[c]	60%	NR	18% RILD
Lasley et al.[21] (2005-2012)	48 Gy in 3 40 Gy in 5	59	[a]33.6 mL (2.0-107.3)	A: 64% B: 36%	18%	16%	A: 91% B: 82%	A: 72% B: 32.7%	A: 44.8 B: 17	Gr 3 + 4: A: 10.5% B: 38%
Kang et al.[23] (2008-2011)	42-60 Gy in 3	47	2.9 (1.3-7.8)	A: 87% B: 13%	11%	100% TACE	94.6%	68.7%	NR	6.4% (4.3% Gr 4)
Takeda et al.[19] (2007-2012)	35-40 Gy in 5	90	2.3 (1.0-4.0)	A: 91% B: 9%	3%	65% (TACE)	96% (3Y)	67% (3Y)	54.7	8.9% CP ↓ 2 p
Moon et al.[22] (2009-2014)	7.5-45 Gy in 3-5	11	3.5 (1.7-6.5)[d]	A: 93% B: 7%	NS	46.7%[d]	82% (1Y)	36% (1y)	20.8[d]	3%
Feng et al.[20] (2010-2014)	23-60 Gy in 5	69	3 cm (0-13)	A: 77% B: 23%	18%	Median 2	95%	NR	NR	7% CP 2 p ↓
Weiner et al.[26] (2012-2014)	40-55 Gy in 5	12	5.0 (1.6-12.3)[d]	A: 88%[d] B: 12%	27%[d]	47%[d]	91% (1Y)	38% (1y)	9.8	46% (8.0% Gr 5 RILD)[d] 35% CP ↓ 2 p[d]
Kim et al.[29] (2012-2015)	36-60 Gy in 4	32	2.1 (1.0-4.5)	A: 88% B: 12%	0	81%	81%	81%	NR	3% CP 2 p ↓
Jang et al.[18] (2012-2015)	45-60 Gy in 3	65	2.4 (1.0-9.9)	A: 64 A 1 B	6%	100% (TACE)	97%	84% 76% (3Y)	NR	2% 2% nonclassic RILD

CP, Child-Pugh; GI, gastrointestinal; HCC, hepatocellular carcinoma; LC, local control; OS, overall survival.

[a]Volume is reported where largest size is not available (mL).

[b]No greater than Gr 3 unless otherwise specified.

[c]Crude rate.

[d]Characteristics for the entire study population if HCC-specific characteristics are not available.

Several points should be made regarding the collective SBRT experience. Although extreme hypofractionation of 6 or fewer fractions can be quite effective for smaller lesions, the dose often has to be reduced for larger lesions to remain within the safe parameters with regard to the surrounding normal tissues. However, one important consequence of this is the relative decrease in the therapeutic ratio of RT. Practically, this means that for large liver tumors, the individualized safe treatment dose in 6 fractions may be too low to control the tumor and is no longer considered ablative. In a prospective protocol limited to lesions of 4 cm in size enrolling 90 patients with HCC with median size of 2.3 cm and receiving doses ranging from 35 to 40 Gy in 5 fractions, Takeda et al.[19] observed excellent 3-year LC of 96% and OS of 67%. This is in contrast to the most recent update of the Princess Margaret experience, which included 102 patients with HCC enrolled in two sequential phase I and II studies of individualized 6-fraction SBRT ranging up to 54 Gy. The tumors were large, with a median size of 7 cm, and 55% had TVT, which often requires a larger treatment field, resulting in the median prescription dose of only 36 Gy. Perhaps, as a consequence the 1-year LC of 87% and median and 1-year OS of 17 months and 55%, respectively. These outcomes were inferior compared with the SBRT trials that excluded large lesions and with proton data where more protracted fractionation schemes are more commonly used (outlined in a later section).[28] A dose-response relationship has been described by some investigators[28,30] and may be size dependent. Another manifestation of the reduced therapeutic ratio associated with extreme hypofractionation is a higher rate of toxicity: accordingly, the rate of grade ≥3 toxicity was high in the Princess Margaret experience with 7 patients dying of treatment-related causes.[28] This underscores the need for using more protracted ablative fractionation schemes with either hypofractionated IMRT or proton beam therapy (PBT) for lesions requiring large treatment fields.

In addition, although SBRT is safe for patients with normal liver function, it is associated with greater risk of classic RILD and nonclassic liver decompensation in patients with cirrhosis, which may be further compounded by toxicity of other liver-directed therapies. The risk of liver decompensation correlates with Child-Pugh (CP) scores[21] (see Chapter 4). Furthermore, an increase in the CP score by 2 points or more within 3 months of SBRT has been shown to correlate with mortality and has become a more sensitive and informative way of reporting hepatic dysfunction.[31] Many protocols limit enrollment to patients with CP B liver disease or use more stringent liver constraints when planning RT for these patients. A more novel approach is to go beyond individualizing RT dose based on a population-based model of normal tissue complication for a given CP class toward a more personalized and rigorous risk-adaptive strategy based on the functional assessment of the individual patient's liver function. The group at the University of Michigan has found that subclinical decline in a patient's liver function after RT could be estimated by assessing indocyanine green (ICG) extraction, which is removed from the circulation only by the liver and thus is a direct measurement of dynamic liver function.[20,32] Using ICG retention at 15 minutes as a direct biomarker of liver function, they adapted the planned 5-fraction SBRT course midway through the course of therapy to maintain liver function after the complete course. As a result of the individualized approach, 2-point decline in CP score was seen in 7%, and excellent LC of 95% at 2 years was achieved

for HCC patients.[20] Another direction to explore is imaging markers for spatial assessment of liver function after RT, such as portal venous perfusion changes.

The promising SBRT results provided the basis for an ongoing RTOG randomized controlled trial of SBRT followed by sorafenib versus sorafenib alone (NCT01730937). The study was designed at the time when sorafenib was the standard of care for unresectable patients. Despite recent advances in systemic options that have expanded beyond sorafenib, the trial will answer an important question regarding the benefit of adding effective local therapy to systemic therapy.

Another currently unresolved question is selection of inoperable HCC patients for SBRT (or another ablative RT technology) versus a different liver-directed therapy. While some of the selection is based on anatomic and practical considerations where tumors unsuitable for other modalities are referred to radiation oncology departments, there is a large group of patients who are eligible for multiple options. Several ongoing trials aim to compare SBRT with TACE or RFA. In addition, a combination of low-dose RT with TACE was recently shown to be a safe strategy superior to sorafenib alone,[33] thus setting the stage for future exploration of combination therapy.

Intrahepatic Cholangiocarcinoma (see Chapter 50)

The data on the use of EBRT for IHCC have primarily consisted of heterogeneous single-institution series that often included other biliary or liver malignancies. The Princess Margaret 6-fraction SBRT trial discussed previously included 10 patients with IHCC and reported a median survival of 15 months for that group.[17] A Stanford single-fraction dose escalation SBRT study for liver malignancies ≤5 cm included 5 IHCC among 26 enrolled patients with 2-year OS of 53.6% in primary liver tumors.[34]

The most comprehensive analysis was reported by investigators from MD Anderson and included 79 consecutive patients.[35] The majority of the patients had large tumors with the median diameter 7.9 cm (range, 2.2–17 cm) and had received systemic chemotherapy before radiation. A range of RT doses from 35 to 100 Gy (median, 58.05 Gy) had been used over the study period, in part reflecting changing institutional practice patterns over time and the evolution of the RT delivery techniques. The majority were treated with IMRT, although a minority of patients received PBT or 3D-CRT. The median OS from the time of diagnosis was 30 months and the 3-year OS rate was 44%. A dose-response relationship was noted. Patients treated with doses above the median had 3-year LC and OS rates of 73% and 73%, respectively, compared with 45% and 38% in patients below the median. No significant treatment-related toxicity was noted. This experience was the first to establish that dose escalation beyond a median bioequivalent dose of 80.5 Gy resulted in improved tumor control, less disease-related liver failure, and longer survival than palliative doses of radiation.

PROTON BEAM THERAPY

Proton therapy is a form of external beam radiation therapy that uses charged particles to cause potentially lethal direct DNA damage to tumor cells. The benefit of protons derives from the unique dose distribution in tissue compared with conventional photon beams. When passing through tissue, a proton beam deposits increasing dose slowly until reaching a peak, known as the Bragg peak, at the depth that correlates with its energy. This eliminates the exit dose seen with photons, resulting in a lower integral dose to normal tissues compared with IMRT. Specifically for liver malignancies, this means that the same prescription dose to the tumor can be delivered with greater sparing of the liver parenchyma compared with the photon-based treatments.[36] Because the tolerance of the liver to radiation is related to restricting the lower doses, protons are a particular advantage for larger liver tumors in patients with underlying liver disease and when large doses per fraction are given. The main dosimetric disadvantage of PBT, compared with IMRT, is the wider penumbra, or the beam's edge, making it more challenging to spare nearby sensitive structures where a curved, rather than straight, dose gradient is required.

Although therapeutic PBT dates back to 1950s, the adoption of this radiation modality has become more widespread recently due to technologic advances. Data have emerged to support its use for liver tumors as discussed in the subsequent section. NRG-GI003 (NCT03186898) is a randomized phase III trial evaluating photons versus protons in HCCs larger than 4 cm with an OS endpoint that will direct the impact of protons in HCC. Carbon ion irradiation is another form of particle radiation therapy. In addition to sharing the dose distribution qualities of proton therapy, carbon ions also have a higher linear energy transfer, which results in greater biologic effectiveness, and a smaller penumbra, which combines the physical advantages of photons and protons. However, due to the cost, there are only two carbon ion centers in the world and clinical experience and published data are limited.

Hepatocellular Carcinoma

Much of the early clinical experience with PBT for HCC came from the University of Tsukuba in Japan, where HCC is endemic.[37] The largest retrospective series from the institution

included 318 patients treated from 2001 through 2007. Most were allocated to one of three fractionation schemes based on anatomic considerations with regard to liver hilum and the luminal GI tract, ranging from 66 GyE in 10 fractions to 77 GyE in 35 fractions and previously determined to be equally effective.[38] The majority of the patients had CP A cirrhosis (73.6%) and many (61.9%) had prior liver-directed therapy. OS was 89.5%, 64.7%, and 44.6% at 1, 3, and 5 years, respectively. Survival was affected by CP status with 3- and 5-year survival rates of 69.1% and 55.9%, respectively, for patients with CP A disease and 51.9% and 44.5%, respectively, for patients with CP B disease.

Several prospective trials have been reported (Table 95.2) with 5-year local tumor control rates of up to 90%.[38-44] The first prospective US experience from Loma Linda included 76 patients with relatively advanced disease. Over half of the patients were outside the Milan criteria with a mean tumor size of 5.5 cm.[42] Importantly, 36 and 18 patients had CP B and C cirrhosis, respectively. Patients received 63 GyE in 15 fractions. Median survival times for CP class A, B, and C patients were 34, 13, and 12 months, respectively. Eighteen patients underwent transplantation with 3-year OS of 70%. Specimen analysis from patients undergoing liver transplantation provided intriguing efficacy data: 33% of liver explants showed a pathologic complete response and 39% showed only microscopic residual disease. There were no cases of RILD or other liver function test abnormalities within the timeframe when RILD or nonclassic RILD would be expected. The most significant toxicities encountered were GI complications seen early in the trial in patients with tumors adjacent to luminal organs, and subsequently minimized with modifications in technique.

A recent US multi-institutional phase II study of high-dose hypofractionated PBT for liver tumors included 44 HCC patients with median tumor size of 5.0 cm and TVT present in

---

TABLE 95.2 Prospective Studies of Proton Beam Therapy for HCCO

STUDY	STUDY DETAILS FRACTIONATION SCHEME	N	TUMOR CHARACTERISTICS MEDIAN SIZE, CM (RANGE)	CP CLASS	PRIOR LOCAL THERAPY	2Y LC	OUTCOMES 2Y OS	MEDIAN SURVIVAL, MONTHS	GI TOXICITY GRADE 3[b]
Kawashima et al.[40] (1999-2003) Ph II	76 GyE in 20	30	4.5 (2.5-8.2)	A: 67% B: 33%	37%	96%	66%	41[a]	6
Bush et al.[42] (1998-2006) Ph I/II	63 Gy in 15	76	5.5[c] (0-10+)	A: 30% B: 47% C: 24%	NA	(5y) 80%[d]	70% (Tx) 10%[a] (no Tx) (3Y)	34 (CP A) 13 (CP B) 12 (CP C)	0
Kim et al.[43] (2007-2010) Ph I	60 GyE in 20 66 GyE in 22 72 GyE in 24	27	3.2 (2-7) 2.3 (1.5-5) 2.5 (1.3-6.2)	A: 89% B: 11%	96%	(3y) 71.4%-83.3%	(3Y) 25%-73.3%	38	0
Hong et al.[41] (2009-2015) Ph II	67.5 GyE in 15 58.05 GyE in 15	44	5.0 (1.9-12)	A: 72.7% B: 20.5%	20%	95%	63%	50	0
Bush et al.[44] (2009-ongoing) Ph IIIR	70.2 GyE in 15	69	3.2 (1.8-6.5)	NA	NA	88%	59%	30	NA

CP, Child-Pugh; GI, gastrointestinal; HCC, hepatocellular carcinoma; LC, local control; OS, overall survival; Tx, transplant.
[a]Estimated from Kaplan-Meier curve.
[b]No grade 4 or 5 toxicity was reported.
[c]Mean.
[d]Crude rate.

29.5%. Planned dose was 67.5 GyE in 15 fractions for peripheral tumors and 58.05 GyE in 15 fractions for central tumors. Dose deescalation was allowed for meeting liver constraints. Median dose delivered was 58 GyE (range, 40.5–67.5). LC and OS for this group at 2 years were 94.8% and 63.2%, respectively.[41] Importantly, very few grade 3 toxicities and no grade 4 or 5 toxicities were observed. Worsening CP score (all A to B) was noted in only 3.6%, which compares favorably with the SBRT experience.

The greater ability of PBT to spare the liver parenchyma as manifested by little change in CP scores or presence of nonclassic RILD in the proton experience has been associated with improved survival. In the toxicity analysis of 259 HCC patients treated with PBT at Tsukuba, 9 of 11 patients with a CP score increase ≥2 died from liver failure without tumor progression at 24 months.[45] In a single-institution retrospective comparison of protons versus photons in 133 patients with HCC treated with biologically equivalent ablative doses of RT, proton radiation therapy was associated with improved OS and decreased incidence of nonclassic RILD as compared with photon radiation therapy despite greater prevalence and more advanced cirrhosis in the proton group.[46] In the absence of observed differences in locoregional control, the difference in OS was postulated to result from decreased incidence of posttreatment liver decompensation.

The greater sparing of liver parenchyma associated with PBT is particularly meaningful for patients with very large tumors or significant TVT necessitating a large central field, which make it more challenging to spare uninvolved liver. In a single-institution experience of PBT in 22 patients with large HCCs measuring greater than 10 cm (median, 11 cm; range, 10–14 cm) treated with a median dose of 72.6 GyE in 22 fractions, 2-year LC and OS were 87% and 36%, respectively.[47] Several groups have reported that PBT is an effective and feasible liver-directed modality for patients with TVT.[48–50]

The ongoing NRG Oncology randomized phase III trial of photon versus proton RT (NCT03186898) should help to clarify the role of PBT therapy with regarding to liver sparing. Both 5-fraction SBRT fractionation and 15-fraction hypofractionation are allowed in both arms at the discretion of the treating physician.

A randomized trial of PBT versus TACE, which is currently the most common liver-directed therapy for advanced unresectable HCC, has recently finished enrollment and reported interim results.[44] Thirty-three patients received 70.2 Gy in 15 fractions. There was a trend toward improved 2-year local tumor control (88% vs. 45%, $P = .06$) and progression-free survival (48% vs. 31%, $P = .06$) and a 6-fold reduction in hospitalizations favoring the PBT group. The 2-year survival rate was 59% in both groups, with about one third going on to transplant, which probably served to balance the survival duration between the groups. Although more mature data are needed for

a more definitive assessment, these results provide support for inclusion of PBT in the treatment algorithm for inoperable HCC patients, especially those with poor underlying liver function, large tumors, and TVT.

Intrahepatic Cholangiocarcinoma

Hong et al.[41] reported outcomes for 39 patients with IHCC included on the multi-institutional high-dose hypofractionated PBT protocol. The median size was 6 cm (2.2–10.9 cm). The median dose delivered to the tumor was 58.0 GyE (range, 15.1–67.5 GyE) in 15 fractions, which corresponds to a biologically effective dose of 80.5 Gy. LC and OS at 2 years were 94.1% and 46.5%, respectively, and median survival was 22.5 months.

Unlike HCC, where there are many established liver-directed options, the efficacy of embolic treatment options for inoperable IHCC has not been established, possibly due to the relative hypovascularity of these tumors. As discussed elsewhere in this edition, hepatic artery infusional chemotherapy approaches have effectively led to durable local tumor control and improved survival. Collectively, the ablative RT results discussed in the IMRT section and here compare favorably with other liver-directed therapies for inoperable IHCC (Table 95.3).[41,51–56] Representative intraarterial embolic therapy series summarized in Table 95.3 have reported median OS of 9 to 15 months without an incremental improvement with the use of drug-eluting beads or radioembolization. Radiofrequency ablation has been very effective for the appropriately selected smaller tumors.

CONCLUSION

The technologic advances that have enabled RT dose escalation and contributed to a more comprehensive understanding of radiosensitivity of liver tumors and the safety limits of the normal liver parenchyma have paved the way for a renewed interest in EBRT as a complementary modality to other definitive treatment options for primary liver tumors. More precise treatment delivery enabled by the evolution of image guidance and motion management techniques and the increased conformality of RT treatment planning systems have allowed for the delivery of increasingly higher doses of RT to liver tumors safely. Retrospective and prospective studies using SBRT, image-guided ablative IMRT, and PBT have all shown high rates of LC with limited risks of hepatic decompensation or GI toxicity (Fig. 95.1). The results of ablative radiation doses seem particularly promising for the larger inoperable hepatomas compared with other options. Ongoing and future randomized comparative studies are needed to further define the optimal liver-directed modality for each subgroup of patients.

The references for this chapter can be found online by accessing the accompanying Expert Consult website.

TABLE 95.3   Liver-Directed Local Therapies for Unresectable IHCC

STUDY	TREATMENT MODALITY	N	MEDIAN SIZE, CM (RANGE)	RESPONSE[a]	3Y LC	MEDIAN PFS, MONTHS	3Y OS	MEDIAN OS, MONTHS
Tao et al., 2015[35]	RT (32% proton beam)	79	7.9 (2.2-17)		54%	30	44%	30
		19	6.5 (2.2-17)		78%		73%	NR
	BED > 80.5 Gy	60	8.75 (2.3-15)		45%		38%	27
	BED ≤ 80.5 Gy							
Hong et al., 2016[41]	High-dose proton therapy	38	6.0 (2.2-10.9)		94.1% (2y)	8.4	46.5% (2y)	22.5
Kim et al., 2011[52]	RFA	13	<5	88%	30%[b]	NA	51%	38.5
Kim et al., 2008[51]	TACE	49	8.9	86%	NA	10	30%	12
Kuhlmann et al., 2012[56]	TACE + DEBTACE	26	NA	46%	NA	3.9	NA	11.7
	TACE	10		20%		1.8		5.7
	Chemo	31		71%		6.2		11.0
Ibrahim et al., 2008[55]	Y90	24	NA	95% (86% by EASL)	NA	NA	NA	14.9
Saxena et al., 2010[54]	Y90	25	NA	74%	NA	NA	13%	9.3
Hyder et al., 2013[53]	IAT (all)	198	8.1	87% (82% by EASL)	NA	NA	22%	13.2
	TACE	128						13.4
	DEBTACE	11						10.5
	TAE	13						14.3
	Y90	46						11.3

BED, Biologically effective dose; *DEBTACE*, drug-eluting beads TACE; *EASL*, European Association for the Study of Liver; *IAT*, intraarterial therapy; *IHCC*, intrahepatic cholangiocarcinoma; *NA*, not available; *NR*, not reached; *OS*, overall survival; *PFS*, progression-free survival; *RFA*, radiofrequency ablation; *TACE*, transarterial embolization.

[a]Includes complete response, partial response, and stable disease using RECIST criteria unless otherwise noted.
[b]Estimated from Kaplan-Meier curve.
[c]Only complete and partial response reported.

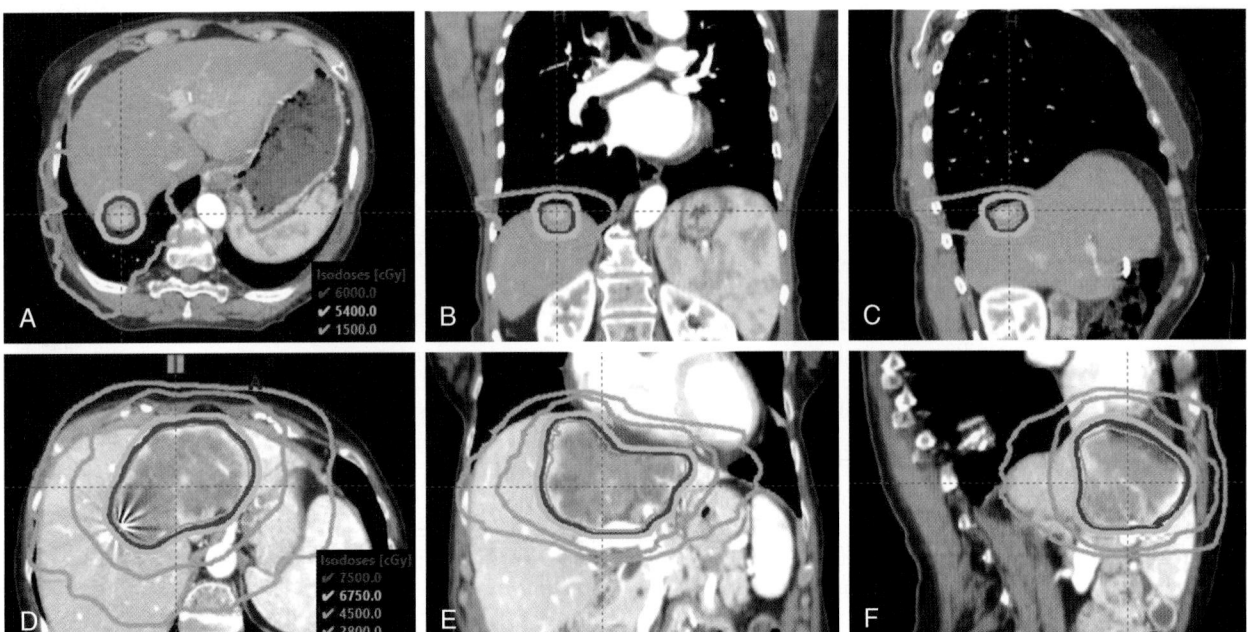

FIGURE 95.1 **Examples of SBRT and hypofractionated ablative IMRT.** Top panel depicts axial **(A),** coronal **(B),** and sagittal **(C)** views of a 3-fraction 6000-cGy SBRT treatment plan for a 1.5-cm segment 7 HCC in a medically inoperable patient. Small size and peripheral location away from luminal GI organs allow for extreme hypofractionation. Bottom panel depicts axial **(D),** coronal **(E),** and sagittal **(F)** views of a 25-fraction 7500-cGy ablative IMRT treatment plan for an 8.2-cm central unresectable IHCC. Proximity to the liver hilum and stomach necessitated longer fractionation. Ablative doses were delivered in both cases: red and green lines indicate 100% and 90% prescription doses showing the steep gradient in each case. Orange line indicates a second, lower prescription dose to cover areas at risk of harboring microscopic disease. The pink line indicates the threshold dose for hepatic tolerance: a sufficient volume of the liver parenchyma must be kept below a safe threshold.

Ablative treatment of liver tumors: Overview

Riccardo Lencioni

Image-guided ablation techniques have evolved considerably during the past 25 years and are increasingly used in the definitive treatment of small primary and secondary liver tumors. Image-guided ablation is recommended as the best therapeutic choice for patients with early-stage hepatocellular carcinoma (HCC)—defined as either a single tumor smaller than 5 cm or as many as three nodules smaller than 3 cm—when surgical options are precluded and is also offered as a first-line therapy, instead of surgery, for patients with very-early-stage tumors smaller than 2 cm[1-3] (see Chapter 91). In addition, image-guided ablation is used to treat limited unresectable hepatic metastatic disease, especially from colorectal cancer.[4]

Image-guided ablation must seek to provide predictable and contiguous cell-lethal ablation zones with a clinically effective, *global ablation margin* in all three planes, also termed *A0* and broadly defined as tumor-free margin of 5 to 10 mm (Fig. 96A.1).[5] Volumetric assessment of the safety margin and image fusion of pre- and post-interventional scans can be used to evaluate local treatment success.[6] When considering tumor ablation, the disease must be targetable, the treatment should be controlled and scalable, unnecessary collateral injury should be avoided, and, because ablation is an in-situ therapy, the lesion should be amenable to noninvasive verification of treatment response. Many interventional and imaging issues contribute to achieving these goals in liver tumor ablation, including ablative technologies, imaging guidance, and manipulation of the tumor setting.

ABLATIVE TECHNOLOGIES

Several methods for focal tumor destruction have been developed and clinically tested. Although radiofrequency ablation (RFA) has been the most popular technique to date, several alternate technologies, including thermal and nonthermal methods, have recently been adopted because they seem to overcome some of the specific limitations of RFA.[7,8]

Radiofrequency Ablation (see Chapter 96B)

Radiofrequency ablation involves the application of high-frequency (375–480 kHz) alternating current to the target tissue by using a needle-like applicator, with cell death resulting from frictional heating. Active tissue heating occurs only within a few millimeters of the exposed tines of the applicator, and larger-volume tissue destruction mainly relies on conductive heating. RFA probes are usually placed under ultrasound or computed tomography (CT) guidance either directly to or iteratively around the tumor to create a confluent ablation zone. Manufacturers of RFA instruments have adapted radiofrequency probes through internal cooling, pulsed application, and expandable multitined probes to overcome this limitation. However, the resultant ablation zone remains sensitive to related convective "heat sumping" to adjacent flowing vessels larger than 3 mm and perfusion-mediated background tissue cooling.

These effects can result in compromised predictability of the ablation zone and, although RFA remains the most clinically prevalent ablation tool, this modality is increasingly superseded by other ablative technologies because of these limitations. A recent development in RFA technology is the introduction of a no-touch technique, which consists of activating, in bipolar mode, multiple electrodes inserted just beyond the tumor margins. This approach has been reported to be especially useful to treat tumors in subcapsular location.[9]

Microwave Ablation (see Chapter 96C)

Microwave ablation (MWA) achieves tissue heating through the point application of electromagnetic microwave radiation from a needle-like probe. These probes essentially contain a broadcast antenna within the "feed point," toward the tip of the device. Most MWA devices are tuned to excite water within soft tissue by "broadcasting" at a frequency of 900 to 2,450 MHz that, by virtue of the inefficient oscillation of polarized water molecules, leads to localized tissue heating throughout an approximate 2 cm tissue sphere around the probe tip. This larger zone of active heating seems much more robust and less compromised by tissue-mediated factors than tissue heating by RFA.[10] However, both RFA and MWA cause tissue vaporization and gas formation, which can obscure imaging of the tumor target during application of treatment. Treatment zones of 3 to 5 cm in diameter can be achieved in five to eight minutes with MWA. More predictable treatment outcomes are attained only through careful iterative or multiprobe techniques and depend on operator experience.[5,11]

Cryoablation (see Chapter 96D)

Cryoablation has been a recognized therapeutic approach for some decades, but the advent of newer, third-generation, 17-gauge argon cryoprobes has led to a clinical resurgence of this technique.[12] The outstanding feature of cryoablation is that tissue destruction is achieved through a phase change in the target tissue, leading to formation of a therapeutic "iceball" and to induction of a *cell-lethal isotherm* of −30° to −40°C within this zone.[13] The iceball itself is readily resolved in all three planes during operative imaging procedures, which provides a well-defined, periprocedural imaging surrogate of the ultimate ablation zone.

Irreversible Electroporation (see Chapter 96C)

Irreversible electroporation (IRE) is a relatively new and reportedly nonthermal ablative technique. This modality involves tissue destruction through millisecond pulses of direct current between monopolar probes carefully placed in parallel within the target tumor. These bursts of current can perforate, or *porate*, the cell by disruption of the electrical potential across the cell membrane; if applied for slightly longer durations, these bursts of current can cause irreversible electroporation of the target tumor cells. IRE seems to spare collagenous or connective

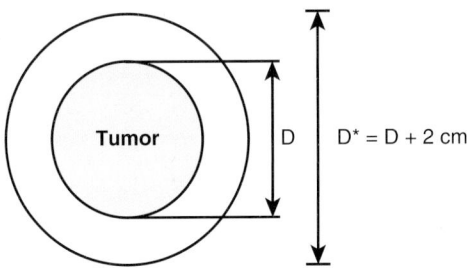

FIGURE 96A.1   Schematic model of thermal ablation. The target diameter of the ablation zone (D*) ideally must be 2 cm larger than the diameter of the tumor that undergoes treatment (D).

tissue structures, such as blood vessels and possibly bile ducts. This intrinsic property proved useful in the complete destruction of awkwardly located perivascular or peribiliary liver tumors. Therefore IRE is currently recommended for unresectable primary and secondary malignancies that are unsuitable for thermal ablation because of proximity to critical structures.[14]

Other Techniques

Extracorporeal-focused ultrasound can achieve small focal zones of tissue destruction, termed *sonications*, of approximately 12 mm × 3 mm within targeted tissues. This technique avoids placement of invasive probes, but the effectiveness of the approach can be limited by intervening bone or gas, and the formation of truly contiguous ablation zones requires complex motion correction and respiratory gating. To date, these issues have effectively restricted oncologic applications. Other tissue-ablative techniques include chemical ablation (e.g., using absolute alcohol [percutaneous ethanol injection] or acetic acid) and laser photocoagulation.[5]

IMAGING GUIDANCE

Image guidance, both in treatment planning and during periprocedural and postprocedural assessments, is critical to ensure

rigorous "surgical" results from ablation techniques (see Chapter 103).

Treatment Planning

Not all tumors are spherical, and many lie adjacent to critical structures. Also, some tumors are poorly accessible by using percutaneously placed ablation devices. These considerations emphasize that all ablation procedures must be carefully planned such that either iterative probe placement or clusters of concurrent probes are meticulously positioned to achieve contiguous ablation zones with adequate treatment margins. A number of preprocedural software packages are under development to improve the preplanning and implementation of treatments (Fig. 96A.2).

Although ablative techniques become more robust, the ultimate ablation zone should become more predictable in a manner analogous to radiotherapy planning. Once probe placements are decided, appropriate treatment dosimetry should permit the prediction of treatment volumes in the substrate organ and with respect to the target tumor mass. Individual imaging strategies can be problematic for tumor targeting; for example, ultrasonography provides real-time multiplanar imaging, but the tumor might be partially obscured by overlying gas or bone. Coregistration of CT or magnetic resonance imaging (MRI) and real-time ultrasonography has been found to be useful in some treatment settings. However, tissues deform during the placement of physical devices, and intraprocedural changes, such as poorly controlled respiration, can modify the target position in a manner that can be difficult to predict mechanically.

Periprocedural and Postprocedural Assessment

The tissue-lethal ablation zone must be assessed during and/or immediately after ablation to determine treatment completion, analogous to pathology evaluation of surgical resection margins. Contrast-enhanced CT or MRI performed at the end of the procedure allows initial evaluation of treatment effects.[15] The typical ablation zone within the liver is observed as a nonenhancing area, with or without a peripheral enhancing rim,

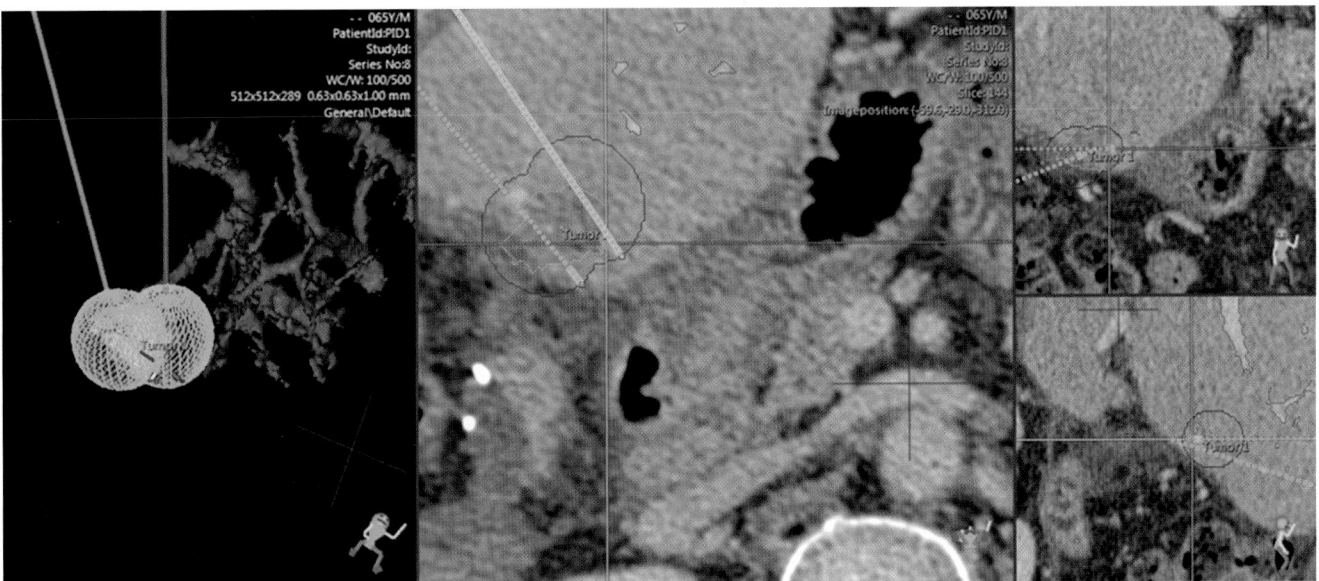

FIGURE 96A.2   Pretreatment assessment of target tumor and expected ablation volumes by using a dedicated workstation (Maxio, Perfint Healthcare) enables accurate planning of the procedure.

TABLE 96A.1   Main Potential Advantages and Disadvantages of Ablative Technologies

	POTENTIAL ADVANTAGES	POTENTIAL DISADVANTAGES
RFA	High rates of local control in tumors 3 cm or smaller Established safety profile Known limitations Experience in combination treatments (HCC) No-touch technique	High rates of incomplete ablation in tumors larger than 3 cm Heat-sink effect ("heat sumping") in perivascular tumors Potential risk of thermal injury to critical structures Variability in RFA devices
MWA	Potential to treat tumors larger than 3 cm more effectively Less impacted by heat-sink effect Ability to activate multiple probes at the same time No grounding pads required	Limited long-term efficacy data (predictability and reproducibility) Limited safety data Potential risk of thermal injury to critical structures (and vessels?) Variability in MWA devices
CRYO	Ability to activate multiple probes at the same time Ability to image the iceball formation	Insufficient clinical data Risk of bleeding Risk of cryoshock
IRE	Potential to treat tumors located in the vicinity of critical structures Heat-sink effect not relevant	Limited indications Neuromuscular blockage and cardiac gating required

CRYO, Cryoablation; *HCC,* hepatocellular carcinoma; *IRE,* irreversible electroporation; *MWA,* microwave ablation; *RFA,* radiofrequency ablation.

which is usually visualized as a concentric but often irregular ring, with smooth inner margins. If observed, this enhancing rim is a transient response to thermal injury that represents initial reactive hyperemia with subsequent giant cell reaction and fibrosis, so it is a benign physiologic response. This benign enhancement in periablational tissues must be distinguished from residual untreated tumor, which can also result in irregular peripheral enhancement at the treatment margin. A potentially distinguishing feature of residual unablated tumor is that the enhancing soft tissue often grows in scattered, nodular, or eccentric patterns, in contrast to the relatively concentric ring associated with benign periablational enhancement that diminishes over time.

TUMOR MANIPULATION

Embolization or localized vascular occlusion can render a tumor more amenable to temperature-based treatment by reducing perfusion-mediated vascular cooling or heat sumping in adjacent flowing vessels[16] (see Chapter 94). In addition, increasing emphasis has been placed on operative technique, on manipulation of the tumor setting, and on tumor location with respect to adjacent temperature-sensitive structures, to avoid collateral injury. Operators are increasingly appreciating that time spent on displacement of adjacent heat-sensitive structures permits the application of a more rigorous and clinically adequate ablation zone. Adjacent bowel can usually be displaced by using generous intraperitoneal fluid instillation, sometimes carbon dioxide insufflation, or careful deployment of intraperitoneal catheter balloons. Caution and careful consideration of treatment dosimetry must be used in ablating tumors in critical locations (e.g., around the perihilar biliary tree) to avoid collateral injury. IRE proved to be useful in this setting.

CLINICAL APPLICATION

The clinical application of each energy-based ablation technology is discussed in the relevant chapters. Currently, there is no accepted algorithm for the use of the different ablative techniques in the treatment of primary and metastatic liver tumors. Further studies are needed to establish whether novel technologies will expand the clinical role of image-guided ablation and improve long-term patient outcomes with respect to RFA. Table 96A.1 provides a critical appraisal of potential advantages and disadvantages of each thermal and nonthermal ablation technology, based on experimental findings and available clinical data. It is important to note that these considerations refer to the general characteristics of each technology. However, significant variability appears to exist among the different equipment and devices within each technology. Therefore, detailed information should be provided concerning technique parameters to enable a comprehensive understanding of the data, critical appraisal of the efficacy, and safety profile of each ablation system. Ultimately, as opposed to a generic indication of the technology, specific information of the recommended techniques and protocols should be implemented in clinical practice guidelines, similar to pharmaceutical treatment regimens.

References are available at expertconsult.com.

Radiofrequency ablation of liver tumors

Patrick D. Lorimer and Anton J. Bilchik

Resection for curative intent is the gold standard for metastatic and primary hepatic tumors where feasible. Resectability, as previously discussed in other chapters, is the result of a coalescence of factors: technical/anatomic feasibility, adequacy of the predicted future liver remnant, and appropriate patient performance status to tolerate major surgery (see Chapter 101A). Liver resections range widely in terms of technical difficulty and risks posed to the patient. This is governed largely by the disease burden and anatomic location of the lesion(s) in question. Though technically feasible in a suitable patient, some resections are prohibitive due to an insufficient future liver remnant (see Chapter 102). Cases of extensive multifocal or bilobar disease present a particular challenge to even the most skilled surgeon. Though techniques such as portal vein embolization and associating liver partition and portal vein ligation for staged hepatectomy (ALPPS) have arisen to optimize the future liver remnant, resectability remains limited by this.[1,2] In select cases, orthotopic liver transplantation for primary hepatic malignancies is an attractive option because it can be curative. Although a viable option that must be considered, transplantation is predicated on donor organ availability and exposes the patient to the potential toxicities of immunosuppressive medications.

Patients with unresectable disease may be candidates for ablative therapies that cause cancerous tissue necrosis by heating (radiofrequency ablation, microwave ablation, laser ablation, high-intensity focused ultrasound), irreversible electroporation (IRE), cooling (cryoablation), or injection of toxic agents (absolute alcohol)[3-10] (see Chapters 96A, 96C, and 96D).

Ablative techniques were initially reported as a treatment option for unresectable malignancies in the 1920s. The destructive potential of heat generated by passage of an electric current through tissue was originally reported by Clark et al.,[11] who described the application of a high-frequency current to cancerous tissues and the resultant thermic effect on that tissue.

During the last three decades, radiofrequency ablation (RFA) has been successfully used in the treatment of unresectable hepatic tumors. In 1990 McGahan et al.[12] demonstrated the efficacy of ultrasound-monitored RFA in fresh bovine liver. Five years later, the first use of RFA in humans to treat small hepatocellular carcinoma (HCC) of the liver was reported.[13] The US Food and Drug Administration (FDA) approved RFA for generic tissue ablation in 1996 and for ablation of unresectable hepatic metastases in 2000. The first randomized trial investigating the efficacy of RFA versus resection in early HCC demonstrated comparable overall survival,[14] although further trials have uncovered discrepancies.[15,16] Table 96B.1 details the long-term survival in recent nonrandomized trials comparing RFA with surgical resection of early HCC. RFA treatment of colorectal liver metastases and intrahepatic cholangiocarcinoma has also been studied, but no data exist from randomized controlled trials (RCTs).[17,18]

Radiofrequency ablation can be performed in the operating room by laparotomy or laparoscopy or in the radiology suite through a percutaneous approach. RFA may be combined with hepatic resection (see Chapters 101 and 102), hepatic artery perfusion (see Chapter 100), or transarterial chemoembolization (TACE) (see Chapter 94) along with systemic therapy, if there are other sites of metastatic disease.[5,38,39] The Society of Interventional Radiology described preferred candidates for RFA as patients with inadequate liver function or comorbid conditions, patients whose tumors have an anatomic distribution not compatible with resection, and those in whom local control of tumor is necessary before transplantation.[40]

RADIOFREQUENCY ABLATION TECHNOLOGY

Radiofrequency ablation destroys tissues by denaturing cell proteins and causing cell death with heat (Fig. 96B.1). Early work in ablation technology demonstrated that the rate of necrosis is exponentially related to the temperature generated within a tissue. Instantaneous cell death occurs at 60°C, a temperature readily achieved with commercially available RFA devices.[41] During RFA, an electric generator propagates a rapidly alternating radiofrequency (RF) current that ranges from 300 to 500 kilohertz (kHz) across an electric circuit formed between the needle electrode and a grounding pad placed on the patient's skin. Resistive heating is generated through intense friction by the Joule effect.[42] The current around the ablation electrode creates a uniform zone of heat that radiates out from the electrode through conduction. The size of the ablation zone is directly related to the impedance of the tissue being ablated. If tissue impedance is low, an expanding spherical zone of ablated tissue is created. The spherical size of the ablated tissue is proportional to the square of the RF current (radiofrequency power density). Between 45° and 100°C, an exponential rise in irreversible coagulative necrosis destroys the tumor without disrupting tissue architecture. Necrosis may be limited by carbonization and charring at ablative temperatures above 100°C (because of increased tissue impedance), convective cooling from nearby blood vessels (the heat-sink effect), and reduced RF power density at longer distances from the heat source.[43,44]

Several companies are currently producing RF electrodes for commercial use in liver ablation. AngioDynamics and Boston Scientific both offer multiarray electrodes and are commonly used. AngioDynamics StarBurst Radiofrequency Ablation System offers real-time temperature monitoring at ablative margins. A variety of percutaneous RFA devices are compatible with multiple imaging modalities (Fig. 96B.2). Flexible trocars allow 90-degree articulation, and ablative fields can reach as large as 7 cm in diameter. The RF3000 Radiofrequency Generator (Boston Scientific) uses impedance to assess end points. The LeVeen Needle electrode (Boston Scientific) has multiple talons in an umbrella-shaped array that allows spherical ablation. An RCT showed that two stepwise hook extension

TABLE 96B.1   Nonrandomized Trials Comparing Radiofrequency Ablation (RFA) and Liver Resection (LR) for Hepatocellular Carcinoma (≤5 cm) With 5-Year Follow-up: 2012 to 2019

STUDY	TREATMENT	RFA TYPE	NO. PATIENTS	TUMOR SIZE (MEAN ± SD, CM)	DISEASE-FREE SURVIVAL (%)	OVERALL SURVIVAL (%)
Wang et al., 2012[19]	LR		208	≤3	50.8	77.2
	RFA	Perc	254	≤3	14.1	57.4
Peng et al., 2012[20]	LR		74	1.1 ± 0.5	40	62.1
	RFA	Perc	71	1.2 ± 0.6	67	71.9
Imai et al., 2013[21]	LR		101	2.14 ± 0.55	46.8	87.5
	RFA	—	82	1.87 ± 0.50	23.9	59.4
Tohme et al., 2013[22]	LR		50	3.07 ± 1.17	34	47
	RFA	Open/lap	60	2.36 ± 0.94	28	35
Desiderio et al., 2013[23]	LR		52	≤3	26.9	46.2
	RFA	Perc	44	≤3	22.7	36.4
Hasegawa et al., 2013[24]	LR		5361	≤3	36.2	71.1
	RFA	Perc	5548	≤3	28.3	61.1
Lai & Tang, 2013[25]	LR		80	2.9 ± 1.1	60	71
	RFA	Lap	31	1.8 ± 0.6	40	84
Wong KM et al., 2013[26]	LR		46	2.1 ± 0.6	53.7	84.6
	RFA	Perc	36	1.9 ± 0.6	14.9	72.8
Peng et al., 2013[27]	LR		91	≤5	33.1	51.9
	RFA	Perc	89	≤5	35.5	55.2
Zhou et al., 2014[28]	LR		21	1.7 ± 0.3	76.2	81
	RFA	Lap/perc	31	1.7 ± 0.4	71	80.6
Iida et al., 2014[29]	LR		15	2.5 ± 0.4	48.6	68.7
	RFA	Perc	33	2.0 ± 1.1	7.2	32.7
Park et al., 2014[30]	LR		129	3.0 ± 1.0	20.6	64.9
	RFA	Open/perc	57	2.3 ± 1.0	—	74
Lei et al., 2014[31]	LR		133	3.9 ± 0.6	58.6	66.2
	RFA	Open/perc	156	3.7 ± 0.5	54.5	66
Gory et al., 2015[32]	LR		52	≤5	51	62
	RFA	Lap/Perc	96	≤5	24	37
Lee et al, 2015[33]	LR		330	—	—	76
	RFA	—	369	≤5	—	66
Santambrogio et al., 2018[34]	LR	Lap	59	2.09 ± 6.7	45	56
		Lap	205	1.91 ± 5.8	20	40
Uhlig et al., 2019[35]	LR		10085	5.1 (3.1–8.1)[b]	—	45.6
	RFA	Mixed	8211	2.8 (2.1-3.9)[b]	—	30.7
Jianyong et al., 2019[36]	LR		72	3.7 ± 0.5	47	48
	RFA	Open	59	3.8 ± 0.5	30	33
Yamashita et al., 2019[37]	LR	Lap	40	2.4 ± 0.9	57[a]	76
	RFA	Mixed	62	2.0 ± 0.6	55[a]	85

Lap, Laparoscopic; *Mixed,* laparoscopic/open/percutaneous; *Perc,* percutaneous; *SD,* standard deviation.

[a]2-year disease-free survival.

[b]SD not provided, range included.

Adapted from Xu Q, Kobayashi S, Ye X, et al: Comparison of hepatic resection and radiofrequency ablation for small hepatocellular carcinoma: A meta-analysis of 16,103 patients. *Sci Rep* 2014;4:7252.

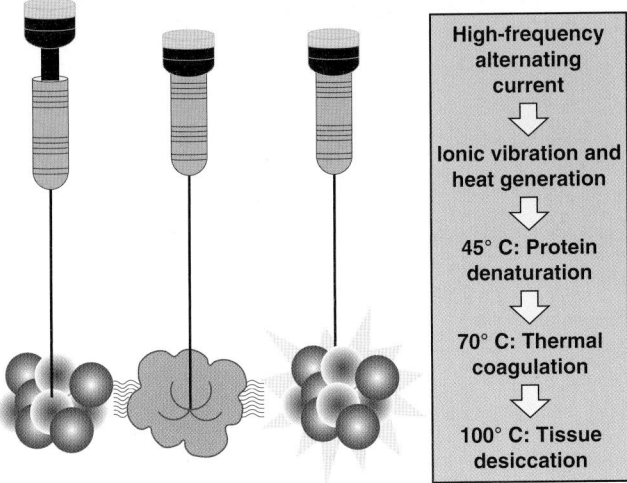

High-frequency alternating current
⇩
Ionic vibration and heat generation
⇩
45° C: Protein denaturation
⇩
70° C: Thermal coagulation
⇩
100° C: Tissue desiccation

FIGURE 96B.1   Schematic of radiofrequency ablation.

techniques that use the 17 gauge LeVeen SuperSlim 30 mm electrode could tailor the ablation field to tumor size and shape.[45] The Soloist single-needle electrode (Boston Scientific) is also available for treating lesions as large as 1 cm in diameter. Covidien offers the Cool-tip RF Ablation System E Series. This system has a touch-screen interface and single or three-pronged electrodes. Internal probe perfusion with cold saline reduces charring and maximizes ablative potential. Concurrent use of three separate electrodes can extend the ablative diameter to 6.5 cm. A temperature probe can be placed in adjacent liver parenchyma to monitor temperature.

RADIOFREQUENCY ABLATION PROCEDURE

Patients who present with primary liver tumors should be evaluated for curative resection or transplantation and discussed in a multidisciplinary conference. Computed tomography (CT), magnetic resonance imaging (MRI), and in some circumstances fluorodeoxyglucose (FDG) positron emission tomography (PET) (see Chapter 18) should be used to verify extent of disease before consideration of resection or ablation.[46]

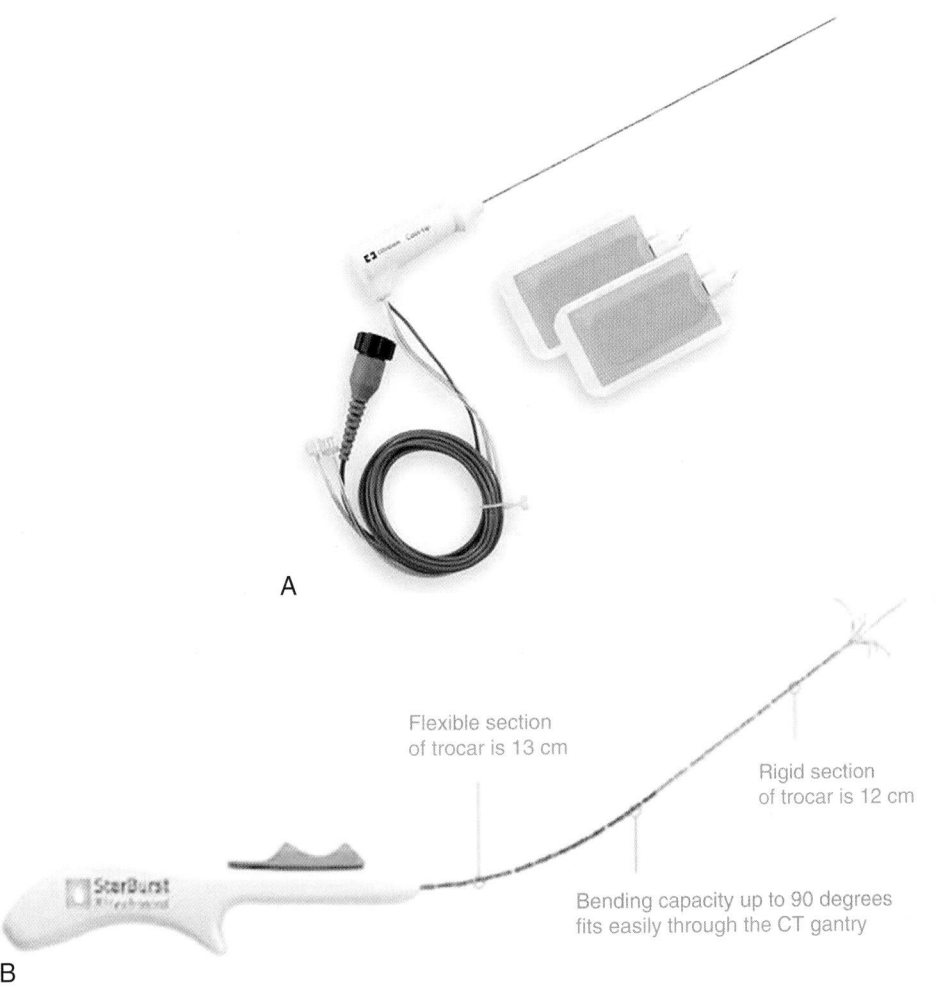

Flexible section of trocar is 13 cm

Rigid section of trocar is 12 cm

Bending capacity up to 90 degrees fits easily through the CT gantry

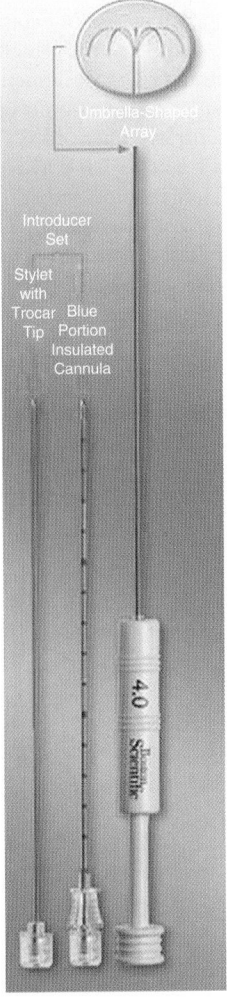

FIGURE 96B.2   A, Cool-tip 17-gauge straight radiofrequency ablation (RFA) trocar. *(All rights reserved. Used with the permission of Medtronic.)* **B,** StarBurst Xli-enhanced Semi-Flex RFA electrode (AngioDynamics); *CT,* computed tomography. **C,** Leveen CoAccess Electrode System (Boston Scientific). (Image provided courtesy Boston Scientific. © 2016 Boston Scientific Corporation or its affiliates. All rights reserved.)

MRI with gadoxetate disodium (Eovist), a gadolinium-based contrast agent with extracellular and hepatocyte-specific properties, is highly sensitive and specific for characterizing metastatic colorectal disease[47] (see Chapter 15). If whole-body imaging techniques reveal extrahepatic sites of metastatic disease, systemic therapy should be considered. Baseline hepatic function should be assessed through laboratory data and the patient's Model for End-Stage Liver Disease (MELD) score, and the Child-Pugh classification should be calculated to determine the severity of disease (see Chapter 4). A thorough history and physical examination are essential to determine patient performance and prior treatment history. If a patient's comorbidities, performance status, tumor location, and either hepatic or systemic burden of disease preclude resection, ablative therapies should be considered.

Radiofrequency ablation can be performed via laparotomy, laparoscopy, or a percutaneous approach. The choice of technique depends on the patient's condition, the number and location of liver tumors, and the skill of the physician performing the ablation. Each approach offers certain advantages and disadvantages that must be weighed to determine the best approach for the individual patient.

Ultrasonography, MRI, or CT imaging is used during RFA to guide the probe into a lesion and monitor the expanding hyperechogenic zone of ablation. Compared with B-mode sonography RFA, contrast-enhanced harmonic sonographic guided RFA has a higher rate of complete ablation and a lower number of treatment sessions (Fig. 96B.3).[48] Contrast-enhanced ultrasound-guided RFA has also been compared with contrast-enhanced CT-guided RFA and found to outperform CT-guided RFA in terms of obtaining a complete ablation.[49] Each ablation should create at least a 5 mm margin of treated normal parenchyma to ensure complete tumor destruction and reduce the risk of local recurrence. Multiple overlapping ablations may be required to completely treat larger lesions and produce the necessary peripheral rim of necrosis (Fig. 96B.4).

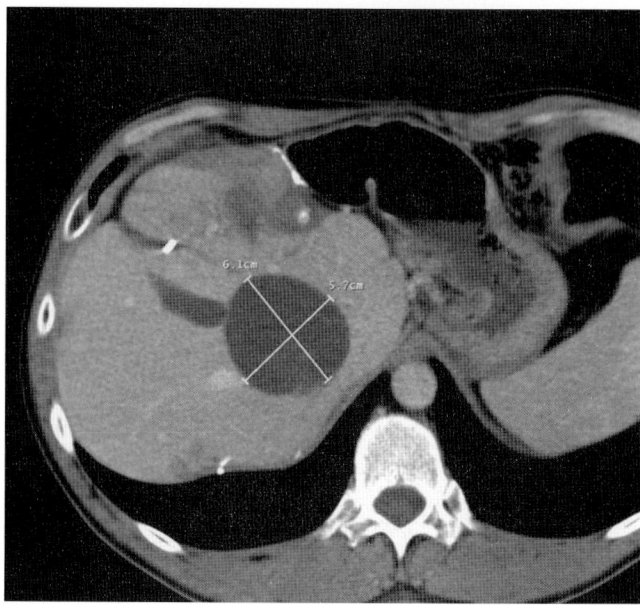

FIGURE 96B.4 Computed tomography scan demonstrating large-volume ablation achieved with multiple overlapping ablation technique.

In such cases, it is prudent to begin with ablation at the most posterior aspect of the lesion as it is not possible to reliably interpret this location with intervening hyperechogenic tissue from ablation. By starting at the posterior aspect of the lesion and moving anteriorly, the treating physician is able to visualize adequate ablation of the entire lesion. Between ablations, the probe should be slowly withdrawn in 2 cm increments to create sequentially overlapping zones of ablated tissue. If target temperatures are not reached, the tines should be withdrawn slightly or rotated approximately 45 degrees to increase temperature within the region of ablation. After ablation, the probe

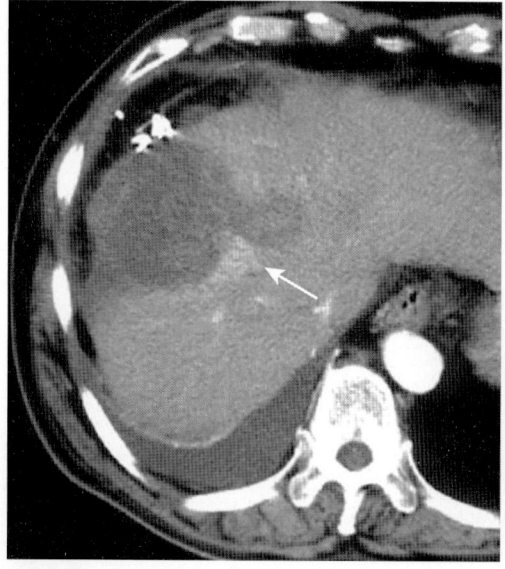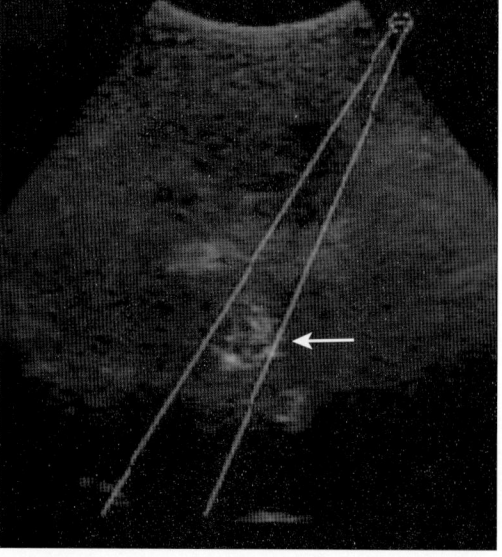

FIGURE 96B.3 Comparison of **left,** early-phase dynamic computed tomography, and **right,** contrast-enhanced ultrasonography, in detecting a 2.0-cm progression of hepatocellular carcinoma after radiofrequency ablation (see Chapter 14). (Reprinted from [Contrast Harmonic Sonography-Guided Radiofrequency Ablation Therapy Versus B-Mode Sonography in Hepatocellular Carcinoma: Prospective Randomized Controlled Trial, Yasunori Minami, Masatoshi Kudo, Hobyung Chung, Toshihiko Kawasaki, Yukinobu Yagyu, Taro Shimono and Hitoshi Shiozaki, the American Journal of Roentgenology title and 188/2, Copyright© 2007, copyright owner as specified in the American Journal of Roentgenology])

tract is cauterized as the RFA needle is slowly withdrawn, to prevent hemorrhage and tumor seeding of the needle tract.

Percutaneous Radiofrequency Ablation

Interventional radiologists perform percutaneous RFA under ultrasound or CT guidance or with a combination of ultrasound, CT, or MRI. The patient is given a local anesthetic, mild sedation is used, and the procedure can be performed in the outpatient setting. Intraprocedural use of contrast-enhanced CT or contrast-enhanced ultrasonographic imaging allows for identification of any areas of inadequate ablation so that additional targeted ablations can be carried out to ensure completeness of ablation.

A percutaneous approach may not be appropriate for hilar tumors proximal to vessels larger than 4 mm given the heat-sink effect and potential for inadequate ablation or for tumors that are near major bile ducts due to complications.[50] Lesions at the periphery of the liver also may be problematic because thermal ablation can injure other visceral structures such as the small bowel, stomach, gallbladder, or transverse colon. Ablation of liver lesions located at the superior aspect of segments II, IVa, VII, and VIII may result in thermal injury to the diaphragm. Techniques to avoid diaphragmatic injury include preablation use of "artificial ascites," or introduction of carbon dioxide between the dome of the liver and the diaphragm.[51,52]

Percutaneous RFA has the advantage of being less invasive and may be preferable in patients unable to undergo surgery.[5] Compared with resection in the setting of very early HCC (<2 cm) and with two or three nodules (≤3 cm), percutaneous RFA has also been found to be more cost-effective.[53]

Open or Laparoscopic Radiofrequency Ablation

Radiofrequency ablation via laparotomy or laparoscopy is performed in the operating room by a surgeon while the patient is under general anesthesia. The initial surgical approach may use diagnostic laparoscopy with intraoperative ultrasound to identify any extrahepatic or intrahepatic disease not detected by preoperative imaging (see Chapter 24). This avoids committing a patient to a larger operation, as the long-term benefit of ablation in the setting of widely metastatic disease is questionable. A thorough intraabdominal survey examining all parietal and visceral peritoneal surfaces, the lesser sac, omentum, and viscera should be undertaken. Careful sonographic examination of the hepatic parenchyma using an articulating laparoscopic ultrasonic probe can identify liver lesions and their proximity to major vascular and biliary structures. To assist in visualizing difficult lesions in the superior or posterior aspects of segments VII and VIII, the patient can be placed in the Trendelenburg position and normal saline instilled in the right upper quadrant; this allows for more clear visualization of the parenchyma where the probe cannot contact the liver due to anatomic constraints.[54] In a study of 308 patients undergoing laparoscopic RFA with intraoperative hepatic ultrasonography, preoperative imaging failed to identify extrahepatic disease in 12% of patients and additional hepatic lesions in 33% of patients.[3] Another advantage of the operative approach is that a Pringle maneuver may be performed to reduce the heat-sink effect associated with ablating lesions near large vessels. RFA may also be combined with formal surgical resection to manage bilateral liver metastases.[55] Typically, larger lesions will be targeted for resection, whereas smaller lesions in the opposite lobe would be candidates for RFA.

Laparoscopy is less invasive than laparotomy and patients often require slightly shorter hospital stays. In some cases, however, a laparotomy is unavoidable due to the location of lesions within the liver and physical limitations of the ultrasound and RFA probe under laparoscopy. Laparoscopy may not be possible if there are multiple adhesions in the abdomen from prior operations or if the tumor cannot be approached safely. In this case, a laparotomy is prudent.

Monitoring and Follow-up

After laparoscopic or percutaneous RFA, patients are either discharged home the same day or admitted to the hospital for a 23-hour observation period. RFA by laparotomy usually requires hospitalization for 3 to 5 days. Postablation hemoglobin levels, leukocyte counts, liver function tests (LFTs), and body temperature are closely monitored. Transient mild elevations in LFTs, core temperature, and leukocyte count are not uncommon and typically normalize within 3 days. Persistent elevation for 5 or more days after RFA may indicate an underlying complication and should prompt further clinical investigation.

Surveillance of the tumor should use both laboratory testing and imaging. Tumor markers such as carcinoembryonic antigen (CEA) for colorectal cancer metastases and α-fetoprotein (AFP) for HCC should be drawn and compared with preablation levels. Contrast-enhanced ultrasound, MRI, CT, or PET may be chosen and should be consistently used during follow-up.[46,56] As there is not a standardized postablation surveillance protocol, the authors recommend postablation clinical follow-up at 1 month with imaging, followed by imaging with the same modality at 3 months, and then quarterly. Periablation enhancement due to inflammation can appear as residual disease, thus necessitating at least a 1-month delay before initial postablation imaging.[57,58] FDG-PET scanning is particularly sensitive in assessing the adequacy of ablation, identifying recurrence at the margin of ablation (Fig. 96B.5), or distinguishing viable tumor from areas of previous surgical or ablative therapy (Fig. 96B.6) (see Chapter 18).

Radiofrequency Ablation of Colorectal Hepatic Metastases

The most common indication for hepatectomy in Western populations is colorectal liver metastases[2] (see Chapter 90). Resection with curative intent remains the treatment of choice but it is only feasible in 15% to 25% of patients.[59] Five-year survival after resection has classically been described as ranging between 40% and 60%.[60-62] A meta-analysis of 13 studies of RFA versus liver resection of colorectal metastases between 2003 and 2011 found that surgical resection was superior to RFA for overall survival and disease-free survival.[63] Despite this, many patients are poor candidates for resection and RFA provides a locoregional alternative.

No randomized trial has yet compared RFA with resection in patients with colorectal hepatic metastases. The forthcoming COLLISION trial is currently recruiting. This randomized, intention-to-treat trial is designed to compare outcomes for patients with colorectal liver metastases undergoing resection or ablation, and is expected to report in late 2022.[16] In a prospective nonrandomized trial, Otto et al.[64] demonstrated comparable 5-year overall survival after RFA versus resection of colorectal liver metastases amenable to surgery (48% vs. 51%, respectively; $P = .961$), although progression was faster after

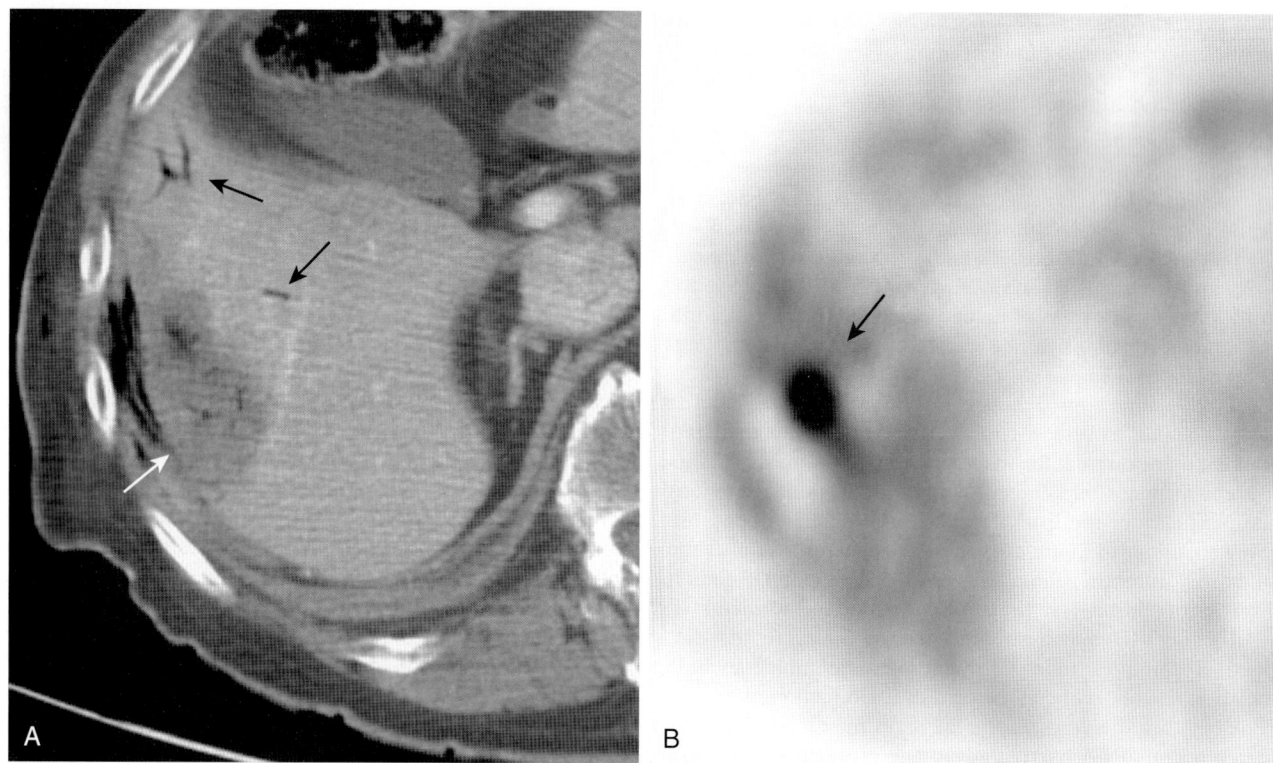

FIGURE 96B.5   **A,** Marginal recurrence not clearly visualized by computed tomography. **B,** Recurrence is clearly identified by positron emission tomography scan (see Chapter 18).

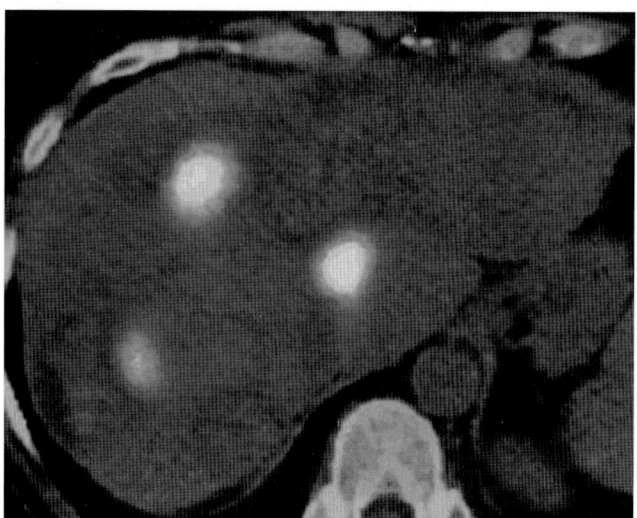

FIGURE 96B.6   Positron emission tomography scan demonstrating areas of viable tumor distinguished from areas of successful ablation (see Chapter 18).

RFA (203 vs. 416 days; P = .017). Other nonrandomized studies have shown varying results (Table 96B.2). A retrospective study of 358 patients compared resection, RFA plus resection, RFA alone, and laparotomy with biopsy.[65] RFA was used for cure when complete resection was not possible. All patient-related and tumor-related factors known to influence outcome were similar among the groups.[65] The rate of recurrence was 84% after RFA alone, 63% after RFA plus resection, and 52% after resection alone (P < .001). Local recurrence (in the area treated) was more common after RFA plus resection (9%) than

RFA alone (5%) or resection alone (2%) (P = .02).[65] The 3-year overall survival was 73% after resection, 43% after RFA plus resection, and 37% after RFA alone. Patients who underwent RFA had a survival advantage versus patients who underwent biopsy with or without chemotherapy.[65]

Another retrospective study comparing resection and RFA concluded that RFA is a safe alternative treatment of smaller metastases.[66] In 226 patients with a solitary colorectal liver metastasis less than 3 cm in size, no difference in overall survival and disease-free survival after RFA versus resection was found. Disease-free survival was, however, diminished when tumors of 3 cm or larger were treated with RFA versus resection.[66] A more recent meta-analysis comparing RFA with resection in colorectal liver metastases demonstrated a 20% higher rate of intrahepatic recurrence overall for lesions treated with RFA, but no difference in extrahepatic recurrence.[17] Decreased overall and disease-free survival were also reported in RFA compared with resection, but patients with RFA also experienced significantly fewer complications.[17]

Most patients with metastatic colon cancer receive systemic treatment (see Chapters 97 and 98). Ruers et al.[71] conducted an RCT to establish the role of RFA and chemotherapy in disease-free survival. A comparison of the treatment of colorectal metastases with chemotherapy alone versus chemotherapy plus RFA found progression-free survival to be improved with RFA (16.8 vs. 9.9 months when treated with systemic therapy alone).[71]

Radiofrequency Ablation of Hepatocellular Carcinoma (see Chapter 89)

Locoregional methods for ablation of HCC that have been compared with RFA in randomized trials include percutaneous

TABLE 96B.2   Five-Year Survival Data for Radiofrequency Ablation (RFA) Versus Liver Resection (LR) of Colorectal Liver Metastases: 2011–2014

STUDY	TREATMENT	NO. PATIENTS	RFA APPROACH	OVERALL SURVIVAL (%)
Kim et al., 2011[66]	LR	278		51.2
	RFA	177	Open	51.1
Lee et al., 2012[6]	LR	25		44.0
	RFA	28	Percutaneous	17.9
Agcaoglu et al., 2013[67]	LR	94		57.5
	RFA	245		17.0
Aliyev et al., 2013[68]	LR	60		56.7
	RFA	44		46.0
Ko et al., 2014[69]	LR	12		66.7
	RFA	17	Percutaneous	37.8
Nishiwada et al., 2014[70]	LR	60		38.4
	RFA	32		40.7

LR, Liver resection; *RFA*, radiofrequency ablation.
Adapted from van Amerongen MJ, Jenniskens SFM, van den Boezem PB, et al. Radiofrequency ablation compared with surgical resection for curative treatment of patients with colorectal liver metastases—A meta-analysis. *HPB (Oxford)*. 2017;19:749–756.

ethanol injection (PEI), cryosurgery, laser ablation, microwave ablation, and RFA (see Chapters 96C and 96D). Giorgio et al.[72] compared PEI and RFA of small HCC in 271 patients enrolled in an RCT. For 3- and 5-year survival and 3- and 5-year recurrence, no significant difference was found between RFA and PEI. PEI did cost significantly less than RFA treatment.[72] RFA offers some notable advantages versus PEI because PEI requires multiple treatments and needle insertion to treat a single lesion, whereas RFA can treat an entire tumor with one or two probe insertions and results in a higher rate of complete necrosis.[73] A separate randomized trial found no differences between RFA and laser ablation of small HCC for complete tumor ablation, time to local tumor progression, and mean overall survival.[74] In an RCT comparing cryoablation with RFA, cryoablation was associated with significantly slower tumor progression during the first 3 years, although overall survival rates out to 5 years were not statistically different.[75] However, compared with cryoablation, RFA has less blood loss, less thrombocytopenia, and a shorter hospital stay.[3] Cryoablation also carries the risk of a significant systemic inflammatory response that can result in renal insufficiency, coagulopathy, hypotension, and death.[76] This response has not been reported with RFA.

Microwave ablation has been retrospectively compared with RFA in the treatment of HCC. In 52 patients, no difference was found between therapies in regard to complete response, rate of unablated disease, and recurrence.[77] Laparoscopic application of either ablative therapy also has no effect on short- and long-term results.[77–79]

Stereotactic body radiation therapy (SBRT) is also being used to treat unresectable HCC[80–82] (see Chapter 95). One multinational retrospective study demonstrated similar outcomes of SBRT compared with RFA, particularly in tumors larger than 3 cm and those lesions close to the diaphragm.[80] At present, SBRT seems to be most useful in patients who are not good surgical candidates.

Clinical outcomes using RFA for HCC have shown promising results. Early trials in RFA for HCC demonstrated a local recurrence rate of only 2.8% at a median follow-up of 31 months for tumors less than 2 cm.[83] A study evaluating 2982 RFA treatments on 1170 primary HCC lesions demonstrated that 5- and 10-year local tumor progression rates were both 3.2%, distant recurrence rates were 74.8% and 80.8%, and overall survival rates were 60.2% and 27.3%, respectively.[84] A recently reported study of percutaneous RFA for solitary HCC smaller than 3 cm demonstrated local recurrence of 20.4% and 25.1% at 5 and 10 years, respectively, with subphrenic and periportal lesions being higher risk for recurrence.[85] The 5- and 10-year overall survival rates were 83.7% and 74.2%, respectively.[85]

Radiofrequency Ablation Versus Resection for Hepatocellular Carcinoma

Meta-analyses still support resection of HCC when possible (Table 96B.3). Prospective randomized trials of RFA versus resection for the treatment of primary liver carcinoma were published in 2010 and 2012.[15,86] In one of the landmark RFA trials, 230 patients who met the Milan criteria (single HCC ≤5 cm or as many as three nodules, each <3 cm) were randomized to resection or RFA.[15] The 5-year overall survival rate and 5-year recurrence rate were 54.78% and 63.48% in the RFA group and 75.65% and 41.74% in the resection group, respectively, both significantly in favor of resection.[15] This contradicts a comparable 2006 study in which 180 patients were randomly assigned with a solitary HCC (<5 cm) to either resection or percutaneous RFA; 4-year overall survival was 67.9% in the RFA group and 64% in the resection group.[14] Local recurrence rates were also similar, and the RFA group demonstrated less morbidity.[14] Another trial comparing percutaneous RFA and resection in 168 patients with small HCC (diameter <4 cm and as many as two nodules) found no significant difference in overall or recurrence-free survival rates between groups out to 3 years.[86] Thus percutaneous RFA may be a suitable alternative for small HCC with limited hepatic involvement (Table 96B.4).

TABLE 96B.3 Meta-Analyses of Radiofrequency Ablation (RFA) in Treatment of Hepatic Tumors, 2012–2020

STUDY	TREATMENT	TUMOR TYPE	STUDIES COMPARED (NO.)	DISEASE-FREE SURVIVAL ANALYSIS (NO. STUDIES) (SIGNIFICANT MODALITY)	OVERALL SURVIVAL ANALYSIS (NO. STUDIES) (SIGNIFICANT MODALITY)
Weng et al., 2012[63]*	RFA vs. resection	CLM	13	RR = 2.227, $P < .001$ (10) (Resection superior)	RR = 1.474, $P < .001$ (12) (Resection superior)
Xu et al., 2012[9]*	RFA vs. resection	HCC	13	OR = 1.68, $P = .02$ (10) (Resection superior)	OR = 0.6, $P = .003$ (10) (Resection superior)
Duan et al., 2013[87]*	RFA vs. resection	HCC	12	OR = 0.54, $P < .00001$ (5) (Resection superior)	OR = 0.46, $P < .0001$ (5) (Resection superior)
Qi et al., 2014[88]	RFA vs. resection	HCC	3	HR = 1.41, $P = .001$ (3) (Resection superior)	HR = 1.41, $P = .02$ (3) (Resection superior)
Cai et al., 2014[89]*	RFA vs. resection	rHCC	6	OR = 3.70, $P = .000$ (3) (Resection superior)	OR = 0.97, $P = .846$ (6)
Wang et al., 2014[75]*	RFA vs. resection	HCC	28	OR = 0.52, $P = .007$ (9) (Resection superior)	OR = 0.68, $P = .03$ (15) (Resection superior)
Xu et al., 2014[90]*	RFA vs. resection	HCC	31	OR = 0.47, $P < .00001$ (20) (Resection superior)	OR = 0.57 (20) (Resection superior)
Yi et al., 2014[91]*	RFA vs. resection	HCC	19	OR = 0.47, $P = .0003$ (14) (Resection superior)	OR = 0.64, $P = .005$ (14) (Resection superior)
Fu et al., 2014[92]*	RFA vs. resection	HCC	5	OR = 0.38, $P = .0005$ (1) (Resection superior)	OR = 0.39, $P = .001$ (1) (Resection superior)
Feng et al., 2015[93]*	RFA vs. resection	HCC	23	OR = 0.50, $P = .001$ (15) (Resection superior)	OR = 0.55, $P < .001$ (18) (Resection superior)
van Amerongen et al., 2017[17]*	RFA vs. resection	CLM	20	OR = 2.20, $P = 0.007$ (9) (Resection superior)	OR = 2.20, $P < 0.00001$ (13) (Resection superior)
Yu et al., 2020[94]*	RFA	HCC	5	RR = 0.77 $P = 0.01$ (Resection superior)	RR = 0.86, $P = 0.43$ (no difference)

*5-year survival.

CLM, Colorectal liver metastases; HCC, hepatocellular carcinoma; rHCC, recurrent hepatocellular carcinoma; RR, risk ratio; OR, odds ratio; HR, hazard ratio.

TABLE 96B.4 Randomized Clinical Trials Examining Radiofrequency Ablation (RFA) Versus Liver Resection (LR) for Hepatocellular Carcinoma

STUDY	TREATMENT	NO. PATIENTS	MORBIDITY (%)	DISEASE-FREE SURVIVAL (%)	OVERALL SURVIVAL (%)
Chen et al., 2006[14,a]	LR	90	55.6	51.6	64.0
	RFA	71	4.2	46.4	67.9
Huang et al., 2010[15,b]	LR	115	27.8	51.3	75.65
	RFA	115	4.3	28.69	54.78
Feng et al., 2012[86,c]	LR	84	21.4	32	74.8
	RFA	84	9.5	42	67.2
Lee et al., 2018[95,b]	LR	26	37.9	44.4	83.4
	RFA	29	26.5	31.2	86.2

[a]4-year survival.

[b]5-year survival.

[c]3-year survival.

Radiofrequency Ablation for Recurrent Hepatocellular Carcinoma

The majority of patients with HCC succumb to liver failure because of intrahepatic recurrence. Salvage resection of locally recurrent lesions is recommended, but often is not feasible because of inadequate hepatic reserve, making RFA an effective therapeutic alternative. A retrospective review of locally recurrent HCC after ablative therapy in 50 patients found no difference in overall survival in patients treated with salvage resection versus salvage RFA, even though the RFA group did have a significantly higher recurrence rate.[96] Also, patients receiving RFA had significantly more impaired liver functional reserve preoperatively, suggesting a selection bias.[96] RFA may be the treatment of choice for carefully selected patients with recurrent hepatic disease, especially in patients with impaired hepatic reserve (Fig. 96B.7).

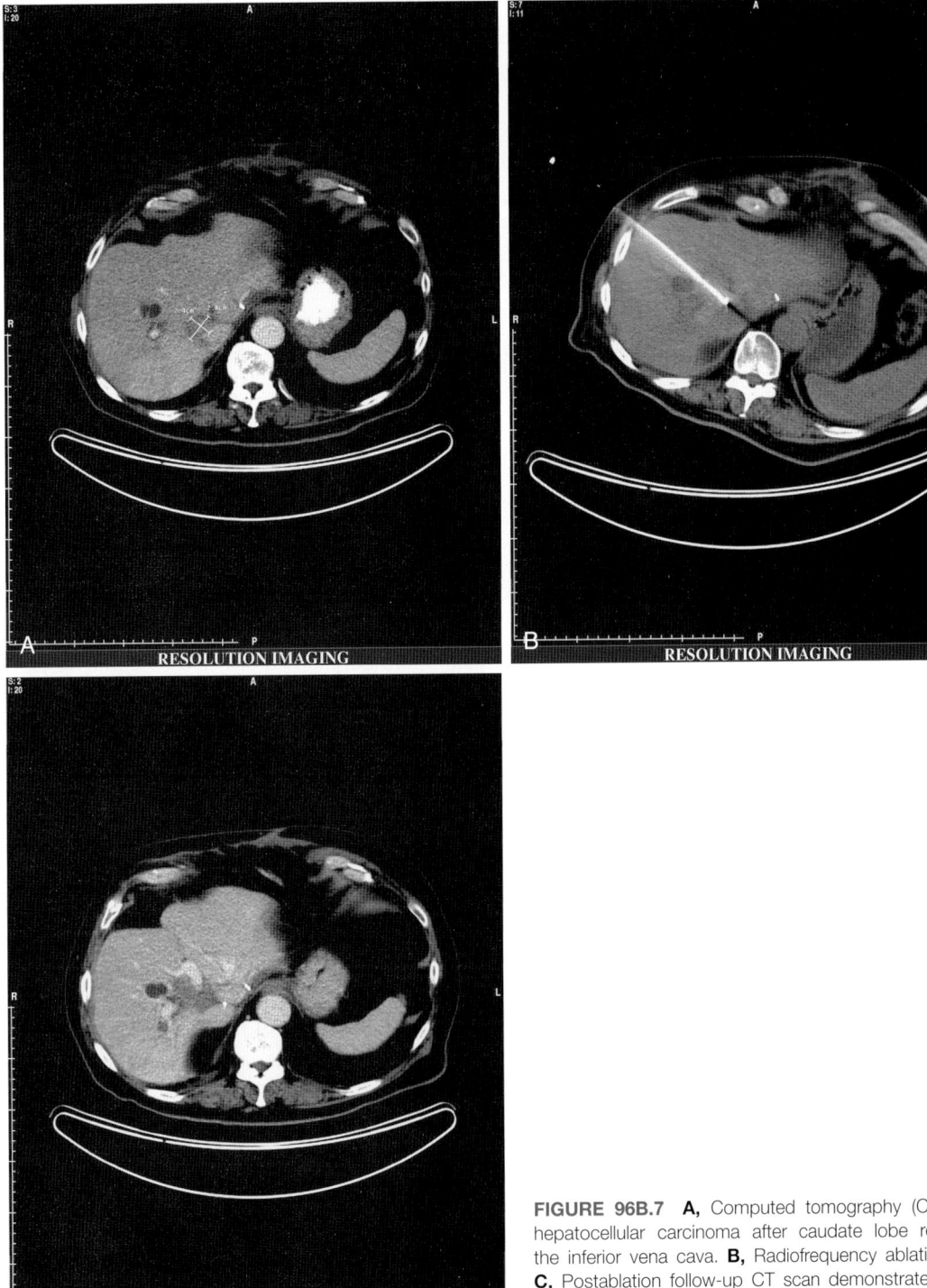

FIGURE 96B.7 A, Computed tomography (CT) scan of recurrent hepatocellular carcinoma after caudate lobe resection adjacent to the inferior vena cava. **B,** Radiofrequency ablation probe placement. **C,** Postablation follow-up CT scan demonstrates hypodensity at the ablation site consistent with successful ablation (see Chapter 14).

Recent European data on use of RFA as salvage therapy for individuals who had previously undergone major hepatectomy demonstrated that, in patients with up to three lesions less than 3 cm in size and no extrahepatic disease, RFA can successfully be used to treat recurrence with similar outcomes to their initial resection in terms of survival and time to recurrence.[97] In other words, ablation as a salvage after resection is an acceptable strategy with fewer complications where patients may not be candidates for or tolerate re-resection.

Radiofrequency Ablation as a Bridge to Transplantation

Transplantation is also a form of salvage therapy for recurrence (see Chapters 105 and 108A). Unfortunately, many patients with HCC succumb to liver failure while waiting for a suitable organ or are removed from the transplant list because of tumor progression. Recurrent intrahepatic HCC within the Milan criteria has been found to have a 60% disease-free survival out to 5 years when treated with transplantation.[98] RFA has effectively been used as a bridge to transplantation. Mazzaferro et al.[99] reported a series in which no patients dropped off the list because of progression when treated with pretransplant RFA. The impact on overall survival, however, is less clear. A prospective study of patients with HCC awaiting transplantation who received RFA showed no survival benefit compared with an observation group.[100]

Radiofrequency Ablation and Intrahepatic Cholangiocarcinoma

Numerous authors have reported successful treatment of unresectable intrahepatic cholangiocarcinoma (ICC) with RFA[101–105] (see Chapter 50). A retrospective study reported a 38.5-month mean overall survival after RFA treatment in seven patients.[106] In the largest retrospective study to date, 36 patients were treated with RFA and had a median overall survival of 60 months (91% 1-year survival, 71% 3-year survival).[107] No RCT exists for the treatment of ICC with RFA (Table 96B.5).

TUMOR RESPONSE AND RECURRENCE

The same imaging modality used before RFA should be used for serial monitoring after RFA to identify recurrence. CT and MRI have traditionally been used to evaluate response rates, but contrast-enhanced ultrasound has recently been shown to be effective in postablation surveillance[49] (see Chapters 14 and 15). Perfluorocarbon microbubbles (Sonazoid) are useful as a contrast agent because they are not trapped by Kupffer cells, therefore allowing differentiation between reactive hyperemia and residual HCC.[110] CT with contrast enhancement may reveal a hypovascular ablation field with a rim of hypervascular inflammatory tissue that fades with time. Recurrences appear as irregular, nonenhancing areas on contrast CT.[49]

Complete and Incomplete Response Rates to Radiofrequency Ablation

Response rates to RFA vary from 48% to 98% across studies, in part because of differences in the size and number of treated

lesions.[83,111] Livraghi et al.[83,111] evaluated RFA in patients with HCC; their 2000 study involving 114 patients with tumors larger than 3 cm revealed a complete response rate of 47.6% and the 2008 follow-up study in 218 patients with solitary tumors of 2 cm or less showed a 97.2% sustained complete response rate. The success rate was lower for infiltrating versus noninfiltrating HCC.[83,111] In studies of RFA treatment of liver metastases, a 91% response rate on follow-up CT at 1 month was achieved in patients with colorectal cancer metastases[112] and a 92% response rate when treating breast metastases.[113]

The approach to RFA will also influence response rates. Curley et al.[114] reported that 6 of 76 patients who underwent percutaneous RFA had an incomplete response, whereas all 34 patients who underwent laparoscopic or open RFA had a complete response. This early difference might be explained by better hepatic imaging with intraoperative ultrasonography during laparoscopy or laparotomy than with transabdominal ultrasonography during percutaneous RFA. A more current study, however, demonstrated a complete response rate of 84.6% percutaneously and 82.5% surgically ($P = .617$) in the treatment of HCC and liver metastases.[115]

Tumor location adjacent to large vessels also influences response rates. Blood flow from large vessels will create a heat-sink effect that cools surrounding tissue and increases the temperature necessary for complete ablation. Further, large vessels are resistant to high temperatures that can damage surrounding tissue. Lu et al.[116] found that porcine vessels smaller than 3 mm thrombosed or necrosed during RFA; those larger than 5 mm were not affected. In a trial evaluating the efficacy of hepatic artery occlusion during RFA, a spherical zone of ablation was also more often achieved when hepatic artery occlusion was used during ablation.[117] This supports the use of a Pringle maneuver to more effectively ablate tumors located near major blood vessels and improve response rates.

Because the gallbladder can also cause a heat-sink effect during ablation, elective cholecystectomy is recommended at ablation to decrease heat-sink and postablation complications. A recent study investigating laparoscopic RFA of HCC revealed a lower complete response to treatment in tumors located near the gallbladder.[118]

Rates of Recurrence at Radiofrequency Ablation Site

Reported recurrence rates are difficult to compare because they may be based on images obtained at different postoperative

---

TABLE 96B.5 Radiofrequency Ablation (RFA) in Treatment of Intrahepatic Cholangiocarcinoma (ICC)

STUDY	TUMOR TYPE	NO. PATIENTS	RFA APPROACH	TUMOR SIZE	SURVIVAL	
					MONTHS	%
Haidu et al., 2012[107]	ICC/RICC	11	Stereotactic	3 cm (median)	60 (median)	71 (3-year)
Fu et al., 2012[108]	ICC/RICC	17	Open/percutaneous	4.4 cm (median)	33 (median)	28.9 (5-year)
Butros et al., 2014[106]	ICC/RICC	7	Percutaneous	2.4 cm (mean)	38.5 (mean)	20 (5-year)
Yousaf et al., 2019[105,a]	ICC/RICC	206	Open/percutaneous	Not reported	8.7-52.4 (median)	16 (5-year)
Giorgio et al., 2019[102]	ICC	34	Percutaneous	3.1 cm (median)	48 (median)	65 (5-year)
Wu et al., 2019[109]	ICC	86	Percutaneous	3.0 cm (median)	Not reported	17.6 (5-year)
Brandi et al., 2020[101]	ICC	29	Percutaneous	>2.0 cm	27.5 (median)	11 (4-year)

RICC, Recurrent intrahepatic cholangiocarcinoma.

[a]Denotes a meta-analysis.

times, and in some cases, with different imaging modalities. We previously reported that tumor size significantly influences local recurrence of metastatic disease, independent of RFA technique employed.[119,120] In a study evaluating 234 patients undergoing RFA for 274 HCC tumors of 2 cm or less, there were 145 cases in which a complete ablation was achieved.[121] Of those, four had local recurrence by year 3 of follow-up.[121] Prior studies found that patients with large tumors, tumor vascular invasion, and hepatic dysfunction had a statistically higher recurrence rate.[122] To date, no study has shown that differences in technique influence the rate of recurrence after a complete response.

COMPLICATIONS OF RADIOFREQUENCY ABLATION

Reported morbidity and mortality rates associated with RFA can be difficult to interpret, in part because technical approaches vary. Some investigators combine RFA with other treatments, such as liver resection, and the addition of a second procedure may inflate the complication rate. Ablation of multiple tumors also increases the risk of complications such as bleeding or bile leak.

Unfortunately, the reporting of morbidities is not standardized and therefore it is inconsistently reported. This is highlighted by reports of complications ranging from 2.9% to 24.5% in some series.[50,123] Variations in patient selection and disease type also confound interpretation of results, because patients with HCC have different comorbid factors than those with colorectal metastases.

Direct complications of RFA include biloma, biliary fistula, ascites, hepatic insufficiency, arteriovenous fistula, portal vein thrombosis, symptomatic pleural effusion, hepatic abscess, pain, diaphragmatic hernia, hemorrhage, hydropneumothorax, pneumothorax, tumor implantation, and thermal injury to surrounding structures.[124] Burns related to grounding pads have also been reported; these can be avoided by proper positioning of the pads, by using a larger number of pads for longer ablations, and by carefully following manufacturers' directions.[125] Other potential complications are surgery related, such as myocardial infarction, cardiac arrhythmias, and pneumonia.

In the largest series to date, Maeda et al.[50] report a 2.92% rate of complications over 11,298 ablations performed in Japan. They report a 0.06% mortality rate and a very low rate of complications.[50] The most frequent complication is hepatic injury, which occurred in 1.31% of patients; extrahepatic organ injury occurred in 0.74% of patients, and hemorrhage occurred in 0.56% of patients.[50]

The following two cases illustrate why RFA should be undertaken only by skilled physicians able to identify and manage its complications and only at centers equipped with appropriate staff and equipment for acute care. Figure 96B.8 shows a bile duct injury (see Chapter 42) caused by RFA of a colorectal cancer metastasis near the porta hepatis. The injury was treated with endoscopic retrograde cholangiopancreatography (ERCP) and biliary stenting. Percutaneous RFA has specific anatomic limitations. The close proximity of the liver dome and the diaphragm increases the risk of diaphragmatic injury. Figure 96B.9 illustrates a diaphragmatic hernia diagnosed 18 months after successful RFA to an HCC in segments IV and VIII. The hernia was primarily repaired after performing a bowel resection for strangulated small intestine.[126] Lesions located at the liver's edge increase the risk of gastrointestinal damage. A multicenter study found that 33% of all mortality was associated with gastrointestinal thermal injury.[127] In an animal model, balloon interposition significantly decreased bowel injury near an ablation zone.[128] If interposition devices are unavailable, consideration of open or laparoscopic RFA instead of percutaneous RFA is recommended for tumors within 1 cm of the liver edge adjacent to bowel.

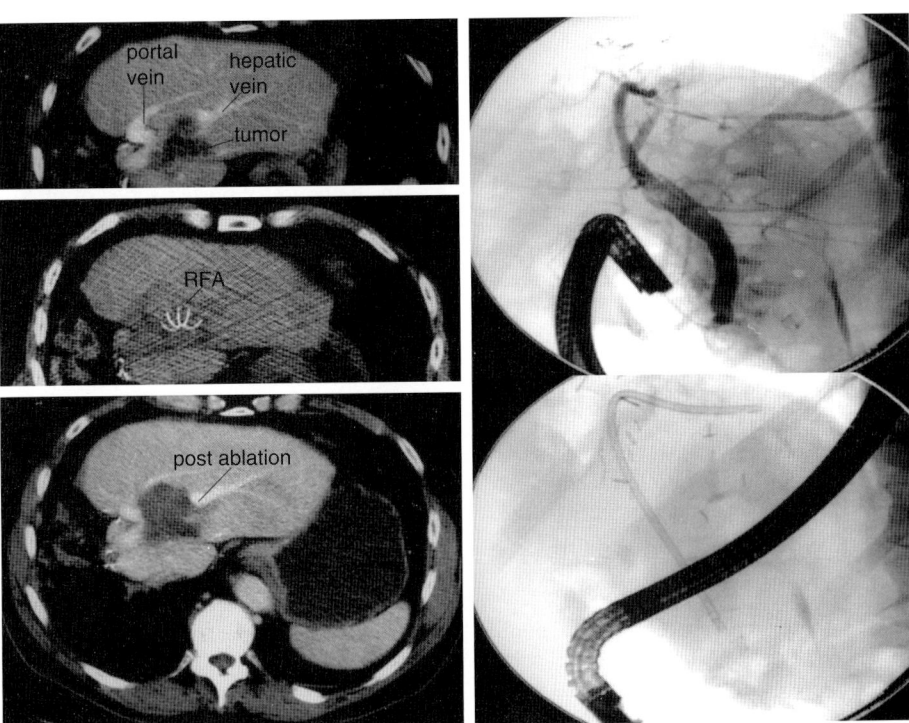

FIGURE 96B.8 Biliary injury after radiofrequency ablation *(RFA)* treated with ERCP and stent placement (see Chapter 42).

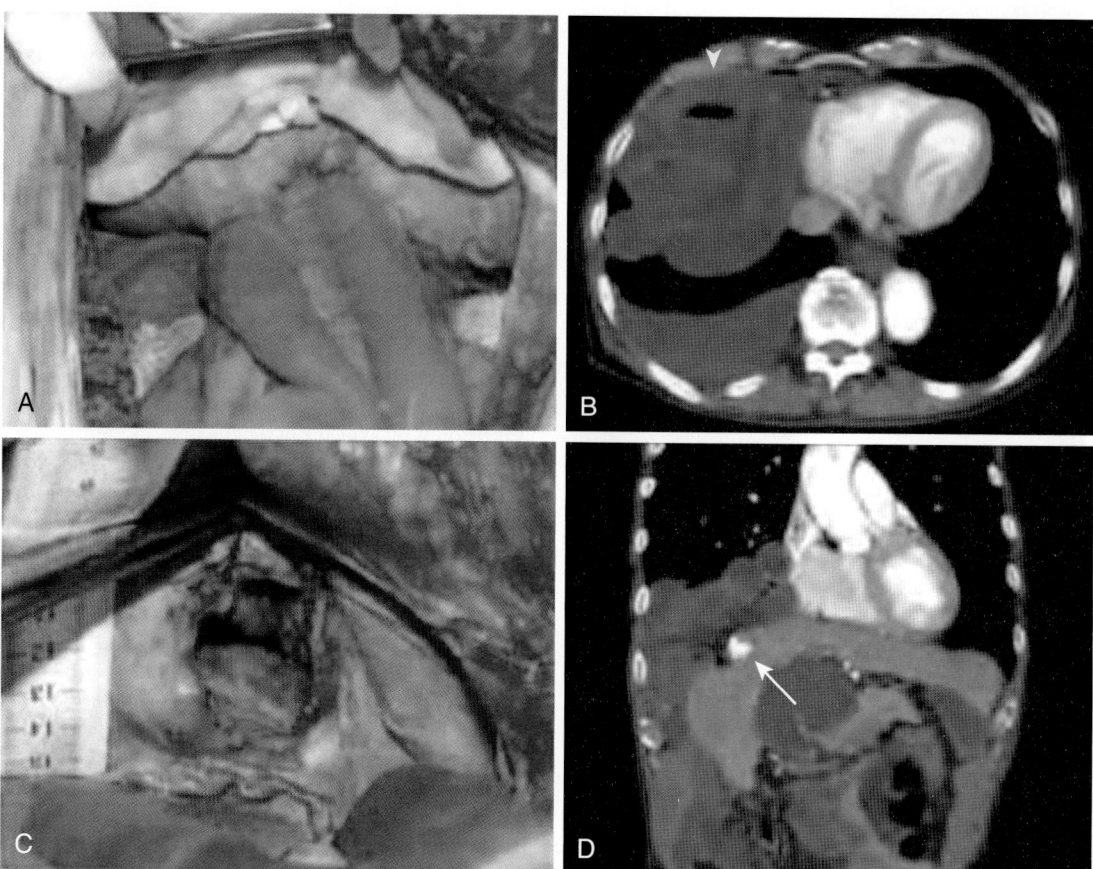

FIGURE 96B.9   Right-sided diaphragmatic hernia after radiofrequency ablation. A, Strangulated bowel. **B** and **D,** Computed tomography scans illustrating dilated loops of small bowel. **C,** Diaphragmatic defect after hernia reduction. (From Nakamura T, et al. Successful surgical rescue of delayed onset diaphragmatic hernia following radiofrequency ablation for hepatocellular carcinoma. *Ulus Travma Acil Cerrahi Derg.* 2014;20[4]:295–299.)

In a 2014 randomized trial comparing complications between percutaneous RFA treatment and hepatectomy in 120 patients with HCC of 3 cm or less, Fang et al.[129] reported only one major complication in the percutaneous RFA group (pleural effusion) but 14 major complications in the hepatectomy group. Albumin and bilirubin levels on day 7 after treatment were also significantly worse in the surgical group compared with patients receiving ablation.[129]

Intrahepatic abscess typically appears approximately 2 weeks after ablation and may necessitate percutaneous or surgical drainage.[130] Low-grade fever and fatigue can occur immediately after RFA and persist for as long as 7 to 10 days; this so-called *postablation syndrome* is normal, but any continued or significant elevation should prompt CT imaging for possible hepatic abscess. The need for prophylactic antibiotics during RFA remains controversial. A recent retrospective single-center study reported one intrahepatic abscess (0.8%) in a cohort not treated with prophylactic antibiotics.[131] Antibiotics should be considered for a patient with a previous biliary enteric anastomosis, uncontrolled diabetes, or large, centralized tumors close to central bile ducts.[131]

Reports of tumor seeding vary from 0.018% to 2.8%.[50,132,133] Risk of seeding is increased if the tumor is a subcapsular, poorly differentiated, primary HCC or is associated with an elevated AFP level. Risk is also increased if multiple needle insertions are required to ablate the lesion successfully.[134] Techniques to minimize tract seeding include adherence to meticulous technique, avoidance of repositioning, and tract ablation on withdrawal.

Injury to bile ducts during RFA can result in biliary stricture, biloma formation, bilioperitoneum, and biliopleural fistula. This occurs most often when ablating hilar tumors or tumors less than 1 cm from a major bile duct[135] (see Chapter 42).

In the largest reported series of intraductal cooling during RFA, cooled (4°C) Ringer's lactate was infused through a catheter after choledochotomy in 13 patients undergoing RFA of tumors within 6 mm of a central bile duct.[136] One patient had a local recurrence, and one had biliary stenosis.[136] Biliary stenting has also been described as a technique to avoid biliary injury during ablation of a tumor near a major bile duct.[120]

CONCLUSION

Radiofrequency ablation can treat primary or metastatic liver tumors operatively or percutaneously with reasonable success and minimal morbidity or mortality. An operative approach allows thorough surveillance for extrahepatic disease in the abdomen, as well as superior evaluation of intrahepatic disease when using intraoperative ultrasound. It also allows for isolation of the liver from adjacent organs that could be injured during ablation and ablation of lesions not anatomically amenable to percutaneous treatment. Conversely, a percutaneous approach is less invasive, has a quicker recovery, employs real-time image-based assessment of the ablation, and can be performed as an outpatient procedure. Although the proximity of a tumor to surrounding structures may limit the success of percutaneous ablation, multiple techniques have been developed to separate the ablation zone from neighboring tissue, minimizing iatrogenic morbidity. Percutaneous ablation should be considered in patients with high-risk, limited hepatic reserve or recurrent disease.

Randomized trials use different inclusion criteria and thus report varying recommendations. When adhering to the Milan criteria, resection allows HCC patients to reach better overall and recurrence-free survival. In smaller lesions, RFA provides therapeutic effects comparable to resection. Until more randomized studies present data to the contrary, resection remains the standard of care for patients with acceptable performance status and resectable disease confined to the liver. RFA is an alternative for those unable to undergo resection because of limited hepatic reserve, bilobar disease, and/or poor performance status. In these

patients, RFA can be very successful with limited risk and durable results. Although RFA provides local control of metastatic colorectal liver metastases, its impact on survival is unclear. Systemic therapy should be used to treat or prevent other sites of metastatic disease.

The field of ablation continues to evolve, with improvements in probe technology leading to higher rates of complete response. Newer probes are now able to tailor the ablation zone to specific tumor sizes and shapes. One possible direction for future growth in the use of RFA comes from the fact that RFA has been documented to produce a more robust immune response than other ablative technologies, something that may prove useful as more and more patients are being treated with immunotherapy drugs. Research on this topic is in its infancy, results are disparate, and in order to get to mainstream clinical use more exploration is required before conclusions can be drawn.[8,137-140]

The references for this chapter can be found online by accessing the accompanying Expert Consult website.

Microwave ablation and irreversible electroporation of liver tumors

Robert CG Martin II and Robert Rickert

OVERVIEW

Each year nearly 1 million liver cancers are diagnosed across the world, making liver cancer the fifth most common cancer in men and ninth in women[1,2] (see Chapter 89). Liver cancer is one of the most fatal cancers, being the second leading cause of cancer death in men and sixth leading cause of cancer death in women.[2] The most common liver cancer remains hepatocellular carcinoma (HCC) (see Chapter 89), a primary liver malignancy and the third most frequent cause of cancer-related death worldwide.[3] Another category is secondary malignancies, also known as metastatic tumors; common metastatic tumors to the liver include colorectal liver metastases (see Chapter 90) and metastatic neuroendocrine tumors (see Chapter 91). There are various treatment options available for these lesions, including liver transplant (see Chapter 105), surgical resection (see Chapter 101), and thermal and nonthermal ablation (see Chapters 94, 96B, and 96D), but surgical resection remains the standard of care for selected patients. Many factors must be taken into account when considering which option is viable for a given patient; for example, when considering MWA the histology of the tumor, the size of the lesion, the patient's comorbidities, the extent of extrahepatic metastasis, and the knowledge of the practicing physician should all be considered.[4] For many patients, resection is not possible.

The thermal and nonthermal ablative techniques, due to their unique physical properties and minimally invasive procedure, have increased the curative ablative treatment options; these techniques can be used when resection is contraindicated.[4] These thermal-based and non–thermal-based techniques are characterized in Table 96C.1. Microwave ablation (MWA) and radiofrequency ablation (RFA) are the two most common thermal ablation techniques used today, but they differ in how they deliver heat, leading to different amounts of tissue destruction between them. As discussed later in this chapter, comparisons between the two techniques have shown similar long-term results, but MWA has the added benefits of resistance to heat-sink effect, higher intratumor temperatures, faster procedure, and larger ablation volumes.[5–7]

PHYSICS OF MICROWAVE ENERGY

MWA achieves heat destruction of tissue through both active and passive heating. The active heating process of microwave energy requires the presence of dielectric molecules, such as water, to function. MWA reaches a much higher operating frequency (2450 MHz) than RFA, which makes it potentially more efficient (rapid temperature) for thermal ablation of solid organs. As a dipole molecule, water is affected by the applied electromagnetic field broadcast by the microwave antenna during the procedure. This is called *dielectric permittivity*. This property allows for dielectric hysteresis, which induces rotation of the dipole molecules and accounts for the efficient amount of heat generated during microwave ablation. One or more molecules are dipoles with unequal electrical charge distribution and they attempt to reorient continuously at the same rate in the microwave's oscillating electric field. As a result of the microwave transmission, the water molecules flip back and forth at a billion times a second leading to this vigorous movement to produce friction and heat, which leads to cellular death via coagulation necrosis. An additional mechanism responsible for heat generation in microwave ablation is ionic polarization, which occurs when ions move in response to the applied electric field of the microwave. The displaced ions cause collisions with other ions, converting this kinetic energy into heat. However, this is the lesser of the two mechanisms that generate the efficient heat from microwave ablation. Microwaves emit nonionizing radiation for heating which produces homogeneous heating within the field regardless of the tissue types; this distinguishes MWA from monopolar RFA in terms of mechanism of heating and makes it a clinically superior method for ablation.[8] The passive phase of microwave heating is by conduction of heat beyond the active heating zone and is susceptible to local tissue factors such as heat and current sinking.

The current frequencies of the commercially available microwave ablation devices are at 915 MHz or 2450 MHz. The reported potential benefit of the 915-MHz microwave is that it could penetrate deeper than the 2450-MHz microwave, which may theoretically yield larger ablation zones. However, the energy deposition is influenced by the dielectric properties of the antenna design.[8] Microwave energy can be generated through a magnetron or solid-state amplifier,[9] and the antenna broadcasts the electromagnetic energy to the target tissue. The coaxial cable consists of an inner and outer conductor with the dielectric material placed between the two layers. At its tip, the outer conductor is stopped to expose the inner conductor for broadcasting the microwave energy. This inner conductor is covered in a ceramic pointed tip for insertion into the tissue and microwave energy can pass freely through the ceramic.

Large ablative volumes via the 2450-MHz system can be created by increasing the power (wattage) and duration of the microwave energy. The ablative size can be manipulated to personalize each procedure to a specific patient. Physical factors that influence the ablative size include the water content of tissue (e.g., normal liver vs. cirrhotic liver vs. fatty liver) and the type of tissue being ablated (e.g., hepatocellular vs. metastatic colorectal vs. metastatic neuroendocrine). Some mechanical factors include the power output of the generator, the type of cable in use, the design of the antenna, the duration of the electrical current, and the number of antennas being used during the procedure.[10]

TABLE 96C.1 Main Potential Advantages and Disadvantages of Each Energy-Based Ablative Technology in Hepatic Tumor Treatment

TECHNOLOGY	POTENTIAL ADVANTAGES	POTENTIAL DISADVANTAGES
RFA	High rates of local control in tumors smaller than 3 cm Established safety profile Known limitations Experience in combination treatments (HCC)—TACE and DEB Widely available	High rates of incomplete ablation in tumors larger than 3 cm Heat-sink effect in perivascular tumors Potential risk of thermal injury to critical structures Variability in RFA devices
MWA	Potential to treat tumors larger than 3 cm more effectively Less affected by heat-sink effect Ability to activate multiple probes at the same time No grounding pads required Efficacy data (predictability and reproducibility) Established safety data	Potential risk of thermal injury to critical structures (and vessels?) Variability in MWA devices
CRYO	Ability to image the ice-ball formation during the procedure	Very limited clinical data Risk of bleeding and cryoshock
IRE	Potential to treat tumors located in the vicinity of critical structures Heat-sink effect not relevant Established patient selection and clinical data	Neuromuscular blockage and cardiac gating required General anesthesia required Multiple probe placement

CRYO, ; *IRE,* irreversible electroporation; *MWA,* microwave ablation; *RFA,* radiofrequency ablation.

LOCAL TISSUE FACTORS THAT AFFECT THERMOABLATION

The success of a thermal ablation procedure depends partly on the local tissue surrounding the lesion to be ablated. Intrinsic factors of a given tissue type, such as dielectric permittivity and electric conductivity, will influence the size and shape of the ablation zone formed during the procedure, as well as how energy is deposited in the target tissue by the thermal source, be it RFA, MWA, or irreversible electroporation (IRE). Box 96C.1 summarizes some of the clinical considerations to take into account when using these techniques.

As discussed in the previous section, microwaves generate heat and subsequent tissue necrosis, based on the generation of an oscillating electric field that causes dipolar molecules, such as water molecules, to flip back and forth generating friction and heat. Not all tissues have the same water content, and some tissues are well perfused by blood vessels containing a rapidly moving stream of blood. Proximity to blood vessels can cause an adverse event called *heat sinking* that occurs when the electric current is too close to the vessel; the blood flow imparts a cooling effect on the adjacent tissue. Heat sinking can lead to incomplete tumor ablation—the tissue near the vessel will not reach the necessary temperature for ablation that surrounding tissue reaches. Similarly, close proximity to the blood vessel will also cause *current sinking*—the vessel causes a distortion of the electric current, which can alter ablation performance. RFA suffers from both of these adverse events due to its method of heat delivery; RFA produces circulating electrical currents that dissipate heat to the surrounding tissue. Heat deposition depends on the electric conductivity of the tissue, which is in turn influenced by water content. Thus MWA is often a better choice for the patient. MWA is still affected by these adverse effects, but much less so; the microwaves generated rely primarily on the dielectric permittivity of the target tissue, and these microwaves will transmit through any tissue, including nearby vasculature or tissue with variable water content, keeping the electric field relatively constant throughout.[11,12] Clinicians should still bear these adverse events in mind during the

BOX 96C.1 Critical Considerations for Clinical Validation of Novel Energy-Based Ablation Technologies in Hepatic Tumor Treatment

- Monopolar RFA is an established technique for the treatment of tumors that are limited in number (3 or less) and size (3 cm or less) and are located 1 cm or more from critical structures and vessels.*
- MWA appears to have potential to improve the rate of complete ablation achieved with RFA in tumors that are larger than 2–3 cm or multiple; device-specific safety and efficacy data, including predictability and reproducibility, are warranted.
- MWA seems to have potential to overcome the limitations of RFA in the treatment of tumors in perivascular location; device-specific safety and efficacy analyses are warranted.
- IRE has demonstrated promise for the treatment of small tumors located in the vicinity of bile ducts and blood vessels; continued efficacy data are warranted given the high demands on targeting of the multiple IRE probes.
- More data are needed to define the potential for other energy-based ablation technologies in the specific field of liver tumor treatment.

*Vessels 3 mm or more in caliber are considered relevant for heat-sink effect.
IRE, Irreversible electroporation; *MWA,* microwave ablation; *RFA,* radiofrequency ablation.

procedure, though, as ablation zone size and shape can never be assumed and must be checked to ensure ablation success.

In addition, dehydration and consequent carbonization can occur when using RFA to treat a given lesion. This will lead to a significantly decreased final ablation volume; the treated tissue, without any remaining water, will block the necessary complete electric circuit from forming and less heat will be generated. At the same time, if the tissue to be ablated is heated too quickly to above 100°C, the intracellular components can vaporize and carbonize; the gas will act as an insulator and prevent proper heat dissipation to the surrounding tissue. Both components will impede complete ablation of the desired lesion. Microwave ablation is not limited by these factors, because, as mentioned, microwaves transmit throughout the tissue more evenly, producing a consistently more uniform ablation.

For these reasons, MWA has gained traction as an excellent option for tumors in close proximity to vital structures. As can be seen in Table 96C.2, authors have compared MWA success rates for tumors near blood vessels, the diaphragm, and in subcapsular locations with less risky locations. Based on the studies listed, we have noted no significant difference in ablation success and recurrence rates for HCC tumors in these various locations when treated with MWA. This reinforces the utility of MWA for liver tumors in challenging locations, although some authors did report increased complications when performing ablations in difficult to access areas.[13,14]

A wide array of MWA systems are available for use (Table 96C.3). On an individual basis, they may use a single probe or multiple probes, use gas-cooling or water-cooling systems, and use different ablation frequencies.[15,16] Many different manufacturers worldwide have produced their own ablation systems, and there are currently many different competing models available. There are limited comparisons available due to the widely varying nature of tumors present and although authors have recently compared systems for individual indications, no clear consensus is present yet. In 2015 Leung et al.[17] found a 4% local recurrence rate for ablations performed with a 915 MHz system and a 12.6% local recurrence rate for ablations performed with a 2.4 GHz system, but the results may have been affected by the fact that the 2.4 GHz system was used for patients with larger tumors, more noncolorectal metastases, and less pretreatment chemotherapy. However, Vogl et al.[18] performed a similar comparison and found a complete ablation rate of 90.2% with 915 MHz and 95.5% with 2.4 GHz, as well as an overall survival of 82.98% at 4 years with 915 MHz, against 92.91% overall survival at 4 years with the 2.4 GHz system. In addition, multiple authors have established the use of the Emprint 2.45 GHz Ablation System for MWA and found it to be safe and effective for a variety of liver tumors, with complete ablation rates ranging from 83% to 100%.[19–21] Hopefully in future years additional comparisons will be performed following the ablation standards established by North and Martin in 2014 and specific indications for particular MWA frequencies can be set.[4]

TECHNICAL CONSIDERATION FOR PERFORMING MICROWAVE ABLATION

Three approaches can be used for MWA: open, laparoscopic, and percutaneous. The underlying principles of any microwave ablative therapy stay the same, but the ability to accommodate and individualize each procedure in accordance with the patient's unique needs is essential to MWA success. The approach chosen should reflect the tumor biology, tumor histology, size of tumor, and segments involved; it is important to target the skill level of the practitioner and tailor the choice to the patient's needs. The goal of any MWA should be complete ablation in greater than 95% of all tumors. Terms such as *cytoreduction, partial ablation,* and *debulking* do not reflect accepted concepts in oncology and are poor substitutes, indicative of bad technique and poor patient selection. Patients should not be "owned" by a physician; the technique used must always be in the patient's best interest regardless of the MWA access.

Surgical resection remains the optimal management for selected patients, based on histology and disease extent. A surgical MWA approach is primarily used when tumor morphology requires multiple ablation therapies; when tumors are located near the dome of the liver, for which percutaneous ablation might cause pneumothorax or damage to the diaphragm; or when the tumor is located near the visceral organs such as the gallbladder, colon, or stomach.[22] If MWA alone is the sole goal in a patient's care, a laparoscopic approach should be performed in most cases. Lesions located anteriorly and not adjacent to a major pedicle can be ablated percutaneously using ultrasound (US) guidance and computed tomography (CT) confirmation. If the lesion is located deep in the liver at the dome, next to a major pedicle, or adjacent to other structures such as the diaphragm or colon, ablation should be performed surgically, either laparoscopically or open, based on the patient's past surgical history, body habitus, and level of the surgeon's laparoscopic ultrasound skill. If an open approach is used, it is best done through a subcostal or midline laparotomy.

Regardless of the approach, the patient is usually positioned supine or in a lateral position on the table. The key to a successful ablation session is adequate exposure of the liver in order to perform a methodic evaluation of the liver by intraoperative US. All eight segments of the liver must be evaluated to ensure no lesions are overlooked (see Chapter 24). After all lesions have been identified, the plane of the needle track should be evaluated to ensure that it does not cross a portal or major hepatic vein pedicle. The type of antenna(s) to deploy should be decided on *before* the operation. All of the 915 MHz systems require at least 2 to 3 probes placed in parallel in order to obtain a similar ablation as a single antenna of the 2450 MHz systems when treating a lesion greater than 2.5 to 3.9 cm in size. Different amounts of power are deposited by the antenna at different frequencies, which leads to different ablation volumes created depending on the antenna used.[18] Considering desired ablation size may also aid in deciding which frequency to use. It is important to make sure that there are not any vital structures within 1.0 to 1.5 cm near the microwave field (Fig. 96C.1). MWA times can vary from 5 minutes to 45 minutes. The deepest lesion is usually treated first; in a staged procedure, the most difficult lesion is treated first.

The need to perform overlapping ablations should be decided before the first ablation. Given the artifact and distortion that occurs during the first ablation, subsequent US imaging can lead to inaccurate second and third needle placements to complete an overlapping ablation. The three-dimensional ablation zone is conceptually difficult to grasp for practitioners, considering that intraoperative US provides only a two-dimensional view.

To further improve MWA technique, authors have developed mathematical models to aid in guidance of MWA. Gao et al.[23] used their model to significantly improve their complete ablation rates for CT-guided MWA from 88.3% in the control group to 97.7% in the model group. Similarly, Mbalisike et al.[24] reported the usage of a robotic guidance system for MWA in 2015, with fewer needle insertions per procedure, fewer needle readjustments, and quicker insertion time present in procedures with the robotic guidance compared with manual.

Further, authors experimented with different imaging modalities during procedures. 1.5T magnetic resonance imaging (MRI) guidance for MWA had a complete ablation rate of 100% in a recent study and 98% in another, with an overall survival of 41.6 months.[25,26] A study comparing the use of ordinary US-guided MWA versus contrast-enhanced US-guided

TABLE 96C.2   Microwave Ablation Studies on Tumor Location

STUDY	NO. OF PATIENTS	HISTOLOGY	WAS ABLATION SUCCESS REPORTED AND DEFINED?	OVERALL SURVIVAL (Y/N) MEDIAN	LOCAL RECURRENCE	LIVER RECURRENCE	MORTALITY	COMPLICATIONS
An et al., 2020[13]	489	489 HCC	Yes, 95.2% in challenging locations vs. 94.9% in nonchallenging locations	At 5 years: Adjacent vital structures 70.5%, gallbladder 76%, hepatic hilar regions 62.9%, major vessel 78.3%, diaphragm 92.8%, capsule 85.3%, nonchallenging location 89.7%	—	—	—	Challenging locations: hemoperitoneum (1), cholangiectasis with jaundice (3), liver abscess (2) Nonchallenging location: large pleural effusion (2)
Dou, 2017	406	406 HCC	Defined, not reported	Vessel group: 98% at 1 year, 82% at 3 years, 46.9% at 5 years Safe group: 98.1% at 1 year, 73.7% at 3 years, 48.2% at 5 years (After PSM)	Vessel group: 6.5% at 1 year, 10.8% at 3 years, 10.8% at 5 years Safe group: 9% at 1 year, 14.3% at 3 years, 14.3% at 5 years (After PSM, LTP)	—	—	Vessel group: pleural effusion (2), tumor seeding (2), abscess (1), thrombosis (1), hemorrhage (2) Safe group: pleural effusion (2), tumor seeding (1), abscess (1), hemorrhage (1)
Li et al., 2015[14]	155	97 HCC, 58 metastases	Yes, 92.2% study group, 94% control group Also 97.1% HCC, 87.5% metastatic tumors	—	17.6% study group, 12.8% control group. 8.9% HCC, 25% metastatic tumors *Recurrence not defined	—	—	Study group: fever (12.2%), abdominal pain (20.4%), pleural effusion (6.1%), nausea and vomiting (14.3%) Control group: fever (2.8%), abdominal pain (3.8%), pleural effusion (4.7%), nausea and vomiting (1.9%)
Liu, 2017	463	463 HCC	Yes, 95.5% subcapsular tumors, 98.3% non-subcapsular	Subcapsular group: 95.7% at 1 year, 90.1% at 2 years, 82.9% at 3 years, 71.1% at 4 years Non-subcapsular group: 98.5% at 1 year, 92.8% at 2 years, 83.2% at 3 years, 73.6% at 4 years	5.4% for subcapsular group, 6.3% for non-subcapsular (LTP here both new lesions and incomplete ablation growth)	—	0% procedure related; 14.7% subcapsular group, 10.4% non-subcapsular group on follow-up	Subcapsular: pleural fluid aspiration (4), peritoneal seeding (1), moderate right upper quadrant pain (30) Non-subcapsular: pleural fluid aspiration (2), abdominal wall seeding (1), moderate right upper quadrant pain (17)
Zhi-Yu, 2017	189	189 HCC	Yes, 98.2%	—	11.1% at 1 year, 18.1% at 2 years, 19.1% at 3 years, 19.9% at 4 years (LTP)	—	—	Pain, postablation syndrome, minimal asymptomatic perihepatic fluid or blood collection

HCC, Hepatocellular carcinoma; LTP, ; PSM,

TABLE 96C.3 Currently Available Microwave Ablation Systems

SYSTEM	DEVICE MANUFACTURER	GENERATOR AND ANTENNA	MAXIMUM GENERATOR POWER (W)	MAXIMUM ANTENNA POWER (W)	MAXIMUM SELECTABLE ABLATION TIME (MIN)	PROPOSED MAXIMUM ABLATION TIME (MIN)	FREQUENCY (HZ)	WATER COOLED?	NO. OF ANTENNAS
A	AngioDynamics	Soleror, Acculis Sulis Vp$_{MTA}$ and Accu2i	180	140	6	6	2.45×10^9	Yes	1
B	HS Hospital Service	HS Amica-Gen and APK14150T19V4	140	100	25	10	2.45×10^9	Yes	1
C	Medtronic	Evident MWA Generator and VT1720	60 per device	45 per antenna	10	10	915×10^6	Yes	1-3
D	Medwaves	Avecure Microwave Generator and 14-15-LH-35	40	32 (modulated)	15	15	$(902-928) \times 10^6$ (modulated)	No	1
E	Perseon	MicroThermX and SynchroWave Antenna	180	60 per antenna	—	—	915×10^6	Yes	1-3
F	Ethicon	NEUWAVE Certus	140	—	—	—	2.45×10^9	No	1-3
G	Vision Medical (formerly Forsea)	MTC-3C	150	—	—	—	2.45×10^9	Yes	1-2
H	Canyon Medical	KY-2000	100	—	—	—	915×10^6 2.45×10^9	Yes	Multiple
I	Alfresa Pharma	Microtaze	70	—	—	—	2.45×10^9	Yes	—
J	Medtronic	Emprint Ablation System	100	—	10	—	2.45×10^9	Yes	1
K	Eco Medical	ECO-100A1	120	—	—	—	2.45×10^9	Yes	—
L	Qi Ya Medical Treatment Facility Limited Company	Model III	120	—	—	—	2.45×10^9	Yes	—

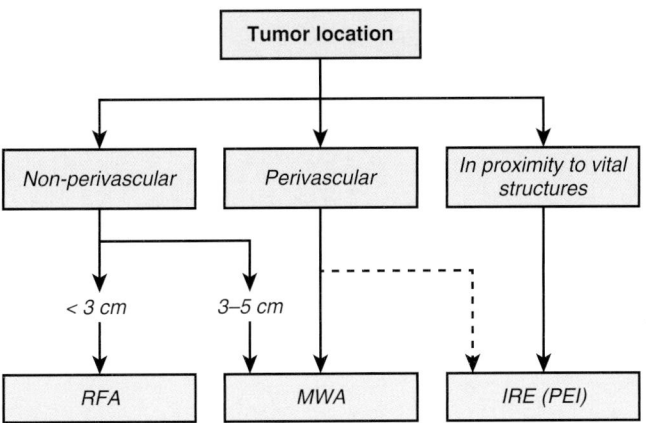

FIGURE 96C.1 Proposed algorithm for the use of the different techniques of image-guided ablation in the treatment of malignant liver tumors. The algorithm assumes a successful completion of the described clinical validation process and takes into account tumor size and location as the main drivers for the choice of the ablation technique. RFA is supposed to remain an accepted option for small (3 cm or less) tumors in nonperivascular locations. MWA is expected to become the preferred modality for ablation of tumors of intermediate size (3–5 cm) or in perivascular locations. Tumors in proximity to vital structures (including vessels) are directed toward nonthermal techniques such as IRE or percutaneous ethanol injection (PEI). The use of PEI is only recommended for small HCC tumors. *IRE,* Irreversible electroporation; *MWA,* microwave ablation; *PEI,* percutaneous ethanol injection; *RFA,* radiofrequency ablation.

MWA found significantly reduced local recurrence of 8% in contrast-enhanced US compared with 16% in ordinary US.[27] In addition, fewer complications, such as pain, intraabdominal hemorrhage, and infection, were noted in contrast-enhanced US MWA.[27] As evidenced by this work, further refinement of MWA protocol can continue to improve outcomes.

Defining the success of the MWA is paramount. Well-established quality parameters were published by North and Martin et al.[4] and agreed on in a multi-institutional review of all clinical papers. They are defined as follows:

- *Ablation success.* Defined as complete eradication of the tumor using high-quality cross-section contrast-enhanced imaging (CT or MRI) within 4 weeks of ablation, specifically disappearance of any intratumoral contrast enhancement as described in modified RECIST criteria (see Chapters 14, 15, and 96B).
- *Local recurrence after ablation.* After confirmation of ablation success (i.e., >4 weeks), local recurrence is defined as evidence for viable tumor at or within 1.0 cm of a prior ablation site for which ablation success was documented. Confirmed by multislice, multiphase dynamic imaging (see Chapters 14 and 15).
- *Nonlocal hepatic recurrence.* Evidence for viable intrahepatic tumor more than 1.0 cm from any prior ablation site at any time interval after ablation.
- *Indications for ablations and morbidity.* The number of patients and the number of tumors with the segments involved should be reported with at least 90-day morbidity follow-up on all ablation cases regardless of access. Morbidity should be reported per established surgical morbidity definitions.[28]

Rate of complete ablation of liver tumors, ablation recurrence defined as recurrent disease within 1 cm of ablation site,

hepatic recurrence at nonablated sites, and morbidity and mortality associated with the procedure should be reported in all clinical MWA studies regardless of access.[8] It is also important to be able to define success shortly after the procedure is performed so any potential corrections can be made. Success can be defined on immediate or 24-hour post-CT scan that demonstrates a zone of ablation encompassing both the tumor and a rim of normal liver tissue approximately 1 cm beyond the tumor in each dimension.[29]

CLINICAL RESULTS OF MICROWAVE ABLATION

Clinical Results for Hepatocellular Carcinoma (see Chapter 89)

In the intervening 25+ years since Seki et al.[30] first reported the application of microwave ablation for hepatocellular tumors, use of MWA has expanded to encompass both primary and metastatic liver tumors, as well as symptomatic hepatic hemangiomas, all of which are discussed below. The utility of MWA has grown such that substantial work has compared its efficacy with other more established treatment methods, such as surgical resection and RFA, as authors look to define the role of MWA in today's surgical practice.

MWA continues to be used successfully for the treatment of hepatocellular carcinoma (Table 96C.4). In recent years many studies have recorded their experience with MWA, with complete ablation rates as high as 100% for tumors less than 5 cm in diameter and 91.7% for tumors greater than 5 cm in diameter.[31] Ma et al.[31] reported a local recurrence rate of 12.9% for MWA of HCC tumors, despite the fact that their study included 72 tumors ≥5 cm in diameter, with a local recurrence rate of 19.7%, raising their overall local recurrence rate. Other authors reported even lower local recurrence rates for HCC; Yin et al.[32] reported a local intrasegmental recurrence rate of 7.3% for CT-guided ablation of HCC tumors with an average diameter of 2.98 cm.

As MWA has grown in prominence, authors have delineated success rates for tumors of varying sizes. Wang et al.[33] reported in 2016 that complete ablation rates at first MWA session decrease as tumors increased in size from ≤3 cm (94.9%) to 3 to 5 cm (93.2%) to greater than 5 cm (81.8%). They also reported that tumor sizes ≤3 cm and 3 to 5 cm have a significant positive correlation with overall survival when compared with tumors greater than 5 cm.[33]

Clinical Results of Colorectal Liver Metastases (see Chapter 90)

MWA is also indicated for treatment of colorectal cancer (CRC). A recent study by Zhou et al.[34] of 295 patients with CRC tumors with an average maximum diameter of 2.9 cm reported complete ablation in 96.6% of patients. They also found a 33-month overall survival, ablation-site recurrence rate of 8.8%, and intrahepatic recurrence rate of 35.9%.[34] Another study by Qin et al.[35] found a slightly higher complete ablation rate of 97.81% for tumors with an average diameter of 1.54 cm, along with 85.9% overall survival at 3 years. Notably, the authors also reported a significantly higher local tumor progression rate for tumors ≥3 cm in diameter: 38.46% versus 4.27% for tumors ≤3 cm in diameter.[35] One additional study reported a median overall survival of 48 months for 70 CRC patients

TABLE 96C.4 Microwave Ablation

STUDY	NO. OF PATIENTS	HISTOLOGY	WAS ABLATION SUCCESS REPORTED AND DEFINED?	OVERALL SURVIVAL (Y/N) MEDIAN	LOCAL RECURRENCE (WITHIN 1 CM OF ABLATION)	LIVER RECURRENCE	MORTALITY	COMPLICATIONS
Baker, 2017	219	Hepatocellular carcinoma (219)	Yes, 97.1%	Yes, 14.8 months	13.9%	34.8%	Overall 38.5%, 30-day mortality 1.8%	Pulmonary (13.7%), renal (14.2%), cardiac/circulatory (3.7%), gastrointestinal (9.6%), infectious (0.9%), other (5.2%)
Kapoor et al., 2020[20]	53	100 lesions: hepatocellular carcinoma (76), CRCLM (18), neuroendocrine metastasis (5), cholangiocarcinoma (3), GIST (1), prostate cancer metastasis (1)	Yes, 83%	Yes, 24.7 months	—	30% (16/53) in different liver segment, 17% in same liver segment	0%	Pneumothorax (2), partial portal vein thrombosis (3)
Ma et al., 2017[31]	433	Hepatocellular carcinoma (433)	Yes, 100% for tumors <5 cm, 91.7% for tumors >5 cm	Yes, 43 months	12.9%	58.9%	1-year (18.5%), 2-year (40.8%), 3-year (58.6%)	Renal insufficiency (6), hepatic encephalopathy (1), adrenal crisis (1), ablation lesion infection (2), ascites (3), pleural effusion (5), hyperbilirubinemia (5)
Perrodin et al., 2019[39]	23	8 Neuroendocrine tumors, 4 breast cancer, 3 sarcoma, 2 non–small cell lung cancer, 6 other	Yes, 97.5%	18 months	10%	29%	—	Major complications (0%), minor complications (12%)
Qin et al., 2019[35]	137	137 CRCLM	Yes, 97.81% of patients	98.1% at 1 year, 90.6% at 2 years, 85.9% at 3 years	16.06%	—	0%	Major complications (3.65%), minor complication (8.03%)
Ryu, 2019	459 (421 after exclusions)	Hepatocellular carcinoma (421)	Not defined, but reported 97.9%	Yes, 5.5 years	8.3%	78.9%	0%	Major: wound infections (8), ascites (5), pleural effusion (4), intra-abdominal abscesses (2), intraabdominal hemorrhages (2)
Wang et al., 2016[33]	221	Hepatocellular carcinoma (221)	Yes, first procedure (91%), second procedure (3.6%)	Yes, 41 months	Out of 209 patients with complete ablation, 16%	Out of 209 patients with complete ablation, 57%	0%	Minor: pleural effusion (5), ascites (2), intraperitoneal hemorrhage (2), hyperbilirubinemia (5), hepatic encephalopathy (1), renal deficiency (6), adrenal crisis (1) Major: pleural effusion (1), hyperbilirubinemia (2), hepatic encephalopathy (1), renal deficiency (3), adrenal crisis (1)

Study	n	Tumor type (n)	Local control	Survival				Complications
Yin et al., 2017[32]	220	Hepatocellular carcinoma (220)	Yes, 92.82%	Yes, 95.45% at 1 year, 89.09% at 2 years	7.3%	15.5%	0%	Hepatalgia (136), transient abnormal liver function (110), fever (68), mild liver subcapsular hemorrhage (4), biloma (2)
Yu et al., 2015[37]	1249	Hepatocellular carcinoma (928), cholangiocarcinoma (14), metastases (307)	No	Yes, 92.7% at 1 year, 81.1% at 2 years, 70.6% at 3 years, 58.9% at 4 years, 51.7% at 5 years	8.6% of patients 4.3% of primary liver tumors, 4.1% of metastatic tumors	—	—	—
Zaidi et al., 2016[40]	53	CRCLM (20), neuroendocrine (10), primary (9), breast (4), ovarian (2), leiomyosarcoma (2), other (6)	Not defined, reported incomplete ablation in 1 of 149 lesions	—	0.7%	13%	—	Small bowel obstruction (1), portal vein and superior mesenteric vein thrombus (1), deep vein thrombus and asymptomatic segmental pulmonary embolism (1), asymptomatic segmental pulmonary embolism (1), postoperative cardiac dysrhythmia (1), postoperative urinary retention (1)
Zhou et al., 2017[34]	295	295 CRCLM	Yes, 96.6%	33 months	8.8%	35.9%	—	Pleural effusion (6), transient fever (136), abdominal pain (63), nausea (25)

CRCLM, Colorectal cancer liver metastasis; GIST, gastrointestinal stromal tumor.

treated with MWA, although the authors did not report recurrence rates.[36]

Clinical Results for Neuroendocrine Tumors (see Chapter 91) and Metastasis From Other Primary Tumors (see Chapter 92)

For tumors of other histology, MWA continues to be used as well (Tables 96C.4 and 96C.5). In a study of 1249 patients, including 307 patients with metastatic tumors to the liver, the local tumor progression rate of metastatic tumors was 4.1% per tumor.[37] Specifically, complete ablation rates with MWA for neuroendocrine tumors has recently been reported at 98.5%, with no reported complications.[38] Perrodin et al.[38] treated 47 neuroendocrine tumors with either surgical resection, MWA, or both, and reported an overall survival rate of 57 months in total, along with a local recurrence rate of 2.1%. Other studies have reported similar complete ablation rates with neuroendocrine tumors comprising a substantial portion of their cases.[39,40]

Clinical Results for Hepatic Hemangiomas (see Chapter 88A)

Recent work has also reported the successful use of MWA for giant hepatic hemangiomas in place of resection with tumors treated up to 15 cm in diameter (Table 96C.6). Microwave ablation offers therapeutic efficacy along with lower morbidity and mortality than other invasive methods, such as surgical resection or minimally invasive methods such as transarterial chemoembolization.[41,42] Tang et al.[43] reported a 93.2% complete ablation rate of 5 to 10 cm hemangiomas with MWA with no recurrences and similar complication rates as surgical resection. Patients were treated with MWA if they met at least the following criteria: diagnosis of giant hepatic hemangioma based on contrast-enhanced CT or MRI and typical clinical symptoms caused by giant hepatic hemangioma such as abdominal pain, nausea, and abdominal fullness.[41,44–46] Tang et al.[43] only used MWA for patients who declined surgical resection. Both 915 MHz and 2.45 GHz microwave ablation systems are reported in the literature, typically either the Vision Medical or Canyon systems.[41,43–46] With local recurrence rates being low and substantial ablation success being very high, this is a newer application of MWA that can broaden its clinical usage.

MICROWAVE ABLATION COMPARED WITH OTHER TECHNIQUES

Microwave Ablation and Surgical Resection

Resection, when technically possible and based on the underlying diagnosis, disease extent, and patients' comorbidities, continues to be the standard of care for patients with liver tumors of all origins. Since 2015 investigators have compared the efficacy of MWA versus surgical resection, although it should be noted that in these studies MWA is often used for tumors where surgical resection is not optimal, biasing any true comparison. For example, Liu et al.[7] found comparable overall survival rates of 99% at 1 year, 97.9% at 3 years, and 82.2% at 5 years for MWA, and 97.1% at 1 year, 88.4% at 3 years, and 80.5% at 5 years for resection. They also reported 4.2% local recurrence rate and 4.7% intrahepatic recurrence rate for resection, compared with 13.8% local recurrence rate and 65% intrahepatic recurrence rate for MWA.[7] However, they did report

higher rates of complications such as blood transfusion (20.3%) and diarrhea (14.6%) for resection compared with MWA.[7] These trends are consistent across other studies, as illustrated in Table 96C.5, with the exception of Chen et al.,[47] who reported overall survival of 50.9 months for MWA and only 36.7 months for resection, along with a local recurrence rate of 5.4% and intrahepatic recurrence rate of 41% in MWA, compared with 13.6% local recurrence rate and 46.1% intrahepatic recurrence rate in resection. Although these conflicting results demonstrate that further studies are needed, we believe these studies show MWA to be a safe and efficacious option for patients who are not candidates for surgical resection.

Microwave Ablation and Radiofrequency Ablation (see Chapter 96B)

Recent studies have also sought to clarify the differences in success, overall survival, and recurrence rates between MWA and RFA, the two most common thermal ablation techniques. In our review we have found MWA and RFA to perform similarly (Table 96C.7). MWA was found to have a statistically significant shorter ablation time 1 (4.21 minutes on average for RFA and 4.41 minutes on average for MWA)[6] and higher rates of overall survival: 99% at 1 year, 94.6% at 3 years, and 79.3% at 5 years for MWA, and 96.4% at 1 year, 80.7% at 3 years, and 68.4% at 5 years for RFA, after propensity score matching of patient groups.[48] Authors reported similar complete ablation rates for both procedures, as well (see Table 96C.7). Differences in these values may be a result of the differences in heat delivery between the techniques.[48]

Microwave Ablation and Transarterial Chemoembolization (see Chapter 94)

Transarterial chemoembolization (TACE) is another minimally invasive technique used in treatment of liver tumors that cuts off a tumor's blood supply, limiting its growth, while delivering a targeted dose of chemotherapy to the tumor. TACE has been used alone or in conjunction with other procedures for treatment of a variety of liver tumors (Table 96C.8). In a direct comparison between TACE and MWA for the treatment of HCC tumors less than 5 cm in diameter, MWA was found to have a complete ablation rate (100%) and higher than TACE (72.4%), as well as superior overall survival than TACE: 96.5% at 1 year, 76.4% at 3 years, and 70.2% at 5 years for MWA, versus 87.8% at 1 year, 59.1% at 3 years, and 43.6% at 5 years for TACE.[49] The complication rates between the two procedures were also similar.[49] Other authors have combined TACE with MWA, which outperformed TACE alone in overall survival, 26.6 months for TACE + MWA, 17.1 months for TACE only, and in complete ablation rate, 58.7% in TACE + MWA, compared with 12.7% in TACE, with similar complication rates.[50]

MICROWAVE ABLATION: SPECIFIC COMPLICATIONS AND FUTURE APPLICATIONS

Despite its less invasive nature, MWA does uniformly heat the entire electromagnetic field, which may damage nearby vital structures and lead to thrombus formation in the hepatic or portal veins, as well as obstruction of bile ducts. Authors also report the occurrence of abscesses, ascites, pleural effusion, and surgical wound infection, among other complications (Table 96C.9).

TABLE 96.5 Microwave Ablation Versus Resection

STUDY	NO. OF PATIENTS	HISTOLOGY	WAS ABLATION SUCCESS REPORTED AND DEFINED?	OVERALL SURVIVAL (Y/N) MEDIAN	LOCAL RECURRENCE	LIVER RECURRENCE	MORTALITY	COMPLICATIONS
Chen et al., 2018[47]	303	303 HCC	Neither defined nor reported	50.9 months for MWA and 36.7 months for resection	5.4% in MWA, 13.6% in resection	41% in MWA, 46.1% in resection	0.8% for MWA at 30 days, 1.5% for resection at 30 days	MWA: abdominal abscess (8.9%), bile leakage (7.1%), surgical wound infection (4.4%), pleural effusion (2.6%), uncontrolled ascites (2.6%), postoperative bleeding (2.6%) Resection: abdominal abscess (3.1%), bile leakage (2.3%), surgical wound infection (7.8%), pleural effusion (10.4%), uncontrolled ascites (5.2%), postoperative bleeding (3.6%)
Chong, 2018	442	442 HCC	Neither defined nor reported	MWA: 98.4% at 1 year, 72.3% at 3 years, 61.3% at 5 years Resection: 95.2% at 1 year, 82.6% at 3 years, 79.6% at 5 years	14.3% for MWA, 0.5% for resection	65% for MWA, 4.7% for resection	0%	—
Liu et al., 2019[7]	1309	1309 HCC	Yes, only patients with complete ablation included	MWA: 99% at 1 year, 97.9% at 3 years, 82.2% at 5 years Resection: 97.1% at 1 year, 88.4% at 3 years, 80.5% at 5 years (after PSM)	13.8% for MWA, 4.2% for resection (after PSM) *Method of evaluating recurrence not defined	35.3% for MWA, 26.9% for resection (after PSM)	13.5% in MWA, 13% in resection group	MWA: fever (12.9%), pain (51.7%), diarrhea (1.7%), vomiting (9.5%), blood transfusion (4.3%), significant pleural effusion (2.6%) Resection: fever (21.2%), pain (32.5%), diarrhea (14.6%), minor ascites (0.5%), vomiting (6.6%), arrhythmia (2.4%), blood transfusion (20.3%), lung infection (3.3%), significant pleural effusion (1.9%), liver failure (0.5%) (after PSM)
Perrodin et al., 2020[38]	47	47 neuroendocrine tumors	Yes, 100% in resection group, 98.5% MWA group	57 months for all patients	2.1%	19.2%	—	MWA: 0 complications Resection: major complications (3), minor complications (11)
Ryu, 2019	551	551 HCC, 188 after propensity score matching	Neither defined nor reported	MWA: 99% at 1 year, 85% at 3 years, 77% at 5 years, 48% at 10 years Resection: 100% at 1 year, 89% at 3 years, 76% at 5 years, 47% at 10 years	7.4% for MWA, 2.1% for resection	51% for MWA, 45% for resection	0%	MWA: intraabdominal abscess (1.1%), ascites (1.1%), pleural effusion (3.4%), cardiac arrhythmia (1.1%), pneumonia (1.1%) Resection: intra-abdominal abscess (3%), bile leakage (1%), wound infection (1%), ascites (1%), portal thrombosis (3%), pneumonia (1%), renal disorder (1%)

Continued

TABLE 96.5 Microwave Ablation Versus Resection—cont'd

STUDY	NO. OF PATIENTS	HISTOLOGY	WAS ABLATION SUCCESS REPORTED AND DEFINED?	OVERALL SURVIVAL (Y/N) MEDIAN	LOCAL RECURRENCE	LIVER RECURRENCE	MORTALITY	COMPLICATIONS
Tinguely et al., 2020[36]	271 (after PSM)	271 CRCLM	Neither defined nor reported	54.7 months in resection group, 48 months in MWA group	—	—	MWA 1% at 30 days Resection 0.5% at 30 days Not PSM	MWA: severe complications (7%) Resection: severe complications (16.4%)
Xu, 2015	90	90 primary liver cancer	Defined, not reported	MWA: 88.89% at 1 year, 66.67% at 2 years, 33.33% at 3 years Resection: 91.11% at 1 year, 68.89% at 2 years, 37.78% at 3 years	20% MWA, 8.89% resection *Method of evaluating recurrence not defined	MWA total recurrence 48.89%, resection total recurrence 44.44%	—	MWA: bile leakage (2.22%), pleural effusion (2.225), postoperative blood loss (2.22%) Resection: bile leakage (6.67%), pleural effusion (6.67%), postoperative blood loss (4.44%)

CRCLM, Colorectal cancer liver metastasis; *HCC,* hepatocellular carcinoma; *MWA,* microwave ablation; PSM..

TABLE 96C.6 Microwave Ablation Hemangiomas

STUDY	NO. OF PATIENTS	HISTOLOGY	WAS ABLATION SUCCESS REPORTED AND DEFINED?	OVERALL SURVIVAL (Y/N) MEDIAN	LOCAL RECURRENCE	LIVER RECURRENCE	MORTALITY	COMPLICATIONS
Chen et al., 2019[41]	131	Hemangioma ≥5 cm	Defined, not reported	—	0%	0%	0%	LMWA group: 21.6% hemoglobinuria, 12.8% fever, 4.3% skin burn, 1.1% pneumothorax ORES group: 21.6% fever, 2.7% biliary leakage, 5.4% wound infection, 2.7% postoperative bleeding
Li et al., 2019[44]	58	Hemangioma ≥5 cm	Yes, 97.7 ± 2.44 in 3D group, 94.5 ± 3.7% in 2D group	—	—	—	0%	3D group: hemoglobinuria 32% 2D group: hemoglobinuria (57.6%), AKI (3.33%)
Liu et al., 2018	49	Hemangioma >4 cm	No	—	—	—	—	Hemoglobinuria (41%), AKI (2%)
Liu et al., 2018	40	Hemangioma >4 cm	No	—	—	—	0%	Hemoglobinuria (37.5%), fever (15%), pleura effusion (5%), AKI (2.5%)
Tang et al., 2019[43]	112	Hemangioma 5-10 cm	Yes, 93.2% in MWA group, 95.6% in surgical resection group	—	0%	0%	0%	MWA group: pain (22.7%), excessive wound exudate (6.8%), low-grade fever (4.5%), coprostasis (13.6%), stomach discomfort (4.5%), AKI (6.8), diaphragmatic hernia (2.3%) Surgical resection group: pain (22.1%), excessive wound exudate (10.3%), cough and dyspnea (4.4%), low-grade fever (5.9%), coprostasis (25%), stomach discomfort (14.7%), incisional hernia (1.5%), seroperitoneum (1.5%), perihepatic effusion (4.4%), pleural effusion (2.9%)
Tang, 2015	46	Hemangioma 5-10 cm	Yes, initial rate 91.5%, total rate 95.7%	—	—	6.5%	0%	Acute renal dysfunction (4.3%), pleural effusion (4.3%), fever/mild pain/transient hepatic dysfunction (78.3%), elevated bilirubin (2.2%)
Wang et al., 2018[42]	12	Hemangioma 10-15 cm	Yes, initial rate 76.9%, total 84.6%	—	—	—	0%	Fever (15.4%), constipation (30.8%), slight wound pain (30.8%), stomach discomfort (7.7%), high bilirubin (53.8%), elevated serum transaminase (100%), elevated serum creatinine (15.4%)

2D, Two-dimensional; *3D,* three-dimensional; *AKI,* acute kidney injury; LMWA, ; ORES,.

TABLE 96C.7 Microwave Ablation Versus Radiofrequency Ablation

STUDY	NO. OF PATIENTS	HISTOLOGY	WAS ABLATION SUCCESS REPORTED AND DEFINED?	OVERALL SURVIVAL (Y/N) MEDIAN	LOCAL RECURRENCE	LIVER RECURRENCE	MORTALITY	COMPLICATIONS
Chong, 2020	93	93 HCC	Yes, 95.7% for MWA, 97.8% for RFA	MWA: 97.9% at 1 year, 67.1% at 3 years, 42.8% at 5 years RFA: 93.5% at 1 year, 72.7% at 3 years, 56.7% at 5 years	—	—	0% at 30 days	MWA: postoperative ileus (1) RFA: ascites (1)
Du et al., 2020[5]	452	452 HCC	Not defined but reported, 88.5% for MWA, 85.5% for RFA	MWA: 92.7% at 1 year, 84.5% at 2 years, 77.5% at 3 years, 72.3% at 4 years RFA: 96.6% at 1 year, 88.5% at 2 years, 83.9% at 3 years, 79.7% at 4 years	48.6% for MWA, 51.3% for RFA	5.5% for MWA, 6.0% for RFA	—	MWA: fever (7), seroperitoneum (1), pain (13), skin burn (3) RFA: fever (10), seroperitoneum (2), pain (13), skin burn (1)
Kamal et al., 2019[6]	56	56 HCC	Yes, 88% first procedure for RFA, 100% after second procedure; 94% first procedure MWA, 100% after second procedure	—	9.1% for both MWA and RFA at 1 year. De novo lesions in 18.2% RFA, 18.2% MWA at 1 year	—	15.3% for RFA, 14.8% for MWA	MWA: pain at the site of intervention (43%), right shoulder pain (14.35), low-grade fever (28.6%), bleeding requiring embolization (3.6%), hematemesis within 24 hours after the procedure (3.6%) RFA: pain at the site of the intervention (43%), right shoulder pain (7.1%), low-grade fever (21.4%)
Liu et al., 2018	562	562 HCC	—	MWA: 99% at 1 year, 94.6% at 3 years, 79.3% at 5 years RFA: 96.4% at 1 year, 80.7% at 3 years, 68.4% at 5 years (after PSM)	13.8% for MWA, 18.7% for RFA (after PSM) (defined as LTP)	—	13.5% for MWA, 18.3% for RFA	MWA: pleural effusion (3) RFA: pleural effusion (4), intraperitoneal hemorrhage (3), pneumothorax (1), hemothorax (1), GI penetration (1), portal vein thrombosis (1), acute biliary pancreatitis (1)
Xu, 2017	460	460 HCC	Yes, 98.3% for MWA, 98.1% for RFA	MWA: 99.3% at 1 year, 90.4% at 3 years, 78.3% at 5 years RFA: 98.7% at 1 year, 86.8% at 3 years, 73.3% at 5 years	9.6% for MWA, 10.1% RFA (defined as LTP)	40.5% for MWA, 47.8% for RFA	0%	MWA: pain, fever, fatigue (65.5%), intestinal perforation (0.3%), persistent jaundice (0.3%) RFA: pain, fever, fatigue (60.4%), persistent jaundice (0.6%)

GI, Gastrointestinal; HCC, hepatocellular carcinoma; LTP,; MWA, microwave ablation; RFA, radiofrequency ablation.

TABLE 96C.8 Microwave Ablation Versus Transarterial Chemoembolization

STUDY	NO. OF PATIENTS	HISTOLOGY	WAS ABLATION SUCCESS REPORTED AND DEFINED?	OVERALL SURVIVAL (Y/N) MEDIAN	LOCAL RECURRENCE	LIVER RECURRENCE	MORTALITY	COMPLICATIONS
Chen, 2017	144	144 HCC	Yes, TACE + MWA complete response 91.7%, TACE complete response 32.3% (after PSM)	TACE-MWA: 100% at 6 months, 91.7% at 1 year, 88.5% at 1.5 years, 88.5% at 2 years TACE: 96.9% at 6 months, 87.2% at 1 year, 81.1% at 1.5 years, 77% at 2 years	—	—	—	TACE + MWA: fever, nausea, vomiting, abdominal pain (77.1%) TACE: fever, nausea, vomiting, abdominal pain (81.3%)
Cui et al., 2019[49]	202	202 HCC	Yes, 100% complete response in MWA, 72.4% in TACE (after PSM)	MWA: 96.5% at 1 year, 76.4% at 3 years, 70.2% at 5 years TACE: 87.8% at 1 year, 59.1% at 3 years, 43.6% at 5 years (after PSM)	—	—	23.3% for MWA, 53.7% for TACE died during follow-up	MWA: hydrothorax (2), ascites (1), liver abscess (1) TACE: liver abscess (1), femoral artery pseudoaneurysm (1)
Zhang, 2018	150	150 HCC	Yes, total response 37.3% at 1 year for TACE, 15.8% at 2 years 47.8% at 1 year for TACE-MWA, 31.8% at 2 years for TACE-MWA	18.5 months TACE + MWA, 14.8 months TACE	—	—	—	TACE + MWA group: iatrogenic pneumothorax (2%), nausea, vomiting (26%), abdominal pain (70%), fever (44%), elevated liver enzyme (24%) TACE group: hypokalemia caused by severe vomiting (1%), severe hepatic dysfunction (2%), GI bleeding (1%), nausea, vomiting (38%), abdominal pain (56%), fever (53%), elevated liver enzyme (25%)
Zheng et al., 2018[50]	258	258 HCC	Yes, complete response 58.7% in TACE + MWA, 12.7% in TACE	26.6 months TACE + MWA, 17.1 months TACE only	TACE+MWA group: 47.8% at 1 year, 78.3% at 2 years, 94.6% at 3 years. TACE group: 74.7% at 1 year. 96.4% at 2 years, 97.6% at 3 years	—	—	TACE + MWA group: liver abscess (1.1%), subcapsular hematoma (1.1%), abdominal pain (68.5%), fever (77.2%), vomiting (39.1%), grade 1-2 myelosuppression (3.2%), self-limiting pleural effusion (8.7%) TACE group: upper GI bleeding (1.2%), biloma with abscess (1.8%), abdominal pain (71.1%), fever (74.1%), vomiting (45.8%), grade 1-2 myelosuppression (3.6%), self-limiting pleural effusion (4.2%)

GI, Gastrointestinal; *MWA*, microwave ablation; *PSM*, ; *TACE*, transarterial chemoembolization.

TABLE 96C.9   Microwave Ablation: Future Directions and Technical Studies

STUDY	NO. OF PATIENTS	HISTOLOGY	WAS ABLATION SUCCESS REPORTED AND DEFINED?	OVERALL SURVIVAL (Y/N) MEDIAN
An et al., 2020[13]	130	130 HCC	Yes, 98.3% in 3D group, 97.1% in 2D group	Yes, 22 months in 3D group, 20 months in 2D group
Berber, 2016	18	7 colorectal, 3 primary liver tumors, 3 neuroendocrine, 2 ovarian cancer, 1 esophageal cancer, 1 leiomyosarcoma, 1 uveal melanoma	Not defined, but 100%	—
Dong, 2019	71	71 HCC	Yes, 87.5% for parallel group, 87% for crossed group	Parallel group: 88.5% at 1 year, 79% at 2 years, 71.8% at 3 years Crossed group: 93.8% at 1 year, 87.5% at 2 years, 87.5% at 3 years
Gao et al., 2016[23]	103	54 colorectal liver metastases, 49 HCC	Yes, 97.7% model group, 85% control group initially; 97.7% model group, 88.3% control group at 1 month	Model group: 33.3 months, control group: 29.8 months
Imajo et al., 2018[19]	21	15 HCC, 5 adenocarcinoma, 1 squamous cell carcinoma	Yes, 95.2%	—
Jia, 2017	56	45 HCC, 8 colon cancer, 3 gastric cancer	Yes, 82.2%	—
Kapoor et al., 2020[20]	53	100 lesions: 76 HCC, 18 colorectal, 5 neuroendocrine, 3 cholangiocarcinoma, 1 gastrointestinal stromal tumor, 1 prostate cancer	Yes, 83%	24.7 months
Lachenmayer, 2019	88	88 HCC	Yes, 96.3%	—
Leung et al., 2015[17]	176	Colorectal metastases 81%, HCC 8.4%, primary biliary cancer 1.7%, noncolorectal metastases 8.9%	Neither defined nor reported	57 months
Lin et al., 2019[25]	35	28 HCC, 4 colonic metastases, 2 rectal carcinoma metastases, 1 gastric carcinoma metastases	Yes, 100%	—
Mbalisike et al., 2015[24]	70	93 tumors: 32 HCC, 3 benign hepatic adenomas, 58 liver metastases	Neither defined nor reported	—
Peng, 2018	99	99 colorectal cancer liver metastases	Neither defined nor reported	—
Tinguely, 2017	51	54 ablations: 28 CRLM, 22 HCC, 2 neuroendocrine tumors, 1 melanoma, 1 carcinoma of adrenal gland	Neither defined nor reported	—
Vogl et al., 2016[18]	221	65 CRCLM, 53 HCC, 57 breast cancer, 5 undifferentiated liver carcinoma, 4 esophageal cancer, 6 cholangiocellular carcinoma, 9 pancreatic carcinoma, 2 bronchogenic carcinoma, 3 cancer of unknown primary, 1 adrenal carcinoma, 5 gastric cancer, 3 choroidal melanoma, 5 ovarian cancer, 1 hemangiopericytoma, 1 cervical carcinoma, 1 Hodgkin's lymphoma	Yes, 90.2% for low-frequency MWA, 95.5% for high-frequency	Low-freq: 98.93% at 1 year, 95.74% at 2 years, 82.98% at 4 years. High-freq: 100% at 1 year, 97.63% at 2 years, 92.91% at 4 years

LOCAL RECURRENCE	LIVER RECURRENCE	MORTALITY	COMPLICATIONS
—	35.5% in 3D group, 49% in 2D group	46.4% in 3D group, 40.4% in 2D group	Major complications: 9.1% 3D group, 9.4% 2D group
—	—	0% at 90 days	0% at 90 days
—	—	20.8% in parallel group, 8.7% in crossed group	—
Model group: 11.6% at 1 year, 23.3% at 2 years, 39.5% at 3 years Control group: 15% at 1 year, 37.9% at 2 years, 51.7% at 3 years(LTP)	—	0%	Model group: small amount of hepatic subcapsular hematoma (2.3%), small sized pulmonary hematoma (2.3%), pneumothorax (2.3%), right shoulder pain (4.7%) Control group: small amount of hepatic subcapsular hematoma (6.7%), small sized pulmonary hematoma (5.0%), pneumothorax (6.7%), right shoulder pain (20%)
0%	—	0%	Takotsubo cardiomyopathy (1), pleural effusion (1), biloma (1)
—	—	—	—
17% (same liver segment)	30.2% (different liver segment)	0%	Chest tube for pneumothorax (2), partial portal vein thrombosis (3)
6.3% after 6 months (LTP)	—	28.4% during follow up period	Ascites decompensation (2), pleural effusion (1), pneumothorax (1), other (2), liver abscess (1)
12.6% for 2.4 GHz, 4% for 915 MHz	38%	0%	Wound infection (12), intraabdominal abscesses (12), noninfected intraabdominal collections including bile leaks (9), gastrointestinal (6), respiratory (5), cardiac (4), bleeding (4), venous thromboembolism (3), miscellaneous (15)
0%	—	—	High fever (2), procedural pain (6), vomiting (1)
—	—	0%	Manual group: 5% Robotic group: 0%
—	58.6%	3.1% overall	—
32% (including 9 patients with concurrent local and intrahepatic recurrences; this is both de novo lesions and progression of incomplete ablations)	32%	2%	Accentuated postoperative pain (2), ascites leak from port side (2), combined port side bleeding and cardiac decompensation (1), urinary tract infection (2), fever of unknown origin (2), wound infection (1), partial thrombosis of left portal vein (1), transfusion due to perihepatic hematoma (1), intrahepatic abscess (1), pleural effusion (1)
			High-frequency group: right shoulder pain (8.7%) All patients: small subcapsular hematoma (3.2%)

TABLE 96C.9 Microwave Ablation: Future Directions and Technical Studies—cont'd

STUDY	NO. OF PATIENTS	HISTOLOGY	WAS ABLATION SUCCESS REPORTED AND DEFINED?	OVERALL SURVIVAL (Y/N) MEDIAN
Vogl et al., 2018[21]	88	ECSEC group (56 lesions): 14 colorectal, 13 breast cancer, 11 HCC, 18 others LF-MWA (20 lesions): 5 colorectal, 3 breast cancer, 5 HCC, 7 others HF-MWA (20 lesions): 4 colorectal, 7 breast cancer, 5 HCC, 4 others	Yes, 100% in ECSEC, 100% in LF-MWA, 95% in HF-MWA	—
Wang, 2020	48	48 HCC	Yes, 100%	—
Weiss et al., 2020[26]	47	17 HCC, 18 colorectal liver metastases, 6 melanoma metastases, 2 uveal melanoma metastases, 1 ovarian cancer metastasis, 1 kidney cancer metastasis, 1 breast cancer, 1 liver sarcoma, 1 mixed adenoneuroendocrine carcinoma, 1 myofibroblastic inflammatory cancer, 1 cancer of unknown primary	Yes, 98%	41.6 months
Yan et al., 2016[27]	100	100 primary liver tumors	Neither defined nor reported	11.7 months in ordinary US group; median overall survival not reached in contrast-enhanced US group.
Yu et al., 2015[51]	29	29 HCC	Neither reported nor defined	100% in immunotherapy group, 80% in control group
Zhou, 2018	30	30 HCC	Neither reported nor defined	—
Ziemlewicz, 2015	75	75 HCC, 3 patients had additional tumors smaller than 1 cm of other origin	Yes, 91.6% primary effectiveness, 94% secondary effectiveness *Ablation success only defined as based on imaging, no details	—

2D, Two-dimensional; *3D,* three-dimensional; ECSEC, ; *HCC,* hepatocellular carcinoma; *HF-MWA,* high-frequency microwave ablation; *LF-MWA,* low-frequency microwave ablation; LTP, ; *US,* ultrasound.

Notably, MWA is frequently found to have lower complication rates than surgical resection, as well as similar rates to RFA procedures, demonstrating the overall high safety of this technique.[5–7]

As MWA has grown in prominence, other therapies have been coupled with MWA to increase its success. Concurrent immunotherapy with MWA for HCC tumors has been shown to increase T-cell counts after combined treatment compared with MWA alone, but long-term results were not statistically significant.[51]

IRREVERSIBLE ELECTROPORATION

Irreversible electroporation (IRE) is a novel, non–thermal-injury ablative technology that utilizes multiple short pulses (70–90 microsecond pulse length) at high voltage (2250–3000 volts) of electrical energy to induce permanent electroporation of the tissue.[52] IRE is the newest ablative technology and was provided 510K indications for use for soft tissue ablation by

the Food and Drug Administration (first 510K in 2006).[53] This ablation technique takes advantage of the electrical potential gradient that exists across cell membranes. This technique was reported as early as the 1750s, but its use for medical purposes dates back only 30 years[54]; it was first developed in conjugation with chemotherapy. Its advantage compared with conventional thermal ablation techniques is its non–thermal-injury delivery mechanism. When properly applied, theoretically, it only affects the target tissue. Proteins, the extracellular matrix, and critical structures such as blood vessels and nerves are all unaffected and left healthy by this treatment.[55] This expands the scope of treatment of lesions near major vascular and biliary structures when compared with conventional thermal-injury ablative techniques. The major disadvantage of IRE is the need for general anesthesia (deep paralysis) for its energy delivery.[56] IRE can be performed with open, laparoscopic, or percutaneous approaches. Repeated reports have demonstrated the advantages of IRE against other thermal ablation techniques, including no heat-sink effect,

LOCAL RECURRENCE	LIVER RECURRENCE	MORTALITY	COMPLICATIONS
3.57% of ECSEC, 5% of LF-MWA, 5% of HF-MWA, at 12 months	42.9% for ECSEC, 50% for LF-MWA, 40% for HF-MWA, at 12 months	16.1% ECSEC group, 15% LF-MWA, 10% HF-MWA	ECSEC group: low grade subcapsular bleeding (1), subcapsular liver abscess (1) 0% HF-MWA, 0% LF-MWA
6.3%	20.8%	0%	Mild pain (16.7%), mild fever (25%), moderate pain (35.4%), moderate fever (18.8%)
8%*Types of recurrences not defined	64%	—	Pneumothorax (1), pleural effusion with dyspnea and partial thrombosis of the portal vein (1), abdominal pain and biliary peritonitis (1), subcutaneous necrosis of extrahepatic applicator tract (2), postablation syndrome (7), postprocedural subcapsular hematoma (1)
16% in ordinary US group, 8% in contrast-enhanced US group	22% in ordinary US group, 6% in contrast-enhanced US group; 10% combination local and distant recurrence in ordinary US group, 2% in contrast-enhanced US group	—	Ordinary US: pain (54%), fever (42%), intraabdominal hemorrhage (16%) infection (24%)Contrast-enhanced US: pain (28%), fever (28%), intraabdominal hemorrhage (6%), infection (4%)
—	7.1% in immunotherapy group, 33.3% in control group	20% in control group at 1 year	Immunotherapy group: fever (42.9%), severe abdominal pain (7.1%)
—	26.67%	—	—
—	26.7%	24% during follow-up period, 1.33% periprocedural	Nonocclusive asymptomatic main portal vein thrombus (1)

tumor-specific immunologic reactions, little impact on the collagen network within treated tissues, and the potential to ablate tumor tissues near large vessels.[57]

PHYSICS OF IRREVERSIBLE ELECTROPORATION

Electroporation is a dynamic phenomenon by which cell membrane integrity is compromised by inducing permanent nanopores using transmembrane electrical distortion.[58] Reversible electroporation has been used as a technique for electrotransfection of genetic material or intracellular drug delivery. When the energy of the pulses is increased above a certain electric field threshold, the permeabilization becomes irreversible resulting in electrolyte disturbances, predominantly calcium, and thus cell death through apoptosis.[59] Immunohistochemistry studies confirm the induction of the apoptotic pathway by electroporation, which will ultimately lead to cell death and necrosis.[60]

Using an electrical field of 2500 V/cm^3, it is postulated that IRE creates nano-sized pores (0.08–0.5 μm) in the cell membrane that are unable to reseal because of the electrical pulse strength and duration that surpasses the cell membrane threshold, permanently damaging the plasma membrane. The nanopores then allow micromolecules and macromolecules to be transported into and out of the cell. With high voltage, cells are unable to compensate for their altered transmembrane ionic concentration differences in which cell death occurs secondary to the disruption of cellular homeostasis.[54]

The area of tissue where the cells have been altered is the ablation zone. Thermal injury ablation techniques have various degrees of damage because of their reliance on passive heat diffusion or degree of water molecule distribution across the ablation area, which can lead to uncertainty in the effectiveness of the procedure. IRE is advantageous because of the well-defined region of tissue ablation. The ablation zone in IRE shows where a cell is either destroyed or not destroyed without any uncertainty.[53] The complete electroporation zone and cell death occurs over weeks and takes 8 to 10 weeks for electroporation efficacy.

LOCAL TISSUE FACTORS THAT AFFECT IRREVERSIBLE ELECTROPORATION

Crucially, proper IRE usage does not damage structures adjacent to the treatment site, making it a safer option for tumors that are not suitable for surgical resection or thermal ablation.[61] IRE does not damage the adjacent extracellular matrix, either, as these structures lack a cell membrane and cannot be affected by IRE; thanks to its method of delivery, IRE does not suffer from the heat-sink effect. In addition, IRE leads to lower rates of complications such as increased bilirubin, portal hypertension, and ascites, because it does not damage nearby vital structures as thermal techniques do.[62]

However, there are complications reported when using IRE near vasculature; Baumler et al.[63] reported thrombosis in 47 of 205 venous structures and vessel narrowing in 20 of 205 venous structures after IRE. An earlier study reported lower complication rates: vessel narrowing in 14 of 191 venous structures and complete or partial portal vein thrombosis in 5 of 191 instances.[64] Low complication rates after IRE use near bile ducts have been reported: narrowing in 8 of 55 bile ducts and dilation in 7 of 55 ducts located near the ablation site.[65] Baumler et al.[63] do state that 13 of their 20 vessel-narrowing incidents spontaneously resolved within 3 months perhaps the vessel narrowing is a temporary venous alteration in the postintervention edematous inflamed liver. Taken in sum, the literature confirms that IRE is a promising and safe method for liver tumor ablation near blood vessels or bile ducts, and future work may reduce these complication rates even further.

TECHNIQUE OF PERFORMING IRREVERSIBLE ELECTROPORATION IN LIVER FOR TUMORS WITH VASCULAR PROXIMITY

The clinical indication for IRE of liver tumors must be made based on (1) tumor biology, (2) tumor size less than 4 cm, (3) tumor location within 5 mm or less of a vital structure that needs to be spared, and (4) the ability to undergo general endotracheal anesthesia. IRE is not a replacement for MWA or RFA. The current commercially available system consists of a computer-controlled pulse generator that delivers a maximum 3000 volts between each probe pair based on the number and spacing configuration of the IRE probes. A minimum of 90 pulses must be delivered that last from 20 to 100 μsec each. The most common pulse length is 70 to 90 μsec, based on the degree of electrical resistance that is encountered. Patient selection is of paramount importance. A multidimensional thin cut (0.7–1 mm) CT scan or contrast-enhanced dynamic MRI must be performed preferably less than 1 month from treatment.[66–68] From those images, a three-dimensional reconstruction can be performed in order to plan (1) number of IRE needles required, (2) needle trajectory, and (3) access—open, laparoscopic, or percutaneous. The tumor dimensions are input into the IRE pulse generator, which will recommend the number and possible spacing of probes needed to create the desired electroporation zone based on a mathematical algorithm. Optimal probe spacing is critical to the safety and efficacy of the device, with the optimal spacing being 1.5 to 2.3 cm. Spacing less than 1.5 cm can lead to a small or ineffective electroporation (called reversible) or thermal damage (defined as >54°C for >10 sec).[69] Probe spacing greater than 2.3 cm will lead to ineffective electroporation. This precision of spacing places the burden on the physician to ensure high-quality US is used during needle placement and to document this spacing. The probes themselves are 19 gauge in diameter and radiopaque to aid in intraprocedural identification of the probe tip.[70] Intraoperative navigation systems should also be considered for physicians without expertise in liver US.[71,72] The pulses delivered from the NanoKnife system are synchronized with the patient's ECG to avoid cardiac arrhythmias.[58]

Every patient is unique in the care and service they need to have a successful treatment. The abilities of each surgeon vary, and their particular skills should be addressed before performing IRE. In summary, factors to consider before performing IRE are the size of the ablation zone, the number of probes needed for the procedure, the distance between the probes, and the length of the active electrode tip. A set procedure plan will lessen the chance for complications or mistakes. After gaining access to the liver, the probes are inserted under continuous US vision to ensure accurate placement, but also to avoid mechanical damage to the hepatic inflow, bile ducts, or hepatic outflow based on the lesion location. Once the probes are in the correct positions, the electrical pulses are delivered from the NanoKnife system.[73] This can last from 10 to 60 minutes.[74] Once the electrical pulses are finished, the patient is closed and is sent into recovery. Detailed procedure-related steps have been presented for hepatic tumors.[75]

In recent years, investigators have also experimented with IRE protocols in search of better outcomes. Beyer et al.[76] found that stereotactic IRE ablation decreased procedure time until the start of the ablation from 104.1 to 55.2 minutes, decreased deviation of IRE electrode placement from the reference electrode from 3.3 to 2.2 mm, decreased total dose-length product of the entire intervention from 4886 to 3510 mGy*cm, and had identical complete ablation results of 100% to manual IRE. Another study evaluated robot-guided IRE using the Maxio system compared with manual IRE and also found similar results to the aforementioned study.[77] Both of these studies were performed with small patient populations and did not record long-term outcome data, but assisted guidance shows promise.

IRE of the liver has well-defined criteria based on ablation recurrence, which is defined as persistent viable tumor indicated by dynamic imaging compared with pre-IRE scan or tissue diagnosis. Ablation success is defined as the ability to deliver the planned therapy in the operative room and at 3 months to have no evidence of residual tumor on cross-sectional imaging of the treating team's choice, such as CT, MRI, or positron emission tomography (PET) (if they had a preoperative PET avid scan).[58,74] Authors also recently compared T1.5 EOB-MRI, contrast-enhanced US, and contrast-enhanced CT for accuracy in evaluating IRE treatment response within 1 week of ablation and found contrast-enhanced US to have the highest specificity of the three in detecting residual tumor or local recurrence at 0.857, compared with 0.643 for EOB-MRI and 0.464 for contrast-enhanced CT[78] (see Chapters 14 and 15). However, another study found similar complete ablation measurement rates between MRI, CT, and contrast-enhanced US at multiple times after ablation.[79] They reported 91.7% complete response in both MRI and contrast-enhanced US and 100% complete response on CT at 1 month; 91.7% complete response for MRI and contrast-enhanced US and 95.3% complete response for CT at 3 months; and 91.7% complete response for all three modalities at 6 months.[79] Based on these results, we cannot make a clear recommendation on which modality to employ most at this time, but we feel confident all three can deliver satisfactory results and we encourage practitioners to use the response criteria established by Martin et al.[80] in 2016 for IRE of pancreatic cancer to determine treatment success.

CLINICAL RESULTS OF IRREVERSIBLE ELECTROPORATION FOR HEPATIC MALIGNANCIES

Current work has continued to demonstrate the effective use of IRE for treatment of HCC, as well as for other primary or metastatic liver tumors (Table 96C.10 and Table 96.C11). IRE complete ablation rates for small liver lesions have reached 100% for HCC tumors with an average diameter of 2.6 cm, and 95.8% for CRC tumors with an average diameter of 2.3 cm.[61,63,81] However, complete ablation rates for larger tumors are lower; another recent article reported 66.6% complete ablation rate for HCC tumors 3.1 to 4 cm, and 25% complete ablation rate for HCC tumors 5.1 to 11.5 cm.[82] Although the number of patients included was low, this study demonstrates that although IRE is safe for medium to large tumors, its efficacy for tumors of that size has room for improvement.

Additional recent studies have compared the effectiveness of IRE versus MWA for treatment of HCC tumors. In 2016 Bhutiani et al.[62] found that IRE had lower complication rates than MWA, lower hospital readmission rates, shorter hospital length of stay, and similar 90- and 180-day treatment success rates to MWA. Another study found that RFA/MWA had similar complication rates to IRE, but higher treatment efficacy.[83] The authors in that work also noted that the tumors ablated with IRE were significantly closer to vital structures than those ablated with MWA/RFA, possibly increasing their IRE complication rates.[84]

The initial IRE use for liver was reported by Cannon et al.[70] with 44 patients undergoing 51 total IRE procedures. Lesions were in proximity to vital structures in 40 (88%) patients. Initial success was achieved in 50 (100%) treatments. Five patients had 9 adverse events, with all complications resolving within 30 days.[70] Local relapse-free survival at 3, 6, and 12 months was 97.4%, 94.6%, and 59.5%, respectively. There was a trend toward higher recurrence rates for tumors over 4 cm (hazard ratio 3.236, 95% confidence interval [CI] 0.585–17.891; $P = .178$).[70] The authors concluded that IRE was a safe treatment for hepatic tumors in proximity to vital structures. A significant inflection point occurred for all tumors greater than 3 cm, with higher local recurrence rates seen.[70] Thus initial recommendation for new use was to start with hepatic tumors that were less than 3 cm in size and in proximity to vital structures.

The true technical report of which tumor locations were appropriate for IRE, especially within the hepatic hilum, was published by Martin et al.[75] Typically, a minimum of 90 pulses is delivered, lasting from 20 to 100 microseconds each. The most common pulse length is 70 to 90 microseconds, with the shorter durations used in cases where high electrical resistance is encountered. The pulse voltages and duration are based on preclinical studies.[59,83,85] Treatment planning is based on three-dimensional preoperative CT scanning in which the tumor dimensions and location of surrounding structures are measured. From the preoperative scan, the tumor dimensions are input

into the pulse generator with a set planned margin. Multiple monopolar probes are used (maximum of 6) with greater numbers of probes needed for larger ablation zones. The maximum effective probe spacing can vary from 1.4 to 2.2 cm. If the probe spacing is either less than 1.4 or greater than 2.2 cm, the effectiveness of the electroporation is reduced and will lead to an incomplete ablation. The maximum probe exposure used in liver IRE is 2 to 2.5 cm exposure. Optimal technique requires the user to place the needle along the longest axis of the tumor—most commonly the caudal to cranial plane (coronal plane)—and then perform sequential pullbacks to achieve both cranial and caudal margins. It is our recommendation not to attempt to perform the "overlapping ablation" technique that was first popularized with RFA, secondary to the fact that IRE therapy induces artifact and human error to ensure precise spacing would lead to a greater incidence of ineffective therapy (i.e., reversible electroporation).

These results were further confirmed by Philips et al.,[74] who reported on an analysis of 150 consecutive patients treated over 7 institutions from September 2010 to July 2012. Patients were chronologically divided into three groups and analyzed for outcomes: group A (first 50 patients treated), group B (second 50 patients treated), and group C (third 50 patients treated).[74] Imaging was performed at the time of IRE therapy, and follow-up imaging to confirm ablation success was performed at 12 weeks and at 3-month intervals. An initial discharge scan was done to evaluate any complications from this new technique and not for treatment efficacy. Ablation recurrence was defined as persistent viable tumor based on dynamic imaging compared with pre-IRE scan or tissue diagnosis. Dedicated body-imaging radiologists at each center, who were not blinded to treatment, made radiologic interpretation of recurrence as defined by the RECIST criteria.[86] When imaging was equivocal, biopsies were obtained at the discretion of the treating physician. A total of 167 IRE procedures were performed, with the majority being for liver (39.5%) and pancreatic (35.5%) lesions.[74] The three groups were similar with respect to comorbidities and demographics. Group C had larger lesions (3.9 vs. 3 cm, $P = .001$), had more numerous lesions (3.2 vs. 2.2, $P = .07$), had more vascular invasion ($P = .001$), underwent more associated procedures ($P = .001$), and had longer operative times ($P < .001$).[74] Despite this, complication and high-grade complication rates were comparable among the three groups ($P = .24$). IRE-attributable morbidity rate was 13.3% (total 29.3%) and high-grade complications were seen in 4.19% of patients (total 12.6%). Pancreatic lesions ($P = .001$) and laparotomy ($P = .001$) were associated with complications.[74] This review represented the single largest review of IRE soft tissue ablation demonstrating initial patient selection and safety. Over time, complex treatments of larger lesions and lesions with greater vascular involvement were performed without a significant increase in adverse effects or impact on local relapse-free survival. This evolution demonstrates the safety profile of IRE and speed of initial IRE users to treatment of more complex lesions, which was greater than 5 cases by institution. IRE is a safe and effective alternative to conventional ablation with a demonstrable learning curve of at least 5 cases to become proficient.

A final review was conducted by Cannon et al.[87] from a prospective, institutional review board–approved evaluation of 107 consecutive patients from 7 institutions; all had tumors that had vascular invasion and were treated with IRE from May

TABLE 96C.10 Irreversible Electroporation

STUDY	NO. OF PATIENTS	HISTOLOGY	WAS ABLATION SUCCESS REPORTED AND DEFINED?	OVERALL SURVIVAL (Y/N) MEDIAN	LOCAL RECURRENCE	LIVER RECURRENCE	MORTALITY	COMPLICATIONS
Bhutiani et al., 2016[62]	55	55 Child-Pugh B (7/8) HCC	Yes, 100% at 90 days for MWA, 100% at 180 days for MWA; 100% at 90 days for IRE, 97% at 180 days for IRE	—	—	—	0%	IRE: high current during procedure (2), increased ascites within 30 days (5), increased ascites within 90 days (2), pleural effusion (5), portal vein thrombosis (1), uncontrolled ascites (1), dehydration (1), liver failure (2) MWA: 30 day AST and ALT 1–4-fold increase (4), 30 day total bilirubin increase (1.5), increased ascites (14), 90 day AST and ALT increase (2), increased ascites (5), pleural effusion (14), portal vein thrombosis (5), uncontrolled ascites (4), dehydration (2), liver failure (5)
Eller, 2015	14	3 HCC, 9 colorectal carcinoma, 1 neuroendocrine tumor, 1 squamous cell carcinoma	Yes, 86%	—	17% of initial 12 successful ablations	—	0%	Arterioportal shunt at needle track (1), intraperitoneal bleeding (1), right side hematohoraces (2)
Fruhling, 2017	30	16 colorectal cancer, 8 HCC, 1 adrenal cancer, 1 midgut carcinoid, 1 neuroendocrine tumor, 2 cholangiocarcinoma, 1 malignant melanoma	Yes, 78.9% at 3 months, 65.8% at 6 months	—	21.1% at 3 months, 34.2% at 6 months	—	0% at 30 days, 3.3% at 4 months	Bile duct dilation and stricture of portal vein and bile duct (1), transient increase in liver transaminases (13), postprocedural pain (7), hematoma (1), shortness of breath (1), tachycardia (1), postoperative function (1), increased blood pressure (1)
Kalra et al., 2019[81]	21	21 HCC	Yes, 100%	—	24%	14.3%	0%	Fever (3), hemoperitoneum (4), pleural effusion (2), pneumothorax (2)
Langan, 2017	40	77 lesions included: colorectal (57), HCC (7), leiomyosarcoma (5), neuroendocrine (4), ampullary (3), cholangiocarcinoma (1)	—	—	13.4%	—	—	Cardiovascular (6), infection (4), paralytic ileus (4), pulmonary embolism (3), hematoma (2), hemorrhage (2), pleural effusion (1), intraoperative cardiac arrhythmia (1), postoperative hepatic vein perfusion defect (1), postoperative hepatic vein thrombosis (1), perihepatic hematoma (1)
Mafeld, 2019	52	20 HCC, 3 cholangiocarcinoma, 28 colorectal, 1 neuroendocrine, 1 pancreatic, 1 breast, 1 GIST, 1 malignant thymoma	Yes, 75%	38 months	—	—	1.9%	Atrial fibrillation (3), minor pain (2), subcapsular hematoma (1), gallbladder perforation with resultant bile leak and peritonitis (1), systemic inflammatory response syndrome (1)
Niessen et al., 2016[90]	34	15 HCC, 12 colorectal liver metastases, 4 cholangiocellular carcinoma, 1 testicular cancer metastasis, 2 neuroendocrine tumor metastases	Yes, 95.4%	—	25.2% at 12 months, mean time to local recurrence was 15.5 months	—	2.94% after 9.8 months	Intraperitoneal bleeding (1), partial thrombosis of portal vein (1), abscess (4), hematoma (6), pneumothorax (2)

Study	N	Tumor Type	Complete Ablation	Follow-Up	Recurrence	Mortality	Complications
Niessen et al., 2017[91]	71	31 HCC, 27 colorectal carcinoma, 4 cholangiocellular carcinoma, 9 other metastases	Yes, 92.2%	26.3 months	31.7%	—	Liver abscess (4), myocardial infarction (1), pneumothorax (2), cardiac arrhythmia (2), hematoma (3)
Schicho et al., 2019[61]	24	24 colorectal liver metastases	Not defined, but 66.7% after first session, 95.8% after second session	26.5 months	—	—	—
Stillstrom, 2019	42	20 colorectal carcinoma, 17 HCC, 6 cholangiocarcinoma, metastases from cholangiocarcinoma, leiomyosarcoma, adrenocortical carcinoma	Not defined, reported incomplete ablation rate of 19%	—	3% at 3 months, 26% at 6 months, 37% at 1 year	0% 30 day mortality	Pneumothorax (3), bleeding (1), liver failure (1), portal vein thrombosis (2), infection (1), brachial plexus injury (3)
Sutter, 2017	58	58 HCC	Yes, 77.3% after first IRE, 89.3% after second IRE, 92% after third IRE	—	20% of completed ablations	3.5%	Group 1: pain (1), transient jaundice (1), asymptomatic gastric fistula (1), pneumothorax (1), partial portal thrombosis (2), transient encephalopathy (1), liver failure (1) Group 2: decompensated chronic bronchitis (1), liver failure (1), death from liver failure (1)
Verloh et al., 2019[84]	164	164 HCC	Not defined, reported 84.3% for RFA/MWA and 67.2% for IRE	—	—	0.9% in MWA/RFA group, 0% IRE group	Grade I classification 9.4% RFA/MWA, grade I classification 19.1% IRE, grade II classification 17.1% RFA/MWA, grade II classification 14.9% IRE, bleeding after RFA (1), pleural effusion after MWA (1), HB drop after IRE (1), partial main portal vein thrombosis after MWA (1)
Zeng et al., 2017[82]	14	8 HCC, 6 cholangiocarcinoma	Yes, 42.8% total, 25% in large tumor size group, 66.6% in medium tumor size group	—	—	—	Large tumor group: elevated intraoperative blood pressure (1), hypokalemia (3), low blood pressure and low WBC count and platelet abnormality (1), abdominal distention (4), limb edema (2) Medium tumor group: elevated intraoperative heart rate (1), hypokalemia (3), low serum albumin (3), low blood pressure (1), stomach pain (1)

ALT, ; AST, ; *HCC,* hepatocellular carcinoma; HB, ; *IRE,* irreversible electroporation; *MWA,* microwave ablation; *WBC,* white blood cell.

TABLE 96C.11 Irreversible Electroporation Near Biliary Ducts and Blood Vessels

STUDY	NO. OF PATIENTS	HISTOLOGY	WAS ABLATION SUCCESS REPORTED AND DEFINED?	OVERALL SURVIVAL (Y/N) MEDIAN	LOCAL RECURRENCE	LIVER RECURRENCE	MORTALITY	COMPLICATIONS
Baumler et al., 2019[63]	87	50 HCC, 7 cholangiocarcinoma, 21 colorectal tumor metastases, 3 mammary carcinoma metastases, 6 others (carcinoma of unknown origin, neuroendocrine tumor)	Neither reported nor defined	—	—	—	—	Thrombosis (47/205 venous structures), vessel narrowing (20/205 venous structures)
Distelmaier, 2017	29	4 breast cancer, 13 colorectal cancer, 2 HCC, 2 cholangiocellular carcinoma, 2 pancreatic cancer, 1 melanoma, 1 mesothelioma, 2 esophageal carcinoma, 1 renal cell carcinoma, 1 gastrointestinal stromal tumor	Yes, 90%	—	7.7% of patients (5% of tumors)	30.8% of patients had needle tract seeding (27.5% of tumors ablated) 17.2% of patients developed tumors elsewhere in liver	—	Subcapsular hematoma (1), hematoma in intercostal space (1), arterioportal fistula (1), mild to moderate cholestasis (5)
Dollinger et al., 2015[64]	43	16 HCC, 4 cholangiocellular carcinoma, 16 colorectal tumor metastases, 2 mammary carcinoma, 1 neuroendocrine tumor, 4 other (testicular tumor, gastrinoma, esophageal cancer, carcinoma of unknown origin)	Neither reported nor defined	—	—	—	—	Vessel narrowing (14/191 venous structures), partial portal vein thrombosis (2/191), complete portal vein thrombosis (3/191)
Dollinger et al., 2016[65]	24	7 HCC, 2 cholangiocellular carcinoma, 10 colorectal tumor metastases, 2 breast carcinoma metastases, 3 others	Neither reported nor defined	—	—	—	—	Elevated bilirubin (3), elevated alkaline phosphatase (1), bile duct lumen dilation (7/55 bile ducts), bile duct lumen narrowing (8/55 bile ducts)

HCC, Hepatocellular carcinoma.

2010 to January 2012. Locally advanced tumors were defined as primary tumor less than 5 mm from major vascular structure based on preoperative dynamic imaging or intraoperative criteria. IRE was used in locally advanced tumors in the liver (N = 42, 40%) and in the pancreas (N = 37, 35%), with a median number of lesions being 2 with a mean target size of 3 cm. IRE-attributable morbidity rate was 13.3% (total 29.3%), with high-grade complications seen in 4.19% (total 12.6%). No significant vascular complications were seen, and of the high-grade complications, bleeding (2), biliary complications (3), and deep vein thrombosis/pulmonary embolism (3) were the most common. Complications were more likely with pancreatic lesions (P = .0001) and open surgery (P = .001). Calculated local recurrence-free survival was 12.7 months with a median follow-up of 26 months censured at last follow-up. The tumor target size was inversely associated with recurrence-free survival (R = 0.81, 95% CI: 1.6 to 4.7, P = .02) but this did not have a significant overall survival impact. The authors were able to conclude that IRE represents a novel therapeutic option in patients with locally advanced tumors involving vital structures that are not amenable to surgical resection. Acceptable to high local-disease control and long local relapse-free survival can be achieved with this therapy in combination with other multidisciplinary therapies.

In the future, IRE has the potential to be an efficacious cancer treatment. More complex treatments of larger lesions and lesions with greater vascular involvement will become available with more research and clinical trials.

IRREVERSIBLE ELECTROPORATION: FUTURE DIRECTIONS AND COMPLICATIONS

Two studies have recently combined IRE with natural killer (NK) cell immunotherapy and noted improved outcomes after combination treatment. Yang et al.[88] noted an increase in overall survival to 23.2 months after IRE-NK combination therapy compared with 17.9 months with IRE alone, as well as higher levels of T and NK cells in the IRE-NK group. Alnaggar et al.[89] likewise found longer overall survival of 10.1 months in their IRE-NK group compared with 8.9 months with IRE alone and observed increased T-cell count in the IRE-NK group compared with the IRE group. The authors also found lower ALT and AST values 1 month after treatment in the IRE-NK group, possibly suggesting immunotherapy aided in improving liver function.[89] The additional immunotherapy may improve immune response and produce additional antitumor effect, leading to improved response rates after treatment (Table 96.C12).

Future work may also seek to decrease complication rates associated with IRE. Due to the challenging nature of tumors treated with IRE, which are often not candidates for surgical resection or MWA/RFA, higher levels of complications may be expected. However, the literature shows that while hematomas, pneumothorax, and vessel thromboses are some of the most common complications following hepatic IRE, complication rates are overall low.[63,81,90,91]

References are available at Expertconsult.com.

TABLE 96C.12 Irreversible Electroporation: Future Directions and Technical Studies

STUDY	NO. OF PATIENTS	HISTOLOGY	WAS ABLATION SUCCESS REPORTED AND DEFINED?	OVERALL SURVIVAL (Y/N) MEDIAN	LOCAL RECURRENCE	LIVER RECURRENCE	MORTALITY	COMPLICATIONS
Alnaggar et al., 2018[89]	40	40 HCC	Yes, complete response 25% in IRE-NK group, 20% in IRE group	10.1 months in IRE-NK group, 8.9 months in IRE group	—	—	0%	Tussis (10), nausea and emesis (5), pain of puncture point (21), fatigue (12), fever (18), transient reduction of intraoperative blood pressure (16), white cell count reduction (13)
Beyer et al., 2016[76]	20	16 HCC, 4 colorectal cancer metastases	Yes, 100% in manual IRE ablation, 100% in robot-assisted IRE ablation	—	—	—	—	0%
Beyer et al., 2017[77]	35	40 lesions: 18 HCC, 18 colorectal cancer metastases, 2 breast cancer metastases, 2 pancreatic cancer metastases	Yes, 94.7% in manual IRE ablation, 100% in robot-assisted IRE ablation	—	—	—	—	0%
Granata, 2015[79]	20	20 HCC	Complete response defined in 91.7%	—	—	—	—	Peripheral arteriovenous shunt (1), segmental dilation of intrahepatic biliary ducts (1)
Granata et al., 2016[79]	20	20 HCC	Complete response defined in 91.7% based on MRI, 100% based on CT	—	—	—	—	Peripheral arteriovenous shunt (1), segmental dilation of intrahepatic biliary ducts (1)
Sugimoto et al., 2017[78]	16	13 HCC, 1 colorectal tumor metastasis, 1 gastric neuroendocrine tumor metastasis, 1 vaginal tumor metastasis	Defined, not reported	—	6.25%	—	—	—
Yang et al., 2019[88]	40	22 HCC, 18 cholangiocarcinoma	Yes, complete response in 16.7% of IRE-NK group, 4.5% of IRE group	23.2 months in IRE-NK group 17.9 months in IRE group	—	0% IRE-NK group 4.5% IRE group	— IRE-NK group — IRE group	IRE group: pain (6), pleural effusion (1), ascites (3), fatigue (3), fever (10). IRE-NK group: pain (4), pleural effusion (4), ascites (4), fatigue (5), fever (11)

CT, Computed tomography; HCC, hepatocellular carcinoma; IRE, irreversible electroporation; IRE-NK, irreversible electroporation with natural killer cell immunotherapy; MRI, magnetic resonance imaging.

Cryotherapy and ethanol injection

Chandrasekhar Padmanabhan, T. Peter Kingham, and Kevin C. Soares

CRYOTHERAPY

Introduction

Hepatic ablative techniques remain an important tool in the armamentarium against both primary and metastatic liver tumors. Liver resection continues to be the gold standard in management; however, ablative therapies are useful for patients with limited disease and compromised liver function,[1-7] and in some cases they can be curative.[8] Because the majority of malignant liver tumors present as unresectable disease, there has been an increased interest in minimally invasive ablative techniques to prolong survival.[9]

Liver failure continues to be a major cause of death in patients with unresected liver tumors, especially in the setting of preexisting liver dysfunction.[10,11] Ablation can be used in combination with parenchymal-sparing resection to control disease progression within the liver. Intrahepatic recurrences are common after liver resection for primary and metastatic malignancies. Hepatic ablation is a useful tool to manage recurrences in liver remnants that are inadequate for re-resection.

The most common modalities of thermal ablation include radiofrequency ablation (RFA; see Chapter 96B), microwave ablation (MWA; see Chapter 96C), and cryoablation (or cryotherapy). One of the original ablative techniques, cryotherapy has largely been replaced by RFA and MWA due to reduced complication rates and improved oncologic outcomes.[12,13]

Patient Population

Hepatocellular Carcinoma (see Chapter 89)

Hepatocellular carcinoma (HCC) is the sixth most common new cancer diagnosis in the world with 841,080 new cases in 2018 and the fourth most common cause of cancer-related death in the world with 781,631 deaths in 2018.[14] Incidence and mortality vary by geographic location with highest incidence and mortality in Eastern Asian and North African countries. Viral hepatitis, mainly hepatitis B, is a key risk factor for HCC and the incidence of hepatitis B mirrors that of HCC.[15] In the United States, hepatitis C is much more common and has likely driven the rising incidence of HCC (see Chapter 68).

HCC is typically preceded by cirrhosis (see Chapter 74), hence a curative resection is typically reserved for those patients with early-stage cancers and preserved liver function.[16] Unfortunately, only 5% to 10% of patients present with resectable disease.[8] Ablation can be curative in early stage disease and as such, ablative techniques are typically used for patients with very early stage HCC (single nodules, <2 cm, Child-Pugh A, ECOG Performance Status: 0) and patients with early stage HCC (up to 3 nodules <3 cm, Child-Pugh A-B, ECOG Performance Status: 0). Survival after ablation in Child-Pugh A patients has been shown to be 50% to 75% at 5 years, paralleling survival after resection.[8]

Metastatic Disease

The most common site of metastatic disease for gastrointestinal malignancies is the liver. Colorectal cancer liver metastases (CRLM) represent the most common metastatic tumors to the liver both in the United States and worldwide (see Chapter 90). Although locoregional therapies for most secondary liver tumors have not translated into a survival benefit, CRLM are the exception.[17-21] Of the 20% to 35% of patients with CRLM who present with metastatic disease confined to the liver, only a fraction are truly candidates for liver resection.[22] Patients who are not candidates for liver resection may be candidates for regional ablative therapies as a means to control their disease. Patients with bilobar CRLM present a unique challenge as their disease may be resectable in a staged fashion. Ablative techniques can be useful in this setting as well in combination with liver resection.

Indications for Cryotherapy

A majority of patients with either primary liver cancers or metastatic liver cancers present with unresectable disease, largely because these tumors are relatively asymptomatic. Disease can be technically unresectable due to tumor involvement of both the right and left portal inflow pedicles as well as involvement of multiple hepatic veins such that any attempt at resection would result in an inadequate liver remnant. Disease can also be unresectable due to oncologic factors such as aggressive tumor biology, extent of disease in the liver and elsewhere in the body, and risk of recurrence, as these reduce the risk of long-term survival and/or cure. Patients with HCC have the added complexity of compromised liver function (cirrhosis, portal hypertension, or both) rendering safe liver resection unfeasible (see Chapter 74). Numerous techniques have been developed to help treat unresectable liver tumors, including chemoembolization, radioembolization, irreversible electroporation, and ablation. Many of these can be used alone, in conjunction with resection, or, in the case of HCC, as bridging therapy for a curative liver transplant.[23] It is important to always keep in mind that ablated liver is nonfunctional and future liver remnant calculations must be adjusted accordingly.

Cryotherapy has been used to treat both primary and metastatic liver tumors. Although mostly of historical significance due to the improved outcomes and lower cost of RFA and MWA,[24] favorable long-term outcomes are still reported.[25] In relation to other ablative techniques, there are no specific absolute indications and contraindications, and which modality to use is dependent on what technology is available and what the proceduralist has the most experience with.

Pathophysiology of Cryotherapy

Neither cryotherapy nor any of the other ablative techniques can distinguish normal liver tissue from neoplastic tissue. Whereas RFA and MWA generate heat to trigger cellular death, cryotherapy, as the name suggests, cools tissue to subzero temperatures, thereby causing tissue necrosis. Cellular death is highly dependent on the rate of cooling, depth of hypothermia, rate of thawing, number of freeze-thaw cycles used, and delayed effects of post-thaw ischemia. When a cryoprobe is inserted into the liver, three overlapping zones of injury develop within the ice ball. Rapid tissue freezing occurs closest to the cryoprobe. The rate of freezing decreases in proportion to the distance from the probe, creating zones of intermediate and slow cooling. Similarly, a gradient of temperature develops in the ice ball, decreasing 3°C/mm to 10°C/mm from −170°C near the probe to just below 0°C at the periphery of the cryolesion. The dynamics of the freezing process cause different mechanisms of injury in these three idealized zones.[26,27]

Cooling Rate

The rate at which the tissue cools directly affects the degree of cell death. Slow cooling results in cellular dehydration whereas rapid cooling induces ice crystallization, which disrupts cellular membranes (Fig. 96D.1). Both slow and rapid cooling induce maximal cell death. Intermediate cooling rates, however, are associated with the greatest degree of cellular survival.

SLOW COOLING RATES. Extracellular and intracellular fluid are composed of varying concentrations of electrolytes, proteins, other macromolecules, and water. Various homeostatic mechanisms maintain iso-osmolarity between the two fluid compartments. The presence of solute in water depresses the freezing point such that supercooling occurs rather than crystallization at below-freezing temperatures.

The actual composition of each fluid compartment differs so greatly that the freezing point of the intracellular compartment is depressed further than the freezing point of the extracellular compartment. Therefore, when tissues are cooled, the extracellular fluid freezes first. When ice forms in the extracellular space, solutes are excluded, making the remaining fluid hyperosmolar. Cellular dehydration occurs as the unfrozen intracellular water flows out of the cell across the osmotic gradient. At a critical level of dehydration, no further fluid can be extracted from the cell because the intracellular macromolecules become concentrated enough to equalize the osmotic gradient across the cell membrane. The ion concentration across the membrane becomes deranged, however, allowing ions to flow into the cell from the hypertonic extracellular fluid to reestablish the Gibbs-Donnon equilibrium. As a consequence of cellular dehydration, the intracellular pH and ion concentrations are altered, proteins denature, and membranes and membrane-bound enzyme systems are disrupted. Some cells will die as a direct result of dehydration, but others require the additional insult provided during the thaw cycle of cryotherapy. When the cryolesion thaws, the extracellular fluid thaws, creating a hypo-osmotic environment. Water flows across the osmotic gradient back into the cells, causing them to swell and ultimately lyse. This type of injury predominates in the slowly cooled zone at the periphery of the cryolesion.

INTERMEDIATE COOLING RATES. With intermediate cooling rates (1°–10°C/min), cells dehydrate as the extracellular fluid turns to ice. The temperature falls fast enough, however, to freeze the intracellular water before cellular dehydration reaches the critical level to produce irreversible cell injury. Intracellular ice formation excludes solutes, increasing the intracellular osmotic concentrations, equalizing the osmotic gradient across the cell membrane, and stopping further cellular dehydration.

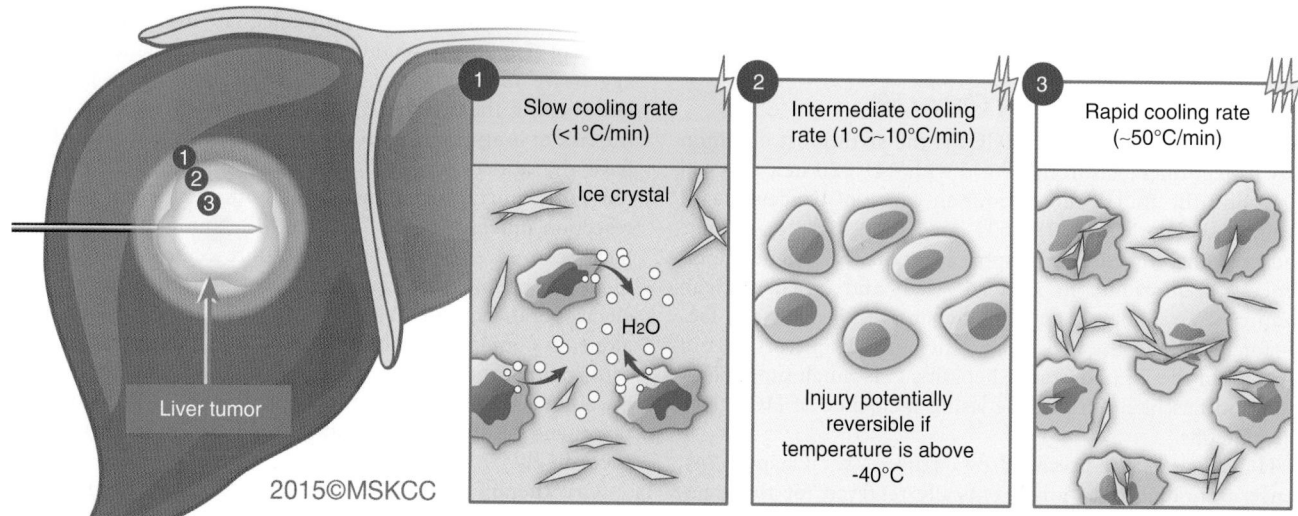

FIGURE 96D.1 **Mechanisms of cell death in different cryoablation zones.** The rate at which the tissue cools directly affects the degree of cell death. Slow cooling results in cellular dehydration whereas rapid cooling induces ice crystallization, which disrupts cellular membranes. Both slow and rapid cooling induce maximal cell death. Intermediate cooling rates, however, are associated with the greatest degree of cellular survival. Thawing of frozen tissues induces cellular damage and is dependent on the rate of thaw. Rapid thawing is associated with increased survival whereas slow thawing is more destructive. (Courtesy of Memorial Sloan Kettering Cancer Center © 2014 Memorial Sloan Kettering Cancer Center. All rights reserved)

As a result, the critical level of dehydration allowing influx of solutes is not reached, protecting the cell from the lethal injury caused by water influx secondary to isotonic rehydration during the thaw cycle. Cells in the zone of intermediate cooling do not suffer the consequences of the cellular dehydration and their survival is improved. Cells located in the intermediate zone may survive, which is a limitation to the efficacy of this therapy.[28]

RAPID COOLING RATES. Rapidly frozen tissue is destroyed by an altogether different mechanism. Cooling rates on the order of 50°C/min, found only in close proximity to the cryoprobe, cause intracellular fluid to freeze before cellular dehydration occurs. Intracellular ice is particularly lethal. Small ice crystals coalesce, causing a physical grinding action that disrupts organelles and cellular membranes. This leads to reproducible and certain cell death.

DEPTH OF HYPOTHERMIA AND TISSUE RESPONSE. Regardless of the cooling rate, temperatures less that −20°C result in extensive tissue injury. Moreover, temperatures below −40°C are lethal for nearly all cells. At these temperatures, intracellular fluid freezes and ice crystals are formed, resulting in irreversible cellular damage as described previously. Unfortunately, only tissues near the cryoprobe reliably reach these temperatures, rendering cryotherapy less consistent at inducing cellular death at the periphery of the ablation zone.

The sensitivity of different tissues to hypothermia varies considerably. Most normal hepatocytes die at −15° to −20°C, whereas at −10°C, most hepatocytes survive. Bile ducts, connective tissue, and vascular structures tolerate slightly lower temperatures than hepatocytes. In contrast, liver tumors tend to require deeper hypothermia to −40°C for complete and reliable cell death. As a general rule, the −40°C isotherm is located approximately three-quarters the distance from the probe to the edge of the ice ball, as seen at intraoperative sonography. To reach this level of hypothermia and obtain reliable ablation at the tumor margin, the ice ball is extended 1 cm beyond the peripheral edge of the tumor.

JOULE-THOMPSON EFFECT. The argon-helium system uses a high-pressure freezing gas (argon) system based on the Joule-Thompson effect. This effect relies on the physical principle that gas changes temperature by expansion through a narrow port into the low-pressure zone that occurs at the tip of a probe. While compressed argon gas passes through the cryoablation needle, the tip is cooled, forming an ice ball that destroys tumor cells. To thaw the tissue, a high-pressure gas (helium) is converted to a warm, low-pressure gas.[29]

Thawing Process

Thawing of frozen tissues induces cellular damage and is dependent on the rate of thaw. Rapid thawing is associated with increased survival whereas slow thawing is more destructive than either rapid or slow cooling. In slowly thawed tissue, the extracellular ice melts before the intracellular ice, briefly making the extracellular fluid relatively hypo-osmolar compared with the intracellular fluid. Free water flows down this osmotic gradient into the cells, causing them to swell and ultimately burst. Simultaneously, the ice within the cell undergoes recrystallization, especially in the temperature range

of −20° to −25°C. Recrystallization is a process during which the ice crystals reform, coalesce, and enlarge, mechanically disrupting the cellular membranes. The effects of thawing are potentiated by allowing the entire lesion to reach ambient temperature slowly and passively.

Repeated Freeze-Thaw Cycles

Repeated freeze-thaw cycles have been shown to increase the certainty of cellular destruction. With each cycle, tissue cooling occurs more efficiently due to the increased thermal conductivity of the frozen tissue and the volume of frozen tissue increases, pushing the border of cellular destruction closer to the periphery of the ice ball.[26] Repeating a freeze-thaw cycle has been shown to increase tissue necrosis to include approximately 80% of the prior frozen volume.

Microvascular Effects

In addition to the direct cellular injury induced by the freeze-thaw cycle as described above, cryotherapy disrupts the microvasculature within the ablation zone, resulting in delayed hypoxia and subsequent necrosis.[30] Freezing at slow cooling rates causes the radius of the sinusoids to increase by a factor of two, which is equivalent to increasing the volume in the intravascular space by a factor of four. The expansion of the vascular space tears the endothelium, exposing and disrupting the underlying basement membrane. Platelet thrombi develop and permeability increases, leading to swelling and microcirculatory failure. The tissues supplied by these damaged vessels become ischemic and necrotic. This mechanism of injury is more important in the intermediate and slow cooling zones, where direct cellular injury by intracellular ice formation or dehydration is not reliable.

Conclusion

Cryotherapy takes advantage of the physiologic changes that occur both in the freeze cycled and thaw cycles to induce cell death within the target ablation zone. The rate of cooling and thawing cycles directly affects the rate of cellular death and repeated freeze-thaw cycles increase the volume of tissue destruction within the ablation zone. Acute cell death occurs secondary to the formation of intracellular ice crystals and cell lysis secondary to changes in osmotic gradients, whereas chronic cell death occurs secondary to ischemic effects from microvascular disruption. For maximal benefit, cryotherapy should be performed with multiple freeze-thaw cycles with a rapid freeze and slow thaw.

Morphologic and Histologic Changes After Cryotherapy

Immediately after thawing, the area of liver treated with cryoablative techniques appears dark red, swollen, and usually well demarcated. Histologic examination reveals congestion of the hepatic sinusoids associated with hemorrhage. There are decreased levels of cellular glycogen and an absolute reduction in the number of mitochondria. With time, the lesion takes on a light-gray color and slowly resorbs during the ensuing weeks. Microscopically, this period correlates with polymorphonuclear cell and macrophage infiltration of the tissue. The cryolesion is progressively replaced with fibrous tissue. There is usually a persistent area of necrosis and fibrosis, but occasionally the lesion is completely resorbed.

Immunology and Cryoablation

Cells within the core of the ablation zone typically undergo necrosis whereas cells in the periphery undergo mitochondrial-mediated apoptosis.[31] Cell death by necrosis is highly immunogenic as it results in the exposure of intracellular antigens to the immune system. Early reports of cryoablation in the 1970s demonstrated regression of prostate cancer metastases after treatment of the primary tumor.[32] Though the exact mechanism was not discernible, the authors implied that a humoral immune response was somehow induced after ablation of the primary tumor.

The immune response generated by cryoablation has been confirmed in preclinical models. In orthotopic mammary carcinoma mouse models, tumor-bearing mice treated with cryoablation were highly resistant to tumor re-challenges compared with mice treated with resection.[33] T-cells isolated from the draining nodal basins of the tumor-bearing mice treated with cryoablation demonstrated high levels of interferon-gamma secretion when presented with tumor antigens. Adoptive T-cell transfer from mice treated with cryoablation into new tumor-bearing mice reduced lung metastases 3-fold compared with T-cell transfer from mice treated with resection. These results suggested a T-cell–dependent immune response induced by cryoablation.[33]

In the modern era, there has been great interest in combining cryoablation with immune checkpoint inhibitors to generate a durable and tumor-specific immune response, especially in malignancies thought not to be immunogenic.[34] Cryotherapy-induced cell death and subsequent release of tumor antigens into the circulation have been shown to promote a cytotoxic CD8[+] T-cell response in preclinical tumor models.[35,36] Isolated case reports and early phase clinical trials have shown promising results. Further studies are warranted, however, to determine the ability of cryoablation to function as an in vivo vaccination tool in solid tumors by eliciting an immune response capable of a systemic antitumor effect.[37]

Operative Technique

Hepatic cryotherapy can be performed by a variety of approaches, including percutaneous, laparoscopic, and open methods. The open approach allows the most flexibility and accuracy but introduces the morbidity that accompanies a laparotomy incision. Cryotherapy at laparotomy is less anatomically limiting than minimally invasive approaches and permits treatment of lesions in areas that are difficult to access by the other methods. Despite these anatomic constraints, minimally invasive cryotherapy approaches are feasible and well described.[25] The technology of laparoscopic instrumentation and percutaneous localization continues to improve for all types of ablation and the role of these techniques continues to increase. With the recent development of argon-helium–based cryotherapy, reported to be less painful, cold-based ablative techniques can be performed under local anesthesia.

Preoperative Preparation

In general, the same preoperative preparations are required before cryosurgery as for liver resection. Careful review of preoperative imaging is essential to define the tumor's location and proximity to major vascular and biliary structures. If multiple tumors are considered for cryoablation, ensuring adequate

nonablated liver remnant is essential. Patients with more than 40% of the liver replaced with tumor are not candidates for cryoablative techniques because it is difficult to ablate such a high volume of tumor, and the perioperative morbidity is prohibitive.

Two devastating complications associated with hepatic cryotherapy are cryoshock syndrome, a complex of severe coagulopathy with resultant disseminated intravascular coagulation and multisystem organ failure, and intraoperative hypothermia. Cryoshock is an extremely rare complication with an incidence ranging from 0.05% to 1%.[25,38] Minimizing ablation volume decreases this risk. Hypothermia can be alleviated by using heated fluid and airway circuits and the use of forced air warming blankets such as the Bair Hugger (Arizant Healthcare, Eden Prairie, MN). Blood products should be available in the rare event of intraoperative bleeding.

Cryotherapy at Laparotomy: Open Cryotherapy

The abdomen is approached through a right subcostal, midline, or bilateral subcostal incision with vertical midline extension. The peritoneal cavity is thoroughly explored to detect extrahepatic metastatic disease. Enlarged lymph nodes, particularly those in the porta hepatis, are evaluated by frozen section. The liver is mobilized from its ligamentous attachments and examined bimanually. With a 5-MHz intraoperative ultrasound transducer, each Couinaud segment of the liver is systematically scanned to determine the extent of disease and its relationship to the hepatic outflow, portal inflow, and biliary structures. Suspicious lesions undergo ultrasound-directed core biopsies for histologic confirmation. All lesions seen on preoperative studies should be confirmed by intraoperative ultrasound or biopsy or both.

When an operative strategy is defined, the porta hepatis is encircled for the possibility of needing the Pringle maneuver during the procedure. The cryoprobe is introduced into the center of each lesion under ultrasound guidance. The placement is sonographically confirmed by viewing the probe in two or three perpendicular planes. In general, it is preferable to introduce the cryoprobe through the anterior surface of the liver while monitoring the introduction of the probe and formation of the ice ball, with the ultrasound transducer placed on the posterior side of the liver. Intraoperative ultrasound allows safe placement of the probe, avoiding injury to major intrahepatic vascular and biliary structures. To minimize tumor spillage and to avoid "cracking" the surface of the tumor, the cryoprobe is optimally inserted through normal liver before entering the tumor.

Depending on the depth of the lesion, either direct introduction of the probe into the tumor or wire-guided, Seldinger-style localization may be used. The Seldinger technique is best used for deep intraparenchymal and nonpalpable tumors. First, the tumor is identified by intraoperative ultrasound; then an echogenic needle is passed into the center of the lesion under ultrasound guidance and subsequently is exchanged for a J wire (Fig. 96D.2A). When the J wire is in place, the tract of the wire is dilated with a coaxial dilator and peel-away sheath. The dilator is withdrawn and the cryoprobe is inserted through the sheath into the center of the tumor. The position of the cryoprobe is evaluated again using ultrasound in two or three different axes. The probe must be placed through the center of the tumor with the tip near the opposite margin to encompass the tumor completely within the cryolesion. Some authors have

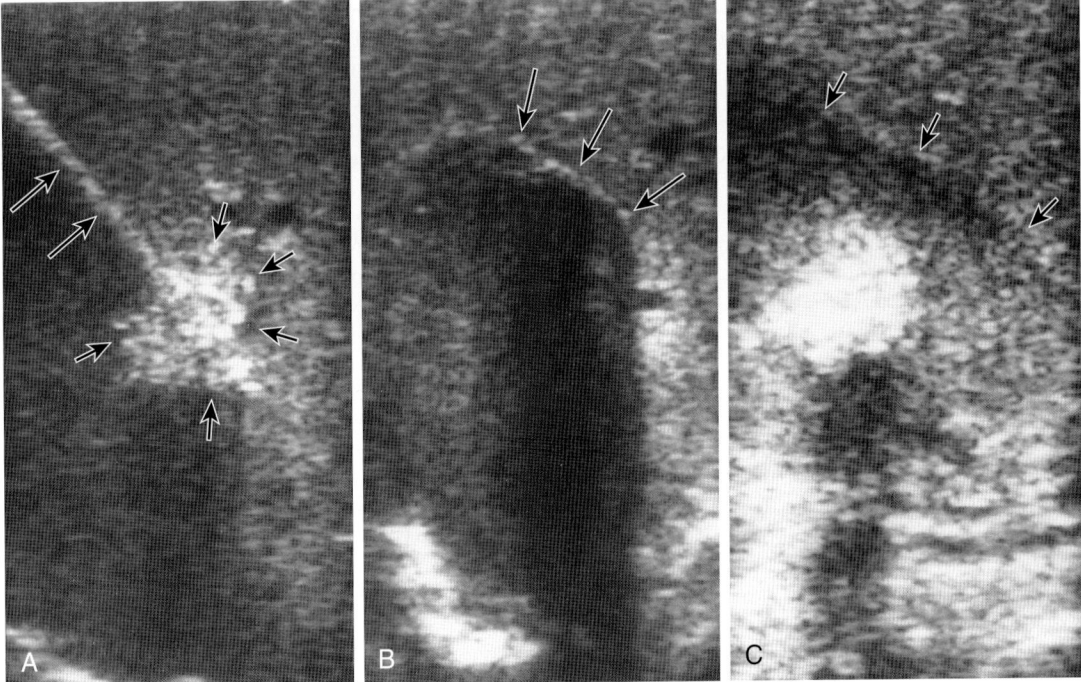

FIGURE 96D.2 **A,** Ultrasound of an echogenic wire-guided localization of an intraparenchymal hepatic metastasis. *Large arrows* indicate the J wire. *Small arrows* indicate the margins of the tumor. **B,** Intraoperative ultrasound of the ice ball. *Arrows* indicate the limits of the freeze front. **C,** Ultrasound of the thawed ice ball showing the halo appearance caused by edema around the ablated tumor. *Arrows* indicate margins of edema.

described the use of combined probes (as many as three) to achieve a greater diameter of the ice ball. Multiple probes, however, can increase procedural morbidity, hence single probes are preferred.[29]

It is crucial to tailor the type of cryoprobe and freezing technique to the size and location of the tumor. The temperature gradient within the cryolesion significantly affects the efficacy of the procedure. The temperature near the probe approximates that of liquid nitrogen, whereas at the periphery of the ice ball, the tissue may be only a few degrees below 0°C. In addition, the rate of cooling is determined by the size of the probe, the flux of refrigerant, and the thermoconductivity of the uninsulated portion of the probe. To achieve maximum tumor ablation, the operator must understand the physical properties of the cryotherapy system.

The system typically uses vacuum-insulated probes and supercooled liquid nitrogen refrigerant and permits the use of four simultaneous and completely independent probe placements. Two probes are available with this system, accommodating different-sized tumors. The 3 mm blunted probe creates a cryolesion 4 cm in diameter, whereas the 8 mm trocar point probe creates a freeze zone of 6 cm. Two 8 mm probes, used in tandem, create a 10 cm cryolesion.[39] Other systems have flat-faced probes that can be applied to a flat surface, creating a hemispheric-shaped cryolesion of 3 to 4 cm, which can be helpful to treat close margins.[40]

Once the trajectory is chosen and appropriate placement of the probes is accomplished, the liver is insulated from surrounding tissues using laparotomy pads, towels, or rubber mats. After the probe is placed and the surrounding tissue protected, the freezing process is started. At −100°C, the probe sticks to the tissue, allowing safe placement of additional probes without

dislodging the first probe. Two or three probes can be placed in the liver at the same time. We do not recommend treating more than three lesions simultaneously because it is difficult to monitor concurrent cryoablations adequately and there is a higher incidence of intraoperative hypothermia. Maximal cooling is then started with real-time ultrasound monitoring of the freezing process. The freeze front is seen as a hyperechoic rim with posterior acoustic shadowing (see Fig. 96D.2B). Cooling continues until the freeze front extends 1 cm beyond the ultrasound margin of the tumor. Typically, the freezing process takes 8 to 15 minutes to complete depending on the efficiency of the cryotherapy system and the size of the tumor. The freeze zone shown by intraoperative ultrasound closely approximates the pathologic and histologic volume of cryonecrosis. After completion of the first freeze cycle, the tissue is allowed to passively thaw. Active rewarming is unnecessary and may adversely influence results. Complete thawing of the tumor may take 20 to 30 minutes, extending the overall operative time. Because cryotherapy failure usually occurs at the periphery of the ice ball, it is necessary only to thaw the most peripheral centimeter of the ice ball before initiating the second freeze cycle. This reduces operative time without compromising clinical efficacy. The second freeze-thaw cycle is accomplished in a similar fashion.

After completion of the second freeze-thaw cycle, the probe is actively rewarmed, allowing it to disengage before the tumor completely thaws. The probe tract is packed with absorbable hemostatic material and gentle pressure is applied to the liver to prevent delayed hemorrhage from the probe tract. Rough handling of the thawing ice ball may cause a cleavage plane to develop at the interface of the ice ball and the normal liver parenchyma, resulting in massive hemorrhage. Generally, the probe insertion tract stops bleeding promptly as the coagulation cascade activates at body temperature. After two freeze-thaw cycles, the treated volume usually remains hyperechoic on ultrasound, whereas the surrounding normal liver becomes hypoechoic due to edema. This gives the treated tumor a "halo" appearance on imaging studies (see Fig. 96D.2C).

Laparoscopic Cryotherapy

Cryoablation can also be performed using minimally invasive approaches. Laparoscopic cryoprobes are 40 cm long and can pass through a 5 mm port. Because the probes are not malleable, expertise in laparoscopic hepatic ultrasound and optimal placement of the working trocars are essential. Patients with lesions in segments VI and VII can be placed in the left lateral decubitus position to maximize exposure of the right upper quadrant. The Seldinger technique described earlier is adapted to facilitate accurate placement of the laparoscopic cryoprobe. The dilators have been modified to make them stiffer than the dilators used in the open procedure. The probe is passed into the sheath, and the sheath is retracted to the liver edge during the freeze-thaw cycles. The cryoablation is completed under laparoscopic vision and ultrasound monitoring. A split-screen image allows simultaneous viewing of the probe and ultrasound image of the developing ice ball. The reported experience with laparoscopic cryotherapy is scant and the patients are highly selected. With the expansion of RFA and MWA and their laparoscopic applications, laparoscopic cryoablation has become less popular.

Postoperative Care

There are typically no special considerations in the postoperative management of patients treated with cryoablation. Fluid shifts tend to be minimal, and standard enhanced recovery protocols can be followed in regard to diet advancement and fluid management. There is usually a transient elevation of the liver enzymes, leukocytosis, thrombocytopenia, and fairly high fevers in the early postoperative period. The increase in liver transaminase levels is related directly to the volume of liver treated and usually resolves within 1 week. Thrombocytopenia occurs in the first few postoperative days, then stabilizes and typically normalizes in 7 to 10 days. Less frequently, the coagulation profile deteriorates with prolonged partial thromboplastin and prothrombin times, and elevation of serum levels of fibrin split products and d-dimer. Clinically significant disseminated intravascular coagulopathy is rare. Pleural effusions are common, as a result of liver mobilization and treatment of areas adjacent to the diaphragm. Most of the early consequences of surgery spontaneously resolve and the hospital stay is generally fewer than 6 days.

Percutaneous Cryotherapy Approaches

Percutaneous approaches for cryotherapy are established but have fallen out of favor with the explosion in popularity of percutaneous RFA and MWA. This approach originally was limited by the large diameter of current cryoprobes, location of the tumors, and accurate radiologic localization. Despite these problems, several moderate-sized series have confirmed the feasibility and safety of this approach.[25,41] Guidance most typically was performed with computed tomography (CT) or ultrasound, but more recently techniques using magnetic resonance imaging (MRI) have been developed.[42]

Postoperative Surveillance of Patients Treated With Cryotherapy

Given the increased risk of recurrence after ablation, it is important to follow a standardized surveillance program. Follow-up typically consists of complete histories and physical examinations, contrast-enhanced CT scans, liver enzymes, and tumor markers. Patients should undergo clinical evaluations every 3 to 4 months for the first 2 years and then every 6 months. Carcinoembryonic antigen (CEA) and α-fetoprotein (AFP) levels usually reach their nadir 4 to 8 weeks after ablation.[43]

Liver CT scans should be obtained at least every 6 months for the first 2 years. It is important to obtain an early CT scan within a few weeks after treatment to be used as a baseline. Successfully treated tumors initially appear larger than the original lesion because of swelling and the additionally treated margin of normal tissue (Fig. 96D.3). Subsequently, the lesion decreases in size and may disappear completely. Gas bubbles may be seen within the necrotic tumor and may be a result of the packed probe tract. These bubbles rarely indicate hepatic abscess and should not be a concern unless there are other signs of sepsis. In 3 to 6 months, the lesions shrink, leaving a persistent area of fibrosis and architectural distortion.

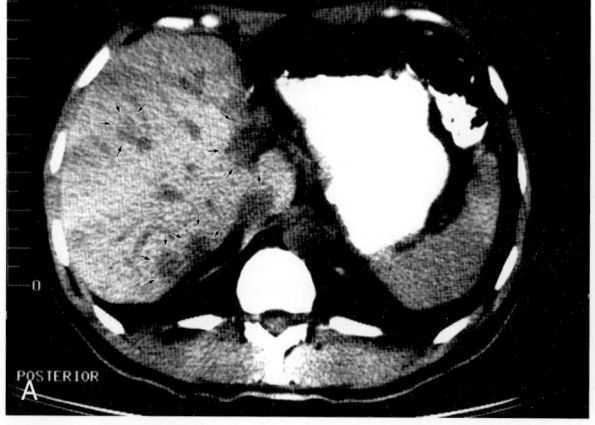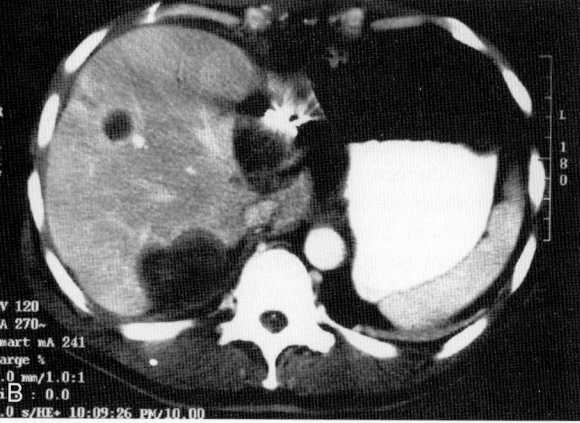

FIGURE 96D.3   A, Pretreatment computed tomography (CT) scan shows multiple liver metastases *(arrows)* in a patient who previously had undergone resection of segments II and III for metastatic disease. **B,** CT scan 7 days after cryotherapy of five metastatic tumors. The area of necrosis is larger than the original lesions (see Chapters 15, 96B, and 96C).

Technical Considerations

Inflow Occlusion

Blood vessels adjacent to liver tumors could act as cold sinks and change the conformation of the ice ball during cryoablation. Some groups have suggested inflow occlusion with the Pringle maneuver to diminish this effect.[44] Preclinical studies in pigs, however, have not confirmed this concern.[45] The relative contraindication of cryoablation near major inflow pedicles and/or draining veins may only be a theoretical one.

Monitoring the Cryolesion

Most proceduralists use ultrasound to monitor cryolesion formation given the relative ease of use and accessibility in operating theatres and interventional radiology suites. One of the major advantages of cryotherapy is the ability to readily visualize the treatment zone and margin of ablation as denoted by the bright leading edge of the ice ball under ultrasound guidance. MRI technology can accurately evaluate temperature gradients within the cryolesion and may also provide accurate quantification of the degree of cellular necrosis. MRI, however, is not nearly as accessible as ultrasound and remains investigational.

Bile Duct Warming

To protect the major bile ducts from the adverse effects of cryotherapy, some surgeons have proposed cannulating the bile ducts to circulate warmed fluids during the cryoablation. At present, the evidence is insufficient (i.e., animal studies and case reports) to support this invasive procedure.[46,47]

Complications of Cryotherapy

Technical complications directly resultant from cryoablation itself include cryolesion fracture, hemorrhage, myoglobinuria, systemic hypothermia, biliary fistula and leak, cryoshock, and death (Table 96D.1). Each of these complications is discussed separately. In addition to the technical complications, the inherent risks of laparotomy, laparoscopy, and percutaneous procedures exist and must not be overlooked when considering cryoablation.

Cryolesion Fracture and Hemorrhage

If the liver capsule is involved within an ablation zone, it can fracture during the thaw phase of cryoablation resulting in

hemorrhage. If the fractured areas are anatomically accessible, bleeding control can be feasible with sutures and hemostatic agents. When fractures are located on the posterior surface of the liver, however, hemostasis can be much more difficult to achieve, particularly during laparoscopic or percutaneous approaches.

After removal of the cryoprobe, hemorrhage through the probe tract is common. Cold temperatures blunt the clotting cascade making pressure and hemostatic agents essential. On occasion, the cryolesion can crack at the interface between normal liver parenchyma and frozen liver parenchyma resulting in catastrophic hemorrhage. A combination of packing, topical hemostatic agents, and transfusion can stop the bleeding, but rarely, conversion to resection may be required. Major bleeding complications have been reported in up to 20% of cryoablation cases, but this was largely during an era of open cryoablation with large probes up to 9 mm in diameter.[24,48] Smaller probes and diligent use of imaging to avoid vascular structures during probe placement minimizes this problem.

Myoglobinuria

Acute kidney injury after cryoablation is a result of myoglobin deposition within the renal tubules. The degree of kidney injury is directly correlated with the size of ablation zone and the number of freeze-thaw cycles. In early studies, myoglobinuria was noted in nearly all patients undergoing hepatic cryosurgery but was cleared after at most 3 days.[49] Intravenous hydration and alkalization of urine was renal protective during these studies.[48] Though the mechanism of myoglobinuria is still unclear, it is postulated that cytokine release during cryoablation may result in skeletal muscle rhabdomyolysis and resultant kidney injury.

Hypothermia

Hypothermia is a rare complication of cryotherapy and is dependent on the number of treated lesions and the proximity of those lesions to the hepatic veins and the inferior vena cava. Intraoperative hypothermia can lead to cardiac depression and/or arrhythmias and coagulopathy. Hypothermia can largely be prevented with the judicious use of warmed intravenous fluids, closed-circulation body warmers, and heating blankets. Most important, the treatment of multiple large lesions simultaneously should be avoided.

Biliary Fistula

Biliary complications occur in approximately 3% of patients undergoing cryoablation.[50] Bilomas and fistulae are more common when superficial lesions are treated. Major biliary strictures are a late complication after cryotherapy and are typically caused by bile duct injury during the freezing process. Cholangitis can occur as a consequence, especially in patients with tumors near the confluence of the right and left hepatic ducts. Long-term studies are lacking to better quantify this risk of bile duct injury and stricture.

Cryoshock

Cryoshock defines the onset of multisystem organ failure and disseminated intravascular coagulopathy after cryotherapy. Approximately 18% of deaths after hepatic cryotherapy can be attributed to cryoshock.[51] In a survey of all groups using cryotherapy, cryoshock was reported in only 21 of 2173 patients undergoing hepatic cryotherapy to treat tumors.[51] The exact

TABLE 96D.1	Complications After Hepatic Cryotherapy: Summary of 869 Patients in 20 Series	
COMPLICATION	**INCIDENCE (%)**	**RANGE (%)**
Cracking of ice ball	19*	1-25
Hemorrhage	3.7	0-13
Coagulopathy	3.8	0-8
Acute renal failure	1.4	0-17
Bile fistula/biloma	2.9	0-10
Intraabdominal abscess	1.7	0-9
Pleural effusion	6.3	4-18
Death	1.6	0-8

*Reported in only 5 of 20 studies.
From Seifert JK, Junginger T, Morris DL. A collective review of the world literature on hepatic cryotherapy. *J R Coll Surg Edinb.* 1998;43:141–154.

pathophysiology that drives cryoshock is unknown but is likely secondary to the release of proinflammatory cytokines such as tumor necrosis factor and interleukins 1, 2, and 6.[52] Experimental studies have suggested the risk of cryoshock is correlated with size of ablation zone and higher concentrations of circulating proinflammatory cytokines.[52,53]

Mortality

Overall mortality for cryotherapy is low (1.5%, range: 0%–8%).[46] In expert hands, the operative mortality for major hepatic resection is similar. The most common causes of death after hepatic cryotherapy are cardiopulmonary in etiology and are not specific to the cryotherapy.[51] The more common treatment-specific causes of death include cryoshock, liver failure, and hemorrhage.

Long-Term Results of Cryotherapy

Hepatocellular Carcinoma

As previously discussed, the majority of HCC cases arise in the setting of liver cirrhosis and compromised liver function, which can be prohibitive for liver resection. Ablative techniques have gained favor for patients with early stage disease who are not candidates for transplantation. Although there are many reports of cryoablation for HCC in the literature, outcomes are difficult to interpret because the endpoints are not consistent. Some studies report the effect of cryotherapy on AFP, others report changes in tumor size by the Response Evaluation Criteria in Solid Tumors (RECIST) or World Health Organization criteria, and others report disease-free and overall survival alone. In addition, many studies report on the effect of cryotherapy combined with other modalities, including resection, chemotherapy, or hepatic artery ligation. Nevertheless, cryotherapy is an effective modality in the management of HCC.

Historically, 5-year actuarial survival for patients with HCC treated with cryotherapy alone was 30%. Survival was shown to be dependent on tumor size such that 5-year actuarial survival for patients with tumors less than 5 cm was 48% whereas 5-year actuarial survival for patients with tumors larger than 5 cm was 25%.[54] A more recent study reported on 1595 patients with 2313 HCC tumors treated with cryoablation alone.[55] The 5- and 10-year survival rates were 25.7% and 9.2%, respectively, with a median survival of 31.8 months. Complete response rates were achieved in 99% of tumors less than 3 cm in diameter, 95% of tumors less than 5 cm in diameter, and 46% in tumors larger than 5 cm.[55] Major complications occurred in only 3.5% of patients, and there were no treatment-related mortalities. Approximately 84% of patients had intrahepatic recurrences, of which 39% were local recurrences and 61% were distant intrahepatic recurrences. The median time to recurrence was 16.1 months.[55]

Liver Metastases

Liver metastases arising from colorectal, lung, pancreas, and stomach primary tumors constitute the most common malignant tumors of the liver. Most cancers that metastasize to the liver do so in combination with extrahepatic dissemination. CRLM, in addition to being the most common metastatic primary malignancy to the liver, are unique because they can present with the liver as the only site of metastatic disease. Fifty percent of patients with primary colorectal cancer will present

with liver metastases within 5 years of diagnosis. Twenty percent of these patients will present with the liver as the only site of metastatic disease, and 25% of patients with liver metastases present with disease amenable to surgical resection. The remaining 75% of patients, however, have unresectable disease but may be candidates for regional therapies to the liver.[19]

The ultimate goal of regional treatment of liver metastases is increased survival. Long-term follow-up of patients after cryotherapy for liver metastases is largely inadequate. Most published studies do not have follow-up exceeding 2 years, and fewer groups have treated enough patients to draw valid conclusions regarding the efficacy of cryotherapy in this setting. Series reporting 3- and 5-year survival rates have been published, but with relatively small numbers. In addition, cryotherapy has been used primarily as a salvage procedure or in combination with other treatment modalities, including resection or hepatic artery ligation or infusion, which obscures the results for cryotherapy alone.[34,39,46,50,54–73]

Most series report median overall survival of about 2 years after cryoablation of liver metastases (Table 96D.2). In 24 patients treated with cryotherapy, regardless of whether the ablation was complete, Ravikumar et al.[74] reported disease-free and overall survival rates of 24% and 63%, respectively. Similarly, Weaver et al.[62] found that 11% of patients were disease free at a mean follow-up of 30 months and 62% of treated patients were alive at 24 months after cryoablation. Seifert and Morris,[50] in a series of 116 patients with colorectal metastases, showed a median survival of 26 months and 13% of patients were alive at 5 years. Other publications have reported 4- and 5-year actuarial survival ranging from 22% to 36%.[46,71,72] Despite the wide variation in outcome with cryotherapy, some patients in each of the series achieved durable survival with this treatment.

Ng et al.[73] reported a series of 293 patients with advanced colorectal liver metastases treated over 20 years. Similar to other published series, the reported overall survival at 5 years was 24.2%. For intrahepatic recurrences after ablation in this series, 23% recurred at the ablation site and 78% at a different site in the liver remnant.[73] The authors described the additional use of cryoablation in patients with liver resection in whom margins were positive, cryoablating the liver edge. They identified four factors that affected survival in univariate analysis: node-positive primary tumor, preoperative CEA level, number of lesions, and adjuvant chemotherapy.[73] Actual follow-up is greater than 5 years for individual patients, suggesting that cryotherapy can be curative in some cases. Based on the worldwide data, it seems that durable local control is achieved in about 20% to 60% of patients treated with cryotherapy (see Table 96D.2).[75]

Comparison With Radiofrequency Ablation, Microwave Ablation, and Irreversible Electroporation

During the last 15 years, RFA (see Chapter 96B) and MWA (see Chapter 96C) have replaced cryotherapy in many centers (Table 96D.3). Pearson et al.[76] prospectively studied the complication and early local recurrence rates in patients with primary or metastatic liver tumors who were treated with cryotherapy or RFA. A 41% complication rate was reported in the cryotherapy group versus 3% in the RFA group ($P <$ .001). The majority of complications in cryotherapy patients

TABLE 96D.2 Survival After Cryotherapy: Review of Published Series

STUDY	TYPE OF TUMOR	NO. OF PATIENTS	TYPE OF TREATMENT	MEDIAN SURVIVAL (MONTHS)	MEDIAN DISEASE-FREE SURVIVAL	OVERALL SURVIVAL
Zhou et al., 1998[75]	HCC	235	C, C + H, C + R	—	—	39.8% (5 yr)
Haddad et al., 1998[56]	CRM, PLC, other	31	C, C + R	18	7	—
Seifert & Morris, 1998[50]	CRM	116	C, C + R, C + H	26	—	13% (5 yr)
Yeh et al., 1997[57]	CRM	24	C, C + R	31	20	85% (3 yr)
Adam et al., 1997[58]	HCC, CRM	34	C, C + R	NR at 16	—	52% (2 yr)
Korpan et al., 1997[59]	CRM	63	C, C + R	—	—	44% (5 yr)
Shafir et al., 1996[60]	CRM, HCC, other	39	C	NR at 14	—	65% (3 yr)
Crews et al., 1997[61]	CRM, HCC, other	40	C	—	—	30% (5 yr)
Weaver et al., 1995[62]	CRM, other	47	C, C + R	22	11% at 30 mo	62% (2 yr)
Wren et al., 1997[63]	HCC	12	C	19	—	—
Ravikumar et al., 1991[39]	CRM, HCC	32	C, C + R	—	24%	63%
Onik et al., 1991[64]	CRM	18	C, C + R	33% at 29	—	—
Lam et al., 1998[65]	HCC	4	C, C + R	1 NED, 3 AWD at 12 to 23	—	—
Lezoche et al., 1998[66]	CRM, other	18	C	78% NED at 11	—	—
McKinnon et al., 1996[67]	CRM, PLC	11	C, C + R	73% at 18	—	—
Heniford et al., 1998[68]	CRM, other	12	C	83% at 11	—	—
Dale et al., 1998[69]	CRM	6	C, C + R	100% at 17	—	—
Sheen et al., 2002[70]	CRM, other	57	C, C + R	22	12	—
Rivoire et al., 2002[71]	CRM	57	C, C + R	—	—	36% (4 yr)
Seifert & Junginger, 2004[46]	CRM	55	C, C + R	—	—	26% (5 yr)
Kerkar et al., 2004[72]	HCC, CRM, other	98	C	33	—	22% (5 yr)
Ng et al., 2012[73]	CRM	293	C, C + R	29	9	24.2% (5 yr)
Niu et al., 2013[34]	HCC	45	C, C + I, I	18	—	—
Rong et al., 2015[55]	HCC	1595	C	31.5	—	25.7% (5 yr)

AWD, Alive with disease; *C,* cryoablation; *CRM,* colorectal metastases; *H,* hepatic artery ligation; *HCC,* hepatocellular carcinoma; *I,* immunotherapy; *NED,* no evidence of disease; *NR,* not reported; *PLC,* primary liver cancer; *R,* resection.

TABLE 96D.3 Characteristics and Comparison of Cryoablation, Radiofrequency Ablation (RFA), and Microwave Ablation (MWA)

	CRYOABLATION	RFA	MWA
Technique			
Mechanisms	Freeze-thaw cycle	Thermal ablation	Thermal ablation
Hemostasis	Packing needle tract with hemostatics	Thermal coagulation of needle tract	Thermal coagulation of needle tract
Clinical Features			
Anesthesia	Local or general	General	General
Tumor sites to be avoided	Adjacent to liver surface (risk of cracking)	Adjacent to diaphragm, gallbladder, bowel, or porta hepatis	Adjacent to diaphragm, gallbladder, bowel, or porta hepatis
Size of ideal treatable tumor	<5 cm	<3 cm	<3 cm
Extratumoral immunologic effect	Yes	No	No
Local recurrence rates	11.9%-59.4%[12,76,77]	2.1%-16.4% (<3 cm)[12,76,77,79,80]	6%-8%[79,80]
Bleeding	1.7%	2.5%	3.4%

were symptomatic pleural effusions and intrahepatic abscesses. Recurrence rates with a median follow-up of 15 months also favored RFA, with a 2% recurrence rate versus 14% for cryoablation ($P < .01$).[76] Comparing percutaneous cryotherapy and RFA in a retrospective group of 64 patients, Adam et al.[12] reported complication rates of 29% for cryotherapy and 24% for RFA patients ($P = .66$), but local recurrence rates were 53% for cryotherapy versus 18% for RFA ($P = .003$). In a retrospective series of colorectal cancer liver metastases, Kingham et al.[77] showed a hazard ratio (HR) of 2.96 ($P < .05$) for local recurrence when comparing RFA and cryoablation. Despite cryoablation's association with higher complication rates, a Cochrane review showed that the quality of cryoablation trials is low, and among 628 papers, only one met quality criteria to be reviewed in that publication.[78]

In the last several years, MWA has been replacing RFA as the first modality of ablative technique for liver lesions largely given its ease of use. Though one study showed an ablation-site recurrence rate of 20% in RFA versus only 6% in MWA patients ($P < .05$),[79] a recent systemic review and meta-analysis comparing MWA with RFA for HCC demonstrated similar outcomes in the percutaneous setting and no difference in complication rate, but reduced local recurrence in the laparoscopic setting.[80]

More recently, irreversible electroporation (IRE) (see Chapter 96C) is being used to treat primary and secondary liver malignancies. This image-guided ablation technique uses high-voltage electric impulses to induce cell death. As this technology does not rely on heat, it is particularly useful for treatment of tumors in close proximity to hepatic veins and portal pedicles.[81–83] IRE can be accomplished via an open, laparoscopic, or percutaneous approach.[83–86] In a retrospective review of 28 patients and 65 treated tumors, the overall morbidity was 3% without any treatment-associated mortalities.[83] Subsequent studies with longer follow-up have demonstrated acceptable efficacy and safety, making this technique useful for small tumors in well-selected patients.[82,87]

ETHANOL INJECTION

Percutaneous ethanol injection (PEI) was one of the first percutaneous ablative techniques introduced in clinical practice. This technique consists of injecting 95% ethanol in liver tumors through a needle to induce coagulative necrosis, fibrous reaction, thrombosis of tumor microvasculature, and tissue ischemia. Ebara et al.[88] reported on a series of 270 patients with small HCC (patients with ≤3 tumors all of which were ≤3 cm in diameter) over a 20-year period. Local recurrence at 3 years was 10%; 3-year and 5-year overall survival was reported at 81.6% and 60.3%, respectively. Factors influencing survival on Cox regression analysis were preprocedure liver function and serum AFP.[88]

A meta-analysis by Weis et al.[89] comparing RFA versus other interventions included six randomized trials with a total of 1088 HCC patients. RFA appeared to be superior to PEI in

regard to local recurrence rates, overall survival, and event-free survival. This analysis also showed similar rates of major complications when comparing these two techniques. PEI trials were conducted mainly in Italy and East Asia. In this meta-analysis, Asian trials demonstrated superior overall survival in RFA patients (HR, 1.95; confidence interval [CI], 1.38–2.75), whereas Italian trials showed no such benefit (HR, 1.24; CI, 0.84–1.83).[89] Pompili et al.[90] reported a series of patients with HCC smaller than 2 cm, comparing RFA and ethanol injection. Although there was not a significant difference in 5-year overall survival (64.7% in ethanol injection vs. 72.9% in RFA), patients receiving ethanol injection had significantly higher local tumor progression (49% vs. 30.1%) and 5-year local recurrence rates (73.3% vs. 49%).[90]

Despite higher long-term recurrence rates and inferior overall survival, PEI has specific indications. Lesions in the liver hilum and close to major vessels are adequate sites for this procedure, where chemical injection can be effectively targeted to the tumor while protecting adjacent structures that would be damaged by thermal ablation. Another modest benefit is that the cost of ethanol injection is approximately 100 times less than the cost of RFA,[91] requiring fewer resources and equipment. Contraindications for PEI include patients with low platelet levels (<40,000), coagulation disorders, portal vein thrombosis, and CTP class C. A limitation of chemical ablation is the need to ensure equal distribution and exposure of the tumor parenchyma to the ethanol. Hard fibrous tumors, such as metastatic adenocarcinoma, can be difficult to penetrate, thus rendering the treatment less effective. Given that, this technique is generally considered for small (<2 cm) HCC where resection or thermal ablation is contraindicated.

CONCLUSION

There is an increasing role for ablation in the management of both primary and metastatic liver tumors as the majority of patients present with unresectable disease and patients who undergo ablative therapies have improved outcomes compared with those managed with palliative strategies. Ablations can be performed safely in patients with significant comorbidities and in patients with marginal liver function. Given high recurrence rates in many series, novel approaches combining systemic and/or other liver-directed therapies are needed to control occult metastases. For now, ablation expands the possible treatments of both primary and metastatic liver malignancies and may improve recurrence-free and overall survival.[92]

In the modern era, cryoablation has largely been replaced by newer technologies, including RFA, MWA, and IRE, due to improved outcomes and reduced morbidity and mortality. However, cryotherapy might again have an expanded role in hepatic ablation if synergistic activity with immunologic-based therapies can be demonstrated.

The references for this chapter can be found online by accessing the accompanying Expert Consult website.

CHAPTER 97

Regional chemotherapy for liver tumors

Louise C. Connell and Nancy E. Kemeny

OVERVIEW

The liver is a unique organ with a rich dual blood supply (see Chapter 2) and serves as a target organ for many tumor metastases. As the portal vein drains the gastrointestinal (GI) tract, malignancies arising from these organs frequently give rise to hematogenous liver metastases. Because colorectal cancer most frequently results in distant metastatic spread to the liver, most hepatic arterial infusion (HAI) chemotherapy studies address outcomes related to colorectal liver metastases (see Chapter 90). Data supporting the use of HAI therapy are presented in this chapter, with a special focus on technical issues related to device placement and drug delivery to the liver.

SYSTEMIC CHEMOTHERAPY

Responses to systemic therapy (SYS) vary with the type of tumor. For example, patients with liver metastases from a breast primary may have high response rates with SYS,[1] in contrast to metastases from a gastric or pancreatic primary tumor. Many chemotherapy trials do not differentiate patients with liver-only metastases to show how this subgroup of patients respond to chemotherapy. In tumors with high response rates, such as breast carcinoma, a reasonable response to SYS is found even in patients with liver metastases, although the response is lower with liver metastases than with soft tissue metastases.[2] In patients with colorectal cancer, the liver is the most common site of tumor dissemination, and liver metastases develop in 60% of patients during the course of their disease[3] (see Chapter 90).

Outcomes related to the use of SYS have improved significantly with the addition of more modern chemotherapeutic agents such as irinotecan and oxaliplatin[4,5] (see Chapter 98) There has since been a positive correlation between the number of cytotoxic drugs used and overall survival (OS), leading to common chemotherapeutic regimens that are now well established. Dual chemotherapeutic regimens are frequently used and incorporate 5-fluorouracil (5-FU) with either irinotecan-based (FOLFIRI) or oxaliplatin-based regimens (FOLFOX), with little difference in efficacy between the two regimens.[6] The choice depends on toxicity, drug availability, and patient preference. Median survival is generally in the 20-month range, with response rates ranging between 30% and 40%. Interestingly, triple-therapy combinations, which include 5-FU, oxaliplatin, and irinotecan (FOLFOXIRI), have been investigated in phase III studies with mixed results when compared with those with FOLFIRI.[7,8] Owing to additional toxicity, this particular combination is not routinely used.

Improved outcomes have been demonstrated with the addition of biologic agents in first-line and subsequent regimens, including drugs targeting vascular endothelial growth factor pathways (bevacizumab) or epidermal growth factor receptor (EGFR) pathways (cetuximab).[9,10] Furthermore, the introduction of molecular tumor biomarker analysis, including *KRAS* and *BRAF*,

has allowed further tailoring of SYS therapy to underlying tumor genotype. For example, *KRAS* gene mutations that arise in codons 12 and 13 render patients resistant to EGFR monoclonal antibody therapy. As such, only wild-type *KRAS* tumors have been treated with cetuximab, with improved response rates versus nonbiologic agents alone in those patients.[6] Similarly, quadruple therapy (addition of a biologic agent to FOLFOXIRI) regimens are being explored, with recent data suggesting benefit for use of FOLFOXIRI plus bevacizumab, particularly, in patients with *BRAF* mutations.[11–13] Median survival with the addition of biologic agents is improved to approximately 24 months, and response rates are increased to nearly 60%.

In terms of second-line therapy, patients generally alternate between oxaliplatin or irinotecan, depending on which agent was initially administered before progression. Although outcomes are equivalent with second-line therapies compared with first-line regimens, responses occur less frequently and with shorter progression-free survival (PFS).[14] Biologic agents are also used in second-line therapy, based on treatment intent, molecular profile, patient factors, and drug factors, with several studies currently underway to evaluate the role of biologic agents as second-line therapies in the treatment of metastatic colorectal cancer.[15,16]

RATIONALE FOR HEPATIC ARTERIAL CHEMOTHERAPY

The rationale for HAI is based on anatomic and pharmacologic principles.

1. Liver metastases are perfused almost exclusively by the hepatic artery, whereas normal hepatocytes derive their blood supply from both portal venous and hepatic arterial flow.[17] After injection of floxuridine (FUDR) into either the hepatic artery or the portal vein, mean liver concentrations of the drug do not differ based on the route of injection; however, mean tumor FUDR levels are significantly increased (15-fold) when the drug is injected via the hepatic artery.[18]

2. The use of drugs that are largely extracted by the liver during first-pass metabolism results in high local concentrations of drug with minimal systemic toxicity. Ensminger et al.[19] showed that 94% to 99% of FUDR is extracted by the liver during the first pass compared with 19% to 55% of 5-fluorouracil (5-FU). FUDR is therefore an ideal drug for HAI, with a 400-fold increase in hepatic exposure with FUDR. The pharmacologic advantage of various chemotherapeutic agents for HAI is summarized in Table 97.1.[20]

3. Drugs with a steep dose-response curve are more useful when given by the intrahepatic route because small increases in the concentration of administered drug result in a large improvement in response. FUDR follows linear kinetics without response saturation at high doses.

4. Drugs with a high total-body clearance are more useful for hepatic infusion. The area under the concentration-versus-time

TABLE 97.1 Estimated Increase in Hepatic Exposure for Drugs Given by Hepatic Arterial Infusion

ESTIMATED INCREASE BY DRUG	HALF-LIFE (min)	HEPATIC ARTERIAL EXPOSURE
Fluorouracil	10	5- to 10-fold
Floxuridine	10	100- to 400-fold
Bis-chloroethyl-nitrosourea	5	6- to 7-fold
Mitomycin C	10	6- to 8-fold
Cisplatin	20–30	4- to 7-fold
Doxorubicin	60	2-fold
Dichloromethotrexate	—	6- to 8-fold

From Ensminger WD, Gyves JW. Clinical pharmacology of hepatic arterial chemotherapy. *Semin Oncol.* 1983;10:176–182.

curve is a function not only of drug clearance but also of hepatic arterial blood flow. Because hepatic arterial flow has a high regional exchange rate (100–1500 mL/min), drugs with a high clearance rate are required.[21] If a drug is not cleared rapidly, recirculation through the systemic circulation mitigates the advantage of intraarterial therapy versus SYS.[22]

5. Another rationale for hepatic arterial chemotherapy, especially for patients with metastatic colorectal cancer, is the concept of a stepwise pattern of metastatic progression.[23,24] This theory states that hematogenous spread occurs first via the portal vein to the liver, then from the liver to the lungs, and then to other organs. Aggressive treatment, either resection or hepatic infusion, of metastases confined to the liver yields prolonged survival for some patients.

The development of an implantable infusion pump allowed the safe administration of hepatic arterial chemotherapy in the outpatient setting.[25] Early trials with an implantable pump and continuous FUDR therapy produced a median response rate of 47%[26] and a median survival of 17 months.[27] To further demonstrate that HAI possessed a therapeutic benefit, several randomized studies were subsequently conducted and are reviewed in detail later.

SURGICAL TECHNIQUE AND OPERATIVE CONSIDERATIONS

Hepatic Artery Pump Placement

The arterial anatomy of the liver varies (Table 97.2),[28–32] with conventional anatomy present in only approximately two thirds of patients[28] (see Chapter 2). Before consideration of pump placement, it is imperative to carefully review available images, including the arteriogram, with the radiologist and formulate a plan for the management of aberrant anatomy. In the past, direct arteriography was required (see Chapter 21), but now excellent definition can be ascertained from computed tomography (CT) angiography. In most cases, a pump with a single catheter can adequately provide access to the entire hepatic arterial inflow. It is best not to place the catheter directly into the hepatic artery, which risks thrombosis of the vessel. Instead, the catheter should ideally be placed into an accessible side branch. The gastroduodenal artery (GDA) is the preferred conduit and provides the most reliable method of catheter implantation.[28] As previously mentioned, cholecystectomy should be performed to prevent chemotherapy-induced cholecystitis. Different surgical incisions have been used for this operation with success, including an upper midline incision, right subcostal incision, or limited right subcostal hockey-stick incision. Perioperative intravenous antibiotic administration before incision and adherence to other surgical care improvement project protocols are recommended.

For patients with unresectable disease, a staging laparoscopy is advisable to rule out occult extrahepatic disease, which, in past experience, was seen in approximately one third of patients,[33] but this figure has certainly declined more recently (see Chapter 24). A thorough examination of the abdomen is performed at laparoscopy and at laparotomy to look for extrahepatic disease.[34] The most common sites of extrahepatic metastases are the peritoneum and portal lymph nodes. A biopsy should be performed if the lymph nodes appear suspicious because nodal involvement precludes use of the pump. The extent of liver involvement should be assessed by using intraoperative ultrasonography. Any radiographically occult hepatic tumors should be noted, and the potential for future resection should be specifically addressed in the operative note.

Conventional Hepatic Arterial Anatomy (see Chapter 2)

A standard cholecystectomy is performed, and the hepatic artery and its branches are circumferentially dissected. The common hepatic artery and the GDA are palpable superior to the body of the pancreas and the first portion of the duodenum. The GDA runs parallel to and lies immediately to the left of the common bile duct, and it is advisable to start by dissecting the common hepatic artery to minimize the risk of injuring the bile duct. The right gastric artery is ligated and divided. The distal common hepatic artery, the entire GDA, and the proximal proper hepatic artery are dissected away from their attachments. It is important to mobilize the full length of the extrapancreatic GDA to

TABLE 97.2 Summary of Reported Prevalence (%) of Hepatic Arterial Anatomic Variants

	DALY et al., 1984[29]	MICHELS, 1966[30]	KEMENY et al., 1986b[31]	CURLEY et al., 1993[32]	ALLEN et al., 2002[28]
	(*n* = 200)	(*n* = 200)	(*n* = 100)	(*n* = 180)	(*n* = 265)
Anatomy					
Normal	70	55	50	63	63
Variant gastroduodenal artery	6	—	9	9	11
Accessory right hepatic artery	4	7	4	1	1
Replaced right hepatic artery	6	12	16	12	6
Accessory left hepatic artery	3.5	8	1	2	10
Replaced left hepatic artery	4	10	16	11	4
Other	5	2.5	1	2	5

From Allen PJ, Stojadinovic A, Ben-Porat L, et al: The management of variant arterial anatomy during hepatic arterial infusion pump placement. *Ann Surg Oncol* 9:875–880, 2001.

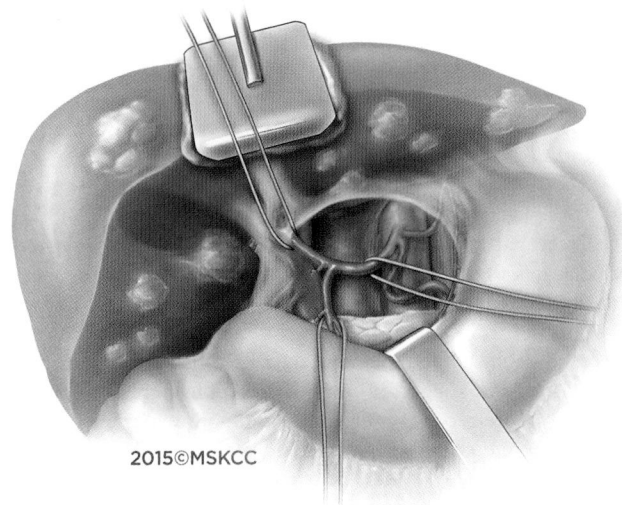

FIGURE 97.1 The common hepatic, proper hepatic, and gastroduodenal arteries are completely mobilized. All branches to the stomach, duodenum, or pancreas are identified and ligated (see Chapter 2).

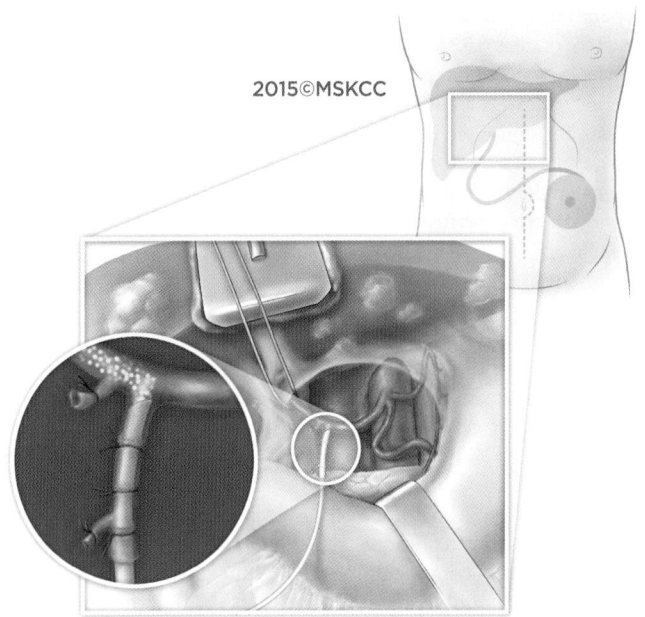

FIGURE 97.2 The infusion pump ideally is placed in the left lower quadrant, away from the liver, to avoid artifacts on subsequent computed tomographic scans. With normal anatomy, the catheter is placed in the gastroduodenal artery and secured with nonabsorbable ties, the right gastric artery is ligated, and the gallbladder is removed.

facilitate insertion of the catheter. Suprapyloric side branches of the GDA are often encountered and must be ligated. Frequently, branches to the pancreas and duodenum arise from many of these dissected vessels, and it is essential to identify and ligate these branches to avoid extrahepatic perfusion of the pancreas, stomach, or duodenum. The common hepatic artery is mobilized 1 cm proximally, and the proper hepatic artery is mobilized approximately 2 cm distally from the origin of the GDA. Branches to the retroperitoneum from the right or left hepatic artery commonly exist and should be ligated. Review of preoperative imaging to detect these branches is important. At this point, a complete circumferential dissection of the common hepatic artery, GDA, and proper hepatic artery should be ensured such that no vessels to the pancreas, stomach, or duodenum remain (Fig. 97.1). The GDA should be temporarily occluded with palpation of the proper hepatic artery to rule out critical retrograde flow to the liver through the GDA secondary to celiac artery disease or stenosis. No attempt to dissect the common bile duct is necessary, which would risk devascularization and ischemic stricturing.

The pump pocket should be created in the lower abdomen so that the pump lies below the waist and avoids contact with the iliac spine and the edge of the ribs. In obese patients, placement of the pump over the ribs should be considered because this may help with postoperative pump access. The pump and catheter should be handled carefully and contact with the patient's skin should be avoided. The catheter is trimmed at a level just beyond the last tying ring and is tunneled into the abdominal cavity. The pump is secured to the abdominal fascia with nonabsorbable sutures. The catheter should be positioned behind the pump to prevent injury by a needle. The GDA is ligated with a nonabsorbable tie at its most distal point, and vascular control of the common and proper hepatic arteries is achieved with vascular clamps or vessel loops. Isolated vascular control of the GDA at its orifice also can be used to avoid occlusion of the hepatic artery (see Chapter 127F).

A transverse arteriotomy is made in the distal GDA, and the catheter is inserted up to, but not beyond, the junction with the hepatic artery (Fig. 97.2). If the catheter protrudes into the

common hepatic artery, turbulence of blood flow can lead to thrombosis of the vessel. Conversely, failure to pass the catheter up to that junction leaves a short segment of the GDA exposed to full concentrations of FUDR without the diluting effect of blood flow, potentially resulting in sclerosis, thrombosis, or late dislodgment. When positioned, the catheter should be secured two or three times with nonabsorbable ties proximal to the tying rings on the catheter. Perfusion of both lobes of the liver and lack of extrahepatic perfusion is confirmed by infusing 2 to 3 mL of half-strength fluorescein through the pump and visualizing it with a Wood's lamp. Half-strength methylene blue injection is an alternative method of ensuring proper perfusion. After the perfusion test, the catheter is flushed with heparinized saline, and the wounds are closed. Antibiotic lavage (bacitracin solution) of the subcutaneous pocket is recommended. There are no data to support continued postoperative administration of antibiotic therapy. Pump infection, however, is a serious complication, and any sign of erythema indicates a wound infection postoperatively that should be treated immediately and aggressively (see Chapter 127F).

Aberrant Hepatic Arterial Anatomy (see Chapter 2)

As discussed earlier, aberrant hepatic arterial anatomy is common, and numerous variations occur. Each anatomic situation is specifically addressed here, but first, general principles in managing variant anatomy are discussed. In analyses of our extensive experience with this operation, the factor most consistently associated with catheter-related complications and decreased durability of the catheter is cannulation of a vessel other than the GDA. The overall preferred technique is placement of the catheter in the GDA with ligation of the isolated variant vessel. This method relies on intrahepatic collateral development and cross-perfusion to the liver fed by the ligated vessel (see Chapter 5). Although concerns have been raised over incomplete hepatic perfusion with this technique, this rarely occurs. In our published experience with this operation for variant anatomy, incomplete hepatic perfusion occurred once in 52 cases. Cross-perfusion may take as long as 4 weeks to occur, and early perfusion scans may be abnormal initially. However, these should be rechecked after a few weeks to assess for complete cross-perfusion because most normalize.[28,32] The only exception to this rule may be patients with central tumors so large that they impede cross-collateralization. Lastly, although cross-perfusion after ligation of aberrant vessels is highly reliable, it has not been proven that this results in equal blood flow for chemotherapy delivery.

Aberrant Origin of the Gastroduodenal Artery

The GDA can arise from the right or left hepatic artery, or there can be a trifurcation in which the GDA, right hepatic artery, and left hepatic artery all arise simultaneously from the common hepatic artery. This anomaly occurs 6% to 11% of the time.[28] In general, it is preferable to place the catheter into the GDA and ligate vessels that are not receiving catheter-directed flow because this is the technique associated with the lowest rate of catheter-related complications.[28,35] In the case of a trifurcation, the catheter should be placed in the GDA, and perfusion should be tested with fluorescein or methylene blue. If bilobar perfusion is adequate, ligation of vessels is unnecessary. If no perfusion to one lobe of the liver is seen at testing, the hepatic artery to that lobe should be ligated, most commonly the left hepatic artery, thereby relying on cross-perfusion of the left liver.

The hepatic arterial tree also may be accessed through the splenic artery just to the left of the celiac axis. The catheter is placed in the splenic artery and maneuvered across the celiac axis to lie freely in the hepatic artery, ending proximal to the bifurcation. The GDA and the right gastric artery are ligated, and the catheter is secured in the splenic artery. This technique is technically difficult because it requires extensive dissection of the celiac axis and manipulation of the catheter across the celiac artery branches. It is also associated with more complications, including thrombosis and extrahepatic perfusion and is therefore rarely used. Another option is retrograde cannulation of the common hepatic artery through the GDA with an attached short, stiff, small-gauge catheter. This technique, however, is also associated with a higher rate of complications, including arterial dissection and thrombosis, and it should be used rarely, if ever.

Accessory Left Hepatic Artery (see Chapter 2)

An accessory left hepatic artery arises from the left gastric artery, crosses the gastrohepatic ligament, enters the liver at the base of the umbilical fissure, and typically supplies segments II and III. The native left hepatic artery, which arises from the proper hepatic artery, also supplies the left liver, typically segment IV in this situation. This abnormality is present in 2% to 10% of cases. The simplest, safest, and most reliable option is to ligate the accessory left hepatic artery and place the pump catheter in the GDA because cross-perfusion is highly reliable. Another option is to use two catheters (or pumps), one in the GDA and one in the accessory left hepatic artery, although this technique is cumbersome and is generally not necessary.

Accessory Right Hepatic Artery (see Chapter 2)

Accessory right hepatic arteries arise from the superior mesenteric artery and run in the portacaval space to supply a portion of the right lobe of the liver. This abnormality is present in 1% to 7% of patients. Accessory and replaced right hepatic arteries

rarely have side branches adequate for cannulation. The preferred technique in this situation is placement of the catheter in the GDA and ligation of the accessory vessel because cross-perfusion is reliable. Placement of a second catheter directly in the accessory vessel is another option but is generally unnecessary and not recommended.

Replaced Left Hepatic Artery (see Chapter 2)

A replaced left hepatic artery arises from the left gastric artery and supplies the left liver, without a native left hepatic artery. This abnormality exists in 4% to 16% of patients. Once again, the preferred technique is to place the catheter in the GDA and ligate the replaced left hepatic artery. Initial reports on this specific situation suggested rates of incomplete cross-perfusion of 40%.[36] More recent reports, including our experience, show that incomplete cross-perfusion is uncommon in this situation and occurred in only 1 of 10 of our patients at last analysis.[28,32] Other techniques, such as placement of catheters in the GDA and in a branch of the replaced left hepatic artery can be considered in patients with bulky disease in the left liver or in those with a large central tumor that may impede cross-perfusion.

Replaced Right Hepatic Artery (see Chapter 2)

A replaced right hepatic artery originates from the superior mesenteric artery, runs in the portacaval space, and supplies the whole right liver. No branches to the right liver originate from the proper hepatic artery, an anatomic situation that occurs 6% to 16% of the time. If the surgeon ligates the replaced right hepatic artery, cross-perfusion from the left hepatic artery occurs almost uniformly.[28,32,36] The catheter should be placed in the GDA, and the replaced right hepatic artery should be ligated. Other techniques have been described, such as placing a second catheter in the replaced right hepatic artery, either directly through a small arteriotomy, because there are no significant side branches from this vessel, or using a vascular graft, but these are rarely indicated. This technique requires that the catheter be trimmed flush just beyond the tying ring and that it be placed such that the ring lies just inside the vessel, and the arteriotomy closed over the ring.

PUMP PLACEMENT AFTER MAJOR HEPATECTOMY

In the event that a pump is placed for adjuvant therapy after hepatectomy, the specific anatomy to the remnant liver must be considered. In general, the best results are obtained if the catheter is placed in the GDA. In the presence of replaced or accessory vessels to the remnant liver, the surgeon must consider the condition of the liver remnant (i.e., steatosis, congestion, and jaundice) and the potential risk of ligating the arterial supply or risking thrombosis by directly cannulating the vessel to the remnant. One option that is often available after a hemihepatectomy is to use the stump of the artery to the resected liver as a conduit for the catheter, if the anatomy allows this. If the arterial anatomy is normal, or if a trifurcation is present at the GDA, there is generally no issue, and the catheter is placed routinely in the GDA. When a variation of the origin of the GDA is present (i.e., off of the right or left hepatic artery), care must be taken to preserve the origin such that the catheter can be placed. For a remnant right lobe, an accessory right hepatic artery generally can be ligated, unless major concerns about the condition of the liver remnant are an issue. In the case of a remnant right lobe and a replaced right hepatic artery, it is generally not recommended to place a pump because it would require direct cannulation of that artery, risking thrombosis, injury, and a higher rate of catheter-related complications in general. For a remnant left lobe, an accessory left artery generally can be ligated. If the remnant left lobe is fed solely by a replaced left hepatic artery, a pump can be placed, but this requires dissection of the left gastric artery and identification of a suitable side branch for the catheter. Special care must be taken to ensure that all branches to the stomach have been properly ligated to prevent extrahepatic perfusion.

POSTOPERATIVE ASSESSMENT

After surgery and before administering chemotherapy, the distribution of arterial perfusion is assessed by a radionuclide pump-flow study (see Chapter 18). A baseline technetium-99m–sulfur colloid scan is obtained to identify the liver contour. Pump perfusion is assessed by infusing ^{99m}Tc-labeled macroaggregated albumin (MAA) through the bolus port of the pump and into the hepatic artery. When the MAA scan produces an image that matches the sulfur colloid liver scan, the pump is perfusing the entire liver as intended. Perfusion of extrahepatic tissues produces ^{99m}Tc signals outside the liver image (Fig. 97.3). Incomplete perfusion of the liver produces an incomplete image on the MAA scan. Malperfusion is discovered in 5% to 7% of cases and often can be corrected by surgical or angiographic intervention to occlude additional hepatic vessels missed at operation.[37] If no additional vessels are seen on angiography for embolization, it is worth repeating the scan in a few weeks to allow sufficient time for intrahepatic collaterals and cross-perfusion to develop.[28]

TECHNICAL COMPLICATIONS OF HEPATIC ARTERY INFUSION PUMP PLACEMENT

Surgical and technical complications of pump placement occur, and the spectrum and frequency of these complications must be understood by the surgeon, the medical oncologist, and the patient before initiating treatment. To assess the risks of insertion and the use of an implantable pump for HAI, we reviewed the charts of all patients who underwent pump insertion for

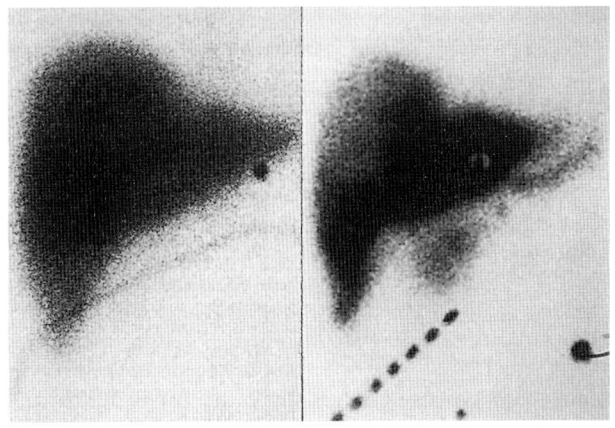

FIGURE 97.3 The liver-spleen technetium-99m–sulfur colloid scan on the left shows the normal liver. The macroaggregated albumin scan on the right shows extrahepatic perfusion to the duodenum and head of the pancreas (see Chapter 18).

unresectable metastases during a 15-year period (1986–2001) at Memorial Sloan Kettering Cancer Center (MSKCC).[35] During this period, 544 infusion pumps were inserted by multiple surgeons for HAI of FUDR alone or in combination with other drugs for patients with isolated unresectable colorectal hepatic metastases. Variant arterial anatomy was present in 205 patients (38%), most of which (82%) involved a single vessel. A colectomy was performed in addition to the pump placement in 136 patients (25%). Operative mortality was low, and 5 patients died within 30 days of the operation (0.9% mortality rate). Early in the series, 2 deaths occurred from hepatic failure secondary to extensive metastatic disease within the liver. We now exclude patients with extensive (>70%) liver replacement from pump placement because of this risk. Generalized operative morbidity unrelated to the pump itself occurred in approximately 25% of patients in our series. The most common complications were prolonged ileus, wound complications, atelectasis, and abscesses.

Pump-related morbidity occurred in 120 patients (22%) and is summarized in Table 97.3. Most of these complications (63%) occurred more than 30 days after pump placement.

TYPE OF COMPLICATION	TOTAL (*N*)	EARLY (<30 DAYS)		LATE (>30 DAYS)	
		n	% SALVAGED	*n*	% SALVAGED
Pump malfunction	6	6	100	—	—
Pocket infection	14	4	50	10	40
Hematoma	1	1	100	—	—
Pump migration	4	1	100	3	33
Catheter occlusion	11	—	—	11	36
Dislodgment	18	—	—	18	11
Erosion	4	—	—	4	0
Arterial hemorrhage	1	1	100	—	—
Thrombosis	33	13	31	20	30
Extrahepatic perfusion	16	9	100	7	57
Incomplete perfusion	12	9	78	3	67
Overall	120	44	70	76	30

TABLE 97.3 Postoperative Pump-Related Complications and Salvage Rates in 544 Hepatic Artery Infusion Pump Placements

From Allen PJ, Nissan A, Picon AI, et al. Technical complications and durability of hepatic artery infusion pumps for unresectable colorectal liver metastases: an institutional experience of 544 consecutive cases. *J Am Coll Surg.* 201:57–65, 2005.

The most common complications (51%) were related to the hepatic arterial system and included thrombosis, hemorrhage, or perfusion abnormalities. Early (<30 days) pump-related morbidity occurred in only 8% of cases, and all of the catheter-related complications occurred after 30 days. Overall, pumps were salvaged from these complications 45% of the time. However, salvage was much more common with early complications (70%) than with late complications (30%). At multivariate analysis, surgeon experience and the use of any vessel other than the GDA were independently associated with pump-related morbidity and pump survival. Pump failure was generally low, recorded at 5% at 6 months, 9% at 1 year, 16% at 2 years, and 26% at 3 years. HAI was discontinued for pump-related complications in only 9% of cases. The performance of a concomitant colorectal resection was not associated with a higher rate of complications.

Extrahepatic Perfusion

Small branches of the hepatic artery to the stomach, duodenum, and pancreas can be missed on preoperative angiography. If small vessels are not divided and ligated, perfusion of the bowel with FUDR produces severe pain and GI ulceration. If the pancreas is perfused, severe pancreatitis will ensue. These complications are potentially lethal, and extrahepatic perfusion should be identified and corrected before starting chemotherapy whenever possible.

If extrahepatic perfusion is seen on the ^{99m}Tc MAA scan, the next step is to perform an angiogram by bolus injection through the pump. The angiogram often demonstrates the vessel responsible for the extrahepatic perfusion. This occasionally is unsuccessful, and a transfemoral celiac or superior mesenteric artery study is needed to identify the problem (Fig. 97.4). More recently, we have proceeded directly to transfemoral angiograms for assessment of patients in whom the perfusion scan shows obvious extrahepatic perfusion. This approach simplifies the process because this procedure can both diagnose the problem and potentially treat it. In our review of 544 cases, 9 patients (2%) were found to have extrahepatic perfusion on the postoperative scan. The cause was identified arteriographically, and, in 7 cases, it was corrected with transarterial embolization or surgical ligation. These patients went on to receive HAI without complication.[35] In a more recent review from our institution, 327 patients who underwent pump implantation between 2008 and 2011 were evaluated to help identify common culprit arterial branches that result in extrahepatic perfusion to determine whether alterations in surgical technique during pump placement may prevent extrahepatic perfusion.[38] There were 24 cases of extrahepatic perfusion. The arterial branch responsible for extrahepatic perfusion perfused the duodenum, pancreas, and/or stomach, and arose from the proper hepatic artery, first-, second-, or third-order hepatic artery branches in 7, 10, 5, and 2 patients, respectively. Most branches beyond the proper hepatic artery causing extrahepatic perfusion originated from the right hepatic artery.

Incomplete Hepatic Perfusion

In nine cases from our series (2%), the postoperative ^{99m}Tc MAA scan showed incomplete perfusion of the liver.[35] Causes included failure to ligate a replaced or accessory hepatic artery and failure to achieve cross-perfusion after ligation of an accessory artery (one case). In every case, the anatomic problem was identified by a side port or transfemoral angiogram. Overall, seven of the nine cases were corrected with embolization or surgical ligation of the accessory vessel, and chemotherapy was administered uneventfully. In the instance of incomplete cross-over perfusion, collateral flow to the remaining liver developed with time. A repeat MAA scan in 4 weeks confirmed the development of collateral blood flow.

Gastroduodenal Ulcers

In rare instances, the ^{99m}Tc MAA scan fails to identify subtle extrahepatic perfusion. The most frequent anomaly is a small branch to the lesser curve of the stomach. Early in our experience, we treated three patients who were clinically shown to have extrahepatic perfusion that was not apparent on ^{99m}Tc MAA scan, even in retrospect. Severe epigastric pain developed in the patients during the first course of chemotherapy, and endoscopy showed large ulcers in the stomach or duodenum. These patients do not respond to standard antiulcer therapy because the cause is not acid hypersecretion but, rather, loss of mucosa in the area perfused with FUDR. The diagnosis is confirmed by angiography, and treatment requires angiography or laparotomy for identification and ligation of the vessel. When the offending vessel has been occluded and the ulcer has healed, chemotherapy can be then safely administered. If a patient experiences unexplained epigastric pain during infusional chemotherapy, the pump should be emptied immediately and refilled with heparinized saline until the cause of the pain can be elucidated.

Arterial or Catheter Thrombosis

Complete dissection and thrombosis of the hepatic artery intraoperatively has been described during pump insertion, but this condition is rare.[35] 13 cases (2%) of acute postoperative arterial thrombosis were noted, but the technical problem leading to thrombosis was uncertain in most of these cases. Of these 13 cases of early thrombosis, 31% were salvaged with anticoagulation or lytic therapy. We also observed that delayed thrombosis of the hepatic artery (20 cases) was more common

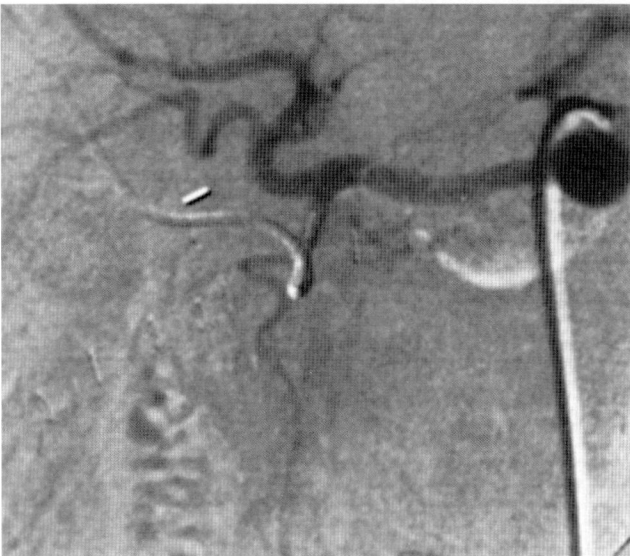

FIGURE 97.4 A transfemoral celiac angiogram shows a vessel arising from the gastroduodenal artery (GDA), which had not been ligated. At operation, this vessel was found to be arising from the posterior aspect of the GDA.

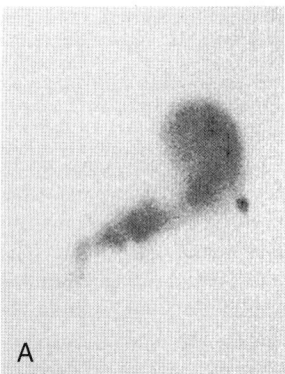

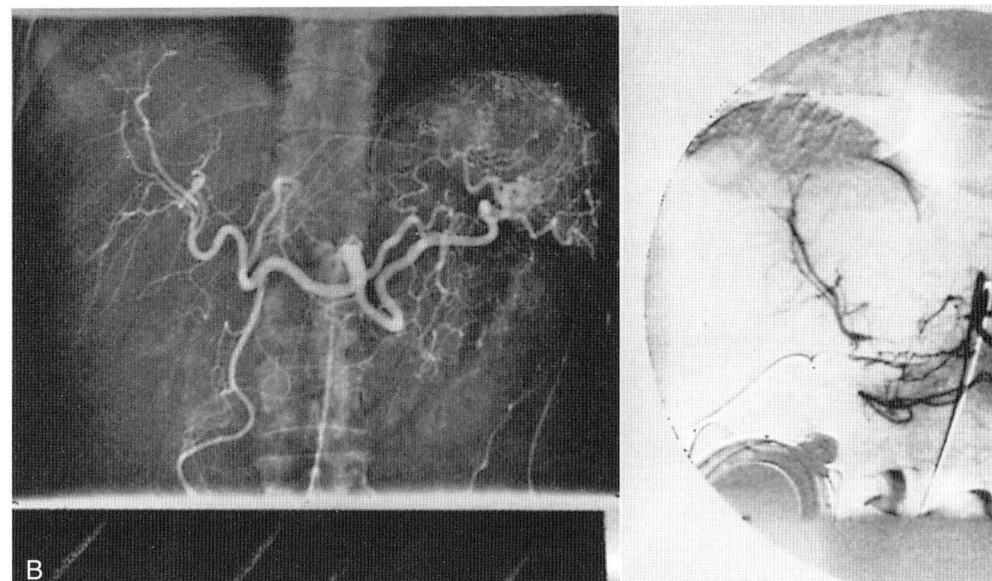

FIGURE 97.5 A, When hepatic artery thrombosis occurs, the macroaggregated albumin scan shows an absence of perfusion of the liver together with perfusion of the spleen, stomach, and pancreas. **B,** Arteriogram before operation shows normal patent vessels *(left),* but postoperative arteriography *(right)* confirms that the artery is thrombosed. The first sign of hepatic artery thrombosis may be abdominal pain occurring with chemotherapy owing to perfusion of the stomach and pancreas. If severe pain occurs during chemotherapy, the first step should be to empty the pump and replace the chemotherapy with heparinized saline.

than acute thrombosis (13 cases). The vasculitis caused by infusional chemotherapy is thought to contribute to late arterial thrombosis. Often, arterial thrombosis manifests as extrahepatic perfusion on ^{99m}Tc MAA scan (Fig. 97.5). Catheter thrombosis was seen only as a late complication, which occurred in 11 cases (2%), and was more likely to be related to technical errors, such as not filling the pump frequently or allowing back bleeding into the catheter during sideport manipulation.

Infectious Complications

Infectious complications associated with any major operation, including pneumonia, urinary tract infections, and wound infections, may occur after laparotomy and pump placement. Because a foreign body is inserted during this operation, particular care must be directed against wound or pump-pocket infections. Technical precautions must be taken in the operating room to limit bacterial contamination of the pump. Postoperatively, any sign of pump-pocket erythema should be treated early and aggressively with parenteral antibiotics.

We have not seen an increased incidence of complications in patients undergoing pump insertion combined with colectomy.

It is preferable to place the pump first, close the pump pocket, exclude the catheter from the rest of the procedure, and then proceed with colectomy, thereby protecting surgical instruments and the operative field from inevitable bowel contamination. The surgeon may also choose to mobilize the bowel initially without transecting the bowel.

Hemorrhagic Complications

Bleeding complications developed in two patients postoperatively. In one case, the patient experienced severe abdominal pain when the pump was injected for the initial ^{99m}Tc MAA scan. On the flow scan, extrahepatic extravasation of ^{99m}Tc was seen. At laparotomy, bleeding from a suprapyloric branch that had been inadequately clipped during the operation was observed. A second patient experienced bleeding into the pump pocket that resulted in a hematoma. Both complications were salvaged, and the pumps were used successfully.[35]

Biliary Sclerosis

In a study by Ito et al.[39] the incidence of biliary sclerosis was 5.5% in patients who received HAI as adjuvant therapy after hepatectomy (16/293 patients) and 2.2% in patients who received HAI with FUDR for unresectable disease (2/100 patients). In their study, the authors noted that the common hepatic duct was the site most frequently affected (87.5%). Biliary sclerosis was associated with abnormal postoperative flow scans, postoperative infectious complications, and larger doses of FUDR. No patient died directly of biliary sclerosis, and median survival was not compromised by the development of biliary sclerosis (see Chapter 42).

Biliary sclerosis is an uncommon complication after HAI that does not compromise survival if adequately salvaged by stenting or dilation and is associated with the dose of intraarterial chemotherapy and postoperative surgical complications. The addition of systemic bevacizumab to HAI FUDR is known to lead to increased biliary toxicity, and these two drugs should never be given concurrently.[40]

MINIMALLY INVASIVE TECHNIQUES FOR PLACEMENT OF HEPATIC ARTERIAL INFUSION PUMPS (SEE CHAPTER 127F)

The necessity of a laparotomy to place HAI pumps has been, and remains, a hurdle for pump chemotherapy. Because a major operation is mandated, many oncologists and patients have been deterred. HAI pump placement requires substantial skill, sophisticated knowledge of upper GI anatomy, and clinical experience, making this operation technically challenging and difficult to perform laparoscopically.

The technique of laparoscopic HAI pump placement should mimic the open operation. Review of the preoperative angiogram remains crucial, and management of aberrant anatomy must be planned in advance. A right subcostal port is placed for retraction of the liver, and a three-port working triangle is created in the left upper quadrant, aimed at the porta hepatis. The dissection and isolation of the vessels is the same as in the open operation. Ultrasonic dissectors are helpful to divide dense lymphatics and keep bleeding to a minimum. Branches to the stomach, duodenum, and pancreas can be clipped or divided with the ultrasonic dissector. Because controlling torn branches can be difficult, patience is crucial.

Once the critical vessels are identified and dissected, the pump pocket is made in the right abdominal wall and the catheter is placed into the peritoneal cavity under laparoscopic visualization. The distal GDA is ligated, and ties are left long for countertraction. Laparoscopic bulldog clamps are used for vascular isolation. A bulldog clamp can be placed on each of the common hepatic artery and proper hepatic artery, or a single clamp may be placed at the orifice of the GDA. A tie is left around the GDA in anticipation of tying the catheter place, and a laparoscopic No. 11 blade is used to create a transverse arteriotomy. Using countertraction on the GDA, the catheter is placed into the GDA, while ensuring the catheter does not extend beyond into the hepatic artery. The catheter is subsequently tied in place. The clamps are carefully removed and hemostasis is ensured. This is followed by intraoperative dye injection to confirm bilobar hepatic perfusion and absence of extrahepatic flow.

Published experience with laparoscopic placement of HAI pumps is largely limited to small cases series.[41–45] The largest series to date was published by Cheng et al.[42] and describes their experience in 38 patients, of whom 24 had additional radiofrequency ablation (RFA), 2 had a laparoscopic partial

hepatectomy, and 1 was converted to laparotomy. The median time in the operating room was 5.5 hours, and the overall results were excellent. There was only one postoperative cardiac-related mortality reported, without pump-related morbidity, and the median hospital stay was 3 days.

The most recent report, a Belgian case series, included 29 patients who underwent laparoscopic catheter placement.[46] Ten patients were noted to have nonconventional anatomy. In those patients, all accessory or aberrant vessels were ligated, and the authors confirmed successful arterial collateralization 3 weeks after the index procedure by using angiography. Mean operative time was only 106 minutes, and median hospital stay was 2 days (1–13 days). Although there were no reported intraoperative complications, one patient with a prior history of partial gastrectomy died 1 week after the procedure as a result of hepatic arterial rupture.

Robotic-assisted laparoscopic pump placement has recently been described.[47] The procedure carries the potential to improve perioperative outcomes but warrants surgical expertise with new costly technology, and it is noted to be technically challenging. Interestingly, no additional reports of robotic-assisted placement have surfaced since the publication of this isolated report.

In a retrospective review of hepatic arterial infusion pump (HAIP) placement surgeries at our institution, there were 45 minimally invasive cases attempted during a 13-year period from 2003 through 2016.[48] Of those, 24 cases were robotic and 21 were laparoscopic procedures. Robotic HAIP placement was associated with a significantly lower conversion rate to open operation than laparoscopic pump placement (17 vs. 67%; $P < .01$). In the robotic series, there were a total of 4 conversions to open pump placement among 24 patients, of which 2 occurred in cases with concomitant hepatic resection. Three of these conversions occurred among the first 12 patients, as familiarity with the robotic procedure was developing. There was a trend toward shorter median length of hospital stay with robotic pump placement compared with open and laparoscopic placement (4 vs. 5 vs. 5 days, respectively; $P = .09$). Complication rates were equivalent among the three groups when concomitant resections were excluded. There can be technical challenges associated with safe dissection and cannulation of the GDA using minimally invasive techniques. Therefore it is crucial that these cases are attempted by surgeons experienced in both laparoscopic surgery and open pump placement at specialized institutions only.

PLACEMENT OF HEPATIC ARTERIAL INFUSION PUMPS USING PERCUTANEOUS INTERVENTIONAL TECHNIQUES

HAIP placement can be done safely by laparotomy with an acceptable morbidity. Poor overall prognosis and the requirement for a laparotomy have discouraged many surgeons and oncologists from using this modality, however. Several groups have worked on alternative placement methods to eliminate the laparotomy "hurdle" (see Chapter 100).

Percutaneous techniques to catheterize the hepatic artery for delivery of intrahepatic chemotherapy have been developed using a variety of peripheral arteries for access (Table 97.4).[49–55] Most of these techniques have been abandoned or are used only by a few specialized groups for the following reasons:

1. The insertion is technically difficult. The technique described by Arai et al.[49,50] requires embolization of the GDA to anchor the catheter. The tip of the catheter remains anchored in the

TABLE 97.4 Peripheral Arteries Used for Catheter Placement in the Hepatic Artery

ARTERY	REFERENCES
Femoral artery	Matsumada et al., 1997[52]
Brachial artery	Cohen et al., 1980[53]
Axillary artery	Arai, 1988[49]; Cohen et al., 1983[54]
Subclavian artery	Arai, 1988[49]; Arai et al., 1997[50]
Hypogastric artery	Arai et al., 1997[50], 1988[49]
Intercostal artery	Castaing et al., 1998[55]; Saldinger & Sandhu, 2004[56]

GDA, and perfusion is achieved through a side hole in the catheter.

2. The insertion site is in a mobile part of the body, such as the arm or the leg, resulting in risk of catheter dislocation or migration.[56]
3. The artery used for access is "essential" for limb perfusion, and any thrombotic complication is potentially limb-threatening (see Table 97.4).

Castaing et al.,[54] attempted to address these shortfalls by using an intercostal artery as conduit. A cutdown was performed over the 10th left rib. The intercostal artery was catheterized and the catheter advanced, under fluoroscopic control, across the aorta into the ostium of the celiac axis, and ultimately into the proper hepatic artery, just beyond the takeoff of the GDA. The catheter was connected to an implantable port located in the left upper quadrant. The study included 35 patients with metastatic lesions to the liver, mainly from colorectal cancer, and 30 patients (86%) underwent successful placement. Placement was not feasible in five patients because of an unsuitable artery. No procedure-associated deaths were reported, no thrombotic complications occurred in either the aorta or hepatic artery, and no dislocations or migrations of the catheter occurred. Follow-up was brief because most of these patients died of their disease, although all of the patients had not responded to previous standard treatments and had advanced disease by the time they underwent catheter placement.

This method possesses clear advantages because of its relative simplicity and the fact that the catheter is attached to an immobile part of the body, thus preventing catheter dislocation. Catheter patency, however, was less than 50% at 4 months, likely as a result of a lack of continuous flow. In addition, the catheter used in Castaing's study[54] is not approved by the US Food and Drug Administration for prolonged indwelling use, thereby limiting application in the United States.

A modification of Castaing's method has been reported to address these issues.[54] A peripherally inserted 3-French (Fr) central catheter was chosen as the indwelling arterial catheter (Arrow International, Reading, PA). We used a 15-mL Codman 3000 constant-flow implantable pump for access and drug delivery (Codman, Raynham, MA). The pump catheter and arterial catheter were connected via a special connector (Arrow International) (Fig. 97.6). Our method used largely similar techniques as described by Castaing[54] but with a few notable differences:

1. A preoperative angiogram was obtained for mapping of the hepatic vessels (Fig. 97.7). The angiogram was saved and used during the procedure as a guide. Accessory hepatic arteries were embolized to optimize pump perfusion, and, if

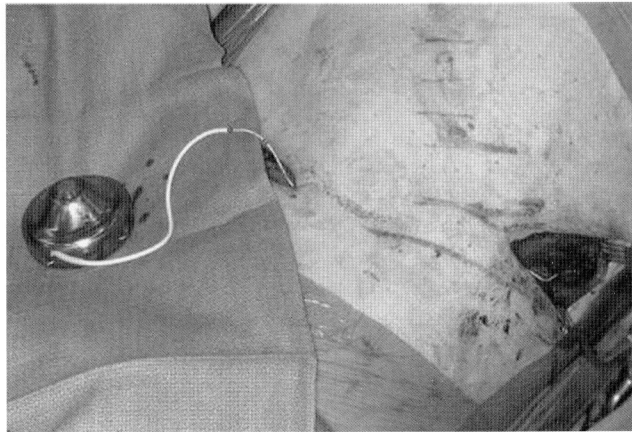

FIGURE 97.6 The indwelling arterial catheter is tunneled from the insertion site at the 11th rib to the left upper quadrant, where it is connected to the catheter of the infusion pump via a connector. The pump is placed into a pocket in the subcutaneous tissue.

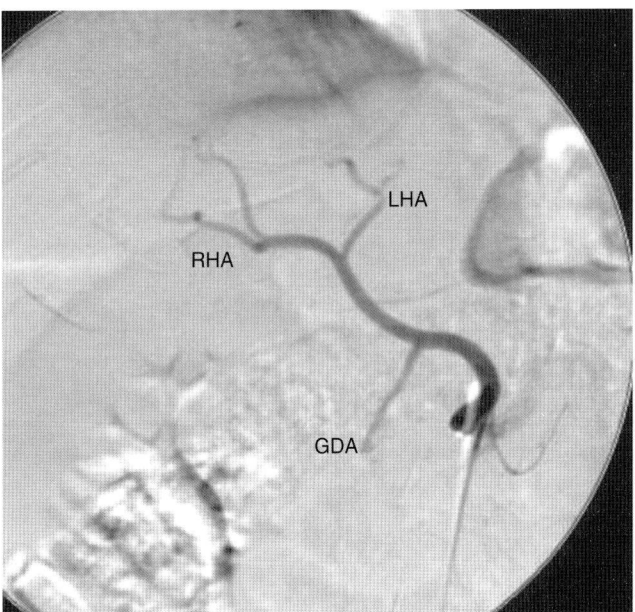

FIGURE 97.7 Transfemoral Celiac Arteriogram Mapping the Hepatic Arterial Anatomy. *GDA*, Gastroduodenal artery; *LHA*, left hepatic artery; *RHA*, right hepatic artery. (See Chapter 2.)

the distance between the GDA and the hepatic bifurcation was deemed too short, the GDA was embolized; that is, if it posed a risk for nondelivery of the target drug.

2. The intercostal artery was accessed by micropuncture, followed by introduction of a sheath. The sheath allowed repeated introduction of wires, should the situation have required this. A guidewire was introduced and placed into the hepatic artery. The 3-Fr catheter was advanced into the hepatic artery, the wire withdrawn, and the catheter was secured (Fig. 97.8). An on-table angiogram was obtained through the catheter to confirm proper placement. We confirmed catheter placement and excluded extrahepatic perfusion the next day with a perfusion scan. The pump was filled on the same day with chemotherapy.

This procedure was performed successfully in four patients with metastatic colon cancer to the liver as part of a feasibility

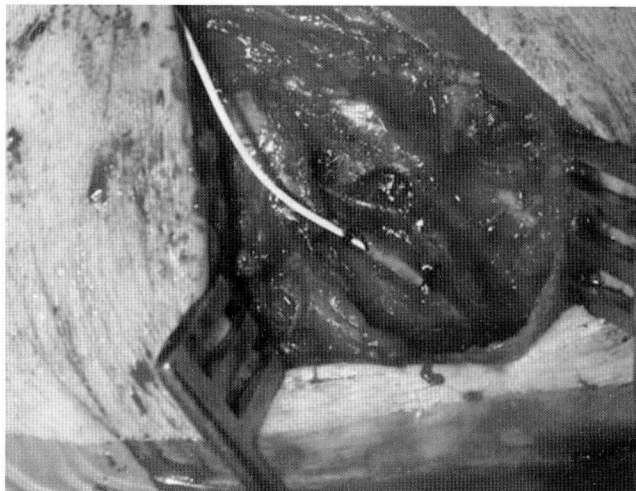

FIGURE 97.8 A 3-French Catheter Secured to the Intercostal Artery. The inferior border of the 11th rib has been exposed, allowing exposure of the intercostal artery and vein.

study. All patients had failed at least two chemotherapeutic regimens and were unresectable; no perioperative deaths or complications were reported. The catheters remained patent until the patients' deaths from progression of disease at 1, 3, 6, and 7 months. The percutaneous placement of HAIPs is a safe method and possesses all the advantages of minimally invasive procedures. Its role in the armamentarium of therapies to treat metastatic colorectal cancer to the liver depends largely on the role of intraarterial chemotherapy for liver tumors.

TOXICITY AND RESPONSE RATES OF HEPATIC ARTERIAL INFUSION THERAPY

The following section discusses toxicity of intrahepatic therapy and approaches to reducing toxicity associated with intraarterial therapy, such as the incorporation of dexamethasone for toxicity abrogation to improve overall outcomes.

Toxicity of Intrahepatic Therapy

Table 97.5 summarizes the GI toxicities noted by investigators using the implantable pump.[26,27,57-64] The side effects of SYS

are almost never observed with HAI, and myelosuppression does not occur with intrahepatic FUDR.[57] Although intrahepatic mitomycin C or bis-chloroethyl-nitrosourea may depress platelet counts, the absolute decrease and frequency of cytopenias are less than with systemic administration. Nausea, vomiting, and diarrhea do not occur with HAI FUDR. If diarrhea does occur, shunting of the chemotherapeutic agent to the bowel should be suspected.[58]

The most common problems with HAI therapy are ulceration and hepatic toxicity.[57,65] Severe ulcer disease results from inadvertent perfusion of the stomach and duodenum with drug via small, unligated branches from the hepatic artery, but this can be prevented by meticulous dissection at the time of pump placement.[65] However, even without radiologically visible perfusion of the stomach or duodenum, mild gastritis and duodenitis can occur. This toxicity can be reduced by careful dose reductions when any GI symptoms arise. Patients are otherwise maintained on proton pump inhibitor therapy during treatment. Hepatobiliary toxicity is the most problematic toxicity seen with HAI. Although some evidence of hepatocellular necrosis and cholestasis has been found on liver biopsy specimens,[66] most studies point to a combined ischemic and inflammatory effect on the bile ducts as the most important cause of this toxicity. The bile ducts are especially sensitive to HAI because their blood supply is derived almost exclusively from the hepatic artery.[67]

In patients with severe toxicity, endoscopic retrograde cholangiopancreatography (ERCP) shows lesions resembling primary sclerosing cholangitis.[63] Because the ducts are sclerotic and nondilated, ultrasound is not usually helpful. In some patients, the strictures are more focal, and they are usually worse at the bifurcation, and drainage procedures by endoscopic or by percutaneous transhepatic intubation may be helpful. Duct obstruction from metastases should be excluded first with liver CT scans.

Close monitoring of liver function tests is crucial to avoid biliary sclerosis. If the serum bilirubin becomes elevated, no further treatment should be given until the bilirubin level returns to normal, and treatment should then proceed with only a small test dose (0.05 mg/kg/day). In patients who cannot tolerate even a low dose for 2 weeks, it may be possible to continue treatment by giving the FUDR infusion for 1 week rather than the usual 2 weeks. At MSKCC, we modify treatment as outlined in Table 97.6.

TABLE 97.5	Hepatic Arterial Floxuridine Infusion With Internal Pump: Toxicity						
REFERENCE	NO. PATIENTS	GASTRITIS (%)	ULCER (%)	AST (%)	ELEVATED SERUM BILIRUBIN (%)	DIARRHEA (%)	BILIARY SCLEROSIS (%)
Niederhuber et al., 1984[59]	70	56	8	32	24	—	—
Balch & Urist, 1986[60]	50	—	6	23	23	0	—
Kemeny et al., 1984[57]	41	29	29	71	22	0	5
Shepard et al., 1985[61]	53	—	20	49	24	—	—
Cohen et al., 1983[54]	50	—	40	10	25	—	—
Weiss et al., 1983[27]	17	50	11	80	23	23	—
Schwartz et al., 1985[62]	23	53	—	77	20	10	—
Johnson et al., 1985[26]	40	−3	8	50	13	0	5
Kemeny et al., 1985[63]	31	17	6	47	—	8	19
Hohn et al., 1989[64]	61	35	2	0	78	11	29

AST, Aspartate aminotransferase.

TABLE 97.6   Dose Modification of HAI of FUDR for Hepatic Toxicity

	ASPARTATE AMINOTRANSFERASE		FUDR (%)
Reference value (ref)	≤50 U/L	>50 U/L	—
Current value	0 to <3 × ref	0 to <2 × ref	100
	3 to <4 × ref	2 to <3 × ref	80
	4 to <5 × ref	3 to <4 × ref	50
	≥5 × ref	≥4 × ref	Hold
If held, restart when:	<4 × ref	<3 × ref	50% off last dose
	ALKALINE PHOSPHATASE		**FUDR**
Reference value	≤90 U/L	>90 U/L	—
Current value	0 to <1.5 × ref	0 to <1.2 × ref	100
	1.5 to >2 × ref	1.2 to 1.5 × ref	80
	≥2 × ref	≥1.5 × ref	Hold
If held, restart when:	<1.5 × ref	<1.2 × ref	25% off last dose
	TOTAL BILIRUBIN		**FUDR**
Reference value	≤1.2 mg/dL	>1.2 mg/dL	—
Current value	0 to <1.5 × ref	0 to <1.2 × ref	100
	1.5 to <2 × ref	1.2 to <1.5 × ref	50
	≥2 × ref	≥1.5 × ref	Hold
If held, restart when:	<1.5 × ref	<1.2 × ref	25% off last dose

Reference value is obtained on the day patient received the last FUDR dose. Current value is obtained at pump emptying or on the day of planned treatment, whichever is higher.
FUDR, Fluorodeoxyuridine; HAI, hepatic arterial infusion.

In earlier trials, cholecystitis occurred in 33% of patients receiving HAI.[68] In more recent series, the gallbladder was removed at the time of catheter placement to prevent this complication and to avoid confusion with other hepatic side effects of chemotherapy.

Approaches to Decrease Hepatic Toxicity

New approaches to decrease the hepatic toxicity induced by HAI FUDR have been studied. Because portal triad inflammation may lead to ischemia and stricturing of the bile ducts, the hepatic arterial administration of dexamethasone decreases biliary toxicity. As previously mentioned, a prospective double-blind randomized study of intrahepatic FUDR with dexamethasone versus FUDR alone was conducted at MSKCC.[69] The response rate in 49 evaluable patients was 71% for those who received FUDR plus dexamethasone versus 40% for those given FUDR alone (P = .03). Survival also favored the FUDR plus dexamethasone group at 23 months versus 15 months for FUDR alone (P = .06). In addition, a trend was noted toward decreased bilirubin elevation in patients receiving FUDR plus dexamethasone compared with the group receiving FUDR alone (9% vs. 30%; P = .07).

A second method to decrease hepatic toxicity is the use of circadian modification of hepatic intraarterial FUDR infusion. In a retrospective nonrandomized study,[70] a comparison of constant (flat) infusion versus circadian-modified HAI of FUDR was conducted in 50 patients. During nine courses of treatment, the patients with circadian-modified infusion tolerated almost twice the daily dose of FUDR. Circadian-modified infusion resulted in 46% of patients having no hepatic toxicity versus 16% after flat FUDR infusion. The authors did not present information on response rates achieved in both groups.

Another approach to decrease toxicity from HAI is to alternate intraarterial FUDR with intraarterial 5-FU. A weekly intraarterial bolus of 5-FU has similar activity to intraarterial FUDR but does not cause hepatobiliary toxicity. However, it frequently produces treatment-limiting systemic toxicity or arteritis with the pharmacokinetic differences previously discussed. Stagg et al.[71] used an alternating regimen of HAI of FUDR and HAI of 5-FU, with a response rate of 51% and median survival of 22.4 months. In contrast to the experience with single-agent HAI of FUDR, no patient had treatment terminated because of drug toxicity. Another report described 57 patients with colorectal cancer with unresectable liver metastases treated with an alternating HAI schedule of FUDR and 5-FU.[72] Biliary sclerosis developed in two patients (3.5%), and 12 (21.1%) had mild transient liver function abnormalities.

Methods to Increase Response Rate

Because systemic combination chemotherapy regimens are more effective than single agents, the potential benefit of multidrug HAI has been evaluated. In an early study using mitomycin C, bis-chloroethyl-nitrosourea, and FUDR, Cohen et al.[73] achieved a 69% partial response rate. In a randomized trial at MSKCC comparing this multidrug regimen with FUDR alone,[74] the response rates were 45% for the multidrug regimen and 32% for FUDR alone in the 67 patients who entered the trial. The median survivals from the initiation of HAI were 18.9 months and 14.9 months. Other trials with FUDR and leucovorin (LV) have produced response rates as high as 62%.[64]

FIRST-LINE HEPATIC ARTERIAL CHEMOTHERAPY IN UNRESECTABLE LIVER METASTASES (SEE CHAPTER 90)

One of the first randomized trials was conducted at MSKCC.[75] Before randomization, patients were stratified for extent of liver involvement by tumor and baseline lactate dehydrogenase level,

TABLE 97.7	Randomized Studies of Hepatic Arterial Infusion (HAI) Versus Systemic Chemotherapy (SYS) for Unresectable Hepatic Metastases						
	HAI			**SYS**			
GROUP (REFERENCE)	**NO. PATIENTS**	**DRUG**	**RESPONSE (%)**	**DRUG**	**RESPONSE (%)**	**P VALUE**	
MSKCC (Kemeny et al., 1987)[75]	162	FUDR	50	FUDR	20	.001	
NCI (Chang et al., 1987)[78]	143	FUDR	42	FUDR	10	.0001	
NCOG (Hohn et al., 1989)[64]	64	FUDR	62	FUDR	17	.003	
City of Hope (Wagman et al., 1990)[79]	41	FUDR	55	FU	20	—	
Mayo Clinic (Martin et al., 1990)[80]	69	FUDR	48	FU	12	.02	
French (Rougier et al., 1992[81])[a]	163	FUDR	44	FU	—	—	
HAPT (Allen-Mersch et al., 1994)[82]	100	FUDR	—	FU or BSC			
German (Lorenz & Muller, 2000)[83]	168	FUDR	43	FU/leucovorin	22	.009	
EORTC (Kerr et al., 2003)[84]	290	FU/leucovorin	22[b]	FU/leucovorin	19	—	
CALGB (Kemeny et al., 2006)[85]	135	FUDR/dexamethasone	47	FU/leucovorin	24	.012	

[a]Patients received SYS only when they became symptomatic (not all received SYS in HAPT).

[b]Responses calculated at single time point (12 weeks).

BSC, Best supportive care; *CALGB*, Cancer and Leukemia Group B; *EORTC*, European Organization for the Research and Treatment of Cancer; *FUDR*, fluorodeoxyuridine; *FU*, follow-up; *HAPT*, Hepatic Artery Pump Trial; *MSKCC*, Memorial Sloan-Kettering Cancer Center; *NCI*, National Cancer Institute; *NCOG*, Northern California Oncology Group.

two factors that have been shown to be important prognostic indicators of survival (Table 97.7).[64,75–85] This prospective randomized trial compared HAI with SYS by using the same chemotherapeutic agent (FUDR), drug schedule (a 14-day continuous infusion), and method of administration (internal pump) in both groups.

Of the 99 evaluable patients, 2 complete responses and 23 partial responses (53%) were observed in the group receiving HAI, and 10 partial responses (21%) were reported in the SYS group (P = .001). Of the patients randomly assigned to SYS, 31 (60%) crossed over to HAI after tumor progression. Of these patients, 25% went on to have a partial response after the crossover, and 60% had a decrease in carcinoembryonic antigen (CEA) levels.

Toxicity differed between the two groups. An increase in hepatic enzymes and serum bilirubin levels occurred in the HAI group. In the SYS group, diarrhea occurred in 70% of patients, and 9% required admission for intravenous hydration. Mucositis occurred in 10% of patients receiving SYS.

The median survival for the HAI and SYS groups was 17 and 12 months, respectively (P = .424). The interpretation of survival in this study is difficult because 60% of the patients in the systemic group crossed over. The patients who did not cross over usually had clots of the hepatic arterial system and had a median survival of only 8 months compared with 18 months for the patients who crossed over to hepatic infusion (P = .04). An analysis of baseline characteristics in the crossover and non-crossover groups revealed no significant differences.

Two subsequent European randomized trials using HAI in this setting have been published. The first was conducted by the Medical Research Council (MRC) and European Organization for the Research and Treatment of Cancer (EORTC) groups, which compared HAI 5-FU/LV with intravenous 5-FU/LV. Crossover from the intravenous line to the HAI arm was not allowed. Of 290 patients randomly assigned, only 66% on the HAI arm received treatment. Response rates were 22% for HAI and 19% for intravenous 5-FU/LV. This trial used subcutaneous ports rather than implantable pumps and had significant catheter-related problems (36% of HAI patients).[84] The median

survival was 14.7 months and 14.8 months in the HAI and SYS groups, respectively (P = .79).

The second European trial was conducted by a German cooperative group that randomly assigned 168 patients with unresectable colorectal liver metastases to HAI of FUDR, HAI of 5-FU/LV, or intravenous 5-FU/LV.[83] Response rates were higher in the two HAI arms, with no significant differences in time to progression, the primary end point, or OS between the arms. Only 70% of patients on the HAI arms actually received the assigned treatment. The study also used ports instead of pumps.

The Cancer and Leukemia Group B (CALGB) completed trial 9481,[85] which compared systemic 5-FU/LV via the Mayo Clinic regimen, considered standard of care at the time of trial design, with HAI of FUDR, LV, and dexamethasone, a regimen that had produced high response rates (78%) and lower toxicity (3% biliary sclerosis) in an earlier phase II study.[86] Another earlier trial randomly assigned patients to HAI of FUDR with or without dexamethasone and demonstrated less biliary toxicity and a trend toward median overall survival (23 months vs. 15 months, respectively, P = .06) in the dexamethasone-containing arm.[69] In CALGB 9481, no crossover was permitted, and a total of 134 patients were randomly assigned. Most patients (70%) had greater than 30% liver involvement, and 78% had synchronous metastases. Of the patients, 97% were chemotherapy naïve. Response rates were higher in the HAI-only group (47% vs. 24%; P = .012), although time to progression was not significantly different (5.3 months vs. 6.8 months; P = .8). Time to hepatic progression was better in the HAI arm (9.8 months vs. 7.3 months; P = .017) and time to extrahepatic progression was better in the SYS arm (7.7 months vs. 14.8 months; P = .029). Median OS was significantly better in the HAI arm (24.4 months vs. 20 months; P = .0034).[85] Resource use, quality of life, and molecular markers of prognosis, such as thymidylate synthase (TS) and *p21* gene expression, were examined prospectively in this study and final analysis of these factors were presented. At 3- and 6-month follow-up, physical functioning was improved in the HAI group. TS levels correlated with survival in HAI patients (24 months if TS >4,

TABLE 97.8 Summary of 1- and 2-Year Survival in Randomized Trials Comparing Hepatic Arterial Infusion (HAI) and Systemic Chemotherapy (SYS)

GROUP (REFERENCE)	SURVIVAL (% ALIVE)				SURVIVAL (% ALIVE)			
	1 YEAR		2 YEARS		1 YEAR		2 YEARS	
	HAI	SYS	HAI	SYS	CROSSOVER	NO CROSSOVER	CROSSOVER	NO CROSSOVER
MSKCC (Kemeny et al., 1987)[75]	60	50	25	20	60	28	25	14
NCOG (Hohn et al., 1989)[64]	60	42	30	20	78	42	40	17
NCI[a] (Chang et al., 1987)[78]	85	60	44	13	—	—	—	—
France (Rougier et al., 1992)[81]	61	44	22	10	—	—	—	—
CALGB (Kemeny et al., 2006)[85]	—	—	51	35	—	—	—	—
Mean	66	49	34	20	69	35	37	15

[a]Excludes patients with metastasis to hepatic lymph nodes

CALBG, Cancer and Leukemia Group B; *MSKCC*, Memorial Sloan-Kettering Cancer Center; *NCI*, National Cancer Institute; *NCOG*, Northern California Oncology Group.

14 months if TS ≤4), but these differences were not significant (P = .17).

A total of 10 randomized phase III trials have been done, most of which demonstrated a higher response rate with HAI versus SYS in patients with hepatic metastases from colorectal cancer (see Table 97.7). Whether this increase in response rate translates into increased survival is controversial. Several factors complicate this issue. Importantly, most of the trials contained relatively few patients and were therefore underpowered to detect significant survival differences. Also, because of early successes with intrahepatic infusion, some of these studies allowed patients in the SYS arm to cross over to the HAI arm after tumor progression on SYS. This crossover may have negated any difference in survival between the two groups. The studies showed a survival advantage for those who received subsequent HAI, with a mean 1-year survival of 69% for the patients who had crossed over from SYS to HAI versus 35% for the patients who did not cross over (Table 97.8). Additionally, some trials included patients with extrahepatic disease, thereby complicating survival analyses in the absence of systemic treatment. Other factors to consider are that some patients randomly assigned to HAI did not receive it but were included in the survival analysis, and an absence of modern toxicity-based dose-titration schema may have resulted in fewer cycles of treatment.

The European studies are difficult to interpret because, in the first two studies, the SYS group received SYS only when they became symptomatic. The two new European studies used ports instead of pumps, which resulted in more technical complications and may have underestimated the efficacy of pump therapy.

Two meta-analyses of the original seven trials were conducted and included more than 600 patients. The Meta-Analysis Group in Cancer (MAGIC)[87] confirmed the increased response rates seen with HAI over SYS (41% vs. 14%). However, survival differences were only deemed statistically significant in the trials that included a control group treated only when symptoms arose. With the statistical methodology used, the authors were unable to include the data from Hohn et al.[64] A second meta-analysis published the same year, however, did incorporate the results from that study and found an absolute survival difference of 12.5% at 1 year (P = .002) and 7.5% at 2 years (P = .026) in favor of HAI.[88] The authors omitted the trial by Allen-Mersch et al.,[82] given the fact that most patients in the SYS

arm of that study received best supportive care only. Furthermore, they analyzed their results to show that, when omitting the data from Rougier et al.,[81] in which, like the study from Allen-Mersch et al.,[82] only half of the patients in the SYS arm received chemotherapy, survival was only statistically significantly higher at the 1-year time point. Nonetheless, factoring only those six studies without crossover, the survival differences at 1 and 2 years were accentuated, and both significantly favored HAI.

As mentioned earlier, CALGB 9481 permitted no crossover, and with the incorporation of dexamethasone, it demonstrated survival with HAI that compares well with published results with modern SYS regimens. However, a recent and well-orchestrated third meta-analysis that accounted for the design flaws discussed earlier examined all 10 randomized trials to date and failed to demonstrate a survival benefit with HAI.[89] This report and the published commentary that followed demonstrated that, although there may be no clear survival benefit in using HAI alone instead of SYS, combining HAI and SYS led to high response rates with acceptable toxicity profiles. The use of combination HAI and SYS to improve overall outcomes is discussed next and underscores the need to examine response and OS data in the context of modern treatment paradigms.

COMBINED HEPATIC ARTERIAL INFUSION AND SYSTEMIC CHEMOTHERAPY

Extrahepatic disease develops in 40% to 70% of patients who undergo HAI. Such metastases can occur even when the patient's hepatic tumors are responding. In many patients, extrahepatic disease is the cause of death. Safi et al.[90] studied whether concomitant SYS reduces the development of extrahepatic metastases in patients who receive HAI. Ninety-five patients were randomly assigned to intraarterial FUDR (0.2 mg/kg/day for 14/28 days) or a combination of intraarterial FUDR (0.21 mg/kg/day) and intravenous FUDR (0.09 mg/kg/day) given concurrently for 14 of 28 days (intraarterial/intravenous). The response rates were 60% for both arms of the study. However, the incidence of extrahepatic disease was significantly less in patients who received the intraarterial/intravenous treatment (56%) compared with intraarterial treatment (79%; P < .01). No significant difference in survival was found between the two groups (P = .08). The results of this trial, as well as the development of improved SYS

TABLE 97.9 Results of Hepatic Arterial Infusion Combined With Systemic Chemotherapy in the Second-Line Setting

DRUG (REFERENCE)	NO. PATIENTS	RESPONSE (%)	MEDIAN SURVIVAL FROM PUMP PLACEMENT (mo)
FUDR + dexamethasone + sideport mitomycin C (Kemeny et al., 2005b)[91]	37	70	20
FUDR + dexamethasone + SYS CPT-11 (Kemeny et al., 2001)[92]	56	74	20
FUDR + dexamethasone + SYS oxaliplatin + CPT-11 (Kemeny et al., 2005)[93]	21	90	28
FUDR + dexamethasone + SYS oxaliplatin + FU/leucovorin (Kemeny et al., 2005)[93]	15	87	22

CPT-11, Irinotecan; *FU,* follow-up; *FUDR,* fluorodeoxyglucose; *SYS,* systemic chemotherapy.

regimens, have underscored the need for further study of combined systemic/intraarterial regimens. Results of some of these studies are presented in Table 97.9,[91-93] and SYS irinotecan and oxaliplatin are discussed in detail later.

Irinotecan is a topoisomerase I inhibitor with proven efficacy in first-line and second-line treatment of metastatic colorectal cancer. The activity of irinotecan is not inhibited by high TS activity[94]; combining systemic irinotecan with HAI may result in improved control of extrahepatic disease. In a phase I study at MSKCC, 46 patients with unresectable liver metastases, 8 of whom underwent cryosurgery, received HAI of FUDR/dexamethasone and systemic irinotecan in escalating doses; all 38 patients who did not undergo cryosurgery were previously treated, and 16 had prior therapy with irinotecan. The regimen was well tolerated, with dose-limiting toxicities of diarrhea and myelosuppression. The response rate was 74%, median time to progression was 8.1 months, and 13 of 16 patients who had previously received irinotecan had partial responses.[92]

Another nonrandomized study used HAI of FUDR with systemic irinotecan as "adjuvant" therapy after cytoreduction (therefore not "true adjuvant") of unresectable hepatic colorectal cancer metastases. The cytoreduction was defined as use of ablative techniques (see Chapter 96), partial resection, or some combination to treat all identifiable sites of disease. Seventy-one patients received "adjuvant" therapy and were compared with a historic control group that received cytoreduction alone. Time to progression was 19 months versus 10 months, and median survival was 30.6 months versus 20 months for HAI versus control groups, respectively.[95] A Japanese group examined HAI of 5-FU and SYS irinotecan in previously treated patients and demonstrated response rates of 76.5%, with median OS of 20 months.[96]

Oxaliplatin is a cytotoxic agent with a mechanism of action similar to that of other platinum derivatives, but it has a different spectrum of activity and toxicity. When combined with 5-FU/LV, clinical response rates have been greater than 50%, with median survival of 16.2 months in untreated patients with metastatic colorectal cancer.[15,97] Preliminary studies that used systemic oxaliplatin-based regimens combined with HAI of FUDR demonstrated the feasibility and safety of this approach and revealed promising early results.[98]

Conversion of Unresectable to Resectable Disease

In an MSKCC phase I study, 36 patients with unresectable hepatic metastases, 89% of whom were previously treated, received HAI of FUDR/dexamethasone and SYS oxaliplatin plus either SYS irinotecan or SYS 5-FU/LV. Both regimens were well tolerated, and response rates for the two groups were 90% and 87% (see Table 97.9).[93] This high response rate for second-line therapy with HAI plus SYS, as well as conversion to resectability, was also demonstrated in a recent MSKCC pooled analysis of phase I data in 49 patients with unresectable liver metastases from colorectal cancer.[99] Patients received HAI of FUDR/dexamethasone, SYS irinotecan, and SYS oxaliplatin, and 98% had bilobar disease, whereas 85% had tumors bordering vasculature. A partial or complete response was reported in 92% (84% partial, 8% complete), and 47% of patients were able to undergo resection, 3 with pathologic complete responses. With a median follow-up of 26 months from time of pump placement, OS was 51 months for previously untreated patients; all 23 patients responded to treatment, and 57% underwent resection. OS was 35 months for previously treated patients; 85% responded to treatment, and 38% underwent resection. This revealed that even in heavily pretreated patients with significant hepatic metastasis, HAI of FUDR can still increase response and resection rates when combined with modern SYS.

Similarly, in a phase II trial of HAI and SYS chemotherapy for patients with unresectable hepatic metastases from colorectal cancer, 49 patients underwent evaluation of the conversion rate from unresectable liver metastases to complete resection as the primary outcome,[100] with 65% of patients having received previous chemotherapy. The median number of metastases was 14. With a regimen of HAI of FUDR and SYS oxaliplatin, irinotecan, and bevacizumab, or SYS irinotecan, 5-FU/LV, and bevacizumab if patients had previously received more than two cycles of oxaliplatin, overall response rates were 76% with 4 complete responders. Conversion to resection was achieved by 23 patients (47%) in a median of 6 months from treatment initiation. Median OS and PFS were 38 and 18 months, respectively, with conversion being the only factor associated with prolonged OS and PFS on multivariate analysis. Resection, as compared with no resection, was associated with 3-year OS of 80% versus 26%, respectively, with 10 patients demonstrating no evidence of disease at the time of publication at a median of 39 months.

Neoadjuvant treatment is a strategy increasingly used in solid-tumor oncology, given the multifaceted rationale that it may enable downsizing and subsequent resectability of tumor burden. Numerous reports have been made that HAI of oxaliplatin, for instance, has shown benefit in response and resectability rates when combined with SYS 5-FU.[101-103] Future randomized trials are needed to confirm the impact that HAI specifically has in these outcomes.

Refractory Disease Setting

For patients who fail first-line chemotherapy, modern systemic chemotherapy agents such as irinotecan alone, irinotecan and cetuximab, and FOLFOX produce response rates ranging from 9% to 22% and a median survival of 14 months or less. In patients who fail first-line and second-line chemotherapy, therapeutic options are very limited. Regorafenib and TAS102 in the refractory setting demonstrate response rates of 1% and 1.6%, respectively, and a median survival of 6.4 and 7.1 months, respectively.[104,105]

In a 2016 study of a heavily pretreated population of patients who had progressed after 5-FU/LV, oxaliplatin, and irinotecan therapies, the response rate was 33%, the median survival was 20 months, and the PFS was 6 months after using HAI plus SYS. Of 57 patients, 19 (33%) had a partial response and 31 (54%) had stable disease.[106]

ADJUVANT HEPATIC ARTERIAL CHEMOTHERAPY AFTER LIVER RESECTION OF COLORECTAL METASTASES

The rationale for the use of adjuvant chemotherapy after resection of liver metastases from colorectal cancer is based on the observation that, although some patients have long-term disease-free survival (DFS) after resection, disease recurrence is common (see Chapter 98). Recurrence may be solely in the liver, it may be extrahepatic and intrahepatic, or it may be solely extrahepatic. An effective adjuvant treatment may have a substantial impact on recurrence and survival. The use of SYS without HAI has been formally tested in this setting. A randomized study by Portier et al.[107] met its primary end point and showed a 5-year DFS of 33.5% for the chemotherapy group and 26.7% for the control group (P = .028). However, the study failed to show a survival benefit with 6 months of adjuvant 5-FU/folinic acid. Because this trial and another phase III study (EORTC) both closed early as a result of slow accrual, their results were pooled and reported together,[108] demonstrating both a lack of DFS and OS statistical significance for 5-FU adjuvant therapy in this setting. When adjusting for poor characteristics in a multivariate analysis, however, an increase in DFS was reported for the group treated with chemotherapy.

In EORTC 40983, using 5-FU plus LV and oxaliplatin (FOLFOX) compared with surgery alone showed no new increase in OS.[109]

Because combining HAI and SYS may be useful in decreasing recurrence, four relatively large randomized trials were conducted in this group of patients (Table 97.10). In the MSKCC study,[110] 156 patients with resected hepatic metastases were randomly assigned to 6 months of systemic 5-FU/LV or systemic 5-FU/LV plus HAI with FUDR. Primary end points were 2-year OS and PFS. A total of 40% of patients received prior adjuvant chemotherapy after resection of their primary colorectal cancer, and 15% had received prior chemotherapy as treatment for metastatic disease. Randomization was performed intraoperatively after complete resection of metastases, and patients were stratified based on number of metastases and prior treatment history. Of enrolled patients, 92% received treatment as assigned. Survival of 2 years was 86% in the combined-therapy group versus 72% for those who received SYS alone (P = .03), with median survivals of 72.2 months and 59.3 months, respectively. In an updated analysis, with all patients followed for a minimum of 6 years (median follow-up, 10.3 years), overall PFS was significantly greater in the combined-therapy group than in the monotherapy group (31.3 months vs. 17.2 months; P = .02). Median survival free of hepatic progression had not yet been reached in the combined-therapy group but was 32.5 months in the monotherapy group (P < .01). Ten-year survival was 41% in the HAI plus SYS group versus 27% in the SYS-alone group, with median survivals of 68.4 months and 58.8 months, respectively (Figs. 97.9 and 97.10).[111] If patients with poor clinical risk scores are considered,[112] their survival is still improved with HAI compared with SYS alone (Fig. 97.11).

Toxicity was increased in the combined group, and 39% of patients required hospitalization for diarrhea, neutropenia, mucositis, or small bowel obstruction, compared with 22% in the monotherapy group (P = .02). Elevated bilirubin was seen in 18% of patients in the combined group. In most patients, the bilirubin returned to normal, but 6% of patients required biliary stents. In the control group, 2% had an elevation in bilirubin, and 2% required biliary stents. No significant difference was found among the groups in therapy-related deaths (one in combined group, two in monotherapy group).

	TABLE 97.10 Randomized Trials of Adjuvant Hepatic Arterial Infusion After Resection of Liver Metastases							
	MSKCC, 1999		**INTERGROUP, 2002**		**GERMAN, 1998[a]**		**GREEK, 2001**	
ARMS	HAI + SYS	SYS	HAI + SYS	CONTROL	HAI (PORT)	CONTROL	HAI + SYS	SYS
n	74	82	53	56	113	113	62	60
Median time to progression (mo)	37.4[b]	17.2	37[c]	18[c]	20[a]	12.6[a]	60%[le]	20%[le]
Median time to hepatic progression (mo)	Not reached[b]	42.7	Not reached	20.2	44.8[a]	23.3[a]	85%[f]	50%[f]
Median overall survival (mo)	72.2	59.3	63.7	49.7	44.8	39.7		
2-year overall survival	86%[b]	72%	62%	53%	62%[c]	65%[c]	92%	75%
5-year overall survival	57%[d]	48%[d]	55%[d]	37.5%[d]	—	—	73%	60%

[a]Results are for treated patients.
[b]Statistically significant difference (P < .05) compared with control group.
[c]Not reported, but calculated based on Kaplan–Meier curves published in original citations.
[d]Updated results.
[le]5-Year disease-free survival.
[f]Hepatic disease-free survival.
HAI, Hepatic artery infusion; MSKCC, Memorial Sloan-Kettering Cancer Center; SYS, systemic chemotherapy.

From Cohen AD, Kemeny NE. An update on hepatic arterial infusional chemotherapy for colorectal cancer. *Oncologist.* 8:553–566, 2003.

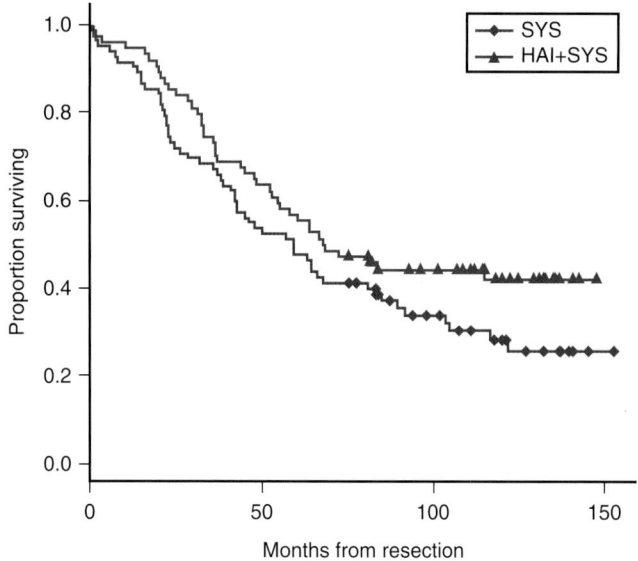

FIGURE 97.9 Updated overall survival from the Memorial Sloan-Kettering Cancer Center trial comparing adjuvant systemic therapy (SYS) with hepatic arterial infusion (HAI) plus SYS.

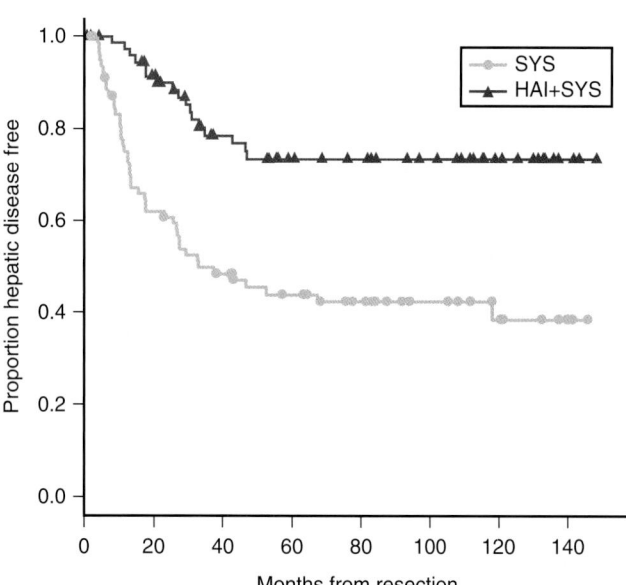

FIGURE 97.10 Updated hepatic disease-free survival from the Memorial Sloan-Kettering Cancer Center trial comparing adjuvant systemic therapy (SYS) with hepatic arterial infusion (HAI) plus SYS.

The Intergroup study[113] randomly assigned 109 patients to resection alone or resection, followed by four cycles of HAI with FUDR and infusional systemic 5-FU, followed by eight more cycles of systemic 5-FU. Patients with more than three liver metastases or extrahepatic disease at laparotomy were excluded, with 80 of 109 patients actually included in the study, which was designed to examine the effect of adjuvant therapy on DFS. When patients were analyzed as treated ($n = 75$), the 4-year DFS (46% vs. 25%; $P = .04$) and 4-year hepatic DFS (67% vs. 43%; $P = .03$) favored HAI versus the control groups. Based on an intention-to-treat analysis, no difference was reported in

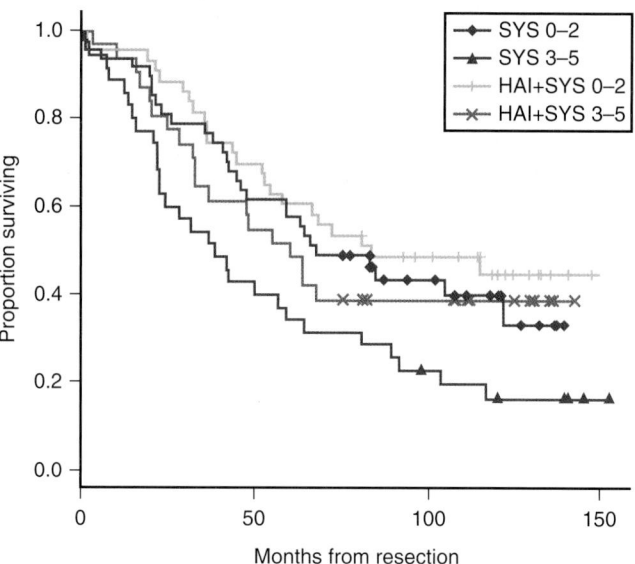

FIGURE 97.11 Survival Stratified by Clinical Risk Score. A score ranging from 0 to 5 was calculated by adding 1 point for the following clinical variables: tumor size >5 cm, tumor number >1, serum carcinoembryonic antigen >200 ng/mL, node-positive primary tumor, and disease-free interval >12 months. *HAI,* Hepatic arterial infusion; *SYS,* systemic therapy. (From Fong Y, Fortner J, Sun RL, et al. Clinical score for predicting recurrence after hepatic resection for metastatic colorectal cancer: analysis of 1001 consecutive cases. *Ann Surg.* 1999;230:309–318.)

median or 4-year overall survival between the groups. Currently, the 5-year survival is 55% versus 37.5% favoring adjuvant therapy (M. Kemeny, Personal communication, 2005). However, this study was not designed to examine OS.

In the German cooperative multicenter study,[114] 226 patients were randomly assigned to resection alone or resection plus 6 months of HAI with 5-FU/LV given as 5-day continuous infusion every 28 days. The study was terminated early because an interim analysis suggested a very low chance of showing a survival benefit with adjuvant therapy. The impact of HAI in this study is difficult to assess because only 74% of patients assigned to HAI received this treatment and only 30% completed it. No difference in time to progression, time to hepatic progression, and median OS were noted in an intention-to-treat analysis. When patients were analyzed "as treated," time to hepatic progression (45 months vs. 23 months) and time to progression or death (20 months vs. 12.6 months) were improved in the HAI arm. Grade 3 or 4 toxicity, including stomatitis, nausea, and vomiting, was noted in 63% of patients who received adjuvant therapy. These findings reflect significant systemic absorption of 5-FU when given via HAI.

A study conducted in Greece on 122 patients used mitomycin C, 5-FU, and interleukin-2 by both HAI and the IV route versus the IV route alone. The 2-year survival was 92% versus 75%, and 5-year survival was 73% versus 60% for the HAI plus SYS group versus the SYS-alone group, respectively. DFS was significantly longer for the HAI plus SYS group, 60% at 5 years versus 20% for the intravenous group ($P = .0012$), and hepatic DFS was 85% versus 50% ($P = .0001$).[115]

The two American studies showed a reduction in hepatic and extrahepatic recurrence for combined HAI plus SYS after surgical resection. Of the two European studies, one showed a significant increase in survival and DFS, whereas the other did not.

In the MSKCC study, 2-year survival after liver resection was significantly improved with combined therapy: 86% compared with 72% with SYS alone. Historic 2-year survivals[78,116–118] for patients treated with resection alone range from 55% to 70%.

Nonrandomized studies of modern chemotherapy regimens (see Chapter 98) combined with HAI of FUDR in the post–liver metastasis resection (adjuvant) setting have been conducted and suggest improved outcomes. Phase I and II trials of adjuvant SYS irinotecan combined with FUDR/dexamethasone in 96 patients showed a 2-year survival of 89% at a median follow-up of 26 months. The dose-limiting toxicities were diarrhea and neutropenia, and all 27 patients treated at the maximum-tolerated dose were alive at publication.[119] A phase I trial of adjuvant HAI of FUDR/dexamethasone with escalating doses of SYS oxaliplatin/5-FU/LV in 35 patients revealed 4-year survival and PFS of 88% and 50%, respectively, at a median follow-up of 43 months. Dose-limiting toxicities of diarrhea and elevated bilirubin each occurred in 8.5% of patients.[120]

A multivariate analysis performed as a part of a recent review of more than 1000 patients showed that post liver metastasis resection HAI was one of the significant factors to improve survival. Median OS was 50 months in those who did not receive HAI and 68 months in those who did ($P = .0001$).[121] Another MSKCC retrospective review to analyze 10-year survival described 612 patients who underwent liver resection from 1985 to 1994 and could be evaluated for 10-year survival. The 10-year OS was 38% for patients who received HAI of FUDR and 15% for those who did not ($P < .0001$).[122] Another MSKCC review retrospectively compared outcomes from 125 patients with metastatic colorectal cancer who received postoperative SYS (FOLFOX or 5-FU plus LV or irinotecan [FOLFIRI]) with 125 similar patients who received only SYS. The 5-year hepatic PFS was 75% in the HAI group and 52% in the SYS group ($P = .0005$), with a median follow-up of 43 months. OS at 5 years was 72% and 52%, respectively.[123] These data favor combination HAI and SYS therapy but underscore the need for randomized studies of modern HAI plus SYS compared with modern SYS alone.

The inclusion of additional agents to HAI regimens has been attempted. In an attempt to evaluate the effect of systemic bevacizumab with HAI, patients were randomly assigned to HAI plus SYS therapy with or without bevacizumab in a randomized phase II trial in patients who had undergone liver metastasis resection.[124] Standardized therapy between the two arms included HAI with FUDR, 5-FU/LV, and oxaliplatin, or irinotecan if oxaliplatin was previously administered. With a median follow-up of 30 months, 4-year survival was 85% and 81%, 4-year recurrence-free survival (RFS) was 46% and 37%, and 1-year RFS was 83% and 71%, for no-bevacizumab versus bevacizumab arms, respectively. Although outcomes were approximately similar to prior HAI with SYS regimens, the inclusion of bevacizumab did not appear to improve survival. In fact, hyperbilirubinemia greater than 3 mg/dL occurred in five patients in the bevacizumab arm, with four requiring placement of biliary stents. The addition of bevacizumab did not seem to increase RFS or survival but instead resulted in increased biliary toxicity.

Interestingly, in an analysis of 203 patients from three prospective studies, systemic bevacizumab was added to HAI FUDR-based chemotherapy to improve outcomes, and biliary toxicity was specifically reviewed.[38] Studies included the adjuvant study discussed earlier, a study comprising patients with unresectable liver metastases who received HAI plus SYS plus bevacizumab,[120] and a study with patients having unresectable intrahepatic cholangiocarcinoma or hepatocellular carcinoma (HCC).[125] In the three respective studies, the incidence of hyperbilirubinemia and need for biliary stent placement were increased by the addition of bevacizumab, but bevacizumab was not associated with improved PFS or OS. Combining bevacizumab elsewhere with HAI has also resulted in high biliary toxicity.[100] Its inclusion cannot be currently recommended in HAI.

In a study validating *KRAS* mutation as a predictor of RFS or OS in patients with resected colorectal liver metastases, 169 patients received adjuvant HAI plus SYS, of whom 118 were *KRAS* wild-type (WT), and 51 had *KRAS*-mutated (MUT) tumors.[126] The 3-year RFS for patients with *KRAS* WT tumors was 46%, compared with 30% for patients with *KRAS* MUT tumors ($P = .005$). The 3-year OS was 95% versus 81%, respectively. Interestingly, *KRAS* was a significant predictor of RFS (hazard ratio [HR], 1.9) on multivariate analysis.

Another recent publication from MSKCC looked at 2368 consecutive patients who underwent liver resection of colorectal metastases; 785 had HAI and 1583 did not. The HAI group of patients had a significantly higher disease burden (i.e., significantly increased clinical risk score) but still had a longer median survival of 67 versus 44 months for those treated with adjuvant systemic chemotherapy alone ($P < .01$).[127] The analysis, which spanned over 21 years from 1992 through 2012, also assessed whether HAI therapy was administered with preoperative modern systemic chemotherapy as a subgroup analysis. The results showed prolonged 5-year OS for patients receiving HAI therapy, compared with those treated without HAI (52.9% vs. 37.9%, $P < .001$), and also greater 10-year OS (38.0% vs. 23.8%, $P < .001$) (Fig. 97.12).

Subgroup analysis demonstrated that independent of receiving modern systemic chemotherapy or not, and regardless of whether HAI was received in the preoperative or adjuvant setting, there remained a significantly greater OS in the HAI arm. For those who received preoperative modern systemic chemotherapy, median OS rates in the HAI arm and the no HAI arm were 77 and 45 months, respectively. For those who did not receive preoperative modern systemic chemotherapy, median OS rates in the HAI arm and the no HAI arm were 55 and 43 months, respectively.

In a study by Buisman et al.[128] published in 2019, the impact of HAIP chemotherapy on hepatic recurrences and survival in patients with resected colorectal liver metastases was evaluated. The study included 2128 patients, of whom 601 patients (28.2%) received adjuvant HAIP and systemic chemotherapy (HAIP + SYS). The overall recurrence rate was similar with HAIP + SYS or SYS (63.5% vs. 64.2%, $P = .74$). The 5-year cumulative incidence of initial intrahepatic recurrences was lower with HAIP + SYS (22.9% vs. 38.4%, $P < .001$). HAIP was an independent prognostic factor for DFS (adjusted HR [aHR], 0.69; 95% CI, 0.60–0.79; $P < .001$), and OS (aHR, 0.67; 95% CI, 0.57–0.78, $P < .001$).

Currently, there are two ongoing randomized clinical trials being conducted to further assess the role of adjuvant HAI after resection of colorectal cancer with liver metastases (CRCLMs). The first is a phase II trial, the so-called PUMP trial, which is being performed in the Netherlands that is planned to evaluate the efficacy of adjuvant HAI FUDR therapy in "low-risk" patients. Low risk for recurrence is defined as no more than two of five of the following factors: disease-free interval less than 12 months, node-positive CRC, more than 1 CRCLM, largest

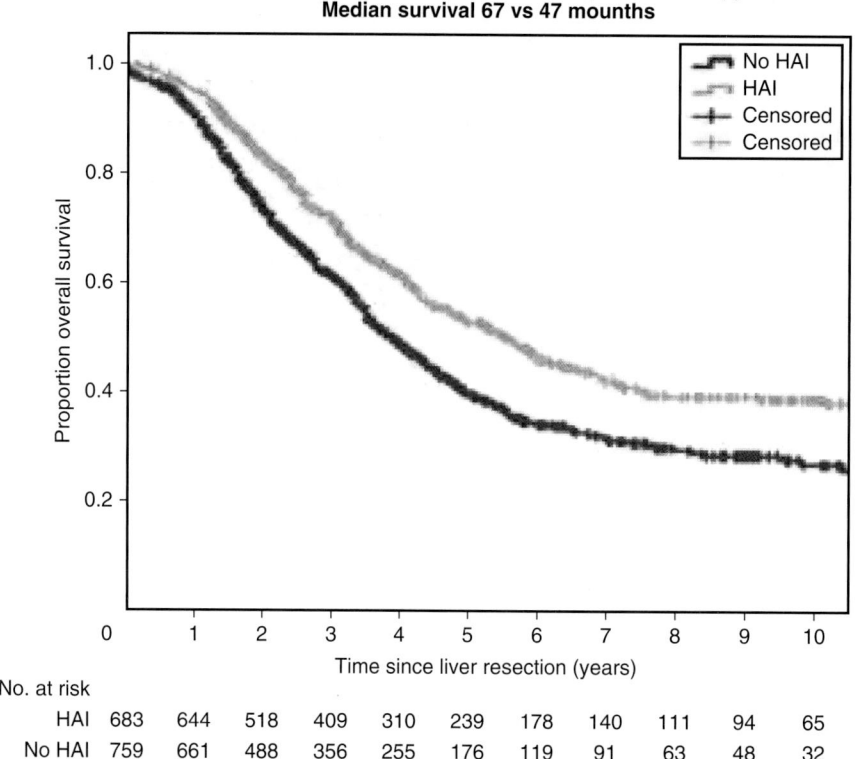

FIGURE 97.12   Survival With HAI and Systemic Chemotherapy Versus Modern Systemic Chemotherapy. (From Groot Koerkamp B, Sadot E, Kemeny NE, et al. Perioperative hepatic arterial infusion pump chemotherapy is associated with longer survival after resection of colorectal liver metastases: a propensity score analysis. *J Clin Oncol.* 2017;35[17]:1938–1944.)

liver metastasis more than 5 cm in diameter, serum CEA above 200 µg/L.[129] Patients are randomized to either resection without any adjuvant therapy or HAI pump placement at time of resection with six cycles of HAI FUDR. The primary endpoint of the study is PFS. Secondary endpoints are OS, hepatic PFS, safety, quality of life, and cost effectiveness. The aim of the study is to corroborate prior results at MSKCC for adjuvant HAI FUDR.[115]

A second study currently underway is a phase II/III trial, PACHA-01, which is comparing adjuvant systemic FOLFOX and HAI oxaliplatin + systemic 5-FU in patients deemed "high risk" for recurrence, defined as having four or more resected CRCLMs in patients who have undergone R0 or R1 resection and/or thermal ablation.[130] The primary objectives are to assess the 18-month hepatic recurrence-free survival in patients treated with HAI oxaliplatin + systemic 5-FU after curative intent surgery, and demonstrate superiority in recurrence-free survival of HAI oxaliplatin compared with systemic oxaliplatin + 5-FU (FOLFOX).

HEPATIC ARTERIAL INFUSION FOR NONCOLORECTAL LIVER METASTASES AND PRIMARY LIVER CANCER

Although liver metastases from noncolorectal cancers are less commonly treated with regional therapy, HAI chemotherapy has been used in cases of breast cancer, HCC, melanoma,[131] bronchogenic carcinoma, and pancreatic cancer. Studies in breast cancer have used numerous HAI agents, including

FUDR, mitomycin/FU/doxorubicin, vinblastine/cisplatin, and cyclophosphamide/etoposide (see Chapter 92) One trial of 15 patients undergoing systemic chemotherapy for refractory metastatic breast cancer tested HAI of FUDR and mitomycin and demonstrated a partial response rate of 53% and OS of 18 months after HAI was begun.[132] FUDR alone and in combination with various cytotoxic agents also has been evaluated in HCC (see Chapter 89), including treatment with mitomycin/interferon/FUDR[133] and LV/doxorubicin/cisplatin/FUDR[134] in 27 patients. In the latter, response rates were 41% to 54%, and median OS was 15 months.

More recent experience with HAI for HCC and intrahepatic cholangiocarcinoma (ICC) (see Chapter 50) at MSKCC was published, showing the correlative and predictive utility of dynamic contrast-enhanced magnetic resonance imaging (DCE-MRI) in 34 patients with unresectable disease treated with HAI of FUDR/dexamethasone. Partial responses were seen in 47%, with median OS of 30 months.[135] One patient in this study responded sufficiently to undergo resection and was found to have had a complete pathologic response. The median duration of response was 1 year, and median time to progression was 7 months. Median follow-up at time of publication was 35 months, and 1- and 2-year survival was 88% and 67%, respectively. Therapy was well tolerated, and DCE-MRI data showed that pretreatment and posttreatment tumor perfusion and permeability parameters correlated with median survival, which may therefore serve as biomarkers of treatment outcome.

The inclusion of HAI with bevacizumab in the treatment of primary liver cancer was previously discussed; however,

17 patients were treated with HAI FUDR-based therapy, followed by systemic bevacizumab for 14 days in a separate report.[136] The addition of systemic bevacizumab induced a reduction in tumor perfusion kinetics that is measurable by DCE-MRI, with a median time to progression of 8.8 months. The changes noted by DCE-MRI appeared to reflect a normalization of the deranged tumor vasculature, resulting in improvement in hypoxia and possibly more effective delivery of cytotoxic drug, ultimately leading to longer time to progression.

In an updated analysis combining findings from the previously discussed studies, Konstantinidis et al.[137] provided long-term outcomes for a total of 44 patients (26 FUDR and 18 FUDR/bevacizumab). At a median follow-up of 29.3 months, 41 patients had died of disease. Partial response was observed by the Response Evaluation Criteria in Solid Tumors (RECIST) study in 48%, and 50% had stable disease. Three patients underwent resection after response, and 82% received additional HAI after removal from the trials. Median survival was similar between the two combined trials (29.3 months in FUDR trial vs. 28.5 months in FUDR/bevacizumab trial). Ten patients survived more than 3 years, of whom 5 survived more than 5 years. The authors concluded that HAI can result in prolonged survival in unresectable ICC.

More recently, a multicenter phase II trial by Cercek et al.[138] assessing HAI FUDR combined with systemic gemcitabine and oxaliplatin (GemOx) in unresectable IHC was published. A response rate of 58% and an excellent disease control rate of 84% in the primary tumor was demonstrated at 6 months. More recently, the combination of intraarterial 5-FU and oxaliplatin also showed some activity in a phase II trial in which 37 patients with locally advanced biliary tract malignancies (32 ICC; 1 EHC; 4 gallbladder cancer) were included. In this trial, the response rate, PFS, and OS were 16%, 6.5 months, and 13.5 months, respectively. Based on this trial, HAI plus systemic chemotherapy appears to be highly active and tolerable in patients with unresectable IHC and further evaluation is warranted.

CONCLUDING REMARKS

HAI offers several advantages. From a pharmacologic standpoint, HAI is more effective than SYS because higher drug levels are achieved at the sites of metastatic disease. Use of agents with high hepatic extraction virtually eliminates the systemic toxicity observed with standard SYS. The 50% to 70% response rate obtained in trials of intrahepatic FUDR therapy has not been matched by any SYS to date. The addition of dexamethasone to FUDR has increased both response rate and survival. Most randomized HAI studies do not clearly evaluate the issue of survival, mainly because a crossover was allowed in many studies. Although HAI may produce GI or hepatic toxicity, this is minimized with proper surgical technique during pump placement, with close monitoring of liver function tests, and with HAI of dexamethasone.

Because the liver is often the initial site of metastatic disease in patients with CRC, early intensive therapy with surgical resection, HAI, or both at a time when the tumor burden is small may prevent the progression of metastases to other sites. HAI is applicable to selected patients with hepatic metastases and may prove to be the best therapy available for them. Administration and delivery of HAI therapy can certainly be complex, which may well explain its relatively infrequent use in the global oncology community to date. It is important to stress the value and inherent need of a dedicated multidisciplinary infrastructure incorporating all aspects of HAI management such as surgical, medical, radiologic, and nursing to run a successful HAI program. In recent years, the potential of HAI therapy is being increasingly acknowledged and more centers in the United States and Europe are emerging as advocates in this specialized treatment, with several phase II and III trials underway currently.

Future directions in the field will involve refining further the patient selection process, including the identification of those patients likely to benefit from HAI through the assimilation of molecular markers as well as the inclusion of increasing data of molecularly driven systemic therapies into clinical trial design. Furthermore, a key component to progressing the field is the establishment of multi-institutional registries comparing combination HAI regimens with not only systemic chemotherapy alone but also with alternative liver-directed treatment approaches (e.g., yttrium-90 radioembolization and transarterial chemoembolization) increasingly used in CRCLMs, in an effort to improve survival, in a patient group with an inherently poor prognosis.

References are available at expertconsult.com.

CHAPTER 98

Systemic chemotherapy for colorectal liver metastasis: Impact on surgical management

Marc-Antoine Allard and René Adam

INTRODUCTION

Over the past decades, the management of colorectal liver metastases (CLM) has been transformed by several improvements in both medical and surgical fields (see Chapters 90, 97, 101, and 102). The development of modern and efficient chemotherapeutic regimens has increased tumor response rates as well as overall prognosis of metastatic patients. A better knowledge of tumor biology has allowed tailoring indications of targeted therapies, thus initiating the era of personalized medicine. From the surgical point of view, technical refinements have pushed the boundaries of resectability while maintaining acceptable surgical risk.

The interplay between surgery and chemotherapy has become the cornerstone of the modern management of CLM, and this "onco-surgical approach" is now recognized as a standard. Therefore understanding the consequences related to chemotherapy is essential to define the most appropriate onco-surgical strategy.

The aim of this chapter is to discuss the impact of systemic chemotherapy on the surgical management of patients with CLM. We discuss the role of chemotherapy in three different clinical situations:

- Initially resectable disease
- Initially unresectable disease with a possibility of resectability in case of good response to conversion chemotherapy
- Definitively unresectable disease

A BRIEF HISTORY OF SYSTEMIC CHEMOTHERAPY IN COLORECTAL LIVER METASTASES

The spontaneous median survival of a metastatic colorectal cancer (CRC) without treatment is 5 months.[1] The past two decades have seen the development of new systemic chemotherapies, reaching around 3 years of median survival with the most recent protocols.

In 1957, 5-fluorouracil (5-FU) was the first chemotherapy authorized in colorectal cancer, but when used alone, its effect was limited, offering a response rate of around 10%. Response rates were doubled after discovering that folinic acid (leucovorin) stabilized the interaction between 5-FU and thymidylate synthase, thereby increasing the effect of 5-FU.[2,3] The modalities of administration (bolus, continuous infusion) were later improved to decrease toxicity without impairing tumor control. De Gramont et al.[4] proposed the LV5-FU2 protocol (biweekly cycles consisting of an intravenous [IV] administration of leucovorin over 2 hours followed by a bolus of 5-FU and a slow IV administration of 5-FU over 2 days), which quickly gained wide acceptance.

The 2000s were marked by the introduction of two major anticancer drugs effective in colorectal cancer: irinotecan and oxaliplatin. Irinotecan (a topoisomerase I inhibitor, transformed after a first hepatic passage into an active metabolite SN38 by a carboxylesterase) demonstrated a benefit in terms of survival in patients resistant to 5-FU. Associated with LV5-FU2, Douillard et al.[5] showed a higher response rate (49% vs. 31%) and a median survival reaching 17 months. This protocol was later simplified to become FOLFIRI (see Chapter 97).

Oxaliplatin is a derivative of platinum salts, which inhibit DNA repair. The first report concerning the high response rate observed with this drug was made in 1990.[6] Then the combination of LV5-FU2 and oxaliplatin (FOLFOX) became a standard by showing better oncologic results compared with LV5-FU2 alone.[7] The sequence FOLFOX followed by FOLFIRI, in the event of resistance, was compared with the reverse sequence in a European trial. The results did not show differences in survival, suggesting that the sequence of the two protocols and their effectiveness were comparable.[8]

The therapeutic armamentarium in metastatic CRC was enriched in 2004 with the development of two monoclonal antibodies directed against an oncogenic activation receptor present on the surface of tumor cells: cetuximab targeting the epidermal growth factor receptor (EGFR) and bevacizumab directed against the vascular endothelium growth factor (VEGF).[9,10] Both targeted therapies combined with FOLFOX or FOLFIRI regimens further improved outcomes in metastatic CRC patients.[9,11] It was later discovered that the efficiency of anti-EGFR was compromised in tumors exhibiting a mutation of KRAS, a protein involved in the transduction of the EGFR. This finding marked the starting point of tailored oncology in CRC.[12,13] Additional mutations of the RAS/RAF pathway conferring resistance to anti-EGFR therapies were later identified, and overall about half of metastatic CRC patients cannot be efficiently treated by anti-EGFR therapies.[14] The efficiency of more aggressive protocols combining three chemotherapeutic agents (oxaliplatin, irinotecan, and LV5-FU2) with bevacizumab was demonstrated in 2010. This aggressive protocol yielded objective response rates of 65% and a median survival of 31 months.[15] The end of the 2010s has seen the impressive results of immunotherapy in tumors with microsatellite instability (MSI-H, about 5% of patients).[16,17] A combination of immune checkpoint inhibitors makes it possible to obtain an objective response in 69% of MSI-H patients with resistant disease to systemic chemotherapy. The evolution of systemic treatment in metastatic CRC over the past decades across main trials is described in Table 98.1.

Evolution of the Definition of Resectability

The first patients who underwent surgical resection for CLM were very selected. Surgery was not considered beyond three lesions or in the presence of concomitant extrahepatic disease.[18]

TABLE 98.1   Main Randomized Trials of First-Line Chemotherapy in Metastatic CRC Since 2000

FIRST AUTHOR (STUDY NAME)	YEAR	NO. OF PATIENTS	RAS/RAF	EXPERIMENTAL ARM (VS. CONTROL ARM)	MEDIAN OVERALL SURVIVAL,* MONTHS	MEDIAN PFS,* MONTHS	OBJECTIVE* RR, %
De Gramont	2000	420		FOLFOX (vs. LV5-FU2)	16.2	9.0	50.7
Douillard	2000	387		FOLFIRI (vs. 5FU-folinate)	17.1	6.7	35
Hurwitz (AVG2107g)	2004	813		Irinotecan 5FU leucovorin (IFL)–bevacizumab (vs. IFL)	20.3	10.6	44.8
Falcone	2007	244		FOLFOXIRI (vs. FOLFIRI)	22.6	9.8	66
Van Custem (CRYSTAL)	2009	1198	KRAS	FOLFIRI-cetuximab (vs. FOLFIRI)	24.9	9.9	47.1
Bokemeyer (OPUS)	2011	337	KRAS-BRAF	FOLFOX4-cetuximab	22.8	8.3	67
Douillard (PRIME)	2013	512	KRAS-NRAS -BRAF	FOLFOX 4-panitumumab (vs. FOLFOX 4)	25.8	10.1	–
Schwartzberg (PEAK)	2014	285	KRAS	FOLFOX6-panitumumab vs. FOLFOX6-bevacizumab	41.3	13.1	64
Heinemann (FIRE-3)	2014	592	KRAS	FOLFIRI-cetuximab vs. FOLFIRI-bevacizumab	28.7	10.0	62
Loupakis (TRIBE)	2014	508		FOLFOXIRI-bevacizumab (vs. FOLFIRI-bevacizumab)	29.8	12	65
Venook (CALGB-SWOG80405)	2017	1074	KRAS	FOLFIRI or FOLFOX6-cetuximab vs. bevacizumab	30.0	10.5	

*Results given for the experimental arms.

With the combined improvements of surgery and chemotherapy, criteria of resectability have been expanded and the current definition is no longer dogmatic but rather pragmatic. The number of lesions and the maximal size of lesions are no longer absolute contraindications for resection. To date, resectability can be defined as the possibility to resect all lesions present at the time of diagnosis while preserving sufficient volume of functional remnant liver.[19] Most groups agree that a safe volume of remnant liver should be at least 25% to 30% of the total liver functional volume (i.e., after subtracting tumor volume) and/or 0.5% of the remnant liver volume to body weight ratio.[19–22]

PREOPERATIVE CHEMOTHERAPY IN PATIENTS WITH UPFRONT RESECTABLE DISEASE

Advantages and Disadvantages of Preoperative Chemotherapy for Upfront Disease

Whether chemotherapy should be given before surgery in patients with upfront resectable disease remains a matter a debate. The advantages of such an approach are as follows:

1. Preoperative chemotherapy makes it possible to test the chemosensitivity of tumors. This enables us to choose appropriate adjuvant chemotherapy and to select good surgical candidates, based on the evidence that progression while on chemotherapy impairs oncologic outcomes.[23]
2. Preoperative chemotherapy may also facilitate resection with tumor-free margins by tumor downsizing and the preservation of normal parenchyma.

Disadvantages include the following:

1. It can be responsible for parenchymal injury of the nontumoral liver, thus increasing the morbidity of resection (see Chapter 69).

2. The radiologic disappearance of small lesions (so-called "missing" metastases) is another drawback because missing lesions on imaging does not mean sterilization of the tumor,[24] and their surgical removal is more challenging and may not even be possible.

A special situation is the one concerning patients with resectable metastases progressing while on chemotherapy. In patients with at least three lesions, 5-year overall survival after hepatectomy was only 8% in patients with progressive disease versus 37% and 30%, respectively, for patients with responding or stable disease, indicating that progression while on chemotherapy should be considered as a relative contraindication for resection.[23] A later analysis from the LiverMetSurvey registry enabled researchers to refine the indications for hepatectomy in a context of tumor progression on chemotherapy. It appears that patients with low CEA (<200 ng/mL) and no more than three lesions, with none of them being larger than 5 cm, experienced 5-year overall survival rates of 53%.[25] This favorable outcome argues in favor of resection in selected patients despite progression.

Upfront Resection Versus Neoadjuvant Chemotherapy: Evidence From the Literature

A randomized trial has compared perioperative FOLFOX versus no chemotherapy in patients with upfront resectable CLM with no more than four lesions.[26] Patients treated by chemotherapy experienced a significantly improved disease-free survival at 3 years (25% vs. 16%) at the cost of a higher morbidity. However, this advantage in disease-free survival did not improve overall survival.[27] The main limitation of this trial was the absence of adjuvant chemotherapy in the control group. Later, three randomized controlled trials (PANTER NCT01266187,

EXPERT UMIN000007787, NCT01035385) have attempted to compare perioperative chemotherapy versus upfront surgery followed by adjuvant chemotherapy, but all have been closed due to low recruitment issues. A retrospective analysis based on the LiverMetSurvey registry showed that preoperative chemotherapy did not yield better results in patients with a single, metachronous metastasis not exceeding 5 cm.[28]

More recently, the strategy "upfront surgery plus adjuvant chemotherapy" was compared with perioperative chemotherapy in patients with upfront resectable liver disease.[29] After adjustment for confounding factors, there was no difference in disease-free survival or overall survival. So far, preoperative chemotherapy does not seem to provide an obvious survival benefit, provided that efficient chemotherapy is given postoperatively. Therefore upfront surgery can be reasonably considered in patients with a limited metachronous disease requiring a low-risk hepatectomy. In contrast, synchronous disease is recognized as a more advanced disease, and in a consensus meeting, most experts agreed to propose preoperative chemotherapy even when disease was resectable.[30] By combining number and maximum size of metastases in the large cohort of the LiverMetSurvey registry, we concluded that the more extensive the disease, is even when initially resectable, the more useful the preoperative chemotherapy is in terms of survival expectancy after liver resection (unpublished data). In our own practice, we consider the use of chemotherapy in case of synchronous metastases and/or in patients with more than three metastases, mainly when the maximum diameter exceeds 3 cm.

Type of Chemotherapy in Upfront Resectable Patients

The two trials (EORTC intergroup trial 40983, new EPOC) that addressed the question of perioperative chemotherapy in patients with resectable CLM have chosen the FOLFOX regimen. However, FOLFIRI was allowed in patients previously treated by adjuvant FOLFOX after resection of the primary tumor in the new EPOC study. Hence, no other regimen can be recommended in patients with resectable disease. The new

EPOC study evaluated the effect of adding cetuximab to FOLFOX in wild-type RAS patients with upfront or suboptimally resectable disease. Surprisingly, the addition of cetuximab to perioperative FOLFOX in a population of wild-type RAS patients was associated with poorer progression-free survival and lower overall survival.[31,32] Differences in tumor biology, selection of a more aggressive disease by cetuximab, and increased number of missing metastases have been advocated to explain this unexpected finding.[33] In any case, the use of cetuximab in resectable patients should be avoided.

PATIENTS WITH INITIALLY UNRESECTABLE BUT POTENTIALLY RESECTABLE DISEASE

Increasing evidence has shown that the prognosis of patients in whom liver disease can be resected is far better than for those treated by chemotherapy only (Fig. 98.1). In addition, patients with initially unresectable disease who were switched to be resected after a major response to chemotherapy have experienced almost similar outcomes as those with upfront resectable disease[34] (Fig. 98.2). These findings have introduced the concept of "conversion chemotherapy" and have led to considering secondary liver resection as a primary endpoint in the strategy of treatment of patients with nonresectable metastases. Therefore the aim of preoperative chemotherapy should be interpreted according to the initial resectability of the liver disease, which highlights the need for a multidisciplinary team approach and a careful assessment of resectability by experienced liver surgeons.

Results of Conversion Chemotherapy

The feasibility of rescue surgery in patients with unresectable disease was first reported by Adam et al. in 2001.[35] In this study, liver surgery could finally be achieved in 13.5% of patients with unresectable disease after initial chemotherapy consisting mainly of 5-FU and leucovorin combined with oxaliplatin. A major finding of this study was the favorable long-term

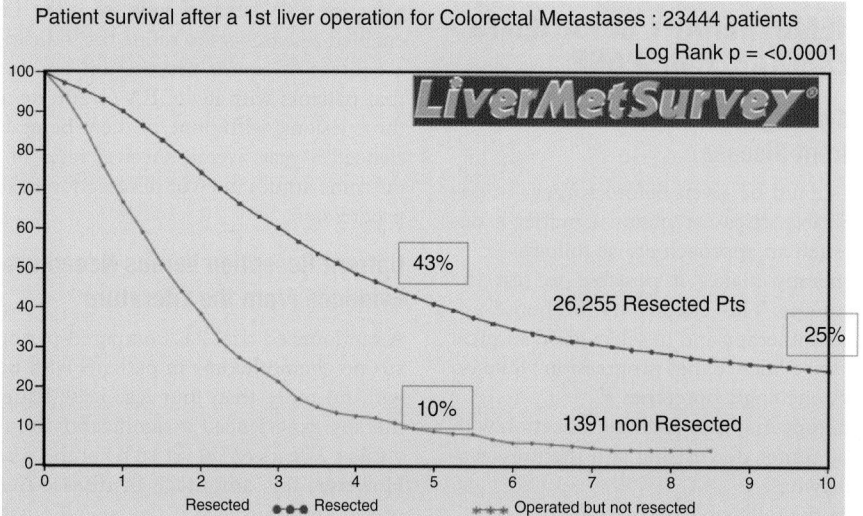

LIVERMETSURVEY : SURVIVAL AFTER LIVER RESECTION
June 2019: 28,208 Pts - 356 centers - 61 countries

Patient survival after a 1st liver operation for Colorectal Metastases : 23444 patients

Log Rank p = <0.0001

LiverMetSurvey

43%

26,255 Resected Pts

25%

10%

1391 non Resected

Resected   ●●● Resected   +++ Operated but not resected

FIGURE 98.1   Kaplan-Meier survival according to resection in patients who underwent surgery for colorectal liver metastases in the LiverMetSurvey registry.

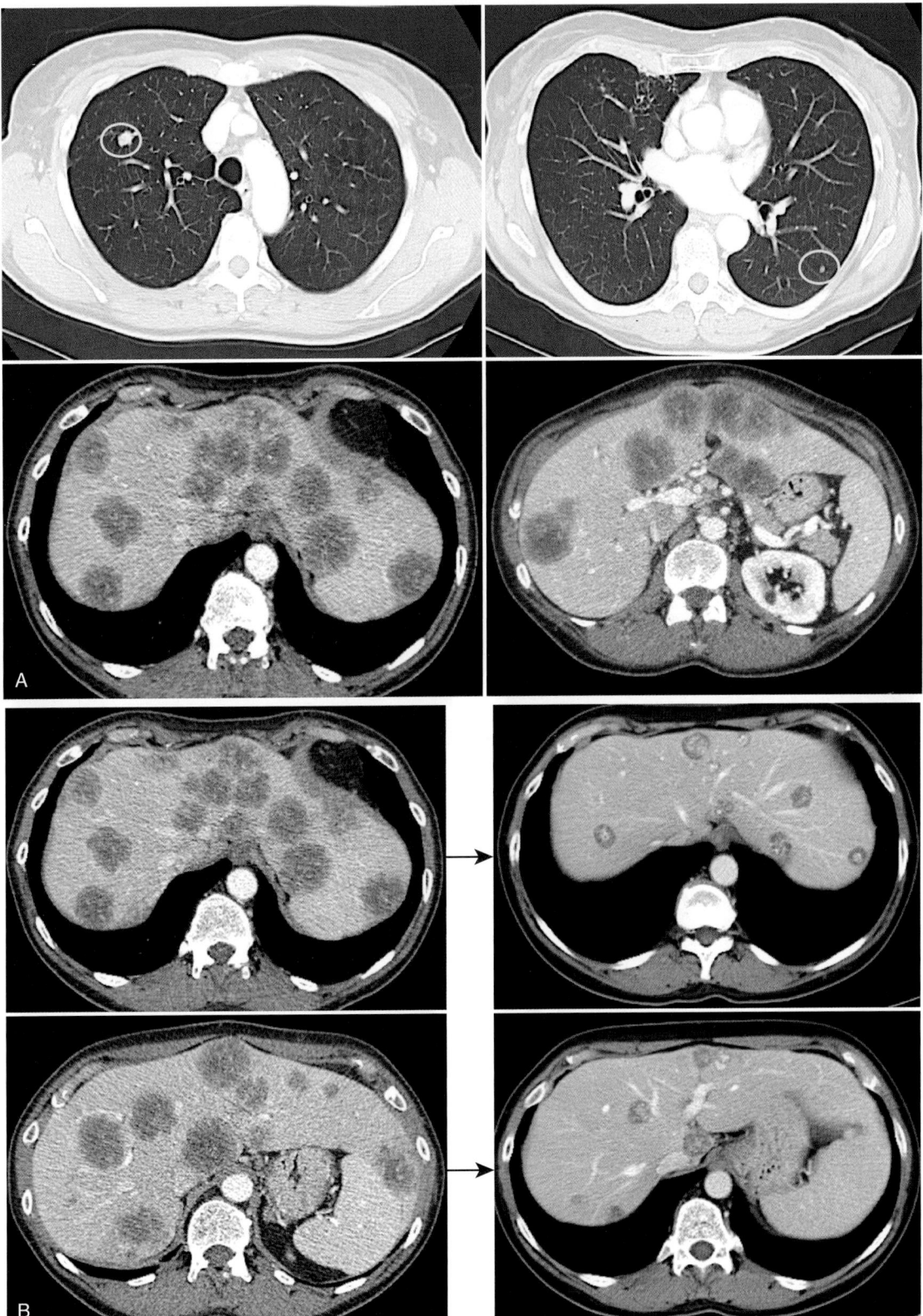

FIGURE 98.2 Illustration of onco-surgical management of a patient with initially unresectable colorectal liver metastases (CLM). A 55-year-old woman was diagnosed with an adenocarcinoma of the upper part of the rectum (KRAS mutation at codon 12) revealed by abdominal pain and asthenia. Initial serum levels of carcinoembryonic antigen (CEA) and carbohydrate antigen 19-9 (Ca19-9) were 499 UI/L and 52,753 UI/L, respectively. CT scan showed multiple bilobar CLM involving all segments and two bilateral lung metastases **(A).** She was first treated by FOLFOX-bevacizumab (12 courses) with a good response **(B).** Chemotherapy was changed to FOLFIRI-bevacizumab (15 courses) because of oxaliplatin-related neurotoxicity. The workup after 2 lines (total of 31 courses) showed an excellent biologic and morphologic response (CEA: 2.7 and Ca19-9: 23;

Continued

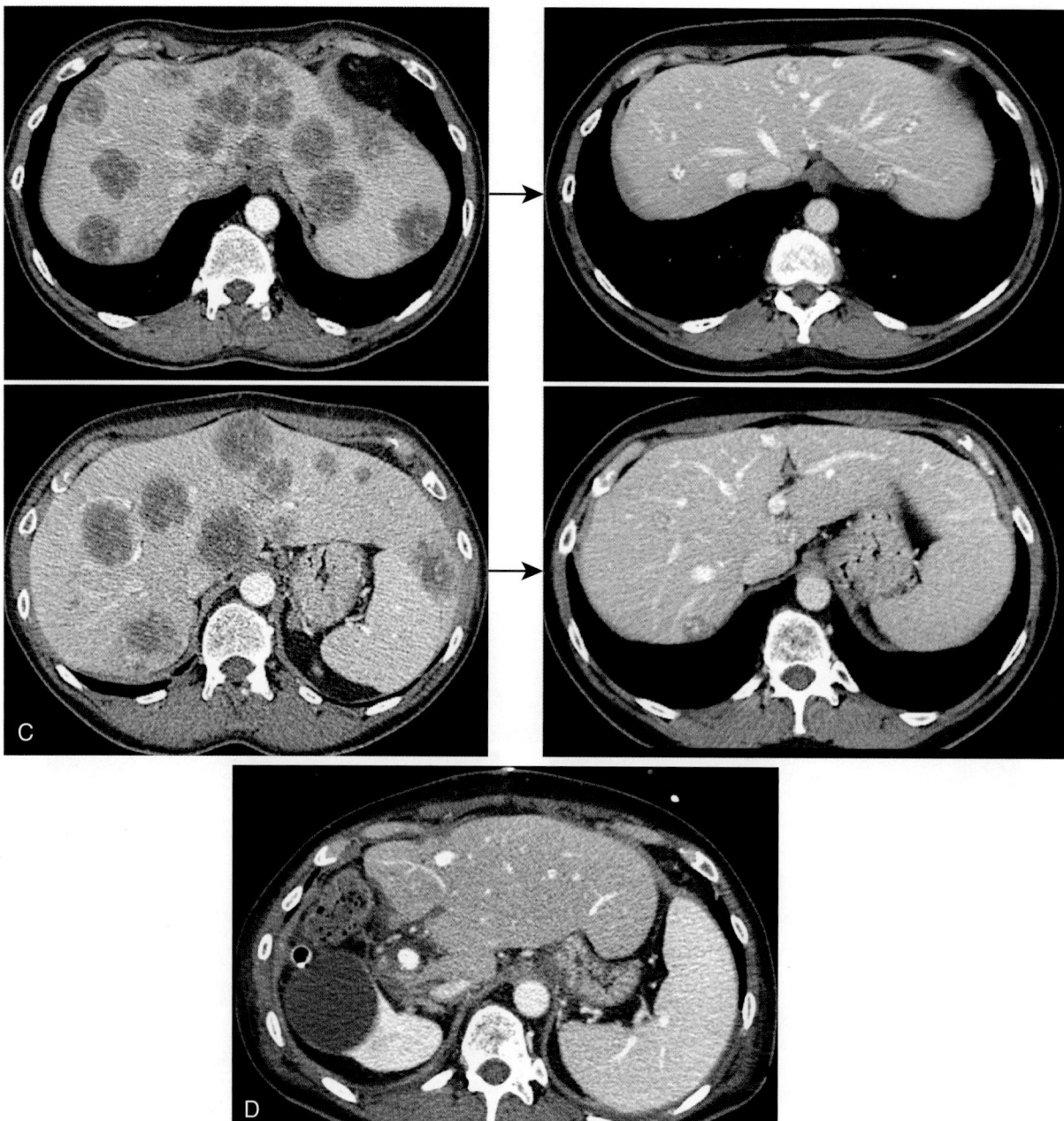

FIGURE 98.2, cont'd **C**). She could finally undergo a two-stage hepatectomy. **D,** The remnant liver after the second stage (extended right hepatectomy). Pathology found 15 nodules with a major pathologic response (average of 10% of remaining viable cancer cells). Further management included resection of rectal adenocarcinoma (pT3N1), resection of two lung metastases, a third hepatectomy for liver recurrence, and two other lines of chemotherapy. The patient is alive with lung and liver recurrence 6 years after the diagnosis of unresectable CLM with extrahepatic disease.

outcome of patients who underwent resection, with 5-year overall survival rates of 33%, close to those of patients with upfront resectable disease.[36] These good results were confirmed by further prospective studies with 5-year survival reaching 46% in the CELIM trial.[37] More recently, the ARCAD-Liver-MetSurvey registry confirmed, on a multicenter prospective international basis, that survival of 4034 patients initially unresectable, but switched to resectability by systemic chemotherapy, was 34% at 5 years versus 46% in 17,988 patients with initially resectable disease (www.livermetsurvey-arcad.org, update December 2019, Fig. 98.3).

Initial Response Rates and Conversion to Surgery

Folprecht et al.[38] showed that the initial response rate to chemotherapy strongly correlates with the chance of resection rate. This association was recently confirmed in a review of the literature including 18 prospective studies.[39] The good correlation between the response to initial chemotherapy and the chance of secondary resection justifies the use of an intensive first-line chemotherapy in patients with unresectable disease and absent or limited extrahepatic disease, for whom secondary resection could be reasonably considered, provided a partial response to chemotherapy. A summary of the main prospective

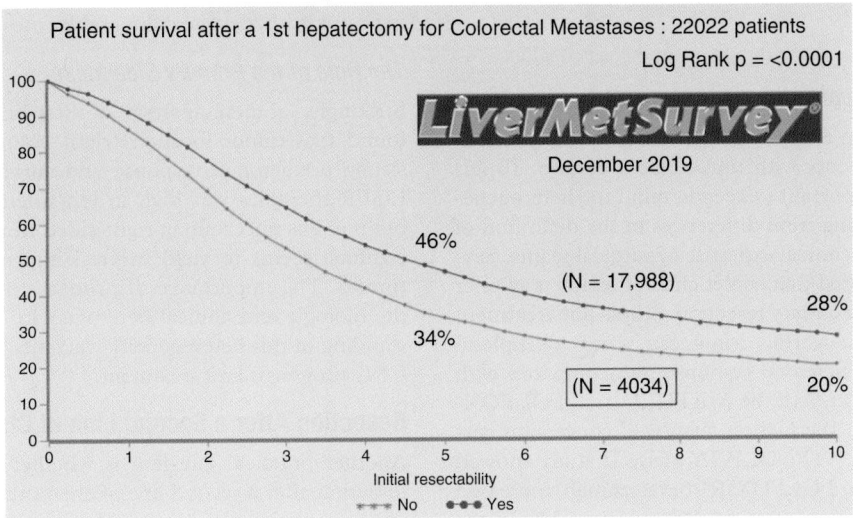

Survival after Liver Resection of Colorectal Metastases
LiverMetSurvey: Resectable vs initially unresectable

FIGURE 98.3   Kaplan-Meier survival in patients resected for colorectal liver metastases from the LiverMetSurvey registry according to the initial resectability of the liver disease.

TABLE 98.2   Main Prospective Randomized Studies (>50 Patients Included) Evaluating Conversion Surgery in Patients With Initially Unresectable Tumors

FIRST AUTHOR (STUDY NAME)	YEAR	NO.	EXPERIMENTAL TREATMENT	CONTROL TREATMENT	CONVERSION SURGERY (EXPERIMENTAL GROUP)	CONVERSION SURGERY (CONTROL GROUP)	INTERPRETATION OF FINDINGS
Folprecht (CELIM)	2010	111 (RAS wild-type or mutant)	FOLFOX6- cetuximab	FOLFIRI- cetuximab	26* (49)	23* (43)	Chemotherapy with cetuximab increases chance for secondary resection
Ychou (METHEP)	2013	125 (RAS wild-type or mutant)	FOLFIRINOX-FOLFOX7-FOLFIRI-HD)	FOLFIRI/FOLFOX4	FOLFIRINOX (66.7%)–FOLFOX 7 (43.3%)–FOLFIRI HD (59.4%)	40%	Higher secondary resection rates after FOLFIRINOX
Gruenberger (OLIVIA)	2015	80 (RAS wild-type or mutant)	FOLFOXIRI-bevacizumab	FOLFOX-bevacizumab	25 (61)	19 (49)	Higher response and resection rates in the FOLFOXIRI-bevacizumab arm
Rivera (PEAK)	2017	170 RAS wt)	FOLFOX6-panitumumab	FOLFOX6 -bevacizumab	12 (14)	9 (11)	No significant difference
Modest (VOLFI)	2019	96 (RAS wild-type)	FOLFOXIRI-panitumumab	FOLFOXIRI	21 (33%)	4 (12%)	The addition of panitumumab to FOLFOXIRI increases the chance for secondary resection
Modest (FIRE-3)	2020	270 (RAS wild-type)	FOLFIRI-panitumumab	FOLFIRI-bevacizumab	13 (10%)	20 (14%)	Lung metastases, BRAF mutation, phosphatase alkalines are predictors of failure of conversion surgery

*R0-R1 radiofrequency ablation.

studies evaluating tumor response rates and conversion surgery in patients with unresectable CLM is given in Table 98.2.

Practical Attitude

Basic Chemotherapy Regimens

In practice, the question is how to maximize the chance of objective response in patients with unresectable disease. To address this point, it is important to keep in mind the heterogeneity across studies resulting from differences in the definition of resectability or in the technical expertise of surgical teams. Several studies have suggested that triplet chemotherapy may offer the highest chance of secondary resection. A first-line treatment combining 5-FU, leucovorin, irinotecan, and oxaliplatin (FOLFOXIRI) allows increased response rate compared with FOLFIRI (60% vs. 34%).[40] In the METHEP trial, FOLFOXIRI was associated with the highest chance of conversion surgery (67% of patients).[41] The OLIVIA phase II study showed that the association of FOLFOXIRI-bevacizumab increased the chance of R0 resection rates to 49% versus 23% in the control group receiving FOLFIRI-bevacizumab.[42] A pooled analysis of studies that used triplet chemotherapy plus bevacizumab has confirmed the favorable results, with overall resection rates of 39%.[43]

Adding Targeted Therapy

To maximize the chance of rescue surgery, the role of targeted therapies in association with modern regimen must be documented. Adding anti-EGFR therapies to chemotherapy proved to be beneficial on survival of metastatic CRC patients.[14,44,45] A Chinese randomized trial showed that cetuximab in addition to either FOLFOX or FOLFIRI was associated with a significant increase of R0 resection rates (26% vs. 7%) in KRAS wild-type patients with synchronous liver-only metastases.[46] A meta-analysis has shown that the resection rates were increased by 60% with the use of EGFR inhibitors.[47] The favorable effect of anti-EGFR therapy on the chance of surgical conversion has been confirmed in a recent review.[39]

Early molecular evaluation of the RAS/RAF mutations in patients with unresectable liver disease is therefore needed. This can be done by using a biopsy of the primary tumor given the high concordance in RAS mutations between primary tumor and liver metastases.[48]

The effect of bevacizumab to improve secondary resectability is less convincing. In a randomized study, there was no increase in the response rates of the group who received bevacizumab in addition to oxaliplatin-based chemotherapy compared with chemotherapy alone.[49] Moreover, conversion rates of patients treated with bevacizumab remained similar to those of patients treated with chemotherapy alone in other comparative studies.[39] This absence of effect might be explained by the specific features of the morphologic response induced by anti-VEGF therapy. Indeed, optimal response to bevacizumab is characterized by homogeneous low attenuation on computed tomography (CT) scan with sharply defined tumor–liver interface, but without shrinkage of the tumor.[50]

Bevacizumab Versus Cetuximab

In metastatic CRC, two randomized trials have compared bevacizumab versus cetuximab in association with modern regimen as first-line treatment in KRAS exon 2 wild-type untreated metastatic CRC patients. Overall survival and response rates were similar in the CALGB/SWOG 80405 trial,[51] whereas the FIRE-3 trial found longer overall survival in the group receiving cetuximab, despite comparable rates of objective response.[52]

The Role of the Primary Sidedness

Strikingly, a meta-analysis of first-line chemotherapy trials found that tumor location (right colon vs. left colon) was a strong predictor of response and survival. The effect of anti-EGFR therapies was high in left-sided RAS wild-type tumor but remains uncertain in right-sided tumor.[53] In contrast, bevacizumab seems to yield survival improvements in right-sided tumors. The importance of primary tumor location illustrates the biologic and clinical heterogeneity of CRC. Better understanding of this heterogeneity warrants future improvements in CRC prognosis and treatment.

Resection After a Second Line of Chemotherapy

Another practical question is whether it is worth attempting resection after a second line of chemotherapy because this situation suggests a more aggressive disease with poorer prognosis. A study based on a large multicenter cohort showed that resection after a second line of chemotherapy offers a similar overall survival compared with patients resected after a single line of chemotherapy, when the disease is controlled by chemotherapy.[54] Resection should not be denied after failure of a first-line regimen provided that tumor control is obtained with a second line.

CHEMOTHERAPY-ASSOCIATED LIVER INJURY (SEE CHAPTER 69)

Numerous studies have explored the relationship between preoperative chemotherapy and histologic injuries to the nontumoral parenchyma.[55] The two most commonly observed lesions are sinusoidal obstruction syndrome (SOS) and steatohepatitis, often referred to as chemotherapy-associated steatohepatitis (CASH).

Sinusoidal Obstruction Syndrome

Sinusoidal obstruction syndrome (SOS) is characterized by damaged endothelial cells that line hepatic sinusoids, leading to partial or complete obstruction of small hepatic veins and ultimately to perisinusoidal fibrosis and nodular regenerative hyperplasia. Clinical manifestations including jaundice, ascites, hepatomegaly, and splenomegaly can be observed, but these severe presentations were described under the term "veno-occlusive disease," mainly after conditioning high-intensity regimen for stem cell hematopoietic transplantation.[56] SOS was rediscovered in metastatic CRC patients treated by oxaliplatin-based chemotherapy.[57] According to the severity of sinusoidal changes, SOS can be graded as mild, moderate, or severe. The most striking feature is the macroscopic appearance of the liver with a marbled aspect and blue tones, named "blue liver" (Fig. 98.4). The occurrence of SOS is related to the oxaliplatin-based regimen, affecting up to 79% of patients.[57] The likelihood of SOS was higher beyond 6 cycles of FOLFOX,[58] whereas a protective effect of bevacizumab against SOS was suggested by several groups.[59–61]

The relationship between SOS and postoperative morbidity has been explored in several studies.[62] The heterogeneity of chemotherapy protocols, the small number of patients, and the nonstandardization of SOS evaluation make it challenging to

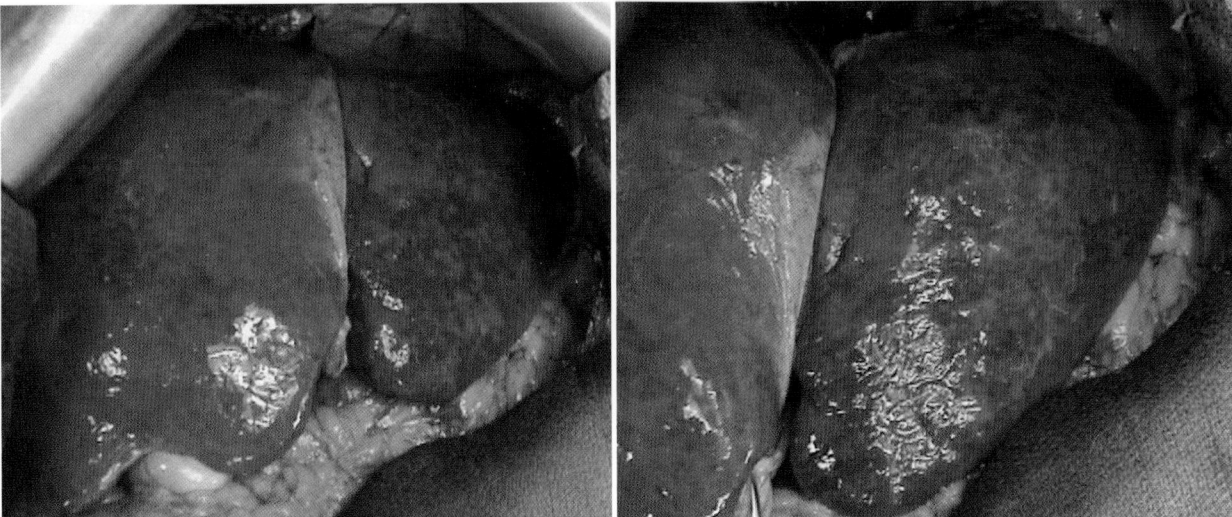

FIGURE 98.4   Intraoperative findings of oxaliplatin-induced sinusoidal obstructive syndrome revealed by the macroscopic aspect of "blue liver."

draw a definitive conclusion on the surgical risk of SOS. However, the risk of liver failure after major hepatectomy appeared to be higher in patients with moderate to severe SOS in several studies[58,63,64] (see Chapters 101 and 102). Besides the impairment of liver function, there is no specific complication that can be related to SOS. However, one report found that the amount of blood loss during hepatectomy was higher in patients with chemotherapy-related liver injury.[65]

For that reason, predicting SOS with noninvasive tools can be helpful for surgical candidates. Most severe forms are easily suspected in the presence of splenomegaly and thrombocytopenia. An aspartate aminotransferase to platelets ratio index (APRI) greater than 0.36 was predictive of severe SOS.[66] Abnormal indocyanine green (ICG) clearance is often found in SOS, with a 4-fold increase in the risk of sinusoidal injury when ICG clearance at 15 minutes is greater than 10%.[67]

Severe forms of SOS observed after hepatic-arterial infusion of oxaliplatin-based chemotherapy resulted in a collapse of ICG clearance, leading to postponing the operation. An interval of 2 to 3 months without oxaliplatin makes normalization of the ICG clearance possible, suggesting the reversibility of lesions induced by oxaliplatin[68] (see Chapter 97).

Chemotherapy-Associated Steatohepatitis

Although steatosis carries a 2-fold higher risk of postoperative complications after major hepatic resection,[69] its link with preoperative chemotherapy is not clearly established[70] (see Chapters 101 and 102).

Histologically, steatohepatitis differs from simple steatosis by the presence of an inflammatory infiltrate and ballooning of hepatocytes.[71,72] The main risk factors are obesity, diabetes, and dysmetabolic syndrome. Steatohepatitis is identified as chemotherapy-related lesions because several studies have suggested a link between steatohepatitis and irinotecan, contrary to isolated steatosis.[73] The group of Vauthey observed the presence of steatohepatitis in 20% of patients treated with irinotecan.[74] Of note, the prevalence of steatohepatitis was higher in overweight patients. These histologic lesions are clinically meaningful because of a higher risk of 90-day mortality after major hepatectomy reaching up to 14%. In addition, fatty infiltration of the liver impairs the diagnostic performance of intraoperative ultrasound and makes the detection of small lesions more challenging.

Pathologic Response to Chemotherapy

Chemotherapy before liver resection offers the opportunity to assess the efficiency of therapy. Numerous studies have demonstrated that pathologic response to chemotherapy (PRC) is a robust predictor of outcomes after hepatectomy for CLM.[75-78] Complete pathologic response, defined by the absence of any viable cancer cells in all resected lesions, is associated with excellent outcomes. However, PRC occurred in less than 5% of cases and cannot be diagnosed preoperatively.[75,78] Small number of lesions, size less than 30 mm, and radiologic response have been identified as predictive factors of PRC, but the predictive value of these factors remains insufficient to ascertain the complete histologic diagnosis and therefore to avoid resection of the metastatic site.

Major pathologic response also yields improved results. A percentage of remaining viable cancer cells below 50% was associated with better disease-free survival.[78] Rubbia-Brandt et al.[79] described a scoring system to assess histologic tumor response, called Tumor Regression Grade (TRG), integrating fibrosis and amount of residual cancer cells. Prognosis after hepatectomy could be stratified according to major, partial, or no histologic tumor regression. The most accurate method for assessing pathologic response remains a matter of debate, but the predictive value of histologic response has been confirmed in all studies.[80]

There is no clear relationship between radiologic response and pathologic response. Some patients may exhibit major radiologic response but minor pathologic response, and conversely. This radiologic and pathologic discordance was observed in up to 40% of patients,[81] but prognosis after resection was driven by pathologic response rather than by radiologic response.

Missing Metastases

Preoperative chemotherapy may lead to complete radiologic response, defined by the disappearance of a metastasis on imaging in about one-third of patients, either as a result of chemotherapy efficacy or more difficult detection due to nontumoral liver changes in relation to chemotherapy.[82] Understanding the underlying meaning of a missing metastasis is crucial because of its implication for clinical practice. Leaving in place or removing the area previously involved by the tumor are the two options when facing disappearing CLM.

Benoist et al.[24] studied 66 CLM that disappeared after chemotherapy based on the CT scan of reevaluation. They found persisting tumor foci or early recurrence when involved areas were left in place in 83% of cases.[24] Their conclusion was that complete response on CT scan does not mean sterilization of the tumor, suggesting that areas of missing metastases should be removed (see Chapter 15).

Small and deeply located missing lesions are problematic because of their related high risk of disappearance after chemotherapy and the subsequent need to resect a large volume of parenchyma to ensure their resection. To make resection easier and limit its extent, fiducial markers can be placed before starting chemotherapy for lesions at risk of disappearance after chemotherapy.[83]

The dogma of "always" resecting missing metastases has been progressively challenged, in particular in patients with initially unresectable disease that become eligible for surgery after conversion chemotherapy. The analysis of 69 missing CLM on magnetic resonance imaging (MRI) in a series of initially unresectable patients revealed that 69% had not recurred after a follow-up of 51 months.[84] However, in this study all patients were treated with adjuvant intraarterial hepatic oxaliplatin. It is likely that these figures could not be extrapolated to systemic chemotherapy, and on a probabilistic policy the recommendation should be to resect as much as possible all the initial metastatic sites.

The importance of optimal quality imaging studies using hepatocyte-specific imaging and contrast-enhanced intraoperative ultrasound should be emphasized. Oba et al.[85] showed that more than half of missing metastases on CT scan can be detected by EOB-MRI and contrast-enhanced intraoperative ultrasound. In this study, among the 110 lesions that remained invisible after EOB-MRI and contrast-enhanced intraoperative ultrasound, remaining tumor or recurrence for those left in place occurred in only 9 cases (8%) (see Chapter 15).

So far, it is not possible to ascertain a fully reliable diagnosis of PRC by imaging. Therefore resection of previously involved areas is still advocated after optimal imaging studies. This decision should be counterbalanced by the technical feasibility and the impact on the volume of the remnant liver. Marker placement for unique, deep, and small lesions can be discussed to preserve liver parenchyma and facilitate further resection after chemotherapy.

CHEMOTHERAPY IN PATIENTS WITH DEFINITIVELY UNRESECTABLE DISEASE

The impact of chemotherapy on surgery is weak in such patients. However, some situations of high response to chemotherapy in young patients with liver-only disease may lead to a possibility of secondary liver resection likely to correspond to a debulking surgery but with an option of a prolonged survival. These unexpected resections (so-called "accidental hepatectomies") are driven by a dramatic and usually quick response to an efficient chemotherapy.

An alternative to partial liver resection is the possibility of liver transplantation in patients with liver-only disease, but with extensive disease to all segments, responding well to chemotherapy and for whom no partial hepatectomy can be curative. Five-year survival in these situations has been proved to be 60% and even 83% in selected and hyperselected patients, respectively[86,87] (see Chapter 105). However, the role of liver transplantation in the armamentarium of patients with CLM remains to be scientifically proved, and a randomized trial currently running in France will definitively respond to this challenging question. The principles and conditions of preoperative chemotherapy are the same as those for conventional surgery.

POSTOPERATIVE CHEMOTHERAPY

There are currently no evidence-based data to recommend routine systemic chemotherapy after hepatectomy for CLM. A pooled analysis of two randomized trials comparing 5-FU–based adjuvant systemic chemotherapy following CLM resection versus surgery alone failed to demonstrate a statistically significant difference in overall survival.[88] A Japanese trial comparing adjuvant oral uracil-tegafur with leucovorin versus surgery alone found a disease-free survival superiority but no difference in overall survival.[89]

Recurrence rates after complete resection of CLM remain high, even when disease is limited.[90] In addition, adjuvant FOLFOX is a validated standard after resected stage III CRC.[91] For that reason, most groups consider that surgery alone in metastatic disease is not recommended. In practice, European, American, and Japanese guidelines recommend adjuvant therapy after CLM resection.[22,92,93]

CONCLUSION

The transformation of prognosis after CLM surgery is largely related to improvements of systemic chemotherapy. Radiologic response to chemotherapy (and, much less frequently, pathologic response to chemotherapy) remains the main determinant of outcomes. High response rates after induction chemotherapy allow secondary resection in a growing subset of patients with liver disease considered as initially unresectable, thus offering a prolonged survival after such an "onco-surgical approach." However, intensive chemotherapy regimens induce specific histologic lesions that may impair the function of the future remnant liver and increase surgical morbidity. Therefore a preoperative evaluation of liver function and identification of indirect signs of chemotherapy-associated liver injury are necessary to prevent postoperative morbidity.

In the modern management of CLM, chemotherapy cannot be dissociated from surgery. This highlights once again the importance of a collaboration among oncologists, radiologists, pathologists, and liver surgeons to propose for each patient a tailored onco-surgical strategy.

The references for this chapter can be found online by accessing the accompanying Expert Consult website.

CHAPTER 99

Advances in systemic therapy for hepatocellular carcinoma

Ghassan K. Abou-Alfa, Imane El Dika, and Eileen M. O'Reilly

OVERVIEW

Hepatocellular carcinoma (HCC) represents a challenging malignancy of global importance (see Chapter 89). It is the fifth most common solid tumor in terms of incidence and the third leading cause of cancer-related death worldwide.[1] Its incidence mirrors that of chronic liver injury, which is predominantly attributable to viral hepatitis infection, both hepatitis B and C (see Chapter 68). Other etiologic factors that cause chronic liver injury and cirrhosis include alcohol; nonalcoholic steatohepatitis (NASH)[2] (see Chapter 69), commonly associated with morbid obesity and diabetes; and other metabolic diseases, for instance, hemochromatosis. The highest incidence of HCC remains in Southeast Asia and sub-Saharan Africa, driven chiefly by hepatitis B viral infection.[3] However, there is continued concern about the rising incidence of HCC in North America.[4] A 3-fold increase in the age-adjusted rates for HCC associated with hepatitis C, from 2.3 per 100,000 between 1993 and 1995 to 7.0 per 100,000 between 1996 and 1998, has been observed. This is most likely explained by the increased incidence of hepatitis C that has been seen in North America during that time period. In an effort to understand the projected incidence of HCC among United States population, a forecast model based on data from the Surveillance, Epidemiology, and End Results (SEER) database and the US census bureau was used.[5] Asians/Pacific Islanders population had the highest incidence of HCC. In the projected period through 2030, a decline is expected with a rise among Hispanic and Black populations. This is mostly attributed to the historically high incidence of hepatitis B virus (HBV) infection among the Asian population, which started to decrease after the introduction of universal vaccination. The majority of HCC cases are attributed to metabolic syndrome and diabetes and this incidence is expected to continue to rise as the obesity epidemic continues. Hispanics and Blacks are among the populations with the highest obesity prevalence. In fact, an analysis of 18 SEER registries[6] showed that in the United States, HCC incidence and mortality has decreased among Asians/Pacific Islanders between the year 2000 and 2010, whereas a higher incidence of HCC was observed among Blacks, Hispanics, and Whites. Hepatitis C virus (HCV) infection constitutes a large proportion of HCC incidence in the United States, and the advent of second-generation direct antiviral therapy is expected to improve the incidence of HCC. Nonetheless the cost of these medications might preclude its widespread use and is a barrier to HCV eradication. A plateauing of HCC cases by 2025 is expected; however, this and other predictions do not necessarily reflect the global incidence and prevalence of HCC. For example, in sub-Saharan Africa, the rate of HBV vaccination remains low, thus a significant decline in HBV-related HCC

cases is not expected. In Europe, HCV was driving the majority of HCC cases, and it is being replaced by alcoholic cirrhosis and nonalcoholic fatty liver disease.[7] HCC incidence and etiology vary by geography, ethnicity, and socioeconomic factors. Global studies are crucial to delineate the intrinsic disease differences (see Chapter 89).

Chemotherapeutic agents, either as monotherapy or in combination, demonstrated a low response rate (RR) and limited survival advantage.[8] The advent of targeted therapies and checkpoint inhibitors, and their demonstrated positive survival impact for patients with HCC, led to an explosion of novel therapeutic approaches and a paradigm shift in the management of advanced HCC cases, with evolving opportunities to explore systemic therapeutic indications in other stages of the disease (e.g., adjuvant and neoadjuvant).

HEPATOCELLULAR CARCINOMA AND CIRRHOSIS: TWO DISEASES IN ONE

A fundamental challenge in HCC is the coexistence of underlying liver injury and hepatic dysfunction as the premalignant environment in the majority of patients. Both the underlying cirrhosis and the tumor itself affect the HCC patient's overall survival (OS; see Chapter 74). Thus there is a need to evaluate the cirrhosis status of patients with liver cancer to guide treatment decisions. The original scoring system, developed by Child in 1964,[9] consisted of three key parameters: jaundice (bilirubin), ascites, and encephalopathy. This scoring system was later updated by Pugh and colleagues,[10] with the addition of hepatic synthetic function assessment by evaluation of serum albumin levels and prothrombin time (Table 99.1). Today this combined score is known as the Child-Pugh score. It remains the most commonly used scoring system for liver cirrhosis (see Chapter 4). The major pitfall of the Child-Pugh score is the lack of inclusion of any parameters relating to the cancer itself, as it was developed in patients who had cirrhosis but not cancer. As such, it is unlikely to be the best predictor of outcome in patients with HCC.

Okuda and colleagues[11] recognized the need for an HCC staging system that incorporated factors related to both the background cirrhosis and the tumor itself and, therefore, designed the Okuda staging system, which encompasses four variables: albumin, bilirubin, ascites, and tumor size defined as a percentage function to the size of the liver (greater or less than 50%). The Okuda staging system served as a platform for more advanced and sophisticated prospective scoring systems that used the Cox proportional hazard regression model. The Cancer of the Liver Italian Program (CLIP) devised a scoring system in patients with HCC, and primarily hepatitis C as the etiologic driver,[12,13] that determined the independent prognostic variables for HCC

TABLE 99.1 Child-Pugh Scoring System

	POINTS		
PARAMETER	1	2	3
Albumin (g/dL)	>3.5	2.8–3.5	<2.8
Bilirubin (mg/dL)	<2	2–3	>3
Ascites	Absent	Slight	Moderate
Encephalopathy	None	I–II	III–IV
PT (INR)	<1.7	1.8–2.3	>2.3
Score	A	B	C
Points	5–6	7–9	10–15

INR, International normalized ratio; PT, prothrombin time.

patients to be the Child-Pugh score plus three additional variables relating to the tumor itself: tumor morphology (assessed by the number of lesions and extent in the liver), presence or absence of portal vein thrombosis, and α-fetoprotein (AFP) level (Table 99.2). Patients with high scores of 4 to 6 were shown to have a median survival of only 3.2 months.

The Chinese University Prognostic Index (CUPI), another scoring system that is based on multivariate analysis, in contrast to CLIP, was developed mainly in patients with hepatitis B–associated HCC.[14] This prognostic index identified bilirubin, alkaline phosphatase, and presence or absence of ascites, in addition to tumor stage based on the tumor-node-metastasis (TNM) staging, and AFP levels, as the most important predictors of outcome. Furthermore, a clinical assessment parameter of presence or absence of symptoms at presentation was incorporated (Table 99.3). An important aspect of the CUPI index is the different weight attributed to the various parameters. The median survival of the highest-risk group was close to 1 month. Other scoring systems include the Groupe d'Étude et de Traitement du Carcinoma Hépatocellulaire (GETCH) staging

system,[15] the Japan Integrated Staging (JIS) score,[16] and the Barcelona Clinic Liver Cancer (BCLC) classification system.[17]

The BCLC was created with the aim of fine-tuning the differences between patients with early-stage disease, which is a feature that the Okuda staging system fails to characterize. However, by the same token, the BCLC staging system had limited permutations for patients with advanced disease and grouped patients with unresectable disease, with Okuda stage I or II, or with Child-Pugh A or B in the exact same category of advanced disease. In a retrospective analysis of patients with advanced HCC reviewed by medical oncologists at Memorial Sloan-Kettering Cancer Center (MSKCC) during a 5-year period, we attempted to identify which of these well-known eight scoring systems would be most valuable in this specific clinical setting.[18] Using a concordance index (c-index), the GETCH, CLIP, and CUPI were the most informative staging systems in predicting survival in patients with advanced HCC. BCLC did not score well in this exercise studying a specific niche of patients with advanced HCC, all of whom fall within the single basket of category C of BCLC that lacks any discriminatory abilities. Other groups have come to the same conclusion regarding BCLC independently.[19] Another liver function assessment model was developed in Japan and several geographic regions, the Albumin-Bilirubin (ALBI) score.[20] As opposed to the Child-Pugh score developed in patients with liver cirrhosis and no HCC, the ALBI score was studied in patients with HCC with a validation cohort of patients with liver cirrhosis only. ALBI score relies solely on objective measures of liver function being albumin and bilirubin, as evaluation of ascites and hepatic encephalopathy can be clinically challenging. The score stratifies patients into three categories and compared well with the Child-Pugh score. Interestingly ALBI score provided further dissection within the Child-Pugh A score, where patients could be dichotomized into two groups with significant survival difference.[21,22]

TABLE 99.2 Cancer of the Liver Italian Program Scoring System

	SCORE		
PARAMETER	0	1	2
Child-Pugh score	A	B	C
Tumor morphology	Uninodular and extension ≤50%	Multinodular and extension ≤50%	Massive or extension >50%
Portal vein thrombosis	No	Yes	
α-Fetoprotein (ng/dL)	<400	≥400	
Score	0	1	2 3 4–6

TABLE 99.3 Chinese University Prognostic Index Scoring System

PARAMETER			WEIGHT (CUPI SCORE)			
Bilirubin (mg/dL)	<1.9	0	1.9–2.8	3	≥2.9	4
Ascites	Present	3				
Alkaline. phosphatase	≥200 IU/L	3				
Tumor-node-metastasis stage	I and II	−3	IIIa and IIIb	−1	IVa and IVb	0
α-Fetoprotein (ng/mL)	≥500	2				
Disease symptoms on presentation	None	−4				
Risk group	Low		Intermediate		High	
Score	−7 to 1		2–7		8–12	

CUPI, Chinese University Prognostic Index Scoring System.

ROLE OF CHEMOTHERAPY IN HEPATOCELLULAR CARCINOMA

Almost every class of chemotherapy has been investigated in advanced HCC.[23] Doxorubicin is one of the most studied drugs in this disease setting. This is partly due to a solitary trial originally reported by Olweny and colleagues in 1975.[24] Many subsequent attempts to try to replicate this high RR have been made, both as monotherapy[25–31] and in combination with other chemotherapeutic agents,[32–36] but to no avail.

Other older and newer chemotherapeutic agents have also been studied in HCC, including cisplatin,[37] etoposide,[35] mitoxantrone,[37] vinblastine,[38] capecitabine,[39] gemcitabine,[40] irinotecan,[41] and paclitaxel,[42] all with reported dismal RRs and no impact on survival.

Although several combination chemotherapy regimens have led to improved RRs, the impact on survival was not marked in the majority of cases.[43–45] A combination of cisplatin, interferon (IFN), doxorubicin, and 5-fluorouracil (5-FU), which became commonly known as PIAF.[46] PIAF was subsequently modified and studied in the outpatient setting.[47] An RR of 26% was observed in this Phase II trial of 50 patients. More importantly, 18% (9 patients) proceeded to surgical resection of their tumor after completion of therapy, and of these resected patients, 4 had pathologic complete responses (CRs) noted in the resected tumor specimen. A randomized trial of PIAF versus doxorubicin followed.[48] This trial revealed the same 21% RR for PIAF, versus 10% for single-agent doxorubicin. The study failed, however, to show any survival advantage in favor of the PIAF combination (8.7 vs. 6.8 months, $P = .83$). Although the study failed to bolster support for the use of PIAF as a conventional palliative treatment option for advanced disease, the regimen remains rarely used for carefully selected patients with potentially resectable tumors as a conversion therapy. A phase III trial of FOLFOX4 (infusional fluorouracil, leucovorin, and oxaliplatin) versus doxorubicin as palliative chemotherapy for advanced HCC was performed in Asia and included 371 patients. The primary end point was OS; secondary end points included progression-free survival (PFS), RR by the Response Evaluation Criteria in Solid Tumors (RECIST) criteria (version 1.0), and safety. At the prespecified final analysis, median OS was 6.40 months with FOLFOX4 (95% confidence interval [CI], 5.30–7.03) and 4.97 months with doxorubicin (95% CI, 4.23–6.03; $P = .07$; hazard ratio [HR], 0.80; 95% CI, 0.63–1.02). It is not until continued follow-up that a true survival benefit of FOLFOX4 was noted (HR, 0.79; 95% CI, 0.63–0.99; $P = .04$). Toxicity was consistent with previous experiences with FOLFOX4; proportions of grade 3 to 4 adverse events were similar between treatments. It is important to note that the doxorubicin dose was only 50 mg/m^2 in this study. Although the study did not meet its primary end point, the trend toward improved OS with FOLFOX4, along with an increased PFS and RR, led to the approval of FOLFOX4 as an accepted standard regimen for advanced HCC in China.[8]

Some of the generally disappointing results seen to date may be explained by the genetic make-up of HCC. HCC is comprised of highly resistant clones of cancer cells.[49] HCC cells carry a high "genetic mutational load," making them less amenable to the destructive cytotoxic actions of chemotherapy.

Floxuridine (FUDR) and dexamethasone administered via hepatic arterial infusion (HAI) was also explored in HCC.[50] Among 8 patients studied, the RR was 25%, and the hepatic

PFS was 9.4 months. HAI will be discussed in more detail in Chapter 97.

In summary, no chemotherapy agent, whether used alone or in combination, has so far shown any real impact on survival in patients with HCC. The emergence of several novel targeted agents and checkpoint inhibitors has changed the treatment paradigm in HCC as a viable option where cytotoxic chemotherapy failed. However, chemotherapy is not necessarily forgotten, as the potential of combining it with targeted therapies may carry a certain promise in HCC, given the success of such a strategy in other solid tumors models.

BIOLOGIC THERAPIES IN HEPATOCELLULAR CARCINOMA

The advent of novel targeted therapeutics in oncology, together with an imminent need in terms of therapeutics for advanced HCC, led to the exploration of several relevant targets in HCC along the signal transduction pathways[51] (Fig. 99.1).

The epidermal growth factor receptor (EGFR) was one of the first and well-studied therapeutic targets in HCC, despite controversial views on the expression of EGFR between HCC and noncancerous diseased liver tissue.[52–54] Efforts evaluating erlotinib,[55] cetuximab,[56,57] lapatinib,[58,59] and a combination regimen of cetuximab in conjunction with gemcitabine-oxaliplatin chemotherapy,[60] did not demonstrate satisfactory outcomes to enhance further investigation. Insulin growth factors (IGFs) are reported to be strong mitogens of HCC, exerting their effect through the IGF-1 receptor (IGF-1R)[61] led ultimately to a phase II study of cixutumumab monotherapy[62] with poor outcome. Rapamycin and everolimus mTOR pathway inhibitors were evaluated preclinically[63] and in clinical trial[64] to no avail. Thus there is no concrete foundation to recommend the routine use of any of the single agents, such as EGFR, mTOR, or IGF-R inhibitors, in the management of HCC.

Tyrosine Kinase Inhibitors

Sorafenib is a small molecule multikinase inhibitor that inhibits the serine/threonine kinase RAF-1 in vitro in addition to both proangiogenic (vascular endothelial growth factor receptor

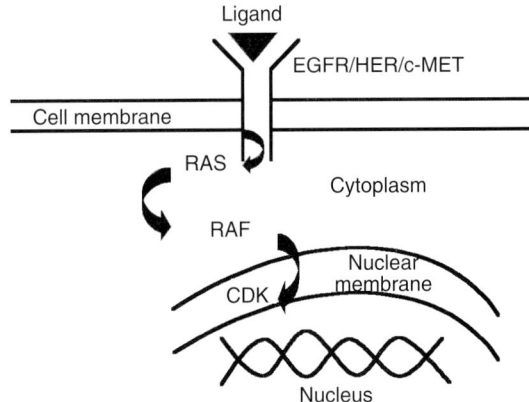

FIGURE 99.1 Potential targets for hepatocellular carcinoma therapy along the signal transduction pathway. *CDK*, Cyclin-dependent kinase; *c-MET*, mesenchymal epithelial transition factor; *EGFR*, epidermal growth factor receptor; *HER*, human epidermal growth factor receptor; *RAF*, rapidly growing fibrosarcoma (serine/threonine protein kinase); *RAS*, rat sarcoma (guanosine triphosphate–binding protein). (See Chapter 9C.)

[VEGFR]-1, -2, -3; platelet-derived growth factor receptor-β [PDGFR-β]) and tumorigenic (RET, FLT3, c-KIT receptor tyrosine kinases [RTKs]).[65]

The initial phase II trial evaluating response to sorafenib in patients with advanced HCC showed an RR of 2% when assessed by conventional RECIST criteria,[66] yet 34% of patients had stable disease for a minimum of 4 months. This was associated with a median time-to-progression (TTP) of 4.2 months and median OS of 9.2 months, both of which compare favorably with historic controls at that time.[48] The main grade 3 to 4 toxicities were fatigue (9.5%), diarrhea (8%), and palmar-plantar erythrodysesthesia (5.1%), known as hand-foot syndrome (HFS). The high rate of stable disease was associated with an observed phenomenon of central tumor necrosis in many patients on the study whose tumors were evaluated by using triphasic computed tomography (CT) scans, including an arterial phase (Fig. 99.2; see Chapter 14). This central tumor necrosis was quantified, and the volume of the tumor it encompassed within was measured by using a computer algorithm for semiautomated delineation of tumors.[67] It was later found that the ratio of the percentage of the described tumor necrosis to the tumor volume correlates with the objective response.[68] This phenomenon is still pending validation and is currently the subject of many prospective correlative studies of ongoing HCC clinical trials.

The signal of improved outcome in this phase II study led to a large, double-blind, randomized phase III trial evaluating sorafenib versus placebo in patients with advanced HCC and Child-Pugh A cirrhosis.[69] with two primary end points: OS and time-to-symptomatic progression (TTSP) using the FHSI8 (Functional Assessment of Cancer Therapy Hepatobiliary Symptom Index 8)-TSP instrument. This pivotal phase III SHARP trial demonstrated an improvement in survival of 10.7 months in the sorafenib group versus 7.9 months for the placebo arm (HR, 0.69; $P < .001$). The second primary end point evaluating for TTSP showed no difference between the two arms ($P = .77$). This observation is limited, however, by the poor understanding of the validity of FHS18-TSP instrument in this setting. In addition, a significant proportion of patients on this study, including 17% with locally advanced tumor BCLC B patients, had an excellent performance status and lacked any symptoms that the FHS18-TSP instrument would otherwise depend on for its measurements. The toxicity profile

was similar to that noted in the phase II study, with grade 3 to 4 diarrhea developing in 8% of patients and 8% experiencing HFS. There were rare bleeding events (<1%), which required caution considering the antiangiogenic nature of sorafenib, similar to other agents in its class (for instance, bevacizumab and sunitinib) that may cause fatal bleeds.[70,71]

A second randomized phase III study evaluating sorafenib in patients with advanced HCC and Child-Pugh A cirrhosis was conducted in the Asia-Pacific geographic area.[72] The study had similar eligibility criteria compared with the SHARP trial yet had two fundamental differences in the design. The study had a 2:1 randomization design, typically done to help encourage accrual, and did not have a predefined primary end point; rather, it looked at several end points. Similar to the SHARP trial, the Asia-Pacific study showed an improvement in survival in favor of sorafenib (6.5 months) versus placebo (4.2 months). This statistically significant improvement ($P = .014$), however, was not of the same magnitude as the SHARP trial, despite a similar HR of 0.68 and 0.69 in the Asia-Pacific and SHARP study, respectively. In an attempt to explain the difference in magnitude of the OS, it was argued that in the Asia-Pacific study, patients were more ill at the time of accrual, compared with the SHARP trial,[73] and had more extensive-stage disease. This observation may partly explain the difference in magnitude of benefit from sorafenib between those two populations, and suggests, in view of the similar HRs, that the benefit for sorafenib was expressed on the survival curve at two different time points in the natural history of HCC: an earlier one in the SHARP trial and a later one for the Asia-Pacific study. Another possible explanation for this numerical difference could be attributed to higher incidence of HBV-related HCC in the Asia-Pacific study population, as opposed to HCV, which was associated with better outcomes with sorafenib.[74]

Patients with unresectable HCC and Child-Pugh A liver function who are eligible for sorafenib based on the SHARP trial encompass no more than 50% of the patients seen in daily clinical practice by medical oncologists.[18] The safety and efficacy of sorafenib in patients with Child-Pugh B or C cirrhosis, who comprise the other 50% of HCC patients, remains a subject of debate. In the phase II study evaluating sorafenib in HCC,[66] 28% of patients had Child-Pugh B cirrhosis, with pharmacokinetic profiles including area under the curve (AUC) and maximum concentration (C_{max}) that were comparable to

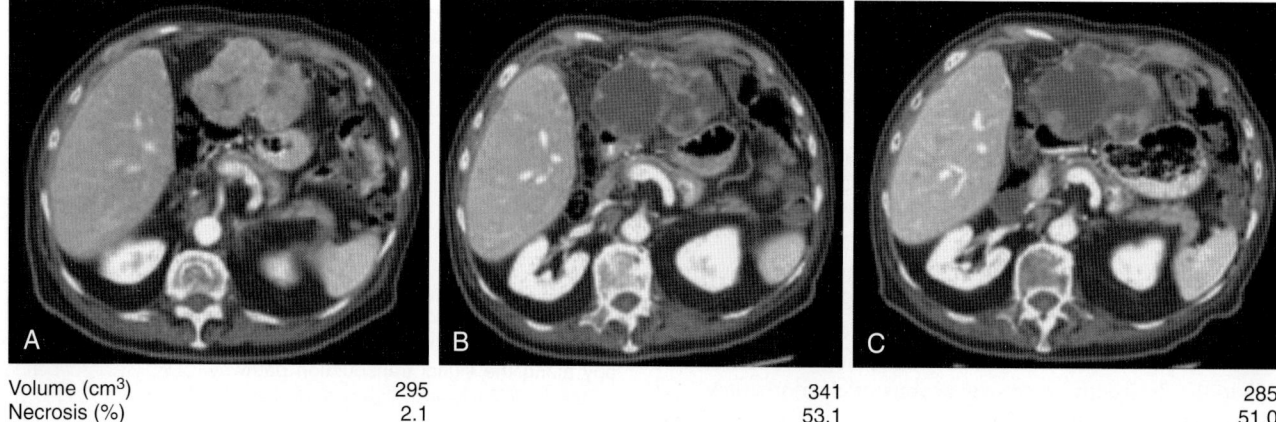

	A	B	C
Volume (cm³)	295	341	285
Necrosis (%)	2.1	53.1	51.0

FIGURE 99.2 (A–C), Baseline and serial follow-up scans demonstrating tumor necrosis in a hepatocellular carcinoma patient. (From Abou-Alfa GK, et al. A phase II study of sorafenib in patients with advanced hepatocellular carcinoma. *J Clin Oncol.* 24[26]:4293–4300, 2006.) (See Chapter 14.)

patients with Child-Pugh A score. The Child-Pugh B patients were, however, noted to have more frequent worsening of their liver function, including elevated total serum bilirubin, worsening ascites, and encephalopathy.[75] In a phase I study evaluating two different dosage regimens of sorafenib in Japanese patients with advanced HCC,[76] geometric means of AUC 0 to 12 and C_{max} were slightly lower in patients with Child-Pugh B cirrhosis compared with Child-Pugh A cirrhosis, despite the lack of any substantial differences in the incidence of adverse events between the two groups. One further study, evaluating sorafenib in 150 patients with a variety of solid tumor malignancies in predefined cohorts with different levels of liver dysfunction helps give some guidance on the optimal use of sorafenib in such patients.[77] Among all the cohorts with higher than normal total bilirubin, the most commonly reported drug-limiting toxicity (DLT) was further elevation of bilirubin. The study suggested the following dosing of sorafenib: 400 mg orally twice per day if bilirubin is below upper limit of normal (ULN), 200 mg orally twice per day for bilirubin up to 1.5 ULN, 200 mg orally once per day for bilirubin 1.5 to 3 times ULN, and to avoid prescribing sorafenib for bilirubin higher than 3 times ULN. These recommendations continue to serve as a clinical guideline until more data are available regarding the safety and efficacy of sorafenib in patients with HCC and Child-Pugh B or C. This would require a randomized study that will allow analysis of the natural history of the disease and means of evaluating worsening cirrhosis in noninvasive ways, but with more predictive measures than simply bilirubin levels.

Lenvatinib, a multiple receptor kinase inhibitor became of interest with HCC-related targeting of angiogenesis (VEGFR 1–3), fibroblast growth factor (FGF) receptor (FGFR 1–4), and PDGFR.[78,79] The REFLECT trial[80] was a multicenter, phase III, open-label, randomized, noninferiority study of lenvatinib versus sorafenib as a first-line therapy in unresectable and metastatic HCC. Nine hundred fifty-four patients were randomized to receive lenvatinib or sorafenib in a 1:1 fashion. Eligible patients had to have Eastern Cooperative Oncology Group (ECOG) performance status of 0 or 1, Child-Pugh A liver function, and adequate organ function. Patients with more than 50% liver involvement, or Vp4 main portal vein invasion (defined as presence of a tumor thrombus in the main trunk of the portal vein or a portal vein branch contralateral to the primarily involved lobe or both lobes) were excluded.[81] The study showed a median survival of 13.6 months (95% CI, 12.1–14.9) for lenvatinib compared with 12.3 months (10.4–13.9) in the sorafenib group (HR, 0.92 [95% CI, 0.79–1.06]), confirming noninferiority as per predetermined statistical design. Secondary end points included TTP, PFS, and objective response rate (ORR). Median TTP was 8.9 months (95% CI, 7.4–9.2) for lenvatinib compared with a TTP of 3.7 months (3.6–5.4) for sorafenib (HR, 0.63 [0.53–0.73], $P < .0001$). Lenvatinib-associated PFS was 7.4 months (6.9–8.8) compared with 3.7 months (3.7–4.6) on the sorafenib arm (HR, 0.66 [0.57–0.77], $P < .0001$). ORR as defined by modified RECIST (mRECIST) was 24.1% (20.2–27.9) for lenvatinib compared with 9.2% (6.6–11.8) in the sorafenib group with $P < .0001$. The improvements in all secondary end points were clinically and statistically meaningful. The difference was consistently noted when using blinded independent imaging review according to RECIST1.1 (18.8% vs. 6.5%, $P < .0001$). This was among the first phase III trials to depend prospectively on mRECIST.[82] The most common observed adverse events were hypertension, diarrhea, decreased appetite for lenvatinib, palmar-plantar erythrodysesthesia, diarrhea, and hypertension in the sorafenib arm. This study confirmed noninferiority to sorafenib and established lenvatinib as another first-line treatment in advanced HCC.

Sunitinib, a multitargeted RTK inhibitor that targets angiogenic pathways, was evaluated as a single agent in patients with advanced HCC in two phase II studies.[70,83] Despite nonreassuring findings, enthusiasm remained regarding the potential therapeutic value of sunitinib in HCC, prompting a phase III clinical trial evaluating sunitinib versus sorafenib in patients with advanced HCC.[84] This study of 1074 patients was terminated early. For sunitinib and sorafenib, respectively, median OS was 7.9 versus 10.2 months (HR, 1.30; one-sided $P = .9990$; two-sided $P = .0014$), and median PFS (3.6 vs. 3.0 months; HR, 1.13; one-sided $P = .8785$; two-sided $P = .2286$) were comparable.

Surprisingly, regorafenib, an oral tyrosine kinase inhibitor, that similarly to sorafenib targets angiogenesis among other cancer pathways with more potent antiangiogenic activity and distinct oncogenic targets,[85] was evaluated as a second-line treatment for patients who have radiologically progressed on sorafenib in the first line. RESORCE was an international phase III, randomized, placebo-controlled, double-blind study. Patients had to have tolerated sorafenib to be included in the RESORCE study.[86] Tolerance to sorafenib was defined as the ability of patients to tolerate the drug for 20 of the last 28 days at a minimum dose of 400 mg per day. Five hundred and seventy-three patients were randomized in a 2:1 fashion. Median duration on prior sorafenib was 7.8 months, and the median interval from progression on sorafenib until start of regorafenib was 1.4 months. Response was assessed by mRECIST criteria. Patients receiving regorafenib had a median OS of 10.6 months (95% CI, 9.1–12.1) versus 7.8 months (6.3–8.8) for patients who received placebo (HR, 0.63 [95% CI, 0.50–0.79]; $P < .0001$). Median PFS was 3.1 months (95% CI, 2.8–4.2) with regorafenib and 1.5 months (1.4–1.6) with placebo. Median TTP was 3.2 months (95% CI, 2.9–4.2) with regorafenib and 1.5 months (1.4–1.6) with placebo. The most clinically relevant grade 3 or 4 adverse events with regorafenib were hypertension, HFS, and fatigue. Authors looked at the collective survival outcomes in patients who received sorafenib followed by regorafenib as an exploratory retrospective analysis of the RESORCE trial.[87] Median OS reached 26 months (22.6–28.1) for patients who received subsequent regorafenib compared with 19.2 months (16.3–22.8) for placebo.

Hepatocyte growth factor (HGF), and its receptor c-MET, which were found to be overexpressed in 33% and 20% of human HCC tissues, respectively,[54] were zoomed in as potential oncologic targets in HCC. c-MET was overexpressed preferentially in early-stage resected HCC, but without effect on outcome as measured by OS.[88] Tivantinib, a tyrosine kinase inhibitor with anti c-MET activity, was studied in both the phase I[89] and phase II setting[90] with encouraging results. In a phase II trial of advanced HCC patients with progression post–first-line therapy, tivantinib therapy led to a median TTP of 2.7 months versus 1.4 months for placebo (HR, 0.43; 95% CI, 0.19–0.97) and a median OS of 7.2 months versus 3.8 months for placebo (HR, 0.38; 95% CI, 0.18–0.81) in those patients with high MET-expressing tumors. Interestingly, high MET expression in the placebo group was associated with shorter OS (median OS, 3.8 vs. 9.0 months), suggesting that MET may also be a prognostic biomarker. Given these data, tivantinib was tested in a randomized phase III multicenter, randomized, placebo-controlled, double-blind clinical study of 340 patients with advanced HCC and excellent hepatic function, who experienced disease progression while receiving sorafenib. Of interest, tivantinib was administered only to patients with high MET expression (defined as >50%; 3 to 4+ expression by immunohistochemistry [IHC]), offering the first example of a trial using an a priori molecular characteristic to enrich for activity in HCC.[91] Median OS was 8.4 months (95% CI, 6.8–10.0) in the tivantinib group and 9.1 months (7.3–10.4) in the placebo group (HR, 0.97; 95% CI, 0.75–1.25; $P = .81$). Cabozantinib fared better. In addition to MET and VEGFR-2, cabozantinib inhibits other tyrosine kinases, including RET, KIT, AXL, and FLT3.[92] It has shown promising efficacy in a cohort of 41 patients with advanced HCC.[93] In 78% of patients, tumor regression was observed by RECIST criteria with a 5% confirmed partial response (PR). The median PFS for the cohort was estimated at 4.2 months. These results led to the phase III CELESTIAL study, a multicenter randomized double-blind placebo-controlled phase III trial in patients whose disease has progressed after at least one and up to two lines of systemic therapy, including sorafenib.[94] Given the molecular intratumoral heterogeneity of HCC (see Chapter 9C), cabozantinib was evaluated in all-comers as opposed to the strategy used in tivantinib. Seven hundred and seven patients were enrolled and randomized in a 2:1 fashion. Patients had a histologically confirmed diagnosis of HCC, Child-Pugh A liver function, ECOG performance status of 0 to 1, and adequate organ function. Patients received cabozantinib at 60 mg orally daily. Cabozantinib was associated with a median OS of 10.2 months compared with a median OS of 8 months with placebo (HR, 0.76; 95% CI, 0.63–0.92; $P = .005$). Median PFS, which was the secondary end point, was superior for cabozantinib over placebo, 5.2 vs 1.9 months (HR, 0.44; 95% CI, 0.36–0.52; $P < .001$). Subgroup analysis showed favorable outcomes with cabozantinib across various etiologic and demographic factors. In the subgroup of patients who received sorafenib as the only prior systemic therapy, median OS was 11.3 months with cabozantinib and 7.2 months with placebo (HR, 0.70; 95% CI, 0.55–0.88). Most common clinically relevant grade 3 or 4 adverse events observed on the cabozantinib arm included palmar-plantar erythrodysesthesia (17%), hypertension (16%), fatigue (10%), and diarrhea (10%).

Antiangiogenics

Bevacizumab, a humanized anti-VEGF monoclonal IgG antibody, has been investigated extensively in patients with advanced HCC. Bevacizumab was studied as monotherapy in 46 patients with advanced HCC at doses of 5 mg/kg or 10 mg/kg every 2 weeks.[71] Median PFS was 6.9 months, and median survival time was 12.4 months. Grade 3 to 5 hemorrhage occurred in 11% of patients, including one death secondary to a variceal bleed. In the initial phase of this study, of 18 patients accrued, 4 patients discontinued therapy because of serious adverse events, including one transient ischemic attack and three serious esophageal bleeding events. The study was thus modified to screen for and manage esophageal varices before enrollment.[95] Another study evaluating single-agent bevacizumab in HCC showed similar results.[96] Among 24 patients evaluable for response, 3 had PR and 13 had stable disease.

Brivanib, a dual inhibitor of VEGF and FGF, showed some promise when tested in the second-line setting in phase II

trials,[97,98] yet failed in a phase III trial of brivanib versus placebo[99] in the second-line setting post sorafenib progression. A phase III randomized study of brivanib versus sorafenib[100] in patients with advanced HCC and no prior systemic therapy failed to meet its primary end point of OS noninferiority to sorafenib (HR, 1.06; 95.8% CI, 0.93–1.22).

Linifanib is a VEGF and PDGF inhibitor.[101] A phase III study failed to show improvement over sorafenib, with a median OS of 9.1 months for the linifanib-treated cohort versus 9.8 months for the sorafenib arm (HR, 1.046; 95% CI, 0.896–1.221).[102]

Ramucirumab, a monoclonal antibody to VEGFR-2, has shown favorable survival data in treatment-naïve patients on a phase II study[103]; however, a randomized placebo-controlled phase III study of ramucirumab after sorafenib failure did not meet its primary end point of OS.[104] This global phase III trial included 565 patients with advanced HCC, BCLC B or C, Child-Pugh A, have documented disease progression on or after discontinuation of sorafenib, and in need of a second-line treatment. Patients were randomly assigned 1:1 to receive ramucirumab (8 mg/kg intravenously [IV]) or placebo every 2 weeks. The OS HR was 0.866 (95% CI, 0.717–1.046; $P = .1391$); median OS was 9.2 months for ramucirumab versus 7.6 months for placebo. Median PFS with ramucirumab and placebo was 2.8 months and 2.1 months, respectively (HR, 0.63; 95% CI, 0.52–0.75; $P < .0001$). In a selected population of 250 patients with baseline AFP greater than or equal to 400 ng/mL (prespecified), OS HR was 0.67 (95% CI, 0.51–0.90; $P = .0059$), with median OS of 7.8 months for ramucirumab versus 4.2 months for placebo, a finding the authors felt warranted further investigation. This led to further exploration of ramucirumab in patients with AFP greater than or equal to 400 ng/ml (REACH2 study).[105] The study randomized 292 patients to receive ramucirumab versus placebo. At a median follow-up of 7.6 months, median OS was in favor of ramucirumab 8.5 months ([95% CI, 7.0–10.6] vs. 7.3 months [5.4–9.1]; HR, 0.710 [95% CI, 0.531–0.949]; $P = .0199$) and PFS was 2.8 months ([2.8–4.1] vs. 1.6 months [1.5–2.7]; (0.452 [0.339–0.603]; $P < .0001$).

The 10-month median OS shown in numerous studies for patients given sorafenib established a ceiling for single-agent antiangiogenic therapy. Newer strategies were badly needed. This started with an effort to tailor treatment for patients with HCC based on disease etiology, ethnic origin, and the molecular profile of individual cancers. While the clinical community explores new approaches for the treatment of advanced HCC, it seems that the inhibition of angiogenesis solely has limitations and that an improved understanding of molecular differences between individual patients with HCC will be needed to advance patient outcomes beyond this approach.[106]

ARGININE METABOLISM

The biosynthesis of arginine depends on the enzymes argininosuccinate synthetase and argininosuccinate lyase. A subset of HCC lacks argininosuccinate synthetase and extract arginine from the circulation.[107] Pegylated arginine deiminase (ADI-PEG 20), an arginine-degrading enzyme, decreases HCC cell viability in vitro and depletes arginine levels and prolongs survival in vivo. ADI-PEG 20 has been evaluated in phase I/II studies[108–110] with mixed yet rather promising results. A randomized phase III study of ADI-PEG 20 versus placebo for advanced HCC patients who have not responded to prior systemic treatment followed.[111] The study included 635 patients with confirmed HCC, who progressed on (70%) or were intolerant to sorafenib (16%). Median OS was 7.8 months for ADI-PEG 20 versus 7.4 for placebo ($P = .88$; HR = 1.02) and median PFS was 2.6 months versus 2.6 ($P = .07$; HR = 1.17).

IMMUNOTHERAPY

One of the first attempts at using immunotherapy was IFN-α2b in a Gastrointestinal Tumor Study Group (GITSG) trial that showed a limited RR of 7%.[112] Several mechanisms of immune escape have been identified in HCC and seem to confer a worse prognosis with a higher likelihood of metastatic disease[113] (see Chapter 10). Early clinical data have demonstrated that immune checkpoint blockade with tremelimumab, a monoclonal antibody to cytotoxic T-lymphocyte antigen-4 (CTLA-4), exerts an antitumor activity in patients with heavily pretreated unresectable and metastatic hepatitis C–related HCC.[114] Tremelimumab at a dose of 15 mg/kg IV every 90 days was administered until tumor progression or severe toxicity. Twenty patients were assessed for toxicity and viral response, and 17 were assessed for tumor response. Most patients were in the advanced stage, and 43% had an altered liver function (Child-Pugh class B). A good safety profile was recorded. A favorable ORR of 17.6% was achieved, and disease control rate (DCR) was 76.4%. TTP was 6.48 months (95% CI, 3.95–9.14). A significant drop in viral load was observed while new emerging variants of the hypervariable region 1 of HCV replaced the predominant variants present before therapy, particularly in patients with a more prominent drop in viral load. This antiviral effect was associated with an enhanced specific anti-HCV immune response.

Preclinical data have suggested that program death receptor-1 (PD-1) and program death receptor-1 ligand (PDL-1) can suppress HCC growth,[115] and, subsequently, several studies investigated these agents in HCC as monotherapy and in various combination.

Preliminary data from a multi-arm expansion study of MEDI4736 (later named durvalumab), an anti–PDL-1 antibody, in patients with advanced solid tumors, including HCC, have shown promise.[116] Nivolumab is a PD-1 receptor inhibitor. A phase I/II study, CheckMate 040,[117] showed that patients receiving nivolumab had a durable ORR of 20% and a relatively favorable safety profile; 91% of responders had a response to therapy that lasted 6 months and 55% of responders had a response that lasted 12 months. A randomized, multicenter, phase III study, CheckMate 459[118] followed. Patients were randomized to receive nivolumab or standard of care sorafenib as first-line treatment. The primary end point of OS was not met. Nivolumab-treated patients had a median OS of 16.4 months versus 14.7 months for the sorafenib-treated patients (HR, 0.85; 95% CI, 0.72–1.02; $P = .0752$). Nivolumab therapy was associated with a higher ORR of 15% compared with 7% with sorafenib. Treatment-related grade 3 to 4 adverse events were 22% with nivolumab and 49% with sorafenib. Pembrolizumab is another anti–PD-1 monoclonal antibody that was evaluated in a phase II, non-randomized, open-label clinical trial (KEY-NOTE-224) for patients with advanced HCC after first-line therapy.[119] The study demonstrated a median PFS of 4.8 months (95% CI, 3.4–6.6); 6-month PFS and OS rates were

43.1% and 77.9%, respectively. DCR was 62% (95% CI, 52–71), with 77% durable response of 9 months; the median duration of response was not reached (3.1–14.6+ months). These results led to KEYNOTE-240, a phase III trial of pembrolizumab and best supportive care versus placebo and best supportive care.[120] Patients with HCC that progressed on first-line sorafenib were randomized in a 2:1 ratio. The study did not meet both primary end points of OS and PFS. Median OS was 13.9 months (95% CI, 11.6–16.0 months) for pembrolizumab versus 10.6 months (95% CI, 8.3–13.5 months) for placebo (HR, 0.781; 95% CI, 0.611–0.998; $P = .0238$). Median PFS for pembrolizumab was 3.0 months (95% CI, 2.8–4.1 months) versus 2.8 months (95% CI, 1.6–3.0 months) (HR, 0.718; 95% CI, 0.570–0.904; $P = .0022$). These data raised the argument for the limited benefit of checkpoint inhibitors when used as a single agent in HCC.

With the advent of immunotherapy as a cornerstone in HCC treatment, special considerations should be taken in patients who are recipients of liver transplant as they are not routinely included in immunotherapy clinical trials. A single-center experience[121] retrospectively evaluated seven patients with metastatic cancer and history of liver transplant who received immune checkpoint blockade. Two patients developed allograft rejection, which occurred within a median time of 20 days. Caution should be practiced when considering immune checkpoint inhibitors in liver transplant patients, with close monitoring and early initiation of treatment in case signs of rejection are suspected.

Combination Therapies

Combination therapies were in the mindset form the start with the continued urgent need for enhancing survival. These were based on the standard chemotherapeutic combinations, followed by the combination of chemotherapy and biologics, immunotherapy, and mix of such combinations.

Sorafenib has also been evaluated in combination with erlotinib.[122] A randomized phase III study evaluated sorafenib plus erlotinib versus sorafenib alone in patients with advanced HCC. The addition of erlotinib to sorafenib did not significantly prolong OS (9.5 vs. 8.5 months; HR, 0.929; 95% CI, 0.781–1.106; $P = .204$) or TTP (3.2 vs. 4 months; HR, 1.135; 95% CI, 0.944–1.366; $P = .91$).[104]

A randomized phase II study evaluated doxorubicin plus sorafenib versus doxorubicin plus placebo in 96 patients with advanced HCC and Child-Pugh A.[123] The primary end point, median TTP, was 9 months for the doxorubicin and sorafenib arm compared with 5 months for the doxorubicin and placebo arms. An exploratory comparison of OS between the two arms showed a significant difference of 13.7 months in favor of doxorubicin and sorafenib versus 6.5 months for doxorubicin and placebo (HR, 0.45; $P = .0049$). A potential synergistic effect between doxorubicin and sorafenib that may explain the improved outcome was suggested. Anthracyclines (e.g., doxorubicin) depend on apoptosis signal-regulating kinase-1 (ASK-1) in exerting their apoptotic effect. In cancer cells, a basic fibroblast growth factor (bFGF)-mediated activation of rapidly growing fibrosarcoma (protein) (RAF-1), a target of sorafenib, may promote a complex between RAF-1 and ASK-1 at the mitochondria level, leading to inhibition of ASK-1 kinase activity and prevention of stress-mediated apoptosis of anthracyclines. Inhibiting RAF kinase activity with sorafenib may release ASK-1 and restore the apoptotic activity of doxorubicin[124] (Fig. 99.3).

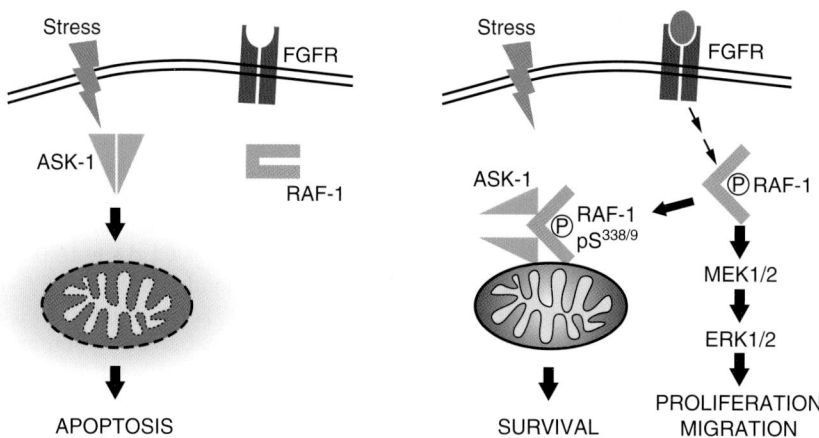

FIGURE 99.3 Role of rapidly growing fibrosarcoma (RAF)-1 in regulation of apoptosis signal-reducing kinase-1 (ASK-1)-mediated apoptosis. At the mitochondria, basic fibroblast growth factor (bFGF)-mediated activation of RAF-1 promotes a complex between RAF-1 and ASK-1, leading to inhibition of ASK-1 kinase activity and prevention of stress-mediated apoptosis. *ERK,* Extracellular signal-regulated kinase; *FGFR,* fibroblast growth factor receptor; *MEK,* mitogen-activated protein kinase/ERK kinase; *P,* phosphorylation; $pS^{338/9}$, phosphorylated $S_{338/9}$ (the active domain). (From Alavi AS, et al. Chemoresistance of endothelial cells induced by basic fibroblast growth factor depends on Raf-1-mediated inhibition of the proapoptotic kinase, ASK1. *Cancer Res.* 67:2766–2772, 2007.) (See Chapter 9C.)

To further explore this hypothesis, CALGB 80802, a large randomized phase III trial evaluating the combination of sorafenib and doxorubicin versus sorafenib alone in the first-line setting, was undertaken.[125] The study included 356 patients with a primary end point of OS. At the planned interim analysis, median OS was 9.3 months (95% CI, 7.3–10.8 months) in the doxorubicin plus sorafenib arm and 9.4 months (95% CI, 7.3–12.9 months) in the sorafenib alone arm (HR, 1.05; 95% CI, 0.83–1.31). The median PFS was 4.0 months (95% CI, 3.4–4.9 months) in the doxorubicin plus sorafenib arm and 3.7 months (95% CI, 2.9–4.5 months) in the sorafenib arm (HR, 0.93; 95% CI, 0.75–1.16. This effort established the lack of benefit from adding doxorubicin to sorafenib.

Several phase II studies have evaluated bevacizumab in combination with cytotoxic chemotherapy,[126–128] with nonencouraging efficacy outcomes on top of bleeding and hemorrhage as the most serious reported adverse events. Bevacizumab has been studied in combination with erlotinib[129] and erlotinib or sorafenib,[130] but this was not pursued further considering limited efficacy and concerning toxicity, including hemorrhage. A phase Ib/II clinical trial[131] explored a combination approach for patients with HCC using the antiangiogenic agent ramucirumab with a MET monoclonal antibody, LY2875358. The dose escalation study included a total of 45 patients with HCC among a total of 97 patients. The best antitumor activity observed on the study was noted in HCC patients with a 6.7% ORR, 60% DCR, and a PFS of 5.42 months (95% CI, 1.64–8.12). Of note, HCC with high MET expression (determined by IHC) showed improved PFS with an approximately 3-fold increase in PFS (8.1 vs. 2.8 months) relative to tumors with low MET expression.

ADI-PEG 20 was explored in combination with other agents, both cytotoxic chemotherapy and sorafenib. After establishing the safety in a phase I study, a phase II trial of ADI-PEG 20 and FOLFOX in patients with HCC was performed.[132] This was an international, single-arm, open-label study.

Similarly, a phase I trial combining ADI-PEG 20 with sorafenib for HCC patients (www.clinicaltrials.gov, NCT02101593) was initiated.

Immunotherapy-Based Combinations

The disappointing low response, coupled with increased toxicity due to the use of high IFN doses, led to testing lower doses in combination with chemotherapy,[133,134] with no reproducible favorable results.[135,136] The preliminary indication of some activity for IFN set the platform for a more intense combination of cisplatin, IFN, doxorubicin, and 5-FU, which became commonly known as PIAF,[46] with negative outcome as detailed above.

COMBINATION OF CHECKPOINT INHIBITORS AND ANTIANGIOGENICS.
There is a potential synergy between antiangiogenic and immune checkpoint pathways. The combination of antiangiogenic therapy and immune checkpoint inhibitors had recently shown clinical efficacy in different tumors.[137] Studies have shown that the tissue hypoxia induced by antiangiogenics may lead to up-regulation of immune checkpoint protein PDL-1, which could potentiate the effects of immunomodulators such as PD-1/PDL-1 inhibitors. The combination of the PDL-1 antibody atezolizumab and bevacizumab was evaluated as part of a phase III trial (IMbrave150) comparing atezolizumab plus bevacizumab to the standard of care single-agent sorafenib in patients with advanced HCC and no prior systemic therapy.[138] This was an open-label phase III study of 501 patients randomized 2:1 to receive atezolizumab 1200 mg and bevacizumab 15 mg/kg every 3 weeks versus sorafenib at the standard dose. Eligible patients had HCC proven either by histology or clinical features according to the American Association for the Study of Liver Diseases (AASLD) criteria, ECOG performance status of 0 or 1, and Child-Pugh score of A. Importantly, patients with autoimmune diseases, coinfection with HCV and HBV, and untreated esophageal varices were excluded. the coprimary end points were OS and PFS. The median follow-up was 8.6 months. OS was significantly longer with atezolizumab–bevacizumab; the 6-months and 12-months OSs were 84.8% (95% CI, 80.9–88.7) and 67.2% (95% CI, 61.3–73.1), respectively, in the atezolizumab–bevacizumab group and 72.2% (95% CI, 65.1–79.4) and 54.6% (95% CI, 45.2–64.0) in the sorafenib group. Median OS for sorafenib was 13.2 months and was not reached for the combination arm (HR, 0.58; 95% CI, 0.42–0.79; *P* < .001). PFS was

improved from 4.3 months with sorafenib to 6.8 months for atezolizumab and bevacizumab (HR, 0.59; CI, 0.47–0.76; $P < .0001$). The ORR reached 27% in the investigational arm versus 12% with sorafenib ($P < .0001$) per RECIST1.1, and 18 patients (5.5%) in the investigational arm had a CR. Serious adverse events occurred more frequently with the atezolizumab–bevacizumab combination compared with sorafenib. The most common grade 3 or 4 adverse event with the combination was hypertension (15%).

COMBINATION OF CHECKPOINT INHIBITORS AND TYROSINE KINASE INHIBITORS. The combination of immune checkpoint blockade and tyrosine kinase inhibitors was evaluated in several solid tumors. The pembrolizumab and lenvatinib combination was initially studied in an open-label phase 1b trial (KEYNOTE-524).[139] Thirty patients with unresectable HCC, BCLC stage C or B not amenable to local therapy, Child-Pugh A liver function, and ECOG performance status of 0 or 1 were included. No patients experienced dose-limiting toxicities. The most common adverse events were decreased appetite and hypertension. The expansion part of the study evaluated both safety and tolerability as primary outcomes and efficacy (as defined by ORR and PFS) using mRECIST criteria as a secondary outcome. The combination therapy showed a favorable safety profile and a historically high ORR of 50% by mRECIST and independent imaging review with a significantly durable response. Duration of response reached 18.7 months. These promising results led to an ongoing phase III trial (LEAP-002) currently testing the use of the pembrolizumab and lenvatinib combination compared with single-agent lenvatinib as front line treatment in patients with advanced HCC (www.clinicaltrials.gov NCT03713593).

MOLECULAR PROFILING AND RESPONSE TO THERAPY (SEE CHAPTERS 9B AND 9C)

In a subgroup analysis of the SHARP trial, it was noted that patients with hepatitis C–related HCC (see Chapter 68) when treated with sorafenib ($n = 93$) had a median survival advantage of 14 months compared with the entire sorafenib-treated group of 10.7 months.[140] This led to a suggestion of a possible positive influence of hepatitis C status on the efficacy of sorafenib. The placebo-controlled hepatitis C group did not have any added survival advantage to the placebo population of the study, proving the lack of any advantage brought on by the HCV itself. Of note, in HCV infection, the virus core proteins result in high basal activity of RAF-1, which itself leads to a sustained response to EGF by hepatocytes, resulting in an increased possibility of neoplastic transformation.[141] A similar observation was noted in a retrospective analysis of the phase II trial evaluating sorafenib in patients with advanced HCC.[66] In this analysis, it was noted that patients who were infected with HCV but not HBV ($n = 13$) had a longer TTP of 6.5 months compared with 4 months ($P = .05$), respectively, for patients infected with HBV ($n = 33$).[142] A similar trend for survival advantage ($P = .29$) for hepatitis C (12.4 months) versus hepatitis B patients (7.3 months) was noted. In contrast, 73% of patients accrued on the Asia-Pacific study had hepatitis B as the underlying etiologic driver for their developed HCC, compared with only 18% of patients in the SHARP trial. This difference in HCC etiology may offer another explanation, or at least a complementary one for the difference in the outcome

magnitude between the two studies. Patients with HBV in the SHARP trial seemed to have similar survival outcomes as the rest of the randomly assigned population. This observation does undermine somewhat the antiangiogenic effect of sorafenib, which remains indicated for all patients with unresectable HCC, irrespective of the etiology of their tumor.

Median OS was similar among Asian (7.7 vs. 8.8 months; HR, 1.21; one-sided $P = .9829$) and hepatitis B–infected patients (7.6 vs. 8 months; HR, 1.10; one-sided $P = .8286$), but was shorter with sunitinib in hepatitis C–infected patients (9.2 vs. 17.6 months; HR, 1.52; one-sided $P = .9835$).[84]

Etiologic-dependent genomic differences in HCC have been observed in several molecular studies[143-145] (see Chapters 9B and 9C). Activating *CTNNB1* mutations are more common in HCV-related HCC compared with HBV-related HCC, and these mutations are associated with a particular *WNT* gene expression profile.[146,147] Sorafenib modulates this transcriptomic signature and leads to HCC growth suppression in preclinical models. HCV has also been shown to upregulate Raf-1, a known sorafenib target.[141] In vitro data have suggested that sorafenib inhibits HCV viral replication directly.[148] Thus it is plausible that patient outcomes with sorafenib and potentially other therapies might be dependent on the specific factors that lead to the development of HCC. However, this has not been proved so far, and all available therapies described previously showed improvement in outcome irrespective of etiologic factors. In a recent report of next-generation sequencing (NGS) in HCC,[149] the predictive effect of oncogenic pathways on response to therapy was observed. A total of 127 tumors were sequenced through a hybridization capture-based NGS assay. The oncogenic PI3K–mTOR pathway alterations were associated with lower DCR (8.3% vs. 40.2%), shorter median PFS (1.9 vs. 5.3 months), and shorter median OS (10.4 vs. 17.9 months) in patients ($n = 81$) treated with sorafenib. For 31 patients receiving immunotherapy, activating alteration in WNT/β-catenin signaling pathway was associated with lower DCR (0% vs. 53%), shorter median PFS (2.0 vs. 7.4 months), and shorter median OS (9.1 vs. 15.2 months). In this study, 24% of patients harbored potentially actionable genetic alterations (FGF19 and MET amplifications). Similarly, other investigators demonstrated that HCC tumors escape the immune system by upregulating β-catenin (CTNNB1) pathway in mouse models. β-Catenin-driven tumors were resistant to anti–PD-1 therapy.[150] However, HCC is a complex occurrence involving genetic, host, and environmental factors.[151] Several steps are concerned in the process from cirrhosis to HCC. Telomere and telomerases are involved in this process and TERT alterations are the most frequent in HCC. It seems that in normal hepatocytes, CTNNB1 activating mutations are involved in tumorigenesis. Genomic profiling enabled a proposal of two major molecular clusters: proliferation, enriched with RAS/MAPK, MET, AKT/MTOR pathway activation and a more aggressive tumor phenotype, and nonproliferation, more enriched with the classic WNT pathway. The predictive value of such classification is yet to be defined.

Tumor suppressor gene TP53 is commonly mutated in HCC. It was shown[152] that HCC patients with TP53 mutations had a shorter OS compared with patients with wild-type TP53 (HR, 1.86; 95% CI, 1.37–2.52; $P < .001$).

In 2004 Lee et al.[153] evaluated the possibility of identifying distinct HCC subtypes. Two different subclasses were identified with different survival outcomes based on gene expression signatures. Cell proliferation markers like proliferating cell nuclear antigen (PCNA); cell cycle regulators such as CDK4, CCNB1, CCNA2, and CKS2; and antiapoptotic genes were more expressed in the poor survival subclass. Furthermore, investigators looked at HCC cases to differentiate molecular signature based on etiology.[154] Genetic expression patterns in HBV-related HCC were different from those with HCV as underlying etiology. CYP2E, AKR1C4, EPHX1, and FMO3 enzymes are known to convert several procarcinogens to activated metabolites and were exclusively expressed in HCV cases. Expression of detoxification enzymes UGT1A1, UGT2B10, and GPX2 was preferential in HBV-related HCC.

The presumptions that such alterations may occur half-hazard, may occur later as the disease evolves, and are not etiology driven are worth investigating further.

NEOADJUVANT AND CONVERSION THERAPY

Conversion therapy as a concept may render some unresectable tumors surgically approachable and may also contribute to better outcome by possibly eradicating microscopic local and systemic disease. This is different from neoadjuvant therapy, which is given to patients considered resectable a priori. Different modalities have been studied in the context of conversion therapy for HCC, but none thus far has been shown to add any survival benefit over surgery alone. Bridging to transplant may be contemplated under the same umbrella, in view of the goal of maintaining or reducing a tumor size to fit within the transplant criteria, for instance, Milan criteria.[155] Recently, a retrospective study looked at the role of radioembolization with yttrium-90 (Y-90) microspheres for patients before liver transplant[156] (see Chapter 94B). Twenty-two patients were treated with Y-90 before liver transplant, 19 of whom were outside of the Milan criteria. Downstaging was observed in 80% of cases. Survival was not different among patients who received Y-90 and those who did not.

Transarterial chemoembolization (TACE) has been evaluated in multiple randomized studies (see Chapter 94A). A randomized trial of one to five TACE applications before surgery (24 patients) versus surgery alone (28 patients) did not confer a benefit as neoadjuvant therapy.[157] TACE had no effect on 33% of the patients who had the intervention, and they either remained with stable disease or experienced progression. No difference was found between the two groups in operative morbidity or mortality rates and pathology staging. The disease-free survival (DFS) rate in the two groups was similar, but the incidence of extrahepatic cancer recurrence was higher in the neoadjuvant group (57% vs. 23%, $P = .03$), and 5-year survival was also significantly worse in the TACE group (30% vs. 60%, $P = .01$).

The experience with transarterial embolization (TAE; without chemotherapy) has not proven any different. In a study that randomly assigned 97 patients to TAE plus surgery versus surgery alone, despite an increased rate of necrosis in the TAE group, the DFS rate did not differ between the two groups (39 vs. 31.1).[158] The experience with Y-90 TheraSpheres (Theragenics, Buford, GA) in the treatment of locally advanced HCC continues to expand[159] (see Chapter 94B).

Chemotherapy-based clinical trials in the conversion therapy setting have lagged in view of the discouraging RRs seen in the advanced-disease setting. This has changed somewhat with the use of the more intense chemoimmunotherapy combination

of cisplatin, IFN, doxorubicin, and 5-FU, also known as PIAF.[46] In the phase II study discussed earlier, of 50 patients with unresectable HCC, 13 (26%) had a PR.[47] Of those 13 patients, 9 (18%) underwent surgical resection, and 4 had a pathologic CR, that is, no viable tumor at surgery. PIAF, however, did not stand the test of a randomized phase III trial[48] versus doxorubicin in the advanced-disease setting. It is important to recall that the PIAF combination carries substantial treatment-related morbidity and mortality. The majority of these excellent-performance status patients had grade 3 or higher hematologic toxicity, and two deaths occurred secondary to neutropenic sepsis. The role of PIAF may therefore be limited to those very thoroughly reviewed cases in a multidisciplinary clinic more so with now currently available alternative approaches.

ADJUVANT THERAPY

Despite the advancements in surgical techniques during the last decade, a high proportion of patients with resected HCC will have recurrence of their disease.[160] In one published series, the recurrence rate after surgical resection was 55% after 26 months' follow-up[161] (see Chapter 101). The experience with liver transplantation has been better, with lower recurrence rates; however, this is a nonrandomized comparison, and transplant patients are more carefully selected and in general have a lower volume of disease[155] (see Chapter 108A). Although liver transplantation eliminates the cirrhotic fertile ground for recurrence,[162] it unfortunately cannot address the need of every individual patient with HCC, because of the limited supply of organs and because of its limited efficacy in anything other than small tumors. Thus the question of adjuvant therapy to reduce the risk of recurrence after surgical resection is important and pressing.

Previously, the lack of active systemic chemotherapy for advanced HCC generally precluded serious consideration of the use of chemotherapy in the adjuvant setting. One very small, randomized study investigated oral carmofur (1-hexylcarbamoyl-5-fluorouracil) versus observation.[163] The study randomized and stratified 67 patients based on their Liver Cancer Study Group Japan staging.[81] The regimen was poorly tolerated and offered no survival advantage for either stage I or II disease. DFS for the stage I patients showed a tangible advantage of 60% versus 30% at 3 years and 50% versus 20% at 5 years ($P = .04$). This trial was suspended prematurely because 56% of the treated patients had unacceptable side effects.

Hepatic arterial chemotherapy, with or without systemic chemotherapy, has also been used in the adjuvant HCC setting (see Chapter 97). An underpowered randomized study combined hepatic arterial epirubicin and systemic epirubicin and carmofur versus no further therapy[164] and showed no survival or DFS benefit. Side effects again led to the discontinuation of therapy in 21% of randomly assigned patients. In addition, a randomized trial of hepatic artery epirubicin versus the same therapy plus oral tegafur showed no difference in survival or rate of recurrence between the two groups.[165] There was no difference in side effects between the two study arms.

TACE, as opposed to bland embolization or simply TAE, was tested in the adjuvant setting (see Chapter 94A). An improvement in DFS was reported in a randomized study of a bolus HAI of Lipiodol containing doxorubicin and mitomycin C versus no adjuvant therapy after surgical resection

(32% vs. 12% at 3 years, $P = .02$).[166] There was, however, no survival advantage reported. Another trial randomly assigned patients to hepatic artery emulsion of iodized oil with cisplatin and IV epirubicin.[167] This trial showed a worse DFS in the treatment group at 3 years (18% vs. 48%, $P = .04$). A third study of TACE versus observation postsurgical resection was able to show a survival advantage in patients defined at risk for residual tumor and thus recurrence.[168] These risk factors included tumor diameter greater than 5 cm, multiple nodules, and vascular invasion. Five-year survival was 44.36% in the adjuvant TACE group versus 37.40% in the control group ($P = .0216$).

More promising data in the adjuvant setting come from the use of transarterial iodine-131 Lipiodol.[169] In a randomized phase II trial that evaluated transarterial ^{131}I-Lipiodol versus no adjuvant therapy postsurgical resection, there was an improvement in DFS in favor of the adjuvant therapy arm of 74% versus 36% ($P = .037$). Three-year OS also improved, occurring in 85% of the treatment group versus 46% of the control group ($P = .039$). A recent update showed the actuarial 5-year DFS in the treatment and control groups to be 61.9% and 31.8%, respectively ($P = .0397$). The actuarial 5-year OS in the treatment and control groups was 66.7% and 36.4%, respectively ($P = .0433$). However, after the seventh year from randomization, the DFS and OS benefits lost their statistical significance.[170] Of note, ^{131}I-Lipiodol is not available in the United States.

Immune modulators have also been tested in the adjuvant setting. These included an attempt at infusing autologous lymphocytes that were cultured with interleukin (IL)-2 and antibodies to CD-3 versus no therapy,[171] HAI of doxorubicin and IL-2 plus an infusion of lymphokine-activated killer (LAK) cells versus hepatic arterial doxorubicin,[172] oral acyclic retinoids versus placebo,[173] and IFN-α versus no therapy.[174] None of those studies reported a survival advantage, except for the retinoid study that showed a survival benefit on further follow-up and 2 years after the study was originally reported.[175] Six-year survival was 74% in the acyclic retinoid group versus 46% in the placebo group ($P = .04$).

Active immunization has also been evaluated in the adjuvant setting for HCC. An HCC vaccine consisting of autologous formalin-fixed tumor (vaccine) tissue fragments (AFTV), biodegradable microparticles containing human granulocyte-macrophage colony-stimulating factor, human IL-2, and tuberculin was tested in a small, randomized trial.[176] Nineteen patients received three intradermal vaccinations at 2-week intervals, beginning 4 to 6 weeks after hepatic resection, whereas 22 patients received no further therapy after surgical resection. In a median follow-up of 15 months, the risk of recurrence in the vaccinated patients was reduced by 81% ($P = .003$). Vaccination significantly prolonged OS by 89% ($P = .01$). AFTV was most effective in preventing recurrence in patients with small tumors. Twelve vaccinated patients showed a positive delayed-type hypersensitivity response, and 92% of those patients were recurrence free at the end of the trial. Adverse effects were limited to grade 1 or 2 skin toxicities, such as erythema, dry desquamation, and pruritus. Again, this is a very small trial that is intriguing, but larger confirmatory data will be required before we can fully assess the merits of this approach.

A more aggressive approach was attempted in a very small pilot study on five patients who, after receiving an orthotopic liver transplant (OLT) for HCC, received a nonmyeloablative preparative regimen of fludarabine combined with total-body irradiation or cyclophosphamide, followed by allogeneic peripheral blood allogenic stem cell transplant (PSCT), which was performed 16 to 135 days after OLT with human leukocyte antigen–matched donors.[177] The aim of the study was to see if a stable mixed donor chimerism could be sustained. This was observed in one of two patients with HCC on the study. Chimerism analysis 36 days post-PSCT showed 100% donor T cells and 90% donor myeloid cells in peripheral blood. This patient was reportedly doing well, albeit with only 10 months follow-up after OLT.

As in other solid-tumor malignancies, when success of a drug is established in the metastatic setting, there is often a move to test for the same approach in adjuvant cases. This was indeed the case for sorafenib. In a multinational phase III trial, 1114 patients with HCC who had undergone surgical resection or locoregional therapy with curative intent were randomly assigned to sorafenib versus placebo. The primary end point of the study of recurrence-free survival (RFS) was not met.[178] Of the 1114 patients enrolled, 81% had resection, 97% were Child-Pugh A, and 46% had a high recurrence risk. The analysis was based on a total of 464 RFS events. No differences in RFS, time to recurrence, and OS were observed. RFS was 33.4 months for the sorafenib group compared with 33.8 months in those patients treated with placebo (HR, 0.940; 95% CI, 0.780–1.134; $P = .26$).

Investigators have used almost every therapeutic modality in a collaborative effort to reduce the risk of recurrence of HCC after surgical resection or transplantation. Although there have been some rare positive outcomes reported, the majority were either part of a very small series or lacked the statistical power to show true evidence of a survival advantage. A phase III randomized trial is currently exploring the role of nivolumab therapy in the adjuvant setting, in patients after curative resection of HCC (www.clinicaltrials.gov, NCT03383458). Until these issues and many others, such as the molecular predictors of recurrence, are answered or identified, there is no standard adjuvant therapy for resected HCC, and adjuvant treatment outside of a clinical trial cannot be supported by available data at this time.

COMBINING LOCAL AND SYSTEMIC THERAPIES

The combination of systemic antiangiogenic therapy and locoregional therapies such as TACE (see Chapter 94A) for the treatment of unresectable HCC is the subject of several ongoing clinical trials. The efficacy and optimal timing of antiangiogenic therapy given in combination with TACE has yet to be established.[179,180] Three approaches have been proposed: a sequential approach, in which TACE is completed and then followed by antiangiogenic therapy; the interrupted approach, in which antiangiogenic therapy is given throughout and only temporarily interrupted around the time of TACE; and the continuous approach, with administration of antiangiogenic therapy intended to inhibit the surge of VEGF that occurs immediately after embolization.[180] Although there is much interest in this combined approach, two randomized studies have failed to show a clinically meaningful improvement in outcome when TACE has been combined with sorafenib. A phase III study examining the sequential approach of sorafenib after TACE in Japanese and Korean patients with unresectable HCC failed to demonstrate prolongation of TTP when sorafenib was administered after TACE. Greater than 50% of patients in the experimental arm started sorafenib more than 9 weeks after TACE, with 73% of the patients requiring dose reduction. The authors concluded that these factors may have influenced the results of their study. Regardless, the findings do not support the use of sequential treatment.[181] A multi-center randomized phase II trial (TACTICS trial) explored TACE with or without sorafenib in 156 patients with unresectable HCC.[182] The primary end point was PFS defined by "time to unTACEable progression," which means that intrahepatic new lesion was not considered tumor progression as long as is amenable to TACE. The addition of sorafenib to TACE translated into a PFS of 25.2 months versus 13.5 months with TACE alone ($P = .006$). The observed PFS advantage in this study cannot be interpreted without taking into consideration that disease progression within the liver was not considered a progression as defined by the study end point. The OS was not evaluable because the number for events was not reached.

The randomized phase II SPACE study evaluated TACE with doxorubicin-eluting beads (DEBDOX) in combination with sorafenib or placebo administered 3 to 7 days before TACE and given continuously. The primary end point, median TTP determined by independent reviewers, was nearly identical in the two arms: 169 days with sorafenib versus 166 days with placebo, although the study of 0.15 (HR, 0.797; 95% CI, 0.588–1.080; $P = .072$). There was no difference in OS (HR, 0.898; 95% CI, 0.606–1.330; $P = .295$).[183]

Recently the ECOG 1208 phase III study evaluating the use of chemoembolization with or without sorafenib (TACE 2 weeks after commencement of sorafenib/placebo) has been stopped because of poor accrual (www.clinicaltrials.gov, NCT01004978). A phase III study of similar design is recruiting patients in the United Kingdom: TACE with DEBDOX performed 2 to 5 weeks after commencing sorafenib or placebo (www.clinicaltrials.gov, NCT01324076).

It is important to note that the combination of local and systemic therapy, although not proven yet as a treatment option in the setting of locally advanced disease, is not justified for use in the metastatic setting. A retrospective analysis of 243 HCC patients treated with hepatic arterial embolization (HAE) at MSKCC during a 7-year period identified 36 patients with metastatic disease on initial diagnosis.[184] Of these, 22 received embolization only, whereas 14 received HAE plus systemic therapy at some time during their whole treatment course. The analysis demonstrated that those patients with metastatic HCC who underwent HAE alone had a median OS of 5.8 months (95% CI, 4.1–11.0), whereas those who received sorafenib with HAE had a median OS of 19.3 months (95% CI, 3.7–66.7). These data suggest that there may be a survival benefit in patients with metastatic HCC treated with transarterial therapies added to systemic therapy that is given at some time during their whole treatment course. A retrospective study compared the safety and efficacy of TACE/TAE compared with HAI using oxaliplatin and 5-FU.[185] Chemotherapy was infused for 3 days every 4 weeks and 46 patients were identified. Median OS was 20.8 months in the HAI chemotherapy group versus 4.0 months in the TACE/TAE group ($P < .001$; HR, 0.17). The HAI group showed higher tumor RRs than the TACE/TAE group (59.1% vs. 22.7%; $P = .014$) and a longer median PFS (9.6 vs. 1.5 months; $P < .001$; HR, 0.09). Understandably, these results should be interpreted cautiously due to the retrospective nature of the study. A phase III open-label randomized controlled trial compared sorafenib alone to sorafenib combined with HAI chemotherapy (SoraHAIC) with FOLFOX administered over 2 days every 3 weeks.[186] 247 patients with locally advanced HCC with confirmed PV invasion were randomized. Median OS was 13.37 months (95% CI, 10.27–16.46) in the SoraHAIC group versus 7.13 months (95% CI, 6.28–7.98) with sorafenib alone (HR, 0.35; 95% CI, 0.26–0.48; $P < .001$). RR was higher in the combination arm, (40.8% vs. 32.46%; $P < .001$). Median PFS was also in favor of the SoraHAIC combination (7.03 [95% CI, 6.05–8.02] vs. 2.6 [95% CI, 2.15–3.05] months; $P < .001$). Grade 3 and 4 adverse events more frequent in the SoraHAIC group included cytopenia and vomiting.

Several studies of combined modality therapy in the setting of locally advanced HCC using modern approaches are currently ongoing.

CONCLUSION

The incidence of HCC is on the rise, especially in developed countries, primarily due to an increased incidence of NASH.[1] Treating HCC implies the understanding and management of both the underlying cirrhosis and the cancer itself. A detailed and thorough understanding of the underlying cirrhosis is imperative as part of understanding the status of the disease and to help identify the appropriate therapies that a physician might recommend.

Other novel therapies and combinations of biologics and chemotherapies continue to be evaluated in advanced HCC and results are awaited. With such a major shift in treatment paradigm the most pressing clinical question remains how to better sequence these available therapies in a patient with HCC. Since sorafenib, the rapid advent of other therapies added lenvatinib as first-line therapy; regorafenib, ramucirumab, nivolumab, pembrolizumab and most recently the ipilimumab/nivolumab combination as second-line therapy; plus cabozantinib as second- and third-line therapy. Atezolizumab plus bevacizumab as first-line therapy, one of many other potential combinations, is disruptive and would pause question about the true and applicable sequences of all those therapies. With this change, will subsequent therapies be moved one step down the line, or will what is currently called first- and second-line options, such as sorafenib, lenvatinib, and cabozantinib, become one mix to pick from? It is clear now that the field is heading toward the combination strategy for eligible patients; however, only time will tell if eventually the long-term outcomes are truly superior compared with sequencing therapies. Data from modern studies will further inform clinicians about potential correlation between etiology (such as HBV, HCV, or NASH), ethnicity, and disease characteristics (portal vein involvement, pattern of metastasis) with outcomes and subsequently which patient will benefit from which combination. Predictive genetic biomarkers are needed to tailor therapy and understand the role for more genetic-targeted approaches. NGS of HCC tumor biopsies should be performed universally and preferably at different times to detect targetable alterations and mechanisms of resistance. Liquid biopsies and measuring circulating tumor DNA might provide the solution for serial genetic testing once this approach is validated.

Finding a better therapy for advanced HCC does not mean only developing better therapeutics, but also having a superior means of assessing the disease. The infiltrative nature of HCC, the poor margination, and its hypervascularity limit the use and benefit of the standard radiologic techniques such as CT and magnetic resonance imaging (MRI). Newer modalities that evaluate the necrosis and dynamic aspects of the cancer are in development and parallel the investigation of novel biologics in the treatment of HCC.

Thus far, neoadjuvant and adjuvant therapies have failed to be proven effective in HCC, but efforts to improve outcomes are still ongoing. The development of systemic therapy is a critical component when managing patients with advanced HCC. How exactly to strategize an optimal treatment approach for advanced HCC, by combining systemic therapy with locoregional techniques, remains a work in progress.

References are available at expertconsult.com.

CHAPTER 100

Isolated hepatic perfusion for unresectable hepatic metastases

James Francis Pingpank, Jr.

Each year, isolated hepatic metastases from a variety of primary malignancies pose a significant clinical dilemma for tens of thousands of patients (see Chapters 90, 91, and 92). For a small percentage of patients, surgical resection or ablation is effective in controlling clinically apparent disease, but for many patients with colorectal, gastrointestinal neuroendocrine tumors, and ocular melanoma, the number of tumors and volume of affected liver render resection and/or ablation incapable of meaningful disease control. In more selected circumstances, metastases arising from tumors of the breast, skin, and soft tissue can be present solely as hepatic disease, with patient quality of life and survival dictated by the ability to control intrahepatic disease. Since the 1950s, strategies designed to focus chemotherapy solely upon liver metastases have been investigated by many researchers at a limited number of institutions around the world, with sequential improvements in safety and efficacy observed with advances in surgical and catheter-based technology. Isolated hepatic perfusion (IHP) has been developed under a series of clinical trials within institutions with experience in regional therapies to the liver, limb, and lung; approaches share a common goal of focused high-dose treatment to the cancer bearing region of the body, while minimizing systemic drug exposure and toxicity. Regional isolation of drug delivery ensures that unaffected tissue avoids drug exposure and potential associated toxicity via complete separation of the regional and systemic circulation, allowing dose escalation of therapeutic agents, limited largely by the tissue tolerance of the perfused organ or limb. For agents with a sharp dose response curve such as melphalan, improved efficacy manifested via increased tumor response can be observed as the absence of bone marrow and gastrointestinal visceral exposure to a drug, allowing dose escalation into more clinically relevant dose levels. For chemotherapeutic agents more traditionally used in the treatment of metastatic colorectal cancer, IHP with oxaliplatin with or without 5-FU, has demonstrated early-stage clinical activity. Based on its unique vascular anatomy (see Chapter 2), the liver is a favorable site for delivery of regional therapy, as complete control of circulatory inflow and outflow can be readily obtained. Additionally, established tumors in liver derive the majority of blood flow from the arterial tree, while the portal vein is maintained as the primary source of nutrient flow to the hepatic parenchyma, allowing intra-arterial delivery to effectively concentrate drug within tumor bearing areas of the liver. Animal models described by Ridge[1,2] demonstrate nearly 100% of blood delivered to tumors arises from the arterial circulation versus 25% to normal liver. The ability to obtain complete vascular isolation also permits the manipulation of acid-base status of the circuit and the delivery of clinically relevant levels of hyperthermia and/or biologic agents, which would otherwise be too toxic or technically impractical to deliver. Additionally, drugs such as melphalan have greater tumor absorption and efficacy in an acidotic environment, conditions easily obtained within a closed perfusion circuit. For patients with multiple hepatic metastases, the likelihood of additional subclinical disease being present within the liver increases with greater tumor volume, and thus treating the entire diseased organ through regional perfusion strategies allows the targeting of micrometastatic disease within the treated organ.

The initial report detailing the clinical use of IHP was published in 1961 by Robert Ausman from the Roswell Park Cancer Center, describing his experience with both a porcine treatment model along with 5 treated patients.[3] In this brief report, evidence of antitumor efficacy was seen in 2 patients after a 60-minutes perfusion with melphalan. Over the ensuing 2 decades, additional small series examining the utility of prolonged hyperthermic perfusions[4] without drug as well as normothermic perfusions utilizing melphalan[5] or mitomycin-C and 5-FU[6] were described by Skibba (Medical College of Wisconsin) and multiple European groups, respectively. The absence of long-term follow-up and the presence of significant toxicity prevented wide-spread adoption of this approach until interest in the field of regional therapy was reignited in 1992 by Lienhard and Lejeune et al. who reported the successful delivery of a combination of melphalan, tumor necrosis factor (TNF), and interferon-α via hyperthermic isolated limb perfusion in a group of 29 patients with advanced extremity sarcoma or melanoma. Clinical results demonstrated a 90% complete response rate in patients with advanced melanoma along with an 80% limb salvage rate in patients with advanced sarcoma.[7] Of equal or greater significance was the demonstration that meticulous surgical technique could result in effective, near complete vascular isolation, with resultant decrease in out of field drug exposure and associated toxicity. When this increased attention to circuit integrity and leak monitoring was applied to the patients undergoing IHP, a similar decrease in systemic toxicity permitted the more widespread investigation of this clinical approach.

In the United States, a significant effort in the development and refinement of vascular isolation-perfusion techniques was initiated by Fraker and Alexander in the Surgery Branch of the National Cancer Institute. Two initial studies examined the utility of TNF alone[8] and TNF plus melphalan[9] regimens for unresectable hepatic metastases in separate phase I, dose escalation trials. TNF alone was associated with coagulopathy at a maximally tolerated dose of 1.5 mg, with minimal antitumor effects. A subsequent trial included alternating dose escalation of TNF and melphalan, establishing maximum tolerated doses of 1.0 mg and 1.5 mg/kg, respectively. This regimen also demonstrated an overall response rate of 75% in patients with unresectable hepatic metastases. Ultimately, TNF was dropped from the treatment regimen when its lack of clear clinical benefit led to its removal from the US market, but the encouraging early results led to IRB approved protocols examining the clinical benefit of melphalan as a single agent administered over a 60-minutes hyperthermic, acidotic perfusion. Subsequently, two sequential studies completed at the University of Pittsburgh have detailed the safe utilization and maximally tolerated doses of oxaliplatin alone[10] and in combination with 5-FU[11] within the 60-minutes IHP circuit.

SURGICAL TECHNIQUE

Preoperative evaluation of patients thought suitable for IHP should include an assessment of the patients overall cardiovascular risk factors, the extent of both intra and extrahepatic tumor malignancy, and an assessment of the liver functional status. Standard preoperative cardiac clearance should include a treadmill stress test, as the induction of veno-venous bypass can lead to the induction of atrial fibrillation in patients so disposed. Hepatic reserve is important to assess (see Chapter 4), as the dose limiting toxicity observed in phase I trials was liver based, and more frequent in patients with greater than 50% of hepatic replacement with tumor or a serum bilirubin over 3 mg/dL. For patients with colorectal cancer and a significant chemotherapy history including either oxaliplatin and/or irinotecan, extensive portal inflammation, hepatic congestion or steatohepatitis must be ruled out via biopsy assessment of the uninvolved hepatic parenchyma. In such patients, it is our practice to obtain a preoperative biopsy of the liver to assess for significant steatohepatitis, periportal fibrosis, and/or hepatic venous sinusoidal congestion. Patients who have had extensive

portal or hepatic venous dissection associated with major hepatectomy should be approached with caution.

IHP is performed under general anesthesia via an upper midline incision, with a right subcostal extension once extrahepatic disease is ruled out. In patients whose primary tumor remains in situ, a full midline incision is indicated to facilitate the resection of the primary colon tumor, with a diverting loop ileostomy created for all patients with left colon or rectal cancer. The presence of extrahepatic disease other than periportal lymphadenopathy or primary tumor amenable to complete resection is a contraindication to perfusion.

Preparation of the liver for perfusion includes completion of cholecystectomy, and full mobilization the liver.[12,13] All lateral attachments are taken down so that the vena cava is fully visualized and all retroperitoneal venous tributaries are taken to ensure there will be no leak of chemotherapy from the isolated segment of the retrohepatic IVC. The duodenum is mobilized, and the vena cava is mobilized from the renal veins to the hepatic veins. The right adrenal vein is ligated and divided, but both phrenic veins are preserved. The common hepatic artery is identified and the gastroduodenal artery (GDA) is mobilized from its origin for a length of 2 cm and will serve as the arterial inflow catheterization site. Nodal tissue in the porta hepatis is dissected to allow clamping of the portal structures, with the hepatic artery clamp proximal to the takeoff of the GDA. Minor accessory right and left hepatic vessels may be ligated, but replaced or accessory arteries of a significant size prepared for cannulation along with the GDA. The extent of vascular dissection and liver mobilization is pictured in Fig. 100.1. After completion of dissection, the patient is heparinized to an ACT

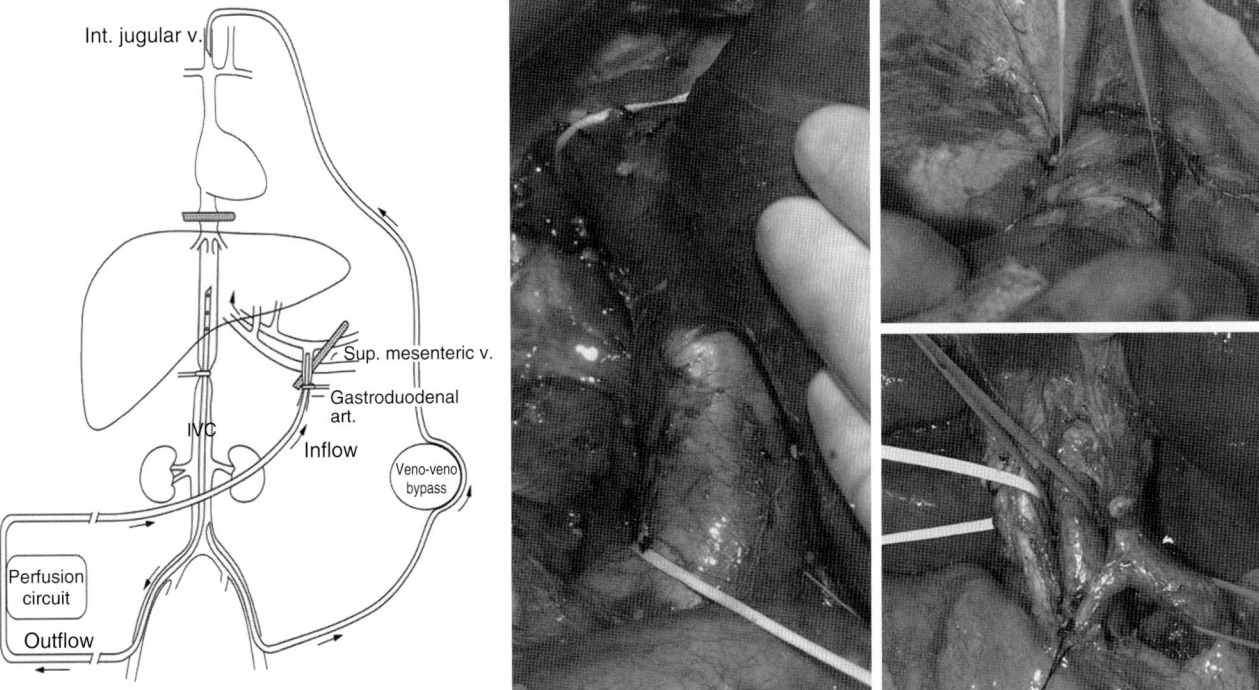

FIGURE. 100.1   Isolated hepatic perfusion (IHP). IHP is accomplished with dual circuits including a veno-venous circuit from the left femoral vein to the right internal jugular vein and a hepatic circuit with inflow via the GDA and outflow through a percutaneously placed IVC catheter collecting the hepatic venous outflow. A complete retro-hepatic dissection, including 360-degree control of the supra-hepatic IVC and completed periportal lymph node dissection and vascular exposure is pictured.

above 400 seconds. An external venovenous bypass circuit is established by placing a cannula into the left femoral vein and advancing it into the infrarenal IVC and then advancing a second cannula through the internal jugular vein into the superior vena cava. This allowed maintenance of the systemic circulation by actively shunting IVC blood during treatment. Once the venous bypass had been established, the IHP circuit is constructed. The GDA is ligated distally. The inflow perfusion cannula for perfusion is positioned in the proximal GDA, and, once secured, a cross clamp was placed across the entire porta hepatis, including the common hepatic artery, bile duct, and portal vein. The perfusion outflow cannula is inserted into the retrohepatic IVC via a percutaneous cannulation of the right femoral vein and a tourniquet is placed around the cannula at the level of the suprarenal infrahepatic IVC. The suprahepatic IVC is then crossclamped, completing the vascular isolation of the liver, and perfusion is initiated. The perfusate consists of approximately 500 mL Ringer's lactate to which 2 units of packed red blood cells are added. Once perfusion is initiated, flow through the isolated circuit is maintained between 400 and 600 mL/min. The routine use of leak monitors has been abandoned as detectable leak is rare in the presence of a stable circuit reservoir,[14] with labile systemic blood pressure or gain/loss in reservoir greater than 100 cc an indication of incomplete liver isolation. Temperature probes are placed into the anatomic right and left lobes of the liver, and the perfusate is heated to maintain hepatic hyperthermia of 40°C. Once hyperthermia is obtained and perfusion parameters are stable, Melphalan (1.5 mg/kg, Ideal Body Weight) is administered into arterial limb of the isolated perfusion circuit over 5 min. The liver is perfused for 1 hour, after which time the circuit is flushed with 2000 cc saline, and 500 cc colloid to flush all chemotherapy from the hepatic vasculature. The portal and suprahepatic IVC clamps are removed allowing native blood-flow to be restored. The GDA is either suture ligated or a hepatic arterial infusion pump is placed. The veno-venous bypass circuit is halted and anticoagulation is reversed with protamine and 2 units of fresh frozen plasma. Once the circuit has been removed, placement of hepatic artery infusion pumps is completed in a standard fashion for patients with colorectal cancer and cholangiocarcinoma. When significant accessory or replaced hepatic vessels are present (see Chapter 2), flow is preserved in the postoperative setting, as the potential ischemia associated with intraoperative ligation is a significant increase in hepatic toxicity. Embolization of accessory or replaced vessels in the interventional radiology suite is performed before discharge, once postperfusion hepatic toxicity has resolved. Postoperative care focuses on the maintenance of normal coagulation profiles and standard fluid resuscitation. Heparin is contra-indicated in the postoperative period as high levels of heparin induced antibodies are common at this time and additional heparin exposure can create an activated thrombotic state.[15] This phenomenon is rare but can lead to devastating consequences if heparin is administered in the early postoperative setting.

Pharmacokinetic analyses performed during early phase IHP trials have demonstrated that complete vascular isolation is routinely achieved, with no detectable levels of melphalan detected in the systemic circulation.[16] A transient significant elevation of aspartate and alanine transaminases was routinely observed but was self-limited and resolved within 7 days. Biliary congestion and cholestatic jaundice are rare when proper patient selection with regard to underlying liver disease

and tumor volume is maintained. Overall operative mortality is 4% across single institution experiences.[13] Operative times and blood loss have decreased with the implementation of less invasive catheterization techniques, with operative times of less than 5 hours and mean operative blood loss less than 500 cc and a length of stay of 4 days.

RESULTS

Colorectal Cancer (see Chapter 90)

The greatest amount of data regarding clinical effectiveness of IHP arise in patients with metastatic colorectal cancer treated at 3 institutions, the Surgery Branch of National Cancer Institute in Bethesda, the Leiden Medical Center in the Netherlands, and the University of Pittsburgh. In a series of 154 patients reported by van Iersel, 105 patients were deemed eligible for IHP at laparotomy. A 50% response rate with a median survival of 11.4 months was reported in treated patients, with improved survival associated with the delivery of adjuvant systemic chemotherapy. The primary site of progressive disease was liver alone (68%) or other organ (18%).[17]

Alexander et al reported a series of 120 patients treated with melphalan based IHP over an 11-year period ending in 2005 at the NCI in Bethesda, MD.[18,19] The majority of patients received melphalan alone ($n = 69$) or in combination with TNF ($n = 41$), with an additional 10 patients receiving TNF alone. The latter small cohort of patients did not appear to show any clinically meaningful benefit from the IHP. Overall, this was a heavily pretreated patient group, with 74 patients having a history of previous systemic or liver directed therapy for their metastatic disease. A median overall survival of 17.4 months was achieved, with a 2-year survival of 34% and an overall response rate of 61%. Five treatment related mortalities were reported, but three of these events were associated with the phase I, dose-escalation portion of the program. A multivariate analysis of factors associated with hepatic progression-free and overall survival demonstrated that a preop CEA <30 ng/mL and the ability to successfully administer postoperative hepatic artery infusion (HAI) therapy with FUdR (see Chapter 97) were associated with significant gains in both outcomes. Of interest, neither response rate nor duration of survival were impacted negatively by a history of previous chemotherapy, contrary to observations made in other second-line approaches. Fig. 100.2 demonstrates the impact of IHP (melphalan) and HAI FUdR for patients with unresectable liver metastases treated with liver perfusion, HAI pump placement, and resection of the primary tumor after being deemed refractory to systemic chemotherapy.

Zeh and Bartlett published a phase I dose escalation trial examining the use of oxaliplatin administered via the IHP circuit with dosing based upon ideal body weight. Dose limiting hepatic veno-occlusive disease was noted at 60 mg/m², establishing the maximally tolerated dose of 40 mg/m², a dose at which minimal hepatic toxicity was observed.[10] Although only 10 patients were included in this report, the Response Evaluation Criteria in Solid Tumours (RECIST) based assessment of overall response at 6 months was 66%. A subsequent phase I dose escalation trial examined the use of oxaliplatin and 5-FU in combination within the IHP circuit, revealing the potential for increased response rates and prolonged disease control in patients with metastatic colorectal cancer.[20]

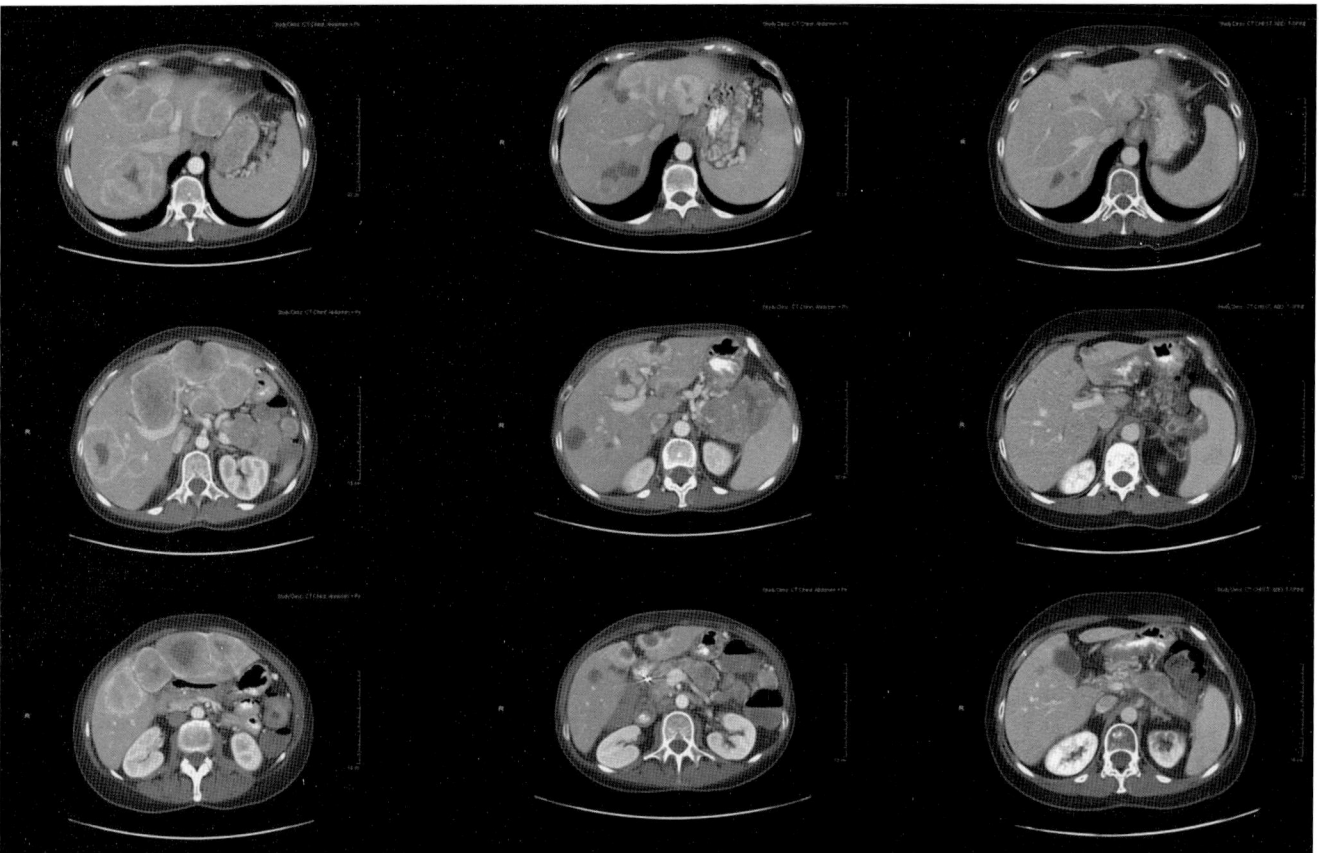

FIGURE 100.2   Response to IHP and hepatic artery infusion (HAI) FUdR. Baseline (pre-IHP) CT scan of a patient with metastatic colon cancer to the liver refractory to systemic chemotherapy pictured on right, 6 weeks after IHP with Melphalan *(middle column)*, and 6 months after HAI FUdR and systemic chemotherapy (see Chapter 15).

Ocular Melanoma (see Chapter 92)

Ocular melanoma has a unique ability to metastasize to the liver in the absence of clinically apparent extrahepatic disease, with liver failure being a significant source of mortality in this patient population. Of the approximately 4000 patients who develop ocular melanoma on an annual basis in the United States, nearly 50% will develop metastatic disease, for 80% percent of whom the liver will be the sole or life-limiting site of spread. The Surgery Branch at the NCI group reported an overall response rate of 62%, including a 10% complete response rate, in 29 patients treated with melphalan alone via the IHP circuit.[21] Overall survival for all treated patients 12 months along with a median progression free survival of 8 months. In those patients who achieved a response by RECIST criteria, the median duration of response was 10 months, with the majority (66%) of patients experiencing hepatic progression as the initial site of progressive disease. Recently, a review of the 103 patients treated at the University of Pittsburgh, demonstrated at similar response rate, with 2- and 3-year survival rates of 31% and 21%, respectively.[20] Transient, self-limited grade 3 or 4 toxicity was observed in 19 patients, with no treatment mortalities. Patient selection criteria limited treatment to individuals with less than 50% hepatic replacement with tumor, and elevations in preoperative LDH was observed as a strong predictor of poor outcome.

Several European groups reported similar experiences in cohorts of patients with metastatic ocular melanoma, including Noter and Rizell, both supporting the results of Alexander et al. Noter and colleagues at the Leiden University Medical Center treated 8 patients with a fixed dose of 200 mg melphalan for 60 minutes, reporting a 50% response rate and median progression-free and overall survival of 6.7 and 9.9 months, respectively. Two-year survival was 37.5%.[22] A larger series of 27 patients with a response rate of 71% and a median overall survival of 12.6 months was reported by Rizell and colleagues.[23] Multiple series consistently report recurrent liver disease to be the greatest threat to patient survival, even after significant treatment responses.

OTHER TUMOR HISTOLOGIES

Phase II trials examining the utility of IHP for patients with advanced gastrointestinal neuroendocrine tumors and primary hepatobiliary tumors were reported by the NCI group. Grover et al described a group of 13 patients with unresectable hepatic metastases from primary gastrointestinal neuroendocrine tumors who were treated with melphalan ($n = 10$), melphalan plus TNF ($n = 2$), or TNF alone ($n = 1$).[24] A single treatment associated mortality was observed as was a response of 50% along with a median overall survival of 48 months. Nine patients with hepatocellular carcinoma and cholangiocarcinoma were treated under the same conditions. Baseline tumor volume was significant with a median percent hepatic replacement of 41%. Overall response rate (all PR) was 66% with a median progression-free and overall survival of 7.7 and 16.3 months, respectively.[25]

PERCUTANEOUS HEPATIC PERFUSION

The greatest weakness of the IHP technology is the inability to repeat the procedure secondary to extensive surgical scarring around the IVC, made more acute by the observation that intrahepatic recurrence is common even after significant clinical responses. First reports of a less invasive technique of liver perfusion were published by Curley et al. in 1993. In this series utilizing percutaneously catheters and hepatic venous filtration, 80% of doxorubicin administered via the hepatic artery was effective filtered from the hepatic venous circulation.[26,27] Ravikumar and colleagues reported a similar series of 28 patients who underwent 58 treatments with either 5-FU or doxorubicin.[28] Neither series established a clear utility for the technology, and further studies were not completed.

A systematic examination of a refined percutaneous hepatic perfusion (PHP) system was initiated at the Surgery Branch of the NCI in 2001, using melphalan in a formal dose-escalation protocol with results published in 2005. The PHP system employs a double balloon inferior vena cava (IVC) catheter system (Delcath Systems, Inc., New York, NY) to isolate hepatic venous outflow and allow high-dose infusion of chemotherapy to the liver. The cephalic balloon blocks the IVC superior to the hepatic veins, while the caudal balloon obstructs the IVC

inferior to the hepatic veins, allowing complete isolation of hepatic venous outflow. The span between the two occlusion balloons consists of a fenestrated segment that feeds into the large, central lumen, which exits the catheter from the proximal end. During the procedure, melphalan is infused through a catheter percutaneously inserted into the hepatic artery. The melphalan perfuses the liver and exits the organ through the hepatic veins. Hepatic venous effluent is collected using the occlusion balloon catheter and melphalan-dosed blood from the central lumen is pumped through an extracorporeal circuit consisting of a centrifugal pump and two activated-carbon filter cartridges arranged in parallel. The filtered blood is returned to systemic circulation via a venous return sheath inserted into the internal jugular vein. Treatments are administered with patients under general anesthesia. The circuit and vascular isolation are detailed in Fig. 100.3.

The completed phase I study reported 28 patients who underwent 74 treatments. Twelve patients were treated in an initial feasibility cohort at 2.0 mg/kg before a 16-patient dose-escalation to 3.5 mg/kg where dose-limiting bone marrow toxicity was observed in 2 of 6 treated patients. Maximum tolerated dose was established at 3.0 mg/kg for a total of 4 planned treatments per patient. Examination of the venous filtration system revealed a consistent 78.5% percent melphalan extraction. At the MTD, grade 3 and 4 hepatic and hematologic (neutropenia and thrombocytopenia) toxicity were observed in 19% and 66% of treated patients, respectively. An overall response rate

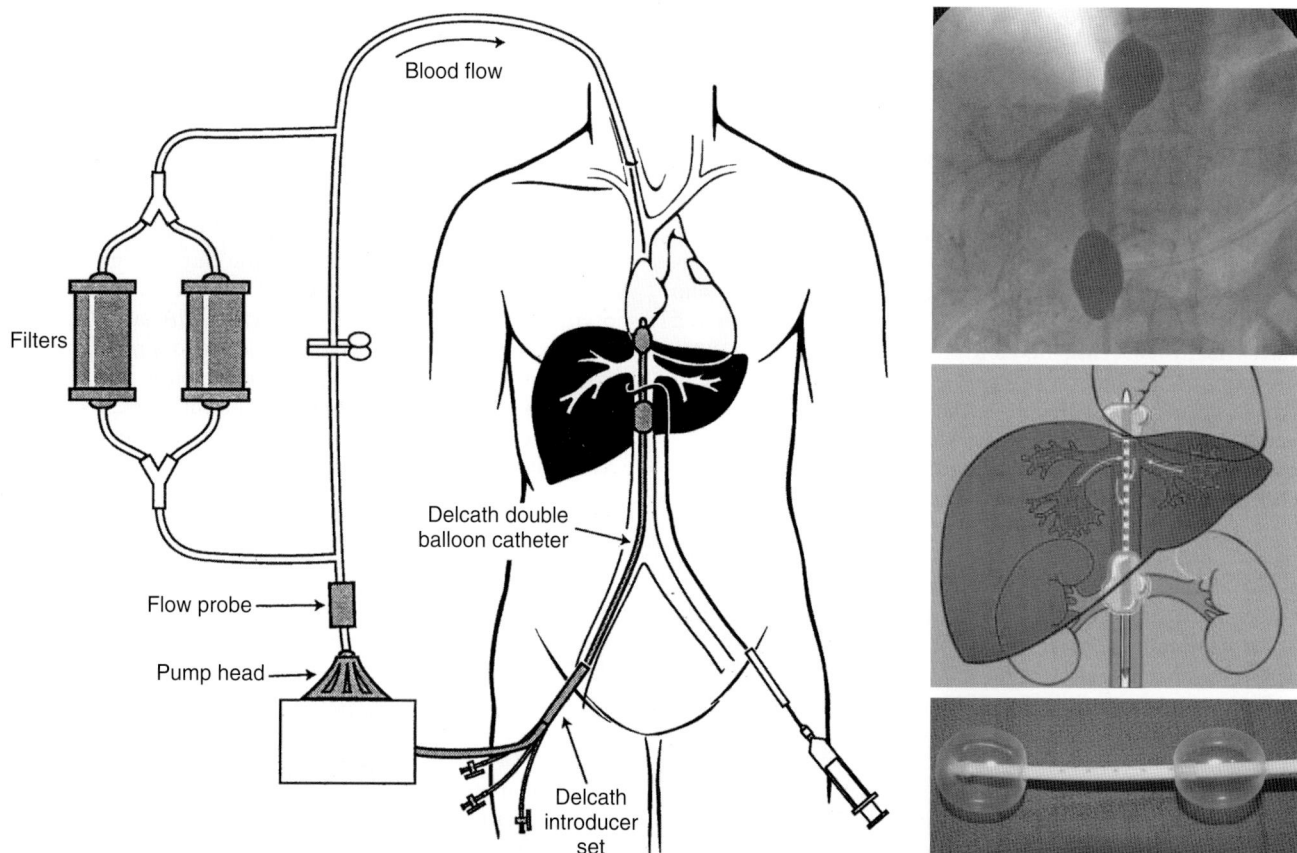

FIGURE 100.3   **Percutaneous hepatic perfusion (PHP).** The PHP circuit allows drug infusion via an arterial catheter in the common hepatic artery with hepatic venous effluent collected and run through parallel activated charcoal filters before return via a right IJ catheter. Complete caval isolation is achieved via a double-balloon catheter placed percutaneously via the right femoral vein.

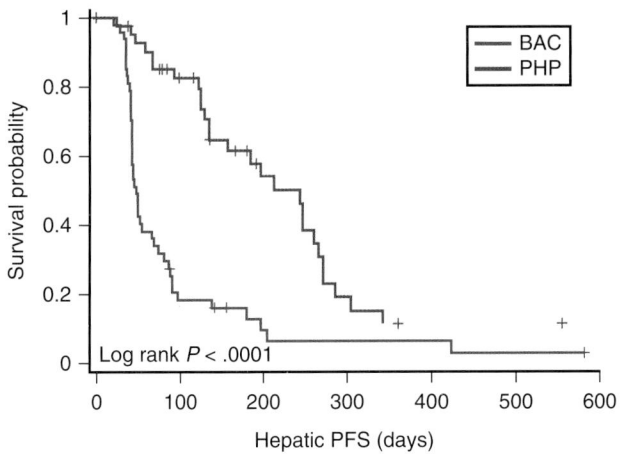

	No. of subjects	Event	Censored	Median survival (95% CI)
BAC	49	88% (43)	12% (6)	49.0 (43.0 68.0)
PHP	44	61% (27)	39% (17)	245.0 (136.0 267.0)

FIGURE 100.4 Impact of PHP on hepatic melanoma metastases. The impact of PHP with melphalan delivered every 4 to 8 weeks compared with standard of care is demonstrated by a significant prolongation of hepatic progression-free survival in the treatment arm.

of 30% was reported across multiple tumor types and all dose levels, with a 50% response rate noted in the 10 patients with metastatic ocular melanoma.[29] Two subsequent trials have been reported including a phase II cohort of 23 patients with metastatic gastrointestinal neuroendocrine tumors. The overall response rate was 79% in the 19 evaluable patients, with median hepatic progression-free and overall survivals of 39 and 40 months, respectively.[30] A recently completed phase III, randomized control trial comparing PHP with melphalan to standard of care for patient with hepatic metastatic melanoma has been reported. The primary endpoint of this trial was hepatic progression-free survival. Ninety-three patients were randomized at 10 institutions, with 27 of 49 patients crossing over from the standard of care arm at hepatic progression. Median hepatic (245 days vs. 49 days, $P < .001$, HR: .301) and overall (186 days vs. 46 days, $P < .001$, HR: .404) progression-free survival were significantly improved on the experimental (PHP) arm of the study (Fig. 100.4). Overall survival was not significantly improved, in part due to the high crossover rate. Overall response rate was 34.1% (15/44) for PHP (15/44) vs. 2.0 %

(1/49) for BAC ($P < .001$).[31] Food and Drug Administration (FDA) approval was not obtained in part due to the lack of a survival benefit secondary to patient crossover along with concerns surrounding systemic drug exposure and bone marrow toxicity which led to creation of a second generation of blood filters.

Multiple institutions have investigated the utility of the second generation of filters associated with the PHP system. A porcine model examined the efficacy of this new system was completed in six animals, with data regarding filter extraction efficacy (melphalan), transfilter pressure gradient, and hematologic toxicity and compared with clinical data from early trials at the NCI, suggesting an improvement in all areas.[32] An ongoing phase III trial in patients with metastatic uveal melanoma to the liver is ongoing and results have yet to be reported. Publications of prospective phase II[33] and retrospective[34,35] series have indicated a potential for equal or mildly improved response rates and survival in patients treated with second generation hemofiltration system with an apparent decrease in toxicity. In these series, response rates for patients with metastatic uveal melanoma have ranged from 42% to 72%, with progression-free and overall survival noted between 6 to 8 and 12 to 19 months, respectively. Overall response rate for patients with metastatic cholangiocarcinoma was 31% in the single reported series, with progression-free and overall survival not documented.

CONCLUSION

Regional hepatic perfusion with high dose melphalan provides an important clinical benefit for patients with diffuse hepatic metastases not amenable to surgical resection. IHP is well tolerated and effective with growing evidence supporting the use of multiple chemotherapeutic agents. PHP has demonstrated efficacy for patients with ocular melanoma but remains a developmental stage technology. Careful patient selection and appropriate use of appropriate systemic chemotherapy is very important for these patients. The characteristics of the nonspecific alkylating agent melphalan make it an ideal candidate for these systems as incremental dose-escalation provides meaningful increases in drug efficacy. The use of additional drugs such as 5-FU and oxaliplatin with known therapeutic benefit against colorectal and primary biliary malignancies is the rational next step in the development of these treatment modalities and is underway at a limited number of centers.

References are available at expertconsult.com.

SECTION II. Neoplastic

E. Treatment: Resection

CHAPTER 101A

Hepatic resection: General considerations

William R. Jarnagin

OVERVIEW

Partial hepatectomy has evolved into the standard therapy for patients with a wide array of localized malignant tumors and highly selected patients with benign disease. Liver surgery is now performed routinely, often with removal of a large amount of liver tissue and/or combined with resection of other organs, with the expectation of a full recovery and an opportunity for long-term disease control in most patients. Although other therapeutic modalities, including chemotherapy, ablation/ embolization, and transplantation, have shown progressive improvement in efficacy for several hepatopancreatobiliary (HPB) diseases, resection remains the single most effective treatment for the large majority of patients. Increasingly, multimodality therapy is employed, with resection playing a central role, extending the traditional limits of surgical treatment.

Reports of hepatic resection date back to antiquity (see the Introduction), but these were typically amputations of a portion of the liver exposed by traumatic injuries. It was not until the report by Lortat-Jacob and Robert of an elective right hepatectomy for malignancy in 1952[1] that the modern era of hepatobiliary surgery began, creating new possibilities to treat a wide range of disorders; however, from that point forward, the initial experience with hepatic resection was inauspicious to say the least. In 1977 Foster and Berman[2] published a multi-institutional summary of hepatic resection surgery in the United States, comprised of 168 resections performed during the preceding 14 years. This report documented a worrisome, unacceptably high operative mortality rate, primarily caused by the inability to control hemorrhage in the operating room and postoperative liver failure.

Since those dismal results were reported, there have been progressive advances in many areas, leading to the improvement in outcome required for hepatic resection to take its place as a mainstream procedure. These advances have come on several fronts, but perhaps most noteworthy has been a greater appreciation of the segmental anatomy of the liver and the willingness and ability of surgeons to pursue segmental hepatic resections based on anatomic principles (see Chapters 2, 102B, and 118B). This change in approach has had a profound effect by not only improving the results of major resections but spurring greater use of parenchyma-sparing sectoral, segmental, and subsegmental resections, such as posterior or anterior sectorectomy or central hepatectomy, rather than right or extended right hepatectomy, respectively. The increased use of

such parenchymal-sparing resection has clearly reduced the risk of perioperative liver failure, and, consequently, morbidity and mortality. Equally important, this change fundamentally altered the approach to patients who require bilobar resections.

Several studies have documented this trend and its downstream effects of reduced blood loss and transfusion rates, hospital length of stay, and operative mortality.[3-5] A more recent analysis of over 4000 resections confirmed these earlier findings and showed continued and marked reductions in operative morbidity and mortality.[6]

Practice changes in other areas, including intraoperative and perioperative management and patient selection (see Chapters 25 and 26), increased the use of enhanced recovery after surgery (ERAS) pathways (see Chapter 27) and improvements in managing postoperative complications, which have all contributed to better outcomes.[7] The use of low central venous pressure (CVP) anesthesia, now widely used, represented a notable change in the previous standard practice of fluid loading before resection. Despite concerns of possible risks of air embolization or disturbance of renal function, both unfounded, low-CVP anesthetic management has been shown to reduce blood loss during the resection because of decreased filling pressures and reduced distension of the hepatic veins, and it does so with no significant untoward effects.[8,9] The advent of accurate noninvasive monitoring systems (i.e., FloTrac, Edwards Lifesciences) has allowed the use of fluid restrictive intraoperative management without the need for central venous catheters, as shown in a recent study of over 3900 patients.[10]

Beyond the technical aspects of partial hepatectomy, surgeons have acquired a better understanding of the impact of resection on the natural history of many diseases, along with a clearer delineation of perioperative risk. Together, this has allowed a much more informed patient selection process, one that has led to resections that more effectively target those patients who are most likely to benefit from surgery (see Chapters 49–51 and 89–93). In this regard, the genetic underpinnings and determinants of outcome have come into clearer focus for many diseases, contributing to more rational treatment allocation and better therapies (see Chapter 9).

Over time, it has become clear that the quality and quantity of the future liver remnant (FLR) are critically important variables in patient selection, especially for major resections (see Chapter 102). Both of these factors have assumed particular relevance for patients with hepatic colorectal metastases, for whom the advent of more active chemotherapeutic agents has led to more frequent treatment before operation (see Chapters 92, 97, and 98). The latter development has greatly altered the landscape of this disease by allowing many more patients, particularly those with very advanced lesions previously considered surgically unapproachable, to undergo potentially curative surgery[11,12]; however, although enhancing the results of resection, such therapy has the potential to cause significant hepatotoxicity and increase the risk of postoperative liver failure.[13] In an effort to mitigate the risks in heavily pretreated patients and those with fibrosis or cirrhosis, preoperative portal vein embolization (PVE), first introduced 30 years ago, has been used with increasing frequency and has emerged as a powerful tool for inducing hypertrophy of the FLR[14] (see Chapter 102C). Preoperative PVE is increasingly combined with venous outflow deprivation, a technique that appears to enhance regeneration of the liver remnant.[15] More recently, the technique known as associating liver partition and portal vein ligation (ALPPS) for staged hepatic resection has evolved as a potentially useful technique in this regard[16] (see Chapter 102D). The procedure is performed in two stages and involves division of the liver parenchyma and the portal vein supplying the portion of liver to be resected (typically a right or extended right hepatectomy); hepatic arterial inflow, hepatic venous outflow, and biliary drainage are maintained. Rapid hypertrophy of the FLR usually occurs after a period of several days, at which time a second operation is undertaken to complete the resection and remove the specimen. Although this approach clearly shortens the time needed for FLR hypertrophy to occur, preliminary experience was associated with significant morbidity and mortality, particularly for hilar cholangiocarcinoma.[17,18] For metastatic colorectal cancer, a recent study showed excellent results in terms of regeneration of the FLR and apparent improvement in postoperative morbidity.

The changing treatment paradigm for hepatic colorectal metastases, with chemotherapy playing an increasingly prominent role (see Chapters 90, 97, and 98), has yet to evolve in other malignant diseases; however, as more effective drugs emerge, it is more than likely that similar changes in practice will be seen in other tumor types. Noted examples are biliary tract cancer, with publication of the ABC-02 trial,[19] the BILCAP trial[20] and the results of a recent study of systemic and regional chemotherapy,[21] and hepatocellular carcinoma, with the increasing number of effective targeted agents (see Chapter 89).

Advances in imaging technology deserve special mention because treatment allocation is critically dependent on high-quality radiographic studies and is continually refined. Radiologic evaluation previously required invasive investigations in many cases; however, complete, noninvasive assessment of the liver, biliary tree, arterial and venous anatomy, and disease extent in the case of malignant disease is now possible (see Chapters 13–19). Indeed, for certain tumors, classic imaging findings are now considered pathognomonic and have supplanted the need for a biopsy.

Specific examples in this regard include liver hemangiomata and focal nodular hyperplasia (see Chapters 14 and 88A) and the guidelines for the diagnosis of hepatocellular carcinoma.[22] Going forward, advances in imaging technology likely to influence the practice of hepatic resectional surgery include computer-aided reconstruction, functional imaging, and intraoperative navigation[23–26] (see Chapters 19, 24, and 103).

Technical progress in other areas, particularly with devices such as vascular staplers and those used to transect the liver parenchyma (see Chapters 101, 102, 118, and 119), are often hailed as major advances; however, although their value should not be dismissed, they cannot overcome poorly conceived or poorly executed operations, and their contribution, compared with the enhancements in other aspects, is relatively modest.

Advances in imaging continue to play a major role in postoperative management, particularly in diagnosing and treating postoperative complications (see Chapter 24). During the last several years, the marked reduction in operative mortality after hepatic resection has seemingly occurred with little more than modest reductions in morbidity. This observation suggests an overall improvement in the ability to salvage patients who experience significant complications.[6] The ready availability of high-quality imaging and a heightened awareness of the breadth of perioperative problems have led to earlier detection of complications. These changes, combined with the ability to manage many problems percutaneously or endoscopically, rather than operatively, have clearly had a major positive impact on perioperative outcomes.

CONCLUSION

This chapter detailed the contemporary approach to hepatic resection for a wide variety of diseases and indications (see Chapters 49–51 and 88–93), and specifically will address major and minor resections for benign and malignant disease of the liver and biliary tract (see Chapters 118 and 119). Later chapters will address parenchymal-sparing techniques (see Chapter 102), technical aspects of partial hepatectomy for living-donor transplantation (see Chapter 121), resection in cirrhotic patients (see Chapter 120), and advances in minimally invasive approaches (see Chapters 127D and E). The latter represents a remarkable evolution in hepatic surgery, and continued technical progress will certainly bring laparoscopic and robotic approaches to resection further into the mainstream. The descriptions herein reflect the current state of the art, built on the collective contributions of many pioneering surgeons over the past several decades, continuing to the present. The techniques and approaches discussed include some element of author bias, but the overriding theme must always be adherence to best principles of hepatic resection surgery, although alternative viewpoints should be considered where appropriate.

References are available at expertconsult.com

Hepatic resection for benign and malignant liver and biliary tract disease: Indications and outcomes

Hop S. Tran Cao, Jean-Nicolas Vauthey and Ryan William Day

INTRODUCTION

A wide variety of diseases affect the liver that can potentially be addressed with hepatectomy. They range from benign and asymptomatic, as in the case of simple liver cysts (see Chapter 88), to premalignant (biliary cystadenomas) and malignant. Malignant tumors can further be classified as primary liver tumors, such as hepatocellular carcinoma (HCC; see Chapter 89) and intrahepatic cholangiocarcinoma (IHC; see Chapter 50), or secondary liver tumors, the most common of which are colorectal liver metastases (Table 101B.1; see Chapters 90–92). Each of these pathologies involves unique considerations including systemic treatments, surgical indications, and surgical approaches. The goal of this chapter is to provide the reader with information regarding each condition and current data regarding both perioperative and long-term outcomes after treatment with hepatectomy. For a more in-depth discussion of individual pathologies referenced in this chapter, please refer to the chapters focused on each subject.

Although there are unique elements to each of the pathologies discussed, there are also commonalities that can be seen across the spectrum of liver diseases when surgical resection is being considered. Anatomic descriptions in this chapter, when applicable, will use the Couinaud classification system of segmental liver anatomy originally described by Claude Couinaud in *La Presse Médicale* in 1954[1] (Fig. 101B.1; see Chapter 2). When referencing types of liver resections, the main distinction in this chapter is largely between anatomic approaches, as described by *The Brisbane 2000 Terminology of Resections,* and parenchymal sparing techniques.[2,3] Operative techniques, such as surgical approaches to parenchymal transection, are beyond the scope of this chapter; for information on this topic, please reference the section on liver surgery techniques (see Chapters 118 and 119).

Preoperative Evaluation

All patients for whom hepatic resection is planned will require evaluation of their baseline liver function. The cornerstone of assessment remains history and physical examination. History should focus on symptoms of liver disease, previous related diagnoses, and thorough social history to identify high-risk behavior. Physical examination should focus on stigmata of underlying liver disease, including the presence of jaundice, hepatomegaly, ascites, and varices. Liver function testing can augment the information obtained through history and physical examination but is often inadequate for discerning underlying liver dysfunction on its own.

Several chronic conditions can compromise liver function, and care should be taken to discern them before performing liver resection. Hepatitis C virus (HCV) and hepatitis B virus (HBV) can both lead to chronic liver inflammation through cycles of viral activation and ultimately progression to decompensated cirrhosis (see Chapter 68). Although merely being infected with viral hepatitis does not appear to increase the perioperative risk associated with hepatic resection, decompensated cirrhosis does (see Chapter 74). Other potential causes of chronic liver disease include chronic alcoholic liver disease, nonalcoholic fatty liver disease, hemochromatosis, primary biliary cirrhosis, primary sclerosing cholangitis, and autoimmune hepatitis. In some cases, the severity of the underlying liver disease can have a larger impact on long-term survival than the characteristics of the malignancy being resected.[4] Importantly, the presence and degree of liver cirrhosis can dictate the extent of hepatectomy that would be considered safe and influence the minimum standardized functional liver remnant (sFLR) required to proceed with liver surgery.[5]

Several scoring systems are used to quantify the extent of liver disease and indirectly select patients for hepatectomy (see Chapter 4). The Model for End Stage Liver Disease (MELD), originally developed to predict 3-month survival in patients with cirrhosis, can be used to predict posthepatectomy liver failure. It may be useful in the determination of hepatectomy versus liver transplantation in patients where both options represent reasonable approaches, and it has been adopted by the United Network for Organ Sharing (UNOS) to prioritize patients awaiting liver transplantation in the United States. However, MELD is not routinely used for calculating standardized future liver remnant (sFLR) thresholds before surgery.[6] Instead, the Child-Pugh-Turcotte (Table 101B.2) score has the advantage of considering clinical manifestations of liver disease when compared with MELD.[7] For patients with Child-Pugh-Turcotte A cirrhosis, an sFLR of greater than 40% is typically required to proceed to hepatic resection. The same threshold applies for those with class B cirrhosis, although these patients are generally not suitable candidates for major hepatectomy. Patients with Child-Pugh-Turcotte C scores are considered poor surgical candidates. By comparison, in the absence of cirrhosis, sFLR greater than 20% is generally deemed adequate for patients with normal liver function. In addition to scoring systems, dynamic measures to calculate liver function are also used. Indocyanine green (ICG) clearance at 15 minutes was first introduced in Japan, and a meta-analysis found that values less than 7.1% are better predictors of posthepatectomy liver failure than either MELD or Child-Pugh-Turcotte score.[8]

In addition to the severity of chronic liver disease, other factors will also need to be considered when determining the optimal sFLR and timing of surgery. Patients who receive 5-fluorouracil-based chemotherapy are at risk for hepatic steatosis; irinotecan-based chemotherapy can cause steatohepatitis, and oxaliplatin is associated with sinusoidal obstruction syndrome (SOS; see Chapter 69). Although steatosis and SOS minimally increase perioperative risks, patients found to have

TABLE 101B.1 Common Benign and Malignant Liver Lesions

MALIGNANT PATHOLOGIES	BENIGN AND PREMALIGNANT PATHOLOGIES
Primary Tumors: Hepatocellular carcinoma (HCC) Fibrolamellar HCC Intrahepatic cholangiocarcinoma Gallbladder cancer Perihilar cholangiocarcinoma	**Benign Lesions:** Hemangioma Focal nodular hyperplasia Hepatic cyst Echinococcal cyst Bile duct hamartoma Angiomyolipoma Regenerative nodule
Secondary Tumors: Colorectal cancer Neuroendocrine tumors Breast cancer Other cancers	**Tumors With Malignant Potential:** Hepatic adenoma Biliary cystadenoma

TABLE 101B.2 Child-Pugh-Turcotte Score Assignment

	POINTS		
FACTOR	1	2	3
Encephalopathy	None	Grade 1 and 2	Grade 3 and 4
Ascites	None	Slight	Moderate
Bilirubin	<2 mg/mL	2–3 mg/mL	>3 mg/mL
Albumin	>3.5 mg/mL	2.8–3.5 mg/mL	<2.8 mg/mL
Prothrombin Time/INR	<4 sec/<1.7	4–6 sec/1.7 to 2.2	>6 sec, >3 points

Child-Pugh-Turcotte A: 5 to 6 points; Child-Pugh-Turcotte B: 7 to 9 points; Child-Pugh-Turcotte C: 10 to 15 points.

INR, International normalized ratio.

steatohepatitis on their resected liver specimen have postoperative 90-day mortality that is significantly increased from 1.6% to 14.7%, with most deaths caused by posthepatectomy liver failure.[9] Additionally, patients with extensive exposure to chemotherapy (>12 cycles) have increased rates of posthepatectomy liver failure with sFLR less than 30%.[10] For this reason, our group reserves major hepatectomy for patients treated with extensive chemotherapy to those whose sFLR is at least 30% (see Chapter 102).

For patients with inadequate sFLR to consider hepatic resection, preoperative volume expansion of the FLR can be attempted via several approaches. Preoperative portal vein embolization (PVE) by interventional radiology is the most commonly employed and best studied method for sFLR augmentation (see Chapter 102C). This procedure is most frequently accomplished with percutaneous vascular access and embolization of the right portal vein, with or without embolization of segment IV branches. After PVE, patients undergo repeat volumetry; those who demonstrate more than 2.0% growth per week (referred to as kinetic growth rate) have a 0% rate of liver

failure in the perioperative period after hepatectomy.[11] This technique can be employed as part of a single stage or two-stage approach to hepatic lesions (Fig. 101B.2).

Associating liver partition and portal vein ligation for staged hepatectomy (ALPPS) is another strategy for patients who do not have adequate sFLR to undergo hepatectomy (see Chapter 102D). In this two-stage operation, patients undergo parenchymal transection and portal ligation at a first-stage operation and then, 1 to 2 weeks later, undergo a second operation to remove the portion of the liver affected by disease. Advocates of this approach point to higher rates of liver hypertrophy and more patients undergoing definitive resection than PVE, whereas detractors note high perioperative mortality rates of 9% in the international ALPPS registry.[12] For more information on PVE and ALPPS, please reference the discussions in Chapters 102C and 102D, respectively.

Although the factors previously discussed are common to all patients undergoing hepatectomy for almost any indication, disease-specific outcome determinants need to be considered as well. This chapter will explore both malignant and benign indications for liver surgery and their associated outcomes.

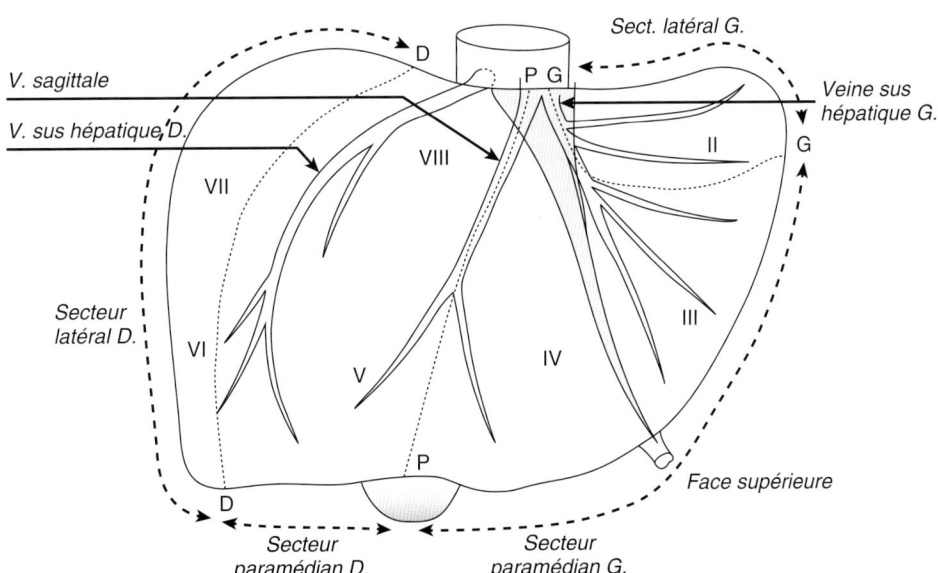

FIGURE 101B.1 Liver segments described by Couinaud. See Chapter 2. (From Couinaud C. [Liver lobes and segments: Notes on the anatomical architecture and surgery of the liver]. *Presse Med.* 1954;62[33]:709-12.)

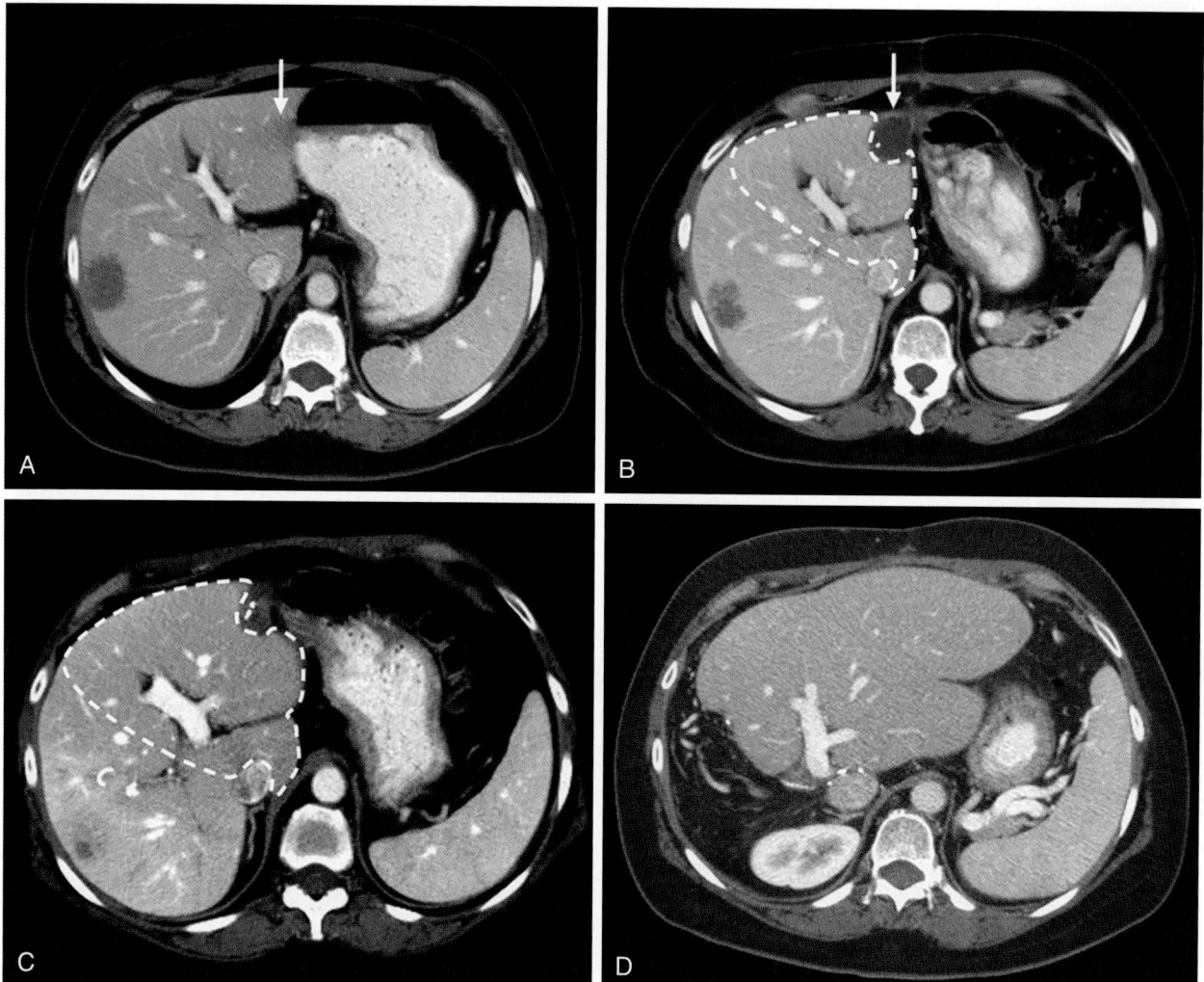

FIGURE 101B.2 A patient who underwent staged approach to volume expansion and complete resection. **A,** Two liver masses were identified at initial diagnosis. **B,** The morphologic response to systemic therapy and planning for portal vein embolization. **C,** Left liver hypertrophy after portal vein embolization. **D,** Complete resection of all metastases including right hepatectomy and partial left hepatectomy. See Chapter 102C.

PRIMARY HEPATIC MALIGNANCIES

Hepatocellular Carcinoma (see Chapter 89)

HCC is the most common primary liver tumor and accounts for roughly 70% of primary liver tumor diagnoses.[13] The incidence of HCC has increased over the last 30 years and is anticipated to continue increasing in the future.[14,15] HCC often occurs in the setting of chronic liver disease and cirrhosis. It is typically diagnosed late in its course, although screening initiatives have led to earlier diagnoses in the last 2 decades.[16] Mortality from HCC remains high and is one of the fastest rising causes of cancer-related deaths.[17] Underlying liver disease, which is the most significant risk factor for HCC, often complicates or precludes aggressive treatment via liver resection and other liver-directed modalities.

HCC has several established risk factors that can be broadly grouped into the following categories:
1. Chronic liver disease
2. Metabolic risk factors
3. Genetic risk factors

These categorizations can help with identification, risk mitigation, and, ultimately, treatment planning.

The most common causes of chronic liver disease in the world are the viral causes of hepatitis, and HBV and HCV are also the two most commonly identified risk factors preceding a HCC diagnosis worldwide[18] (see Chapter 68). HBV is the incident risk factor identified most commonly globally, whereas HCV is the most common in the United States.[19] Patients who have chronic infection with HBV are at risk for developing HCC even in the absence of cirrhosis. Progression to cirrhosis further increases the risk of developing HCC, with reported rates of 1% to 8% per year.[20,21] With the introduction of combination treatment with sofosbuvir and ledipasvir, HCV now represents a potentially modifiable risk factor.[22] Similarly, HBV vaccination presents another opportunity to address a potentially modifiable target.

Nonalcoholic fatty liver disease (NAFLD) is the fastest rising cause of chronic liver disease in the world and the most frequent chronic liver disease in the United States (see Chapter 69). NAFLD can progress to nonalcoholic steatohepatitis (NASH).[23]

It represents a crossover between metabolic diseases and chronic liver disease because of the implication of insulin resistance.[24] NAFLD/NASH do not appear to increase risk of HCC on their own but instead confer additional risk with progression to cirrhosis.[25] Alcohol intake similarly does not appear to be related to carcinogenesis outside of the setting of cirrhosis. Diabetes is another modifiable metabolic risk factor for HCC development. In one meta-analysis, diabetes was associated with up to a 2.5 times greater risk of HCC.[26] Additionally, there is some evidence that use of metformin can decrease HCC prevalence in both diabetics and nondiabetics with metabolic syndromes.[27,28]

Genetic disorders have been associated with increased prevalence of HCC. These include hemochromatosis, an autosomal recessive disorder of inborn iron metabolism, which is strongly associated with HCC, particularly once progression to cirrhosis has occurred.[29] Additionally, alpha-1 antitrypsin deficiency, primary biliary cirrhosis, and Wilson disease have all been associated with a less profound risk of progression to cirrhosis and HCC development[30] (see Chapters 74 and 89).

The diagnosis of HCC is largely dependent on imaging and may be established on the basis of imaging characteristics alone in cirrhotic patients. Under screening protocols for at-risk individuals, initial findings of a mass on liver ultrasound should lead to follow-up cross-sectional imaging. The combination of arterial hyperenhancement and early contrast washout in the venous and/or delayed phases is highly suggestive of HCC, and in high-risk patients, there is no need for routine biopsy in the presence of these computed tomography (CT)/magnetic resonance imaging (MRI) findings.[31] In fact, these imaging findings make up part of the Liver Reporting & Data System (LI-RADS), a standardized reporting system developed by the American College of Radiology to apply consistent terminology and facilitate communication between clinicians when dealing with patients at risk of developing HCC (Fig. 101B.3; see Chapter 14).

Once a diagnosis of HCC is established, a wide array of treatment options is available that must consider both tumor and underlying liver characteristics. There is no single consensus ideal staging algorithm to dictate treatment of HCC, although the Barcelona Clinic Liver Cancer and American Joint Committee on Cancer (AJCC) TNM systems are the most widely used. Two prior consensus statements from the Americas Hepato-Pancreato-Biliary Association (AHPBA) have counseled against routine use of either system for all patients.[32,33]

Often the etiology and severity of the underlying chronic liver disease will direct a patient toward and away from individual treatment modalities. In many patients with localized disease, the severity of their underlying liver disease may preclude the

CT/MRI diagnostic table

Arterial phase hyperenhancement (APHE)		No APHE		Nonrim APHE		
Observation size (mm)		< 20	≥ 20	< 10	10–19	≥ 20
Count additional major features:	None	LR-3	LR-3	LR-3	LR-3	LR-4
• Enhancing "capsule" • Nonperipheral "washout" • Threshold growth	One	LR-3	LR-4	LR-4	LR-4 / LR-5	LR-5
	≥ Two	LR-4	LR-4	LR-4	LR-5	LR-5

LR-4 / LR-5   Observations in this cell are categorized based on one additional major feature:
• LR-4 – if enhancing "capsule"
• LR-5 – if nonperipheral "washout" **OR** threshold growth

A

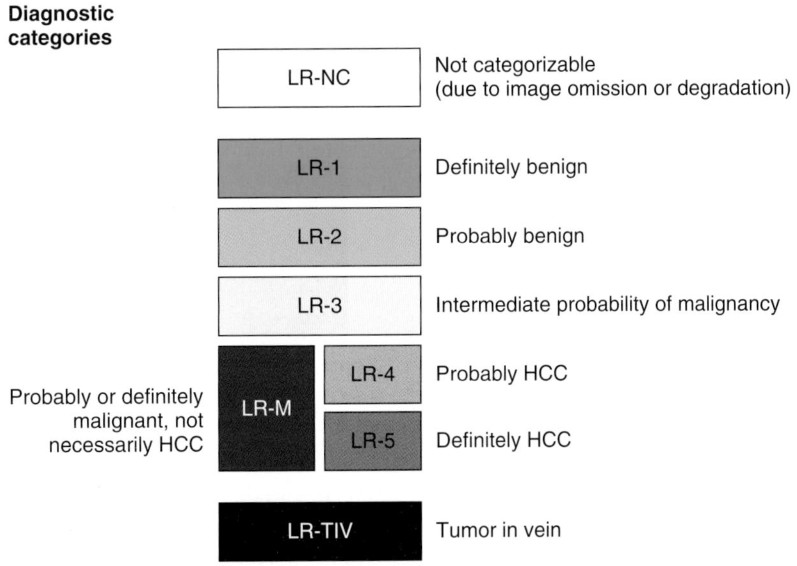

Diagnostic categories

LR-NC	Not categorizable (due to image omission or degradation)
LR-1	Definitely benign
LR-2	Probably benign
LR-3	Intermediate probability of malignancy
LR-4	Probably HCC
LR-5	Definitely HCC
LR-M (Probably or definitely malignant, not necessarily HCC)	
LR-TIV	Tumor in vein

B

FIGURE 101B.3 AND 3B   Liver Reporting and Data System (LI-RADS) standardized diagnostic system developed by the American College of Radiology. See Chapter 14. *CT,* Computed tomography; *MRI,* magnetic resonance imaging.

safe performance of liver resection, which may otherwise have been a good option. For patients who are not eligible for resection, transplantation is the treatment of choice should criteria be met because it would address both the cancer and the underlying diseased liver condition (see Chapter 105). Ablation represents another potentially curative option but is best reserved for small tumors (see Chapter 96). When surgery is considered, preoperative selection of patients should focus on the likelihood of disease being confined to the liver, anatomic constraints of resectability, and limits of underlying liver dysfunction.

Resection should be considered in patients who have disease confined to the liver and with normal underlying liver function or compensated liver cirrhosis. Evidence of portal hypertension, including presence of ascites, splenomegaly with associated thrombocytopenia, or varices and/or a recanalized umbilical vein (Fig. 101B.4), or other signs of decompensated cirrhosis will render most patients ineligible for resection-based therapy (see Chapter 74). All patients with known liver disease should undergo evaluation with a validated system such as the Child-Turcotte-Pugh or MELD systems. If the status of the patient's liver disease is unclear from these systems, or when concern persists for portal hypertension despite reassuring liver function tests, direct hepatic vein-portal vein gradient can be measured to assess the presence and degree of portal hypertension.

Patients who have signs of decompensated cirrhosis with refractory ascites, hepatorenal syndrome, hepatopulmonary syndrome, or spontaneous bacterial peritonitis should not be considered for resection. Similarly, only patients with Child-Pugh-Turcotte class A cirrhosis should be considered for major resection. Based on these clinical criteria, in the absence of portal hypertension and with adequate sFLR, approximately 5% to 10% of patients with cirrhosis and HCC will be eligible for resection.[34] In these patients, resection is relatively safe, with perioperative mortality of 2% and transfusion rates of 10%.[35] After successful resection, cirrhotic patients with HCC can expect 5-year survival rates up to 50% to 70%.[36]

For patients who are not suitable candidates for hepatic resections, other available treatment modalities include systemic therapy (see Chapter 99), radiofrequency ablation (RFA; see Chapter 96B), microwave ablation (see Chapter 96C), percutaneous alcohol injection (see Chapter 96D), bland embolization (see Chapter 94A), trans-arterial chemoembolization (TACE; see Chapter 94A), transarterial radioembolization (TARE) with yttrium-90 (Y-90; see Chapter 94B), stereotactic body radiation therapy (SBRT; see Chapter 95), proton beam irradiation (see Chapter 95), and liver transplantation (see Chapters 105 and 108A). These therapies are often used in conjunction with one another and sometimes as strategies for local control to bridge to transplant or resection. They are covered in greater detail in the chapters dedicated to HCC treatment.

Several randomized controlled trials (RCTs) have compared RFA and liver resection for small, potentially resectable HCC.[37,38] These trials focused on different populations, and all but one showed inferiority of RFA to surgery. Subsequent meta-analyses of these trials found that RFA is inferior to surgery for patients who can undergo liver resection.[39–41] One meta-analysis included patients who had HCC less than 2 cm and were Child-Pugh Class A with or without cirrhosis. It showed similar 1-year overall survival (OS) but demonstrated that resection was associated with improved 3- and 5-year OS[39] (see Chapter 96B).

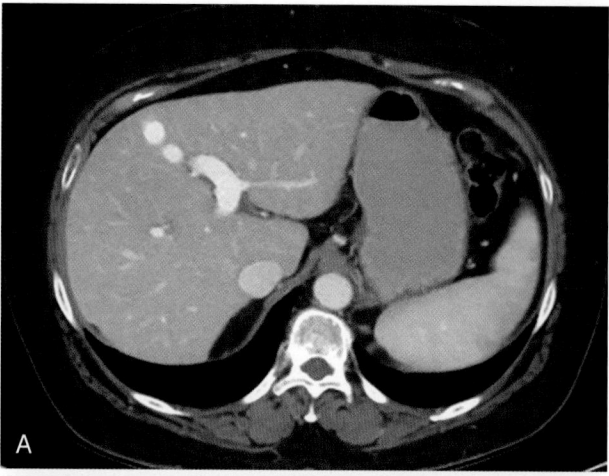

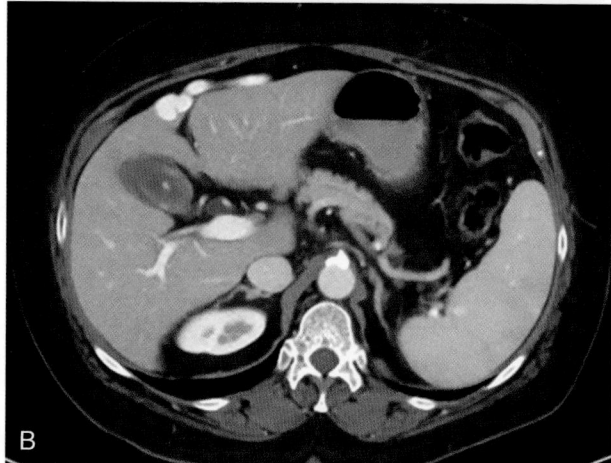

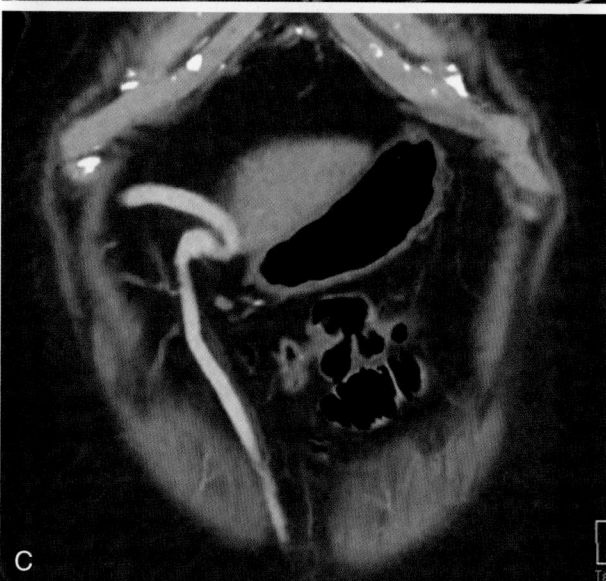

FIGURE 101B.4 Recanalized umbilical vein as a manifestation of portal hypertension on cross-sectional imaging. *HCC,* Hepatic cholangiocarcinoma.

For tumors that are larger than 2 cm but less than 5 cm, RFA is generally discouraged because of incomplete coverage of the ablation zone. The question shifts instead to the type and extent of surgical resection, with several studies investigating the question of anatomic versus nonanatomic resection. In this regard, meta-analyses on the topic have reached different conclusions. One early meta-analysis showed similar OS for both approaches but with decreased rates of local intrahepatic recurrence and early postoperative recurrence in the anatomic resection group. Morbidity and mortality were similar between the two approaches.[42] A more recent meta-analysis contradicted these findings and showed that anatomic resection was associated with disease-free survival (DFS) benefits at 1, 3, and 5 years. Additionally, the meta-analysis showed improved OS at 5 years.[43] Our group recommends anatomic resection for HCC when feasible.

Historically, surgeons have been reticent to approach large (>5 cm) and giant (>10 cm) HCCs surgically because of concerns for both poor short-term operative outcomes and long-term survival outcomes. More recent reports, however, have indicated that surgery can be safe in well-selected patients with perioperative mortality less than 3%.[44] Long-term outcomes in recent case series have also been encouraging, with 5-year survival ranging from 29% to 53% for tumors greater than 5 cm and 27% to 35% for tumors greater than 10 cm.[45] TACE has previously been recommended for these patients, but a recent comparison indicated that surgical resection is associated with superior survival.[46] With improving surgical technique and perioperative pathways, we do not recognize a tumor size limit for surgical resection and offer this option to patients whenever possible. It should be noted that TACE or TARE may represent good initial treatments before surgical resection by offering a window into the tumor biology.

Macrovascular invasion is one of the strongest predictors of poor survival in HCC and is associated with intrahepatic and extrahepatic metastases (see Chapter 89). Additionally, portal vein and hepatic vein thromboses, when present, can significantly increase the operative morbidity and mortality of hepatectomy, which approaches 8% in these patients. In this setting, survival tends to be poor, regardless of the treatment approach. Median survival for patients with macrovascular invasion managed with best supportive care is 5 months and stretches to 6 months with sorafenib. One multicenter surgical series was able to demonstrate 10% 5-year survival for patients who underwent surgical resection, with an 11-month median survival.[47]

For patients who are not eligible for resection but still fulfill the Milan criteria, liver transplantation is an option.[48] The original report from which the Milan criteria were developed showed 75% OS at 5 years and recurrence-free survival of 83% for patients who underwent transplantation for HCC. Since that time, 70% has become the benchmark OS at 5 years after liver transplantation for HCC. After concerns that the Milan criteria may be too restrictive, various centers adopted less restrictive guidelines, including the University of California San Francisco (UCSF) criteria that expanded transplant criteria for HCC (Table 101B.3). When compared, neither set of criteria was predictive of improved survival[49] (see Chapter 108A).

In patients who undergo successful resection of their primary HCC, about half will recur within 2 years. Median survival after recurrence is less than 2 years.[50] At the time of recurrence, only 5% to 30% of patients will be eligible for salvage resection. Many patients will undergo other strategies for local control, including RFA, TACE, TARE, and systemic chemotherapy. Patients who have liver-only recurrences are potentially eligible for salvage liver transplant. Those who do undergo salvage liver transplant have comparable 1-, 3-, and 5-year survival to primary liver transplant for HCC (100%, 95%, 85%,

TABLE 101B.3   Milan and UCSF Criteria for Liver Transplant for HCC

Milan Criteria (Mazzaferro et al., 1996)	Single tumor ≤ 5 cm *or*
	2–3 tumors none exceeding 3 cm, *and*
	No vascular invasion or extrahepatic spread
UCSF Criteria (Yao et al., 2001)	Single tumor ≤6.5 cm *or*
	2–3 lesions, none exceeding 4.5 cm with total tumor diameter ≤8.5 cm, *and*
	No vascular invasion or extrahepatic spread

HCC, Hepatic cholangiocarcinoma; *UCSF*, University of California San Francisco.

respectively) but are more likely to develop tumor recurrence (28% vs. 15.6%).[51] For further information on HCC, please refer to Chapter 89.

Intrahepatic Cholangiocarcinoma
(see Chapters 50 and 118)

IHC is a relatively rare cancer. It is the second most common primary liver malignancy and accounts for 10% to 20% of primary liver cancer diagnoses. Among cholangiocarcinomas, IHC is the least common and is thought to represent 5% to 10% of all cholangiocarcinoma diagnoses, although this relative percentage might be rising with the growing incidence of this condition. For the purposes of this chapter, IHC is treated as a distinct entity from perihilar cholangiocarcinoma. Despite their similar histology, these malignancies have different biologies, treatment options, and outcomes.

In the United States, the overall incidence of IHC is low at 0.95 cases per 100,000; it can be up to 100 times more frequent in East Asian countries. The incidence in America has risen over the past several decades, mostly with new diagnoses at early stage disease.[52] Epidemiologically, the rise in the incidence of IHC has nearly mirrored a corresponding decline in the rate of cancers of unknown primary (CUPs), suggesting that IHC might have previously been misidentified as CUP. At the same time, there appears to be a true increase in the incidence of IHC that is possibly related to the epidemic of metabolic syndrome. Risk factors for IHC include viral hepatitis, cirrhosis, primary sclerosing cholangitis (PSC), NAFLD, parasitic infection (*Clonorchis sinensis* and *Opisthorchis viverrini*), and diabetes.[53] Like other biliary cancers, incidence also increases with age.

Patients with cholangiocarcinoma at extrahepatic sites are likely to develop jaundice as a presenting symptom. For IHC, jaundice is less common, whereas right upper quadrant pain, weight loss, or incidental discovery are more likely. The majority of cases are diagnosed via cross-sectional imaging for the mass-forming morphology. Typical features on CT imaging are a hypodense lesion with rim enhancement during both arterial and portal venous phases. When no mass is apparent on imaging, other highly suggestive findings include unexplained biliary dilation and liver atrophy.[54] On MRI, IHCs appear hypointense on T1-weighted imaging and hyperintense on T2-weighted imaging. Cross-sectional imaging is also useful for staging and may demonstrate suspicious lymph nodes, intrahepatic spread, or carcinomatosis (see Chapter 14).

In addition to imaging abnormalities, patients may have laboratory abnormalities including elevated levels of alkaline phosphatase. Bilirubin is usually normal in patients with IHC. Tumor markers including carcinoembryonic antigen (CEA), carbohydrate antigen 19-9 (CA19-9), and alpha-fetoprotein (AFP) should be monitored and can point to other potential etiologies, including colorectal liver metastases with CEA elevation and HCC with elevated AFP. Markedly elevated CA19-9 can be indicative of more advanced disease, and levels over 100 U/mL have been associated with worse DFS after surgical resection.[55] Tumor markers alone are insufficient for establishing a diagnosis of IHC however.

Accurately staging patients with IHC is important when considering curative-intent surgery. Patients who are found to have extra-regional distant metastases or invasion of critical structures not amenable to resection are not candidates for surgery. In the absence of these features, staging laparoscopy may still be indicated in the presence of high-risk features such as suspicious lymph nodes, multifocal nodules, and/or high serum CA19-9.[56] Up to a third of these patients will be found to have occult peritoneal disease or intrahepatic metastases at the time of exploration.

In patients where there is no contraindication to surgery and an adequate sFLR can be maintained after R0 resection, surgery is the only potentially curative therapy. In patients undergoing surgery for IHC, R0 resections are obtained only 75% of the time.[57] Large primary tumor size, locally advanced disease, or invasion of critical structures are risk factors for positive margins. Surgeons may be tempted to undertake more extensive and extended resection to achieve R0 resections, but margin status must be balanced against the likelihood of surgical complications. Indeed, postoperative complications have been found to be an independent predictor of worse long-term outcomes, which correlate with the severity of the complications.[58]

Lymphadenectomy during surgical resection for IHC remains controversial. Although there is no definitive evidence that lymphadenectomy is associated with improved survival, it does allow for more accurate disease staging. The information gained has been shown to direct decision making regarding adjuvant therapy and refine prognostication. Lymphadenectomy identifies positive nodes up to 30% to 40% of the time, which is associated with decreased median survival.[59] For these reasons, consensus statements, including the National Comprehensive Cancer Network (NCCN) guidelines, recommend routine lymphadenectomy at the time of hepatectomy for IHC.[56,60] Despite these recommendations, some controversy remains, with a recent meta-analysis showing no difference in OS or recurrence but increased postoperative morbidity associated with lymphadenectomy[61] (see Chapter 50). At our institution, we routinely perform lymphadenectomy for the purpose of accurate disease staging.

In patients who undergo curative-intent hepatectomy, disease stage is an important prognostic consideration. Five-year survival ranges from 90% for resected stage IA IHC to 16.2% for stage IIIB using the AJCC 8th edition staging system (Table 101B.4).[62] In addition to stage, microvascular invasion, perineural invasion, and surgical margins have been associated with worse prognosis.[63] Several nomograms have been developed that consider other factors including tumor size and number, vascular invasion, and tumor markers to further refine prognostication after hepatectomy.[64–67]

Local recurrence is the most frequent pattern of disease recurrence, even with R0 resection after hepatectomy. Up to two-thirds of patients with IHC will experience recurrence

TABLE 101B.4 Survival by AJCC 8th Edition Stage for Patients With Intrahepatic Cholangiocarcinoma

STAGE	% OF DIAGNOSES	% 5-YEAR SURVIVAL	95% CI 5-YEAR SURVIVAL
IA	5.1	90.0	47.3–98.5
IB	6.1	50.6	19.9–75.0
II	12.5	55.1	34.5–71.7
IIIA	7.4	49.7	16.6–76.2
IIIB	68.9	16.2	9.5–24.5

AJCC, American Joint Committee on Cancer; CI, confidence interval.

Adapted from Spolverato G, Bagante F, Weiss M, et al. Comparative performances of the 7th and 8th editions of the American Joint Committee on Cancer staging systems for intrahepatic cholangiocarcinoma. *J Surg Oncol.* 2017;115(6):696–703.

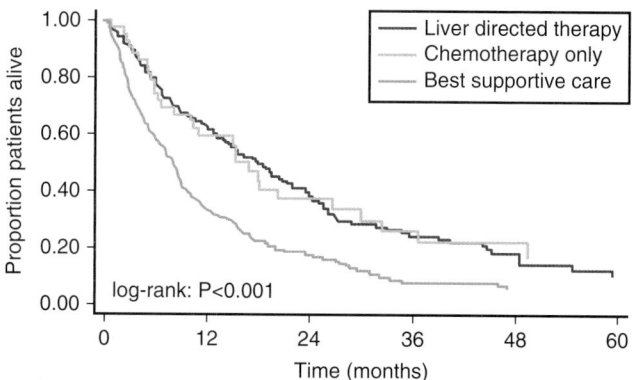

FIGURE 101B.5 Recurrent intrahepatic cholangiocarcinoma overall survival by type of treatment. See Chapter 50. (From Spolverato G, Kim Y, Alexandrescu S, et al. Management and outcomes of patients with recurrent intrahepatic cholangiocarcinoma following previous curative-intent surgical resection. *Ann Surg Oncol.* 2016;23[1]:235–243.)

within 2 years of surgery.[68] Although recurrent tumors are associated with worse outcomes, patients who can be salvaged with repeat hepatectomy see increased median survival from 11.1 months to 26.7 months.[69] Among patients who cannot undergo salvage hepatectomy, median survival is shortest for patients who receive best supportive care at 8 months and increases to 16.8 months with systemic therapy and 18 months with liver-directed therapy (Fig. 101B.5).

Data for adjuvant therapy in resected IHC remain sparse. To date, only one RCT has been completed on this subject that has demonstrated a survival benefit with adjuvant therapy. In the BILCAP trial, which included all bile duct and gallbladder cancers, patients randomized to the capecitabine arm after resection had significantly longer OS compared with those in the observation arm (53 months vs. 36 months) on a predetermined per-protocol analysis (Fig. 101B.6), as well as longer DFS (24.4 months vs. 17.5 months).[70] Large retrospective series have also suggested a benefit to adjuvant therapy, especially for patients with lymph node positive disease and advanced T-stage with gemcitabine-based regimens.[71] On the other hand, the PRODIGE 12 trial failed to demonstrate a benefit to adjuvant gemcitabine and oxaliplatin for resected biliary tract cancers (including 88 patients with IHC) compared with observation[72] (see Chapter 50).

For patients with unresectable disease, there is a well-defined role for both systemic therapy and liver-directed treatment

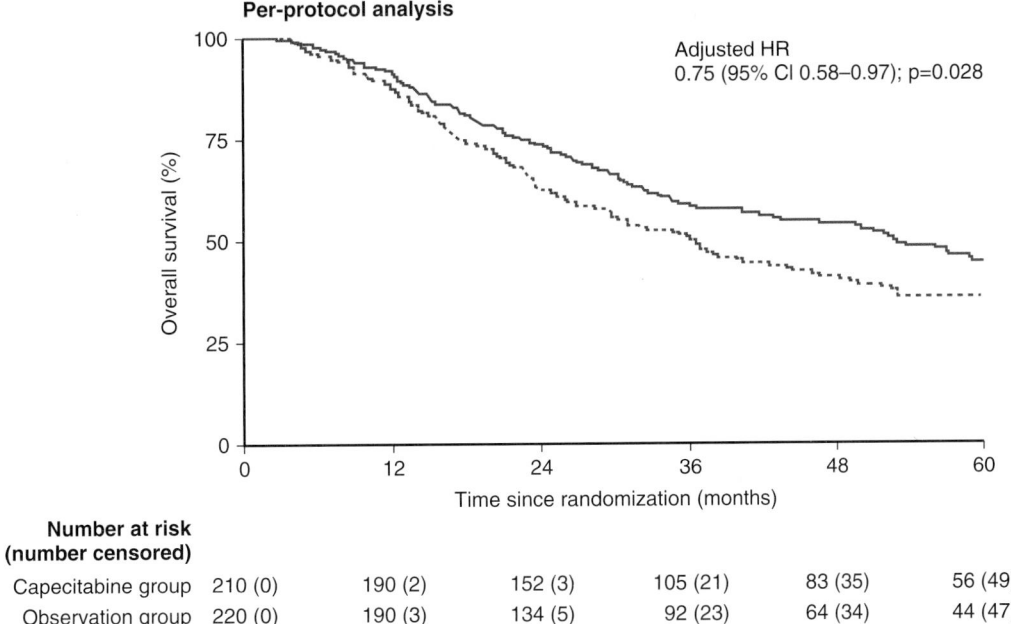

Per-protocol analysis

Adjusted HR
0.75 (95% CI 0.58–0.97); p=0.028

**Number at risk
(number censored)**

	0	12	24	36	48	60
Capecitabine group	210 (0)	190 (2)	152 (3)	105 (21)	83 (35)	56 (49)
Observation group	220 (0)	190 (3)	134 (5)	92 (23)	64 (34)	44 (47)

FIGURE 101B.6   Recurrence-free survival after adjuvant treatment with capecitabine in resected biliary tract tumors. *CI,* Confidence interval; *HR,* hazard ratio. (Reprinted with permission from Elsevier (The Lancet, 2019, 20, 663-673))

strategies besides hepatectomy. The ABC-02 trial showed improvement in OS (11.7 months vs. 8.1 months) and progression-free survival (PFS; 8 months vs. 5 months) for gemcitabine and cisplatin versus gemcitabine alone.[73] Liver-directed therapies including hepatic artery infusion (HAI), TARE with Y-90, TACE, and drug-eluting bead TACE (DEB-TACE) have all been identified as potential local control strategies. In one meta-analysis, HAI was associated with the best survival outcomes and response rates compared with Y-90 and TACE.[74] For further information on IHC, please refer to Chapter 50.

Gallbladder Cancers (see Chapters 49 and 119A)

Gallbladder cancer is the most common biliary tract cancer worldwide, although its incidence in the Unites States is low.[75] It is endemic in certain geographic areas of the world and among some ethnic groups in countries in Asia and South America.[76] Gallbladder cancer is unusual in that it is the only primary liver or biliary cancer with a higher incidence in women than in men. It is an aggressive malignancy with an exceedingly poor prognosis and often presents at advanced stages. Diagnosis at an early stage often occurs in the setting of an incidental finding on cholecystectomy performed for what is thought to be a benign indication. For this reason, surgical therapy for gallbladder cancer often occurs in a staged fashion.

Before curative-intent surgery for gallbladder cancer, accurate staging is of utmost importance. Two paradigms begin to emerge in the treatment of gallbladder cancer: patients who are diagnosed incidentally at the time of cholecystectomy for presumed cholecystitis or symptomatic cholelithiasis and patients who are diagnosed with gallbladder cancer before surgical resection. In both scenarios, characteristics of the primary tumor such as T-stage and molecular analysis can provide insights about future therapies. Lymphatic spread is common and even patients with T2 disease can have lymph node involvement more than 40% of the time.[77]

Incidental Diagnosis

Patients who are found to have incidental T1a tumors resected with negative margins on cholecystectomy are felt to be cured, and extended resection does not increase long-term survival. These tumors are associated with low rates of lymph node metastases of less than 5%.[78] For individuals with T1b tumors, which penetrate the muscle layer, most guidelines and retrospective analyses favor more extensive resection.[79] The need for completion radical or extended cholecystectomy, which includes partial hepatectomy of the gallbladder bed and regional lymphadenectomy, is supported by the 15% rate of nodal involvement with T1b disease.[80] Decision analysis shows a potential survival benefit to extended resection despite equivalence in small retrospective series.[81]

For patients with T2 disease, aggressive surgery can have marked effects on long-term survival. Series have shown increased long-term survival with extended resection versus simple cholecystectomy, a finding that is also demonstrated in large population-based registries, including the Surveillance, Epidemiology, and End Results (SEER) database.[82] T2 tumors have higher rates of positive margins and local recurrence when simple cholecystectomy is performed and these patients should undergo completion radical cholecystectomy to realize the survival benefit of patients who are identified preoperatively.[83] Those with T3 and T4 tumors are unlikely to be discovered incidentally because the tumor extends outside the confines of the gallbladder. When that is the case, however, patients with T3 tumors will have residual disease in more than 77.3% of cases in one retrospective study.[84]

Even in this re-operative setting, use of minimally invasive techniques has been shown to be safe and feasible to achieve a complete regional lymphadenectomy and hepatectomy and may be aided by the use of fluorescence angiography and cholangiography for surgical navigation (Fig. 101B.7).

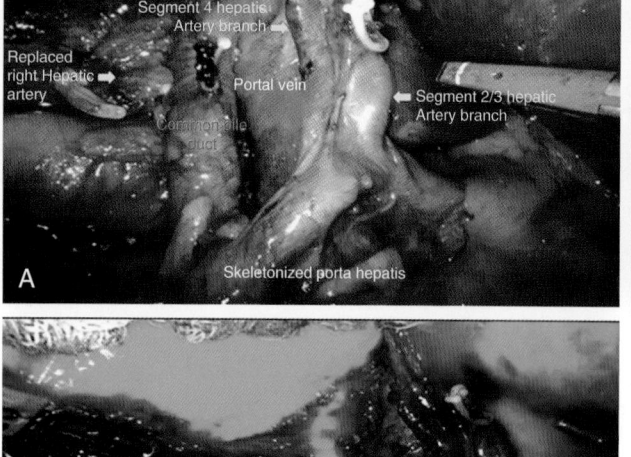

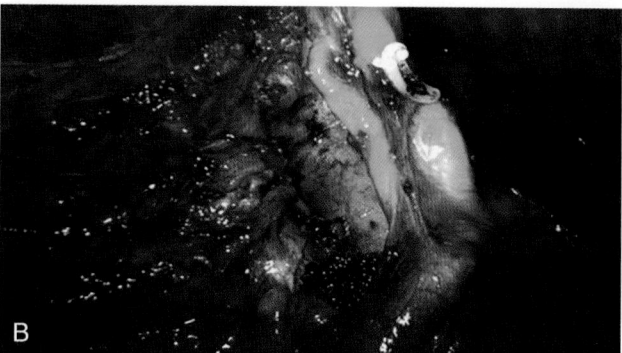

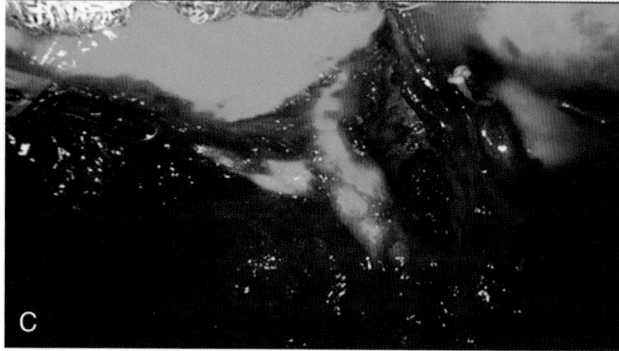

FIGURE 101B.7   Demonstration of fluorescence imaging in **(A)** skeletonized porta hepatis **(B)** with fluorescence angiography early after indocyanine green (ICG) injection and **(C)** fluorescence cholangiography 20 minutes after ICG injection with demonstration of cystic duct stump (*yellow arrow*).

Preoperative Diagnosis

Patients who are diagnosed with gallbladder cancer before surgery should undergo imaging to determine the possibility of spread and ultimately staging laparoscopy if the cancer is thought to be resectable. Liver metastases, peritoneal metastases, malignant ascites, distant lymphatic spread, extensive involvement of the hepatoduodenal ligament, and/or encasement of the hepatic artery or portal vein are contraindications to proceeding with definitive surgical resection. Staging laparoscopy is an important tool for determining resectability and avoiding nontherapeutic laparotomy because up to a quarter of patients who are thought to be resectable based on imaging alone will have findings precluding resection on staging laparoscopy[85] (see Chapter 24).

T3 tumors perforate the gallbladder serosa and/or invade the liver or another adjacent organ. For these patients, extended resection is warranted to achieve a margin negative resection and may require en bloc resection of the involved organ. T4 disease may be apparent on preoperative imaging or at the time of exploration; in well-selected patients, surgical resection may be possible, although major vascular invasion is a terrible prognostic sign and precludes resection. For further discussion on the extent of lymphadenectomy and extent of resection, please refer to Chapter 119A.

Perioperative outcomes depend on the type of resection performed. Simple cholecystectomy is well tolerated with little in the way of mortality, whereas radical resection has historically been associated with mortality rates as high as 5%. Morbidity and mortality rates are correlated with resection extent and are higher when bile duct excision and major hepatectomy are required to clear disease (see Chapters 102 and 119A). Given their greater rates of complications, these aggressive maneuvers should only be used as needed to achieve negative margins because their routine application has not been shown to confer any survival benefit.[86] Similarly, anatomic resection of segments IVB and V has been shown to have increased morbidity without survival benefit when compared with nonatomic (2-cm rim) resection.[86]

If radical resection is attempted and negative margins are achieved, the most frequent site of recurrence is distant disease as opposed to locoregional recurrence. This reflects the aggressive biology of the tumor and potentially points to a role for adjuvant therapy in advanced cases. There is a dearth of information regarding optimal regimens and timing. Patients with gallbladder cancer were included in the BILCAP trial, where adjuvant capecitabine was shown to improve survival in the aggregate per protocol analysis.[70] Although capecitabine did not appear to be associated with a clear survival benefit for gallbladder cancer on subset analysis, the study was not intended nor powered to answer this specific question. Combination gemcitabine and cisplatin is frequently used in the setting of unresectable disease and is another potential option, although level I data to support this regimen are still lacking. The ongoing ACTICCA-1 RCT is investigating this combination, with the control arm having recently been changed from observation to capecitabine in response to the BILCAP trial.

OS in gallbladder cancer is poor because of a combination of aggressive biology and advanced stage at diagnosis in most patients. T-stage is a surprisingly good discriminator of OS absent other criteria in gallbladder cancer because more advanced T-stage is directly correlated with higher rates of advanced disease.[87] Additionally, in patients with T2 tumors, the location of the tumor seems to impact OS. Tumors located on the peritoneal side of the gallbladder, designated T2a in AJCC 8th edition, have higher 3- and 5-year survival versus those on the hepatic parenchymal side (T2b; 73.7% vs. 52.1% and 64.7% vs. 42.6%, respectively; Fig. 101B.8).[87] Beyond staging, for patients who undergo curative-intent resection, positive margins,

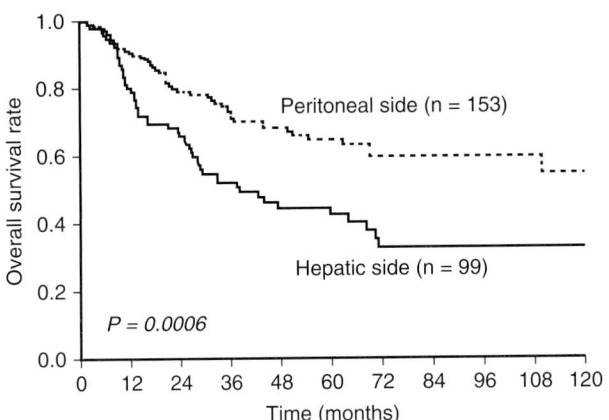

FIGURE 101B.8 Prognostic influence of tumor location after resection of T2 gallbladder cancer. See Chapter 49. (From Shindoh J, de Aretxabala X, Aloia TA, et al. Tumor location is a strong predictor of tumor progression and survival in T2 gallbladder cancer: An international multicenter study. *Ann Surg.* 2015;261[4]:733–739.)

lymph node metastasis, poor pathologic differentiation, and the presence of ascites have all been associated with worse OS.[88] Common bile duct involvement of the primary tumor is also associated with worse OS in some analyses.[89] Several nomograms have been developed to help predict survival, with some specifics regarding geographic areas reflecting a potential difference in disease biology.[90] One robust model developed from the SEER database identified T-stage, lymph node metastases,

CA19-9, surgical margin, tumor grade, and the presence of high-risk features including lymphovascular and perineural invasion as factors that can be used to determine prognosis (Fig. 101B.9).[91] For further information regarding gallbladder cancer, please see Chapter 49.

Perihilar Cholangiocarcinoma
(see Chapters 51 and 119B)

Perihilar cholangiocarcinoma used to be the most common biliary tract cancer, although its incidence appears to be on the decline recently. These tumors arise in the area of the biliary bifurcation extending from the second-order biliary radicals down to the cystic duct junction with the common hepatic duct. Approximately 7000 new cases are diagnosed each year in the United States and the incidence has remained stable or has decreased in the past several decades. Known risk factors for the development of perihilar cholangiocarcinoma are similar to other biliary tract cancers and include primary sclerosing cholangitis, hepatolithiasis, and parasites (*Clonorchis sinensis* and *Opisthorchis viverrini*). Despite these known risk factors, the majority of cases are sporadic with no identified antecedent.[92]

There are three main subtypes of extrahepatic (including perihilar) cholangiocarcinoma: sclerosing, nodular, and papillary. Most patients present with the nodular or sclerosing subtypes, which correspond to mass-forming and periductal infiltrating lesions as they progress. Least commonly, patients will present with the papillary form, which tends to have an endobiliary growth pattern and carries a more favorable prognosis.[93] In one series of patients with resected perihilar cholangiocarcinomas, disease-specific survival for papillary tumors was longer

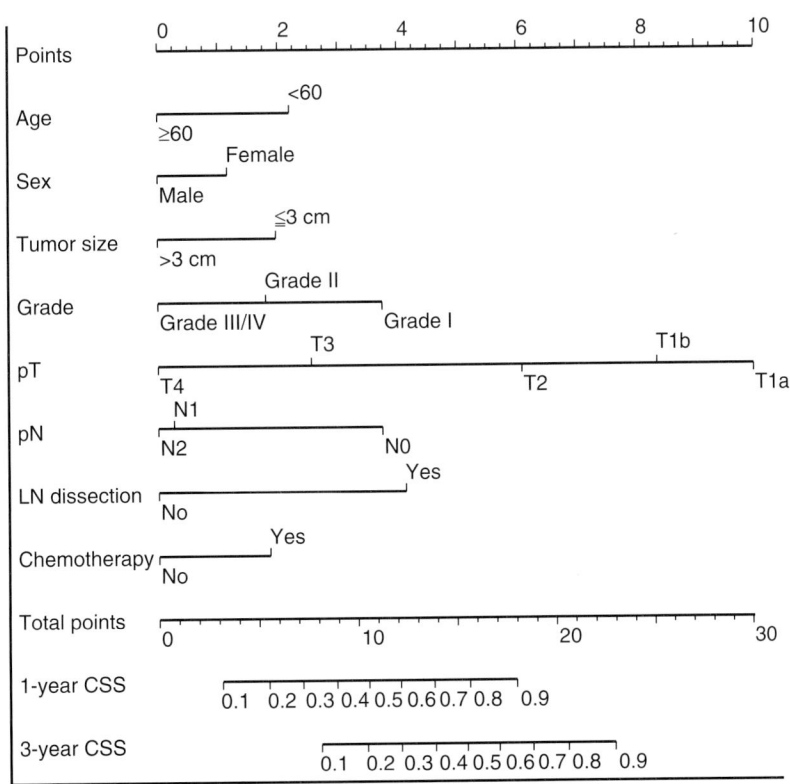

FIGURE 101B.9 Postoperative prognostic model for patients with nonmetastatic gallbladder cancer. (From Zhang W, Hong HJ, Chen YL. Establishment of a gallbladder cancer-specific survival model to predict prognosis in non-metastatic gallbladder cancer patients after surgical resection. *Dig Dis Sci.* 2018;63[9]:2251–2258.)

at 55.7 months compared with nodular-sclerosing lesions at 33.5 months.[94] It is not uncommon for overlapping features to be present in the same tumor.

Most patients present with jaundice or other biliary symptoms including cholangitis. These, however, tend to manifest late in the disease process, such that patients frequently present with locally advanced disease or distant spread.[95] Rarely, patients are identified incidentally on imaging performed for other purposes. Historically, late presentation has led to poor survival and inability to resect patients who present with perihilar cholangiocarcinoma.

Initial evaluation of patients identified with perihilar cholangiocarcinoma should focus on discerning which patients may benefit from surgical resection. Cross-sectional imaging can include CT, MRI, and magnetic resonance cholangiopancreatography (MRCP; see Chapter 16). The goal of these investigations should be to determine whether there is distant disease, which would preclude resection, and to define both the longitudinal and radial extent of the tumor for surgical planning. Which imaging modality is employed will depend on local expertise and preferences; however, in patients with obstructive jaundice at diagnosis, initial imaging evaluation should be appropriately performed before biliary decompression because intervention such as stent can cause inflammatory changes in the surrounding biliary tract, making it difficult to evaluate the extent of tumor spread precisely. Laboratory investigations should include liver function tests and CA19-9. When patients present with jaundice, CA19-9 may not be accurate and should typically be measured after decompression of obstructive jaundice. After biliary decompression, patients who have persistently elevated CA19-9 greater than 90 U/mL are highly likely to have a malignant cause of their biliary obstruction.[96]

Because most patients present with obstructive jaundice, many will undergo a pretreatment biliary drainage procedure. In addition to the relief of obstructive jaundice via stenting, endoscopic retrograde cholangiopancreatography (ERCP) also provides opportunities for visualization of the biliary tract and pathologic confirmation via brushings and fine-needle aspiration (FNA) of any suspicious lymph nodes. Unfortunately, conventional cytology frequently yields indeterminate results but accuracy can be increased with the addition of fluorescent in situ hybridization (FISH).[97] Direct cholangioscopy can also be used to assist in defining the extent of disease to better inform operative planning and guide biopsy (see Chapters 20 and 30). Nevertheless, ERCP should be used with caution, given the difficulty

associated with accurate stent placement. The endoscopic approach to decompressing a proximal may lead to misplacement of stents, incomplete drainage, and/or cholangitis, which can complicate management. For many patients, the percutaneous approach may be preferred (see Chapters 51B and 52).

Because of their location at or around the bifurcation of the right and left hepatic ducts, perihilar cholangiocarcinomas almost universally require major hepatic resection to achieve negative margins (see Chapter 119B). Surgical treatment for perihilar cholangiocarcinoma is largely determined by the Bismuth-Corlette classification (Fig. 101B.10). It may be possible to treat type I and II lesions with bile duct resection and reconstruction without the need for parenchymal resection. Type III tumors, however, will necessitate major hepatic resection. In rare instances, type IV tumors can be addressed at highly specialized centers with resection, although liver transplantation may offer a better alternative (see Chapter 108B).

When major hepatic resection is considered for perihilar cholangiocarcinoma, several factors will dictate whether resection can be safely achieved. Often, preoperative classification systems such as the Blumgart classification can be used to further delineate the likelihood of resectability.[98] Indeed, the interplay between laterality and extent of disease involvement of the hepatic duct, the portal vein, the hepatic artery, and the degree of atrophy of the hepatic lobe in relation to one another is critical in determining resectability (Table 101B.5).[98]

Perioperative mortality from resection of perihilar cholangiocarcinoma is largely related to infections and liver failure and appears to have diminished over the last 30 years with better understanding of liver physiology and appreciation for the future liver remnant (FLR). Patients who experience perioperative liver failure from inadequate FLR or postoperative bile leaks are at much greater risk for mortality in the perioperative period. For this reason, perihilar cholangiocarcinomas present unique challenges to the surgeon. Perihilar cholangiocarcinomas often spread along bile ducts further than is appreciated on preoperative imaging. Surgeons must weigh the benefit of "chasing" negative margins along the bile duct with increasingly high-risk biliary reconstructions that place the patient at high risk for perioperative morbidity and mortality. The two strongest predictors of postoperative liver failure–related death for perihilar cholangiocarcinoma in one retrospective study were preoperative cholangitis (odds ratio [OR] 7.5) and FLR volume less than 30% (OR 7.2).[99] Because of biliary obstruction, these patients frequently have impaired regenerative capacity of the

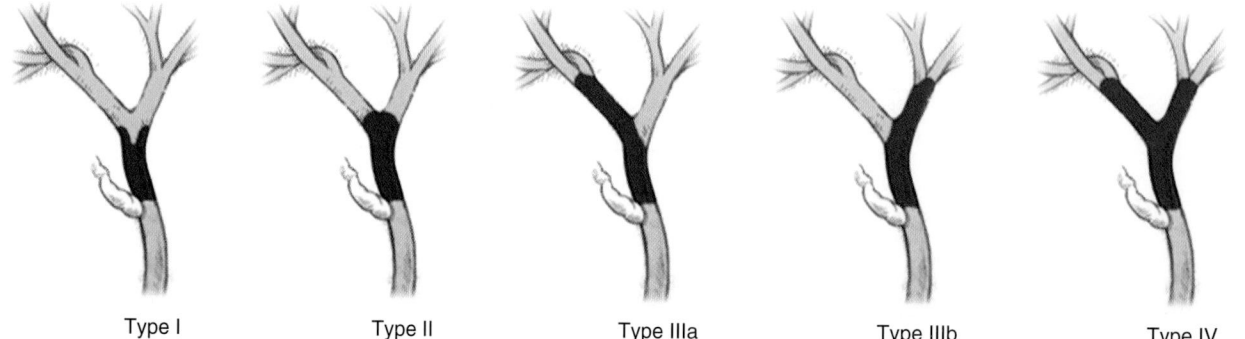

Type I   Type II   Type IIIa   Type IIIb   Type IV

FIGURE 101B.10   Bismuth-Corlette classification of Perihilar cholangiocarcinoma. See Chapter 51. (From Blechacz B. Cholangiocarcinoma: Current knowledge and new developments. *Gut and Liver.* 2017;11[1]:13–26.)

TABLE 101B.5 Blumgart Classification of Perihilar Cholangiocarcinoma

STAGE	CRITERIA (ALL STAGES INVOLVE THE BILIARY CONFLUENCE)
T1	± unilateral extension to second-order biliary radicles
T2	± unilateral extension to second-order biliary radicles with ipsilateral portal vein involvement ± ipsilateral hepatic lobar atrophy
T3	bilateral extension to second-order biliary radicles OR
	unilateral extension to second-order biliary radicles with contralateral portal vein involvement OR
	unilateral extension to second-order radicles with contralateral hepatic lobar atrophy OR
	main or bilateral portal vein involvement

TABLE 101B.6 Scoring System for Predicting Early Recurrence of Type IV Perihilar Cholangiocarcinoma After Curative Surgery

FACTOR	SCORE
CA19-9	
<200 (U/mL)	0
≥200 (U/mL)	1
Resection Margin	
R0	0
R1	1
AJCC N stage	
0	0
1	1
2	2
Lymphovascular invasion	
Absent	0
Present	1

AJCC, American Joint Committee on Cancer; *CA19-9,* carbohydrate antigen 19-9.

liver.[100] For this reason, strategies to augment the FLR and a low threshold for biliary decompression before surgery are warranted[99] (see Chapters 52 and 102).

In recent years, liver transplantation has become a viable option for patients with perihilar cholangiocarcinoma. When otherwise unresectable disease is present, highly selected patients (e.g., tumor mass visible on cross-sectional imaging, < 3 cm in greatest diameter, no regional or peritoneal involvement) can undergo treatment with neoadjuvant chemoradiotherapy and subsequent liver transplantation.[101] Recent studies have shown 5-year DFS rates of 65% to 70% when this approach is used in highly selected patients, similar to other oncologic indications for liver transplantation.[102] Additionally, in patients who meet the Mayo Clinic selection criteria previously mentioned, liver transplantation was found to be associated with superior 5-year OS when compared with surgical resection in a recent multi-institutional retrospective series (64% vs. 18%)[103] (see Chapter 108B).

The most common long-term failure of disease control is local recurrence after surgical resection. Rarely, local recurrences are isolated and may be addressed surgically; frequently, however, even when distant disease is not evident on imaging, it will be encountered if exploration is attempted. This recurrence pattern influences adjuvant treatment strategies. Capecitabine is now established as a standard of care adjuvant therapy for resected biliary tract cancers based on the BILCAP trial, although its effect size for perihilar cholangiocarcinoma was rather disappointing. Nevertheless, it should be noted that the study was not powered to evaluate perihilar cholangiocarcinoma alone.[70] Locoregional control may be improved by the addition of adjuvant radiation. In both Eastern and Western series, local recurrence rates and OS rates are improved by the addition of adjuvant chemoradiation.[104,105]

When patients can undergo margin-negative resection, which often requires the addition of hepatectomy to biliary resection, 5-year survival rates may exceed 50%. The major prognostic factors for both disease recurrence and survival include margin status, vascular invasion, and lymph node metastases, which are largely reflected in the TNM staging system. Scoring systems have been developed to help predict patients at highest risk for recurrence after resection (Table 101B.6),[106] and recently a nomogram has been developed based on data from SEER that allows for several survival comparisons to be developed (Fig. 101B.11), reaffirming the relationship between disease stage and prognosis.[107]

Perihilar cholangiocarcinoma continues to present a unique challenge for hepatobiliary surgeons. It is best addressed in a multidisciplinary fashion, starting from diagnosis all the way through treatment and surveillance. The presentations are nuanced and often require careful evaluation of radiographic studies and complex decision making with regards to surgical and systemic therapy. For further information on perihilar cholangiocarcinoma, please refer to Chapter 119B.

SECONDARY HEPATIC MALIGNANCIES

The disease processes that can result in secondary hepatic metastases are too numerous to count. In this chapter, we review the three most common to be considered for resection: colorectal cancer (far and away the single most common), neuroendocrine tumors, and, to a much lesser extent, breast cancer. This review is not meant to be an exhaustive list of all secondary liver tumors for which resection may be appropriate presently or in the future with the development of increasingly effective systemic therapies.

Colorectal Liver Metastases (see Chapters 90 and 118)

Colon cancer is one of the most frequent malignancies affecting patients in the United States and throughout the world. Approximately 50% of patients who are diagnosed with primary colon cancer will experience hepatic metastases at some point in their disease course, whether they present synchronously or metachronously. The liver is the most common site of spread for colorectal cancer, and colorectal liver metastases (CRLMs) are the number one indication for liver surgery in the United States.

Patients who present with CRLM should be evaluated by a multidisciplinary team to map out the best treatment course; critically, they should be evaluated by a liver surgeon before systemic therapy is initiated. All patients will require high-resolution cross-sectional imaging with CT or MRI to assess disease burden and anatomy (see Chapter 15). Positron emission tomography (PET/CT) may be useful for detecting extrahepatic metastases, although its routine use for staging and preoperative planning is not established. Its use does not supplant the need for other high-resolution cross-sectional imaging (see Chapter 18). All patients will also require evaluation of any

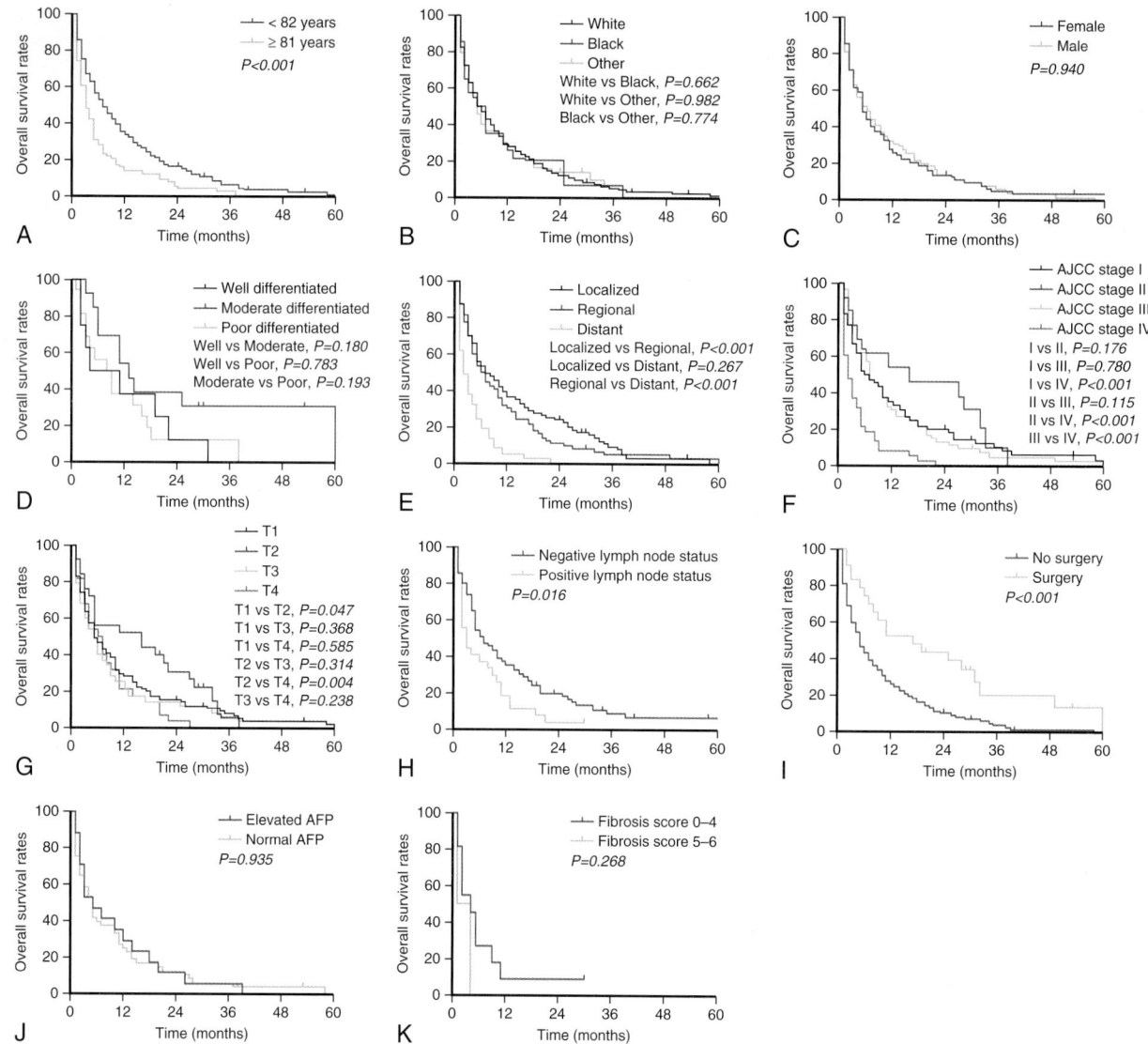

FIGURE 101B.11 Kaplan–Meier curve of overall survival in Klatskin tumor patients stratified by **(A)** age at diagnosis; **(B)** race; **(C)** sex; **(D)** primary tumor differential grade; **(E)** Surveillance, Epidemiology, and End Results (SEER) historic stage; **(F)** American Joint Committee on Cancer (AJCC) stage; **(G)** primary tumor size; **(H)** lymph node status; **(I)** surgery for primary tumor; **(J)** alpha-fetoprotein (AFP) level; **(K)** fibrosis score. See Chapter 51. (From Qi F, Zhou B, Xia J. Nomograms predict survival outcome of Klatskin tumors patients. *PeerJ*. 2020;8:e8570.)

underlying liver disease with a thorough history and examination. Those who have abnormal liver function tests (LFTs), ascites, cirrhosis, or other signs of liver disease will likely require further interrogation of the status of their liver condition to assess candidacy for localized therapy, including surgery.

Historically, contraindications to hepatectomy for CRLM included more than three liver metastases, portal lymph node involvement, small-volume lung metastases, and inability to achieve 1 cm margins. These contraindications have all been challenged in the era of modern liver surgery and many of them have been abandoned altogether. Advances in systemic therapy and in operative technique, along with a better understanding of tumor biology and molecular profiling, have all made CRLM increasingly treatable.

The main factors to consider when contemplating liver resection for CRLM are tumor-specific and anatomic. The biology of the patient's malignancy is important to consider for both planning of systemic therapy as well as accurate prognostication. Several mutational pathways have been identified in colorectal cancer that impart deleterious effects on survival, including *RAS*, *SMAD4*, *BRAF*, TP53, and *APC/PIK3CA*. In one study, patients with *RAS* wild-type disease had a median survival of 71 months after resection of CRLM versus 48 months for patients with *RAS* mutations. Individuals with *RAS* and *TP53* co-mutations saw further decrease in survival to a median of 41 months after resection.[108] Knowledge of these mutations can help guide the use of appropriate systemic therapy, operative planning, consideration of ablation and/or surgical margins, or the decision to proceed with nonoperative local control therapies.

Anatomic considerations are largely confined to whether the patient will have adequate FLR remaining after the operation to avoid postoperative liver insufficiency and/or failure (see Chapter 102). The minimum FLR needed will vary based on the quality of liver and presence of underlying liver disease. Factors involved in determination of required FLR include patients' liver volumes and body surface area, chronic liver disease, and exposure to chemotherapy. In general, the estimated minimum FLR is 20% for patients with a normal liver, 30% for patients with mild liver dysfunction (including chemotherapy-associated liver injury), and 40% for patients with cirrhosis. Strategies for liver expansion in patients with inadequate FLR include PVE, hepatic artery embolization and/or hepatic vein embolization (HVE), radioembolization (Y90), and ALPPS. Details about these techniques can be found in other chapters.

Most individuals who present with synchronous or metachronous metastatic disease will be candidates for systemic therapy before surgical resection, but this remains an area rife with controversy. Systemic therapy has a well-established role in converting patients with unresectable disease to potentially resectable disease (see Chapters 97 and 98). Patients who can successfully undergo resection after conversion enjoy long-term survival benefits over those who do not convert to resectability.[109] Similarly, HAI pumps have also been used in combination with systemic oxaliplatin or irinotecan and have been shown to downstage patient's disease into resectability.[110]

The use of chemotherapy in potentially resectable patients can allow for the natural history of disease to be observed before resection, shrink tumors to limit the extent of resection, and increase the odds of R0 resection. The European Organisation for Research and Treatment of Cancer (EORTC) intergroup trial 40983 randomized patients to perioperative 5-fluorouracil and leucovorin with oxaliplatin and showed improved 3-year PFS at 42.4% compared with 33.2% in patients who underwent surgery alone. This came at the cost of an increase in perioperative morbidity from 16% to 25%. There was no difference in OS after a median follow-up of 8.5 years.[111,112] Advocates of upfront surgery and those of perioperative chemotherapy both point to this trial as supporting their point of view, and significant controversy remains regarding the need for and timing of systemic chemotherapy in the setting of resectable oligometastatic CRLM (see Chapter 98).

One potential drawback to administration of systemic chemotherapy before liver resection is chemotherapy-induced hepatotoxicity (see Chapter 98). Regimens containing oxaliplatin or irinotecan have been implicated in steatohepatitis, vascular injury, and sinusoidal dilation syndrome (nodular regenerative hyperplasia). In patients who receive oxaliplatin, nearly half experience some degree of sinusoidal dilation and in those who receive irinotecan, approximately 10% will experience steatosis or steatohepatitis. Both findings have been associated with increased perioperative morbidity. This increase in morbidity was especially significant when the interval between completion of chemotherapy and surgical resection was less than 4 weeks, or when the number of cycles of chemotherapy received was greater than 8.[113,114] Additionally, some data suggest that the addition of bevacizumab may temper the severity of oxaliplatin-induced sinusoidal injury.[115,116]

Another challenge to the neoadjuvant chemotherapy approach is the phenomenon of disappearing liver metastases. In patients who receive at least four cycles of preoperative chemotherapy, 5% to 25% will experience disappearing metastases, lesions that are no longer detectable on cross-sectional imaging or on intraoperative assessment.[117] Importantly, although radiographic disappearance may predict pathologic complete response, 33% of these disappeared lesions will have residual disease on pathologic evaluation.[118] One strategy to mitigate disappearing liver metastases is the placement of fiducial markers before the initiation of chemotherapy.[119] Although it is not always possible to delineate which lesions will, in fact, disappear, at our center we routinely place fiducials for tumors less than 2 cm that are not capsular or subcapsular and would not routinely be part of a planned anatomic resection (see Chapter 15).

Up to 20% of patients with colorectal cancer will be diagnosed with synchronous liver metastases at the time their primary colorectal cancer is discovered. These patients have decreased 5-year survival rates after resection when compared with those with metachronous presentations.[120] For patients with straightforward presentations of their primary cancer and synchronous low-volume liver disease, proceeding straight to surgery is an acceptable strategy per NCCN guidelines, although the majority of patients with this presentation will receive neoadjuvant systemic therapy.[121] One review of the Liver-MetSurvey International Registry showed patients treated with a neoadjuvant approach and those treated with upfront surgery followed by adjuvant chemotherapy had similar 5-year survival rates; however, patients who did not receive any systemic therapy had worse DFS and OS.[122] The data support the idea that patients who are more likely to experience perioperative morbidity from extensive primary or liver resections should receive neoadjuvant chemotherapy so that complications do not prevent them from return to intended oncologic therapy and the resulting poorer oncologic outcomes.[123]

When dealing with synchronous presentations, clearly defining the optimal sequencing of primary resection and liver resection remains a challenge. There is no "one size fits all" approach that can be applied to all patients; instead, characteristics of the patient, treating institution and practitioners, as well as of the tumors themselves will have to be considered. A symptomatic primary tumor will often mandate early intervention. For instance, patients who have obstructing or near-obstructing primary colonic tumors will likely be better served with the conventional approach whereby the primary tumor is resected first followed by delayed liver resection (unless the CRLM is amenable to a straightforward partial hepatectomy), often with systemic therapy administered in between. This approach can palliate symptoms but carries the risk of progression in the liver. Many patients managed with the conventional approach never make it to liver resection.[124] The reverse strategy, which addresses the liver-based disease first, is often appropriate in the setting of low-risk primary tumors and extensive liver disease. Using this treatment approach, patients are more likely to complete the entire sequence of care than the conventional pathway.[125] Increasingly, combined colorectal and liver resection is performed during the same operation. Cumulative morbidity and mortality rates for well-selected patients are lower than staged procedures, and oncologic outcomes are similar. A meta-analysis of the liver first, conventional, and combined approaches showed that oncologic outcomes, including survival, were not different.[126]

Several prognostic scoring systems have been devised that factor in preoperative, intraoperative, and postoperative characteristics and can stratify survival by these variables.[127,128] These systems range from simple scoring systems to complex nomograms and multiplicative indices that are not possible to calculate by hand. Some of these models have been maintained and updated as new predictive measures, such as mutational status, have evolved. These tools can be helpful when counseling patients and caregivers about the benefits of a surgical or other therapeutic approach.

The potential permutations of size, number, and distribution of CRLM are near infinite and a full discussion of potential surgical approaches to different lesions is beyond the scope of this chapter. In the past, anatomic liver resections, including major hepatectomies, had been more prevalent and routinely offered, especially when dealing with multiple tumors. In recent years, recognition of patterns of liver-based recurrence have prompted interest in parenchymal-sparing techniques that focus on multiple nonanatomic resections to preserve functional liver. Several studies have shown similar rates of R0 resection, liver recurrence-free survival, and OS for parenchymal-sparing hepatectomy when compared with anatomic resection, with the benefit of increased salvageability in the event of liver-based recurrence, with improved survival.[129-131] In some cases, parenchymal-sparing resections can be taken to extremes to preserve liver, including the use of novel techniques like transverse hepatectomy and "tunnel" procedures (Fig. 101B.12).[132] Despite this evolution, there remains a robust role for anatomic resections when dictated by patient anatomy or disease.

Bilobar liver metastases remain one of the most challenging scenarios facing surgeons in the management of CRLM. Historically, bilobar disease was a contraindication to surgical intervention, but with advances in surgical and interventional radiology techniques, it has become increasingly manageable. Frequently, two-stage hepatectomy can be used, in combination with portal vein embolization to clear bilobar disease (see Chapter 102). This consists of a first stage wherein disease in the left liver is cleared with partial hepatectomies, followed by PVE to the right liver. After adequate hypertrophy of the left liver (which has been cleared of tumors), the patient then undergoes a right hepatectomy. Alternative approaches for clearance of bilobar disease include ALPPS, but the long-term oncologic effects of ALPPS versus PVE remain unknown currently. The judicious use of ablative techniques in addition to resection can expand the options in dealing with more widespread intrahepatic dissemination of CRLM (see Chapter 96). HAI may also play a role in converting unresectable disease to resectability, although this is accomplished in only a small minority of patients.

Historically, the optimal margin for CRLM was quoted as 1 cm. Several large case series have challenged this surgical

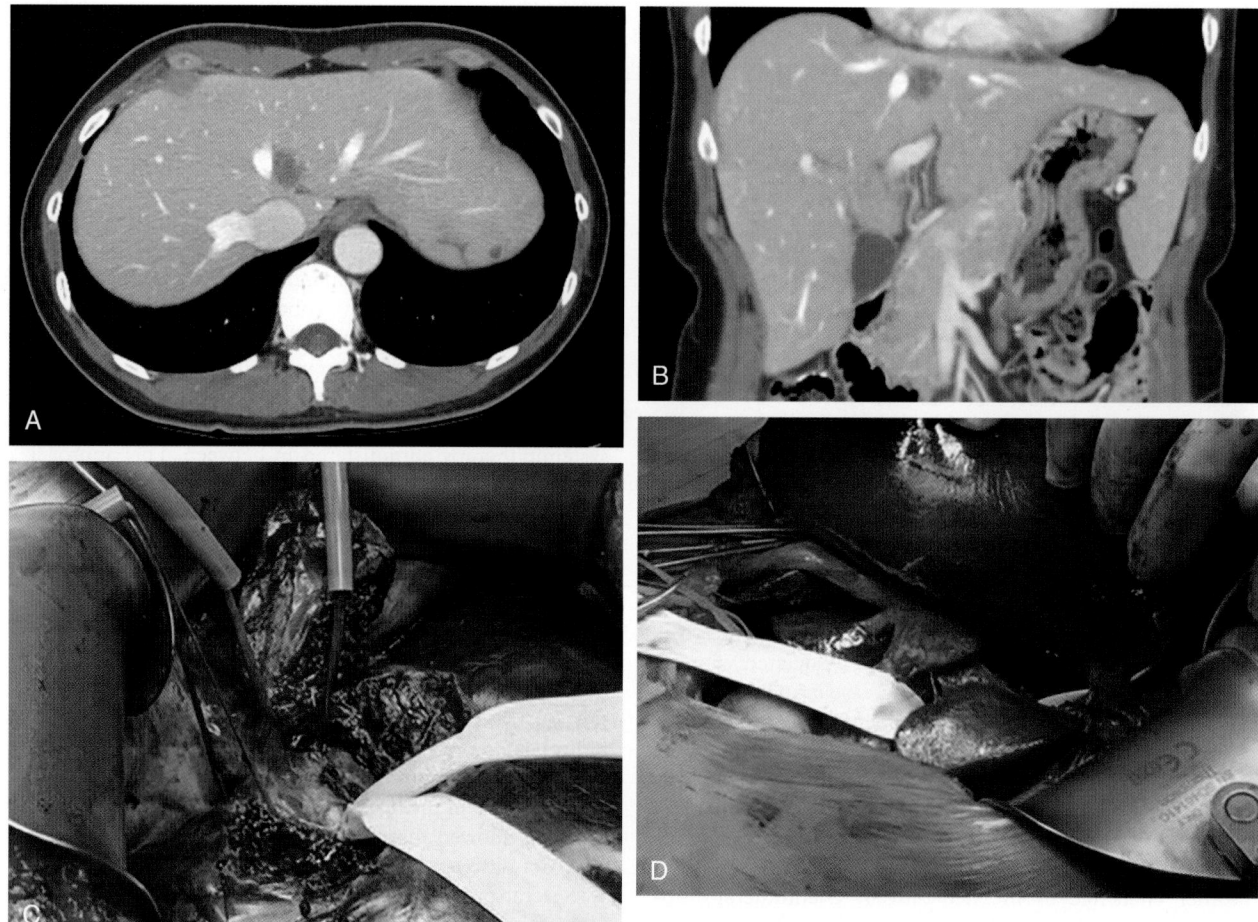

FIGURE 101B.12 **A,** Axial and **(B)** Coronal formats of computed tomography (CT) scan from a 52-year-old woman with a colorectal metastasis in segment IVA intimately involving the middle hepatic vein and extending toward the superior aspect of the paracaval caudate. Intraoperative photos demonstrate **(C)** the right middle and left hepatic veins isolated in Rummel tourniquets with dissection off of the inferior vena cava (IVC) and reflected cephalad (Sp). A Penrose drain has been advanced along the IVC as part of a hanging maneuver. The tunnel was created through division of the ligamentum venosum. **(D)** A medial to lateral view: The tunnel is formed by creating a hepatectomy between the left lateral sector (LLS) and the caudate lobe (CL) to facilitate dissection. See Chapter 15.

dogma and have shown that R0 resection of 1 mm or greater can achieve similar rates of DFS and OS.[133,134] There has also been some recognition that R1 margins, particularly when associated with vessels that would otherwise necessitate further resection leading to sacrificing of large liver volumes, may be acceptable in some circumstances.[135] Re-resection of R1 margins to achieve R0 margins has not shown to decrease liver-based recurrence, and when intrahepatic recurrences do occur, the pattern tends to be disseminated throughout the liver and not necessarily along the previous positive margin.[136]

For patients who have received neoadjuvant chemotherapy before resection, there is growing recognition that tumor viability impacts not only local recurrence rates but also OS. Complete pathologic response to preoperative chemotherapy is one of the strongest predictors of long-term survival after hepatectomy (Fig. 101B.13).[137] Unfortunately, this information is not available until after resection is completed. There has been some effort to correlate pathologic response with imaging-based morphologic criteria with some success, although this remains a weaker correlative than pathologic data.[138]

The consideration for adjuvant therapy in patients who undergo resection of metachronous disease is not dictated by level I evidence; instead, it is largely inferred from treatment of primary colorectal cancer where node-positive disease benefits from adjuvant chemotherapy.[139] For this reason, it is important to consider the context of the patient's disease and prior treatment regimens. In patients with metachronous disease who are naïve to systemic therapy, it is reasonable to administer adjuvant chemotherapy, particularly in patients with unfavorable prognostic criteria. For patients who have received previous therapy, the role of additional chemotherapy is less clear. RCTs to date have largely shown increases in DFS with adjuvant chemotherapy, but those results have paradoxically translated into similar or even decreased OS[112,140,141] (see Chapter 98).

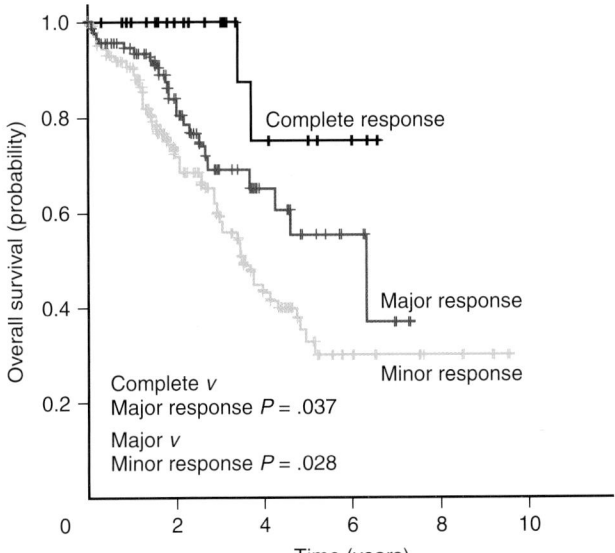

FIGURE 101B.13 Overall survival for colorectal metastases stratified by degree of pathologic response. See Chapter 90. (From Blazer DG, 3rd, Kishi Y, Maru DM, et al. Pathologic response to preoperative chemotherapy: A new outcome end point after resection of hepatic colorectal metastases. *J Clin Oncol.* 20 2008;26[33]:5344–5351.)

Similar to systemic adjuvant therapy, HAI of cytotoxic chemotherapy has also been shown to increase DFS (see Chapter 97). HAI has previously been shown to improve OS when compared with infusional 5-fluorouracil, but it is unknown whether that benefit would remain when compared with modern doublet and triplet chemotherapy.[142] Additional barriers to the more widespread use of HAI include its limited availability at few centers and need for specialized expertise.

There are a wide variety of clinical scenarios for patients with metastatic colorectal cancer. This remains one of the most clinically diverse areas of practice within liver surgery. Many valid approaches to these patients are available and require the engagement from a multidisciplinary team. Ongoing trials and active development of new therapies are likely to continue to reshape the landscape of available therapeutic options for CRLM in the near future. For further information on colorectal liver metastases, please refer to Chapter 90.

Gastroenteropancreatic Neuroendocrine Tumors
(see Chapters 91 and 118)

After metastatic colorectal cancer, the most common secondary malignant tumors treated with liver resection are gastroenteropancreatic neuroendocrine tumors (NETs). The incidence of NETs has more than doubled in the last two decades and metastatic disease is encountered in 10% to 34% of patients at the time of diagnosis. Another 38% will go on to develop metastatic disease during their treatment.[143] Liver is the dominant site of metastasis, and multifocal liver disease is the dominant pattern of spread. Liver metastases are the main cause of mortality in patients with metastatic NET.

Symptoms from NETs can be vague or nonexistent based on the primary site of disease, leading to late presentation. NETs can be broadly classified according to whether they produce hormones or not as functional and nonfunctional tumors. Some functional tumors are not symptomatic until they are metastatic, either because of small burden of disease or metabolism of hormones by the liver. Functional hormones frequently produced by NETs include gastrin, insulin, serotonin, vasoactive intestinal peptide, glucagon, and somatostatin.

In addition to functional status, grade is another important biologic factor to consider when selecting therapy for patients with NET liver metastases. The natural history for G1 (Ki-67 index up to 2%) and G2 (Ki-67 index 3%–20%) tumors is that of an indolent course with mean OS of 8.1 years from symptom onset.[144] G3 (Ki-67 index > 20%) tumors, on the other hand, have been shown to have worse prognosis, with a median OS of 5 months in the metastatic setting and consequently less clear treatment guidelines.[145] The European Neuroendocrine Society (ENETS) publishes separate guidelines for G1/G2 and G3 tumors, and for metastatic G3 tumors, recommends against surgical resection, debulking, or ablative strategies for liver metastases.[146] Subsequently, a retrospective case series showed that in highly selected patients, there may be a benefit in OS with surgery, particularly for patients with lower Ki-67 of 21% to 54% and those who receive adjuvant systemic therapy.[147] There may exist grade heterogeneity between primary tumor and liver metastases, between liver lesions, and even between biopsies of the same lesion; in this scenario, patients are classified according to the more aggressive feature because even one G3 lesion on biopsy predicts significantly worse PFS.[148]

For patients with G1 or G2 NET liver metastases, surgical resection has been shown to increase OS and symptom control.

The goals of surgery will depend on the distribution of disease. A useful framework to help guide this discussion was reported by Frilling et al.[149]:

Type I: Single metastasis of any type
Type II: Isolated metastatic bulk accompanied by smaller deposits
Type III: Disseminated metastatic spread, with both liver lobes always involved, single lesion of varying size, and virtually no normal liver parenchyma

Lesions that fit the definition of type I are frequently approached with curative-intent hepatectomy. Some patients with type II disease can also achieve an R0 curative-intent hepatectomy but are more likely to require strategies for volume expansion and staged operations. For type II patients for whom R0 resection cannot be achieved, treatment with debulking and local control strategies may be the next best option; this can be employed in some type III patients as well. Select patients with types II and III disease who are unable to be cured by liver resection may be eligible for liver transplantation as an alternative therapy with curative intent.[150]

Preoperative imaging underestimates the disease burden of NETs by approximately 50% when compared with analysis of explanted specimens, frequently missing less than 2-mm metastases.[151] Patients who are planning to undergo curative-intent surgery are found to have more extensive disease and only undergo R0 resection a median of 63% of the time in one meta-analysis.[152] Undergoing curative-intent surgery is associated with improved survival, which is likely reflective of lower disease burden.[153] Even when hepatectomy is undertaken with curative-intent, 50% to 94% patients will ultimately develop intrahepatic recurrence by 5 years.[154,155]

In patients who are not eligible for curative-intent surgery, surgical debulking is another option. This approach has been shown to provide relief from symptomatic metastases, increasing symptom control to 86% versus 64% with medical therapy alone.[156] There is debate in the literature about the optimal target volume for resection. Some published experiences use the threshold of 90% of liver-based disease being resected for effective debulking, whereas others have used a lower threshold of 70%. Debulking 70% or more of the disease has been shown to improve PFS (3.2 years vs. 1.3 years) and OS.[157] Interestingly, 90% cytoreduction showed improved PFS when compared with less than 90% (3.8 years vs. 1.5 years) but was not associated with improvement in OS.[157] Our group tries to clear disease in the liver whenever possible but refrains from engaging in radical hepatectomies that result in high-risk morbidities.

Ablative therapies are frequently used to treat NETs in individuals who will not tolerate liver resection. Additionally, it is also used as an adjunct therapy when all disease is unable to be cleared by surgery. The largest impediment to ablative therapy is that many NET liver metastases are larger than 3 cm and are inadequately addressed by ablation alone, and in the setting of substantial unresectable bilobar disease, ablation alone is contraindicated. When ablation can be employed as sole therapy, median survival is 11 years with only a 6.3% recurrence rate.[158] This is likely reflective of small tumors and low overall tumor burden. In patients who undergo combined modality treatment with surgery and completion ablation, median survival is lower and recurrence rates are much higher, a function of more advanced disease.[156] In a meta-analysis comparing modalities, liver resection is associated with higher rates of symptom relief and longer OS than nonsurgical regimens.[153] When surgery is compared with intra-arterial therapy, surgery improved median survival (123 months vs. 34 months) and 5-year survival (74% vs. 30%). The survival benefit of surgery was especially pronounced in patients who had symptomatic tumors.[159]

It is unclear if the tumor's primary organ site plays a role in prognosis. A large retrospective single-institution study identified small bowel NETs as having better OS than pancreatic NETs (OR 0.5) in patients who had liver metastases.[160] A subsequent multi-institutional retrospective review showed similar results, but the difference in survival did not persist after propensity score matching.[161] A recently published, externally validated nomogram identified primary tumor location as one of four variables that were predictive of DFS (Fig. 101B.14).[162]

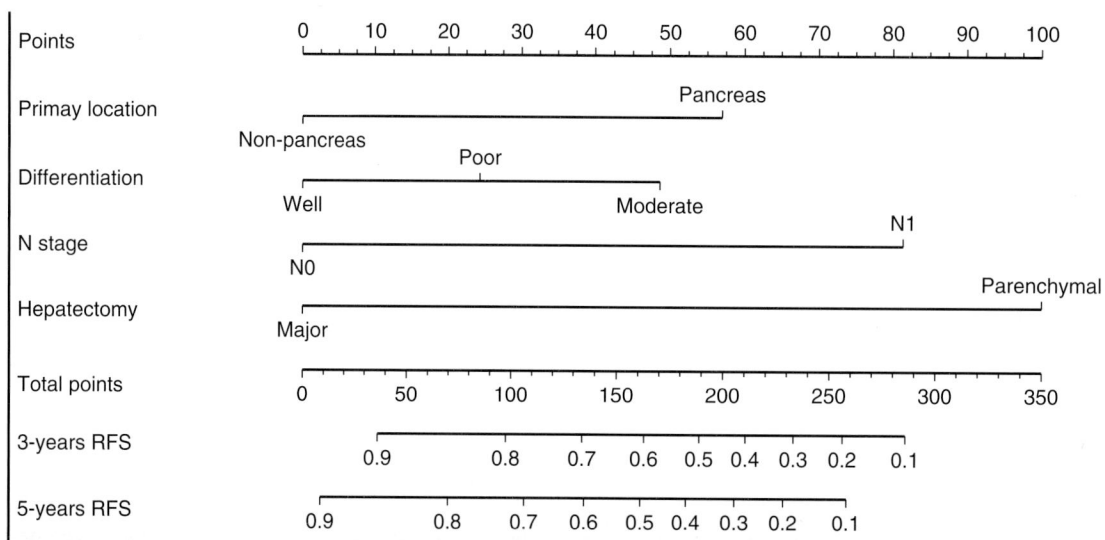

FIGURE 101B.14 Prognostic nomogram predicting the 3 and 5-year recurrence-free survival rates of patients with neuroendocrine liver metastasis. See Chapter 91. (From Xiang JX, Zhang XF, Weiss M, et al. Multi-institutional development and external validation of a nomogram predicting recurrence after curative liver resection for neuroendocrine liver metastasis. *Ann Surg Oncol.* 2020;27[10]:3717–3726.)

The other factors in the nomogram included tumor differentiation, nodal disease, and type of liver resection (major vs. parenchymal sparing). It is unclear if anatomic resection provides better margin control for NETs or if parenchymal sparing approaches are a surrogate for more extensive disease based on this analysis.

The evidence for neoadjuvant and adjuvant systemic therapies in metastatic NET liver metastases comes from small retrospective case series. Peptide receptor radionuclide therapies have successfully been used to downstage some unresectable NET liver metastases into resectability.[163] Reports of adjuvant therapy have been less encouraging, with one retrospective study finding no difference in PFS or OS for patients who received streptozotocin-5FU versus observation after resection of NET liver metastases.[164] A full discussion regarding systemic treatment of NET is beyond the scope of this chapter.

Orthotopic liver transplantation has been used in some patients with extensive bilobar disease that would otherwise be considered unresectable (see Chapter 108B). Despite having a more indolent disease process than other indications for liver transplantation, such as HCC, IHC, or perihilar cholangiocarcinoma, patients with NET liver metastases who undergo liver transplantation have historically had disappointing survival. A report of the UNOS dataset from 1988 to 2013 found that 5-year survival was only 49% with 39% graft survival at 5 years for patients with NET liver metastases.[165]

Metastatic Breast Cancer (see Chapters 92 and 118)

Breast cancer is the second leading cause of cancer-related death in women. In the United States, there are more than 250,000 new diagnoses of breast cancer and 42,000 deaths each year. There are a wide variety of metastatic presentations in metastatic breast cancer and median survival from diagnosis is 17 to 24 months.[166] Systemic therapy is the primary treatment modality for most patients with metastatic breast cancer, but there is some evidence that patients with low disease burden can be treated aggressively with resection. Approximately 10% of patients who have metastatic breast cancer will present with isolated hepatic metastases and, depending on underlying liver function and distribution of disease, may be eligible for local therapies, including hepatectomy.[167]

Historically, metastatic breast cancer was primarily treated with palliative chemotherapy and best supportive care. Patients who had metastases to the liver did worse than patients with metastatic disease at other sites, and overall had poor prognosis with median survival of 4 to 11 months.[168] In the last 30 years, with significant improvements in systemic therapy options, liver-directed therapy has been offered with increasing frequency to patients with metastatic breast cancer. When selecting patients with liver metastases for resection, it is important to consider hormone receptor status and the patient's response to systemic therapy, in addition to traditional considerations of underlying liver disease and FLR.

Unfortunately, no RCTs have been completed for hepatectomy in metastatic breast cancer and survival data is largely from retrospective studies that likely suffer from significant selection bias. Patients who undergo successful liver resection have a median survival of 35.1 months with 5-year survival of 33%. Median DFS is 21.5 months with 18% DFS at 5 years.[169] The most common pattern of recurrence after hepatectomy is liver-only, and some patients will be eligible to undergo repeat hepatectomy or other local therapies as salvage. Less commonly, patients will have both liver and systemic recurrence, and systemic recurrence alone is the least common recurrence pattern.[170] For patients undergoing hepatectomy, factors associated with poor prognosis included positive margins and hormone receptor–negative disease.[171] Additionally, our group has recently analyzed breast cancer liver metastases based on luminal classification[172] and reported that HER2-enriched subtype was associated with prolonged PFS in patients who underwent hepatectomy for breast cancer liver metastases.[173]

Similarly, there has been no RCT that compares hepatectomy with other local-control therapies. A recent meta-analysis found that RFA had inferior DFS and OS when compared with hepatectomy but that significant heterogeneity existed in the published retrospective literature.[174] TACE has also been investigated as an alternative method of local control but, again, significant heterogeneity exists in the literature. Reported OS for TACE ranges from 7.3 to 47.0 months and DFS from 2.0 to 17.0 months.[175]

Treatment algorithms have not been as clearly defined for breast cancer liver metastases as colorectal or neuroendocrine surgery but likely represent the next frontier in potentially curative surgery for metastatic liver disease. It is reasonable to consider patients for liver resection if they have low-volume oligometastatic disease to the liver and favorable hormone-receptor status and R0 resection is achievable.

BENIGN AND PREMALIGNANT HEPATIC LESIONS (SEE CHAPTERS 88 AND 118)

This portion of the chapter will focus on benign and premalignant hepatic lesions. This review is not meant to be exhaustive but rather will cover the most common lesions and those that frequently indicate resection.

Hepatic Hemangiomas

Hepatic hemangiomas are the most common benign liver tumors and the second most common liver tumors after metastases. Their true incidence is difficult to ascertain but has been reported to range from 0.4% to 20% of the general population.[176] These lesions are thought to be congenital in nature, arising from epithelial cells, and typically have a cavernous vascular space when examined histologically and therefore may be referred to as cavernous hemangiomas. Hepatic hemangiomas are benign, and the vast majority are asymptomatic and require no intervention, even when they are "giant" hemangiomas (>10 cm; Fig. 101B.15). They are usually discovered incidentally on abdominal imaging or during workup of another liver-related pathology.

Rarely, hemangiomas may cause symptoms that warrant intervention. Giant hemangiomas pushing on the stomach may cause early satiety. Surgeons should be wary of pain as a sole indication for operation because the vast majority of patients with abdominal pain are found to have another underlying cause.[177] In addition to these chronic presentations, patients with giant hemangiomas may experience hemorrhage, rupture, or Kasabach-Merritt syndrome (acquired thrombocytopenia secondary to consumptive coagulopathy) that are indications for intervention.

For patients who are truly symptomatic, hepatic resection can be undertaken to relieve symptoms. Although both anatomic resection and enucleation have been described in the treatment of hemangiomas, the latter has been shown to result

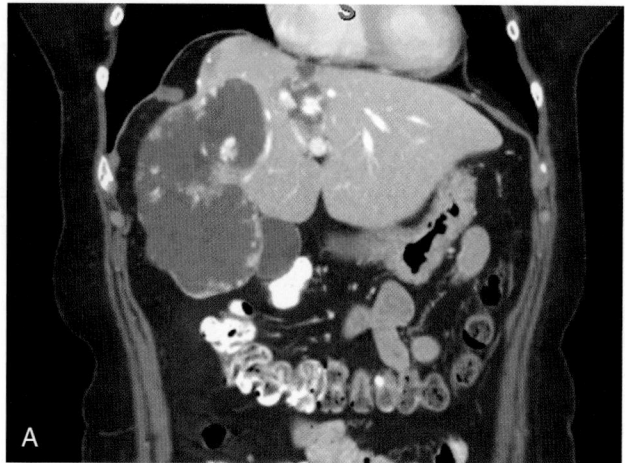
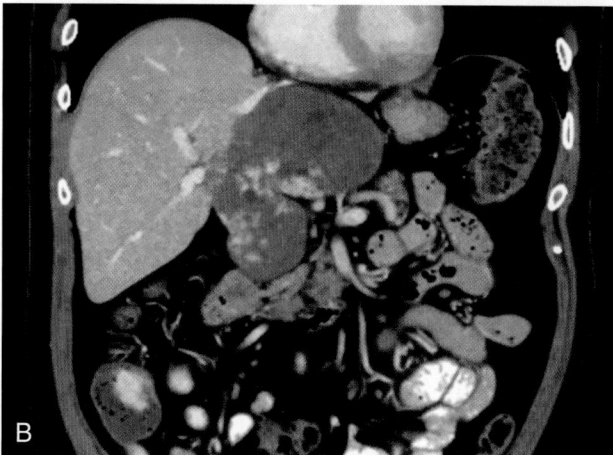

FIGURE 101B.15 Computed tomography (CT) imaging from two asymptomatic patients with giant hemangiomas. **A,** A 61-year-old woman with multiple hemangiomas, including a giant 16-cm hemangioma that occupies most of the right liver. **(B)** A 70-year-old man with incidentally diagnosed giant hemangioma growing from the caudate lobe. See Chapter 14.

in lower rates of blood loss and bile leak while preserving normal liver parenchyma.[178] One exception is centrally located lesions, which may be more difficult to approach with enucleation.[179] For patients at high risk for bleeding with surgical intervention because of difficult lesion locations and large hemangioma size, preoperative transarterial embolization has been shown to decrease need for intraoperative blood products and may also serve as standalone treatment for cavernous hemangiomas.[180] For patients who undergo successful surgery, recurrence of the hemangioma is exceedingly rare with few reported cases in the literature.[181] Although there are reports of alternative nonoperative treatments including RFA, radiation therapy, and others, outcomes data remain limited and they should be reserved for patients with absolute contraindications to surgical therapy.[182,183]

Hepatic Adenomas

Hepatic adenomas are rare, solid liver lesions also termed hepatocellular adenomas. They are more common in women than men and are associated with exposure to estrogens, either endogenous or exogenous. They are also associated with anabolic androgen use, obesity, and glycogen storage disorders. Unlike hemangiomas, adenomas may undergo malignant transformation. Adenomas can be solitary or multiple, and when more than 10 lesions are present, in the absence of risk factors, the condition is termed liver adenomatosis.[184,185]

The largest risk factor for adenoma development is exposure to estrogens, most commonly from pregnancy or oral contraceptives. The increase in adenoma size has a dose-dependent relationship with oral contraceptives. Stopping oral contraceptives is associated with regression of adenomas and can be a valid treatment strategy alone.[186] Similarly, adenomas are associated with anabolic steroid use and cessation may also lead to regression (Fig. 101B.16).

Distinct subtypes of hepatic adenomas have been described that have different associated risks, including malignant degeneration. The most common subtype is inflammatory adenoma (HCA-I) and is associated with obesity and NASH (see Chapter 69). The second most common subtype is HNF1α (HCA-H) mutated hepatocellular adenoma, which is associated with a mutation in the estrogen receptor. The third subtype is associated with mutation in the β-catenin gene (HCA-B). HCA-B is associated with an increased risk of malignant transformation, particularly when lesions are larger than 5 cm in size.[187] Finally, the unclassified variant (HCA-U) covers adenomas that do not fit the other categories.

The risk of rupture, bleeding, and malignant transformation of adenomas is not insignificant, prompting a different management approach than other benign liver tumors. The clinical presentations of hepatic adenomas range widely, from small asymptomatic lesions found incidentally to large tumors presenting with acute life-threatening rupture. The risk of spontaneous rupture and bleeding is especially significant when tumor size exceeds 5 cm.[188] A diagnosis of adenoma can usually be established with cross-sectional imaging (CT or MRI) alone without the need for biopsy (see Chapter 14). This is because adenomas have characteristic features on imaging that include sharp, nonlobulated margins and partial enhancement on contrast-enhanced CT scans. On MRI, these tumors are mostly hyperintense on T1-weighted images. They appear heterogeneous and show differential findings on T2-weighted images.[189] Occasionally, a biopsy is needed when the diagnosis is unclear on imaging and to help distinguish between pathologic subtypes

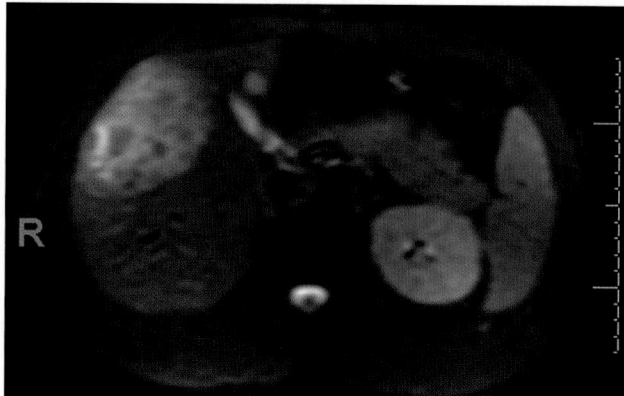

FIGURE 101B.16 Magnetic resonance imaging (MRI) of a 39-year-old man who developed a giant adenoma (9.5 cm) and several smaller adenomas after anabolic steroid use. The largest lesion was resected and found to be a beta-catenin adenoma. The remaining tumors regressed after steroid cessation. See Chapter 14.

for risk stratification. Larger lesions may present with elevations in gamma-glutamyltransferase (GGT).

Large reviews have shown that the risk of rupture for tumors less than 5 cm is virtually nonexistent. Large tumor size is also associated with malignant transformation, again with 5 cm marking a threshold above which the risk is significantly increased, regardless of subtype. Additional factors that increase the risk of malignant transformation include male sex, which is associated with a 6-fold to 10-fold higher risk; the β-catenin adenoma subtype; anabolic steroid use; recent oral contraceptive use; and glycogen storage diseases. On the other hand, the number of adenomas does not represent a risk factor for malignant transformation or for rupture or hemorrhage.

Patients at high risk for complications can be selected for resection. Male patients should undergo resection for any hepatic adenoma because of the increased risk of malignant transformation. In female patients, other risk factors need to be considered and there is a potential for nonoperative management, particularly in patients with small tumors (<5 cm) who can stop oral contraceptives. These tumors can be followed with imaging alone. Even tumors greater than 5 cm can be shrunk by cessation of oral contraceptives and observed with response or proceed to resection if they fail to regress. Any patients with symptoms can be offered resection for palliation, but the risk of intervention should be balanced against the severity of symptoms. Patients with multiple adenomas should be managed based on symptoms or the size of the largest tumor and not the number of lesions.

In those patients who cannot be safely observed, hepatic resection is the gold standard. Because they are benign, adenomas can be resected without the need for wide margins and via any approach that can deliver a safe outcome, whether it be minimally invasive or open, parenchymal sparing or anatomic. In patients who present with adenomas that have already ruptured, the mortality associated with immediate surgical intervention may exceed 8%. Instead, transarterial embolization can be used to temporize bleeding before proceeding to surgical resection (see Chapter 21). This strategy has been associated with lower blood loss, postoperative complications, and length of stay.[190] Adenomas are unlikely to recur after surgical resection except in the case of a liver field defect, which is most commonly encountered in individuals with glycogen storage disorders. In this scenario, continued recurrence may necessitate proceeding to liver transplantation as definitive management. In patients who do not undergo resection for hepatic adenomas, continued surveillance with imaging is warranted.

Focal Nodular Hyperplasia

Focal nodular hyperplasia (FNH) is the second most common benign liver lesion after hemangiomas. It is approximately twice as common as hepatic adenomas and is 3 to 8 times more likely to be present in women.[191] It is a polyclonal lesion that is made up of vascular abnormalities often around a central scar without any potential for malignant transformation.[192] Although some patients present with vague abdominal symptoms such as pain or early satiety, most have no symptoms, and lesions are found incidentally on cross-sectional imaging.

The diagnosis of FNH can be established by characteristic imaging features (see Chapter 14). When CT scan is performed, FNH will typically appear hypointense or isointense to liver parenchyma. After contrast administration, the lesion will become hyperintense compared with liver parenchyma with a

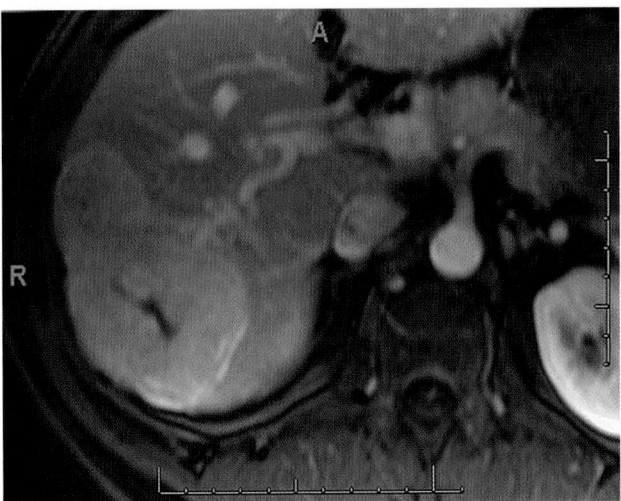

FIGURE 101B.17   T1 magnetic resonance imaging (MRI) of a patient with a benign focal nodular hyperplasia with characteristic central scar. See Chapter 14. (From Tran Cao HS, Marcal LP, Mason MC, et al. Benign hepatic incidentalomas. *Curr Probl Surg.* 2019;56[9]:100642.)

nonenhancing central scar. On washout and delayed imaging, the lesion will be hypointense or isointense, but the central scar may enhance. On MRI, the lesion will appear hypointense or isointense on T1-weighted imaging and hyperintense on T2-weighted imaging. The central scar is hypointense on T1 imaging (Fig. 101B.17) and hyperintense on T2 imaging.[193,194] When CT and MRI are inconclusive, a gadoxetic-acid-enhanced MRI (Gd-EOB-DTPA-MRI) can be used to secure a diagnosis with high sensitivity and is the diagnostic approach taken at our center.[195] If a diagnosis is unable to be secured with noninvasive imaging, percutaneous biopsy can be performed and should include the central scar. Microscopic examination of the scar revealing bile ductules is pathognomonic.

Once the diagnosis of FNH has been secured, most patients can be reassured. On subsequent imaging, FNH may fluctuate in size, but this is of little consequence in the asymptomatic patient. There is no role for estrogen avoidance, unlike hepatic adenomas.[196] The most common indications for surgical resection are diagnostic uncertainty followed by symptom palliation.[197] Surgical approaches to FNH vary widely in the literature and will depend on the size and anatomic location. Parenchymal sparing approaches can be frequently used for FNH with only a minority of patients requiring major hepatectomy. Enucleation is generally not recommended because of the vascular nature of FNH. In patients who undergo resection, morbidity is low at 14% and mortality is exceedingly rare.[197] Given the benign nature of FNH, recurrence is not typical after resection and is rarely reported.

In summary, FNH is a frequently encountered benign liver lesion. Most patients can be diagnosed by imaging and managed nonoperatively. The patients who do require operative intervention are typically for diagnostic uncertainty or symptoms and tolerate hepatectomy well with good outcomes.

Liver Cysts (see Chapters 73 and 88B)

There are several cystic conditions of the liver that span the spectrum of benign to malignant diseases. Treatment of liver cysts is similarly diverse and can range from observation to hepatectomy to liver transplant. This portion of the chapter will seek to review the most common cystic diseases of the liver, indications for surgical resection, and the outcomes from the surgical resection.

Simple Hepatic Cysts

Simple hepatic cysts are the most common liver cysts in the general population. They are more common with advanced age and female sex, with a 3 to 1 ratio for women to men. Simple cysts are estimated to be present in 2% to 18% of the population.[198] They can be solitary or frequently multiple; the presence of more than 20 simple hepatic cysts is defined as polycystic liver disease. Simple cysts contain serous fluid and have no connection to the intrahepatic bile ducts. They are benign and present no risk of malignant transformation.

Most simple cysts are asymptomatic and are found incidentally on abdominal imaging performed for other reasons. Once identified, they do not require further investigation or intervention. The female preponderance is even more pronounced when it comes to symptomatic simple cysts, with a 10 to 1 ratio over men.[199] Simple hepatic cysts may be associated with a wide range of symptoms, and many of them are related to compression of adjacent structures. Compression of bile ducts can lead to jaundice, that of hepatic veins can cause Budd-Chiari syndrome, and extrinsic compression of the stomach can cause early satiety. Another symptom may be pain related to intracystic hemorrhage or possibly stretching of the liver capsule.

For symptomatic patients, intervention is warranted. The evidence for aspiration with or without a chemical sclerosing agent is mixed with largely retrospective studies. Most reports agree that the procedure is technically simple with low complication rates and generally successful in achieving initial size reduction. However, many cysts will recur with this approach and there is a risk of infection.[199] Additionally, some patients cannot tolerate instillation of the sclerosing agent because of intractable pain with the procedure.[200] One systematic review compared sclerotherapy with laparoscopic fenestration and found similar rates of recurrence and complications.[201]

Operative approaches to simple hepatic cysts are varied and include open and minimally invasive approaches. Intraoperative techniques include cyst fenestration by excision of the cyst wall (Fig. 101B.18), subtotal cyst resection, or even parenchymal sparing and anatomic hepatectomy. Long-term follow-up after surgical treatment of simple hepatic cysts shows recurrence ranging from 4% to 41%, although techniques and follow-up varied amongst reports.[202,203]

Polycystic Liver Disease (see Chapter 73)

Polycystic liver disease (PLD) is defined as the presence of more than 20 simple liver cysts.[204] The condition can occur in isolation or as a manifestation of autosomal dominant polycystic kidney disease (ADPKD). PLD is frequently progressive with continued growth over time, with 2.4% to 7.4% increase in liver volume per year, which may lead previously asymptomatic individuals to become symptomatic during observation.[205] Young (<48 years old) female patients are most likely to develop symptoms that necessitate intervention.[205]

Although symptoms are generally similar to simple hepatic cysts, individuals with PLD can have more advanced presentations because of overall compressive effects that can cause portal hypertension from venous outflow obstruction or portal vein obstruction. Similarly, inferior vena cava obstruction has also been

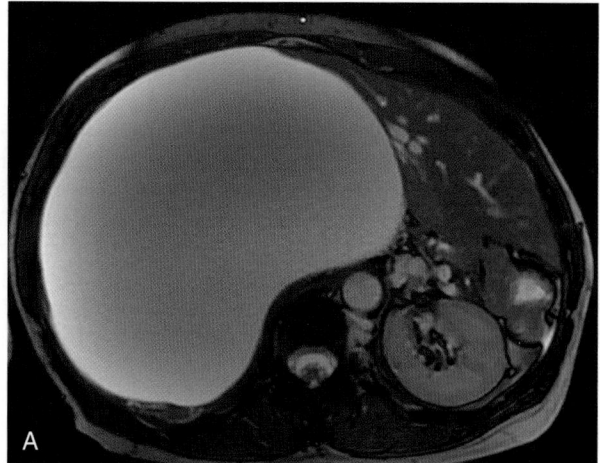
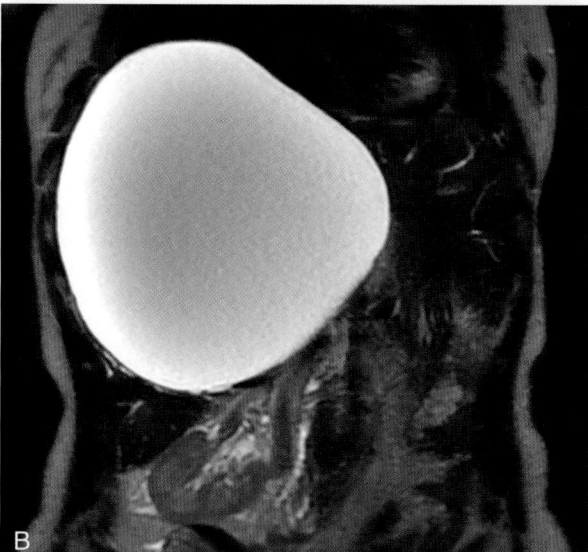
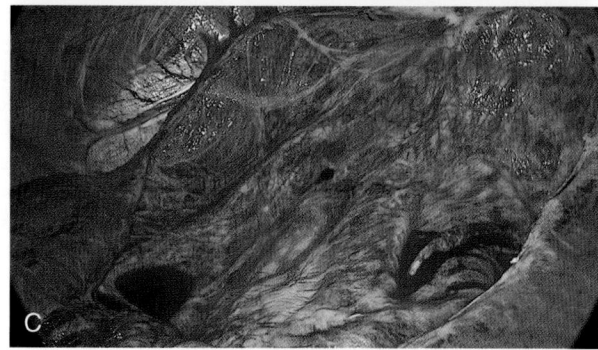

FIGURE 101B.18 A 55-year-old woman with a giant cyst measuring 20 × 20 × 17 cm occupying the right liver and causing mass effect by displacing the left liver and resulting in gastric outlet obstruction on **(A)** T1 axial magnetic resonance imaging (MRI), **(B)** T1 coronal MRI, and **(C)** after laparoscopic fenestration of the giant cyst. The hepatic veins can be seen coursing in the chronically compressed and thinned out right liver behind the remaining cyst wall. *LHV,* Left hepatic vein; *MHV,* middle hepatic vein; *RHV,* right hepatic vein. See Chapter 14.

described, which can lead to worsening renal function because of increased renal vein pressures. This is of particular concern in patients who already have some degree of renal impairment from ADPKD.

Classification systems for PLD largely focus on the amount of involved liver in the case of the Gigot classification of PLD (Table 101B.7) or identifying patients who will benefit from hepatic resection and transplantation as in the Schnelldorfer classification of PLD (Table 101B.8).[206,207] Multiple pharmacologic treatments have been investigated including somatostatin analogs, mammalian target of rapamycin (mTOR) inhibitors, ursodeoxycholic acid, and others, but the strongest evidence is for somatostatin analogs. A pooled analysis of 3 RCTs showed a 2.9% to 8% reduction in liver volume compared with placebo with octreotide.[205]

When intervention is indicated, only the largest or most symptomatic cysts need be addressed. Like simple hepatic cysts, aspiration and sclerosis is an option when there are large dominant cysts that are thought to be responsible for a patient's symptoms. Unfortunately, in this population, recurrence of cysts has been described in up to 80% of patients with this approach.[208] Cyst fenestration, excision, or hepatic resection by open or minimally invasive approach is effective at treating symptoms in the majority of patients but will still lead to recurrence of symptoms and/or cyst progression in up to a quarter of patients.[209]

For patients with severely compromised liver function and diffuse disease without adequate uninvolved liver, liver transplantation presents another therapeutic option. Historically, liver transplantation for polycystic disease was associated with significant perioperative morbidity (41%) and mortality (5%), likely representing the advanced disease necessary to be eligible for transplantation. Patients who require liver-only transplantation have better survival at 5 years versus those who require simultaneous liver and kidney transplantation (92% vs. 80%).[209]

Echinococcal Cysts (see Chapter 72)

Echinococcal cysts are also known as hydatid disease and are secondary to ingestion of tapeworm eggs from the *Echinococcus granulosus* parasite. The definitive hosts for the parasite are dogs with sheep acting as an intermediate host. Once ingested, the eggs release larvae in the small intestine, which enter blood or lymphatics. They subsequently become trapped in the liver, which leads to cyst formation. The liver is the most common site, but lung, brain, and other viscera can also be affected.

Patients with echinococcal cysts can be asymptomatic for several years, but the most common presentation is right upper quadrant pain that may be associated with other symptoms like nausea and fever. More uncommon presentations are related to cyst rupture, causing fever, pruritis, or even anaphylaxis. Biliary presentations such as cholangitis may also be seen with rupture or erosion into the biliary tract.[210] Diagnosis is secured through a combination of serologic markers and cross-sectional imaging. Screening tests include hemagglutination, latex agglutination, and enzyme-linked immunoassay (ELISA) for specific antigens have high sensitivity but low specificity. Confirmatory consist of arc-5 immuno-electrophoresis and immunoblotting using parasite-specific agents and have nearly 100% specificity.[210] The Casoni skin test is only of historical import because of its low sensitivity.[211] Cross-sectional imaging can reveal characteristic findings of calcified cystic walls, daughter cysts, and multiple cysts. Additionally, cross-sectional imaging can help with interventional planning (see Chapter 14).

Treatment of echinococcal cysts is accomplished with the combination of antiparasitic drugs and interventional procedures. The anthelminthic drugs albendazole and mebendazole should be started before surgery to inactivate parasites, lowering the risk of anaphylaxis, prevent secondary infection, and soften cyst walls before surgery. For patients who are ineligible to undergo interventional procedures, continued systemic therapy can help to prevent morbidity from *E. granulosus* infection. When combined with surgery, perioperative treatment with antihelminthic agents can decrease recurrence rate to 1%.[212] Surgery in these patients is classically described as pericystectomy, resection of the cyst with a small rim of hepatic tissue. Both open and laparoscopic techniques have been described and a meta-analysis comparing the approaches showed no difference in postoperative complications, mortality, recurrence, or cure rate.[213] Before cyst resection, frequently sterilization procedures are frequently undertaken where ethanol or hypertonic saline is injected into the cyst to prevent anaphylaxis from spillage (Fig. 101B.19).[194] This surgical approach has less morbidity when compared with external drainage, simple closure, and marsupialization (17.9% vs. 36.5%).[214] Additionally, external drainage carries a high rate of recurrence when compared with more aggressive surgical procedures like pericystectomy and hepatic resection.

There is a viable nonsurgical alternative for the treatment of echinococcal cysts, percutaneous aspiration-injection-reaspiration (PAIR). The procedure is performed under imaging guidance: The cyst is penetrated with a needle and aspirated and a sterilizing agent is injected followed by repeated aspiration. The steps are repeated until there are no parasites present on immediate histologic examination.[215] Contraindications to this approach include patients with superficial cysts that are at risk for intraabdominal rupture, cysts with direct biliary erosion,

TABLE 101B.7 Gigot Classification of Polycystic Liver Disease

	NUMBER OF CYSTS	CYST SIZE	REMAINING AREAS OF NONCYSTIC LIVER PARENCHYMA
Type I	<10	Large (>10 cm)	Large
Type II	Multiple	Small, medium	Large
Type III	Multiple	Small, medium	Few

TABLE 101B.8 Schnelldorfer Classification of Polycystic Liver Disease

	SYMPTOMS	CYST CHARACTERISTICS	AREAS OF RELATIVE NORMAL LIVER PARENCHYMA	ISOSECTORAL PORTAL VEIN OR HEPATIC VEIN OCCLUSION OF PRESERVED SECTOR
Type A	Absent or mild	Any	Any	Any
Type B	Moderate or severe	Limited number with large cysts	>2 sectors	Absent
Type C	Severe (or moderate)	Any	>1 sector	Absent
Type D	Severe (or moderate)	Any	<1 sector	Present

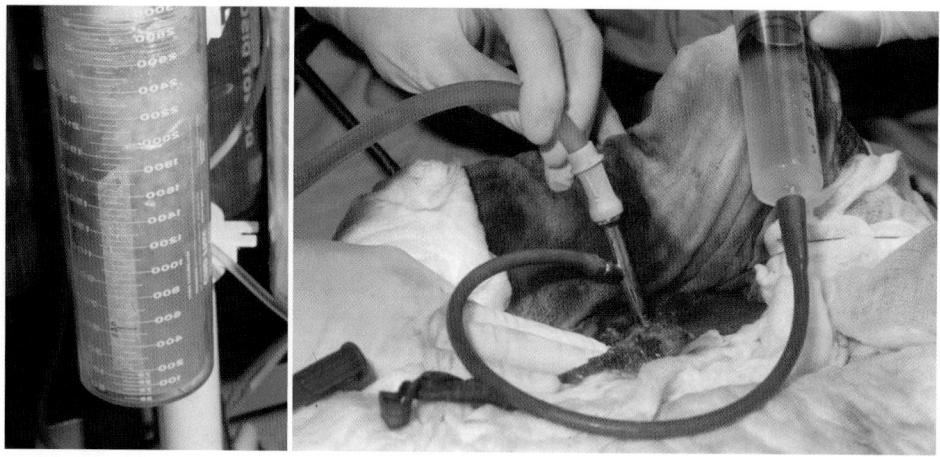

FIGURE 101B.19 Aspiration of echinococcal cyst content and infusion of hypertonic saline. (From Tran Cao HS, Marcal LP, Mason MC, et al. Benign hepatic incidentalomas. *Curr Probl Surg.* 2019;56[9]:100642.)

and calcified cysts that are unable to be penetrated with a needle.[216] A meta-analysis compared PAIR with laparoscopic resection and showed that PAIR has lower mortality rates (1.1% vs. 1.8%) but higher rates of recurrence (5.0% vs. 3.9%).[217] Overall, both procedures are safe with low rates of recurrence and the appropriate approach must be considered in the context of the patient and disease presentation.

Other benign cystic lesions of the liver include Caroli disease, liver abscess, biloma, bile duct hamartomas, and intrahepatic pseudocysts. Their discussion is beyond the scope of this chapter; please refer to Chapter 88 for further information.

Mucinous Cystic Neoplasms (see Chapter 88B)

Mucinous cystic neoplasms bridge the gap between benign, biliary cystadenoma, and malignant biliary cystadenocarcinoma. These entities exist on a continuum and are classified based on the highest degree of microscopic architectural distortion. Biliary cystadenoma is more common and accounts for approximately 5% of hepatic cysts.[218] It is considered a premalignant lesion which may progress to biliary cystadenocarcinoma, although the pathway of malignant transformation remains unknown. Biliary cystadenoma is more common in female patients and is often found to have ovarian-type stroma with estrogen and progesterone receptors.[219]

Biliary cystadenomas, in contrast to other benign hepatic cysts, tend to grow to large sizes with reports of 15-cm to 30-cm cysts regularly found in the literature. Like other benign hepatic cysts, they can be asymptomatic and found on incidental imaging or present with vague abdominal symptoms related to increased size and compression from cyst growth. Diagnosis is difficult with radiographic imaging alone and often requires multiple modalities, including MRCP, which can be useful for demonstrating biliary connections. Many times, these lesions cannot be distinguished from biliary cystadenocarcinomas and ultimately percutaneous FNA may be helpful in establishing a definitive diagnosis. Biliary cystadenomas frequently have a thinner wall, whereas biliary cystadenocarcinomas tend to be thicker and more irregular and will often have CEA elevation in aspirated fluid.[220]

The presence of biliary cystadenoma is an indication for surgical management. Malignant transformation of biliary cystadenomas is estimated to occur 10% to 20% of the time.[221]

Additionally, biliary cystadenoma is often difficult to differentiate from biliary cystadenocarcinoma preoperatively. Nonoperative (cyst aspiration, sclerotherapy) and minimalistic surgical approaches (cyst fenestration, partial resection, and narrow margin excision) have been described but lead to recurrence 80% to 100% of the time.[222,223] Even when patients can undergo more extensive resection with wide margins, recurrence still occurs 5% to 20% of the time for unclear reasons.[223] Large lesions with liver atrophy, centrally located biliary cystadenomas, and bilobar disease may be unresectable via traditional methods and patients can be considered for liver transplantation.

By comparison, biliary cystadenocarcinomas should always be approached by formal hepatectomy because of the risk of inadequate resection of a malignant entity. Most data regarding biliary cystadenocarcinomas are small case reports, but long-term survival (2.5–13 years) is reported with formal resection.[224] The effects of systemic therapies and other treatment strategies like external beam radiation are poorly understood for this entity.

Cystic Hepatocellular Carcinoma

HCC is the most common primary tumor of the liver as previously discussed. Cystic presentations of HCC and fibrolamellar HCC are rare but have been described.[225] Although treatment does not vary from that discussed for HCC, recognition that cystic lesions may indeed be HCC in the right clinical context is of critical importance (see Chapter 87).

Cystic Liver Metastases

In addition to the causes of cystic liver lesions above, metastases from several different primary organ sites can present with cystic metastases. Greater than 50% of cystic liver metastases are secondary to a colorectal primary, but other sites, including kidney, prostate, and gastrointestinal stromal tumors (GIST) and neuroendocrine tumors, have been described. The ability to surgically approach these tumors and subsequent outcomes will vary widely depending on innumerable factors but that is beyond the scope of this chapter. The most critical factor is including cystic liver metastases as part of the differential diagnosis for multiple cystic lesions of the liver (see Chapter 87).

References are available at expertconsult.com.

Parenchymal preservation in hepatic resectional surgery: Rationale, indications and outcomes

Aslam Ejaz, Jordan M. Cloyd, and Timothy M. Pawlik

INTRODUCTION

Advances in patient selection, surgical technique, and perioperative management have improved the outcomes of patients undergoing hepatic resection in recent years. As a result, the utilization of liver resection for patients with both benign and malignant disease has increased worldwide[1,2] (see Chapter 101A). Marked improvements in operative and anesthetic techniques, improved patient selection, and the emergence of hepatobiliary surgery have reduced mortality rates following liver resection from over 20% to under 2% by experienced surgeons at high-volume centers.[3] In addition, there is now a better understanding of liver anatomy, an enhanced knowledge of tumor biology, improvements in diagnostic imaging technology, and more effective systemic and liver-directed therapies for hepatic malignancies. These advances have facilitated personalized surgical approaches based on individual patient anatomy and tumor biology.

A parenchymal-sparing approach to hepatic resection has emerged as a novel method of optimizing the amount of normal hepatic tissue in order to minimize the risk of postoperative liver insufficiency and maximize the potential for liver-directed therapies in the future.[4] The principle behind parenchymal-sparing hepatectomy (PSH) is to maximize the future liver remnant (FLR) by removing the minimal tissue necessary to achieve optimal oncologic outcomes. In contemporary practice, this principle is most frequently equated with techniques involving resection of one or more liver segments rather than an entire hepatic "lobe." Anatomic resections, such as *segmentectomy* or *sectionectomy*, are often used in parenchymal-sparing approaches. Obtaining adequate tumor clearance can also be achieved by more limited nonanatomic resections, termed variously *nonanatomic, atypical,* or *wedge* resections.[5,6]

This chapter reviews the rationale and indications for PSH for various primary and secondary hepatic malignancies. The short- and long-term outcomes of PSH are reviewed here; the technical aspects of surgical approach are reviewed in Chapter 118B.

TERMINOLOGY

Modern surgical liver anatomy is based on the Brisbane classification, which separates the liver into 8 Couinaud segments and 4 anatomic sections (right posterior, right anterior, left medial, left lateral) (see Chapter 2). Nevertheless, confusion persists regarding terminology to describe the extent of hepatic resection including major/minor, wedge, nonanatomic, and PSH.[7] Traditionally, hepatic resections were categorized as either "major" (≥3 segments) or "minor" (<3 segments) based on the number of resected segments. This designation does not represent technical complexity; in fact, some traditionally "major" resections (e.g., left hepatectomy) can be technically less demanding than certain "minor" resections (e.g., right posterior sectionectomy). Resections are also commonly classified as "anatomic" or "nonanatomic" where

anatomic resection refers to excision of an entire liver segment with its anatomic pedicle. The term *parenchymal-sparing hepatectomy* can be applied to either situation as it refers to a technique that maximally preserves healthy liver tissue. Whereas the term *wedge resection* connotes a nonanatomic minor resection, the term *parenchymal-sparing hepatectomy* does not imply whether the resection is anatomic or nonanatomic. Figure 102A.1 illustrates various parenchymal-sparing and anatomic resection options based on tumor location. Table 102A.1 lists the nomenclature proposed for various parenchymal-sparing operative procedures.[8–10]

DETERMINING "ANATOMIC" RESECTION MARGINS

Ahn et al.[11] have demonstrated that tumors are not always located in the center of a segment; sometimes they are located within proximity to multiple portal branches. In these cases, an anatomic segmentectomy may not be oncologically sufficient, but at the same time, resection of multiple segments or hemihepatectomy may be unnecessarily extensive. For example, for a small tumor located on the ventral or dorsal aspect of segment VIII, a classic anatomic segment VIII resection may represent an overly extensive surgery and may not be feasible in patients with underlying liver disease because segment VIII can account for almost one quarter of total liver volume.[12] Instead, systematic resection of either the ventral or the dorsal portion of segment VIII may be considered an oncologic surgical approach that maximizes the safety of hepatic resection. These considerations have led some authors to redefine "anatomic resection" as a surgical maneuver that removes the territory of one or more third-order portal branches.[13]

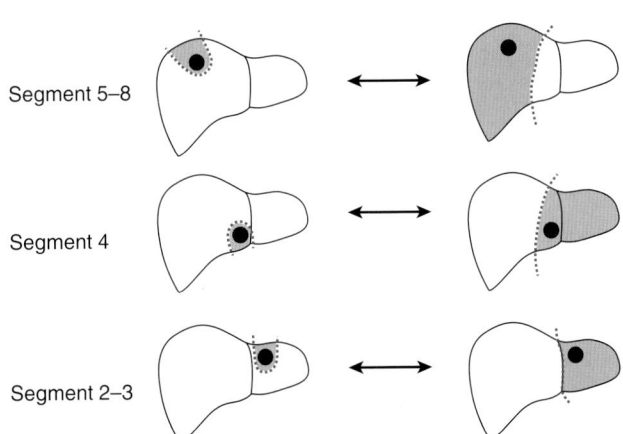

FIGURE 102A.1 Parenchymal-sparing and anatomic resection options for various hepatic lesions. (From Mise Y, Aloia TA, Brudvik KW, et al. Parenchymal-sparing hepatectomy in colorectal liver metastasis improves salvageability and survival. *Ann Surg.* 2016;263[1]:146–152.)

TABLE 102A.1 Proposed Nomenclature for Commonly Performed Open and Laparoscopic Parenchymal-Sparing Hepatectomies, Stratified by Technical Difficulty

TYPE OF RESECTION	SEGMENT(S) RESECTED
Grade 1 (Low Complexity)	
Peripheral wedge resection	Any isolated segment
Left lateral sectionectomy	S2 and S3
Grade 2 (Medium Complexity)	
Right posterior sectionectomy	S6 and S7
Grade 3 (High Complexity)	
Right anterior sectionectomy	S5 and S8
Central hepatectomy	S4, S5, S8
Right inferior bisegmentectomy	S5 and S6
Right superior bisegmentectomy	S7 and S8
Central anterior bisegmentectomy	S4b and S5
Central posterior bisegmentectomy	S4a and S8
Left medial sectionectomy	S4a and S4b

MHV, Middle hepatic vein; *RHV,* right hepatic vein.
Adapted from Alvarez and Kawaguchi et al.[8–10]

Several innovative diagnostic techniques have been developed to assist in the reliable identification of hepatic segments and subsegmental anatomy. Intraoperative ultrasound (IOUS) is certainly critical for any hepatobiliary surgeon (see Chapter 24). In addition, novel near-infrared fluorescent imaging techniques using intrabiliary or intravascular injection of indocyanine green (ICG) paired with fluorescent imaging systems allow for intraoperative visualization of biliary and vascular anatomy and can aid surgeons in defining their intended resection plane with high accuracy.[14,15] A recently revisited technique, described as early as 1985, uses IOUS-guided dye injection of the portal venous branch feeding a tumor, in order to accurately delineate the extent of tumor-bearing parenchyma that should be resected.[11,16] In a series of 65 segmentectomies performed for hepatocellular carcinoma (HCC), Ahn et al.[11] noted that 45% of resected tumors were fed by two or more segmental portal branches, with almost one-quarter having a complex pattern of portal venous supply. In all these cases, portal venous dye injection allowed the surgeon to establish a precise resection plane based on tumor–portal vein relationships. The authors were able to perform a limited nonanatomic resection while maintaining oncologic resection principles.[11] Importantly, the long-term disease-free survival (DFS) and overall survival (OS) rates reported by this group were comparable with those reported by other series.[11,17]

Despite the technically demanding nature of some of these techniques, the specialized equipment needed, and the additional time and training that may be required, these maneuvers enhance real-time identification of liver anatomy and facilitate anatomic-based parenchymal-preserving resections that are oncologically sound.

RATIONALE FOR PARENCHYMAL-SPARING SURGERY

Mitigating the Risk of Posthepatectomy Liver Failure Through Parenchymal-Sparing Techniques

The primary rationale for parenchymal-sparing techniques is that maximizing the *volume* of liver remaining after a planned resection also maximizes *functional* parenchyma, which is highly predictive of postoperative morbidity, mortality, and liver dysfunction.[18,19] Resections removing up to 80% of functional parenchyma can be safely

performed in the setting of normal liver function.[19] However, an FLR of at least 40% is often necessary in patients with underlying liver disease, such as cirrhosis, steatohepatitis, chemotherapy-induced liver injury,[20] or in the setting of biliary obstruction and jaundice.[21] The relationship between liver volume and liver function is not static, particularly in the setting of underlying liver disease, where parenchymal-sparing techniques are often indicated. Accurate calculation of the volume and function of the FLR is imperative in order to determine resectability, discuss perioperative risk with the patient, and predict postoperative outcomes. The degree to which the underlying liver disease constitutes an absolute versus relative contraindication to hepatic resection depends on the anticipated volume and function of liver remaining after resection. Quantitative measures of liver function, including ICG clearance[22] and lidocaine conversion tests,[23] can assist in preoperative planning. Systematic measurement of liver remnant volume and careful assessment of liver function have improved the safety of major resections (see Chapter 4).

Several studies have found a decreased risk of posthepatectomy liver failure (PHLF) after hepatic resection through parenchymal-sparing techniques, particularly in patients with impaired liver function. Fisher et al.[24] reported a large, retrospective, multi-institutional study of almost 600 patients undergoing formal right hepatectomy versus a parenchymal-sparing right posterior sectionectomy for benign and malignant disease; a right posterior sectionectomy was associated with a significantly lower rate of PHLF (1% vs. 8.5%), as defined by hyperbilirubinemia or significant ascites. These findings were confirmed by other studies associating extent of liver resection with increased rates of PHLF.[25,26] To that end, parenchymal-sparing techniques maximize the liver volume and liver function after resection and subsequently decrease the risk of PHLF compared with more extensive resections.

Parenchymal-Sparing Techniques Minimize the Physiologic Impact of Liver Resection

In addition to maximizing the functional FLR, parenchymal-sparing techniques may also reduce the risk of postoperative complications through other mechanisms. Regardless of FLR volume, intraoperative bleeding can result in postoperative hepatic compromise. Multiple studies have shown a relationship between intraoperative blood loss and poor outcomes after major hepatic resection, including in-hospital and postoperative mortality[27] and intraabdominal sepsis.[28] Compared with major hepatectomy, PSH has been associated with less perioperative blood loss, less intensive care unit (ICU) admission, shorter hospital stay, and lower mortality.[29] Redaelli et al.[30] retrospectively reviewed 77 classic anatomic hepatectomies and 90 parenchymal-sparing resections for primary and secondary malignancies of the liver performed over 7 years at a single institution and similarly noted a significant decrease in blood loss and transfusion, ICU utilization, and hospital stay for patients who underwent a parenchymal-sparing resection. The authors specifically noted a higher rate of biochemical liver insufficiency, encephalopathy, and sepsis in the classic resection group; this physiologic advantage of parenchymal-sparing hepatic resection persisted when the analysis was confined to noncirrhotic patients.[29] With regard to the risk of blood loss and bile leak, a systematic review of 2505 patients undergoing hepatectomy for colorectal liver metastasis (CRLM) found that PSH was comparable with anatomic resection with regard to estimated blood loss, length of stay, and OS.[31] Given the heterogeneity of these case series, it is difficult to quantify the true physiologic benefit of parenchymal-sparing techniques. Table 102A.2 summarizes findings from these and other observational studies.[24,29,30,32]

TABLE 102A.2 Perioperative Outcomes After Major Hepatectomy or Parenchymal-Sparing Hepatectomy

SERIES	YEARS INCLUSIVE	COMPARISON GROUPS	OPERATIVE TIME (MIN)	ESTIMATED BLOOD LOSS (ML)	PATIENTS TRANSFUSED	HOSPITAL LENGTH OF STAY (DAYS)	INTENSIVE CARE USE	MORBIDITY	LIVER DYSFUNCTION	MORTALITY
Jarnagin et al., 2002[29]	1991-2001	<3 segments (n = 468) vs. ≥3 segments (n = 667), hepatectomy only		508 ± 30 vs. 995 ± 42	31% vs. 55%	7.7 ± 0.2 vs. 11.1 ± 0.4	2.3% vs. 6.9%	31% vs. 49%		0.9% vs. 3%
		<3 segments (n = 221) vs. ≥3 segments (n = 447), complex hepatectomy[a]		653 ± 51 vs. 1159 ± 59	34% vs. 66%	9.1 ± 0.4 vs. 12.6 ± 0.4	4.5% vs. 12.6%	41% vs. 57%		0.5% vs. 6.7%
Redaelli et al., 2002[30],[b]	1993-2000	Tissue-preserving (n = 90) vs. formal (n = 77) resection	221 (70-550) vs. 313 (105-540)	965 (100-6000) vs. 1850 (200-12000)		15 (5-69) vs. 20 (6-115)	1 day (1-14) vs. 2 days (1-36)	27% vs. 34%	9% vs. 26%[c] (encephalopathy, 7% vs. 19%)	2.2% vs. 5.1%
Fisher et al., 2013[24]	2000-2012	Right posterior sectionectomy (n = 100) vs. right hepatectomy (n = 480)[d]		697 vs. 713	19% vs. 17%	7.5 vs. 8.3		42% vs. 42%	1% vs. 8.5%[e]	3.0% vs. 5.2%
Mise et al., 2016[32]	1993-2013	PSH (n = 156) vs. anatomic resection		100 vs. 200				Major morbidity: 3.2% vs. 6.3%		0% vs. 0.7%

a Including one or more additional hepatic or extrahepatic procedures, including additional hepatic wedge resections or enucleations to organ resection, bile duct resection, or vascular reconstruction.

b Data presented as median and range.

c Biochemical definition of liver dysfunction based on hyperbilirubinemia, elevated serum ammonia, and prothrombin time prolongation.

d Right hepatectomy was defined as resection of segments 5–8 with or without caudate lobectomy and right posterior sectionectomy as resection of segments 6 and 7 with ligation of the posterior branch of the right portal pedicle with or without division of the right hepatic vein.

e Defined as postoperative hyperbilirubinemia or presence of significant postoperative ascites.

Parenchymal-Sparing Techniques Preserve Oncologic Outcomes

In addition to demonstrating the safety of parenchymal-sparing techniques for resection of primary and secondary hepatic malignancies, it is imperative that PSH maintains the oncologic principles to minimize the risk of local recurrence and to optimize long-term outcomes. There were initial concerns that PSH resulted in a higher rate of margin positivity compared with hemihepatectomy and trisectionectomy.[33] Recent data, however, have demonstrated the oncologic safety of PSH for patients with CRLM and neuroendocrine liver metastasis (NELM).[31,34] Though slightly more controversial, an anatomic segment-oriented resection for HCC and intrahepatic cholangiocarcinoma (ICC) has also been demonstrated to be an oncologically acceptable approach.[35,36]

Colorectal Liver Metastasis (see Chapter 90)

The histologic appearance of CRLM favors a parenchymal-sparing approach; CRLM are histologically well-circumscribed micrometastases in the surrounding liver parenchyma, are rare and primarily found at the immediate tumor border, and satellitosis and Glissonian sheath extension are uncommon, suggesting that extended resections beyond a 1-cm margin are unnecessary.[37,38]

In an early study by Kokudo et al.,[39] the authors found that OS in patients with CRLM did not differ based on whether the patient underwent anatomic or nonanatomic (wedge) resection. In a subset analysis of patients with unilobar disease, the authors noted an ipsilateral intrahepatic recurrence rate of 19.6% after wedge resection and suggested that more extensive hepatic resection in these patients would have been unnecessary (i.e., would not have prevented disease recurrence) in four of five patients.[39] In a subsequent study by Pawlik et al.,[5] the authors identified 557 patients who underwent hepatic resection for CRLM over a 15-year period from a multi-institutional database established by three major hepatobiliary centers. The series included patients who underwent an extended hepatectomy (18%), hemihepatectomy (39%), and lesser nonanatomic resections (43%). Patients were classified into four subgroups according to the width of the resection margin: positive (tumor <1 mm from surgical margin) or negative (by 1–4, 4–9, or at least 10 mm); with a median follow-up of 29 months, 40% of patients experienced a recurrence.[5] A positive resection margin resulted in worse DFS, but sites and incidence of recurrence were similar among patients with a negative margin of resection, regardless of the width of the margin. The 1-, 3-, and 5-year OS rates after resection of CRLM were 97%, 74%, and 58%, respectively, and there was no significant difference in OS among patients with a negative margin, regardless of the width of the margin or extent of hepatic resection (Fig. 102A.2).[5]

In a separate study by Zorzi et al.,[40] oncologic outcomes were examined in a subset of patients undergoing less than a hemihepatectomy and those undergoing a wedge resection. The incidence of isolated intrahepatic recurrence after a wedge resection was 14% compared with 9% after an anatomic resection ($P = .2$).[40] Similar to Pawlik et al.,[5] there were no differences in overall recurrence, patterns of recurrence, or OS after resection of CRLM treated with anatomic versus wedge resection.[40] Recurrence at the surgical margin was more common in patients who had a positive resection margin regardless of the type of resection, but margin positivity was equivalent between

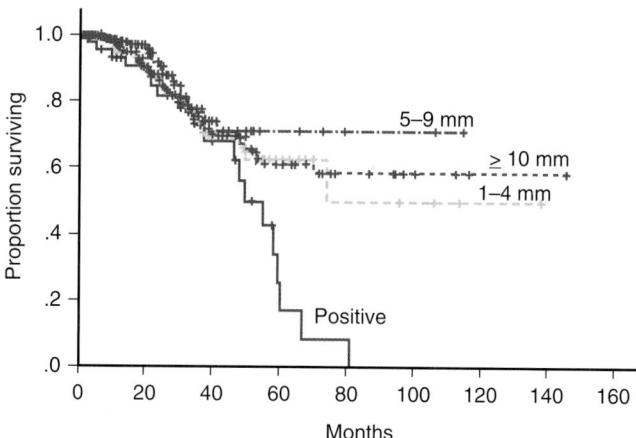

FIGURE 102A.2 Survival after hepatic resection of colorectal liver metastases, stratified by margin status. Median survival was 49.6 months in patients with positive margins and was not yet reached in patients with negative margins ($P = .005$). No significant difference in survival was seen in patients with a negative surgical margin, regardless of the width of the margin (all $P > .5$). (From Pawlik TM, Scoggins CR, Zorzi D, et al. Effect of surgical margin status on survival and site of recurrence after hepatic resection for colorectal metastases. *Ann Surg.* 2005;241[5]:715–722, discussion 722–724.)

the groups.[5] These results were confirmed in a recent systematic review of 12 studies encompassing 2505 patients undergoing resection for CRLM.[31] The authors found no difference in length of stay, R0 resection rates, and OS for patients undergoing PSH for CRLM compared with those who received an anatomic resection.[31]

These findings have been challenged by more recent studies evaluating surgical margin width and recurrence in the CRLM patient population. In a systematic review and meta-analysis of 11,147 CRLM patients, Margonis et al.[41] found that a resection margin of at least 1 cm was associated with improved DFS and OS. In a separate study by Sadot et al.,[42] the authors found that a negative margin resection was the most important factor related to long-term survival irrespective of margin width. The authors argue that the biologic behavior of the tumor, rather than margin width and surgical technique, are the likely main drivers of the survival differences seen between groups.[42] However, this has also been debated as separate studies have found differing results with regard to the impact of PSH versus anatomic resection among patients with aggressive KRAS-mutated tumors.[43,44] Though still debated, it appears that margin negativity and tumor biology, as opposed to margin width or extent of resection, primarily drive local oncologic outcomes and support the use of PSH for patients with CRLM.

Neuroendocrine Liver Metastasis (see Chapter 91)

Hepatic resection of NELM is associated with improved long-term OS, as well as for patients with CRLM.[45] In patients with NELM, multiple groups have demonstrated the importance of surgical resection on long-term DFS and OS.[46,47] According to results compiled from 29 studies of hepatic resection for neuroendocrine tumors, the most important factors affecting OS in the setting of NELM are histologic grade, the presence of extrahepatic disease, and a macroscopically incomplete resection.[48] Interestingly, several studies have found that R1 margin status is not associated with worse outcomes.[46,49] This lack of prognostic impact of a microscopically positive margin status may be due to the relative expansive or well-encapsulated behavior of neuroendocrine metastases versus the more infiltrative nature of other liver malignancies. In this context PSH approach is preferable for NELM because it showed similar long-term outcomes.[50]

Intrahepatic Cholangiocarcinoma (see Chapter 50)

The surgical approach to patients with intrahepatic cholagiocarcinoma (ICC) involves hepatic resection with negative margins and a portal lymphadenectomy. R0 resection margins are achieved in 46% to 98% of cases and vary dramatically by institution, due to factors such as surgeon experience, pathologic evaluation, and patient selection.[51-53] A multi-institutional analysis of 434 patients undergoing resection for ICC found that negative margin resection, but not margin width, was predictive of survival.[54] This is likely due to the fact that several other tumor-related factors, such as lymph node involvement, multifocality, and vascular invasion, appear to be more predictive of survival than extent of hepatic resection. These findings were echoed by Li et al.,[36] who used a propensity score-matched analysis and found that a PSH was similar to anatomic resection for patients with ICC. Given the aggressiveness of ICC and the controversial data related to margin status and width, the use of PSH should be considered when technically feasible, as it does not appear to affect long-term oncologic outcomes.

Hepatocellular Carcinoma (see Chapter 89)

In contrast to patients with CRLM and NELM, anatomic resections that remove the hepatic segment defined by tumor-bearing tissue have traditionally been advocated in patients with hepatocellular carcinoma (HCC).[55] HCC has a proclivity to invade portal tributaries, hence some investigators have proposed that anatomic resections are oncologically necessary.[56] In a retrospective review of 210 hepatic resections for HCC over 7 years, Hasegawa et al.[57] reported superior DFS and OS among 84 patients with an anatomic segmentectomy and subsegmentectomy compared with 54 patients with limited, nonanatomic resections. In this study, 5-year DFS and OS were 67% and 28%, respectively, in the segmentectomy and subsegmentectomy group, compared with 35% and 16% in the group of patients undergoing limited resection. However, patients undergoing nonanatomic resections were more likely to have cirrhosis and had worse liver function (as measured by ICG R15).[57]

In 2008 Eguchi et al.[58] reported long-term results from the Liver Cancer Study Group of Japan, which has been conducting nationwide surveys of patients with primary liver cancer since 1969. The authors studied 5781 patients with solitary HCC who had either an anatomic resection ($n = 2267$)—defined by the complete resection of a portal territory containing a tumor (as indicated by Glissonian method or dye puncture)—or a nonanatomic hepatectomy ($n = 3514$; securing at least 5-mm surgical margin). With a median follow-up of over 2 years, DFS (40% vs. 34% at 5 years) and OS (34% vs. 29% at 10 years) appeared to favor anatomic resection.[58]

Given the inherent biases of retrospective studies, some have questioned whether an uncompromising anatomic resection is strictly necessary to achieve oncologic goals.[6,11] Indeed, a meta-analysis of 18 observational studies including over 9000 patients undergoing anatomic versus nonanatomic resection of HCC found that survival differences observed between anatomic and nonanatomic resection were largely explained by worse liver function in the nonanatomic resection group.[35] Conversely, Zhou et al.[59] analyzed 16 studies encompassing 2917 patients and found that patients undergoing nonanatomic resection had worse OS and DFS than those undergoing an anatomic resection. Patients undergoing an anatomic resection, however, had a lower incidence of cirrhosis and more favorable hepatic function compared with those undergoing nonanatomic resection, which may have affected the findings.

Although the literature regarding anatomic versus PSH for HCC is controversial, the role of PSH for minimizing PHLF and enabling future liver-directed therapies remains sound. In a retrospective review of 20 hemihepatectomies and 29 PSH for HCC, Redaelli et al.[30] reported that patients with equivalent tumor stage undergoing segmental resection had better OS than those undergoing formal resection (median survival: 42 vs. 29 months), postulating that the difference could be attributed to a better preservation of liver function with PSH. Others have demonstrated similar DFS and OS rates after PSH versus hemihepatectomy and more extensive resections.[60,61] More recently, Famularo et al.[62] evaluated long-term oncologic outcomes of 455 patients undergoing resection for HCC. The authors found that PSH resulted in equivalent outcomes compared with anatomic resection, and survival was largely driven by measures of liver function (cirrhosis) and tumor biology (microvascular invasion and satellitosis). Taken together, these data suggest that an anatomically based parenchymal-sparing approach should be considered when feasible for patients with solitary HCC, as more extensive operations do not appear to confer an oncologic survival advantage. Table 102A.3 and Fig. 102A.3 summarize data addressing oncologic outcomes in parenchymal-preserving versus classic or extended resections in CRLM and HCC.

Parenchymal-Sparing Techniques Maximize the Patient Population Eligible for Curative-Intent Surgery

In general, curative-intent surgical resection offers the best long-term survival for patients with primary and secondary hepatic malignancies. Unfortunately, many patients with malignant hepatic tumors are not candidates for resection due to underlying liver disease or the extent of hepatic tumor burden. This includes patients whose liver function will not permit a formal hepatic resection and those with bilateral disease or anatomically challenging lesions such as those deep, centrally located, or involving or threatening major vessels.

In a report by Kokudo et al.[39] among patients undergoing PSH for CRLM, 90% of patients who had tumor recurrence in the hepatic lobe ipsilateral to their original surgery were resectable in a second operation. Conversely, recurrences were less likely to be resectable (20%) among those who initially underwent a more extensive operation. Similarly, Zorzi et al.[40] reported that 43% of patients with CRLM had multiple metastases and 12% of these underwent more than one wedge or anatomic resection in their case series. Although the authors did not comment on the number of patients who would have been ineligible for surgery if parenchymal-sparing techniques had not been employed, this report and others suggest that a large number of patients benefit from techniques that preserve liver parenchyma and/or allow multiple synchronous resections or staged operations.[32,40,63]

TABLE 102A.3 Overall Survival (OS) After Resection of Colorectal Liver Metastasis (CRLM) and Hepatocellular Carcinoma (HCC) According to Anatomic vs. Nonanatomic ("Wedge") Parenchymal-Sparing Resection Strategies

SERIES	TUMOR PATHOLOGY	YEARS INCLUSIVE	N	1-YEAR OS	3-YEAR OS	5-YEAR OS	10-YEAR OS	P
Anatomic vs. Nonanatomic Parenchymal-Sparing Techniques								
Kokudo et al., 2001[39]	CRLM	1980-1999						
Nonanatomic			78	98%	57%	40%		.64
Anatomic			96	90%	58%	46%		
Zorzi et al., 2006[40]	CRLM	1991-2004						
Nonanatomic			72	100%	83%	61%		.15
Anatomic			181	95%	72%	60%		
Hasegawa et al., 2005[57]	HCC	1994-2001						
Nonanatomic			54	93%	66%	35%		.01
Anatomic			156	95%	84%	66%		
Eguchi et al., 2008[58]	HCC	1994-2001						
Nonanatomic						62%	34%	.05
Anatomic						66%	29%	
Parenchymal-Sparing (PS) Techniques vs. Classic or Extended Resections								
Redaelli et al., 2002[30]		1993-2000						
Classic resection	CRLM		28	40%				NS
PS technique	CLRM		25	62%				NS
Classic resection	HCC		20	36%				NS
PS technique	HCC		29	62%				NS
Mise et al., 2016[32]		1993-2013						
Classic resection	CRLM		144			64%		NS
PS technique	CRLM		156			62%		NS
Famularo et al., 2018[62]		2001-2015						
Classic resection	HCC		177				20%	NS
PS technique	HCC		177				17%	NS

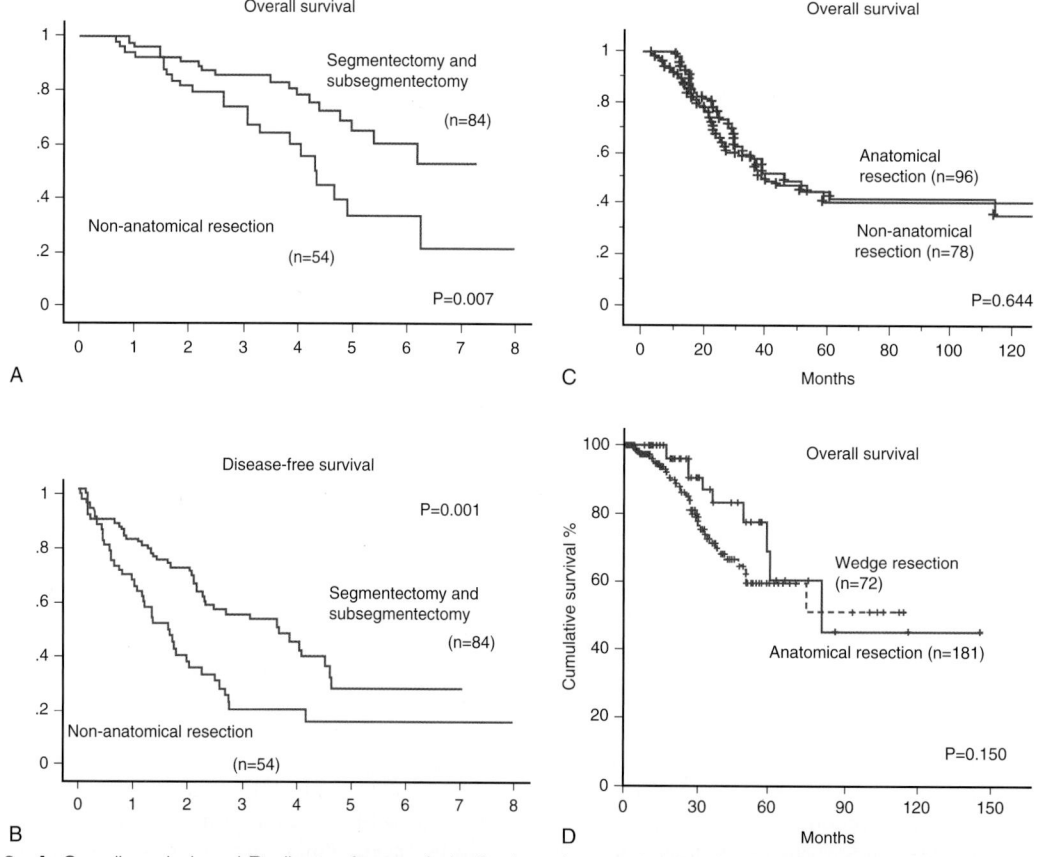

FIGURE 102A.3   A, Overall survival, and **B,** disease-free survival, after hepatic resection for single hepatocellular carcinoma, stratified by type of resection. **C** and **D,** Overall survival after hepatic resection for colorectal liver metastases, stratified by surgical procedure. (**A** and **B** from Hasegawa K, Kokudo N, Imamura H, et al. Prognostic impact of anatomic resection for hepatocellular carcinoma. *Ann Surg.* 2005;242 [2]:252–259; **C** from Kokudo N, Tada K, Seki M, et al. Anatomical major resection versus nonanatomical limited resection for liver metastases from colorectal carcinoma. *Am J Surg.* 2001;181[2]:153–159; and **D** from Zorzi D, Mullen JT, Abdalla EK, et al. Comparison between hepatic wedge resection and anatomic resection for colorectal liver metastases. *J Gastrointest Surg.* 2006;10[1]:86–94.)

Parenchymal-Preserving Techniques Allow for Repeat Hepatectomy for Recurrent Disease

Although the liver has a substantial regenerative capacity, patients who have undergone a prior major resection frequently have insufficient hepatic parenchyma left to allow a second extensive operation. Thus a more conservative initial resection maximizes the potential for repeat hepatectomy if new lesions develop.[45] This is important because salvage/repeat hepatectomy is associated with improved survival compared with nonsurgical techniques.[32,64,65] In a report by Mise et al.,[32] patients undergoing PSH for CRLM more frequently underwent repeat hepatectomy than those who initially underwent a non-PSH (68% vs. 24%). Furthermore, the authors noted that patients in the PSH group had improved 5-year survival in the case of tumor recurrence.[32] Similarly, Matsumura et al.[66] found that 81.5% of patients who initially underwent PSH for CRLM were able to undergo a repeat hepatectomy if recurrence occurred. By using parenchymal-sparing techniques, higher preservation of normal liver tissue allows for second salvage operations in the case of tumor recurrence, which in turn results in improved oncologic outcomes.

TECHNICAL CONSIDERATIONS FOR PARENCHYMAL PRESERVATION (SEE CHAPTER 118B)

To ensure an oncologic appropriate resection, real-time image guidance is critical. One technique employs the use of IOUS to facilitate "radical but conservative" resections of anatomically challenging hepatic tumors that preserve the maximum amount of liver while still satisfying principles of radical resection of tumor-bearing portal tributaries.[6] IOUS allows for intraoperative adjustment of the surgical approach based on accurate intraoperative staging and detailed visualization of the tumor in relation to hepatic vasculature.[67] Superficial easily accessible tumors represent the optimal indication for PSH, but deep-placed tumor resections can also be safely performed.[68]

In addition to IOUS, other novel image guidance techniques are emerging that facilitate anatomic-based PSH by determining the tumor-bearing region of liver parenchyma, including methylene blue counter staining, ICG fluorescence imaging, and Glissonian "pedicle-first" techniques.[69] Standard perioperative considerations are also critical for improving the outcomes of patients undergoing PSH. Minimizing intraoperative blood loss through the use of low–central venous pressure anesthesia and the use of hemostatic devices are important. Furthermore, use of techniques such as minimally invasive surgery[70] and the Pringle maneuver[71] has shown improvements in perioperative outcomes for patients undergoing hepatectomy. Finally, local therapies such as intraoperative or planned postoperative ablation are adjuncts to parenchymal preservation and can further increase patients' eligibility for surgery[72] (see Chapter 96). This use of postoperative "completion ablation"—percutaneous ablation after hepatic resection—has been shown to be effective and potentially expand the population eligible for surgical resection among patients with advanced disease.[73] A complete description of technical aspects of PSH is included in Chapter 118B.

CONCLUSION

A parenchymal-sparing approach to liver resection for primary and secondary malignancies should be the preferred approach when feasible. PSH diminishes the physiologic impact of surgery, reduces complication rates, enhances postoperative recovery, minimizes the risk of PHLF, and increases the surgical salvageability for intrahepatic recurrence. These benefits apply to cirrhotic and noncirrhotic patients alike, hence broaden the population eligible for surgical therapy for liver cancer. When appropriately applied, parenchymal-sparing techniques result in oncologic outcomes equivalent to those after major hepatic resection and should be considered a necessary part of the oncologic surgeon's practice. Successful application of the parenchymal-sparing principle and utilization of parenchymal-sparing techniques are enhanced by sophisticated preoperative and intraoperative imaging techniques, a deeper understanding of liver anatomy, and the application of advanced surgical techniques. In the near future, PSH may cease to be a label for special-intent surgery and instead become the rule in order to maximally preserve non–tumor-bearing liver tissue in all patients undergoing resection for hepatic malignancy.

References are available at expertconsult.com.

Segment-oriented anatomic liver resections: Indications and outcomes

Cornelius A. Thiels and Alice C. Wei

OVERVIEW

Segment-oriented hepatectomy is defined as the removal of one or more of the eight anatomic segments of the liver. The techniques of segment-oriented anatomic liver resection are based on the pioneering work of Claude Couinaud, who identified intrahepatic anatomy by creating vascular and biliary casts of the liver[1] (see Introduction and Chapter 2) Couinaud established that the liver is subdivided into eight autonomous segments, each having its own biliary drainage and vascular inflow and outflow. Anatomic resection was originally described by Lortat-Jacob and Robert in 1952 and subsequently by Pack and Miller (1961) and McBride and Wallace (1972).[2-4] Because each liver segment has individual function, each segment can be removed without affecting the others.[5,6] Segment-oriented liver resection is now a refined technique that allows safe removal of liver disease while preserving normal liver parenchyma (see Chapter 118B).

Driven largely by the increased surgical management of colorectal cancer liver metastasis (CRCLM), there has been a significant increase in the use of nonanatomic, parenchymal-sparing liver resection in the past 2 decades.[7,8] However, segmental liver resection remains indicated in a variety of situations. The ability to resect one or more segments, rather than the entire lobe, allows parenchymal preservation in patients with diseased parenchyma or in repeat resection patients with limited residual volume. In addition, anatomic resection facilitates the removal of tumor-bearing biliary and portal tributaries, which may help eradicate any tumor that has spread along these structures and improve oncologic outcomes for select tumors. Finally, in specific situations, segmental resection may be technically more feasible and safer than nonanatomic parenchymal-sparing liver resection. This chapter will provide an overview of indications, important technical and anatomic considerations when performing segmental resections, and technical aspects of various segmental liver resections.

Segmental Resections for Hepatocellular Carcinoma
(see Chapters 89 and 101B)

Surgery remains the treatment of choice for hepatocellular carcinoma (HCC). However, high recurrence rates after curative-intent R0 hepatectomy have prompted ongoing research to determine the optimal extent of resection.[9] HCC appears to spread via the portal pedicles, and therefore removal of tumor-bearing portal tributaries by a segmental approach may better eradicate intrahepatic metastases in the vicinity of the primary tumor.

It is hypothesized that oncologic outcomes may be improved with anatomic resections over nonanatomic resections for patients with HCC.[10,11] Multiple independent series have reported better overall and disease-free survival with an anatomic approach.[12-18] However, there are conflicting data, with other studies identifying no outcome differences between anatomic and nonanatomic resection.[19,20] Although the literature lacks randomized data, a meta-analysis of 16 observational studies including 2917 patients with HCC (1577 anatomic and 1340 nonanatomic resections) found anatomic resection to be superior to nonanatomic resection in terms of overall and disease-free survival.[21] An updated meta-analysis of 25 observational studies (10216 patients) also demonstrated a 5-year survival advantage for patients undergoing anatomic resection compared with nonanatomic resection, with no difference in morbidity between the two groups.[22] Nevertheless, achieving a balance between parenchymal-sparing and radical oncologic clearance remains of utmost importance in HCC patients with cirrhosis. Segmental liver resection is a bridge between major hepatectomy and nonanatomic resection, and can preserve liver volume and functional reserve in order to minimize postoperative liver insufficiency.[10,18]

In situations in which anatomy is unsuitable or when the residual liver would be at high risk of complications after an anatomic resection, nonanatomic resection must be used. In recent years there has been an increasing effort to determine the ideal resection margin in HCC. Although some institutional series have found that narrow resection margin (<1 cm) was not associated with worse oncologic outcomes,[23-25] a meta-analysis[26] and multi-institutional series[27] have demonstrated improved survival with wide margins. A prospective randomized trial examining wide (2 cm) versus narrow (1 cm) resection margins for solitary HCC demonstrated improved overall survival in the wide margin cohort, including in the subset of patients with tumors less than 2 cm.[28] In addition, an international multi-institutional analysis of patients with T1 HCC undergoing negative-margin hepatectomy demonstrated that wide resection margins (>1 cm) were associated with decreased local recurrence.[29] However, in this series, wide resection margin was not associated with lower recurrence rates in the subset of patients undergoing anatomic resection (80% of the overall cohort), suggesting that a narrower margin may be sufficient when performing an anatomic resection.[29] Recently, an institutional series of 2508 consecutive patients who underwent liver resection for solitary hepatitis B virus–related HCC demonstrated improved oncologic outcomes with wide margins (>1 cm); however, a survival advantage was seen only in patients with microvascular invasion.[30]

Segmental Resections for Colorectal Liver Metastases
(see Chapters 90 and 101B)

Despite early reports of improved outcomes with anatomic resection for CRCLM,[31,32] subsequent studies failed to confirm this observation. Current data support parenchyma-sparing nonanatomic resection in the vast majority of patients.[33-36]

Resections are designed to encompass the tumor as well as an adequate margin of nontumor liver. Recent series have subsequently confirmed the safety, and even oncologic benefit, of parenchymal-sparing nonanatomic resection for most CRCLM when technically feasible.[37–40] A parenchymal-sparing approach is also supported in patients with multifocal or bilobar lesions.[41] Thus anatomic resections are largely reserved for patients with multiple or large tumors in contiguous segments. Even when anatomic resection is needed, parenchymal-sparing principles can be applied by using segmental/bisegmental resection instead of hemihepatectomy. This is particularly beneficial in patients who are heavily pretreated with chemotherapy, given the association among chemotherapy, steatohepatitis, and hepatic sinusoidal congestion.[42,43]

The molecular profile of colorectal cancer may influence resection planning. Mutations in *KRAS* are the most commonly studied in CRCLMs (occur in 15%–50% of patients) and are associated with aggressive clinical behavior and early recurrence.[44–46] Margonis et al.[47] found that that nonanatomic resection was associated with worse disease-free survival in patients with *KRAS*-mutated tumors compared with patients undergoing anatomic resection (10.5 vs. 33.8 months). Another study by Brudvik et al.[48] reported that *KRAS* mutations were independently associated with higher rates of positive margins compared with patients with wild-type tumors. Similarly, *BRAF* mutations in tumors are seen in approximately 10% of patients with colorectal cancer and are associated with early recurrence after resection.[46,49] However, there are limited data on how *BRAF* mutations affect outcomes after resection, likely because of its rarity and association with poor prognosis.[44]

Other Indications for Segmental Resections

Beyond a biologic rationale, anatomic considerations are also important indications for segmental resection. For example, segmental resection is commonly used when there is tumor invasion of a major portal pedicle or hepatic vein. Segmental resection also may be indicated for biliary tumors or in the setting of stone disease or biliary strictures. In select situations, segmental resection may also be more technically feasible and safer than a nonanatomic approach. Deeply seated lesions, such as in segments IVa or VIII may benefit from the formal vascular control afforded by an anatomic approach to better manage bleeding, particularly when a large parenchymal transection surface is involved. An anatomic resection may also minimize the risk of bile leak resulting from an orphan bile duct, which occurs when a biliary radical is separated from its draining biliary system in a nonanatomic resection. However, data to support these potential benefits are limited because most series report an overall equivalent complication rate between colorectal cancer patients undergoing anatomic and nonanatomic resections.[8,50] An exception to this, however, is hepatic insufficiency, which is lower in patients undergoing parenchymal-sparing nonanatomic approaches compared with major hepatectomies.[51] Living donor liver transplantation is also an indication to perform a segmental liver resection, which often involves a left lateral sectionectomy (see Chapter 121).

LIVER ANATOMY (SEE INTRODUCTION AND CHAPTER 2)

The current understanding of the segmental anatomy of the liver has come from the original 1952 descriptions of Couinaud.[1,52,53] These segments have evolved to become the standard for hepatic nomenclature. The Brisbane terminology eliminated confusing terminology of "lobes" and "sectors" used in the American, European, and Japanese descriptions of liver anatomy.[54] The terms *hemiliver* (first-order division), *section* (second-order division), and *segment* (third-order division) are not interchangeable, providing universal terminology for better communication among liver surgeons.

The first-order divisions are *right liver* (segments V through VIII) and *left liver* (segments II through IV), or *hemiliver,* the boundary of which lies along Cantlie's line marked by the path of the middle hepatic vein (MHV) from the middle of the gallbladder fossa to its termination in the inferior vena cava (IVC) (Fig. 102B.1). The second-order division into liver sections is based on hepatic arterial supply and biliary drainage. The sections are derived from the primary divisions of the major right and left portal triads. The right hemiliver is divided into sections known as the *right anterior* (segments V and VIII) and *right posterior* (segments VI and VII), separated by the right hepatic vein (RHV). The left hemiliver is divided into *left lateral* (segments II and III) and *left medial* (segments IVa and IVb) sections by the umbilical fissure and falciform ligament. Together, segments II and III are often erroneously referred to as the "left lateral segment." The third-order division, segments I through VIII, is defined by hepatic arterial supply and biliary drainage. The axial plane is at the level of the intersection of the hepatic veins and the axial plane of the bifurcation of the portal vein (Table 102B.1 and Fig. 102B.2).

Biliary and vascular variations are common and should be anticipated in segmental resections (see Chapter 2). Mapping of vital vascular and biliary structures before resection facilitates high-quality surgery. Biliary and arterial anomalies are most common, with up to 50% of patients having nonstandard biliary anatomy and approximately 30% of patients having a major arterial variant. Major anatomic variants (e.g., a right posterior sectoral biliary duct draining into the left hepatic duct) and common hepatic arterial abnormalities should be identified on preoperative imaging and considered before performing any resection. However, there are also less common minor variants that must be considered when performing resections of isolated segments (discussed further later). A more comprehensive list of anatomic variants that may have an

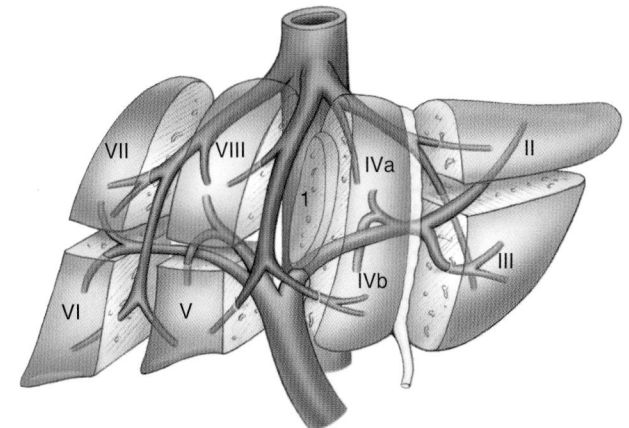

FIGURE 102B.1 Diagram depicting the relationship of the eight liver segments with the major hepatic veins and portal veins of the idealized liver (see Chapter 2).

TABLE 102B.1	Anatomic Boundaries of Each Liver Segment		
SEGMENT	VERTICAL BOUNDARY	HORIZONTAL BOUNDARY	OTHER
I	Middle of IVC		Posterior to PV
II	Left of left PV (falciform)	Cephalad to left HV	
III	Left of left PV (falciform)	Caudate to left HV	
IVa	Right of left PV (falciform) Left of middle HV	Cephalad to bifurcation of PV	
IVb	Right of left PV (falciform) Left of middle HV	Caudate to bifurcation of PV	
V	Right of middle HV Anterior to right HV	Caudate to bifurcation of PV	
VI	Posterior to right HV	Caudate to bifurcation of PV	
VII	Posterior to right HV	Cephalad to bifurcation of PV	
VIII	Right of middle HV Anterior to right HV	Cephalad to bifurcation of PV	

HV, Hepatic vein; *IVC,* inferior vena cava; *PV,* portal vein.

impact on the safety and feasibility of segmental resections can be found in Chapter 2.

PREOPERATIVE PLANNING

Assessment of the suitability of segmental resection requires precise mapping of the vascular and biliary anatomy and associated variants. This is typically achieved using preoperative computed tomography (CT) and/or magnetic resonance imaging (MRI) (see Chapters 14 through 16). With the appropriate protocols for arterial and venous enhancement, third- and fourth-level vascular structures can be accurately defined, and most major anatomic variants can be identified preoperatively and planned for accordingly. Angiography and ultrasound are occasionally used when additional details of hepatic anatomy are required for surgical planning. In addition to high-quality preoperative imaging, many surgeons use intraoperative ultrasonography (discussed further later).

In recent years, numerous computer-assisted surgical planning software programs have become available. It has been proposed that these technologies can improve patient selection, operative planning, identification of variant anatomy, and better delineate resection margins. These programs typically involve three-dimensional reconstructions of the liver that can be manipulated preoperatively and even intraoperatively.[55] Systems include MeVIS imaging system (MeVisLab, Bremen, Germany), Vital's Vitrea Enterprise Imaging (Canon Group Company, Minnetonka, Minnesota), Myrian XP-Liver (Intrasense, Paris), and Synapse 3d (Fujifilm, Tokyo). Three-dimensional printed models of the liver have also been made to aid in preoperative planning, but to date they are primarily used for surgical education and training.[56] Finally, augmented reality has been proposed to improve intraoperative navigation.[57] Although these technologies continue to evolve, data remain limited on whether they improve outcomes over current best practice.

GENERAL OPERATIVE PRINCIPLES

Preoperative assessment, preparation, and mobilization for liver resections are described in Chapters 4, 26, and 118). Volumetric analysis should be performed in patients with potentially

UPPER SLICES OF THE LIVER

LOWER SLICES OF THE LIVER

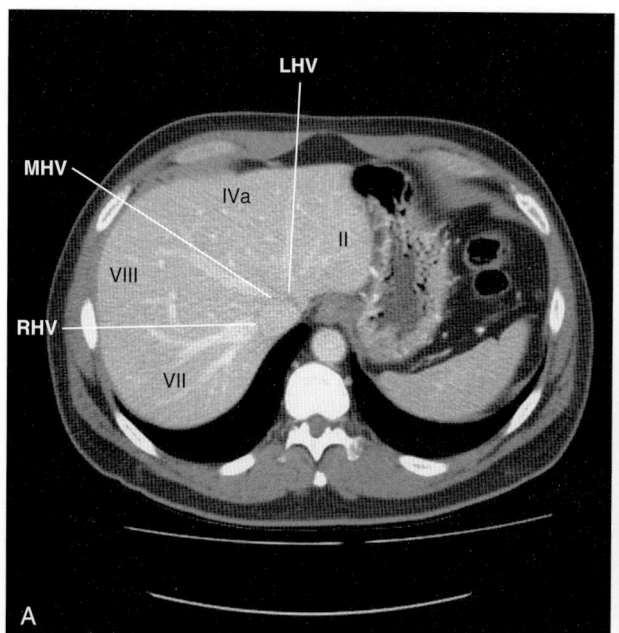

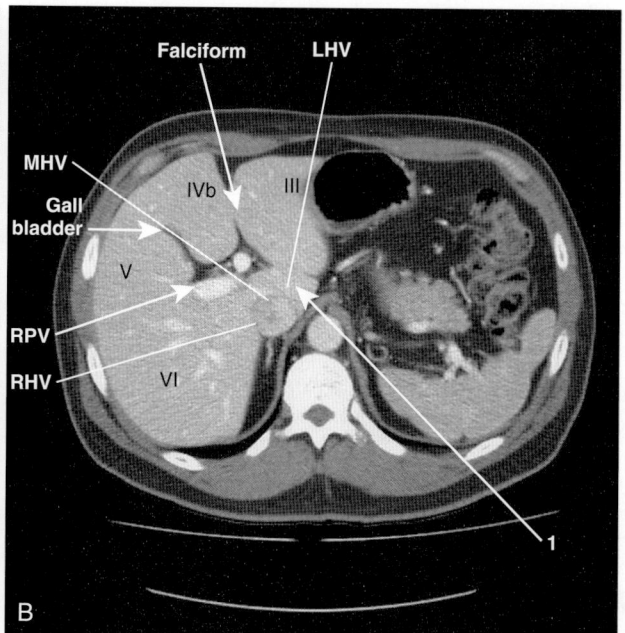

FIGURE 102B.2 **A,** Axial computed tomography (CT) image through the upper liver, demonstrating the anatomic boundaries of segments II, IVa, VIII, and VII. **B,** Axial CT image through the lower liver, demonstrating the anatomic boundaries of segments I, III, IVb, V, and VI. *LHV,* Left hepatic vein; *MHV,* middle hepatic vein; *RHV,* right hepatic vein; *RPV,* right portal vein (see Chapter 2).

marginal residual liver volume and function and is discussed in Chapters 4, 102C, and 102D.

Intraoperative Assessment (see Chapter 24)

Intraoperative assessment of the liver requires correlation of the findings at inspection and palpation of the mobilized liver with those from preoperative imaging. Although intraoperative ultrasound was initially advocated as a mean to confirm preoperative findings and identify unexpected findings in the liver,[58] with the increased precision of preoperative imaging, ultrasound seldom alters the procedure.[59] However, intraoperative ultrasound remains an essential tool for intraoperative, dynamic, and real-time mapping of intraparenchymal anatomy and the relationship among tumor, vital structures, and transection lines.

It is imperative to precisely identify the surgical margin of the hepatic segment being removed when performing anatomic resections. Dye injection directly into the portal branches feeding a target segment to delineate segments has been used for many years.[60] However, the duration of staining is short and the boundary of the target hepatic segment can only be marked on the surface of the liver. Similarly, when the boundary is demarcated by ischemia, it is also only clearly evident on the surface of the liver. Therefore many institutions have begun using near-infrared fluorescence imaging with indocyanine green (ICG) (PINPOINT, Novadaq, Mississauga, Canada), which is amenable to open and laparoscopic procedures. The software for ICG fluorescence is also integrated into the da Vinci robotic system (Intuitive, Sunnyvale, CA), enabling real-time visualization via ICG in robotic cases. ICG fluorescence has been in use for many years, and it is a safe intraoperative tool for identifying major hepatic arteries and the common bile duct. More recently, ICG fluorescence also has been proposed for intraoperative navigation as a modality to improve the feasibility and safety of segmental resections.[61] This can be done by either division of the inflow vessels followed by intravenous injection or via direct injection of the target portal branch.[62] Superselective intraarterial hepatic injection of ICG for segmental resections also has been proposed.[63]

Minimally Invasive Segmental Liver Resections (see Chapter 127D)

The majority of hepatopancreaticobiliary centers now perform minor liver resections, including peripheral wedges and left lateral sectionectomies, using a minimally invasive approach. In recent years, the use of minimally invasive approaches for more complex segmental resections has increased. Many centers perform minimally invasive segmental resections of segments II, III, V, and VI in selected patients. However, despite growing success with these techniques, minimally invasive segmentectomies are often considered more difficult than major hepatectomies. More complex minimally invasive resections, including segment I, IVa, VII, and VIII are considered more difficult.[64-66] Ban et al.[67] developed a scoring system to preoperatively predict the difficulty of various laparoscopic liver resections. This system is based on various factors, including tumor size, extent of liver resection, tumor location, proximity to major vessels, and severity of fibrosis and may aid in appropriate selection of patients for minimally invasive resection according to the surgeon's skill level.[66] Lastly, techniques, including intraoperative ultrasound, ICG fluorescence, and an extrahepatic Glissonian approach,[68,69] are particularly useful for more difficult minimally invasive resections. Additional information on minimally invasive segmental resections can be found in Chapters 127D and 127E.

Transection Techniques

There are at least two philosophies of liver transection, which result in distinct surgical techniques and styles. The first is that blood loss from the transected liver is minimized by speed, external compression, vascular occlusion (outflow and/or inflow),[70,71] and the use of surgical interventions to stop bleeding (e.g., cautery, sutures, and tissue glues). The second is that blood loss is best minimized by prevention of injury to vascular structures, using transection techniques that dissect structures from the surrounding parenchyma as understood and anticipated by preoperative imaging and planning. A variety of transection techniques have been developed and these techniques can be successfully applied to each philosophy of liver transection. There is no clear dominant method, and a working knowledge of more than one transection technique is beneficial (see Chapter 118).

The crush clamp method of liver transection is used at many centers.[72-74] This allows for precise, controlled transection of the liver parenchyma and identification of intrahepatic structures. Similarly, a Cavitron Ultrasonic Surgical Aspirator (CUSA; ValleyLab, Boulder, CO) or a Helix Hydro-Jet dissector (ERBE USA, Marietta, GA) can also provide selective destruction of liver parenchyma with relative sparing of denser fibrotic tissue, such as hepatic veins and portal triads. Inflow and outflow vascular occlusion may be added to these techniques for better hemostasis. Because there is no evidence to clearly support the superiority of any specific technique,[75] the transection method for any particular operation should depend on the surgeon's expertise.

These techniques are often used in conjunction with traditional surgical techniques, such as cautery, suture ligation, and clips, as well as advanced devices such as linear cutting staplers, computer-controlled bipolar cautery (LigaSure, Covidien, Boulder, CO), saline-linked radiofrequency monopolar devices (Dissecting Sealer, Metronic, Dublin, Ireland), saline-linked radiofrequency bipolar devices (Aquamantys, Metronic, Dublin, Ireland), or the argon beam coagulator (Force GCU Systems, ValleyLab). Radiofrequency ablation (Habib; AngioDynamics, Latham, NY) has been proposed as a mechanism for reducing blood loss without the need for vascular exclusion maneuvers,[76] but this has not been widely adopted because of a variety of safety concerns and limitations.[77,78] Numerous energy-based instruments now exist to facilitate minimally invasive parenchymal transection, including the ultrasonic dissector (Harmonic ACE, Johnson & Johnson, New Brunswick, NJ or Sonicision, Medtronic, Dublin, Ireland), computer-controlled bipolar cautery (LigaSure, Covidien), saline-linked radiofrequency monopolar device (Dissecting Sealer, Metronic, Dublin, Ireland), ultrasonic surgical aspirator (CUSA Excel+ System, integra lifesciences Plainsboro Township, NJ), and the combined ultrasonic and bipolar device (Thunderbeat, Olympus, Tokyo).

Pretransection vascular control is used by many surgeons for anatomic delimitation and hemostasis.[70,71] Hepatic artery and portal vein inflow control to those segments being resected facilitates the resection with reduction of blood loss, by defining the line of division between ischemic segments to be removed and the well-perfused remnant liver. Pretransection occlusion of inflow to the segments to be resected before outflow results in better hemostasis. Ligation of the inflow to sectors of the right hemiliver (VI-VII and V-VIII) or to the segments of the left lobe (II, III, IVa, and IVb) can be performed either by entering the Glissonian capsule to identify and divide the hepatic artery (HA) and portal vein of interest,[79] or by the extra-glissonian technique.[69,80] In the latter, the sectional or segmental portal pedicle is encircled in the plane between the Glissonian capsule and the liver parenchyma. In this method, the duct, artery, and vein of interest can be transected en masse by suture or with a linear stapler.

PROCEDURES

Important considerations for monosegment and bisegment resections will be discussed in the following sections. See Part 10 for a detailed description of hepatic resections.

Segment I Resection

Segment I lies behind to the left and posterior to the portal bifurcation and receives inflow predominantly from the left portal vein (PV) and the left hepatic artery (see Chapter 2) The biliary drainage of segment I is variable; segment I bile duct runs in the hilar plate and enters the posterior aspect of either the left or right hepatic duct. Although these ducts most commonly (78% of patients) drain into both right and left hepatic duct systems, drainage solely into the left or right hepatic ductal system occurs in 15% and 7% of patients, respectively.[81] Segment I rests on the IVC, and most of its outflow drains directly into the IVC by a series of fragile veins. Venous drainage of segment I into the IVC can range from one to nine veins.[82] Tumors arising in the caudate lobe are closely related to the posterior aspect of the left hepatic vein (LHV) and MHV. This "critical oncologic margin" is a decisive factor in the choice between an isolated caudate resection and a left hepatectomy, including the caudate lobe, with or without the MHV.

The falciform ligament is dissected in a cephalad direction, until the anterior and left surface of the suprahepatic vena cava has been isolated. The LHV is identified, and the left triangular ligament is divided from left to right. As the dissection is carried medially, care should be taken to avoid injury to any low-entering phrenic veins and the LHV. The fissure for the ligamentum venosum, the *caudate groove*, is identified by retracting segments II and III to the right, and the hepatogastric ligament is incised (see Chapter 118).

For large tumors, the right liver should be mobilized to fully expose the caudate lobe from the right side as well. The resection can usually be performed from the left, although some large tumors may require an anterior approach. Peritoneal reflection onto the IVC in the lesser sac is incised, which allows some retraction of segment I, and occasionally the left side of the IVC is exposed through some or all of its length. The small bridge of liver between segments I and VI is also divided. To obtain further mobility and reduce the chances of a traction injury to the hepatic veins, the ligamentum venosum is ligated and divided in the superior aspect of its fissure, as it enters the posterior aspect of the LHV or MHV. The inflow vessels are ligated as they emerge from the posterior aspect of the PV and HA. Often, two distinct paired PV branches enter segment I.

The dissection of segment I from the IVC then continues in a cephalad direction, dividing several thin-walled veins that drain segment I into the IVC. A large, dominant vein of segment I is often present 1 to 2 cm below the MHV and LHV confluence. Some of the venous branches between segments VI and VII and the IVC may be divided to provide adequate mobilization of the caudate off the IVC. Usually, very few vascular structures are found in this plane, although segment I duct and hilar plate tissue should be anticipated anteriorly. During parenchymal

transection, the fissure for the ligamentum venosum is sometimes encountered and may need to be divided again. Dissection continues to its completion at the apex of segment I beneath the confluence of the hepatic veins. Alternatively, an anterior approach has been described for very large segment I tumors.

Segment II or III Resection

Given the discrepancy between PV supply and biliary drainage and also given the difficulty of preserving LHV drainage, combined segment II and III resection (left lateral sectionectomy; Fig. 102B.3) is often safer and more feasible than isolated resection of segments II or III. When either of these segmentectomies is being planned, the plane of resection is by either side of the LHV (left and posterior for segment II resection, right and anterior for segment III resection). The inflow is approached on the left side of the falciform ligament by incising the peritoneal reflection onto the liver and identifying the segment II or III portal pedicles. Once the inflow is stopped, the line of parenchymal transection becomes prominent between the ischemic segment to be resected and the normally perfused residual segment (see Chapter 118).

Combined Resection of Segments II and III

The left lateral section is mobilized by division of the falciform ligament and the left triangular ligament (Fig. 102B.4). The

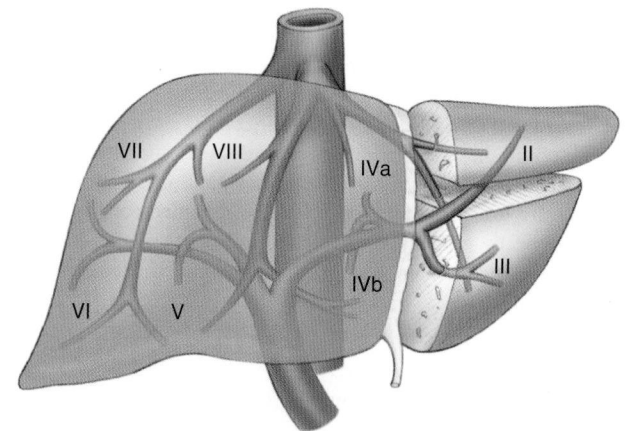

FIGURE 102B.3 Diagram of the planes of transection for resection of segments II and III or segments IV, V, VI, VII, and VIII (extended right hepatectomy) (see Chapters 2, 101B, and 118).

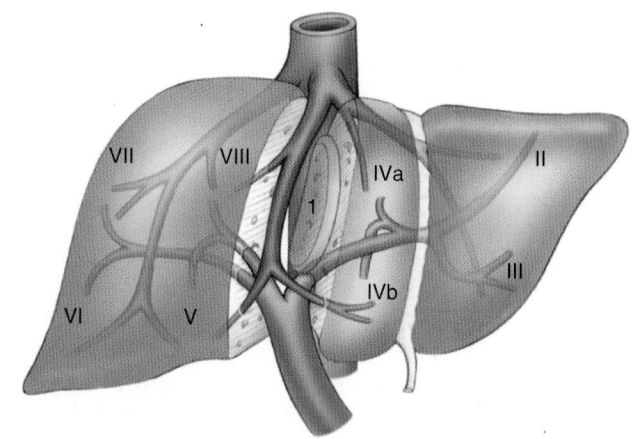

FIGURE 102B.4 Diagram of the planes of transection for a right or a left hepatectomy (hemihepatectomy) (see Chapters 2, 101B, and 118).

LHV typically joins the MHV in an intrahepatic position, and isolating the LHV extrahepatically can be difficult. The extrahepatic portion of the LHV can be lengthened by dividing the fibrous tissue to the left of the IVC down to the level of the fissure for the ligamentum venosum, which is then ligated and divided as it enters the posterior aspect of the LHV. This allows encircling of the LHV, if its IVC junction is separate from the MHV. Otherwise, the isolation of the LHV is delayed until completion of the parenchymal transection. When performing left lateral sectionectomy, the presence or absence of a segment IV fissural vein (vein of the umbilical fissure) must be considered. If it is in the plane of resection, it can be preserved or removed, but its location should be noted to prevent bleeding during transection.

The inflow to segments II and III is usually isolated during transection of the parenchyma to the left of the falciform ligament. Occasionally, pedicles to segments II and III can be identified and encircled outside the liver in the left side of the portoumbilical fissure. The plane of parenchymal transection follows the falciform ligament. As the liver is divided, the portal structures to segments II and III will become apparent, and these can be electively ligated and divided. Once this is done and the parenchyma surrounding the LHV has been dissected, the vein also can be ligated and divided. The transection is completed by dividing the parenchyma anterior to the caudate lobe in the fissure for the ligamentum venosum. The blood supply to the caudate emerges from the PV and left HA at the level of the umbilical fissure, and these vessels should be identified and preserved before parenchymal transection (see Chapter 118).

Segment IV Resection

Isolated resection of segment IV or IVa alone is relatively uncommon. Segment IV is limited posteriorly by the hilar plate and IVC, on the right by the falciform ligament, and on the left PV and MHV. Inflow and biliary drainage to segment IV come left to right from the left-sided portal structures in the base of the falciform ligament (the "comeback" branches from the left PV). Sometimes, aberrant right anterior and posterior sectional ducts cross in this position; these should be preserved during resection. Outflow from segment IV is predominantly to the MHV, but occasionally a separate draining vein along the line of the falciform ligament (scissural vein) goes directly to the suprahepatic IVC or to the terminal part of the LHV or MHV (see Chapter 2).

Once the falciform ligament has been divided, with identification of the termination of the hepatic veins, the arterial and venous inflow can be divided. By incising the peritoneal reflection on the right of the falciform ligament, the segment IVa and IVb pedicles can be isolated, encircled, and divided; the lines of transection become demarcated on the surface of the liver along Cantlie's line

Resection continues at the base of segment IV off the anterior surface of the hilar plate. Care must be taken to avoid excessive use of cautery in the hilar plate, because the bile duct bifurcation and left hepatic duct lie immediately behind this area. Parenchymal transection commences on the right side of the falciform ligament with identification of portal pedicles to segments IVa and IVb (see Chapter 118). These may arise from a common trunk and occasionally there are more than two, but this is usually seen on preoperative imaging.

Transection continues superiorly to the level of the suprahepatic IVC to the junction of the LHV and MHV. The veins usually join within the liver at this point before insertion into the IVC, and in this case, dissection terminates inferior to this

point. Care should be taken to identify significant venous tributaries from segment IV into the LHV, which may not be identified on preoperative imaging. The dissection of the right side is along Cantlie's line to the left of the MHV. Several tributaries to the MHV, the IVa and IVb veins, will need to be identified and ligated. Once the medial border of the hilar dissection has been reached, the parenchymal transection is done in a transverse plane to complete the separation of segment IV.

Segment V Resection

The bifurcation of the right portal pedicle into anterior and posterior pedicles may be intrahepatic, and primary ligation of these pedicles is difficult, especially for segment VIII; therefore some parenchymal transection along Cantlie's line toward the pedicle is required before its division to allow demarcation of either segment V or VIII. Isolated segment V resection begins with division of the liver on the undersurface up the center of the gallbladder fossa and anteriorly along Cantlie's line halfway up toward the IVC. The parenchyma is then divided in a plane to the left of the RHV, which extends on the undersurface of the liver along the incisura dextra (Rouvière's sulcus) to the free edge and anteriorly halfway toward the IVC. This posterior plane is quite coronal and usually results in a large, exposed area of parenchyma. The resection is completed by connecting the two vertical transection lines by division of the parenchyma horizontally from anterior to posterior immediately below the level of PV division (see Chapter 118).

Segment VIII Resection

Isolated segment VIII resection is a very challenging procedure because no external demarcation of this segment is apparent. The initial landmark is Cantlie's line with parenchymal transection on the right side of the MHV. The segment VIII pedicle, which corresponds to the ascending division of the right anterior sectional pedicle, can be isolated either at this point, after division of the liver, or by dividing the liver between segments IV and V in the horizontal plane along the level of the PV bifurcation. This latter maneuver is useful because it allows for demarcation of the right-sided resection margin, which is on the left side of the RHV. This horizontal transection should follow the coronal plane of the RHV, which requires intraoperative ultrasound guidance.

The parenchymal division of the right-sided resection margin continues superiorly; using the termination of the RHV as a landmark, there is often only 1 to 2 cm of liver at the upper margin of the transection between the RHV and MHV. Care must be taken during the right-sided parenchymal division to adhere to the correct transection plane, because this plane takes about a 45-degree angle from the vertical. This allows resection of segment VIII while avoiding injury to the RHV. Segment VIII resection is completed by separating the remaining parenchyma off the deep attachment to the IVC, although this should have been mostly completed during mobilization (see Chapter 118).

Combined Resection of Segments V and VIII

Segments V and VIII compose the right anterior sector. The combined resection of segments V and VIII requires division of the right anterior sectional portal triad with left-sided parenchymal division along Cantlie's line along the right side of the MHV; the right-sided parenchymal division is in the coronal plane of the left side of the RHV. The anterior sectoral pedicle may be encircled from outside the liver, either anteriorly or posteriorly, and it is divided en masse with a linear cutting stapler, or it may be identified during the parenchymal transection along Cantlie's line at the base. Early division of inflow provides demarcation of the ischemic parenchyma, which facilitates identification of the planes of parenchymal transection (see Chapter 118).

Segment VI Resection

The right posterior sectional pedicle can be identified in the incisura dextra of Ganz (Rouvière's sulcus), which corresponds to the horizontal fissure lateral to the gallbladder fossa. The segment VI/VII branch of the right HA can usually be isolated extraparenchymally; however, the segment VI/VII portal branch, which corresponds to the posterior division of the right portal branch, is more difficult to isolate. Therefore the pedicle for an isolated resection of segment VI or VII is usually approached within the liver during parenchymal transection (Fig. 102B.5). Isolated segment VI resection commences with an oblique transection line along the incisura dextra in the inferior surface of the liver and anteriorly halfway toward the IVC, following the posterior side of the RHV (Fig. 102B.6). The horizontal plane of resection is at the level of the PV bifurcation. The descending

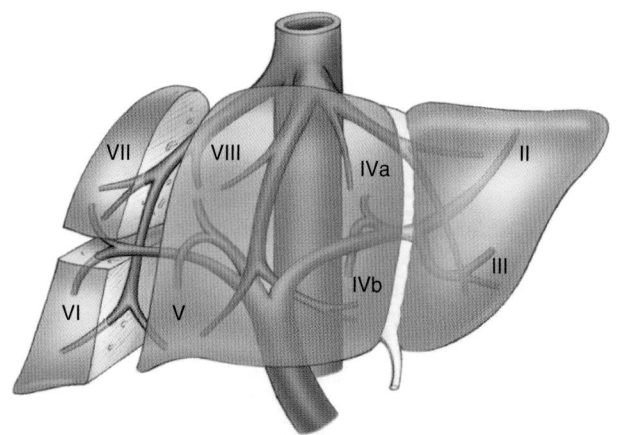

FIGURE 102B.5   Diagram of the planes of transection for resection of segments VI and VII or segments II, III, IV, V, and VIII (extended left hepatectomy) (see Chapters 2, 101B, and 118).

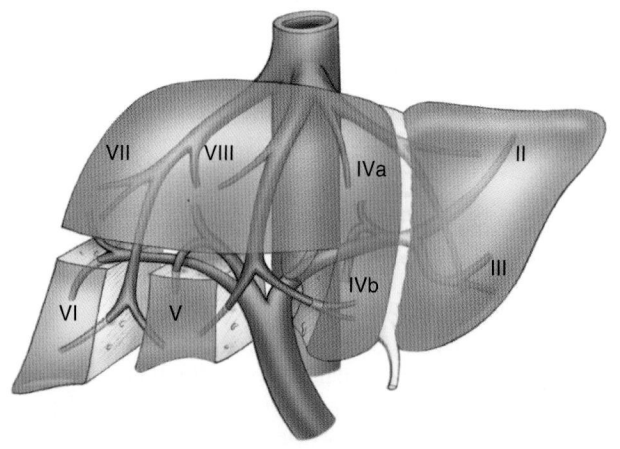

FIGURE 102B.6   Diagram of the planes of transection for resection of segments V and VI (see Chapters 2 and 118).

branches of the right posterior sectional portal triad are encountered about two-thirds of the way through the dissection. The resection is completed by taking a horizontal transection plane through the posterior surface of the liver lateral to the RHV (see Chapter 118).

Segment VII Resection

An isolated segment VII resection commences with the horizontal transection line just above the PV bifurcation; this line is congruous with the horizontal resection line for a segment VI resection (see Fig. 102B.5). The resection continues medially to the lateral margin of the RHV. During the horizontal resection, the ascending right posterior sectional branches can be isolated and divided, which will allow for demarcation of the medial aspect of the resection. The vertical transection line runs obliquely through the liver lateral and posterior to the RHV (see Chapter 118).

Combined Resection of Segments VI and VII

This right posterior sectionectomy is a procedure often considered as an alternative to a right hepatectomy, especially in patients with diseased parenchyma (see Fig. 102B.5). Identification of the right posterior sectional pedicle may be possible from outside the liver. Early division of the inflow facilitates the identification of the transection margins. Otherwise, the segment VI and VII HA and PV may be divided separately, leaving the transection of the VI and VII duct and plate for later, during the parenchymal transection. The plane of transection posterior to the RHV is coronal and results in a relatively large surface area of cut parenchyma, which requires specific attention for hemostasis and biliostasis (see Chapter 118).

Combined Resection of Segments V and VI

Resection of segments V and VI is frequently performed. The vertical plane of transection is along Cantlie's line on the right side of the MHV from the edge of the liver to halfway up toward the IVC (see Fig. 102B.6). The horizontal plane of transection is at the level of the PV. The portal pedicles to segments V and VI are usually divided during the parenchymal transection, which requires full mobilization of the right liver from the diaphragm with division of segment VI and most, if not all, of the segment VII hepatic veins on the anterior surface of the IVC. The transection starts in the middle of the gallbladder fossa and extends along Cantlie's line up to the level of the right portal pedicle. Then, with a dissection to the left, the horizontal plane of transection is developed from the top of the vertical plane. The segment V portal pedicle may be identified at the base and divided, followed by division of the segment VI pedicle posteriorly. From right to left, the horizontal dissection plane reaches the RHV.

ACKNOWLEDGMENTS

Sincere thanks to Dr. Charbel Sandroussi and Dr. Paul D. Greig for their original contributions to this chapter in previous editions.

References are available at expertconsult.com.

Preoperative portal vein embolization: Indications, technique, and results

Junichi Shindoh

INTRODUCTION

Portal vein embolization (PVE) is the most common portal flow modulation procedure performed preoperatively to reduce the risk of extensive liver resection in patients with a small anticipated future liver remnant (FLR).[1–4] PVE redirects portal blood flow to the intended FLR and is expected to produce a shift in hepatic functional reserve resulting from atrophy of the embolized liver and compensatory hypertrophy of the FLR (see Chapters 5 and 6). PVE can reduce perioperative morbidity and allow for safe, potentially curative hepatectomy for patients previously considered ineligible for resection because of a small anticipated FLR[3,5,6] (see Chapters 101, 102A, and 102B). Therefore PVE is currently performed at many hepatobiliary centers worldwide before major hepatectomy. In this chapter, indications, technical details and clinical outcomes of PVE are reviewed and discussed.

EVALUATION OF THE FUTURE LIVER REMNANT VOLUME TO PREDICT THE SAFETY OF MAJOR HEPATECTOMY

The safety of extensive liver resection is highly dependent on the net functional reserve of the FLR. The FLR[6–10] volume and the regenerative capacity of the liver[11,12] are important predictors of postoperative morbidity and mortality after major hepatectomy. Therefore systematic volumetry and estimation of hepatic functional reserve are needed to assess the risk of major hepatectomy (Fig. 102C.1).

Systematic Volumetry

A previous anatomic study revealed that only 25% of patients would have a sufficient FLR volume (i.e., >20% of the estimated standard liver volume) for safe extended right hepatectomy; the same study revealed that 90% of patients would have a sufficient FLR volume for right hemihepatectomy (Fig. 102C.2).[13] Thus routine volumetry using a validated method is recommended, especially in patients for whom extended right hepatectomy is being considered.

For volumetric calculations, the FLR volume should be calculated as the absolute volume of the fully functioning part of the liver after resection; in other words, the part of the liver that will have adequate inflow and outflow. When a hepatic vein draining a specific part of the liver is removed, the corresponding part of the liver will become congested and will atrophy as a result of losing its normal function.[14,15] Therefore, in calculating the FLR volume for patients undergoing extended right hepatectomy, in which the middle hepatic vein will be removed or compromised, segment IV volume should not be included. This is because in the absence of middle hepatic vein drainage, most of segment IV will become congested and lose its normal function unless an anatomically significant umbilical fissure vein or a segment IV vein directly draining into the left hepatic vein is present.

Minimal Future Liver Remnant Volume Required for Safe Liver Resection

Several methods have been described to evaluate the risk of major hepatectomy based on the volume of the FLR. In Japanese high-volume centers, volumetry is currently performed using three-dimensional (3D) image reconstruction systems (Fig. 102C.3), which allow direct measurement of the liver parenchymal volume per se, excluding vascular structures and tumors; they provide reliable results based on semiautomatic calculations of the vascular territories.[16] Conventionally, the minimum FLR volume required was calculated on the basis of the functional reserve of the liver determined by the indocyanine green (ICG) clearance test,[17] and recent reports have clarified that an estimated ICG clearance rate of the FLR (ICG-Krem) of 0.05 or greater is predictive of the maximum limit of liver resection.[18,19] Overall, it is important to obtain a reliable result for the required FLR volume when determining the surgical indications based on the safety limit for hepatectomy. Although the 3D simulation technique mentioned earlier has recently been reported to allow precise volumetry of the liver and direct measurement of the metabolic function of the liver through an ICG clearance test and is a reliable method, the limitations of this approach include the requirement of high-quality thin-slice CT images for the 3D image reconstruction and ICG clearance test is not always available in many countries.

At The University of Texas MD Anderson Cancer Center, the standardized FLR (sFLR) volume is used to evaluate regeneration after PVE and to estimate the surgical risk. The sFLR is defined as the measured FLR volume divided by the estimated total liver volume (TEL)[20] (Fig. 102C.4). At MD Anderson Cancer Center, the FLR volume is obtained from 3D reconstruction of the CT images of the FLR. TEL is estimated using a formula that relies on the linear correlation between the total liver volume and body surface area (BSA),[21] as follows:

$$\text{TEL (cm}^3) = -794.41 + 1267.28 \times \text{BSA (m}^2)$$

This method of estimating the FLR has several advantages: (1) It avoids direct 3D computed tomography measurement of the portion of the liver to be removed, which might not reflect adequate hepatic function (dilated bile ducts, hypertrophy from steatosis, or atrophy from cirrhosis). (2) It avoids the cumulative error associated with the measurement of multiple tumors that need to be subtracted from the total liver volume. (3) It is based on the actual hepatic physiologic needs of the individual patient as reflected in the patient's BSA. (4) The standardization corrects for patient size: small patients need a small liver remnant, and large patients need a large liver remnant.

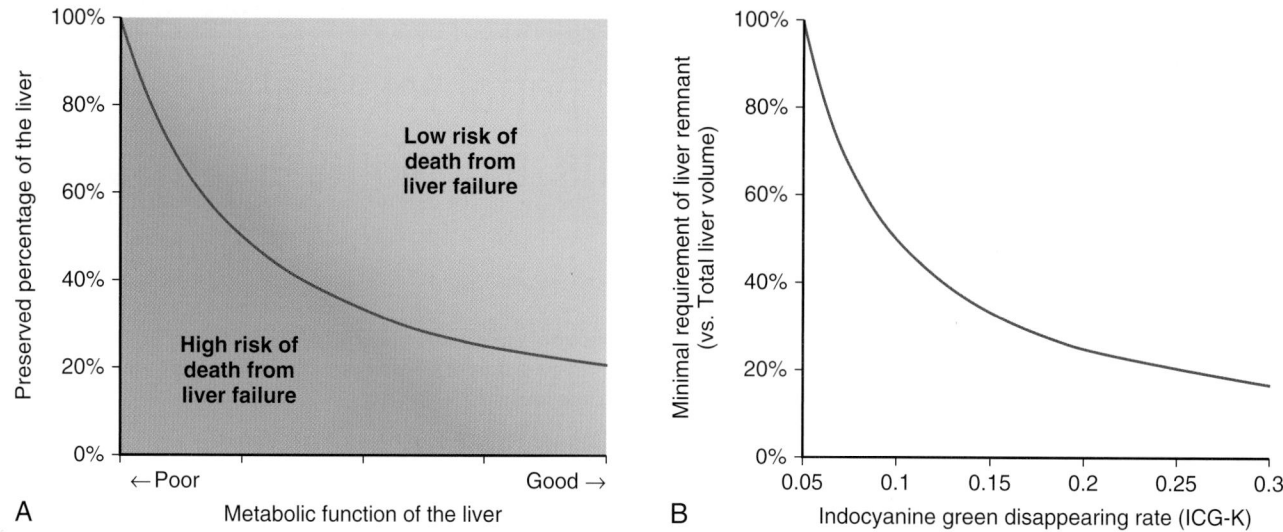

FIGURE 102C.1 The risk of postoperative hepatic insufficiency and death from liver failure has empirically been defined by the percentage of the liver remnant after surgery determined according to the metabolic function of the underlying liver **(A).** The estimated minimal requirement for future liver remnant volume calculated from the indocyanine green disappearance rate (ICG-K) according to expanded Makuuchi's criteria clearly shows a similar threshold curve for the risk of mortality after hepatectomy **(B).** (Kobayashi Y, Kiya Y, Sugawara T, et al. Expanded Makuuchi's criteria using estimated indocyanine green clearance rate of future liver remnant as a safety limit for maximum extent of liver resection. *HPB.* 2019;21[8]:990–997.)

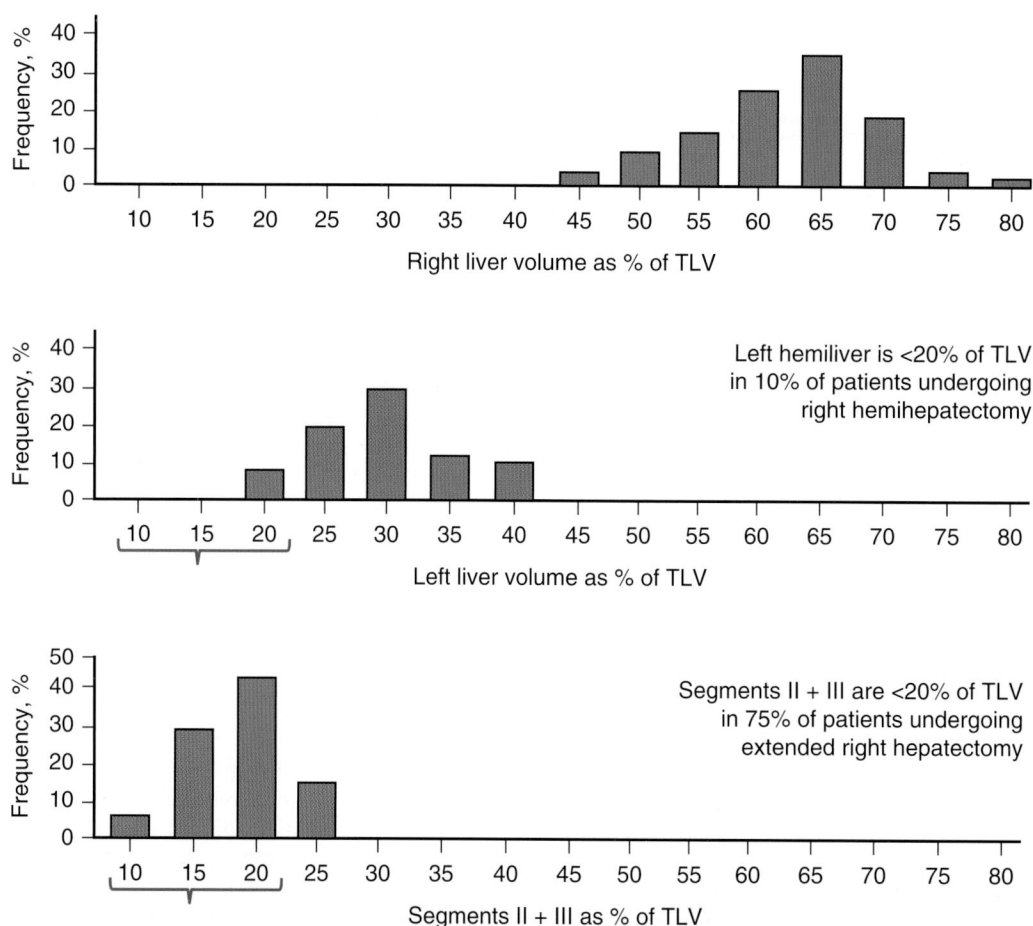

FIGURE 102C.2 **Distribution of patients by future liver remnant volume according to type of major hepatectomy.** *TLV,* Total liver volume. (Adapted from Abdalla EK, Denys A, Chevalier P, et al. Total and segmental liver volume variations: implications for liver surgery. *Surgery.* 2004;135:404–410 with permission.)

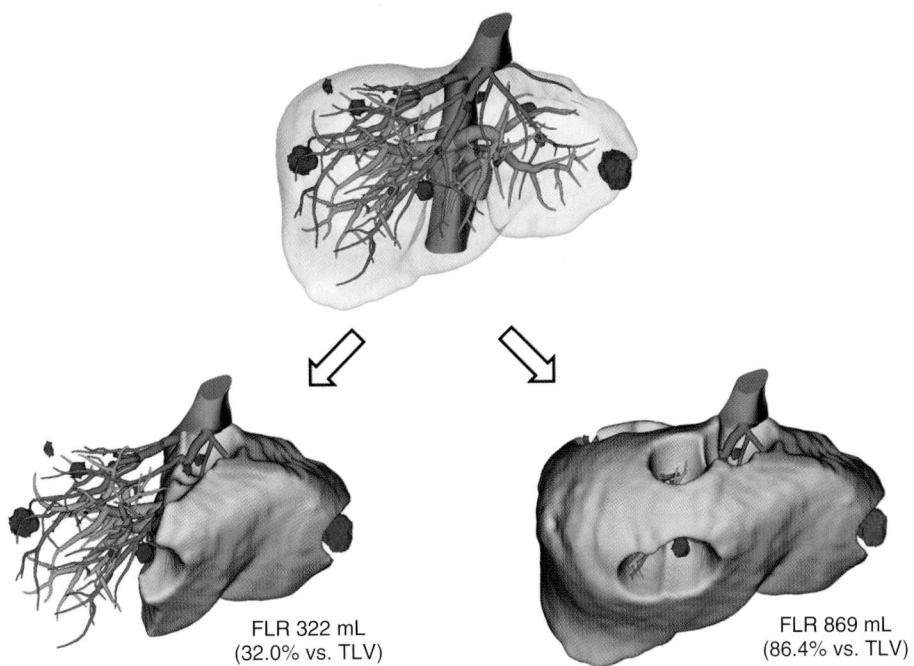

FIGURE 102C.3 **Surgical planning using a three-dimensional simulation software.** For a patient with 12 colorectal liver metastases, various types of resections were tested on the three-dimensional virtual hepatectomy simulator. Direct measurement of the liver remnant volume in each procedure enables risk assessment of surgical procedure as a part of the preoperative workup enabled a precise assessment of the risk associated with the surgical procedure. *FLR*, Future liver remnant; *TLV*, total liver volume. (Courtesy Dr. Takamoto, National Cancer Center Japan.)

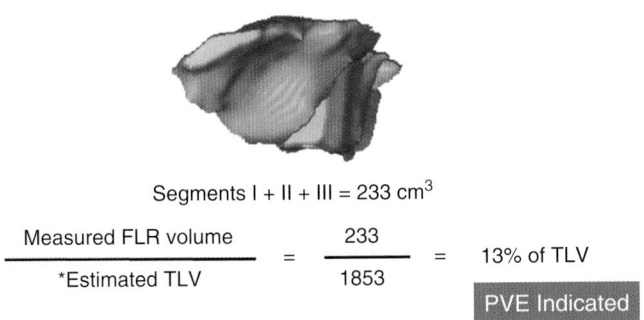

FIGURE 102C.4 **Measurement of standardized future liver remnant (sFLR) volume to estimate the risk of extended hepatectomy.** Total liver volume *(TLV)* can be estimated on the basis of body surface area according to the formula: Estimated TLV = −794.41 + 1267.28 × Body surface area (m²).[21] The estimated TLV can then be used to calculate the sFLR, which allows for a comparison of outcome between patients. *PVE*, Portal vein embolization.

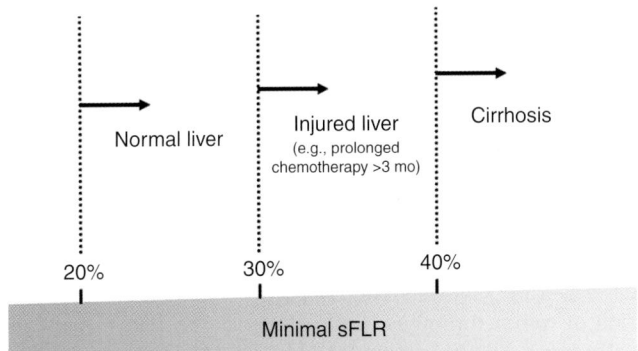

FIGURE 102C.5 Minimal standardized future liver remnant *(sFLR)* required to avoid postoperative hepatic insufficiency.[7–9,22]

In a series of 301 patients without chronic liver disease or hepatic injury undergoing extended right hepatectomy, an sFLR of less than 20% was a risk factor for postoperative liver insufficiency and 90-day postoperative mortality.[7] However, functional reserve per liver volume depends on the quality of the hepatic parenchyma. Therefore different sFLR cutoff values apply for safe liver resection in patients with hepatic injury or chronic liver disease. Patients with chemotherapy-induced liver injury after prolonged chemotherapy (e.g., >3 months) require an sFLR of approximately 30%, and patients with cirrhosis require an sFLR of at least 40%.[8,9,22] (Fig. 102C.5)

INDICATIONS AND CONTRAINDICATIONS FOR PORTAL VEIN EMBOLIZATION

PVE should be considered when the FLR or sFLR is not large enough to permit safe hepatectomy given the quality of the patient's underlying liver and the planned extent of surgery.

There are two absolute contraindications for PVE: established portal hypertension and extensive tumor thrombus of the ipsilateral portal vein. For patients with mild subclinical portal hypertension, PVE is not always contraindicated. However, PVE may increase portal vein pressure and worsen the clinical symptoms associated with portal hypertension (e.g., esophageal bleeding). Therefore considerable attention should be given to patients requiring PVE who have clinical evidence of portal hypertension.

TECHNICAL ASPECTS OF PORTAL VEIN EMBOLIZATION

Access Routes to the Portal Venous System

PVE can be performed by any of three standard approaches: the transileocolic venous approach, transhepatic contralateral approach (percutaneous portal vein access via the FLR), and transhepatic ipsilateral approach (percutaneous portal vein access via the liver to be resected). It is important to note that the approach to the portal vein is chosen at the discretion of the operator, and the decision may be based on multiple factors, including the extent of the embolization and surgery, the operator's preference for a specific embolic agent, tumor burden within the liver, and the operator's level of experience with one technique over another.[23]

Transileocolic Venous Approach

The transileocolic venous approach was the first approach described for performing preoperative PVE.[4] This technique is performed at laparotomy by direct cannulation of the ileocolic vein and introduction of a catheter into the portal system for embolization. This approach is usually adopted when additional treatment is needed during the same surgical exploration, when a percutaneous approach is not considered feasible, or when an interventional radiology suite is not available.[24,25] The disadvantages of the transileocolic venous approach are the need for general anesthesia and laparotomy, with their inherent risks, and the reliance on imaging equipment available in the operating room, which is often inferior to imaging equipment available in most modern interventional radiology suites. Therefore, because minimally invasive techniques have become favored and because interventional radiology equipment—imaging equipment, catheter systems, and embolic agents—has become more advanced, the indications for the transileocolic venous approach are currently limited.

Percutaneous Transhepatic Contralateral Approach

The percutaneous transhepatic contralateral approach was first described by Kinoshita and colleagues[26] to slow the progression of tumor thrombus within the portal system in patients with hepatocellular carcinoma (HCC). Modifications of this technique were later developed for the purpose of causing FLR hypertrophy (Fig. 102C.6A).[2,27] The percutaneous transhepatic contralateral approach requires ultrasound-guided percutaneous puncture, using an 18- or 22-gauge needle, of a peripheral portal branch, preferably segment III accessed via the subxiphoid route. Because access is gained through the FLR, care is taken to limit the number of punctures, and the most peripheral branch is targeted to avoid damage to the central structures.

Accessing the portal vein can be challenging with the contralateral approach when segment IV embolization is indicated. To ensure adequate distance between the portal entry point and the segment IV branches, the operator must perform the puncture in a branch of the left lateral liver, usually from the Rex recess. Segment IV embolization is performed after right PVE has rendered the segment IV branches more visible and dilated; however, a puncture in the Rex recess makes catheterization difficult, owing to the sharp angle of the vein and the risk of losing access. Segment III is often easier to access than segment II, and sonographic guidance in the axial plane makes it easy to differentiate segment II from segment III and the Rex recess. Because segment III branches arise in front of segment II branches within the Rex recess, catheterization of segment IV branches may be easier after puncture of segment III branches. After complete occlusion of the targeted portal branches is achieved, the access catheter to the portal vein is removed. Because the catheter entry site is in the FLR, embolic material is not used to seal the puncture tract.

The major advantage of the contralateral approach over the ipsilateral approach is that catheterization of the right portal branches is technically easier because the operator does not have to contend with awkward angles. In addition, embolization is performed with the catheter pointed toward the direction of portal venous flow. It must be acknowledged, however, that with the use of reverse-curve catheters, PVE can also be performed safely in the direction of portal venous flow with the ipsilateral approach.[28] Some authors report that the contralateral approach allows better visualization of the embolized portal branches on the final portogram[29]; however, other authors have found that with a modified ipsilateral approach, the image quality of the final postembolization portogram is similar between the ipsilateral and contralateral approaches.[28]

The main drawback of the contralateral approach is that it requires introducing instruments into the left hepatic parenchyma during catheterization of the portal venous branches supplying the FLR, which may injure the FLR parenchyma and/or the left portal vein.[3] If there are complications after PVE, these may involve the FLR and make the planned surgical resection more difficult or, in some cases, impossible.

Percutaneous Transhepatic Ipsilateral Approach

The percutaneous transhepatic ipsilateral approach was first described by Nagino and colleagues[30] and is now advocated by many other investigators.[31–34] With this approach, access is obtained through the portal branches within the tumor-bearing liver (see Fig. 102C.6B). A distinct advantage of the ipsilateral approach is that no instruments are introduced into the FLR. The ipsilateral approach also allows for straightforward catheterization of segment IV branches, should embolization of segment IV be required.

Puncture of the anterior segment of the right portal vein is preferred because use of this segment is associated with a lower complication rate[35]; however, catheterizing the right portal branches can be challenging owing to the sharp angles of the right portal veins (see Chapter 2), which often necessitate use of reverse-curve catheters or balloon occlusion catheters with multiple lumina.[30,36]

In Nagino's modification of the ipsilateral approach (see Fig. 102C.6C), the right anterior portal vein is punctured using sonographic guidance, and a 6-Fr sheath is introduced into the right portal venous system.[36] To make this procedure feasible, the authors designed two types of 5.5-Fr triple-lumen balloon catheters. The first type of catheter, "type 1," was designed with one lumen connected to the balloon and two lumina connected to the catheter tip. The second type of catheter, "type 2," had two separate lumina opening proximal to the balloon, and the balloon was used to prevent any backflow of embolic material. Both catheters had two separate lumina so that fibrin glue and iodized oil could be injected simultaneously. To facilitate resection and reduce the risk of left and/or main portal vein thrombosis, the authors advocated leaving patent a proximal right portal vein segment at least 1 cm long. Depending on the portal

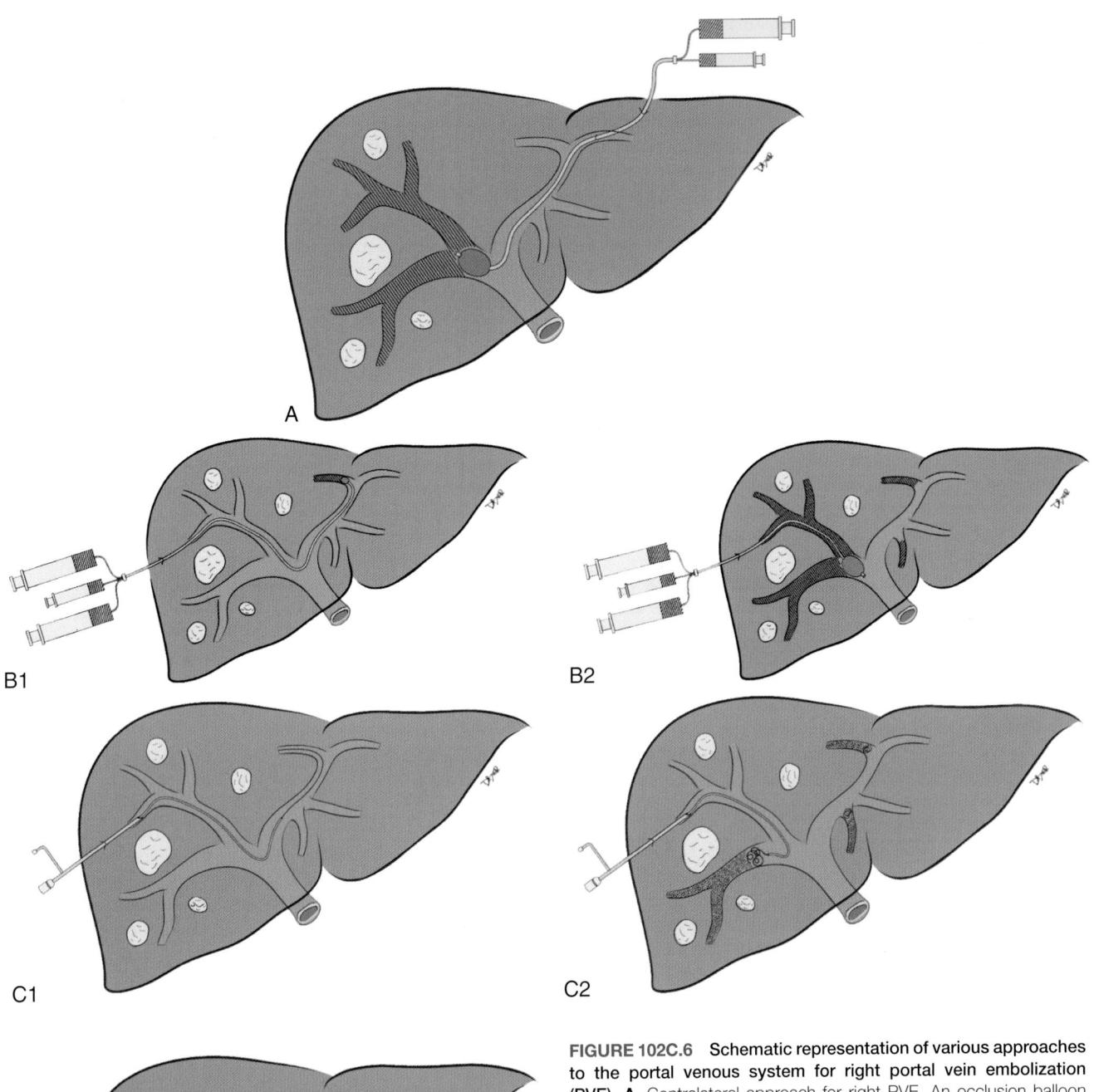

FIGURE 102C.6   Schematic representation of various approaches to the portal venous system for right portal vein embolization (PVE). **A,** Contralateral approach for right PVE. An occlusion balloon catheter is placed through the left lobe into the right portal branch, and the embolic agent is delivered in the antegrade direction. **B,** Ipsilateral approach for right PVE extended to segment IV as described by Nagino et al. Different balloon catheters are used for antegrade embolization of segment IV veins **(B1)** and for retrograde delivery of the embolic agent into the right portal venous system **(B2). C,** Modification of the ipsilateral approach for right PVE extended to segment IV. **C1,** A 6-Fr vascular sheath is placed in the right portal branch. An angled 5-Fr catheter is placed into the left portal system with coaxial placement of a microcatheter into a segment IV branch. Particulate embolization is performed followed by placement of coils until all the branches are occluded. **C2,** After segment IV is completely occluded, a 5-Fr reverse-curve catheter is used for right PVE. **C3,** After the right and segment IV portal veins are completely occluded, the access tract is embolized with coils to prevent subcapsular hemorrhage.

vein anatomy and whether the proximal right portal vein needed to be spared, type 1 or type 2 catheters were used for embolization. The type 1 catheter was used for embolization of branches distal to the catheter tip, whereas the type 2 catheter was used for embolization of branches proximal to the catheter tip, as mandated by each patient's portal vein anatomy. Unfortunately, these specialized balloon catheters were not available outside Japan.

In the early 2000s, Madoff and colleagues[31,32] described a technique using angiographic catheters commercially available worldwide. Under sonographic guidance, a 22-gauge Chiba needle (Neff Percutaneous Access Set; Cook Medical, Bloomington, IN) is used to puncture a distal branch of the right portal system. Subsequently, a 5-Fr or 6-Fr vascular sheath is advanced over a guidewire into the right portal vein branch to aid with subsequent catheter exchanges. Flush portography is performed with a 5-Fr angiographic flush catheter placed within the main portal vein just above the splenic vein–superior mesenteric confluence. Anteroposterior and craniocaudal projections are obtained as needed to delineate the portal anatomy.

When embolization of the right portal vein is extended to segment IV (Fig. 102C.7), segment IV embolization should be performed first.[32] This sequence is advocated because of the potential difficulty of exchanging catheters through a previously embolized right portal venous system and because embolic material could be dislodged from the right liver during subsequent treatment of segment IV, which is usually embolized with a 3-Fr microcatheter placed coaxially through a selective end-hole 5-Fr angiographic catheter. Early on, polyvinyl alcohol particles (Contour SE Microspheres; Boston Scientific, Natick, MA) were the embolic agent of choice.[31] Polyvinyl alcohol was administered in a stepwise fashion: first, smaller particles (355–500 µm) were used to occlude the distal branches; then larger particles (up to 1000 µm) were used to occlude more proximal branches. Larger particles were not used until the forward portal blood flow was considerably reduced. Additional embolization was then performed with the larger particles, until near-complete stasis was achieved. Later, with the introduction of spherical embolic agents, tris-acryl gelatin microspheres (EmboGold Microspheres; Biosphere Medical, Rockland, MA) became the embolic agent of choice.[32] Tris-acryl gelatin microspheres ranging from 100 to 700 µm in diameter are administered in a stepwise fashion, similar to the method used for administering polyvinyl alcohol particles. After particulate embolization is complete, platinum microcoils (Boston Scientific) are placed within the proximal segment IV branches to further reduce portal blood inflow that could lead to recanalization.

For right PVE, the working catheter is usually exchanged for a 5-Fr reverse-curve catheter (Sos-2, Simmons-1, AngioDynamics, Latham, NY) to enable safe delivery of the particulate embolic agent. Reverse-curve catheters are chosen for their ease of manipulation into the right portal branches, given the severe angles that must be navigated in the right portal tree with the ipsilateral approach. As with segment IV embolization, smaller particles are used first to occlude the distal, smaller portal branches, and larger particles are used later to occlude the more proximal, larger portal branches. After near-complete stasis is achieved, 0.035- or 0.038-inch embolization coils (Gianturco, Cook Medical) are placed within the secondary portal branches to further reduce portal inflow that could lead to recanalization. A final portogram is obtained with the flush catheter positioned within the main portal vein to assess the completeness of the embolization. At the end of the procedure, the access tract is embolized with coils and/or absorbable gelatin compressed sponge to minimize the risk of bleeding at the liver puncture site.

Optimal Extent of Embolization

The optimal extent of PVE is a subject of considerable debate.[37] Currently, at most centers where PVE is performed to prepare patients for extended right hepatectomy, only branches of the right portal vein are occluded, and the segment IV portal veins are left patent.[2,38] This approach does result in some FLR hypertrophy, but the maximal stimulus for FLR hypertrophy is derived from full diversion of the portal flow to segments II and III.[36,39–41] Although leaving the segment IV portal veins patent leads to hypertrophy of segment IV, this is undesirable for an extended right hepatectomy, because of the increased morbidity associated with a larger area of intraoperative parenchymal transection across this hypertrophic segment.[41]

Nagino and colleagues[36] were the first to show that left lateral bisegment hypertrophy is greater after right PVE extended to segment IV (50% increase in the FLR volume) than after right PVE alone (31% increase in the FLR volume, $P < .0005$). Recent studies have supported Nagino and colleagues' conclusions and shown that extending PVE to segment IV does not increase PVE-associated complications.[39,40,42,43] Because segment IV embolization has been shown to be advantageous, the ipsilateral approach for right PVE extended to segment IV has been further refined, which has led to improved FLR hypertrophy and better operative outcomes.

Another potential benefit of extending right PVE to include segment IV is that the entire tumor-bearing liver is systematically embolized (i.e., right PVE for right hepatectomy, right PVE extended to segment IV for extended right hepatectomy) to reduce the risk of tumor growth that may result from increased portal blood flow and delivery of hepatotrophic factors.[3,11,44] Investigators from a large academic cancer center recently evaluated 112 patients in whom the entire tumor-bearing liver was systematically embolized, and reported that they found no increase in the median tumor size during the waiting period.[11] In contrast, two small studies have reported potential tumor growth within the nonembolized liver after PVE.[45,46] In these series, however, the patients had not undergone arterial embolization or received preoperative chemotherapy before PVE. Therefore it could not be proven that the tumor growth accelerated because of PVE.

Sequential Arterial Embolization and Portal Vein Embolization

In 2004, Aoki and colleagues[47] described their experience with the use of sequential transcatheter arterial chemoembolization followed within 2 weeks by PVE in 17 patients with HCC (see Chapter 94A). The authors' justification for this approach was 3-fold. First, the livers of most patients with HCC are compromised by underlying liver disease such that the liver's regenerative capacity after hepatic resection is weakened, making it hard to predict whether adequate FLR hypertrophy can be achieved after PVE. Second, arterioportal shunts often found in cirrhotic livers and HCC may limit the effectiveness of PVE. Third, since most HCCs are hypervascular, supplied largely by arterial blood flow, termination of portal flow induces compensatory augmentation in arterial blood flow (i.e., "arterialization of the

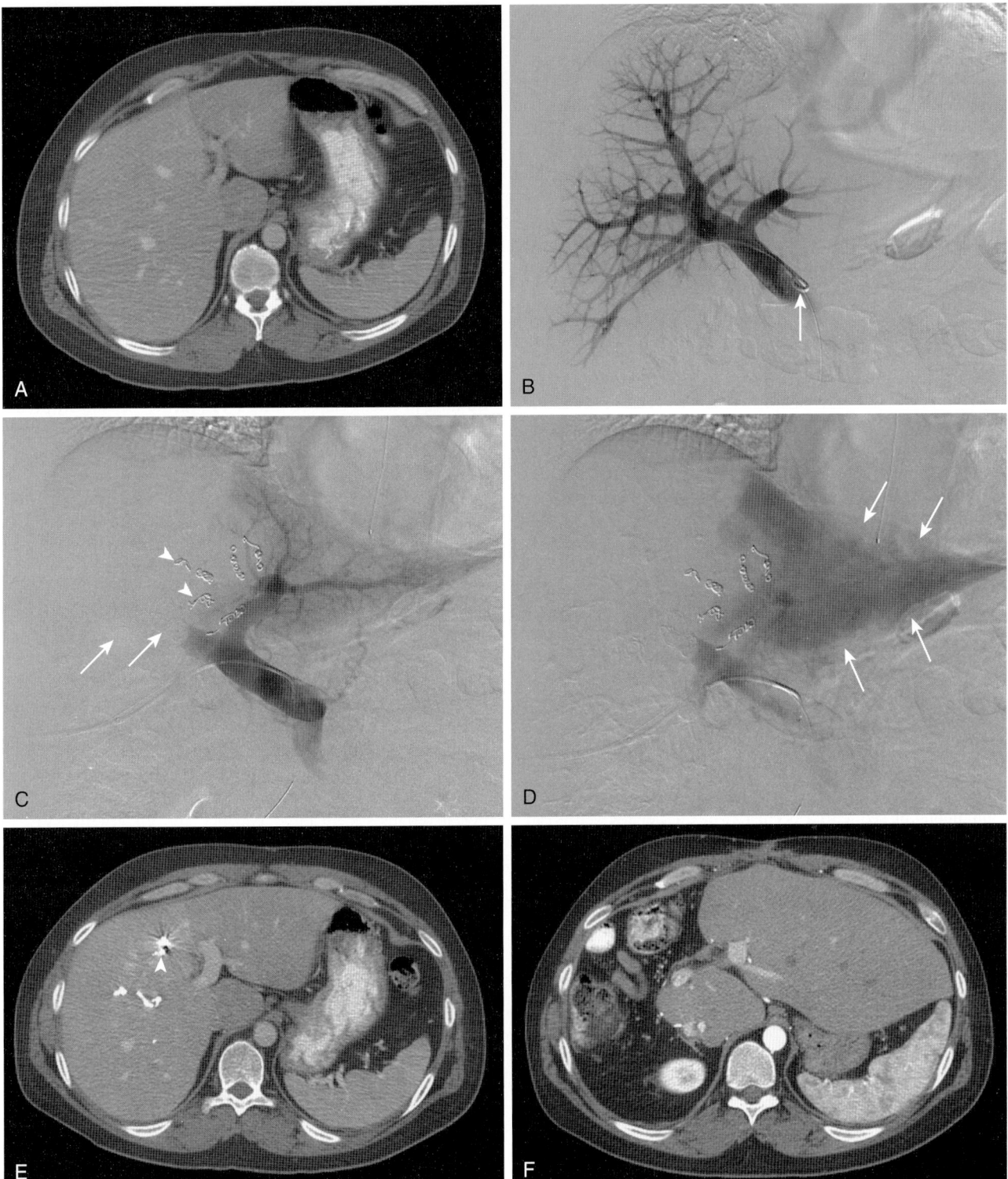

FIGURE 102C.7   A 38-year-old man with metastases in the liver from colorectal cancer underwent transhepatic ipsilateral right portal vein embolization with particles and coils extended to segment IV before extended right hepatectomy. **A,** Contrast-enhanced computed tomography (CT) scan of the liver shows a small left lateral liver (ratio of future liver remnant to estimated total liver volume [FLR/TEL], 16.9%; *shaded area*). **B,** Anterior–posterior flush portogram from the ipsilateral approach shows a 6-Fr vascular sheath in a right portal vein branch and a 5-Fr flush catheter *(arrow)* in the main portal vein. **C,** Postprocedure portogram shows complete occlusion, with particles and coils, of the portal vein branches to segment IV *(arrowheads)* and the right liver *(arrows)* with continued patency of the veins supplying the left lateral liver. **D,** A portogram obtained later confirms persistent flow to the left liver *(arrows)*. **E,** Contrast-enhanced CT scan performed 4 weeks after portal vein embolization shows hypertrophy of the left lateral liver (FLR/TEL is now 27.2% [degree of hypertrophy, 10.3%]) with rounded margins *(shaded area)*. A coil within segment IV *(arrowhead)* and coils within the right liver are seen. **F,** Contrast-enhanced CT scan of the liver performed after successful extended right hepatectomy shows hypertrophy of the liver remnant.

liver") in the embolized segments that may lead to rapid tumor progression after PVE.

Aoki and colleagues[47] used sequential chemoembolization and PVE to prevent tumor progression during the interval between PVE and planned hepatectomy and to improve the efficacy of PVE by chemoembolizing arterioportal shunts. The combined procedures were found to be safe and to induce sufficient FLR hypertrophy within 2 weeks, and they caused no worsening of the basal hepatic functional reserve and no increase in tumor progression. Importantly, when the explanted livers were assessed, tumor necrosis was profound, but there was no substantial injury to the noncancerous liver. Based on these findings, the authors encourage the aggressive use of sequential arterial chemoembolization and PVE in patients with large HCC and chronically injured livers.

More recently, a French group reported on the use of sequential chemoembolization and PVE in 36 patients with HCC and chronic liver disease before right hepatectomy.[48] In this study, 18 patients underwent chemoembolization followed by PVE 3 to 4 weeks later, and the remaining 18 patients underwent PVE alone. PVE was well tolerated in all patients, and the mean increase in FLR volume was significantly higher for patients in the combined chemoembolization and PVE group than in patients who underwent PVE alone ($P = .022$). Patients who underwent sequential chemoembolization and PVE also had a higher incidence of complete tumor necrosis (83% [15/18] vs. 6% [1/18]; $P < .001$) and a higher 5-year disease-free survival rate (37% vs. 19%; $P = .041$). Given the risk of hepatic infarction, the authors recommended that the two procedures be separated by at least 3 weeks to reduce procedure-related morbidity.

Liver Venous Deprivation: Simultaneous Hepatic Vein Embolization With Portal Vein Embolization

Another potential procedure to enhance hypertrophy of FLR is simultaneous or sequential occlusion of the hepatic vein(s) in addition to the portal vein (PVE+HVE).[49,50] Recently, Kobayashi et al.[51] reported their experiences of simultaneous hepatic vein embolization with PVE, termed "liver venous deprivation (LVD)." In this study, 21 patients underwent LVD leading to a superior degree of hypertrophy (DH) (8.5% vs. 5.6%) and kinetic growth rate (KGR) (2.0% vs. 1.4%) compared with 39 patients undergoing PVE alone without increased incidence of per procedural complications. Despite the faster rate of hypertrophy, whether HVE should be performed routinely or selectively after failure of PVE remains unclear. However, given the encouraging results reported by Kobayashi et al., LVD could be a potential choice of preoperative hemodynamic modulation, especially for patients presenting with very small FLR before planned extended hepatectomy.[52]

DEGREE AND SPEED OF HYPERTROPHY AND RISK OF POSTOPERATIVE HEPATIC INSUFFICIENCY

In a review of 358 patients reported by investigators at MD Anderson Cancer Center, PVE was completed successfully at the first session in 350 patients (97.8%), and the median FLR regeneration rate was 50.3% (interquartile range, 27.0%–77.8%) at a median of 32 days after PVE (range, 5–385 days).[53] Of the 358 patients in the series, 282 (78.8%) proceeded to surgery, and 76 (21.2%) were unable to undergo surgical

resection because of interim disease progression ($n = 44$, 12.3%), insufficient FLR regeneration ($n = 13$, 3.6%), or medical comorbidities ($n = 19$, 5.3%).

It has been widely accepted that post-PVE sFLR volume is a sensitive predictor of postoperative hepatic insufficiency. However, recent studies have confirmed that regeneration capacity and speed of regeneration also independently predict short-term surgical outcomes in patients undergoing PVE for small FLR. Ribero and colleagues[11] reported that DH in sFLR volume after PVE (DH defined as the change in sFLR volume from before to after PVE divided by the sFLR volume before PVE) was significantly associated with surgical outcomes. DH greater than 5% after PVE in combination with an sFLR volume greater than 20% predicted good postoperative outcomes with high specificity and sensitivity in patients with normal liver function (Fig. 102C.8). Our group recently found that the KGR, defined as DH at initial volume assessment divided by number of weeks elapsed after PVE, further sensitively predicts the risk of postoperative hepatic insufficiency. KGR greater than 2.0% per week is strongly associated with low risk of postoperative morbidity and mortality irrespective of the sFLR (Fig. 102C.9) or timing of initial CT evaluation after PVE (Fig. 102C.10).[12] These results were validated by Leung and colleagues,[54] who reported that both DH and KGR were strong predictors of postoperative hepatic insufficiency.

COMPLICATIONS OF PERCUTANEOUS PORTAL VEIN EMBOLIZATION

For PVE, as for all transhepatic procedures, potential complications include subcapsular hematoma, hemoperitoneum, hemobilia, arterioportal shunts, arteriovenous fistula, pseudoaneurysm, portal vein thrombosis, transient liver failure, pneumothorax, and sepsis.[29,35] Kodama and colleagues[35] compared complication rates between the contralateral and ipsilateral approaches to the portal venous system in 47 patients who underwent PVE. The overall rate of complications associated with percutaneous PVE using either approach was 14.9%. Complications occurred in 2 of 11 patients (18.1%) who underwent contralateral PVE and in 5 of 36 patients (13.9%) who underwent ipsilateral PVE. This difference was not statistically significant. The following complications were found in this patient cohort: two subcapsular hematomas, two pneumothoraces, one inadvertent arterial puncture, one pseudoaneurysm (in a patient who also had a subcapsular hematoma), one case of hemobilia, and one portal vein thrombosis. The authors stressed that given the potential for injury to the FLR with the contralateral approach, the ipsilateral approach should be tried first.

Di Stefano and colleagues[29] later reported on 188 patients who underwent PVE performed using the contralateral approach. These authors reported that only one patient experienced a major complication (complete portal vein thrombosis) directly related to the contralateral approach that precluded the planned surgical resection. Two other patients experienced inadvertent migration of embolic material into the FLR that required intervention; one needed a portoportal graft during hepatic resection because of portal vein thrombosis. On CT imaging, another 10 patients were found to have embolic material in nontargeted portal venous branches.

In 2012 our group reviewed 358 patients who underwent PVE at MD Anderson Cancer Center and reported that complications occurred in 14 patients (3.9%); complications

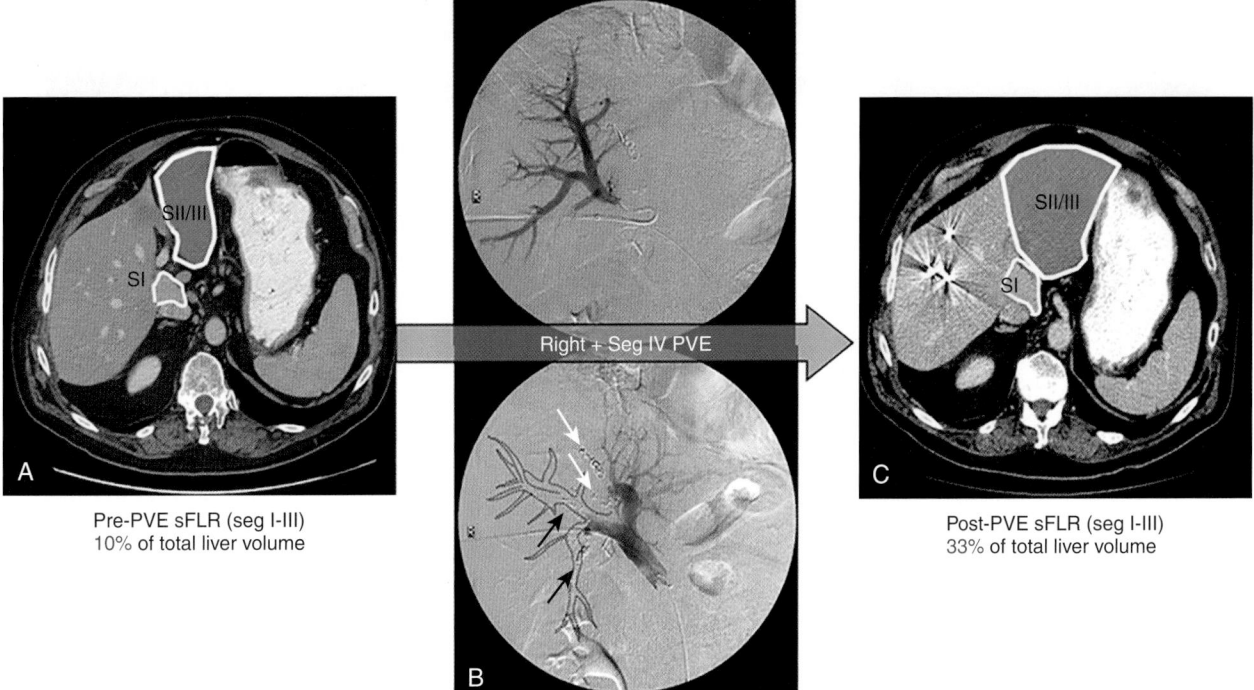

Pre-PVE sFLR (seg I-III)
10% of total liver volume

Right + Seg IV PVE

Post-PVE sFLR (seg I-III)
33% of total liver volume

FIGURE 102C.8 Representative images from contrast-enhanced computed tomography of the liver before **(A)** and after **(C)** right portal vein embolization (PVE) extended to segment IV resulting in increase of the sFLR from 10% to 33% (degree of hypertrophy, 23%). **B,** Portogram captured during PVE shows contrast in the right portal vein and its branches before PVE *(top image)* and contrast in the main and left portal veins except segment IV branches after PVE *(lower image)*. Coils in segment IV branches are marked with *white arrows,* and the embolized right portal vein is outlined with *dashed lines. Black arrows* indicate anterior and posterior branches of the right portal vein.

included portal vein thrombosis ($n = 8$, 2.2%), coil misplacement ($n = 3$, 0.8%), subcapsular hematoma ($n = 2$, 0.6%), and esophageal bleeding ($n = 1$, 0.3%).[53] The authors concluded that in an adequately selected population, PVE can be performed safely with minimal procedural complications.

CLINICAL OUTCOMES

Short-Term Surgical Outcomes

In the MD Anderson Cancer Center series, 62 of 240 patients (25.8%) developed major complications after major or extended hepatectomy after PVE, and 9 patients (3.8%) died of liver failure within 90 days. As compared with patients who did not die within 90 days after surgery, those who died of liver-related causes were older, more likely to be males, and more likely to have received preoperative chemotherapy and had a significantly smaller sFLR, significantly lower DH, and significantly lower KGR after PVE. Although the number of high-risk patients with livers exposed to preoperative systemic therapy has increased, the overall complication rates have decreased over time: the major complication rate was 27.7% in 1995 to 2000 versus 21.4% in 2010 to 2012, the hepatic insufficiency rate was 10.6% in 1995 to 2000 versus 2.9% in 2010 to 2012, and the 90-day liver-related mortality rate was 4.1% in 1995 to 2000 versus 2.9% in 2010 to 2012.

Recently, our group demonstrated that atrophy of the liver after extensive chemotherapy for colorectal liver cancer metastases (CRCLMs) is associated with a decrease of the hepatic functional reserve and may increase the risk of postoperative

morbidity.[55,56] This phenomenon seemed to be associated with an increased incidence of sinusoidal injury in the liver parenchyma after chemotherapy, and was significantly correlated with hepatic dysfunction in both the medical and surgical cohorts that had received chemotherapy for colorectal cancer. In such a high-risk group of patients, however, Omichi et al.[57] demonstrated that KGR 2.0% or greater achieved after PVE mitigates the deleterious effects of hepatic atrophy after extensive chemotherapy, reducing the risk of postoperative hepatic insufficiency to almost zero.

Long-Term Surgical Outcomes

Hepatocellular Carcinoma (see Chapter 89)

Information about the impact of preoperative PVE on the long-term prognosis of patients with HCC is rather scarce.[22,58–61] However, it has been shown that there is no difference between patients who required PVE and those who did not require PVE in either disease-free survival rates or overall survival rates. In an MD Anderson Cancer Center series, the postoperative mortality rate was 0% in patients who underwent liver resection after PVE and 18% among patients operated on up front. The 5-year survival rate was 72% in the PVE group and 54% in the non-PVE group, although the difference was not significant; there was no difference between groups in the 5-year disease-free survival rate.[58]

Biliary Tract Cancer (see Chapter 51)

Makuuchi et al.[4] reported encouraging short-term outcomes for patients with hilar cholangiocarcinoma in their initial study

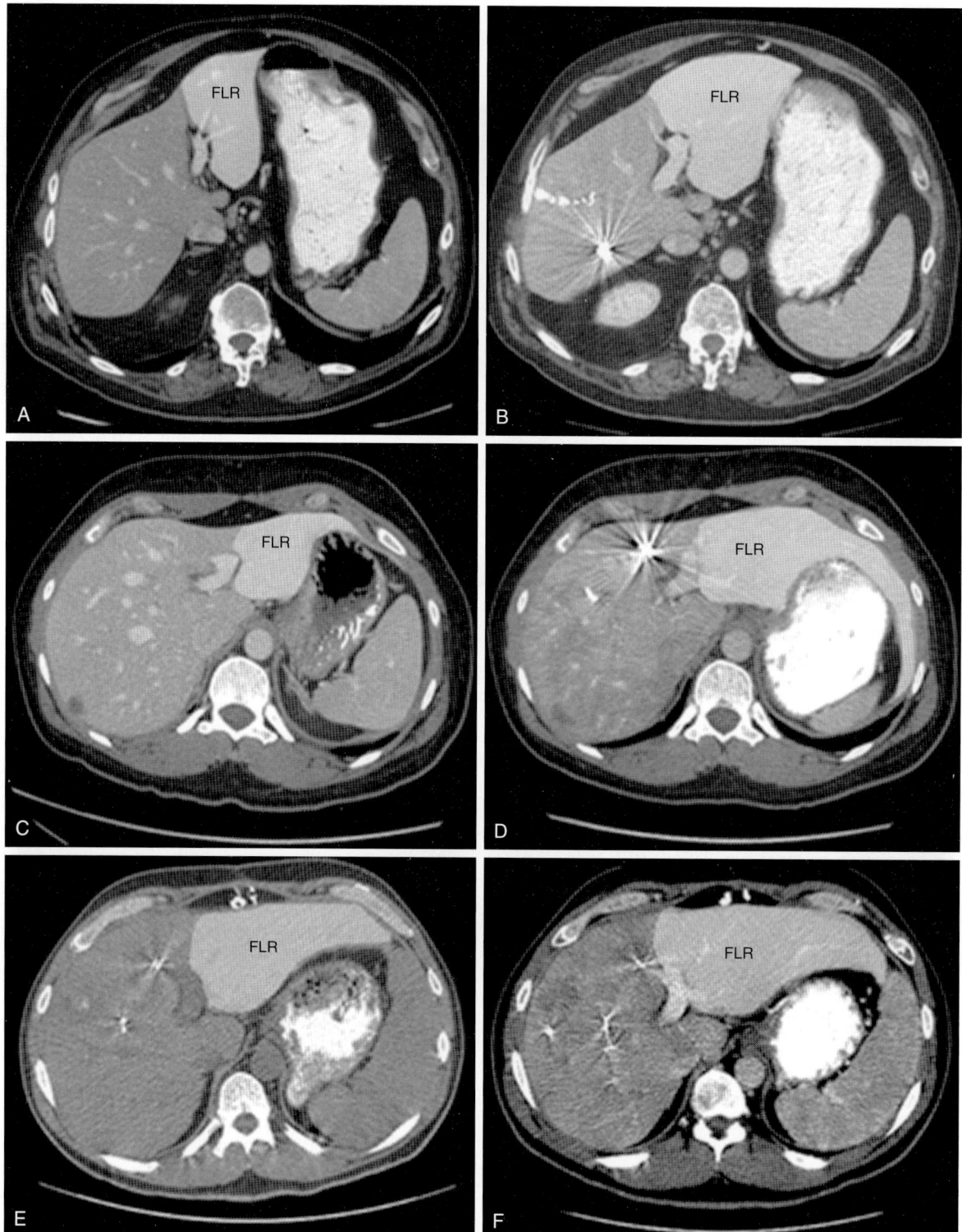

FIGURE 102C.9 Examples of the clinical utility of kinetic growth rate (KGR). All patients had standardized future liver remnant (s*FLR*) volume 30% or greater and degree of hypertrophy (DH) 7.5% or greater (suggested eligibility criteria for resection); however, KGR was a more accurate predictor of outcome. **A** and **B,** A 60-year-old man. **A,** On the basis of the initial computed tomography (CT) scan, sFLR was estimated at 9%. **B,** Final CT 35 days after right portal vein embolization (PVE) extended to segment IV indicated an sFLR of 33%, DH of 24%, and KGR of 4.8% per week. The patient had an uneventful postoperative course. **C** and **D,** A 37-year-old woman. **C,** On the basis of the initial CT scan, sFLR was estimated at 15%. **D,** Final CT 35 days after right PVE extended to segment IV indicated an sFLR of 30%, DH of 15%, and KGR of 3.0% per week. The patient had an uneventful postoperative course. **E** and **F,** A 43-year-old man. **E,** On the basis of the initial CT scan, sFLR was estimated at 23%. **F,** Final CT 70 days after right PVE extended to segment IV (additional waiting time was required to attain adequate remnant volume) indicated an sFLR of 31%, DH of 8%, and KGR of 0.3% per week (determined after first CT 28 days after PVE). The patient died of postoperative liver failure. (From Shindoh J, Truty MJ, Aloia TA, et al. Kinetic growth rate after portal vein embolization predicts posthepatectomy outcomes: toward zero liver-related mortality in patients with colorectal liver metastases and small future liver remnant. *J Am Coll Surg.* 2012;216:201–209 with permission.)

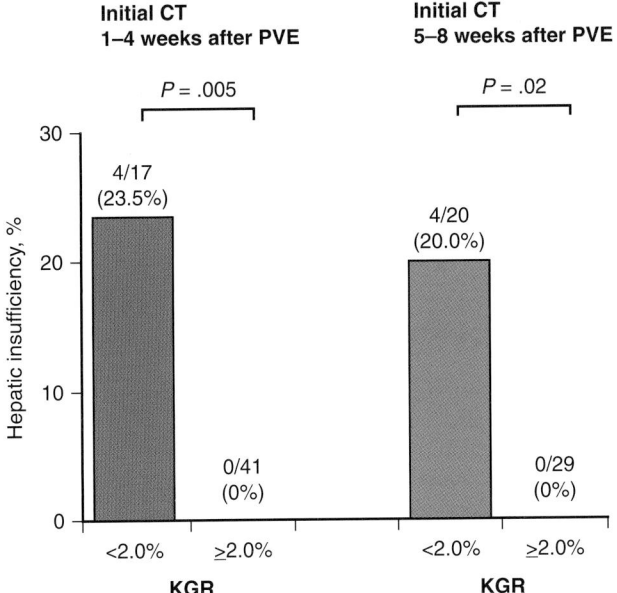

FIGURE 102C.10 Kinetic growth rate and risk of postoperative hepatic insufficiency. Timing of initial volumetric evaluation does not influence the predictive value of kinetic growth rate *(KGR)* for hepatic insufficiency when measured within 8 weeks after portal vein embolization. *CT*, Computed tomography; *PVE*, portal vein embolization.

on PVE. Since then, PVE has been widely used in patients requiring extended hepatectomy for biliary tract cancers. In a series of 494 patients who underwent PVE before planned extended hepatectomy for biliary tract cancers,[62] Ebata and colleagues[62] reported that 372 patients (75.3%) underwent successful surgical resection after PVE and 24 of these patients (6.5%) died of postoperative complications. The 5-year overall survival rate was significantly better for patients with cholangiocarcinoma (39%) than for patients with gallbladder cancer (23%).

Colorectal Liver Metastases (see Chapter 90)

Wicherts and colleagues[63] analyzed 364 patients who underwent a major hepatectomy for CRCLMs and found that PVE increased resectability and that patients who were able to undergo resection after PVE had significantly higher 3-year and 5-year survival rates (44% and 21%, respectively) than those whose disease remained unresectable. Similarly, our group has recently reported that among 139 patients who required PVE before extended right hepatectomy for CRCLMs 87 patients (62.6%) were able to proceed to surgery, and these patients had

long-term outcomes similar to those of 123 patients who did not require PVE before surgery. The 5-year overall survival rates for patients requiring and not requiring PVE were 42% and 38%, respectively ($P = .45$), and the 5-year disease-free survival rates were 19% and 22%, respectively ($P = .45$).[64]

Outcomes in Patients With a Very Small Future Liver Remnant

A landmark study reported in 2009 showed that PVE can allow patients with an initial sFLR 20% or less to experience a postoperative course similar to that of patients with a larger initial sFLR volume and that the true sFLR cutoff value for safe surgery in a normal liver is 20%.[39] In a recent study on outcomes of right PVE plus segment IV embolization in 144 consecutive patients with liver tumors with very small liver remnant volumes (ratio of liver remnant to body weight less than 0.5%), percutaneous PVE was successfully performed in 141 patients (97.9%), and adequate regeneration was obtained in 139 of these patients (98.6%); the median ratio of liver remnant to body weight was 0.33% before PVE and 0.52% after PVE ($P < .0001$), representing a per-patient median regeneration of 62% at a median of 34 days after PVE. Of the 144 patients in the series, 104 (72.2%) underwent curative resection and 40 (27.8%) were not able to undergo resection because of short-interval disease progression ($n = 27$, 18.8%), insufficient liver regeneration ($n = 5$, 3.5%), or medical comorbidities ($n = 8$, 5.6%). Rates of major morbidity, hepatic insufficiency, and 90-day liver-related mortality were 33.0%, 12.5%, and 5.8%, respectively.[42] In this report, PVE plus segment IV embolization compared favorably to the ALPPS procedure (associating liver partition with portal vein ligation for staged hepatectomy), which was associated with worse morbidity (40%) and mortality (12%).[65] Therefore, because of its ability to select patients with a resectable liver and its superior safety and efficacy profiles, right PVE plus segment IV embolization and interval surgery should remain the standard of care for patients with a very small FLR.[66]

CONCLUSION

PVE is a safe and effective technique to reduce the risk of extensive hepatectomy. Currently, the ipsilateral percutaneous transhepatic approach is the most used procedure, and sufficient regeneration of the FLR can be expected with minimal procedural complications in an adequately selected population. Operators must pay particular attention to the technical aspects of PVE, aberrant portal venous anatomy, and treatment strategies to ensure the best outcomes of PVE for patients.

References are available at expertconsult.com.

CHAPTER 123

Associating liver partition and portal vein ligation for staged hepatectomy: Indications and outcomes

Karl J. Oldhafer and Thomas M. Van Gulik

The associating liver partition and portal vein (PV) ligation for staged hepatectomy (ALPPS) procedure is a modification of the two-staged liver resection combining two established surgical techniques: right portal vein ligation (PVL) and in situ splitting of the liver (ISS).[1,2] The first large series introducing this novel technique of two-stage hepatectomy was published as a multicenter experience of German surgeons.[3] Dr. Hans Schlitt initiated the concept of ALPPS in 2007 when he explored a patient with hilar cholangiocarcinoma resectable by right trisectionectomy.[4] However, because of the patient's long-standing cholestatic condition and small size of the future liver remnant (FLR), Schlitt abandoned the resection and instead performed a hepaticojejunostomy for drainage of the FLR after dividing the liver and ligating the right PV. Computed tomography (CT) scan on postoperative day 9 revealed a dramatic hypertrophy of the FLR of about 90% that was not previously observed. Schlitt and his group called this procedure "right portal vein ligation with in situ splitting."[4] Later the acronym ALPPS was introduced and is now accepted worldwide.[5]

The ALPPS concept was received favorably by the surgical community and rapidly adopted by some groups.[6-9] Further experience confirmed that the volume increase after ALPPS was more rapid compared with PVL or portal vein embolization (PVE; see Chapter 102D) in the regular setting of two-stage resection, allowing resection of the diseased part of the liver within 1 to 2 weeks after the first stage. The rate of complete tumor resection has been shown to be higher after ALPPS than after two-stage hepatectomies, including PVE and PVL.[10] At the same time, however, the high postoperative morbidity and mortality rates reported for ALPPS raised concerns and sparked a controversy over the benefits and risks of the ALPPS procedure.[11,12] In recent years, improved patient selection, increased experience, and modifications in operative techniques (e.g., partial ALPPS) have resulted in significant improvements in morbidity and mortality. However, definitive evidence for a long-term benefit in survival after ALPPS is still lacking. In this chapter, we describe the ALPPS procedure in regard to indications, surgical management, and results.

INDICATIONS

The ALPPS technique has been used for almost all liver tumors[13] with the same indications used for two-stage liver resection or PVL/PVE. The main indication to date is bilateral colorectal cancer liver metastases (CRCLMs; see Chapters 98 and 102C); in fact, most cases of ALPPS have been performed for this indication.[14,15] Currently, CRCLM is the most promising indication, especially for bilobar metastases.[16,17] In a recent study dealing with patients from the international ALPPS registry, it has been shown that more than 15% of ALPPS procedures were done in patients who may have had no indication for

a two-stage hepatectomy.[18] Thus a tendency for potential overuse of ALPPS was observed. Hepatocellular carcinoma (HCC; see Chapter 89) typically arising in the cirrhotic liver (see Chapter 120) also has been resected by ALPPS.[19,20] Data from Asia are convincing but probably not reproducible elsewhere; thus these data must be interpreted with caution.

ALPPS for perihilar (PHC) and intrahepatic (IHC) cholangiocarcinoma is vigorously discussed in the surgical community, with no final agreement and a tendency to be very cautious in these indications[21] (see Chapters 51 and 119B). The reason for caution is the reported high mortality.[13,22] However, in some selected cases of cholangiocarcinoma, ALPPS may be the only operative option; it is important to remember that the first successful case was performed in a patient with PHC. If ALPPS is used in PHC, preoperative biliary drainage is advised.

The ALPPS procedure may be considered in any patient needing major liver resection in whom the FLR is deemed to be insufficient during preoperative workup (see Chapters 101, 102B, 102C, and 119B). When an extreme volume gain is needed, ALPPS could have an advantage over the other methods. Otherwise, when only minimal hypertrophy is necessary, PVE is the better approach in view of its lower morbidity and mortality rates. In case of tumor load in the FLR, ALPPS or classic two-stage hepatectomy is more appropriate than PVE because the FLR can be cleared of tumor during the first stage.[10] Additionally, ALPPS should be considered in every patient in whom PVE or the classic two-stage approach is not feasible or has failed ("rescue ALPPS").[23,24] Because of the higher morbidity and mortality rates, some authors advise primarily to attempt PVE and then proceed with ALPPS only when the hypertrophy response of the FLR has proved insufficient.[25]

The combination of ALPPS with additional procedures, such as resection of the colorectal primary tumor, has been performed and represents a potential indication, although caution is advised in view of the increased surgical risk.[26] Extrahepatic metastases, severe portal hypertension, high anesthesiologic risk, and medical contraindications to major hepatectomy constitute clear contraindications to performing this procedure, similar to other complex surgical procedures.

ASSESSMENT OF FUTURE LIVER REMNANT

Assessment of FLR volume is a key determinant in planning for ALPPS; it must be performed before surgery and reevaluated before the second stage. The most widely used method is CT volumetry using thin sections (1–2 mm), preferably carried out by a radiologist together with a liver surgeon. Three-dimensional (3D) reconstructions are used to calculate the nontumorous liver volume, tumor volume, and FLR volume (see Chapters 102A, 102B, and 102C). The limits for safe hepatic resections are usually considered from 20% to 40%,

TABLE 102D.1 Degree of Hypertrophy After Stage 1 of ALPPS Procedure

SERIES	NO. PATIENTS	INTERVAL STAGE (MEAN DAYS)	DEGREE OF HYPERTROPHY (%)
Schnitzbauer et al., 2012[3]	25	9	74
Knoefel et al., 2013[33]	7	6	63
Li et al., 2013[34]	9	13	87.2
Nadalin et al., 2014[13]	15	10	87.2
Torres et al., 2013[9]	39	14.1	83
Robles Campos et al., 2014[35]	22[a]	7	61
Alvarez et al., 2015[36]	30	6	89.7
Hernandez-Alejandro et al., 2015[37]	14	8	93
Wanis et al., 2017[38]	58	8 (median)	91
Serenari et al., 2018[39]	26	10 (median)	99

[a]Associating liver tourniquet and portal ligation for staged hepatectomy (ALTPS).

ALPPS, Associating liver partition and portal vein ligation for staged hepatectomy.

depending on the quality of liver parenchyma (fibrosis, steatosis, chemotherapy-related liver injury). On the practical level, the lower limit for FLR volume is set at 20% in patients with a normal liver, 30% to 35% in patients with chemotherapy-related liver injury, and 40% in patients with chronic liver disease.[27–29] Alternatively, the more personalized standardized FLR (sFLR) volume or the ratio of FLR volume measured by CT volumetry and body weight ratio (BWR) are used.[30–32] Cutoff values for proceeding to stage 2, usually after 7 to 14 days, are sFLR greater than 30% (BWR >0.5%) or 40% (BWR >0.8%) depending on parenchymal quality. Table 102D.1 summarizes degree of hypertrophy of FLR reported after stage 1.[33–39] Especially in patients with hepatic comorbidities, CT volumetry may be unreliable as a predictor of function of the FLR. CT can then be complemented with an additional, quantitative liver function test such as hepatobiliary scintigraphy using technetium-99m mebrofenin.[22,40–45] This functional test has been used as a predictor of insufficient functional hypertrophy after PVE, identifying patients who are potential candidates for upfront ALPPS.

SURGICAL TECHNIQUE

Anatomic Aspects

Most postoperative vascular and biliary complications of the ALPPS procedure can be attributed to either technical problems or failure to recognize anatomic variations. Knowledge of surgical anatomy and the implications of anatomic abnormalities is essential (see Chapter 2). High-quality imaging before stage 1 therefore is crucial to map out the hepatic and biliary anatomy. Because most frequently an extended right hepatectomy will be performed, the anatomic variations of the PV are relevant, such as PV trifurcation with separate entries of the right anterior and posterior sectional branches, as reported in 15% to 26% of studied populations.[46] When an anterior sectional PV originating from the left PV is missed during surgery, deportalization of the right liver lobe will be incomplete,

resulting in reduced hypertrophy of the FLR. This variation is especially important in partial ALPPS. Intraoperative ultrasound at the end of stage 1 can help avoid this technical failure. An undivided PV at the hilum is rare but represents an absolute anatomic contraindication to ALPPS.

Postoperative bile leakage is largely responsible for the high morbidity after ALPPS. The source of the leak is often found to be from the segment IV bile ducts. According to the Smadja and Blumgart classification,[47] there should be no increased risk of biliary problems in type A (normal anatomy) or type B (trifurcation) bile duct variations when a right trisegmentectomy is planned. Type C (aberrant drainage of the right anterior or right posterior sectoral hepatic ducts into the common hepatic duct) and type D (aberrant drainage of right anterior or right posterior sectoral hepatic duct into the left hepatic duct) variations have a potential higher risk of developing biliary complications after stage 1. Type E (absence of hepatic duct confluence) variation carries a greater risk of damage to the left bile duct during stage 2[47] (see Chapter 2). Regarding biliary complications in general, it is worth mentioning that dissection at the hilum should be minimized to preserve the arterial vascular plexus, which supplies blood to the bile duct system. Intraoperative cholangiography during stage 1 has the potential to define the biliary anatomy at the liver hilum and to identify anomalies. This is helpful to minimize the incidence of postoperative biliary complications.

Anomalies of the arterial system are also common and influence the outcome, especially the arterial supply of segment IV (see Chapter 2). Segment IV normally obtains its arterial supply from the left hepatic artery, so there is a risk of dividing the segment IV artery during partition when a right trisegmentectomy is planned. In these cases, loss of the segment IV artery at stage 1 carries a high risk of necrosis of segment IV. For this reason, it is advantageous when the segment IV artery is coming from the right hepatic artery; this is a common variant. In case of preservation of segment IV, the artery to segment IV should be preserved. Concerning hepatic venous drainage, multiple patterns of the ramifications of hepatic veins exist. In ALPPS the middle hepatic vein (MHV) is of special interest because it receives tributaries from segment IV on the left and from segments V and VIII on the right. The MHV should not be transected during stage 1 (unless it is infiltrated by tumor), in order to maintain optimal venous outflow of the FLR and the deportalized lobe.

Surgical Aspects

The ALPPS procedure typically consists of two stages. In stage 1, the tumor-bearing lobe of the liver is deportalized, while preserving ipsilateral arterial perfusion, and parenchymal transection is undertaken. At the same time, the FLR is cleared of tumor in case of bilateral involvement. In stage 2, the hepatic artery and the bile ducts of the deportalized part of the liver are taken down along with the corresponding hepatic veins, this allows the specimen to be removed. Different types of ALPPS have been reported (Table 102D.2).[23,33–35,48–54] Partial ALPPS represents one of the more recent modifications of the technique. It has been shown that transection of only 50% of liver parenchyma resulted in similar effects on hypertrophy but with a significant reduction in perioperative morbidity.[55] A classic complete transection down to the inferior vena cava seems to be necessary only in patients with a risk of tumor progression into the FLR during the interstage period.

TABLE 102D.2 Different Types of ALPPS Procedures

TYPE (STUDY)	PORTAL VEIN	LIVER PARENCHYMA	COMMENTS
ALPPS	Ligation	Complete transection	Classic technique
Partial (p-) Partial ALPPS[50]	Ligation	Incomplete transection (>50% of transection surface)	Reduction of morbidity
ALTPS[a,35]	Ligation	Partial transection and occlusion by tourniquet	Reduction of morbidity
RALPP[b,51]	Ligation	Complete, radiofrequency-induced necrosis	Reduction of morbidity
Hybrid ALPPS[52]	Portal vein embolization	Complete, surgical	Helpful when right portal vein is compromised by the tumor
Mini ALPPS[53]	Intraoperative portal vein embolization	Partial parenchymal transection	Reduction of morbidity
Partial TIPE[c] ALPPS[54]	Transileocolic portal vein embolization	Partial parenchymal transection	Reduction of morbidity

[a]Associating liver tourniquet and portal ligation for staged hepatectomy.

[b]Radiofrequency-assisted liver partition with portal vein ligation.

[c]Transileocecal portal vein embolization.

Open surgical technique is the most largely adopted approach, although other laparoscopic variants have been reported very early after introduction of ALPPS.[56–58] In a large series on laparoscopic stage 1 in ALPPS, a stage 2 completion rate similar to the open approach has been reported, with no complications of CD 3a or greater (Clavien-Dindo classification), no mortality, and a significantly shorter hospital stay compared with that with open ALPPS.[59] Complete robotic ALPPS also has been performed.[60,61] The standard ALPPS procedure for a right trisegmentectomy is described in the following section.

Stage 1

First, the parenchyma is assessed macroscopically; when necessary, a biopsy is taken from the nontumorous liver. The right liver is mobilized by dissecting all ligaments. Retroperitoneal adhesions are dissected and the vena cava exposed.[62,63] Resectability is confirmed using intraoperative ultrasound.

Lymphadenectomy of the hepatic pedicle is advised both for oncologic/staging reasons and for better identification of the hilar structures. The right PV branch is either divided and sewn over or divided using a vascular stapler. During parenchymal dissection, all portal and biliary segment IV branches are divided and closed. Supplying or draining structures to segment I are divided only when resection of the caudate lobe is necessary. Subsequently, total or, preferably, partial parenchymal dissection is performed using the anterior approach (Fig. 102D.1) possibly with "hanging liver" maneuver, using an ultrasound dissector or LigaSure and bipolar coagulation.[64] Biliary and arterial structures and venous drainage of the right liver segments to be resected are left intact. Finally, the right hepatic artery and the right bile ducts are tagged with vessel loops to facilitate their identification during stage 2 (Fig. 102D.2).[8,65] To detect biliary leaks, a "white test" may be performed with a T-tube in the common bile duct (CBD) or a catheter in the cystic duct. After liver partition, the resection plane can be covered by a piece of plastic bag or with a hemostatic patch to prevent adhesions between the planes.[66] The main disadvantage of using a plastic bag or sheet during stage 1 is that if stage 2 cannot be performed for any reason, the patient will still require a reoperation to remove the foreign body. The question of whether the MHV should be divided during stage 1 is under debate. In the original paper by Schnitzbauer and colleagues,[3] the MHV was divided in only 3 of 25 patients. The disadvantage

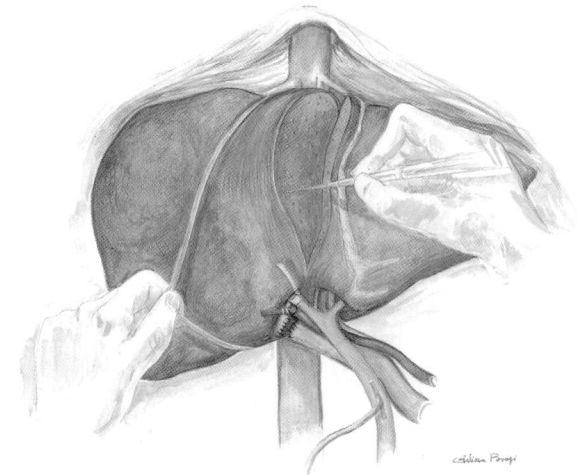

FIGURE 102D.1 Stage 1 of associating liver partition and portal vein ligation for staged hepatectomy. Ligation and transection of right portal vein, together with liver parenchyma transection through an anterior approach (hanging maneuver). Identification tags are used in the form of colored loops; T-tube is inserted. (Illustration by Mrs. Giuliana Brogi.)

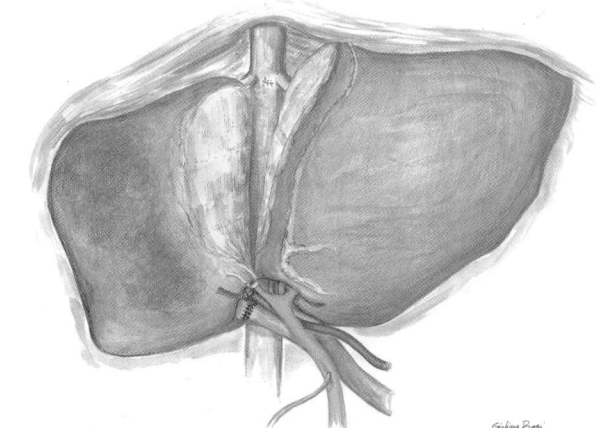

FIGURE 102D.2 Results After stage 1 of associating liver partition and portal vein ligation for staged hepatectomy. Volumetric reduction of deportalized right liver, with hypertrophy enhancement of future liver remnant. The deportalized liver is working as an auxiliary liver. Fibrin sponge on cut liver surfaces avoids bleeding and is a good alternative to plastic sheet/bag. (Illustration by Mrs. Giuliana Brogi.)

of cutting the MHV during stage 1 is insufficient venous drainage and congestion of the FLR. With partial ALPPS, the MHV is preserved. Tumor excisions in the left lateral segments during stage 1 may be necessary to render the FLR tumor free. Finally, at least one drain is placed near the resection surface.

Interval Phase

One week after the operation, an abdominal CT scan is performed, and the FLR volume, total liver volume (TLV), and volume gain are calculated. Cutoff values for proceeding to stage 2 are sFLR greater than 30% (BWR >0.5%) or 40% (BWR >0.8%) depending on parenchymal quality. The usual waiting time between stage 1 and 2 is 7 to 14 days.

Stage 2

Excision of the deportalized lobe is performed during stage 2, completing the extended hemihepatectomy. Because local anatomy may be modified as a result of FLR hypertrophy with displacement of the hepatic pedicle, caution is advised with dissection during stage 2.

The right hepatic artery and right bile ducts are ligated and cut. The right (and possibly the middle) hepatic vein is divided near its junction with the vena cava (Fig 102D.3). Remaining parenchymal bridges of liver parenchyma are divided if present. Intraoperative cholangiography may be performed to check for biliary continuity. This strategy is feasible not only for extended right hemihepatectomy but also for a left hemihepatectomy or for a central ALPPS (Fig. 102D.4).

Pathophysiologic Aspects

Although liver regeneration has been an area of research for several decades, the mechanism by which the superior hypertrophy response is achieved in ALPPS is largely unknown, because the atrophy–hypertrophy complex after unilateral PV occlusion is poorly understood[67–70] (see Chapters 5 and 6). First, the in situ split in ALPPS adds to deportalization of the ipsilateral lobe by cutting off any portal collateral communications that may reperfuse the ipsilateral lobe and render portal

venous occlusion less efficient.[71,72] Second, the surgical trauma of parenchymal transection results in the release of cytokines that enhance the process of liver regeneration.[73] However, although the deportalized liver lobe is deprived of portal blood, compensatory hyperperfusion by the ipsilateral hepatic artery occurs; this maintains oxygen supply and function of the deportalized liver. While hypertrophy of the FLR develops, the sustained metabolic function prevents the patient from contracting liver failure until the FLR has gained sufficient volume and stage 2 of ALPPS can be carried out. It has been shown that neoadjuvant chemotherapy had no negative effect on growth of FLR.[74] Several animal models of ALPPS that will help clarify these issues have been developed.[75–77]

RESULTS

In the beginning, one of the most discussed and controversial aspects of ALPPS was the reported high morbidity and mortality rates. The most frequent complications of ALPPS are still posthepatectomy liver failure, biliary fistulae, infected collections, and sepsis. In the first report on ALPPS, Schnitzbauer and colleague[3] described, according to the Clavien-Dindo classification, 50 complications in 16 patients and in-hospital mortality in 3 of 25 patients. These data triggered an intensive debate about the safety of the procedure.[78] Although several subsequent reports confirmed the high morbidity and mortality, others reported better outcomes with acceptable mortality rates in single-center studies.[36,37] Table 102D.3 summarizes the data from series with more than 12 cases. Increased experience and a number of technical details might have contributed to improved results: accurate 3D volumetric calculation, application of partial ALPPS, use of colored plastic loops during stage 1, intraoperative cholangiography, white test to detect biliary leaks at the end of stage 1, and maintenance of the MHV whenever possible.[*]

In the first report of the International ALPPS Registry, which included about 202 patients, the perioperative 90-day mortality was 9%.[79] Severe complications, including mortality (CD grade >IIIa), were 28%. Red blood cell transfusion, duration of stage I surgery greater than 300 minutes, and age greater than 60 years were identified as significant risk factors. Based on a growing experience with complications after ALPPS, many recommendations were made to reduce the surgical morbidity and mortality.[83] In a recent study from the ALPPS registry a continuous drop in early mortality (from 9% to 4%) and complication (above CD3b) rate (25%) after stage 2 was described in centers performing more that 10 ALPPS procedures in 33 years.[55] The indication for ALPPS is also an important factor.[84] Patients undergoing ALPPS because of primary liver cancer have more severe complications than patients with CRLM.[13]

Although the primary objective of ALPPS is to avoid liver failure after hepatectomy in patients with small FLR, postoperative liver insufficiency is the leading cause of death and severe complications after ALPPS (see Chapter 28). Posthepatectomy liver failure occurs even when the volume of the FLR is considered sufficient.[22] Thus the rapid gain in liver volume does not directly correlate with the increase in liver function in all cases; regional liver function tests are needed. The ALPPS

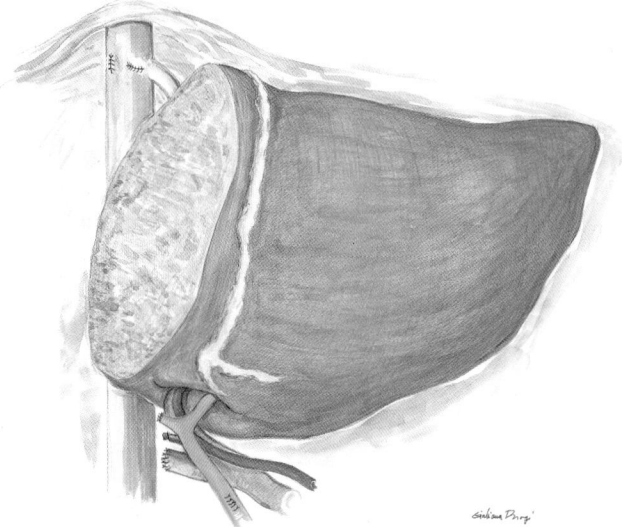

FIGURE 102D.3 Final results after stage 2 of associating liver partition and portal vein ligation for staged hepatectomy. Deportalized liver is removed, and future liver remnant is able to replace the complete liver function. (Illustration by Mrs. Giuliana Brogi.)

---

*References 35, 44, 55, 66, 65, 79–82.

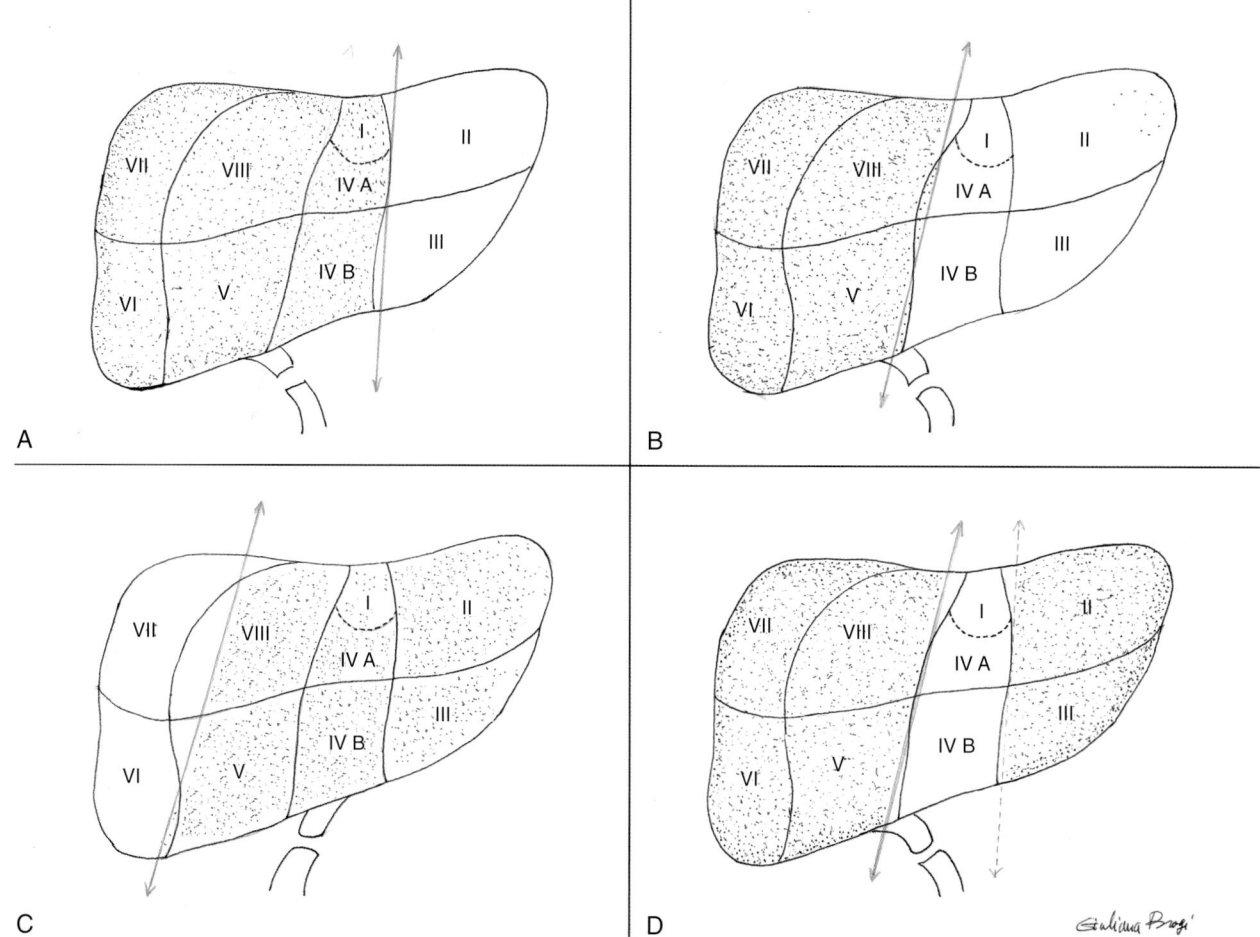

FIGURE 102D.4 Schematic representation of four technical variants of associating liver partition and portal vein ligation for staged hepatectomy (ALPPS). **A,** Original strategy of right trisectionectomy. The future liver remnant (FLR) is represented by segments II, III, and I. The right portal vein is ligated and the split is right of the falciform ligament. **B,** Standard right ALPPS. The FLR is represented by segments I, II, III, and IV. The right portal vein is ligated, and the split is along Cantlie's line. **C,** Left ALPPS. Segments VI, VII, and I represent the FLR after left trisectionectomy. The left portal vein is ligated, and the split is left of the border of segments VI/VII. **D,** Central ALPPS. The FLR is represented by segments IV and I. During the first stage, a left lateral bisegmentectomy combined with right portal vein ligation is performed. The split is along Cantlie's line. During the second stage, a right hemihepatectomy is performed. (Illustration by Mrs. Giuliana Brogi.)

TABLE 102D.3 Morbidity and Mortality After ALPPS[a]

SERIES	NO. PATIENTS	30-DAY MORTALITY (%)	90-DAY MORTALITY (%)	MORBIDITY AFTER STAGE 1(%)[b]	MORBIDITY AFTER STAGE 2 (%)[b]
Schnitzbauer et al., 2012[3]	25	0	12	44[c]	
Torres et al., 2013[9]	39	12.8[c]		59[c]	
Schadde et al., 2014[79]	202	2	9	40[c]	
Hernandez-Alejandro et al., 2015[37]	14	0	0	0	21
Alvarez et al., 2015[36]	30	0	6.6	30	33.3
Truant et al., 2015[32]	62	12.9[c]		22.6	32.2
Björnsson et al., 2016[80]	23	0	4		39[c]
Olthof et al., 2017[81]	70		7.5	11.1	28.5
Wanis et al., 2017[38]	58		0[d]		37[c]
Serenari et al., 2018[39]	26	0	0	23.1%	19.2%

[a]Published series (n ≥12).

[b]Clavien-Dindo classification grade ≥IIIA.

[c]No differentiation between stage 1 and stage 2.

[d]In-hospital mortality.

ALPPS, Associating liver partition and portal vein ligation for staged hepatectomy.

TABLE 102D.4   Long-Term Outcomes After ALPPS for Colorectal Cancer Liver Metastases

YEAR	SERIES	CRCLM	MEDIAN FOLLOW-UP	RECURRENCES (%)	OVERALL SURVIVAL			
					1-YEAR (%)	2-YEAR (%)	3-YEAR (%)	5-YEAR (%)
2014	Schadde et al., 2014[79]	141	NS	NS	76	63		
2015	Alvarez et al., 2015[36]	19	NS	NS	82			
2015	Ratti et al., 2015[17]	12	12	NS	92			
2016	Björnsson et al., 2016[80]	23	22.5[a]	18 (82)	83	59		
2017	Olthof et al., 2017[85]	70				62		
2017	Wanis et al., 2017[38]	58	35	37 (79)	93	66	50	
2018	Serenari et al., 2018[39]	26	21.5	20 (76.9)	83.4		48.9	
2019	Linecker et al., 2019[86]	213	NS	NS	84	66	54	34

[a]Median follow up after stage 2

ALPPS, Associating liver partition and portal vein ligation for staged hepatectomy; *CRCLM,* colorectal cancer liver metastasis; *NS,* not specified.

Registry also found that the vast majority of lethal outcomes occur after stage 2; thus patient selection after stage 1 and timing of stage 2 seem to be crucial. Patients can undergo stage 2 when they are in adequate clinical condition, when they do not have a relevant surgical complication, and when the liver function tests are at least near normal.[32] This means that stage 2 should not always be performed in the first 2 weeks, although the risks of increasing the interval between the two stages are related to a more difficult stage 2. In general, posthepatectomy liver failure remains the most severe complication after major liver surgery and ALPPS.

Since ALPPS is a novel technique and has been employed for many different indications, long-term results are still needed. CRCLM represents the main indication today for ALPPS.[14,16] Table 102D.4 summarizes data about long-term outcomes after ALPPS for CRCLM. In series with more than 10 patients, overall 1-year survival ranged from 76% to 93%.[†] One report showed a survival rate of 62% at 2 years.[79] Recent data on 3-year overall survival showed a rate of about 56%.[87] However, many patients have shown early recurrence during the first 12 months and analysis of disease-free survival found a mean recurrence time of 9 months, interestingly with 40% of patients showing extrahepatic recurrence earlier than intrahepatic recurrence.[88] Data from other studies seem to confirm that early recurrence is not a rare event, with disease-free survival ranging from 50% to 67% after 1 year.[17,36,39] The ALPPS procedure not only stimulates liver regeneration, resulting in a dramatic hypertrophy of the FLR, but also enhances tumor proliferation.[89,90] This increased tumor growth also has been observed in patients undergoing PVE or classic two-stage hepatectomy.[78,91,92] The only randomized, controlled trial (Ligro-Trial) so far showed no difference between ALPPS and two-stage hepatectomy with regard to perioperative complications.[93,94] ALPPS, however, resulted in a better resection rate. This trial clearly showed that ALPPS at least for CRCLM, was as safe as two-stage hepatectomy. However, a recent systematic review and meta-analysis still revealed higher mortality and morbidity rates in ALPPS than in two-stage hepatectomy, but liver related mortality was similar.[95]

CONCLUSION

The ALPPS technique is a two-stage liver resection enabling resection in patients who are otherwise unresectable because FLR volume is too small. The hypertrophy response is fast and exceeds the volume increase reported after PVE; thus stage 2 ALPPS can be performed in 7 to 14 days. The increased morbidity and mortality rates initially reported after ALPPS have decreased with increased institutional experience and application of partial ALPPS; rates are now comparable with the rates accepted for traditional extended liver resections. ALPPS does not replace conventional two-stage resection or PVE, but rather provides an additional method when these techniques are not expected to result in sufficient hypertrophy. When the hypertrophy response after PVE or PVL proves to be insufficient, an additional "rescue ALPPS" can be performed. The main challenge for the future is to confirm that ALPPS does not increase cancer progression, in order to further exploit its potential in the treatment of patients with unresectable liver tumors. ALPPS is now well established in the technical armamentarium of hepato-pancreato-biliary surgeons, although issues such as optimal technique and selection of tumor entity are still under investigation.

[†]References 17, 36, 38, 39, 55, 79–81, 85, 86.

References are available at expertconsult.com.

CHAPTER 103

Adjuncts to hepatic resection: From ultrasound guidance to new oncologic and technical horizons

Guido Torzilli, Guido Costa, Jacopo Galvanin, Fabio Procopio

INTRODUCTION

Adequate oncologic margins and enough future liver remnant (FLR) with proper inflow and outflow are the pillars for any successful strategy in liver surgery (see Chapter 101). Given that tumor-free margin remains the mainstream of any oncologic surgery, liver regeneration has been considered the most suitable path to address successfully both surgical radicality and safety for advanced oncologic liver involvement. By treating the diseased part to hypertrophy, the FLR has been a practical translation from the 1990s[1,2] to now[3] (see Chapter 102C). Nevertheless, the failure of portal vein (PV) embolization (PVE) to obtain an adequate FLR has limited this approach both for colorectal liver metastases (CLMs) and hepatocellular carcinoma (HCC).[4,5] Thus a temporary debulking surgery splitting into two operations the organ clearance with or without PVE was proposed for multiple bilobar CLM: the two-stage hepatectomy (TSH).[6,7] The relatively high dropout because of tumor progression between the two procedures induced some authors to shorten the interval between them by combining in the first operation the right PV ligation, the clearance of the left liver, and the division of the two hemilivers, creating the so-called *associated liver partition and PV ligation for staged hepatectomy* (ALPPS)[8,9] (see Chapter 102D). The surgical community has learned from the ALPPS procedure that the liver division together with the PV ligation can boost liver regeneration, resulting in a faster and larger grow. However, mortality and morbidity remain relatively high.[10] Refinements in technique and variants will probably contribute to a better position for this approach among those available.[11] Liver venous deprivation (LVD) followed by major hepatectomy is the most recently described approach aimed at enhancing liver regeneration (see Chapter 102C). Simultaneous occlusion of PV inflow and hepatic vein (HV) outflow seems safe and efficient in terms of FLR increase and consequent limitation of patient dropout, but the results need further validation, particularly in cirrhosis.[12] All of these solutions enhance the FLR by means of major vessel amputation, reducing the chance of redo surgery in case of relapses. Indeed, it seems somehow obvious that fewer remnant vascular structures reduce the options available for technical solutions for tumor clearance.

On the other hand, it appears reasonable that in a three-dimensionally complex organ, like the liver is, featured by the capacity to regenerate and then significantly tolerate tissue deprivation, there should be room for systematizing more technical solutions between major liver resection and peripheral parenchymal-sparing resection. In early 2000, the so-called "radical but conservative policy" was introduced[13,14] based on the guidance of intraoperative ultrasound (IOUS). This approach aimed to challenge conservatively the deeply located lesions, leveraging on the organ anatomy as a sort of path for systematizing the new procedure and offering otherwise unfeasible solutions, a path that has conducted to the IOUS and vessel-guided parenchyma-sparing hepatectomies.[15,16]

THE PILLARS

Intraoperative Ultrasound (see Chapter 24)

Imaging techniques have been introduced as aids for surgeons in performing liver resection. In fact, since the early 1980s, IOUS has been used in hepatic surgery, initially in patients with liver cirrhosis.[17] Since then, ultrasound (US) guidance has been progressively applied to deal with complex tumor involvement of the liver up to the aforementioned "radical but conservative" approach[13,14,18] as a reliable alternative to major hepatectomy.[19–21] IOUS allows for an accurate definition of the relationship between the tumor, the portal branches, and the HVs. Disclosing precisely the tumor-vessel relationships is relevant for planning the type of resection. IOUS easily allows the surgeon to recognize if a tumor is separated by some normal parenchyma from the vessel, is in contact with the vessel without invading its wall, or is invading the vessel wall. In addition, IOUS can assist in determining the presence of proximal bile duct dilation and whether it is associated with a tumor thrombus. IOUS helps also in the estimation of the circumferential extent of the tumor-vessel contact, which opens to the technical scenarios discussed later.[22]

Equipment

Suitable probes should be sterilizable to be used in direct contact with the targeted organ, then eliminating the artifacts created by an US sterile cover. Efficient systems for sterilizing IOUS probes, such as hydrogen peroxide gas-plasma technology (Sterrad; ASP, Rome, Italy), are now available.

High-frequency echoprobes (7.5–10 MHz) are often recommended to perform IOUS because they allow a higher spatial resolution than those operating at lower frequencies (3.5–5 MHz). However, lower frequency probes are also useful, at least for the initial exploration, providing a better panoramic view that helps compensate for the lower spatial resolution (Fig. 103.1). In the scenario in which a superficial nodule is slightly visible on IOUS but is not palpable, particularly in a cirrhotic liver, a surgical glove filled with sterile water can be positioned between the probe and the liver surface, making the lesion more visible (Fig. 103.2). In this situation, indocyanine green (ICG) fluorescence has further provided helpful insights.[23]

Crucial points to be evaluated when a probe is selected are its shape and volume. Indeed, an optimal probe should represent the best compromise among (1) the size, which should be small enough to facilitate handling in deep and narrow spaces; (2) the US scanning window, which should be large enough to enable the widest area of exploration at once; and (3) the

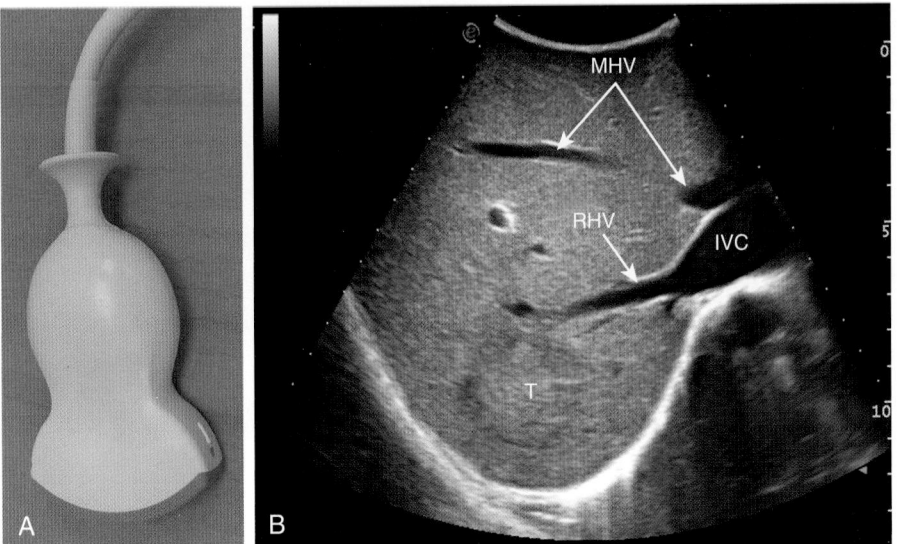

FIGURE 103.1   **A,** Convex probe for percutaneous exploration used intraoperatively for an initial overview. The relatively low frequency allows visualization of deep structures, although it offers some degree of spatial resolution. **B,** Appearance of a convex probe scan. In one scan, it is possible to visualize the liver with a tumor *(T)* and to recognize the middle hepatic vein *(MHV)*, the right hepatic vein *(RHV)*, and the retrohepatic inferior vena cava *(IVC)*.

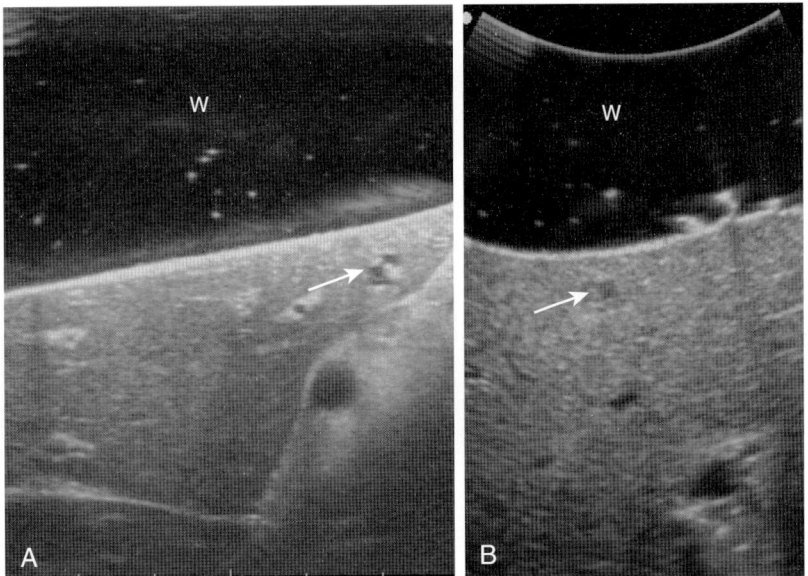

FIGURE 103.2   For better exploration of the superficial structures, a glove filled with deaerated water *(W)* is positioned in between the probe and the targeted surface. The *arrows* indicate two 1-mm lesions superficially located, a simple cyst **(A),** and a small colorectal liver metastasis **(B).**

adherence with the surface of the target organ, which should be good enough to enable adequate stability during handling and for avoiding gas interposition and artifacts that may compromise organ exploration.

The most frequently used probes are the T-shaped (Fig. 103.3), interdigital, and microconvex probes (Fig. 103.4). The microconvex probe represents the best compromise among all the previous requirements. Indeed, the T-shaped probe, although it remains more stable and is associated with higher image resolution, has a lower ratio between lateral length and US scanning window than the microconvex probe. More recently, linear transducers with enlarged scanning windows combine the stability of the linear probes and their higher image resolution with larger scanning

windows and a limited volume (Fig. 103.5). When probes are evaluated, another aspect that should be considered is the feasibility and ease of use for surgical maneuvers, such as the selective intrahepatic vessel compression mentioned later.

Color Doppler imaging, and particularly more sensitive color-flow modes, have progressively assumed greater roles in the intraoperative evaluation of inflow and outflow of the liver (Fig. 103.6) and assessment of flow modifications during surgical maneuvers. This provides crucial data for allowing surgical strategies that would not otherwise be feasible.

Contrast-enhanced IOUS (CE-IOUS) is now an established application of US[24] and IOUS systems should be equipped accordingly (Fig. 103.7).

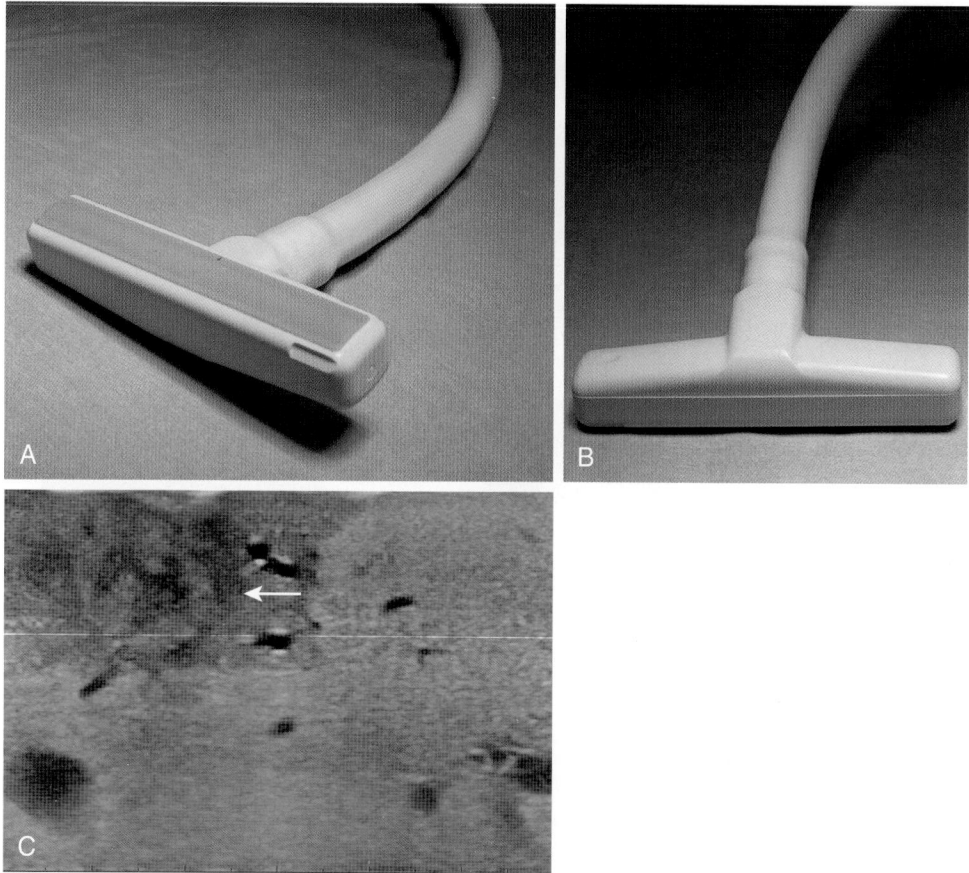

FIGURE 103.3   From left to right, the scanning side of a T-shaped echoprobe, the reverse side, and the scanning area: a small metastatic lesion is shown *(arrow).* This high-frequency echoprobe (7.5–10 MHz) features high resolution but low ultrasound penetration.

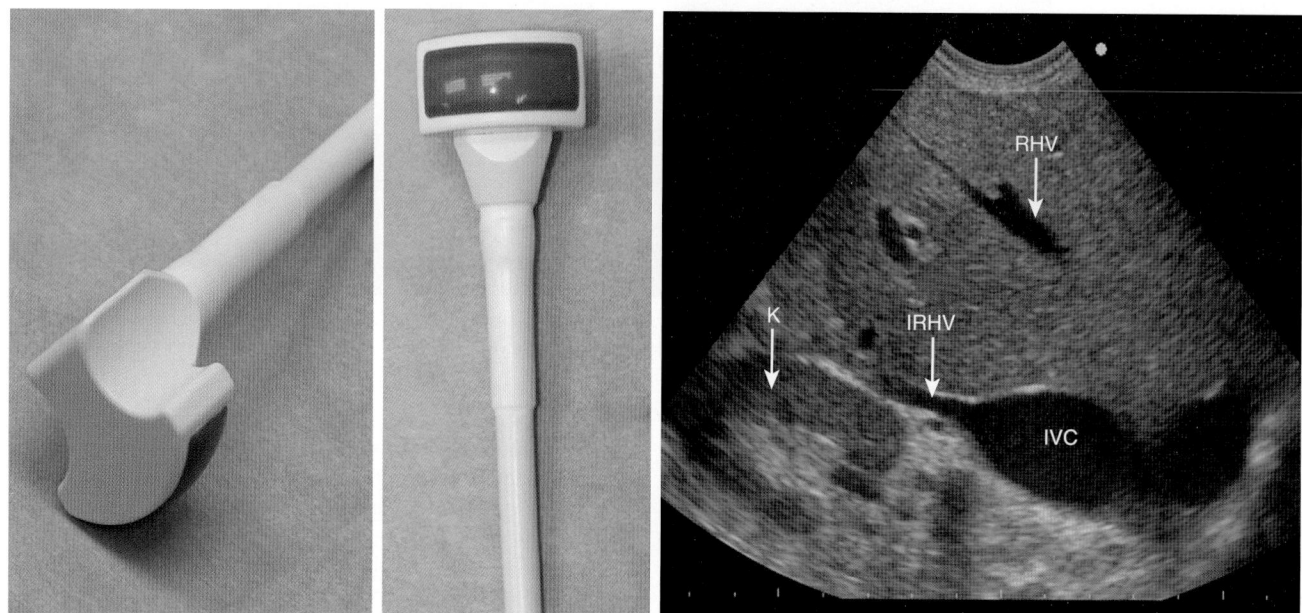

FIGURE 103.4   From left to right, the microconvex echoprobe, the scanning side of the probe, and the scanning area is shown. This wide-range frequency echoprobe (2–7 MHz) makes it possible in one scan to visualize the liver with a tumor, in which the right hepatic vein *(RHV),* an inferior right hepatic vein *(IRHV),* and the right kidney *(K)* are recognizable. *IVC,* Inferior vena cava.

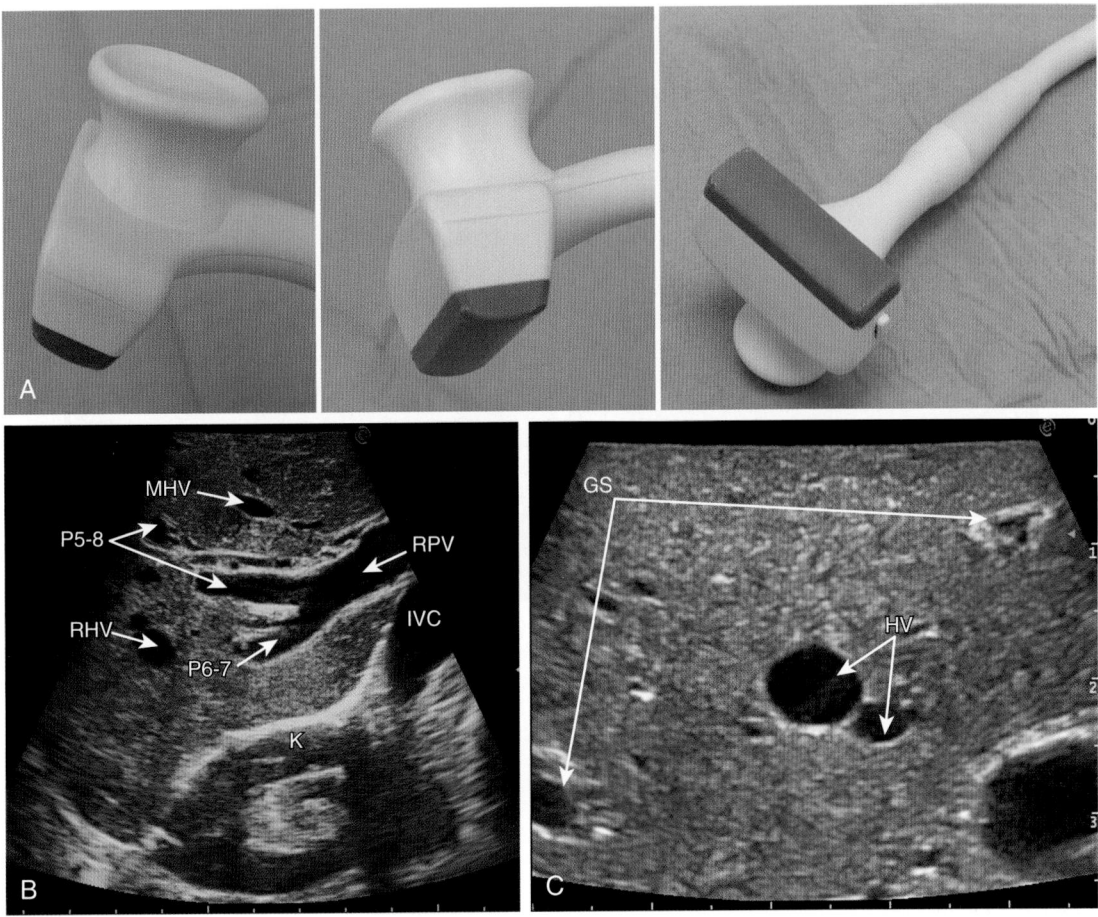

FIGURE 103.5   This intraoperative linear probe **(A)** (Esaote SpA, Genova, Italy) features a trapezoidal scanning area **(B)** mimicking the scanning window of a convex probe: This probe combines the stability of a linear transducer, the wideness of the scanning window of a convex probe, and the resolution of a high-frequency transducer. It was designed also for allowing ultrasound-guided compression maneuvers. Indeed, its shape allows ergonomic placement of the surgeon's finger *(arrows)* to facilitate handling. *GS*, Glissonean sheath; *HV*, hepatic vein; *K*, Kidney; *IVC*, inferior vena cava; *MHV*, middle hepatic vein; *P5-8*, portal branch to segments V and VIII; *P6-7*, portal branch to segments VI and VII; *RHV*, right hepatic vein.

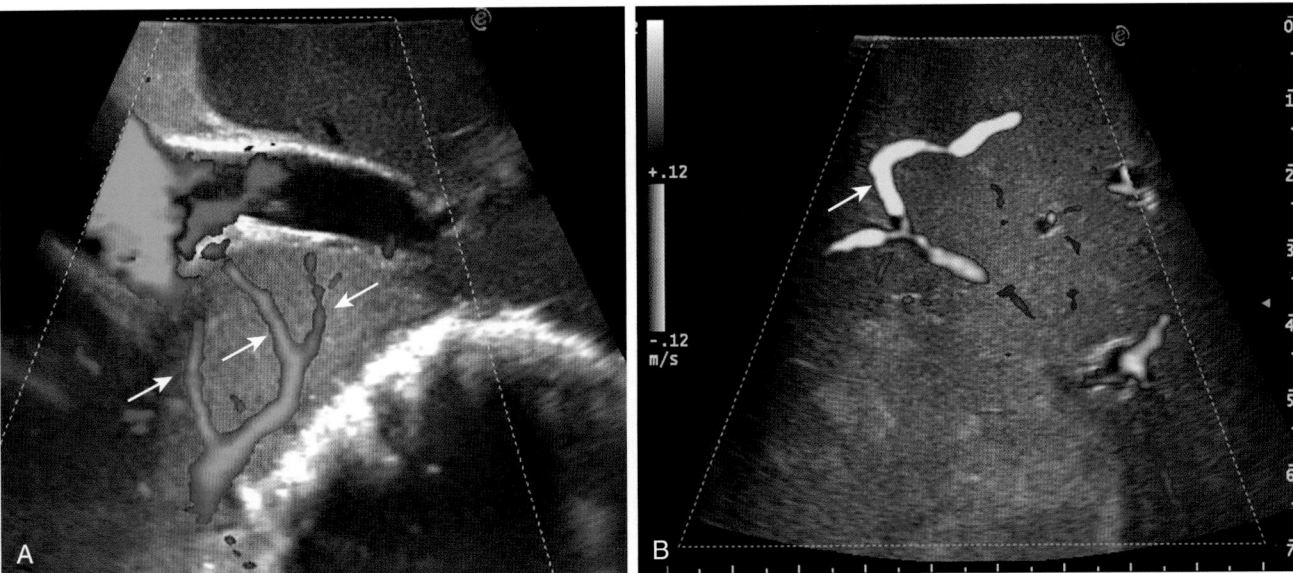

FIGURE 103.6   The appearance of the liver, once the exploration is carried out under the color flow intraoperative ultrasound (CF-IOUS) mode, a more sensitive modality compared with color Doppler for analyzing the blood flow. This increases the sensitivity and allows precise mapping of the slow-motion flow as shown in these pictures; tiny vessels *(arrows)* are clearly depicted.

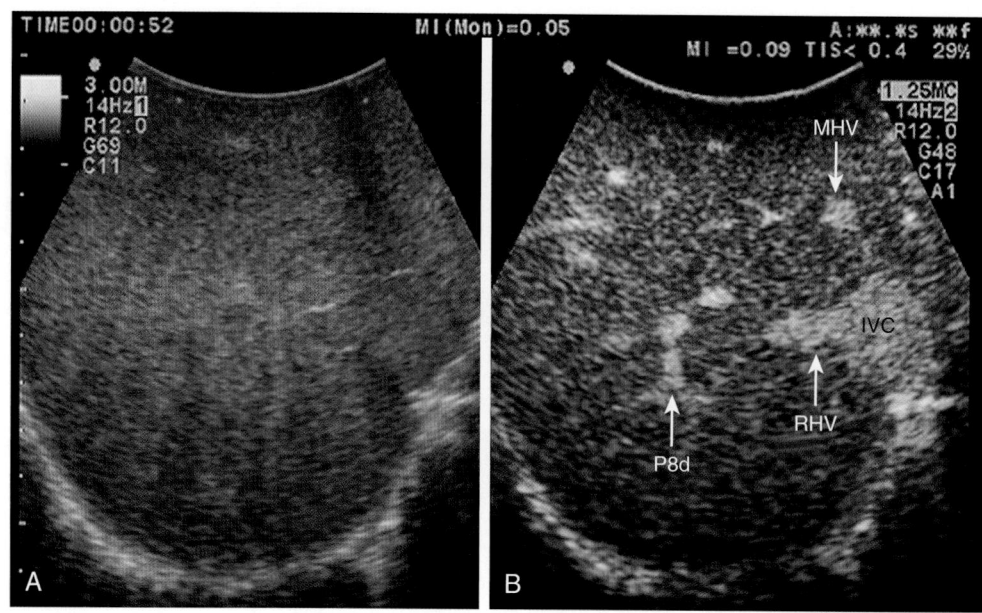

FIGURE 103.7   The appearance of the liver at intraoperative ultrasound (IOUS) using contrast enhancement. **A,** B-mode conventional modality is shown on the ultrasound (US) system screen simultaneously with the contrast-enhanced image shown in **B. B,** Liver is shown at 52 seconds after injection of contrast (time appears in the left upper corner in **A**). The vessel and parenchymal enhancement are shown; both portal branches and hepatic veins are filled with contrast. On the upper right corner of the image, *MI* refers to the mechanical index, which should be less than 0.1 so as not to break the microbubbles and to allow the contrast effect of real-time enhancement at ultrasound. *IVC,* Inferior vena cava; *MHV,* middle hepatic vein; *P8d,* portal branch to segment VIII dorsal; *RHV,* right hepatic vein.

Preparation for Liver Exploration

First, it must be stressed that the surgeon in charge of the surgical procedure should carry out the IOUS, rather than assistants, radiologists, or technicians. This is because to provide the most meaningful benefit for the patient and finalization of surgical strategy, the IOUS with US-guided maneuvers and operation should be performed by the same person.

The US system should be positioned opposite to the first operator, who must be able to simultaneously view both the screen and the operative field (Fig. 103.8) unless the operating room (OR) is equipped with multiple screens placed across the surgical field. The screen must be large enough to allow optimal visibility at that distance, and the lights should be positioned with caution not to interfere with the visibility of the US screen. A transparent, sterile covering pad should be available to handle the keyboard directly.

After the abdominal cavity is entered, liver mobilization, division of the round and falciform ligaments, and division of adhesions to free the anterosuperior and inferior surfaces of the liver should be performed before liver exploration with IOUS. Adhesions from the tumor to other organs or structures should not be manipulated because they may represent areas of tumor infiltration; in this situation, IOUS can help by excluding or confirming tumor invasion, which could change the surgical strategy.

For wide exposure of the liver surface, the round ligament can be pulled for traction, allowing tracing of the portal branches and the HVs. The probe should be managed by using enough pressure to ensure good contact with the liver surface but not so much as to compress the intrahepatic vascular structures, particularly the HVs.

IOUS Semiology

Solid knowledge of the liver anatomy is required to perform IOUS properly (see Chapter 2). For surgical anatomy, the Brisbane terminology is considered here.[25]

Exploration starts from the Glissonean branches following the portal pedicles at the sectional, segmental, and subsegmental

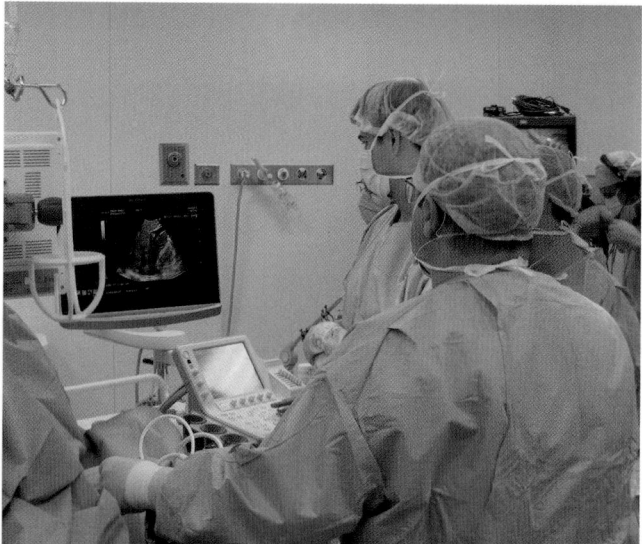

FIGURE 103.8   The ultrasound system positioned in the operating room: The operator is facing the screen while the keyboard is managed by the first or second assistant in the event a sterile pad is applied or, as in this case, by a member of the team who is not scrubbed in.

levels, then defining precisely the anatomic location of the IOUS target. Initially, Glissonean pedicles (GPs) can be followed by positioning the probe horizontally, grossly between the cross-margin of segments IV, V, and VIII, to visualize the first order bifurcation (Fig. 103.9). The first-, second-, and third-order Glissonean branches then can be followed in a right-to-left clockwise manner (right GP, right anterior, right posterior, left GP, pedicle to segment IV superior/inferior, segment III, and segment II), just tilting the probe upward and downward, and/or rotating it on its perpendicular axis (Fig. 103.10). Because of the existence of the Glisson capsule, the GPs, which include PV branches, arteries, and bile ducts, have thicker vessel walls compared with the HVs and thus appear at IOUS as echo-free zones surrounded by a thicker, hyperechogenic layer (Fig. 103.11A). Furthermore, other parallel, thinner vascular structures are visible, which are the arteries (Fig. 103.12); the bile ducts of the Glissonean triad are also visible (Fig. 103.13). In principle, however, distinction between HVs and portal branches should be based not only on their appearance but also, and mainly, on their anatomy. Indeed, in the cirrhotic liver, as already mentioned, the vessel wall of the HV could be thicker (see Fig. 103.11B) and not easily differentiated from a peripheral portal branch. Further, cross-sectional scanning could give the wrong impression of two vessels running parallel within a Glissonean sheath, whereas they are the IOUS representation of two branches of an HV scanned just before their confluence (see Fig. 103.5C).

The appearance of the bile ducts on IOUS is worth mentioning because of their peculiarity. Although normally appearing as thin, echo-free zones in the Glissonean triad (see Fig. 103.13), once dilated, the bile ducts appear as more evident echo-free zones with a serpiginous path (Fig. 103.14). The element that is difficult to recognize in the IOUS study of the bile ducts is their segmental anatomy; the confluence of sectional and segmental ducts is closer to the hilum compared with the bifurcation of the portal branches (Fig. 103.15). As a result, it is possible to visualize more than one segmental bile duct with one scan, and with enough US background, IOUS can allow exact definition of the bile duct anatomy, not only in pathologic conditions but also in the normal state. This ability also allows for assessment of variations in the normal anatomy, such as confluence of the right posterior sectional bile duct into the left hepatic duct (Fig. 103.16), which is clearly critical information, particularly if a left hepatectomy is planned.

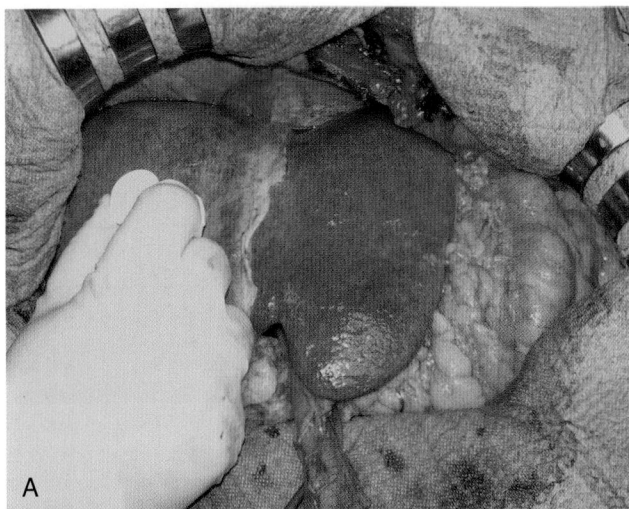

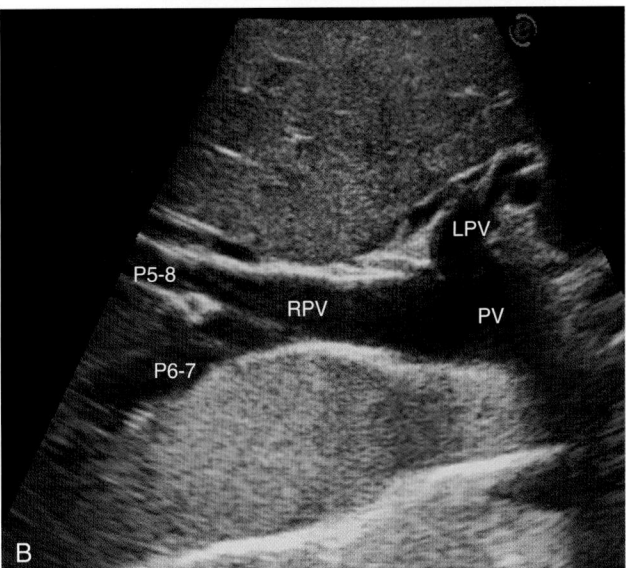

FIGURE 103.9   **A,** Liver exposed for initial exploration, once the falciform ligament has been cut; the surgeon is handling a probe. **B,** Typical branching pattern of the portal branches with the portal branch to right anterior section *(P5-8)* and to the right posterior section *(P6-7)* originating from the right portal vein *(RPV)*. *LPV,* Left portal vein; *PV,* portal vein.

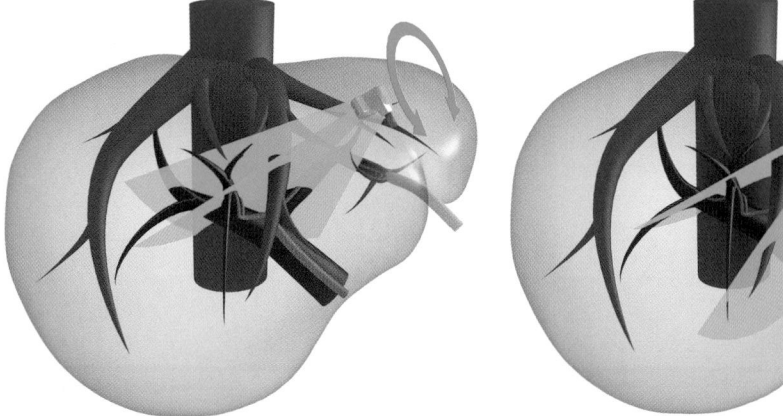

FIGURE 103.10   In these two schemas are shown the axis along which the probe is moved for initial liver exploration carried out by following Glissonean sheaths and hepatic veins.

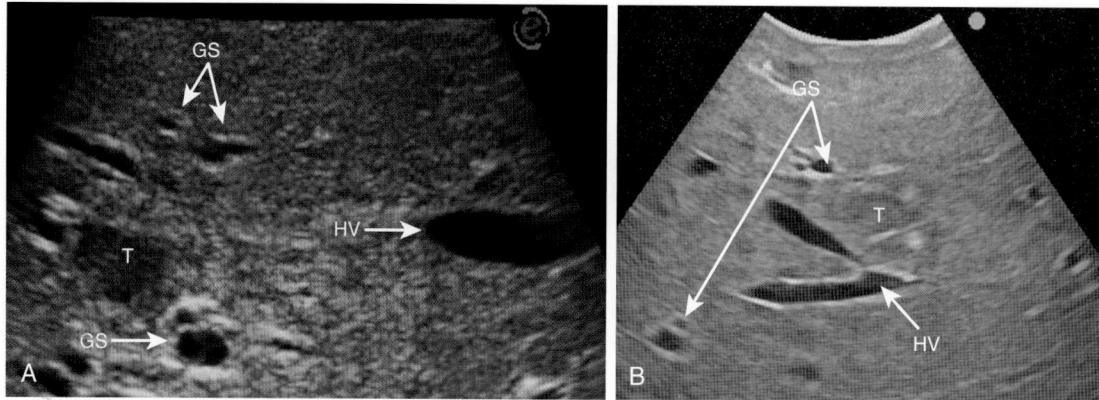

FIGURE 103.11   A, The Glissonean sheath *(GS)* and hepatic vein *(HV)* in a normal liver have a different wall thickness on intraoperative ultrasound. The GS is represented by at least two anechoic *(black)* structures, representing the artery and the portal vein; the bile duct is always seen in the case of the first- and second-order branches, which are often disclosed, particularly when dilated in the case of a more peripheral GS. **B,** In the cirrhotic liver, HVs have a thickened wall that mimics the wall of a GS; the anatomic landmarks and the inclusion of various structures together allow their proper differentiation. *T,* Tumor.

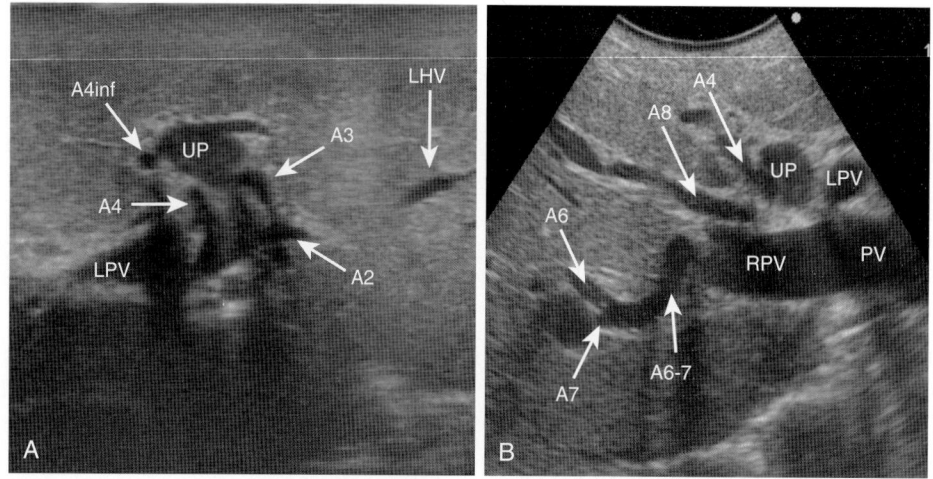

FIGURE 103.12   Arterial branching pattern in the left **(A)** and right **(B)** hemiliver. *A2,* Arterial branch to segment II; *A3,* arterial branch to segment III; *A4,* arterial branch to segment IV; *A4inf,* arterial branch to segment IV inferior; *A6,* arterial branch to segment VI; *A7,* arterial branch to segment VII; *A6-7,* arterial branch to the right posterior section; *A8,* arterial branch to segment VIII; *LHV,* left hepatic vein; *LPV,* left portal vein; *PV,* portal vein; *RPV,* right portal vein; *UP,* umbilical portion.

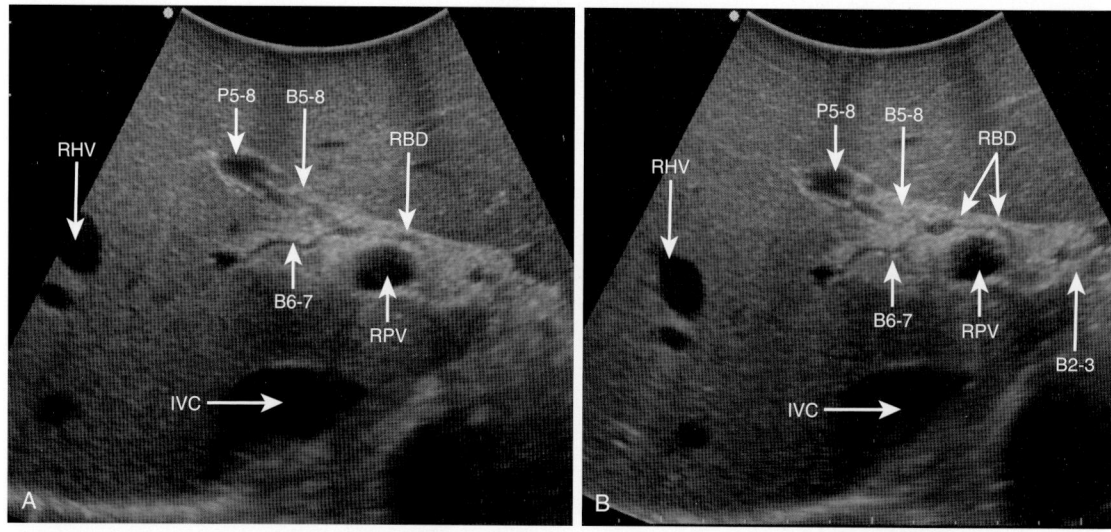

FIGURE 103.13   The biliary branching pattern in the right hemiliver **(A),** and partially the left **(B).** *B2-3,* Bile duct to segments II and III; *B5-8,* bile duct to right anterior section; *B6-7,* bile duct to right posterior section; *LPV,* left portal vein; *MHV,* middle hepatic vein; *P5-8,* portal branch to right anterior section; *RBD,* right bile duct; *RHV,* right hepatic vein; *RPV,* right portal vein.

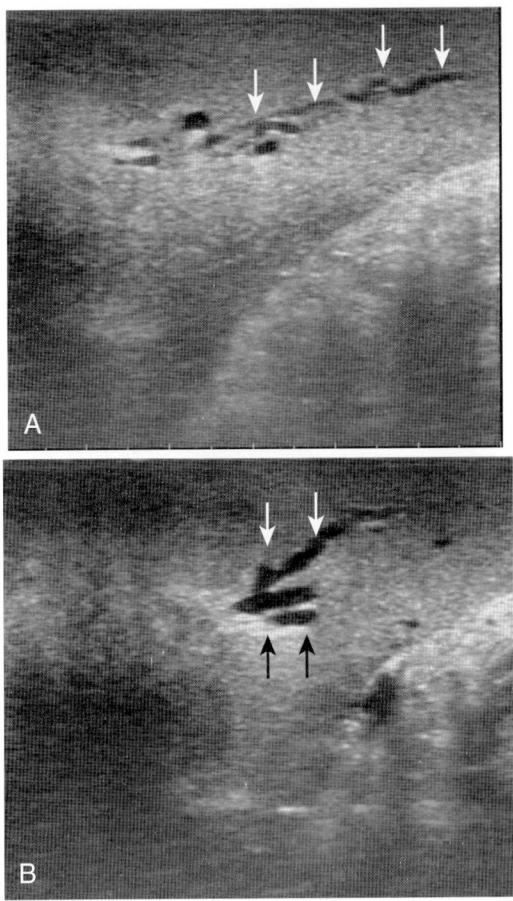

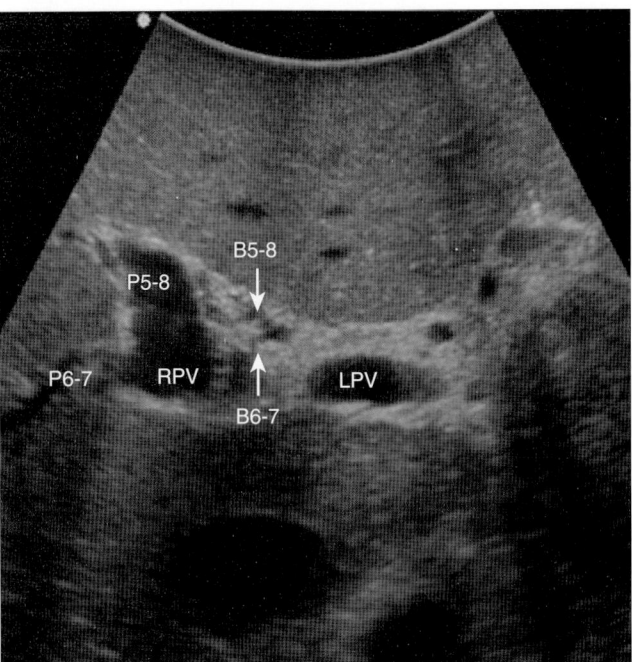

FIGURE 103.15 Centripetal branching pattern of the bile duct compared with that of the portal vein. *B5-8,* Bile duct to right anterior section; *B6-7,* bile duct to right posterior section; *LPV,* left portal vein; *P5-8,* portal branch for right anterior section; *P6-7,* portal branch to right posterior section; *RPV,* right portal vein.

FIGURE 103.14 **A** and **B** show the dilation of segmental bile ducts, which assumes a serpiginous path *(arrows).*

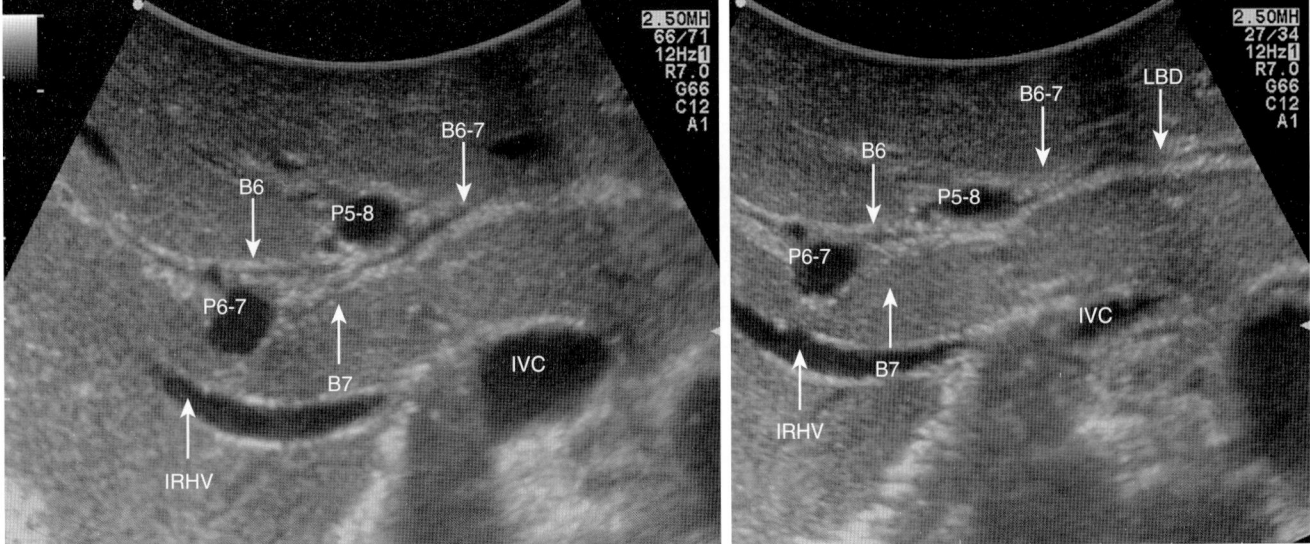

FIGURE 103.16 **A,** The confluence of the segmental bile ducts of segments VI *(B6)* and VII *(B7)* into the sectional bile duct of the right posterior section *(B6-7)*; **B,** B6-7 is flowing into the left bile duct *(LBD)* as shown in this figure. *IRHV,* Inferior right hepatic vein; *IVC,* inferior vena cava; *P5-8,* portal branch for right anterior section; *P6-7,* portal branch to right posterior section.

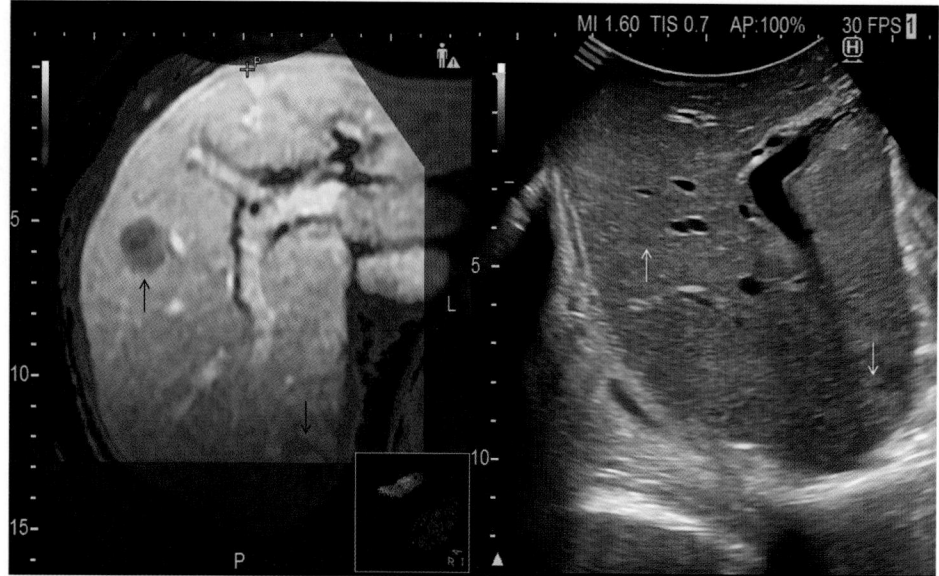

FIGURE 103.17 Matching the computed tomography (CT) images *(left side of the image)* obtained before chemotherapy and uploaded in the ultrasound system before the operation, with those of intraoperative ultrasound (IOUS; *right side of the image*) at surgery allows us to locate the disappeared colorectal liver metastases *(black arrows in the CT image, white arrows in the IOUS image)*.

The three main HVs are readily identified at their junction with the inferior vena cava (IVC) as visualized once the portal tree has been entirely explored. The left HV (LHV) appears in between the GPs for segment II and III. Following it upward, the LHV at the hepatocaval confluence is visualized, and when the probe is gently withdrawn, the HV paths can be traced into the liver. As mentioned, HVs appear as echo-free zones in the liver parenchyma, and the vessel wall is invisible or appears as a thin, hyperechogenic line (see Fig. 103.11A). The walls of HVs can be thicker in the cirrhotic liver, and their lumen can be thinner, as a result of the stiffness of the diseased liver (see Fig. 103.11B).

Diagnosis and Staging

Despite the improvement of preoperative imaging,[26] IOUS remains the gold standard for detection and differentiation in liver surgery. Indeed, although palpation still plays a fundamental role,[27] in the case of HCC growing in a cirrhotic liver, or in those patients having had previous liver resection, the firm and irregular hepatic surface makes tumor detection difficult. Up to now, more than 10% of patients have additional intraoperative findings provided by laparoscopic US or IOUS.[28] In the setting of CLM, the problem is sometimes the opposite because with the more efficient systemic treatment extensively used preoperatively, it is not rare to have it assist with the disappearance of some lesions that are anyhow frequently not visible but viable[29] (see Chapters 15, 90, 101, and 118). In this sense, real-time intraoperative fusion imaging could represent a useful tool.[22] Indeed, the possibility to couple in real time the previously uploaded images of the computed tomography (CT) or magnetic resonance imaging (MRI) performed before the systemic therapies with the real-time IOUS scans enables the detailed recognition of the areas in which the disappeared lesions were located (Fig. 103.17).

Given all of that, characterization of any new lesion detected intraoperatively remains crucial. The only nodule that can be easily featured at IOUS is the small hemangioma because it displays a typical US pattern, and when compressed, it changes in shape because of its compressibility (Fig. 103.18; see Chapter 14). Elastography allowing lesion differentiation based on tissue stiffness expressed on the IOUS screen by different colors may further help in this sense (Fig. 103.19).[30,31] Regenerative nodules

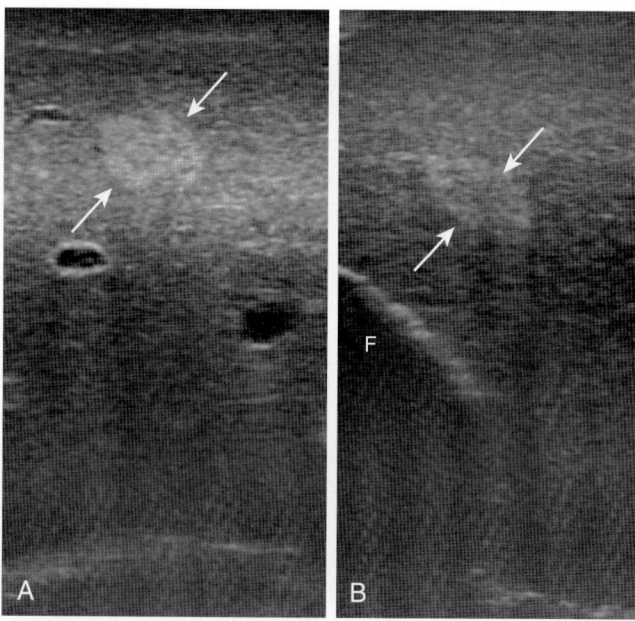

FIGURE 103.18 Test for diagnosing a hemangioma. **A,** Hemangioma *(arrows)* with hyperechoic *(bright)* pattern compatible with this type of lesion, although not specific enough. **B,** Once compressed under intraoperative ultrasound (IOUS) guidance, the lesion modifies its shape *(arrows)*; this finding together with its echogenicity leads to the diagnosis of hemangioma. *F,* Finger. (See Chapters 14 and 88A.)

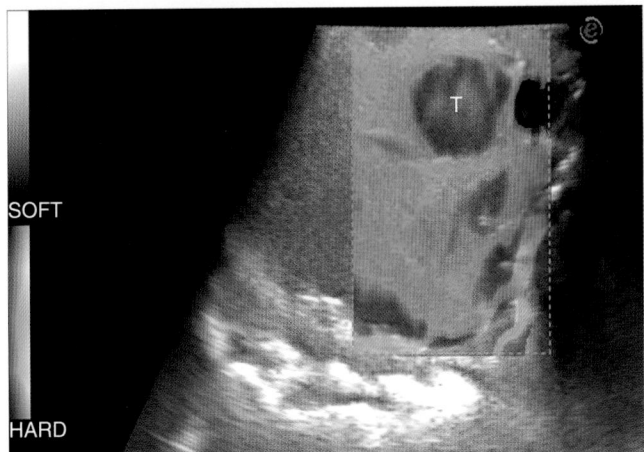

FIGURE 103.19 Potential value of elastography in estimating the tissue stiffness, relating it to a color scale disclosed on the left of each image. Tumor *(T)* as it appears at elastography; the tumor appears blueish, according to its higher stiffness compared with the surrounding liver parenchyma.

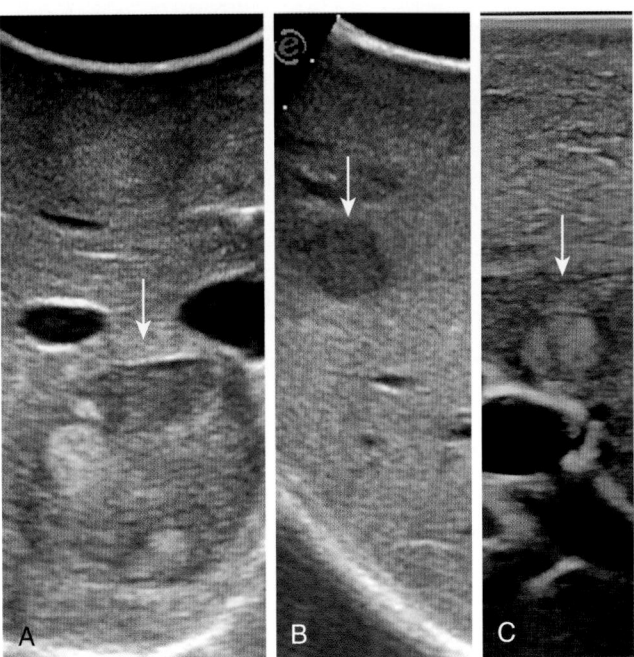

FIGURE 103.21 **A,** Nodule *(arrow)* with a mosaic pattern on intraoperative ultrasound (IOUS). **B,** Nodule *(arrow)* with a hypoechoic dark pattern at IOUS. **C,** Nodule *(arrow)* with a hyperechoic bright pattern at IOUS.

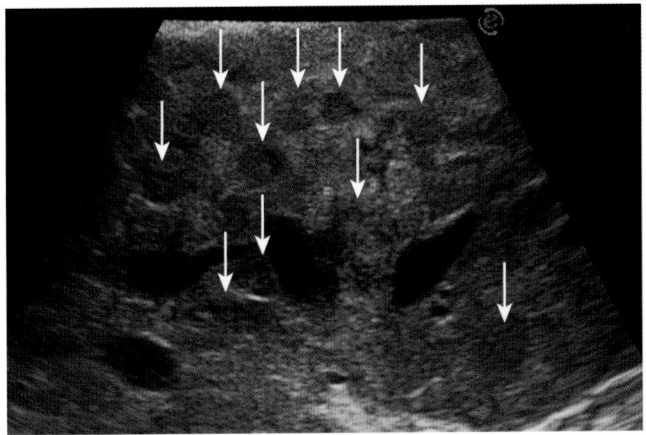

FIGURE 103.20 Cirrhotic liver with an inhomogeneous pattern as a result of the presence of an uncountable number of hypoechoic *(dark)* nodules mimicking tumors.

in cirrhotic patients operated for HCC is a relevant issue for lesion characterization. In this sense, IOUS may risk overestimating the HCC stage (Fig. 103.20). Indeed, except for those nodules with a mosaic pattern evident on US (Fig. 103.21A), of which more than 80% are malignant, only the minority are hypoechogenic (dark; see Fig. 103.21B) and hyperechogenic (bright; see Fig. 103.21C), meaning they are neoplastic.[32,33] CE-IOUS as described in the next paragraph plays a relevant role in the nodule differentiation and detection.

Contrast-Enhanced IOUS

In 2004 CE-IOUS was introduced (see Fig. 103.7) both for characterization and detection of liver lesions[34] (see Chapters 14, 15, and 24). Since then, several studies with different contrast agents have shown that CE-IOUS enhances tumor detection, despite the progress of preoperative imaging[26] and preventive IOUS exploration.[34–42] It has been feasible to differentiate between HCC and a dysplastic nodule-using vascular contrast

agent such as Sonovue. A classification of the enhancement pattern of lesions seen at CE-IOUS has been established, upon which the surgical decision making is established[36] (Fig. 103.22). In brief, any pathologic lesion will appear as hypoechogenic at the late phases, with or without full enhancement (Fig. 103.23) or inner vascularity (Fig. 103.24) during the arterial phase, and should be removed. More recently, using a vascular and postvascular contrast agent (Sonazoid), patterns of enhancements seem linked to the overall and recurrence-free survival and even to some gene expression profiling featured by poorer prognosis.[43]

Using Sonovue, the improvement of the detection of CLM in all patients undergoing liver resection, which was initially sustained,[35,37,38–40] have been further confirmed.[44] Indeed, CLM, in the late phase, which lasts from 2 to 5 minutes after injection, remains unenhanced and black in comparison with the surrounding enhanced liver parenchyma: the so-called "black-hole effect" (Fig. 103.25). Thankfully, CE-IOUS has allowed us to detect 9% additional nodules in our experience.[37] This increment in sensitivity appears to have particular relevance in the absence of a bright liver[45] and in the presence of multiple isoechoic CLM: these last conditions represent those with the higher risk of missed lesions with simple IOUS[46] (Fig. 103.26). In contrast, for those presenting with hypoechoic CLM in a bright liver, visibility is generally optimal on IOUS (Fig. 103.27). Also, CE-IOUS with Sonazoid proved to increase CLM detectability.[47] Both Sonovue and Sonazoid appear to increase the detectability of those CLM that disappeared after chemotherapy at preoperative imaging,[48,49] despite the improvement of the preoperative imaging with the advent of liver-specific MRI contrast agents.[50] CE-IOUS and hepatospecific MRI are rather complementary; a recent analysis has shown that CLM disappearance both at preoperative hepatospecific MRI and Sonazoid is associated with a high probability of CLM having truly disappeared.[51]

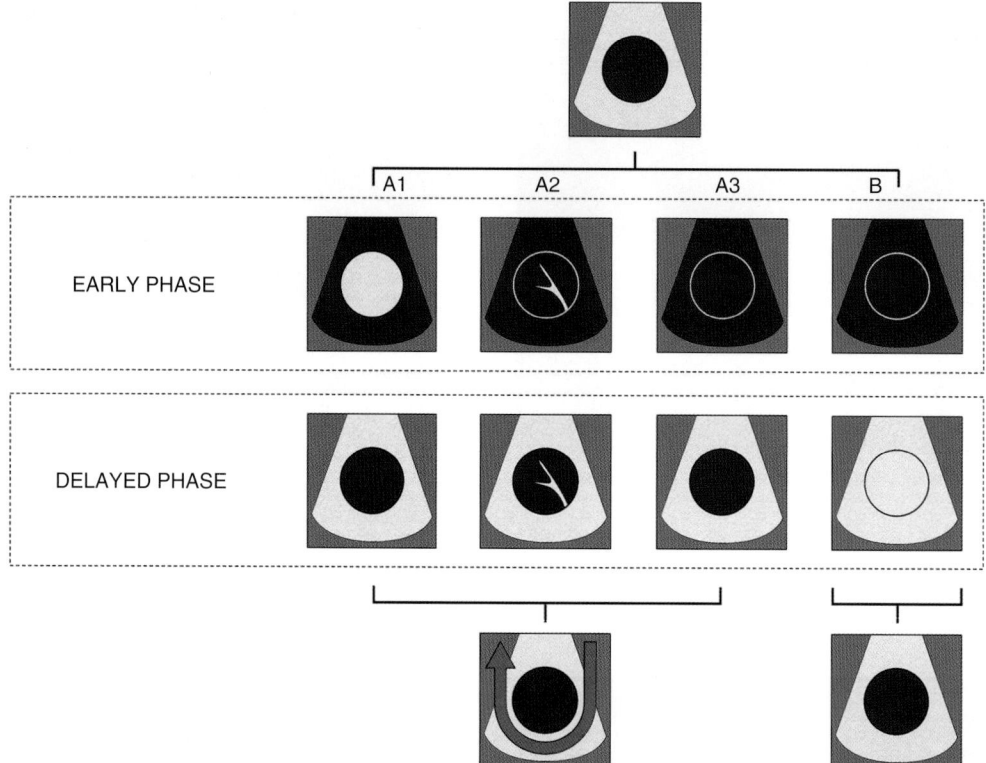

FIGURE 103.22 Classification of pattern of enhancement with contrast-enhanced intraoperative ultrasound (IOUS) of those lesions detected at IOUS and during surgery for hepatocellular carcinoma. Lesions with a class A pattern of hypervascular enhancement in early phase *(A1-A2)* or a hypoechoic pattern in the delayed phases *(A1, A3)* must be resected; inversely, lesions showing a class B pattern of enhancement (disappearance during contrast phases) are not removed.

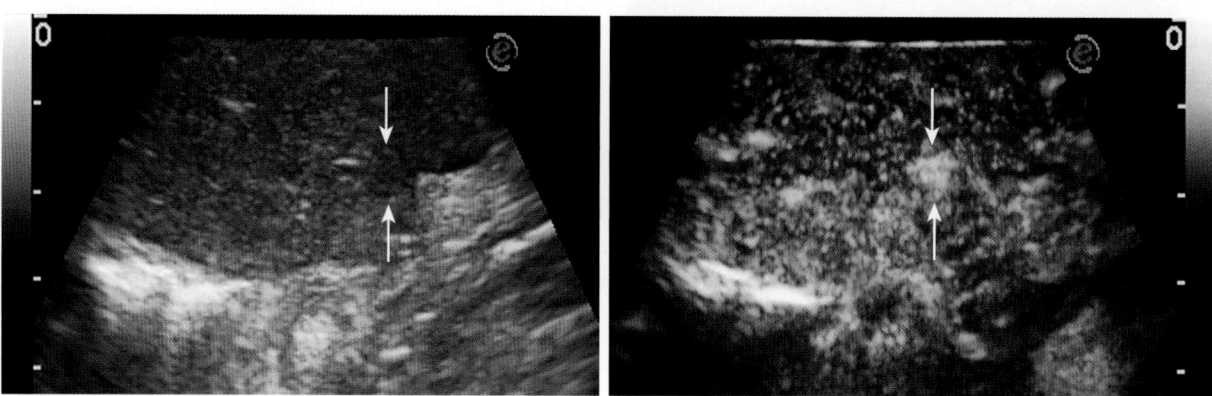

FIGURE 103.23 A, *Arrows* indicate a lesion. **B,** At early phase, the same lesions *(arrows)* show intranodular enhancement becoming hyperechoic, which allow its classification as an A1 nodule.

Caution should be used in patients with CLM who have coexisting liver cysts, which may appear like the CLM along the delayed phases of contrast enhancement. However, the cysts should have been already mapped based on the preoperative imaging and identified at exploration with conventional IOUS. Although liver cysts at unenhanced IOUS have an anechoic content and a posterior echo (Fig. 103.28), however, tiny CLMs can also assume a hypoechoic pattern with posterior echo mimicking that of small cysts (Fig. 103.29). Therefore any new black hole detected in the liver in locations where no cysts

were detected should be considered suspicious for malignancy (see Chapters 14, 15, and 24).

The impact of CE-IOUS in modifying the surgical strategy is strongly influenced by the attitude of the surgeons.[52] Given the capability of CE-IOUS to improve tumor detection, for the liver clearance, the confirmation of the predicted strategy depends on the possibility of including the new lesions within the planned resection area; this is often a subjective decision based on surgical attitude and expertise.[46] Then, despite new findings by CE-IOUS, it is not obvious to assist in a modified surgery;

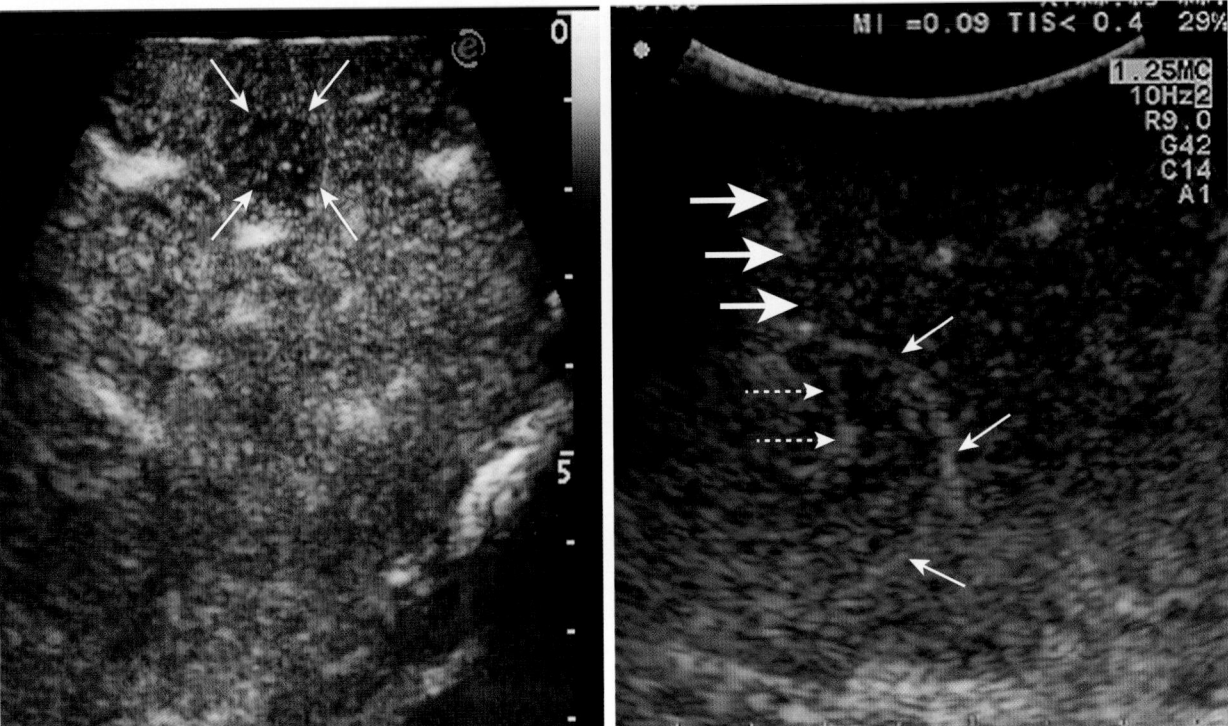

FIGURE 103.24   On the left, *arrows* indicate a lesion at early enhancement, which shows intranodular, hyperechoic (bright) spots, and for that is classified as an A2 nodule. On the right, a lesion at early enhancement, showing a feeding artery *(thick arrows)*, an artery describing a basket surrounding the nodule *(arrows)*, and an artery which run within the tumor *(dashed arrows)*; also, this lesion can be classified as A2.

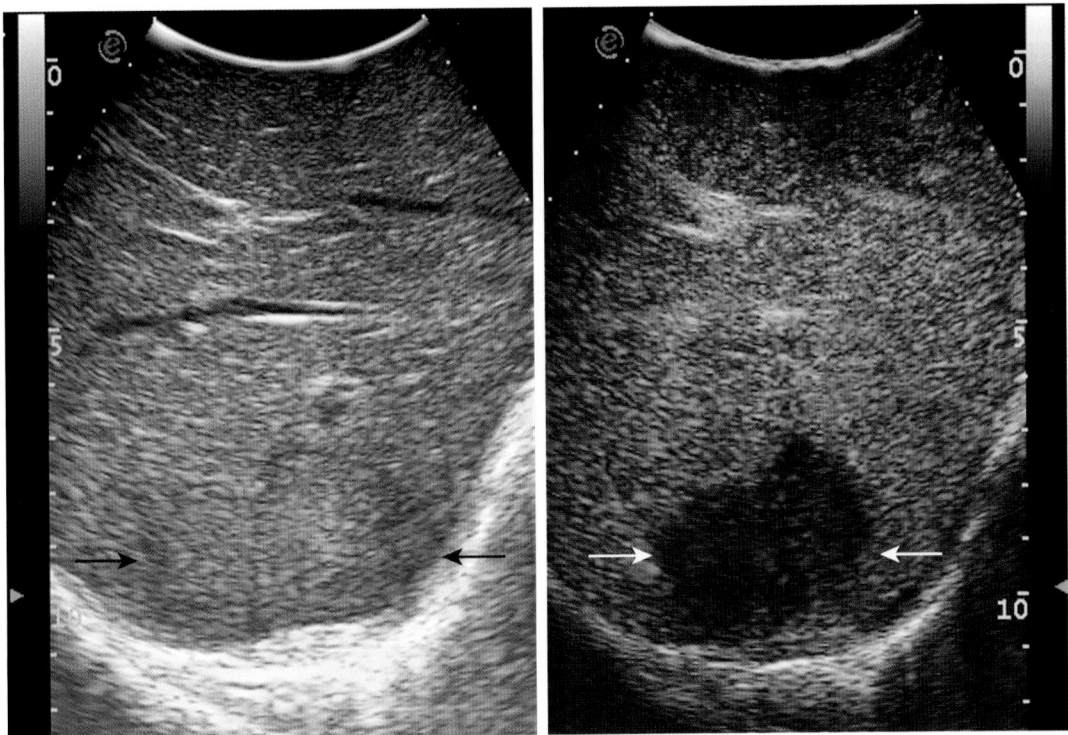

FIGURE 103.25   On the left this relatively large metastatic lesion is substantially isoechoic *(black arrows)* compared with the surrounding liver parenchyma. On the right, during portal phase, the lesion is clearly visible *(white arrows),* showing the so-called "black hole" effect.

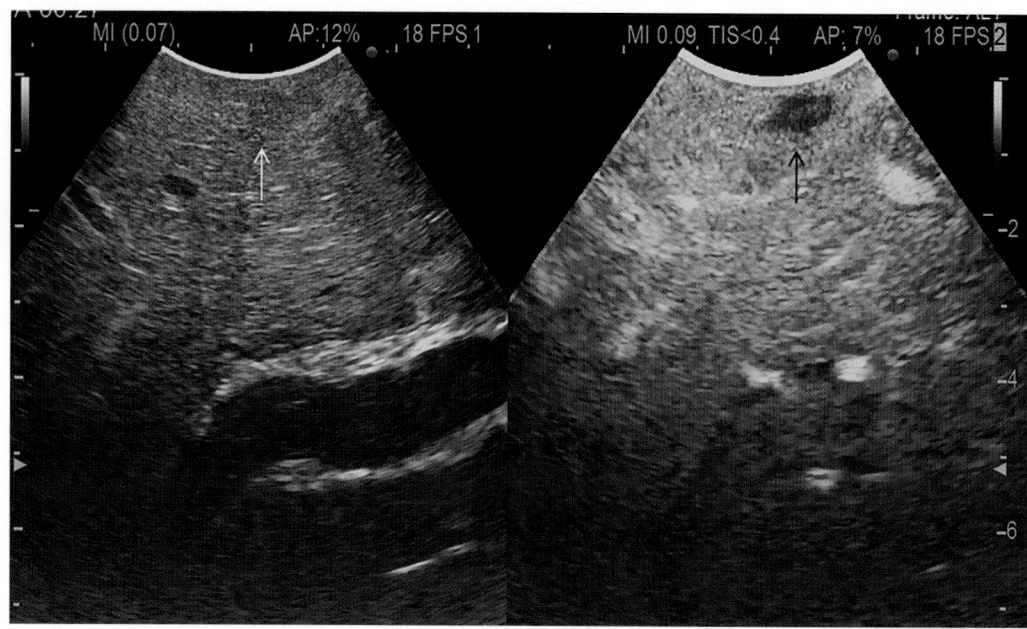

FIGURE 103.26   On the left a small metastatic lesion is isoechoic *(white arrow)* and almost invisible. On the right, during portal phase, the lesion is clearly visible *(black arrow),* showing the so-called "black hole" effect.

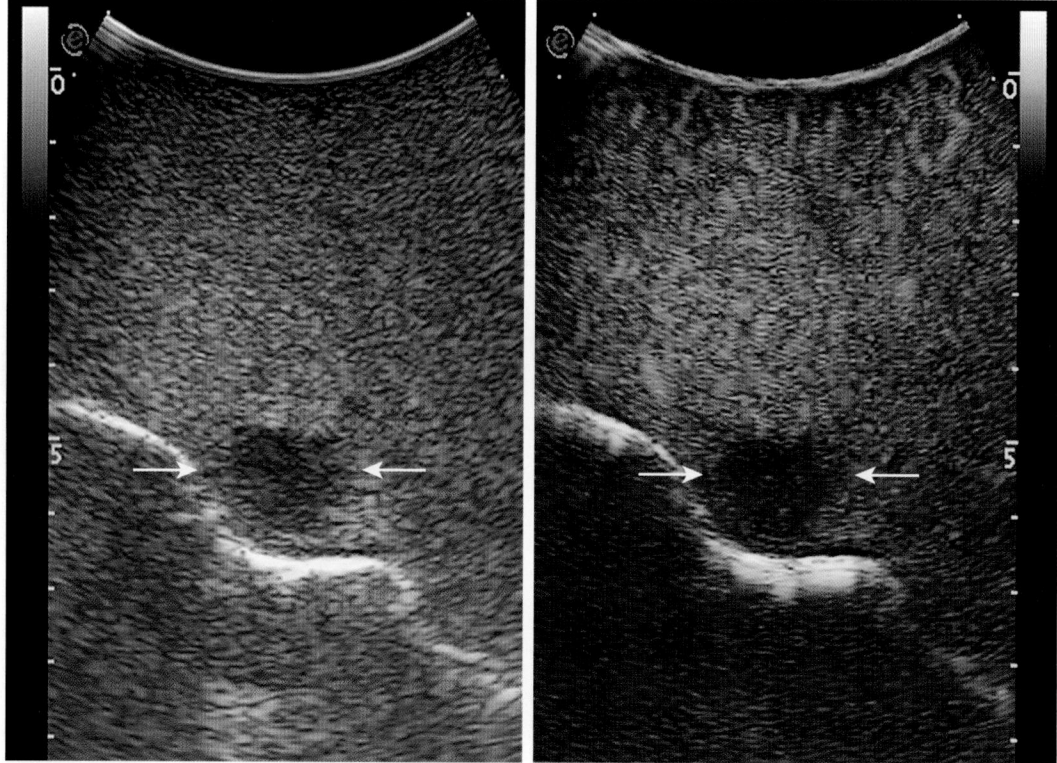

FIGURE 103.27   On the left a small metastatic lesion *(arrows)* in a "bright" *(fatty)* liver assumes a hypoechoic pattern well visible at intraoperative ultrasound (IOUS). On the right, it can be appreciated how the increment in terms of increased visibility of the lesion *(arrows)* during contrast-enhanced (CE)-IOUS is almost nil (see Chapter 14).

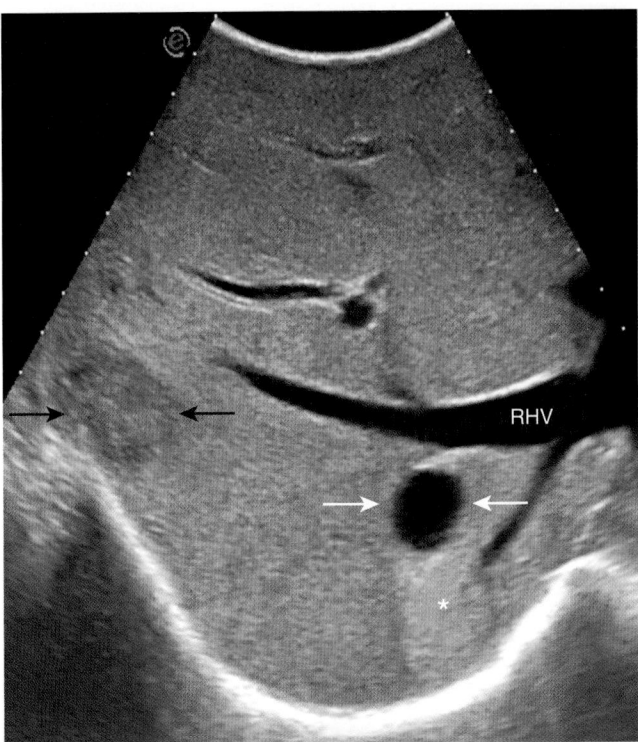

FIGURE 103.28   A small, simple hepatic cyst *(white arrows)* and a small metastasis *(black arrows)*; the cyst is featured by a posterior echo *(asterisk)* and an echo-free *(black)* content, which is not the case of the metastasis. *RHV*, Right hepatic vein. (See Chapter 14.)

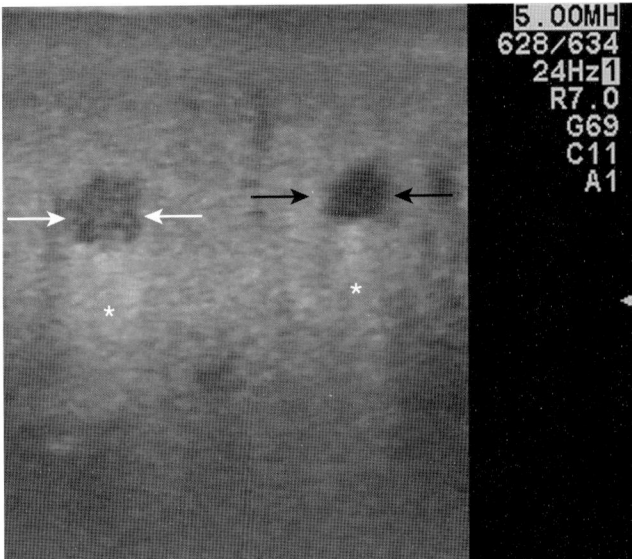

FIGURE 103.29   A small, simple hepatic cyst *(black arrows)* with its typical posterior echo *(asterisk)* and the echo-free *(black)* content. The white arrows show an ipoechoic solid lesion corresponding to colorectal metastases. (See Chapters 14 and 15.)

however, this element, being basically subjective, does not diminish the value of this specific diagnostic tool.

Still, concerning the resection guidance, CE-IOUS has provided some additional tricks to the surgeon for improving technical performances, such as the intraparenchymal profiling of

the liver segments using Sonazoid, which aids in resection of HCC in an anatomic fashion.[53]

From a technical standpoint, as mentioned, visual effects could last up to 5 minutes after injection, which can be repeated for global reassessment, or to assess the arterial phase enhancement of identified lesions for their characterization. With vascular and postvascular phase agents, detection of malignant lesions can appear up to 20 to 25 minutes post-injection in the hepatospecific phase.[41,47,54,55] Irrespective of the contrast agent used, high doses should be avoided because this limits US penetration in all phases.

IOUS-Guided Surgical Maneuvers

ANATOMIC RESECTIONS BY IOUS-GUIDED GLISSONEAN COMPRESSION. These resections are performed by following exactly the planes that divide hemilivers, sections, segments, and subsegments (see Chapters 101 and 118). Technical requirements for accomplishing truly anatomic sectionectomies and formal major hepatectomies are uniformly accepted and could be divided into two modalities: one based on the dissection of the vascular elements at hepatic hilum and one based on blunt encirclement from the hepatic hilum of the hemiliver or sectional pedicles. Conversely, an anatomic segmental and subsegmental resection demands the recognition of the feeding GP, its harboring, and the related area perfused. Segmentectomy and subsegmentectomy are mainly selected for removing HCC given the oncologic requirement of removing the tumor in an anatomic fashion and the need for sparing parenchyma for the frequent association of this tumor with a diseased liver (see Chapter 102). The first procedure described in this area was the systematic segmentectomy devised in the early 1980s,[17] which consists of puncture of the portal branch feeding the tumor and subsequent injection of dye; more recently, ICG fluorescence has been substituted for the dye injection.[56,57]

Initially used for tumors located in the left hemiliver,[58] GP compression has been successfully extended in its application to any segmental location[59,60] and for sectionectomies.[61,62] For HCC, this approach has proven its oncologic suitability both in terms of long-term local control and overall survival.[63]

Segmentectomies and Subsegmentectomies. Conceptually, the procedure can be summarized as shown in Figure 103.30. In practice, once the feeding GP is identified at IOUS (Fig. 103.31A), it is compressed by using the IOUS probe on one side of the liver and the finger on the opposite side, confirming the proper compression by IOUS real-time control (Fig. 103.32; see also Fig. 103.31B); in this way, it is possible to induce a transient ischemia of the portion of the liver distal to the compression site. This portion can be marked with electrocautery, the compression is released, and the resection is carried out (see Fig. 103.31C and Fig. 103.32). This technique is simple, fast, noninvasive, not dependent on the vessel diameter, and, most importantly, reversible, with the possibility of modifying the site of compression if necessary. More recently, ICG intravenously injected by the anesthesiologist once the compression has been started has allowed us to further enhance the demarcation with a counter-fluorescence of the area to be spared, overcoming those situations of nuanced demarcation (Fig. 103.33).[64]

The compression can be also used in a counter-compression manner, borrowing from the counterstaining technique proposed by Takayama and colleagues[65] for defining the adjacent segmental margins. For segments such as I and IV superior, for

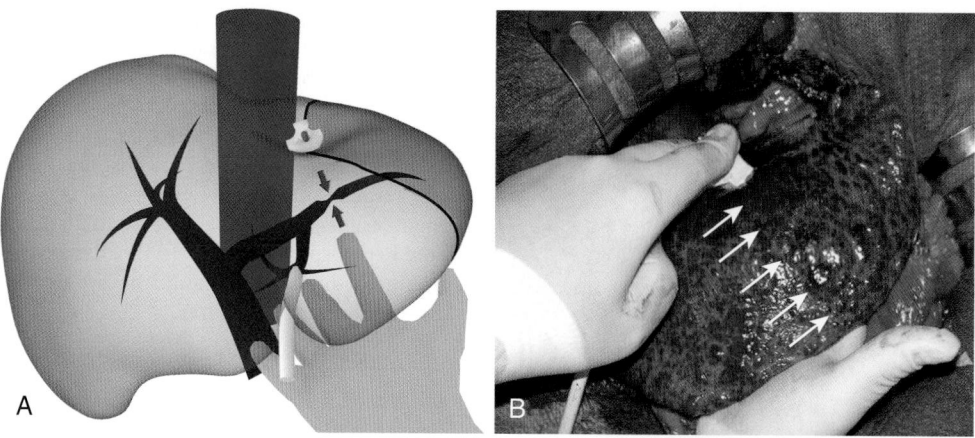

FIGURE 103.30 For segmentectomy by means of compression, the feeding portal branch is identified and compressed at the point targeted by intraoperative ultrasound (*red arrows in* **A**), resulting in discoloring of the segmental area (*white arrows in* **B**), which in this way can be marked with the electrocautery and selectively removed.

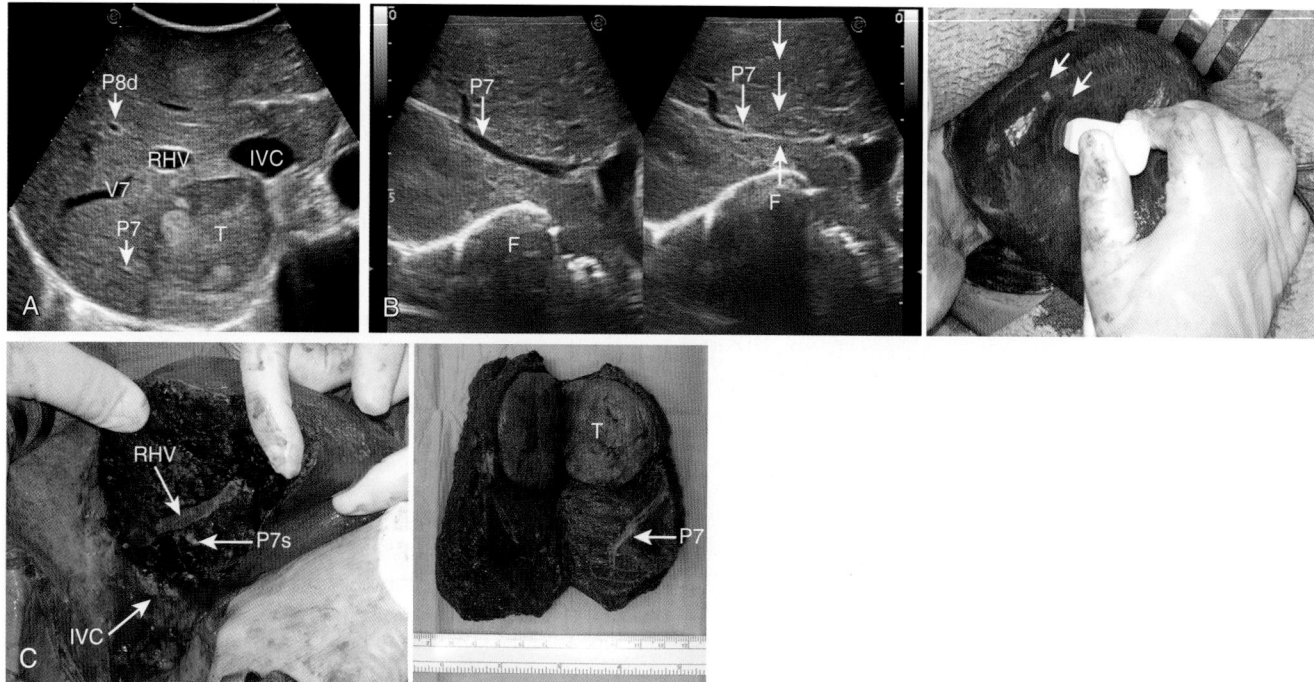

FIGURE 103.31 **A,** This intraoperative ultrasound (IOUS) scan shows the portal branch (*P7*) feeding the tumor in segment VII. **B,** From left to right, once identified under IOUS guidance, P7 compression is carried out (*arrows*) by means of the probe and the surgeon's finger (*F*) positioned on the opposite side as shown on the right: The segmental area results then discolored (*arrows*). **C,** On the left, the liver after anatomic resection of segment VII showing the right hepatic vein (*RHV*) and the stump of P7 (*P7s*) on the cut surface as landmarks of a true anatomic segmentectomy; on the right, the specimen showing the tumor (*T*) and P7. *IVC,* Inferior vena cava; *P8d,* portal branch to subsegment VIII dorsal; *V7,* hepatic veins draining segment VII.

which direct compression of the feeding portal branch is difficult if not unfeasible, compressing the adjacent segmental branch allows for definition of their segmental margins.[59]

In the event of HCC with tumor thrombus in the feeding portal branch, staining and compression techniques could not be performed to demarcate the segment. In such cases, intravenous (IV) injection of ICG performed by the anesthesiologist once the proper hepatic artery is selectively clamped at the hepatic hilum enables the demarcation of the segmental margin by counter-fluorescence.[66]

Right Posterior Sectionectomy. As for segmentectomies, the demarcation of the sectional area to be removed is advocated. Among methods proposed for obtaining this demarcation, extrahepatic isolation of the right-sided sectional pedicles consists of careful and meticulous skeletonization of each sectional arterial and portal branch.[67] Alternatively, the three GPs in their surrounding fibrous sheath could be encircled as a whole, with or without the use of a hepatotomy incision.[68] As an alternative to these established techniques, the compression technique could be applied.[62] The hepatic pedicle is encircled with a tourniquet but not dissected.

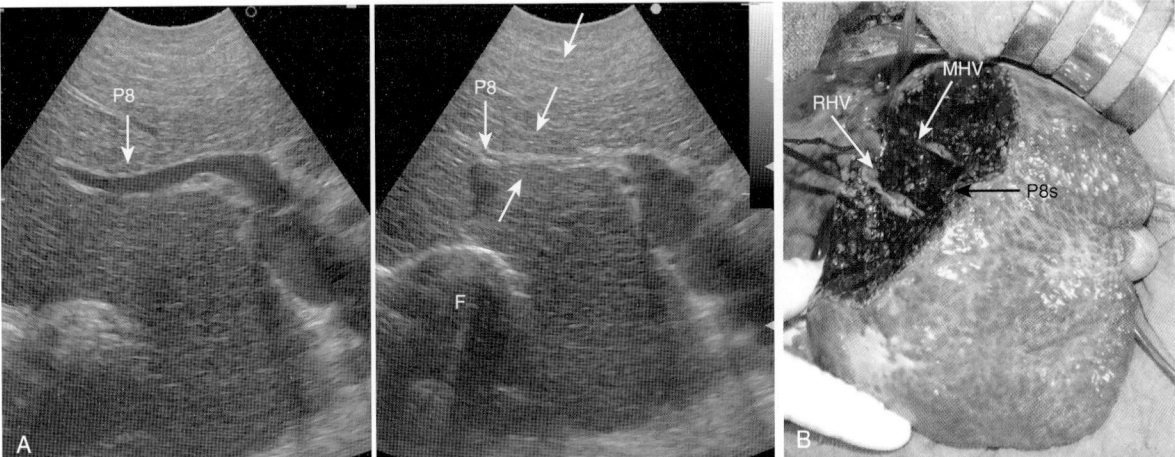

FIGURE 103.32   From left to right, intraoperative ultrasound (IOUS) scan shows the portal branch *(P8)* feeding the tumor in segment VIII, which is compressed under IOUS control *(arrows)* with the probe and the surgeon's finger *(F)* positioned on the opposite side; on the right, the liver after resection of segment VIII, showing the right hepatic vein *(RHV)*, the middle hepatic vein *(MHV)*, and the stump of P8 *(P8s)* on the cut surface as landmarks of a true anatomic segmentectomy.

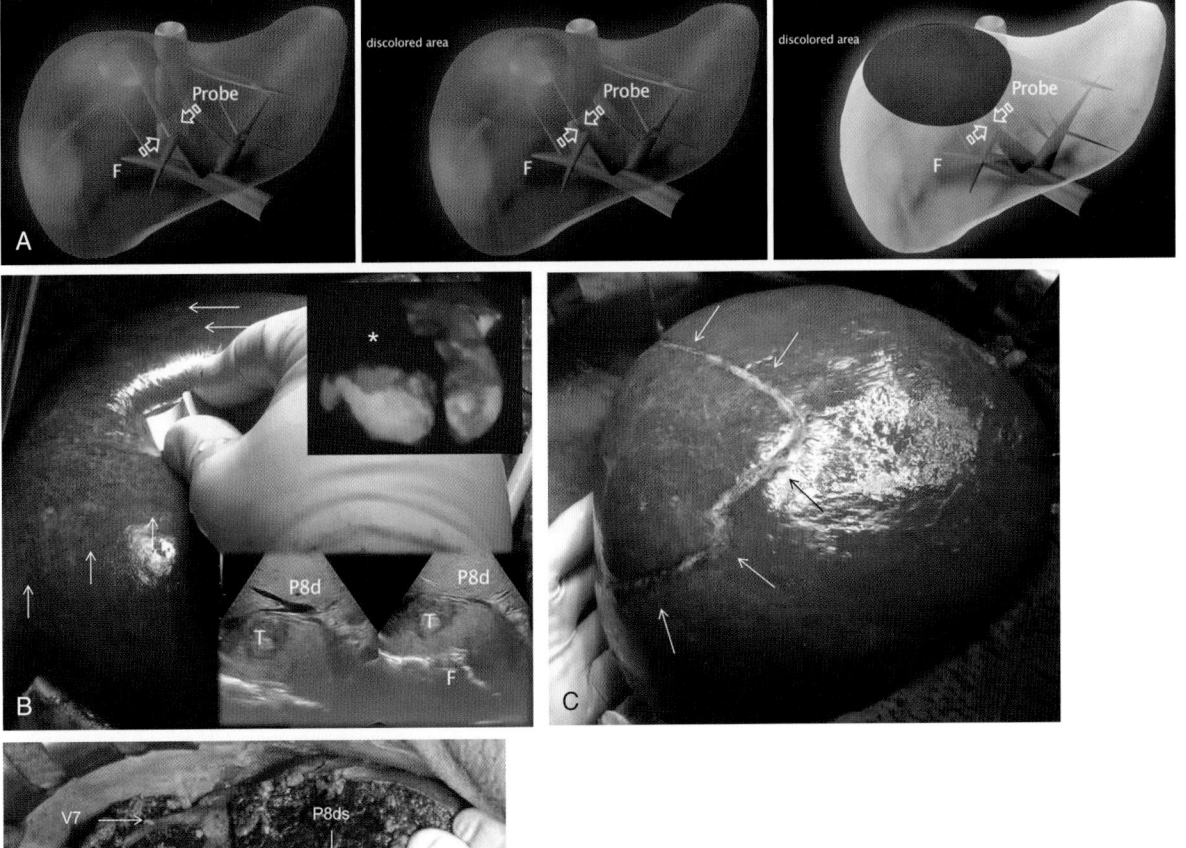

FIGURE 103.33   A, From left to right, the schema shows the compression technique with indocyanine green (ICG) counter-fluorescence, featured by the identification of the pedicle *(left)*, its compression with parenchyma discoloring *(center)*, the ICG-enhanced contrast between the compressed segment, and the rest of the liver *(right)*. **B,** Under intraoperative ultrasound (IOUS) guidance *(right-inferior box)*, portal pedicle to subsegment VIII dorsal *(P8d)* compression is carried out *(arrows)* with the probe and the surgeon's finger *(F)* positioned on the opposite side; compression results in discoloration of the subsegment *(white arrows)*, emphasized *(white asterisk)* by the ICG intravenous injection carried out by the anesthesiologist, which enhances the adjacent parenchyma *(right-upper box)*. **C,** Arrows indicate the defined resection area marked on the liver surface with the electrocautery. **D,** Cut surface at the end of the segment VIII dorsal resection showing the right hepatic vein *(RHV)* with its branch draining segment VII *(V7)*, and the stump *(P8ds)*.

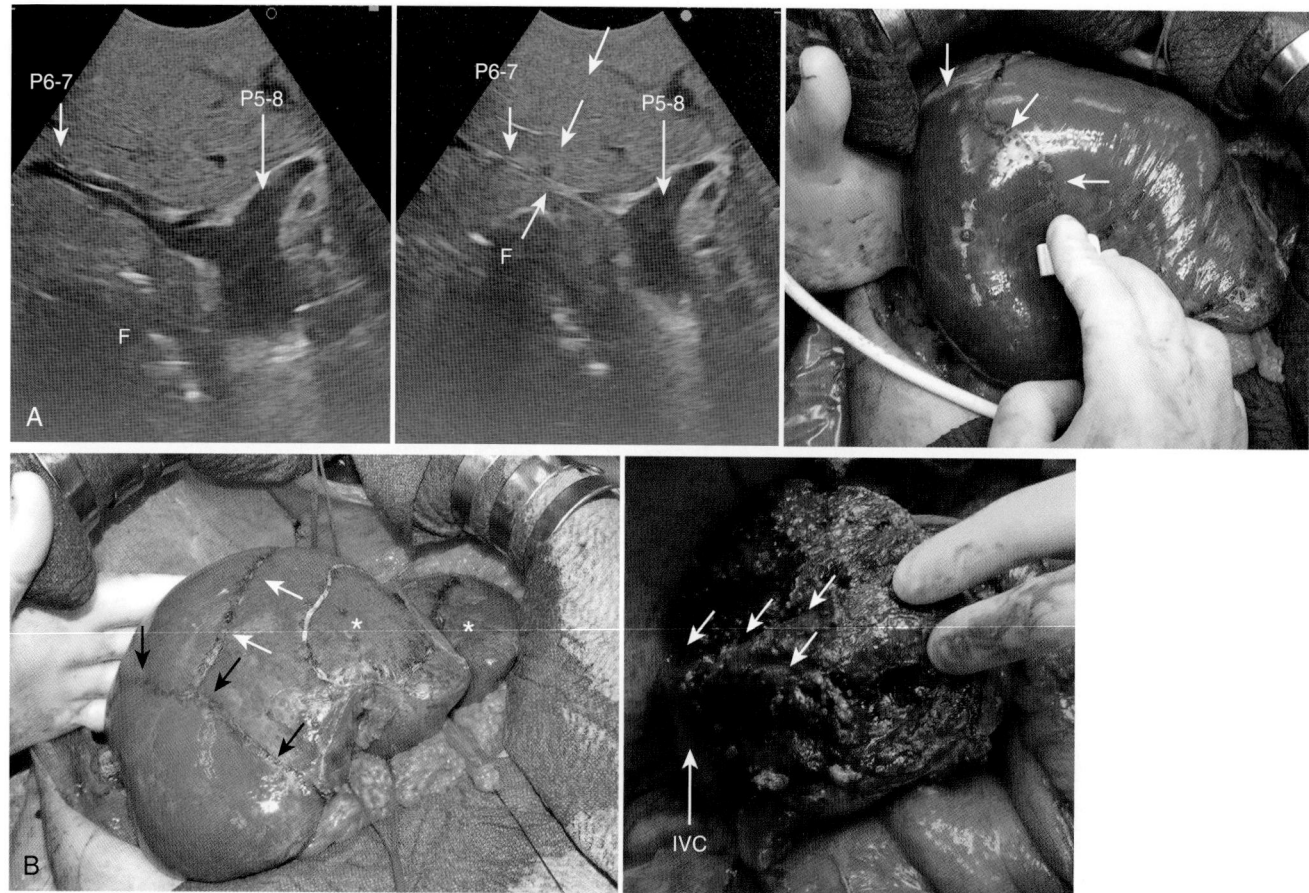

FIGURE 103.34   A, From left to right, the intraoperative ultrasound (IOUS) scan shows the sectional portal branches for the anterior *(P5-8)* and posterior *(P6-7)* sections; to disclose the margins of the right posterior section in the eventuality of a right posterior sectionectomy, under IOUS guidance, P6-7 compression is carried out *(arrows)* with the probe and the surgeon's finger *(F)* positioned on the opposite side; compression results in discoloration of the right posterior section to be removed *(arrows)*, and the area is marked with electrocautery. **B,** In this case carrier of multiple bilobar colorectal metastases, an atypical extension to segment VII *(white arrows)* of the area to be resected corresponding to the right posterior section *(black arrows)* was needed, as were associated other resections areas in the left hemiliver *(asterisks)*; the cut surface previously of the liver at the end of the extended right posterior sectionectomy: Arrows indicate the right hepatic vein *(RHV)* fully exposed. *IVC,* Inferior vena cava.

At IOUS, the portal pedicle for the right posterior section (segments VI and VII) is identified as well as the branches for segments VI and VII; the level targeted for compression is then decided (Fig. 103.34). The surgeon's nondominant hand is positioned behind the right hemiliver, and the probe is positioned with the dominant hand to show the sectional portal branch at the level of interest, which corresponds to the most distal portion of the vessel in relation to its origin but proximal to the tumor to be removed.

The surgeon next uses the fingertips of the nondominant hand and the IOUS probe as instruments to compress the liver bilaterally at the targeted position, resulting in compression of the sectional portal branch in the previously identified tract. When there is no common sectional pedicle to segments VI and VII, compression is applied to the respective segmental portal pedicle as previously described. This maneuver is constantly monitored in real time by IOUS by means of the probe used for compression, and compression is maintained until the surface of the right posterior section lateral to the compression site starts to discolor (see Fig. 103.34A). At this time, the assistant marks the discolored area with the electrocautery device, and the compression is released. In this way, a three-dimensional (3D)

plane has been drawn on the liver surface that passes through portal branch at the level of compression; liver resection is then carried out following this plane (see Fig. 103.34B).

For right posterior sectionectomy, the demarcation could be emphasized adopting the counter-fluorescence technique, as described for segmentectomies.[64]

Right Anterior Sectionectomy. Similarly, as for the right posterior section, the hilar dissection or the encirclement of the sectional GPs are the most commonly adopted techniques for defining the resection area in a fully anatomic manner. The counter-compression technique has also been applied for this purpose.[61] The portal pedicle feeding the right posterior section (segments VI and VII) is identified at IOUS, and the level targeted for compression is then detected just after its origin from the right portal branch (see Fig. 103.34A). Demarcation of the right posterior section is carried out as previously described. To demarcate the left-sided demarcation line, the left PV (LPV) is identified at IOUS, and the level targeted for compression is then identified just past its origin from the main PV. LPV compression is performed and is released once Cantlie's line becomes evident by left hemiliver discoloration, and it is demarcated with electrocautery. Once the right anterior section is defined, resection can be performed.

In this case, the ICG fluorescence could play a relevant role as well. Counter-compression of the right posterior GP is carried out: the right anterior section and the left hemiliver become fluorescent and the right-sided dissection plane margin becomes more evident.[64] In the event of a tumor thrombus occluding the right anterior portal branch, as described for the segmentectomy, the counter-fluorescence can be realized just by clamping the proper hepatic artery and intravenously injecting the ICG (Fig. 103.35).

ANATOMIC RESECTIONS BY EXTRAPARENCHYMAL SELECTIVE CLAMPING OF THE GLISSONEAN PEDICLE (SEE CHAPTER 102B).

The segmental portal branches to segment IV are generally divided into two groups, those for the superior and those for the inferior portion, but the most common branching pattern can be recognized in only half of patients.[70] As an alternative to the compression or staining techniques, the segment IV branches can be approached by dissecting the umbilical portion. Once exposed, the vessel can be encircled with a suture then pulled, under IOUS control, to verify that the branch that moves on the US machine screen is the one to the inferior portion of segment IV. Clamping that branch should allow segment IV inferior demarcation, which, upon pedicle ligation and division, can be removed selectively; this is an application of the so-called "hooking technique."[71] The superior portion of subsegment IV could be resected by clamping the portal branch to the inferior portion because it is identified with the hooking technique; the discolored subsegment IV inferior caudally, the plane that includes the middle HV (MHV) laterally (as seen on IOUS), and that marked by the falciform ligament medially delimit the area to be resected.

LIMITED RESECTIONS (SEE CHAPTER 102).

Selection of an anatomic or nonanatomic resection for HCC, although a controversial issue,[72–77] is leaning in favor of the anatomic approach.[56,63,78,79] In contrast, limited resection is commonly accepted as an oncologically proper approach for CLM.[80] For limited resections, IOUS guidance plays a fundamental role as well. Indeed, although there is no need to identify exactly the area of the liver fed by the portal branch to be ligated, IOUS guidance allows us to tailor the resection area unless it results smooth and warrants enough resection margin in respect to the liver anatomy and the oncologic requirements. In practice, once the tumor is identified on IOUS, the surgeon can mark the border of the lesion and that of the area to be removed on the surface of the liver with electrocautery under IOUS control. To perform this maneuver, the flat and thin tip of the electrocautery device is positioned between the probe and the liver surface. This results in a shadow on the IOUS image that runs deep just below the electrocautery (Fig. 103.36A). In this way, it is possible to define the position of the electrocautery device with the tumor edge and consequently to mark the nodule profile on the liver surface with electrocautery and select the safer edge for the incision. The adequacy of the marked edge can be further checked with IOUS because the air trapped between the probe and the irregular surface of the demarcation line drawn with electrocautery on the liver surface can be visualized on IOUS and are similar to the images that result from electrocautery (Fig. 103.37).

Additionally, with the probe positioned on the liver surface at the site of the resection margin previously drawn, the surgeon can use a fingertip to push at the opposite edge of the resection area so that the profile of the resection area is visualized on IOUS (see Fig. 103.36A). Consequently, structures between the fingertip and the tumor edge can be precisely estimated, the resection area can be marked on the liver surface, and the dissection plane is visualized. Once the resection area is drawn on the liver surface, the main target to be obtained is such that at the end of the dissection, the cut surface is oriented smooth and regular (see Fig. 103.36D).

LIVER PARENCHYMA DISSECTION.

The main advantage of IOUS-guided resection is that it modifies the traditional way to dissect the liver tissue, which was originally done on vertical planes to avoid the tumor exposure on the cut surface. IOUS allows the surgeon to follow the dissection plane in real time, to see it constantly in relation to the tumor edge, and then to modify its direction when needed. This is because the dissection plane can be visualized on the IOUS image, which appears as an echogenic line because of the entrapment of air bubbles and clots between facing cut surfaces (see Fig. 103.36B). If the dissection plane is not clearly visible, it can be better visualized by inserting plain gauze (see Fig. 103.36B) between facing surfaces. These techniques allow the surgeon to keep the proper dissection plane and recognize an improper one early. In this way, it is possible to carry out a rounded trajectory of the dissection plane around the tumor, avoiding tumor exposure, its eventual disruption, and potentially cancer seeding, as well as allowing the surgeon to spare important vascular structures. This results in more conservative but radical treatments and in a lower rate of major hepatectomies.

The artifacts that may appear on IOUS sometimes mask structures critical to the dissection plan, such as portal branches, which should be either ligated or preserved. For this reason, to better visualize the targeted point where the portal branch should be divided, the "hooking technique" has been devised.[81] When the Glissonean sheath is exposed and skeletonized, it is encircled with a stitch. Under US control, the stitch hooking the exposed vessel is then gently pulled up, which stretches the portal branch slightly; this traction point is demonstrated clearly by IOUS (see Fig. 103.36C). If the exposed portal branch is not clearly visible because it has collapsed, the portal triad is unclamped. If the target site is correct, the portal branch is ligated and divided, and resection is completed under IOUS guidance. Conversely, if the exposed vessel was not the targeted one, it is spared, and unnecessary sacrifice of further liver parenchyma is avoided.

A practical example of using the hooking technique is during ventral or dorsal subsegmentectomy of segment VIII. The portal trunk to this segment may show bifurcation in its dorsal branch and ventral trunk near the origin of the portal vessel to segment V. In this situation, there is the risk of ligating and dividing the portal branch of segment V, instead of the planned subsegmental branch of segment VIII, and necrosis of segment V may occur. Under IOUS control, the hooking technique enables the identification of the branch, which was encircled, and then the surgeon can decide with certainty whether to ligate it.

The hooking technique is also useful with tumor thrombus in portal branches.[13] Once the portal branch is skeletonized, it is encircled with a stitch, which is gently pulled up under IOUS control; this traction stretches the portal branch slightly, and the traction point is demonstrated clearly by IOUS (Fig. 103.38). If the traction point is not at the level of the tumor thrombus, it is possible to ligate the portal branch and proceed with the liver resection, ensuring that the thrombus will not migrate because of surgical manipulation.

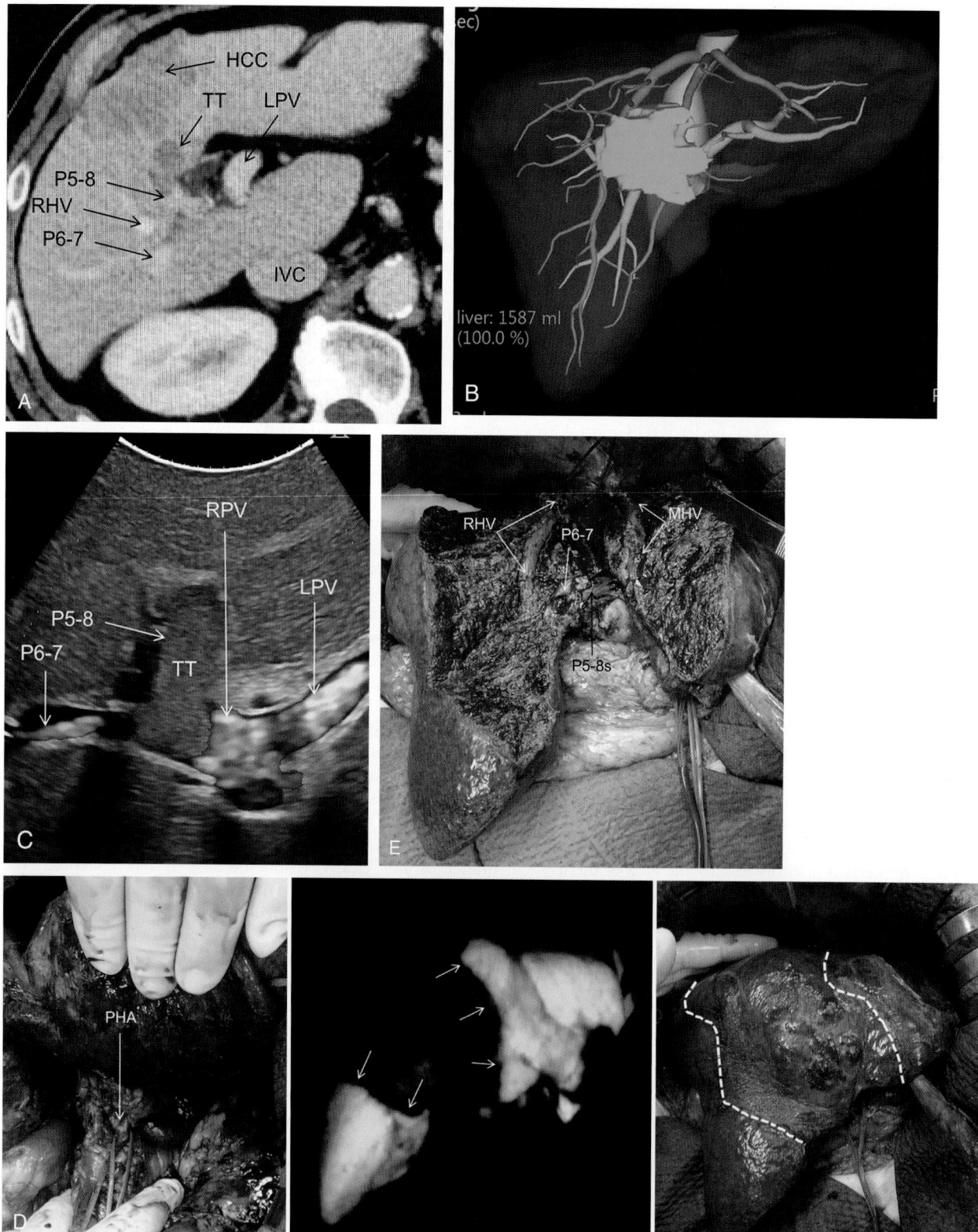

FIGURE 103.35   A, Computed tomography (CT) slice showing a hepatocellular carcinoma *(HCC)* with infiltrative growing pattern with a tumor thrombus *(TT)* occupying the portal pedicle to the right anterior section *(P5-8; see Chapter 14).* **B,** Virtual cast based on the CT images with the lesion in green. **C,** IOUS image of the TT occluding P5-8 and bulging into the right portal vein *(RPV).* **D,** From left to right, isolation of the proper hepatic artery *(PHA),* which is clamped before indocyanine green (ICG) intravenous injection carried out by the anesthesiologist; after clamping the PHA and injecting ICG, the right anterior section remains dark *(white arrows)* while the area beside the liver enhances and the resection area is marked *(white dotted lines).* **E,** Resection is carried out, exposing both the right *(RHV),* and the middle hepatic vein *(MHV)*; the right posterior Glissonean pedicle *(P6-7)* is preserved, and P5-8 is resected *(P5-8s)* after having cleared by means of peeling off technique of the right portal vein.[69] *IVC,* Inferior vena cava

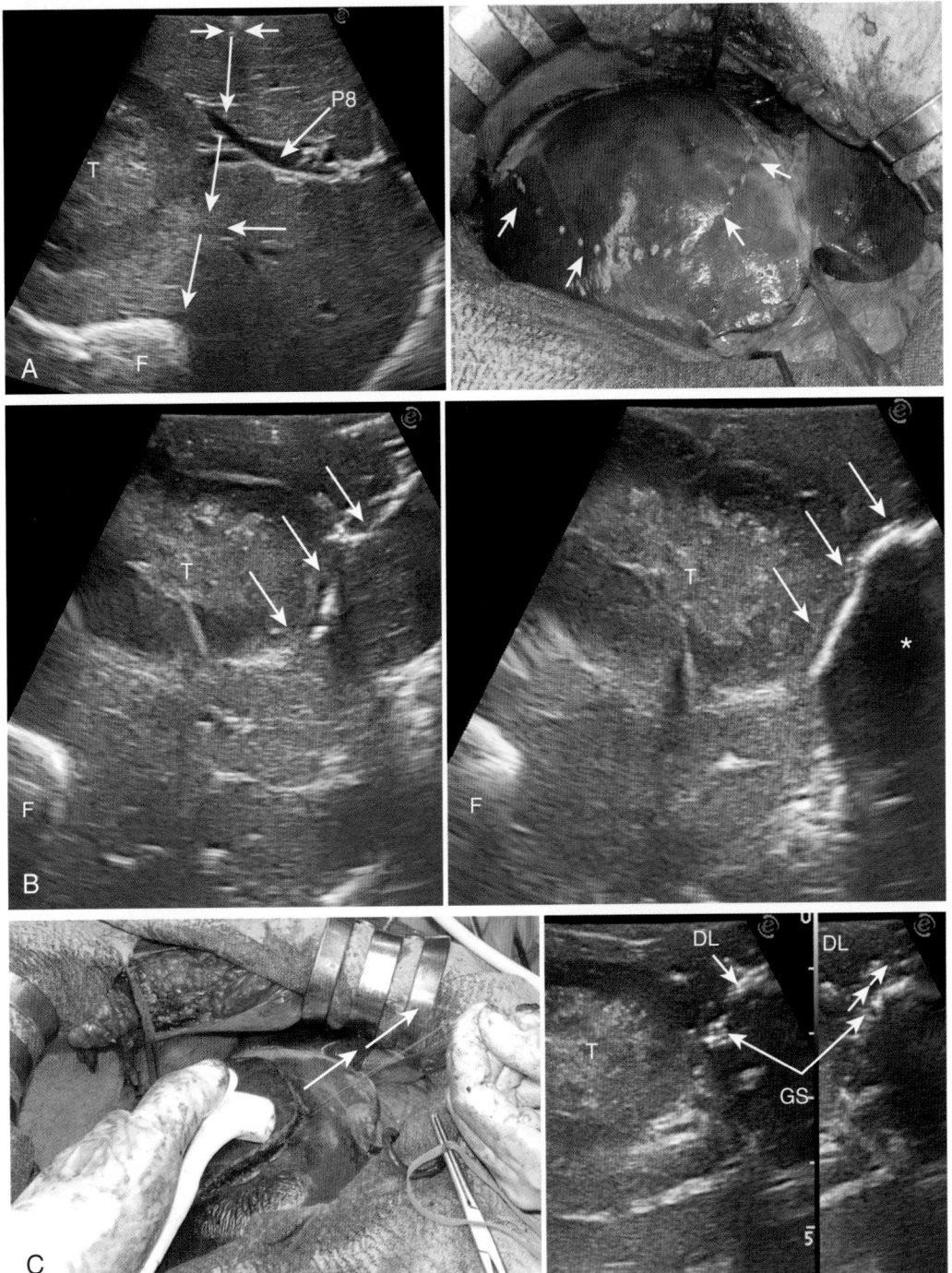

FIGURE 103.36   A, On the left, both the shadow generated by the electrocautery *(thick arrows)* and the profile of the surgeon's finger *(F)* are visualized, and the surgeon can draw an ideal dissection plane *(arrows)* that can be followed as shown on the right once the resection area is marked using these landmarks *(arrows).* **B,** Dissection is carried out and followed by intraoperative ultrasound (IOUS) just targeting the surgeon's fingertip *(F)*; the dissection line is visualized, as shown on the left, taking stock of the air and clots trapped between the faced cut surfaces *(arrows)*, or, as shown on the right, by using a gauze interposed between the faced cut surfaces *(arrows)*. The first method makes less evident the dissection line, while the second, although making the dissection line clearer, masks with its posterior echo (*) the deeper structures. **C,** Once during dissection a vessel is encountered and encircled with suture, its discrimination between a vessel that should be preserved or divided can be done by adopting the so-called "hooking technique." Particularly in the case of the bifurcation between portal branch to segment V and segment VIII, the encircled vessel is pulled up by the stitch *(arrows)* and at intraoperative ultrasound (IOUS) the visualization of the traction point makes sure which vessel is the one encircled, then it is preserved or divided, accordingly.

Continued

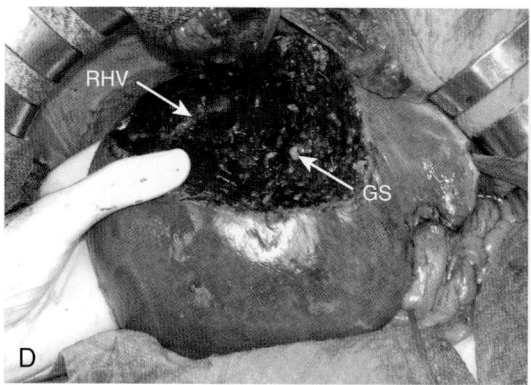
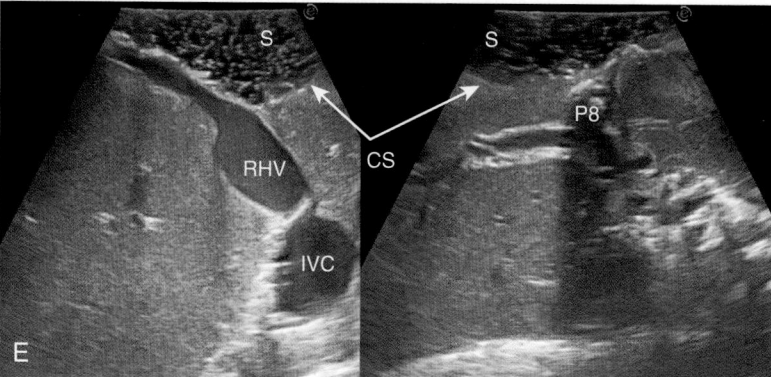

FIGURE 103.36, cont'd   D, The cut surface at the end of the resection showing the right hepatic vein *(RHV)* exposed, and the ligated Glissonean sheath *(GS)* of the limited resection with exposure of the tract of the MHV, which was in contact with the lesion. **E,** The cut surface *(CS)* of the end of the resection can be checked at IOUS for verifying the eventual presence of residual disease by putting some saline on it *(S)*. *DL,* Dissection line; *IVC,* inferior vena cava; *P8,* portal branch to segment VIII.

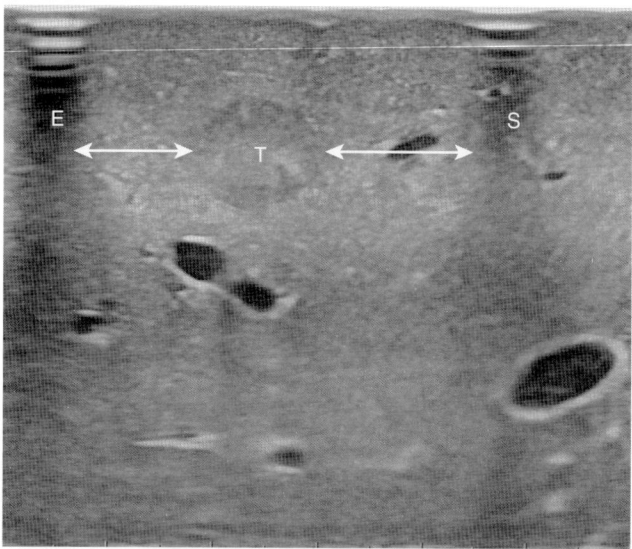

FIGURE 103.37 Intraoperative ultrasound shows both the electrocautery *(E)* and the scar *(S)*. A vertical shadow is generated that allows verification of the proper margins of resection in relation to the tumor *(T)* location *(arrows)*.

During liver dissection, the backflow bleeding from the HVs is an important source of blood loss, and it is one of the most important factors in determining the short- and long-term outcome; therefore limiting the backflow bleeding from the HVs is a priority in liver resections. A US-guided technique is simple and effective for backflow bleeding control.[82] Once the hepatocaval confluence is exposed anteriorly (Fig. 103.39), dissection proceeds until the surgeon's fingertip is able to compress the targeted HV at its caval confluence; the effectiveness of this maneuver is checked by color flow (CF)–IOUS (Fig. 103.40).

POSTRESECTIONAL CONTROL. After nodule removal, IOUS offers two options for specimen handling. The "water bath" technique consists of real-time control of the proper resection of the targeted nodule, verifying its complete inclusion in the specimen removed from the liver (Fig. 103.41).[83] The second option

involves checking the cut surface, which is refilled with saline to avoid the artifacts generated by the residual air bubbles and clots (Fig. 103.42; see also Fig. 103.36E).

In patients who require major resection, color Doppler IOUS allows the proper positioning of the remnant liver such that there is no partial occlusion or turbulence of the inflow and outflow in terms of velocity and waveform (Fig. 103.43).[84]

INTRAOPERATIVE CHOLANGIO-ULTRASOUND. Intraoperative US can be used to delineate the intrahepatic bile duct anatomy and its variants even when not dilated (Fig. 103.44; see Chapters 2 and 16). CE-IOUS may also play a role in this sense because it provides a negative image of the biliary tree compared with the enhanced surrounding liver parenchyma. On the other hand, bile duct injury during major hepatectomy occurs in 8% of patients and in 22% of left-sided major resections and can be life threatening[85] (see Chapters 28, 42, 101, and 118). Bile duct injury can be reduced by performing intraoperative cholangiography, which still represents the gold standard for studying the biliary tract anatomy and for guiding reconstruction in cases of bile duct resection. Furthermore, with the advent of living-donor transplantation, it is the standard reference for validating preoperative imaging.[86] However, IOUS could have a role in the study of the biliary tree for checking its integrity and the proper drainage after bile duct resection.[22]

Intrahepatic Biliary Tree Integrity. It is crucial to confirm biliary tree integrity after suspicion of damage during surgical dissection to avoid postoperative morbidity and the resulting need for invasive procedures and even redo surgery. This can be done by using a simple, self-made contrast agent that can be visualized on IOUS, thereby providing a real-time intraoperative cholangio-ultrasound (IOCUS). The contrast agent consists of a compound of air and saline, the respective amount of which varies from that of pure air (Fig. 103.45) to that representing the same amount of saline and air. The latter should be the preferred method for examining anatomic detail, although similar anatomic information can be provided with the injection of pure air. Indeed, once the air is injected slowly, its progressive mixture with the bile juice provides anatomic details too (Fig. 103.46A). In contrast, when air is injected under pressure, a parenchymatous effect is obtained (see Fig. 103.46B), which is useful for checking the integrity of the biliary tract draining a specific portion of the liver. Nonetheless,

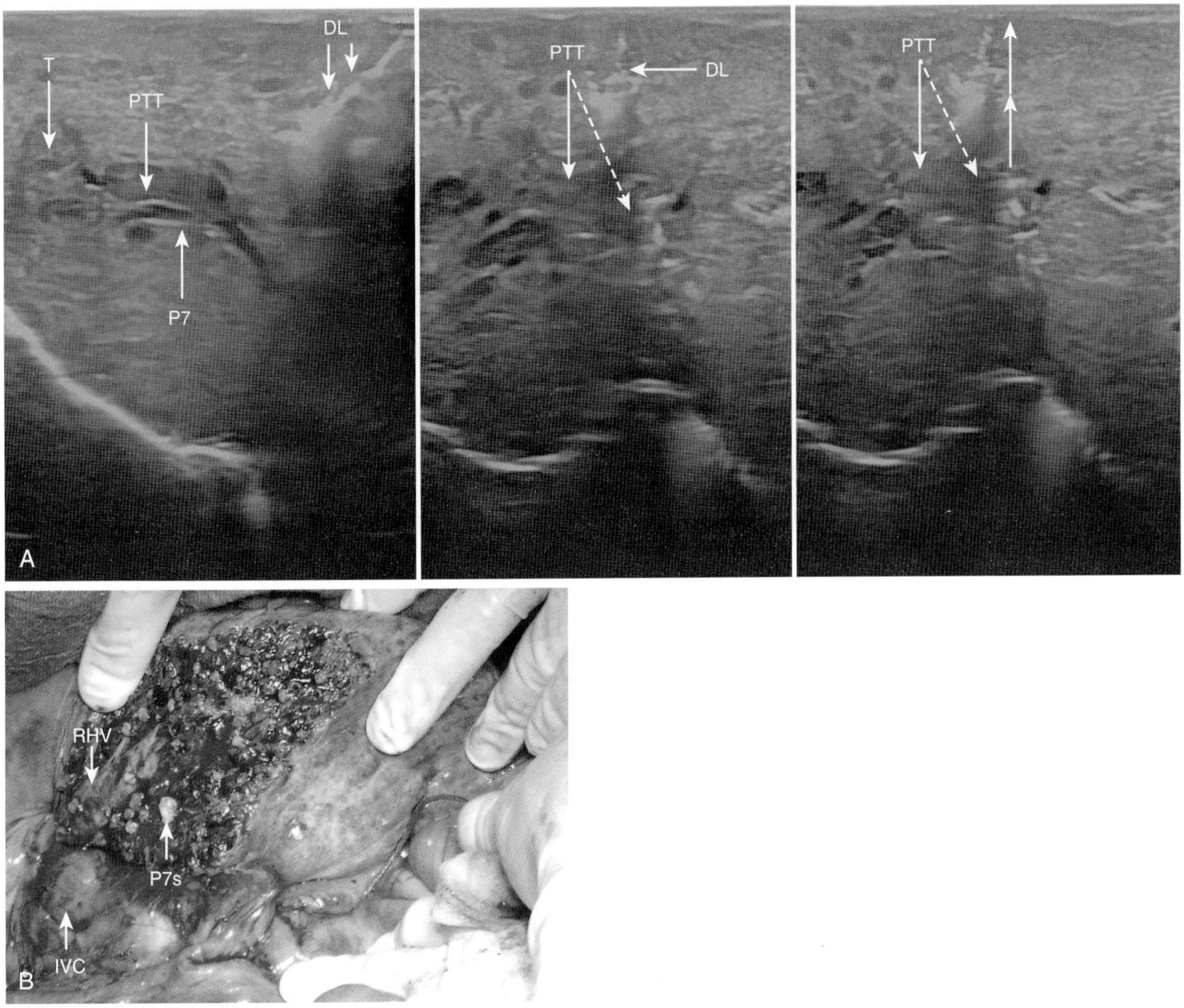

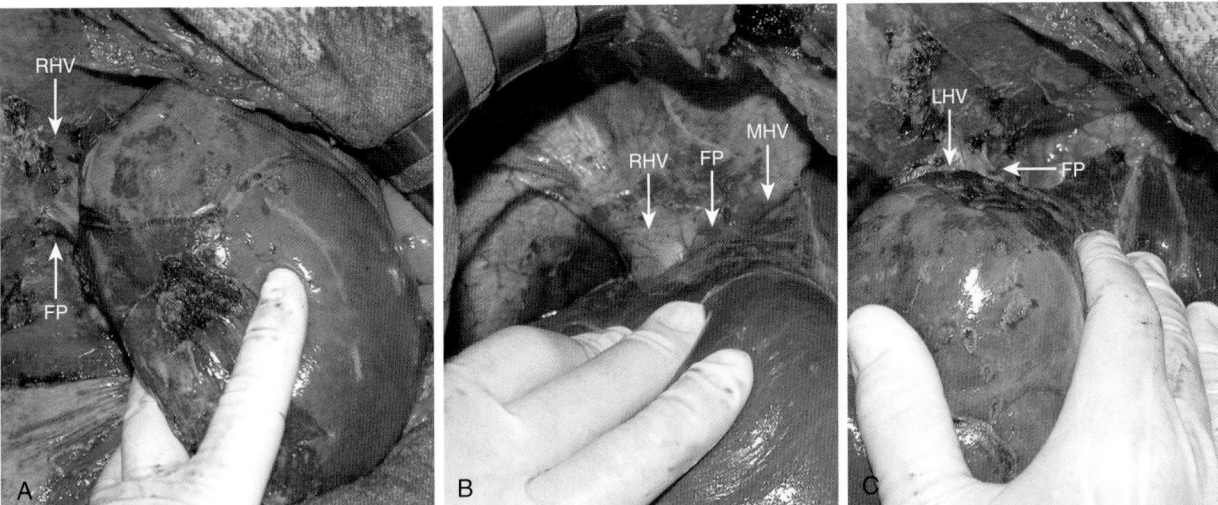

FIGURE 103.38   **A,** From left to tight, a tumor thrombus *(PTT)* in the portal branch to segment VII *(P7)* is visualized at intraoperative ultrasound (IOUS) and progressively reached through the dissection line *(DL)*; once P7 has been achieved and encircled with suture, it is pulled up and the level of the encirclement with respect to the PTT is confirmed by the traction *(dashed arrows).* **B,** Once the integrity of the PTT is confirmed by the previously shown hooking maneuver, the resection is carried out and at the end the cut surface shows the full exposure of the right hepatic vein *(RHV)* and the stump of P7 *(P7s). IVC,* Inferior vena cava; *T,* tumor.

FIGURE 103.39   From left to right, the hepatocaval confluence preparation for intraoperative ultrasound–guided compression maneuvers on the right hepatic vein *(RHV)*, the middle hepatic vein *(MHV),* and the left hepatic vein *(LHV). FP,* Fingertip position.

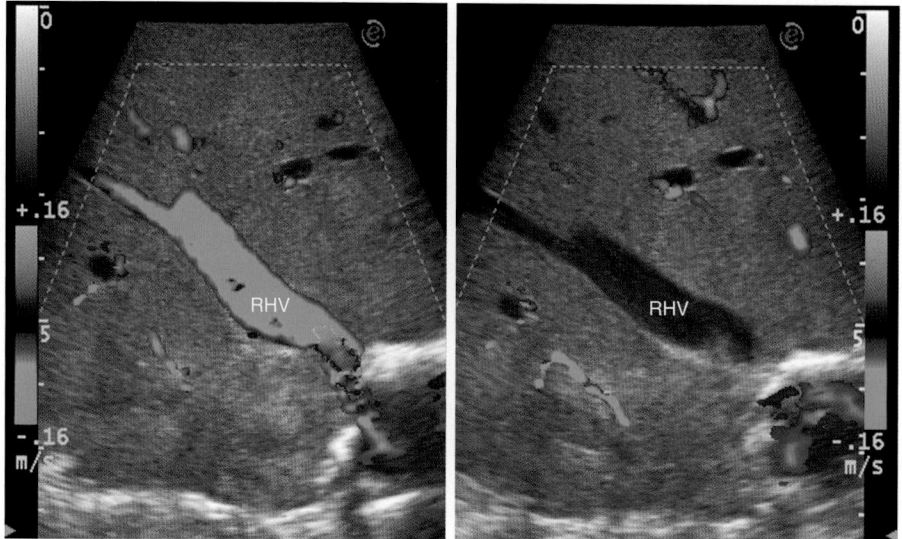

FIGURE 103.40 Once the vein, in this case the right hepatic vein *(RHV),* to be compressed is visualized at color-flow intraoperative ultrasound (IOUS), the compression results in the disappearance of the color flow inside the compressed vein.

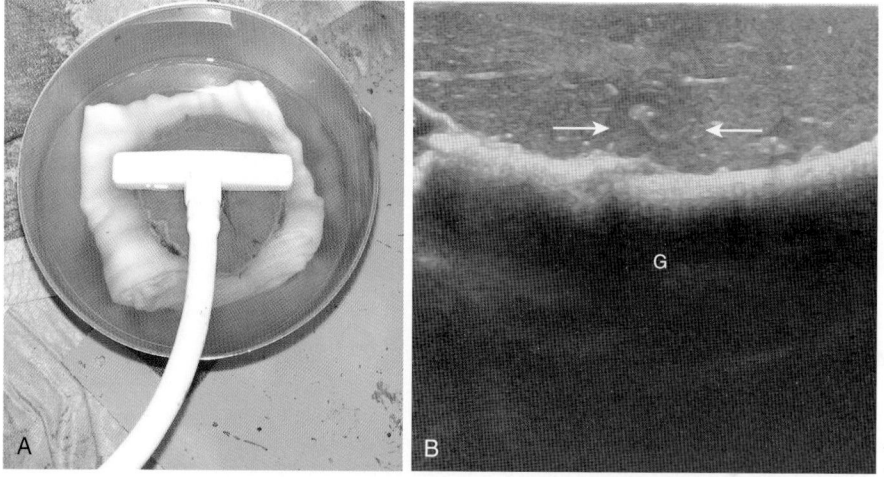

FIGURE 103.41 From left to right, the water-bath technique for checking the surgical specimen; the inclusion of the targeted nodule *(arrows)* is confirmed at intraoperative ultrasound (IOUS). *G,* Gauzes.

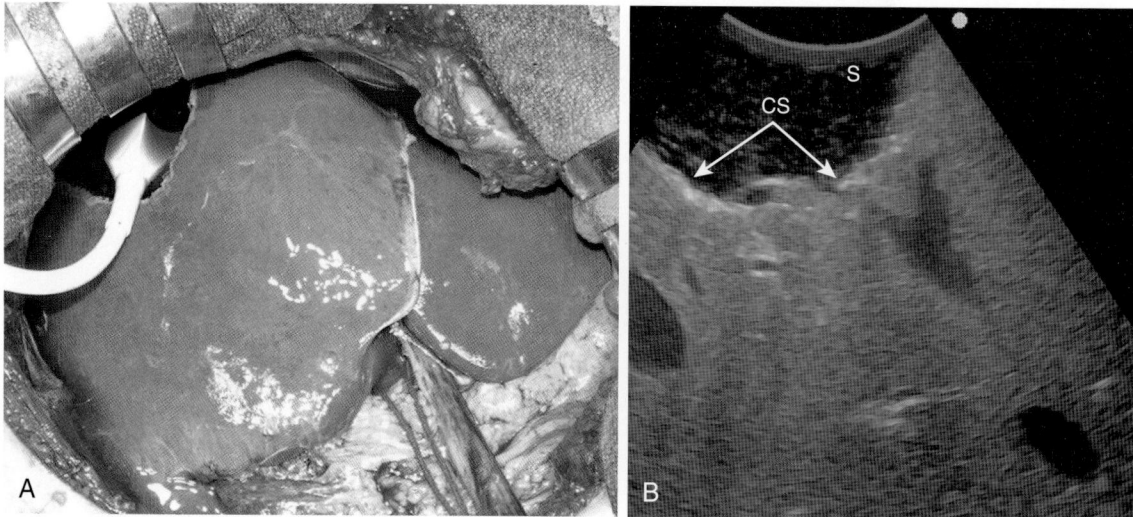

FIGURE 103.42 For further control, particularly if the inclusion of the lesion in the specimen is not confirmed, the cut surface *(CS)* filled with saline *(S)* can be explored with intraoperative ultrasound (IOUS).

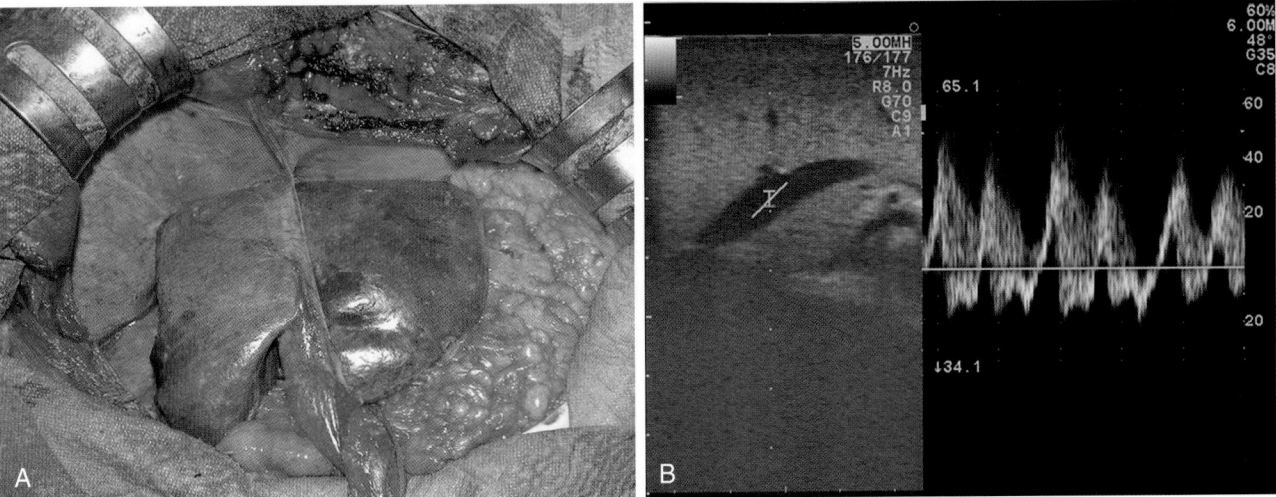

FIGURE 103.43 If a right hepatectomy is carried out **(A),** the proper repositioning of the remnant liver is performed using color Doppler to see whether the proper outflow is obtained with a triphasic wave pattern as shown **(B).**

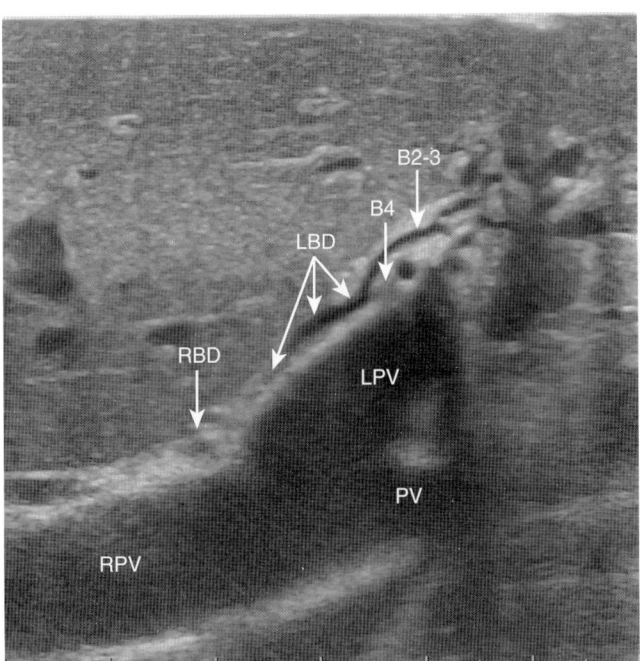

FIGURE 103.44 Intraoperative ultrasound (IOUS) per se could provide anatomic details of the intrahepatic biliary tree even if not dilated by taking stock of the main anatomic feature of it, which has a centripetal bifurcation pattern: herein, are recognizable in a single scan the right biliary duct *(RBD),* the left bile duct *(LBD),* the one draining the segment IV *(B4),* and the one draining segments II and III *(B2-3). LPV,* Left portal vein; *PV,* portal vein; *RPV,* right portal vein.

the injection of air in the biliary tree is anyhow useful also to rule out the presence of bile leaks on the cut surface: the so-called "air-leak test."[87]

Proper Drainage of Bile Duct Stump. The proper biliary drainage of the remnant liver once a bile duct has been resected is critical. This is particularly true in patients operated on for perihilar cholangiocarcinoma. To verify drainage, IOCUS in a parenchymatous phase can be used for identifying undrained liver segments (Fig. 103.47).

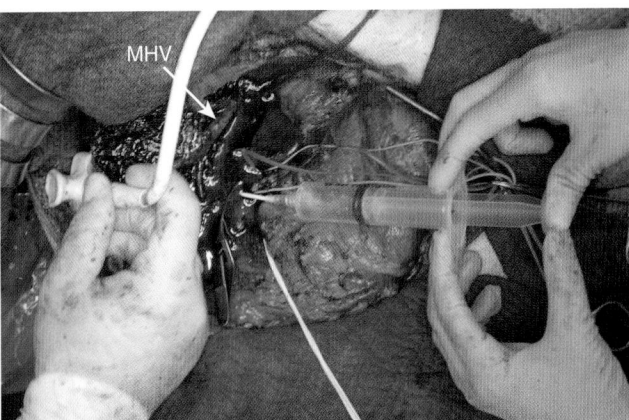

FIGURE 103.45 Injection of air into the stump of the left hepatic duct after the accomplishment of the left hepatectomy. *MHV,* Middle hepatic vein. (See Chapter 24.)

Vessel-Guided Hepatectomy

The Tumor and the Intrahepatic Vessels

Major intrahepatic vessels, namely GPs and HVs, are key structures distinguishing different parts of the liver (see Chapter 2). GP and HV are separated by the liver parenchyma not just by the Glissonean sheath, and the vein wall respectively, but also by the *Laennec* capsule as the IVC itself is.[88] With these premises, detaching a tumor from the intrahepatic vessel (R1vasc) rather than from the liver parenchyma (R1par) could be considered. The encouraging preliminary findings featuring similar recurrence risk of R1vasc and R0 surgery, initially for HCC,[13,14] and subsequently for CLM, and even mass-forming cholangiocarcinoma (MFCCC),[89] confirmed the initial impression. More recently, larger series for CLM[90] and HCC[91] support clinically the reliability of R1vasc, which conversely could not be confirmed for MFCCC.[92] This last finding further sustains the peculiarity of an aggressive growth pattern of MFCCC[93] for which the R1vasc should be limited just to patients otherwise unresectable. Possibly, further investigation may disclose which subgroup of MFCCC is more prone to recur. For now, despite

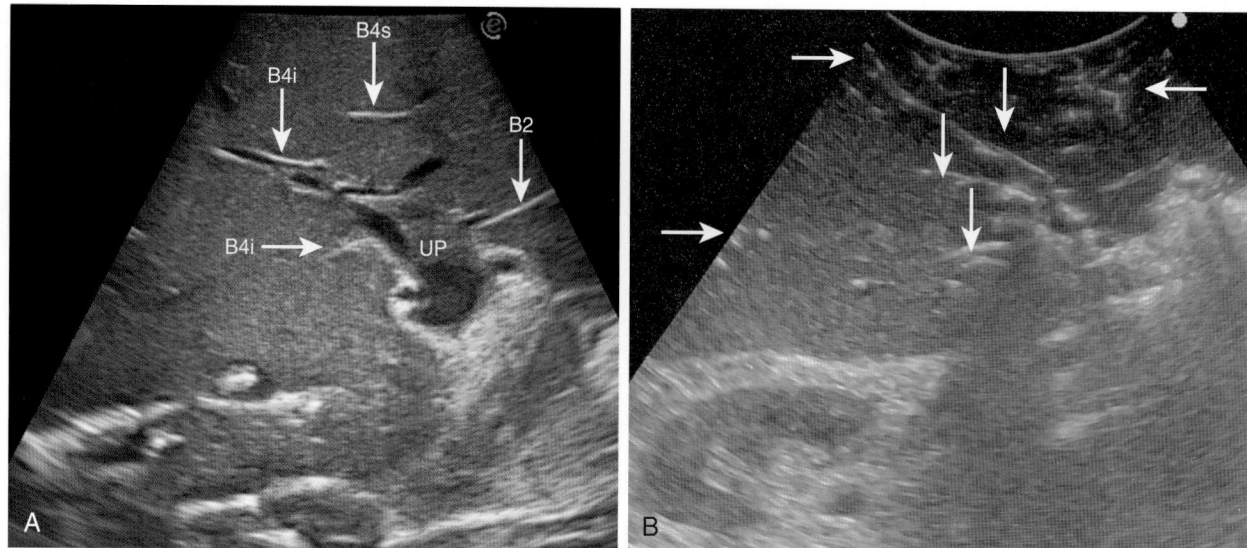

FIGURE 103.46 A, Once the air is injected slowly, and then it mixes with the bile juice, the anatomy of the biliary tree can be detailed at intraoperative ultrasound cholangiography; in this image, the bile ducts draining segment II *(B2)*, segment III *(B3)*, subsegment IV inferior *(B4i)*, and subsegment IV superior *(B4s)* are visualized. **B,** If the injection is carried out more rapidly, the parenchyma with all the peripheral bile ducts appear evident *(arrows)*. *UP,* Umbilical portion.

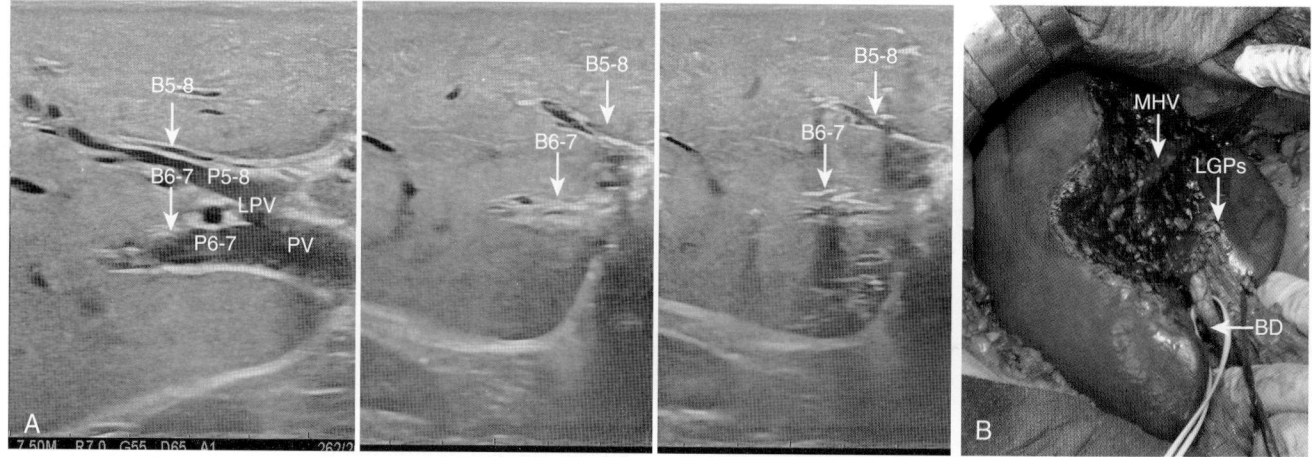

FIGURE 103.47 A, From left to right, the intraoperative ultrasound cholangiography carried out without contrast injection in which it can be recognized the anatomy disclosing the portal branch to the right anterior section *(P5-8)*, originating from the left portal vein (LPV): Bile ducts draining right anterior section *(B5-8)*, and the right posterior one *(B6-7)* are evident; once air is injected into the stump of the left bile duct after its division, having the pedicle still clamped (Pringle maneuver), B6-7 and B5-8 are enhanced confirming the integrity of the right sided intrahepatic biliary tree. **B,** The cut surface at the end of the left hepatectomy. *LGPs,* Left Glissonean pedicle stump; *LHV,* left hepatic vein; *P6-7,* portal branch to the right posterior section.

its limited suitability, challenging R1vasc in MFCCC patients can widen the therapeutic options in conditions otherwise not amenable to other alternatives.

Schematically the R1vasc policy according to the type of tumor removed is represented in Figure 103.48.

TUMOR IN CONTACT WITH GLISSONEAN PEDICLE. The GP may be spared even when an encapsulated HCC or a CLM is in contact. The integrity of the vessel wall can be appreciated with IOUS, and lack of involvement can be further confirmed by the absence of bile duct dilation (Fig. 103.49). Bile duct dilation, presence of tumor thrombus, and invasion of the vessel wall

usually require pedicle division (Figs. 103.50 and 103.51). In these conditions, an R1vasc resection could not be carried out and extension of the hepatectomy should be pursued for complete tumor clearance.

TUMOR IN CONTACT WITH HEPATIC VEIN. Similar to the GP, the HV may be spared when in contact with an encapsulated HCC or a CLM. The integrity of the vessel wall can be appreciated on IOUS (Figs. 103.52 and 103.53). Given the integrity of the vessel wall, contact extension less than two-thirds of the vein circumference at IOUS would allow the HV sparing (Figs. 103.54 and 103.55A,B,F). In any event, in the case of partial infiltration of the HV wall, a

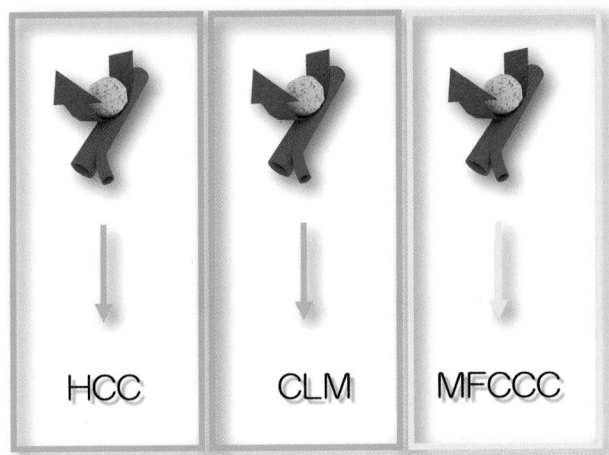

FIGURE 103.48   This schema visually emphasizes the oncologic suitability of R1vasc in the case of hepatocellular carcinoma *(HCC)* and colorectal liver metastases *(CLM)*, whereas in the case of mass-forming cholangiocarcinoma *(MFCCC)*, it is considered just in case of otherwise unresectability.

partial resection with reconstruction by direct suture or patching can still allow preservation of the original venous outflow; this was the case in more the one-third of our patients with colorectal liver metastases in contact with HV at the caval confluence.[94]

The Outflow

Sometimes R1vasc surgery may not be possible. In the event that the infiltrated major vessel would be a first- or second-order GP, there may be no alternative to removing the involved liver parenchyma together with the infiltrated vessel. Inversely, for the HV, major parenchymal removal should not be considered as inevitable. Several authors have shown the feasibility of grafting an infiltrated HV to spare parenchyma and expand the FLR. Technically sophisticated, HV grafting is possible but associated with high morbidity and mortality[95] (see Chapter 122);

recently, Urbani et al. combined this attitude to R1vasc surgery successfully.[96] Makuuchi et al. in the 1980s suggested the possibility of parenchymal-sparing surgery despite invasion of HV at caval confluence just profiting of the accessory HV as a thick inferior right HV (IRHV),[18] which is present in 15% to 20% of patients.[97] In 2010 we showed that in the presence of tumor-HV contact not amenable to detachment at the caval confluence, a compensatory circulation between the adjacent HVs could almost always be detected.[98] These communicating veins (CVs), once recognized and preserved, can still spare liver parenchyma[94] (Fig. 103.56; see also Fig. 103.55C–F). Given that, an extension of the resection to the liver parenchyma theoretically drained by the HV to be resected is considered only if one of the following US signs is absent:

- Presence of accessory HVs at IOUS, such as an inferior right HV (IRHV; Fig. 103.57)[18] in the presence of an invasion at the caval confluence of the right HV.
- CF-IOUS showing hepatopetal blood flow in the feeding portal branch (Fig. 103.58) once the HV to be resected is clamped[14] by encirclement or finger compression of the vein extrahepatically.[82]
- CVs connecting adjacent HVs, which are more easily detectable using CF-IOUS (Fig. 103.59A; see also Figs. 103.55E and 103.56B).[98]

The Anarchist Anatomic Resections

It has been herein discussed how IOUS guidance is an indispensable tool for driving parenchyma-sparing surgery. Results with R1vasc surgery and the existence and reliability of CV in the event of compromised outflow have added a bit more to that. IOUS, R1vasc, and CV constitute the pillars for something different: the vessel-guided hepatectomies. According to this policy, the surgeon intentionally challenges the major vessels and their exposure and lets them drive the course of the liver resection. Sparing the main GPs and the main HVs allows the surgeon to keep the core of the organ cleared by the tumors and getting towards the core of the liver becomes something to be pursued. Technically, this means searching for pedicles, either GP or HV, just a few millimeters below the liver surface, and

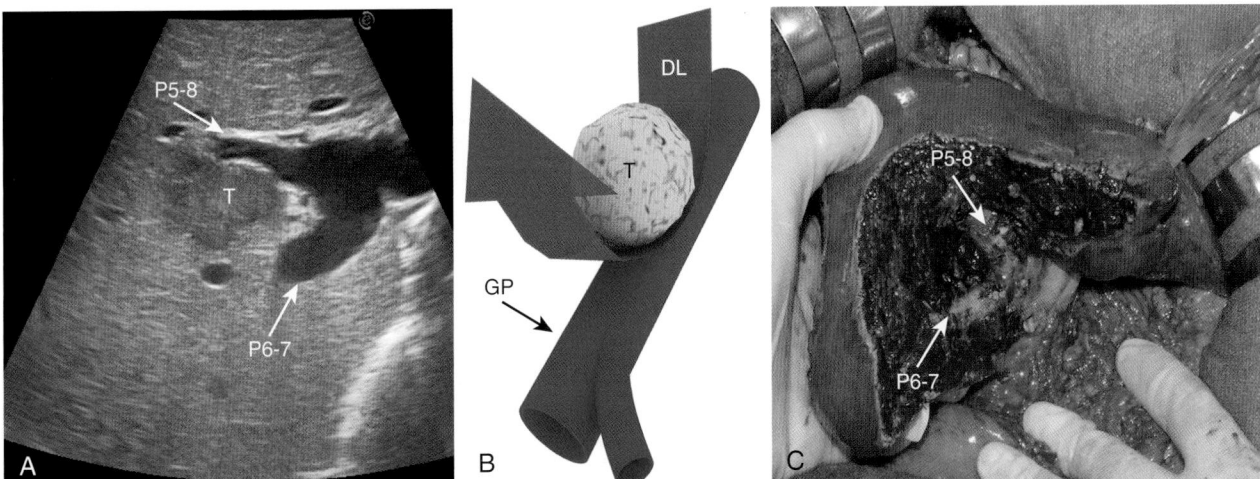

FIGURE 103.49   A, The intraoperative ultrasound (IOUS) shows a tumor *(T)* located in contact with the portal vein branch to the right anterior section *(P5-8)* and to that to the right posterior section *(P6-7).* **B,** The tumor-vessel relations can be classified as shown in the schema. **C,** A parenchyma-sparing resection preserving both P5-8 and P6-7 is then carried out. *DL,* Dissection line; *GP,* Glissonean sheath.

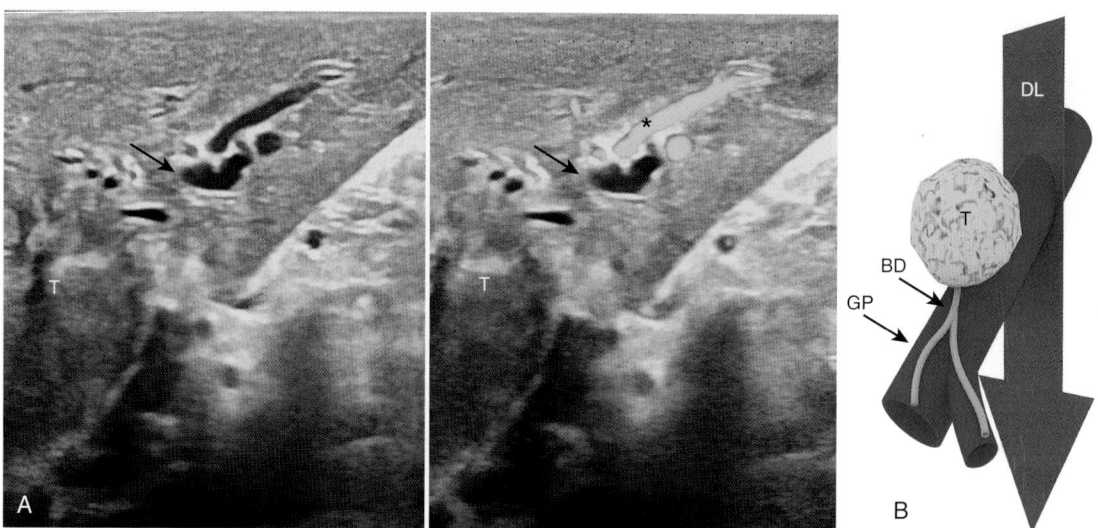

FIGURE 103.50   **A**, On the left, the intraoperative ultrasound (IOUS) shows a tumor *(T)* provoking dilation of the bile duct *(arrows)*, which appears, on the right, as serpiginous and without color filling (*) at color-flow IOUS. **B**, The tumor-vessel relations can be classified as shown in the schema. *BD*, Bile duct; *DL*, dissection line; *GP*, Glissonean pedicle.

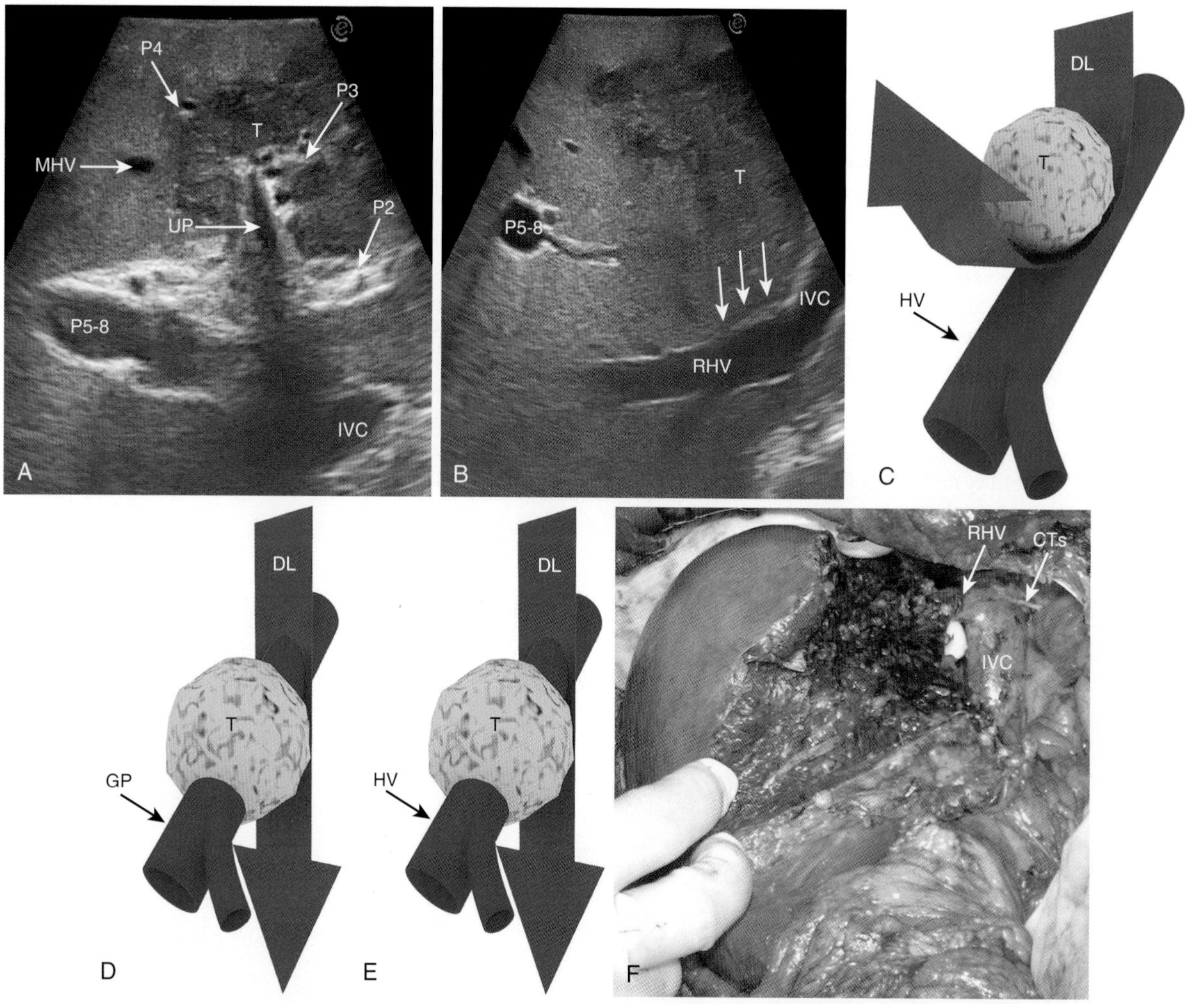

FIGURE 103.51   **A**, The IOUS shows a tumor *(T)* surrounding and encircling the umbilical portion *(UP)*. **B**, The same tumor invades both the middle *(MHV)* and the left hepatic veins and achieves in contact *(arrows)* with the right hepatic vein *(RHV)*. **C–E** show the schemas of the three tumor-vessel relations simultaneously present in this case, which are representative of contact with the hepatic vein *(HV)*, invasion of the Glissonean pedicle *(GP)*, and invasion of a HV, respectively. **F**, A left extended hepatectomy including segments I and VIII and sparing segment V was carried out. *CTs*, Common trunk stump; *DL*, dissection line; *IVC*, inferior vena cava; *P2*, portal branch to segment II; *P3*, portal branch to segment III; *P4*, portal branch to segment IV; *P5-8*, portal branch to the right anterior section.

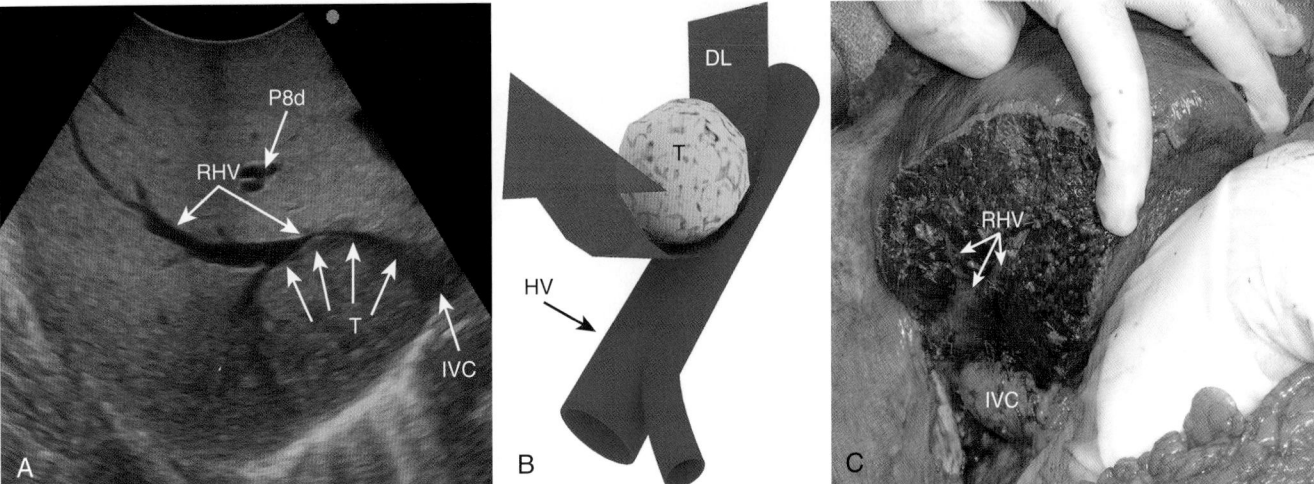

FIGURE 103.52   A, The intraoperative ultrasound (IOUS) shows a tumor *(T)* in contact *(arrows)* with the right hepatic vein *(RHV)*. **B**, The schema shows the type of tumor-vessel relation as classified at IOUS and the recommended approach. **C**, A segment VII resection was carried out exposing the RHV on the cut surface. *DL*, Dissection line; *HV*, Hepatic vein; *IVC*, Inferior vena cava; *P8d*, Portal branch to sub-segment VIII dorsal.

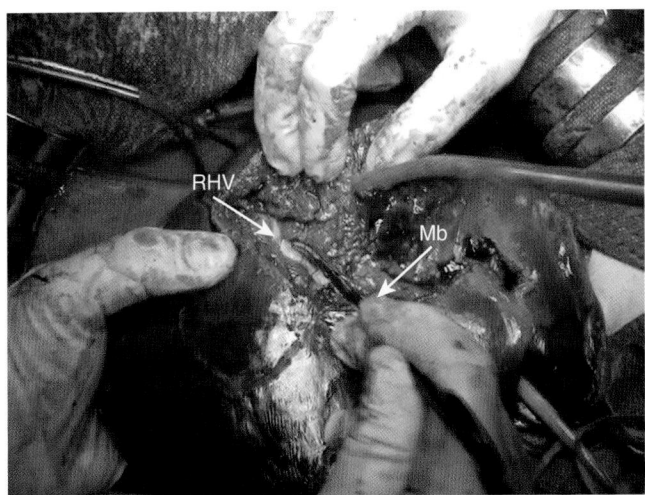

FIGURE 103.53 The method for dissection of a detachable tumor-vessel relation: The Metzenbaum *(Mb)* scissors can be bluntly used for this purpose. *RHV*, Right hepatic vein.

then proceeding with the dissection being driven by them; thereby, the liver guides the surgeon (see Fig. 103.59F). Following vessels from the surface to the deep parenchyma requires an anatomic approach but with infinite trajectories according to the selected vessel and consequently infinite solutions, maximizing the parenchyma sparing by not just challenging the complexity of the liver but being guided exactly by such complexity. Recognizing and tracking peculiarities such as accessory veins and CVs can further expand technical solutions in case of unsuitability of R1vasc surgery.

Vessel-guided hepatectomies can be used when recognizing the liver anatomy and its variations with IOUS, when challenging liver anatomy pursuing R1vasc, and when profiting of liver anatomy disclosing the CV. Interacting with the liver anatomy, the tumor and surrounding structures, and the consequent rearrangements (see Fig. 103.59A,D,F) can result in the implementation of

surgical options (Fig. 103.60)[21,22] and in an increase in salvage-ability in case of relapse.[94,99] Sculpturing rather than simply dividing the liver has induced a revision of the concept of minor and major hepatectomy,[100] suggesting a new dictionary of liver surgery to be written.

SYSTEMATIC EXTENDED RIGHT POSTERIOR SECTIONECTOMY. Systematic extended right posterior sectionectomy (SERPS) is a surgical technique that allows for sparing of part of the right anterior section in the presence of the tumors shown in Figure 103.61.[19]

Eligibility Criteria. Patients suitable for SERPS are those with tumors showing one of three conditions:

1. Invasion of the right HV (RHV) within 4 cm of the hepatocaval confluence with other lesions involving segment VI and eventually segment VII (see Fig. 103.61A).
2. Invasion of the RHV within 4 cm of the hepatocaval confluence without other lesions involving segment VI, without an inferior RHV (IRHV), and with hepatofugal portal blood flow on CF-IOUS in the portal branch to segment VI (P6) when the RHV is clamped if not already occluded (see Fig. 103.61B). In the presence of an IRHV, or in its absence, when the flow direction in P6 remains hepatopetal, resection of segments VII and VIII together with the RHV is carried out,[18] rather than SERPS. Therefore SERPS is applied as an alternative to resection of segments VII and VIII in patients who do not have proper outflow for segment VI once the RHV is divided.
3. Evident contact with the right anterior Glissonean sheath and a relationship with the right posterior section, with at least one of the following features: contact with the right posterior section and proximal bile duct dilation or Glissonean wall invasion (see Fig. 103.61C).

Procedure. In the first two conditions, extension to the right anterior section is tailored to guarantee complete removal of the tumor and a dissection line is drawn on the left side of the RHV, which is also resected (see Fig. 103.61A–B). Flow direction in the right anterior portal branch at CF-IOUS is estimated as previously described once the RHV is clamped if it is not occluded (Fig. 103.62). The right anterior pedicle is not necessarily

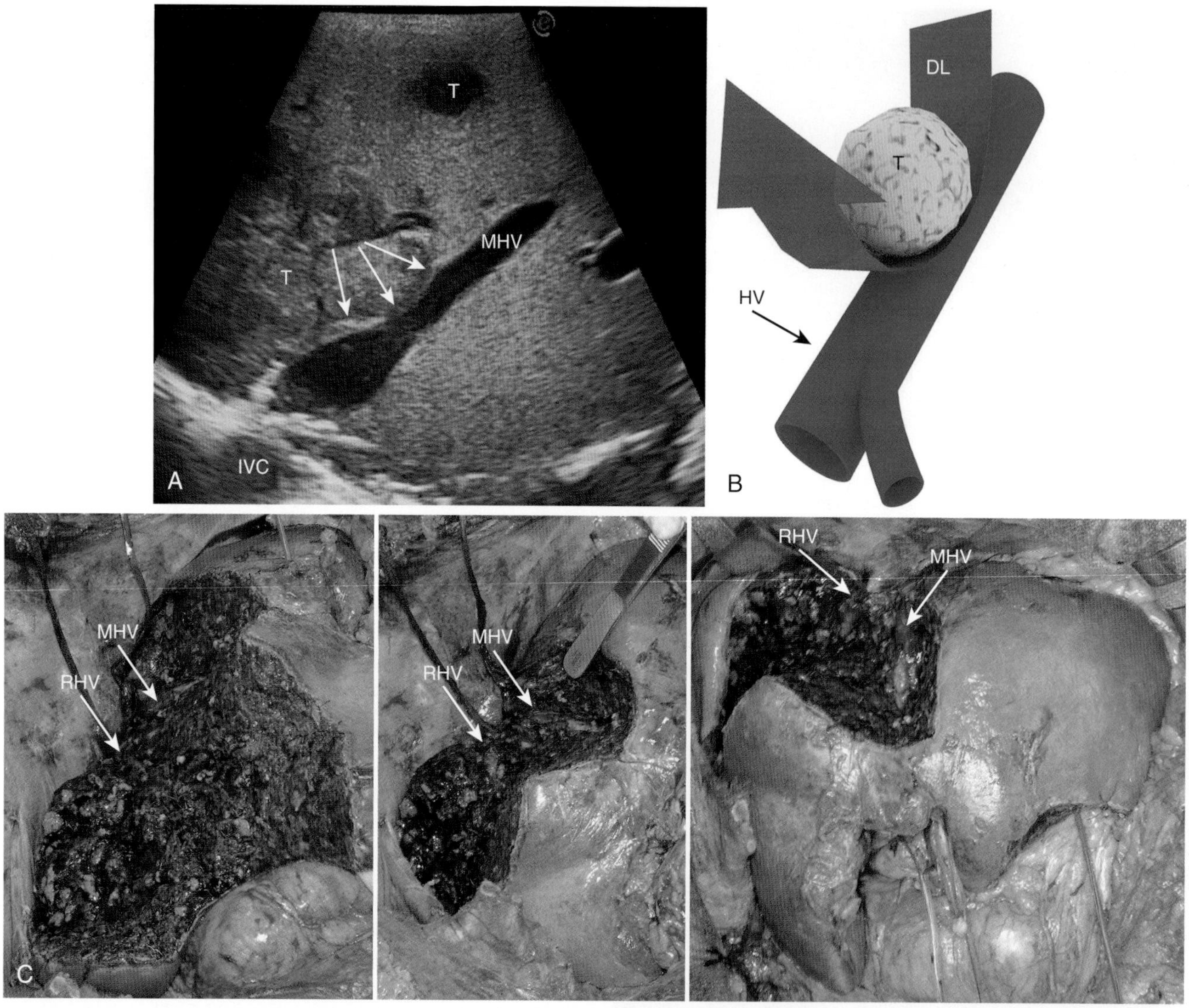

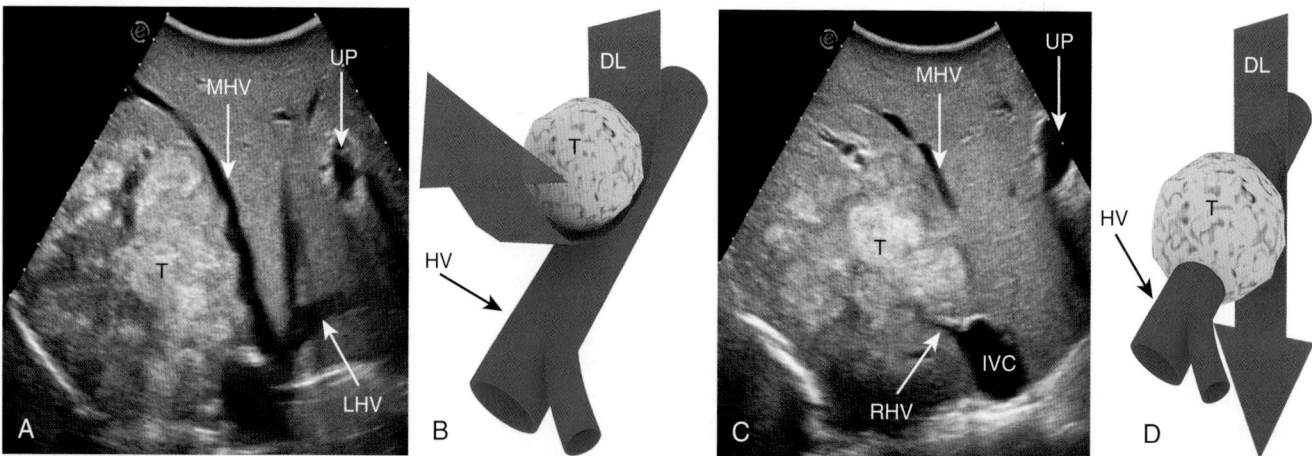

FIGURE 103.54 **A,** The intraoperative ultrasound (IOUS) shows a tumor *(T)* in contact *(arrows)* with the middle hepatic vein *(MHV)* in a patient carrier of multiple colorectal liver metastases. **B,** The schema shows the type of tumor-vessel relation as classified at IOUS and the recommended approach. **C,** Resection of segments IV superior, VII, and VIII, extended partially to segments V and VI, was carried out with exposure of both the right hepatic vein *(RHV)* and the MHV. *DL,* Dissection line; *HV,* hepatic vein; *IVC,* inferior vena cava.

FIGURE 103.55 At intraoperative ultrasound (IOUS) **(A)** a large tumor *(T)* in contact with the middle hepatic vein *(MHV)* in a patient carrier of multiple colorectal liver metastases is visualized. The schema **(B)** shows the type of tumor-vessel relation as classified at IOUS and the recommended approach. At IOUS **(C)** the same tumor invades the right hepatic vein *(RHV)* at its caval confluence *(IVC)*.

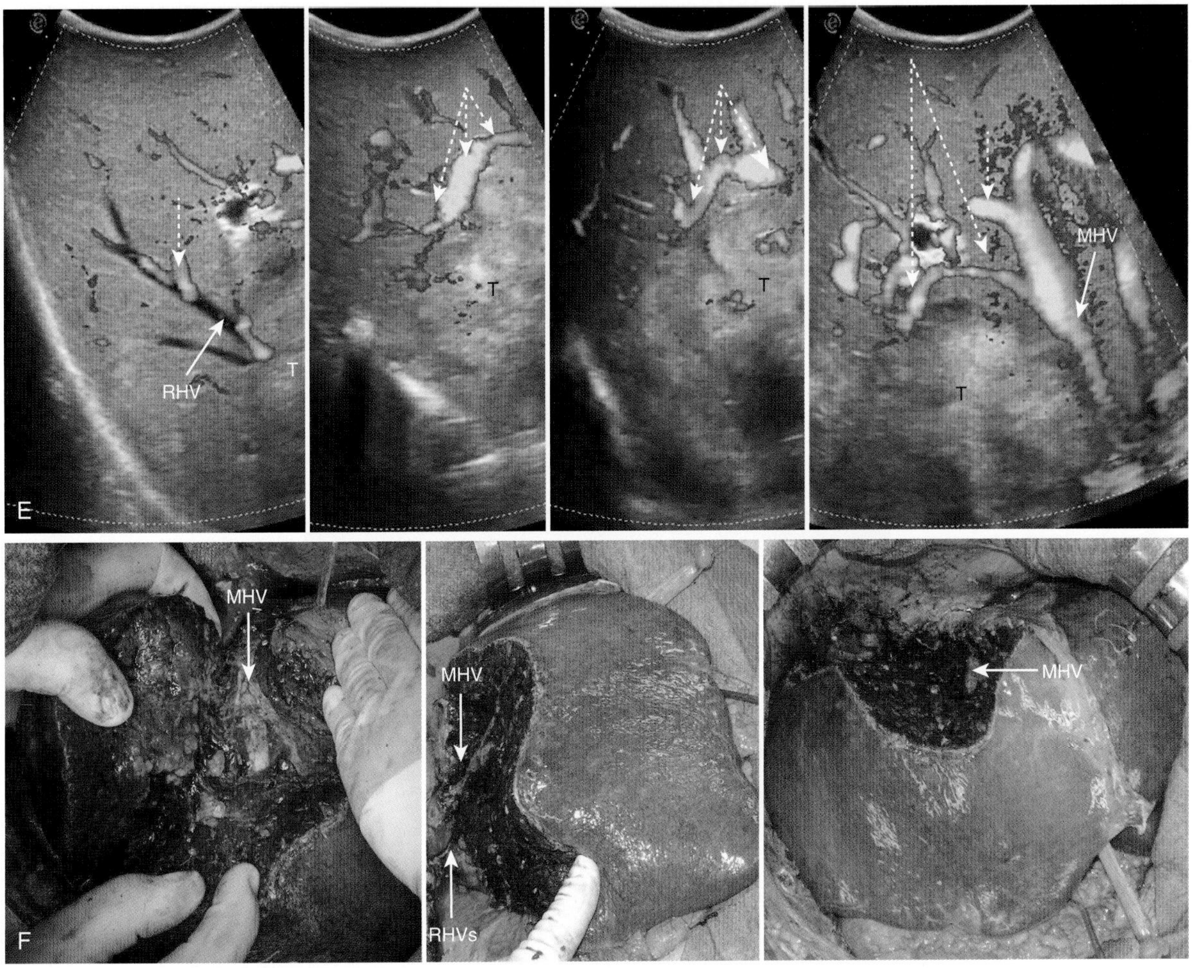

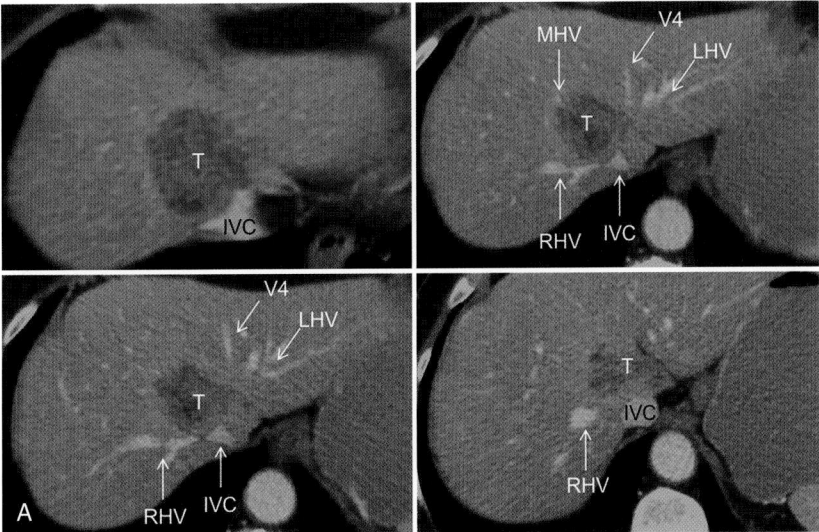

FIGURE 103.55, cont'd   The schema **(B)** shows the type of tumor-vessel relation as classified at IOUS and the recommended approach. The color-flow IOUS shows the existence of communicating veins *(dashed arrows)* connecting the RHV before its neoplastic occlusion and the MHV: The red/blue colors indicate the flow direction *(toward the probe if red; the opposite when blue)*. The operation **(F)** consists of a so-called "mini-upper trans-versal hepatectomy" in which from left to right the MHV has been detached from the tumor as shown in Fig. 103.53, and the RHV has been resected. *DL*, Dissection line; *HV*, Hepatic vein; *RHVs*, Right hepatic vein stump; *UP*, Umbilical portion.

FIGURE 103.56   A, Computed tomography (CT) image of a tumor *(T)* occupying segments VIII, IV superior, and I; the tumor is in contact at caval confluence with the right hepatic vein *(RHV),* and with the confluence of the hepatic vein draining the segment 4 *(V4)* and the left hepatic vein *(LHV);* the middle hepatic vein *(MHV)* flows into the tumor.

Continued

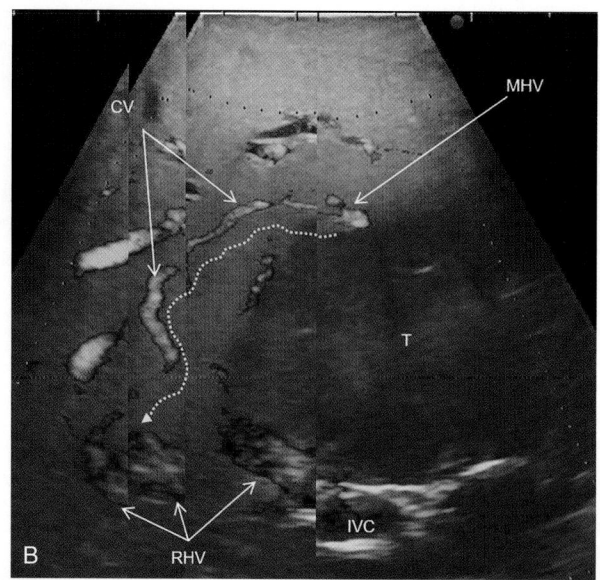

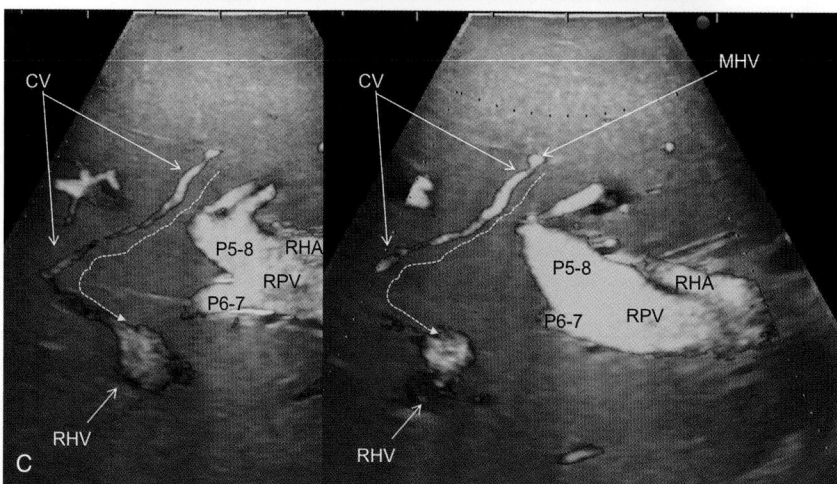

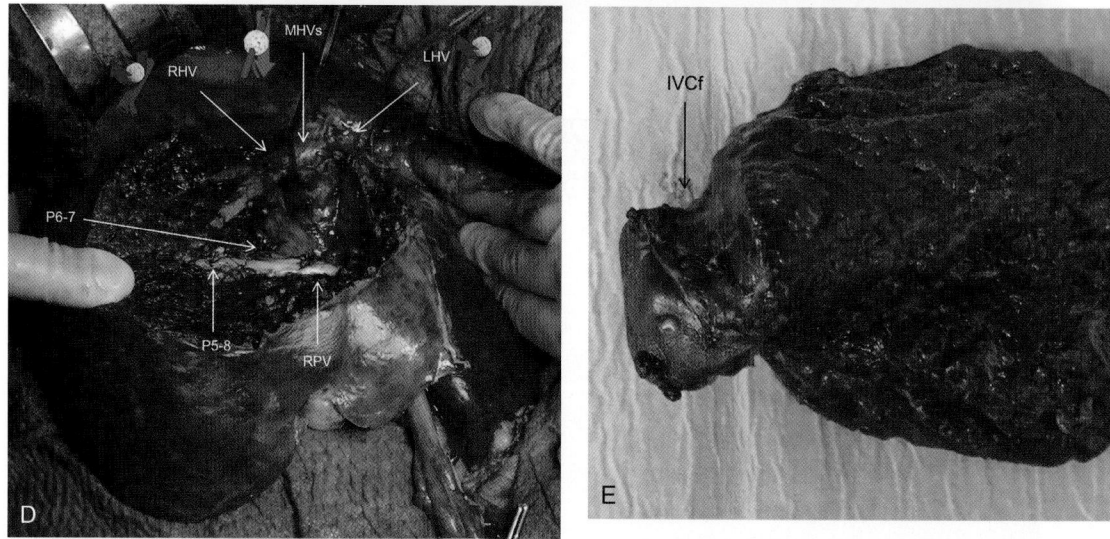

FIGURE 103.56, cont'd   **B**, A communicating vein *(CV)* between the RHV and the MHV as disclosed in a color-flow intraoperative ultrasound (IOUS): CV trajectory and flow direction are emphasized by the yellow-dotted arrow. **C**, Color-flow IOUS disclosure of another CV between the RHV and the MHV: CV trajectory and flow direction are emphasized by the yellow-dotted *arrow*, which should be followed, shifting the sight from right to left. **D,** Panoramic view of the cut surface; notably, the primary and secondary Glissonean sheaths are exposed in their upper and posterior aspects, as the inferior vena cava *(IVC),* the stump of the middle hepatic vein *(MHVs),* the right hepatic vein *(RHV),* and the left hepatic vein *(LHV).* **E,** The specimen after removal. *IVCf,* Inferior vena cava fossa; *P5-8,* portal branch to the right anterior section; *P6-7,* portal branch to the right posterior section; *RPV,* right portal vein.

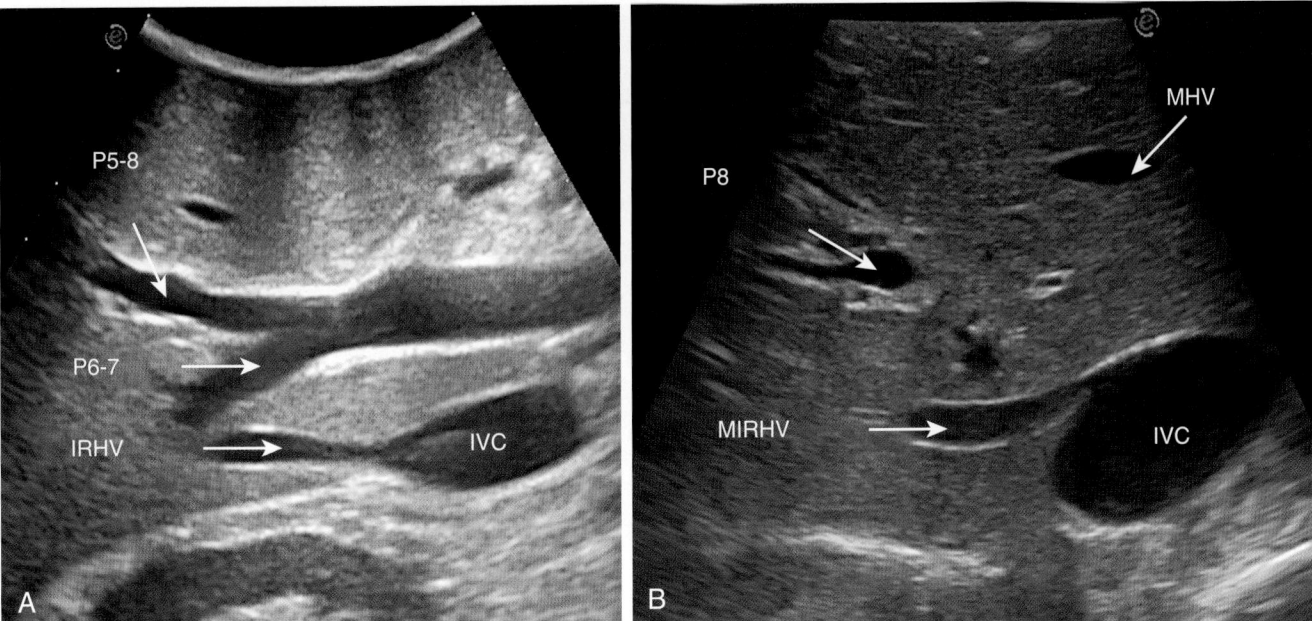

FIGURE 103.57   A, Intraoperative ultrasound (IOUS) appearance of a thick inferior right hepatic vein *(IRHV)* that typically runs behind the right-sided first- and second-order portal branches. **B,** The middle inferior right hepatic vein *(MIRHV),* which usually runs more cranially and medially compared with the route of the IRHV. *IVC,* Inferior vena cava; *MHV,* middle hepatic vein; *P8,* portal branch to segment VIII; *P5-8,* portal branch to the right anterior section; *P6-7,* portal branch to the right posterior section.

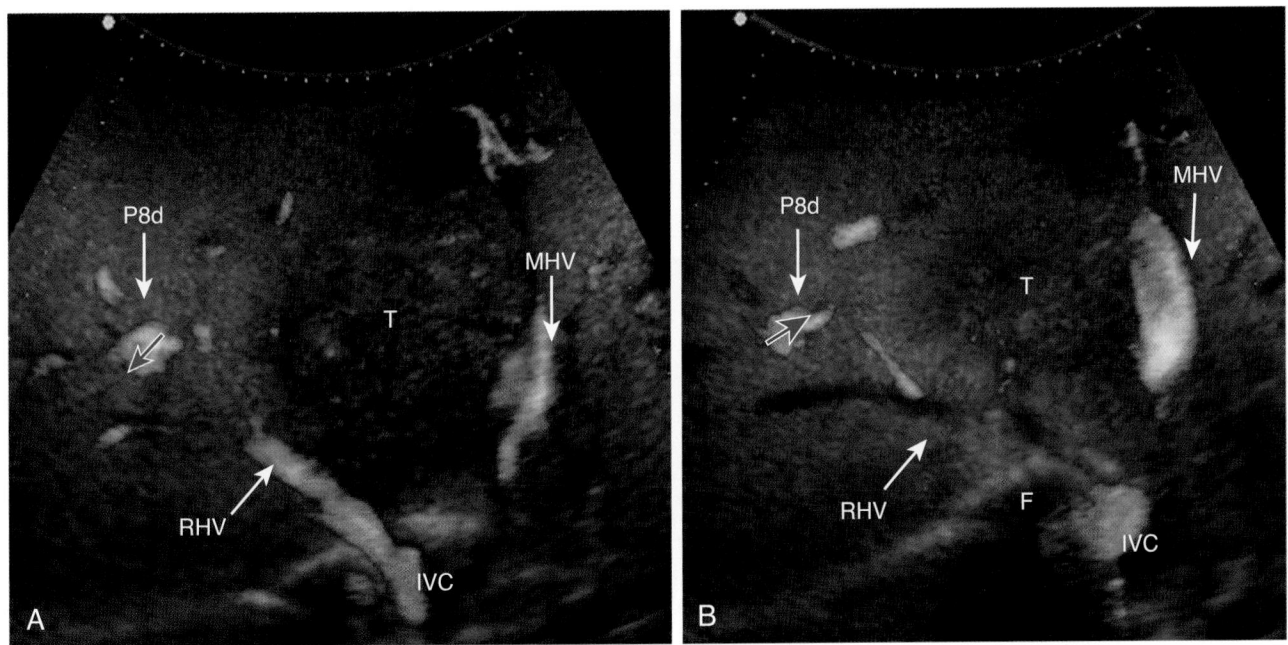

FIGURE 103.58   A, Hepatopetal flow direction *(blue arrow)* at color-flow intraoperative ultrasound (IOUS) of the portal branch to the dorsal portion of segment VIII *(P8d).* **B,** When finger compression *(F)* is applied to the right hepatic vein *(RHV)* at its caval confluence, the flow direction in P8d becomes hepatofugal *(red arrow). IHV,* Inferior vena cava; *MHV,* middle hepatic vein; *T,* tumor.

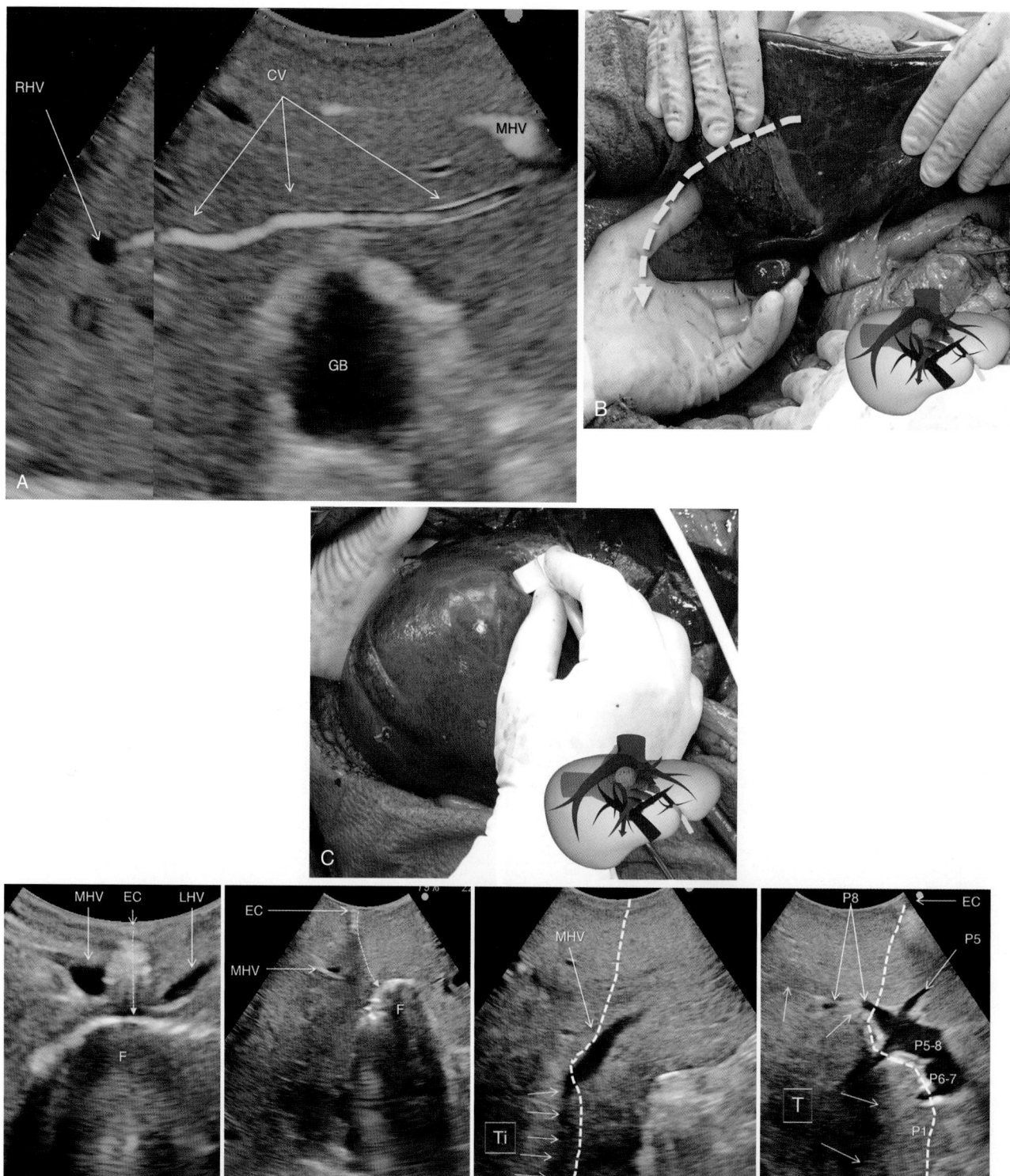

FIGURE 103.59   **A,** A communicating vein *(CV)* between the right hepatic vein *(RHV)* and the middle hepatic vein *(MHV)* as disclosed by a color-flow intraoperative ultrasound (IOUS): CV trajectory and flow direction are emphasized by the yellow-dotted arrow. **B,** Complete liver mobilization and the fingertips of the nondominant hand gripping the Arantius ligament; the yellow-dotted arrow indicates the repositioning of the liver over the surgeon's hand as disclosed by the superimposed schema. **C,** The IOUS probe positioned to identify the optimal dissection plane connecting the anterior surface of the liver and the surgeon's fingertips positioned as shown in the overlapped schema. **D,** From left to right, the definition of the left, mid-left, and mid-right dissection margins; the left sided shows the planned dissection line *(yellow-dotted arrow)* connecting the electrocautery *(EC)* with the finger-tip *(F)*, at caval confluence, and just passing in between the middle hepatic vein *(MHV)* and left hepatic vein *(LHV)*; the mid-left discloses the trajectory *(yellow-dotted arrow)* connecting the EC and the F; the mid-right, the planned dissection line to be followed to expose at first and then to pass through the MHV, which results infiltrated *(yellow arrows)* by the tumor *(Ti)*; the right-sided, the planned dissection line to be followed to expose the dorsal portion of the right anterior Glissonean pedicle *(P5-8)*, then surfing over the surface of the root of the right posterior one *(P6-7)*.

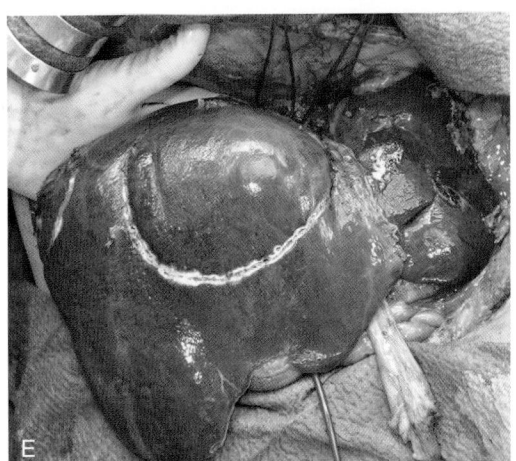

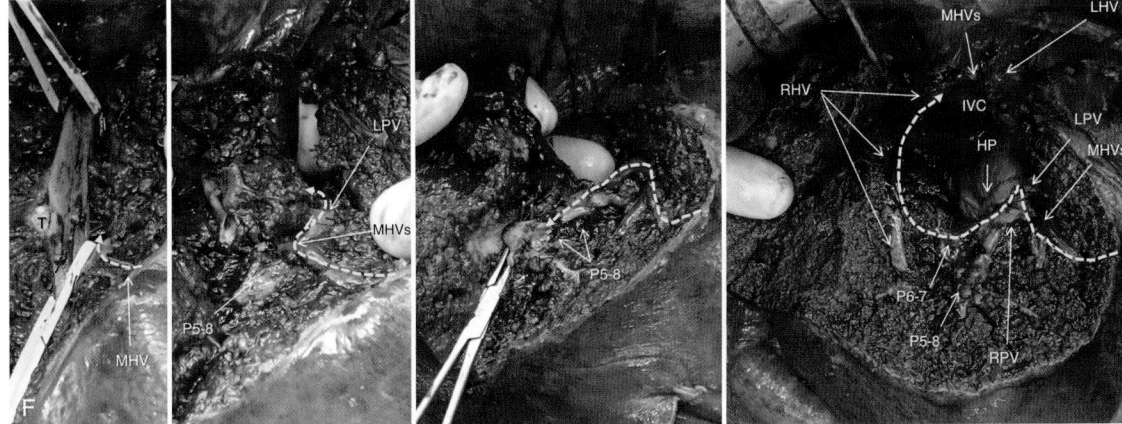

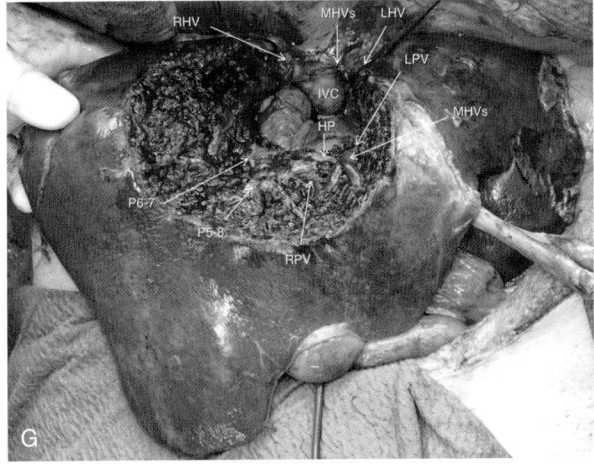

FIGURE 103.59, cont'd E, The resection area as disclosed (arrows). **F**, From left to right, liver dissection discloses just under the surface a peripheral branch of the MHV, which is gently exposed being driven to the main trunk, which is resected because infiltrated; then the dissection proceeds following the left Glissonean pedicle (LPV) appearing just beneath the resected MHV; facilitated by the tilting of the right-sided parenchyma by the surgeon's nondominant hand, dissection proceeds surfing over the LPV, the dorsal portion of P5-8 is progressively exposed, and the pedicles to the segment VIII are divided; finally the root of the P6-7 and the RHV are exposed and resection is concluded as a result of the trajectory just described and visually disclosed by the yellow-dotted arrows. **G**, The liver tunnel with MHV resection is finalized. *HP*, Hepatic pedicle; *IVC*, inferior vena cava; *MHVs*, MHV stump; *RPV*, right portal vein.

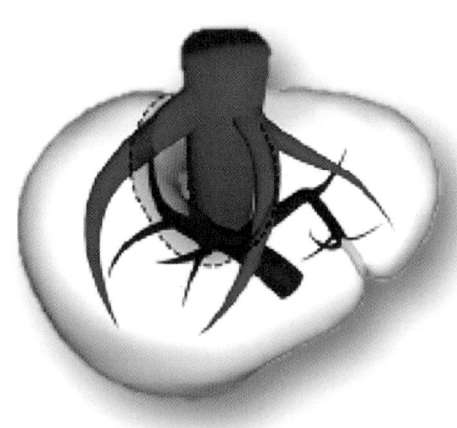

FIGURE 103.60 Schemas of some of the procedures based on the R1vasc concept and the detection when needed of the communicating veins]. **A,** Limited resection with tumor detachment at caval confluence. **B**, Systematic extended right posterior sectionectomy. **C**, Rollercoaster procedure; mini-mesohepatectomy. **D**, mini-upper transversal resection in absence of an inferior right hepatic vein or a segment 6 draining middle hepatic vein. **F1**, Right-sided upper transverse resection. **F2**, left-sided upper transverse resection. **G,** Total upper transverse resection. **H1**, Liver tunnel with middle hepatic vein resection. **H2**, Liver tunnel without middle hepatic vein resection.

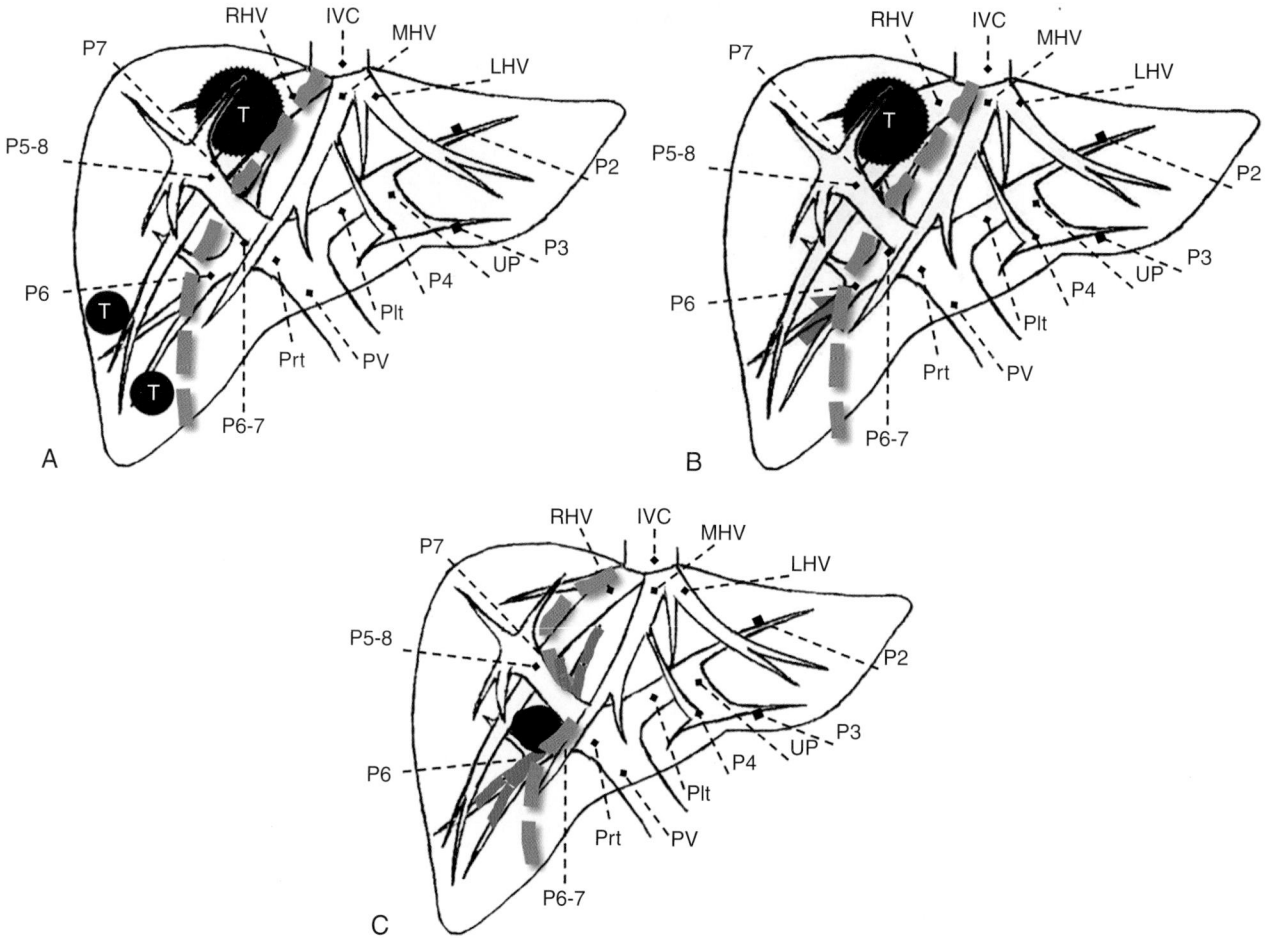

FIGURE 103.61 Eligibility criteria for systematic extended right posterior sectionectomy (*SERPS*). In all circumstances, at color-flow intraoperative ultrasound (IOUS), hepatopetal portal blood flow *(arrows)* has to be evident in the main portal branch to the right anterior section *(P5-8)*, once the right hepatic vein *(RHV)* is clamped, if not already occluded. **A,** Presence of vascular invasion of the RHV at the hepatocaval confluence (within 4 cm) with other tumors *(T)* in segment VI. **B,** Presence of vascular invasion of the RHV at the hepatocaval confluence (within 4 cm) without tumor in segment VI but with hepatofugal portal blood flow *(arrow)* in the portal branch to the right posterior section *(P6-7)*, once the RHV is clamped, if not already occluded. **C,** Presence of vascular invasion of the right posterior portal branch *(P6-7)* or biliary dilation of sectional branches *(dB6* and *dB7)*, with tumor *(T)* in contact with the P5-8 without signs of biliary dilation. *IVC,* Inferior vena cava; *LHV,* left hepatic vein; *MHV,* middle hepatic vein; *PV,* portal vein.

exposed on the liver cut surface. In the third condition, the extension of the resection into the right anterior section is tailored to preserve most of the parenchyma of segment VIII, the tract of the RHV at the hepatocaval confluence, and the left portion of segment V without division of the right anterior pedicle, which is exposed on the cut surface (see Fig. 103.61C).

MINI-MESOHEPATECTOMY. Mini-mesohepatectomy (MMH) represents an alternative to the conventional mesohepatectomy in patients with tumors that invade the MHV at its caval confluence. MMH consists of a limited resection, including the tract of the invaded vein without reconstruction while sparing segments IV inferior and V in Figure 103.63 and as described in the next section.[101]

Eligibility Criteria. Patients suitable for MMH are those with tumors that have macroscopic signs of vascular invasion of MHV at hepatocaval confluence on preoperative imaging and IOUS (Fig. 103.64A).

Procedure. Mobilization of the right and left hemiliver is tailored based on the size of the lesion and its cranial extension toward the MHV-caval confluence. As a rule, mobilization of

the liver to obtain the encirclement of the HVs at the caval confluence should be recommended. For planning an MMH (see Fig. 103.64), the following findings should be assessed by CF-IOUS:

1. Detection of CVs between the MHV and RHV and/or LHV and/or IVC. This is accomplished initially without clamping of the MHV. If no CVs are seen, the MHV is clamped to increase the probability of detection (see Fig. 103.64B).
2. If no CVs are evident at CF-IOUS, reversal of flow in the peripheral portion of the clamped MHV should be confirmed: This finding suggests the existence of CVs with the adjacent HVs (see Fig. 103.64C).
3. Hepatopetal flow in the residual portion of the central segments (IV, V, and VIII) also suggests the existence of CVs with the adjacent HVs (see Fig. 103.64D).

If none of these findings is confirmed, and especially if hepatofugal flow direction in portal branches to segments V and/or IV inferior is detected, the hepatectomy should be extended to the area fed by those portal branches.

Either the posterior wall of the MHV or the portion of the tumor involving the paracaval section is used as a deep landmark

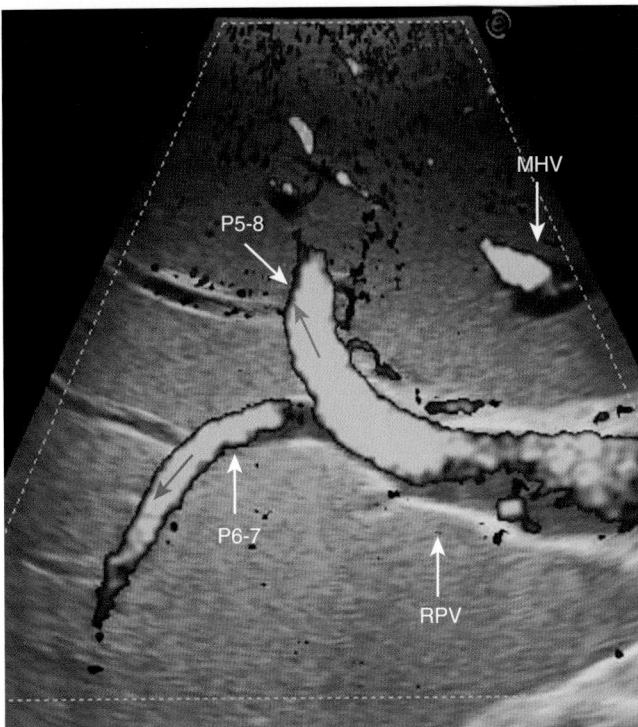

FIGURE 103.62 Direction of hepatopetal blood flow *(arrows)* into the right-sided sectional portal branches *(P5-8* and *P6-7)*, as it appears at color-flow intraoperative ultrasound (IOUS). *MHV*, Middle hepatic vein; *RPV*, right portal vein.

for delineating the resection area. A crucial point for proper performance of the MMH in the presence of a CV is to delineate a dissection plane that does not interrupt the vein.

TRANSVERSE HEPATECTOMIES. For tumors involving more than one and up to all three HVs at the hepatocaval confluence, the choice must be made between vascular reconstruction and unresectability. In 1987 Makuuchi reported that once the presence of a thick IRHV is evident on preoperative imaging and/or IOUS, resection of the tumor together with the RHV is

feasible without carrying out a formal right hepatectomy, limiting the liver parenchyma removed to only segments VII and VIII. This was the first paper showing how an anatomic variant can allow a surgical procedure that previously was not considered feasible.[18] Taking into account the pioneering experience of Makuuchi, both SERPS and MMH have been released, and we have further proceeded with the transverse hepatectomies, which could be classified according to the resection or detachment of the HVs and in the event of resection by the number of HV sacrificed.

Transverse Hepatectomy Without HV Resection

Rollercoaster Hepatectomy. These are transverse hepatectomies with one to multiple tumors in contact with at least two HVs at hepato-caval confluence; contact should be characterized by full detachability of the tumor from the HV or at worst partial resection of the HV wall (Fig. 103.65).[102]

Transverse Hepatectomy With HV Resection. These are transverse hepatectomies for tumors in no detachable relation with one or more HVs at hepato-caval confluence in the presence of an IRHV and CVs (Fig. 103.66A–B) or just CVs (see Fig. 103.66C–D). The tumor could lie over the hilar plate with contact but no invasion of the right and left portal branches (Fig. 103.67A) and eventually over the segmental portal branches to the antero-inferior segments. The following subtypes can be recognized:

Mini-upper Transverse Hepatectomy. This involves resection of SVIISVII-VIII with the RHV (right mini-upper; see Fig. 103.60E) or SII-IVs with the LHV (left mini-upper). For the right-sided, the outflow of SVI is provided by an IRHV,[18] by branches of the MHV,[22] or by CVs between the RHV and the MHV[103] (Fig. 103.68). For the left-sided, the outflow of SIII is provided by CVs between the LHV and the MHV.[22]

Right Upper Transverse Hepatectomy. This involves resection of SVII-VIII-IVs and partial or total of SI with the RHV and the MHV (see Fig. 103.60F1). The outflow of SIVi-V-VIVI is provided by the IRHV and CV or CVs only, among the RHV stump, the MHV stump, and the LHV[104] (see Figs. 103.66 and 103.67).

Left Upper Transverse Hepatectomy. This involves resection of SII-IVs-VIII and the cranial portion of SI paracaval with the LHV and the MHV (see Fig. 103.60F2). The outflow of segments IIIVVIII-IVi-V is provided by CVs among the LHV, and MHV stumps and the RHV and an IRHV is present[22].

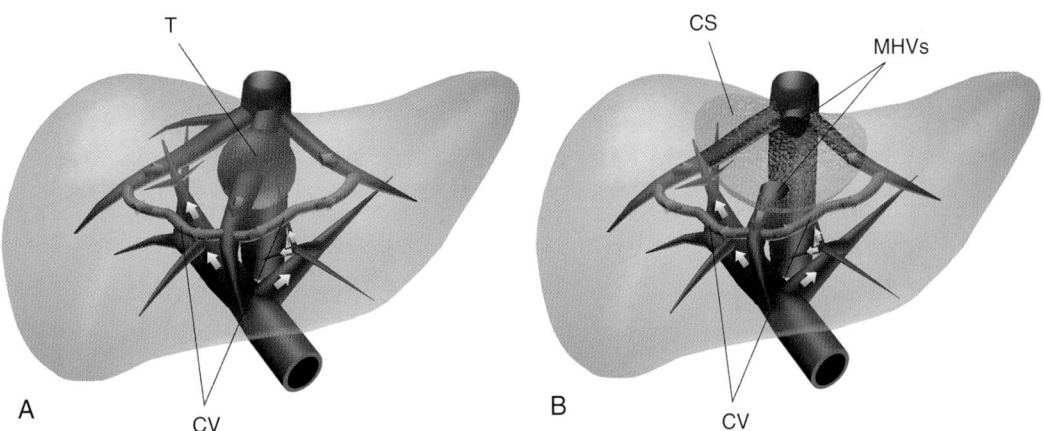

FIGURE 103.63 These schemas are showing the pattern of presentation of a tumor invading the middle hepatic vein *(MHV)* in which communicating veins *(CV)* exist between the MHV itself and one or both the adjacent hepatic veins allowing the blood to be drained by that vein *(red arrows)* **(A)** and allowing a limited resection denominated mini-mesohepatectomy **(B).** *CS,* Cut surface; *MHVs,* middle hepatic vein stump.

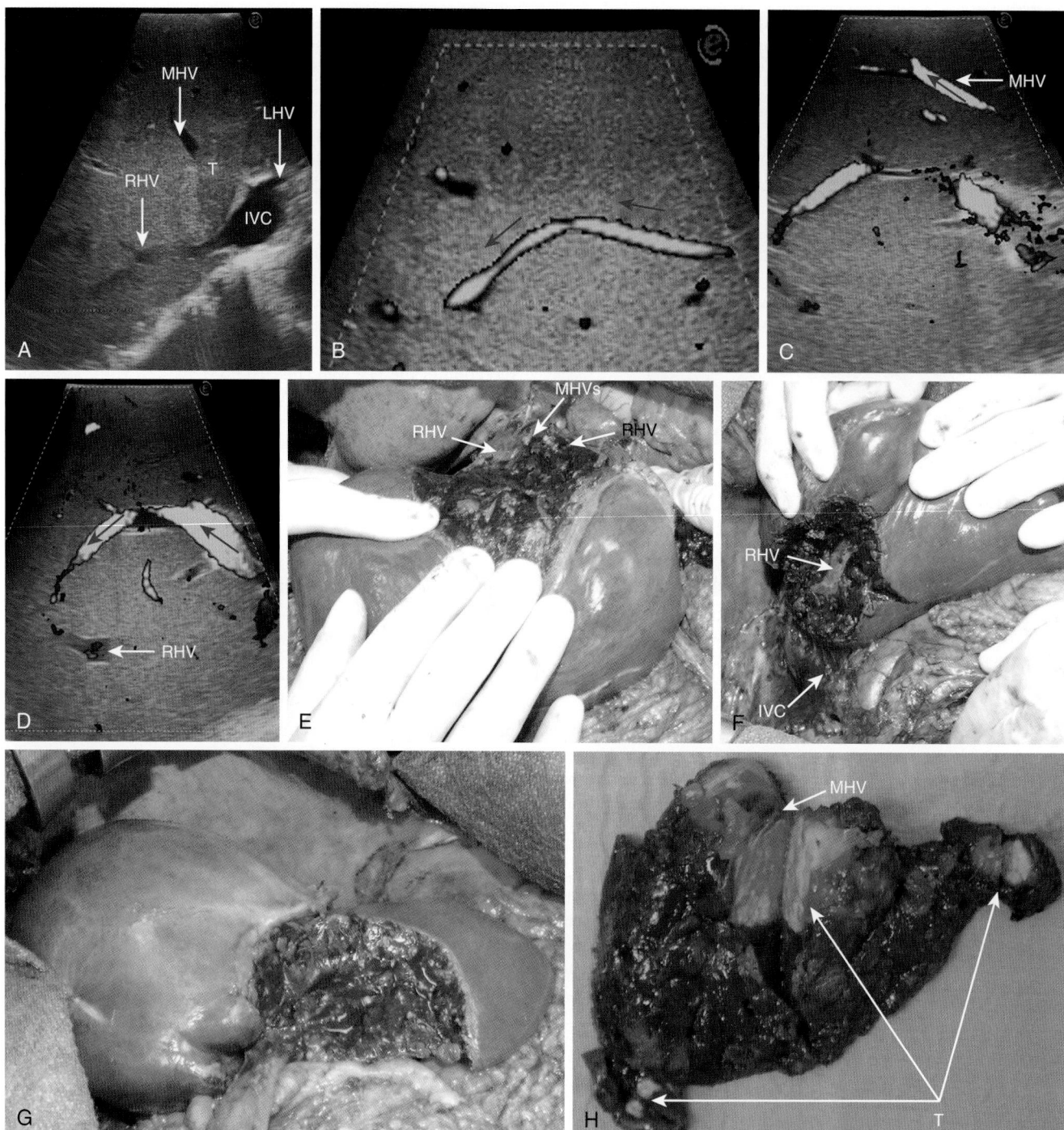

FIGURE 103.64 Surgical treatment of a patient with colorectal liver metastases *(CLM)* invading the middle hepatic vein *(MHV)* at caval confluence and receiving a mini-mesohepatectomy *(MMH)*. **A,** Intraoperative ultrasound (IOUS) appearance of the CLM. The isoechoic tumor *(T)* is invading the MHV and is also in contact with the right hepatic vein *(RHV)* and the left hepatic vein *(LHV)*. **B,** The communicating vein is evident at color-flow (CF)-IOUS: Colored arrows indicate the flow direction. **C,** Reversal blood flow into the MHV: A *red arrow* indicates the flow direction. **D,** Hepatopetal blood flow into the portal branches to right anterior section *(P5-8)*: Colored arrows indicate the flow direction. **E–G,** The liver after removal of the multiple CLMs: The RHV is exposed both in the MMH resection area **(E)** and in the one shown in **F**, in which it appears its posterior surface. **H,** The resected specimen of the MMH in which are evident the tract of MHV removed and 3 CLM. *MHVs,* MHV stump.

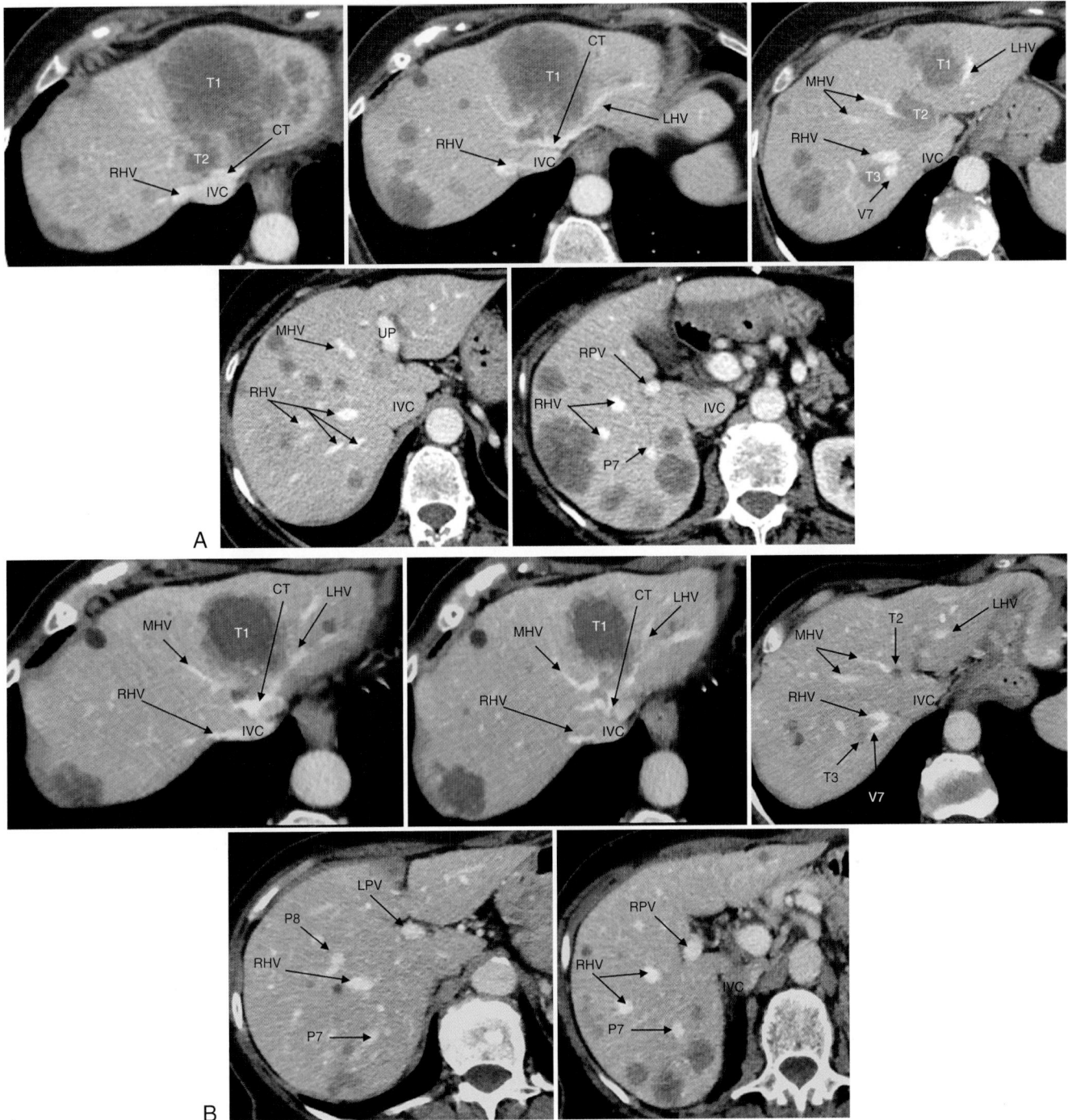

FIGURE 103.65   Surgical treatment of a patient with multiple bilobar colorectal liver metastases *(CLM)*. **A,** Prechemotherapy computed tomography (CT) showing scattered bilobar CLM with a confluent group of them *(T1* and *T2)* in extensive contacts with the left hepatic vein *(LHV),* the common trunk *(CT),* and the middle hepatic vein *(MHV),* and another one *(T3)* in contact with the right hepatic vein *(RHV)* at the level of the confluence of the main trunk with the one draining the segment 7 *(V7).* **B,** Preoperative CT after partial response to chemotherapy with reduction of all the contacts between the CLM and LHV, CT, MHV, and RHV.   *Continued*

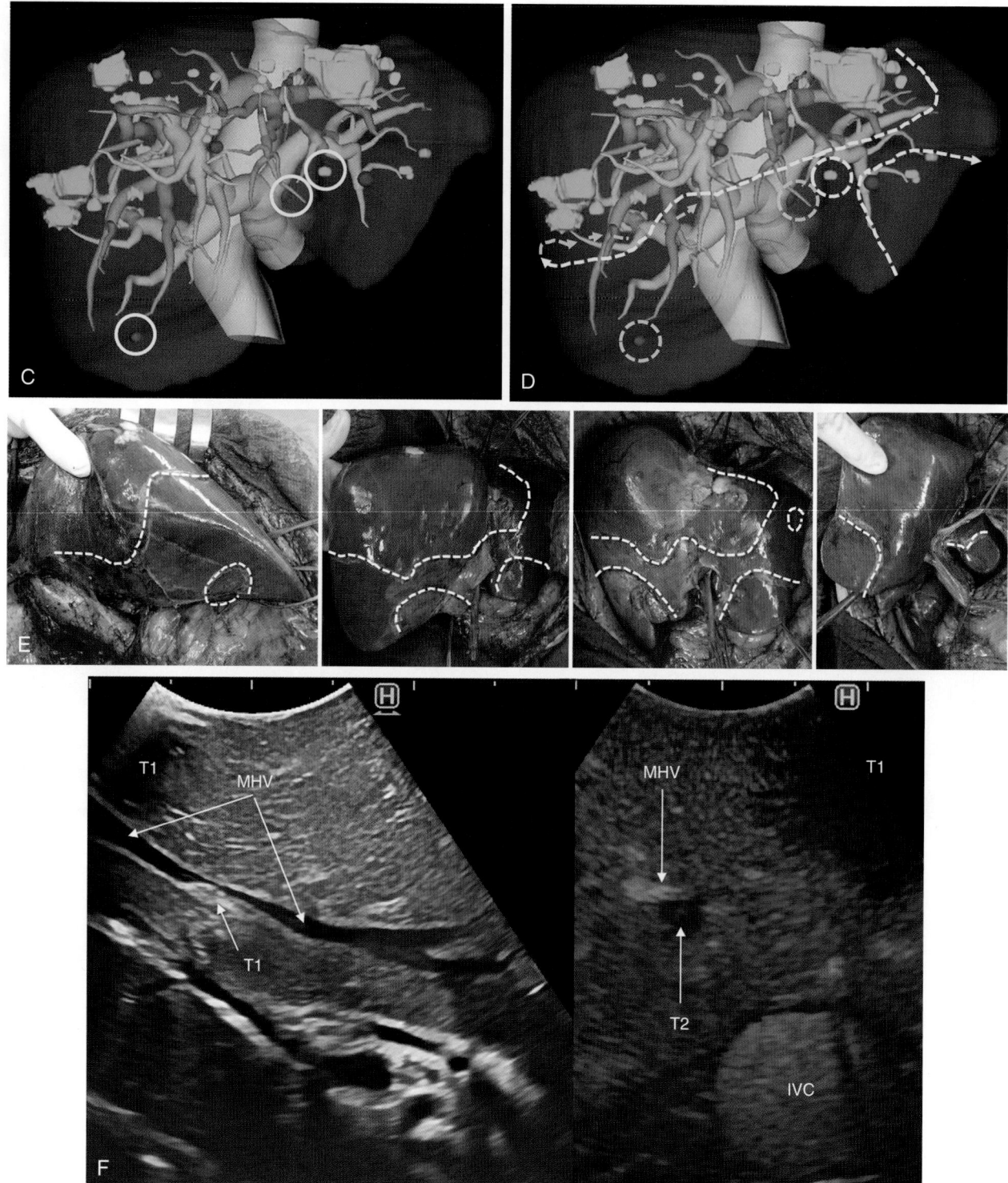

FIGURE 103.65, cont'd   C, The liver cast is built according to the preoperative CT: Areas delimited by yellow-dotted lines group the lesions included in four recognizable clusters, while in circles, those CLM which should be removed in separated resection areas (*in green, the still visible lesions, and in pink those no longer visible*). **D**, *Yellow* (anterior) and *orange* (posterior) *dotted lines* indicating the dissection planes base on the clusters disclosed in **C**; the red circles are highlighting those in close adjacency with major vessels (*MHV and Glissonean pedicle, P5-8*) or most peripheral *(compound points)*. **E**, The resection areas drawn on the liver surface. **F**, On the left, IOUS image of the lesion in contact with the MHV (T2), which is better visualized at CE-IOUS as shown on the right side.

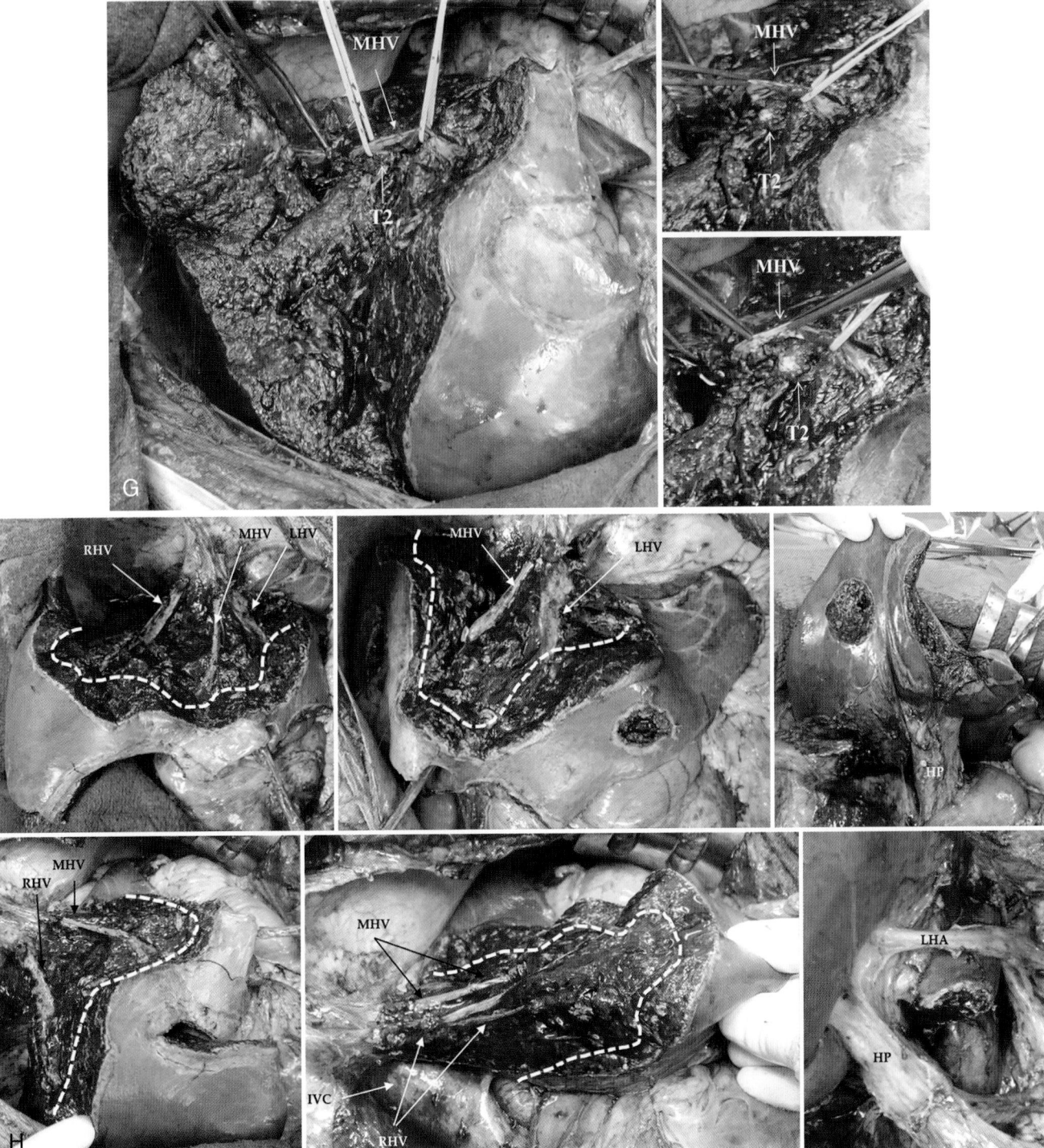

FIGURE 103.65, cont'd   **G**, The MHV is skeletonized and cranially and caudally to the lesion (T2); the latter is detached from the posterior surface of the MHV with partial resection of its wall as shown in the right-upper part of the figure, whereas in the lower-right portion, the MHV after reconstruction by direct suture is disclosed. **H**, Multiple resections with the dissection trajectories shown by the *white-dotted lines*. *HP,* Hepatic pedicle. *IVC,* inferior vena cava. *LHA,* left hepatic artery; *P7,* Glissonean pedicle for segment VII.

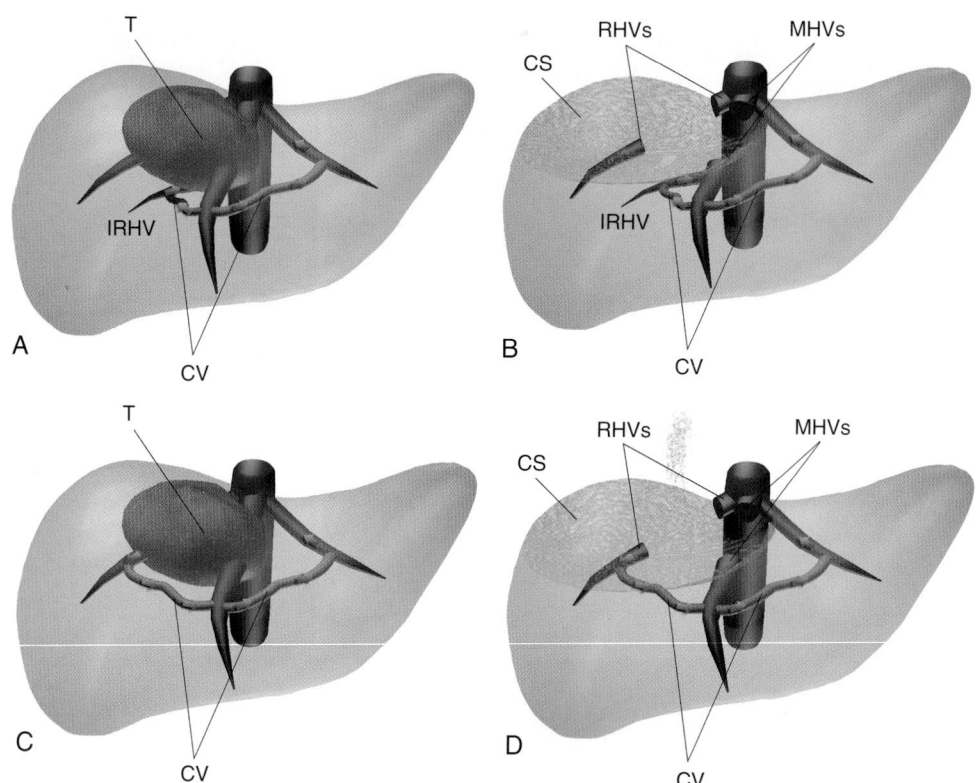

FIGURE 103.66 **A,** The schema is representing the condition suitable for an upper transverse hepatectomy *(UTH),* which is based on the recognition and respect of the communicating veins *(CV).* **B,** The schema of the cut surface *(CS)* at the end of the resection. **C,** The schema is representing a further condition suitable for an UTH, which is based on the recognition of just the communicating veins *(CV)* in the absence of an IRHV. **D,** The schema of the cut surface *(CS)* at the end of the resection. *MHVs,* Middle hepatic vein stumps; *RHVs,* right hepatic vein stump.

Total Upper Transverse Hepatectomy. This involves resection of IIIVVIIVIIISII-IVs-VII-VIII with section of the RHV, the MHV, and the LHV in presence of an IRHV and CVs among the liver-side stumps of the HVs, which warrantee the outflow of SIII-IVi-V-VIVI[22,105] (see Fig. 103.60G).

Procedure. The IOUS study in these patients should precisely map the accessory veins, IRHVs, and CVs, specifically describing all the suitable connections between two adjacent HVs (see Fig. 103.68C) or an HV and the IVC. In the absence of accessory veins as part of the vicariant outflow drainage, the caval plane can fully be freed (see Fig. 103.67C). Adequate exposure and mobilization should allow for positioning of the nondominant hand at the posterior aspect of the defined dissection plane. For all these reasons, a J-shaped thoracophrenolaparotomic access is frequently used in these circumstances, particularly for the right-sided resections. The direct view to the hepatocaval plane favored by this incision allows proper mobilization of the liver from the caval plane; in the event of an IRHV, this approach facilitates mobilization without sectioning the vein root. Furthermore, traction and handling of the portion of the liver to be removed is better controlled, reducing any excessive strain on the structures. The access, mobilization, inflow/outflow mapping, and IOUS guidance allow for removal of a relatively small and almost completely diseased part of the liver while preserving the vast majority of the functioning liver parenchyma with adequate inflow and outflow (see Figs. 103.67C,D and 103.68F,G). The proper identification and preservation of an IRHV and the CVs can make the removal of all the superior liver segments and the three HVs feasible.[22]

LIVER TUNNEL. The liver tunnel[99,106] procedure represents an extension of the MMH,[101] with or without removal of the MHV, and includes the total removal of segment I (Fig. 103.69; see also Figs. 103.56, 103.59, and 103.60H).

Eligibility Criteria. Patients eligible for this approach are those with tumoral involvement at various degree of segments VIII, IV superior, and I. There could be contacts between the tumor or the tumors with the MHV, the LHV, and the RHV at caval confluence, and similarly with the right and the left first- and second-order portal branches. The MHV could be invaded or not by the tumor at its caval confluence, in presence of CVs between the MHV, the RHV, and/or the LHV (Fig. 103.70; see also Figs. 103.56 and 103.59).

Liver Tunnel Without Resection of the Middle Hepatic Vein. This involves limited or anatomic resection of segment VIII or IV superior associated with removal of segment I, sparing of the MHV, and IVC exposure (Figs. 103.71 and 103.72; see also Fig. 103.60G2.)

Liver Tunnel With Resection of the Middle Hepatic Vein. This involves limited or anatomic resection of segment VIII or IV superior with section of MHV and complete removal of segment I. The outflow of segments V and IV inferior is provided by CVs between the MHV and the RHV and/or LHV (see Figs. 103.56, 103.59, 103.60G1 and 103.70).

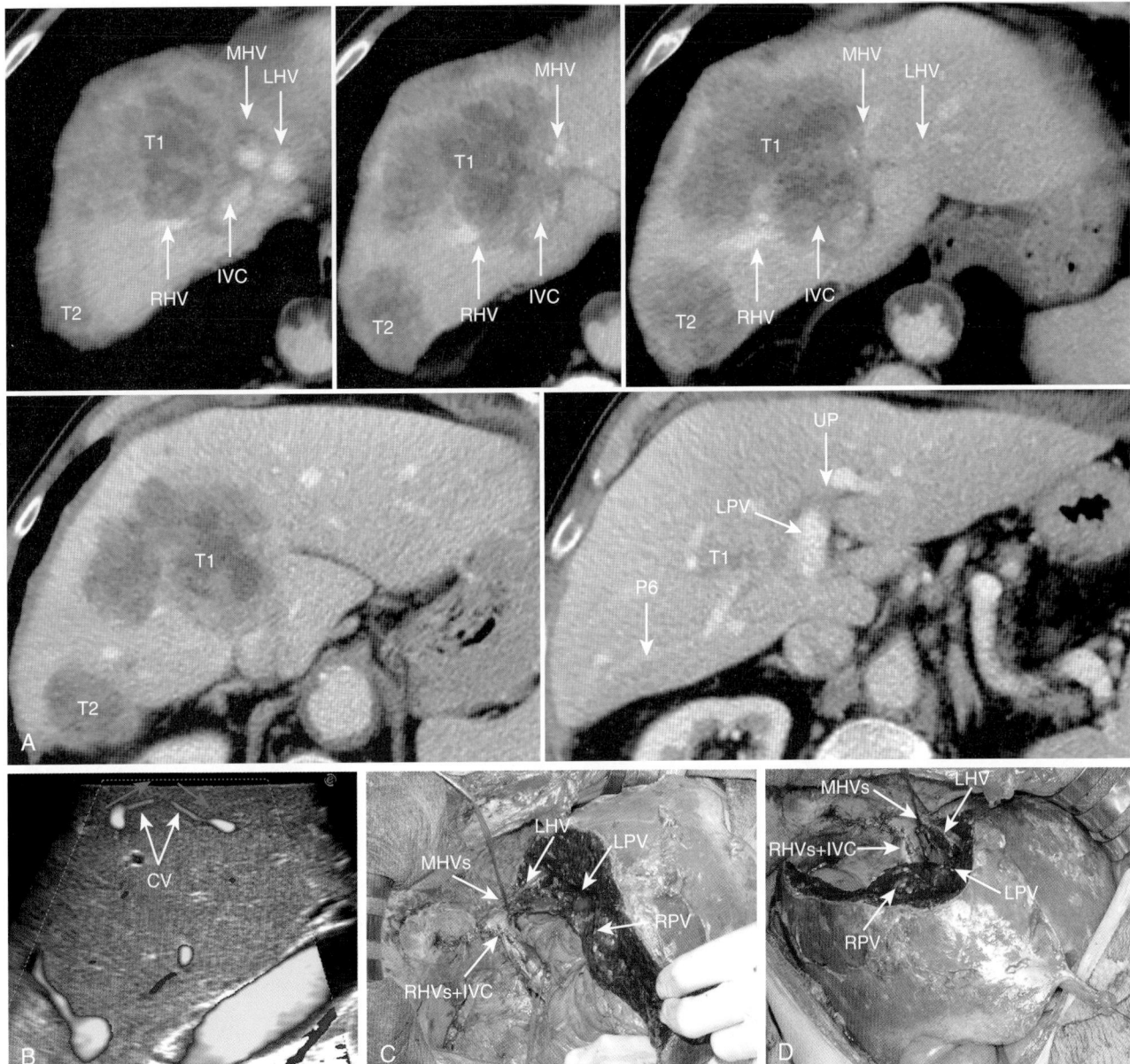

FIGURE 103.67   A, From left to right and from top to bottom, these pictures shows the computed tomography (CT) of a patient having a condition suitable for the so-called "upper transverse hepatectomy" because the right (RHV) and middle hepatic vein (MHV) are involved by a large colorectal liver metastases (T1), which has a wide contact with the left hepatic vein (LHV), in the absence of an inferior right hepatic vein (IRHV). The tumor is bulging over the hilar plate. **B,** The communicating veins (CV) are recognized at color-flow intraoperative ultrasound (CF-IOUS). **C–D,** The cut surface shows the left (LPV) and the right portal branch (RPV), the LHV, which was detached from the tumor, removing part of its wall and reconstructing the vein by direct suture; the RHV (RHVs), and MHV (MHVs) stumps are also shown; the inferior vena cava (IVC) was partially resected and the IVC reconstructed by direct suture because of tumor infiltration.

Procedure. Complete mobilization of the liver must be accomplished with full detachment of the retrohepatic IVC. Once the anterior surface of the hepatocaval confluence is exposed, the resection area is drawn under IOUS guidance by targeting the relationship between the tumor, the HV, and the dorsal and posterior surfaces of the GP facing this complex portion of the liver (see Figs. 103.59 and 103.71B). The surgeon's nondominant hand fingertips grip the Arantius ligament, shifting at IOUS almost on the same axis as the MHV and the Arantius ligament itself (Figs. 103.59B,C and 103.71C). Dissection is started from the low-medial side of the resection area, with the nondominant hand positioned between the posterior surface of the liver and the IVC (see Fig. 103.59F). In the event of MHV resection, this procedure is carried out as described in Figure 103.59F. The dissection then moves toward the posterosuperior aspect of the left GP, then to the right GP and the dorsal portion of the portal branch to segments V and VIII. The RHV is then exposed, following its course toward the IVC until resection is completed (see Figs. 103.69F–G, 103.70B, and 103.71D,E).

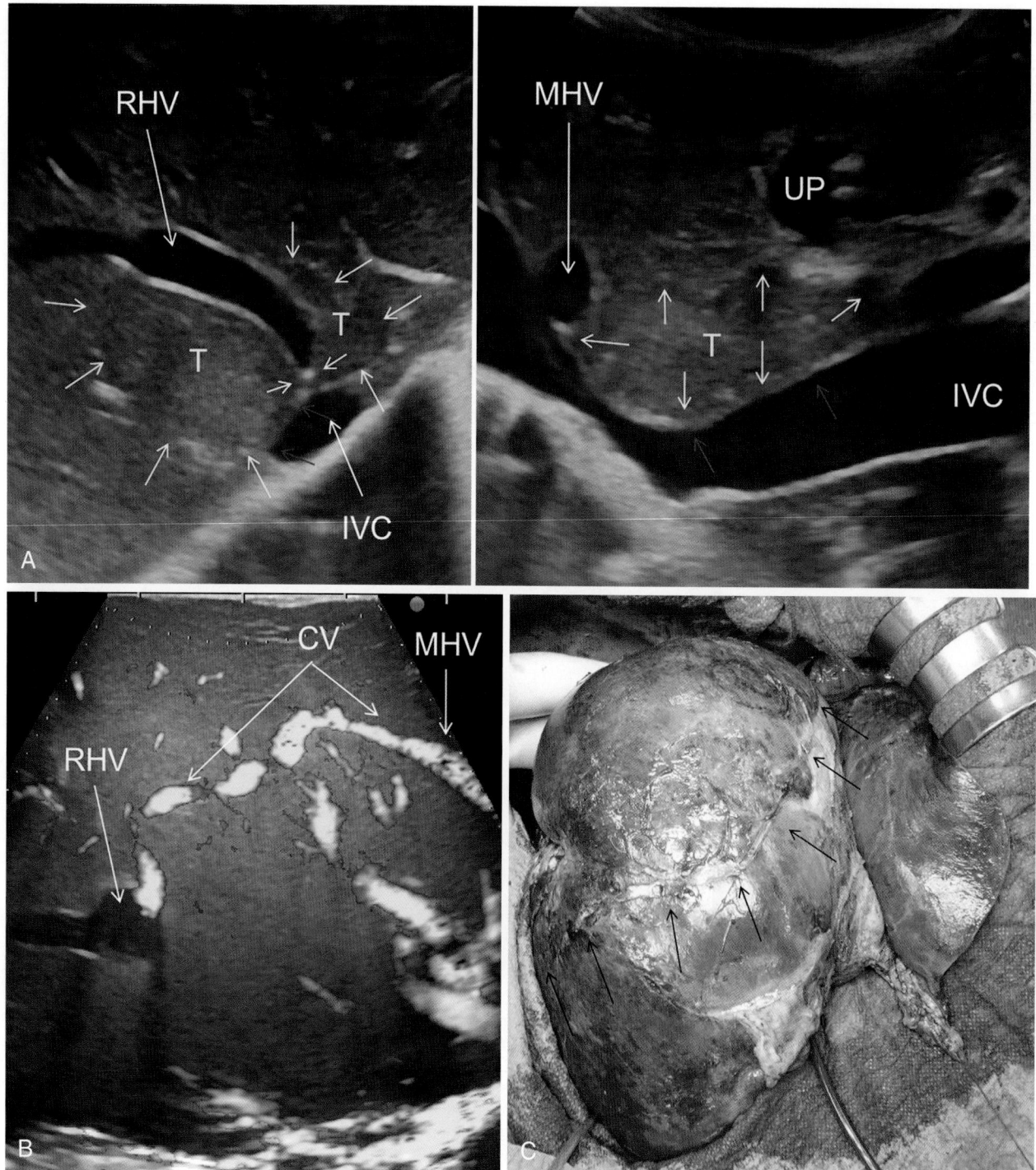

FIGURE 103.68 **A,** From left to right, intraoperative ultrasound (IOUS) scan showing a isoechoic tumor (*T*) at caval confluence invading the right hepatic vein *(RHV)* and in infiltrative contact with the inferior vena cava *(IVC)*: The red arrows delimited the IVC wall where the echogenicity shifts from the usual hyperechoic pattern to the hypoechoic one as the tumor. **B,** Color-flow IOUS shows a communicating vein *(CV)* between the middle hepatic vein *(MHV)* and the RHV. **C,** The front view of the resection area *(arrows).*

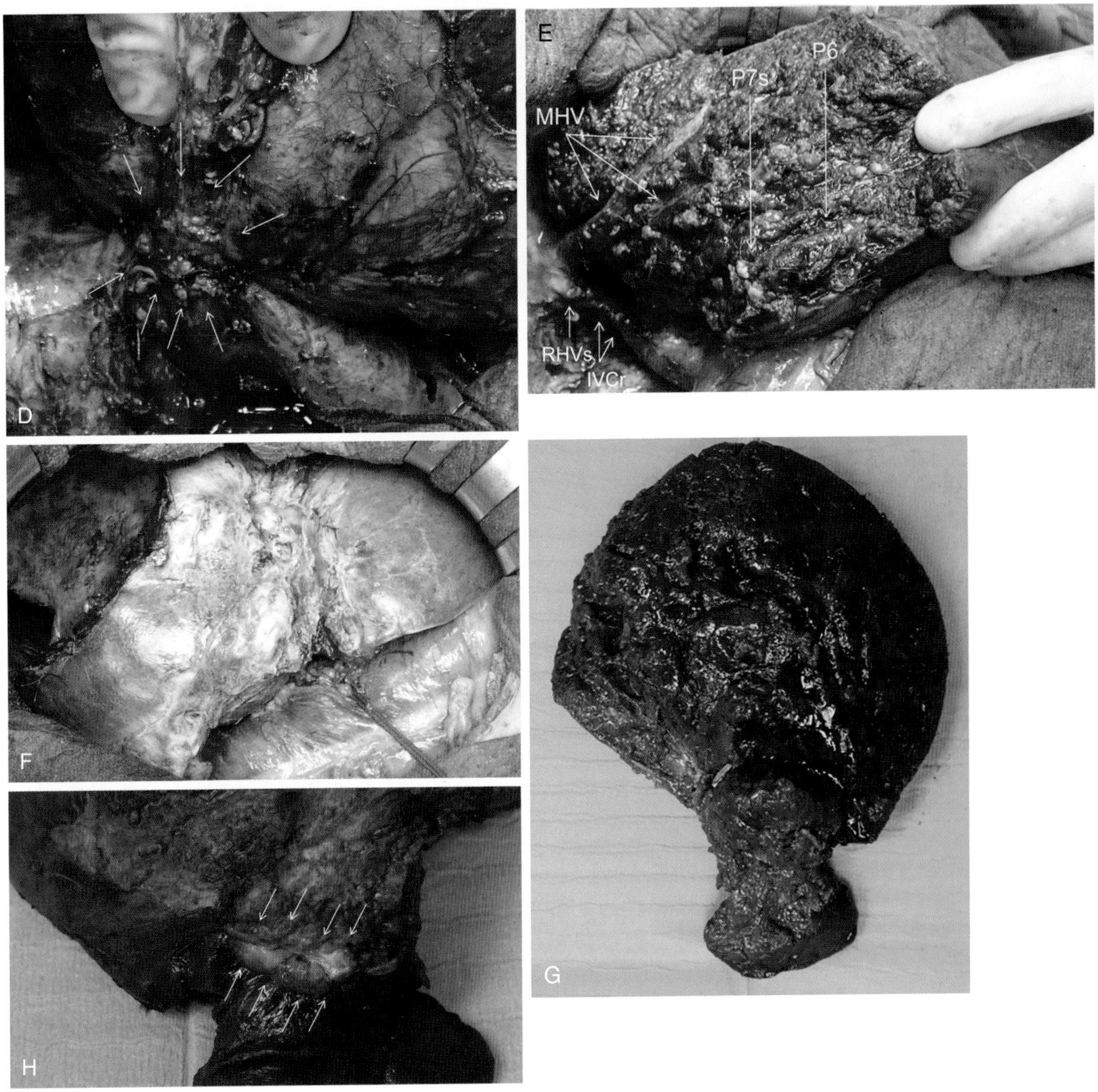

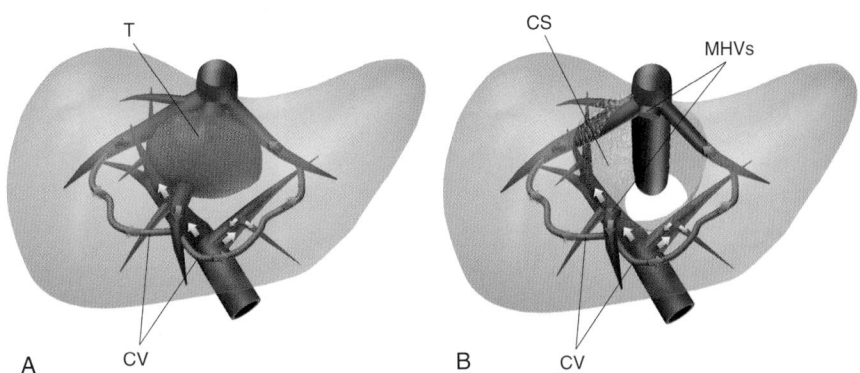

FIGURE 103.68, cont'd D, The area in which the tumor invades both RHV and IVC *(arrows).* **E,** Mini-upper transversal hepatectomy with RHV resection and IVC partial resection with reconstruction by direct suture. **F,** Frontal view of the resection from which is evident the sparing of liver tissue. **G,** The specimen, which includes segments I, VII, and VIII. **H,** The specimen with detailed by *arrows* the portion of IVC wall resected because infiltrated. P6, Glissonean branch to segment VI; *P7s,* stump of the Glissonean pedicle to segment 7; *UP,* umbilical portion.

FIGURE 103.69 A, The typical tumoral condition demanding a liver tunnel: the tumor is occupying the segments 1,4, and 8 at the caval confluence invading the middle hepatic vein and presenting communicating veins (CV) allowing the blood flow to shift *(red arrows)* toward the right and left hepatic veins; **B,** Liver tunnel at the end of the resection which included also the middle hepatic vein.

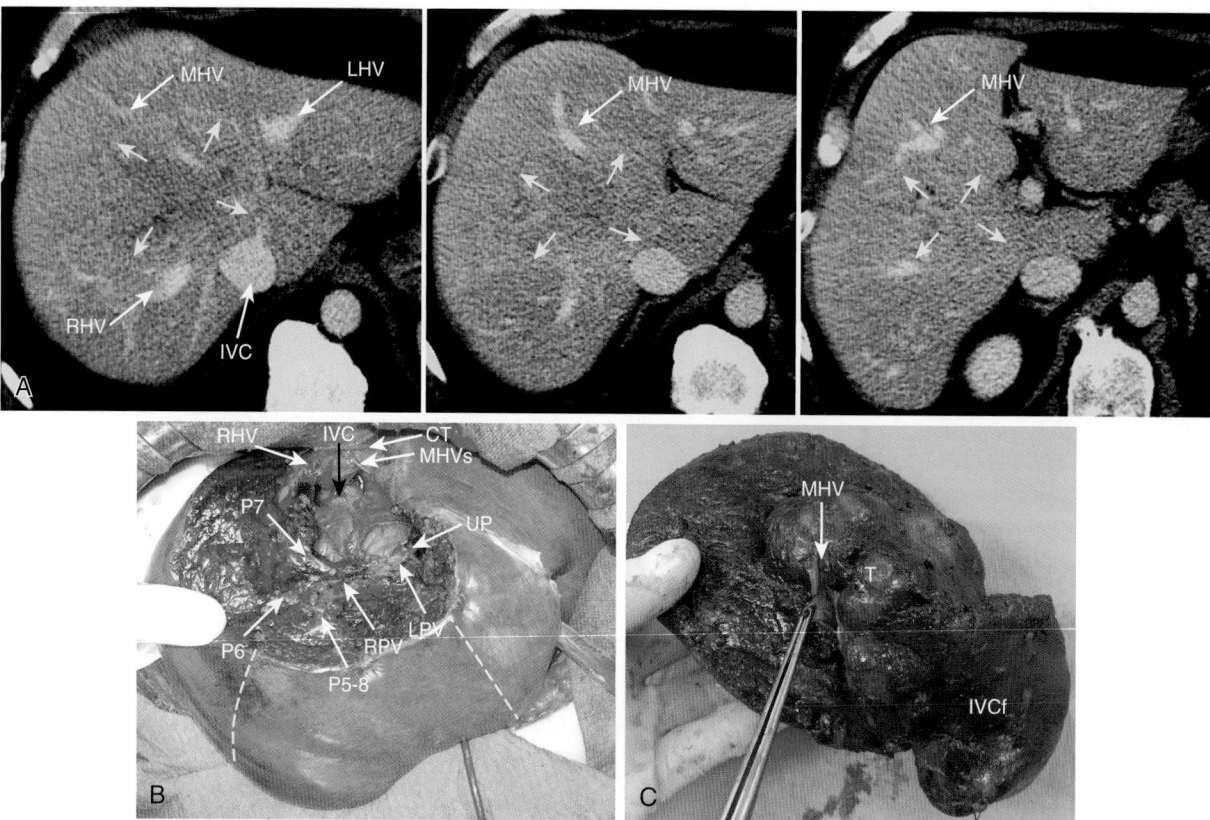

FIGURE 103.70 **A,** Computed tomography (CT) image of a tumor (*T* and *yellow arrows*) occupying segment VIII, IV superior, and I. **B,** A panoramic view of the cut surface from beyond and from the bottom; notably the primary and secondary Glissonean sheaths are exposed in their upper and posterior aspects, as the inferior vena cava *(IVC),* the common trunk *(CT)* with the stump of the middle hepatic vein *(MHVs),* and the right hepatic vein *(RHV);* in yellow dashed lines, the area theoretically drained by the resected MHV. **C,** The specimen after removal that includes the resected portion of the MHV. *CT,* Common trunk; *IVCf,* inferior vena cava fossa; *LHV,* left hepatic vein; *LPV,* left portal vein; *P6,* portal branch to segment VI; *P7,* portal branch to segment VII; *P5-8,* portal branch to the right anterior section; *RPV,* right portal vein; *UP,* umbilical portion.

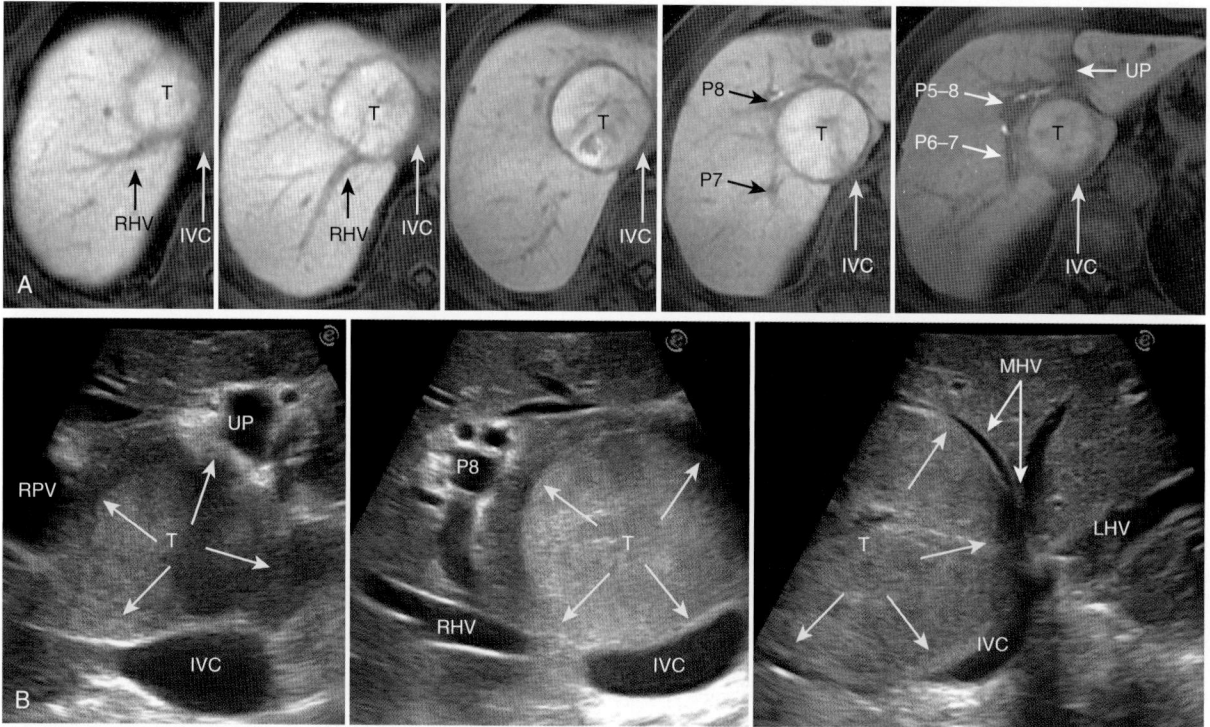

FIGURE 103.71 **A,** Magnetic resonance image (MRI) of a hepatocellular carcinoma (HCC; *T*) occupying segment VIII and I.

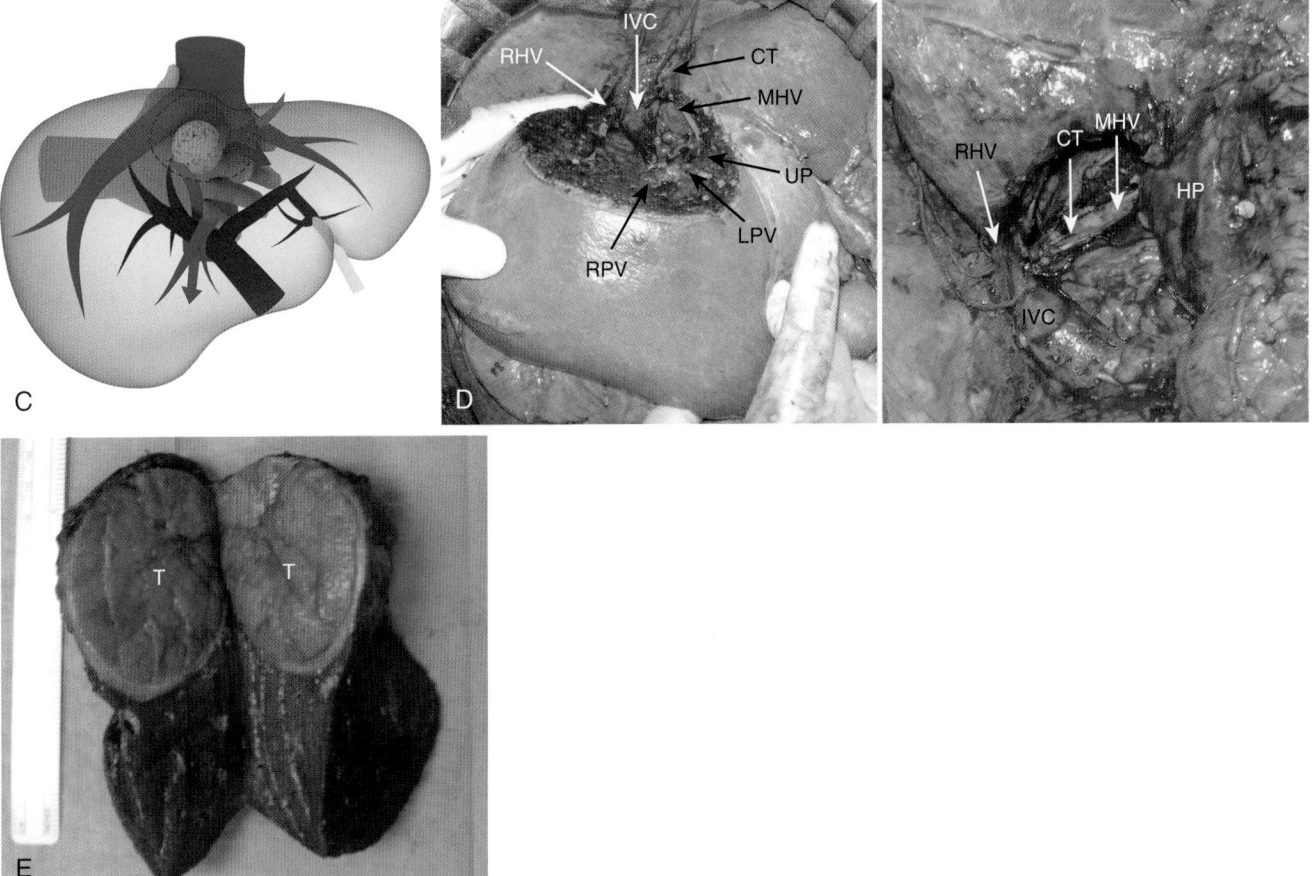

FIGURE 103.71, cont'd   B, Intraoperative ultrasound (IOUS) image of the same HCC occupying segment. VIII and I. **C**, This schema shows the role of the surgeon's left hand in aiding resection guidance in this complex procedure: After full mobilization of the liver by disconnecting all the short hepatic vein, the left hand stays in between the inferior vena cava and the posterior surface of the liver; the surgeon's left hand fingertip pulls to the right the caudate lobe by gripping the Arantius ligament; in this way, the dissection plane from the supero-anterior liver surface to the Arantius ligament passing in between the tumor and the middle hepatic vein *(MHV)* becomes straight *(right-sided red arrow)*; **D**, From left to right, a panoramic view of the cut surface from beyond and from the bottom; notably, the primary and secondary Glissonean sheaths are exposed in their upper and posterior aspects, as the inferior vena cava *(IVC)*, the MHV, and the right hepatic vein *(RHV)*. **E**, The specimen after removal. *CS*, Cut surface; *CT*, common trunk; *CV*, communicating vein; *HP*, hepatic pedicle; *LHV*, left hepatic vein; *LPV*, left portal vein; *P6-7*, portal branch to the right posterior section; *P5-8*, portal branch to the right anterior section; the dissection lines *(red arrows)* followed for removing this lesion; *RPV*, right portal vein; *UP*, umbilical portion.

PARENCHYMA-SPARING MAJOR HEPATECTOMIES. The procedures mentioned, derived from the combination of IOUS and vessel guidance, have been often used in combination with other resections in patients with bilobar metastases. Combining them and associating them with other minimal procedures (i.e., rollercoaster resections featured by tumor vessel detachment and/or transverse hepatectomies or a liver tunnel or a mini-mesohepatectomy) with simple limited resections results as a sum of parenchyma-sparing procedures, which more or less could be assimilated to major hepatectomies.[16] The only difference between the conventional major hepatectomies and these parenchyma-sparing major hepatectomies is that the first imply vessel amputation, whereas the others are based exactly on the opposite. Maintenance of the liver scaffold and the main vessel harboring of the organ are the pillars, while removing liver tissue in an amount that is comparable with that removed for any right or even extended right/left hepatectomy. The basic principles for performing such procedures are essentially:

1. Recognition of suitable clusters of lesions: The possibility of grouping the lesions in recognizable clusters able to optimize the ratio between normal and diseased tissue removed, which is crucial for performing these kinds of procedures (see Fig. 103.65C–E).

2. Identification of the compass points of each cluster of lesions: These are represented by the deepest lesion and those lesions in contact or close adjacency with the major intrahepatic vessels (Fig. 103.73; see also Fig. 103.65C,D).

TRICKS AND TIPS. To achieve the planned resection strategy as safely as possible using the aforementioned procedures, and particularly for the parenchyma-sparing major hepatectomies, some tools, tricks, and tips are needed.

Virtual Cast. An accurate preoperative estimation of the FLR is a key factor for a successful hepatectomy. The manual plotting of resection areas on each CT/MRI scan (so-called "hand-trace technique") still remains the gold standard for assessing the liver volume. The planning of anatomic hepatectomy using this method can be relatively easy to perform, and a certain degree of accuracy in the volume estimation can be achieved.[107,108] The introduction of 3D simulation modalities

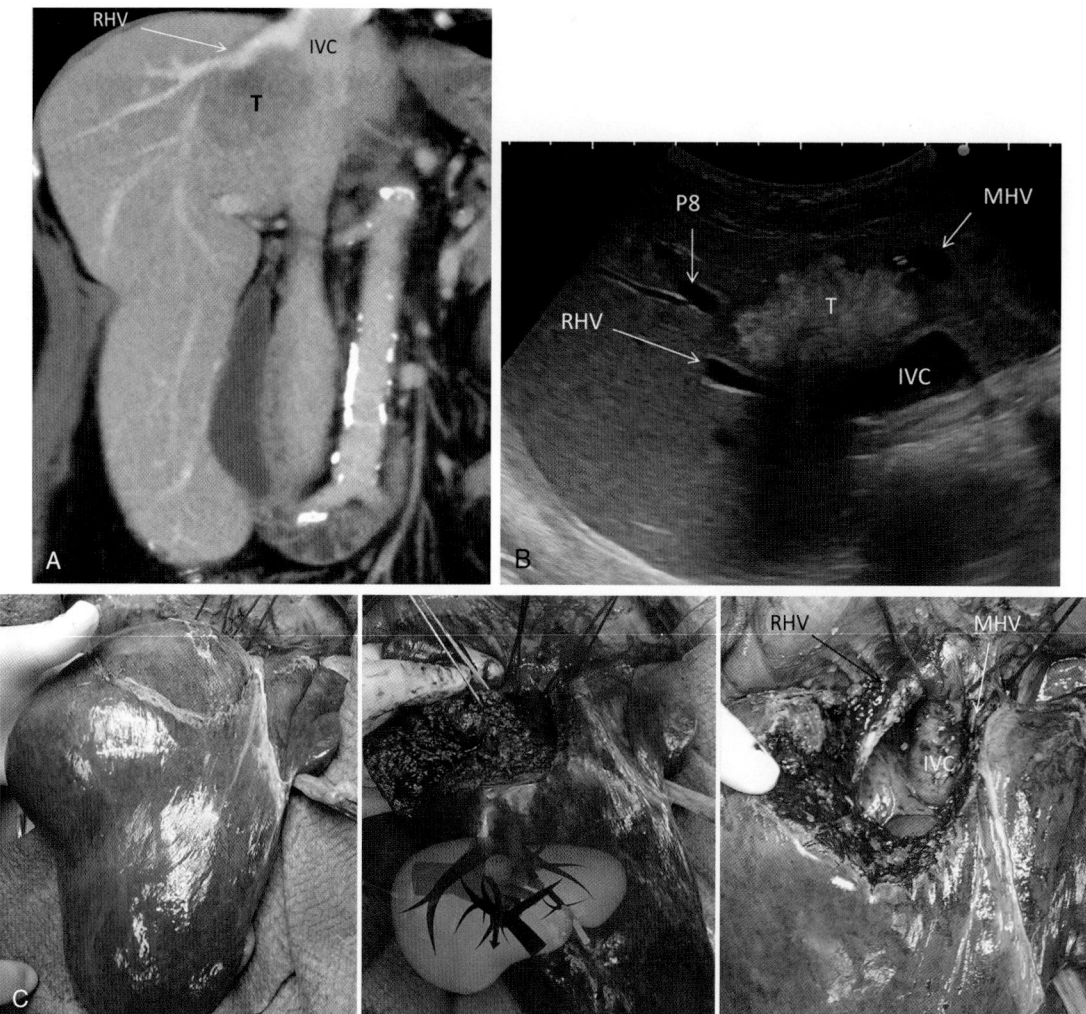

FIGURE 103.72   A, Computed tomography (CT) showing colorectal liver metastases (CLM; *T*) in contact with the inferior vena cava *(IVC)* and the right hepatic vein *(RHV)*. **B,** At intraoperative ultrasound (IOUS), the tumor position dorsal to the Glissonean pedicle for segment VIII *(P8)* and in contact with the middle hepatic vein *(MHV)*, the RHV, and the IVC is well evident. **C,** The liver is fully mobilized and resection is carried out, having the surgeon's nondominant hand placed in front of the IVC and behind the liver gripping the caudate lobe as shown in the overlapped schema. At the end, a liver tunnel with MHV sparing has been performed.

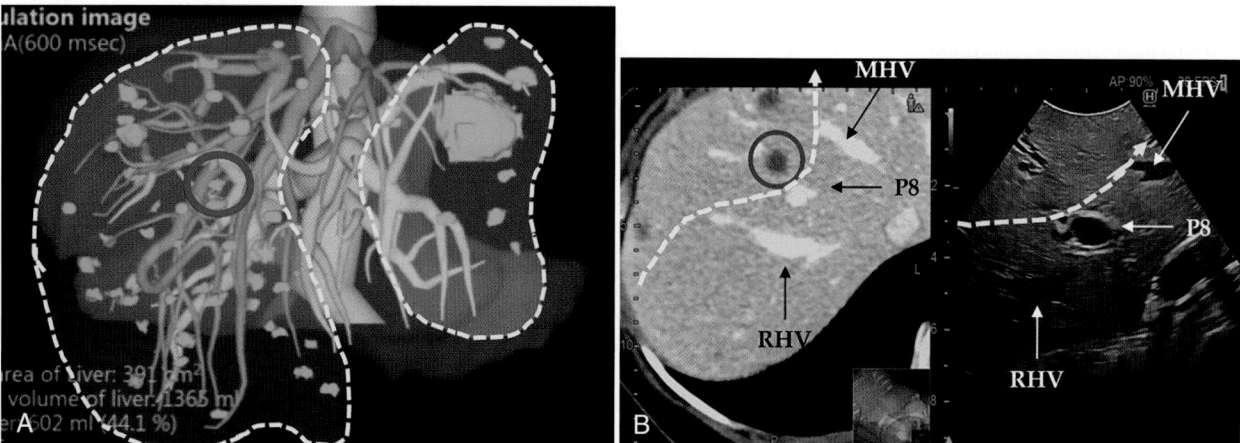

FIGURE 103.73   Surgical treatment of a patient with multiple bilobar colorectal liver metastases *(CLM)*. **A,** Prechemotherapy cast showing areas delimited by yellow-dotted lines, which are grouping the two recognizable clusters; the red circle is highlighting the deepest lesion of the largest cluster *(compound point)*. **B,** At fusion imaging, matching in real time the scans of the prechemotherapy computed tomography (CT) with the intra-operative ultrasound (IOUS) allows us to target the deepest lesion *(red circle)* visible at CT but not at IOUS: With this crucial compound, it is possible to delineate the cluster as grouped on the 3D.

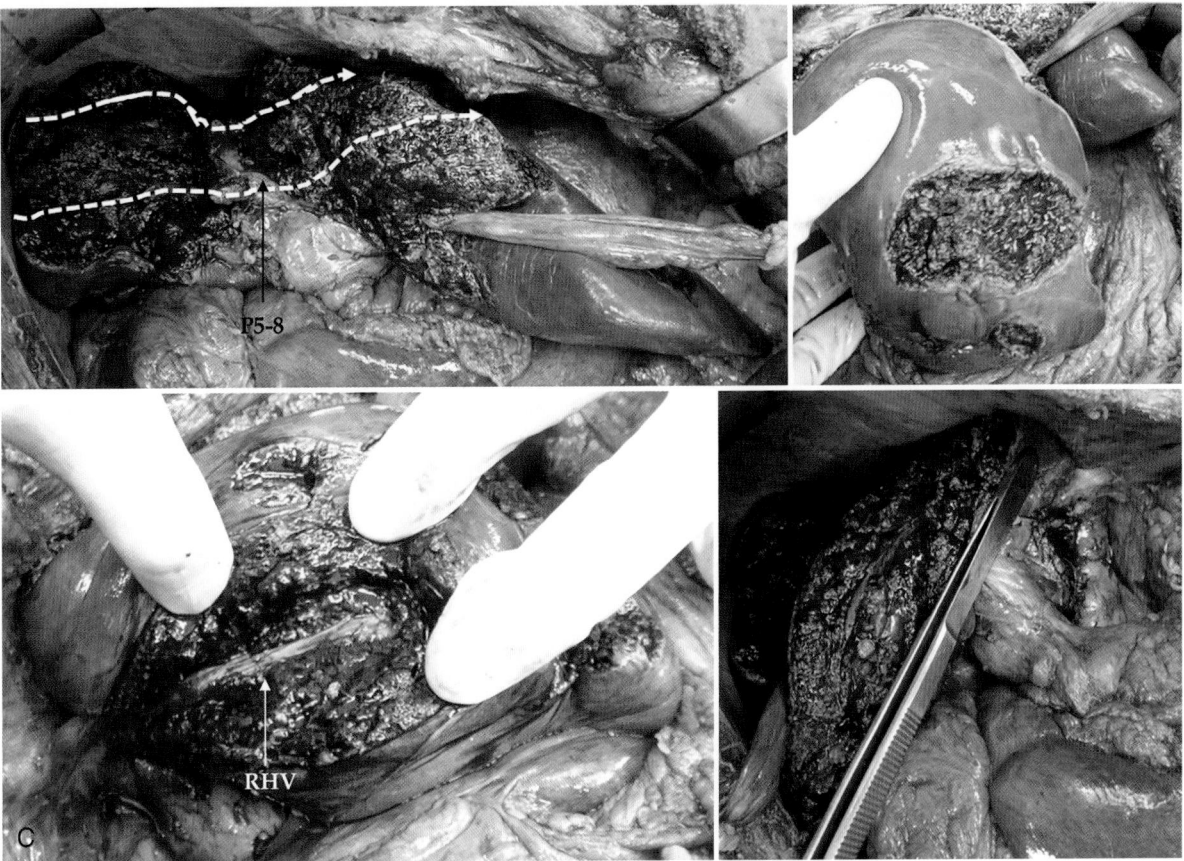

FIGURE 103.73, cont'd   **C**, Resection is carried out, completely removing 83 CLM.

has standardized the FLR estimation in the anatomic resections by computing the modality, limiting the operator dependence of the hand-trace technique and also speeding up the process.[109–111]

Things become more complex when the resections have a multiplanar path and once they are multiple. For such a condition, the hand-trace estimation of FLR becomes unfeasible, although for complex parenchyma-sparing resection, intraoperative findings may impact the surgeon decision making, resulting in a modified strategy, and a reliable preoperative estimation of the FLR according to the previous planning could serve as a reliable baseline. Recently, we demonstrated the reliability of 3D virtual cast in predicting the FLR exclusively in patients with bilobar and deep-located CLMs.[112] A minimal difference between the pursued and real FLR, with a slight preoperative underestimation (median error rate was −0.6%) was disclosed. The intraoperative "adjustment" of the planned surgical procedure, aiming to maximize the parenchyma-sparing in these patients, could partially explain a minimal and negligible difference. For sure, 3D virtual cast applied in the peculiar setting of parenchyma sparing major hepatectomies for multiple bilobar CLM resulted in increased safety and as a consequence could act as a further element favoring its standardization and ultimate diffusion (Figs. 103.74B and 103.75B; see also Figs. 103.65C–D and 103.73A).

Fusion Imaging. In the surgical treatment of multiple bilobar CLM, whatever the planned procedure, a precise definition of the liver involvement should be recommended before starting any neoadjuvant therapy. Indeed, measurement of the treatment response and disclosure of any CLM disappearance are the most relevant issues to be defined after systemic treatment and before surgery. CLM disappearance at the preoperative imaging does not compulsorily mean a real vanishing of any vital residual tumoral tissue other than their removal should be pursued. As mentioned, in the event that surgical strategy would consist in a single session of parenchyma sparing-major hepatectomy, the identification of the clusters' compass points represents one of the pillars. This becomes essential in those conditions featured by multiple CLM disappeared after chemotherapy. For this reason prechemotherapy imaging assumes a crucial role because it may act as a standard of reference for disclosing any CLM and particularly those acting as compass lesions, and eventually disappeared. The fusion imaging feature of advanced US systems matches in real-time any preoperative imaging, even prechemotherapy CT or MRI, with the IOUS resulting in simplified and low-cost solutions for intraoperative navigation in these particular circumstances (see Figs. 103.73B and 103.74C). For this purpose, the probes should be equipped with adapters for sensor allocation as shown in Figure 103.76.

Fusion imaging provides a further advantage for surgeons. Indeed, IOUS scans are simultaneously shown on the same screen with the CT or MRI scans for that particular patient. This facilitates the surgeon's interpretation of IOUS images, which may help in speeding up the learning curve (Fig. 103.77).

Mobilization of the Liver. The aforementioned procedures are still reserved to the open approach given the 3D complexity of the dissection for the complex and often multiple tumor-vessel

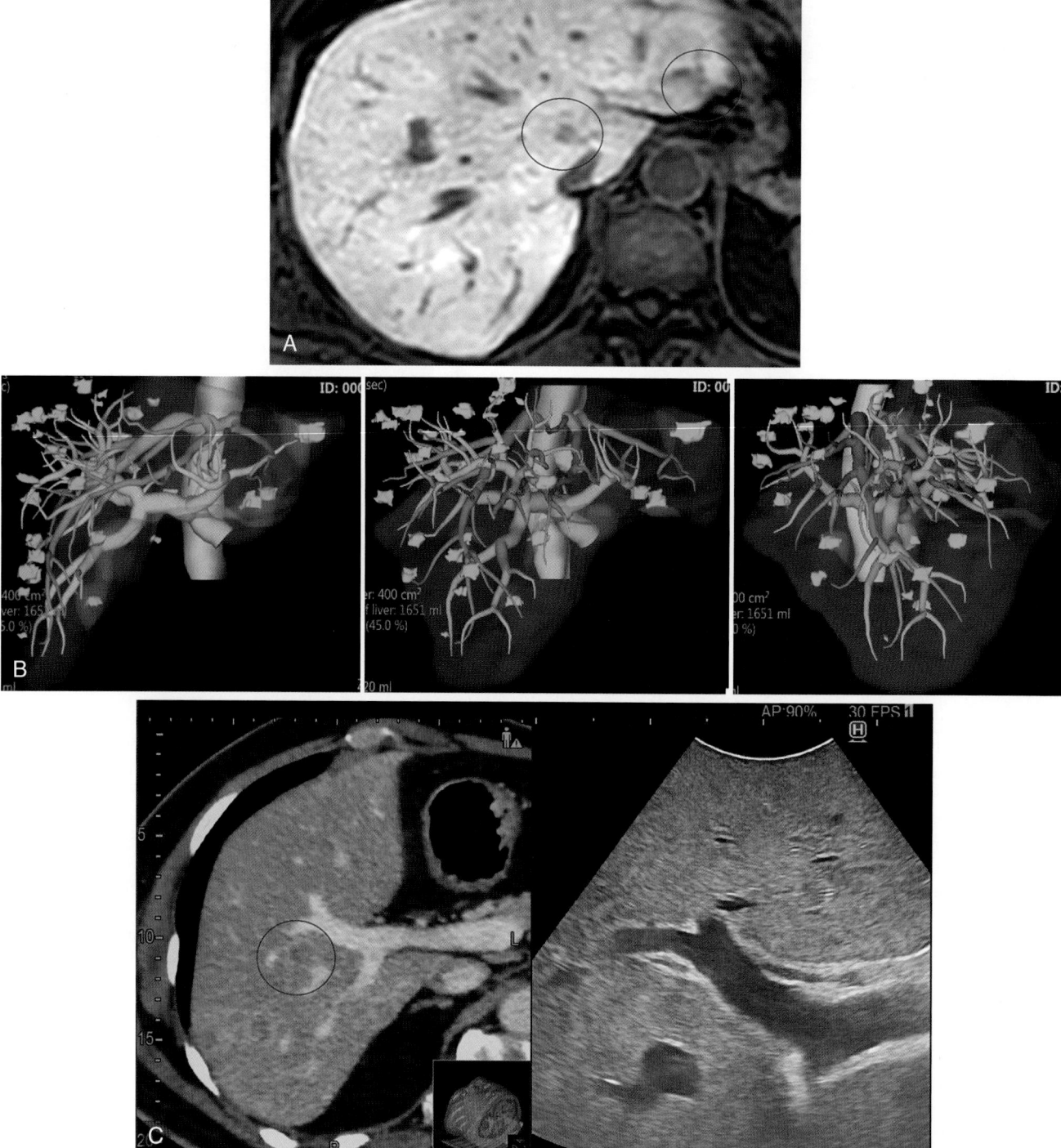

FIGURE 103.74 Surgical treatment of a patient with multiple bilobar colorectal liver metastases *(CLM)*. **A,** At preoperative magnetic resonance, just two lesions are visible *(red circles)*. **B,** The prechemotherapy cast showed multiple bilobar CLM *(green nodules)*; herein, it is shown from three different perspectives. **C,** At fusion imaging, matching in real time the scans of the prechemotherapy computed tomography (CT) with the intraoperative ultrasound (IOUS) allows us to target the deepest lesion *(red circle)* visible at CT but not at IOUS, disclosing its relations with the major vessels: With this crucial compound, it is possible to delineate the dissection line *(black-dotted arrows)* focused on the vessels as a landmark to remove the area inclusive of all the lesions *(red and yellow circles)*.

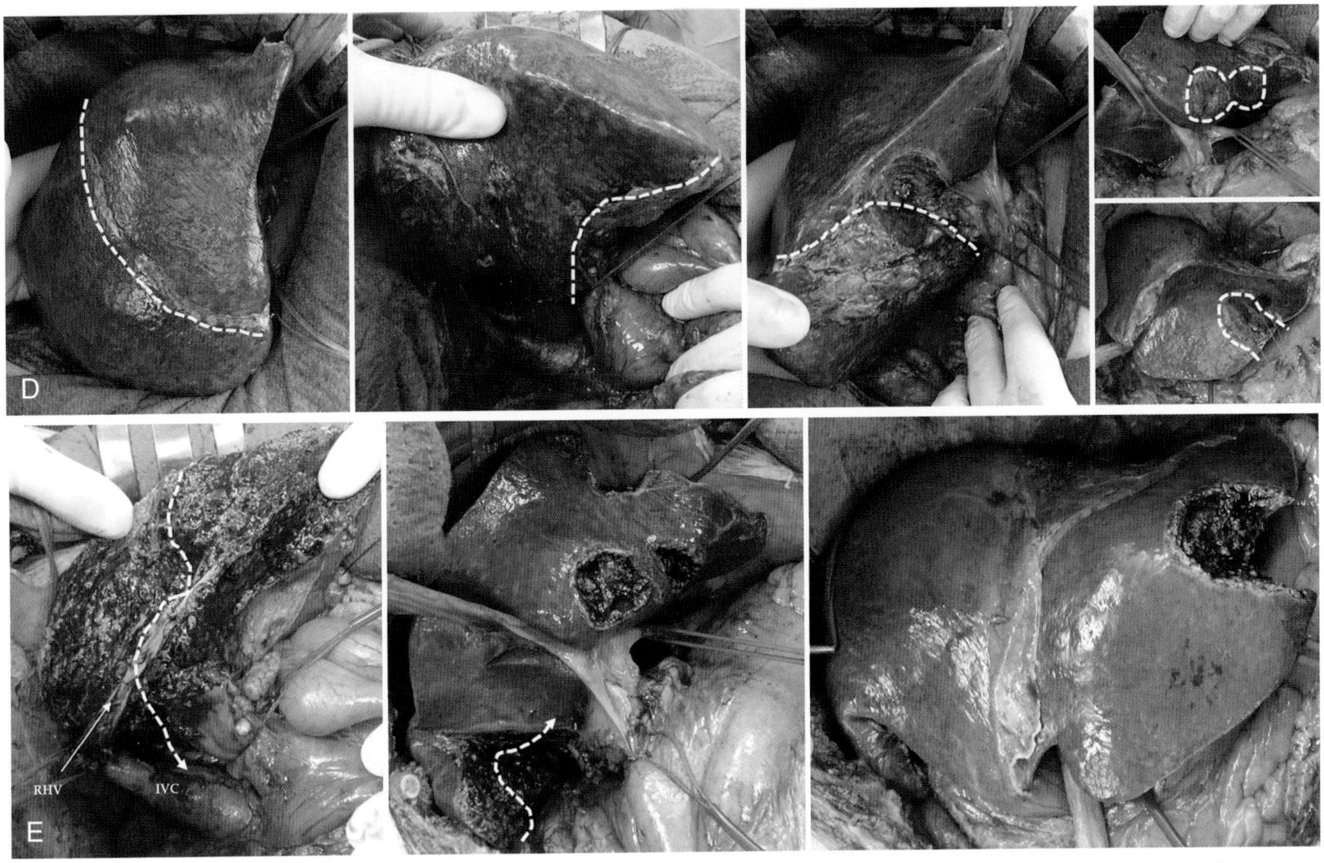

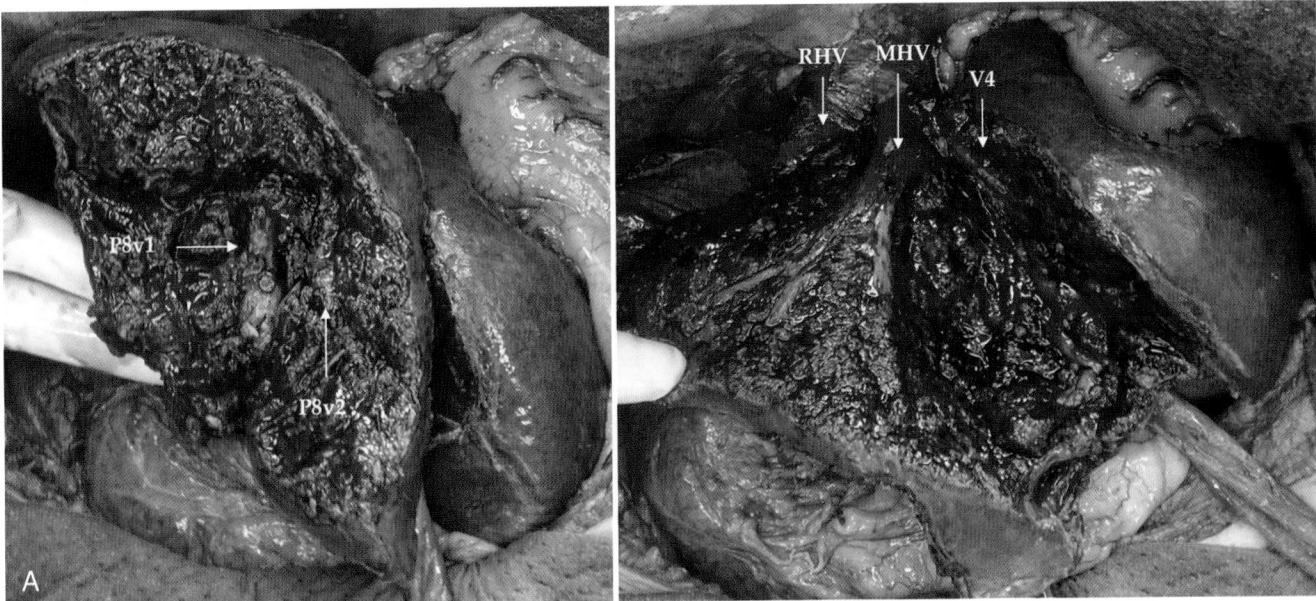

FIGURE 103.74, cont'd   D, The resection areas were drawn on the liver surface and highlighted by the white-dotted lines. **E,** Cut surfaces at the end of the procedure; the white-dotted arrows correspond to the planned dissection. *P6-7,* Portal branch to the right posterior section; *P5-8,* portal branch to the right anterior section; *P8d,* portal branch to segment VIII dorsal; *P8v,* portal branch to segment VIII ventral; *RHV,* right hepatic vein.

FIGURE 103.75   Surgical treatment of a patient with multiple bilobar colorectal liver metastases *(CLM)* recurring after removal of 36 CLM a year and a half before. **A,** The images of the cut surfaces after the first operation.   *Continued*

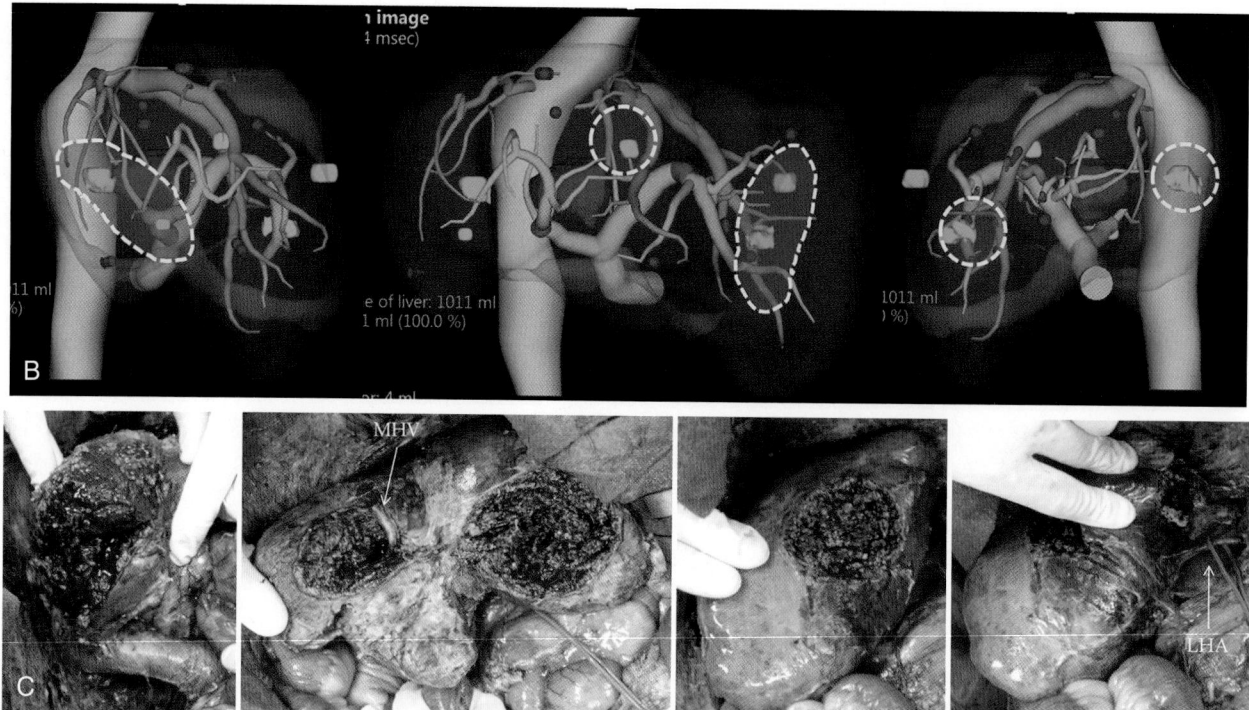

FIGURE 103.75, cont'd   B, Preoperative cast showing globally six lesions (in green, whereas those in pink are cysts) with areas delimited by yellow-dotted lines. C, Resection areas at the end of the operation with one R1vasc procedure to remove a lesion in contact with the middle hepatic vein (MHV). P8v1 and P8v2, portal branches to segment VIII ventral; RHV, right hepatic vein; V4, scissural vein.

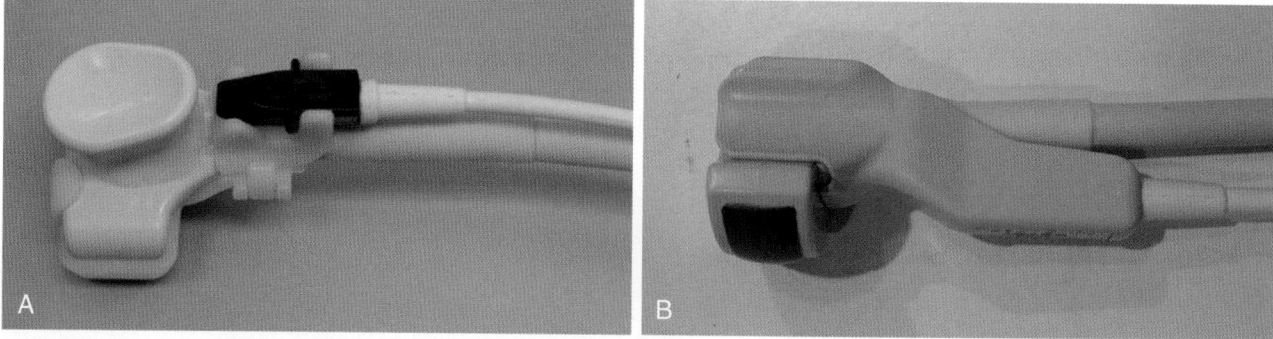

FIGURE 103.76   From left to right, this image shows probes with the adapter for sensor allocation: The sensors allow the ultrasound system to recognize the position of the probe and to match the related scan with the uploaded images of the preoperative computed tomography (CT) or magnetic resonance imaging (MRI; see Fig. 103.77).

relations. In this setting, other than tools (virtual cast and IOUS), oncologic principles (R1vasc), and anatomic features (CV), adequate preparation of the surgical field is essential, which implies adequate incision and liver mobilization. A J-shaped laparotomy is usually performed, and a J-shaped thoracophrenolaparotomy is carried out when the tumor is in the paracaval portion or at the hepatocaval confluence; control of the HVs at this level could be difficult with an abdominal incision only.[113,114] In particular, the surgeon handling of the specimen is critical once liver dissection approaches the hepatocaval confluence and specimen removal is almost accomplished, but the chest has not been opened.

For right-sided segmentectomies, subsegmentectomies, or sectionectomies, the bare area is dissected and the right hemiliver mobilized, until the surgeon's nondominant hand is positioned

behind the hemiliver to support it and is passing over the resection area established by IOUS (Fig. 103.78). As a general principle, there should be enough space to allow the surgeon's fingertip to hang the liver but not place excessive traction, potentially causing injury to the preserved short HVs, which if damaged could lead to critical bleeding. Slight mobilization of the right hemiliver, just dividing the triangular ligament and partially or completely dividing the bare area, will assist in the exposure of lesions located in segments V, VI, and segment VII inferior (Fig. 103.79). Conversely, the right side of the retrohepatic IVC is reached for lesions located in the dorsal portions of segments VII and VIII (Fig. 103.80). If the lesion is in the superior portion of segment VII or the dorsal portion of section VIII—that is, close to the hepatocaval confluence, in the last 4 cm—but it is not in contact with the HVs, and if an anatomic segmental approach is not

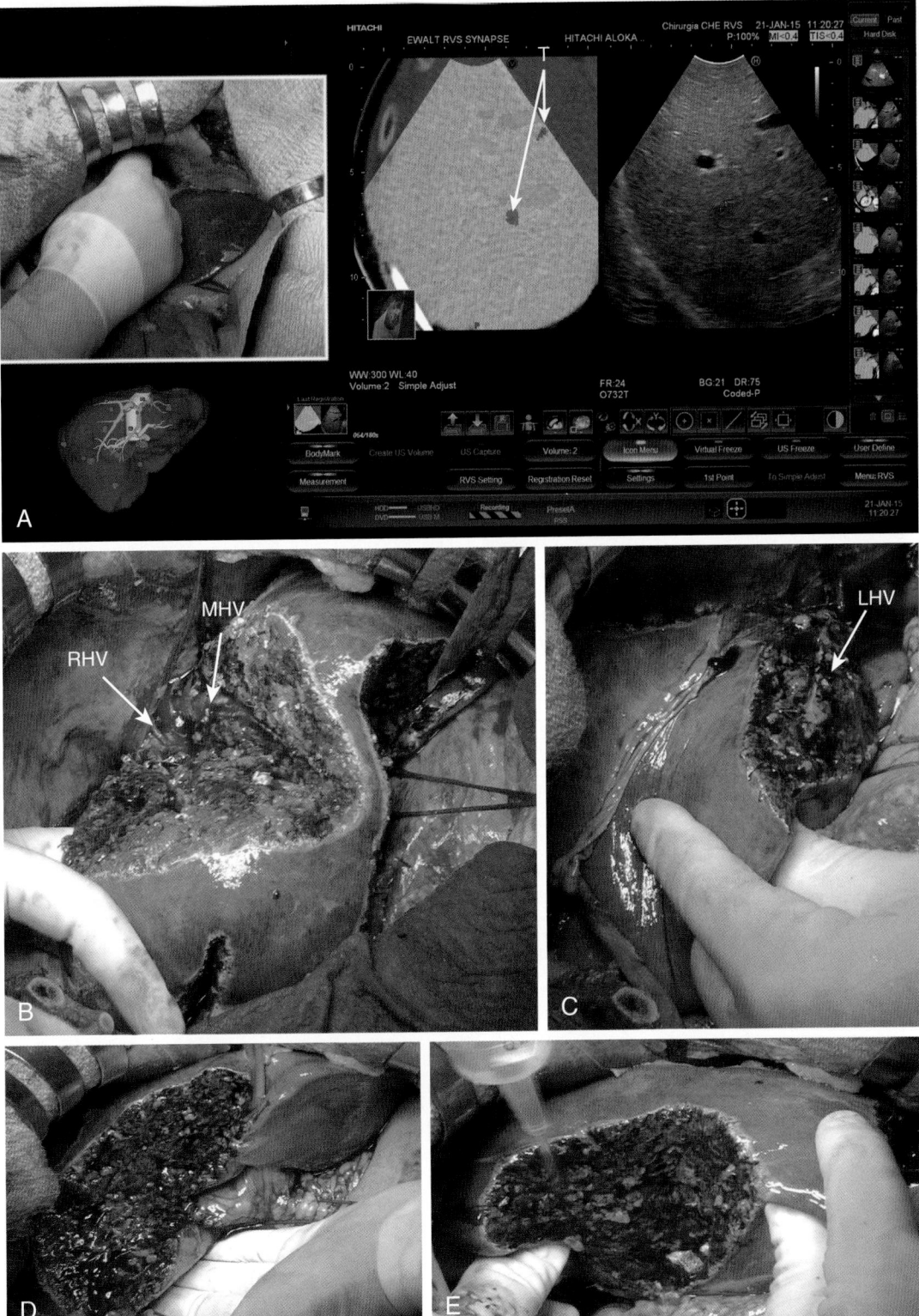

FIGURE 103.77   A, Matching the computed tomography (CT) images at the center of the picture obtained before chemotherapy and uploaded in the ultrasound system before the operation, with those of intraoperative ultrasound (IOUS; *right side of the image*) at surgery (*the probe exploring the liver on the left side of the image*) allows us to locate the disappeared colorectal liver metastases (colored in the CT images for being further highlighted). At the bottom left is the virtual cast of the liver with all the lesions to be removed. **B–E,** The cut surfaces after the IOUS-guided removal of 18 lesions.

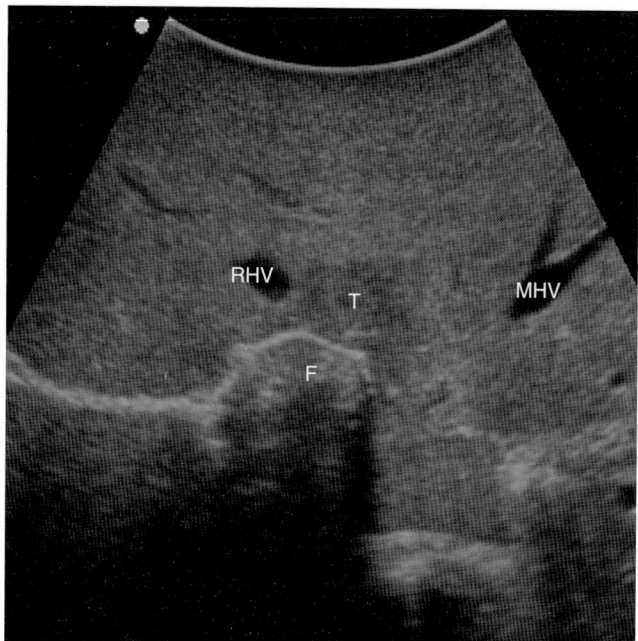

FIGURE 103.78 Intraoperative ultrasound shows the surgeon's finger-tip *(F),* which can be positioned over the left edge of the tumor *(T),* located in the paracaval portion of segment I. This means that the mobilization is probably almost complete. *MHV,* Middle hepatic vein; *RHV,* Right hepatic vein.

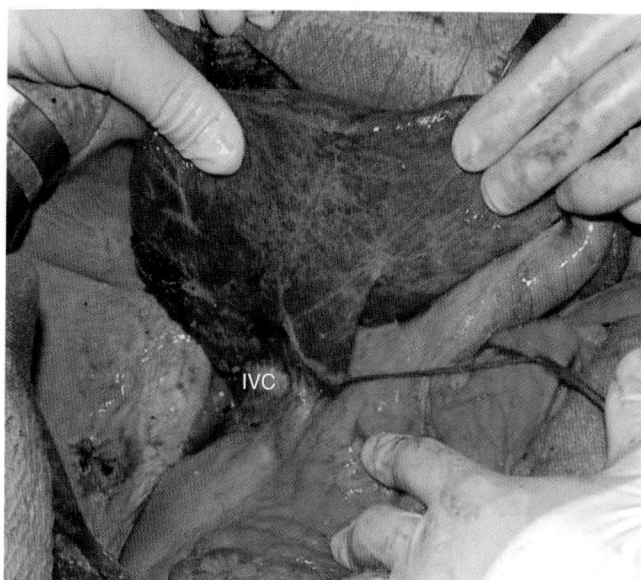

FIGURE 103.79 Mobilization of the right hemiliver just showing the inferior portion of the right-sided anterolateral aspect of the retrohepatic inferior vena cava *(IVC).*

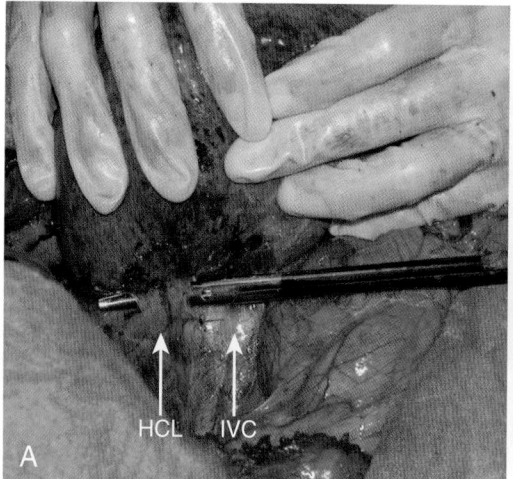 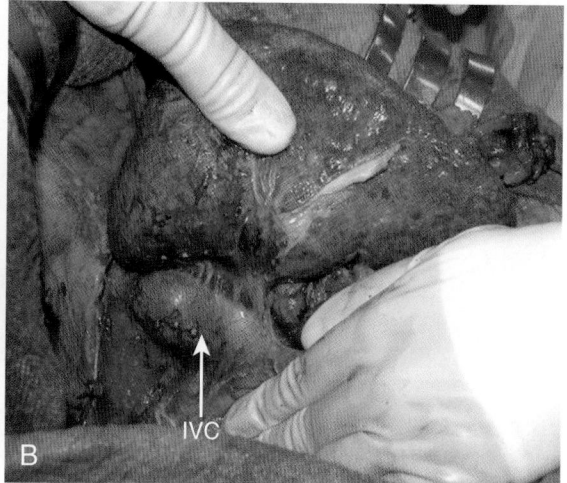

FIGURE 103.80 A, Dissection of the hepatocaval ligament *(HCL)* from the inferior vena cava *(IVC)* with scissors. **B,** This pattern of mobilization allows exposure of the right-sided anterolateral aspect of the retrohepatic IVC.

required, the hepatocaval ligament is not divided, and only the space between the RHV and the MHV is dissected to allow fingertip insertion. The caval confluence of the RHV is recognized by following the course of the right inferior phrenic vein, which flows near the RHV at this level and is a constant landmark (Fig. 103.81).[115]

If the lesion is still right sided but contacts an HV at its caval confluence, or if it involves the paracaval portion of segment I, liver mobilization includes division of the retrohepatic caval ligament and exposure of the retrohepatic IVC. This proceeds until the area to be resected is under control of the surgeon's nondominant hand, with the surgeon's fingertip reaching over the most distal portion of the planned dissection plane, including the complete detachment (Fig. 103.82).

For segment II and III segmentectomies or subsegmentec-tomies, the left triangular ligament and the left coronary ligament are divided, and with the surgeon's nondominant hand, the left liver is handled. For lesions located in the superior portion of segment IV at the hepatocaval junction without contact with the LHV or MHV, the mobilization combines those described for lesions at segment VII (inferior) and those in the left liver. In the case of contact with HVs, their selective encirclement at the caval confluence and eventually exposure of the retrohepatic IVC are performed.

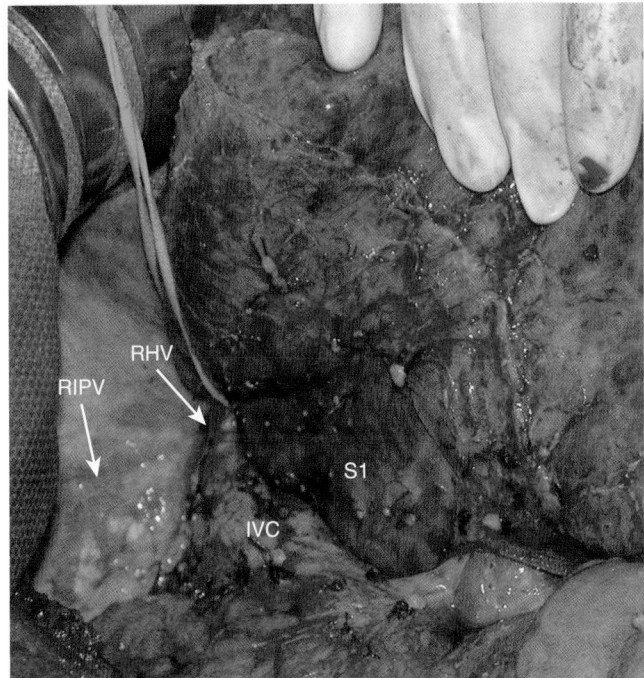

FIGURE 103.81   Full mobilization of the liver from the retrohepatic inferior vena cava (*IVC*) and the right inferior phrenic vein (*RIPV*), which has a trajectory indicating the confluence of the right hepatic vein (*RHV*) into the IVC. *S1*, Segment I.

CONCLUSION

Parenchyma-sparing surgery is often synonymous with limited resections for small superficial tumors ("cherry-picking surgery") or minor anatomic resections for selected deep-located lesions. Herein, hopefully, we have shown parenchyma-sparing surgery to be a reliable solution for complex liver involvement. In the event of multifactorial complexity as high disease burden, both in size and number, and multiple major tumor-vessel

relations, parenchyma-sparing surgery could still be an option and result in a major but different hepatectomy. Some major technical and oncologic issues represent the backbone of this path. First, IOUS guidance, more recently with the aid of preoperative 3D virtual cast, lets the surgeon identify clusters of tumors to be grouped in resection areas and then removed accordingly. That can be performed through a complex multiplanar dissection trajectory, which can be determined preoperatively and determined under real-time intraoperative control (see Fig. 103.65). Second, the possibility to detach tumors from major intrahepatic vessels whenever IOUS excludes infiltration, resulting in oncologically suitable solutions at least for CLM and HCC,[89–91] is the other factor that has moved toward the completion of this policy. Third, CVs among main HVs once recognized and preserved guarantee an adequate outflow to liver parenchyma even after main HV resection. This further element involves the triad of factors representative of a policy in which the liver anatomy, and in particular its vascular architecture, once determined through IOUS, becomes the driver for the surgeon to realize a different paradigm of parenchyma-sparing surgery spelled out as parenchyma-sparing major hepatectomy.

A policy enabled limiting conventional major hepatectomy with vessel amputation in less than 1% of patients with tumors involving one or more HVs at the caval confluence,[94] and limited to 3% of right hepatectomies and 7% of left in patients with multiple bilobar CLM, with up to 83 lesions removed at once (see Fig. 103.73). Preserving the liver scaffold increased the salvageability in case of relapse (see Fig. 103.75).[22,99] Sculpting rather than just resecting the organ also pushes for reconsidering the concept of minor and major hepatectomy,[100] implementing if not rewriting the dictionary of liver surgery. A safer clinical outcome after major tissue deprivation in a vessel-guided hepatectomy fashion compared with that after major resections through conventional vessels amputation should also deserve some consideration.[100,116,117] ALPPS has been shown to be associated with an increment in liver volume, which does not translate one to one with liver function.[118] Parenchyma-sparing major hepatectomy keeping the organ scaffold even after removal of a large

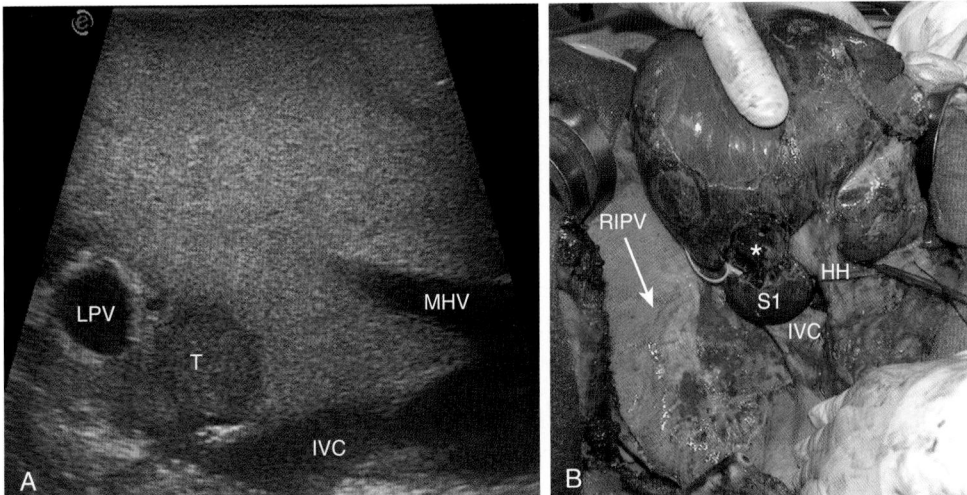

FIGURE 103.82   **A,** Intraoperative ultrasound image of a lesion (*T*) located in the paracaval portion of segment I. **B,** For its removal by means of a limited resection (*asterisk*), full mobilization of the liver from the retrohepatic inferior vena cava (*IVC*) is carried out. *LPV,* Left portal vein; *HH,* hepatic hilum; *MHV,* middle hepatic vein; *RIPV,* right inferior phrenic vein; *S1,* segment I.

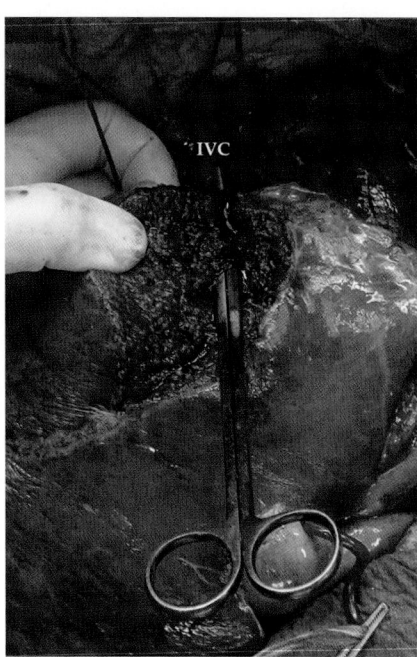

FIGURE 103.83 **A,** Metzenbaum scissors used for tunneling the plane between the liver parenchyma and the anterior face of the middle hepatic vein up to its caval confluence. *IVC,* Inferior vena cava.

and workshops accordingly. Comparably, its partial applicability to the concept of minimal access liver surgery that currently attracts large investments of the health industry stands in stark contrast to the visibility within the surgical community of robotics and laparoscopic techniques. The latter are as yet more prone to perform even staged procedures rather than complex parenchyma-sparing resection featured by multiplanar dissection.[119] The coexistence and merging of the parenchyma-sparing IOUS and vessel-guided surgery and MALS attitudes could and should be the challenge for the near future, yet the focus needs to remain on safety, oncologic radicality, salvageability of the surgical approach in case of recurrence, and, of course, quality of life.

In term of training, in our own experience, a young surgical team (mean age of 36 years) could independently cover on a yearly basis up to 80% of surgical procedures as herein described within 5 to 6 years of the learning curve.[15] A critical point could be the tutorship but that is the case with any kind of innovative approach.

In summary, the policy described in this chapter uses the IOUS and the main intrahepatic vessels as drivers for dissection and tumor clearance. It provides by following the intrahepatic vessel then respecting the organ anatomy a greater degree of freedom than any "anatomic" approach based on vessel amputation only (i.e., right/left hepatectomies, sectionectomies, and segmentectomies). Moreover, it introduces new oncologic concepts, such as R1vasc surgery, which make suitable surgery previously considered unfeasible as in case of bilateral tumor-vascular contact. It indicates the possibility of conservative surgery, even amputating HVs at caval confluence by disclosing the constant existence of CVs in these circumstances and emphasizing their role in guaranteeing the outflow. It increases the safety by saving the liver scaffold, which suggests a more physiologic regeneration, perhaps avoiding a small for size syndrome by acute vessel amputation. Finally, it enhances the salvageability in case of relapse, warranting more technical solutions once the liver scaffold is preserved.

For all these reasons, parenchyma-sparing IOUS/vessel-guided resections should enter in the armamentarium of every hepatic surgeon. The present and future challenge should be to train young surgeons to make this approach fully established in the practice of hepatic surgery. If so, parenchyma-sparing complex and even major hepatectomies will no longer sound like a paradox but like an option.

References are available at expertconsult.com

amount of liver tissue, as it happens in the case of multiple complex resections for bilobar colorectal liver metastases, has shown a low rate of liver failure.[116,117] Milder regeneration of the liver by preserving the liver scaffold compared with that evident after major amputation of the organ may not be just a suggestion.

Despite the strengths of this policy, implementation into a wider clinical practice remains to be demonstrated. As a technically sophisticated procedure, it is first and foremost based on the surgeon-skill resources rather than on technology. Essentially, ignoring the 3D virtual cast, anyhow based on a computer and a software, all that is basically needed is a US probe, a Kelly clamp, and a pair of Metzenbaum scissor (Fig. 103.83; see also Fig. 103.53). The procedure cost is comparably low and the clinical applicability potentially wide. However, the absence of any highly technologic equipment makes the interest from the health industry relatively low, and thus there is a reduced attention and fewer sponsored opportunities for training

PART 8

Liver and Pancreas Transplantation

I. General

II. Indications

SECTION I. General

CHAPTER **104**

Liver and pancreas transplantation immunobiology

Andrew S. Barbas, Michael E. Lidsky, and Allan D. Kirk

Allotransplantation, defined as the transfer of tissues between genetically nonidentical individuals, has evolved into a highly successful therapy for end-stage organ failure in the modern era. However, unless some modification of the recipient immune system is made, transplanted organs are invariably destroyed through a process broadly known as *rejection.*

Over the last several decades, the ability to manipulate the immune response has become increasingly selective and less morbid. Through a general understanding of alloimmunity and the unique properties of the liver and pancreas, transplantation results have steadily improved.[1,2] This chapter provides a synopsis of the principles governing immune management of liver and pancreatic transplant recipients, highlighting agents and strategies available for clinical use.

GENERAL CONSIDERATIONS: SPECIFICITY AND CONTEXT

Allograft rejection is mediated by the normal elements of the physiologic immune system but arises in response to the non-physiologic practice of *solid organ transplantation.* As with most immune responses, rejection requires a specific *recognition* event combined with a *context* that signifies that this recognition warrants a response (see Chapter 10).

Immune recognition is mediated through one of two types of lymphocyte receptors: the T-cell receptor (on the surface of T cells) or the immunoglobulin (Ig) receptor (on the surface of B cells). Immune specificity is dictated by the ability of these receptors to bind a complementary epitope. In the setting of transplantation, the recipient immune system recognizes specific molecules present on the surface of graft cells, known as *major histocompatibility complex* (MHC) molecules. In humans, these proteins are also referred to as human leukocyte antigens (HLAs). MHC molecules arise from a cluster of highly polymorphic genes on chromosome 6, with tens of thousands of different MHC alleles identified in humans. Graft MHC molecules serve as the primary immune targets after transplantation, as described further in the chapter.

The context of an immune response is governed through another set of receptors known as *costimulation receptors.* Broadly speaking, these receptors provide signals that determine whether antigen recognition should evoke an immune response and whether that response should be aggressive or attenuating. These receptors are also involved in the mechanisms of response termination, ensuring that immune responses are contained within physiologic parameters. By separating the signals

for specificity and context, the immune response to pathogens, and allografts, can be tightly regulated and finely manipulated.

Typically, the ligands for costimulation receptors are most prominently expressed on antigen-presenting cells (APCs), including dendritic cells and macrophages, which play a central role in initiating and sustaining an immune response. The interactions between APCs and lymphocytes usually take place in lymphoid organs, such as the spleen or lymph nodes. The requirement for APCs and the necessity for secondary lymphoid organs provide additional opportunity for regulation and reduce the risk of autoimmune responses.

PHYSIOLOGIC IMMUNITY

The immune system evolved to protect the body from pathogens, not to mediate transplant rejection. Although alloimmunity and physiologic immunity differ, it is critical to understand the components of the alloimmune response in their physiologic roles (see Chapter 10).

The immune system is organized into two complementary arms, innate and acquired. The *innate immune system* is activated by heterogeneous molecular patterns derived from either microbial products (for example, lipopolysaccharide [LPS]) or tissue damage arising from sterile inflammatory states including ischemia, necrosis, and trauma.[3-6] The *acquired immune system* subsequently recognizes and eliminates pathogens in a specific manner through antigen presentation and recognition. Both systems interact to maintain overall homeostasis. Typically, innate responses generate localized inflammation at sites of injury and are less overtly regulated. In contrast, acquired immune responses lead to carefully regulated destruction of antigen-expressing tissue. The regulatory checks on acquired immunity prevent autoimmunity and uncontrolled lymphocyte proliferation. It is important to recognize that the acquired immune system is tailored for each individual based on their unique MHC makeup. Evolutionarily, this diversity reduces the chance that a particular pathogen can evade all individuals within a population. However, this also means that an individual's acquired immune response may be deleterious when exposed to foreign MHC in the setting of allotransplantation.

Innate Immunity

The cellular components of the innate immune system include dendritic cells, macrophages, neutrophils, and natural killer cells. These cells are activated by binding of either microbial by-products (pathogen-associated molecular patterns [PAMPs]) or products of sterile tissue injury (damage-associated molecular patterns [DAMPs]) to pattern-recognition receptors located in both intracellular and cell surface compartments. Perhaps the most well-described pattern-recognition receptor is the Toll-like receptor (TLR). This highly conserved family of receptors responds to PAMPs associated with microbial infection, including LPS as well as DAMPs generated by cell death, including high mobility group box-1 (HMGB1).[7] Interestingly, the TLRs expressed in the liver differ from those expressed in the periphery and tend to be less responsive to ambient LPS.[8] This is likely an adaptation to portal bacteremia and is thought to make the liver more tolerant of minor perturbations that would evoke an innate response in other organs. It is important to note that innate immune receptors are conserved between individuals and do not demonstrate the polymorphic nature of MHC as described previously.

Binding of PAMPs and DAMPs to innate immune receptors initiate signaling cascades resulting in generalized inflammation and activation of complement.[3,4,9] Of particular relevance in transplantation, ischemia-reperfusion injury and associated cell death results in the release of multiple DAMPs derived from different subcellular compartments including the nucleus (extracellular DNA, HMGB1) and mitochondria (mitochondrial DNA, reactive oxygen species). Recently, greater attention has been paid to the effects of DAMP-mediated inflammation on both early graft injury and function and the connection with the subsequent adaptive immune response.[10,11]

The complement system acts as the primary mediator of cytolysis, and the by-products of complement help link the innate and acquired immune responses.[12,13] Platelets have also been increasingly recognized as serving an innate immune role through the release of chemotactic proteins and other immunostimulatory molecules.[14]

Acquired Immunity

Specific recognition is the hallmark of the acquired immune system. The immense structural diversity of the lymphocyte receptors (T-cell and B-cell receptors) facilitates recognition of a vast array of antigens. Furthermore, initial antigen recognition induces physiologic change in the lymphocyte, lowering the threshold for activation in response to subsequent encounters. This phenomenon underlies the concept of *immunologic memory*, which results in a more rapid (anamnestic) response to subsequent antigen encounters.[15] T-cell receptors (TCRs) bind peptide antigens that have been processed and presented in combination with MHC. B-cell Igs bind antigens in their native conformation and can be secreted in soluble form as circulating antibodies that act remotely.

Cellular Immunity

Understanding the unique nature of the TCR is fundamental to understanding its function.[16,17] T cells, formed in the bone marrow and fetal liver, migrate to the thymus during development, where they undergo rearrangement of the DNA that encodes the TCR.[18] Each gene rearrangement results in the generation of a TCR with specificity generally restricted to one epitope, although some cross-reactivity can occur with similar epitopes. The sum of all random TCR gene rearrangements generates TCRs with approximately 10^9 unique specificities. If such a vast array of T cells was to be released immediately into the periphery, they would mediate widespread and fatal autoimmune processes. Accordingly, the process of thymic selection eliminates those T cells likely to induce autoimmunity.[19,20]

The initial phase of thymic selection occurs through the interaction of cortical thymic epithelial cells with the cohort of developing T cells. These T cells express the accessory cell surface markers CD4 or CD8, which facilitate stronger binding interactions between the TCR and MHC. If T-cell binding does not occur to the self MHC molecules presented by the thymic epithelium, the T cells are eliminated because they are unable to interact with self MHC molecules, which is required for normal immune surveillance and function. This process is known as *positive selection*.

Positive selection produces a repertoire of T cells capable of recognizing and binding to self MHC, which is critical for normal functioning in the periphery. However, this step does not distinguish T cells with normal affinity from those with inappropriately strong affinity to self MHC, which would predispose to autoimmunity. To eliminate cells with a high risk of autoimmune recognition, the developing T cells then move into the thymic medulla, where either CD4 or CD8 expression is lost. If binding to self MHC in the medulla results in a high-affinity interaction, these T cells are also eliminated, a process known as *negative selection*. Therefore, after this step the majority of T cells released from the thymus bind to self MHC but fail to become activated in the absence of additional costimulatory molecules. This process is imperfect, and autoreactive cells occasionally escape thymic selection, contributing to disease processes such as primary sclerosing cholangitis (see Chapters 10 and 41), autoimmune hepatitis (see Chapters 10 and 68), and type 1 diabetes. However, the bar for activation remains high and thus limits the risk of autoimmunity. For example, a single interaction of TCR and antigen-bearing MHC is inadequate to trigger T-cell activation; rather, approximately 8000 TCR-MHC interactions over the course of several hours are needed to initiate activation,[21-23] which further limits the likelihood of autoimmunity. Costimulatory molecules greatly alter this need for redundancy, as discussed subsequently.

T cells are further distinguished by the accessory cell surface molecules CD8 and CD4 that influence the cell types that they are capable of interacting with and their roles in the immune response.[24,25] CD8[+] T cells, known as *cytotoxic T cells*, bind to cells expressing class I MHC molecules. This binding interaction is facilitated by CD8 stabilization of TCR-MHC class I ligation. All parenchymal cells express class I MHC and display internal cellular peptides within the binding groove of this molecule. Cytotoxic T cells recognize diseased or infected parenchymal cells and activate cytolytic mechanisms. T-cell killing can occur through either calcium ion (Ca^{2+})-dependent secretory mechanisms or Ca^{2+}-independent direct cell contact mechanisms.[26]

CD4[+] T cells, also known as helper T cells, interact with APCs expressing MHC class II including dendritic cells, macrophages, and activated endothelial cells. This interaction is mediated by CD4 stabilization of TCR-MHC class II ligation. MHC class II displays peptide fragments that have been phagocytized from the extracellular space.[27,28] Interestingly, resting sinusoidal endothelial cells of the liver are capable of presenting antigen to T cells, making the liver an organ with considerable ability to evoke or suppress an immune response.[29] The interaction between CD4[+] T cells and APCs influences subsequent activation of CD8[+] T cells.[30,31] This process is mediated through upregulation of cell surface molecules on APCs known as *costimulation receptors*. Thus while APCs act as initiators of an immune response, they require CD4[+] T cells to activate the primary effector arm of the acquired immune system mediated by CD8[+] T cells.

An additional subset of T cells, regulatory T cells (Treg), further limit promiscuous immune responses. Treg cells have the ability to suppress cytokine secretion, adhesion molecule expression, and costimulatory signaling. The most extensively studied population of Treg cells express CD4 and CD25, the high-affinity α-chain of the interleukin (IL)-2 receptor.[32] Animal models suggest that these cells play a critical role in controlling immune activation.[32,33] The prevailing evidence suggests that Treg cells are responsive to established inflammation, rather than serving a prophylactic role in preventing inflammation. However, harnessing the power of Treg cells to quell counteradaptive immune responses such as rejection is an ongoing area of research in autoimmunity and alloimmunity.[34]

Humoral Immunity

B cells recognize antigen in its native, unprocessed form.[35] When antigen binds to two cell surface antibody receptors, the antibodies are brought together in a process known as *cross-linking*, stimulating B-cell proliferation and differentiation into an antibody-secreting plasma cell. The activation threshold for a resting B cell is relatively high, and similar to TCR recognition, costimulation can lower this threshold substantially.[36] B cells also have the ability to internalize antigen bound to surface immunoglobulins and process them for presentation to T cells along with costimulation molecules.[37]

Antibody structure is determined in the bone marrow through mechanisms similar to those that govern the generation of TCR diversity in the thymus.[18,38] Five different heavy-chain loci (μ, γ, α, ε, and δ) on chromosome 14 and two different light-chain loci (κ and λ) on chromosome 2, each with V, D, and/or J, and C regions, are brought together randomly by the RAG1 and RAG2 apparatus to form a functional antigen receptor.[39] The basic antibody structure consists of two identical heavy chains and two identical light chains. The type of heavy chain dictates the Ig class: IgM, IgG, IgA, IgE, or IgD. The overall structure of the antibody results in two identical antigen-binding sites and a common region, the Fc portion. Bound antibody triggers activation of the complement cascade.[40] In addition, most phagocytic cells have receptors for the Fc portion of IgG, allowing them to actively engulf antibody-coated cells.

Unlike the TCR, B-cell immunoglobulin loci undergo several forms of alteration after stimulation to improve the functionality of the secreted antibody. *Isotype switching* is the process of shifting from the initial heavy-chain IgM to one of four types to improve function and specialization of the secreted antibody. IgG is the most significant soluble mediator of opsonization and is the dominant antibody produced in response to alloantigen. IgA is important in mucosal immunity, IgE is involved in mast cell–mediated immunity, and IgD is primarily cell bound. After a B cell is activated, the specific D and J regions of the heavy- and light-chain genes undergo random alterations of the antigen-binding site. The resultant B-cell clones have altered antigen affinity, and this process is termed *affinity maturation*.[41] Clones that have higher affinity for the target antigen have a selective survival advantage and form the basis for a more vigorous response on reexposure to the antigen.

Evolving Cellular Composition With Age

A hallmark of immunity is the ability to adapt based on prior immune experience, such that initial immune responses are less robust than anamnestic responses. As humans age, immune experience grows, manifesting in an observed loss of naive

T and B cells and a commensurate accumulation of cells expressing a memory phenotype. This transition is accentuated by physiologic thymic atrophy, which slows the production of naive T cells.[42] In fact, the pool of available naive T cells is a function of thymic involution and the ongoing conversion to memory and senescent CD8 T cells.[43] This transition with aging imparts a significant effect on the immune system that is particularly evident in elderly persons but measurable in most people by the fourth decade of life.[44–46]

By using established markers of resting naive T cells and memory cell activation, four T-cell subpopulations have been described that appear to differ in terms of their degree of antigen experience, prior activation history, and migratory capabilities.[47] These can be defined as naive T cells, effector memory T cells, central memory T cells, and terminally differentiated effector cells. During the last decade, numerous surface markers have been used to assess the myriad differentiation pathways seen after antigen exposure, and it is now clear that the lymphocyte repertoire is dynamic over time.[48] Although it is beyond the scope of this chapter to define the specifics of this migration from naiveté to experience, it should be recognized that each individual's immune repertoire is a product of both their inherited molecular makeup and their prior immune exposures. This is increasingly important because many of the molecules targeted in transplantation, particularly costimulatory molecules, are altered with immune experience such that optimal immune management is likely to require cognizance of these changes.

Mediators of Context: Costimulation and Cytokines

Isolated TCR binding with an MHC-peptide complex or antibody ligation with an antigen is not usually sufficient for naive lymphocyte activation. Receptor-ligand pairs on T and B cells and APCs, known as *costimulation receptors*, determine the character of the T-cell response (Fig. 104.1).[49–51] The type of costimulatory signal received by the lymphocyte determines whether the cell will become activated, remain quiescent, die, or become resistant to subsequent immune stimulation.

The biology of T-cell costimulation is substantially more developed than that of B-cell costimulation. Examples of T-cell costimulation receptors include CD28 and CTLA-4 (CD152). CD28 promotes T-cell activation and leads to the expression of CTLA-4, which then promotes downregulation of the T-cell response; thus activation typically begets deactivation. The B7 molecules CD80 and CD86, found on APCs, are the ligands for CD28 and CTLA-4. Although B7 molecules can bind to either receptor, their affinity for CTLA-4 is much greater; when B7 is in limited supply, the higher-affinity interaction with CTLA-4 predominates. Because B7 molecules are not expressed by normal tissues, CD8$^+$ T-cell interaction with class I self MHC does not elicit a proliferative response; instead it reinforces quiescence of autoreactive T-cell clones.

Although the mechanisms of costimulation have not been completely elucidated, it is known that binding of CD28 allows more efficient T-cell signal transduction. Through CD28-B7 interactions, the number of binding events required to trigger activation of a T cell decrease from 8000 to 1500.[22,23] In contrast, when CTLA-4 binds B7, the T cell becomes incapable of producing IL-2 during the encounter and even in subsequent interactions.[52] The CD19-CD21 complex provides comparable control of antigen receptor binding for B cells.[36]

Additionally, costimulation is mediated through another pair of receptors: CD40, found on dendritic cells, endothelium,

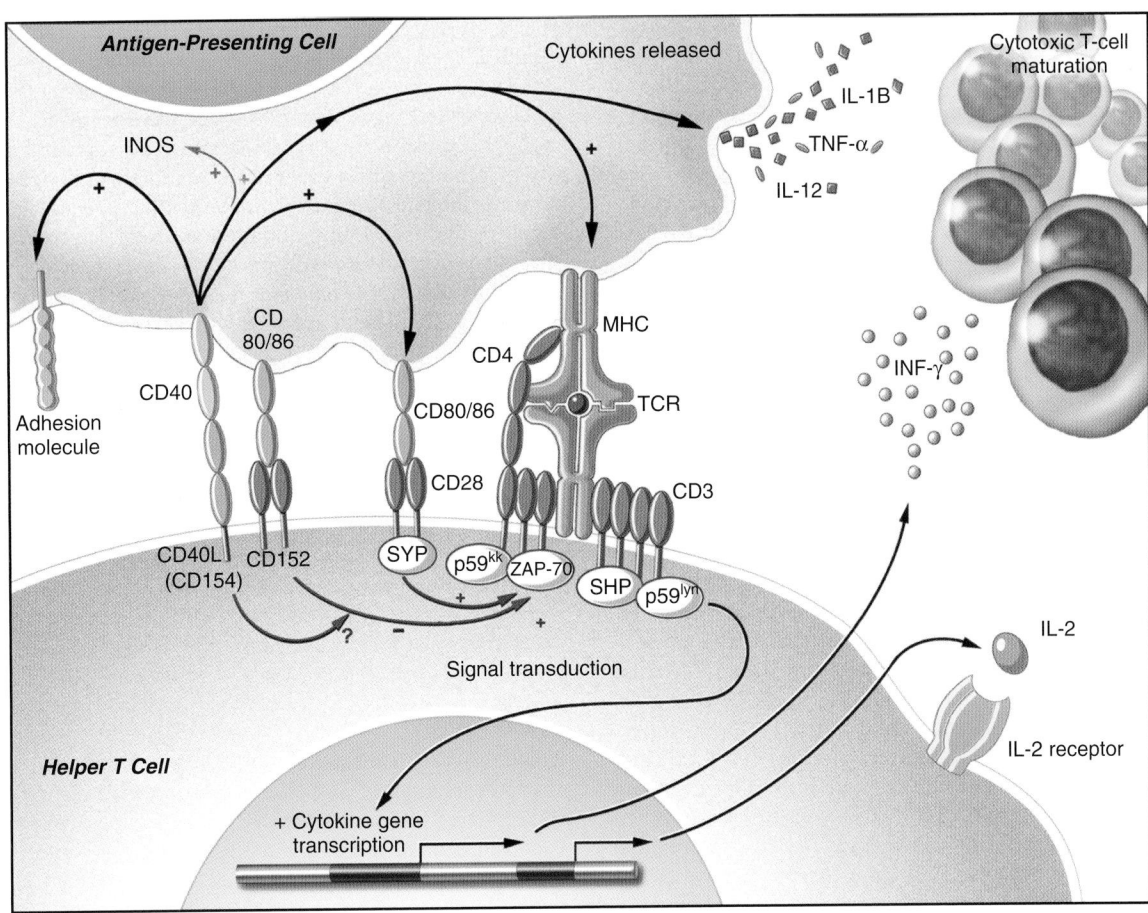

FIGURE 104.1 **T-cell interactions with an antigen-presenting cell (*APC*).** The T-cell receptor *(TCR)* is bound to class II major histocompatibility complex *(MHC)* with the CD4 accessory molecule stabilizing the interaction. Depicted are selected costimulatory molecule interactions and the resultant effects on cytokine secretion and signal transduction. For example, CD40 ligation on the APC results in the induction of many critical APC functions, including increased MHC and B7 expression and cytokine secretion. Increased B7 expression allows CD28-positive regulation to override the negative regulation of CD152 (CTLA-4). This potentiates TCR signal transduction through CD3 and results in interferon *(IFN)*-γ and interleukin *(IL)*-2 synthesis. IFN-γ, along with APC-secreted cytokines, promotes cytotoxic T-cell maturation. IL-2 promotes T-cell proliferation in an autocrine fashion. *INOS,* Inducible nitric oxide synthetase; *TNF,* tumor necrosis factor (see Chapter 10); *SYP,* synaptophysin; *ZAP70,* Zeta-chain-associated protein kinase 70; *SHP,* Src homology region 2 domain-containing phosphatase.

B cells and other APCs, and CD154 on T cells and platelets.[53-57] The ability of APCs to stimulate a cytotoxic T-cell response is greatly augmented by the effects of CD40 binding. After CD40 ligation, activating cytokines are released and B7 molecules are upregulated.[58,59] CD154 is upregulated after TCR ligation and provides positive feedback to the APC. In addition, CD154 is found in and released by activated platelets at sites of endothelial injury.[56] Therefore sites of trauma that recruit platelets create an environment of activating costimulatory molecules, thereby bridging the innate and acquired immune systems.[60]

Direct cell-to-cell contact is not the only means by which immune cells communicate. Soluble mediators of communication known as *cytokines,* or *interleukins,* are polypeptides that are released from many cells; they can either activate or suppress adjacent cells,[61] and the pattern of cytokine expression is thought to influence the resultant type of T-cell response.[62,63] Once activated, T cells have been described by one of several cytokine-secretion phenotypes. T cells that promote cytotoxic responses are characterized by expression of IL-2, IL-12, IL-15, and interferon (IFN)-γ and are called *helper T type 1* (Th1) cells; T cells that promote humoral or eosinophilic responses are

characterized by secretion of IL-4, IL-5, IL-10, and IL-13 and are called *helper T type 2* (Th2) cells. More recently, additional cytokine lineages have emerged; the most relevant to this chapter is the Th17 lineage, involved in gut immunity and driven by IL-6, IL-23, and transforming growth factor (TGF)-β.[64]

In addition to cytokines, other soluble mediators of inflammation are capable of promoting increased blood flow and improved exposure of an area of injury to innate and acquired immune elements. Some suggest that the APCs of the liver are more efficient in generating Th2 responses, which may be a mechanism by which liver allografts avoid late cellular rejection.

TRANSPLANT IMMUNITY

T-cell responses to allogeneic organs are largely the result of nonphysiologic TCR-MHC interactions. During development, T cells are initially selected to bind to self MHC and are then eliminated if that binding event leads to activation. However, this sequence of events does not preclude the survival of cells that, through chance, bind to the MHC molecules of another individual, perhaps with high affinity. The discrepancies between self TCR selection and allo-MHC interactions form the basis for most transplant recognition. This nonphysiologic recognition provides the foundation for an antagonistic immune response but does not mandate it in the absence of additional contextual requirements such as expression of costimulatory molecules. Thus alloimmunity is more likely than autoimmunity, but also requires costimulation and innate immune activation to elicit a physiologic immune response.

Most of the significant sequence polymorphism of MHC is located in the areas of the molecule that interact with the TCR, and individual variation in the sequence at the MHC-TCR interface defines alloreactivity. The lack of recipient T-cell thymic education with donor MHC leads to a high frequency of alloreactive peripheral T cells. Many of these cells are cross-reactive with antigen encountered during prior viral exposures, or even with autoantigens in the case of autoimmune disease. This is known as *heterologous immunity* and results in a situation whereby recipients have allospecific memory without having prior exposure to the alloantigen.[65,66] Thus a person's immune response to a donor is the composite product of the individual's MHC makeup and past immune exposures. This can lead to vigorous early rejection in apparently nonsensitized recipients.

T cells recognize alloantigen through their TCR in two distinct pathways. First, in the direct pathway, *donor* APCs expressing donor MHC and costimulatory molecules migrate from the graft and bind to recipient T cells, leading to activation. Conversely, in the indirect pathway, *recipient* APCs phagocytize and process alloantigens derived from the graft and present them bound to self MHC.[67] In the case of transplanted organs, surgical trauma and ischemia exacerbate the potential for T-cell activation by causing an upregulation of class I and II MHC molecules.[68] Moreover, adhesion and costimulation molecules are upregulated in the perioperative period.[69,70]

Initial T-cell binding to donor cells is nonspecific, mediated by adhesion molecules upregulated during donor cell activation.[71] CD40 on donor APCs and endothelial cells is important in mediating cell activation in this setting via CD154 on T cells and activated platelets.[56] Following nonspecific adhesion, MHC recognition occurs in the relatively high costimulatory environment induced by surgical trauma and ischemia.[70] Once alloreactive T cells are activated, they secrete cytokines, including IL-2 and IFN-γ, and they stimulate APCs to secrete IL-12.[61,72,73] The resultant cytokine milieu recruits more T cells to the site of injury and potentiates clonal expansion. Secretory perforin/granzyme mechanisms and cell contact–dependent Fas mechanisms are involved in T-cell cytotoxicity within the graft, resulting in graft destruction.[74] Although acute rejection is the result of T-cell activation, antibody responses accompany many episodes. Cellular and soluble components of immunity mediate multiple distinct clinical rejection syndromes through cytokine-mediated toxicity, cellular cytotoxicity, and direct effects of antibody and complement.

Clinical Rejection Syndromes
Hyperacute Rejection

Hyperacute rejection (HAR) is caused by a donor-specific antibody that exists at the time of transplantation as a result of prior exposure to donor antigens or to antigens with cross-reactivity. It develops precipitously within minutes to hours after graft reperfusion. Typically, HAR is avoided by confirming ABO compatibility and performing a crossmatch by using techniques that detect donor-specific antibodies. When clinically relevant donor-specific antibodies are detected, graft survival is significantly decreased for most organ types.[75] However, the liver has long been regarded to be relatively resistant to HAR, and crossmatching is often done only retrospectively.[76] Interestingly, the rates of acute rejection and graft survival are similar whether there is a positive or negative crossmatch; however, this does not hold true for ABO-incompatible liver allografts.[77] A detailed discussion of antibody-mediated rejection (AMR), specific to liver allografts, continues later.

Unfortunately, the pancreas does not exhibit such resistance to HAR, and a positive crossmatch represents an absolute contraindication to pancreas transplantation. Although high-titer antibodies mediate rapid and dramatic graft injury, chronic exposure to lower-titer antibody results in more insidious graft damage, particularly in the case of the pancreas. The role of chronic alloantibody in liver transplantation remains controversial but likely mediates some degree of graft injury over time. Autoantibody directed against nonpolymorphic determinants of a graft is increasingly recognized as detrimental in pancreas transplantation, with recurrent β cell–specific autoimmunity responsible for at least some late graft loss after pancreas transplantation.[78] Recurrent autoimmunity is also relevant in autoimmune hepatitis.[79]

Acute Rejection

Acute rejection is most common between 4 days and 6 months after transplantation, and rejection that occurs during this time is considered *early acute rejection;* acute rejection after 6 months is considered *late acute rejection.* Liver allografts undergo acute rejection at a rate of approximately 24% to 47%,[80-82] whereas pancreas allografts in the modern era (after 1995) undergo acute rejection at a rate of approximately 15% to 30%.[2] These observed differences in rejection rate may be attributed to the use of less immunosuppression in liver transplant recipients but may also reflect the greater sensitivity of serum liver function test (LFT) measurements and relative ease of liver graft biopsy in establishing the diagnosis.

In both organs, acute rejection evolves during days to weeks. After activation by either direct or indirect allorecognition, T cells infiltrate the allograft and initiate organ destruction through cytolysis and endothelial and ductular damage. Much of the acute graft dysfunction is likely mediated through the effects of macrophage-derived inflammatory cytokines that hinder parenchymal function without necessarily causing cell death.[83] Thus prompt treatment has the potential to quell the rejection before direct T cell–mediated cytotoxicity. Usually, acute liver allograft rejection is also accompanied by graft and peripheral eosinophilia.[84]

Early detection of acute rejection is critical to facilitate intervention before permanent T cell–mediated parenchymal damage occurs; therefore unexplained hepatic dysfunction should prompt a graft biopsy in the absence of any mechanical concerns (vascular inflow or biliary obstruction). In the case of pancreas allografts, often no direct biochemical evidence of rejection is present. If the pancreas transplant was performed in the setting of a simultaneous pancreas-kidney (SPK), rejection of the kidney precedes or signals concomitant pancreas rejection in approximately 80% of cases. In isolated pancreas transplants, fever, abdominal pain, allograft tenderness, and elevations in serum amylase or lipase may be signs of rejection; however, many rejections occur without early signs or symptoms.[85] Hyperglycemia is a late complication in pancreas rejection because acinar cell rejection precedes that of β-cells.

Prompt recognition of acute rejection is imperative because prolonged rejection allows for recruitment of multiple arms of the immune system and consequently results in decreased efficacy of antirejection therapies directed against T-cell responses. T cell–specific therapies can resolve acute rejection episodes in most cases, and corticosteroids are the first-line agent. Typically, early acute rejection episodes have a negative impact on the long-term survival of an allograft, although the liver is relatively resistant to this effect, perhaps because of an increased regenerative capacity.[86] In fact, even late acute rejection in liver transplantation has not been shown to influence long-term graft function.[87] This greatly contrasts with both early and late acute rejection episodes in pancreas transplantation, which have repeatedly been shown to be deleterious to long-term graft survival.[88,89]

Chronic Graft Loss

The causes of chronic graft loss remain poorly characterized.[90] Although frequently referred to as *chronic rejection,* it is likely mediated by a combination of both immune and nonimmune etiologies. Evolving over months to years, chronic graft dysfunction remains resistant to conventional immunosuppressive therapies. Regardless of the transplanted organ, it is characterized by fibrosis with modest lymphocytic infiltration. Monocytic and dendritic cell infiltrates predominate, and destruction of epithelial and endothelial structures is progressive.

Many aspects of chronic graft loss are related to early events after transplantation, such as ischemic injury. In the liver, chronic graft loss manifests as *ductopenia,* or *vanishing bile duct syndrome,*[91] typically defined as a condition wherein less than 50% of portal triads contain bile ducts.[92] The rate of chronic graft loss is much lower for liver grafts than other organs, likely because of the ability of the liver to regenerate after subtle injury. In the modern era, as many of the technical challenges of pancreas transplantation have been overcome, chronic graft loss has become more prevalent[93]; a significant portion may be associated with recurrent autoimmune diabetes.

Antibody-Mediated Rejection

In addition to the rejection syndromes described earlier, recent emphasis has been placed on the humoral immune system and AMR. Although historically, liver allografts have been thought to be resistant to HAR,[94] more contemporary data suggest that a positive crossmatch indicating the presence of donor-specific alloantibodies (DSAs) may place recipients at increased risk for early graft injury and failure.[95] O'Leary and colleagues[96] recently summarized the consensus opinion, noting that antibody-mediated damage to liver allografts is perhaps more common than previously accepted. DSAs, especially those that are high titer and remain present after transplant, put the graft at risk. AMR of liver allograft in the immediate 90 days after transplant is 10-fold higher in DSA-positive patients than in those with a negative crossmatch (10% vs. 1%). However, identifying which patients are at risk, and why, remains a considerable challenge.

When transplanted simultaneously, liver allografts have a protective effect on renal allografts, especially those with preformed class I DSA in a low to moderate titer.[97] This is likely mediated through a competitive absorption of the antibody, reducing its availability to bind to the kidney. With these findings in mind, novel diagnostic strategies are crucial to identify relevant and significant DSAs that have deleterious effects on liver allografts. This information can help identify patients in whom untoward long-term consequences may be likely to develop.[96] Additionally, for those who will experience rejection, future endeavors should aim to identify patients who may have improved outcomes from alternate immunosuppressive regimens, and those who will be more likely to respond to treatment.

IMMUNOSUPPRESSION

To date, no single agent has been discovered that effectively prevents allograft rejection, although liver transplant recipients can often be eventually weaned to a single-drug regimen. Similarly, immunosuppressive agents that limit rejection also increase susceptibility to infection and malignancy. Thus far no immunosuppressant is allograft specific; therefore the rational selection of immunosuppressants involves the use of multiple synergistic agents to prevent rejection without simultaneously crippling defense against pathogens. Typically, liver allografts require less immunosuppression than other organs.[98] This has been attributed to the unique APCs in the liver, the sheer size and antigenic load of the liver, and its regenerative capacity. Indeed, studies indicated that 10% to 20% of liver transplant recipients can eventually be withdrawn from all immunosuppressive agents over time.[99] It is important to note that no immunosuppressive regimen has clearly been established as superior; thus the regimens chosen remain variable from one transplant center to another.

The immune system is most likely to reject an allograft in the perioperative period due in part to the surgical trauma and ischemic injury associated with transplantation; therefore the most intense immunosuppression is generally administered in the first few weeks following transplantation. In some cases, a high-intensity immunosuppressive agent is given at the time of transplantation, a practice described as *induction therapy.*[100] These strategies typically consist of T cell–depleting agents that, while effective, are too toxic to be administered as maintenance therapy. Conversely, maintenance immunosuppression is less potent but can be administered daily to prevent acute rejection. Finally, agents used to halt ongoing rejection episodes are known as *rescue agents.* Figure 104.2 shows the sites of action of various immunosuppressive agents.

Corticosteroids

Corticosteroids have been a mainstay of transplant immunosuppression for decades.[101] At low doses, glucocorticosteroids, typically prednisone or methylprednisolone, are used as maintenance immunosuppression; at higher doses, they can be used as rescue therapy. Although corticosteroids are ineffective as monotherapy to prevent rejection, they have been effectively combined with other agents to improve graft survival. Unfortunately, the desirable immunosuppressive effects of corticosteroids are counterbalanced by their contribution to transplant morbidity; therefore many ongoing efforts have sought to minimize or eliminate glucocorticosteroid use for maintenance immunosuppression. Many centers now rapidly wean liver allograft recipients off corticosteroids. In contrast, most pancreas programs rely on low-dose steroids indefinitely, although steroid-free regimens are increasingly being used.[102–104]

The immunosuppressive mechanism of glucocorticosteroids was elucidated long after its clinical introduction.[105,106] After nonspecific cytoplasmic uptake, steroids bind to an intracellular receptor, enter the nucleus as a receptor-ligand pair, and increase

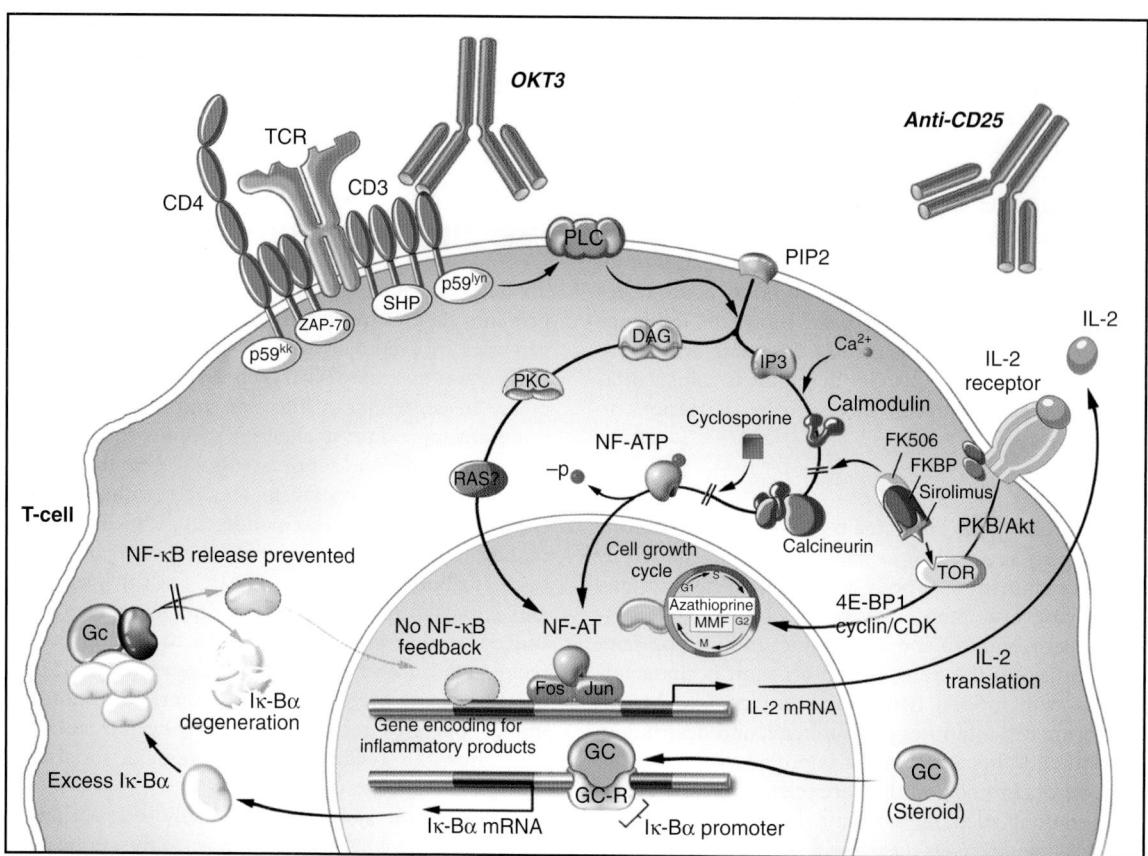

FIGURE 104.2 T-cell receptor (*TCR*) signal transduction and the sites of action of various immunosuppressants. TCR signal transduction proceeds through Ca^{2+}-dependent dephosphorylation of the nuclear factor of activated T cells (*NF-AT*), which enter the nucleus and, in conjunction with nuclear factor kappa B (NF-κB), facilitates cytokine gene expression. Cyclosporine and tacrolimus (*FK506*) both inhibit signal transduction by blocking the ability of the calcineurin-calmodulin complex to potentiate NF-AT dephosphorylation. The autocrine activity of interleukin (*IL*)-2 facilitates entry into the cell cycle and cell division. Sirolimus inhibits IL-2 receptor signal transduction by blocking the interactions of macrolide-binding protein (*FKBP*). Mycophenolate (*MMF*) and azathioprine prevent cell cycling by altering nucleic acid metabolism. Corticosteroids upregulate inhibitor of kappa light polypeptide gene enhancer in B cells (*Iκ-Bα*) synthesis and inhibit the ability of NF-κB to enter the nucleus. Monoclonal antibodies bind T-cell surface molecules and alter key interactions necessary for T-cell function. *CD,* Cluster of differentiation; *CDK,* cyclin-dependent kinase; *4E-BP1,* 4E binding protein 1; kinase alpha; *OKT3,* muromonab CD3; *PIP2,* phosphatidylinositol diphosphate; *PKC,* protein kinase C; *PKB/Akt,* protein kinase B/AKT; *PLC,* phospholipase C; *TOR,* target of rapamycin (see Chapter 10); *ZAP,* Zeta-chain-associated protein kinase; *SHP,* Src homology region 2 domain-containing phosphatase; *GC,* Glucocorticoid; *GC-R,* Glucocorticoid receptor; *DAG,* diacylglycerol; *NF-ATP,* nuclear factor of activated T cells, phosphorylated; *IP3,* Inositol tri-phosphate

the transcription of several genes, notably *IκBα*. This protein binds to and inactivates nuclear factor kappa B (NF-κB), an important transcription factor involved in T-cell/APC activation and cytokine production.

The NF-κB pathway is an important amplification step in the T-cell and APC response, and blockade of this pathway results in diverse effects. Corticosteroids decrease IL-1, tumor necrosis factor (TNF)-α, and IFN-γ transcription and also decrease MHC upregulation. Inhibition of phospholipase A_2 results in blockade of the entire arachidonic acid cascade, and steroids mute the entire inflammatory process and decrease the costimulatory environment. Corticosteroids also promote apoptosis of activated T cells and limit the signal transduction of many innate immune receptors, such as the TLRs.

Antiproliferative Agents

Azathioprine

The antimetabolite azathioprine (AZA) was the first immunosuppressant used in solid organ transplantation.[107,108] AZA undergoes hepatic conversion to 6-mercaptopurine (6-MP) and then subsequently to 6-thio-inosine-monophosphate (6-tIMP). These derivatives alkylate DNA precursors and inhibit DNA synthesis. In addition, they can introduce chromosomal breaks and interfere with DNA repair mechanisms. AZA works on all rapidly dividing cells; consequently, bone marrow, hepatic, and gastrointestinal toxicity are limiting factors. As monotherapy, AZA is ineffective and is rarely found in modern immunosuppressive regimens.

Mycophenolate Mofetil

Since 1995, mycophenolate mofetil (MMF) has been an approved immunosuppressant for use in adults.[109] MMF is a morpholinoethyl ester of mycophenolic acid (MPA), a noncompetitive, reversible inhibitor of inosine monophosphate (IMP) dehydrogenase with improved bioavailability. MMF prevents a critical step in RNA and DNA synthesis by blocking the formation of guanosine monophosphate (GMP) by IMP dehydrogenase. In all cells except lymphocytes, there exists a "salvage pathway" for GMP formation. This crucial difference makes MMF a relatively lymphocyte-specific immunosuppressant. MMF blocks the proliferation of T and

B cells and inhibits the formation of donor-specific antibody. Its introduction has dramatically improved the success of pancreas transplantation; therefore it is used as an adjuvant immunosuppressive agent in most pancreas centers.

In liver transplantation, the use of MMF has continued to gain favor because it allows a reduction in calcineurin inhibitors, the cornerstone of most immunosuppressive regimens. Presumably, this reduction mitigates the deleterious effects calcineurin inhibitors have on renal function in hepatic and pancreatic transplant recipients.[110] MMF combined with low-dose calcineurin inhibitors and corticosteroids has also proved successful in decreasing episodes of acute rejection.[111] Its chronic use is typical in pancreas transplantation, and MMF plays at least a temporary role in most liver transplant regimens.

Calcineurin Inhibitors

Cyclosporine

Cyclosporine A (CyA) is a cyclic undecapeptide isolated from the fungus *Tolypocladium inflatum Gams*.[112,113] Its introduction revolutionized solid organ transplantation, extending the field beyond kidney transplantation. The mechanism of action of this T cell–specific immunosuppressant is mediated through cyclophilin (Cn) binding. The CyA-Cn complex binds to the calcineurin-calmodulin complex and prevents de-phosphorylation and activation of nuclear factor of activated T cells (NF-AT), a regulator of transcription. Blockade of NF-AT prevents IL-2 gene transcription. In addition, TGF-α transcription is unregulated, and other genes critical for T-cell activation are altered.[114,115] These and other effects may be responsible for the toxicity of CyA. Primarily, CyA blocks TCR signal transduction but does not inhibit costimulatory signaling.[116] The effects of CyA can be overcome with high levels of IL-2; therefore once IL-2 is present in the graft, as in the case of ongoing rejection, CyA is rendered ineffective. Consequently, CyA is used as a maintenance immunosuppressant but has no role in rescue therapy.

CyA nephrotoxicity is a primary consideration in its long-term use. Through a TGF-α–mediated mechanism, CyA decreases renal blood flow by as much as 30%.[114,115] Increased transcription of endothelin also activates the renin-angiotensin pathway, leading to hypertension, and these effects of CyA may also delay resolution of hepatorenal syndrome in liver transplant recipients. CyA may also lead to neurologic side effects, hypertrichosis, and malignancy.[117] In addition, metabolism of CyA through cytochrome P450 enzymes leads to multiple drug interactions.

Tacrolimus

Kino and colleagues first demonstrated the immunosuppressant effects of tacrolimus in 1987,[118] and it has become the mainstay of most liver and pancreas transplant regimens. Tacrolimus is a macrolide antibiotic produced by *Streptomyces tsukubaensis*. As with CyA, tacrolimus blocks NF-AT activation and its downstream effects.[119] The intracellular target of tacrolimus is FK-binding protein (FK-BP). Like CyA, tacrolimus increases TGF-α transcription and therefore shares similar toxicities.[114,115] Although tacrolimus is 100 times more potent than CyA in preventing IL-2 and IFN-γ transcription, its toxicities limit the dose to approximately 1% of CyA. In addition to its use as a maintenance agent, tacrolimus has been shown to have efficacy at high doses in reversing liver rejection episodes.[120]

Compared with CyA, tacrolimus has more pronounced neurologic side effects, most commonly headaches and tremors. Tacrolimus use also results in a higher rate of post-transplant type 2 diabetes, although it has fewer cosmetic side effects. Tacrolimus has been shown to be superior to CyA in preventing acute rejection episodes, reducing the number of steroid-resistant acute rejections and improving long-term graft and patient survival. For these reasons, tacrolimus has replaced cyclosporine as the first-line calcineurin inhibitor used in both liver and pancreas transplantation in most centers.[121] Because tacrolimus is metabolized by cytochrome P450 enzymes, drug interaction concerns are similar to those with CyA. In recent years, many liver transplant recipients have been successfully weaned to tacrolimus monotherapy, but this trend has not been seen in pancreas transplantation.

Undoubtedly, calcineurin inhibitor therapy represents the current standard of care in solid-organ transplantation. The powerful immunosuppressive properties of these drugs have certainly revolutionized and improved both allograft and patient survival, and they have made liver and pancreas transplantation viable, long-term therapeutic options. However, these agents are associated with a host of side effects that have necessitated the development of alternative immunosuppression strategies involving the minimization or elimination of calcineurin inhibitors.

mTOR Inhibitors

Sirolimus and Everolimus

Sirolimus and everolimus are macrolide antibiotics developed from *Streptomyces hygroscopicus*.[122–124] Like tacrolimus, these agents bind to the immunophilin FKBP12, also known as the mammalian target of rapamycin (mTOR). Unlike tacrolimus, these agents do not affect calcineurin activity.[125–127] The primary effect of mTOR inhibitors is to inhibit IL-2 receptor signal transduction rather than blocking NF-AT nuclear translocation; therefore T cells are rendered incompetent against the proliferative effects of exogenous IL-2,[128] but they are still capable of IL-2 gene transcription.

Because of the increased toxicity associated with calcineurin inhibitor–based immunosuppression, including renal insufficiency, drug-induced diabetes, and neurotoxicity, efforts have been made to reduce exposure to such agents by the use of alternative agents. In this context, the principal manner in which mTOR inhibitors are used in transplantation is as an adjunct or alternative to calcineurin inhibitors. However, in certain clinical situations, mTOR inhibitors are favored due to their unique anti-cancer effects. In particular, mTOR inhibitor use in patients transplanted for hepatic malignancies has been investigated over the last decade.[129–131] A meta-analysis of five studies investigating the use of sirolimus in patients transplanted for hepatocellular carcinoma demonstrated a benefit compared with calcineurin inhibitors, manifested by lower recurrence rate, longer recurrence-free survival, and longer overall survival.[132]

In terms of efficacy in preventing rejection, mTOR inhibitors are generally viewed as inferior to calcineurin inhibitors. A multicenter, prospective, randomized Phase II trial was conducted to determine the safety and efficacy of sirolimus combined with reduced-dose tacrolimus immediately after liver transplantation.[133] Limited to primary, liver-alone transplant recipients, patients were randomly assigned to receive conventional-dose tacrolimus (FK trough, 7–15 ng/mL) or reduced-dose tacrolimus

(FK trough, 3–7 ng/mL) combined with sirolimus (15 mg loading dose followed by 5 mg titrated for trough of 4–11 ng/mL). Although it was hypothesized that the combined regimen would result in improved efficacy, defined as reduced acute rejection and graft loss, the opposite was observed and the study was terminated early. The sirolimus arm was associated with a significantly lower survival at 24 months after transplant (22 vs. 9 deaths) and significantly higher graft loss (26.4% vs. 12.5%). These findings contributed to the US Food and Drug Administration black-box warning for sirolimus administration in the first 28 days after liver transplant, with untoward results thought to be secondary to an increased risk of hepatic artery thrombosis. Thus its use in liver transplantation remains limited to trial-based conversion regimens.

An open-label, prospectively randomized trial investigated such a conversion strategy in liver transplant recipients.[134] With the understanding that calcineurin inhibitors, while resulting in improved patient survival, are associated with nephrotoxicity, this study evaluated the safety, efficacy, and tolerability of sirolimus conversion compared with continuing calcineurin inhibition. Graft survival was greater than 93% at 12 months, similar in both arms. However, biopsy-confirmed acute rejection was significantly higher in the sirolimus-conversion arm. Additionally, cumulative treatment failure at 72 months was almost twice as frequent in the sirolimus-conversion group (48.3% vs. 26.7%), while failing to preserve renal function versus calcineurin inhibition alone, demonstrated by similar glomerular filtration rate (GFR) between treatment arms. Treatment-related adverse events were also more common in sirolimus-conversion patients, including infectious processes in the first 12 months after treatment initiation. These data are somewhat limited, however, because of high cumulative treatment discontinuation rates.

The other common mTOR inhibitor, everolimus, was prospectively investigated for liver transplantation.[135] With the primary end point set as the composite efficacy failure rate of treated biopsy-proven acute rejection, graft loss, and death, and a secondary end point as renal function, patients were randomly assigned 30 days after transplant to receive either everolimus with reduced-dose tacrolimus, standard tacrolimus alone, or tacrolimus cessation. The latter arm was discontinued early due to increased rejection. In the remaining arms, biopsy-proven acute rejection was significantly less frequent 2 years after randomization in the everolimus/reduced-tacrolimus arm (6.1% vs. 13.3%). Additionally, patients in the everolimus cohort had better preservation of their renal function. Although the results suggest that combination regimens, including calcineurin and mTOR inhibitors, are beneficial, the overall literature remains mixed. Therefore combination and conversion strategies designed to minimize calcineurin inhibitor–associated toxicities should still be considered and investigated.

Antilymphocyte Agents

Antilymphocyte agents are frequently used in pancreas transplantation as induction agents.[136,137] Their use in liver transplantation is sparse because of the relatively reduced immunogenicity of liver grafts.

Antilymphocyte/Antithymocyte Globulin

A polyclonal antilymphocyte globulin (ALG) is produced by inoculating an animal, such as a horse or rabbit, with human lymphocytes and then collecting the serum and purifying the resultant IgG. This preparation contains antibodies with multiple epitope specificities directed against lymphocytes and other cell antigens.[138,139] In the United States, the most common immunogen is thymocytes, and the resultant polyclonal antibody is rabbit antithymocyte globulin (RATG). These agents promote T-cell depletion through opsonization and complement-mediated lysis.[139] They also have multiple nondepletional effects that inhibit T-cell activation and function, such as cross-linking costimulation and adhesion molecules and blocking TCR signal transduction through internalization of other cell surface receptors.

Both ALG and RATG can be used as induction and rescue agents. The primary function of these agents is to reduce the number of primary effector cells below the threshold required for acute rejection and to allow for slow repopulation after the immediate post-transplant period. Although RATG is generally well tolerated, side effects include thrombocytopenia, increased viral disease, and transient cytokine release.

OKT3

Unlike polyclonal antibody preparations, monoclonal antibodies have single-target epitope specificity. Muromonab CD3, better known as OKT3 (Orthoclone OKT3; Ortho Pharmaceuticals, Raritan, NJ), is a murine antibody directed against the CD3 signal transduction subunit of the TCR; it was the first monoclonal antibody approved for clinical use.[140,141] OKT3 mediates its effects by binding to CD3 and causing internalization of the TCR complex, thereby preventing antigen recognition.[141,142] OKT3 also opsonizes T cells, causing their activation and degranulation. This exhausts the cell, making it ineffective as an effector, but it also leads to OKT3's primary side effect, cytokine release syndrome.[143] Cytokine release can result in profound hypotension, pulmonary edema, and cardiac depression. Because of the relatively toxic side effect profile and the availability of other agents that accomplish the same purpose, OKT3 is no longer manufactured.

Anti–interleukin-2 Receptor α-Chain Monoclonal Antibodies

The high affinity α-subunit of the IL-2 receptor (CD25) has been the target of two monoclonal antibodies, daclizumab and basiliximab. CD25 is required for clonal naive T-cell expansion and is therefore an attractive target for specific elimination of activated T cells.[144] Unlike OKT3, binding of the target epitope does not result in cytokine release. Thus administration is generally well tolerated, although the antirejection effect is similarly modest. Daclizumab was discontinued for use in the United States and Europe, and basiliximab is used in approximately one-third of all pancreas and liver transplant centers.

Costimulation Blockade

As detailed earlier, T cells not only require presentation of peptides in the context of self MHC, but also require a second signal or costimulatory interaction to produce an effective and appropriate immune response (see Fig. 104.1). This is particularly true of naive T cells that have never encountered antigen. Both the CD154-CD40 and the CD28-CD80/86 pathways have been targeted in solid-organ transplantation with agents specifically designed to prevent these potentiating signals. Although promising in nonhuman primate trials, a drug targeting the CD154-CD40 pathway was abandoned after thromboembolic complications were reported. Although intense research continues pursuant to this pathway, the development of CD28-CD80/86–specific agents has advanced to the clinic.

In renal transplantation, the costimulatory antagonist belatacept, a high-affinity fusion protein specific for the B7 molecules

CD80 and CD86 on APCs, demonstrates similar efficacy to cyclosporine with respect to patient and graft survival, but with superior renal function and cardiac outcomes.[145–149]

Compared with viral antigen, the response to alloantigen is generated primarily from immature T cells and evokes a greater T-cell response, in part because of greater cytokine production.[150] These naive T cells express CD28, the primary target of belatacept, but CD28 tends to be lost with cell maturation. Whereas the calcineurin inhibitor tacrolimus inhibits both naive and mature T cells, belatacept is primarily effective against immature T cells that are activated in the presence of alloantigen. Conversely, it is relatively ineffective against mature T cells activated in response to virus. Therefore belatacept's ability to block the immune response, in particular to alloantigen, was based on two criteria: the preservation of its target, CD28, with an immature T-cell response involving naive T cells.

With its demonstrated efficacy and improved toxicity profile in renal transplantation and known action on naive CD28$^+$ T cells in response to alloantigen, belatacept was tested in de novo liver transplant recipients in a Phase II trial.[151] The 260 patients were randomly assigned into five treatment arms, including two groups receiving different dosages of belatacept. Unfortunately, this study was terminated early, after only 12 months of follow-up, because of a significantly higher number of patients in the belatacept groups experiencing acute rejection, graft loss, or death. Ongoing studies are indeed essential to determine the role of belatacept in liver and pancreas transplantation.

Minimization of Maintenance Immunosuppression

The benefit of organ replacement with transplantation comes with the burden of chronic maintenance immunosuppression. Recently, numerous efforts have been made to decrease the amount of immunosuppression given to transplant recipients. The basic strategies pursued in clinical and preclinical trials include minimization of maintenance immunosuppression through aggressive induction protocols, withdrawal of immunosuppression after the initial post-transplant period, and experimental strategies to facilitate immunologic tolerance.

The strategy involving use of depletional agents such as RATG to reduce the requirement for maintenance immunosuppression continues to gain acceptance. Alemtuzumab is a CD52-specific antibody that rapidly depletes T cells and, to a lesser degree, B cells and monocytes from the circulation and from secondary lymphoid organs. It is approved for treatment of lymphoid malignancies and is investigated off-label in transplantation. Alemtuzumab has been used with low-dose tacrolimus to prevent rejection in liver transplant recipients.[152,153] Similar efforts have been made using antithymocyte globulin induction therapy.[154] Alemtuzumab depletion has also been used in pancreas transplantation,[155] and this strategy has been used effectively in kidney transplantation.[156–158]

IMMUNOSUPPRESSION WITHDRAWAL AND OPERATIONAL TOLERANCE

Steroid withdrawal can be achieved in approximately 85% of liver transplant recipients at 3 months without a significant increase in acute rejection rates[159] and has the benefit of avoiding the numerous side effects associated with chronic glucocorticosteroid use. Although attempts to withdraw corticosteroids in patients receiving pancreas transplants have been less successful, with appropriate patient selection, as many as 70% of pancreas transplant patients may be amenable to steroid withdrawal.[160]

A modest percentage of liver transplant recipients can be completely withdrawn from all immunosuppressive agents.[161–165] Although the periods of follow-up in withdrawal studies vary greatly and the long-term incidence of chronic rejection and graft loss has not been defined, some recipients clearly are capable of spontaneously accepting liver allografts. The challenge remains to establish criteria for appropriate withdrawal from immunosuppression and to identify those individuals in whom drug withdrawal is a safe strategy. At present, the best predictor of successful drug withdrawal is long-term rejection-free survival on low-dose immunosuppression. Liver transplant recipients receiving single-drug therapy for more than 10 years are 10 times more likely to be withdrawn successfully compared with patients in the first 3 years after transplantation.

From its conception,[166] *acquired allospecific tolerance* has been defined as the ability to maintain a functional allograft and an intact immune response without the need for therapeutic drugs. Numerous strategies have been attempted in reaching this goal, but to date, prospective attempts to create broadly applicable, reliable, and durable tolerance in human liver transplant recipients have failed, with rare anecdotal exceptions. No prospective studies have been performed for pancreas transplantation. Ongoing strategies include the manipulation of costimulation signals, depletional approaches, and techniques designed to induce *mixed chimerism*, a state in which elements of both the donor and the recipient immune system persist in one individual.[167–169]

Both clinical and genetic factors have been investigated with regard to operational tolerance.[99] Clinical parameters (e.g., age, gender, immunosuppression regimen, cell counts) were not predictive of tolerance and did not correlate with tolerant-related genetic profiles. However, there is evidence that signatures of recipient gene expression or other biologic parameters can identify a pro-tolerant signature in liver transplantation patients.[99,163] From peripheral blood lymphocytes of 80 transplant recipients and 16 healthy patients without transplant, a signature of 24 genes was found to correlate with tolerance in liver graft recipients. The majority of these targets are associated with natural killer (NK) and γδTCR$^+$ T cells, from which the transcriptional (mRNA) profiles could be used to predict which liver transplant patients might be operationally tolerant.

The inability to reach operational tolerance may be secondary to virally induced alloreactive memory.[65,66] This theory of heterologous immunity suggests that T-cell memory is the direct result of previous immunologic exposure, resulting in response to unrelated antigens.[170] In a murine model, Adams identified memory T cells (CD8$^+$), in response to prior viral exposure, to be responsible for the immune response targeted at alloantigen. Achieving a critical threshold of such T cells produced an environment favoring rejection. Furthermore, this barrier to tolerance secondary to prior immune encounters was abated with NF-κB inhibition combined with costimulation blockade, allowing for antigen-specific tolerance. Strategies such as this may provide opportunities for future clinical trials, with the goal of altering the immunologic milieu toward one that is operationally tolerant.

If heterologous immunity is indeed responsible for resistance to attaining tolerance, pediatric liver recipients should be more successful in becoming operationally tolerant, given their likely exposure to fewer viral and other cross-reactive antigens. A prospective, multicenter pilot study enrolled 20 children receiving liver grafts from parental donors into a prolonged immunosuppression withdrawal program.[171] Maintained on single-agent immunosuppression at enrollment, these patients underwent a stepwise immunosuppressant reduction during a minimum of 36 weeks, with scheduled graft biopsies; 60% met the primary end point of operational tolerance, defined as no immunosuppression for 1 year without evidence of rejection. A longer interval between transplantation and withdrawal of immunosuppression correlated with attaining tolerance (median, 100.6 vs. 73 months), as did less inflammation and lower C4d scores on primary biopsy. Given that no deaths occurred, and that patients who failed complete withdrawal were able to maintain graft function with increased or reinitiation of immunosuppression, attempts at immunosuppressant withdrawal in this patient population may be reasonable.

Withdrawal of immunosuppression in transplant recipients must be monitored closely. First, biochemical markers, including aspartate transaminase (AST), alanine transaminase (ALT), alkaline phosphatase (ALP), γ-glutamyl transpeptidase (GGT), and bilirubin, may indicate rejection, but these are often insensitive. Second, graft biopsy may be performed to evaluate for rejection and parenchymal injury.[172,173] Although graft biopsy remains the most sensitive test to evaluate for rejection, it is costly, inconvenient, and potentially injurious. Moreover, histopathologic changes are not always clear. Benefits, however, include early detection of subclinical rejection.[174] Biopsies obtained before immunosuppression withdrawal, associated with successful weaning, demonstrate reduced portal inflammation, decreased CD3[+] and CD8[+] T cells with increased CD45RO[+] lymphocytes, and minimal C4d complement deposits.[171,175] Based on these previous findings, the Banff Working Group recommends graft biopsy before immunosuppression withdrawal to evaluate for histopathologic changes conducive to reduced immunosuppression and perhaps operational tolerance, with attention to portal inflammation, centrizonal and perivenular inflammation, bile duct changes, parenchymal fibrosis, and arteriopathy.[172] If these criteria are favorable, weaning of immunosuppression may be attempted, and serial biopsies should be performed to reevaluate the success of withdrawal.

Many have speculated that liver recipients are more likely to become tolerant than other allograft recipients, and indeed the emerging results from immunosuppression withdrawal trials suggest this to be the case. Reasons cited include the unique APCs in the liver, the liver's regenerative capacity, its sheer antigenic bulk, and its tendency to seed the recipient's body with donor hematopoietic cells, perhaps overwhelming the recipient immune system into a state of clonal exhaustion.[176] Tolerance attempts in liver transplantation are likely to continue in the coming years, and their results will be critically evaluated. In contrast, the pancreas has been considered an immunogenic organ with little capacity to regenerate or deal with immune insults. As such, pancreas allograft tolerance is much less likely to be achieved in the near future with the current strategies available.

The references for this chapter can be found online by accessing the accompanying Expert Consult website.

CHAPTER **105**

Liver transplantation: Indications and general considerations

James Neuberger

The first human orthotopic liver transplant was carried out by Starzl in 1963. In the subsequent two decades, only a relatively small number of patients received grafts, usually those who were moribund with end-stage disease, and survival results were disappointing. However, with increasing surgeon experience and confidence, better anesthesia, and improved microbiologic and immunologic treatments, results started to improve. Increasingly more patients were grafted, with a major increase in the number of transplant centers. In both Europe and the United States, more than 7000 procedures are performed annually. Results are such that many centers are currently reporting 1-year survival rates greater than 90% in elective cases.

It is difficult to identify any one cause for the increase in transplant success. The contribution of better surgical and anesthetic techniques (see Chapters 106 and, 125), improved postoperative care (Chapters 26, 106, and 111), and availability of better immunosuppressive agents (Chapter 104) have all contributed to the improvements in survival. There is also a better understanding of indications and contraindications for the procedure, and patients are now generally referred for transplantation at a stage when they are likely to have the greatest chance of success. However, the increasing success of liver transplantation and the reduction in contraindications have meant that the number of potential recipients is increasing, while the number of donors in many countries is either remaining static or falling. The increasing discrepancy between supply and demand means that the mortality of patients awaiting a transplant is increasing; the patients often wait longer, so they are sicker; and the chance of survival decreases while resource utilization increases. Increasing the donor pool by using split livers, organs from selected donors after circulatory death (DCD), donors with higher risk profiles, and organs from living donors, and a better understanding of the contraindications to grafts and the use of machine perfusion both to evaluate graft function and intervene to improve graft function have had a significant impact but have not met the need.

Different healthcare administrations have adopted a variety of approaches to provide a transparent approach to selection and allocation that balances the needs for equity, utility, need, and benefit. In North America and many European countries, the method of allocation is based on need with a focus on reducing the risk of death on the waiting list (see Model for End-Stage Liver Disease [MELD] score; see Chapter 4). In almost all cases, this has resulted in the reduced mortality of patients awaiting liver transplantation without an appreciable effect on survival after transplantation, although with an increase in resource utilization. Increasingly, organs are allocated according to benefit rather than need (that is, the estimated difference in survival with and without transplantation). Also, those responsible for allocation policies are looking at quality of life (QOL) as an additional measure on which to base allocation. Nonetheless, there remains a need to define futility, that is to identify those patients, whether referred for listing or actual transplant candidates, when transplantation is futile. Transplant units and liver units must make palliative care an option in such cases.

The shortage of deceased donors has stimulated the use of livers from living donors. Limitations include the risks to the donor; even after careful evaluation, the risk of donor death is approximately 1 in 250 (risk depends on lobe[s] removed), and morbidity is approximately 30%,[1] although a lack of obligatory reporting and national registries in many countries makes it difficult to assess the true risk. In general, the indications for transplantation in recipients of living donor livers mirror those for deceased donation, although some centers are expanding the indications, especially for liver cancer and alcohol.

GENERAL INDICATIONS AND CONTRAINDICATIONS

In general, the indications for transplantation are relatively easy to define, although the application of these principles is often much more difficult. The two broad indications for grafting are

1. A survival benefit from transplant (compared with nontransplant) and
2. $\Theta O\Lambda$ (because of the liver disease) unacceptable to the patient.[2]

However, where organs are allocated solely on the basis of need, such as to those with intractable symptoms, there may be a very long wait for transplantation unless there is access to living donors where there is targeted allocation.

Transplantation should be considered for an individual patient with the following (Box 105.1):

- A survival benefit as evidenced by MELD score of greater than 17 (see Chapter 4)
- Signs of decompensation, including ascites, encephalopathy, and renal impairment (see Chapters 77 and 78)

BOX 105.1   Indications for Referral for Consideration of Liver Transplantation in Adult Patients With Cirrhosis

Symptoms
Hepatic decompensation
Increasing ascites unresponsive to medical/diet therapy
Recurrent variceal bleeding
Spontaneous bacterial peritonitis

Side Effects of Liver Disease
Increasing osteopenia
Hepatopulmonary syndrome
Portopulmonary hypertension
Intractable ascites
Intractable encephalopathy
Development of hepatocellular carcinoma
Muscle wasting and increasing frailty

Biochemical Markers
MELD Score >17
Serum albumin <30 g/dL
Serum bilirubin >50 μmol/L for parenchymal disease
Serum bilirubin >100 μmol/L for cholestatic disease

MELD, Model for End-Stage Liver Disease.

- Liver cell cancer for which other measures are considered less effective (see Chapters 89 and 108A)
- Hepatopulmonary or portal pulmonary hypertension (see Chapters 74, 78, and 79)
- Intractable pruritus
- Intractable encephalopathy

Development of any of these criteria does not necessarily mean that transplantation is indicated, but merely that it should be considered.

Absolute contraindications to liver transplantation include the following:

- The patient is not fit enough to withstand surgery (e.g., because of advanced cardiac or pulmonary disease).
- The patient is unlikely to survive the procedure (e.g., active sepsis).
- Survival after transplantation may be too short to justify the risks of transplantation (e.g., with metastatic disease).
- The postoperative QOL may be unacceptable to the patient (e.g., severe intractable depression).
- Surgery is technically not possible (e.g., patients with extensive venous thromboses).
- The patient does not choose to undergo the operation.

Relative contraindications to transplantation include the following and are discussed below:

- *Age:* Few centers have an upper age limit, but older age is a risk factor for poor outcomes.
- *Obesity:* Those with body mass index (BMI) greater than 40 kg/m² have a poorer outcome.
- *Cholangiocarcinoma:* Considered only in highly selected patients in agreed protocols with chemotherapy and irradiation because of early recurrence (see Chapters 51 and 108B).
- *Metastatic colon cancer:* It is available in selected centers (see Chapter 90).
- *Chronic or refractory active infections:* Depending on type of infection and whether amenable to cure with available therapy.

- *Poor social support:* Despite full interventions that will adversely impact on graft or patient survival, particularly in biologically older patients with anticipated prolonged recovery after transplant.
- Ongoing tobacco use or illegal drug use.
- Active alcohol use.
- Frailty.

In 2019, in the United States, there were 8372 liver transplants from deceased donors and 524 from living donors (https://optn.transplant.hrsa.gov/data/view-data-reports/national-data/#). During that year, 1179 died awaiting a graft and 1186 were removed as they had become too sick. As of April 30, 2020, there were 12,706 patients awaiting a transplant in the United States.

There have been many changes in the demographics of transplantation. The proportion of patients grafted for alcoholic liver disease and nonalcoholic fatty liver disease (NAFLD; see Chapter 69) is rising.

- The proportion of patients grafted for cholestatic diseases is falling and the number of patients being grafted for hepatitis C virus (HCV) infection is falling because of the success of effective treatment (see Chapter 68).
- The use of living donors (see Chapters 109 and 121) has not made a significant impact on the number of transplants in Europe and North America. However, living liver donation remains a major source of activity in many Asian and Far Eastern countries.
- Use of organs from DCD, in contrast to living donors, has been increasing (see Chapter 109). Rates are lower in the United States (about 5%) than in United Kingdom, where the proportion of DCD is about 30%. These livers may develop ischemic cholangiopathy months after transplantation.
- Σplitting livers allows two transplants from a single donor. Criteria for splitting are well established. Use of split livers has greatly reduced the mortality of patients on the paediatric waiting list

GENERAL CONSIDERATIONS

Malnutrition and Frailty (see Chapters 26 and 27)

Malnutrition is a common finding in end-stage cirrhosis, with a prevalence of up to 60%[3] (see Chapter 26) (see Box 105.1; Box 105.2). Malnutrition in these patients has many causes: the disease itself, poor intake, dietary restrictions (often inappropriate in those with encephalopathy), and malabsorption (which itself has many causes). Hyperammonemia will also increase sarcopenia. Malnutrition and sarcopenia are associated with increased susceptibility to infection and poor healing.

Although there is no convincing evidence that improving the nutritional state will alter the outcome of liver transplantation, it seems prudent to optimize nutrition: the use of branch-chain amino acid and vitamin supplementation remains uncertain.

It has been recognized that frailty is a strong predictor not only of outcome in those with cirrhosis but also for survival and QOL after transplant and as the risk of acute cellular rejection. Frailty is a multidimensional construct that represents the end manifestation of derangements of multiple physiologic systems leading to decreased physiologic reserve and increased vulnerability to health stressors.[4] Investigation of frailty has largely focused on physical frailty, which includes functional performance, functional capacity, and disability. It is recommended

Acute Liver Failure
Multisystem disorder in which severe acute impairment of liver function with encephalopathy occurs within 8 weeks of the onset of symptoms and no recognized underlying chronic liver disease

Subacute Liver Failure (Late-Onset Hepatic Failure)
Chronic Liver Disease
Cirrhosis which may be due to
Fatty liver disease
- Alcohol
- Nonalcohol related

Chronic viral hepatitis B
Chronic viral hepatitis C
Primary biliary cholangitis,
Primary sclerosing cholangitis
Autoimmune hepatitis
Genetic hemochromatosis
Wilson disease
α_1-Antitrypsin deficiency
Congenital hepatic fibrosis and other congenital or hereditary liver diseases
Secondary biliary cirrhosis
Liver Tumors
Hepatocellular carcinoma
Unresectable hepatoblastoma (without active extrahepatic disease)
Unresectable benign liver tumors with disabling symptoms
Hepatic epithelioid hemangioendothelioma

Variant Syndromes, Metabolic Diseases, and Other Indications
Intractable pruritus
Hepatopulmonary syndrome
Cirrhotic cardiomyopathy
Familial amyloidosis
Primary hypercholesterolemia
Polycystic liver disease
Recurrent cholangitis
Nodular regenerative hyperplasia
Hereditary hemorrhagic telangiectasia
Glycogen storage disease
Ornithine transcarbamylase deficiency
Primary hyperoxaluria
Maple syrup urine disease
Porphyria
Amyloidosis
Alagille's syndrome
Progressive familial intrahepatic cholestasis
Caroli syndrome

that all liver transplant candidates should be assessed at baseline and longitudinally using a standardized frailty tool, which should guide the intensity and type of nutritional and physical therapy in individual liver transplant candidates.[5] Both the optimal tool for assessment and management of frailty are uncertain[6]: simple scores such as the Charlson Frailty Index, Karnofsky performance scale, and the Liver Frailty Index (hand grip, balance, and chair stands) have been used. A recent meta-analysis[7] found 11 exercises improve VO2 peak, anaerobic threshold, 6-minute walk distance, muscle mass/function, and QOL in patients. Improvements were greater with a combination of aerobic and resistance exercises at moderate-high intensity.

Thus both malnutrition and frailty are markers of a higher mortality both before and after transplantation. Neither marker should be used as an absolute contraindication to transplantation. If accepted for transplantation, the time awaiting an offer of a graft should be used to improve both frailty and malnutrition. Formal dietetic advice and, where appropriate, nutritional supplementation and home-based exercise regimens are likely to benefit both well-being and outcome after transplant.

Obesity

Obesity, especially associated with metabolic syndrome, is increasingly common, and NAFLD is an increasing indication for liver transplant (see Chapter 69). The data on the effect of obesity on outcome are conflicting, in part because of the careful selection and assessment and the difficulty in distinguishing the effect of obesity itself with the associated conditions of diabetes, cardiovascular disease, and other comorbidities. Most studies indicate that transplantation can be done safely in those with a BMI up to 40 kg/m^2.[8] Some centers undertake bariatric surgery in the peritransplant period, although the timing and risks and benefits remain uncertain.[9]

Psychological Assessment

Transplantation is associated with major psychological stress, both for the patient and the family. More than half of liver transplant candidates have a wide range of psychological health problems.[10] However, full psychological and psychiatric assessment of all potential transplant candidates is rarely undertaken as routine practice. However, psychiatric assessment of potential liver transplant recipients is becoming increasingly common in clinical practice. Risk factors associated with a poor outcome include
- Mood disorders,
- Lack of social support,
- Substance misuse, and
- Alcohol dependence.[11]

Chronic poor health, possibly associated with subclinical encephalopathy and future uncertainties, makes it difficult sometimes to predict the patient's outcome accurately. When the patient has a history of psychiatric illness, expert assessment by a multidisciplinary team is required because some people with psychiatric illness not responsive to therapy or with a history of recurrent episodes of self-harm may not be suitable candidates for transplantation. It is not unreasonable to withhold from transplantation patients who, despite optimal treatment and support, are likely to have an unacceptable QOL.[12] The transplant team should also assess the likelihood of noncompliance (irrespective of cause), and when noncompliance, despite full social and other types of support, is likely to lead to graft loss, it is acceptable to exclude the patient from listing. This is a particular issue in adolescents and those in their early 20s; the use of transitional and handover clinics together with newer technologies may mitigate this problem.[13]

Tobacco Use

Ongoing tobacco use is associated not only with an increased risk of cardiovascular and lung diseases and cancer (before and after transplantation), but also increased morbidities.[14] Some centers will withhold listing from those who continue to smoke cigarettes or do not comply with nicotine withdrawal programs.

Illicit Drug Use

As with tobacco users, some centers will exclude from transplantation those with active illicit drug use and those who fail to engage in withdrawal treatment. Such patients may have other codependencies. However, in contrast to those who use tobacco, outcomes are not worse in those who have or are using marijuana and other illicit drugs.[15] Those who are well stabilized on methadone as opioid replacement therapy should not be excluded and generally should continue on a stable dose. Outcomes are good although perioperative management may be a challenge.

Age

There is no agreed upper age limit, but increasing age is associated independently with mortality after transplant.[16] The concept of biologic age has superseded that of chronologic age, although the former cannot readily be defined or quantified. Outcomes of carefully selected patients over age 70 are encouraging, although older age does remain an independent predictor of survival both before and after transplantation.[17]

Previous Abdominal Surgery

The presence of adhesions, especially in the patient with portal hypertension, adds considerably to the difficulties of surgery and may affect outcome, especially when this involves surgery to the biliary tree.

Infection

Active bacterial, fungal, or protozoal sepsis is an absolute contraindication to transplantation. Once appropriate therapy has been instituted, however, the patient is a suitable candidate for the procedure.

Human Immunodeficiency Virus

Although early studies showed patients with HIV infection fared poorly (Rubin et al., 1987), with the introduction of highly active antiretroviral therapy (HAART), the natural history of HIV infection has been greatly altered. The majority of those with HIV infection who develop end-stage liver disease have HCV coinfection, and current treatments for HCV have also affected the need for liver transplantation. An analysis of the European and North American Registries showed that from 2008 to 2015, around 1% of recipients were HIV infected with a declining proportion with HCV infection. Outcomes have improved over time.[18] Indications are becoming better defined[19] and include (1) end-stage liver disease, (2) low or undetectable levels of HIV RNA, (3) no AIDS-defining complication, and (4) CD4 count greater than 200 cells/μL.

Cardiovascular Disease

As with other diseases, the prognosis of patients with cardiovascular diseases will dictate whether liver replacement is an appropriate therapy. Cardiac disease is common in liver transplant candidates and an important cause of perioperative and postoperative disease. There are many causes of cardiac dysfunction, including the cardiovascular disease, valvular disease, cardiomyopathies due to causes such as cirrhotic cardiomyopathy (CCM), metabolic diseases such as amyloidosis, hemochromatosis, and toxins as alcohol. Tools to assess the degree of cardiac disease and to define those where transplantation is not indicated are lacking.[20]

Multivessel Moderate to Severe Coronary Artery Disease

Coronary artery disease (CAD) is present in 15% of patients with end-stage liver disease.[21] Preoperative assessment of cardiovascular status is, at best, imprecise; no clear guidelines are available to define limits below which grafting is unsafe. All candidates should undergo at least echocardiography not only to detect abnormalities of the heart muscle and valves, but also to seek evidence of pulmonary hypertension. When evidence of possible ischemic heart disease is found, patients should have a stress test, such as dobutamine-stimulated or adenosine-stimulated echocardiography and myoscintigraphy. Functional testing of cardiac reserve may be helpful, but there is no clear indication of when transplant is contraindicated. If there is significant coronary artery stenosis (>70%), then revascularization should be considered before transplantation. Surgery carries a significant risk in those with cirrhosis and stenting may be a preferable option. A staged rather than simultaneous approach may be preferable.

Cirrhotic Cardiomyopathy

CCM is defined as the presence of systolic and diastolic dysfunction and electrophysiologic abnormalities.[22] The diagnosis is based on contemporary Doppler/echocardiography measurements or quantitative magnetic resonance imaging (MRI). CCM is characterized by a high output state at rest with impaired ability to increase contractility at stress, diastolic dysfunction, and electromechanical abnormalities.[23] Patients are often asymptomatic and cardiac dysfunction may not be apparent until the perioperative and postoperative period because the low peripheral resistance associated with arterial vasodilation of the splanchnic circulation decreases left ventricular afterload. However, CCM is difficult to diagnose using the traditional cardiovascular imaging modalities. The role of other imaging modalities, such as cardiac magnetic resonance (CMR), may help in the diagnosis of CCM.[24] Although features of CCM may improve after transplantation, the condition remains an important contributor to early death post-transplant.

Respiratory Function

Routine screening of patients with chest radiograph, electrocardiogram (ECG), lung function tests, and measurement of peripheral oxygen saturation will usually identify those with pulmonary problems. Additional investigations include arterial blood gases (both lying and standing to detect hepatopulmonary syndrome [HPS]) and on 100% oxygen (to detect shunting), high-resolution computed tomography (CT), contrast-enhanced echocardiography, and isotope-labeled macroaggregated albumin lung scan. Pulmonary angiography and right-sided heart catheterization may be indicated, as suggested by the clinical and simple investigations. Arterial hypoxemia (oxygen saturation <92% or arterial oxygen pressure <70 mm Hg) may be found in up to 70% of patients with liver disease. Causes of this hypoxemia include ventilation/perfusion mismatch, diffusion limitation, alveolar hypoventilation, shunt, and a diffusion/perfusion abnormality. Furthermore, pulmonary dysfunction is present in up to 2% of patients with advanced liver disease. The presence of significant pulmonary disease is usually apparent on history and examination, but sometimes significant pulmonary disease may be cryptic.

The many possible causes for pulmonary abnormalities include the following:

- Diseases unrelated to the liver disease (e.g., smoking)

- Effects associated with the liver disease (e.g., α_1-antitrypsin deficiency)
- Respiratory conditions associated with the liver disease (e.g., fibrosing alveolitis associated with primary biliary cirrhosis [PBC])
- Effects of the liver disease on the respiratory function (e.g., effects of ascites causing pleural effusion or simple lung compression)
- HPS
- Portopulmonary hypertension (PPH)

Hepatopulmonary Syndrome

HPS (see Chapters 74, 77, and 78) is both an indication and contraindication for liver transplantation. HPS, which may be detected in up to one-third of transplant candidates, results from intrapulmonary microvascular dilation in the setting of chronic liver disease and/or portal hypertension and leads to arterial deoxygenation. The diagnosis requires demonstration of the triad of the presence of liver disease and/or portal hypertension, an elevated room air alveolar arterial oxygen gradient ($\geq$15 mm Hg or $\geq$20 mm Hg in patients >64 years old), and evidence of intrapulmonary vascular dilatations. The diagnosis is suggested by showing orthodeoxia (a fall in arterial blood oxygen when standing). Intrapulmonary shunting is demonstrated either by contrast echocardiography or by 99mTC macroaggregated albumin (MAA) lung-brain perfusion scanning. HPS improves after transplantation in the majority of patients but may take 6 months or more to improve and there is no association between the severity of the HPS and the severity of cirrhosis. Thus HPS may be an indication for liver replacement, even in the presence of otherwise good liver function. Severe HPS characterized by a preoperative PaO$_2$ less than 50 mm Hg alone or in combination with an MAA shunt scan of greater than 20% is a good predictor of increased mortality after liver transplantation. An association between HPS and CCM remains uncertain.

Portopulmonary Hypertension

Diagnostic criteria for portopulmonary hypertension (PPH) include presence of liver disease (resulting in portal hypertension) and an elevation of the mean pulmonary artery pressure (MPAP) greater than 25 mm Hg. PPH is not correlated with the severity or etiology of portal hypertension. PPH is detected in less than 10% of transplant candidates. Mild PPH (MPAP <35 mm Hg) is usually of little concern, but moderate (MPAP >35 mm Hg) and severe PPH (MPAP >45 mm Hg) are predictors of increased mortality after transplant. The diagnosis is made by exclusion of other causes of pulmonary hypertension (such as pulmonary emboli, intrinsic lung disease, and left heart failure). The initial screening is with contrast-enhanced echocardiography to estimate right ventricular systolic pressure (RVSP), but right heart catheterization is needed to confirm the diagnosis, which requires an MPAP greater than 35 mm Hg in association with an elevated pulmonary vascular resistance (PVR) greater than 240 dyn-s/cm$^-$5 and a pulmonary wedge pressure less than 15 mm Hg. Vasodilator therapy should be tried in those with severe PPH, and liver transplant can be considered if the MPAP can be reduced to less than 35 mm Hg and PVR to less than 400 dynes-s/cm$^-$5. Drugs that have been used include endothelin receptor antagonists (such as bosentan), phosphodiesterase type-5 inhibitors (such as sildenafil), and prostanoids (such as epoprostenol), either as monotherapy or in combination therapy. Sildenafil monotherapy or in combination with prostacyclins is commonly used, but these are not all licensed for this indication (see Chapters 74, 77, and 78).

Coexisting Disease

The presence of coexisting disease may affect the decision to offer the patient a liver graft, because the prospects of recovery are adversely affected, or because long-term survival may be reduced.[25]

Diabetes mellitus is often found in patients with chronic liver disease, especially in those with HCV infection. This may result from the insulin intolerance associated with advanced liver disease and thus will resolve after successful transplantation. Concerns with diabetic patients center on the microvascular complications. Those with insulin-dependent diabetes have a worse outcome after transplant.[26] Evidence of proliferative retinopathy, diabetic nephropathy, or autonomic neuropathy, as evidenced by simple tests such as abnormal beat-to-beat variation on Valsalva maneuver or postural hypotension, may be relative contraindications for transplantation. Other contraindications include diabetic gastroparesis. The presence of advanced microvascular disease puts the patient at risk of major autonomic disruption during the procedure, and survival of such patients is relatively poor.[27]

Hyponatremia is a common finding in patients with advanced chronic liver disease and occurs usually as a consequence of injudicious diuretic therapy or because of the reduced free water clearance. Grafting patients with severe hyponatremia (serum sodium <120 mmol/L) has shown that there is an increased risk of central pontine myelinolysis.[28] Significant hyponatremia should be corrected before transplantation by simple water restriction and, if appropriate, stopping diuretic therapy, or if more rapid correction is required, use of renal support. The role of aquaretics may be helpful in this situation.[29]

Vascular thromboses are not uncommon in patients with chronic liver disease. These may occur because of the cirrhosis itself or as part of an associated underlying thrombotic tendency (e.g., myeloproliferative disease associated with Budd-Chiari syndrome, presence of lupus anticoagulant, protein C or S deficiency, impaired fibrinolysis). In early series, portal vein thrombosis was considered a contraindication to transplantation, but it is now appreciated that this is no longer the case, and portal venous inflow to the graft can be provided by the superior mesenteric vein or even a splenic vein. It is only in rare patients with extensive venous thrombosis, and when it is impossible to provide a suitable portal supply to the graft, that transplantation may be currently contraindicated.

Renal disease may result from hepatorenal syndrome or intrinsic kidney damage (see Chapters 77 and 78). In hepatorenal syndrome, there is no structural damage to the kidney, and once satisfactory liver function is reestablished, the kidney will function normally. Therefore, although the prognosis may be reduced in the presence of advanced renal insufficiency, the hepatorenal syndrome is not an absolute contraindication to transplantation. However, in the patient with coexisting advanced renal disease, it may be advisable to consider combined liver and kidney transplantation. Renal function remains a major predictive factor for survival after transplantation, as well as the risk for renal impairment.[30] Whether pretransplant correction of renal parameters (e.g., by dialysis) is associated with an improved survival is uncertain.

Combined liver and kidney transplantation may be considered for patients with the following:

- Liver failure and end-stage kidney disease (excluding hepatorenal syndrome)
- Liver failure and chronic kidney disease, with glomerular filtration rate (GFR) less than 30 mL/min
- Liver failure with chronic kidney disease, with renal histology showing greater than 30% fibrosis or 30% glomerulosclerosis or other renal disease (such as polycystic kidney disease)
- Liver failure and acute kidney injury, with serum creatinine greater than 2.0 mg/dL, and renal support for at least 8 weeks

Past history of malignancy is a relative contraindication to transplantation, because the effect of surgery and resulting immunosuppression may predispose the patient to early recurrence of the tumor.[31] The Israel Penn Tumor Registry has identified tumors that carry a high risk of recurrence after transplantation (Box 105.3).[32,33] Caution must be used when following these recommendations, however, because the registry relies on voluntary reports rather than a systematic review. Most centers will offer transplantation when the risk of recurrence is less than 10% at 5 years. Colorectal cancer (18.8%), nonmelanoma skin cancers (23.5%), thyroid carcinoma (25%), oral squamous carcinoma (33%), vulvovaginal cancers (33%), and breast carcinoma (33%) are associated with a greater than 10% risk after liver transplantation.[34] Only in exceptional cases should patients with these extrahepatic malignancies be considered suitable candidates for transplantation.

Bone Disease

Many patients with chronic liver disease will have bone disease. The prevalence of osteomalacia, caused by vitamin D malabsorption, is low and can readily be corrected by parenteral administration of vitamin D. Osteoporosis, however, is a much greater problem and is particularly seen in female patients with chronic cholestatic disease. In many cases, successful transplantation will halt or retard the progression and may even improve bone mineralization.[35] The presence of severe osteoporosis may result in additional complications if there is significant thoracic or lumbar vertebral collapse or the presence of fractures. The development of severe osteoporosis is a rare indication for transplantation.

SPECIFIC DISEASES

Fulminant Hepatic Failure (see Chapters 77, 78, and 107)

Liver transplantation is an effective form of therapy for patients with fulminant hepatic failure (FHF), that is, the presence of encephalopathy occurring within 8 weeks of the onset of symptoms in a patient with previously normal liver (Box 105.4).[36] FHF requiring transplant accounts for less than 5% of liver transplants. In patients with severe FHF and grade IV hepatic encephalopathy, the mortality approaches 80%. Common causes of FHF include acetaminophen (paracetamol) overdose, viral infections (hepatitis A, B, E, and rarely C), drug and xenobiotic toxicity (including herbal remedies), Wilson disease, and liver diseases of pregnancy.

Patients with FHF experience early multiorgan failure and require intensive supportive therapy. The common causes of death are cerebral edema, multiorgan failure, sepsis (bacterial or fungal), cardiac arrhythmia or arrest, and respiratory failure.[37]

Patients with FHF pose a difficult problem because there is a very narrow window between the time when it is apparent that the patient's survival is likely to be poor in the absence of transplantation and the onset of irreversible complications that preclude a successful outcome. Several groups have now published prognostic factors, and based on those, criteria are available for super-urgent transplant (see Box 105.4).[38,39] The King's College Hospital model has been validated in other centers and found to be robust. With advances in the medical management of patients with FHF, these prognostic factors likely require modification. Contraindications to transplantation in FHF include the onset of irreversible complications. Thus the development of irreversible cerebral edema, characterized by prolonged elevation of intracranial pressure (ICP), as documented on intracerebral pressure monitoring, or by the presence of fixed, dilated pupils for more than 6 hours, precludes transplantation. Active sepsis is also a contraindication.

One of the best guides to progression is given by serial estimation of the prothrombin time (PT)[40] or factor V levels,[41] because in the absence of extraneous blood products, these best represent the synthetic function of the liver. Initial improvement in PT followed by deterioration suggests the presence of sepsis, which should be actively treated before transplantation. The patient remains at risk for complications of increased intracerebral pressure for as long as 48 hours after successful transplantation.

Because of the prognostic importance of clotting parameters, patients with FHF should not be given clotting factors until the decision for transplantation has been made, unless there are pressing clinical reasons. Once the decision for transplantation has been made, clotting should be normalized as much as possible given the constraints of volume replacement and avoidance of the complications of intracerebral edema. The

---

BOX 105.3   Effect of Immunosuppression on Tumor Recurrence[a]

Low Recurrence Rates (0%-10%)
Incidentally discovered renal tumors
Lymphoma
Testicular carcinoma
Uterine carcinoma
Cervical carcinoma
Thyroid carcinoma

Intermediate Recurrence Rates (11%-25%)
Uterine body carcinoma
Wilms tumor
Colon carcinoma
Breast carcinoma
Prostate carcinoma

High Recurrence Rate (>26%)
Bladder carcinoma
Sarcomas
Melanoma
Symptomatic renal carcinomas
Myelomas
Nonmelanoma skin cancers

[a]This list is derived from patients undergoing renal transplantation and should be used only as a guide when applied to those patients.
From Penn I. The effect of immunosuppression on pre-existing cancers. *Transplantation.* 1993;55:742–747.

BOX 105.4 Current Transplant Criteria in United Kingdom for Registration as a Super-Urgent Transplantation for Fulminant Hepatic Failure (2020)

Category 1 Etiology: Acetaminophen Poisoning
pH <7.25 more than 24 hours after overdose and after fluid resuscitation

Category 2 Etiology: Acetaminophen Poisoning
Coexisting prothrombin time >100 seconds or INR >6.5, and serum creatinine >300 µmol/L or anuria, and grade 3-4 encephalopathy

Category 3 Etiology: Acetaminophen Poisoning
Significant liver injury and coagulopathy following exclusion of other causes of hyperlactatemia (e.g., pancreatitis, intestinal ischemia) after adequate fluid resuscitation: arterial lactate >5 mmol/L on admission and >4 mmol/L 24 hours later in the presence of clinical hepatic encephalopathy.

Category 4 Etiology: Acetaminophen Poisoning
Two of the three criteria from category 2 with clinical evidence of deterioration (e.g., increased ICP, FiO_2 >50%, increasing inotrope requirements) in the absence of clinical sepsis

Category 5 Etiology: Favorable Non-Acetaminophen Etiologies Such as Acute Viral Hepatitis or Ecstasy/Cocaine-Induced ALF
The presence of clinical hepatic encephalopathy is mandatory and prothrombin time >100 seconds, or INR >6.5, or any three from the following:
- Age >40 or <10 years
- Prothrombin time >50 seconds or INR >3.5
- Any grade of hepatic encephalopathy with jaundice to encephalopathy time >7 days
- Serum bilirubin >300 µmol/L

Category 6 Etiology: Unfavorable Non-Acetaminophen Etiologies Such as Seronegative or Idiosyncratic Drug Reactions
Prothrombin time >100 seconds, or INR >6.5, or in the absence of clinical hepatic encephalopathy, INR >2 after vitamin K repletion and any two from the following:
- Age >40 or <10 years
- Prothrombin time >50 seconds or INR >3.5
- If hepatic encephalopathy is present then jaundice to encephalopathy time >7 days
- Serum bilirubin >300 µmol/L

ALF, Acute liver failure; *ICP*, intracranial pressure; *INR*, international normalized ratio.
From https://nhsbtdbe.blob.core.windows.net/umbraco-assets-corp/17399/pol195.pdf. Accessed April 2020.

ability to give large volumes of fluid may be limited by impaired renal function, but the presence of renal support will allow fluid therapy to be stopped sooner.

Because many of the extrahepatic manifestations of FHF may be the result of large amounts of necrotic tissue, some centers have advocated a two-stage procedure in which the failed liver is removed and the patient remains anhepatic until a suitable graft can become available.[42] Although after hepatectomy the patient's condition may well improve, there are few convincing data at present to suggest that this beneficially affects outcome. However, such a procedure may be indicated in a patient who is rapidly deteriorating, and a graft has been found, but logistic conditions may enforce some delay before the graft can be successfully performed.

One of the dilemmas in considering liver transplantation in patients with acute liver failure is that if the liver does recover, a complete return to normal structure and function is likely. The use of auxiliary transplants (e.g., auxiliary partial orthotopic liver transplantation [APOLT]) or partial transplants (see Chapter 125) may allow the earlier use of liver grafting as a safety net; if the patient's liver does recover, the donor liver can be removed or allowed to atrophy, and the patient can return to a life of good liver function free of immunosuppression. The use of artificial liver support devices (see Chapter 80) remains uncertain, but systems such as the molecular absorbent recirculation system (MARS) may offer a bridge.[43]

Patients in whom FHF develops as a consequence of acetaminophen (paracetamol) overdose pose a special problem. Patients with a long history of psychiatric disease that is unresponsive to full intervention and support or with a history of recurrent overdose are not usually appropriate candidates. Many of the patients with acetaminophen overdose have taken the overdose on an impulse because of a relatively trivial problem, and it is usually appropriate to offer these patients transplantation. In contrast, if the overdose is taken because of long-term social or domestic problems, even after successful grafting the patient may return to identical problems with the additional burden of a liver transplant and its consequences, thus grafting in such patients may not be appropriate.

Variants of Acute Liver Failure
Subacute Liver Failure

In some patients, the natural history is a subacute illness (or late-onset hepatic failure), with fluctuating encephalopathy that may develop days or weeks after onset of a hepatitis-like illness. This may be seen in middle-aged women and with no obvious precipitating factors.[44] These patients have a very poor prognosis without transplantation.

Fulminant Autoimmune Hepatitis

Fulminant autoimmune hepatitis (AIH) refers to patients with FHF in association with serologic markers of AIH, including increased serum immunoglobulins and high-titer autoantibodies. Whether this represents a form of classic AIH is unclear; response to corticosteroids is disappointing, and the decision to offer transplant should not be delayed (see Chapter 68).

Metabolic Diseases

A number of metabolic diseases, accounting for less than 5% of liver transplants in adults, may be corrected by liver transplantation (Table 105.1; see Chapter 74). In some cases, where the metabolic defect arises in the liver, transplantation will correct that defect. Hepatocyte transplantation and auxiliary transplantation may become suitable alternate approaches.

Correction of the metabolic abnormality is seen, for example, with Wilson disease or hemophilia. In other conditions, such as some types of hypercholesterolemia, the metabolic defect occurs within the liver, but the heart is the major organ affected. Some centers have advocated the use of liver transplantation to prevent the onset of severe CAD. When the patient already has cardiac disease, combined heart and liver transplants may be performed. Similar considerations apply to hyperoxaluria requiring liver and kidney replacement. Equally, porphyria is an indication for transplantation in selected patients but should be accompanied by stem cell transplant as the

TABLE 105.1 Inborn Errors of Metabolism That Have Been Treated by Liver Transplantation

LIVER AFFECTED	OTHER ORGANS ALSO AFFECTED
α₁-Antitrypsin deficiency	Primary hyperoxaluria
Wilson disease	Crigler-Najjar syndrome
Protoporphyria	Primary hypercholesterolemia
Tyrosinosis	Niemann-Pick disease
Tyrosinemia	Sea-blue histiocyte disease[a]
Galactosemia	Hemophilia A and B
Glycogen storage disease types I and IV	Protein C deficiency
Byler disease	Protein S deficiency
Hemochromatosis[a]	
Cystic fibrosis	
Gaucher disease[a]	
Urea cycle enzyme deficiencies	

[a]May recur after transplantation.

condition is not "cured" by liver transplant alone.[45] In other conditions, such as hemophilia, for which alternative therapies are available, such as replacement with factor VIII, transplantation should only be considered with extensive liver disease, as may occur with HCV infection transmitted by blood products. The possibility of recurrence of the metabolic disease should not necessarily be considered a contraindication to transplantation. Thus, although the consequences of genetic hemochromatosis may recur after transplantation, organ damage can be prevented by early recognition and treatment. Similarly, in erythropoietic protoporphyria, the disease is likely to recur after transplantation, but the morbidity of disease may be delayed by appropriate treatment with cholestyramine. Thus, in these patients, the decision to offer transplantation needs to be taken with a view to the benefits obtained, and the indications remain similar to those in patients with other liver diseases.

Budd-Chiari Syndrome

The role of liver transplantation in patients with Budd-Chiari syndrome remains uncertain (see Chapter 86). There may be underlying thrombotic disorders, such as protein C or S deficiency, factor V Leiden mutation, lupus anticoagulant, polycythemia, or myeloproliferative disorders; some of these will be corrected by transplantation, whereas others will carry the risk of complications such as malignant transformation. The early use of anticoagulants and interventional radiology, especially transjugular intrahepatic portosystemic shunting (TIPS), have changed the management of these patients[46] (see Chapter 85). In general, transplantation should be considered only when portal decompression has failed (or is not feasible) or there is established cirrhosis.

Other Indications

Other indications for transplantation are shown in Boxes 105.3 and 105.4. Polycystic liver disease (see Chapter 73) is an indication in a small proportion of patients; transplantation may be considered an option when the enlarged liver results in severe and constant pain and when the enlarged liver impacts on the stomach and so leads to poor nutrition. In general, transplantation is indicated when the liver reaches into the pelvis.[47] For

those with combined liver and kidney involvement, dual transplantation may be indicated.

Transthyretin amyloidosis (ATTR) is characterized by progressive impairment of neurologic and cardiac function because of deposition of misfolded transthyretin. Liver transplantation has a place in highly selected patients and the resected liver is sometimes used in a domino procedure.[48] However, there are newer agents such as TTR tetramer stabilizers, TTR silencers, and fibril disruptors that might reduce the need for transplantation in this group of patients.

Chronic Liver Disease

In many respects, patients with chronic liver disease pose the most difficult problems in regard to transplantation (see Chapter 74). The main concern lies not primarily with whether the patient is a suitable candidate for transplantation, but rather in deciding on the *appropriate time* to offer the patient the procedure. On the one hand, the fitter the patient, the greater the probability of surviving the procedure; on the other hand, the patient's life will have been shortened if the procedure is unsuccessful. If transplantation is offered too late, the chances of success are reduced (see Chapter 79), although the quality of the donor liver remains a major factor in predicting outcome.

Broadly speaking, there are two major indications for transplantation in patients with chronic liver disease: poor QOL and poor estimated length of life. Assessment of QOL is often difficult because a QOL that is unacceptable to one person may be acceptable to another. Furthermore, it is often difficult to disentangle the effects of borderline encephalopathy and depression associated with the knowledge of chronic liver disease from the effects of the tiredness and lethargy caused by the liver disease itself. Some patients do adopt the "sick role" and, even after successful transplantation, either the patient or the family is reluctant for the sick role to be abandoned. However, although intractable pruritus is a valid indication for transplantation if all other measures for treatment are unsuccessful, lethargy often fails to improve and thus is not, in itself, an indication[49]; it is important to exclude extrahepatic disorders, such as coexistent myxedema, or therapy that may cause the lethargy.

Most centers consider transplantation as appropriate when the estimated length of life in the absence of transplantation is limited to 1 year. In practice, in many patients, this is difficult to assess. Generally, the diseases run a predictable course, although the patient's life may be threatened by unpredictable events such as sepsis or variceal hemorrhage. For this reason, timing of transplantation remains an inexact science. A further feature to be considered is that many factors predicting poor survival in patients with cirrhosis are different than those that predict outcome after transplantation. The use of prognostic models has helped in defining variables that predict outcome, but these suffer from disadvantages. First, most prognostic models are defined from retrospective studies that use patient data at referral or at a certain point in the course of the illness. It may be inappropriate to reapply these models sequentially unless time-dependent models are used. Second, models provide data for populations, and their application to an individual is limited by the relatively wide confidence intervals. Nonetheless, the Child-Pugh (CP) score is not a useful guide, although it may not be sufficiently detailed for estimation of short-term survival, and the Pugh score does use semi-quantifiable parameters (such as ascites), which adds concern to the generalization of this model. The MELD score is also a useful marker of short-term prognosis and may be more accurate than the CP score.[2,50,51] There have been a variety of suggested variations in the MELD score, such as MELD-Na (which includes serum sodium) but the MELD score remains the most used tool[52] (see Chapter 4).

Development of hepatic decompensation is a useful clinical marker of a poor prognosis. Box 105.3 provides indications for consideration of transplantation.

The development of complications may often precipitate referral for transplantation. Thus the development of severe ascites, spontaneous bacterial peritonitis, recurrent variceal hemorrhage, and intractable encephalopathy are all indications that hepatic reserve is limited. Both the CP and the MELD score are relatively poor prognostic guides to survival after grafting. However, data suggest that transplantation of a patient without malignancy who has a MELD score less than 12 is associated with a reduction in survival at 1 year compared with continued observation.[53]

Other centers have concentrated on functional tests of the liver (see Chapter 3). Thus, although the aminopyrine breath test (MEGX test) and galactosamine elimination clearance have their advocates, none has added greatly to clinical or serologic assessment or has been applied widely, and these tests are now rarely used.

Primary Biliary Cholangitis (see Chapter 74)

A number of prognostic models have been developed, including both static and time-dependent ones. These are helpful in defining variables that predict survival both in the absence of transplantation and after transplantation From these models, an estimate of survival can be made However, these models must be used with some care because the confidence intervals are relatively wide, and any information derived from such models must be made in conjunction with clinical judgment. Ursodeoxycholic acid (UDCA), at a dose of 13 to 15 mg/kg/day is associated with a significant delay to the time of transplantation, especially in those who show a significant biochemical response to UDCA. Obeticholic acid, as a second-line treatment, may well further reduce the need for transplantation. Indications are clearly set out in North American and European guidelines.[54,55]

Indications for liver transplantation for patients with PBC are similar to those with other forms of chronic liver disease. Patients should be referred for liver transplant evaluation in the setting of decompensated cirrhosis, a MELD score greater than 15, total bilirubin greater than 6 mg/dL (American Association for the Study of Liver Diseases [AASLD] Guidelines) or between 3 and 5 mg/dL (European Association for the Study of the Liver [EASL] Guidelines), or a Mayo risk score greater than 7.8.

Transplantation in patients with PBC may also be indicated for intolerable and intractable pruritus. However, it is important that all therapies for pruritus are considered before transplantation is considered. The therapeutic options are increasing: cholestyramine is the mainstay, but trials of rifampicin, naltrexone, sertraline (unlicensed indications), and, in exceptional cases, either plasmapheresis or MARS should be considered before transplantation is offered to those with good liver function (see Chapter 78). There are many causes for lethargy in patients with PBC; depression is common and often responds to antidepressant medication. However, although lethargy improves somewhat after transplantation, it rarely resolves,

so lethargy alone, in the absence of other indications, should not be considered an indication for transplant.[56] Celiac disease is found in 3% of patients with PBC and, if unrecognized and untreated, may cause lethargy. Low levels of antibodies to gliadin are common in patients with liver disease, so the syndrome should be tested for by measuring anti-endomysial or anti-transglutaminase antibodies and a small bowel biopsy taken when these antibodies are present. Coexisting myxedema should be excluded by measuring serum thyroid-stimulating hormone (TSH) and Addison disease tested for if appropriate. Sometimes the pruritus usually disappears within 2 to 3 days after surgery.

PBC does recur in the allograft; this is likely to be at a slow rate and should not preclude transplantation. Other extrahepatic manifestations of PBC will not be affected.

Primary Sclerosing Cholangitis (see Chapter 41)

In contrast to PBC, the natural history of primary sclerosing cholangitis (PSC) is less clear and predictable and accounts for approximately 6% of all transplants (see Chapter 41). For many patients, the disease runs a fluctuating course with exacerbations and remissions that may be caused by episodes of spontaneously occurring bacterial cholangitis. Underlying these fluctuations in liver function, there is a persisting and relentless progression toward liver failure. As with other chronic liver diseases, serum bilirubin and serum albumin remain useful markers of progression, and prognostic models will help in timing the procedure. The CP and MELD scores are as reliable as the Mayo model.[57] The AASLD Guidelines[58] and UK Guidelines[59] recommend that the indications for referral for patients with PSC are broadly similar to those for other indications. However, the decision to transplant is more problematic as worsening jaundice may respond to endoscopic therapy of dominant strictures or treatment of cholangitis. The development of cholangiocarcinoma (see later) will add further to the challenges of timing of listing. The incidence of cholangiocarcinoma in PSC is up to 1.5% a year, with a prevalence of 6% to 13% and a lifetime risk of up to 20%.

Most cases of PSC are associated with inflammatory bowel disease, usually ulcerative colitis. Patients with PSC and colitis are at increased risk of colonic cancer compared with those with colitis alone. Because the cancers tend to be in the ascending colon, a full colonoscopy is recommended in all potential transplant candidates to exclude colonic neoplasia and to assess the degree of colitis. Quiescent colitis is not a contraindication to transplantation, but active colitis should be treated before transplantation. When surgical treatment is required to control the colitis, this can safely be done at the transplant procedure. Colectomy either before or during transplantation confers a protective effect against recurrent PSC in subsequent grafts[60]; however, the benefit is currently not considered sufficiently strong to advise prophylactic colectomy.

PSC is a premalignant condition, with the patient at increased risk for cholangiocarcinoma in any part of the biliary tree and a cancer may develop in as many as 20% of patients with PSC, especially in smokers (see Chapters 50 and 51). Bile duct dysplasia may identify a group of patients at special risk, but this is still controversial. It is often difficult to be certain whether a sudden deterioration in the patient is caused by the development of cholangitis (see Chapter 43), the natural history of the disease, or the development of cholangiocarcinoma (see Chapters 50 and 51). Methods of detection of cholangiocarcinoma are often unrewarding: serum markers such as carcinoembryonic antigen (CEA) are relatively nonspecific and insensitive; elevated levels of CA19-9 may be more helpful but are not specific.[61] Other tumor markers have insufficient sensitivity and specificity[62] for clinical use. Tumor markers are often elevated in those with advanced liver disease and ascites. Imaging techniques, including CT, MRI, ultrasound, and angiography, are often unreliable and miss even quite large tumors. Although the presence of dilated intrahepatic bile ducts may be a useful sign of cholangiocarcinoma, it also is too insensitive and nonspecific for routine use.

The biliary tree can usually be well visualized by magnetic resonance cholangiopancreatography (MRCP)(see Chapter 16), which provides images almost as good as those obtained at endoscopic retrograde cholangiopancreatography (ERCP); however, MRCP does not allow tissue to be taken for histology or cytology. ERCP may be helpful if combined with brushing and biopsy of strictures and bile cytology with fluorescent in situ hybridization. Although the specificity is high, the sensitivity is relatively low, and ERCP is not without risk of precipitating severe cholangitis. Directed percutaneous biopsy or aspiration cytology again may give a positive diagnosis, but negative findings do not exclude the possibility of cholangiocarcinoma. It must be emphasized that ERCP in the presence of advanced PSC may lead to sudden deterioration, presumably caused by the introduction of biliary sepsis. If a cholangiocarcinoma is known to be present before transplantation, survival is poor. Thus most centers believe the patient who is known to have cholangiocarcinoma should not be considered for transplantation. However, a very small proportion of patients with cholangiocarcinoma may benefit from an aggressive approach with neoadjuvant chemoradiation before orthotopic liver transplantation[63,64] (see later and Chapter 108B).

Currently, there is no effective medical treatment for PSC, and the role of UDCA is uncertain. Surgical intervention may be helpful, although endoscopic dilation or stenting should usually be considered only in the presence of a single dominant extrahepatic stricture. The use of biliary diversions and biliary reconstruction is associated with a poorer outcome after transplantation. Analysis of the Mayo Clinic database suggested that the prognostic markers for patients with PSC after transplantation included disease severity, previous biliary or shunt surgery, concurrent bile duct cancer, and presence of inflammatory disease.[65] Our own analysis confirms these observations although we did find that although ulcerative colitis was associated with a better outcome, Crohn disease was associated with an adverse outcome (Neuberger et al., 1999).

Therefore, because PSC is a premalignant disease and cholangiocarcinoma is usually difficult to detect, patients with PSC should be considered earlier for transplantation and, during the course of their illness, biliary surgery avoided if possible.

Alcoholic Liver Disease

Selected patients with alcoholic liver disease are excellent candidates for transplantation, and this is becoming an increasing indication for transplantation. Initial concerns that these patients would continue to drink alcohol to excess, comply poorly with follow-up, and be unreliable with taking their immunosuppressive medication have by and large not been substantiated. Other concerns were that the extrahepatic alcohol-associated damage may affect heart, brain, pancreas, and bone marrow. In 1988, Starzl and colleagues[66] reported an estimated survival of more than 70% in 41 patients transplanted for alcoholic liver disease; only two returned to alcohol abuse and subsequently died. The survival rates of these patients were similar to other patients with cirrhosis. Nonetheless, a decreasing body of opinion takes the view that, because alcoholic liver disease is a self-induced injury, and in view of the expense of the procedure and the limited supply of donor organs, such candidates should not be considered. In the view of most transplant units, however, this is not considered appropriate because patients with alcoholic liver disease are not necessarily alcohol dependent. A large number of self-induced diseases exist, and it would be no more appropriate to deny a patient with alcohol-induced liver disease transplantation because it is self-induced than to deny treatment for a broken limb in a rugby player or mountain climber. Furthermore, current evidence suggests that public opinion is becoming more supportive for the use of organs for selected patients with alcohol use disorders

In addition to the usual criteria for transplantation and contraindications to the procedure, other specific factors need to be considered for patients with alcoholic liver disease. The first is the effect of abstinence, which improves survival in patients even in those who have shown signs of decompensation. Although those who are seen with variceal hemorrhage or severe ascites often see only limited benefit after abstinence from alcohol, those with mild ascites or other complications may have significant improvement in both quality and quantity of life once they abstain from drinking.[67] A period of abstinence is helpful, in part to ensure that the liver will not recover to such an extent that transplantation is no longer required, but also to identify the reason for the excessive drinking and initiate appropriate measures to reduce the risk of recurrence after transplantation. Therefore the period of abstinence must be considered in the light of the patient's condition, and transplantation should be offered to the patient who has remained abstinent since being so advised. There is no evidential basis for a fixed period of abstinence.[68]

It is recommended that the candidate with alcoholic liver disease be carefully evaluated by a multidisciplinary team that includes clinicians expert in substance abuse.[69] A number of prognostic models have been proposed including the Michigan alcoholism prognostic scale, the high-risk alcoholism relapse, the "Alcohol Relapse Risk Assessment," and the Stanford Integrated Psychosocial Assessment for Transplantation. Factors that are associated with sobriety include social integration as evidenced by a spouse or partner, stable home and work environment, insight into the disorder, and absence of failed rehabilitation attempts or preexisting psychiatric disorders. Some centers require the potential candidate to sign a contract to agree to remain abstinent. Although this has clearly no legal validity, it does provide a clear understanding that the patient has committed to abstinence both before and after transplantation.

Alcoholic Hepatitis

The role of transplantation in patients with alcoholic hepatitis (severe hepatitis characterized by high serum bilirubin and prolonged clotting) is more difficult to define than in those with alcoholic liver disease (see Chapter 68). Those with encephalopathy and renal failure have a dismal prognosis. There is usually insufficient time to evaluate the patient's background, and the outcome after transplantation is usually poor. Early treatment with corticosteroids may be effective in some patients.

The initial study in 2011 by Mathurin and colleagues[70] reported that, in highly select patients with advanced disease and no response to medical therapy, reasonable outcomes can be achieved. Selection criteria were strict and included

- No prior episodes of alcoholic hepatitis,
- Lille scores ≥ 0.45 or rapid worsening of liver function despite medical therapy,
- Supportive family members,
- No severe coexisting conditions, and
- A commitment to alcohol abstinence.

Outcomes after transplantation were reasonable (77% at 6 months) compared with 27% in those who were not transplanted; 2 of the 26 transplanted patients returned to alcohol. Since this landmark publication, other centers have started to transplant patients with severe alcoholic hepatitis, with broadly similar outcomes to those observed by Mathurin.[71]

There is increasing clarity about the role of medical therapies in supporting those with alcoholic hepatitis (such as corticosteroids and newer agents). There are several prognostic models, such as the Lille model, Maddrey Discriminant Function, Glasgow Alcoholic Hepatitis Score, ABIC (age, serum bilirubin, international normalized ratio, and serum creatinine) and MELD,[69] which may help identify those with a poor outcome with medical therapy. In recent years, the boundaries for transplantation in those with alcoholic hepatitis are slowly expanding. Outcomes are still relatively short term and the place of liver transplant in these patients is evolving.

Patients with alcoholic hepatitis therefore have a greater need for a multidisciplinary approach to evaluation. On the physical side, in addition to the routine workup, the extrahepatic effects of alcohol should be assessed, and those with advanced alcoholic cardiomyopathy or pancreatitis may not be suitable on these grounds.

Patients with alcoholic liver disease thus are certainly potential candidates for transplantation and, as such, do require appropriate referral for consideration.

Hepatitis A and Hepatitis E Viral Infection

Rarely, acute hepatitis A virus (HAV) infection is an indication for liver transplantation, and the indications are those listed earlier for FHF. A few patients have recurrent infection in the graft, but this is of little clinical significance.[72] Hepatitis E virus (HEV) infection, another rare cause of FHF, may persist after liver transplant; patients should be monitored and if HEV persists, offered appropriate treatment[73] (see Chapter 68).

Hepatitis B Viral Infection

Patients with hepatitis B virus (HBV) infection can be considered for transplantation either because of FHF or because of chronic liver disease, accounting for less than 5% of transplants (see Chapter 68). Of those with FHF, the conventional criteria apply as previously indicated. Because it is thought that the liver failure in these patients is caused by the rapid clearance of viral-infected hepatocytes, most patients at transplantation are HBV DNA negative, and, as such, the disease recurs less frequently than in those with chronic HBV infection.

However, different considerations apply to patients with chronic liver disease. Those who are HBV DNA positive at transplantation are much more likely, if untreated, to have recurrence of disease after transplantation, and this is associated with a significantly poorer outcome.[74] Thus patients with high HBV DNA positivity before transplantation should, where

feasible and safe, be offered antiviral treatment before transplantation. The introduction of effective antiviral therapy has significantly reduced the need for liver transplantation. Treatment should be given to achieve HBV DNA negativity.[75] Nucleos(t)ide analogs, such as entecavir or tenofovir, are currently recommended, as both drugs appear safe in decompensated liver disease and lead to HBV-DNA negativity within 1 year in up to three-quarters of patients. A higher dose of entecavir (1 mg) is recommended for decompensated cirrhosis and side effects should be monitored carefully. The NA dose must be adjusted according to kidney function. Studies of safety and efficacy of tenofovir alafenamide (TAF) in patients with decompensated cirrhosis are lacking, but this may be an alternative, particularly in patients with renal impairment. Pegylated interferon is contraindicated in patients with decompensated liver disease.

Treatment with hepatitis B immune globulin and oral antiviral agents is usually continued after transplant, but the optimal regimen remains uncertain.

Patients coinfected with hepatitis D virus remain a challenge. Although interferon is effective in some patients, its use in those with decompensated cirrhosis remains problematic.

Hepatitis C Viral Infection

Indications for transplantation for those with HCV-cirrhosis, with or without alcohol-associated liver disease or associated hepatocellular carcinoma (HCC) are as for those without HCV (see Chapter 68). The impact of effective direct-acting antiviral agents (DAAs) has dramatically reduced the need for transplantation for those infected with HCV. HCV RNA positivity at the time of transplant is associated with infection of the graft; the subsequent rapid onset of cirrhosis and graft failure meant that patient and graft survival was significantly reduced compared with those with other causes of cirrhosis. Now that increasing numbers of patients with HCV-related cirrhosis are RNA negative at transplantation, it is probable that long-term graft and patient survival will be similar to other causes for cirrhosis. The use of DAA in those with cirrhosis is covered by standard guidelines (see, for example,[76]). Ideally, treatment should be offered before the onset of decompensation. Indeed, the response to treatment in some has meant that the patient could be removed from the transplant list.[77] In contrast, treatment in those with decompensated liver disease (and therefore potential transplant candidates) and the use of protease inhibitor–containing regimens should be considered with extreme caution due to potential toxicity. Options include treatment deferral to the post liver transplant period; indeed, the chance of receiving a graft would be increased if the recipient were to agree to accept an organ from a deceased donor who also carries the virus. The optimal time and regimen for treating HCV infection after transplant remains uncertain: some argue for institution of DAA once the patient and graft are stable and healthy, whereas others advocate awaiting the onset of early fibrosis. Patients with hemophilia and HCV infection pose few special problems. Although liver transplantation will correct the defect in hemophilia, this in itself is not an indication for liver transplantation. Many patients will have contracted HCV through contaminated blood products. Provided the patient is supported with adequate amounts of the appropriate blood products, liver transplantation poses no major problem, and many patients will not need support beyond 72 hours.[78]

Hepatocellular Carcinoma

HCC may occur in a noncirrhotic liver, but in Western populations, it more often arises in those with cirrhosis and accounts for as many as 30% of transplants (see Chapters 89 and 108A). Several approaches to the treatment of HCC have been adopted,[79,80] including chemotherapy (see Chapter 99), resection (see Chapters 101 and 102), transarterial embolization/radio-embolization/chemoembolization (TACE) (see Chapter 94), injection with ethanol (see Chapter 96D), cryotherapy (see Chapter 96D), radiofrequency ablation (RFA; see Chapter 96B), microwave ablation (see Chapter 96C), and transplantation (see Chapter 108A), and newer approaches such as immunotherapy. As newer and more effective agents become available, the algorithm for managing HCC will evolve.[81]

There are very few well-conducted, prospective randomized trials of treatment, and most reports are based on select patients and compared with historic controls. It must also be remembered that in patients with HCC that arises in a cirrhotic liver, the optimal treatment for these cancers will depend not only on the natural history of the HCC, but also on the severity, prognosis, and extent of the liver disease. The questions that continue to challenge include the following:

- Where is the place of transplantation in light of the alternative regimens?
- What are the biomarkers (such as α-fetoprotein [AFP]) that indicate futility of transplantation?
- What is the role of downstaging?
- How far does the number and size of tumors seen on imaging reflect spread?
- What is the pretransplant role of genomic, molecular, or histologic markers in defining indications?
- What is the impact of immunosuppression after transplant, especially with a mammalian target of rapamycin inhibitor (mTORi)?

For most patients with HCC, transplantation offers the only prospect of long-term survival (see Chapter 108A). Given the current shortage of donor organs, guidelines must be agreed on to determine the indications and contraindications for liver replacement. The recent EASL Guidelines[82] recommended liver transplantation for those patients whose tumors are unsuitable for resection but within the Milan criteria.[83]

These criteria are a single tumor less than 5 cm in diameter, or in those with multiple tumors, no more than three tumors, all less than 3 cm in diameter. It should be noted that this retrospective analysis was based on only 48 patients. Extrapolation for these observations to current practice must be done with caution because imaging techniques have improved, so more lesions are being detected. Equally, it is clearly not the size of the tumor per se that is important, but that the size reflects the likelihood of tumor microinvasion and spread, and thus the risk of recurrence after transplant (not strictly "recurrence," but persistence). Indeed, other groups have suggested that these criteria are too strict and should be expanded. Thus the San Francisco group has suggested that the indications should be expanded to include either a solitary tumor 6.5 cm or less in diameter or three or fewer nodules with the largest lesion 4.5 cm or less and a total tumor diameter of 8 cm or less.[84] The EASL Guidelines recommended that patients with tumors initially outside the Milan criteria but that reached the criteria after downstaging can be considered for transplantation and those with tumors that are outside the Milan criteria should be transplanted only in the context of agreed protocols.

Vascular invasion and extrahepatic spread are currently both contraindications for.

In general, the restriction of access to transplantation to some of those with HCC is because of the gap between the need for transplantation and availability of suitable organs. Many patients with HCC outside the Milan criteria would benefit from transplantation in terms of survival but would not benefit enough. Whether indications for transplant with cadaver donor livers should be the same as for living donor livers is controversial, but most units accept that indications for deceased donor transplants should be the same for living donor organs.

Other markers include serum AFP, which is a moderately useful serum marker. The absolute level of AFP used as a contraindication to transplantation is not certain, but many centers will exclude transplantation in patients with an AFP greater than 1000 ng/mL.[85] The rate of AFP increase may also be a useful guide to identify those tumors that are unlikely to be "cured" by transplantation. As previously indicated, molecular markers may provide a valuable guide to prognosis, but data are not sufficiently sensitive or validated at this time. Evaluation also involves multiphasic CT or MR examination, whereas others may use contrast-enhanced ultrasound to evaluate the tumor (see Chapter 14).

The role of liver biopsy to establish the diagnosis of HCC or assess the biologic characteristics needs to be considered.[86] Because of the risk of tumor seeding (around 1%) along the needle biopsy track,[87] biopsy should be considered when the diagnosis is uncertain from imaging and serology or when the specimen will be used for prognostic purposes. The clear cell variant of HCC is often difficult to distinguish from pancreatic and renal neoplasm. In contrast, in a patient with known cirrhosis, a primary space-occupying lesion, and rapidly increasing serum AFP, the diagnosis is fairly certain, and percutaneous biopsy would only increase the risk of metastasis and should be avoided. The role of "liquid biopsies" is uncertain but probably has little place in this context.[88]

If accepted for transplantation, those with T1 tumor should be regularly monitored with serum AFP and imaging for at least every 3 months.[89] For those with T2 stage HCC, AASLD suggests bridging to transplant in patients listed for liver transplantation within OPTN T2 (Milan) criteria to decrease progression of disease and subsequent dropout from the waiting list. However, there was insufficient evidence to suggest any preferred form of therapy. As with the EASL Guidelines (2018), those who have T3 tumor may be considered for liver transplant if, after downstaging the tumor, it is within Milan criteria.

Consideration should be given to the use of immunosuppression after transplantation. The evidence for a survival benefit of mTORi (sirolimus and everolimus) is limited,[90] but it may be of benefit to a small degree in selected patients.

Fibrolamellar and other primary liver tumors arising in a noncirrhotic liver may be an indication for transplantation if unresectable and there is no evidence of spread outside the liver (see Chapter 108B).

Cholangiocarcinoma

As previously indicated, cholangiocarcinoma is usually regarded as a contraindication to transplantation because the recurrence rates are high (see Chapter 108B). Thus, in 1998 Jeyarajah and Klintmalm[91] reported a 1-year patient survival of 53% but a 3-year disease-free survival rate of only 13%. Recent analyses by Goldaracena and colleagues[63] and Machairas and coworkers[92] found that, for hilar cholangiocarcinoma, 5-year overall survival was between 21% and 56%; most of the patients had undergone the Mayo Clinic protocol (or a minor modification). This consists of a combination of external beam and transcatheter radiation with intravenous 5-fluorouracil. Features suggesting a dropout from the protocol were CA19-9 greater than 500 U/mL, a mass greater than 3 cm, malignant brushing or biopsy, and MELD score greater than 20. The overall survival for those transplanted for hilar cholangiocarcinoma were much worse (less than 40%), although not all received adjuvant treatment. However, those with small and incidentally found cholangiocarcinoma can do quite well.[93] In 2020 Cambridge and associates[94] did a meta-analysis of 20 studies of the outcomes after transplantation for patients with unresectable perihilar cholangiocarcinoma. They did not find any prospective randomized studies. The pooled 1-, 3-, and 5-year overall survival rates following transplant without neoadjuvant therapy were 71%, 48%, and 32 %, respectively; when neoadjuvant chemoradiation was completed, survival rates were 83%, 66%, and 65% respectively. Pooled recurrence after 3 years was 24% with neoadjuvant chemoradiation and 52% without. However, in one recent nonrandomized study[64] patients with locally advanced, unresectable intrahepatic cholangiocarcinoma, without extrahepatic disease or vascular involvement, underwent gemcitabine-based chemotherapy and those with at least 6 months of radiographic response or stability were listed for liver transplantation. Of the 21 patients referred for evaluation, 12 were accepted and 6 patients underwent liver transplantation. All patients received neoadjuvant chemotherapy while awaiting liver transplantation. Overall survival was 100% at 1 year and 83.3% at 5 years. Three patients developed recurrent disease at a median of 7.6 months

The role of transplantation compared with resection remains uncertain[95] but, where there is underlying liver disease (such as sclerosing cholangitis), transplantation should be considered in those with a small (<2 cm) intrahepatic tumor. Thus, for most centers and in most countries, transplantation for known cholangiocarcinoma is a contraindication and should be restricted to those with unresectable cancer and after completion of neoadjuvant chemoradiation. The advent of newer and more effective agents, such as checkpoint inhibitors, may allow a subgroup of patients to benefit sufficiently from transplantation to justify access to this limited resource.[96]

Secondary Liver Cancers

With few exceptions, transplantation is not usually indicated for metastatic malignancy because of the high rate of recurrence. The major exceptions are carcinoid and other neuroendocrine tumors (see Chapter 91) and colorectal metastases (CRM: see Chapter 90).

Neuroendocrine Tumors

Because long-term results are sometimes good, with rapid symptomatic relief, liver transplantation may be indicated. A multidisciplinary approach is required for optimal management.[97] Guidelines from the European Neuroendocrine Society (ENETS)[98,99] suggest the following indications for liver transplant:

- Well-differentiated NET with Ki-67 proliferation index less than or equal to 10%
- Primary tumor removed at least 6 months before transplantation
- Less than 50% liver involvement or less than 75% liver involvement in patients with refractory hormonal symptoms

- Stable disease for at least 6 months
- Age less than 55 years
- Diffuse unresectable disease confined to the liver with robust extrahepatic exclusion (gallium-68 positron emission tomography/CT, etc.).

Colorectal Metastases

The role of liver transplantation in CRM is unclear as yet. A few centers in Europe, notably the University of Oslo, have shown an overall survival advantage over unresectable patients with liver-limited disease managed with chemotherapy only. The recent update[100] analyzed their experience. Their earlier trial had shown liver transplantation provided an overall survival of 60% (SECA-I). Risk factors for death were CEA greater than 80 µg/L, progressive disease on chemotherapy, size of largest lesion greater than 5.5 cm, and less than 2 years from resection of the primary tumor to transplantation. In their second study (SECA-II), colorectal cancer patients with nonresectable liver-only metastases determined by CT/MRI/positron emission tomography scans, an interval from diagnosis to transplant greater than 1 year, and at least 10% response to chemotherapy were included. At a median follow-up of 36 months, Kaplan-Meier overall survival at 3 years was 83%, and disease-free survival was 35%. Recurrence was mainly slow-growing pulmonary metastases amenable to curative resection. The use of liver transplant for this group of patients is largely a reflection of the availability of organs for transplantation and the need of potential recipients. However, recurrence rates suggest a need for better patient selection and treatment sequencing optimization.[101]

PEDIATRIC TRANSPLANTATION

The medical indications for liver transplantation in children are essentially similar to those in adults (see Chapters 76 and 110). Additional indications include growth retardation and the development of metabolic bone disease. The most common indication for transplantation in children remains disorders of the biliary system, most often biliary atresia (see Chapter 40). The procedure of portoenterostomy may be effective in some children if performed early, but if performed after 2 months, the chance of a successful outcome is limited. Thus, if bile drainage is not established soon after surgery, the child should be considered for transplantation rather than the surgeon making further attempts to reconstruct the bile duct system to establish bile flow. Other disorders of the biliary tree that may require transplantation include Alagille syndrome, Byler disease, and nonsyndromic intrahepatic biliary hypoplasia. Disorders of metabolism are the next most common indications for transplantation and include Wilson disease, tyrosinemia, glycogen storage disease, galactosemia, and Gaucher syndrome.

ASSESSMENT OF PATIENTS FOR LIVER TRANSPLANTATION

When the patient is referred for liver transplantation, it is important to confirm the diagnosis of the liver disease, assess the indications for liver transplantation, and assess any conditions that may preclude transplantation or add to the risk of the procedure. The patient and family should be counseled about the benefits and risks of surgery (see Chapter 106). Along with a thorough history, examination, and review of histology, the investigations required will depend on the medical condition. Some chronic liver diseases are associated with extrahepatic diseases; thus primary biliary cholangitis and AIH are associated with thyroid disease, celiac disease, and Addison disease. These should be excluded because untreated myxedema, for example, may lead to lethargy and, if corrected, may obviate the need for transplantation.

In patients with chronic liver disease, in addition to complete blood count, assessment of clotting, renal function tests, and liver function tests, it is important to check viral status for HAV, HBV, HCV, HIV, and cytomegalovirus (CMV). Some centers will also screen for evidence of infections that may be activated by immunosuppression (such as tuberculosis, human herpes virus [HHV]-8, and other viruses). In patients who are not immune to hepatitis A and B, it is worthwhile to offer immunization before transplantation; there have been occasional reports of HBV acquired during the transplant procedure through an infected organ or infected blood.

In patients with established cirrhosis, ultrasound of the liver and serum estimations of serum AFP should be performed to check for HCC. In patients with a possible history of tuberculosis, tests should be directed to determine the presence of previous infection, and in such cases, our practice is to give isoniazid and pyridoxine for the first 6 months after transplantation. Additional blood tests will be determined by the nature of the disease and include autoantibodies, immunoglobulins, copper studies, and α_1-antitrypsin phenotypes, as appropriate, along with crossmatching.

Cardiopulmonary function is difficult to assess. ECG, echocardiography, and simple lung function tests may be adequate to recognize pathology requiring further investigation. If appropriate, in a patient with possible ischemic heart disease, for example, further investigations should proceed with an echocardiogram, exercise ECG test preceding thallium scanning, and coronary angiography or other imaging, as indicated. Measurement of arterial blood gases is important and, if the arterial oxygen is low, it is important to repeat these after exercise and after giving 100% oxygen, to provide some guidance as to the extent of intrapulmonary shunting.

Radiologic investigations consist primarily of a chest radiograph and ultrasound scan of the liver, biliary tree, pancreas, spleen, and vessels. If patency of the portal vein is uncertain, angiography (direct, CT, or MR) is done, also to assess the presence of splenic superior mesenteric vein patency. Some units do not routinely perform CT or MRI unless there is a suggestion of malignancy. In patients with sclerosing cholangitis, as indicated earlier, investigation of the biliary tree may be indicated. This may reveal undiagnosed cholangiocarcinoma, but, where possible, endoscopic evaluation should be avoided as this may result in an episode of cholangitis. Most patients with PSC have colitis, and although this is usually mild and often clinically inapparent, it is important to screen for active disease and cancer in such patients before surgery. In particular, those with a long history of pancolitis require full investigation by colonoscopy. This procedure, however, is not without risk, especially in those with ascites. In the presence of significant dysplasia, it may be sensible to consider early colectomy because the additional effect of immunosuppression may further increase the risk of colon cancer.

Routine psychiatric evaluation is not indicated unless there is a history of psychiatric disease that may preclude successful rehabilitation. A dental examination is usually required, and any carious teeth are usually removed before transplantation. Patients are routinely assessed by the anesthetist before receiving a transplant.

CONSENT

During the assessment is a good time to ensure the candidate understands not only the benefits of transplants but also the risks and the implications. Because of the increasing shortage of organ donors, surgeons are using increasingly marginal organs. Patients must understand and accept such risks as inadvertent transmission of infection (viral, bacterial, other), cancers, metabolic disorders, and autoimmune diseases, and the implications of having a graft associated with higher risk, such as a split liver or DCD graft. Patients' understanding of risk is variable and ensuring fully informed consent usually involves time and presentation of risks and benefits in multiple formats (oral, printed, electronic). Although the decision for transplantation rests with the patient, it is important to include the family in discussions because their cooperation and understanding are essential for successful rehabilitation after transplantation. Consent should be obtained when the patient is listed and should be confirmed immediately before transplantation.

MANAGEMENT OF PATIENTS AWAITING TRANSPLANTATION

In general, patients should be maintained as fit as possible while awaiting a transplant. Vitamin deficiency should be corrected, and the patient should adopt a high-protein, high-calorie diet. The presence of encephalopathy should not exclude a high-protein diet, and other methods should be used to control hepatic encephalopathy, such as use of lactulose and, if necessary, metronidazole, rifaximin, or neomycin. Where appropriate, candidates should be given a program of activity to maintain or improve physical status.

Candidates should have their immunization history reviewed and immunization offered as indicated. In particular, live or attenuated vaccines, which are contraindicated in the immunosuppressed patient after transplantation, should be considered at this time. It is reasonable to offer nonimmune patients immunization with hepatitis A and B vaccines. Any infection should be rigorously sought and actively treated.

The presence of ascites itself may be an indication for treatment, because not only do these patients remain catabolic, but they also are at risk for spontaneous bacterial peritonitis. Patients with ascites should be treated with prophylactic antibiotics, such as ciprofloxacin or amoxicillin/clavulanate, which are not only efficacious and cost-effective, but also without major risk of developing bacterial resistance. In those with severe ascites resistant to therapy with diet and diuretics and requiring repeated episodes of paracentesis, there is a role for TIPS (see Chapters 79 and 85). The role of such shunts before transplantation remains uncertain; although effective in reducing portal hypertension, and thus improving ascites and risk of variceal hemorrhage, insertion carries the risk not only of sepsis but also of perforation and portal vein thrombosis.

Patients with grade II or III varices or a prior history of variceal bleeding should be given either pharmacoprophylaxis (with propranolol or carvedilol) or should be in a banding program (see Chapters 80 and 81). TIPS is valuable in selected patients (see Chapter 85).

Patients with PSC should be monitored for cholangiocarcinoma or bowel cancer, and those with HCC should have their tumor burden reviewed. This is usually done in the context of other therapies. As indicated earlier, the time on the waiting list can be used to adopt measures to reduce tumor spread and growth.

Finally, it is important to avoid therapy that will exacerbate the liver disease. In particular, nonsteroidal antiinflammatory drugs should be avoided because of the risks of inducing gastric hemorrhage, renal failure, and fluid retention. Drugs such as opiates that result in constipation and sedative drugs should also be avoided because of the risk of precipitating encephalopathy. Diuretics must be used with care and renal function carefully monitored; renal failure is associated with a poor outcome after transplantation and hyponatremia with the development of central pontine myelinolysis.

For those with alcohol use disorders, many centers will adopt a program of regular alcohol screening, by measurement of alcohol in breath, blood or urine, or ethanol metabolites in hair. Similar considerations apply to those with a history of illicit drug use. For those with tobacco use (if not contraindicated), the time on the waiting list should be used to support abstinence.

The transplant clinicians need to remain in close contact with the patient so that problems can be detected and treated early. Although the waiting time for transplantation increases, patients will deteriorate and may experience complications precluding a successful outcome, or the probability of survival may become too small for transplantation to proceed. With the increasing shortage of donor organs, transplant clinicians need to consider those criteria that suggest a patient should be removed from the transplant list.

References are available at expertconsult.com.

CHAPTER 106

Liver transplantation: Perioperative anesthetic considerations

Andrea Vannucci and Ivan Kangrga

INTRODUCTION

The Global Observatory on Donation and Transplantation[1] estimates that more than 35,000 liver transplantations are performed annually worldwide, but the number of patients on the waiting list continues to exceed donor organ availability. Because of the continuous donor shortage, dramatic changes in recipient and donor selection have emerged in the past decade, leading to an amplification of clinical challenges for perioperative liver transplant physicians. United Network for Organ Sharing data from the 2018 Scientific Registry of Transplant Recipients (https://www.srtr.org/reports-tools/srtroptn-annual-data-report/) show that patients older than 65 and those with a Model for End-Stage Liver Disease (MELD) score equal to or higher than 30 are more frequently transplanted and that prevalence of obesity and diabetes among transplant recipients has increased markedly over the past 10 years.[1] In addition, combined kidney and liver transplants are also performed more often than in previous years, and extended-criteria donors are increasingly used, including donation after cardiac death (see Chapters 105 and 109).

Despite the increasing medical complexity, overall graft and patient outcomes have continued to improve. According to the US Organ Procurement and Transplantation Network (OPTN)/Scientific Registry of Transplant Recipients (SRTR) 2018 Annual Data Report Health and Human Services (HHS)/Health Resources and Services Administration (HRSA), graft survival rates of patients transplanted with a cadaveric graft are about 92% at 1 year for transplants performed in 2017, 84% at 3 years for transplants performed in 2015, and 76% at 5 years for transplants performed in 2013.

These encouraging figures, achieved by experienced transplant teams, have resulted from the progressive advancement and standardization of surgical and anesthetic techniques[2] and the adoption of a systematic approach to quality improvement (QI) and patient safety in this demanding multidisciplinary area of healthcare.[3–6] With current trends of transplanting older and sicker recipients[7] and the expanded use of marginal donor organs, patient outcomes critically depend on accurate and timely perioperative assessment and medical management by an anesthesiology consultant, among others.

COVID-19 Pandemic

The COVID-19 pandemic, named for the illness caused by the SARS-CoV-2 virus, has been spreading across the world since the end of 2019 and has challenged the (liver) transplantation system worldwide, resulting in a temporary decrease of transplant activities.

This epidemic presents multiple issues for liver transplant centers: (1) the straining of resources (limited intensive care unit [ICU] bed and equipment availability); (2) the concerns for the risk of nosocomial COVID-19 infection in recipients, and the possibility of transmitting the disease to healthcare workers; and (3) the recognition that COVID-19 may manifest with hepatic signs and symptoms common to other forms of acute hepatitis, mandating that patients presenting with newly elevated serum liver enzymes undergo a comprehensive differential diagnostic process.[8] The orthotopic liver transplantation (OLT) community has responded to these challenges by creating "COVID-19 protocols," which often include screening for both donors and recipients before liver transplant[9]; the use of "good-quality graft," which will likely result in expeditious recipient recovery and discharge from hospitals[8]; and the use of telemedicine to minimize the need for bringing in OLT candidates for transplant evaluation and recipients for routine follow-up visits.[8]

It is too soon to draw any conclusions on the effectiveness of these measures to support clinical activities and protect patients and healthcare team members. Liver transplant centers should therefore continue to use caution and closely monitor their performance and clinical outcomes.

PREOPERATIVE ANESTHETIC ASSESSMENT

Liver transplantation is the definitive treatment for acute and chronic irreversible liver failure; for syndromes not manifesting with end-stage liver disease (ESLD), including polycystic liver disease and metabolic diseases; for some malignancies confined to the liver; and for cholestatic liver diseases. Of accepted contraindications to OLT, those of particular interest to anesthesiologists include severe cardiopulmonary conditions, such as symptomatic coronary artery disease (CAD), severe systolic dysfunction, advanced cardiomyopathy, severe valvular heart disease, severe pulmonary hypertension, sustained intracranial pressure greater than 50 mm Hg, and uncontrolled sepsis.[10] More recently, the impact of frailty on liver transplant outcomes has been recognized and the use of standardized tools to assess frailty in the evaluation of liver transplant candidates has been recommended.[11] As part of a multidisciplinary transplant team, anesthesiologists should participate in the evaluation of candidate recipients. A 2012 United Network for Organ Sharing (UNOS) bylaw mandates that transplant centers appoint a Director of Liver Transplant Anesthesia and establish the directorship criteria, based largely on recommendations by the American Society of Anesthesiologists. This decision by UNOS was motivated by the evidence that standardized care by a dedicated and experienced liver transplant anesthesia team may influence key quality and safety outcomes and resource utilization, including blood transfusion, length of mechanical ventilation, and duration of ICU and hospital stay.[12–14] An anesthetic evaluation is part of a multidisciplinary team approach to assess suitability for transplant, optimize medical management, and design an individualized perioperative treatment plan. Efforts based on a machine-learning approach are ongoing to develop predictive models for perioperative mortality of cadaveric liver transplant recipients at the time of their initial evaluation.[15] For patients, whose comorbidities present a prohibitive operative risk, alternative treatments should be considered[16,17] (see Chapter 105).

Central Nervous System

Hepatic encephalopathy (HE) is a progressive but potentially reversible syndrome of the central nervous system (CNS) associated with variable degrees of brain edema. Presentation ranges from subclinical to coma. HE is an overt or covert manifestation of cirrhosis in up to 80% of cirrhotic patients, and it is a defining sign and main cause of death in acute liver failure (ALF)[18,19] (see Chapters 77, 78, and 105). Based on the etiology, the American Association for the Study of Liver Diseases (AASLD)[20] recognizes that *type A* is associated with ALF, *type B* with a transjugular intrahepatic portosystemic shunt (TIPS), and *type C* with cirrhosis. Based on the severity of neurologic impairment, HE ranges from unimpaired to minimal (grade 0) to coma and brain death (grade 4). Because presence and severity of HE is of prognostic significance, including impaired brain recovery post-transplant, experts have called for its inclusion into the MELD score[21] (see Chapter 4).

The pathophysiology of HE is complex and incompletely understood.[22] Evidence supports the central role of ammonia, which bypasses first-pass liver clearance via portosystemic shunting. Ammonia crosses the blood–brain barrier (BBB) and promotes astrocyte and neuronal swelling by increasing intracellular glutamine content and creating osmotic imbalance. Transported to the mitochondria, glutamine contributes to production of reactive oxygen species (ROS) and activation of mitochondrial transition permeability pore and various kinases, resulting in cytotoxic swelling. Increased ammonia levels have been shown to alter cerebral blood flow and brain glucose utilization.[19,22–24] High arterial and brain levels of ammonia in ALF correlate well with cerebral edema and increased intracranial pressure (ICP), with consequent high risk of mortality from brain herniation and hypoxia.[25]

Multiple other endogenous mediators have been implicated, including benzodiazepine- or γ-aminobutyric acid (GABA)–like agonists and neurosteroids acting on $GABA_A$ receptors, ROS, inflammatory cytokines, hyponatremia, and manganese.[26] Other evidence implicates neuroinflammation, including activation of microglia and proinflammatory cytokines and as a cause of altered permeability of the BBB leading to vasogenic edema and accumulation of ammonia in the brain.[22,27,28] Low-grade brain edema, evident on advanced magnetic resonance imaging (MRI) and positron emission tomography (PET) imaging, is associated with increased interstitial water caused by BBB breakdown and seems to be more common in chronic liver disease (CLD) than initially appreciated.[19] ICP remains mostly normal in part because of the neuronal loss.

In cirrhosis, HE has a slow onset, a progressive course, and only partial responsiveness to therapy. Significant cerebral edema typically does not develop, and a precipitating event (e.g., infection, excessive dietary protein, dehydration, gastrointestinal [GI] bleeding) can be often identified. TIPS, a known risk factor, is associated with 30% of new or worsening encephalopathy. In addition to correction of any precipitating factors, treatment includes nonabsorbable disaccharides, which reduce the intestinal production and absorption of ammonia; antibiotics that target urease-producing bacteria; ornithine and acarbose; benzodiazepine receptor antagonists; and probiotics. Minocycline, an agent with potent central anti-inflammatory properties, reduces neuroinflammation, brain edema, and encephalopathy in liver failure, as does the anti–tumor necrosis factor (TNF) agent etanercept.[27] The molecular absorbent recirculating system (MARS) and therapeutic plasma exchange (TPE) improve hemodynamics and grade of HE in ALF and acute-on-chronic liver failure, with TPE also improving survival in ALF, but more studies need to be done.[29]

The hallmarks of HE in ALF are cerebral edema and increased ICP. Both are life-threatening complications of grade 3 and 4 encephalopathy. Treatment includes several general and specific interventions aimed at promoting cerebral perfusion pressure (CPP) above 60 mm Hg (Table 106.1); this is achieved by maintaining the mean arterial pressure (MAP) and reducing ICP to below 20 mm Hg by reducing brain edema. Grade 3 or 4 HE requires endotracheal intubation for airway protection. Mild hyperventilation temporarily relieves brain hyperemia, but prolonged hyperventilation is not beneficial and may cause CNS ischemia. Mannitol is effective in reducing ICP in the short term, but prophylactic use is not recommended. N-acetylcysteine treatment may also prolong transplant-free survival in ALF unrelated to paracetamol/acetaminophen toxicity.[30,31]

The role of ICP monitoring is controversial because it is associated with a high risk of bleeding in this patient population and little data exist to support its role in improving patient outcomes. ICP monitoring has been recommended in ALF[32] and comatose patients with computed tomography (CT) evidence of brain edema.[22] A noninvasive alternative to ICP monitors is transcranial Doppler (TCD) sonography. By measuring blood flow velocities in middle and anterior cerebral arteries and calculating resistance and pulsatility indexes, TCD allows serial estimates of cerebral blood flow in the setting of impaired autoregulation and developing brain edema.[33] In a small series of ALF patients, the feasibility of intraoperative TCD to assess main cerebrovascular hemodynamic parameters was recently demonstrated,[34] but more studies are needed to ascertain the value of intraoperative TCD in OLT.

TABLE 106.1 Management of Encephalopathy and Elevated Intracranial Pressure in Acute Liver Failure

GENERAL MEASURES	SPECIFIC INTERVENTIONS
Head elevation to 30 degrees	Endotracheal intubation for grades 3 and 4 hepatic encephalopathy
Judicious (restrictive) fluid management	Hyperventilation: limited, temporary benefit
Judicious if any sedation	N-acetylcysteine, if ALF is due to acetaminophen
Cerebral perfusion pressure > 60 mm Hg	Renal replacement therapy: CVVHD
Osmotic diuresis, hypertonic saline	ICP monitoring (>10% bleed); transcranial Doppler
Empiric: antibiotics, antivirals, disaccharides	Hypothermia: mild, bridge to transplantation

ALF, Acute liver failure; *CVVHD,* Continuous venovenous hemodialysis; *ICP,* intracranial pressure.

Mild to moderate hypothermia (32°C–35°C) reduces brain ammonia and cytokine levels and in part restores cerebrovascular autoregulation and brain glucose metabolism. Although experimental evidence provides a strong rationale, only limited clinical data on efficacy and safety of hypothermia in humans with ALF are available, and future studies are warranted.[22,30,35]

Cardiovascular System

Cardiovascular complications are responsible for the majority of nongraft morbidity and mortality in the early post-OLT period[36] (see Chapter 111). Common clinical problems that impact postoperative outcomes include hyperdynamic circulation, CAD, and nonischemic cirrhotic cardiomyopathy.[37]

Hyperdynamic Circulation

Patients with ESLD develop high cardiac output state and systemic hypotension secondary to reduced systemic vascular resistance (SVR) and abnormal distribution of central, splanchnic, and peripheral circulation (i.e., the splanchnic steal).[38] The compensatory mechanisms include activation of the sympathetic system and the renin-angiotensin-aldosterone axis that may result in organ hypoperfusion such as kidney hypoperfusion. Importantly, the low SVR may mask compromised cardiac function because of cirrhotic cardiomyopathy that is common in ESLD[39] and may progress to heart failure under the demands of liver transplant surgery.[40] Understanding the pathophysiology of hyperdynamic circulation is critical to successful intraoperative management of OLT candidates (see Chapters 77, 78, and 105).

Coronary Artery Disease

Incidence of CAD in OLT candidates is reported in up to 37% of decompensated liver disease patients, with nonalcoholic steatohepatitis (NASH) as a leading etiology.[41,42] Although historically, significant mortality and morbidity were reported in patients with CAD,[43] revascularization and newer management strategies seem to allow for better outcomes.[44,45] Safadi and colleagues (2009)[46] reported that history of stroke, CAD, postoperative sepsis, and increased interventricular septal thickness were markers of adverse perioperative cardiac outcomes, whereas use of perioperative β-blockers was significantly protective. Pretransplant troponin T, a sensitive troponin assay, has proved to be a strong predictor of post-transplant cardiovascular events.[47]

National guidelines exist for cardiac evaluation of OLT candidates.[41] Symptoms and functional capacity are not the key indicators for testing because exertional intolerance is a common feature of ESLD that may conceal cardiac pathology. Dobutamine stress echocardiography (DSE) is recommended as an initial screening test recognizing that it has low sensitivity and negative predictive value in ESLD patients.[48] Cardiac catheterization is indicated if CAD cannot be confidently excluded.[10] Left-sided heart catheterization is associated with higher risk of minor complications but can be performed safely in candidates for OLT.[49]

Cardiopulmonary exercise testing with measurement of maximum aerobic capacity and ventilatory or aerobic threshold (e.g., the 6-minute walk test) can predict post-OLT outcomes. Although an attractive concept, this methodology is not widely adopted because it requires specialized equipment, staff training, and time.[36,50]

Computed tomography (CT) detection of coronary calcification is a sign of possible ischemic heart disease in asymptomatic patients. Severe coronary calcification, indicated by a coronary calcium score greater than 400,[51] predicted cardiovascular complications occurring within 1 month after OLT in a study by Kong et al.[52] Stress cardiac magnetic resonance (MR) is suitable in OLT candidates because of its higher sensitivity and specificity for CAD then DSE, and inclusion of functional cardiac assessment and noncardiac imaging (liver MRI) in the same session.[53]

Cirrhotic Cardiomyopathy

Nonischemic cirrhotic cardiomyopathy is characterized by blunted systolic function and diastolic dysfunction, chronotropic incompetence, and electrophysiologic alterations, often manifesting as prolonged QTc interval.[39] Diastolic dysfunction is associated with severity of the postreperfusion syndrome[54] and development of post-transplant heart failure.[55] Structural myocardial abnormalities, left atrial enlargement, and hypodynamic state ensue with progression of cirrhosis, independent of etiology.[56]

Diagnosis is based primarily on advanced echocardiographic and radiologic imaging (e.g., myocardial performance index, MPI/Tei index; speckled echocardiography assessing global longitudinal strain; cardiac MRI), and elevated levels of brain natriuretic peptide.

Pathophysiologic hallmarks of nonischemic cardiomyopathy are down-regulation and desensitization of β-adrenergic receptors, myocardial fibrosis, myocyte hypertrophy, and ion-channel defects. Medical treatment is based on sodium restriction and administration of β-blockers and aldosterone antagonists; liver transplantation can reverse this condition.[57,58]

Nonischemic cardiomyopathy can also manifest as a complication of the primary disease such as ethanol abuse, amyloidosis, hemochromatosis, and Wilson disease. When present, dilated and hypertrophic cardiomyopathy rarely reverts to normal after OLT (see Chapters 77, 78, and 105).

Pulmonary System

As many as 70% of patients with CLD have respiratory problems, which manifest as impaired respiratory mechanics and gas exchange.[59] Most pulmonary comorbidities are independent from liver disease, but for a few exceptions such as α_1-antitrypsin deficiency and cystic fibrosis.[60] Pulmonary evaluation includes history and physical examination, radiologic studies, arterial blood gases (ABGs), and pulmonary function tests. Right-sided heart catheterization is indicated when clinical or echocardiographic evidence suggests significant pulmonary hypertension.

Portopulmonary Hypertension

Portopulmonary hypertension (PPH) is a specific type of pulmonary artery hypertension. It involves increased pulmonary vascular resistance (PVR) and portal hypertension with or without advanced liver disease. From 2% to 10% of patients with cirrhosis are affected by PPH.[60] The physiologic mechanism is multifactorial and incompletely understood, but hyperdynamic circulation, imbalance between pulmonary vasodilators (nitric oxide and prostacyclin) and vasoconstrictors (endothelin-1 and thromboxane), and proliferative pulmonary arteriopathy all play a role in the genesis of this syndrome.[61]

Diagnosis requires the presence of portal hypertension, mean pulmonary artery pressure (mPAP) greater than 25 mm Hg, PVR greater than 240 dynes/sec/cm^{-5}, and pulmonary artery occlusion pressure less than 15 mm Hg.[62] Other causes of pulmonary hypertension (e.g., high flow state, volume overload, chronic obstructive pulmonary disease [COPD]) should be ruled out. Right-sided heart catheterization is indicated if right ventricular (RV) systolic pressure is higher than 50 mm Hg on echocardiography[62]; the severity of PPH is then classified as *mild* (mPAP 24–34 mm Hg), *moderate* (mPAP 35–44 mm Hg), or *severe* (mPAP $\geq$ 45 mm Hg)[10] (see Chapters 77, 78, 79, and 105).

Medical optimization is indicated before transplantation, and treatment is based on vasodilators that frequently have side effects that limit their applicability.[63] Prostaglandins (intravenous [IV] epoprostenol or inhaled iloprost), phosphodiesterase inhibitors (sildenafil), and endothelin-1 antagonists (bosentan, macitentan) are often used in combination therapy. Most liver transplant centers do not transplant patients with an mPAP greater than 50 mm Hg or PVR greater than 240 dynes/sec/cm^{-5}. Current recommendations suggest offering OLT to recipients who respond to medical therapy and with mPAP of 35 mm Hg or less.[10,64] Post-OLT outcomes such as hospital length of stay (LOS) and 1-year survival were comparable in liver transplant (LT) recipients with normal mPAP and those with mPAP ranging between 35 to 50 mmHg after treatment.[65]

Hepatopulmonary Syndrome

Hepatopulmonary syndrome (HPS) is a vascular disorder characterized by hypoxemia secondary to pulmonary capillary vasodilation (up to 100 μm) in patients with liver disease. The estimated incidence in patients with cirrhosis is between 5% and 30%.[62] The natural course of HPS is characterized by poor survival, especially in patients with arterial oxygen partial pressure (PaO$_2$) less than 50 mm Hg: median survival without LT is approximately 24 months.[66] The pathologic feature of HPS is gross dilation and an increase in the number of the pulmonary precapillary and capillary vessels[62,67] leading to a ventilation-perfusion mismatch. The symptoms are platypnea and dyspnea, with or without orthodeoxia. Pulse oximetry (O$_2$ saturation less than 96%) is a useful screening test. The diagnosis is confirmed with ABGs (resting PaO$_2$ < 80 mm Hg or PA-aO$_2$ gradient >15 mm Hg, or 20 mm Hg in patients older than 65), contrast-enhanced echocardiography, or macroaggregated albumin lung perfusion scan. The echocardiographic signature is a positive bubble test with a delay of four to six beats indicating transpulmonary shunt. No effective medical therapy exists for HPS, and LT is the only treatment. Severe HPS (PaO$_2$ < 50 mm Hg on room air) is associated with increased perioperative mortality, complexity of peri-transplant management, but overall favorable long-term outcomes in survivors.[66,68–71] The 2016 International Liver Transplant Society Practice Guidelines recommend the following postoperative interventions: early extubation to minimize the risk of ventilator-associated pneumonia; 100% oxygen administration to maintain O$_2$ saturation greater than 85%; avoidance of fluid overload; and inhaled nitric oxide to improve oxygenation[62] (see Chapters 77–79 and 105).

Hepatic Hydrothorax

Hepatic hydrothorax is defined as a pleural effusion greater than 500 mL not caused by cardiac or pulmonary diseases in a patient with cirrhosis.[61] A diaphragmatic defect allowing passage of ascites from the peritoneal to the pleural cavity is considered the main mechanism leading to this complication. Pleural effusions are symptomatic in 5% to 10% of patients with ESLD,[72] and the main respiratory impairment is hypoxemia secondary to atelectasis and shunting; chest radiograph confirms the diagnosis. Treatment is based on medical management of ascites with sodium restriction and diuretics, paracentesis, and possible placement of a TIPS.[73] In cases of refractory hydrothorax, pleurodesis and diaphragmatic repair can be considered; thoracentesis is generally performed only in emergency situations because avoidance of tube thoracostomy is preferred. Chest tube placement should be avoided but use of a pleural catheter with intermittent decompression may stave off the need for hospitalization (see Chapters 77–79 and 105).

Chronic Obstructive Pulmonary Disease and Smoking

COPD is common and often undiagnosed in candidates for LT, except for patients with known α$_1$-antitrypsin deficiency. In a prospective study involving several US academic centers, 18% of OLT candidates had COPD, and 80% of those patients had not been previously diagnosed. Older age and smoking were significant risk factors. The impact of moderate COPD on perioperative outcome in liver transplantation is not well defined.[74] Severe COPD was found associated with a complicated postoperative course and worse long-term survival.[75] A recent national observational study from Spain[76] including 14,970 OLT recipients showed that COPD patients had significantly lower rates of infection and other complications, and lower in-hospital mortality than those without COPD (4.07% vs. 8.91%).

Hemostasis in End-Stage Liver Disease

The traditional view that ESLD is a hypocoagulable state has been revised (see Chapters 77 and 78). The current concept emphasizes complex disturbances of procoagulant, anticoagulant, and fibrinolytic pathways and platelet function, that result in *rebalancing* of the hemostatic system.[77,78] The resulting fragile, rebalanced state can be easily tipped towards hypocoagulability and bleeding or towards hypercoagulability and thromboembolism. Importantly, the latter is still an often-underestimated risk in ESLD.[79]

Understanding the hemostatic system in ESLD is essential to perioperative coagulation management and optimization of blood-product transfusion practices, which are related to morbidity and mortality in LT.[80,81] Deficiency in primary hemostasis is caused by quantitative and qualitative platelet changes.[82] Mild to moderate thrombocytopenia is common. Causes are splenomegalic platelet sequestration in portal hypertension, impaired megakaryocytopoiesis from reduced production of thrombopoietin by the cirrhotic liver, folic acid deficiency in alcoholic cirrhosis or acute hepatitis C infection, and reduced platelet half-life related to autoantibodies. Evidence for impaired platelet aggregation and adhesion in cirrhosis is controversial. The proposed mechanisms are complex and multifactorial, including the role of two potent endothelium-derived platelet inhibitors, nitric oxide, and prostacyclin. More recent work suggests that the functional capacity of platelets in cirrhosis may be preserved, suggesting that the main defect in primary hemostasis is thrombocytopenia. A compensatory mechanism for the deficient platelet function in cirrhosis is an increase in endothelium-synthesized von Willebrand factor (vWF), because of deficiency in ADAMTS-13, a vWF cleaving protease that is reduced in cirrhosis. The upregulated vWF promotes adhesion of platelets to injured endothelium and may explain the poor correlation between platelet number and bleeding time.[80] Thrombocytopenia, as low as 60 × 10^9 per liter, is sufficient to preserve thrombin generation at a level equivalent to the lower limit of normal.[77]

The liver synthesizes all procoagulant factors except for vWF, which is synthesized by the endothelium. Factor VIII is synthesized by hepatocytes but also by nonhepatic sinusoidal endothelial cells. Reduced levels of coagulation factors are observed in acute and chronic liver disease. Several factors—II, VII, IX, and X—are vitamin K-dependent and exist in plasma as inactive precursors when vitamin K is deficient in decreased absorption (cholestasis) or antagonism (warfarin). In ALF, plasma concentrations of coagulation factors with the shortest half-life (factor VII, 4–6 hours; factor V, 12 hours) decrease first, followed by those with a longer half-life. Exceptions are factors VIII and vWF, which may be elevated in chronic and acute liver disease because of inflammatory cytokine-mediated upregulated extrahepatic production. Fibrinogen is usually well preserved: its decrease is a mark of advanced cirrhosis or ALF. Even when levels are normal, fibrinogen is often functionally aberrant because of impaired fibrin polymerization. The result is an abnormal thrombin time (TT), despite normal international normalized ratio (INR) and partial thromboplastin time (PTT).

The deficiency in procoagulant factors is, at least in part, offset by decreased production of anticoagulants, including proteins C and S, antithrombin, and heparin cofactor II. Proteins C and S are vitamin K dependent and may be deficient in cholestatic disease, and although genetic deficiency of these two proteins is rare, such deficiency is found in both Budd-Chiari syndrome and portal vein (PV) thrombosis. Antithrombin is synthesized by hepatocytes and endothelium, deficiencies are usually mild, and thromboembolic complications are rare.

All proteins involved in fibrinolysis are synthesized by the liver except tissue plasminogen activator (tPA) and plasminogen activator inhibitor type 1 (PAI-1). Consequently, reduced levels of liver-synthesized factors—plasminogen, plasmin inhibitor, thrombin activatable fibrinolysis inhibitor (TAFI), and factor XIII—are found in both ALF and chronic liver failure. Cirrhosis is classically associated with hyperfibrinolysis, whereas patients in ALF may have hypofibrinolysis because of increased production of PAI-1. The expert viewpoint emphasizes that balance of profibrinolytic and antifibrinolytic factors in liver disease is often restored, and the role of hyperfibrinolysis in bleeding is limited.[77] Increased levels of fibrinogen degradation indicators—d-dimers, plasmin-antiplasmin and thrombin-antithrombin complexes, thrombin fragment F1+2—could be explained by delayed clearance by the diseased liver. Coagulation tests, such as prothrombin time (PT) and activated PTT (aPTT) are used to assess the severity of synthetic dysfunction, and PT-INR is a part of the Child-Turcotte-Pugh (CTP) and MELD prognostic indexes.[83] As tests of in vivo coagulation function, PT-INR and PTT are conceptually deficient because they measure only the procoagulant pathway and ignore the anticoagulant function. The seminal observation that thrombin generation in cirrhotic patients is close to normal[84] may, in part, explain why PT-INR and PTT are poor predictors of bleeding in cirrhosis and liver transplantation.[80,81] Viscoelastic tests, thromboelastography (TEG, Haemonetics Corporation, Braintree, MA) and rotation thromboelastometry (ROTEM; Pentapharm, Munich, Germany) have the advantage of assaying whole-blood clot formation and lysis, including the platelet contribution, but do not incorporate the endothelial component (see Intraoperative Monitoring, later). Importantly, these assays allow for easy recognition of hypercoagulable states (Fig. 106.1).[81]

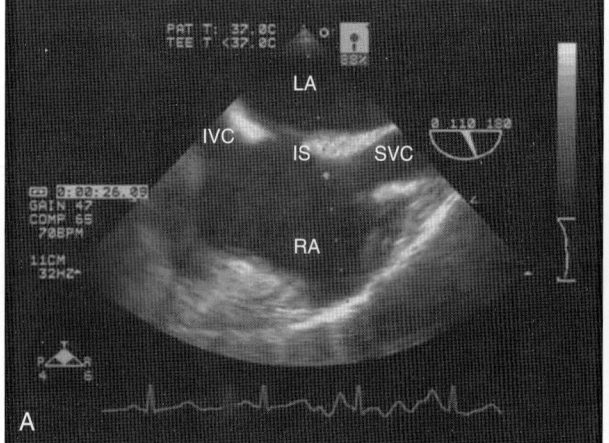

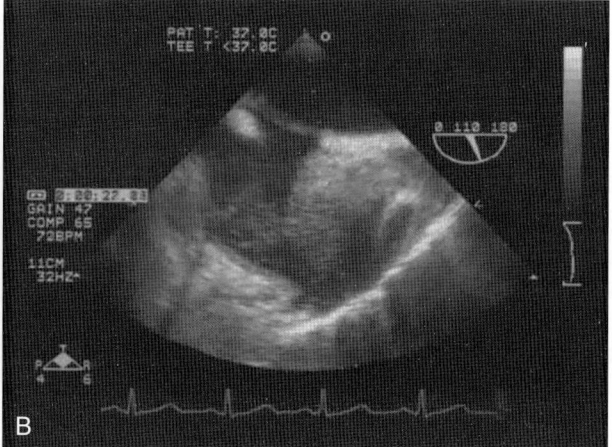

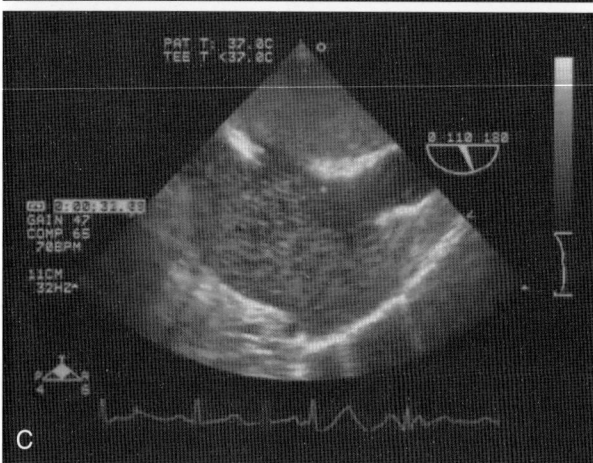

FIGURE 106.1 Intraoperative transesophageal echocardiography (TEE) in a patient with hepatopulmonary syndrome and intrapulmonary shunting demonstrates a positive bubble study. **A,** Midesophageal bicaval view. **B,** Bolus of contrast injectate (agitated saline-blood mixture) is visible entering the right atrium via the superior vena cava *(SVC)* following an injection through the central venous port. **C,** Several heartbeats later, the injectate is present in the left atrium *(LA),* indicating transpulmonary passage. *RA,* Right atrium; *IS,* interatrial septum; *IVC,* inferior vena cava.

Renal System

Renal failure confers increased risk of death to cirrhotic patients, both while on the waiting list and after LT.[85] Even mild renal disease increases the risk of cardiovascular and all-cause mortality.[86] Implementation of the MELD score in 2002 has prioritized patients with renal failure waiting for a liver transplant, resulting in reduced overall mortality on the transplant list.[87] *Hepatorenal syndrome* (HRS) is a specific type of functional renal failure in patients with decompensated cirrhosis (see Chapters 77 and 78). It is marked by renal vasoconstriction and a severe reduction in glomerular filtration rate (GFR < 30 mL/min) but only minimal histologic abnormalities.[88,89] The primary pathophysiologic process is a circulatory disturbance: portal hypertension facilitates translocation of bacteria from the intestinal lumen into the mesenteric lymph nodes and induces production of inflammatory cytokines and local vasodilators, such as nitric oxide, carbon monoxide, and endogenous cannabinoids. Resulting splanchnic vasodilation decreases the overall SVR and activates several compensatory mechanisms. The initial response is hyperdynamic and includes tachycardia, increased cardiac output, low SVR, and hypotension. With progression of cirrhosis, sympathetic and renin-angiotensin vasoconstrictor systems are activated and temporarily maintain arterial blood pressure (BP), but they also cause renal vasoconstriction and hypoperfusion. Activation of nonosmotic hypersecretion of arginine vasopressin, aimed at preserving circulatory volume, results in retention of solute-free water with attendant hyponatremia, edema, and ascites. HRS is almost invariably associated with ascites and rarely develops in its absence. Onset of HRS is often triggered by a discrete event, such as spontaneous bacterial peritonitis, use of nonsteroidal antiinflammatory drugs (NSAIDs), or hypovolemia because of diuretic use, GI bleeding, or fluid losses. Recently, inflammation has emerged as an important determinant in the development of HRS.[90] Until recently, serum creatinine (SCr) values above 1.5 mg/dL (133 μmol/L) were used to define renal insufficiency in cirrhosis.[88,91] In 2012 the definition of acute renal failure (ARF) was updated and replaced by acute kidney injury (AKI).[92] AKI is a syndrome with multiple possible etiologies. In 2015 a revised definition of AKI in cirrhosis was proposed, with a new "dynamic" scoring system called International Club of Ascites (ICA)-AKI[93]; AKI is diagnosed by an increase in absolute SCr of more than 0.3 mg/dL or by a 1.5- to 2-fold increase from baseline. Three categories of increasing severity are defined by levels of SCr or initiation of renal replacement. In the presence of AKI, it is important to differentiate acute tubular necrosis (ATN) from the "classical" hepatorenal syndrome because the therapeutic approach is different, even if the two entities are currently considered a continuum. Vasoconstrictors (such as terlipressin) are not indicated for the treatment of ATN.[90]

Measurement of SCr remains the primary test of renal function despite its well-known limitations. GFR and creatinine clearance are more accurate but less practical tests when repeated assessments are needed. Other tests measure serum and urinary electrolytes, fractional sodium excretion (FeNa), albumin, osmolarity, sediment, and biologic markers. No specific diagnostic test exists for HRS. Rather, diagnosis is based on the presence of liver disease, a precipitating factor, and FeNa less than 1%, signifying preserved tubular reabsorption; however, the latter test is invalidated in the presence of diuretics. Still, recent investigations have suggested that several urine biomarkers may have a diagnostic and prognostic value in cirrhotic patients with AKI. Neutrophil gelatinase-associated lipocalin

(NGAL), interleukin (IL)-18, and albumin appear particularly promising in cirrhotic patients. NGAL and IL-18 are associated with tubular renal injury, whereas albumin is associated with glomerular injury. More specifically, NGAL and IL-18 levels are much higher in patients with ATN than in those with HRS-AKI of prerenal, hypovolemia-induced AKI.[94]

General treatment measures are aimed at preventing infection, in particular subacute bacterial peritonitis; maintaining adequate intravascular volume; and avoiding nephrotoxic agents. Circulatory volume losses, often the result of large-volume paracentesis or a GI bleed, are best treated with albumin or, if indicated, by blood products and not with crystalloids, to avoid retention of solute-free water. The main pharmacologic approach uses vasoconstrictors, including a selective vasopressin V1 receptor agonist (e.g., terlipressin) or α-adrenergic agonists (e.g., norepinephrine, midodrine). Vasoconstrictors in conjunction with albumin are only modestly beneficial but are the best medical therapy currently available. Placement of a TIPS improves renal function and GFR and reduces sympathetic and renin-angiotensin-aldosterone axis activation in about 60% of patients.[95] No advantage in survival has been demonstrated in patients with refractory ascites treated by TIPS compared with repeated paracentesis and intravascular volume replacement with albumin. Renal replacement therapy (RRT) offers a bridge to transplant, but the optimal RRT method in HRS and the benefit to patient outcomes are not known.[88,96] Continuous venovenous hemodialysis (CVVHD) seems to be hemodynamically the most favorable form of RRT.[97,98] CVVHD can be used to effectively control intravascular volume, pH levels, and solutes (Na, K, SCr, urea, ammonia). In addition, it corrects sodium in a time-controlled fashion, which is particularly relevant to minimize the risk of CNS demyelination in patients with hyponatremia. LT is the treatment of choice for patients with cirrhosis and HRS.[95] About 90% of patients with HRS recover kidney function after successful LT. The remaining 10% do not recover their kidney function and require prolonged RRT and eventual kidney transplantation. Listing criteria for simultaneous liver and kidney transplant, based on OPTN guidelines, include factors such as duration of AKI and RRT and evidence of CKD.

Enhanced Recovery Protocols

Enhanced recovery after surgery (ERAS), first published in colorectal surgery,[99] pertains to a highly coordinated, multidisciplinary surgical patient care continuum, driven by evidence-based protocols and best practices (see Chapter 27). The continuum spans from preoperative medical and nutritional optimization, prehabilitation to offset frailty, and standardization of intraoperative surgical and anesthetic care to postoperative care, including analgesia, early removal of drains and tubes, early mobilization, and rehabilitation. Benefits of ERAS pathways are well documented in several surgical specialties and include improved outcomes and patient satisfaction and reduced LOS and cost.[100] Most transplant centers have well-developed protocols that incorporate individual ERAS elements (e.g., the use of regional techniques for analgesia),[101] but published evidence of a comprehensive ERAS program in LT is limited.[102,103] A small single-center randomized controlled trial (RCT) demonstrated decreased blood loss and transfusion requirements[104] and another small pilot study demonstrated a decrease in ICU and hospital stay with no other outcome differences.[103] It is increasingly recognized that the concept of

ERAS has been applied safely and effectively across surgical subspecialties and that it should be adopted in OLT through center-specific standardization of care.

INTRAOPERATIVE MONITORING

Central Nervous System Monitoring

Bispectral Index (BIS) monitoring assesses anesthetic depth based on processed encephalography (EEG). Patients with HE have a lower baseline BIS index (i.e., a slow EEG), and this decrease is proportional to the degree of HE.[105,106] Intraoperative studies using BIS have demonstrated that appropriate depth of surgical anesthesia can be achieved with lower concentrations of inhalational anesthetics in OLT candidates with HE. A good correlation has been demonstrated between the severity of liver disease and a lower requirement for inhalational anesthetics.[105,107] The underlying mechanisms of CNS inhibition in HE are multifaceted and incompletely understood (see earlier). Use of BIS (or raw EEG, which requires additional expertise) to guide intraoperative anesthetic management during OLT prevents excessive use of inhalational agents and may help minimize anesthetic-induced vasodilatation, hypotension, cerebral hyperemia, and hemodynamic instability[108] (see Chapter 25).

TCD ultrasonography allows continuous noninvasive monitoring of cerebral hemodynamics in a variety of clinical conditions. A recent study in patients with ALF undergoing OLT demonstrated the feasibility of an intraoperative multimodal TCD approach to assessing cerebrovascular hemodynamics.[34] The main cerebral hemodynamic parameters, including noninvasive ICP, CPP, cerebral autoregulation, and pulsatility index were all markedly impaired.[34] Validation and utility of TCD in OLT will need to be confirmed in larger studies. Near-infrared spectroscopy (NIRS) is a noninvasive tool for assessing regional cerebral oxygenation. NIRS has been used in OLT, but the utility of this modality in intraoperative management must be still proved.[26,109]

Hemodynamic Monitoring

Hemodynamic management is a cornerstone in the perioperative care of LT patients, but no consensus has been reached on the standards of hemodynamic monitoring.[110] Continuous invasive arterial pressure monitoring may be the only ubiquitously used hemodynamic monitor in OLT. Commonly used radial artery pressure may underestimate the true aortic pressure, particularly during periods of hypotension or when high doses of vasopressors are used. A femoral arterial line reflects central aortic pressure with higher fidelity and consistently records higher systolic pressures than the radial artery. Because of this discrepancy, some centers routinely use both femoral and radial arterial lines.[111] The pulmonary artery catheter (PAC) has long been the mainstay of hemodynamic monitoring in LT; however, the clinical utility of PACs has been questioned because of criticism that its invasiveness is not justified by improved outcomes and that measured pressures are not good estimates of ventricular preload. Although several less invasive technologies have emerged, PACs are still advocated by many for OLT,[111] but there is consensus on its utility in managing patients with PPH.[112] Newer, less invasive hemodynamics monitors have been used in OLT for several years. The PiCCO system (Pulsion Medical Systems, Munich), LiDCO device (LiDCO Group, London), and Flo-Trac/Vigileo (Edwards Lifesciences, Irvine, CA) are among the most often reported monitoring systems. Although performance varies across these devices,[113] none has demonstrated a good agreement with PAC or superiority.[114] Transesophageal echocardiography (TEE) has gained acceptance in LT,[110] with use in large-volume centers reported in up to 80% of cases.[111] TEE provides different but complementary information to that provided by PACs. Standard TEE examination, according to the phases of LT surgery, has been proposed, and advantages of TEE in this patient population have been discussed.[115] Figure 106.1 presents TEE detection of a transpulmonary shunt as a positive bubble test in a patient with HPS. The main advantages of TEE are that it provides continuous, real-time visualization of cardiac structures and dynamic function. TEE is a superior modality for estimating ventricular volume status, global left ventricular (LV) contractility and ejection fraction, RV function, segmental wall motion abnormalities, and septal motion. Doppler modalities allow for interrogation of transvalvular flows (Fig. 106.2), dynamic LV outflow obstruction, intracardiac shunts, and diastolic function.[55,115,116] In addition, TEE is the only intraoperative monitor that allows an instantaneous diagnosis of pulmonary vein,

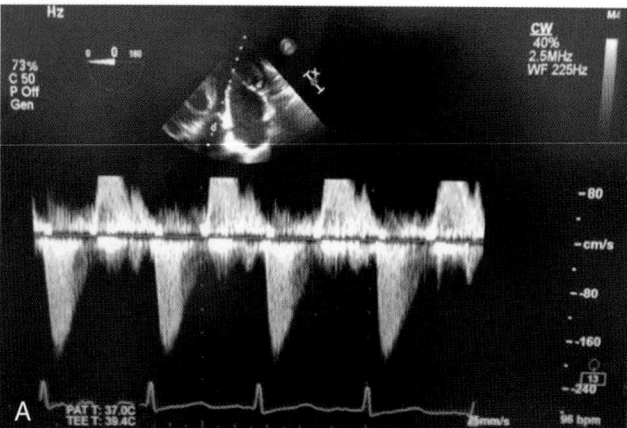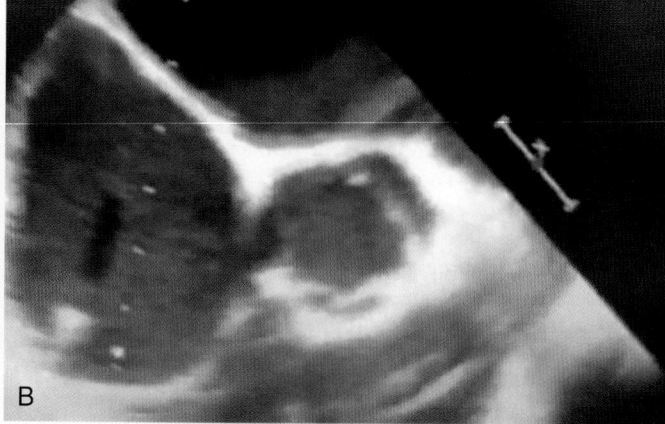

FIGURE 106.2   Intraoperative transesophageal echocardiography (TEE) in a patient with hyperdynamic circulation. **A,** Deep transgastric view demonstrates high continuous-wave Doppler velocity (>2 m/sec) across the aortic valve. **B,** Midesophageal short-axis view shows normal opening of the aortic valve, ruling out aortic valve stenosis.

inferior vena cava (IVC), TIPS, or intracardiac thrombus,[117–120] pericardial or pleural effusion, LV outflow tract obstruction, and Takotsubo's cardiomyopathy.[121,122] In addition to requiring significant training and resources, TEE has several disadvantages worth considering.[123] A common concern in the LT population is the risk of rupture of gastroesophageal varices. Although rare,[124,125] this complication does emphasize the need for careful risk/benefit assessment of this monitoring modality in each individual recipient. It is prudent to withdraw the TEE probe from the stomach during surgical gastric retraction, making transgastric views inaccessible during most of the procedure. Another disadvantage is that TEE is not adept at providing and trending traditional numerical data (e.g., cardiac output), which are readily provided by the PAC. Visual assessments used in TEE are also highly operator dependent. As suggested, there are no cardiovascular monitors suitable for all clinical situations,[112] and anesthesiologists should be familiar with advantages and limitations of a wide range of tools; this is particularly relevant during OLT. Nevertheless, we believe that TEE is an essential monitoring and diagnostic tool in LT anesthesia.[126]

Monitoring of Hemostasis

Conventional tests of hemostasis, PT and PTT, have several important limitations.[78,81,127] First, these assays use plasma samples devoid of platelets. Thus the contribution of activated platelets and endothelium to the coagulation process is not assessed by these tests. Second, PT and PTT measure only the activity of procoagulant factors. When PT is modified to include also anticoagulant factors, thrombin generation in cirrhotic patients is not different from normal controls.[84] An important practical shortcoming of the laboratory PT and PTT is a long turnaround time, typically about 45 minutes. Alternatively, point of care (POC) PT and PPT assays are quick (5–15 minutes), cartridge-type, whole-blood tests offered by several manufacturers. An acceptable agreement of such assays with plasma-based tests has been reported in OLT,[128] suggesting their utility for intraoperative hemostatic management. Activated clotting time (ACT) should be a part of the POC battery because with the reperfusion of the graft, a massive dose of unfractionated heparin is flushed into the circulation. ACT may help guide the use and dosing of protamine.

Both TEG and ROTEM are real-time POC assays that measure viscoelastic properties of whole-blood clot formation and lysis. Both technologies have been used to drive transfusion algorithms,[129–133] but the effect on outcomes has not been demonstrated. TEG measures time to onset and rate of clot formation, tensile strength, and rate of lysis (Fig. 106.3). Treatment of samples with an intrinsic pathway activator, kaolin, shortens clot formation, whereas addition of heparinase dissects the effects of exogenous heparin from intrinsic heparinoids.

ROTEM generates five assays, four of which can be run concurrently, that test different aspects of coagulation. Ex-TEM and in-TEM assess the extrinsic and the intrinsic pathway, respectively. Fib-TEM allows for the assessment of the contribution of fibrinogen, and indirectly platelets, to the maximal clot firmness. Hep-TEM enables detection of the effects of circulating heparin, and ap-TEM, in presence of fibrinolysis, assesses the potential response to antifibrinolytics. ROTEM is very useful in determination of poor tensile clot strength caused by combined platelet and fibrinogen deficiency, and it is a reliable method for detecting hypofibrinogenemia or dysfibrinogenemia, both common in liver disease.[134]

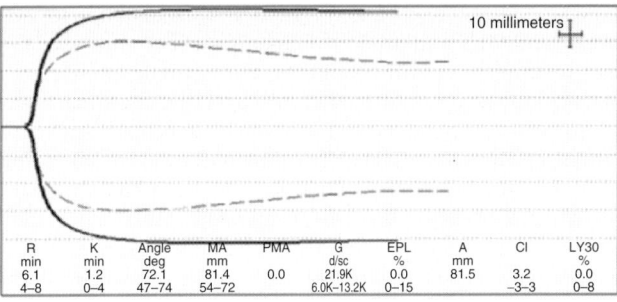

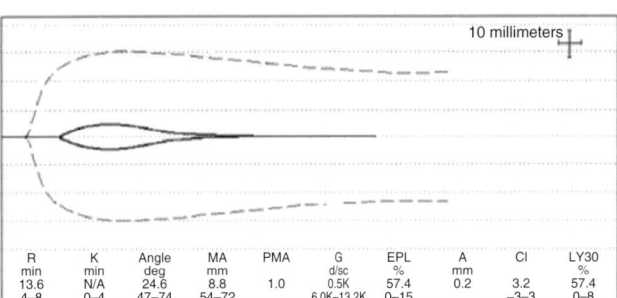

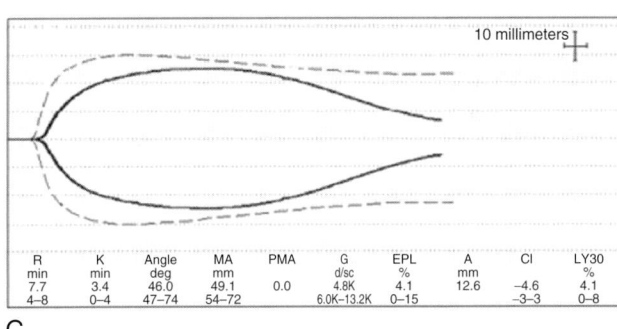

FIGURE 106.3 Intraoperative thromboelastogram (TEG) recordings from three orthotopic liver transplantation patients with different hemostatic derangements. In each panel, a "normal" TEG trace, generated by the instrument, is presented with an interrupted line. **A,** Hypercoagulable state in a patient with primary biliary cirrhosis. **B,** Postreperfusion TEG shows profoundly suppressed clot formation and marked fibrinolysis. **C,** Mild hypocoagulability and fibrinolysis in a patient with hepatitis C.

Both TEG and ROTEM are quick and superior monitors of hypercoagulability, fibrinolysis, and therapeutic effects of antifibrinolytics. The main conceptual deficiency of the two monitors is the inability to evaluate endothelial function. It is worth emphasizing that although both instruments plot clot formation similarly, TEG and ROTEM do not generate the same results when analyzing blood without exogenous activation and are not interchangeable.[135,136] Monitoring and management of hemostasis remain great challenges in OLT, and it has been well established that blood loss and blood-product transfusion are an important cause of morbidity and mortality.[80] Adherence to an algorithm-driven transfusion practice may reduce unnecessary perioperative blood and blood-component transfusion, but no consensus has been reached on what constitutes standard intraoperative monitoring of hemostasis or a standard hemostatic intervention. Difficulties stem from the incomplete understanding of complex coagulation abnormalities in liver disease and OLT and from the limitations of currently available tests to emulate in vivo conditions. For example, preoperative coagulation tests do not predict intraoperative bleeding,[81] and transfusion requirements are lower when abnormal coagulation parameters are not corrected by infusion of fresh frozen plasma (FFP) because blood loss in OLT is related more to PV pressure and surgical bleeding than to coagulopathy. Most importantly, these findings emphasize the need for careful interpretation of coagulation tests within the clinical context (e.g., clinical evidence of coagulopathy and bleeding) rather than relying on interventions formulated solely on the basis of test results.[127,137]

Metabolic Monitoring

Glucose Control

ESLD is associated with impaired glucose control; hypoglycemia is common in ALF, whereas hyperglycemia because of peripheral insulin resistance and metabolic syndrome are common in CLD (see Chapter 26). Factors that contribute to acute intraoperative hyperglycemia are routine administration of corticosteroids and response to surgical stress. Retrospective studies have shown association of a higher incidence of infections, graft rejection, and 1-year mortality with poor perioperative glucose control.[138–140] Another study demonstrated the effectiveness and safety of close, protocol-driven POC post-transplant monitoring and management of blood glucose levels.[141] In a small single-center prospective RCT, there was no difference in 1-, 3-, and 5-year patient and graft survival between the strict and conventional (80–120 vs. 180–200 mg/dL) intraoperative glucose management,[142] suggesting that conventional glycemic management is a reasonable and achievable perioperative goal. The importance of intraoperative glycemic control and its association with postoperative glycemic management and outcomes cannot be overemphasized.

Electrolytes

Electrolyte monitoring is done as POC testing, usually on an hourly basis and when indicated, such as to optimize electrolyte balance immediately before graft reperfusion. Hyperkalemia is ominous and may cause fatal arrhythmias, particularly after reperfusion.[143] Independent predictors of hyperkalemia are the number of red blood cells units (RBCs) transfused and higher initial values, especially in acidemic patients with renal insufficiency.[144] Ionized calcium levels predictably decrease with blood-product and albumin administration. Low-serum sodium is a hallmark of advanced cirrhosis and an independent predictor of mortality on the transplant waiting list[145,146] and addition of serum sodium levels to MELD score improves its predictive value (MELD-Na+).[147] Intraoperative sodium levels are elevated by administration of normal saline-based fluids and particularly by sodium bicarbonate. A large increase in serum sodium during OLT has been associated with worse short-term outcomes.[148] An important concern is that rapid correction of serum sodium levels may cause pontine demyelination.[149] Recent studies have highlighted that demyelination may involve both central pontine as well as extrapontine areas and led to a renaming of this nosologic entity that is now known as osmotic demyelination syndrome (ODS).[150] ODS occurs in 1.1% of LT recipients with severe hyponatremia (serum sodium < 125 mEq/L); it manifests with multiform neurologic manifestations, from mild dysarthria to quadriparesis and "locked-in" syndrome; it can be prevented

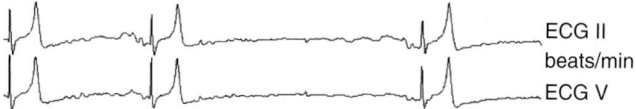

FIGURE 106.4 A two-lead intraoperative electrocardiogram (ECG) recorded on the operating room monitor shortly after reperfusion shows profound bradycardia and tall T waves. Such changes are not uncommon in the period immediately following graft reperfusion.

by a rate of correction of up to 8 to 10 mEq/L in the first 24 hours and up to 18 mEq/L in the first 48 hours.[150]

Temperature Monitoring

Monitoring of core temperature is usually achieved with an esophageal probe, bladder probe, or PAC. Although hypothermia is common during OLT,[151] surprisingly little has been reported on temperature management in OLT, especially considering that hypothermia is a key sign of liver failure and a significant problem during surgery. Well-known detrimental effects of hypothermia include impaired wound healing and coagulation and increased risk of infectious complications. A recent study[152] showed that "...the lowest [intraoperative] temperature was at 5 min after reperfusion" and that hypothermia was associated with increased bleeding, increased amount of intraoperative transfusion, prolonged intubation, and higher 30-day bacterial infection rate. An acute decrease in central temperature results from the cold perfusate returning to the heart after graft reperfusion. This precipitous hypothermia contributes to postreperfusion hemodynamic instability and bradyarrhythmias that may progress to cardiac arrest (Fig. 106.4).[143] The hypothermic insult can be partially mitigated by achieving upper limit normothermia in the pre-reperfusion period; thus the value of continuous temperature monitoring and interventions to ensure normothermia cannot be overemphasized. A special circumstance is deliberate mild hypothermia, which acts by decreasing brain metabolism and mediators of oxidative stress; thus mild hypothermia is an accepted treatment of increased ICP in ALF.[153,154]

INTRAOPERATIVE MANAGEMENT

Hemodynamic, Fluid, and Transfusion Management
(see Chapter 25)

Hemodynamic and fluid management and blood transfusion are critically related and should be considered together. Excessive fluid administration may result in increased pressure in the IVC, PV, and collateral veins, contributing to blood loss during liver dissection, hemodilution of coagulation factors and platelets, and tissue edema (see Chapter 25).[155] Conversely, inadequate intravascular volume repletion may result in hemodynamic instability and organ hypoperfusion and kidney damage.[156] Whereas the low central venous pressure (CVP) strategy may be possible in select patients with normal kidney function and good cardiovascular reserve, targeting low CVP may be detrimental in patients with diastolic dysfunction or dynamic LV outflow obstruction.[55,116,157] Restrictive fluid and transfusion management based on POC laboratories result in marked reduction in blood product administration, including transplantation without transfusion and better outcomes.[158–162] A recent systematic review of seven RCTs testing fluid management strategies in LT recipients[163] suggested that intraoperative fluid restriction may reduce pulmonary complications, duration of mechanical ventilation, and blood loss, without negatively affecting AKI.

CVP is not a reliable index of preload, so volumetric assessment with TEE or dynamic indexes is a superior approach to guiding fluid management.[112,115]

Hypotension is common during all phases of OLT, but little is reported on the impact of intraoperative hypotension on long-term patient outcomes. De Maria and colleagues (2013)[164] reported increased 30-day mortality and graft failure in recipients who sustained periods of intraoperative hypotension with MAP below 50 mm Hg.

Scant evidence is available to provide guidance regarding the choice of intraoperative vasopressors. Agents are chosen based on their pharmacologic properties and side effects.[165] Frequently used agents are phenylephrine, norepinephrine, and vasopressin. Of note, vasopressin-1 and α_1-adrenergic agonists are useful in preserving renal function in HRS[88,166]; vasopressin reduces splanchnic blood flow, which may reduce bleeding from portal collaterals during the dissection phase but may also impede PV flow during the neohepatic phase.[167,168]

Most centers use a combination of crystalloids and colloids for fluid replacement. Studies highlighted concerns regarding the use of artificial colloids, suggesting deleterious effects on renal function and coagulation, as assessed by TEG.[169,170]

Severe pulmonary hypertension (PVR > 240 dynes/sec/cm^{-5}) is associated with high perioperative mortality and is a contraindication for proceeding with LT. In moderate PPH with preserved RV function, the goal of intraoperative management is to lower PVR and promote myocardial contractility and organ perfusion. General measures include increasing FiO$_2$, avoiding hypercapnia and acidosis, and using pulmonary vasodilators. Inhalational pulmonary vasodilators, nitric oxide, and prostacyclin exert minimal systemic effects. In contrast, IV vasodilators cause more pronounced drop in systemic blood pressure and preload, may compromise right-sided heart perfusion, and may inhibit platelet aggregation.[171] Milrinone and dobutamine are used as inotropes and pulmonary vasodilators but with caution because they also cause systemic hypotension. Pulmonary pressure management is particularly challenging in the postreperfusion period because of ensuing acidosis, hypothermia, sudden volume load, and ventricular hypocontractility. TEE is essential to monitor and manage RV contractility and preload. Pulmonary vasodilators are weaned gradually to avoid rebound pulmonary hypertension. It has been recommended that the extubation be delayed if inhalational vasodilators agents are needed.[172,173]

After MELD implementation, more patients with renal insufficiency present for OLT. Renal failure is associated with increased short- and long-term mortality after OLT and often requires intraoperative and postoperative RRT.[98,174] Intraoperative renal protection strategy is based on the maintenance of adequate intravascular volume and renal perfusion. No specific renoprotective agents have proved effective, but it is reasonable to maintain perfusion pressure with vasopressin and adrenergic agonists, also effective in HRS. Surgical techniques that preserve vena caval flow, such as a piggyback technique, favor better renal outcomes. Intraoperative RRT is feasible and has proved safe and successful in maintaining electrolyte and fluid balance and potentially improving outcomes after LT.[98,175] A recent single-center review[176] of patients undergoing OLT between

2004 and 2016 found that preoperative anemia was associated with increased odds of postoperative AKI.

Markers of renal injury, such as neutrophil gelatinase–associated lipocalin, are useful in predicting and assessing post–LT AKI.[177-179]

The administration of RBCs, FFP, and platelets has been associated with increased mortality.[82,159,180] Threshold-based strategies may help decrease the need for blood transfusion in OLT.[181] However, no universal thresholds have been accepted for transfusing RBCs, FFP, and platelets, and practice differs among various centers and clinicians. POC testing, including TEG and ROTEM, have been used to define transfusion algorithms.[127]

The use of intraoperative blood salvage has recently regained favor because it helps minimize allogenic blood transfusions without negatively impacting other clinical outcomes, even in recipients with liver malignancies.[182] Average blood-product requirements have decreased dramatically over the past 2 decades, and now OLT can often be performed without transfusion.[80,183]

Although it would be useful to prospectively identify patients at high risk of major bleeding, factors predictive of higher transfusion requirements are still debatable. Low pretransplant hemoglobin and high MELD are better predictors than previous abdominal surgery, prolonged INR, and low platelet counts.[183,184] In a retrospective study,[185] the authors found that lowering the CVP by phlebotomy (7–10 mL/kg body weight) was associated with lower odds of significant blood loss and of transfusion of 2 or more RBC units.

The selective use of antifibrinolytic agents in the presence of persistent fibrinolysis is indicated, but routine prophylactic use of these agents is controversial.[186]

No consensus exists regarding the choice of any specific antifibrinolytic agent, dose, or time of administration; therefore monitoring of fibrinolysis and early detection of hypercoagulability are of critical importance. The prevailing view is that TEG/ROTEM may best provide such information, and TEE may be useful for detection of intracardiac clots adhering to the central lines.

Tranexamic acid has been shown to reduce transfusion requirements without increasing the risk of thromboembolic events.[187] Prophylactic use of activated factor VII has been associated with increased incidence of vascular thrombosis,[188] but as a rescue treatment, it is associated with reduced mortality.[189]

Cryoprecipitate, a source of factors I, VIIIc, and of vWF; fibrinogen concentrate; and prothrombin complex concentrates that contain vitamin K–dependent factors II, VII, IX, and X are increasingly used as an alternative to FFP. The advantages of these products over FFP are smaller fluid volume, lower risk of infectious complications, and standardized dosing.[80,190]

Ventilation Management

Mechanical ventilation should optimize respiratory gas exchange and maintain lung volumes and capacities to facilitate early postoperative extubation because prolonged mechanical ventilation after OLT has been associated with increased mortality and graft loss.[191] Preexisting respiratory comorbidities, such as ascites and hydrothorax, must be considered when setting the ventilatory parameters. Although not much is reported about the ventilation in OLT, it seems reasonable to adopt a protective ventilatory strategy to prevent atelectasis and avoid high, nonphysiologic tidal volume and high peak airway pressures.[192-194]

Multiple factors can cause increased pulmonary capillary permeability and predispose the lungs to interstitial edema. Positive end-expiratory pressure (PEEP) is a rational tool to prevent lung edema, and a PEEP of up to 10 mm Hg has proved safe in maintaining hemodynamics and graft perfusion after cadaveric and living-donor OLT.[195–197]

A high fraction of inspired oxygen may be required to modulate pulmonary vascular resistances in case of pulmonary hypertension or maintain oxygenation in HPS.

CRITICAL INTRAOPERATIVE EVENTS

Postreperfusion Syndrome and Refractory Hypotension

Postreperfusion syndrome (PRS), first described by Aggarwal and colleagues in 1987,[198] was originally defined as a decrease in systemic arterial pressure to less than 70% of the pre-reperfusion value or a mean BP below 60 mm Hg within 5 minutes of liver reperfusion and lasting at least 1 minute. The low systemic BP is associated with an increase in PVR and central pressures and occasionally with bradycardia, which could progress to asystole.[199] Other authors proposed similar definitions based on hemodynamics,[200–203] and one proposed an expanded concept that, in addition to unstable hemodynamics, included postreperfusion fibrinolysis requiring administration of antifibrinolytics.[204] Depending on the reporting center, significant PRS is evident in 25% to 55% of patients, an acknowledgment that the incidence depends on the definition. In a significant percentage of patients undergoing LT, reperfusion can be complicated by bradycardia that is resistant to chronotropic agents and asystole that requires cardiopulmonary resuscitation.[143]

The mechanisms behind bradycardia and reperfusion syndrome are not yet fully understood. Several possible factors have been indicated, such as the release of vasoactive substances from the liver graft or the recipient gut—potassium, prostanoids, bradykinin, ILs—along with hypovolemia, hypothermia, or small air or thrombotic emboli.[201,205] In a multivariable logistic regression analysis, Paugam-Burtz and colleagues (2009)[203] found that absence of portocaval shunt and duration of cold-ischemia time were independent predictors of PRS. Other authors suggest an association between PRS, patient hypothermia, and liver graft macrosteatosis.[206,207]

PRS is associated with adverse outcomes, including an increase in blood loss and transfusion requirements, and higher incidence of postoperative allograft loss. Common preventative interventions include pretreatment with chronotropic and vasoconstrictor agents[206,208] and optimization of temperature, pH, and electrolytes.

The occurrence of ischemia-reperfusion injury is well recognized, but its exact relevance to PRS is not fully understood. Therapeutic approaches that use nitric oxide, prostaglandin E_1, and various antioxidants aimed at mitigating the inflammatory response and cellular cascade triggered by the ischemia-reperfusion are undergoing clinical evaluation.[209] Methylene blue and hydroxocobalamin have been used in treatment of postreperfusion vasoplegia, a refractory hypotension resistant to catecholamines.[210–214] Their likely mechanism is scavenging NO and H2S. Evidence is limited to case reports and small series demonstrating improved BP and reduction in vasopressor requirements.

Recent investigations of machine liver graft perfusion have demonstrated, among other benefits, lower incidence of PRS with both normothermic and hypothermic perfusion protocols.[215]

Intracardiac Thrombosis and Pulmonary Embolism

Intracardiac thrombosis (ICT) and pulmonary embolism are rare but potentially catastrophic complications of OLT. Intravascular clots are frequently adherent to central venous lines or TIPS.[117,119,216] Some ESLD diagnoses, such as NASH, primary biliary cirrhosis, or primary sclerosing cholangitis, are associated with hypercoagulability despite increased INR. However, the potential for thrombosis in the tenuously rebalanced coagulation system in ESLD is frequently underestimated.

The incidence of ICT has been reported in the 0.4% to 6.2% range.[216–218] In the largest to date and best documented single-center review (528 patients, routine use of TEE), the incidence of ICT was 4.2% with 45% mortality.[219] This study identified higher MELD, longer warm ischemia time, and high donor body mass index (BMI) as variables associated with ICT. Conversely, administration of IV heparin before IVC cross-clamping was protective. Although earlier studies have implicated antifibrinolytics in development of ICT,[220] no study to date has demonstrated a significant link between antifibrinolytics and ICT,[216,219] including a large propensity-matched cohort (734 patients) specifically aimed at efficacy and safety of tranexamic acid in OLT.[187] We advocate for a judicious use of tranexamic acid limited only to treatment of persistent postreperfusion fibrinolysis. Insufficient evidence exists with regards to the risk from the surgical approach such as venovenous bypass and type of caval cross clamping.

The most common initial presentation of intraoperative pulmonary embolism (PE) is systemic hypotension with a simultaneous increase in pulmonary pressure[220] and a decrease in end-tidal carbon dioxide, progressing often to pulseless electrical activity. A preventive strategy is based on routine use of TEE, identification of hypercoagulable conditions with TEG/ROTEM, avoidance of unnecessary prophylactic administration of antifibrinolytics,[186] and judicious use of IV heparin.

TEE is critical for early diagnosis and immediate treatment and can improve outcomes.[219] Treatment is based on hemodynamic support, thrombolysis, and/or clot evacuation. Examples of successful resuscitation with intraoperative administration of recombinant tPA and/or extracorporeal membrane oxygenation (ECMO) have been reported,[221,222] but mortality rates from massive PE or ICT remain high.

Paradoxical embolus is a possible complication when an anatomic or functional atrial septum defect is present. Such a complication is more likely to occur in pediatric recipients and in the early postreperfusion period, when right atrial pressure may exceed left atrial pressure. It is worthwhile to rule out such a defect during pretransplant evaluation and to possibly plan for percutaneous closure when the defect size is significant and unlikely to heal.

Air embolism, a simultaneous laceration of a large vein, such as the IVC or hepatic veins, and a low CVP allow active entrainment of air into the central circulation. A disconnect in the venovenous bypass circuit can also lead to air entrapment in the central circulation.

SPECIAL SITUATIONS

Acute Liver Failure

ALF is defined as a severe liver dysfunction causing encephalopathy and coagulopathy (INR > 1.5) within 24 weeks of the onset of symptoms in patients without previous liver disease; it is considered *fulminant,* if it develops in less than 2 to 4 weeks[223] (see Chapters 77 and 78). ALF accounts for just over 8% of all LTs and carries a 1-year survival around 80%.[224] *Acute-on-chronic liver failure* is a newly described syndrome characterized by an acute decompensation of cirrhosis and multiorgan disorder, including liver, kidney, brain, and circulatory failure, and poor survival (28-day mortality, 30%–40%).[225]

Increased ICP and severe coagulopathy are the hallmarks of ALF and are also the main perioperative challenges. Because cerebral edema is the most common cause of death in ALF, control of intracranial hypertension and maintenance of adequate CPP are critical intraoperative tasks. Widely accepted minimal goals are ICP less than 25 mm Hg and CPP 60 to 70 mm Hg or higher. Continuous invasive monitoring of ICP is ideal for guiding management, but it is associated with a high risk of bleeding. ICP typically rises during the dissection phase and peaks after reperfusion. A simultaneous drop in MAP makes postreperfusion the most critical period for management of CPP. A protocol that included intraparenchymal ICP monitoring, maintenance of CPP greater than 60 mm Hg, hyperventilation (Pco_2 at 30–35 mm Hg), mannitol and 3% saline, mild hypothermia (33°C–34°C), and a high dose of pentobarbital titrated to ICP effect resulted in favorable neurologic outcomes in a small series of ICU and LT patients.[226] The current viewpoint favors a multifactorial approach, involving support of respiratory, circulatory, and renal function together with interventions to prevent intracranial hypertension and metabolic and infectious complications.[227]

No RCTs or consensus statements are available that stipulate the safety and efficacy of different types of ICP monitors or specific management protocols during LT, but it is increasingly recognized that clinically meaningful inferences may require multimodal approaches, including brain tissue oxygen monitoring and microdialysis[228] or monitoring of cerebral hemodynamics using TCD.[34,229] Interventions aimed at management of CPP are outlined in Table 106.2.

Despite profound coagulation abnormalities in ALF (Box 106.1), serious bleeding is rare during LT because ALF patients have minimal or no portal hypertension.[230] No evidence-based protocols have been outlined for correcting coagulopathy in ALF, but it is recognized that prophylactic administration of FFP and other products simply to correct PT is not justified. However, correction of coagulopathy is an important consideration before placement of an ICP transducer. Whole-blood assays (TEG, ROTEM) and clinical assessment are more useful guides for intraoperative treatment of coagulopathy. A major limitation of FFP is the potential for volume overload aggravating brain edema and causing transfusion-related acute lung injury (TRALI). Cryoprecipitate is typically considered when the fibrinogen level falls below 100 mg/dL. Activated recombinant factor VII (rFVIIa), prothrombin, and fibrinogen concentrates are advantageous because of the low volume, but their optimal use remains to be determined. Antifibrinolytics should be considered if clinically significant fibrinolysis is found. Both high-dose corticosteroids given during the anhepatic period may be protective against brain edema but, in conjunction with a functioning graft, may cause hyperglycemia in the neohepatic phase. Because hyperglycemia has an adverse effect on ischemia-reperfusion brain injury, plasma glucose should be kept in the normal range, and continuous infusion of insulin is often required. Restoration of liver function by the functioning graft gradually eliminates encephalotoxins and improves metabolic homeosta-sis, which eventually leads to reduction of brain edema and normalization of ICP and CPP.

Combined Liver-Kidney Transplantation

With the introduction of MELD, the percentage of simultaneous liver and kidney transplantation has been increasing, to 8.2% of all LTs in the United States in 2019.[231] Although combined transplantation should be reserved only for patients with irreversible renal failure, reliable predictive factors for reversibility are sometimes difficult to define.[232] Current criteria

TABLE 106.2 Early Complications After Liver Transplantation

TYPE	COMPLICATION
Pulmonary	TRALI/ARDS, pneumonia, pleural effusions, persistent shunting
Cardiovascular	CHF, hypotension, myocardial ischemia, arrhythmias
Renal	ATN, hepatorenal syndrome, CNI nephrotoxicity
Metabolic	Hyperglycemia/diabetes mellitus, electrolyte abnormalities
Neurologic	Persistent encephalopathy, seizures, posterior leukoencephalopathy, central pontine myelinolysis
Infectious	Wound infections, seromas, intraabdominal abscess, sepsis
Abdominal	Surgical bleeding or bleeding as a result of coagulopathy
Vascular	Hepatic artery or portal vein stenosis/thrombosis, IVC obstruction
Biliary	Biliary stricture or leaks
Rejection	Cellular rejection
Immunosuppressant toxicity	Seizures, kidney failure

ARDS, Acute respiratory distress syndrome; *ATN,* acute tubular necrosis; *CHF,* congestive heart failure; *CNI,* calcineurin inhibitor; *IVC,* inferior vena cava; *TRALI,* transfusion-related acute lung injury.

BOX 106.1 Hemostatic Abnormalities in Liver Disease

Anticoagulant
Thrombocytopenia
Impaired platelet function (?)
Reduced hematocrit
Upregulated NO[a] and prostacyclin[a] inhibit platelets
Low levels of coagulation factors II, V, VII, IX, X, and XI
Vitamin K deficiency
Hypofibrinogenemia, dysfibrinogenemia
Decreased factor XIII, TAFI
Elevated levels of tPA,[a] decreased PAI-1[a]

Procoagulant
Elevated factor VIII[b] and von Willebrand factor[b]
Decreased proteins S and C and antithrombin III[†]
Decreased plasminogen and α_2-antiplasmin

[a]Extrahepatic synthesis.
[b]Extrahepatic and intrahepatic synthesis.
NO, Nitric oxide; *PAI-1,* plasminogen activator inhibitor type 1; *TAFI,* thrombin activatable fibrinolysis inhibitor; *tPA,* tissue plasminogen activator.
Data from Lisman T, Leebeek WG. Hemostatic alterations in liver disease: A review on pathophysiology, clinical consequences, and treatment. *Dig Surg.* 2007;24:250–258.

recommended by OPTN in 2017 differ depending on whether it is CKD or AKI. CKD criteria include GFR of less than or equal to 60 mL/min for at least 3 months with recent GFR of less than or equal to 30 mL/min or on hemodialysis, and metabolic disease (hyperoxaluria, etc.). AKI criteria are dialysis for more than 6 weeks and GFR of less than or equal to 25 mL/min for more than 6 weeks documented every 7 days.

An analysis of 4275 cirrhotic patients with renal failure from the OPTN database demonstrated an overall significantly higher liver allograft and patient survival rate in recipients with HRS who underwent a combined kidney-liver transplant compared with those with LT alone.[233] Liver allograft survival was superior in combined transplant patients irrespective of whether they received dialysis. LT alone was a significant risk factor both for graft loss and mortality. In addition, prevalence of post-transplantation renal failure was higher for up to 3 years in patients who received an LT only.[233] The better outcomes of recipients of simultaneous liver and kidney transplant can be explained by an immunologic advantage provided by the liver to the kidney graft.[234]

Patients presenting for combined liver and kidney transplantation present an anesthetic challenge. Electrolyte abnormalities and metabolic acidosis may mandate preoperative hemodialysis, whereas hyperkalemia greater than 5.5 mmol/L and hyponatremia less than 120 mmol/L are typically considered prohibitive to transplantation. Intraoperative monitoring of preload and strategies for judicious volume administration and correction of electrolyte abnormalities are essential. Hyperkalemia is common and should be managed aggressively by maintaining a normal pH and administering insulin and glucose, inhaled β-adrenergic agonists, and furosemide, if urine output is preserved. Banked blood is a major source of potassium; ideally, it should be washed, and units with the longest remaining shelf life should be preferentially used.

Intraoperative continuous RRT is possible, and it is routinely used in some centers.[98] Although the kidney transplantation part may prompt a somewhat more liberal fluid regimen, goals for both OLT and kidney transplantation should be maintenance of a normal-range preload to allow optimal stroke volume and organ perfusion.

Donation After Cardiac Death (see Chapter 109)

The use of liver grafts from donation after cardiac death (DCD) has historically been at 5% to 6% of all LTs because of concerns of graft failure, primarily because of ischemic cholangiopathy (IC).[235] Recent evidence shows that by optimizing recipient selection and minimizing cold ischemia time, comparable outcomes between DCD and donation after brain death (DBD) donors can be achieved.[235,236]

DCD LT is associated with increased cost and resource utilization[3,237,238] because of higher complexity of perioperative anesthetic and surgical care. Historically, the use of DCD has been associated with increased prevalence of post-reperfusion syndrome; coagulopathy, including hyperfibrinolysis; electrolyte and hemodynamic instability; need for postoperative mechanical ventilation; multiorgan support and ICU stay; and inferior graft survival.[239,240]

Intra-arterial tPA flush used in DCD donor grafts decreases the incidence of ischemic biliary complications and improves 1-year survival, without evidence of increased transfusion requirements.[241] Other strategies to improve DCD outcomes include a rapid recovery technique by experienced procurement teams, premortem cannulation techniques, ex vivo organ perfusion, and minimization of cold- and warm-ischemia time.[242] DCD grafts and extended criteria donors are increasingly recognized as a valuable resource, and with selective and judicious use, they can produce satisfactory results.[243]

Living-Donor Liver Transplantation
(see Chapters 109 and 121)

In 2019, in the United States, 524 of 8896 (5%) of all LTs were performed with the graft from a living donor: 5.3% (445) of all adult and 14.3% (79) of all pediatric OLTs.[244] Living-donor liver transplantation (LDLT) may provide significant long-term benefits such as decreased death on waitlist and excellent post-transplant outcomes.[245]

Because the survival of recipients of a living graft is similar to that of cadaveric graft recipients,[246,247] the current modest proportion of living versus deceased donors is mainly driven by a justified concern for donor morbidity and mortality and cost.[247,248] The main goal of anesthetic management of living donors is to preserve graft perfusion and prevent donor complications. During OLT, challenges for the anesthesiologist depend more on the recipient's characteristics and comorbidities than on the donor category.

Retransplantation

The most common reasons for retransplantation are primary nonfunction, recurrence of viral hepatitis, acute or chronic rejection, and thrombosis of the hepatic artery[249,250] (see Chapter 111). The interval between the primary transplantation and retransplantation (early vs. delayed retransplantation) depends on the etiology of the graft failure. More than 14,000 liver retransplantations have been performed since the inception of the UNOS registry—about 8% of all OLTs since 1988. A declining trend toward the need for retransplantation is apparent; for example, in 1988, the retransplantation rate was 24.5%, whereas in 2019, the rate was only 3.8% of all LTs.[231]

The survival rate for retransplanted patients is historically lower than for primary transplant recipients: at 1 year, the survival is 68.7% versus 83.3%; at 5 years, it drops to 46% versus 67.4%.[246] With appropriate recipient selection, better outcomes are possible, and 1- and 5-year survival rates have been reported as high as 78% and 67%, respectively, with retransplantation.[249] General agreement has been reached on two points: whole graft should be used in adults,[249] and retransplantation should not be undertaken with extended-criteria donors.[251,252]

The current modest results emphasize the need for strategies to improve retransplantation survival. In particular, a strong interest has been shown in the development of valid predictive criteria.[251,252] For example, according to Kitchens et al. and Berumens and Hemming,[251,252] patients who require mechanical ventilation, those who have advanced renal failure, and patients of advanced age have worse outcomes and should not be considered for retransplantation. MELD score has prognostic value in retransplantation; patients with lower scores have better outcomes than those with MELD scores of more than 25.[251,252]

Anesthetic challenges depend on the overall recipient condition on the day of surgery and time elapsed because the primary transplant, difficult vascular access, a need to support liver and coagulation function, increased blood loss, and a higher requirement for blood-product transfusions[253] may complicate intraoperative management. Main causes of mortality after retransplantation are bacterial infection, multisystem organ failure, bleeding, and recurrence of disease.[249,251,252]

Pediatric Transplantation (see Chapter 110)

Main indications for LT in the pediatric population include biliary atresia (32%) and metabolic/genetic conditions (22%), followed by ALF (11%), cirrhosis (9%), neoplasm (9%), immune-mediated liver and biliary injury (4%), and other conditions (13%).[254,255] More than 17,700 OLTs have been performed since 1988 in patients younger than 18 years, the majority carried out in patients younger than 5 years (65%).[244]

Age at Transplantation and Survival

Age at transplantation mainly depends on the specific etiology of the liver disease. Historically, age at transplantation was one of the main factors that determined survival, and infants used to have poorer outcomes than older children; however, with recent improvement of surgical techniques and better overall perioperative care, 1-year infant survival is over 86%, similar to that of older children after OLT.[244] Renal dysfunction remains a frequent post-liver transplant complication because of nephrotoxicity of calcineurin inhibitors (CNIs).[256]

Recipient Selection

Organ allocation to pediatric recipients in the United States is based on the Pediatric End-Stage Liver Disease (PELD) score, developed based on data derived from a database of children with ESLD, to predict mortality on the waiting list; it considers bilirubin, INR, serum albumin, age, and the child's height and weight. Additional PELD points are awarded for specific risk factors not taken into account in the original PELD equation, such as presence of HPS, metabolic diseases, and liver tumors.[254]

Type of Surgical Graft

Whole, reduced, and split grafts from both cadaveric and living donors have been used to maximize the number of pediatric LTs performed and to minimize the risk of patients dying while on the waiting list.[257]

Intraoperative Anesthesia Challenges

Multifactorial hypoxemia is sometimes present, possibly related to HPS, whereas PPH is usually present only in children affected by Alagille syndrome. Cuffed endotracheal tubes should be used to guarantee effective mechanical ventilation in the presence of high airway pressures. Most children undergoing LT have preserved kidney function, but they are at high risk of developing hypoglycemia.

Vascular Access

Two large-bore IV catheters are usually sufficient for fluid and blood administration. Arterial catheters are usually placed in the upper limbs; a femoral line may produce unreliable values once the surgeon clamps the aorta to build an arterial conduit. The length of the central venous line catheter must be appropriate for the body size of the patient, and PACs are rarely used because of size issues.

It is important to note that children are at increased risk of intraoperative hypothermia and active maintenance of temperature is critical to prevent dysrhythmias, clotting abnormalities, and possible wound infections.

The most common complications of a pediatric OLT are hepatic artery thrombosis, surgical bleed, and biliary complications.[257] Thrombosis of the hepatic artery may lead to a graft loss

and need for retransplantation. Keeping the hematocrit between 25% and 30% to prevent excessive blood viscosity and avoiding overcorrecting coagulation function are common protective strategies. Administration of aspirin or alprostadil in the immediate postoperative period has been reported to blunt platelet activity.[258]

POSTOPERATIVE INTENSIVE CARE
(SEE CHAPTERS 26 AND 111)

Transfer of care to the ICU team should be smooth, following a structured hand-off process to ensure continuation at the same level of monitoring and care as in the operating room (OR). The main goals of the early postoperative period are maintenance of homeostasis and timely recognition and treatment of complications, including infections and acute rejection. The risk of developing early postoperative complications depends on the patient's preoperative condition, quality of the graft, and appropriateness of care.[259] Because mortality after OLT is highest in the immediate perioperative period, high-quality postoperative care is paramount.[159]

Early Extubation

Prolonged mechanical ventilation after OLT is associated with worse outcomes[191] and considerable efforts have been directed toward early extubation.[260] Safe immediate (in the OR) or early (in the ICU) postoperative extubation of most LT patients has been reported by many centers. A large review and meta-analysis suggests that early extubation may confer shorter ICU and hospital stay without increased morbidity and mortality.[261] The exact criteria and recipients who may benefit from early extubation remain a matter of debate. Great variability in rates of extubation and complications between centers reflect differing center-specific patterns of practice and physician experience.[262] Multiple studies agree that encephalopathy is a strong predictor of the need for prolonged ventilation. Volume of blood transfused and RRT are less consistent predictors and may be only indirect markers of poor graft function, severity of illness, and a lack of standardized intraoperative protocols.[260] A study suggested that serum lactate of 8.2 mmol/L or less and RBC transfusion of fewer than 7 units are compatible with early extubation after OLT.[263]

No randomized studies are currently available that demonstrate the positive impact of early extubation, but possible outcome and cost benefits have been suggested.[264]

Early extubation is the initial step of the fast-tracking protocol, with the goal of avoiding ICU admission with attendant cost savings but without compromising patient safety. An experienced transplant center reported fast tracking in majority of OLT recipients, emphasizing the importance of patient selection, teamwork, and adequate resources on the surgery floor.[265,266]

Early Medical Complications (see Chapter 111)

Pulmonary complications that include pneumonia, acute respiratory distress syndrome (ARDS), TRALI, and pleural effusions are common in the immediate postoperative period. These complications occur in over 50% of patients after OLT and lead to hypoxemia, prolonged mechanical ventilation, and decreased survival.[267–270] Pneumonia is the most frequent postoperative infection in patients after OLT, and it carries a high mortality. ARDS may be complicated by fluid overload, and the risk of TRALI increases with the number of transfusions. Pleural effusion promotes atelectasis and contributes to impaired respiratory exchange. When mechanical ventilation is required, protective approaches should be employed.[194] The addition of PEEP may be effective in improving oxygenation; PEEP up to 10 cm H_2O does not affect perfusion of the liver graft, as assessed by Doppler.[196]

Cardiac complications are common in the early postoperative period occurring in up to 8% of cases at 30 days and 11% at 90 days.[271] Cardiovascular death was the leading cause of 30-day mortality in a review of the 2002 to 2012 OTPN database, accounting for 42% of all deaths.[272] Most common diagnoses include arrhythmias, congestive heart failure, and myocardial infarction.[55,272,273] Cardiac complications are associated with worse outcomes, prolonged hospital and ICU stay, and readmissions.[274,275] Cirrhotic patients continue to exhibit hyperdynamic circulation during the first hours or days after OLT. Arterial hypotension and the need for vasopressors are common. With the graft functioning and no evidence of surgical complications, the hemodynamics tend to normalize, which allows downgrading of invasive monitoring and of hemodynamic support. ECMO is increasingly recognized as a rescue strategy in patients with cardiopulmonary failure that is considered transient.[276]

Maintenance of kidney perfusion pressure is paramount because AKI is common (17%–95%) and is associated with increased ICU LOS and mortality.[277] The causes of post-OLT acute renal failure are multifactorial and include preexisting renal dysfunction, HRS, perioperative acute tubular necrosis, and CNI nephrotoxicity. RRT is necessary in 5% to 35% of patients who develop postoperative AKI and is associated with decreased survival.[278] Preventing the occurrence of new injury and managing preexisting kidney dysfunction are priorities in the postoperative care of OLT recipients.[277]

Endocrine and metabolic complications are common in the early post-transplant period. Surgical stress, corticosteroid administration, and CNIs contribute to early post-transplant hyperglycemia, which frequently evolves to diabetes mellitus and hypertension. Diabetes occurs in up to 30% of post-transplant patients, and hypertension is seen in over 50%. Hyperglycemia requires an IV insulin regimen and improves as corticosteroids are tapered; hypertension should be treated aggressively to prevent cardiovascular complications. Neurologic complications have been reported in 30% to 50% of LT recipients.[279-281] Such complications contribute to longer ICU and hospital stay and may result in long-term poor quality of life. The most common neurologic complications are of metabolic-toxic etiology, including encephalopathy, seizures, osmotic demyelination syndrome, and poorly understood posterior reversible encephalopathy. The most common nonmetabolic complications are intracranial hemorrhage, infections, and ischemic stroke. The etiology is multifactorial and includes poor graft function, use of corticosteroids and possibly CNIs, infection and systemic inflammatory response, electrolyte imbalance, and embolic events.

Meticulous perioperative neurologic assessment and quick recognition of neurologic impairment are essential. Specific therapeutic modalities are limited (i.e., tapering steroids, exchanging CNIs), but when applied in a timely manner, they may improve outcome. In addition, a key factor of neurologic improvement is the recovery of graft function.

Infections, occurring in up to 80% of OLT recipients,[282] are the second most common cause of 30-day mortality after OLT, accounting for about 28% of deaths.[272] Many infections that occur in the first days after transplantation are related to the surgery itself, such as wound infections, seromas, and perigraft fluid collections. Postoperative and opportunistic infections are common in the immunocompromised and debilitated transplant patients. In the immediate post-transplant period, nosocomial bacterial infections dominate; 1 to 6 months after transplant, viral and fungal infections are most common, followed by community-acquired pathogens at later stages of recovery. Such infections may lead to sepsis and multiorgan failure and therefore require a high level of suspicion. Routine postoperative prophylactic protocols include broad-spectrum antibacterial, antiviral, and antifungal agents.

The incidence of corticosteroid-resistant rejection has been steadily decreasing, with about 4% of late mortality being attributed to chronic rejection.[283] Cellular rejection is suspected with increasing serum transaminases and normal hepatic vascular Doppler studies, and diagnosis is confirmed with liver biopsy. However, early episodes respond well to boluses of corticosteroids and rarely lead to graft failure.

Surgical Complications (see Chapter 111)

Surgical complications may result in prolonged ICU and hospital stay, reoperation, increased resource utilization, and worse outcomes.

Postoperative hemorrhage is primarily a clinical diagnosis that can be confirmed by abdominal imaging techniques. It occurs in 10% to 15% of OLT recipients. It is important to quickly diagnose surgical hemorrhage, which may not always be easy because of persisting coagulopathy. Hemodynamic instability and transfusion of more than 4 to 6 units of packed RBCs over a 24-hour period are usually an indication for surgical re-exploration.[284]

Early vascular complications include hepatic artery and PV stenosis or thrombosis and venocaval obstruction or kinking. Poor graft function and protracted elevation of liver enzymes point to a vascular complication; however, the diagnosis is made based on a bedside vascular Doppler and can be confirmed with conventional or MR angiography. Hepatic artery thrombosis occurs in 2.5% to 10% of adult patients and in 5% to 20% of children; PV thrombosis is much less common (0.3%–2.2%), and flow obstruction at the level of the infrahepatic and suprahepatic vena cava occurs in 1% to 2%.

All vascular complications require urgent surgical intervention. If vascular repair is delayed, the ensuing graft failure may necessitate retransplantation. Many vascular complications have been successfully treated using various endovascular approaches, including percutaneous angioplasty, stent placement, or thrombolysis.[285]

Biliary complications occur in about 10% to 40% of patients after LT.[284,286] Stricture of the biliary tree accounts for most of the complications, but biliary leak is a more common early complication. The most severe manifestations of biliary leak are peritonitis and sepsis, but asymptomatic bilomas are also a common presentation. The diagnosis of the leak is based on percutaneous transhepatic cholangiography or endoscopic retrograde cholangiopancreatography. Ultrasound and CT scan are useful in diagnosis of biliary dilations caused by obstruction, bile collections, or abscesses. Treatment of biliary obstruction includes percutaneous balloon dilation and drainage or surgical revision. Treatment of biliary leaks involves percutaneous transhepatic drainage, a technically difficult alternative to surgical repair.[259] Nonanastomotic leaks and leaks secondary to hepatic artery thrombosis are particularly ominous because they are less amenable to percutaneous repair and often require retransplantation.[285]

References are available at expertconsult.com.

CHAPTER 107

Liver transplantation in patients with fulminant hepatitis

Jessica Lindemann and Maria B. Majella Doyle

Acute liver failure (ALF), formally known as fulminant hepatic failure, is a rare and devastating condition characterized by the development of encephalopathy and impaired synthetic liver function (international normalized ratio [INR] > 1.5) occurring within 26 weeks of acute-onset jaundice and elevated transaminases (see Chapters 77 and 78). Stemming from a broad range of etiologies, ALF is the direct result of the overwhelming death of hepatocytes exceeding the regenerative capacity of the liver. ALF is a potentially life-threatening condition, presenting most often in a patient without cirrhosis or preexisting liver disease. The immediate cause of death in 35% of ALF patients is brain herniation from increased intracranial pressure (ICP), and most other deaths are secondary to severe refractory hypotension resulting from supervening sepsis and culminating in multi-organ failure.[1] The most prevalent causes of ALF include viral hepatitis, drug-induced liver injury, autoimmune liver disease, and shock or hypoperfusion, although many cases have no discernible cause[2] (see Chapters 68, 77, and 78). ALF can also involve marked activation of systemic inflammation, followed by the development of a secondary immune response, increased risk of infection, and subsequent progression to multi-organ dysfunction and death.[3] Additional complications in patients with ALF include renal failure, hypoglycemia, metabolic acidosis, pancreatitis, and cardiopulmonary distress. Left untreated, the prognosis is poor, with mortality rates of approximately 30% to 35%, with 20% to 25% of patients requiring emergency liver transplantation (LT), and 40% to 45% of patients able to survive spontaneously because of advances in intensive care management.[4–6]

The incidence of ALF is low, developing in fewer than 10 cases per 1 million persons per year in the developed world. Because of this low frequency and patient heterogeneity, supportive care for these patients has often been anecdotal, with limited level 1 evidence to guide management. However, certain strategies have become well established and their benefits widely proven. Rapid recognition of ALF followed by adequate specialized management remains mandatory to improve survival.

INITIAL RECOGNITION AND MANAGEMENT IS KEY TO PROGNOSIS

In patients with clinical or laboratory evidence of acute hepatitis, initial evaluation should begin with a thorough history to elucidate any potentially contributing factors followed by careful physical examination to identify subtle alterations in mentation and to rule out evidence of stigmata of chronic liver disease. Prothrombin time (PT) and INR should be monitored and if abnormal (PT prolongation of ≥ 4–6 seconds, INR ≥ 1.5) with the presence of encephalopathy, hospitalization is mandatory for frequent clinical and laboratory monitoring, preferably within an intensive care unit (ICU; see Chapters 26 and 77).

Prompt referral to a specialized liver unit and rapid medical intervention with specific therapies in certain etiologies can prevent progression and improve survival.[7] Immediate contact with a transplant center should occur once altered mental status develops because clinical deterioration may be very rapid. Under ideal circumstances, transfer to a transplant center should occur when the patient has grade I or II hepatic encephalopathy (HE; Box 107.1) and is still clinically stable because within hours HE may progress, intracranial hypertension (ICH) may develop, and clinical instability may ensue, rendering the patient nontransferable because of a high risk of brain herniation.

Sedation should be avoided because it may mask the signs of worsening HE or cerebral edema. In patients who are severely agitated, short-acting benzodiazepines may be given with caution. Opioids must be avoided because they can decrease the seizure threshold. Antiemetics can also deteriorate mental status and should be avoided. Replacement therapy for thrombocytopenia and/or prolonged PT is recommended only in the setting of hemorrhage or before invasive procedures.[8–9] Overall coagulation homeostasis, as measured by thromboelastography (TEG), is normal even in patients with a greatly elevated INR, making spontaneous bleeding uncommon.[10] Additionally, serial evaluation of laboratory coagulation variables is critical for prognostic purposes, so administration of coagulation factors or plasma should be strictly limited. Nephrotoxic drugs and radiologic contrast agents should also be minimized because renal failure often complicates ALF and has a strong prognostic impact.

Efforts to determine the specific etiology of ALF should be initiated as early as possible to guide management decisions. Early initiation of specific etiologic therapy, when possible, can be lifesaving. The etiology of liver failure is recognized as one of the best prognostic indicators of ALF and plays an important role in the decision to proceed with LT. Early laboratory screening in these patients should focus on determining the severity of ALF and include routine chemistries, arterial blood gases (ABGs), complete blood count (CBC), and blood typing. Etiologic screening should include viral serologies, circulating acetaminophen (APAP) level, screens for other drugs and toxins, tests for Wilson disease, autoantibodies, and pregnancy tests for women (Box 107.2). Considering the frequency of drug toxicity involved in ALF, a careful drug history should include all prescription and nonprescription drugs, herbs, and dietary supplements taken during the past year, duration involved, and recent quantity ingested. All nonessential medications should be discontinued.[11] In patients with suspected or known APAP overdose, early (within 4 hours of ingestion) activated charcoal may be useful for intestinal decontamination. N-acetylcysteine (NAC) should also be given as soon as possible, although it may still be of value even 48 or more hours after ingestion.[12,13]

Despite extensive evaluation of the etiology of ALF, the cause remains elusive in approximately 15% to 40% of cases, even though the incidence of cryptogenic disease is declining.[14] Data suggest that in 20% of these patients, ALF might be attributable

---

BOX 107.1 West Haven's Criteria for Hepatic Encephalopathy

Grade 0
Lack of detectable changes in personality or behavior
No asterixis

Grade I
Trivial lack of awareness
Euphoria or anxiety
Shortened attention span
Impaired performance of addition
Asterixis may present

Grade II
Lethargy or apathy
Minimal disorientation for time or place
Inappropriate behavior
Subtle personality
Slurred speech
Impaired performance of subtraction

Grade III
Somnolence to semi-stupor but responsive to verbal stimuli
Confusion
Gross disorientation
Asterixis is usually absent

Grade IV
Coma (unresponsive to verbal or noxious stimuli)

From Mullen KD. Review of the final report of the 1998 Working Party on definition, nomenclature, and diagnosis of hepatic encephalopathy. *Aliment Pharmacol Ther.* 2007;25(Suppl 1):11–16.

BOX 107.2 Etiologies of Acute Liver Failure

Viral
Hepatitis A virus
Hepatitis B virus
Hepatitis D virus
Hepatitis E virus
Herpes simplex virus
Varicella-zoster virus
Human herpesvirus 6
Epstein-Barr virus
Cytomegalovirus
Parvovirus B19
Adenovirus

Drugs
Acetaminophen/paracetamol
Tetracyclines
Isoniazid
Halothane
Antiepileptic agents
Nonsteroidal antiinflammatory drugs

Microvesicular Steatosis
Fatty liver of pregnancy
Reye syndrome

Vascular
Ischemic hepatitis (shock liver)
Acute Budd-Chiari syndrome
Veno-occlusive disease

Toxins
Amanita mushrooms
Chlorinated solvents
White phosphorus
Herbal products
Cocaine, ecstasy, methamphetamine

Miscellaneous
Wilson disease
Malignant infiltration (breast cancer, lymphoma, small cell lung cancer, and melanoma)
Autoimmune hepatitis

Indeterminate Origin
Unknown

---

to undiagnosed APAP overdose.[15] When etiologic diagnosis remains elusive after extensive initial evaluation, liver biopsy through a transjugular approach may be appropriate to identify a specific cause that might impact treatment strategy, such as malignant infiltration precluding transplantation, autoimmune hepatitis, certain viral infections, and Wilson disease.[16,17]

ETIOLOGY OF ACUTE LIVER FAILURE

ALF can affect patients of all ages because of a wide variety of causes (see Box 107.2). Etiologies vary in adults compared with infants and children,[5,18,19] and the relative frequency of etiologies show geographic and temporal variations[20,21] related to epidemiologic, socioeconomic, and cultural differences. As a result, ALF is less common in the developed world than in developing countries. In the United States (US) and Western Europe, APAP overdose has become the most common cause of ALF.[14] This was demonstrated in data from the US over a 17-year period where APAP overdose represented nearly half of all ALF cases, followed by non-APAP related drug-induced liver injury.[22] Similarly, APAP overdose remains a common cause of ALF in the United Kingdom (UK), even after introduction of legislation to reduce the size of over-the-counter APAP packets.[21] Unfortunately, in the rest of the world, acute viral hepatitis is still the predominant etiologic factor in ALF, especially in pediatric series (see Chapters 105 and 110).

Viral Hepatitis

Globally, hepatitis A and E infections account for the majority of ALF cases in developing countries, with mortality greater than 50%. ALF is estimated to develop in less than 1% of patients with hepatitis A and in 1% of patients with acute hepatitis B.[23,24] ALF caused by hepatitis B is more common in some Asian and Mediterranean countries. Data from Sudan,[25] Bangladesh,[26] Mexico,[27] and India[28–30] report prevalence of viral hepatitis among ALF patients to be as high as 27% to 94%, including hepatitis A, B, D, E, and hepatitis A with E. Improved sanitation, vaccine programs, and better regulation of blood products have reduced the incidence of ALF caused by viral hepatitis in the US and in Western European countries.[31,32] In addition, ALF has been described in association with herpes simplex virus (HSV), varicella-zoster virus (VZV), Epstein-Barr virus (EBV), adenovirus, and cytomegalovirus (CMV), in both immunocompromised and immunocompetent patients[33] (see Chapters 77 and 78).

Drug-Induced Liver Injury

Although ALF only occurs in a small fraction of cases of drug-induced liver injury, these patients require high resource use and have relatively poor outcomes.[34] Data from the US Acute Liver Failure Study Group (ALFSG), a multicenter network established in 1998 to gather data prospectively on all forms of ALF, has shown that drug-induced liver injury accounts for nearly 50% of ALF cases in the United States.[35] Drug toxicity may be dose dependent and predictable, as with APAP, or idiosyncratic and unpredictable, as with other medications. In a recent analysis of 1033 patients enrolled through 2007, APAP toxicity accounted for 46% of cases, followed by indeterminate origin (15%) and idiosyncratic drug reactions (12%).[36] The clinical pattern of presentation of APAP toxicity is different in the UK than in the US, where half of cases result from unintentional overuse of APAP-containing compounds for pain or fever relief at therapeutic doses, mainly by patients with ongoing alcohol abuse.[14,37] Other compounding factors, including obesity, a nutritionally depleted state, or concurrent use of medications known to induce the cytochrome P450 system, such as anticonvulsants, may result in a "therapeutic misadventure" and unintentional overdose.[38] Risk of death is directly related to substantial drug ingestion over hours or days, rather than at a single time point.

Idiosyncratic drug-induced liver injury is much rarer, even among patients exposed to potentially hepatotoxic medication, and few patients have progression to ALF.[39] Factors such as an older age, increased serum transaminases and bilirubin levels, and coagulopathy are associated with an increased risk of death.[40,41] It is important that ingredients of nonprescription medications be determined whenever possible. Strict inquiry should also include herbal preparations, weight loss agents, and other nutritional supplements.[11]

MANAGEMENT OF THE PATIENT WITH ACUTE LIVER FAILURE (SEE CHAPTER 77)

As a result of the rarity of patients with ALF, the heterogeneity of etiologies, variable levels of disease severity, and different access to LT, ALF is extremely difficult to study. Randomized controlled trials (RCTs) for ALF are limited[42] and optimal management remains poorly defined, center specific, and mostly opinion based. The basis of management should focus on three main objectives: (1) determination of etiology to provide specific treatment in selected cases; (2) prevention, recognition, and early treatment of complications that could lead to multi-organ system failure and death; and (3) assessment of prognosis for distinguishing patients who have a chance to improve spontaneously from those who will require LT and should be urgently listed (see Chapter 79).

Specific Etiologic Treatment

Specific treatments are limited and should be delivered as early as possible (Table 107.1). In APAP overdose, the role of NAC administration in limiting liver injury is through repletion of hepatic glutathione, which neutralizes *N*-acetyl-p-benzoquinone imine (NAPQI), the toxic metabolite of APAP metabolism.[43] NAC has been shown to be effective and safe in large case series[44-46] and a small, controlled trial.[47] There appears to be a treatment benefit even when doubt exists about timing, dose ingested, or plasma concentration of acetaminophen.[37,48] Intravenous (IV) NAC is preferred because of alterations in mental

TABLE 107.1 Etiology-Specific Treatments in Acute Liver Failure (ALF)

ALF ETIOLOGY	TREATMENT
Herpes simplex virus or varicella zoster virus	Acyclovir, 30 mg/kg daily intravenously (IV)
Acetaminophen/paracetamol	*N*-acetylcysteine: Oral: 140 mg/kg load, followed by 70 mg/kg every 4 hours IV: 150 mg/kg load in 15–60 min, followed by 12.5 mg/kg hourly for 4 hours, then 6.25 mg/kg/hr
Autoimmune hepatitis	Prednisone, 40–60 mg/day orally
Hepatitis B	Lamivudine, 100–150 mg/day, or entecavir
Hepatitis D	Lamivudine, 100–150 mg/day, or entecavir
Acute fatty liver of pregnancy/HELLP	Delivery
Mushroom poisoning (*Amanita phalloides*)	Penicillin G, 300,000 to 1 million units/kg/day IV Silibinin (milk thistle, not available in the United States), 30–40 mg/kg/day IV or oral for 3–4 days

status and the potential side effects of nausea and vomiting; however, oral therapy is an option for patients with mild or no HE. Other side effects include diarrhea, fever, and, in rare cases, hypotension and anaphylaxis.[49,50] Duration of NAC administration should be determined by clinical improvement (resolution of HE, improving coagulopathy, declining transaminases) or outcome (death or LT) rather than by time or serum APAP levels.

NAC also has beneficial effects on systemic hemodynamic parameters, provides substrates for hepatic adenosine triphosphate (ATP) synthesis supporting mitochondrial energy metabolism, and improves oxygen delivery to peripheral tissues.[51,52] Consequently, NAC has been evaluated as a treatment for other forms of ALF unrelated to APAP overdose. Lee and colleagues evaluated 173 patients with non-APAP-induced ALF randomly allocated to receive either IV NAC or placebo.[53] There was no benefit in 21-day survival, although transplant-free survival and 1-year post-transplant survival were improved. Furthermore, in the subgroup of patients with grade I or II HE, survival at 1 year was significantly better in those who received NAC than in all other individuals.

With the exception of prompt delivery once the mother has been stabilized in women with acute fatty liver of pregnancy or HELLP, there are insufficient data to recommend evidence-based therapies for ALF secondary to other etiologies. However, several etiology-specific measures based on experience, the relative innocuousness of the measures, and the high mortality associated with ALF have been suggested (see Table 107.1).

In autoimmune hepatitis, whether the use of corticosteroids can prevent transplantation or death is still not clearly defined, and there is much concern over the risk of septic complications. Corticosteroid therapy may still be considered, particularly in patients with early stages of the disease and coagulopathy with mild encephalopathy, starting with prednisone at 40 to 60 mg/day. However, consideration for LT should not be delayed while awaiting response to corticosteroid therapy (see Chapters 10, 77, and 68).

In patients with HBV-associated ALF, nucleos(t)ide analogues should be considered for treatment, although evidence of efficacy is still equivocal.[54] Even if not clearly beneficial, antiviral treatment should be given for prevention of post-transplant recurrence in ALF candidates for transplantation. In patients with documented or suspected cases of HSV or VZV as the cause of ALF, acyclovir (5–10 mg/kg every 8 hours) should be given for at least 7 days[55,56] or until herpes infection has been excluded (see Chapter 68).

In patients with known or suspected mushroom poisoning after *Amanita phalloides* ingestion, early administration of activated charcoal that binds to amatoxin is associated with improved survival. Administration of penicillin G and silibinin are accepted antidotes and should be administered despite a lack of RCTs proving their efficacy while the patient is listed for transplantation because this procedure is often the only life-saving option for these patients.

Patients in whom Wilson disease is the likely cause of ALF should be promptly evaluated for transplantation because fulminant presentation of the disease is uniformly fatal.[57] Plasma exchange to remove large amounts of copper in a short period may act as a temporizing measure.[58] Use of chelation therapy plays no role in the management of ALF secondary to Wilson disease (see Chapter 77).

Budd Chiari syndrome resulting in ALF is associated with a poor prognosis and should be managed initially with therapeutic anticoagulation followed by evaluation for endovascular intervention (see Chapter 86). In patients with ALF caused by hepatic ischemia, treatment is directed to reversal of the underlying cause of ischemia, which may include severe congestive heart failure, drug-induced hypotension, sepsis, and hypoxia.[11,59] LT in these patients is seldom indicated.[11]

PREVENTION, RECOGNITION, AND EARLY TREATMENT OF COMPLICATIONS

Initial symptoms in patients with ALF are usually nonspecific, including fatigue, malaise, nausea/vomiting, anorexia, right upper quadrant tenderness, pruritus, and jaundice.[60] When the metabolic and detoxification function of liver become impaired, the signs of ALF emerge, including jaundice, encephalopathy, coagulopathy, hemodynamic instability, acute lung injury/acute respiratory distress syndrome (ARDS), renal failure, sepsis, and metabolic disturbances.

Hepatic Encephalopathy

HE is a major defining criterion of ALF in the adult population (see Chapters 77 and 78). Children, particularly younger children, do not demonstrate classic features of HE, which has resulted in a revision of the definition of ALF for this specific patient population to include pediatric patients with advanced coagulopathy (INR ≥2.0), regardless of their mental status.[61] Neurologic findings in patients with ALF are variable, ranging from minimal changes in behavior to coma. Severity of HE can be graded into four stages according to the New Haven criteria (see Box 107.1 and Chapter 106). Overall prognosis for patients with only grade I or II HE is good, whereas that for patients with grade III or IV HE is much poorer. Irreversible neurologic damage is uncommon in ALF, but neuropsychiatric disturbances may persist, and warrant follow-up after recovery of liver function.[62]

The severity of HE is related to the occurrence of cerebral edema and ICH. Cerebral edema is a devastating consequence of ALF and may be associated with a decrease in intracerebral perfusion, along with the potential risks of brainstem herniation and death.[63] Cerebral edema is uncommon in patients with grade I or II HE, but it is present in 25% to 35% of those with grade III HE and in approximately 75% of those with grade IV HE.[64] Cerebral edema can also lead to ischemia and hypoxic injury to the brain. Usually, cerebral ischemia occurs when the cerebral perfusion pressure (CPP)—mean arterial pressure (MAP) minus ICP—falls below 40 to 50 mm Hg. The presence of the classic signs of elevated ICP (systemic hypertension, bradycardia, irregular respiration) carries a poor prognosis. These late manifestations, which may be absent or difficult to detect, are not a reliable guide for therapeutic intervention.

The incidence of ICH is variably reported, although it appears to be progressively less frequent. Data from 3300 patients seen at a single tertiary liver center showed that the proportion of patients with ICH fell from 76% in 1984 to 1988 to 20% in 2004 to 2008 ($P < .0001$). In those who developed ICH, mortality decreased from 95% to 55% ($P < .0001$). This mirrored a decrease in the admission markers of disease severity and most likely reflects earlier illness recognition, improved intensive care, and use of salvage LT.[31]

Seizure activity is common in ALF, further increases ICP, and should be expeditiously treated with phenytoin or short-acting benzodiazepines.[11,65] Seizures can be difficult to detect clinically, especially when patients are intubated, as demonstrated in a trial that investigated subclinical seizure activity with electroencephalography and found 32% of patients were affected.[66] Two RCTs in patients with ALF and advanced HE came to different conclusions with regard to the efficacy of phenytoin in seizure prevention and survival.[66,67] Evidence to support prophylactic treatment in patients with high-grade HE caused by ALF is lacking and therefore prophylactic phenytoin is not recommended.

Although precise pathogenic mechanisms of HE in ALF remain unclear, there is evidence that both systemic and local inflammation, as well as circulating neurotoxins, particularly ammonia, play a pivotal role. Cytotoxic and vasogenic cerebral edema have been implicated in ALF, with experimental data favoring cytotoxic mechanisms.[68] Classic theories involve the development of astrocyte swelling and cerebral hemodynamic derangements, characterized by high cerebral blood flow and failure of cerebral autoregulation in response to changes in MAP.[69,70] Loss of cerebral autoregulation of blood flow has been related to the rapid occurrence of electrolyte disorders in ALF, in contrast to cirrhosis or even in subacute liver failure, in which the mechanisms of osmotic regulation are still active. Cerebral edema is more prevalent among patients with hyperacute liver failure compared with subacute disease, probably as a result of the rapid accumulation of glutamine that overwhelms the mechanisms of compensatory expulsion of organic osmolytes from the astrocytes. High serum ammonia concentrations (>150–200 µmol/L) also increase the risk of cerebral edema, although the relationship between ammonia and ICP is not linear.[71–73]

Recent work suggests a central role of proinflammatory cytokines (tumor necrosis factor [TNF]-α, interleukin [IL]-6, IL-1β) in patients with uncontrolled ICP, indicating activation of the inflammatory cascade in the brain.[74] Dysregulation of cerebrovascular tone as a result of the inflammatory response causes cerebral hyperperfusion, which may result in cerebral edema, ICH, and HE.[75] Variables predictive of progression of

ICH and HE are the Model for End-Stage Liver Disease (MELD) score, alone or in combination with ammonia levels, age, requirement for vasopressors and renal replacement therapy, and the presence of infection and/or systemic inflammatory response syndrome (SIRS).[71,76] There is also evidence emphasizing the importance of free-radical formation occurring at a mitochondrial level as the potential mediator of cellular dysfunction induced by ammonia neurotoxicity.[77]

Basic interventions for the management of cerebral edema should be applied universally in patients with high-grade HE. These include elevation of the head of the bed to 30 degrees, except if CPP falls below 30 mm Hg, in which case the patient should preferably be put in the supine position. The neck should be maintained in a neutral position with endotracheal intubation and mechanical ventilation in grade III to IV HE, painful stimuli should be minimized, and arterial hypertension adequately controlled.[78] In agitated patients, propofol is a reasonable choice for sedation because it may protect from ICH. Factors that increase ICP need to be avoided and include hypercapnia, hyponatremia, frequent movements, neck vein compression, fluid overload, fever, hypoxia, coughing, sneezing, seizures, and endotracheal suctioning. Fever increases ICP and should be vigorously treated with cooling measures. Hypo-osmolality, specifically hyponatremia, should be avoided and corrected immediately. Spontaneous hyperventilation, which occurs regularly in patients with ALF and results in mild hypocapnia, promoting cerebrovascular constriction should not be inhibited.[79,80] However, $PaCO_2$ levels less than 30 mm Hg can worsen cerebral ischemia and cause rebound cerebral edema.[81] Therefore a $PaCO_2$ of between 30 and 40 mm Hg should be targeted.[82] In ALF patients at high risk for cerebral edema, including serum ammonia greater than 150 μmol/L, grade III to IV HE, acute renal failure, or vasopressor requirement to maintain arterial pressure, prophylactic induction of hypernatremia with hypertonic saline targeting a sodium level of 145 to 155 mEq/L is recommended.[11]

Because the most accepted pathogenetic theory of HE is the increased production of nitrogenous substances in the gut lumen, medical management of cerebral edema in a patient with ALF has focused on reducing the generation and absorption of these products through orally administered lactulose and/or nonabsorbable antibiotics (e.g., rifaximin). However, the ability of these modalities to lower the risk of cerebral edema in patients with ALF has not been tested. Further, the utility of oral lactulose in this setting is controversial[83] and may even have detrimental effects,[31,84] increasing gaseous distension of the bowel, favoring aspiration in patients with advanced HE, and fostering intravascular depletion. Also, lactulose may affect the surgical field by increasing bowel distension during LT. Continuous venovenous hemofiltration or intermittent hemodialysis for clearance of ammonia in cases where the serum ammonia level is three times the upper limit of normal or if the patient has high-grade HE has been recommended.[85] However, the recommendation is by expert opinion only as data on outcomes are limited.

The monitoring of ICP by using an intracranial sensor is controversial.[63,86] Its use has been recommended in centers with expertise in ICP monitoring in patients with grade IV HE or in patients with grade III HE that is rapidly progressing, given the difficulty in accurately following increased ICP based on clinical examination only. Currently, ICP monitoring is used by more than half of transplantation programs in the US and worldwide.[87,88] Major complications are bleeding and infection. Complication rates vary among the different types of catheters used. There is a growing body of evidence to support the use of intraparenchymal monitoring, with several small studies reporting symptomatic intracranial hemorrhage rates of between 0% and 7%.[89-92] However, the use of ICP monitoring in patients with ALF remains contentious and the local expertise with each catheter should be considered when choosing a specific procedure. In all cases, insertion should be done cautiously, and coagulation defects should be corrected before such a procedure. Alternative noninvasive modalities are being evaluated but have thus far not been proven to be reliable methods for measuring ICP. In the absence of ICP monitoring, frequent neurologic evaluation is recommended to identify early evidence of ICH.

A computed tomography (CT) scan of the head is recommended in patients with progression of HE or who experience an abrupt change in mental status, and before ICP monitor placement, to rule out any other rare intracranial pathology, especially bleeding. Therapy should be targeted toward maintenance of the ICP below 20 mm Hg and the CPP above 60 mm Hg.[11]

The development of ICH despite prophylactic measures should prompt urgent treatment. First-line therapy includes increasing blood osmolality, either with a mannitol bolus (0.5–1.0 g/kg body weight) and/or hypertonic saline boluses, which draw water from swollen astrocytes back into the intravascular space. When renal failure with oliguria is present, mannitol can be deleterious, so continuous venovenous hemofiltration or hemodialysis with polyacrylonitrile membranes is performed to decrease hyperkalemia, fluid overload, and ICP.

If no response or relapse of ICH is observed after mannitol administration, alternative measures include the use of hypertonic saline boluses, induction of therapeutic hypothermia, sedation with propofol,[93] short-acting barbiturates,[94] or IV boluses of indomethacin.[95] Indomethacin perfusion (25 mg IV for every peak of ICP) has been shown to normalize CPP and ICP, probably through direct arteriolar constriction of cerebral vessels.[96] Induction of moderate hypothermia to a core body temperature of 34°C to 35°C is useful in treating uncontrolled ICH as a bridge to LT.[97-100] There is concern over potential deleterious effects of hypothermia on the risk of infection, coagulation disorders, cardiac arrhythmias, and liver regeneration rates.[101] In patients with ICH refractory to all medical measures, total hepatectomy has been advocated to remove the major source of the proinflammatory cytokines that contribute to cerebral hemodynamic derangements.

Coagulopathy

In addition to neurologic changes, coagulopathy is also a major criterion of ALF, resulting from inadequate hepatic synthesis and increased consumption of clotting factors (see Chapters 77 and 78). There is also reduced clearance of both activated factors and factor inhibitor complexes, as well as quantitative and qualitative platelet dysfunction.[102] However, serum concentrations of thrombopoietin do not correlate with platelet counts,[103] and the pathogenesis of thrombocytopenia remains unclear. Affected patients characteristically have low fibrinogen and low levels of factors II, V, VII, IX, and X, resulting in the prolongation of PT and partial thromboplastin time (PTT).[104]

Although low-grade fibrinolysis and intravascular coagulation may occur, these syndromes are difficult to distinguish from the changes caused by failure of hepatic synthesis alone.[105] In patients with ALF, 81% had moderate (INR 1.5–5), 14%

severe (INR 5–10), and 5% very severe (INR >10) coagulopathy. Certain etiologies are associated with greater severity of coagulopathy, whereas ALF in fatty liver of pregnancy presents the least severe coagulopathy.[106]

Despite evidence of a bleeding diathesis in patients with ALF, spontaneous bleeding is unusual, most common in the gastrointestinal (GI) tract (8%). Spontaneous intracranial bleeding is exceedingly rare (<1%) in the absence of an ICP monitor. The incidence of upper GI bleeding in ALF patients has been shown to be decreased by gastric acid suppression with IV histamine-2 receptor antagonists.[107] Therefore prophylaxis with IV histamine-2 blockers, proton pump inhibitors, or sucralfate as a second-line agent is recommended for prevention of gastric acid–related GI bleeding associated with stress.[11]

Vitamin K should be routinely administered for patients with ALF because vitamin K deficiency for this patient population has been reported.[108] Prophylactic administration of fresh frozen plasma (FFP) is not recommended because it has not been proven to influence mortality, can interfere with assessment of liver function, and may worsen cerebral edema.[109] FFP is only indicated in the setting of active hemorrhage or before invasive procedures. Use of recombinant human factor VIIa (rFVIIa) has been evaluated in small pilot studies[91,110–112] and was associated with improvement or normalization of PT and bleeding control, although risk of secondary thrombosis has been reported.[113] It has also been suggested that the combination of rFVIIa with FFP is superior to FFP alone in correcting coagulopathy, with an additional beneficial effect on morbidity and mortality.[114] Larger controlled studies are still required. It has become acceptable to administer rFVIIa before invasive procedures with a high risk of bleeding (e.g., transjugular liver biopsy, ICP monitor placement) in circumstances in which FFP has failed to correct PT/INR to an acceptable level, or the patient has become volume overloaded.

Routine administration of platelets to correct thrombocytopenia is not recommended and the threshold for platelet transfusion in patients with ALF has not been studied. If invasive procedures are required and/or for patients who develop significant bleeding, transfusion to a platelet count of at least 50,000/mm³ has been recommended.[11,102] In follow-up of ALF patients, serial determinations of INR and factor V provide useful prognostic information.

Infections

Patients with ALF have enhanced susceptibility to infections and sepsis because of deficient opsonization caused by a reduction in factors such as fibronectin, opsonins, and chemoattractants, including components of the complement system[115] (see Chapters 77 and 78). Additionally, patients have an increase in bacterial translocation, white blood cell dysfunction, Kupffer cell dysfunction, and a high requirement for invasive procedures. It has been emphasized that mediators as a part of SIRS induces a compensatory anti-inflammatory response, resulting in a true immunosuppressive state, favoring infection and the development of sepsis.[3] The impact of infection in ALF is significant because it inhibits hepatic regeneration, induces progression of HE and renal failure, reduces the successful rate of LT, and increases multi-organ failure. Bacteriologically proven infection has been recorded in up to 80% of patients with ALF and fungal infection in 32%, predominantly with *Candida* species. The most common sites of infection are the respiratory tract (47%), urinary tract (22%), bacteremia with (12%) or

without (15%) a recognized infecting source, and indwelling catheters (4%). Gram-positive organisms, mainly streptococci and *Staphylococcus aureus*, predominate in ALF, suggesting that entry through the skin is more important than intestinal entry, the pathway of gram-negative organisms.[116] Leukocytosis and fever are frequently absent (<50%), and a high index of suspicion for active infection should surround the worsening of HE, renal function, or clinical status. Periodic surveillance cultures and chest radiographs have been strongly recommended to detect bacterial and fungal pathogens as early as possible.

Prophylactic antibiotic regimens have shown little benefit.[76,117] However, a low threshold for starting appropriate antibiotics or antifungals should be maintained. Administration of antibiotics should be started promptly when infection or the likelihood of impending sepsis is high, surveillance cultures reveal significant isolates, there is clinical progression of HE or renal failure, refractory hypotension is present, or when any component of SIRS develops.[84] Broad-spectrum coverage for gram-positive and gram-negative bacteria, such as with a third-generation cephalosporin, should be chosen with consideration of patient-specific isolates from surveillance cultures and historical hospital-specific isolates or antibiograms. Vancomycin is specifically recommended in all patients with possible IV catheter–related sepsis or risk factors for infection with methicillin-resistant *Staphylococcus aureus*. An antifungal agent also is recommended in any patient without prompt improvement in signs of infection or persistent fever after initiation of antibacterial agents.[84] A finding of disseminated fungemia is predictive of a poor prognosis.[118]

Hemodynamic Complications

ALF is characterized by a hyperdynamic circulation with high cardiac output, low MAP, and low systemic vascular resistance (see Chapters 77, 78, and 106).[119] Increased nitric oxide (NO) production and cyclic guanosine monophosphate (cGMP) may be involved in these hemodynamic disturbances. Generalized systemic vasodilation is not limited to the splanchnic circulation, as typically occurs in patients with chronic liver disease.[120,121] Because of poor oral intake, transudation of fluid into the extravascular space, and GI bleeding (when present), most patients with ALF are volume-depleted and require initial fluid resuscitation and maintenance of adequate intravascular volume on presentation. The treatment of hypotension should involve IV infusion of normal saline initially, changed to half-normal saline containing 75 mEq/L sodium bicarbonate if acidotic, before considering the use of vasopressors.[122] Patients with ALF may have such greatly deranged circulation that volume status becomes difficult to assess; thus placement of monitoring devices to provide information about changes in hemodynamic parameters may be helpful because management of fluid balance can be complicated by elevated ICP and renal dysfunction. After adequate fluid replacement and treatment of infection and sepsis if present, vasopressors may also be required to maintain an adequate MAP (≥75 mm Hg) and to ensure sufficient CPP. The MAP should be maintained in a narrow range to achieve a CPP of 60 to 80 mm Hg to prevent cerebral hypoperfusion and to minimize further cerebral hyperemia. Vasopressin or its analogue terlipressin can be added to potentiate the effects of norepinephrine in refractory cases but should be used cautiously in severely encephalopathic patients with ICH. Patients with persistent uncorrectable hypotension after volume repletion and vasopressor administration should be evaluated for adrenal insufficiency, which occurs frequently in this setting and can be corrected with a stress dose of hydrocortisone, 200 to 300 mg/day in divided doses.[123] Total hepatectomy has been advocated based on anecdotal references as a terminal salvage therapy in patients with severe refractory circulatory dysfunction.

Acute Renal Failure

The incidence of acute renal failure in ALF is as high as 50% to 80% when an increase in creatinine concentrations is taken as a diagnostic criterion, and oliguria is a common finding.[109,124-126] However, normal creatinine concentrations do not exclude the presence of acute renal failure and therefore the true incidence of renal compromise is probably underestimated. Acute renal failure resembling hepatorenal syndrome (HRS; see Chapters 77, 78, and 106) is multifactorial in the setting of ALF and results mainly from two different situations. First, direct nephrotoxic effects of some etiologies of ALF, as observed with APAP,[127] nonsteroidal antiinflammatory drugs (NSAIDs), or *Amanita* mushroom intoxication,[128,129] usually result in acute tubular necrosis. Second, patients may present with dehydration or experience renal failure that resembles the HRS of cirrhosis, resulting in acute tubular necrosis caused by ischemia from hypotension. The pathogenesis remains unclear, even though the marked reduction in renal blood flow and glomerular filtration rate (GFR) is similar to renal perfusion changes in cirrhosis, with pronounced renal arteriolar vasoconstriction caused by loss of systemic vascular resistance, activation of compensatory vasoconstrictor systems, and reduced renal prostaglandin excretion. However, ALF has distinctive hemodynamic features and only rarely is the degree of portal hypertension in ALF comparable to that of HRS in patients with cirrhosis.[130] Mean reported hepatic venous pressure gradients for patients with ALF and renal dysfunction is significantly lower compared with patients with cirrhosis and HRS (14 vs. 21 mm Hg).[130,131] In addition, development of abdominal compartment syndrome, caused by ascites, intra-abdominal hemorrhage, or severe abdominal and gut wall edema, is a common cause of renal impairment in ALF.

Early recognition of renal failure has important clinical implications, and once established, it is usually progressive and associated with increased mortality.[132-134] Treatment options without transplantation are limited, and preventive measures are restricted to early identification, maintenance of adequate hemodynamics, early diagnosis and adequate treatment of infection, and avoidance of nephrotoxic agents (i.e., NSAIDs, aminoglycosides). Worsening renal failure needs to be addressed early with renal replacement therapy to correct intravascular fluid overload, electrolyte disorders, and acidosis. Potential triggers for initiation might be low urine output, a rise in creatinine levels more than 0.3 mg/dL over baseline, or rise in serum ammonia above 150 μmol/L.[122]

Continuous rather than intermittent modes of renal replacement are usually preferred to avoid abrupt shifts in solute concentrations that can result in increased ICP.[135,136] Additionally, most patients with ALF tolerate intermittent hemodialysis poorly as a result of circulatory instability.[137]

Pulmonary Complications

Recently, with improved critical care and judicious use of IV fluids, the incidence of acute lung injury has decreased from 30% to approximately 20%.[124,138] ARDS is not uncommon and may involve severe multi-organ dysfunction, particularly a requirement for vasopressors.[139] Impaired gas exchange, leading to hypoxemia and mixed acidosis, may favor progression of hepatic encephalopathy.[70,140] Mechanical ventilation may be required to ensure oxygenation and to secure the airway in patients who progress to grade III HE. However, caution should be used to maintain the lowest level of positive end-expiratory pressure (PEEP) that achieves adequate oxygenation because high levels may exacerbate cerebral edema and hepatic congestion.[124] In patients with APAP intoxication, acute lung injury and ARDS can occur in one-third of patients and cause intractable hypoxemia that may contribute to death (see Chapters 77, 78, and 106).[79]

Metabolic Disturbances

Common metabolic abnormalities in ALF include acid-base and electrolyte disorders, hypophosphatemia, and hypoglycemia. Among acid-base disorders, hypocapnia with mixed alkalosis is common in the early stages, occurring in more than 50% of patients.[141] As ALF progresses, patients typically evolve to metabolic acidosis with respiratory alkalosis. ALF is a catabolic state characterized by a negative nitrogen balance and an increased resting energy expenditure. Patients are particularly prone to hypoglycemia as a result of hepatocyte necrosis that generates glycogen depletion, as well as defective glycogenolysis and gluconeogenesis (see Chapters 77 and 78).

Rapid development of hypoglycemia, which can confound HE, should be managed with continuous IV glucose infusion.[142] However, hyperglycemia should be avoided because it may contribute to poor ICP control. Metabolic homeostasis should be carefully maintained and overall nutritional status, as well as phosphate, glucose, potassium, and magnesium levels, should be frequently monitored and supplemented.[18] Low systemic blood pressure and poor systemic microcirculation result in a buildup of lactate, a complication that may be exacerbated by the lack of lactate metabolism in the failing liver. Correction of hyperlactatemia is important because it can affect circulatory function and aggravate cerebral hyperemia. Enteral nutrition should be administered early whenever possible, avoiding excessive free-water that can result in hypo-osmolality and worsen cerebral edema. There is no firm evidence that branched-chain amino acids are superior to other enteral preparations.[133,143] Severe protein restriction should be avoided, and a normal protein intake of approximately 1 g/kg/day is reasonable in most cases.[144] If enteral feeding is contraindicated, parenteral nutrition remains an option.

DISTINGUISHING PATIENTS WHO WILL IMPROVE SPONTANEOUSLY FROM THOSE WHO WILL NEED LIVER TRANSPLANTATION

Deciding when to proceed with LT is the most challenging aspect of management in ALF. Orthotopic LT (OLT) remains the only definitive treatment for patients with proven irreversible liver injury who are unable to achieve sufficient hepatic regeneration. Approximately half of patients admitted with ALF will receive an LT worldwide.[145] The decision to proceed with LT depends on the identification of patients with no medical or psychiatric contraindications who have no chance to recover before the development of complications that render the procedure futile because of irreversible brain injury, multi-organ failure, or sepsis. There is only a very narrow window for the application of OLT to avoid unnecessary transplants in patients who would spontaneously recover and to avoid LT in those who would not survive.[146]

ALF accounts for approximately 8% of LT activity in Europe and the US.[147,148] Unfortunately, currently available prognostic scoring systems do not adequately predict outcome or determine candidacy for LT. It has been recognized that among patients listed for LT for ALF, 15% to 20% will recover spontaneously without need for grafting and approximately 15% to 25% will die or be removed from the waiting list because of disease progression.[35,149,150] It is likely that some patients with ALF are transplanted needlessly, although data for "overtransplantation" rates are lacking.[33] Generally, the highest rate of spontaneous transplant-free survival is observed in patients with hyperacute liver failure, whereas the worst survival is observed in slowly evolving disease (subacute liver failure).[151]

Prognostic Factors

Several prognostic indicators have been suggested to allow early identification and listing of those patients who would otherwise not survive without LT. The most important factors include the degree of HE, age, and etiology of ALF, reflecting the relevance of the severity of hepatic injury and the likelihood of reversal of the underlying process. Spontaneous recovery is more likely in patients with grade I or II HE (65%–70%; see Chapter 106), whereas a higher degree of HE on admission represents a significant independent variable of poor outcome, with recovery in less than 20% of patients who progress to coma.[133]

Outcome in children is more favorable (see Chapter 110).[152] In the series of Dhiman and colleagues, the survival rate in patients older than 50 years was lower than in younger patients.[153] However, ages younger than 10 and older than 40 years are also considered adverse markers of outcome. The lowest survival rate (33%) corresponds to patients older than 65 years, probably related to more comorbidities and less APAP intoxication. Reevaluating outcome in older patients, Schiodt and colleagues observed superior overall survival (OS) in younger compared with older patients (67.9% vs. 48.2%; $P < .001$), yet no significant differences were demonstrated in spontaneous survival among both groups, suggesting that hepatic regeneration is preserved in elderly patients, which is in accordance with the rise in α-fetoprotein (AFP) levels that is similar in both populations.[154]

The likelihood of spontaneous recovery is not uniform and depends on the etiology of the insult. In a study of 315 patients listed for LT, spontaneous survival was higher in patients with hepatitis A virus (HAV) infection (43%), followed by APAP overdose (31%), hepatitis B virus (HBV) infection (8%), indeterminate origin (7%), and other drug-induced ALF (0%).[155] More recent data evaluating prognosis of indeterminate liver failure showed no significant difference with other etiologies.[156] In other series, the same favorable prognosis corresponds to APAP overdose, HAV infection, and pregnancy-related ALF but not to patients with an indeterminate cause, non-APAP-related ALF, HBV infection, autoimmune hepatitis, Wilson disease, or Budd-Chiari syndrome.[5,157]

Several other variables have been identified as potential predictors of prognosis, including severity of coagulopathy, PT/INR ratio, arterial ammonia levels, high body mass index (BMI),[158] and genetic polymorphisms.[159] AFP levels, arterial ketone body ratio, arterial pH, hyperbilirubinemia, renal dysfunction, serum phosphate level, the presence of SIRS,[160,161] surrogate markers

of cell death, and the extent of parenchymal necrosis on biopsies have also been proposed to predict probability, although their predictive accuracy has not been well validated.

The chronologic evolution of the clinical course of ALF, estimated by the interval between onset of jaundice and encephalopathy, has also proven to be predictive of clinical features and outcome.[141] Bernuau and colleagues have made the distinction between *fulminant* (interval <2 weeks) and *subfulminant* hepatitis (interval 2 weeks to 3 months),[162] whereas the group at King's College Hospital (KCH) in London has defined three groups of patients: those seen with *hyperacute* liver failure (development of HE within 7 days after jaundice), *acute* liver failure (7–28 days), or *subacute* liver failure (28 days to 3 months).[151] Hyperacute presentation is more frequently associated with hepatitis A or APAP overdose, whereas idiosyncratic drug reactions usually present with a delayed-onset clinical course. Cerebral edema is more frequent in hyperacute liver failure, but it is rare in subfulminant disease. In contrast, manifestations of portal hypertension with ascites and renal failure are much more common in patients with subfulminant liver failure. The cessation of liver cell destruction, rather than the occurrence of liver regeneration, appears to be the most critical variable governing outcome.[163] The protracted course in patients with subfulminant presentation is associated with persistence of elevated transaminases, suggesting persistence of liver cell destruction.

Independent coagulation factor activities are significant indicators of prognosis. Several small studies have implicated factors V and VII as potential prognostic markers.[164-166] Plasma protein actin-free Gc globulin, a member of the extracellular scavenger system synthesized by the liver, was decreased in patients who died or required LT for ALF and correlates with poor survival.[167]

Serum AFP levels increase in patients undergoing rapid liver regeneration, and increasing levels indicate a better prognosis.[168] More recently, a high level of soluble CD163 (from activated macrophages) has been proposed to predict mortality in patients with ALF.[169] Interestingly, Volkmann and colleagues found that caspase activation (which increases IL-6 and TNF-α levels) is associated with spontaneous recovery.[170] Detectable liver atrophy has been classically associated with a poor prognosis. Yamagishi and colleagues reported that the ratio of estimated to standard liver volume (SLV) reflected the prognosis of patients with ALF.[171] They investigated the usefulness of the ratio of CT-derived liver volume to the calculated SLV to establish a new prognostic formula to predict the course of ALF. The sensitivity was 94.1% and specificity 76.9%, but the findings of this small study need to be confirmed in a larger series.

Prognostic Scores

In an attempt to identify patients who are likely to benefit from LT, several models have been developed combining diverse prognostic factors to improve accuracy (see Chapter 4). Unfortunately, many of these models are methodologically flawed and subject to bias.[172] The King's College Criteria[133] are based on a retrospective cohort of 588 patients with medically managed ALF and were later validated in a prospective study of 175 patients. The criteria are widely used to assess the severity of ALF and the potential variability of prognosis, with a sensitivity of 68% to 69% and specificity of 82% to 92% (Box 107.3). The King's College Criteria are etiology based, with predictors stratified according to whether ALF was secondary to APAP ingestion. In patients with APAP-induced ALF, a pH less than 7.3 at 24 hours or more after overdose is an indication for LT (after appropriate volume replacement and correction of hypothermia). Otherwise, LT should be considered in the presence of all three of the following factors: PT greater than 100 seconds, grade III/IV HE, and serum creatinine greater than 300 µmol/L. In non-APAP-related ALF, the decision is based on the presence of at least three of the criteria listed in Box 107.3.[133,173] Addition of arterial lactate levels[174] and serum phosphate concentrations[175] in patients with APAP-induced ALF has been proposed to improve sensitivity of the criteria and identifies patients in need of earlier OLT. Generally, the King's College Criteria are useful in predicting death, but the absence of these criteria is not predictive of survival.

The Clichy/Villejuif criteria were initially developed in a cohort of French patients with acute HBV infection.[176] A serum factor V level of less than 20% in patients younger than 30 years or less than 30% in any patient with grade III to IV HE predicted mortality with a positive predictive value of 82% and a negative predictive value of 98%.[164,176,177] Factor V level measurements are less readily available than the measures in the King's College Criteria, and subsequent studies have shown these criteria to be less accurate than the King's College Criteria in predicting outcome.[178,179]

In patients with non-APAP-induced ALF, the MELD score has been proposed as a significant predictor of OS, whereas patients with ALF of other etiologies experienced a high rate of spontaneous recovery that was independent of MELD score.[180] Other studies suggest MELD scores obtained on admission may be helpful to establish the optimal timing for pre-OLT evaluation and listing.[181] In a recent systematic review and meta-analysis comparing the ability of the King's College Criteria and the MELD score to predict hospital mortality in patients with ALF, the King's College Criteria was found to be more accurate for patients with APAP-induced ALF, whereas the MELD score was more accurate for patients with non-APAP-induced ALF.[182] Overall pooled estimates of sensitivity and specificity for the King's College Criteria were 59% (95% confidence interval [CI] 56%–62%) and 79% (95% CI 77%–81%),

respectively, and for the MELD score were 74% (95% CI 71%–77%) and 67% (95% CI 64%–69%), respectively. The authors note there was significant heterogeneity among the 23 included studies and conclude that neither prognostic tool is optimal for predicting mortality in patients with ALF.

Other systems, such as the Acute Physiology and Chronic Health Evaluation (APACHE) II score and Sequential Organ Failure Assessment (SOFA),[183] have also been used to determine the prognosis in ALF. In a study of 87 patients, the sensitivity and specificity of the King's College Criteria, MELD score ($\geq$32), and APACHE II (cut-off scores of 8.5–18.5) and APACHE III (cut-off scores of 80–90) scores were determined and were unsatisfactory for all prognostic systems.[184]

Rutherford and colleagues developed a prognostic index (ALFSG index) for ALF based on the level of M30 (a cleavage product of cytokeratin-18 caspase, indicative of apoptotic hepatocyte cell death).[185,186] The ALFSG index is a prognostic model created using stepwise logistic regression, which predicted need for LT or death in ALF combining three classes of variables: clinical (coma grade), laboratory (INR, serum bilirubin, phosphorus), and a marker of apoptosis (M30). This model has a sensitivity of 85.6% and specificity of 64.7%. The ALFSG index is broadly applicable across the many etiologies of ALF. The contribution of a marker of hepatocyte apoptosis to outcome supports consideration of caspase inhibitors to treat ALF.

Currently available prognostic scoring systems do not adequately predict outcome or determine candidacy for LT. Reliance entirely on these guidelines is thus not recommended.[11] Whether or not patients are listed for LT, they should be monitored for the many complications of ALF while they progress to the point of recovery, death, or LT. Likewise, patients listed for LT may develop complications that preclude this intervention or may occasionally show unexpected signs of recovery before a donor organ becomes available. In this dynamic process, the final decision on LT is made when an organ is available.

PROGNOSIS

Contraindications to LT, such as substance abuse, suicidal ideation, psychiatric disorders, uncontrollable sepsis, and other organ system involvement (irreversible brain damage, extrahepatic malignancy, cardiovascular failure requiring >1 µg/kg/min norepinephrine infusion, ARDS requiring Fio_2 >60% and PEEP >12 cm H_2O) should be identified and patients excluded from consideration for LT (see Chapter 105). Neurologic limits to LT are controversial, although evidence of brain death, uncontrolled systemic sepsis, and hemodynamic instability from multi-organ failure are considered absolute contraindications for LT.

Survival rates at 1 year of patients undergoing OLT for ALF range between 61% and 76% and are 7% to 15% less than in patients transplanted for chronic end-stage liver disease.[147,187] This occurs in part because of the extreme emergency conditions often encountered and when LT is achieved, patients eventually die because of the poor condition at the moment of LT (i.e., brain damage, sepsis, or multi-organ failure) or because of the use of marginal or ABO-incompatible (ABO-I) donor organs.[188,189] After the first year, this trend is reversed, and ALF patients have a better long-term survival. The retransplantation rate in patients with ALF is higher because of the use of marginal or ABO-I organs, leading to increasing rates of acute rejection, primary graft nonfunction, and intrahepatic biliary strictures. In the KCH experience of more than 3300 patients treated between 1973 and 2008, the hospital survival rate increased from 16.7% to 62.2%. There was an improvement in survival after LT, from 66% to 86%, and transplant-free survival also increased to 48%. This improved survival was most apparent in APAP-related ALF and absent in cases of indeterminate causation.[190]

There is evidence that the effects of neurologic and infectious complications of ALF extend into the post-transplant period, given the gap in survival rates in ALF compared with elective LT. The contribution from neurologic causes to mortality rates was 13% in a single-center UK study.[191] The European Liver Transplant Registry (ETLR) and United Network for Organ Sharing (UNOS) data attribute death to infection in 18% to 24% of cases, with an additional 5.6% linked to fungal infection in the UNOS study.[148,192]

PREOPERATIVE MANAGEMENT
(SEE CHAPTERS 26 AND 106)

Once the need for an LT is established, organ allocation systems generally give patients with ALF very accelerated priority, and as a consequence, the majority of patients are transplanted within 4 days of being placed on the waiting list.[193] The primary goal while awaiting liver availability is to maintain all other organ function and correct any reversible physiologic abnormalities. As previously described, etiology-specific therapy should be initiated, MAP should be maintained at 75 mm Hg or greater to achieve a CPP of at least 60 mm Hg, GI acid-suppression prophylaxis and vitamin K should be administered, electrolyte and metabolic abnormalities should be corrected, and infection surveillance should be continued.

INTRAOPERATIVE CONSIDERATIONS
(SEE CHAPTERS 25 AND 106)

In 1993 Ringe and colleagues described the two-stage total hepatectomy with a temporary portacaval shunt as a procedure carried out in patients who have "toxic liver syndrome" with cerebral edema or multi-organ failure.[194] The patient is left anhepatic and subsequently undergoes LT. Although this extreme procedure can be lifesaving for ALF patients with toxic liver syndrome, it is exceptional.[195] The physiologic basis for its success in case reports is related to a decrease in the serum concentration of circulating proinflammatory cytokines (IL-1, IL-6, TNF-α) after hepatectomy.[196]

Specific intraoperative considerations in ALF include severe coagulopathy, hemodynamic instability, a potentially elevated ICP, and the absence of portal hypertension. Without portal hypertension, total clamping of the inferior vena cava (IVC) and the portal vein (PV) is poorly tolerated. Therefore it is often necessary to perform venovenous bypass or to preserve the IVC using the "piggyback technique." Additionally, performing a temporary portocaval anastomosis facilitates liver mobilization without changing the hemodynamic state that could otherwise increase the ICP (see Chapters 84, 124, and 125).

Careful anesthetic management of the patient is necessary: the operating table should be positioned at 30 degrees and variations in ICP should be carefully controlled; measures to avoid an increase in ICP should be taken to protect the brain.

ICP monitoring should be maintained for 24 hours after LT because ICP may increase after surgery.[197] Longer monitoring is required in cases of poor graft function. Given the urgency of this procedure, marginal donors (steatotic livers, livers from nonheart-beating deceased donors, ABO-mismatched grafts) are often accepted, thus increasing the risk of poor function or primary nonfunction.

ABO-I LT has been considered to be a formidable challenge in LT surgery because of the increased risk of infection, antibody-mediated rejection, and consequent vascular and biliary complications. The main reason for poor survival was anti-A or anti-B antibody–mediated rejection, which induced a high incidence of hepatic necrosis and intrahepatic biliary complications.[198] Shen and colleagues from China described a new treatment consisting of rituximab (a novel monoclonal anti-CD20 antibody that depletes B cells and prevents antibody production)[199] and IV immunoglobulin (IVIG) alone.[200] A total of 35 patients with ALF received ABO-I livers and were compared with 66 patients who received ABO-compatible livers; the 3-year cumulative patient survival and graft survival rates were 83.1% and 80.0% and 86.3% and 86.3%, respectively ($P > .05$). The final decision on when to use an ABO-I graft depends on the transplant team.

LIVING-DONOR LIVER TRANSPLANTATION

Although it is generally agreed that recipient disease indications for living-donor liver transplantation (LDLT) should be similar to deceased-donor liver transplantation (DDLT), ALF is a controversial indication for several reasons. First, initial reports showed inferior outcomes with LDLT in highly urgent situations. Second, in countries where deceased organ donation is well developed, recipients have a higher chance of receiving a graft on time (high priority on the list). Finally, there are serious concerns regarding donor coercion in such urgent situations and the limited time for thorough evaluations could increase the risk for donors (see Chapter 109).

The use of LDLT for children with ALF has gradually gained acceptance because the lifesaving potential of the procedure far outweighs any ethical concerns.[201,202] Expansion of LDLT to adult patients with ALF has been reported.[203,204] However, both donor risk and the ethical risk of coercion are concerns in this situation because most potential donors are likely to be brothers, sisters, children, or spouses, who are influenced by the imminent death of the patient. On the other hand, compared with DDLT grafts, live-donor grafts offer some advantages: (1) early transplantation of ALF patients, (2) better graft function, and (3) shorter cold-ischemia time.

There is growing evidence to refute the suggestion that partial grafts from living donors are marginal and may result in inferior outcomes for high-urgency patients with ALF. Urrunaga and colleagues examined post-transplant outcomes of adults with ALF undergoing LDLT and DDLT in the United States, analyzing Organ and Procurement and Transplantation Network (OPTN) data for adults with ALF listed as status 1 who underwent LDLT ($n = 21$) or DDLT ($n = 2316$).[205] No strong evidence could be found that the survival probabilities for adults with ALF who underwent LDLT were inferior to those who underwent DDLT. Although this report describes the largest US study of patients receiving LDLT for ALF, the number of patients is small, representing only 0.9% of all patients transplanted for ALF. We suggest that if deceased-donor livers are unavailable, LDLT is an acceptable option in experienced centers for adults with ALF.

Yamashiki and colleagues from Japan reported the largest cohort of patients undergoing LDLT for ALF (n = 209).[206] The outcome was excellent and included 1-, 5-, and 10-year patient survival rates of 79%, 74%, and 73%, respectively. Patient age was associated with short- and long-term mortality after LT, whereas ABO-I affected short-term mortality and donor age affected long-term mortality. Previous studies from Korea and Hong Kong include series with less patients but show similar results.[207,208]

Although used in elective adult LT, liver grafts from donation after cardiac death donors are more susceptible to poor initial function, and most centers are reluctant to consider their use in the situation of ALF, where good initial function is imperative.

AUXILIARY LIVER TRANSPLANTATION

Auxiliary partial OLT (APOLT) has been used in ALF as a bridge to survival without the need for lifelong immunosuppression (see Chapters 78 and 109). The precise indications have not yet been determined but are molded by two important considerations: the ability of the native liver to regenerate to normal morphology with time and the absence of a clinical need for the immediate benefits of total removal of the diseased liver. In general, candidates for APOLT are patients younger than 40 years with fulminant hepatitis resulting from HAV, HBV, or APAP toxicity.[209] Proponents of auxiliary transplantation for ALF claim that in most cases, had the patient survived, the native liver would have recovered. If true, then removal of the entire native liver during LT for ALF eliminates any such recovery and unnecessarily commits the patient to the lifelong risks of immunologic rejection and immunosuppression.[210,211]

When sufficient regeneration of the native liver is evident, immunosuppression can be discontinued according to two options: (1) abrupt discontinuation, which often results in severe and symptomatic rejection, or (2) progressive tapering of immunosuppression, with the aim of inducing a slowly progressing chronic rejection and subsequent atrophy of the graft. The second approach is preferred by most groups.[212,213] Removal of the auxiliary graft should not be attempted.

Quaglia and colleagues described the evolution of histologic changes in native livers after APOLT for ALF.[214] In as many as 62.5% of patients, the native liver regenerates to full recovery. In all such patients, immunosuppression can be reduced, and in the vast majority (80%), it can ultimately be suspended. APAP toxicity, in particular, is an excellent indication for APOLT, with full native liver recovery occurring in 100% of surviving patients with an auxiliary graft. In general, the hyperacute syndromes are more likely to regenerate to normal morphology when regeneration does occur. In seronegative hepatitis and the subacute syndromes, regeneration may occur, but it does so at the risk of significant fibrosis.

Lodge and colleagues proposed a new approach for patients with ALF caused by APAP overdose fulfilling King's College Criteria for "superurgent" LT.[215] This new approach consists of a subtotal hepatectomy followed by auxiliary transplantation with a whole liver (AWOLT) and a gradual withdrawal of immunosuppression after recovery. The results of 13 patients treated with this approach compared with 13 patients who had undergone OLT in the same period were similar in morbidity and mortality but better in terms of quality of life because the AWOLT patients did not need long-term immunosuppression.

Auxiliary OLT as a bridge to survival without the need for lifelong immunosuppression is an exciting concept but only occurred in 2% of patients from 2004 to 2009.[148] Although the technique may be considered in the setting of limited organ supply, it remains controversial with limited data to support positive outcomes.[11]

LIVER SUPPORT DEVICES

Extracorporeal liver support devices have been advocated to replace liver function in ALF patients either as a bridge to recovery or until LT can be performed (see Chapter 80). The complexity of metabolic, synthetic, detoxifying, and excretory hepatic functions, however, makes adequate extracorporeal hepatic support a reasonable but difficult-to-achieve goal. At present, liver support systems are not recommended outside of clinical trials and their future in the management of ALF is still unclear. Currently available liver support systems involve artificial systems that provide detoxification support only and bioartificial systems that use cellular material, providing detoxification and, in theory, additional synthetic support to the failing liver. For further details regarding liver support devices, see Chapter 78.

CONCLUSION

ALF, previously known as fulminant hepatic failure, is a dramatic clinical disorder that puts a healthy patient in a potentially deadly condition. Improvements in intensive care management have optimized survival, and nontransplant survival rates have improved significantly for APAP-related, non-APAP/drug-associated, and viral etiologies. In many ALF patients, however, the only definite treatment is still emergency LT. Several therapies, with the goal of maintaining the patient in good clinical condition as a bridge to transplantation, have shown promise and should be further evaluated. RCTs are difficult to perform within this context, given the rare and complex nature of ALF, but may be useful whenever therapies prove effective in individual cases. One of the most important strategies in this area should be to avoid ALF in the first place. Further public health measures in Europe and the US should be implemented, directed at the prevention of drug-induced liver injury and the reduction of excessive alcohol consumption. In developing countries, enhanced efforts aimed at reducing enteric spread and increasing immunization against viral hepatitis infections will reduce the incidence of ALF.

References are available at expertconsult.com

Liver transplantation for hepatocellular carcinoma

Garrett Richard Roll and John Paul Roberts

Cancer of a solid organ is an uncommon indication for organ transplantation, but hepatocellular carcinoma[1] (HCC) is an important exception to that general rule (see Chapters 89 and 105). HCC is the most common tumor treated with whole-organ transplantation, and it is listed as the primary indication in approximately 25% of liver transplantations (LTs).[2] The existing treatment options for HCC include hepatic resection, local ablation, or LT, and, in the last 20 years, LT has become the therapy of choice for early-stage malignancy in the setting of cirrhosis. The literature lacks randomized controlled trials (RCTs) regarding the treatment of HCC; therefore most centers base their practice guidelines on local experience, retrospective data, theoretic decision analyses, and the availability of treatment options.

Ever since the first LT was performed in a patient with HCC in the 1960s, recurrence has been a concern. Before the late 1990s, LT for HCC carried high recurrence rates, and the 2-year survival was only approximately 30%. The poor outcomes were the result of the consensus at that time to treat smaller tumors with liver resection and more advanced disease with LT. Discouraging results plagued LT for HCC, until it was noted that subgroups of patients with smaller tumors who underwent LT achieved better outcomes.[3]

A group from Milan, Italy, conducted a prospective trial, published in 1996, in which patients with smaller tumors achieved 4-year survival rates of 75%, equivalent to the survival for non-HCC patients who underwent transplantatio,[4] and similar results were seen in the United States.[5] Resultant changes in patient selection, dictated by these *Milan criteria*, allowed similar results to be reproduced at other centers,[6,7] and the United Network of Organ Sharing (UNOS) adopted these criteria in 1998 and gave priority for transplantation to HCC patients.[8] This priority, coupled with the rise in patients with hepatitis C virus (HCV), in whom HCC frequently develops, fueled the rapid expansion of this indication for transplantation. This chapter discusses LT for HCC, concentrating on its unique pathophysiology and how it relates to diagnosis and dictates therapy.

HEPATOCELLULAR CARCINOMA (SEE CHAPTER 89)

HCC is the fourth most common cause of cancer-related death and accounts for 80% of liver cancers worldwide[9] and is the fastest rising cause of cancer death in the United States.[10] This disease develops in the setting of cirrhosis in more than 90% of cases.[11] The risk of HCC development in patients with cirrhosis from any cause is approximately 2.0% to 6.6% per year versus 0.4% for patients with viral hepatitis without cirrhosis[12–16] (see Chapters 9B and 9C).

The incidence of HCC was previously rising for decades,[17–22] but even with the widespread use of direct-acting antivirals (DAAs), it does not appear that HCV will be eliminated in high-income countries for another 30 years.[23] Despite the reduced incidence of HCV, there are still a large number of patients who have lived with HCV cirrhosis for 20 to 30 years and are aging, and they are at risk for developing HCC.[24] It is hoped that the introduction of vaccination for hepatitis B virus (HBV)[25] and the success of the DAA for HCV will decrease the incidence of HCC. Despite the potential decrease in HCC related to viral diseases, the epidemic of obesity and resultant nonalcoholic fatty liver disease (NAFLD) can be expected to generate at-risk cirrhotic patients for the foreseeable future (see Chapters 69, 74, and 89). The overall survival (OS) in patients with HCC varies dramatically from 2 months to greater than 60 months,[9] highlighting the importance of an in-depth understanding of this cancer and the options to treat it.

Biology of Hepatocellular Carcinoma (see Chapters 9B and 9C)

An understanding of the biology of HCC is critical to assist in clinical decision making about surveillance and treatment. Although the molecular biology of HCC remains to be fully elucidated, the close association between cirrhosis and the development of HCC is clear.[26] Viral hepatitis, chronic alcohol use, and NAFLD (see Chapter 105) are the most common causes of cirrhosis in the Western world. NAFLD, an unfamiliar diagnosis as recently as the early 1980s, is now present in 17% to 30% of Americans,[27] progressing to nonalcoholic steatohepatitis (NASH) in 32% to 37%[28–30] and then to cirrhosis in 5% to 24%.[30,31] The development of cirrhosis in patients with NAFLD is driven by repetitive liver injury from lipid peroxidation, fatty acid toxicity, mitochondrial impairment, and oxidative stress, and 2.6% of patients with NASH cirrhosis develop HCC per year.[32] A rough calculation, on the conservative side (330,000,000 Americans $\times$ 17% $\times$ 32% $\times$ 5% $\times$ 2.6%) yields 23,337 people developing HCC from NASH cirrhosis every year. This is to be compared with the prevalence of HCV in the US population of 0.9% (or 2.3 million people),[33] and an expected rate of HCC development in this population over 30 years is about 1% to 3%.

Viral infection with HBV and HCV lead to cirrhosis by different mechanisms (see Chapters 9B). HBV induces transgene activation, oncogene transcription, and loss of tumor suppressor genes as a result of viral DNA integration into the host genome.[34–37] HCC will develop in as many as 30% of patients with chronic HBV without cirrhosis.[38] HCV does not integrate into the host genome but rather leads to chronic inflammation through continued viral replication.[39] This rapid hepatocyte turnover in the presence of oxidative stress drives the development of multiple dysplastic nodules.

Unlike what has been found in some other cancers, no sequential progression of genetic defects has been identified that leads to the development of HCC. Instead, a variety of genetic alterations are usually seen, broadly grouped into events that occur either early or late in the development of a tumor.

Genetic alterations that lead to inhibition of the insulin-like growth factor II receptors are considered early mutations.[40] Loss of heterozygosity of a variety of genes, often of tumor suppressor genes such as *TP53*, is a late event in the development of neoplasia[41,42] (see Chapters 9B and 9C).

Clinically Relevant Aspects of Hepatocellular Carcinoma Pathogenesis

The clinician must understand three aspects of HCC pathogenesis: (1) the influence of cirrhosis on HCC development, (2) arterial recruitment of the tumor, and[43] the tendency for HCC to invade portal vein (PV) branches (see Chapters 14 and 89).

First, HCC most often develops in the context of cirrhosis, and the biology of HCC is related directly to the environment found in the cirrhotic liver (see Chapters 9B, 9C, and 74). Repeated insult causes chronic inflammation driven by tumor necrosis factor (TNF)-α; transforming growth factor (TGF)-β; and interleukin (IL)-1 from Kupffer cells, endothelial cells, and hepatocytes (see Chapters 9B and 9C). This inflammation stimulates nodular regeneration with bridging fibrosis. Rapid cellular turnover in this regenerative environment leads to low-grade dysplastic nodules that contain only mild atypia and then to high-grade dysplastic nodules with at least moderate atypia.[44] Eventually, a small percentage of these high-grade dysplastic nodules will go on to develop microscopic foci of HCC before becoming frank carcinoma.[45] Evidence suggests that tumor cells may even secrete IL-6 and TNF-α, directly contributing to the inflammatory microenvironment by activating Toll-like receptors.[46]

Because of the diffuse nature of the liver injury, multiple tumors can develop at the same time. If a focus of HCC is removed, recurrence is most often at a distant site (Fig. 108A.1).[47] This second tumor at the distant site is most likely a second primary tumor. Because most of the second lesions are found within a few years of treatment of the primary lesion, the tumor was most likely present when the first tumor was treated but was too small to be detected. The occurrence of synchronous and metachronous lesions in the same organ suggests the entire cirrhotic organ has the potential for neoplastic conversion, similar to the genetic defect in the colon in familial adenomatous polyposis, which leads to multiple cancers; this situation is referred to as a *field defect*.

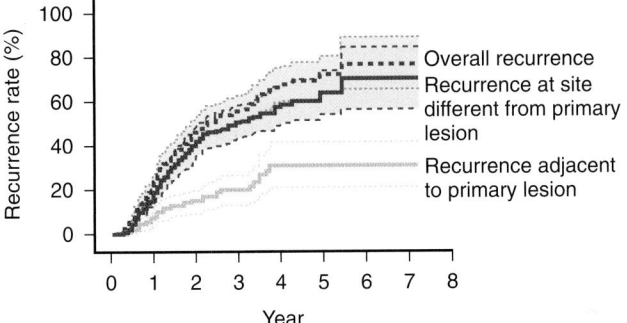

FIGURE 108A.1 Recurrence of hepatocellular carcinoma after ablation most often occurs at a site distant from the primary tumor, suggesting a second tumor was present at the time of treatment that was too small to be detected. (From Koike Y, Shiratori Y, Sato S, et al. Risk factors for recurring hepatocellular carcinoma differ according to infected hepatitis virus - An analysis of 236 consecutive patients with a single lesion. *Hepatology*. 2000;32[6]:1216–1223.)

Second, there is a clinically relevant difference in blood supply between foci of HCC and low-grade dysplastic nodules, which derive most of their blood supply from the PV. Histopathologic evaluation of high-grade dysplasia and HCC demonstrates the tumor being fed by branches of the hepatic artery that are not paired with the other structures of the portal tract, a process called *arterial recruitment* or *neoangiogenesis*. The resulting hepatic artery dominance in blood supply produces the characteristic hyperdense appearance of HCC that is used to identify tumors during the arterial phase of contrast imaging[48,49] and it allows for treatment by selective hepatic artery embolization.

Lastly, HCC is known to invade vascular structures, typically the PV but also hepatic veins (HVs) and, less frequently, the biliary tree (see Chapters 14 and 89). The development of vascular invasion appears to be a key step in the metastatic potential of the tumor, and the risk of PV invasion seems to be directly related to size and differentiation status of the tumor.[50] Venous invasion is such a strong predictor of metastatic disease that tumor size and tumor number can be thought of as surrogate markers for vascular invasion.

The likelihood of microvascular and macrovascular PV invasion has implications for treatment decisions; for example, evidence of venous invasion on imaging or biopsy rules out transplantation because the probability of recurrence is unacceptably high. It is this risk of recurrence with large or multiple tumors that resulted in the poor outcomes with early attempts at LT for HCC, and it is the reason why patients with small tumors are selected for transplantation.

Hepatocellular Carcinoma Screening

Patients with HCC presenting as symptomatic disease have a 0% to 10% 5-year survival rate,[15] so a screening program that identifies early disease can have a major impact on treatment outcomes (see Chapter 89). HCC meets the World Health Organization (WHO) criteria for performing screening,[51] and an RCT showed that screening for HCC reduces mortality.[52] An effective screening program evaluates patients at risk for disease, using a highly standardized and relatively inexpensive test with a high sensitivity. A screening program is used if the cost of screening a large population is less than the benefit of early detection of the disease in a small number of individuals in that population. Several decision-analysis and cost-efficiency models for HCC screening suggest that the ability of a screening program to decrease mortality while remaining cost-effective depends on the inclusion of patients with an incidence of HCC of at least 1.4% to 1.5%.[53–55] Box 108A.1 lists patients who should be included in a screening program. Screening for HCC in patients with cirrhosis from NASH, α1-antitrypsin deficiency, and autoimmune hepatitis is not considered mandatory,[56] but most centers include these patients in their screening population. Consensus on screening patients with NASH that do not have cirrhosis is lacking.

The most used serum tumor marker to detect HCC has been α-fetoprotein (AFP), produced by normal fetal hepatocytes and by tumor cells, but not by healthy, mature hepatocytes. AFP has traditionally been used for diagnosing HCC, predicting outcome after resection, and screening for recurrence postoperatively.[57] The normal range of AFP in the serum is 10 to 20 ng/mL; an absolute value of 20 ng/mL was used as the screening cutoff, but this yields a sensitivity of only about 64%, making it a poor screening test.[58] Moreover, normal AFP levels vary widely across ethnic backgrounds,[59] and the test has a lower positive predictive value (PPV) in patients with acute viral hepatitis or cirrhosis from a viral cause.[59,60]

In patients with a liver mass, a concomitant serum AFP greater than 200 ng/mL carries a very high PPV,[58] but because of its unacceptably low sensitivity and specificity, the American Association for the Study of Liver Disease (AASLD) recommended that serum AFP no longer be used as a screening tool, although it still plays a diagnostic role.[61] Using an absolute value greater than 400 ng/mL is considered diagnostic regardless of the patient's ethnic background or the cause of their liver disease.

A serum AFP greater than 1000 ng/mL is a strong predictor of vascular invasion, and 5-year survival after LT in patients with AFP over 1000 ng/mL is approximately 50% compared with 80% in patients with AFP less than 1000 ng/mL.[62] For that reason, AFP greater than 1000 ng/mL is a contraindication to LT at most centers, and a rate of AFP increase greater than 7.5 ng/mL per month portends worse outcome.[63] There has been a suggestion that chemoembolization of liver tumors with subsequent reduction in AFP from greater than 1000 to less than 500 results in satisfactory outcomes.[64] Research is ongoing to identify better serum markers for screening, diagnosis, and prognostication, and possible candidate compounds include AFP-L3 and des-γ-carboxy prothrombin, circulating tumor cells and cell-free DNA, and the neutrophil-to-lymphocyte ratio.[61,65–74]

Ultrasound (US) is the most widely used radiologic screening tool (see Chapter 14). It has a sensitivity of 65% to 85% and specificity greater than 90% when used as a screening test.[75] Although the performance of US in patients with cirrhosis is not as well-defined,[1,76–79] and the test is operator dependent, US remains superior to any widely available serologic screening test. A large, prospective RCT in China suggests that surveillance of high-risk individuals with US and serum AFP testing every 6 months reduces HCC-related mortality by close to 40%, even though patients were offered only resection and not transplantation. Screening compliance was only approximately 60%, however, and may have dampened the reduction in mortality.[52,80] Combined AFP and US surveillance increases sensitivity[81] but raises the cost, and using both tests increases the rate of false-positive results from 5% for AFP alone to 7.5% for combined screening,[82] especially if a nodule is present.[79] It is clear that further RCTs are needed, but based on the available information, the AASLD recommends screening patients at risk for HCC with US alone every 6 to 12 months.[61] Evaluation of serum AFP can be added to US in the event of concerns regarding operator influence, but the use of AFP as the lone surveillance tool is discouraged.

Early HCC can be difficult, if not impossible, to distinguish from cirrhotic nodules by US, but any suspicious nodule less than 1 cm should be evaluated for stability by repeat US at 3- to 6-month intervals for as long as 2 years. All 1- to 2-cm nodules should be investigated with a dynamic contrast-enhanced (CE) imaging modality—computed tomography (CT; see Chapter 14), magnetic resonance imaging (MRI; Chapter 14), or US—although contrast-enhanced US (CEUS) has not yet been adopted in the United States.

The sensitivity of US screening for HCC is reduced in obese patients.[48] Another frequently used radiologic surveillance tool is CT scanning.[43,83,84] Although the use of CT is commonplace, the radiation exposure to a patient from screening every 6 to 12 months is considerable, and its use as a screening tests has only been modeled.[85] Also, cross-sectional imaging tests are the diagnostic tests used to confirm HCC, and the screening test should be different from the confirmatory test. The American College of Radiology (ACR) published the Liver Imaging Reporting and Data System[86] to standardize the categorization of liver lesions in patients with cirrhosis based on the arterial phase hyperenhancement, lesion diameter, washout during the venous phase, presence of a capsule, and threshold growth, which are HCC characteristics first observed during CT scanning.[87,88]

The use of MRI with or instead of CT has been slowly increasing ever since MRI proved sensitive at detecting HCC in patients with cirrhosis.[89] MRI with gadolinium-based or iron oxide–based contrast as a screening test is not well studied, but meta-analysis of single-center reports suggests this modality is 95% to 98% specific for HCC in patients with cirrhosis, whereas CT scanning is 86% to 90%.[86] Moderate signal strength on T2-weighted images is specific for HCC because dysplastic and regenerating nodules are not hyperintense on T2, unless they have infarcted, which can occur. Delayed venous phase hypointensity with concomitant delayed enhancement of the rim of the lesion is also a feature specific to HCC.[90] More abbreviated MRI protocols without T2 and diffusion-weighted imaging (DWI) are also being considered because they appear to correctly characterize 93% to 96% of lesions.[91] Similar to CT, characterization of small nodules with MRI can be difficult because small lesions are frequently isointense on T2.[92] Gadoxetic acid increases the sensitivity of MRI for lesions less than 2 cm in single-center reports at specialized centers to 92% to 95%, with a specificity of 96% to 98%.[93] It remains to be seen whether CE MRI is cost-effective as a screening tool for HCC, but it may prove to be marginally superior to CT for characterization of known small hypervascular lesions in patients with cirrhosis.

A nodule that is 2 cm or larger and hypervascular with PV washout on a single dynamic imaging study, or a 1- to 2-cm nodule on two such confirmatory studies, is treated as HCC. If the results are contradictory, a biopsy of the lesion should be obtained.[61] If the lesion is larger than 2 cm and has a typical appearance on a single dynamic imaging study, or if it is found in concert with a serum AFP level higher than 200 ng/mL, biopsy is not required. Biopsy should be performed on any 1- to 2-cm lesion in any patient without cirrhosis who has risk factors for HCC. Biopsies should be read by expert pathologists, and patients with negative biopsy results should undergo US or CE imaging every 3 to 6 months and should be rebiopsied if the characteristics of the lesion change.[61] Biopsy results that suggest a high risk for progression to HCC include *dysplastic nodules*, both low and high grade[94]; *small and large cell change*, formerly called "small cell dysplasia" and "large cell dysplasia" (International Consensus Group for Hepatocellular Neoplasia [ICGHN], 2009; International Working Party, 1995); and *dysplastic foci*, defined as atypia outside of a dysplastic nodule (ICGHN, 2009).

TREATMENT OPTIONS

HCC is not responsive to traditional cytotoxic chemotherapeutic agents. A phase III clinical trial showed that sorafenib, an oral multikinase inhibitor of the vascular endothelial growth factor (VEGF) receptor, the platelet-derived growth factor receptor, and Raf kinase prolonged the median survival (10.7 vs. 7.9 months) and the time to radiologic progression (5.9 vs. 2.8 months) in patients with advanced HCC versus placebo[95] (see Chapter 99). Additionally, immunotherapy is evolving rapidly and has shown promise in patients with advanced HCC, but local ablation/embolization (see Chapters 94, 95, and 96), hepatic resection (see Chapters 101 and 102), and LT (see Chapter 105) are still the best options available for patients with early-stage disease to achieve a cure.

Treatment decisions should be based on three factors: (1) extent of local disease, (2) underlying liver disease, and[43] (3) local organ availability. Patients whose liver disease is Child-Turcotte-Pugh (CTP) class A (see Chapter 4, 5, and 102) who have early-stage HCC are candidates for treatment with the goal of long-term survival free of HCC. Unfortunately, because of the advanced biologic activity of the cancer, 80% to 90% of patients will present at a later stage too advanced for surgical resection or transplantation.[96] Those patients with advanced disease or patients with poor functional status should be offered a combination of sorafenib, immunotherapy, locoregional therapies, and/or palliative care.

In the rare patient without cirrhosis, no evidence of venous invasion or metastatic disease, and tumor burden limited to one lobe, resection should be considered. Conversely, resection of part of a cirrhotic liver invariably leaves scattered dysplastic nodules behind. The tumorigenic cytokine milieu that bathes the remaining dysplastic nodules puts the patient at risk for the development of a second primary tumor. In addition to these de novo tumors, some researchers have suggested recurrence is more frequently the result of microscopic dissemination of the primary tumor at treatment.[97,98] Astoundingly, the risk of developing recurrence after resection for HCC in patients with cirrhosis is approximately 35% at 1 year,[99] 40% to 50% at 3 years,[47,100,101] and as high as 70% at 5 years,[4,26,102,103] making the history of a previous HCC the greatest risk factor in the development of a new primary HCC.

It is this high risk of recurrence that has driven LT as a method to remove the entire precancerous liver to prevent the development of subsequent lesions. The results of LT have improved dramatically in the last 25 years, in large part because of better patient selection, and currently the recurrence rate ranges from 11% to 18%. The mortality rate after liver resection for HCC is 1% to 7%, and the major cause is decompensated liver failure.[104-110] Given the risks of HCC recurrence and postoperative liver failure after resection, some controversy exists regarding the best treatment strategy in patients with limited disease and adequate hepatic function. Although sufficient hepatic reserve can usually be determined, no method is currently available to determine whether a patient will be among the 60% to 70% to recur within 5 years, or if they will remain recurrence free.

The current 5-year benchmark is 70% survival in patients with HCC undergoing LT,[111] but the long waiting time experienced in some regions must also be considered in the decision of resection versus transplantation. The risk of tumor progression while awaiting LT must be balanced against the risk of recurrence. If waiting times are relatively long in a given region, this may favor liver resection because a prolonged waiting time risks tumor progression that may exclude the patient as a candidate for any surgical treatment.

A decision analysis from 2000 compared primary resection and salvage transplantation for recurrence versus primary LT in patients with small tumors.[112] Theoretic decision models use multiple variables, so the weight of any single variable is difficult to determine, but the authors concluded that wait times shorter than 6 months favored LT, and those longer than 12 months favored primary liver resection. Another early decision analysis compared the projected survival benefit from LT with resection in patients with small HCCs.[113] The authors noted that the magnitude of the survival benefit relied heavily on the amount of time spent on the waiting list. They concluded that if the waiting period exceeded 6 to 10 months, the survival benefit gained from removal of the field effect is overwhelmed by the risk of progression while waiting, and resection becomes the preferred therapy (Fig. 108A.2). Although this analysis did not include the costs or clinical effects of locoregional therapy, it offers insight into how extended waiting times increase the relative benefit of resection (see Chapter 101) and locoregional therapy (Chapters 94–97). The most recent cost-effectiveness analysis comparing LT to liver resection using a Markov cohort model found that LT is cost effective when 5-year survival is greater than 87% in the Unites States.[114]

The possibility of mitigating the risk of progression with a locoregional therapy while awaiting a transplantation has been suggested. Whether locoregional therapy offers a measure of disease control while awaiting LT is not clear. Maddala and colleagues examined 54 patients with HCC treated with an average of three transarterial chemoembolization (TACE) sessions before LT at a median of 211 days.[115] Eight patients dropped off the waiting list, two for non-HCC reasons and six from HCC progression. Of the six with progression, two developed extrahepatic metastases, two developed PV invasion, and two had intrahepatic progression. Interestingly, these events all occurred within 4 months of listing. The short period between initiation of therapy and discovery of disease progression would suggest the disease had spread much earlier, and neither resection nor transplantation would have been helpful.

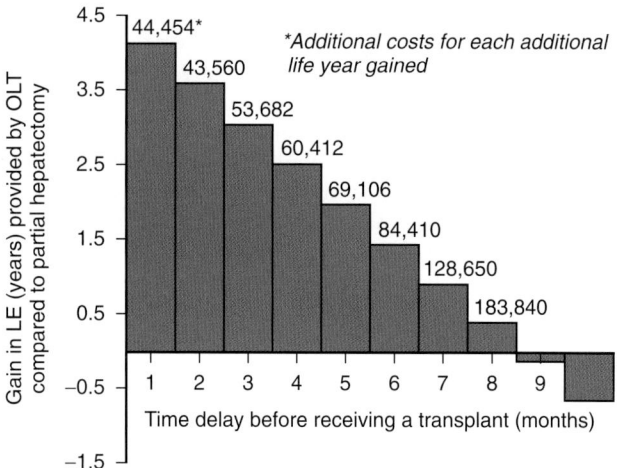

FIGURE 108A.2   Mean gain in life expectancy *(LE)* and marginal cost-effectiveness ratios provided by orthotopic liver transplantation *(OLT)* compared with partial hepatectomy *(vertical axis)* as a function of different time delays before receiving a transplant *(horizontal axis)*. (From Sarasin FP, Giostra E, Mentha G, Hadengue A. Partial hepatectomy or orthotopic liver transplantation for the treatment of resectable hepatocellular carcinoma? A cost-effectiveness perspective. *Hepatology.* 1998;28[2]:436–442.)

In a small study of 20 patients (median of two treatments, mean time to transplantation of 343 days), Hayashi and colleagues found that seven patients whose tumors were within Milan guidelines dropped off the waiting list: two for causes unrelated to HCC, one for decompensation, and the other five for increased intrahepatic disease.[116] The time to exclusion for HCC was less than 6 months in four of five patients, and no patients experienced HCC after LT at a mean follow-up of 2.9 years.

Another strategy is to prioritize, or fast-track, patients to have them receive a transplant as soon as possible without pretransplant treatment. Although this may be the most reassuring strategy for patients, it takes away the ability to observe the tumor biology in time. A subset of patients with newly diagnosed HCC will have very unfavorable tumor biology, and even if transplanted shortly after diagnosis, they are likely to experience rapid recurrence. A reasonable amount of time on the waiting list may, in fact, be beneficial, allowing tumor biology to unfold such that very aggressive disease will become obvious in short-term follow-up, thereby avoiding a futile procedure. Patients with small tumors that fall within the Milan criteria have approximately a 10% risk of recurrence, which corresponds reasonably well to the percentage of patients with tumors that have aggressive histologic characteristics.[6] Fast-tracking such patients likely would significantly increase recurrence rates. One series examining this issue showed that recurrence rates were significantly higher in patients who were fast-tracked and in patients who underwent living-donor liver transplantation (LDLT) compared with patients who had longer waiting times.[117] Patients with small but aggressive tumors are seen infrequently, but fast-tracking yields unacceptably high recurrence rates in the more common patient, with tumor burden close to the limits of or beyond the Milan criteria.[4,6,103,118] It has also been suggested that fast-track prioritization is not cost-effective.[119] Unfortunately, no stated guidelines have been established, but it appears that even for LDLT, a waiting time

of approximately 6 months is appropriate.[120] Patients with a large tumor burden that is initially outside transplant criteria can be treated until the tumor is within criteria, but these patients must then wait before undergoing deceased-donor transplant in the United States under UNOS policy derived from this understanding of tumor biology.

There is clearly a subset of patients with HCC with low risk of disease progression while on the waiting list. In 398 consecutive patients with stage T2 HCC listed for LT at University of California–San Francisco (UCSF), competing risk regression determined the overall risk of being dropped from the waiting list because of tumor progression or death to be 9.4% at 6 months and 19.6% at 12 months. A subgroup of patients had a significantly lower risk of tumor progression. Regression analysis defined this lower-risk subgroup as patients with a solitary tumor measuring 2 to 3 cm, AFP level of 20 ng/mL or less after the first locoregional therapy, and complete radiologic response to the initial locoregional therapy. Patients in this low-risk subgroup experienced 1- and 2-year probabilities of dropout of only 1.3% and 1.6%, respectively, whereas the risk of dropout was 21.6% and 26.5% at 1 and 2 years, respectively, in all other patients with HCC on the waitlist ($P = .004$).[121]

Radiofrequency (RFA) has also been reported to provide good results in patients who undergo subsequent transplantation (see Chapter 96B). Mazzaferro and colleagues reported 50 patients who underwent a single ablation session and then waited an average of 9.5 months before LT.[122] Apparently, there were no waiting list dropouts, and at a median follow-up of 22 months, only two patients had cancer recurrence. Lu and colleagues reported 52 patients who underwent RFA, most frequently in isolation (mean sessions 1.46).[123] After 12 months, three patients had dropped out at a mean of 11 months, and two patients had extrahepatic disease; in all, 41 patients underwent transplantation, and none had HCC recurrence at a mean follow-up of 15 months. For small tumors, it has been suggested that RFA may be equivalent to resection for long-term disease control, with a lower risk of postoperative liver decompensation,[124] but further trials with long-term outcome data are required.

Since the description of the Milan criteria in 1996, transplant centers have grappled with the concept of transplant for cancer, more recently attempting to identify the optimal waiting time in patients with HCC. Two recent studies address this issue using regional waiting list disparities in the United States. Samoylva and colleagues compared recurrence rates in patients with HCC waiting more than 120 days for transplant to patients waiting less than 120 days. The risk of recurrence was 40% lower in patients waiting more than 120 days for transplant.[125] Halazun and colleagues described outcomes from 10 years of transplanting 10,728 patients with HCC who were given HCC priority points.[126] The authors compare HCC waiting list and OS of recipients who experienced a long versus a short waiting time (7.6 months vs. 1.6 months). Although the risk of death awaiting transplant was higher in the patients with a longer waiting time (8.4% vs. 1.6%; $P < .0001$), 5-year survival after transplant was higher in the recipients who waited longer for transplant (75% vs. 67%; $P < .0001$). Multivariate analysis identified shorter waiting time as a predictor of worse survival (hazard ratio [HR], 1.545; confidence interval [CI], 1.375–1.736; $P < .0001$). A good oncologic response to locoregional therapy while waiting for LT portends a lower recurrence,[127] as do the ability to control the rise of serum AFP, termed the AFP response, and an AFP slope increase of less than 7.5 ng/mL/mo.

Given the limited side effect profile and success of DAA therapy, many patients with HCV complicated by HCC are undergoing HCV treatment before LT. Treatment of HCV with DAAs does not appear to increase the risk of mortality or HCC recurrence after LT in an international multicenter intent-to-treat analysis.[128]

In summary, resection and ablation are viable options for patients with small tumors without cirrhosis and for patients with cirrhosis and preserved liver function (normal bilirubin and wedged hepatic vein pressure gradient < 10 mm Hg) in regions with very long waiting times. LT is appropriate for patients with tumors that fall within the selection criteria and in those with small tumors but poor liver function. There is a subgroup of patients with HCC defined by solitary tumor measuring 2 to 3 cm, an AFP level of 20 ng/mL or less after the first locoregional therapy, as well as a complete radiologic response to the initial locoregional therapy, who are at a very low risk to drop off the waiting list because of tumor progression. Finally, some waiting time before transplant allows the biology of the tumor to declare itself, and rushing patients to transplant likely worsens long-term survival, and these observations have resulted in the institution of a 6-month waiting time interval from the time of diagnosis before access to deceased-donor LT in the United States (see next section).

Indications for Transplantation (see Chapter 105)

An unlimited supply of organs and money would allow for a liberal policy of transplantation for patients with HCC confined to the liver; but resources are limited, so efforts must be made to allocate organs to those recipients with a high likelihood of long-term survival. Recurrence risk is clearly higher in patients with more advanced disease, and the size and number of nodules in the patient's explanted liver is directly correlated with the risk of HCC recurrence.[4,6]

Based on these observations, selection criteria have been developed. The primary set of selection criteria are the Milan criteria, created to allocate organs to patients with HCC who would have a similar chance for long-term survival as patients without HCC (Fig. 108A.3).[4] To allocate scarce organs in such a way that all recipients have an acceptable chance for long-term survival, patients with HCC are currently evaluated for suitability based on three factors: (1) tumor size in centimeters, (2) number of radiologically evident tumors, and[43] (3) evidence of PV invasion or extrahepatic disease. These factors are a crude but somewhat effective method for predicting overall tumor biology and subsequent risk of recurrence.

Preoperative staging, as outlined by UNOS, includes a triple-phase CT scan of the abdomen to quantify intrahepatic disease burden,[129] and a scan should be done of the chest to look for extrahepatic disease. This can also be accomplished with MRI of the abdomen and a noncontrast CT of the chest.[115,130] Unfortunately, these imaging modalities—the gold standard for HCC imaging—understage about 20% of patients[131] and can sometimes also overestimate actual tumor burden. When explant or resection pathologic correlation is used to confirm the diagnosis, CT scan is only 37% to 75% sensitive at detecting HCC in a cirrhotic liver,[92] and MRI with gadoxetic acid-enhanced and DWI is 68% to 97%,[132] although they remain the gold standard for diagnosis and preoperative staging. Bone scintigraphy was used in the past to locate extrahepatic disease but is no longer used because of low sensitivity and specificity.

In the United States, the modified tumor-node-metastasis (TNM) staging system of the American Liver Tumor Study Group (ALTSG) is used to allocate livers from deceased-donors to patients with HCC awaiting transplantation (Table 108A.1; UNOS, 2004) to ensure that all patients who receive an organ have a reasonable chance at long-term survival. The original transplantation criteria from the mid-1990s, the Milan criteria, are equivalent to stage I or II of this TNM classification system. Using these criteria, recurrence is between 4% and 16%, and 5-year survival is 71% to 75%.[6,7,133] Patients whose disease falls outside the ALTSG criteria for stage II disease, and thus outside the Milan criteria, may be at higher risk for recurrence.

In February 2002, the Model for End-Stage Liver Disease (MELD) scoring system was implemented (see Chapter 4). As part of this system, priority was given to patients with TMN stage T1 and T2 HCC in an effort to combat the risk of tumor progression in patients awaiting a transplant. The prioritization was revised in 2004 to no longer include T1 tumors, so that only patients with T2 tumors receive priority listing to prevent over-allocation of organs to patients with HCC, and because approximately 30% of patients with presumed HCC (a single lesion ≤2 cm with arterial enhancement) were found to have no tumor in their explant.[134]

It has been suggested that the Milan criteria are too restrictive and that the size criteria are somewhat arbitrary. Several centers have extended their criteria to include highly selected stage III patients who are expected to have a tolerable rate of recurrence.[135-140] A recent retrospective analysis of 1556 patients undergoing transplantation at 36 centers included 1112 patients with tumor burden exceeding the Milan criteria on post-transplant pathologic review. Of these, 283 patients had no evidence of microvascular invasion with tumor burden as large as 7 cm in largest diameter or as large as seven nodules, and this subset of patients achieved a 5-year survival of 71%.

The UCSF criteria—single tumor smaller than 6.5 cm, maximum of three total tumors with none larger than 4.5 cm, and cumulative tumor size smaller than 8 cm (see Table 108A.1)—represent a modest expansion of the Milan criteria and have been validated at other centers. One such evaluation, a retrospective review of preoperative imaging and explant pathology, looked at 467 transplantations performed during a 20-year period and found similar 5-year survival in patients meeting the Milan criteria and the UCSF criteria by explant pathology (86% vs. 71%) and preoperative imaging (79% vs.

Milan Criteria

Single lesion, not >5 cm   **Up to 3 lesions, none >3 cm**

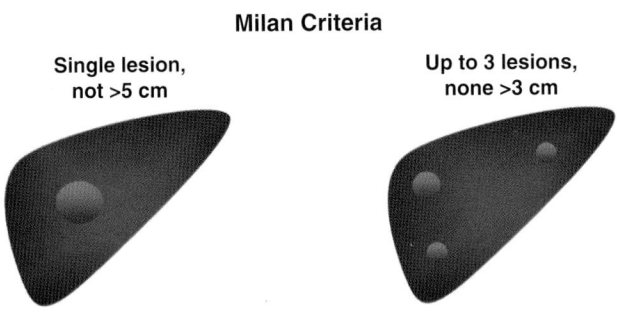

FIGURE 108A.3 Milan selection criteria for transplantation call for either a single lesion 5 cm or smaller or two to three lesions 3 cm or less, equivalent to stage T1 and T2, respectively, of the American Liver Study Group modified tumor-node-metastasis classification system.

TABLE 108A.1 American Liver Tumor Study Group Modified TNM Staging and the University of California–San Francisco Staging Criteria

MODIFIED TNM		UCSF CRITERIA	
TRADITIONAL STAGE	TUMOR BURDEN	STAGE	TUMOR BURDEN
T1	One nodule ≤1.9 cm		
T2	One nodule 2 to 5 cm or two to three nodules all ≤3 cm		
T3	One nodule >5 cm or two to three nodules, at least one >3 cm	IIIa	One nodule 5.1 to 6.5 cm, two to three nodules, all ≤4.5 cm, or total diameter ≤ 8 cm
		IIIb	One nodule >6.5 cm, two to three nodules, of which one is ≥4.5 cm, or they have a total diameter >8 cm
T4a	Four or more nodules, any size		
T4b	T2, T3, or T4a plus gross intrahepatic portal or hepatic vein involvement as indicated by CT, MRI, or ultrasound		

CT, Computed tomography; MRI, magnetic resonance imaging; TNM, Tumor-node-metastasis.

Modified from Yao FY, Ferrell L, Bass NM, et al. Liver transplantation for hepatocellular carcinoma: Expansion of the tumor size limits does not adversely impact survival. Hepatology. 2001;33(6):1394–1403.

64%). Survival for patients with tumors beyond UCSF criteria was less than 50% at 5 years.[135]

This discussion highlights the point that tumor burden is only a surrogate for vascular invasion and microscopic metastatic disease, which, along with extrahepatic disease, limits the effectiveness of LT. Because many centers have reported equivalent survival of highly select patients outside the Milan criteria, and with the advent of downstaging, this topic has taken on widespread debate. In 2017 UNOS changed the criteria to allow patients with HCC outside the Milan Criteria a pathway to LT, termed *downstaging*. Under these new criteria, a patient with a single lesion between 5 cm and 8 cm, or with two or three lesions with one between 3 cm and 5 cm and a total tumor diameter less than 8 cm, or four to five lesions each less than 3 cm with a total tumor diameter less than 8 cm are eligible for downstaging. These patients undergo downstaging with locoregional therapy and are eligible for transplant if they have T2 lesions after downstaging.

Another consideration is the impact of MELD exception points for patients with cancer or the selection of patients with liver failure as a result of benign disease. In regions with long waiting times, if patients with tumor burden beyond the Milan criteria are transplanted, organs are taken away from patients with liver failure from other causes. Volk and colleagues examined the issue of acceptable outcome risk for transplantation of patients with HCC compared with using the organ in a patient without HCC. On a national basis, they found that expansion of the Milan criteria would significantly increase waiting list mortality, unless 5-year post-transplant survival for the expanded criteria recipients exceeded 61%.[141] The authors also showed a dramatic difference in the effect of a policy change based on transplant region. This regional variability appeared to result from dramatic differences in the risk of death for patients without HCC because the MELD score at transplantation of non-HCC patients was quite low in some regions. In regions where the risk of death of the non-HCC patients without transplantation is low (low MELD score at LT), the HCC criteria could be expanded to allow transplantation in the HCC patients with a post-transplant survival in the HCC patients of 25%, which would mean that patients could have very large tumors or more than four or five tumors. This is compared with the need for criteria for transplantation in HCC patients that resulted in a post-transplant survival of 70% in

regions where there was a greater need for transplantation (higher MELD scores) in the non-HCC population. This wide variation in outcome suggested that changes in national policies would have a variable effect, depending on the region. In 2019, after much debate, UNOS implemented liver allocation based on acuity circles replacing the median MELD at transplant in the DSA or region with the median MELD at transplant within the acuity circle surrounding the transplant center. Patients with HCC are listed for LT with an initial exception score of 6. Six months later, the exception score is increased to the median MELD at transplant minus 3, where it remains.

Waiting List Screening for Hepatocellular Carcinoma

Patients awaiting LT are cirrhotic and therefore at risk for HCC, so longer wait times can affect survival. The average waiting time for LT is extremely variable and is based on ABO blood group, progression of liver failure, and geographic location even after allocation changes geared toward parity. The mean waiting time in the United States varied widely (from <6 months to >18 months)[142] before the 2019 UNOS allocation changes. Despite the allocation policy working toward parity, there are likely still differences between regions, and for patients with prolonged waiting times, it is important to screen patients with CT or MRI of the abdomen every 3 to 6 months while they await transplantation.

Pre-transplant Management of Patients With Hepatocellular Carcinoma (see Chapter 106)

Unfortunately, RCTs to evaluate different treatment options for patients awaiting LT have not been completed. The sole published series followed patients undergoing surveillance without local therapy and showed a high rate of dropouts from the waiting list because of tumor progression or progression of liver failure during the period of the study.[103] This report, combined with the understandable anxiety felt by patients and caregivers observing unhindered tumor progression, compelled most centers to offer cancer-directed treatment for patients awaiting transplantation. Retrospective data suggest that cancer-directed therapy should be used if the expected waiting time exceeds 6 months.[61]

Options for pre-transplant locoregional control include TACE (see Chapter 94A), transarterial radioembolization

(TARE) with y90[143] (see Chapter 94B), ablation with microwave (see Chapter 96C) or RFA (see Chapter 96B), percutaneous cryotherapy and ethanol injection (see Chapter 96D), or some combination of these modalities. TACE is used by many centers because it offers locally effective treatment with a low risk of complications. Three studies support the argument that TACE may help reduce attrition from the pre-transplant waiting list.[115,144] These data include patients with variable waiting times and follow-up periods, but they suggest that pre-transplant TACE is associated with a dropout rate of only 2% to 14%, with the possible added benefit of a lower post-transplant recurrence rate (8%–10%).

A decision analysis evaluated the waiting list interval associated with the greatest impact of neo-adjuvant TACE (i.e., greatest reduction in the dropout rate) and showed the greatest benefit in patients transplanted within 4 to 9 months.[145] The authors reported that when waiting time was less than 4 months, waiting list attrition was similar in treated and untreated patients (20% vs. 34%; $P = .08$), and when waiting times exceed 9 months, dropout rates re-equilibrated (33% vs. 46%; $P = .06$). TARE is becoming a commonly used alternative to conventional TACE. In a recent meta-analysis, TARE offered better overall survival, and improved oncologic outcome when compared with TACE.[146] The patient characteristics to suggest which of these two therapies is optimal before LT are not well characterized because this decision varies based on tumor location, tumor number and size, degree of synthetic liver dysfunction and portal hypertension, response to previous treatments, local expertise, and expected weighting time.

No studies have described percutaneous ethanol injection (PEI)[147] as a sole treatment in patients awaiting transplantation, although several studies suggest it is a safe and reliable component of multimodal therapy for tumors smaller than 3 cm.[148–150] PEI uses a small needle that reduces the risk of tract seeding to 0.6%. Some authors have suggested that pretreatment with arterial embolization to disrupt intratumoral septa facilitate the ethanol diffusion and may therefore improve the efficacy of subsequent ethanol injection.[151] PEI requires several sessions when used as primary treatment for unresectable HCC, and prospective evidence supporting it as a neoadjuvant therapy is lacking; as a result, the trend has been toward other treatment methods. A meta-analysis reported that RFA is superior to PEI in the treatment of small HCC with respect to survival and cancer-free survival at 1, 2, and 3 years; tumor response; and risk of local recurrence.[152] Recurrence is more common in patients with tumors larger than 4 cm, and in 95%, it occurs within 6 months and at a site distant from the primary tumor.[153] This again suggests that tumor size is only a surrogate marker for microscopic metastatic spread and neoplastic potential of the remaining dysplastic nodules.

RFA induces tissue necrosis by delivering heat at the tip of one or several electrodes. Major complications occur in less than 10% of patients, and mortality is less than 1%.[152] This strategy is at least as efficacious as PEI for tumors smaller than 2 cm but requires fewer treatments, and RCTs suggest that RFA improves survival.[54,154,155] Given these data, RFA was the preoperative treatment of choice for tumors larger than 2 cm,[61] and more recently TARE is used in these patients as well.

Downstaging

Two observations have fueled the current debate about the proper selection criteria for transplantation in patients with HCC. First, not all tumors of the same size carry the same risk of recurrence. Second, it is well documented that some patients outside the Milan criteria will benefit from LT.[156] This has led to efforts to select patients with more advanced disease, but with favorable tumor biology, who might benefit from LT.[129] The process of downstaging disease to within Milan criteria may be a mechanism for identifying such patients. This approach allows treatment of the tumor, and concomitant selection of patients with favorable tumor biology, by excluding patients who do not respond to locoregional ablative therapy, and it allows time for unfavorable biology to manifest.

A prospective intention-to-treat analysis evaluated 61 highly select patients with tumor stage exceeding T2 who underwent tumor-directed therapy before transplantation. The study included patients with one lesion larger than 5 cm but smaller than 8 cm; those with two to three lesions, with one lesion larger than 3 cm but smaller than 5 cm, with a total diameter less than 8 cm; and those with four to five lesions, all smaller than 3 cm with a total diameter less than 8 cm.[156] An interval of at least 3 months was required between treatment and transplantation. Downstaging was successful in 70% of patients, with the remaining patients dropping out, usually from disease progression. The 1- and 4-year post-transplant survival rates were 96% and 92%, respectively, suggesting that carefully selected patients with disease exceeding the Milan criteria can be downstaged with excellent post-transplant outcome. A recent update from the same authors compared outcomes of 118 patients undergoing downstaging with 488 patients listed for LT with T2 tumors: 54% of patients received LT after downstaging and 90.8% of patients were recurrence-free at 5 years compared with 88% in the T2 group ($P = .66$). The 5-year intention-to-treat survival was 56.1% in the downstaging group versus 63.3% in the T2 group ($P = .29$).[157]

It is important to note that the median time between the first treatment and transplantation was 8.2 months in the Yao and colleagues' study and 9.8 months in the update. It is this waiting time that appears to allow tumor biology to manifest; patients with more biologically aggressive tumors dropped out during the waiting period, allowing selection of lower-risk patients for transplantation.[156] A review of downstaging reinforced the concept that an aggressive downstaging protocol is a selector of tumor biology rather than a modulator of tumor behavior.[158] The UCSF protocol for downstaging of patients initially exceeding the Milan criteria was adopted by UNOS in 2017 (Box 108A.2).

A rising serum AFP while on the waiting list suggests aggressive tumor biology, especially if there is concomitant radiologic evidence of tumor progression after locoregional therapy. A multicenter European study found that AFP rising at a slope greater than 15 ng/mL/month was the best predictor of recurrence after transplant for patients both inside and outside the Milan criteria.[159] A recent large multicenter cohort of 4359 LT recipients with HCC that underwent LT analyzed the success of downstaging.[160] Of the 789 patients with HCC initially beyond Milan criteria, 465 were downstaged and underwent LT. The patients who required downstaging and were able to make it to LT actually had better 5-year overall survival (71.3% and 68.2%) and recurrence free survival (64.3 and 59.5%,) compared with the patients that were always within Milan criteria, further supporting the concept that response to therapy over time is the most valuable prognostic indicator of tumor biology. The role of systemic therapy

---

BOX 108A.2 University of California–San Francisco Downstaging Protocol for Patients Initially Outside the Milan Criteria

Inclusion Criteria for Downstaging

One tumor >5 cm and ≤8 cm

Two or three lesions, at least one >3 cm but ≤5 cm, and total tumor diameter ≤8 cm

Four or five lesions, all ≤3 cm, and total diameter ≤8 cm

No evidence of vascular invasion by imaging

Criteria Defining Success of Downstaging by Imaging

Tumor size and number meeting UNOS T2 criteria *or*

Complete tumor necrosis by imaging without suggestion of residual tumor

Criteria Defining Treatment Failure

Death from any cause before liver transplantation

Exclusion from liver transplantation

Recurrence of hepatocellular carcinoma after liver transplantation

Additional Guidelines

A minimum follow-up period of 3 months is required before liver transplantation, with concomitant imaging studies that meet the "success" criteria.

Approval must be obtained by the regional UNOS review board for priority listing for deceased-donor liver transplantation after successful downstaging.

Patients can undergo living-donor liver transplantation if a donor is available and imaging studies meet the selection criteria.

Patients with liver decompensation after downstaging are not eligible for liver transplantation unless the above criteria are met.

In patients treated with resection as a downstaging procedure, the presence of microvascular invasion in the resection specimen is a contraindication to liver transplantation.

UNOS, United Network for Organ Sharing.

Modified from Yao FY, Kerlan RK, Jr., Hirose R, et al. Excellent outcome following down-staging of hepatocellular carcinoma prior to liver transplantation: An intention-to-treat analysis. *Hepatology.* 2008;48(3):819–827.

in concert with locoregional therapy before LT may be evolving but is not thoroughly studied. Two RCTs showed that the addition of sorafenib did not reduce waitlist dropout and possibly increased the rate of biliary complications after transplant.[161,162] Currently, approximately 1% of patients receive sorafenib before LT.[163] Since 2017 immunotherapy with checkpoint inhibitors (CPIs) seems to be quickly changing the landscape of treatment for advanced HCC,[164] as atezolizumab and bevacizumab combination therapy is likely to become the standard of care in the near future. CPIs have not yet been studied in patients with early or mid-stage HCC. The role of these therapies in the neoadjuvant setting before LT is not defined, but clearly CPI exposure in the peritransplant period results in significantly increased risk of graft loss from rejection, as high at 54% in a small review of patients with liver or kidney transplant.[165]

Technical Aspects of Liver Transplantation in Hepatocellular Carcinoma (see Chapter 125)

LT for HCC presents some technical challenges that need special consideration. The most important consideration is to perform the operation based on well-established oncologic principles, involving clear surgical margins and avoiding tumor seeding during the procedure to ensure the lowest recurrence

rate. The tumor should be handled as little as possible, using the so-called "no-touch technique," until the lympho-vascular pedicle has been ligated. Hepatic artery ligation at the beginning of the hepatectomy can theoretically limit tumor dissemination during the dissection; however, no available evidence suggests that such an approach lowers the post-transplant recurrence risk.

The transplant surgeon should be aware of prior therapy because during RFA or biopsy, the needle tract and the diaphragm may be seeded with tumor. If a limited amount of diaphragmatic seeding is identified during the native hepatectomy, it is reasonable to perform a diaphragmatic resection with primary repair at hepatectomy. Primary repair of the diaphragmatic defect is usually sufficient, and tube thoracostomy is not required. Diffuse seeding should preclude LT.

Immune suppression after transplant is an important variable in the risk of HCC recurrence. Doses of corticosteroids and antimetabolites have not been found to be independent predictors of recurrence. Alternatively, high calcineurin inhibitor (CNI) levels after transplant, especially tacrolimus trough levels greater than 10 ng/mL or cyclosporine trough more than 300 ng/mL in the first month after transplant, have been associated with higher 5-year recurrence rates compared with patients with lower CNI trough levels (27.7% vs. 14.7%).[166] In a systematic review of 3666 patients, mammalian target of rapamycin (mTOR) inhibitors used in patients with greater tumor burden and more vascular invasion achieved lower rates of recurrence than patients receiving CNIs (13.8% vs. 8.0%, $P < .001$). It is important to note the follow-up periods for the patients treated with mTOR inhibitors were considerably shorter.[167] A prospective international RCT of 525 LT recipients with HCC compared mTOR-free immunosuppression versus conventional maintenance immunosuppression with the addition of an mTOR inhibitor. This trial showed that the addition of an mTOR inhibitor modestly improved recurrence-free survival up to 5 years after transplant (64.5% vs. 70.2%, respectively), although the data is challenging to interpret because of a significant amount of crossover between the treatment groups during the trial. It is notable, however, that the effect on recurrence-free survival was most pronounced in the patients with lowest projected risk of HCC recurrence rather than patients with the highest risk.[168] A follow-up study suggests that early addition of an mTOR and minimization of calcineurin inhibitor may result in less long-term renal dysfunction.[169]

Predicting and Screening for Tumor Recurrence

The propensity of HCC to recur after surgical therapy has spurred investigations of potential biomarkers that might help improve patient selection (see Chapter 9B, 9C, and 89). Formalin-fixed tissue was used for genome-wide expression profiling of the normal tissue surrounding a focus of HCC, and a reproducible expression signature was seen that correlated well with survival.[147] Even with the diversity of genetic events that lead to HCC, specific regions of loss of heterozygosity have been identified that could be used to quantify a patient's risk of HCC recurrence.

Efforts have been made to identify markers of extrahepatic tumor spread to avoid transplantation in the face of unrecognized extrahepatic disease. One attempt has been to find evidence of malignant cells in the bone marrow of patients with HCC as a method to predict recurrence or survival,[170] although this practice is not routinely performed.

A multivariate analysis of 136 patients undergoing hepatectomy for HCC reported that low AFP mRNA levels identified by real-time quantitative polymerase chain reaction (PCR) correlated with patient survival and disease-free survival.[171–173] Patients with negative AFP mRNA had 97% survival at 1 year and 91% survival at 3 years versus 86% and 56%, respectively, in patients with positive AFP mRNA ($P < .0001$). Similarly, 1- and 3-year disease-free survival rates were 73% and 45% in patients with negative AFP mRNA versus 55% and 26%. Although not widely used, these tests may help quantify risk of recurrence and could have implications for organ allocation and the effectiveness of LT for cure.

Screening all patients with imaging and serum AFP after transplant is not cost effective, but evidence-based data guiding post-transplant screening of certain populations is quickly growing. Screening high-risk patients, as defined by adverse histopathologic characteristics in the explanted liver, is a more promising and potentially cost-effective strategy.[174] Moreover, because 70% to 75% of recurrence occurs within the first 2 years after transplantation, screening during this time is the most critical and is most likely to have the greatest yield.[175,176] Recently a prognostic score was developed to identify what patients would benefit from post-transplant screening based on the presence or absence of microvascular invasion on the explant pathology, the serum AFP at time of LT, and the sum of the largest viable tumor diameter and number of viable tumors on explant,[177] which was later validated on the UNOS database.[178]

Once patients experience recurrence after transplantation, therapeutic options are somewhat limited. In approximately 40% of patients with recurrence, the HCC recurs at extrahepatic sites, and chemotherapy is generally ineffective, leading to a median survival of only 8.7 to 21.3 months.[4,179] Recurrence that occurs within 2 years portends a much worse outcome.[180] TACE and TARE are commonly used treatment modalities that have prolonged survival somewhat.[181] A subset of approximately 10% of patients with recurrence can be expected to achieve long-term survival after resection.[131] The use of sorafenib in this situation has shown limited success,[179] and immunotherapy with CPIs may have oncologic efficacy but risks severe rejection and graft loss,[165] so it is generally avoided.

Salvage Transplantation

To better maintain the pool of donor organs, some have argued that primary liver resection should be first-line therapy for patients with preserved liver function and solitary HCCs smaller than 5 cm, and salvage transplantation can be offered to patients who experience recurrence that falls within the Milan criteria. In 2003, Poon and Wong evaluated survival and recurrence after resection of potentially transplantable small HCCs.[182] They concluded that in patients with preserved liver function (CTP class A) with small solitary HCCs, primary resection achieved 5-year survival of 70%, comparable to reported survival after primary transplantation for similar-size tumors. To apply salvage transplantation, screening must be diligent to find those who recur. Screening after resection with US every 3 months would be an important aspect of any treatment strategy using salvage transplantation for treatment of recurrence. The hope is that if patients recur, they will do so with transplantable disease within the Milan criteria.

Two early studies addressed the issue of outcome after salvage transplantation but reached opposing conclusions. The first was a retrospective analysis of 358 patients with cirrhosis and HCC who underwent either transplantation ($n = 195$) or resection ($n = 163$, of whom 98 were transplant candidates at therapy); those patients with recurrence after resection underwent salvage transplantation ($n = 17$). The authors reported lower operative mortality rate (2% vs. 28%), lower recurrence rate (18% vs. 54%), and higher 5-year post-transplant survival (61% vs. 41%) and disease-free survival (58% vs. 29%) for patients who underwent LT compared with patients who underwent resection and then had salvage LT for recurrence.[183]

The results of this study suggest that resection and salvage transplantation produced worse outcomes, but this was not supported by the second study of 88 patients with disease meeting the Milan criteria who underwent LT versus 18 who underwent resection followed by salvage transplantation for recurrence.[184] The authors reported no difference in morbidity (51% vs. 56%), 30-day mortality (5.7% vs. 5.6%), 3-year survival (82% vs. 82%), 5-year survival (59% vs. 61%), or recurrence after primary LT versus salvage transplantation ($n = 3$ vs. 1).

Reasons for the discordant results could be the differences in time to salvage transplantation, patient selection, or operative technique of liver resection between the studies (27% underwent a transthoracic resection in the latter study). Another issue limiting the comparability of these two studies is that 7 of the 18 patients who underwent "salvage transplantation" in the latter study did not have recurrence but were transplanted for deterioration of liver function or because of pathologic findings in the resection specimen. Also, the theoretic transplantability of patients with recurrence after resection seems to be different than the actual transplantability documented by many centers. Although Poon and colleagues describe an optimistic rate of patients with recurrence who would theoretically be transplantable after resection (79%),[185] the percentage of patients who have undergone salvage transplantation, documented in the literature, is 1% to 30%.[103,186] Recently, Lee and colleagues described experience with 114 patients with HCC recurrence after liver resection, showing that the presence of microscopic PV invasion and the presence of a satellite nodule at resection were risk factors for HCC recurrence after transplant.[187] More recently an intention-to-treat analysis identified MELD greater than 10 and the absence of neoadjuvant TACE, a complication-free recovery from resection and T1 to T2 disease at the time of liver resection as predictors of success with salvage LT.[188]

Reports of recurrence after salvage vary widely, from 5% to 54%.[184,189–191,188] Currently, the efficacy of resection followed by salvage transplantation for recurrence is limited by the difficulties that attend screening for recurrence, prolonged waiting times, and a shortage of donor organs, but it may be a viable option for patients with HBV without cirrhosis who have a single lesion.

Future Perspectives

LT for HCC has been shown to offer long-term survival and recurrence-free survival for patients with cirrhosis, but the shortage of donor organs is likely to perpetuate interest in resection and salvage transplantation. Currently, no consensus exists about an optimal method to select patients for transplantation after resection, which may be offered to patients with documented recurrence, but a more proactive strategy might improve outcomes.

One strategy is to use the well-established histopathologic findings of microvascular invasion or multiple nodules unseen on preoperative imaging[14,192–195] to select patients at high risk for recurrence after resection. Identification of these findings in the resection specimen could initiate listing for LT.[196] This strategy may select for patients who are at risk for early recurrence to undergo transplantation,[197,198] thus selecting a population who is likely to recur, even if they do undergo LT. The concern with this strategy is that patients whose explant specimens after LT demonstrate vascular invasion are at increased risk for extrahepatic disease.

Another possible strategy takes advantage of recent advances in gene-expression profiling of fixed liver tissue, from the liver parenchyma away from the tumor, to reliably predict risk of late (de novo) recurrence by quantifying the field defect.[147] Using this technology, gene-expression profiling could theoretically select the population with a field defect that places them at high risk for late recurrence; this group might be targeted for transplantation, while allowing those with low risk for late recurrence to have resection and to be followed.[199] Although this strategy offers some promise, it remains investigational.

Yet another strategy is treatment of all patients with HCC with locoregional therapy and downstaging while monitoring for lack of radiographic HCC progression. This finding, combined with low post-treatment serum AFP that does not rise more rapidly than 15 ng/mL/month, could be used to select candidates for whom transplantation offers a low risk of recurrence. Relatively low CNI trough levels after transplant and use of mTOR inhibitors are likely to decrease recurrence.

Even with the improvements in overall and cancer-free survival in the last 20 years, many areas of HCC treatment require RCTs, such as preoperative screening, postoperative surveillance, and downstaging protocols. Nontransplant therapies (e.g., re-resection, RFA, TACE, TARE, PEI) need to be evaluated against salvage transplantation for patients with recurrence. Lastly, systemic therapeutic options for patients with advanced HCC are improving, but the role of these treatments in patients undergoing LT is yet to be defined.

The references for this chapter can be found online by accessing the accompanying Expert Consult website.

Liver transplantation for nonhepatocellular malignant disease

Timucin Taner, Charles B. Rosen, Julie K. Heimbach, and Gregory J. Gores

OVERVIEW

Liver transplantation (LT) is considered standard of care for select patients with hepatocellular carcinoma (HCC) arising in the setting of cirrhosis (see Chapter 108A). The role of LT in treatment of other malignancies arising in the liver such as hilar and intrahepatic cholangiocarcinoma (CCA), hepatic epithelioid hemangioendothelioma (HEHE), or tumors metastatic to the liver such as neuroendocrine cancer (NEC) and colorectal cancer (CRC) continues to evolve. Herein we review the results of LT for these malignancies—specifically hilar and intrahepatic CCA, metastatic NEC, HEHE, and metastatic CRC—with an aim to suggest guidelines for the application of LT in the treatment of these diseases.

HILAR CHOLANGIOCARCINOMA (SEE CHAPTER 51)

CCA, the second most common primary malignant tumor of the liver, arises from the cholangiocytes of the intrahepatic and extrahepatic bile ducts. The incidence of this tumor has been estimated at 3000 to 5000 cases per year,[1,2] and the prevalence of intrahepatic disease appears to be on the rise.[3] CCA can arise within the liver, in the perihilar location, or along the extrahepatic bile duct (see Chapters 50 and 51). CCA has three growth patterns: (1) *mass-forming tumors* are usually intrahepatic, (2) *sclerosing tumors* arise in the perihilar and extrahepatic bile ducts, and (3) *polypoid tumors* grow within the major intrahepatic and extrahepatic ducts. Surgical extirpation has been the standard treatment for all three tumor types.

The treatment of hilar CCA has been most troublesome because of the difficulty achieving a tumor-free (R0) margin of resection. Radical resection with partial hepatectomy has been shown to improve survival[4] for patients with hilar CCA, but few patients come to medical attention with disease amenable to complete resection. Indeed, fewer than 30% of patients are candidates for resection at diagnosis because of either bilateral liver involvement, encasement of hilar vascular structures, involvement of sectoral bile ducts, and/or underlying liver disease, such as primary sclerosing cholangitis (PSC; see Chapter 41). LT appeared promising for the treatment of intrahepatic and hilar CCA; LT affords a radical resection, is not limited by bilateral ductal or vascular involvement, and treats underlying liver disease.

EARLY EXPERIENCE WITH LIVER TRANSPLANTATION

Unfortunately, early experiences with LT for the treatment of CCA were uniformly poor. LT for both hilar and intrahepatic CCA was fraught with high recurrence rates and poor patient survival. The Cincinnati Tumor Registry reported a large multicenter analysis for patients transplanted from 1968 to 1997, wherein 1-, 3-, and 5-year patient survival rates were only 72%, 48%, and 23%, respectively.[5] The recurrence rate was 51% with a median time to recurrence of only 9.7 months. Local recurrence within the allograft was the most common initial site of recurrence (47%) followed by distant metastases to the lung (30%). Recurrence of tumor portended an extremely poor prognosis, with a median survival of only 2 months. Adjuvant therapy was not found to be beneficial, and no difference was reported in the survival rate of known tumors versus incidental tumors found at the time of orthotopic liver transplantation (OLT); results were poor for both intrahepatic and hilar tumors.

A multitude of retrospective studies have confirmed these findings. A Spanish multicenter study reported similar results for 59 patients who underwent OLT for CCA from 1988 to 2001[6] and found 5-year survival was 30% with a 53% recurrence rate for 39 patients with hilar CCA. Results were equally poor for 23 patients with intrahepatic CCA, for which 5-year survival was 42%, and the recurrence rate was 35%. Similarly, a Scandinavian study reported a 5-year survival of 30% after OLT in a PSC population with early-stage CCA.[7]

Several centers have reported their outcomes with incidental tumors discovered in patients undergoing transplantation for chronic liver disease. Ghali and colleagues (2005)[8] reviewed the Canadian experience from 1996 through June 2003 and identified 10 cases, 8 arising in patients with PSC. Most of these tumors had favorable characteristics that included small size (<1 cm) and absence of perihepatic lymph node involvement; 90% were well differentiated, and 60% arose in the extrahepatic or hilar ducts. Despite the favorable characteristics, 3-year survival was only 30%. Only the University of California–Los Angeles (UCLA) has reported reasonable survival outcomes in incidental CCA detected in the explant after OLT.[9] Ten patients with incidental CCA had a 5-year survival of 87%, which was comparable to PSC patients without CCA, although pathologic characteristics were not included in the paper. As with all other experiences, the 4 patients transplanted with known CCA had poor outcomes, and none were alive at 5 years.

A more radical approach with cluster abdominal transplantation reported by the University of Pittsburgh had equally poor results: a 3-year survival of 20% and a 57% recurrence rate.[10] A similar experience was recently reported by Neuhaus' team in Berlin.[11] Sixteen patients with CCA were treated by combined LT and pancreatoduodenectomy (PD) between 1992 and 1998, and results were compared with those achieved for 8 patients who did not undergo PD, which at the time of LT was associated with significantly higher morbidity than transplantation alone. Long-term survival (>4 years) was achieved in only 3 of 20 patients without lymph node–involvement who survived the perioperative period. Neuhaus and colleagues concluded that "there is no good evidence that more radical resections alone are able to markedly improve long-term results."

With uniformly poor results of LT for these tumors, intrahepatic and hilar CCA became widely recognized as absolute contraindications for LT. Both intrahepatic and hilar CCA are best treated by resection; unresectable disease has a prohibitively high recurrence rate after transplantation and warrants additional or palliative therapy.

NEOADJUVANT THERAPY AND LIVER TRANSPLANTATION

Despite the overall poor results with LT alone, some patients with favorable hilar CCA, such as those with negative resection margins and no regional lymph node metastases, did benefit from transplantation.[12] In addition, a small group of patients at Mayo Clinic treated with primary radiotherapy and chemosensitization alone, without resection, had 22% 5-year survival.[13] Based on the known palliative efficacy of radiotherapy for CCA—and knowledge that CCA resection failures are usually because of locoregional recurrence rather than distant metastases[14]—the transplant team at the University of Nebraska pioneered a strategy of high-dose neoadjuvant brachytherapy and chemotherapy followed by LT[15] for patients with unresectable hilar CCA.

The initial Nebraska protocol used high-dose intrabiliary brachytherapy, 6000 cGy, followed by daily intravenous (IV) 5-fluorouracil (5-FU) until OLT. Patients underwent operative staging when a donor liver became available for transplantation. At operation, the patients were assessed for extrahepatic metastases or regional lymph node involvement. Either finding precluded transplantation, and the donor liver was reallocated to another patient. Seventeen patients received neoadjuvant brachytherapy: 2 patients died from disease progression, and 4 were found to have extrahepatic disease at exploration; 11 patients underwent transplantation. Median survival after transplantation was 25 months; 5 (45%) were alive and disease-free at a median of 7.5 years (range, 2.8–14.5 years) after transplantation, 2 patients died from recurrent disease, and 4 patients died from perioperative complications. Overall survival was 30% for the 17 patients 5 years after the start of neoadjuvant therapy.

MAYO CLINIC EXPERIENCE

The transplant team at the Mayo Clinic embraced the concept pioneered by the team at the University of Nebraska and implemented a protocol in 1993 through a collaborative effort of medical and radiation oncologists, hepatologists, and surgeons. The general concept is that neoadjuvant therapy and LT should provide the best possible control of local disease. The rationale for the protocol is based on several factors: (1) the known CCA tumor response to high-dose radiotherapy; (2) hepatotoxicity of radiotherapy is obviated by LT; (3) LT achieves radical resection, including removal of residual disease after neoadjuvant therapy; (4) LT is not limited by underlying liver disease (PSC), vascular involvement, or concern about intrahepatic extension of disease; (5) neoadjuvant therapy before operative staging and transplantation might avoid tumor dissemination

during operation; and (6) careful patient selection with operative staging before LT could exclude patients with advanced disease and regional lymph node metastases that are destined to develop distant metastatic disease.

Inclusion and Exclusion Criteria

Criteria for protocol enrollment are designed to select those patients least likely to develop metastatic disease, most likely to respond to neoadjuvant therapy, and who have a high probability for survival after transplantation. Appropriate patients include those with early-stage hilar CCA determined to be unresectable or those who have underlying PSC because CCA arising in the setting of PSC has a very poor natural history after standard resection[16] (see Chapters 41 and 51).

Criteria for anatomic unresectability include bilateral segmental ductal extension, encasement of the main portal vein (PV), unilateral segmental ductal extension with contralateral vascular encasement, and unilateral atrophy with either contralateral segmental ductal or vascular involvement. Because of the difficulty of assessing extent of disease along the bile duct, especially in the setting of PSC, no longitudinal limits exist for bile duct involvement (see Chapters 41, 51, and 119B).

Original criteria required that hilar CCA not extend lower than the cystic duct, but it was subsequently found that early CCA arising in PSC with unsuspected common bile duct (CBD) involvement found at transplantation was amenable to transplantation with PD; however, patients with CCA extending below the cystic duct on cholangiography are excluded because they have larger tumors that are more likely to abut the PV and be less amenable to complete extirpation during transplantation.

Vascular encasement of the hilar vessels is not a contraindication to transplantation. The upper limit of tumor size is 3 cm in radial diameter (perpendicular to the biliary duct at the site of origin) when a mass is visible on cross-sectional imaging studies, and there must be no evidence of intrahepatic or extrahepatic metastases by chest computed tomography (CT), abdominal CT or magnetic resonance imaging (MRI), ultrasonography, or bone scan. Endoscopic ultrasound (EUS) is performed before neoadjuvant therapy to exclude patients with regional lymph node metastases.

The Mayo Clinic protocol specifically excludes patients with evidence of intrahepatic or extrahepatic metastases or gallbladder involvement. Surgical intervention and any type of transperitoneal biopsy or fine-needle aspiration have emerged as absolute contraindications to enrollment. These procedures result in an unacceptable rate of peritoneal seeding, which has been discovered during operative staging or recurrence after transplantation (unpublished data). Candidates must have no active infections or medical conditions that preclude either neoadjuvant therapy or OLT. These exclusion criteria are quite restrictive and select for patients with early-stage disease. Indeed, a recent review of 732 patients with CCA in the Netherlands found that 154 (21%) patients had potentially resectable disease, 335 (46%) patients had regional lymph node or distant metastases, and only 84 (11%) met tumor criteria. Of those 84 patients, only 34 (5% of the total number of CCA patients) were deemed to have been potential candidates as the others were above their age limit of 70 years.[17]

Tumor Diagnosis

Diagnostic criteria for neoadjuvant therapy and LT require a malignant-appearing stricture on cholangiography and either visualization of a mass on cross-sectional imaging at the site of the stricture, cytologic or histologic confirmation of CCA by transluminal brushing or biopsy, elevation of carbohydrate antigen (CA19-9) greater than 100 U/mL in the absence of acute bacterial cholangitis, or polysomy by fluorescence *in situ* hybridization (FISH). Patients with indeterminate diagnostic criteria—such as FISH trisomy (7 or 3), dysplasia from brushings, FISH polysomy in the absence of a malignant-appearing stricture, or a malignant-appearing stricture in the absence of a mass lesion are followed closely with repeat endoscopic retrograde cholangiography (ERCP) with brushings, cross-sectional imaging, and laboratory testing. Patients with PSC and multifocal FISH polysomy are especially of concern because over 80% of these patients develop CCA within 3 years.[18]

Neoadjuvant Therapy

Neoadjuvant therapy is administered by external beam radiation (40–45 Gy), followed by transcatheter radiation (20–30 Gy) with iridium wires. Wires are placed preferentially by ERCP and percutaneous transhepatic cholangiography (PTC) when ERCP is technically not possible. Occasionally, brachytherapy is not possible, and a comparable dose of radiation is administered as a localized boost. IV 5-FU is administered for chemosensitization during radiation therapy, and capecitabine is administered afterward, while patients await transplantation.

Staging Operation

All patients undergo operative staging before OLT. Operative staging includes a thorough abdominal exploration with careful palpation of the liver to identify small, previously undetected intrahepatic metastases, biopsy of any suspicious nodules, and excision of a proximal proper hepatic artery lymph node (at the takeoff of the gastroduodenal artery) and a pericholedochal lymph node (posterior to the CBD just superior to the pancreas). The caudate process and retrohepatic vena cava are assessed for suitability of a caval-sparing hepatectomy, which is necessary for recipients of living-donor liver grafts. Extrahepatic or intrahepatic metastases, lymph node involvement, or locally extensive disease preclude transplantation. Survival for patients with these findings beyond a year is very rare. The staging operation was initially performed through a right subcostal incision with extension along the future LT incision as necessary. During the past decade, most procedures have been accomplished by hand-assisted laparoscopy using a smaller, right subcostal incision and several separate port insertion sites. The staging procedure is initiated as a laparoscopic survey of the abdomen followed by placement of a hand port to facilitate palpation of the liver and perihepatic region and excision of the hepatic artery and pericholedochal lymph nodes. Seprafilm (Sanofi-Aventis, US, LLC) has been used to try to prevent adhesions for patients that stage negative and are awaiting deceased-donor liver transplantation (DDLT).

Timing of the staging operation depends on the possibility of living-donor liver transplantation (LDLT) or the anticipated waiting time for DDLT. The staging procedure is performed 1 to 2 days before LDLT or as time nears for DDLT. Patients with underlying cirrhosis from PSC or liver dysfunction from cholestasis are at risk for decompensation after the staging procedure. Liver decompensation may lead to an increase in a patient's calculated Model for End-Stage Liver Disease (MELD) score and advance their position on the deceased-donor waiting list, but it also leads to an increase in perioperative morbidity

and mortality. Unfortunately, only supportive care is possible for those patients who decompensate after a positive staging operation, and few survive the perioperative period. An occasional patient is too sick to undergo operative staging as a separate operation, usually because of liver decompensation with a high MELD score or medically refractory ascites. Operative staging can be done when a donor liver becomes available, but this approach requires close coordination with the donor organ procurement organization (OPO) and arrangements for a back-up patient in the event that the findings of the staging procedure preclude LT.

Before 2003, 30% to 40% of patients had findings during the staging operation that precluded LT. EUS-guided aspiration of regional nodes (not the primary tumor) was implemented to exclude patients with lymph node metastases before initiation of neoadjuvant therapy. Initial findings from 47 patients identified 8 (17%) with metastases.[19] No morphologic features of the lymph nodes were found at EUS that predicted microscopic disease. Thus it is important to sample the regional lymph nodes even if they appear benign on endoscopic ultrasound. Since routine use of EUS was implemented in 2003, the percentage of patients with a positive staging exploration has been reduced to 20% overall, 14% for patients with CCA arising in PSC, and 26% for patients with CCA arising de novo. EUS avoids the morbidity and mortality of high-dose neoadjuvant therapy and prevents an unnecessary operation for patients destined to fall out at operative staging.

Liver Transplantation

The technical difficulty and nuances of transplantation for patients with CCA and neoadjuvant radiotherapy exceed those of standard OLT (see Chapter 125). Hilar dissection is avoided to prevent tumor manipulation and to reduce the possibility of intraoperative dissemination. There is typically extensive scar tissue in the hepatoduodenal ligament because of the neoadjuvant therapy and the previous staging procedure, which can make the dissection very difficult. The irradiated native hepatic artery is avoided during transplantation with a deceased-donor liver, and arterial inflow is established with a segment of deceased-donor iliac artery sewn to the infrarenal aorta. This approach was initially applied to LDLT but unfortunately resulted in an unacceptable rate of hepatic artery thrombosis. Better results have been achieved using the native artery, which is sewn directly to the living-donor artery despite prior radiation therapy. Use of the irradiated artery is associated with more frequent hepatic artery stenosis and thrombosis, but surveillance with Doppler ultrasound effectively enables early detection and intervention if problems arise.

The CBD is transected as close to the pancreas as possible, and it may be possible to enucleate a short segment of additional CBD from the head of the pancreas. The margin is submitted for frozen section examination. Microscopic tumor involvement at this margin occurs in 10% to 15% of patients with PSC but rarely with CCA arising de novo. The possibility of PD is discussed with all PSC patients before initiation of neoadjuvant therapy. Bilioenteric continuity is restored with a standard Roux-en-Y hepaticojejunostomy (living-donor graft) or choledochojejunostomy (deceased-donor graft).

The PV may be somewhat brittle and fragile because of the neoadjuvant therapy, and an injury may be difficult to control. The PV is divided as low as possible and is not dissected free up into the hilus of the liver. Despite low division, the deceased-donor PV is almost always long enough for an end-to-end anastomosis. A segment of a deceased-donor iliac vein is often used as an interposition graft between a living-donor right or left PV and the native vein during LDLT. We used to think it was important to insert a short vein graft for living-donor right livers to enable intervention after transplantation (discussed later), but a graft is now used only when necessary to make up the distance between the donor and recipient PVs.[20] A caval-sparing hepatectomy is performed in most cases, and the donor suprahepatic vena cava is sewn to the left/middle hepatic vein trunk or the retrohepatic cava during DDLT; the right or left/middle hepatic vein trunk is reconstructed in an end-to-end fashion during LDLT along with implantation of infrahepatic and caudate veins larger than 0.5 cm and reconstruction of segment V and VII veins if necessary. If there is concern for tumor extension into the caudate, which is usually detectable during the staging operation, the retrohepatic cava is excised, and the donor retrohepatic vena cava is sewn to the suprahepatic and infrahepatic

cavae as an interposition graft, usually with use of portovenous and venovenous bypass.

Results

Three hundred seventy-six patients were enrolled in the Mayo Clinic protocol from 1993 through 2019 (Fig. 108B.1A). Fifty-four patients died, became too debilitated for transplantation, or had disease progression before operative staging. Twelve patients underwent transplantation at other centers, and five were receiving neoadjuvant therapy and/or awaiting operative staging. Three hundred five patients underwent operative staging, and 58 patients (19%) had findings precluding transplantation. After staging, 6 patients died or developed disease progression precluding transplantation, 1 patient was awaiting transplantation, and 3 patients underwent transplantation at other centers. The remaining 237 patients underwent transplantation, 155 with deceased-donor grafts, 81 with living-donor grafts (15 left liver; 66 right liver), and one with a domino familial amyloid donor graft. The patient outcomes

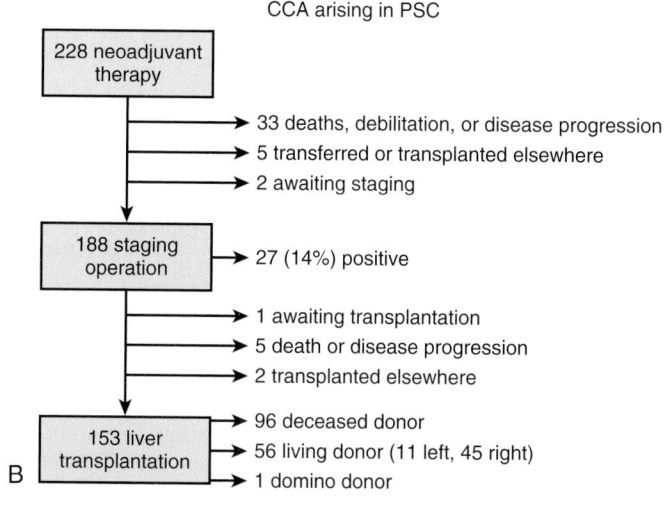

FIGURE 108B.1   **A,** Mayo Clinic Cholangiocarcinoma Treatment Protocol, all patients. (Courtesy Mayo Clinic.) **B,** Mayo Clinic Cholangiocarcinoma Treatment Protocol, cholangiocarcinoma (CCA) arising in primary sclerosing cholangitis (PSC). (Courtesy Mayo Clinic.) **C,** Mayo Clinic Cholangiocarcinoma Treatment Protocol, cholangiocarcinoma (CCA) arising de novo. (Courtesy Mayo Clinic.)

moving through the protocol are shown separately for patients with CCA arising in PSC (see Fig. 108B.1B) and CCA arising de novo (see Fig. 108B.1B).

Overall patient survival from enrollment in the protocol (intention-to-treat analysis) was 52% (± 3%) at 5 years and 44% (± 3%) at 10 years after the start of neoadjuvant therapy (Fig. 108B.2A). Survival for patients with underlying PSC (*n* = 228) was 58% at 5 years and 51% (± 4%) at 5 and 10 years compared with 41% (± 5%) and 32% (± 5%) for patients with de novo CCA (*n* = 148; see Fig. 108B.2B). Survival after transplantation was 68% (± 3%) at 5 years and 60 (± 4%) at 10 years for the entire group (Fig. 108B.3A). Patients with underlying PSC (*n* = 153) had 5- and 10-year survival of 74% (± 4%) and 67 (± 4%) compared with 58% (± 6%) and 47% (± 6%) for patients with de novo CCA (*n* = 84; see Fig. 108B.3B).

Eighty-six patients have died after transplantation: 13 from surgical complications within a year after transplantation; 56 from recurrent cancer (median intervals – 28 months after transplantation and 9 months after detection of recurrence); and 32 from unrelated causes more than a year after transplantation including 4 from other cancers (thyroid, uterine, colon,

and unknown adenocarcinoma 11 years after transplantation and PD).

Recurrence and Prognostic Factors

Sixty-three of the 237 patients (27%) who underwent OLT developed recurrent disease at a median of 18 months and a mean of 24 months (range, 3–80 months) after OLT. The most frequent locations for recurrence were abdominal (70%), chest and mediastinum (16%), and bone (6%; Table 108B.1).

The Mayo group reviewed their experience in 2012 with an aim to identify clinical and pathologic predictors of protocol dropout and recurrence after transplantation.[21] At that time, 199 patients had begun neoadjuvant therapy, 62 dropped out because of staging findings or disease progression, 6 underwent transplantation or were transferred to other centers, and 131 had undergone transplantation. The median follow-up was 2.6 years (0–17.8 years). Twenty-six patients (20%) had documented recurrences at a median of 23 months after transplantation. Clinical characteristics found to be predictive of protocol fall-out included: mass of at least 3 cm, CA19-9 level greater than 500 U/mL, cytology, or histology confirmation of CCA, and a calculated MELD score greater than 20. Clinical

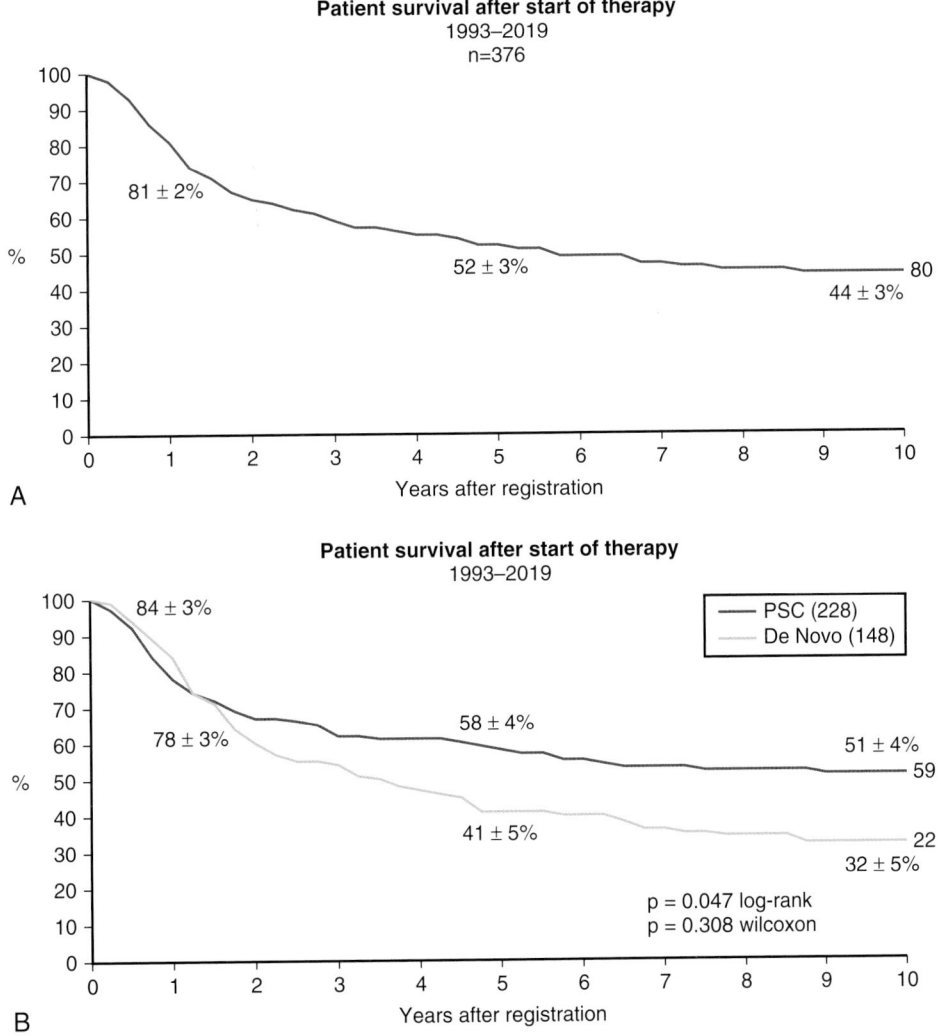

FIGURE 108B.2 A, Mayo Clinic protocol: Survival after start of therapy, all patients. (Courtesy Mayo Clinic.) **B,** Mayo Clinic protocol: Survival after start of therapy, cholangiocarcinoma (CCA) arising in primary sclerosing cholangitis (PSC) and CCA arising de novo. (Courtesy Mayo Clinic.)

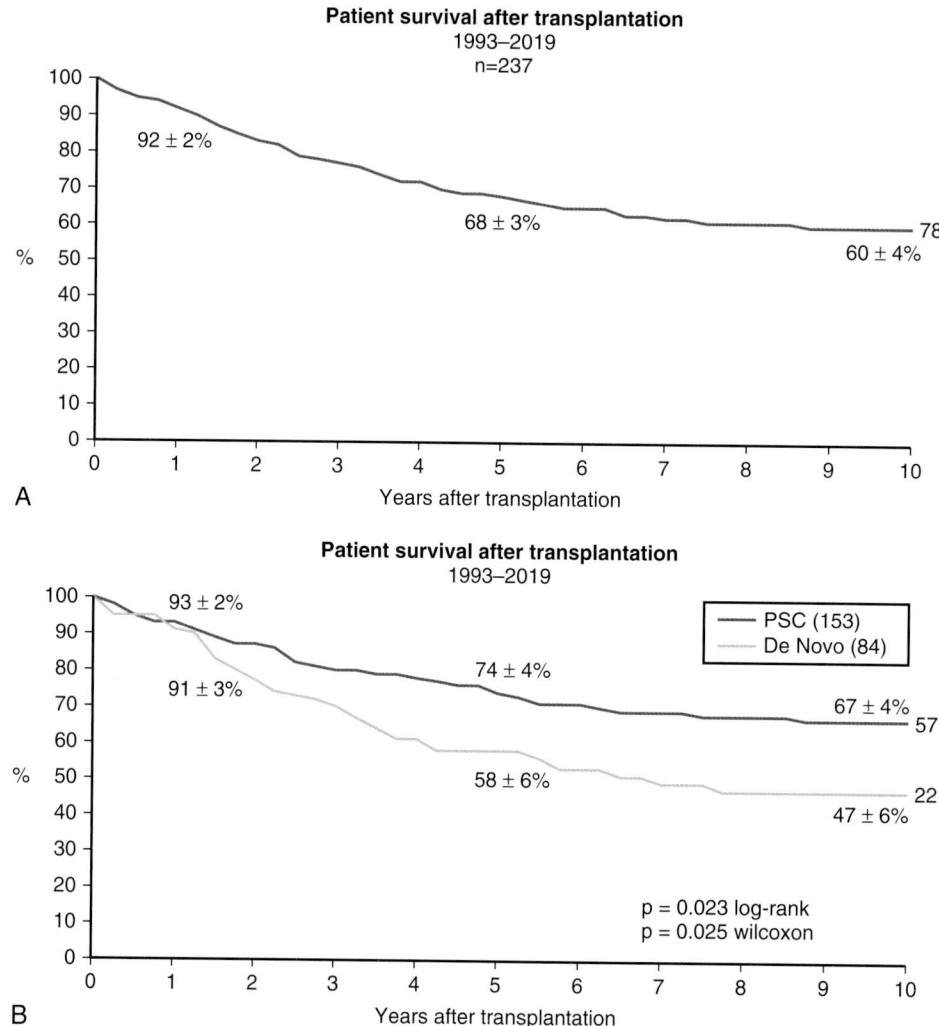

FIGURE 108B.3 **A,** Mayo Clinic protocol: Survival after transplantation, all patients. (Courtesy Mayo Clinic.) **B,** Mayo Clinic protocol: Survival after transplantation, cholangiocarcinoma (CCA) arising in primary sclerosing cholangitis (PSC) and CCA arising de novo. (Courtesy Mayo Clinic.)

TABLE 108B.1	Cholangiocarcinoma Recurrence After Transplantation	
SITE	TIME (MO)	STATUS (MO)
Regional	7, 10, 14	Dead at 10, 17, 18
	14, 15, 17, 65	Alive at 21, 16, 24, 67
Peritoneal	15	Alive at 23
	22, 25, 27	Dead at 29, 41, 43
Chest	18, 24	Alive at 36, 48
	22, 30, 40	Dead at 24, 30, 64
Bone	7, 8, 55	Dead at 37, 10, 84
	47	Dead at 48
Miscellaneous	34	Alive at 37
	47	Dead at 48
Mean time to recurrence was 25 months.		

factors identified as predictors of recurrence after transplantation included elevation of CA19-9 at the time of enrollment, PV encasement, and presence of residual cancer in the explanted liver. The presence of residual cancer was the most significant of these three factors. When matched for tumor characteristics, there was no difference in risk for recurrence between patients with CCA arising in PSC and those with CCA arising de novo. An updated review of patients undergoing LDLT for hilar CCA demonstrated that residual tumor found in the explant was associated with significantly worse outcomes, whereas underlying liver disease (e.g., PSC) or vascular/biliary complications did not influence outcomes.[20]

Pancreatoduodenectomy and Transplantation

Approximately 10% (13 of 146, excluding 7 patients that underwent planned en bloc PD) of PSC patients with hilar CCA have been found to have CBD involvement during transplantation. Three patients underwent re-excision of the CBD within the head of the pancreas, and all three developed recurrent cancer. The other 11 patients underwent PD. The addition of a PD greatly increases the technical complexity of transplantation and has a significant impact on postoperative morbidity and mortality (see Chapter 117A). The Mayo Clinic experience includes 20 patients that underwent combined OLT and PD: 7 that had en bloc hepatopancreatoduodenectomy for preoperatively recognized CBD involvement and 13 because of findings on frozen section of the transected CBD (12 malignancy, 1 high-grade dysplasia). Five-year survival was only 38%

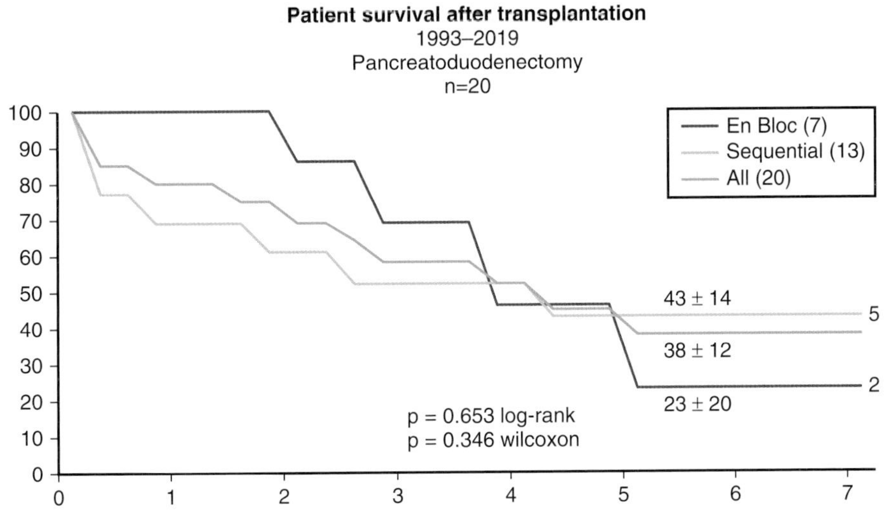

FIGURE 108B.4 Patient survival after combined pancreatoduodenectomy and liver transplantation. (Courtesy Mayo Clinic.)

($\pm$ 12%; Fig. 108B.4), much less than the 74% ($\pm$ 4%) 5-year survival for all patients with CCA arising in PSC. Six of the 13 (46%) patients that underwent sequential PD because of CBD involvement and 1 of the 7 (14%) that underwent en bloc PD developed recurrent cancer, and there was no difference in survival between those patients that underwent sequential versus planned en bloc PD (see Fig. 108B.4). Combined OLT-PD is also associated with higher morbidity.[22] Biliary and pancreatic leaks are especially troublesome with combined OLT-PD using living-donor liver allografts, and we have recently modified our technique for reconstruction using the proximal jejunum for the pancreas anastomosis (standard reconstruction) and a separate Roux-en-Y jejunal limb for the biliary anastomosis.[23] The results of combined OLT-PD remain marginal, and the procedure should be performed with great caution and only for patients with microscopic CBD involvement or technical issues arising in favorable situations.

Vascular Complications

Vascular complications are much more common after transplantation for CCA than after other indications because of the neoadjuvant therapy[20,24] (see Chapter 111). Use of the irradiated native common hepatic artery is avoided during DDLT in lieu of a deceased-donor iliac artery graft from the infrarenal aorta. This strategy was initially implemented in LDLT but resulted in an unacceptable rate of acute hepatic artery thrombosis. Subsequently, the native hepatic artery has been used for arterial inflow in LDLT; this strategy reduced early hepatic artery thrombosis, but it is associated with a 20% late (after 2 weeks) stenosis/thrombosis rate. Likewise, there is also a 20% rate of late PV stenosis (with or without thrombosis) after DDLT and a 30% rate after LDLT. The Mayo Clinic team has routinely used a segment of deceased-donor iliac vein as an interposition graft during LDLT. Use of the graft is often necessary to bridge the gap between the recipient PV (which is divided as low as possible) and the living-donor allograft right or left PV. Use of the graft also allows better placement of a transhepatic PV stent should the patient develop portal stenosis; the added length allows the stent to be positioned within the iliac vein graft such that it does not obstruct the right anterior or right posterior PV branch within the liver allograft. Stenoses

after LDLT with portal interposition grafts have always involved the native PV and its anastomosis with the interposition graft and not the donor PV. We recently reported, however, that use of an interposition graft is associated with an increased risk for PV stenosis,[20] and we now only use a graft when necessary to bridge a gap between the donor and recipient PVs.

All patients undergo Doppler US and contrast CT examination 4 months after transplantation. These imaging studies enable detection of an asymptomatic stenosis that is usually amenable to angioplasty with or without stent insertion. Arterial complications are treated by a transarterial approach, and portal complications are treated by a transhepatic approach.

Medical and Neoadjuvant Complications

The effect of neoadjuvant radiotherapy on the liver is profound. Widespread necrosis is found in the hilus with necrotic debris in the major ducts; thus pre-transplant infectious complications related to neoadjuvant therapy are very common and require continuous care and frequent hospitalization for patients awaiting transplantation. Nearly all patients have one or more episodes of cholangitis with occasional development of intrahepatic abscesses. Cholecystitis is treated nonoperatively with antibiotics, although severe cases may require endoscopic placement of a cystic duct stent or percutaneous cholecystostomy. Several patients have developed gallbladder necrosis with rupture that required emergency operations. Gastritis, duodenitis, and poor gastric emptying are also common and can persist after transplantation, which can lead to difficulties with nutrition. Several patients have required operative intervention for duodenal perforation or life-threatening hemorrhage from duodenitis and peptic ulceration.

CCA patients are hypercoagulable and at risk for deep venous thrombosis (DVT) and pulmonary embolism, as observed with other types of malignancies. Thus they receive DVT prophylaxis whenever hospitalized for nonbleeding complications and especially during the perioperative periods after operative staging and transplantation.

Key Questions

Despite the success reported by the Mayo Clinic, the results remain controversial. Key questions fueling controversy pertain to (1) accuracy of diagnosis before neoadjuvant therapy, (2) efficacy of the protocol, (3) whether transplantation for CCA is an appropriate use of donor organs, (4) whether these patients warrant prioritization for deceased-donor liver allocation, and (5) whether transplantation after neoadjuvant therapy should be used for patients with potentially resectable CCA in lieu of standard resection. These questions were identified in earlier versions of this chapter and continue to be subject to ongoing analysis.

Diagnostic Accuracy

The protocol diagnostic criteria allow for enrollment of patients without pathologic confirmation of CCA. It is indeed probable that some patients who did not have CCA were treated with neoadjuvant therapy and LT; although these patients would favorably affect the results, their impact is not significant. Furthermore, it would be difficult to require pathologic confirmation of disease before treatment. Pathologic confirmation is notoriously difficult for hilar CCA, and a large proportion of patients treated without it are subsequently confirmed by findings at the staging operation or transplantation. In 2012 the Mayo Clinic team reported that pathologic confirmation of CCA before therapy was achieved in 45 of 87 (52%) PSC patients and 22 of 49 (45%) de novo patients that underwent transplantatio.[25] Pretreatment pathologic confirmation was associated with significantly worse 5-year survival after start of therapy for PSC patients (50% vs. 80%, $P = .001$) but not for de novo patients (39% vs. 48%, $P = .27$). Pre-treatment pathologic confirmation was associated with worse 5-year survival after transplantation for PSC patients (66% vs. 92%, $P = .01$) but not for de novo patients (63% vs. 65%, $P = .71$). The difference in the PSC patients was not because of recurrent cancer. Absence of pre-treatment pathologic confirmation did not result in less detection of residual CCA in the explanted livers nor in less recurrence after LT. It would thus be difficult to deny treatment to patients who fulfill the diagnostic criteria but do not have pathologic confirmation of CCA.

Efficacy

Intention-to-treat analysis of the Mayo Clinic experience demonstrates 52% and 44% 5- and 10-year survival (split PSC and de novo). These results have been corroborated by several large multicenter studies and smaller single-center experiences. Twelve large-volume US transplant centers, reported 53% 5-year survival for 287 patients (including 193 from Mayo Clinic).[26] This study added validation to the Mayo Clinic exclusion criteria; the study included several patients that had tumors larger than 3 cm in radial diameter that adversely affected survival. The US Extrahepatic Biliary Malignancy Consortium includes three centers (Emory University, University of Wisconsin, and Washington University) that together have accrued experience with 70 patients transplanted for CCA. Their results are similar to those reported by Mayo Clinic; 53% survival at 5 years with a similar ration between patients with CCA arising in PSC and de novo CCA.[27] A recent meta-analysis of published worldwide experiences has also corroborated the efficacy of transplantation and confirmed the significant benefit afforded by neoadjuvant therapy.[28] Most of the patients included in these series had unresectable disease, either because of technical considerations and/or underlying PSC, such that no other potentially curative treatment was available for them. All of these results clearly exceed the natural history

of untreated de novo CCA, which has a 50% to 90% mortality rate at 1 year.[17,29,30] In the latter study, 34 patients with a diagnosis of CCA in the Netherlands were determined to have had unresectable disease and would have been eligible for transplantation based on the Mayo Clinic criteria. The median survival for these patients that did not undergo transplantation was only 13 months. It is well established that survival for patients with CCA arising in the setting of PSC is dismal.[16]

The standard surgical treatment for hilar CCA arising de novo is resection with partial hepatectomy, en bloc excision of the extrahepatic duct, and radical lymphadenectomy. After complete extirpation of tumor, 5-year survival after an R0 resection ranges from 30% to 45% (see Chapters 51 and 119B).

The Mayo protocol has achieved comparable results with patients having unresectable de novo CCA, with 5-year survival of 37% for 107 patients after the start of neoadjuvant therapy and 5-year survival of 37% for 64 patients after transplantation. Furthermore, these results clearly demonstrate the efficacy of neoadjuvant therapy because 43% of patients with pathologic confirmation before neoadjuvant therapy had neither residual disease in the explant nor a recurrence after transplantation.[25]

Appropriate Use of Donor Organs

The results achieved with LT for CCA after neoadjuvant therapy and operative staging are comparable to results achieved with LT for other malignant, chronic, and acute liver diseases such as PSC, hepatitis C, and HCC.[31] Because patients with CCA arising in the setting of PSC and those with unresectable CCA arising de novo have no other potentially curative treatment options, we have advocated that LT is an appropriate use of both deceased-donor and living-donor livers. There is a significant difference in the 5-year survival after transplantation for patients who developed hilar CCA in the setting of PSC (74 ± 4%; $n = 153$) versus those patients with de novo cancer (58% ± 6%; $n = 84$), and this difference is even greater with LDLT (75.9% vs. 47.5% 5-year survival).[20] The lower survival outcome after transplantation for de novo hilar CCA patients will need to be carefully monitored to ensure appropriate allocation and use of both deceased and living-donor liver allografts.

It is important to assess both survival after start of neoadjuvant therapy and survival after transplantation. Survival after start of neoadjuvant therapy is an "intention-to-treat analysis" and demonstrates efficacy of treatment. Survival after LT is important for assessment of donor liver utilization.

Deceased-Donor Allocation and Prioritization

As CCA emerged as a valid indication for LT, allocation of deceased-donor livers became highly controversial (see Chapter 109). Mayo Clinic Rochester is within United Network of Organ Sharing (UNOS) Region 7, and that region's review board members agreed to MELD score exception guidelines shortly after the implementation of MELD for liver allocation in 2002. MELD score exceptions were given to patients who successfully completed neoadjuvant therapy and had no evidence of metastases at operative staging. The initial adjustment was a score of 20, matching that of HCC at the time and was increased in parallel to the score schedule for HCC, but at 6-month rather than 3-month intervals, as was done for HCC.

Additional aims of the guidelines were to determine the risk of disease progression in patients awaiting transplantation and to retain incentives for use of living liver donors and use of extended criteria donors. The Mayo Clinic transplanted 42 patients between September 2002 and January 2006, with a median staging-to-transplant interval of 114 days. After transplantation, 1 of 21 patients with an interval less than 114 days developed recurrent disease, whereas 4 of 21 patients with an interval greater than 114 days developed recurrent disease (92% ± 7% vs. 56% ± 19% disease-free 2.5-year survival). Although the difference was not statistically significant because of the small number of patients, the results suggested that prolongation of waiting time led to an increase in recurrent disease after transplantation (unpublished data). A group of transplant surgeons and physicians met as an ad hoc MELD Exception Study Group in March 2006 to review the available data for the treatment of hilar CCA with neoadjuvant therapy followed by OLT.[32] The group concluded that sufficient data existed to justify priority for patients enrolled in clinical trials that used neoadjuvant therapy provided that (1) transplant centers submit formal patient care protocols to the UNOS Liver and Intestinal Committee; (2) candidates satisfy accepted diagnostic criteria for CCA and are considered to be unresectable on the basis of technical considerations or underlying liver disease, such as PSC; (3) tumor mass, when visible on cross-sectional imaging studies, is less than 3 cm in radial diameter; (4) imaging studies to assess patients for intrahepatic and extrahepatic metastases are repeated before interval score increases; (5) regional hepatic lymph node involvement and the peritoneal cavity is assessed by operative staging after completion of neoadjuvant therapy and before transplantation; and (6) transperitoneal aspiration or biopsy of the primary tumor is avoided because of the high risk of tumor seeding associated with these procedures. The group also concluded that prioritization of patients with biliary dysplasia to avoid progression to CCA was not justified. In 2009, UNOS adopted these MELD exception criteria, and the score adjustment is identical to that for HCC, with score increases at 3-month intervals. With the most recent changes in UNOS liver allocation policy, hilar CCA patients meeting UNOS criteria are granted MELD exception scores equivalent to 3 points less than the listing transplant center's median MELD score of the time, with no further escalation while on the waiting list. We are now re-assessing the risk for patients to fall-out of the treatment protocol, and preliminary data suggest that the risk for protocol fall-out (before, during, or after the staging operation) is 45% (± 5%) for patients with de novo CCA and 43% (± 5%) for patient with CCA arising in PSC at one year after the start of treatment (censoring those patients that underwent transplantation at the time of transplantation) (unpublished results). We also have preliminary (unpublished data) that suggests that early transplantation (with waiting times less than 4 months) have more recurrent CCA after transplantation. This finding is similar to results with LT for HCC, which led to a change in the UNOS MELD score exception guidelines for HCC that now require a 6-month interval of observation before a MELD score exception.

Resection Versus Transplantation

Because results with the Mayo protocol equal or exceed the results achieved with resection, it would seem reasonable to consider neoadjuvant therapy and LT in lieu of resection for patients with potentially resectable disease. We retrospectively compared results for patients treated by potentially curative resection and neoadjuvant therapy and LT at the Mayo Clinic

between 1993 and 2004.[33] Although no statistically significant difference in survival was found between the two groups, a strong trend was seen toward better survival in the group treated with neoadjuvant therapy and LT (see Chapters 51 and 119B).

Since that time, the Mayo group has accrued a larger experience with LT for patients with unresectable de novo CCA, and the results with the protocol show an overall survival of 58% (± 6%) at 5-years after the start of neoadjuvant therapy. A prospective trial of resection versus transplantation once considered impractical because of the large number of patients that would be necessary to show a significant difference in survival is now underway in France. It is important to recognize that crossover between the resection and transplant treatment arms is not possible. Patients treated with neoadjuvant therapy are not amenable to resection. The effect of high-dose neoadjuvant therapy on the underlying liver and bile duct is profound (Fig. 108B.5A–B) and precludes biliary reconstruction because of widespread intrahepatic duct necrosis. Patients found to be unresectable at operation are not appropriate for subsequent neoadjuvant therapy and transplantation. Results with resection are also improving with increasing experience and technical innovation; Neuhaus and colleagues (1999, 2003)[34,35] demonstrated excellent 5-year survival using vascular reconstruction

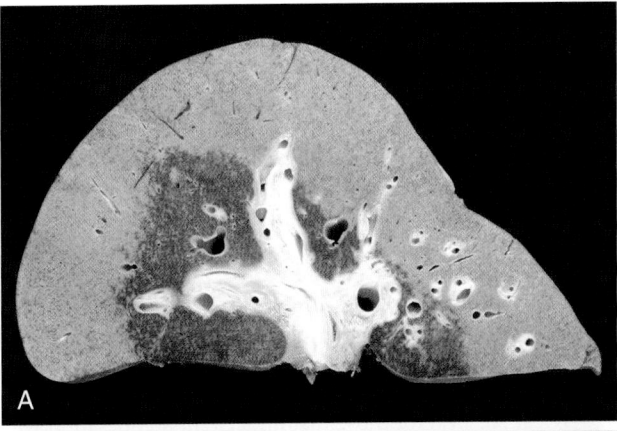

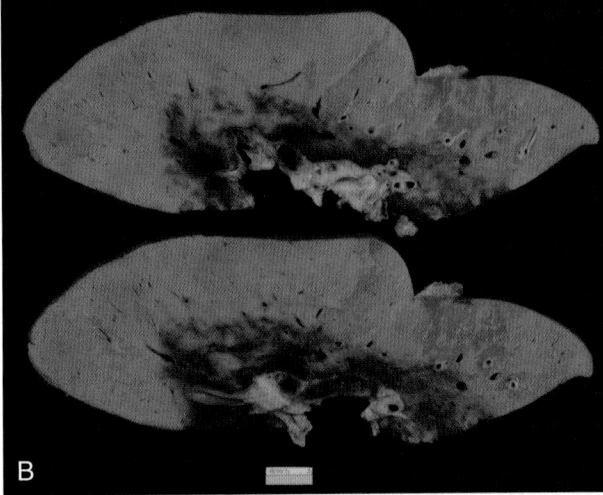

FIGURE 108B.5 A, Explanted liver after neoadjuvant therapy showing radiation effect. (Courtesy Mayo Clinic.) **B,** Explanted liver after neoadjuvant therapy showing duct necrosis and intraductal debris. (Courtesy Mayo Clinic.)

with extended hepatectomy.[36] Nagino and colleagues have achieved exceptional results with a large experience[37] even for patients with advanced disease beyond the criteria for neoadjuvant therapy and transplantation.[38]

The early report by Rea et al. in 2005[33] included patients with both PSC and de novo hilar CCA. Our group published an updated retrospective review that only included de novo cancer from 1993 to 2013. The goal was to determine if potentially resectable or borderline resectable patients would be better treated with neoadjuvant therapy and OLT ($n = 90$) versus resection ($n = 124$). Overall survival at 1, 3 and 5 years was 90%, 71%, and 59% for OLT and 81%, 53%, and 36% for resection ($P = .003$). However, no difference was found between the two groups when adjusting for patient age, lymph node metastases, and tumor size. Subset analysis in patients with Bismuth-Corlette IV hilar CCA were found to have a statistically significant worse survival than patients undergoing OLT ($P = .039$; $n = 40$). These data suggest that clearly resectable de novo hilar CCA should be treated with resection and that borderline resectable patients with Bismuth-Corlette type IV patients are probably best treated with OLT.[39]

The US Extrahepatic Biliary Malignancy Consortium (10 centers, including 3 that have experience with neoadjuvant therapy and LT for patients with CCA) conducted a review of their experience to compare results of neoadjuvant therapy and transplantation to resection.[27] Three hundred four patients were treated at the 10 centers between 2000 and 2015; 234 underwent resection and 70 were enrolled in the neoadjuvant therapy and transplantation protocol (the largest published experience not including the Mayo Clinic). Intention-to-treat analysis demonstrated improved survival for patients enrolled in the neoadjuvant therapy protocol compared with resection (53% vs. 17% 5-year survival), and 5-year survival after transplantation was 64%. They concluded that for patients with CCA meeting transplant criteria (other than unresectability), that resection was associated with substantially decreased survival compared with transplantation. An accompanying editorial,[40] however, emphasizes that the results (41% 5-year survival for patients that began neoadjuvant therapy versus 27% 5-year survival for those that underwent an operation with intent to achieve resection) only show a difference of 14%. Although the difference is statistically significant, the results with resection are slightly lower than results commonly reported in the literature. The main issue, however, is whether this benefit (even if it is as large as a 14% improvement in survival) is large enough to justify use of deceased or living-donor liver. It is also suggested that surgeons deciding between the two treatment options should estimate survival after resection by multiplying survival results achieved with R0 resection with an estimated likelihood of achieving and R0 resection. Patients likely to have an R0 resection should undergo resection and those with a lower likelihood of having an R0 resection should undergo neoadjuvant therapy and LT.

Summary—Hilar Cholangiocarcinoma

Neoadjuvant therapy followed by OLT for the treatment of hilar CCA achieves excellent results for highly selected patients with early-stage disease. The results compare favorably to survival after OLT for chronic liver disease and for HCC. Neoadjuvant therapy with subsequent LT has emerged as the treatment of choice for patients with unresectable hilar CCA or

hilar CCA arising in the setting of PSC. Long-term outcomes of de novo cancer undergoing OLT will require further scrutiny to ensure appropriate allocation of liver grafts to these patients. Success requires careful patient selection with adherence to protocol and operative staging before OLT. Neoadjuvant therapy introduces considerable morbidity and unique complications not usually encountered with transplantation alone, and these challenges highlight the need for a multidisciplinary team that includes hepatologists, interventional radiologists, gastroenterologists, radiation and medical oncologists, and transplant surgeons to achieve success.

INTRAHEPATIC CHOLANGIOCARCINOMA AND MIXED HCC/CCA

Intrahepatic CCA (see Chapter 50) has long been recognized as a contraindication for LT. Liver resection is the only available potentially curative treatment, but few patients have disease amenable to resection and survival after resection is low. Nevertheless, some patients with intrahepatic CCA do undergo LT, either for known small intrahepatic CCA or because they were thought to have HCC. Sapisochin and colleagues reported 65% 5-year survival for patients with intrahepatic CCA less than 2 cm in diameter compared with 45% survival for patients with larger tumors in a large international multicenter study.[41] Likewise, a similar study from Mayo Clinic Florida assessed outcomes for patients with an initial diagnosis of HCC that were found to have intrahepatic CCA or mixed tumors in the explanted liver after transplantation.[42] Forty-four of 618 (7%) patients transplanted with primary liver cancer were found to have CCA in their explanted livers. Twelve of these patients were considered to have early CCA (less than 2 cm and thought to be HCC), and their survival was compared with 319 patients with HCC that were within Milan criteria. Five-year patient survival was 63.6% for those with CCA compared with 70.3% for HCC ($P = .25$). Similar results have been reported for patients with small mixed HCC-CCA tumors as reported in a literature search study[43] and a series matched with HCC.[44] The latter study also demonstrated that patients with mixed HCC-CCA that are low grade and only have well to moderate differentiation do as well as patients with HCC with similar pathology after transplantation.

Hong and colleagues at UCLA reported encouraging results for a series of patients with hilar and intrahepatic CCA that received various neoadjuvant therapies before transplantation.[45] Inspired by this experience and results achieved with neoadjuvant therapy and LT for hilar CCA, a collaborative team effort by Methodist Hospital and MD Anderson in Houston has attempted a similar strategy for the treatment of patients with intrahepatic CCA.[46] The Methodist – MD Anderson team developed a protocol for patients with locally advanced, unresectable intrahepatic CCA. They excluded patients with extrahepatic disease or vascular involvement. Patients received neoadjuvant gemcitabine-based chemotherapy and were required to have a minimum of 6 months of radiographic response before being considered for LT. Twelve of 21 patients referred for evaluation were enrolled in the protocol and 6 patients underwent LT. Three patients developed recurrent disease 6 to 9 months (median 7.6 months) after LT with 80% patient survival and 50% disease-free 5-year survival. These results have encouraged others to consider similar trials, both for patients with unresectable disease and for patients with small cancers because of the marginal results achieved with resection.

METASTATIC NEUROENDOCRINE CANCER (SEE CHAPTERS 65 AND 91)

Gastroenteropancreatic neuroendocrine cancers (NECs) are a rare, diverse group of tumors with an incidence of 1 to 2 cases per 100,000 per year with a slight female predominance.[47] These tumors are characteristically indolent in nature and are frequently found to be metastatic at the time of diagnosis. The liver is the most common site for metastases, and widespread hepatic dissemination resulting in liver failure is the leading cause of death in these patients.[48] Fortunately, these cancers are often confined to the liver for protracted periods of time with 5-year survival of 13% to 54% even without treatment.[49–51]

Various therapeutic options have been used for NEC with hepatic metastases; such treatments include transarterial chemoembolization (TACE; see Chapter 94A), radiofrequency (RFA and cryoablation (see Chapters 96A and 96D), systemic chemotherapy (see Chapters 65 and 91), peptide receptor radionuclide therapy (see Chapters 65 and 91), cytoreductive resection, surgical resection (see Chapters 101, 102, and 118), and LT. Surgical extirpation with an R0 resection is the most effective therapy for metastatic NEC confined to the liver; however, only 10% to 57% of these tumors are amenable to complete resection.[48,52–57]

LT is an option for treatment of patients with a low probability of achieving adequate debulking. The goals of LT are to (1) achieve palliation by alleviating symptoms for patients with functioning NEC; (2) achieve palliation by delaying death caused by tumor replacement of the liver, taking advantage of the slow progression and the time it will take to replace the new liver with tumor, "resetting the clock"; and (3) achieve a cure. LT is highly effective at relieving symptoms for patients with functioning NEC. There are several single-center[55,58–60] and multicenter[61–63] studies reporting 36% to 90% patient survival at 5 years. A systematic review of all single-center, multicenter, and registry data studies to date found that disease recurrence after LT ranges from 31.3% to 56.8%.[64] Disease-free survival is only 20% to 77% at 5 years, and tumor recurrence after 5 years is common. Five-year overall survival is 63%. Several clinical factors such as liver involvement exceeding 50% of the liver mass and pancreatic origin of NEC, as well as tumor biology (Ki-67 index over 10%) are associated with worse outcomes after LT.

Widespread acceptance of OLT as a reasonable option for the treatment of this disease remains limited and controversial (see Chapter 105) for multiple reasons that include the scarcity of deceased-donor organs available for OLT and the availability of other treatment modalities that can also provide palliation. Furthermore, reliable selection criteria have not been identified, and long-term data are limited because of the low incidence of the disease. Most importantly, it remains difficult to determine the actual benefit derived from OLT because of the protracted course of metastatic disease and unknown natural history of disease for those patients selected as candidates for transplantation. However, based on available data, the Organ Procurement and Transplantation Network (OPTN) in the US has established a guidance document for a select group of patients with metastatic NEC to the liver meeting Milan criteria[55] to be granted MELD exception points for

liver allocation (http://optn.transplant.hrsa.gov/resources/by-organ/liver-intestine).

The Mayo Clinic developed a protocol in 2002 designed to assess efficacy of LT for patients with metastatic NEC confined to the liver and regional hepatic lymph nodes.[65] The clinical inclusion/exclusion criteria are summarized in Box 108B.1. Each patient was screened for locally recurrent and extrahepatic disease with chest, abdomen, and pelvic CT scans, bone scan, and somatostatin receptor scintigraphy within 60 days of preliminary registration for transplantation. Prior treatment modalities did not exclude patients, as long as they did not technically prohibit OLT. Patients were observed for 6 months after resection of the primary NEC to exclude extrahepatic disease progression. Reevaluation for metastatic disease before LT was performed every 4 months via laboratory tests, tumor marker assays, and abdominal imaging studies. Extrahepatic metastases were excluded via operative staging with laparoscopy before OLT.

The results were published with short follow-up. Since that time, 25 patients with metastatic NEC have undergone transplantation at the Mayo Clinic, with 74% patient survival and 44% disease-free survival at 5 years (unpublished data). Consistent with information in the literature, patients with carcinoid tumors fared slightly better than those with islet cell tumors originating in the pancreas. In summary, LT effectively alleviates symptoms for patients with diffuse, functioning NEC liver metastases. LT may improve patient survival for those destined to

---

BOX 108B.1 Mayo Clinic Transplantation Selection Criteria for Patients With Metastatic Neuroendocrine Carcinoma

Inclusion Criteria

1. Histologic confirmation of NEC (liver primary vs. metastatic disease confined to the liver)
2. Unresectable hepatic disease involving both lobes
3. Complete resection of the primary NEC or single dominant liver NEC believed to be a primary lesion
4. Absence of extrahepatic disease with the exception of regional lymph nodes resectable as part of standard liver transplantation
5. At least a 6-month interval from resection of primary NEC and transplantation without extrahepatic disease progression
6. Patient deemed suitable for liver transplantation, meeting all United Network for Organ Sharing listing criteria

Exclusion Criteria

1. Prior nonselective hepatic artery embolization unless approved by the transplant surgeon (only for living-donor transplantation)
2. Rectal NEC
3. Anaplastic or poorly differentiated (grade 3 or 4) tumor
4. Right atrial pressure > 15 mm Hg
5. Known pregnancy
6. Other factors that preclude transplantation, including severe comorbidities, infection, or other malignancies

Other

1. Patients are staged with computed tomographic scan of the chest, abdomen, and pelvis; bone scan; and somatostatin receptor scintigraphy scan
2. All patients undergo open or laparoscopic staging celiotomy
3. Patients are reevaluated every 4 months with abdominal imaging to evaluate for extrahepatic disease progression

NEC, Neuroendocrine cancer

succumb to liver replacement by tumor, but no studies actually demonstrate efficacy nor has any study evaluated the potential for improvement in quality of life.[66] Recurrence is common after transplantation, and results with metastatic gastrinoma and glucagonoma are poor, so transplantation should not be done for these types of tumors. Recent studies have attempted to clarify the indications and optimal timing for transplantation,[62,66,67] but these guidelines remain controversial and ill defined.

METASTATIC COLORECTAL CANCER (SEE CHAPTER 90)

CRC is one of the most common malignancies in the world, and approximately half of the patients are diagnosed with metastases at the time of presentation. The liver is the most frequent site of CRC metastasis, and unfortunately curative resection of the liver metastases is possible in only about 20% of patients. LT provides the theoretical opportunity to achieve an R0 resection by replacing the whole liver for patients with unresectable metastases. The initial results with LT for metastatic CRC were poor. Five-year survival was less than 20% because of perioperative mortality and disease recurrence. These results led to discontinuation of LT for patients with unresectable CRC metastases. With improvements in perioperative care, imaging techniques and advances in chemotherapy, the University of Oslo group rejuvenated interest in LT. In 2006, they initiated the SECA-I (SEcondary CAncer) trial, a pilot study designed to investigate the efficacy of LT in the treatment of unresectable CRC metastases.[68] The Oslo group transplanted 21 patients with unresectable CRC metastases. All patients had completed radical excision of the primary tumor, received at least 6 weeks of chemotherapy, and underwent perioperative staging to assess perihepatic lymph nodes for metastatic disease before LT. Although patient survival exceeded expected survival for patients treated with chemotherapy (60% at 5 years), 19 of 21 patients developed metastases or local recurrence 2 to 24 months (median 6 months) after LT. Four clinical factors were associated with worse overall survival: maximal tumor diameter above 5.5 cm, time from resection of primary tumor less than 2 years, carcinoembryonic antigen (CEA) levels exceeding 80 μg/L at the time of transplantation, and progression of metastatic disease on chemotherapy. These four factors were used to establish the Oslo score (0–4), which correlated with survival.

The SECA-II trial, by the same group, used a more stringent set of criteria in 15 patients treated with LT for unresectable metastatic CRC.[69] They selected patients with at least a 1-year interval between diagnosis and LT and at least a 10% response to chemotherapy and reported 5-year actuarial survival of 83% (and 3-year disease-free survival of 35%). Analyzing their cumulative experience (both SECA-I and SECA-II trials), they found that the 5-year survival of patients with an Oslo score of 0 to 2 was 67%, compared with 17% for those with a score of 3 to 4, with a median follow-up of 85 months. In a multicenter European experience of 12 patients with unresectable CRC metastases, LT achieved 50% 5-year survival, with a median follow-up of 26 months.[70] Notably, in all three studies, most patients had disease recurrence.

These recent results demonstrate that LT can provide good outcomes in patients with unresectable liver metastases from CRC. Data from both Oslo series show that patients with less of a tumor burden, less aggressive disease behavior, and more

favorable prognostic factors fare better than other patients.[71] Although the Oslo group's adoption of more restrictive selection criteria led to better patient survival, it is not known whether these same selection criteria would affect patient survival if transplantation were not available. Currently, experience with transplantation for metastatic CRC is too limited and follow-up is too short to support wider adoption of LT for this indication. Resectability of CRC liver metastases and patient survival with and without resection continues to improve with advances in chemotherapy and ablative therapy. Acceptance of metastatic CRC as an indication for LT will require more stringent comparison of patients treated with the multitude of modalities now available, and several trials in the United States and Europe are currently underway.

HEPATIC EPITHELIOID HEMANGIOENDOTHELIOMA (SEE CHAPTER 87)

HEHE, first described in 1982, is a rare neoplasm that originates from vascular endothelium and has unpredictable malignant potential.[72] Ishak and colleagues (1984)[73] first reported liver involvement in a series of 32 patients with HEHE, which arises between the second and ninth decades with 3 to 2 female predominance.[74] The etiology of HEHE remains elusive, although a multitude of conditions have been proposed to contribute to its development; these conditions include viral hepatitis, liver trauma, oral contraceptives, primary biliary cirrhosis, alcohol consumption, and exposure to vinyl chloride, asbestos, and Thorotrast.[74–79]

The most common clinical manifestations of HEHE are right upper quadrant pain, hepatomegaly, and weight loss. Weakness, anorexia, epigastric mass, ascites, nausea, jaundice, and fatigue are additional symptoms. Up to 25% of these lesions are detected as incidental findings.[74,77]

Two variants of HEHE have been described, *nodular* and *diffuse*. In actuality, the variants represent early- and late-stage disease. The *nodular type* is seen early with a highly variable number of 1- to 12-cm lesions arising throughout the liver. The lesions are typically hypodense on CT scan with high-density contrast uptake in the periphery. Individual nodules increase in size by spreading along the hepatic veins or PVs, and they eventually coalesce to form diffuse peripheral lesions. The CT appearance of the later *diffuse type* is typically a large, slow-growing lesion resulting from coalescence of smaller lesions. Flattening of the capsule may occur because of fibrosis, peripheral enhancement of contrast may be seen with many hypervascular central lesions, and hypertrophy of the unaffected segments of the liver may be apparent.[80–82]

Definitive radiographic diagnosis of the HEHE is usually not possible, especially in the nodular form, because of the similarity of this tumor with primary epithelial liver tumors and hepatic metastases. In a review of 434 cases of HEHE, most patients (87%) had multifocal disease involving both lobes of the liver at the time of presentation. Extrahepatic disease at diagnosis was common (36.6%) with involvement of the lung (8.5%), regional lymph nodes (7.7%), peritoneum (6.1%), spleen (3.2%), and diaphragm (1.6%).[74]

Histologically, HEHE may resemble other conditions such as venoocclusive disease, CCA, hemangioma, angiosarcoma, and metastatic signet ring cell carcinoma.[83] Furthermore, immunohistochemical staining may suggest a tumor of neuroendocrine origin. Histologic findings are consistent with epithelioid or histiocytoid morphology and intracytoplasmic lumina containing red blood cells. Immunohistochemical staining is positive for factor VIII–related antigen and endothelial cell markers (CD31, CD34) and negative for mucin, bile, CEA, and α-fetoprotein. Ultrastructural findings are characterized by a well-developed basal lamina, pinocytotic vesicles, and Weibel-Palade bodies.[73,74,77]

Treatment of HEHE is difficult. Resection is often not possible because of the presence of multifocal bilobar disease at the time of diagnosis. In the review by Mehrabi and colleagues (2006)[74], only 9.4% of patients were amenable to resection. Patient survival was 100% at 1 year and 75% at 5 years. For many patients, observation alone is reasonable because progression may be extremely slow, if it occurs at all. Others have reported poorer results[84] and have suggested that resection should be limited to patients presenting with unilobar, liver-confined disease.[85]

LT is an option for patients with extensive intrahepatic disease. Several series have reported outcomes equivalent to those for LT for other diagnoses. A multicenter Canadian experience with 11 patients reported 5-year survival of 82% with a 36.4% recurrence rate.[86] A query of the UNOS database identified 110 patients who underwent OLT for HEHE in the United States between 1987 and 2005.[87] Patient survival was 80% and 64% at 1 and 5 years. In their survey of the available literature, Mehrabi and colleagues (2006)[74] reported 1- and 5-year patient survival of 96% and 54.5%, respectively, after OLT.

The European Liver Transplant Registry (ELTR) reported a large series of transplantation for patents with HEHE in 2007[88] and updated this experience in 2017.[89] The initial report demonstrated 93%, 82% and 72% patient survival and 90%, 82%, and 64% disease-free survival at 1, 5, and 10 years after transplantation. A larger updated analysis of the ELTR was published in 2017 that studied 149 patients who underwent LT between 1984 and 2014. One-, 5- and 10-year patient survival was 88.6%, 79.5%, and 74.4%, respectively. Disease-free survival was 88.7%, 79.4%, and 72.8%.[89] Thirty-seven (24.8%) patients developed disease recurrence after a median time of 18 months after transplantation. The authors found 3 factors associated with increased risk of disease recurrence after transplantation: macrovascular invasion, involvement of hilar lymph nodes, and a short interval (less than 120 days) between diagnosis and transplantation. The authors postulate that a waiting time longer than 3 months allows observation of the disease process to avoid futile transplantation for patients with aggressive tumors or a hepatic angiosarcoma, and they suggest a mandatory waiting time that would also permit the administration of neoadjuvant therapy. It is important to rule out hepatic angiosarcoma (which is difficult to differentiate from HEHE by histology) because all patients with hepatic angiosarcoma developed recurrences within 6 months and none survived more than 2 years. The authors recommended tumor biopsy before transplantation to detect macrovascular invasion and regional lymphadenectomy at the time of transplantation. They did not feel as though the difference in survival between patients with and without regional lymph node involvement (65.4% vs. 84.2% long-term disease-free survival) was large enough to consider regional nodal involvement to be a contraindication to transplantation. The authors developed a scoring system using these three factors (macrovascular invasion, regional lymph node metastases, and waiting time less than 120 days) to stratify patients' risk of tumor recurrence, which could be applied to patient selection and/or adjuvant

therapy and immunosuppression management decisions after transplantation. They also demonstrated that extrahepatic disease (present in 26.8% of patients) did not significantly affect outcome (71.6% vs. 82.2% 5-year and 61.4% vs. 76.5% 10-year survival for those with and without extrahepatic disease; $P = .25$).

The Mayo Clinic reviewed its experience with 30 patients treated for HEHE between 1984 and 2007[90] and found a 2 to 1 female predominance with a mean age at diagnosis of 46 years (range, 21–79 years). The diagnosis of HEHE was confirmed in all cases by immunohistochemical staining for factor VIII–related antigen, CD31, and CD34. Patients were divided into groups based on the number and size of nodules present within the liver: half had 10 or fewer nodules, and half had more than 10 nodules; the largest lesion was smaller than 5 cm in 43%, it was 5 to 10 cm in 30%, and it was larger than 10 cm in 27% of cases. Extrahepatic disease was present at diagnosis in 37% of patients ($n = 11$). Sites of metastases included lung ($n = 8$), peritoneum ($n = 2$), bone ($n = 2$), brain ($n = 1$), and skin ($n = 1$), and one-third of the patients had multiple sites of extrahepatic involvement.

Therapeutic management included OLT ($n = 11$), primary resection ($n = 11$), systemic chemotherapy ($n = 5$), and no medical treatment ($n = 3$). Median follow-up was 41.6 months (range, 0–243), and in this time, 12 deaths (40%) were reported: 1 patient died within 2 years of primary resection, 6 patients died after OLT (1 month to 11 years), and 5 patients treated nonsurgically died 1 month to 4 years after diagnosis. Patient survival after primary resection at 1, 3, and 5 years was 100%, 86%, and 86%, respectively, compared with 91%, 73%, and 73%, respectively, for patients treated with OLT. Patient survival after nonoperative management was 57%, 43%, and 29% at 1, 3, and 5 years, respectively. Disease-free survival after primary resection was 78%, 62%, and 62% at 1, 3, and 5 years, compared with 64%, 46%, and 46% after OLT. Although no significant differences were seen in patient survival ($P = .128$) or disease-free survival ($P = .405$), patients who underwent primary resection had significantly fewer tumor nodules and less diffuse liver involvement compared with those who underwent OLT ($P = .004$).

Morphologic features associated with prolonged disease-free survival were nodular disease pattern ($P = .01$) and largest hepatic lesion 10 cm or smaller ($P = .003$). Patients with 10 or fewer tumor nodules showed a trend toward better survival ($P = .052$). Factors associated with decreased overall patient survival were tumor size larger than 10 cm ($P = .0007$, hazard ratio [HR], 10.97; 95% confidence interval [CI], 2.76–43.68), more than 10 nodules ($P = .023$; HR, 5.83; CI, 1.27–26.8), diffuse disease pattern ($P = .0076$; HR, 8.14; CI, 1.75–37.91), and involvement of more than four liver segments ($P = .041$; HR, 4.92; CI, 1.06–22.77). The presence of extrahepatic disease did not have an impact on patient survival ($P = .5$).

The Mayo Clinic findings demonstrate that primary resection and LT achieve comparable survival for patients with HEHE. Resection is favored for patients with 10 or fewer lesions, involvement of four or fewer liver segments, and disease amenable to complete extirpation of tumor. Transplantation is recommended for those with more than 10 lesions, involvement of more than four liver segments, and unresectable disease.

These experiences support HEHE as an indication for LT, especially for patients with unresectable disease, absence of macrovascular involvement, and a period of observation demonstrating favorable tumor behavior. Results achieved with LT are comparable to those achieved for other indications, even for patients with limited, non–life-threatening, extrahepatic disease.

SUMMARY

LT is appropriate therapy for selected patients with malignancies other than HCC. Excellent results have been achieved for patients with unresectable hilar CCA and hilar CCA arising in the setting of PSC. Success requires rigorous adherence to protocol with careful selection of patients with early-stage disease confined to the hilus along with neoadjuvant chemoradiotherapy and operative staging to exclude patients with regional lymph node metastases. LT without prior neoadjuvant therapy is rarely successful and should not knowingly be performed for patients with CCA.

The role of LT in the treatment of intrahepatic CCA remains unknown. Patients that undergo transplantation for HCC within transplant criteria and are found to have intrahepatic CCA or mixed tumors instead of HCC have a less favorable prognosis than those with HCC, but transplantation is still beneficial with a reasonable chance for prolonged survival. Trials are underway studying the efficacy of neoadjuvant therapy and LT for larger, unresectable intrahepatic CCA, and transplantation for intrahepatic CCA should at this time only be done in the setting of an investigational protocol.

The role of LT in the treatment of metastatic NEC remains unclear. Experience to date shows that most patients develop recurrent disease; however, transplantation may prolong survival by delaying death from tumor replacement of the liver. Because of the indolent nature of the disease, survival beyond 5 years is achievable, but the actual benefit—that is, the difference in survival with and without transplantation—remains unknown. Even more controversial is the role of LT in the treatment of metastatic colorectal cancer. Careful patient selection helped to achieve 83% 5-year actuarial survival in the pioneering work performed by the University of Oslo group. However, the recurrence rate remains high, and the results will need to be replicated by ongoing clinical trials.

LT achieves results comparable to resection for patients with HEHE, and transplantation should be considered for patients with more than 10 nodules, involvement of more than four liver segments, or tumors not amenable to resection. As with other malignancies, a period of observation before transplantation allows an assessment of disease behavior and an opportunity to administer neoadjuvant therapy, which may lessen the likelihood of futile transplantation.

References are available at expertconsult.com

Orthotopic liver transplantation: Standard donation after brain death, donation after cardiac death, and live donor – indications and outcomes

Teresa C. Rice, Fangyu Zhou, and William C. Chapman

Since the initial descriptions of successful deceased donor liver transplantation (LT) in the 1960s by Dr. Thomas Starzl (see Chapter 125), there has been tremendous change and growth in the field of transplantation. Advancements in organ preservation, immunosuppression, perioperative management, and refinements in surgical technique have contributed to an increased number of patients undergoing LT and growing indications for the procedure (see Chapter 105). For many patients with end-stage liver disease (ESLD), LT represents the only viable treatment modality. LT is an excellent option as curative therapy for early-stage hepatocellular carcinoma (HCC; see Chapter 108A) and in select cases of cholangiocarcinoma (CCA; see Chapter 108B), with good long-term outcomes. The obesity epidemic has led to a rapidly increasing number of patients with nonalcoholic steatohepatitis (NASH) listed for transplant.[1–3] Direct-acting antiviral therapy has altered the outcome of LT for hepatitis C virus (HCV) and allowed for the use of organ donors who are HCV antibody-positive.[4,5] Overall, patient survival after LT continues to improve and currently is 93% at 1 year, 87% at 3 years, and 80% at 5 years.[6]

Despite remarkable advancements in the last 50 years in the field of LT, limitations persist. Notably, there is a relatively fixed pool of cadaveric organ donors with a growing number of new waiting list registrations. Techniques implementing the use of donation after cardiac death, living-donor liver transplantation (LDLT), and ex-vivo normothermic liver perfusion may extend the benefit of LT to more patients awaiting transplantation.

This chapter presents a broad overview of LT, including common criteria for recipient and donor selection (see Chapter 105), common postsurgical complications (see Chapter 111), and outcomes related to LT and the underlying etiology of ESLD. Specialized techniques including LT and hepatectomy in LDLT are addressed in Chapters 121, 125, and 128.

DEMAND FOR LIVER TRANSPLANTATION

For many patients with irreversible acute and chronic liver disease and cirrhosis, orthotopic LT (OLT) represents the only curative treatment option, regardless of etiology (see Chapters 105 and 107). Despite increasing acuity, 5-year patient survival after LT has increased from less than 50% to greater than 80% over the last 50 years.[7] The improvement in patient survival has contributed to the expanded indications for LT and concomitant increase in the number of patients referred and listed for transplantation (see Chapter 105). The consequence of this success is the persistent disparity between the number of potential recipients awaiting LT and the number of available donor organs.

In 2019, 8896 LTs were performed in the United States, the greatest number of LTs performed in a single year, and a 41% increase from 10 years ago.[6] LDLT increased 31% compared with 2018, accounting for 524 LTs.[6] However, there is also continued growth in the number of waiting list registrations, with 12,767 new registrations in 2019 (Fig. 109.1).[6] The donor-to-recipient disparity leads to longer waiting times and worsening medical status. The severity of liver disease at time of listing has increased as measured by a higher first active Model for End-Stage Liver Disease (MELD) score[6,7] (see Chapter 4). The proportion of patients receiving LTs with MELD scores of 35 or higher has doubled in the last decade, representing greater than 10% of LT recipients.[6,8] Despite this, there has been a decline in peak pre-transplant mortality rate over the last 5 years from 17.9 per 100 waiting list years in 2014, to 12.4 per 100 waiting list years in 2019 because of improvements in perioperative care.[6] The most dramatic improvement in pre-transplant mortality was observed among patients with HCV, reflecting the efficacy of direct-acting antiviral therapy.

Organ Allocation and Listing

The process by which potential recipients are listed for LT has undergone extensive revisions to optimize equitable and just allocation of a scarce resource. Before 2002, potential recipients were prioritized based on the Child-Turcotte-Pugh (CTP) scoring system (Table 109.1), time on the waiting list, and patient location (intensive care unit [ICU], hospitalized, ambulatory). Waiting lists grew under this system, and it became evident that these parameters were inadequate measures of disease severity.[9] In 1999 the Institute of Medicine proposed that a continuous disease severity score based on medical urgency over waiting time could improve the allocation of cadaveric livers for LT.[10] This resulted in the adoption of the MELD criteria to assess necessity for LT and determine waiting list priority (Table 109.2). As shown in Figure 109.2, the use of MELD criteria for predicting mortality from ESLD results in an appropriate correlation between severity score and actuarial survival at 3 months. Survival benefit analysis of LT recipients stratified by MELD score demonstrates that the risks involved in transplantation are equivalent or less than the risks associated with remaining a transplant candidate on the waiting list with a MELD score greater than 15[11] (see Chapter 4).

Special considerations, or exceptions, for subsets of patients with liver disease are ongoing. At the time the MELD score was adopted, patients with HCC and early cirrhosis were prioritized on the waiting list, when they would potentially benefit most from LT (see Chapter 108A) and before progression of tumor

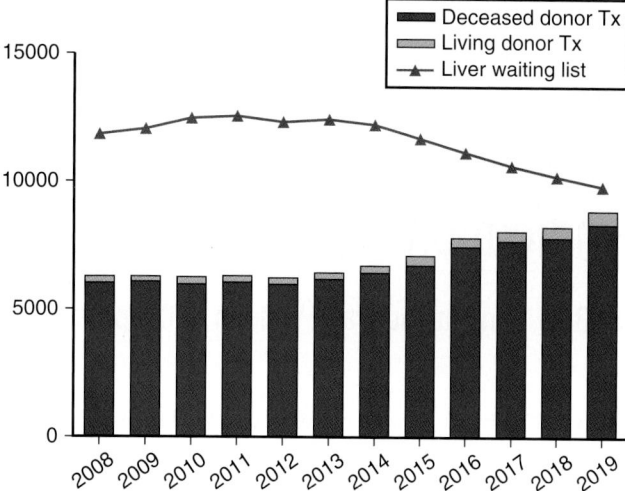

FIGURE 109.1 Persistent disparity between patients on the waiting list and recipients of deceased-donor and living-donor allografts. The number of patients awaiting a liver transplant at year's end decreased after the introduction of the Model for End-Stage Liver Disease (MELD) and the pediatric MELD allocation system. *Tx,* Treatment. (Data from the Scientific Registry of Transplant Recipients [SRTR], 2019 *OPTN/SRTR Annual Report.*)

TABLE 109.1 Child-Turcotte-Pugh Classification

	POINTS		
	1	**2**	**3**
Encephalopathy	None	1 or 2	3 or 4
Ascites	Absent	Slight	Moderate
Bilirubin (mg/dL)	1–2	2–3	>3
Albumin	>3.5	2.8–3.5	<2.8
Prothrombin time (seconds prolonged)	1–4	4–6	>6

TABLE 109.2 Predicted Mortality According to the Model for End-Stage Liver Disease Score[a]

SCORE	NO. PATIENTS	MORTALITY RATE (%)	DEATH OR REMOVAL FROM LIST BECAUSE OF ILLNESS (%)
<9	124	1.9	2.9
10–19	1800	6	7.7
20–29	1098	19.6	23.5
30–39	295	52.6	60.2
≥40	120	71.3	79.3

[a]$R = (0.957 \times \text{Log}_e[\text{creatinine mg/dL}] + 0.378 \times \text{Log}_e[\text{total bilirubin mg/dL}] + 1.120 \times \text{Log}_e[\text{INR}] + 0.643) \times 10.$

INR, International normalized ratio.

Modified from Wiesner R, Edwards E, Freeman R, et al. Model for end-stage liver disease [MELD] and allocation of donor livers. Gastroenterology. 2003;124(1):91–96.

burden, which would eliminate LT as a therapeutic option. Guidelines exist for awarding exception points for other liver disease–related conditions whose severity and associated risk of mortality are not captured by the calculated MELD score, including hilar CCA, hepatopulmonary syndrome, portopulmonary hypertension, cystic fibrosis, hepatic artery thrombosis after LT, pediatric hepatoblastoma, inborn errors of metabolism,

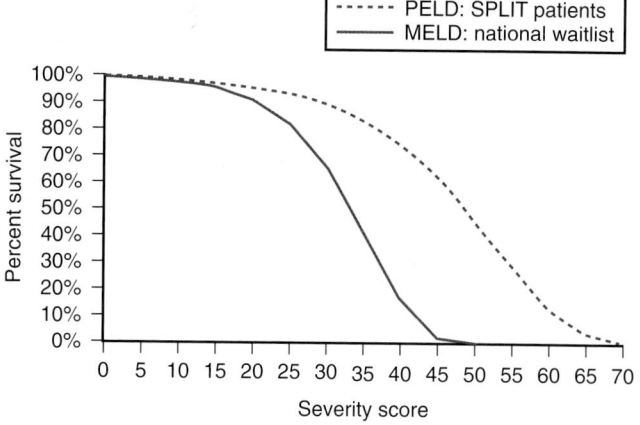

FIGURE 109.2 Correlation between Model for End-Stage Liver Disease (*MELD*) and the pediatric MELD *(PELD)* score and patient mortality. *SPLIT,* Studies of Pediatric Liver Transplantation. (Freeman RB Jr, Wiesner RH, Harper A, et al. The new liver allocation system: Moving toward evidence-based transplantation policy. *Liver Transpl.* 2002;8:851–858.)

familial amyloidosis, and primary hyperoxaluria (see Chapters 51, 77, 78, 105, and 110). However, the process is highly variable by region.[12–14]

In the last decade, disparities in deceased-donor transplant rates because of geographic location continued to grow within the United States, leading to the implementation of new liver allocation policy and establishment of the National Liver Review Board to optimize outcomes for liver candidates while simultaneously maintaining good organ stewardship. Based on donor-specific-areas throughout the United States, the median MELD at time of transplant varied significantly. The greatest median MELD at time of transplant was reported in New York at 39 and the lowest in Arkansas at 19.[6,15] To address these disparities, the Organ Procurement and Transplantation Network (OPTN) implemented a new distribution system that emphasizes the medical urgency of LT candidates and the distance between donor and recipient hospitals. This went into effect in February 2020 and while statistical modeling project lower waitlist mortality, its effects on LT remain to be determined. Nonetheless, because of the limited supply of donor organs, appropriate recipient and donor selection is critical to improve resource utilization and long-term outcomes.

RECIPIENT SELECTION

Common indications for LT (see Chapter 105) include portal hypertension (as manifested by variceal bleeding), ascites, encephalopathy, hyperbilirubinemia, hepatic synthetic dysfunction, and lifestyle limitations. Alcohol-related liver disease and NASH continue to rise, representing the two most common diagnoses of ESLD requiring LT. Malignancy, in particular HCC, is a growing indication for LT, accounting for 6.7% of LT in 2002 and 14% in 2019[6,16] (see Chapter 108). Five years ago, viral hepatitis was the most common etiology of liver failure resulting in LT, accounting for 25% of transplants (see Chapter 68). However, with the use of direct-acting antiviral agents, the proportion of LTs performed for HCV has declined dramatically and now only accounts for 7.3% of transplants as seen in Figure 109.3.[6] Biliary atresia is the most common

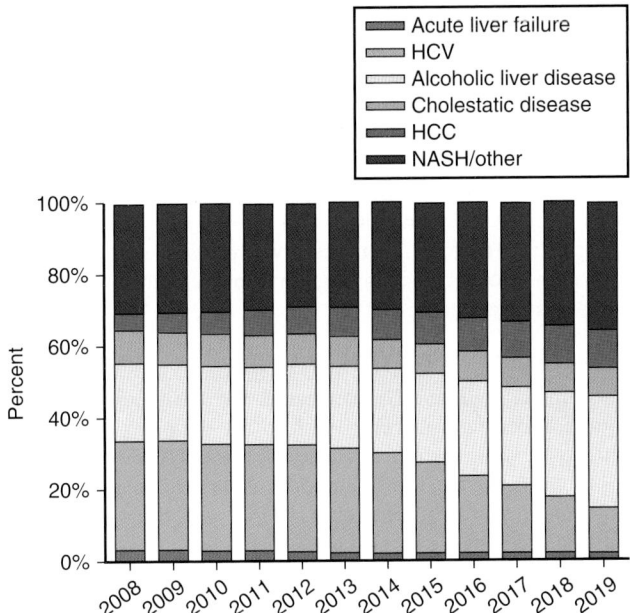

FIGURE 109.3 **Percent of liver transplants performed by etiology of liver disease.** With the advent of direct acting antiviral agents, hepatitis C virus *(HCV)* continues to decline. Meanwhile with the ongoing obesity epidemic, transplantation for nonalcoholic steatohepatitis *(NASH)* cirrhosis is rising. (Data from the Scientific Registry of Transplant Recipients [SRTR], 2019 *OPTN/SRTR Annual Report.*)

BOX 109.1 **Contraindications to Orthotopic Liver Transplantation**

Absolute
Advanced cardiopulmonary disease
Extrahepatic malignancy
Uncontrolled sepsis
Active substance abuse
ABO incompatibility

Relative
Hemodynamic instability
Severe hypoxia (except with hepatopulmonary syndrome)
Human immunodeficiency virus infection
Refractory psychiatric disorders
Absence of adequate social support

---

indication for LT in patients younger than 18 years (see Chapter 110).[6] The rising incidence of NASH coincides with an increase in obesity (body mass index [BMI] ≥ 30) and prevalence of diabetes among transplant recipients over the last decade.[6,17] It is anticipated that the obesity epidemic will present new challenges to the transplant community with a rise in NASH and NASH-related HCC, exacerbating the demand for LT while simultaneously reducing the availability of suitable organ donors with non-steatotic livers[2,18,19] (see Chapter 69).

Few true, absolute contraindications to LT exist that uniformly portend a poor patient outcome (Box 109.1). Advanced cardiopulmonary disease, known extrahepatic malignancy not meeting oncologic criteria for cure, uncontrolled systemic sepsis from a source originating outside the liver, acquired immunodeficiency syndrome (AIDS), and ongoing or recent substance abuse are absolute contraindications.[20,21] Many relative

contraindications are conditions that are expected to improve after successful LT. Examples include severe hemodynamic instability requiring multiple pharmacologic agents to maintain perfusion, extreme pulmonary hypertension, or severe hypoxia uncorrected by conventional intensive care measures in the context of hepatopulmonary syndrome. Other relative contraindications to LT are extensive mesenteric venous thrombosis, morbid obesity, psychiatric disorders uncontrolled by conventional means, absence of a suitable social support network, and extremes of age[22,23] (see Chapter 105).

Advancements in surgical technique and medical supportive care have expanded LT candidacy to subsets of recipients and conditions formerly considered to be absolute contraindications, including portal vein (PV) thrombosis (PVT), human immunodeficiency virus (HIV) infection, and advanced age. Although obesity is not a contraindication to LT, several authors have shown that BMI greater than 40 is associated with significantly reduced 5-year patient and graft survival.[17,24,25] Further, severe morbid obesity is associated with increased length of stay (LOS), risk of infectious complications, and posttransplantation malignancy.[17] These patients pose long-term challenges in dosing immunosuppressive medications affected by appropriate dosing weight. Given these consequences, many centers have incorporated interventions to combat obesity in transplant recipients including nutritional education, exercise regimens, and bariatric surgery.[2,17,24,25]

Transplantation for HIV is an example of a relative contraindication that is site-specific. With the advent of highly active antiretroviral therapy (HAART), HIV has become a chronic condition such that patients may begin to suffer the morbidity and mortality of other diseases, including ESLD. Patients with HIV may be considered for LT if their CD4 T-cell count is greater than 200 and their HIV RNA viral load is less than 50 copies/μL within 12 months before LT. Additionally, patients with HIV have the option of receiving an organ from an HIV-infected organ, according to the HIV Organ Policy Equity Act, enacted in 2013.[21]

The average age of LT recipients continues to rise. Nearly 70% of LT are performed for patients older than 50 years, and 20% were older than 65.[26] With an aging population, thorough screening for medical comorbidities typically found in older populations, such as lifestyle-limiting cardiopulmonary disease, systemic vascular disease, and chronic renal insufficiency, is crucial to successful LT. Although septuagenarians have lower 5-year patient survival (70.8%) compared with those less than 60 (80.7%), survival of LT recipients, regardless of age, surpasses those denied LT.[26] When appropriately selected, older patients with ESLD can benefit from LT.[27,28]

DONOR SELECTION

With fewer contraindications to LT and a growing list of potential recipients, there is a well-established demand for donors. Optimizing donor selection and management is critical to reducing this disparity. An optimal deceased donor is generally considered an otherwise healthy, hemodynamically stable, young individual who sustained an irreversible cerebral insult resulting in brain death. Restricting use to these "ideal donors" fails to meet the needs of an expanding waiting list. With increasing demand, transplant centers are turning to marginal liver allografts from extended-criteria donors (ECDs) and donation after cardiac death (DCD).[29,30] The acceptance of these more marginal allografts are associated with higher risks of primary nonfunction, early graft dysfunction, biliary complications, and decreased long-term graft survival.[29,31,32] Thus the surgeon must make an assessment to determine suitability of a particular donor for a specific recipient.

Numerous donor and recipient characteristics associated with graft and recipient outcomes have been evaluated, but comparisons can be difficult given variable clinical factors and severity of underlying liver disease. When considering donors, special consideration must be given to recipient selection because a patient with higher MELD or increased comorbidities may not tolerate a period of slow graft function or ischemia reperfusion to the same extent as a healthier, low MELD recipient. In 2006, a donor risk index (DRI) was derived to help quantify and stratify allografts by predicted failure risk.[33] Risk factors associated with graft loss include increased donor age, DCD, use of split grafts, Black donors, shorter donors, death because of cerebrovascular accident (CVA), and causes of brain death other than trauma or anoxia.[33] Experience with the DRI demonstrated use of high-risk donor livers is associated with increased relative risk of allograft failure and development of complications including hepatic artery thrombosis (HAT), biliary complications, and survival in selected subsets.[33,34] However, there are limitations of the DRI statistical modeling that cannot capture the patient's overall health status and frailty.[33,34]

Donor Age

With an aging population, there has been a growing need to consider organs from elderly donors. Carefully selected older donor allografts (including septuagenarians and octogenarians) have been used with good success.[35–37] It is important to note the presence of atherosclerosis, steatosis, or fibrosis that may affect the recipient. Limiting cold ischemia time and degree of steatosis are hypothesized to be important in optimizing the results of transplantation from older donors. Further, accepting an older donor is associated with lower 5-year mortality as compared with those who declined the same donor and waited for another organ offer (23% vs. 41%).[35] Therefore age alone should not exclude a potential donor when matched to an appropriate recipient.

Steatosis

The obesity epidemic not only challenges the transplant community with a rapidly growing number of potential recipients with NASH cirrhosis but also has the potential to limit donors with nonsteatotic livers, further exacerbating the disparity in organ donation. When encountering a graft with a fatty appearance, biopsy and the histologic determination of fat content may help guide use of steatotic livers.[38] Histologically, microvesicular steatosis is characterized by numerous small lipid droplets in the cytoplasm without any alteration in the position of the nucleus. Macrovesicular steatosis describes the presence of large lipid droplets within hepatocyte cytoplasm that displaces the nucleus. Microvesicular steatosis has minimal effect on allograft function. However, allografts with increased macrovesicular steatosis are characterized by poor microcirculation, depleted ATP-energy stores because of impaired capacity for mitochondrial recovery, and an increased inflammatory response after more severe ischemia-reperfusion injury.[39,40] Overall, this results in impaired recovery and regenerative capacity and poorer graft function.[41] Moderate (30%–60%) and severe (>60%) macrovesicular steatosis is associated with early graft

dysfunction and primary nonfunction with rates as high as 35% and 15%, respectively.[42] When carefully selected, liver allografts with up to 40% macrosteatosis may be used in select groups of recipients with similar 5-year graft survival as compared with livers with mild macrosteatosis.[38,43] Although patient survival is not affected, grafts with moderate steatosis have been associated with increased resource use including increased transfusions, longer hospital stays, and prolonged ICU course.[44] Among these donors, it is necessary to minimize other risk factors, such as cold ischemia time, to improve recipient and graft outcomes (see Chapter 105).

Donors With Positive Viral Serology

The opioid epidemic has increased the availability of organ donors, albeit with increased risk to the recipient of potential hepatitis C transmission. Historically, use of HCV+ donors has raised concern that transplantation would result in aggressive recurrent disease in the recipient. The introduction of novel oral-direct acting antiviral (DAA) agents for HCV continues to alter the field of LT.[6,45,46] Several studies have demonstrated that use of HCV+ donors into HCV+ recipients is safe, with long-term outcomes comparable to HCV– allografts, in the absence of severe inflammation or fibrosis.[47–49] The use of these organs is not associated with inferior graft or patient survival.[50] The proportion of HCV+ recipients receiving HCV+ livers has increased from 6.9% in 2009 to 16.9% in 2015 and the rate of discard of HCV+ livers continues to decline.[6,46] Nucleic acid testing (NAT) has expanded the donor pool as well. There is growing literature in the use of HCV Ab+/NAT- donors into HCV seronegative recipients. Development of HCV viremia in the recipient is treatable with standard of care direct acting antivirals with no difference in graft loss or mortality.[51] From 2017 to 2019, 9.0% of LTs were from donors with HCV Ab+.[6] Among LT recipients without a history of HCV, 4.2% received a liver from an HCV Ab+ donor.[6] For the first time, the percentage of recipients willing to accept an HCV+ organ has surpassed those who declined HCV+ organs, attributed to successful medical advancements in antiviral therapy.[6]

The use of donors with serologic markers for past HBV infection have potential for use and expansion of the donor pool. Grafts from hepatitis B core antibody positive donors may be offered to potential recipients using protocols that incorporate immunoglobulin therapy and antiviral therapy for both HBV positive and negative recipients with comparable survival.[52–54]

Donation After Cardiac Death

Another source of allografts is from DCD, formerly referred to as non-heart-beating donation. These organs are from donors who have sustained an irreversible, catastrophic illness without hope for meaningful recovery but do not meet criteria for brain death. In the DCD setting, life support is withdrawn, and the donor is observed until time of death, which is declared by a nontransplant physician. From cessation of circulation, an additional 2- to 5-minute waiting period is mandated before organ retrieval is initiated. It is important to note that 10% of potential donors do not die within 2 hours of withdrawal of support; these patients are not candidates for subsequent organ donation and are transferred back to the ICU and allowed to expire.[55] Circulation is unlikely to resume after 2 minutes of complete cessation; a minimum waiting period of 2 minutes is required, and a 5-minute interval between cessation of circulation and declaration of death before organ retrieval is strongly encouraged.[56] Unlike DBD donors, allografts from DCD donors have increased warm ischemia time that begins with withdrawal of life support, includes the progressive hypoxia and hypoperfusion, until declaration of death and initiation of cold preservation. This prolonged warm ischemia time increases the risk for delayed graft function, primary nonfunction, and biliary complications related to ischemic cholangiopathy.[29,55,56]

After the concept of brain death became widely accepted in 1968 with the Harvard Neurologic Definition and Criteria for Death, use of DCD organs fell out of favor. DCD organ transplantation was reintroduced in the 1990s with improvement in preservation and procurement techniques. The percent of deceased donors liver transplants in the United States that are DCD has grown form 1% in 1996 to 8.5% in 2019.[6] In 2000, Reich et al. published the first successful series of controlled DCD LT with excellent outcomes including 100% patient and graft survival and no arterial thrombosis or biliary complication during an 18 month follow-up period.[57] Since then, numerous larger studies have published their experiences. In 2003 the University of Pennsylvania was the first to report a higher incidence of biliary complications, in particular ischemic cholangiopathy, because of sensitive biliary epithelium that are susceptible to prolonged warm ischemia time and more severe ischemia reperfusion injury.[58] Ischemic cholangiopathy is often associated with the need for hospital readmissions, prolonged antibiotic use, endoscopic and percutaneous biliary drainage procedures, and abscess formation.[29,58-60] Additionally, it may progress to graft loss, need for re-transplantation, or even death.[29,59,60]

Another major complication of DCD recipients is an increase in renal insufficiency. Despite normal preoperative creatinine and glomerular filtration rate (GFR), recipients of DCD organs more frequently develop acute kidney injury (AKI; 14.7% vs. DBD 7.3%) and need for dialysis (up to 40% of DCD recipients).[29,61] This is thought to be related to the increased reperfusion injury associated with DCD allografts.

Consequently, there has been interest in identifying suitable DCD donors and recipients to minimize associated morbidity and mortality. Use of standardized DCD protocols with strict selection criteria has led to excellent results, comparable to DBD donors at select institutions.[29,62,63] Donor age less than 50 years, weight less than 100 kg, warm ischemia times less than 30 minutes, and cold ischemia times less than 10 hours are associated with improved graft and patient survival.[32,63,64] Given that older donors are more susceptible to biliary ischemia, some suggest against use of DCD donors more than 50 years old. Recipient risk factors such as older age, re-transplantation, serum creatinine greater than 2.0 mg/dL and life support before LT are associated with inferior patient and graft outcomes. In general, donor, recipient, and surgical variables that minimize ischemia time and its associated affects are associated with more favorable outcomes because the donor graft is protected against additional ischemia.[63,65-67] Mayo Clinic established a relationship that with each minute increase in declaration of death to cross clamp, there is an associated 16.1% increased odds of ischemic cholangiopathy.[63] Similarly, prolonged cold ischemia times are associated with increased risk of graft failure such that each hour increase in cold ischemia time was associated with 6% higher graft failure rate. Cold ischemia time between 6 and 10 hours was associated with a 64% higher graft failure risk compared with cold ischemia time less than 6 hours.[66] Given the associated morbidity and mortality with

ischemic cholangiopathy, protocols to minimize biliary complications have been implemented at some institutions. Tissue plasminogen activator (TPA) injection into donor hepatic artery may lower the risk of biliary complications by minimizing thrombus formation in the peribiliary microcirculation.[68] Flushing of the biliary system and using less viscous preservation solution may provide some benefit as well.[69]

DCD donors provide an additional option for donation when DBD is not feasible. Acceptance of these organs is not without risk, but careful technique, standardized protocols, and patient and recipient selection may help to mitigate associated complications. An area of ongoing interest and future development is the use of normothermic ex vivo machine perfusion. This has the potential of reducing the ischemia-reperfusion injury and associated complications identified in the setting of DCD liver transplantation. Altogether, further investigation and optimization potential donors and recipients may help to expand the donor pool.

Living-Donor Liver Transplantation

An alternative to cadaveric donation is the use of living donor allografts. The first adult-to-adult LDLT in the United States was reported in 1998,[70] and use has fluctuated since then. Initially, numbers of LDLT rose with a peak in 2001, representing approximately 10% of all LTs, but they currently represent 5.3% of LTs performed.[6] LDLT is appealing because it allows for a more elective transplantation after optimizing the health of the recipient, reduces cold-ischemic times, and potentially expedites waiting times. However, the risk of morbidity and mortality to an otherwise healthy donor is notable. Donor hepatectomy remains a technically demanding surgical procedure with higher complication rates than seen in living kidney donation[71] (see Chapter 121). Refinements in technique are critical to optimizing donor safety, which remains of utmost concern. Despite inherent risks to the donor, right hepatic lobe LDLT has become an important option in the management of liver disease. Details of the donor operation, open and minimally invasive, are described in in Chapters 121 and 128.

In 2002, the Adult-to-Adult Living Donor Liver Transplantation (A2ALL) consortium was developed and funded by the National Institute of Health. It consisted of nine transplant institutions experienced in performing LDLT and sought to provide accurate information on outcomes for both donors and recipients.[72] The results of this can help guide and educate surgeons and patients when considering LDLT versus deceased-donor LT (DDLT) because one must consider the potential risk to an otherwise healthy donor versus benefit to a recipient and likelihood of receiving a DDLT before disease progression.

Despite initial reports suggesting worse outcomes in LDLT, a trend has been seen toward improved graft and overall patient survival in the United States in the last 10 years.[72-74] This is particularly evident when compared with waiting for a deceased donor or remaining on the list without a transplant. The reduction in mortality is greatest in centers with increased experience with LDLT.[75] A learning curve has been described with increased graft and patient loss with the first 15 to 20 cases at a single institution.[76] When considering appropriate candidates, one must take into account the unique components of LDLT. Compared with DDLT, LDLT recipients have a slightly higher complication rate and receive a smaller graft. This may not be acceptable for decompensated patients with more advanced liver disease.

In the setting of acute liver failure (ALF), recipients typically have sufficiently high MELDs such that deceased donor livers are available for transplantation because these recipients are of highest allocation priority (see Chapter 107). Additionally, potential living donors may struggle to complete a thorough evaluation and consideration of donation without unnecessary risks in the short interval. As a result, LDLT is rarely performed for ALF in the United States to avoid unnecessary risks to a donor. Nonetheless, the A2ALL group demonstrates that LDLT in this setting is an acceptable option with comparable survival to DDLT at 5-year follow-up if criteria for donation are met. Among recipients of LDLT in the setting of ALF, there were no observed deaths while waiting for transplantation.[77]

Recipient complications and re-transplantation rates are higher in the setting of LDLT compared with DDLT. LDLT recipients have a higher rate of technical complications, including biliary leaks, biliary strictures, HAT, and PVT.[78] In contrast, complications related to graft issues or ischemia reperfusion are more common in DDLT recipients. Ascites, pulmonary edema, intra-abdominal bleeding, and cardiac complications occur more frequently in DDLT. Once a complication occurs, time to resolution is comparable between LDLT and DDLT[78] (see Chapter 111).

With regards to long-term outcomes, the A2ALL consortium showed 10-year survival was 70% for LDLT and 64% for DDLT based on 1427 liver recipients (with 964 LDLT).[74] For all recipients, a diagnosis of PSC was associated with improved survival, whereas dialysis and older recipient/donor age were associated with worse survival. A higher MELD was also associated with increased graft failure.[74] Recipient diagnosis, age, disease severity, and presence of renal failure should all therefore be taken into account when considering appropriateness for LDLT. Overall, LDLT has been shown to improve survival in patients with lower MELD scores, decreases waitlist mortality, and has good long-term outcomes.[74,76–78]

Living donation is unique in that an otherwise healthy donor undergoes surgery; therefore minimizing morbidity and mortality of the donor is critical (see Chapter 121). Donor evaluation is comprehensive and includes a donor advocate, history and physical, cardiac clearance, psychosocial evaluation, and delineation of donor anatomy. Details of this complete evaluation are published elsewhere.[79,80] During the donor evaluation, graft size is an important consideration. Small-for-size syndrome, or early allograft dysfunction, is characterized by the presence of jaundice or coagulopathy without technical complications. This is most frequently associated with grafts smaller than 0.8% graft weight to recipient body weight or less than 40% of standard liver volume.[81,82] This is reported to occur in up to 19% of LDLT grafts.[82] Risk factors include use of left lobe grafts, small size, high preoperative bilirubin, high portal perfusion pressure, increased donor age, and increased donor BMI.[81–83] Recipients who develop small-for-size syndrome are at increased risk for graft loss within 90 days.[83]

Meticulous surgical technique and completion of appropriate donor evaluation are critical to ensure donor safety and minimize morbidity and mortality. Nonetheless, up to 40% of living liver donors experience a complication. A cohort of 760 living donors enrolled in the A2ALL consortium provides a comprehensive assessment of donor complications.[71] Commonly reported complications include bacterial infection (12.5%), biliary infection (9.7%), incisional hernia (5.6%), pleural effusion (5.3%), psychological distress (4.1%), and aborted hepatectomy (2.7%).[71] Although mortality is low, it is not nonexistent, with a reported rate of 0.4%.[71] These results should be provided to potential donor candidates as part of their comprehensive evaluation and informed consent process. As the role of LDLT continues to evolve, continued efforts to optimize donor and recipient selection and operative technique will be critical for program and patient success.

Machine Perfusion

Advancements in organ preservation techniques is an ongoing area of research to expand options for organ donation. Static cold storage (SCS) at 4°C is the standard method of preservation of liver allografts. Although metabolic activity is reduced, anaerobic metabolism continues, leading to adenosine triphosphate (ATP) depletion with accumulation of lactic acid, cell swelling, and cell death. If prolonged, SCS can exacerbate ischemia-reperfusion injury and intensify complications such as primary nonfunction, early allograft dysfunction, biliary strictures, and ischemic cholangiopathy. Alternate methods of preservation have been successful in kidney transplantation, with improved graft and patient outcomes. In 2009, Guarrera et al. reported the first human trial using machine perfusion in liver allografts.[84] Machine perfusion allows for an influx of nutrients and oxygen while flushing pro-inflammatory cytokines, reducing ATP depletion, and mitigating the effects of ischemia reperfusion injury associated with SCS.[84–86] Placement of a liver on machine perfusion and subsequent monitoring can be seen in Figures 109.4 and 109.5. Initial reports demonstrated lower serum injury markers and mean hospital LOS, fewer biliary complications, and reduced rates of graft dysfunction.[84]

Since the initial report demonstrating safety and feasibility, others have sought to use machine perfusion with marginal or extended-criteria donor livers. In these early studies, machine perfusion has shown protection of early and late allograft injury in DCD donors, fewer biliary complications, and reduced hospital LOS.[87–89] Machine perfusion allows for assessment of

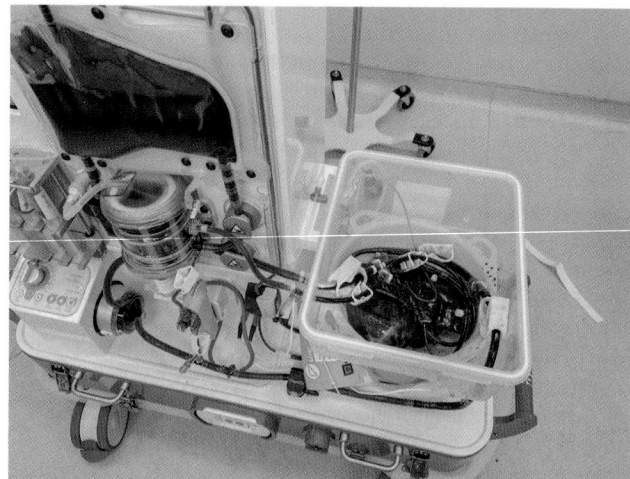

FIGURE 109.4 **Depiction of a liver perfusion device in use at Washington University in St. Louis.** OrganOx is an example of normothermic machine perfusion in which a procured liver is placed on the pump and continuously perfused with oxygenated blood and nutrients while allowing for assessment of parameters to estimate allograft viability.

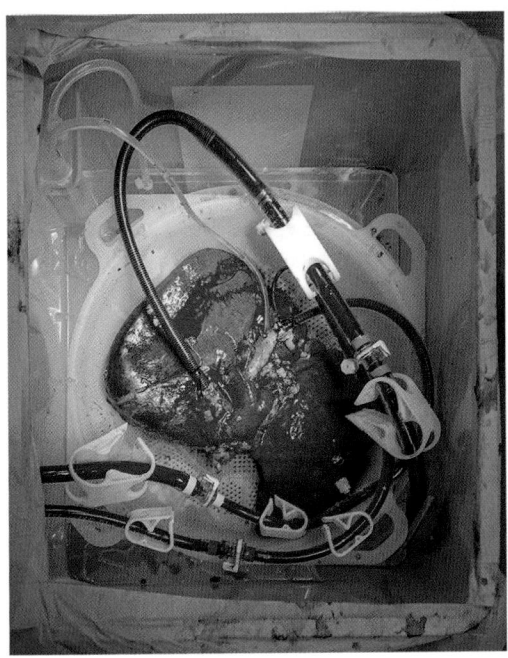

FIGURE 109.5 An example of a liver that has been cannulated and placed on the pump for monitoring.

allograft viability using markers of bile production, biliary chemistry, and lactic acid levels.[90,91] Aspartate transaminase (AST) and alanine aminotransferase (ALT) are cytoplasmic enzymes used as markers of hepatocyte injury present in the effluent perfusate, and, notably, early studies have demonstrated a reduction of AST and ALT, suggesting improved graft function.[92] Hepatic arterial and PV pressure and resistance measure may provide early measures of graft viability and function as well.[89]

In a randomized trial of 220 LTs, machine perfusion was associated with 50% lower level of graft injury. Importantly, these results were achieved with improved organ utilization (e.g., lower discard rates) and longer preservation time when compared with SCS.[86] With growing use of marginal donors, increased prevalence of steatotic livers poses a challenge to transplantation.[93] There is a need to identify methods to optimize these donors so that steatotic organs may be suitable for transplantation. In 2017, of the 4346 steatotic livers recovered, 50.6% were discarded.[93] There is some suggestion that machine perfusion with selected perfusates may be able to enhance liver function of steatotic livers and increase intracellular lipid metabolism and reduce macrovesicular steatosis.[41,94] Continued advancements in machine perfusion may help reduce waiting list mortality and continue to improve patient and graft outcomes.

OPERATIVE TECHNIQUES

The first published description of human LT was by Starzl and colleagues in 1963 at the University of Colorado[95] (see Chapter 125). In this seminal paper, the dismal outcomes of three LT recipients were described, including one intraoperative death from uncorrectable coagulopathy and two survivors at 7 and 22 days. In addition to the pioneering conceptual framework and implementation of LT, the advanced techniques

included grafts from non–heart-beating donors, venovenous bypass in the recipients, choledochocholedochostomy, and coagulation monitoring via thromboelastography (TEG). Many of these concepts remain or have re-entered the realm of LT more than 50 years after their initial description. Details of the operative procedure, including DDLT and living related-LT are discussed in Chapters 121, 125, and 128.

OUTCOMES

Modifications in surgical technique, immunosuppression, and perioperative care have led to reductions in morbidity and mortality after LT. Nonetheless, premature graft loss and reduced patient survival may result from technical problems (such as HAT or biliary stricture), immune-mediated rejection, or recurrent liver disease (viral, autoimmune, extrahepatic metabolic disease).[96] Recipients are also at risk for increased cardio- and cerebrovascular disease, malignancy (de novo or donor-acquired), and infectious complications (see Chapter 111).

Patient Survival

Long-term outcomes after LT continue to improve as a result of refinements in organ procurement and preservation, recipient selection, surgical and anesthetic techniques, perioperative care, and long-term immunosuppression. Currently, overall patient survival after LT continues to improve and currently is 93% at 1 year, 87% at 3 years, and 80% at 5 years.[6] Agopian et al. analyzed 30 years of experience at a single center and noted that recipients in the post-MELD era are older, more likely to be hospitalized, have increased MELD, and more likely to require renal replacement therapy (RRT). Despite this apparent increase in acuity, patient survival has increased as compared with pre-MELD era.[7] In a review of the Scientific Registry of Transplant Recipients (SRTR) database, factors identified to predict death among highest acuity (MELD ≥40) included mechanical ventilation pre-transplant, re-transplantation, increased recipient or donor age, DCD, and increased cold ischemia time.[97]

Graft Outcomes

Among DDLT recipients, graft failure occurs in 8.9% at 1 year, 15.2% at 3 years, and 21.6% at 5 years.[6] Outcomes are similar for LDLT recipients, with graft failure occurring in 7.1% at 1 year, 13.8% at 3 years, and 23.7% at 5 years.[6] Among DDLTs, 5-year graft survival rates exceed 75% for all age groups, except those age older than 65 years and for all BMI categories except those less than 18.5 kg/m². In 2019, 5-year graft survival for livers donated after DCD donation are lower than for those receiving livers after DBD donation (72.6% vs. 77.1%).[6] Graft survival rates for DDLTs with HCV were comparable to other etiologies of liver disease, which may point to the effectiveness of oral DAA agents for HCV introduced in 2013 (see Chapter 111).

Primary Nonfunction

Primary nonfunction is defined as early graft failure after LT in the absence of identified technical complications. Clinical presentation varies, but patients display signs consistent with liver failure, including altered mental status, hemodynamic instability, worsening acidosis, elevated transaminases, coagulopathy, and ensuing multiorgan failure. The reported incidence of primary nonfunction varies between 1% and 7% of all LTs.[98–100] Re-transplantation is the treatment of choice and should be performed as soon as possible after the initial transplant to minimize complications and progression of multi-organ failure.

The etiology of primary nonfunction is unclear but is likely multifactorial. Factors reported as associated with nonfunction include prolonged cold- and warm-ischemic times, donation after cardiac death, intraoperative systemic hypotension (mean arterial pressure [MAP] < 40 mm Hg), significant donor steatosis, and recipient factors such as PVT, renal failure, dependence on life support, and status 1 listing.[7,99,101,102] Severe macrosteatosis is associated with increased risk of graft failure. However, donors with moderate steatosis may have acceptable risks for appropriate candidates without other risk factors for primary nonfunction[99,103] (see Chapter 111).

Hepatic Artery Thrombosis

HAT can be divided into early and late presentations with distinct etiologies, clinical manifestations, and treatments. There is no formal consensus, but early HAT is often defined as occurring within the first 1 to 2 months after LT with a mean incidence of 2.9% in adults and as high as 9% in pediatric populations.[104,105] The ischemic injury that ensues from early HAT carries a high risk of graft loss and patient mortality (53% and 33%, respectively).[104] Technical, donor, and recipient factors contribute to an increased risk of HAT.[104–106] Donor factors may include small-caliber vessels, aberrant anatomy that requires complex arterial reconstruction, use of aortic conduits, or donor-recipient mismatch for cytomegalovirus (CMV) seropositivity. Pre-transplant recipient PVT and hypercoagulable states are associated with early HAT and may benefit from use of anticoagulation.[107]

Although early HAT may be asymptomatic, it may present as fulminant hepatic necrosis evidenced by severely increased transaminase levels and impaired hepatic synthetic function. Alternatively, it may present as ischemic necrosis of the bile ducts. The hepatic artery is the sole blood supply to the donor bile duct; therefore early HAT often presents with bile leak, cholangitis, or sepsis. Duplex ultrasound is diagnostic in most cases of HAT in adults, although visceral angiography remains the gold standard.[105,108] If diagnosis is prompt, emergency exploration with attempted thrombectomy and revascularization may salvage the graft, although this is usually not possible.

Some reports suggest that endovascular procedures—intra-arterial thrombolysis, percutaneous transluminal angioplasty, and endoluminal stenting—can be successful in hepatic arterial revascularization.[109] However, a majority of patients eventually require re-transplantation. Although re-transplantation improves patient survival over arterial revision or thrombolysis in the first year, there is no significant advantage in long-term survival.[109] Early HAT within the first week after LT is an indication for relisting as a status 1 candidate. These candidates benefit from use of ideal donors to minimize potential morbidity and mortality.

Late HAT is typically more indolent, frequently because a previously undiagnosed stricture allows for collateral circulation to develop. Clinical presentation may be asymptomatic or may result in recurrent bacteremia, perihepatic abscess, biliary leak, biliary strictures, or cholangitis.[109,110] Contributing factors are active tobacco abuse; coagulation abnormalities, such as

factor V Leiden; CVA as donor cause of death; donor death after 50 years; recipient CMV positivity; and use of donor iliac interposition graft.[110–112]

Treatment may be attempted with endoscopic or percutaneous biliary decompression, stenting, or even systemic anticoagulation. Re-transplantation is required less often for late HAT than for early HAT. Although LT is associated with high bleeding risks, there is a new paradigm of "rebalanced hemostasis" that can lead to hypercoagulability.[113] Postoperative antiplatelet therapy may reduce the rate of late HAT in high-risk patients,[114] and it has become our practice to prescribe daily aspirin (81 mg) for all patients (see Chapter 111).

Hepatic Artery Stenosis

Hepatic artery stenosis (HAS) without thrombosis is also a recognized complication of LT, with an incidence of 4% to 11%.[115,116] Initial presentation typically includes a mild increase in transaminase levels with or without associated graft dysfunction or biliary complications. Doppler US demonstrates increased resistance in hepatic arterial flow and is often diagnostic, but confirmation by arteriography is the gold standard. Therapeutic options include angioplasty with or without stenting. Primary patency of small caliber donor arteries may be improved with the use of drug-eluting stents[116] (see Chapter 111).

Portal Vein Thrombosis

PVT occurs with an incidence less than 2% in adult recipients and 10% in pediatric recipients.[109,117] (see Chapters 110 and 111). PVT adversely affects overall survival after LT.[109] Low portal flow, small-diameter veins (<5 mm), preexisting PVT in the recipient, donor-recipient vessel size mismatch, and the use of vascular grafts for reconstruction are known risk factors for PVT.[118] PVT is typically symptomatic, and patients can present with acute hepatic failure or with the sequelae of portal hypertension, such as increasing ascites, splenomegaly, and variceal hemorrhage.[109] Diagnosis is made using duplex ultrasound or contrast-enhanced computed tomography (CT) portal venography.

Depending on the timeliness of diagnosis and the acuity of the patient, several treatment options exist. In patients with fulminant hepatic failure from PVT, re-exploration and attempted portal revascularization may be performed. These patients sometimes require re-transplantation, particularly in the rare setting of combined PVT and HAT (total absence of hepatic inflow). The use of a portocaval shunt to augment flow through the reconstructed PV has been described,[119] as has transjugular intrahepatic portosystemic shunt (TIPS) in conjunction with thrombolytics.[120,121] Systemic anticoagulation may be sufficient in patients with preserved graft function.[109] Symptoms of portal hypertension but preserved graft function often can be managed medically with standard therapies for ascites in combination with variceal banding or sclerotherapy; however, the graft salvage rate with these alternative strategies is typically much less than 50%[109] (see Chapter 111).

Portal Vein Stenosis

PV stenosis, in contrast to PVT, is frequently diagnosed on routine screening ultrasound in asymptomatic patients. The most common area of stenosis is the extrahepatic PV anastomotic site. Narrowing of the main PV diameter by more than 50%, presence of a poststenotic jet, or lack of visualized flow on Doppler imaging are diagnostic. Many stenoses can be managed endovascularly with percutaneous transhepatic balloon angioplasty and stenting[122] (see Chapter 111).

Biliary Complications

Biliary complications are the most common post-LT complication, affecting up to 34% of LT recipients[123,124] Patients with HAT, acute rejection, living-donor allografts, and DCD livers are at higher risk for biliary complications.[123-125] Historically, Roux-en-Y choledochojejunostomy was associated with higher complication rates than choledochocholedochostomy;[126] however, this remains a controversial topic in transplantation techniques. All patients found to have a biliary complication should undergo ultrasound to evaluate for HAT as a contributing factor.

Biliary strictures occur twice as frequently as anastomotic biliary leaks and can be classified as *anastomotic* or *nonanastomotic (ischemic cholangiopathy)*.[127] Most anastomotic strictures are managed endoscopically with balloon dilation and stenting (see Chapters 30 and 111). Ischemic cholangiopathy more often results from bile duct ischemia or an immune response, appears later, affects multiple sites, tends to be more difficult to manage, and is rarely amenable to endoscopic treatment (see Chapter 31). Nonanastomotic strictures are associated with a higher rate of graft failure requiring re-transplantation.[59,127] A multidisciplinary approach to diagnosis and management of biliary complications is necessary and can result in higher patient and graft survival rates.

In an asymptomatic patient with stable liver function, biliary complications can often be managed nonoperatively. Bilomas should be drained percutaneously under ultrasound or CT guidance, and small leaks or duct mismatch may be managed with endoscopic stent placement across the anastomosis.[128] Major leaks or total disruption usually requires operative conversion to a choledochojejunostomy or hepaticojejunostomy, an option that can result in long-term biliary patency.[127] Patients who suffer biliary complications have prolonged ICU stays and higher readmission rates with increased morbidity and hospital costs.[123] Careful donor and recipient selection with attention to meticulous technique may help reduce associated morbidity (see Chapter 111).

Infection

Infection is the most common cause of death after LT at all time points,[97,129] causing 28% of all deaths in LT patients (see Chapters 10 and 111). LT recipients possess several high-risk features including immunosuppressant regimens, prolonged hospitalization, malnourishment, chronic illness, dialysis, blood-product transfusions, and lengthy and complex surgical procedures.[130,131] The risk is further increased by the comorbidities of diabetes and morbid obesity, which are consistently increasing in the recipient population.[130,132] Recognition and diagnosis of infection can be complicated by the relative paucity of symptoms because of use of immunosuppressive agents and steroids. Fever is frequently absent and only 50% develop leukocytosis in the setting of bacteremia[133]; therefore clinicians must maintain a high index of suspicion because delay in diagnosis can result in graft loss and mortality. Appropriate antimicrobial prophylaxis can reduce the postoperative infection rate by more than half, depending on the pathogen. Box 109.2 shows the current prophylactic regimen used at Washington University in St. Louis.

Bacterial pathogens are the most common infectious agent in the early postoperative period, and the proportion of post-LT

BOX 109.2 Antimicrobial Prophylaxis for Liver Transplantation Patients at Washington University in St. Louis

Bacterial
Routine use of broad-spectrum antibiotics on-call to operating room, continued for 24 hours postoperatively.

Fungal
Fluconazole (Diflucan, 200 mg daily) for 14 days postoperatively in high-risk patients

Pneumocystis carinii
Trimethoprim-sulfamethoxazole (Bactrim/Septra SS) for 1 year postoperatively.
Pentamidine (Pentam) or dapsone for patients with sulfa sensitivity

Viral
High-Risk
Donor CMV+/recipient CMV−: valganciclovir, 900 mg daily for 3 months, then 450 mg daily for 9 months.

Intermediate-Risk
(D+/R+ or D−/R+): valganciclovir 450 mg daily for 6 months

Low-Risk
(D−/R−): acyclovir, 200 mg twice daily for 3 months

CMV, Cytomegalovirus.

---

infections caused by bacteremia has increased significantly with improved prophylaxis for viral and fungal pathogens.[134] The prevalence of specific pathogens varies among transplant centers. Although gram-negative bacilli remain frequent causes of postoperative infection after LT, gram-positive cocci, such as methicillin-resistant *Staphylococcus aureus* (MRSA) and vancomycin-resistant enterococci (VRE), have become increasingly prevalent at many transplant centers.[133,135] MRSA bacteremia develops in 25% of LT patients, with colonization of indwelling vascular catheters accounting for approximately half the cases.[136] Other sources of post-LT bacteremia include, in decreasing order of frequency, pneumonia, biliary infections, abdominal sources infections, and surgical wound infections.[137]

CMV is the most common viral pathogen encountered, although incidence of CMV infection has declined as a result of improved prophylaxis regimens.[138] The highest risk occurs in the first 3 months after LT, correlating with higher levels of immunosuppression.[139,140] CMV donor positive, recipient negative patients are at highest risk (44%–65%) of de novo CMV infection. The International CMV consensus guidelines recommend 3 months of antiviral prophylaxis for these high-risk patients.[141] Active CMV infection may manifest as a viral syndrome or tissue invasive disease and increases the incidence of acute rejection and HAT.[142] Pre-emptive therapy with valganciclovir reduces the incidence of CMV disease with end-organ damage in LT recipients. Ganciclovir-resistant CMV has been observed in 20% of solid-organ transplant recipients, with presentation typically observed late in the first year.[143] Cellcept and calcineurin inhibitors appear to increase the risk and severity of CMV infection.[144,145] Therefore immunosuppression dose reduction or modification is necessary while treating post-LT CMV.

Invasive fungal infections are most commonly caused by *Candida, Aspergillus,* and *Cryptococcus* with an incidence of 5% to 9% in LT patients.[146] Candidiasis is the most frequently encountered fungal infection. Risk factors for invasive candidiasis include the use of prophylactic antibiotics to prevent spontaneous bacterial peritonitis, need for RRT, morbid obesity, pre-LT bariatric surgery, post-LT bile leaks, LDLT, and re-transplantation.[147,148] Patients with invasive fungal infections have increased mortality, prolonged hospital stays, and incur excessive increased costs.[146,149] Guidelines from the American Society of Transplant and Infectious Disease Society of America currently recommend targeted antifungal prophylaxis based on risk stratification.[150] Limiting antifungal coverage to targeted therapy versus universal prophylaxis has no difference in LT outcomes with equivalent rates of mortality and rejection.[150]

Infection with the protozoan *Pneumocystis carinii* occurs in 3% to 11% of LT patients in the absence of prophylaxis.[151] Because T-cell immunity is the primary defense against *P. carinii*, prolonged use of corticosteroids or muromonab-CD3 monoclonal antibodies and active CMV infection increase the risk of infection. Trimethoprim-sulfamethoxazole offers highly effective prophylaxis at low cost with minimal side effects. Prophylaxis generally is continued during the first 12 months after LT when the risk of *P. carinii* infection is highest[151] (see Chapter 111).

Rejection

Rejection can be a major hurdle to long-term survival after LT (see Chapter 111). Within 1 year of transplant, 12.3% of LT recipients experience at least one episode of acute rejection, most often among younger recipients.[6] Previously reported to occur in 40% to 70% of LT patients,[152] the development of novel immunosuppressive regimens has reduced the lifetime rejection rate to less than 20%.[153] Long-term management of immunosuppression should aim to suppress immune responses while minimizing adverse effects. This is an individualized process that must account for recipient characteristics, etiology of liver disease, and evidence of prior rejection. The University of Pittsburgh experience shows that immunosuppression can be withdrawn successfully in almost one-third of patients,[154] although there is wide variability in minimization protocols across institutions.[155]

Symptomatic patients with acute liver rejection may present with signs of fever, malaise, or right upper quadrant abdominal pain. Liver functions will invariably be elevated in the presence

of rejection and often detected before physical symptoms. T cell-mediated rejection (TCMR) is characterized by T-cell infiltrates with decreased populations of other inflammatory cells. Histologic grading is standardized based on the Banff working group on liver allograft pathology with assessment of portal inflammation, bile duct inflammation/damage, and venous endothelial inflammation.[156] The international LT society consensus statement recommends early TCMR be treated with an increase in calcineurin inhibitors. Moderate and severe TCMR should be treated with pulse steroid therapy and an increase in maintenance immunosuppression. For those who fail to respond, use of antibody-depleting therapy (antithymocyte globulin) may be necessary. Repeat biopsy may be useful to assess response to therapy. Late TCMR is associated with reduced graft survival.[157] Additional histologic findings include interface hepatitis, plasma cell infiltrates, and perivenulitis.[156] Biopsy-proven antibody mediated rejection (AMR) is rare. A diagnosis of acute AMR requires classic histologic features, C4d+ vascular staining, circulating donor-specific antibody (DSA), and exclusion of other causes.[158] Mild, acute AMR should be managed with steroid boluses. Moderate to severe AMR can include plasmapheresis and intravenous immunoglobulin (IVIG) and consideration of anti-B cell agents.[159] Standardized histopathologic evaluation of acute and chronic rejection using the Banff schema allows objective decision making and facilitates comparisons of natural histories among patients (Tables 109.3 and 109.4). Chronic rejection may require re-transplantation (see Chapter 111).

Renal Failure

Renal failure is common among LT recipients, with approximately 15% of patients requiring transient RRT post-LT[160] and up to 25% developing stage 4 chronic kidney disease (CKD) within 5 years.[161] Pre-LT AKI is predictive of post-LT CKD, which is associated with increased mortality and cardiovascular events.[162] Donor factors associated with AKI include advanced age, steatosis, DCD donors, and prolonged warm and cold ischemia times.[162] Normothermic or hypothermic machine liver graft machine perfusion may help to attenuate ischemia reperfusion injury and lower rates of AKI.[87] Recent reports using novel serum biomarkers, such as neutrophil gelatinase-associated lipocalin (NGAL), as markers of ischemia-reperfusion

---

TABLE 109.3 Rejection Activity Index From the Banff Schema for Acute Hepatic Rejection

CATEGORY	CRITERIA	SCORE
Portal inflammation	Mostly lymphatic inflammation involving a minority of the triads	1
	Expansion of most triads by a mixed infiltrate containing lymphocytes, neutrophils, and eosinophils	2
	Marked expansion of most or all triads by a mixed infiltrate containing numerous blasts, with spillover into periportal parenchyma	3
Bile duct damage	Minority of ducts infiltrated by inflammatory cells, with only mild reactive changes in epithelial cells	1
	Most or all ducts infiltrated by inflammatory cells, with occasional degenerative duct changes, such as nuclear pleomorphism, disorder polarity, and vacuolization	2
	As above, with most or all ducts showing degenerative changes	3
Venous endothelial inflammation	Subendothelial lymphocytic infiltration of some portal or hepatic venules	1
	Subendothelial infiltration involving most or all portal or hepatic venules	2
	As above, with perivenular inflammation extending into surrounding parenchyma and associated hepatocyte necrosis	3

This index has a range from 0–9, classified as follows: 0–3, minimal acute rejection; 4–6, mild acute rejection; 7–9, moderate to severe acute rejection.

Modified from the Banff Consensus. Schema for grading liver allograft rejection: An international consensus document. *Hepatology* 1997;25:658–663.

TABLE 109.4 Banff Schema for Chronic Hepatic Rejection

STRUCTURE	EARLY CHRONIC REJECTION	LATE CHRONIC REJECTION
Small bile ducts (<60 μm)	Degenerative changes involving most ducts: increased nuclear-to-cytoplasmic ratio, nuclear hyperchromasia, uneven nuclear spacing, ducts partially lined with epithelium	Degenerative changes in remaining bile ducts
	Bile duct loss in <50% of portal tracts	Bile duct loss in >50% of portal tracts
Terminal hepatic venules	Intimal/luminal inflammation	Focal obliteration
	Lytic zone 3 necrosis and inflammation	Variable inflammation
	Mild perivenular fibrosis	Severe (bridging) fibrosis
Portal tract hepatic arterioles	Occasional loss involving <25% of portal tracts	Loss involving >25% of portal tracts
Large perihilar hepatic artery branches	Intimal inflammation, focal foam-cell deposition	Luminal narrowing by subintimal foam cells and fibrointimal proliferation
Large perihilar bile ducts	Inflammation damage, focal foam-cell deposition	Mural fibrosis
Other	"Transition" hepatitis with spotty necrosis of hepatocytes	Sinusoidal foam cell accumulation, marked cholestasis

Modified from Demetris A, Adams D, Bellamy C, et al. Update of the International Banff Schema for Liver Allograft Rejection: Working recommendations for the histopathologic staging and reporting of chronic rejection: An international panel. *Hepatology* 2000;31:792–799.

injury and early AKI are being investigated and may help guide clinical decision making in the future.[163,164] The use of calcineurin inhibitors (CNIs) is associated with increased risk of renal failure because of renal artery vasoconstriction and development of thrombotic microangiopathy. CNI-related kidney injury is dose dependent; therefore strategies that minimize or withdrawal CNI may have some benefit for renal recovery. Renal-sparing alternatives, including the use of mechanistic target of rapamycin (mTOR) inhibitors in combination with low-exposure CNI therapy, has shown promising results, with improved estimated GFR in patients receiving mTOR inhibitors with low-exposure CNI versus standard CNI dosing at 3 years after transplant.[165] Given the reduction in mortality with post-LT AKI, recognition of risk factors is key to rapid implementation of nephroprotective strategies (see Chapter 111).

DISEASE-SPECIFIC CONSIDERATIONS AND OUTCOMES

Patients undergoing transplantation for specific disease processes often have unique considerations that may contribute to recovery as well as morbidity and mortality and are briefly discussed here.

Alcoholic Cirrhosis

Alcoholic cirrhosis is one of the leading indications for LT in the United States.[6] Most centers require a minimum interval of abstinence of 6 months before listing. However, there is conflicting data on whether this accurately predicts rates of recidivism.[166] Overall recidivism rates are reported to range from 10% to 30% and are associated with decreased graft and patient survival.[167,168] Strategies to reduce rates of relapse are necessary to preserve allografts.

In the setting of severe alcoholic hepatitis, the Lille model can be used to identify patients unlikely to respond to medical treatment. These patients have a high predicted mortality of 70% in 6 months.[169] Mathurin et al. demonstrate that in severe alcoholic hepatitis, those who received LT had improved survival of 77% versus 23% with low rates of recidivism, challenging the 6-month rule and suggesting that with appropriate selection, LT may be an acceptable treatment.[170] These patients

have excellent outcomes of 94% survival at 1 year and 84% at 3 years[171] (see Chapters 105 and 107).

Nonalcoholic Steatohepatitis

Cirrhosis secondary to NASH is a rapidly increasing indication for LT, and the most common liver disease in the United States (see Chapters 69 and 74). Additionally, there is a growing prevalence of steatosis and NASH among donor allografts. Morbidly obese recipients are at increased risk for post-LT metabolic syndrome, infectious complications, and renal failure after LT,[172,173] although overall survival rates are similar to patients without NASH.[174] Recurrent NASH is a commonly reported phenomena after LT. Independent risk factors for graft steatosis after LT include diabetes, hypertension, hyperlipidemia, alcoholic cirrhosis as the primary indication for LT, and pre-transplant graft steatosis.[175] The prevalence of dyslipidemia, hypertension, and insulin resistance increase post-LT because of effects of immunosuppression. Reduction of steroids and minimization of use of calcineurin inhibitors may be considered to reduce complications of metabolic syndrome[172] (see Chapter 106). Use of bariatric surgery at the time of LT or postoperatively has the potential to improve obesity-associated comorbidities and abrogate the incidence of graft steatosis.[2] Although optimal timing of bariatric surgery is unclear,[176] those who underwent combined LT and sleeve gastrectomy maintained a higher percentage of total body weight loss, lower prevalence of hypertension, insulin resistance, and steatosis.[177]

Primary Sclerosing Cholangitis

Primary sclerosing cholangitis (PSC) is a chronic cholestatic liver disease characterized by inflammation and fibrosis of intra- and extra-hepatic bile ducts and is frequently associated with inflammatory bowel disease (typically ulcerative colitis)[178] (see Chapter 41). Medical therapies exists but have no long-term effect on survival or disease progression. Ultimately, LT is recommended for patients who have developed complications of ESLD or recurrent cholangitis because of chronic biliary obstruction. When performing LT, any remaining recipient biliary duct tissue is at risk for fibrotic change. Therefore biliary reconstruction is typically performed with a Roux-en-Y choledochojejunostomy. Outcomes for PSC are excellent, with

5-year patient survival rate greater than 87%.[179] The risk for CCA is increased in patients with PSC, occurring in 10% to 20% of cases.[180] Risk factors for CCA include alcohol, tobacco use, and duration of inflammatory bowel disease (IBD).[181] A carbohydrate antigen (CA)19-9 greater than 100 U/mL has 75% sensitivity and 80% specificity in identifying PSC patients with CCA[181] (see Chapters 41 and 51). Endoscopic retrograde cholangiopancreatography (ERCP) with brushings may be used for diagnosis with polysomy detected by fluorescence *in situ* hybridization (FISH) to improve diagnostic yield.[182] Acute cellular rejection occurs at increased risk in the setting of PSC and result in reduced patient and allograft survival. Unfortunately disease recurrence is estimated to occur in 10% to 20% of recipients, with mean time to recurrence at 4 years.[183,184]

Hepatitis C Virus

Formerly, HCV was the most common indication for LT performed in the United States (see Chapter 68). The introduction of DAA regimens has transformed therapy for HCV infection because it is highly effective and well tolerated.[185] Attaining a sustained virologic response with therapy, as defined as an undetectable RNA level 12 weeks after completion of therapy, is associated with improved survival and reduced need for transplantation and incidence of HCC.[186] The success of DAA is reflected in the declining need of LT for HCV.[6] Additionally, it has led to a paradigm shift and consideration of HCV+ liver allografts as a step to expand the donor pool, as described previously in this chapter. In 2017 the American Society of Transplantation Consensus conference concluded that use of HCV+ donors into HCV viremic recipients is safe, if the donor biopsy shows less than stage 2 fibrosis.[50] Several studies have demonstrated successful use of HCV+ donors into HCV seronegative recipients.[4,51] Post-LT patient and graft survival are comparable to seronegative donors.[51] Use of DAA therapy in the recipients has been successful in attaining sustain virologic response with good outcomes.

Hepatocellular Carcinoma

HCC was one of the first documented indications for LT[187] and is currently the third most common diagnosis for LT[6] (see Chapters 89 and 108A). The use of LT for patients with HCC is based on the oncologic premise that best outcomes will be achieved with the most complete extirpation of disease. Total hepatectomy allows for complete resection of tumors and removes potential future sites of tumor formation in the diseased remnant liver. This is discussed in detail in Chapter 108A. In their landmark series examining LT for HCC, Mazzaferro et al.[188] obtained a 75% 4-year actuarial survival using specific guidelines in highly select patients. Subsequently termed the *Milan criteria* for LT, patients under this protocol were offered LT if they had a solitary tumor less than 5 cm in diameter or no more than three nodules, each less than 3 cm in diameter (stage II). Largely as a result of this report, the United Network for Organ Sharing (UNOS) adopted these criteria for listing potential recipients with HCC,[189] limiting LT to patients with stage I (single tumor as large as 2 cm in diameter) or stage II disease. Several centers have extended LT to patients with tumors exceeding the Milan criteria and have met with varying degrees of success. The University of California–San Francisco (UCSF) criteria permit LT for patients with solitary tumors smaller than 6.5 cm diameter, fewer than three tumors, and a maximum diameter less than 4.5 cm or total cumulative diameter less than 8 cm.[190] MELD exception points are awarded on a routine basis to patients with stage II HCC. Excellent results have been achieved in patients with HCC, with reported 5-year survival after LT for HCC of generally 60% to 75%.[191]

Locoregional therapy (LRT), such as ablation, chemoembolization, or radioembolization of tumors is employed as a down-staging or bridging therapy in the pre-transplant setting (see Chapters 89, 94, 96, and 108A). An argued benefit of waiting time before transplant is that it allows observation of tumor biology or aggressiveness. In 2020, a Multicenter HCC Transplant Consortium demonstrated that patients receiving LRT, achieving a complete pathologic response results in lower post-LT recurrence and superior survival at 1, 3, and 5 years. Predictors of complete pathologic response were younger age, lower MELD and AFP, and more likely to have tumors within Milan criteria.[192] Identification of these factors may help guide LRT and transplant strategies to improve cancer outcomes.

Cholangiocarcinoma

Surgery remains the only potentially curative treatment for hilar CCA; however, survival remains poor, ranging from 20% to 40% at 5 years.[193] Surgical resection is feasible in less than 30% of patients because patients often present with advanced disease[194] (see Chapters 51 and 119B). Patients with PSC, a known risk factor for CCA, are often poor candidates for resection because of concurrent cirrhosis (see Chapter 41). Although early reports of the use of LT for treatment of CCA was associated with 5-year survival rates of 30%, more recently, surgeons at the Mayo Clinic have reported successful results using strict treatment protocols for performing LT in patients with localized, node-negative hilar CCA, with the use of neoadjuvant chemoradiation, staging laparotomy, resection to negative margins, and LT[195] (see Chapter 108B). Using these or similar protocols, 5-year survival rates of 72% have been achieved in a highly select group of patients, including many of whom had PSC.[196,197] Retrospective analysis revealed improved outcomes for patients enrolled in the Mayo protocol compared with those of patients undergoing major hepatic resection.[197] However, neoadjuvant therapy is associated with higher rates of arterial and venous complications after transplantation.[198]

CONCLUSION

Successful management of LT patients requires a multidisciplinary approach. Outcomes have continued to improve over the past 5 decades. The success can be attributed to the following:

1. Organized regional and national networks designed for the early identification of potential organ donors and rapid procurement in select candidates
2. Improved surgical and anesthetic techniques, allowing previous obstacles to LT to be overcome (e.g., PVT, severe coagulopathy)
3. Novel antirejection and antimicrobial agents, with increasing emphasis on achieving minimal immunosuppression in the shortest time possible
4. Increased vigilance for the occurrence of acute complications after LT, with the development of rapid screening tests for HAT, PVT, and primary nonfunction

As the only treatment option and potential cure for thousands of patients, LT will continue to be offered for the foreseeable future. Methods for expanding the donor pool and recent revisions to the allocation process may help ease the shortage of suitable hepatic grafts. In recent years, the use of well-tolerated and successful DAA agents for HCV has drastically altered the makeup of the transplant candidate list and donor pool. However, we are encountering new challenges with NASH and increased steatotic donor livers in the setting of the growing obesity epidemic. Future research and efforts to optimize selection, augment use of marginal grafts, and consider machine preservation techniques may help expand the limited donor liver allograft supply and mitigate the demand for transplantation while improving recipient outcomes.

References are available at expertconsult.com.

CHAPTER 110

Liver transplantation in children: Indications and outcomes

Ola Ahmed and Adeel S. Khan

HISTORIC OVERVIEW

Thomas Starzl attempted the first human liver transplantation (LT) in 1963 in a 3-year-old child with biliary atresia (BA; see Chapter 125). Unfortunately, the child died in the operating room from uncontrollable hemorrhage.[1] Just a few years later, however, Starzl successfully performed eight LTs in eight children. In contrast to his first attempt, all survived the operation and half survived for more than 1 year postoperatively.[2] Since those heroic beginnings 5 decades ago, advances in immunosuppression, surgical technique, anesthesia, and critical care have made LT an effective, reliable, and lifesaving procedure that is performed every day at LT centers throughout the world. In children with end-stage liver disease (ESLD), LT has become the accepted therapy, and its use is limited only by the availability of suitable grafts.

In 2018, 8250 adult and 563 pediatric LTs were performed in the United States alone.[3] Currently, approximately 13,046 registrations exist on the LT waiting list, and 1046 of the candidates are younger than 17 years of age.[4] Potential recipients such as infants, toddlers, and young children are limited in graft choice partly because of the narrow options of available graft sizes as they face unique challenges unbeknownst to an adult population. Historically, the lack of size-matched organ availability, coupled with the disproportionate number of adults on the waiting list, has significantly disadvantaged children awaiting transplantation. This challenge still remains in the modern era with 30% of organs refused because of size mismatch.[5] Recent evidence reported that nearly half of pediatric deceased-donor organs are allocated to adult patients.[6] Despite this obvious disadvantage, children with ESLD can deteriorate quickly and cannot afford to spend too much time awaiting transplantation when compared with adults. An infant with decompensated liver disease from cirrhosis typically cannot survive on a waiting list for more than a few months or years. Currently, children aged 1 to 5 years make up the largest age group on the waiting list (31%) and patients younger than 1 year constitute the single age group majority (23%).[3] In addition, the shortage of pediatric donors and size-matched organs contributes to longer waiting times, which translates to an increased mortality in children on the transplant waiting list. In the earlier days of LT, as many as 50% of children on the waiting list would die before they could receive a transplant.[7] Encouragingly, pre-transplant mortality has decreased in all age groups and has since improved to a 10% mortality on the pediatric LT waiting list.[3,5] Despite this progress, the waiting list mortality for children younger than 1 year continues to exceed that of any other adult or pediatric age group, estimated at 17.1 deaths per 100 waitlist-years.[3,4,8]

INDICATIONS (SEE CHAPTER 105)

Box 110.1 lists common indications for pediatric LT, largely falling into two categories: cholestatic and noncholestatic. The classic and most common indication for LT is still ESLD; however, the rates of multiorgan transplants inclusive of LT have also increased. Liver-kidney and liver-pancreas-intestine candidates accounted for 2.5% and 12.6% of pediatric LT candidates in 2018[3] (see Chapter 112).

Cholestatic Indications

BA is a progressive, inflammatory, and fibrosing cholangiopathy of unclear pathogenesis (see Chapters 1 and 40). It occurs in 1 in 8000 to 18,000 live births, and although rare, the majority of affected children eventually develop ESLD, making it account for approximately 35% of indications for all pediatric LTs.[3,8,9] Most children with this disease lack an extrahepatic biliary tree, resulting in impaired bile flow, conjugated hyperbilirubinemia, acholic stools, and hepatomegaly. The hepatic parenchyma becomes congested, and progressive damage leads to secondary biliary cirrhosis. As a result, BA can lead to severe and intractable consequences such as malnutrition, recurrent cholangitis, and worsening portal hypertension, further expanding the indications for LT. Moreover, extrahepatic manifestations of disease, such as hepatopulmonary syndrome and portopulmonary hypertension, may further complicate the course and count as additional indications to proceed to LT.[9] A portoenterostomy, also known as the *Kasai procedure*, may yield some clinical improvement and remains the first-line treatment.[10] Clinical success of the procedure is best judged by the reinstatement of the biliary system, with good bile flow and jaundice clearance at 3 months correlating with transplant-free survival rates ranging from 75% to 90% at 10 years.[9,11] For this reason, children should be evaluated early for bile flow restoration because approximately 70% to 80% of children with BA eventually require LT, making it the most common indication for LT among all pediatric age groups.[3,12]

Alternative causes of cholestasis in children include primary sclerosing cholangitis (PSC; see Chapter 41); idiopathic neonatal hepatitis; infection by both viral and bacterial pathogens (see Chapter 70), including toxoplasmosis and syphilis; progressive familial intrahepatic cholestasis (Byler disease); metabolic and genetic diseases; familial arteriohepatic dysplasia (Alagille syndrome); choledochal cysts (see Chapter 46); and ischemia-reperfusion injury.[13] Regardless of the various etiologies, impaired bile flow and the resultant cholestasis may ultimately progress to cirrhosis in all the aforementioned instances.

Long-term parenteral nutrition in pediatric cases of intestinal failure has also been implicated in intrahepatic cholestasis and has

Cholestatic Hepatic Failure
Biliary atresia
Primary sclerosing cholangitis
Alagille syndrome
Byler disease
Total parenteral nutrition–induced liver failure
Idiopathic disease

Infectious Hepatic Failure
Viral infection, such as with hepatitis A, B, or C
Toxoplasmosis
Syphilis
Bacterial infection

Genetic or Metabolic Hepatic Insufficiency
α_1-Antitrypsin deficiency
Cystic fibrosis
Wilson disease
Glycogen storage disease
Tyrosinemia
Primary hyperoxaluria
Hereditary hemochromatosis
Crigler-Najjar syndrome
Neoplastic hepatic primaries
Hepatoblastoma
Hepatocellular carcinoma

Extrahepatic Diseases
Hemophilia
Familial hypercholesterolemia

Other Causes of Hepatic Failure
Autoimmune hepatitis
Budd-Chiari syndrome
Toxicity
Giant arteriovenous malformation

been associated with the risk of cirrhosis. Peden et al. were the first to report the potential association in 1971 in a premature infant receiving total parenteral nutrition.[14] The infant developed progressive hyperbilirubinemia, eventually succumbing to worsening symptoms and passing away on the 71st day of life. Fortunately, the incidence and mortality from parenteral nutrition–associated cholestasis and cirrhosis has decreased significantly.

Noncholestatic Indications

Noncholestatic indications for pediatric LT include liver failure secondary to infectious, metabolic, genetic, and neoplastic etiologies (see Chapters 68, 87, and 93). Although less frequent in children than in adults, postnecrotic liver cirrhosis is an indication for LT in approximately 10% of pediatric patients and commonly results from viral hepatitis or idiopathic cryptogenic cirrhosis.[15]

Inherited Metabolic Disorders

Metabolic liver diseases are genetic disorders that lead to the production of aberrant transport proteins or enzymes and altered metabolic pathways. These inborn errors of metabolism, such as α_1-antitrypsin (AAT) deficiency or Wilson disease, may cause direct injury to the liver and result in liver failure, with or without injury to other organs. Specific dietary restrictions may attenuate liver injury when combined with medications to eliminate toxic metabolites, enhance residual enzyme activity, or replenish downstream products hampered by the metabolic block in question.[16] In some instances, however, if left untreated, abnormal liver metabolism, including urea cycle disorders or oxalosis, may lead to end-stage damage consequently facilitating concomitant multiorgan damage. Although their prevalence has remained static overtime, such diseases still account for approximately 13% of all pediatric LTs[3,16] (see Chapters 105 and 107).

ALPHA-1 ANTITRYPSIN DEFICIENCY. AAT deficiency is a genetic disorder that leads to the defective production of the serine protease α_1-antitrypsin, an enzyme produced in the liver to protect the lungs from neutrophil elastase. The abnormal protein accumulates in the liver and can result in extensive hepatic damage, although the mechanism of injury remains unclear. This may manifest as neonatal jaundice and acholic stools, particularly in the first week of life, and ultimately progresses to cirrhosis and a need for LT in childhood.[17] Augmentation therapy in the form of synthetic AAT has some utility in the treatment of AAT deficiency–related emphysema by slowing lung decline; however, effective therapeutic strategies have not been proven in hepatic disease.[18] Novel therapeutic approaches are under development such as stimulating autophagy and using siRNA technology but are still in the early experimental phase and no clinical success in human models has been ascertained.[19,20] Further research is still warranted in the molecular pathobiology of AAT and, for the time being, LT is the most viable option for AAT-related cirrhosis in children (see Chapters 105 and 106).

WILSON DISEASE (HEPATOLENTICULAR DEGENERATION). Wilson disease is an inborn error of copper metabolism characterized by defective copper excretion and the accumulation of toxic amounts in the liver, basal ganglia, kidney, and cornea, which may lead to the characteristic Kayser-Fleischer rings. The defect is located on chromosome 13 and is inherited in an autosomal recessive manner, affecting 1 in 50,000 births. The process of copper excretion is not well developed in newborns, and normal newborns may often show hepatic copper concentrations similar to patients diagnosed with Wilson disease.[21] The copper excretory pathway begins to function more effectively within the first year of life and any failure or impairment in the process ultimately leads to the pathologic accumulation of copper at birth, which can progress into adult life. Initial disease presentation within pediatric patients occurs between the ages of 9 to 13, on average. Early symptoms are nonspecific and include lethargy, anorexia, vague abdominal pain, and weight loss. Some patients are seen with asymptomatic hepatomegaly and others with fulminant hepatic failure.[22] Consequently, LT is often indicated for acute liver failure or decompensated cirrhosis. One of the difficulties in management is identifying who may benefit from surgery and in an attempt to address this issue, a group from King's College have devised a prognostic index score by analyzing data from their pediatric cohort. The calculation combines aspartate aminotransferase (AST), albumen, bilirubin, international normalized ratio (INR), and white cell count and has shown considerable accuracy when compared with other validated scoring systems and offers a reliable adjunct to patient selection[23,24] (see Chapters 105).

Urea Cycle Disorders

Some metabolic diseases, such as urea cycle disorders, Crigler-Najjar syndrome, and familial hypercholesterolemia, do not result in primary liver disease but cause extrahepatic impairment as a result of dysfunctional hepatic gene products or metabolites that affect distant organs. Urea cycle defects (UCDs) result in the accumulation of nitrogenous waste products and, in some instances, severe and lethal hyperammonemia. Two diseases within this group of disorders are described by their respective enzyme deficiencies: carbamyl phosphate synthetase (CPS) deficiency and ornithine trans-carbamylase (OTC) deficiency. Three others are described by the primary metabolite that accumulates in affected individuals: citrullinemia, argininosuccinic aciduria, and argininemia. Epidemiologic data predicts that 114 newborns with UCDs are born each year in the United States of whom 26% present with hyperammonemia during their first month of life; the disease is reported to carry a neonatal mortality rate as high as 26%.[25]

Although still in early phases of experimentation, hepatocyte transplantation may provide a bridge to surgery in children with severe UCDs[26]; however, LT offers the only "cure" in hepatic disease. Based on United Network for Organ Sharing (UNOS) pediatric transplantation data of patients between 2002 and 2012, 5.4% of LTs were for UCDs. Transplant outcomes vary with patient age and higher 5-year graft and patient survival rates are seen in older children with UCDs: 78% and 88% in children younger than 2 years old and 88% and 99% for children 2 years old or older, respectively.[27]

Crigler-Najjar Syndrome

Crigler-Najjar syndrome is a rare genetic disorder caused by mutations of the gene that codes uridine diphosphate glucurono-syltransferase-1, resulting in unconjugated hyperbilirubinemia.[28] The disorder is inherited in an autosomal recessive manner, affecting 1 in 1,000,000 births and two phenotypes are described, type 1 being the most lethal form.[28] Untreated neonates develop a condition of severe neuronal damage and *kernicterus* ultimately leading to severe disability or death in advanced stages.[29] Intensive phototherapy and plasmapheresis are potential therapeutic options, but, LT remains the main definitive treatment.[29,30] Despite undergoing LT, neurologic sequelae in patients are oftentimes irreversible and, for this reason, the optimal timing of LT is debatable.[29]

Familial Hypercholesterolemia

Homozygous familial hypercholesterolemia (HFH) is a rare but life-threatening disease caused by mutations in the gene that codes the low-density lipoprotein (LDL) receptor.[31] The receptor may be defective or completely absent, and affected individuals have dramatically elevated plasma cholesterol levels, leading to accelerated atherosclerosis, childhood coronary artery disease, and premature death from myocardial infarction.[32] LT as a treatment for familial hypercholesterolemia was first performed by Starzl in 1983 on a 6-year-old girl who also received a heart transplant.[33] LDL receptors are primarily found in hepatocytes and, therefore, LT corrects these conditions by providing the required cellular machinery to synthesize the correct gene product or metabolite.[28,31] Anecdotally, auxiliary hepatic transplantation has been performed in these circumstances; a segmental resection of the native liver is performed (right hemihepatectomy), and a segmental section of a donor liver is implanted (right hemiliver transplant).[34] This is in contrast with AAT deficiency, which has the potential to progress into hepatocellular carcinoma (HCC) and, hence, precludes auxiliary LT and mandates total hepatectomy.

Cystic Fibrosis

Cystic fibrosis (CF) is an autosomal recessive multiorgan disorder and is one of the most common lethal inherited diseases affecting the White population, with a frequency of 1 in 2000 to 3000 live births.[35] Although management of these patients continues to improve, CF liver disease (CFLD) is increasingly recognized as a significant cause of morbidity and mortality in patients with CF and is now considered the third leading cause of death in patients.[36] The median age of CFLD diagnosis is 10 to 11 years with up to 90% diagnosed before the age of 20.[37] Approximately 5% to 10% of CF patients will progress to cirrhosis, which further complicates portal hypertension, nutritional deficits, and pulmonary decline. LT remains a viable option for decompensated cirrhosis and the complications of portal hypertension in the pediatric cohort, with 1- and 5-year survival rates approaching 90% and 85%, respectively.[38] Transplantation not only assists with nutritional and functional status but in some instances may deter lung decline.[38] A significant number of patients with CFLD may be helped with an isolated LT or a concomitant liver and lung transplantation; however, the debate is ongoing in the literature regarding the timing of LT in these patients.[39] If isolated LT is considered, it should ideally be performed before the development of end-stage lung failure and when pulmonary function is still preserved (forced expiratory volume [FEV] >50%).[40]

Budd-Chiari Syndrome

Although more common in adult patients, chronic Budd-Chiari syndrome with severe hepatic congestion and focal areas of liver fibrosis or cirrhosis may be an indication for LT in older children and accounts for less than 1% of cases[41] (see Chapter 86). This typically presents with ascites, hepatomegaly splenomegaly, and, less commonly, variceal bleeding.[42] Pre-transplant evaluation is imperative to recognize predisposing prothrombic states, present in up to two-thirds of children,[41] and underlying diseases such as myeloproliferative disorders, primary hepatic protein deficiencies—of proteins C and S, antithrombin III, and activated protein C resistance—or secondary protein deficiencies, such as increased intestinal protein loss in inflammatory bowel disease. Up-to-date long-term outcome data after LT in pediatric patients is lacking; however, survival is likely impacted by the underlying cause of Budd-Chiari syndrome.

Fulminant Hepatic Failure

Fulminant hepatic failure (FHF) is associated with a mortality rate greater than 70% (see Chapter 107). It is essential to transfer children with FHF to a transplant center immediately for management, urgent evaluation, and listing for LT. Because cerebral edema develops rapidly, careful monitoring and intensive supportive care are required. Mild elevation of intracranial pressure (ICP) may be managed acutely by hyperventilation and elevation of the patient's head, although maintenance likely requires strict sodium (hypernatremia), osmolar, and intravascular volume control. Placement of an ICP monitor should be considered, but regardless, attention to maintenance of cerebral perfusion pressure (CPP) is paramount. Transplantation evaluation in patients with signs of cerebral edema is urgent because this may lead to irreversible brain damage or death. Poor prognostic factors for LT in children with FHF include age younger than 10 years, liver disease other than viral hepatitis, grade II or III hepatic encephalopathy, coagulopathy (prothrombin time [PT] >30 seconds, INR ≥2.55), and increasing jaundice (bilirubin ≥10 mg/dL).[43–45] A review of the UNOS data showed significantly reduced 5-year patient and graft survival in children with acute liver failure (ALF) compared with patient and graft survival rates in children transplanted for BA (73% and 59% vs. 89% and 78%, respectively).[46,47]

Malignancy

Liver tumors account for less than 3% of all indications for pediatric LT[3] (see Chapter 89 to 93). Hepatoblastoma, HCC, and fibrolamellar HCC represent the most frequent tumors. In contrast to adults with viral hepatitis or alcoholic liver disease, the predisposing factors for malignant liver tumors in children are more often metabolic disorders, such as AAT deficiency, BA, tyrosinemia, or glycogen storage disease.[48] In patients without cirrhosis, hepatic resection is the treatment of choice, if the tumor meets criteria for resectability. LT should be considered in the case of unresectable tumors confined to the liver.[49] Transplantation is also indicated in patients with advanced cirrhosis or HCC meeting Milan criteria and in some instances demonstrates more superior outcomes than resection and chemotherapy.[50] Rarely, giant arteriovenous malformations and benign liver tumors—when they replace the whole liver, or when they have the potential for malignancy (e.g., hepatic adenomatosis or multiple adenomas in glycogen storage disease; Fig. 110.1)—may be indications for total hepatectomy and LT.[51,52]

EVALUATION OF THE POTENTIAL TRANSPLANT RECIPIENT

A multidisciplinary evaluation of a child with decompensated liver disease should be completed with the involvement of surgeons, hepatologists, nurses, anesthesiologists, psychologists, and social workers. Early referral to a transplant center allows maximum time to develop a management strategy and to optimize pre-transplantation clinical status. In 2018 children between the ages of 1 and 5 years old (31%) and 11 years or older (29.9%) formed the largest subgroup on the pediatric waiting list, followed by infants less than 1 year old (23.7%) and the 6 to 10 year age group (15.3%).[3] The timing of LT is crucial; late referral of patients with significant hepatic complications and malnutrition can result in considerable perioperative morbidity, mortality, and a poorer outcome. The expected waiting time on the transplant list may vary based on the geographic region, and this should be taken into account.[53] As of data collected on December 2018, over 67% of pediatric patients had been waiting for transplantation for less than 1 year.[3] Over 60% of pediatric LT recipients were not hospitalized before surgery and up to 18.5% of patients were in intensive care between 2016 and 2018 pre-transplantation.[3] In infants younger than 2 years who weigh less than 10 kg, maintaining metabolic and nutritional support is often challenging. Ideally, children should be considered for LT before the onset of complications of malnutrition, such as weight loss and growth failure.[54] With chronic liver disease, prolonged clotting times, intractable ascites, recurrent variceal bleeding secondary to portal hypertension, and recurrent cholangitis with severe cholestasis are all indications for LT.

The prognosis after LT for chronic liver disease is influenced by preoperative comorbidities. The advent of the Pediatric End-Stage Liver Disease (PELD) and Model for End-Stage Liver Disease (MELD) scores has allowed for better prediction of mortality and progression of liver disease while awaiting LT (see Chapter 4). The pertinent factors in the PELD score are the INR, total bilirubin, serum albumin, age younger than 1 year, and weight or length less than 2 standard deviations (SD) from the mean for age and sex.[55] The PELD score is used for patients younger than 12 years, and the scores range from a negative value (−10) to 50. Adolescents aged 13 to 18 years are allocated organs based on the MELD score, similar to adults. Box 110.2 presents the formulas for calculating MELD and PELD scores. In the United States, between 2016 and 2018, the most common PELD score at transplant was 30 or higher (41.6%), with 9.3% of children having a PELD score less than 15.[3] Pre-transplant mortality has continued to decrease for all age groups to 6.5 deaths per 100 wait-list years in 2017 to 2018, with the highest rates for candidates less than 1 year at 17.1 deaths per 100 wait-list years in 2017 to 2018 and lowest for the 6 to 10 year age group at 3.6 deaths.[3] Consideration should be given to referring these young and small infants to pediatric specialty centers that have expertise with these challenging cases

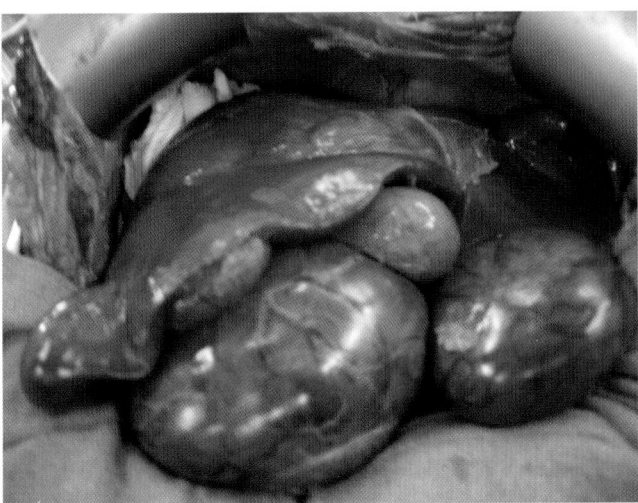

FIGURE 110.1 Multiple giant adenomas in an explanted liver.

BOX 110.2	MELD and PELD Calculations

MELD

$$10 \times [0.957 \, ln(Creatinine \, [mg/dL]) + 0.378 \, ln(Total \, bilirubin \, [mg/dL]) + 1.120 \, ln(INR) + 0.643]$$

PELD

$$10 \times [0.480 \times log_e(Bilirubin \, [mg/dL]) + 1.857 \times log_e(INR) - 0.687 \times log_e(Albumin \, [g/dL]) + 0.436 \, (if \, the \, patient \, is < 1 \, year \, old) + 0.667 \, (if \, the \, patient \, has \, growth \, failure \, [<2 \, SD])]$$

The resulting score is rounded to the nearest whole number.

INR, International normalized ratio; *MELD*, Model for End-Stage Liver Disease; *PELD*, Pediatric End-Stage Liver Disease; *SD*, standard deviation.

Significant changes in the waiting list structure have been observed by comparing the periods before and after the introduction of the MELD and PELD scores.[56] There was a significant decrease of patients in the emergency category (46%–26%) and reduced waiting-list mortality (21%–17%). There were no differences in 1-year patient survival between the pre-score and post-score eras.

CONTRAINDICATIONS

One of the main challenges in organ transplantation is the scarcity of donor organs, particularly in the pediatric population. It is absolutely imperative for transplant teams to identify which children need urgent transplantation and who will benefit the most. Small size and young age are no longer contraindications, and many transplants for BA are now done in infants who weigh less than 10 kg.[57] Absolute contraindications are clinical circumstances that consistently lead to poor patient and graft outcomes[58]. The few absolute contraindications to pediatric LT include uncontrolled systemic sepsis, severe cardiopulmonary conditions, irreversible brain edema, and extrahepatic malignancy (Box 110.3).

PEDIATRIC LIVER TRANSPLANTATION— TECHNICAL CHALLENGES

Combined with the scarcity of donors, another challenge in pediatric LT is the technical complexity of implantation. The shortage of donor organs has motivated surgeons to develop innovative techniques in an effort to expand the donor pool, particularly for pediatric transplantation. Initially, adult cadaveric livers were made smaller by removing the right hemiliver (segments V–VIII) and medial section of the left hemiliver (segments IV and I) to enable grafting of the left lateral section (segments II and III) into small recipients. In this way, the size restrictions imposed on any particular donor-recipient combination could be overcome. The application of reduced-size grafts led to a shift of cadaveric livers to children and small adults, but it did not increase the total graft pool. Various other techniques have been proposed to overcome the restrictions of size mismatch and of inserting a whole liver (Fig 110.2). Living-donor (LDLT), split liver, and reduced-size LT have not only contributed to expanding the donor pool but offer favorable outcomes when combined with astute patient selection[59–62] and have been one of the most exciting and challenging advances recently in LT. The encouraging outcomes seen in

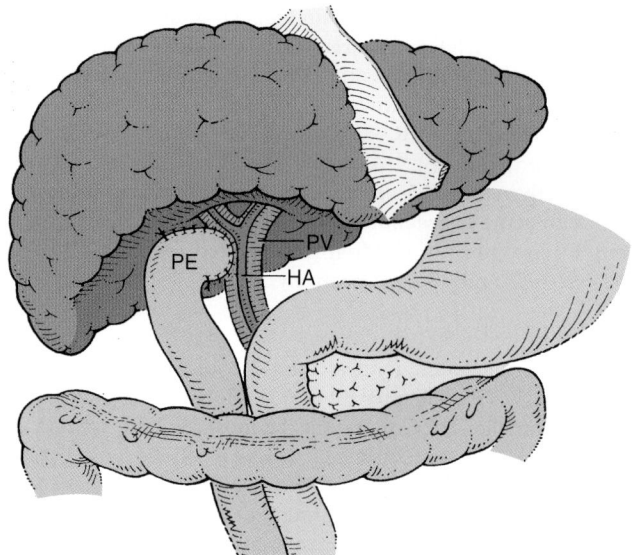

FIGURE 110.2 Recipient hepatectomy. The hilum is examined carefully, and a previous portoenterostomy *(PE)* is taken down. The portal vein *(PV)* and hepatic artery *(HA)* are divided high in the porta hepatis. (See Chapter 125.)

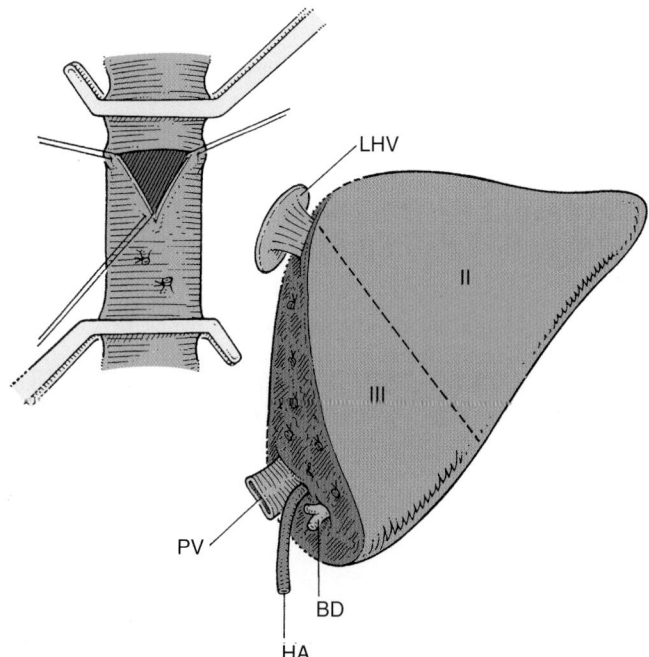

FIGURE 110.3 The most frequently used segmental graft uses segments II and III of the left liver. The recipient's inferior vena cava *(IVC)* is preserved, and the left hepatic vein *(LHV)* is sutured to a large triangular venotomy cut on the anterior aspect of the IVC. The portal vein *(PV)*, hepatic artery *(HA)*, and bile ducts *(BD)* are depicted before anastomosis. (See Chapter 125.)

BOX 110.3	Contraindications to Pediatric Liver Transplantation

Absolute
Uncontrolled systemic sepsis
Irreversible brain edema
Uncorrectable symptomatic heart defects
Nonreversible pulmonary hypertension
Extrahepatic malignancy

Relative
Portomesenteric thrombosis
HIV-positive status
Severe psychosocial impediments

HIV, Human immunodeficiency virus.

reduced-size and split-liver transplantation facilitated the development of additional techniques for using liver segments from living donors for pediatric grafts (Fig 110.3). With increasing experience, donations from living-donor livers are no longer confined to left lateral sections or left hepatic lobes but have expanded to include full right hepatic lobe grafts, which con-

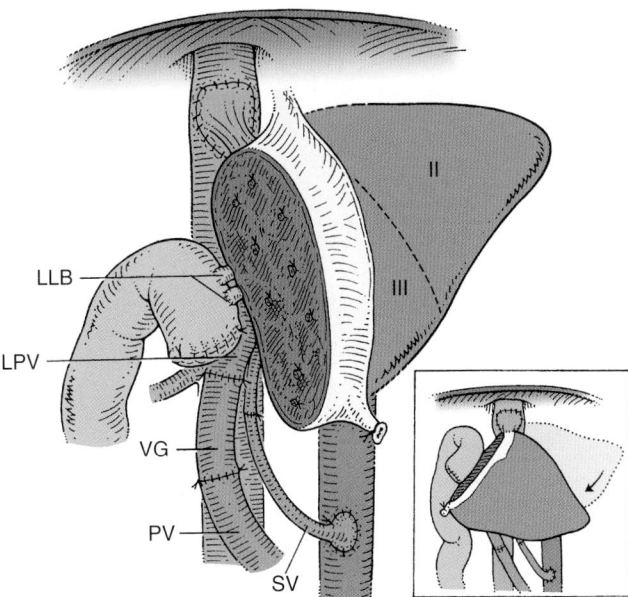

FIGURE 110.4 Completed recipient implantation. The variant with two bile ducts is depicted. Interposition grafts are used for the hepatic artery and the portal vein to ensure adequate length. *Inset,* Final position of the graft after abdominal closure. *LLB* represents segment II and III bile ducts; *LPV,* left portal vein; *PV,* portal vein; *SV,* saphenous vein graft to hepatic artery from aorta; *VG,* vein graft. (See Chapter 125.)

tributes to the adult organ pool as well. Progressive improvements in surgical technique have evolved such that now the left lateral section and the right trisegment graft can each be used separately, meaning that a single liver can potentially be divided and transplanted into two recipients: one child and one adult (Fig 110.4). With this innovative technique, continued efforts in expanding the pediatric donor pool do not necessarily have to disadvantage adult recipients. Except in unusual circumstances, the use of a reduced-size liver allograft in which the remnant is discarded is rarely justified. Between 2016 and 2018, nearly 40% of pediatric candidates received partial or split LTs.[3] The use of reduced-size liver grafts declined from 26.1% to 20.2% of pediatric LTs during the last decade, but, during this same time, the use of split-liver allografts increased to 19.2%[3,63] (see Chapters 109, 121, and 125).

POSTOPERATIVE MANAGEMENT AND COMPLICATIONS AFTER PEDIATRIC LIVER TRANSPLANTATION

In the immediate postoperative period, monitoring graft function is achieved by evaluating acid-base status, blood glucose, mental status, coagulation time, liver enzymes, and cholestasis parameters. Doppler ultrasound is frequently performed to ascertain the patency of hepatic vessels, particularly the hepatic artery. Prolonged mechanical ventilation has been shown to be associated with significant perioperative complications in both adult and pediatric LT recipients. Recent studies have advocated early or even immediate extubation in the operating room after transplantation.[64,65]

Primary nonfunction (PNF) of the graft occurs in less than 5% of patients and no effective cure exists other than immediate re-transplantation.[66,67] PNF carries a high mortality, with

only one-third of affected children surviving. The incidence of PNF is lower after LDLT and in situ split-LT and is thought to be related to decreased cold-ischemia times. Contributing factors for PNF are thought to include cause of donor death, technical surgical complications, time spent in the intensive care unit (ICU), and hyperacute rejection. For pediatric recipients, re-transplantation with a reduced-size graft from a cadaveric donor or a living donor may offer emergency options (see Chapter 121 to 123).

The most frequent complication after LT is hemorrhage, which may occur during the transplant procedure or in the immediate perioperative period.[54] Periodic, serum hemoglobin, drain output, and bedside parameters are important. Bleeding intensity is oftentimes greater in cases of reduced LTs because of the raw surface of the graft, which may bleed.[66] If a child becomes unstable or hypotensive postoperatively, it is prudent to re-explore immediately. Judicious use of intraoperative and perioperative blood transfusion is recommended, given the well-reported detrimental effects of liberal blood transfusion in critically ill adult and pediatric patients.[64] The use of the protease inhibitor aprotinin (Trasylol) and an antifibrinolytic agent such as aminocaproic acid (Amicar) or tranexamic acid (TXA) may help reduce diffuse bleeding, but the debate continues concerning the potential increased risk of arterial thrombosis after their use.[64]

Hepatic artery thrombosis (HAT) is the most common vascular complication in pediatric orthotopic LT (OLT) and is a major cause of early graft failure and re-transplantation.[68] Previously published rates of HAT were over 25% but more recent large series report rates ranging from 5% to 19%.[64,69] This may present as ALF, biliary fistulas, fevers, or deranged liver enzymes.[66] Decreases in the incidence of HAT are attributed to enhanced surgical techniques and perioperative care. Careful anticoagulation, rheologic management, and improved anti-rejection strategies may also diminish the risk of HAT. Doppler ultrasound, used routinely intraoperatively in some units or with a low threshold based on clinical indication, is essential for early diagnosis and possible thrombectomy and revascularization.

Pediatric recipients are at a greater risk for developing vascular-related complications when compared with adult patients (Fig 110.5).[69] Another devastating complication is portal vein thrombosis (PVT), occurring less frequently than HAT but still in the range of 3% to 8% of all pediatric OLTs,[54] and the incidence is increased with segmental grafts. This may manifest as liver failure, variceal bleeding, encephalopathy, or an asymptomatic increase in liver enzymes.[66] Similar to HAT, graft rejection or preservative injury with swelling of the liver increases the risks for PVT.[68] Large-for-size transplantation is another risk factor for PVT, and accurate preoperative planning and patient selection are needed to avoid this possibility. Early PVT rarely may be treated successfully by emergency thrombectomy and revascularization. Late PVT with complications of portal hypertension may be an indication for re-transplantation.[69] Portal vein stenosis (4%–8%), IVC stenosis (<1%), and hepatic vein stenosis (2%) are other vascular complications of surgery (11%–20%) and have seen a decrease in incidence with improved surgical methods and perioperative care[69,70] (see Chapter 111).

Biliary strictures are one of the most common complications of segmental OLT (12%–50%) and are more common in children weighing less than 10 kg, resulting in significant morbidity and mortality.[71] In partial grafts, the biliary complication rate

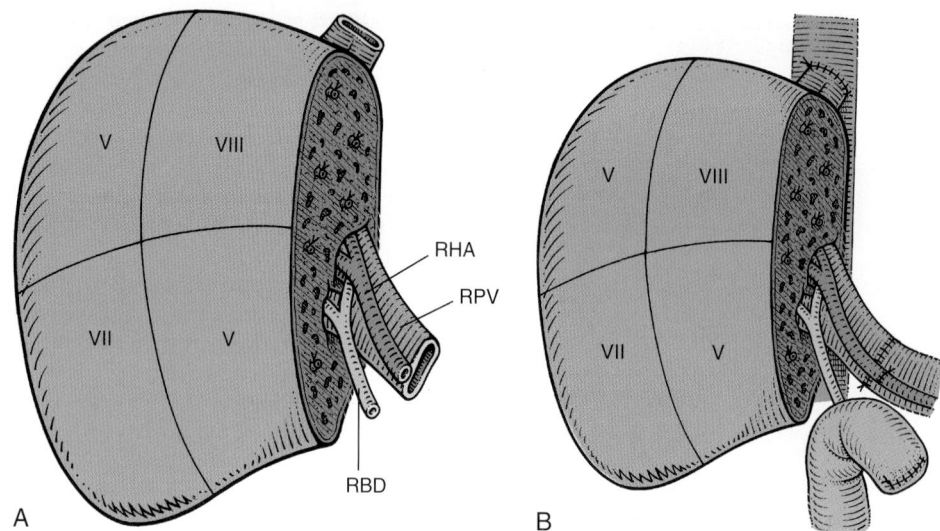

FIGURE 110.5 **A,** Right graft from a living donor with short hilar structures and a short right hepatic vein *(RHV).* **B,** Completed recipient implantation of a right graft. *RBD,* Right bile duct; *RHA,* right hepatic artery; *RPV,* right portal vein.

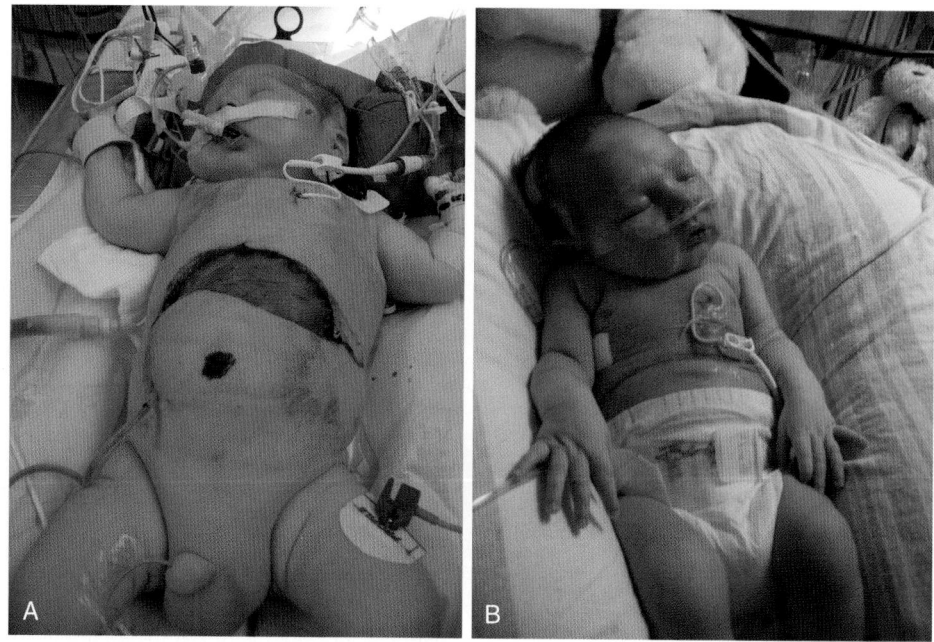

FIGURE 110.6 A, Temporary abdominal closure, using a prosthetic patch, after transplantation of a left lateral section graft into a neonate. B, The patch is reduced in size over several days and is finally removed altogether, and the abdomen is closed.

can be as high as 40%. It is important to recognize biliary complications early and to treat them aggressively because they can account for approximately 8% of late graft loss in pediatric OLTs.[72,73] With widespread use of endoscopic and percutaneous radiologic intervention, such as transhepatic and endoscopic balloon dilation and stenting, the need for surgical reintervention and reconstruction has significantly decreased in recent years[74] (see Chapter 111).

Many children who undergo LT have had a prior portoenterostomy and are at risk for iatrogenic bowel injury because of the adhesiolysis during native hepatectomy. A high index of suspicion and early repeat laparotomy with primary closure of any perforation are crucial to prevent systemic complications

of sepsis. Many children have compromised pulmonary function before the transplant procedure because of significant arteriovenous pulmonary shunting, pulmonary infections, or pleural effusions. Postoperatively, respiratory problems may worsen because of diaphragmatic splinting or temporary right hemidiaphragm paralysis, right-sided pleural effusion, pulmonary edema secondary to perioperative fluid shifting, or atelectasis. In children with high intra-abdominal pressure secondary to a relatively large liver, a tension-free temporary closure of the abdomen with a prosthetic graft (patch) is advisable[75–77] (Fig. 110.6). This abdominal wall graft may be reduced in size during several days, similar to when an abdominal wall silo is used in newborns with gastroschisis.

Peritransplant impairment of renal function is common but is usually reversible.[78] This may occur secondary to electrolyte imbalances and fluid shifts during and after surgery. Reduction or temporary cessation of nephrotoxic immunosuppressive medications (e.g., cyclosporine or tacrolimus) may help to improve renal function. Less than 5% of children need temporary dialysis after transplantation, unless this was already a pretransplantation requirement.

Septic complications and infections are lifelong risks in an immunocompromised patient and are a frequent cause of morbidity and mortality in pediatric patients.[79] Perioperative infections have been closely linked to malnutrition particularly in children and thus lies the emphasis of nutritional optimization and rehabilitation at the time of transplantation. In the initial postoperative course, bacterial infections with *Enterococcus faecalis, Pseudomonas* species, and *Staphylococcus aureus* are most common, often related to central venous lines or bacterial translocation from the gut.[80] Increasing problems are encountered with antibiotic-resistant organisms such as *Staphylococcus, Klebsiella,* and *Enterococcus.* The presence of gram-negative organisms and *Candida* species in the peritoneal fluid after transplantation could be suggestive of bowel perforation or biliary leak. Pediatric patients are also vulnerable to viral infections after transplantation and recent reports suggest that only 20% to 30% of children have a completed immunization schedule before transplantation.[81] Viral infections, which usually occur in children immunologically naive to cytomegalovirus (CMV) or Epstein-Barr virus (EBV) before transplantation, typically manifest approximately 6 weeks after transplantation and may be effectively treated with ganciclovir.[82] Fungal infections are also relatively frequent in patients with acute hepatic failure, the most common agent being *Candida albicans.* For this reason, prophylactic oral antifungal medication such as fluconazole may be administered especially during the first few weeks after transplantation[66] (see Chapter 106 and 111).

IMMUNOSUPPRESSION

Improved immunosuppressive strategies have led much of the progress in pediatric LT and treatment regimens are constantly in development, even as new drugs become available. Adherence and compliance with a strict medical regimen are vital to ensure promising long-term outcomes and in the pediatric context both the child and family must play an active role. Nonadherence to medication is estimated in 35% to 50% of adolescents and is a common and devastating cause of rejection in those receiving LT.[83]

Baseline immunosuppression consists of a corticosteroid and a calcineurin inhibitor (tacrolimus or cyclosporine) and are discussed in detail in Chapters 105 and 106. The management of immunosuppressive medication is oftentimes more challenging in infants and young children for several reasons. First, unlike adults, doses in children are usually weight based and because suspensions may vary, parents must be educated to remember specific concentrations rather than volume.[81] Second, medications may be unpalatable especially for young children and parents may need to develop creative ways to avoid medication refusal.[81] In instances of poor medication uptake, nasoenteric or percutaneous tube feeding may be indicated to ensure accurate administration.[81]

In the early postoperative period, immunosuppressive drug levels should be maintained at a higher level to avoid rejection in which incidences peak between the fifth and tenth postoperative day.[66] Paradoxically, elevated drug levels can result in severe graft edema with subsequent arterial vein thrombosis or PVT, so drug levels are tapered with time and most children can be weaned off the corticosteroid component within 1 year. Recent studies have shown excellent graft survival in pediatric OLT recipients maintained on tacrolimus (Prograf) monotherapy and this was associated with high levels of patient satisfaction.[84] In addition to improved compliance, reduced immunosuppression is also associated with decreased infection rates, improvements in renal function and optimized growth rates. Complete withdrawal of immunosuppressants in children several years after transplantation has been reported, with no significant detrimental effect on graft function[85]. A prospective multicenter pilot trial looking at complete immunosuppression withdrawal and subsequent allograft function was conducted on 20 pediatric LDLT recipients of parental donors. Of the 20 patients, 12 (60%) met the study endpoint of maintaining normal allograft function for a median of 35.7 months after discontinuing immunosuppression therapy.[86] The results of the Phase 2 iWITH trial (NCT01638559) will hopefully delineate some of the issues with immunosuppressive withdrawal in pediatric patients and detail the feasibility of this.

LONG-TERM OUTCOMES OF PEDIATRIC LIVER TRANSPLANTATION

Pediatric patient outcomes have continued to improve with parallel advances in surgical technique, perioperative care, and immunosuppressive regimens. The application of split-liver grafts and LDLT has helped alleviate some of the pressure on the donor pool. In 2018, nearly half of pediatric donors were from living relatives and 19.2% of all LTs were split-liver grafts.[3] Overall 5-year patient survival is reported to be 88.4% and varies from 87.2% in the 1 to 5 year age group to 92.2% in those aged 6 to 10 years.[3] When disease etiology is considered, patient survival is most superior in those with BA and metabolic diseases and worse in transplantation for hepatoblastoma.[3] Other factors impacting survival in pediatric patients are PELD scores less than 25, graft-weight-body-weight-ratios (GWBWR) less than 3%, patient weight greater than 7 kg, renal function, and mechanical ventilation.[78,79,88] Similar to patient survival, 5-year graft survival is also influenced by age: 80.3% in patients younger than 1 year, 80.5% for ages between 1 and 5 years, 87.3% in the 6 to 10 year age group and 82.7% for ages 11 to 17 years.[3] Predictors of graft survival include warm ischemia time, re-transplantation, and patient weight.[87]

There is an emerging focus on long-term and social issues that may arise secondary to the improved survivorship in pediatric transplantation. A multicenter North American study of 167 children who survived beyond 10 years post-LT scored consistently lower in all aspects of health-related-quality of life (HRQOL) including psychosocial health and school functioning.[88] Children undergoing LT are also more likely to repeat or be held back a school year. Although early patient referral to specialist pediatric units are critical decisive factors influencing the success of transplant, a multidisciplinary approach with several specialists is also essential to ensure improved functional, social, and emotional outcomes for a complex disease and management paradigm.

CONCLUSION

LT remains the only curative option for ESLD and is a lengthy process for the transplant patient. Continued innovation and medical research have resulted in improved outcomes over the past few decades, but challenges remain as a result of a small donor pool and a complex procedure that is only performed in select institutions. Efforts to overcome this have focused on increasing LDLT, which not only leads to the relief of organ shortage but also offers the advantage of careful timing and performance of LT under elective conditions. Although this strategy may minimize waiting times in children, the ultimate goal of the successful pediatric transplant center should be to decrease waiting list mortality while maintaining excellent post-transplant outcomes. This is most often accomplished using a strategy that uses all donor types.

The references for this chapter can be found online by accessing the accompanying Expert Consult website.

CHAPTER 111

Early and late complications of liver transplantation

Hunter B. Moore and James J. Pomposelli

Liver transplantation (LT) has evolved from a high-risk procedure with significant morbidity and mortality to a standard treatment for patients with liver failure. Patients who undergo successful liver replacement have 1-year and 5-year survival rates that exceed 85% and 70%, respectively (see Chapters 105–110). Despite this dramatic improvement in outcome, a significant percentage of patients experience life-threatening complications that can result in the need for reoperation.

Recent changes in the treatment of liver disease have begun to shift the demographics of transplant recipients. Hepatitis C cirrhosis has historically been the main indication for LT in Europe and North America, but with effective antiviral therapy, nonalcoholic steatohepatitis (NASH) is quickly becoming the most common indication.[1] The rapid increase in NASH resulting in decompensated liver failure is expected to surpass the number of effectively treated viral hepatitis with an anticipated increase in end-stage liver disease (ESLD)–related deaths by 178% by 2030.[2] The obesity epidemic has had a 2-fold effect impacting LT complications. The first is increasing the demand for livers, and the second is increasing the prevalence of fatty liver disease in potential organ donors. Fatty liver disease has resulted in an increased number of discarded liver from brain-dead donors,[3] while increasing the number of transplanted liver grafts with a higher degree of macrosteatosis.[4] Although the survival rates with macrosteatosis greater than 30% are comparable to donors with less fatty liver disease, the postoperative complication rates of postreperfusion syndrome (PRS), early allograft dysfunction (EAD), and postoperative dialysis and the need for a second operation are markedly increased.[5] Furthermore, the LT recipients are going to have a higher frequency of obesity, in which a body mass index (BMI) greater than 30 is associated with an increased rate of postoperative cardiopulmonary complications and longer intensive care unit (ICU) stays.[6] Although expertise in the procedure grows, surgeons will have to perform LT in patients who previously were considered poor candidates for surgery and will have to use more marginal donor livers.

Surgical techniques to increase the donor pool include reduced-size grafts, split-liver grafts. With these liver parenchymal–splitting operations has come a new series of complications unique to these procedures.[7,8] The incidence of hepatic artery thrombosis (HAT), bile leaks, and stricture is at least two times higher in patients who receive living-donor grafts compared with those who receive cadaveric grafts. There is a learning curve for reducing these complications as well.[9] Another major complication after LDLT is the *small-for-size syndrome* (SFSS), characterized by hyperbilirubinemia, coagulopathy, and encephalopathy observed shortly after transplant.[10,11] The terminology of SFSS is becoming a historic term as early allograft dysfunction (EAD) has become a more appropriate

term to describe graft dysfunction after transplant because graft size is not the only factor for slow return of hepatic function in LDLT[12] and cadaveric donors.[13] Despite a higher morbidity rate in recipients of living-donor grafts, patient and graft survival are similar or superior to those observed with deceased donors.[14]

This chapter reviews common early and late complications encountered during and after LT. Because complications after LT represent a continuum, most can occur at any time after surgery.

PROCUREMENT INJURY TO THE GRAFT

The process of organ transplantation begins with identification of a suitable organ for a particular recipient. When an organ is identified, procurement teams are dispatched for recovery of various organs. In general, the liver procurement team dictates the conduct of dissection below the diaphragm, and the cardiac team works in concert with the thoracic team, if lungs and heart also are to be recovered. Because the infradiaphragmatic dissection takes considerably longer than the thoracic dissection, careful planning is required to minimize cold-ischemia time for the heart and lungs, which is more time sensitive. The heart procurement team stays in contact with the recipient heart team to minimize total ischemic time.

Under ideal conditions, the conduct of the operation is orderly and well controlled; however, a patient who progresses to brain death rapidly can show cardiac instability and can be difficult to manage. This situation can result in an expedited operation in which perfusion cannulae are hastily placed, and organ procurement rapidly follows. During such events, identification of appropriate anatomy is difficult, and technical errors are more likely to occur.

To increase the number of organs available, donation after cardiac death (DCD) has gained popularity since the 1990s.[15] It was estimated that DCD organs could increase the organ donor pool by 10% in 2010.[16] According to United Network for Organ Sharing (UNOS) data, the percent of DCD donors from 2010 to 2019 has increased from 6% to 11% of all donors in the United States, supporting high utilization. In this form of donation, a patient who is deemed hopeless but has not met criteria of "brain death" is allowed to die naturally after removal of supportive measures. After a period of 2 to 5 minutes (dependent on hospital policy) of asystole, organs can be procured for transplantation. Despite the various periods of hypotension and warm ischemia that develop, DCD outcomes have been mixed but generally acceptable. In liver grafts procured from DCD donors, there were concerns for increased biliary strictures and worse long-term graft survival,[17] but a more modern assessment supports comparable outcomes to brain-dead donors with appropriate donor selection.[18] The management of ischemic cholangiopathy will be discussed in a future section. With the use of normothermic regional perfusion[19,20] and normothermic machine perfusion,[21] the incidence of this feared complication is believed to have become much less common.

Injuries during liver procurement occur in roughly 20% to 30% of organ donors.[22,23] These injuries can be broken down into parenchymal injuries, vascular injuries, and bile duct injuries. The most common major injury during liver procurement is aberrant hepatic artery ligation and division.[23] This injury occurs by failure to recognize a replaced or accessory right or left hepatic artery during hilar dissection or by unintentional division during organ removal. The frequency of these aberrant arterial anatomy is described in a 1000 donor case series by Hiatt et al.,[24] in which a replaced/accessory right occurred in roughly 10% of donors, with a similar frequency for left replaced/accessory arteries, and 3% had dual replacement arteries. Despite the lower frequency of the nontraditional vascular anatomy of the liver, hilum–replaced left and right arteries represent two-thirds of all vascular injuries during procurement.[23] Such injuries are serious because segments of the liver are not perfused during recovery and usually require reconstruction on the back table before reimplantation. Injuries to these arteries are associated with a high rate of early HAT (30%) and subsequent need for re-transplantation.[23] The management of HAT is discussed in a later section.

Injuries to the liver parenchyma during graft removal are the most common form of minor liver injury during graft removal. These minor injuries often can be treated with topical hemostatic, cautery, or liver stitch. These injuries can also occur during graft implantation. Parenchymal injuries are associated with long operative times and increased blood loss but do not have an impact on long-term graft function.[25] The more infrequent complication is an injury to the bile duct that can be because of stripping vascular supply or cutting the duct too short. These injuries can be managed by Roux-en-Y biliary reconstruction[23] and typically not associated with graft loss.

Other donor factors that can contribute to morbidity to the organ recipient in relationship to the donor operation include prolonged cold-ischemia time. Grafts that have more than 12 hours of cold ischemia are at an increased risk for graft loss and complications.[26] Additionally, macrosteatosis greater than 30% is also associated with poor early graft function.[5] High BMI donors are used less commonly for liver grafts.[27] Bedside biopsy and procurement biopsy can help improve high BMI donor liver utilization without increased risk to the recipient by confirming the percent of macrosteatosis. It is estimated that macrosteatosis greater than 30% is only prevalent in 21% of high BMI donors[27] and that the majority of these donors can be used for LT. Visceral adipose tissue makes the technical aspects of liver procurement more challenging and time consuming. To minimize dissection-related injuries, some authors suggest the en bloc method of removing abdominal organs with back-table dissection after procurement.[28] Regardless of the technique used, attention to detail and identification of the appropriate anatomy can help avoid graft procurement injury.

PERIOPERATIVE MANAGEMENT OF COAGULOPATHY AND BLEEDING

Patients with ESLD come to the operating room (OR) with a spectrum of coagulation abnormalities. The adaptive changes in coagulation related to ESLD are a combination of pro and anti-coagulants with derangements of fibrinolysis in which individuals are prone to both massive hemorrhage or life-threatening thrombosis.[29] This can be compounded by portal hypertension[30] and adhesions from prior abdominal surgery.[31] The combination of these two conditions results in a significant challenge for the surgeon and anesthesiologist. Patients who have undergone previous operations are at particular risk because prolonged lysis of adhesions may greatly increase the duration of the operation, create additional raw surface areas for bleeding, and lead to derangements in temperature and fluid homeostasis. The net result is worsening coagulopathy, which creates a vicious cycle during the procedure.

Preoperative assessment of the patient's coagulation status can help guide anesthesia and the surgical team for patients' risk of massive bleeding in the OR. Attenuating blood loss has been proposed to improve long-term outcomes after LT. Blood loss during surgery has an incremental increase in postoperative complications and decrease in graft survival.[32] In addition, blood utilization in LT is under close scrutiny with the historical reputation of this surgery draining the blood banks. An early report from Stazl in the 1980s estimated that 3% to 9% of all blood products in the Pittsburgh central blood bank were used for LT.[33] A proposed threshold for excessive bleeding in LT is more than 10 units of red blood cells (RBCs).[34] Viscoelastic testing (thrombelastography [TEG] and rotational thrombelastography [ROTEM]) have been used in this setting to predict massive transfusion. A TEG maximum amplitude has been demonstrated to be associated with massive transfusion with a higher performance than INR and MELD.[35] ROTEM has also been demonstrated to outperform conventional assays in predicting nonsurgical bleeding after LT.[36]

Preemptive treatment of coagulopathy before the OR is often not indicated for mild to moderate derangements in coagulation. Hemostatic blood products such as platelets are believed to be rapidly sequestered by the spleen based on historic data.[37] Plasma transfusions can result in exacerbation of venous hypertension and can paradoxically increase bleeding. Although controversial, the early use of prothrombin complex concentrate (PCC) has been associated with reduced blood loss during LT.[38] PCC corrects INR while not requiring the volume of plasma. However, PCC has been associated with life-threatening thrombotic complications[39] and conservative use is advised until the results of ongoing clinical trials are released. Regardless of the institution's treatment plan for addressing presurgical coagulopathy, high-risk patients warrant careful intraoperative planning, including mobilization of the blood bank and the use of cell saver for autologous blood transfusion.

With evolving measurements of coagulation in LT, it has now been appreciated that there are a cohort of LT recipients who present to surgery with a hypercoagulable profile. Cirrhosis has recently been appreciated to be an independent risk factor for deep vein thrombosis (DVT) in hospitalized patients.[40] NASH is associated with an even higher risk of thrombotic complications.[41] Conventional coagulation measurements do not capture this hypercoagulable state in LT.[42] An elevated preoperative TEG maximum amplitude (clot strength) has been associated with a 5-fold risk of early HAT.[43] This unmeasured hypercoagulability associated with HAT was attributed to the operating surgeon.[44] Although there are no guidelines on managing preoperative hypercoagulability in LT recipients, we have adopted the use of intraoperative heparin bolus after hepatic artery anastomosis in selected recipients (particularly LDLT with PSC of HCC) that have high clot strength (MA >65) on early intraoperative TEG results.

Improvements in surgical techniques and better patient selection have led to the performance of LT without the need for blood transfusion in selected patients. The advent of the transjugular intrahepatic portosystemic shunt (TIPS) can significantly lower portal hypertension preoperatively and may help to reduce blood loss during transplantation; however, a misplaced TIPS in the vena cava or portal vein can be a life-threatening complication during LT. In these situations, TIPS removal is difficult and may lead to massive hemorrhage if vascular control of the native vessels cannot be achieved. Temporary portocaval shunts can also be used to decompress the portal circulation during hepatectomy.[45]

In the presence of severe portal hypertension and underlying coagulopathy, the infusion of fresh frozen plasma, cryoprecipitate, and antifibrinolytic agents can help with hemostasis during LT. These modalities cannot supplant the need for sound surgical technique with adequate control of all surgical bleeding sites. During surgery it is essential to have good communication with the anesthesiology team regarding blood loss assessment of coagulopathy. We have begun to use a scoring system[46] as a tool to communicate with anesthesia for when a patient warrants coagulation assessment for moderate coagulopathy and empiric transfusions for uncontrolled coagulopathy.

An important transition in hemostasis management occurs when the native liver is removed and the new graft undergoes early reperfusion. It has been well appreciated since the origins of LT that recipients develop a hyperfibrinolytic state (excessive clot degradation from elevated levels of tissue plasminogen activator [t-PA]) when the native liver is removed.[47] However, after reperfusion, the majority of patients correct their fibrinolytic state.[48] This is likely because of the rapid clearance of t-PA by the liver, which has a half-life of 5 minutes in humans because of multiple hepatic endothelial receptors.[49] A lack of clearance of t-PA after graft reperfusion can be associated with massive bleeding,[50] which is also exacerbated by metabolic disturbances.[51] In these scenarios, the use of antifibrinolytics may be of value to improve hemostasis control. Bleeding observed after reperfusion may be related to poor initial graft function but also has been related to the release of heparin and heparin-like substances from the graft.[52] Protamine administration is rarely used, and this heparin effect can often be mediated by plasma transfusion. When medical strategies fail to halt reperfusion fibrinolysis, temporary intra-abdominal tamponade with laparotomy packs provides the most conservative management, with temporary vacuum-pack closure and plans for subsequent reexploration. If the graft functions well and the patient responds to core temperature warming and continued resuscitation, packs usually can be removed within 24 to 48 hours. Prophylaxis against intra-abdominal sepsis with parenteral antibiotics is of unproven benefit but may be prudent in the patient with immunosuppression.

After reperfusion in grafts that demonstrate good function, de-escalation of hemostatic blood products is warranted. TEG and ROTEM have comparable performance for monitoring of coagulation during LT.[53] Routine use of both TEG[54] and ROTEM[55] have been associated with using less plasma during surgery in randomized clinical trials (RCTs) but are not associated with a reduction in RBC transfusions. Almost all LT recipients will develop inhibition of their fibrinolytic system 2 hours

after reperfusion.[48] This fibrinolysis shutdown persists beyond postoperative day 1 in the majority of LT patients. With a lack of capacity to break down endogenous clots, it is essential to not overtransfuse recipients during this time frame. Fibrinolysis shutdown has been associated with decreased graft survival and postoperative thrombotic complications.[56] Platelet transfusions have been associated with decreased survival after transplantation,[57] which has been attributed to the development of postoperative lung injury.[58]

The decision to transfuse hemostatic blood products on LT patients postoperatively should be guided predominantly by clinical judgement with laboratory confirmation of stable hemoglobin levels. Failure to identify coagulopathy will result in a return trip to the OR. There are no definitive thresholds for transfusions. Our group, however, uses a target hemoglobin of 10 to promote platelet margination[59] to optimize hemostasis with thrombocytopenia; platelet transfusion for an absolute platelet count of less than 30,000, or TEG MA 50 in patients with dropping hemoglobin; and plasma transfusion for TEG R time greater than 10 minutes or INR greater than 2 with dropping hemoglobin, and cryoprecipitate for a Clauss fibrinogen less than 100 or TEG angle less than 55 if hemoglobin is dropping. Patients with normal coagulation parameters and dropping hemoglobin should prompt concerns for surgical bleeding. Our group often used the threshold of more than 6 hours of RBC postoperative bleeding as an indicator for the need to return to the OR.

EARLY ALLOGRAFT DYSFUNCTION AND PRIMARY NONFUNCTION

Numerous conditions can interfere with the initial function of the allograft after LT, including donor-related, procurement-related, and recipient-related factors. Donor-related factors that can affect graft function adversely include hemodynamic instability, poor nutritional status, extremes of age, drug toxicity, and steatosis. There is a spectrum of graft dysfunction after LT ranging from early allograft dysfunction (EAD) to the most extreme, primary nonfunction (PNF). Patients with PNF require relisting for transplantation, and the mortality rate can be as high as 50% even after re-transplantation.[60] PNF occurs in 2% to 6% of LTs[61] and because the patients do not retain hepatic function, clinical manifestations are often not subtle, including altered mental status, persistent acidosis, hypoglycemia, coagulopathy, and hemodynamic instability. A major risk factor for PNF is steatosis of the donor liver[60] in addition to female donor, older donor, and long cold and warm ischemia times.[61] Laboratory values concerning for PNF include serum transaminase levels greater than 8000 IU/L within the first 24 to 48 hours in association with diminished bile and urine output. In our practice, postoperative trends in the serum bilirubin and international normalized ratio (INR) have been the most reliable predictors of graft function and outcome. Laboratory studies drawn immediately after surgery serve as the baseline; serum bilirubin and INR should plateau and then trend toward normalization within days with good graft function; any increase in the serum bilirubin and INR portends a worse prognosis and may represent PNF, especially if this occurs rapidly. An elevated INR that neither increases nor decreases may suggest primary graft dysfunction; recovery usually occurs with time, if no additional insults occur, such as infection or rejection.

There are numerous biomarkers and tests that can be performed to assess graft function after transplanatation[62]; however, there is no definitive test that can differentiate slow graft function that will improve over time from PNF for patients that are extremely sick in the immediate postoperative period. In addition to trends in the bilirubin and INR, a clinical assessment can be helpful in identifying patients with graft dysfunction or nonfunction. Resolution of hepatic encephalopathy, adequate urine production, and absence of metabolic acidosis are reassuring in the early postoperative period. In patients who have received significant quantities of blood products, the development of metabolic alkalosis may be a sensitive indicator of early graft function.[63] Such indicators are based on the ability of the liver graft to process citrate in the administered blood products to bicarbonate[64]; failure to metabolize citrate to bicarbonate may reflect early allograft dysfunction.

In patients with progressive graft dysfunction or nonfunction, early consideration for relisting with a higher urgency (status 1) may be the only way to salvage the patient and prevent mortality. Similar to patients that experience hypoglycemia with acute liver failure,[65] death usually occurs within hours. In this situation, aggressive metabolic supportive measures are needed to prevent bleeding complications, maintain acid-base status, and prevent permanent brain injury from cerebral edema or a coagulopathic bleed.

PNF, as previously mentioned, is at the extreme of graft dysfunction after transplant. EAD is a broader term that captures LT recipients who do not necessarily require re-transplantation but have less favorable outcomes. EAD occurs in roughly 25% of recipients[66,67] and is associated with up to a 7-fold increased risk of early graft loss and 10-fold risk of mortality after transplant.[13] Although clinical gestalt for slow graft function is made after reperfusion of the liver, the time frame for diagnosis of EAD with objective laboratory data is commonly calculated at 7 days after LT.[13] Risk factors for EAD in adults include high levels of macrosteatosis, donor location, donor weight, DCD donor, recipient obesity, recipient HCC, severity of postreperfusion syndrome, warm and cold ischemia time, operative time, and the amount of transfused fresh frozen plasma.[68–70] Because EAD presents a spectrum of graft dysfunction after surgery, newer definitions of EAD have included a continuous variable termed the model for early allograft function (MEAF), which can grade the severity of dysfunction and ranges from 1 to 10 based on postoperative day 3 laboratory values.[71] Each increase in MEAF score was associated with progressively lower graft survival time. There are numerous other definitions of EAD in the literature that have variances in how well they perform.[72] We currently prefer to use the Othoff et al.[13] definition because of its simplicity and agreement between LDLT and cadaveric liver recipients.

In LDLT, graft size was an initial concern for development for EAD. SFSS can be a significant cause of live-donor graft dysfunction and graft loss, but additional evidence has suggested the importance of pressure and flow as major contributors of the syndrome rather than size alone.[73,74] With subsequent work, it has been demonstrated that a graft to body weight ratio of 0.8 can be transplanted successfully.[75] A key prognostic factor for good graft function with smaller-sized livers is achieving a portal systemic gradient less than 15 mm Hg.[76] Most recently, EAD serves as a better predictor for long-term graft function than small graft size.[12] Increasing age of the donor, the BMI of the donor, left liver grafts, and enlarged spleen in the recipients are risk factors for LTLD EAD.[12]

EAD has been proposed as an appealing target to improve graft outcomes,[77] yet specific mechanisms driving this process remain unclear.[77,78] There has been one successful RCT targeting EAD. In this study, 65 patients were randomized to steroids or standard of care if they met the EAD definition of a bilirubin greater than 10 on postoperative day 7.[79] The steroid intervention group received methylprednisolone intravenously once daily for 5 days. Both arms of the trial received 250 mg of oral ursodeoxycholic acid three times a day for this duration. At the end of 2 weeks, the treatment arm had lower alkaline phosphatase levels, low bilirubin levels, and shorter hospital length stay. There were not reported increased rates of infections or other steroid-related complications.

VASCULAR COMPLICATIONS

Hepatic Artery Thrombosis

Vascular complications are a major source of morbidity and graft loss in LT patients, especially those who receive live-donor grafts. Arterial complications, of which HAT is the most common, account for 64% to 82% of the vascular complications encountered.[80] The overall incidence of HAT is 1.6% to 8% in various adult series, but it can be 15% to 26% in pediatric patients.[81,82] The incidence of HAT in LDLT varies widely and is influenced by the type of graft, surgeon experience, and donor anatomy. Risk factors for HAT include donor cytomegalovirus (CMV) positivity in a CMV-negative recipient, prolonged operating time, redo LT, arterial conduit, variate arterial anatomy, and low surgical volume.[83] Preoperative transarterial chemoembolization (TACE) has been associated with complications related to the hepatic artery[84] but not specific to HAT.

HAT is divided into early and late forms. The time cut off for early HAT remains an academic debate and can range from 7 to 100 days. Regardless, UNOS policy defines early HAT as lasting less than 7 days with an AST of greater than 3000 and INR greater than 2.5 or acidosis (arterial PH < 7.3 or lactate > 4) to qualify for status 1A. Early HAT of less than 14 days regardless of other factors qualifies the recipients as a MELD 40.[85] An attempt at revascularization should be conducted in the setting of early HAT because salvage is possible, and the alternative is re-transplantation, which uses another organ and the timing remains of an offer for the organ is indeterminate. Alternatively, late HAT will typically present as a biliary complication or identified incidentally on imaging for an alternative indication. Bilomas are the most common presenting symptom of late HAT and can be salvaged with percutaneous drainage and antibiotics.[86] Late HAT has a lower frequency than early HAT and tends to have a better prognosis with a lower rate of requiring re-transplantation. Asymptomatic individuals can often be overserved and followed for biliary complications. Risk factors for late HAT include CMV infection and variant arterial anatomy.[86]

Doppler ultrasound (US) is the best screening method for HAT and should be used liberally in the first 2 weeks after transplantation with any change in graft function or significant elevation in bilirubin or transaminases. Because collateral blood flow through the gastroduodenal artery can result in a false-negative result, care must be taken to establish arterial flow within the hepatic parenchyma. In cases of suspected HAT revealed by US, confirmation should be made by celiac

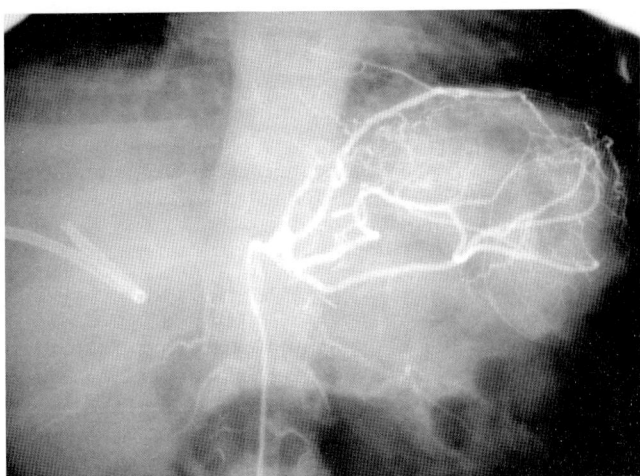

FIGURE 111.1   **Hepatic artery thrombosis.** The patient experienced a rapid increase in serum transaminases in the early postoperative period. Ultrasound could not locate an intrahepatic arterial signal. Celiac arteriography shows left gastric and splenic arterial flow and fails to show any contrast in the liver. This is consistent with intimal dissection of the entire common hepatic artery. The T-tube within the common bile duct is visible.

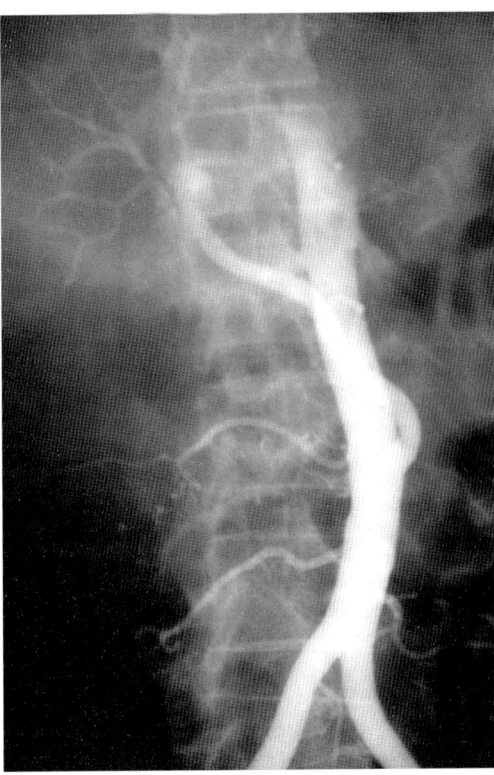

FIGURE 111.2   **Hepatic artery reconstruction.** With early diagnosis of hepatic artery thrombosis, immediate reconstruction with a donor iliac artery allograft can be performed. In this case, the iliac artery graft is anastomosed between the infrarenal aorta and liver allograft common hepatic artery.

arteriography (Fig. 111.1), multiphase computed tomography (CT), or operative exploration. Failure to make a rapid diagnosis can result in hepatic necrosis and graft loss.

Intimal dissection of the recipient hepatic artery down to the origin of the celiac axis is a common cause of intraoperative HAT. In these cases, immediate reconstruction with a donor iliac allograft is indicated (Fig. 111.2). Under no circumstances should the patient leave the OR without a completely revascularized graft. When a donor iliac allograft is unusable or unavailable, an autogenous saphenous vein graft should be used. Rarely, an artificial conduit made from Dacron or expanded polytetrafluoroethylene can be used.

The clinical presentation of HAT observed postoperatively ranges from a completely asymptomatic patient with minimal alterations in liver function to a critically ill patient with fulminant hepatic necrosis. A more common presentation of HAT is with postoperative biliary complications, including leaks and stricture formation. Treatment for HAT in the early postoperative period is the same, whether symptoms are present or not; rapid reestablishment of arterial inflow should be attempted, which generally requires urgent operation with arterial reconstruction by using a donor iliac artery allograft or autogenous graft material. Some authors have attempted thrombolysis using fibrinolytics followed by stent placement,[87] but this is not common practice and durable successful results remain limited.[84] Most often, hepatic artery intimal dissection is not amenable to thrombolytic therapy, and attempts at systemic thrombolysis waste valuable time and resources and worsen outcome. The majority of patients (50%–70%) will ultimately require re-transplantation.[88]

Portal Vein Thrombosis/Stenosis

Portal vein thrombosis (PVT) observed before surgery was previously considered an absolute contraindication to orthotopic LT (OLT). Although this problem no longer precludes successful LT, its presence may substantially increase the surgical complexity and perioperative morbidity. Depending on the patient population, PVT can be found in 5% to 25% of LT

recipients.[89] The severity of thrombosis ranges greatly between patients. Portal vein inflow is essential for successful LT and imaging with duplex of CT before implant can be an invaluable resource for intraoperative planning. Scoring systems have been created for intraoperative planning. An example is from Yerdel et al.[90] in which grade 1 is less than 50% PVT, 2 is greater than 50% with minimal superior mesenteric vein (SMV) obstruction, 3 is 100% PVT, and 4 is 100% PVT with SMV thrombosis. The authors advocate that intraoperative thrombectomy can be used for grades 1 and 2, a jump graft can be used for grade 3, and grade 4 is a relative contraindication to transplant unless bypass is achievable to a nonmesenteric venous source. Reconstruction of the portal can be accomplished using a donor iliac vein allograft anastomosed between the SMV and liver allograft portal vein. Successful reconstructed inflow for grade 4 has been reported in more than 75% of patients but is prone to stenosis.[91] Living-donor grafts that have relatively short portal vein segments can be difficult to reconstruct, and some institutions consider PVT an absolute contraindication to LDLT.

PVT observed after transplantation is a rare complication that can occur in the immediate postoperative period, usually for technical reasons, such as incomplete thrombectomy or twisting of the anastomosis. Early PVT has a poor prognosis with a mortality rate of 50%, predominantly because of later complications after attempted repair.[92] Risk factors for early PVT include postoperative platelet transfusions, RBC transfusion, and PVT before transplant.[92] PVT observed several months to years after transplantation usually results from intimal hyperplasia with gradual cavernous transformation with collaterals. A high index of suspicion is needed to make the diagnosis. Accumulation of ascites, splenomegaly, or the presence of varices after transplantation should prompt investigation. Early thrombosis is best treated with reoperation, thrombectomy, and systemic anticoagulation. Partial PVT can alternatively be approached with systemic heparinization and followed with serial ultrasounds to evaluate for regression. The treatment of late thrombosis and portal vein stenosis has been reported to be increasingly successful with interventional procedures with angioplasty, stent placement, and anticoagulation.[93] Selective shunting procedures can sometimes be considered in the setting of control variceal hemorrhage with adequate liver function.

Inferior Vena Cava Obstruction

Inferior vena cava (IVC) obstruction is a rare complication that occurs in 1% of patients after LT.[94,95] Historically, the donor IVC was anastomosed with the suprahepatic and infrahepatic IVC. The *piggyback transplantation*, with the anastomosis of the donor suprahepatic IVC to the confluence of the recipient middle and left hepatic veins, leaving the recipient IVC in situ, has become increasingly popular. The piggyback technique has been associated with reduced blood loss, shorter warm ischemia times, and lower rates of acute kidney injury after LT.[96] However, there have been reported concerns for an increased rate of outflow obstruction because of anastomotic strictures or kinking at the hepatic veins,[97] which tend to have high frequencies in LTLD[98] pediatric LTs.[99]

Early after transplant, high outflow obstruction can be confused with increased central venous pressure (CVP) because of high volume resuscitation manifesting as DGF, ascites, and peripheral edema. This nonanatomic source of outflow obstruction can be treated with diuretics when tolerated by the patient, targeting CVP below 11.[99] When CVP has been ruled out as a source of venous outflow obstruction, the patients can be evaluated with venography of the vena cava with segmental pressures above and below the anastomosis. A gradient of more than 10 mm Hg in the setting of clinical symptoms of lower extremity edema, ascites, and slow hepatic function can warrant intervention, which often includes angioplasty. Later-onset anastomotic stenosis can be treat with repeat angioplasty and stenting with durable long-term results.[96]

An additional cause of outflow obstruction includes thrombosis. Treatment of IVC thrombosis usually depends on the cause. Direct surgical removal is difficult in a critically ill patient and requires extensive mobilization of the right colon and small bowel mesentery to facilitate exposure. Nonoperative management of IVC thrombosis was successful in our experience and that reported by others.[100] Our experience suggests that a more conservative management algorithm that uses invasive radiologic procedures and systemic anticoagulation can treat this complication satisfactorily. Thrombolytic therapy can also be adjunctive in resolving "fresh" thrombus formation.

In some cases, high-grade venous outflow obstruction cannot be corrected, and TIPS may be used as a bridge to mediate ascites and bleeding complications for patients that are candidates for re-transplantation.[101] However, the use of TIPS posttransplantation is associated with accelerated decline in hepatic function and is not a durable therapy because the patient will progress to need another LT. An additional cause of symptoms that can mimic outflow obstruction includes veno-occlusive disease sinusoidal obstruction syndrome (VOD/SOS). This disease process is believed to be related to acute rejection and drug toxicity, which often occurs months after transplant. VOD/SOS was originally described in bone marrow transplants and has more recently been identified as a rare cause of liver failure after transplantation.[102] VOD/SOS is diagnosed via liver biopsy and demonstrates fibrous obliteration of the small hepatic veins. The most effective treatment in bone marrow patients is Defibronate.[103] Success with LT recipients is not as clear, and the medication that activates the fibrinolytic system poses a risk of bleeding. Alternative strategies include steroids, increasing immunosuppression, and TIPs as a last-line therapy.[104]

BILIARY COMPLICATIONS

Biliary tract complications related to bile duct reconstruction previously were considered the Achilles heel of LT, but improvements in operative technique have greatly reduced these complications. Nevertheless, bile duct obstruction and leaks are the cause of approximately half of all technical failures after LT and require reoperation in 10% to 20% of patients.[105,106] In general, recipients of living-donor grafts have an incidence of biliary complications approximately two times higher than recipients of cadaveric grafts.[107] HAT is associated with biliary complications and may partly explain the increased incidence among living-donor graft recipients.

Biliary Leaks

The reported incidence of biliary leaks after LT varies widely, from 10% to 50%.[108] Leaks are observed most often at the site of choledochal anastomosis or the choledochal T-tube insertion site. Leaks at the insertion site are observed most frequently at tube removal and occur in as many as 25% to 40% of patients.[109,110] Most of these patients can be managed conservatively with a short course of analgesics and antibiotics. To minimize this risk, many surgeons today prefer not to place stents.

In our practice, rather than using a conventional T-tube, we stent our choledochal anastomosis with a 5 French (F) pediatric feeding tube placed through the cystic duct stump, which is secured with a hemorrhoidal band and polydioxanone suture (PDS). In theory, the hemorrhoidal band obliterates the lumen of the preformed tract at stent removal, usually 6 to 8 weeks postoperatively. Anastomotic leaks encountered in the early postoperative period are related to technical errors, tension at the anastomotic site, or ischemic necrosis after HAT.

The bile ducts of living-donor or split-liver grafts can be reconstructed with a duct-to-duct (choledochocholedochostomy) or Roux-en-Y hepaticojejunostomy. The leak rate is similar in both types of reconstructions.[111] Signs and symptoms related to biliary leaks include bilious fluid in drains (biliary fistula), abdominal or shoulder pain or both, increased serum bilirubin, nausea, vomiting, and fever. Diagnosis can be confirmed by cholangiography if a choledochal tube is in place; otherwise, endoscopic retrograde cholangiography (ERC) or percutaneous transhepatic cholangiography (PTC) can be performed. We favor ERC because treatment with endoscopic stent placement can be readily achieved without the risk associated with the indwelling transhepatic catheters used during PTC. Large biliary leaks resulting in bile collections adjacent to the liver require percutaneous drainage.

Larger leaks and those associated with ischemic necrosis require surgical revision with Roux-en-Y hepaticojejunostomy. The development of early postoperative leaks is associated with late stricture formation, and lifelong surveillance by the surgeon is warranted.

Biliary Stricture or Obstruction

Biliary obstruction (stricture) occurs in approximately 7% to 15% of patients after LT.[110,112] As with leaks, the site of obstruction aids in determining the cause. Anastomotic stricture accounts for 50% of obstruction cases and can occur early in the postoperative period, secondary to edema, or later, as a result of compromised blood supply (Fig. 111.3). Biliary strictures usually present within weeks but may occur years after transplantation. Two types of biliary obstruction usually are found: anastomotic and nonanastomotic. Nonanastomotic obstruction or stricture can be caused by or associated with bile duct ischemia or sludge and debris that can accumulate in the biliary system after transplantation (Fig. 111.4).

The diagnosis of biliary stricture or obstruction is suggested by an obstructive pattern on routine liver function tests. Typically, patients are seen with constitutional symptoms of rigor, fever, headache, and fatigue. Occasionally, patients are seen with severe symptoms of cholangitis and sepsis. Because patients with "mild" signs and symptoms also may reflect the presence of any number of serious conditions—acute rejection, HAT, CMV infection, or recurrent disease—diagnosis can be difficult. To ascertain the correct diagnosis rapidly, a series of diagnostic studies that include abdominal US, cholangiography, and liver biopsy are obtained immediately after the onset of abnormal clinical signs and symptoms.

Regardless of the method used to reestablish the biliary continuity, the most common site of a biliary stricture in the posttransplantation setting is at the biliary anastomosis. Technical error during reconstruction is an important causative factor, but the patency of the hepatic artery also should be assessed, particularly in pediatric recipients. Other factors that have been implicated in

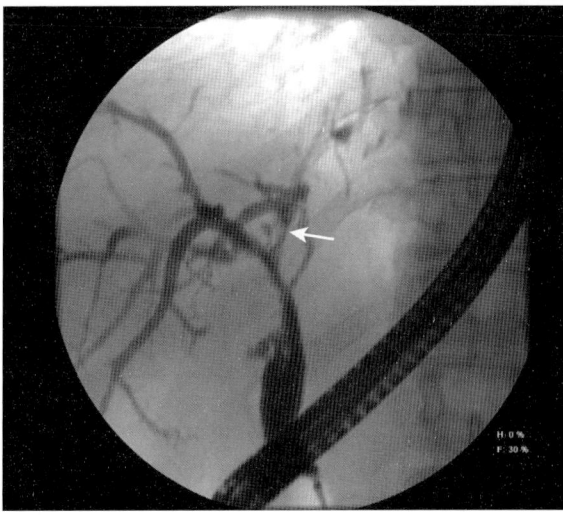

FIGURE 111.4 Nonanastomotic biliary stricture *(arrow)* observed from ischemic injury to a liver graft in a patient who received a liver from a donor who died of cardiac death rather than brain death. Donation after cardiac death, rather than after brain death, is an attempt to expand the organ donor pool, but such grafts are more prone to ischemic injury problems such as bile duct stricture. (See Chapter 109.)

the development of biliary stricture include ABO incompatibility,[113] prolonged preservation times,[114] recurrent rejection,[115] viral infections,[116] and recurrence of primary ductal disease that can occur in up to 50% of recipients at long-term follow-up.[117]

Biliary reconstruction after LDLT is by Roux-en-Y hepaticojejunostomy or duct-to-duct anastomosis. Anastomotic leak or stricture is generally two times more common after LDLT versus cadaveric LT.[118] Nonanastomotic strictures (NAS) can occur in the hilar region or intrahepatically. As with anastomotic strictures, thrombosis of the hepatic artery or one of its branches should be suspected. NAS also have been reported in association with chronic ductopenic rejection, ABO blood group incompatibility, and as a result of ischemia-reperfusion injury associated with allograft preservation, especially in grafts from DCD donors.[114]

After appropriate fluid resuscitation and antibiotic coverage, we recommend ERC to confirm the diagnosis and to implement treatment with immediate stenting if possible. Failure to cross the stricture through endoscopic means requires PTC or surgical revision with Roux-en-Y hepaticojejunostomy. Intrahepatic strictures are best treated with percutaneous balloon dilation. Rarely, long-term stents are needed to achieve a satisfactory outcome.

ISCHEMIC CHOLANGIOPATHY

Ischemic cholangiopathy represents a spectrum of NAS in LT that tends to be diffuse. The main causes of ischemic cholangiopathy include ischemia reperfusion injury, immune mediate injury, and bile salt injury.[119] The major risk factors of ischemic cholangiopathy include HAT and DCD donors. Ischemic cholangiopathy can be broken down into clinical and subclinical cholangiopathy based on laboratory assessment and cholangiography. Subclinical cholangiopathy often can be observed and with minimal effect on long-term outcomes. However, within the clinical cholangiopathy score, there is a rapidly progressive form associated with necrosis that warranted urgent re-transplantation.

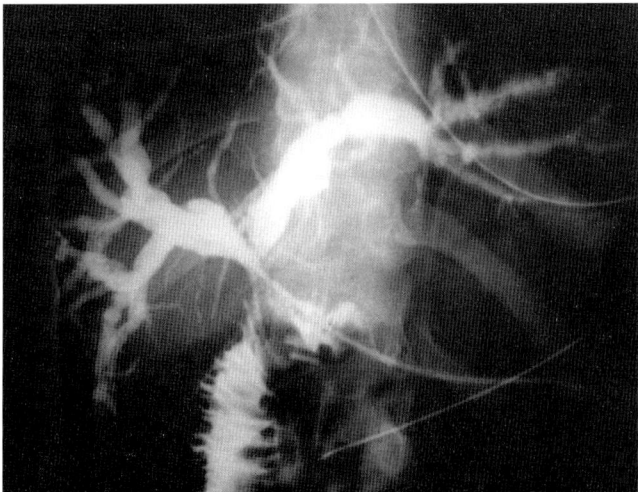

FIGURE 111.3 Biliary stricture. This patient had a previously created Roux-en-Y hepaticojejunostomy and now has an anastomotic stricture. Note the dilated intrahepatic ducts. Percutaneous access of the Roux-en-Y limb affords the ability to make the diagnosis and treat with balloon dilation. Using this technique, placement of transhepatic catheters is avoided.

Additional types of more indolent forms include multifocal progressive stenosis and centrifugal progressive stenosis. The last form of clinical cholangiopathy includes hilar confluence abnormalities. The combination of laboratory abnormalities and cholangiogram abnormalities is associated with a marked reduction in graft survival at 5 years.[120] There are no effective treatments for ischemic cholangiopathy aside from treating focal strictures as discussed in the previous section. These can be managed on repeat interventions and enable the patient to avoid transplantation. Ultimately, the best strategy is to avoid ischemic cholangiopathy altogether. This has been proposed by tissue plasminogen activator (tPA) treatment in DCD donors, which has demonstrated a reduction in ischemic cholangiopathy and improved graft survival.[121] Newer strategies include machine perfusion of high-risk donors, which has demonstrated promising results in reducing biliary complications after LT in several clinical trials.[122]

RENAL DYSFUNCTION

Renal dysfunction is observed to some degree in almost every patient who undergoes LT.[123] Early renal dysfunction usually is characterized by a period of oliguria with a transient increase in serum creatinine but can also manifest as anuria with acute renal failure. Risk factors include preexisting renal dysfunction and primary graft nonfunction. In patients with normal preoperative serum creatinine and good initial graft function, the usual mechanism is prerenal azotemia secondary to periods of hypotension and hypovolemia during the operative procedure. An additional insult to renal function can be incurred by the administration of nephrotoxic agents, especially the calcineurin inhibitors (CNIs) cyclosporine and tacrolimus; renal failure induced by CNIs occurs in approximately 5% of transplanted patients.[124,125]

Although the etiology of renal failure in transplant patients can be multifactorial, long-term exposure (dose/time) to CNIs is a clear risk factor. As a result, there has been increasing interest in automatic dose reduction in patients many years after transplantation and in those showing signs of progressive renal dysfunction. Another strategy to reduce calcineurin renal toxicity has been substitution of the immunosuppressive regimen by drugs that do not cause renal dysfunction, such as the mammalian target of rapamycin (mTOR) inhibitors (e.g., sirolimus, everolimus).

Sirolimus (rapamycin) is a macrocyclic antibiotic originally developed as an anticandidal and antitumor agent.[126] It is often used for renal sparing but has the disadvantage of increasing the risk for dyslipidemia and impaired wound healing. The impaired wound healing may be related to alterations in vascular endothelial growth factor (VEGF) and may explain the apparent benefit of sirolimus in reducing cancer formation in patients.[127] Because sirolimus has been associated with early HAT after LT, the manufacturer recommends waiting at least 4 weeks after transplantation before initiating therapy.

Post-transplantation renal failure so acute as to require dialysis is uncommon, unless the patient is diagnosed with preexisting hepatorenal syndrome or severe hypotension, and hemorrhage is encountered during surgery that results in acute tubular necrosis. In our experience, dialysis for these patients is best performed with continuous venovenous hemodialysis using a dedicated, large-bore, double-lumen venous access device. Recovery of normal renal function usually is achieved within 2 weeks, if no other metabolic stress is incurred.

FLUID AND ELECTROLYTE DISTURBANCES

Fluid and electrolyte disturbances and alterations in acid-base status are universal after LT. Preoperative protein-calorie malnutrition and ESLD lead to derangements in total body water and electrolyte balance that are worsened initially by the metabolic stress of surgery and massive fluid and blood-product resuscitation. The rapidity of recovery depends largely on the patient's renal and liver allograft function postoperatively. For a patient with stable postoperative renal and liver graft function, minimal metabolic manipulation is required to correct such derangements.

The early development of metabolic alkalosis secondary to metabolism of citrate in blood products is a favorable sign of graft function but can be serious if alkalemia develops. In this situation, judicious replacement of chloride in the form of normal saline or hydrogen chloride is warranted.

Excess total body water and excess sodium are best treated with gentle diuresis with furosemide. Careful repletion of potassium should be instituted, but it must be monitored closely in the setting of medications such as tacrolimus, which tends to increase serum potassium levels. Derangements in serum calcium, magnesium, and phosphorus are common in patients with cirrhosis, and levels should be repleted to avoid neurologic, skeletal, and cardiac muscle dysfunction.

ACUTE CELLULAR REJECTION

In the early days of LT, the importance of rejection was overshadowed by technical complications. As surgical technique has evolved, with concomitant improvement in graft preservation, rejection has taken on greater clinical importance. *Acute cellular rejection* is defined as an acute deterioration in allograft function associated with specific histologic changes in the liver allograft. These changes include a mixed inflammatory cell infiltrate, predominantly lymphocytes, that involves the portal triads and disrupts the biliary, hepatic artery, and portal venous endothelia.[128]

The incidence of acute rejection is approximately 45% (range, 24%–80%), depending on the series reported. Although acute rejection has little to no impact on mortality, significant morbidity results in increased hospitalization and higher overall costs.[129,130] In the early stage, most patients are asymptomatic, but a variety of clinical signs and symptoms may develop that include fever, abdominal pain, malaise, fatigue, and poor appetite.

The earliest laboratory indicator of acute rejection is elevated bilirubin level, which may be associated with a modest increase in alkaline phosphatase and transaminase levels. Prothrombin time (PT) and serum albumin levels are usually unaffected. Because laboratory measurements are neither sensitive nor specific for acute cellular rejection, liver histology obtained from a percutaneous biopsy specimen remains the standard for the diagnosis of cellular rejection.

The initial treatment for acute cellular rejection depends on the degree of rejection based on histologic evaluation based on the Banff score.[131] Mild rejection (rejection activity index [RAI] <4) can be treated with increasing calcineurin inhibitor, but moderate (RAI 4–6) and severe (RAI >7) RAI should be treated with high-dose pulse corticosteroids, which are successful in approximately 80% to 90% of cases.[132] Use of other induction immunosuppressive agents, such as antithymocyte globulin (thymoglobulin) does not improve the rates or graft survival rates of LT patients when used as an induction agent[133] but can be used as an adjunct in steroid-resistant antibody-mediated rejection (AMR).

Unlike acute rejection, chronic rejection in LT is associated with reduced graft survival.[134] There are no effective treatments of chronic rejection, which occurs in roughly 10% of all LTs.[134] With chronic ductopenic rejection rarely occurring in the first 2 months after LT, *ductopenic rejection* is defined as loss of bile ducts in more than 50% of portal tracts, when 20 or more portal tracts are available for evaluation, and is diagnosed on the basis of histologic criteria.[135] Early ductopenia is associated with a high mortality rate.[134] In addition, arteriopathy has been described, which affects large and medium-sized arteries, characterized by foam cell infiltration of the intima. The most important manifestation of chronic rejection, the term *ductopenic rejection* is used synonymously with the histologic description *vanishing bile duct syndrome*. The only effective treatment for this problem is re-transplantation.

AMR represents a rare form of immunologic complications after LT. The overall rate of AMR is estimated to be 1% of all LTs but is increased to 5% in patients with positive donor-specific antigen (DSA). AMR is diagnosed with C4D-positive stained biopsies.[136] The treatment of AMR is plasmapheresis, intravenous immunoglobulin (IVIG), and a B-cell–depleting medication, such as rituximab.[131] AMR is a relatively newly appreciated phenomena in LT and ongoing work on long-term outcomes after effective treatments is ongoing. There is also concerns that AMR is underdiagnosed and a rising DSA level post-transplant could be a cause of occult liver fibrosis over an extended period of time.[137] However, this remains an area of debate and a standardized treatment based on post-transplant DSA has not been established.

INFECTION

With few exceptions, all patients who undergo transplantation are committed to lifelong immunosuppressant therapy to prevent graft rejection. Inadequate immunosuppression can result in graft loss, whereas injudicious use of immunosuppression can result in life-threatening infection or development of post-transplant lymphoproliferative disease (PTLD). A tenuous balance exists between the proper amount of immunosuppression to prevent rejection and minimization of the risk for nosocomial and opportunistic infection. Despite better understanding of the immune response and proliferation of more selective immunosuppressive agents, approximately two-thirds of transplant patients experience at least one episode of serious infection, which accounts for more than half of the observed mortality associated with LT.[138]

Risk factors for postoperative infection after LT include those incurred from the donor, recipient, and intraoperative course: donor and recipient viral status, underlying medical comorbidities, and nutritional status all can contribute. Prolonged surgery with massive blood loss, prolonged ischemia time, and violation of the gastrointestinal (GI) tract also are risk factors for nosocomial infection.

Bacterial infections tend to occur within the first month after LT and vary from center to center. Early risk factors include prolonged operating time, indwelling catheters, biliary obstruction, PVT, and poor graft function. In addition, vascular ischemia, recurrent hepatitis C virus (HCV) infection, patient exposure to resistant organisms, and chronic rejection and hyperglycemia can

contribute to nosocomial infection.[139,140] Common bacterial pathogens include gram-negative organisms found in the bile (*Escherichia coli*, *Enterobacter* and *Pseudomonas* spp.) and gram-positive organisms (*Staphylococcus aureus*, coagulase-negative staphylococci, group D streptococci). Rarely, *S. aureus* can result in the development of toxic shock syndrome in the early postoperative period. *Listeria*, *Nocardia*, and *Legionella* are uncommon but significant pathogens.

Viral infections are common in immunocompromised patients after transplantation. In addition to the more common viral infections described here, other equally important but less common viral infections can be devastating to immunocompromised transplant patients; these include human immunodeficiency virus (HIV), adenovirus, influenza, and respiratory syncytial virus (RSV). In addition, transplant patients are at risk for acquiring viral hepatitis from infected organs, blood transfusions, and illicit drug use.

CMV is the most important infection observed in organ transplant patients. An asymptomatic infection in the general population, CMV attains significant potential severity in immunosuppressed transplant recipients and is the most important pathogen in clinical transplantation.[141] CMV disease usually occurs 30 to 50 days after transplantation, with clinical manifestations that include fever, malaise, arthralgia, leukopenia and thrombocytopenia, hepatitis, interstitial pneumonitis, enterocolitis, and disseminated disease. Differentiation between *CMV disease* and *CMV infection* is clinically important: *CMV disease* is defined as a histologically evident invasive CMV infection or a positive CMV culture from deep tissue specimens—liver biopsy, endoscopic mucosal biopsy or brushing, bronchoscopic mucosal biopsy or brushing—in the setting of clinical manifestation. The presence of positive blood, body fluid, or serologic tests is insufficient to establish the diagnosis of CMV disease. Liver biopsy with immunostaining using a monoclonal antibody against CMV antigen enables early diagnosis. Common histologic findings include hepatocyte necrosis, parenchymal microabscesses, and a magenta-colored intranuclear inclusion surrounded by a clear halo, the so-called *owl's eye nucleus*.

Risk factors for CMV disease include a seronegative recipient who received an organ from a seropositive donor, the use of anti-lymphocyte antibody therapy (particularly OKT3), and re-transplantation. In general, the level of immunosuppressive therapy influences manifestation of CMV infection. Chronic CMV infection with persistent CMV replication within hepatocytes is associated with cholestatic hepatitis and vanishing bile duct syndrome.[142]

Patients who manifest CMV disease are treated with a reduction, if possible, of the immunosuppressive regimen, particularly tapering of the corticosteroid dose. For years, intravenous (IV) ganciclovir had become the mainstay of therapy and is safe and effective for prophylaxis and treatment. Occasionally, foscarnet is required as an alternative in cases of ganciclovir resistance, but it is less well tolerated and can be nephrotoxic.

Prophylaxis against CMV disease using oral and IV ganciclovir after transplantation has been effective. Other prophylaxis regimens using IV ganciclovir plus oral acyclovir for 3 months after LT or oral acyclovir used alone have been less successful.[143,144] Using oral valganciclovir in the prevention and treatment of mild CMV infection has been demonstrated to be as effective as IV ganciclovir. Because of the effectiveness of oral valganciclovir, most transplant centers have switched to prophylactic regimens that range from 3 to 6 months of daily oral treatment (450 or 900 mg, depending on renal function). Side effects are minimal, but leukopenia can occur. Late-onset CMV disease remains a potential problem, especially in patients on higher doses of immunosuppression and in high-risk groups, whose donor was CMV positive when the recipient was CMV negative (CMV D+/R–).

Herpes simplex virus (HSV) seropositivity is present in most patients undergoing LT. HSV infection observed postoperatively usually is related to immunosuppression-induced reactivation. Herpesvirus infection usually manifests as a mild mucocutaneous oral or genital disease that responds to acyclovir treatment; however, prompt recognition is important to prevent progression to lethal disseminated disease or fulminant hepatitis with coagulopathy, disseminated intravascular coagulation, and death. Graft involvement is diagnosed by a characteristic histologic picture on liver biopsy.

Epstein-Barr virus (EBV) belongs to the herpes family, and infection in a transplant patient is characterized by a mononucleosis-like syndrome that differs from that observed in the normal host by the absence of a heterophil antibody response and the infrequency of pharyngitis or splenomegaly.[145] The clinical significance of EBV infection in an LT patient is related to its role in the pathogenesis of PTLD, the development of which is thought to reflect the unrestricted proliferation of B cells stimulated by EBV infection.[145] The incidence and treatment for established PTLD are discussed later.

Opportunistic infections also are frequently encountered. The incidence of clinically significant fungal infection is 20% to 25% in LT recipients. Risk factors for fungal infection include poor nutrition status, re-transplantation, bacterial infection with prolonged antibiotic use, high doses of immunosuppression, and biliary reconstruction using Roux-en-Y hepaticojejunostomy.

Invasive fungal infection can occur in 1% to 3% of LT patients and is associated with a high mortality rate.[146,147] There are several risk factors (operative time >11 hours, re-transplant, creatinine >3.0, CMV infection, MELD > 30, fulminant hepatic failure, prolonged ICU stay) that have been associated with increased odds of developing a postoperative fungal infection.[148,149] Retrospective data support that prophylactic antifungals have a role in reducing postoperative invasive fungal infections.[147] High-risk patients at our institution are started on prophylactic Eraxis at the time of surgery and continued on this medication until hospital discharge. If the suspicion of invasive fungal infection is high in the postoperative period, every effort should be made to obtain histologic or culture evidence to establish early diagnosis. Emerging evidence supports that prophylaxis in combination with early detection and treatment of invasive fungal can reduce mortality from historic rates of near 100% mortality to less than 20% mortality.[150] *Candida* is the most common fungal infection that can be acquired by inhalation and colonizes the airways or may already be colonized in the recipient's biliary tract.[151] *Aspergillus*, the second most frequent fungal pathogen, is angioinvasive and tends to disseminate to the central nervous system (CNS) and can cause infarcts and cavitation in the lungs.[149] The incidence of invasive aspergillosis is approximately 1% in LT recipients, with a mortality rate close to 100% despite adequate treatment.[152]

Infection by *Cryptococcus neoformans* usually occurs months to years after transplantation and affects approximately 0.25% of LT patients. Because signs and symptoms may be subtle, delayed diagnosis is common. Symptoms that bring the patient to medical attention include changes in mental status, headache,

and fever. In our experience, one patient was seen initially with lesions in the CNS and large, cavitating masses in the thorax that required operative removal. Coccidiomycosis is another form of rare fungal infection that is endemic to the southwest. It has been our practice to give organ recipients from this region long-term fluconazole prophylaxis after transplant.

Pneumocystis carinii pneumonia was previously a common pathogen in the immunocompromised host. With the introduction of routine use of prophylaxis with daily low-dose oral trimethoprim/sulfamethoxazole (TMP/SMX) for 6 to 12 months, or aerosolized pentamidine in patients intolerant to TMP/SMX, the incidence of *P. carinii* pneumonia has decreased dramatically. Because prophylaxis has been so effective, *P. carinii* pneumonia has occurred almost exclusively in patients who do not receive prophylaxis. Given the low morbidity associated with the prophylactic regimens, no patient should be excluded.

Legionella pneumophila is an uncommon cause of pneumonia in patients after LT. As in the normal host, the source of legionellosis is usually the water supply. Traditionally, treatment of *Legionella* pneumonia has been with erythromycin, but quinolones also have proved effective and have the advantage of not interacting with immunosuppressive agents such as cyclosporine or tacrolimus.

POST-TRANSPLANTATION LYMPHOPROLIFERATIVE DISORDER

PTLD is a life-threatening complication of chronic immunosuppression.[153] Lymphoproliferative disorders have been strongly associated with the replication of EBV in B cells induced by enhanced immunosuppression; this has been observed primarily in patients who have received more than one course of polyclonal antilymphocyte globulin or monoclonal OKT3.[154] An association with CMV infection also has been noted. The incidence of PTLD varies from 1% to 3% among LT recipients, and prognosis depends on the histologic characteristics of the tumor. Polyclonal PTLD is treatable with discontinuation of immunosuppression with relatively low risk of rejection.[155] Monoclonal PTLD is more difficult to treat and can result in death. Antibody against CD20 represents a novel approach in treating monoclonal PTLD, with favorable outcome.[155] The clinical presentation of PTLD varies and includes fever, malaise, and lymphadenopathy with or without tonsillitis. In addition, GI bleeding, perforation, or obstruction; hepatocellular dysfunction; and CNS manifestations, such as seizures, mental status changes, and focal neurologic symptoms, also have been described.

Lymphoproliferative disorders occurring after LT have characteristics distinct from the lymphoproliferative disorders that occur in the general population. Non-Hodgkin lymphoma accounts for 65% of lymphomas in the general population, compared with 93% in transplant recipients. These tumors are mostly large-cell lymphomas, and most are of the B-cell type. Extranodal involvement is common and occurs in approximately 70% of cases.

Treatment of polyclonal PTLD consists of reduction of immunosuppressive medications and antiviral therapy. Patients with monoclonal PTLD and patients with polyclonal disease that does not respond to reduced immunosuppression have been treated with radiation, chemotherapy, and occasionally surgical resection. Therapy using monoclonal antibody against CD20 shows promising results for patients with monoclonal PTLD.[156]

ACUTE IMMUNOSUPPRESSIVE DRUG TOXICITY

Immunosuppression after transplantation must achieve a balance between the beneficial effects of the drugs in preventing or reversing rejection and the dangers of excess immunosuppression with the development of acute toxicity symptoms, nosocomial infection, and lymphoproliferative disorders. The most common agents used for immunosuppression in LT patients are the CNIs cyclosporine and tacrolimus, with or without corticosteroids. Azathioprine was used frequently in the past, especially in those patients who received triple-drug therapy. Mycophenolate mofetil has essentially replaced azathioprine in the immunosuppression regimen after liver and kidney transplantation. After the initiation of immunosuppressive therapy, development of infection and acute toxicity are usually seen early during treatment, whereas lymphoproliferative disorders and other malignancies are long-term sequelae, as previously discussed.

The side effect profiles of cyclosporine and tacrolimus are similar and include GI disturbances, headache, and tremor. Gingival hyperplasia and hirsutism are encountered frequently during cyclosporine and corticosteroid treatment, whereas glucose intolerance is reported more often with tacrolimus than cyclosporine therapy. Hyperkalemia, hyperuricemia, hypophosphatemia, and hypomagnesemia are manifestations of renal tubular dysfunction and usually can be controlled by adjusting the dose according to drug levels. Nephrotoxicity is the most clinically significant adverse effect of both drugs and manifests as acute azotemia. This effect is largely reversible after reducing the dose of the drug and providing adequate hydration. Occasionally, progressive chronic renal disease can develop in as many as 5% of patients, which is usually irreversible and may require renal replacement therapy or renal transplantation.[124] Other renal effects of cyclosporine include chronic tubular dysfunction and, rarely, hemolytic uremic syndrome.

The mycophenolate mofetil side effect profile includes GI disturbances (e.g., nausea, vomiting, diarrhea) and may increase certain postoperative infections.[157] These symptoms are not uncommon in many early transplant patients, and it may be difficult to differentiate the cause, although drug toxicity is usually inferred. Alternative forms of the drug may be helpful, as well as dose modification or discontinuation.[158]

RECURRENT HEPATITIS

In patients in whom cirrhosis develops secondary to chronic hepatitis B virus (HBV) infection, the recurrence rate, as evidenced by signs of viral replication (HBV e-antigen–positive or positive titers of HBV DNA), is approximately 80% to 90% in the first year. Given the almost universal recurrence of HBV antigenemia in the early postoperative period, some authors have questioned the utility of liver replacement in these patients. With the advent of hepatitis B immunoglobulin (HBIG) and other adjuvant therapies, such as interferon and lamivudine, to prevent recurrent disease, transplantation now is routinely offered to patients with chronic HBV infection, with excellent results.

Recurrent HCV infection is universal after LT. In 90% of patients, HCV can be confirmed on routine biopsy. Of these, 60% have mild hepatitis, whereas 30% develop a more severe pattern, as seen on histologic examination. In patients with severe recurrent HCV, cirrhosis develops in 20% within 5 years if untreated. The advent of improved HCV medications, with almost 100% cure rates, has significantly improved the outlook for patients with HCV infection who are waiting for or have received an LT.

BONE DISEASE

Almost all patients who undergo LT have some degree of hepatic osteodystrophy, especially those with primary biliary cirrhosis.[159] The mechanism seems to vary according to the underlying disease. The causes are multifactorial and include corticosteroid therapy, bed rest, and cholestasis. Osteoporosis is particularly common 3 to 6 months after LT; however, by the end of the first year after transplantation, patients start gaining bone density. This late improvement is probably because of a reduction in corticosteroid therapy use and the resolution of the pre-transplantation condition that was deleterious to skeletal health. Atraumatic bone fractures are more frequent within the first 6 months after LT because of the extensive bone loss that occurs during this period. Avascular necrosis and vertebral body collapse may also occur, especially in those maintained on corticosteroid therapy.

NEUROPSYCHIATRIC COMPLICATIONS

Severe neuropsychiatric changes can occur after LT. In addition to the acute neurophysiologic changes associated with fluid and electrolyte shifts during the perioperative period, anxiety and depression are common psychiatric conditions observed in many transplant patients. Seizures, altered levels of consciousness, and CNS infections are infrequent but are significant causes of morbidity and mortality. Encephalopathy observed after LT may be related to poor initial graft function, but it is more often multifactorial in etiology. Metabolic derangements, hypoxia, sedation, and drug interactions all can contribute.

Neurologic signs and symptoms associated with immunosuppression toxicity related to cyclosporine and tacrolimus include tremors, headaches, and seizures. These can be avoided by close monitoring of drug levels. High-dose corticosteroids can result in emotional lability or mania. Any patients seen with new neuropsychiatric symptoms should have a cranial CT scan and lumbar puncture to rule out other causes of mental status changes, such as intracerebral bleeding or an infectious etiology.

HYPERTENSION AND HYPERLIPIDEMIA

Common sequelae of immunosuppression are the development of hypertension and hyperlipidemia in the post-transplantation period.[160] Although patient survival improves, the consequences of these conditions have greater importance on long-term prognosis. Hypertension is observed in approximately 70% of LT recipients at 1 year, and almost 40% of patients manifest metabolic syndrome with diabetes, sustained hypercholesterolemia, and hypertriglyceridemia during the same period.[161] The pathophysiology of post-transplantation hyperlipidemia is complex. Rapamycin immunosuppression does not cause glucose intolerance, but it can lead to hyperlipidemia, problems with wound healing, and mouth ulcers.[162] Omega-3 fatty acids found in fish oil can reduce hypertriglyceridemia significantly. In our experience, oral supplementation with over-the-counter fish oil capsules providing 1 to 2 g of Eicosapentaenoic acid (EPA) and docosàhexaenoic acid (DHA) has shown a dose-response reduction in serum triglycerides.

Because most fish oil supplements are 30% to 55% EPA and DHA, multiple capsules may be needed. Given the additional risk of coronary artery and peripheral vascular disease, aggressive therapy with dietary changes, exercise, and medication is indicated.

CONCLUSION

LT is a lifesaving treatment modality for patients with ESLD. The wide range of comorbidities that develop preoperatively contributes significantly to the development of postoperative complications. Aggressive use of immunosuppression is successful in preventing rejection in many cases, but therapy can be complicated by the development of life-threatening neoplasms.

Recent trends favor significant reduction of immunosuppression with time and early withdrawal of corticosteroids, once the mainstay of immunosuppressive regimens. The reduction of immunosuppression in select patients and early withdrawal of steroids have significantly reduced morbidity and life-threatening complications.

Positive outcomes after LT require a multidisciplinary team approach that includes surgeons, transplant coordinators, hepatologists, and internists to maintain constant surveillance for the inevitable complications that arise. Early diagnosis with rapid treatment provides the best opportunity for disease-free survival.

References are available at expertconsult.com.

CHAPTER 112

Whole organ pancreas and pancreatic islet transplantation

Niraj M. Desai and James F. Markmann

Type 1 diabetes mellitus (DM), formerly known as "juvenile diabetes," is characterized by hyperglycemia resulting from the nearly complete destruction of insulin-producing β-cells of the pancreatic islets of Langerhans. The loss of β-cells is the result of a T lymphocyte–mediated autoimmune attack that typically occurs during childhood or early adolescence. Insulin replacement can lead to acceptable control of blood glucose levels; however, affected individuals are subject to various secondary microvascular complications that include cardiac disease, stroke, retinopathy and blindness, nephropathy and renal failure, peripheral and autonomic neuropathy, and amputation.[1] Although tight glycemic control has been shown to decrease the number of diabetes-related secondary complications, it is associated with an increased number of dangerous hypoglycemic episodes.[2]

Transplantation therapy for type 1 diabetes was developed as an alternative to insulin administration with the added theoretic benefit of reducing or eliminating the development of secondary complications of the disease by providing superior glycemic control. Both whole-organ pancreas and isolated pancreatic islets are being transplanted into select individuals with type 1 diabetes. Whole-organ pancreas transplantation is an established and widely available therapy that has been available for decades. Clinical islet transplantation is an approved therapy in several European countries and Canada. In the United States, registration studies have been completed and the first Biologics License Application for islets was just recently approved by the Food and Drug Administration (FDA).[3,4] This step forward will allow islet transplantation to become a clinically available therapy in the United States.

WHOLE-ORGAN PANCREAS TRANSPLANTATION

History and Early Results

On December 20, 1893, P. Watson Williams grafted three pieces of sheep pancreas into the subcutaneous tissues of a child with diabetes; the child died three days later of unrelenting diabetic ketoacidosis.[5] This first attempt to treat diabetes with transplantation, although unsuccessful, was followed by several decades of animal experimentation in which investigators developed the methods necessary to perform a vascularized pancreas transplant and subsequently used it as a model to study diabetes and glucose homeostasis.

The first clinical vascularized pancreas transplant was performed on December 17, 1966, by William Kelly and Richard Lillehei at the University of Minnesota. The patient had temporary insulin independence but eventually required graft removal and ultimately died of postoperative complications.[6] The early experience with pancreas transplantation that followed at Minnesota and at a few other centers was characterized by some technical success, but no graft functioned beyond 1 year, and consequently the enthusiasm for this procedure waned.

During 1975, only six pancreas transplants were performed worldwide. However, the introduction of cyclosporine as an immunosuppressive medication and further technical refinements allowed for improved outcomes after pancreas transplantation, such that throughout the 1980s and early 1990s, the number of pancreas transplants increased dramatically. By 2004, almost 1500 pancreas transplants were performed in the United States. However, since that peak year, the number has declined with fewer than 1000 pancreas transplants in the United States in 2020.

Indications and Patient Selection

Most patients who undergo pancreatic transplantation have both type 1 DM and renal failure. In these individuals, pancreas transplantation is either performed with a simultaneous kidney transplantation (SPK; 86% of US pancreas transplants in 2020) or are pancreas after kidney transplant (PAK). The precise glucose control achieved by the pancreas transplant protects the transplanted kidney from recurrent diabetic nephropathy[7] and is beneficial from an overall quality of life perspective. In a small proportion of patients with diabetes that is very brittle and difficult to manage, but with preserved renal function, pancreas transplantation alone (PTA) may be indicated. It should be noted that SPK and PAK recipients require immunosuppressive therapy to protect both the kidney and the pancreas from rejection, whereas in the case of PTA recipients, the initiation of immunosuppression is solely for the pancreas. This difference becomes important when weighing the risk versus the benefit for each category of recipient.

One notable change in pancreas transplantation has been the inclusion of some patients with type 2 diabetes and kidney failure as candidates for a simultaneous pancreas and kidney transplant. This group includes individuals that meet a traditional definition of type 2 diabetes and individuals that have maturity-onset diabetes of the young (MODY). Carefully selected patients with type 2 diabetes that have a body mass index (BMI) of 30 or less can undergo a successful simultaneous pancreas and kidney transplant, provided they meet listing criteria and have an insulin requirement that is below 1 to 1.5 units per kilogram per day.[8] In the past, very few patients with type 2 diabetes underwent an SPK; however, in recent years nearly 20% of patients on the pancreas waiting list are individuals with type 2 diabetes.[9]

Potential pancreas recipients are carefully screened for contraindications to transplantation, such as an ongoing infectious process or malignancy. These candidates almost always have medical comorbidities because of secondary complications from diabetes; as a result, a thorough assessment of a candidate's cardiovascular status is essential. Cardiac contraindications to pancreas transplantation include the presence of uncorrected coronary artery disease, significantly decreased ejection fraction, or myocardial infarction within the preceding 6 months. Recipient age is also important, and in most programs, recipients older than 60 years of age are not considered candidates because of an increased risk of perioperative complications coupled with the uncertainty of long-term benefit in the setting of life expectancy compromised by comorbidities.

Donor Operation (see Chapter 126)

Selection of an appropriate deceased pancreas donor includes standard donor selection criteria. In addition, a bias exists toward using organs from younger, leaner, and more hemodynamically stable deceased donors. Donors with hemodynamic instability or those that require high doses of vasopressors are considered at higher risk for graft failure and graft-related complications. In addition, pancreata with significant steatosis are usually avoided because they are associated with a greater likelihood of postoperative complications, such as pancreatitis, peripancreatic fat necrosis, and infection. Based on these selection criteria, which are relatively stringent compared with those applied to the liver or kidney, only a fraction of deceased donors are deemed suitable for whole-organ pancreas donation. In the United States, there were 12,588 deceased donors during 2020. Of these, only 962 pancreata were transplanted (7.6%), compared with 8415 livers (66.8%) and 17,583 kidneys.

The procurement of the pancreas is often performed concurrent with the liver procurement, requiring careful delineation of the blood supply to the liver to ensure that both organs can be removed and safely transplanted (see Chapter 109). In the majority of cases, variation in vascular anatomy should not preclude the transplantation of both organs. Initial dissection involves entering the lesser sac by division of the gastrocolic ligament to expose the anterior surface of the pancreas. Visual inspection is an essential element to the pancreas procurement process to assess the organ for the presence of infiltrating fat or hematoma that might preclude transplantation. The porta hepatis is carefully dissected, with division of the common bile duct and the gastroduodenal artery. In addition, the common hepatic, proximal left gastric, and proximal splenic arteries are all dissected free of surrounding nerve and lymphatic tissues. Further mobilization of the pancreas includes a Kocher maneuver to free the head and division of the lienophrenic and lienocolic ligaments to mobilize the body and tail. Of note, the spleen is left in continuity with the pancreas. The duodenum is decontaminated by flushing the lumen with povidone-iodine solution through a nasoduodenal tube by many but not all centers performing this procedure.

After the patient has been systemically heparinized, the abdominal aorta is ligated at its bifurcation and is cannulated in a retrograde direction for perfusion. The liver team may elect to place a cannula for portal perfusion through the inferior mesenteric vein. The supraceliac aorta is cross-clamped, the vena cava is vented, and the abdominal organs are flushed in situ with preservation solution, typically University of Wisconsin (UW) solution, at 4°C. In addition, topical cooling with saline slush is standard. Some centers prefer that only arterial flush is performed or that the portal flush is limited to avoid increased portal pressure during the flushing period.

Once the organs have been adequately flushed, the liver and pancreas are either separated in situ and removed individually from the donor, or both organs are removed *en bloc* and divided

at the back table. In the in situ separation situation, the liver is removed first by dividing the portal vein approximately 1 cm cephalad to the superior margin of the pancreatic head (at the level of the coronary vein) and dividing the splenic artery 5 mm beyond its origin, thus preserving the entire celiac axis with the liver.

Next, removal of the pancreas proceeds. The proximal duodenum just beyond the pylorus and the distal duodenum are divided with a gastrointestinal (GI) anastomosis (GIA) stapler. The small bowel and colonic mesentery that lies inferior to the pancreas is divided, and the superior mesenteric artery (SMA) is divided at its origin from the aorta. Long segments of donor iliac vessels are removed to use for vascular reconstruction during back-table preparation of the pancreas.[10]

Back-Table Preparation of the Pancreas (see Chapter 126)

Relative to other solid organs, the pancreas requires more extensive preparation before implantation into the recipient. This back-table preparation is performed in ice-cold preservation solution to minimize any further ischemic injury to the organ. The duodenum is often shortened with a GIA stapler, being careful to exclude any gastric tissue and also being careful not to compromise the opening of the ampulla of Vater. The small bowel mesentery in the donor is shortened by firing a stapler across this mesentery and then reinforcing the staple line with a running vascular suture. The spleen is removed by dividing the vessels in the splenic hilum, being careful not to injure the tail of the gland. Finally, the arterial inflow to the graft must be reconstructed because the organ has two major sources of blood supply that are not in continuity: the splenic artery supplies the body and tail, and branches of the SMA supply the head.

In most instances, arterial reconstruction can be performed using the donor iliac artery as a bifurcated Y graft. The internal iliac artery is joined to the splenic artery, and the external iliac artery is joined to the SMA. The common iliac artery of the donor Y graft can then be anastomosed to the recipient iliac artery, serving as the arterial inflow to the pancreas. In rare instances, it is necessary to create a portal vein extension graft on the back table using donor iliac vein; however, this technique should be avoided if possible because it may increase the risk of venous thrombosis of the pancreas graft.

Recipient Operation (see Chapter 126)

The techniques used for transplanting the pancreas have evolved significantly during the past few decades. Partial segmental grafts that contained only the body and tail were once common but are rarely used today. Exocrine secretions were once managed by pancreatic duct ligation or by injection of a polymer that would cause duct obliteration; however, exocrine secretions are now routinely handled by internal drainage, either through the intestinal tract or the urinary tract. Throughout most of the 1980s and 1990s, drainage of the pancreatic secretions into the recipient bladder was the favored form of exocrine drainage. This technique is technically straightforward and convenient for monitoring organ function by measurement of amylase levels in the urine; however, problems with cystitis, urethritis, hematuria, bicarbonate loss, and dehydration are all associated with bladder drainage. These complications necessitate surgical revision to enteric drainage in as many as 20% to 30% of bladder-drained pancreas recipients.[11] Based on these issues, and on the lower rejection rates observed with newer immunosuppressive medications, the majority of transplant centers now perform enteric drainage of the exocrine secretions. This enteric drainage is either directly into a loop of jejunum in a side-to-side manner or into a Roux-en-Y jejunal limb.

The venous drainage of the graft is to the systemic circulation, through the iliac vein or inferior vena cava (IVC), or to the portal circulation. Portal venous drainage has the theoretic advantage of delivering insulin in a more physiologic manner because insulin undergoes a "first pass" through the liver, and the hyperinsulinemia that results from systemic drainage is avoided.[12] Also, an immunologic advantage of portal drainage has been observed in several experimental studies, in which the delivery of foreign antigen to the portal system results in diminished antidonor immune responses. Despite these potential advantages, no demonstrable difference has been found in outcomes between human transplants drained by the portal vein and those drained by a systemic vein.[13] Although systemic venous drainage is how the majority of pancreas transplantations are performed, the portal venous approach can be very useful in situations where systemic drainage is impossible or complicated.

There are two common locations in the abdomen where the transplant is placed based on the type of venous drainage planned: either in the pelvis (usually on the right side) for systemic venous drainage or in the mid-abdomen for portal venous drainage. When the graft is placed in the pelvis, the donor portal vein is anastomosed to the external iliac vein, the common iliac vein, or the distal IVC. In this pelvic position, the graft can be oriented with the duodenum in an inferior orientation, if bladder drainage is planned (Fig. 112.1A), or with the duodenum in either the superior (see Fig. 112.1B) or inferior position, if enteric drainage is planned. Alternatively, for portal venous drainage, the pancreas is placed in the midabdomen below the transverse colon with the duodenum oriented superiorly. The portal vein of the pancreas is anastomosed in an end-to-side manner to the superior mesenteric vein, found at the base of the transverse colon mesentery (Fig. 112.2). Enteric drainage for exocrine secretions must be used with the portal venous drainage technique. With either venous drainage technique, the donor arterial conduit to the pancreas graft is anastomosed in an end-to-side manner to the recipient common or external iliac artery.

Complications

The major complications after pancreas transplantation are generally technical. Pancreas graft thrombosis, arterial or venous, is more frequent after pancreas transplantation than after other solid-organ transplants, with a reported incidence of 5% to 10%. Thrombosis typically occurs within the first week after transplantation and likely reflects the relatively low blood flow through the organ. In most cases of thrombosis, graft removal is necessary.[14] Early pancreatitis occurs in 10% to 20% of patients and is largely a reflection of ischemic damage to the gland during donor demise or preservation, and reperfusion injury. Hyperamylasemia and graft edema are characteristic, and graft pancreatitis is usually treated with octreotide. Leakage at the

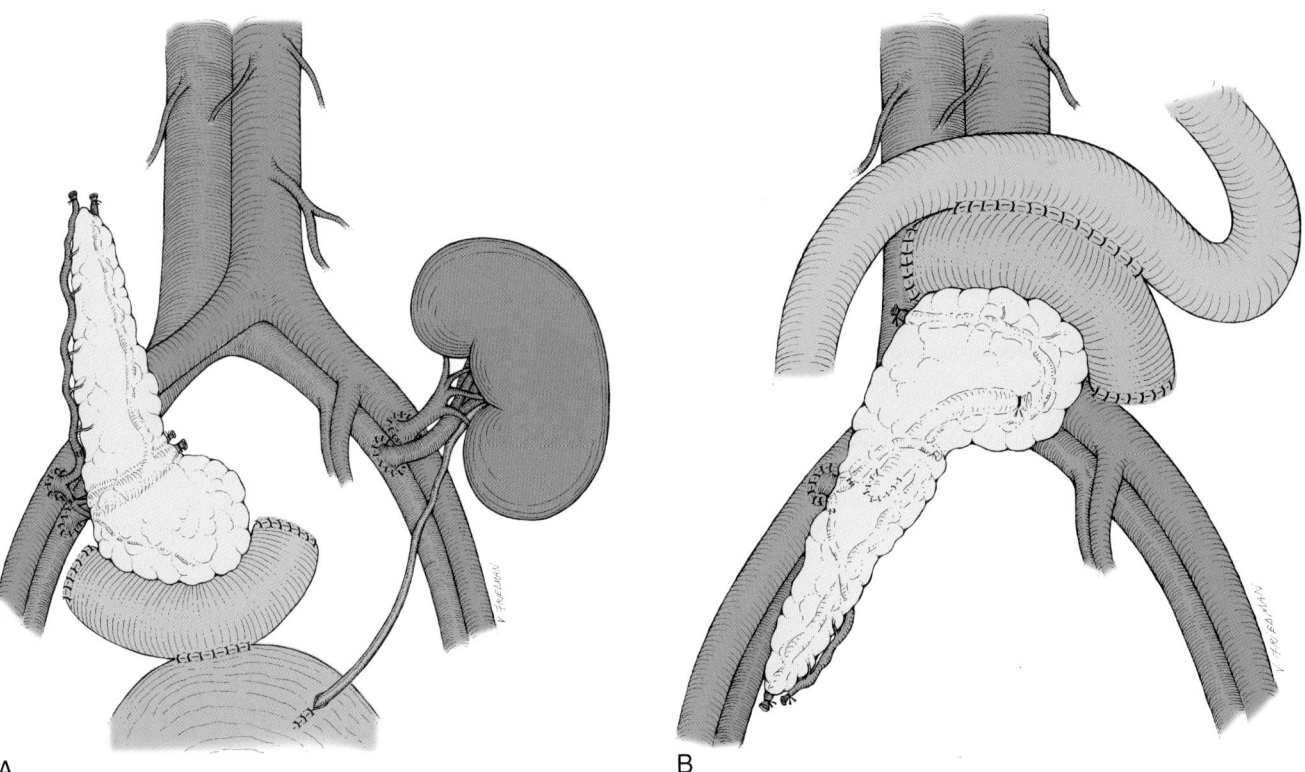

A   B

FIGURE 112.1 **Whole-organ pancreas transplantation with systemic venous drainage.** The pancreas is placed in the right pelvis with anastomosis of the donor iliac artery Y graft to the recipient iliac artery to provide arterial inflow to the graft and anastomosis of the donor portal vein to the recipient iliac vein for venous drainage. Simultaneous kidney transplantation can be performed using the left-sided iliac vessels. **A,** The duodenum is oriented in the inferior direction to allow anastomosis to the bladder *(shown)* or to the small intestine *(not shown).* **B,** Alternatively, the duodenum is oriented superiorly for anastomosis to the intestine.

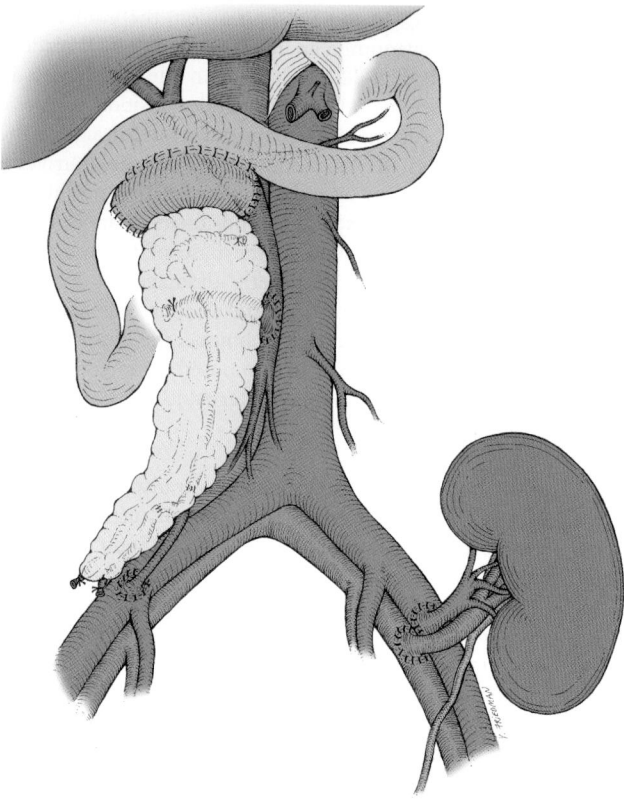

FIGURE 112.2 **Whole-organ pancreas transplantation with portal venous drainage.** The pancreas is placed in the midabdomen with anastomosis of the donor portal vein to a major branch of the superior mesenteric vein and anastomosis of the donor iliac artery Y graft to the recipient iliac artery. The duodenum is oriented in the superior direction for anastomosis to the intestine. A simultaneous kidney transplant can be performed using either the left iliac (shown) or right iliac vessels.

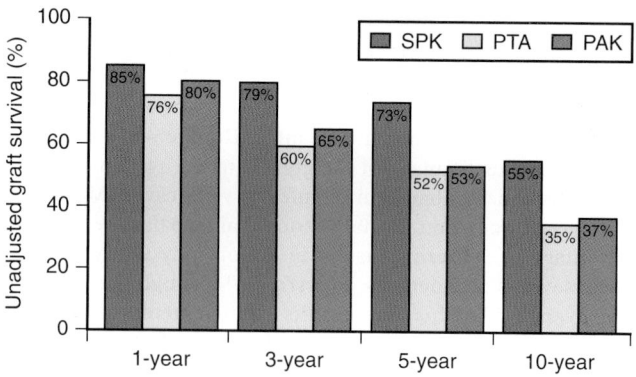

Death is included as an event.

FIGURE 112.3 Pancreas graft survival rates (unadjusted) at 1 year, 3 years, 5 years, and 10 years after whole-organ transplantation by transplant category. PAK, Pancreas transplantation after a successful kidney transplantation; PTA, pancreas transplantation alone; SPK, Simultaneous pancreas and kidney transplantation. (Modified from Axelrod DA, McCullough KP, Brewer ED, Becker BN, Segev DL, Rao PS. Kidney and pancreas transplantation in the United States, 1999-2008: the changing face of living donation. Am J Transplant. 2010;10 [4 Pt 2]:987–1002.)

site of pancreatic exocrine drainage is another early complication, with management dictated by the method of drainage. Bladder-drained transplants with a small leak at the duodeno-cystostomy can be managed by Foley catheter drainage of the bladder, allowing the site of leakage to heal with time. Enteric-drained transplants with a leak at the duodenojejunostomy will often result in peritonitis and usually require operative intervention to control the leak.

Rejection after pancreas transplantation was once common. Pancreas rejection is often difficult to diagnose, and a variety of indicators are used to help make the diagnosis. These include tenderness over the area of the pancreas allograft, increased serum amylase and lipase, decreased urinary amylase excretion (if bladder drainage is used), biopsy of the pancreas, and hyperglycemia. It is noteworthy that hyperglycemia is a late indicator of rejection, and endocrine function of the pancreas is difficult to salvage once hyperglycemia has occurred. If SPK transplantation is performed, renal allograft dysfunction can often assist with the diagnosis of pancreas rejection because the rejection process may occur concomitantly in both organs. As a result of the high incidence of rejection and the difficulty in making the diagnosis, pancreas transplant recipients usually receive potent induction immunosuppression with a T cell–depleting agent and maintenance therapy with tacrolimus, mycophenolate mofetil, and corticosteroids (see Chapter 104).

The total amount of immunosuppression pancreas recipients receive is among the highest of any solid-organ transplant recipient. As a result, they are more likely to experience the complications of immunosuppressive therapy, including infection with opportunistic bacteria, viruses, and fungi; malignancy; GI complications; and more. The high incidence of these complications makes effective prophylaxis strategies important (see Chapter 104).

Results

Patient and graft survival after pancreas transplantation have improved significantly in recent years. Depending on the type of transplant—SPK, PAK, or PTA—patient survival is approximately 97% to 99% at 1 year and 90% to 92% at 5 years after transplantation (Fig. 112.3). The definition of pancreas graft failure was refined in recent years, resulting in changes to overall graft failure rates. Although there is some variation in graft survival based on the category of pancreas transplant being performed, overall pancreas graft survival is approximately 95% at 90 days after transplantation and exceeds 90% at one year after transplantation. These results reflect an improvement over historic graft survival rates that should carry through to further time points from the time of transplantation.[9]

The impact of a successful pancreas transplant on the complications associated with diabetes mellitus is debated. Because successful transplantation restores euglycemia and normal hemoglobin A_{1c} levels, most proponents argue that diabetic complications should cease and perhaps reverse. Neuropathy appears to stabilize and slowly improve after pancreas transplantation, whereas retinopathy progression slows after several years of graft function. The development of diabetic nephropathy in the transplanted kidney of SPK and early PAK recipients appears to be prevented by successful pancreas transplantation. In PTA recipients, diabetic nephropathy appears to stabilize after transplantation[16]; however, the renal benefit to PTA recipients is likely outweighed by the detriment to renal function caused by the immunosuppressive agents, specifically tacrolimus and cyclosporine. The recent introduction of non-nephrotoxic regimens and new agents on the horizon will hopefully address this problem.

Risk/Benefit Considerations

As discussed previously, evidence suggests that successful pancreas transplantation can retard and, in some cases, reverse the secondary complications of diabetes. Despite this evidence, the procedure is considered appropriate for only a select subset of patients with type 1 diabetes because of its invasive nature, compared with insulin therapy, and the potential for significant surgical complications; however, most important in risk/benefit consideration is the need for lifelong immunosuppression. These issues are of utmost importance in pancreas transplantation and play an essential role in both the donor and the recipient selection processes.

One analysis evaluated the survival benefit of pancreas transplantation by examining a large transplant database to compare the survival of pancreas recipients with patients listed for transplantation who did not receive a transplant. Using this study design, the two patient groups were ensured to be as similar as possible. Because the indications, risks, and benefits differ, depending on whether the patient had underlying renal failure, the analysis was stratified based on whether the patient was listed for or transplanted with an SPK, PAK, or PTA.[17] This analysis revealed a marked survival benefit for those patients who received a combined pancreas and kidney transplant with a 57% *reduction* in mortality rate observed during 4 years, compared with similar patients who remained on the waiting list.

In contrast to the clear survival benefit of SPK transplantation, the PAK and PTA recipients experienced an increased mortality after transplantation. During the 4-year follow-up period, PAK recipients experienced a 42% *increase* in mortality rate, and PTA recipients experienced a 57% *increase* in mortality rate compared with the comparable group of patients who remained on the waiting list. A conceptually similar analysis challenged the survival disadvantage of PAK and PTA.[18] Again, as expected, the SPK procedure conferred a marked survival advantage; however, unlike the Venstrom study, no survival disadvantage was evident in PAK or PTA transplant recipients.

There are two important caveats to these risk/benefit studies by Venstrom and Gruessner. First, the impact of pancreas transplantation on quality of life was not evaluated in these nonrandomized retrospective analyses and would likely heavily favor the group with successful PAK and PTA recipients; whether this factor would outweigh any survival disadvantage in the short term, and the cost of these complex procedures remains an open question. Critical outcome measures lacking from these studies are the long-term impact of successful pancreas transplantation on the secondary complications of diabetes and impact on patient quality of life. As previously noted, evidence suggests that diabetic nephropathy, neuropathy, and retinopathy may be positively impacted by the long-term restoration of normoglycemia conferred by transplantation; however, these studies have not included well-controlled trials with large numbers of patients.

These results substantiate the marked clinical benefit observed in patients who undergo the SPK procedure.[19] Importantly, the relative contribution of the transplanted kidney versus the transplanted pancreas to overall patient survival has not been differentiated in a controlled study. This issue is significant given the marked patient survival benefit that has been attributed to kidney transplantation alone that is most pronounced in patients with diabetes.[20]

A retrospective database analysis lends important insight into the role of pancreas graft function in overall patient survival.[21] This analysis examined outcomes in individuals on the SPK waiting list who underwent either an SPK transplant or transplantation of the kidney alone. Recipients of an SPK transplant who had pancreas allograft function 1 year after transplantation had significantly greater patient survival at 7 years (89%) compared with SPK recipients who lost their pancreas transplant within the first year after transplantation (74%) or recipients who underwent a kidney transplant alone from either a living donor (80%) or a deceased donor (65%).

Although the survival benefit for SPK recipients is clear, the survival benefit for PAK and PTA recipients has not been conclusively demonstrated.[22] The same analysis by Weiss demonstrates improved patient survival at 5 years for diabetic recipients who underwent a PAK compared with kidney transplantation alone, although this did not reach statistical significance and was subject to selection bias. A single-center report demonstrates excellent outcomes 3 years after PAK, in which both patient and graft survival are similar to SPK recipients.[23] In this report, PAK recipients had a 90% pancreas allograft, 92% kidney allograft, and a 92% patient survival 3 years after PAK transplantation, compared with 83% pancreas allograft, 86% kidney allograft, and 88% patient survival in SPK recipients. If these excellent PAK outcomes persist with further follow-up and can be replicated at other centers, it is reasonable to assume that a survival benefit to PAK could be demonstrated in future data analyses.

Currently, the strongest conclusion that can be drawn is that PAK transplants should be performed in carefully selected recipients who failed optimal medical management who have well-preserved kidney allograft function and that these procedures should be performed at transplant centers with excellent outcomes. The field remains dynamic because of improvements in surgical technique and perioperative care and the introduction of new immunosuppressive agents with more favorable safety profiles. However, improving outcomes with pancreatic islet transplantation and more sophisticated device technology may ultimately challenge the need to perform whole-organ pancreas transplantation for the treatment of type 1 diabetes, especially in those not already obligated to lifelong immunosuppression for the care of a renal transplant.

PANCREATIC ISLET TRANSPLANTATION

History and Early Results

The original descriptions in rodents of successful islet isolation[24] and subsequent transplantation[25] led to great excitement in the medical community, based on the hope that this cellular therapy might be applied to patients with type 1 diabetes. Although the ability to gain normal glucose control in diabetic rodents with an islet transplant was first described decades ago,[26] translating this success to humans has been difficult. Starting in 1974, several centers attempted human islet transplantation, with 445 recipients receiving islets between 1974 and 2000. Most of these recipients also received a kidney transplant, either before or at the same time as the islet transplant. Analysis of the reported cases between 1990 and 2000 demonstrated that only 19% of patients were off insulin for more than 1 week, and at 1-year follow-up, only 11% of recipients were insulin independent.[27]

These discouraging results were attributed to a number of factors, including the possibility that recurrent autoimmunity was causing progressive islet damage after transplantation because the diabetes in these recipients was from autoimmune beta cell loss. Support for this hypothesis came from a series of patients at the University of Pittsburgh who underwent upper abdominal exenteration, including total pancreatectomy and hepatectomy, followed by whole-organ liver and islet allotransplantation. In this group of 11 patients who did not have autoimmune diabetes, six (55%) exhibited sustained insulin independence, a success rate far greater than what had been achieved in type 1 DM recipients.[28]

Islet Autotransplantation

Autotransplantation of pancreatic islets was developed for patients with chronic pancreatitis, in whom total pancreatectomy provided the best option for treatment. Surgically induced diabetes is generally brittle, characterized by an absence of both insulin and counterregulatory hormones, and accompanied by a high rate of long-term morbidity. Treatment involves processing of the surgically removed pancreas in the islet isolation facility, followed by infusion of either purified islets or crude pancreatic digest into the liver by the portal vein.

The success rate in recipients of autotransplantation after total pancreatectomy has historically been better than in those who received allogeneic islets for the treatment of type 1 diabetes. The largest reported series is from the University of Minnesota; from 1977 to 2011, 409 patients with chronic pancreatitis (see Chapter 58) underwent total, near total, or completion pancreatectomy with islet autotransplantation. Sutherland and colleagues (2012)[29] achieved a 90% rate of graft function and a 30% rate of insulin independence at 3 years after the procedure; the rate of success correlated closely with the yield of islets from the removed pancreatic tissue after digestion and processing. This group previously reported higher rates of successful islet autotransplantation in patients who had no prior surgery or only a prior Whipple procedure, whereas those who had a prior Puestow procedure or distal pancreatectomy had lower chances of success.[30] Similar results have been reported from the University of Cincinnati in a series of 166 patients; 27% of patients were insulin independent 5 years after the procedure.[31] Interestingly, both of these groups infused unpurified pancreatic digests, and the islets had not undergone the additional purification step routinely performed during deceased-donor pancreas processing for islet allotransplantation. In patients who undergo total pancreatectomy and islet autotransplant, overall improvement in quality of life and reduction in chronic pain are also important.[32] A multicenter study is underway that aims to evaluate patient selection and timing for total pancreatectomy and islet auto transplantation such that optimal post-treatment outcomes can be achieved.[33]

The Edmonton Protocol and Beyond

Interest in allogeneic islet transplantation exploded when investigators at the University of Alberta, Edmonton, Canada, reported that, for the first time, diabetes in patients could be consistently reversed by isolated islet transplantation.[34] It was hoped the long-awaited cure for type 1 diabetes had arrived. The Edmonton Protocol approach relied on a novel immunosuppression regimen

that completely avoided corticosteroids and used a unique combination of induction therapy with an interleukin (IL)-2 receptor antibody and maintenance therapy with sirolimus and tacrolimus (see Chapter 104). The rationale for this combination was based on the goal to avoid agents with known β-cell toxicity. Although this drug combination was likely an important factor in the trial's success, perhaps of even greater impact was the large number of islets that patients received; Edmonton investigators achieved transplantation of a greater islet mass than prior trials, by using two or three infusions per patient, acquired sequentially from different deceased donors.

Although previous trials in the late 1990s had often achieved partial success with single infusions of islets, as evidenced by a reduced insulin requirement and increased C-peptide levels, in no trial had the further step been taken to retransplant such patients to increase the net islet mass.[35] In the Edmonton series, patients who showed evidence of partial success from the first infusion received an additional infusion or two, until they had accumulated a sufficient islet mass to gain insulin independence. In general, this occurred when a threshold of 8000 to 10,000 islets per kilogram of recipient body weight had been infused.

After the landmark report by the Edmonton investigators, the next decade saw almost 500 recipients receiving islet transplants distributed among approximately 40 centers worldwide.[36] In the first concerted effort to replicate the provocative results of the Edmonton Protocol, a multicenter trial sponsored by the Immune Tolerance Network enlisted 10 centers in North America and Europe to each perform four islet transplants using the Edmonton regimen.[37] Despite a diligent attempt to ensure uniformity in technique among centers, the rate of success varied dramatically, and depended in part on the extent of experience at the transplanting site. At the three most experienced centers, reversal of hyperglycemia was routinely achieved. However, less experienced teams gained insulin independence in only a fraction of cases (~20%). Thus, although these results confirmed the efficacy of Edmonton's approach, they also revealed the exacting nature of the technique and demonstrated the inherent difficulty in replicating an identical protocol at all centers.

Numerous single-center reports have now corroborated the results of the Edmonton Protocol,[38,39] and although this protocol represented a tremendous leap forward for the field, the Edmonton results also defined the major problem that remains: the need for islets procured from multiple deceased donors to gain insulin independence in a single recipient. This requirement greatly increases costs and represents a distinct disadvantage when compared with whole-organ transplantation. However, it should be remembered that the pancreata used for isolated islet transplantation are organs that were declined for whole-organ transplantation and thus represent a net addition of transplanted patients. These organs are generally inferior to those used in whole-organ transplantation, and improved results may be achieved if islet transplantation candidates had access to the best organs.

The need for such a large number of islets to achieve insulin independence in clinical transplantation was unexpected in light of the finding that as little as 10% of the total islet mass can maintain normoglycemia after partial pancreatectomy. Because the total islet mass in healthy individuals is estimated at 1 to 2 million, transplanting only 200,000 islets should regain normoglycemia in the majority of recipients with diabetes.

Instead, accumulating evidence from the islet transplant studies by the Edmonton and other investigators suggests that for an average individual, 700,000 to 1,000,000 islets are required. The almost two-thirds loss of potency after transplantation has not been fully explained in patients, but experimental data from small-animal studies indicate that the majority of transplanted islets fail to engraft.[40] Understanding and overcoming the loss of islet mass during the engraftment phase have been an important focus of ongoing clinical trials in islet transplantation. Some centers have reported improved success at gaining insulin independence with islets from a single donor by refining the Edmonton approach.[39,41,42] An even more impressive result was reported in patients that received polyclonal antithymocyte globulin (Thymoglobulin) for induction therapy. In a series of 10 consecutive patients treated with Thymoglobulin, 9 were rendered insulin independent with a single infusion of islets.[41] Collectively, these studies suggest that insulin independence can be achieved consistently with single-donor islet infusions under highly optimized conditions.

A second obstacle in performing islet transplantation is that the durability of function is less than that with whole-organ pancreas grafts. In an early report by Edmonton investigators with follow-up of their ongoing series of islet transplant recipients,[43] fewer than 25% of patients remained free from exogenous insulin administration at 3 years (Fig. 112.4B). Although a disappointing result, more encouraging was the observation that more than 85% of these patients had evidence of some islet graft function by C-peptide measurement (see Fig. 112.4A) and that even a low level of function was sufficient to prevent severe hypoglycemic events (SHEs). Recognizing that glycemic control and freedom from SHEs can be effectively addressed with a partially functioning graft, two recent multicenter trials were based on this principle. Both of these trials were developed and conducted through the NIH sponsored Clinical Islet Transplant Consortium (CIT), and both were pivotal phase III trials seeking to set the stage for FDA approval of islets. These trials were an essential step in setting the stage for allogeneic islet transplantation to be reimbursable by Medicare and private insurers, and the key to allow for widespread clinical application in the United States.

The first CIT trial (CIT-07) enrolled patients with normal renal function and type 1 diabetes complicated by poor glycemic control and severe hypoglycemic events despite optimal medical management of diabetes.[3] The second (CIT-06) targeted patients who required a kidney transplant for diabetic nephropathy.[4] In this cohort, the risk/benefit considerations are simplified since the candidates for islets are already obligated to lifelong immunosuppression to support their kidney. Both trials were highly successful, meeting pre-specified metrics from the FDA that would allow for islet transplantation to become an approved therapy.

Complications and Risk/Benefit Considerations

Demonstrating that the procedure is safe for the recipient has been important in the early trials of isolated islet transplantation. The most feared potential complications include bleeding and portal vein thrombosis (PVT). More recent studies such as the CIT trials demonstrate a significant bleeding rate at 5% or less when performed by an interventional radiologist gaining access to the portal vein via a percutaneously placed transhepatic catheter and releasing the islets into the portal system.[44] Alternatively, the procedure can be performed via a small laparotomy to gain access to a small mesenteric vein, through which a catheter can be advanced into the main portal vein for islet

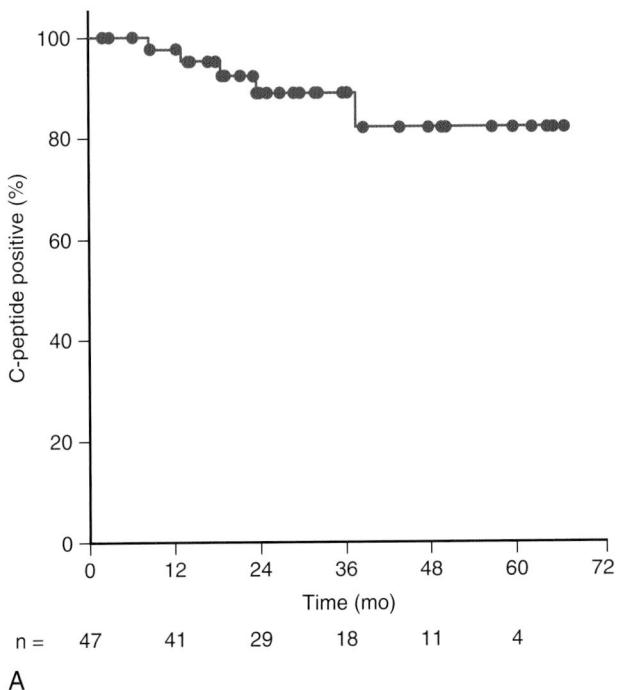

A

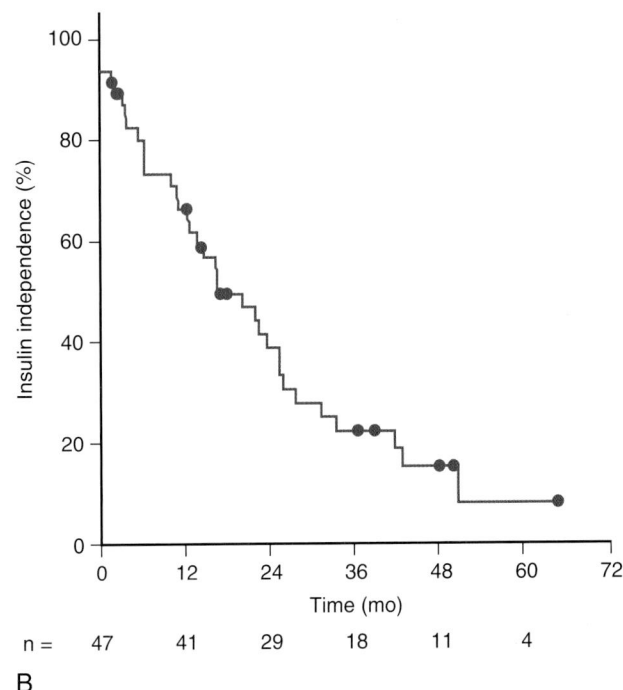

B

FIGURE 112.4 Islet graft survival rates following isolated islet transplantation at the University of Alberta, Edmonton, Canada. **A,** Survival analysis for islet function as documented by C-peptide secretion over time, demonstrating 85% graft survival at 3 years. **B,** Survival analysis for insulin independence with time, demonstrating that fewer than 25% of patients are free from exogenous insulin therapy at 3 years. (From Ryan EA, Paty BW, Senior PA, et al. Five-year follow-up after clinical islet transplantation. Diabetes. 2005;54[7]:2060–2069.)

infusion.[45] The small vein is then ligated, essentially eliminating the potential for hemorrhage. The operative approach allows anticoagulation to be administered without the risk of bleeding from a puncture site in the hepatic parenchyma, although it usually requires a general anesthetic. The Edmonton experience in 65 patients demonstrates that bleeding occurred in more than 20% of recipients, most of whom required either transfusion or surgical intervention. Main PVT, the most potentially troublesome complication of portal islet infusion, has fortunately been extremely rare (<1%); however, in the Edmonton experience, 7% of recipients had evidence of segmental PVT that resolved without sequelae.[43]

The relative safety advantage of islet transplantation compared with whole-organ pancreas transplantation was clearly evident in a comparison of the two approaches.[46] In this study, major complications that included bleeding that required transfusion and reoperation were more common in the whole-organ group, although a number of minor complications were frequent in the islet transplant group, including immunosuppression-related toxicity (mouth ulcerations, edema), periportal hepatic steatosis, and mild liver function test abnormalities. Table 121.1 provides a comparison of the major advantages and disadvantages of whole-organ pancreas and isolated islet transplantation.

Islet transplantation also incurs the risk of infusion-related infection. This complication is minimized by screening potential donors for infection, administering prophylactic antibiotics to the recipient, and assessing the islet preparation for bacterial contamination by microscopic examination and endotoxin testing. As with all forms of transplantation, the need for chronic immunosuppression carries a risk of opportunistic infection and a small but discernible risk for the development of malignancy, especially lymphoma and skin cancer. Similarly, exposure of the recipient to allogeneic tissue may induce an immune response in the recipient and generate cytotoxic antibodies against the HLA antigens of the donor. This exposure may be especially detrimental in islet recipients who receive transplants from multiple donors, thereby broadening their antigenic exposure. The presence of anti-HLA antibodies could hamper future attempts at islet transplantation, and more importantly, of lifesaving organs such as the kidney (see Chapter 104).

One of the most common and concerning potential complications of islet transplantation is calcineurin inhibitor–associated nephrotoxicity. Chronic renal failure in the setting of nonrenal solid-organ transplantation is well described, with an approximate 10% to 20% incidence at 10 years.[47] Similar results in islet transplant recipients would represent a particularly morbid complication given the well-established detrimental impact of renal failure on survival in the diabetic population.[48,49] In the CIT-07 trial in islet patients without a renal transplant, there was a small decrement in renal function observed. In the CIT-06 trial in patients post-renal transplant, a slight fall in GFR was transient and recovered to baseline at two years.

As mentioned previously, the CIT trials can secure a place for islet transplantation as a standard therapeutic modality in the United States. For isolated islet transplantation to gain equal footing with or to surpass whole-organ pancreas transplantation as the preferred therapy for patients with diabetes, a number of conditions will need to be met. First, improvements must occur so that reversal of diabetes is readily accomplished with the islets from a single donor in the majority of cases. This will require not only advances in isolation techniques that allow greater recovery of healthy islet tissue but will also require a greater understanding of the events early after transplantation that are responsible for engraftment of only a fraction of the delivered islet mass.[36] Second, clarification is needed of the immunologic and physiologic mechanisms that contribute to islet dysfunction over time and lead to the need for reinstitution of low doses of exogenous insulin in many islet transplant patients.

Future Directions in Islet Transplantation

Despite the promise of islet transplantation and the advances over the last 10 years, there are significant hurdles that precluded widespread application and competing therapies that show promise. The primary hurdle over the decades has been that unlike many other countries around the world, allogeneic islet transplantation was not yet reimbursed by insurance because it lacked FDA approval. It was expected that FDA approval would follow quickly after completion of the CIT trials in 2017; however, it was not until early 2021 that a biologic license agreement was finally awarded to a startup company to manufacture islets for clinical application. It appears that many of the academic medical centers who participated in the CIT trials were reluctant to assume the potential risks of being an islet manufacturer and the costs of application for a Biologic License Agreement from the FDA to allow commercial production of an islet cell product. Having a company approval for islet manufacture opens the door to widespread application for this cell therapy.

Because of the risks associated with long-term immunosuppression, islet transplantation is largely limited to a small subset of individuals with type 1 diabetes who have the most severe disease, with poor glycemic control and problems with severe hypoglycemia. This limitation could be overcome by nontoxic immunosuppression or the ability to safely develop immune tolerance to avoid the long-term immunosuppression regimen. Although several interesting technologies are under study (islet encapsulation, regulatory cell therapy, mixed chimerism induced tolerance, and potentially tolerogenic biologics), none appears on the near horizon.

At the same time, tremendous progress has been made on mechanical insulin delivery and continuous glucose sensing. The latter allows patients suffering from severe hypoglycemic events to be notified by an automatic alarm when their glucose falls below a predetermined threshold. When successful, the risk of hypoglycemia is markedly attenuated, thus removing one of the primary indications for islet transplantation. In parallel, a closed loop pump may ultimately provide near physiologic insulin and glucagon delivery through sophisticated computer algorithms. This will potentially address the other major indication for islet and pancreas transplantation, poor glycemic control, all without the risks of chronic immunosuppression. It should be made clear, however, that patients are unlikely to ever feel "cured of their disease" while attached to a mechanical pump and sensor; such devices require maintenance, calibration, and close attention by the user.

For this reason, the field remains hopeful for a biologic cure with minimal or no immunosuppression. Two leading candidates for this role are xenogeneic islets and stem cell–derived islets, both with the potential to provide a limitless β-cell supply. Xenogeneic islets from porcine donors have been studied for many years, and several cases have been transplanted to human recipients. Although some attempts have demonstrated some function as measured by c-peptide levels, no patients have had their diabetes reversed. The reasons for failure of pig islet transplantation in humans is poorly defined, but it is safe to assume that a potent xenoresponse is a major factor. Recent developments in gene editing using CRISPR technology may provide a solution through genetic modification of pigs to reduce their vulnerability to xeno-antibody mediated damage.

In parallel, recent technologic developments have achieved successful differentiation of human stem cells to islet-like cell clusters. This can be accomplished with induced pluripotent stem cells (iPS) or from embryonic stem cells (ES) and potentially other stem cell sources. Although the cells do not perfectly replicate insulin secretion of native human islets, when tested ex vivo, there is evidence that they may differentiate further in vivo post-transplant. Two companies have active clinical trials underway using embryonic stem cell–derived endocrine cells to treat patients with type 1 diabetes and hypoglycemia unawareness. One trial place the endocrine cells within a device and surgically implanted into the subcutaneous space of recipients (NCT03163511). A second clinical trial infuses embryonic stem cell–derived endocrine cells directly into the patient's liver via the portal circulation (NCT04786262).

Because ES-derived islet-like cells are from another individual, they are allogeneic and subject to immune-mediated rejection like allogeneic human islets from a deceased donor. For this reason, immunosuppression will be required and thus may incur all the restrictions on target populations as detailed for allogeneic islets. It is yet to be determined whether stem cell–derived islets will benefit immunologically from the fact that they consist of a pure endocrine population and lack immunogenic antigen preventing cells and endothelial cells found in allogeneic islets. If so, it is conceivable that less immunosuppression will be required than for deceased donor islets.

There are several theoretical solutions to the allogeneic barrier. One that has received considerable recent attention because of improved technology is gene editing to reduce the expression of cell surface proteins such as HLA molecules or to add immunoprotective molecules. This approach can theoretically be applied to pluripotent stem cells and to allogeneic and xenogeneic islets. Much work is still needed to determine the required gene edits and their safety.

An alternative approach could be personalized medicine generating islets from iPS derived from the intended recipient. The generated islets would be genetically identical to the recipient and immunosuppression to prevent rejection would not be required. However, unlike the "one size fits all" approach of ES-derived cells, iPS islet may require a separate manufacturing process with optimization, as well as a separate regulatory pathway for each patient; the exorbitant associated costs of this approach have to date deterred industry interest. Another consideration with iPS-derived islet cells is that these cells would appear immunologically identical to native islets. Because type 1 diabetes is autoimmune in nature, the same immune process that destroyed the native islets can destroy iPS-derived islets; thus some level of immunosuppression may still be needed (see Chapter 104).

SUMMARY

This is an exciting time for the field of β-cell replacement. The role of whole pancreas and allogeneic islet transplantation in the treatment of diabetes will likely be challenged in the next 10 years. No matter the ultimate outcome of these evolving technologies, it seems likely that effective care of diabetic patients will only improve in the next decade, and perhaps there will be true cure for this devastating disease.

Ultimately, derivation of β-cells from xenogeneic or stem cell sources promise to provide a limitless supply of transplantable β-cells. The ongoing clinical trials of allogeneic islet transplantation will provide a critical foundation for these future therapies by defining the optimal site for implantation, the best means to monitor survival, and the most conducive immunosuppression that avoids autoimmune and alloimmune damage without pharmacologic β-cell toxicity.

References are available at expertconsult.com.

PART 9

Hepatobiliary Injury and Hemorrhage

CHAPTER 113

Injuries to the liver and biliary tract

Woon Cho Kim and Lucy Kornblith

INTRODUCTION

The majority of hepatobiliary injuries are managed nonoperatively, supported by tenets of patient selection, appropriately timed adjunct interventions, and careful monitoring. The liver is a well-vascularized solid organ (see Chapter 5), making hemorrhage a common cause of mortality in severe trauma. Therefore, in hemodynamically unstable patients or clinically deteriorating patients, timely surgical intervention for hemorrhage control is critical. Hepatobiliary injuries associated with blunt and penetrating mechanisms include a wide range of injury patterns: deep parenchymal disruptions, hemorrhage from veins and arteries, major juxtahepatic venous injuries, and extrahepatic and intrahepatic biliary injuries. This chapter presents the current approach to hepatobiliary injuries from the perspective of a trauma surgeon, recognizing that treatment of complex hepatobiliary trauma requires a multidisciplinary approach. The principles and techniques of both nonoperative and operative management of hepatic and extrahepatic biliary tree trauma are reviewed with an emphasis on the fundamental differences between emergency and elective hepatobiliary operations.

EVOLUTION OF MANAGEMENT OF HEPATOBILIARY TRAUMA

The evolution of the management of hepatic trauma during the last century reflects the progression of the discipline of trauma surgery overall.[1,2] The approach to hepatic trauma in the early 1900s was largely expectant management, which for severe liver injuries was uniformly fatal.[1] Controlling hepatic inflow via manual compression of the hepatoduodenal ligament was first described by Dr. James Hogarth Pringle in 1908 for hepatic hemorrhage[3]; this technique has become known as the Pringle maneuver. Although less often appreciated, Dr. Pringle also described packing around the liver and kidney to stop solid organ hemorrhage in the same series of patients.[3] Halsted modified the technique further by placing rubber sheets between the packs and the liver to protect the parenchyma from adhering to the packs[4] (see Introduction).

Decades later, World War II and post-war civilian trauma experiences stimulated development and use of more aggressive surgical strategies, including formal resection, debridement of devitalized liver, selective hepatic artery ligation, and perihepatic drainage.[1] These approaches emphasized operative treatment of hepatic trauma by way of hemorrhage control. Several series in the 1960s and 1970s reported successful application of formal anatomic resections with portal triad control.[5–7] Selective hepatic artery ligation was popularized during this era as a way to control initial massive hemorrhage and prevent delayed bleeding,[8,9] although associated high infection rates raised concern with this technique.[10,11] Direct repair of injuries to perihepatic veins was addressed by the development of the atriocaval shunt,[12] but mortality from such devastating injuries remained high.[13,14]

Perihepatic packing fell out of favor during this era of early aggressive surgical interventions; however, it was repopularized in the 1990s with recognition of the importance of damage control surgical and resuscitation techniques. The term "damage control" was first defined by Dr. Michael Rotondo as a way to rapidly control hemorrhage and contamination, allowing for resuscitation and deferment of definitive reconstruction until physiologic optimization.[15] Before this, perihepatic packing was only used in limited series to control hemorrhage when definitive operative interventions failed. A landmark study by Lucas and Ledgerwood described perihepatic packing in devastating juxtahepatic venous injury,[16] and Calne and colleagues described packing to temporize massive liver hemorrhage for safe transfer to referral centers.[17] In a sentinel paper from Feliciano and colleagues, packing was advocated as a rescue maneuver to tamponade diffuse coagulopathic liver bleeding in patients otherwise deemed nonsurvivable.[18] A series of reports followed, suggesting a "paradigm shift" away from aggressive operative interventions and resections for hepatic trauma.[19,20] In aggregate, the realization that major hepatic resection in trauma is ill-advised[21] developed out of an understanding that severe trauma and extensive surgery lead to irreversible physiologic insult, hypothermia, coagulopathy, and death.[22–24]

Another dramatic shift in treatment of hepatic trauma ensued with the introduction of computed tomography (CT) and alternative modes of hemorrhage control by angiography and endovascular embolization (see Chapters 21, 94A, 115, and 116).[1] These shifts supported an approach of nonoperative management (NOM) with selective operative interventions. It was the advancement of NOM of solid organ injuries in hemodynamically stable children[25] that encouraged a similar strategy in adults. In 1990, Knudson and colleagues reported on 52 patients with major hepatic injuries successfully managed nonoperatively with careful surveillance.[26] Several reports subsequently demonstrated the safety and efficacy of NOM of hepatic injuries in adults with both blunt and penetrating mechanisms.[1,2,20,27–36] However, these shifts highlighted the importance of patient selection for the success of NOM of hepatic trauma, and for interventional techniques to manage the sequelae of major hepatic trauma. Reliance on adjuncts, including angiographic embolization of hepatic arterial bleeding, endoscopic biliary decompression, delayed laparoscopic drainage, and percutaneous debridement and drainage of liver necrosis and abscess (see Chapters 21, 30) added to the armamentarium for treatment of hepatic trauma.

ANATOMY AND CLASSIFICATION OF HEPATIC TRAUMA

From a trauma surgeon's perspective, the surgical anatomy (see Chapter 2) has to do with the anatomic location of injury and the mechanism of injury and hemodynamic status of the patient. The

TABLE 113.1 American Association for the Surgery of Trauma Liver Injury Classification (1994 Revision)

GRADE[a]	INJURY TYPE	INJURY DESCRIPTION
I	Hematoma	Subcapsular, <10% surface area
	Laceration	Capsular tear, <1 cm parenchymal depth
II	Hematoma	Subcapsular, 10%-50% surface area Intraparenchymal, <10 cm in diameter
	Laceration	1-3 cm parenchymal depth, <10 cm in length
III	Hematoma	Subcapsular, >50% surface area or expanding; ruptured subcapsular or parenchymal hematoma Intraparenchymal hematoma >10 cm or expanding
	Laceration	>3 cm parenchymal depth
IV	Laceration	Parenchymal disruption involving 25%-75% of hepatic lobe or 1-3 Couinaud segments within a single lobe
V	Laceration	Parenchymal disruption involving >75% of hepatic lobe or >3 Couinaud segments within a single lobe
	Vascular	Juxtahepatic venous injuries; i.e., retrohepatic vena cava/central major hepatic veins
VI	Vascular	Hepatic avulsion

[a]Advance one grade for multiple injuries, up to grade III.

American Association for the Surgery of Trauma (AAST) liver injury scale offers an anatomic classification for radiologic imaging or for direct visualization during exploration (Table 113.1 and Fig. 113.1).[37] Typically, AAST grade I to II liver injuries are considered mild, grade III moderate, and grade IV to V severe. Patients with grade VI hepatic avulsion injuries rarely survive to undergo further therapy. Based on the AAST classification, the World Society of Emergency Surgery (WSES) 2020 guidelines added the patient's hemodynamic status to the injury classification (Table 113.2).[36]

Diagnosis of Hepatic Trauma

Abdominal ultrasound, as part of the focused assessment of sonography in trauma (FAST) exam, was validated by Dr. Grace Rozycki in the 1990s as an alternative to identifying hemoperitoneum[38] as a noninvasive alternative to diagnostic peritoneal lavage (DPL).[39] This was of value because although DPL was sensitive, it resulted in many negative or nontherapeutic laparotomies, including in the setting of low-grade hepatic injuries that did not warrant an operation. Point-of-care FAST is used to rapidly triage the need for emergent laparotomy when performed in hemodynamically unstable patients with blunt abdominal injuries.[40] Positive findings, however, cannot determine the source of blood or grade of injuries.

CT scan has become the gold standard for diagnosing solid organ injury in hemodynamically stable patients. Intravenous (IV) contrast–enhanced CT scan of the abdomen gives a rapid assessment of liver injury grade, other solid organ injuries, and degree of hemoperitoneum (see Chapter 14). Further, it can provide evidence of concurrent bowel injury, and the trajectory of penetrating wounds that can help tailor further interventions.

Nonoperative Management of Hepatic Trauma

In this section, we will review the core principles of NOM of hepatic trauma (Box 113.1), highlighting subtle differences between blunt and penetrating injuries. Most patients with liver injuries, regardless of mechanism, who are hemodynamically stable and without diffuse peritonitis or signs of concurrent bowel injury can be safely observed and treated nonoperatively.[1,28,41] Recent series of severe liver injuries (AAST 4 or 5) demonstrate that 90% to 93% of patients who underwent NOM had successful management of complex hepatic trauma, with variable adjunctive early angiographic embolization.[29,31,32]

NOM of hepatic trauma can help avoid unnecessary laparotomies and associated risks,[42] including anesthesia-associated complications, iatrogenic injury, longer recovery and hospital stays, and longer-term adhesive small bowel obstruction and incisional hernias.[43–45] However, the advantages of NOM go beyond simply avoiding an operation. Richardson and colleagues suggested that hepatic-specific trauma mortality improved by adapting the NOM strategy.[27] In fact, although nonoperative observational approaches for liver injuries increased over the past 25 years, mortality drastically decreased.[27]

However, with this, the concept of patient selection became paramount in successful NOM of hepatic trauma. Patients considered for NOM must be hemodynamically stable without signs of concurrent intestinal injuries, regardless of the grade of injury or patient age. Hemodynamically unstable patients, or those with peritonitis, should be taken urgently for laparotomy. Patients undergoing NOM should also be considered for nonsurgical adjunctive therapies, including angiographic embolization, percutaneous drainage, and endoscopy for biliary drainage (see Chapters 16, 20, 21, 30, 31, and 94A). Delayed laparoscopy for bile leak or hematoma may also be considered.

Nonoperative Management of Blunt Hepatic Trauma

The overall success rate of NOM in blunt hepatic trauma is high.[20,32,46] Higher grades of injury carry a greater risk of failure of NOM. Patients with minor to moderate hepatic injuries (AAST 1–3 or WSES 1–2) have success rates near 100%,[32,47] and those with severe injuries (AAST 4–5, WSES 3) have success rates of 83% to 94%,[29,32] aided by early hepatic angiographic embolization (see Chapters 21, 94A, 115, and 116).

NOM is centered on early CT evaluation of liver injuries, and heightened vigilance with repeated clinical reassessment for early signs of active hemorrhage. Therefore, for moderate to severe injuries, patients typically require close hemodynamic monitoring and frequent hemoglobin checks in the intensive care unit. As it stands, there is insufficient data to suggest a standard of care for duration of monitoring, frequency of laboratory checks, time to enteric diet initiation, duration of activity restriction, and safe time for chemical prophylaxis for venous thromboembolism.[30,36] However, frequent abdominal examinations are paramount during the observational period, and any clinical deterioration, particularly with signs and symptoms of active hemorrhage, necessitates reassessment and consideration of angiogram or urgent operation. Therefore consensus supports that NOM should only be considered in environments that allow continuous monitoring, serial clinical evaluations, transfusion, and have access to angiographic embolization adjuncts and an operating room with trained surgeons available.[30,36]

One must also be on alert for missed injuries in patients undergoing NOM for hepatic trauma. Severe solid organ injury is associated with concomitant visceral injury, and failure of

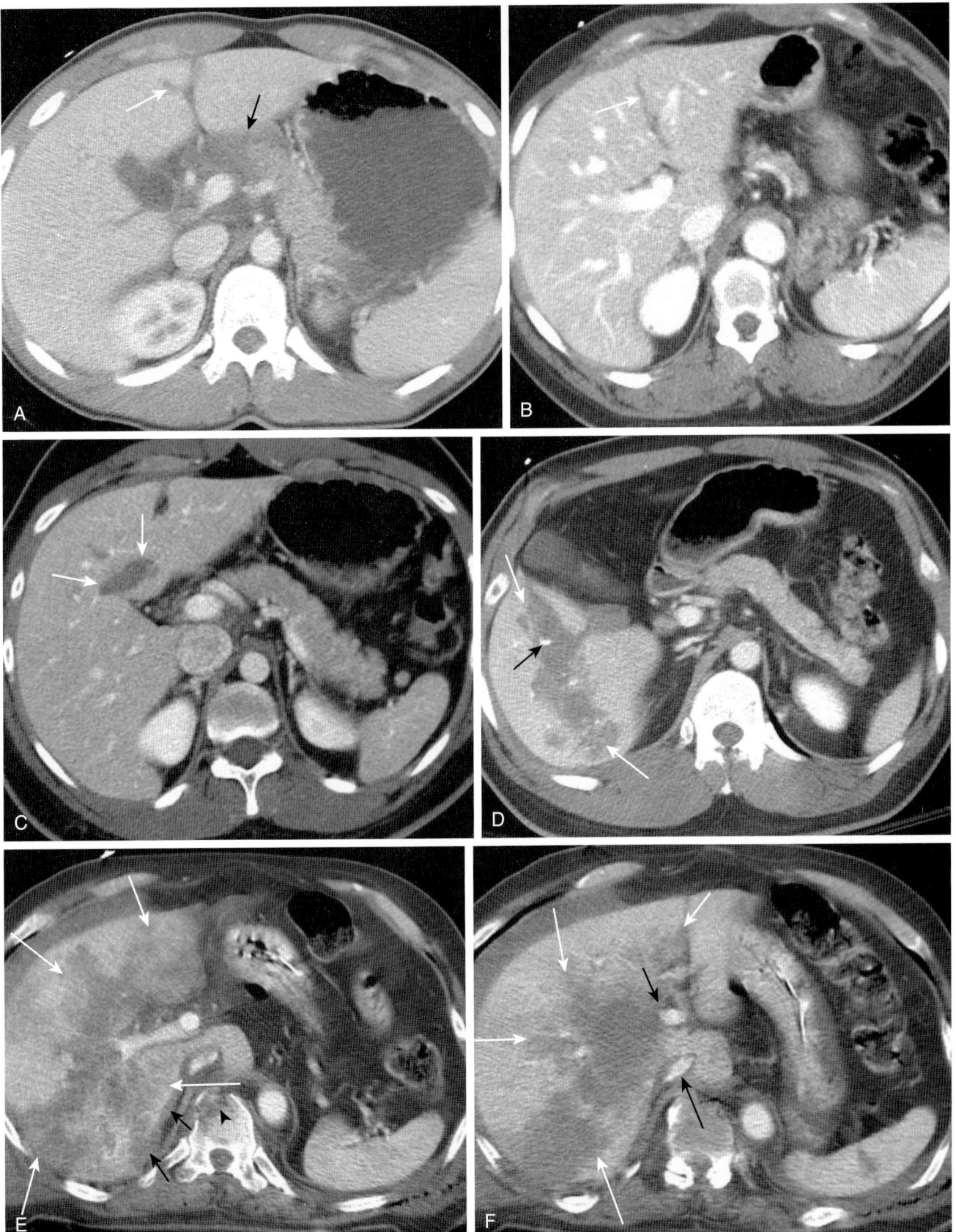

FIGURE 113.1 **Computed tomographic image of hepatic trauma according to the AAST liver injury scale.** **A,** Grade I injury. **B,** Grade II injury. **C,** Grade III injury. **D,** Grade IV injury. **E,** Grade V injury. **F,** Grade VI injury. (Courtesy Dr. R. Thoeni.)

TABLE 113.2 World Society of Emergency Surgery Liver Injury Classification (2020)

	WSES GRADE	AAST	HEMODYNAMIC
Minor	WSES grade I	I-II	Stable
Moderate	WSES grade II	III	Stable
Severe	WSES grade III	IV-V	Stable
	WSES grade IV	I-VI	Unstable

AAST, American Association for the Surgery of Trauma; *WSES,* World Society of Emergency Surgery Liver Injury.

BOX 113.1 Core Principles of Nonoperative Management of Hepatic Trauma

1. NOM is recommended in hemodynamically stable patients with blunt and penetrating hepatic trauma regardless of grade.
2. NOM is considered only after excluding concurrent intestinal injuries.
3. NOM is limited to environments where continuous monitoring, serial clinical evaluations, transfusion, angiographic embolization, and an operating room for urgent laparotomy are available.
4. Patients with hemodynamic instability and peritonitis require urgent operative intervention for hemorrhage control.
5. Intravenous contrast-enhanced computed tomographic scan of the abdomen is the diagnostic modality of choice for evaluating hepatic trauma, and repeat imaging should be guided by the patient's clinical status.
6. Adjunctive therapies, such as angiographic embolization, percutaneous drainage, endoscopy/endoscopic retrograde cholangiopancreatography, and laparoscopy are important adjuncts to NOM.

NOM, Nonoperative management.

timely recognition of intestinal injury can be catastrophic.[48] Although CT enables earlier diagnosis of visceral injury, it is notoriously not sensitive for hollow viscous injury, missing up to 20% of intestinal perforations.[49]

Nonoperative Management of Penetrating Hepatic Trauma

As with blunt hepatic trauma, hemodynamic stability and absence of other operative abdominal injuries are requirements of successful NOM of penetrating injuries to the liver. Historically, mandatory laparotomy was the predominant management strategy for all penetrating wounds of the abdomen. Derived from the experience of blunt hepatic trauma, NOM is becoming an acceptable management option in certain penetrating injuries as well. However, as with blunt trauma, patient selection is paramount, especially in high-energy penetrating mechanisms. The majority of abdominal gunshot wounds (GSWs) still require an immediate exploration, in up to 60% to 80% in modern series.[50,51] Approximately 7% to 15% of patients undergoing NOM for abdominal GSW require a delayed laparotomy.[52,53] Despite this, successful NOM has been reported with both GSW and stab wounds to the liver.[50,51,54-56]

In the absence of an immediate indication for surgery, a CT scan is extremely helpful for visualizing the projectile trajectory, determining the degree of liver injury, and diagnosing associated abdominal injuries, including hollow viscous and other solid organ (kidney, spleen, or pancreas) injuries.[50,57,58] Physical

examination is important, as any clinical changes may prompt an urgent operation, angiography, or further imaging for diagnosis and management of delayed infectious or biliary complications. For this reason, as for blunt hepatic trauma, NOM of penetrating hepatic trauma should be performed only in resource-rich environments.[36]

Failures and Complications of Nonoperative Management of Hepatic Trauma

There is no consensus regarding identifying predictors of failure of NOM for hepatic trauma, whether it be grade of injury, concurrent solid-organ injury, neurologic status, presence of contrast blush on CT scan, or age older than 55 years.[30,31,47,59-61] Yet, several experiences demonstrate that failed NOM requiring a delayed operation has higher mortality,[29,44,47,62] and recurrent or delayed hemorrhage is a common cause of failure of NOM.[36] Given failure of NOM is uncommon but potentially life-threatening, early recognition of hypotension, tachycardia, decline in hematocrit, or new-onset abdominal pain is critical.[20] There is no consensus on how much blood loss or transfusion mandates intervention, whether operatively or angiographically,[30] but patients who demonstrate shock or hemodynamic instability should be taken to the operating room emergently for exploration.

Rarely, hepatic artery pseudoaneurysm after a significant hepatic trauma can rupture and decompress into the adjacent biliary tree, causing hemobilia (see Chapters 115 and 116).[63,64] These patients tend to present weeks to months after the initial trauma with jaundice, abdominal pain, and upper gastrointestinal bleed.[64] Timely angiographic evaluation and embolization can be extremely effective.[65]

Missed hollow viscous injury is a devastating complication of NOM and requires a high index of suspicion. In an intubated and sedated patient, physical examination alone may not be reliable to detect peritonitis. Signs of a missed bowel injury can be subtle changes in the abdominal exam, vital signs, laboratory abnormalities, or derangement from the expected clinical trajectory, all of which should prompt a repeat CT scan or exploration in search of a missed injury. Box 113.2 lists other complications of NOM. Biliary and infectious complications are common, especially after the initial angiographic embolization.[66] Symptomatic lesions can be addressed with adjunctive therapies that are discussed in the following sections.

Adjunctive Therapies of Nonoperative Management of Hepatic Trauma

Patients undergoing NOM often require adjunctive procedures, including angiographic embolization, image-guided percutaneous drainage, endoscopic retrograde cholangiopancreatography

BOX 113.2 Complications of Nonoperative Management of Hepatic Trauma

Delayed or recurrent hemorrhage
Hepatic artery pseudoaneurysm
Biliary complications: bile leak, biliary fistula, bile peritonitis, hemobilia
Infectious complications: hepatic abscess, intraabdominal abscess
Hepatic necrosis
Missed hollow viscous injury
Abdominal compartment syndrome

(ERCP) (see Chapters 16, 20, 21, 30, 31, and 94A), and in some instances, delayed laparoscopy for drainage of bilomas or hematomas.[2,29,31] Necessitation of adjunctive procedures are not "failures" of NOM; rather, they are adjuncts to successful control of hemorrhage and bile leak.

Angiographic embolization is a useful adjunct in NOM of hepatic trauma (see Chapters 21, 94A, 115, and 116). Evidence suggests that liberal use of angiographic embolization is safe and effective to prevent delayed hemorrhage,[67,68] although the standard timing of this is unclear. Advanced injury grading, contrast extravasation, pseudoaneurysm, and large hemoperitoneum on CT scan alone do not mandate angiography,[69,70] but early angiographic embolization should be strongly considered in patients who transiently respond to resuscitation as a first-line therapy for hemorrhage control.[71] Angiographic embolization can also be used postoperatively after a damage control operation to further control devastating injuries.[72]

Image-guided percutaneous drainage plays a key role in NOM of liver injuries. Patients undergoing angiographic embolization are susceptible to developing ischemic complications such as hepatic necrosis, hepatic abscesses, and bile leaks.[66,72,73] Gallbladder infarct and necrosis are well described after right hepatic artery embolization[73,74] (see Chapter 94A). Although a number of these patients require surgical exploration for hepatic resection or washout, most patients with complex liver injuries warrant a discussion with the interventional radiologist for percutaneous drainage as source control. Many patients with high-grade liver injuries often require multiple percutaneous drains for biliary source control (Fig. 113.2), resulting in prolonged hospital stay, and in some instances, delayed exploration.[72] Persistent high-output bile drainage may indicate injury to a segmental or lobar bile duct, and ERCP with biliary decompression is helpful to control these persistent biliary fistulas (see Chapters 20 and 30).[75]

Percutaneous drainage of major hepatic necrosis is not without complication. There are no universally accepted ways of managing major hepatic necrosis of complex liver injuries; benefits and risks of delayed hepatic resection versus multiple percutaneous drains is a field of ongoing debate, and the decision to operate should be determined by an experienced surgeon.[76]

Finally, delayed laparoscopy is a helpful tool for evacuating bile peritonitis or hematoma once successful control of hemorrhage is achieved.[77] This minimally invasive procedure can help inspect the liver surface and drain perihepatic collections under direct vision. Superficial loculations can be carefully lysed, with great caution to avoid disrupting the hemostatic injured area of the liver.

Follow-Up Surveillance and Imaging

Routine follow-up imaging may not be necessary in most cases of hepatic trauma. Serial clinical evaluation and hemoglobin measurement are important. Although there are no clear standard protocols for follow-up and monitoring,[78] persistent fever, abdominal pain, jaundice, acute hemoglobin drop, and gross derangement of transaminases should prompt repeat imaging for sources of biliary sepsis or hemorrhage.[36]

OPERATIVE MANAGEMENT OF PATIENTS WITH HEPATIC TRAUMA

Patients with hemodynamic instability and peritonitis should be considered for exploratory laparotomy regardless of the injury mechanism. General principles of damage control apply, where rapid hemorrhage control, bile leak management, and enteric spillage control take priority during the index surgery. Immediate availability of universal and type-specific blood is mandatory, with early activation of massive transfusion protocols.[79] Exploratory laparotomy is conducted through a generous midline incision for adequate exposure, followed by rapid evisceration of the small bowel and packing of all four abdominal quadrants. Communication with anesthesia providers is key. If major juxtahepatic vena caval or hepatic venous injury is identified, femoral venous lines should be clamped, and adequate supradiaphragmatic IV access is obtained to allow resuscitation with concurrent hemorrhage control.[80] Once adequate resuscitation and hemostasis are present with packing in place, coordinated removal of packs and examination of individual quadrants is appropriate. In the case of major hepatic injury, the right upper quadrant should be the last to be unpacked and explored.

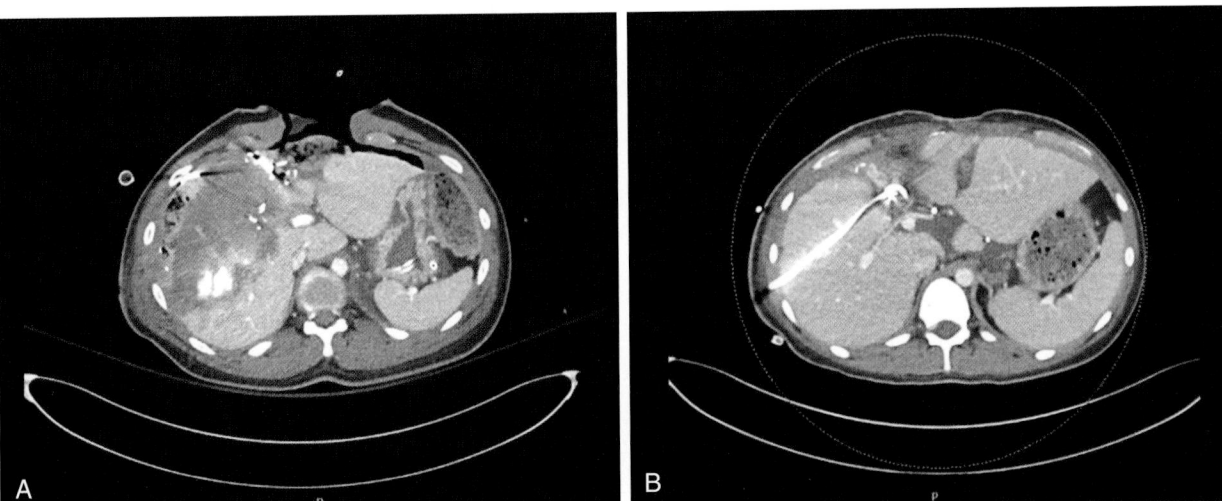

FIGURE 113.2 **Computed tomographic image of a patient with complex liver injury requiring operative and nonoperative interventions.** **A,** Immediate postoperative image after perihepatic packing, right hepatic arterial ligation, and right hepatic arterial branch angioembolization. **B,** Interval scan with percutaneously placed drains for hepatic abscesses and bilomas.

Operative Techniques (see Chapters 101, 118, and 120)

Superficial, Low-Grade Injury

Minor bleeding from grade I and II liver injuries can be managed by manual compression or packing alone. Other simple hemostatic techniques include the use of electrocautery, bipolar devices, or argon beam coagulation to achieve local hemostasis along raw parenchymal surfaces.[81] Topical hemostatic agents can be useful adjuncts. Once bleeding is controlled, these superficial lacerations can be approximated using "liver sutures" if necessary, which are classically heavy chromic catgut sutures on a large blunt needle. For deeper lacerations, placing a healthy portion of omentum and suturing to the liver capsule can serve a similar purpose.

Packing of Deep Hepatic Parenchymal Injury

In the case of major hemorrhage from high-grade liver injuries, manual compression and perihepatic packing can be life-saving maneuvers to temporize bleeding.[36,82] This technique aims to achieve hemostasis by compressing the fractured parenchyma between packs placed above and below. Perihepatic packing must be performed systemically and quickly. First, the surgeon's hands reapproximate the lateral edges of the liver to compress the right and left lobes back to normal anatomy. Simultaneously, the liver is directed posteriorly to tamponade potential venous bleeding.[80] Packs are then placed around the liver to achieve the same effect.

Placing the packs too tightly can compress the inferior vena cava (IVC) and impede venous return to the heart. When this occurs, packs must be removed gradually to identify the degree of packing that achieves hemostasis without causing excessive IVC compression and decreased venous return. If the perihepatic packing alone controls the massive hemorrhage, one may choose to leave the packs in place for a planned removal in 1 to 2 days, or as soon as the associated physiologic derangements and coagulopathies are reversed.[1,83] Some authors suggested using commercially available kaolin-impregnated hemostatic packs in addition to laparotomy packs during damage control operations.[84] Although these products have excellent safety profiles in prehospital wounds[85] and swine models with large liver injuries,[86] their clinical use as perihepatic packing has not been extensively studied.

Although perihepatic packing has been a widely popularized technique of damage control, mesh wrapping techniques in which absorbable mesh is tightly wrapped to reapproximate the shattered liver parenchyma have been reported with successful results in complex liver injuries.[87,88] The major benefit is that using absorbable material theoretically prevents the need for a mandatory reoperation.

It is important to note that packing is an excellent method to control diffuse ooze from venous bleeding, but often is not effective for arterial hemorrhage.[1] Therefore postoperative angiographic embolization (see Chapters 21, 94A, 115, and 116) should be considered in (1) stable patients with contrast blush on postexploration CT scan or (2) those with uncontrolled suspected arterial bleeding despite surgical attempts at hemostasis.[36,89] Immediate postoperative angiography with selective embolization in severe hepatic trauma can be life-saving adjuncts that have been shown to improve mortality.[90,91]

Hepatic Inflow Control

If perihepatic packing fails to control bleeding, the next step is to perform a Pringle maneuver.[80] A surgeon's finger is placed through the foramen of Winslow, posterior to the hepatoduodenal ligament. Another window is created in the gastrohepatic ligament, where an atraumatic clamp can be applied to isolate and compress the porta hepatis. Alternatively, the hilum can be occluded using an umbilical tape and Rummel tourniquet, or a double-looped vessel loop tightened with a large clamp.[80] Intermittent hepatic inflow occlusion is preferred over continuous occlusion if feasible; 15 minutes of clamp time followed by 5 minutes of flow is considered safe in elective hepatic resection[92] for up to 120 minutes.[93] The degree of liver ischemia and perfusion injury from portal clamping is difficult to assess in trauma, which may be confounded by ongoing hypotension.

As a general rule, a Pringle maneuver should only be applied to control major bleeding.[80] This maneuver can be both therapeutic and diagnostic for identifying the source of hepatic bleed. Occluding the inflow will cease bleeding from a hepatic arterial or portal venous source. If bleeding continues despite portal occlusion, this represents back bleeding from the juxtahepatic vena cava or hepatic veins, which necessitates more aggressive operative approaches discussed later. Further, bleeding from aberrant hepatic arteries should be considered in these situations.[36]

Other Techniques for Deep Liver Lacerations

Other techniques have been described performed in conjunction with a Pringle maneuver inflow occlusion. Hepatic debridement and finger-fracture hepatotomy performed under inflow occlusion can help isolate bleeding vessels in deep lacerations.[80,94] Selective vascular ligation can be then be performed using surgical clips and fine sutures. For bleeding involving the left lateral segment, stapled segmentectomy can achieve rapid hemostasis.[80,95] For superficial bullet or knife tracts, stapled tractotomy can expose the injured vessel for ligation.[96] For penetrating trauma with deep tracts into the liver parenchyma not responsive to packing, balloon tamponade can be a helpful technique.[81] A balloon device can be improvised by inserting a red rubber catheter into a 1-inch Penrose drain with both proximal and distal ends secured with heavy silk ties (Fig. 113.3).[97] Alternative techniques have been described using a Sengstaken-Blakemore balloon[98] (see Chapter 81). The balloon device is inserted into the tract and inflated with sterile saline to achieve a tamponade effect. The balloon can be removed during the take back operation.

Delayed Resection versus Serial Debridement

Major hepatic necrosis, a common complication after angiographic embolization (see Chapter 94A) of complex hepatic trauma, can be a conundrum for a trauma surgeon.[72] Early anatomic resection (see Chapters 101 and 102) during index surgery is associated with poor outcomes and death in trauma patients in hemorrhagic shock. Delayed resection of the injured tissue is a safe option once the patient survives life-threatening hemorrhage and is optimized for a planned reoperation. Compared with percutaneous or operative serial debridement, delayed anatomic resection is known to reduce morbidity, the number of procedures required, and length of stay.[76] Deep hepatic lacerations involving the bulk of the liver warrant consideration of early resection. Staying true to the damage control principles described earlier, many trauma surgeons have avoided exploring deep hepatic lacerations in the critically ill, opting instead for reapproximating the liver parenchyma. Although this technique works in some situations, this is not always ideal, as it can lead to internal hemorrhage, abscess, or biliary complications that may need definitive management.[80]

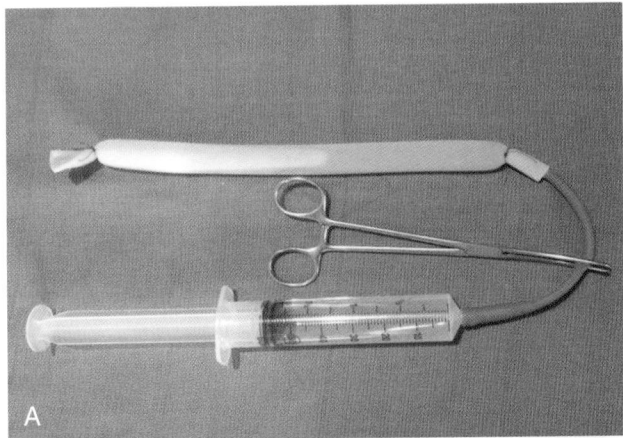

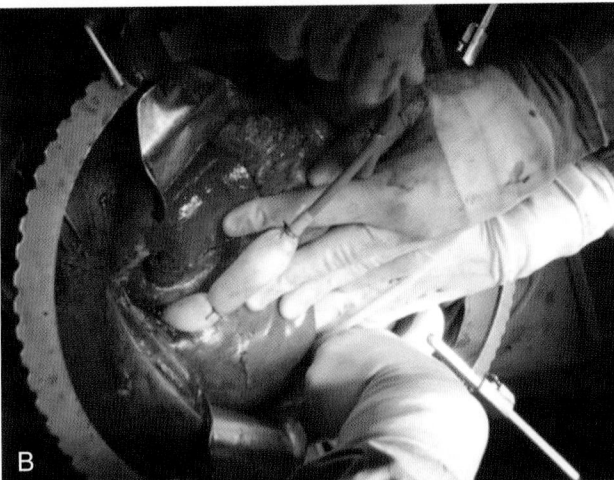

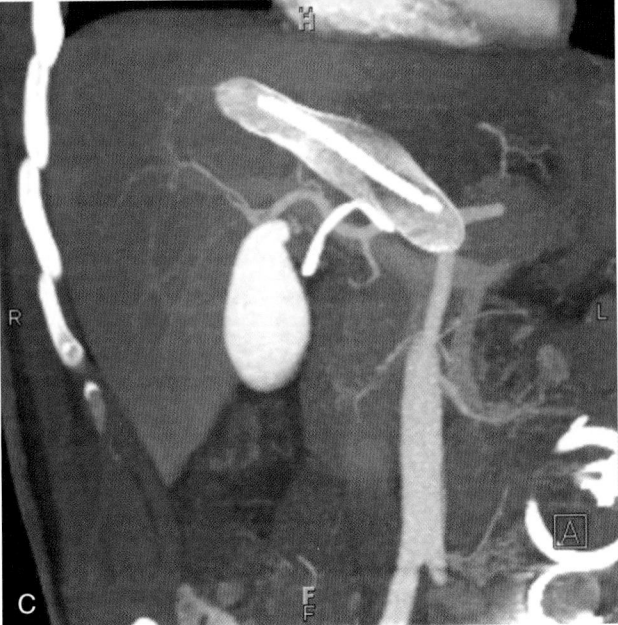

FIGURE 113.3 **Intrahepatic balloon tamponade using Penrose drain and red rubber catheter. A,** Balloon device consists of 1-inch Penrose drain and 12-French red rubber catheter. **B,** Balloon device deployed within the penetrating hepatic injury tract. **C,** Balloon device deployed in a computed tomography image. (Courtesy Dr. E. Haut.)

A minimalist approach is generally safest, as aggressive attempts to explore deep lacerations for hemorrhage control may exacerbate bleeding and rapid physiologic deterioration in a critically ill patient. Perihepatic packing, when successful, is the best approach, and immediate postoperative angiographic embolization can be a life-saving adjunct in the acute period.

Hepatic Arterial Injury

Injury to the proper hepatic artery should be repaired primarily if possible (see Chapter 122). If repair is not feasible and the patient is too unstable to undergo angiographic embolization, selective hepatic artery ligation is a viable option.[36,80] When the right hepatic artery is ligated, cholecystectomy (see Chapter 36) has been recommended to avoid subsequent gallbladder necrosis[80]; however, in the nontrauma setting, for embolization of liver tumors, gallbladder necrosis is rare, occurring only in the setting of errant injection of embolic material into the cystic artery.

Portal Venous Injury

Injury to the portal vein should also be repaired primarily if possible (see Chapter 122). Main portal vein ligation is ill-advised because of a high risk of developing liver necrosis and bowel edema and necrosis.[36] In this scenario, perihepatic packing is preferred to ligation of segmental or subsegmental branches.[36]

Bleeding From the Juxtahepatic Vena Cava and Hepatic Veins

When juxtahepatic vena caval or hepatic venous injury is suspected, there are three viable surgical options: (1) tamponade with perihepatic packing, (2) direct repair (with or without hepatic isolation; see Chapter 122), and (3) lobar resection (see Chapters 101 and 118).[36] In most cases, tamponade with perihepatic packing is the safest option.

Two types of juxtahepatic venous injury patterns are described.[99] Buckman type A injuries are major hepatic venous injuries from extensive parenchymal disruption, where bleeding is seen through the injured liver.[99] Rapid manual compression and perihepatic packing can typically contain and tamponade low-pressure venous bleeding. The Pringle maneuver should be attempted. Applying posterior and inferior traction of the falciform ligament to compress the IVC with the liver mass can help tamponade the bleed.[80]

Buckman type B injuries are extraparenchymal and involve a large defect of the retrohepatic IVC. Massive bleeding can be seen pooling around and posterior to the liver. It is associated with disruption of the suspensory ligaments and the diaphragm, which typically help contain the venous bleeding.[99] Compression, perihepatic packing, and the Pringle maneuver alone may not stop the bleeding in these situations. Although these injuries are rare, when this is suspected, a rapid mobilization of the hemiliver is made to expose the retrohepatic IVC.[80] A side-biting vascular clamp can help control the IVC bleed and allow for primary repair. If this is insufficient, complete occlusion proximal and distal to the injury is performed in a technique known as complete vascular isolation.[80,100] Partial hepatectomy may be required for hemorrhage control and IVC exposure in some cases[101]; however, any major resection in acute hemorrhagic shock should be cautioned because of high mortality.[99]

Various techniques of hepatic exclusion and shunts have been described for direct vascular repair (see Chapter 122). A venoveno bypass is a described but rarely used method.[36,80] The atriocaval shunt is by far the most well-known technique for vascular isolation (Fig. 113.4).[12] After performing a median sternotomy

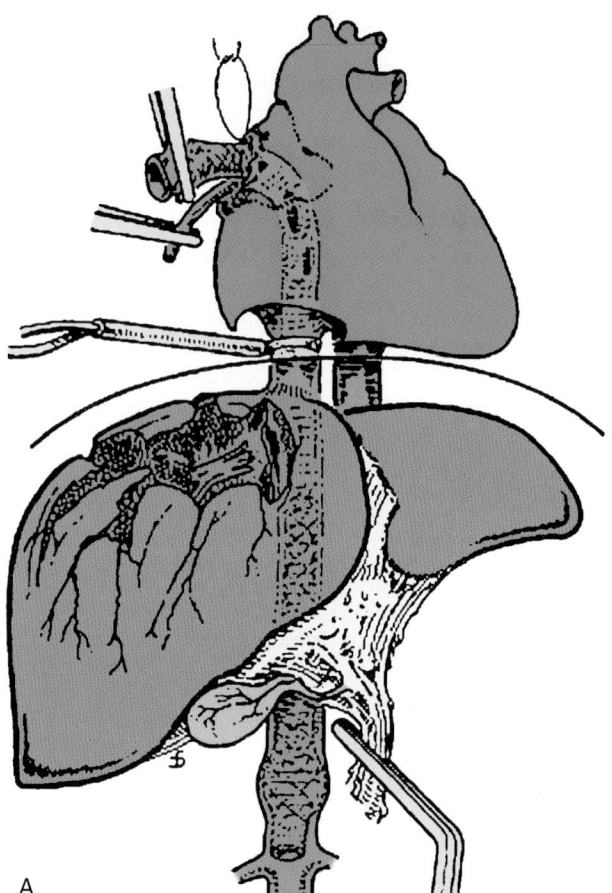

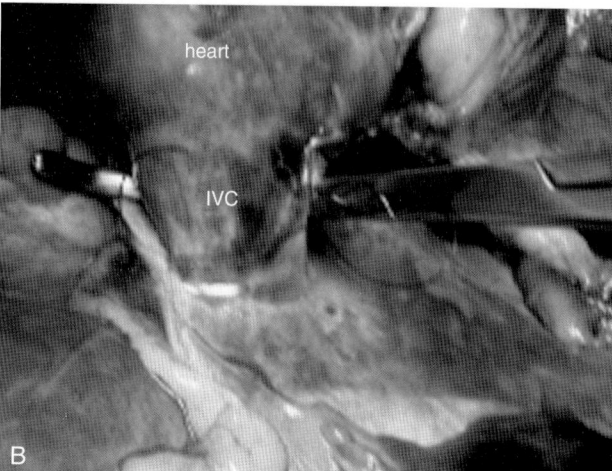

FIGURE 113.4 **Atriocaval shunt.** IVC, Inferior vena cava.

or a resuscitative thoracotomy, a chest tube is inserted through the right arterial appendage and threaded down the IVC near the renal veins. Rummel tourniquets are used to tighten around the IVC and the stent near the pericardium and just above the renal veins. This maneuver shunts the venous return to the heart while bypassing the injured caval segment, enabling the surgeon to repair the vein. It is a technically difficult technique with high mortality, often complicated by the fact that the decision to perform the shunt occurs later in the operation when other options have failed.[36]

Vascular isolation of the injured liver is always challenging. Cross-clamping the vena cava is generally poorly tolerated by the hypovolemic patient. This can be a technically difficult maneuver as well. Although the infrahepatic cava can be more easily isolated while performing the Pringle maneuver, dissection of the infradiaphragmatic suprahepatic vena cava can be challenging, especially for the emergency surgeon who infrequently operates in this region. Even in the most experienced hands, mortality rates in liver injuries requiring shunting are reported to be over 88%.[1]

In recent years, resuscitative endovascular balloon occlusion of the aorta (REBOA) catheter has been utilized in hemorrhage control. Concurrently, a resuscitative endovascular balloon occlusion of the vena cava (REBOVC) can be inserted through the femoral venous catheter to occlude the retrohepatic vena cava. The goal of this maneuver is to obtain proximal and distal control of the retrohepatic vessel injury using the two REBOVC

catheters, ultimately achieving hepatic exclusion using a hybrid endovascular/open approach with the Pringle maneuver.[102]

In rare cases of hepatic avulsion or total crush injury, liver transplant (see Chapter 105) has been described in the literature.[103] Extracorporeal support for trauma-induced hepatic dysfunction is available in limited centers.[104]

Urgent versus Planned Reoperation

In the setting of damage control techniques, indications for urgent reoperation in patients with hepatic injury are (1) continued hemorrhage, (2) abdominal compartment syndrome, and (3) missed injury. Incomplete hemostasis of the original injury is a common cause of urgent reoperative intervention, followed by missed injury, iatrogenic complications, or diffuse coagulopathy.[105] Rebleeding from hepatic injury may be difficult to control, and mortality is high. Vigilance in recognizing early signs of bleeding is crucial for timely interventions.

Patients with extensive abdominal injury, especially with concurrent large-volume resuscitations, are at higher risk of developing abdominal compartment syndrome. In these cases, an urgent decompressive laparotomy is necessary with temporary abdominal closure.

Planned reoperation is an integral part of managing hepatic trauma after the initial damage control laparotomy. In general, the patient is reexplored 24 to 48 hours after the initial operation, once hemodynamic stability is achieved. Although the data are not robust, early (<24 hours) removal of perihepatic packing is associated with increased bleeding, whereas leaving the packs beyond 72 hours increases infectious risks.[106,107]

Extreme care should be taken when removing perihepatic packing. This should be done slowly with ample amounts of warm irrigation to avoid excessive tearing of the raw surfaces of the liver that can cause rebleeding. Any additional bleeding can be addressed with the argon beam coagulator or other forms of local hemostatic techniques. If there is gross necrosis visible, further nonanatomic debridement can be considered with local wide drainage. Ongoing bleeding should prompt repacking. It is important to avoid aggressive attempts at hemostasis or surgical resection, as an injured liver can be edematous and friable, making it more susceptible to bleeding and iatrogenic injury.

Extrahepatic Biliary Injury

Extrahepatic biliary injury is rare, seen in only 0.1% of adult trauma.[108,109] Isolated injury to the extrahepatic biliary system is even rarer, as it is typically associated with concurrent liver, pancreas, and duodenum trauma (see Chapter 114).[110] The AAST and WSES classifications of injuries are presented in Table 113.3.[110,111] Although rare, delayed, or missed injuries to the biliary tree can lead to morbid complications. CT scan can be a useful diagnostic tool in hemodynamically stable patients. FAST or DPL are not reliable ways to diagnose extrahepatic biliary tree injury. Hepatobiliary iminodiacetic acid (HIDA) scans (see Chapter 18) are not advisable in the setting of acute trauma because of long scan times and limited resource availability.[110]

NOM of extrahepatic biliary injuries can be considered in the absence of other abdominal injuries requiring surgery as long as the patient remains hemodynamically stable. However, this strategy does require serial examination, ability to repeat imaging, and availability and low threshold to offer advanced endoscopic and percutaneous interventions for biliary decompression.[110]

Similar to hepatic injuries, hemodynamically unstable patients must undergo rapid surgical exploration. Many of the extrahepatic biliary tree injuries are found intraoperatively. For isolated gallbladder injury, cholecystectomy (see Chapter 36) is the treatment of choice.[109] However, in an unstable coagulopathic patient with extensive blood loss or significant liver injury, it may be unwise to perform a complete cholecystectomy during the initial damage control surgery, as it creates a further surface for hemorrhage. In this case, a tube cholecystostomy for bile control may be a safer option (see Chapter 35).

Small lacerations of the extrahepatic biliary ducts can be managed with primary closure with absorbable suture and external drainage. Primary closure over T-tube can be considered as well.[112] For moderate to severe injuries (AAST IV–V, WSES II–III), hepaticojejunostomy or choledochojejunostomy ultimately must be considered[109,113] (see Chapter 32). For patients with multiple injuries undergoing initial damage control procedures, extrahepatic biliary injury can be stabilized with drainage, and further definitive reconstruction should be performed in a staged approach.[110] For intrapancreatic bile duct injury, primary ductal repair over T-tube or duodenal diversion can be considered.[113] Hepatic or pancreatic resections are reserved for extreme circumstances in which biliary reconstruction is not possible[109] (see Chapter 114).

Failure of NOM in extrahepatic biliary injuries should warrant an evaluation for hepaticojejunostomy.[110] Long-term sequelae of biliary strictures can be managed with ERCP and stent placement (see Chapter 30)[114]; however, failed endoscopic

TABLE 113.3 American Association for the Surgery of Trauma (1994 Revision) and World Society of Emergency Surgery (2019) Classification of Extrahepatic Biliary Injury

GRADE	AAST[a]	INJURY DESCRIPTION	WSES
Minor	I	Gallbladder contusion Portal triad contusion	I
	II	Partial gallbladder avulsion from liver bed; cystic duct intact Laceration or perforation of the gallbladder	
	III	Complete gallbladder avulsion from liver bed Cystic duct laceration/transection	
Moderate	IV	Partial or complete right hepatic duct laceration Partial or complete left hepatic duct laceration Partial common hepatic duct laceration (≤50%) Partial common bile duct laceration (≤50%)	II
Severe	V	>50% transection of common hepatic duct >50% transection of common bile duct Combined right and left hepatic duct injuries Intraduodenal or intrapancreatic bile duct injuries	III

[a]Advance one grade for multiple injuries, up to grade III.
AAST, American Association for the Surgery of Trauma; *WSES,* World Society of Emergency Surgery Liver Injury.

management should undergo hepaticojejunostomy reconstruction[115] (see Chapter 32).

CONCLUSION

NOM of hemodynamically stable patients with hepatobiliary trauma, from both blunt and penetrating mechanisms, has become the standard method of care. With this approach, patient selection is important. These patients require close monitoring and early utilization of adjunctive therapies to manage the sequelae and complications.

Hemodynamically unstable patients require emergent exploration, although most patients with significant hemorrhage can and should be managed with perihepatic packing to allow resuscitation and hemostasis. A hybrid approach with perioperative angiographic embolization can be life-saving. Rarely, a patient with a juxtahepatic vena caval injury will not respond to packing or hepatic inflow control. In this situation, an early decision to achieve proximal and distal vascular control of the liver is essential. Even in the most experienced hands, mortality for significant juxtahepatic vena caval injuries remains high.

Isolated injuries to the extrahepatic biliary tract are uncommon. Hemodynamically unstable patients should be managed with damage control techniques, and definitive reconstructions of the biliary tract should only be undertaken when the patient is stable.

The references for this chapter can be found online by accessing the accompanying Expert Consult website.

CHAPTER 114

Pancreatic and duodenal injuries

Michael Farrell and Andre Campbell

INTRODUCTION

Injuries to the pancreas and the duodenum are some of the most feared injuries in trauma. Because of the location of the pancreatoduodenal complex (PDC) and the surrounding structures, even simple injuries are complicated and have the potential of major long-term consequences (see Chapter 2). In this chapter, we will review the history of pancreatic and duodenal injuries, as well as current recommendations for diagnosing and managing injuries through a variety of approaches, ranging from nonoperative to damage control techniques. Throughout this discussion, it is imperative to remember that success in managing injuries to the PDC depends on having a high index of suspicion and using safe operative principles.

HISTORY

Injuries to the PDC were originally described in autopsy observations. The first reported blunt pancreatic injury was published by Travers in 1827.[1] By the early 1900s, there were only 45 reported cases, but this quickly grew in the 1920s after Walton described distal pancreatectomy (see Chapter 117B).[2] Although many modifications have been made to this procedure over the last 100 years, the principles hold true: adequate exposure, hemostasis, and wide drainage.

As often is true in trauma surgery, we did see a reduction in pancreatic mortality through the experience of war. Only a handful of reports are available for pancreatic injuries in the Civil War and World War I, but by World War II, there were 62 reported duodenal injuries with an associated 56% mortality. In the Korean War, the number of cases decreased to 9 cases, but the mortality improved to 22%.[3] Duodenal injuries have been notoriously difficult to manage throughout history. The earliest reported series of traumatic duodenal ruptures came from Berry and Giuseppi,[4] who reported 29 patients with duodenal injuries, all of whom died. The largest series of military-related duodenal injuries to date came from World War II, which identified 118 cases and described an associated 56% mortality.

Despite high levels of motor vehicle collisions and penetrating trauma, pancreatic and duodenal injuries remain rare. A review of the United Kingdom's Trauma Audit and Research Network database found that PDC trauma occurs in 0.32% of cases, with a male-to-female ratio of 2.5:1.[5] Unfortunately, these cases are often lethal, with a reported mortality of approximately 20% in both pancreatic and duodenal trauma, irrespective of the mechanism.[5] This high rate of mortality is often due to exsanguination secondary to injuries of other organs.[5] One-third of patients with an injury to the pancreas or the duodenum will have a concomitant injury, with 58% having an injury to the stomach, 57% having an injury to the liver (see Chapter 113), and 35% having a vascular injury.[6] Variables associated with predicting mortality include increased age, increased injury severity score, and hemodynamic compromise

SURGICAL ANATOMY OF THE PANCREAS AND DUODENUM: A TRAUMA SURGEON'S PERSPECTIVE

The pancreas and the duodenum are uniquely situated in that they are both surrounded by critical structures and both are not immediately accessible. It is the complexity of their structures that requires a detailed anatomic understanding of both the pancreas and duodenum (see Chapter 2) separately, and as the combined PDC.

The duodenum is a mostly retroperitoneal structure that begins at the pylorus and extends to the ligament of Treitz. The second portion of the duodenum contains the ampulla of Vater, which is where the pancreatic ducts enter the duodenum to allow the flow of pancreatic fluid and bile. The proximal pancreas consists of the head, uncinate process, and neck. The head of the pancreas is held within the C loop of the duodenum. The uncinate process extends to the left behind the superior mesenteric vessels. The distal pancreas consists of the body and tail; the body of the pancreas rests over the aorta, and the tail of the pancreas extends to the splenic hilum.

The vasculature of the pancreas and duodenum is robust (see Chapter 2). The PDC is fed by the gastroduodenal, superior mesenteric, and splenic arteries, with substantial collateralization. The gastroduodenal artery branches into the superior pancreaticoduodenal artery, which further divides into anterior and posterior branches. The inferior pancreaticoduodenal artery is a branch from the superior mesenteric artery, and it also subdivides into anterior and posterior branches. There are multiple variations to the blood supply (see Chapter 2), with 15% to 20% of patients having a replaced right hepatic artery from the superior mesenteric artery.[7] The splenic artery runs posterior to the pancreas along the length of the body and tail. All of these vessels originate in close proximity to each other, which can make controlling hemorrhage difficult in the setting of a devastating trauma.

DIAGNOSIS OF PANCREATIC AND DUODENAL TRAUMA (IMAGING AND GRADING)

The initial workup in any trauma situation begins with the primary and secondary assessment as described in the American College of Surgeons Advanced Trauma Life Support (ATLS) course.[8] Even with the trauma evaluation algorithm taught in ATLS, it is essential to have a high level of suspicion when assessing for pancreatic and duodenal injuries. If the patient is hemodynamically unstable, and the source of distress based on physical examination is intraabdominal, the patient should be explored immediately. If the patient is hemodynamically stable or the source of distress is unclear, it is reasonable to consider additional imaging. In the trauma setting, the first imaging available will often be a chest x-ray or a focused abdominal sonography for trauma (FAST) examination. The FAST examination is an ultrasound that looks for free fluid in the right upper quadrant, left upper quadrant, and pelvis and signs of pericardial effusion or tamponade.[8] The FAST will often be of limited value for diagnosing pancreatic and duodenal injuries because of their retroperitoneal location.[9] If the imaging is grossly positive and the patient is hemodynamically unstable, this should be taken as sufficient evidence to proceed to the operating room for exploration. Additionally, penetrating abdominal trauma that violates the fascia also requires exploration.

In patients who are hemodynamically stable and have experienced blunt trauma, it is reasonable to pursue additional imaging. Missed injuries may result in significant morbidity and mortality.[10] Findings suggestive of a duodenal injury include wall thickening greater than 4 mm, lack of wall continuity, periduodenal fluid, fluid in the right anterior pararenal space, diminished bowel-wall enhancement, and extraluminal air or contrast.[11] Multidetector computed tomography (MDCT) imaging is 98% accurate for stomach and duodenal perforations.[12] The FAST examination has mostly replaced diagnostic peritoneal lavage (DPL), but some do consider DPL a helpful adjunct in an otherwise stable trauma patient with unexplained findings on computed tomography (CT). In this situation, DPL can be as high as 100% sensitive for bowel injuries.[13] More commonly, diagnostic laparoscopy or exploratory laparotomy are used in these cases.[14]

Pancreatic injuries are more complicated to identify. Overall, CT imaging has a sensitivity of 70% to 95% for detecting pancreatic injuries.[15] With MDCT, imaging accurately identified the grade of pancreatic injury in 91% of patients.[16] MDCT imaging has the greatest sensitivity in the detection of main duct injuries and is 97.9% sensitive in the parenchymal phase and 100% sensitive in the portal venous phase at identifying pancreatic duct injuries. This suggests that the portal venous phase is the best contrast phase to assess the pancreas in the setting of blunt trauma[15] (see Chapter 17).

The management of pancreatic injuries is primarily based on pancreatic duct involvement. Consequently, it is imperative that the status of the duct be assessed in patients where there is a concern for injury, such as those with parenchymal lacerations with moderate peripancreatic fluid.[14] In patients who are hemodynamically stable, endoscopic retrograde cholangiopancreatography (ERCP) or magnetic resonance cholangiopancreatography (MRCP) (see Chapters 17 and 30) may be of

value.[17,18] ERCP allows for an intervention to be completed at the same time as diagnosis; however, ERCP is an invasive procedure with its own risk of complications and it may miss injuries to nearby structures. MRCP is noninvasive and may be used to assess additional structures, but it does not offer a means to intervene. The sensitivity of MRCP can be enhanced with the addition of secretin stimulation.[19]

Some patients will require surgical intervention before imaging is available. In this case, it is important to assess the duodenum and pancreas intraoperatively. Later, how to best visualize the duodenum and pancreas will be discussed, but the principal goals are to mobilize the duodenum to facilitate a circumferential evaluation and to fully visualize the pancreas to assess for any obvious ductal injury. If there is any concern for a ductal injury, it is reasonable to proceed with an intraoperative fluoroscopic cholecystocholangiograph. This may be performed by inserting an angiocatheter into the gallbladder and injecting 20 to 30 mL of water-soluble contrast. The visualization may be made easier by mixing methylene blue with the contrast material. Intravenous morphine can also be used to promote contraction of the sphincter of Oddi to help visualize the pancreatic ducts.[20] An intraoperative ERCP also may be considered if the patient is hemodynamically stable. Historically, pancreatograms were obtained by creating an enterotomy in the duodenum to cannulate the ampulla of Vater; however, this has fallen out of favor and is not recommended by the American College of Surgeons (ACS). However, one scenario in which the pancreatogram is still supported by the ACS is if the distal pancreas is already injured, in which case is reasonable to cannulate the distal duct for a contrast or methylene blue study.[20]

The American Association for the Surgery of Trauma (AAST) has provided a grading system for the pancreas and the duodenum.[21] This grading system is helpful in operative decision making, as well as prognostication (Tables 114.1 and 114.2). Serial laboratory tests may be of value for individuals with potential pancreatic injuries but for whom imaging was not definitive and a reliable examination cannot be followed. In these cases, serum amylase and lipase should be obtained at admission and trended every 6 hours.[14] A normal initial serum lipase has a negative predictive value of 99.8%, but it is greatly limited in its ability to predict injuries, with a positive predictive value of only 3.3%.[22] Persistently elevated or rising serum

TABLE 114.1	Pancreatic Injury Scale			
GRADE[a]	TYPE OF INJURY	DESCRIPTION OF INJURY	ICD-9	AIS-90
I	Hematoma	Minor contusion without duct injury	863.81-863.84	2
	Laceration	Superficial laceration without duct injury		2
II	Hematoma	Major contusion without duct injury or tissue loss	863.81-863.84	2
	Laceration	Major laceration without duct injury or tissue loss		3
III	Laceration	Distal transection or parenchymal injury with duct injury	863.92/863.94	3
IV	Laceration	Proximal[b] transection or parenchymal injury involving ampulla	863.91	4
V	Laceration	Massive disruption of pancreatic head	863.91	5

[a]Advance one grade for multiple injuries up to grade III. 863.51, 863.91: head; 863.99, 862.92: body; 863.83, 863.93: tail.

[b]Proximal pancreas is to the patient's right of the superior mesenteric vein.

AIS, Abbreviated Injury Score; *ICD,* International Classification of Diseases.

From Moore EE, Burch JM, Francioise RJ, et al. Staged physiologic restoration and damage control surgery. *World J Surg.* 1998;22:1184–1190.

TABLE 114.2 Duodenum Injury Scale

GRADE[a]	TYPE OF INJURY	DESCRIPTION OF INJURY	ICD-9	AIS-90
I	Hematoma	Involving single portion of duodenum	863.21	2
	Laceration	Partial thickness, no perforation	863.21	3
II	Hematoma	Involving more than one portion	863.21	2
	Laceration	Disruption <50% of circumference	863.31	4
III	Laceration	Disruption 50%-75% of circumference of D2	863.31	4
		Disruption 50%-100% of circumference of D1, D3, D4	863.31	4
IV	Laceration	Disruption >75% of circumference of D2	863.31	5
		Involving ampulla or distal common bile duct		5
V	Laceration	Massive disruption of duodenopancreatic complex	863.31	5
	Vascular	Devascularization of duodenum	863.31	5

[a]Advance one grade for multiple injuries up to grade III.

AIS, Abbreviated Injury Score; *ICD, International Classification of Diseases; D1,* first position of duodenum; *D2,* second portion of duodenum; *D3,* third portion of duodenum; *D4,* fourth portion of duodenum.

From Moore EE, Burch JM, Francioise RJ, et al. Staged physiologic restoration and damage control surgery. *World J Surg.* 1998;22:1184–1190.

amylase and lipase levels, however, have a combined 100% specificity and 85% sensitivity for predicting pancreatic injury and may be of some value.[23]

OPERATIVE EXPOSURE OF INJURIES TO THE PANCREAS AND DUODENUM

Once it is determined that a patient needs operative exploration, the patient should be taken emergently/urgently to the operating room. The patient should be placed in a supine position and should be broadly prepped, typically from the neck to mid-thighs. It is important to have excellent communication between the surgical and anesthesia teams, because significant hemodynamic changes may occur with the release of hemoperitoneum on entry into the abdomen and when entering the lesser sac. A trauma laparotomy is customarily through a midline approach. It is imperative that the surgeon be prepared to pack all four quadrants and control any major bleeding. The full approach of a trauma laparotomy and damage control techniques are beyond the scope of this chapter, but the surgeon should then proceed in a systematic approach with the goals of hemostasis, stopping and potentially fixing gross contamination, and completing a full exploration of the abdomen.

Specifically, for pancreatic and duodenal trauma, the operative management begins with a thorough inspection of the structures anterior to them. Attention should be paid to assess the distal stomach, pylorus, and gastrohepatic ligament for signs of bile stainage. The transverse colon should be elevated to assess for a hematoma at its base that may indicate an injury to the pancreas or the third or fourth portion of the duodenum. Consideration of nonoperative management in stable patients will be discussed later, but it is worth noting that once in the operating room, any hematomas to the duodenum or pancreas warrant inspection.

A Kocher maneuver is used when there are signs of trauma to the head/neck of the pancreas or the C-loop of the duodenum (see Chapter 117A). This technique separates the lateral peritoneal attachments of the duodenum, and it should be extended distally onto the duodenum. In situations in which additional visualization is required, a right-sided medial visceral rotation (Cattell-Braasch maneuver) can further expose the midline of the

retroperitoneum (zone 1) while also showing the right lateral retroperitoneal (zone 2) structures. This maneuver is completed by mobilizing the white line of Toldt from the cecum up to and including the hepatic flexure. Through the combination of the Kocher and Cattell-Braash maneuver, the entire duodenum and the majority of the pancreas should be able to be visualized. It does, however, have limited exposure of the duodenal-jejunal junction. This occurs at the ligament of Treitz, and it can be easily visualized by dividing the ligament of Treitz.

The pancreas lies in the lesser sac. To fully assess the anterior portion of the pancreas, one can divide the gastrocolic omentum. By simply moving the stomach superiorly the peritoneal coverage of the pancreas can be seen and sharply divided. In this position, the entire anterior pancreas can be assessed. The posterior pancreas is best visualized with an Aird maneuver. This is completed by sharply taking down the lienophrenic and lienocolic ligaments. The spleen is then grasped and delivered into the operative field, with the pancreatic tail. The combination of the Kocher and Aird maneuvers allow for complete exposure of the anterior and posterior portions of the pancreas.

MANAGEMENT OF INJURIES TO THE PANCREAS

The management of pancreatic injuries depends on two main factors: the hemodynamic status of the patient and the grade of injury. If a patient is not hemodynamically stable enough to tolerate a prolonged procedure, damage control techniques should be implemented.

In the absence of additional injuries, hemodynamically stable patients with grade I and grade II injuries often can be managed nonoperatively. The majority of the available research on nonoperative management of pancreatic trauma has focused on the pediatric population. From these studies, we have observed that approximately 90% of patients will be successful with nonoperative management.[24–26] Nonoperative management is similar for pediatric and adult patients, and the exact treatment approach depends on hemodynamic stability, clinical presentation, and associated injuries.[14] Mild injuries discovered in the operating room are often able to be managed with wide drainage and hemostasis.[14,27]

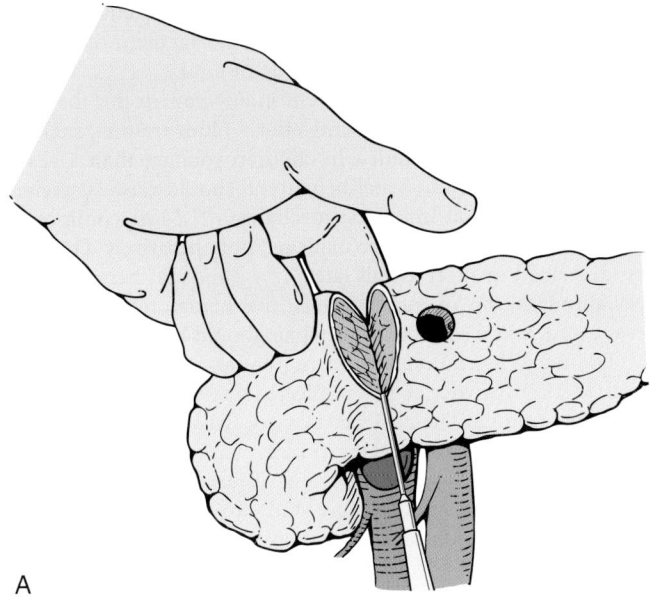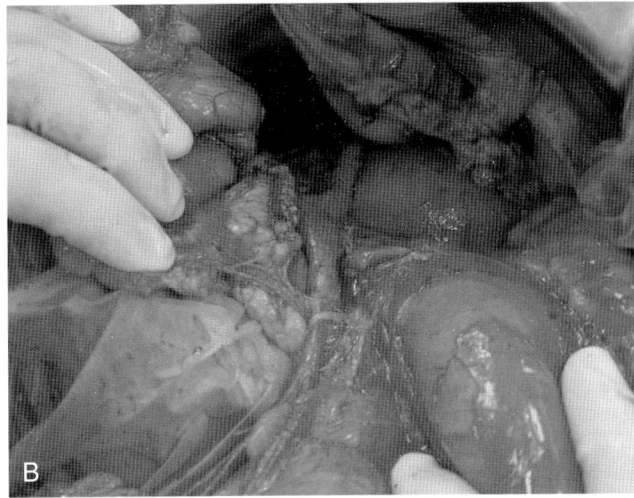

FIGURE 114.1 **A,** Division of pancreas to expose portal vein. **B,** Portal vein injury with distal pancreatectomy and splenic preservation.

Grade III pancreatic injuries are distal and are often managed with a distal pancreatectomy (Fig. 114.1) (see Chapter 117BA). There is no difference in the rate of complications between a stapled distal pancreatectomy and a scalpel resection that is over-sewn. A stapled approach is commonly performed because of consideration of time in the operating room, but both approaches are safe.[28] In the trauma situation, a distal pancreatectomy often should be accompanied by a splenectomy because of the significant risk of vascular compromise or splenic injury. That said, if the surgeon elects not to perform a splenectomy, careful attention must be paid to assess for any injuries from the initial trauma and from the pancreatectomy. After transection of the pancreas, the duct should be visualized and suture ligated, as this has been associated with decreased leak rates.[29] This step is less of a concern if a stapler is used for the pancreatectomy, but the duct still warrants consideration before closure of the abdomen. Similarly, wide drainage should be left in place at the time of closure.

Grade IV injuries are those that lacerate the pancreas proximal to the superior mesenteric vein or those that involve the ampulla of Vater. It is often best to perform damage control techniques in these patients. Considerations in these situations include packing, suture ligation, and completing a pancreatectomy. Pancreaticoduodenectomy (see Chapter 117AA) for trauma, also known as the "trauma Whipple" is an often discussed but rarely used technique. Thompson et al.[30] presented the largest single-center case series in 2013 that included 15 patients over a 15-year period.[30] In this cohort, 80% of patients first required a damage control surgery because of acidosis, hypothermia, and coagulopathy. The operative time for patients who received a damage control procedure was 243 ± 112 minutes compared with 460 ± 98 minutes in patients who had a pancreatectomy completed at the initial operation. The overall mortality was 13%, which is the lowest reported mortality in the available literature for the "trauma Whipple" procedure. The authors suggest this success was in part related to the high usage of damage control techniques at the first operation. Alternatives to the

pancreaticoenteric anastomosis include total pancreatectomy with islet cell autotransplantation (see Chapter 112A) and ductal ligation with preservation of the distal pancreas. Institutional capabilities must be considered with these options. Further discussion of the technical aspects of these procedures is beyond the scope of this chapter.

There are risks and benefits of parenchymal preservation and parenchymal resection. Specifically, preservation of damaged pancreas may result in fistula formation, secondary hemorrhage, and wound complications. Alternatively, resection could result in pancreatic insufficiency (see Chapter 3A).[31] It is important to consider the risk-versus-benefit ratio in each scenario. In general, an accepted approach is to use close-suction drainage for proximal pancreatic injuries that are not devastating in nature. Distal injuries without duct involvement may also be managed with closed-suction drainage. If there is any ductal involvement or if the injury is severe, it should be managed with a distal pancreatectomy (see Chapter 117B).[32]

Pancreatic Injuries in the Stable Patient

Nonoperative management may be considered in hemodynamically stable patients with isolated grade I or grade II pancreatic injuries. These patients must be expectantly observed in a facility that has urgent endoscopic, interventional radiologic, and surgical intervention availability. Serum amylase and lipase should be obtained at admission and trended every 6 hours.[14] Decreasing enzyme levels have been correlated with predicting success of nonoperative management.[33] The specific management of these patients must be individualized. Some will likely require percutaneous drainage, whereas others may benefit from endoscopic drainage or may not require drainage at all. In one retrospective study, ERCP with stent placement allowed 25% of patients to be managed nonoperatively.[17] We recommend keeping the patient initially nil per os and, based on clinical judgement, determine how best to advance nutrition (see Chapter 26). The more significant the injury, the higher the likelihood that the patient will fail nonoperative management.

Postoperative Pancreatic Complications

Postoperative pancreatic complications (see Chapter 28) are very common when the procedures are performed for trauma. It is the responsibility of the surgeon to anticipate the complications so as to minimize the morbidity associated with them. The most common complication is the formation of a pancreatic fistula (see Chapter 117A).[14] This occurs approximately 20% of the time and is defined as persistent pancreatic drainage after postoperative day 3, with the amylase level greater than three times that in the serum.[34] Drains should be left in place at the time of abdominal closure, and we recommend keeping the drains in place until the output is minimal when the patient is tolerating an oral diet. If a pancreatic fistula does develop, the drain should be left in place. Most patients can be fed through the drainage, but some patients will require parenteral nutrition to decrease pancreatic stimulation (see Chapter 26). Somatostatin analogues may also decrease the volume in high-output fistulas, which will make them more likely to resolve. In a Cochrane study, the rate of fistula formation decreased by 34% when somatostatin analogues were used.[35] Approximately 95% of all fistulas will resolve with drainage and time. Success is even higher for those fistulas with less than 200 mL/day output.[36] If the leak persists, or there is concern for missed injury, it is reasonable to consider an ERCP with stent and sphincterotomy.[17] The ERCP does require manipulation of the recent traumatized tissue, and the risks of complications are higher in this population than normal. Therefore it should be completed only by experienced providers and in situations in which the benefits truly outweigh the risks.[37,38] There is limited literature available to help guide this decision but what is published suggests a high rate of success. A single retrospective study of 1550 ERCPs completed by a single provider for patients with high-output fistulas (>200 mL/day) or persistent fistulas (failure to resolve within 30 days), described a 100% success rate with fistula resolution.[39]

The development of postoperative fevers and leukocytosis should raise concern for the development of an intraabdominal abscess (see Chapter 28). Abscesses are often best diagnosed with CT imaging. Once identified, most will be amenable to drainage by interventional radiology. A short course of antibiotics may be warranted, but prolonged antibiotics are usually not required after obtaining source control.

Pancreatic pseudocysts are more common in patients treated with nonoperative management. Pseudocyst formation is cited to occur in approximately 10% to 20% of all cases. When stratified, approximately 20% of patients treated with nonoperative management will develop pseudocysts, compared with 5% in patients treated with operative management.[40,41] A CT scan is often the initial diagnostic imaging test (see Chapters 17 and 28), but both ultrasound and endoscopic ultrasound (see Chapter 22) also can be used to follow the progression of the pseudocyst. In asymptomatic patients, no intervention is required. However, in patients who develop symptoms, drainage procedures, including percutaneous drainage, ERCP, or cystgastrostomy, are reasonable considerations (see Chapters 22, 28, and 30).[14,40]

Operative Management of Injuries to the Duodenum

Duodenal injuries are complicated by the potential for additional injuries to surrounding structures. Postoperative complications in this area can have long-lasting effects on the patient's morbidity and mortality. As previously described, duodenal injuries are graded on a scale of I to V and are subdivided into hematoma and laceration injuries. The management of duodenal injuries is dependent on the grade of injury.

Duodenal hematomas can occur in any patient but they are classically seen in young patients after a blunt trauma, such as an isolated handlebar injury. In children younger than 4 years of age, an isolated duodenal hematoma should raise suspicion for a nonaccidental traumatic mechanism.[42] Most commonly, duodenal hematomas can be managed nonoperatively. This will be described in more detail later. If a duodenal hematoma is visualized in the operating room, the hematoma should be evacuated, and a seromuscular repair should be completed.

Duodenal lacerations always require an operative intervention. In 1980, Snyder et al.[43] published a review of 247 cases of duodenal trauma. The goal was to assess what type of intervention was required for specific injury patterns, and the study estimated that 80% of all duodenal injuries can be managed with a primary repair. The same study assessed which surgical repairs required additional protection. This work was before the AAST grading, so Snyder et al.[43] considered mild pancreatic injuries to be stab wounds and those injuries that presented within 24 hours and involved less than 75% of the circumference of the third or fourth portion of the duodenum, provided there was no injury to the biliary system. The study concluded that patients with mild pancreatic injuries were best treated with a simple repair that did not require additional protection. The AAST grading scale would classify these injuries as grade I or II, and both Snyder et al. and the AAST recommend a primary repair of the injuries. This repair can be completed in either a stapled, single-layer suture, or double-layer suture approach. The success of these repairs depends on factors similar to those seen in other areas. Namely, the length of repair, degree of intramural edema, amount of tissue loss, amount of tension, and severity of associated injuries/contamination will all contribute to the outcome of the repair. As minor grade I and II lacerations are typically simple repairs, they do not require additional protection.[20,43]

Snyder et al.[43] classified blunt injuries or gunshot injuries that involved more than 75% of the circumference of the duodenum as severe injuries. Severe injuries also included any injury involving the first or second portion of the duodenum, or if the patient presents more than 24 hours after the initial trauma. Snyder et al. recognized that severe injuries did require a protective repair. Similarly, the AAST recommends that these injuries be managed with either a primary repair, resection, and anastomosis, or Roux-en-Y duodenojejunostomy. Additionally, it is recommended to protect these repairs with either a decompressive or diversion procedure.

There are numerous decompressive procedures that can be used in duodenal trauma. One early method described is the three-tube technique. This involves inserting (1) gastrostomy or gastroduodenostomy tube, (2) retrograde duodenostomy tube placed through a jejunostomy, and (3) a second jejunostomy tube that can ultimately be used for feeding. This approach avoids an additional injury to the duodenum, which is why a simple tube duodenostomy has fallen out of favor.[20]

Diversion procedures include duodenal diverticularization and pyloric exclusion. Duodenal diverticularization involves decompressing the stomach with a gastrostomy tube and diverting biliary and pancreatic secretions with a T-tube.[44] This essentially creates a low-output fistula that can be managed over many weeks. Alternatively, pyloric exclusion requires obstructing

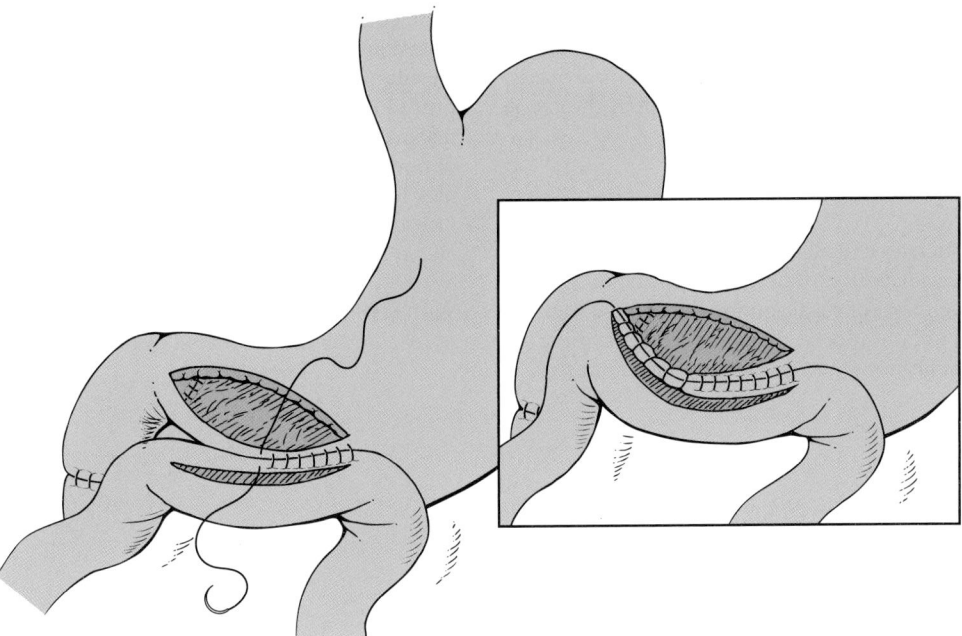

FIGURE 114.2   Pyloric exclusion showing occlusion of the duodenum just distal to the pylorus followed by a gastrojejunostomy.

the pylorus with either a noncutting stapler or suturing the pylorus closed through a gastrotomy (Fig. 114.2).[45,46] No matter the approach of closing the pylorus, it will spontaneously reopen in approximately 6 weeks. To allow for gastric drainage, a gastrojejunostomy is created. The jejunal limb should be created with sufficient length to prevent reflux. The creation of a gastrojejunostomy does leave the patient at risk for developing marginal ulcers. A vagotomy may help further reduce the risk of ulceration, but the risk of significant bleeding is rare and as the pylorus will spontaneously reopen, a vagotomy is not routinely required.[45,46] The theory behind the pyloric exclusion procedure is that any duodenal repair will have sufficient time to heal by the time the pylorus reopens.[20,45,46] The limitations of either diversion procedure is that they both rely on the primary duodenal repair, and neither actually improve the durability of the repair. In a 10-year retrospective review on the use of pyloric exclusion, it was found that the procedure did not improve clinical outcomes, and there was a trend toward a higher overall complication rate.[47] As a consequence of this deficiency, if these procedures are used, external drainage should be left in place for additional protection.

The Roux-en-Y and loop duodeno-jejunostomy procedures are alternatives to duodenal diverticularization and pyloric exclusion. In both of these procedures, the jejunum is brought proximally and used to directly repair the duodenum. This allows the duodenum to be debrided and minimizes the concerns of luminal compression. Additionally, this limits the risk of tension and the development of delayed ischemia at the suture line.

It is worth noting that although the previously mentioned trauma Whipple may be necessary for devastating injuries to the pancreas or proximal duodenum, the patient should be optimized before committing to a prolonged and complicated procedure (see Chapter 117A) It is often in the patient's best interest to complete a damage control initial procedure. Devitalized tissue should be resected, and wide drainage should be left in place at the time of the initial procedure. If able, a nontraumatic clamp

can be placed on the bile duct in the first procedure to allow it to dilate in preparation for the repair at the subsequent surgery. The patient should be resuscitated to correct for coagulopathy, acidosis, and hypothermia before considering returning to the operating room. If a staged approach is possible, it is best for the trauma Whipple to be completed by a surgeon who regularly performs the procedure.

Duodenal Injuries in the Stable Patient

Duodenal hematomas in an otherwise stable patient can be managed expectedly. These injuries most commonly manifest with symptoms of abdominal pain and nausea or vomiting. The majority of research on duodenal hematomas is in the pediatric population, which has a median duration of symptoms of 1.25 days.[48] It is possible that hematomas will progress over the course of hours to days, but they will often resolve within 7 to 14 days.[48,49] If obstructive symptoms have not improved after 14 days, repeat CT should be done to re-evaluate the obstructive process. It is incredibly rare that a patient will require a surgical intervention for an isolated hematoma, but it can be treated with either an open or laparoscopic approach.[50]

Postoperative Duodenal Complications

A leak from the duodenal suture line can be a devastating complication. Fortunately, it is rare.[47] Leakage of bile or any deviation from the expected postoperative course should trigger a workup for possible duodenal leak. A CT scan with contrast is the imaging of choice, because it will help with the diagnosis and treatment planning. If the leak is controlled with a drain, it is reasonable to consider keeping the patient nil per os and treating as a controlled fistula. Most of these injuries will close spontaneously with appropriate drainage and nutritional support (see Chapter 26). An uncontrolled leak requires an urgent re-exploration. Unfortunately, these injuries can be difficult to manage, and often the only reasonable treatment approach is inserting a mushroom tipped catheter (i.e., Mallinckrodt tube) into the hole and leaving wide regional drainage. Late discovery of a duodenal leak in a septic patient is also an indication for operative intervention. If the leak is discovered relatively early, a diversion procedure may be of benefit, but often the tissue quality limits aggressive intervention.[51]

CONCLUSION

Injuries to the pancreas and duodenum are uncommon but pose significant risk for both morbidity and mortality. It is essential to have a high level of suspicion for any of these injuries. The overall goal is to fully address the injury while planning for the expected complications and preventing any unnecessary damage to surrounding structures. This often requires a multi-staged approach, with the first procedure focusing on immediate life-threatening injuries. After stabilization, a second-look procedure provides an opportunity for definitive repair. In most instances, simple damage-control techniques will be the better option than heroic operations. Still, management of these complex injuries requires a thorough understanding of the anatomy (see Chapter 2), as well as sound technical expertise in pancreaticoduodenal surgery and damage control techniques.

The references for this chapter can be found online by accessing the accompanying Expert Consult website.

CHAPTER 115

Aneurysm and arteriovenous fistula of the liver and pancreatic vasculature

Max E. Seaton and Vikas Dudeja

INTRODUCTION

A wide variety of lesions may affect the liver and pancreatic vasculature. These lesions range from common to exceedingly rare, and they can be acquired or congenital. Some are harmless, whereas others have a high risk of causing morbidity and mortality. In this chapter, we discuss splanchnic artery aneurysms and pseudoaneurysms, arterioportal fistula (APF), hemangiomas, portal vein (PV) anomalies and aneurysms, congenital portosystemic shunts (CPS), and pancreatic arteriovenous malformations.

SPLANCHNIC ARTERY ANEURYSMS AND PSEUDOANEURYSMS

Pathophysiology and Epidemiology

Splanchnic artery aneurysms are aneurysms involving the celiac, superior mesenteric, and inferior mesenteric arteries and their branches (see Chapter 2). These aneurysms are frequently referred to as visceral artery aneurysms; however, this term includes renal artery aneurysms as well. A true aneurysm is a dilation of an artery greater than 1.5 times its expected diameter that involves all three layers of the vessel wall.[1] The most common etiology of aneurysm is atherosclerosis, but rare causes include fibromuscular dysplasia, Marfan syndrome, Ehlers-Danlos syndrome, polyarteritis nodosa, systemic lupus erythematosus, scleroderma, and mycotic aneurysms because of septic emboli from infective endocarditis.[2,3] In the early twentieth century, mycotic aneurysms were much more common and were associated with infective endocarditis, but these are uncommon now in industrialized nations after the development of effective antibiotics.

In contrast, a pseudoaneurysm (or "false aneurysm") is caused by disruption of the intimal and medial layers of the vessel wall and is contained only by the adventitial layer or perivascular tissue.[1] Iatrogenic injury from endovascular or surgical procedures are common causes of pseudoaneurysm, and rare causes include trauma and vasculitis (see Chapters 113 and 114). Pancreatitis is another common cause of splanchnic pseudoaneurysms (see Chapters 55–58); in one series, it was the etiology in 86% of cases.[3]

Based on autopsy and angiographic studies, the incidence of splanchnic artery aneurysms is between 0.1% and 2%.[4] In a recent large series, 77% of aneurysms were true aneurysms, 15% were pseudoaneurysms, and 8% were indeterminate.[5] The majority are located in the splenic artery (SA; 60%) followed by the hepatic artery (HA; 20%), with a small percentage located in the superior mesenteric artery (5%), the celiac artery (4%), and smaller celiac branches (4%).[6] Approximately one-third of patients with a splanchnic artery aneurysm have a concomitant aneurysm elsewhere. Thus patients who are found to have a splanchnic artery aneurysm should be screened for other abdominal, thoracic, intracranial, and peripheral aneurysms.[7] The main risk of splanchnic artery aneurysms is their potential to rupture and cause life-threatening hemorrhage that is challenging to control.

Computed tomography (CT) angiography is the diagnostic test study of choice (see Chapter 21). Three-dimensional (3D) vascular reconstructions of CT images are often helpful if intervention is being considered (see Chapters 13, 14, and 17). This imaging modality can characterize the lesion and provide useful information for operative planning, such as collateral blood supply, and in the case of HA aneurysm (HAA), information on the patency of PV flow. Magnetic resonance (MR) angiography is another option if iodinated contrast is contraindicated because of allergy or other reasons.

Splenic Artery Aneurysms and Pseudoaneurysms

True SA aneurysms (SAAs) are the most common splanchnic artery aneurysms. The majority (80%) are asymptomatic and discovered incidentally. True SAAs are seen more frequently in females than males, in a 4 to 1 ratio.[8] Pregnancy and portal hypertension are both associated with an increased risk of SAA, either through structural alterations in the arterial wall in response to hormonal changes or through increased wall stress from portal congestion. There have been more than 100 case reports of ruptured SAAs during pregnancy,[9] and rupture is associated with high maternal and fetal mortality rates of 75% and 95%, respectively.[10]

The majority of true SAAs are incidental findings on cross-sectional imaging or angiograms. Three-quarters of aneurysms are located in the distal artery, and 20% are located in the middle third of the vessel. Some SAAs have calcifications of the aneurysm wall that are likely because of arterial wall degradation rather than underlying atherosclerosis. Calcifications are common in the walls of ruptured aneurysms and therefore should not be considered a sign of aneurysm stability.[11] In a large series by the Mayo Clinic,[8] median age at the diagnosis of SAA was 61 years. Seventy percent of aneurysms were less than 2 cm, 22% were 2 to 3 cm, and 8% were greater than 3 cm.

SA pseudoaneurysms are less common than true SAAs and are usually associated with trauma, infection, or inflammation. The most common etiology of SA pseudoaneurysm is pancreatitis complicated by pseudocyst formation (see Chapters 55–58). In one report, 7% of patients with a pancreatic pseudocyst had an associated SA pseudoaneurysm.[12]

Hepatic Artery Aneurysms and Pseudoaneurysms

Unlike SAAs, HAAs have a 2 to 1 male predominance. The median age at presentation is 60 years, although HAA can be

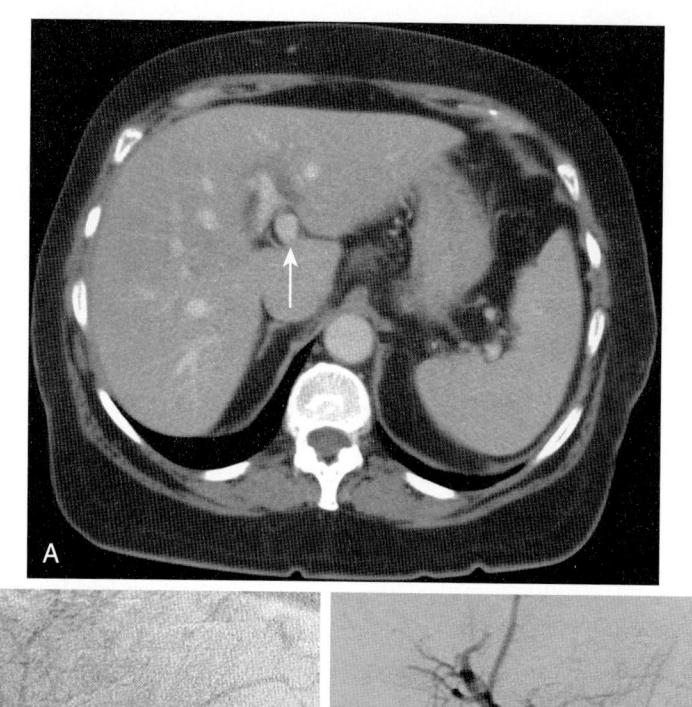

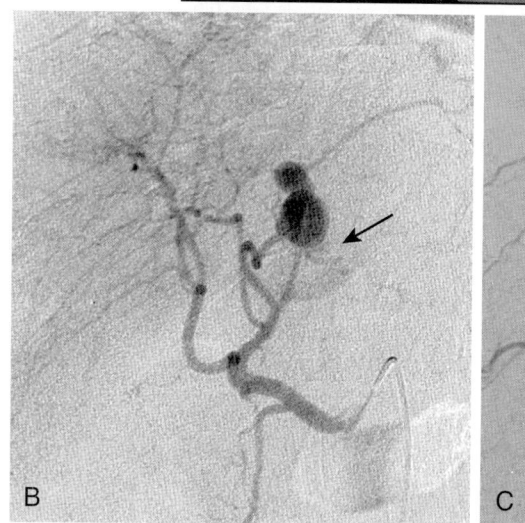

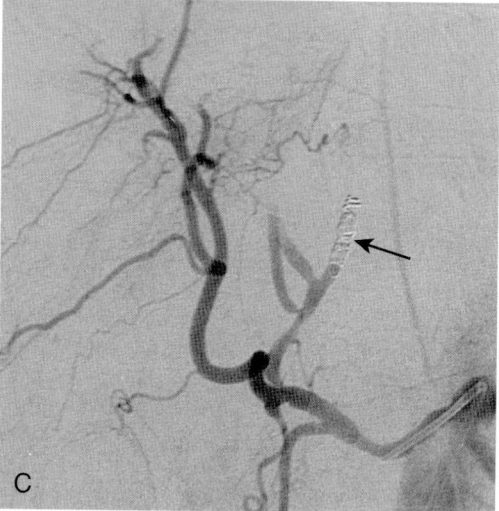

FIGURE 115.1   Hepatic artery aneurysm. A, Axial enhanced computed tomographic (CT) image shows a 2-cm aneurysm of a segment II branch of the left hepatic artery. **B,** Digital subtraction fluoroscopy image from subselective catheter angiography of the common hepatic artery. Note active extravasation *(black arrow)* from the bilobed aneurysm, which was subsequently embolized. **C,** After embolization with gelfoam and microcoil placement in the aneurysm *(black arrow)*; angiography confirmed its exclusion from the hepatic circulation. (See Chapters 14 and 21.)

seen at any age, including in children. HAAs are most frequently solitary (80%) and extrahepatic (Fig. 115.1). The most common sites for HAA are the common hepatic (63%), right hepatic (28%), and left hepatic (5%) arteries.[13,14] Although accounting for only one-fifth of visceral aneurysms, HAAs are thought to have the highest risk of rupture. It is difficult to determine the true rupture rate, but reports in the literature range from 18% to 44%.[13,14]

Pseudoaneurysms account for approximately 50% of all aneurysms affecting the HA. They are usually associated with pancreatitis, trauma, or iatrogenic injuries from percutaneous, endovascular, or surgical procedures (see Chapters 55–58, 113, 114, and 116). They have been reported after numerous types of surgeries, including laparoscopic cholecystectomies, pancreaticoduodenectomies, liver resections, and liver transplants (LTs).

Presentation

The majority of splanchnic artery aneurysms are asymptomatic and are diagnosed incidentally on cross-sectional imaging.

However, a substantial proportion are symptomatic, and 15% to 30% present with rupture,[5] which has an associated mortality ranging from 7% to 30%.[5,15] In a large retrospective study of 233 patients with visceral artery aneurysms, 27% presented with symptoms such as abdominal pain, vomiting, chest pain, or gastrointestinal (GI) bleeding.[5] Fifteen percent presented with a rupture, and all were symptomatic at the time of rupture. Anemia was a common sign at presentation, occurring in 54% of symptomatic patients and in all patients with a rupture.[5] The risk of presenting with a rupture was substantially higher for pseudoaneurysms compared with true aneurysms (76% vs. 3%, respectively).[5] Among patients who presented with a rupture, 78% had a pseudoaneurysm. There was no difference in size between ruptured and nonruptured aneurysms (mean diameter 1.5 cm vs. 1.6 cm, respectively), although the diameter of the aneurysm is often difficult to determine after it has ruptured. This suggests that size is not a reliable marker for rupture.[5]

Rupture can occur into the peritoneum, retroperitoneum, or adjacent structures. Patients may present with severe hypotension with hemoperitoneum or GI bleeding. Rupture of an SAA can be accompanied by sudden onset of sharp abdominal pain in the epigastrium or left upper quadrant and left shoulder pain (Kehr sign). Occasionally, these patients will present with abdominal pain followed by hemodynamic instability 6 to 96 hours later. This "double-rupture" phenomenon is caused by initial bleeding with tamponade in the lesser sac, followed by subsequent delayed intraperitoneal hemorrhage.[16,17] Alternately, an SAA can erode into the stomach, colon, or pancreatic duct, resulting in GI bleeding, or into the PV, resulting in a splenic APF. Extrahepatic HAAs usually present with free rupture into the peritoneum. Intrahepatic aneurysms can rupture into the biliary system, resulting in hemobilia (see Chapter 116). Patients with hemobilia may present with Quincke's triad of jaundice, right upper quadrant pain, and upper GI hemorrhage, although less than 35% of hemobilia cases present with all three of these signs and symptoms.[18]

Indications for Interventions

Emergent intervention is required for all ruptured aneurysms. Management of nonruptured aneurysms is less clear because splanchnic artery aneurysms are relatively rare, and there are no randomized control trials supporting particular management strategies.[19] Nevertheless, in 2020, the Society of Vascular Surgeons published clinical practice guidelines based on expert opinion and a systematic review of 80 observational studies.[19] Treatment for nonruptured pseudoaneurysms, regardless of size or location, is recommended because of the high risk of rupture. Nonruptured true SAAs of any size in women of child-bearing age should be treated because of the high risk of rupture and associated high mortality. In addition, true SAAs that are symptomatic or more than 3 cm should be treated. True SAAs that are stable, asymptomatic, and less than 3 cm can be observed with annual CT angiograms or ultrasound (US).

True HAAs should be treated if they are symptomatic, more than 2 cm, or enlarged by more than 0.5 cm per year. In addition, a true HAA should be repaired, regardless of size, if it is associated with a vasculopathy, vasculitis, or positive blood cultures. If a true HAA is less than 2 cm and asymptomatic, it can be observed with annual CT angiograms (see Chapters 14 and 17). All aneurysms of the superior mesenteric, gastroduodenal, and pancreaticoduodenal arteries should be treated, regardless of size, because of the high risk of rupture.[19] The European Society for Vascular Surgery has published similar recommendations.[7]

Endovascular and Surgical Interventions

Treatment of visceral artery aneurysm can be divided into *acute* management of ruptured aneurysms or *elective* management of large, growing, or symptomatic lesions. When intervention is indicated, the purpose is to exclude the aneurysm from the circulation to prevent it from rupturing, while maintaining perfusion to the distal tissues. Options include endovascular procedures such as embolization, coiling, or stenting; or surgical procedures such as ligation or excision of the aneurysm with primary repair or interposition grafting.[20] In the elective setting, endovascular procedures are preferred, and they have become the most common type of intervention on splanchnic aneurysms.[19,20] Endovascular procedures are also commonly used for ruptured aneurysms in the emergent setting. In one retrospective study that included 37 patients with ruptured visceral artery aneurysms, 87% were managed with an endovascular intervention, with no periprocedural deaths and a 30-day mortality rate of 5%.[5]

After an endovascular intervention on a true aneurysm, surveillance imaging at 3-year intervals is recommended.[7] Surveillance after endovascular treatment of a pseudoaneurysm is only needed if the underlying etiology persists.[7]

Interventions for Splenic Artery Aneurysms

Endovascular techniques, including embolization and stent graft placement, are the gold standard for managing SAAs. Between 1980 and 2017, 68% of interventions on SAAs were performed with the endovascular approach.[20] Embolization of SAAs with narrow necks can be achieved through embolization of the artery proximal to the aneurysms using coils, Gelfoam, glue, thrombin, or Amplatzer vascular plug. In lesions with good collateral flow, the efferent arterial flow can be temporarily occluded with a balloon or embolized to enhance aneurysm thrombosis.[21] Technical success rates greater than 90% have been reported, particularly in lesions in the proximal or middle splenic artery. Recanalization requiring re-intervention may occur in 10% to 12.5% of cases; technical factors associated with incomplete embolization include large-neck, distal, or intrasplenic lesions and tortuosity of the splenic artery. A post-embolization syndrome characterized by fever, abdominal pain, ileus, and pancreatitis may occur in up to 30% of patients. Stent graft placement has the advantage of excluding the aneurysm while preserving flow in the splenic artery. Size, location, and arterial tortuosity may contribute to the successful placement of stent grafts, which is often most appropriate for proximal lesions. Distal and intrasplenic aneurysms may be difficult to embolize, are associated with a higher risk of splenic infarction, and, in certain cases, may be best approached with splenectomy.[16,21]

Elective operative management of SAs should be considered in lesions not amenable to endovascular transcatheter approaches. Surgical options include proximal and distal artery ligation and aneurysm resection. Laparoscopic approaches to SAA may be considered in elective cases.[22] In cases of severe hemodynamic instability, proximal control may be obtained through placement of a proximal splenic, celiac, or supra-celiac aortic clamp. Exposure of the SA can be rapidly obtained through an anterior approach by division of the gastrocolic omentum. The SA can then be ligated, and a splenectomy performed if needed.

Overall, mortality rates for both endovascular and surgical intervention are low and not statistically different.[20] Nevertheless, patients who present with a ruptured SAA that requires open surgery have a 20% to 30% perioperative mortality.[23,24]

Interventions for Hepatic Artery Aneurysms

Similar to SAAs, the majority of HAAs are managed with endovascular techniques. Between 1980 and 2017, 64% of reported interventions on HAAs were performed with the endovascular approach.[20] This proportion is likely much higher in recent years. With any intervention, efforts should be made to preserve arterial supply to the liver to avoid biliary ischemia and other sequelae. The presence of replaced or accessory HA supply (see Chapter 2) should be noted and may permit arterial perfusion after embolization or ligation of other branches. Similarly, occlusive approaches to lesions of the common HA, proximal to the origin of the gastroduodenal artery, can be considered because hepatic flow may be maintained based on collateral supply from the superior mesenteric artery.[25]

Angiography (see Chapters 21 and 116) should be considered in hemodynamically stable patients with suspected HAA rupture, although surgery may be indicated in cases of hemo-dynamic instability or when the source of bleeding is unknown. Flow-diverting stents have the advantage of excluding or reducing flow in the aneurysm while maintaining flow in the HA. Deployment of covered stents may be challenging in lesions close to bifurcation points in the HA. Recent publications have indicated that successful stent deployment can result in aneurysm thrombosis in greater than 90% and size reduction in more than 80% of cases, with low rates (<10%) of main vessel thrombosis.[26] If deployment of a flow-diverting stent is not possible, embolization of the afferent and efferent arteries on either side of the HAA can be achieved using catheter-based placement of embolic coils, resulting in thrombosis of the aneurysm in the vast majority (>90%) of cases. Intrahepatic aneurysms can be coil embolized.[19] Complications of HAA embolization related to loss of arterial supply to the liver and bile ducts can include gallbladder ischemia, hepatic abscess, and secondary biliary cirrhosis.[27] If a large intrahepatic aneurysm is embolized, resection of the involved liver lobe (see Chapter 101) may be needed to avoid hepatic necrosis.[19]

Surgical ligation can be considered in HAA located in the common HA. Alternatively, lesions detected emergently at the time of rupture associated with hemodynamic instability may be treated with ligation to obtain vascular control. Aneurysm resection remains the mainstay of elective surgical treatment (see Chapter 122). Options for arterial reconstruction after ligation or resection include end-to-end anastomosis and autologous or prosthetic interposition graft. Autologous interposition grafts using saphenous or left renal vein have been described, as well as arterial reconstruction using the gastroduodenal or splenic arteries. Prosthetic aortohepatic grafts can be used in the absence of sepsis or contamination.

Elective repair of HAA is associated with a mortality rate of up to 5%, whereas mortality of emergent repair of ruptured aneurysms ranges from 22% to 33%.[13,28] There is no significant difference in short- or long-term mortality between the endovascular approach and surgery, although the need for re-intervention is higher with the endovascular approach.[20]

Other Splanchnic Artery Aneurysms

All true aneurysms and pseudoaneurysms of the superior mesenteric artery should be repaired or treated with endovascular stenting.[29] Aneurysms of the gastroduodenal or pancreaticoduodenal arteries should be coil embolized or ligated.[19]

ARTERIOPORTAL FISTULA

APF is an anomalous communication between the splanchnic arterial system and PV system. APFs can be intrahepatic or extrahepatic and can be acquired or congenital (see Chapters 5, 74, and 76). The severity and nature of symptoms often depend on the location, size, and flow through the fistula, as well as the resistance in the liver to the increased portal blood flow. The most common symptoms result from the development of presinusoidal portal hypertension because of the high-pressure arterial flow into the portal vasculature. This can result in GI bleeding and ascites (see Chapters 74, 76, and 79–81). Heart failure can develop as a result of decreased systemic vascular resistance with a compensatory increase in cardiac output. Diarrhea and malabsorption can occur secondary to intestinal ischemia caused by mesenteric venous congestion or arterial steal syndrome.[30,31] Because of their proximity to the PV within the liver and porta hepatis, the majority of APFs arise from the HAs (65%), with the splenic and superior mesenteric arteries less often involved (~10% each).[31] The most common etiologies for APF include trauma (28%; see Chapters 113 and 114), iatrogenic causes (16%; see Chapters 23, 28, 31, 52, 85, and 96), congenital (15%), and erosion of splanchnic aneurysms (14%).[31]

Acquired Arterioportal Fistula

Acquired APF can occur after trauma, endovascular procedures, surgery, and splanchnic aneurysms. They can occur spontaneously in association with cirrhosis or hepatic malignancy. Because of the proximity of the HA and PV structures in the portal triad, injury to one or both vessels can result in the establishment of a fistula between the two (Fig. 115.2). A review

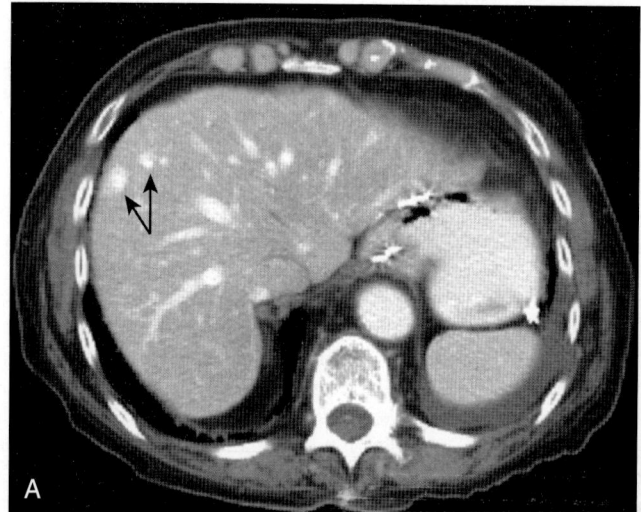
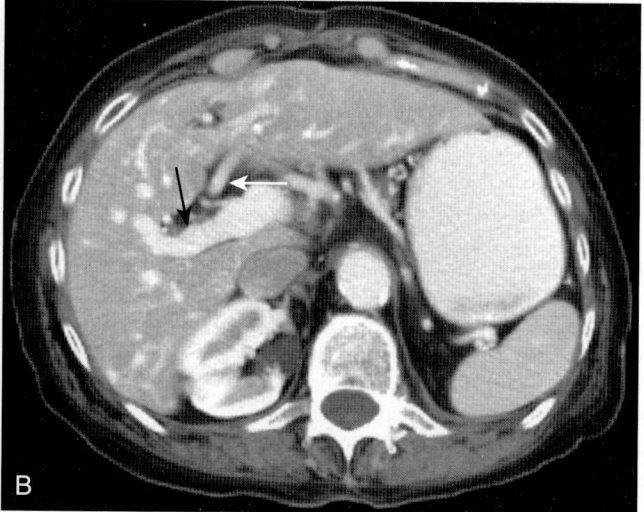

FIGURE 115.2   Hepatic arteriovenous malformations (AVMs). A, Axial enhanced computed tomography (CT) image in the portal venous phase shows multiple peripheral, rounded, hyperattenuation lesions *(black arrows),* predominantly in the right lobe. They were continuous with abnormal, enlarged portal veins and compatible with AVMs. Previous upper abdominal surgery is also evident. **B,** More caudal axial CT image shows enlargement of the left portal vein *(black arrow)* and hepatic artery *(white arrow).* (See Chapter 14.)

of post-traumatic APFs demonstrated that they are usually associated with penetrating trauma (97%) compared with blunt injuries, with 79% of cases associated with gunshot wounds and 17% with stab wounds[32] (see Chapters 113 and 114).

Acquired APFs can be subclassified into Type 1 and Type 2.[33] Type 1–acquired APFs are small peripheral intrahepatic fistulas that have minimal physiologic sequelae, and they are commonly iatrogenic. They may occur after interventional hepatic procedures, including liver biopsy (see Chapter 23), percutaneous ablation of liver lesions (see Chapter 96), transjugular intrahepatic portosystemic shunting (TIPS; see Chapter 85), and transhepatic biliary procedures (see Chapters 31 and 52). Okuda and colleagues[34] performed hepatic arteriograms 1 month after procedures and demonstrated a 5.4% incidence of APFs after liver biopsy, 3.8% after percutaneous transhepatic cholangiography, and 26.2% after transhepatic biliary drainage. Hellekant (1976)[35] identified APFs in 52% of patients 1 week after liver biopsy, which subsequently decreased to 10% after 3 weeks. These observations indicate that although APFs may be common after interventional liver procedures, many of these are small and will resolve without further intervention. They should be followed with Doppler US, and if they persist for longer than 1 month or are symptomatic, they can be embolized.[33]

Type 2 APFs are large intrahepatic or extrahepatic fistulas that cause presinusoidal portal hypertension and hepatoportal sclerosis.[33] These APFs are usually associated with major penetrating trauma or erosion of an SAA into the portal system. Because of the high prevalence of symptoms with Type 2 APFs, treatment is recommended.

Congenital Arterioportal Fistula

Congenital APFs account for 10% to 15% of all fistulae involving the splanchnic arteries and are associated with hereditary telangiectasias, arteriovenous malformations (AVMs), and aneurysms. They are classified as Type 3 APFs.[33] Congenital APFs are frequently multiple and bilateral; the symptoms and age at presentation depend on the degree of shunting and the number of fistulae. Complex APFs often present before 2 to 3 years of age with symptoms of portal hypertension and bleeding. Mesenteric ischemia caused by venous congestion often precedes the development of portal hypertension and can manifest with diarrhea, malabsorption, weight loss, and failure to thrive. Rarely, APFs in young infants may result in congestive heart failure caused by persistence of the ductus venosus, although this is more common with arteriovenous fistula (AVF).

Hereditary hemorrhagic telangiectasia (HHT), commonly known as Osler-Rendu-Weber disease, is an autosomal dominant disorder (Online Mendelian Inheritance in Man [OMIM] #187300) resulting from mutations in genes encoding endoglin (*ENG*, HHT type 1) or activin receptor type II–like kinase 1 (*ALK-1*, HHT type 2). Both genes code for endothelial cell transmembrane proteins, and therefore mutations in *ENG* and *ALK-1* are thought to produce imbalances between anti- and pro-angiogenic factors. Clinically, HHT is characterized by cutaneous telangiectasias, visceral AVMs, spontaneous and recurrent epistaxis, and a family history of the disease. Approximately 75% of HHT patients will have AVMs involving the liver, predominantly in HHT type 2 patients with *ALK-1* mutations, and including fistulae to the PV (APF) and systemic venous (AVF) circulation (see Chapter 21; Fig. 115.3). Only 8% of HHT cases will have symptomatic complications of AVMs, which include high-output cardiac failure, portal hypertension, and biliary necrosis.[36] Treatment of symptomatic HHT is directed at decreasing flow through shunts and can be accomplished through angiographic embolization, surgical ligation, or resection resulting in decreased cardiac output.[37] LT is considered curative for HHT patients with symptomatic liver AVMs and is recommended earlier in the disease course before cardiac decompensation occurs.[38] A phase 2 clinical trial involving 25 patients suggested that anti-vascular endothelial growth factor (VEGF)

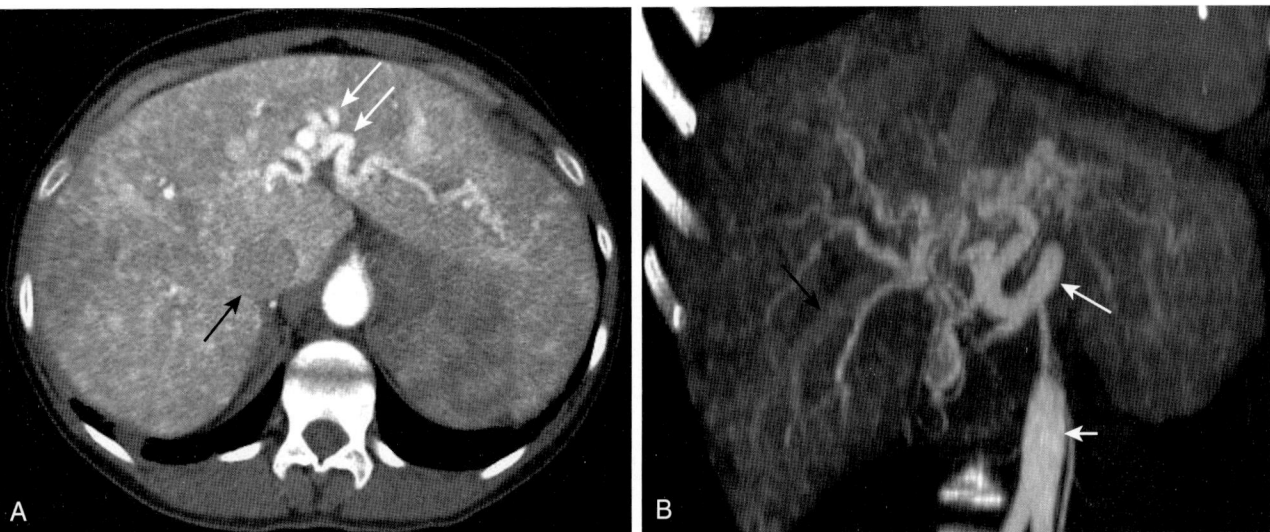

FIGURE 115.3   Hereditary hemorrhagic telangiectasia (HHT). A, Arterial-phase axial computed tomography (CT) image shows hepatomegaly and diffusely abnormal parenchyma with multiple arterial-hepatic venous malformations. Note distended hepatic arteries in the left lobe *(white arrows)*. The unopacified inferior vena cava is also distended because of the abnormal communications *(black arrow)*. **B,** Coronal oblique maximum intensity projection (MIP) image shows enlarged hepatic artery proper *(long white arrow)* with multiple enlarged intrahepatic branches. Part of the distal abdominal aorta is also seen *(short white arrow)*. Note the accessory segment VI hepatic vein *(black arrow)*, opacified in the arterial phase as a result of arteriovenous shunts. (See Chapter 14.)

monoclonal antibody, bevacizumab, may be effective in normal-izing cardiac output and reducing symptoms in HHT patients with hepatic AVMs.[39] Nevertheless, there has been a reported case of systemic thrombosis (pulmonary emboli, right atrial thrombus, and right HV thrombus) in a patient 3 months after starting bevacizumab, so it should be used with caution.[40]

Management of Arterioportal Fistula

Transarterial embolization (TAE; see Chapters 21 and 116) is considered the first-line therapy for type 2 APFs, with surgical ligation or resection reserved for cases that either fail or are not suitable for TAE. Treatment of congenital APFs (Type 3) is often required because of symptoms and can include TAE, hepatic arterial ligation, resection, transplantation, and anti-VEGF ther-apy.[31,33,41] Several types of embolic agents have been described, including detachable coils, detachable balloons, Gelfoam parti-cles, isobutyl cyanoacrylates, n-butyl cyanoacrylate glue, Amp-latzer vascular plugs, polyvinyl alcohol, microspheres, and sclerosants. Careful planning and selection of embolic technique are required, especially in larger hepatic and mesenteric fistulae, because of the risk of venous thrombosis from the passage or migration of thrombogenic material into the venous system or arterial ischemia from non-target embolization.[41,42] Splenoportal embolization can usually safely be performed without concern for splenic ischemia because of the presence of collateral flow through the short gastric vessels. TAE is frequently successful in eliminating flow across the shunt and improving PV pressures. Repeat TAEs may be required in cases of multiple or complex APFs. Embolization of the PV segment may also be required.[43]

Surgical management is reserved for APFs that either fail TAE or are deemed unsuitable for embolization because of high flow or large fistula diameter and the risk of nontarget embolization or portal thrombosis. Surgical approaches to APFs can include ligation or resection. Ligation is preferred over resection in many cases because of decreased complexity, blood loss, and morbidity, although the risk of end-organ isch-emia should be considered. For this reason, ligation should be used very selectively in mesenteric fistulae or HA fistulae in patients with limited hepatic reserve (see Chapter 4). Hepatic resection can be considered in patients with large APFs that have failed, or are not amenable to, embolization. Hepatic transplantation has been described for patients with APFs and limited hepatic reserve, as well as in patients with complex bilateral congenital fistulae.[38]

HEMANGIOMA

Hepatic hemangiomas are benign tumors of mesenchymal ori-gin and are the most common benign liver tumors[44] (see Chapter 88A). Incidence in Western populations is estimated at approximately 2%. The majority of lesions are asymptom-atic, with detection an incidental result of the increasing prevalence of cross-sectional imaging modalities. A female preponderance is well-established at a ratio of approximately 5 to 1.[45] Hemangiomas can occur in all age groups from in-fancy to late adulthood, but most are detected between the fourth and sixth decades.

Histologically, hemangiomas are composed of masses of ir-regular blood vessels, and some consider these to be "congenital hamartomas." Although the etiology remains unclear, cortico-steroids,[46] estrogen therapy, and pregnancy[47,48] are thought to contribute to the growth of hemangiomas.

Clinically, hemangiomas can be part of well-recognized syn-dromes, including Klippel-Trenaunay-Weber, Kasabach-Merritt, Osler-Weber-Rendu, and von Hippel-Lindau. The hemangioma itself can be responsible for the clinical condition, mandating eradication of the lesion. In Kasabach-Merritt syndrome, for example, coagulopathy can be attributed to thrombocytopenia and intravascular thrombosis stimulated by the giant hepatic hemangioma.[49]

The vast majority of hemangiomas are asymptomatic and are identified incidentally (Fig. 115.4). Rare symptoms that can be attributed to these lesions include abdominal pain or full-ness, biliary obstruction, GI hemorrhage from hemobilia[50] (see Chapter 116), high-output cardiac failure as a result of massive shunting, pyrexia of unknown origin,[51] and abdominal mass. Size and number of lesions correlate with the likelihood of symptoms, with pain as a result of thrombosis, and subsequent

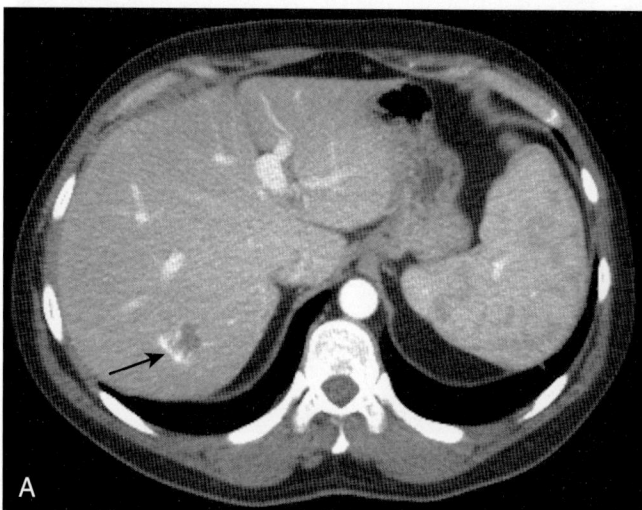
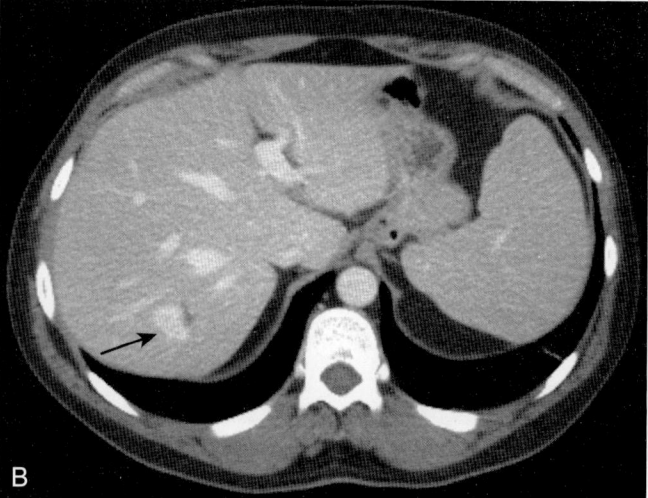

FIGURE 115.4 **Hepatic hemangioma. A,** Arterial-phase axial computed tomography (CT) image shows typical early peripheral puddling of contrast *(black arrow)* in a 2-cm segment VIII hemangioma. **B,** Portal venous–phase image from the same study shows typical progressive filling with contrast in the hemangioma. (See Chapters 14 and 88A.)

infarction or hemorrhage into larger lesions being a common phenomenon. Nonspecific abdominal pain often leads to the imaging modality that identifies the hepatic lesion; however, it is often difficult to attribute the symptom to the hemangioma. Pressure effects on adjacent viscera can result in nausea or early satiety but usually only in the case of massive lesions. Compression of the inferior vena cava (IVC) with resultant lower-limb edema has also been reported. Spontaneous rupture of giant hemangiomas is vanishingly rare but can occur. More often, but still infrequently, hemangioma rupture can result from abdominal trauma.[52,53]

The investigation of hepatic hemangioma is important because the differential diagnosis includes angiosarcoma, hepatocellular carcinoma (HCC), and vascular metastases (see Chapters 87, 89, 91, and 92), as well as benign entities such as cysts, adenomas, focal nodular hyperplasia, and regenerative nodules (see Chapter 88A). The gold standard imaging modality is magnetic resonance imaging[54] (MRI), but contrast-enhanced CT (CECT), US,[55] single-photon emission CT,[56] and technetium scintigraphy are all helpful (see Chapters 13–15 and 18). The combination of MRI with CT can yield excellent sensitivity, and radiologic diagnosis is now sufficiently accurate that biopsy is neither necessary nor recommended. Hepatic arteriography has been supplanted by newer, noninvasive modalities. Laboratory tests may be helpful to rule out malignant lesions. Normal values for α-fetoprotein (AFP), carcinoembryonic antigen (CEA), and carbohydrate antigen (CA)19-9 are reassuring in this context. Occasionally, thrombocytopenia may be seen with massive hemangiomas from platelet sequestration. *Hemangiomatosis* is a rare condition in which the hepatic parenchyma is replaced by hemangiomatous lesions (Fig. 115.5). Hemangiomatosis does not have a distinct border and can often be found at the border of giant hemangiomas (see Chapter 88A).

Management of hemangiomas requires accurate imaging to confirm the diagnosis. After diagnosis, follow-up imaging at 6 or 12 months to confirm stability of size and appearance is usually sufficient to exclude alternate diagnoses. Surveillance imaging thereafter is rarely required; however, the presence of atypical imaging features, multiplicity of lesions, large size (>10 cm), new-onset abdominal pain, or ongoing estrogen or hormone therapy should mandate surveillance. In these patients, annual imaging is adequate. Sclerosis of hemangiomas can be seen, but this radiologic diagnosis should be approached with caution because several malignancies can have a similar appearance.

Resection is rarely indicated but may be considered selectively in several settings (see Chapter 101B). Resection may be considered when the diagnosis of malignancy cannot be excluded despite a thorough and exhaustive radiologic evaluation. Similarly, rapidly growing or severely symptomatic lesions should be removed.[57] Nevertheless, the confident identification of a hemangioma as the cause of abdominal pain or other symptoms can be difficult. Large lesions (>10 cm) represent a management dilemma. Proponents of resection suggest it is warranted to avoid risks of spontaneous or post-traumatic rupture or high-output cardiac failure, but evidence suggests that each of these outcomes is rare. Also, in the absence of symptoms, it is difficult to advocate resection, particularly when major hepatectomy may be required. For symptomatic lesions, however, it is reasonable to propose resection, and the full range of surgical options may be employed, including laparoscopic or open approaches, nonanatomic resection, and major hepatectomy (see Chapters 101, 102, 118, 127D, and 127E). LT (see Chapter 105) is rarely used but has good outcomes in selected cases.[58] Nonsurgical methods have been employed with success, including radiofrequency ablation (see Chapter 96B)[59], microwave ablation (see Chapter 96C),[60] and transarterial embolization (TAE; see Chapter 94).[61] External beam radiation therapy is rarely used because it is not curative and has adverse effects, such as radiation hepatitis. Medical therapies are rarely employed, but avoidance of exogenous estrogen or corticosteroids is recommended. Initial reports suggested that

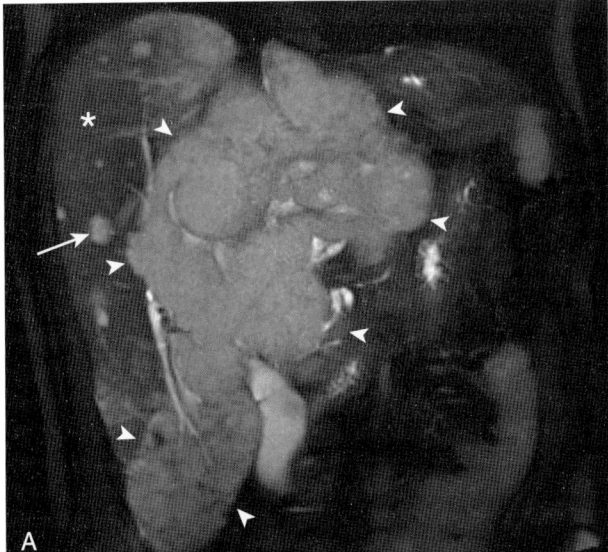
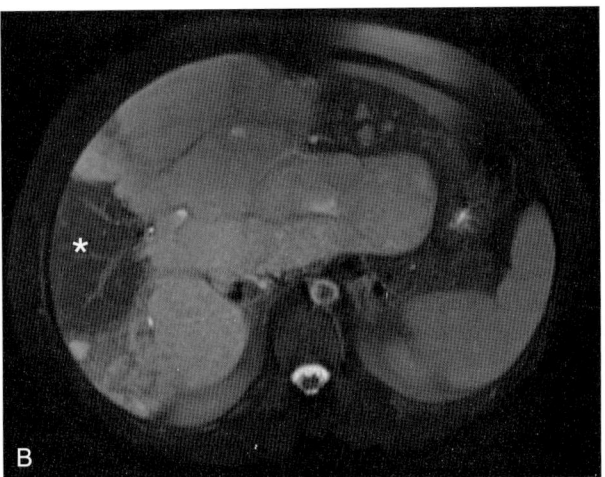

FIGURE 115.5 **Hepatic hemangiomatosis. A,** Coronal T2-weighted HASTE (Half Fourier Acquisition Single Shot Turbo Spin Echo) magnetic resonance (MR) image shows hepatomegaly with hemangiomatosis. There is replacement of much of the hepatic parenchyma by multiple T2 hyperintense lobulated masses *(white arrowheads)*, which are infiltrating around vessels without invading them. Additional discrete hemangiomas are seen more peripherally *(white arrow)*. Unaffected liver has normal low T2 signal intensity *(asterisk)*. **B,** Axial T2-weighted HASTE MR image again demonstrates extensive infiltrative T2 hyperintense lobulated masses. Normal low T2 signal intensity is seen in the unaffected hepatic parenchyma *(asterisk)*. (See Chapters 14 and 88A.)

antiangiogenic therapies, such as bevacizumab and kinase inhibitors (e.g., sorafenib), may be effective, but a subsequent study found no evidence to support this.[62] Malignant transformation of a hepatic hemangioma has never been reported, and there is minimal risk of recurrence after complete surgical resection.

Congenital and Infantile Hepatic Hemangiomas

Two types of hemangiomas occur in infants: congenital hemangiomas and infantile hemangiomas. Both types can usually be diagnosed with Doppler US. The lesions may be unifocal or multifocal and on Doppler US can appear either hypoechoic or hyperechoic. Smaller lesions are homogenous, whereas larger lesions are heterogeneous with areas of calcifications, cystic spaces, and fibrosis.[63] Liver MRI is recommended if the Doppler US is nondiagnostic.

Congenital hemangiomas develop in utero and are fully formed at birth (see Chapters 1 and 88A). There are three subtypes based on their involution pattern: rapidly involuting congenital hemangiomas (RICH), which involute by 2 years of age; partially involuting congenital hemangiomas (PICH); and noninvoluting congenital hemangiomas (NICH).[63] In contrast, infantile hemangiomas proliferate from birth until 6 to 12 months of age and gradually involute until 3 to 9 years of age.[63] Infantile hemangiomas are distinguished histologically by expression of the glucose transporter 1 (glut-1) protein, although histologic confirmation is rarely required.[63] Both congenital and infantile hemangiomas are usually asymptomatic but in rare instances can cause severe complications.[64] Congenital hemangiomas can cause high-output cardiac failure, thrombocytopenia, and hypofibrinogenemia. Infantile hepatic hemangiomas can cause high-output cardiac failure, consumptive hypothyroidism, liver failure, and abdominal compartment syndrome.[63] Oral propranolol is now first-line therapy for infantile hemangiomas that need treatment and was approved for this indication by the Food and Drug Administration (FDA) in 2014.[65] In the past, corticosteroids were considered the primary treatment, but propranolol has been shown to have a superior safety profile. There are also case reports of successful treatment with drug combinations, such as sirolimus, corticosteroids, and propranolol.[66]

VENOUS ABNORMALITIES

Development of the fetal liver commences in the fourth week of gestation (see Chapter 1); the venous structures develop based on three major venous systems of the fetal circulation: the cardinal, vitelline, and umbilical veins. The systemic venous system develops from the anterior and posterior cardinal veins, whereas the afferent (portal) system arises from the vitelline and umbilical veins. The system gradually develops by processes of vascular coalescence and cellular differentiation that culminate in separate arterial and venous conduits. Congenital intrahepatic shunts are rare anomalies characterized by abnormal communication between the HA system, PVs, hepatic veins, or systemic veins as a result of disordered embryologic development about the fifth gestational week.

The right and left vitelline veins pass around the duodenum and enter the septum transversum (primitive liver), where they are broken up into sinusoids by the developing liver parenchyma before draining into the sinus venosus. The left vitelline vein then involutes, and blood from the right vitelline vein is distributed to both sides of the liver. The right and left umbilical veins begin with two branches; one drains directly into the sinus venosus, and the other enters into the hepatic sinusoids. The umbilical vein branches into the sinus venosus and eventually involutes, directing all blood toward the liver.[45,67]

The PV develops from persistence of the superior aspect of the right vitelline vein, the retroduodenal communication between the veins, and the inferior aspect of the left vitelline vein, giving the PV its S-shaped configuration. The PV drains into the portal sinus, which gives rise to the intrahepatic portal circulation. The IVC originates from the sinus venosus and the infradiaphragmatic anastomosis of the vitelline veins.[67]

Congenital Portal Vein Anomalies

Congenital anomalies of the PV are relatively common compared with other vascular abnormalities of the pancreas and liver. Variations in embryologic development yield several dominant patterns that can have implications for the surgeon (see Chapters 1 and 2). In particular, living-donor LT (LDLT) and major hepatic resection require accurate identification of the PV anatomy (see Chapter 118). The prevalence of PV variants is reportedly as high as 35%.[68,69] Trifurcation and origin of the right posterior pedicle as the first branch of the main PV are particularly common variants. Rarely, a single right PV will supply the entire liver.[70–73] These anatomic variants are typically asymptomatic, but a few rare anomalies can have clinical implications.

PV duplication is a rare anomaly resulting from atypical fusion of the superior and inferior mesenteric veins. The resulting duplicated PV runs in a variable preduodenal course to join the right PV. The splenic vein runs posteriorly behind the pancreas, receiving the coronary vein, then turning anteriorly and terminating in the left PV.[74] The separate channels may communicate to form a single PV, but this is not always the case. This arrangement can cause duodenal obstruction requiring bypass. Portal hypertension resulting in formation of varices may also occur, but the mechanism is unclear.

The *preduodenal PV anomaly* is a well-recognized radiologic finding[75] and is typically associated with any of a number of developmental variations of the spleen, pancreas, heart, gut rotation, and IVC.[70,76–78] An important, albeit rare, cause of gastric outlet obstruction in pediatric populations, preduodenal PV anomaly has also been reported in adults.[79] It is also of further significance in the adult population because its presence, and the associated derangement of the mesentericoportal confluence, can complicate the surgical approach to the pancreas.

PV agenesis was first described by Abernethy in 1793. The spectrum of malformations that bears his name, the clinical consequences, and treatment options are discussed in detail later. Outcomes depend on the specific type of malformation and the presence or absence of congenital heart disease and liver disease.[80]

Portal Vein Aneurysms

PV aneurysms (PVAs) represent 3% of all venous aneurysms and are the most common visceral aneurysm.[72,81,82] However, overall PVAs are uncommon vascular lesions.[83] Because of the rarity of these aneurysms, their natural history is not well understood, and management recommendations are based on case reports and small case series. The normal diameter of a PV is less than 1.5 cm in noncirrhotic patients and less than 1.9 cm in cirrhotic patients, so a PV diameter greater than 2.0 cm is considered aneurysmal.[84] PVAs can have either a saccular or fusiform morphology. The majority of PVAs are extrahepatic, with approximately 25% located at the confluence of the main PV, 20% located in the splenic vein, and 20% located at the bifurcation of the main PV.[85] Approximately 20% are intrahepatic, and approximately 20% of patients have multiple PVAs.

PVAs can be congenital or acquired. Congenital PVAs likely arise from a diverticulum resulting from an incompletely regressed right vitelline vein[86] (see Chapter 1). Acquired PVAs frequently arise because of portal hypertension, which causes intimal thickening and medial hypertrophy followed by medial fibrosis and weakening of the vessel wall.[86,87] Nevertheless, PVAs are rare even among patients with portal hypertension, so it is possible that an inherent weakness in the PV wall is required for the aneurysm to develop.[86] Other causes of acquired PVAs include pancreatitis (see Chapters 54–58), trauma (see Chapters 113 and 114), and invasion of the PV by a malignancy (see Chapter 87).[83] Approximately 40% of PVAs have no identifiable cause so are believed to be congenital, and 45% are associated with portal hypertension and cirrhosis.[85]

Most PVAs are asymptomatic and are incidental findings on imaging.[85] Nevertheless, they may present with GI bleeding, PV thrombosis, and mass effect on surrounding structures, such as the common bile duct, duodenum, and IVC.[83] The risk of rupture is low because it is a low-pressure system, but there have been case reports of this complication.[88] Hematologic abnormalities are also frequently associated with PVA and may be causative.[85] Thrombosis may be observed in the lumen of the aneurysm and may warrant treatment. The concern arises particularly when associated with liver disease because the aneurysm may predispose to thrombosis with severe clinical consequences. The demonstration of calcification within the PV wall indicates recurrent thrombosis and mandates therapy.[89] Many of these lesions are identified incidentally on cross-sectional imaging and are usually asymptomatic. The best imaging modalities to diagnose and characterize PVAs are Doppler US, contrasted CT scan, and MR angiography.

Small and asymptomatic PVAs without evidence of liver disease or worrisome features, such as calcification, can be safely observed with serial imaging[83] to identify progression or complication.[90] In one case report, a 6-cm aneurysm was followed for over 10 years and remained stable.[86] Nevertheless, surgery or other interventions should be considered if the lesion is symptomatic, thrombosed, enlarging, at high risk of rupture, or greater than 3 cm in diameter.[91] Approximately 20% of PVAs require an intervention.[83] Surgical options for patients without portal hypertension include aneurysmorrhaphy or aneurysmectomy.[83] For patients with portal hypertension, a portocaval or mesocaval shunt can be performed to decrease pressure in the aneurysm (see Chapters 83 and 84).[83] If the patient receives an LT, the aneurysm may be resected during that surgery.[83] Therapeutic options for thrombosis in PVA include anticoagulation, either as prophylaxis or for management of thrombosis,[92,93] and various percutaneous therapeutic approaches in the form of transhepatic thrombectomy and/or intraarterial thrombolysis.[83]

Congenital Portosystemic Shunts

CPS is a developmental abnormality resulting from the diversion of portal blood from the liver into the systemic circulation (see Chapters 1 and 76). Its occurrence is probably explained by the role of the vitelline veins in the development of both PVs and the IVC. The first description of CPS was from John Abernethy at St. Bartholomew's Hospital, London, based on the postmortem examination of a 10-month-old female who had died of unknown causes. The infant was noted to have a PV that terminated in an end-to-side anastomosis with the IVC, along with an enlarged HA, dextrocardia, and transposition of the great vessels.[94]

Previously, CPS was detected in children with other associated anomalies or in adults as a result of shunt complications. The expanding use of neonatal and pediatric Doppler US has led to an increase in the detection of asymptomatic CPS in children. Complications of CPS are related to decreased blood flow to the liver and systemic delivery of portal blood directly into the circulation. Hepatic atrophy has been reported as a result of reduced blood flow, oxygenation, or supply of hypertrophic factors (e.g., insulin, glucagon). Histologic evaluation of liver tissue in CPS reveals absent portal venules, periportal fibrosis, arterialization, and bile duct proliferation. An increased prevalence of benign liver lesions (e.g., focal nodular hyperplasia, adenomas, regenerative nodules, ciliated foregut cysts) has been reported, as well as an increased risk of HCC and hepatoblastoma. Elevated blood ammonia and galactose levels can be seen from direct delivery of splanchnic blood into the systemic circulation without metabolic clearance by the liver. If left untreated, CPS can lead to pulmonary hypertension, hepatopulmonary syndrome (HPS), and hypoxemia.[45,67]

As a result of its original description, CPS may be referred to as an "Abernethy malformation." Several classification schemes for CPS have been proposed, the most common proposed by Morgan and Superina[95] and refined by Lautz and colleagues.[96] Type 1 CPS consists of an end-to side shunt between the PV and IVC with no intrahepatic portal flow. Type 2 anomalies are side-to-side H shunts with some preservation of portal flow to the liver; this type is further classified based on the location of the shunt from the right or left PV (Type 2a; Fig. 115.6), the main PV (Type 2b), or the mesenteric, splenic, or gastric veins (Type 2c).[67] Limitations of this classification are that it is mainly descriptive, and some patients with Type 1 CPS may in fact have small, hypoplastic intrahepatic PV structures within the liver that can be demonstrated with balloon occlusion of the shunt. Recently, Blanc and colleagues[97] proposed a new classification based on anatomy, as well as a surgical approach based on the location of the shunt, the status of the intrahepatic PV system, and operative approach.

Closure of CPS is indicated to either treat or prevent complications. The ductus venosus usually closes within the first 3 weeks of life, but spontaneous closure of persistent patent ductus venosus and intrahepatic CPS above the PV bifurcation (Type 2a) may be seen up to 1 year after birth.

Pretreatment assessment of CPS includes transjugular or transfemoral venography to document the shunt. This is followed by balloon occlusion of the shunt close to its anastomosis with the IVC, with evaluation of the existence and status of intrahepatic PV flow and portal pressures. The finding of portal pressures below 30 mm Hg with occlusion of the CPS indicates that shunt ligation can be attempted with a low risk of splanchnic venous congestion. Angiographic occlusion of shunts using plugs, stents, or coils can be performed (see Chapters 21, and 116), although use of these approaches is often limited in cases of short, wide shunts because of the risk of plug or coil migration.[67]

Traditional management of Type 1 CPS is LT (see Chapters 105 and 110) because these shunts cannot be closed without developing severe portal hypertension. LT has been described for Type 1 CPS associated with refractory encephalopathy, biliary

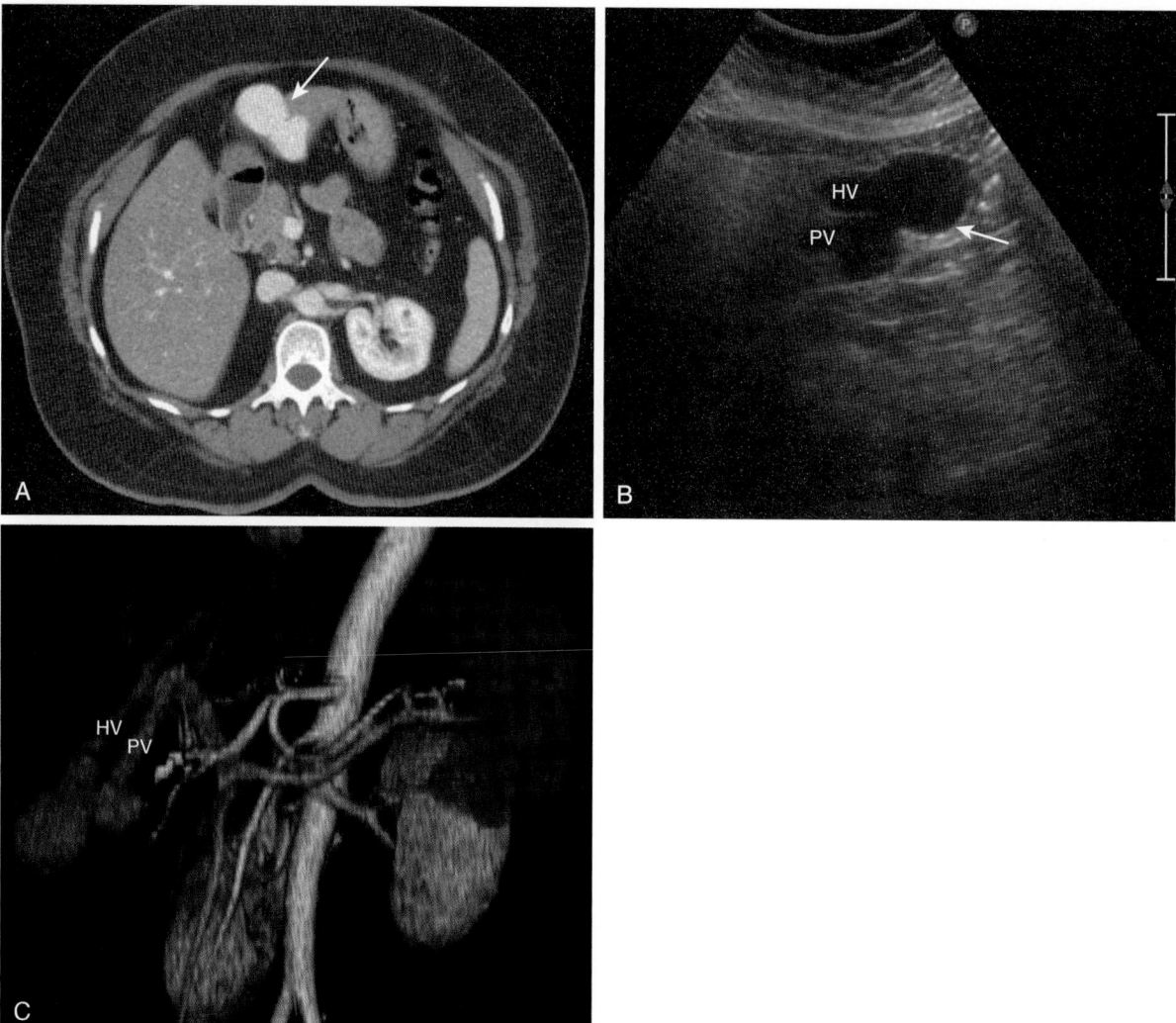

FIGURE 115.6   Congenital portosystemic shunts. A, Large spontaneous hepatoportal venous shunt. Axial portal venous–phase enhanced computed tomography (CT) image shows large bilobed varix *(white arrow)* inferiorly in segment III. A left portal branch and left hepatic vein branch both communicated with the lesion, consistent with a hepatoportal venous shunt. **B,** Sagittal gray-scale ultrasound image depicts subcapsular varix *(white arrow)* at the inferior aspect of segment III, which communicates with portal vein branch *(PV)* and hepatic vein branch *(HV)*. Color Doppler showed turbulent flow in the cystic mass, and venous waveforms were recorded in both the communicating branches. **C,** Three-dimensional reconstructed image demonstrates large shunt between segment III portal vein and left hepatic vein branch. (See Chapter 14.)

atresia, HPS, or as a prophylactic measure before the onset of symptoms. PV reconstruction can be challenging in these patients, with the graft PV anastomosed to the divided shunt in an end-to-end or end-to-side manner with subsequent partial or complete shunt ligation.[67,98] Blanc and colleagues[97] described the management of five patients with end-to-side CPS without LT using a two-stage operative approach, with banding of the shunt as a first-stage procedure to allow development of the intrahepatic PV system, followed by delayed occlusion or ligation of the shunt once appropriate hepatic flow had developed. Extrahepatic portosystemic shunts (Type 2c) between distal PV branches and the systemic circulation (mesocaval, splenorenal, mesoiliac), H-type shunts, intrahepatic shunts (Type 2a), and persistent patent ductus venosus can be treated with one-stage ligation without significant hemodynamic consequences.

Side-to-side CPS (Type 2b) can be managed by ligation, caval partition, or a two-stage banding approach, depending on the anatomy or the shunt and pattern of blood flow with trial fistula clamping and occlusion. Intraoperative evaluation of side-to-side CPS involves placing a vascular clamp across the shunt with Doppler venous US assessment of flow in the IVC and PV. The clamp is progressively moved from the anterior toward the posterior aspect of the IVC until occlusion of the shunt is demonstrated, with good portal and caval flow without bowel congestion. Once this is achieved, the shunt and IVC are partitioned at the site of the vascular clamp. In cases where the shunt cannot be successfully divided in one stage, a band or ligature is placed around the shunt to decrease flow and promote development of intrahepatic portal flow.[97]

PANCREATIC ARTERIOVENOUS MALFORMATIONS

Pancreatic AVMs (PAVMs) are rare lesions, the identification of which has increased significantly with the increasing utility of non-invasive imaging. Accurate data regarding prevalence are difficult to obtain because many lesions will not progress to clinically significant entities, but it has been reported that PAVMs represent 1% to 5% of GI tract AVMs.[99,100] Congenital lesions account for 80% to 90% of cases, and the original case report described such a case in a patient with Osler-Weber-Rendu syndrome[101] (see Chapter 1). Acquired lesions are typically the result of inflammation, malignancy, or trauma and even occur after transplantation.[102,103] Anatomically, AVMs may occur in any portion of the gland and can be associated with extrapancreatic AVMs. The most common location is the head (40%–50%), followed by the body and tail (>30%) and entire gland (>14%).[104–106]

Clinically significant lesions most frequently present with GI hemorrhage, which may be secondary to variceal bleeding as a result of portal hypertension, duodenal erosions, or hemorrhage into the pancreatic or bile ducts.[106–108] Hemorrhage can be severe, mandating emergency intervention. Less frequently, patients may present with abdominal pain or jaundice, or rarely pancreatitis, although many are asymptomatic.[99,109,110] Radiologic imaging characteristics have been well described,[104,107–109] and lesions are well demonstrated by CECT, MRI, US, and angiography (see Chapters 13, 17, and 21).

Several management approaches to PAVM have been described. Radiation therapy has been used for extensive lesions affecting the entire gland, with good short-term and intermediate-term results.[111,112] Resection, including pancreaticoduodenectomy, distal pancreatectomy, and even total pancreatectomy (see Chapters 117A–C), has been reported.[108,109,113] Embolization has been recommended before surgical resection to reduce bleeding.[114,115] However, given the increased facility of endovascular approaches, surgical therapy should be reserved for larger or refractory lesions. Numerous reports have demonstrated the efficacy of catheter-based modalities in effecting definitive resolution of PAVM, but recurrence rates can approach 30%[103,116] (see Chapter 114).

References are available at expertconsult.com.

CHAPTER 116

Hemobilia and bilhemia

Tahsin M. Khan and Jonathan M. Hernandez

INTRODUCTION

Hemobilia and bilhemia are clinical phenomena that arise from admixing of blood and bile due to anomalous connection between the bloodstream and biliary tract.[1-3] In general terms, a fistula between the hepatic arterial supply and the bile ducts can lead to blood invading the biliary tree, leading to hemobilia. Similarly, aberrant connection between the biliary tract and the portal or hepatic venous supply can result in hemobilia, or in bile entering the bloodstream and systemic circulation leading to bilhemia. This reverse flow of bile into the circulatory system is facilitated by high biliary ductal pressures, such as in the case of obstructive jaundice, and the low-pressure venous system. Although rare, these conditions can be clinically significant and lead to major morbidity and mortality if not identified and rectified appropriately.[4,5] The epidemiologic and therapeutic landscape for hemobilia/bilhemia has shifted over time, but awareness of the pathophysiology, etiology, and clinical manifestations is key to early diagnosis and effective management of these disorders.[2,6,7]

PATHOPHYSIOLOGY AND CLINICAL MANIFESTATIONS

The pathophysiology of hemobilia/bilhemia pertains directly to the dual blood supply of the liver and the intimate relationship between bile ducts and blood vessels within the hepatic parenchyma (see Chapters 2 and 5). Briefly, the liver receives 25% of its total blood flow (and 30%–50% of its oxygen content) from the hepatic artery, with the portal venous system accounting for the remainder. Importantly, the hepatic arterial system is the sole source of blood supply to the intrahepatic bile ducts. The hepatic arterioles, portal venules, and bile ductules exist in close proximity within the hepatic parenchyma.[8] In the context of hemobilia, any aberrant fistulous connection between either the arterial and biliary system (and to a lesser extent portal/venous and biliary system) can lead to blood leaving the high-pressure arterial system and translocating along a pressure gradient to enter the lower pressure biliary system. The bleeding can arise from anywhere along the intrahepatic and extrahepatic biliary tract, or the liver parenchyma itself. Blood then courses through the biliary ductal system to enter the gastrointestinal tract. As such, significant hemobilia will classically manifest as upper gastrointestinal bleeding. In the context of indwelling biliary drains, the bleeding may also manifest as blood per the drainage system itself.[9] Additionally, the hemorrhage may lead to formation of blood clots in the biliary tract (given the propensity of blood to precipitate away from bile due to difference in composition and viscosity), thereby leading to biliary obstruction (see Chapter 8).[10] This in turn can manifest as right upper quadrant pain and jaundice. Indeed, this trifecta of signs and symptoms—upper gastrointestinal hemorrhage, jaundice, and right upper quadrant abdominal pain—are collectively designated as *Quincke's triad* of hemobilia, originally described in 1871.[11] Gastrointestinal bleeding can either be melena or frank hematemesis in 90% or 60% of cases, respectively, and pain is seen in 70% of cases and jaundice in 60%. Though all three findings may comanifest in only 22% to 35% of patients with hemobilia, any combination of gastrointestinal bleeding with jaundice or right abdominal pain, especially in the context of a history of hepatic trauma or instrumentation, should raise suspicion for hemobilia.[7] In addition to pain and jaundice, the blood clots, if left unaddressed, can also lead to choledocholithiasis (see Chapter 33), cholangitis (see Chapter 43), cholecystitis (see Chapter 34), and pancreatitis (see Chapters 54–58), depending on where they come to rest within the biliary tree.[10,12-19] Laboratory abnormalities associated with hemobilia include findings of anemia and elevated liver enzymes (particularly bilirubin and alkaline phosphatase) based on the severity and chronicity of the disease. For reference, the average laboratory values for a series of 37 patients with hemobilia included hemoglobin of 10.6 g/dL (range 7.3–15.8 g/dL), aspartate aminotransferase (AST) of 353 IU/L, alanine aminotransferase (ALT) of 243 IU/L, alkaline phosphatase of 834 IU/L, γ-glutamyl transferase (GGT) of 385 IU/L, and total bilirubin of 10.5 mg/dL.[20]

Bilhemia, on the other hand, arises from the reverse flow of bile into the systemic circulation, typically through abnormal conduits into the portal or hepatic venous systems.[5,21-24] As mentioned previously, this problem is exacerbated by concomitant biliary obstruction (see Chapter 8), which can increase the pressure within the biliary system over that of the venous system.[25] The symptoms of bilhemia typically manifest as rising serum bilirubin levels without a corresponding rise in liver function tests.[26] Thus, much like in obstructive biliary diseases, bilhemia can result in jaundice. The more feared consequence of bilhemia is septicemia secondary to flow of infected bile into the sterile bloodstream.[27] Bilhemia should therefore be part of the differential diagnosis alongside more common disorders, such as cholangitis (see Chapter 43), in septic patients with rising direct serum bilirubin levels.

ETIOLOGY

Advances in the management of hepatobiliary trauma (see Chapters 113) and minimally invasive hepatobiliary procedures (see Chapter 127) have led to a shift in the common etiologies of hemobilia and bilhemia (Fig. 116.1).[2,6,7] Accidental hepatic trauma was historically the most common cause, but most instances of hemobilia/bilhemia are now iatrogenic secondary to percutaneous or endoscopic diagnostic and therapeutic interventions (see Chapters 23, 30, 31, 52, 85, and 96), malignancies (see Chapters 50, 89, and 90–93), inflammatory and infectious conditions (see Chapters 44, 45, and 70–72), and vascular anomalies (see Chapter 115).

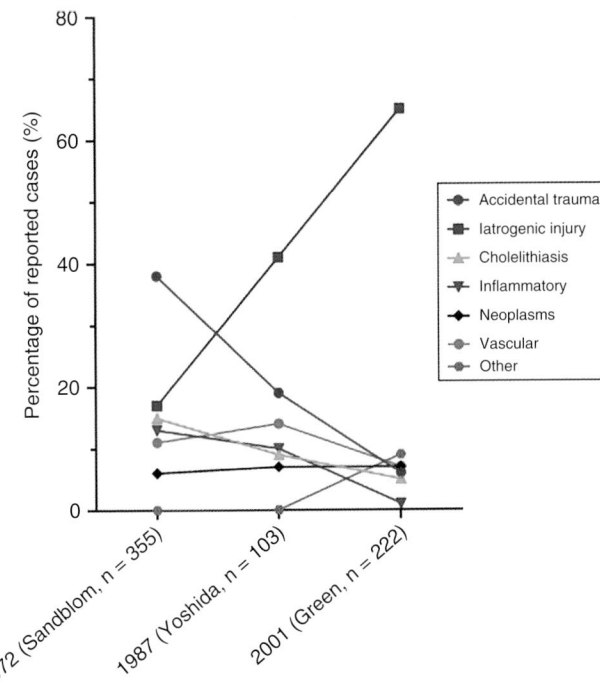

FIGURE 116.1 Changing etiology of hemobilia over time. Historically, accidental trauma was the most common cause, but this has been replaced by iatrogenic trauma in recent years. (Data from Sandblom P. *Hemobilia (Biliary Tract Hemorrhage): History, Pathology, Diagnosis, Treatment.* Thomas; 1972; Yoshida J, Donahue PE, Nyhus LM. Hemobilia: review of recent experience with a worldwide problem. *Am J Gastroenterol.* 1987;82[5]:448–453; Green MH, Duell RM, Johnson CD, Jamieson NV. Haemobilia. *Br J Surg.* 2001;88[6]:773–786.)

Iatrogenic Injuries

Iatrogenic injuries are now thought to account for over 70% of all cases of hemobilia (see Fig. 116.1; also see Chapters 23, 30, 31, 52, 85, and 96). The most common injury is that to the hepatic artery (see Chapter 5), which leads to hemorrhage and formation of anomalous connection to the biliary tract (Fig. 116.2). The highest risk of injury is associated with percutaneous transhepatic biliary drainage (PTBD) and percutaneous transhepatic cholangiography (PTC) (see Chapters 52), which is estimated to be between 1% and 2% (Table 116.1). PTBD is associated with the highest incidence given the utilization of larger bore needles, multiple catheters, and placement of indwelling drains.[28,29] The size of needle used to access appears to affect hemobilia rates, with smaller (21-gauge) needles associated with fewer instances of hemobilia compared with 18-gauge needles.[30–32] The impact of approach side (right vs. left biliary tree) is less clear; an earlier series demonstrated no influence on left- vs. right-sided approach,[28] although more recent studies have found higher global rates of bleeding with either left- or right-sided approach.[33,34] Finally, a nondilated biliary tree (making for a smaller target) and chronic portal vein thrombus (leading to more collateral vessels) are also thought to increase the risk of bleeding complication from PTBD/PTC.[35]

Compared with PTBD/PTC, percutaneous liver biopsies (see Chapter 23) performed for diagnostic purposes carry a lower risk of hemobilia, between 0.005% and 0.2%.[36–38] The risk of hemobilia may be higher in patients with chronic liver disease who may harbor coagulopathies that increase risk of bleeding. For instance, Seeff et al.[37] have demonstrated elevated international normalized ratio (INR) and thrombocytopenia to be associated with increased risk of hemobilia. Finally, case reports of hemobilia and bilhemia resulting from placement of transjugular intrahepatic portosystemic shunts (TIPS) also exist (see Chapter 85).[39–41]

Endoscopic procedures have also been shown to cause hemobilia. In general, the most common bleeding complication from endoscopic retrograde cholangiopancreatography (ERCP) (see Chapters 30) involves hemorrhage secondary to sphincterotomy, which has an incidence of 2%; the incidence of hemobilia specifically was noted to be 0.5% in a series of 400 patients.[42–44] In most cases this blood flows a short distance from the cut papilla into the duodenal lumen, but in rare instances it may reflux into the biliary tree itself. Risk factors for ERCP-related hemobilia parallel those associated with any

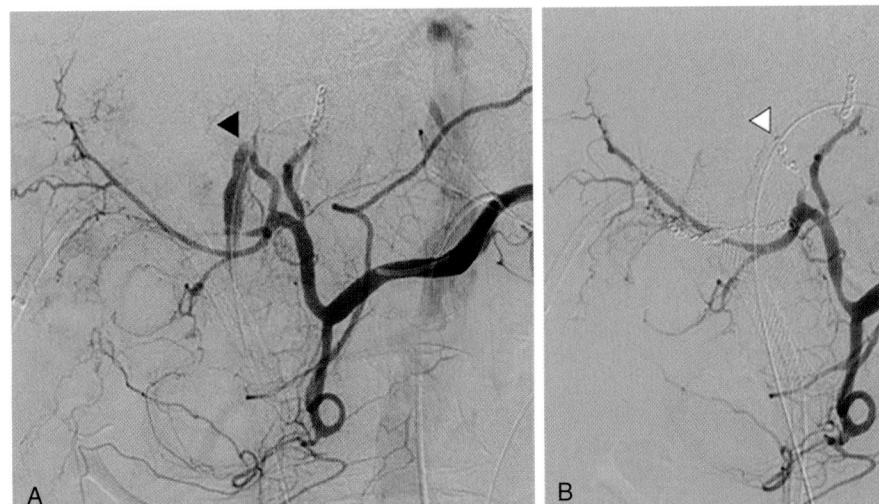

FIGURE 116.2 **Hemobilia in a patient with biliary drainage.** Subtraction images from angiogram demonstrating contrast extravasation into the biliary tree *(black arrowhead)* suggesting fistulous connection at the level of the right hepatic artery **(A).** Postembolization angiogram demonstrates no further contrast extravasation at previous fistula *(white arrowhead,* **B)** (see Chapter 115). (Photographs courtesy of Memorial Sloan Kettering. All rights reserved.)

TABLE 116.1 Risk of Hemobilia from Iatrogenic Procedures and Accidental Trauma

PROCEDURE	RISK (%)
Percutaneous transhepatic cholangiography	1–2
Percutaneous transhepatic biliary drainage	1–2
Percutaneous liver biopsy	0.005–0.2
Percutaneous radiofrequency ablation	0.5
Endoscopic retrograde cholangiopancreatography with sphincterotomy	0.5
Surgery	
Laparoscopic cholecystectomy	0.16
Liver transplantation	1.2
Accidental trauma	0.2–3

bleeding after endoscopy and include variables such as coagulopathy, variant anatomy (see Chapter 2), vascular anomalies, and the invasiveness and complexity of the biliary intervention being performed (e.g., balloon dilation or biopsies obtained within the biliary tract).[35,45] Similarly, endoscopic ultrasound–guided biopsies of hepatopancreaticobiliary lesions can also lead to hemobilia as a rare complication.[46,47]

The incidence of hemobilia after surgical procedures appears to be rare, with most instances being associated with injury to the right hepatic or cystic arteries. In the early days of minimally invasive surgery, laparoscopic cholecystectomy (see Chapter 36) was associated with increased incidence of injury to hepatic artery leading to subsequent pseudoaneurysms and fistula formation with biliary tract and presentation of hemobilia (see Chapter 115). Although isolated cases of hemobilia following laparoscopic cholecystectomy are still being reported,[48] the overall incidence of vascular injury after laparoscopic cholecystectomy is rare (0.16%).[49] It must be noted, however, that most instances of hemobilia after surgical intervention involve the initial formation of a vascular pseudoaneurysm that subsequently erodes into the adjacent biliary tree.[50–53] As such, presentation of hemobilia after surgical injury may be delayed from the time of index operation.[54] Furthermore, hemobilia can also result from open hepatobiliary surgery, including pancreaticoduodenectomy (see Chapter 117) and liver transplantation (see Chapter 111).[55,56] A case series by Park et al.[57] reported spontaneous hemobilia in 33 out of 2701 liver transplant cases (1.2%). Emergent liver transplant, alcoholic cirrhosis, and body mass index less than 24.5 were factors associated with spontaneous hemobilia in this series.[57]

Finally, percutaneous radiofrequency ablation (RFA) of tumors (see Chapter 96B) can be associated with hemobilia.[58,59] This frequency has been reported to be around 0.5%; however, in one series of 195 patients undergoing computed tomography (CT)–guided RFA, the rate of hemobilia was noted to be as high as 8%.[60] Factors associated with hemobilia in this series included more than 1 tumor being treated, a central puncture tract and puncture through the hepatic hilum, needle puncture length, and low platelet count.[60] Although the cause of hemobilia after RFA is thought to be due to simultaneous puncture of both the arteries and hepatic trees during access to the target lesion, the thermal spread associated with this procedure and subsequent injury to surrounding tissue are also suspected to play a role.

Accidental Trauma

Once the most common cause of hemobilia, traumatic hepatic injury (see Chapter 113) is now thought to account for less than 5% of cases of hemobilia (see Fig. 116.1). Nevertheless, given that the liver is the most commonly injured organ during blunt trauma (in ~25% of cases), traumatic hemobilia remains an important clinical entity affecting anywhere between 0.2% and 3% of all patients with major liver injury.[61–63] Hemobilia after hepatic trauma typically arises secondary to deep parenchymal injury, whereby damaged blood vessels and bile ducts may drain into a deep cavity of parenchymal damage resulting in the mixing of blood and bile. Alternately, blunt trauma may result in formation of arterial pseudoaneurysms that could subsequently encroach into the biliary tree secondary to ongoing inflammation and healing (Fig. 116.3) (see Chapter 115). Of note, in both these scenarios, hemobilia results from a gradual process and may thus manifest weeks to months after the initial trauma.[64,65] More immediate hemobilia, on the other hand, may result from penetrating injuries to the liver in which both blood vessels and biliary structures get transected during the index insult. Although such penetrating injuries typically necessitate immediate operative intervention, the vast majority of hepatic trauma (up to 80%) are treated nonoperatively in recent times. Reassuringly, no significant association between nonoperative management and increased incidence of hemobilia has been established.[66,67] For instance, in a series of 135 adult patients with hepatic trauma managed nonoperatively, only 2 (1.5%) developed hemobilia. In a similar series of nonoperative pediatric liver trauma patients, the rate of hemobilia was just 1 in 185 (0.5%).[68,69]

Neoplasms

Primary (e.g., hepatocellular carcinoma [see Chapter 89], cholangiocarcinoma [see Chapters 50 and 51], gallbladder cancer [see Chapter 49]) and secondary (i.e., metastatic [see Chapters 90–92]) hepatobiliary tumors account for 5% to 10% of all hemobilia cases (see Fig. 116.1).[7,20] Hemobilia arises when these lesions gradually grow and invade into the biliary tree, and as such, the rate of bleeding associated with tumors is generally indolent. The risk of bleeding can be increased, however, because these tumors tend to have enhanced vascular supply and be surrounded by friable tissue owing to local tumor-related inflammatory and microenvironmental changes. Benign lesions (see Chapter 48), such as gallbladder polyps, biliary cystadenomas, or choledochal cysts, can also lead to hemobilia,[70–73] but this is uncommon. Of note, hemobilia may be the initial presenting sign in cases of hepatobiliary malignancies, as evidenced by case reports.[74–76] As such, a thorough search for occult malignancies should be performed in instances of unexplained hemobilia. Finally, the treatment of hepatobiliary malignancies itself can also lead to hemobilia. In addition to percutaneous RFA described previously, therapies such as transarterial chemoembolization, chemotherapy, and small molecule kinase inhibitors (sorafenib) all have been reported to cause isolated cases of hemobilia.[77–79]

Vasculopathy and Coagulopathy

Vascular malformations account for around 10% of all hemobilia cases, and hepatic artery aneurysms, either spontaneous or secondary to iatrogenic/accidental trauma as discussed previously, are the most common vascular culprit (see Chapter 115).[80] Nontraumatic, spontaneous causes of arterial aneurysms include those associated with atherosclerotic disease (30%), polyarteritis

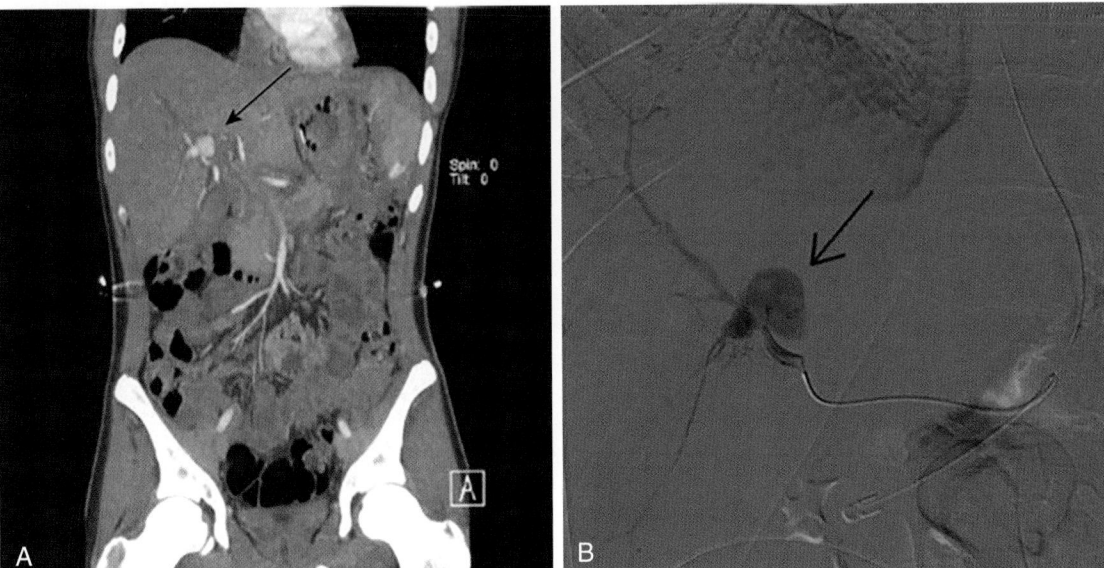

FIGURE 116.3 **Hepatic vascular injury from blunt trauma.** Contrast-enhanced computed tomography **(A)** (see Chapter 13) and angiogram **(B)** (see Chapters 21 and 115) demonstrating pseudoaneurysm of right hepatic artery *(arrows)* following accidental blunt trauma. (From Schouten van der Velden AP, de Ruijter WM, Janssen CM, Schultze Kool LJ, Tan EC. Hemobilia as a late complication after blunt abdominal trauma: a case report and review of the literature. *J Emerg Med.* 2010;39[5]:592–595.)

nodosa, fibromuscular dysplasia, or mycotic aneurysms.[81–88] Hemobilia from the rupture of an arterial aneurysm is typically massive and clinically significant with high mortality rate if not treated emergently. Fortunately, visceral arterial aneurysms are uncommon and affect only 0.1% to 2% of the population, out of which only 20% are hepatic arterial aneurysms.[80,89] Other infrequently reported vascular malformations that can cause hemobilia include angiodysplasia, arteriovenous malformations, and hemangiomas.[90–93] Hemobilia in the context of mixed connective tissue disorder, systemic lupus erythematosus, hemophilia, and platelet disorders such as Bernard-Soulier syndrome have all been reported.[94–100]

Inflammatory and Infectious Conditions

Acute and chronic inflammation leading to hemobilia has been described for both infectious and noninfectious causes. The most common noninfectious cause is gallstones (see Chapter 33), which, when causing prolonged biliary ductal obstruction, can lead to a chronic inflammatory process culminating in penetration of the stones into the biliary vasculature adjacent to the affected bile ducts, thereby leading to hemobilia.[101] Interestingly, historical accounts of gallstone disease have reported rates of microscopic hemobilia in 25% of cases with gallbladder stones and 33% with common duct stones.[102] Though much rarer than the other manifestations of gallstone disease such as cholecystitis (see Chapter 34) or obstructive jaundice, significant hemobilia caused by gallstones can be associated with high mortality rates. Moreover, acute and chronic inflammation associated with both calculous and acalculous cholecystitis can also lead to formation of fistulae between arterial and biliary tracts leading to hemobilia.[103–106]

Liver abscesses and invasion and infection of the biliary tract by parasites can also lead to hemobilia (see Chapters 45, 70, 71, and 72).[107–110] Liver flukes and roundworms such as *Clonorchis sinensis, Fasciola hepatica,* and *Ascaris lumbricoides* have all been implicated in hemobilia.[111–114] In addition, *Echinococcus* infections

can also cause hemobilia secondary to local inflammation, causing vascular and biliary damage adjacent to areas of hydatid cyst growth.[115]

DIAGNOSTIC MODALITIES

The diagnostic and management algorithm for hemobilia is contingent on the suspected cause of bleeding. The armamentarium available to diagnose hemobilia includes endoscopy, angiography, and conventional noninvasive imaging modalities (see Chapters 16, 20, 21, 30, and 52). Although ultrasound and nonangiographic CT imaging can reveal stigmata of bleeding (e.g., clotted blood and hematoma), these modalities have low specificity for hemobilia, and thus a high index of clinical suspicion should also be exercised. Of these, angiographic interrogation of suspected bleeding vessels remains the "gold standard" (see Chapter 21). Typically, angiography is undertaken in a systemic manner by cannulating the branches of celiac trunk, followed by the hepatic arterial branches and, if needed, the superior mesenteric artery. Passage of intravascular contrast into the biliary tract, frank extravasation, presence of pseudoaneurysm, or arteriovenous fistula to the portal venous system should raise suspicion for hemobilia[116] (see Chapter 115 and Figs. 116.2 and 116.3). An added benefit of angiography is that it can be both diagnostic and therapeutic, as coil embolization or stenting of the bleeding vessels can be performed via the same vascular access and cannulation. Like direct angiography, CT angiogram (see Chapter 13) can also be employed based on the concept of contrast extravasation into biliary tree to diagnose hemobilia. An added benefit of CT angiography is that it can provide simultaneous information regarding the intraabdominal organs as well. It must be kept in mind that the ability of both direct and CT angiography to detect bleeding is contingent on the rate and presence of active bleeding at the time of study. As such, the possibility of a false-negative study must be entertained while interpreting these results.

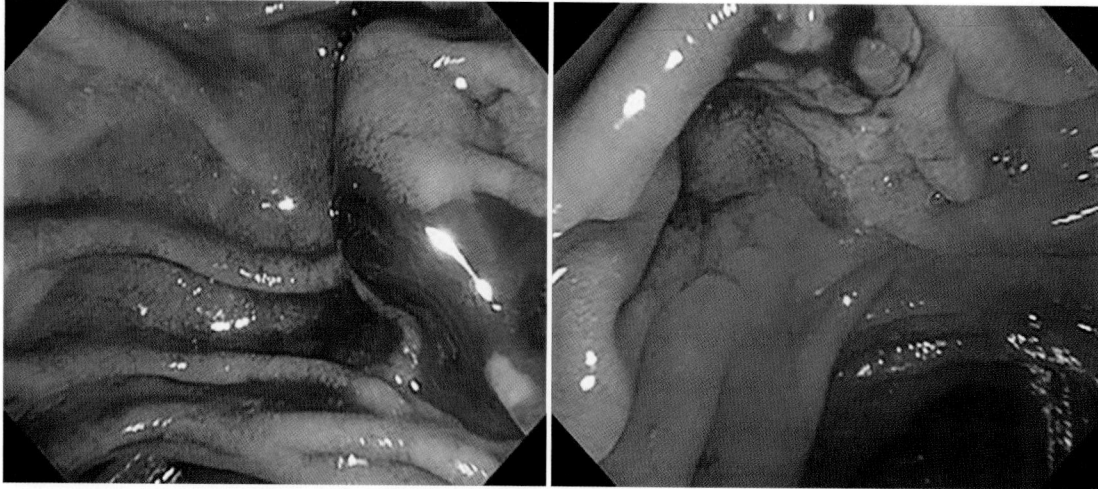

FIGURE 116.4 Blood emanating from ampulla of Vater during endoscopy signifying bleeding in the biliary tract, that is, hemobilia (see Chapter 30). (Photographs courtesy of Memorial Sloan Kettering. All rights reserved.)

Direct visualization of the duodenal lumen/papillary ampulla via endoscopy, or interrogation of the biliary tree endoscopically via endoscopic retrograde cholangiopancreatography (ERCP) (see Chapters 20 and 30), can also be used to diagnose hemobilia. Visualization of blood extravasating from the ampulla is a telltale sign of hemobilia during endoscopy, and any filling defect in the biliary tract can hint at the presence of blood clots[20] (Fig. 116.4). Indeed, ERCP can help remove such blood clots and restore biliary flow, which is an important treatment consideration in hemobilia.[117,118] Additionally, ultrasonography using endoscopic probes (i.e., endoscopic ultrasound [EUS]) can also be employed to detect hemobilia (see Chapters 22 and 30).[119,120] Given that most diagnostic algorithms for suspected upper gastrointestinal bleeding necessitate upper endoscopy, this modality should be freely employed in suspected cases of hemobilia as well. Moreover, ERCP may be the sole means to detect occult cases of bilhemia, as these typically involve portal or hepatic venous vasculature and therefore will not become apparent in arteriography. In bilhemia, contrast extravasation from the biliary tract into the venous system during endoscopy will be the classic diagnostic finding.

Other, less common, diagnostic modalities include abdominal ultrasound or magnetic resonance cholangiopancreatography (see Chapter 16). Both these modalities are beneficial in that they are noninvasive, but their ability to directly detect hemobilia is limited at best. Both ultrasound and magnetic resonance cholangiopancreatography (MRCP) can reveal stigmata of hemobilia, such as dilated biliary ducts caused by obstructive blood clots or vascular pseudoaneurysms (see Chapter 16).[121,122] MRCP can also provide a detailed view of the intrahepatic and extrahepatic biliary tree and thus identify any potential site of injury. Nevertheless, these modalities should be considered secondary to direct angiography, upper endoscopy, and contrast-enhanced axial imaging in the diagnosis of hemobilia.

MANAGEMENT

The guiding principles of hemobilia management are (1) stopping the bleeding and (2) clearing any biliary obstruction and restoring bile flow. Additionally, adequate resuscitation of the

bleeding patient, and treatment of any sequelae of biliary obstruction (if present), such as cholangitis, cholecystitis, and pancreatitis, must also be emphasized (see Chapters 34, 43, and 54–58). Minor hemobilia (i.e., those with limited bleeding without associated hemodynamic changes) can often be managed conservatively, for instance by readjusting the positioning of indwelling biliary catheters or correcting underlying coagulopathy. The urgency and degree of invasiveness of any therapeutic intervention for major hemobilia depend on clinical factors, such as the rate of blood loss, hemodynamic stability, and suspected source of bleeding. In the most drastic cases, surgical ligation of bleeding vessel, resection of hepatic segment with biliary obstruction (see Chapters 101 and 102B), or exploration of the bile duct (see Chapter 32) to retrieve clots may be necessary.

Endovascular interventions (see Chapters 94 and 115) using transarterial chemoembolization or vascular stenting remain the most successful approach to treat hemobilia, and should be considered as the therapeutic modality of choice once diagnosis is confirmed (see Fig. 116.2).[123] The choice of embolic material ranges from physical coils to embolic agents such as thrombin, gelfoam, polyvinyl alcohol, or n-butyl-2-cyanoacrylate particles.[124–127] Embolization should be attempted as selectively as possible, with nonselective embolization of the left or right hepatic artery being reserved when other options are limited. The success rate of arterial embolization techniques approach 100% and are generally well tolerated, owing to the dual blood supply of the liver and intrahepatic arterial collaterals between the right and left hepatic arterial systems. However, ischemic injury of the bile ducts, which derive all their blood supply from the hepatic arterial system, may occur and is a serious side effect of embolization techniques (see Chapter 5). Patients with compromised portal venous flow (e.g., those with cirrhosis, portal or hepatic vein thrombosis, or liver transplant recipients) should be approached cautiously, as they are particularly susceptible to such ischemic sequelae of arterial embolization.[45] To this end, occlusion of areas of vascular injury using covered endovascular stents has emerged as a possible alternative to embolization.[128,129] These stents can have a tamponade effect at the site of bleeding/defect in the blood vessel, while still allowing for blood flow distally through the artery. They are particularly useful if the bleeding source is a proximal lesion within the left or right hepatic artery territory. In general, successful tamponade by stenting is achieved using stents that are slightly larger in diameter than the target vessel (by 10%–20%) and have an approximately 10 mm "landing zone" of robust, uninjured endothelium on either side of the defect in the vessel wall.[130] Placement of stents, much like embolization, should be carried out by versed interventional radiologists or vascular surgeons.

Concurrent with endovascular treatment modalities, endoscopic interventions also play a key role in the management of hemobilia and bilhemia. For one, endoscopy can also be used to treat select cases of bleeding, such as those secondary to sphincterotomy, wherein endoscopic epinephrine injection, coagulation, or clipping may be performed on the suspect vessel (typically a branch of the superior pancreaticoduodenal artery).[131] Additionally, endoscopy can also be used to place biliary stents and thus occlude the fistula and prevent further inflow of blood into the biliary tract (see Chapter 30).[132–135] Perhaps the most unique utility of endoscopy, however, is the ability to clear blood clots and thus relieve biliary obstruction that may result from hemobilia and, if untreated, can result in obstructive jaundice, cholecystitis, or cholangitis.[136] In the context of bilhemia, given the limited option for coiling or stenting of the portal and hepatic venous system, the management strategy focuses on relieving biliary obstruction and thus reducing intraductal pressures to help reverse the active flow of bile into the venous system and thus allow for the fistula to heal with time.[137–139] Endoscopy therefore remains the treatment modality of choice in this setting, although if endoscopy fails, percutaneous biliary drainage may also be attempted.

Surgical intervention, popularized in the early 1900s and historically considered the treatment of choice, has now been relegated to salvage situations when endovascular or endoscopic interventions fail to control bleeding, or when the patient is too hemodynamically unstable to tolerate minimally invasive procedures.[31,140,141] The principle of surgical intervention is ligation of the offending bleeding vessel or resection of pseudoaneurysm; however, in cases where this vessel cannot be adequately identified, ligation of the right or left hepatic artery itself can also be an option (albeit one with a much higher risk of subsequent ischemic injury to liver). In a series published in 2014, surgical intervention carried a success rate of 90% in controlling massive hemobilia, albeit with a 10% mortality rate.[142] The other, perhaps more appropriate, use of surgery is for cases where the etiology of hemobilia itself merits surgical intervention, such as in cases of neoplastic processes where resection of tumor may be the only valid method to control hemobilia and offer a definitive intervention for the underlying process.

The references for this chapter can be found online by accessing the accompanying Expert Consult website.

PART 10

Techniques of Pancreatic and Hepatic Resection and Transplantation

Pancreaticoduodenectomy

Peter J. Allen

OPERATIVE APPROACH

Pancreaticoduodenectomy (PD) is one of the few remaining operations where major morbidity rates hover in the range of 25% and the 90-day mortality rate remains in the 2% to 4% range, even under the care of the highest-volume surgeons at the highest-volume centers. This chapter will describe an approach to the exploration, resection, and reconstruction of patients undergoing PD with the understanding that multiple techniques have been shown to be equally as effective and with the recognition that individual steps of the procedure may—and should—be performed in a different order depending on the nature and location of the abnormality. Although I am the sole author on this chapter, my use of the terms "we" and "our" is to recognize that this approach is derived from my current and former mentors and colleagues (namely, Murray Brennan, Leslie Blumgart, William Jarnagin, and Michael D'Angelica) and from other pancreatic experts in centers at which I have had the privilege to collaborate (namely, Johns Hopkins Hospital, Massachusetts General Hospital, University of Verona, and University of Heidelberg).

This chapter will focus on the specific technique of open PD. Minimally invasive approaches (laparoscopic and robotic) are described in a later chapter (see Chapter 127). Minimally invasive PD has been developed over the past 20 years; however, more than 95% of these operations continue to be performed with an open technique. The data published to date suggest that a minimally invasive approach to PD can be performed safely with equivalent outcomes to the open approach in very select high-volume centers that have a team dedicated to this endeavor.

Exploration and Assessment of Distant Metastatic Disease

Exploration of the abdomen should be initially performed to rule out subradiographic metastatic disease, which would be a contraindication to resection. The use of staging laparoscopy (SL) for patients with adenocarcinoma of the pancreas is subject to individual surgeon preference and institutional experience (see Chapters 24 and 62). Reports have suggested that SL is currently performed routinely, selectively, or never.[1] The yield of SL will decrease as the quality of cross-sectional imaging increases. Our current approach is to perform SL in a selective fashion, on a case-by-case basis. Indications for SL include a concerning feature on preoperative imaging or a significantly elevated carbohydrate antigen (CA) 19-9 level.[2] The degree of elevation in CA 19-9 that warrants SL is variable among different studies and ranges from 130 to 250 U/mL. Attention should be paid to the status of the biliary tree at the time of CA 19-9 evaluation because biliary obstruction can increase the CA 19-9 level.

When SL is not felt to be necessary, the operation should begin with a limited upper midline incision. The initial incision should be small to do a visual and manual inspection for metastatic disease, particularly when operating for cancer. Careful inspection of the liver and peritoneal surfaces should be performed, and targeted liver ultrasound should be considered for any liver parenchymal abnormalities (see Chapter 24). Once metastatic disease is ruled out, the incision should be extended to whatever length is needed to perform and complete the operation safely for that individual patient.

Mobilization and Assessment of Local Resectability

For more information, see Chapter 2.

Once retractors are applied, a wide Kocher maneuver is performed to the level of the aorta and the left renal vein, including mobilization of the ligament of Treitz from the patient's right side. To facilitate this maneuver, the transverse mesocolon is mobilized off of Gerota's fascia and the head of the pancreas, allowing for dynamic and manual retraction of the transverse colon and its mesentery caudally to optimize exposure. This enables an assessment of the retroperitoneum and relationship of the mass with the superior mesenteric artery (SMA; Fig. 117A.1). During the Kocher maneuver, there is no routine oncologic reason to enter Gerota's fascia of the right kidney or to remove posterior aortocaval lymph nodes. Both of these maneuvers may increase specific risks of the operation, such as lymphatic leak, and provide no proven oncologic benefit.[3] Care should be taken to avoid the right gonadal vein as it enters the inferior vena cava (IVC) because this vein is thin walled and if injured will result in brisk bleeding.

At this time, the SMA can also be inspected from the ligament of Treitz and dissected on its right lateral surface to exclude any tumor infiltration. This approach has been termed the *artery-first approach* (Fig. 117A.2) and may help with assessment of SMA involvement early in exploration.[4] We do not routinely perform this particular maneuver because high-quality preoperative imaging and careful palpation in the operating room are typically adequate for excluding gross SMA involvement.

After Kocherization, access to the lesser sac should be achieved through dissection of the greater omentum off of the transverse colon. Some surgeons may enter the lesser sac by directly dividing the omentum near the gastroepiploic vessels. Although this may seem to be the more direct and technically easier approach, it will result in an ischemic distal omentum as the branches from the gastroepiploic arcade are divided. In an obese patient with significant omental bulk, this ischemic tissue is at risk for postoperative infection, particularly in the setting of postoperative pancreatic leak. An additional advantage to lifting the omentum off the transverse colon to enter the lesser sac is that the healthy perfused omentum can be later used as a vascularized flap to cover the pancreatic and biliary anastomoses, and gastroduodenal arterial (GDA) stump, at the conclusion of the operation.

Careful dissection in the avascular plane between the hepatic flexure and the duodenum and extension of the Kocher

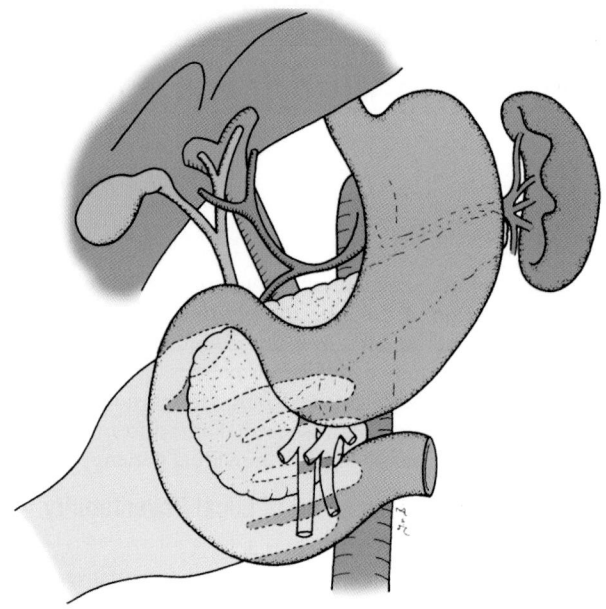

FIGURE 117A.1 Adequate Kocherization to facilitate assessment of the retroperitoneum and the relation of the tumor to the vascular structures.

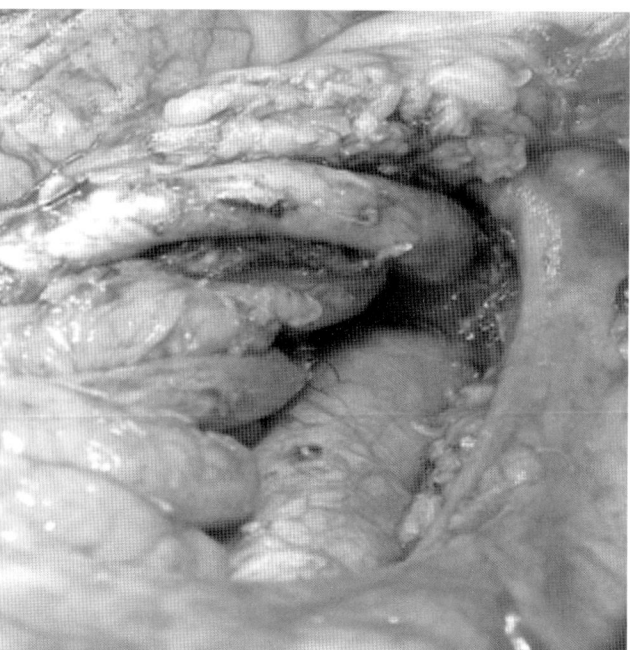

FIGURE 117A.2 Artery-first approach. The superior mesenteric artery is dissected, and infiltration of the artery is ruled out as one of the first steps of the operation.

maneuver separates the third part of the duodenum from the colonic mesentery. The avascular plane between the gastro-epiploic and middle colic veins is divided as it leads to the superior mesenteric vein (SMV) at the inferior edge of the pancreas. Several small crossing vascular branches may be encountered and should be prospectively divided. The gastro-epiploic vein may be ligated at this point; however, reserving this until after the pancreatic neck has been divided can make this maneuver more efficient. The SMV is now identified, and

early development of the tunnel between the pancreatic neck and SMV and portal vein (PV) confluence should be achieved.

Once the inferior border of the pancreas and SMV have been identified, attention should be turned to the supraduodenal compartment. While retracting the stomach anteriorly and inferiorly, the gastrohepatic ligament should be incised from the lesser curve of the stomach to the origin of the right gastric artery (RGA). The RGA should then be retracted anteriorly and the avascular tissue between the GDA and RGA incised. This maneuver will expedite the division of the RGA. The common hepatic artery is reliably identified by removing the lymph node that sits anterior to it, known as the "common hepatic artery lymph node." This node has been referred to by some as "the node of importance" because its involvement with disease may have some prognostic value in patients with pancreas cancer.[5,6] Regardless, it should generally be removed and sent for pathologic evaluation, but it should not be used as a determinant of proceeding with resection. The GDA can then be encircled and clamped to ensure a preserved pulse in the right and left hepatic arteries. This excludes misidentification of the GDA or a tight celiac artery stenosis that makes hepatic arterial inflow dependent on retrograde flow from the GDA. Once it is deemed safe to divide the GDA, it is ligated and divided.

There are two points worth emphasizing around the ligation of the GDA. First, one must be prepared for "what to do" if the pulse within the hepatic artery is lost, or diminished, when the GDA is clamped. Careful preoperative assessment of high-quality contrast enhanced imaging is essential (see Chapter 17). Clinically significant celiac stenosis and retrograde GDA flow is typically evident on preoperative imaging through arterial collateralization around the pancreatic head or an enlarged GDA. In this setting, attempts should be made to divide the fibrotic attachments resulting in the stenosis; however, in our experience, this rarely results in a normal pulse. Even after clamping (and subsequent division), intraoperative duplex ultrasound will generally identify continued flow in the hepatic artery, and in this setting we proceed with resection. The second consideration is how critically important GDA ligation is to minimizing the morbidity and mortality of PD. GDA stump blowout is a significant contributor to postoperative mortality and has been reported in as many as 6% of patients.[7] Because of this, a variety of tissue coverage techniques (falciform ligament, omentum) to protect this site of ligation from infection and leak have been recommended.[8,9] In general, we perform triple ligation of the GDA stump (tie, suture ligation, and clip) and will attempt to place omentum over the stump at the end of the case.

Ligation of the GDA exposes the anterior surface of the PV lying below. The anterior surface of the PV is dissected free, and the lateral border is identified. The lateral portal lymph nodes are mobilized away from the bile duct and brought down toward the duodenum to be included in the specimen. With the PV in view, the bile duct is encircled. In 10% to 15% of patients, a replaced or accessory right hepatic artery will course just posterior and lateral to the bile duct. Attention must be paid to assessing for this, and it should generally be preserved if present. In the absence of jaundice, however, either an accessory or replaced right hepatic artery can typically be safely ligated and resected, if indicated for oncologic reasons. This, however, should be avoided in the setting of jaundice because of the possible complication of postoperative right liver necrosis.

At this point, there should be a final assessment of the pancreatic neck and overall resectability. Before proceeding, many surgeons will create a tunnel behind the pancreatic neck to ensure that the vein is uninvolved, or if it is involved, that safe resection can be performed (see section on transection). Our approach is to attempt creation of the tunnel when the vein does not appear to be involved on preoperative imaging. Nevertheless, when PV resection and reconstruction is either possibly or definitely going to be required, it may not be safe to complete this tunnel without some division of the pancreas. In this latter circumstance, one must often determine whether PC reconstruction can be safely performed without creating a complete tunnel. This assessment of the pancreatic neck, and PV, is critical and can be subtly difficult. Intraoperative consultation with senior partners should be considered when there is not complete clarity on the extent of vascular involvement. Good decisions come from experience, and experience comes from making bad decisions.

Resection

Once deemed resectable, a cholecystectomy is performed, usually in an anterograde fundus-down technique. In patients with preoperative biliaryobstruction, the gallbladder can be distended and inflamed. Sometimes emptying the gallbladder of its contents can facilitate its dissection and removal. As the gallbladder is separated from the liver, the cystic artery and duct are identified and ligated. Care should be taken to avoid any iatrogenic injury to the right hepatic artery, which usually runs posterior to the common hepatic duct (see Chapter 2).[10] Some will leave the gallbladder attached and divide the common hepatic duct, whereas others will ligate the cystic duct and later divide the common bile duct. In the setting of pancreatic cancer, where a positive bile duct margin is generally not an issue, our approach is to ligate the cystic duct and then later divide the bile duct. In the setting of cholangiocarcinoma of the distal bile duct, however, our approach is to leave the gallbladder attached and later divide the common hepatic duct to achieve a negative margin.

Once the gallbladder is removed, the stomach is transected with two fires of a gastrointestinal stapler (GIA stapler) just distal to the incisura. Whether or not to resect or preserve the pylorus is a question that has resulted in more than eight clinical trials over three decades with over 1000 patients being prospectively evaluated. These studies have demonstrated no difference in outcome, and therefore any debate over an advantage or disadvantage to pylorus preservation is an exercise of opinion rather than an exercise in evidence-based medicine.[11,12] If preservation of the pylorus is planned, the right gastric and right gastroepiploic arteries are divided 2 cm beyond the pylorus, and the duodenum is skeletonized. The duodenum is divided and the stomach, along with the omentum, is packed away in the left upper quadrant.

At this time, attention is directed toward dividing what remains of the ligament of Treitz and jejunal transection. The body wall retractors are adjusted to expose the ligament of Treitz and the jejunum is then transected. The location of transection chosen, particularly the distance from ligament of Treitz, is partly affected by the planned route of the biliary-pancreatic limb for reconstruction, namely, via the ligament of Treitz or through the transverse mesocolon. The site of transection should allow for ample mesenteric mobility to enable a tension-free anastomosis for biliary and pancreatic reconstruction. Once the jejunum is transected, the mesentery is divided close to the bowel on the specimen side down to the level of the

root of the mesentery and the uncinate process of the pancreas. Because of the potential for postoperative hemorrhage from the proximal jejunal mesentery, it is our practice to control these vessels with the LigaSure device in combination with clips. The ischemic jejunal limb is then rotated under the ligament of Treitz to the right upper quadrant.

In preparation for pancreatic neck transection, the tunnel over the PV is fully developed. A Penrose drain or vessel loop can be placed into this tunnel to encircle the neck when possible (Fig. 117A.3); alternatively, a renal pedicle clamp can be used to guide the transection. Hemostatic sutures are placed at the superior and inferior borders of the pancreas on each side of the planned transection plane, being careful not to include the pancreatic duct. These sutures serve to ligate the superior and inferior pancreatic vessels running longitudinally in the pancreatic parenchyma and to decrease bleeding from the cut surface after transection. The superficial portions of the pancreas can be divided with electrocautery to minimize bleeding, but the deeper gland, especially the pancreatic duct, should in general be divided sharply with a scalpel. Division of the bile duct is typically reserved for this point in the operation to minimize the duration of bile drainage into the right upper quadrant, especially in preoperatively stented patients. Some will place a clamp on the distal bile duct to further minimize the spillage of bile. At this time, the SMV-PV is dissected away from the pancreas and tumor. Any small venous branches are controlled with clips, ties, or a coagulation device.

Once the vein is completely freed, attention is directed toward the SMA dissection. Releasing posterior attachments of the specimen to the retroperitoneum facilitates the dissection along the right lateral plane of the SMA. Once the specimen's attachments are isolated to the lateral aspect of the SMA, the dissection is completed along this plane to remove the specimen. During this step, the specimen that comprises the pancreatic head, duodenum, and proximal jejunum is retracted to the patient's right, and the position of the SMA is continuously assessed to avoid any injury. Aided by gentle retraction of the SMV toward the patient's left, the anterolateral aspect of the SMA is completely skeletonized of its investing tissues. This can be done by making

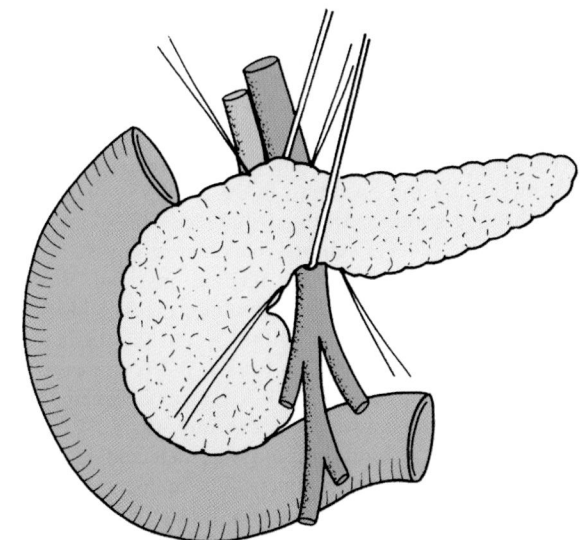

FIGURE 117A.3 Full development of the pancreatic neck may allow for safe passage of a Penrose drain or clamp anterior to the portal vein.

small windows in the tissue and sealing it with either ties, clips, or a coagulation device, such as the LigaSure. Clips can be used in combination with a coagulation device as well, especially on the inferior pancreaticoduodenal artery. A stapled transection should typically be avoided, particularly when there is concern regarding the oncologic margin.

If venous resection is required, the dissection along the SMA should be performed first to leave the venous resection as the last step. This minimizes clamp time on the PV and allows for more expeditious proximal and distal venous control. Also, control and often ligation of the inferior mesenteric vein, splenic vein, and left gastric vein is necessary to isolate the SMV-PV before doing a venous resection. Once the specimen is removed, hemostasis is ensured, and the operative field is washed with warm fluid before proceeding to the reconstruction phase.

Vascular Resection

For more information, see Chapter 122.

More than 30 years ago, Fortner at Memorial Sloan Kettering reasoned that a more radical resection might improve survival by enhancing tumor clearance, and, specifically, that tumor adherence to the PV or SMV, previously regarded as a criterion of unresectability, could be overcome by en bloc resection of the involved vessels.[13] Randomized evaluation of portal and SMV resection in patients with tumors adherent to these vessels is difficult because considerable variation in the interpretation of adherence and technique is likely, and thus no randomized controlled trial (RCT) evaluates this topic. Our approach to vascular resection is that when it is confirmed to be safe, it is reasonable to perform, and thus PV resection and even isolated hepatic arterial resection are deemed appropriate in carefully selected patients. We do not consider routine SMA resection and reconstruction appropriate because the most recent review of the literature revealed a 20% operative mortality rate and an 11-month disease-specific survival.[14]

Data published on venous resection and reconstruction are typically favorable, however. A systematic review evaluated 52 manuscripts with 6333 patients in whom pancreatic resection was performed for pancreatic cancer; 1646 of these patients (26%) underwent synchronous portal and SMV resection.[15] The median number of resections per publication evaluated was 82, and of those, 23 patients underwent portal and SMV resection. The proportion of portal and SMV resections per publication varies widely, ranging from 2% to 77%, which mirrors the various treatment approaches to pancreatic cancer in different institutions today. Within this systematic review, there is information on the operation in 39 studies with 1334 patients. The operations performed included PD (71%), total pancreatectomy (24%), subtotal pancreatectomy (3%), and distal pancreatectomy (2%). The median operation time was 513 minutes (range, 168–1740 minutes), median blood loss was 1750 mL (range, 300–26,000 mL), and the median time for PV occlusion was 20 minutes (range, 7–302 minutes). The perioperative mortality rate was 5.9%, varying between 0% and 33%, and the postoperative morbidity rate was 42%, ranging from 9% to 78%. Venous invasion was detected in 64% of all PV and SMV resection specimens. The median survival was 13 months (range, 1–109 months) after PV and SMV resection. The 1-, 3-, and 5-year overall survival rates of 1351 patients undergoing PV and SMV resection were 50%, 18%, and 8%, respectively.

The assessment of pooled data is substantially influenced by the quality of each institutional report. The standards of perioperative care, surgical technique, and adjuvant therapy have developed and improved dramatically. The wide variations in outcome parameters observed, including perioperative death, operative time, and blood loss, reflect the immense heterogeneity in the experience of each institution. Despite a potentially increased perioperative morbidity, long-term survival remains comparable to patients undergoing PD without vein resection.[16] Furthermore, as surgical expertise continues to improve, particularly in high-volume centers performing pancreatic resection, perioperative morbidity and mortality rates reported for pancreatic resections with PV or SMV resection are often reported as similar to those without it.[17–19] Thus venous involvement should not be a contraindication to resection if technically feasible, and, when in your own hands at your own institution, has acceptable morbidity and mortality.

The exact technique of portal vein reconstruction depends on the extent of involvement. In patients with less than 1 to 2 cm of involvement that is not circumferential, an interposition graft is generally not necessary. When this approach is performed, however, adequate mobilization before venotomy is important because the defect should almost always be closed horizontally in an effort to decrease narrowing of the lumen. When a larger extent of vein resection is required, then interposition with autologous vein (typically saphenous) or prosthetic is appropriate.[20] Historically, there was concern over the use of prosthetic for PV reconstruction not only because of the long-term patency of these materials in venous reconstruction but also because of their tendency to infection, particularly in the setting of pancreatic leak. Recent data have suggested that the use of prosthetic has a low risk for infection and similar long-term patency rates (approximately 75% at 1–2 years) as autologous vein.[21] After reconstruction most surgeons will consider the use of either aspirin or warfarin as a means of prolonging patency, although there are no data to support such an approach.

In summary, resection of the PV and SMV should be performed when adherence or infiltration of the tumor is present because perioperative morbidity, mortality, and long-term survival are similar to those patients in whom an R0 resection can be performed without vein resection. The degree and extent of venous resection is individualized to the degree and extent of tumor involvement and the patient's anatomy. These patients should be considered as having borderline resectable disease and thus should normally undergo some form of preoperative therapy (see Chapter 62). In contrast, arterial involvement is a poor prognostic factor with regard to both short-term and long-term outcomes. Although resection of the SMA is sometimes technically feasible, no data suggest that this leads to any improvement in the patient's long-term survival, and reported perioperative mortality is high.

Multivisceral Resections

The utility of resection of contiguously involved structures for locally advanced pancreatic cancer has been addressed in several reports.[22,23] In fact, about 35% of patients present initially with locally advanced pancreatic cancers with involvement of surrounding structures and organs. This is most often a phenomenon of pancreatic adenocarcinoma of the body or tail because these tumors are generally detected later and have therefore reached a greater size than cancers of the pancreatic head at the time of diagnosis. Although several reports in the past showed that morbidity of extended resection was increased and survival benefit limited, some have demonstrated that en bloc resection of contiguously involved organs can be performed safely in well-selected patients.[23] In the referenced paper from Sasson, no difference was reported with regard to perioperative morbidity (35%) and mortality (3%) compared with patients undergoing a standard resection. Although operative time is longer because of the extended resection, which can include mesocolon, colon, adrenal glands, liver, and stomach, blood loss and hospital stay have not been reported to be significantly different from what is observed after a standard procedure. The primary goal of the extended procedure must be an R0 (margin negative) resection because this is an important predictor of long-term survival.[24] Because it pertains primarily to left-sided (body/tail) cancers, the survival rate after resection of the mesocolon and colon, as well as the stomach, is not significantly decreased compared with a standard procedure and exceeds that of patients who do not undergo resection at all. In a series of more than 100 patients with multivisceral resections, the authors showed that perioperative mortality rate and long-term outcome were similar to those of patients undergoing standard resections but that the morbidity was increased.[22,23]

Lymphadenectomy

The rationale for performing an extended lymphadenectomy is that studies have confirmed positive lymph nodes outside the confines of a standard dissection.[25] Even for small cancers, lymph nodes in the para-aortic region, between the celiac trunk and the origin of the inferior mesenteric artery (see Chapter 2), can harbor metastases; it has been suggested that these should be removed en bloc with the primary tumor.[26] This approach of extended lymphadenectomy is most popular in Japan, where retrospective data on this approach have shown improved survival and similar morbidity and mortality.[27]

What constitutes an extended lymphadenectomy is still widely debated. In an attempt to standardize the definition, a consensus conference on the surgical treatment of pancreatic cancer took place in Castelfranco Veneto, Italy.[28] This consensus statement provided a standardized definition of the variable extent of lymphadenectomy using the Japanese Pancreas Society's terminology for lymph node stations to define which lymph nodes should be removed to constitute a certain procedure. The three types of lymphadenectomy during PD were named *standard, radical,* and *extended radical,* depending on which nodal stations were removed. For cancers of the body or tail, two different procedures were identified: standard and radical.

Six prospective nonrandomized studies have been published on this topic as well. A prospectively conducted study in which the decision to perform a standard or extended lymphadenectomy was made based on the clinical status of the patient revealed no significant differences in perioperative mortality rate and long-term survival but did show a trend toward a better outcome in the standard lymphadenectomy group.[29] This may be because of selection bias, (i.e., there may have been a higher percentage of patients with advanced-stage tumors in the extended lymphadenectomy group). Furthermore, extended lymphadenectomy was associated with an increased rate of severe diarrhea in the early postoperative phase. Gazzaniga and colleagues showed that morbidity, mortality, and long-term survival were similar between standard and extended lymphadenectomy.[30] Studies from Capussotti and colleagues confirmed the results of the previous reports

with unchanged morbidity, mortality, and survival rates between the two groups.[31] Four RCTs have been conducted to assess the value of an extended lymphadenectomy and were summarized in a meta-analysis.[3,32-35] Interestingly, these four level I studies are from centers on three different continents. The first study by Pedrazzoli and colleagues did not reveal any differences with regard to morbidity, mortality, and survival between the standard and extended lymphadenectomy groups. The extended lymphadenectomy included removing lymph nodes from along the aorta, the inferior and superior mesenteric arteries, and the celiac trunk. A subgroup analysis performed retrospectively revealed a significantly prolonged survival for node-positive patients who received an extended lymphadenectomy. This finding has been debated at length because its validity from a retrospectively performed subgroup analysis is dubious.

The largest study on this subject enrolled 294 patients; it was published in 2002 and updated in 2005 by Yeo and colleagues.[3] The authors randomized 294 patients into standard and extended lymphadenectomy arms after intraoperative frozen sections confirmed tumor-negative margins. However, the study encompassed heterogeneous tumor types, and only 57% of the patients included in the study had tumors that were of pancreatic origin, thus making interpretation of the survival data difficult. Nevertheless, perioperative mortality and long-term survival rates were similar between the two groups, although there was a significant increase in morbidity in the extended lymphadenectomy group (43% vs. 29%; $P < .01$). Much of the morbidity was related to higher rates of delayed gastric emptying and pancreatic fistula.

Based on these data, it should be concluded that extended lymphadenectomy is not routinely indicated. Additional studies from the Mayo Clinic and from Japan supported the same conclusions (i.e., that extended lymphadenectomy is associated with increased morbidity but not improved survival).[32,34] In summary, none of the RCTs, except for a retrospective subgroup analysis within the study by Pedrazzoli and colleagues, showed any survival benefit for extended lymphadenectomy, whereas overall morbidity was increased, with diarrhea and delayed gastric emptying, in particular, occurring more frequently. Furthermore, both Yeo and colleagues and Farnell and colleagues report a reduction in quality of life in the extended lymphadenectomy group, primarily because of high rates of postoperative diarrhea with subsequent development of malnutrition (see Chapter 29). Therefore the current standard for pancreatic head tumors remains PD without extended lymphadenectomy.

Reconstruction
Pancreaticojejunostomy

A pancreatic leak is the major cause of procedure-related death (see Chapter 28). Simply occluding the pancreatic duct and not creating an anastomosis has been shown to result in higher fistula rates in addition to increasing the risk for pancreatic exocrine and endocrine insufficiency.[36] Thus drainage of the pancreatic remnant to the gastrointestinal (GI) tract remains a crucial step in successful recovery. It is thus not surprising that the pancreatoenteric anastomosis has intrigued surgeons, motivating them to search for a more reliable technique to avoid this complication. Many techniques have been described, and the literature will continue to report novel techniques that promise to be even safer. However, more so than the choice of the variant used, successful management of a pancreatic anastomosis is most dependent on the surgeon's concentration on meticulous execution of the chosen technique.[37] For as long as the basic tenets of a safe anastomosis are met—namely, careful handling of the pancreatic tissues, a tension-free adaptation, good perfusion, and no distal obstruction—any pancreatoenteric anastomotic technique can have excellent outcomes.

The most common structure to which the pancreas is connected is the jejunum. This can be performed by invaginating the transected pancreas into the end of the jejunum, the so-called *dunking procedure,* or the pancreatic duct can be directly sutured to a separate opening in the jejunum, the so-called *duct-to-mucosa technique.* The technique of pancreaticojejunal anastomosis—whether end-to-side or end-to-end, duct-to-mucosa or dunking—does not seem to significantly influence the anastomotic leak rate. Another organ to which the pancreas can be connected is the stomach, and proponents of pancreatogastrostomy (PG) have cited various reasons to choose this method. For one thing, it is easier to perform given the close proximity of the stomach to the pancreas. For another, the anastomosis is less prone to ischemia because of the rich gastric perfusion.[38] Because the exocrine enzymes enter an acidic environment, it was once thought that the leak rate would be lower because the enzymes do not get activated, but this hypothesis has not proven true. In a prospective RCT comparing pancreaticojejunostomy (PJ) with PG, the leak rates were not significantly different (PJ, 11%; PG, 12%).[39] When reviewing the numerous prospective RCTs that have evaluated anastomotic technique, one must remember that these trials typically have randomized patients between the "institutional norm" and a technique that the surgeons are not as familiar with. It should therefore not be surprising that the institutional norm is the technique that is generally found superior or at least equivalent.

We prefer to construct a duct-to-mucosa PJ in an end-to-side fashion with a retrocolic jejunal limb as originally described by the Editor Emeritus (LHB) of this textbook.[40] Before starting the anastomosis, the jejunum is brought to the right upper quadrant. This can be accomplished via the ligament of Treitz or through a defect in the mesocolon just to the right of the middle colic vessels. We prefer the latter because the jejunal limb is theoretically less vulnerable to obstruction in the face of a local recurrence. The pancreatic remnant should be mobilized off the splenic vein for approximately 2 cm. The previously placed hemostatic sutures before neck transection are used to slightly elevate the gland away from the venous confluence. The anastomosis is performed in two layers. The first layer consists of transpancreatic horizontal mattress sutures placed through and through the pancreas approximately 1 cm proximal to the cut transection edge. We use 3.0 polydioxanone (PDS) sutures for this layer. It may be helpful to straighten the needle to allow for a perpendicular path of the suture through the gland. It is important to start 1 to 2 cm away from the edge anteriorly and also to exit the gland posteriorly the same distance away from the transection edge. The reconstruction is started on the inferior edge of the gland. The suture is passed through the pancreas anterior to posterior. Next, a seromuscular horizontal mattress suture is placed through the jejunal limb, longitudinally oriented and halfway between the mesentery and anti-mesenteric bowel, approximately 3 cm away from the stapled transected edge of the jejunum. The suture is then passed again through the pancreas, entering the posterior surface and exiting the anterior surface, again keeping 1 to 2 cm away from the cut edge. This,

in effect, creates a horizontal mattress-type suture between the full thickness of the pancreas and the biliopancreatic limb (Fig. 117A.4). In most cases, the pancreas will accommodate two or three such stitches inferior to the pancreatic duct and two or three superior. A probe should be placed in the pancreatic duct to protect it from being occluded while placing the horizontal mattress sutures. The needles should be left on each suture because this stitch will be used for the final anterior layer to complete the anastomosis.

Once this initial layer is complete, attention is turned toward the duct-to-mucosa inner layer. The pancreatic duct is approximated to a small full-thickness enterotomy in the jejunum with PDS; 4.0 PDS is sufficient for most cases, although 5.0 or 6.0 may be more appropriate in certain cases, depending on the size of the duct. The enterotomy should be placed approximately 1 cm away from the line of horizontal sutures to allow for a tension-free duct-to-mucosa adaptation. Normally, four to six sutures are able to be placed to fully approximate the duct to jejunum, with two at the corners and one to two placed anteriorly and posteriorly. It is helpful to place and tie the posterior suture first to more easily visualize the duct for the remaining stitches (Fig. 117A.5).

Once the duct to mucosa anastomosis is completed, the previously placed 3.0 PDS sutures are used to complete the final

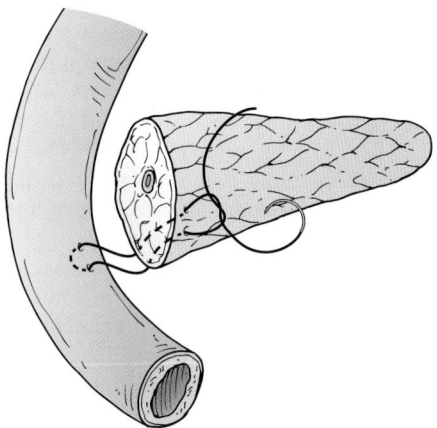

FIGURE 117A.4 Full-thickness 3.0 Vicryl horizontal mattress stitch through the pancreas and seromuscular layer of jejunum.

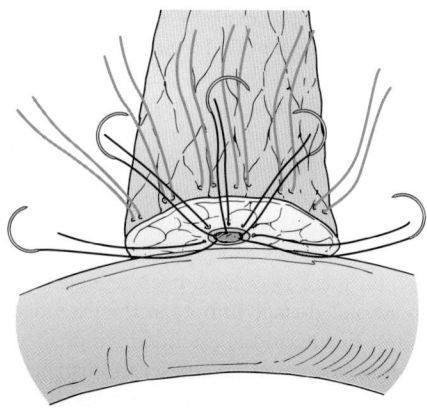

FIGURE 117A.5 The corner and anterior row stitches placed in the pancreatic duct to tent the duct open to facilitate placement of the posterior row.

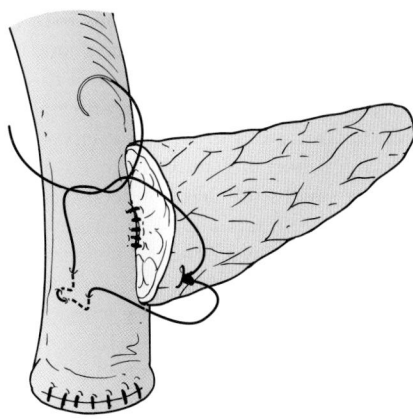

FIGURE 117A.6 After completion of the duct-to-mucosa layer, the Vicryl sutures are tied down. The inferior-most suture is placed in a vertical fashion in the jejunum, and then a second horizontal bite is taken to allow the jejunum to fold over the anterior surface of the pancreas.

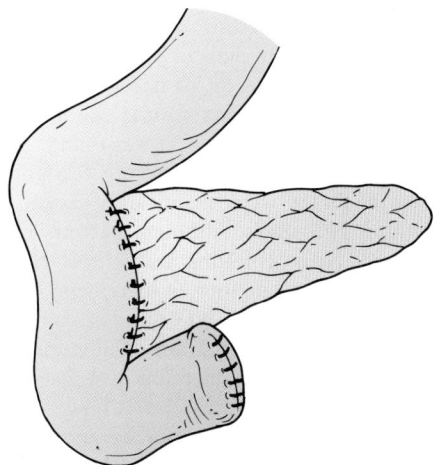

FIGURE 117A.7 The completed pancreaticojejunostomy. None of the duct-to-mucosa sutures should be visible once the anterior row is complete, and the jejunum is folded over the anterior surface of the pancreas.

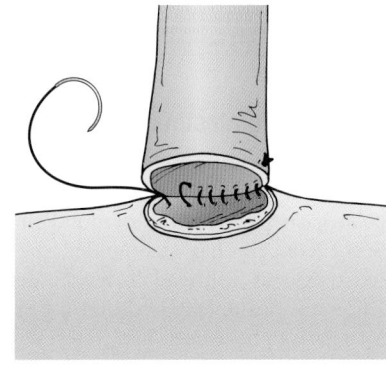

FIGURE 117A.8 Posterior suture row of the bilioenteric anastomosis in a continuous fashion.

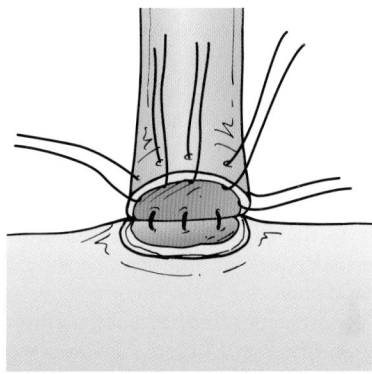

FIGURE 117A.9 Interrupted suture technique for bilioenteric anastomosis showing completed posterior row with corner and anterior bile duct sutures in place.

anterior row of the anastomosis. Each suture is tied down, starting with the inferior edge of the pancreas. For the most inferior stitch, the suture is placed in a vertical fashion through the jejunum about 1 cm inferior to the pancreatic edge, guiding the needle anteriorly. A second bite is then taken through the jejunum in a horizontal mattress fashion, far enough away from the pancreas to allow the jejunum to fold over the anterior surface of the pancreas (Fig. 117A.6). When tying these knots, it is imperative to tie the jejunum down to the pancreas. These horizontal mattress sutures are continued, working from the inferior edge to the most superior stitch. The last stitch is placed in a mirror image to the first inferior stitch (i.e., two bites in the jejunum, with the first one in a vertical fashion followed by a horizontal mattress stitch directed back toward the pancreas). These vertical stitches serve to wrap the jejunum around the inferior and superior edge of the pancreas. Once all the horizontal mattress sutures are tied down, the inner layer PDS sutures should not be visible, and the anastomosis is complete (Fig. 117A.7).

The end-to-side technique allows the adaptation of the jejunal opening to the specific requirements of the pancreatic remnant.

Separate duct-to-mucosa adaptation also keeps the duct orifice open, thereby ensuring the unobstructed flow of pancreatic secretions through the anastomosis. We do not use pancreatic stents.

Bilioenteric Anastomosis

The bilioenteric anastomosis has less variability in its construction and is less likely to experience leak or fistula. It can be fashioned with a continuous or interrupted technique, depending on the size of the bile duct (see Chapter 32). The authors normally use a 4.0 PDS suture to construct the biliary anastomosis. For a continuous technique, a single-layer full-thickness anastomosis is constructed. The posterior layer is completed first by starting at the 3 o'clock position and stopping at the 9 o'clock position (Fig. 117A.8). A second suture is then used to complete the anterior layer to prevent a purse-stringing of the anastomosis.

If an interrupted technique is chosen, which is the preferred technique for small bile ducts less than 5 mm in diameter, the anterior row and corner sutures are first placed in the bile duct. This serves to hold the duct open to facilitate construction of the posterior row, similar to the discussion for the PJ. A small enterotomy is made in the jejunum, approximately 6 to 8 cm away from the PJ. The posterior bile duct sutures are then placed and passed through full-thickness jejunum as well. Once all sutures are placed, the posterior row is tied down such that the knots are on the inside of the anastomosis (Fig. 117A.9). The anterior row and corner sutures are then passed through full-thickness jejunum. Once all sutures are placed, the anterior row is tied down, starting with the corner stitches and working toward the 12 o'clock position, with the knots tide outside of the anastomosis.

Reconstitution of Gastrointestinal Continuity

Depending on whether a classic PD or pylorus-preserving PD (PPPD) is performed, the reconstruction phase ends either with an antecolic gastrojejunostomy or duodenojejunostomy, respectively. Some concern has surrounded the question of whether an intact pylorus will lead to higher delayed gastric emptying (DGE) rates postoperatively after a PPPD; however, this controversy seems to have been laid to rest with the results of several RCTs to which we have previously alluded. Therefore, based on evidence available in 2004, it is apparent that pylorus preservation does not increase the frequency of DGE.[41]

The technique used to reconstitute GI continuity may have an impact on the incidence of DGE, however. One group speculated that a retrocolic reconstruction predisposes the jejunal limb to venous congestion and bowel edema, which can consequently slow recovery of jejunal peristalsis at the duodenojejunostomy.[42] Postoperative gastroparesis may also lead to temporary gastric distension, which can lead to angulation of the anastomosis because it lies relatively fixed through its retrocolic position.[41] Additionally, the close proximity of the duodenojejunostomy to the PJ may also predispose to DGE in the event of a small PJ leak or transient postoperative remnant pancreatitis. Opponents to these theories have suggested that an antecolic reconstruction may actually predispose the stomach to angulation or torsion.[43] Some feel that the risk of DGE caused by local inflammation is reduced by placing the duodenojejunostomy in the infracolic compartment through a separate mesenteric window, away from the pancreatic and biliary anastomoses, which lie in the supracolic compartment.

Regardless of whether a classic PD or PPPD is performed, we routinely perform an antecolic end-to-side duodenojejunostomy or gastrojejunostomy about 50 cm downstream from the hepaticojejunostomy, using the transverse colon and omentum to shield the anastomosis away from the PJ. The anastomosis is constructed in a single layer using monofilament absorbable 3.0 PDS sutures in a continuous fashion.

Abdominal Drains and Nasogastric Tubes

Intraperitoneal drainage of the biliary and pancreatic anastomoses with the intention of controlling leakage of biliary, lymphatic, or pancreatic secretions has been recommended for decades. Such a practice has been prophylactic in nature, and the reason for it stems more from surgical dogma than level 1 evidence. The first RCT that addressed the benefit of drains after pancreatic resection was conducted at Memorial Sloan-Kettering and found that placement of drains did not translate into a reduction in surgical morbidity.[44] Rather, a significantly higher proportion of patients randomized to the drain group developed intraperitoneal sepsis, fluid collection, or fistula. Similarly, a randomized trial of 438 patients from Heidelberg showed no difference in postoperative fistula or fistula-related complications between those who received a drain or not, and

in-hospital mortality was 3% in both groups.[45] To the contrary, a multi-institutional study was conducted and prematurely closed at an early interim analysis because of the findings of a significantly higher morbidity and 90-day mortality rate in the group that did not receive a drain (mortality 12% vs. 3%).[46] The extremely high mortality rate in the no-drain group reported in this very small study has not been seen by others. We do not routinely place drains after PD because the results of two large RCTs do not show a benefit. The studies do not show clear harm with drain placement, and thus selective use of drains is certainly reasonable. For those who are not comfortable with the prospective randomized data demonstrating the lack of benefit from drain placement, a middle ground of "early drain removal" has become popular. In a prospective RCT by the Verona group, early drain removal by postoperative day 3 was associated with decreased rates of pancreatic fistula.[47] Regardless of whether drains are placed or not, the postoperative management of all patients should include early cross-sectional imaging and intervention for evidence of undrained pancreatic collection (see Chapter 28). Failure to rescue and subsequent mortality after PD and pancreatic leak can often be attributed to late intervention on early signs of sepsis.

A meta-analysis on the need for nasogastric (NG) decompression has also refuted dogma around routine NG decompression after PD.[48] In their report, it was found that fever, atelectasis, and pneumonia were significantly less common, and days to first oral intake were significantly fewer, in patients managed without NG tubes. Although patients may develop abdominal distension or vomiting without an NG tube, this does not necessarily translate into an increase in complications or length of stay. Furthermore, NG tubes are omitted in most enhanced recovery pathway programs. The authors currently leave an NG tube in place on the night of surgery and remove it on the morning of postoperative day 1; however, a trend toward omitting NG tube decompression as part of an enhanced recovery postoperative management protocol is being observed (see Chapter 27).

SUMMARY

The surgical technique and operative outcomes for patients undergoing PD have made significant advances since being reported by Allan Whipple in 1935.[49] Patients may anticipate operative mortality rates of approximately 1% at high-volume centers, and median lengths of stay of approximately 7 days. There has been no single advance, approach, or technique that has resulted in this improvement but rather incremental and thoughtful investigation by a series of surgeon-researchers over decades. Randomized data have not shown any single approach to be superior, and we would encourage every surgeon to develop the approach to this operation that works best for their patients, who undergo resection at their hospital.

The references for this chapter can be found online by accessing the accompanying Expert Consult website.

Distal and central pancreatectomy

John M. Creasy, Peter J. Allen, and Michael E. Lidsky

Open central (segmental) pancreatectomy is also described in detail and remains an alternative for benign, indolent, or premalignant lesions in the pancreatic neck, when an enucleation is not feasible and a lymphadenectomy not required. This technique preserves normal pancreatic tissue and function and does not include a splenectomy but requires two planes of transection in the pancreas, leading to potential for increased morbidity. We advocate stapled or sutured closure of the proximal pancreatic stump and reconstruction of the distal pancreas with a dunking, invaginating pancreaticogastrostomy. In selected patients, open central pancreatectomy remains a viable option to preserve pancreatic and splenic function and also avoid an extended pancreatectomy.

OVERVIEW

Technical refinements have facilitated a more individualized, disease-directed approach for patients undergoing pancreatectomy. This chapter focuses on some of these surgical techniques, as well as pertinent perioperative considerations for patients subjected to open distal and central pancreatectomy. Specifically, this section details approach, exposure, and technical nuances that facilitate safe and effective surgical resection of lesions located with the neck, body, and tail of the pancreas.

Previous chapters (see Chapters 54–63, 65) have outlined the definition, classifications, pathogenesis, clinical aspects, diagnostic assessment, and management of acute pancreatitis, chronic pancreatitis, and periampullary and pancreatic tumors, including pancreatic cancer and cystic and endocrine tumors, and will not be discussed here. Preoperative workup and perioperative management (including anticoagulation, antibiotics, preoperative biliary drainage, octreotide analogues, and enhanced recovery pathways) are detailed in Chapters 12, 13, 25, 27, and 62. Management of short-term and long-term complications and subsequent surveillance after resection are described in preceding chapters (see Chapters 28 and 62).

RESECTIONAL TECHNIQUES

Open Distal Pancreatectomy

The surgical procedure of choice for a tumor arising in the body or tail of the pancreas is a distal pancreatectomy. This operation entails the removal of that portion of the pancreas extending to the left of the superior mesenteric vein and does not include the duodenum and distal bile duct (see Chapter 2). The pancreas is usually divided anterior or to the left of the superior mesenteric vein (SMV)-portal vein (PV) trunk, the exact line of transection depending on the location of the tumor. When feasible and without compromising a margin negative resection, attempts should be made to preserve pancreatic parenchyma and function. Because of advances with minimally invasive surgical techniques, laparoscopic and robotic resections are now

commonly performed, even for pancreatic adenocarcinoma (see Chapter 127).[1-3] However, there remains a role for open distal pancreatectomy in certain clinical situations. At our institution, laparotomy for distal pancreatectomy remains the ideal approach for bulky pancreatic adenocarcinomas, those with potential for vascular involvement or multivisceral resection, tumors that are proximal and directly overlying the SMV-PV trunk, or significant varices. A thorough review of cross-sectional imaging provides a preoperative assessment regarding vascular involvement (see Chapters 13 and 17); however, intraoperative ultrasound can be used to confirm this suspicion and guide safe resection (see Chapter 24). Intraoperative ultrasound allows for identification of landmark anatomy and the direct location and extent of the tumor, and surgeons must be skilled in the application of this technology. It is imperative that surgeons do not compromise the oncologic outcomes and thus require proficiency in both laparoscopic and open left-sided pancreatic resections.

Technique

The abdomen may be entered through either a midline laparotomy or a limited upper midline incision with a left subcostal extension. Our preference is the left subcostal incision because of the exposure this provides in the left upper quadrant, especially in patients with a large body habitus. In thin patients with adequate distance from the xiphoid to the umbilicus, however, a midline laparotomy can be used. A wound protector may be used, especially for cases that involve multivisceral resection, and we use a Bookwalter (or occasionally Thompson) retractor for exposure. After a thorough examination of the peritoneal cavity, the gastrocolic ligament is divided sufficiently with mobilization of the splenic flexure, which allows for full visualization of the pancreas to its tail and the hilum of the spleen. The short gastric vessels are then divided. Care should be taken to preserve the gastroepiploic arcade. The point of pancreatic division is selected in the proximal normal pancreas, and the overlying peritoneum is divided along the superior and inferior borders of the pancreas. If necessary, intraoperative ultrasonography is performed to confirm the anatomic landmarks and location of the tumor (see Chapter 24).

Once the pancreas has been adequately exposed, attention should be paid to the three structures (splenic artery, splenic vein, and pancreatic parenchyma) that will be divided (Fig. 117B.1). These may be divided in any sequence, depending on the location of the lesion, the patient's anatomy, and whether or not splenic preservation is being considered. The exact method for pancreatic transection and stump closure has been the subject of much debate. Sharp transection with pancreatic duct suture ligation and over-sewing of the stump has been a frequently reported technique; however, division of the gland with a stapling device, with or without the use of staple reinforcement (i.e., SeamGuard, Gore Medical, Flagstaff, AZ), has also been reported. There is no evidence that one technique is consistently superior, and both

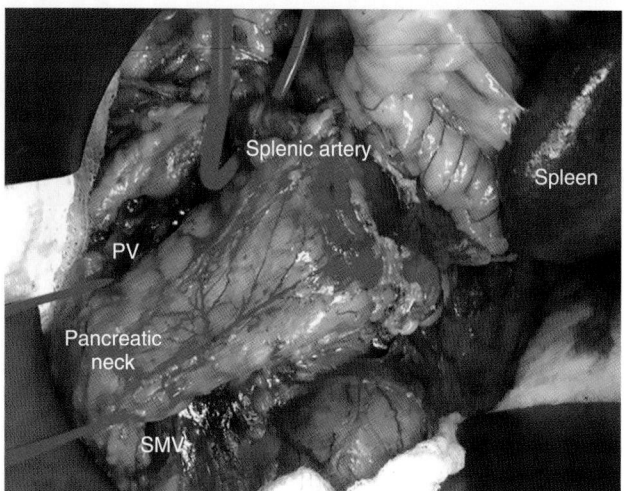

FIGURE 117B.1 Intraoperative photograph demonstrating exposure and isolation of the pancreatic neck and splenic artery.

techniques for management of the pancreatic remnant will be reviewed.

The splenic artery, which runs along the cephalad border of the pancreas (see Chapter 2), should generally be identified and controlled proximal to the lesion, if not near its origin. When feasible, the splenic artery should be divided before the splenic vein to avoid splenic engorgement. Before dividing the splenic artery, the artery should be temporarily occluded and the proper hepatic artery palpated to ensure that the common hepatic artery is not inadvertently ligated. If a pulse remains after occluding the vessel, the proximal splenic artery is then typically divided with an endovascular stapler. Alternatively, the artery may be divided between ties and clips, with or without proximal suture ligation. When feasible, the ideal splenic artery stump is long enough to facilitate coil embolization in the event of postoperative hemorrhage. The splenic vein may be divided with the endovascular stapler or by suture ligation. Care must be taken not to narrow the SMV, and a long splenic vein stump without flow should be avoided. Leaving a long splenic vein stump without flow (such as an intact inferior mesenteric vein) may increase the likelihood of developing thrombus within the stump that can propagate into the SMV and PV, compromising small bowel outflow.

Once the pancreas has been divided and the splenic vasculature ligated, the body and tail of the pancreas are completely mobilized out of the retroperitoneum along the superior and inferior aspects of the gland. Lastly, the spleen is then mobilized anteromedially by dividing the attachment to the lateral side wall and diaphragm, including any remaining splenocolic ligament, and the specimen is removed from the operative field.

Management of the Pancreatic Remnant

Pancreatic fistula remains the most common surgery-related complication after distal pancreatectomy, with rates ranging from approximately 10% to 35% in the literature (see Chapter 28).[4-7] Many techniques have been described in the literature with regard to the management of the residual transected pancreatic parenchyma and the divided pancreatic duct to lower the risk of leak. These include direct duct ligation, enteric drainage, prolamine injection, sealing with fibrin glue, mesh reinforcement, and transection with linear stapling devices.[8] The plethora of surgical

strategies described in the literature simply highlights the fact that no single technique has been convincingly shown to consistently reduce the incidence of pancreatic leak.

When the pancreas has a soft texture and is not too thick, the pancreas may be transected with a linear stapling device (Fig. 117B.2). This device gives a staple line consisting of a triple row of closely placed staples. Our preference is to employ a stapler designed for moderate to thick tissues. Many centers use a reinforced stapler (SeamGuard, Gore Medical, Flagstaff, AZ), although the data regarding this technique are variable.[8,9] In instances where the gland is thick and fibrotic, the pancreas should be transected with cautery or a scalpel; the pancreatic duct should be identified and closed under direct vision with a figure-of-eight absorbable suture (PDS; Fig. 117B.3A), and the resection margin closed with interrupted horizontal mattress PDS sutures (see Fig. 117B.3B). At our institution, we additionally place a running-locking suture along the length of the transected parenchyma (see Fig. 117B.3C). A European multicenter randomized trial comparing the stapled and sutured techniques did not show any difference in pancreatic fistula rates.[10] A recent meta-analysis reported that selective closure of the pancreatic duct resulted in fewer severe pancreatic fistula, but the overall differences between the suture and stapling technique were small.[11] The most recent International Study Group on Pancreatic Surgery (ISGPS) consensus guidelines do not recommend one technique over the other, and surgeons should make individualized decisions and be comfortable with both methods.[12] Regardless of the technique chosen, the authors believe that use of a well-vascularized omental flap to cover the transection edge is valuable in preventing and/or controlling a pancreatic fistula.

Splenic Preservation

Conventionally, the spleen has been removed *en bloc* when performing a distal pancreatectomy. This was believed to be necessary because of the close relationship of the splenic artery and vein to the body and tail of the pancreas (see Chapter 2).[13] Furthermore, this was thought to be technically simpler than trying to preserve the spleen. Splenic preservation can be performed either with the division of the splenic artery and vein or with preservation of the entire length of both vessels. The paramount prerequisite in the former surgical approach is preservation of the gastrosplenic vessels to ensure splenic perfusion and venous drainage. The incidence of infectious complications that require intervention has been reported to be significantly higher in patients undergoing concomitant splenectomy.[13] The long-term infectious risk, however, in an adult population undergoing splenectomy that receives the appropriate vaccines is negligible. Schwarz et al. found that patients undergoing resection of pancreatic adenocarcinoma with a splenectomy had a median actuarial survival of 12.2 months compared with 17.8 months in patients who did not have a splenectomy.[14] This association of reduced survival and splenectomy is also evident in patients undergoing resection for gastric and colon cancer. Although there is potential immune-based etiology for this observation, the need for splenectomy is likely a surrogate for extent of disease and biologic aggressiveness of the tumor. Nevertheless, based on the available evidence, we concur with Conlon et al. that splenic preservation may be attempted in patients with low-grade malignancies or other more indolent tumors of the pancreatic body/tail, but that splenic preservation may compromise oncologic clearance

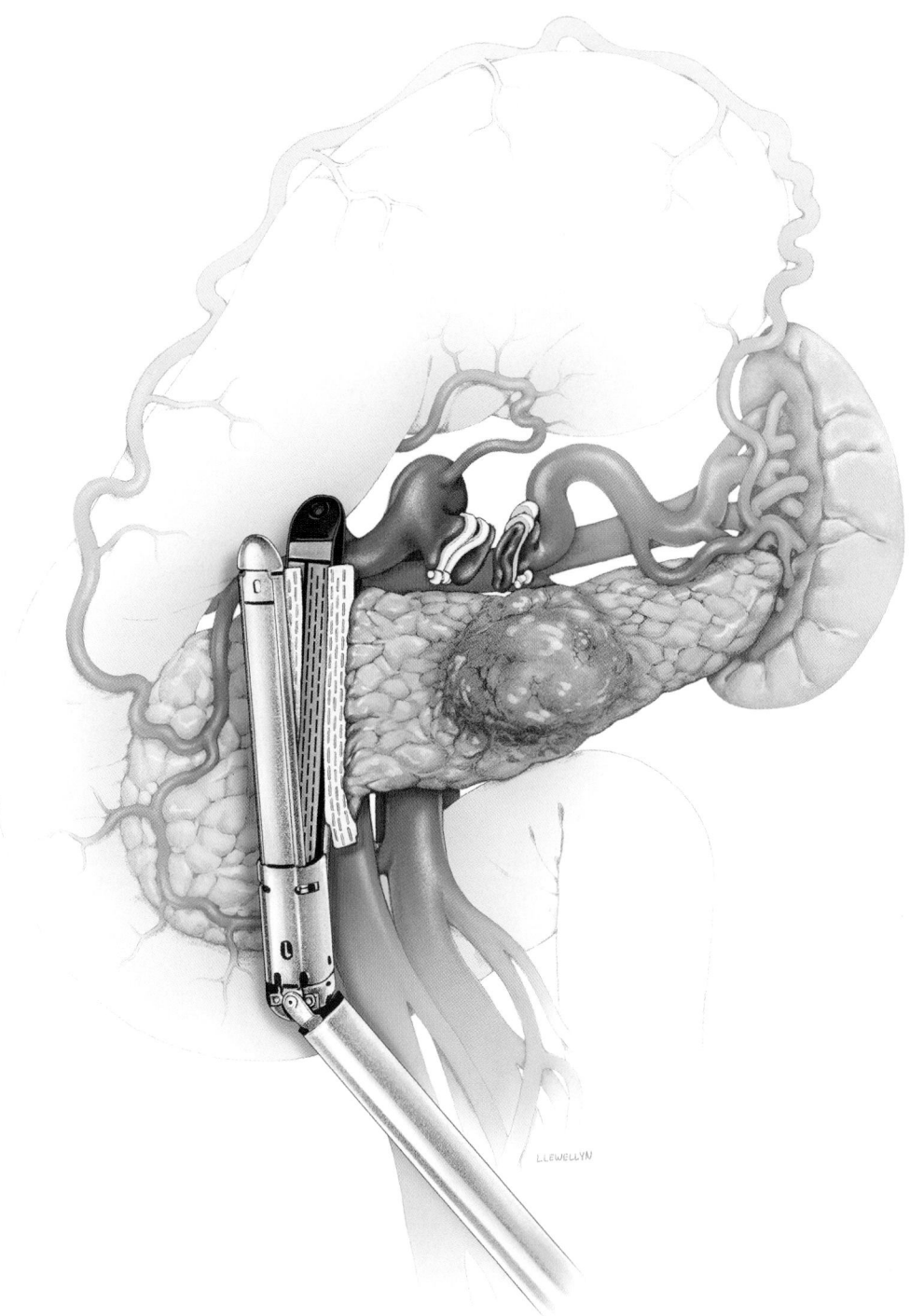

FIGURE 117B.2 Transection of pancreatic parenchyma with linear, reinforced stapler.

and staging if performed for pancreatic adenocarcinoma, and thus should not be performed.[15]

If the case is appropriate for splenic preservation and such a route is selected, our preference is to attempt to preserve the splenic artery and splenic vein to reduce the risk of splenic necrosis and abscess formation, because splenic perfusion based solely on the short gastric vessels alone has been shown to be potentially inadequate.[16] At the point of planned transection of

the pancreas, the gland has to be dissected free from the splenic artery and vein. After division of the pancreas, the distal stump is elevated with traction sutures and rotated gently to the patient's left. Multiple small, short branches of the splenic artery and vein are then identified and clipped serially with hemostatic clips and cut. An energy coagulation device can be used instead of, or along with, clips as well. The dissection proceeds from the proximal to distal pancreas, until the tail of the pancreas can be

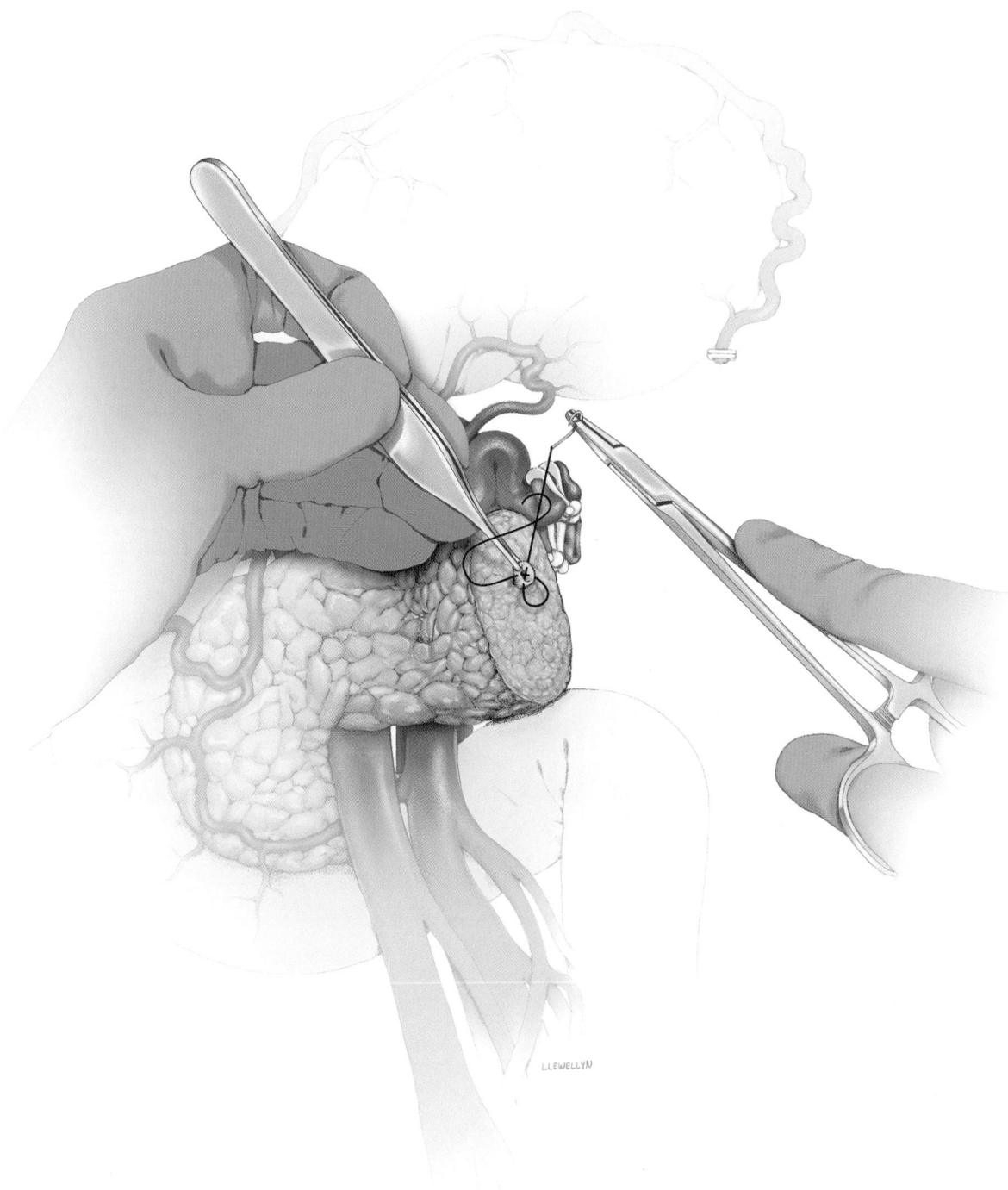

A

FIGURE 117B.3   A, Identification and closure of the pancreatic duct under direct vision with figure-of-eight absorbable suture.

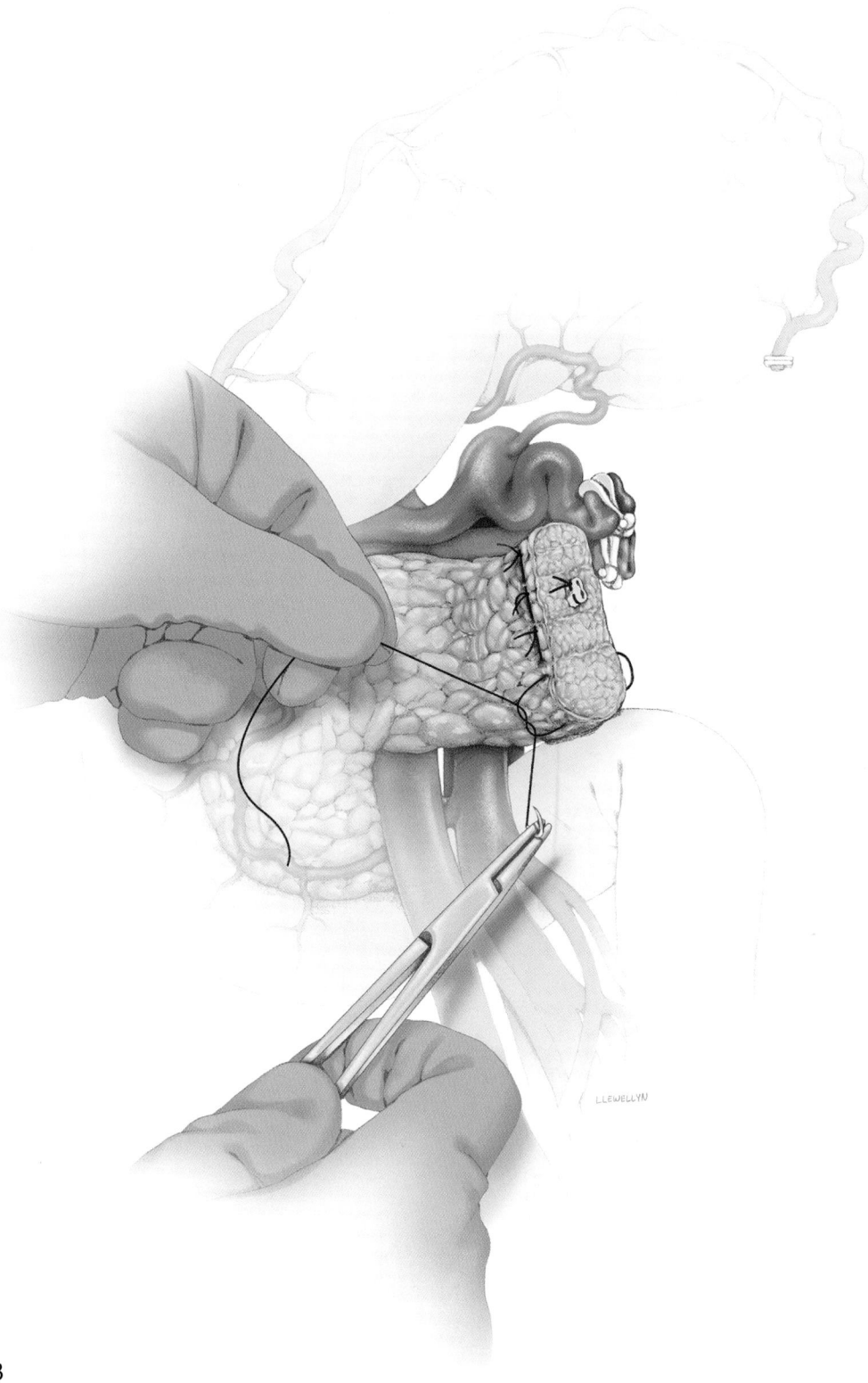

B

FIGURE 117B.3, cont'd   B, Suture closure of the pancreatic remnant with interrupted horizontal mattress sutures. One of the sutures encompasses the pancreatic duct.

Continued

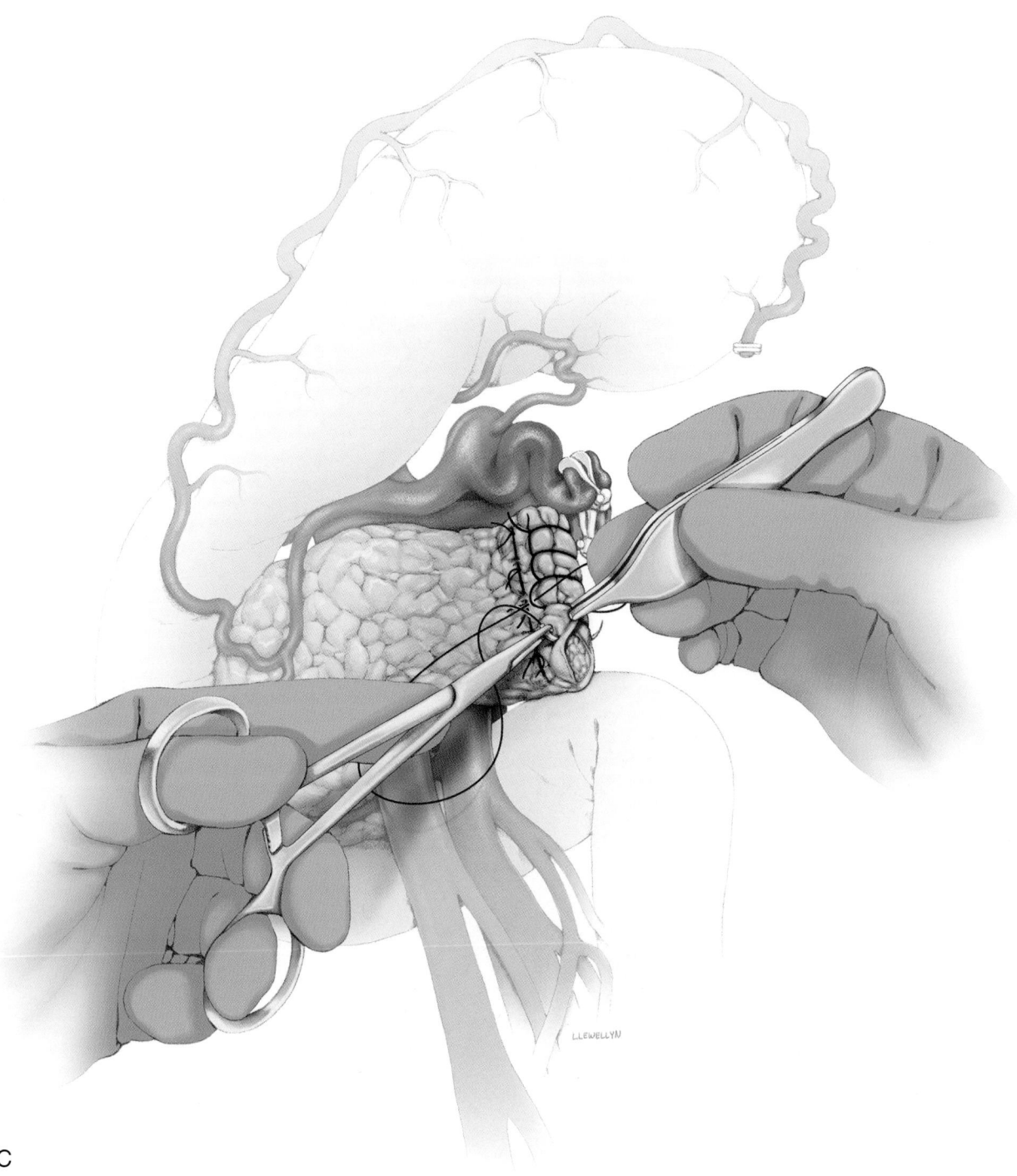

C

FIGURE 117B.3, cont'd C, Additional suture closure performed with a running-locking suture along the length of the transected parenchyma.

separated from the splenic hilum. This separation of the splenic vein from the pancreas can only proceed in the direction toward the spleen because the vein has already branched into small vessels that can easily be injured at the level of the splenic hilum. Any vessel injury can be repaired by suturing with monofilament 5.0 vascular sutures. If attempts at hemostasis of such vascular injuries are unsuccessful, we divide the splenic pedicle. We avoid mobilizing the spleen medially into the operative field because this step is unnecessary and carries the risk of iatrogenic splenic injury. If the vessels need to be divided because of intraoperative bleeding or inability to separate the pancreas, and a decision needs to be made to allow the spleen to perfuse on the short gastric vessels or to just convert to a splenectomy, then we prefer the latter.

Segmental (Central) Pancreatectomy

In 1959 Letton and Wilson were the first to describe the technique of segmental, or central, pancreatectomy for two cases of traumatic transection of the pancreatic neck.[17] After a central segmental resection, the proximal stump was oversewn, and a Roux-en-Y jejunal limb was constructed and anastomosed to the distal stump. Pancreatic surgeons were quick to recognize the versatility of this procedure and have since adapted it to the treatment of benign, indolent, or premalignant lesions of the pancreas situated in the pancreatic neck because a lymphadenectomy is not included as part of this procedure. Benign or low-grade tumors arising from this region present a unique challenge. Conventionally, if the lesion is small, enucleation may be the optimal strategy. If the lesion measures more than 2 cm, however, or when it is situated deep within the parenchyma such that damage to the pancreatic duct becomes a real risk, the surgeon may have to resort to either an extended distal pancreatectomy or pancreaticoduodenectomy (PD; see Chapter 117A) to remove the lesion. Such operative strategies for a small lesion come at the cost of a significant loss of normal pancreatic tissue, along with the inherent risk of morbidity and mortality that accompanies such extended pancreatectomies.

Segmental, or central, pancreatectomy represents an organ-preserving extirpation technique that offers the advantages of avoiding the morbidity and mortality associated with PD (see Chapter 117A); preserving splenic function by avoiding splenectomy, which often accompanies distal pancreatectomy; and preserving maximal pancreatic endocrine and exocrine function.[18] Perhaps the most beneficial attraction seems to be the excellent preservation of endocrine function. This is not surprising because the risk of diabetes is proportional to the extent of resection and length of follow-up observation.[19] On the other hand, the prime concern when performing a central pancreatectomy is whether pancreatic fistula rates are significantly higher because of two possible sources of pancreatic leakage (i.e., a pancreatic stump and an anastomosis). In the literature, the frequency of pancreatic leak after segmental pancreatectomy ranges from 14% to 30%, similar to what is reported for a distal pancreatectomy. In 1998 Iacono et al. succinctly summarized the prerequisites that allow segmental pancreatectomy to be considered as a reasonable approach: (1) small lesions (<5 cm in diameter) that are (2) benign or low-grade malignant tumors, (3) located in the neck or its contiguous portion, and (4) a distal pancreas stump of at least 5 cm in length.[20] A critical adjunct is the availability of frozen-section examination to confirm that the lesion is benign or indolent and to verify a free resection margin (see Chapter 59).[21]

Technique

A midline laparotomy is performed and the lesser sac is entered, facilitating exposure of the anterior aspect of the pancreas. Adhesions between the posterior surface of the stomach and the pancreas are divided. This is followed by intraoperative pancreatic ultrasonography to better delineate the lesion and to exclude concomitant lesions that may necessitate a change of plan. The pancreas is then elevated off the SMV-PV trunk. Stay sutures are placed in the superior and inferior pancreatic margins to indicate the proximal and distal limits of division and to aid in the subsequent dissection of the pancreas from the splenic vein. The pancreas is then divided proximally, either with a vascular stapler, cautery, or sharply with a scalpel, at least 1 cm to the right of the lesion. If divided with cautery or sharply, the duct is isolated and oversewn and the proximal stump is closed with interrupted horizontal mattress sutures and a running-locking suture, as described above. The distal stump is then gently retracted toward the left to allow the cautious and tedious process of freeing the splenic vein from the posterior surface, controlling all the fine venous tributaries lying between the splenic vein and the pancreas. The splenic artery is also dissected free from the gland. The pancreas should be mobilized off the splenic vessels for at least a distance of 2 to 3 cm to the left of the planned distal transection plane to facilitate reconstruction. The pancreas is then divided distal to the lesion with cautery or a scalpel, and the specimen is sent for analysis and margin assessment.

Our typical technique of reconstruction of the distal stump is to fashion a pancreaticogastrostomy using a dunking, invagination technique. The site of the anastomosis is selected and marked along the posterior wall of the stomach, being careful to account for the space needed for the pancreas to be flipped anteriorly inside the stomach. A 3.0 PDS suture is used to approximate the posterior wall of the stomach just to the left of the planned anastomotic site to the anterior capsule of the pancreas, approximately 2 cm away from the transection edge (Fig. 117B.4A). Next, four to six traction sutures, two to three on each side of the duct, are placed along the pancreatic transection edge (see Fig. 117B.4B). Either 3.0 Vicryl or PDS sutures are used for this step. A blunt probe is inserted in the pancreatic duct during placement of the sutures to prevent inadvertent occlusion. The sutures are then placed together on a single hemostat. A small posterior gastrotomy is then made to the right of this suture line, limiting it to about 75% of the width of the pancreas to allow a snug fit of the pancreas inside the stomach (see Fig. 117B.4C). A point anterior gastrotomy is then made, and a clamp is passed through the anterior gastrotomy and through the posterior gastrotomy to grab the traction sutures. The traction sutures are used to pull the pancreas inside the gastric lumen (see Fig. 117B.4D). These sutures are held on tension to maintain the pancreas inside the stomach while seromuscular sutures on the stomach are placed to the right of the gastrotomy to approximate the posterior capsule of the pancreas to the stomach. There are no sutures approximating the mucosa of the stomach to the pancreatic duct. The anterior gastrotomy is then closed, which can usually be accomplished with a single absorbable stitch. This technique allows the pancreas to be dunked inside the stomach in a tension-free manner. Alternatively, a Roux-en-Y jejunal limb can be used to drain the distal pancreatic remnant. The anastomosis is fashioned as previously described for a PD (see Chapter 117A).

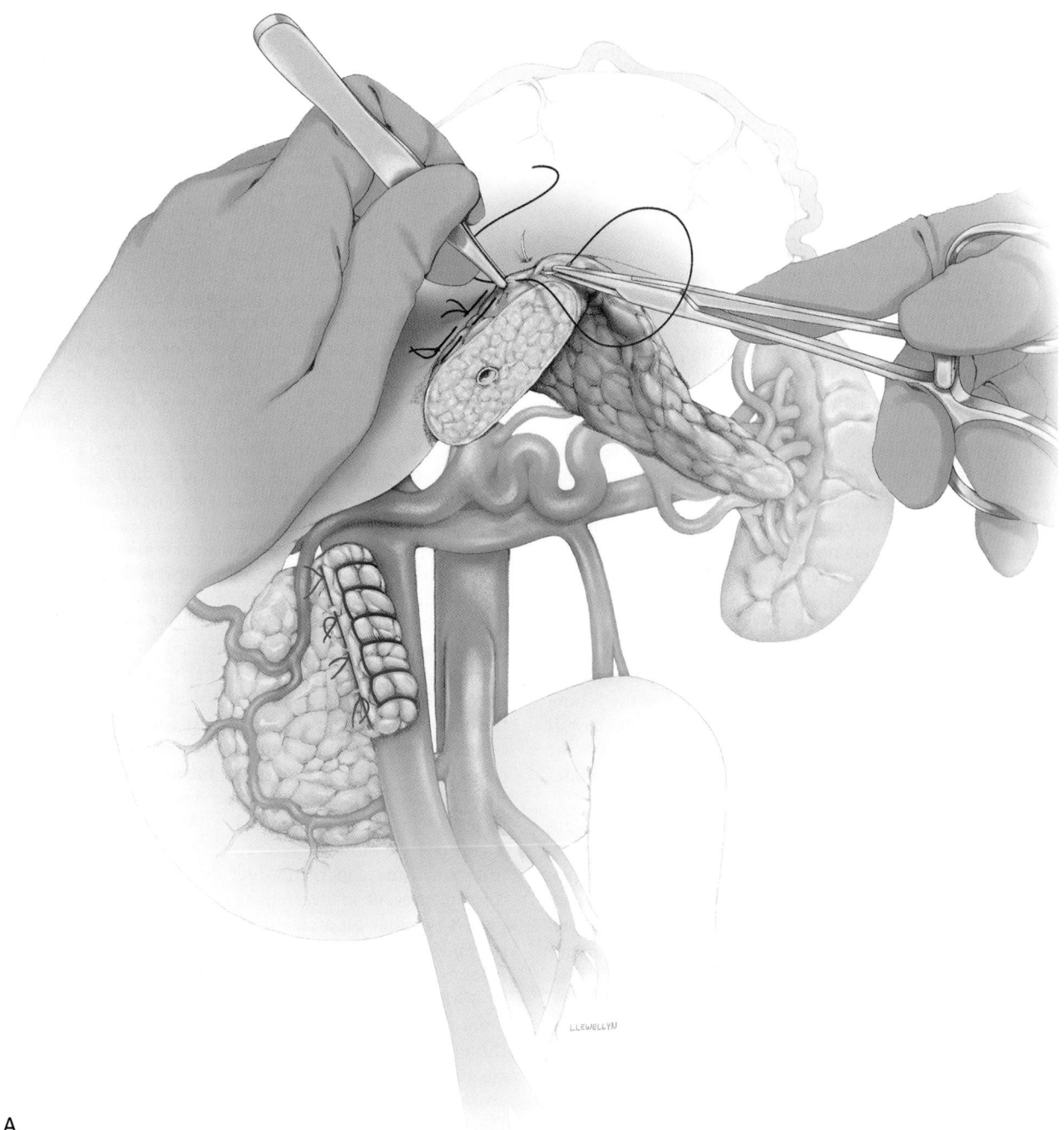

A

FIGURE 117B.4   A, Absorbable suture is used to approximate the posterior wall of the stomach to the anterior capsule of the pancreas, approximately 2 cm away from the transected edge.

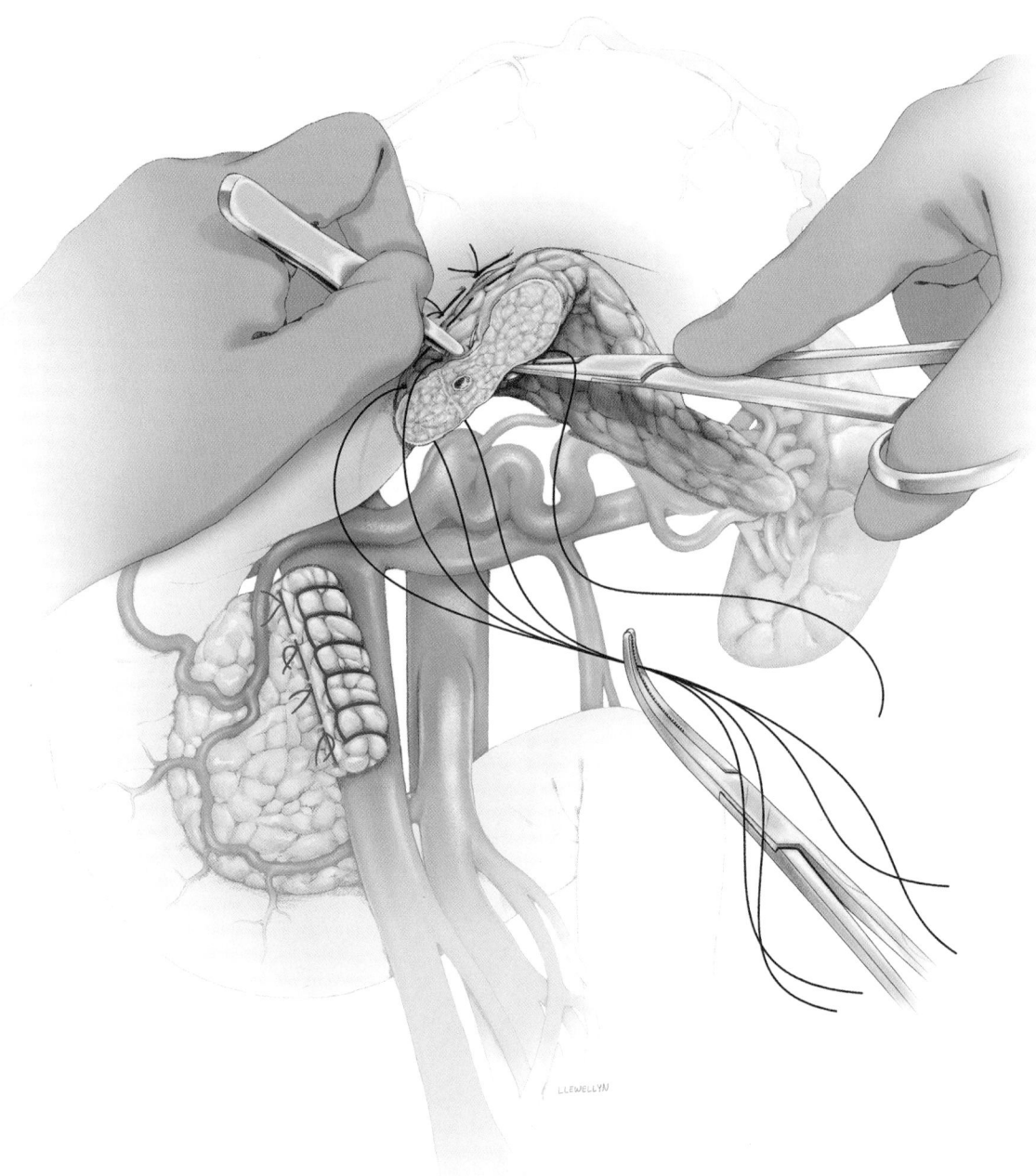

B

FIGURE 117B.4, cont'd B, Full-thickness traction sutures are placed through the transected edge and collected together on a hemostat, with careful attention to avoid injuring or narrowing the pancreatic duct.   *Continued*

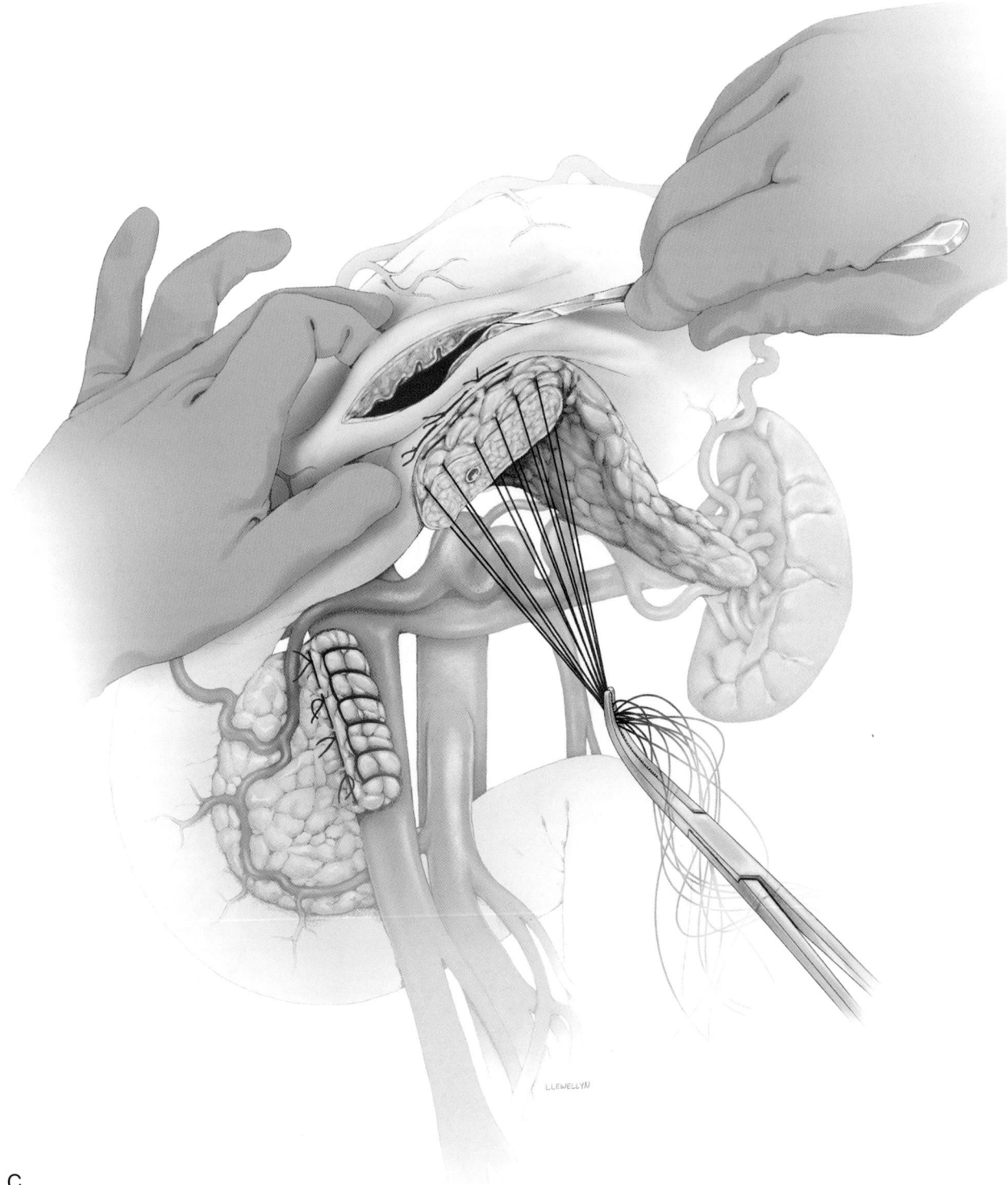

C

FIGURE 117B.4, cont'd C, A posterior gastrotomy is made, limiting it to approximately 75% of the width of the pancreas to allow a snug fit of the pancreas inside the stomach.

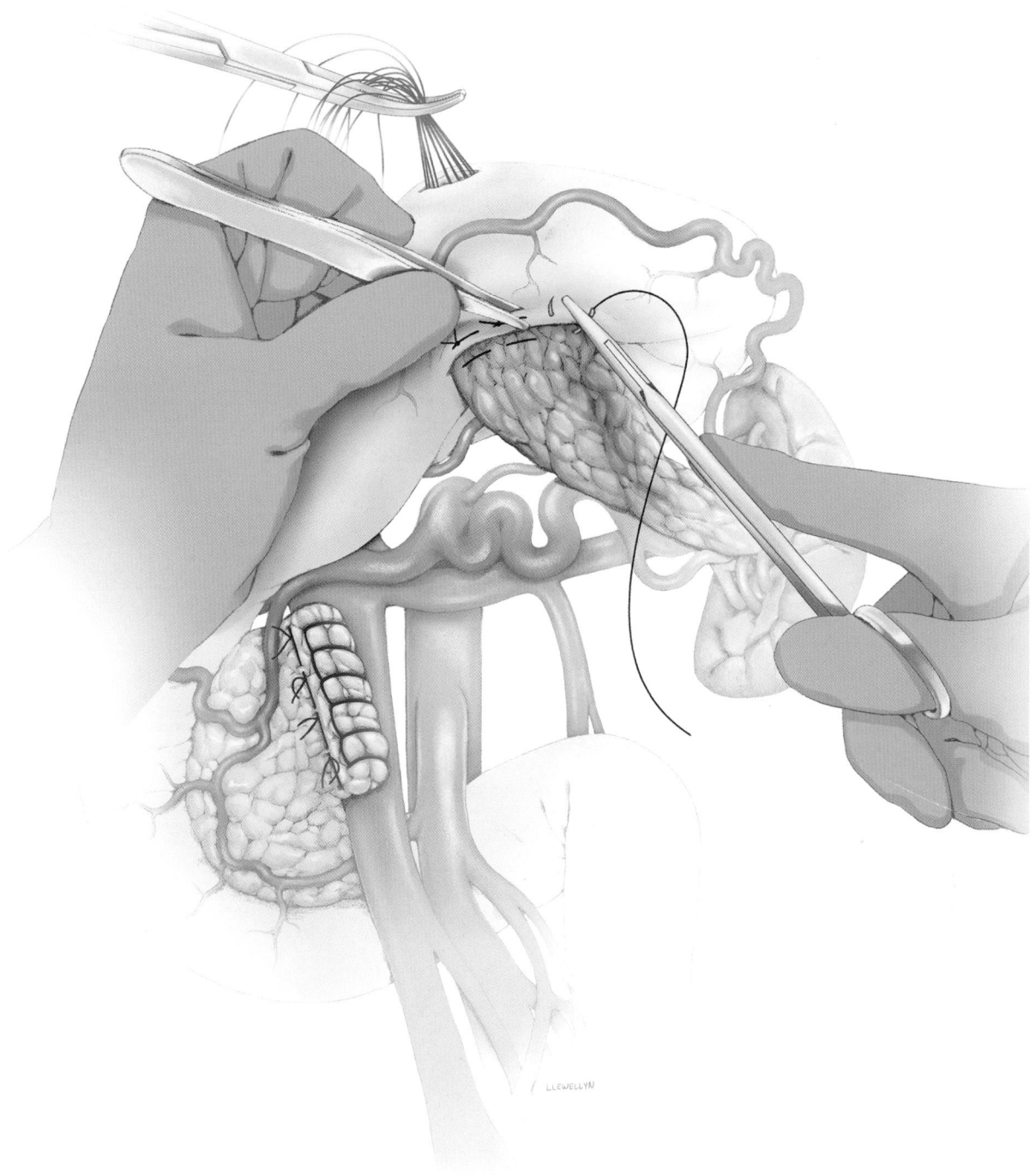

D

FIGURE 117B.4, cont'd   **D,** Anterior pinpoint gastrotomy is made, and a clamp is passed through the anterior and posterior gastrotomies to grab the traction sutures and pull the pancreas inside the stomach. These traction sutures are kept on tension while seromuscular sutures are placed from the posterior capsule of the pancreas to the stomach.

CONCLUSION

Pancreatic resection has evolved from a procedure synonymous with high mortality rates and poor quality of life for the survivors to one that is now recognized as the standard of care for pancreatic pathology because of its vastly improved safety profile and efficacy. Modern pancreatic resection is one in which the extent of resection, including the decision to perform the operation through an open approach, can be tailored to the individual needs of the patient, based on the disease process and its extent. These improvements in overall outcome are a result of advances in surgical technique, patient selection, perioperative care, and diagnostic imaging, just to name a few.

The management of patients with pancreatic diseases is best done with a multispecialty approach, with the surgeon in a central and coordinating role.

Pancreatic resection is now an accepted form of therapy for a large spectrum of pancreatic diseases, both benign and malignant. In sharp contrast with the nihilistic views that permeated the profession during the 1970s, the medical profession and patients alike have now recognized that pancreatic resection is a worthwhile undertaking.

The references for this chapter can be found online by accessing the accompanying Expert Consult website.

Danielle K. DePeralta and Matthew J. Weiss

INTRODUCTION

Total pancreatectomy is associated with significant metabolic consequences secondary to the loss of exocrine and endocrine function. Resultant brittle type III diabetes can be difficult to manage and result in severe recurrent hypoglycemia in some patients. Outcomes after total pancreatectomy for pancreatic adenocarcinoma (PDAC) are particularly poor, and this operation is rarely indicated in this setting.[1-3] More appropriate indications include chronic, recurrent acute, or hereditary pancreatitis, as well as main duct intraductal papillary mucinous neoplasm (IPMN) involving the entire gland (see Chapters 53, 56, 58, and 60; Box 117C.1).[4,5] Islet auto transplant is offered at select centers and may be considered, particularly for benign disease. With advances in pancreatic enzyme supplementation and insulin management, total pancreatectomy can be performed safely with acceptable quality of life in appropriately selected patients.[6,7]

PREPARATION

Proper preoperative planning is the backbone for success (see Chapters 12, 25–27; Box 117C.2) In addition to appropriate cardiopulmonary and medical work-up, extensive counseling regarding the endocrine and exocrine consequences of total pancreatectomy is necessary. The patient should be followed closely by the endocrinology team in the perioperative period. Indications and goals of surgery must be discussed extensively to ensure the patient is able to make an informed decision. This discussion is tailored to indication and will vary considerably between patients undergoing surgery for benign versus malignant processes. Auto islet cell transplantation is gaining acceptance, and this should also be considered, particularly for patients with benign disease.

On the morning of surgery, a thoracic epidural, arterial line, and Foley catheter are placed. Radiology images are displayed. A single preoperative dose of antibiotics and a prophylactic dose of heparin are administered. Sequential compression devices are placed on bilateral lower extremities and a hard-stop time out is performed.

POSITIONING, INCISION, AND EXPOSURE

The patient is positioned supine with the arms at 90 degrees (or tucked at the side) with careful attention to padding all pressure points. The abdomen is prepped widely. Diagnostic laparoscopy is performed if indicated (see Chapter 24). In most cases, a midline incision provides adequate exposure, but some prefer a bilateral subcostal incision. The abdominal cavity is carefully inspected to ensure there are no benign or malignant processes that would preclude resection. A self-retaining retractor is used to gain exposure to the entire peritoneal cavity. The resection portion of the case combines the techniques previously discussed for pancreatoduodenectomy (PD; see Chapter 117A) and distal pancreatectomy (see Chapter 117B). It should be noted that patients with chronic and recurrent acute pancreatitis often have a particularly hostile operative field, and the surgeon must have significant experience operating in this setting.

KOCHER MANEUVER, ENTRY OF LESSER SAC, AND IDENTIFICATION OF SUPERIOR MESENTERIC VEIN

The resection begins with a generous Kocher maneuver to expose the left renal vein and aorta. The hepatic flexure is mobilized. The omentum is dissected free from the transverse colon. The lesser sac is carefully inspected and the attachments between the pancreas and the stomach are divided. This can be challenging in patients with pancreatitis depending on the extent of surrounding inflammation. Specifically, the transverse colon mesentery may be fused to the anterior surface of the pancreas and posterior surface of the stomach and meticulous dissection is needed to avoid devascularization of the transverse colon, injury to the stomach, or significant hemorrhage. The middle colic and gastroepiploic veins are encountered toward the head of the pancreas and commonly join to form a gastrocolic trunk, which can be followed to the superior mesenteric vein (SMV). Ligation of the gastrocolic trunk and other draining tributaries prevents unintentional traction injury and bleeding during the remainder of the dissection. Bleeding encountered during dissection of the gastroepiploic vein, gastrocolic trunk, or SMV can be controlled by placing the left hand behind the head of the pancreas/duodenum and compressing the SMV/portal vein between the thumb and left fingers. A carefully placed Prolene stitch can typically control SMV bleeding. Specific attention should be paid to avoid narrowing or occluding the SMV. Careful dissecttion allows exposure of the SMV, which can be traced to the inferior border of the pancreas.

DISTAL PANCREAS DISSECTION AND SPLENECTOMY

The retroperitoneal reflection between the inferior border of the pancreas and transverse mesocolon is divided to mobilize the entire length of the gland from the neck to the tail. The splenic flexure is mobilized, and the short gastric vessels are ligated and divided. The peritoneal attachments to the spleen are divided and the spleen is mobilized medially out of the left upper quadrant and dissection continues to the level of the takeoff of the splenic artery. The splenic artery is divided at its origin from the celiac trunk and the splenic vein is divided at the level of the portal vein. Depending on the location of the inferior mesenteric vein, this tributary may be spared. The coronary vein can serve as an anatomic landmark (see Chapter 2) coursing between the common hepatic and splenic arteries and frequently can be spared.

Splenic preservation can be considered, particularly for benign disease. This will require dissection of the pancreatic tail

Benign
- Chronic pancreatitis after exhausting other options
- Recurrent acute pancreatitis after exhausting other options
- Hereditary pancreatitis

Premalignant
- Intraductal papillary mucinous neoplasm with inability to clear margin

Malignant
- Pancreatic adenocarcinoma with inability to clear margin (rarely, after careful consideration)
- Completion pancreatectomy for new/recurrent premalignant or malignant neoplasm
- Completion pancreatectomy for uncontrolled pancreatic leak after partial pancreatectomy after exhausting other options (extremely rare)

BOX 117C.2   Preoperative Checklist

- Goals of surgery discussion
- Endocrinology evaluation
- Postsplenectomy vaccines
- Consideration of auto islet cell transplantation if appropriate
- Consideration of diagnostic laparoscopy for malignant disease
- Preoperative antibiotics
- Thromboembolism prophylaxis

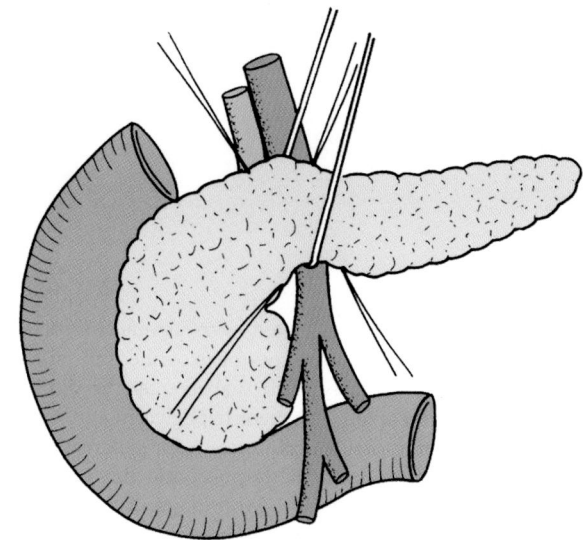

FIGURE 117C.1   A tunnel beneath the pancreas connecting the portal vein and superior mesenteric vein (SMV) is completed and a Penrose drain or umbilical tape is used to assist with retraction.

out of the splenic hilum while preserving the left gastroepiploic and short gastric vessels. Alternatively, the splenic artery and vein may be preserved and the posterior surface of the pancreas can be dissected off of these structures.[8–10]

PORTAL DISSECTION

Once the infrapancreatic and splenic dissection is completed, attention is turned to the suprapancreatic dissection. Cholecystectomy is performed (see Chapter 36). Aberrant vascular anatomy should be identified in advance on preoperative imaging (see Chapters 2 and 13). The gastrohepatic ligament is opened widely. The station 8, or common hepatic artery lymph node, is usually a good marker of the hepatic artery. The common hepatic artery is traced distally to identify the right gastric artery, which is divided between silk ties. This typically exposes the gastroduodenal artery (GDA), which is either suture ligated or divided with a 35 mm vascular stapler. Before division of the GDA, the left and right hepatic arteries are identified and the GDA is occluded with a bulldog or spoon clamp to ensure hepatic inflow is not compromised. This confirms that the anatomy has been correctly identified and that the GDA has not been mistaken for the proper or common hepatic artery. It also confirms that hepatic inflow is not dependent on retrograde flow through the GDA from the superior mesenteric artery (SMA), as may be the case in severe celiac stenosis. In cases of aberrant arterial anatomy with a common hepatic trunk from the SMA, the common hepatic artery will travel behind that pancreas with the SMV and will be visualized posteriorly and to the left of the GDA. If this is the case, it may be easier to identify the proper hepatic artery and GDA and trace those structures posteriorly to the common hepatic artery.

Division of the GDA reliably exposes the portal vein immediately posterior. Dissection along the anterior and medial border of the bile duct continues, and the bile duct is isolated with a vessel loop. Isolation of the bile duct is performed from medial to lateral to avoid inadvertent injury to the portal vein. Careful attention is paid to ensure there is not a replaced or accessory right hepatic artery tracing behind and lateral to the bile duct. The bile duct is divided and sent for frozen if the operation is for a malignant indication. If a stent was placed preoperatively, this is sent for gross pathology and the bile duct is swabbed for culture. A bulldog clamp is placed on the proximal bile duct and the handle is oriented laterally to avoid it from interfering with the ongoing dissection. Once the portal dissection is complete, the tunnel beneath the pancreas connecting the portal vein and SMV is completed (Fig. 117C.1). Depending on the indication for total pancreatectomy, the pancreatic neck may be divided followed by dissection of the uncinate process off of the SMA as is performed in PD (see Chapter 117A). This will result in two specimens and is the most commonly employed method of total pancreatectomy. In cases where division of the pancreatic neck is not appropriate, the specimen may be resected *en bloc*. En bloc resection can be technically challenging, and we find that it is safest and most efficient to fully mobilize the entire specimen, lift the left pancreas out of the operative field and to the patient's right side, and complete the uncinate dissection as discussed later. The duodenum or the stomach is divided at the discretion of the surgeon. There is some data to suggest better nutritional outcomes and quality of life in patients that undergo pylorus preserving total pancreatectomy compared with classic total pancreatectomy.[11,12]

JEJUNAL AND UNCINATE RESECTION

The jejunum is divided approximately 10 cm distal to the ligament of Treitz. The mesentery is divided along the surface using an energy device. The dissection should proceed immediately adjacent to the jejunum to avoid unintentional bleeding from the jejunal mesentery. The ligament of Treitz is fully mobilized

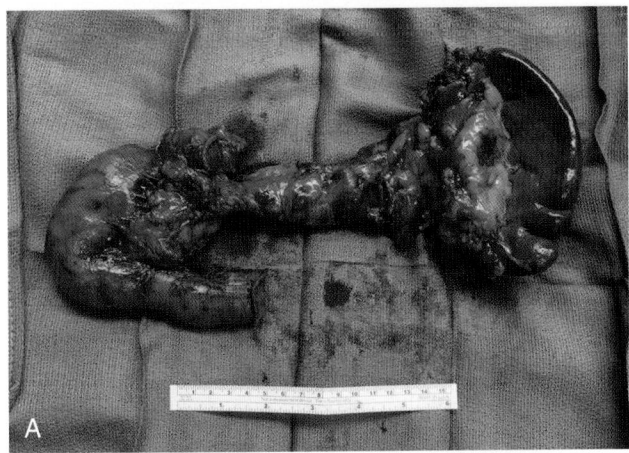

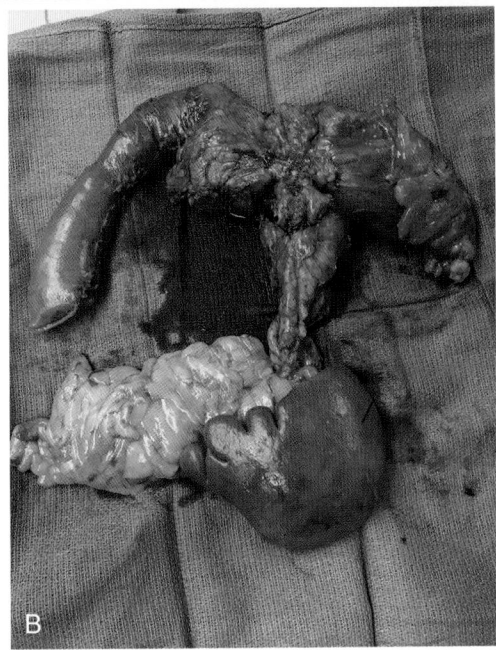

FIGURE 117C.2 **A,** Total pancreatectomy resection specimen with pylorus preservation and en bloc splenectomy performed in chronic pancreatitis. Islet autotransplantation was performed. **B,** Total pancreatectomy resection with antrectomy and en bloc splenectomy in patient with chronic pancreatitis. Islet autotransplantation was performed.

and the jejunum is passed through the defect. If the specimen is to be removed en bloc, the remaining uncinate dissection is best performed by lifting the left pancreas out of the operative field toward the patient's right side. This will expose the retropancreatic portal vein and SMA. Extreme care is taken to avoid avulsing the remaining venous tributaries to the portal vein. These are divided with clips, ties, or a 35 mm vascular stapler as appropriate. Once the pancreatic head is fully mobilized off of the portal vein, a vein retractor is used to apply gentle leftward traction on the portal vein. This exposes the SMA nicely, which is skeletonized to free the remaining attachments to the uncinate process and retroperitoneum. Branches are divided as appropriate using an energy device, ties, clips, or a 35 mm vascular stapler. The specimen is passed off the field (Fig. 117C.2), margins are sent for frozen section as appropriate, and absolute hemostasis is ensured.

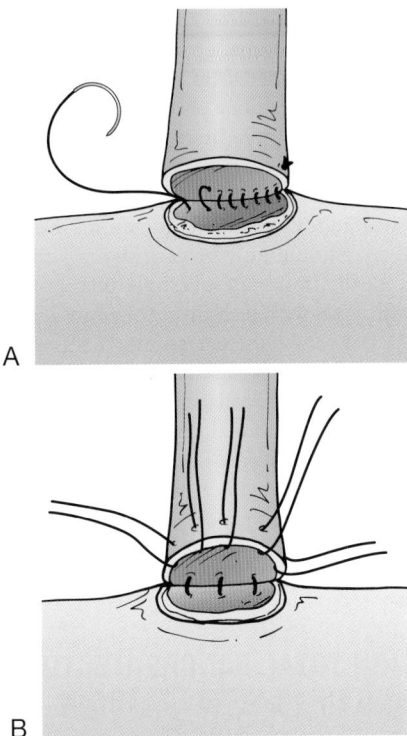

FIGURE 117C.3 **A,** Posterior wall biliary anastomosis. **B,** Anterior wall biliary anastomosis.

RECONSTRUCTION

A small defect is created in the transverse mesocolon, to the right of the middle colic vessel and the jejunal limb is delivered into the upper abdomen. The staple line is oversewn. An end-to-side hepaticojejunostomy is created (see Chapter 32). If the bile duct is dilated, a running anastomosis is created. The posterior layer is fashioned with PDS suture. The bowel is opened with needle point electrocautery and a second posterior layer of interrupted Vicryl sutures to ensure the mucosa is appropriately incorporated is created. (Fig. 117C.3A). The anterior layer is performed with a second PDS suture. If the bile duct is small or particularly thin walled, then an interrupted anastomosis is created with PDS or Vicryl sutures (see Fig. 117C.3B). Approximately 30 cm downstream, an antecolic duodeno- or gastrojejunostomy is created. This is handsewn with 2 layers of PDS. The jejunum is tacked to the defect in the right colon mesentery with interrupted silk sutures. The defect at the ligament of Treitz is close with silk sutures. A single 19 round Blake drain in placed behind the biliary anastomosis. Hemostasis is again ensured. We frequently place an incisional wound vac, especially in cases with prior instrumentation of the biliary tree.[13]

A handful of centers have reported acceptable outcomes with either a laparoscopic[14] or robotic[15,16] approach for total pancreatectomy (see Chapter 127). Minimally invasive total pancreatectomy should be limited to high-volume centers with significant experience in minimally invasive pancreatic surgery.

ISLET CELL TRANSPLANTATION

Total pancreatectomy with islet auto transplantation was first performed in 1977 at the University of Minnesota for a patient with refractory chronic pancreatitis. The goal of islet cell transplantation is to prevent, or at least mitigate, the consequences of type III diabetes by restoring beta cell function (see Chapter 112). Refractory chronic pancreatitis, recurrent acute pancreatitis, and hereditary pancreatitis are generally accepted indications for total pancreatectomy with islet auto transplantation (see Chapters 53, 56, and 58).[4,17] Some centers have advocated for expanded indications, but this remains controversial and should only be considered at highly specialized centers, ideally under an investigational protocol.

Either pylorus preservation or antrectomy is acceptable in most cases.[18] After total pancreatectomy, the specimen is delivered to a laboratory with experience in islet isolation. The pancreatic duct is infused with collagenase and islets are harvested. Depending on the institutional resources and expertise, islets may be processed on or off site. Once available, they are infused into the portal circulation, either during the same operation or percutaneously as a staged procedure. Portal pressures should be monitored closely and not exceed 25 cm H_2O. Increased portal pressures during delivery increase the risk of portal vein thrombosis.[19]

COMPLETION TOTAL PANCREATECTOMY IN THE SETTING OF POSITIVE MARGIN

This continues to be an area of significant debate. In the setting of main-duct or multifocal IPMN, the patient should be counseled preoperatively that this disease represents a field defect and that the entire gland may be at risk (see Chapter 60). Generally, the morbidity of total pancreatectomy outweighs the prophylactic pancreatectomy. Nevertheless, several scenarios warrant total pancreatectomy in fit patients, including diffuse main duct involvement, multifocal disease in high risk patients, and persistent high-grade dysplasia at the pancreatic resection margin. It is our practice to send frozen section in these cases. If the margin returns as high-grade dysplasia, we attempt to clear this margin. If there is persistent high-grade dysplasia at the resection margin, total pancreatectomy is performed if

there are no contraindications.[20,21] If the patient is not appropriate for total pancreatectomy or there is low-grade dysplasia at the resection margin, long-term surveillance is our approach, as it is with all patients with IPMN.

Pancreatic adenocarcinoma at the resection margin is a poor prognostic indicator and is likely a marker of aggressive biology (see Chapter 62). When performing a Whipple for adenocarcinoma, we send the pancreatic neck margin for frozen section analysis and make every attempt to clear this margin but avoid a total pancreatectomy whenever possible. There is conflicting evidence as to whether frozen section analysis with clearance of the pancreatic neck margin is associated with improved survival.[1,22,23] Outcomes after total pancreatectomy for adenocarcinoma are poor and this operation is rarely indicated, even in the setting of a positive resection margin after partial pancreatectomy.[2,24]

POSTOPERATIVE CARE (SEE CHAPTERS 26–28)

The patient is monitored in the intensive care unit overnight and started on an insulin drip. A nasogastric tube is typically left in place and removed on the morning of postoperative day one. The Foley catheter is removed once it is no longer necessary for urine output monitoring. The patient is slowly advanced to a diabetic diet over the coming days and endocrinology assists with dosing of long- and short-acting insulin. The epidural catheter is removed once the patient is tolerating a full liquid diet. Pancreatic enzymes are administered as the patient begins to increase their oral intake. The surgical drain is removed assuming it is nonbilious. Nutrition and diabetes education is paramount. The patient is discharged home once all criteria are met and is evaluated frequently as an outpatient by the surgical, endocrinology, and nutrition teams.

The references for this chapter can be found online by accessing the accompanying Expert Consult website.

Transduodenal resection of the papilla of vater

Chandrasekhar Padmanabhan, and William R. Jarnagin

INTRODUCTION

First described by Samuel Collins in 1685 and later by Abraham Vater in 1720,[1] the ampulla of Vater is a papillary structure in the second portion of the duodenum in which the common bile duct and the pancreatic duct converge just before draining into the duodenal lumen (Fig. 117D.1; see Chapter 2). The most common benign neoplasms of the ampulla of Vater are villous and tubulovillous adenomas (see Chapter 59). Autopsy studies in the 1930s and 1940s identified ampullary adenomas in 0.04% to 0.12% of individuals.[2,3] Although they are classified as benign tumors, they are truly premalignant lesions with the potential to transform into adenocarcinomas.[4–6] In addition, ampullary adenomas harbor occult dysplasia or adenocarcinoma in as many as 60% of cases.[7]

Patients with sporadic adenomas typically present later in life; however, patients with polyposis syndromes, such as familial adenomatous polyposis syndrome and MUTYH-associated polyposis syndrome, present much earlier in life. Approximately 30% to 50% of ampullary neoplasms present with painless jaundice,[4,5,7–9] but increased use of screening protocols has identified an increasing number of patients with asymptomatic ampullary neoplasms. Duodenoscopy, endoscopic ultrasound (EUS), and endoscopic retrograde cholangiopancreatography (ERCP) remain the diagnostic modalities of choice but distinguishing between adenoma and adenocarcinoma is extremely unreliable because the false negative rate for ampullary biopsy ranges between 25% to 60%.[10]

It is generally accepted that pancreaticoduodenectomy (PD) is the operation of choice for ampullary adenocarcinoma because of a higher margin negative resection rate and resultant lower recurrence rates, adequate lymph node staging, and the elimination of the need for surveillance endoscopy[7] (see Chapters 62 and 117A). Survival is better for ampullary adenocarcinoma than for any of the other periampullary adenocarcinomas and is largely dependent on lymph node status; five-year survival ranges from 64% to 80% for patients with node negative disease and 17% to 50% for patients with node positive disease.[11–23] Rate of lymph node metastases are 6% to 10% in pT1 ampullary adenocarcinomas but approach 50% in pT2 and pT3 tumors.[24,25]

Although PD remains the treatment of choice for ampullary adenocarcinoma, optimal management of benign ampullary neoplasms remains controversial. Complete resection remains the only way to ensure the absence of high-grade dysplasia or occult adenocarcinoma within an ampullary adenoma. Given this, some have argued that PD should be performed in all cases. Higher recurrence rates after local excision are also cited by those in favor of PD. Farnell et al. reported recurrence after transduodenal excision (TDE) of villous adenomas of 32% at 5 years and 43% at 10 years.[26] This is comparable to the 46% recurrence rate after TDE reported by Galandiuk

et al.[4] Others have suggested, however, that TDE is an adequate form of treatment because it is associated with reduced operative time, reduced inpatient postoperative stay, and decreased morbidity and mortality rates when compared with PD.[10,27] Local recurrences, when benign, can typically be salvaged with re-excision.[10,28,29]

Over the past 30 years, endoscopic ampullectomy has had an increasing role not only in the diagnosis of but also in the management of ampullary adenomas (see Chapter 30). First reported in the literature in the 1980s, initial experiences with endoscopic ampullectomy reported periprocedural complication rates of approximately 25% and recurrence rates of approximately 25% to 50%.[30,31] More recent series have reported a periprocedural complication rate of approximately 20% with recurrence rates ranging from 10% to 30%.[32,33] Piecemeal excision is associated with a recurrence rate of 54.3% versus 26.2% for en-bloc resection.[34] Much like recurrences after TDE, recurrences after endoscopic can typically be salvaged with repeat endoscopic resection.[32]

Regardless of the chosen approach, the presence of high-grade dysplasia on pathology after TDE or surgical ampullectomy is associated with invasive adenocarcinoma in the final specimen in 50% to 60% of cases.[35,36] Although endoscopic findings such as induration and rigidity of the papilla on probing, ulceration, and a submucosal mass effect are suggestive of underlying malignancy, they are certainly not conclusive.[7] Given this, PD should be considered if high-grade dysplasia or adenocarcinoma is identified.

TECHNIQUE

Laparotomy is made and a thorough abdominal exploration is performed to ensure there is no metastatic disease. If no metastatic disease is identified, the hepatic flexure of the colon is mobilized and a generous Kocher maneuver is performed to the level of the aorta to elevate the second portion of the duodenum from the retroperitoneum (see Chapter 117A). Stay sutures are placed and a lateral duodenotomy is performed using electrocautery (Fig. 117D.2A). To facilitate identification of the bile duct, a cholecystectomy may be performed with placement of a trans-cystic cholangiocatheter into the common bile duct and out of the ampulla. This can be very helpful when the bile duct is not dilated. Needle-point tip electrocautery is then used to excise the ampulla (see Fig. 117D.2B). Excision begins at the 11 o'clock position and continues down through the duodenal mucosa until the bile duct is identified. A 5-0, absorbable, monofilament suture is then placed full thickness through the bile duct and out the duodenum to oppose the wall of the bile duct to duodenal mucosa. This dissection is continued in a clockwise fashion, placing interrupted sutures to approximate the bile duct to the duodenal mucosa. The pancreatic duct will be encountered at

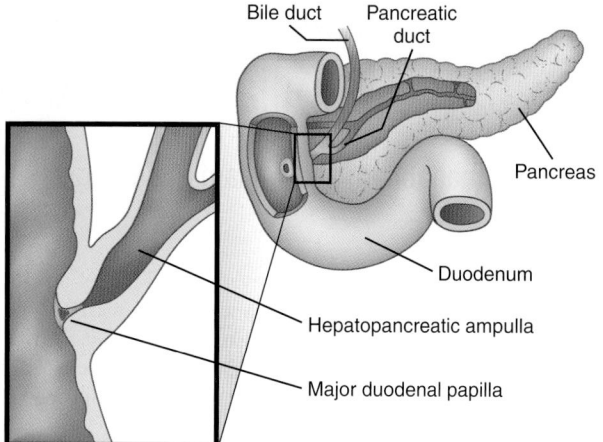

FIGURE 117D.1   The ampulla of Vater is a papillary structure in the second portion of the duodenum in which the common bile duct and the pancreatic duct converge just before draining into the duodenal lumen. (From Mamadievich RZ, Suratovich OF, Dekhkanovich DT. Gross and microscopic anatomy of the Vater papilla (hepatopancreatic ampulla) in animals with and without gall bladder. *Am J Med Sci.* 2020;10[1]:55–58.)

approximately the 2 o'clock position and is sutured to the duodenum in the same manner as described for the bile duct. If the pancreatic duct cannot be identified, intravenous secretin can be administered to facilitate pancreatic secretions and subsequent identification of the duct. The dissection is continued circumferentially until the mass is completely excised. The specimen should be carefully oriented for the pathologist to facilitate frozen-section examination. The opposing walls of the pancreatic duct and the common bile duct should be approximated with interrupted monofilament, absorbable sutures as depicted in Fig. 117D.2C. All sutures are tied, fully approximating the bile duct and the pancreatic duct to the medial duodenal wall (see Fig. 117D.2D). There is typically a mucosal defect adjacent to the anastomosis because the duodenal mucosal defect is typically larger than the circumference of the bile duct and pancreatic ducts. This defect is closed with interrupted sutures (Fig. 117D.3). The lateral duodenotomy is closed in a transverse fashion to avoid narrowing the lumen. A pedicled omental flap can be placed over the closure and a drain can be left at the discretion of the operating surgeon.

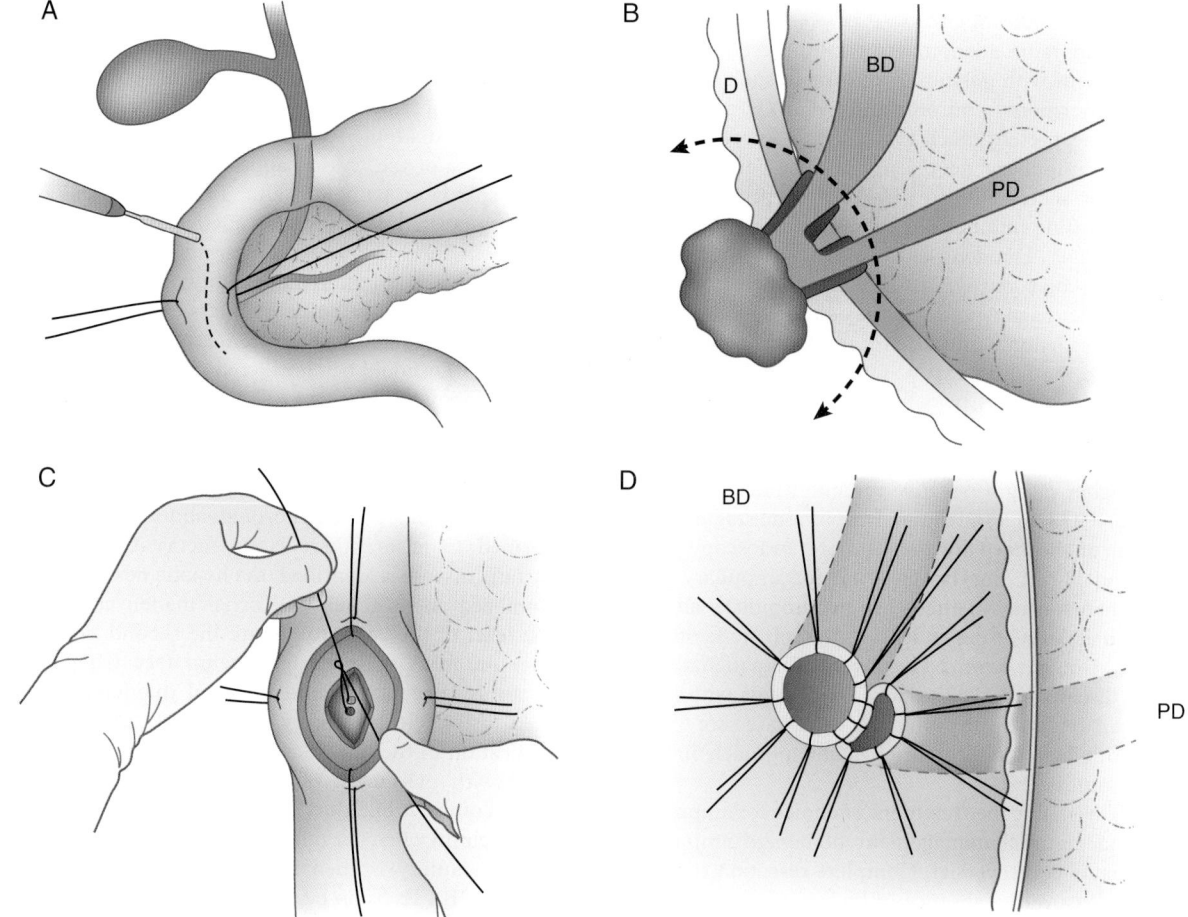

FIGURE 117D.2   **A,** After a generous Kocher maneuver, stay sutures are placed as depicted and a lateral duodenotomy is performed using electrocautery. **B,** Cross-sectional depiction of the ampullary region. Ampulla is excised with a margin depicted by the dotted line such that the bile duct *(BD)* and pancreatic duct *(PD)* orifices are identified separately. The former is typically identified at the 11 o'clock position and the latter is typically identified at the 2 o'clock position. Interrupted, absorbable, monofilament sutures are placed as the ampulla is excised but not tied. **C,** Once the ampulla has been excised, the opposing walls of the BD and PD are approximated with interrupted, absorbable, monofilament sutures. **D,** All sutures are tied, thereby approximating the walls of the BD and PD to the duodenal mucosa. (**A** and **C,** From Kaiser J, Contin P, Strobel O. Enucleation and transduodenal surgical ampullectomy for pancreatic and periampullary neoplasms: How I do it. In: Tewari M., ed. *Surgery for Pancreatic and Periampullary Cancer.* 2018. Springer. **B,** From Lee JW, Choi SH, Chon HJ, et al. Robotic transduodenal ampullectomy: A novel minimally invasive approach for ampullary neoplasms. *Int J Med Robot.* 2019;15[3]:e1979.)

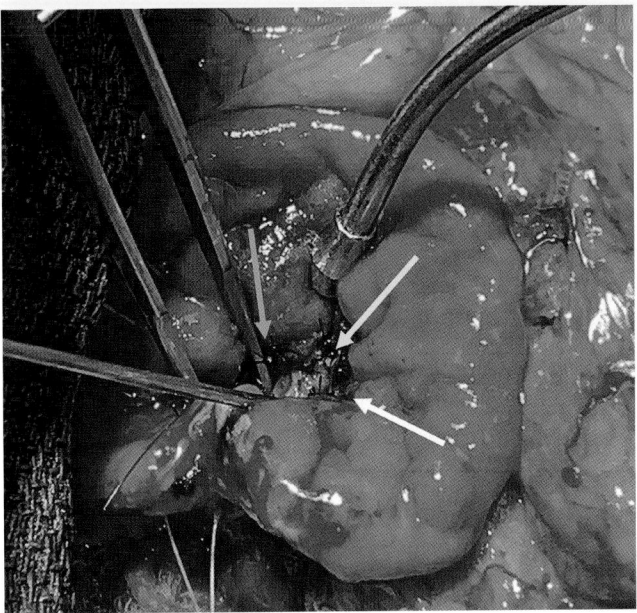

FIGURE 117D.3 Completed ampullectomy. Bile duct (*blue arrow*) and pancreatic duct (*yellow arrow*) have been approximated to the duodenal mucosa with interrupted, absorbable, monofilament sutures. Resultant defect in duodenal mucosa has been closed with interrupted sutures (*white arrow*). (Photograph courtesy Dr. Kamran Idrees MD, Department of Surgery, Vanderbilt University Medical Center.)

CONCLUSION

The management of ampullary neoplasms has evolved over the last 30 years. Because the morbidity and mortality after PD has dramatically improved in the modern era, the authors favor its use in the management of ampullary neoplasms given the high incidence of high-grade dysplasia and occult adenocarcinoma. TDE can still be performed in certain instances where PD cannot be performed.

The references for this chapter can be found online by accessing the accompanying Expert Consult website.

Major hepatectomy and extended hepatectomy

Brett L. Ecker and Michael I. D'Angelica

INTRODUCTION

Major hepatectomy is typically defined as a resection of three or more contiguous hepatic segments. Most commonly, this definition encompasses right and left hemihepatectomies and extended left and right hepatectomies. Extended hemihepatectomies can include a small subsegmental portion of the adjacent parenchyma or a more formal "trisectionectomy" where the adjacent segments (i.e., segment IV for a right sided resection, or segments V/VIII for a left sided resection) are included in the resection. Further, the caudate lobe may be included in any of these resections.

The term *major hepatectomy* is an appropriate description of these operations given that they are technically challenging and are associated with significant rates of postoperative morbidity. Among the spectrum of liver resections, these operations are associated with the highest rates of postoperative morbidity, including postoperative hepatic failure and other life-threatening complications. This chapter reviews the technical aspects of these operations. Operations requiring biliary or vascular resection (see Chapters 118A to 119A and 119B) or operations for living donor hepatectomy (see Chapter 121) are not covered in this chapter. Although this chapter does not focus on minimally invasive hepatic resections (see Chapter 127E), the same principles apply to a major hepatic resection regardless of surgical approach.

INDICATIONS

Major hepatectomy is most commonly indicated for malignant tumors of the liver and biliary tree (see Chapters 89–92 and 101). Rarely, large symptomatic or premalignant benign tumors are indications for a major hepatectomy (see Chapters 88 and 101). It should be stressed that in the contemporary era, a diagnostic hepatic resection for an indeterminate liver mass is rarely indicated—particularly with modern imaging and access to accurate pathology from percutaneous biopsy (see Chapters 13–15 and 23). Last, some less common indications for major hepatectomy include en bloc resections of perihepatic tumors (e.g., diaphragm, adrenal, retroperitoneum, stomach, duodenum), as well as management of certain benign conditions, including infections of the liver or biliary tree (see Chapter 11), trauma, and complex bile duct injuries (see Chapter 113).

In a sense, major hepatectomy should be an operation of last resort. Whenever possible, parenchymal-sparing operations that remove less liver tissue should be the operation of choice (see Chapters 102 and 118B). The reason for this is simple: Although parenchymal-sparing resections can be more challenging, the removal of less hepatic parenchyma is consistently associated with less postoperative morbidity. Specifically, removal of three or fewer segments of liver rarely results in liver failure, which is

the most life-threatening complication of hepatic resection.[1] Therefore a major hepatectomy should only be performed when the pathology involves inflow and outflow vessels that mandate removal of a hemiliver or more. It is often difficult to decide between parenchymal-sparing resections and major resections; it is therefore incumbent on the surgeon to weigh the risks (morbidity) and benefits (completeness of resection) of either approach.

The hepatic surgeon should also have a good sense of volume of hepatic parenchyma. In general, right-sided major hepatic resections are the largest volume resections. Typically, the right hemiliver encompasses approximately two-thirds of the liver and the right liver combined with segment IV can occupy over 80% of the liver. Left hemiliver resections, even when somewhat extended, are relatively low-volume resections. The volume of the right posterior sector is variable but the majority of left trisectionectomies leave a future liver remnant (FLR) of over 30%. Since it is the volume of residual liver parenchyma that is directly responsible for posthepatectomy morbidity,[2] the surgeon should have a sense of these relative volumes and the resources to directly measure the relative volume of the planned hepatic resection (see Chapters 4 and 102).

PREOPERATIVE PLANNING

Workup of specific diseases is covered in other chapters (see Chapter 12). For major hepatic resections, however, is it mandatory to have high-quality, multiphasic (arterial and portal venous phases) cross-sectional imaging to assess the extent of disease, vascular proximity, and anatomic variation (see Chapter 13). The surgeon should be able to assess the branching patterns of the hepatic veins, portal veins, and hepatic artery, as well as specific issues related to the proximity of the pathology being treated. Both magnetic resonance imaging and computed tomography (CT) can provide the necessary level of detail for preoperative planning, and each has specific advantages in different clinical scenarios.

Biliary anomalies are relatively common and preoperative recognition of specific branching abnormalities is important (see Chapter 2). The most common biliary anomalies involve right sectoral ducts draining either to the left bile duct or as low insertions into the common hepatic/bile duct. Therefore imaging of the biliary tree is most relevant for left-sided major resections so as to be prepared for right sectoral ducts that may be injured during a left hepatectomy. It can be argued that hilar branching of the biliary tree should be known in every case, but it is not often relevant in right-sided major resections. Classically, magnetic resonance cholangiopancreatography (MRCP) with gadolinium contrast is the imaging study of choice to assess the biliary tree (see Chapter 20), but MRCP with Eovist contrast and specific CT protocols can also be used to delineate biliary anatomy[3] (see Chapter 16).

Assessments of overall liver function and the size and function of the FLR are critical when planning major hepatic resections. Details of the assessment and management are covered in other chapters (see Chapters 4, 101, and 102). The Child-Pugh scoring system is a simple, easily obtainable, and clinically useful measure of hepatic function. However, it is critical to also assess patients for evidence of portal hypertension (see Chapters 5 and 74), which is not included in the Child-Pugh criteria and can be present even in the face of normal synthetic function. Portal hypertension can result from chronic liver disease or extensive treatment with systemic chemotherapy, and can often be diagnosed by virtue of readily available clinical findings such as splenomegaly, thrombocytopenia, and evidence of varices. In general, large-volume resections should only be performed in patients with Child-Pugh A liver function and no evidence of portal hypertension, as the presence of either major synthetic dysfunction or portal hypertension portends prohibitive operative risk.[4] Direct measurement of FLR volumes should be liberally assessed, even when the future liver remnant appears adequate. FLR volumes of less than 25% to 30% are associated with a significant risk of posthepatectomy liver failure,[2] with even higher volume thresholds in patients with chronic liver disease or chemotherapy-related hepatic injury.[5] Strategies to increase both the volume and function of the FLR such as portal vein embolization must be considered when volumes are not adequate (see Chapter 102C). Assessment of absolute changes in volume and the kinetics of such growth are very good markers of liver function and improve the safety of major resections.[6]

RELEVANT ANATOMY (ALSO SEE CHAPTER 2)

Hepatic Artery

The common hepatic artery typically branches off the celiac axis, coursing to the right along the superior border of the body of the pancreas (see Fig. 2.37). After giving off an inferior branching gastroduodenal artery and then the right gastric artery (with somewhat variable origins), the proper hepatic artery then branches into the right and left hepatic artery. The proper hepatic artery can be of variable distance and may not exist at all with an immediate bifurcation after the gastroduodenal artery. In its typical course, the left hepatic artery runs cephalad along the left border of the porta hepatis toward the base of the umbilical fissure. The distal left hepatic artery most commonly branches at the base of the umbilical fissure into a segment IV and a left lateral section branch (segments II and III). Alternatively, the segment IV branch can arise off of the proximal right hepatic artery where it runs into the right border of the umbilical fissure. In this case, the apparent "left hepatic artery" only supplies the left lateral section. The right hepatic artery courses cephalad, to the right, and typically (90%) posterior to the common hepatic bile duct. Alternatively, when the right hepatic artery runs anterior to the common hepatic duct (10% of patients), it is the most anterior structure in the right side of the porta hepatis. Branching of the right hepatic artery into sectoral branches often occurs outside of the hepatic parenchyma—proximal to the invagination of Glisson capsule—and can be dissected and encircled in the porta hepatis if necessary.

Anomalies of the hepatic arterial system are common. Replaced vessels originate from a branch other than the hepatic artery and completely replace the blood supply to a hemiliver. Accessory vessels originate from a branch other than the hepatic artery and supply a portion of a hemiliver in conjunction with the standard arterial inflow. Most commonly, replaced and accessory right hepatic arteries originate from the superior mesenteric artery and course posteriorly along the right side of the porta hepatis lateral to the portal vein. Most commonly, replaced and accessory left hepatic arteries originate from the left gastric artery and run through the gastrohepatic ligament, where they enter the liver at the left side of the base of the umbilical fissure. The common hepatic artery can also be replaced to the superior mesenteric artery where, most commonly, it runs cephalad and anteriorly between the portal vein and the common bile duct, entering the anterior portion of the porta hepatis. Right and left hepatic arteries can also originate proximal to the gastroduodenal artery from the common hepatic artery. It is important to realize that nearly any branching pattern is possible, and this anatomy should be known from preoperative imaging and anticipated at surgery (see Chapters 2 and 13–15).

Portal Vein

The portal vein forms from the confluence of the splenic vein and superior mesenteric vein. From its origin, the portal vein courses toward the liver posteriorly and to the right within the porta hepatis. At the base of the liver between the caudate lobe and the base of segment IV, the portal vein most commonly splits into a long transverse, leftward running left portal vein and a shorter, more cephalad coursing right portal vein. The first branches of the right and left portal vein are those to the caudate lobe; these must be identified before encircling the right or left portal vein. The caudate branch off of the right portal vein arises proximally and supplies the caudate process. The left portal vein gives off a significant caudate branch that supplies the left side of the caudate just before curving into the umbilical fissure, adjacent to the insertion of the ligamentum venosum. There are small segment IV portal vein branches that branch superiorly off of the transverse portion of the left portal vein and are visualized when completely mobilizing the left portal vein or when lowering the hilar plate. The left portal vein typically branches into the segments of the left liver intrahepatically. The right portal vein most commonly gives off an anterior and posterior sectoral branch, which can be dissected in the porta hepatis.

There are numerous anomalous branching patterns that must be anticipated by careful review of preoperative imaging (see Figs. 2.38–2.43). The posterior sectoral branches often originate without a common posterior sectoral portal vein. In 5% to 10% of patients, an early branching posterior sectoral vein directly off the main portal vein will be followed by the right anterior sectoral branch and left portal vein. In the most dangerous situation (albeit very rare; <1%), a single branch enters the substance of the liver; after giving off a right portal vein (or separate origins of right anterior and posterior sectoral branches), it courses to the left yielding the left portal vein. With a single vein in the porta hepatis, it can be easy to mistakenly divide the whole portal venous anatomy during a major hepatectomy in this situation. In addition to these anomalies, there are innumerable variations on branching patterns that need to be anticipated (see Chapter 2).

Preservation of portal venous inflow is critically important for postoperative liver regeneration, particularly for major resections. Compromise of portal venous inflow in any meaningful way can result in postoperative liver failure.

Bile Duct

The common bile duct is located anteriorly along the right border of the porta hepatis. The common hepatic duct is defined as the duct cephalad to the variable insertion of the cystic duct. Relevant to dissection in the porta hepatis is the fact that the biliary tree is supplied by hepatic artery branches that run along the lateral borders of the duct (3 and 9 o'clock branches). Since the function and viability of the ductal wall is reliant on this arterial inflow, skeletonization of the biliary tree along its lateral aspects can result in ischemia with the potential for strictures or necrosis. The bile duct branches into a long, left bile duct that courses transversely along the base of segment IV where it enters the umbilical fissure and gives off segmental branches to the left liver. The right bile duct runs into the substance of the right liver at the base of the cystic plate and is short with early branching into sectoral/segmental branches. Similar to the portal vein, both the right and left bile ducts provide biliary drainage to the caudate lobe. Left-sided caudate branches drain into the left bile duct, whereas branches from the caudate process/right side of the caudate drain into the right bile duct. Myriad biliary branching anomalies exist (see Fig. 2.25); the most relevant to major hepatectomy include sectoral branching of right branches into the left bile duct. A relatively common anomaly involves the right posterior or anterior sectoral duct entering the left bile duct. These left-sided insertions of right sectoral ducts are particularly relevant for left-sided major resections, as it can be easy to injure, narrow, or ligate right-sided biliary branches. Sectoral branches can also exit the liver and insert into the common hepatic/bile duct as low entry sectoral ducts. Unexpected encounters with these anomalous sectoral branches can be confusing during major hepatectomy and may require biliary exploration and/or cholangiogram to determine the exact anatomy in order to proceed with safe resection (see Chapters 20 and 24). In general, and whenever possible, it is safest to divide and ligate biliary branches intrahepatically to ensure protection of the contralateral bile duct branches. Contralateral biliary injuries during major hepatectomy can be a source of catastrophic morbidity.

Hepatic Veins

Understanding and anticipation of venous anatomy is critical to the performance of a safe major hepatectomy (see Figs. 2.2 and 2.3). Bleeding from major hepatic veins and their branches is the most common source of significant hemorrhage during major hepatectomy. Further, venous injuries, especially when incurred during low–central venous pressure anesthesia, can result in significant air embolus (see Chapter 25). It is therefore critical for the surgeon to understand not only the typical venous anatomy, but the anatomy of each specific case. Also, compromise of hepatic venous outflow can result in postoperative hepatic failure.

There are three major hepatic veins that course through the scissurae of the liver within the intrahepatic sectoral planes. The right hepatic vein courses in the right scissura between the right anterior and posterior sector. The middle hepatic vein runs in the main scissura between the right and left hemilivers. The left hepatic vein runs in the left scissura between segment II posteriorly and segments III and IV anteriorly within the left liver. The left and middle hepatic vein commonly join as a single common branch of varying length before entering the vena cava, but may also enter the suprahepatic cava as separate branches.

The right hepatic vein typically branches to the right giving off major segmental venous branches to segment VI and VII and does not typically give off major branches to the anterior sector. Occasionally, one (or multiple) inferior right hepatic vein(s) may be present, which drains segment VI into the inferior portion of the retrohepatic vena cava. In this case, the main right hepatic vein is small and only drains segment VII. The middle hepatic vein provides the principal drainage of the anterior sector via dominant branches to segment VIII and V. The middle hepatic vein typically has only small branches to the left to segment IV, but this varies. When dividing the liver in the principal plane during a right or left hemihepatectomy, one should anticipate on which side of the vein the transection will proceed and the relevant branches that will be encountered. The left hepatic vein, once beyond the posterior aspects of segment IV, courses between segment II and III. A segment II branch often enters the left hepatic vein proximally and can have a somewhat extrahepatic course along the posterior aspect of the left lateral section. Distal to the segment II branch, the left hepatic vein serves as the dominant drainage of segment III. An umbilical vein is nearly always present and courses anterior to the umbilical fissure between segments III and IV and provides additional drainage to segments III and IV. Most commonly, the umbilical vein drains into the left hepatic vein, but can drain into the middle hepatic vein or enter into the confluence of the left and middle hepatic vein as a trifurcation. It bears repeating that venous anatomy, in detail, should be known for every case from preoperative imaging and anticipated during parenchymal transection (see Chapters 2 and 13–15).

Vena Cava

The vena cava borders a groove along a central strip of the posterior aspect of the liver. To the right, this abuts the posterior aspects of segments VI and VII. To the left it abuts the caudate lobe. At the cephalad portion of the retrohepatic cava, there is a ligament (known as the caval ligament) of fibrous tissue with varying amounts of hepatic parenchyma that wraps from the posterior aspect of segment VII around the posterior aspect of the cava to attach to the left border of the caudate lobe on the left side of the cava forming a sling around the cava (Fig. 118A.1). Dissecting, controlling, and dividing this ligament is essential to expose the upper portion of the retrophepatic cava and the right hepatic vein laterally and for mobilization of the caudate lobe. The retrohepatic cava arises just above the renal veins and given its relative cephalad location, the right renal vein can be fairly close to the inferior border of the liver. The vena cava provides varying small- and medium-sized draining branches from the posterior aspect of the liver (mainly the caudate lobe) and when dissecting the liver off the cava, these branches require control and ligation. Some of these branches can be of sufficient size to require suture control or division with a stapler. As mentioned, an inferior right hepatic vein, when present, drains into the retrohepatic cava. The right adrenal vein is rarely encountered during hepatectomy because it drains posteriorly to the right along the right side of the cava. Rarely, branches from the adrenal vein can drain directly into the liver and can be encountered while mobilizing the liver. There are rarely posterior branches from the vena cava along its retrohepatic portion. The major hepatic veins drain into the vena cava just above the liver where the cava pierces the diaphragm to enter the right atrium. Before entry into the chest, the left and right phrenic veins—which course along the peritoneal side of the diaphragm—enter the left and right side of the cava just above the hepatic

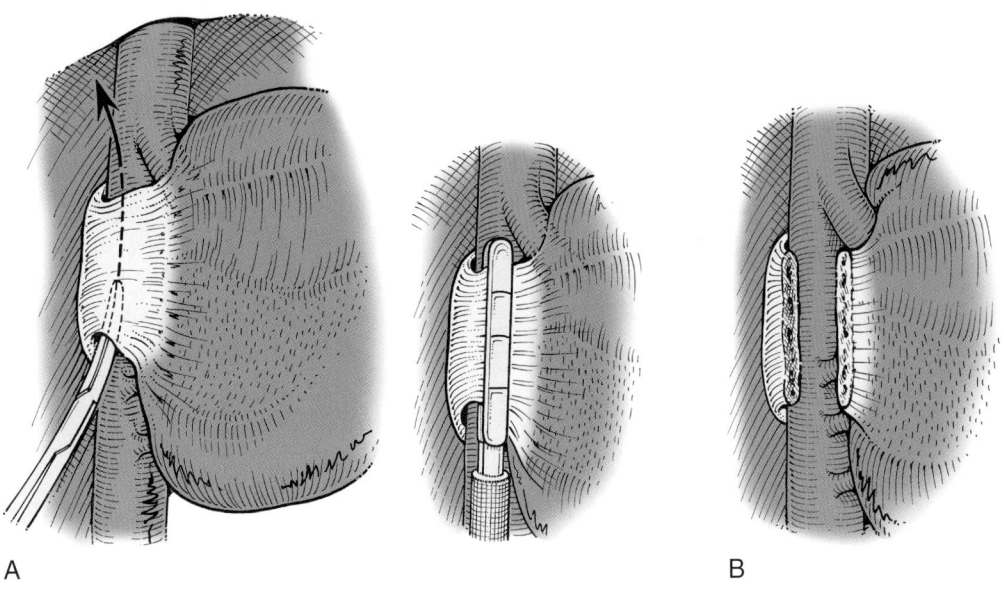

FIGURE 118A.1   **A,** The ligament also may be mobilized, and a clamp is passed beneath it *(left)*. It is divided with the Endo GIA (Covidien) vascular stapler *(right)*. **B,** The retrohepatic IVC is fully exposed.

veins. Less commonly, the phrenic veins can drain directly into the right and left hepatic veins.

Intrahepatic Segmental Branching Patterns

Once the hilar vessels enter the liver substance, they are invaginated by Glisson capsule (visceral peritoneum of the liver) and form intrahepatic sectoral/segmental branches, which we will refer to as "pedicles." Variation of pedicular branching patterns is the rule; thus knowledge and anticipation of these patterns, guided by preoperative imaging, is essential. The left inflow pedicle forms at the base of the umbilical fissure. From within this fissure, the first branch to the left lateral section is a cephalad branch to segment II and then, more distally, a branch to segment III anteriorly. There are often small additional branches to the left lateral section. Occasionally, there is a single pedicle that splits into segment II and III branches intrahepatically. Although we conveniently refer to segment IV as having A and B segments, branching to such segments does not exist. There are typically multiple inflow pedicles to segment IV coming from the transverse portion of the left inflow vessels (along the base of segment IV), as well as the more dominant branches originating from within the umbilical fissure. The main right inflow pedicle is typically short, or even nonexistent, and branches into an anterior and posterior sectoral pedicle. Most commonly, the anterior pedicle runs as a large dominant pedicle cephalad and to the right to segment VIII. Along the way, the anterior pedicle typically gives off multiple small segment V branches. There is not a dominant segment V pedicle typically. Segment VIII reliably branches into a ventral and dorsal branch. The dorsal branch often arches superiorly over the right hepatic vein. The posterior sectoral pedicle is often short and sometimes nonexistent. Segment VI and VII branches commonly arise proximally. Segment VI runs in the fissure of Gans (also known as the Sulcus of Rouvier) and can usually be seen in this fissure on the surface of the liver. Segment VII runs cephalad and posteriorly where it remains posterior to the right hepatic vein straight into segment VII.

Perihepatic Ligaments/Attachments

Since major hepatic resections require mobilization of the liver by division of its ligaments, the perihepatic attachments must be familiar to the surgeon (Fig. 118A.2). The ligamentum teres runs along the abdominal wall and terminates at the falciform ligament anterior to the liver. The ligamentum teres carries the obliterated umbilical vein and a small branch of the hepatic artery. Division of this and the falciform ligament cephalad begins to expose the left and right coronary/triangular ligaments, which cover the hepatic veins. The right triangular ligament is typically broad and must be divided along a plane between the right liver and the diaphragm. Division of this ligament with rotation of the liver to the left begins to expose the vena cava and right side of the caval ligament. The left triangular ligament is thin and lies just inferior to the left phrenic vein. Though typically avascular, small phrenic veins draining into the segment II vein can occasionally be encountered. Division of the left triangular ligament mobilizes the left lateral section up to the left hepatic vein. The ligamentum venosum (Fig. 118A.3; also see Figs. 2.11 and 2.12) runs from the left portal vein along the border between the left lateral section and the caudate lobe at the insertion of the gastrohepatic ligament and then enters the left hepatic vein. Division of the ligamentum venosum near the left hepatic vein (usually accompanied by mobilization of the superior portion of the caudate) is essential to expose the posterior aspect of the left and middle hepatic veins and allows encircling of these veins extrahepatically. The caval ligament is mentioned earlier in this chapter.

Caudate Lobe

Knowledge of the anatomy of the caudate lobe is essential to understanding major hepatic resections (see Figs. 2.11 and 2.12 and Fig. 118A.3). The vascular inflow, biliary drainage,

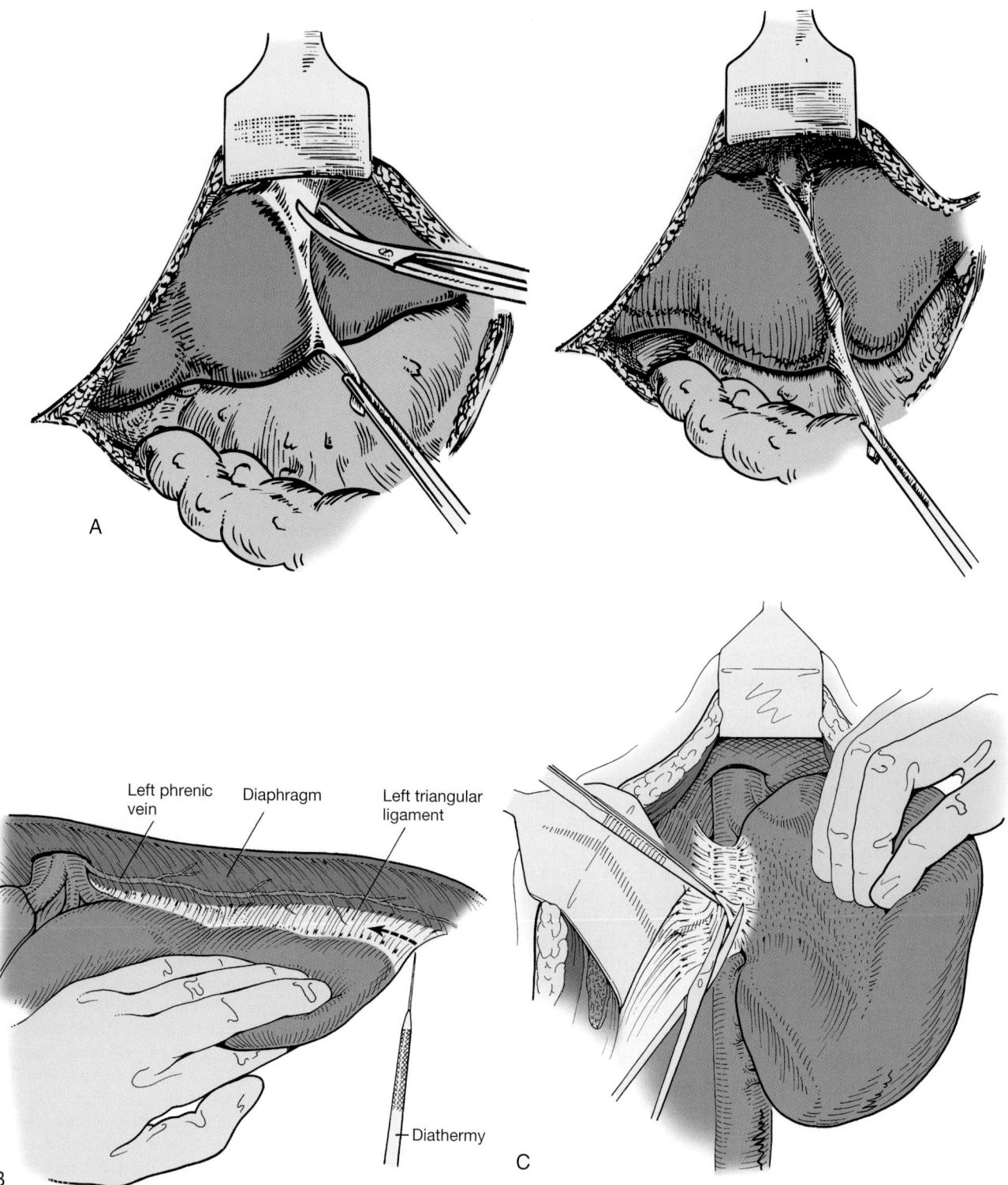

FIGURE 118A.2   A, The ligamentum teres is secured, and division of the falciform ligament is begun. The falciform ligament is divided backward to expose the suprahepatic inferior vena cava (IVC). **B,** The left triangular ligament is exposed and divided with cautery. Care should be taken not to injure the left phrenic vein. **C,** Incision of the peritoneal reflection of the right triangular ligament allows mobilization of the right liver. The exposure is deepened to display the right lateral margin of the IVC.

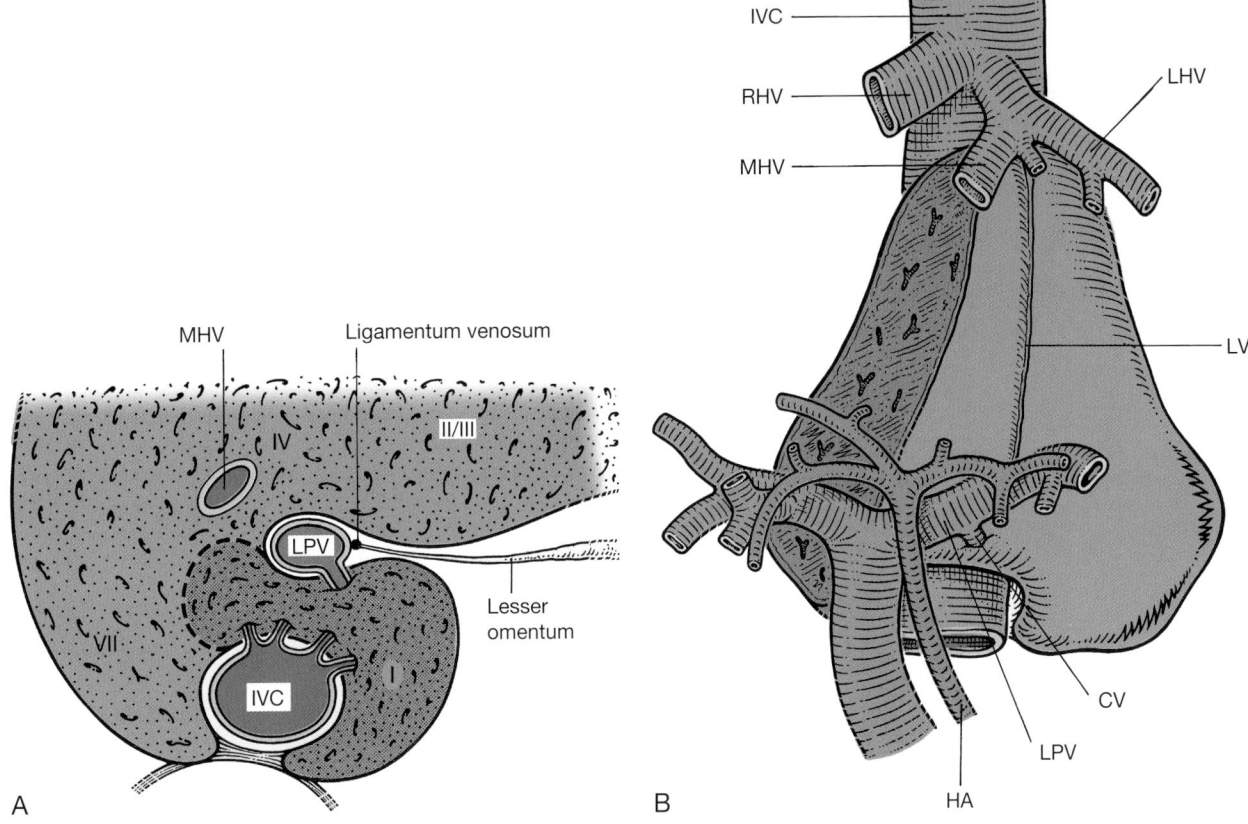

FIGURE 118A.3 **A,** Cross-sectional sketch shows caudate lobe anatomy at the level of the porta hepatis. Note the principal caudate branch of left portal vein *(LPV)*. Note the position of (1) the lesser omentum and ligamentum venosum; (2) middle hepatic vein *(MHV)*, which separates segments IV and V and is close to right portion of caudate lobe; and (3) the posterior ligamentous band joining segments I and VII. **B,** The relationships of the caudate lobe are illustrated. The caudate lies anterior to the inferior vena cava *(IVC)* but posterior to the portal venous structures; the caudate lobe has a right portion. Blood supply to the caudate lobe is mainly from the caudate branch *(CV)* of the LPV. This branch may arise from the main trunk of the portal vein in some cases. *HA,* Hepatic artery; *LHV,* left hepatic vein; *LV,* ligamentum venosum; *RHV,* right hepatic vein.

and venous outflow anatomy are described earlier. The caudate lies between the rest of the liver and the vena cava except for the rightmost aspects of the right hemiliver. For example, the anterior sector of the liver does not border the cava but rather lies anterior to the caudate lobe. The right side of the caudate, called the caudate process, lies adjacent to the posterior border of the right inflow pedicles and division of this tissue is critical for exposure of the right inflow pedicle(s). The left liver also lies anterior to the caudate and therefore does not abut the vena cava except for the small portion near the hepatic veins superiorly. Tumors involving any portion of the caudate often mandate a major hepatic resection en bloc with the caudate. This involves complete mobilization and division of inflow vessels. For right hepatectomies that include the caudate, the caudate should be mobilized such that it can be completely placed on the right side of the cava.

Positioning, Retractors, and Incision

The patient is positioned supine with the arms out laterally to provide peripheral vascular access. Table positioning during a major hepatectomy can be very valuable. Most commonly, the patient can be kept in the reverse Trendelenburg position to drop the abdominal viscera and expose the liver. Right- or left-sided rotation throughout the case should be used liberally, as

these maneuvers can help with exposure of different parts of the liver. Many incisions can be used for major hepatectomy (Figs. 118A.4 and 118A.5). The most common incision involves a generous right subcostal incision, which in most cases should involve a midline superior extension to the xyphoid process (i.e., hockey stick incision). It is sometimes necessary to extend a hockey stick incision to the left as a bilateral subcostal incision (i.e., Mercedes type incision). Although this extension is rarely necessary, it can be helpful in patients with large tumors that cannot be completely mobilized. A midline incision is a useful incision when a combined resection with another, more inferior organ is required. A midline incision is adequate for left-sided resections but can make it difficult to reach the right aspect of the right liver, particularly for obese patients. Another consideration is whether extension into the right chest is necessary with a thoracoabdominal incision. Though rarely necessary, extension to the right chest with division of the diaphragm allows for enhanced exposure of the superior aspects of the cava and can be valuable in cases of caval injury or with large right-sided tumors obscuring caval exposure. The thoracoabdominal incision can be a J-type incision or an extension of the Mercedes or hockey stick incision into the chest. Retractors for major hepatectomy are numerous and vary by institution and/or individual. The essential part of retraction

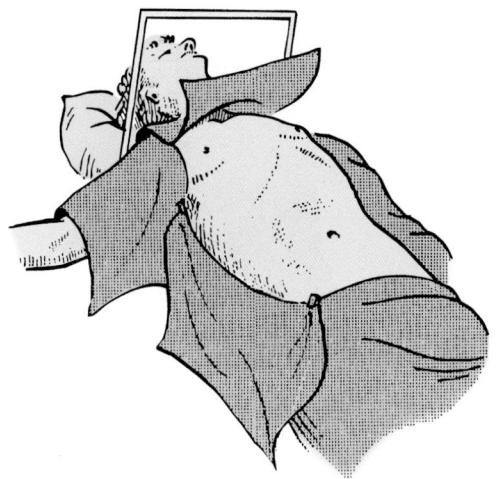

FIGURE 118A.4 Position of the patient on the operating table. Note the wide exposure of the abdomen and chest. The cross bar later holds a large retractor, used to elevate the costal margin.

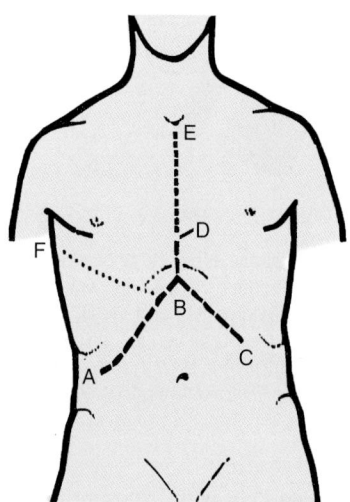

FIGURE 118A.5 Incisions used for partial hepatectomy. *ABCD,* Mercedes type incision. *DE,* Median sternotomy. *F,* Right thoracic extension. Most often, an extended right subcostal incision *(ABD)* is adequate. In many patients, a midline incision with good lateral retraction is sufficient.

is cephalad retraction of the costal margin at an approximately 45-degree angle. Other helpful areas of retraction include lateral retraction of the right chest wall and inferior retraction of the lower abdominal viscera.

GENERAL CONSIDERATIONS (INFLOW, OUTFLOW, PARENCHYMAL TRANSECTION, ORDERING)

The principal steps of a major hepatectomy can be broken up into four different phases: mobilization, inflow control, outflow control, and parenchymal transection. The order of these steps can vary but some general principles apply. Except for rare cases (e.g., anterior approach to right hepatectomy; see later in this chapter), mobilization is the first step in order to have easier access to the perihepatic vasculature and the liver itself. Outflow division should not be performed before inflow

control, as this results in congested liver parenchyma and venous bleeding. Inflow vessels can be taken extrahepatically or in their intrahepatic location as pedicles. Extrahepatic control of inflow vessels with a hilar dissection provides the advantage of early vascular control to the liver to be resected. Division of the inflow as intrahepatic pedicles can be approached in two ways. One way is to divide the liver parenchyma in the plane of transection down to the pedicles of interest. Another approach to pedicle ligation that does not require parenchymal transection is the use of hepatotomies around the inflow pedicle(s). Unless the location of a tumor mandates extrahepatic dissection, the approach to the inflow vessels is at the discretion of the surgeon, as there has been no demonstrable difference in outcomes between these two techniques.[7] The outflow vessels can be taken extrahepatically as they enter the cava or intrahepatically after division of the liver. The advantage to early extrahepatic venous division before parenchymal transection is a further level of mobilization and early control of potential bleeding from the involved vein. At times, the location of pathology or difficulty in extrahepatic dissection makes it preferable to divide parenchyma back to the hepatic vein insertions, where they can be taken just as they exit the liver.

Safe and controlled parenchymal transection is a critical skill for the liver surgeon. Notwithstanding the myriad techniques for parenchymal transection, the details of which are beyond the scope of this chapter, there are certain universal principles for parenchymal transection. The goal of parenchymal division is to dissect through parenchyma in order to expose the anticipated anatomy (based on preoperative imaging), which allows for appropriate control and division of inflow and outflow structures. Hepatic transection should be a dissection, not a frantic effort to control hemorrhage. Likewise, the use of coagulating energy devices should not be an excuse to blindly coagulate while splitting liver tissue. The use of intraoperative ultrasound is also a critical skill for the liver surgeon (see Chapters 24 and 103). Ultrasound is used to document vascular proximity and vascular patency/flow, identify occult lesions (although this is uncommon with modern imaging), and identify relevant intrahepatic structures that guide hepatic division. Portal clamping with a Pringle maneuver is not necessary for all cases, but it has been shown to be safe in many trials.[8,9] A Pringle maneuver should be prepared for all liver resections so that it is ready to be employed as necessary. There should be a low threshold to transect under Pringle control if bleeding is an issue or blood obscures visualization or dissection. In general, intermittent clamping is preferred to prevent portal venous congestion.

If the dissection has gone well, there should be minimal bleeding from the raw liver surface beyond the expected minor oozing. Major bleeding from vascular branches (most commonly the middle hepatic vein) may require suture repair. In general, the first move is simple compression for a few minutes, which often controls minor venous bleeding. There are numerous topical hemostatic agents and coagulation devices that can assist with hemostasis. Whatever method is used, care should be taken not to substantially injure contralateral structures, which can occur with deep sutures or excessive use of energy devices. It is well worth the surgeon's time to meticulously inspect the liver surface for bleeding and/or bile leaks. Some advocate for routine testing for bile leaks (e.g., air cholangiogram, see Chapter 24), but this has not been proven effective in randomized trials. Small bile leaks can be controlled with fine suture repair. In general, drains are not recommended based on randomized trials[10,11]; however, if there is ongoing bile leakage, it is advisable to leave a drain in the operative bed.

It should be stressed that there are many ways to perform a major liver resection, and this will necessarily result in differences in technique, ordering of steps, and specific technical maneuvers. This is the essence of the art of surgery. Next, specific operations are discussed and should be interpreted as general concepts. Variation in technique and order of maneuvers should be individualized and adapted to the specific situation in each case.

SPECIFIC OPERATIONS

Right Hemihepatectomy

The right liver is mobilized by first dividing the ligamentum teres and falciform ligament. The right coronary and triangular ligaments are then divided back to the hepatic veins. The right phrenic vein is an easily visualized landmark that drains to the cava in close proximity to the right hepatic vein and helps identify this structure before its dissection. The dissection should proceed to the origin of the right and middle hepatic vein, deliberately dissecting the groove between these veins. Once the anatomy of the right hepatic vein is visualized, the liver is turned to the left and inferiorly to expose the broad right triangular ligament, which is divided to expose the bare area of the right liver. From this position, the right triangular ligament should be divided as much as feasible approaching the caval ligament and vena cava. Next, the base of the right liver is retracted superiorly and the kidney is retracted inferiorly. From here the inferior border of the right triangular ligament is visualized and divided from the cava around toward the prior dissection. It is critical during this dissection to cut more than you retract as the peritoneal reflections are stronger than the liver parenchyma and it is easy to tear liver tissue along these reflections, leading to unnecessary hemorrhage. The liver should now be quite mobile, and it is now retracted off the vena cava to the left. The right adrenal gland is dissected off the liver and dropped back into the retroperitoneum. It is noteworthy that sometimes the adrenal is adherent to the liver and requires deliberate dissection to drop it off the liver. Occasionally, parts of the adrenal are left attached to the liver and obtaining hemostasis of the divided adrenal gland is necessary. At this point, the superior border of the caval ligament and the lateral aspect of the vena cava/right hepatic vein are dissected. Then, dissection along the anterior border of the cava commences from inferior to superior, controlling and dividing the retrohepatic caval branches until the inferior border of the caval ligament is encountered. Inferior right hepatic veins are taken at this time. The space between the caval ligament and the lateral border of the vena cava/right hepatic vein is now dissected—most effectively with a curved blunt clamp (see Fig. 118A.1). Once the ligament is encircled and it is clear that the cava/right hepatic vein are protected, the caval ligament is divided. It is convenient to divide this ligament with a vascular load stapler. There are typically more caval branches from the liver between the caval ligament and the base of the right hepatic vein and dissection, control, and division of these veins commences up until the base of the right hepatic vein is exposed. Now a tunnel between the right and middle hepatic vein is created for control of the right hepatic vein. This tunnel is a relatively wide and avascular plane that can be dissected with a combination of dissection

from above (started earlier) and below. The plane curves anteriorly when approached from below. The right hepatic vein is then encircled for division at a later time. If there is difficulty exposing and/or encircling the right hepatic vein, it can be approached intrahepatically during transection of the liver. It is, however, advisable to have the right hepatic vein controlled early if at all possible.

At this point, attention is turned to the inflow. The hilar plate should be lowered with an incision in the peritoneal reflection at the base of segment IV (see Chapter 32). Small branches from the portal vein may be encountered here requiring control. This maneuver serves to drop the left bile duct away from the rest of the dissection thereby protecting it. In the case of extrahepatic vascular control (Fig. 118A.6), the dissection starts with a cholecystectomy (see Chapter 36) and retraction of the cystic duct stump to the left. This pulls the biliary tree to the left, exposing the right hepatic artery in the groove between the bile duct and portal vein. If the right hepatic artery is anterior (which should be known based on preoperative imaging), it can be dissected and encircled anterior to the bile duct in the porta hepatis. Once the right hepatic artery is encircled, it is prudent to clamp it and make sure that a pulse is palpable at the base of the umbilical fissure in the left hepatic artery. It is not necessary to dissect all the arterial anatomy in the porta in the majority of cases. The right hepatic artery is then divided and from its most common location posterior to the bile duct, the proximal artery is retracted to the left, acting as a sling to pull the biliary tree further to the left. In the case of an accessory or replaced right hepatic artery, these vessels are dissected more posteriorly along the right side of the porta hepatis as described earlier. Next, the portal vein is dissected exposing the main, right, and left portal vein. This requires retraction of the biliary tree anteriorly and to the right. A vein retractor can be helpful for this exposure. It is critical to see the anatomy of both the right and left portal vein. With careful dissection right on the plane of the vein, the right portal vein is dissected. A branch to the caudate process is nearly always present and should be identified and ligated. Alternatively, the branch can be taken with the right portal vein if encircled proximal to this branch. Once the right portal vein is encircled (with clear visualization of the main and left portal vein) it should be clamped and demarcation noted. It is also prudent to document portal flow to the left liver with Doppler ultrasound. If the bile ducts will be taken inside the liver, the right portal vein does not necessarily have to be divided. It can simply be tied off arresting vascular flow to the right liver. It is good practice to divide the right bile duct inside the liver within the pedicles to maximize distance from the left bile duct. It cannot be overstated how important it is to protect the left bile duct during right-sided resections. If pathology mandates division of the liver within the porta hepatis, the right portal vein is divided and the right bile duct is identified and either divided now or once the liver is transected. It is advisable to divide the right bile duct sharply and probe the left and main bile duct to ensure patency. If there are any concerns about patency of the left bile duct, there should be a low threshold to perform cholangiography (see Chapter 24). Once the inflow is taken, the right hepatic vein is taken at its origin. This provides complete vascular control of the right liver and additionally provides an additional degree of mobilization off of the vena cava. Alternatively, the right hepatic vein can be taken at the end of parenchymal transection.

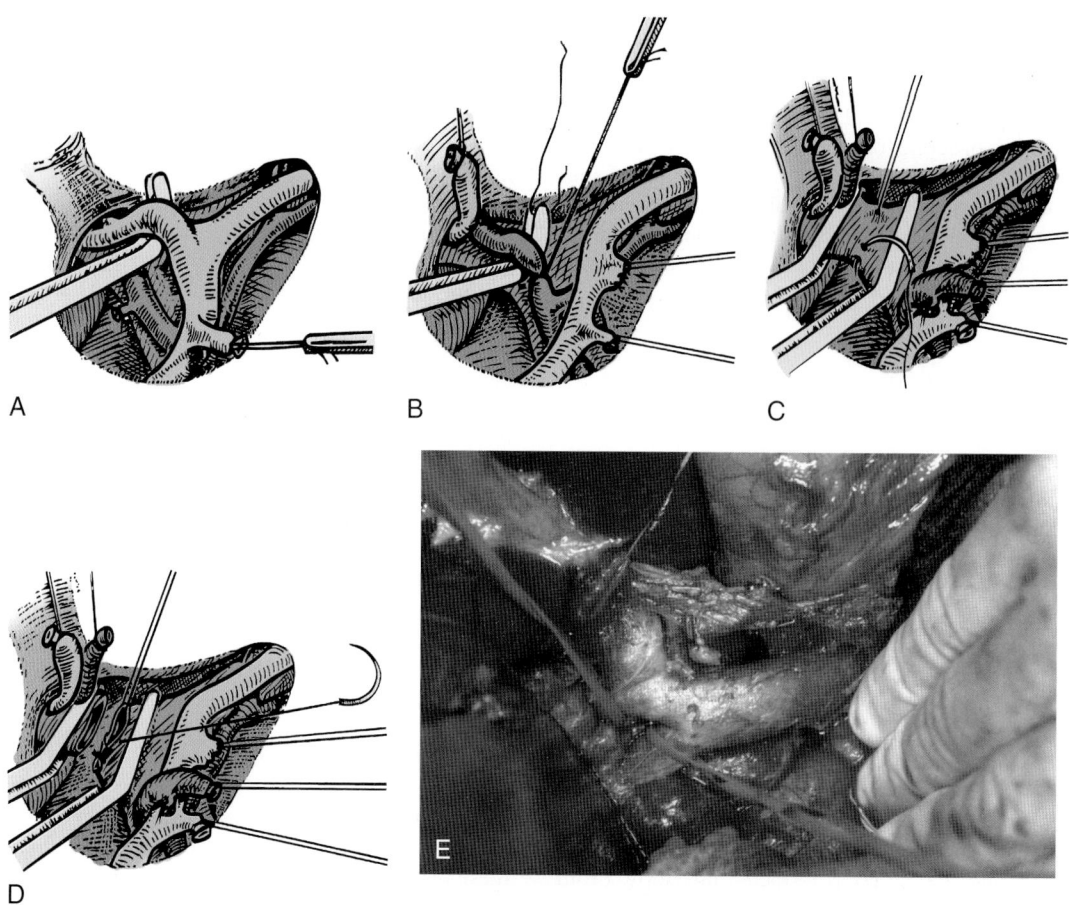

FIGURE 118A.6   A, The right hepatic duct is dissected (now, more often than not, we leave the right hepatic duct for intrahepatic control during parenchymal transection; see text). The confluence of the hepatic ducts and the origin of the left hepatic duct are shown. **B,** The right hepatic duct has been affixed with absorbable suture material, divided, and ligated or oversewn. Alternatively, it may simply be divided under direct vision and then oversewn. In any event, the suture is held and retracted toward the left. Traction on the sutures attached to the cystic duct and the right hepatic duct stump allows retraction of the common hepatic duct and common bile duct to the left and assists display of the vessels beneath. The right hepatic artery is dissected, ligated, and divided, usually to the right *(as shown)* but sometimes to the left of the common hepatic duct. **C,** The right portal vein (PV) is dissected, and forceps are gently passed beneath it. Special care is taken not to damage the first branch of the right PV, which comes off early and posteroinferiorly. This branch is sought initially and ligated and divided or avoided. Straight-bladed vascular clamps are applied to the right PV. Note the retaining sutures that secure the vein before division. **D,** The vein is divided, and its proximal stump is oversewn using a vascular suture. The distal stump is affixed with 3-0 polyglactin 910 (Vicryl) suture and ligated. Light traction on the cystic duct, right hepatic duct stump, and right hepatic artery assists display. **E,** Photograph illustrates dissection of the PV and its branches, seen from the patient's right. The main PV gives rise to the anterior and posterior sectoral or sectional branches independently; both of these are surrounded by blue vessel loops. The left PV and the anterior right sectional vein arise at the same point. It is important to recognize this variant anatomy and to identify all branches during dissection.

The inflow can also be taken as a pedicle within the parenchyma of the liver. There are two approaches to pedicle ligation: an anterior approach and a hepatotomy approach (Fig. 118A.7). The anterior approach to pedicle ligation is performed by splitting the liver parenchyma in the principal plane toward the inflow, and encircling the main right pedicle or the sectoral pedicles at their origin. In the hepatotomy approach, flanking incisions are made in the caudate process and the base of the gallbladder fossa and using a finger or blunt-angled clamp the pedicles are encircled. The middle hepatic vein and its branches to segment V typically drape over the right inflow pedicle and must be anticipated during these maneuvers. Flow to the left liver should be ensured before division of the pedicles.

An anterior approach without mobilization has also been described.[12] This has been studied in patients with large right-sided hepatocellular carcinoma. The falciform ligament is divided to expose the hepatic veins above the liver, but no mobilization of the coronary or triangular ligaments is carried out. The vascular inflow to the right liver is divided extrahepatically, and then the liver is split in the principal plane down through the inflow to the vena cava. Only at this point are the right hepatic vein, retrohepatic caval branches, right caval ligament, and then the right triangular ligament taken. This anterior approach can also be approached with what is referred to as a hanging maneuver,[13] in which a large clamp is used to dissect the caval space between the liver and cava from its infrahepatic location up to and between the middle and right hepatic vein. The clamp is replaced with a soft drain or tube, which is then used as a guide for the parenchymal resection. This anterior approach can be helpful for large right-sided tumors.

Parenchymal transection is the last step. Since the middle hepatic vein is the plane between the right and left liver, it is

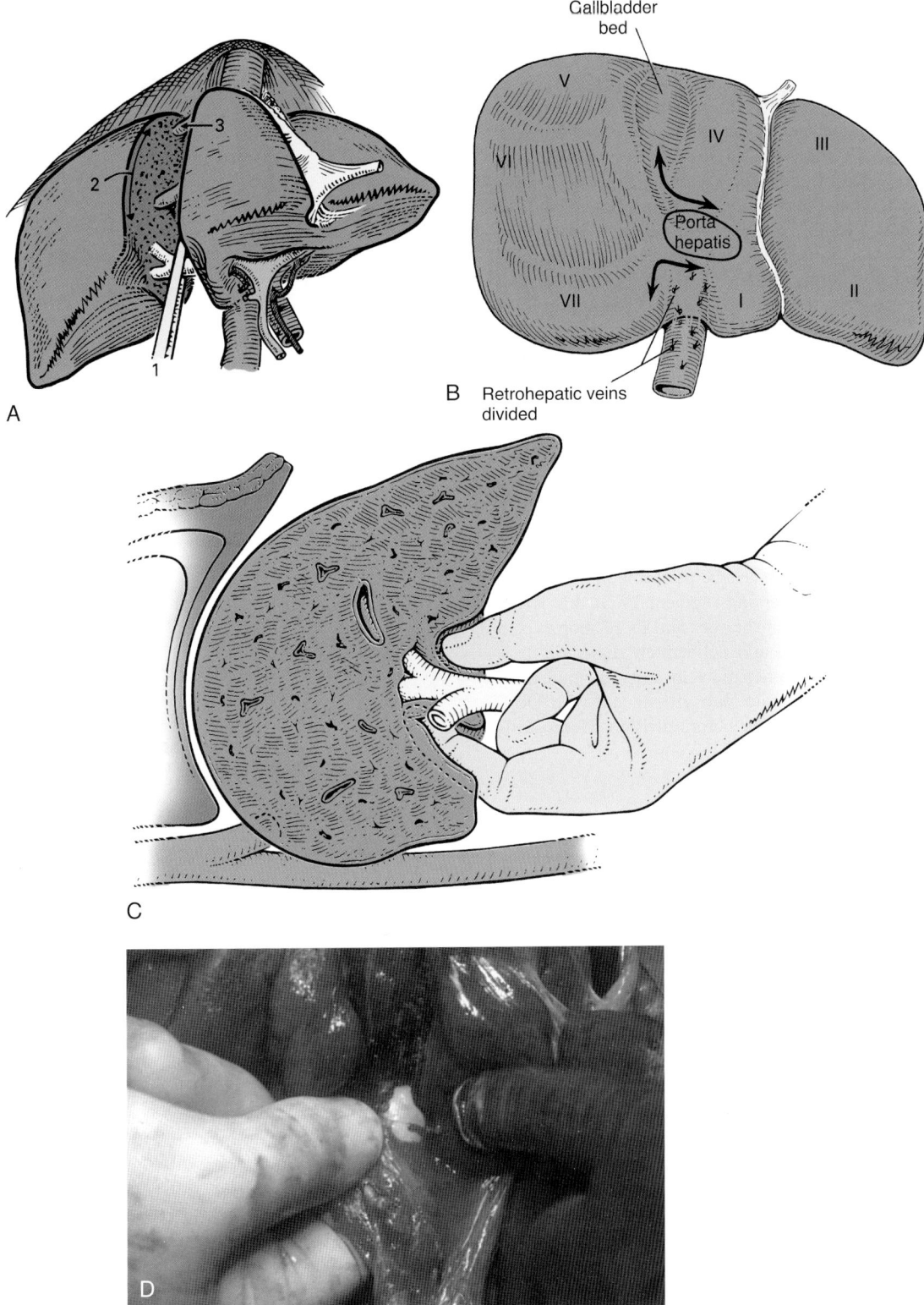

FIGURE 118A.7 A, Intrahepatic control of the portal pedicles *(1)* followed by parenchymal transection *(2)* with subsequent intrahepatic control of the hepatic veins *(3)*. **B,** Approach to the right portal pedicle. The liver has been mobilized from the inferior vena cava by division of the retrohepatic veins lying behind the caudate process. Hepatotomies have been made in the region of the gallbladder fossa and the caudate process. The *curved double-headed arrows* indicate the sites of the hepatotomies above and below the porta hepatis. The approach in the caudate process is essentially a posterior approach. **C,** Illustration shows digital isolation of the right pedicle. **D,** Photograph illustrates insertion of the index finger through a hepatotomy in the caudate lobe, where it merges with the base of the gallbladder fossa to isolate the right portal pedicle.

critical to decide which side of the middle hepatic vein the dissection will proceed and, if it is to be on the left, where the middle hepatic vein will be divided. It is preferable to preserve the middle hepatic vein by dissecting along its right side, in order to maximize venous drainage of the remnant. As the transection commences, the middle hepatic vein is identified and branches to segment V are taken. These segment V branches are typically draped over the anterior sectoral pedicle and once there is adequate visualization, the right inflow pedicles (or main right inflow pedicle) are exposed. An incision is then made in the caudate process and the pedicle(s) are encircled and divided while ensuring distance from the left inflow and bile duct. This should be the method for biliary division in most cases. Flow to the left liver should be ensured throughout. The transection commences along the middle hepatic vein toward the cava. Branches to segment VIII should be carefully anticipated, dissected, encircled, and divided. The most common sources of hemorrhage are injuries to these branches or the middle hepatic vein itself. The transection continues to the base of the right vein and through the posterior aspect of the liver to complete the resection. If the right hepatic vein was not taken before parenchymal transection it has to be approached at the end of parenchymal transection either intrahepatically or at its origin. A right hepatectomy can also be performed to the left of the middle hepatic vein preserving segment IV. If this is the case, the level of transection of the vein and its relationship to branching should be planned and deliberately dissected. It is prudent to clamp the middle hepatic vein at its planned transection point and observe venous flow grossly and with Doppler ultrasound from the left liver before division. Hemostasis and biliostasis are then ensured.

Extended Right Hepatectomy and Right Trisectionectomy

This operation, in general, follows the steps for a right hepatectomy as detailed previously. An extended right hepatectomy encompasses part of segment IV and removes at least some of the middle hepatic vein. A right trisectionectomy removes all of segment IV and the middle hepatic vein at its origin. From an inflow perspective, the additional steps involve taking the segment IV inflow vessels. This is most easily accomplished within the parenchyma during parenchymal transection to the right of the umbilical fissure, by taking the segment IV inflow as intrahepatic pedicles (Figs. 118A.8 and 118A.9). If mandated by the proximity of pathology, dissection can take place within the umbilical fissure. In this scenario, it is of obvious importance to ensure that inflow vessels and bile duct branches to segments II and III within the umbilical fissure are preserved.

From an outflow perspective, how and where the middle hepatic vein will be divided should be planned preoperatively. The most effective method of middle hepatic vein division is from within the liver. This approach is often necessary because the origin of the middle hepatic vein is located intrahepatically where it joins the left hepatic vein. For an extended resection, the level of division of the middle hepatic vein to be transected should be decided upfront and dissected intrahepatically with specific attention to the location of venous branches to segments V and VIII. For a more formal trisectionectomy, the middle hepatic vein is typically taken at or near its origin. The origin of the middle hepatic vein can be identified during hepatic transection with careful attention to protect the left

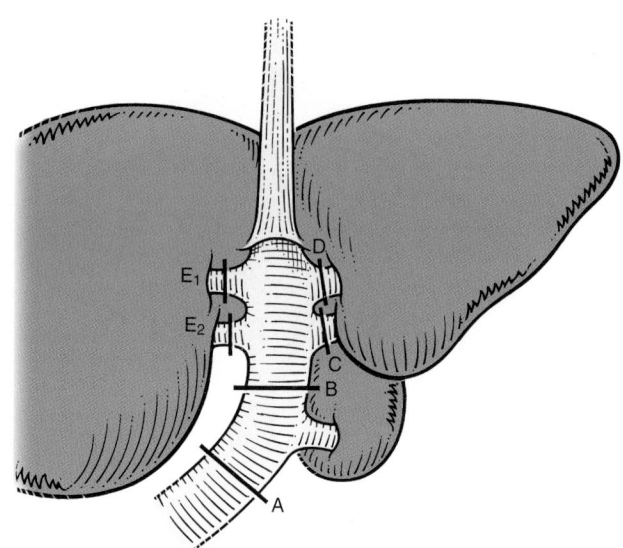

FIGURE 118A.8 Distribution and points of division of pedicles at the base of the left liver. *A,* Pedicle to left liver including segment I. *B,* Pedicle to left liver, sparing segment I. *C,* Pedicle to segment II. *D,* Pedicle to segment III. *E₁,* Pedicle to segment IVb. *E₂,* Pedicle to segment IVa.

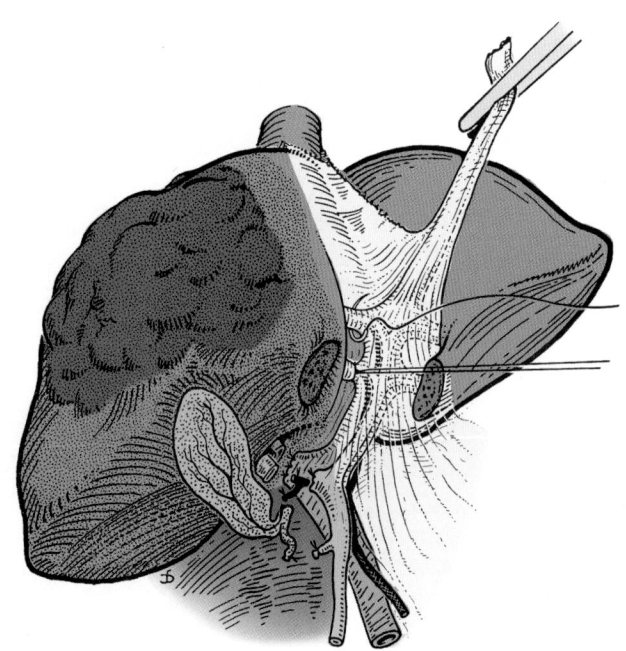

FIGURE 118A.9 Feedback vessels from the left portal triad may be secured in the parenchyma just slightly to the right of the falciform ligament. This dissection must be within the umbilical fissure in the event of adjacent tumor in segment IV, but this is more safely carried out within the liver tissue just to the right of the falciform ligament. Preliminary suture ligation within the umbilical fissure may be performed as illustrated. This procedure deprives segment IV of its blood supply.

hepatic vein and its insertion into the vena cava through the common channel. When taking the middle hepatic vein, it is prudent to clamp and without inflow occlusion observe the venous drainage of the left lateral section grossly and by Doppler ultrasound. The middle hepatic vein can also be dissected extrahepatically, although this is not typically necessary and is only possible if the branching of the left and middle hepatic vein occurs extrahepatically or there are separate origins of these veins. Once the right hepatic vein is divided, the right border of the middle hepatic vein can be more easily visualized, dissected, and encircled. This is rarely needed, and it is best to have good exposure of the suprahepatic cava before this maneuver. The umbilical vein, which most commonly drains into the left hepatic vein, should also be identified and preserved. If the umbilical vein drains instead into the middle hepatic vein, this must be addressed specifically with plans to preserve or take it with protection of the left hepatic vein. The importance of avoiding injury to the left hepatic vein during these operations cannot be overstated: Injury, narrowing, or occlusion of the left hepatic vein is a severe life-threatening injury, as this injury (if not reconstructed/repaired) disrupts nearly all of the venous outflow from the liver.

The parenchymal transection, as noted, requires identification of the segment IV inflow and middle hepatic vein. The other key issue for these operations is that the transection requires a sharp right turn at the base of segment IV. The transection for these operations does not continue as a straight line as this would proceed directly into the left inflow. This can be an awkward dissection but is critical to protect the left-sided inflow/biliary drainage.

Left Hepatectomy

Mobilization of the left liver is more straightforward compared with the right liver. This is because the left liver lies anterior to the caudate lobe, and does not abut the vena cava except for its superior-most border where the left and middle hepatic vein enter the cava. To mobilize, first the ligamentum teres and falciform ligament are divided back to the hepatic veins. The groove between the middle and right hepatic vein should be identified and exposed, as this marks the superior border between the right and left liver. The common channel between the middle and left hepatic vein is dissected an exposed. Then the lateral border of the common channel is defined. The left triangular ligament is then divided from lateral to medial, up to the previously identified lateral border of the left hepatic vein/common

channel. Care should be taken to identify and avoid injuring the left phrenic vein, which will course along the diaphragm and enter the cava near the left hepatic vein. With the left lateral section retracted to the right, the lesser omentum is divided and the ligamentum venosum is divided just before its entry into the left hepatic vein. This exposes a narrow plane just inferior to the hepatic veins and superior to the caudate lobe. It can be helpful to incise the peritoneal attachments along the superior border of the caudate to expose this space. If feasible, the left and middle hepatic veins should then be controlled at their origins in an extrahepatic location (Fig. 118A.10).

With a combination of dissection from above and below the liver, a tunnel encircling the left and middle hepatic vein is developed and these vessels are encircled. When there are separate origins of the left and middle hepatic vein they can be encircled separately with this dissection. Due to anatomic or tumor-related anatomic constraints, this dissection can be tedious and—at times—dangerous. Thus it is also reasonable to divide the veins after transecting the liver back to their origins. It can be helpful to mobilize some of the right liver to better expose the anatomy for a left hepatectomy and this should be employed if there are any difficulties.

Once the left liver has been mobilized and the hepatic veins dissected, attention is drawn to the inflow. Extrahepatic control of inflow vessels is preferable for a left hepatectomy because they are more easily accessible than on the right (Fig. 118A.11). To begin, a cholecystectomy is performed (see Chapter 36) and anatomy of the common bile and hepatic duct are noted. Then the left side of the porta hepatis is dissected. The most anterior structure is the left hepatic artery, which is dissected along the left border of the porta hepatis and encircled. The branching of the right and left hepatic artery is dissected in order to confirm anatomy and protect the right hepatic artery. Additionally, deliberate dissection of the proximal right hepatic artery will help identify any branches to segment IV originating from the right, which is a common finding. If there is a replaced or accessory left hepatic artery these are identified within the lesser omentum as it courses toward the base of the umbilical fissure. Before

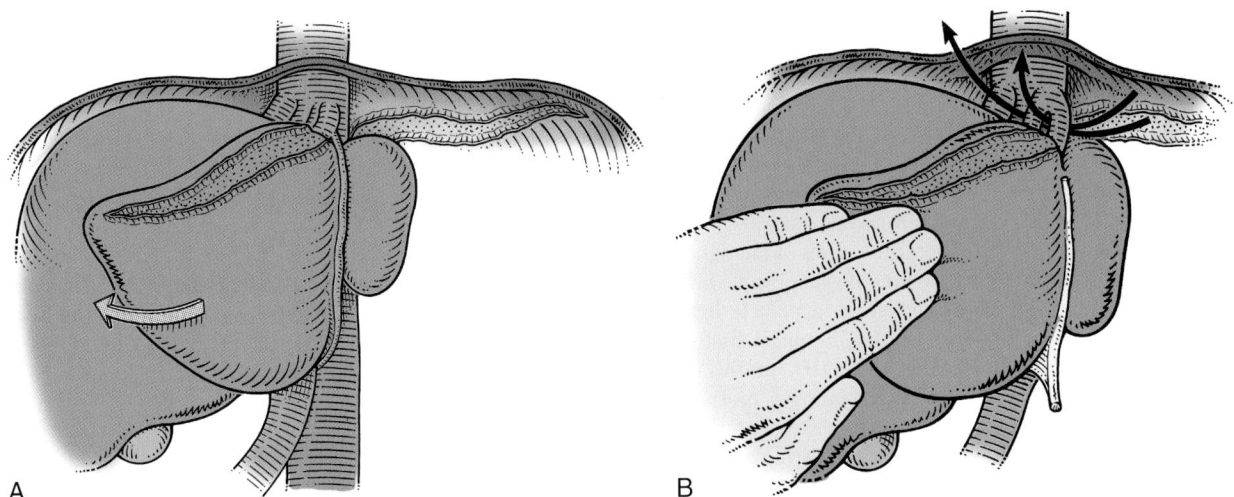

FIGURE 118A.10 Approach and dissection of the left and middle hepatic veins, applicable to left hepatectomy and extended left hepatectomy. **A,** The left lateral section (segments II and III) is completely mobilized from the diaphragm and turned to the right. The gastrohepatic ligament is divided, and the line of the ligamentum venosum is exposed. **B,** The ligamentum venosum is divided. This maneuver allows the exposure of the window between the vena cava and the left hepatic vein. By dissection in this space, it is possible to dissect free the left and middle hepatic veins separately or together *(black curved arrows)*. The left and middle hepatic veins are clamped, divided, and oversewn or divided with the Endo GIA vascular stapler.

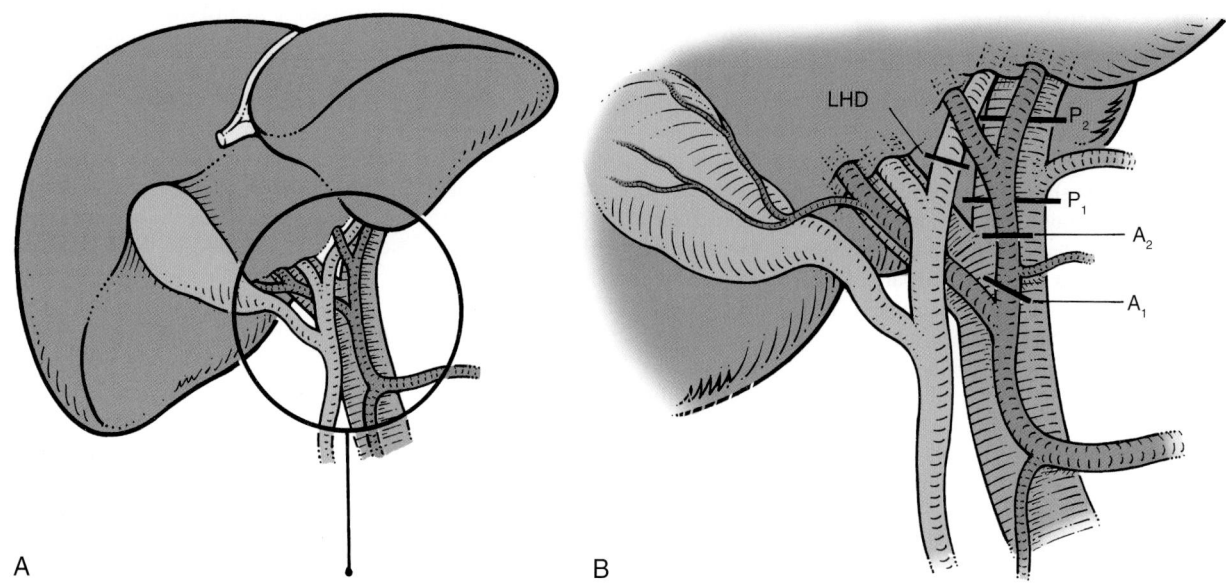

FIGURE 118A.11   A, Dissection for left hepatectomy at the base of the umbilical fissure. **B,** Left hepatic duct *(LHD)* is divided at the base of the umbilical fissure. A_1, Point of division of left hepatic artery (LHA) for concomitant removal of caudate lobe; A_2, point of division of LHA for left hepatectomy; P_1, point of division of left portal vein (LPV) for left hepatectomy and caudate resection; P_2, point of division of LPV for left hepatectomy alone.

dividing the left arterial inflow, it is prudent to test clamp and ensure a pulse remains on the right side of the porta hepatis. The arteries are then ligated and divided, exposing the underlying main and left portal vein. With retraction of the biliary tree and stumps of the left hepatic artery(s), the right, left, and main portal veins are dissected. The caudate branch off the left portal vein is identified and should be protected. Just beyond this toward the liver is the insertion of the ligamentum venosum into the left portal vein. The left portal vein is best encircled in the space between the caudate branch and the ligamentum venosum, thus preserving portal flow to the caudate. Small portal branches to segment IV should be sought and controlled to avoid injury during this dissection. The left portal vein is then clamped, and demarcation and right portal flow are documented grossly and by Doppler ultrasound. The left portal vein is then ligated and divided if necessary. Due to the common anatomic variation of right sectoral ducts draining into the left bile duct, it is best practice to divide the left bile duct in the left main pedicle to maintain distance from any right-sided biliary branches. If tumor proximity mandates division of the left duct in the porta hepatis, a dissection of the duct and any branches is carried out. This left biliary dissection can be carried out early in the porta or after splitting the liver. Protection of the right bile duct and aberrant right sectoral branches of is of obvious importance. The left inflow can also be taken as a pedicle ligation through hepatotomies at the base of the umbilical fissure or through an anterior approach (see Fig. 118A.7B), but this is less often helpful for left-sided resections as the inflow is more easily dissected. Once the inflow is taken, the left (or left and middle) hepatic vein(s) can be taken at its origin. This is most easily accomplished with a vascular stapler. If there are any concerns about taking veins at this point, this can be done at the end of parenchymal transection once the liver has been split back to these veins.

Next, parenchymal transection commences. Similar to a right hepatectomy, the surgeon must determine whether this dissection will take place to the left or to the right of the middle hepatic vein, and—if to the right—where the middle hepatic vein will be transected. During this transection, it is important to note (based on imaging and intraoperative ultrasound) the origin of the umbilical vein so as to avoid injuring it. The transection through the principal plane starts from the anterior surface and heads toward the plane of the ligamentum venosum, preserving the underlying caudate lobe. In the plane to the left of the middle hepatic vein, there are not typically dominant branches—although the umbilical vein proximally can originate from the middle hepatic vein. If the transection is occurring to the right of the middle hepatic vein, the same segment V and VIII venous branches mentioned earlier for a right hemihepatectomy must be anticipated and controlled accordingly. If the hepatic veins have not been taken early, the liver is split back to their origin and they are taken at the end, either intrahepatically or at their insertion into the vena cava. When the bile duct is being taken intrahepatically, the liver is split down to the base of the umbilical fissure, where the left inflow pedicle can be encircled (and ligated and divided) after making a hepatotomy at the posterior aspect of segment II. If the bile duct must be taken in the porta hepatis and has not been encircled, it can be exposed after dividing the liver. Identification of any aberrant draining sectoral branches is critical before dividing the left bile duct. If there is any concern, the bile duct can be divided sharply and probed; there should be a low threshold to perform a cholangiogram (see Chapter 24). Hemostasis and biliostasis are ensured.

Extended Left Hepatectomy

An extended left hepatectomy includes the left liver along with an incomplete portion of segment V and/or VIII. The parenchymal transection, by definition, is to the right of the middle hepatic vein for at least some of its course. The mobilization and inflow/outflow control are the same as a left hepatectomy except that it is preferable for this operation to have extrahepatic control of the left and middle hepatic vein before parenchymal transection. If this is not feasible or safe, the liver can be split back to the space between the middle and right hepatic vein and the veins can be taken after parenchymal transection. The specific extent of the anterior sector to be resected must be planned and specifically dissected. Some or all of segment V or VIII can be taken, depending on the individualized anatomy of each case. The inflow anatomy to these segments (i.e., which branches will be taken and which branches will be preserved) is critical to plan. An ill-advised extension of a left hepatectomy into anterior sectoral pedicles without an appropriate parenchymal resection can leave ischemic liver behind and increase the risk of postoperative morbidity. The inflow vessels to the resected portion of anterior sector are taken intrahepatically during parenchymal transection, whereas the inflow to the left liver is taken as described earlier. While approaching the inflow and outflow in the resected anterior sector, it is prudent to clamp and test perfusion to the portions of liver to be left behind before division in order to ensure complete resection of the parenchyma supplied. Intraoperative ultrasound guidance can also be critical in these somewhat atypical transection planes (see Chapters 24 and 103).

Left Trisectionectomy

A left trisectionectomy is a challenging operation that removes the left liver en bloc with segment V and VIII of the right liver (Figs. 118A.12 and 118A.13). By definition, the left and middle hepatic veins are taken at their origin. Complete mobilization of the liver is advisable for this operation using the techniques for the right and left liver described earlier. The three hepatic veins should be dissected at their origin and it is preferable to encircle the left and middle hepatic veins at their insertion into the cava.

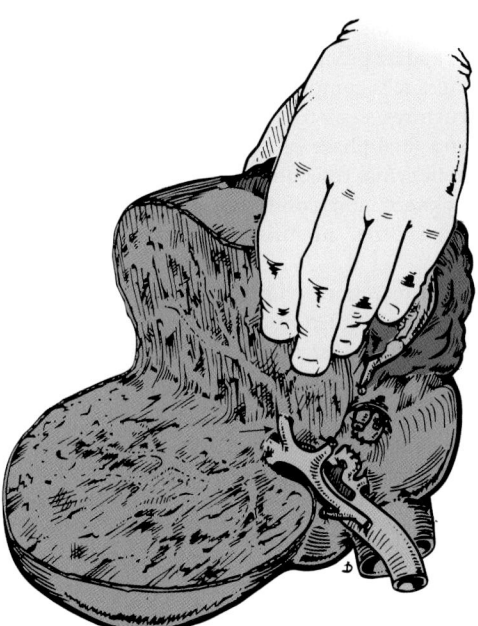

FIGURE 118A.12 Extended left hepatectomy. The liver tissue is entered for the parenchymal transection just anterior to the estimated lower limit of the right scissura. This plane of dissection is followed, with the operator working toward the base of the gallbladder fossa and the point of entry of the right hepatic duct into the liver substance. The anterior sectional vessel of supply and the bile ducts are identified in the liver substance *(arrow)* and can be ligated.

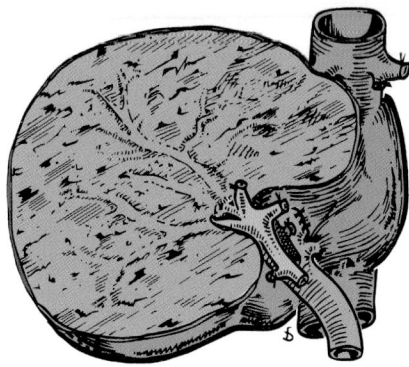

FIGURE 118A.13 The liver substance is removed anterior to the posterior sectional ducts and vessels, and the upper part of this parenchymal dissection runs just anterior to the right hepatic vein and involves control of the middle and left hepatic vein. After resection, the right posterior sectional portal triad can be seen branching on the surface of exposed liver tissue.

It is not necessary to encircle the right hepatic vein but its insertion should be visible, as a critical element to this operation is preservation of the right hepatic vein. The inflow and outflow control for the left liver is as described earlier. There are two options for taking the right anterior sectoral inflow. Preferably, when tumor proximity allows, it is advisable to take the anterior sectoral inflow as a pedicle inside the liver. This pedicle can be taken by encircling it through hepatotomies or after splitting the liver in the right scissura (plane of the right hepatic vein) to the base of the pedicle. Alternatively, dissection in the porta hepatis can identify the anterior sectoral portal and arterial branches, although this can be a tedious dissection and risks injury to the posterior sectoral vessels. Taking the inflow early will show demarcation and help the surgeon identify where to start the transection, but this is not necessary. The transection is marked by the plane of the right hepatic vein, which can be identified by ultrasound (see Chapters 24 and 103). When the inflow is taken during this operation, regardless of technique, it is critical to assess flow grossly and by Doppler ultrasound to ensure that the posterior sector is well perfused. If inflow to the anterior sector is taken in the porta hepatis, it is still advisable—when feasible—to take the anterior sectoral bile duct within the liver. This will ensure distance from the right posterior sectoral duct.

The parenchymal transection plane for this operation is to the left of the right hepatic vein ultimately heading toward the ligamentum venosum. There are usually no dominant leftward branches off the right hepatic vein. Of note, the dorsal inflow branch to segment VIII usually feeds an area of parenchyma superior and to the right of the right hepatic vein, and this should be anticipated and resected so as not to leave ischemic liver behind. The transection curves to the left, anterior to the intrahepatic caudate, toward the base of the anterior sectoral pedicle. Once the anterior sectoral pedicle is divided and the left inflow has been taken, the left and middle hepatic veins can be taken at their origin. Alternatively, the vein can be taken at the end of the parenchymal transection. After division of the anterior sectoral pedicle the transection curves to the left to base of segment IV, and the left biliary tree is taken with the pedicle of the left liver at the base of the umbilical fissure. The left bile duct can be taken extrahepatically if the tumor mandates this approach, but it is preferable to take it within the main left pedicle to minimize the chance of any contralateral biliary injury. This operation is best thought of as preservation of the posterior sector and the right hepatic vein, and every maneuver is taken with this in mind. Liberal use of intraoperative ultrasound (see Chapter 103), test clamping vessels, and careful transection are critical throughout this operation.

En Bloc Caudate Resection

A number of clinical scenarios mandate an en bloc caudate resection with a major hepatectomy. Hilar cholangiocarcinoma (see Chapters 51B and 119B) and large tumors extending into the caudate are the most common indications for a combined major hepatectomy with caudate resection. Understanding the typical and individual anatomy of the caudate is critical in every case.

A critical element to caudate resection is complete mobilization of the caudate from the cava (Figs. 118A.14 and 118A.15). For right-sided resections, this means that the caval dissection continues to the left dissecting the caudate off the cava. Ultimately, the caval ligament at the left side of the caudate must be divided and is best approached after first mobilizing and retracting the left lateral section. For left-sided resections, it is possible to divide the left side of the caval ligament and mobilize the caudate from the cava completely from the left; however, right-sided mobilization is helpful in some cases. Retrohepatic caval branches are serially dissected and divided between clips or ties. There is commonly a large branch centrally that often requires suture control or stapler division.

As described earlier, the inflow and biliary drainage of the caudate originate proximally from both right and left main branches. For right-sided resections, the inflow to the left side of the caudate must be taken at the base of the umbilical fissure, where the branches arise from the left portal vein and hepatic artery. Small biliary branches are also encountered here and controlled with ties or clips as necessary. Once the inflow to the left caudate is taken, the caudate should be mobilized such that it can be placed on the right side of the vena cava. When taking

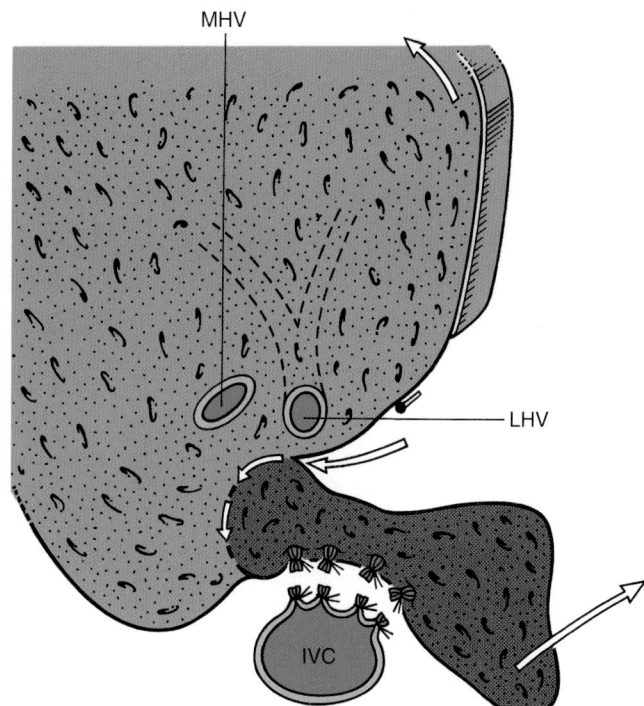

FIGURE 118A.15 Parenchymal phase of dissection *(arrows)*. Note proximity of the left hepatic vein *(LHV)* and middle hepatic vein *(MHV)*. The right portion of the caudate lobe lies just to the left of the MHV. *IVC,* Inferior vena cava.

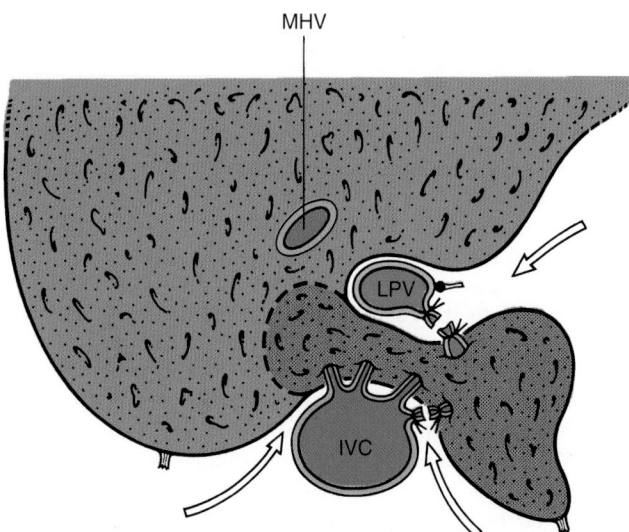

FIGURE 118A.14 Lines of approach *(arrows)* to free the caudate lobe. The lesser omentum has been opened, and the caudate branch of the left portal vein has been tied. The ligamentous attachments of the caudate lobe posteriorly have been opened, and dissection of the retrohepatic caudate veins can be approached from the right or left side. *IVC,* Inferior vena cava; *MHV,* middle hepatic vein; *LPV,* left portal vein.

the right portal vein, the branch to the caudate process must be taken along with it. A right hepatectomy is performed as described previously, except that when the transection approaches its posterior extent, the caudate lobe is retracted to the right and included in the resection as the transection proceeds to the left of the caudate process. It is of obvious importance to ensure that the caudate is completely free of the cava and the left-sided inflow structures so as to avoid injury to them during this retraction and final phase of the transection. The final elements of the parenchymal resection for a right and caudate resection can be awkward and confusing, and it is prudent to move slowly with specific attention to preserving the contralateral structures.

Left-sided resections with the caudate are somewhat more intuitive than right-sided resections because the majority of the caudate is a left-sided structure. The caudate mostly lies to the left, and—depending on the situation—the caudate process can be preserved for a combined left and caudate resection. Mobilization is as described previously, but with the caudate mobilized, the origins of the left and middle hepatic veins are more easily exposed, facilitating extrahepatic control. The inflow to the left portion of the caudate is taken by dividing the inflow proximally, ensuring that the caudate vessels are included. A left and caudate resection mandates biliary dissection in an extrahepatic location; the biliary anatomy must be elucidated and the left duct taken proximally in the porta hepatis. The duct can be taken sharply and probed to confirm anatomy and patency of the main and right bile ducts. Again, if there is any concern, there should be a low threshold to perform a cholangiogram (see Chapter 24). Right sectoral ducts draining into the left bile duct should be identified and preserved if it all possible—otherwise biliary reconstruction may be necessary.

SUMMARY

Major hepatic resections can be technically difficult and morbid operations. These operations require extensive mobilization of the liver and expertise in its working anatomy. Vascular control and preservation of contralateral structures are critical, as failure of these maneuvers can result in hemorrhage and/or ischemia of the remnant liver, liver failure, or even death. Anatomic variation is common, and each case must be individualized and technique appropriately adapted. In general, these are operations of last resort and should only be performed when mandated by the underlying pathology, such as large tumors and central tumors involving vasculature. Parenchymal-sparing resections are much preferred, whenever possible, as the risk of major morbidity and liver failure is significantly lower. Extensive training and experience are critical, both to guide judgment regarding when to use a major hepatic resection and the technical skill to successfully navigate their performance.

The references for this chapter can be found online by accessing the accompanying Expert Consult website.

Segmental resection

Camille Stewart, Kelly J. Lafaro, and Yuman Fong

INTRODUCTION

Liver resection plays an increasingly important role in the management of benign as well as primary and metastatic liver tumors (see Chapters 50, 51B, 88, 89, and 90–93). Historically, the high morbidity and mortality of liver resections limited their use. However, over time, the morbidity and mortality of liver resections have decreased due to advances allowing for reduced intraoperative blood loss and preservation of liver parenchyma with the adoption of segment-oriented liver resection.[1-3] Resection of individual segments or sectors of the liver rather than an entire lobe allows for maximal conservation of normal liver parenchyma while optimizing oncologic outcomes (see Chapters 102A and 102B).[4-7] Parenchymal preservation is especially important in patients with underlying hepatocellular dysfunction or limited future residual volume. Advances in understanding the liver anatomy (see Chapters 2 and 102B) and improvements in radiographic technology (see Chapters 2, 13–15, and 19) are the basis of segmental liver surgery.

GENERAL PRINCIPLES

Anatomy and Terminology (see Chapter 2)

Lortat-Jacob et al.[8] reported one of the first anatomic liver resections for cancer in 1952. Following this, Claude Couinaud solidified the current understanding of the segmental anatomy with his comprehensive descriptions of the segmental anatomy of the liver.[9-11] Using vascular and biliary casts of the liver, Couinaud determined that it comprised eight segments, each with its independent vascular inflow and outflow, as well as biliary drainage (Fig. 118B.1). His work supported the idea that it is possible to remove individual segments without disrupting the remaining liver. This idea that each segment could be resected independently was further confirmed by Bismuth in 1982.[12,13] These segments have evolved to become the standard for hepatic nomenclature; however, there has been significant variation in the terminology of liver anatomy between America, Europe, and Japan. The Brisbane 2000 Terminology of Hepatic Anatomy and Resection aimed to eliminate this variation and standardize terminology.[14] This consensus proposed three orders of division: *hemiliver* (first-order division), *section* (second-order division), and *segment* (third-order division), which are not interchangeable, thus providing universal terminology for better communication among liver surgeons. Operations described in this chapter are those at the second- and third-order divisions (Table 118B.1).

Precise knowledge of the surgical anatomy of the liver is imperative to perform segmental liver resections (see Chapter 2). The first-order divisions are *right liver* (segments V through VIII) and *left liver* (segments I through IV), or *hemiliver*, the boundary of which lies along Cantlie's line marked by the path of the middle hepatic vein (MHV), from the middle of the gallbladder fossa to its termination in the inferior vena cava (IVC) (Fig. 118B.2). The second-order division into liver sections is based on hepatic arterial supply and biliary drainage.

The sections are derived from the primary divisions of the major right and left portal triads. The right hemiliver is divided into sections known as the *right anterior* (segments V and VIII) and *right posterior* (segments VI and VII), separated by the right hepatic vein (RHV). The left hemiliver is divided into *left lateral* (segments II and III) and *left medial* (segments IVa and IVb) sections by the umbilical fissure and falciform ligament. The third-order division, segments I through VIII, is defined by hepatic arterial supply and biliary drainage. The axial plane is at the level of the intersection of the hepatic veins and the axial plane of the bifurcation of the portal vein. When considering a segmental resection, it is important to identify common biliary, arterial, and portal venous anomalies on preoperative imaging that may affect the technical approach (Fig. 118B.3) (see Chapters 2, 13, and 102B).

Difference Between Segmental Resections Defined by Hepatic Venous or Portal Venous Anatomy

When planning a segmental resection, the surgeon must choose to follow either hepatic venous outflow or portal pedicle inflow to guide a segmental resection. It turns out the two are largely overlapping but not the same.

The anatomy used to guide segmental resection varies based on tumor histology and geographic region of the surgeon's practice (see Chapters 2 and 102B). Within Asia, hepatocellular carcinoma is the more common tumor resected by the liver surgeon, largely due to higher rates of hepatitis B infection.[17] Hepatocellular carcinomas tend to metastasize via tumor seeding along the portal veins (see Chapter 89).[18,19] As such, the segments as defined by the portal inflow are resected. This may be performed with a so-called "Glissonian pedicle approach" in which the portal inflow is identified by dissecting it out and ligating it, and then parenchymal transection proceeds by following the intersegmental plane marked by the vascular color change.[20] Portal venous dye has also been used to demarcate liver segments intended for resection[21] (Fig. 118B.4). This technique is performed by identifying the portal veins in question using intraoperative ultrasound (IOUS) (see Chapters 24 and 103), and then injecting them with 5 mL of 1% methylene blue or 0.8% indigo carmine. This segmental injection of dye is most easily performed when the tumor is fed by a single portal vein branch.[21] Once the liver parenchyma is stained, it is marked off using electrocautery, and a "systematic segmentectomy" may proceed, during which the hepatic veins are exposed and preserved.[21] This technique may be especially helpful for

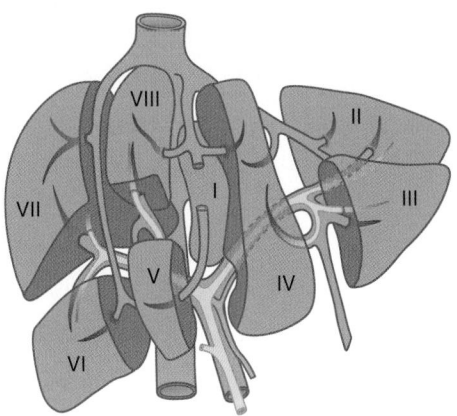

FIGURE 118B.1 Schematic of the liver segments and their relationships to the hepatic and portal veins[15]. It should be noted that the portal veins are used as borders between segments 4A and 4B, between segments 5 and 8, and between segments 6 and 7. The left hepatic vein is what divides segments 2 and 3. The Middle hepatic vein separates the right and left lobes of the liver. The right hepatic vein separates the right anterior section from the right posterior section. From Elsevier: Dudeja V, Ferrantella F, Fong Y. The Liver. In: Townsend C, Beauchamp D, Evers M, Mattox K, eds. Sabiston Textbook of Surgery. 20 ed. Philadelphia, PA: Elsevier; 2020:1425–1488.

TABLE 118B.1	Segmental Resections of the Liver		
ANATOMIC TERM	ALTERNATIVE	TERM FOR SURGICAL RESECTION	SEGMENTS
Second-Order Divisional Resections			
Right anterior section	Right anterior sector	Right anterior sectionectomy	5, 8
Right posterior section	Right posterior sector	Right posterior sectionectomy	6, 7
Left medial section	Segment 4	Segmentectomy 4	4
Left lateral section	Left lateral segment	Left lateral sectionectomy	2, 3
Third-Order Divisional Resections			
Segments 1-8		Segmentectomy 1-8	
Atypical Resections			
Bisegmentectomy 5, 6; 7, 8		Bisegmentectomy	5, 6; 7, 8
Segments 4, 5, 6	Central hepatectomy	Mesohepatectomy	4, 5, 8

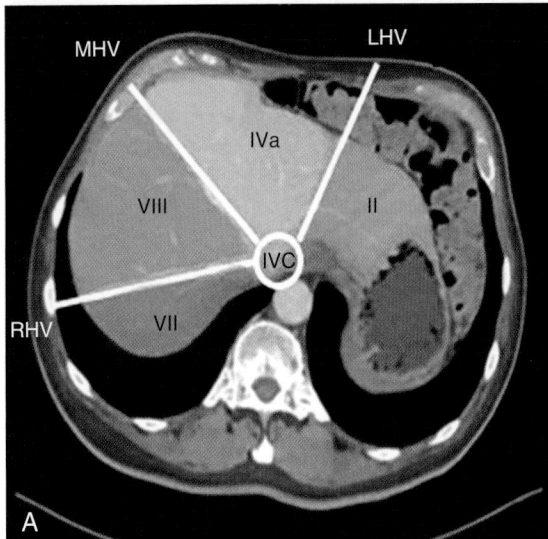

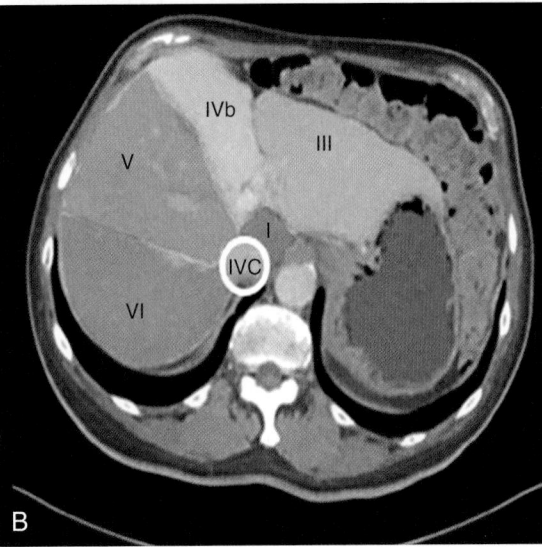

FIGURE 118B.2 The segments of the upper liver **(A)** and of the lower liver **(B)** are shown.

segments VII and VIII, which can be challenging due to their deep vascular pedicles and a relative absence of surface anatomic landmarks.[21]

An alternative methodology for performing a segmental liver resection is to follow the major hepatic veins during transection (Fig. 118B.5), ensuring complete resection of entire segments using hepatic veins as boundaries. The tumor type most commonly resected in the Western world is metastatic colorectal cancer (see Chapter 90). Traditionally, anatomic resections were advocated for metastatic colorectal cancer because of the high likelihood of a positive margin for wedge resections. In a classic series from Johannes Scheele, wedge resections were associated with a positive margin rate of 19%.[22] This is likely due

to the difficulty in judging margins of the tumor deep in the parenchyma. Wedge resections are also complicated by the fact that the transection line tends to fracture at the interface of the hard colorectal tumor and soft normal liver. Following the hepatic veins during a segmental resection evolved to assist the surgeon in achieving a negative margin. A recent meta-analysis of more than 2500 patients undergoing resection for colorectal liver metastases concluded that both margin status and overall survival were similar between the wedge and anatomic resections.[23] This is likely due to expertise of surgeons at present for choosing to use either wedge or segmental resections to achieve a low rate of margin positivity.

Another reason for choosing a hepatic venous based resection is the failure of IOUS to identify tumors. Many patients who have had a lot of neoadjuvant chemotherapy develop fatty liver or chemotherapy-associated steatohepatitis (CASH) (see Chapters 69 and 98).[24] The liver becomes hyperechoic and the hyperechoic tumors become indistinguishable from the surrounding liver. Following the hepatic veins (see Fig. 118B.5) allows the liver surgeon to best avoid a positive margin or leaving cancer behind.

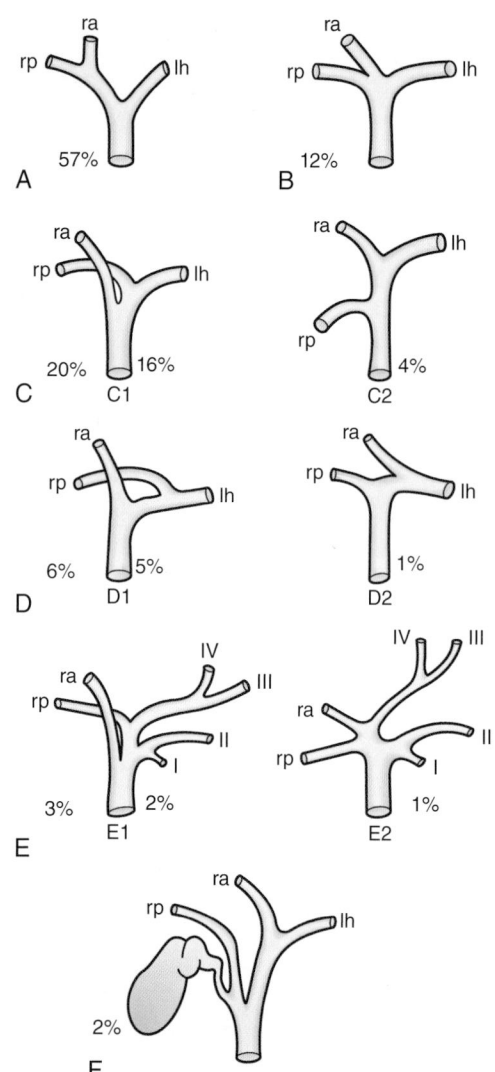

FIGURE 118B.3 Intra-hepatic biliary anatomy and known anatomic variations by frequency[16]. The anatomy described under A is the most common, conventional anatomy. (From Elsevier: Dudeja V, Ferrantella F, Fong Y. The Liver. In: Townsend C, Beauchamp D, Evers M, Mattox K, eds. Sabiston Textbook of Surgery. 20 ed. Philadelphia, PA: Elsevier; 2020:1425–1488.)

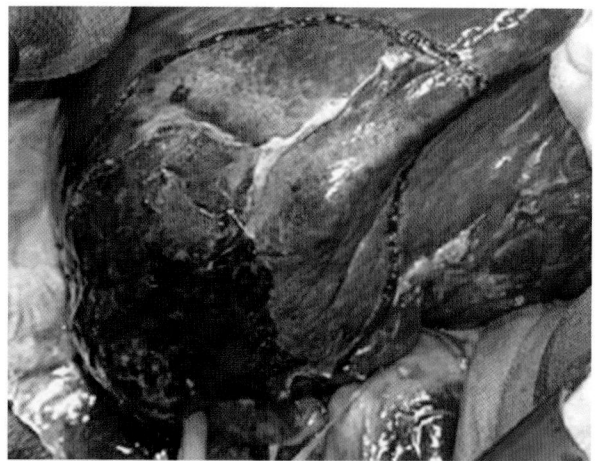

FIGURE 118B.4 Use of portal dye technique for systematic segmentectomy.[21]

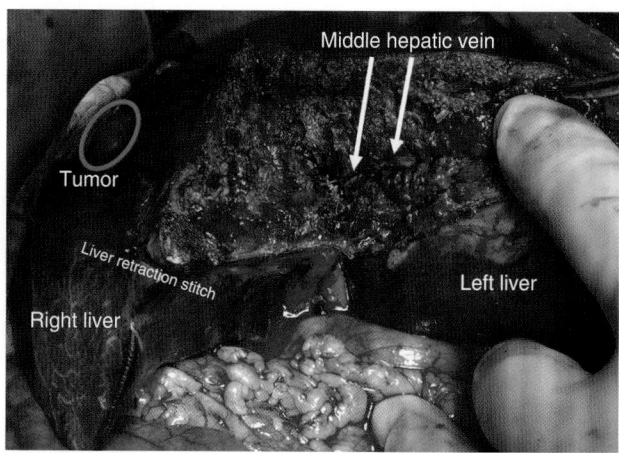

FIGURE 118B.5 Anterior approach to right hepatectomy—initial transection. The transection line follows Cantlie's line/the principle plane, just to the right of the middle hepatic vein. 1-0 chromic suture is used to facilitate retraction of the left and right liver as it is being divided.

Conditions That Should Be Treated by Nonanatomic Resections

Symptomatic benign liver cysts or tumors of low malignant potential should be surgically addressed with liver-sparing techniques including enucleation or nonanatomic parenchymal sparing resection (see Chapters 88 and 91). Enucleation can be used for most benign liver lesions, including symptomatic liver cysts, hemangiomas, adenomas, cystadenomas, and focal nodular hyperplasia, or for hydatid cysts of the liver.

Well-differentiated neuroendocrine tumors separate well from the surrounding liver (see Chapter 91). They require almost no margin and have low local recurrence even when enucleated.

Preoperative Scanning

Imaging is performed both to stage patients to determine the appropriateness of resection and to allow anatomic technical planning for the resection (see Chapters 12–16, 24, and 102B).

Scanning for Staging

The first consideration when patients are being referred for segmental liver resection is the oncologic appropriateness. For most primary and metastatic disease to be resected from the liver, the best staging is afforded by computed tomography (CT) scan of the chest in conjunction with either a triphasic CT or magnetic resonance imaging (MRI) of the abdomen and pelvis. A CT of the chest even without contrast offers the most sensitive detection of pulmonary metastases. An MRI offers the best detection and characterization of liver lesions regardless of parenchymal liver disease, including fatty liver and cirrhosis. Of note, subcentimeter pulmonary nodules found on chest imaging should not necessarily preclude hepatic resection, especially in the setting of colorectal liver metastases.[25] Depending on the primary tumor, a positron emission tomography (PET) scan may also be considered.

Diagnostic laparoscopy (see Chapter 24) may be performed in certain select cases where a laparotomy is planned to identify patients with subradiographic metastatic disease to avoid unnecessary incision and prolong recovery after nontherapeutic laparotomy.[26] The tumors with the highest diagnostic yield from laparoscopy include cholangiocarcinoma[27] and gallbladder cancer.[28]

Scanning for Surgical Planning

Cross-section scanning by CT or MRI allows direct visualization of the arterial, portal, and hepatic venous anatomy for surgical planning (see Chapters 13–16). There are many intrahepatic portal anatomic variations (see Chapter 2). Typical portal anatomy is present in approximately two-thirds of patients, with variations present in one-third[29] (see Fig. 118B.3). Anatomic understanding is crucial and is greatly facilitated by studying the patient's imaging with either MRI or CT that includes portal venous and venous contrast phases.

Interpretation of imaging can be further facilitated by three-dimensional (3D) reconstructions, which can be generated from two-dimensional (2D) imaging including CT and MRI (see Chapter 13).[30] Surgeons are better able to localize liver tumors on models after viewing 3D reconstructions, as compared with 2D scans.[31] These 3D reconstructions may also enable faster surgical planning with trainees and greater concordance with staff on surgical planning.[32] Products such as 3D Slicer[33] exist as free open-source software. Companies and commercially available software also exist that create 3D graphical liver models, including TeraRecon (Foster City, California, USA), Materialise Mimics (Leuven, Belgium), and Visible Patient (IRCAD, Strasbourg, France).

Software providing 3D CT reconstructions of the liver allows the surgeon to view the anatomy dynamically and identify the relationship of the tumor with the segmental hepatic venous outflow and portal venous inflow. One technique for preoperative planning is to first determine which hepatic veins require resection and at what level for an adequate margin, and then to consider the portal triads that need to be included as a basis for the segmental resection.

More sophisticated software programs allow virtual surgical resection of the liver, which can be used to determine the appropriate plane of transection, taking into account the minimum resection margin and residual liver volume. Some of the available systems include the MeVIS imaging system (MeVisLab, Bremen, Germany), Myrian XP-Liver (Intrasense, Paris), Synapse 3D (Fujifilm, Tokyo), IQQA-Liver (EDDA Technology, Princeton, NJ), and Hitachi Image Processing System (Hitachi Medical Corporation, Nishinomiya, Japan). Furthermore, some of these systems have been extended to facilitate real-time, image-guided resection by coupling the preoperative images of the virtual liver to real-time liver and instrument tracking systems. These advances offer significant potential for increased precision of preoperative planning for segment-oriented liver resections and intraoperative application to facilitate image-guided surgery. However, limited data currently exist on their use in liver surgery and whether they are an improvement over current best practice.

OPERATIVE APPROACH

Segmental liver resections are currently performed using open as well as minimally invasive techniques, including laparoscopy and robotics. Minimally invasive techniques are increasingly being adopted, which can lead to decreased length of hospitalization.[34] When performing minimally invasive liver surgery, this author's preference is to use a robotic surgical system to overcome some of the limitations of laparoscopy.[35,36]

For patients with disease concentrated in a segment and an additional deep central lesion, a minimally invasive segmental resection with additional ablation of the deep lesion can be considered to avoid a major or extended hepatectomy in select cases. The following technical considerations, however, will focus on an open operative approach, which still often is necessary. Indications and technical considerations for minimally invasive liver surgery are discussed in further detail elsewhere (see Chapter 127).

Patient Positioning

For open segmental liver resections, the patient should be placed in the supine position. The authors prefer to have arms tucked. Arms are tucked for two reasons. The first is that this gives the greatest flexibility for table-mounted retractor placement and assistant positioning. The second is that these operations may take several hours to complete, and leaving the arms out may produce perioperative upper extremity nerve traction injuries through arm hyperabduction.[37] In general, a large-bore IV is placed in each arm, and the arterial line is also placed when necessary before tucking the arms. This author rarely uses central lines and will monitor central venous pressure (CVP) for low CVP anesthesia by liver ultrasound inspection of hepatic veins (see Chapters 24 and 25). The patient is placed in a Trendelenburg position to allow for maximum venous return to the heart in the setting of low venous vascular volume to optimize cardiac output while keeping CVP low.

The abdomen is prepped from nipples to pubis, and laterally down to the surgical table. Drapes should be placed to enable maximum exposure to the abdomen. Lights are positioned so that one is directly over the operative field, and a second is positioned angled over the right shoulder of the primary surgeon and between the surgeon and the assistant. Two suctions should be available so that one is always available to both the surgeon and the assistant.

Exposure and Mobilization for Open Resection

For an open segment-oriented liver resection, operative exposure can be achieved through a variety of incisions, which should take into account the patient's body habitus and tumor location. The choice of incision is almost always determined in order of importance by (1) body habitus, (2) location of the liver, (3) location of the lesion, and (4) history of prior incisions. In a thin, tall patient, almost any resection can be performed through a long midline incision. In a patient with a high body mass index or a liver high in a barreled chest, a transverse extension of the incision is almost always needed.

A midline incision is usually adequate for left-sided lesions. This incision affords the option to extend the incision laterally at the level of the umbilicus to a point midway between the costal margin and anterior superior iliac spine (L-incision). Other common incisions include the right subcostal with midline extension cephalad ("hockey stick") or a bilateral subcostal incision with midline extension cephalad ("Mercedes" incision) or without ("Chevron" incision). Occasionally for posterior lesions, a thoracoabdominal incision may be required, although it can often be avoided using a transverse extension of a midline incision with appropriate costal margin retraction. Of note, trifurcated incisions such as the chevron incision are associated with higher ascitic leak and hernia formation.[38]

Retraction

Excellent retraction cephalad is essential, thus the best retractors for liver surgery generally have a crossbar across the patient's chest. The authors' preference is a Thompson retractor (Thompson

Surgical Instruments, Traverse City, MI). A bilateral crossbar (hinged or unhinged) is positioned approximately 15 cm above the skin and 10 cm superior to the apex of the incision. A single crossbar is then positioned on the patient's right, with the angle of the bar toward the patient's body and the short end of the bar toward the patient's head. Subcostal retractors connected to a micro-adjustable clip-on ratchet is used on the right and left costal margins. Retractors positioned on the left and right inferior aspects of the wound provide lateral retraction. If a long midline incision is chosen, a Balfour retractor may assist in even-tensioned lateral retraction.

Other suitable retractors include the Omni-Tract (Omni-Tract Surgical, St. Paul, MN) or the Iron Intern (Automated Medical Products, Edison, NJ). The Bookwalter (Codman, Raynham, MA) retractor may be adequate, especially for left-sided segment-oriented resection, but we find that it provides inadequate exposure for right posterior lesions.

If diagnostic laparoscopy is not performed (see Chapter 24), a minimal incision should be made first and systematic inspection of the entire abdominal cavity performed to check for metastatic disease in (1) peritoneal lining, (2) diaphragms, (3) lesser omentum, (4) portal-caval lymph nodes, (5) hepatic artery lymph nodes, and (6) celiac axis lymph nodes. If possible, the lower abdomen should also be inspected, but this may be difficult in patients who have had previous surgery. Extensive lysis of adhesions to inspect the pelvis is not necessary and reliance on adequate preoperative imaging is acceptable.

Liver Mobilization

In open hepatectomy, after the laparotomy and general inspection of the abdomen, the liver is mobilized by transection of the ligamentum teres and division of the falciform ligament cephalad to the subdiaphragmatic inferior vena cava (IVC) (see Chapter 2). A long silk tie should be left on the ligamentum teres to use as a handle for manipulation of the liver or fixed cephalad to the retractor to provide additional exposure to the undersurface of the liver and hepatic hilum. The falciform ligament is transected using Bovie electrocautery to identify the origins of the hepatic veins. At this point, visual and manual palpation inspection of the liver should be performed. The bare area in the lesser omentum should be divided to expose the caudate lobe (segment I) for inspection and palpation. Care should be taken during this step to identify and avoid an anomalous left hepatic artery, arising from the left gastric artery. IOUS may be used to identify any lesions that are not seen on preoperative cross-sectional imaging that would prevent proceeding with resection or change the operative plan. See Chapter 103 for more details on IOUS.

Mobilization of the left and right lobes may be performed either before or after pedicular dissection, which is at the discretion of the surgeon. Mobilization of the left liver requires division of the left triangular ligament. Laparotomy pads should be placed posterior to segment II to protect the esophagus, cardia of the stomach, and spleen during division of the triangular ligament. The superior vena cava (SVC) and left hepatic vein should become visible. Care should be taken to identify the path of the left phrenic vein to protect it.

Mobilization of the right liver requires division of the falciform ligament to expose the extrahepatic right hepatic vein. Early identification of the vein allows the surgeon to avoid injury to it during lateral mobilization. Next, division of the right triangular ligament is performed (Fig. 118B.6). The peritoneal

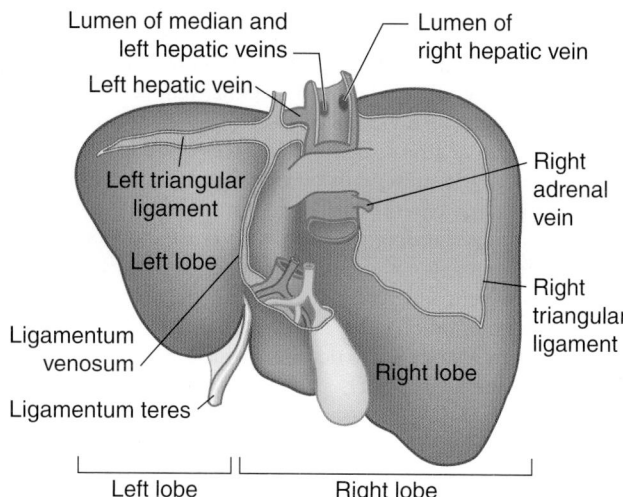

FIGURE 118B.6 Posterior hepatic anatomy including ligaments requiring division during liver mobilization[16] (see Chapter 2).

reflection at the edge of the triangular ligament is incised laterally and division of the anterior layer of the coronary ligament, as it reflects from the diaphragm onto segment VIII, and the posterior layer of the coronary ligament that reflects onto segment VI is developed. The liver is mobilized off the right hemidiaphragm, thereby exposing the bare area of segments VI and VII. The right adrenal gland is separated from segment VI, and the retrohepatic IVC is identified. This allows the liver to be rotated to the left and access the posterior segments.

If the tumor is noted to be adherent to the diaphragm, it can be separated if there is an adequate transection plane or the area resected, and diaphragm repaired primarily. It is particularly important to be careful during dissection of the tendinous portion of the diaphragm. Here, the diaphragm is only one layer thick, and errant dissection especially with the Bovie will produce a pneumothorax. Pneumothorax may lead to contamination of the chest with tumor in cancer cases and bacteria in contaminated cases. The diaphragm could also billow downwards obscuring the operative field.

Thus all defects in the diaphragm should be repaired immediately if possible. Diaphragmatic repair is performed using nonabsorbable running sutures. Typically, the author sutures each corner and runs the two sutures to the middle where they are tied. Before tying the suture, a red rubber catheter is threaded through the defect, and the anesthesiologist is asked to perform a Valsalva maneuver. The rubber catheter is then quickly pulled out of the defect as the suture is being tied down.

If the segments to be resected contain a tumor in proximity to the vena cava, the dissection must proceed posteriorly and medially until the IVC is visualized and ultimately completely exposed. A pair of closed Metzenbaum scissors can be used to gently push toward the vena cava to create this plane. The small venous branches draining from the back of the liver to the vena cava must then be divided (Fig. 118B.7). Failure to divide all small venous attachments to the IVC may result in future tearing of these veins and hemorrhage that is difficult to control. Ligation of these vessels can be performed using metal clips, silk ties, or a bipolar vessel sealer. The authors prefer ties over clips in the region of the major hepatic veins since clips may interfere with stapled transections of the hepatic veins and may lead to misfiring of the stapler (Fig. 118B.8).

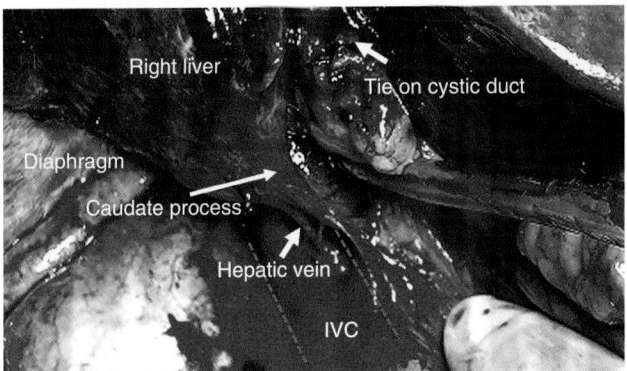

FIGURE 118B.7 Mobilization of the right liver with exposure of the short hepatic veins. The inferior vena cava (IVC) trajectory is marked with *dotted blue lines*. Note the large inferior hepatic vein draining the caudate process to the vena cava.

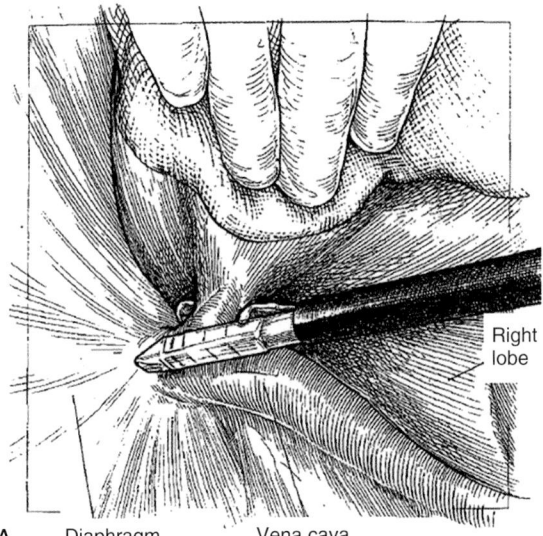

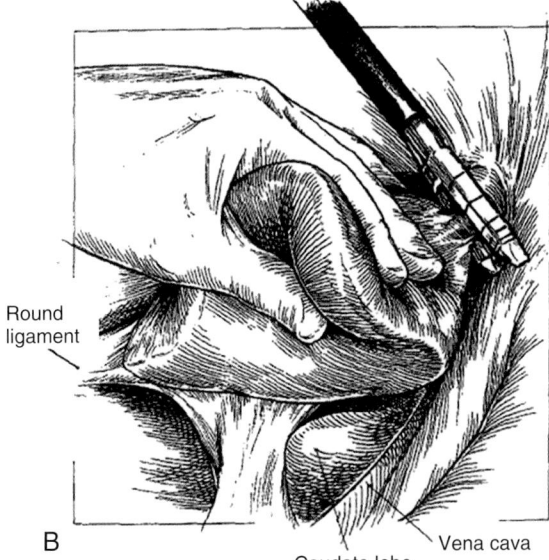

FIGURE 118B.8 Stapled ligation of the **(A)** right hepatic vein and **(B)** the left hepatic vein.[39] (From Fong Y, Blumgart LH. Useful stapling techniques in liver surgery. *J Am Coll Surg.* 1997;185[1]:93–100.)

Special mention must be made of the perforator veins behind the caudate process (see Fig. 118B.7). This is the bridge of liver tissue belonging to segment VI that bridges this segment and the caudate lobe. If a large inferior right hepatic vein is present (as it is in 21% of patients, often draining segment VI),[40] it usually lies behind the caudate process (see Chapter 2). This can be ligated during mobilization, or one may elect to leave it in place as the primary drainage for the remaining right-sided parenchyma. There may also be a tongue of liver tissue that passes from the back of the right lobe of the liver around the vena cava to the caudate on the left. In others, this structure may only be ligamentous and has been called the dorsal ligament, Makuuchi ligament, hepatocaval ligament,[41] or the caudate-caval ligament.[42] This tissue may contain vasculature and can be divided using a stapler. To do this, the liver is retracted medially, and a stapler is passed from below, parallel to the inferior vena cava.

The left liver mobilization begins by dividing the lesser omentum along the inferior edge of segment III. This usually is avascular, but if present, a replaced or accessory left hepatic artery will run in this plane. A laparotomy pad is placed under segment II, with a portion extending beyond the edge of the liver. This is to help protect the esophagus and stomach, which are just to the left of the IVC. The left hand is used to retract the left liver downward, and electrocautery is used to divide the loose attachments of the left triangular ligament in a lateral to medial fashion until the white of the laparotomy pad is visualized. As dissection proceeds medially, attention should be paid to the takeoff of the left hepatic vein, which again can be identified by tracing the drainage of the left phrenic vein on the diaphragm.

Methods of Liver Transection (also see Chapters 102B and 118)

There are several instruments that can be used during parenchymal transection of the liver, and several techniques to use these instruments. The authors' preference is to use cautery through the liver capsule and then to "Kelly crush-clamp" the liver parenchyma, followed by using the electrothermal bipolar vessel sealer to seal and divide the remaining small intrahepatic vasculature (Fig. 118B.9A). Monopolar electrocautery, set to coagulation fulgurate at 50 to 70 Watts, is used to divide the liver capsule approximately 25 mm in depth. One jaw of a curved Rochester-pean is then advanced along the transection line, capturing approximately 25 to 50 mm thickness tissue at a time within its jaws. The pean is gently advanced until it cannot advance further without resistance; this resistance usually represents a vessel at the tip of the instrument. If there is immediate resistance, the jaws of the pean are opened slightly to include the vessel in the clamp or closed slightly to slide over it. The pean is then slowly closed to utilize the crush-clamp technique. In essence, the pean separates the soft liver parenchyma, revealing the remaining small vessels, biliary channels, and larger pedicles. Once exposed, these structures can be secured and divided by using a variety of techniques that include simple and economic methods of clips and suture ligation. Alternatively, the vessels can be divided using the bipolar vessel sealer (LigaSure; Valleylab, Boulder, CO) or staplers (see Fig. 118B.9).

However, a variety of more complicated devices can also be used for parenchymal transection, including a saline-linked radiofrequency ablation bipolar sealer (Aquamantys, Medtronic,

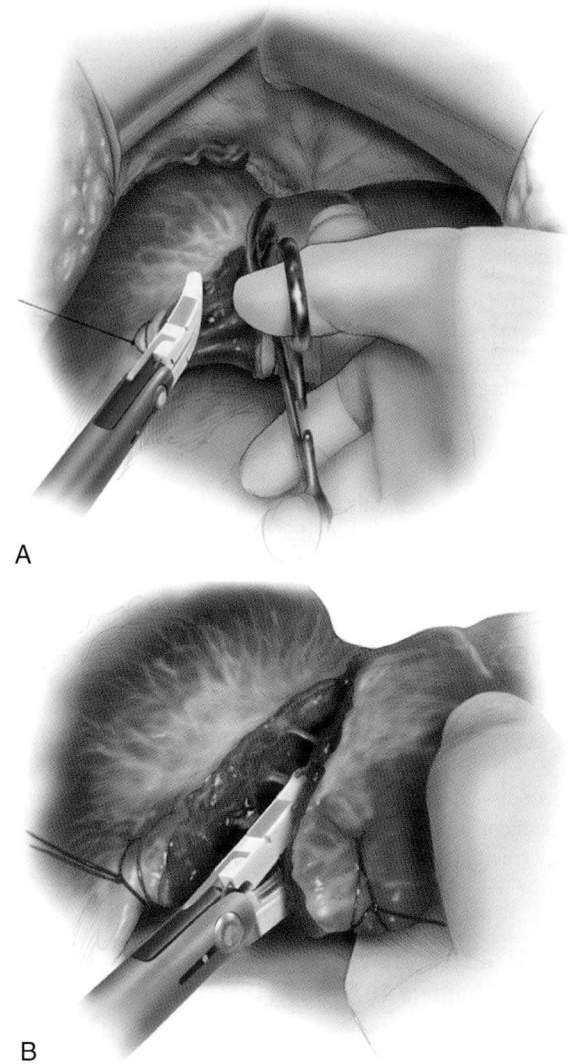

A

B

FIGURE 118B.9 Bipolar-assisted, Kelly crush technique of parenchymal transection. Traditional Kelly crush dissection of the liver parenchyma is performed **(A)**. The soft hepatocytes are bluntly dissected. After visualization of blood vessels and bile ducts, all vessels smaller than 5 mm are ligated with the LigaSure vessel sealer **(B)**. (From Patrlj L, Tuorto S, Fong Y. Combined blunt-clamp dissection and LigaSure ligation for hepatic parenchyma dissection: postcoagulation technique. *J Am Coll Surg.* 2010;210[1]:39–44.)

Minneapolis, MN) or ultrasonic shears (Harmonic Shears, Johnson & Johnson, New Brunswick, NJ). These devices have all been used with reported success.[43–45] Dissection technique using tools such as the Cavitron Ultrasonic Surgical Aspirator (CUSA; Valleylab, Boulder, CO) or Helix Hydro-Jet dissector (ERBE USA, Marietta, GA) facilitate a precise, controlled transection of liver parenchyma and allow the dissection of intrahepatic structures while minimizing blood loss through prevention of injury to small vascular structures within the parenchyma.[46] Techniques that use destructive hemostatic control include the use of linear cutting staplers, in-line radiofrequency ablation (Habib; Angiodynamics, Latham, NY), and bipolar cautery (Gyrus; Gyrus ACMI, Southborough, MA; and LigaSure; Covidien, Boulder, CO). Pretransection extrahepatic vascular control is used by many surgeons to facilitate adequate

oncologic margin as it will provide anatomic delimitation and decrease bleeding.[47,48]

Early occlusion of the hepatic venous outflow of any segments being resected may reduce the risk of venous tumor emboli. Occlusion of the hepatic artery and portal vein to those segments being resected facilitates the procedure with reduction of blood loss by defining the line of division between ischemic segments to be removed and the well-perfused remnant liver. Pretransection occlusion of the inflow of the segments to be resected before outflow results in better hemostasis and avoids congestion of the liver.

Vascular Inflow and Outflow Control

Occlusion of the inflow to sectors for major hepatectomy is described in detail in Chapter 118A. The surgeon may also choose to apply intermittent inflow occlusion using a Pringle maneuver to control blood flow to the remnant liver. Ideally, this inflow occlusion should be limited to periods of 15 minutes followed by at least 5 minute periods of relief to restore perfusion to the remnant and to avoid bowel edema.[49] However, total vascular isolation using a Pringle maneuver may require fluid loading or use of pressors during the 15-minute period of occlusion, which are often avoided using the selective vascular control techniques described earlier. The use of low CVP and selective vascular control have acceptable blood loss and comparable blood transfusion rates in comparison with total vascular control and therefore should be used when possible.

It is also our preference to staple intrahepatic portal pedicles. Once a portal pedicle is dissected free, an umbilical tape is passed. A right-angle dissector may then be slid down on the umbilical tape, compressing the soft liver parenchyma so that the portal pedicle is visible. Upward traction is then placed on the portal pedicle using the umbilical tape, and a 30 mm white staple load is passed, and then fired. Hepatic veins are more delicate than the portal pedicles; for this reason, a silk suture is used instead to encircle the vein once it is dissected out. Hepatic veins may then be tied, oversewn, or stapled in a similar fashion.

Control of Hepatic Venous Drainage (see Chapter 188A)

Liver segments reside between the three primary hepatic veins, but liver segmental resection will often necessitate the division of these hepatic veins. When performing segmentectomy and sectionectomy, typically the portal pedicle inflow is divided before the hepatic vein outflow. This is to prevent hepatic congestion during surgery and to limit blood loss. One may decide, however, to gain early control of the hepatic veins, so that they can be clamped down quickly if bleeding occurs during surgery. After complete mobilization of the liver, the hepatic veins should be discernable at the superior-most aspect of the liver, which can be identified by following the falciform ligament posteriorly. The right hepatic vein is found by tracing the right phrenic vein medially on the diaphragm towards the IVC. Isolation of the right hepatic vein is obtained by retracting the liver to the left and using a blunt right-angle dissector from superior to inferior, through the fossa between the right and middle hepatic veins, sliding above and parallel to the IVC. A silk tie or vessel loop is passed to maintain this channel, and the right vein can then later be tied off, over-sewn, or stapled. To transect the right hepatic vein with a stapler, the liver is retracted to the left, and a stapler is passed from below, toward the base of the heart and parallel to the IVC (see Fig. 118B.8).

The left hepatic vein is identified by tracing the left phrenic vein medially on the diaphragm toward the IVC. It should be noted that the middle and left hepatic veins are fused at the IVC in 70% of patients.[50] The trajectory of the middle hepatic vein follows from the center of the gallbladder bed to the IVC, the so called "principle plane," also known as Cantlie's line (see Fig. 118B.6). Gentle dissection is performed using a blunt right-angle dissector from above, in the fossa between the right and middle hepatic veins. This is brought toward the left, to encircle the trunk of both the middle and left hepatic veins, and a silk tie or vessel loop is passed around them. To transect the left hepatic vein, the liver is retracted by grasping the left lateral lobe inferiorly and laterally to enable visualization of the junction of the left and middle hepatic veins from below, which is dissected free. This may require ligation of the ligamentum venosum to visualize the hepatic veins from below. A stapler is passed from right to left to help ensure only the left vein is divided (see Fig. 118B.8).

PROCEDURES (ALSO SEE CHAPTER 102B)

See Chapter 2 for anatomic details related to specific resections and Chapter 118A for techniques regarding lobectomy, hepatectomy, and extended hepatectomy.

Left-Sided Liver Resections

Segment I (Caudate Lobe) Resection

Segment I of the liver, the caudate lobe, lies between the portal vein and the IVC, with venous drainage through many small hepatic veins directly into the IVC (Fig. 118B.10). Its portal inflow is from both the right and left portal veins[51] but typically is primarily via the left portal vein.[42] Of note, the inflow from the right usually arises from the right portal pedicle and travels via the caudate process. Smaller tumors may be approached from the left, whereas larger tumors may be better accessed from the right, from both sides, or by splitting the liver through the principal plane. As mentioned in the description of mobilization, there may also be a tongue of liver tissue that passes from the back of the right lobe of the liver around the vena cava to the caudate on the left. In this scenario, present in up to 50% of patients, the caudate completely encircles the IVC,[52] whereas in others this structure may only be ligamentous. When there is significant retrocaval parenchyma, a right-sided approach is often necessary. This tissue can be divided using a stapler, by retracting the right liver to the left and passing a stapler from below, parallel to the IVC.

RIGHT-SIDED APPROACH. To begin a caudate resection, the primary caudate portal inflow is identified at the inferior aspect of the caudate lobe. The caudate portal pedicle branch is at the base of the umbilical fissure and is the first branch coming off of the left portal pedicle (see Fig. 118B.10A). This can be identified by lowering the hilar plate, that is, incising the veil of peritoneum overlying the portal structures as they enter the parenchyma of the liver. The ligamentum teres is retracted to the right to expose the left side, and in the base of the umbilical fissure, one can often see the caudate branch take off from the left portal pedicle without further dissection. A right-angle dissector is used to encircle the portal pedicle, which is then stapled or oversewn.

Mobilizing the right liver allows the safest approach to ligation of retrocaudate vessels entering the vena cava. Division of

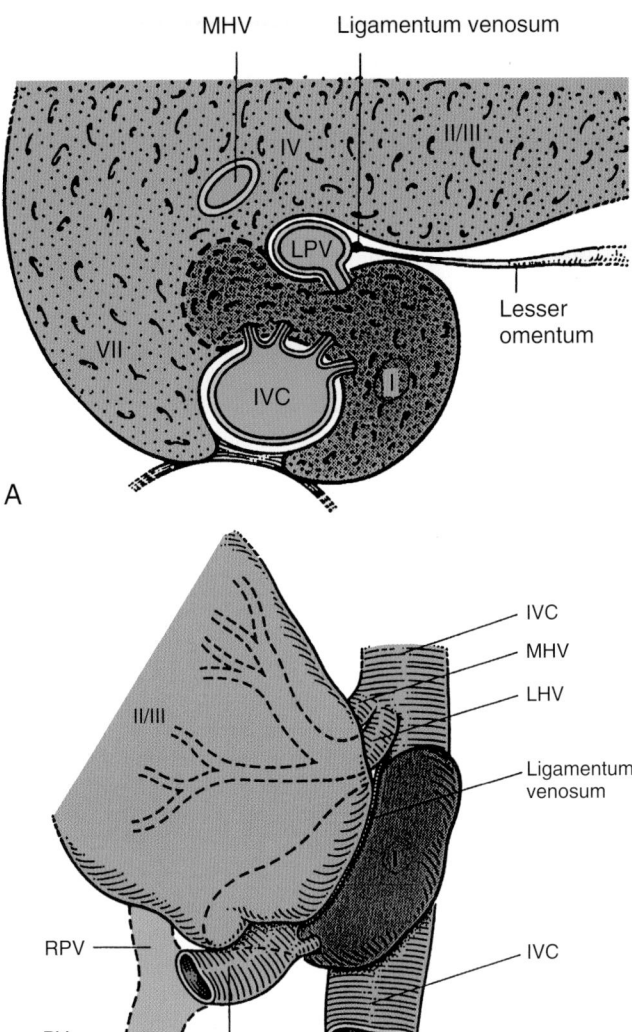

FIGURE 118B.10 Cross-sectional anatomy of the caudate lobe anatomy at the level of the porta hepatis.[52] **(A)** Unaltered planes. **(B)** The lesser omentum has been opened, and the left liver is retracted to the right. The ligamentus attachments posteriorly can be divided to facilitate approach from the left or the right (see Chapter 2). *IVC,* Inferior vena cava; *I,* caudate lobe/liver segment 1; *II/III,* liver segments 2 and 3; *IV,* liver segment 4; *LHV,* left hepatic vein; *LPV,* left portal vein; *MHV,* middle hepatic vein; *PV,* portal vein; *RPV,* right portal vein; *VII,* liver segment 7. (From Bartlett D, Fong Y, Blumgart L. Complete resection of the caudate lobe of the liver: technique and results. *Br J Surg.* 1996;83[8]:1076–1081.)

the caudate veins occurs during the mobilization of the right hepatic lobe described earlier, in a caudal to cranial manner. This is performed serially until the major hepatic vein trunks are reached. In practice, the liver is often flipped back and forth until the vena cava is entirely cleared. At this point, there will be vascular demarcation of the caudate lobe.

Once the caudate veins are cleared, parenchymal transection may proceed. For tumors in the inferior caudate, the parenchyma is divided from superior to inferior, left to right, parallel, and just lateral to the IVC. For more superior caudate tumors, the transection may proceed from inferior to superior, right to left, and starting just to the left of the ligamentum teres at the caudate process. Once the caudate process is divided, the caudate is retracted toward the left, and parenchymal transection proceeds superiorly. The transection line itself always slants from the left hepatic vein to the right portal vein and will be clear from the vascular demarcation. Bridges of tissue to segment VIII (between the IVC and the middle hepatic vein) and segment IV (between the middle hepatic vein and the left portal vein) will need to be divided. Throughout the transection, attention should be paid to the location of the middle hepatic vein given its proximity. At the top of the caudate, there is usually a large venous tributary draining directly into the left hepatic vein or the left and middle vein junction. Identification of this tributary is essential to prevent hemorrhage.

It should be noted that coded descriptions of multisegment hepatic resections do not automatically include the caudate lobe, so this should be specifically included in the name of the procedure.

LEFT-SIDED APPROACH. The falciform ligament is dissected in a cephalad direction until the anterior and left surface of the suprahepatic vena cava has been isolated. The left hepatic vein (LHV) is identified, and the left triangular ligament is divided from left to right taking care to avoid injury to any low-entering phrenic veins and the LHV. The left lobe of the liver can then be rotated to the right. The fissure for the ligamentum venosum, the *caudate groove*, can then be identified. To obtain further mobility and reduce the chances of a traction injury to the hepatic veins, the ligamentum venosum is ligated and divided in the superior aspect of its fissure, as it enters the posterior aspect of the LHV or MHV.

For smaller tumors, particularly in noncirrhotic livers, isolated caudate resection can usually be performed from the left. Mobilization of the caudate lobe involves complete division of the gastrohepatic omentum and dorsal caudate-caval ligament which lies posterior to the IVC and allows some additional retraction of segment I. The small bridge of liver between segments I and VI (caudate process) is also divided with care to ligate the caudate process pedicle as it exits from the right main pedicle to feed the caudate process and the right side of the caudate lobe.

The dissection of segment I from the IVC then continues in a cephalad direction, dividing several thin-walled veins that drain segment I into the IVC using suture ligation or clips moving from the left to right. These veins are fragile and meticulous dissection is imperative. A large vein from segment I is often present 1 to 2 cm below the confluence of the MHV and LHV and must be divided. This exposure may not be possible with a bulky tumor and care must be taken to not injure the MHV posteriorly, which can result in significant hemorrhage. To prevent this, the MHV and LHV may be dissected and isolated extrahepatically as discussed in Chapter 118A. Once segment I is mobilized, the thin parenchymal bridge between the caudate groove and the posterior transection line is divided. This plane is usually avascular; however, the segment I duct and hilar plate tissue should be anticipated anteriorly. During parenchymal transection, the fissure for the ligamentum venosum is sometimes encountered and may need to be divided a second time. Dissection continues to its completion at the apex of segment I beneath the confluence of the hepatic veins.

If, during an attempted left-sided approach to a caudate resection, there is compromised exposure, the approach should be converted to a right-sided mobilization to provide better exposure. Some of the venous branches between segments VI

and VII and the IVC may need to be divided from the right to provide adequate mobilization of the caudate off the IVC (see Chapter 2).

ANTERIOR APPROACH. If the tumor is large, superior, and close to the hepatic veins, or is in a cirrhotic liver that cannot be rotated for right-sided mobilization (see Chapter 120), the caudate parenchymal transection alternatively can be approached anteriorly, by completely dividing the liver in half just to the right of the middle hepatic vein, along the edge of segment IV. This technique enables direct visualization of the major hepatic veins, preventing inadvertent injury.

In these situations, some surgeons advocate obtaining suprahepatic and infrahepatic control of the IVC with vessel loops before parenchymal transection, to help mitigate bleeding from hepatic veins.[41]

After splitting the liver in half, the caudate lobe is at the base of the hepatotomy. Parenchymal transection then proceeds from superior to inferior following the right hepatic and middle veins around the caudate lobe. Should the hepatic veins be injured during this dissection, they can be repaired using 4-0 polypropylene suture. As dissection proceeds inferiorly, the division of the portal pedicle into the right and left branches is visualized. These are dissected free and are ligated. At this point, the only remaining attachments are to the IVC. The caudate lobe is carefully retracted to visualize the caudate veins to the IVC, which are isolated and ligated. Once the tumor is resected, the split liver can be reapproximated using sutures.

Segment II or III Resection

Isolated resection of segment II or III may be performed when it is necessary to preserve as much of the left lateral section as possible. Left liver mobilization is performed as described above by ligation of the left triangular ligament.

Splitting the liver parenchyma medial to the left portal pedicle within the umbilical fissure allows visualization of the segment III pedicle. Ligation of this pedicle with a suture or a stapler will allow the demarcation of segment III. Parenchymal transection along the demarcation line coming from left to right will allow facile resection of segment III. Care must be taken during this transection to protect the left hepatic vein (see Chapter 2).

Given the discrepancy between portal vein supply and biliary drainage, and given the difficulty of preserving LHV drainage, combined segment II and III resection (left lateral sectionectomy) is safer and more feasible than isolated resection of segment II alone. However, in the setting of bilateral liver resections or patients with tenuous liver function, it may be necessary to perform an isolated segment II resection. The segment II portal pedicle should be identified in the umbilical fissure above the caudate branches. Ligation of this pedicle delineates the parenchyma of segment II to guide parenchymal transection.

Combined Resection of Segments II and III: Left Lateral Sectionectomy

The left lateral sectionectomy is a common operation that can be completed easily via an open or minimally invasive approach (see Chapter 127D). The left lateral section is mobilized by the division of the falciform ligament and the left triangular ligament. The extrahepatic portion of the LHV can be lengthened by dividing the fibrous tissue to the left of the IVC down to the level of the fissure for the ligamentum venosum, which is then ligated and divided as it enters the posterior aspect of the LHV. This allows a clamp to be passed around the LHV and encircle it. This may not be possible if the LHV joins with the MHV intraparenchymally, in which case isolation of the LHV is delayed until completion of the parenchymal transection.

The liver is retracted cranially using the silk tied to the end of the falciform ligament. There may be a bridge of liver tissue crossing between segments III and IV. If present, a right-angle dissector is used to encircle this parenchyma, which is divided. A large right-angle dissector is then used within the umbilical fissure to control segment III and then segment II pedicles. Umbilical tapes are passed around each to protect the main left portal pedicle during ligation of the segment II and III pedicles. Parenchymal transection proceeds along a plane 5 mm to the left of the ligamentum teres, with vessels and portal structures divided as they are encountered. Parenchymal transection directly along the falciform ligament itself risks injury to the segment IV pedicle. Once the parenchyma is divided, only the LHV remains, which can be stapled or oversewn. Alternatively, the LHV can be ligated right after ligation of the segment II and III portal pedicles.

Of note, the blood supply to the caudate emerges from the portal vein and left hepatic artery at the level of the portoumbilical fissure, and these should be identified and preserved before the parenchymal transection (Figs. 118B.10 and 118B.11).

Segment IV Resection

Segment IV is divided into two subsegments based on portal inflow pedicles (see Chapter 2). Isolated resection of segment IV or IVa alone is possible but uncommon; however, segment IVb may be resected alone or in combination with an extended right hepatectomy. Segment IV is limited posteriorly by the hilar plate and IVC, on either side by the left portal pedicle, and the MHV. Inflow and biliary drainage to segment IV come from left to right from the left-sided portal structures in the base of the

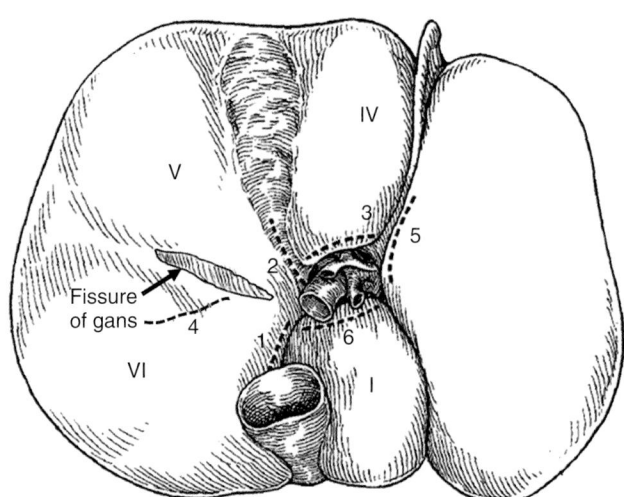

FIGURE 118B.11 Sites for hepatotomy to enable intrahepatic portal pedicle control, when the liver is retracted cephalad to view the posterior surface.[39] Hepatotomies 2 and 4 allow isolation of the right anterior pedicle. Hepatotomies 1 and 4 allow isolation of the right posterior pedicle. Hepatotomies 1 and 2 allow isolation of the right main portal pedicle. Hepatotomies 3 and 5 allow isolation of the left portal pedicle. (From Fong Y, Blumgart LH. Useful stapling techniques in liver surgery. *J Am Coll Surg.* 1997;185[1]:93–100.)

falciform ligament. Sometimes, aberrant right anterior and posterior sectional ducts cross in this position, which must be preserved during resection. Outflow from segment IV is predominantly to the MHV, but occasionally a separate draining vein (scissural vein) goes directly to the suprahepatic IVC or the terminal part of the LHV or MHV.

The falciform ligament should be divided to the level of the suprahepatic IVC to expose the base of the hepatic veins. The hilar plate should then be lowered to release the portal structures from the base of segment IV. By incising the peritoneal reflection on the right of the falciform ligament, the segment IVa and IVb pedicles can be isolated, encircled, and divided; the lines of transection become demarcated on the surface of the liver along Cantlie's line.

Parenchymal transection commences just to the right side of the falciform ligament to avoid injury to the umbilical portion of the left portal vein. This will lead to identification of the portal pedicles to segments IVa and IVb. These pedicles may arise from a common trunk, and occasionally there are more than two, which is usually appreciable on preoperative imaging.

Transection continues superiorly to the level of the junction of the LHV and MHV at the suprahepatic IVC. The veins usually join within the liver at this point before insertion into the IVC, and in this case, the dissection terminates inferior to this point, and often outflow control is not obtained until the liver is divided. Care should be taken to identify venous tributaries from segment IV into the LHV. The dissection of the right side is along Cantlie's line to the left of the MHV. Several tributaries to the MHV, the IVa and IVb veins, will also need to be identified and ligated. Once the medial border of the hilar dissection has been reached, the parenchymal transection is done in a transverse plane to complete the separation of segment IV to detach it from segment I posteriorly (see Fig. 118B.10).

Right-Sided Liver Resections

Before engaging in a right-sided liver resection, the gallbladder should be removed to permit unimpeded access to the gallbladder bed and the base of the right portal pedicle, which lays directly behind it (see Chapters 36 and 118A). Rouviere's sulcus, also known as the fissure of Ganz,[53] is visible in 68% to 90% of individuals.[53] The junction of the right anterior and posterior pedicles usually lies deep within the medial extent of this sulcus.[54] Control of portal pedicles can be performed either extrahepatically or intrahepatically with appropriately placed hepatotomies (see Fig. 118B.11). The decision to obtain extrahepatic or intrahepatic control is made based on the location of the tumor to be excised, with preference given for obtaining control further away from the tumor to maximize the likelihood of a negative margin, which is paramount.

Segment V Resection

Isolated segment V resection begins with the division of the liver on the undersurface up the center of the gallbladder fossa and anteriorly along Cantlie's line halfway up toward the IVC. The parenchyma is then divided in a plane to the left of the RHV, which extends on the undersurface of the liver along the fissure of Ganz to the free edge and anteriorly halfway toward the IVC. This posterior plane is quite coronal and usually results in a large exposed area of the parenchyma. The resection is completed by connecting the two vertical transection lines by division of the parenchyma horizontally from anterior to posterior immediately below the level of PV division (Fig. 118B.12).

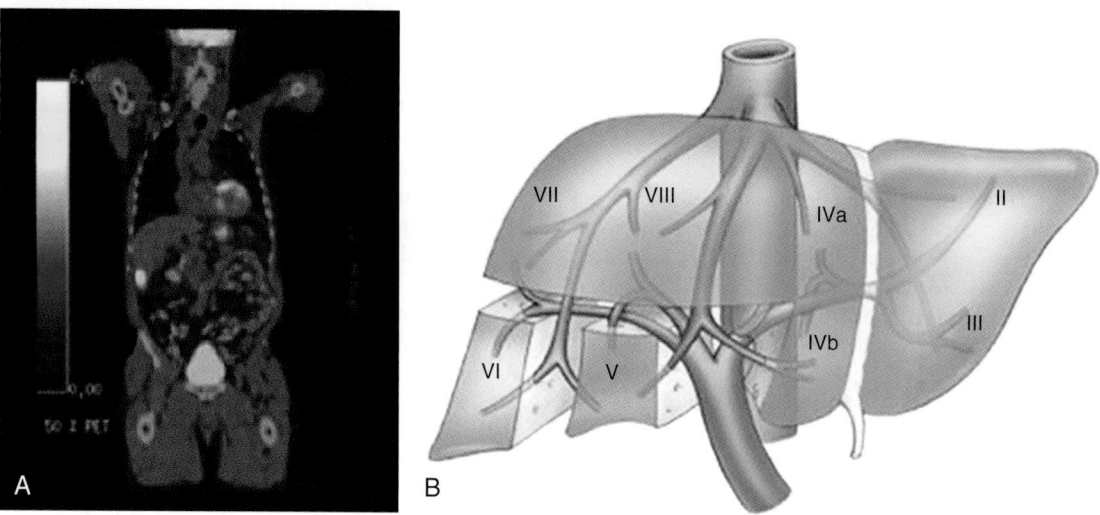

FIGURE 118B.12 The planes of dissection for segments 5 and 6. Tumors in segment 6, as identified by PET scanning in **(A),** are easily resected. The horizontal plane of dissection is along the right portal pedicle **(B)** (see Chapter 2).

Segment VIII Resection

Due to the challenging nature of an isolated segment VIII resection, the primary indications are narrow including a small, solitary metastasis or focal hepatocellular carcinoma (HCC) in a patient with cirrhosis (see Chapter 120). This resection is challenging since there is no external demarcation of this segment and no easy way of controlling the inflow pedicle early. The initial landmark is Cantlie's line with a parenchymal transection on the right side of the MHV. The segment VIII pedicle, which corresponds to the ascending division of the right anterior sectional pedicle, can be isolated either at this point, after division of the liver, or by dividing the liver between segments IV and V in the horizontal plane along the level of the portal vein bifurcation. This latter maneuver is useful because it allows for demarcation of the right-sided resection margin, which is on the left side of the RHV. This horizontal transection should follow the coronal plane of the RHV, which requires IOUS guidance (see Chapters 24 and 103).

Alternatively, an anatomic resection may more simply proceed by following the hepatic veins (see Chapter 2). The middle hepatic vein runs along the principle plane/Cantlie's line, from the IVC to the center of the gallbladder bed. The lateral parenchymal edge will follow the RHV, which can be identified at the apex of the liver. An IOUS is used to follow the veins inferiorly and can be traced with electrocautery to direct future parenchymal transection (see Chapters 24 and 103). After electrocautery is applied to the liver surface, the ultrasound is used to view the marking, which appears as an area of hyperintensity at the top of the ultrasound image. The ultrasound confirms the electrocautery marks in relation to the tumor being transected, to further ensure a negative margin. The liver capsule is further divided using electrocautery, and then parenchymal transection proceeds until the portal pedicle is encountered. A right-angle dissector is used to encircle the pedicle, an umbilical tape is passed, and then the portal pedicle is stapled or oversewn.

Segment V and VIII Resection (Right Anterior Sectionectomy)

Segments V and VIII compose the right anterior sector. For intrahepatic control of the right anterior portal branches to segments V and VIII, the liver is retracted cephalad, so that the inferior surface of the liver is visible. A hepatotomy is made along the base of the gallbladder bed through the cystic plate. A large right angle is used to dissect toward the trajectory of the right anterior portal pedicle mentioned earlier (see Fig. 118B.11, from incision 2 to incision 4). Once the branch point of segment V and VIII is in view, a right-angle dissector is used to free the segment desired for division. An umbilical tape is passed around the segment pedicle. The right angle is then slid down on the umbilical tape, compressing the soft liver parenchyma around the right anterior portal pedicle so that it is clearly visible. The umbilical tape is then pulled up to provide traction for the passage of either a stapler or two clamps to enable oversewing. The division of hepatic parenchyma continues using a pean and bipolar vessel sealer. This will follow the margin of vascular demarcation just to the right of the middle hepatic vein.

Alternatively, the bifurcation of the right portal pedicle into anterior and posterior pedicle can be identified intraparenchymally (Fig. 118B.13). Due to the intrahepatic bifurcation, parenchymal transection along Cantlie's line and splitting the liver along the principal plane facilitate the identification of the right anterior pedicle. Early ligation of the base of the cystic plate allows mobility of the junction of the anterior and posterior pedicles for safe dissection. Parenchymal transection toward the pedicle is required before its division to allow demarcation of either segment V or VIII (see Fig. 118B.13). The segment V pedicle emerges anteriorly and runs anteroinferiorly, and the segment VIII pedicle emerges posteriorly and runs superiorly. The horizontal plane of transection for an isolated segment V or VIII resection runs through the liver at the level of the portal vein bifurcation, with segment V below and segment VIII above this line. The medial and lateral limits of the resection are the MHV and RHV, respectively.

Segment VI Resection

Segment VI resection is relatively uncomplicated due to its anterior position and distance from the major pedicle. An oblique transection line along the fissure of Gans on the inferior surface of the liver and anteriorly halfway toward the IVC, following the posterior side of the RHV can be used. The horizontal plane

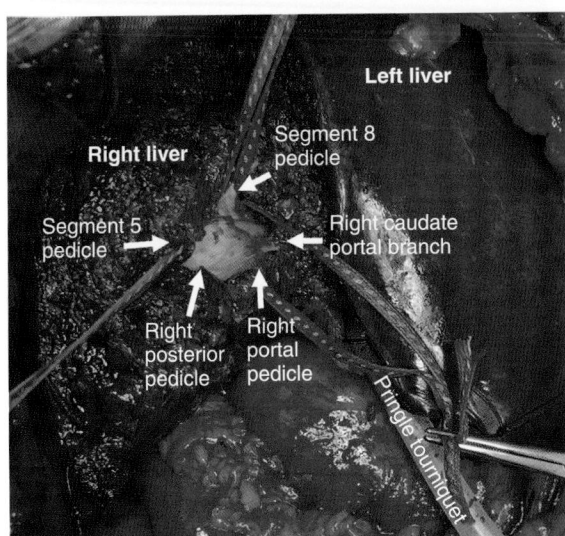

FIGURE 118B.13 Anterior approach to right hepatectomy—identification of portal pedicles. The portal pedicles are viewed after the majority of the parenchyma has been transected. Umbilical tape is placed around the pedicles to facilitate upward traction for placement of a stapler.

of resection is at the level of the portal vein bifurcation. Inflow control is obtained by ligating the descending branches of the right posterior sectional portal triad which are encountered about two-thirds of the way through the dissection. One must take care to preserve the portal supply to segment VII if it originates from the right posterior pedicle. The resection is completed by taking a horizontal transection plane through the posterior surface of the liver lateral to the RHV. The RHV can be sacrificed for an isolated segment VI resection (see Fig. 118B.12). This resection can also be performed by a minimally invasive surgery approach (see Chapter 127D).

Segment VII Resection

An isolated segment VII resection is not commonly performed unless there are circumstances where a right posterior sectionectomy is not appropriate given baseline liver function. However, it is useful for small hepatocellular carcinomas in segment VII of cirrhotic patients. It is more difficult than a segment VI resection due to the posterior trajectory of the inflow and the location up against the right diaphragm. A horizontal transection line just above the portal vein bifurcation should be continued medially reaching the lateral margin of the RHV, which should be preserved. During the horizontal parenchymal transection, the ascending right posterior sectional branches can be isolated and divided, which will allow for demarcation of the medial aspect of the resection. The vertical transection line runs obliquely through the liver lateral and posterior to the RHV. The RHV should be spared in an isolated segment VII resection to allow for adequate drainage of segment VI unless there is an inferior accessory RHV on preoperative or intraoperative imaging.

Combined Resection of Segments VI and VII (Right Posterior Sectionectomy)

A right posterior sectionectomy is an alternative to a formal right hepatectomy, especially in patients with underlying hepatic dysfunction. Identification of the right posterior sectional pedicle may be possible extrahepatically or with a perihilar hepatotomy in the fissure of Gans. The pedicle should be

clamped to demarcate the posterior section followed by early division to facilitate the identification of the transection margins. The RHV could be encircled to allow occlusion during parenchymal transection and can be sacrificed if necessary. In 25% of patients, there is an accessory RHV with direct drainage into the IVC.[55,56] The plane of transection posterior to the RHV is coronal and results in a relatively large surface area of cut parenchyma, which requires specific attention for hemostasis and biliostasis.

For intrahepatic control of the right posterior portal branch to segments VI and VII, the liver is retracted cephalad, so that the posterior aspect of the liver is visible. If there is a clear fissure of Gans, a right-angle retractor can be used to encircle the right posterior pedicle without a hepatotomy. Otherwise, hepatotomies can be made just inferior to where the right anterior portal pedicle is expected, and along the lateral border of the caudate lobe (see Fig. 118B.11, from incision 4 to incision 1). Once the pedicle is encircled, an umbilical tape is passed. A similar methodology as above is used to identify the portal branch point of segments VI and VII. Once the portal pedicle is divided, parenchymal transection follows to the right of the RHV and will be demarcated on the liver surface due to devascularization.

Atypical Resections
Combined Resection of Segments V and VI

Resection of segments V and VI is frequently performed. The right liver must be mobilized from the diaphragm with division of segment VI and VII hepatic veins on the anterior surface of the IVC. The vertical plane of transection is along Cantlie's line on the right side of the MHV from the edge of the liver in the middle of the gallbladder fossa to approximately halfway toward the suprahepatic IVC to the level of the right portal pedicle. The horizontal plane of transection is at the level of the portal vein (see Fig. 118B.12). Then, with a dissection to the left, the horizontal plane of transection is developed from the top of the vertical plane. The segment V portal pedicle may be identified at the base and divided, followed by division of the segment VI pedicle posteriorly. The horizontal parenchymal dissection plane continues to the RHV, which should be preserved if possible.

Combined Resection of Segments VII, VIII

This resection is rarely performed and involves removal of the top of the right liver. Indications would be for tumors directly on the RHV. This resection relies on effective venous drainage of the lower right liver (segments V, VI) directly into the vena cava from short hepatic veins or through large, lower accessory veins.[40] This resection is particularly relevant for patients with cirrhosis, where saving every bit of functional liver parenchyma is important (see Chapters 74 and 120).

Parenchymal transection usually starts just to the right of the MHV. Once inferior to the tumor by an adequate margin, parenchymal transection then angles directly to the right. The right liver is retracted to the left, and control of the RHV is obtained. In this resection, often, no mobilization of the lower right lobe is performed to preserve venous drainage.

Resection of Segments IV, V, and VIII: Mesohepatectomy/Central Hepatectomy

This resection is also infrequently performed and is indicated primarily for large central tumors where a formal extended right or left hepatectomy will not leave enough residual liver. It involves removal of the gallbladder, segments IV, V, VIII, and hepatic vein en bloc. It requires ligation of inflow from both the right and left portal pedicles making it technically challenging. Segment I may also be resected especially in the case of a hilar cholangiocarcinoma (see Chapter 119B).[57]

The liver must be completely mobilized and the RHV, MHV, and LHV identified as they enter the IVC (see Chapter 118A). After cholecystectomy, the hilar plate is dropped down from the base of segment IV by dividing the areolar tissue between the bifurcation of the common hepatic duct and the liver. Early identification and division of the right anterior portal pedicle demarcates segments V and VIII and identifies the lines of transection on the right side of the liver. The inflow pedicle to segment IVb may be controlled outside the liver within the umbilical fissure. However, more often the segment IVa and IVb pedicles are divided during the parenchymal transection. One must be careful not to ligate the left main portal vein. The right anterior sectional pedicle may be controlled using the Glissonian extrahepatic approach, or the segment V and VIII pedicles may be ligated during the transection.

The boundaries of transection on the left are to the right of the falciform ligament and the umbilical fissure, and that of the right-sided plane is to the left side of the RHV. The coronal transection plane is above the hilum and anterior to the right posterior sectional portal pedicle.

The parenchymal transection begins to the right of the falciform ligament. The portal pedicles to segments IVa and IVb are ligated and divided as they come back from the left-sided portal structures. This transection plane is carried cephalad toward the MHV-LHV junction. Care must be taken to ensure that the LHV is not injured or inadvertently divided. The deeper portions of the left-sided dissection plane are best left until the right-sided parenchymal transection is complete. The right-sided transection plane is to the left of the RHV, angled approximately 45 degrees from the horizontal and vertical planes.

The right-sided parenchymal transection begins to the right of the gallbladder fossa and is directed anteriorly toward the right middle groove and posteriorly toward the incisura dextra. Care must be taken to remain anterior to the right posterior portal pedicle and not to injure the RHV. At the base of this transection plane, the right anterior sectional portal pedicle or the individual segment V and VIII pedicles are divided, if they were not controlled earlier. Before division, a test clamping is advisable to ensure that the right posterior portal pedicle is not accidentally encircled. The dissection continues until the upper aspect of the left and right transection margins meet, and then the MHV is divided to complete the resection. For large tumors, care must be taken to avoid the left hepatic duct as you come down to the base of the liver. Because of the large surface of the cut liver and the proximity to the hilar plate, these resections are more prone to bleeding and bile leak and may be covered with an omental flap.

Management of Intraoperative Bleeding (see Chapter 25)

Bleeding from the liver can come from the inflow (hepatic artery or portal vein) or the outflow (hepatic veins). In general, bleeding from outflow is the most troublesome. To minimize outflow bleeding, the most important maneuver is maintaining low CVP (<5 mm Hg) before and during the liver parenchymal transection.[58] The efficacy and tolerability of this technique were demonstrated in a case series of 496 liver resections at Memorial Sloan Kettering Cancer Center, in which only 3% of patients developed a persistent increase in their serum creatinine postoperatively.

Clamping the extrahepatic portal triad, known as the Pringle maneuver, is an effective maneuver for decreasing inflow bleeding.[59] This can easily be performed using a Rumel tourniquet and a timer. Originally described by James Hogarth Pringle in 1908 for the management of hepatic bleeding due to trauma,[60] the efficacy of this maneuver for limiting blood loss during hepatectomy was later demonstrated in a randomized controlled trial.[59] In this study, the Pringle maneuver was applied during parenchymal transection for 20 minutes at a time, with 5-minute breaks, until the liver resection was completed.[59] Some groups leave the Pringle on for the entire duration of parenchymal transection. The esteemed group at the University of Hong Kong has found that the Pringle maneuver can be applied even in cirrhotic livers for over an hour.[61]

The practical steps in tracking down and solving an active bleed start with clamping the extrahepatic portal triad. If bleeding continues, the source is likely from the hepatic veins. If the source of bleeding is a visible perforation in a hepatic vein, this can be addressed with a 3-0 or 4-0 polypropylene figure-of-eight suture. Alternatively, mattress stitches tied on the liver capsule are highly effective in stopping venous bleeding from vessels that have retracted into the parenchyma. The two edges of the split liver can also be "closed" to facilitate tamponade. Oxidized regenerated cellulose can also be tied down onto the cut edge to buttress the suture and to encourage hemostasis.

For mild surface bleeding without a clear source, one may choose to paint the cut liver edge with monopolar electrocautery, an argon beam coagulator, or application of a bipolar sealer, or to lay down a sheet of oxidized regenerated cellulose. For mild bleeding, packing a laparotomy pad and allowing platelets and the coagulation cascade to do their jobs often solves the problem.

Intraoperative Hepatobiliary Navigational Tools

There has been an effort to develop tools that can be used intraoperatively to provide feedback to the surgeon regarding the position of the transection line versus the lesion of interest and major vasculature (see Chapter 103). This is to decrease the likelihood of a positive resection margin, lower the risk of vascular injury, and increase the volume of preserved normal hepatic parenchyma.[30]

One class of devices involves using fluorescent dyes to see tumors, blood vessels, or bile ducts. The most employed of these utilize near-infrared fluorescence (NIRF) imaging with indocyanine green (ICG). ICG is an NIRF dye with a peak spectral absorption around 800 nm that is delivered intravenously and can be visualized when stimulated by polarized light. After injection of approximately 2.5 mg of ICG, the agent rapidly binds to albumin, and in this way highlights vasculature with a half-life of 2 to 5 minutes.[62] ICG is selectively taken up by hepatocytes and then excreted unchanged into bile approximately 45 minutes after injection.[63,64] ICG is taken up and retained preferentially by primary hepatic tumors compared with parenchyma,[65] and preferentially trapped within CK7-positive hepatocytes compressed by metastatic tumor.[66] Therefore primary liver tumors appear bright, and metastases have a bright rim.[67] ICG has been shown to identify more and smaller metastases than CT, MRI, intraoperative palpation, and IOUS,[68,69] and does not add significant time to the surgical procedure.[70]

Another class of devices uses 3D reconstructions of preoperative scans and overlays the images onto the surgical anatomy for anatomic guidance (see Chapter 103). Two navigational systems have also predominated the literature in this area: the CAS-One surgical system (CAScination AG, Bern, Switzerland) and the Explorer Liver system (Analogic Corporation, Peabody, MA, USA). The use of the CAS-One system for intraoperative liver navigation entails CT 3D reconstructed image registration with intraoperatively identified landmarks. This is performed using an optically tracked pointer tool visible to a system camera overhead. The model is then viewed on a bedside screen. Instruments are tracked by attaching a similar tool used for registration, monitored by the overhead camera, and viewable on the bedside screen.[71] In one study, 78% of surgeons believed that detection of at-risk structures was improved after using this system.[71] Another system that has been studied for this purpose but is no longer available is the Explorer Liver system (Analogic Corporation, Peabody, MA, USA). This system used CT 3D reconstructed image registration and infrared optically tracked tools. A tracked stylus was used to trace portions of the liver, and a tracked ultrasound further assists with identification of tumors. This method was applied in 50 patients, and with the tracked ultrasound, the surgical plan was adjusted in 5 of 50 (10%) patients.[72] These are nascent technologies that have not entered the mainstream but are mentioned here as methodologies for segmental liver resection likely to be used in the future.

Drainage of the Abdominal Cavity

Multiple studies have suggested that hepatic resection should be performed without intraoperative drainage catheter placement when possible (see Chapter 27). This was first suggested by Franco in 1989,[73] in a prospective study of 61 consecutive patients, and confirmed by a large prospective randomized control trial by Fong et al. in 1996.[74]

A drain should be considered in four select cases. The first case where drainage catheter placement should be considered is ongoing biliary leakage from the cut surface of the liver that cannot be controlled with clips or sutures. The second situation is when a diaphragmatic resection is performed. In that situation, if there is a bile leak, it would be better drained through an abdominal drain than have it fistulize through the chest via a chest tube. The third indication is an infected field. Fourth would be in patients with chronic obstruction of the bile duct where many dilated bile ducts are at the cut edge.

If a drainage catheter is indicated, it would be preferred to drain it without suction to a gravity bag. If suction is used, a low-pressure bulb suction should be used and not high-pressure suction that may dislodge sutures and ties.[75]

The references for this chapter can be found online by accessing the accompanying Expert Consult website.

Hepatic resection for biliary tract cancer: Gallbladder cancer

Nicole M. Nevarez, Michelle R. Ju, and Adam C. Yopp

INTRODUCTION

Although gallbladder cancer is rare, accounting for just 1.2% of all global cancers,[1] it is the most common biliary tract malignancy, making up 80% to 95% of all biliary cancer diagnoses[2] (see Chapter 49). Gallbladder cancer occurs most often in patients in their fifth decade of life and has a significant female predominance, with females affected 3 to 4 times as often as males.[3] Although the underlying pathogenesis of gallbladder cancer is unknown, several risk factors have been identified that share a common characteristic of gallbladder inflammation,[4] including gallstone disease,[5,6] gallbladder polyps,[7] primary sclerosing cholangitis,[8] and chronic infections with organisms such as *Salmonella typhi*[9,10] and *Helicobacter bilis*[11,12] in endemic areas (see Chapters 9E and 49).

Gallbladder cancer portends dismal prognosis as 70% to 90% of cancers are diagnosed at an advanced and thus noncurative stage.[13] Median overall survival is 6 months, with a 5-year survival rate of just 5%.[14] Systemic therapies have limited effectiveness, and surgical resection remains the only potentially curative therapy. Although surgery is the only potentially curative treatment option, survival following surgery is highly variable, ranging from 10% to 100% at 5 years depending on disease stage and extent of resection[15–17] (see Chapters 9E and 49). In this chapter, we discuss the surgical management of gallbladder cancer, management of port site recurrences, and timing of re-resection for incidentally discovered gallbladder cancer following routine cholecystectomy.

SURGICAL MANAGEMENT OF GALLBLADDER CANCER

Incidentally Diagnosed Gallbladder Cancer

More than half of gallbladder cancers are incidentally diagnosed during evaluation and treatment for presumed benign biliary disease[18,19] (see Chapters 12, 34, and 49). A diagnosis of malignancy is either made intraoperatively or, more commonly, postoperatively based on histopathologic examination of the cholecystectomy specimen.

In patients with incidentally diagnosed gallbladder cancer recognized intraoperatively during cholecystectomy (see Chapters 34 and 36), a frozen section biopsy should be performed to obtain pathologic confirmation of malignancy and to determine the extent of disease.[20] If gallbladder cancer is confirmed, no further dissection is recommended and surgery should be aborted. Prior recommendations were for completion of a curative-intent resection based on surgeon comfort, but current National Comprehensive Cancer Network (NCCN) guidelines recommend cessation of the procedure, to obtain a proper staging workup, and referral of the patient to an experienced hepatobiliary center for further evaluation and definitive resection.[21] The rationale for this strategy is that residual disease (a non-R0 resection) at the initial operation despite an R0 resection is associated with outcomes equivalent to stage IV gallbladder cancer.[20,22]

When gallbladder cancer is incidentally diagnosed postoperatively on pathologic examination of the specimen, accurate confirmation of pathologic stage is of utmost importance in guiding further treatment strategies. Consideration should be given to having the specimen re-evaluated by a hepatobiliary pathology specialist to confirm pathologic staging.[21]

Whether a diagnosis of gallbladder cancer is made intraoperatively with cessation of further dissection or incidentally, postoperatively following cholecystectomy, all patients should undergo an extent of disease staging workup consisting of dynamic contrast-enhanced imaging, either computed tomography (CT) or magnetic resonance imaging (MRI) of the abdomen and pelvis plus chest CT (with or without contrast) (see Chapters 13 and 16). The role of fluorodeoxyglucose positron emission tomography (FDG-PET) in incidentally found gallbladder cancer is not well defined (see Chapters 18 and 49). A report in 63 patients with incidentally found gallbladder cancer found that in only 13% of patients did acquisition of FDG-PET imaging change management due to identification of metastatic disease.[23] Tumor markers including serum carcinoembryonic antigen (CEA) and/or cancer antigen (CA) 19-9 are also often obtained; however, although used as a prognostic biomarker, there are few data to suggest increased sensitivity or specificity compared with high-resolution imaging in the identification of metastatic disease.[24,25]

Staging Laparoscopy

Due to the high prevalence of metastatic disease and the lack of palliative surgical options in gallbladder cancer, a staging laparoscopy should be routinely performed[21,26–28] to identify occult liver, peritoneal, and lymph node metastases (see Chapters 24 and 49). Agarwal et al.[29] reported that laparotomy can be avoided in 56% of patients with unresectable gallbladder cancer with the use of staging laparoscopy. Furthermore, Butte et al.[22] demonstrated that although disseminated disease in incidentally found gallbladder cancer was an infrequent event, the likelihood of metastatic disease correlated with increasing T-stage, positive margin at initial cholecystectomy, and increasing tumor grade. Given the low risks of diagnostic laparoscopy and the benefits of avoiding a necessary laparotomy in the presence of disseminated disease, diagnostic laparoscopy should be routinely performed in all patients undergoing re-resection or primary resection of gallbladder cancer.

To perform a staging laparoscopy, entry into the abdomen is obtained with a Veress needle, an optical trocar, or an open cutdown method based on surgeon preference. A thorough

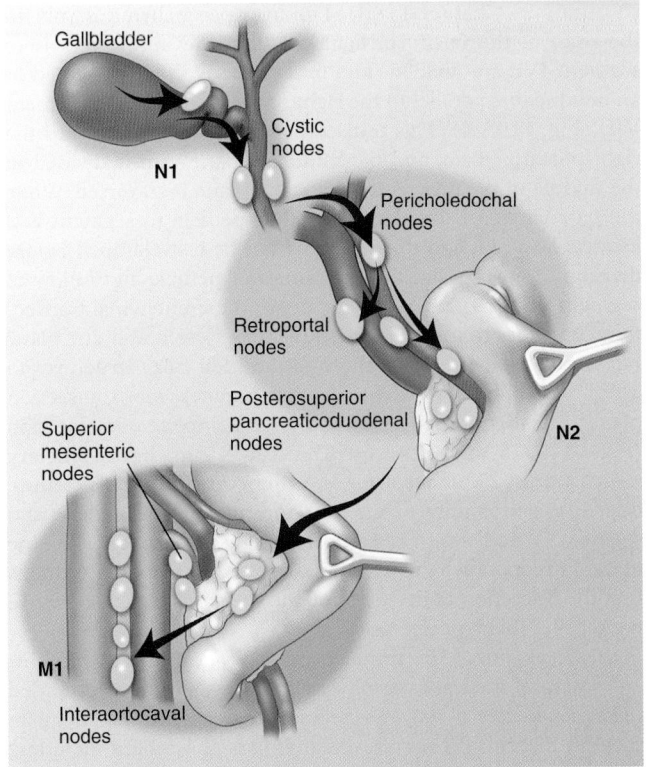

FIGURE 119A.1 The lymph node basins and their respective roles in staging in gallbladder cancer. (From Qadan M, Kingham TP. Technical aspects of gallbladder cancer surgery. *Surg Clin North Am.* 2016;96[2]: 229–245. doi:10.1016/j.suc.2015.12.007)

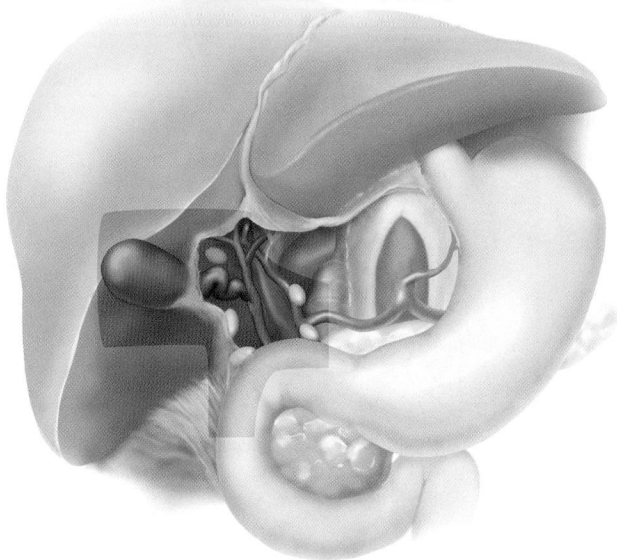

FIGURE 119A.2 Illustration of a radical cholecystectomy, which includes a cholecystectomy, a segment IVb/V partial hepatectomy, and a hepatoduodenal lymphadenectomy. (From Qadan M, Kingham TP. Technical aspects of gallbladder cancer surgery. *Surg Clin North Am.* 2016;96[2]:229–245. doi:10.1016/j.suc.2015.12.007)

inspection of both the visceral and parietal peritoneum in the abdomen and pelvis and the greater omentum is performed to identify metastatic lesions. If any suspicious areas are identified, frozen section biopsy is performed. A Kocher maneuver is performed reflecting the second portion of the duodenum and pancreatic head medially exposing the retropancreatic and aortocaval lymph nodes, which are inspected for abnormalities indicating N2 lymph node involvement (Fig. 119A.1). If metastatic disease in the form of either peritoneal carcinomatosis, omental deposits, or N2 lymphadenopathy is identified, long-term outcomes following surgical resection are rare and thus the procedure is complete with no further resection. If no metastatic disease is identified, the operation proceeds according to operative intent, based on underlying cancer stage.

Surgical Treatment of Incidentally Found Early Stage Gallbladder Cancer (T1 and T2) (also see Chapter 49)

In T1a gallbladder cancer there is absence of muscular layer invasion as tumor cells are limited to the lamina propria, therefore simple cholecystectomy without lymph node dissection is appropriate (see Chapter 36). This can be performed using minimally invasive approaches (laparoscopically/robotically, see Chapters 127A and 127D) or an open approach. Historically, an open approach was preferred in cancer operations; however, Feng et al.[30] demonstrated that patients with Tis and T1a gallbladder cancer who underwent laparoscopic simple cholecystectomy had 100% 5-year survival, indicating favorable oncologic outcomes in laparoscopic resection. A simple cholecystectomy performed for gallbladder cancer is similar to a cholecystectomy performed for benign biliary disease; however, a few important differences must be

considered. First, avoiding iatrogenic gallbladder perforation is imperative, as bile spillage is associated with a significantly higher risk of port site metastases (12.3% vs. 5.1%; $P = .035$) and local recurrences (22% vs. 11.7%; $P = .034$) with a nonsignificant trend toward a lower rate of peritoneal carcinomatosis (12.1% vs. 15.1%).[31] Using a laparoscopic retrieval bag for specimen extraction can also decrease the risk of port site recurrences in general but especially if the gallbladder is perforated.[32]

In T1b and T2 tumors, simple cholecystectomy fails to offer optimal oncologic benefit compared with radical resection, consisting of re-resection of the hepatic bed (partial hepatectomy of segments IVb/V) and hepatoduodenal lymphadenectomy (Fig. 119A.2). In both T1b and T2 tumors, simple cholecystectomy is associated with 5-year survival rates of 20% to 40% compared with 70% to 90% following radical resection.[33] Both incidence rates of residual disease within the hepatic parenchyma and lymph node metastatic disease are associated with advanced T stage. In T1b tumors, residual hepatic disease incidence of 10% and lymph node metastatic disease of 10% to 20% is associated with locoregional recurrence rates of 20% to 50%. Furthermore, in T2 tumors, hepatoduodenal lymph node metastatic disease has been reported in 30% to 60% of patients.[34–36]

Surgical Treatment of Incidentally Found Advanced Stage Gallbladder Cancer (T3 and T4)

T3 tumors invade through the visceral peritoneum of the gallbladder with direct extension into the liver or an adjacent organ, and although they are treated in a similar fashion as T1b and T2 tumors, the extent of resection to ensure a negative surgical margin is often greater and can encompass an extensive hepatic resection, bile duct resection, and/or concomitant adjacent organ resection. T3 tumors have a higher incidence of residual disease and metastatic lymph node involvement compared with T1b and T2 tumors, 36% and 46%, respectively.[37] T4 tumors encompass the main portal vein or hepatic artery and/or two or more adjacent organs, and the perioperative morbidity of extensive vascular reconstruction generally precludes

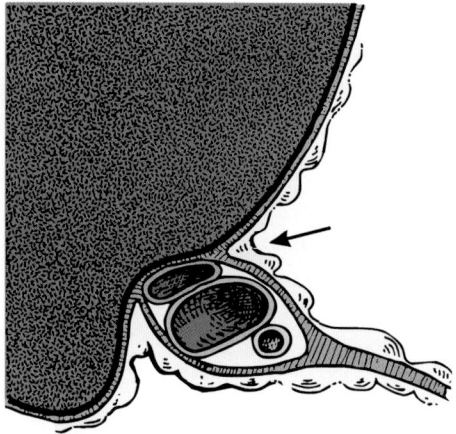

FIGURE 119A.3 **The hilar plate.** An important initial step of a partial hepatectomy of segment IVb/V is lowering of the hilar plate, which includes separating segment IV from the portal triad (see Chapter 103).

upfront surgical resection and is unwarranted. The role of neoadjuvant chemotherapy and chemoradiation therapy in advanced gallbladder cancer is discussed further in Chapter 49.

Extent and Technique of Hepatic Margin Resection (also see Chapters 49 and 118)

Extent of hepatic resection in incidentally found gallbladder cancer is predicated on the extent of underlying tumor involvement and ranges from a segment IVb/V partial hepatectomy to an extended right hepatectomy. The goal of the hepatic resection is to ensure that residual parenchymal disease is completely resected and operative planning is aided through the review of preoperative axial imaging and intraoperative ultrasonography (IOUS) (see Chapter 24). The use of IOUS is particularly important as vascular anatomy including middle hepatic vein branches can be accurately delineated ensuring controlled hepatic parenchymal transection and minimization of blood loss.

In a partial hepatectomy involving segments IVb/V typically the resection begins by lowering the hilar plate (Fig. 119A.3) to avoid injury to the left bile duct, exposure and control of the vessels within the umbilical fissure, and parenchymal dissection to the right of the falciform ligament and along the principal

scissura (see Chapter 118B). The liver parenchyma is split to the right of the falciform ligament, and the inflow vessels to segment IVb are divided. The liver tissue is then transected in an oblique line parallel to the right scissura to preserve segment VIII (Fig. 119A.4). This transection is then carried toward the right portal pedicle, and the middle hepatic vein is divided in the middle of the liver as the principal plane is traversed. While the parenchyma is divided, the inflow pedicle to segment V is located, secured, and divided. This can be test-clamped before division to ensure that the right anterior pedicle and inflow to segment VIII are preserved. The depth of parenchymal transection continues to include the gallbladder fossa and cystic plate, but it must remain above the right and left hilar structures to avoid any injury. The right and left parenchymal transection planes are then joined at this level to complete the resection (Figs. 119A.5 and 119A.6). Meticulous care ligating biliary radicles must be undertaken at all junctures in the procedure due to the proximity of the anterior right portal pedicle and segment IV pedicles to avoid postoperative biliary leak. The use of the intraoperative Pringle maneuver and postoperative drains is at the discretion of the surgeon, but there is a lack of evidence warranting their routine use.[38,39]

If the extent of the tumor burden is such that there is involvement of the right portal vein or artery, a right or extended right hepatectomy may be necessary to ensure an adequate surgical margin. Preoperative planning is paramount including determination of future liver remnant size to reduce perioperative morbidity and mortality (see Chapter 4). The use of neoadjuvant therapy in these instances where major anatomic hepatic resections are contemplated is warranted to assess underlying tumor biology and to avoid unnecessary surgical resections (see Chapter 49). The technical details of right hepatectomy and extended right hepatectomy are discussed further in Chapter 118A.

Concomitant solid organ resection including the colon and duodenum in well-selected patients with no evidence of disseminated disease, usually following a period of neoadjuvant therapy to better assess underlying tumor biology, is reasonable.

Extent and Technique of Lymphadenectomy

Due to T-stage correlation with lymph node metastases, portal or hepatoduodenal lymphadenectomy is routinely performed,

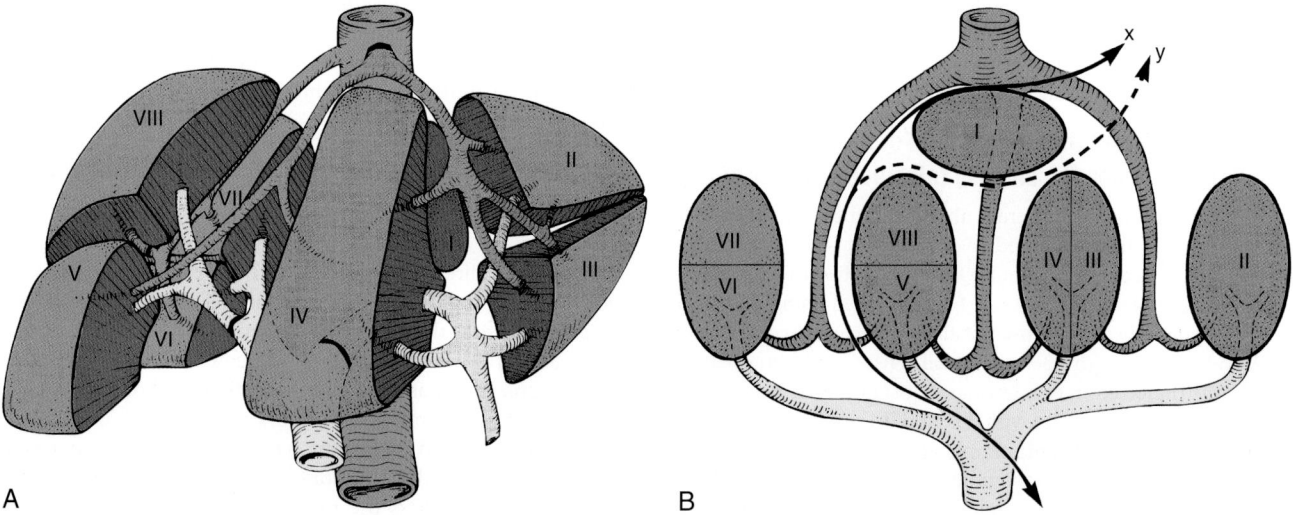

A

B

FIGURE 119A.4 **A,** Illustration showing the segments of the liver. **B,** Illustration of an extended left hepatectomy. The solid line labeled *x* and dotted line labeled *y* indicate the removal and preservation, respectively, of the caudate lobe in an extended left hepatectomy (see Chapter 2).

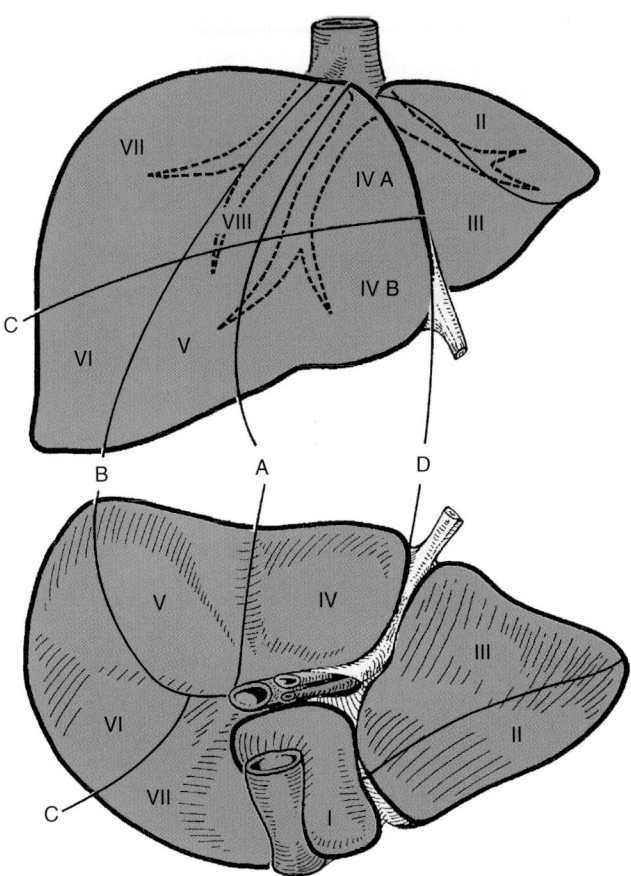

FIGURE 119A.5 **Lines of resection for excision of various segments.** Resection of segments VIb and V are bordered by *B, C,* and *D* (see Chapter 2).

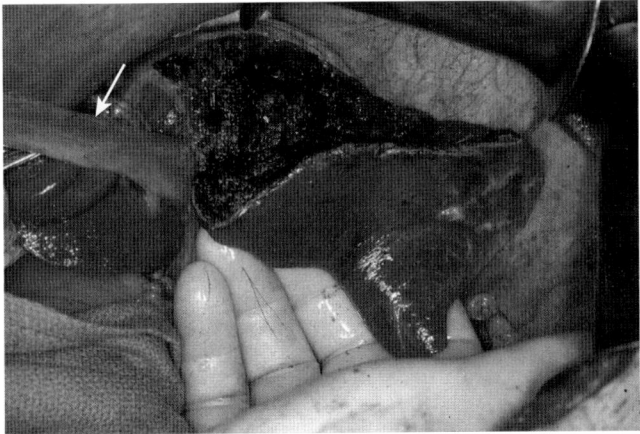

FIGURE 119A.6 **Segment III resection.** The *arrow* indicates the ligamentum teres.

in addition to hepatic resection in T1b-stage tumors and greater. Lymph node dissection includes retrieval of N1 lymph nodes, located in the gastrohepatic ligament, retroduodenal space, and hepatoduodenal ligament at the porta hepatis (see Fig. 119A.2). The procedure begins by performing a thorough Kocher maneuver mobilizing the duodenum, allowing for

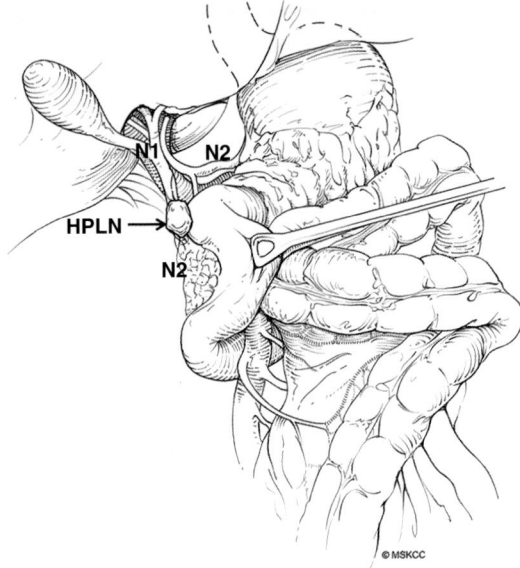

FIGURE 119A.7 The highest peripancreatic lymph node, which lies between the N1 and N2 lymph node basins. (From Kelly KJ, Dukleska K, Kuk D, et al. Prognostic significance of the highest peripancreatic lymph node in biliary tract adenocarcinoma. *Ann Surg Oncol.* 2014;21[3]:979–985. doi:10.1245/s10434-013-3352-4)

resection of the lymphatic tissue along the common bile duct near the pancreatic head. The highest peripancreatic lymph node, at the junction of the common bile duct and superior border of the pancreas, delineates between N1 and N2 nodal basins and has been demonstrated to be prognostic of disease-specific and recurrence-free survival[40] (Fig. 119A.7). At this point, enlarged lymph nodes within the aortocaval and retropancreatic basins should be sampled intraoperatively via frozen specimen pathologic assessment and if deemed malignant, further dissection should cease as this is consistent with M1 disease. The peritoneum is sharply incised overlying the structures of the porta hepatis, identifying and resecting the lymphatic tissue and identifying the common hepatic artery, common bile duct, and main portal vein. The common bile duct and then the common hepatic duct is completely cleared of lymphatic tissue anteriorly from the base of the liver to the superior border of the pancreatic head. Using the cystic duct stump for retraction, the common bile duct is retracted medially to allow for dissection of the lymphatic tissue posterior and lateral of the common bile duct and anterior to the portal vein. At the end of the dissection, the anterior surface of the portal vein is visible and all the lymphatic tissue around the common and proper hepatic artery and common bile duct is resected (Fig. 119A.8).

Based on the American Joint Comittee on Cancer (AJCC) eighth edition, a minimum of six lymph nodes is indicative of an adequate nodal staging[41] and has been associated with improved survival outcomes. Fan et al.[42] demonstrated an association of a survival benefit with pathologic examination of six lymph nodes compared with one to five lymph nodes. Furthermore, Ito et al.[43] concluded that disease-specific survival of patients with N0 gallbladder cancer is based on a total lymph node count (TLNC); less than six was significantly worse than that seen in N0 patients with a TLNC greater than six (24 vs. 41 months, $P < .001$). Sahara et al.[44] and Tsilimigras et al.[45]

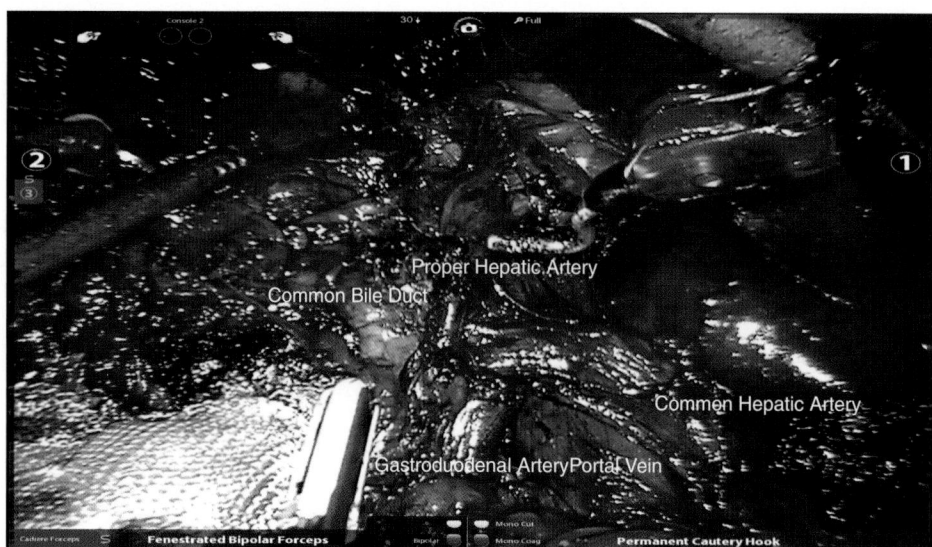

FIGURE 119A.8 The view at the completion of a hepatoduodenal lymphadenectomy showing the skeletonized common bile duct, common (and proper) hepatic artery, and the anterior surface of the main portal vein.

determined that small lymph node yield resulted in lower therapeutic index for surgery and higher hazard of death, respectively. Additionally, it is not recommended to extend the lymphadenectomy to include the N2 lymph node basin as this is associated with increased perioperative morbidity with a lack of survival benefit.[46]

Extent of Extrahepatic Biliary Tree Resection

Extrahepatic biliary tree resection should not be routinely performed as it has not been demonstrated to improve outcomes in gallbladder cancer, rather increasing perioperative morbidity. Tumoral involvement of the cystic duct stump margin is confirmed early during the definitive surgical resection through intraoperative frozen section biopsy. If the cystic duct stump margin is consistent with malignancy, a bile duct resection with division of the bile duct at the level of the duodenum may be necessary to obtain negative surgical margins. Reconstruction of the biliary tree is completed using a Roux-en-Y hepaticoje-junostomy[21,26,28,47,48] (see Chapter 32). Furthermore, routine common bile duct resection is not warranted solely for the purpose of acquiring more lymph nodes as it has not been shown to improve lymph node yield.[48]

Management of Surgical Port Sites (also see Chapter 49)

In patients with incidentally discovered gallbladder cancer following laparoscopic cholecystectomy, there is a potential risk of occult tumor seeding at port sites. This may be exacerbated by spillage of bile or gallstones during the initial cholecystectomy, and port site recurrences are estimated to occur in approximately 17% to 19% of patients.[49,50] Because of this high percentage, historically, port site excision during re-resection for gallbladder cancer was advocated. However, recent studies have called into question this dogma, citing increased morbidity of port site excision with no survival advantage.[50]

A 2017 multicenter analysis from the US Extrahepatic Biliary Malignancy Consortium examined 266 patients with incidentally discovered gallbladder cancer, 73% of whom underwent curative re-resection over 15 years at 10 institutions.[51] Of the patients who underwent re-resection, 24% received port

site excision. There were no differences in 3-year overall survival between groups that did versus did not undergo port site excision. Furthermore, distant disease recurrence rate was identical between the two groups (80% for port site excision vs. 81% for no excision; $P = 1.0$). As port site recurrences are considered a harbinger of systemic disease and best treated with nonlocalized therapy such as local excision, routine resection of port sites during reexploration for gallbladder cancer is not advised.

Timing of Re-resection

Although the current recommendation is to perform radical re-resection in select patients with incidentally discovered gallbladder cancer, the optimal time interval for re-resection following initial cholecystectomy has been debated[18] in a recent retrospective review of 207 patients with incidentally discovered gallbladder cancer who underwent reoperation, divided patients into three time intervals from date of original cholecystectomy to date of reoperation: less than 4 weeks, 4 to 8 weeks, and greater than 8 weeks. After adjusting for clinicopathologic and surgical factors, patients who underwent radical re-resection between 4 and 8 weeks had the longest median overall survival (40.4 months vs. 17.4 months for <4 weeks and 22.4 months for >8 weeks; $P = 0.03$). An intentional period of delaying radical re-resection is paramount to ensuring that careful evaluation of residual disease and metastatic spread is undertaken, as well as to observe the underlying tumor biology. Although there is a possibility of delaying definitive re-resection to such a length as to compromise outcomes, a recent study has demonstrated that the median time from incidentally found gallbladder cancer following cholecystectomy to radical re-resection is 52 days, within the 4- to 8-week timeframe.[37]

Nonincidental Gallbladder Cancer

Currently, approximately half of all patients who present with gallbladder cancer are detected incidentally during or after elective or emergent cholecystectomy. Previous studies have demonstrated that compared with incidentally found gallbladder cancer, patients diagnosed with nonincidental gallbladder cancer had worse median overall survival when adjusted for clinicodemographic variables and tumor staging.[18,52,53] Likely the differences in survival are secondary to worse tumor biology in nonincidentally found gallbladder cancer and more wide-ranging patient signs and symptoms of malignancy. Although the diagnostic workup for both incidentally and nonincidentally found gallbladder cancer is similar (see Chapter 49), due to theoretical worse underlying tumor biology (see Chapter 9E), neoadjuvant therapy is proffered in nonincidentally found gallbladder cancer before definitive resection as described previously.

Jaundice

The presence of obstructive jaundice in a newly diagnosed patient with gallbladder cancer is seen as sign of advanced disease due to likely invasion of the extrahepatic biliary tree (see Chapters 8 and 49). Historically the presence of obstructive jaundice as an initial symptom precludes surgical resection[62] in a landmark study, demonstrated in a cohort of 82 patients who presented with jaundice-associated gallbladder cancer that only 4 patients underwent surgical resection with a negative margin. In a matched cohort of 158 nonjaundiced patients the median disease-specific survival was 16 months, compared with 6 months with no disease-free survivors at 2 years in the jaundiced cohort. Recent data have demonstrated that although jaundice is associated with worse survival, when adjusting for N status, liver invasion, and resection margin, jaundice is not an independent predictor of poor outcome.[54] Given the relatively poor prognosis of obstructive jaundice in a newly diagnosed patient with gallbladder cancer, careful patient selection is warranted before radical surgical resection. Likely following endoscopic or percutaneous decompression of the biliary tree, a period of neoadjuvant chemotherapy is warranted to further determine the tumor biology before resection.

Minimally Invasive Techniques in Gallbladder Cancer Resection

Historically, development and implementation of either laparoscopic or robotic assisted surgical techniques for curative treatment of gallbladder cancer has been hindered due to concerns over higher risk of intraperitoneal cancer dissemination, port site recurrences, and inadequate hepatic parenchymal resection or lymphadenectomy.[55–57] Although minimally invasive surgical (MIS) techniques are becoming increasingly used in oncologic resections in other hepatic and pancreatobiliary malignancies (see Chapter 127), its use in gallbladder cancer resection has only recently been recognized. Recent studies have demonstrated that MIS techniques for extended cholecystectomy are associated with similar oncologic outcomes as seen in open procedures.[58–61] Briefly, our preference is to use a robotic assisted approach with the patient in a lithotomy position with the assistant surgeon standing between the patient's legs. Robotic port placement is shown in Figure 119A.9. We begin the procedure by performing a thorough IOUS of the liver as described in Chapter 24. Before performing hepatic resection we perform the hepatoduodenal lymphadenectomy to allow for better visualization during the subsequent liver resection (Figs. 119A.10 and 119A.11). The principles of MIS techniques for radical cholecystectomy, hepatic resection, and hepatoduodenal lymphadenectomy should be similar to open procedures and are discussed in Chapters 127D and 127E.

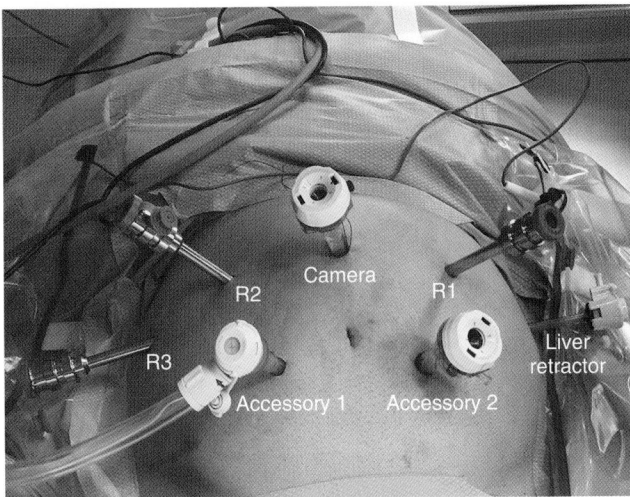

FIGURE 119A.9 Port placement for a robotic assisted radical cholecystectomy with segment 4b/5 hepatic resection with hepatoduodenal lymphadenectomy (see Chapter 127).

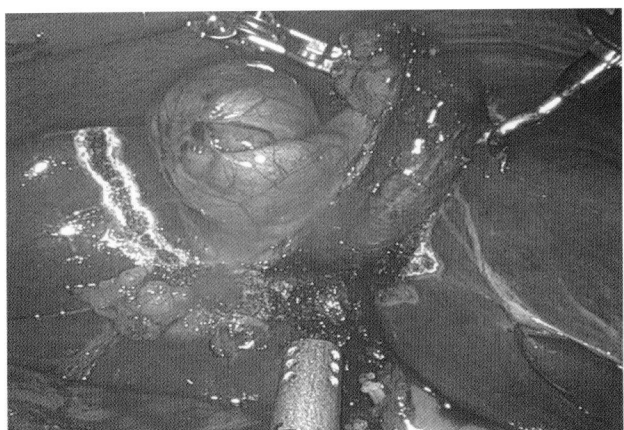

FIGURE 119A.10 The proposed resection margins of the segment IVb/V partial hepatectomy in an incidentally diagnosed gallbladder cancer with the gallbladder already removed.

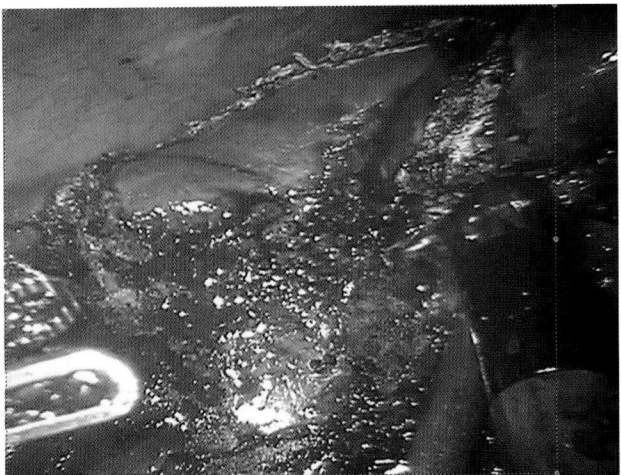

FIGURE 119A.11 The proposed resection margins of a segment IVb/V partial hepatectomy in a nonincidentally diagnosed gallbladder cancer as the gallbladder is still present.

CONCLUSION

Current recommendations for the surgical management of gall-bladder cancer include simple cholecystectomy for stage ≤T1a, radical cholecystectomy for stage T1b to T2, and radical chole-cystectomy with possible adjacent organ resection for stage T3. Although overall prognosis of gallbladder cancer is poor, im-provements have been made in identifying high-risk patients, preoperative staging accuracy, and patient selection for surgical resection. Recognizing patients with potential gallbladder cancer at an early stage is key to improving prognosis, since surgical resection at an early stage provides the best chance of long-term survival. The use of neoadjuvant chemotherapy before radical surgical resection is often recommended to further delineate tumor biology. Open or minimally invasive techniques of resec-tion are used at the discretion of the surgeon and have similar oncologic results.

The references for this chapter can be found online by accessing the accompanying Expert Consult website.

Hilar cholangiocarcinoma: Standard and extended resections of perihilar cholangiocarcinoma

Takashi Mizuno, Tomoki Ebata, and Masato Nagino

OVERVIEW

Perihilar cholangiocarcinoma[1,2] is a devastating disease because the majority of patients are diagnosed with advanced disease at initial presentation. At the present time, surgical resection offers the only possibility of cure for this disease, and achieving tumor-free surgical margins is one of the main goals of resection. Hilar bile duct resection with or without limited hepatectomy has been performed previously but is likely to result in positive margins, yielding unsatisfactory long-term outcomes. Recent advances in surgical techniques (see Chapters 51 and 118), additional understanding of tumor pathology (see Chapter 47), and improved presurgical management (see Chapters 25 and 26) have driven hepatobiliary surgeons to perform hemihepatectomy with bile duct resection as a standard procedure.[3–6] In addition to standard resections, more extended procedures have been challenged to increase the resectability of the intractable malignancies in specific centers: hepatic trisectionectomy[7,8] (see Chapter 118A), combined resection with reconstruction of the hepatic inflow vascular structures[9–14] (see Chapter 122), and hepatectomy combined with pancreatoduodenectomy (hepatopancreatoduodenectomy [HPD]).[15,16] The rarity and variety of this disease, however, frequently preclude an accumulation of surgical expertise. This chapter particularly describes technical details not only of standard resections but also of the aforementioned extended resection procedures, introducing several anatomic variations that are possibly associated with technical difficulties during surgery.

PREOPERATIVE RADIOLOGIC EVALUATION FOR SURGICAL SUCCESS (SEE CHAPTER 51B)

Precise knowledge of the anatomy of the segmenta hepatis, hepatic inflow and outflow vessels, and biliary channel is crucial for a successful surgery and for avoiding inadvertent intraoperative injury of the vessels to be preserved (see Chapter 2). Multiplanar reformation three-dimensional images reconstructed from images taken during dynamic enhanced multidetector-row computed tomography (CT) help not only identify the ramification pattern and running course of the hepatic arteries and portal vein but also evaluate the presence or absence of vascular involvement (see Chapter 13).[17,18] When CT images are taken before biliary drainage in patients with obstructive jaundice, the anatomic relationship between the vasculatures and dilated biliary trees is also identifiable.[19] The anatomic relationship among the hepatic arteries, portal veins, and bile ducts should also be precisely evaluated because the anatomy of the hilar vasculature differs from case to case.

STANDARD RESECTION

Standard resection for perihilar cholangiocarcinoma involves either a right or a left hemihepatectomy, caudate lobectomy, bile duct resection, and lymph node dissection followed by bilioenteric anastomosis. Perihilar tumors originate either from the large bile ducts (right hepatic duct, left hepatic duct, biliary confluence, or upper bile duct) or from the hepatic parenchyma adjacent to the hilum.[20,21] The tumors frequently invade the portal structures and the bile ducts of the caudate lobe. Preoperative imaging often underestimates tumoral infiltration in the caudate lobe; therefore a caudate lobectomy is required for curative resection of perihilar cholangiocarcinomas. Standard resections are indicated for Bismuth type I, II, and III perihilar cholangiocarcinomas without macrovascular invasion, and the resection typically proceeds in the following sequence: (1) lymphadenectomy with division of the distal bile duct; (2) vascular division of the hemiliver in the hepatic hilum; (3) mobilization of the hemiliver and caudate lobe to be resected; (4) liver parenchymal transection; and (5) division of the proximal intrahepatic bile duct.

Several types of incisions are used for laparotomy, and the authors preferentially use the upper midline incision cephalad up to the xiphoid process with the right transverse incision reaching the anterior axillary line (reverse L incision). The transverse incision is extended to the left anterior axillary line (reverse T incision) in some overweight patients as an alternative approach to gain a better surgical view. After checking for intra-abdominal distant metastasis and/or peritoneal dissemination, the curve of the duodenum is mobilized by the Kocher maneuver to evaluate the periaortic lymph nodes for staging.

LYMPHADENECTOMY WITH DIVISION OF THE DISTAL BILE DUCT

The main goal of this procedure is to achieve a negative margin at the distal bile duct and thorough lymph node dissection of the following regional lymph nodes: hilar, cystic, choledochal, portal, hepatic arterial, and posterior pancreaticoduodenal. A sufficient number of lymph nodes needs to be retrieved for accurate staging because recent studies have demonstrated that the number of lymph nodes examined is associated with survival, particularly for node-negative patients.[22–24] The authors prefer to start regional lymphadenectomy by opening the lesser sac to display the lymph nodes cranioventral to the common hepatic artery. The lymph nodes are detached from the pancreas and flipped up cranially to expose the common hepatic artery and its bifurcation into the gastroduodenal artery and proper hepatic artery (Fig. 119B.1). Retraction of

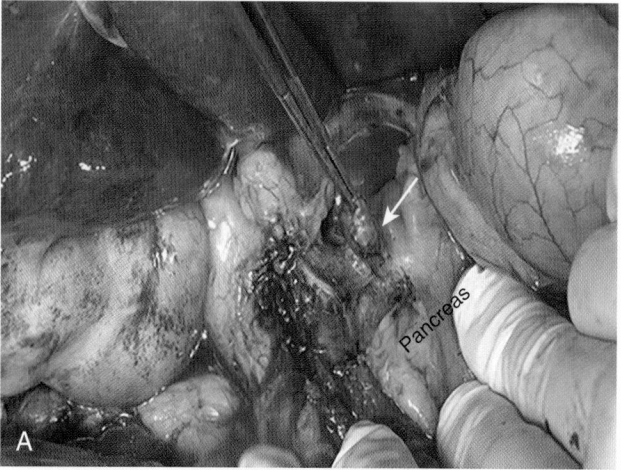

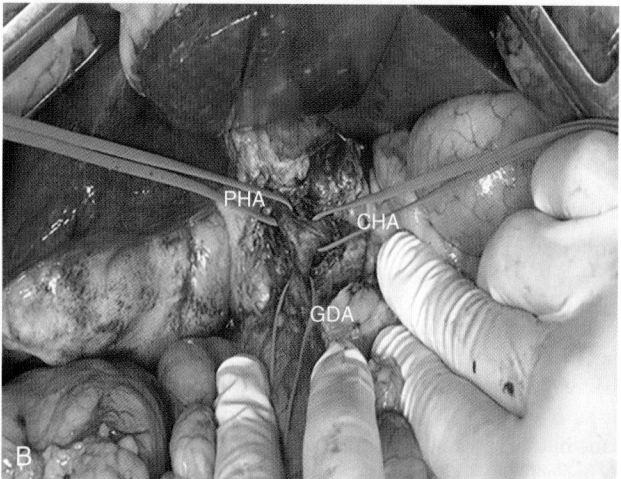

FIGURE 119B.1 Standard resection of perihilar cholangiocarcinoma. **A,** Lymph nodes cranioventral to the common hepatic artery *(white arrow)* are flipped up cranially to expose the common hepatic artery. **B,** The common hepatic artery *(CHA)*, gastroduodenal artery *(GDA)*, and proper hepatic artery *(PHA)* are isolated and taped for lymph node dissection.

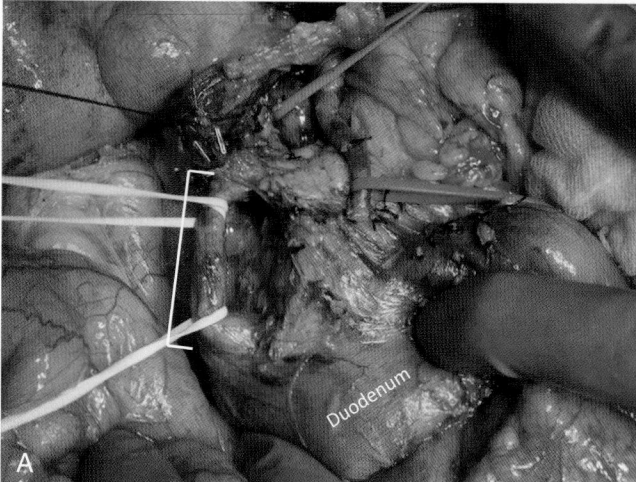

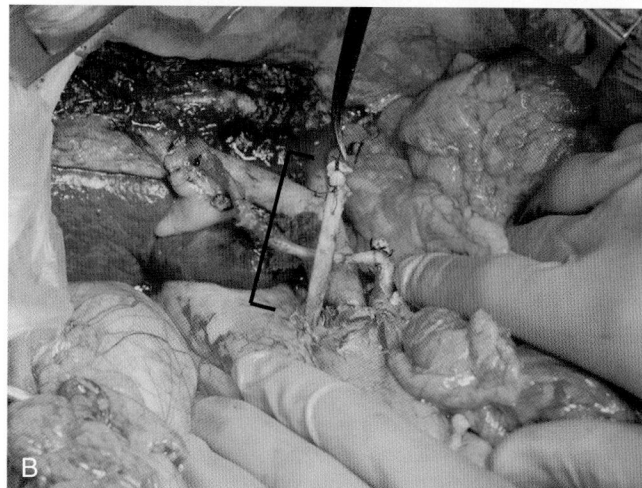

FIGURE 119B.2 Standard resection of perihilar cholangiocarcinoma. **A,** The intrapancreatic duct *(white bracket)* is widely isolated from behind the pancreas. The distal resection line can be set near the duodenum. **B,** Additional resection of the intrapancreatic bile duct when the distal duct stump has cancer involvement. The avulsion of the intrapancreatic bile duct *(black bracket)* provides an additional 4 cm in margin length.

the gastropancreatic fold to the left provides a better surgical view for lymph node dissection and avoids inadvertent injury of the left gastric artery. Next, the covering visceral peritoneum on the hepatoduodenal ligament is cut at the superior aspect of the duodenum, and the duodenal bulb is pulled down to isolate and cut the common bile duct (CBD) at the entry of the pancreatic head as far away from the tumor edge as possible to allow for a satisfactory ductal margin length. The stump of the CBD is closed with sutures, and the distal bile duct margin is submitted for frozen section examination. If the distal margin is positive according to the frozen section examination, additional resection of the intrapancreatic bile duct is possible[25] (Fig. 119B.2). The portal vein is identified and taped posteriorly between the dissected CBD and the proper hepatic artery that was taped beforehand. Then, the posterior pancreaticoduodenal lymph nodes are detached from the posterior surface of the duodenum and pancreas head, and several tiny vessels leading to the lymph nodes are cautiously ligated and cut. The lymph nodes dorsal to the portal vein and common hepatic artery are dissected in conjunction with the posterior pancreaticoduodenal lymph nodes. Finally, lymph node dissection

around the pancreatoduodenum and the common hepatic artery is completed.

After the aforementioned lymph node dissection, the peritoneum of the hepatoduodenal ligament is opened upward to the hepatic hilum, and lymph nodes in the hepatoduodenal ligament are completely dissected. The authors prefer to cut the covering peritoneum just in front of the proper hepatic artery to facilitate isolation of the artery and its bifurcation into the right and left hepatic arteries and divide connective tissue in front of the portal vein to expose and isolate the main portal vein successively.

DIVISION OF THE HILAR VASCULAR STRUCTURES

Right Hepatectomy (see Chapter 118A)

During right hepatectomy, the left hepatic artery (supplying segments II and III), middle hepatic artery (supplying segment IV), and left portal vein are isolated and detached from the hilar plate, and the right hepatic artery and portal vein are ligated and cut at the origin. For vascular division of the hepatic arteries, the left and middle hepatic arteries are isolated upward to the base of the umbilical fossa after dividing the right hepatic artery. The left hepatic artery commonly runs into the umbilical fossa to the left of the elbow of the left portal vein and in front of the ligamentum venosum. In contrast, the middle hepatic artery (the hepatic artery supplying segment IV) normally originates from the proper, right, or left hepatic artery and traverses the left portal vein into the umbilical fossa to the right of the elbow of the left portal vein. Small arterial branches supplying the caudate lobe that possibly originate from the left and middle hepatic artery at the hepatic hilus need to be cautiously ligated and divided.

For the portal vein, the right portal vein is cut at the bifurcation, and several small portal branches to the caudate lobe originating from the transverse portion of the left portal vein are ligated and cut cautiously. The ligamentum venosum is dissected left posteriorly to the elbow of the left portal vein, and the transverse portion of the left portal vein is fully detached from the hilar plate. Finally, division of the hilar portal vein is completed. Sufficient detachment of the middle hepatic artery and the transverse portion of the left portal vein from the hilar plate is mandatory because the future cut line of the left hepatic bile duct will be just to the right on the cranial side of the umbilical portion of the left portal vein and next to the hepatic entry of the middle hepatic artery and because the resection line of the proximal bile duct depends on the extent of these dissections at the hilum (Fig. 119B.3A).

Left Hepatectomy (See Chapter 118A)

During left hepatectomy, the right hepatic artery and right portal vein are isolated and detached from the hilar plate, and the middle and left hepatic arteries and left portal vein are ligated and cut at the origin. Regarding vascular division of the hepatic arteries, one problem is that the right hepatic artery normally runs just behind the hilar tumor and is susceptible to involvement. When involvement of the right hepatic artery is confirmed during the procedure, combined resection of the hepatic artery is considered, if possible (see "Combined Vascular Resection"). After division of the left and middle hepatic arteries and cystic artery, the right hepatic artery is detached from the posterior wall of the hilar bile duct, and the dissected CBD is flipped up and retracted cranioventrally. The artery is then isolated distally toward the bifurcation of the right hepatic artery into the right anterior (RAHA) and posterior hepatic (RPHA) arteries and toward the hepatic entry of the arteries. The RAHA normally runs into the hepatic entry between the right anterior portal vein and right hepatic bile duct, and, in contrast, the RPHA runs into the hepatic entry at Rouviere's sulcus, far from the hilar bile ducts. Therefore the RAHA needs to be cautiously isolated because of its close proximity to the right hilar ducts (see Fig. 119B.3B). In a minority of cases, however, the RPHA or its branch separates from the right hepatic artery and runs along the left side of the RAHA and cranially to the right portal vein (supraportal type, combined type). In such cases with an anomalous RPHA, the RPHA needs to be cautiously isolated because of its close proximity to the right hilar ducts and the RAHA[26] (Fig. 119B.4).

For the portal vein, the left portal vein is cut at the portal bifurcation, the small portal branches to the caudate lobe originating from the right portal trunk are ligated and cut cautiously, and

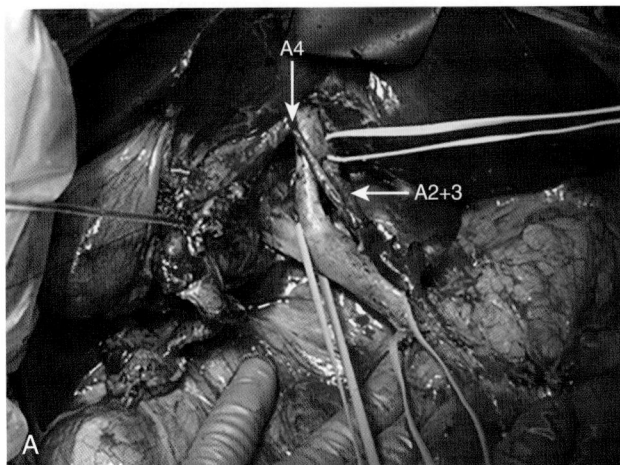

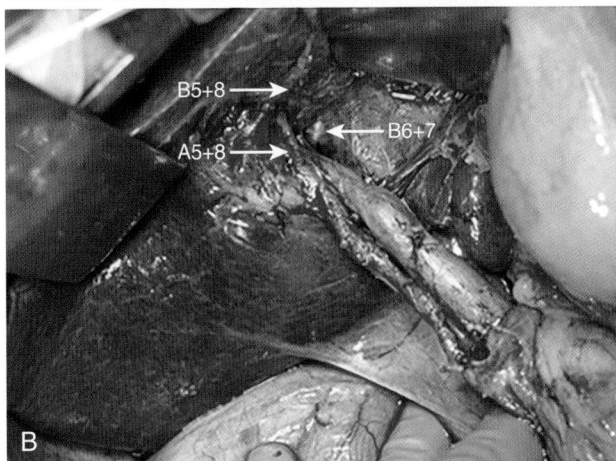

FIGURE 119B.3 A, Hilar dissection during right hepatectomy. The left hepatic artery and the left portal vein are freed from the left biliary ductal system. Arantius' duct is identified with yellow tape; the right portal vein *(with blue tape)* is about to be divided. **B,** Hilar dissection during left hepatectomy. The right anterior hepatic artery *(A5+8)* and the right portal vein are freed from the right biliary ductal system. The numerals indicate the hepatic segment according to the Couinaud classification. *A,* hepatic artery; *B,* bile duct.

the right portal trunk is isolated from the hilar plate toward the hepatic entry. Then, division of the hilar vascular structures can finally be completed. Detachment of the RAHA and right portal vein or right anterior portal vein from the ductal system as proximally as possible is mandatory because the future cut line of the hepatic bile duct margin will be just cranial to the right portal vein or right anterior portal vein and RAHA and because the resection line of the proximal bile duct depends on the extent of these dissections at the hilum (see Fig. 119B.3B).

MOBILIZATION OF THE HEMILIVER AND CAUDATE LOBE (SEE CHAPTERS 102A AND 118B)

Techniques for liver mobilization are similar to formal right or left hepatectomy except that the hemiliver is mobilized together with the caudate lobe. The authors prefer to mobilize the hemiliver and caudate lobe only from the right side in right-sided hepatectomy and from the left side in left-sided hepatectomy, preserving the collateral artery branches from the phrenic

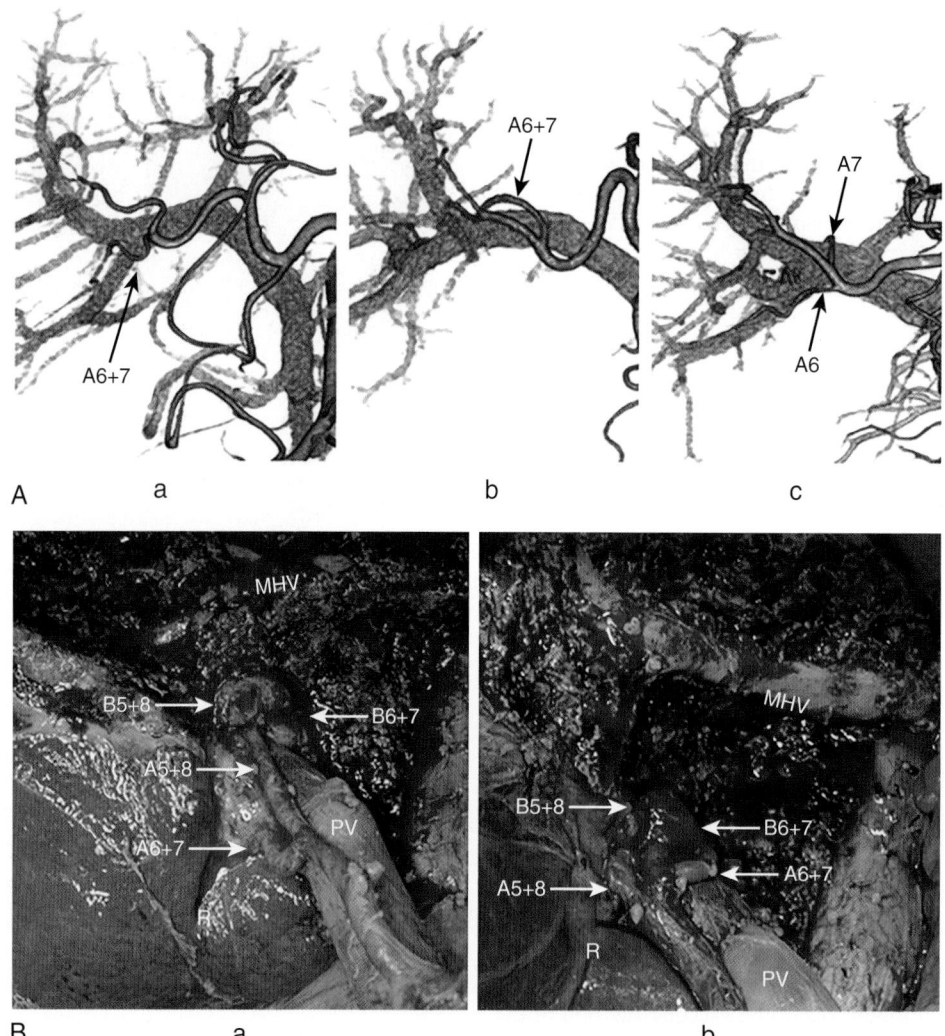

FIGURE 119B.4 Anatomic variations of the right hepatic artery. **A,** Computed tomography arteriography and portography showing the three types of the right posterior hepatic artery. The right posterior hepatic artery *(A6+7)* normally runs caudally to the right portal vein (**a**), although in a minority of cases, the anomalous right posterior hepatic artery (**b**) or its branch (**c**) runs cranially to the right portal vein. **B,** Photographs of completed left hemihepatectomies with caudate lobectomy and extrahepatic bile duct resection, paying special attention to the right posterior hepatic artery. The right posterior hepatic artery *(A6+7)* normally runs to the right of the right anterior *(A5+8)* hepatic artery and into Rouviere's sulcus (**a**); in contrast, the abnormal right posterior hepatic artery *(A6+7)* runs to the left of the right anterior hepatic artery *(A5+8)* between the bile duct and portal vein. The numerals indicate the hepatic segment according to the Couinaud classification. *A,* hepatic artery; *B/BD,* bile duct; *MHV,* middle hepatic vein; *PV,* portal vein; *R,* Rouviere's sulcus. (A, from Yoshioka Y, Ebata T, Yokoyama Y, Igami T, Sugawara G, Nagino M. "Supraportal" right posterior hepatic artery: An anatomic trap in hepatobiliary and transplant surgery. *World J Surg.* 2011;35[6]:1340–1344.)

artery and/or the adrenal artery to the remnant liver as much as possible. The caudate lobe is detached from the anterior surface of the inferior vena cava (IVC), and a number of short hepatic veins are ligated and divided. On the upper side of the IVC, the thin, band-like connective tissue bridging both edges of the caval groove in which the IVC is embedded, known as the IVC ligament, is carefully dissected. The ligamentum venosum connecting the confluence of the middle and left hepatic veins is cut at the distal end. In right-sided hepatectomy, dissection of the right hepatic vein facilitates a better surgical view for mobilization of the caudate lobe. In left-sided hepatectomy, the caudate lobe is fully detached from the anterior part of the IVC, the right border of the IVC is exposed, and the common trunk of the middle and left hepatic veins is taped (Fig. 119B.5).

LIVER PARENCHYMAL TRANSECTION (SEE CHAPTERS 102A AND 118A)

As the hepatic artery and portal vein to the hemiliver to be resected are controlled, the right and left liver are demarcated on the liver surface because of discoloration of the hemiliver to be resected. The transection line on the liver upper surface is aligned with the demarcation line, projected through a plane running from the medial margin of the gallbladder bed to the left of the IVC posteriorly. The transection line on the liver undersurface is different between right and left hepatectomy: it is along the medial margin of the gallbladder bed on the liver edge to the right of the base of the umbilical fossa in right hepatectomy and along the craniomedial margin to the

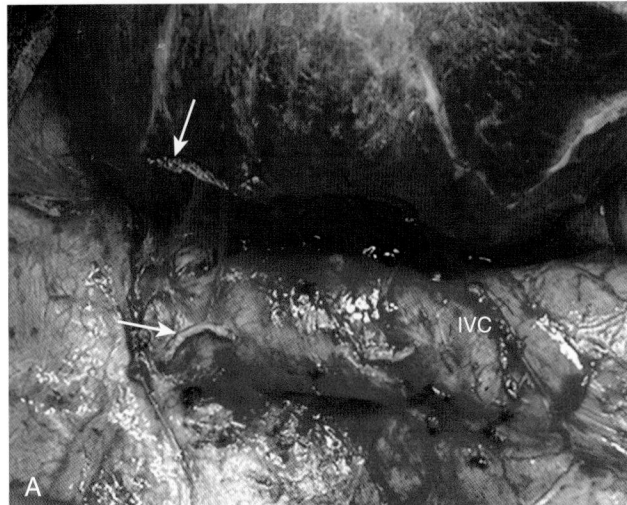

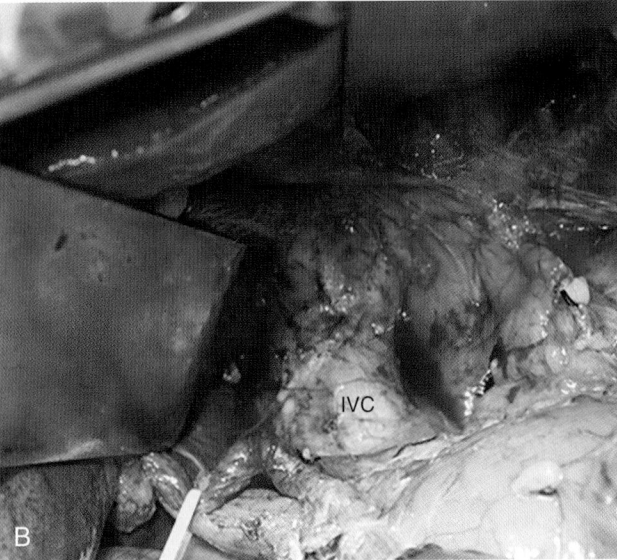

FIGURE 119B.5 Mobilization of the hemiliver together with the caudate lobe. **A,** Right hemihepatectomy. The right hepatic vein has already been cut *(white arrows)*. **B,** Left hemihepatectomy. The right border of the inferior vena cava is fully exposed. *IVC,* Inferior vena cava.

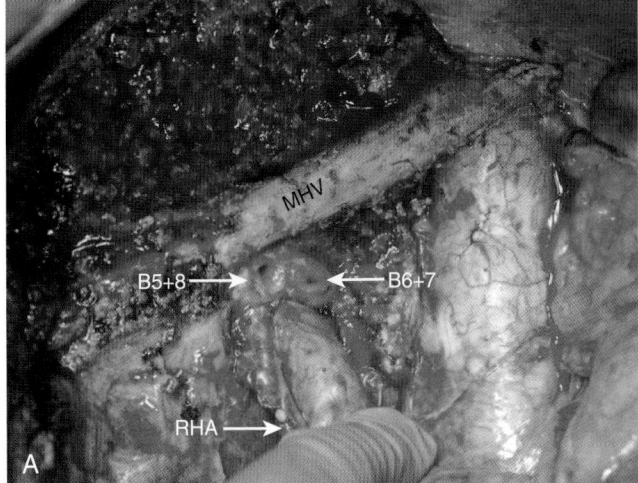

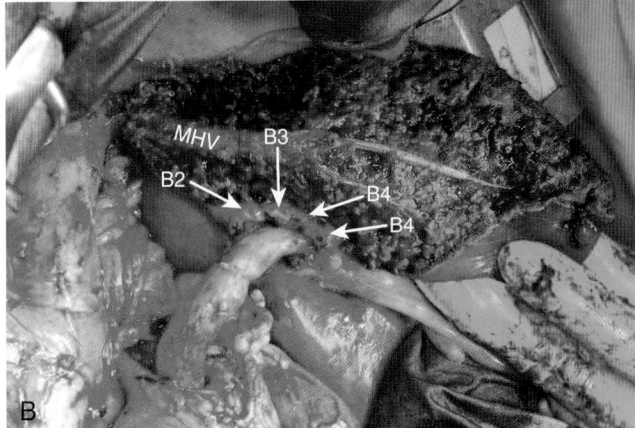

FIGURE 119B.6 Photographs of a completed hemihepatectomy with caudate lobectomy and extrahepatic bile duct resection. **A,** Left hemihepatectomy; *RHA,* right hepatic artery. **B,** Right hemihepatectomy. The numerals indicate the hepatic segment according to the Couinaud classification. *B,* Bile duct; *MHV,* middle hepatic vein.

hepatic entry of the right anterior hepatic duct in left hepatectomy. For parenchymal transection, the authors prefer to use a cavitron ultrasonic surgical aspirator (CUSA) or an instrument to facilitate the fracture technique under intermittent hepatic inflow vessel clamping for 15 or 20 minutes at 5-minute intervals.

Liver parenchymal transection is first performed along the aforementioned demarcation line, and the middle hepatic vein is exposed and preserved towards the hepatic venous confluence until the transection reaches the confluence of the middle hepatic vein. Second, the direction of transection is turned to the left just ventrally to the ligamentum venosum in right hepatectomy, and the direction is turned posteriorly toward the right edge of the IVC in left hepatectomy. Finally, the intrahepatic bile ducts are isolated and dissected to the right side of the umbilical portion of the left portal vein in right hepatectomy and cranially to the right portal vein or the right anterior portal vein in left hepatectomy (Fig. 119B.6).[6,8]

RECONSTRUCTION

After removal of the specimen, several orifices of the bile ducts can be identified at the proximal stump. These orifices may be separate and distant from each other and sutured for unification if possible. Bilioentelic continuity is re-established by Roux-en-Y hepaticojejunostomy (see Chapter 32).[27] The jejunal limb is cut approximately 20 to 30 cm on the anal side from the Treitz ligament and brought through the mesocolon to traverse in the lesser sac between the pancreas and stomach to reach the hepatic hilum (retrocolic-retrogastric route). This route is preferentially used because the jejunal limb easily reaches the intrahepatic bile duct stump irrespective of the thickness of the transverse mesocolon and greater omentum.[28] Bilioenteric anastomosis is performed with mucosa-to-mucosa alignment, either by continuous or interrupted sutures using 5-0 absorbable monofilament sutures. External stents, which are inserted through the stump of the jejunal limb, may not always be necessary; however, the authors prefer to employ these stents because they facilitate anastomosis and help with postoperative biliary decompression and prevent severe obstructive cholangitis.

EXTENDED RESECTION

Hepatic Trisectionectomy (See Chapter 118A)

In patients with Bismuth type IV tumors, R0 resections are difficult to achieve by standard hepatectomy because of bilateral second-order biliary radicle involvement. Bismuth and colleagues[29] proposed in 1992 that tumors considered type IV based on his classification system were unresectable, and surgeons have followed this "dogma" for a long time. This concept is no longer valid because either a left or "anatomic" right hepatic trisectionectomy allows for R0 resection with negative proximal margins in many patients with type IV tumors.[7,8,30] Several techniques for hepatic trisectionectomy are similar to those for standard resection; however, the approaches for dividing the hilar vascular structures and hepatic parenchymal transection are different and require special technical expertise. In addition, minor but important anatomic variations in the hilar vasculature should be noted to ensure a successful surgery because misidentification and/or inadvertent injury of the portal vein and hepatic artery may cause serious ischemia in the remnant liver, leading to fatal postoperative hepatic insufficiency, especially after trisectionectomy.

Right Trisectionectomy

Techniques for lymphadenectomy and liver mobilization in anatomic right trisectionectomy are similar to those in right hepatectomy (see Chapter 118A). To divide the hilar vascular structures, unlike for right hepatectomy, the hepatic artery and portal branches supplying segment IV are divided, as well as the right hepatic artery and right portal vein.[7,30,31] The hepatic artery supplying segment IV (known as the middle hepatic artery) normally originates extrahepatically from the left, right, or proper hepatic artery and is divided at the origin. In contrast, the left hepatic artery normally originates from the proper hepatic artery, runs the leftmost in the hepatoduodenal ligament and enters the umbilical fossa to the left of the umbilical portion of the left portal vein. In a minority of cases, however, an anomalous common trunk of the artery supplying segments II, III, and IV runs into the hepatic entry to the left or right of the base of the umbilical portion of the left portal vein. The anomalous common trunk ramifies into the hepatic arteries to segment IV and to segments II and III cranially to the umbilical portion of the left portal vein in the umbilical fossa.[32,33] In such cases, the hepatic artery supplying segment IV is ligated and divided by opening the umbilical fossa, and the artery supplying segments II and III needs to be cautiously detached from the hilar plate behind the umbilical portion of the left portal vein.

For the portal vein, the umbilical portion of the left portal vein is exposed by dissecting the serosa on the right side of the umbilical fossa to isolate the portal branches supplying segment IV at the origin after dividing the right portal vein and detaching the transverse position of the left portal vein from the hilar plate. Next, small portal branches arising from the cranial side of the umbilical portion are carefully ligated and divided, and the umbilical portion of the left portal vein is rotated to the left. Then, the proximal side of the ligamentum venosum is ligated and divided cranially to the elbow of the left portal vein. Finally, the cranial side of the umbilical portion is completely detached from the umbilical plate.[7,30,31] With this procedure, the left hepatic duct can be resected approximately 10 mm beyond the confluence compared with that in a "classic" right hepatectomy. Consequently, the incidence of negative proximal ductal margins in patients with Bismuth type IV tumors with right-sided predominance increases from 57% with right hepatectomy to 89% with anatomic right trisectionectomy.[30]

After vascular division, the left medial and lateral sectors are demarcated on the liver surface by discoloration of the left medial sector. The transection line on the liver upper surface aligns with the demarcation line and projects through a plane running from the round ligament anteriorly to the left of the IVC posteriorly. The liver parenchyma is transected along the demarcation (on the left side, not the right side of the falciform ligament), and the root of the middle hepatic vein is dissected at the confluence of the left hepatic vein. Next, as the umbilical portion of the left portal vein is retracted to the left, the bile ducts of the left lateral sector are divided on the left side of the umbilical portion of the left portal vein proximal to the confluence of the bile ducts from segments II and III. Before dissecting the bile ducts, the bile ducts should be reconfirmed to be sufficiently detached from the left lateral sectional branches of the left portal vein and left hepatic artery to avoid injury to the vessels (Fig. 119B.7).

Left Trisectionectomy

The techniques for lymphadenectomy and liver mobilization in left trisectionectomy are similar to those in left hepatectomy (see Chapter 118A). To divide the hilar vascular structures, unlike in left hepatectomy, the hepatic artery and portal vein supplying the right anterior sector need to be dissected, in addition to dissection of the left and middle hepatic artery and the left portal vein.[8] The right posterior portal vein is detached from the hepatic hilus, after division of the portal branches to the caudate lobe. As mentioned in the section on left hepatectomy (see "Left Hepatectomy"), the RPHA normally bifurcates from the right hepatic artery and runs caudally to the right portal vein and into the liver at Rouviere's sulcus. In a minority of cases, however, the RPHA or its branch runs cranially to the right portal vein (supraportal or combined type; see Fig. 119B.4A).[26] In such cases of an RPHA anomaly, the RPHA is likely to run to the left of the RAHA near the origin and into the hepatic entry between the right portal vein and hilar bile ducts. Therefore the artery should be cautiously detached from the hilar bile ducts as the right anterior portal vein is cut at its origin. After controlling the hepatic vasculature to the liver to be resected, the demarcation between the right anterior and posterior sectors emerges on the liver surface.

After mobilizing the left liver and caudate lobe off the IVC from the left side, the liver parenchyma is transected along the demarcation line. This parenchymal transection is slightly more complicated than that in other hepatic resections for the following reasons. First, left trisectionectomy is an uncommon procedure, accounting for less than 5% of all procedures in several large series. Second, the right intersectional plate (right portal scissure or right portal fissure) is not always flat, and the right anterior sector overhangs cranially to the right posterior sector in some cases. Third, there are no clear landmarks on the transection surface because the right hepatic vein does not always emerge on the transection surface.[34-37] Because of these complexities, parenchymal division can become a time-consuming component and is likely to result in increased intraoperative blood loss. In addition, the transection might follow the wrong direction dorsally to the cranial part of the right hepatic vein.

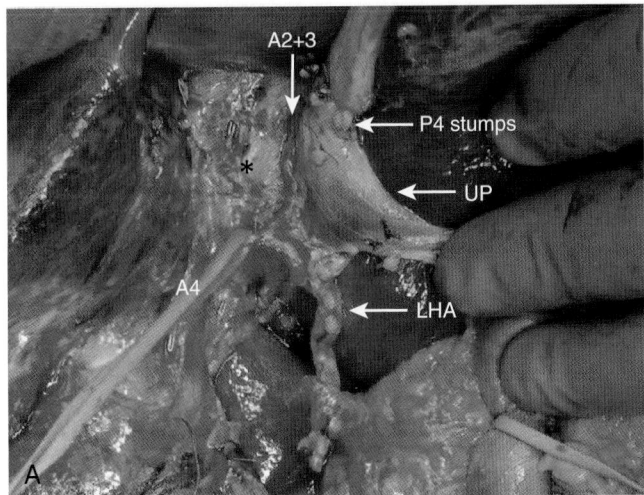

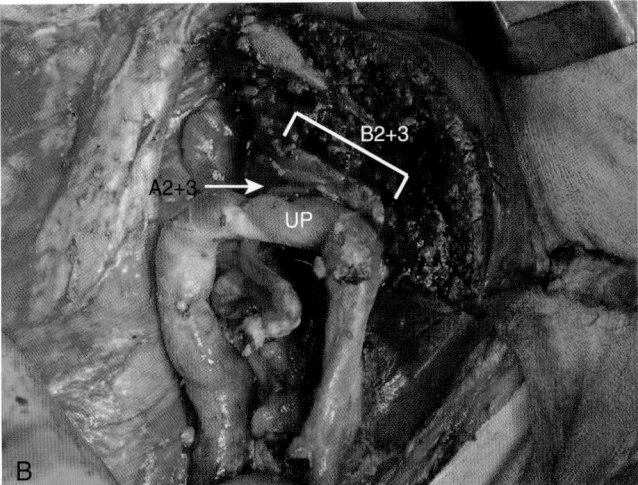

FIGURE 119B.7 Right hepatic trisectionectomy with caudate lobectomy and extrahepatic bile duct resection. **A,** The umbilical portion of the left portal vein *(UP)* is completely mobilized from the umbilical plate (*). The hepatic artery supplying segment IV *(A4)* ramifies from the common trunk of the artery *(A2+3+4)*; the feeding artery of the left lateral segment *(A2+3)* is also freed from the umbilical plate. Note that *A2+3+4* runs into the hepatic entry to the left of the base of the umbilical portion of the left portal vein, and the *A4* separates cranially to the umbilical portion of the left portal vein in the umbilical fossa. **B,** Photograph of the completed procedure. The proximal bile duct *(B2+3)* was resected at the left side of the umbilical portion of the left portal vein.

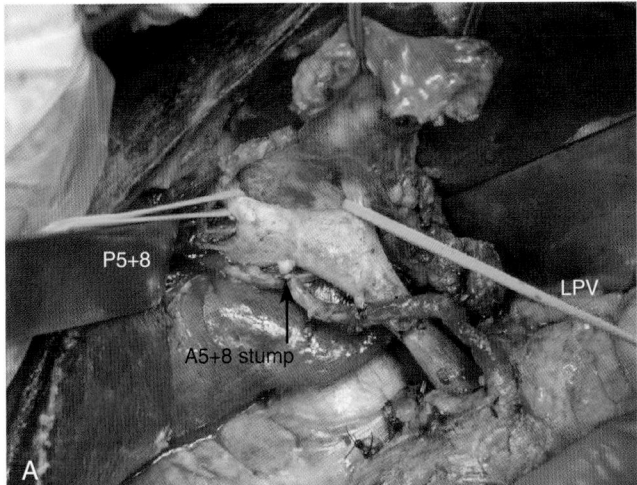

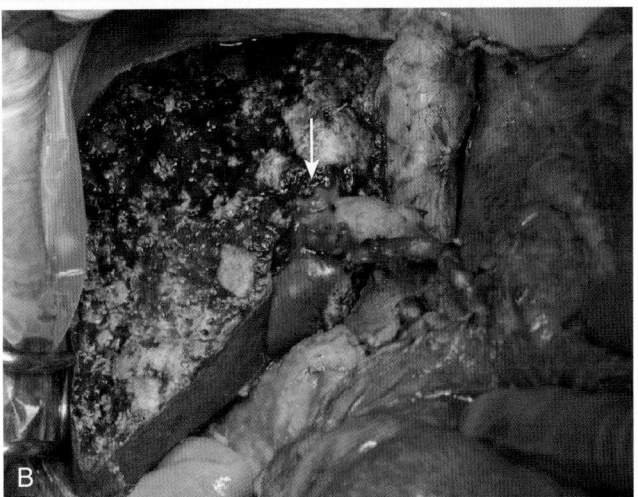

FIGURE 119B.8 Left hepatic trisectionectomy with caudate lobectomy and extrahepatic bile duct resection. **A,** The left portal vein *(LPV)* and right anterior portal vein *(P5+8)* are isolated with blue tape. The right anterior hepatic artery *(A5+8)* was already divided. **B,** Photograph of the completed procedure. The *white arrow* indicates the stump of the right posterior sectional bile duct.

COMBINED VASCULAR RESECTION (SEE CHAPTER 122)

In advanced cases, perihilar cholangiocarcinomas are likely to involve contiguous hepatic inflow vascular structures because of anatomic closeness, and resections with negative surgical margins are often precluded because of vascular involvement of the hepatic arteries and portal veins.[39] With the refinement of surgical techniques, such advanced tumors can be removed by using combined hepatectomy with vascular reconstruction, providing a chance for complete tumor eradication with negative surgical margins.[9–12] Combined vascular resection includes three different modes for resecting the hepatic inflow vasculature: portal vein resection alone, hepatic artery resection alone, and simultaneous resection of the portal vein and hepatic artery. To ensure a successful surgery, not only detailed preoperative radiologic evaluations of the vascular anatomy and involvement but also delicate operative techniques for vascular isolation are mandatory.

The hepatic parenchyma is, therefore, cautiously transected, preserving the right hepatic vein as the only drainage vein from the liver remnant.

After completing liver transection, the right posterior bile duct is divided at the craniodorsal side of the right posterior portal vein. In a minority of cases, the right posterior bile duct or its branch runs ventrally and caudally to the right portal vein and can be divided before liver resection.[38] In this procedure, the right posterior bile duct could be resected approximately 7 mm beyond the confluence (compared with a "classic" left hepatectomy). The percentage of negative proximal ductal margins in patients with Bismuth type IV tumors with a left-sided predominance increases by 13% with this approach (97% in left trisectionectomy vs. 84% in left hepatectomy; Fig. 119B.8).[8]

Portal Vein Resection

Portal vein resection is combined with hepatectomy and trisectionectomy because the bifurcation of the portal trunk, including the right and left portal trunk, is vulnerable to tumor involvement. This combined vascular resection method is widely performed in major centers, and its clinical benefit has been validated in many studies.[10,13,14] Technically, segmental portal vein resection is much easier to perform with right-sided hepatectomy than with left-sided hepatectomy because the transverse portion of the left portal vein is longer than that of the right portal trunk.[10] When portal vein involvement is suspected in the preoperative radiologic workup or during surgery, the resectability and reconstructability of the portal vein need to be evaluated early during resection. Specifically, isolating the portal vein distal to the involvement is one of the keys to a successful surgery because it determines the reconstructability of the portal vein (Fig. 119B.9A). To obtain a safe margin for reconstruction, the distal end of the transverse portion of the left portal vein is isolated in right-sided hepatectomy, the right portal vein

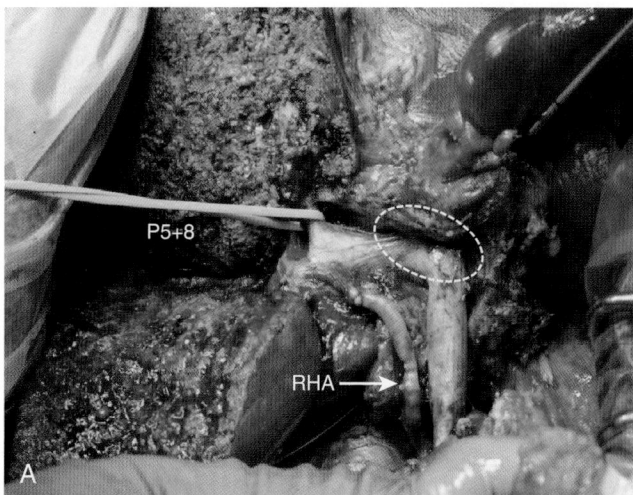

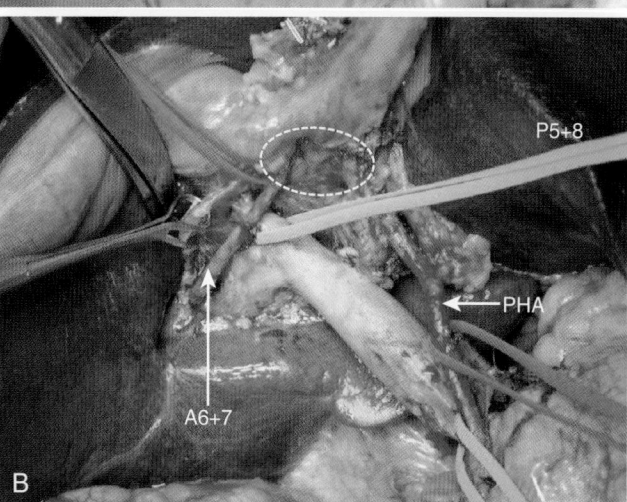

FIGURE 119B.9 Intraoperative findings of vascular invasion *(dashed circles)* during left hepatic trisectionectomy. **A,** The portal vein is involved bilaterally. **B,** The right hepatic artery is involved. The numerals indicate the hepatic segment according to the Couinaud classification. *A,* Hepatic artery; *P;* portal vein; *PHA,* proper hepatic artery; *RHA,* right hepatic artery.

just proximal to the bifurcation that runs into the right anterior and posterior portal vein is isolated in left hepatectomy, and the right posterior portal vein is isolated at Rouviere's sulcus in left trisectionectomy. Several portal branches to the caudate lobe are carefully ligated and divided to isolate those portal branches.

Resection and reconstruction of the portal vein is preferentially performed at the final step of the resection, immediately after removing the specimen because the surgical view becomes optimal for vascular clamp placement and suturing. Segmental resection followed by direct end-to-end anastomosis is used in most cases, but wedge resection followed by direct suture closure or patch graft repair is possible as an alternative if the involved area is sufficiently small. After segmental resection, a direct end-to-end anastomosis is performed using a continuous intraluminal suture in the posterior wall and an extraluminal over-and-over suture in the anterior wall with 5-0 or 6-0 nonabsorbable sutures. If not possible, interposition of an autogenous vein graft is recommended because it reduces the tension of the reconstructed portal vein and avoids the complications associated with post-reconstruction, such as bleeding from the anastomosis, portal vein thrombosis, and stenosis. The left renal vein, external jugular vein, and external iliac vein can be used for the autogenous vein graft; the authors prefer to use a right external iliac vein graft because this vein has a similar diameter to the portal vein, and compared with other autogenous vessels, a greater length can be harvested (Fig. 119B.10).[40,41] For harvesting, the external iliac vein is extraperitoneally approached by placing another lower pararectal incision.

Hepatic Artery Resection

Because the left hepatic artery runs along the leftmost portion of the hepatoduodenal ligament and the right hepatic artery crosses the upper bile duct, right-sided perihilar tumors rarely involve the left hepatic artery. In contrast, left-sided tumors occasionally involve the right hepatic artery. Therefore major hepatectomies with resection and reconstruction of the hepatic artery are predominantly applied in left-sided hepatectomies. The adoption of combined hepatic artery resection for biliary cancers has been controversial because of conflicting results in previous studies[14,42]; however, the authors recently reported a relatively lower mortality rate of 4% and 5-year overall survival of 27% in a large number of patients.[12] When involvement of the hepatic artery is suspected in the preoperative radiologic workup or during surgery, the resectability and reconstructability of the hepatic artery needs to be evaluated early during resection. Specifically, isolation of the right hepatic artery during left hepatectomy and that of the RPHA during left trisectionectomy distal to the involvement is key to a successful surgery because it mostly determines the reconstructability of the artery (see Fig. 119B.9B). Because the RPHA normally runs caudally to the right portal vein and distant from the hilar tumor at the hepatic entry, the artery is safely isolated, and the covering peritoneum cuts in front of Rouviere's sulcus. As mentioned in the sections on left hepatectomy and left trisectionectomy (see "Left Hepatectomy" and "Left Trisectionectomy"), the RPHA or its branch runs cranially to the right portal vein in a minority of cases. In such cases of an anomalous RPHA, the RPHA needs to be isolated posteriorly to the right posterior portal vein; however, isolation of the artery is highly technically demanding.

Resection of the hepatic artery is performed at the final step of hepatic parenchymal transection after dissecting the proximal bile ducts and immediately before removing the specimen. When

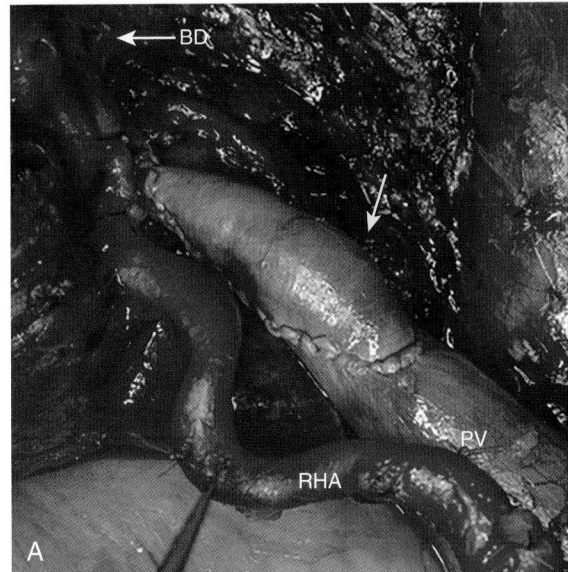

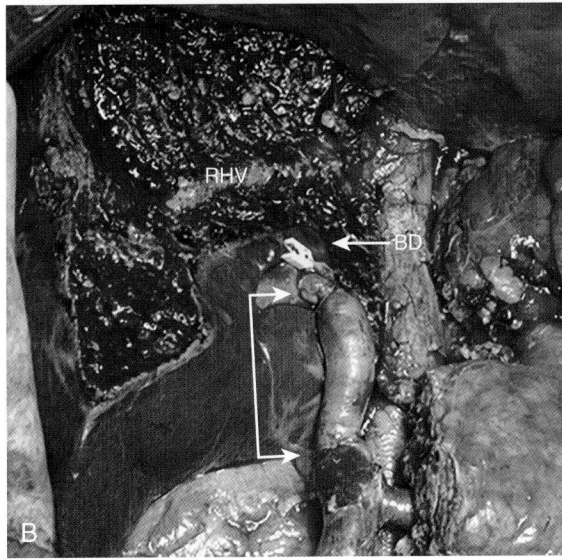

FIGURE 119B.10 Photographs of a completed portal vein reconstruction. **A,** The portal vein was reconstructed using a patch graft *(yellow arrow).* **B,** The portal vein was reconstructed using right external iliac vein graft interposition *(white arrow). BD,* Bile duct; *PV,* portal vein; *RHA,* right hepatic artery; *RHV,* right hepatic vein.

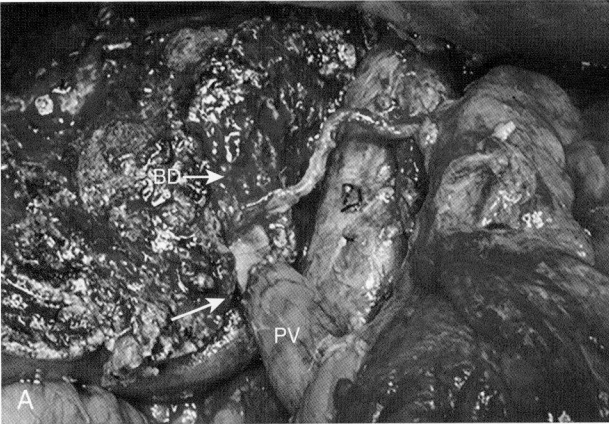

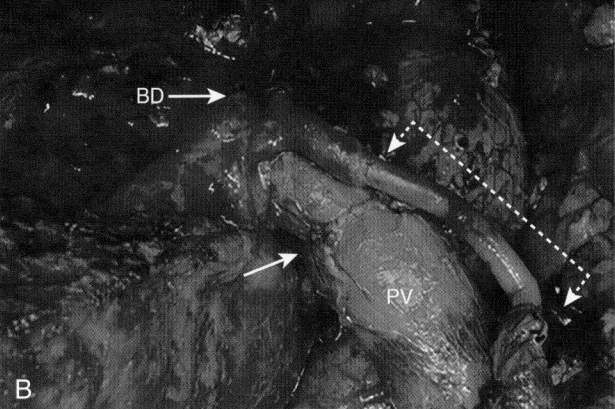

FIGURE 119B.11 Photographs of a completed hepatic artery reconstruction. **A,** The right posterior hepatic artery was reconstructed using the rotated left hepatic artery originating from the left gastric artery *(white arrow).* The portal vein was resected and reconstructed simultaneously *(black arrow).* **B,** The right hepatic artery was reconstructed using radial artery graft interposition *(white dotted arrow).* The portal vein was resected and reconstructed simultaneously *(black arrow). BD,* Bile duct; *PV,* portal vein.

Simultaneous Resection of the Hepatic Artery and Portal Vein

Simultaneous resection of the hepatic artery and portal vein is the most technically demanding combined vascular resection procedure and is predominantly applied in left-sided hepatectomies. Vascular resection followed by reconstruction is preferentially performed during the final step of the resection, and reconstruction of the hepatic artery is performed after reconstruction of the portal vein. Vascular resection and reconstruction techniques have already been detailed for each combined vascular resection approach with reconstruction (Fig. 119B.12).[11]

HEPATOPANCREATODUODENECTOMY (SEE CHAPTER 117A)

HPD is a multivisceral resection defined as a combined resection of the extrahepatic bile duct, portion of the liver, pancreatic head, and duodenum.[43] The main purpose of HPD for biliary tract cancers is to remove the entire extrahepatic biliary system, encompassing the bile duct from the ampulla of Vater up to the hilum and gallbladder. Most HPDs include hemihepatectomy or extended hepatectomy. HPD can be proposed as a treatment option for perihilar cholangiocarcinomas with the following modes of spread:

the hepatic arteries perfusing the future resected liver have not been divided because of involvement, preservation of the hepatic venous outflows from the future resected liver until the division of the hepatic artery avoids excessive congestion of the specimen. In such conditions, resection and reconstruction of the hepatic artery before hepatic parenchymal transection is an alternative option, if possible. The hepatic artery is reconstructed under a microscope using 9-0 or 10-0 monofilament nonabsorbable sutures, and end-to-end anastomosis is possible in most cases. When direct end-to-end anastomosis is not possible, the distal cut end of the hepatic artery is anastomosed with other visceral arteries, and/or alternatively, the radial artery or greater saphenous vein graft is interposed between the proximal and distal cut end of the hepatic artery (Fig. 119B.11).[11,12] Prophylactic anticoagulation therapy is not typically administered during the postoperative period.

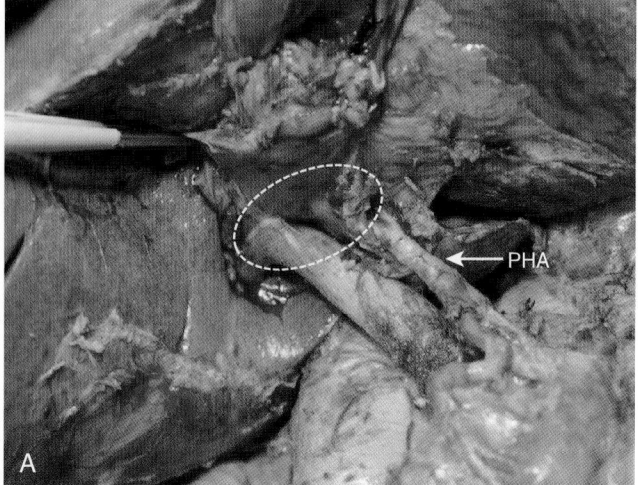

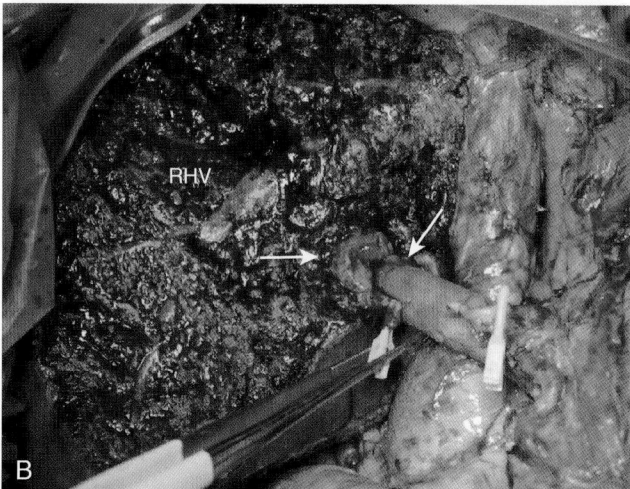

FIGURE 119B.12 Left hepatic trisectionectomy with simultaneous resection and reconstruction of the portal vein and hepatic artery. **A,** The portal vein and right hepatic artery are grossly involved. **B,** Photograph of the completed procedure. The forceps indicate the stump of the right posterior hepatic artery, which is to be reconstructed. The *large and small white arrows* indicate the cut stump of the right posterior bile duct and the portal vein anastomosis, respectively. *PHA,* Proper hepatic artery; *RHV,* right hepatic vein.

(1) a diffusely infiltrating tumor in the entire extrahepatic bile duct, (2) a perihilar tumor exhibiting downward superficial spreading, (3) a middle tumor infiltrating the right hepatic artery and pancreatic head at the advancing margin, (4) a perihilar with bulky nodal metastasis in the pancreatoduodenal region, (5) multiple bile duct tumors, and (6) unexpected cancer involvement of the distal ductal stump.[16,43,44] HPD is primarily applied in cases of a laterally spreading configuration representing modes 1, 2, and 6. Although HPD for biliary cancer remains controversial and is the most challenging operation, this procedure is the only means of treating cholangiocarcinomas with extensive spread that are otherwise unresectable; HPD is the fourth "standard" procedure, after hepatectomy, bile duct resection, and pancreatoduodenectomy (PD; see Chapter 117).[16] It must be emphasized that, in the face of such extensive disease, the benefits of HPD are not universal but are rather limited to patients with favorable tumor biology; careful patient selection is therefore critical.

Although HPD includes several variations of hepatectomy types, this complex procedure basically follows the following

sequence: (1) PD, (2) upward lymph node clearance at the hepatoduodenal ligament with vascular division, (3) mobilization of the ipsilateral hemiliver including the caudate lobe, (4) liver parenchyma transection, and (5) division of the intrahepatic bile duct. Technically, this PD-first approach is rational, useful, and easier to perform than other sequences. In some exceptional cases, a hepatectomy-first procedure might be recommended.[45] For reconstruction, a modified Child's method is preferentially employed, in which the pancreatic stump, the intrahepatic bile duct, and the stomach/duodenum are anastomosed to the Roux-en-Y jejunal limb, in that order. Placement of an external stent for pancreatojejunostomy is routinely employed because the remnant pancreas has a soft parenchymal texture with a nondilated pancreatic duct (Fig. 119B.13).

References are available at expertconsult.com.

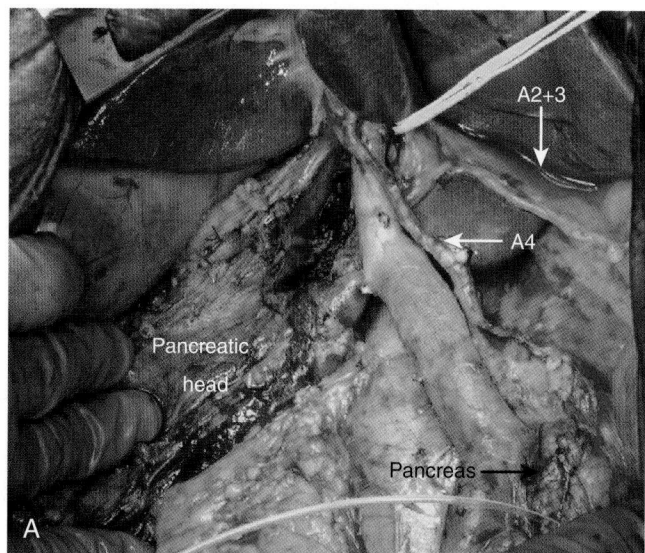

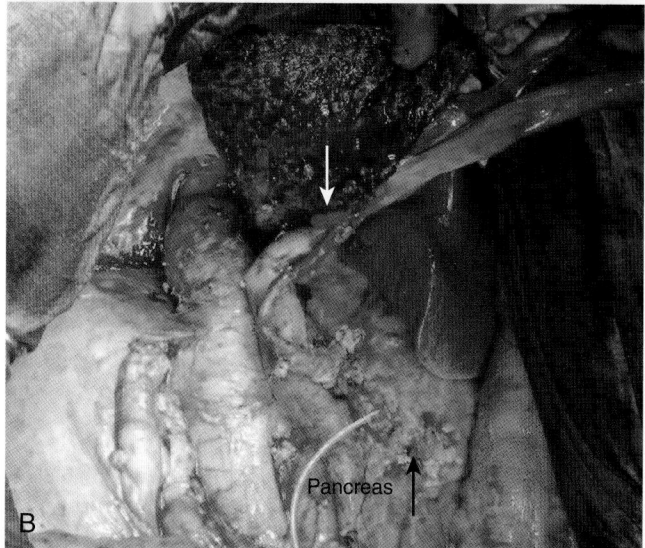

FIGURE 119B.13 Hepatopancreatoduodenectomy (HPD) with right hemihepatectomy. **A,** Completed pancreatoduodenectomy and hilar dissection. Arantius' duct is encircled with yellow tape. **B,** Photograph of the completed HPD. The *arrow* indicates the proximal ductal cut stump. The numerals indicate the hepatic segment according to the Couinaud classification; *A,* hepatic artery.

CHAPTER 120

Hepatic resection in cirrhosis

Norihiro Kokudo, Nobuyuki Takemura, and Kiyoshi Hasegawa

INTRODUCTION

Local tumor control is still the most important consideration in the treatment of hepatocellular carcinoma (HCC), which is the most common diagnosis associated with hepatic resection in the setting of cirrhosis. Because liver resection can completely remove cancerous tissues, it is theoretically regarded as a curative treatment for HCC (see Chapter 89). Patients with HCC often have injured liver tissue or cirrhosis (Fig. 120.1A–B), and this factor should be taken into consideration when deciding on a therapeutic strategy for patients with HCC (see Chapters 68, 69, 74, and 101B). Liver transplantation is an ideal treatment for early-stage HCC (see Chapters 105 and 108A), especially lesions meeting the Milan criteria[1] and/or other expanded criteria for liver transplantation[2-4] because all injured liver tissues with the potential to undergo carcinogenesis and the existing HCC can be removed. However, a severe graft shortage has sometimes made hepatic surgeons select liver resection as a first-line therapeutic strategy for HCC rather than liver transplantation. The safety of liver resection has been established, with a present mortality rate of 2% to 5%,[5-9] even in patients with liver cirrhosis.[10-12]

Prevention of any further deterioration in liver function is a second priority in the treatment of HCC. However, liver resection can be associated with significant blood loss and therefore remains technically demanding. To prevent fatal complications, such as liver failure, careful patient selection and meticulous perioperative management are essential (see Chapters 4 and 26). Because the extensive removal of noncancerous liver parenchyma should be avoided as much as possible, accurate evaluation of the liver volume to be removed and what to preserve is important when deciding on an appropriate procedure (see Chapter 4).

This chapter describes general aspects of liver resection for HCC in patients with cirrhosis, including surgical indication, perioperative management, and surgical techniques, especially focusing on the surgical techniques.

SURGICAL INDICATION

Liver Functional Reserve (see Chapter 4)

In Eastern countries, the indocyanine green retention rate at 15 minutes (ICG R15) is regarded as an important tool for assessing what liver volume to remove accurately.[13-15] Especially in Japan, criteria consisting of the ICG R15 value, ascites, and jaundice ("Makuuchi's criteria") are widely used for decisions regarding surgical indications and to estimate tolerable resection volumes in cirrhotic patients[16] (Fig. 120.2).

In patients with uncontrollable ascites even after use of diuretics and/or a serum total bilirubin level constantly higher than 2.0 mg/dL, liver resection is absolutely contraindicated (see Chapters 77 and 79). When the serum total bilirubin level is 1.1 to 1.9 mg/dL, tumor enucleation or the resection of a small part of the liver is possible. If the level is 1.0 mg/dL or less, the surgical procedure can be determined based on the ICG R15 value. If the ICG R15 value is normal (<10%), a major hepatectomy (i.e., right hemihepatectomy, left trisegmentectomy, and central bisegmentectomy) may be feasible (see Chapter 118A). In patients with a slightly injured liver (ICG R15 of 10%–19%), a one-third resection (left hemihepatectomy, or right lateral or paramedian sectionectomy) can be performed, but major hepatectomy would be associated with high risk. In patients with ICG R15 of 20% to 29%, a one-sixth resection corresponding to a left lateral section or one segment defined by Couinaud is possible. If ICG R15 is more than 30%, only a limited resection can be considered.

Torzilli and colleagues[17] applied the previous criteria to 107 consecutive patients (59.8% cirrhosis) undergoing liver resection for HCC. As a result, the mortality and morbidity rates were 0% and 26.2%, respectively. According to a report investigating the relationship between preoperative liver function and postoperative complications in 127 patients with HCC, the ICG R15 value was confirmed to be the most significant factor for the prediction of mortality.[18] Recently, some of the refined and expanded Makuuchi's criteria are proposed with the accurate estimation of the remnant liver volume.[19,20]

Tumor-Related Factors

In general, a single and small HCC is a good indication for resection; however, multifocal and large lesions can also be treated by resection, providing satisfactory long-term outcomes[21-23] (see Chapter 89 and 101B). For advanced HCC with vascular invasion, liver resection can also offer acceptable results[24-28] compared with the use of a molecular targeted agent (Sorafenib; see Chapters 89 and 99),[29] which is recommended in the treatment algorithm of the Barcelona Clinic Liver Cancer (BCLC) group.[30] Although this algorithm is considered to be the treatment standard worldwide, several investigators have objected to this algorithm, especially in regard to the extent of restrictions placed on the surgical indications.[31-33] Consequently, several additional treatment algorithms are now available.[34-36]

Portal Hypertension (see Chapter 74)

Portal hypertension, which was usually defined as a hepatic venous pressure gradient of 10 mm Hg or larger, can be practically diagnosed by the presence of esophageal varices and/or a platelet count of less than 100,000/μL in association with splenomegaly. In 1996 Bruix and colleagues reported that liver resection for HCC in patients with portal hypertension led to a high incidence of postoperative liver decompensation of as

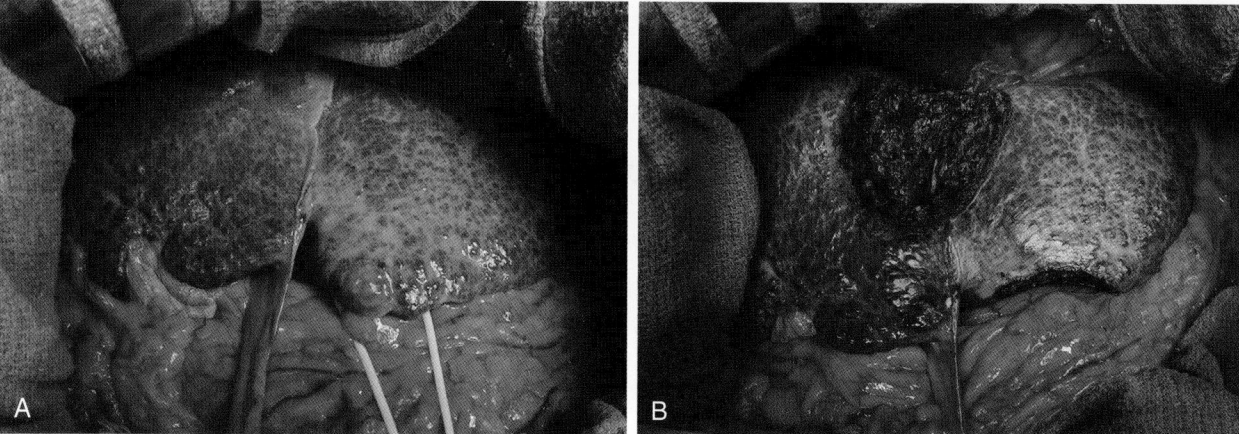

FIGURE 120.1   Appearance **(A)** and cut surface **(B)** of the liver in patients with cirrhosis.

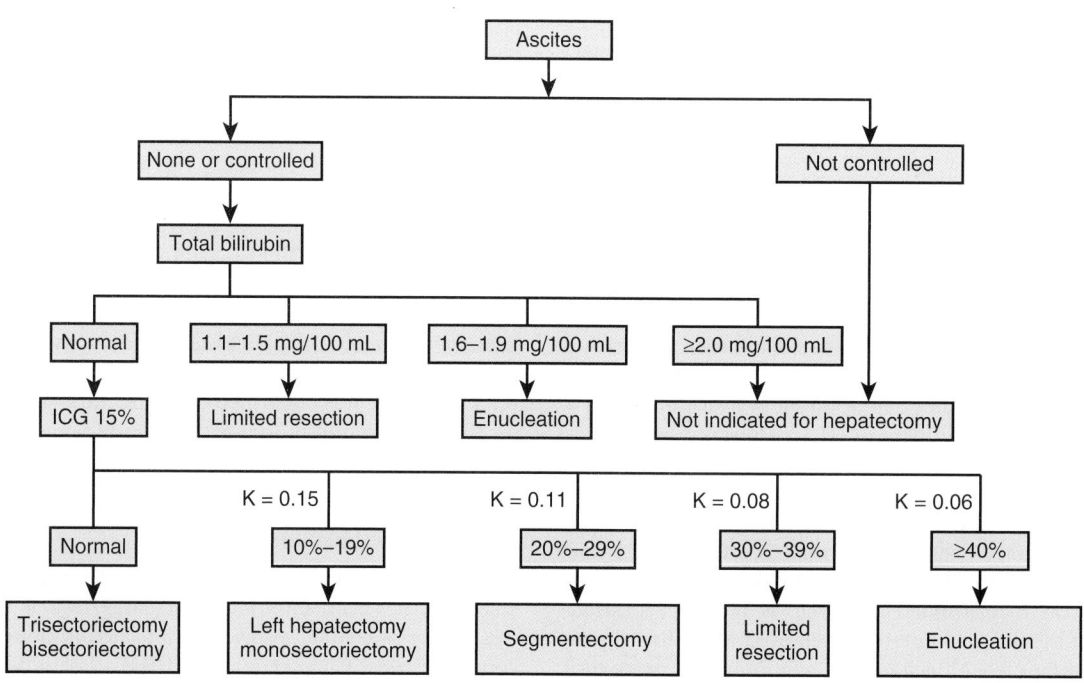

FIGURE 120.2   Decision tree for selection of the operative procedures in patients with hepatocellular carcinoma. Note: The term *sectionectomy* is now preferred for tri-, bi-, mono-"sectionectomy." *ICG,* Indocyanine green. (From Makuuchi M, Kosuge T, Takayama T, et al. Surgery for small liver cancers. *Semin Surg Oncol.* 1993;9:298–304.)

much as 73%,[37] and their group recently published meta-analysis comparing prognosis after hepatectomy with and without portal hypertension, which concluded that portal hypertension increases the risk for mortality and clinical decompensation after surgery for HCC.[38] Based on these results, the American and European guidelines concerning the management of HCC suggested that the presence of portal hypertension may be a contraindication for liver resection, and this recommendation is now widely accepted worldwide.[30,39,40]

Indeed, the prognosis for patients with portal hypertension after hepatectomy for HCC is considered relatively poor compared with that of patients without portal hypertension; however, several investigators have reported satisfactory long-term outcomes after hepatectomy for patients with portal hypertension who were not eligible for liver transplantation.[11,21,31,32,41]

Because comparable outcomes are difficult to obtain with other nonsurgical treatments, the surgical indications for HCC associated with portal hypertension should be discussed further. Discussion of the indication for hepatectomy in patients with portal hypertension should be based not on the comparison with or without portal hypertension among the patients who underwent hepatectomy[38] but on the comparison with or without surgical treatment among the patients who have portal hypertension. Consequently, the BCLC guidelines may need to be modified in terms of the role of surgery.[33]

PERIOPERATIVE MANAGEMENT IN PATIENTS WITH LIVER CIRRHOSIS (SEE CHAPTERS 26 AND 79)

Diuretics

To prevent refractory ascites and edema, the routine administration of spironolactone (aldosterone inhibitor) is recommended, especially in cirrhotic patients, because secondary hyperaldosteronemia is caused by a low degradation of aldosterone through liver metabolic dysfunction.[42] The dose of spironolactone can be approximately decided based on the preoperative ICG R15 value; for example, 100 mg/day and 200 mg/day of spironolactone should be used in patients with ICG R15 values of less than 20% and more than 20%, respectively.[17] If the ascites is uncontrollable, administration of furosemide is a better choice, with an initial dose of 10 or 20 mg/day.

MANAGEMENT FOR PORTAL HYPERTENSION

If liver resection is scheduled in a patient with portal hypertension, careful preoperative evaluation and management are mandatory. Gastrointestinal endoscopy (see Chapters 79 and 80) is necessary to evaluate the presence or absence of varices of the esophagus and stomach, which are frequently associated with liver cirrhosis. If found, esophageal varices with a high risk of rupture, such as those with a red color sign, should be treated before surgery using endoscopic ligation or sclerotherapy[11,43] (see Chapter 80). Hassab's operation (devascularization around the upper stomach with a splenectomy) should be considered for gastric varices with a high risk of rupture. In patients with thrombocytopenia (platelet count <50,000/μL) caused by hypersplenism, which is a major symptom of portal hypertension, a splenectomy is recommended before liver resection to reduce the risks of intraoperative blood loss and postoperative liver failure.[11,44,45] Strategies for the indication of perioperative prophylactic management for portal hypertension[11] are shown in Figure 120.3.

SURGICAL TECHNIQUES

Inflow and Outflow Occlusion (see Chapter 118)

Because ischemia-reperfusion injury was once viewed as a critical form of damage to the liver, neither inflow nor outflow occlusion was applied during liver parenchymal division. Thus liver resection was inevitably associated with a large loss of blood, which sometimes led to liver failure and death. In the early 1980s, the hemihepatic vascular occlusion method[46] was devised, and the total inflow occlusion (Pringle maneuver[47]) became widely used. These inflow occlusion methods contributed to a marked reduction in blood loss. The usefulness of Pringle maneuver was confirmed by a randomized controlled trial (RCT) performed in Hong Kong.[48]

Total vascular exclusion was performed for a time,[49–51] but because of the complexity of the procedure and the risk of postoperative liver dysfunction, it is now used infrequently.[52,53] Clavien and colleagues[54] found that 10 minutes of ischemic preconditioning by inflow occlusion significantly improved postoperative liver function. The superiority of intermittent inflow occlusion versus continuous or total occlusion is now widely accepted[55,56] and is an indispensable technique for improving the safety of liver surgery.

Intraoperative Ultrasound (see Chapter 103)

Intraoperative ultrasound (IOUS), first introduced in the field of liver surgery in the late 1970s by Makuuchi, enables liver surgeons to grasp the location of tumors and anatomic structures.[57,58] Using IOUS, the safety of liver resection has been remarkably improved, especially in patients with cirrhosis, because a limited resection to minimize the loss of liver parenchyma is possible under IOUS guidance. IOUS is also useful for the detection of occult HCCs, which cannot be detected using preoperative imaging modalities.[59,60] The ability of this modality to detect structures has been further improved by using contrast media, such as perfluorobutane microbubbles (Sonazoid; GE Healthcare, Norway).[61–63] IOUS will continue to be indispensable for liver surgery.

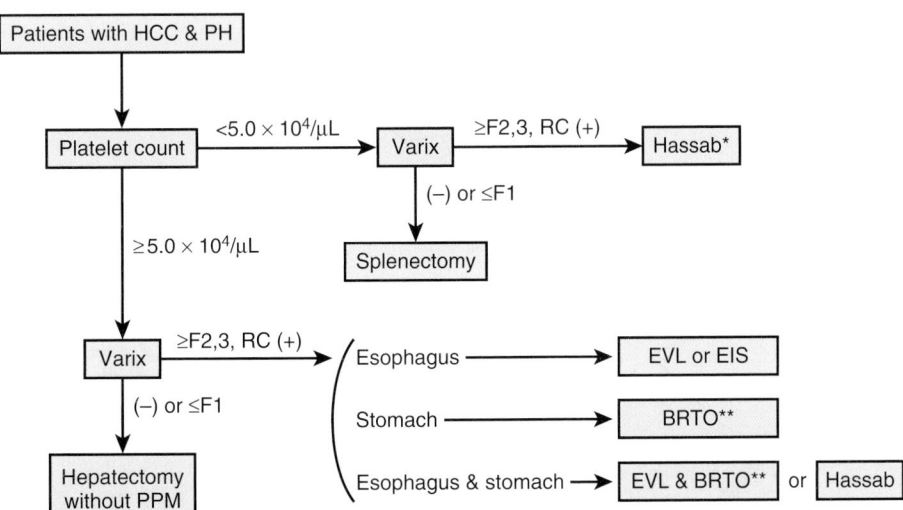

FIGURE 120.3 **Strategies for indication of PPM.** *On occasion, EVL and splenectomy or BRTO and splenectomy could be performed. **BRTO has been indicated since 1999. *BRTO,* Balloon-occluded retrograde transvenous obliteration; *EIS,* endoscopic injection sclerotherapy; *EVL,* endoscopic variceal ligation; *HCC,* hepatocellular carcinoma; *PH,* portal hypertension; *PPM,* perioperative prophylactic management. (From Takemura N, Aoki T, Hasegawa K, et al. Hepatectomy for hepatocellular carcinoma after perioperative management of portal hypertension. *Br J Surg.* 2019;106[8]:1066–1074).

Anatomic Resection (see Chapters 101, 102A, and 102B)

HCC has a unique biologic characteristic in that it tends to spread intrahepatically and to metastasize through the portal venous system.[64] Because even a small HCC may be associated with portal venous invasion, which is correlated with worse prognosis, surgeons should consider removing potential intrahepatic metastases whenever possible. On the other hand, major hepatic resection should be avoided, especially in cirrhotic liver, because of the high risk of postoperative critical liver failure. To overcome this pitfall, anatomic resection, in which the entire segment fed by the tumor-bearing portal branches is completely and systematically removed, is a reasonable surgical procedure for preventing recurrence via this pathway (see Chapter 102B).

Anatomic subsegmentectomy was first proposed by Makuuchi and colleagues.[64] Depending on the size and location of the tumor, the resection of a complete Couinaud segment, part of a segment, or more than one segment extending to the adjacent region can be performed. Figure 120.4 illustrates the procedures used in this technique.[64] First, a blue dye (indigo carmine) is injected into the portal venous branch bearing the tumor under IOUS guidance (see Chapter 103). From the liver surface, a portal branch is manually punctured distal to the point of ligation, and the stained surface of the liver is marked with electric cautery, followed by parenchymal dissection. The hepatic veins should be exposed longitudinally on the dissected surface after complete resection in an anatomic subsegmentectomy (Fig. 120.5).[65] ICG is another useful staining material that can be used instead of indigo carmine. ICG is illuminated by near infrared light, and it emits fluorescence with a peak wavelength of about 840 nm, which lies within the range of absorbance spectra of hemoglobin (<600 nm) and water (>900 nm). The wavelength of ICG excited by near infrared light is not visible to the human eye; therefore the ICG fluorescence system equipped with interferential filters is applied to obtain the fluorescence images[66–70] (Fig. 120.6). Anatomic subsegmentectomy is technically difficult to perform, especially for segments IV, VII, and VIII, because these locations are surrounded by major vascular structures and do not necessarily present with a flat dissection plane[71] (see Chapter 102B).

To date, several studies have shown that anatomic resection is superior to nonanatomic resection.[72–80] As long as the liver function is adequate, anatomic resection is strongly recommended as the surgical procedure of choice for HCC. Anatomic hepatic resection has been recently applied in laparoscopic hepatectomy.[66,81,82]

Laparoscopic Liver Resection

Laparoscopy currently plays a major role in the field of abdominal surgery, enabling minimally invasive procedures to be performed (see Chapter 127A). Laparoscopic liver resection for HCC was initially applied as a treatment option for peripheral HCC. The 2008 Louisville consensus statement of 45 experts proposed that the most suitable candidates among HCC patients for laparoscopic liver resection are those with solitary lesions measuring 5 cm or less in diameter and located in peripheral segments.[83] The second consensus conference in Morioka in 2014 concluded that minor laparoscopic resection had become standard practice and that major laparoscopic resection was still considered innovative and in the exploration phase.[84] Recently, the indication for laparoscopic liver resection has been expanded not only to limited resection for the tumor in the deep part of the liver parenchyma[85] but also to major hepatectomy.[86,87] The procedures of the laparoscopic liver resection are described elsewhere (see Chapters 127A, 127D, and 127E).

Laparoscopic resection may be more useful for HCC, especially in patients with cirrhosis, because of its smaller destruction of the abdominal wall, lesser need for liver mobilization, and lower demand for intravenous (IV) fluid replacement because of the minimization of unnecessary fluid loss during

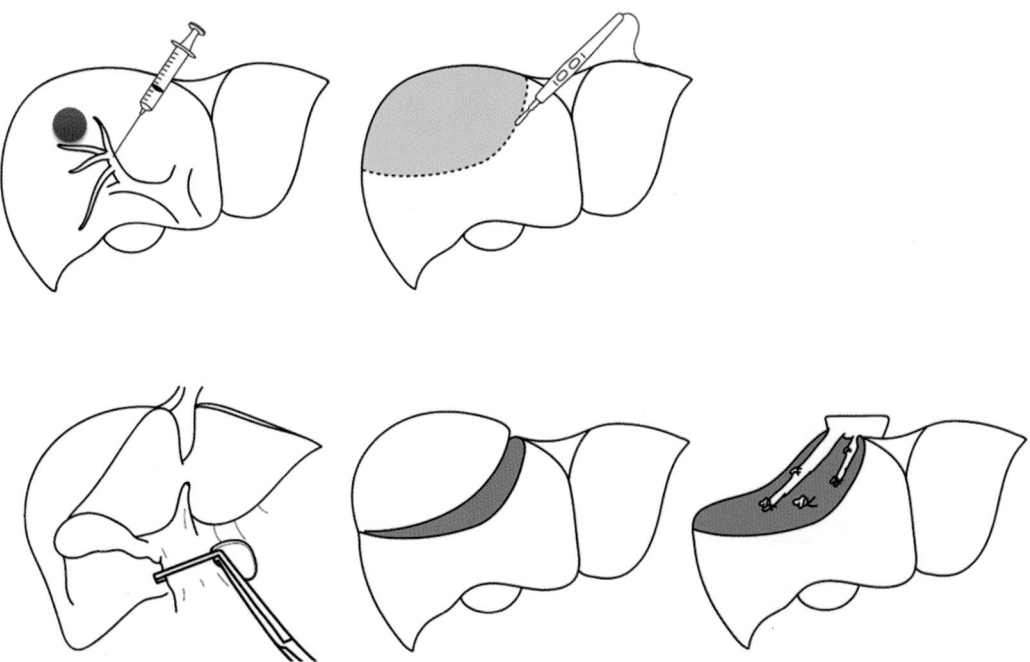

FIGURE 120.4 **Procedures for anatomic resection of HCC.** *HCC,* Hepatocellular carcinoma. (From Makuuchi M, Hasegawa H, Yamazaki S. Ultrasonically guided subsegmentectomy. *Surg Gynecol Obstet.* 1986;161:346–350.)

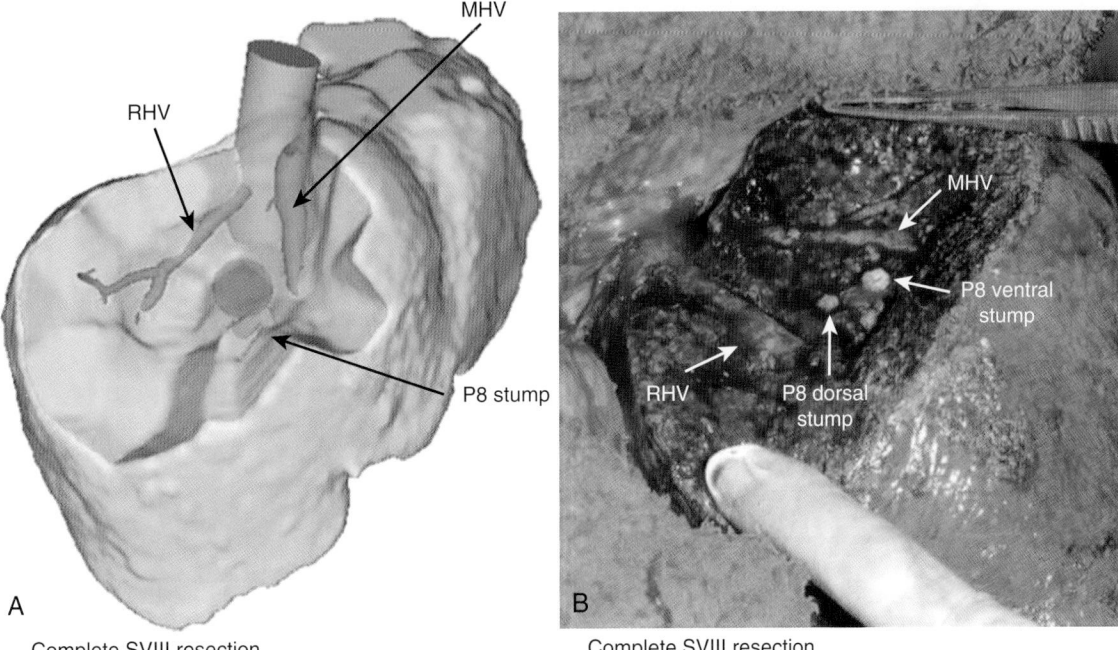

FIGURE 120.5 Dissected surface after complete resection of liver segment VIII (SVIII). *MHV,* Middle hepatic vein; *RHV,* right hepatic vein; *P8,* portal vein branch of SVIII.

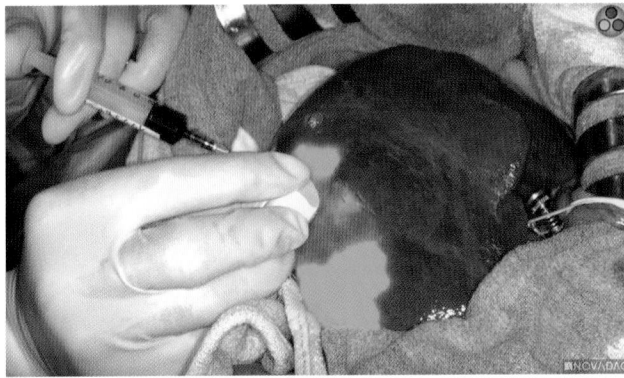

FIGURE 120.6 ICG fluorescent anatomical hepatectomy. *ICG,* Indocyanine green retention.

the operation compared with open liver resection. Fluid accumulation in the third space is also likely to be reduced, resulting in a decreased risk of prolonged postoperative ascites and shorter hospital stay.[86,88–93]

Surgical Devices for Liver Parenchyma Division (see Chapters 101, 102A, 102B, and 118)

Usually, liver parenchyma division consists of two procedures: crushing of the liver parenchyma to detect vessels and their subsequent occlusion. Various types of surgical devices for liver parenchyma division have been developed for one or both procedures. Through the introduction of inflow occlusion, refinements to operative techniques, and the development of surgical devices, the amount of blood loss has been significantly reduced to improve the safety of liver resections. Clamp crushing with forceps combined with ligation remains the standard[94,9] because it is a simple, inexpensive, and useful method. However,

some surgical devices have been developed that are known to reduce operative time and blood loss.

Clamp Crushing

Originally, the surgeon's fingers were used to crush the liver parenchyma, but Pean forceps are now used.[94,95] With forceps, the surgeon removes the parenchyma and identifies the vessels (Glisson triads, hepatic vein) by feeling the structures through the tip of the forceps. The identified vessels are ligated with a string and divided. This method has the advantage of avoiding tissue injury, but experience is needed to make the fullest use of this method. As a crushing device, Pean forceps with blunt tips are preferred for use. In patients with liver cirrhosis, liver parenchyma is hard, so it is easy to crush liver parenchyma using forceps with relatively thin tips not opened too much (Fig. 120.7).

Ultrasonic Dissector

An ultrasonic dissector, the Cavitron Ultrasonic Surgical Aspirator (CUSA), is a device used to crush the liver parenchyma, remove crushed tissues, and expose fibrous tissues (Glisson triads, hepatic vein), with an ultrasonic vibration at its tip. The vessels must be exposed so that they can be occluded with ligation or sealing, as with the conventional clamp-crushing method. Simultaneously, the ultrasonic dissector supplies saline from the tip to wash the surgical field, which is aspirated through the tip to maintain an adequate field of vision. Modified versions that can be attached to an electrocautery device or ultrasonic scalpel are also now available.

For division of cirrhotic liver, the vibration width of the tip must be set wider, but this can make it more difficult to separate vessels because the thin vessels are more easily injured than in normal liver tissue. The CUSA has become one of the standard surgical devices for liver parenchyma transection.[96]

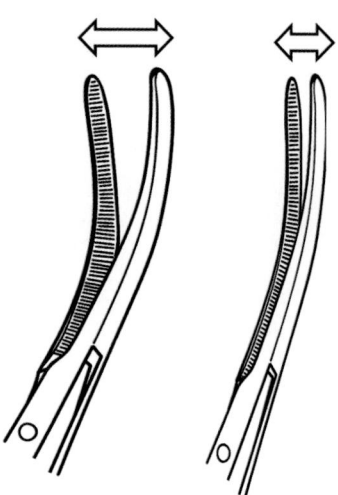

FIGURE 120.7 Blunt-tip Pean forceps and the opening for normal liver parenchymal crushing *(left)* and relatively thin-tip Pean forceps and the opening for cirrhotic hard liver parenchymal crushing *(right)*.

Vessel-Sealing System

Using bipolar electrothermal energy, a vessel-sealing system can seal the vessel wall by denaturing the collagen and elastin in the wall and completely occluding the blood vessel. During liver parenchyma division, the vessel-sealing system can easily occlude vessels exposed by clamp crushing or an ultrasonic dissector. Thus the use of the vessel-sealing system can shorten the liver transection time and reduce the amount of blood loss.[97–101]

By improving the energy generator, the sealing power can be strengthened while minimizing damage to adjacent tissues to increase the sealing speed and certainty. In the current type, the shape of the tip has been made thinner and shorter than the previous type, and scissors are built into the tips to enable the vessels to be cut immediately after sealing. Although clamp crushing itself is possible with the tip of the vessel-sealing system, Pean forceps enable a better feel and vessel exposure in our experience.

Automatic Suture Device (Vascular Stapler)

For laparoscopic liver resection, an automatic suture device is now an indispensable tool frequently used to cut the Glisson triads and hepatic vein.[102] A vascular stapler is first applied to resect hepatic vein during hepatectomy.[103,104] Figueras et al. applied this device to cut the Glisson pedicle with the Glissonean approach.[105] When using a stapler to cut the Glisson triads, attention should be paid to avoid accidental injury of the bile duct confluence. The Glisson triads should be cut with the stapler on the peripheral side as far as possible.[105] Nowadays, some surgeon applied this vascular stapler for liver parenchymal resection and it was called *stapler hepatectomy*.[106] Stapler hepatectomy might reduce the parenchymal transection time[107]; however, it has the risk of hepatic vein avulsion injury, especially in patients with cirrhosis because hemostasis even from thin hepatic vein is sometime difficult.

Anterior Approach

Before liver parenchyma transection, mobilization of the liver is usually done using the conventional approach, which enables a liver surgeon to control bleeding easily.[108,109] For example, in right hepatectomy (see Chapter 118A), the right hemiliver should be fully mobilized through dissection from the right

adrenal gland and extrahepatic division of the right hepatic vein.[110] A thoracophrenolaparotomy is a good option to safely complete mobilization of the right liver. However, several surgeons recommend the anterior approach, in which liver parenchyma division is done before the mobilization, especially when a liver tumor is large.[111] They believe the anterior approach may avoid the risks of massive bleeding from hepatic vein avulsion, prolonged ischemia in the remnant liver, and spillage of cancer cells into the systemic circulation. In an RCT, Liu and colleagues[112] found that the anterior approach for a right hepatectomy had beneficial effects on operative and survival outcomes for patients with HCC. However, Ishizawa and associates[113] reported that the conventional approach would have the advantage of preventing critical bleeding during liver transection, although the anterior approach can be an effective alternative when difficulty is encountered during liver mobilization. Further investigation is needed to address this problem.

Belghiti and colleagues[114] proposed the *hanging maneuver,* in which surgical tape is placed between the liver and the anterior surface of the inferior vena cava (Fig. 120.8A) and lifted to allow the liver to be suspended during division of the liver parenchyma (see Fig. 120.8B). As an option to the anterior approach,

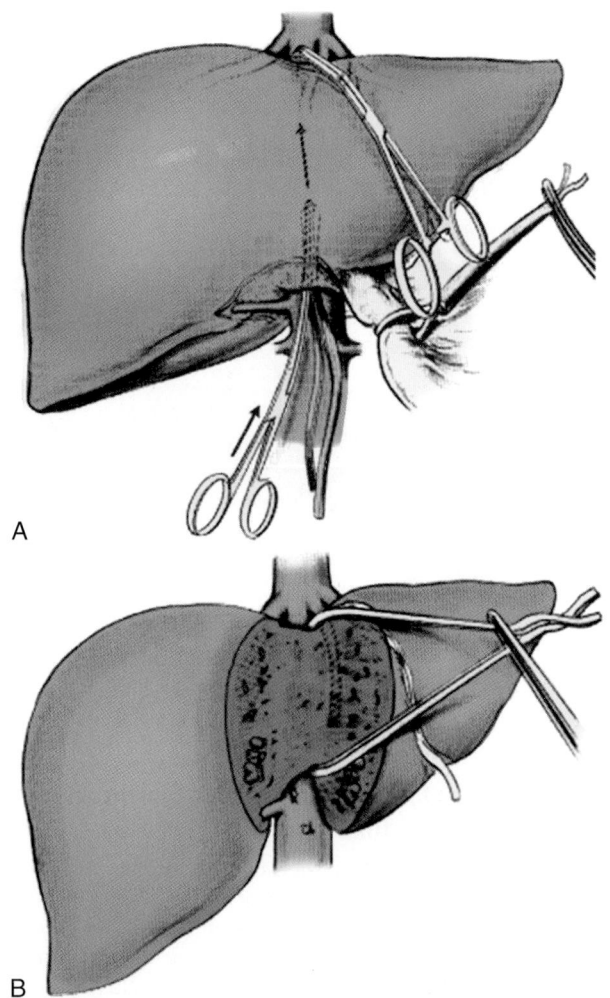

FIGURE 120.8 Hanging maneuver. **A,** Forceps is inserted in front of the inferior vena cava (IVC) from the caudal side of the liver. **B,** Tape is placed between the liver and IVC and lifted up during liver parenchymal transection. (From Belghiti J, Guevera O, Noun R, et al. Liver hanging maneuver: A safe approach to right hepatectomy without liver mobilization. *J Am Coll Surg.* 2001;193:109–111.)

this maneuver can reduce blood loss by compressing the liver parenchyma, making it easier to determine the proper direction of the parenchymal division. The hanging maneuver also allows the mobilization of the right liver to be avoided during a right hemihepatectomy, especially with a large liver tumor. Although this maneuver is associated with a risk of injury to the short hepatic veins, it has been widely applied to liver transection for left hepatectomy[115] and left caudate lobectomy[116] (see Chapter 118A). Despite insufficient evidence, the hanging maneuver is now regarded as a useful surgical technique and has been applied in laparoscopic liver resection.[117,118]

Hepatic Vein Reconstruction (see Chapter 122)

In liver resection for a malignant tumor, hepatic venous reconstruction is also recommended if the functional volume of the residual liver is insufficient.[19] In most patients with HCC, which is likely to demonstrate expansive growth, it is usually relatively easy to detach the HCC from the hepatic vein, even if closely attached to each other. However, if the HCC is a mixed or sclerosis type, detachment may be difficult because of tumor invasion. In such cases, reconstruction techniques using an autologous vein graft obtained from the resected liver specimen are useful, as reported for metastatic liver tumors.[119–120] According to Kawaguchi and colleagues,[121] a congestive area may be functional (corresponding to approximately 30%–40% of normal liver without congestion) to some degree, but these findings are being investigated further.

CONCLUSION

The safety and feasibility of liver resection for HCCs are now established, even in patients with cirrhosis and portal hypertension. This has been achieved by the recent significant progress in preoperative evaluation, surgical techniques, surgical devices, and perioperative management.

The references for this chapter can be found online by accessing the accompanying Expert Consult website.

CHAPTER 121

Resection technique for live donor transplantation

See Ching Chan and Sheung Tat Fan

Living-donor hepatectomy is a major surgical operation performed on a healthy person only for the benefit of a recipient who requires liver transplantation (see Chapters 105, 125, and 128). In 1989 Strong (1999)[1] performed donor left hepatectomy and removed segment IV of the liver on the back table before implantation of segments II and III into a pediatric recipient. In 1990 Tanaka et al.[2] improvised using a right liver graft for a pediatric recipient because of unexpected precarious donor left hepatic arterial anatomy. Living-donor liver transplantation (LDLT) using left liver for adults was first performed by Makuuchi in 1993.[3] The first case of right liver adult LDLT was performed by Fan in 1996.[4] A priori, the right liver graft included the middle hepatic vein (MHV) to address the problems of small-for-size syndrome by providing good venous outflow of the right anterior section. The first seven recipients who underwent right LDLT all had acute liver failure before the transplantation; one died of candidiasis, and the other six survived.[5] Subsequently, semiurgent and elective cases were accepted.

DONOR WORKUP

Donor workup is started after indication for LDLT for the potential recipient is established (see Chapter 105). The workup helps evaluate whether the donor will be psychologically and physically healthy in the long term after recovery from the organ donation. In a stepwise manner, expedience is achieved without omission.[6] Only individuals of good health who have reached the age of consent are accepted.[7]

Step 1

A detailed medical history is taken to identify comorbidities, if any. A body mass index of 30 kg/m^2 or more (27 kg/m^2 for Asians)[8] raises the concern for fatty liver and obesity-related comorbidities. Blood group compatibility is verified. Carriers of the human immunodeficiency virus, hepatitis B virus, or hepatitis C virus (see Chapter 11) are denied liver donation. Although a status of hepatitis B core antibody positivity by itself does not preclude liver donation, it mandates lifelong prophylaxis with lamivudine or entecavir in the recipient.[9]

Step 2a

A psychological assessment is performed to verify the potential donor's knowledge of the operation to be performed and coping abilities. The donor should have adequate knowledge of donor and recipient morbidity, mortality, and survival and should be apprised of the urgency of the transplant.

Step 2b

Chest radiographs are taken, and an electrocardiogram is performed. Computed tomography (CT) of the liver under sodium bicarbonate cover[10] is also performed, and maximum-intensity projections (MIPs) of the hepatic veins (HVs) and portal veins (PVs) are produced (see Chapters 13 and 14). Volumetry of the donor liver by the Heymsfield method[11] measures the volume of the right liver and left liver (for pediatric recipients, segments II and III), using the MHV as a demarcation line on the plane between the right and left liver (Fig. 121.1) (see Chapters 4, 101, and 102). Attenuation of the liver parenchyma in comparison with the spleen on the plain film is appraised for detection of fatty change. HV anatomy (see Chapter 2) is determined by the axial cuts in the venous phase and by MIPs for easier appreciation. The presence of any inferior right HVs allows anticipation at operation of either preservation or division. Attention to the presence of the segment IVb HV or segment III HV draining into the MHV calls for a more caudal division of the MHV, to preserve adequate drainage of segment IV of the remnant left liver.[12] The right, left, and segment IV hepatic arteries are also illustrated by three-dimensional reconstructions for images obtained during the arterial phase.

Step 3

Liver biopsy is performed in selective donors and after genuineness and suitability of the potential donor is ascertained. Steatosis (see Chapter 69) of up to 15% for right liver donors and 20% for left liver donors are acceptable.

Step 4

Informed consent is obtained from the donor and the donor's relative. Donor and recipient morbidity and mortality risks are stated explicitly.

SIDE AND SIZE OF GRAFT

The graft–to–standard liver volume ratio[13,14] is crucial in LDLT. A ratio of more than 35% is required for a predictable recipient success.[15] However, a 20% overestimation of the right liver graft size based on CT volumetry is usually given a conversion factor of 1.19 g/mL.[13,14] Because the left liver is usually one-third the size of the total liver, for a donor with a body size no larger than the recipient, the left liver is usually less than 35% of the recipient standard liver volume. For an individual with a larger left liver/right liver ratio, the left liver may be large enough for donation. It is worth noting that in left LDLT, a gram-to-gram equivalence of graft is not applicable, and a left liver graft of the same size as the right is less efficacious probably because the left liver graft is more likely subject to compression injury when the recipient's abdominal cavity is not large enough to accommodate the graft.[16]

For right liver donation, the liver donor should have a remnant left liver of at least 30% of the total liver volume. For a pediatric

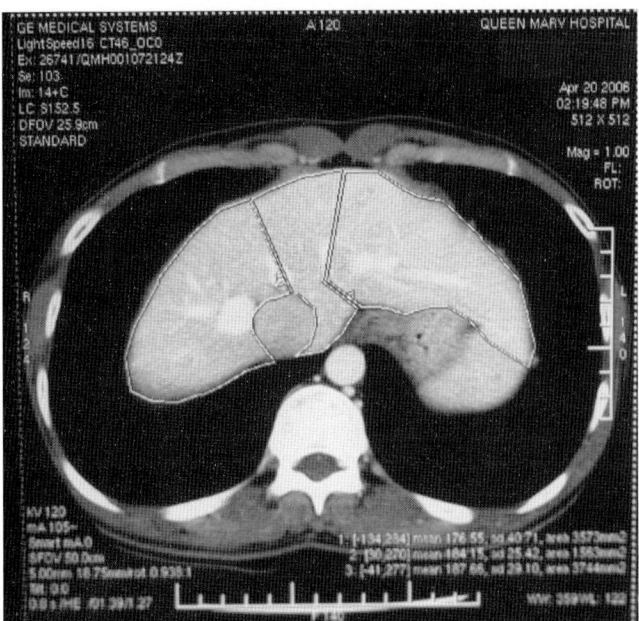

FIGURE 121.1 Volumetric analysis of the donor liver on computed tomography (see Chapter 102).

recipient, a liver graft of 3% of the body weight is optimal; however, the graft size is lowered to 2% of the body weight for older children and teenagers, because a graft of more than 5% of body weight predisposes to hypoperfusion. In such cases, graft reduction to even a monosegment may be necessary.[17]

DONOR RIGHT HEPATECTOMY (SEE CHAPTER 118)

Exposure

The donor is placed supine on the operating table, with care to avoid pressure sores over the occiput, heels, and sacrum. The position of the donor must be optimal for the surgeon and first assistant to face the operative field directly, unhindered by the metal bars of the upper hand retractor or those used to set up a fence between the surgeon and anesthetist.[18] Access is gained through a right subcostal incision, with upper midline extension. The ligamentum teres is ligated and divided, and the falciform ligament is taken down. The two curved blades of the Bookwalter retractor (Codman and Shurtleff, Raynham, MA) pull the rib cage laterally and anteriorly to open up the aperture made by the costal margins. In donors with a narrow costal angle, excising the xiphoid process may improve access to the suprahepatic inferior vena cava (IVC) and the roots of the HVs. Following careful laparotomy, intraoperative ultrasonography (IOUS) is performed to study the junction of the left hepatic vein, MHV, and IVC (see Chapters 24 and 103). The relation of the segment IVb HV to the MHV, already known from CT, is ascertained by IOUS. This also registers the flow characteristics of the hepatic arteries, HVs, and PVs for reference throughout the operation.

Isolation of Major Vessels and Parenchymal Transection

The triangle of Calot is dissected, and the cystic artery is divided between ligatures. The gallbladder is dissected from its fossa, and the cystic duct is cannulated with a 3.5-Fr Argyle

catheter (Tyco Healthcare, Mansfield, MA). The cystic duct is then severed at the site of catheter insertion for delivery of the gallbladder. Next, the peritoneum overlying the right hepatic duct (RHD) is divided for identification. A large metal LigaClip (Ethicon Endo-Surgery, Cincinnati, OH) is put on the liver capsule at the planned line of division of the RHD, 3 to 4 mm away from the hepatic duct confluence. The biliary anatomy is then demonstrated by operative cholangiogram with undiluted contrast under fluoroscopy with a C-arm (see Chapter 24). The image quality of the cholangiogram can be improved by temporary gentle occlusion of the distal common bile duct (CBD) with an atraumatic vascular clamp (Featherlight Bulldog Clamp; Geister, Tuttlingen, Germany) (Fig. 121.2). To avoid devascularization of the donor distal CBD, care must be taken not to dissect more tissue than necessary for application of the clamp; the clamp must be removed once the cholangiogram is finished. The supine donor will have the right posterior sectional duct demonstrated first, followed by the right anterior sectional duct and then the left ducts.[19] A variant PV, but not hepatic artery, anatomy is frequently associated with a variant bile duct anatomy (see Chapter 2). An infraportal right posterior bile duct is more common in donors with a variant PV anatomy.[20] The parallax technique executed by rotation of the C-arm to the right clarifies the anteroposterior (AP) position of the right anterior and posterior sectional ducts. This also provides the true AP view of the biliary system. A marking is made with reference to the LigaClip on the liver capsule with diathermy for the line of division of the RHD.

Hilar dissection is continued to isolate the right hepatic artery (RHA) and right PV. The space between the RHA and RHD should not be disrupted, to preserve the RHD blood supply. To gain an entire length of the right PV, branches to the caudate lobe are ligated and then divided. It is important to note that a sizable branch from the right PV may represent vessels supplying segment VI, which should be preserved (Fig. 121.3). Temporary

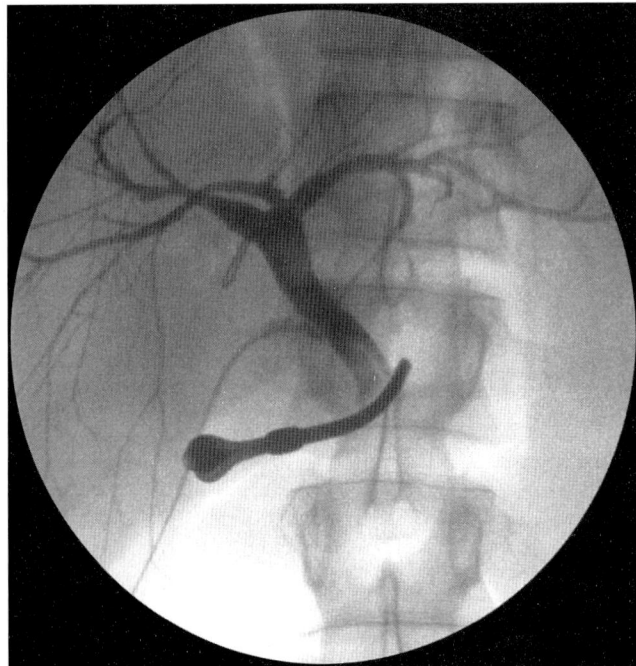

FIGURE 121.2 Operative cholangiogram with metal clip marking the planned line of division of the right hepatic ducts.

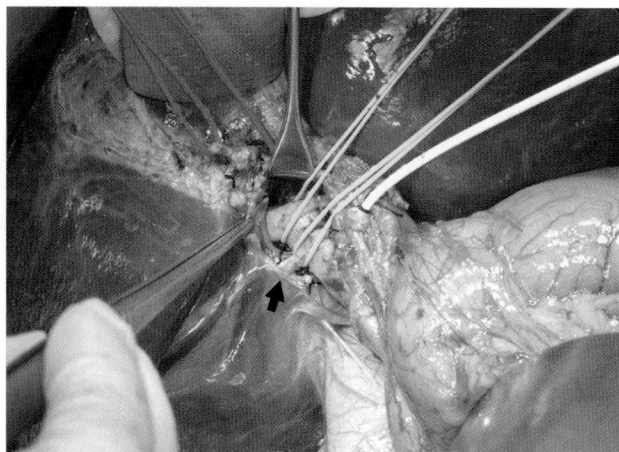

FIGURE 121.3   Hilar dissection with isolation of the right hepatic artery and right portal vein. The branch of portal vein supplying segment VI was preserved *(arrowhead)* (see Chapter 118).

right liver inflow control is performed to mark the line of transection along the Cantlie line with electrocautery (Fig. 121.4). The line on the inferior surface of the liver is just to the left of the gallbladder fossa, joining the planned line of division of the RHD marked earlier.

The right triangular ligament is then taken down, leaving the Gerota fascia intact. In a normal donor liver, the right adrenal gland can often be freed from the liver with careful dissection using electrocautery. Minor bleeding from the right adrenal gland is controlled by the argon beam coagulator, and more severe bleeding is addressed by plication with sutures. Short HVs on the right side of the midline of the IVC are divided between ligatures and plicated as required. Inferior right hepatic veins larger than 5 mm are preserved for anastomosis with the IVC in the recipient (Fig. 121.5).

In contrast to hepatectomy for neoplasm (see Chapters 101 and 118), continuous inflow control during liver transection is not practiced. Although the Pringle maneuver with intermittent reperfusion of the liver, which is adopted by some centers, has been shown to result in less blood loss in the donors, the difference did not reach statistical significance.[21] Possible explanations

for this are that bleeding from the HV tributaries is not controlled by inflow occlusion, and there is bleeding during the 5-minute reperfusion interval. Another potential advantage of the Pringle maneuver is downregulation of the apoptosis pathway by ischemic preconditioning for grafts with long cold ischemic time[22]; however, this has been associated with poorer initial graft function, as shown by a prospective trial in deceased donor liver procurement.[23] For adult LDLT, prolonged cold ischemia should not be an issue, because graft delivery matches the explantation of the native liver. In addition, a low central venous pressure can be attained through good rapport with the anesthetist, and this lowered central venous pressure has proved effective in reducing blood loss.[24] Elevating the head and the trunk by 10 to 15 degrees, complete muscle relaxation of the donor, and cautious use of an ultrasonic dissector are also helpful in reducing blood loss without inflow control.

After mobilization of the right liver from its posterior attachments, a full-thickness suture at the liver edge on both sides of the Cantlie line helps open up the transection plane by the weight of hemostats. The placement of the laparotomy pad behind the right liver renders the transection plane more vertical, but not so excessively as to compromise retraction of the liver during transection. Liver parenchymal transection is started with electrocautery or energy source for the first 1 to 2 cm of parenchyma between segments V and IVa. The rest of the liver transection is done using the Cavitron Ultrasonic Surgical Aspirator (CUSA; Valleylab, Boulder, CO); it exposes the left side of the MHV, the main trunk of which lies at two-thirds the depth from the superior surface of the liver.[25] Terminal branches of the middle hepatic vein may be encountered early at division of the liver near the gallbladder fossa. The terminal branch can be exposed and traced to the main trunk subsequently. At a frequency of 23 kHz, the CUSA is set at an amplitude of 60% for the normal donor liver, and irrigation with normal saline continues at about 4 to 6 mL/min. The liver parenchyma is disrupted by cavitation of the aerosol. When the dissector is set at lower amplitudes, the operator tends to bring the instrument into direct contact with the liver parenchyma, which will damage small, friable vessels. Suction is set to a moderately high level, just enough to provide a clear operative field. Electrocautery incorporated into the CUSA allows diathermy of vessels less than 1 mm in diameter. Should the segment IVb HV insert

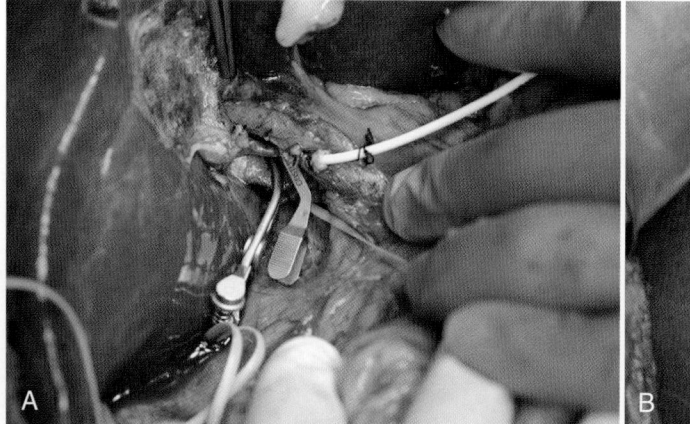
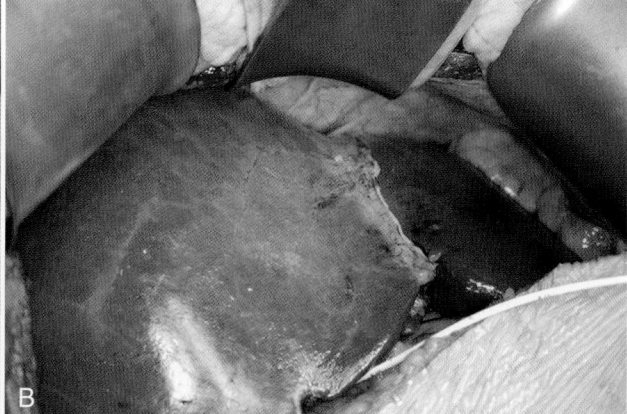

FIGURE 121.4   **A,** Temporary hemiinflow control with vascular clamps applied to the right hepatic artery and right portal vein. **B,** Cantlie's line is revealed after temporary hemiinflow control.

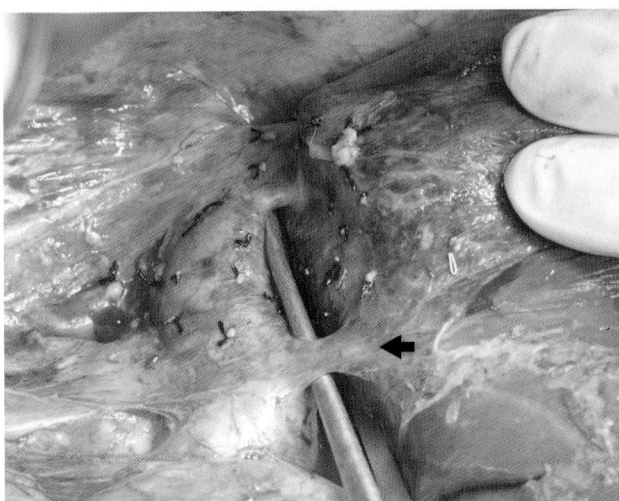

FIGURE 121.5 The inferior right hepatic vein is isolated and preserved (arrowhead).

into the MHV, transection is stopped to preserve this vein for adequate drainage of the left liver.[12] Identification of the segment 4b HV is facilitated by early and complete exposure of full course of the middle hepatic vein.

At the liver hilum, the right portal pedicle containing the RHD is also dissected, with minimal use of the CUSA. Excessive use of CUSA may denude the RHD from its blood supply. The line of division already marked and verified by operative cholangiogram is followed, and any RHDs are severed with scissors tangential to the transection plane, which is often quite horizontal. The RHD stump is repaired by 6/0 polydioxanone continuous suture, and an operative cholangiogram is performed to confirm the patency of the left and main bile ducts (Fig. 121.6). Liver parenchyma dorsal to the MHV and the caudate lobe are

transected, until the IVC is exposed. Lifting up of the caudate lobe with a cotton-tape or right-angled forceps facilitates the transection, and care must be taken to dissect in a definable plane between the liver capsule and the IVC.

Graft Delivery

To have short cold ischemic time, the graft is not delivered until the recipient is ready for explanting of the native liver. Graft delivery starts with application of a clamp onto the proximal RHA, distal to the segment IV hepatic artery. The RHA is then divided with scissors, and the right PV is divided between the vascular clamps, applied at a right angle to the course of the main PV. The MHV, RHV, and if present the inferior RHV are controlled with the vascular stapler (TA 30; Tyco Healthcare) before its division by scissors. To avoid stricture of the PV, the right PV stump is sutured in a transverse manner with 6/0 Prolene continuous back-and-forth sutures. Biliary leakage and patency of the remnant left hepatic duct (LHD) are checked with intraoperative cholangiogram and dilute indigocarmine instillation (see Chapters 24 and 125); the indigocarmine in the bile ducts must be flushed away by normal saline. The cystic duct is ligated with 2/0 Vicryl, and the remnant left liver is maintained in the anatomic position by reconstitution of the falciform ligament with nonabsorbable sutures (Fig. 121.7). The healthy part of round ligament is also anchored onto the abdominal wall by nonabsorbable suture. Otherwise, the left liver may rotate into the right subphrenic cavity, causing kinking of the left hepatic vein, liver congestion, and liver failure. Patency of the vessels is verified with IOUS (see Chapter 103). The hepatic flexure of the colon and the corresponding portion of the greater omentum are allowed to ascend into the right subphrenic space for prevention of adherence of the small bowel to the transection surface of the remnant left liver. Care must be exercised to prevent small bowel going around the hepatic flexure into the right subphrenic cavity. The abdomen is closed without drainage.[26]

The outcomes of donor right hepatectomy, including the MHV, have improved with accumulation of experience (see Chapter 109). In our consecutive series of 200 donor right hepatectomies, all including the MHV, the operation time was shortened, and blood loss decreased with maturity of these techniques.[27] The skill is also transferable to newer surgeons,

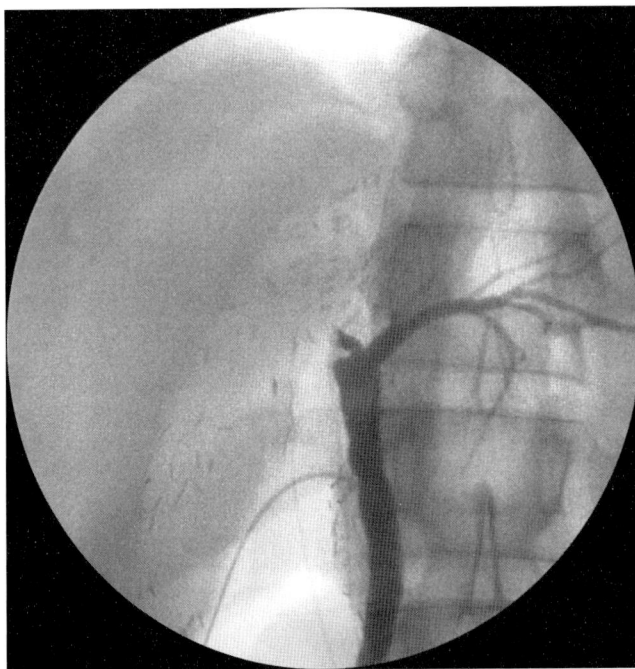

FIGURE 121.6 Operative cholangiogram confirms patent left and main ducts.

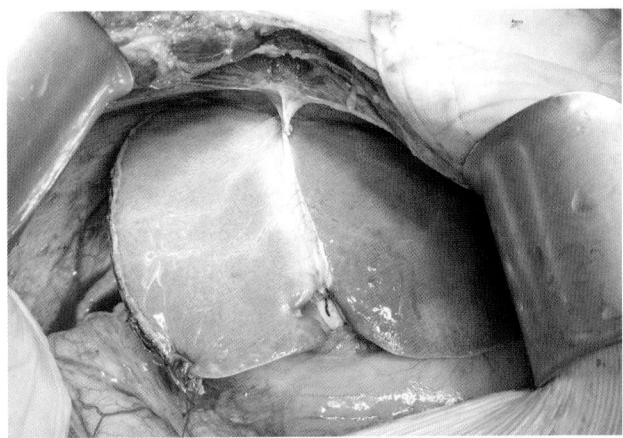

FIGURE 121.7 Remnant left liver is prevented from dropping into the right subphrenic space by suturing the falciform ligament.

and with good surgical outcomes under the guidance from experienced trainers.[28]

INCLUSION OF MIDDLE HEPATIC VEIN

An area of ongoing controversy in right LDLT is whether or not to include the MHV (see Chapter 2). Deleterious effects of no drainage to segments V and VIII include severe venous congestion and necrosis of these segments.[29] The decision to exclude the MHV requires demonstration of collaterals between segment V and VIII tributaries and the RHV.[30]

Researchers at Kyoto University devised an algorithm that includes the MHV when the graft is MHV dominant, or graft-to-recipient weight is less than 1%, and in all cases the remnant left liver is larger than 35%.[31] Chang Gung Memorial Hospital includes the MHV when graft to estimated standard liver volume is 50% or less, or when the segment V and VIII HVs are large and the RHV is small.[32] Researchers at Tokyo University observed congestion of segments V and VIII of the graft after temporary clamping of the RHA before determining venous interpositional grafting.[33]

We include the MHV in all right liver grafts for the simplicity and familiarity of the technique.[34] Irrespective of the venous drainage pattern of segment IV of the remnant left liver, the segment IVb HV is preserved. Utmost care is needed for its preservation, when it drains into the MHV.[12] On the back table, the outflow capacity is guaranteed by venoplasty of the MHV and RHV into a single cuff. The venoplasty would allow a more expedient HV to the IVC anastomosis and higher outflow capacity of the right liver graft.[35]

DONOR LEFT HEPATECTOMY (SEE CHAPTER 118)

For a donor with a low body mass index, an upper midline incision can provide adequate access for the procedure (Fig. 121.8). The left coronary ligament is taken down, and adequate mobilization of the left liver requires division of the ligamentum venosum or Arantius ligament between ligatures. The LHD, which may have a short extrahepatic course, is marked by a large metal clip, and the planned line of division is verified by cholangiogram under fluoroscopic guidance. Special attention is given to identify an insertion of the right posterior sectional duct into the LHD (Fig. 121.9). In this situation, the LHD can only be divided to the left of the right posterior sectional duct. The middle hepatic artery (MHA) should be preserved, when it arises from the left hepatic artery (LHA). An MHA that is not large and arises from the RHA can usually be sacrificed, and segment IV will be supplied adequately by collaterals from the LHA. A replaced LHA arising from the left gastric artery allows a good length of isolated artery (Fig. 121.10). Temporary inflow control of the LHA and PV by the vascular clamp reveals Cantlie line. Liver transection is to the right of the MHV by CUSA. A low insertion of the segment VIII HV into the MHV calls for caution in the final part of the liver transection; this segment VIII vein should be preserved for venous outflow of the right anterior section of the remnant right liver, and inadvertent damage of the vein results in torrential bleeding. When compared with donor right hepatectomy also including the MHV, blood loss is more significant and the operation time longer, likely the result of a larger liver transection surface.[16]

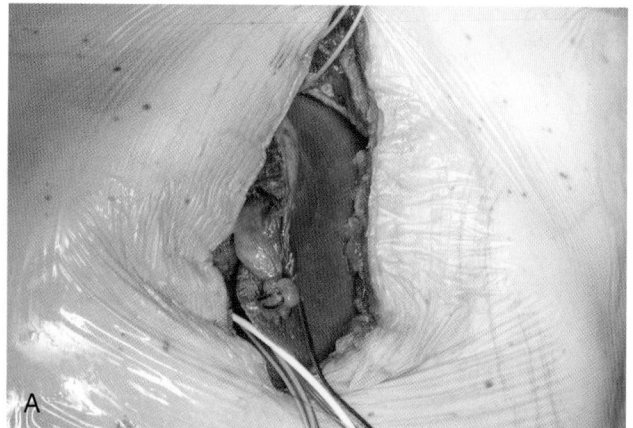
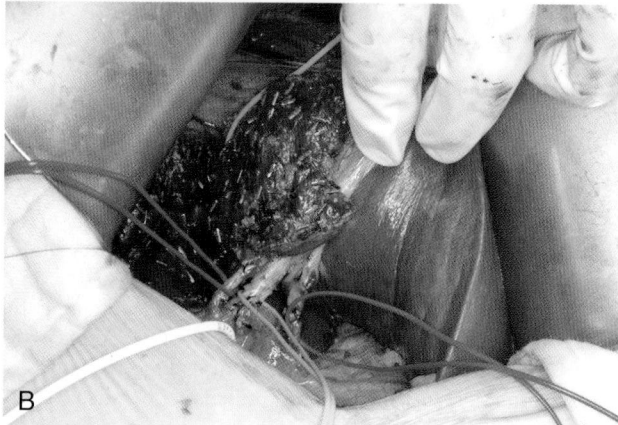

FIGURE 121.8 **A,** Upper midline incision for donor left hepatectomy. **B,** Adequate exposure for hilar dissection and liver transection gained by widening the aperture of the costal angle.

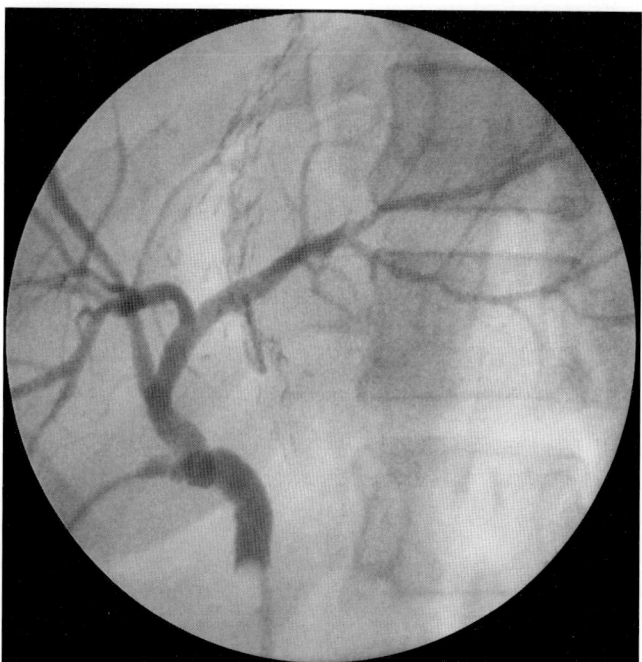

FIGURE 121.9. Operative cholangiogram with a large metal clip marking the planned line of division of the left hepatic duct.

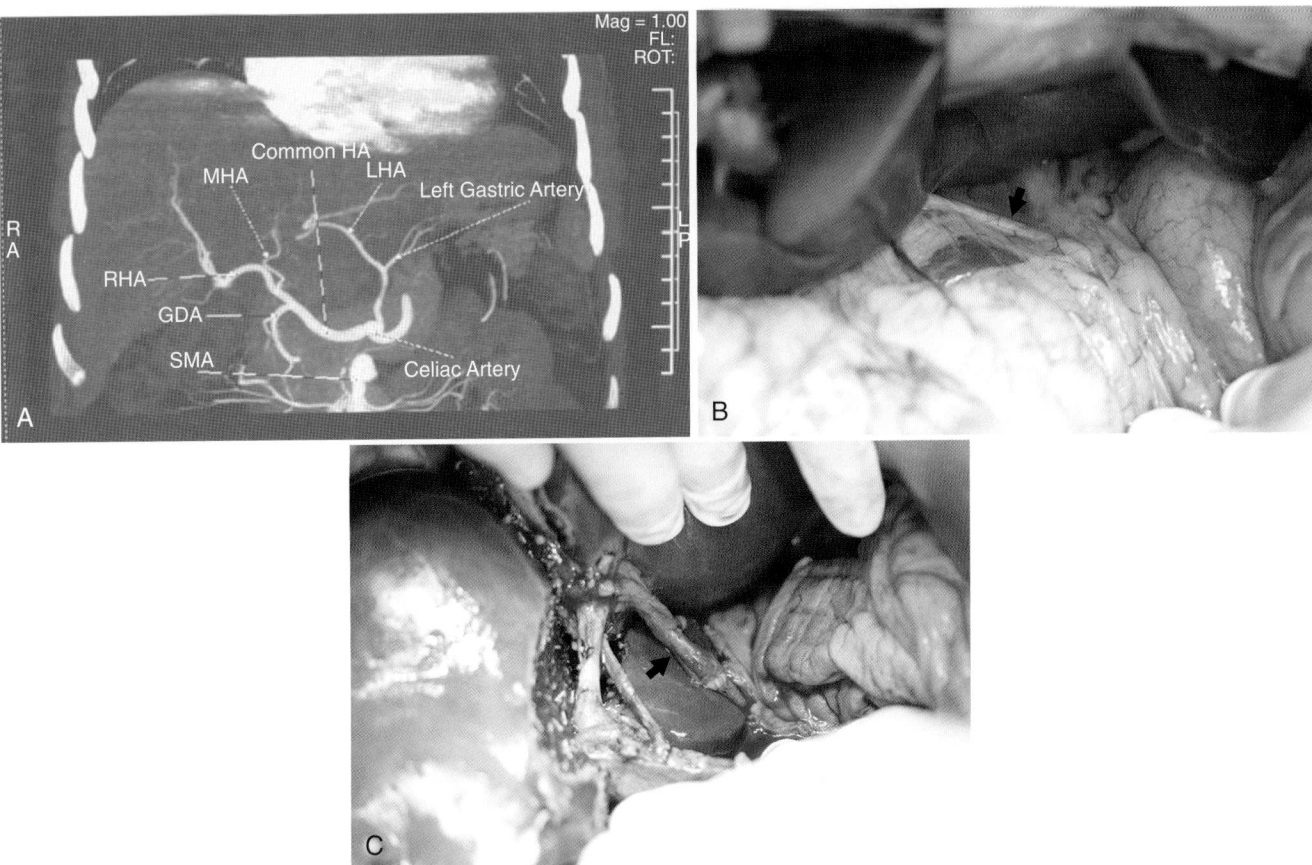

FIGURE 121.10 A, Computed tomography with reconstruction of the hepatic arteries *(HA)* of a donor with the replaced left hepatic artery *(LHA)*. **B,** The replaced LHA is visible in the lesser omentum *(arrowhead)*. **C,** The replaced LHA is isolated and preserved *(arrowhead)*. *GDA,* Gastroduodenal artery; *MHA,* middle hepatic artery; *RHA,* right hepatic artery; *SMA,* small mesenteric artery. (See Chapters 2 and 14.)

SEGMENT II AND III DONOR HEPATECTOMY (SEE CHAPTER 118)

Generally, exposure and hilar dissection are similar to donor left hepatectomy. After isolation of the LHA and left PV, an operative cholangiogram is obtained (see Chapters 24 and 125), with a large metal clip to mark the planned line of division of the LHD. Special attention still must be paid to the location of the right posterior sectional duct, which may insert into the LHD. If the MHA that supplies segment IV arises from the LHA, and enough length is distal to it, it can be preserved; otherwise, it is sacrificed, and the entire LHA is included in the graft. An MHA that arises from the RHA is most favorable and need not be isolated. The liver transection line is about 1 cm to the right of the falciform ligament. The pedicles supplying segment IV are isolated, ligated, and plicated before division, whereas the caudate lobe is often not included into the graft, because the upper abdomen of the recipient often has limited space. The caudate vessels and bile ducts are ligated and divided and plicated if necessary.

ANATOMIC ANOMALIES OF THE DONOR (SEE CHAPTER 2)

Besides inadequacy of size and proportion of the donor liver, occasional anatomic anomalies of the donor liver may preclude liver donation. When a major segmental branch of the right PV arises from the left PV intrahepatically, both right and left

hepatectomy become too hazardous for the donor, so such a finding contraindicates donation. On the other hand, in the case of trifurcation of PV branches, if these are extrahepatic, donor operation is still feasible (Fig. 121.11A). However, the right anterior and posterior branches of the PVs require venoplasty to conform into a single cuff before graft implantation (Fig. 121.11B). If the two branches are too short to merge into one, the portion of the recipient's PV at the bifurcation can be used as an interpositional graft (Fig. 121.11C). These are done on the back table. The segment III or IVb HV could at times drain into the MHV (Fig. 121.12A and B); however, MHV-to-RHV venoplasty is still feasible (Fig. 121.12C). Only in the case of a very caudal insertion of the segment III and IVb HV to the MHV (Fig. 121.13A and B) do the latter and the segment VIII HV need to be divided caudally. This is to preserve the venous outflow of segment III and segment IV of the remnant left liver of the donor. The MHV and the segment VIII HV are merged by venoplasty (Fig. 121.13C). A Gortex vascular graft is then used to provide adequate length for anastomosis with the RHV to form a single luminal outflow (Fig. 121.13D) for anastomosis with the recipient IVC. Such vascular reconstruction is easier with the availability of ABO-compatible deceased-donor iliac arteries. The segment VIII HV and the MHV could be reconstructed with iliac artery branches and the common iliac artery for anastomosis with the RHV (Fig. 121.13E).

Biliary tract anomalies occasionally render a liver graft unsuitable, as in the case of multiple small branches in the graft.[36]

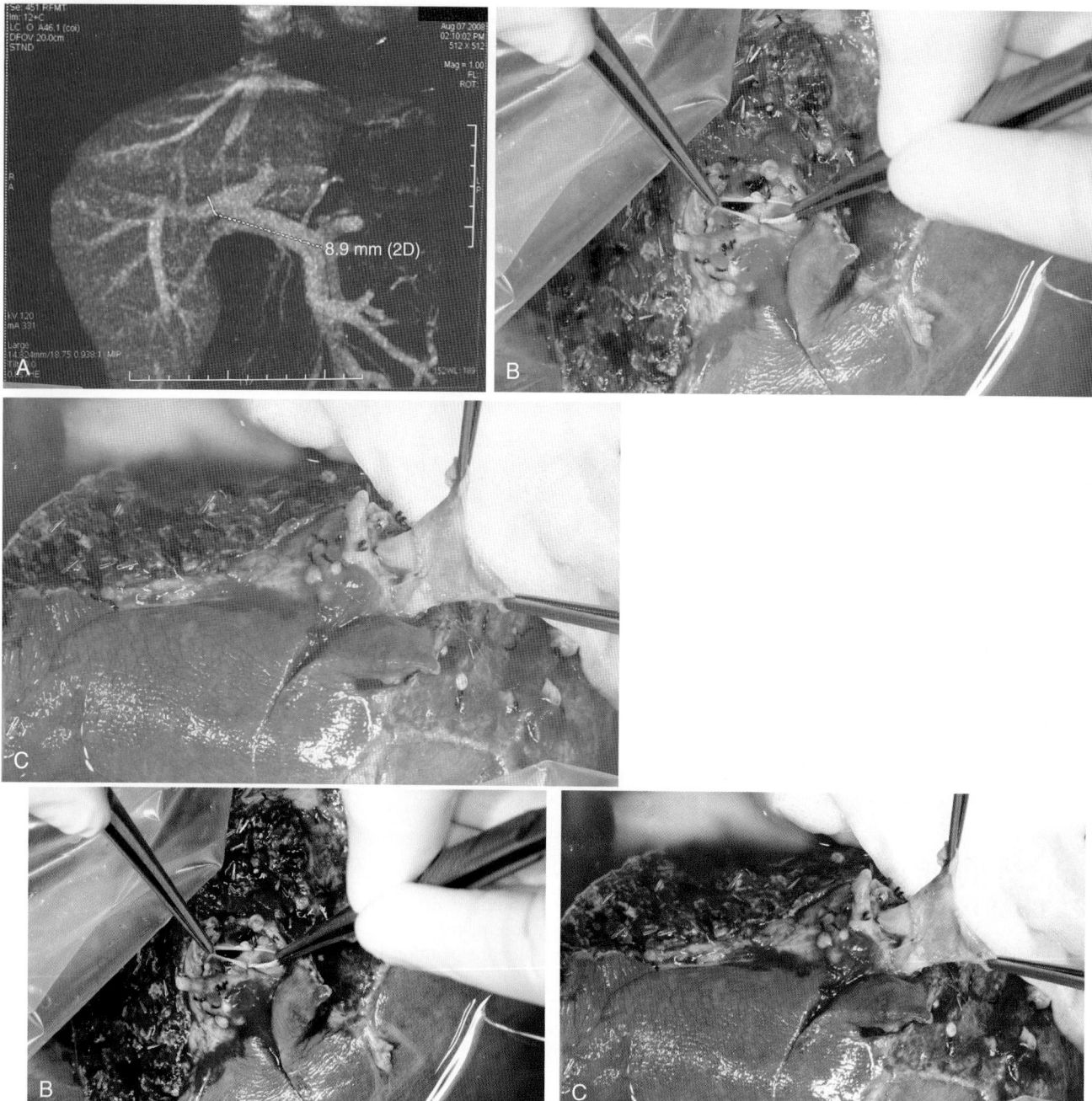

FIGURE 121.11 A, Computed tomography with reconstruction of the portal veins of a donor with separated right anterior and posterior portal vein branches. **B,** Venoplasty of the right anterior and posterior portal vein branches. **C,** Interpositional portal vein from the recipient sutured to the right portal vein branches.

LIVER GRAFT BACK-TABLE PROCEDURE: PERFUSION AND TRIMMING (SEE CHAPTER 125)

To shorten the cold ischemic time, the right liver graft is not delivered until the recipient is almost ready for graft implantation. Once delivered, the graft is flushed with three times the graft volume of a cold solution of histidine-tryptophan-ketoglutarate (HTK; Dr. Franz Köhler, Chemie GmbH, Alsbach-Hähnlein, Germany), while being immersed in an ice-sludge basin on the back table. The right PV is cannulated and adapted to the vein wall with fingers and not ligature (Fig. 121.14A).[37] The right liver graft with separate right anterior and posterior PVs requires simultaneous flushing with two cannulae (Fig. 121.14B). The RHA is flushed with 100 drops of HTK solution through a 21-Fr angiocatheter by gravity (Fig. 121.14C). Inadvertent damage to the artery intima can result in unrecoverable graft loss. The right anterior and posterior sectional ducts are also flushed with cold HTK solution to minimize duct damage during preservation. The graft is weighed and transferred to another basin with cold HTK solution. Venoplasty of the MHV with the RHV of the graft is then performed.[35] Even though the MHV and the RHV are often at a distance of up to 2 cm (Fig. 121.15A), they can be drawn together for fashioning of a single venous cuff (Fig. 121.15B).[38]

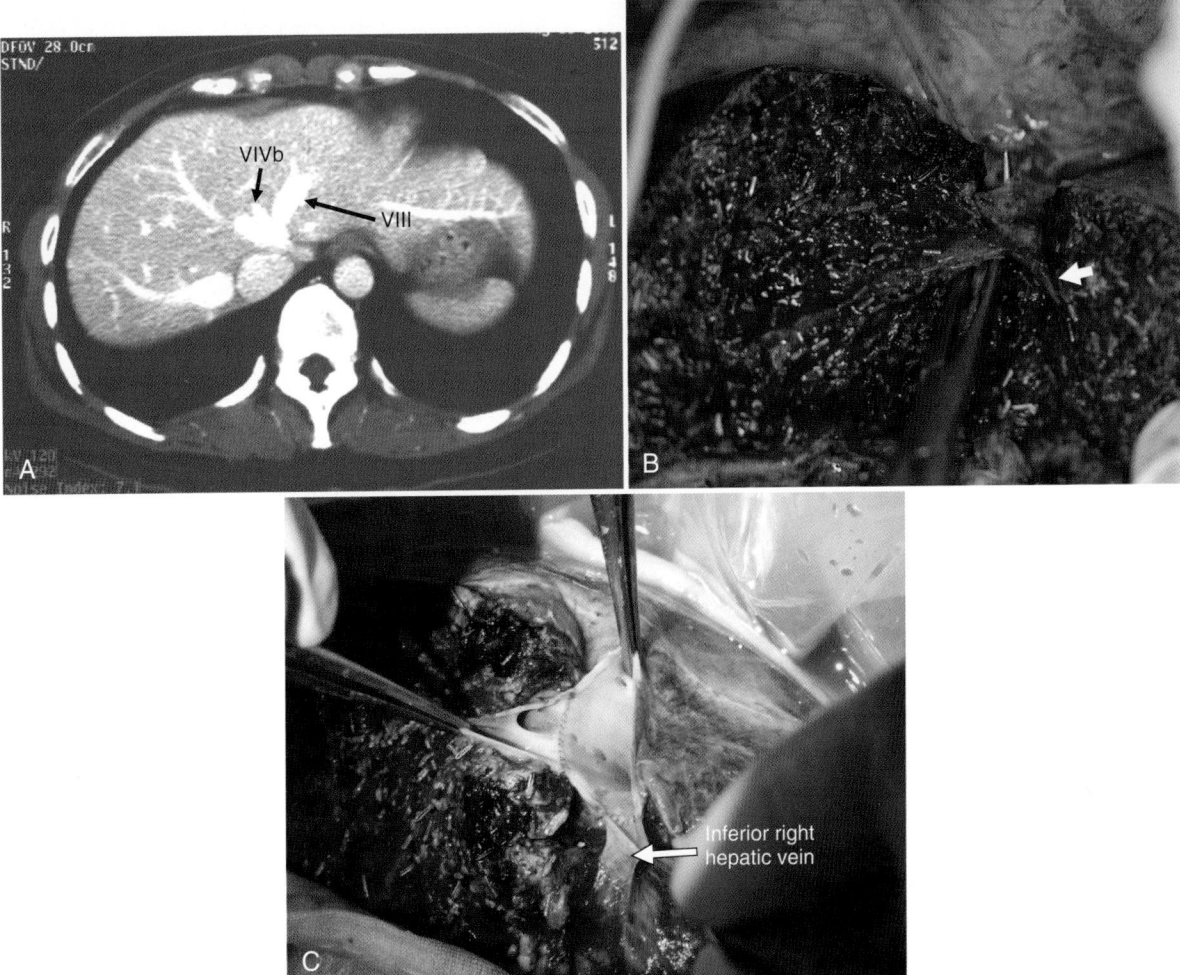

FIGURE 121.12 A, Computed tomography of a donor with segment III and IVb hepatic vein draining into the middle hepatic vein. **B,** The segment III and IVb hepatic vein is preserved during liver transection *(arrowhead).* **C,** Venoplasty of the right, middle, and inferior right hepatic veins into a single cuff.

Often misled by planar schematic drawings, some have a false perception of the inadequate length of the MHV wall portion of the venoplasty for anastomosis to the IVC. In practice the IVC, which is tubular, with a venotomy made over the RHV stump, faces the venoplasty of the MHV and RHV. The portion of the recipient IVC, between the RHV and MHV, also makes up for the deficit in length on the MHV not included in the graft, to preserve the segment IVb HV for venous drainage of the remnant left liver of the donor.

For the left liver graft and the segment II and III graft, if the MHV and the segment II and III vein are separate, they are merged into an equilateral triangle with a single cuff with an apex point to the left by venoplasty. This facilitates HV-to-IVC anastomosis in the recipient. Only with a very low insertion of the segment IVb HV to the MHV is the latter divided caudal to the former. The MHV is reconstructed with artificial vascular graft[39] or deceased donor vessels. The iliac vein is preferred for ease of handling.[40]

The graft is weighed and the weight recorded. The percentage of graft to standard liver volume is calculated, and the graft is then immersed in ice sludge.

DONOR POSTOPERATIVE CARE

Donor hepatectomy, both right and left, is a major surgical procedure undertaken on a healthy volunteer, and meticulous postoperative care should be provided by the healthcare professional (see Chapters 26 and 27). Postoperatively, the donor is transferred to the intensive care unit for close monitoring of hemodynamics and respiratory function (see Chapter 26). Early mobilization and institution of chest physiotherapy minimize the risks of deep vein thrombosis (DVT) and chest infection. Infiltration of wound by local anesthetic before wound closure may reduce wound pain and need of narcotic. The donor will also receive a 6-week course of proton pump inhibitor for peptic ulcer prophylaxis.[27] Female donors receiving hormone replacement therapy and those taking oral contraceptives require aggressive prophylaxis against DVT.

DONOR MORTALITY AND MORBIDITY

Donor safety is fundamental to LDLT (also see Chapter 109). As the application of LDLT has been extended from the child

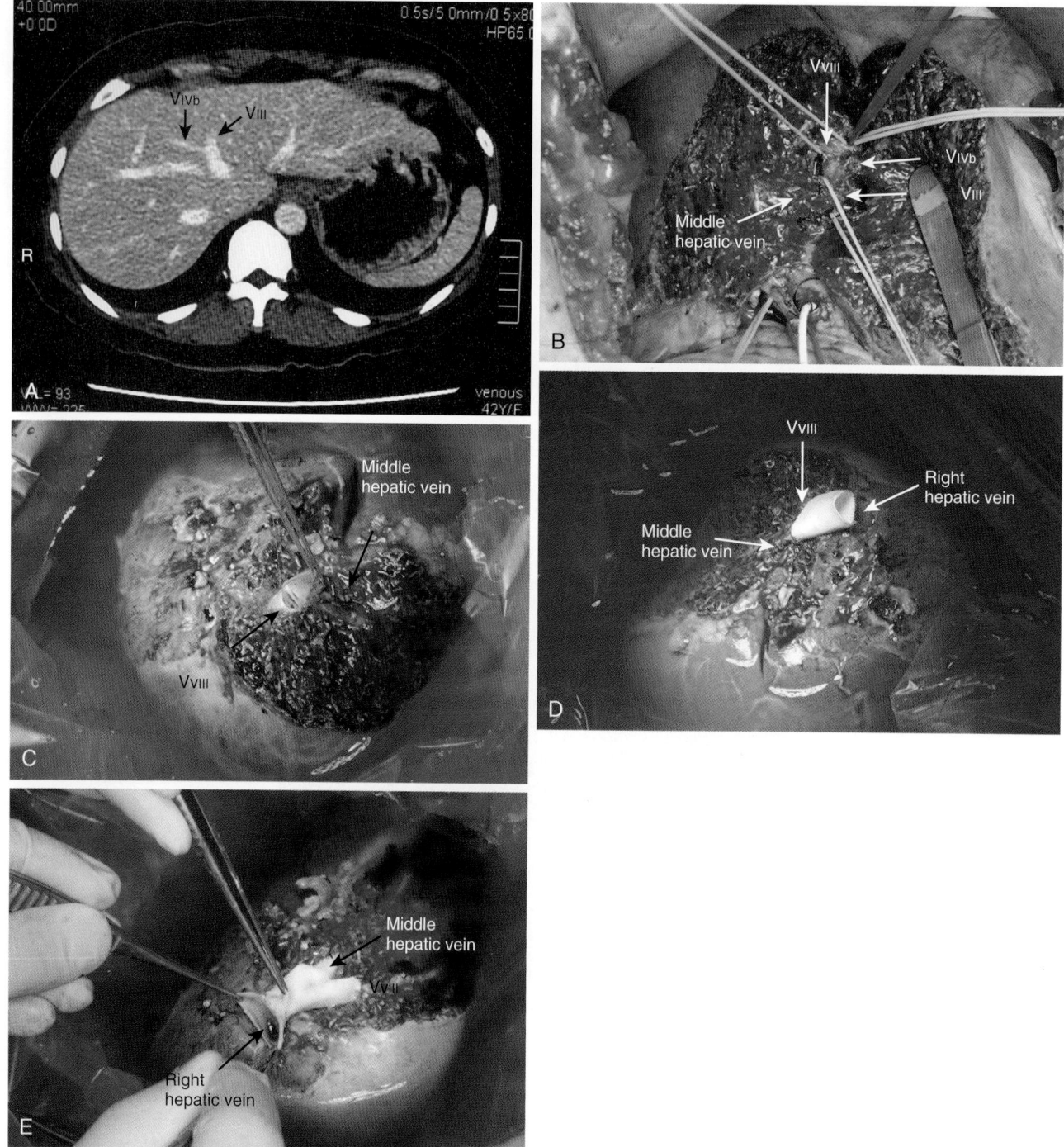

FIGURE 121.13   A, Low insertion of the segment III and Vb hepatic veins to the middle hepatic vein. **B,** Isolation of the segment VIII, III, IVb, and middle hepatic veins. **C,** Merging of the segment VIII and middle hepatic veins by venoplasty using 6/0 Prolene continuous suture. **D,** The single-cuffed segment VIII and middle hepatic veins are merged with a Gore-Tex interpositional graft, which is then merged with the right hepatic vein. **E,** Reconstruction is made with a deceased donor iliac artery graft for segment VIII and middle hepatic veins.

(see Chapter 110) to the adult, and from using the left liver to using the right, the dilemma between recipient success and donor risk has been highlighted. The reported overall complication rate of donors is about 20% but has been reported as high as 67% in one series.[41] A unified system of complication reporting[42] may narrow this range. Although even one donor death is too many, there are at least 19 known donor deaths.[43] The estimated mortality for donor right and left hepatectomy is 0.1% and 0.5%,

respectively,[44] although mortality is lower in a multicenter series in Japan.[45] In achieving a 5-year recipient survival rate of 80%, it takes one donor life to save 160 recipients. Less tangible are the quality of life changes of the donor in comparison to the predonation state.[46] The long-term biologic consequences of donor hepatectomy are not fully known. Nevertheless, decreases in white cell count, platelet counts, and elevation of liver transaminases are demonstrable even 2 years after right liver donation.[47]

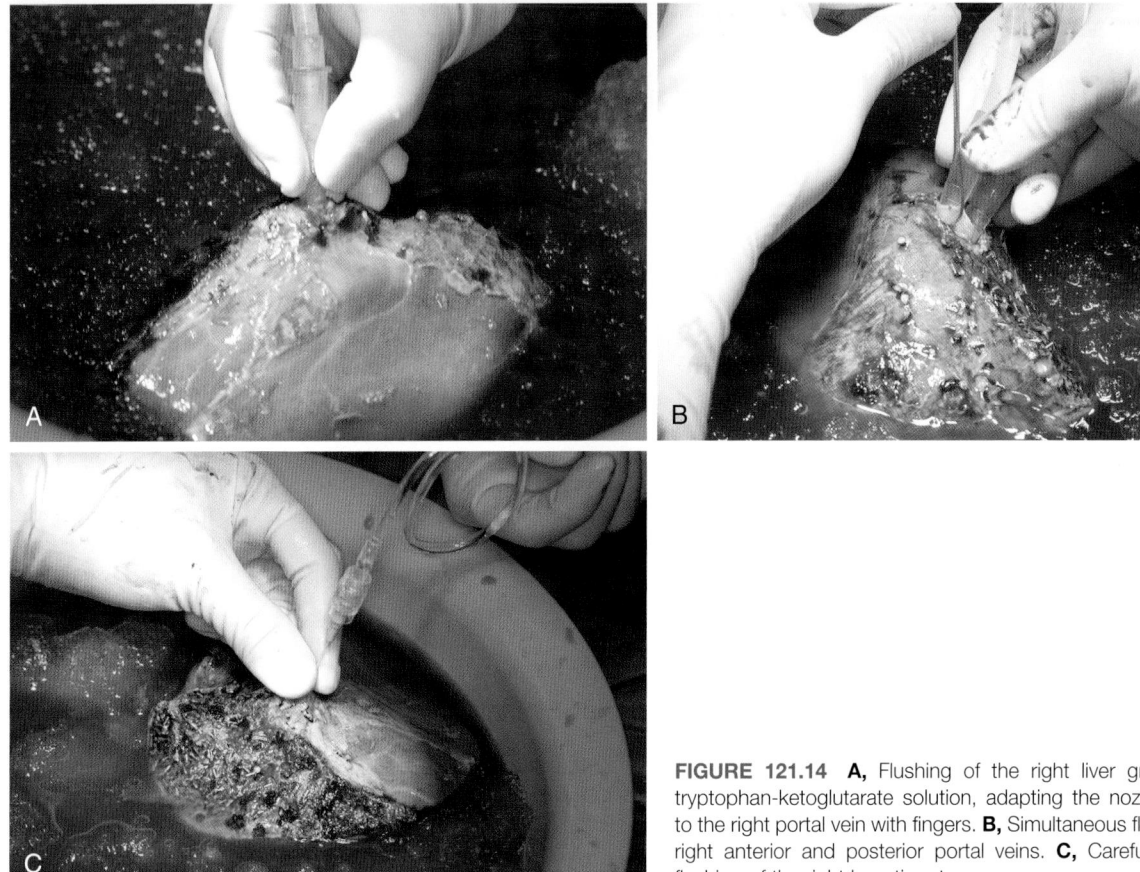

FIGURE 121.14 **A,** Flushing of the right liver graft with histidine-tryptophan-ketoglutarate solution, adapting the nozzle of the cannula to the right portal vein with fingers. **B,** Simultaneous flushing through the right anterior and posterior portal veins. **C,** Careful cannulation and flushing of the right hepatic artery.

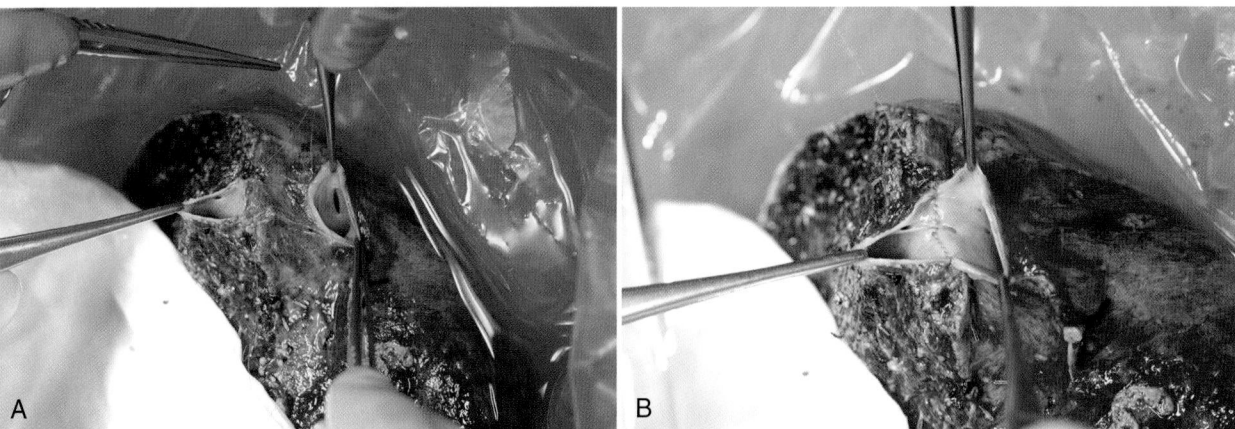

FIGURE 121.15 **A,** Right and middle hepatic veins with a significant distance. **B,** Merging of the right and middle hepatic veins into a single triangular cuff with minimal tension.

CONCLUSION

Although donor mortality after LDLT remains a reality, reducing donor mortality and morbidity and improving recipient survival strengthen the justification for LDLT. With accumulated experience, a smaller liver graft suffices in saving a recipient's life,[48] and thus left LDLT becomes more applicable.[49] However, reducing donor risk should not increase recipient mortality.[50] Donor hepatectomy is an ethical challenge once viewed by the medical community and society with caution and

skepticism.[1,51,52] Donor procedures can only be partially justified by the benefit to a recipient who has no other treatment options. Our common ground is the commitment to provide care of the highest standard to the living liver donor and to perform donor operations in experienced centers.[53] This is the only way to maintain the highest quality and to decrease donor mortality and morbidity.

References are available at expertconsult.com.

CHAPTER 122

Vascular reconstruction techniques in hepato-pancreato-biliary (HPB) surgery

Pietro Addeo and Philippe Bachellier

Over the three last decades, advances in liver surgery have included extensive experience in living and deceased donor-liver transplantation (see Chapters 105 and 125), induction of liver hypertrophy by interventional radiology (portal vein embolization and radioembolization) (see Chapters 94B and 102C) or surgical techniques (associating liver partition and portal vein ligation for staged hepatectomy) (see Chapter 102D), and increased use of neoadjuvant chemotherapeutic drugs to downstage liver disease (see Chapters 97 and 98).

The combination of these medical and surgical advances has led surgeons to push the limits of tumor resectability. The presence of vascular invasion, which can be a common finding in advanced liver tumors, is now not considered as a contraindication for surgery if a radical resection can be reasonably performed with acceptable postoperative morbidity and mortality rates. The risk and benefits of such extended liver resections combined with vascular resection should be balanced against the survival offered by medical treatment. In some cases, the increased perioperative risk of these resections is justified in selected patients undergoing an R0 resection.[1-4] Vascular invasion, however, either of the vessel wall or as a tumoral thrombus, reflects an aggressive tumoral behavior and is a poor prognostic factor. Tumoral thrombosis of the portal vein (PV) and hepatic vein (HV) occurs more often with hepatocellular carcinoma (HCC) and intrahepatic cholangiocarcinoma (ICC) and represents one of the prognostic factors predictive of poor survival.[5,6] Indeed, tumoral invasion of the vascular wall occurs more frequently with adenocarcinoma, notably for ICC and metastatic tumors.[7]

Liver resection in the presence of vascular invasion requires meticulous preoperative preparation for surgery. First, the need for extensive vascular clamping requires appropriate study of the function (indocianine green retention test, functional scintigraphy) and the volume (three-dimensional volumetry) of the future liver remnant (see Chapters 4 and 102). Second, the presence of vascular venous invasion and thrombosis, mainly of the inferior vena cava (IVC) and HVs, promotes the progressive development of intrahepatic venous shunts, which are sources of profuse bleeding during liver transection.[8] These collaterals should be extensively mapped preoperatively and surgical strategy should be adapted to decrease intraoperative bleeding.[9] Third, segmental resection of the involved vessels (vena cava, PV, HV, and hepatic artery) might require vascular interposition grafts. The length and the type of these grafts should be planned preoperatively and grafts should be rapidly available in the operating room. Accurate study of preoperative imaging is of paramount importance in this regard in order to plan the length of the resected vessels and the vascular graft. Fourth, given the bulkiness of some tumors and the need for caval replacement, the use of total vascular exclusion with an extracorporeal venovenous bypass (VVB) can be very common. Specific experience with this technique and the use of VVB is then mandatory before attending these complex procedures. Finally, vascular resection should be performed by well-trained surgeons who should have extensive expertise in both liver surgery and vascular resection to afford the complexity of these resections and give patients the lowest risk of postoperative mortality. In the absence of this experience, patients requiring these complex surgeries should be addressed to tertiary centers experienced in vascular resection during liver surgery (see Chapters 101A and 101B).

RESECTION AND RECONSTRUCTION OF THE INFERIOR VENA CAVA

Generalities

Different types of vascular infiltration of the IVC can be encountered in routine practice. For general rules one can differentiate (1) macrovascular venous invasion as direct extension of a tumoral thrombus into the caval vein, which is frequent in case of renal cell carcinomas, adrenocortical carcinomas, and HCCs; and (2) invasion of the caval venous wall (most frequently seen in ICC and colorectal liver metastasis).[3,4,7,10,11] Based on radiologic examination, tumoral invasion of the IVC can be classified into three groups according to venous segment involved: segment I, infrarenal; segment II, interrenal and suprarenal up to but not including the three hepatic veins; and segment III, suprahepatic with possible intracardiac extension. According to this radiologic classification, clinical symptoms may range from leg edema to life-threatening Budd-Chiari syndrome[12] (see Chapter 86).

Preoperative prediction of histologic IVC invasion remains difficult to assess even with improvements in preoperative imaging and intraoperative exploration by an experienced surgeon. With IVC resection, true histologic vascular wall involvement has been reported to range from 22% to 72% according to different series.[10,11,13,14] In many cases, however, attempts to separate the tumor from the IVC wall, even without histologic involvement, can result in tumoral rupture or sudden entry into the IVC. This occurs frequently in ICC, which can have a desmoplastic reaction between the tumor and IVC wall.[10] Some preoperative computed tomography (CT) findings have been identified as highly suspicious of IVC invasion, such as compression of more than 50% of caval circumference,[15] presence of a peaked deformity of the IVC wall, and extent of the IVC circumference attached to the tumor greater than 25% compared with the whole IVC circumference[7] (see Chapters 14 and 15). The development of large collateral veins between the origins of the hepatic veins mainly in the inferior liver segments is a reliable indirect sign of venous obstruction at the level of the hepatic vein confluence and should be systematically identified before surgery.[16]

Hepatectomy with caval resection should be planned preoperatively and the incidental discovery of caval invasion should remain a rare event. Some basic rules should be used as a guide to such extended resections. Full vascular control below and above the liver of the inferior vena cava as well as the control of the hepatic pedicle and of an eventual accessory left hepatic artery should be the rule. Very often, the presence of a bulky tumor and/or venous thrombus makes liver mobilization difficult and/or risky. In such conditions control of the IVC above the liver should be performed as high as possible without liver mobilization. Different intrapericardial transabdominal approaches of the IVC have been described (see later in this chapter). For parenchymal transection an anterior approach is mostly used and recommended.[17] The presence of venous compression and/or obstruction enhances the development of intrahepatic venous collateral shunts, which can be the source of massive bleeding during parenchymal transection. One should not be reluctant to perform total vascular exclusion (TVE) to reduce bleeding and speed up the procedure. The use of VVB can also reduce the hemodynamic consequences of TVE and provides stability for a longer period.

Control of the Inferior Vena Cava

Resection and reconstruction of the IVC at the time of liver resection requires control of the IVC below and above the liver. Control of the IVC below the liver is easily achieved just below segment I and above the renal veins by a large right angle directed from right to left. On the contrary, control of the IVC above the liver varies according to the extent and location of IVC involvement. The extension of the abdominal incision to the sternum or the thoracic cavity will be determined by the need for controlling the IVC into the thoracic cavity or the need for placing a cardiopulmonary bypass. As a general rule, when the segment of the IVC involved by the tumor is below the hepatic veins, an abdominal incision is sufficient to achieve safe control of the IVC above and below the liver.

A classic method of controlling the IVC entails control of the IVC above the liver after full liver mobilization and ligation of the inferior diaphragmatic veins bilaterally, as described for liver transplantation.[13] This approach could be hazardous in the presence of tumors encasing the hepatocaval confluence, tumoral thrombosis of the retrohepatic IVC, and bulky tumors. In these circumstances, several approaches have been described to achieve safer control of the suprahepatic IVC, either directly into the pericardium by a sternotomy or by a purely abdominal approach. A transabdominal transdiaphragmatic approach to the suprahepatic IVC can often be achieved without the need for sternotomy. The isolation of the suprahepatic IVC can be obtained into the intrapericardial or extrapericardial space (see Chapter 118A).

For the transabdominal transdiaphragmatic intrapericardial approach to the suprahepatic IVC, three different approaches have been described. A first approach entails a transverse incision of the bilateral diaphragm just below the pericardial cavity and then sectioning the bottom of the pericardium.[18] A second approach consists of dissecting off the central tendon of the diaphragm circumferentially. The falciform ligament is divided with cautery, and the incision is continued around each portion of the divided falciform ligament to the right superior coronary ligament. The left triangular ligament and the central diaphragm tendon are dissected until the supradiaphragmatic intrapericardial IVC is identified. The dissection has to be circumferential

so that the intrapericardial IVC can be encircled below or above the confluence into the right atrium.[19] A third approach entails the isolation of the IVC through a transdiaphragmatic pericardial window. After mobilizing the left liver, the diaphragm and bottom of the pericardium are vertically incised, and the intrapericardial IVC is isolated.[20] These approaches are mainly used when, for technical or oncologic reasons, clamping of the IVC must be performed close to the right atrium. Although all these approaches avoid sternotomy, the opening of the pericardium increases right ventricular end-diastolic and end-systolic volumes, resulting in diminished right ventricular ejection fraction. In addition, postoperative pericardial effusion, constrictive pericarditis, and cardiac tamponade can develop.[21] Pericardial drainage should be the rule every time that the pericardium is opened (see Chapter 118A).

Two additional transabdominal transdiaphragmatic extrapericardial approaches to the IVC can be used as alternatives to the previous techniques. The first includes dissecting the diaphragm from the pericardium just below the xiphoid process, cutting the diaphragm vertically toward the IVC, and then taping the IVC after dissecting the fusion space between the pericardium and the diaphragm.[21] In the second approach, after opening the posterior part of the falciform ligament and lowering the liver, the IVC is isolated in the same space while making a 5- to 7-cm transverse incision of the diaphragm 2 to 3 cm above the vena cava foramen. The dissection between the diaphragm and the inferior side of the pericardium allows identification of the IVC that can be taped.[22] In both approaches, the diaphragm must be closed at the end of the procedure.

Clamping Procedures and Inferior Vena Cava Resection

Generally, there is no need to perform TVE of the liver if the part of the IVC involved by the tumor is below the hepatic veins. In such circumstances, parenchymal transection is performed first under intermittent inflow occlusion if necessary.[23] Once the IVC is exposed, portal inflow occlusion is released, the patient is volume-loaded, and clamps are placed above and below the area of tumor involvement (Fig. 122.1). Resection of the retrohepatic IVC will be performed en bloc with the liver tumor. Positioning the clamps below the hepatic vein allows perfusion of the remnant liver by the hepatic pedicle and minimizes ischemia time. With lateral involvement of the IVC below

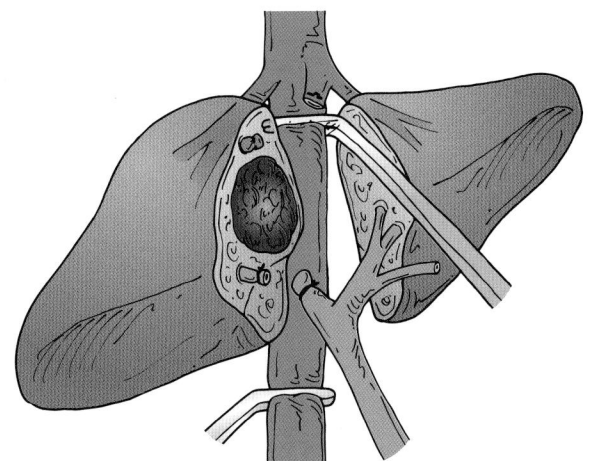

FIGURE 122.1 Clamps placed above and below the area of tumor involvement on the inferior vena cava.

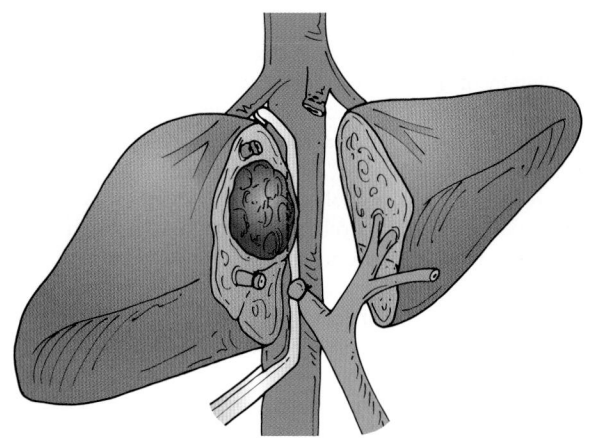

FIGURE 122.2   A single clamp applied tangentially to the inferior vena cava to preserve vena caval flow in the case of lateral wall involvement.

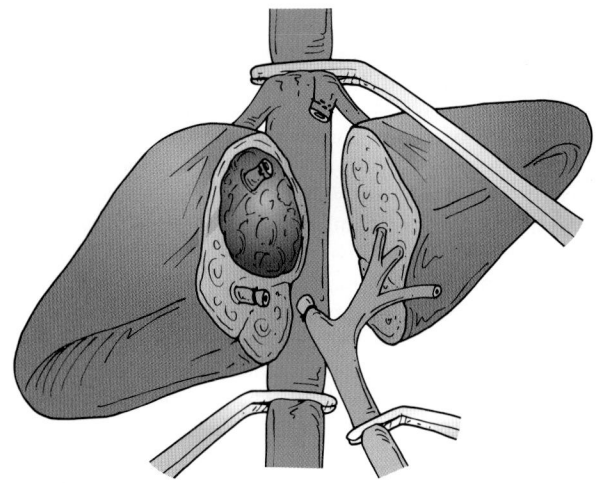

FIGURE 122.4   Clamps positioning for classical total vascular exclusion (TVE) of the liver.

the hepatic veins, a single clamp may be applied tangentially to the IVC to preserve the caval flow (Fig. 122.2). These two techniques cannot be applied when the tumor involves the hepatocaval confluence or there is tumoral thrombotic extension along the vena cava. In such cases, two different approaches may be applied: TVE with preserved liver remnant perfusion[24] and standard TVE with or without an active VVB and in situ cold perfusion of the liver.[2,10,13]

Total vascular exclusion with preserved liver remnant perfusion can be used where there is synchronous involvement of the IVC and any of the hepatocaval confluences with at least one hepatic vein free of tumor.[24] The suprahepatic IVC is taped just below the diaphragm, the common trunk of the left and middle hepatic veins is dissected, and a previously deployed suprahepatic tape is rotated to the right side between the vena cava and common trunk. This isolates the right hepatocaval confluence and juxtahepatic vena cava, leaving the common trunk and the rest of the IVC free. The infrahepatic IVC is clamped, and for the suprahepatic IVC, a clamp is placed obliquely to occlude the right hepatocaval confluence and juxtahepatic vena cava (Fig. 122.3). When the right side of the hepatocaval junction is uninvolved, this procedure can be used in patients with left-sided neoplasms by

reversing the caval tape to the left side.[25] The remnant liver receives complete inflow with uninterrupted outflow through the uninvolved hepatocaval confluence, the patency of which is maintained. This procedure has the potential disadvantage of incomplete vascular control during parenchymal transection in the presence of large veins from the caudate lobe, which leads to backflow venous bleeding. This problem can be overcome by associated resection of segment I.

For classic TVE, control of the IVC above and below the liver and control of the hepatic pedicle are performed as previously described. Once these structures have been clamped, parenchymal transection is performed by the anterior approach. The portion of the liver and involved IVC is then removed, allowing improved access for reconstruction of the IVC (Fig. 122.4). Performance of TVE induces a decrease of 40% to 50% in the cardiac index and may be not well tolerated in some patients.[26] The duration of TVE that a healthy liver can safely tolerate varies among series, ranging from 30 to 120 minutes. Ischemia/reperfusion injury and the subsequent risk of liver failure are the main limitations of standard TVE performed under continuous warm liver ischemia. For this reason, when liver ischemia is expected to exceed 1 hour, the use of hypothermic perfusion through the PV is recommended.[26] This technique is also beneficial in severe hepatic injury (prolonged preoperative chemotherapy, cholestatic liver) requiring complex hepatectomy with IVC resection to prevent postoperative fatal liver failure. Although most patients tolerate TVE, the use of VVB can be considered when the total time of TVE is expected to exceed 1 hour.[26] Hemodynamic intolerance to TVE is characterized by a decrease in mean arterial pressure greater than 30% or a decrease in cardiac index greater than 50%.[27] In such conditions, the use of a VVB reduces the time pressure, maintains stable systemic hemodynamics without the need for fluid overload, and prevents kidney and splanchnic venous congestion.[2] For the in situ hypothermic perfusion of the liver associated with VVB, the right femoral and left axillary veins are surgically cannulated or directly punctured under ultrasound guidance. The portal system will be cannulated through the inferior mesenteric vein, if available. TVE and VVB complete the preparation for hypothermic perfusion. The PV is clamped and a small purse-string suture placed on the anterior wall of

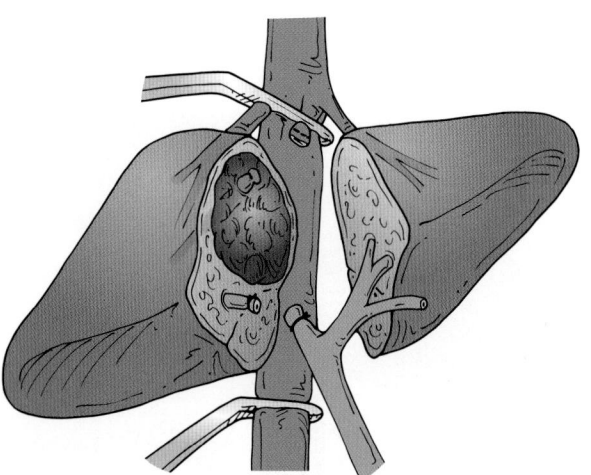

FIGURE 122.3   The infrahepatic vena cava is clamped, and a clamp is placed obliquely on the suprahepatic inferior vena cava to occlude right hepatocaval confluence and juxtahepatic vena cava.

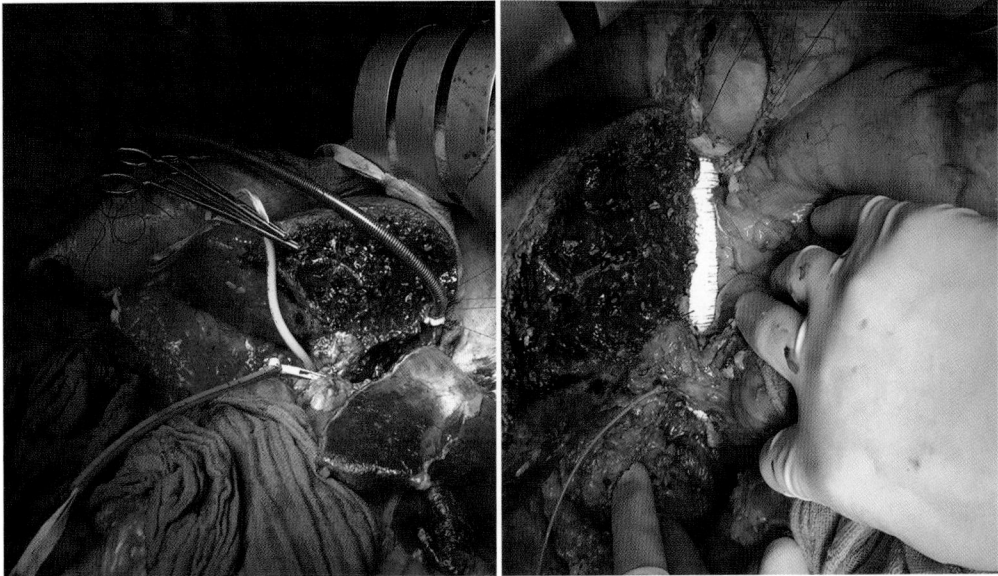

FIGURE 122.5 Intraoperative view of a left hepatectomy extended to the segment 1 and the inferior vena cava (IVC) under total vascular exclusion and venovenous bypass. **A,** The suprahepatic IVC has been isolated via an intrapericardial approach. The right hepatic vein has been isolated during the parenchymal transection and is connected to the venovenous bypass in order to avoid in-situ cooling. **(B)** The inferior vena cava has been replaced by a PTFE prothesis with reimplantation of the right hepatic vein.

the PV above the clamp. A venotomy is done at the same site and the PV cannulated with a Silastic catheter above the portal clamp. TVE is completed and the liver perfused through the portal system with preservation solution at 4°C.[2,13,26,27] A cavotomy is always performed just above the IVC clamp to enable the drainage of the perfusate by a 30-Fr cannula. This is done to prevent spilling the cold perfusate in the peritoneal cavity, which decreases the patient's core temperature. Isolation and ligature of the right adrenal vein and diaphragmatic veins should always be performed before proceeding to TVE, to avoid continuous bleeding into the operative field.

An alternative to the techniques described entails the ex vivo liver resection procedures. Originally described by Pichlmayr et al. (1988),[28] the liver is removed from the body and perfused. The caval and portal flows are maintained through the VVB, and the liver resection is performed on the back table in a bloodless field, allowing reconstruction to be performed under ideal conditions. The main drawback of this technique is represented by the necessity of adding portal, arterial, and biliary reconstruction to caval reconstruction, with potentially significant morbidity. The reported experience with this technique remains limited, and its use should be considered with caution.[10,29] An alternative approach is to use the antesitum approach, where the portal triad structures are left intact (although clamped), and the IVC is divided above and below the tumor. This allows the liver to be rotated up to the surface of the operative field, which permits improved access for IVC reconstruction.[30,31] More recently, in cases of tumoral involvement of the IVC at the hepatocaval confluence requiring inferior vena cava replacement with reimplantation of the hepatic vein of the future liver remnant, one alternative technique can be proposed instead of in situ cooling and TVE. This technique can be considered as a variant of the antesitum technique[30] and entails parenchymal transection (with or without pedicular clamping) up to the hepatic vein to be reconstructed. This hepatic vein is sectioned and cannulated, and the patient is put on an extrahepatic venous bypass. In this technique, the need for

in situ cooling is avoided and the liver maintains its natural perfusion[32] through the hepatic pedicle and its drainage via the hepatic vein through the VVB (Fig. 122.5).

Inferior Vena Cava Reconstruction

With complete obstruction of the IVC, the necessity of reconstruction is debated. Simple ligation can be sufficient after resection of the infrarenal IVC (segment I) and/or retrohepatic IVC (segment II) when the right kidney is resected. In these circumstances, collateral circulation from the left kidney via the genital, middle capsular, and reno-azygo-lumbar veins can provide adequate kidney venous drainage.[12,33] Some authors have reported that edema of the lower limbs after IVC ligation is generally transitory and well tolerated.[33] However, others have suggested that pressure monitoring must be performed to rule out venous hypertension during clamping, specifying that a venous pressure greater than 30 mm Hg indicates caval reconstruction.[12] When the right kidney is not resected, the right renal vein should be reimplanted because collateral venous systems at that level generally are not sufficient.

Reconstruction of the IVC after segmental or tangential resection of the retrohepatic IVC is generally performed after liver resection as the last step of the procedure. However, some authors have described the resection of the IVC before liver resection to obtain a more controlled parenchymal transection.[34] When a tangential resection has been performed, the reconstruction can be achieved by primary closure or patch repair. Resection of more than 50% of IVC diameter makes patch reconstruction always necessary to avoid severe stenosis; autologous or synthetic patches can be used. Some authors offer alternative techniques to avoid use of patch, consisting of primary suturing of a longitudinal lateral defect of the IVC in the transversal approach, as for pyloroplasty.[35] Prosthetic replacement is used for segmental resection of the IVC or as an alternative to patch use when more than 50% of IVC diameter has been resected.[1] The ringed, 18- to 20-mm-diameter Gore-Tex graft is currently the graft of choice for replacing the IVC

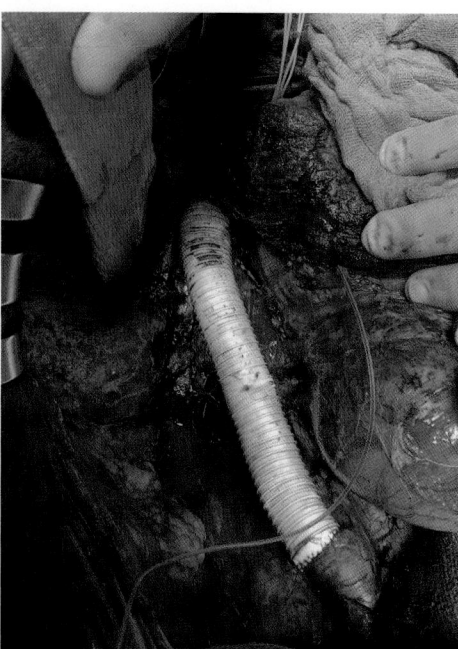

FIGURE 122.6 Intraoperative view of an en-bloc right hepatectomy with right nephrectomy and a long inferior vena cava (IVC) resection. The IVC has been replaced by a 20-mm diameter long Gore-Tex prosthesis with direct left renal vein reimplantation.

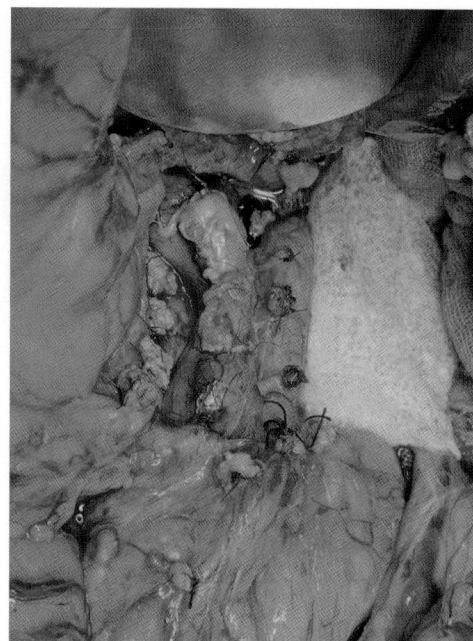

FIGURE 122.7 Intraoperative view of a peritoneal patch used for reconstructing a lateral resection of the spleno-mesenetericoportal venous confluence during a left splenopancreatectomy.

because of its resistance to compression to pressure from surrounding viscera and prevention of respiratory collapse that might favor thrombosis (Fig. 122.6). Its main drawback is possible infection, as already reported.[36] An omental or muscular wrap placed around the synthetic graft has been employed to reduce risk of infection.[37] Another advantage of this graft is its high rate of patency, and current experience recommends only long-term aspirin maintenance.[10] Other authors have described replacement of the IVC by cryopreserved autologous or heterologous venous graft.[38,39] Cryopreserved heterologous grafts have the main advantage of not requiring anticoagulation, although the long-term outcomes of this type of graft have been characterized by a high rate of midterm thrombosis when used in liver transplantation.[40] Recently a new alternative to synthetic materials has been represented by the use of autologous periotoneal patches.[41] In animal studies peritoneal patches have been showed the capability of neoendothelialization.[42] These peritoneal patches can be rapidly harvested anywhere in the abdominal cavity and they do not need long-term anticoagulation.[43] Generally, the peritoneal patch is harvested on the right diaphragm or the right kidney and the peritoneal side is sutured to the vascular wall (Fig. 122.7). Intimal eversion is preferred as a vascular suturing technique to minimize the risk of thrombosis. The main advantages of using peritoneal patches is the unlimited availability, low cost, and easiness to suture. However, the long-term complications of this technique (fibrosis, stenosis, thrombosis) are not yet fully available.

HEPATIC VEIN RESECTION AND RECONSTRUCTION

Tumors in the central or posterior portion of the liver may extend to involve the hepatic veins, making resection using standard techniques difficult (see Chapter 89). Sacrifice of one or two hepatic veins can be one of the technical options, provided that collateral circulation is present. For example, a tumor located in the superior segments of the right liver (VII,VIII, IVa) may require resection of the right hepatic vein (RHV) alone or in combination with the middle hepatic vein (MHV) (see Chapter 118A). This is possible when adequate outflow from segment VI can be maintained through a large inferior hepatic vein or intrahepatic collaterals (Fig. 122.8).[44] However, a large inferior hepatic vein that drains all of segment VI is present in 20% to 24% of patients,[45] and the RHV needs to be reconstructed in case of absence of a right inferior hepatic vein.[46]

In rare cases, all three hepatic veins can be resected when a large inferior RHV draining segments V and VI is present.[47] Experience in living-donor liver transplantation has shown that

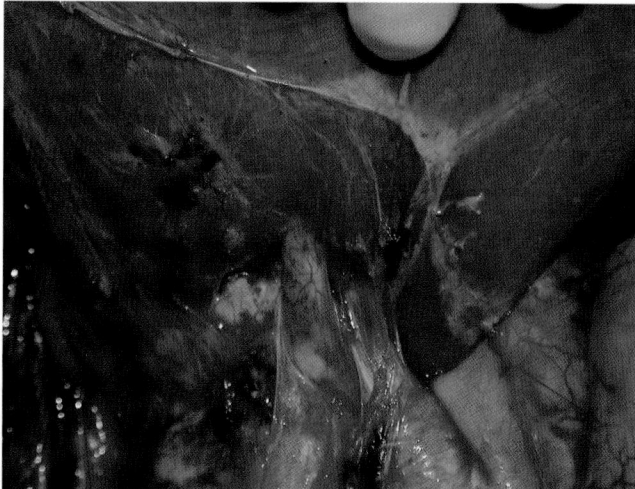

FIGURE 122.8 Intraoperative view of a large Makuuchi vein draining segment VI (see Chapter 2).

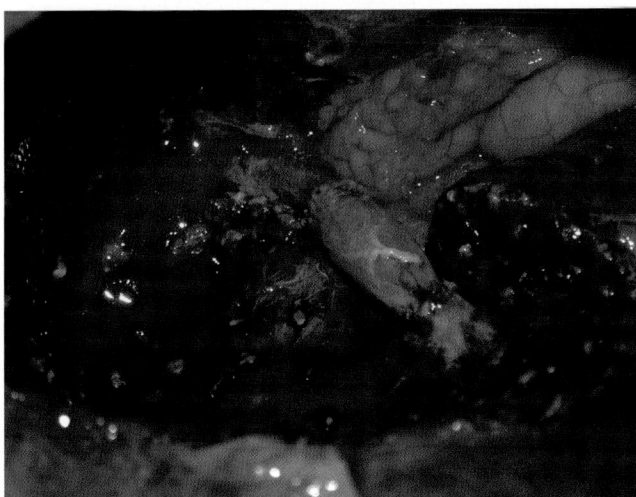

FIGURE 122.9 Intraoperative view of resection of segments II and IVa with the middle and left hepatic veins. The left hepatic vein has been reconstructed using a left renal vein graft.

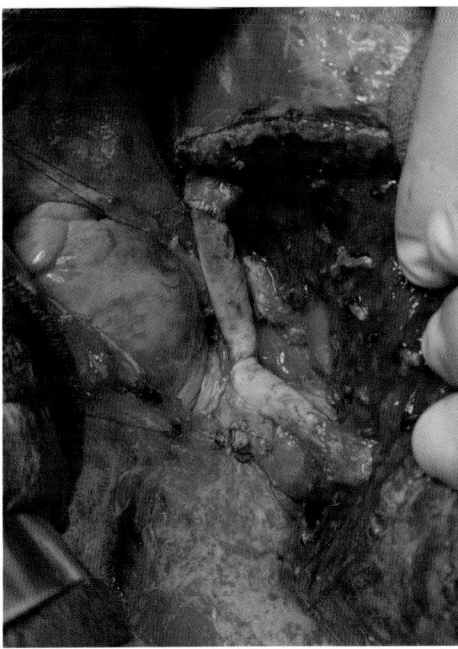

FIGURE 122.10 Intraoperative view of a long segmental resection of the middle and left hepatic vein into the liver parenchyma. Vascular replacement has been achieved by interposing a cryopreserved saphenous graft between the two veins' stumps (end to-end anastomosis) and the anterior face of the inferior vena cava (side-to-side anastomosis).

venous congestion of the remnant liver caused by outflow impairment has detrimental effects on liver regeneration and causes graft dysfunction. To decrease the risks of venous congestion, in right liver living-related liver transplantation, all venous branches greater than 5 mm in diameter are generally reimplanted in the recipient IVC.[48,49]

After resection, different techniques and materials can be used for reconstruction. A simple venoplasty and autologous/heterologous patches can be used for a lateral defect of the major hepatic veins. Autologous materials such as portal and hepatic veins from the resected specimen can be used and have the advantage of not requiring additional procedures in the patient.[45,50] Alternatively, saphenous, left renal, jugular, ovarian, and external iliac conduits can be used (Fig. 122.9).[51,52] With segmental resection of hepatic veins, the left renal vein, iliac, or tubulized saphenous graft can be used and anastomosed directly to the IVC or the stump of the hepatic vein.[51,53] In the case of multiple resections or resection of a long segment of hepatic vein, cryopreserved saphenous and/or iliac grafts can be used for reconstructing the hepatic vein confluence. Parenchymal transection will allow the surgeon to find the trunks of the hepatic veins in the parenchyma and a segment of a saphenous graft can be interposed between the hepatic veins stump into the liver and the IVC directly (Fig. 122.10).

When autologous grafts are not available, polytetrafluoroethylene (PTFE) grafts (8 mm) can be used.[1] The main advantage of these grafts is the wide range of diameters and lengths that are available. However, potential disadvantages are the risk of infection and long-term stricture and thrombosis.[1]

One alternative is direct reimplantation of the distal stump of a hepatic vein on its orifice over the IVC, as described for the MHV after right hepatectomy (Fig. 122.11), or direct reimplantation of the MHV on the left hepatic vein in a limited resection of the superior part of segment IV (Fig. 122.12).[54] This is called the "digging technique," in which an additional atypical resection of part of segment IVa is done, "digging" around the distal end of the MHV to further mobilize the liver and to achieve, with an upward lifting of the remnant liver, a tension-free end-to-end reconstruction of the MHV (see Fig. 122.12).

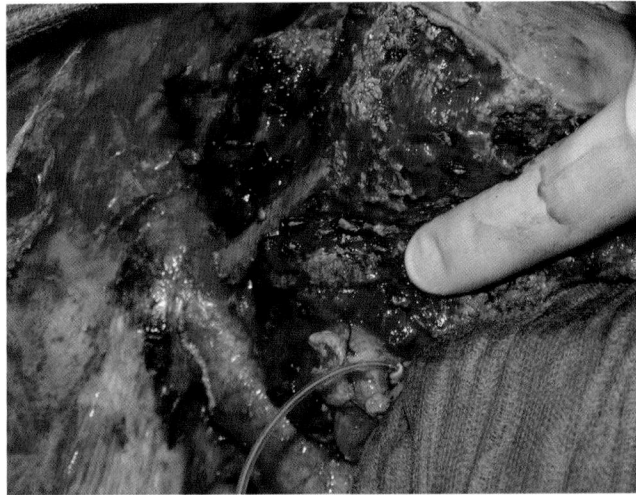

FIGURE 122.11 Intraoperative view of the "digging technique" (see text).

In cases of resection of the RHV along with segments VII and VIII of the liver, parenchymal transection is generally performed with intermittent occlusion of the portal inflow. The origin of the RHV is dissected over the IVC, and the intrahepatic RHV is dissected into the hepatic parenchyma more than 1 cm to allow safe clamping. The parenchymal transection is completed, leaving the specimen attached to the IVC by the RHV. Portal flow is then reestablished, and segment VI is carefully observed for signs of venous congestion. The origin of the RHV is next clamped over the IVC, and resection and reconstruction of the RHV are performed under selective right pedicular clamping.[46]

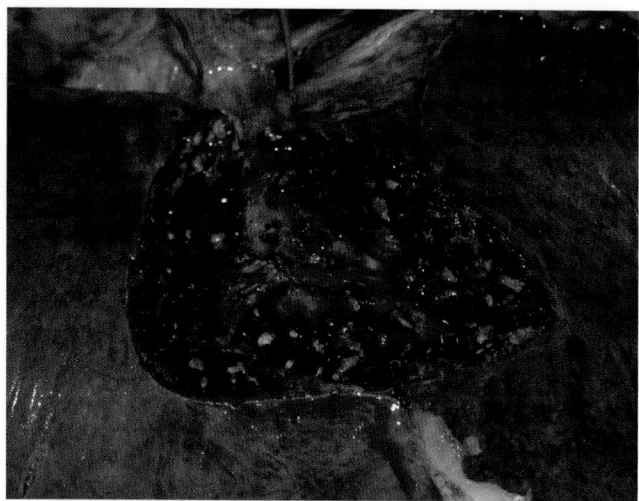

FIGURE 122.12 Intraoperative view showing direct reimplantation of the middle hepatic vein over the left hepatic vein after resection of a colorectal liver metastasis infiltrating the middle hepatic vein.

In cases of tumoral lesions involving the hepatic veins and the IVC, two different approaches can be used. The first is used when there is simultaneous IVC and hepatic vein involvement without portal structure involvement and entails division of the hepatic parenchyma toward the IVC under portal inflow occlusion. Therefore clamps are placed below the tumor on the IVC and above the hepatic vein. The IVC is then transected above and below the tumor, allowing the liver and involved portion of the IVC to be rotated up onto the surface of the operative field. The resection is completed in an in vivo, ex situ position, allowing repair or reimplantation of the hepatic veins.[30,46] In cases of simultaneous involvement of the IVC, hepatic veins, and portal structures, the only approach that can be used is the ex vivo technique.[28]

PORTAL VEIN RESECTION AND RECONSTRUCTION

Metastatic or primary liver cancer can be associated with infiltration of the PV system. Hepatocellular carcinoma tends to diffuse through the PV with tumoral thrombus (see Chapter 89). The presence of portal vein tumor thrombus (PVTT) in patients with HCC is one of the most significant factors for a poor prognosis. In patients undergoing resection of gross PVTT in the portal trunk and first-order branches (main right or main left PV), the 3-year and 5-year survival rates were 15% to 28% and 0% to 17%, respectively.[55-58]

Since tumor thrombus derived from HCC rarely infiltrates the PV wall, thrombectomy represents a viable treatment option. Inoue et al. (2009)[59] reported no differences in survival in patients with macroscopic PVTT undergoing a thrombectomy or PV resection. Thrombectomy should be performed before mobilization to minimize the intraoperative migration of the tumor thrombus into the future liver remnant. During resection of the right liver, parenchymal division should precede thrombectomy to expose the root of the portal branch, enabling a broader surgical field. Hilar cholangiocarcinoma (see Chapter 51), intrahepatic cholangiocarcinoma (see Chapter 50), and colorectal liver metastases can invade the PV bifurcation. Despite recent advances in diagnostic imaging techniques, PV invasion is still a relatively frequent operative finding. Surgeons should suspect invasion if they find severe adhesions between the tumor and the PV bifurcation. In these situations, combined resection and reconstruction of the bifurcation are necessary to obtain a negative surgical margin. Hilar cholangiocarcinoma is prone to perineural and lymphatic spread, and because of its anatomic location, infiltration or severe adhesions to the PV bifurcation frequently occur (see Chapter 51B). Usually, PV resection has been carried out when the vein is adherent to the tumor and cannot be freed. However, even with negative histopathologic margins, local or peritoneal recurrence may occur during the follow-up period. One possible reason for recurrence is microscopic dissemination of cancer cells during PV dissection in the hilar region, where the bile duct involved lies very close to the PV. Indeed, the distance between the tumor and the outer layer of the PV adventitia is less than 1 mm, even without portal infiltration. Ebata et al. (2003)[60] reported that intraoperative macroscopic diagnosis of PV infiltration, regardless of microscopic diagnosis, was a significant prognostic factor, suggesting that tumoral exposure might occur during dissection regardless of the presence of microscopic infiltration. Based on these findings, Neuhaus et al. (1999)[61] developed a "no-touch technique" for right-sided hilar cholangiocarcinoma, combining an extended right hepatectomy and caudate lobectomy with a systematic PV bifurcation resection. This technique avoids the dissection of the right hepatic artery, which can easily be infiltrated by the tumor, and obtains a wide tumor-free biliary margin, since the left hepatic duct measures up to 5 cm. These authors reported significant 5-year survival of 65% using this technique for right-sided hilar cholangiocarcinoma.[61] More recent data showed 87%, 70%, and 58% survival at 1, 3, and 5 years, respectively, after hilar en bloc resection, significantly better than the 79%, 40%, and 29% survival reported after standard right hepatectomy for similar-stage disease,[62] although it must be emphasized that these data are retrospective and uncontrolled (see Chapters 101 and 118A).

With improvements in surgical technique and perioperative care, PV resection is now performed in 10% to 40% of hilar cholangiocarcinoma resections.[63,64] PV resection has not been associated with an increase in morbidity or mortality in subgroup analyses, including studies from high-volumes centers after 2007.[65] The Nagoya Group[66] showed in a large study on PV resection for hilar cholangiocarcinoma that vascular resection did not increase the postoperative morbidity and mortality of liver resection for hilar cholangiocarcinoma. The overall survival of patients who underwent resection with vascular resection (median, 30 months) was shorter than that of those who underwent resection without vascular resection (median, 61 months; $P < .0001$); however, it was longer than that of those who did not undergo resection (median, 10 months; $P < .0001$).

Technically, resection of the left portal vein (LPV) during right and extended right hepatectomies is easier because of its long extrahepatic length and the ready access to the vein within the umbilical fissure beyond the limit of the tumor. LPV resection can be performed early in the operation or at the end of parenchymal transection as the last step.[67,68] The latter option has the advantage of avoiding the risk that surgical maneuvers after PV reconstruction might produce tension on the venous anastomosis with consequent disruption. There is generally no need for interposition graft when resecting the LPV, but

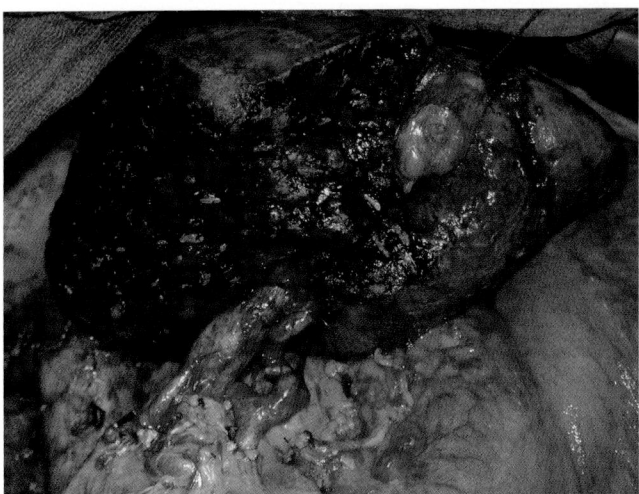

FIGURE 122.13 Intraoperative view of an extended right hepatectomy to segments IV and I by the no-touch technique, with resection and reconstruction of the portal vein bifurcation. A blue-inked line has been drawn on the main portal vein and left portal vein before resection to avoid twisting of the two ends.

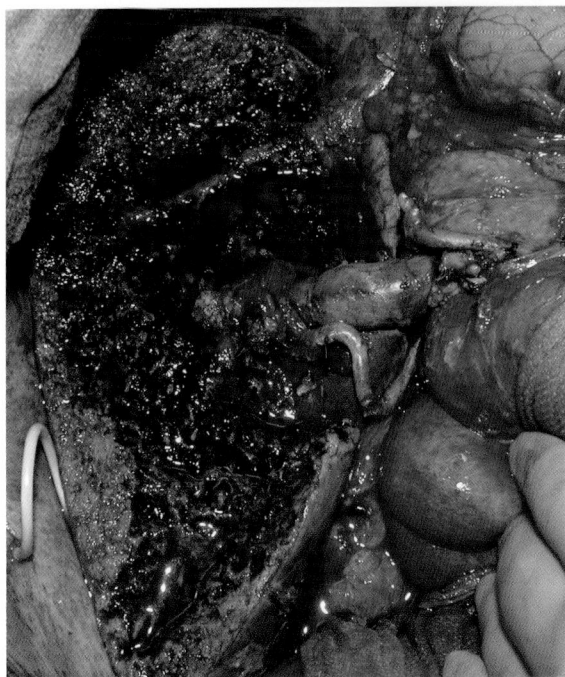

FIGURE 122.14 Intraoperative view of a left trisectionectomy extended to segment I with portal vein bifurcation resection and reconstruction for a left-sided hilar cholangiocarcinoma.

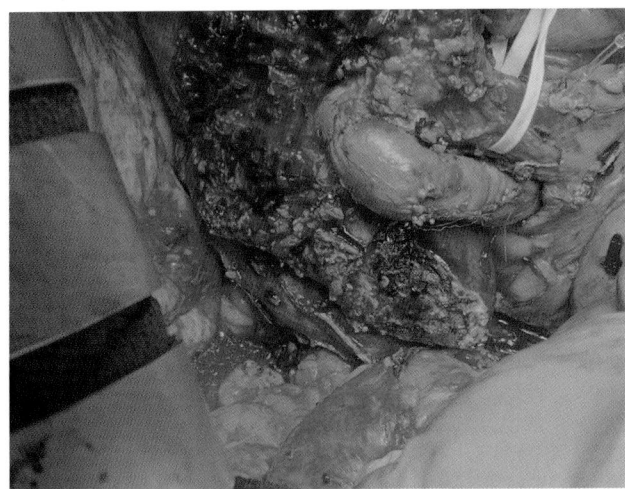

FIGURE 122.15 Intraoperative view of portal vein reconstruction during an extended right hepatectomy for hepatocellular carcinoma. A saphenous tube has been interposed between the main portal trunk and the left portal branch into the liver parenchyma.

systematic right colon and mesenteric root mobilization should be performed to facilitate a tension-free anastomosis between the main portal vein (MPV) and LPV. A continuous suture is used, and an oblique cut of the LPV is performed to minimize discrepancies of caliber. Twisting of the two ends can be avoided simply by drawing a longitudinal line on the MPV and LPV before resection (Fig. 122.13). We refer to this line for end-to-end anastomosis to maintain the axis of the reconstructed vessels.[67] The anastomosis starts by putting the stay sutures on the left and right sides, and the posterior and anterior wall suturing is performed in continuous fashion. A 5-mm growth factor is used to facilitate the vessels' expansion.

Resection of the right portal vein (RPV) after left or extended left hepatectomy can be more technically challenging because the RPV is short and bifurcates early (see Chapter 2). The limits of RPV resection are the point where the first-order branches of the RPV can be safely controlled with vascular clamps (Fig. 122.14). Technical principles are the same as used for LPV resection. However, with resection up to the main RPV, there is considerable discrepancy between the MPV diameter and the sectional branches, which requires technical adjustments such as anastomoses with interrupted sutures.[69] If the length of the PV resected exceeds 6 cm, an interposition graft is needed. Autologous (left renal, iliac, or jugular vein)[45,51,52] or heterologous (10-mm PTFE graft) grafts can be used for these reconstructions.[1]

In case of massive invasion of the left portal vein, a "Rex recess approach" for the resection of a right-sided hilar cholangiocarcinoma can be performed. This technique, which further expands the no-touch concept, has been developed to extend the left margin of the resection to the right side of the left hepatic artery. The LPV is exposed within the Rex recess with its segmental veins. A Satinsky vascular clamp is applied behind the segmental vein, the PV bifurcation is resected, and an end-to-side anastomosis is created between the main portal trunk and the ventral part of the Rex recess PV using an interposition graft (iliac vein).[70]

Alternatively, cryopreserved saphenous grafts can be used for reconstructing the portal vein as described in living-donor liver transplantation. To this aim, those grafts are opened longitudinally and rolled around a 10/20 cc syringe making a venous tube. Transverse and longitudinal edges are sutured together with 6/0 sutures. Venous tubes are used to replace long segments of the portal vein (Fig. 122.15).

As a rule, in patients with vascular (venous and/or artery) reconstruction, we use curative anticoagulation (intravenous heparin) during the first postoperative week. Computed tomography of the abdomen is performed during the first postoperative week to assess permeability of reconstructed vessel. Long-term anticoagulation is not needed and patients are taken on aspirin on the long-term.

HEPATIC ARTERY RESECTION AND RECONSTRUCTION

The role of hepatic arterial resection in liver surgery remains controversial because of its technical complexity. Hilar cholangiocarcinoma (see Chapter 51B) and cancer of the gallbladder neck (see Chapter 49) are more prone to invade the region of the right hepatic artery (RHA) bifurcation, and most of these patients are more likely treated by a major right hepatic resection. However, RHA resection can be required in cases of left-sided hepatic resection for hilar cholangiocarcinoma because the RHA is wedged between the tumor and the PV at the hilum.[71] Initial reports of hepatic artery resection showed dismal results due to high rates of anastomotic dysfunction.[72] In addition to the high operative mortality, 3-year survival was 0%.[73,74] However, the progress achieved in living-donor liver transplantation (see Chapter 104) helped lower the operative mortality of such extended procedures by using microsurgical techniques. Nagino et al. (2010)[75] reported only a 2% operative mortality and 5-year survival of 30.3% in 50 consecutive patients undergoing simultaneous arterial and venous resection. In this series, arterial anastomoses were performed under operating microscope by microvascular surgeons. The same group updated their results in a report of 146 cases with HA resection and reconstruction. There was a 4% mortality and a remarkable 13% rate of arterial complications.[66] Most of the arterial resections were performed for left-sided hilar cholangiocarcinomas because the right hepatic artery is in the vicinity of the tumor in the hilar plate. Arterial resection combined with extended left hepatectomy increases the radicality of resection of a left-sided Klatskin tumor.[66] The two main technical factors for a safe arterial reconstruction are (1) resection and reconstruction of the hepatic artery at the end of the liver transection, to preserve the arterial blood flow to the remnant liver parenchyma for as long as possible and to avoid accidental breakdown of the anastomotic site, and (2) use of an appropriate reconstruction method according to the length and position of the hepatic arteries. After resection, a direct end-to-end anastomosis or interposition graft using saphenous vein, radial artery, or left gastric artery is most often used.[75] The site of proximal implantation can be the proper hepatic artery or, in the case of short vessels, the right renal artery.[76] In an extensive procedure associated with resection of the proper or common hepatic artery, arterial reconstruction can be performed by using a reversed splenic artery, which is anastomosed in end-to-end fashion to the hepatic artery stump, as described for liver transplantation.[77] Alternatively, arterial reconstruction can be performed between a reversed gastroduodenal–right gastroepiploic artery and the distal hepatic artery stump (Fig. 122.16).[78,79] Although resection and reconstruction of the hepatic artery are generally performed at the end of the procedure as the last step, another alternative is preexcisional hepatic artery reconstruction.[80,81] This procedure provides the potential benefit of providing an arterial anastomosis that satisfies the surgeon before performing the resection and an opportunity to abandon the procedure if not feasible. However, major concern with this procedure is that manipulation of the liver during resection may disrupt the arterial anastomosis.

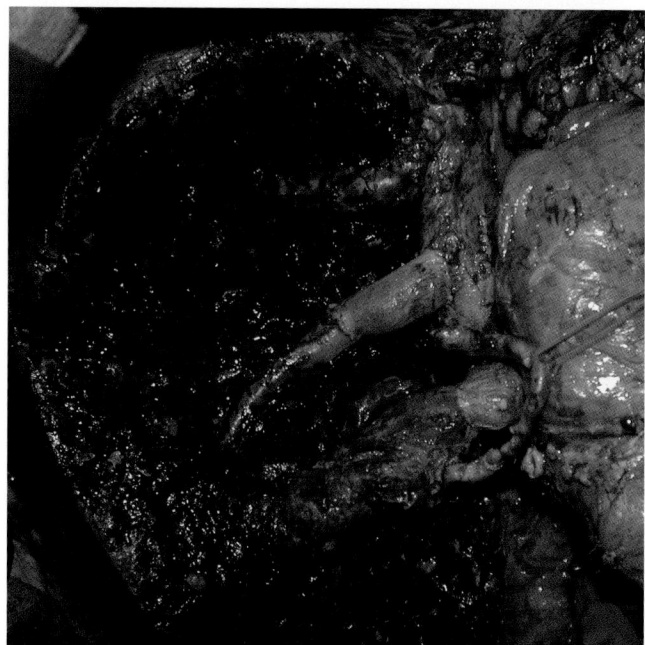

FIGURE 122.16 Intraoperative view of a left trisectionectomy extended to segment I with portal vein bifurcation resection and reconstruction, resection of the right hepatic vein, and resection of the proper hepatic artery. Two hepatic veins draining segments VI and VII have been reconstructed using a left renal vein graft and a tubulized saphenous graft implanted directly into the inferior vena cava. The hepatic artery has been reconstructed by rotating the right gastroepiploic artery, which has been anastomosed, to the posterior branch of the right hepatic artery.

The arterial anastomosis may be impossible to perform due to technical reasons, and simple arterial resection of a liver remnant is followed by bile duct necrosis and liver abscess. Portal vein arterialization (PVA), described as a salvage procedure for dearterialized grafts, could represent a possible alternative in these cases.[82] PVA entails direct anastomosis between the hepatic artery and the PV in an effort to increase both portal pressure and portal oxygenation saturation to preserve viability of the remnant liver and bile ducts. Complications associated with PVA include hyperbilirubinemia and hemorrhage due to portal hypertension. To limit the flow through the fistula, the artery adjacent to the shunt is cuffed with a wrap-around Gore-Tex patch at its creation, and most often, embolization of the artery is done to close the fistula once collateral circulation has developed.[83,84] PVA has been reported as successful in 60% of patients in whom arterial resection for hilar cholangiocarcinoma failed.[85]

CONCLUSION

Hepatectomy associated with vascular resections can be performed with limited morbidity and mortality in tertiary referral centers for hepatopancreatobiliary surgery. This approach is justified in select patients presenting with primary or secondary liver tumors invading liver vessels, because of the lack of therapeutic alternatives and the poor outcomes of nonsurgical management. These complex procedures require extensive experience in liver and vascular surgery.

References are available at expertconsult.com.

Associating liver partition and portal vein ligation for staged hepatectomy (ALPPS): Techniques

Hauke Lang, Fernando A. Alvarez, and Eduardo de Santibañes

BACKGROUND

The liver's amazing capacity to regenerate is unique in the human body and has captivated mankind since ancient civilizations, as in the Greek myths of the giant villain Tityus and the heroic Titan Prometheus[1] (see Introduction). Twenty-seven centuries later, physicians have achieved the ability to use and manipulate such regenerative capacity, not to torture as it was lucubrated in the past, but to treat and eventually cure oncologic liver diseases (see Chapter 6). The most recent surgical innovation to catalyze an accelerated liver hypertrophy, which has motivated debates among liver surgeons for the last decade, is now widely known by the acronym ALPPS (Associating Liver Partition and Portal vein ligation for Staged hepatectomy)[2] (see Chapter 102D). This technique is basically a two-stage strategy to induce rapid and massive future liver remnant (FLR) hypertrophy, thus reducing the usual time interval between stages to 1 or 2 weeks, and allowing resection of liver tumors otherwise functionally irresectable (Fig. 123.1).

The first ALPPS was performed somewhat incidentally by Prof. Hans J. Schlitt from Regensburg, Germany, in September 2007.[3] The scenario occurred in a 49-year-old female patient with hilar cholangiocarcinoma scheduled for a right trisectionectomy. The original procedure consisted of a right portal vein (PV) transection combined with simultaneous complete in situ splitting of the liver along the falciform ligament. The middle hepatic vein (MHV) was taken down but the hepatic artery (HA) still was untouched both to the right and to the left side. Having completely transected the liver, the FLR seemed to be critical and not sufficient for adequate postoperative liver function. Therefore the plan for resection was canceled at this point of the operation. Instead, after dividing the left hepatic duct at the basis of the umbilical fissure a Roux-en-Y hepaticojejunostomy to the left lateral lobe was performed to decompress the biliary tree of segments II and III. The central stump of the left hepatic duct was closed and the operation stopped without removing the tumor. A computed tomography (CT) scan performed 1 week later showed an almost doubling in volume of segments II and III assigned to be the FLR. Hence the decision to return to the operating room was made, and trisectionectomy plus resection of the hilar bifurcation was completed on day 9 after the initial surgery. Postoperative course was uneventful without any signs of liver insufficiency, but the patient developed early tumor relapse. A similar technique—with minor modifications—was then applied in two subsequent patients with colorectal liver metastases (CRLM) and intrahepatic cholangiocarcinoma (ICC). This new approach, originally termed *in situ-split liver resection*, was soon adopted by other hepato-pancreato-biliary (HPB) centers in Germany. In 2011, at the 9th congress of the European-African Hepato-Pancreato-Biliary Association (E-AHPBA) in Capetown, South Africa, a first report of 5 cases (in the abstract of 3 cases) was presented by the group from Mainz, Germany.[4] One year later, and 5 years after the pioneering operation, a multicenter inaugural report with 25 "in situ-split liver resections" from 5 German HPB groups in Regensburg, Mainz, Göttingen, Gießen, and Tübingen was published in *Annals of Surgery*.[5] In this paper, a 74% FLR hypertrophy after a median of 9 days and a 100% resection rate were reported in otherwise irresectable tumors due to a too-small FLR. As the term *in situ-split* was already used for the partition of the liver in segmental liver transplantation, Eduardo de Santibañes and Pierre Clavien suggested that this new procedure be termed *ALPPS* (for *Associating Liver Partition and Portal vein ligation for Staged hepatectomy*).[2] The increasing interest in the ALPPS concept and the great passion involved in its development prompted the creation of the International ALPPS Registry in 2012 (founding members P. A. Clavien, H. Lang, and E. de Santibañes) to collect data on this new procedure from centers all over the world (https://www.ALPPS.net).

This innovative technique, which pushed the limits of resection in a dimension that had never been thought to be possible before, led to an almost euphoric wave among HPB surgeons worldwide.[6] With the introduction of ALPPS as a modification of standard two-stage hepatectomy (TSH), a breakthrough in hepatic surgery seemed to be reached allowing an almost 100% resection rate in tumors otherwise considered irresectable due to an insufficient FLR volume (Fig. 123.2; see Chapter 102D). In selected cases, median hypertrophy rates of 160% and up to 250% were reported, permitting even the resection of all but one liver segment, the so-called monosegment ALPPS.[7] This important finding even challenged one of the basic rules in liver surgery, as functional resectability is traditionally supposed to require the preservation of at least two contiguous Couinaud's segments with intact vascular inflow, outflow, and biliary drainage. However, the initial hype surrounding this new technique soon slowed down in the face of a very high initial perioperative surgical risk (12% mortality in the inaugural multicenter German experience), and some opinion leaders in HPB surgery raised concerns claiming that the increase in resectability in ALPPS was bought at the expense of a loss of safety.[5,8] After analyzing initial data from the ALPPS Registry, it was found that the vast majority of deaths occurred after stage 2 and that posthepatectomy liver failure (PHLF) was paradoxically the main cause of poor outcomes, even when theoretically sufficient FLR volumes had been achieved.[9,10] At the same time reports from Belgium, France, and Italy demonstrated that post–stage 1 complications grade ≥3b (according to Clavien/Dindo)[11] were significant predictors of post–stage 2 mortality.[12,13] Potential risk factors for an unfavorable outcome were in particular post–stage 1 biliary fistula or infected and/or bilious peritoneal fluid at stage 2. In particular, pre–stage 2 bilirubin

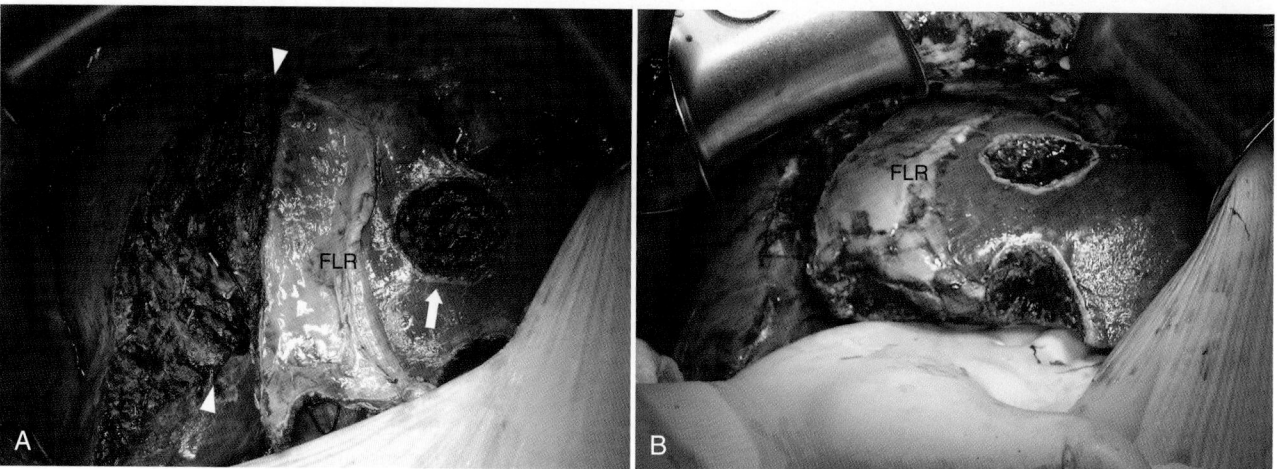

FIGURE 123.1 Surgical photographs of the ALPPS procedure in a patient with bilateral colorectal liver metastases. **A,** Stage 1 showing multiple resections in the future liver remnant *(FLR) (arrow)* and the splitting of the liver parenchyma *(arrowheads)*. **B,** Massive hypertrophy of the cleaned-up FLR 7 days after stage 2.

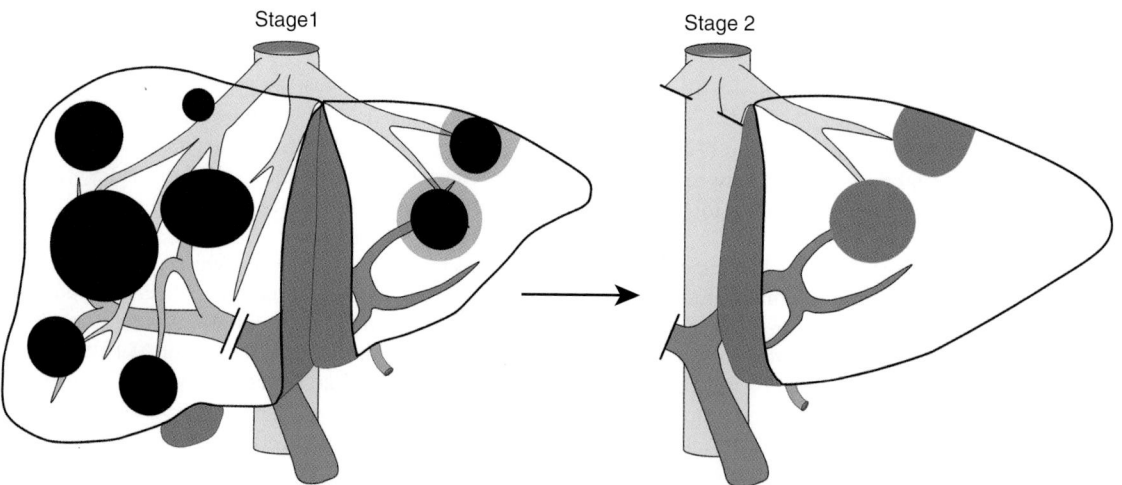

FIGURE 123.2 Diagram detailing both stages of ALPPS. Stage 1 comprises the division of the right portal vein, the resection and/or ablation of tumors in the FLR if present, and the splitting of the parenchyma according to the future resection type. Stage 2 involves division of the right hepatic artery, right bile duct, and right venous drainage to allow resection of the tumor-bearing liver.

and creatinine levels were found to be determinants for the outcome after ALPPS.[10,14] In the following years, with better knowledge of these risk factors and a rising learning curve, several improvements of the classic ALPPS technique evolved.[15] The modifications addressed anatomic and diagnostic aspects as well as the surgical technique itself. Anatomically, special attention was paid to the vascularization and biliary drainage of segment IV (see Chapter 2) in order to avoid ischemia/necrosis or bile leakage. Further on, the importance of the venous drainage of segment IV became evident. The concept of preserving the MHV during stage 1 finally led to the development of "partial ALPPS" through incomplete parenchymal transection, which was soon associated with better perioperative outcomes and equivalent FLR hypertrophy.[16,17] One of the most promising ALPPS innovations aiming to reduce the trauma during stage 1 was to avoid surgical manipulation of the hepatic hilum by replacing surgical portal vein ligation (PVL) by portal vein embolization (PVE; see Chapter 102C), also known as "hybrid

ALPPS."[18] More recently, the combination of partial parenchymal transection and simultaneous intraoperative PVE was named "mini ALPPS."[19] With the introduction of mini ALPPS, not only a modification of the ALPPS procedure but an entire change of paradigm was accomplished. In contrast to classic ALPPS, the surgical extent and the associated trauma of stage 1 were dramatically reduced, and the main surgical steps were performed during the stage 2 operation. Only shortly after the introduction of ALPPS, the first reports on minimally invasive approaches also appeared (see Chapter 127).[20,21] Initial results were encouraging, and the aforementioned technical variations for the open procedure such as partial or mini ALPPS were also applied successfully in the laparoscopic setting.[22] In 2016 the first case reports on robotic ALPPS appeared.[23] Technically, the robotic approach is feasible but needs further evaluation. All these technical refinements and a better patient selection led to a stepwise reduction of overall perioperative morbidity and mortality rates of ALPPS (Fig. 123.3).[24,25]

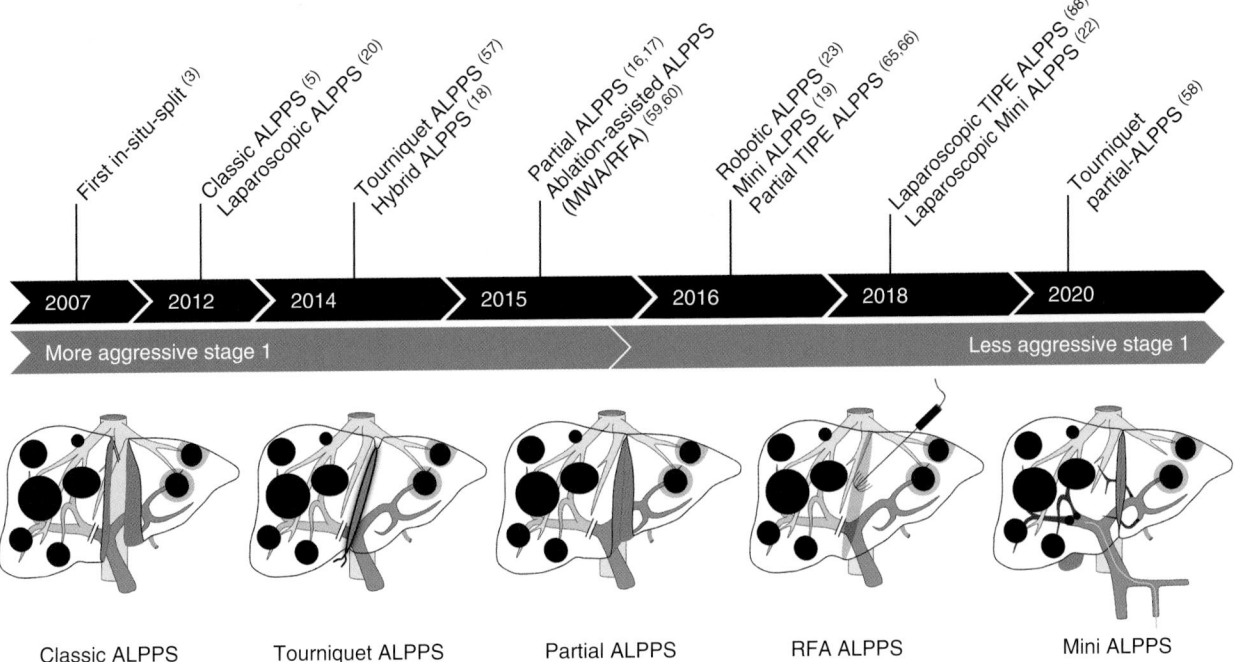

FIGURE 123.3 Timeline of ALPPS development including its most important technical variations.

So far, ALPPS has become a feasible and safe strategy in experienced hands and well-selected candidates, representing a promising option to be included in the multidisciplinary armamentarium to increase resectability in patients with locally advanced liver tumors, especially those suffering from colorectal liver metastases (see Chapters 101 and 102D). Current evidence seems to indicate that this novel short-interval staged hepatectomy has arrived to stay, with the celebration of the "first consensus meeting" in 2015,[12] a "10th anniversary" meeting in 2017,[26] and over 1250 patients currently enrolled in the ALPPS International Registry (https://www.ALPPS.net).

ANATOMIC CONSIDERATIONS (ALSO SEE CHAPTERS 2 AND 102D)

The main components of ALPPS, no matter which technique or modification is used, are the following: (1) the interruption of PV circulation, (2) the manipulation of the liver parenchyma along the transection line, and (3) the two stages of the operation. The ALPPS concept is based on a complete portal venous devascularization of the tumor-carrying liver but with preservation of the arterial blood flow as well as an intact vascularization including biliary drainage of the FLR. Consequently, precise anatomic knowledge is crucial (see Chapter 2).[12,26] Due to the high proportion of vasculobiliary variants, preoperative imaging is mandatory to assess not only the FLR, but all individual anatomic details (see Chapters 4 and 13). This is quite important, particularly when tumor structures alter normal anatomy, a situation frequently encountered when treating patients with advanced liver tumors.

Hepatic Artery

At stage 1, the preservation of arterial inflow to both sides, future remnant and specimen, is crucial. Lesions to the HA or occlusion may cause necrosis and failure of the procedure.

The most common arterial variants are a replaced or accessory right and/or left arteries (see Chapter 2).[27–29] In right trisectionectomy, at stage 1 operation, special attention has to be paid to the "middle HA" and to branches supplying segment IV (Fig. 123.4). The middle HA runs extrahepatically in about two-thirds of cases, originating from either the right or the left HA. In about one-third of cases the middle HA comes from the left HA in the umbilical fissure. The preservation of the perfusion to segment IV is imperative in ALPPS stage 1 to avoid ischemic complications.

Portal Vein

The interruption of specimen-side portal inflow is a key of the ALPPS procedure. PV anatomic variants mainly refer to the right side (see Chapter 2).[30,31] It is useful to distinguish a single PV branching or trifurcation from truly abnormal configurations (Fig. 123.5). Missing and not interrupting a portal branch during ALPPS stage 1 can occur in trifurcation, but is more likely in true aberrant branches, for example, a right anterior sectorial portal branch from the left branch (type C and particularly type D intraparenchymal branching; according to Nakamura).[30] On the left side there is a relatively constant number of portal branches to segments II and III (usually one single branch to segment II and either a single, double, or triple branch to segment III) and a variable number (up to 5–9) of branches to segment IVa and IVb.

Hepatic Vein

The venous drainage runs via the right, middle, and left hepatic veins (HVs), with the middle and left forming a common trunk in about 90% of the cases before entering the vena cava.[30,32] A typical variation of the right side is the presence of an inferior right hepatic vein (IRHV) draining segment VI, which usually is much smaller than the right hepatic vein (RHV) but occasionally may have the same or an even larger size (see Chapter 2).[33]

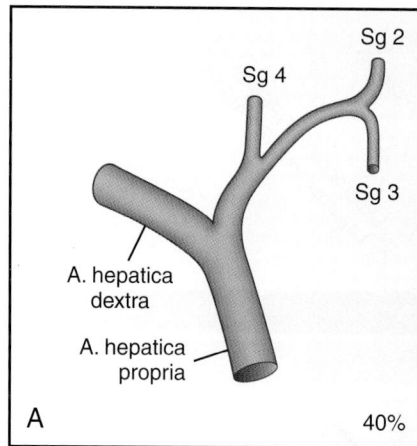
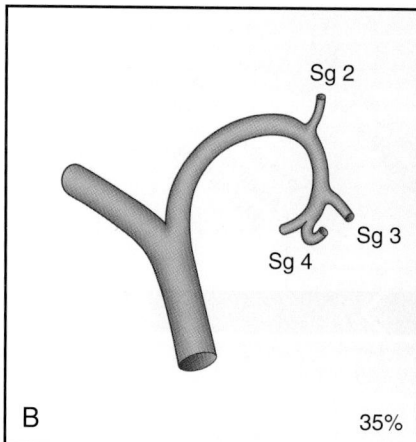
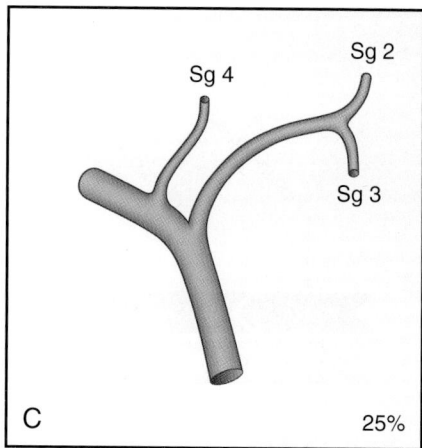

FIGURE 123.4 Arterial vascularization variants of segment (Sg) IV. **A,** Sg IV artery originating early from the left hepatic artery (40%). **B,** Sg IV artery originating from the left hepatic artery in the umbilical fissure (35%). **C,** Sg IV artery originating from the right hepatic artery (25%) (see Chapter 2). (From Expertise Allgemein- und Viszeralchirurgie Leber und Gallenwege Herausgegeben von: Wolf Otto Bechstein und Andreas Anton Schnitzbauer. Thieme Verlag 2018 © Thieme)

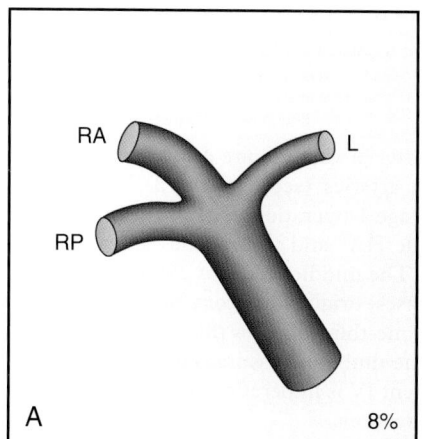
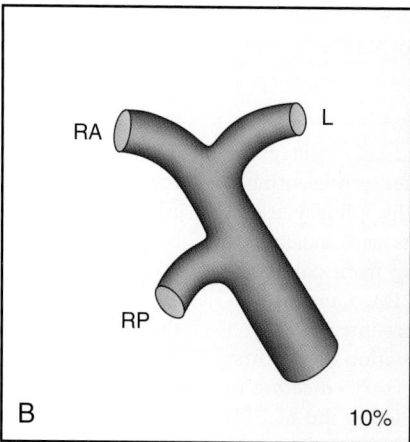
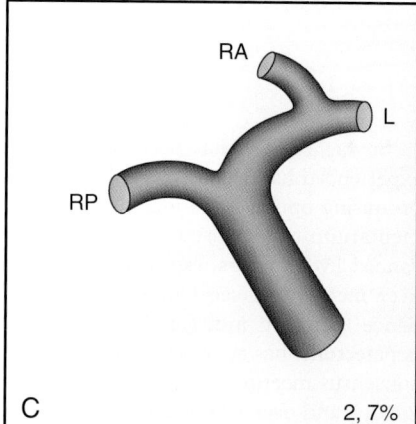

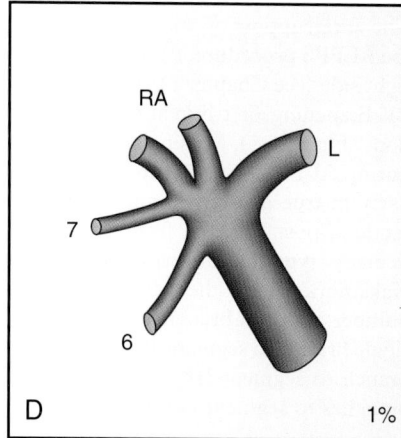
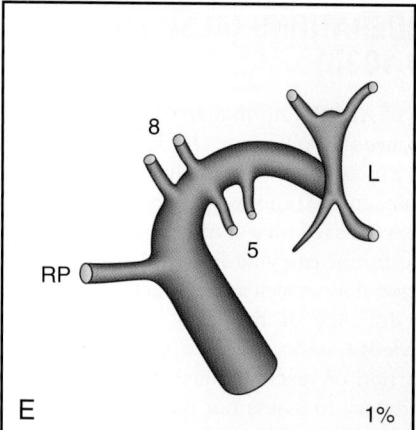

FIGURE 123.5 Variants of the portal vein trunk. **A,** Trifurcation (8%). **B,** Early origin of the right-posterior (RP) branch (10%). **C,** Right-anterior (RA) branch from the left (L) branch (2.7%). **D,** Separate segmental branches of the right anterior and posterior portal branches (1%). **E,** Complex anatomy with a single nonbifurcating portal vein (1%) (see Chapter 2). (From Expertise Allgemein- und Viszeralchirurgie Leber und Gallenwege Herausgegeben von: Wolf Otto Bechstein und Andreas Anton Schnitzbauer. Thieme Verlag 2018 © Thieme)

The MHV may show tremendous variations in size and also draining areas. Regularly, the MHV drains about 20% to 30% of total liver volume, mainly parts of segment IVa and IVb and segments V and VIII. A dominant MHV may drain up to 50% of the liver with contributions also from segment VI, and rarely from segment III. In ALPPS for right trisectionectomy, preservation of the MHV outflow at stage 1 may be crucial, in particular in case of a dominant MHV.

The venous drainage of the left lateral segments is quite constant with a common stem of the segment II and III veins as left hepatic vein (LHV). The rare case of a segment III HV draining into the MHV must be considered. This potentially risky constellation requires the preservation of the proximal MHV in continuity with the aberrant HV at stage 2. Special attention has to be paid also to an intersectional vein running in line with the falciform ligament. This vein usually empties into the LHV but rarely it may enter the MHV.

Bile Duct

The biliary tree shows multiple variations with regard to division and course of bile ducts (BDs) (Fig. 123.6).[30,31] A precise knowledge of bile duct anatomy (see Chapter 2) is of utmost importance as biliary complications are a major source for postoperative morbidity and mortality in ALPPS.[9,13] Anatomic variations of the left biliary system usually refer to distribution and localization of segmental BDs. A single left hepatic duct is present in 98% of cases (Fig. 123.7). In about two-thirds of cases a segment IV BD separate from segment II/III ducts is present. In about one-fourth of cases there is a common segment IV and III and a separate segment II BD, and much less frequently a common segment II and IV BD and a separate segment III duct. Of special relevance are crossing right BDs. A right-posterior BD entering the left hepatic duct is present in about 5% of cases, and a right anterior draining in the left system in only 1%. Even more rare, left hepatic ducts (either segment II or IV ducts or both) cross to the right side.

Patient Selection and Preoperative Assessment

All patients with locally advanced liver tumors could be considered eligible for ALPPS on a case-by-case basis within a multidisciplinary tumor board if an insufficient FLR considering volume and function is present (see Chapters 4 and 102D). Despite the fact that ALPPS was originally proposed and applied for any type of liver tumor, ALPPS for CRLM remains the indication of choice, being the most frequent and with the largest amount of data available (Fig. 123.8).[10,12,26] Recent data from the ALPPS Registry indicate that patients with CRLM are among those that most benefit from this approach, especially if they are younger than 67 years (see Chapter 90).[14] In addition, the recently published Scandinavian LIGRO Trial demonstrated that ALPPS for patients with CRLM offers higher resectability, equal safety, and better long-term results compared with standard TSH.[34,35]

In general, preoperative workup and staging does not differ from that of other major liver resections for patients bearing malignant liver tumors. This includes state-of-the-art imaging (multislice CT scan and/or magnetic resonance imaging [MRI]) of the chest, abdomen, and pelvis using triphase contrasted acquisitions, adding three-dimensional (3D) reconstruction for surgical planning whenever possible (see Chapters 13–15).[36] Liver volumetry including both total liver volume (TLV) and

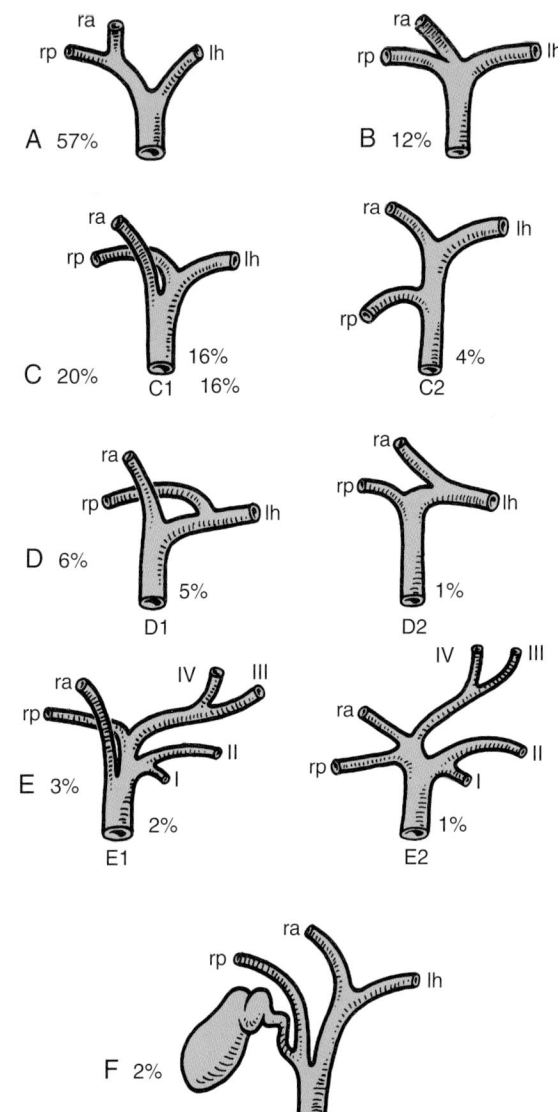

FIGURE 123.6 Variations of segment IV biliary drainage (see Chapter 2). (From Jarnagin WR, ed. *Blumgart's surgery of the liver, biliary tract and pancreas.* 6th ed. Philadelphia: Elsevier, 2016.)

FLR volume is mandatory before major liver resections (see Chapters 4–6). The TLV could be calculated either by imaging-based volumetry or using the following formula: $-794.41 + 1267.28 \times$ body surface area.[37] On preoperative CT scan or MRI-based volumetric planning, an FLR of less than 30% of TLV in healthy livers or less than 40% in patients with cholestasis, macrosteatosis, fibrosis, or long-course chemotherapy is generally used to define FLR inadequacy.[38] If preferred, an FLR-to–body weight ratio less than 0.5% could also be used to determine an insufficient FLR volume in patients with normal liver, less than 0.8% when abnormal liver parenchyma is present, or up to less than 1.4% in cirrhotic livers.[39,40] Imaging and precise individual anatomic details are evaluated, together with volumetry, in all-in-one computerized analyses. Correlation of CT volumetry with liver function and postoperative outcomes, even when based on 3D reconstruction, are, however, not always

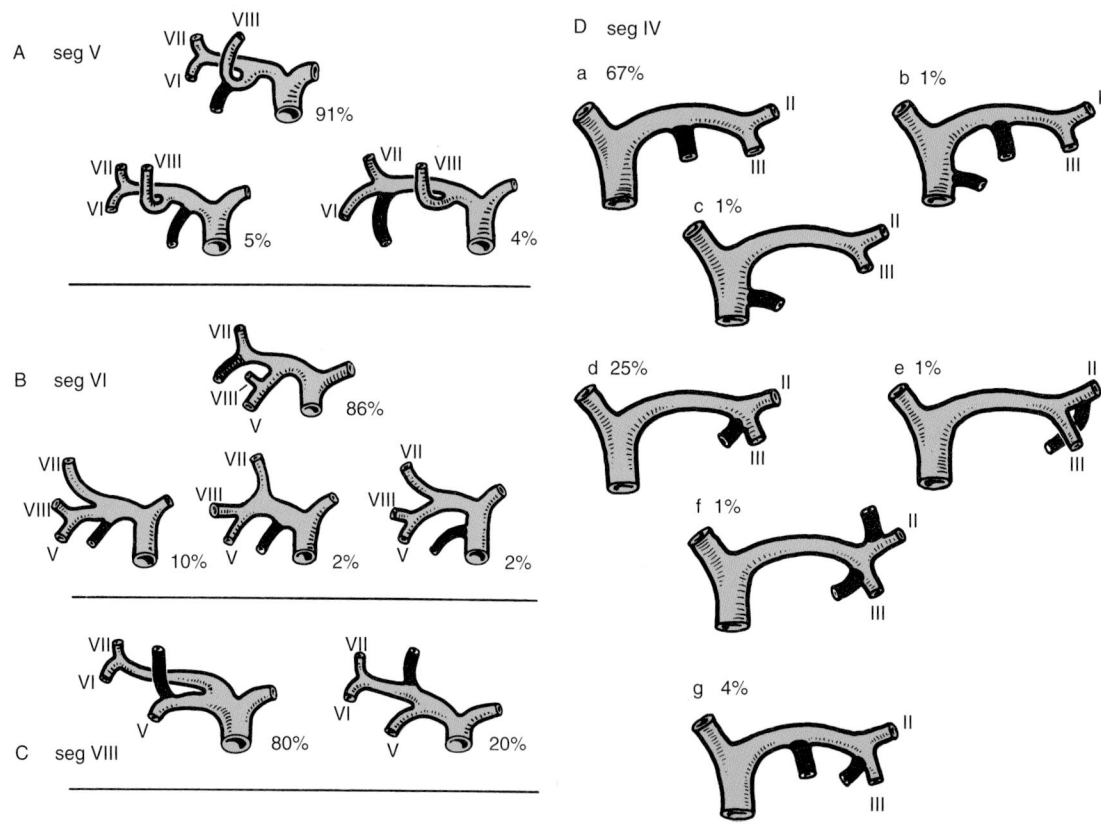

FIGURE 123.7   Main variations of the hepatic duct confluence (see Chapter 2). (From Jarnagin WR, ed. *Blumgart's surgery of the liver, biliary tract and pancreas.* 6th ed. Philadelphia: Elsevier, 2016.)

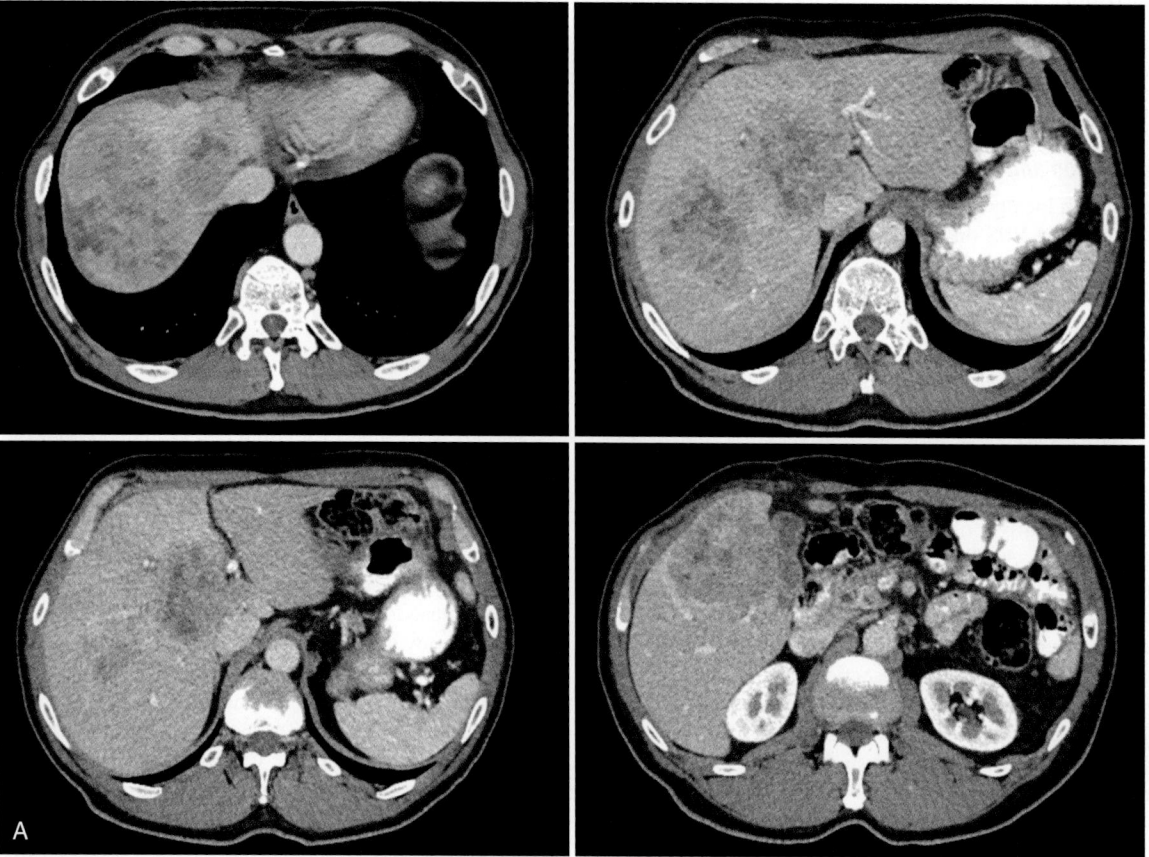

FIGURE 123.8   **Preoperative planning and technique of classic ALPPS in a patient with colorectal liver metastases. A,** Baseline multislice CT scan showing initially irresectable disease with three huge colorectal metastases in segments I and IV to VIII.

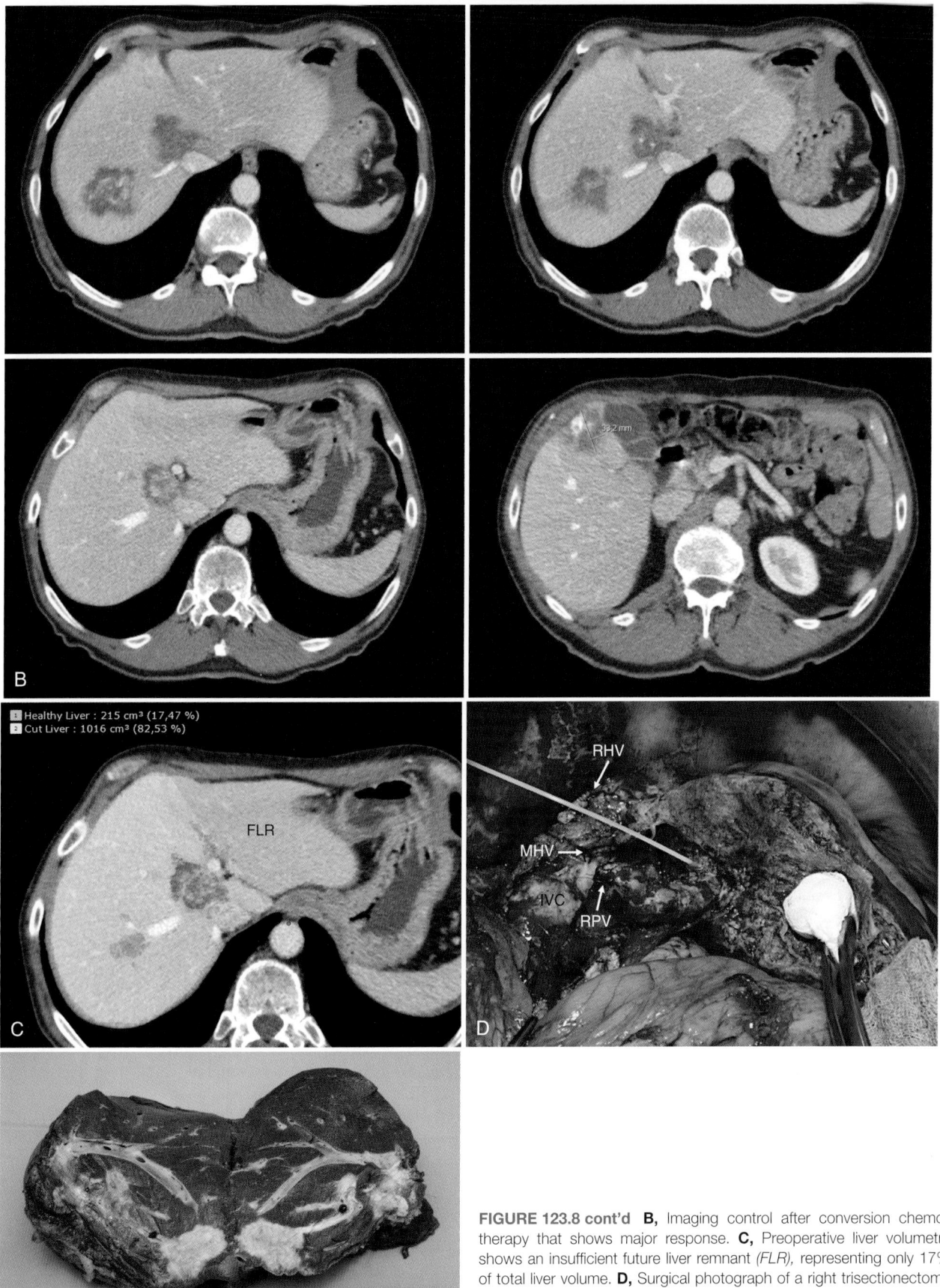

FIGURE 123.8 cont'd B, Imaging control after conversion chemotherapy that shows major response. **C,** Preoperative liver volumetry shows an insufficient future liver remnant *(FLR),* representing only 17% of total liver volume. **D,** Surgical photograph of a right trisectionectomy with bile duct resection and hepaticojejunostomy at stage 2 of a classic ALPPS. **E,** Surgical specimen with an R0 resection of the right tumor-bearing liver. The patient is alive and disease-free 30 months after stage 2 (status quo: July 2020). *IVC,* Inferior vena cava; *MHV,* middle hepatic vein; *RHV,* right hepatic vein; *RPV,* right portal vein.

consistent.[41,42] FLR volume does not necessarily reflect function, the more as hepatocyte function might be impaired by an underlying parenchymal damage. Therefore nuclear imaging techniques such as 99mTc-galactosyl serum albumin scintigraphy or 99mTc-mebrofenin hepatobiliary scintigraphy (HBS) have recently gained wider acceptance as they are capable of measuring both volume and sectorial FLR function, therefore potentially identifying patients at higher risk for PHLF.[41–44] The group from the Academic Medical Center (AMC) in Amsterdam proposed an FLR function cutoff corrected for the body surface area of 2.7%/min/m² using anterior projections only, able to predict PHLF in patients submitted to major hepatectomy regardless of the type and severity of parenchymal liver disease.[41,44]

Despite the aforementioned criteria to generally indicate preoperative liver volume remodeling, in order to get the best from the ALPPS concept, it has been proposed to further restrict it to patients with an insufficient FLR and at least one of the following: (1) a tumor margin close to the FLR or its vascular pedicles; (2) bilobar disease with contraindication for PVE as single-stage strategy; (3) the need for a large hypertrophy (>65%) in an extremely small FLR; (4) an HBS FLR uptake rate less than 1.7/min/m², where it is unlikely to reach sufficient FLR function after PVE; or (5) the failure of PVE/PVL, where isolated parenchymal transection has proven to induce further and sufficient FLR hypertrophy.[12,16,26,45] Over the years this last one, also known as "rescue ALPPS," has become an unquestioned indication for ALPPS.[46]

SURGICAL TECHNIQUE (ALSO SEE CHAPTER 102D)

Briefly, as originally described the technique consists of right portal vein ligation or transection combined with in situ splitting of liver parenchyma along the right side of the falciform ligament during stage 1 operation.[2,5] Completion surgery with resection of the tumor-carrying hepatic lobe is performed at the surgeon's discretion once FLR sufficiency has been ensured, usually within 2 weeks after stage 1. This approach is characterized by an aggressive and time-consuming first surgical procedure followed by a somewhat shorter and simpler second procedure.[47] This philosophy has been adopted by most centers as the "classic ALPPS" technique. Although not surprisingly the initial ALPPS procedure referred to a right trisectionectomy ± segment I, as in standard hepatic resections FLR is smallest when leaving segments II and III only, and other authors later presented the "right hepatectomy ALPPS" and the "left hepatectomy or left trisectionectomy ALPPS."[48] Recent data from the ALPPS registry show that more than 30% of ALPPS procedures refer to right hepatectomy, and a few cases also to left or extended left hepatectomy.

Classic ALPPS and Partial ALPPS

Stage 1 operation begins with a careful exploration of the entire abdominal cavity, and a careful palpation and ultrasound of the FLR are mandatory (see Chapter 103). If there are lesions in the FLR, complete resection of all tumors in the FLR is performed. The liver is completely mobilized and the caudate lobe freed from the vena cava. If the gallbladder is present and there is no gallbladder cancer, cholecystectomy may be performed in stage 1 to provide exposure for and facilitate right portal dissection (see Chapter 36). Subsequently, the PV of the diseased

hemiliver is divided and total (up to the inferior vena cava) parenchymal transection is carried out, most frequently as for a future right liver resection (Fig. 123.9). In some occasions, even if technically more difficult, one could opt to first transect the liver parenchyma and then to take down the PV. If this strategy is selected, it is important to first perform a trial clamping of the right PV to check for patient hemodynamic instability due to portal hyperperfusion in a too small left lobe or with insufficient venous outflow, which could contraindicate PV division. With regard to the parenchymal splitting according to the resection type, the case of a right trisectionectomy deserves special consideration. Although in the original description all portal, arterial, and biliary segment IV branches were supposed to be identified and ligated along the right rim of the round ligament,[5] early in the development of ALPPS it became evident that segment IV vascularization was crucial for the success of ALPPS (Fig. 123.10). Although all small portal branches running into segment IVa and IVb should be taken down to ensure complete portal flow interruption, and the same is true for segment I portal branches if the caudate lobe belongs to the future specimen, special attention needs to be taken to preservation of segment IV arterial blood supply to avoid ischemia with the risk of necrosis and infection. To prevent such complications, an anatomic intraglissonian dissection at the umbilical groove is recommended to preserve segment IV arterial supply and biliary drainage.[26] In line with this concern, although the original version included taking down the MHV whenever encountered at the transection line, one of the earliest technical improvements has been to avoid MHV division at the entry into the common trunk with the LHV. Later, the preservation of the MHV and parts of the surrounding tissue at stage 1 finally led to the concept of "partial ALPPS" (Fig. 123.11).[16] On principle, by reducing the depth of transection this approach also reduces the risk of involuntary section of segment IV bile ducts within glissonian pedicles emerging from the right side of the umbilical fissure during right trisectionectomy, and consequently reducing the risk of biliary leaks.[49] It has been shown that the transection of at least 50% of liver parenchyma in nonfibrotic patients results in similar effects on the velocity and extent of hypertrophy as in classic ALPPS, but with a significant reduction in perioperative morbidity.[17,50] Therefore complete transection of the liver parenchyma during stage 1 could be considered mandatory only in those cases with a risk of invasion of the tumor into the FLR in between both stages due to close proximity of the tumor to the FLR. Given that the tumor-carrying liver will remain during the interval period, meticulous liver partition with equal care to both cut surfaces must be performed, ensuring a correct closure of all vasculobiliary structures. After completing the liver transection and PVL, the confirmation of complete deportalization of the tumor-carrying liver by intraoperative ultrasound (IOUS) is of paramount importance to help avoid technical failures (see Chapters 24 and 103), typically related to a PV variant that might lead to ligation of only the right posterior portal branch. Briefly, with regard to "left trisectionectomy ALPPS," in this case the left portal vein and only the right anterior portal branch are ligated at the hepatic pedicle during stage 1, and the parenchymal transection is carried out between the right anterior and posterior sectors preserving the glissonian pedicles of segments V and VIII to avoid ischemic complications, as for segment IV in right trisectionectomy. At the end of the procedure, it is advisable to perform a transcystic hydraulic

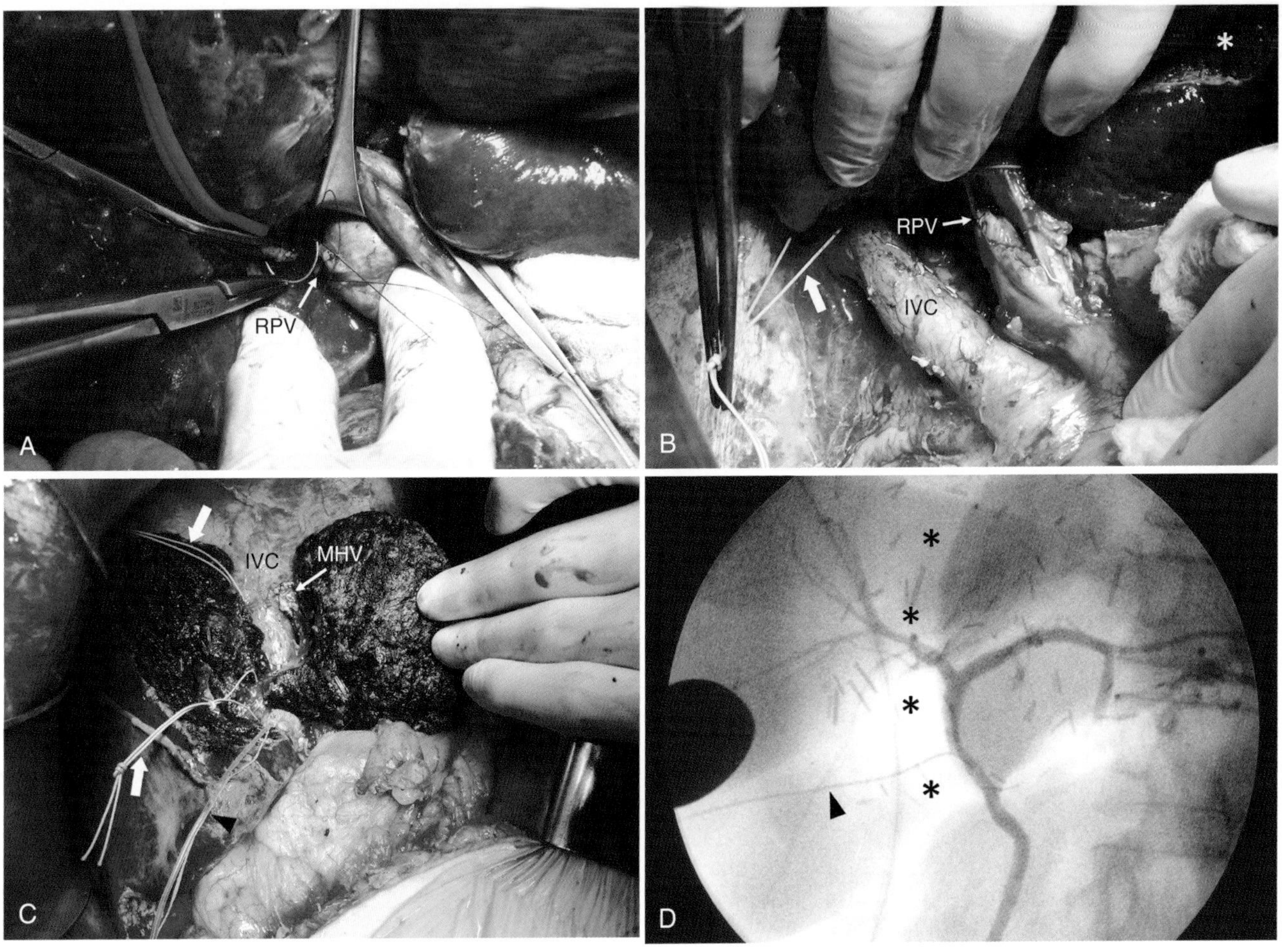

FIGURE 123.9 **Surgical photographs of classic ALPPS stage 1. A,** The right portal vein *(RPV)* is sectioned and sutured. **B,** After cholecystectomy *(white asterisk)* and RPV division, the liver is completely mobilized and the caudate lobe freed from the inferior vena cava *(IVC)*. A light blue tie is left behind as a vascular tag to mark the right hepatic vein *(arrow)*. **C,** The liver parenchyma has been totally divided up to the IVC and the middle hepatic vein *(MHV)* has been taken down and sutured. Light blue vascular tags were left to mark the right main glissonian vasculobiliary pedicle and the right hepatic vein *(arrows)*. **D,** Transcystic intraoperative cholangiogram performed with catheter *(arrowhead)* shows an intact biliary tree and no evidence of biliary leaks. The liver partition is radiolucent *(black asterisk)* with multiple titanium clips in both cut surfaces.

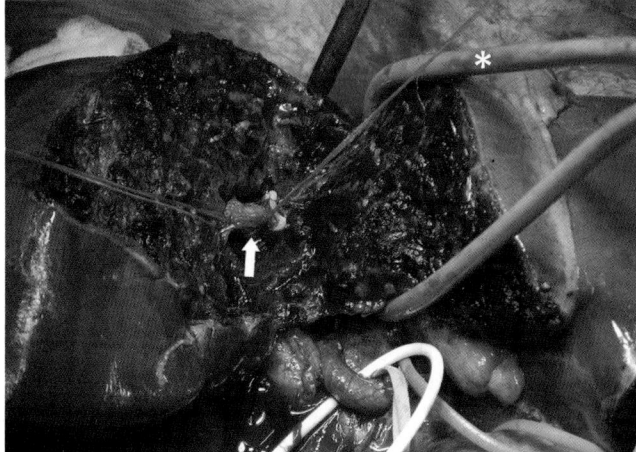

FIGURE 123.10 Surgical photograph during stage 1 of a classical ALPPS for a future right trisectionectomy. A glissonian segment IV pedicle *(arrow)* emerging from the right side of the umbilical fissure is ligated for total parenchymal transection using the hanging maneuver *(asterisk)*. The ligation of this glissonian pedicles is currently considered risky and unnecessary in right trisectionectomy ALPPS.

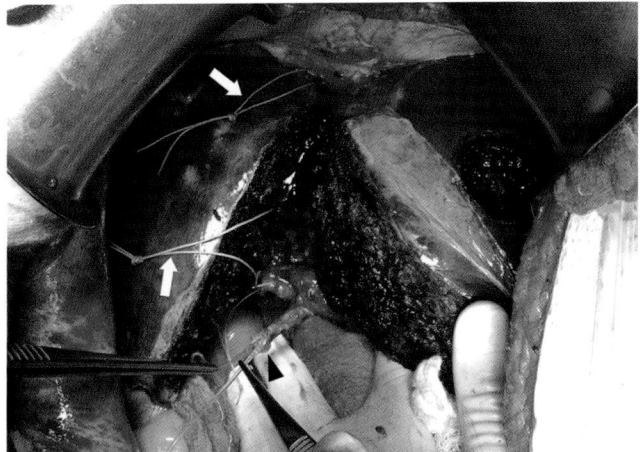

FIGURE 123.11 Surgical photograph during stage 1 of a partial ALPPS. About 50% splitting of liver parenchyma was performed along the right side of the falciform ligament as for a future right trisectionectomy. Light blue vascular tags were left behind to mark the right main glissonian vasculobiliary pedicle and the right hepatic vein *(arrows)*. The cystic duct is cannulated for a transcystic hydraulic test and cholangiography *(arrowhead)*.

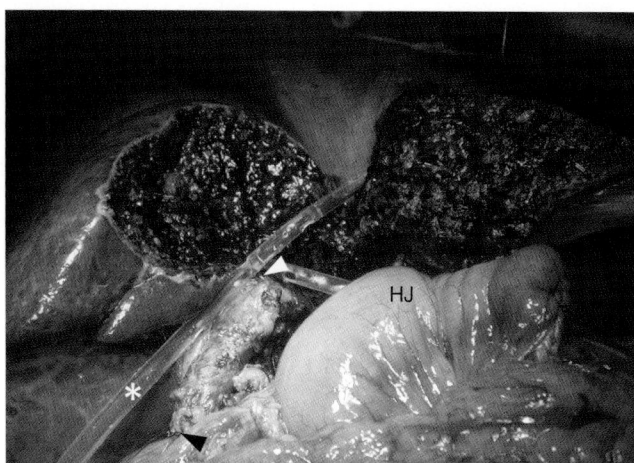

FIGURE 123.12 Surgical photograph showing a hepaticojejunostomy *(HJ)* performed at ALPPS stage 1 in a patient with a Klatskin tumor. An abdominal drain is left between both cut surfaces *(asterisk)* after careful suture of the central stump of the left hepatic duct *(white arrowhead)* and the main bile duct *(black arrowhead)*.

test, an air-bubble or "white" test (e.g., use of propofol), and sometimes cholangiography (see Chapter 24) to prevent postoperative biliary leaks, which have been recognized as an important determinant of morbidity and mortality in ALPPS.[9,10,12,13] Some authors even have suggested to place a T-tube in order to decompress the biliary tree, trying to do everything to avoid bile leakage. However, T-tubes also may be associated with some morbidity, so it is not generally recommended. Bile duct ligation to the future specimen should not be performed as it might lead to cholestasis, infection, and bile leaks. The biliary tree should be manipulated as little as possible during stage 1 operation. Therefore necessary reconstructions, such as hepaticojejunostomy with a Roux-en-Y loop, should be performed at stage 2 operation if possible. In rare cases when biliary decompression of the FLR has not been performed before stage 1 operation, biliary reconstruction can also be performed at stage 1 operation (see first ALPPS). In such a case, careful suture of the central stump of the hepatic duct has to be performed (Fig. 123.12). Given that liver atrophy and contralateral hypertrophy may frequently change the porta hepatis anatomy after stage 1, hindering intraoperative anatomic orientation, it is strongly recommended to mark tumor-carrying liver vasculobiliary structures with silk ties or vessel loops to facilitate their identification during stage 2.[12] Finally, with the aim of minimizing adhesions, bleeding, and trauma during stage 2, either placement of a silastic bag between the two liver parts or other surface-sealing materials not necessarily requiring removal has been suggested. Today most surgeons prefer a hemostatic sheet, but good results have also been reported without the use of any material. Before closure, two drains are placed in the abdominal cavity, one in between the transection lines and the other in the right subphrenic space (Fig. 123.13).

Stage 2 operation starts with a careful exploration after releasing adhesions and performing an extensive washout of the abdominal cavity. An intraabdominal swab is taken for microbiologic analysis to orient antibiotic therapy if ever needed. The hilar structures of the diseased hemiliver are recognized by identifying the vascular tags around them (Fig. 123.14).

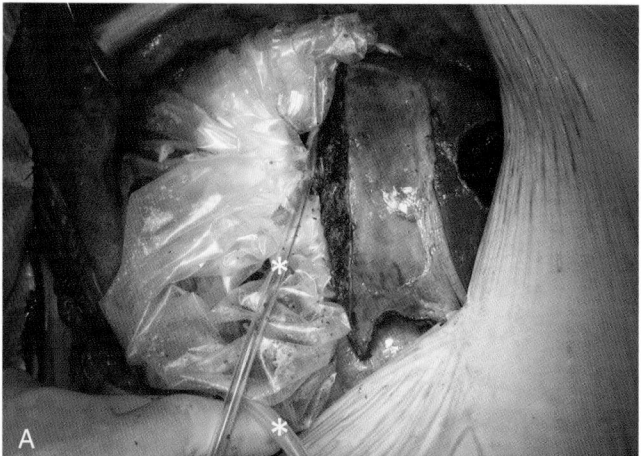

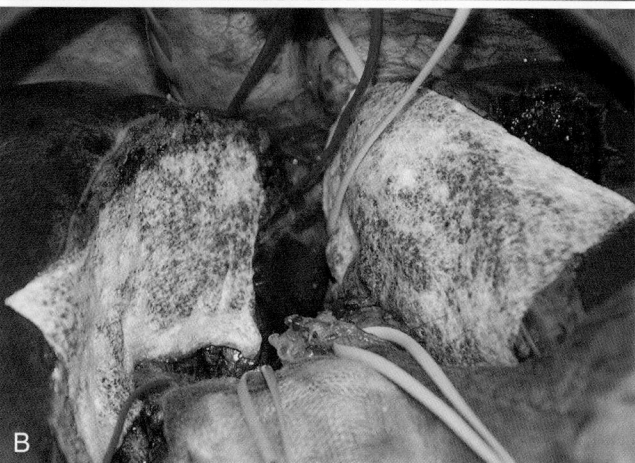

FIGURE 123.13 Surgical photograph at the end of stage 1 in a classic ALPPS. **A,** Two drains are placed in the abdominal cavity before closure, one between the transection surfaces and the other in the right subphrenic space *(asterisks)*. Given that this patient was operated on in 2012, the diseased hemiliver had been left inside a plastic bag. Currently, with the advent of safer technical variations using the anterior approach, this maneuver has been abandoned. **B,** Both cut surfaces are covered with hemostatic sheets to prevent adhesions, which may cause severe bleeding at stage 2.

The resection of the tumor-bearing lobe may be facilitated using staplers for vascular structures and glissonian pedicles. IOUS to check perfusion of the liver (see Chapters 24 and 103), if necessary, thorough check of the remaining liver parenchyma, and a careful positioning of the FLR including refixation of the falciform ligament should be performed. Finally, it is strongly recommended to perform an intraoperative test to find bile leaks.

Monosegment ALPPS

The "monosegment ALPPS" is defined as a liver resection leaving a remnant constituted of 1 single segment ± segment I, considering segment I as an accessory segment.[7] Although segment IV has been subdivided into subsegments IVa and IVb for practical reasons, it is considered by the aforementioned definition as one segment in agreement to Couinaud's anatomy. The first approach to monosegment ALPPS was therefore introduced in 2015 by the group from the Hospital Italiano de Buenos Aires, who preserved only segments I and IV as FLR after performing a left lateral sectionectomy at stage 1 and

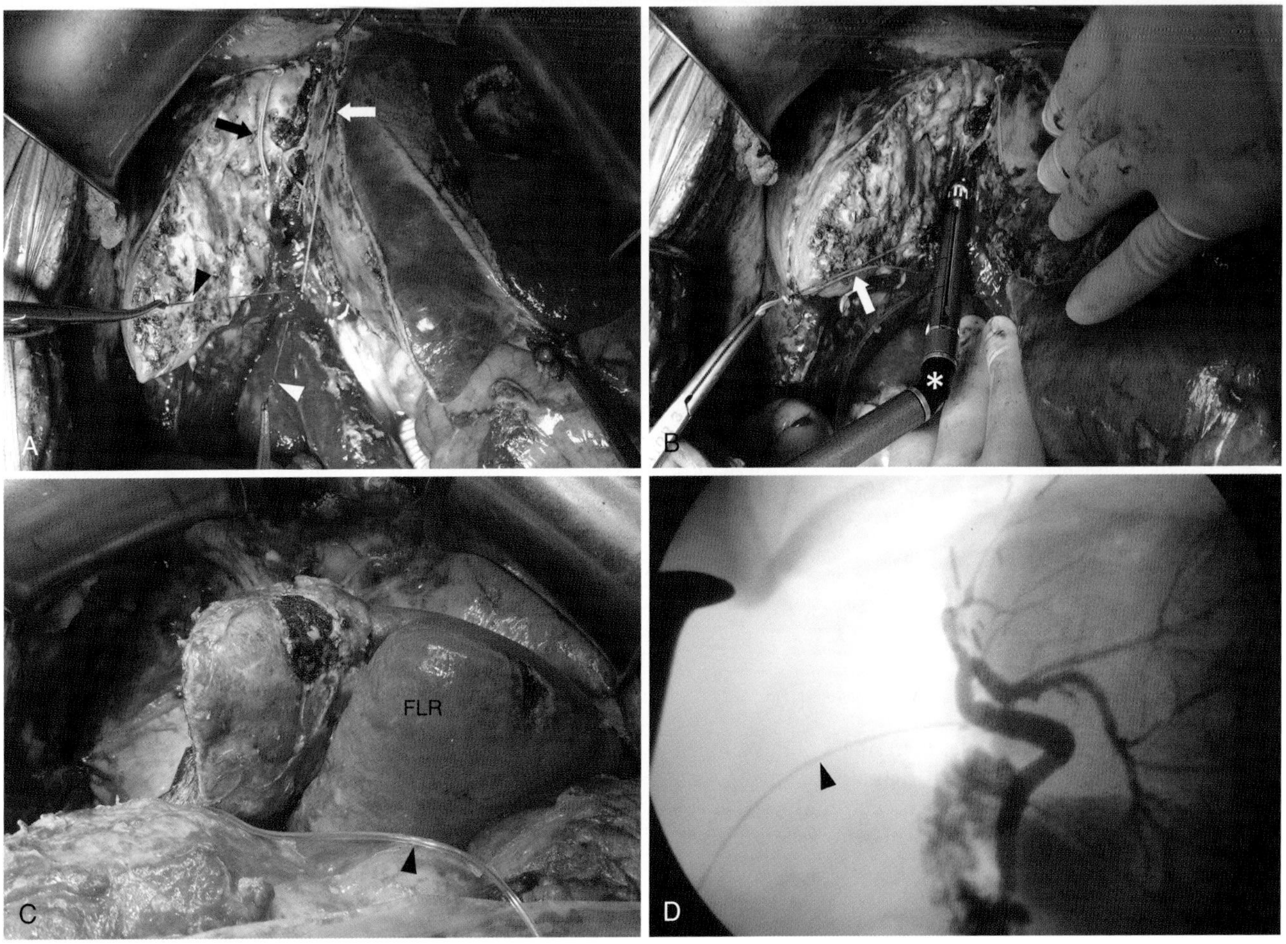

FIGURE 123.14 Surgical photograph at the beginning of stage 2 in a partial ALPPS. **A,** Once lax adhesions between both hemilivers have been broken up with blunt dissection, light blue vasculobiliary tags are easily recognized in the depth of the parenchymal groove marking the right hepatic vein *(black arrow)*, the right main glissonian vasculobiliary pedicle *(white arrow)*, the right hepatic artery *(black arrowhead)*, and the cystic duct *(white arrowhead)*. **B,** Intraparenchymal glissonian division of the right main glissonian vasculobiliary pedicle *(white arrow)* using a vascular stapler *(asterisk)*. **C,** A hypertrophied future liver remnant *(FLR)* is seen after resecting the right tumor-bearing liver. Transcystic catheter for hydraulic test *(arrowhead)*. **D,** Final intraoperative cholangiogram to check the integrity of the biliary bifurcation and to rule out biliary leaks (see Chapter 24).

a right hepatectomy at stage 2 for extensive bilateral CRLM (Fig. 123.15).[51] Subsequently other surgeons reported safely leaving behind other single segment remnants when applying the ALPPS approach.[7] Monosegment ALPPS overcomes left and right trisectionectomy, which are the most extensive liver resections according to the terminology introduced by the IH-PBA Brisbane nomenclature,[52] and is thus a novelty in liver surgery. Although there are some anecdotal reports of monosegment FLRs before the ALPPS era, this were usually the final result of either multiple rehepatectomies or of TSH leaving segment IV after a very long interval.[53,54] Four feasible and safe resection types have been reported: "S2 ALPPS" with segment III resection in stage 1 (Fig. 123.16), followed by a right trisectionectomy in stage 2; "S3 ALPPS" with resection of segment II leaving the LHV skeletonized during stage 1 followed by a right trisectionectomy in stage 2; "S4 ALPPS" with removal of the left lateral segment during stage 1, followed by a right hepatectomy during stage 2; and "S6 ALPPS" in those patients who have an anatomic variation with an IRHV draining segment VI.[7] This last variation is the most challenging, which includes the ligation of the left and right anterior portal branches at the hepatic pedicle during stage 1, followed in stage

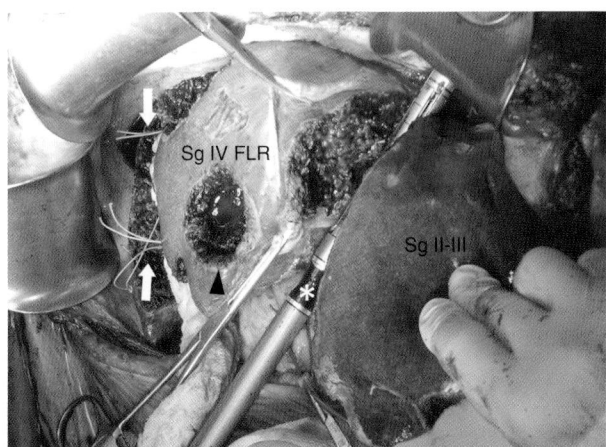

FIGURE 123.15 Surgical photograph during stage 1 of a monosegment IV ALPPS in a patient with extensive bilateral colorectal liver metastases. Liver partition has been performed at the level of the Cantlie's line and light blue vasculobiliary tags have already been left behind *(arrows)*. After segment *(Sg)* IV cleanup *(arrowhead)*, a left lateral sectionectomy is performed using vascular staplers. The future liver remnant *(FLR)* comprises only segments IV and I.

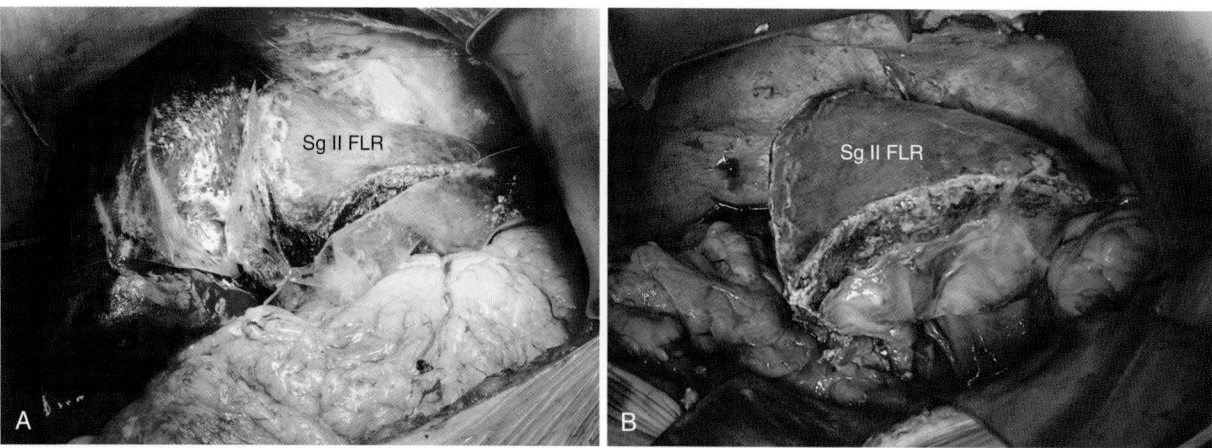

FIGURE 123.16 Surgical photographs of monosegment II ALPPS. **A,** End of stage 1 after resection of segment *(Sg)* III. Plastic sheets have been placed to avoid adhesion formation. **B,** A hypertrophied segment 2 future liver remnant *(FLR)* is seen at the end of stage 2 after right trisectionectomy extended to segment I.

2 by transection of all three HVs and left trisectionectomy extended to segment VII.

TECHNICAL VARIATIONS

During the development and exploration stages of this surgical innovation,[55] different technical variations to the classic ALPPS, focused on the method of parenchymal transection, the method of PV occlusion, and the surgical approach itself, have been introduced with the aim of improving ALPPS outcomes (Table 123.1).[15] Indeed, the use of less invasive techniques in stage 1, which will be described later in this chapter, has been recently confirmed as an independent factor related to a decreased mortality in the ALPPS Registry.[24] To allow comparability of data, the founding members of the International ALPPS Registry have recently suggested a "consensus" terminology to harmonize reports.[56]

Tourniquet ALPPS, Microwave ALPPS, and Radiofrequency ALPPS

Some authors have replaced transection during stage 1 by various different techniques to achieve a functional partition through the liver. The first of these modifications was introduced by Robles et al.[57,63] from Murcia, Spain, by the application of a tourniquet around the liver in a parenchymal groove of 1 cm in the future transection line (tourniquet ALPPS). The tourniquet has to be passed as per the hanging maneuver, in front of the IVC and between the RHV and MHV or between the MHV and LHV depending on the resection planned, but most important between the parenchyma and the right or left portal pedicle using an extraglissonian approach to prevent occlusion of the HA and BD.[57] In this technique it is paramount to knot the tourniquet tightly enough to completely occlude interlobar circulation, which has to be checked with IOUS. Others have proposed to replace parenchymal transection by using radiofrequency or microwave ablation (radiofrequency ALPPS and microwave ALPPS) to create a liver partition through a "necrotic groove."[58,59] Ablation splitting of the liver is performed under IOUS guidance above the major intrahepatic glissonian pedicles, usually ranging from 40 to 60 mm in depth.[64] Both radiofrequency ALPPS and microwave ALPPS can be performed with minimum invasiveness, either by laparoscopic or percutaneous approach.[58,59,64,65] All these approaches have shown to provide a similar hypertrophy of the FLR as classic ALPPS, but with less complications and mortality, even comparing favorably with standard approaches such as TSH or PVE. The REBIRTH trial has shown that radiofrequency ALPPS produced a significantly greater increase in liver volume and within a much shorter time period than PVE, without increased morbidity and mortality.[64] Likewise, a recent propensity score matched analysis demonstrated a higher hypertrophic efficacy and resectability rate for the tourniquet ALPPS compared with TSH, with comparable safety and oncologic outcomes.[66]

TABLE 123.1	Main Surgical Characteristics of Stage 1 for Each of the Main Technical Variations of ALPPS				
TECHNIQUE	**PORTAL VEIN OCCLUSION**	**PARENCHYMAL INTERRUPTION**	**LIVER MOBILIZATION**	**HEPATODUODENAL LIGAMENT DISSECTION**	**CHOLECYSTECTOMY**
Classic ALPPS[3,5,47]	Ligation/division	Complete transection	Full mobilization	Yes (complete)	Yes
Tourniquet ALPPS[57]	Ligation/division	Tourniquet	Anterior approach	Yes (right side)	Yes
Hybrid ALPPS[18]	Interval percutaneous PVE	Partial transection	Anterior approach	Yes (left side)	No
Partial ALPPS[15,16]	Ligation/division	Partial transection	Anterior approach	Yes (right side)	Yes
MWA/RFA ALPPS[58,59]	Ligation/division	Thermal local ablation	Anterior approach	Yes (right side)	Yes/no
Mini ALPPS[19]	IO transmesenteric PVE	Partial transection	Anterior approach	No	No
Partial TIPE ALPPS[60,61]	IO transileocecal PVE	Partial transection	Anterior approach	No	No

ALPPS, Associating liver partition and portal vein ligation for staged hepatectomy; *IO,* intraoperative; *MWA,* microwave ablation; *PVE,* portal vein embolization; *RFA,* radiofrequency ablation; *TIPE,* transileocecal portal embolization.

Hybrid ALPPS

Following the trend to less invasiveness, the ligation of the PV and portal venous branches to the tumor-carrying liver may also be replaced by PVE (see Chapter 102C). The substitution of PVL by PVE during the interval period is known as "hybrid ALPPS."[18] Although this modification was introduced in 2014 to treat patients with gallbladder carcinoma infiltrating the right PV, it has spread to other entities with right liver hilum compromise. Avoiding portal pedicle dissection during stage 1 is in line with the "no-touch" oncologic principle and facilitates stage 2 by generating fewer adhesions and easier identification of hilar vascular and biliary structures. In addition, using PVE instead of PVL is also a useful alternative in patients with PV variants, where the right anterior branch could be missed during PVL or located far cranial making surgical occlusion technically demanding.[67]

Mini ALPPS

The concept of "mini ALPPS" was first presented by the group from the Hospital Italiano de Buenos Aires during the First ALPPS International Consensus Meeting at Hamburg in February 2015.[19] This alternative incorporates in a single procedure the virtues of (1) partial parenchymal transection, (2) intraoperative transmesenteric PVE, and (3) "no-touch" oncologic rules (strictly avoiding portal pedicle dissection and liver mobilization), with the aim of maximally reducing the surgical impact of stage 1 to promote rapid patient recovery and to facilitate stage 2 (Fig. 123.17).[19] With the introduction of mini ALPPS not only a modification of the ALPPS procedure but an entire change of paradigm was accomplished. In contrast to classic ALPPS, the surgical extent and the associated trauma of the stage 1 operation were dramatically reduced

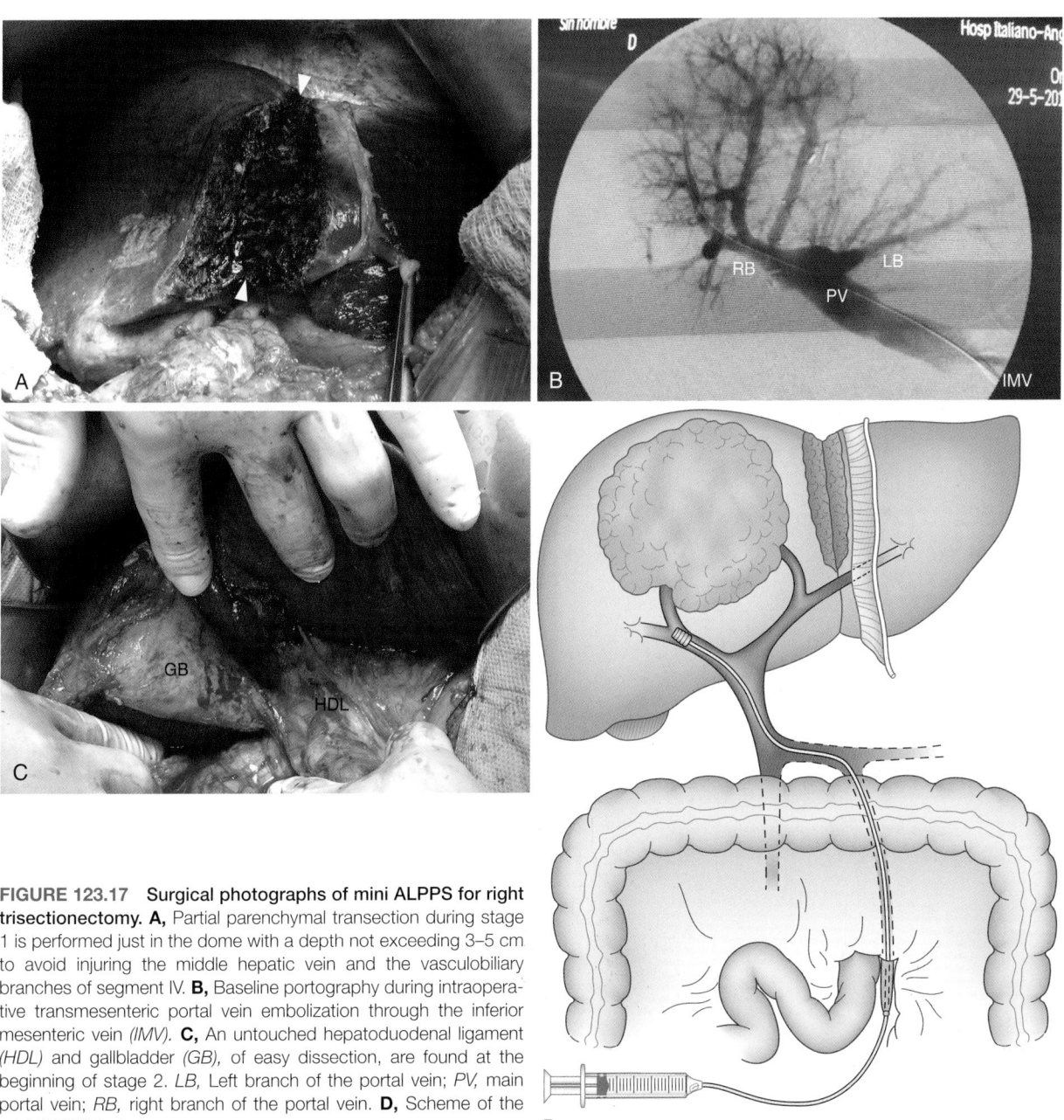

FIGURE 123.17 **Surgical photographs of mini ALPPS for right trisectionectomy. A,** Partial parenchymal transection during stage 1 is performed just in the dome with a depth not exceeding 3–5 cm to avoid injuring the middle hepatic vein and the vasculobiliary branches of segment IV. **B,** Baseline portography during intraoperative transmesenteric portal vein embolization through the inferior mesenteric vein (IMV). **C,** An untouched hepatoduodenal ligament (HDL) and gallbladder (GB), of easy dissection, are found at the beginning of stage 2. *LB,* Left branch of the portal vein; *PV,* main portal vein; *RB,* right branch of the portal vein. **D,** Scheme of the mini ALPPS technique.

while the main surgical steps were performed at stage 2. As such, this new concept is not restricted to tumors with right liver hilum infiltration as the hybrid ALPPS, but to any patient undergoing ALPPS.

Although similar, the mini ALPPS offers some advantages with respect to the hybrid ALPPS. The drawbacks of performing PVE postoperatively instead of intraoperatively are mainly the potential risk of injuring the left PV (ipsilateral approach preferred if possible) or the FLR through the percutaneous puncture (particularly in patients with a cleaned-up FLR) and the necessity of undergoing three procedures with general anesthesia. Moreover, the hybrid ALPPS as originally described

includes the dissection of the left side of the portal pedicle to recognize the FLR PV and HA, which is strictly avoided in mini ALPPS to facilitate stage 2 due to fewer adhesions, which is specifically advantageous if for any reason the stage 2 has to be delayed. Although the first cases of mini ALPPS were performed in an open fashion, intraoperative transmesenteric PVE was soon adapted for a laparoscopic approach, applying an innovative technique for laparoscopic-assisted percutaneous cannulation of the inferior mesenteric vein (IMV) using a 5-Fr introducer and the Seldinger technique, adding the benefits of a minimally invasive approach (Fig. 123.18).[22] Finally, a recent technical variant of the mini ALPPS using transileocecal portal

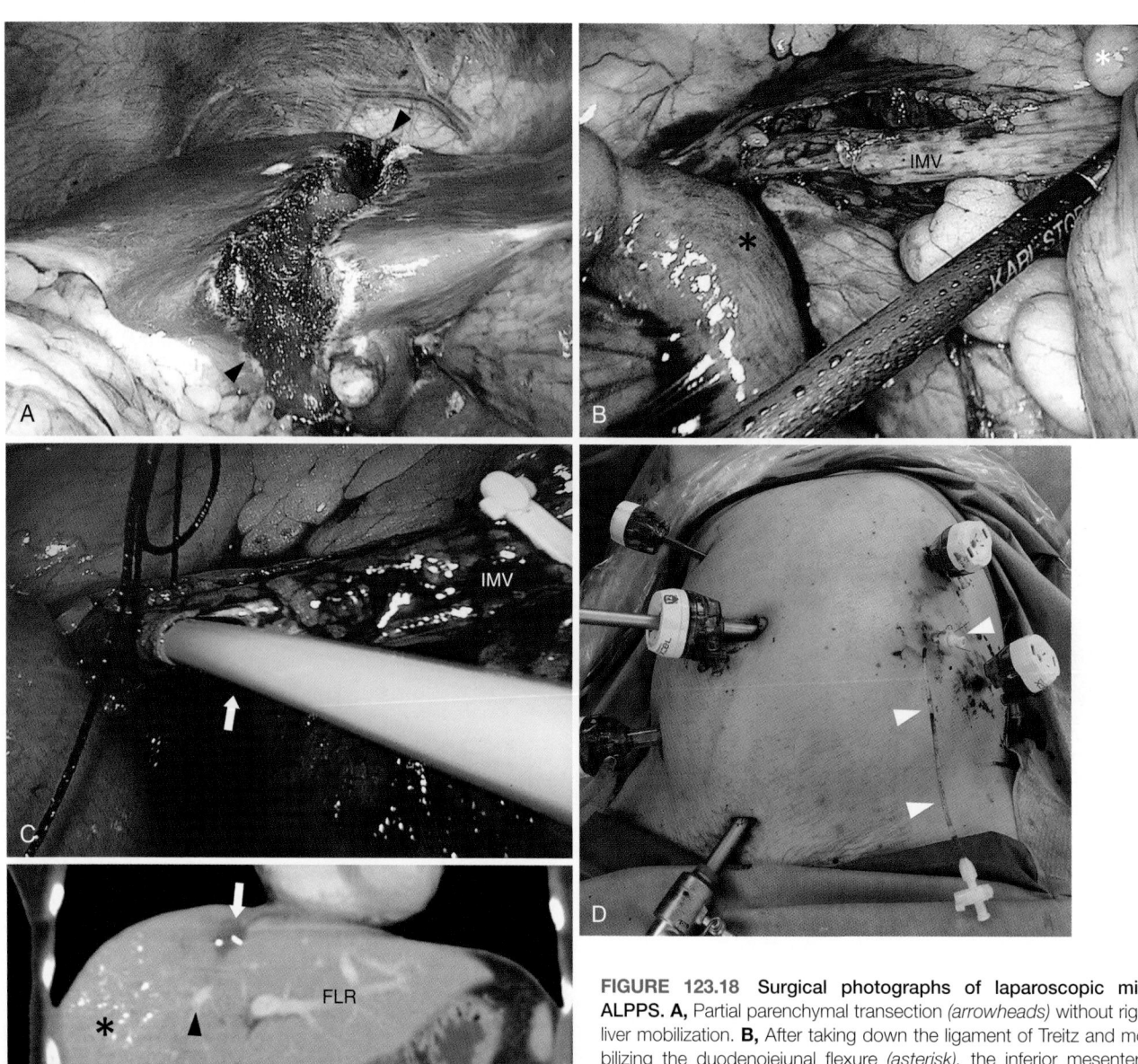

FIGURE 123.18 Surgical photographs of laparoscopic mini ALPPS. **A,** Partial parenchymal transection *(arrowheads)* without right liver mobilization. **B,** After taking down the ligament of Treitz and mobilizing the duodenojejunal flexure *(asterisk),* the inferior mesenteric vein *(IMV)* is individualized. **C,** Laparoscopic-assisted percutaneous cannulation of the IMV with a 5-Fr introducer *(arrow)* after permanent distal occlusion with a polymer locking ligation system and proximal transitory occlusion with a strong silk. **D,** Trocars disposition in the abdomen and percutaneous insertion of the introducer sheath in the left flank *(arrowheads).* **E,** Interval volumetric CT scan shows future liver remnant *(FLR)* hypertrophy, the partial liver partition groove *(arrow)* with preservation of the middle hepatic vein *(arrowhead),* and embolization material in the right portal branches *(asterisk).*

embolization (TIPE) instead of transmesenteric portal embolization, known as "partial TIPE-ALPPS," has been proposed by a Japanese group from Tokyo.[60,61] Although both technical modifications of the ALPPS principle could be performed by laparoscopy, the mini ALPPS seems more appealing as the IMV can be easily found and exposed just left lateral to the ligament of Treitz after pulling the transverse colon upward, whereas the partial TIPE-ALPPS would need a McBurney incision in the abdomen regardless. Given that surgery and PVE are performed simultaneously during the same anesthesia, both techniques (mini ALPPS and partial TIPE-ALPPS) require an interventional radiology suite prepared for any major abdominal surgery, including laparoscopy (hybrid angiography/operating room).

Laparoscopic ALPPS

Based on the several proven benefits of minimally invasive surgery over open surgery (see Chapter 127A), different authors have demonstrated that pure laparoscopic ALPPS applied for either one or both stages is feasible and safe, especially for the aforementioned less invasive technical variations.[21] The preliminary experience from São Paulo and others demonstrates so far a tendency toward less morbidity, mortality, and length of hospital stay of laparoscopic ALPPS compared with open ALPPS.[21,62] As for open surgery, stage 1 includes the exploration of the abdominal cavity and IOUS through a 4- to 6-trocar approach.[22,62] If necessary, nonanatomic resections can be performed in the FLR using laparoscopic IOUS as guidance. The PV is either ligated with a nonabsorbable suture or polymer locking ligation system as per the classic ALPPS, or embolized in the mini ALPPS technique. Subsequently, parenchymal transection is carried from caudal to cephalad using a combination of the various energy sealing devices available—ultrasonic dissectors, bipolar forceps, clips, and even stapler transection for larger vessels—depending on the surgical team experience and preference.

In experienced hands, the stage 2 procedure can also be performed laparoscopically using the same surgical ports. The right liver is fully mobilized off the retroperitoneum, diaphragm, and inferior vena cava. The right glissonian pedicle is divided with an endostapler. Staplers are also used to transect the right and in some patients the middle HVs followed by removal of the specimen inside a large plastic bag through a suprapubic incision.

INTERVAL MANAGEMENT AND TIMING OF STAGE 2

Patient management during the interval period between both surgical stages is key for the successful application of ALPPS (see Chapter 28). Morbidity and mortality during ALPPS have been associated in most series with inappropriate patient selection, unsuitable timing of the second stage, and errors in clinical judgment due to the lack of experience with the application of a new technique.[9,10]

Given that remnant liver volume is a known predictor of PHLF,[68,69] most authors have defined FLR sufficiency during the interval period based in volume rather than function, simplifying postoperative functional assessment between both stages to daily clinical evaluation and liver function blood tests (see Chapter 4). However, the results obtained from such functional evaluation could be misleading as it provides total liver

function assessment, which in this scenario includes also the functional capacity of the diseased hemiliver that will be removed. Moreover, the fact that mortality occurs more frequently after stage 2 due to PHLF indicates that the established volumetric criteria being used to judge FLR sufficiency before reoperation might not be adequate, particularly when taking into account that these volume measurements are applied to a fast-growing parenchyma.[14] Volume may increase rapidly, and as such precede functional recovery.[42] Even though previous studies have observed proliferative and architectural changes at the histologic level accompanying macroscopic FLR hypertrophy in ALPPS (see Chapter 6),[70] rapid volumetric increase may not be immediately followed by an equal increase in function, as recently suggested by histologic findings showing initial edema and hepatocyte immaturity in nontumorous FLR parenchyma within the first 2 weeks of regeneration.[71] This discrepancy between volume increase and the high rate of PHLF suggests the necessity to assess liver function in addition to volume. From the various more sophisticated liver function studies available (HIDA test, galactose elimination capacity, the indocyanine green test, or the LiMAx test), HBS is undoubtedly the most promising (see Chapter 4).[41-45] Combining HBS with SPECT-CT offers quantitative information regarding segmental liver function and therefore provides an accurate measure of FLR function (Fig. 123.19).[44] Sequential measurements of HBS are useful in assessing the functional response to ALPPS over time, and by doing so, it is helpful in timing stage 2 operation. Even though there is agreement that stage 2 should be postponed until a satisfactory function has been reached, the key question yet not fully answered is how good the FLR function has to be in this particular scenario in order to avoid PHLF. One option is waiting until the FLR uptake rate has reached the $2.7/min/m^2$ cutoff proposed by the AMC group in Amsterdam,[41] and the other is to use the more recently developed measure proposed by the Hospital Italiano de Buenos Aires (HIBA) using modern HBS assessment (Gmean and SPECT analysis) called the "HIBA index," with a cutoff value of greater than 15%.[72] These practical cutoffs are of paramount importance to avoid futile indication of ALPPS stage 2. Another method to better assess functional recovery and to reduce the risk for PHLF is the assessment of FLR volume increase over time, called kinetic growth rate (KGR). A recent report from the ALPPS Registry has shown that a KGR cutoff point of less than 4.1% per day also predicts PHLF after stage 2.[73]

Even though the feasibility of ALPPS to remove tumor in a short period of time is very high, the initial 1-week interval dogma has been penalized in several series with high complication rates and mortality. It is therefore important to remark that although ALPPS is indeed a two-stage procedure, the stage 2 should be delayed or even abandoned in case of compromised clinical status, active complications, abnormal liver function tests or a Model for End-stage Liver Disease (MELD) score greater than 10, in order to avoid mortality.[9,10,12] Gathering data from the ALPPS Registry, a statistically validated "risk score" was created in 2016 to predict the individual risk of 90-day and/or in-hospital mortality either upfront or before stage 2, and therefore assist proper patient selection and optimal determination of whether and when to proceed safely with stage 2 surgery.[14,74] Particularly, the pre–stage 2 model includes the pre–stage 1 score, interstage complications ≥3b, serum bilirubin pre–stage 2, and serum creatinine pre–stage 2, with a predicted futility risk of 5%, 10%, 20%, and 50% for patients

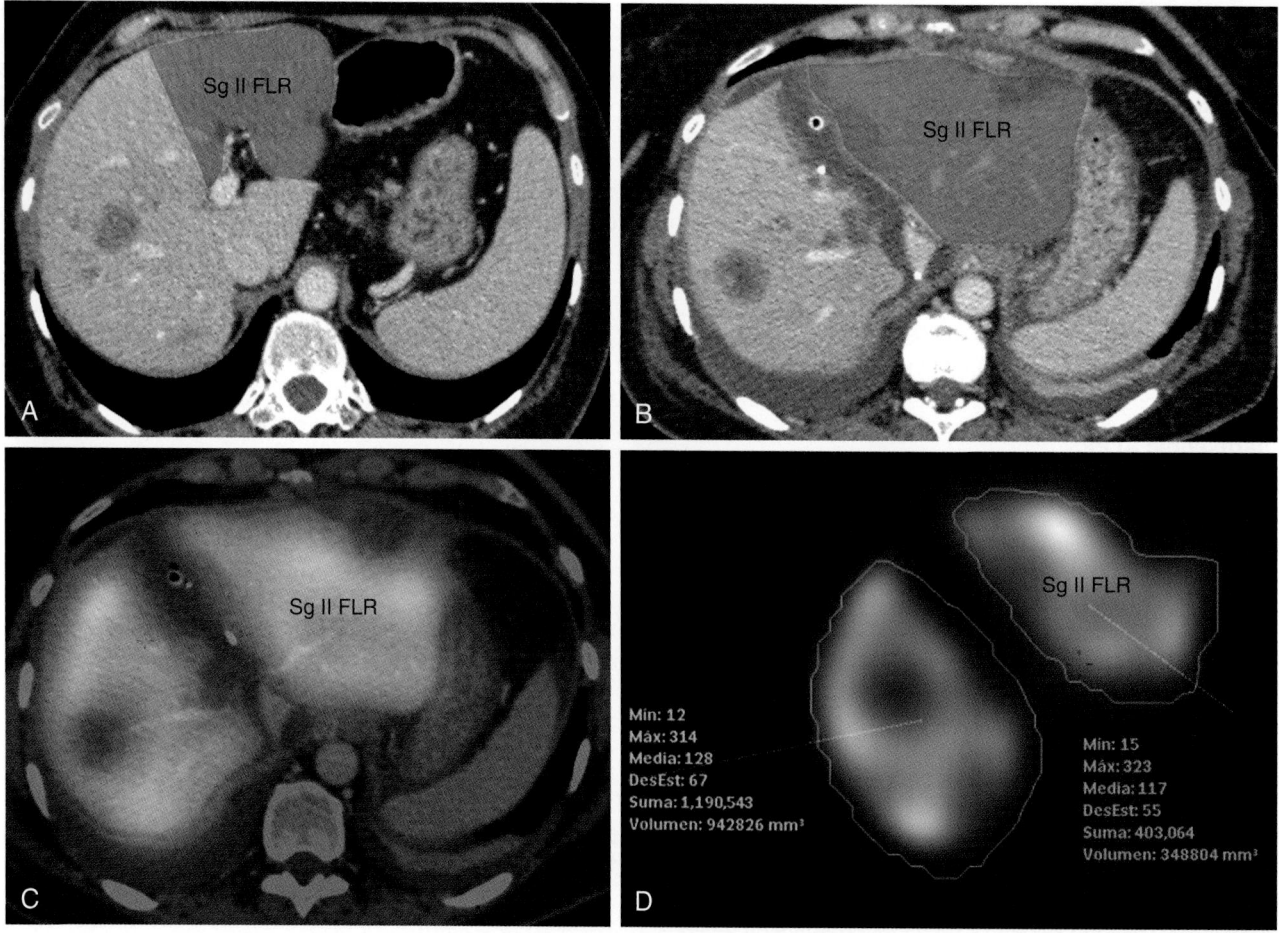

FIGURE 123.19 Perioperative assessment of the future liver remnant *(FLR)* in a patient with bilateral colorectal liver metastases in whom a monosegment II ALPPS was being planned (see Fig. 123.17). **A,** Preoperative baseline CT volumetry depicts the segment *(Sg)* II FLR. **B,** Interval CT volumetry demonstrates a 170% hypertrophy of the segment II FLR 6 days after first stage. **C,** Interstage regional FLR function assessment merging CT scan with 99mTc-mebrofenin hepatobiliary scintigraphy (HBS). Volumes of interest around the FLR and the deportalized liver are manually outlined using single-photon emission computed tomography (SPECT) images linked to the contrast-enhanced CT scan as a reference. **D,** Combination of HBS with SPECT analysis offers quantitative information regarding 3-dimensional regional distribution of liver function, which therefore provides an accurate measure of FLR function.

with scores of 3.9, 4.7, 5.5, and 6.9, respectively.[14] Bearing this in mind, in cases where the patient is in good condition but FLR sufficiency has not been achieved, the patient can be discharged home and readmitted for stage 2 once FLR sufficiency and a low risk score have been achieved during periodic outpatient evaluation (Fig. 123.20).

ALPPS FOR SPECIAL INDICATIONS

The International ALPPS Registry (https://www.ALPPS.net) currently comprises about 1250 cases (June 2020), CRLM being by far the most frequent indication for this procedure, with almost two-thirds of cases. Recent data from the ALPPS Registry has consistently shown CRLM as the best indication for ALPPS (see Chapter 90), with perioperative morbidity and mortality profiles comparable with those of conventional major hepatectomies.[10,14,24] Furthermore, experience at high-volume centers has demonstrated a 3-year overall survival and disease-free survival of 50% and 13%, respectively, with a patient-reported quality of life similar to that of the general population.[75] However, the strongest evidence to support the use of ALPPS in CRLM comes from a recently published Scandinavian LIGRO trial comparing ALPPS with PVL- or PVE-TSH.[34,35] In accordance with previous retrospective studies, the first report from this randomized clinical trial demonstrated a higher resectability rate in ALPPS compared with TSH (92% vs. 57%; $P < 0.0001$), without increasing positive surgical margins (23% vs. 43%; $P = 0.11$), severe complications (43% vs. 43%; $P = 0.99$), or 90-day mortality (8.3% vs. 6.1%; $P = 0.68$).[34] In addition, ALPPS allowed the surgical rescue of more than half (57%) of failures in the TSH group. Regarding oncologic outcomes, the most interesting result from the last report of the LIGRO trial was that ALPPS not only was not associated with a higher rate of rapid recurrences than PVE within 1 year, but it offered improved median survival compared with TSH (46 vs. 26 months; $P = 0.028$).[35,76] The survival data must be viewed with caution, however, because the study was not powered to analyze this endpoint.

Although presence of CRLM is the best-established indication for ALPPS, there are some large series about ALPPS only for hepatocellular carcinoma (HCC) and, to a much lesser extent, for biliary cancer, which are more controversial and will be discussed later in this chapter.

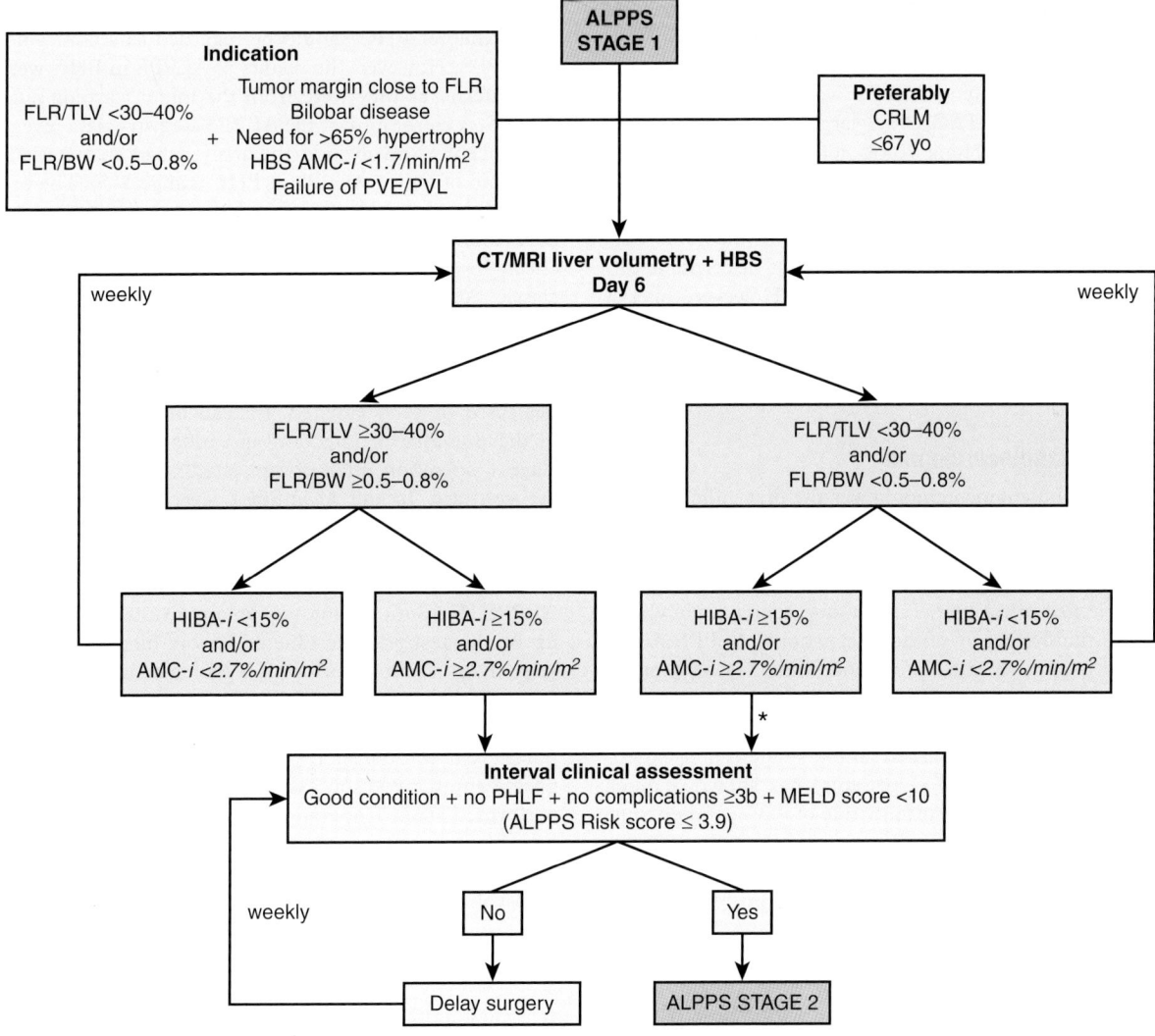

FIGURE 123.20   Flowchart algorithm illustrating the selection and management approach for patients undergoing ALPPS. Although there is a lack of strong evidence to support undertaking stage 2 in such a clinical scenario, retrospective evidence seems to indicate that future liver remnant (FLR) functional sufficiency is more important than volumetric sufficiency. *AMC-i,* Academic Medical Center in Amsterdam; *BW,* body weight; *CRLM,* colorectal liver metastases; *CT,* computed tomography; *HIBA-i,* Hospital Italiano de Buenos Aires index; *HBS,* hepatobiliary scintigraphy; *MELD,* Model for End-stage Liver Disease; *MRI,* magnetic resonance imaging; *PHLF,* posthepatectomy liver failure; *PVE,* portal vein embolization; *PVL,* portal vein ligation; *TLV,* total liver volume.

ALPPS for Hepatocellular Carcinoma

Surgery for HCC is often challenging due to an underlying liver cirrhosis with concomitant portal hypertension and/or impaired hepatic function (see Chapters 89, 101B, and 120). As such, ALPPS seems to be an attractive approach to increase resectability. However, a first report from the ALPPS registry with 35 ALPPS for intermediate-stage HCC revealed a 90-day mortality of 31%.[77] Much better results came later from the Hong Kong University with a 6.5% mortality rate and, with smaller numbers, from San Camillo Forlanini in Rome with a 5.8% mortality rate.[78,79] In particular, the Hong Kong group outlined strict criteria for which patients with hepatitis-related HCC were good candidates for ALPPS (FLR volume <30%, Child A cirrhosis, indocyanine green clearance rate <20% at 15 minutes, platelet count >100 × 10^9/L, and no total right PV thrombosis).[78] Although the degree of FLR hypertrophy in fibrotic/cirrhotic livers appeared somewhat less than in

noncirrhotic livers—in the initial report there was a volume gain of the FLR after 8 days of a little more than 50%—the 90-day mortality rate of 7.7% was encouraging.[80] Of note, in chronic liver disease complete parenchymal transection seems to be associated with a more rapid hypertrophy of the FLR than partial ALPPS. Therefore the Hong Kong group reserves partial ALPPS only for right trisectionectomy or for tumors located between the right posterior section and the caudate lobe.[78] The "anterior approach," with or without the "hanging maneuver," which has been demonstrated to improve operative and survival outcomes compared with the conventional approach for large (>5 cm) HCC in the right liver,[81,82] has also proven to be feasible and safe in ALPPS to reduce tumor manipulation and help liver transection in experienced hands.[78–80,83]

A recent single-center study from Fudan University, China, analyzed the outcome of classic ALPPS in 45 patients with locally advanced otherwise unresectable HCC. The in-detail analysis revealed that the severity of liver disease was inversely correlated with the degree and velocity of hypertrophy. With overall 1- and 3-year survival rates of 64% and 60%, the survival of patients undergoing ALPPS was significantly better than of those receiving TACE.[84] A large retrospective series from the University of Hong Kong comparing ALPPS with PVE in HCC demonstrated that ALPPS conferred higher hypertrophy and resectability rates (97.8% vs. 67.7%; $P <$0.001), with comparable postoperative and long-term oncologic outcomes regardless of tumor stage, and without discernable difference in the pattern of tumor recurrence.[78] However, this last group recommends ALPPS only when the FLR is less than 30%, whereas PVE when the FLR is between 30% and 40%, or for patients with medical comorbidities that preclude two major surgeries.[78]

ALPPS for Cholangiocarcinoma

Although hilar cholangiocarcinoma was the first indication for ALPPS, malignant biliary tumors (see Chapter 51) seem to be the Achilles' heel among indications for ALPPS. Data of ALPPS for biliary malignancies reveal the highest perioperative risk.[9,10,14] For intrahepatic cholangiocarcinoma (ICC; see Chapter 50) the first study of the international ALPPS Registry reported 8 patients and the second study 1 year later reported 13 patients with a 90-day-mortality rate of 13% and 15%, respectively.[9,10] As observed in other tumor entities, not surprisingly the recently published largest single center experience with ALPPS in ICC (14 patients) has shown a much better safety profile, with a mortality rate of 8.3%, and encouraging 3-year and median overall survival figures, being 64% and 4.2 years, respectively.[85] Moreover, a recent multicenter study using the data of the ALPPS registry on 102 patients showed a drop in 90-day mortality rate from 40% before 2012 to 7% in 2017 and 2018, with a 97% resectability rate, 85.3% R0 resection rate, and a better survival than chemotherapy only for otherwise irresectable solitary ICC.[86] These preliminary data suggest that there could be groups of patients with ICC that might benefit from ALPPS, especially considering that opposite to HCC, ICC usually arises in noncirrhotic livers and therefore may be more suitable for such a radical surgical treatment (Fig. 123.21). However, as for HCC, a threshold of FLR per body weight of 0.8% (or 40% of total liver volume) is recommended in patients with ICC waiting for the stage 2 operation. In the future, the role of neoadjuvant downsizing therapies and aggressive surgical treatment strategies will have to be put together for reevaluation in the multimodal treatment concepts for ICC.

With regard to perihilar cholangiocarcinoma (PHC; see Chapter 51B), the risk of perioperative complications is even higher, most probably due to the presence of at least partially devascularized/necrotic liver parenchyma in combination with potentially infected bile and biliary leakage. In 2017 Olthof et al.[87] compared data from the international ALPPS Registry to data of PVE and right trisectionectomy for PHC from two experienced HPB centers, the Academic Medical Center (AMC) in Amsterdam and the Memorial Sloan Kettering Cancer Center (MSKCC) in New York, in a case-matched fashion. Data were devastating, with a perioperative mortality rate of 48% in the ALPPS group (vs. 24% in the matched group with similar, small FLR volumes) and a median survival of 6 months only after ALPPS versus 29 months in the

matched controls ($P = 0.048$). At that point, the question arose whether PHC should be regarded as a contraindication to ALPPS. However, the results of ALPPS in PHC were probably inferior as they were from the initial learning curve with ALPPS. A closer look at the ALPPS Registry data revealed that the 23 centers involved in the analysis had an experience with a median of only 1 ALPPS in PHC (range 1–5). The presented ALPPS results were therefore based on the accumulation of data from at least 50% of centers having first and single experiences. In addition, many of the results had been obtained by classic ALPPS procedures, which undoubtedly raised the chances for improvement. Clearly, ALPPS was performed with the intention to improve resectability by rapid increase of FLR, but to do so, some principles of surgery for PHC were neglected or even violated. Instead of avoiding an operation in the presence of infection and inflammation, the excessive stage 1 operation often complicated by biliary leakage led to the contrary. In the meantime, several substantial improvements based on gathered knowledge and subsequent technical modifications had been developed with the aim to reduce morbidity and mortality, in particular mini ALPPS and hybrid ALPPS.[18,19] Both techniques obtain a suitable growth of FLR in the shortest possible time and avoid hilar dissection during stage 1. In a first report with 3 patients suffering from PHC, Sakamoto et al.[61] presented an alternative to the mini ALPPS procedure using a transileocecal instead of a transmesenteric portal vein embolization (TIPE ALPPS). In 2018 Balci[88] reported another two successful applications of TIPE ALPPS but performed stage 1 operation laparoscopically. Until these less invasive technical refinements are standardized, the widespread use of ALPPS in PHC cannot be recommended outside expert high-volume centers.

SUMMARY

It is now more than 10 years since Hans Jürgen Schlitt from Regensburg, Germany, performed the first ALPPS procedure. In 2012 the first report on 25 so-called in situ splits was published as a novel surgical technique to rapidly induce liver hypertrophy. However, early enthusiasm was hampered by initial high perioperative morbidity and mortality rates, as well as by early and rapid disease recurrence. Continuous efforts to improve patient selection, to optimize timing of stage 2, and to refine operative technique, aiming first and foremost to minimize the trauma of stage 1, have led to reduced morbidity and mortality rates in experienced centers. This short-interval staged strategy has become a milestone in HPB surgery as the ultimate advance to accelerate liver hypertrophy and allow complete tumor resection in selected patients with otherwise unresectable tumors.

As with every operation, in particular for ALPPS, it is true that the most essential decision is the indication of when to use it (see Chapter 102D). ALPPS certainly does not replace other techniques such as PVE or standard TSH, but may allow tumor resection in selected patients without any other surgical option left or who might mostly benefit from ALPPS instead of other strategies. The ALPPS procedure performed in low-risk patients, defined by younger age, high-volume center, and favorable tumor type such as CRLM (benchmark cases),[89] has reached standard outcome measures accepted for major liver surgery, with higher resectability rate, equivalent safety, and

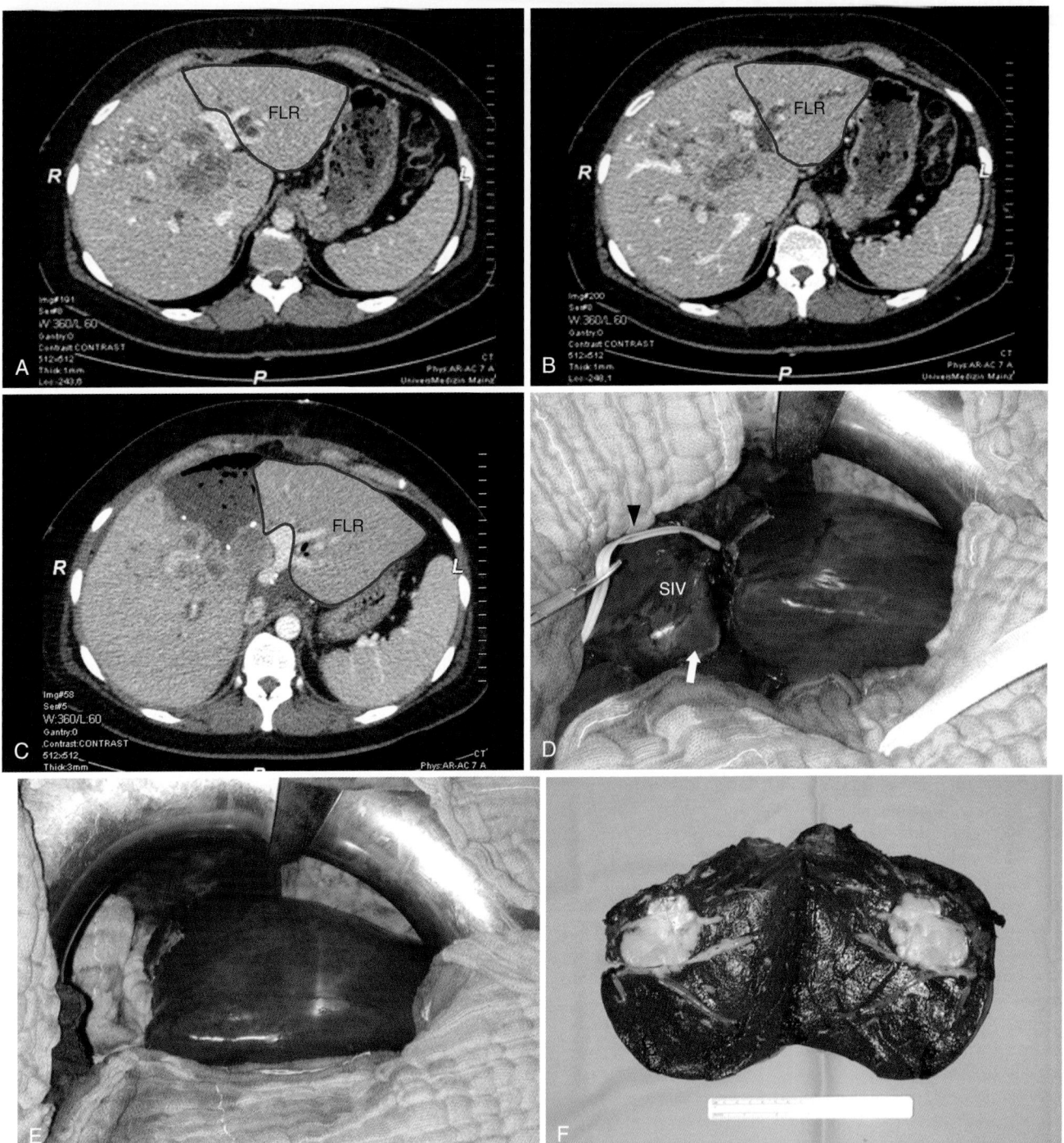

FIGURE 123.21 Classic ALPPS in a patient with intrahepatic cholangiocarcinoma. A and **B,** Baseline CT scan showing a small future liver remnant *(FLR)* and the tumor compromising the biliary bifurcation with intrahepatic bile duct dilation. **C,** Interval CT scan shows FLR hypertrophy. **D,** Surgical photograph at the beginning of stage 2 shows ischemic suffering of SIV *(arrow)* and vascular tag *(blue vessel loop)* marking the right hepatic vein *(arrowhead)*. **E,** Surgical photograph of stage 2 showing the FLR after completion of the right trisectionectomy. **F,** Surgical specimen with an R0 resection of the right extended liver. The patient is alive and recurrence-free 10 years and 11 months after ALPPS (status quo: July 2020).

encouraging survival compared with standard TSH. Although initial results in HCC and PHC were disappointing, technical refinements and better patient selection may enable in the near future the use of ALPPS to treat patients suffering from an otherwise irresectable tumor of these challenging entities. As such, ALPPS is a welcome novel asset that has finally earned its place in the armamentarium of successful therapies for extensive tumor disease of the liver in the hands of experienced hepatobiliary surgeons.

The references for this chapter can be found online by accessing the accompanying Expert Consult website.

CHAPTER 124

Ex vivo and in situ hypothermic hepatic resection

Chaya Shwaartz, Allan Hemming, and Ian D. McGilvray

Liver surgery techniques and liver imaging are constantly evolving, allowing for ever more detailed planning of surgical strategy and complex liver resections. The development of living-donor liver transplantation (LDLT; see Chapter 121) has led to a comfort and familiarity with a variety of techniques that are immediately applicable to complex, nontransplant liver surgery. The same techniques that are routinely used in LDLT, such as resection and reconstruction of vascular and biliary structures, are now more frequently being considered for the resection of hepatic tumors by surgeons experienced in both liver resection and transplantation techniques (see Chapters 122 and 125).

The principal difficulty of vascular reconstruction during hepatic resection is the necessary period of hepatic ischemia, although the liver can tolerate moderate periods of ischemia surprisingly well. During standard liver resections, the use of hepatic inflow occlusion is often used during the parenchymal transection to control blood loss (see Chapter 101). When combined with a low central venous pressure (CVP), inflow occlusion can result in a relatively bloodless transection of the liver. Ischemic preconditioning, meaning intermittent hepatic inflow occlusion, seems to protect the liver from subsequent ischemic injury[1,2] and is performed by applying a Pringle maneuver for 10 minutes, then reperfusing the liver for at least 10 minutes before reapplying inflow occlusion. The mechanisms by which ischemic preconditioning protects the liver from subsequent ischemia have not been fully elucidated, but even longer periods of ischemia are relatively well tolerated. The normal liver can tolerate 60 minutes or more of continuous inflow occlusion and warm ischemia,[3,4] but patients with cirrhosis or altered liver function from biliary obstruction or prolonged chemotherapy may tolerate significantly less ischemic insult before sustaining irreversible injury[5]; the same may be true of older patients.[6] Even with normal liver function, the risk of irreversible liver damage after prolonged periods of continuous ischemia is significant.

Nevertheless, there are many cases where vascular reconstruction mandates that a bloodless field be maintained for longer time periods than the surgeon (or the liver) may find acceptable. For example, tumors that involve the retrohepatic inferior vena cava (IVC) or the hepatic veins (HVs) may require total vascular isolation for a significant period of time. Total vascular isolation may increase the degree of ischemic injury to the liver more than inflow occlusion alone because there is some evidence that backward diffusion of HV blood into the liver attenuates ischemic injury.[7] In most cases, however, the procedure can be planned such that most of the hepatic parenchymal division is performed without total vascular exclusion, and caval clamping is reserved for the relatively short time that is required to deal with the IVC or HVs.

Most complex liver tumor resections can be done without the need for ex vivo liver resection or in situ cold perfusion, even when the tumor involves hepatic vascular structures (see Chapter 122). Tumors that involve hilar vessels usually can be approached by temporary occlusion of the hepatic artery (HA) or portal vein (PV) with relatively short ischemic times and without caval or HV isolation. When the HA *and* PV require reconstruction, it may be possible to do the reconstructions in sequence, maintaining oxygenated hepatic flow through one vessel or the other. Additionally, involvement of the IVC can often be approached with venous side-clamping, by exclusion of the cava while maintaining hepatic outflow (when the infrahepatic cava can be clamped below the insertion of the HVs), or by short-term total liver vascular isolation with or without veno-venous bypass. A minority of patients will have lesions that seem truly unresectable by any conventional technique. In general, these are cases where the vascular reconstruction is complex and is predicted to take a considerable length of time or where the transection of the liver is simply too dangerous to undertake in situ or without total vascular exclusion (as in an acute Budd-Chiari syndrome; see Chapter 86). The classic example is lesions that are centrally placed and involve all three main HVs, with or without involvement of the retrohepatic IVC. These few patients who require complex reconstruction of venous outflow may benefit from ex vivo or in situ hypothermic perfusion of the liver with hepatic resection and vascular reconstruction. The main advantages of this technique are better access to the tumor, minimizing ischemic injury to the future liver remnant using cold preservation, and higher likelihood of a complete R0 resection. At least theoretically, however, ex vivo liver resection surgery may increase vascular and biliary complications because of the need for re-anastomosis. There is a common concern that tumors requiring extensive liver resection are biologically advanced with an unfavorable prognosis, which may question the justification of a major surgery such as ex vivo liver resection. In our experience, however, good long-term survival rates have been achieved.

Experience with ex vivo and in situ cold perfusion liver resections is limited to a few high-volume liver surgery and transplantation centers throughout the world. In this chapter, we try to simplify the description of the techniques involved; we stress the importance of patient selection, preoperative evaluation and planning, intraoperative decision making, and postoperative care that can take place only in highly specialized and experienced centers. We have also collected a series of online educational videos that highlight many of the key points made in this chapter. These videos were created as part of the Toronto Video Atlas of Surgery (www.TVASurg.ca).

HISTORY OF HYPOTHERMIC PERFUSION AND EX VIVO TECHNIQUES

Fortner and colleagues (1974) were the first to describe the use of hypothermic perfusion during liver resection to protect the liver from ischemic injury in a series of 29 patients.[8] Technical improvements in liver surgery over the next two decades, along with a growing understanding of the liver's ability to tolerate normothermic ischemia, made the use of hypothermic perfusion unnecessary in most cases. Over the same period, liver transplantation (LT) had been applied to technically unresectable primary and secondary liver malignancy with dismal results.[9] Although the procedure was technically feasible, transplantation for large, unresectable primary liver tumors, especially for metastatic lesions, resulted in the rapid recurrence of malignancy, either in the new liver or elsewhere, shortly after transplantation (see Chapter 108).

In response to patients with unresectable tumors who were considered inappropriate for LT, Pichlmayr and associates (1988) developed hypothermic perfusion with ex vivo liver resection.[10] During ex vivo liver resection, the liver is removed completely from the body and perfused with cold preservation solution on the back table. The liver resection is performed on the back table in a completely bloodless field such that reconstruction of HV outflow can be performed under ideal conditions. Because morbidity and mortality rates from this procedure are relatively high, in situ and ante situm hypothermic perfusion techniques have been explored.

In this chapter, we describe the procedure and role of three techniques: in situ hypothermic liver perfusion, ante situm hypothermic liver perfusion, and ex vivo liver resection. These techniques overlap tremendously, and all mirror aspects of LDLT (see Chapters 109 and 121).

Both in situ and ante situm hypothermic perfusion do not necessarily require HA and/or biliary reconstruction. Hence the risk for vascular and biliary complications may be lower compared with ex vivo liver resection. However, the exposure with ex vivo liver resection is outstanding and this method can permit even parenchymal hypothermic perfusion (although not if the HV outflow is clotted, a real risk in the setting of a tumor that has led to an acute Budd-Chiari syndrome).

When applied, both in situ and ante situm hypothermic perfusion are performed using standard liver resection mobilization techniques (see Chapter 101). In these cases, the liver is placed in total vascular isolation and a cold perfusion is instituted through the PV or potentially through the HA. The hilar structures are left otherwise intact. The main difference between these two methods is that in ante situm hypothermic perfusion, the suprahepatic IVC (often with the cava below the HVs) is divided and the liver rotated anteriorly and counterclockwise to allow improved access to the area of the liver and IVC at the HV confluence.

IN SITU HYPOTHERMIC PERFUSION

The aim of in situ hypothermic perfusion is to provide a bloodless operative field together with hypothermic cellular protection, to permit prolonged and accurate dissection either for liver resections that necessitate vascular isolation of the liver or during the period of vascular reconstruction itself. Of the three surgical techniques outlined in this chapter, in situ hypothermic perfusion is the most straightforward from a theoretical point of view, but the exposure of the IVC and HVs can be very awkward and the vascular reconstructions, as a result, are often quite tricky.

Hannoun et al. (1993) presented their retrospective study of 34 patients who underwent major liver resection with a single period of vascular occlusion exceeding 1 hour.[11] Importantly, all patients included in the study had a normal liver remnant.

The authors concluded that continuous vascular occlusion (normothermic ischemia) during major liver resection is a useful maneuver that may be performed safely on normal hepatic parenchyma for up to 90 minutes. Liver cooling such as topical refrigeration or hypothermic perfusion was not used. However, the authors advocated for hepatic vascular exclusion with in situ hypothermic perfusion of University of Wisconsin (UW) preserving solution whenever the foreseen complexity of the hepatectomy suggested that vascular occlusion might exceed 120 minutes.

In 1996 the same group showed that these techniques can be successfully applied in patients with underlying liver disease (more sensitive to ischemic damage) that require liver resection. They showed that cooling of the hepatic parenchyma allows for major hepatic resection in patients with liver disease using vascular exclusion for longer than 1 hour without increased morbidity or mortality.[5] Azoulay and colleagues (2005) compared the results of liver resection performed under in situ hypothermic perfusion with standard total vascular exclusion of the liver for less than 1 hour and for longer than 1 hour in terms of liver tolerance that was assessed by the peaks of aspartate transaminase (AST) and alanine transaminase (ALT) postoperatively, liver function (assessed by peak bilirubin and the prothrombin [PT] level), renal functions (assessed by peak of creatinine), postoperative morbidity, and mortality. In the patients that had total vascular exclusion without in-situ hypothermic perfusion, a veno-venous bypass was instituted for hemodynamic intolerance, occurring in 4 of 33 patients undergoing total vascular exclusion for less than 1 hour and 5 of 16 patients that had total vascular exclusion for longer than 1 hour. They demonstrated that hypothermic perfusion of the liver is associated with better tolerance to ischemia in the setting of total vascular isolation of any duration. Further, they showed that hypothermic perfusion of the liver is associated with better postoperative liver and renal function and lower morbidity compared with total vascular exclusion of more than an hour. They also showed that the size of the tumor, the need for PV embolization, and a planned vascular reconstruction were predictive factors for longer liver resection (>1 hour). These predictive factors should be taken into account when considering the need for hypothermic perfusion of the liver.

Total vascular exclusion of the liver, including the clamping of the portal triad, the IVC above and below the liver, is indicated for tumors involving or adjacent to the IVC and/or the confluence of the HVs into the IVC. To perform in situ cold perfusion as originally described by Fortner et al. in 1974, the liver is mobilized as for total vascular isolation with control of the suprahepatic IVC, infrahepatic IVC, and the portal structures. In their description of the procedure, the gastroduodenal artery is isolated and cannulated. The PV was cannulated either via a venotomy or via the branch of the lobe that was to be resected. These cannulae were kept patent with a slow infusion of Ringer's lactate at room temperature. The common HA and PV are clamped proximal to the cannulae. The infrahepatic IVC and suprahepatic IVC are separately occluded by vascular clamps and a cavotomy is made immediately inferior to the liver for placement of a catheter to drain the perfusate. Ringer's lactate solution, chilled to 4°C and with 5 mg/L heparin, is used for the cold perfusion. In this original description of in situ hypothermic perfusion, the authors universally used veno-venous bypass, and the entire hepatic parenchymal transection was performed after cold perfusion of the liver. If IVC or HV resection was required during resection of the tumor, the hepatic hypothermia was extended for a longer period of time, allowing for the safe reconstruction of the vascular structures.

The standard use of veno-venous bypass (cava and/or portal) reduces the time pressure involved in these cases and the gut edema associated with prolonged portal clamping. However, in our experience, most patients tolerate total vascular isolation without the need for veno-venous bypass. In some of the series described, a veno-venous bypass was performed routinely.[3] If a veno-venous bypass is used, a sufficient length of the PV is dissected out (3–4 cm) for insertion of a perfusion catheter and the PV cannula for veno-venous bypass. Before clamping, the patient receives a bolus of at least 5000 U of heparin intravenously (IV). The infrahepatic IVC is clamped and the patient is placed on the caval portion of veno-venous bypass. It is generally advisable to isolate, ligate, and divide the right adrenal vein before clamping the infrahepatic IVC. A portal clamp is placed relatively superiorly on the PV with bypass instituted below this clamp. The portal cannula can be inserted, directed down toward the superior mesenteric vein (SMV) after complete PV division or by dividing just the anterior wall of the PV and sliding the cannula down the back wall. An alternative approach, although not part of the original description—and our preferred method—is to place a temporary biologic graft onto the anterior wall of the SMV and cannulate the graft.

Full veno-venous bypass is started. The liver side of the PV is cannulated with the perfusion solution tubing, and the HA is clamped. The suprahepatic IVC is clamped, and a transverse venotomy is created in the infrahepatic IVC just above the lower caval clamp. Cold perfusion of the liver is begun with preservation solution, and the effluent is suctioned from the venotomy in the infrahepatic IVC to prevent excessive body cooling (Fig. 124.1).

Possible cold preservation solutions include histidine-tryptophan-ketoglutarate (HTK) and UW solution.[12,13] The liver resection proceeds in a bloodless field with excellent visualization of intrahepatic structures. The liver can be cooled continuously throughout the parenchymal transection by slow infusion of cooling solution, or it can be cooled intermittently every 30 minutes by bolus infusion. At completion of the liver resection, the liver should be flushed of the cold preservation solution; this can be done by flushing the PV with cold 5% albumin before restoring flow to the liver or by allowing the initial 300 to 500 mL of venous effluent from the reperfused liver to be vented out the infrahepatic cava venotomy after reperfusion before removing the suprahepatic cava clamp. Next, the portal bypass cannula is removed, and the PV is repaired or reanastomosed if divided. If the liver has been flushed with 5% albumin, the infrahepatic venotomy is closed, and the suprahepatic cava clamp is removed to assess HV bleeding, which should be controlled if present. PV and HA inflow are reestablished.

If the liver is warm-flushed with the initial blood flow through the liver, the sequence is slightly altered to prevent flushing cold, high-potassium effusate into the cardiac return. If a warm-flush technique is used, portal flow is established with the suprahepatic cava clamp in place and the effluent vented though the cava below the suprahepatic clamp, whether through a venotomy or a caval anastomosis that has been deliberately left loose. The initial 300 to 500 mL of blood is suctioned, the venotomy or anastomosis is secured, and the suprahepatic cava

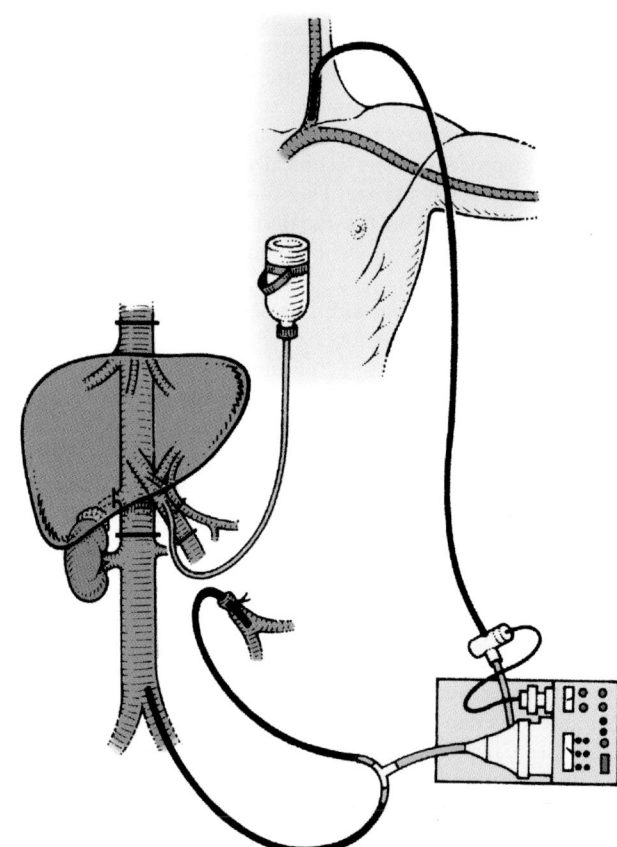

FIGURE 124.1   In situ cold perfusion. The patient is placed on venovenous bypass, and a cold perfusion solution is infused through the portal vein and vented through a venotomy in the infrahepatic inferior vena cava.

clamp is removed. An alternative to this method described is to cold-flush the liver with 5% albumin, which allows for the sequential removal of clamps with separate assessment of HV and portal bleeding on reperfusion, but this method is somewhat time-consuming. The patient is decannulated from caval bypass if veno-veno bypass has been used.

The advent of LDLT, combined with the more frequent use of the anterior approach to liver resection[14] and improved parenchymal transection techniques, have improved the ability to divide the liver parenchyma and dissect along the HVs without the need for extensive periods of inflow occlusion.[14] Hence we try to do most of the parenchymal transection while avoiding inflow occlusion. Only rarely do we use in situ perfusion as previously described with total liver occlusion for the complete liver transection (the exception being cases where the HV outflow is severely compromised, and the parenchyma is very congested as a result). In patients in whom a single HV or the IVC requires reconstruction, most of the parenchymal transection can be performed without inflow occlusion under low-CVP conditions. As the parenchymal transection nears completion, total vascular isolation is applied to enable division and reconstruction of the vascular structures. This practice results in significantly shorter periods of hepatic ischemia and allows a different method of applying in situ cold perfusion that is simpler and generally does not require veno-veno bypass (see Videos: https://pie.med.utoronto.ca/TVASurg/project/extrighthep-insitu/, https://pie.med.utoronto.ca/TVASurg/project/extlefthep-insitu/, https://pie.

med.utoronto.ca/TVASurg/project/extlefthep_cavalresection_cormatrix/).

In this technique, the liver is mobilized as for total vascular isolation. The PV is dissected to the right and left branches, and perfusion tubing is placed into the main PV. One option is to cannulate the PV branch on the opposite side of the liver to be removed (Fig. 124.2). The branch is divided, maintaining portal flow to the side of the liver to be left in but allowing access for cold perfusion. Alternatively, the anterior wall of the main PV can be used as a site of cannula insertion (Fig. 124.3). As much of the hepatic parenchyma as possible is divided under

low CVP conditions, maintaining hepatic perfusion until it becomes necessary to divide the vessels (HV and/or IVC) that require reconstruction.

At this point, the patient is volume-loaded, inotropes are started as necessary, and clamps are placed sequentially on the infrahepatic IVC, PV, HA, and suprahepatic IVC. If only the HV requires reconstruction, caval flow can be maintained by placing a clamp tangentially down onto the IVC across the HV orifice, partially occluding the IVC (Fig. 124.4). The anterior wall of the IVC or HV is incised, and cold perfusion of the liver is instituted through the portal cannula. Only the side of the liver remaining in place is perfused. The vessels are transected, and the specimen is removed. The vessels, HVs, or IVC can be reconstructed in a bloodless field without undue pressure of time (Fig. 124.5). Before completing the anastomoses, the liver can be flushed with cold 5% albumin or flushed with 300 to 400 mL of PV blood with the vena caval clamps still in place, at which point the PV clamp is reapplied, the caval venotomy closed, and all clamps removed. Because of the shorter ischemic periods involved with this technique, we do not generally use veno-venous bypass; even longer periods of total vascular isolation do not necessarily require veno-venous bypass.[15-19]

Of the three procedures described in this chapter, in situ hypothermic perfusion is the least complicated from a theoretical point of view. However, a real caution is that the IVC/HV reconstructions can be very awkward because of the angles involved. This surgical technique demands experience and should be limited to high-volume centers with LT experience. In 2015, Azoulay and colleagues published their experience with this procedure including 77 liver resections performed using standard total vascular exclusion with hypothermic portal perfusion and veno-venous bypass.[20] Although only 33 cases required vascular reconstruction, the 90-day mortality rate was 19.5%. They also identified independent predictors of mortality, including age-adjusted Charlson Comorbidity Index (CCI) of 3 or more, tumor size 10 cm or more, and the presence of 50/50 criteria.[21] The overall 5-year survival rate in their cohort was

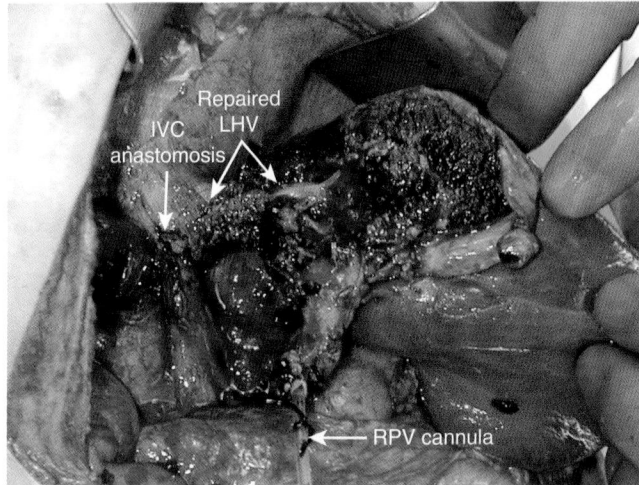

FIGURE 124.2 A portal cannula is inserted in the right portal vein *(RPV)* branch to allow in situ perfusion of the remaining segments II and III in an infant undergoing resection for hepatoblastoma. Cold perfusion allows resection of the inferior vena cava *(IVC)* and resection and repair of the medial aspect of the left hepatic vein *(LHV)* to be done in a controlled fashion.

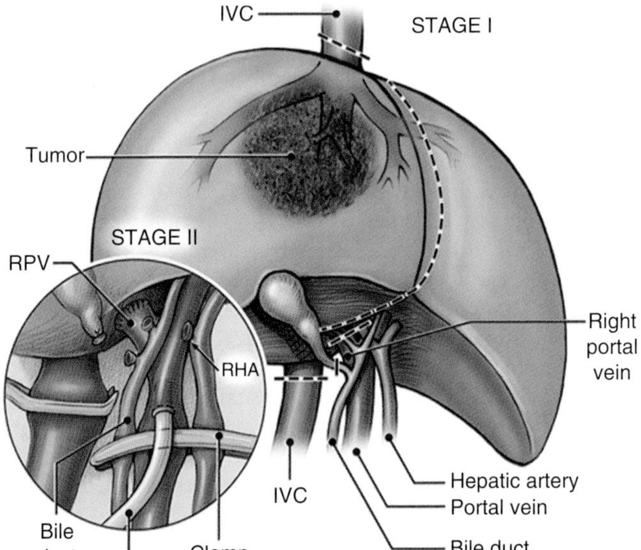

FIGURE 124.3 The anterior wall of the portal vein above the portal clamp can also be used for cannulation and cold perfusion. *IVC,* Inferior vena cava; *RHA,* right hepatic artery; *RPV,* right portal vein.

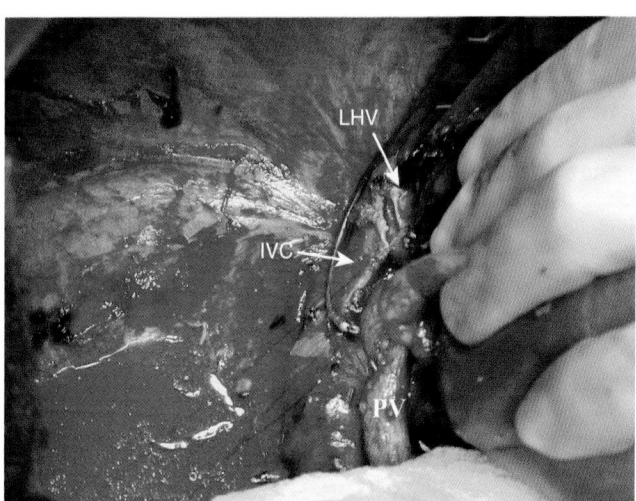

FIGURE 124.4 A vascular clamp can be placed tangentially on the inferior vena cava *(IVC)*, occluding the implantation site of the hepatic vein but allowing maintenance of cava flow. This maneuver may allow in situ perfusion to be performed without the need for veno-venous bypass. *LHV,* Left hepatic vein; *PV,* portal vein.

STAGE III

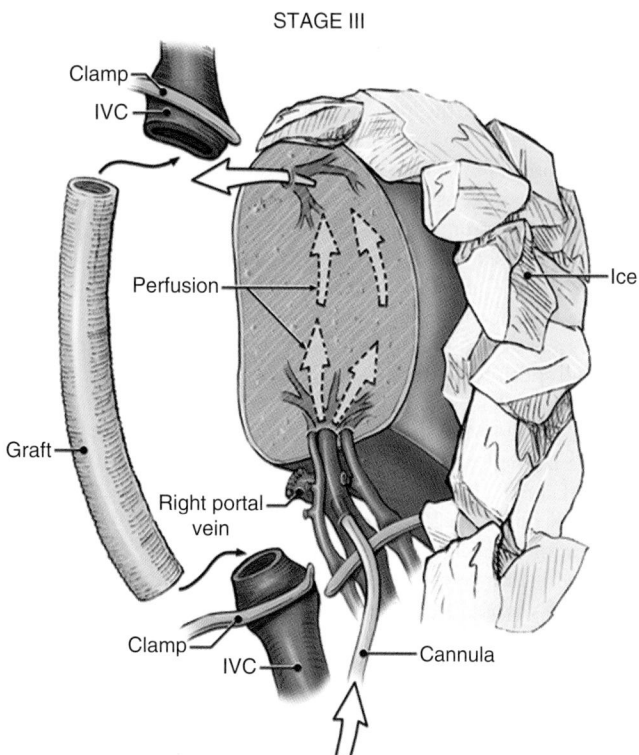

FIGURE 124.5 Continuous cold flushing of the remnant liver allows resection and reconstruction of the hepatic vasculature without time pressure. *IVC,* Inferior vena cava.

30.4%. We strongly believe that the identification of preoperative predictors for mortality should be taken into account when selecting patients for this complex surgery.

ANTE SITUM PROCEDURE

Of the three techniques outlined in this chapter, the ante situm technique is by far the least frequently used. The ante situm technique of liver resection can be used when resection of the IVC and HVs is expected to be difficult and when improved access to the HVs and IVC is required. To improve the access to the posterior side of the liver avoiding the division of the portal triad, Hannoun et al (1991) designed this technique in which the suprahepatic (+/- infrahepatic) cava is divided, allowing rotation of the liver anteriorly to permit the liver to be essentially exteriorized while connected only by the hepatic pedicle.[22] During the procedure the future remnant liver is perfused with a preservation solution via the PV or HA. The liver is then resected with the involved HVs, and the remnant HV(s) is/are reimplanted into the vena cava.

This technique combines in situ hypothermic perfusion with separation of the suprahepatic IVC. Dividing the suprahepatic cava—with the liver fully mobilized as for a bicaval LT—allows for better mobilization of the liver posteriorly by rotating the liver anteriorly towards the abdominal wall. We have used this technique when combined IVC–HV reconstruction is required. The ante situm technique uses the same technique as in situ cold perfusion, with several caveats. The suprahepatic IVC requires more extensive dissection to achieve enough length to clamp, divide, and subsequently reanastomose. Greater exposure of the suprahepatic cava can be obtained by dividing the

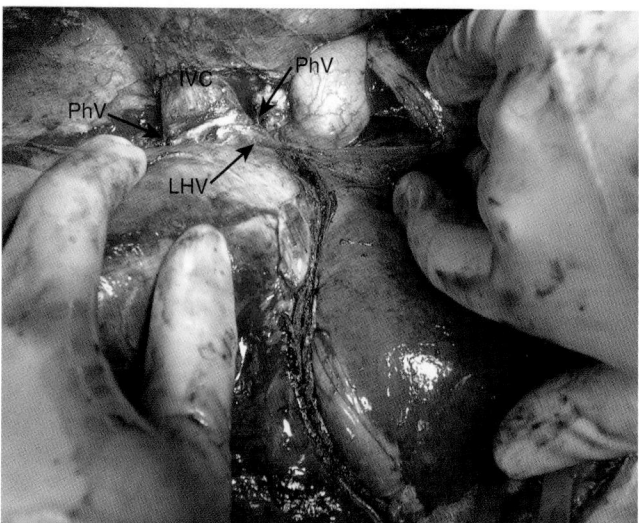

FIGURE 124.6 The phrenic veins *(PhV)* are divided, and the suprahepatic inferior vena cava *(IVC)* is dissected away from the diaphragm to allow adequate length for placement of a suprahepatic cava clamp. This allows for division of the suprahepatic vena cava with enough length to allow reanastomosis. *LHV,* Left hepatic vein.

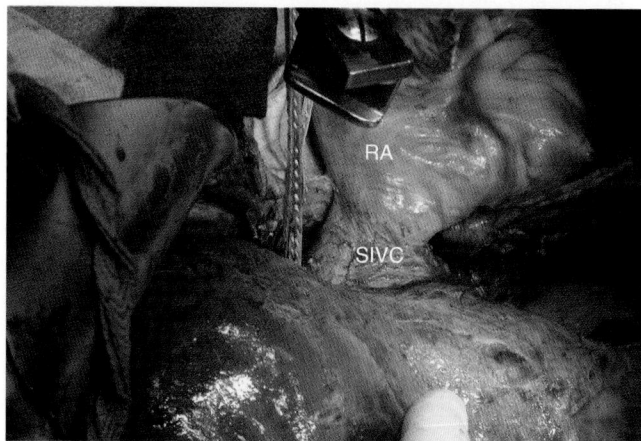

FIGURE 124.7 The addition of a median sternotomy provides excellent exposure to the suprahepatic inferior vena cava *(SIVC)* and confluence of the hepatic veins. *RA,* Right atrium.

phrenic veins and gently dissecting the IVC away from the diaphragm (Fig. 124.6). When using this technique, we frequently also open the pericardium directly anterior to the IVC and mobilize the intrapericardial vena cava and lower atrium; alternatively, a sternotomy provides excellent exposure of the entire area (Fig. 124.7). Nevertheless, we try to avoid sternotomy when possible because of the additional morbidity.

Control of the intrapericardial cava allows for placement of the upper clamp on the vena cava or caudal right atrium within the pericardium as a primary option or as a secondary option in case technical difficulties arise with placement of the original suprahepatic cava clamp. We perform as much of the liver transection as possible without inflow occlusion before cold perfusing the liver. Veno-venous bypass is generally recommended for this procedure; however, many patients tolerate IVC clamping without difficulty, particularly if the anesthesiologist volume loads the patient and institutes appropriate inotropic support (vasopressin is useful in this situation). Cold perfusion is instituted as originally described for in situ perfusion, although the perfusate is vented through the suprahepatic IVC once the suprahepatic cava is divided. Dividing the suprahepatic IVC allows the liver to be rotated forward toward the abdominal wall, enabling greater access to the area immediately around the IVC–HV junction (the hepatocaval confluence; Figs. 124.8 and 124.9).

If further access is required, the infrahepatic IVC can be divided, allowing the liver to be rotated completely up towards the abdominal wall, and the liver can be rotated around the portal axis counterclockwise so that the posterior aspect of the liver faces anteriorly and to the patient's left (See Video: https://pie.med.utoronto.ca/TVASurg/project/antesitum/). With this technique, we have found that continuous, slow cold perfusion is required after the initial flush to prevent excessive warming of the liver. As a rule, the liver is first flushed with about 1 L of ice-cold preservation solution wide open, with the bag suspended at shoulder height. After the initial bolus, the infusion rate is slowed to about half of the original rate. Care is taken to suction the vented perfusate to avoid its systemic absorption.

The liver transection is completed, dividing the HV within the liver and resecting the origin of the IVC–HV junction en bloc with the tumor. If extension grafts are required, vascular reconstruction can be performed; the HV anastomoses, which are the most tenuous, are performed while the liver is rotated onto the abdominal wall. The liver is replaced, and the caval anastomosis is performed. The liver can be flushed with 5% albumin before reperfusion, or it can be flushed with warm portal blood, as previously described.

The ante situm approach gives better access to the IVC–HV junction than does simple in situ cold perfusion. The exposure is usually not as good as with a complete ex vivo approach. The

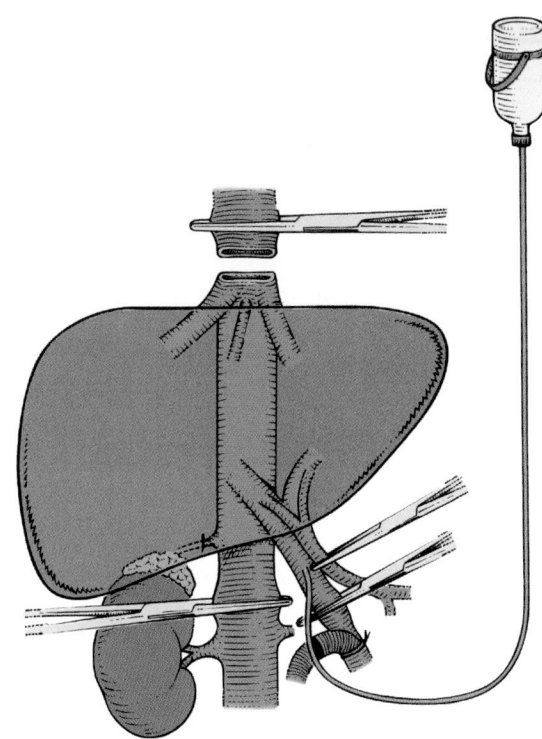

FIGURE 124.9 Veno-venous bypass can be used during ante situm perfusion. If more exposure is required to the retrohepatic inferior vena cava (IVC) than is provided by dividing the suprahepatic IVC alone, the infrahepatic IVC also can be divided, allowing the liver to be rotated completely up onto the abdominal wall.

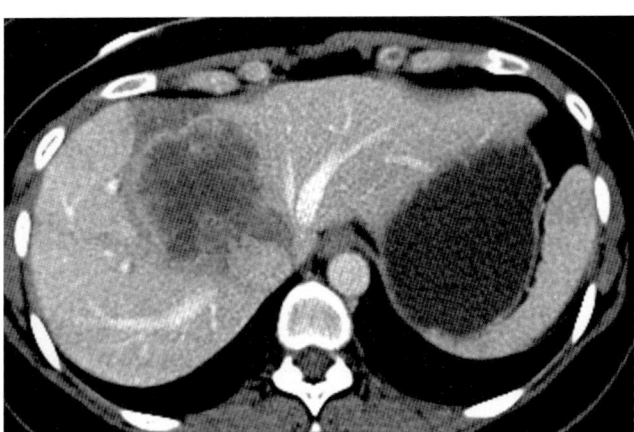

FIGURE 124.10 Computed tomographic scan showing a cholangiocarcinoma centered on all three hepatic veins at the junction of the inferior vena cava. Right portal structures were also involved. A right trisegmentectomy with reconstruction of the left hepatic vein was planned.

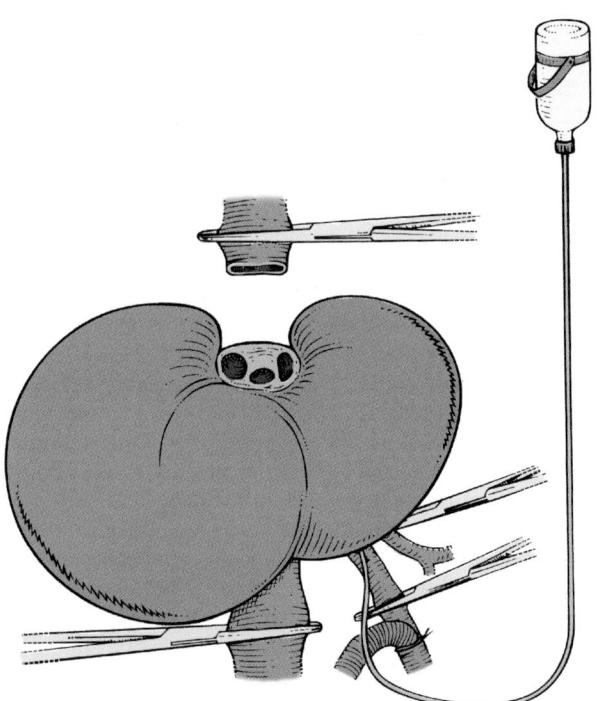

FIGURE 124.8 Ante situm cold perfusion. The suprahepatic inferior vena cava (IVC) is divided, allowing the liver to be rotated forward so the region of the hepatic vein–IVC confluence can be better visualized.

advantage to the ante situm approach is that biliary and HA anastomoses are not required, reducing the ischemic time to the liver and reducing the potential for complications resulting from these additional anastomoses. Only rarely does this technique need to be applied, but it can be considered when the HV/IVC junction needs to be resected en bloc and all three HVs reconstructed to the side of a graft or cava (Figs. 124.10–124.12; see Videos: https://pie.med.utoronto.ca/TVASurg/project/extlefthep-insitu/, https://pie.med.utoronto.ca/TVASurg/project/antesitum/).

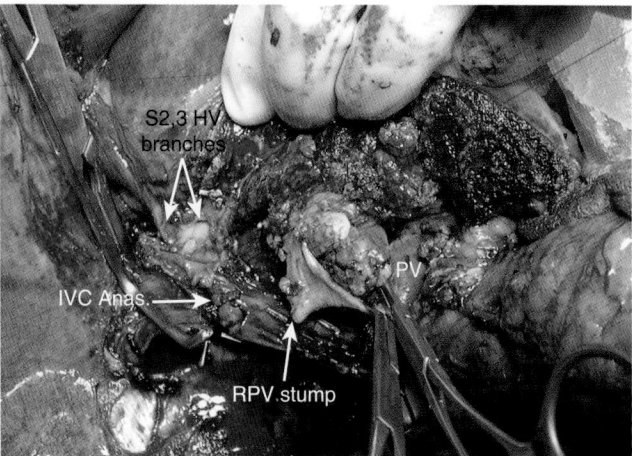

FIGURE 124.11 Ante situm procedure. Parenchymal division along a right trisegmentectomy plane was performed crossing into segments II and III superiorly. A cannula was placed in the stump of the right portal vein *(RPV)* for cold perfusion with University of Wisconsin (UW) solution. A short segment of the inferior vena cava (IVC) at the level of the hepatic veins and the first 3 cm of the left hepatic vein origin were resected, and the liver was rotated anteriorly. The IVC was reconstructed end to end with the left hepatic vein reimplanted above the cava anastomosis. *IVC anas.,* IVC anastomosis; *S2,3 HV,* segments II and III hepatic vein branches; *PV,* portal vein.

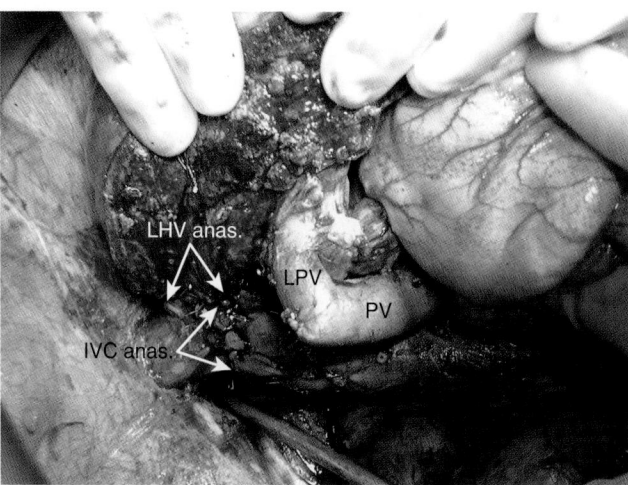

FIGURE 124.12 Ante situm procedure. Reimplanted segments II and III from Figure 124.11. The left hepatic duct was reconstructed later using a Roux-en-Y limb. *IVC anas.,* IVC anastomosis; *LHV anas.,* left hepatic vein anastomosis; *LPV,* left portal vein; *PV,* portal vein.

EX VIVO LIVER RESECTION

Although the techniques previously described can be applied to the majority of patients with difficult HV or vena caval reconstruction, patients who have tumors that involve the IVC and HVs that require complex venous repair; patients with combined, complex HV and hilar involvement; or patients in whom the HV outflow is severely compromised may be candidates for ex vivo resection. During ex vivo resection, the liver is completely removed from the patient and perfused with cold preservation solution on the back table. The hepatic resection is performed in a bloodless field, and vascular reconstructions are performed before reimplanting the remnant liver into the patient (see Videos: https://pie.med.utoronto.ca/TVASurg/project/extlefthep_exvivorppv/, https://pie.med.utoronto.ca/TVASurg/project/exvivo_167resection/).

Patient Selection and Preoperative Workup

In principle, any patient with liver malignancy that is unresectable by other means can be assessed for ex vivo liver surgery. In practice, almost all liver resections can be performed without the need for an ex vivo approach, whether or not hypothermic perfusion of the liver is required. Patients with tumors that involve the IVC–HV junction requiring complex and prolonged vascular reconstruction or patients with combined vascular involvement of the HVs and hilar structures may benefit from a planned ex vivo approach. Other patients who may benefit are those with involvement of all three HVs and some degree of venous outflow obstruction, in whom attempts to mobilize the liver off the IVC or initiate liver transection without vascular isolation would result in massive hemorrhage. In these patients, early removal of the liver to the back table facilitates the procedure. One of the benefits of planning the ex vivo approach—or for that matter, planning any of the hypothermic perfusion techniques—is that at surgery, what initially was thought to be unresectable by any method short of complete removal of the liver may be found to be resectable with a less complex procedure.

General assessment of the patient is like that for LT, with particular assessment of cardiac risk factors. A detailed history should be taken including cardiovascular (CV) risk factors, previous CV disease, history of smoking, or peripheral vascular disease and hypertension. In patients older than 50 or with any cardiac abnormality, a functional stress test is performed. Failure to achieve the target heart rate can be an issue in the elderly population because of arthritis and should be addressed with radioisotope assessment such as dobutamine stress echocardiogram. Any significant cardiac abnormality is a contraindication.

In 2001, Melendez et al. showed that the combination of two factors in the following list led to a very high mortality risk in patients undergoing major liver resection: preoperative cholangitis, elevated serum creatinine, elevated serum bilirubin, more than 3 liters of operative blood loss, and vena cava resection.[23] Therefore even mild renal dysfunction of creatinine level greater than 1.3 mg/dL should be considered a contraindication for such an extensive procedure as ex vivo liver resection. Furthermore, as previously mentioned, Azoulay et al. showed that among the variables available before surgery, the age-adjusted CCI of 3 or more and the maximum size of the tumor of 10 cm or more were independent risk factors of 90-day mortality.[20] Other studies showed that the presence and number of comorbidities such as CV, renal, and pulmonary diseases were independent predictors for mortality after major liver resection. Hence ex vivo liver resection should be attempted only in otherwise healthy, well-selected patients.

Preoperative imaging is crucial for staging the tumor and for assessing its position in relation to HV anatomy (see Chapters 14 and 15). Our current standard is triphasic spiral computed tomography (CT) with three-dimensional (3D) reconstructions to assess the liver anatomy and tumor position and CT of the chest and pelvis to rule out metastatic disease. In some instances, magnetic resonance imaging (MRI) is required, including MR angiography and MR venography, particularly when all three HVs are involved and some degree of venous obstruction is present, preventing adequate flow of contrast material into the HVs during CT. With the combination of CT and MRI, and the present availability of 3D reconstruction, invasive angiography is almost always unnecessary. Contrast-enhanced ultrasound provides a dynamic view of the relationship of the tumor to the HVs and IVC and is particularly useful for estimation of the extent of tumor invasion of vascular structures. A positron emission tomography (PET) scan is considered to assess for otherwise undetected extrahepatic disease and is used in selected cases.

Remnant liver volume assessment can be performed as for extended hepatectomy (see Chapter 102C). In a standard liver resection, assuming normal liver function, 25% of total liver volume (TLV) after resection is considered adequate for resection without the need for preoperative PVE. One caveat is that patients who have undergone or are undergoing prolonged and aggressive preoperative chemotherapy may require more liver volume because of chemotherapy-induced steatohepatitis (see Chapters 69 and 98). With cold preservation and reperfusion, additional ischemic injury occurs beyond that during standard liver resection. We have arbitrarily chosen a projected liver remnant of 40% of TLV as a cutoff for consideration of preoperative PVE in patients who require extended hepatectomy and may need complex vascular reconstruction with cold-perfusion techniques.[18,19,24]

Accurate imaging of the intrahepatic architecture is critical to assess the possibilities for reconstruction. In a systematic review,[25] the authors showed that 3D printed liver models demonstrate hepatic anatomy and tumors with high accuracy.[25] The 3D models can assist with preoperative planning and may be used in the simulation of surgical procedures for the treatment of malignant hepatic tumors. 3D imaging techniques occasionally may reveal unusual anatomy that makes vascular reconstruction unnecessary, such as the presence of a large inferior HV that makes reconstruction of the main right HV unnecessary. Alternatively, anatomy may be discovered that requires additional reconstruction, such as a large segment VI vein that drains into the middle HV.[26]

Anesthesia

The participation of a multidisciplinary team in ex vivo liver surgery is of the highest importance. Optimized anesthetic management of circulation and hemodynamic stability, coagulation function, and patient's core temperature is essential. Anesthetic management during ex vivo liver surgery is a rapidly growing field that evolves dramatically over time while using the knowledge from transplant surgery (see Chapter 106).

The maintenance of hemodynamic stability during surgery is crucial for surgical success and lower complication rates. Liver surgery in general is associated with large fluid shifts that can affect the hemodynamic stability of the patient. Blood loss during surgery, hypovolemia, vascular clamping, intraoperative visceral exposure, and ischemic time can all contribute to the hemodynamic instability of the patient. Usually, the most challenging part of the operation in that aspect is on occlusion of the PV and the IVC as well as on the reperfusion of the liver. One of the key components is using vasoactive agents as early in the case as possible to maintain the stability of the patient. Even when using vasoactive agents early, however, there are

multiple factors that can influence the degree of hemodynamic changes during the surgery such as the habitus of the patient and the collateral circulation of the IVC as well as different sensitivity to vasoactive agents.

Before vascular reconstruction, sufficient infusion of blood products and albumin should be given according to the patient's coagulation state. Additionally, before vena cava clamping, appropriate doses of vasoactive agents should be given to decrease the excessive changes in the hemodynamic state of the patient. Most patients lack sufficient collateral circulation. Communication between the surgeon and the anesthesiologist is extremely important at this stage of the procedure, and a test clamp should take place before clamping of the IVC and the PV. During vascular reconstruction the vasoactive drug doses will be adjusted to ensure that the hemodynamic parameters met the needs of the patient. Moreover, before reperfusion the dose is adjusted again to prevent pulmonary edema.

Maintaining patient temperature is a key component of anesthesia management. There are major heat losses during ex vivo surgery that include the induction of anesthesia, while the patient is exposed and prepared, during the anhepatic phase, and at the time of reperfusion. Hypothermia can cause platelet dysfunction and coagulopathy, slowing of cardiac conduction system, and coronary vasospasm. Routine methods of thermal regulation include use of forced-air warming blankets, warming of all fluids, heated humidifier, placing the patient on heated gel pads during surgery, and maintaining an ambient room temperature as warm as tolerated.

In addition to standard monitoring for liver resection, a Swan-Ganz catheter is inserted for hemodynamic monitoring and assessment of blood temperature in the pulmonary artery (PA). Access for veno-venous bypass, which originally was achieved by cutdowns, has been simplified by percutaneous insertion techniques.

Most cases begin with maintenance of low CVP, as is standard for most liver resections, because most cases do not proceed to ex vivo techniques. When an ex vivo approach is chosen, percutaneous catheters are placed in the internal jugular vein or in the subclavian vein and in the exposed portion of the infrarenal cava for the caval portion of the bypass circuit. At that time, the patient can be volume loaded. The portal limb of the circuit (if chosen) is placed directly into the PV by the surgeon. Alternatives include inserting the portal cannula through the inferior mesenteric vein (this vein can then be ligated at the time of cannula removal) or placing a temporary biologic graft onto the anterior aspect of the SMV and cannulating the graft.

In an ex vivo procedure, the anhepatic phase generally lasts from 2 to 4 hours, and attention must be paid to coagulation during this period. Similar to LT, we give fresh frozen plasma (FFP) or albumin to meet volume requirements during this time and minimize the use of crystalloid. Glucose levels are monitored, and constant glucose infusion is required.

As with LDLT, on reperfusion of the cold autograft, the temperature of the PA blood can precipitously drop. For LT and ex vivo liver resection, we continuously monitor the PA blood temperature (via the Swan Gantz line) and manually compress the portal inflow temporarily, when the temperature decreases to less than 35°C. Portal occlusion for 10 seconds or so allows the PA blood temperature to increase to 36°C, after which portal compression is released. The maneuver is repeated as many times as may be required over the course of reperfusion. PA blood temperature usually decreases to 32°C to 33°C without portal compression on reperfusion. In our experience, avoiding this precipitous drop in PA blood temperature seems to reduce the cardiac dysfunction that occurs on reperfusion of the liver.

Surgical Procedure

Pichlmayr and Hauss described the procedure of ex vivo liver resection in the second edition of this textbook; they appropriately described the procedure in terms similar to LT. The following description of the technique is taken largely from Pichlmayr's original description with some minor modifications. The procedure involves three phases:

(1) Assessment of resectability and removal of the liver
(2) Liver resection and vascular reconstruction on the back table
(3) Reimplantation of the liver autograft

As with the preceding discussion, many of the recommendations are applicable to any of the three hypothermic perfusion techniques described in this chapter.

Assessment of Resectability and Removal of the Liver

An initial assessment of resectability is undertaken by laparoscopy or a limited abdominal incision to assess for peritoneal disease that would preclude proceeding with resection. Even after a negative laparoscopy, we perform a limited abdominal incision and assess the abdominal cavity. Patients undergoing these procedures often have had previous abdominal operations, and the laparoscopic exploration can be limited. Further, it is not uncommon to have a negative laparoscopy only to find additional small lesions in the liver or peritoneal spread that are a contraindication to proceeding.[27,28] A variety of approaches are satisfactory and mostly depend on surgeon preference and the surgical retractor in use. We usually prefer to lengthen the incision to some variation of a bilateral subcostal incision with or without a midline extension. Alternatively, a midline laparotomy with a horizontal right extension can be used; either approach can be combined with a midline sternotomy for the sake of exposure of the hepatocaval confluence. Intra-abdominal adhesions should be divided to have a better access to the liver and to assess the primary tumor site and the peritoneal surfaces.

The liver is assessed for resectability. The indication for ex vivo resection is usually involvement of the HVs, with or without IVC involvement, and the liver may be quite congested as a result of obstructed venous outflow. Therefore care must be taken not to injure the liver during mobilization: Any small breach of the liver capsule becomes an outflow route for the obstructed venous flow, and bleeding can be torrential. Venous congestion of the liver is not a contraindication to resection because the planned resection should relieve the venous outflow obstruction. Large tumors may restrict the ability to rotate the liver without undue tension; in these cases, it is prudent to make an early decision regarding ex vivo resection before attempting to elevate the liver off the IVC. A midline sternotomy can also be useful in these cases.

The liver should be fully mobilized to better assess the tumor and the uninvolved liver. Intraoperative ultrasound is used to assess the level of vascular involvement and to confirm vascular anatomy originally identified on preoperative imaging.

If a decision is made to proceed with an ex vivo approach, the following steps are performed:

1. The hilar structures are prepared. The arterial anatomy is dissected and an appropriate site is chosen for planned division usually just above the common HA–gastroduodenal artery junction. If aberrant arterial anatomy is evident, an alternative site may be required depending on the anatomy and the portion of the liver that remains after the resection. In most cases, to preserve small arterial communications to the biliary plate and tree, the artery is not dissected high into the hilum. If the tumor involves the hilar structures (perihilar cholangiocarcinoma), the artery must be dissected far enough to determine that there is a usable, tumor-free portion of the respective HA branch to reconstruct. The PV is identified and the common bile duct (CBD) is encircled without skeletonization. A cholecystectomy is performed, the CBD is reflected off the PV, taking care to preserve its blood supply, and the neural and lymphatic tissue around the PV is cleared. It can be useful to sling each of the portal structures separately. Both the PV and the HA should be dissected and mobilized so they can be clamped individually to maximize the length for subsequent anastomoses. This dissection should be applied when evaluating for resectability and can be done without commitment to any irreversible steps.

2. The infrahepatic IVC is dissected down to the level of the renal veins and encircled. Planned vascular clamp placement is immediately above the renal veins, although division of the vena cava may be substantially more cephalad. The right adrenal vein should be ligated and divided, and small caudate veins should be divided if accessible. The large size of the tumor may make access to the caudate veins difficult, in which case they can be addressed on the back table.

3. The liver is freed from surrounding attachments. This can be challenging because the liver is often congested because of chronic venous obstruction. If the tumor is infiltrating the diaphragm, this area should be resected en bloc with the tumor.

4. The suprahepatic IVC is prepared. The phrenic veins are divided bilaterally, allowing the diaphragm to be dissected away from the IVC and providing an increased length of intra-abdominal IVC for subsequent clamping and reconstruction. Currently, we also open the pericardium directly anterior to the IVC and loop the intrapericardial IVC, or we use a midline sternotomy. Control of the intrapericardial IVC allows placement of the clamp on the vena cava within the pericardium as a primary option for very large tumors, or as a secondary option in case technical difficulties arise with placement of the original suprahepatic IVC clamp.

5. Clamp placement, subsequent transection lines, and the need for vascular conduits for reconstruction are assessed; alternatives for reconstruction are contemplated before removing the liver. HV branches may be reconstructed using HV or PV segments from the side of the liver to be resected or from autologous vein grafts, such as superficial femoral vein, proximal left renal vein, gonadal vein, or saphenous vein panel grafts. Cryopreserved femoral or iliac vein grafts can be used for reconstruction of long segments of HVs or IVC, although long-term patency is currently unclear. Alternatively, the IVC can be replaced with a 19-mm ringed polytetrafluoroethylene (PTFE; Gore-Tex) tube graft. Planning for these eventualities should occur before placement of clamps and removal of the liver.

6. Percutaneous access of the internal jugular vein and femoral vein/infrarenal cava is achieved, the IVC is clamped, and the cava portion of the bypass is started. The PV is clamped just below the bifurcation, and the portal cannula is inserted

down toward the SMV and secured. The PV is completely transected approximately 1.5 to 2 cm below the bifurcation, and the portal flow is added to the bypass circuit, while the liver continues to be perfused by arterial blood. An alternative to PV clamping, especially when the cava is to be reconstructed in full, is to clamp the PV, reconstruct the cava with a graft, and then perform a temporary portacaval shunt, often with a length of Dacron graft.

7. The CBD is transected sharply approximately 1 to 1.5 cm below the bifurcation. To permit a duct-to-duct anastomosis on reimplantation, we do not ligate either end; alternatively, the duct can be stapled and the stapled ends resected at reimplantation (see Video: https://pie.med.utoronto.ca/TVASurg/project/exvivo_167resection/); the latter technique has the advantage of avoiding bile leakage while the rest of the case continues. The common HA is clamped and transected. The suprahepatic IVC is clamped either below the diaphragm or within the pericardium, and the suprahepatic IVC is transected, far enough away from tumor to provide an adequate oncologic margin but close enough to leave room to perform the suprahepatic cava anastomosis at reimplantation. If the vena cava has been freed of its posterior attachments before clamp placement, the infrahepatic IVC is divided as cephalad as possible, and the liver is removed and placed in an ice bath. Cold perfusion through the PV and HA is initiated on the back table. As with any hypothermic perfusion technique, cold perfusion can be with either HTK or UW solution. If the retrohepatic IVC has not been previously freed up because of the large tumor size and difficulty with access, the liver can be cold perfused through the PV after the suprahepatic IVC is divided. The liver is rotated forward, as in the ante situm approach, and the retrohepatic IVC is freed of attachments. The infrahepatic IVC is divided, and the liver removed and placed in the ice bath. Once the portal and systemic veno-venous bypass has been established, the patient should remain stable for several hours.

8. Bleeding is controlled and the bypass circuit assessed (Fig. 124.13). Flows of 2 to 6 L/min can be achieved on total bypass. The abdomen is loosely packed and covered, and attention is turned to the back table. Again, an alternative to the bypass circuit that should be considered is to reconstruct the vena cava with a length of ringed PTFE (or similar) graft and perform a temporary portacaval shunt, with (see Video: https://pie.med.utoronto.ca/TVASurg/project/exvivo_167resection/) or without (see Video: https://pie.med.utoronto.ca/TVASurg/project/extlefthep_exvivorppv/) another graft.

An alternative method can be performed in patients with complex HV involvement without IVC tumor involvement. If access allows, the liver can be completely mobilized off the retrohepatic IVC until it is suspended only by the HVs. The hilar structures are divided as for standard ex vivo resection, but the patient is not placed on bypass. A vascular clamp is placed partially across the IVC, occluding the HV orifices but allowing cava flow to remain uninterrupted. The HVs are transected, and the liver is removed and cold-flushed on the back table. A temporary portacaval shunt is constructed (Fig. 124.14), decompressing the enteric circulation; this option avoids bypass, but it can be used only when there is no IVC involvement and when the IVC can be preserved in situ. It is worth assessing whether the tumor can be dissected away from the IVC in most patients

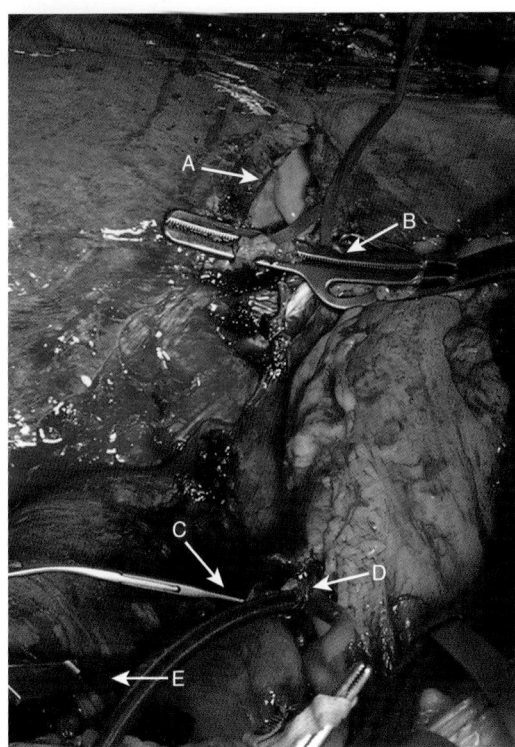

FIGURE 124.13 The liver has been removed, and the patient is on the veno-venous bypass circuit. **A,** Opening in pericardium to control intrapericardial inferior vena cava (IVC). **B,** Vascular clamp on suprahepatic IVC. **C,** Vascular clamp on hepatic artery. **D,** Portal cannula in portal vein. **E,** vascular clamp on infrahepatic IVC.

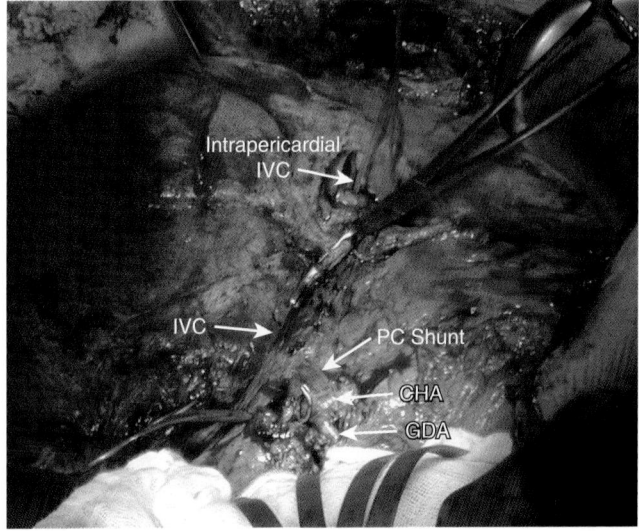

FIGURE 124.14 A temporary portacaval (PC) shunt is constructed, allowing a prolonged anhepatic phase without the need for veno-venous bypass. The intrapericardial inferior vena cava (IVC) has been encircled. CHA, Common hepatic artery; GDA, gastroduodenal artery.

because preoperative imaging can be inaccurate in determining true IVC involvement.[29]

Hepatic Perfusion and Preservation

After it is removed from the patient, the liver is placed immediately in an ice bath and perfused with preservation solution through the PV. We use either UW or HTK solution. After the initial 500 to 1000 mL of solution has been flushed through the liver, the effluent from the IVC should be clear. The HA and biliary tree are also flushed with another 100 mL or so of preservation solution, and the liver is immersed in cold UW solution. The exact accepted time to the reimplantation of the liver is not known; however, up to 4 hours has been associated with good results.[30–33]

Ex Vivo Liver Resection

Hilar structures are dissected out and divided. Great care must be taken not to divide segmental arteries that supply portions of the liver that are to remain because their caliber is too small to reconstruct with confidence. Main segmental divisions of the PV usually can be repaired and reconstructed. Parenchymal transection can be performed using a variety of techniques, including ultrasonic (Cavitron ultrasonic surgical aspirator [CUSA]) and water-jet dissection or even sharp division with a knife without fear of blood loss during the back table dissection. Small bile ducts and vessels are ligated or oversewn and large HVs are sharply cut and assessed later for reconstruction (Figs. 124.15–124.18). Great care must be taken to ligate or clip all visible vessels or ducts to avoid significant bleeding at reperfusion.

A key advantage of the ex vivo approach is the ability to extend the resection to obtain negative margins while providing the necessary time and exposure for complex reconstructions. The resection margin should not be compromised to minimize the subsequent complexity of vascular reconstruction. At completion of the resection, it is helpful to flush the PV, HA, and

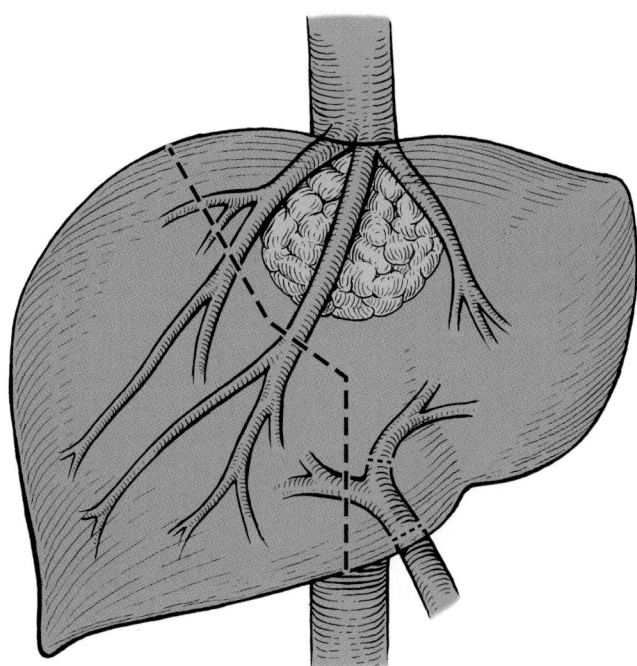

FIGURE 124.16 The planned hepatic transection line for the tumor shown in Figure 124.15. Multiple hepatic vein branches require reconstruction.

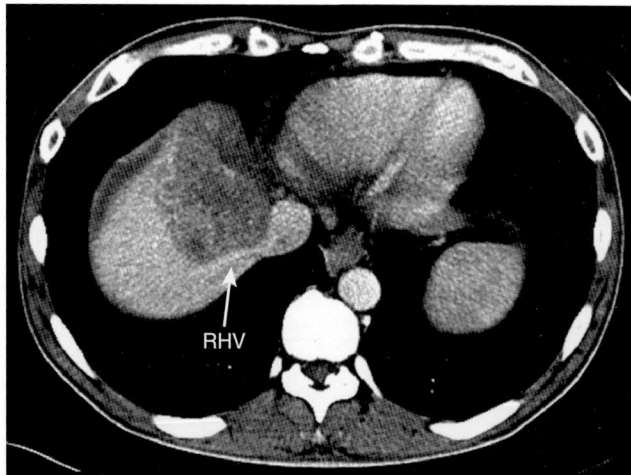

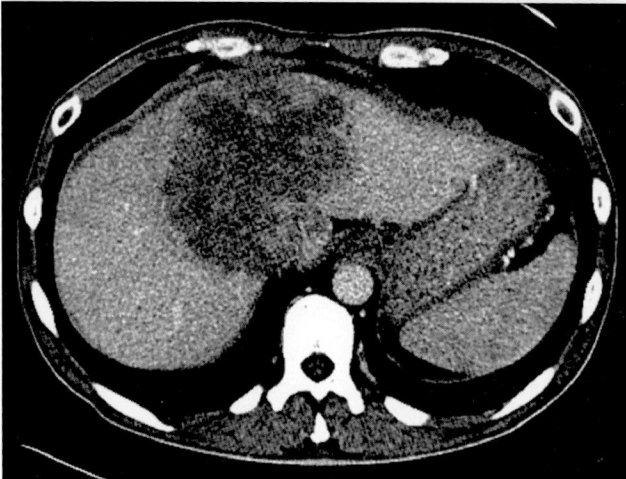

FIGURE 124.15 A single colorectal metastasis *(arrow)* involving all three hepatic veins. *RHV,* Right hepatic vein.

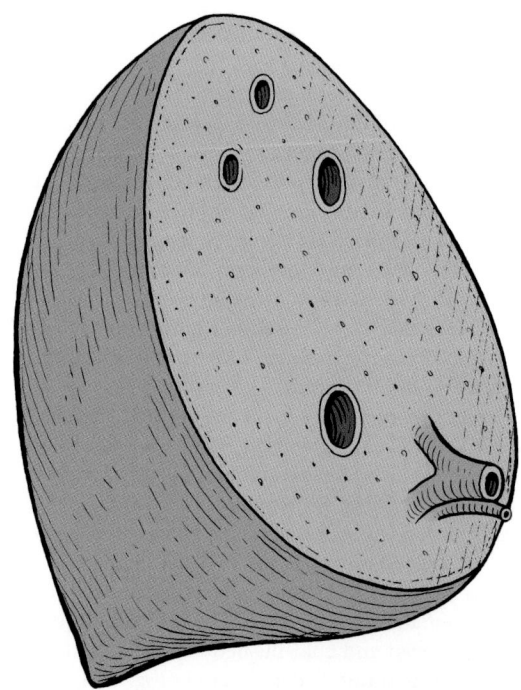

FIGURE 124.17 Back-table transection of the liver results in multiple branches of the right hepatic vein requiring reconstruction. A large segment VI branch that enters the middle hepatic vein also requires reimplantation.

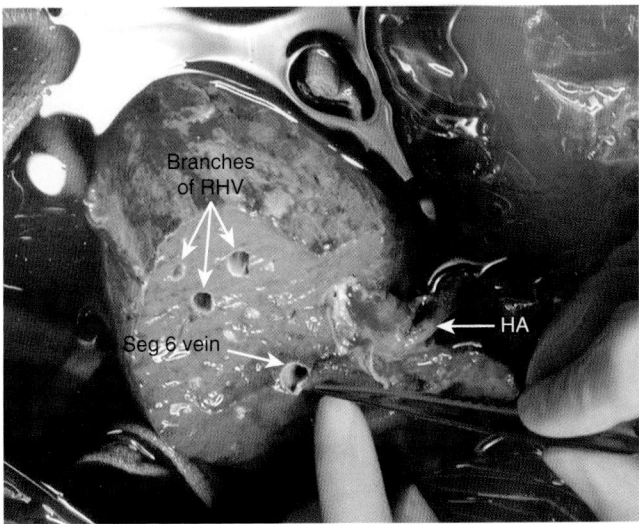

FIGURE 124.18 Completed transection on the back table. *HA,* Hepatic artery; *RHV,* right hepatic vein; *Seg 6,* segment VI.

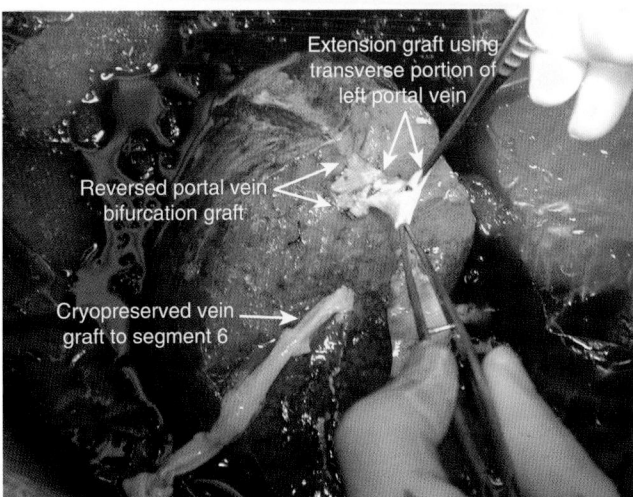

FIGURE 124.19 Joining two of the three right hepatic vein branches together and implanting the resulting two orifices into the reversed portal vein bifurcation taken from the patient's hilum allows reconstruction of the right hepatic vein branches. The transverse portion of the left portal vein is added to allow the graft to reach the inferior vena cava (IVC) without tension. A cryopreserved femoral vein graft is used to extend the segment VI vein to the IVC.

CBD with cold preservation solution to identify leaks from the cut surface of the liver that can be repaired before reimplantation. Fibrin glue (or similar hemostatic agents) may be sprayed on the cut surface of the liver to minimize bleeding.

Hepatic Vein and Inferior Vena Cava Reconstruction

The main reason for ex vivo hepatic resection is extensive involvement of the IVC or HVs by tumor. Complex HV reconstruction, with or without IVC reconstruction, is the raison d'être for ex vivo liver resection. The three main HVs and their major branches are relatively thick-walled and straightforward to reconstruct, even several centimeters from their merging with the IVC. For reconstructions of HVs transected relatively close to the IVC, the liver parenchyma can be trimmed back such that direct reimplantation of the HV into the IVC or the IVC replacement can be performed.

Multiple HV orifices may be sutured together and reimplanted into venous conduits (Figs. 124.19–124.21; see Video: https://pie.med.utoronto.ca/TVASurg/project/extlefthep_cavalresection_cormatrix/). The farther away from the IVC that the HV is transected, the thinner the HV wall, and the more difficult it is to reimplant the vein directly into the IVC. The use of extravenous patches to reduce tension should be considered, similar to LDLT. We have harvested the PV bifurcation, reversed it, and used it to reconstruct multiple HV branches into a single outflow vessel on several occasions.[34] Grafts of saphenous, superficial femoral, internal jugular, and cryopreserved vein all have been used to reconstruct HVs.[35–39] In addition, segments of uninvolved HV from the side of the liver resected can be salvaged and used for grafts or patches.

Venous grafts should be kept as short as possible, and great care must be taken to place the grafts such that they do not kink. For extension grafts, the HV-graft anastomosis is performed first with subsequent reimplantation of the graft into the IVC. One alternative to consider before choosing an extension graft is whether the liver remnant can be rotated on its inflow pedicle such that the HV orifice is brought to lie directly against the caval graft; this avoids the issue of kinking of a venous extension graft. Surprisingly large distances can be

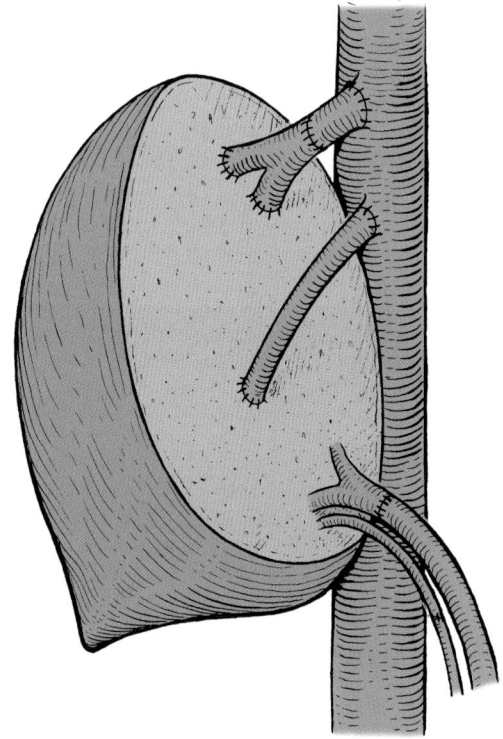

FIGURE 124.20 The prepared autograft is reimplanted into the patient as diagrammed. Reimplantation is done in similar fashion as for living-donor right liver transplantation.

bridged in this manner (see Video: https://pie.med.utoronto.ca/TVASurg/project/seg8resection/).

An important issue is how to reconstruct the vena cava. The resected IVC can be replaced with an autologous vein graft or prosthetic graft. Replacement of the IVC with an autologous vein is superior to a prosthetic graft in terms of infection and

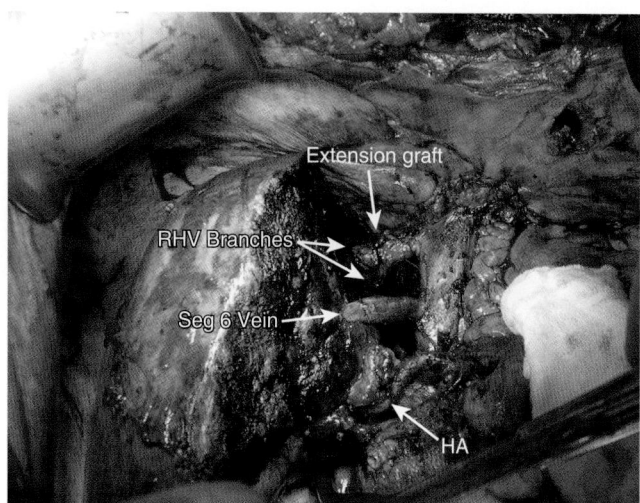

FIGURE 124.21 The reimplanted liver as in Figure 124.20. *HA,* Hepatic artery; *RHV,* right hepatic vein; *Seg 6,* segment VI.

thrombosis; however, that can sometimes be technically impossible when a longer segment of the IVC should be replaced. If possible, it is best to reimplant the HVs into native IVC. Frequently, a large portion of IVC initially removed with the liver can be salvaged and moved superiorly, with the HVs reimplanted into this newly situated portion of IVC. A ringed 19-mm Gore-Tex tube graft can be used to make a composite cava graft with the Gore-Tex graft placed inferiorly. Alternatively, a section of the IVC remaining in the patient immediately above the renal veins can be harvested and used as the segment of IVC into which the HVs are reimplanted. A ringed

19-mm Gore-Tex tube graft is used to replace the segment of IVC immediately above the renal veins. In some circumstances, it is necessary to reimplant the HVs directly into a relatively stiff artificial graft that is replacing the IVC (see Videos: https://pie.med.utoronto.ca/TVASurg/project/antesitum/, https://pie.med.utoronto.ca/TVASurg/project/exvivo_167resection/). In this situation, it is important to make a larger opening in the Gore-Tex than one might expect and to triangulate the anastomosis to prevent anastomotic stricturing.[40] Alternatively, a larger opening in the stiff Gore-Tex can have a cuff of either vein graft or bovine pericardium placed to allow a more pliable implantation of fragile HVs (Figs. 124.22–124.26).

At completion of the back-table reconstruction, the final result is an autograft similar in size to a reduced-size or split-liver allograft (Figs. 124.27–124.30). Total cold ischemic time is usually 2 to 4 hours, which is well within acceptable limits, when comparing cold ischemic times for split-liver or reduced-size LT.

Reimplantation and Reperfusion

Reimplantation is similar to reduced-size LT or LDLT (see Chapter 125). The suprahepatic IVC anastomosis is performed first. If an artificial venous graft has been used to reconstruct the IVC, it is shortened such that it does not kink on implantation. When the back wall of the infrahepatic IVC anastomosis has been completed, the PV is flushed with 500 mL of cold 5% albumin, which is vented through the infrahepatic cava anastomosis. The infrahepatic IVC anastomosis is then completed. The cold rinse washes the UW solution out of the liver before reperfusion because this solution contains high levels of potassium and adenosine, which can cause dramatic cardiac dysfunction or arrest if allowed into the circulation on reperfusion. As previously described, an alternative to cold-flushing the liver

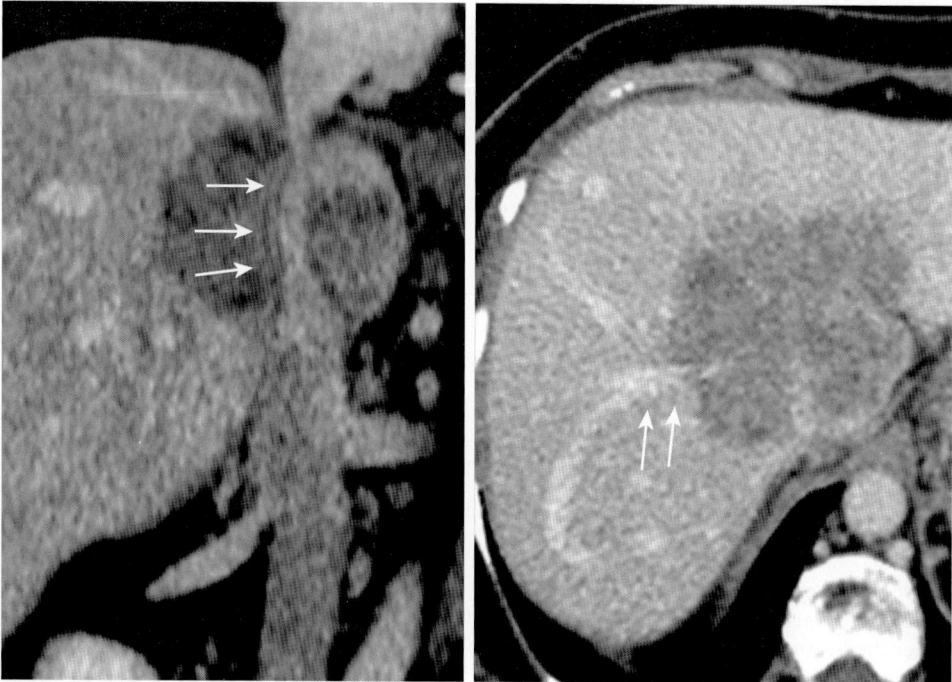

FIGURE 124.22 Computed tomographic images of a centrally placed cholangiocarcinoma that encases the inferior vena cava *(three arrows)* and extends to a trifurcation of the right hepatic vein *(two arrows)*.

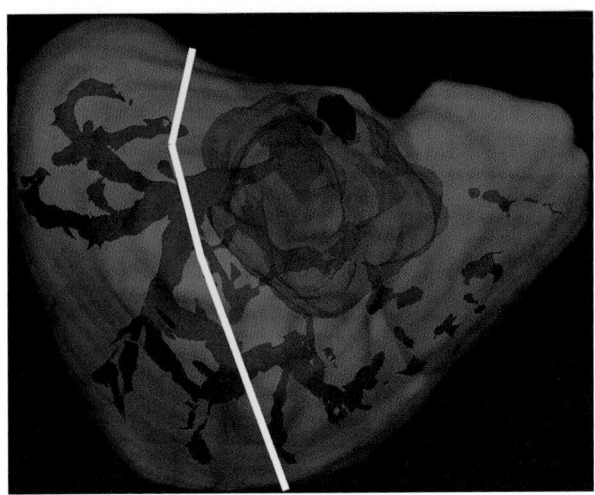

FIGURE 124.23 Three-dimensional reconstruction of proposed transection line shown in Fig. 124.22. Note that the resection will include the retrohepatic inferior vena cava as well as transect the right hepatic vein at the trifurcation.

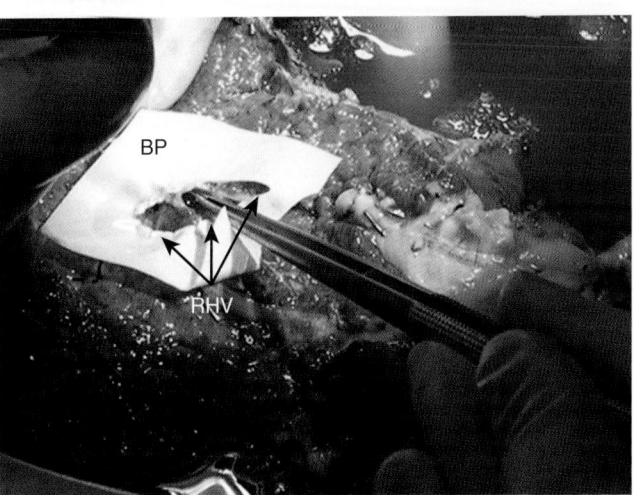

FIGURE 124.25 The liver from Figure 124.24 has been divided on the back table after ex vivo cold perfusion. The three branches of the right hepatic vein *(RHV)* have been sutured together and a cuff of bovine pericardium *(BP)* used to extend the outflow tract.

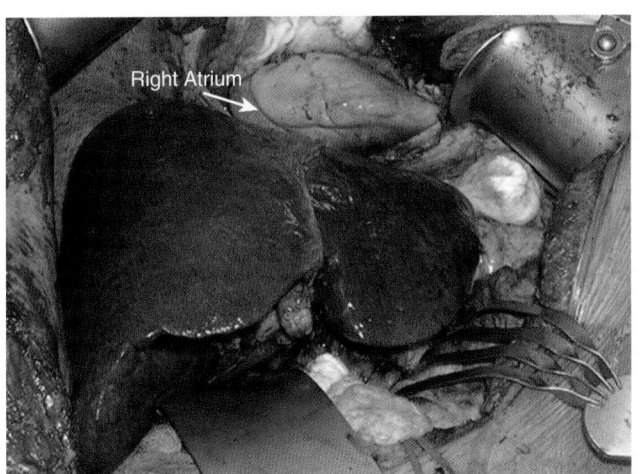

FIGURE 124.24 Patient from Figure 124.22. A median sternotomy has been performed to improve access to the suprahepatic inferior vena cava. Note the venous congestion in the liver secondary to outflow obstruction.

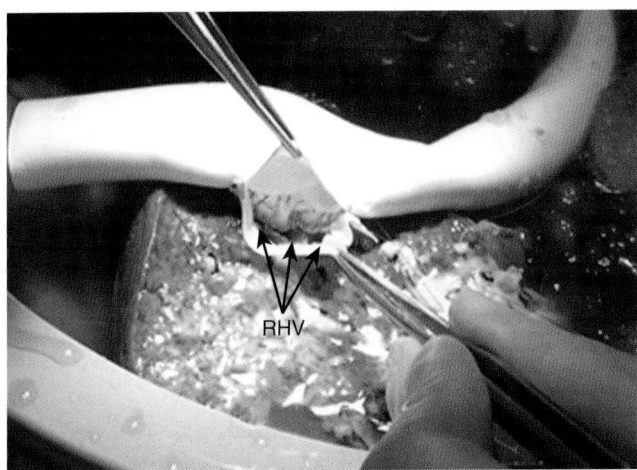

FIGURE 124.26 The liver from Figure 124.25 with the right hepatic vein branches *(RHV)* sutured to the bovine pericardium cuff, which is then reimplanted into a 20-mm Gore-Tex graft.

before reperfusion is to leave the lower cava anastomosis open until after portal reperfusion, venting the initial 300 mL or so of blood before removing the suprahepatic cava clamp.

After the infrahepatic cava anastomosis is performed, the portal limb of the bypass circuit is clamped and removed from the PV; the PV anastomosis is then performed. Next, the suprahepatic IVC clamp is removed and the liver allowed to back-perfuse through the HVs. Any major bleeding is controlled before reestablishing the portal flow. The PV clamp is removed and the liver reperfused. Any bleeding from the cut surface of the liver is controlled, and the patient is taken off veno-venous bypass.

Finally, the arterial anastomosis is performed and the liver reperfused with arterial blood; total warm ischemic time ranges from 20 to 40 minutes. After hemostasis has been achieved, the biliary anastomosis is performed. In the first few ex vivo liver

resections that we performed, our preference was to perform a Roux-en-Y choledochojejunostomy, but our more recent cases have involved duct-to-duct anastomoses (see Video: https://pie.med.utoronto.ca/TVASurg/project/exvivo_167resection/). This experience mirrors our larger experience with right lobe LDLT.

Postoperative Course

Postoperative care is similar to any major liver resection or LT. We follow a protocol of enhanced recovery. Postoperatively the patients are admitted to a step-down unit or intensive care unit as necessary. Ultrasound with Doppler assessment or a CT scan with IV contrast is performed on postoperative day 1 to assess liver blood flow. Day 1 transaminase levels in the 200 to 1000 IU/L range are standard but return to near normal in 1 week. Hyperbilirubinemia as well as coagulopathy (higher international normalized ratio [INR] levels) is common, and

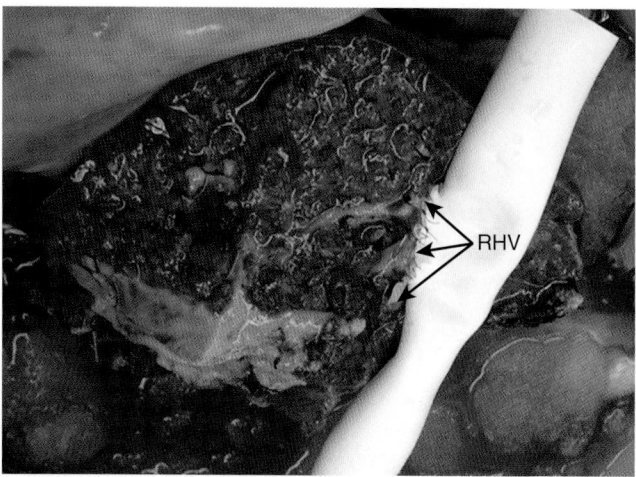

FIGURE 124.27 The liver from Figure 124.26 with back-table reconstruction completed. Note the three branches of the right hepatic vein *(RHV)*.

it seems to vary inversely with the size of the liver remnant.[19] Hyperbilirubinemia by itself is not concerning, if other markers of liver function are improving.

An early sign that the autograft is functioning is the return of lactate levels to baseline in the first 12 to 24 hours after surgery. Maintenance of coagulation parameters, in particular PT or INR, suggests recovery of liver function. It is sometimes necessary, however, to give vitamin K and/or FFP for the first few days to maintain an INR target less than 2.[41] Hypophosphatemia can occur between postoperative days 1 and 3 as the liver regenerates, and it may be so profound as to require constant IV replacement. Without much evidence as to its effectiveness, we have used low-dose IV heparin (500 U/hr) perioperatively, and we attempt to maintain the hematocrit between 30% and 35%. Patients will receive a prophylactic dose of low-molecular-weight heparin for completion of 30 days. Additionally, patients who have artificial venous caval grafts are started on low-dose aspirin before discharge and this is maintained for life, although

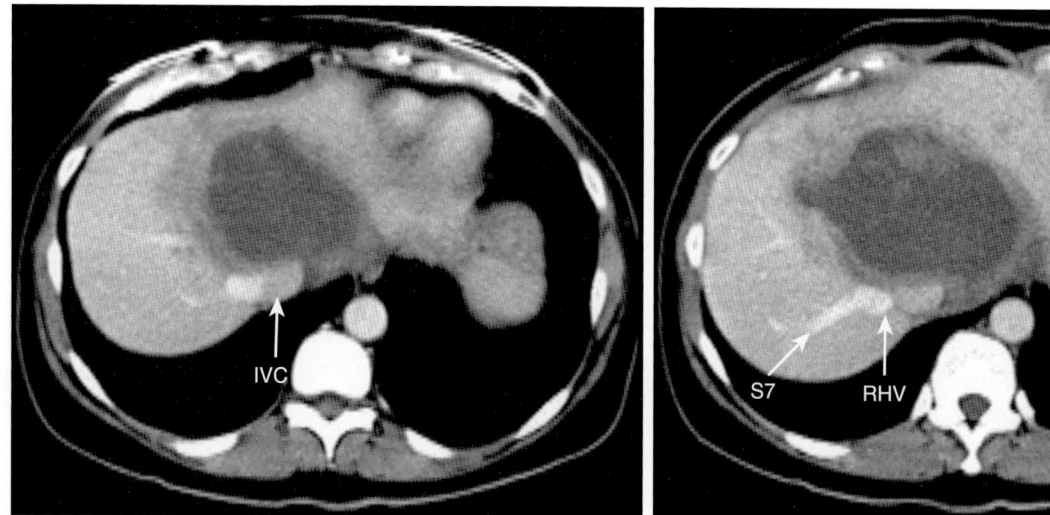

FIGURE 124.28 Computed tomographic images showing a large, centrally placed tumor. *IVC,* Inferior vena cava; *RHV,* right hepatic vein; *S7,* segment VII hepatic vein branch.

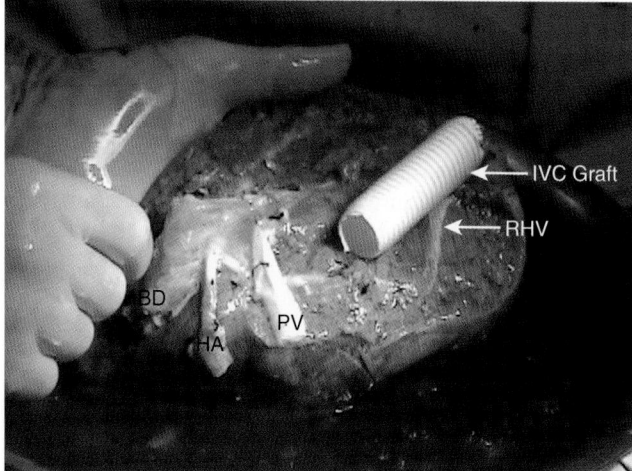

FIGURE 124.29 Ringed Gore-Tex graft has been used to reconstruct the inferior vena cava *(IVC)* on the back table for the case in Figure 124.28. *BD,* Bile duct; *HA,* hepatic artery; *PV,* portal vein; *RHV,* right hepatic vein branch.

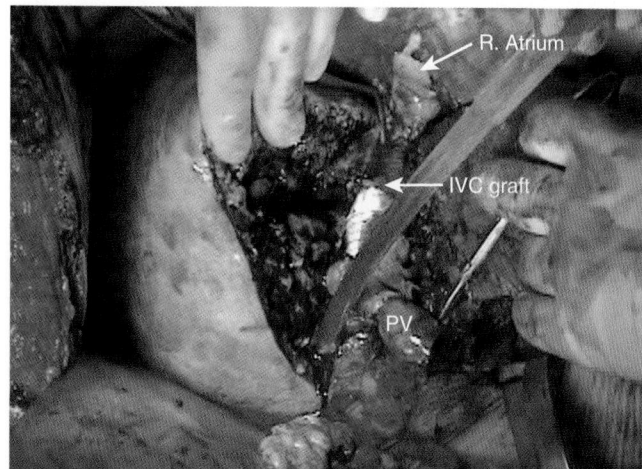

FIGURE 124.30 Case from Figure 124.29 reimplanted at time of initial perfusion through the portal vein *(PV). IVC graft,* Inferior vena cava ringed Gore-Tex graft; *R. Atrium,* right atrium.

there are no data regarding the need for long-term anticoagulation or antiplatelet medication. In our practice, all patients that undergo vascular reconstruction have postoperative imaging to rule out early thrombosis.

There are a few specific complications related to these procedures. HA or PV thrombosis and stenosis can occur and should be suspected if there is a sudden rise in liver enzymes (especially ALT) postoperatively. Ultrasound Doppler or an urgent CT angiography should be performed with low threshold. We recommend full-dose anticoagulation in case thrombosis occurs, especially more than a week from surgery. In the case of venous anastomotic stenosis, the use of balloon angioplasty or endovascular stents is highly efficient. There are few reports of compression of a Dacron IVC graft by the regenerated liver that presented as acute Budd-Chiari syndromes. In these cases, endovascular stent placement resulted in resolution of the symptoms. We have not encountered this complication in our practice; however, when we previously used Dacron IVC graft, it tended to sclerose and ultimately occlude, probably because of the relatively lower pressure in the IVC. However, that was usually asymptomatic because of collateral venous development. Currently, we use ringed PTFE grafts for that purpose and have not encountered this issue with these grafts.

Biliary strictures can happen with any duct-to-duct anastomosis and should be approached in the standard fashion with endoscopic retrograde cholangiopancreatography (ERCP)/percutaneous transhepatic cholangiogram (PTC) stent or balloon dilatation (see Chapter 42).

Graft infection is a potential complication of these procedures. Perioperative antibiotic prophylaxis is important, and avoiding an enteric opening (e.g., by performing a choledochocholedochostomy rather than a choledochoenterostomy) may reduce the risk of graft infection. However, PTFE graft-associated sepsis is rarely reported also in the LDLT when used as a graft for HV reconstruction.[42-44]

Current Role of Ex Vivo Liver Resection

The role of such an extensive procedure in advanced malignancies is open for discussion. Although about three decades have passed since Pichlmayr and colleagues described the first ex vivo liver resection, relatively few surgeons have attempted the procedure.[10] Since the last edition of this textbook about 5 years ago, there have been few additions to the literature besides small case series, although larger series have been updated.[45-48] Ex vivo resection remains an extremely rare procedure and can still be accurately described as "pushing the limits" of what can be done in liver surgery. The largest reported series from Pichlmayr's own group consists of only 22 patients.[33] A major reason for this technique not being adopted is that the two other techniques described in this chapter, in situ and ante situm hepatic hypothermic perfusion, can be applied to the great majority of difficult vascular reconstructions, with the important exception of tumors involving both hilar structures and the HV/IVC and tumors that have caused

an acute Budd-Chiari picture. Also, the ex vivo technique requires a surgeon familiar with advanced techniques in liver resection and LT, which restricts the procedure to relatively few individuals. Many patients who may be candidates for ex vivo resection are deemed unresectable by competent hepatic surgeons and are not referred. Perhaps the most compelling reason for the lack of adoption of this technique is the relatively high risk/benefit ratio. Most of the literature on ex vivo liver resections has been case reports that describe aspects of technique, and long-term follow-up is not available. Even in well-selected patients, perioperative mortality is 10% to 30%. By contrast, the perioperative 30-day mortality for patients undergoing in situ or ante situm hepatic hypothermic perfusion with vascular reconstruction is reported at 10% or less.[3,15,18,43,49] Azoulay and colleagues reported a perioperative mortality to 90 days of 19.5%, with an overall 5-year survival of 30%.[49] In a recently reported series,[50] the authors included 23 patients with hepatocellular carcinoma that underwent ante situm hepatic resection.[50] They reported a 4% 90-day mortality rate, compared with previous studies that showed a 90-day mortality rate ranging from 11% to 20%. Long-term survival after ex vivo liver resection is also poor: at best, 5-year survival for ex vivo resections performed for malignancy is 15% to 30%. In Oldhafer's series, the six patients who underwent ex vivo resection for colorectal metastases had a median survival of 21 months, although it might be expected that the general improvement in survival after resection for colorectal metastases seen over the last decade would apply to ex vivo liver resections as well.[33]

Notwithstanding the previous considerations, undoubtedly the occasional patient is cured by this aggressive procedure. One patient with resection for cholangiocarcinoma in Oldhafer's series was alive and disease free at 3.5 years after resection, whereas one of our own patients who underwent ex vivo resection for HCC was alive and disease free more than 5 years after the operation.[51] Many patients may benefit by being considered for ex vivo liver resection simply because a surgeon qualified to perform an ex vivo resection realizes that the resection can be done using a less aggressive technique, such as in situ cold perfusion or standard vascular reconstruction.

It is also true that liver surgery is constantly evolving, and what is considered questionable today may become a mainstream technique in the future. Even standard liver resection for malignancy was considered of questionable worth several decades ago. Improvements in surgical technique and perioperative care transformed liver resection for malignancy from a technique that many thought bordered on lunacy into an accepted therapy. Further advances in surgical technique, along with advances in adjuvant oncologic therapies, may do the same for ex vivo liver resection. Currently, it seems reasonable to consider highly selected patients for ex vivo liver resection on a case-by-case basis in centers with expertise in both hepatic resection and LT, particularly LDLT.

References are available at expertconsult.com.

CHAPTER 125

Techniques of liver replacement

John A. Goss, Roberto Lopez, J. Wallis Marsh, and James Pomposelli

HISTORIC OVERVIEW

The multiple steps by which liver replacement became the treatment of choice for several liver and biliary diseases were summarized in 2002.[1,2] The basic operation was developed in dogs during the years 1958 through 1960 and first attempted clinically in 1963 under azathioprine-prednisone immunosuppression. The first humans to have prolonged survival were reported in 1969.[3] However, it was not until the availability of cyclosporine in the 1980s that orthotopic liver transplantation (OLT) became accepted worldwide as effective therapy. The results improved again with the advent of tacrolimus in the 1990s.

Factors other than immunosuppression have contributed to the success of liver replacement, including improved patient selection and pretransplantation management, noninvasive diagnostic techniques, new antibiotics, and advances in anesthetic and perioperative critical care. However, perfection of the donor and recipient operations was the crucial factor on which all else ultimately depended.

The First Case

The operative report from the world's first human liver transplant is included, for the sake of historic preservation (Fig. 125.1). The operation took place in Denver, Colorado, in 1963 in a child with biliary atresia (see Chapter 40). It is apparent from the operative description that many great strides have been made in the intervening years; at the same time, it is equally apparent that in some respects, not much has changed. It should be remembered when reading this historic document that central venous access catheters and rapid infusion devices had not yet come into use.

DONOR OPERATION

The use of multiple organs from a single deceased donor became practical with the development of standard procurement methods in the early 1980s. Subsequently, the University of Wisconsin (UW) and histidine-tryptophan-ketoglutarate (HTK) preservation solutions made storage of hepatic allografts relatively safe for 12 to 18 hours. The availability of this much time has allowed widespread sharing of livers while permitting an accurate assessment of the allograft by histologic and metabolic criteria.

Standard Liver Procurement

In the standard procurement technique, a midline incision is made from the suprasternal notch to the pubis to expose the abdominal and thoracic organs of potential interest (Fig. 125.2). After verification that the liver has a normal consistency and color, the left triangular and coronary ligaments are incised, allowing the left lobe to be retracted anteriorly and to the right. This retraction exposes the upper part of the gastrohepatic

ligament, which contains the left gastric artery (LGA) and the arterial supply to the liver. If an anomalous left hepatic arterial branch originates from the LGA (Fig. 125.3), it must be preserved in continuity with the main LGA (see Fig. 125.3, *inset*). When present, this anomalous left hepatic arterial branch is almost always present just posterior to the vagus nerve branch as it courses from the lesser curvature of the stomach through the gastrohepatic ligament to the liver.

The right colon is mobilized by division of its peritoneal attachments and continues across the retroperitoneum inferiorly; the large and small bowel are then reflected superiorly and toward the left upper quadrant. Kocherization of the duodenum is performed, allowing exposure of the distal aorta and inferior vena cava (IVC). The dissection continues superiorly on the anterior surface of the aorta to the left renal vein. The superior mesenteric artery (SMA) is found immediately superior and anterior to the vein. If simultaneous pancreas retrieval is planned, the SMA is encircled with a vessel loop that can be used to stop the infusion of the perfusate to avoid hyperperfusion of the pancreas. The ligament of Treitz is identified and serves as a landmark to identify the inferior mesenteric vein (IMV), which can easily be dissected from the mesocolon in preparation for aortic cannulation.

The largest branch of the celiac axis is usually the common hepatic artery (see Chapter 2). The right gastric artery (which is small and often difficult to identify or absent) and gastroduodenal artery are ligated and divided (see Fig. 125.3). After ligation of the left gastric, right gastric, and gastroduodenal arteries, the subsequent dissection of the common bile duct (CBD) and portal vein (PV) is rendered relatively bloodless. The CBD is transected near the duodenum, and the gallbladder is incised and irrigated with saline, which avoids autolysis of the extrahepatic and intrahepatic bile duct epithelium during storage. The PV is now dissected inferiorly to the confluence of the splenic and superior mesenteric veins (Fig. 125.4).

After completing the hilar dissection, the aorta is encircled superiorly, where it passes through the diaphragm and inferiorly just proximal to its distal bifurcation. After total-body heparinization with 300 IU/kg, cannulae for infusion are placed into the IMV and distal aorta (see Fig. 125.4). When all procurement teams are ready, the aorta is cross-clamped at the diaphragm or in the chest by the abdominal surgeon (see Fig. 125.4) while the thoracic surgical team clamps the ascending aorta. Moderately rapid infusion of cold preservation solution is started into the portal circulation and aortic cannula. Congestion of the various organs is prevented by an incision in the suprahepatic IVC at the level of the right atrium, which allows the blood and perfusate to drain into the pericardium or right chest (see Fig. 125.4). The abdominal cavity is filled with ice slush while the preservation solution perfuses the abdominal organs.

In adults, the liver is usually perfused with 2 L of HTK or UW solution through the IMV (or rarely through the splenic

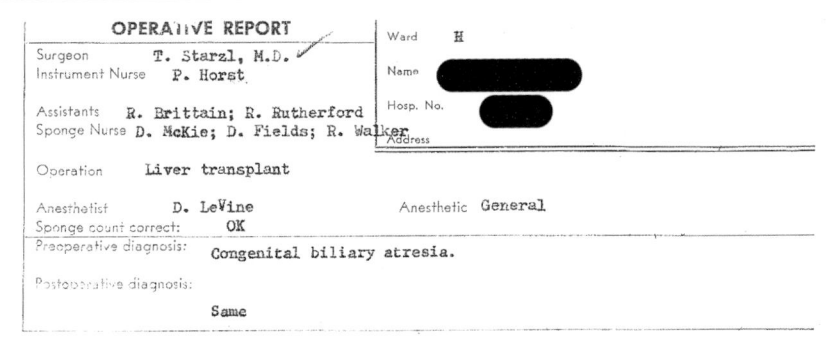

OPERATIVE REPORT

Surgeon   T. Starzl, M.D.
Instrument Nurse   P. Horst

Ward   H

Name ▬▬▬

Hosp. No. ▬▬▬

Assistants   R. Brittain; R. Rutherford
Sponge Nurse   D. McKie; D. Fields; R. Walker

Address

Operation   Liver transplant

Anesthetist   D. LeVine   Anesthetic   General
Sponge count correct: OK

Preoperative diagnosis: Congenital biliary atresia.

Postoperative diagnosis:
     Same

This three-year-old boy was born with biliary atresia and had been explored previously. At the time of the original operation, shortly after birth, no biliary ducts could be found. The child had portal hypertension and a very protuberant abdomen, and had been known to have ascites in the past. It had been planned for some time to perform a hepatic transplant/in preparation, a thymectomy was previously done by Dr. Waddell.

On the day of operation, an emergency call came from the operating room that another child, 2 years of age, had had a cardiac arrest during treatment of a malignant brain tumor. Edward Solis was then rushed to the operating room, while a team headed by Dr. Thomas L. Marchioro prepared to harvest the liver.

The child, ▬▬ was anesthetized with fluothane anesthesia and a large bore needle placed in a vein of the arm. A thoraco-abdominal incision was then made through the eighth right intercostal space and extending transversely down across the abdomen and then back up to the left costal margin. The operative wound was exceedingly difficult to keep dry during the deepening of the incision because of numerous collateral veins secondary to the portal hypertension. Upon entering the abdomen and chest it was found that a piece of ileum was tightly adherent to the liver. This was dissected off with considerable difficulty, chiefly to multiple hemorrhagic areas, both on the detached bowel and on the under surface of the liver. The portal triad was almost inaccessible at this time because of the tedious dissection necessary to reach it.

At this time, word was passed from the donor room that the pumping system for perfusion of liver had failed and that it would be necessary to act with the utmost expedience to remove the child, ▬▬ liver. The triangular ligaments were then cut and the liver removed with considerably less than pains-taking care for hemostasis. When this had been completed, the portal triad which had not previously been dissected was cut across using a Potts clamps to control all incoming structures to the liver. Potts clamps were also placed in the vena cava, above and below the liver, and the liver then removed. Just prior to doing this, a siliconized plastic shunt was placed in the femoral vein, and later on to the jugular vein in the neck to allow blood to by-pass the occluded part of the cava. Because of the presence of numerous varices, it was not necessary to do this for the portal vein. It should be mentioned that just before removing the liver, it was noticed that the needle had become disengaged from its position in the arm, and that the transfusions which had been given up to this point had all been passing out upon the table. The other jugular vein was immediately cut down and a large polyethylene tube placed in this area to allow rapid transfusion.

At any rate, the liver was then removed and the donor liver brought in from the opposite room. The upper vena caval anastomosis was then performed, using continuous 00000 arterial suture. The cuff of upper vena caval was inadequate but a satisfactory anastomosis was obtained. The lower vena caval anastomosis was next performed, and blood allowed to pass back through the liver by this route. The transected portal triad was then brought into approximation with the hepatic artery, and these structures sewed in an end-to-end fashion. Upon release of the clamps, the liver immediately assumed a good color, and despite the hectic circumstances of the transplant, it was initially thought that a good result would be obtained. However, after about 15 or 20 minutes, it was noticed that all raw surfaces were profusely bleeding. A sample was sent down to Dr. Kurt Von Kaulla, and the report came back that there were extremely high titres of fibrinolysin and low titres of fibrinogen in the submitted blood. The next 5 or 6 hours were spent in a desperate effort to control hemorrhage, using literally thousands of sutures and ties, but the hemorrhagic diathesis could never satisfactorily controlled. The child had a cardiac arrest at about 6:00 p.m. which was successfully reverted with cardiac massage and during the ensuing 2 to 3 hours, several more arrests occurred. Finally, at approximately 8:00 p.m. with the advent of the final cardiac arrest, the child was pronounced dead.

Thomas E. Starzl, M.D.

FIGURE 125.1 Facsimile of the world's first human liver transplant performed in Denver, Colorado, in 1963.

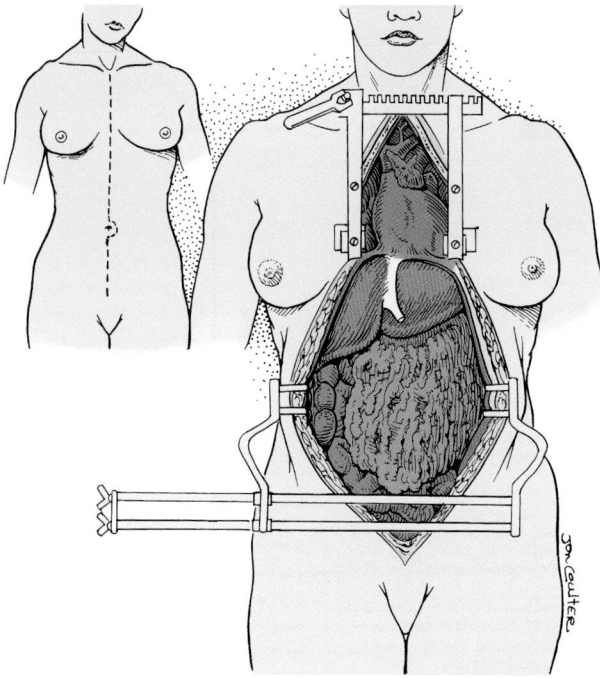

FIGURE 125.2 Exposure for multiple organ retrieval in the deceased donor.

vein if the IMV is too difficult to cannulate); either 8 L of HTK or 3 L of UW solution are infused through the aorta (smaller volumes for children). Alternatively, 8 L of HTK or 3 L of UW solution can be infused solely through the aorta. (The perfusion can also be done solely through the aorta if the portal venous system cannot be cannulated.) Once the liver has been removed from the abdominal cavity, the PV is flushed in an expedited

manner with 2 L of HTK or 1 L of UW solution or until the effluent is clear. When the liver becomes cold and blanched and the heart and lungs have been removed, the hepatectomy is completed. The remaining dissection must be performed expeditiously but methodically. If the celiac axis is to be retained with the allograft, a proximal segment of its splenic arterial branch should also be conserved for potential reconstruction of an anomalous hepatic artery (see later in this chapter).

The most common hepatic artery anomaly is an aberrant right hepatic artery (RHA) originating from the SMA, usually within its first 2 cm, traveling posterior to the PV (Fig. 125.5) (see Chapter 2). If the pancreas is to be discarded, the anomalous retroportal artery can be kept in continuity with the SMA and excised from the aorta (see Fig. 125.5, *inset*); its origin can be incorporated into a Carrel patch shared with the origin of the celiac axis. If the pancreas is being procured, the accessory RHA can be divided to the right of the duodenum and reimplanted into the gastroduodenal or splenic artery stump on the back table.

The liver now remains attached primarily by the vena cava above and below the liver. The vena cava below the liver is transected above the entry of the renal veins (Fig. 125.6). The vena cava above the liver is transected with a surrounding rim of diaphragm that will be excised on the back table. The retrohepatic IVC is dissected free from the attached tissues, including ligation of the right adrenal vein and posterior lumbar tributaries. (These steps can also be done on the back table.) Once the cross-clamp is applied, the retrohepatic IVC can be retrieved in continuity with the liver and surrounding tissue, including the superior half of the right adrenal gland. The liberated liver is immediately placed in a bag filled with chilled preservation solution and surrounded by an outer second bag, all packed in ice (Fig. 125.7); the CBD is flushed with HTK or UW preservation solution before packaging the liver.

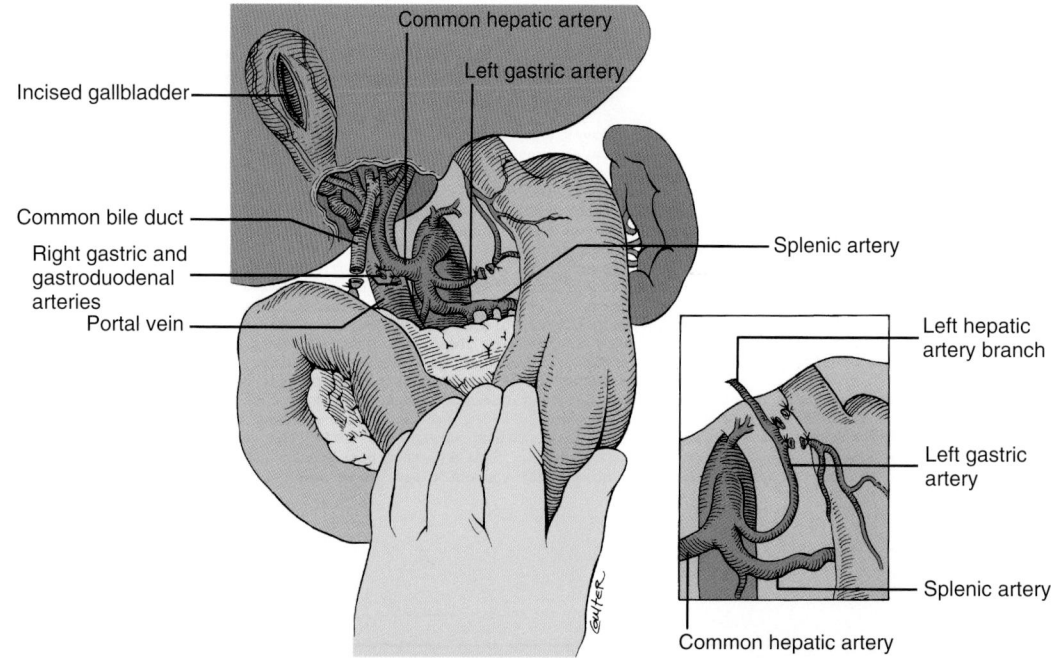

FIGURE 125.3 Normal hepatic arterial anatomy (see Chapter 2). The liver arterial supply shown here is entirely from the common hepatic artery. *Inset,* A common anomaly in which all or part of the left hepatic lobe arterial supply is from the left gastric branch of the celiac axis. The anomalous branch must be preserved. During the hilar dissection, the common duct is divided distally, and the gallbladder is incised to flush the biliary tree.

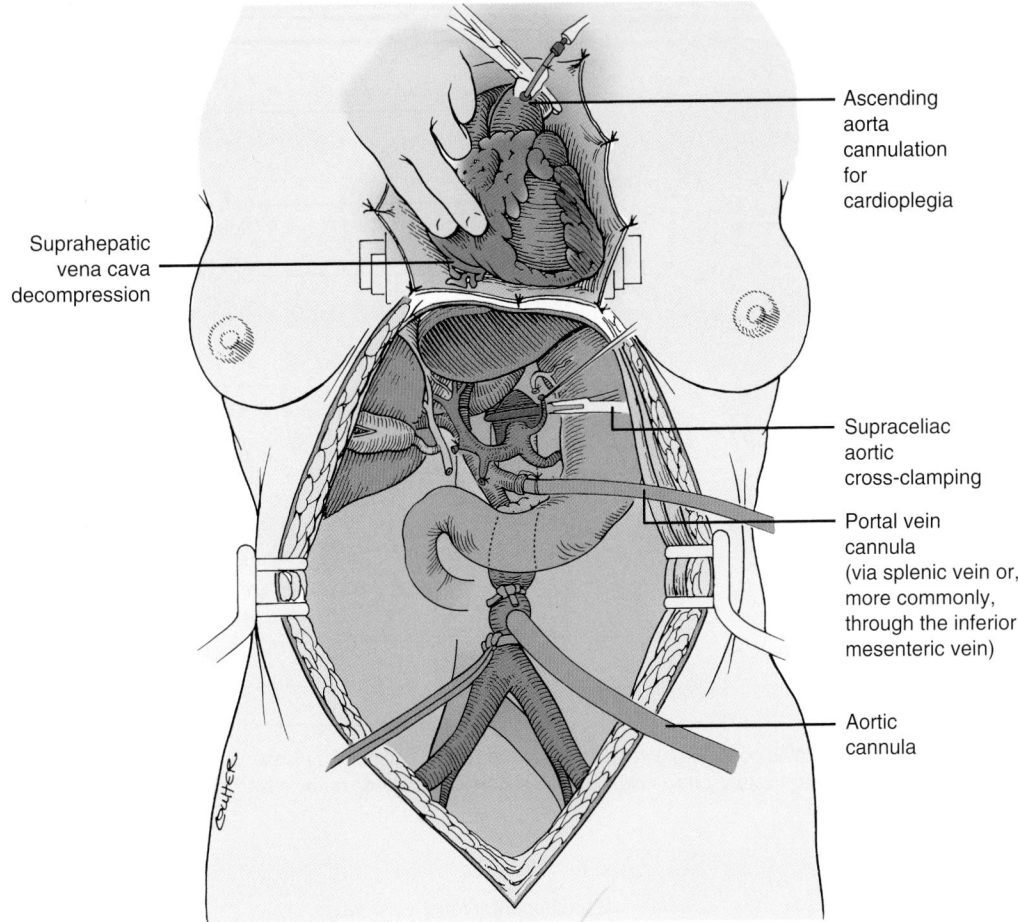

FIGURE 125.4 In situ perfusion technique used when the heart, kidneys, liver, and other viscera are removed from the same donor. University of Wisconsin (UW) or histidine-tryptophan-ketoglutarate (HTK) preservation solution is infused into the inferior mesenteric vein or splenic vein and distal aorta with simultaneous venting of the suprahepatic inferior vena cava into the pericardium. Note the aortic cross-clamp above the celiac axis. The cannulation and cross-clamping of the thoracic aorta for infusion of a cardioplegia solution also are shown (see Chapter 109).

Rapid Procurement

Use of the standard technique in stable donors has allowed the training of relatively inexperienced surgeons in the performance of a donor hepatectomy. When the technique is mastered, faster methods can be applied electively or, if required, by urgent clinical circumstances. With the rapid techniques, little or no preliminary dissection is done except for encirclement of the supraceliac aorta and cannulation of the IMV (or, rarely, the splenic vein) and terminal aorta (Fig. 125.8). If the heart and/or lungs are to be removed, the cardiothoracic surgeon proceeds as if other organs are not to be harvested but gives warning before the circulation is stopped.

At the moment the cardiothoracic surgeon is ready to cross-clamp the thoracic aorta, the supradiaphragmatic IVC should be vented. The abdominal aorta is cross-clamped above or just below the diaphragm, and an infusion of cold preservation solution is infused through the IMV and distal aorta (see Fig. 125.8). The amount of preservation fluid with the rapid technique is approximately the same as that used for the standard method (see earlier discussion). Again, as an alternative, the liver can be flushed only through the aorta and then flushed through the PV ex situ as previously described. When the liver becomes cold, the infusions are slowed. In the

now bloodless field, the main vessels of the celiac axis can be quickly dissected, and the hilar dissection can be completed in a matter of minutes.

The PV is cleaned inferiorly to the junction of the splenic and superior mesenteric veins, and these two tributaries are divided. As in the standard method, the surgeon must promptly exclude the possibility of a retroportal RHA originating from the SMA, as well as other arterial vascular anomalies (see Chapter 2). The hepatectomy is then completed. The kidneys, which are excised only after the liver has been removed from the field, are kept cold throughout by the placement of ice slush into the abdomen and by the slow, continuous intraaortic infusion of the preservation solution. By performing all dissections in the bloodless field, it is possible to remove multiple organs (heart, liver, pancreas, and both kidneys) in approximately one-half hour. Procurement of the intestine adds only a few additional minutes.

Super-Rapid Procurement

In an arrested donor or donation after cardiac death (DCD), an even quicker procedure can be used to procure satisfactory organs (see Chapter 109). This method can also be applied in countries that do not have "brain death" laws or under special

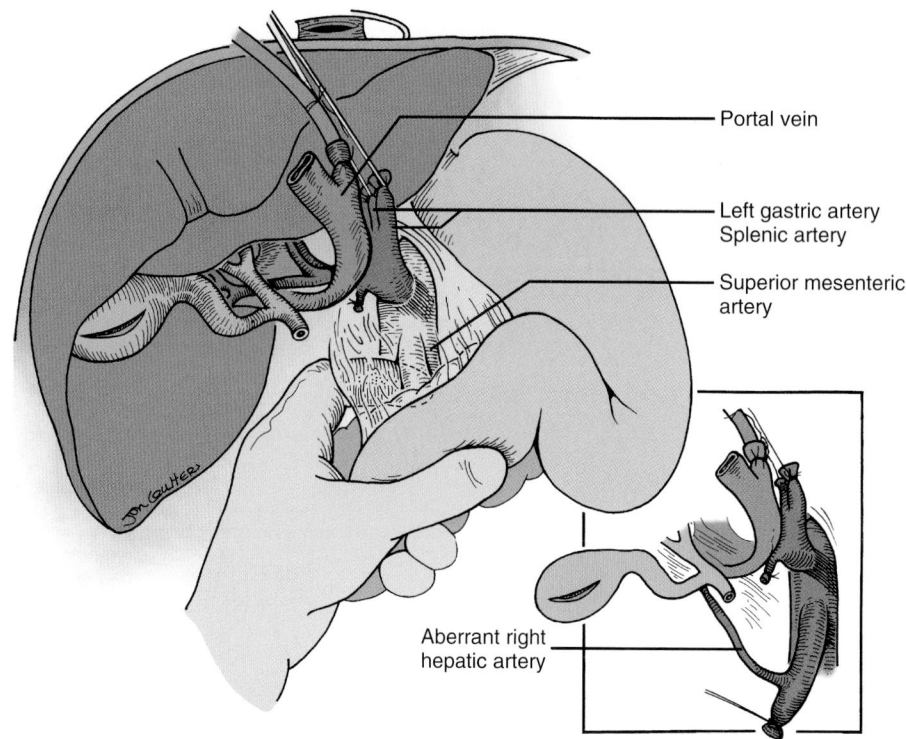

Portal vein

Left gastric artery
Splenic artery

Superior mesenteric
artery

Aberrant right
hepatic artery

FIGURE 125.5   Retraction of the liver and its portal structures to the right and performance of a Kocher maneuver free up the duodenum and head of the pancreas. An anomalous right hepatic artery, originating from the superior mesenteric artery *(inset)* just posterior to the portal vein, is sought and can be palpated behind the portal vein.

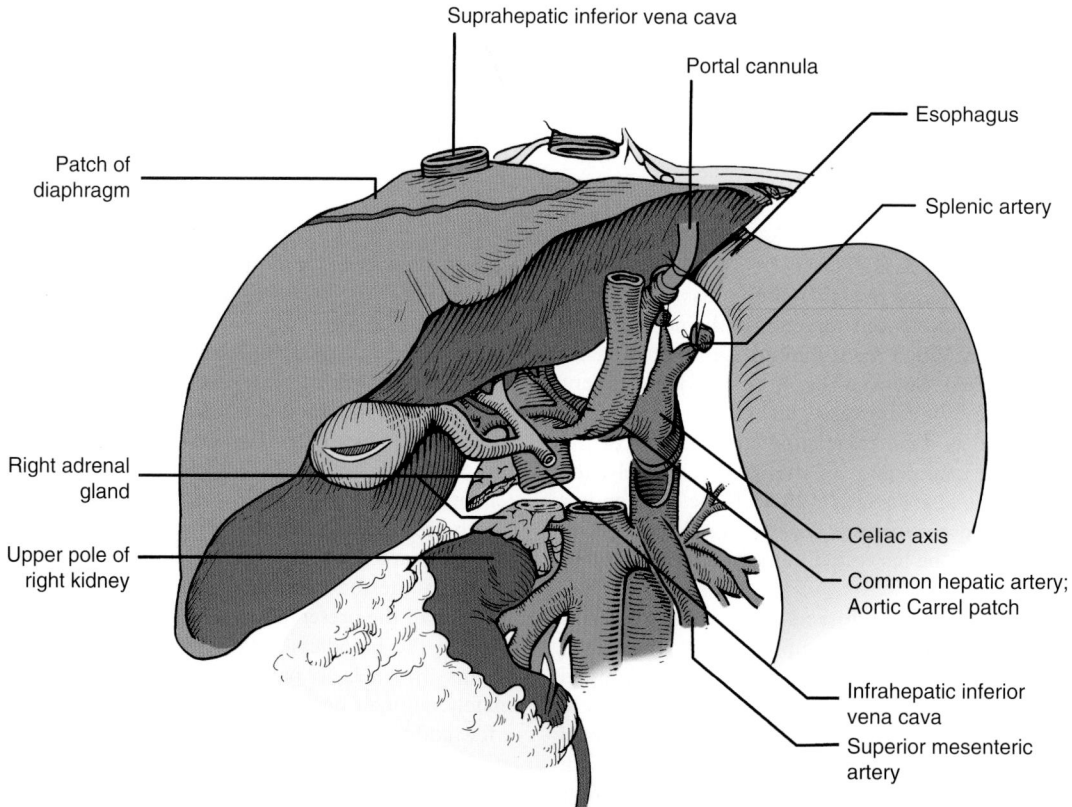

Suprahepatic inferior vena cava

Portal cannula

Esophagus

Patch of
diaphragm

Splenic artery

Right adrenal
gland

Upper pole of
right kidney

Celiac axis

Common hepatic artery;
Aortic Carrel patch

Infrahepatic inferior
vena cava

Superior mesenteric
artery

FIGURE 125.6   The suprahepatic vena cava has been transected, with inclusion of a generous patch of diaphragm on the liver side. The infrahepatic vena cava is divided just above the origin of the renal veins, and the celiac axis is removed with a Carrel patch of anterior aorta. If an anomalous right hepatic artery originates from the superior mesenteric artery (SMA), the origin of the SMA may be included in the Carrel patch (see also Fig. 125.10A).

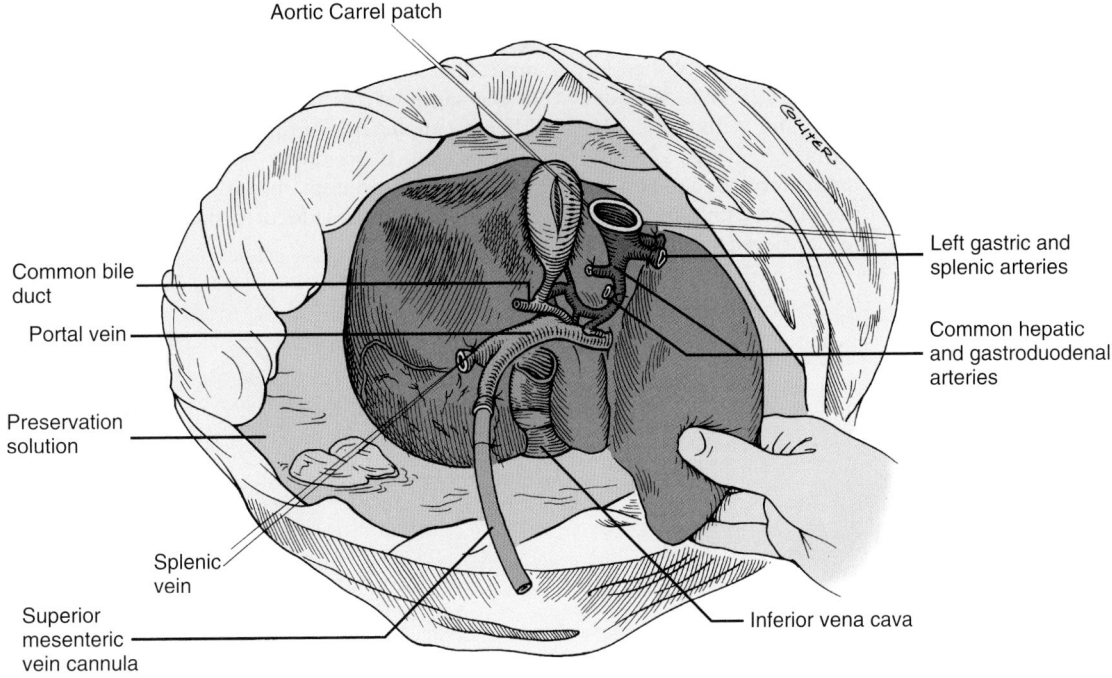

Aortic Carrel patch

Common bile duct

Portal vein

Preservation solution

Splenic vein

Superior mesenteric vein cannula

Left gastric and splenic arteries

Common hepatic and gastroduodenal arteries

Inferior vena cava

FIGURE 125.7 The liver allograft is placed in a basin containing iced preservation solution for back-table preparation. The vascular cuffs are debrided of excess tissue, and any needed arterial reconstruction is performed (see also Fig. 125.10).

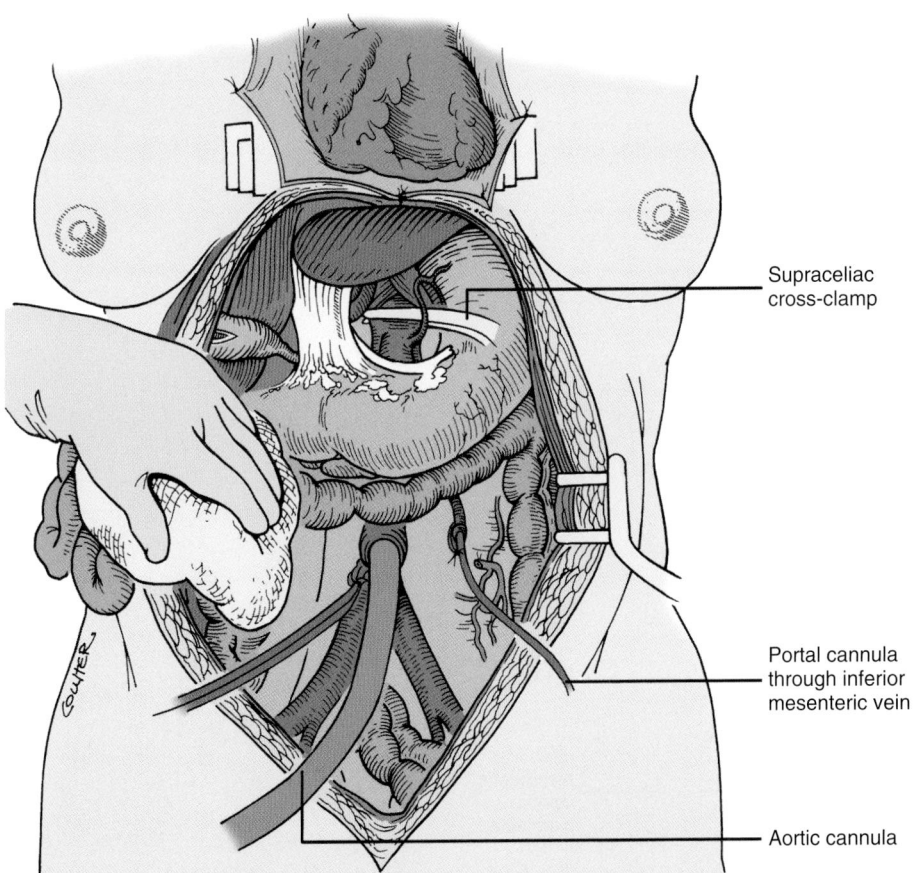

Supraceliac cross-clamp

Portal cannula through inferior mesenteric vein

Aortic cannula

FIGURE 125.8 Rapid technique of organ retrieval in which the initial dissection is limited to the exposure needed for the insertion of perfusion cannulae in the inferior mesenteric vein and distal aorta. If only the abdominal organs are to be used, the aorta can be cross-clamped above or below the diaphragm.

legal or religious circumstances. Here, cooling requires urgent cannulation and cold-fluid infusion into the distal aorta; with practice, cannulation of the IMV can also be accomplished for a simultaneous in situ portal flush (Fig. 125.9A). Sternum splitting, thoracic aortic cross-clamping, and venting the IVC for venous decompression are performed (see Fig. 125.9B); quick clamping of the root of the mesentery should be performed to direct the perfusate to the celiac trunk and renal systems if the pancreas has not been retrieved. Cannulation

and perfusion of the portal venous system can be deferred until after the various organs are at least partially cooled intra-arterially (see Fig. 125.9C). The various dissections are done in the same way as with the standard and rapid techniques. Effective application of this method requires an extremely high level of skill. If the donor hospital's DCD protocol does not allow for intravenous heparinization before procurement, the heparin can be added to the initial bags of preservation solution.

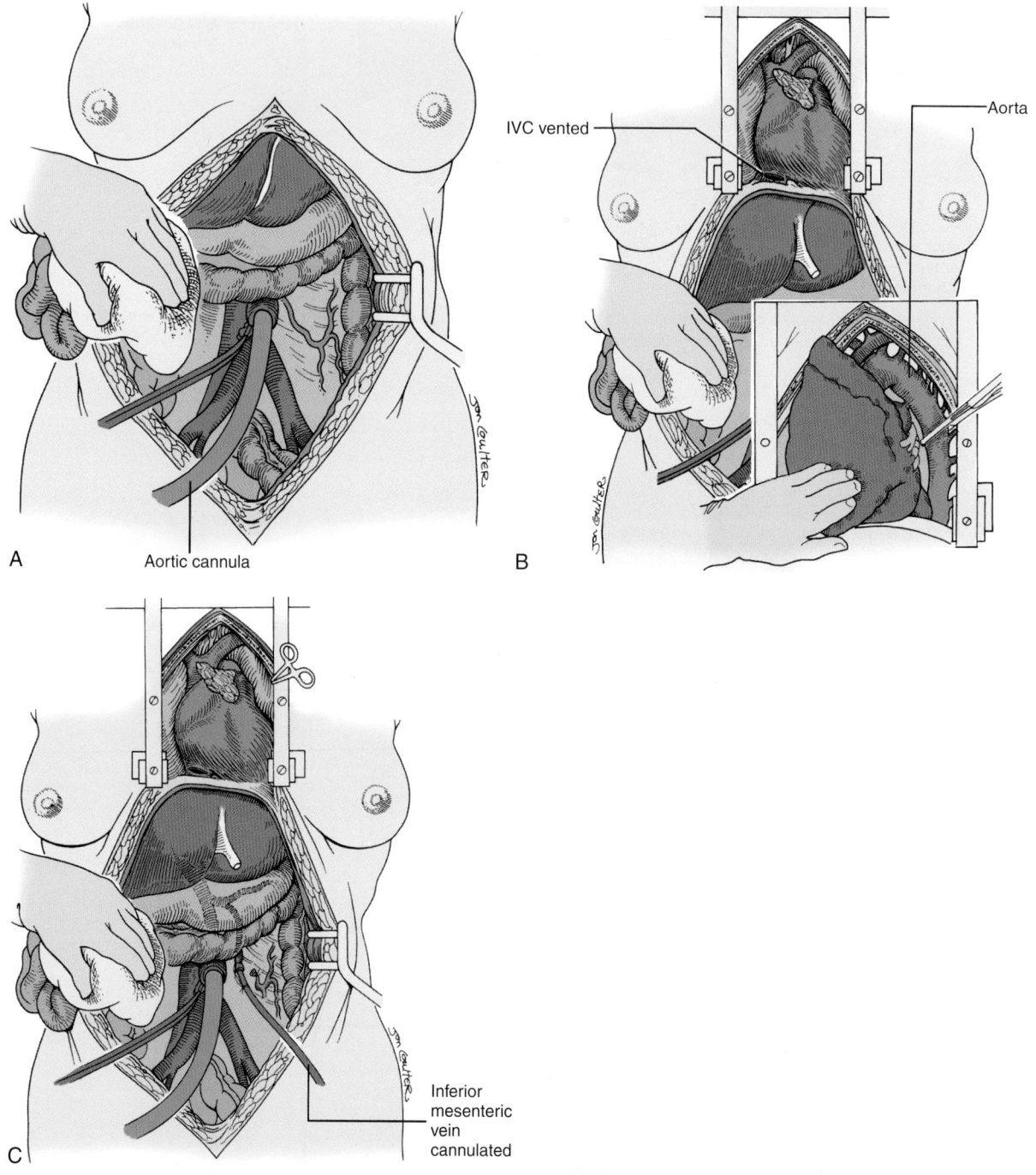

FIGURE 125.9   The super-rapid technique used for unstable donors for whom time is insufficient for exposure; placement of perfusion cannulae is shown. **A,** Midline abdominal incision is used to cannulate the aorta and begin infusion. **B,** The sternum is split to expose the pericardium and thoracic aorta. The suprahepatic inferior vena cava *(IVC)* is incised and vented into the chest, and the descending thoracic aorta is cross-clamped *(inset).* **C,** The inferior mesenteric vein is cannulated and perfused only after steps **A** and **B** are completed.

Back-Table Surgery

No matter which procurement method has been used, further preparation of the liver is performed on the back table before delivering it to the recipient surgeon. The liver should be kept cold by submerging it in a basin containing ice-cold preservation solution surrounded by an outer bag containing sterile ice slush (see Fig. 125.7). Back-table preparation includes the following:

1. Dissection and removal of extraneous tissue (diaphragm, adrenal gland, lymph node, pancreatic, peripancreatic, and ganglionic tissue)
2. Preparation of cuffs of the suprahepatic and infrahepatic vena cava, cleaning of the PV and hepatic artery, and inspection of the bile duct
3. Verification of secure ligatures on small retrohepatic caval, PV, and hepatic arterial branches
4. Ensuring the continuity and integrity of all major structures that must be anastomosed to the companion recipient structures

Failure to have the liver completely ready for implantation can result in irreversible damage or make it impossible to complete the recipient operation. Several methods of back-table vascular reconstruction have been designed to repair technical accidents or to accommodate aberrant vessels or congenital anomalies. A common reason for back-table reconstruction is the presence of an anomalous RHA originating from the SMA (Fig. 125.10).

Liver, Pancreas, and Intestine Procurement From the Same Donor

The pancreas and intestine can be retrieved independently or together with the liver. Before starting the procurement, the operation should be discussed among all surgeons involved. Considerations include organ priority, type and amount of preservation solution to be used, presence of aberrant hepatic arteries, length of PV, and a decision about which organ retains the celiac axis or SMA (see Chapter 126).

An important step in any deceased-donor operation is the removal and storage of long segments of the donor iliac arteries and veins, as well as other arteries and veins. These vessels can be used as vascular conduits to reconstruct the blood supply of the individual organs. With increased experience, it is rare to see any of the abdominal visceral organs discarded for purely technical reasons.

RECIPIENT OPERATION

The recipient procedure has three phases, which may be long and physically demanding. The first phase involves removal of the native liver, almost always in the face of portal hypertension (see Chapters 74 and 79). The second phase is the anhepatic phase, which involves the vascular anastomoses and implantation of the donor liver allograft. The third phase requires the achievement of hemostasis and biliary reconstruction.

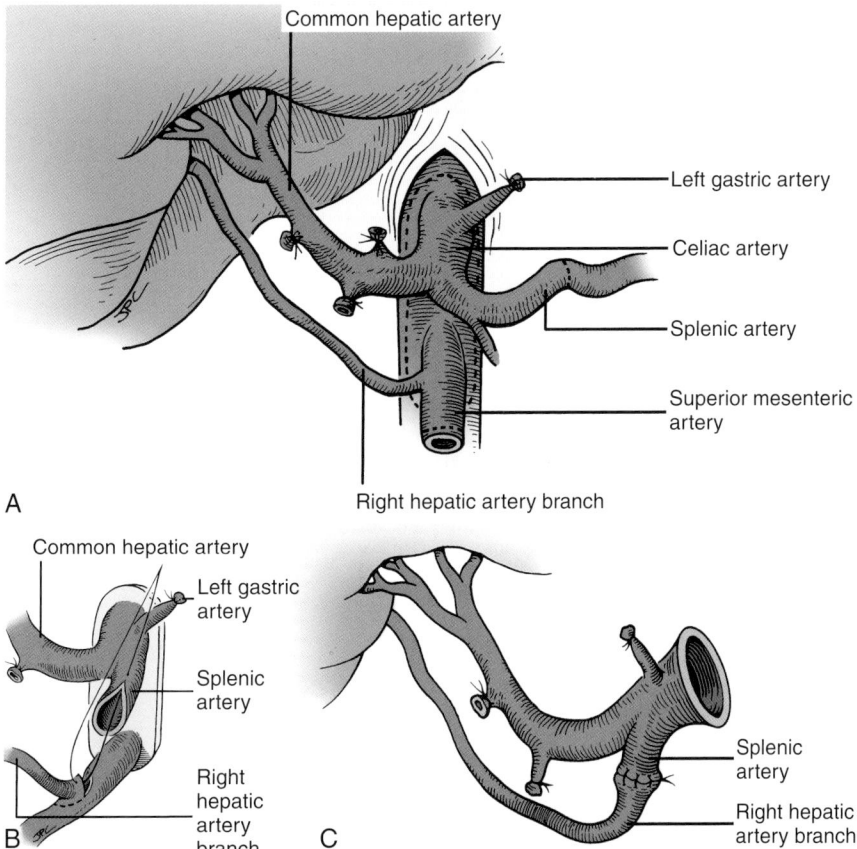

FIGURE 125.10 Examples of reconstruction of an anomalous arterial supply to the liver. **A,** The origins of the celiac axis and superior mesenteric artery are removed from the anterior aorta in a common Carrel patch. **B** and **C,** An anomalous right hepatic artery is anastomosed to the allograft splenic artery, leaving only the origin of the celiac axis for anastomosis in the recipient (see Chapter 2).

Abdominal Incision and Exposure

The exact location of the incision may be influenced by previous right upper quadrant and abdominal surgery. A bilateral subcostal incision is most often used, extending on the right to just beyond the midaxillary line and on the left to the lateral edge of the rectus muscle, with an upper midline extension and excision of the xiphoid process (Fig. 125.11). If exposure of the distal aorta is required for reconstruction of the hepatic arterial supply, the subcostal components can be extended (thoracic extensions are rarely needed). The upper midline extension is usually unnecessary in pediatric patients. Massive hepatomegaly, extensive prior abdominal surgery, or other factors may mandate the selection of a more extensive incision. In patients who require concomitant splenectomy or interruption of a prior splenorenal shunt, the incision may need to be extended to the left subcostal region.

Intraoperative Determination of Surgical Strategy

There is no single best way to carry out OLT. When exposure has been obtained, it is important to assess the intraabdominal pathology and decide on the technical approach that best fits the circumstances. A surgeon who insists on following the same

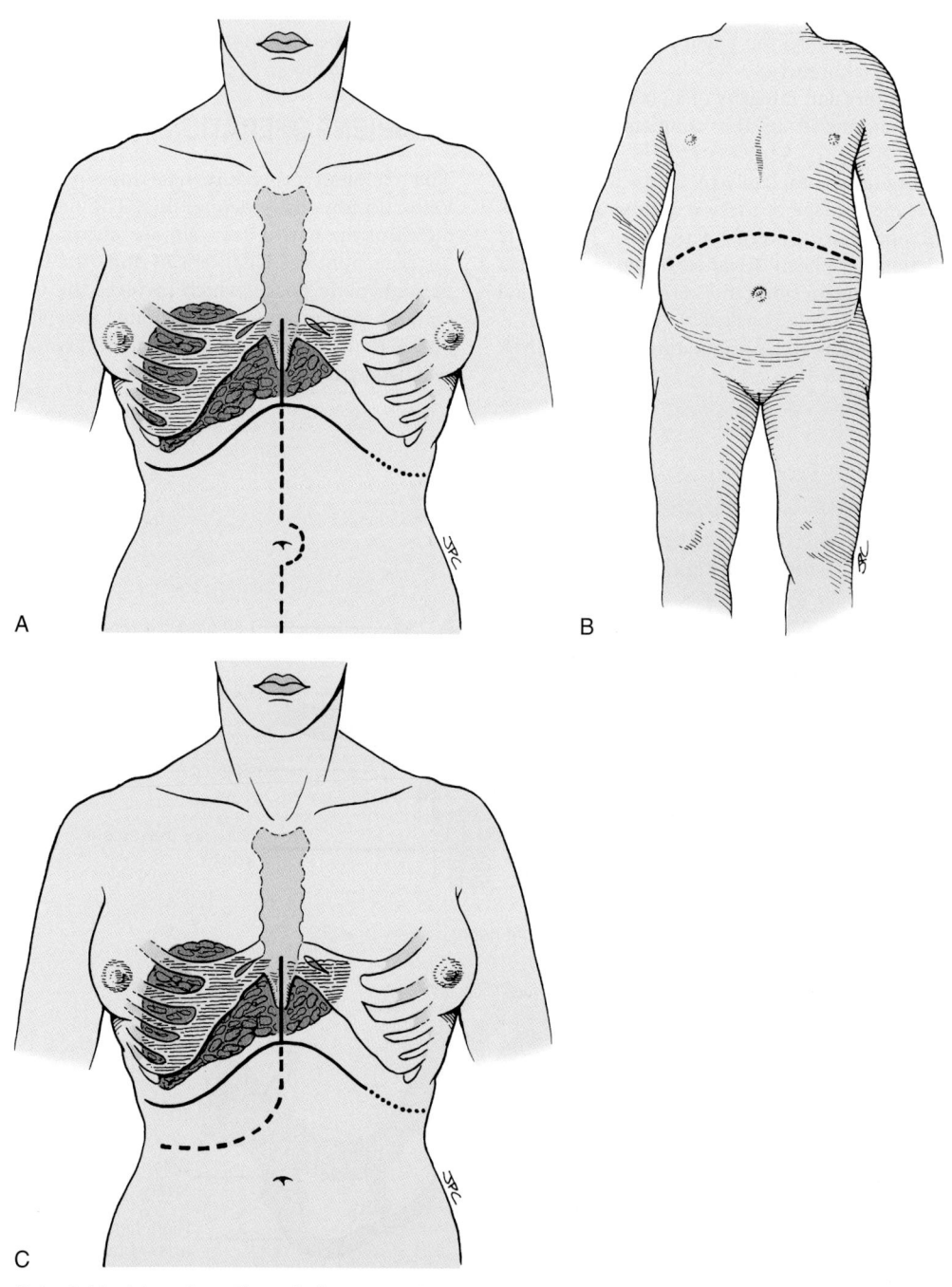

FIGURE 125.11   Potential incisions for orthotopic liver transplantation. A, Bilateral subcostal incision with potential superior or inferior extensions. **B,** Inverted half-moon incision sometimes used in infants and small children. **C,** Simple subcostal incision that may be converted to a hockeystick incision by an upper midline extension, which may include xyphoid resection.

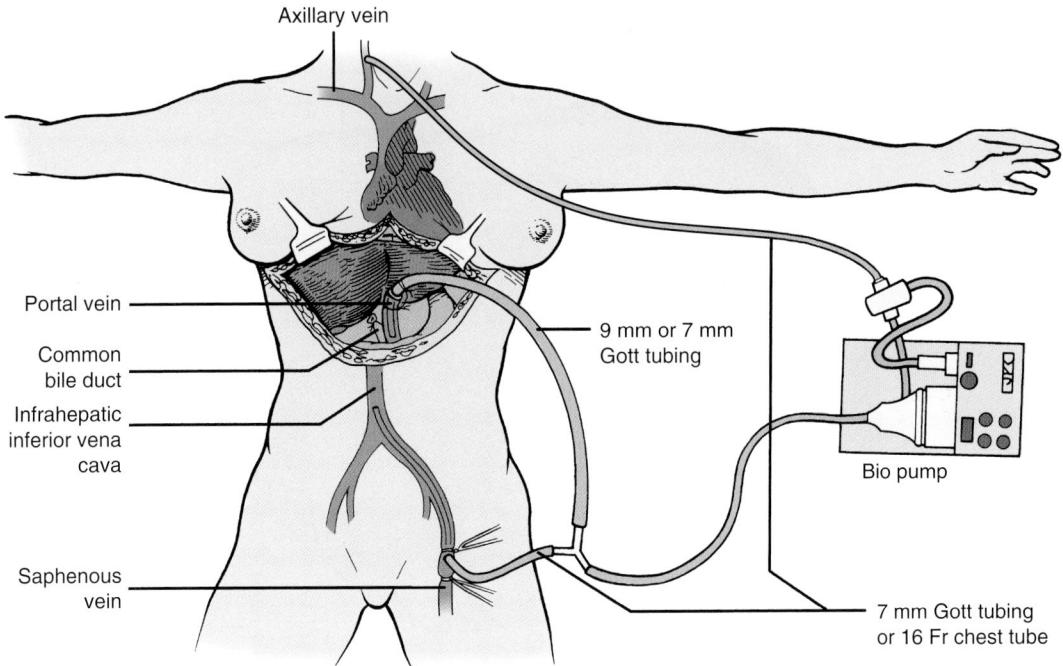

FIGURE 125.12 Pump-driven venovenous bypass used to decompress the systemic and splanchnic venous beds during the anhepatic phase of liver transplantation. The groin and venous return cannulae, when used, are usually placed percutaneously in the left groin and right neck.

steps in unvarying order for all liver recipients will experience unnecessary hardship. The following is a description of the basic components of the recipient operation, with particular emphasis on variations of host hepatectomy.

When the abdomen is entered, no matter how dense the adhesions, an effort should be made to find a plane of dissection just outside the liver capsule, because, although easier and faster, subcapsular dissection can result in disastrous hemorrhage. This is especially true in retransplantation where vascularized adhesions can cause massive bleeding.

Hilar Dissection

Following adhesiolysis and initial mobilization of the native liver, the hepatogastric and hepatoduodenal ligaments are dissected and skeletonized. If a replaced or accessory left hepatic artery is present, it is ligated. The hepatoduodenal ligament is dissected, and the right and left hepatic arteries and cystic and common hepatic ducts are ligated as close to the liver as possible to retain length. The PV is then skeletonized at the level of the bifurcation, and this skeletonization is then carried proximally until a sufficient length is obtained to allow safe clamping. Branches encountered during this skeletonization require ligation. This dissection can be complicated by previous biliary surgery and/or PV thrombosis. If needed, venovenous bypass can be initiated with cannulation of the PV at this time or later (see Chapter 2).

Venovenous Bypass

The most critical stage of the recipient operation is the native hepatectomy and anhepatic phase, during which time the diseased liver is removed and replaced with the allograft. Clamping of the PV and IVC during this period results in splanchnic and lower body systemic venous hypertension. This can lead to increased blood loss, hemodynamic instability, and posttransplant renal insufficiency (particularly in adults). Therefore a

pump-driven venovenous bypass system, used without recipient heparinization, was refined at the University of Pittsburgh to allow splanchnic and systemic blood to return to the heart by way of an inflow cannula placed in the axillary vein (Fig. 125.12).[4–7] This technique permitted the native hepatectomy and implantation of the donor liver to be performed with significant reductions in blood loss, intestinal edema, and postoperative renal failure.

Infants and children weighing less than 15 kg tolerate venous occlusion reasonably well. Currently in adults, experienced surgeons use bypass selectively. When necessary, the cannulae are often placed percutaneously in the femoral and internal jugular veins, thereby obviating the need for cutdowns as previously required. If bypass is not routine, the decision for or against its use should be made as early as possible. The decision can be aided by test occlusion of the IVC and PV. If the test is conducted after preliminary dissection of the portal triad and after the triangular and coronary ligaments are divided, it is also possible to evaluate the extent to which bleeding from raw surfaces can be anticipated without bypass. Alternatively, a temporary end-to-side portocaval shunt can be constructed to prevent mesenteric congestion. The shunt can be created by using a small segment of donor iliac vein or Gore-Tex to retain the full length of the recipient PV and for ease of creating the shunt. The portocaval shunt should be placed on the IVC as inferiorly as possible so that its location does not interfere with placement of the vena caval clamp.

Host Hepatectomy With or Without Vena Cava Removal

Once the hilar dissection has been completed the liver is devascularized and now can be excluded from the circulation by cross-clamping the vena cava or hepatic veins above and vena cava below the liver (Fig. 125.13A). The diseased allograft with or without a segment of retrohepatic IVC can be "peeled" out, working from the hilum up or from the diaphragm down. If the

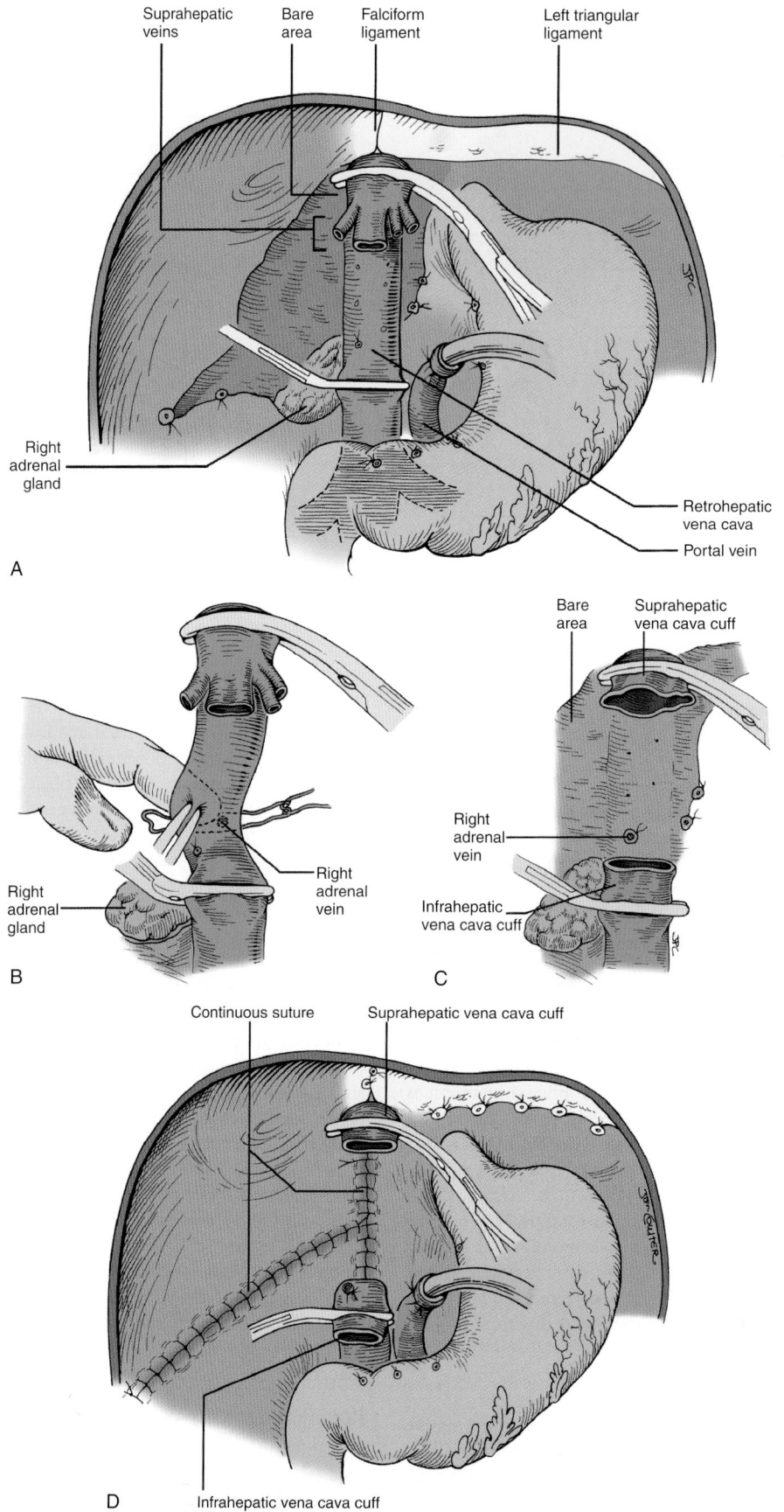

FIGURE 125.13   **Completed recipient hepatectomy on venovenous bypass. A,** With preservation of host retrohepatic vena cava. Note the hepatic vein cuffs. **B,** as in **A,** but with an injury to the right adrenal vein, which is being ligated. **C,** The retrohepatic vena cava has been included in the hepatectomy, necessitating ligation of its tributary lumbar veins and the right adrenal vein. **D,** Closure of the bare area to provide hemostasis. Bleeding from the bare area is more severe if the retrohepatic cava is removed or thrombosed because of the loss of venous drainage.

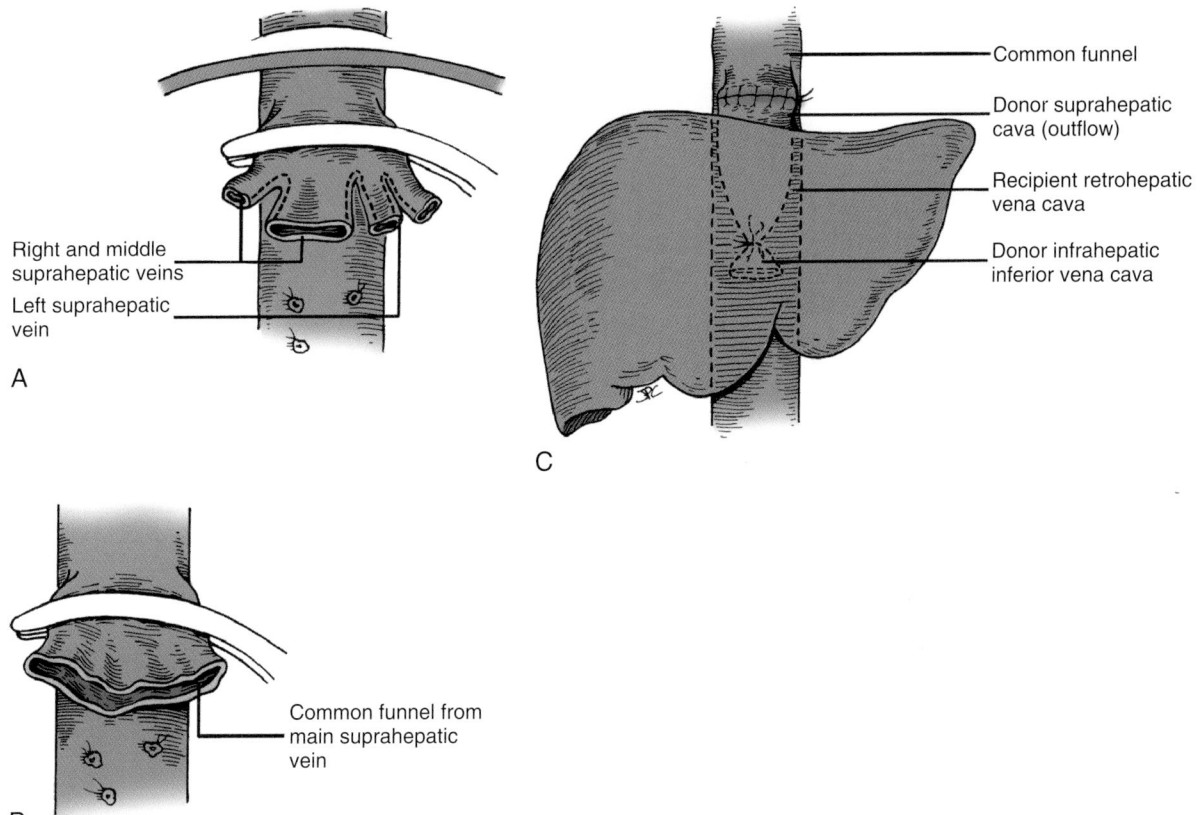

FIGURE 125.14 The piggyback method of allograft implantation with a conserved retrohepatic vena cava. **A** and **B,** Creation of an outflow cloaca from two or more hepatic veins. **C,** Completed anastomosis between the host hepatic veins and the suprahepatic vena cava of the allograft. The inferior end of the allograft vena cava is ligated.

IVC is part of the specimen, this requires an obligatory ligation of the right adrenal vein (see Fig. 125.13B and C). Other systemic venous tributaries to the IVC must be also be ligated. Because of regional venous hypertension in the right-sided bare area, it may be necessary to obtain hemostasis by suturing the bleeding areas, closing or oversewing the edges of the exposed bare areas with a continuous suture, or using such devices as the LigaSure (Covidien, Mansfield, MA) or the monopolar or bipolar sealer (see Fig. 125.13D).

Many of the problems encountered with inferior vena caval clamping can be circumvented if the host retrohepatic IVC is preserved (Fig. 125.14). Separation of the diseased liver from the IVC is performed, retaining the stumps of one or more of the host hepatic veins (see Fig. 125.14A) for eventual receipt of the allograft's venous outflow (see Fig. 125.14B and C); this is known as the *piggyback method* of liver transplantation.[8] Maintaining IVC flow during the anhepatic phase of the transplant can help ensure hemodynamic stability and eliminate the need for venovenous bypass. In addition, the extent and depth of the retroperitoneal dissection are reduced.

The piggyback method is by far the most common currently used method and can be performed with or without venovenous bypass. The procedure is easier to perform on bypass because the liver can be much more easily rotated and retracted superiorly when the hilar structures are no longer in continuity. However, placing the patient on bypass obviates one of the main reasons to perform the piggyback procedure—avoiding venovenous bypass.

The piggyback method requires nothing more than dividing the short hepatic veins in the retrohepatic space from the caudate lobe inferiorly to the main hepatic veins superiorly. Surprisingly, the number and size of short hepatic veins can vary tremendously (see Chapter 2). Two of the most challenging components of the piggyback procedure are dividing the often hypertrophied caudate lobe superiorly where typically it completely surrounds and envelops the vena cava just below the major hepatic veins and isolation and division of an accessory right hepatic vein. Occasionally, a large vein may be within the left side of the caudate, draining directly into the IVC. If a plane can be developed between the caudate and IVC, it is safest to divide these veins and the caudate with a vascular stapler.

Alternative Approaches to Hepatectomy

In many cases, hepatectomy with or without inclusion of the retrohepatic IVC is uncomplicated; however, dissection of the liver hilum is sometimes difficult or impossible because of scarring or the presence of varices. In these situations, the suprahepatic IVC can be approached first. After transecting the suprahepatic IVC, removal of the liver can be done from the top down, approaching the hilar structures from the posterior surface of the liver (Fig. 125.15). If it is not possible to clamp the hepatic veins on the liver side, bleeding can be minimized by placing the fingers into the hepatic veins and retrohepatic IVC or by squeezing shut the venous outflow of the liver.

Alternatively, the IVC below the liver can be used as a "handle" to extract the liver from bottom to top, with cross-clamping or

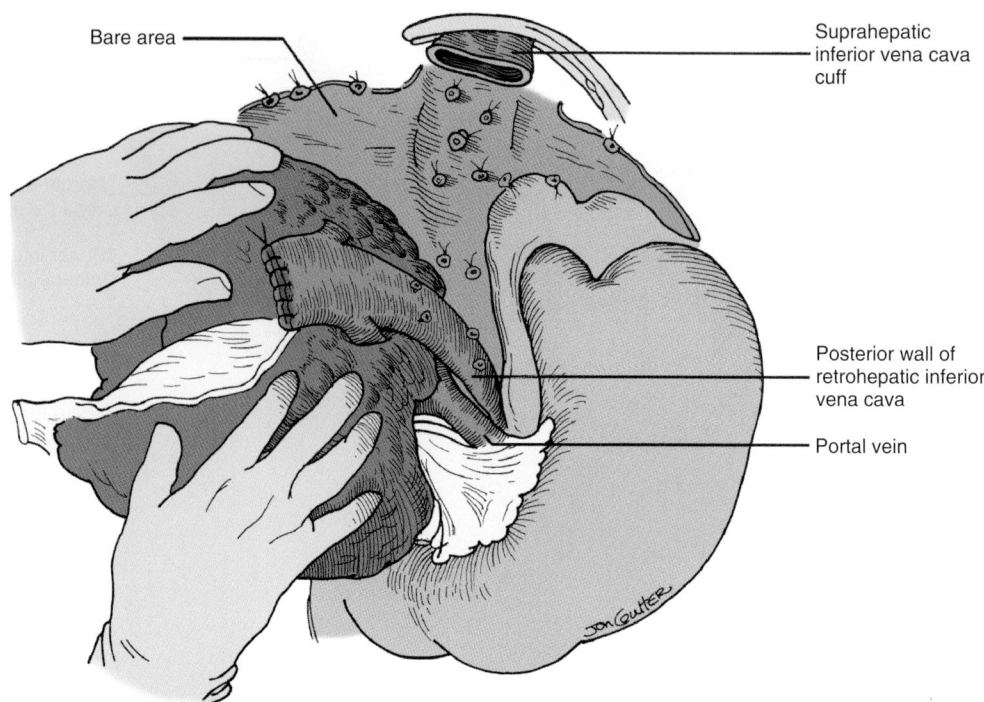

FIGURE 125.15 Removal of the recipient liver from top down.

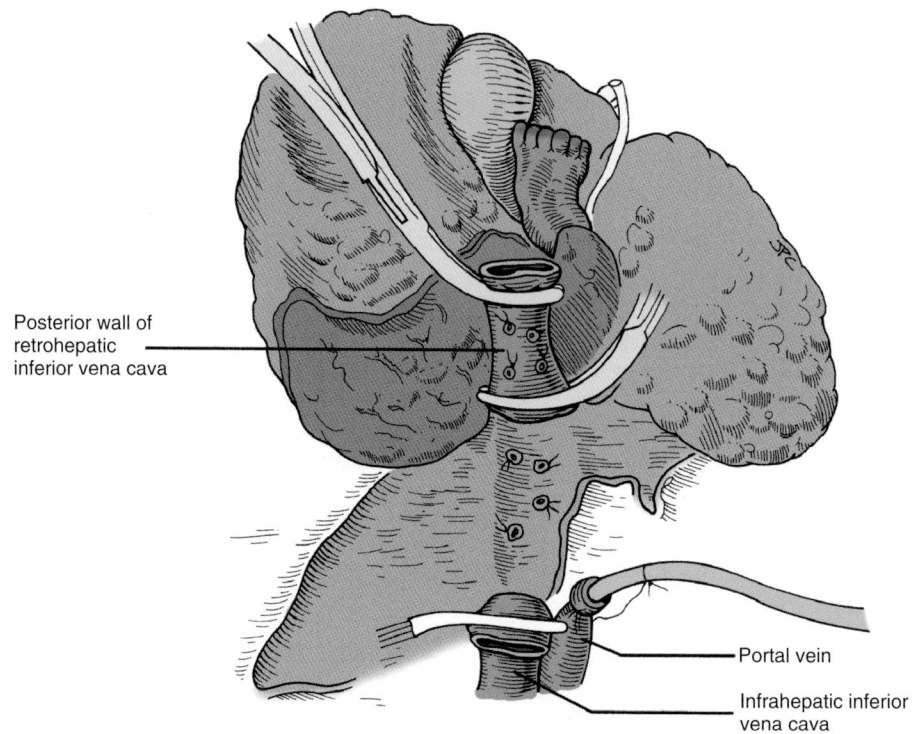

FIGURE 125.16 Removal of the recipient liver from bottom up.

transection of the hilar structures at the earliest possible opportunity (Fig. 125.16). Finally, if adhesions are present that block access to the upper and lower vena cava, the liver can be split in half in a superior-inferior direction, exposing the anterior surface of the retrohepatic IVC from inside the liver (Fig. 125.17). Once bleeding from the raw surfaces is controlled, the two hepatic halves are stripped away from the surrounding structures, ligating

the short hepatic veins from inside the liver from medial to lateral. All these variations are made easier by venovenous bypass.

Access to the upper vena cava can often be difficult, especially in retransplantation. In such cases, it is sometimes advantageous to open the central tendon of the diaphragm and clamp the IVC at its junction with the right atrium. This can be performed in almost all cases without splitting the sternum.

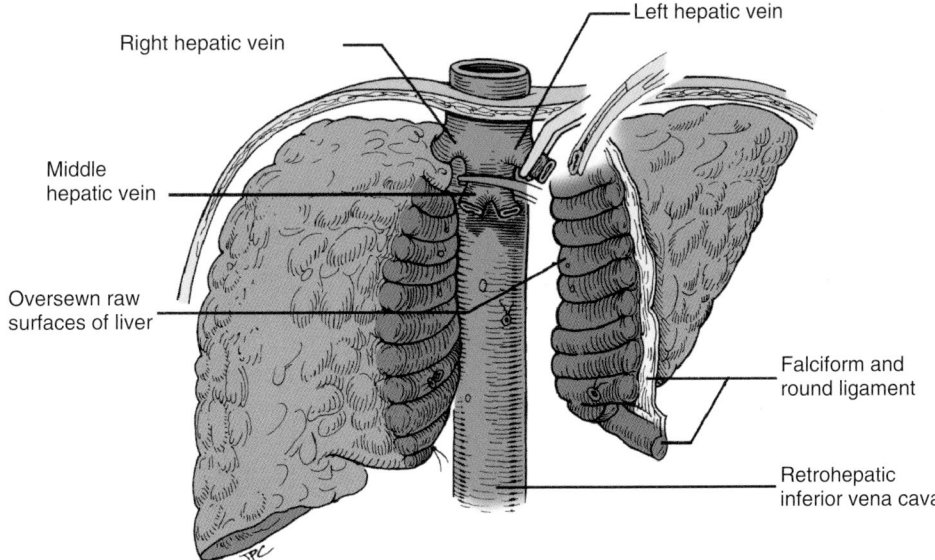

Right hepatic vein

Left hepatic vein

Middle hepatic vein

Oversewn raw surfaces of liver

Falciform and round ligament

Retrohepatic inferior vena cava

FIGURE 125.17   Splitting hepatectomy technique. The split is facilitated by inserting a finger along the relatively vein-free anterior midsurface of the retrohepatic vena cava. The correct plane must be determined carefully by finger probing before any pressure is applied.

The first step of this maneuver is to dissect the pleura and pericardium away from the back of the sternum. Then the pericardium is opened at its most superior border. Great care must be taken because the ventricle will be very close to the pericardium and can easily be injured. Once opened, the easiest method is to place a tonsil or similar clamp into the pericardium, directing it posteriorly; the pericardium is then opened over the clamp with cautery. The incision in the pericardium is directed in a straight line from anterior to posterior until the area of the IVC is reached; the incision is then directed to the patient's right to avoid injury to the intrapericardial vena cava.

Once the pericardium has been opened, the IVC becomes accessible. The heart is lifted superiorly, and a vascular clamp is placed across the intrapericardial vena cava. It is best to use a slightly angled clamp that should be directed not perfectly anteroposteriorly but more inferosuperiorly. A straight anteroposterior approach rarely gives complete occlusion of the IVC. Once clamped, it is useful to pass an umbilical tape through the rings of the handle of the clamp to retract the clamp superiorly; the clamp is stabilized by clamping the umbilical tape to the drapes or retractor. If this is not done, the movement of the clamp generated by the beating heart is distracting and obscures the suprahepatic IVC.

Vascular Anastomoses

It is important to have the surgical field as completely prepared for implantation as possible before the new liver is brought from the back table. The first allograft vessel to be anastomosed is always the suprahepatic vena cava. If host hepatectomy has included removal of the retrohepatic IVC, the anastomosis is an end-to-end, suprahepatic-to-suprahepatic IVC connection at the diaphragm (Fig. 125.18A). With the piggyback operation, in which the host vena cava is conserved, the donor suprahepatic IVC is anastomosed to a cuff of host hepatic veins (see Fig. 125.14B) or by a side-to-side anastomosis between the two vena caval segments (not shown). The recipient structure(s) receiving the donor suprahepatic IVC can be the cuff of all three hepatic veins, the

right hepatic vein alone, or the junction of the middle and left hepatic veins.

The order of the other vascular anastomoses may vary. With the piggyback technique, the infrahepatic IVC of the allograft is usually ligated or stapled before bringing the allograft into the operative field (though some surgeons prefer to vent through this structure during reperfusion). When the host caval segment has been excised, the infrahepatic vena cavae are usually next anastomosed (see Fig. 125.18B), followed by removal of the recipient from the portal (but not systemic) bypass and subsequent PV anastomosis (see Fig. 125.18C) (although the PV anastomosis may be performed before the infrahepatic vena caval anastomosis). An experienced surgeon may prefer to perform the arterial anastomosis before the PV reconstruction or may complete all four anastomoses before unclamping. These decisions are influenced by the anatomic and physiologic circumstances in the individual case, including the efficiency with which the bypass system has functioned and the degree of venous hypertension when bypass is not used.

In all cases when the preservation solution used is UW, it is imperative before reperfusion to flush the UW solution from the allograft. Flushing is done through the portal cannula, either on the back table before beginning implantation or in situ before beginning the PV anastomosis. After its passage through the microvasculature of the allograft, the infusate is vented from the IVC to avoid distention of the liver. The main objective of the flush is to rid the liver of high-potassium preservation solution (UW). Failure to perform this flush can result in hyperkalemic cardiac arrest or dysrhythmias; this step is not necessary if HTK solution is used for preservation.

All venous anastomoses are usually performed with continuous suture. To avoid anastomotic strictures, particularly of the portal anastomosis, special techniques were developed because polypropylene (Prolene) suture glides freely through tissue. A "growth factor" (often equal to at least the diameter of the PV) is left by tying the continuous suture at a considerable distance above the vessel wall.[9] After flow is restored through the anastomosis, the excess polypropylene recedes

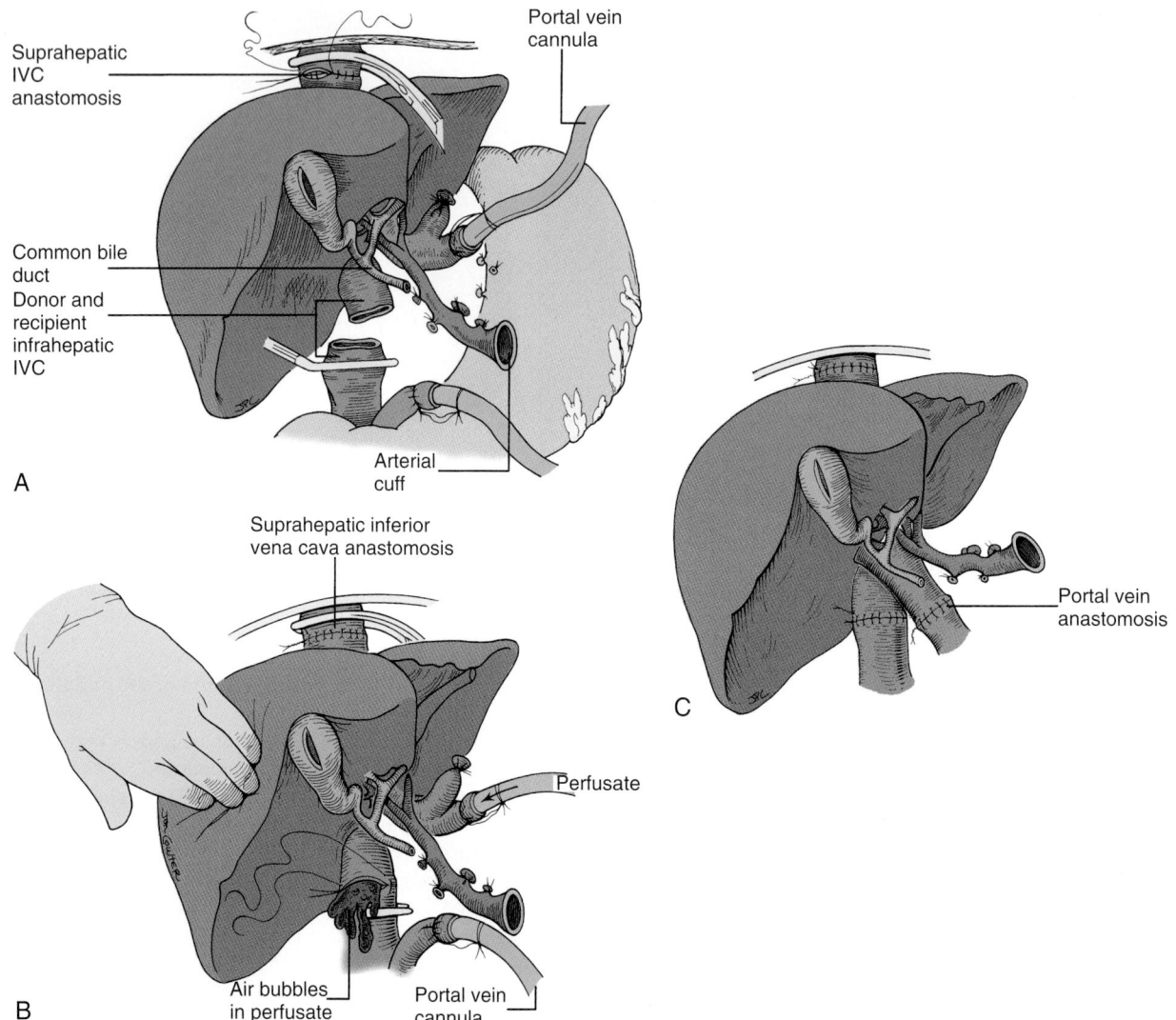

FIGURE 125.18   Implantation steps. A, Suprahepatic inferior vena cava *(IVC)* anastomosis. **B,** Infrahepatic IVC anastomosis. Before completing the anastomosis, the portal vein (PV) is infused with cold albumin or electrolyte solution when UW solution is used as the preservative. This allows air and potassium-rich preservation fluid to be removed. (Alternatively, the liver can be flushed on the back table, and heparinized saline can be used to remove air before completion of the PV anastomosis.) **C,** The PV anastomosis after removal of the bypass cannula.

back into the vessel and redistributes itself throughout the circumference of the suture line (Fig. 125.19), thereby allowing the anastomosis to "grow" or expand to its full circumference. If leaks develop, these are readily controlled with additional interrupted sutures.

Rather than being whimsical, variations of the order and details of revascularization frequently are mandated by anatomic anomalies or by pathologic factors, including PV thrombosis, which once contraindicated liver transplantation until techniques were developed to deal with it. Declotting a thrombosed PV may be possible (Fig. 125.20A) by inserting a clamp or cotton peanut retrograde into the PV and extracting the clot. If inadequate portal inflow remains, bypass of the thrombus may be necessary. Iliac or other veins from the donor may be used as interposition grafts (see Fig. 125.20B) or as mesoportal jump grafts (see Fig. 125.20C). A mesoportal graft may be anastomosed end-to-side to the superior mesenteric vein and tunneled through the transverse mesocolon anterior to the pancreas to reach the hepatic hilum for end-to-end anastomosis to

the donor PV (see Fig. 125.20C). In the most desperate of cases, the PV inflow can be supplied by a portion of the flow through the IVC by means of an end-to-side portocaval shunt. The vena cava above the anastomosis is typically purposefully narrowed to force antegrade flow through the shunt; otherwise the shunt will result in the typical retrograde blood flow out of the liver.

Numerous techniques have also been used to restore the hepatic arterial supply. The ideal reconstruction when the allograft and recipient have normal arterial anatomy is end-to-end at the level of the recipient common hepatic artery (Fig. 125.21). If anomalies, vascular injuries, or pathologic changes are present in the donor or recipient blood vessels that preclude effective rearterialization in the standard manner, grafts obtained from the donor can be used (see Fig. 125.21B and C). The arterial graft usually originates from the infrarenal aorta but can be placed on the recipient celiac trunk or supraceliac aorta as well (Fig. 125.22). In unusual circumstances, other sites of origination are also possible (e.g., splenic artery or right iliac artery).

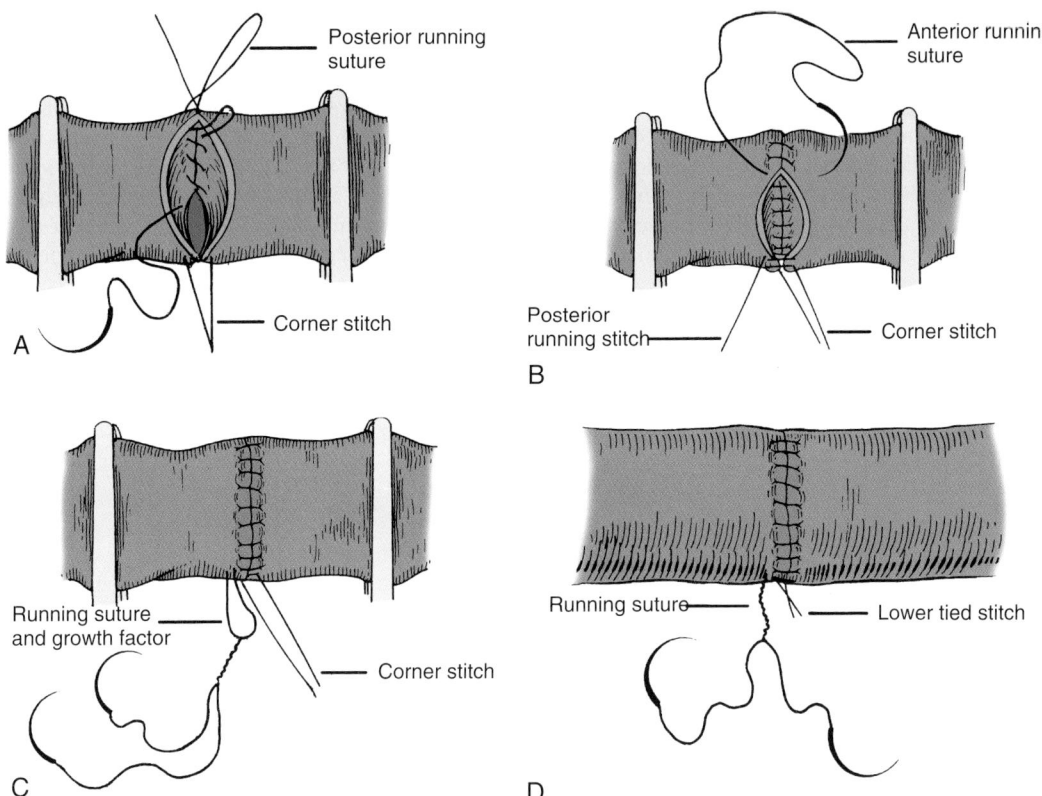

FIGURE 125.19 Technique of venous anastomosis. **A,** Traction sutures are placed at each corner. One end of the far suture is brought to the inside and run in continuous fashion to approximate the back wall. **B,** The other end of the far suture is used from the outside to approximate the anterior wall. **C,** The continuous suture is tied away from the vein wall to allow for a "growth factor." The near corner suture is tied next to the running suture to prevent separation of the vessel. **D,** The excess suture is automatically drawn into the vessel by vessel expansion, allowing the circumference to expand when blood flow is restored.

Biliary Tract Reconstruction

Good hemostasis must be achieved before the biliary reconstruction is performed. If the recipient duct is disease-free and there is a reasonable size match between the donor and recipient ducts, an end-to-end anastomosis is performed with or without a T-tube (Fig. 125.23) (see Chapter 42). The anastomosis usually is performed with 8 to 10 interrupted absorbable sutures, such as 6-0 or 7-0 polyglycolic acid (PGA), or with a continuous suture if the ducts are large enough. Because the integrity of the anastomosis depends primarily on an adequate arterial blood supply to both the donor and recipient ducts, minimal dissection is performed in the periductal tissues. If a T-tube is used, a small purse-string suture is placed around the T-tube exit site to prevent bile leakage, and the T limb is brought out through a stab incision on the lateral side of the recipient duct. An alternative to T-tube placement that also allows for posttransplant cholangiography is placement of a transcystic duct tube, secured to the cystic duct with an absorbable suture and a sterile hemorrhoid band that closes the cystic duct on removal (see Chapter 32).

If the recipient duct is diseased or otherwise inadequate for anastomosis, a choledochojejunostomy is performed. A 40 cm Roux-en-Y limb of proximal jejunum is brought to the hepatic hilum (antecolic or retrocolic); the donor duct is then anastomosed end-to-side to the jejunal limb with an interrupted or continuous 6-0 or 7-0 absorbable PGA suture with or without a stent (see Fig. 125.23, *inset*). When used, the stent is secured

in place with a rapidly absorbable suture, with the assumption that the stent will later pass spontaneously through the intestinal tract. Occasionally, however, the stent is retained and must be pushed into the bowel by an interventional radiologist or removed by push enteroscopy. Rarely does the stent require removal at laparotomy.

PEDIATRIC CONSIDERATIONS

As previously indicated, the optimal approach to liver transplantation varies based on several factors, especially in the pediatric recipient. The surgeon must consider the patient's size/age, underlying disease process, anatomic vascular anomalies or complications, and allograft type.

Recipient Exposure and Hepatectomy

Most pediatric recipients can be transplanted through a bilateral Chevron incision without a midline component as the pediatric abdominal wall is easily retracted to optimize exposure. In addition, most pediatric recipients do not have difficulty with hemodynamic instability during the anhepatic phase and therefore do not require venovenous bypass, piggyback technique, or temporary portocaval shunting.

The pediatric hilar dissection is unique in that the most common indication for transplantation is biliary atresia, and most patients will have had a Kasai procedure within the first 2 months of life (see Chapter 40). During the hilar dissection, the portoenterostomy is left attached to the liver, and the Roux limb is divided just distal to the anastomosis with an endovascular stapler, thereby avoiding dissection of the cirrhotic liver. It is not uncommon for the child with cholestatic liver disease to have hepatic arterial anomalies that will need to be dissected sufficiently to ensure adequate arterial inflow to the allograft. In the cholestatic pediatric patient the PV is frequently small, narrowed, and thickened, resulting in minimal flow. During the hilar dissection the PV needs to be dissected proximally to a point where soft, normal-appearing vein can be used for the anastomosis to the donor PV. In many cases this requires dissection to the junction of the splenic and superior mesenteric veins, with the portal venous anastomosis being performed at this level. To reach this site it is usually necessary to dissect the hepatic artery proximally to the origin of the splenic artery (which can safely be divided) to gain access to the celiac trunk where strong arterial inflow is present. It is also usually beneficial to remove the enlarged periportal lymph nodes, which obstruct access to the hepatic arterial circulation as well as the proximal PV. Care must be taken and attention paid to the hepatic hilum and hepatoduodenal ligament of the child, as a small number of children will have a preduodenal PV that must not be injured or inadvertently ligated.[10]

Following the hilar dissection and depending on the allograft type, the vena cava can either be clamped above and below the liver or preserved using the standard piggyback

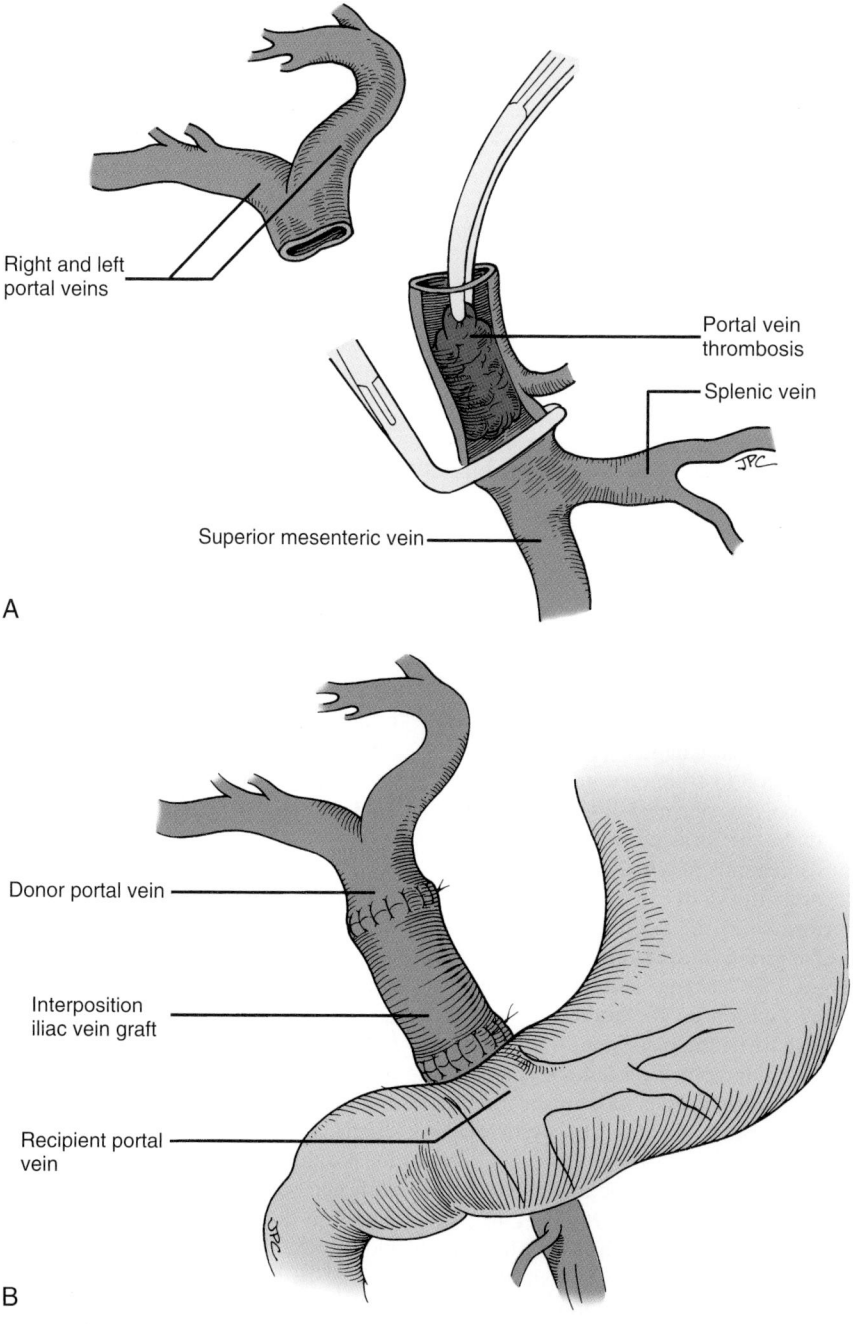

Right and left portal veins

Portal vein thrombosis

Splenic vein

Superior mesenteric vein

A

Donor portal vein

Interposition iliac vein graft

Recipient portal vein

B

FIGURE 125.20 Management of recipient portal vein (PV) abnormalities. A, Removal of thrombus. **B,** Use of an interposition donor vein graft to bridge the gap between donor PV and the confluence of the mesenteric and splenic veins.

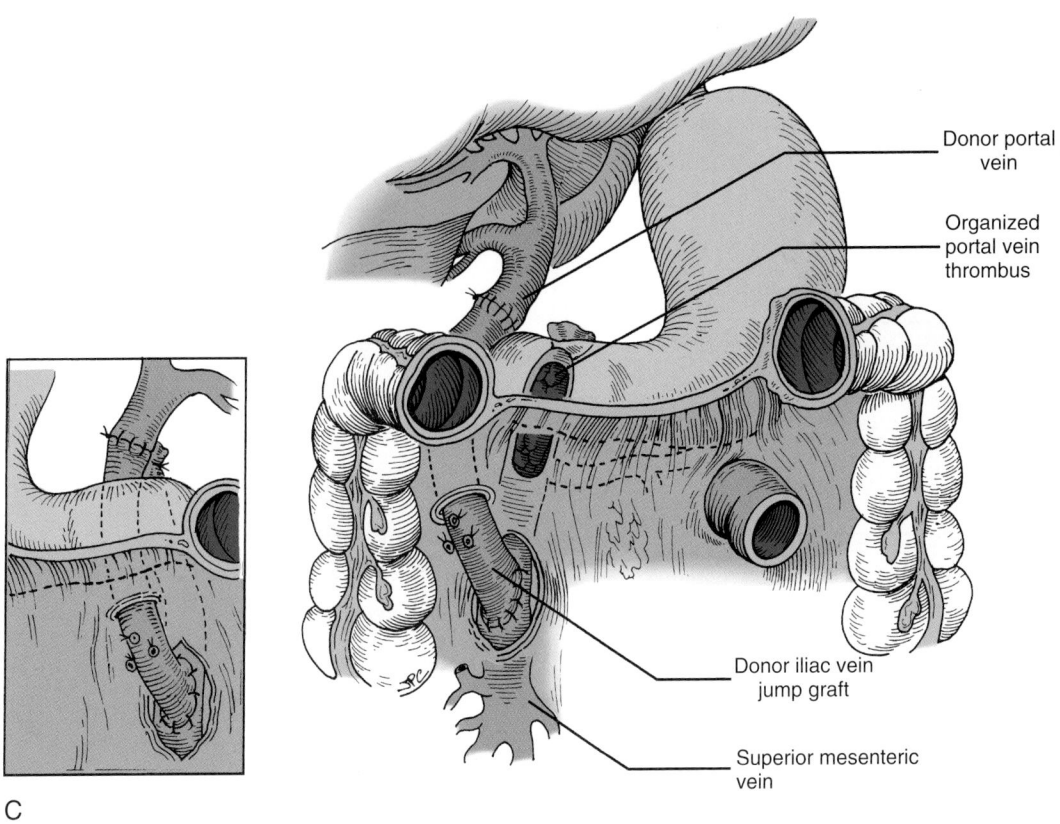

Donor portal
vein

Organized
portal vein
thrombus

Donor iliac vein
jump graft

Superior mesenteric
vein

C

FIGURE 125.20 cont'd   C, Donor vein jump graft from the host superior mesenteric vein to the allograft PV. The jump graft is tunneled through the transverse mesocolon anterior to the pancreas to the hepatic hilum. The graft can be anterior or posterior *(inset)* to the stomach (see Chapter 2]).

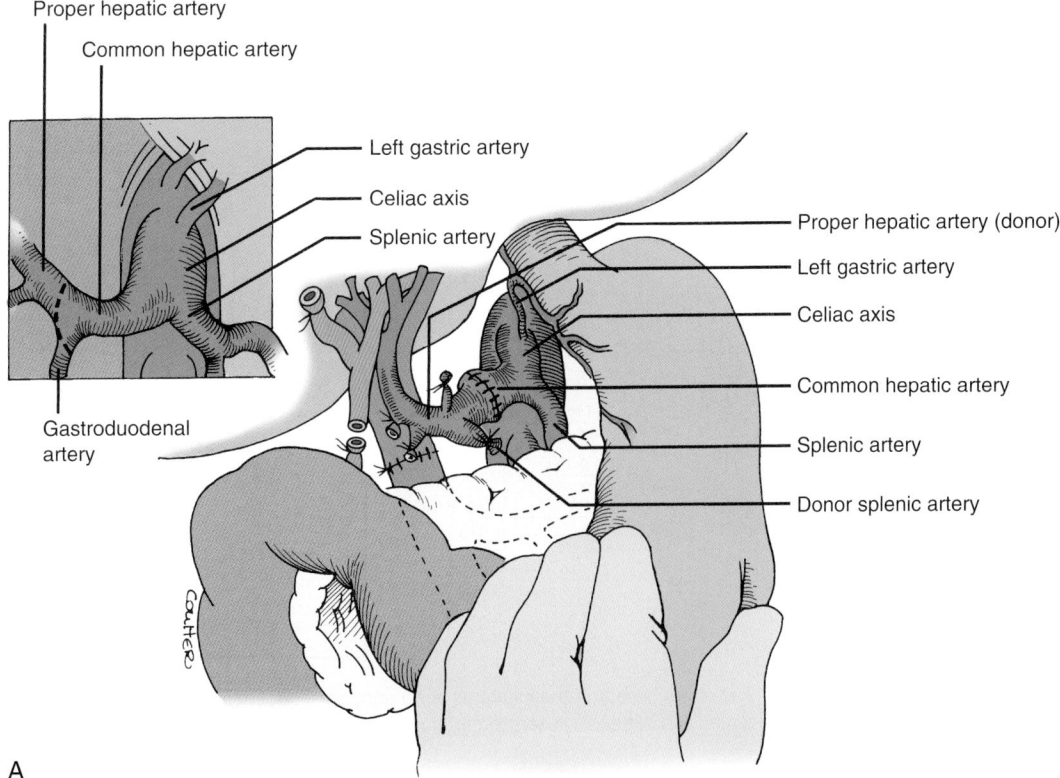

Proper hepatic artery

Common hepatic artery

Left gastric artery

Celiac axis

Splenic artery

Proper hepatic artery (donor)

Left gastric artery

Celiac axis

Common hepatic artery

Splenic artery

Donor splenic artery

Gastroduodenal
artery

A

FIGURE 125.21   Hepatic artery reconstruction. A, The most common reconstruction in which the allograft celiac trunk is anastomosed to the recipient common hepatic artery at the level of the recipient gastroduodenal artery. With discrepant sizes, the circumference of the recipient vessel can be increased, as shown in the *inset.*   *Continued*

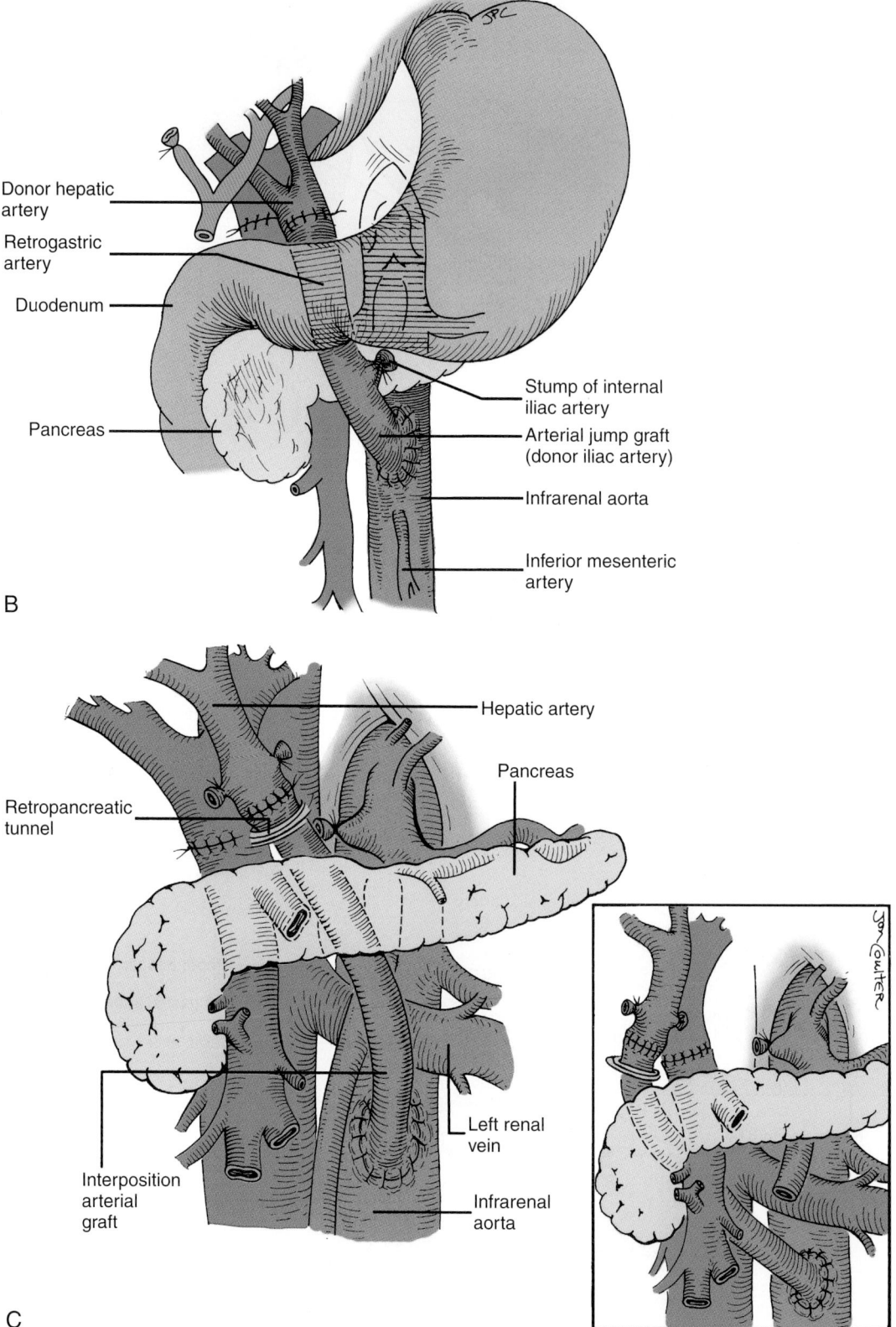

Donor hepatic artery

Retrogastric artery

Duodenum

Pancreas

Stump of internal iliac artery

Arterial jump graft (donor iliac artery)

Infrarenal aorta

Inferior mesenteric artery

B

Hepatic artery

Pancreas

Retropancreatic tunnel

Left renal vein

Interposition arterial graft

Infrarenal aorta

C

FIGURE 125.21 cont'd B, Jump graft of donor iliac artery based off the infrarenal aorta and tunneled anterior to the pancreas. **C,** Rarely used alternative retroperitoneal tunnel posterior to the pancreas and superior mesenteric artery.

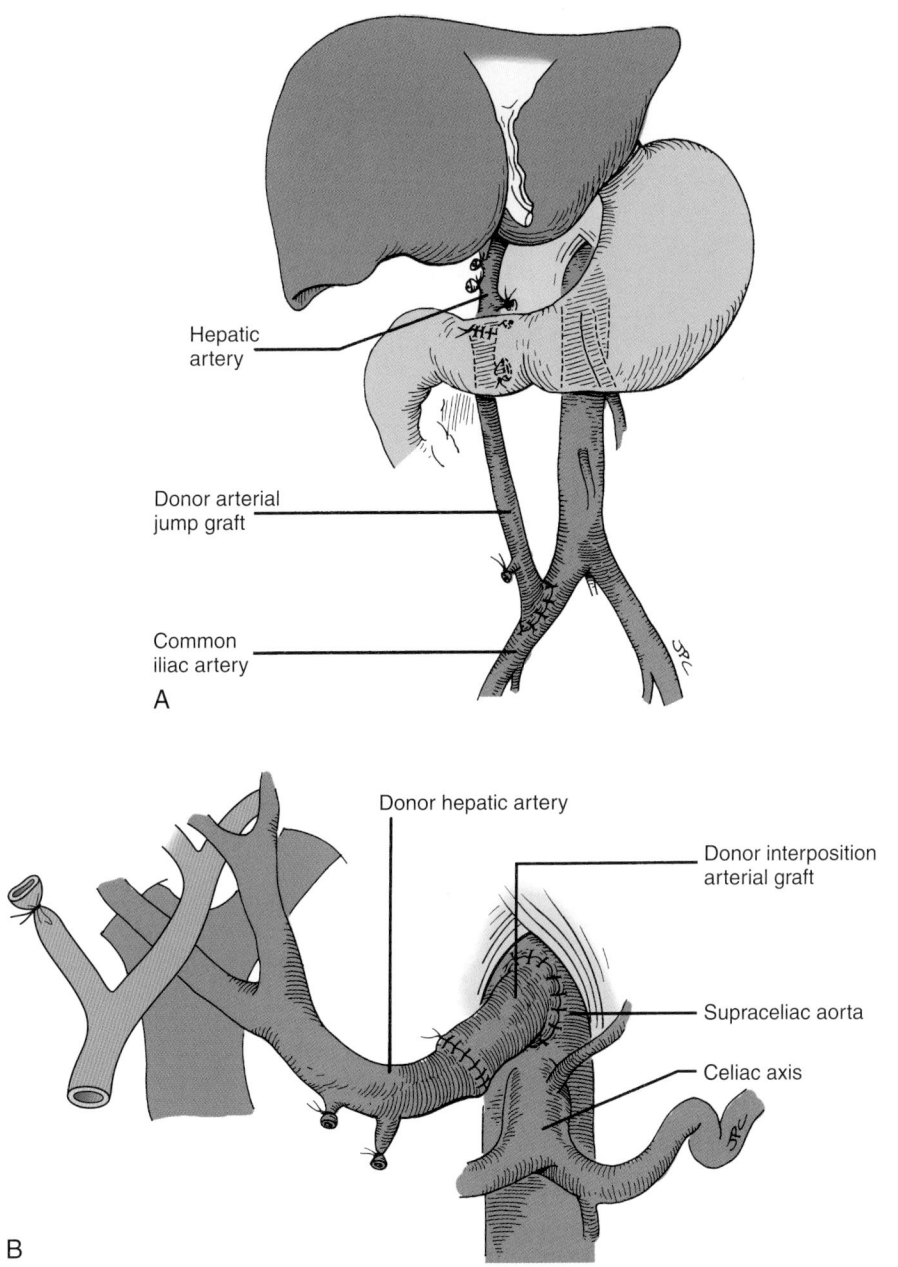

FIGURE 125.22   Other originating sites for an arterial jump graft.   **A,** Host iliac artery. **B,** Supraceliac aorta.

dissection. In the child with an interrupted IVC the liver can be lifted anteriorly and superiorly, with a vascular clamp being placed across the confluence of hepatic veins before removing the native liver.[7]

Implantation of the Liver Allograft

In both the standard and piggyback procedures, the vena caval anastomoses are often performed by running the posterior wall and interrupting the anterior wall to prevent venous stricturing and to allow growth between the sutures. In the child with an absent retrohepatic vena cava, the infrahepatic vena cava of the donor liver is closed and the suprahepatic vena cava of the donor is anastomosed end-to-end to the recipient confluence of hepatic veins.

The portal venous anastomosis is likewise often performed by running the posterior wall and interrupting the anterior wall,

again to prevent strictures and to allow future growth of these structures with the child. It is important to make sure this portal venous anastomosis is performed as proximally as possible, without tension, to utilize the best vein available and maximize portal venous flow. The preduodenal PV is handled in the same manner as the anatomically normal PV. If needed, a portal venous extension graft can be created from donor iliac vein.[11] This is frequently needed in the child who receives a technical variant allograft that only possesses a left PV.

Following the venous anastomoses the liver is reperfused while keeping in mind that in the child with congenital heart disease the air and debris in the donor liver must be vented into the abdomen to avoid it inadvertently entering the arterial circulation. Therefore the clamps are removed in reverse order, and the final three to five suprahepatic vena caval sutures are not tied until it is believed that the air and debris have been

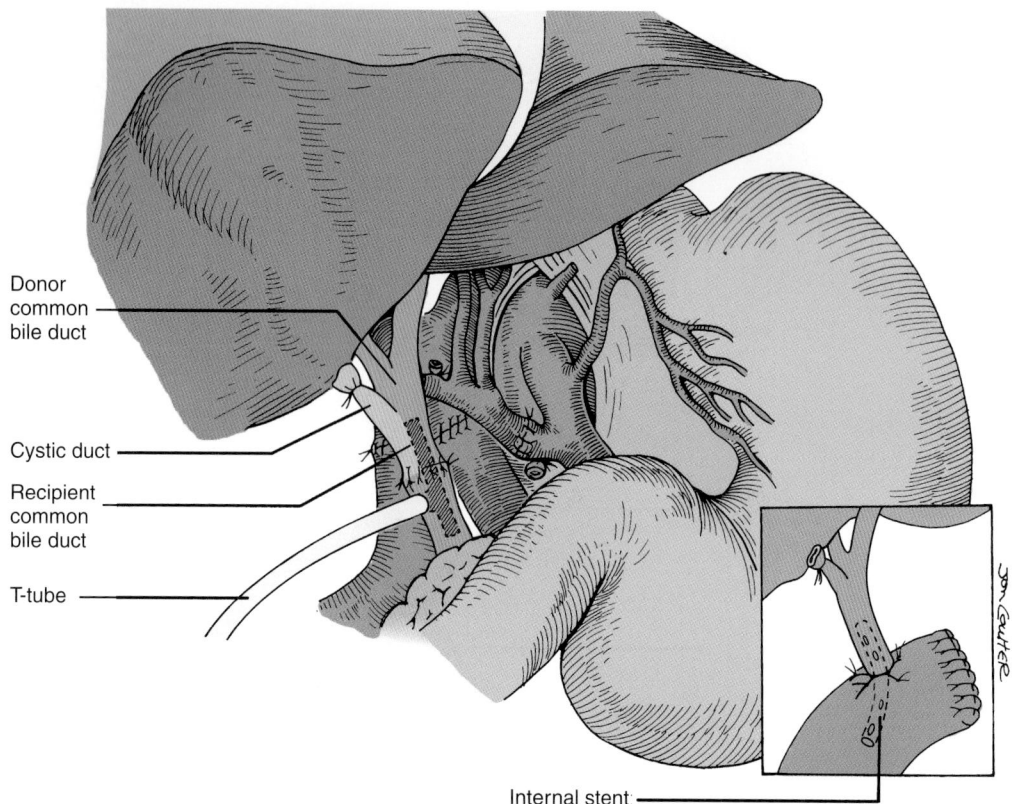

Donor common bile duct

Cystic duct

Recipient common bile duct

T-tube

Internal stent

FIGURE 125.23 **Biliary tract reconstruction with end-to-end anastomosis over a T-tube.** If duct reconstruction is not feasible or is contraindicated, the allograft duct is anastomosed to a Roux-en-Y limb of host jejunum *(inset)*.

cleared. Once this condition is met the suprahepatic clamp is removed and reperfusion is completed. At this point in children less than 20 kg, and in children with metabolic liver disease, heparin is initiated at 5 units/kg/hour titrated to maintain a prothrombin time (PTT) of 55 to 60 seconds to prevent vascular thromboses.[12]

Following reperfusion the hepatic arterial anastomosis is performed as proximally on the celiac trunk as possible using interrupted sutures to maximize arterial inflow. If needed, the celiac trunk can be skeletonized and all branches divided. In the event that hepatic arterial flow is still not adequate or in the child with aberrant arterial anatomy not suitable for use, an arterial conduit is placed on the aorta in either the supraceliac or infrarenal position using donor iliac artery in an end-to-side manner.

The biliary reconstruction is via a Roux-en-Y hepaticojejunostomy with internal stent in children less than 10 kg, in those without a suitable biliary tree, and in the child receiving a technical variant allograft. If the biliary tree can be used it is preferable to perform a choledochocholedochostomy with interrupted absorbable sutures.

In the child receiving a technical variant allograft it is important to reapproximate the falciform ligament of the donor and recipient to prevent the allograft from falling into the vacant right upper quadrant, causing allograft thrombosis.[13] An additional option is to suture the falciform ligament to the abdominal wall for the same purpose.

One final consideration in the pediatric patient is closure of the abdomen. Unfortunately, it is difficult to find a size-matched allograft at the optimal transplant time for small children. In addition, children can have marked anasarca and bowel edema, adding to the limited abdominal domain. Therefore in some patients the abdominal domain is compromised to the point that the abdominal wall fascia may need to be left open or a patch of Gore-Tex placed temporarily to prevent the abdomen from being too tight, resulting in respiratory compromise and pressure on the liver allograft vascular components. In many cases peak inspiratory pressure and ventilation volume can be used to assist in the determination of increasing abdominal pressure.

Cadaveric Technical Variants

The scarcity of pediatric donors and the constraints of size matching often prohibit transplantation of a whole donor liver into a child or small adult. Since 1980 the option of using a partial liver has been utilized at most large transplant centers with results equal to or approaching those achievable with whole-allograft liver transplantation.

Due to the ongoing shortage of allografts suitable for small adults and children, it is not infrequent that the allograft must be technically altered so that a portion may fit. It is important to keep in mind that the goal of performing technical variant procurements is to create two transplantable allografts thereby maximizing the use of the cadaveric liver.

In Situ Split—Right Trisegmental and Left Lateral Segments

The most common technical variant allografts are the in situ split right trisegmental and left lateral segment allografts benefiting both a child and adult.[14] The in situ split is performed by the initial mobilization of the liver, as well as dissection of the aorta, inferior mesenteric vein, and vena cava as described for a standard liver procurement. When determining that the liver is divisible and size appropriate, it is important to understand the hepatic arterial anatomy to determine how the hepatic artery will ultimately be divided.

If a replaced or accessory left hepatic artery is present the hepatogastric ligament is maintained; if not the ligament is divided. The junction of the left and middle hepatic veins is identified and the plane above these veins is developed to assist in the parenchymal division of the liver and left hepatic vein. The hepatoduodenal ligament is dissected as far to the left as possible to avoid damaging the blood supply to the biliary tree. The left hepatic artery is dissected from its origin into the umbilical fissure and ultimately to its entrance into the left lateral segment. Care is taken to avoid injury to any of the vascular or biliary structures. The origin of the right hepatic artery is also identified to assist in the final division of the two allografts.

The left PV is dissected free of all surrounding tissue from the portal bifurcation into the umbilical fissure; special attention is paid to the small branches entering the caudate lobe and segment 4 as they must be ligated and divided to free the left PV from these portions of the liver. In the umbilical fissure the branches from the left hepatic artery and left PV entering segments 4a and 4b are ligated and divided, while the branches entering segments 2 and 3 are preserved. When this dissection is completed the initial parenchymal transection is performed approximately 1 cm to the right of the falciform ligament (Fig. 125.24). This location is chosen with the hope of encountering a single left hepatic duct. This transection is carried into the umbilical fissure between the ties of the previously ligated left hepatic arterial and PV branches. When the left hepatic duct is reached it is sharply divided with scissors. The left hepatic duct on the right trisegmental allograft is oversewn. The parenchymal transection then continues up to the level of the left hepatic vein. The liver is then infused with preservative solution via the portal venous and arterial systems and the whole liver removed. On the back table the liver is infused with 1 additional liter of preservation solution, and the two liver allografts are separated by dividing the left hepatic vein at its insertion into the vena cava, the right hepatic artery

near its origin from the proper hepatic artery, and the left PV just distal to its origin at the PV bifurcation. The two liver allografts are then packaged and transported to their respective transplant centers.

If the liver has a replaced left hepatic artery, the left gastric artery is divided from the celiac trunk and the celiac trunk remains with the right trisegmental allograft (see Chapter 2). If the liver has a replaced right hepatic artery, the celiac trunk stays with the left lateral segmental allograft, and the replaced right hepatic artery or replaced right hepatic artery plus SMA stay with the right trisegmental allograft.

In Situ Split—Right and Left Hepatic Lobes

The liver allograft may also (though less frequently) be divided into right and left hepatic lobes. The initial dissection proceeds as for a standard liver procurement. After isolating all vascular structures and determining that the size is appropriate for two adults, the gallbladder is removed and an intraoperative cholangiogram is performed to rule out aberrant biliary anatomy. The hepatoduodenal ligament is dissected, identifying and isolating the right and left hepatic arteries, the left and right PVs, and the biliary bifurcation. The right and caudate lobes are then dissected free of the vena cava by ligating and dividing the short hepatic veins. The space between the right and middle hepatic veins is developed and a vessel loop is passed between the right and middle hepatic veins superiorly and between the bifurcation of the right and left hilar structures inferiorly. This creates the "hanging liver," and the liver parenchyma can then be divided along Cantlie's line. Care must be taken at the hepatic hilum not to injure any of the vascular or biliary structures. If a large accessory right hepatic vein (usually >1 cm) is encountered, it must be preserved for reimplantation.

Following the parenchymal transection, the liver is perfused with preservative solution via the portal and arterial systems, removed from the body, and flushed on the back table with 1 additional liter of preservation solution via the PV. The liver is then divided into a left and right lobe hepatic allograft by dividing the right hepatic vein at its insertion into the vena cava. If an accessory right hepatic vein is present, it is also divided at its insertion into the vena cava. The left PV is divided at its origin from the portal bifurcation, and the right hepatic artery is divided at its origin from the proper hepatic artery. Replaced right and left hepatic arteries can be handled as outlined previously.

Back-Table Reconstruction of the Technical Variant Allograft

The initial back-table preparation of the technical variant allograft proceeds as outlined previously. However, specific reconstructive techniques need to be employed to make both liver allografts transplantable.[15]

The *left lateral segment* allograft only requires a single modification consisting of placing an iliac vein extension graft onto the left PV, making the anastomosis to the proximal recipient PV easier. This also provides the additional length needed to reach the splenic vein/SMV junction. The left hepatic vein, left hepatic duct, and celiac trunk do not require reconstruction.

The *right trisegmental* allograft requires that the defect in the left vena cava be closed without stricturing the middle hepatic vein; this utilizes a patch of iliac vein sutured with running Prolene suture. The orifice of the left PV is closed using Prolene sutures; the right hepatic artery is reconstructed using an iliac arterial graft to provide the required length using interrupted Prolene sutures. The external iliac artery is preferred for this

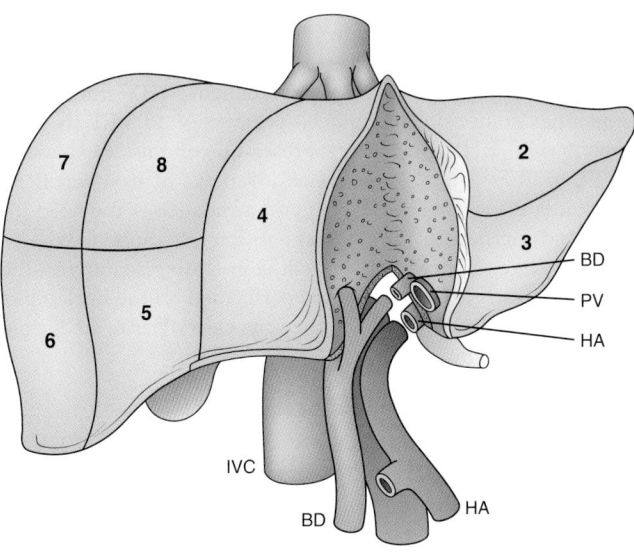

FIGURE 125.24 **Right trisegmental and left lateral segment split.** Numbers represent Couinaud segments. *BD,* Bile duct; *HA,* hepatic artery; *IVC,* inferior vena cava; *PV,* portal vein.

reconstruction as it frequently is size-matched to the right hepatic artery.

The *left lobe* allograft requires closing the orifice of the right hepatic vein and placing an iliac vein extension graft onto the left PV as described previously.

The *right lobe* allograft requires that the orifice of the left PV be closed without structuring, and an external iliac arterial extension graft be placed onto the transected right hepatic artery as outlined previously.

Implantation of the Technical Variant Liver Allograft

The *left lateral segment* allograft requires that the donor left hepatic vein be anastomosed to the confluence of the recipient middle and left hepatic veins in an end-to-end fashion. The posterior wall is commonly sutured in a running manner, and the anterior wall is performed in an interrupted fashion to avoid stricture and to allow future growth with the child. The portal venous and arterial anastomoses are performed as previously described. The biliary reconstruction requires an end-to-side hepaticojejunostomy, usually with an internal stent.

The *right trisegmental, left lobe, and right lobe* allografts are implanted as previously outlined for the whole-allograft transplant procedure.

LIVING DONOR ALLOGRAFT IMPLANTATION (SEE CHAPTER 121)

Right Lobe Live-Donor Transplantation

Live-donor liver transplantation using right lobe allografts is a surgical innovation that is still evolving as further understanding is gained of the interrelated effects of allograft size, portal and hepatic artery blood flow/pressure, and patient disease severity on outcome. Surgeons have performed right lobe implantation with or without incorporating the middle hepatic vein of the donor (extended right hepatectomy). Arguments for including the middle hepatic vein are to improve venous outflow; however, larger resections may pose more risk for the donor.[16–19] For this chapter we restrict discussion to formal right hepatic lobes *without* incorporating the donor middle hepatic vein.

Because no live-donor allografts have the native vena cava attached, the recipient hepatectomy must spare the vena cava, using the piggyback technique. Surgical incisions that may be used include bilateral subcostal (clamshell) or a bilateral subcostal incision with an upper midline extension (inverted "T," Chevron or Mercedes). Alternatively, to spare cutting the left rectus muscle, a right subcostal incision with a vertical midline extension can also be used (hockey stick or Lexus).

Since there is a significant relationship between portal flow, portal pressure, patient disease severity, and outcome, it may be useful to measure portal venous pressure and flow early and again after allograft reperfusion to determine whether "inflow modification" (splenic artery ligation, hemiportocaval shunt, splenectomy) is required to help prevent early allograft dysfunction or "small-for-size syndrome" (SFSS).[20–22] Some surgeons perform a temporary portocaval shunt to minimize blood loss, maintain hemodynamic stability during hepatectomy, and avoid the need for venovenous bypass. If high portal pressure and/or flow are present, especially in the setting of an anticipated small allograft (<0.8 allograft weight to body weight

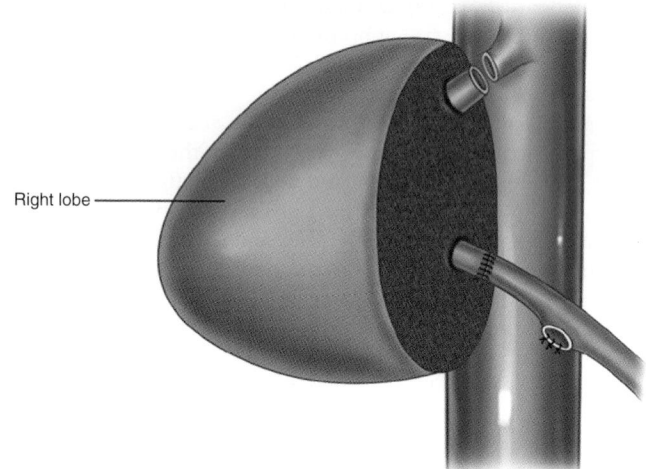

FIGURE 125.25 Standard side-to-side portocaval shunt.

ratio), preemptive inflow modification may be required. In these cases, a side-to-side shunt (Fig. 125.25), a hemiportocaval shunt (HPCS) using recipient right PV (Fig. 125.26), or a 6-mm polytetrafluoroethylene (PTFE) conduit (Fig. 125.27) can be performed during hepatectomy and taken down later if necessary. Criteria providing guidance as to when to perform inflow modifications are not well established but should be considered when absolute portal pressure is greater than 20 mm Hg, portal venous gradient (absolute portal pressure minus central venous pressure) is greater than 12 mm Hg, hepatic artery flow is less than 100 mL/min, or post-reperfusion portal flow is greater than 2.5 mL/gram allograft weight. Due to the hepatic artery buffer response, low hepatic artery flow in the setting of high portal venous flow or pressure (absent technical problems) supports performing inflow modification.

To maximize donor safety, many advocate leaving the middle hepatic vein (MHV) with the donor remnant liver. With this approach, allografts with significant anterior hepatic venous branches (segments V, VIII) may require reconstruction on the back table. Techniques vary widely, from using autologous saphenous vein, IMV, cryopreserved iliac artery allografts anastomosed directly to the vena cava or recipient MHV stump, or a sequential composite technique (segment V to VIII to right hepatic vein [RHV]) using cryopreserved conduit or expanded PTFE grafts[23] (Fig. 125.28). The advantage of using artificial conduit is the relatively low cost and avoidance of the need for a morbid incision in the recipient to harvest saphenous vein. When a large segment VIII branch is in close proximity to the RHV, side-to-side anastomosis is performed on the back table, and then direct anastomosis to the vena cava is performed using anterior venotomy.

Recipient Right Lobe Allograft Implantation

Implantation begins with anastomosis of the donor RHV to either the recipient RHV orifice or an anterior venotomy on the vena cava below the level of the hepatic veins. In both cases, complete caval clamping is unnecessary when using side-biting vascular clamps and maintains recipient hemodynamics. The advantage of the anterior caval venotomy is that it brings the allograft lower in the operative field, closer to the hilar vessels, and avoids the need to perform cavoplasty or other remedial

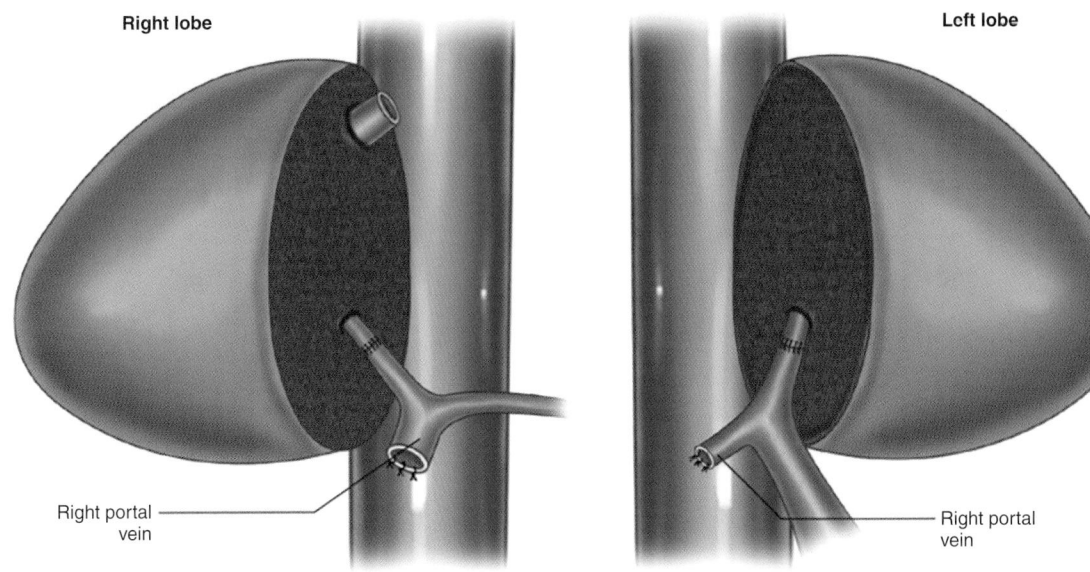

FIGURE 125.26 Hemiportocaval shunt (HPCS) using right branch of the recipient portal vein.

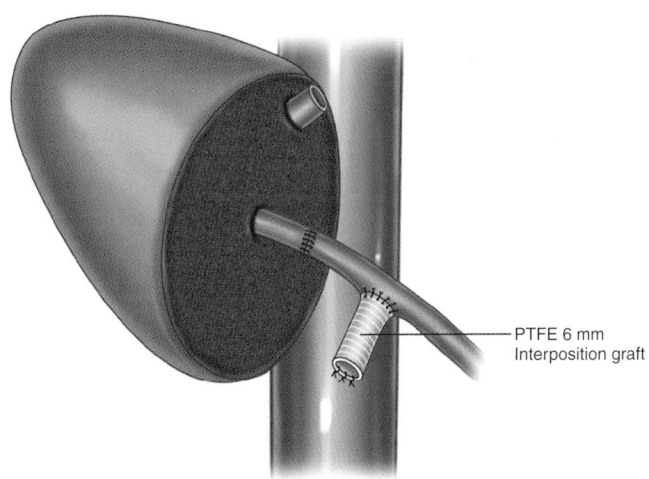

FIGURE 125.27 Hemiportocaval shunt (HPCS) using a 6-mm polytetrafluoroethylene (PTFE) conduit.

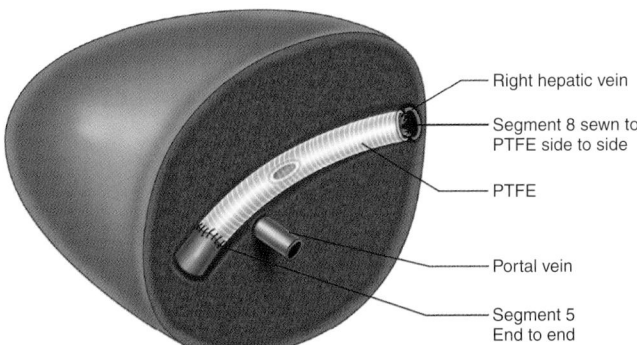

FIGURE 125.28 Sequential composite anterior segment reconstruction can be used to create a single outflow conduit when segment V and VIII need to be reconstructed. Iliac artery allograft or 6-mm PTFE conduit can be used.

procedures. Leaving this anastomosis temporarily untied before reperfusion allows for flushing of the allograft to remove preservation solution or stagnant portal blood and expands the anastomosis before securing it. After reperfusion, the anastomosis is tied and caval clamps removed.

The technique for PV reconstruction is similar to the procedure for deceased-donor transplants, but care must be taken to avoid closing the posterior segment branch when division is near the bifurcation. Generally, the back wall of the anastomosis is sewn from the inside and everted to create good intima-to-intima apposition (Fig. 125.29). A small amount of "growth factor" (see Fig. 125.19) when tying the suture allows for expansion of the anastomosis and avoids narrowing.

Hepatic artery reconstruction is best performed with interrupted fine suture under high-power loupe magnification, although some prefer to use a microscope (Fig. 125.30). Recipient hepatic artery thrombosis (HAT) caused by intimal dissection can be salvaged with a recipient arterial conduit, such as a redundant loop of splenic artery, gastroduodenal artery, gastroepiploic artery, or an interposition graft. Dissection of the hepatic artery into the allograft is generally not salvageable and requires retransplantation. Hypercoagulable states diagnosed in the recipient with thromboelastography or rotational thromboelastometry may benefit from perioperative heparin and/or aspirin therapy.

Biliary reconstruction can be performed in a similar fashion to deceased-donor allografts with either duct-to-duct or Roux-en-Y hepaticojejunostomy (see Chapter 42). In cases where there are separate anterior and posterior bile ducts, the right anterior duct can be reconstructed with a duct-to-duct anastomosis, whereas the right posterior duct can be reconstructed with a Roux-en-Y hepaticojejunostomy. To avoid compression of the hilum, the Roux limb can be passed in a retrocolic and retrogastric fashion (Fig. 125.31). Some surgeons prefer routine use of biliary stents, whereas others are selective or never use them. Patients with cholangiocarcinoma or severe dysplasia throughout the biliary tree may require en bloc resection of the

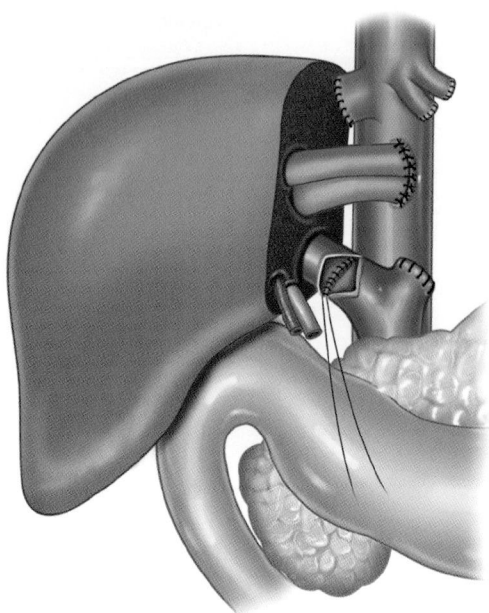

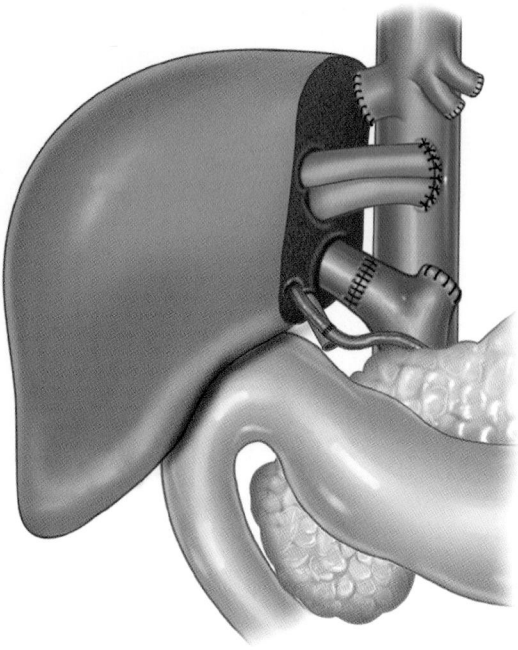

FIGURE 125.29   Portal vein reconstruction is standard and should evert the back wall of the anastomosis to avoid rough, as shown. Care must be taken to avoid inadvertent closure of the posterior segmental branch if portal vein division is near the anterior/posterior bifurcation. In this case, a double portal vein was reconstructed by resecting the recipient portal vein bifurcation from the explanted recipient liver and performing reanastomosis on the back table, with 90-degree rotation from horizontal to vertical on the donor graft to avoid twisting with implantation.

FIGURE 125.30   Hepatic artery reconstruction is best performed using interrupted sutures and high-power magnification. Some surgeons use 4.5× loupe magnification, but others use a microscope aid.

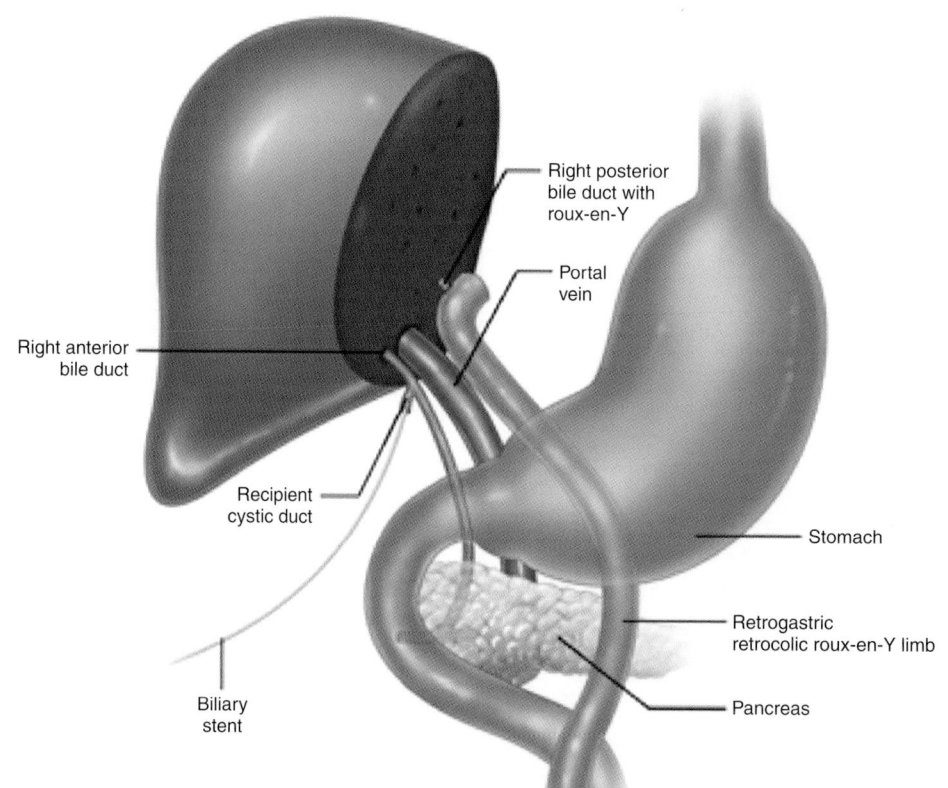

Right posterior
bile duct with
roux-en-Y

Portal
vein

Right anterior
bile duct

Recipient
cystic duct

Stomach

Retrogastric
retrocolic roux-en-Y limb

Pancreas

Biliary
stent

FIGURE 125.31   **Choledochocholedochostomy using recipient native common bile duct to the right duct of the allograft.** The recipient cystic duct stump can be used to place a 5-Fr pediatric feeding tube to be used as a biliary stent for postoperative imaging. In cases where there are separate anterior and posterior bile ducts, the right anterior duct can be reconstructed with a duct-to-duct anastomosis, whereas the right posterior duct can be reconstructed with a Roux-en-Y hepaticojejunostomy. To avoid compression of the hilum, the Roux limb can be passed in a retrocolic and retrogastric fashion.

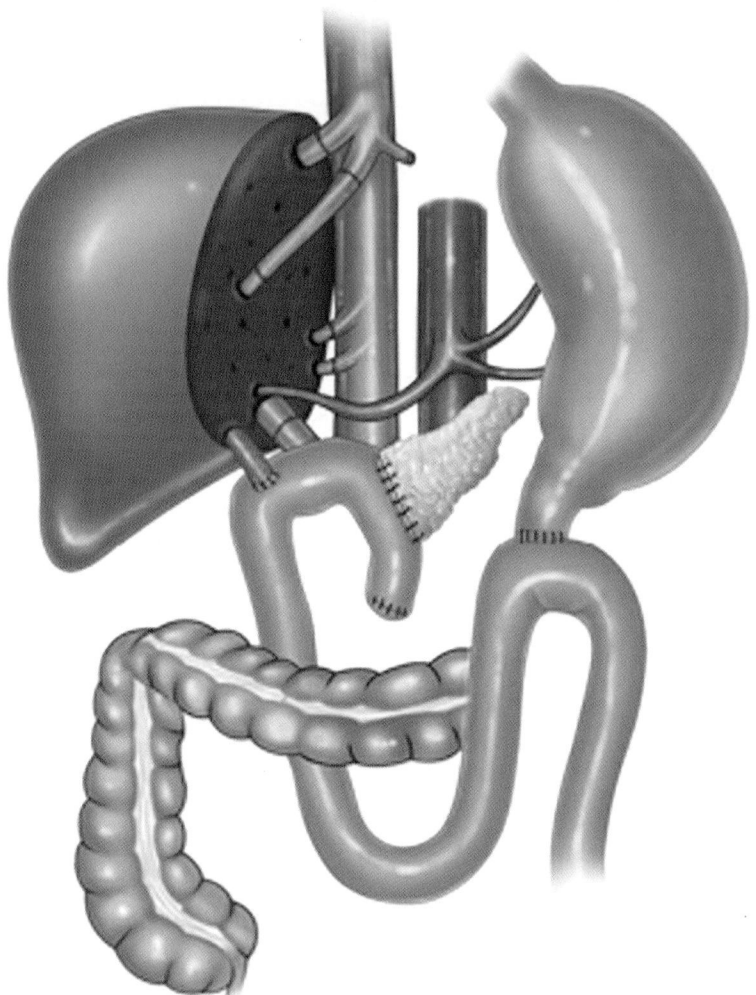

FIGURE 125.32 Reconstruction after combined live-donor liver transplant and pancreaticoduodenostomy for a patient with cholangiocarcinoma or severe dysplasia throughout the biliary tree.

entire biliary tree. In these cases, combined liver transplant and Whipple pancreaticoduodectomy may be required (Fig. 125.32) (see Chapters 51 and 108B). To qualify patients must undergo neoadjuvant chemoradiation.

Left Lobe Live-Donor Transplantation

Left lobe live-donor liver transplantation is useful for smaller adults and/or children. Left lateral segment liver transplant is reserved for babies. In very small babies, these left lateral allografts may need to be further reduced to accommodate the abdominal compartment. The advantage of left lobe live-donor transplant is the lower complication rate in the donor, but this may come at the cost of potentially worse outcome in the recipient. "Healthier" cirrhotic patients with minimal portal hypertension may tolerate a smaller allograft than sicker individuals who require larger allografts.

Recipient Left Lobe Allograft Implantation

Unlike the right lobe allograft, the left hepatic vein (LHV) drainage of the allograft is best performed to the LHV of the recipient due to the closer proximity to the hilar vessels. In addition, the cephalad angle of the left lobe allograft outflow lines

up more precisely to the recipient middle and left hepatic vein stumps. Similar to the right lobe allograft, this anastomosis is left temporarily untied for eventual flushing of the liver and to allow for full expansion.

Portal vein and hepatic artery reconstruction are performed in a similar fashion to the right lobe allograft or deceased-donor liver transplant. Palpable thrill in the hepatic artery portends good flow and good outcome. The patient should not leave the operating room unless the surgeon is satisfied with all vascular anastomoses confirmed by intraoperative ultrasound, flow probe, or handheld Doppler probe. Faith-based surgery relying on hope or prayer is a recipe for bad outcomes. Reperforming an anastomosis during the index operation is much more effective than later allograft removal and retransplant.

In summary, live-donor liver transplantation using either right or left lobe liver allografts is a safe and effective treatment for patients with end-stage liver disease. Like all surgery, good outcomes require technical acumen, sound judgment, and attention to detail.

The references for this chapter can be found online by accessing the accompanying Expert Consult website.

CHAPTER 126

Techniques of pancreas transplantation

Santosh Nagaraju, John A. Powelson, and Jonathan A. Fridell

INTRODUCTION

Diabetes mellitus is associated with extensive morbidity and mortality and represents a significant medical, financial, and emotional burden on society. Long-term diabetes mellitus is frequently associated with cardiovascular, cerebrovascular, peripheral vascular, neurologic, renal, and ophthalmologic complications.[1] Diabetes remains the leading cause of renal failure (44% of new cases every year) and increases the risk of mortality in uremic patients.[1] Despite marked improvements in the medical management, poor glycemic control, hypoglycemic unawareness, and secondary complications of diabetes remain common. Pancreas transplantation not only results in insulin independence but also potentially slows down progression of or reverses some of the secondary complications of diabetes. Pancreas transplantation is currently only offered to select diabetic patients who meet the strict qualifying criteria. In this chapter we present a brief history, indications and types of transplants, donor selection, recipient evaluation, surgical techniques and complications, immunosuppression, and outcomes.

HISTORY OF PANCREAS TRANSPLANTATION (ALSO SEE CHAPTER 112)

In 1922 the team of Banting, Best, and Collip successfully used pancreatic extracts in the treatment of diabetes mellitus; the purified substance was called insulin.[2] Four decades later, in 1966, William Kelly and Richard Lillehei performed the first human simultaneous pancreas and kidney transplantation at The University of Minnesota.[3] The pancreas allograft included the distal segment with ligation of the pancreatic duct and was placed in the left lower quadrant with the kidney on the right. The entire celiac axis was included and the superior mesenteric vein and portal vein were used as a bypass from the external to common iliac veins in order to improve venous flow. The patient immediately became independent of insulin and dialysis but died after 2 months due to sepsis and rejection. By 1969 the same team reported on their subsequent series of 13 grafts.[4] This series included the whole pancreas placed again in the left lower quadrant with celiac arterial inflow and portal venous outflow into the left iliac vein. In the first few transplants, the exocrine secretions were exteriorized via a duodenostomy.[4] Subsequently, the graft duodenum was anastomosed to the recipient jejunum. In this early era, David Sutherland and the team from Minnesota also performed the first successful living donor partial pancreas transplantation, which was also the first successful extrarenal living donor organ transplant.[5]

Pancreas transplantation in this period was plagued with graft losses due to technical complications such as vascular thrombosis, death with a functioning graft, and lethal complications related to exocrine pancreatic drainage. Immunosuppression and organ preservation were in their infancy, so rejection and ischemia reperfusion injury precipitating severe allograft pancreatitis and dysfunction were common. Progress in the field of transplantation was greatly influenced by the development of better organ preservation techniques such as Collins' solution in 1969,[6] the University of Wisconsin (UW) solution in 1989,[7] and improved immunosuppressive medications such as the calcineurin inhibitors (CNIs) cyclosporine and tacrolimus (see Chapter 104). Due to the high graft failure rate, the concept of draining the exocrine secretions into the urinary system was proposed by Sollinger et al.[8] at The University of Wisconsin (duodenal patch) and by Nghiem and Corry[9] at The University of Iowa (duodenal bubble). This technique had the advantages of eliminating an enteric anastomosis and providing more information about allograft function because the amount of amylase secreted by the pancreas could be measured in the urine. Unfortunately, bladder drainage was also associated with complications such as cystitis, metabolic acidosis, dehydration, reflux pancreatitis, and urethritis. More recently, with continued improvement in surgical techniques for the retrieval, preparation, and transplantation of the allograft, enteric drainage has again become the surgical procedure of choice at most transplant centers for whole organ pancreas transplantation. Pancreas transplant outcomes have also improved over the decades with excellent graft survival and function. The 1-year patient survival and pancreas graft function rates are 97.4% and 91.3% for simultaneous pancreas and kidney transplants, 97.9% and 86% for pancreas after kidney transplants, and 97% and 85.7% for pancreas transplants alone, respectively.[10] The international 5- and 10- year patient survival rates for simultaneous pancreas-kidney transplant (1984–2009) are 90% and 76%, respectively. Pancreatic allograft survival rate is 73% at 5 years and 56% at 10 years; kidney survival rate is 81% at 5 years and 62% at 10 years.[10]

INDICATIONS AND TYPES OF PANCREAS TRANSPLANT (SEE CHAPTER 112)

Pancreas transplantation is traditionally performed in diabetic patients who do not produce insulin. Although it is commonly indicated for type 1 diabetes mellitus, the distinction between type 1 and type 2 diabetes mellitus is becoming less clear. Type 1 diabetics may continue to produce a detectable C-peptide level but inadequate insulin in order to maintain euglycemia, and type 2 diabetics may lose enough β-cell mass that they develop undetectable C-peptide levels.[11] Also, as C-peptide is primarily metabolized in the kidney, levels in end-stage renal disease (ESRD) patients can be disproportionately high and may not be representative of the actual functioning β-cell mass.[12]

It is critical to balance the long-term risk of remaining diabetic versus the risks of a pancreas transplant that includes the risk of the operation itself as well as the risks of immunosuppression (see Chapter 104)—including opportunistic infections and malignancy, some of which may be life threatening. Generally, the risk of remaining diabetic is less than the risks of immunosuppression, so most diabetics would not qualify for a pancreas transplant. However, candidates for a kidney transplant for end-stage diabetic nephropathy require immunosuppression anyway, so the trade-off between immunosuppression and diabetes is greatly lessened in those patients.

For this reason, the most frequent form of pancreas transplant is simultaneous pancreas and kidney transplantation (SPK) for ESRD secondary to diabetic nephropathy in a type 1 diabetic patient. Pancreas after kidney transplantation (PAK) is offered if the candidate has already received a functioning kidney graft or if there is a potential living donor for the kidney. In diabetic patients with preserved renal function, a pancreas transplant alone (PTA) without a kidney transplant would be considered only for immediately life-threatening complications of diabetes such as hypoglycemic unawareness, frequent severe hypoglycemia, hyperglycemia or ketoacidosis, incapacitating clinical and emotional problems with exogenous insulin therapy, failure of medical management in preventing acute complications, or insulin allergy.[13]–15 PTA may also be indicated following total pancreatectomy for nonmalignant disease where the candidates typically manifest a particularly brittle form of diabetes (type 3c diabetes) as theirs is a deficiency of all pancreatic hormones, not just insulin.[16,17] These patients also exhibit pancreatic exocrine insufficiency, which typically resolves following pancreas transplantation with a proximal enteric drained pancreas allograft. PTA has been reported for treatment of generalized allergy to human insulin.[13] Pancreas transplantation can achieve complete reversal of glycogen hepatopathy in certain cases.[18] Simultaneous liver-pancreas transplantation[19] and simultaneous lung-pancreas transplantation[20] have also been successfully accomplished in recipients with cystic fibrosis, and provide both endocrine and exocrine function.

Per current US Organ Procurement and Transplantation Network (OPTN) policy,[21] to qualify for registration for a pancreas transplant, each candidate must meet one of the following requirements:

- Be diagnosed with diabetes
- Have pancreatic exocrine insufficiency
- Require the procurement or transplantation of a pancreas as part of a multiple-organ transplant for technical reasons (e.g., a multivisceral transplant)

To qualify for a combined kidney-pancreas registration, each candidate registered on the kidney-pancreas waiting list must be eligible for the pancreas waitlist and for the kidney waitlist (measured or calculated creatinine clearance or glomerular filtration rate [GFR] less than or equal to 20 mL/min). These patients would also be eligible for a pancreas after kidney were they to have a living donor for the kidney. Waiting time for pancreas begins on the date the candidate is first registered as a candidate on the waiting list. For a combined kidney-pancreas, the candidate begins to accrue waiting time once the candidate has met all of the following conditions: registered for a kidney-pancreas; qualifies for kidney (GFR <20 mL/min or started regular dialysis); and is on insulin.[21] If the patient is on dialysis before listing, the start date for waiting time is back-dated to the date of initiation of dialysis.

Type 2 diabetes was once considered an absolute contraindication to pancreas transplantation, but this is no longer the case. Chakkera et al.,[22] Light et al.,[23,24] and others have shown that insulin secretion and sensitivity improve over the long term in type 2 diabetics who undergo SPK. The percentage of type 2 diabetic (per center reporting) recipients in the United States has increased from 2% in 1995 to 7% in 2010 and then 11.7% in 2015.[25,26] Although poorly understood, it is thought that the transplanted pancreas can overcome insulin resistance. Criteria for selection of type 2 diabetics for pancreas transplantation are essentially the same as for type 1 diabetics, but daily total insulin requirement should not be excessive (perhaps <1 unit/kg/day), and patients should make efforts to lose weight if they are obese.[12,27]

Simultaneous Pancreas and Kidney (SPK) Transplantation

SPK is the most commonly performed combination. Due to kidney allocation policies that favor local but do not mandate regional and national sharing of the kidney with the pancreas, the majority of these transplants require a local suitable donor for both organs, leading to a typically longer waiting time for the combined operation. Patient survival with SPK is clearly superior compared with survival on maintenance dialysis or on the transplant waiting list.[28] SPK also prolongs patient survival beyond the survival advantage associated with kidney transplantation alone from either a deceased or living donor, although this may take up to 4 years to become evident.[29] Quality of life is significantly improved after SPK, with the elimination of hypoglycemia, hyperglycemia, insulin dependence, glucose monitoring, dietary restrictions, and other metabolic abnormalities.[30,31] Long-term insulin independence is achieved in the majority of patients receiving SPK.[32] SPK does not reverse macrovascular disease but it does slow down the progression of cerebrovascular disease, cardiovascular disease, and peripheral vascular disease.[33] Improvements in diabetic neuropathy, as manifested by improvements in nerve conduction velocities and muscle action potentials, have been reported.[34,35] Retinal lesions may improve or normalize after SPK, as manifest by improved visual acuity and decreased vitreous hemorrhage.[36]

Pancreas After Kidney (PAK) Transplantation

PAK transplantation involves kidney transplantation, most frequently from a living donor, followed by subsequent deceased donor pancreas transplantation from a separate donor. PAK transplantation requires two separate operations; there is therefore the inherent risk of undergoing a second course of anesthesia, and the risk of a separate incision. Moreover, the kidney and pancreas allografts will be from separate donors; as a result, the organs may behave independently from an immunologic perspective. Despite this, patient survival is nearly identical to that of an SPK recipient. There are several likely explanations. The PAK transplantation is a shorter operation, and the patient is not uremic at the time of surgery. Also, the patient is already on baseline immunosuppression, which may provide an immunologic advantage. PAK allows one to preempt or shorten the duration of dialysis as well as prevent complications that can occur while waiting for a deceased donor kidney transplant.[37] It is possible to entirely eliminate the second surgery by doing both the living donor kidney transplant and the deceased donor pancreas transplant simultaneously[38]; this eliminates the need for a second course of induction immunosuppression and potentially may provide the best results. The disadvantage of this approach is the necessity to set up a living donor retrieval operation on short notice and the extra resources required to run an extra operating room, potentially at inopportune times.

Even today, pancreas transplantation is frequently considered only a life-enhancing rather than a life-saving procedure. However, abundant evidence indicates that, similar to kidney transplantation, successful pancreas transplantation, in the long term, is clearly life-extending in all three recipient categories. The University of Wisconsin published their experience with 1000 kidney-pancreas transplantations with 22-year follow-up.[29] In this report, patient survival following transplantation of both a kidney and a pancreas was dramatically superior to all other options for type 1 diabetic uremic patients, particularly cadaveric renal transplantation and dialysis (Fig. 126.1). Although not evident for the first 4 to 5 years, with the extended follow-up in this particular study, patient survival following SPK was remarkably superior to that of type 1 diabetic uremic recipients undergoing living donor renal transplant alone, supporting the fact that freedom from diabetes has a clear survival advantage. If the patient ultimately comes off dialysis and insulin, there is a greater patient survival advantage compared with remaining diabetic but free from renal failure.[39] This situation would best be accomplished through immediate living donor kidney transplantation if available followed by PAK transplantation. Additionally, if a kidney pancreas recipient receives a living donor kidney, there would be one more standard criteria kidney available for the deceased donor kidney transplant list. A recent study from the OPTN Pancreas Transplant Committee also indicated that the best long-term renal allograft survival was achieved with the combination of a living donor kidney transplant followed by a pancreas.[40]

Pancreas Transplant Alone (PTA)

Only 8% of all pancreas transplants are performed as PTA.[41] Improved insulin therapy options and pump technologies combined with concern regarding outcomes after PTA has led to a steady decline in the number of PTAs. PTA is associated with higher rejection rates, a higher incidence of chronic rejection, and higher rates of PTLD.[42] Potential explanations for these issues include the typically younger age and the absence of uremia in the patient population, both of which may contribute to a more virile immune system compared with recipients undergoing pancreas transplantation with a kidney. PTA graft survival has continued to improve despite the fact that potential candidates are getting older, more obese, and more sensitized and have more longstanding diabetes. Graft survival is 97% at 1 year and 85.7% at 5 years, comparable to that for SPKs and PAKs.[43]

Living Donor Distal Pancreas Transplantation

There is limited experience with living donor distal pancreas transplantation. The two prominent series, one from the United States and another from Japan, have reported favorable 1-year and 3-year graft survival. They also reported higher technical failure rate but lower rejection rate when compared with deceased donor transplants.[44,45] The prevalence of type 2 diabetes is less than 3% in nonobese donors, and there is not an increased risk of type 1 diabetes. This option is optimal for highly sensitized recipients with an appropriately matched donor and who would otherwise face the longest wait times—assuming a suitable cadaveric recipient is ever identified—and potentially

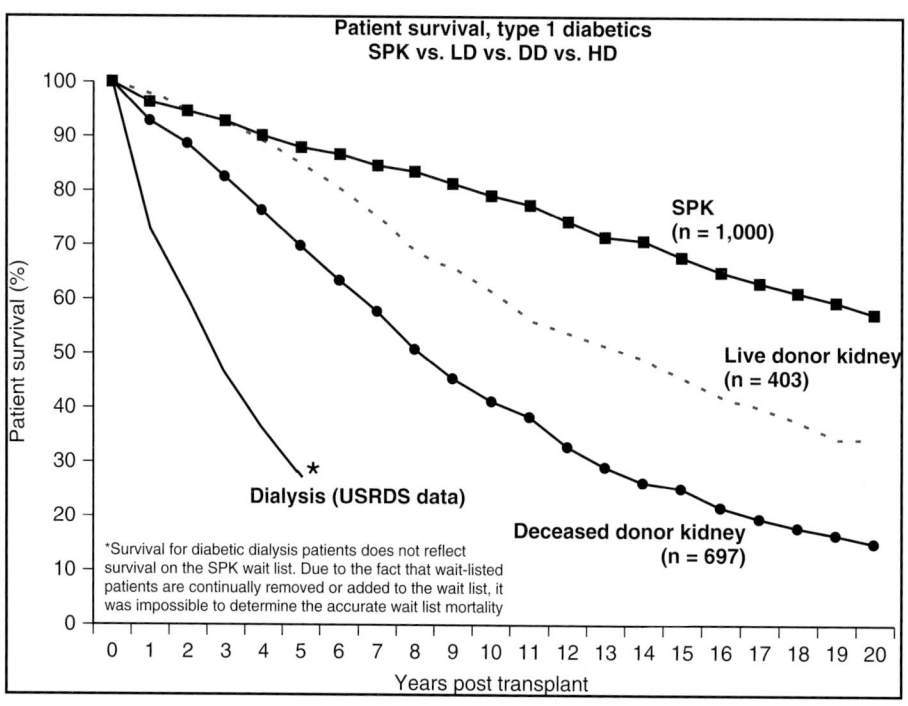

FIGURE 126.1 This graph demonstrates patient survival in type 1 diabetic patients comparing dialysis (United States Renal Data System [USRDS] data), deceased-donor kidney transplantation, live-donor kidney transplantation, and simultaneous pancreas and kidney (SPK) transplantation. Of note, this was a large number of SPK transplants (1000) with 22-year follow-up. Kidney transplantation of any sort in recipients with type 1 diabetes mellitus significantly improves survival compared with remaining on dialysis. Note the significantly improved patient survival in SPK recipients compared with all other types of kidney transplantation, including living donor renal transplantation, which manifests beyond 4 years after transplantation. (From Sollinger HW, Odorico JS, Becker YT, et al. One thousand simultaneous pancreas-kidney transplants at a single center with 22-year follow-up. *Ann Surg.* 2009;250:618–630.)

poorer outcomes. Using a living donor also allows recipient preconditioning and, even though no pancreas transplant has been performed in this setting, increased use of living donor distal pancreas transplantation could even allow for paired donation in certain circumstances.[46]

EVALUATION OF THE PANCREAS TRANSPLANT RECIPIENT (SEE CHAPTER 112)

Type 1 diabetes is frequently diagnosed at a young age and is associated with ESRD at an earlier age compared with other etiologies. There is an increasing trend in the incidence of diabetes and obesity, and with current trends toward increased longevity, there is an increase in the age of candidates referred for pancreas transplantation as well. With the high incidence of gastroparesis in this patient population, there are also many candidates who present malnourished, wasted, and frail. Rather than mandating a strict age or body mass index (BMI) cutoff, it is better to evaluate the recipient for cardiovascular, cerebrovascular, and peripheral vascular comorbidities and decide on a case-by-case basis.[47,48] As they are all diabetic, pancreas transplant candidates have at least one major risk factor for cardiac and vascular disease. Coronary artery disease is associated with 20% 1-year mortality in SPK and PAK recipients. All pancreas transplant candidates should be evaluated for modifiable cardiac conditions and long-term expected survival. Recipients who are older, have had diabetes for more than 25 years, have a smoking history, or are on dialysis should undergo cardiac catheterization, as noninvasive stress test results in these patients have a high incidence of being falsely negative.[49] The remainder of the potential pancreas transplant candidates may undergo a noninvasive stress test with cardiac catheterization if the stress test is positive for coronary ischemia. It may be desirable, however, to avoid contrast administration in patients who are not yet on dialysis or who have significant residual renal function. Coronary artery disease that is not amenable to revascularization is a contraindication to transplantation. Iliac and peripheral arterial pulses should be assessed in all patients. If there are any concerns, calcification and atherosclerosis of the iliac vessels can be evaluated with a computed tomography angiogram (CTA) of the abdomen and pelvis. Severe bilateral iliac or lower-extremity arterial disease or large abdominal aneurysms that are not amenable to intervention are relative contraindications to transplantation, although transplantation may still be accomplished in some cases with arterial reconstruction using donor iliac artery vessels.[50] Recipients with a carotid bruit or high cerebrovascular risk should get a carotid Doppler.

Absolute contraindications to pancreas transplantation include current active infections, malignancy, substance abuse, uncontrolled psychiatric issues, ongoing noncompliance, and shortened life expectancy (life expectancy should at least be greater than the wait time for pancreas ± kidney organ offer). In addition, home oxygen dependence, uncontrolled asthma, severe chronic obstructive pulmonary disease (forced expiratory volume in 1 second [FEV1] <25%), uncorrectable pulmonary hypertension, and frequent lower respiratory infections are absolute pulmonary contraindications. Effective screening tests (such as the Berlin Questionnaire) should be employed to identify patients at high risk for obstructive sleep apnea; these patients should undergo a sleep study for evaluation. All female candidates should have a Papanicolaou (Pap) smear, and those above age 40 should have a screening mammogram. Male patients above 40

should also have a prostate-specific antigen screen. As per guidelines, patients aged 50 and above should be evaluated with a colonoscopy. All patients should also have a gastric emptying study to evaluate for diabetic gastroparesis as this is a very common issue within the diabetic population referred for a pancreas transplant and the most common indication for readmission after transplant. The authors recommend a hypercoagulable workup for all recipients because postoperative thrombosis is a major concern in all cases.

DONOR SELECTION (SEE CHAPTER 112)

Donor selection is critical in pancreas transplantation. Better long-term graft function is associated with donation after brain death, younger age (between 10 and 40 years of age), BMI less than 30 kg/m², and cause of brain death other than cerebrovascular event.[51-53] The Pancreas Donor Risk Index (PDRI) was developed to better predict pancreas allograft survival after transplant and includes 10 donor and one transplant characteristic. The donor factors include donor sex, age, black race, Asian race, BMI, cause of death, creatinine, height, and donation after circulatory death (DCD) status. The transplant factors include pancreas preservation time and an interaction between PAK and the donor cause of death.[54] Another tool used to help predict the likelihood that a donor pancreas will be suitable for transplant is the preprocurement pancreas suitability score (P-PASS). This score takes into consideration the age of the donor (<30, 30–40, >40 years), BMI, intensive care unit stay, cardiac arrest, serum sodium, serum amylase, lipase, need for noradrenaline or dopamine, or dobutamine in the donor. The individual factors were given weighted points and a tally of less than 17 was deemed as a suitable donor. Donors with P-PASS ≥17 were considered suboptimal and three times more likely to be declined.[55] Neither PDRI nor P-PASS has proven to be an absolute prognosticator for donor selection. In fact, excellent outcomes can be achieved with pancreas grafts with individual donor issues such as from DCD donors, older donors,[56] and higher BMI donors[57] when ischemia times are minimized and multiple risk factors rather than individual risk factors per se are avoided.[58]

Finally, pancreases with extensive fibrosis/calcification, intralobular fat (as opposed to peripancreatic fat, which is considered acceptable in many cases), obvious trauma or hematomas, and extensive edema should be discarded.[59] There are no reliable markers for pancreatic ischemia reperfusion injury; the focus should be on minimizing cold ischemia times and increasing post-reperfusion blood flow. Pancreas allografts refused before retrieval by many centers may still be imported and successfully transplanted without affecting survival results, as long as their appearance is acceptable.[60]

SURGICAL TECHNIQUE

The surgical aspects of pancreas transplantation are not just limited to the recipient surgery alone. In fact, an ideal pancreas transplant starts with meticulous procurement, pristine backbench preparation of the allograft, and an immaculate implantation of the organ (also see Chapter 112).

Procurement of the Pancreas From the Deceased Donor

Retrieval of the pancreas from the donor is a critically important step in orchestrating a successful pancreas transplant.

Adequate exposure through a midline incision from the suprasternal notch to the symphysis pubis with either division of the lateral abdominal walls (to form a cruciate incision) or with a wide Balfour retractor is made. Pancreas procurement is usually in conjunction with a liver or a multiorgan procurement. A right medial visceral rotation through a combination of Cattell-Braasch maneuver and an extended Kocher maneuver is performed to expose the infrahepatic vena cava, renal veins, abdominal aorta, and superior mesenteric artery (SMA) (see Chapter 117C). Exposure and mobilization of the pancreas is begun by careful dissection of the gastrohepatic ligament up to the portahepatis, division of the gastrocolic ligament along the greater curvature of the stomach, and ligation and division of short gastric vessels in the gastrosplenic ligament. This provides an excellent view of the pancreas to assess the characteristics of the gland such as the overall appearance, fat content, edema, fibrosis, visible injuries or hematomas, or abnormalities. Mobilization of the spleen by division of lienocolic and lienophrenic ligaments and using the spleen as a handle facilitates careful dissection and subsequent mobilization of the pancreas from the tail toward the head. This technique minimizes handling and potential injury to the pancreas. The portahepatis is then dissected to identify and encircle the gastroduodenal artery (GDA) and bile duct (see Chapters 117A and 117C). The arterial anatomy is further delineated to expose the common hepatic artery, the splenic artery (SA), and the left gastric artery origins (see Chapter 2). The bile duct is ligated at the superior margin of the duodenum. The infrarenal aorta is then cannulated retrograde after systemic heparinization (100 U/kg) and the supraceliac or thoracic aorta is clamped to isolate the abdominal vasculature. The organs are then flushed with a cold preservation solution with concomitant surface cooling with ice slush. The stapling of the small intestine is preferably delayed until after flushing the organs with cold preservative solution, although some surgeons do staple the proximal duodenum just distal to the pylorus in the warm phase. The distal staple division is across the fourth portion of the duodenum or the proximal jejunum. Some groups use a decontamination protocol with povidone-iodine with or without antibiotics and antifungals through a nasoenteric tube. There is no conclusive evidence of any benefits from the decontamination of intestine in the context of enteric drainage. The root of the small bowel mesentery is divided either with a stapler or serial ligation at a good length (at least 2 cm) away from the head of the pancreas so as to avoid injury by inclusion of the inferior pancreaticoduodenal artery into the staple line. The GDA is divided just above the duodenum with the distal end ligated. The splenic artery is divided close to its celiac origin and the SMA is cut with an aortic cuff. The SMA and SA are tagged with a fine monofilament suture to help identify their location because they tend to retract after division. In cases where an accessory or aberrant right hepatic artery is identified arising from the SMA (10%–17% of donors) (see Chapter 2), a cuff of SMA can be retained with the liver or the aberrant hepatic artery can be divided as it passes behind the donor duodenum and pancreas and reconstructed on the liver backbench with anastomosis to the GDA. Since the portal vein is shared between the liver and the pancreas, it is imperative to divide the portal vein so that an adequate length of the portal vein remains available with the pancreas. This is done ideally by dividing it midway between the lower margin of the liver and the upper margin of the pancreas or at least at the level of the coronary (left gastric) vein.

In situations involving intestinal graft procurement, the SMA is shared between the two grafts. A detailed knowledge of the anatomy of the artery is necessary to recognize the various branches arising from the SMA (see Chapter 2). The inferior pancreaticoduodenal artery is vital for maintaining the arterial supply to the head of the pancreas and must be preserved with the pancreas graft. One way of achieving this is to follow the middle colic artery proximally to its origin from the SMA, which usually represents the ideal site for transection of the SMA. The first jejunal branch is usually preserved with the intestinal graft; it can, however, be sacrificed to obtain an adequate length of the SMA for the pancreas and the intestine graft. The superior mesenteric vein (SMV) is dissected distally to the point where there is only a single vessel. Additional length on the SMA and SMV for the intestinal graft is obtained by dissection into the root of the mesentery sacrificing the first jejunal branches or by donor vessels sewn to the SMA and SMV.

Procurement of a pancreas during donation after circulatory death (DCD) is a more challenging process due to the need to achieve cannulation and infusion of cold preservative solution very quickly after declaration of death (see Chapter 109). The principles, however, are the same, without the luxury of meticulous dissection before flushing. The organs can be procured en bloc with the spleen and liver, and then the liver and pancreas can be separated on the back table. Alternatively, they can be separated in situ depending on the comfort level of the procuring surgeon. The experience of the procuring surgeon is a major factor in determining the suitability of a pancreas from a DCD donor for transplantation.

Back-Table Preparation of the Pancreas Allograft (also see Chapter 112)

The preparation of the allograft pancreas on the backbench is crucial as it gives the transplant surgeon a final opportunity to assess the organ, manage any inadequacies or complications from the procurement itself, and plan the implantation. The back-table preparation of the pancreas allograft is a vital step that begins with careful inspection of the pancreas for organ preservation, texture, fatty infiltration, fibrosis, hematomas, visible vascular anomalies, injury, and so on. Usually the inferior mesenteric vein is ligated during the procurement, and the inferior margin of the pancreas is well dissected including ligation of the lienocolic ligament. The spleen is separated from pancreatic tail on the back table by careful ligation of vessels as close as possible to the spleen, taking care not to injure the tail of the pancreas. Meticulous dissection and ligation can avoid hematomas and bleeding from the pancreatic tail after reperfusion. Dissection along the superior margin of the pancreas is not advocated, as the SA, being tortuous in its course and frequently extrapancreatic, is at risk for inadvertent injury. Next the duodenum/jejunal loop is mobilized by careful dissection and ligation of small vessels running between the mesentery and the distal duodenum. The length of the duodenal segment also is dependent on the type of exocrine drainage planned. Usually bladder drainage dictates a shorter segment (4–6 cm) of duodenum than enteric drainage. The small bowel mesentery, which has been stapled across about 2 cm or more away from the head and uncinate process of the pancreas, is reinforced with a running horizontal mattress stitch with a nonabsorbable monofilament suture such as 4-0 polypropylene. Alternatively, many groups propose dissection of the mesentery and individually ligating the blood vessels with double-suture ligation of the SMA and the middle colic artery. The arterial inflow reconstruction to the graft is done using the donor iliac vessels as a Y-graft. The allograft SA and SMA are anastomosed to the internal and external iliac arteries, respectively. Alternate techniques described involve anastomosis of the SA to the side of the SMA, use of an interposition graft between the SA and the SMA, and anastomosis of the SA to the distal end of the SMA in the root of the mesentery.

Recipient Surgery—Pancreas Transplantation

The recipient surgery is begun with a midline incision to enter the peritoneal cavity. The variables in implantation technique involve the venous and exocrine drainage techniques, both of which have two different options. For venous drainage (endocrine drainage), the donor portal vein can be anastomosed to either the systemic circulation (via the external or common iliac vein or the vena cava) or to the portomesenteric venous system, usually via the superior mesenteric vein or a branch. Drainage into the portal circulation results in first-pass metabolism of insulin in the liver resulting in a normal insulin level, whereas systemic drainage bypasses the liver initially and results in higher insulin levels in the circulation. Although portal drainage is more physiologic in theory, long-term graft survival, patient survival, and metabolic effects have not shown any major benefit over systemic drainage.[61] The choice of drainage thus lies entirely with the surgeon, with systemic venous drainage being by far the most common practice.

In the early days of pancreas transplantation, bladder drainage of exocrine secretions was more prevalent.[8,9] This technique has the advantages of eliminating an enteric anastomosis and providing additional information regarding allograft function by monitoring urinary amylase as well as access for possible biopsy. Unfortunately, bladder drainage was also associated with complications such as cystitis, metabolic acidosis, dehydration, reflux pancreatitis, and urethritis. Enteric drainage of the exocrine pancreatic secretions is now the standard of practice, although bladder drainage remains a viable option. Enteric drainage accounts for almost 85% of all pancreas transplants. The technique of enteric drainage requires creation of an anastomosis between the duodenum on the allograft and the native intestine. Native proximal jejunum is preferred as distal jejunal anastomosis is more prone to diarrhea from poor absorption of pancreatic secretions and is inaccessible to endoscopy. Different variations have been tried such as the commonly used side-to-side anastomosis about 45 cm distal to the ligament of Treitz, construction of a roux-en-Y limb for the pancreas drainage, duodenoduodenal anastomosis, and duodenogastric anastomosis.[62–64] The latter two techniques are touted to confer the benefit of the allograft being accessible for monitoring and treatment through endoscopy, endoscopic ultrasound, and endoscopic retrograde cholangiopancreatography. The disadvantage to such a proximal anastomosis is the complexity of allograft pancreatectomy, which would require managing a duodenotomy or gastrostomy. Most surgeons perform a hand-sewn intestinal anastomosis. An alternative way of doing this using an end-to-end anastomotic stapling device was developed by Fridell et al.[65] and was shown to be a safe, fast, and easier approach than the classic hand-sewn technique with reduced risk of spillage and contamination. With a head-up orientation, it is essential that the mesenteric defect created behind the anastomosis be closed by approximation of the native peritoneum around the allograft duodenum in order to prevent internal hernia and volvulus.[66]

In the case of SPK, the kidney is then transplanted by anastomosis of the renal vessels to either the contralateral or ipsilateral external iliac vessels as in a standard kidney transplantation. The site of pancreas implantation in systemic drained SPK transplantation varies among centers. The initial practice was to place the kidney on the left side and the pancreas on the right to the external iliac vessels with the head of the pancreas oriented downward to allow for bladder drainage. With time, it has become more common to implant the pancreas with the head up to facilitate enteric drainage, although enteric drainage is certainly possible with the head-down technique. As such, the site of venous implantation has also moved cranially up the venous system and is now frequently performed directly to the vena cava. Ipsilateral implantation of the pancreas and the kidney on the right side, with systemic venous and enteric exocrine drainage of the pancreas, was first reported in 2004 by Fridell et al.[67] (Fig. 126.2). The advantage of this approach is that the left iliac system is preserved as virgin territory for future use were the recipient to require another kidney.

The sequence of transplantation also varies from center to center. Pancreas followed by kidney shortens the ischemia time for the more sensitive pancreas allograft, renders the patient euglycemic at the time of kidney implantation, and provides better operative exposure for the difficult pancreatic anastomoses. However, since pancreas transplant involves an enteric anastomosis, it makes the field potentially contaminated for the kidney transplant. Also, the presence of the pancreatic tail in the pelvis adds a degree of complexity to the kidney transplantation. There is also concern that the pancreas flow may be jeopardized while exposing for the kidney allograft implantation. Performing the kidney transplant first allows the pancreas

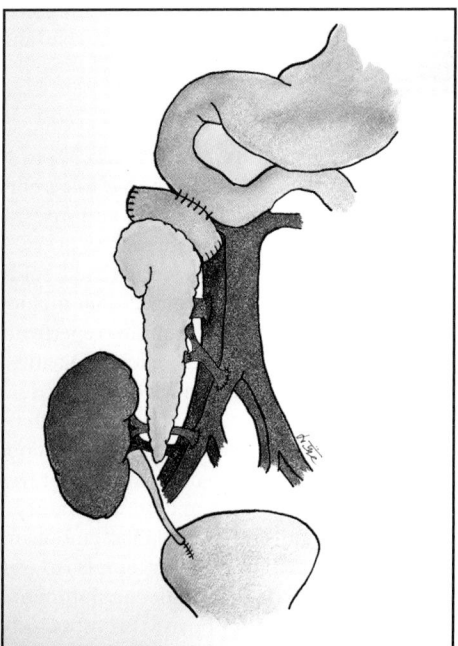

FIGURE 126.2 This is an image demonstrating ipsilateral placement of a simultaneous pancreas and kidney transplant with systemic venous and enteric exocrine drainage. The pancreas transplant is performed initially followed by the kidney transplant. Venous drainage for the pancreas allograft can be performed to either the proximal common iliac vein or to the inferior vena cava. (From Fridell JA, Shah A, Milgrom ML, et al. Ipsilateral placement of simultaneous pancreas and kidney allografts. *Transplantation.* 2004;78[7]:1074–1076.)

transplant portion to be performed in a setting where the patient is making urine, but again care must be taken to avoid malposition of the kidney vasculature while the pancreas is implanted. Either order of implantation is acceptable.

Postoperative admission to the intensive care unit is preferred for close monitoring with frequent blood sugar checks, urine output monitoring, and adequate fluid and electrolyte replacements (see Chapter 26) as well as for monitoring of induction immunosuppression (see Chapter 104). Hyperglycemia is an early indicator of graft problems, and many surgeons have a low threshold for evaluating the graft for perfusion or thrombosis.[68] Ultrasound with Doppler is most commonly used to evaluate blood flow to the grafts because it is immediately available and portable. The timing of the initial ultrasound study is unclear and varies as per surgeon/program preference or protocol, sometimes done as early as in the operating room before waking up from anesthesia.[69] However, early recognition of graft thrombosis is important as it may be amenable to graft thrombectomy and salvage.[68] Emerging data have suggested a role for the use of contrast-enhanced ultrasonography to assess vascular perfusion of the allograft immediately after transplant.[69] There is substantial variation in practice of use of systemic anticoagulation in the immediate perioperative period with heparin.

SURGICAL COMPLICATIONS (ALSO SEE CHAPTERS 28 AND 112)

The technical failure rate in pancreas transplantation is 7% to 9%; the reexploration rate is as high as 35%. Of all early graft losses, 70% are due to technical failures.[70,71] Complications after pancreas transplantation include graft thrombosis, hemorrhage, acute severe allograft pancreatitis, enteric leaks, surgical site infections, intestinal obstruction due to adhesions, or rarely internal herniation of bowel behind the enteric anastomosis with obstruction.

Pancreas Graft Thrombosis

The incidence of pancreas graft thrombosis is 3% to 10%. Risk factors include donor age, donor death due to cerebrovascular accident, donor hemodynamic instability and massive volume resuscitation, suboptimal pancreas organ recovery, preservation and ischemia reperfusion injury, increased cold ischemia time, and isolated pancreas transplantation including PAK and PTA.[72] Other risk factors include reperfusion injury and allograft pancreatitis and CNI toxicity. Diagnosis can be made with ultrasound, CTA, radionucleotide scintigraphy, and conventional angiography. Treatment is most often allograft pancreatectomy, particularly with occlusive thrombosis of the donor portal vein. This is required in order to prevent hemodynamic compromise and systemic inflammatory response from the infarcted organ and pulmonary embolism for systemically drained grafts. However, attempts to salvage the pancreas graft can be made with anticoagulation and thrombolysis for nonocclusive thrombosis, thrombectomy for occlusive thrombosis, and distal graft pancreatectomy for thrombosis limited to the splenic artery or vein. Prevention strategies include atraumatic procurement, low preservation solution flush volumes/pressures, decreased ischemia time, and perhaps low intensity perioperative anticoagulation (although this is controversial). Variations in surgical techniques such as use of a diamond patch from donor vena cava or fence angioplasty of portal vein using donor vena caval patch have been

described.[73,74] Our preference is to keep the donor portal vein as short as possible by transecting as near as possible to the confluence of the splenic vein and the superior mesenteric vein to prevent any lateral kinking that may predispose to thrombosis. The most important aspect of management of this graft-threatening complication is early diagnosis and immediate intervention, which can allow a graft salvage rate of 45% for complete thrombosis.[68]

Bowel Obstruction

As with any abdominal operation, there is a risk of intestinal obstruction from the development of adhesions. The pancreas situated in the retroperitoneum is particularly prone to development of adhesions to loops of intestine. It is our practice to place a lubricating product such as Seprafilm on the front of the pancreas allograft in the retroperitoneum to help prevent adhesion formation. Although rare, if the pancreas is placed with the head oriented cranially and with a proximal jejunal enteric anastomosis, it is possible for bowel to herniate behind the allograft pancreas leading to obstruction (Fig. 126.3). A high index of suspicion and prompt evaluation with an oral contrasted CT scan or a CT enteroclysis may be helpful in early decision making in order to prevent a catastrophic outcome.[66]

Wound and Intraperitoneal Infections and Fistulae

Superficial infections are benign and easily treated. Deep space infections usually occur in the first month and are associated with a high rate of graft loss and increased mortality. Approximately 30% of intraabdominal infections are associated with an anastomotic leak. Diagnosis is most often confirmed via CT scan. Localized infections can be treated with percutaneous drainage. Leaks in enteric-drained pancreases frequently resolve with percutaneous drainage[75] but may occasionally need surgical intervention and may even mandate allograft pancreatectomy; leaks in bladder-drained pancreases can be managed conservatively with percutaneous drainage and a Foley bladder catheter. Addition of oral pancreatic enzyme supplementation may decrease pancreatic exocrine secretion and accelerate healing in these cases.

Graft Pancreatitis

Allograft pancreatitis may be related to ischemia reperfusion injury, prolonged ischemia time, hypotension/hypoperfusion, medication toxicity, or donor issues. Amylase and lipase correlate poorly with severity of allograft pancreatitis and CT scan of the abdomen and pelvis may be necessary (see Chapters 17, 54, and 55). Treatment would include cessation of oral intake and bowel rest (total parenteral nutrition may be required in select cases). Addition of oral pancreatic enzyme supplementation may also be helpful. Reflux pancreatitis in cases of bladder-drained pancreas transplants is treated with Foley catheter placement and other measures to decrease urinary retention; recurrent pancreatitis in such cases is an indication to convert to enteric drainage.

Bleeding

Bleeding is the most frequent indication for relaparotomy but is only responsible for 0.3% of graft losses. Postsurgical bleeding or anticoagulation-associated bleeding is usually salvageable; however, bleeding from an arterial pseudoaneurysm must be urgently ruled out by CT or percutaneous angiography of the iliac arterial system (see Chapter 28). Endovascular management is

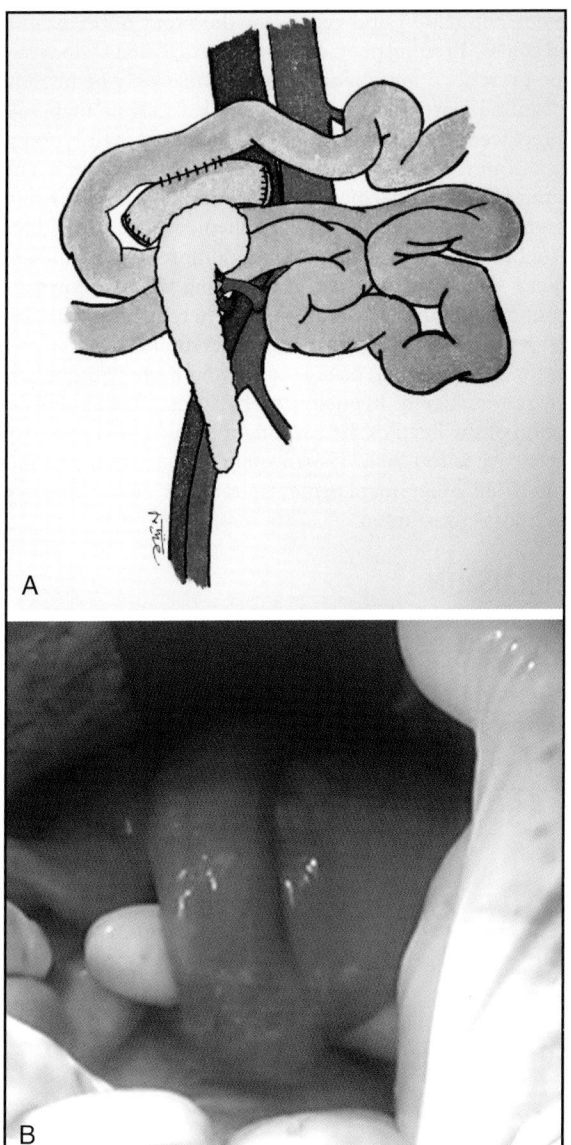

FIGURE 126.3 This illustration **(A)** and photograph **(B)** demonstrate the potential retropancreatic internal hernia defect, which could be a source for bowel obstruction, volvulus, intestinal infarction, or disruption of the enteric anastomosis. It is prudent to close this defect using the reflected peritoneal edge that was incised during mobilization of the colon and intestine at the beginning of the operation. (Adapted from Agarwal A, Maglinte DD, Goggins WC, et al. Internal hernia after pancreas transplantation with enteric drainage: an unusual cause of small bowel obstruction. *Transplantation.* 2005;80[1]:149–152.)

preferred for pseudoaneurysms (see Chapter 115), although graft salvage is usually not possible with this approach.[76] Similarly, enteral bleeding from the enteric anastomosis or hematuria for bladder-drained allografts can be managed expectantly initially but may require endoscopy if the enteric anastomosis is proximally placed, cystoscopy for bladder-drained allografts, or rarely laparotomy. Late gastrointestinal bleeding may be investigated initially with push enteroscopy with visualization of the enteric anastomosis, but failure to identify a source may indicate a herald bleed from an arterioenteric fistula. Urgent CT or percutaneous arterial angiography of the iliac arterial system is essential to rule out this potentially life-threatening complication,

and an endovascular approach with stent placement covering the origin of the donor iliac artery Y graft is potentially lifesaving in these cases.[76]

Immunosuppression (also see Chapter 104)

With the introduction of the CNIs cyclosporine and tacrolimus, acute rejection of the pancreas allograft has become much less common. The use of lymphocyte-depleting antibodies such as rabbit antithymocyte globulin or alemtuzumab for induction has further improved short-term survival. Dual maintenance therapy with mycophenolic acid and CNI has markedly enhanced long-term graft and patient survival. The combination of CNI and mammalian target of rapamycin inhibitors such as sirolimus or everolimus appears also to be an effective alternative, particularly in the setting of rapid steroid withdrawal, with excellent graft survival and low rejection rates.[77] For maintenance therapy, more than 80% of SPK patients receive tacrolimus and mycophenolate mofetil. Steroids are used in about 60% of recipients; however, there has been recent interest and an increasing trend toward steroid avoidance.[78] The combination of CNI and sirolimus appears to be safe and effective in the setting of rapid steroid withdrawal, with excellent graft survival and low rejection rates.

Complications and Side Effects of Immunosuppression (see Chapters 104 and 112)

Most pancreas transplant recipients will have an infection in the first year. Infection is the second most common cause of readmission in the first 3 months and the most common cause of readmission over the long term. Early infections are due to reactivation of preexisting disease, transplant wound infections, urinary tract infections, and infected intravenous catheters. Late infections include opportunistic infections, chronic viral illnesses, and community-acquired infections. Preexisting diabetic neuropathy/peripheral vascular disease can make patients susceptible to infections of the feet, and superficial infections can progress to deep-tissue infections and osteomyelitis.[79] Cytomegalovirus infection in pancreas transplants can be tissue invasive (24%) and have adverse effects on patient and graft survival.

BK virus, a type of Polyoma virus, is frequently seen in immunosuppressed patients. BK virus nephropathy of the transplanted kidney in SPK or PAK recipients is a reversible cause of renal allograft failure, when recognized early. The cornerstone of management of viral infections in transplant recipients involves reduction of immunosuppression.[80,81]

The most common cancers that occur in transplant patients are skin cancers. Post-transplant lymphoproliferative disorders (PTLDs) are the second most common cancers; non-Hodgkin's lymphoma is the most common PTLD. PTLDs in SPK may be more common than or comparable with kidney alone transplants; the risk of death is low (<0.6%) because treatment is effective, particularly with the use of rituximab for CD20-positive cancers. Other cancers that have been reported in pancreas transplants include hepatocellular cancer due to hepatitis B or C and papillomavirus-associated cancers of the cervix/vulva/perineum, as well as sarcoma in allograft pancreas.[82] Age-related cancer screening, sun screen, pelvic examinations, and barrier contraception are recommended.[79]

LONG-TERM COMPLICATIONS OF DIABETES

Long-term diabetes mellitus is frequently associated with cardiovascular, cerebrovascular, peripheral vascular, neurologic, renal, and ophthalmologic complications. Some of these complications, such as microvascular disease, nephropathy, and retinopathy, improve with improved glycemic control.[83] Some of the others, such as gastroparesis and autonomic neuropathy, may have a large impact on the postoperative course after pancreas transplantation.

Gastroparesis has a considerable impact on the quality of life in diabetics. It is prudent to screen for undiagnosed gastroparesis in pancreas transplant candidates as issues with nausea and vomiting after transplant can lead to extended hospital stays and frequent readmissions. Medical management with prokinetic agents is limited mostly to metoclopramide as other available agents are either not approved in the United States (cisapride and domperidone) or interact with the immunosuppression medications, particularly tacrolimus (erythromycin). Ideally, postoperative narcotic usage should be minimized through use of nonnarcotic analgesic alternatives such as transversus abdominal plane blocks.[84] Some of the narcotic impact on colonic function can be mitigated through use of medications such as methylnaltrexone or alvimopan. Endoscopic pyloric injection of botulinum toxin can ameliorate symptoms for short periods of time, but repeated therapy is often needed. Newer endoscopic approaches such as gastric per-oral endoscopic (pyloro) myotomy (G-POEM) have reported successful resolution of symptoms of gastroparesis, but long-term data are lacking. Surgical interventions including gastric electrical stimulator placement, pyloroplasty, gastrojejunostomy, and subtotal gastrectomy have been described with mixed results.

Autonomic neuropathy usually manifests as orthostatic hypotension and may be particularly troublesome after SPK where diuresis of the new kidney and high-volume intravenous fluid replacement complicate the picture. It has been suggested that this phenomenon may be specific to the pancreas transplant recipient population and related to the rapid normalization of blood sugars. Pretransplant antihypertensive medications should not be prescribed automatically and should only be introduced with caution, particularly if the patient is receiving high-volume fluid replacements. In fact, in order to support their blood pressure, it is not unusual for postoperative pancreas recipients to require additional pharmacotherapy such as midodrine, fludrocortisone, pyridostigmine, methylphenidate, or droxidopa to control blood pressure fluctuations. Compression garments and adequate salt intake also aid in balancing venous return to the heart and maintaining volume status, thereby improving orthostasis. It may be necessary to tolerate supine hypertension in order for the patients to be able to stand upright without becoming symptomatically hypotensive. In some cases, a 30-degree elevation of the head of the bed might be indicated if the supine hypertensive is too high. If orthostatic hypotension remains resistant to all other management strategies, home intravenous fluids may be warranted.

CONCLUSION

Pancreas transplantation has come a long way since the first attempts in 1966. With advances in surgical technique, improvements in immunosuppression, and effective diagnosis and management of immunologic events after transplantation, patient and graft survival are excellent and continue to improve. A national initiative is needed to reinvigorate SPK, PAK, or PTA as the preferred transplant options for both type 1 diabetics and type 2 diabetics with or without chronic kidney disease stage V or dialysis dependence.[85]

The references for this chapter can be found online by accessing the accompanying Expert Consult website.

Minimally invasive techniques in HPB surgery: Laparoscopic and robotic: General principles and considerations

T. Peter Kingham

Hepato-pancreato-biliary (HPB) surgery has traditionally lagged other surgical fields in application of minimally invasive techniques. In urology, gynecology, and colorectal surgery, for example, both laparoscopic and robotic approaches are frequently used for the most common procedures performed by surgeons in these fields. Because of the complexity of many HPB resections, uptake has been slower. In the past 10 years, however, with the growth of robotic surgery and expansion of laparoscopic surgery, this is beginning to change. Randomized control trials have now demonstrated significant improvements in outcomes such as length of stay for some minimally invasive surgery (MIS) HPB procedures.[1]

The general principles of MIS techniques for HPB surgery mirror and expand on those of open HPB surgery: appropriate selection of patients, training, and knowledge of anatomy. Appropriate selection of patients is vital to successful outcomes for MIS HPB procedures. For liver resections there are several published guidelines that demonstrate a stepwise approach to selecting patients for MIS liver resection.[2] Cases early in a surgeon's learning curve can be in easily accessible segments of the liver (such as segment III) and later in a career can be highly complex areas (such as segment VII). Attention to selecting patients for MIS liver resections has altered the idea of major and minor liver resections for MIS cases, as some smaller resections (segment VII) are more complex than larger resections (left hepatectomy). The same MIS specific selection criteria exist for MIS pancreas resections. When starting an MIS pancreaticoduodenectomy program, for example, it is patients with a dilated pancreas duct and no vascular involvement who are ideal candidates.

Appropriate training is a major challenge because the learning curves for MIS HPB cases are often steep. For current trainees, many training programs do not have adequate volume for trainees to leave their training ready to perform complex MIS HPB cases. Instead, the focus for training should be in the foundations of HPB surgery to build a comfort level with HPB surgery in general, and as much MIS training as possible. This gives the trainee an adequate foundation to continue their growth as an MIS surgeon in their early career years. For surgeons already in practice, there are different learning curves: open to MIS and laparoscopic to robotic. Each is different and depends on the surgeons open surgery comfort level and volume of open and MIS cases. The challenge of broadening and improving training is one of the major topics confronting the field of HPB surgery. This was evident in a trial of laparoscopic versus open pancreatoduodenectomy.[3] There was an association between the laparoscopic technique and more complication-related deaths, along with no difference in time to functional recovery. It is possible that advances in real-time and virtual simulation can play a role in addressing current and future training needs.

Knowledge of anatomy, although important for open HPB procedures, is even more vital in MIS approaches, given less/no tactile feedback, inability to manually palpate structures, sometimes extreme patient positioning, and alteration of normal visual cues. In addition, intraoperative ultrasound is more challenging to perform and interpret in MIS cases. Given the wide availability of videos for both laparoscopic and robotic cases, there is an immense global library to assist surgeons in building the virtual three-dimensional models needed to successfully navigate MIS HPB cases.

The next chapters address the technical considerations of performing HPB procedures, with many chapters highlighting the MIS approach. These are a useful starting point for surgeons interested in broadening their HPB surgery skills.

Minimally invasive distal and central pancreatectomy

Shiva Jayaraman and Brittany Dalia Greene

INTRODUCTION

Minimally invasive distal and central pancreatectomies are well accepted as safe and effective surgical approaches for the management of left-sided pancreatic lesions.[1,2] Several variations exist in the minimally invasive techniques, which will be detailed in this chapter. The indications and outcomes for minimally invasive compared with open approaches are addressed elsewhere (see Chapters 117B and 127).

LAPAROSCOPIC DISTAL PANCREATECTOMY

The two most common approaches for pancreatic mobilization in minimally invasive distal pancreatectomy are the medial and lateral approaches. A retrospective cohort study of 43 patients compared the medial and lateral approaches and demonstrated shorter operative times and less blood loss with the lateral approach, with no significant differences in rate of successful splenic preservation or rate of conversion to an open procedure.[3] The choice of approach may depend on the lesion or anatomic factors intraoperatively. The techniques described in this chapter can be used in conjunction with one another to facilitate safe and optimal resection depending on the circumstances of the case.

Patient Positioning and Port Placement

The right lateral decubitus position is the most favorable positioning because of its excellent exposure (Fig. 127B.1).[3] The patient may also be secured in a modified right lateral decubitus in a 15- to 30-degree decubitus position for a more centrally located lesion.[2] In these positions, gravity aids in retraction to facilitate exposure of the pancreas body and tail.[3] With the bed flexed to expose more of the abdomen, the bed is tilted right side down. This position, combined with Reverse Trendelenburg will maximize gravity exposure of the tail and body of the pancreas.[3] Left-side down tilting of the bed will flatten the patient to near supine and improve exposure of the neck of the pancreas and access to the portal vein–superior mesenteric vein (SMV) trunk.[2] Alternatively, the patient can be positioned in the French position, supine on a split-leg operating table, allowing an assistant to work from between the patient's legs.[4]

The surgeon works from the patient's right side. The procedure generally requires four to five trocars, as demonstrated in Fig. 127B.1, and a 30-degree laparoscope. A 10-mm supraumbilical port, offset 1 cm to the left and cephalad, is the camera port. Two 5-mm ports are placed in the epigastrium, one along the left lateral costal margin, and a 12-mm port at the left midclavicular line, in line with the camera port at the supraumbilical level.

Exposure of the Pancreas

Start with mobilizing the splenic flexure of the colon to facilitate exposure of the inferior edge of the pancreas (see Chapters 117B and 117C). Begin with the lateral attachments of the proximal descending colon, dividing along the white line of Toldt, then around the splenic flexure. Bluntly separate the plane between the mesocolon and Gerota's fascia. Once completely mobilized, gravity will retract the colon down and medially, away from the left upper quadrant (Fig. 127B.2). Divide short gastric vessels using an energy device, from caudad from cephalad. Enter into the lesser sac near the splenic hilum and divide the gastrocolic ligament from lateral to medial, which facilitates the stomach to medialize and the transverse colon to drop down, while avoiding dangling tissue from obscuring the view of the pancreas.[5]

If the stomach remains an impediment to optimal exposure of the pancreas, gastric suspension can be achieved in several ways. A mechanical retractor, such as the Nathanson liver retractor, can be set up to retract the stomach. An assistant with a grasper may be used for the duration of the dissection. Alternatively, the "stomach roll-up technique" may provide steady retraction, by rotating the stomach on its longitudinal axis and suspending it upwards toward the abdominal wall. In this technique, the falciform is divided and an Endoloop is used to ligate the round ligament. The round ligament and Endoloop are passed through the lesser sac, deep to the stomach, then out through the anterior abdominal wall with a suture passer device.[6]

Mobilization of the Pancreas

After the pancreas is exposed, begin dividing the peritoneum along the inferior border of the pancreas, from lateral to medial (see Chapters 117B and 117C). Vascular structures, including the inferior mesenteric vein and the SMV at its confluence with the splenic vein, are useful landmarks that are encountered along the inferior border of the pancreas (see Chapter 2). To aid in recognition of the SMV, the right gastroepiploic vein can be identified and followed into the SMV. These structures serve as landmarks for the extent of medial mobilization. Direct visualization of the lesion is important to guide the choice of site for pancreatic transection. The spleen may be medialized en-bloc with the pancreas by dividing its ligamentous attachments.

During mobilization, it may be difficult to visualize the index lesion. Indeed, some lesions may not be directly visible at all. Laparoscopic intraoperative ultrasound is a helpful tool to identify occult lesions (see Chapter 24). Ultrasound can also be used to confirm margins of a visible lesion before pancreatic transection.

Medial Approach to Laparoscopic Distal Pancreatectomy
Continued Mobilization and Resection

With the pancreas exposed as previously described, identify the optimal site of planned transection with division of the peritoneal attachments along the inferior border of the pancreas from

Port & Surgical Positioning

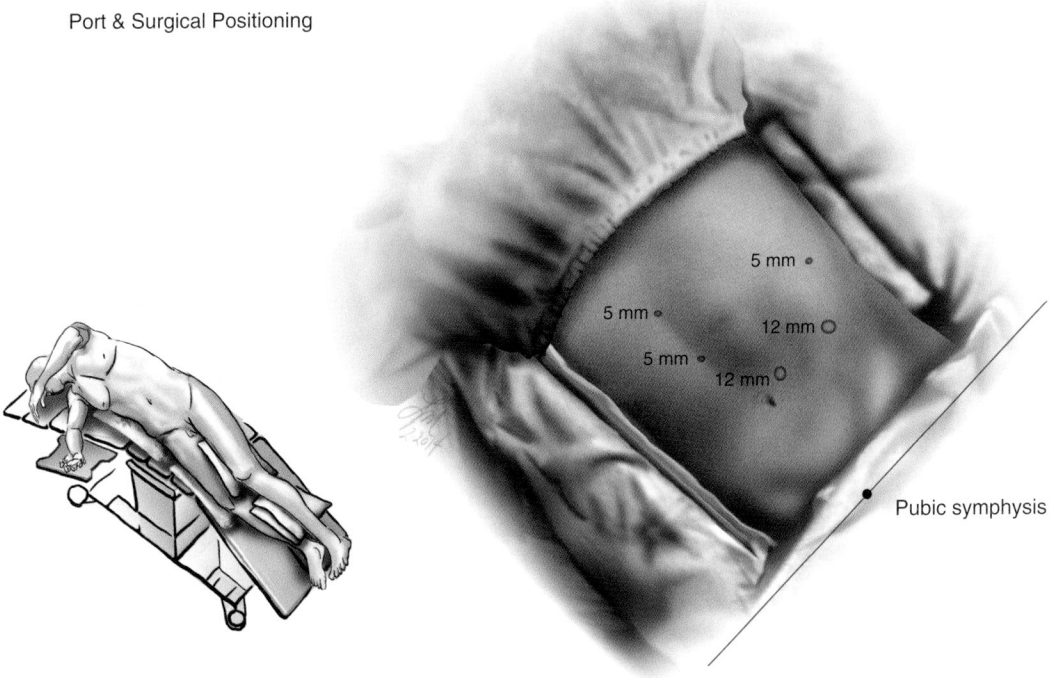

© 2014 Shiva Jayaraman. Illustrated by Laura Maaske

FIGURE 127B.1 Port placement and patient positioning for laparoscopic distal pancreatectomy. (Courtesy Dr. Shiva Jayaraman.)

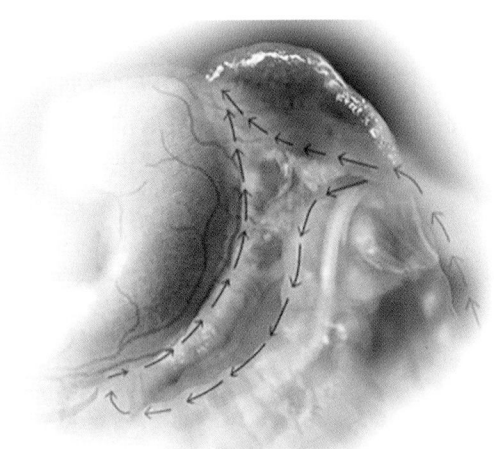

FIGURE 127B.2 Dissection plane for exposure of pancreas for distal pancreatectomy. (Courtesy Dr. Shiva Jayaraman.)

lateral to medial (see Chapter 117B). Then, develop a retropancreatic tunnel, elevating the pancreas off of the retroperitoneum, such that a Penrose drain or vessel loop can be passed through the tunnel, around the pancreas. The approach to the splenic vessels depends on the extent of planned pancreatic resection and whether or not splenic preservation is being attempted. If the transection site is to the left of the celiac axis, the splenic artery and vein can be transected en-bloc with the pancreas. If the pancreas gland is too thick to accommodate a stapler for en-bloc transection, the parenchyma of the pancreas may be thinned using an energy device to accommodate the stapler fitting across the gland and the vessels.[7] If the transection site is at the neck, the tunnel must be developed between the pancreas and SMV–

portal vein trunk.[8] The pancreas should be encircled independently, separate from any vessels. Dissect the inferior and posterior pancreas off the splenic vein and identify the splenic artery. It is crucial to identify the junction of the splenic artery with the celiac trunk and hepatic artery (see Chapter 2). After transection of the pancreas, additional mobilization posterior to the splenic vessels will facilitate division of the vascular pedicle, if indicated. Visualize the pancreatic transection line and remain to the left of that staple line, to divide the splenic artery and vein with a vascular stapler. This landmarking ensures the hepatic artery is protected. As an additional safety check, the splenic artery can be occluded and a Doppler ultrasound performed on the porta to confirm hepatic artery patency before division of the splenic artery (see Chapter 24).

Elevate the transected distal pancreas toward the anterior abdominal wall. Working from medial to lateral, develop the plane between the posterior surface of the pancreas and Gerota's fascia, preserving the left adrenal gland in the retroperitoneum. The left renal vein will course in proximity to the dissection plane and caution should be exercised to ensure it is not damaged. Progressing laterally, the spleen is reached. Divide the splenorenal and splenophrenic ligaments with an energy device to liberate the spleen and distal pancreas.

Lateral Approach to Laparoscopic Distal Pancreatectomy

Continued Mobilization and Resection

The peritoneum along the inferior border of the pancreas is divided as previously described. The peritoneal attachments of the superior border of the pancreas are separated next. If spleen is to be preserved, identify the tip of the tail of the pancreas at the splenic hilum, elevate it, and dissect the pancreas off of the splenic vessels, dissecting from lateral to medial, dividing small branches of the splenic vessels to the pancreas with an energy device (Fig. 127B.3).[5] Alternatively, if splenectomy is to be performed, divide the inferior, lateral, and superior splenic attachments and elevate the pancreas with the spleen, posterior to the splenic vessels, dissecting from lateral to medial, to develop a plane between Gerota's fascia and the posterior surface of the pancreas. Once mobilized well beyond the lesion, divide the pancreas parenchyma and the splenic vessels, either separately or en-bloc as previously described, with the laparoscopic stapler.

Stapler Choice and Technique for Pancreatic Transection

The choice of stapler may be tailored to the characteristics of the pancreas parenchyma and whether vasculature is included. A 4.8 mm staple height is most commonly used for pancreas parenchyma in isolation. Shorter stapler height (e.g., 2.5–3.5 mm) is suitable when the parenchyma is thin and vessels are excluded.[2] A reinforced staple line may be selected for parenchymal transection.[2] If there are concerns about the seal of the staple line of the pancreatic stump, consider buttressing the staple line with a synthetic sealant patch.[9] Alternatively, the staple line can be oversewn with transpancreatic sutures (see Chapter 117B).

The stapler should be closed in a very slow, gradual, stepwise fashion to avoid shearing through the parenchyma.[2] Automatic powered liner staplers are preferable to manual staplers because they fire at a steady pace while the surgeon holds the stapler still, minimizing any sawing motions through the delicate parenchyma.[2] Multiple firings of a 60-mm linear stapler may be required for complete transection.

Splenic vessels are often ligated separately from parenchymal transection, especially the splenic artery when transection occurs close to the celiac axis (see Chapter 117B). Some equipoise exists regarding the safety of dividing the splenic vein en-bloc with the pancreatic parenchyma. A pancreatic fistula after distal pancreatectomy could result in enzymatic degradation to the staple line of the splenic vein stump, leading to intra-abdominal hemorrhage. A multicenter randomized controlled

trial is underway to address the safety of splenic vein resection with pancreatic parenchyma, compared with separated resection after isolation of the parenchyma in distal pancreatectomy (COSMOS-DP trial).[10]

Extraction

Place the specimen within an endoscopic retrieval bag, oriented such that the transected border of the pancreas faces the opening of the bag.[2] Extract the pancreas first, then morcellate the spleen with a finger fracture technique or using ring or sponge forceps at its hilum to facilitate extraction through a small incision.[2] For larger specimens, a Pfannenstiel incision may be used to extract the specimen.[3] Alternatively, the 12-mm supraumbilical trocar site can be extended several cm for extraction.[2] A Pfannenstiel incision may be preferable. In the colorectal literature, the Pfannenstiel is associated with lower rates of incisional hernia than midline extraction sites.[11,12]

Completing the Procedure

Close the fascia of the extraction site then re-insufflate. Inspect the pancreatic staple line to ensure adequate hemostasis. Reinforce the staple line with clips or sutures if needed for any hematoma. Routine drain placement is not recommended for most minimally invasive distal pancreatectomies. Drains may be associated with increased morbidity, longer hospital stay, higher pancreatic fistula rates, and more readmissions.[13] If drains are placed, evidence supports early removal, based on drain fluid amylase concentrations on postoperative days 1 and 3, in addition to the quality of effluent and volume (see Chapter 28).[14]

SPLENIC PRESERVATION

Two surgical approaches to spleen preservation (see Chapter 117B) are detailed in the following sections. In a comparative study of patients undergoing laparoscopic spleen-preserving distal pancreatectomy, the rate of spleen conservation was significantly higher in patients who had intention-to-treat splenic vessel preservation. When splenic vessel injury occurred or difficulties were encountered during dissection, conversion to Warshaw technique resulted in splenic salvage for a large portion of the patients.[15] A recent systematic review and meta-analysis of the two technique suggests shorter operative time and lower blood loss with the Warshaw technique, at the expensive of higher rates of perigastric varices and splenic infarction.[16]

Splenic Vessel Preservation Technique

This technique requires sparing of the splenic artery and vein (Fig. 127B.4). Although more technically challenging, it assures adequate blood supply to the spleen. The splenic artery and vein are isolated from the pancreas and dissected off with an energy device to control small branching vessels that supply the pancreas.[15] This dissection of the splenic vessels off the pancreas can be performed medial to lateral, or lateral to medial, as previously described.

Warshaw Technique

This technique, first described by Warshaw in 1988, involves ligating the splenic artery and vein with preservation of the short gastric and left gastroepiploic vessels (Fig. 127B.5). Caution must be exercised when dividing the gastrocolic ligament

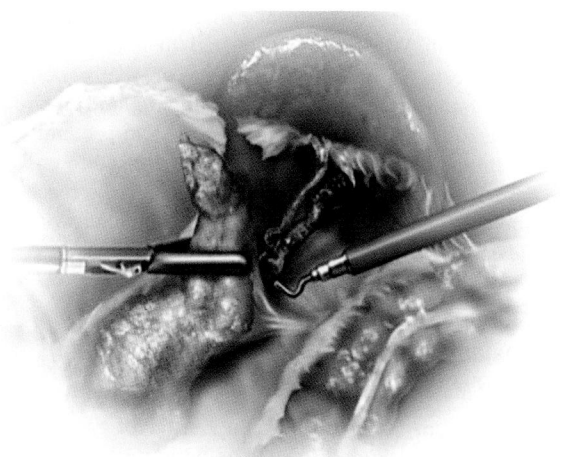

FIGURE 127B.3 Mobilization of pancreas off of splenic vessels. (Courtesy Dr. Shiva Jayaraman.)

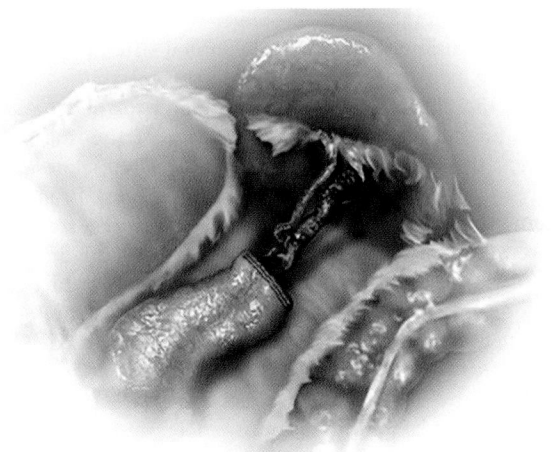

FIGURE 127B.4 Spleen-preserving distal pancreatectomy with vessel preservation. (Courtesy Dr. Shiva Jayaraman.)

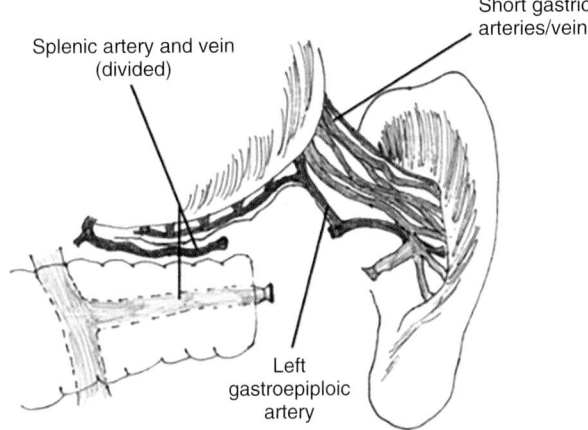

FIGURE 127B.5 Warshaw technique of spleen-preserving distal pancreatectomy with ligation of the splenic artery and vein and preservation of the short gastric and left gastroepiploic vessels. (Courtesy Dr. Andrew L. Warshaw and Dr. Cristina R. Ferrone.)

to preserve the vessels. During pancreatic transection, the splenic artery and vein are divided. The vessels are divided again as they exit the pancreatic tail to enter the splenic hilum.[17] Upon completion of the resection, assess adequacy of splenic perfusion by inspecting the spleen's colour and quantifying areas of clear demarcation. Localized infarction is tolerable if it involves less than half the spleen surface.[18] The Warshaw technique has a very low risk of postoperative splenic infarction as evidenced in a series of 158 patients over 23 years; of those patients, only 1.9% required reoperation for splenectomy, and there were no clinically relevant long-term adverse events observed.[18]

CENTRAL PANCREATECTOMY

Laparoscopic central pancreatectomy is less frequently performed and less well-described in the literature compared with laparoscopic distal pancreatectomy.[19–21] Central pancreatectomy requires reconstruction of the pancreatic duct, which is more technically challenging than the resection without reconstruction of a distal pancreatectomy (see Chapter 117B).

The patient should be positioned in lithotomy or split legs, so that the surgeon may stand between the patient's legs for the reconstruction. Port placement is demonstrated in Fig. 127B.6. A laparoscopic fixed liver retractor may be used to improve exposure. Initial exposure and mobilization of the pancreas is similar to that previously described for a laparoscopic distal pancreatectomy, with mobilization of the splenic flexure, division of the gastrocolic ligament, and dissection along the inferior border of the pancreas from lateral to medial.

Extend the pancreas mobilization medially to the pancreatic neck. Develop a retropancreatic window to expose the confluence of the SMV and splenic vein. Place an umbilical tape around the pancreas through the retropancreatic tunnel to aid in retraction. Identify and preserve the common hepatic and gastroduodenal artery. Perform the medial transection of the pancreas with a stapler. Retract the distal pancreas anteriorly and separate it from the splenic vessels with an energy device for the lateral extent necessary to obtain an adequate margin.

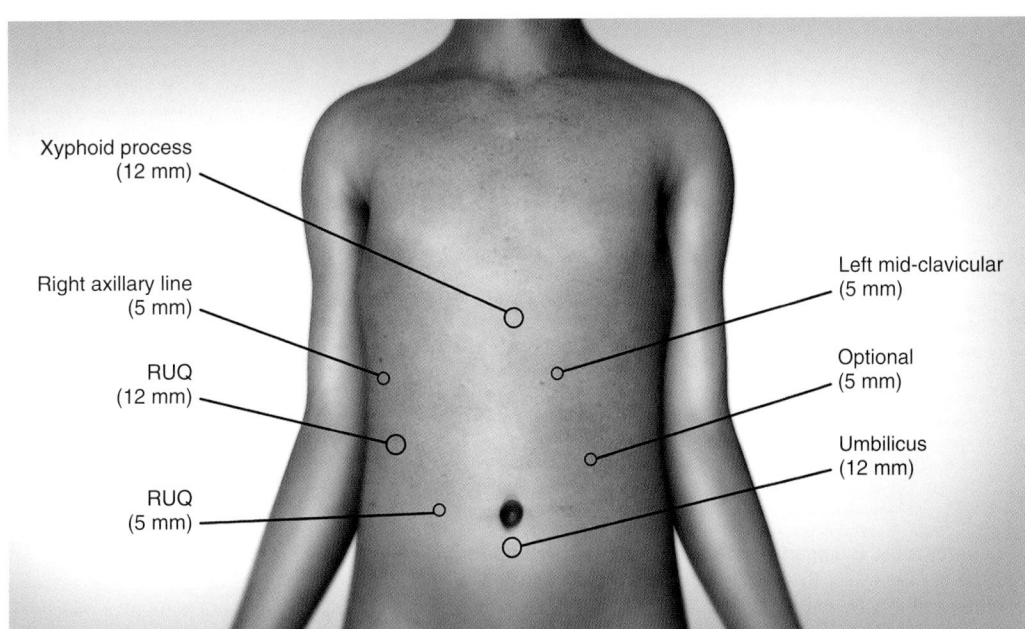

FIGURE 127B.6 Port placement for laparoscopic central pancreatectomy. (Copyright Toronto Video Atlas of Surgery.)

Divide the distal pancreas with an energy device or electrocautery. Place the central pancreas specimen into an endoscopic retrieval bag. Additional mobilization of the distal pancreas may be required to relieve tension on the pancreatic remnant for reconstruction.

RECONSTRUCTION (SEE CHAPTERS 117A AND 117B)

Anastomosis must be performed to establish continuity between the main pancreatic duct of the distal pancreas and the alimentary tract. The options for reconstruction include a laparoscopic pancreaticojejunostomy or pancreaticogastrostomy. Likely because of its scarce performance, no comparative studies exist on the optimal reconstruction after laparoscopic central pancreatectomy. Pancreaticogastrostomy is technically simpler to perform and may be necessary when the main pancreatic duct is very small or not identified.[20]

Laparoscopic Pancreaticojejunostomy (Blumgart Technique; see Chapter 117A)

This technique is inspired by the open Blumgart pancreaticojejunostomy,[22,23] with modifications to facilitate its execution within the constraints of laparoscopy. The goal of the Blumgart style pancreaticojejunostomy is to create an invagination within the small bowel that encapsulates the remnant pancreas with a duct-to-mucosa anastomosis located on the antimesenteric side of the bowel (Fig. 127B.7).[23,24] Develop a Roux-en-Y jejunal limb and bring it up to the pancreatic remnant in a retrocolic fashion, to the right of the middle colic vessels. Line up the antimesenteric side of the bowel with the cut edge of the distal pancreas.

To begin, place an interrupted 3-0 braided absorbable transpancreatic suture through the full thickness of the pancreas to the seromuscular layer of the antimesenteric jejunum, parallel to the long axis of the jejunum.[24] Full-thickness suture through the pancreas prevents tearing of the pancreas

and relieves tension on the duct-to-mucosa anastomosis. Place an additional seromuscular jejunal stitch perpendicular to the long axis of the bowel to "turn the corner."[24] This helps buttress the corner of the pancreas gland to the small bowel serosa, further securing the outer layer of the anastomosis. Advance the suture back through the full thickness of the pancreas and tie it down, leaving the needle on. Proceed with placement of additional transpancreatic sutures, securing the pancreas to the jejunum, from cranial to caudad, until the level of the pancreatic duct.[24] In an open procedure, all sutures of the posterior wall would be placed first, followed by the duct-to-mucosa anastomosis. Because of limited exposure and dexterity in a laparoscopic field, in contrast to the open technique, the duct-to-mucosa anastomosis is completed before placement of additional transpancreatic sutures.[20]

Create an enterotomy in the jejunum, directly opposite to the pancreatic duct. The duct-to-mucosa anastomosis incorporates the pancreatic duct, parenchyma, and full-thickness of the jejunum. The anastomosis typically requires four to six interrupted sutures, placed at 3, 6, 9, and 12 o'clock positions, beginning at 6 o'clock, and ending with the 12 o'clock position, with a 5-0 monofilament suture. Drive the suture from in-to-out on the duct, and out-to-in on the jejunum at the 3, 6, and 9 o'clock positions, and from out-to-in on the duct and in-to-out on the jejunum for the final 12 o'clock position.[24] Tie and cut each suture as progressing through the duct-to-mucosa anastomosis.

Place additional transpancreatic sutures to pull the small bowel posterior to the pancreas, partially creating the small bowel invagination. The same principle of "turning the corner" applies to the final posterior wall suture to buttress the cut surface of the pancreas against the serosa.[24] The seromuscular edge of the jejunum is rolled over onto the pancreatic parenchyma and the anterior wall is completed with the transpancreatic interrupted sutures, using the saved needles from the posterior wall. The "turning the corner" stitches are again performed at the caudad and cranial most stitches of the anterior wall.[24]

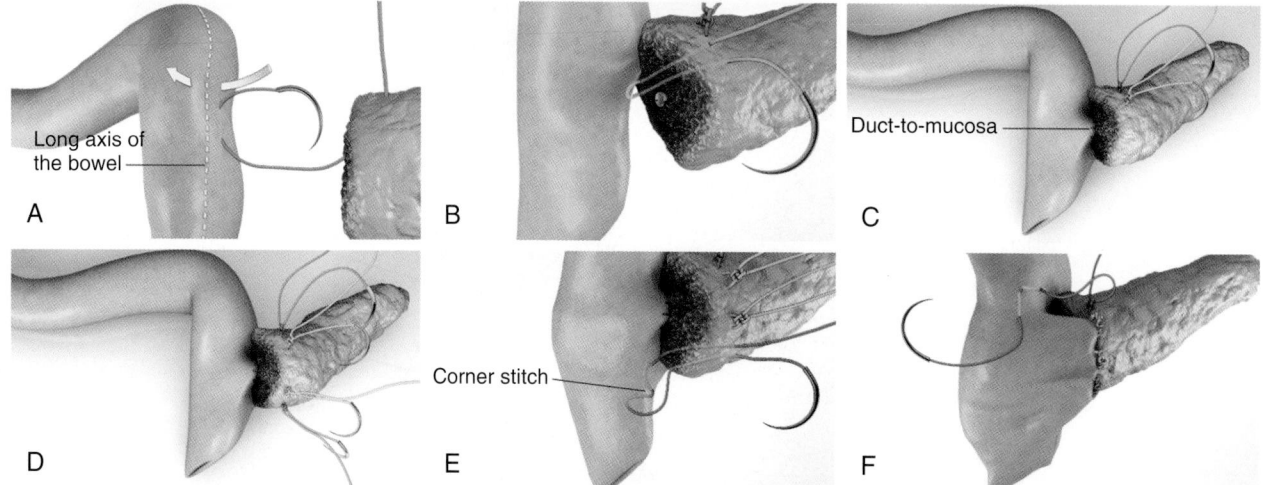

FIGURE 127B.7   **Laparoscopic Blumgart pancreaticojejunostomy. A,** Transpancreatic suture through full-thickness pancreas to seromuscular jejunum, with a "turn the corner" stitch. **B,** Additional transpancreatic sutures placed until pancreatic duct. **C,** Duct-to-mucosa anastomosis created next. **D,** Remainer of transpancreatic sutures placed. **E,** Placement of "turn the corner" stitch to buttress cut surface of pancreas against jejunum. **F,** Completion of anterior wall with saved needles from posterior wall, completely invaginating the cut edge of pancreas within the jejunum. (Courtesy Toronto Video Atlas of Surgery.)

Pancreaticogastrostomy (see Chapters 117A and 117B)

Place transpancreatic stay sutures along the superior and inferior borders of the pancreas. Create a posterior gastrotomy with an energy device. Place a purse-string full-thickness suture around the entire gastrotomy.[25] Prepare a second, smaller gastrotomy through the anterior stomach. Introduce a grasping instrument through the anterior then posterior gastrotomies, then grasp and pull the transpancreatic stay sutures to invaginate the pancreas remnant into the stomach. Once the pancreas is suitably pulled through, tie down the previously placed purse-string tightly (Fig. 127B.8).[25] Two transpancreatic sutures can be placed to further secure the pancreas within the stomach, taking care to avoid the pancreatic duct (Fig. 127B.9). Close the anterior gastrostomy in the usual fashion.[26]

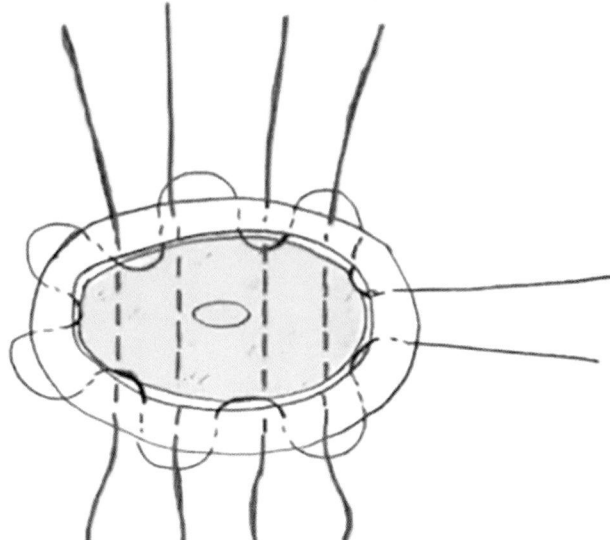

FIGURE 127B.9 Laparoscopic pancreaticogastrostomy. Additional transpancreatic sutures placed to secure pancreas within the stomach, avoiding the pancreatic duct. (Courtesy Dr. Julie Hallet.)

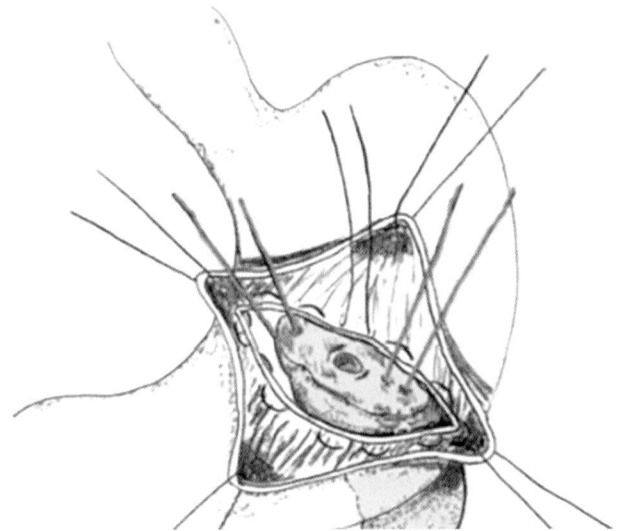

FIGURE 127B.8 Laparoscopic pancreaticogastrostomy. Transpancreatic stay sutures pulled through the posterior gastrotomy and purse-string along gastrostomy tightly tied down to secure the pancreatic remnant invaginated into the stomach. (Courtesy Dr. Julie Hallet.)

ROBOTIC APPROACHES TO MINIMALLY INVASIVE DISTAL AND CENTRAL PANCREATECTOMY

Robotic approaches have been used for both distal and central pancreatectomy.[27,28] The techniques and principles of exposure, mobilization, resection, and reconstruction are very similar to those described in this chapter.[28] A robotic approach may provide improved dexterity compared with the laparoscopic approach. This may be more beneficial for central pancreatectomy, which requires a more technically challenging reconstruction; however, comparative data is lacking. The choice of approach should be based on surgeon experience and resources.[8]

The references for this chapter can be found online by accessing the accompanying Expert Consult website.

Minimally invasive pancreaticoduodenectomy

Patricio M. Polanco and Herbert J. Zeh III

INTRODUCTION

Since its initial description by Codevilla in 1898, through the first procedure performed by Kauch in 1909 and the two-stage procedure described by Whipple in 1935, the pancreaticoduodenectomy (PD) technique has evolved significantly over the last decades to become a common and safe procedure in pancreatobiliary surgery (see Chapters 62 and 117A).[1–3] Currently, PD is executed routinely with low morbidity and mortality rates when performed in experienced high-volume centers.

As in many other fields of surgery, minimally invasive approaches have revolutionized gastrointestinal and hepato-pancreato-biliary (HPB) operations (see Chapter 127A). The overall advantages of minimally invasive surgery include less pain, less use of pain medications, less blood loss, fewer wound complications, shorter length of stay, and earlier recovery, among others.[3] Currently, minimally invasive distal pancreatectomy (laparoscopic or robotic) has become widely used for pancreatic body and tail tumors[4] (see Chapter 117B). Yet, given the complexity of PD (see Chapter 117A) and the steep learning curve for laparoscopic and robotic approaches, the adoption of these minimally invasive techniques has been slow for complex HPB surgery. Another aggravating factor for its implementation has been the cost associated with acquiring equipment for minimally invasive surgery, including the robotic system platform.

Laparoscopic PD was initially used by Gagne and Pomp in 1994, and the first robotic PD was performed by Giulanotti in 2001, and since then minimally invasive PD (MIPD) use has steadily increased across the globe.[5–7] The increased use of minimally invasive techniques has highlighted the potential advantages of laparoscopic and robotic pancreas surgery and motivated a critical review of the current relevant data by experts in the field. The review was an international multi-institutional effort that resulted in recently published evidence-based guidelines for minimally invasive pancreatic resection that were endorsed by the most relevant international societies of HPB surgery.[8]

The aim of this chapter is to describe indications, patient selection, technique, and outcomes associated with MIPD. This chapter will cover the basic aspects of the laparoscopic approach but will focus on robotic MIPD given the trend of modern minimally invasive techniques, the rapid growth of robotic programs globally, and the expertise of our group.

INDICATIONS

Current indications for MIPD are similar to those of the open approach (see Chapters 62 and 117A) and include any peri-ampullary tumor, including pancreatic adenocarcinoma (see Chapters 59, 61, and 62), pancreatic neuroendocrine tumors (see Chapter 65), distal common bile duct cancer (see Chapter 47), duodenal masses (see Chapter 63), and ampullary tumors (see Chapter 62), among others. Depending on the surgeon's expertise, there are just a few absolute contraindications for the minimally invasive approach.

Our group and others have reported using robotic PD in patients with borderline and locally advanced tumors where portal vein resections and repair are needed (see Chapters 62, 117A, and 122).[9,10] For surgeons at the early stages of their learning curve, we do not recommend the use of minimally invasive approaches when major vascular resections are anticipated. To assess these and other anatomic considerations, high-quality preoperative imaging is paramount to determine mesenteric vessel involvement before proceeding with MIPD (see Chapter 17). Specifically, we recommend a multiphasic computed tomography scan or magnetic resonance imaging during an early arterial and portal vein phase. For patients with locally advanced tumors where superior mesenteric artery or hepatic artery resection and reconstruction is anticipated, we recommend the open technique (see Chapter 117A). Another potential contraindication includes patients who are unable to undergo pneumoperitoneum due to CO_2-retaining conditions. Previous upper abdominal operations, a high body mass index, and multiple comorbidities are not considered absolute contraindications. Yet adequate patient selection is highly encouraged in every case. A high level of minimally invasive technical skills should not replace critical clinical acumen and surgical planning. At our institution, all pancreas and periampullary tumors are discussed preoperatively in a multidisciplinary fashion that includes the opinions of specialized HPB surgeons.

OPERATIVE TECHNIQUE

Robotic Pancreaticoduodenectomy

Our group favors the use of the robotic approach for MIPD over the laparoscopic technique because it overcomes most of the limitations of the latter. The robotic platform offers improved instrument articulation, elimination of tremor, improved dexterity (allowing surgeons to dissect or suture with both hands/arms), enhanced camera angles, and three-dimensional visualization.[11,12]

Our technique and outcomes for robotic PD (RPD) have been previously described and reported.[11–14] First, it is important to describe the operating room (OR) setup and patient position. After general endotracheal intubation, the patient is placed supine on a split-leg table with both arms tucked on the sides (Fig. 127C.1). The split-leg table allows the bedside assistant surgeon to stand between the patient's legs in an ergonomic position. Adequate patient padding for arms and legs, including popliteal and elbow support, is crucial to prevent pressure points, nerve

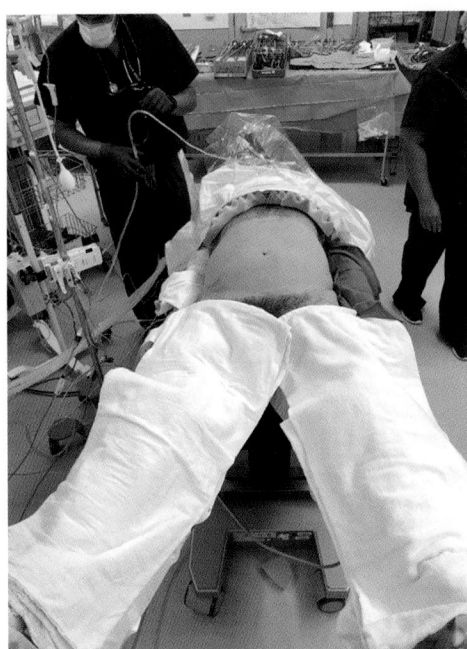

FIGURE 127C.1 Patient positioning and padding.

surgical arm cart to come over the patient's head if a da Vinci Si System (Intuitive Surgical) is used. The OR setup can vary according to room size and disposition (Fig. 127C.2).

Once the abdomen is prepped and draped, we create a pneumoperitoneum through the insertion of a 5-mm optical separator (later exchanged for an 8-mm robotic trocar) in the left upper quadrant. A Veress needle technique or open pneumoperitoneum creation are also acceptable. The trocar placement is depicted in Fig. 127C.3. For the Si System, we propose using a 10-mm camera port, three robotic arm ports in the upper abdomen (one on the patient's left side and two on the right side), two assistant ports in the lower abdomen (5 mm on the right and 15 mm on the left), and a 5-mm liver retractor port. For the da Vinci Xi System, all four robotic trocars can be 8 mm in size. Later in the surgery, the left lower quadrant assistant port site is extended to a 4- to 5-cm incision to extract the specimen.

With robotic ports in place, the robotic arms are docked coming above the patient's head and upper torso (Fig. 127C.4) if a da Vinci Si System is used. During the dissection phase of the operation, we use a gentle robotic grasper in the patient's far right side and a fenestrated bipolar grasper as the right medial instrument, and a robotic (surgeon's "left hand") hook dissector or scissors in the patient's left side (surgeon's "right hand"). During the reconstruction, the fenestrated bipolar and hook instruments are exchanged for robotic needle drivers.

We standardized our RPD technique in eight major surgical steps: identification/preparation of the jejunal limb, colon and duodenal mobilization, portal triad dissection, cholecystectomy,

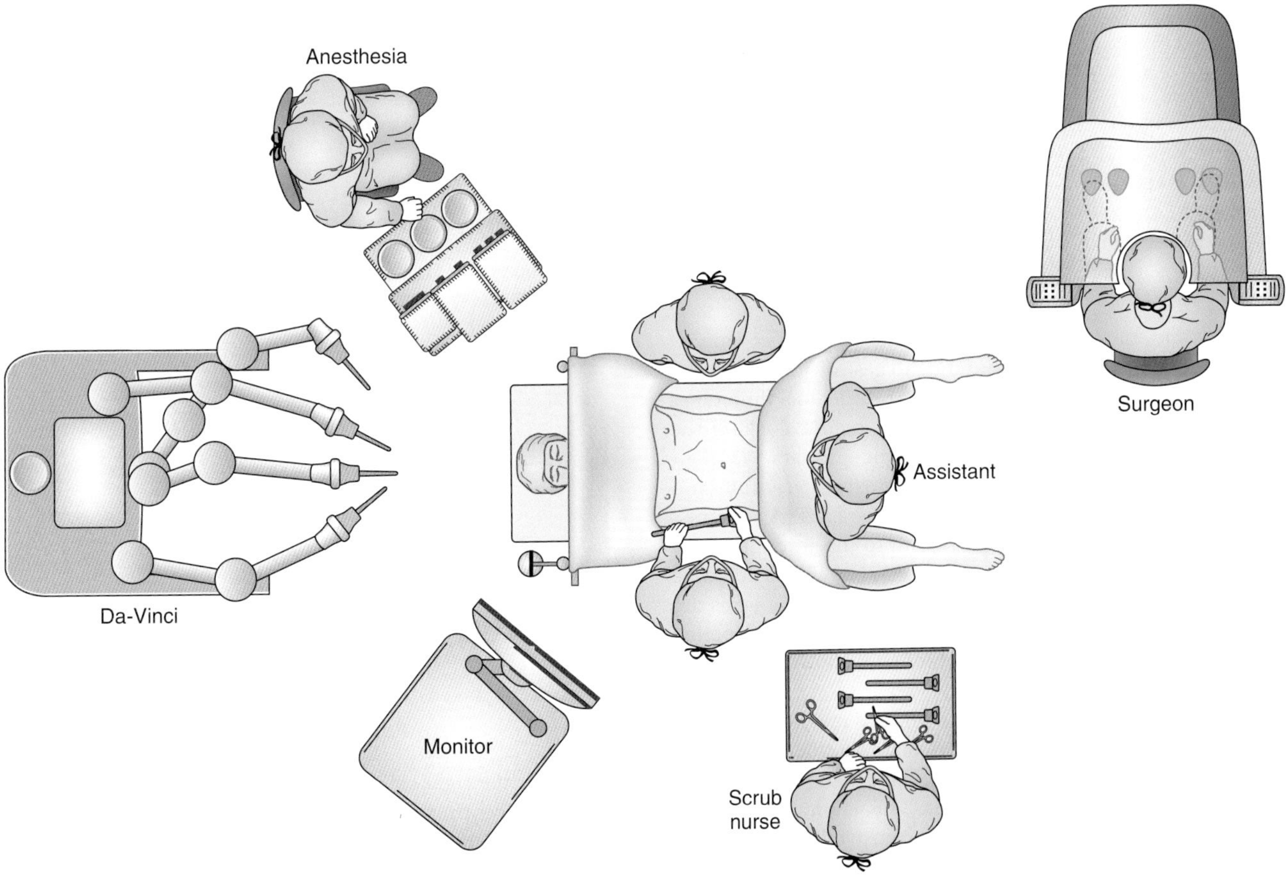

compression, and skin injuries. Cushioned strapping across the chest and individual legs with Velcro belts or surgical cloth tape is recommended to prevent patient and legs from sliding off. The OR table is often rotated 90 degrees to allow a robotic

FIGURE 127C.2 Operating room setup for robotic Whipple using the da Vinci Si System (Intuitive Surgical, Sunnyvale, CA).

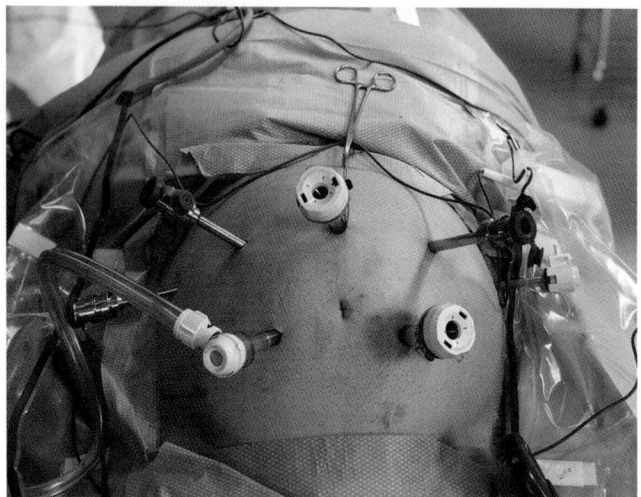

FIGURE 127C.3 Intraoperative photo of port placement.

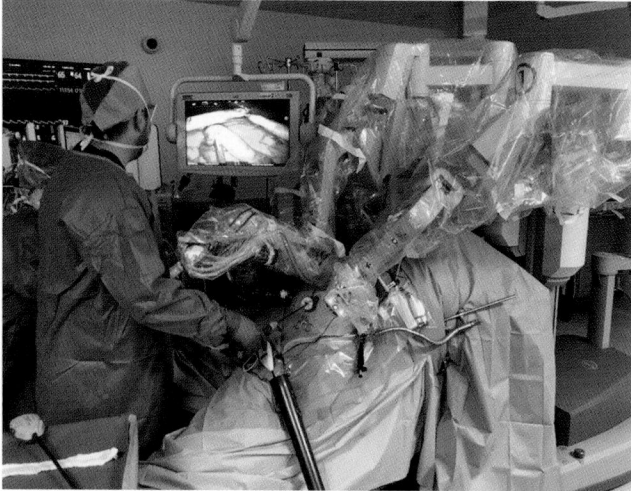

FIGURE 127C.4 Robotic arms docked over patient's head when using the da Vinci Si System (Intuitive Surgical, Sunnyvale, CA).

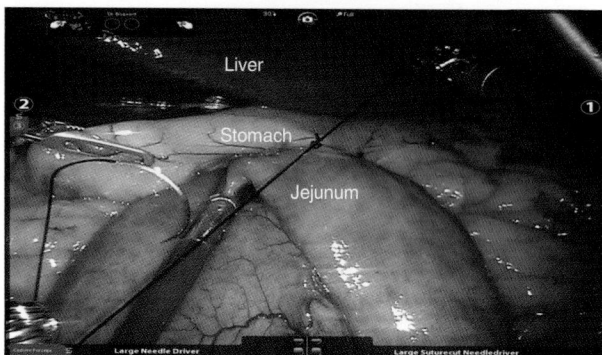

FIGURE 127C.5 Identification and stitching of jejunal limb to stomach for later reconstruction.

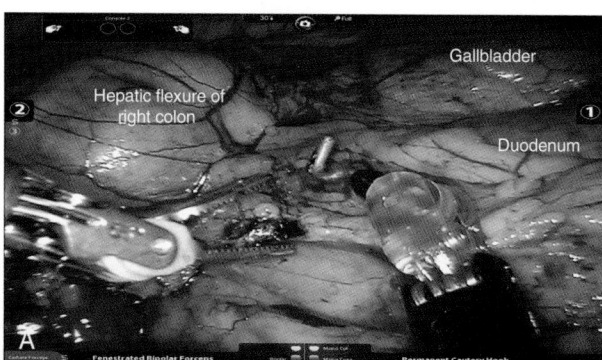

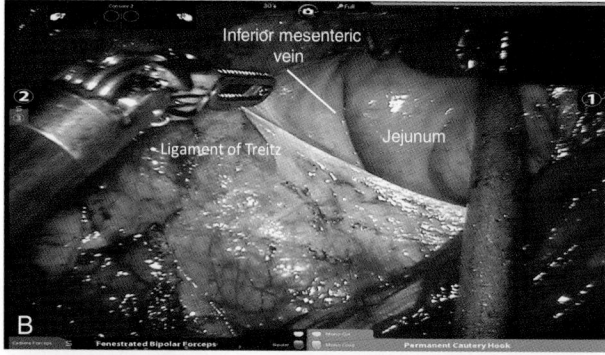

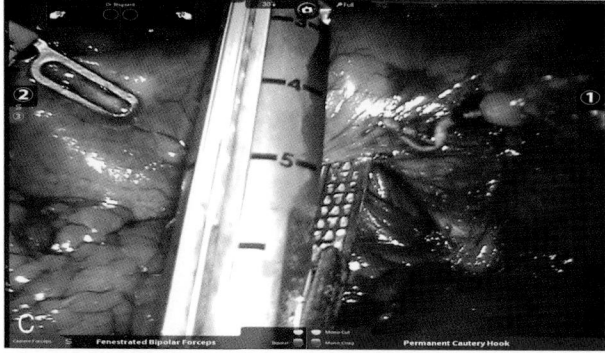

FIGURE 127C.6 Mobilization of right colon **(A)** and duodenum, with dissection of ligament of Treitz **(B)** and division of proximal jejunum **(C)**.

uncinated and retroperitoneal dissection, pancreaticojejunostomy, hepaticojejunostomy, and duodeno/gastrojejunostomy.

The step of *identification/preparation* of the jejunal limb takes place immediately after trocar placement before docking the robotic arms. With atraumatic laparoscopic graspers, we identify the ligament of Treitz (LOT) and proximal jejunum and run the bowel distally up to 100 cm from the LOT. A seromuscular 3-0 silk stitch securing the jejunum to the anterior aspect of the gastric body wall is placed (Fig. 127C.5). This could be done laparoscopically or robotically after the robotic arms are docked. This step facilitates the setup of the reconstruction phase when gastrojejunostomy or duodenojejunostomy is created (see Chapter 117A).

The *mobilization* step includes a complete medial rotation of the right colon dividing the gastrocolic, gastroepiploic, and hepatic flexure attachments of the proximal transverse colon as well as the right Toldt's fascia planes. This allows exposure of the duodenum and completion of an extensive Kocher maneuver separating the duodenum and pancreas from their lateral and medial attachments (also see Chapter 117A). We divide the

LOT from the right side of the mesenteric vessels, allowing the pulling of the proximal jejunum through its native anatomic defect (Fig. 127C.6). The proximal jejunum is then divided with a laparoscopic linear gastrointestinal stapler approximately 10 cm from the LOT. We then divide the distal aspect

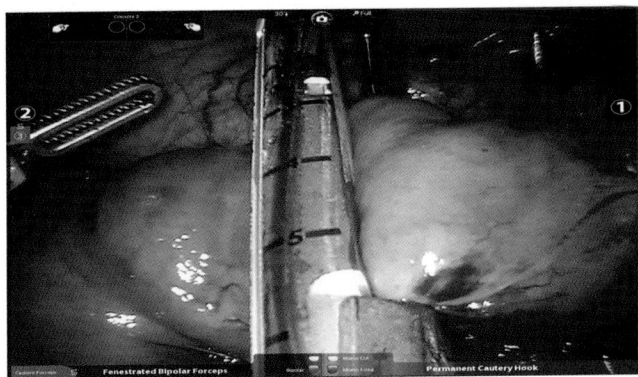

FIGURE 127C.7 Stapling and division of first portion of duodenum (pylorus preserving).

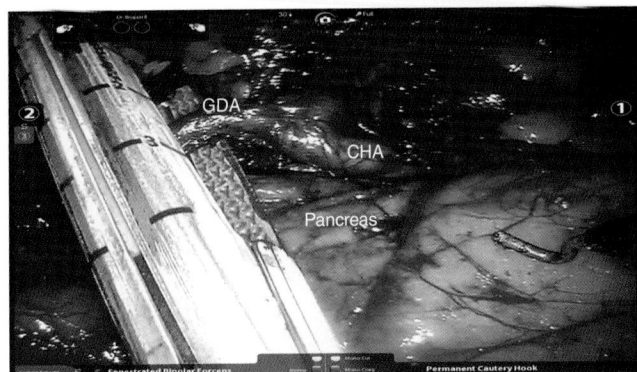

FIGURE 127C.9 Stapling of gastroduodenal artery *(GDA)*.

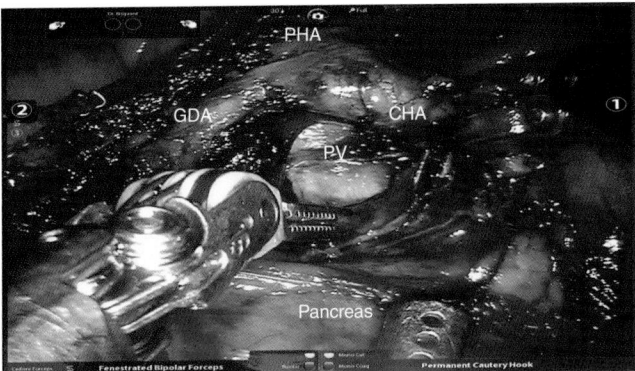

FIGURE 127C.8 Suprapancreatic dissection of common hepatic artery *(CHA)*, gastroduodenal artery *(GDA)*, and portal vein *(PV)*.

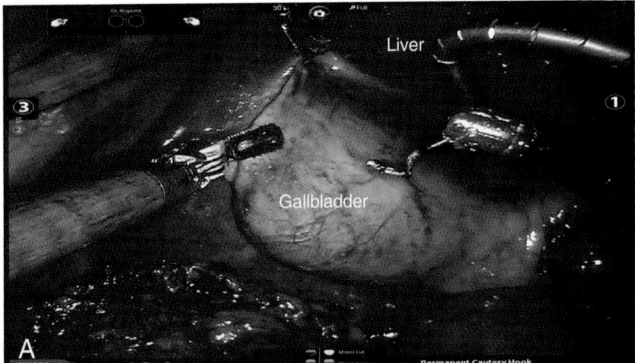

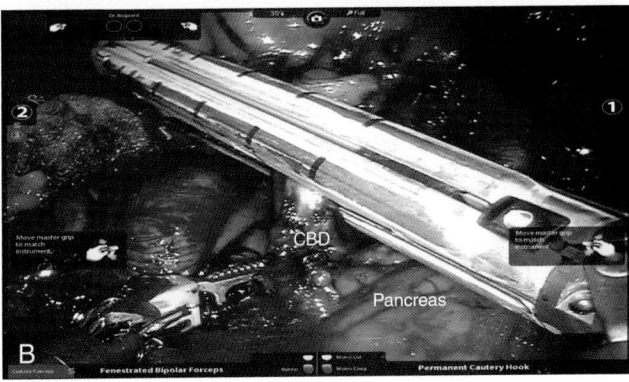

FIGURE 127C.10 Robotic cholecystectomy **(A)** and common bile duct division **(B)**.

of the gastrocolic ligament to enter the lesser sac. The right gastric and gastroepiploic arteries are also dissected and divided. Once the lesser omentum is divided and the distal stomach is circumferentially dissected, it can be divided (classic technique) with a laparoscopic or robotic linear gastrointestinal stapler (Fig. 127C.7). Alternatively, the proximal first portion of the duodenum can be circumferentially freed up and divided (pylorus-preserving technique).

The *porta hepatis dissection* begins with the dissection of the hepatic artery node off the common hepatic artery (also see Chapter 117A). Once this lymph node is removed, we dissect the common hepatic artery and the gastroduodenal artery (GDA) on the superior border of the pancreas neck. In the posterior aspect of the triangle formed by these three structures (see Chapter 2), we identify and dissect the anterior aspect of the portal vein and its suprapancreatic portion (Fig. 127C.8).

The GDA is dissected and later divided (also see Chapter 117A) with the 45-mm linear vascular stapler (Fig. 127C.9). We then extend the dissection to the common bile duct. The medial and lateral aspects of the common bile duct are dissected, bringing down all the lymph nodes from the periportal and portocaval area toward the side of the future surgical specimen.

A *cholecystectomy* is then performed in a top-down fashion with the robotic hook cautery (Fig. 127C.10A) (see Chapter 36). Once the common bile duct is circumferentially dissected, we divide it with a gastrointestinal linear stapler to prevent bile leakage during the rest of the surgery (Fig. 127C.10B). If the RPD

is performed for proximal or middle-portion cancer of the common bile duct, we prefer a sharp division with robotic scissors, and the duct margin is sent for frozen sectioning.

We then turned the attention to the inferior border of the pancreas, identifying the superior mesenteric vein (SMV) (see Chapter 2). We create a tunnel underneath the pancreas neck and anterior to the SMV and the splenoportal junction with gentle blunt and cautery dissection (Fig. 127C.11) (see Chapter 117A). The pancreas is divided with robotic scissors and monopolar energy except for the pancreatic duct, which is cut sharply with no energy (Fig. 127C.12).

Our last portion of the resection phase involves the *uncinate process* and posterior retroperitoneum dissection (see Chapter 117A). We free up the uncinate process of the SMV with monopolar robotic scissors or hook dissection. Larger veins can be

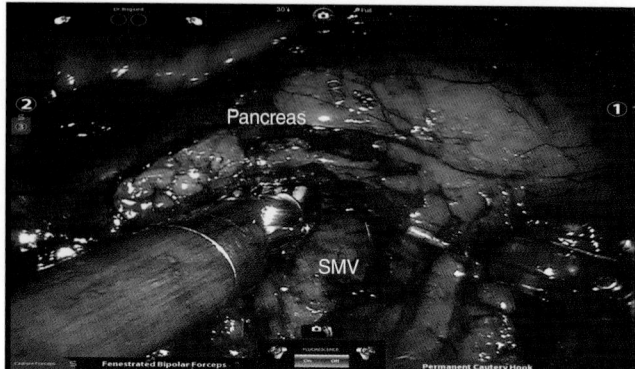

FIGURE 127C.11 Creation of retropancreatic tunnel. *SMV*, Superior mesenteric vein.

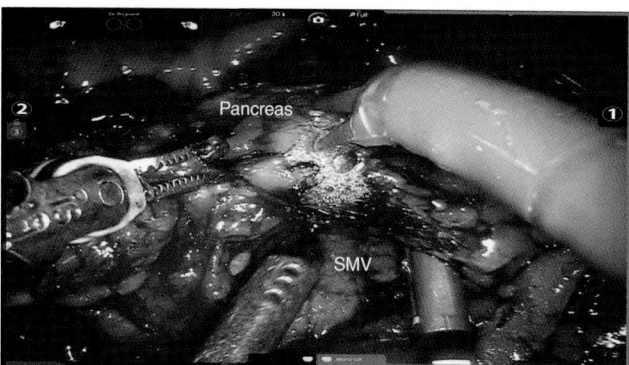

FIGURE 127C.12 Pancreas transection. *SMV*, Superior mesenteric vein.

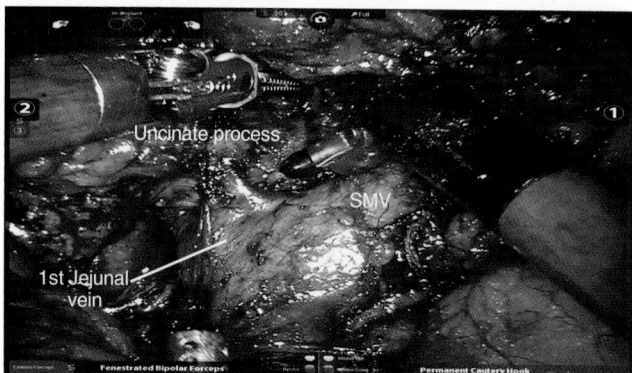

FIGURE 127C.13 Uncinate process dissection. *SMV*, Superior mesenteric vein.

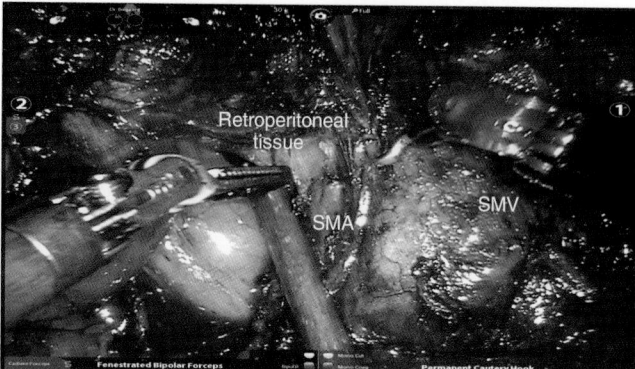

FIGURE 127C.14 Retroperitoneal dissection with dissection and preservation of superior mesenteric artery *(SMA)* and superior mesenteric vein *(SMV)*.

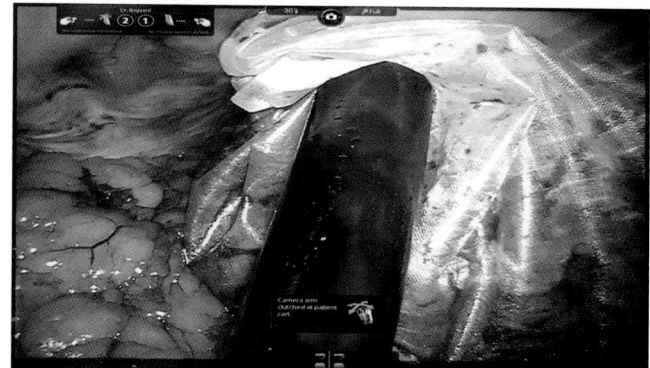

FIGURE 127C.15 Specimen extraction in plastic bag.

divided with a robotic or laparoscopic vessel sealer. The uncinated and pancreas head is rotated clockwise (cephalocaudal axis) to dissect the superior mesenteric artery (SMA), identifying the first jejunal vein as well as the junction of the gastroepiploic toward the portal vein. The first jejunal vein is dissected off the uncinate process. Occasionally, this vein needs to be divided with the vessel sealer depending on the location and extension of the tumor. Dissection continues by separating the uncinate process and the retroperitoneal tissue of the SMA (Fig. 127C.13). Pancreaticoduodenal veins are identified, dissected, and divided with a vessel sealer as well. The last portion of the retroperitoneal tissue of the SMA is divided with the robotic hook cautery and/or vessel sealer (Fig. 127C.14).

The duodenum-pancreas specimen and gallbladder are placed into an endoscopic large bag. The 15-mm utility bedside assist port in the left lower quadrant is extended to 4 to 5 cm and the specimen bag is removed (Fig. 127C.15). A small gel wound protector is placed in the extraction site and the 15-mm laparoscopic trocar is reintroduced.

We then proceed with the *reconstruction* portion of the surgery. We start by creating a *pancreaticojejunal duct to mucosa anastomosis* in a modified Blumgart technique (see Chapters 117A and 127B). We use three 2-0 silk transpancreatic (anterior to posterior) toward a posterior row of the small bowel and back through the pancreas (posterior to anterior). These stitches are tied sequentially (Fig. 127C.16A). Needles are kept in place since these are used for the anterior row. We then proceed with a duct to mucosa anastomosis with interrupted stitches of 5-0 PDS (Fig. 127C.16B). After a posterior row is created, a 4- or 5-French pancreatic duct stent is often used in small ducts through the anastomosis, confirming patency and to facilitate anterior row stitch placement (Fig. 127C.16C). The anterior row to the anastomosis is completed with 5-0 duct to mucosa stitches (Fig. 127C.16D) followed with anterior seromuscular stitches with the previously placed 2-0 silks (Fig. 127C.16E).

A *hepaticojejunal anastomosis* is then created. After removal of the stapled line of the common bile duct, a hepaticojejunal anastomosis is constructed with interrupted 5-0 PDS sutures for cases with small or thin wall ducts. If the hepatic duct is wide and thick walled, running sutures with absorbable 4-0 barbed sutures can be considered (Fig. 127C.17).

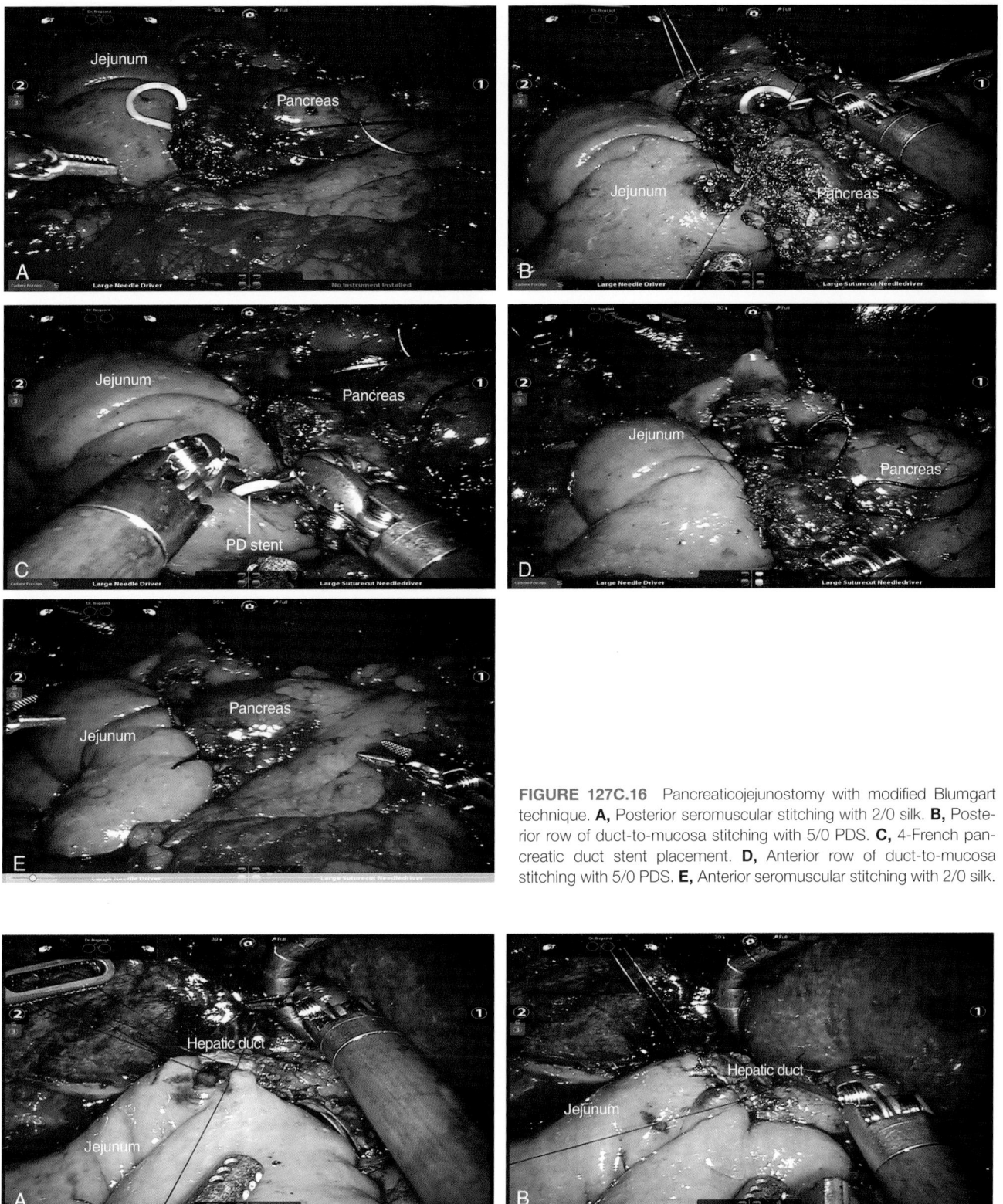

FIGURE 127C.16 Pancreaticojejunostomy with modified Blumgart technique. **A,** Posterior seromuscular stitching with 2/0 silk. **B,** Posterior row of duct-to-mucosa stitching with 5/0 PDS. **C,** 4-French pancreatic duct stent placement. **D,** Anterior row of duct-to-mucosa stitching with 5/0 PDS. **E,** Anterior seromuscular stitching with 2/0 silk.

FIGURE 127C.17 Hepatojejunostomy with interrupted stitches of 5/0 PDS. **A,** Posterior row. **B,** Anterior row.

A *gastrojejunal* or *duodenojejunal* anastomosis is then created with the loop of bowel previously identified and stitched to the stomach during the first *identification/preparation* step. This stitch is now cut and the marked loop of jejunum is set up for the anastomosis with another 3-0 silk stay suture. A duodenojejunal anastomosis is created with a two-layer running suture of 4-0 absorbable barbed sutures in an end-to-side fashion. A gastrojejunostomy is created in the same fashion with a 3-0 absorbable barbed suture. The inner layer is done in a running Connell fashion (Fig. 127C.18). We routinely create a pedicled falciform

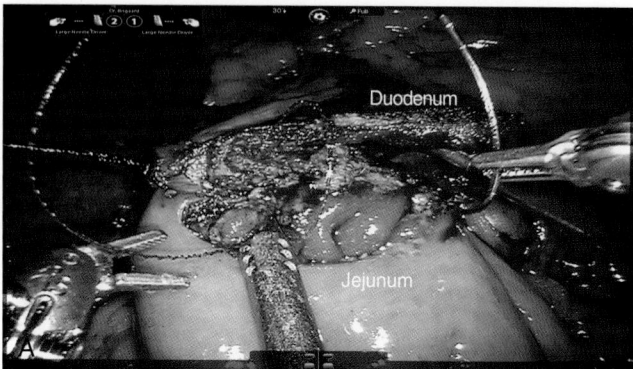

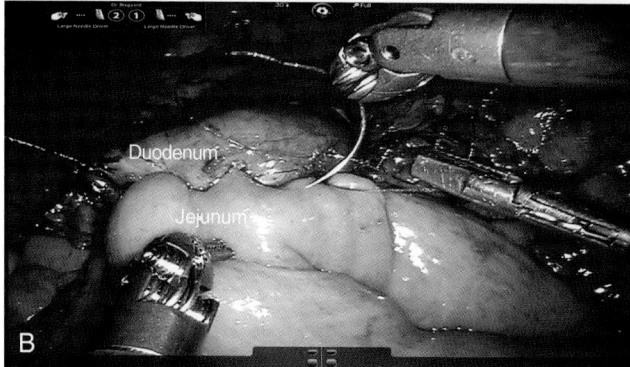

FIGURE 127C.18 Duodenojejunostomy with two layers of running 4/0 barbed absorbable suture. **A**, Posterior row. **B**, Anterior row.

ligament flap and place it carefully over the GDA stump. Based on its anticipated risk of leak, one or two (anterior and posterior) 19-French drains are placed through the right upper quadrant port. Trocars are removed under direct visualization. The 10-mm camera port is closed with 0 Vicryl and an endoscopic needle passer, and the utility port/extraction site incision is closed with interrupted stitches of 0 Vicryl. The skin is closed with 4-0 monofilament absorbable suture and skin glue or sterile adhesive dressing.

We do not routinely admit our patients to intensive care units but instead send them to a regular ward with telemetry monitoring. However, this will depend on the patients' comorbidities and hospital protocols. We use an enhanced recovery after surgery (ERAS) pathway for all our patients as it has been shown to decrease the use of pain medication, shorten the length of stay, and decrease the hospital costs (see Chapter 27).[15]

Laparoscopic Pancreaticoduodenectomy

Several groups have reported their technique for totally laparoscopic PD (LPD).[16–19] After standard antiseptic techniques, patients are preferably positioned in supine split-leg table position, allowing surgeons mobility at different stages of the operation. Most surgeons recommend a minimum of 4 to 6 trocars placed in a semicircle in the upper abdomen facing the duodeno-pancreas region. After ruling out peritoneal disease or metastatic tumor implants, surgery proceeds in a fashion similar to the robotic and open approach. Except for specific patient/surgeon variations, LPD dissection steps include the following: mobilization of the right colon, an extensive Kocher maneuver, division of the LOT, mobilization of the proximal

jejunum, a circumferential dissection and division of the gastric antrum or duodenum with a linear stapler, dissection of the hepatic artery, dissection/stapling of the GDA, dissection of the pancreas neck, retropancreatic tunnel creation, division of the pancreas neck, cholecystectomy, dissection/division of the common bile duct, and a caudal to cranial dissection of the uncinated process and posteromedial margin of the pancreas head off the SMA and SMV. Depending on the surgeon's preference, this dissection can be carried out with a laparoscopic ultrasonic dissector or laparoscopic vessel sealer. Reconstruction techniques vary among surgeons, but most recommend a single-layer hepatojejunostomy (interrupted or running), a two-layer duct-to-mucosa pancreatojejunostomy, and an antecolic gastro/duodenojejunostomy in two layers.

Although some authors have reported hybrid procedures of laparoscopic dissection and open reconstruction through small laparotomies, we believe these hybrid approaches undermine the benefits of the minimally invasive techniques for the patient and limit the improvement of surgical skills and the surgeon's learning curve.

PERIOPERATIVE OUTCOMES

Multiple large institutional series of MIPD, systematic reviews, meta-analyses, and at least two randomized trials of LPD versus OPD have now shown that the minimally invasive approach for Whipple procedures is safe and feasible when performed by pancreas surgeons with expertise in laparoscopic and robotic techniques.

Acknowledging the issue of reporting and selection bias, multiple researchers have consistently shown in systematic reviews and meta-analyses that MIPD is associated with reduced blood loss, reduced hospital stays, and longer operative times when compared with the open technique. The perioperative morbidity, pancreas-specific complications (i.e., pancreatic fistulae and delayed gastric emptying; see Chapter 28), and mortality seem similar in both approaches.[20–24] In a propensity-matched analysis using the pancreas-targeted American College of Surgeons National Surgical Quality Improvement Program, we found that fully minimally invasive PD was associated with a lower prolonged length of stay and decreased wound complications and transfusions.[25]

Palanivelu et al.,[26] in a small, single-center randomized trial comparing LPD versus OPD (32 patients in each arm), found that LPD offered a shorter length of stay compared with OPD. There was no significant difference in the other perioperative outcomes. In another single-center randomized trial of 66 patients, Poves et al.[27] showed that LPD was associated with a shorter length of stay and fewer severe complications. In spite of these encouraging results for MIPD, the most recent randomized trial comparing LPD versus OPD has raised concerns and caution regarding implementation of LPD as well as surgeons' experience with, and the learning curve for, the procedure. The LEOPARD-2 study by van Hilst et al.[28] was a multicenter patient-blinded randomized controlled trial that was closed prematurely due to a 90-day mortality rate of 15% (3/20 patients) in the LPD group. Although no statistically significant differences in outcomes was found between approaches, this study highlights the challenges of adopting a laparoscopic technique for PD. Moreover, whenever a prospective comparison of open versus minimally invasive techniques is attempted, the comparison should account for surgeons' experience and proficiency.

Currently, few surgeons worldwide have overcome their learning curve for MIPD (laparoscopically or robotically).

Our group and collaborators have documented and reported the perioperative outcomes of the largest cohort in RPD. The 10-year experience of clinicians at the University of Pittsburgh with 500 consecutive PD cases was recently published.[14] In this series, major complications (Clavien score of >2) occurred in less than 24% of patients, clinically relevant postoperative pancreatic fistula (CR-POPF) was experienced by 7.8% of patients, 30- and 90-day mortality rates were 1.4% and 3.1%, respectively, and the median length of stay was 8 days. These results highlight that optimal outcomes can be obtained when structured implementation of a robotic pancreas surgery program is adopted in a high-volume institution. In a propensity-matched analysis comparing 405 OPD with 460 RPD patients, Cai et al.[29] reported that the robotic approach was associated with significantly less CR-POPF (7% vs. 16%). Other retrospective propensity-matched analyses and a large database analysis have corroborated the association of RPD with a decreased rate of CR-POPF.[30,31]

Currently, no randomized controlled trials comparing robotic versus the open approach have been performed. Similarly, prospective randomized trials comparing the robotic versus the laparoscopic approach are not available. Although both RPD and LPD are safe and feasible depending on surgeon experience and training, we believe that RPD may allow the completion of more complex pancreatic surgeries, including vascular resections and reconstructions in locally advanced tumors. We suggest this based on our experience, clinical observations, and reported findings of significantly lower conversion rates for RPD (11%) when compared with LPD (27%) in a national cohort of patients.[32]

ONCOLOGIC OUTCOMES

The authors of recent international evidence-based guidelines critically reviewed the current data to address the question of whether MIPD should be used for the treatment of periampullary tumors and pancreatic adenocarcinoma (see Chapters 59 and 62). Based on the available data, the experts agreed that minimally invasive and open approaches are both valid for patients with malignancies and do not have differences in perioperative outcomes and survival.[8] This conclusion is based largely on retrospective single-center reports and large national database analysis.[33–37]

A recent systematic review and meta-analysis that included 18 nonrandomized trials with 13,639 patients with periampullary tumors allocated to RPD (n = 1593) or OPD (n = 12,046) showed that lymph node retrieval and R0 resections were similar in both groups.[38] Although most of the studies in this review suggest comparable oncologic results, in a single-center series of patients with pancreatic adenocarcinoma undergoing surgery at the Mayo Clinic (108 LPD compared with 214 OPD), Kendrick and collaborators found that patients undergoing LPD had longer progression-free survival likely due to shorter hospital stays, faster recovery, and less delay in adjuvant chemotherapy receipt.[33] Although no prospective studies have compared the laparoscopic versus the robotic approach in such patients, we have reported no significant differences in oncologic outcomes (margin status, examined lymph nodes, and overall survival) when comparing RPD versus LPD in a US national cohort of 1623 patients with pancreatic adenocarcinoma.[39]

LEARNING CURVE AND TRAINING

PD, whether performed open or as a minimally invasive procedure, is one of the most challenging procedures in gastrointestinal surgery. As described previously, the surgery entails an extensive dissection of relevant anatomic structures followed by complex and delicate reconstructive anastomosis. Literature suggests that MIPD should be limited to experienced pancreas surgeons in high-volume centers given the long learning curve and the difficulty of the procedure.[37,40,41]

Several groups have tried to address the issue of the LPD learning curve and some have defined benchmarks for training and proficiency. A retrospective study of the first 150 LPD patients of three experienced laparoscopic surgeons suggested that at least 30 cases are needed to overcome the initial learning curve.[42] In a Chinese multicenter/multisurgeon series of 1029 of patients who underwent LPD, thresholds of 40 and 104 cases were found to be relevant to decrease operative time, blood loss, and hospital stay.[43] We believe that these studies underestimate the actual number of cases needed to achieve proficiency, as many of them do not account for factors such as the surgeons' prior experience with open pancreatobiliary operations, the interaction of hospital versus surgeon volume, and trainee participation in the procedures, among others.

In spite of numerous attempts to identify factors affecting its implementation and learning curve, LPD remains a challenging technique with limited widespread adoption. Considering that LPD was first described almost three decades ago, only a few centers across the world have documented experience with the technique and an established training program for it.

The learning curve of the robotic approach for PD has also been studied and described by our group and others. Boone et al.[44] described thresholds of 20, 40, and 80 cases to decrease the rate of conversions, blood loss, and operative time, respectively, in a series of the first 200 RPD cases at the University of Pittsburgh. Other authors have corroborated similar findings for the RPD learning curve.[45–47]

Yet, while thresholds and benchmarks are important, the question of how to achieve proficiency and develop safe training programs to reach these benchmarks remains an issue. Based on our initial experience at a high-volume center with a surgical oncology/HPB fellowship program, we have advocated for deliberate and structured training for robotic HPB surgery. Hogg et al.[48,49] have reported the experience of a proficiency-based training program for safe implementation of RPD. The proposed training model developed by Hogg et al.[48,49] includes the following essential steps: (a) mastery of the instrument, (b) mastery of handling tissues, (c) mastery of the procedures, (d) mastery of psychomotor performance, and (e) decision making and judgment. This translates into five training curricula/evaluations that are steps toward proficiency in robotic surgery: a virtual reality simulation curriculum, an inanimate biotissue curriculum, a video library training curriculum, intraoperative evaluation, and skills maintenance with ongoing assessment.

Despite some skepticism regarding the implementation of a robotic surgery training program for RPD, doing so has been shown to be safe and feasible. Rice et al.[50] evaluated the association of mentorship and a formal proficiency-based skills curriculum with learning curves in a series of 514 RPD cases completed by three generations of surgeons. Conversion rates, operating times, and blood loss decreased across generations without a concomitant rise in adverse patient outcomes, suggesting that a proficiency-based curriculum coupled with mentorship allows for the safe introduction of less-experienced surgeons to RPD without compromising patient safety.

Although training in minimally invasive complex HPB surgery remains an evolving and controversial topic, the rapid growth of this technique and development of newer technologies call for further investigations in how to safely implement it into pancreas surgery.

The references for this chapter can be found online by accessing the accompanying Expert Consult website.

Minimally invasive segmental hepatic resection

Bjørn Edwin, Davit L. Aghayan, and Åsmund Avdem Fretland

INTRODUCTION

When hepatobiliary surgeons consider what treatment is best for a patient with a tumor in the liver, several questions must be answered. What kind of tumor is it, which resection margin is necessary, is the liver sick or healthy, is the liver remnant sufficient, is there more than one tumor, did the patient undergo surgery before? When these questions and others have been answered, the surgeons can decide what operation is suitable (see Chapters 4, 87, 101, and 102). And the answer to that final question might be different from continent to continent, country to country, or even surgeon to surgeon. Some have a strong tradition for hemihepatectomy, some prefer ablation, some do anatomic resections, and some prefer non-anatomic resections (Fig. 127D.1).

Historically, a hemihepatectomy was the operation of choice for most liver surgeons (see Chapters 101 and 118A). To safely control inflow and outflow of the part to be resected ensured a safe division of the often-treacherous liver parenchyma, where large vessels not revealed by preoperative scans could hide. With the development of imaging and anesthesiology and surgical techniques, a range of possibilities opened up, and the surgeons could begin to tailor operations for each patient.[1] Oncologic treatments have evolved that allow better biologic control of disease (see Chapters 65, 91, 92, 96, 97, 98, and 99), thus opening the door for re-resections in patients who already had parts of the liver removed.[2] Thus parenchyma preservation has become increasingly important, and surgeons developed ways to perform parenchyma preserving resections (see Chapter 102).[3,4] Segmental hepatectomy, or parenchyma-sparing liver surgery, can be performed by removing either anatomic segments of the liver, or by removing parts of the liver not defined by Couinaud's segments but by the tumor, which makes the operation necessary (see Chapters 102B and 118B).[5–7]

Most centers worldwide currently use parenchyma-sparing liver resection whenever possible (see Chapters 101 and 102).[8–10] Its role and advantages over formal hepatectomies have been well studied. The idea is to remove the tumor in an oncologically adequate way, while preserving as much healthy liver parenchyma as possible. Parenchyma-sparing liver resections require in-depth knowledge of liver anatomy (see Chapter 2) and experience in intraoperative ultrasound (see Chapters 24 and 103). Patient-specific 3D models may be helpful.

Parenchyma-sparing liver surgery can be performed by two strategies: segment-oriented (anatomic) or tumor-oriented (non-anatomic or atypical resections).[11,12] In anatomic resections (see Chapters 102B and 118B), the surgeon first dissects and divides the vessel supplying the relevant part of the liver from the hilum and then resects the devascularized area of the liver. In atypical resections (see Chapter 102A), the tumor is resected with a necessary margin by approaching the tumor supplying vessel from the surface. In our practice, atypical resections are dominant. We find it faster and easier to approach the tumor supplying vessels from the surface rather than from the hilum of the liver, especially when removing tumors that affect several liver segments. Resecting the tumor from the surface is especially suited for colorectal liver metastases (see Chapter 90), while anatomic resections may be more suitable for hepatocellular carcinoma (HCC) (see Chapter 89) because of segmental spread of metastases. However, the atypical approach can be suitable also for smaller hepatocellular carcinomas and in cases where the future liver remnant is small.[13]

After the first in the early 2000s, parenchyma sparing liver surgery has been described by several authors. A parenchyma-sparing strategy is associated with fewer postoperative complications, equivalent cancer-related outcomes, and a higher feasibility of future resections (see Chapter 102A).[14]

This chapter reviews the surgical technique of laparoscopic atypical segmental hepatectomy.

GENERAL PRINCIPLES

Imaging

Standard preoperative radiologic work-up in our practice is computed tomography (CT) of chest and abdomen (see Chapters 13, 14, and 15). For colorectal liver metastases, it is sufficient with portal venous phase of high quality, while multiple phases are necessary to assess primary tumors. In addition, we always do magnetic resonance imaging (MRI) with a liver specific contrast agent because this sometimes finds small metastases not visible on CT. Close collaboration with the radiology department is essential to ensure high quality imaging, especially for liver MRI. Positron emission computed tomography (PET-CT) is in our practice mostly used to identify extrahepatic disease in situations where we are in doubt if the patient will benefit from surgery. Contrast enhanced ultrasound is occasionally used to clarify the diagnosis of a tumor (see Chapter 18).

Three-dimensional (3D) reconstructions are useful in pre- and intraoperative settings, and we believe that, in the future, it will be used routinely. These patient-specific 3D models can provide a better spatial understanding to create the optimal resection plan (Fig. 127D.2).

Equipment

A wide range of laparoscopic equipment is available in the market. Most surgeons have different preferences; however, it is important that the surgical team has found the optimal list of instruments and the whole team is familiar with setup and functioning of equipment to avoid any disturbance during the operation. It is important that the center has a back-up of equipment if something needs to be replaced. A tray with instruments for open surgery must be available in the operating theater.

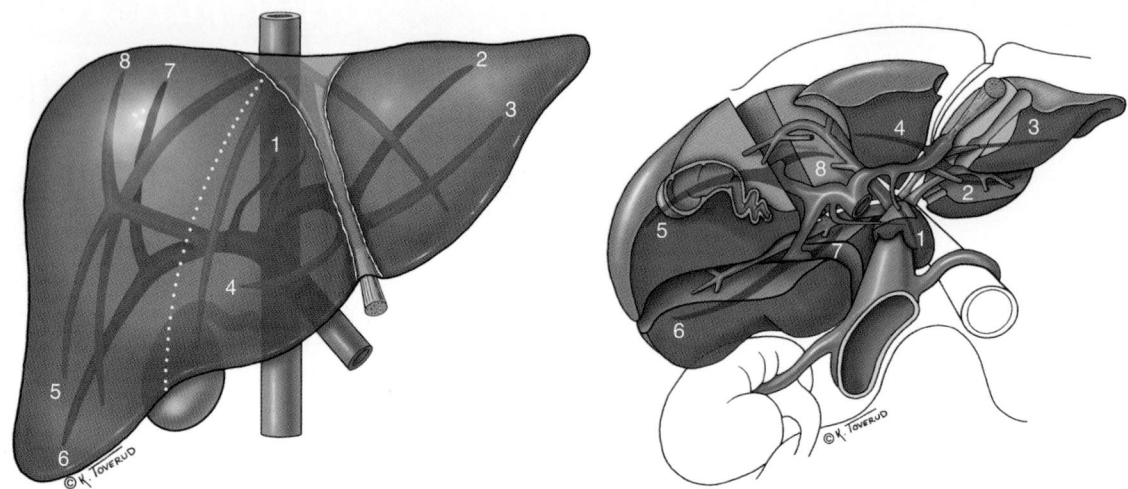

FIGURE 127D.1   Liver anatomy and the laparoscopic view of the liver segments. (Courtesy of Kari C. Toverud CMI.) (see Chapter 2).

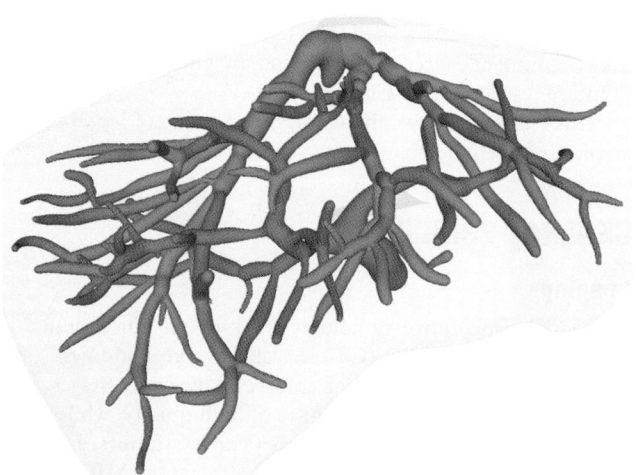

FIGURE 127D.2   Segmented liver based on CT scan images. (Courtesy of Egidijus Pelanis.)

Laparoscope

We prefer a 10 mm, 30-degree laparoscope because it enables parallel visualization from a port placed lateral to the working port ("camera on the shoulder") without conflicting with the working instruments of the operating surgeon. It also makes it possible to look around corners, which is useful when visualizing a resection line or when dissecting a large vessel.

A flexible laparoscope could further improve visualization, especially in posterior segments.

A 3D laparoscope can be useful in specific settings, especially complex tasks like suturing, but it is not a necessity. High-quality 4K cameras and large screens may give similar or even greater advantages.

Intraoperative Ultrasound

The use of intraoperative ultrasound with color doppler function is crucial in both open and laparoscopic surgery (also see Chapters 24 and 103). When learning laparoscopic liver surgery, performing laparoscopic ultrasound is mandatory. It helps clarify the liver anatomy, the tumor location, and the distance of the tumor from large vessels. Occasionally, it reveals new

tumors. Moreover, it helps orientation and to control resection lines and margins. Ultrasound probe manipulation during a laparoscopic procedure is more difficult than in open surgery, especially when examining in the posterosuperior segments. Appropriate liver mobilization and moving the probe between different trocars facilitates this task.

Surgical Instruments

Bipolar vessel sealing device. These devices are widely used in different surgical subspecialties including liver surgery. They facilitate performing parenchyma transection and hemostasis at the same time. The function of these devices is based on compression pressure and powerful radiofrequency energy causing contraction of collagen and elastin between opposing vessel walls. We prefer a straight jaw bipolar device (e.g., LigaSur dolphin tip) because its tip is very suitable for dissection

Ultrasonic sealer/dissection device. These devices are similar to bipolar sealers and provide simultaneous cutting and coagulation but are based on heat created by longitudinal vibration of the blades. The sealing of the vessels with thin wall (e.g., hepatic veins) is not so effective with this type of instruments because the vibrations might tear the fragile vessel wall apart.

Monopolar and bipolar cautery. This is usually used for marking resection lines on the liver surface and performing hemostasis, respectively. Bipolar forceps can also be used for clamp-crushing during the parenchyma transection. A bipolar forceps is a very versatile tool frequently used by many liver surgeons.

Ultrasonic Aspirator. Ultrasonic aspirators are very useful tools that can be used in addition to the clamp-crush technique to dissect intrahepatic vessels, when performing parenchyma transection.

Laparoscopic Suture. Suturing is one of the complex tasks in laparoscopic surgery. In laparoscopic liver surgery, we prefer to use barbed sutures with a pledget as an anchor, especially when suturing in the liver parenchyma. Other sutures are also useful, depending on the surgeon's preference.

Endo-Clips. We use both metal and polymer clips (Hem-o-Lok). The metal clips are suitable for smaller vessels and bile ducts. They save space and can be used as a secondary security. Polymer clips are in comparison safer, as they lock tight on the vessel, and can therefore be used to ligate larger vessels.

Endo-staplers (mainly vascular). These devices allow division of large vessels. They come with an articulating cartridge and straight or curved tips, making it easier to slide beneath difficultly positioned vessels. In addition to vascular stapling, endo-staplers can be used as an alternative method of parenchyma transection. This technique makes transection faster; however, this type of parenchyma transection is blinded, and one always should ensure that the transection area is free of vessels and bile ducts that supply or drain the remnant liver.

Laparoscopic liver retractors. Single or multiple use retractors provide support and retraction of the liver, thus facilitating access to the resection area. To succeed with laparoscopic liver surgery, it is necessary to have a retractor that the whole operative team is familiar with.

Pringle Maneuver

Hepatoduodenal ligament clamping or Pringle maneuver (see Chapter 118) is used to temporarily reduce or stop the blood flow to the liver, thus decreasing the blood loss during the parenchyma transection. The anesthesiologist should be asked to notify surgeons every five minutes after clamping. We usually use 15 minutes clamping and 5 minutes reperfusion and try to avoid clamping more than 120 minutes in total.

Several methods of performing the Pringle maneuver have been described; however, we have adopted two analogous methods to preform the Pringle maneuver:

1. **Internal.** After exposure of the hepatoduodenal ligament and opening the pars flaccida of the gastro-hepatic ligament, the porta hepatis is surrounded by a vessel loop passed behind the hepatic pedicle through the foramen of Winslow and fixed with a Hem-o-Lok clip (Fig. 127D.3). The vessel loop can be tightened when needed by pulling it up with a grasper. It simply surrounds and subsequently ties the hepatoduodenal pedicle to hang it and facilitate the Pringle maneuver, if necessary.

2. **External.** Instead of vessel loop, a cotton tape is passed through the foramen of Winslow, around the porta hepatis. The ends of the cotton tape are pulled with a grasper through a 5 mm port trocar placed laterally on the left side. Then, the 5 mm trocar is replaced by a 16-Ch suction catheter that is pushed inside the abdominal cavity up to the level of the hepatic pedicle, while the external end of the cotton tape and catheter remains outside of the patient so that the tourniquet can be tightened from outside (Fig. 127D.4).

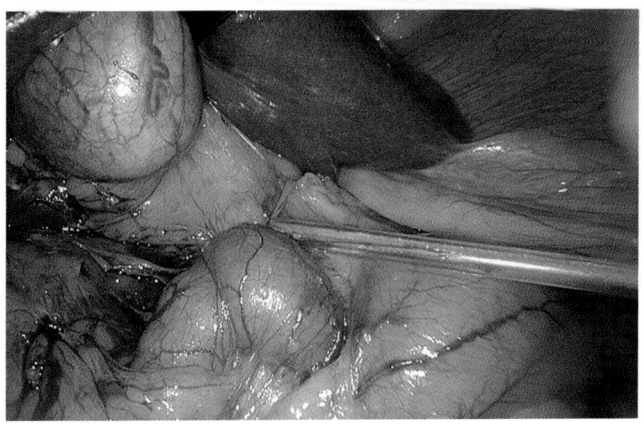

FIGURE 127D.4 External Pringle maneuver.

SURGICAL TECHNIQUE ("CAULIFLOWER" TECHNIQUE)

To simplify the understanding of our technique, we have performed an MRI of a cauliflower and segmented it. This exemplifies the surgical anatomy of the liver (see Chapter 2), and it demonstrates selective removal of segments and subsegments using the "from surface to the pedicle" technique (Fig. 127D.5).

Positioning

The patient is placed in the supine position (anterolateral segments) or in the 30- to 45-degrees with the right side up (posterosuperior segments), which helps achieve gravity-facilitated retraction. The surgeon usually stands on the patient's right side, in some cases to the left side (Fig. 127D.6). The French position (surgeon standing in between patient's legs), is also an option, although not used by our group.

Incisions, Pneumoperitoneum and Trocar Placement

Pneumoperitoneum is established by open technique (in our hands safer than Verres needle), and intra-abdominal carbon dioxide gas pressure is set in a range from 12 to 15 mm Hg. A 30-degree laparoscope and 5 and 12 mm trocars are used.

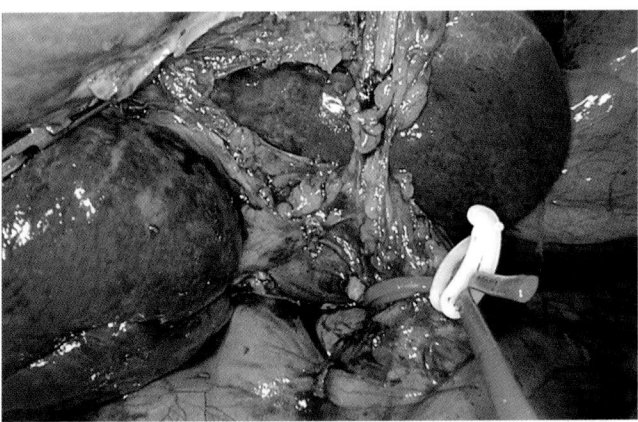

FIGURE 127D.3 Internal Pringle maneuver.

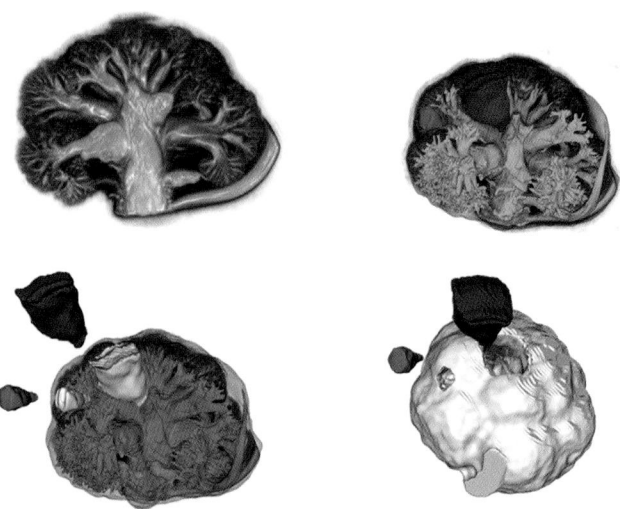

FIGURE 127D.5 Cauliflower segments. (Courtesy of Egidijus Pelanis.)

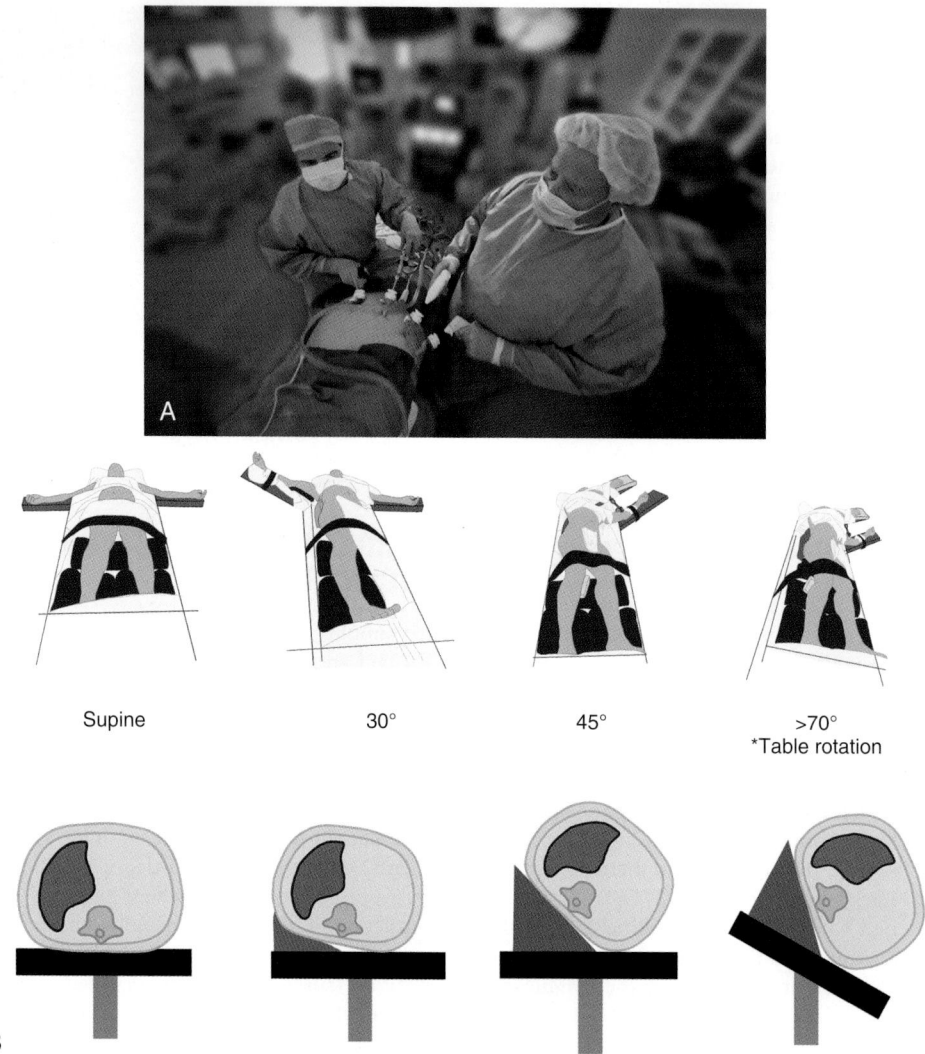

Supine   30°   45°   >70°
*Table rotation

FIGURE 127D.6 Patient positioning for resections in different segments. **A,** Supine position (segments 1 to 4). **B,** 30-degree right side (segments 5 to 8). **C,** 45-degree right side up and arm across the body (segment 7 and posterior part of the segment 6). **D,** >70-degree right side up (same position as 45 degree with rotated table), for extreme access to posterosuperior segments.

In general, we use trocar formations as illustrated, but the trocar formations can be moved around. After pneumoperitoneum and placement of the first trocar, the liver and the abdominal cavity is visualized with the camera. Based on the liver size and position, size of the abdomen and the planned resection area, trocar placement is decided. The number of trocars depends on the lesion location and patient body build (Fig. 127D.7). Usually four trocars and one additional for Pringle are sufficient, but one should not hesitate to place extra trocars if needed. However, increasing the number of trocars may also increase the risk for intraoperative incidents.

Use of Intraoperative Ultrasound

After establishment of pneumoperitoneum and trocar placement, the liver is thoroughly examined with laparoscopic ultrasound to define exact tumor localization and its relation to the vascular anatomy (see Chapters 24 and 103) (Fig. 127D.8).

Liver Mobilization

Proper liver mobilization (also see Chapter 118) is important, especially when performing resection in the posterior segments

and in the upper part of segment 2. Together with appropriate patient positioning, it improves visualization by bringing the resection area into the working space (gravity facilitated retraction).

Left Lobe Mobilization

The procedure is started by dividing the left triangular, the round, the falciform, and the coronary ligaments. The coronary ligament is divided until the left hepatic vein and the suprahepatic vena cava are exposed.

Right Lobe Mobilization

We start first with dividing right triangular and lateral part of the coronary ligaments. Short hepatic veins to the inferior vena cava are sealed individually with a bipolar vessel sealer. Ligation is an option, but it can be dangerous to use metal-clips on these short vessels because they may fall off. We recommend using endo-staplers on larger short veins.

Next, the falciform ligament is divided (we try to spare the round ligament) and the liver is gently pushed downward using a retractor. The coronary ligament is divided until the suprahepatic vena cava and the right hepatic vein are exposed. The

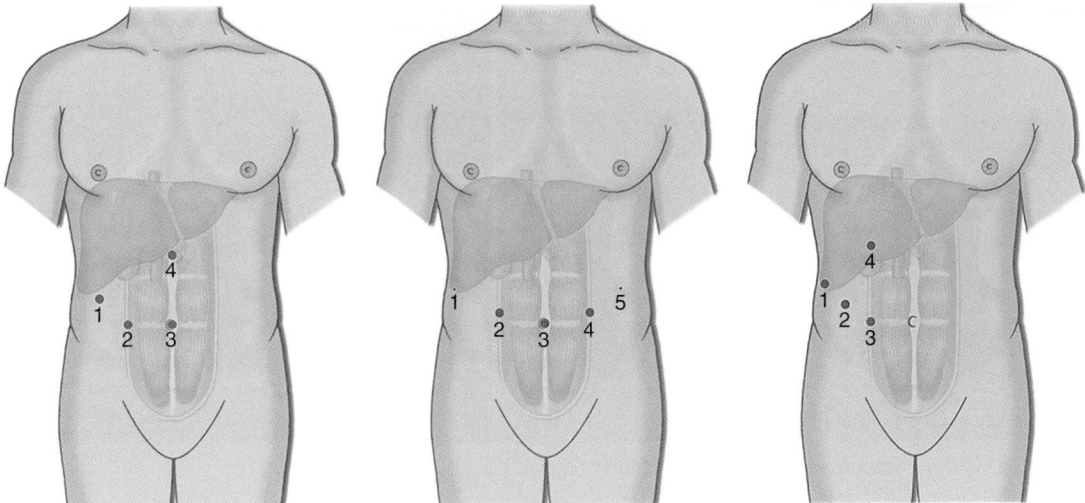

FIGURE 127D.7 Trocar placement for resections in different segments. **A,** L-shaped midline: resections in segments 5 to 8. **B,** Curved left: resections in segments 1 to 4. **C,** L-shaped pararectal: segment 7 and posterior part of the segment 6. (Courtesy of Kari C. Toverud CMI.)

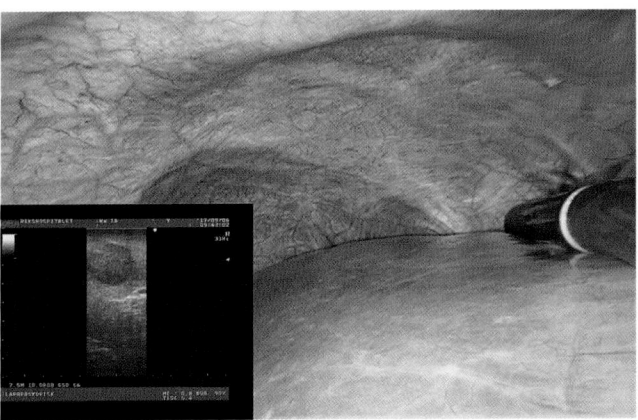

FIGURE 127D.8 Tumor exposure using intraoperative ultrasound.

right liver is then totally mobilized from ligamentous (coronary and triangular) attachments.

Resection Plan

The resection plan is created based on preoperative liver imaging and intraoperative ultrasound (see Chapters 13, 14, 15, 24, and 103), taking into account the tumor size, the distance from the vessels, possible resection margin, and both inflow and outflow of the resection area. The resection line is marked at the liver surface by electrocautery and followed-up with ultrasound examination to clarify the resection margin. Cautery marks give black shadows that mark the transection line, and show the distance from the tumor (Fig. 127D.9). A linear laparoscopic ultrasound probe is preferable over curved probe. The linear probe makes the resection planning easier.

We aim to create straight lateral lines, parallel with the portal tree and aligned with the surgeons two trocars. The anterior line is usually slightly curved. The posterior line can be marked, with the help of ultrasound, after transecting the anterior and lateral lines. It can be useful to mark the posterior line to avoid transecting too much behind the tumor in the liver when passing beneath the tumor.

Transection Techniques (also see Chapter 102B)

We transect the parenchyma with a bipolar vessel sealer in combination with an ultrasonic aspirator for larger resections.

The transection line follows the cautery marks on the liver surface. The resections are guided by repeated ultrasonography to ensure a tumor free margin and to look for portal branches. This reduces remnant liver ischemia and prevents bile leakage. We always try to avoid leaving peripheral bile ducts with no connection to the central bile tree (Fig. 127D.10).

The hepatic branches should also be identified and dissected selectively to avoid outflow occlusion in the liver remnant. However, bridge veins are often present, and these will frequently compensate for outflow occlusion. Vessels in the resection line are divided using the energy device, clips, and laparoscopic linear staplers, depending on the size of the vessels. The aspirator should be used to skeletonize larger vascular structures before they are divided. After completing the liver resection, a thorough visual examination and hemostasis of the resection bed is essential to minimize the risk for postoperative hemorrhage and bile leakage (see tips and tricks section). The resection bed may be covered by a hemostatic patch.

Another method or in addition to ultrasonic aspirator is the modified clamp-crushing. The jaws of the energy device are used to crush parenchyma with or without activating it. This allows the identification of vascular structures without damaging them so that they can be divided selectively. Activation of the instrument depends on deepness of the transection line. In the superficial parts, activation can be used with cutting, while deeper in the parenchyma, activation should be used with caution and without applying the knife. In contrast to superficial transection, where one can use clamp-crushing, deep in the parenchyma where larger vessels and bile ducts are present, the use of an aspirator in combination with a bipolar vessel sealer is recommended. Clamp-crushing with bipolar vessel sealer can be used but with caution.

Extraction, Drainage, and Closure

All lesions are extracted using an endoscopic retrieval bag. We tend to remove specimens through an extension of trocar incisions in the midline (usually the first trocar incision), but a

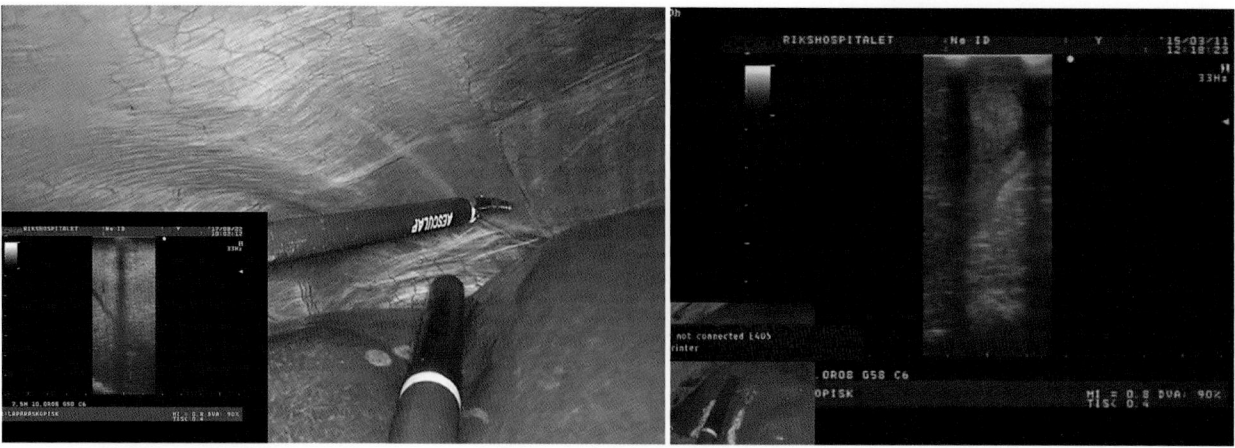

FIGURE 127D.9 Resection planning with ultrasound. Black shadows from the cautery are easily visible on ultrasound.

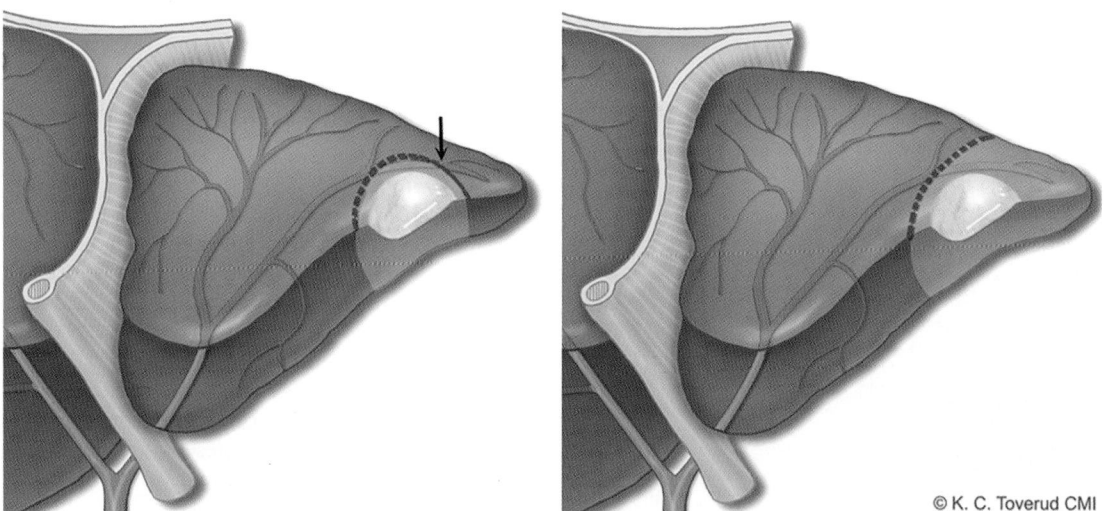

© K. C. Toverud CMI

FIGURE 127D.10 Reducing risk for bile leak. (Courtesy of Kari C. Toverud CMI.)

Pfannenstiel incision is a good option in the absence of adhesion in the lower part of abdomen. We recommend closing the fascia of trocar incisions located in the midline and the one used for extraction. In thin patients, it is recommended to suture the fascia in all incisions.

We rarely use abdominal drains but prefer to leave one if there is a risk for bile leakage (e.g., signs of bile on the resection bed, or after suturing the bile ducts) (see Chapter 118). Drains can be used in case of large resection surfaces.

Tips and Tricks
Keep Patient Dry and CVP Low

Low central venous pressure (CVP) should be achieved before parenchyma transection, which helps reduce the risk for bleeding (see Chapters 25 and 118). Low CVP can be achieved by patient positioning, fluid restriction, ventilation management, and vasodilators use. Close surgeon-anesthesiologist collaboration is important. We operate with a pneumoperitoneum of 12 mm Hg. In case of venous bleeding, we increase the pressure up to 15 mm Hg and rarely 18 mm Hg. In our experience, CO_2 embolism is a small clinical problem (high solubility

of CO_2), but anesthesiologists should be aware of the increased intraabdominal pressure and monitor the end-tidal CO_2 levels. Reducing the airway pressure of the patient (usually by turning off positive end-expiratory pressure on the respirator) may also limit bleeding by reducing pressure in the hepatic veins.

Ensuring the Resection Margins

If one is in doubt of the resection margin when approaching the tumor, ultrasound is of great value (see Chapters 24 and 103). Modern ultrasound equipment can visualize the resection line, but it can be helpful to place a Surgicel® or similar hemostat (Fig. 127D.11), or a metal instrument to clarify the margins by visualizing shadow between tumor and resection bed.

Visualization and Mobilization

Proper liver mobilization (see Chapter 118) before starting the resection is important, especially in posteriorly located tumors. However, unnecessary mobilization can lead to adhesions that may complicate future repeat resections. A rule of thumb is that both the operator's instruments must be able to reach the posterior part of the resection line.

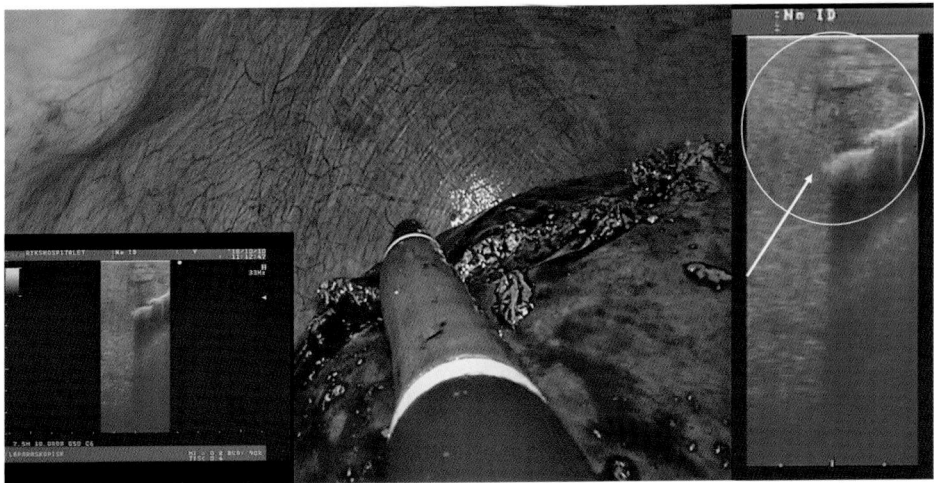

FIGURE 127D.11 Clarifying resection margin. The arrow points to Surgicel® in the resection margin.

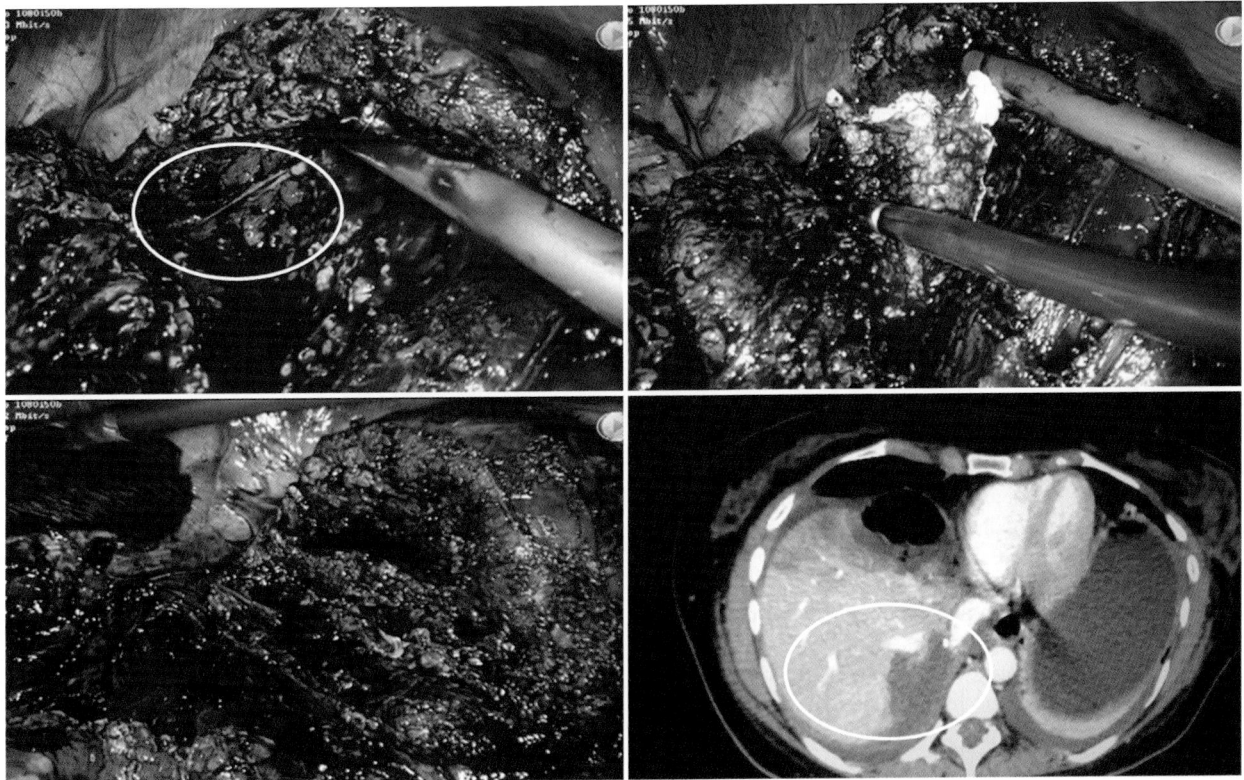

FIGURE 127D.12 Venous bleeding handling with a hemostatic patch. Postoperative CT scan.

Managing Intraoperative Bleeding

A Pringle maneuver is always useful to control the situation and decide what is the best option for repair. Increasing the intraabdominal pressure could have a similar effect but is less efficient. Most bleedings during liver resection will be effectively controlled by compression and patience. If compression is not sufficient, bipolar diathermia directly on the bleeding vessel, or monopolar diathermia applied in a circular pattern around the bleeding vessel can be helpful. Larger bleedings from the portal veins must often be sutured, In that case we prefer a barbed suture with a pledget. Hepatic veins can be more difficult to suture and hepatic bleedings can often be stopped with a hemostatic patch (Fig. 127D.12) because it is a low-pressure system.

Handling Bile Leak

A meticulously placed suture is in our experience the best way to control a bile leak. If the duct can be lifted and visualized, a well-placed clip is a good option.

Teamwork

A well-functioning and well-informed operating team are essential. The World Health Organization (WHO) surgical safety checklist[15] is always used in our operating theatres. The time out at the beginning of the operation is important to collect the focus of the team and address any questions or uncertainty. The surgeons must be respectful leaders and always pay attention to their communication style and behavior to ensure the functionality of the team.

SPECIFIC CASES (EXAMPLES)

Left Lateral Sectionectomy (also see Chapter 118B)

This operation is described here because it is a very suitable procedure to start learning laparoscopic liver surgery. This procedure gives basic understanding and training before beginning with more advanced hepatectomies (e.g., learning how to do dissection and mobilization) and experience with working laparoscopic liver instruments (e.g., aspirator, dissecting instruments) and laparoscopic ultrasound.

The patient is placed in the supine position. The operating surgeon stands to the patient's right side. When teaching a less experienced surgeon this procedure, the expert can stand on the left side and be in complete control, while the trainee can perform most of the operation from the right side.

After establishment of pneumoperitoneum and trocar placement (see Fig. 6B), the left lobe is mobilized by dividing the triangular and coronary ligaments up to the ligamentum venosum Arantii and the left hepatic vein using a bipolar vessel sealing device. The falciform, a part of the right coronary and the rest of the left coronary ligaments, is then dissected to visualize the confluence of the inferior vena cava and the left hepatic vein. The round ligament is then divided and can be used as a handle to facilitate the parenchymal transection. The Pringle maneuver is usually not necessary. The liver parenchyma is then transected ("opening the book") parallel to the falciform ligament with the bipolar vessel sealing device. After dissecting the Rex recesses (to avoid damaging the portal branch to segment 4) and exposing the portal branch to segment 3, it is dissected between clips or with a linear endo-stapler without skeletonizing it. Thereafter, the parenchymal transection is continued to the portal branch of segment 2, which is dissected by the same technique. The resection is continued up to the left hepatic vein, which is sectioned by an endo-stapler.

As an alternative, the pedicle to segments 2 and 3 can be easily divided with one endo-stapler after the liver parenchyma is transected from the liver surface. This approach is faster, but it does not provide the same training for young surgeons.

Tumor Located in Segment 8

Segment 8 is considered one of the more difficult segments for laparoscopic liver surgery. However, the lower parts of segment 8 are easily accessible and smaller tumors in this area are in our view suitable for surgeons learning laparoscopic liver surgery.

In this case, we presented a patient with a large metastasis in segment 8, close to the right hepatic vein, and a right hemihepatectomy was considered. But after re-evaluation, an atypical, *R1 vascular* resection (detaching from the vessel) was preferred, which is oncologically sufficient[16] (Fig. 127D.13).

Trocars are planned as illustrated. The surgeon stands on the right-side using trocars 1 and 2, the camera is in trocar 3, and the assistant's instrument in trocar 4. The umbilicus is opened, and a pneumoperitoneum of 12 mm Hg is established (Fig. 127D.14).

After examining the abdominal cavity for carcinomatosis, we perform laparoscopic ultrasound and mark the resection lines with monopolar cautery. The resection is planned so that the feeding portal vein is found in the lower medial part. That allows early control of the pedicle supplying the resected part. The shape of the resection follows the affected pedicle peripherally and respects pedicles to the liver remnant (Fig. 127D.15).

The parenchyma is opened with a bipolar scaler, first the two lateral lines and then the anterior line. It is crucial that the parenchyma is opened perpendicularly to the surface. This is most easily achieved by angling the lower jaw of the instrument slightly away from the tumor. If one is not careful with this, the resection line could easily come too close to the tumor. Using the aspirator—or clamp-crush technique—the anterior and lateral lines are opened. Lateral lines are continued cranial to the tumor. Then, the anterior and lateral lines are opened further to reach the intentional plane beneath the tumor. It is important to make the corners between anterior and lateral lines free dissected, so that the specimen can be lifted up, and the plane beneath the tumor can be created. Double sealing and a Pringle maneuver are useful in this part, to simplify the dissection and avoid bleeding.

The pedicle supplying the tumor will be found in the lower, medial part and must be dissected carefully. Ultrasonic aspirator and dissector are used to skeletonize the pedicle. It should be ensured that there are no branches posteriorly

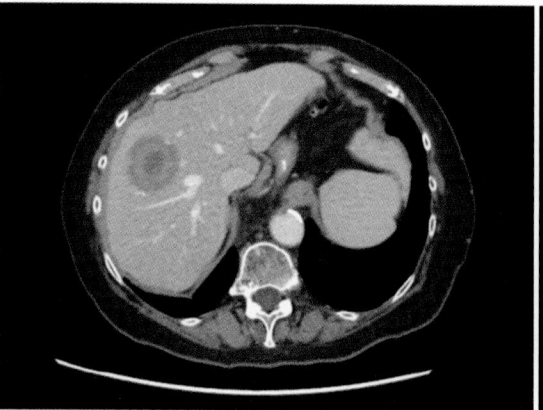
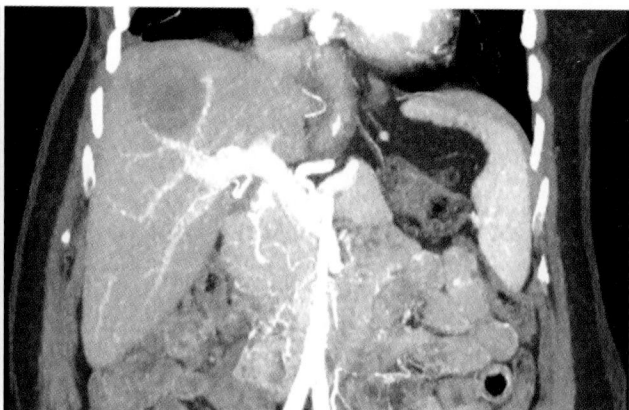

FIGURE 127D.13   CT scan with a tumor located in segment 8.

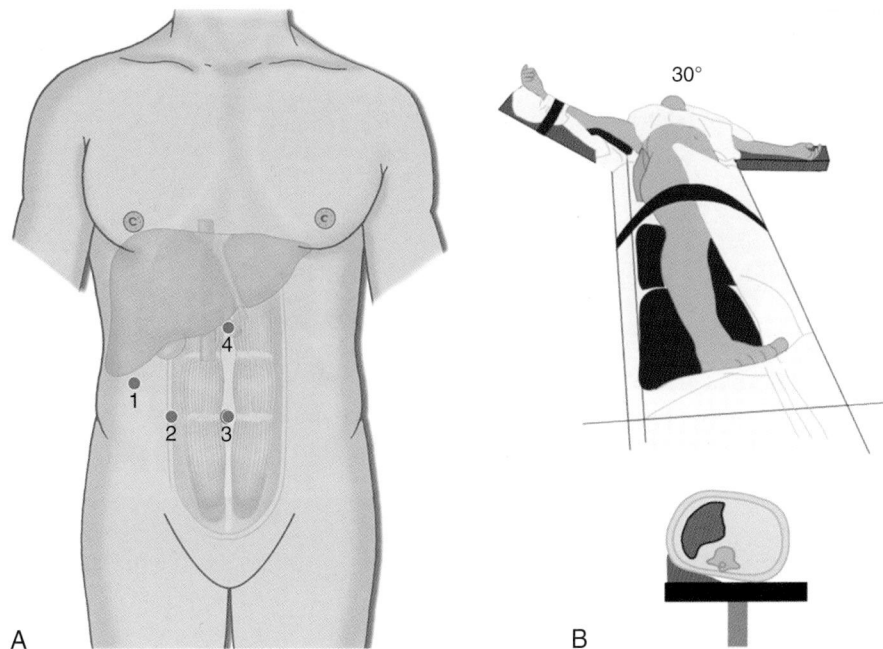

FIGURE 127D.14 A and B, Trocar placement and patient positioning for resection in segment 8. (Part A: Courtesy of Kari C. Toverud CMI; Part B: Courtesy of Egidijus Pelanis.)

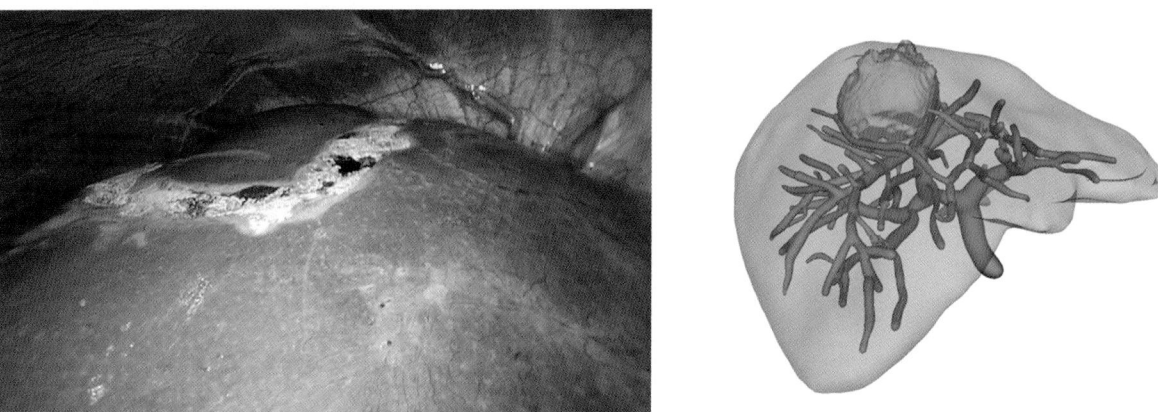

FIGURE 127D.15 Marked resection lines and 3D segmented liver with the tumor. (Courtesy of Egidijus Pelanis.)

before a suitable clip is placed, and the vessel is cut using the sealer (Fig. 127D.16).

Close attention must be paid to further dissection below the tumor. Ultrasound is performed to ensure the margin. The easiest way to dissect the specimen off the hepatic vein is to dissect very close to it and follow it cranially until the tumor is free. The aspirator is of great value here.

Finally, the posterior line of the resection is divided with a combination of sealer and aspirator. It is usually beneficial to do this from both sides, pulling the now rather mobile specimen in the contralateral direction. Trocar 4 will be helpful for managing the posterior line. After completing resection, the specimen removed with the help of retrieval bag and the resection bed is examined (Fig. 127D.17).

Tumor Located in the Posterior Part of Segment 7

Segment 7 is technically demanding to approach laparoscopically and requires a significant experience. An experienced assistant is of great value because appropriate retraction of the liver is necessary to reach most of the segment. We here present a patient with a colorectal metastasis in segment 7 close to the vena cava.

The patient is placed with right side 45 degrees up, right arm across body. If necessary, the table can be tilted until the patient's right side is almost 90 degrees up (Fig. 127D.18). Pneumoperitoneum is established using open technique through an incision just lateral to the rectus abdominis muscle. We always avoid the muscle to prevent accidental damage to the epigastric vessels.

The surgeon operates with trocars 1 and 2, the camera is in trocar 3 and the assistant uses a retractor in trocar 4 (we prefer an endo-retract, fan-shaped, with three fingers). An extra 5 mm trocar laterally and subcostal is often very useful.

The right lobe is completely mobilized to the vena cava, and we never encircle the right hepatic vein. Short vessels are divided with the bipolar sealer, we always make sure we get a

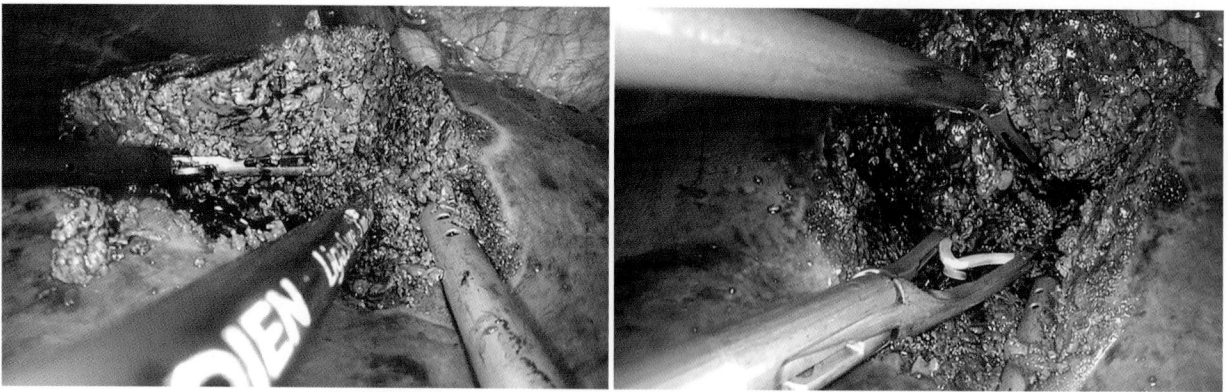

FIGURE 127D.16 Parenchyma transection and inflow control.

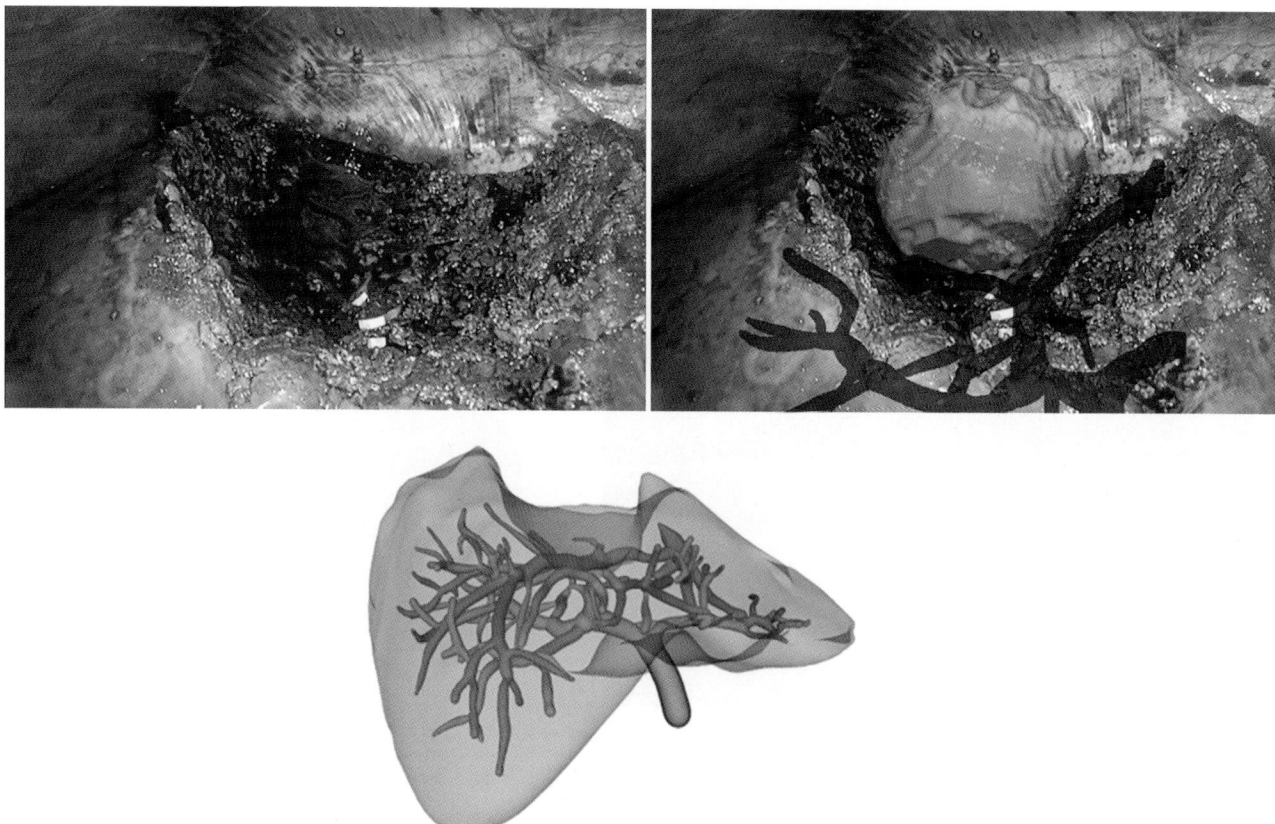

FIGURE 127D.17 Resection bed with augmented tumor and pedicle. Segmented liver based on postoperative CT scan. (Courtesy of Egidijus Pelanis.)

double seal with a certain distance to the cava. We avoid applying clips on short vessels, due to the risk of falling off. If in doubt we cut the sealed vessel with scissors. We divide the falciform and coronary ligaments while we normally spare the round ligament. The assistant must pay attention, so appropriate traction is put on the tissue while avoiding potentially disastrous damage to vena cava and short veins (Fig. 127D.19).

When the liver is completely mobile, the tumor is located using ultrasound. Resection lines are marked as described previously. The retractor is crucial to the next steps of the operation. The optimal position is usually parallel to the superior longitudinal resection line, pressing the liver gently to the left. In this way, the tumor will be nicely presented to the surgeon, and a difficult location is made far easier (Fig. 127D.20).

Pringle is mandatory. The parenchyma is divided as described in 4.3. The anterior line is transected first; then lateral lines are taken. When the anterior line and the lateral lines are opened, the combination of the traction of the left instrument and liver retractor will allow the tumor to gradually "fall out" of the liver ("open the book"). Afterward, the deeper parts of the resection line can be visualized and feeding and draining vessels can be safely identified and divided creating the intentional plane beneath the tumor (Fig. 127D.21).

Hemostasis is ensured. We usually put a hemostatic patch on resection beds close to the cava.

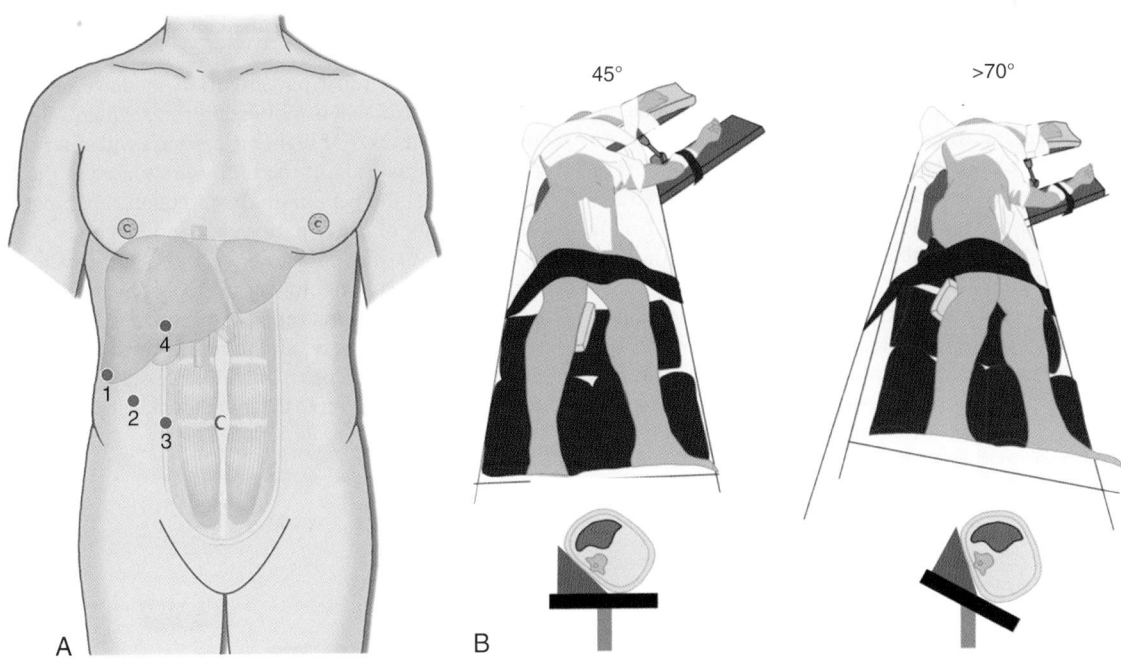

FIGURE 127D.18 A and B, Trocar placement and patient positioning for resection in segment 7. (A, Courtesy of Kari C. Toverud CMI; B, Courtesy of Egidijus Pelanis.)

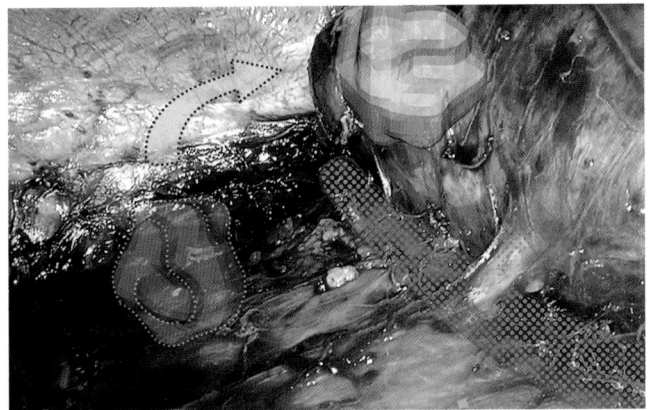

FIGURE 127D.19 Mobilization of the right liver lobe and tumor exposure (marked in yellow). Uncovering of the inferior vena cava, the short vein (marked in blue). (Courtesy of Egidijus Pelanis.)

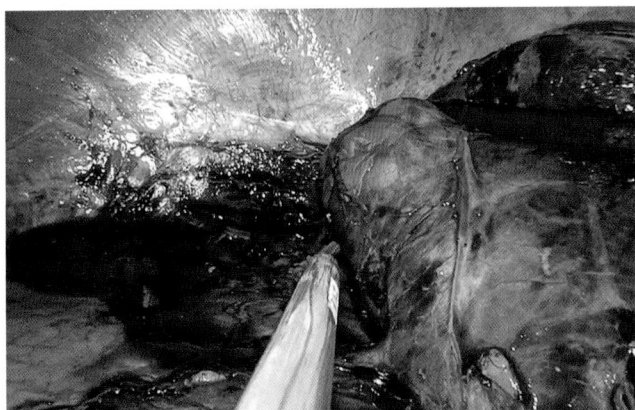

FIGURE 127D.20 Facilitated visualization of the resection area. (Courtesy of Egidijus Pelanis.)

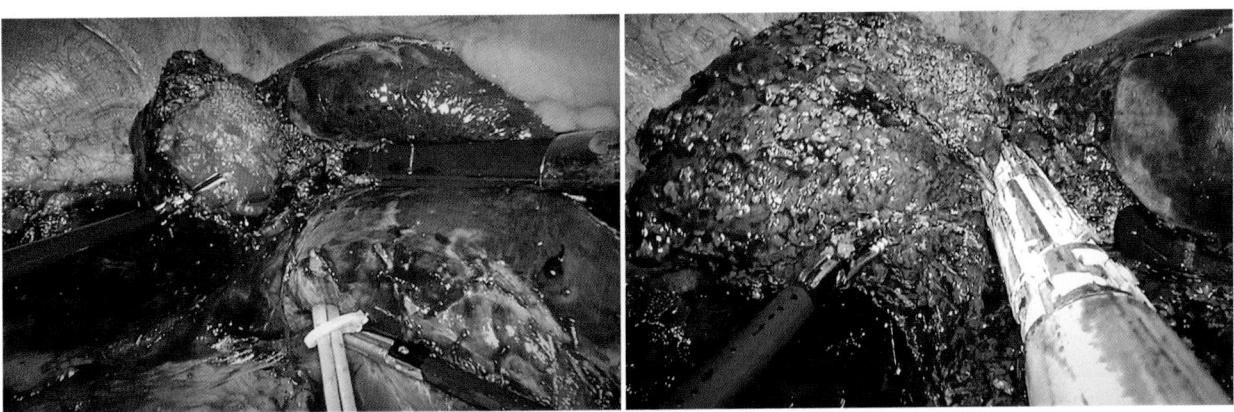

FIGURE 127D.21 Gravity facilitated resection. Parenchyma transection. Inflow and outflow control.

Tumor Located in Segment 1

The resection in segment 1 can be demanding but is usually accessible with the correct approach. The patient is placed in a supine position the first trocar is placed in the umbilicus (3) and then two pararectal trocarsed on both sides (2 and 4). An additional trocar is placed laterally on the right side (1). The camera is usually placed in trocar 3, while the assistant retracts the liver from trocar 4. This allows the surgeon to stand on the right-hand side in a comfortable position, operating through trocars 1 and 2 (Fig. 127D.22).

We start with opening the pars flaccida. The left portion of segment 1 (Spiegel's lobe) is then visible, and accessible for ultrasound examination. If the tumor is solely situated in this part (Fig. 127D.23), it can easily be resected with the bipolar sealing device using either the clamp-crush technique or combining with an aspirator.

The surgeon must pay attention to short veins to the cava that will appear when mobilizing the segment, and the portal vein to the left part of segment 1, which will enter the specimen from the cranial side. If the tumor is situated in the cranial part of segment 1, the person on the resection side must be aware of the proximity of the hepatic vein confluence.

Tumors in the paracaval or right part (caudate lobe) of segment 1 are more complex to resect (Fig. 127D.24). In these cases, right lobe mobilization is useful. A 12 mm trocar in the upper midline will be helpful to retract the liver. Lifting the hilum and segment 4/5 will often provide access. Performing a cholecystectomy without dividing the cystic duct will allow the assistant to

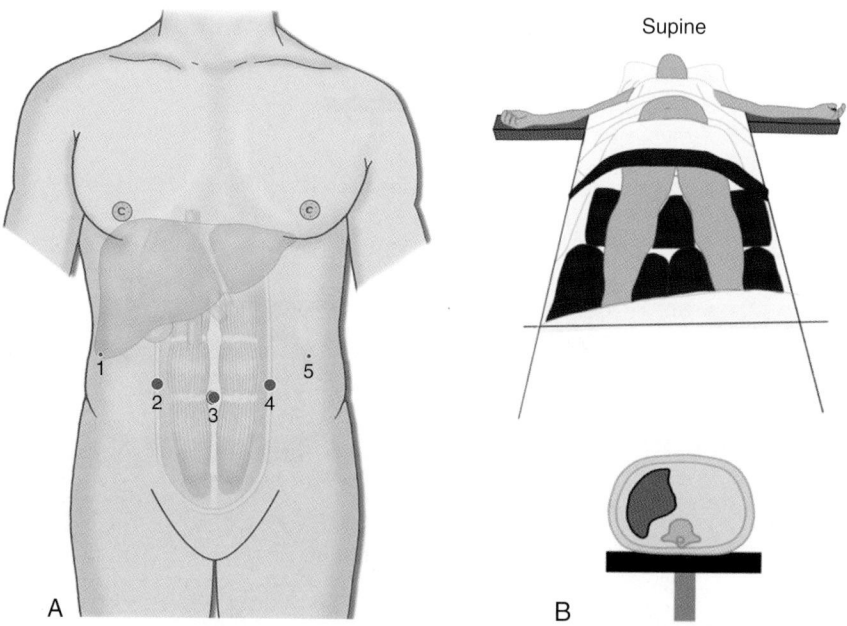

FIGURE 127D.22 A and B, Patient positioning and trocar placement for caudate resection. (A, Courtesy of Kari C. Toverud CMI; B, Courtesy of Egidijus Pelanis.)

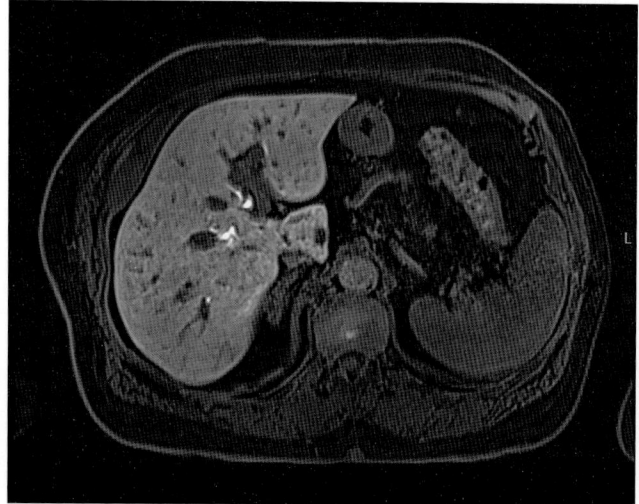

FIGURE 127D.23 MRI picture of tumor located in Spiegel's lobe ion in segment 1.

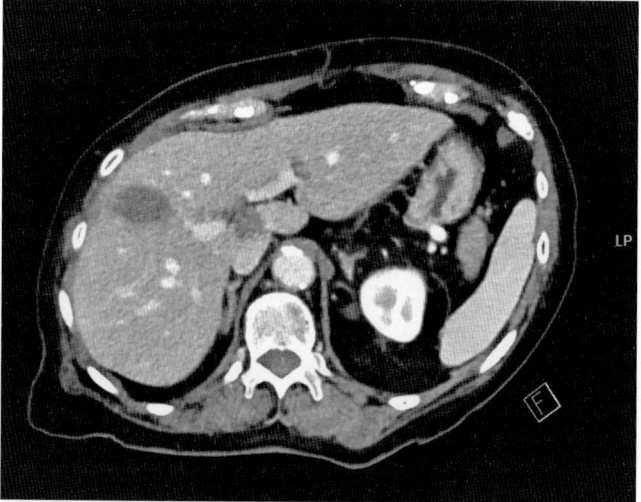

FIGURE 127D.24 CT scan of tumor located in the paracaval/caudate lobe.

retract the hepatoduodenal ligament cranially and to the left so that the tumor can be safely dissected free from the portal vein confluence.

PREVENTING AND HANDLING POSTOPERATIVE COMPLICATIONS (SEE CHAPTERS 27 AND 28)

In Oslo, patients follow a fast-track protocol focused on preoperative information, early feeding, mobilization, and return to normal life. If the patient can follow these principles, postoperative monitoring is usually not necessary, except with daily measurement of hemoglobin, electrolytes, liver function tests. and inflammation markers. Patients get pain relief with paracetamol, nonsteroidal antiinflammatory drugs, and opioids (if needed). Optimal pain relief is necessary for compliance to the fast-track protocol. Patients are routinely given proton pump inhibitors to prevent gastric or duodenal ulcers and low-molecular weight heparin for 30 days to prevent deep venous thrombosis. Patients get a single dose of oral antibiotics preoperatively.

Laparoscopic atypical resections have a relatively low postoperative complication rate.[9] The most common complication that requires postoperative intervention is infected fluid collections (see Chapter 28). These usually occur in the resection bed after 7 to 10 days. In the OSLO-COMET trial, 4 of 129 laparoscopic patients needed a drain because of this complication.[17] Because patients normally stay in hospital only 1 to 3 days, we inform them that symptoms of infected fluid collections can occur after they come home. If they get fever, abdominal pain, or similar, they are instructed to contact their local doctor and if blood tests indicate infection, they are admitted to hospital for a CT scan. If antibiotic treatment does not resolve the infection, an ultrasound-guided drain is placed.

Because patients are kept dry during surgery, we sometimes see postoperative atrial fibrillation that usually resolves with fluid therapy. After larger resections we monitor the liver remnant with lactate and INR daily, and the threshold is low for a postoperative CT scan in case of abnormalities. Many patients have undergone abdominal surgery previously, and bowel injury after adhesiolysis is a dreaded complication. Contamination from bowel perforation combined with a raw wound surface on the liver rapidly can evolve to a sepsis that can be hard to treat. We therefore have a low threshold to re-laparoscope patients where there is suspicion of bowel injury.

FUTURE PROSPECTS

At this moment, laparoscopic parenchyma sparing liver surgery is documented in randomized controlled trials and is well

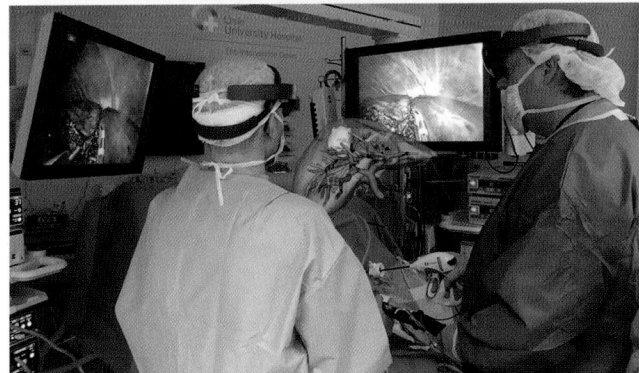

FIGURE 127D.25 Intraoperative use of head mounted mixed reality device. (Courtesy of Egidijus Pelanis.)

established in expert centers worldwide.[8] The next step is to provide training programs to young surgeons and liver surgeons not experienced with laparoscopy. Recent Dutch data suggest that it is difficult to reproduce results from randomized controlled trials (RCTs) on complex laparoscopic surgery to real world practice,[18] and structured training programs, proctoring, and auditing is the best way to achieve this.

We recommend that all hospitals that want to start laparoscopic liver surgery take on training programs. It is also useful if the whole surgical team can travel to an expert center to learn the setup, from patient positioning to central venous pressure. It is vital to the success of the surgery that the whole setup be transferred. Close contact with a mentor when planning the first independent procedures is helpful.

Patient specific 3D models are valuable tools in the preoperative planning of liver surgery.[19] Commercially available software can create models from thin slice CT images, and although no optimal solution exists at the moment, the solutions improve steadily. Head mounted mixed reality devices can improve visualization further (Fig. 127D.25).[20] An attractive addition would be navigated instruments that could be seen in the model in real time.[21] At the moment, no segmentation tool can update the position of the liver in real time while navigating instruments, but several research groups are working to solve this issue. Hybrid operating theatres with intraoperative imaging equipment is necessary to progress this research field.

The references for this chapter can be found online by accessing the accompanying Expert Consult website.

CHAPTER 127E

Laparoscopic major and complex liver resection

Chady Salloum and Daniel Cherqui

The increasing use of laparoscopic procedures has been driven by the ability to perform surgery through small rather than large incisions, with reduced postoperative pain and enhanced recovery. This began with laparoscopic cholecystectomy (see Chapter 36) introduced in 1988 and almost universally adopted within 2 years, although without a proper randomized controlled trial (RCT), because its advantages appeared evident to surgeons, physicians, and patients. The transient increase in bile duct injuries emphasized the learning curve and paramount importance of proper training with innovative procedures. Laparoscopic surgery was soon extended to more complex procedures and has become standard practice for most upper gastrointestinal (GI) and colorectal procedures. New surgical skills made this possible, including complex dissection and suturing techniques, as well as the development of new, highly efficient technologies such as enhanced video equipment, electrosurgical devices, and staplers.

Liver resection, a stand-alone procedure (i.e., without reconstruction or anastomosis required), could be considered an excellent candidate for the laparoscopic approach[1,2] (see Chapter 127A). However, it has remained an area of resistance for several years, with much slower adoption than other laparoscopic procedures, because of the perceived risks of uncontrollable bleeding and oncologic inadequacy (tumor seeding, margins). Another reason for delayed development has probably been the lack of training of established liver surgery experts to advanced laparoscopy. Indeed, laparoscopic liver resections (LLRs) are difficult procedures requiring expertise in both liver surgery and advanced laparoscopy. Mastering simple laparoscopic procedures, such as cholecystectomy, is clearly insufficient, and the "open" liver surgeon must learn a new set of skills. Conversely, being an expert laparoscopic surgeon without a background in indications and techniques for liver surgery is clearly insufficient as well.

Over the past 20 years, several teams worldwide have explored laparoscopic liver surgery. A recent comprehensive review of the literature compiled more than 9000 reported cases.[3] Less than 20 centers reported series of more than 100 LLRs. It must be acknowledged that RCTs comparing open and laparoscopic liver surgery are difficult to perform because of the large samples required, which are difficult to accrue. Unlike other procedures, such as colon resection for cancer, liver resection is less often performed. Also, it addresses various diseases, including primary and secondary liver cancer and normal or diseased underlying liver, and there are many types of resection, including major and minor hepatectomies, with various procedures according to tumor type and location in the liver segments (see Chapters 118–120). The results of RCTs of LLR addressing one disease or one procedure will be difficult to generalize to variable types of diseases or resections.

Available literature consists of case series, case-matched comparative studies, and meta-analyses. Reported cases consist mainly of minor resections in favorable locations (segments II to VI). However, major and more complex resections (anatomic resections, difficult locations) are now more frequently reported.[4–6] Two comprehensive reviews of the literature showed a rise in the proportion of major resection from 15% in 2009[7] to 30% in 2015.[3] Laparoscopic major hepatectomy remains a relatively challenging operation since first reported in 1997.[9] Its development has been slow and the first documented series with more than 10 cases were not published until after 2004.[9–11] Laparoscopic major liver resection is currently perceived as the most complex of all laparoscopic procedures and should be performed only by a team of surgeons experienced in both laparoscopic and hepatobiliary surgery. The high tendency of morbidity and postoperative liver failure after major liver resection limit its clinical application in the field of laparoscopic operation. Moreover, underlying liver diseases such as viral hepatitis with cirrhosis sharply increase the surgical difficulty[12] (see Chapters 74 and 120). Right liver resections have always been performed in the conventional manner, and they were initially considered unsuitable for laparoscopy; however, an increasing number of laparoscopic right liver resections have been reported.[10,13,14] The recommendations from the Second International Consensus on Laparoscopic Liver resection still consider a laparoscopic major hepatectomy an innovative procedure that "is still in an exploration or learning phase (IDEAL 2b) and has incompletely defined risks..." and "...should continue to be introduced cautiously."[15] The first European Guidelines Meeting on laparoscopic liver surgery, held in Southampton in 2017,[16] suggest that the feasibility, reproducibility, and implementation of left and right hepatectomies is sufficiently different that they should be considered separately. For left hepatectomy, compared with an open approach, laparoscopic approach appears to be associated with reduced blood loss, morbidity, and hospital length of stay (LOS) with comparable operative times, completeness of resection, and mortality. For right hepatectomy, in experienced hands, a laparoscopic approach appears to be associated with reduced hospital LOS and blood loss with comparable mortality and completeness of resection, in comparison to open surgery. It must be recognized, however, that these data are derived from retrospective studies, which are associated with significant bias related to patient selection.

Meta-analyses of retrospective comparative series have suggested several short-term advantages of the laparoscopic approach over open surgery, such as decreased pain, bleeding, transfusions, morbidity, and hospital LOS.[3,17] Surgical margins and long-term survivals were not inferior.[3] Other studies suggested identical oncologic outcomes compared with open surgery.[18] Interestingly, no study found any disadvantage to the laparoscopic approach.

Currently, the vast majority of hepatopancreatobiliary (HPB) centers practice laparoscopic minor resection, including left lateral sectionectomy and peripheral wedge resections (see Chapters 118B and 127D). A smaller number of teams are using the laparoscopic approach for formal right or left hepatectomy. An even smaller number have reported complex anatomic resection, including difficult locations (e.g., segmentectomy VII or VIII, anterior or posterior sectionectomy).[19–24] Proportion of resections using the laparoscopic approach varies among centers and ranges from 10% to over 90%; our present rate is 35% of all liver resections. The percentage of resections for benign lesions has remained stable over our experience, whereas the percentage of resections for malignant tumors continues to increase gradually.

TERMINOLOGY AND DEFINITIONS

In 2008 the first expert consensus meeting on laparoscopic liver surgery was held to discuss the international position on LLR. In the resulting Louisville Statement,[25] they agreed on three procedural definitions: pure laparoscopy, hand-assisted laparoscopy, and hybrid technique. Pure laparoscopy applies to complete mobilization and resection through laparoscopic ports, with an incision for specimen extraction only. Hand-assisted laparoscopy applies to the elective placement of a hand port to assist the operation, with transection performed under video laparoscopic view and extraction of tumor through the hand port incision. Hybrid technique refers to a procedure in which laparoscopy, with or without hand assistance, is used for liver mobilization, whereas resection is performed under direct vision through a small incision. According to a comprehensive international review performed by Nguyen and colleagues,[7] 75% of reported laparoscopic resections were pure laparoscopic, 17% were hand-assisted procedures, and 2% used the hybrid technique. In addition, 4% were conversions to laparotomy or hand-assisted procedures, with the remaining 2% using less common techniques, such as a thoracoscopic approach.

Considerable debate arose at the Second International Laparoscopic Liver Consensus Conference,[15] regarding the terminology and definitions of laparoscopic major hepatectomy versus "degree of difficulty." For example, isolated laparoscopic resection of segment VII or VIII as a single segment might be defined as a minor hepatectomy using the classical definition of Couinaud, but the degree of difficulty for these operations minimally invasively is very high. A novel difficulty scoring system for laparoscopic liver resections has been proposed.[26]

Laparoscopic resections should be categorized no differently than open resections. Based on Couinaud and Brisbane 2000 terminology of liver anatomy and resections,[27] segments II, III, IVb, V, and VI are most amenable to laparoscopic resection[25] (see Chapter 2). Isolated resection of tumors located in posterior-superior liver (segments I, IVa, VII, and VIII) and major hepatectomy have been reported[20,24,28,29] (see Chapter 127D). However, these operations are technically more challenging and should be reserved for expert surgeons who are able to extend the limits after safe mastery of segments II to VI laparoscopic resections. In the comprehensive review by Ciria and colleagues,[3] the majority (70%) were minor resections (two segments or less), including nonanatomic wedge resections and left lateral sectionectomies (20% each). Anatomic segmentectomies and sectionectomies, classified as minor by the amount of resected liver, are complex resections reported mainly by Asian surgeons and accounted for 13% and 5% of the cases, respectively. Major resections, consisting of three or more segments, accounted for 24% of the cases, with right and left hepatectomies representing 13% and 11%, respectively. Anecdotal extended hepatectomies were reported, and 6% were unspecified.

INDICATIONS

Indications for LLR should be categorized no differently than open resections (see Chapters 101, 118, and 127A). It must be emphasized that the potential benefits of a minimally invasive resection must not lead to an increase in the indications outside the guidelines or to resection of lesions for the purpose of providing a definitive diagnosis. Specifically, the laparoscopic approach should not be used to resect incidental, asymptomatic lesions convincingly recognized by patient history, imaging, and tumor markers to be benign and without harmful potential, including cysts, hemangiomas, and focal nodular hyperplasia. Also, laparoscopic resection should not be performed for the purpose of diagnosis when lesions are safely amenable to percutaneous biopsy.

Indications for LLR rely on the same guidelines as open liver surgery. Cases should be discussed at multidisciplinary tumor boards. Once the indication for resection has been established, the feasibility of the laparoscopic approach should be evaluated. The extent of resection; the size, location, and number of lesions; and proximity to the major vessels are important factors in determining when laparoscopic resection is appropriate (Table 127E.1). The selection criteria of patients are crucial for successfully performing right or left hepatectomy

TABLE 127E.1 Predictors of Difficulty of Laparoscopic Liver Resection		
FACTOR	EASY	DIFFICULT
Tumor size	<5 cm	>5 cm
Tumor depth	Superficial/pedunculated	Deep
Tumor location	Segments II, III, IVb, V, VI	Segments I, IVa, VII, VIII
Tumor number	Single	Multiple
Distance from hepatic hilum, proximal hepatic veins, or inferior vena cava	>1 cm	<1 cm
Surgeon experience	<25 cases	>25 cases
Liver background	Normal	Injured
Extent of resection	Lateral sectionectomy Peripheral wedge resection	Right/left hepatectomy Anatomic segmentectomy Sectionectomy (2 segments) Extended resection Donor hepatectomy

BOX 127E.1   Indications and Contraindications for Laparoscopic Major Hepatectomy (Three Segments or More)

Indications

The same as open resection for malignant neoplasms and select benign lesions
Lesions < 10 cm

Relative contraindications (can be considered in selected cases)

Lesions near the inferior vena cava, hilum, or major hepatic veins
Early gallbladder cancer and early intrahepatic cholangiocarcinoma
Coagulopathy or thrombocythemia
Biliary reconstruction required
Previous upper abdominal surgery
Lesions > 10 cm

Absolute contraindications

Advanced gallbladder cancer
Advanced intrahepatic cholangiocarcinoma
Hilar cholangiocarcinoma
Portal hypertension (only parenchymal-sparing procedures in patients with portal hypertension)
Vascular reconstruction required
Inability to obtain a surgical margin that would otherwise be possible in an open resection
Patient unable to tolerate pneumoperitoneum

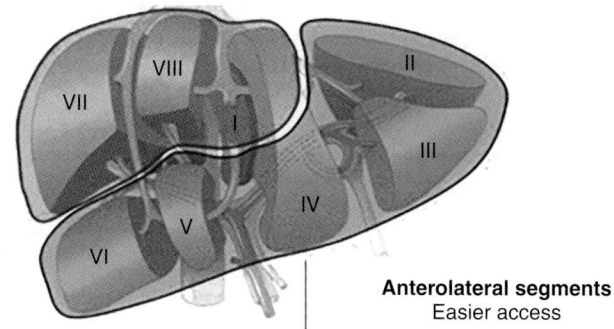

Posterosuperior segments
Difficult access

Anterolateral segments
Easier access

FIGURE 127E.1   Easy locations: segments II to VI (favorable because facing the scope). Difficult locations: segments I, IVa, VII and VIII (difficulty related to access and proximity of hepatic veins and IVC).

(Box 127E.1). Liver function is a determinant regardless of the technique and surgical skills (see Chapter 4). Patients with decompensated liver function are often associated with a vulnerable body condition, which may lead to intraoperative bleeding and anesthetic accident. Thus a Child A score must be achieved preoperatively. No major vascular invasion is essential for radical operation. It is challenging to perform laparoscopic operation in patients with a large subcapsular tumor. The limited space and mobilization of the liver may cause the tumor to break up and spread. The status of the underlying liver should also be considered. Although patients with benign disease have an underlying normal liver (see Chapter 88), patients with malignant disease usually have some degree of liver injury (see Chapters 68, 69, and 74). About 90% of patients with hepatocellular carcinoma (HCC) have a background of chronic liver injury, with chronic hepatitis B or C infection (see Chapter 68), alcohol, and nonalcoholic steatohepatitis (see Chapter 69) being the most common causes. In addition, a significant proportion of patients with colorectal liver metastases increasingly have some degree of liver disease from chemotherapy-induced injury (see Chapter 69). This should be taken into consideration for the laparoscopic approach. The surgical difficulty is highly subjective and influenced by not only tumor and patient factors but also the surgeon's experience. It is important to increase skills gradually according to experience level before performing more complex procedures.

TUMOR SIZE AND LOCATION

The most favorable lesions for laparoscopic resection are solitary tumors less than 5 cm and located in peripheral liver segments II to VI[25] (Fig. 127E.1). Such cases are recommended as initial procedures when initiating an LLR program. Pedunculated

tumors located at inferior or left lateral liver even greater than 5 cm are also favorable to laparoscopic resection. The laparoscopic approach should be considered the standard approach for left lateral sectionectomy[17,25,30] (see Chapter 127D). Peripheral wedge resections are also considered easy procedures. Tumor size itself is no longer an absolute contraindication for LLR.

The complexity of each major hepatectomy procedure differs widely and the number of segments alone does not convey the complexity of a resection. To this end, Lee et al.[31] recently reported that the complexity of open liver resections should not be classified based on whether the resection is "major or minor" but instead based on the extent of the liver resection. The classification divides open liver resection procedures into three complexity groups: low, medium, and high. In this system, a left lateral sectionectomy is classified as low complexity. Left hepatectomy, right hepatectomy, and right posterior sectionectomy are considered medium complexity, and right anterior sectionectomy and central bisectionectomy are considered high complexity. Kawaguchi et al.[32] proposed another classification system of laparoscopic liver resection according to their surgical difficulty. This classification provides levels of difficulty: grade I (the beginning and least complex level, which includes wedge resection and left lateral sectionectomy), grade II (the intermediate level, which includes anterolateral segmentectomy and left hepatectomy), and grade III (the advanced level, which includes posterosuperior segmentectomy, right posterior sectionectomy, right hepatectomy, central hepatectomy, and extended left/right hepatectomy). The rates of overall morbidity and major complications increased significantly with a stepwise increase from grade I to III. Laparoscopic major resections are now well-standardized procedures.[28,33–35] As they gain wider acceptance, these resections will require a higher level of training and experience.

More difficult cases include lesions located at the posterosuperior liver (segments I, IVa, VII, and VIII) and lesions in proximity to major vessels or the hepatic hilum. The laparoscopic field for posterosuperior liver resection lies in the deep area of the subphrenic rib cage and may be overlaid by the side of the diaphragm and abdominal wall. These cases should be restricted to experienced centers, but such resections are increasingly reported[20,24,29] and may involve a more extensive resection by laparoscopic approach than would otherwise be necessary to avoid an open approach. An example would be a laparoscopic right hepatectomy for a posterior lesion that could be resected by a more limited, open segmentectomy or posterior sectionectomy (see Chapter 118B). For each patient, the surgeon must weigh the risks and benefits of the laparoscopic and open techniques with the benefits of parenchymal preservation.

TUMOR PATHOLOGY

As previously emphasized, the availability of minimally invasive techniques should not lead to extending the indications for resection of benign lesions (see Chapter 88) with no harmful potential. The observed trend has been toward a higher proportion of benign disease being treated laparoscopically because these pathologies are more amenable to a minimally invasive approach because of a higher incentive in young patients, and no margins are required.

The main indications for LLR are, as in open surgery, primary liver and biliary cancer (see Chapters 49, 50, 51, and 89), selected patients with metastatic liver cancer (see Chapters 90, 91, and 92) and highly selected patients with symptomatic benign liver lesions (see Chapter 88). Principles of oncologic resection are essential. Surgical margins should not vary between open and laparoscopic resections. If there is concern that an adequate margin cannot be obtained laparoscopically, but it is technically feasible by an open approach, the open approach should be indicated. In this respect, bilobar disease, especially in the case of colorectal liver metastases, is considered a contraindication to the laparoscopic approach by most teams because of the risk of missing some lesions or performing an inadequate oncologic procedure (see Chapter 90). Recently, Okumura et al.[36] reported that laparoscopic two-stage hepatectomy for bilobar colorectal liver metastases is safe and feasible with favorable surgical and oncologic outcomes compared with open two-stage hepatectomy. Perihilar cholangiocarcinoma or gallbladder cancer are also considered contraindications to the laparoscopic approach because of the complexity of biliary and possible vascular resections/reconstructions, as well as the necessary radical dissection of hilar lymph nodes (see Chapters 49, 51A, and 51B).

Interestingly, HCC occurs mainly in patients with cirrhosis, which is the most common single reported indication for LLR, representing more than 50% of those for malignancy[3,7] (see Chapters 74, 89, and 120), whereas in most open liver resection series, colorectal liver metastases form the majority of cases (see Chapter 90). The main reason that HCC appears more amenable to a laparoscopic approach is that screening programs allow a diagnosis of early HCC in patients with known liver disease (i.e., small solitary nodules). A major issue with liver resection in cirrhotic patients, even minor procedures, is postoperative decompensation, including liver failure and ascites (see Chapters 74 and 120). Our group observed that LLR was very well tolerated by cirrhotic patients.[37] In particular, we observed less postoperative ascites than previously experienced after open surgery, probably because the abdominal wall and its collateral venous drainage are better preserved.

This was confirmed by several authors and in meta-analyses.[38–40] It seems that laparoscopy itself may offer some protection from postoperative decompensation. Reasons may include less fluid requirement, avoidance of long abdominal incisions with muscle division, better collateral preservation,

less manipulation, and less respiratory impairment. Recognition of the efficacy and safety of LLR for HCC has led to increased numbers of cases performed, especially in patients with peripheral tumors less than 5 cm.[6,38–42]

Almost 50% of our laparoscopic experience has been with patients who have chronic liver disease.[4] These patients typically require longer operations and more pedicle clamping, but globally they have a better recovery than their open counterparts.[3] In our experience, however, colorectal liver metastases (see Chapter 90) have been less amenable to a laparoscopic approach. This is the result of our referral base consisting mainly of bilobar or difficult-to-resect liver metastases.

SAFETY AND BENEFITS

Laparoscopic liver resection appears to provide the benefits that laparoscopy has offered to patients undergoing many other abdominal operations. Case-control studies have demonstrated lower morbidity,[37,38,40] shorter length of hospitalization,[43–52] less operative blood loss,[4,43,45,46,48,53–55] reduced transfusion requirements,[43,46,49] a reduced need for analgesia and quicker return to oral consumption,[44,56] and fewer postoperative adhesions.[57,58] Studies have demonstrated decreased costs when accounting for shorter operative time and LOS.[43,46,59] The mortality rates in these studies are at least equivalent to those of large case series of open liver resections. In their review of 463 published articles on LLR, Ciria and colleagues[3] concluded a cumulative mortality rate of 0.4%. This compares favorably to the 0% to 5.4% reported in the open-resection literature from high-volume centers. Of 37 deaths, the cause of death was attributed to bleeding, sepsis, or liver failure. There were no reported intraoperative deaths. A 10.5% morbidity rate was reported, with a range of 0% to 50% across studies. Liver-specific complications accounted for 4% and included bile leaks, transient liver failure and ascites, and abdominal collections. The remaining 6% were complications common to all operations, including but not limited to hemorrhage, wound infection, hernia, bowel injury, intra-abdominal fluid accumulation, and urinary or respiratory tract infections. Fretland et al.[60] reported the first single-center RCT (OSLO-COMET study) in patients with colorectal liver metastases who underwent minor parenchyma sparing liver resection and successfully demonstrated the safety of laparoscopic liver surgery and its superiority compared with the open approach regarding postoperative morbidity. Another RCT, the ORANGE II PLUS trial (NCT01441856) comparing the early outcomes of right and left hepatectomy either by laparoscopy or open route, is still active and its results are not yet known.

Tozzi et al.[61] compared laparoscopic versus open approach for right and left hepatectomy using a propensity score matching analysis and concluded that laparoscopic major hepatectomies are safe and feasible procedures allowing a similar complication rate with a shorter LOS and diminished postoperative pain with respect to the standard approach. Laparoscopic right hepatectomy is associated with a longer operative time but less blood loss and shorter LOS than open right hepatectomy.[62] Bleeding control was superior possibly because of improved intraoperative magnification for surgical manipulations, use of new coagulation devices, and the pressure associated with the pneumoperitoneum that may have helped decrease bleeding during liver parenchymal transection. Yoh et al.[63] compared the short-term outcomes between laparoscopic right hepatectomy using the caudal approach and open right hepatectomy with the anterior approach and liver hanging maneuver. Perioperative blood loss and transfusion rates, overall and symptomatic pulmonary complication rates, and hospital LOS were significantly lower in the laparoscopic group, but operation time was significantly longer. In their meta-analysis comparing clinical outcomes of laparoscopic versus open right hepatectomy for liver tumors, Hong et al.[64] showed that no significant difference was observed between the two groups in portal occlusion, rate of R0 resection, transfusion rate, mild complications, and postoperative mortality. Intraoperative blood loss was significantly lower and LOS was shorter in the laparoscopic group compared with the open group. The disadvantage of laparoscopy was the longer operating time.

As a consequence of decreased adhesions formed after an initial laparoscopic resection, reoperations such as repeat hepatectomy and liver transplantation can often be performed more easily with less blood loss, reduced transfusion requirements, and reduced operation time than after an initial open hepatectomy.[4,37,57,58] Another potential advantage of quicker recovery after the laparoscopic approach is the possibility of increased and earlier access to chemotherapy.[65]

Barriers to the wide acceptance of laparoscopic hepatic surgery—such as threat of gas embolism, violation of oncologic principles, and significant risk of bleeding—have not been apparent in the literature.[66] In addition, studies have consistently demonstrated that operative safety and postoperative morbidity improve with experience.[7] When comparing our early and late groups, we found statistically significant reductions in operative time (from 210 to 150 minutes), blood loss (from 300 to 200 mL), conversion (from 16.9% to 2.4%), and morbidity (from 17.2% to 3.4%). We used the technique of cumulative sum analysis (CUSUM) to determine when the learning curve reached a statistical plateau, based on conversion rate in minor hepatectomies, and this was found to be at 60 cases.[67] Cai et al.[68] showed a learning curve for four different well-defined laparoscopic hepatectomy procedures in a single-center experience. On average, 15 to 30 cases for left hepatectomy, 43 cases for left lateral sectionectomy, 35 cases for nonanatomic liver resection, and 28 cases for segmentectomies were necessary. Hasegawa et al.[69] demonstrated that a major laparoscopic liver resection could be safely introduced for a surgeon with an experience level of at least 60 minor laparoscopic liver resection. Nomi et al.[70] reported that 45 major laparoscopic liver resections were required before operating times were reduced. For Chan et al.,[71] by overcoming the learning curve at the 25th laparoscopic major hepatectomy, more pure laparoscopic hepatectomies could be performed. Using this as the cutoff, operative time, need for Pringle, blood loss, and transfusion requirement were brought down with more proficient resection. In a literature review,[72] a steep learning curve of 45 to 60 cases is necessary for laparoscopic major hepatectomy. Nitta et al.[73] compared outcomes between the first 21 and second 21 cases of laparoscopic-assisted major liver resections using the hanging technique and found a decrease in estimated blood loss, shorter LOS, and no difference in complications. The report from the national clinical database in Japan[74] concluded that among the major laparoscopic liver resection procedures, a left hepatectomy could be a good option for a standard practice. This concept was also reported by other studies.[33,75–77] Laparoscopic left hepatectomy has a lower potential risk of bleeding from the inferior vena cava than laparoscopic right hepatectomy because dissection between the inferior vena cava and the liver is not needed. The parenchymal transection area of left hepatectomy is smaller compared with right hepatectomy or posterior sectionectomy. The parenchymal transection along the Cantlie's line is easier than that of the right intersectional plane because of both the lower risk of disorientation and the lower bleeding risk because of the lower hepatic venous pressure.

Additional benefits of laparoscopy include better cosmesis and improved maintenance of the sensorimotor integrity of the abdominal wall. Despite these favorable results, it is important to acknowledge that these findings are mostly from nonrandomized studies and that laparoscopic cases remain highly selected for their potential for success. It can be inferred from the colorectal and bariatric literature that these benefits are real.

ONCOLOGIC OUTCOMES

Initial fears over tumor seeding or adverse oncologic outcomes have not been substantiated. With regard to margins, recurrence, and overall and disease-free survival, comparable results between open and laparoscopic resections have been well demonstrated in the literature.[7,18,66,78–80] In a meta-analysis of 446 laparoscopic liver resections and 556 open hepatectomies, including HCC and colorectal liver metastases, Parks and colleagues[18] found no difference in tumor-free margin status, disease-free survival, and overall survival between laparoscopic and open liver resection for liver malignancies. In a multi-institutional Japanese study, Takahara et al.[74] showed that there were no significant differences in overall survival and disease-free survival between laparoscopic and open liver resection for HCC. Guro et al.[81] compared the surgical outcomes of major laparoscopic liver resection (67 patients) and open liver resection (110 patients) for HCC: the 5-year overall survival rate and the 5-year disease-free survival rate were similar in both groups. Yoon et al.[51] compared laparoscopic versus open right hepatectomy for HCC in patients with cirrhosis with a propensity score matched analysis: there were no significant differences between the laparoscopic and the open groups regarding 2-year disease-free and overall survival rates. Kim et al.[82] compared the outcomes of laparoscopic versus open left hepatectomy for HCC using propensity score matching: the disease-free survival and the overall survival were not different in the two groups. Rhu et al.[83] compared the outcomes of laparoscopic versus open right posterior sectionectomy for HCC using the propensity score matched analysis and showed no differences in both disease-free survival and overall survival. In a systematic review and meta-analysis, Ciria et al.[84] reported that laparoscopic liver resection for HCC is feasible and offers improved short-term outcomes for patients with Child-Pugh A cirrhosis, solitary tumors, and minor resections, with comparable long-term outcomes (5-year overall and disease-free survival) as the open approach. The same results have been demonstrated for both HCC and colorectal metastatic disease in several case-control studies.[85–89] Laparoscopic resection of other metastatic tumors has been reported in small series, mainly breast cancers and melanomas. Further, port-site metastases and peritoneal dissemination have not occurred with the use of closed-bag methods for specimen extraction. Resection of HCC as a bridge to future transplantation should also be a consideration[41,58] (see Chapters 105 and 125). As such, parenchyma-sparing procedures should be promoted in anticipation of repeat operative needs (see Chapter 102).

SURGICAL TECHNIQUE

General Principles

Imaging

High-quality imaging with vascular reconstruction is necessary to understand a patient's hepatic arterial, portal, and venous vascular anatomy (see Chapters 2 and 13–15). Three-dimensional (3D) reconstructions are also very useful in that setting. Review of recent magnetic resonance imaging (MRI), computed tomography (CT), and angiography is essential for planning the operation.

Equipment

All laparoscopic equipment must be state of the art and in good working order, and nursing staff should be familiar with the proper setup and functioning of equipment so as not to occupy the surgeon's attention during the operation at critical moments. The center should have an adequate backup supply of cameras, monitors, insufflators, electrical surgery generators, cables, tubings, and laparoscopic instruments. A set of conventional instruments for open surgery should be readily available in case of need for conversion.

We prefer a 10-mm, 30-degree laparoscope for its versatile imaging. A flexible laparoscope is also helpful for better view, especially in posterior areas of liver.

Recently, 3D video laparoscopic equipment has become available. Velayutham et al.[90] reported that the use of 3D vision reduces total operation time in laparoscopic resection, but their study included a majority of minor resection (75%). Kawai et al.[91] reported the results of 75 consecutive laparoscopic right hepatectomy: 45 cases were performed with two-dimensional vision, and 30 cases with 3D vision. Total operative time and right hepatic pedicle dissection time was significantly shorter in 3D group. Liver parenchyma transection time was also shorter in 3D group although not significant. There was no significant difference in liver mobilization time, intraoperative bleeding/transfusion, and postoperative complications. Although it has not yet been shown to improve outcomes in prospective RCTs, its supporters report enhanced quality of vision and suturing, recognition of dissection plane, and liver parenchymal transection. Our initial experience with these devices supports these statements.

As in open surgery, low central venous pressure (CVP) anesthesia along with a low tidal volume is recommended to reduce hepatic vein bleeding during transection[92] (see Chapter 25). An advantage of the laparoscopic approach is the hemostatic effect of pneumoperitoneum, the pressure of which is usually above CVP. This requires close surgeon-anesthesiologist collaboration. A carbon dioxide (CO_2) insufflator to maintain a pneumoperitoneum of approximately 12 mm Hg is used. Some authors recommend temporarily increasing pneumoperitoneum, up to 15 mm Hg or higher in case of bleeding. This may help with controlling venous bleeding but may increase the risk of gas embolism. Because of high solubility of CO_2, the risk of clinically relevant gas embolism is low, but surgeons and anesthesiologists should remain vigilant, especially in the context of low CVP. Optimized CO_2 insufflation systems (Airseal) maintain a stable pneumoperitoneum pressure by providing an adapted debit response to a slight change in intra-abdominal pressure. This device also can improve the visual field by constantly removing smoke, allowing it to operate at a lower pressure compared with conventional CO_2 insufflators. Some smoke aspiration devices are available and are useful adjuncts.

Hand-assisted laparoscopy can be used for lesions in difficult-to-approach areas or as needed to facilitate the procedure or obtaining hemostasis. A gas-tight hand port is placed, and the incision is later used for extraction of the specimen. Some experts suggest introducing the hand port in advance at the site of the future extraction so that in case of bleeding, the surgeon can put a hand inside to fix the problem without delay.

Positioning

Patient positioning is very important. For left-sided resections, we recommend placing the patient in a supine position with the lower limbs apart on a split-leg table, sometimes referred as the "French position" (Fig. 127E.2). The surgeon stands between the patient's legs with assistants at each side. The scrub nurse and instruments are positioned lateral to the patient's leg or behind the surgeon. Ideally, two monitors should be available at the patient's head so that the surgeon, assistants, and scrub nurse have good visual access (Fig. 127E.3). For right-sided resections except isolated resections of segment VII, the patient is placed in an hybrid lateral decubitus (left lateral decubitus position with right arm elevated and split leg; Fig. 127E.4). For lesions located in segment VI, the surgeon and one assistant can stand on the patient's ventral side, with the scrub nurse opposite at the patient's legs. For tumors in segment VII, we recommend a full left lateral decubitus with the surgeon standing behind the patient's back to obtain a better view and direction to operate (Fig. 127E.5). The monitor towers are positioned across from the surgeon. Advantages of the left lateral decubitus position are facilitation of mobilization of the right liver by gravity and having the scope facing the posterior segments. The table can also be tilted to the right or left to create space necessary according to various stages of the operation. In all cases, reverse Trendelenburg position allows the bowel to drop into the lower abdomen and can help vision and exposure.

Incisions, Exploration, and Exposure

The open technique is preferred to the Veres needle in gaining access to the peritoneal cavity. For the patient with liver cirrhosis (see Chapters 74 and 120), special attention should be paid to the collateral veins around the umbilicus, which should be sought on

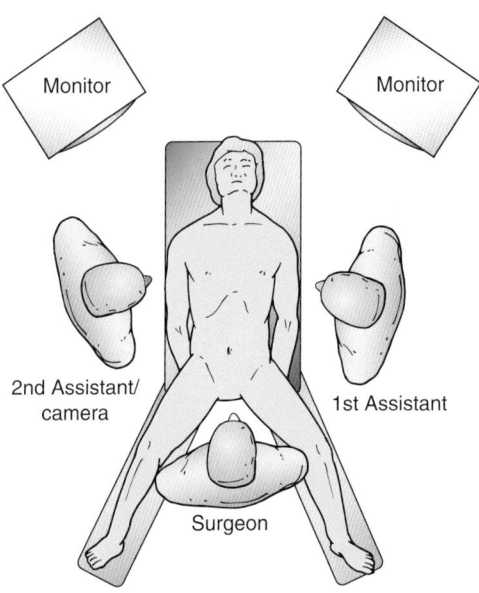

FIGURE 127E.2 Split-leg position.

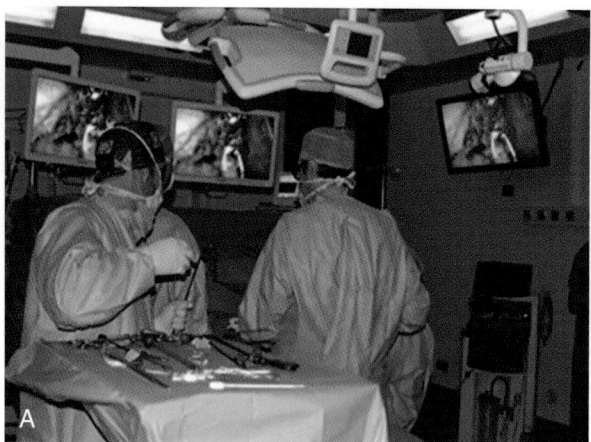
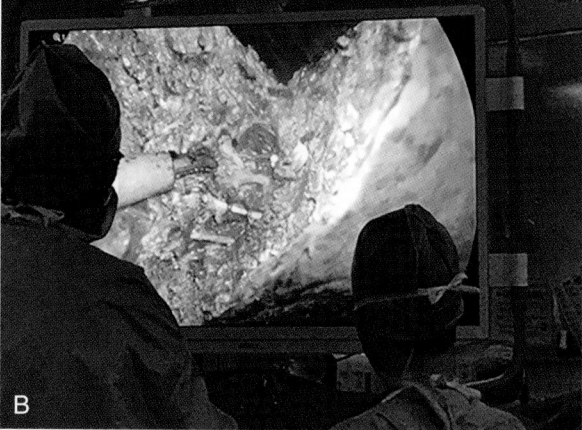

FIGURE 127E.3 Operating room setting of laparoscopic liver resection. **A,** Global view with multiple screens. **B,** 4K wide-screen immersion

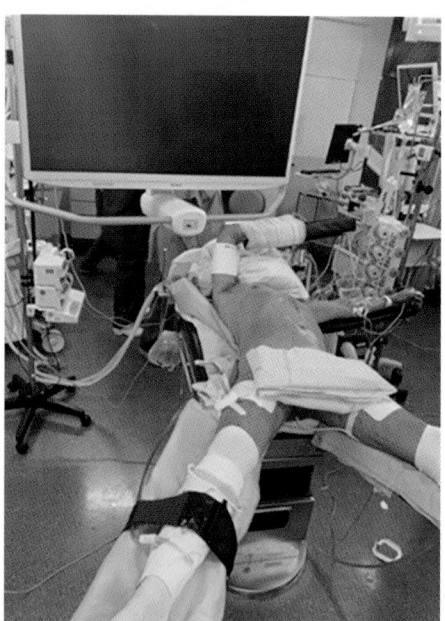

FIGURE 127E.4 Partial left lateral position for right-sided resections.

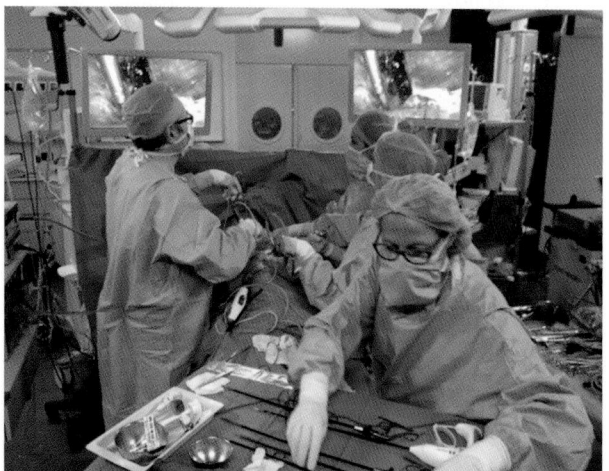

FIGURE 127E.5 For tumors in segment VII, surgeons can stand behind the patient's back to obtain a better view and direction to operate.

preoperative imaging, with shifting of port placement away from these collaterals when present. The following ports are placed under direct laparoscopic vision, with incisions sized to accommodate the necessary trocars (Fig. 127E.6). The median trocar is the camera port, the paramedian ports are the working ports, and the most lateral right and left ports are for retracting assistance. Care should be taken not to place the ports too far from the costal margins because pneumoperitoneum will increase the distance, especially in older males. This may create a problem of instrument length in reaching the liver dome. This is particularly true when using the Cavitron Ultrasonic Surgical Aspirator (CUSA, Integra Lifesciences, USA). For segment VI and VII resections, four or five ports are usually used (Fig. 127E.7). Transthoracic trocars at the right lateral intercostal space are proposed by some surgeons for manipulation of the liver dome area, especially the junction of right hepatic vein and inferior vena cava (IVC).[70]

After a thorough inspection of the peritoneal cavity for ascites, carcinomatosis, and signs of portal hypertension, attention is turned to the liver for signs of superficial lesions, steatosis, cholestasis, cirrhosis, or other gross pathology. Laparoscopic ultrasound is crucial, and a thorough knowledge of liver anatomy (see Chapter 2) and both B-mode and Doppler ultrasonography is mandatory for accurate laparoscopic liver resections[93] (see Chapters 24 and 103). The round ligament is divided close to the abdominal wall. This prevents a dangling remnant that might obstruct the view or soil the tip of the scope. Then, the falciform ligament is divided along its length to the insertion of the hepatic veins into the vena cava. The round ligament, along with the gallbladder remnant, can be used as "handles" for manipulation of the liver.

To anticipate hepatic hilum occlusion, the pars flaccida is opened, and an instrument is passed behind the hepatoduodenal ligament to encircle it with a tape. The tape is then extracorporeally inserted through a short rubber tube to serve as a tourniquet, and it is returned to the abdomen (intracorporeal Pringle maneuver; Fig. 127E.8) or externalized and passed through a catheter (extracorporeal Pringle maneuver; Fig. 127E.9). We currently prefer extracorporeal Pringle maneuver. If pedicle clamping is to be used, we favor 15 minutes of clamping the pedicle flow interrupted by 5 minutes of release. Although we do not routinely clamp the pedicle, this should be regarded as another safety tool in the arsenal of surgeons because even mild parenchymal bleeding may obscure visualization. Liberal use of

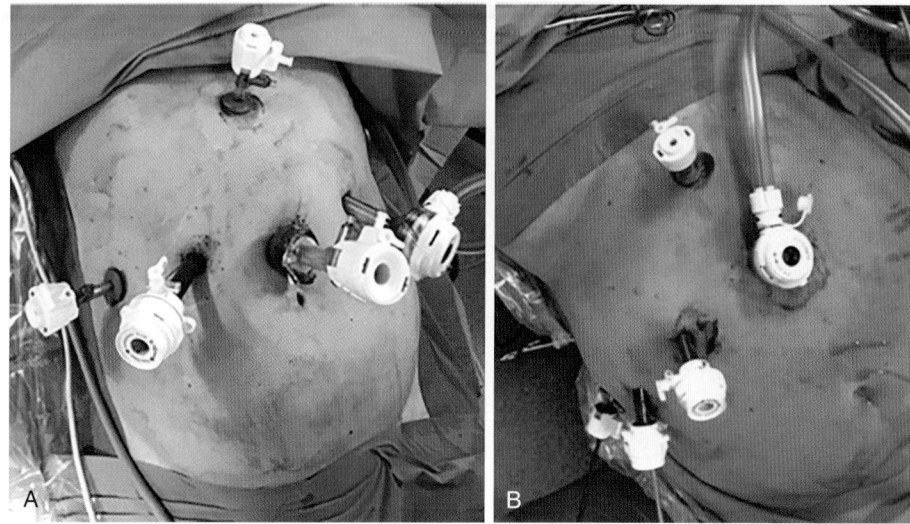

FIGURE 127E.6 Trocars in split-leg position. **A,** Left-sided resections. **B,** Right-sided resections.

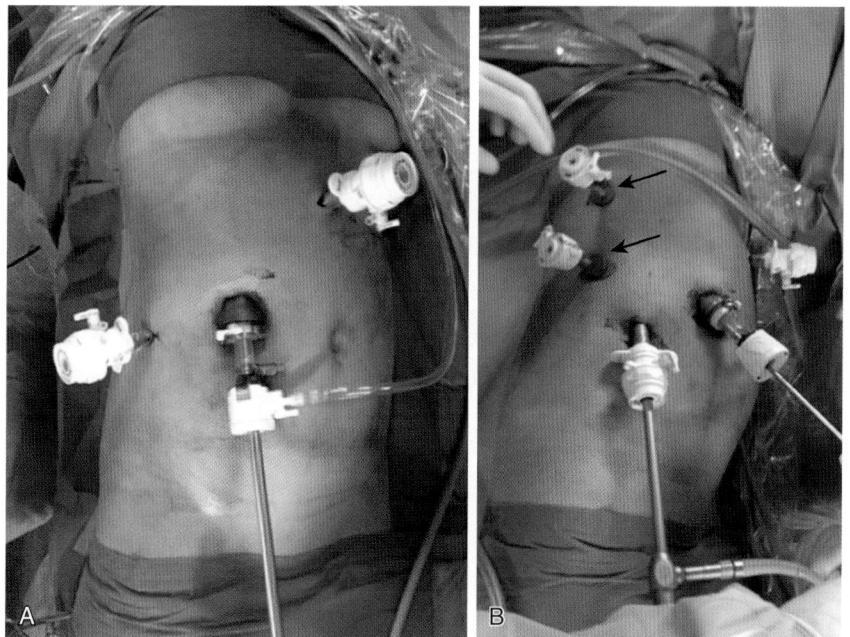

FIGURE 127E.7 Trocars in full left lateral decubitus position. **A,** Initial trocars. **B,** Additional trocars at intercostal space *(arrows)*.

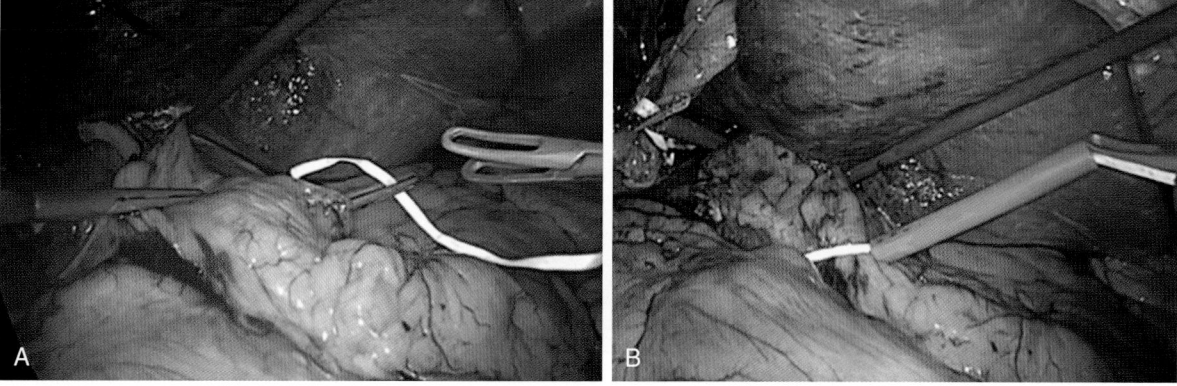

FIGURE 127E.8 Pringle maneuver in laparoscopic liver resection; preparation and locking of tourniquet. **A,** Umbilical tape passed behind hepatic pedicle from right-side port. **B,** Rubber tube used to prepare tourniquet.

Continued

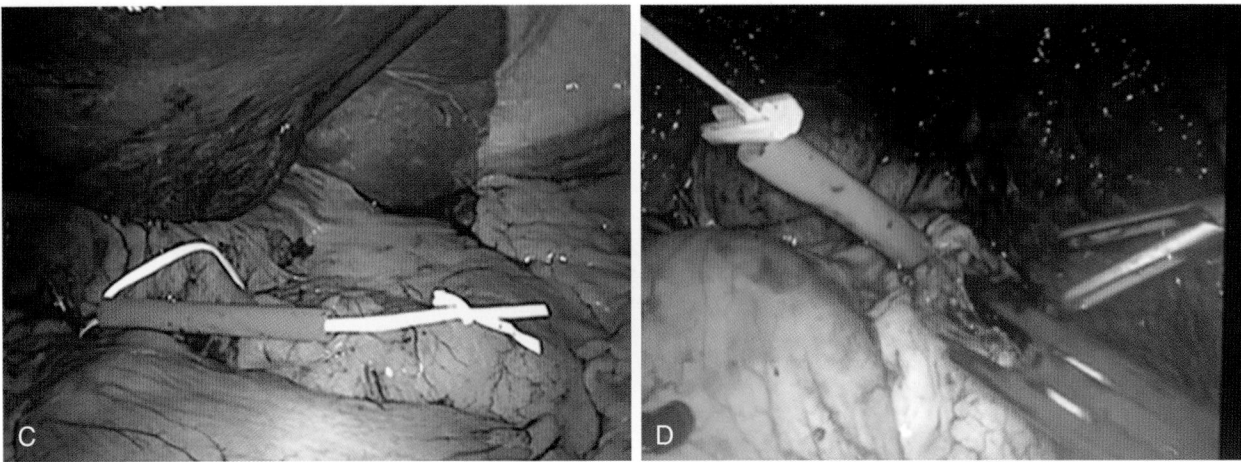

FIGURE 127E.8, cont'd **C,** Tourniquet ready. **D,** Inflow occlusion is obtained by locking the tourniquet with a locked clip.

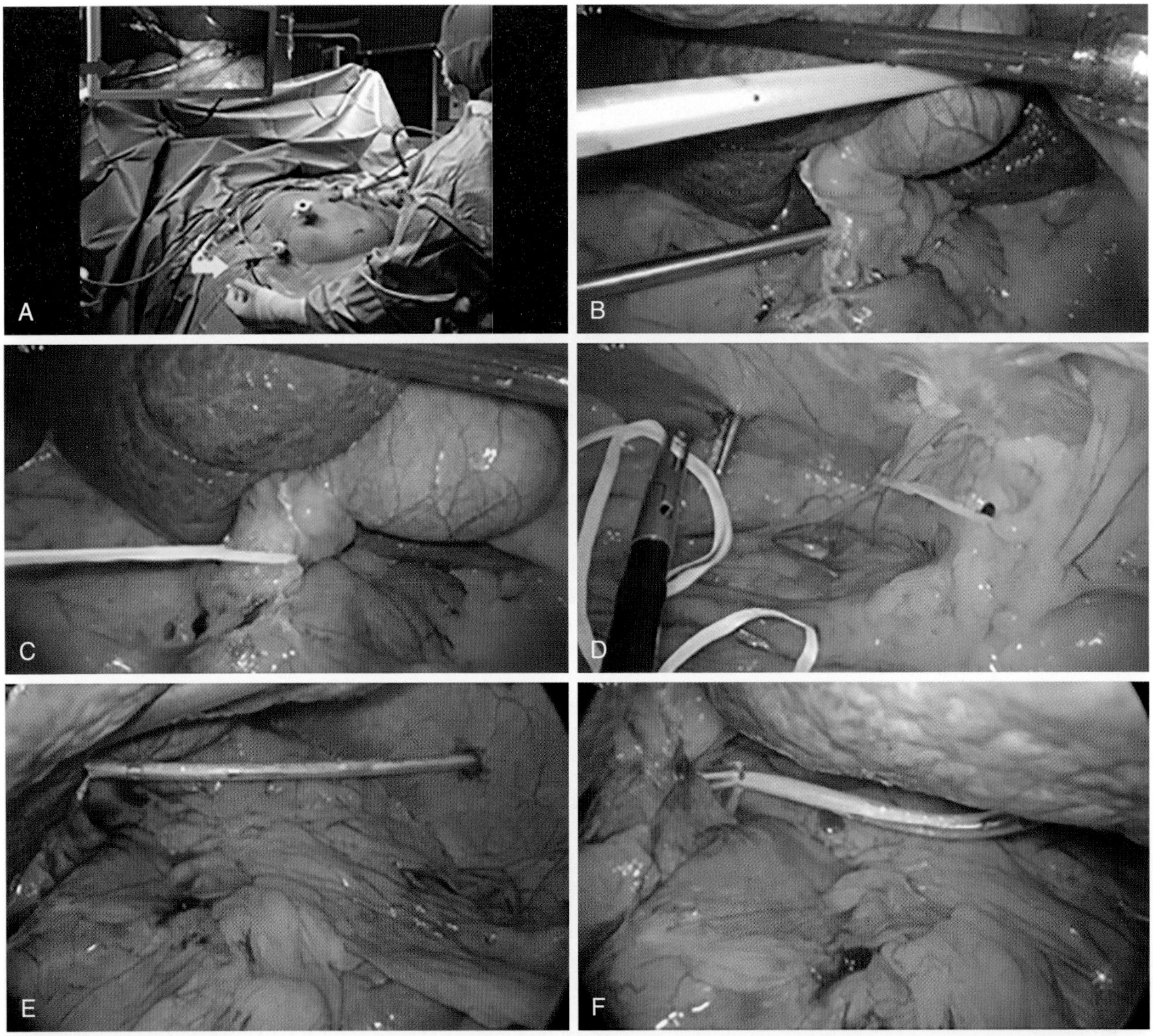

FIGURE 127E.9 **Extracorporeal Pringle maneuver. A,** From the trocar inserted on the right flank *(yellow arrow)*, a grasper *(red arrow)* is passed behind the hepatoduodenal ligament to place an 80-cm long cotton tape around it. **B–E,** The tape is directly externalized through the skin in the left or right flank according to the procedure. A soft tube is passed over the tape used as tourniquet.

on-demand intermittent inflow occlusion, meticulous technique, pneumoperitoneum, and low CVP anesthesia are very effective for limiting blood loss during LLR.

Transection Techniques
(see Chapters 101A, 101B, and 127D)

Transection is a critical time in both open and laparoscopic resection but possibly more so in the latter. Continuous suction interferes with pneumoperitoneum pressure, and bleeding control by compression or suture is more difficult than in open surgery. Consequently, prevention rather than treatment of bleeding is paramount in laparoscopic surgery. The superficial 2 cm of the liver parenchyma contains only small vessels that can easily be managed. Larger vessels are located deeper, especially fragile hepatic veins, whereas inflow pedicles are more solid and surrounded by a Glisson sheath. Therefore deeper transection requires identification of large vessels and avoidance of blind maneuvers.

The transection line is outlined along the liver capsule with monopolar diathermy based on preoperative imaging, knowledge of hepatic anatomy, laparoscopic ultrasonography, or demarcation lines when inflow pedicles are interrupted. Whereas in open surgery the clamp-and crush method is a useful and inexpensive transection technique, newer technologies such as energy devices and staplers are required for laparoscopic operations. Several instruments are available, and individual surgeons have developed preferences and habits with specific instruments because of their history and access. There is no evidence that one device is better than another, and the choice should left to the surgeon's preference. The energy devices are mainly divided into three classes: (1) ultrasonic shears (Harmonic ACE, Ethicon Endo-Surgery, Cincinnati, OH, USA; Sonicision, Covidien, Mansfield, MA), (2) bipolar vessel sealant (LigaSure, Covidien; Enseal, Ethicon Endo-Surgery), and (3) combined ultrasonic and bipolar device (Thunderbeat; Olympus, Tokyo). The energy devices are effective for transecting the superficial 2 cm of liver parenchyma (Fig. 127E.10). For dissection of deeper parenchyma, prior identification and selective hemostasis of larger vessels is recommended. We recommend the use of an ultrasonic aspirator (e.g., CUSA, Integra, Plainsboro, NJ; Fig. 127E.11), although some surgeons do not use it.[70]

Subsequently, vascular and biliary structures less than 5 mm are coagulated and transected using an energy device or bipolar diathermy, or closed by clips. Vessels and bile ducts 5 to 10 mm

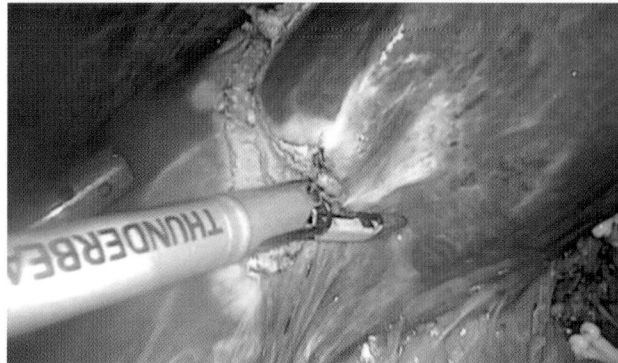

FIGURE 127E.10 Energy devices are effective for transecting the superficial 2 cm of liver parenchyma.

in size are ligated with plastic locking clips (Hem-o-lok, Teleflex Medical, Research Triangle Park, NC; Lapro-Clip, Covidien) and then divided. Laparoscopic linear staplers (Endo GIA, Covidien; Echelon Endopath, Ethicon Endo-Surgery) are used for larger vessels. The stapler can be applied to segmental portal pedicles or to isolated large portal or hepatic veins. It can also be used for division of the right or left bile duct surrounded with hilar plate during hemihepatectomy. The stapler should never be forced closed over a thick tissue mass, and excessive tissue length should not be squeezed into the jaws; such maneuvers risk misfiring, which can lead to difficult-to-control bleeding. Rather, further dissection should be performed until the tissue fits effortlessly within the stapler. Before stapling the right or left portal vein branch near the bifurcation, flow to the opposite pedicle should be confirmed for safety. Some surgeons perform parenchymal transection with repeated application of linear staplers,[94] but we do not favor this technique, which although quicker, lacks precision and may lead to severe bleeding. We prefer meticulous parenchymal dissection to completely visualize intrahepatic vessels and bile ducts, believing that blind application of the linear stapler is a risky technique.

Extraction, Drainage, and Closure

All lesions should be extracted without fragmentation using an endoscopic-protective plastic bag. Small lesions can be removed through extension of trocar incisions. Larger specimens

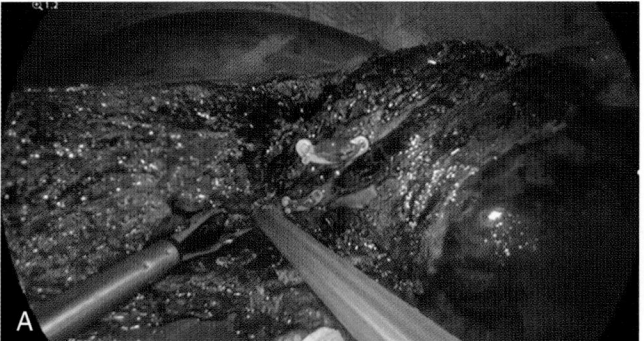 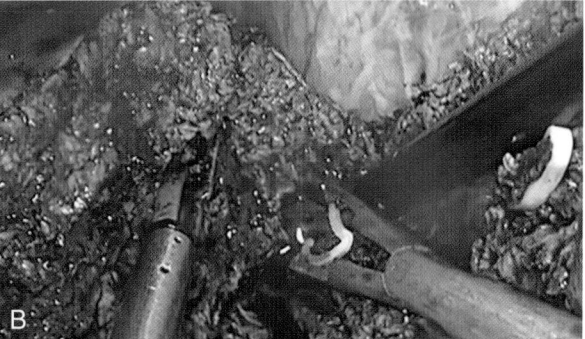

FIGURE 127E.11 **A,** For dissection of deeper parenchyma, prior identification and selective hemostasis of larger vessels are advised. We routinely use the Cavitron Ultrasonic Aspirator (CUSA). **B,** Hemostasis is achieved through bipolar cautery or clips, according to the size of the vessels. Staplers are used for portal pedicles and main hepatic veins.

are usually removed through a 5- to 8-cm suprapubic Pfannenstiel incision without muscle section. Specimens can also be removed through preexisting McBurney or midline incision or through hand-port incision. The extraction incision should fit the size of the specimen to retrieve. It should not be underestimated, so as to allow easy extraction and avoid rupture of the protective bag. The fascia layers are then reapproximated, the pneumoperitoneum is reintroduced, and the operative site is lavaged and examined for hemostasis and possible bile leak.

The use of abdominal drainage depends on surgeon preference (see Chapters 118 and 127D). It is often used in case of major resections and should be avoided in cirrhotic patients. The fascia of ports sites of 10 mm or more should be closed. The skin of the extraction and port-site incisions is closed with absorbable subcuticular sutures.

Conversion to Laparotomy

Conversion rates to laparotomy in the literature range from 0% to 55%. Dagher et al.[28] reported 1184 laparoscopic major hepatectomies carried out from 1996 through 2014 in 18 world centers. The open conversion rate was 10%. Hwang et al.[95] reported data from 265 laparoscopic major hepatectomies coming from 12 surgical centers from 2001 through 2011 in Korea. Open conversion was necessary in 17 patients (6.4%). Cauchy et al.[96] investigated the conversion rate during laparoscopic major hepatectomies describing a correlation between postoperative complications and intraoperative conversion, defining as patients at risk those with high body mass index (BMI), large lesions, and biliary reconstruction. The most cited reasons for conversion are hemorrhage, poor progress of operation, oncologic or margin uncertainty, adhesions, and anatomic difficulties.[7] Bleeding is the most common cause. The rate of conversion is reduced with proper patient selection, and it decreases with time and experience.[67] Conversion should not be considered a failure and should be performed without hesitation when a patient's well-being is at risk.

Hemorrhage may be brisk or continuous and slow. Arterial bleeding usually is easily controlled with instruments used to compress or grasp the vessel while clips or sutures are applied. Hepatic venous branches are the most common source of hemorrhage, and bleeding from these veins may be more difficult to manage because of vessel fragility and retraction.[67] Some advocate temporarily elevating the pneumoperitoneum pressure and decreasing the tidal volume of ventilation to decrease the bleeding from the hepatic vein, providing time and a clear view to control the bleeder.[22] Injury to the IVC may lead to massive bleeding. Although this is a more resistant vessel that can be sutured, excellent visualization is required before embarking on IVC dissection. Significant bleeding should be managed laparoscopically, or at least temporarily, because shock may ensue by the time the laparotomy is performed. This is a matter of urgent decision making by the surgeon, close collaboration with the anesthesiologist, and, above all, mastering of the advanced laparoscopic techniques required to embark on these procedures, such as intracorporeal suturing.

Continuous slow bleeding may occur during parenchymal transection and may be caused by elevated CVP, fragile liver parenchyma, or inappropriate technique. This slows the procedure and often interferes with visualization. In such situations, intermittent portal triad clamping (total or hemi-Pringle maneuver) is recommended, but if conservative measures are ineffective to manage the bleeding, conversion to laparotomy should be performed without delay.

Insufficient exposure, proximity to major vessels, and inability to obtain appropriate margins are a few of the reported difficulties that may cause failure to progress, although this may also be the result of a more difficult or dangerous dissection or transection than was anticipated. Failure to progress or oncologic uncertainty should lead to early conversion, so as to avoid futile lengthening of surgery. In a multicenter review of 2861 cases, Halls et al.[97] reported that patients who require conversion have longer operations with higher blood loss, a longer LOS, increased frequency and severity of complications, and higher 30- and 90-day mortality. Patients who had an elective conversion for an unfavorable intraoperative finding had better outcomes than patients who had an emergency conversion secondary to an unfavorable intraoperative event.

SPECIFIC HEPATECTOMY PROCEDURES
(SEE CHAPTERS 118A, 118B, AND 127D)

Left Hepatectomy

Patient is positioned supine in a split leg table in a reverse Trendelenburg position with five upper abdominal ports: three 12 mm ports and two 5 mm ports (Fig. 127E.12). The 12-mm ports allow an easy change of the instruments to provide the opportunity to use linear stapler with both the right and left hands. Intraoperative ultrasonography is performed routinely to delineate the size and extent of liver tumor, to discover the relationship between the liver tumor with major vessels, and to plan the plane of parenchymal transection. We begin with division of the falciform and left coronary ligaments to mobilize the left lobe. The lesser omentum is checked to verify the presence of an accessory or replaced left hepatic artery originating from the left gastric artery and then sectioned close to the Arantius groove. A cholecystectomy is performed, but the gallbladder is left partially attached to liver so that it may be grasped and retracted superiorly and to the right.

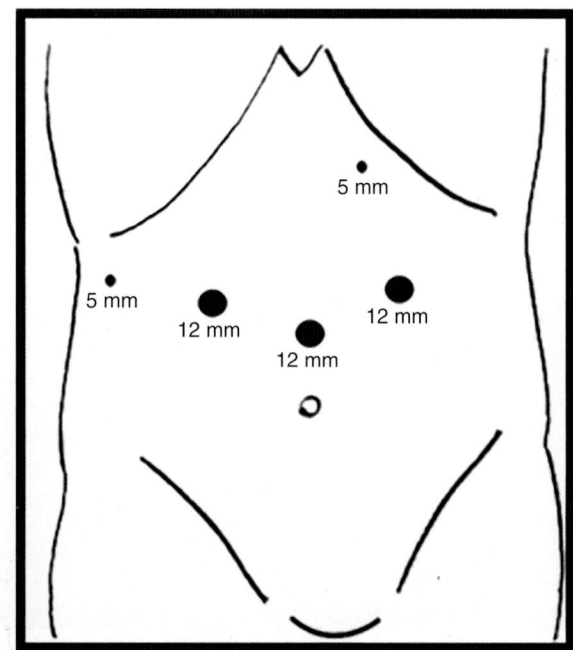

FIGURE 127E.12   Schema for trocar placement in laparoscopic left hepatectomy.

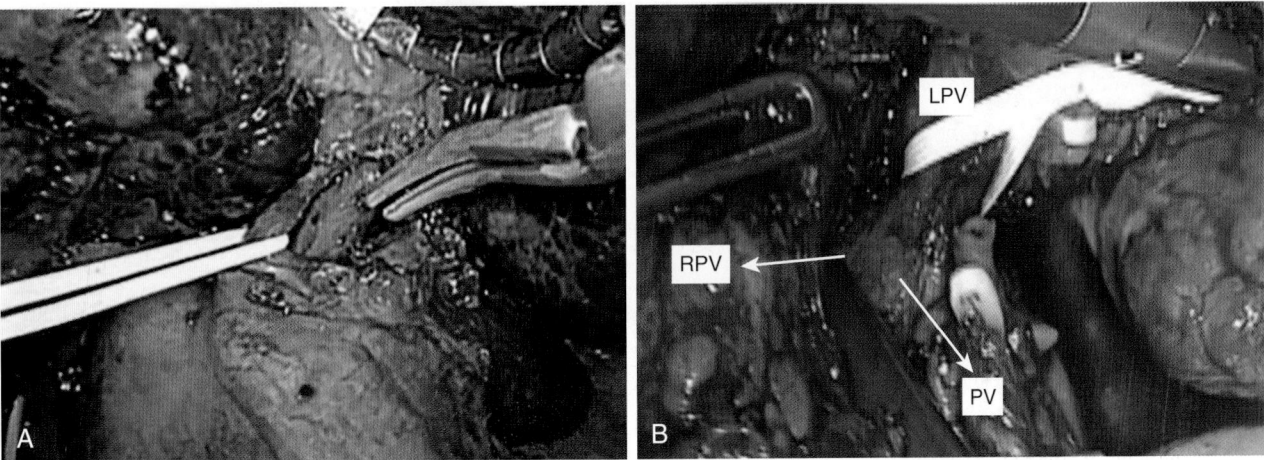

FIGURE 127E.13 **Dissection of left hepatic pedicle. A,** Left hepatic artery. **B,** Left portal vein *(LPV). PV,* Portal vein; *RPV,* right portal vein; (see Chapter 2).

The liver is lifted upwards by two forceps, one on the stump of the round ligament and the other on the gallbladder. Then we begin dissection by incising the peritoneum of the left hepatic pedicle, using endoscopic scissors, right-angled forceps, and bipolar diathermy first identifying and dividing the left hepatic artery between locking clips (Hem-o-loks; Fig. 127E.13A). An arterial branch for segment IV can also be identified and divided. The next step consist of dissection of the left portal vein, which is separated from the surrounding lymphatic tissue upwards and then downwards and is controlled with an umbilical tape. Care must be taken to identify the right portal vein before dividing the left branch (see Fig. 127E.13B). The left portal vein is then divided using locking clips or vascular staplers. The left hepatic artery and left portal vein can be clamped and eventually divided intraparenchymally. The inflow occlusion of the left liver delimits the plane that intersects the gallbladder and IVC fossae, known as the midplane of the liver. A tape is placed around the portal triad and passed through a 16 French (F) rubber drain to be used as a tourniquet for Pringle maneuver. The clamping of the portal triad can be done intracorporeally or extracorporeally (see Figs. 127E.8 and 127E.9). We believe that a routine Pringle maneuver (see Chapters 118A, 118B, and 127D) during parenchymal transection that reduces blood loss is more beneficial than the theoretical risk of liver ischemia because of clamping. The Arantius duct is divided from the left hepatic vein, and the dorsal aspect of the left and middle hepatic vein root is exposed. Dividing the Arantius ligament and retracting its cephalad stump can facilitate the isolation and encirclement of the left hepatic vein or the common trunk between the left and middle hepatic veins. This procedure facilitates secure intraparenchymal dissection of the left hepatic vein once the parenchymal dissection is almost complete. Accidental injury to the left inferior phrenic vein, which may cause postoperative hemorrhage, should be detected intraoperatively and be reliably controlled. Parenchymal transection is performed along the line of demarcation between left and right liver using harmonic scalpel (Thunderbeat, Olympus Co, Tokyo, Japan) for the superficial parenchyma and the laparoscopic CUSA for deeper parenchymal transection. The hemostasis is achieved by using monopolar energy on the CUSA, bipolar diathermy, and Thunderbeat. We use hemostatic clips if the vessels are larger than 7 mm. Intermittent clamping (15 minutes of clamping followed by 5 minutes of unclamping) is used when necessary. As the transection progresses, we find branches of the middle hepatic vein, which are controlled and divided. Although exposing the middle hepatic vein on the cutting plane is not absolutely required oncologically, it is very useful as a landmark to perform appropriate and safe hepatectomy without disorientation during dissection of liver parenchyma. The next step is the dissection and division of the left bile duct. We prefer to divide the duct with scissors (sharp division; Fig. 127E.14). The biliary stump is closed using clip or suture. To mobilize the left lobe from the segment I, we use a linear stapler for dividing the Arantius fissure. Parenchymal transection continues cranially, until it reaches the insertion of the left hepatic vein into the vena cava, at which point it is divided with the linear stapler (Fig. 127E.15). After completion of the hepatic parenchymal transection, a supra-pubic incision is made and a specimen bag is inserted into the abdominal cavity to collect and extract the specimen. The supra-pubic incision is closed and the abdomen is reinsufflated. The raw surface of the liver is carefully examined to obtain good hemostasis and biliostasis by also applying stitches if necessary (Fig. 127E.16). Drainage is not obligatory. Fascia of port sites greater than 10 mm are closed and all skin incisions are closed with subcuticular sutures.

With the extrahepatic glissonian approach, a small incision is made in the capsule above the left portal pedicle. A second

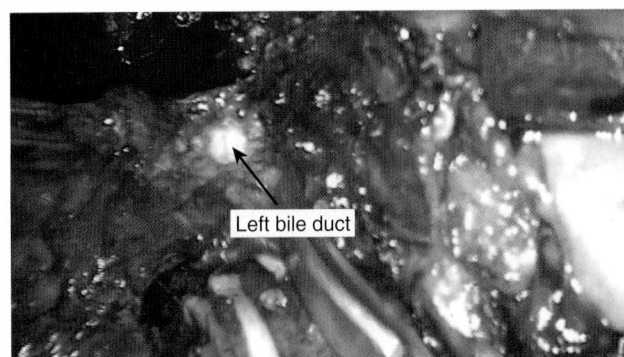

FIGURE 127E.14 Intraparenchymal identification of the left bile duct. It can be encircled and clipped or cut with scissors (sharp division).

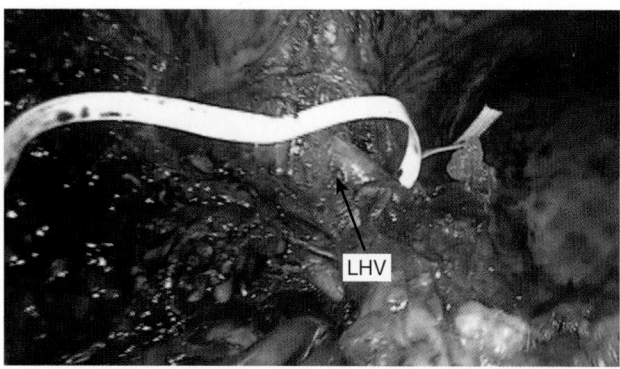

FIGURE 127E.15 After completion of parenchymal transection, the left hepatic vein is controlled with a cotton tape before its division with a vascular stapler.

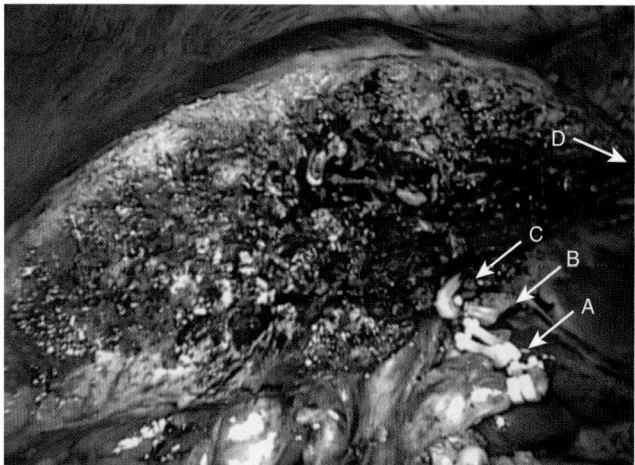

FIGURE 127E.16 View of completed left hepatectomy using extrahepatic division of left hepatic artery and portal vein and transparenchymal division of bile duct. **A,** Divided left hepatic arteries with locking clips. **B,** Divided left portal vein by linear stapler. **C,** Transparenchymally divided left bile duct with locking clip. **D,** Divided hepatic vein by linear stapler.

incision is made just above the Arantius ligament. Retracting the caudal stump of the Arantius ligament, which is attached to the left portal vein, can facilitate the isolation and encircling of the left glissonian pedicle. A blunt instrument "Goldfinger" is inserted to isolate the left pedicle. The instrument is passed above the hilar plate and below the liver parenchyma to encircle the pedicle with a cotton tape. Care must be taken not to include the pedicle of segment I. The posterior sectional bile duct is sometimes joined to the left hepatic duct. Therefore the left glissonian pedicle should be encircled left to the Spiegel branch to avoid right bile duct injury during en bloc transection of the left glissonian pedicle. This approach is very useful in encircling the left extrahepatic glissonian pedicle even in cirrhotic cases. In fact, it may be useful in patients with liver cirrhosis (see Chapters 74 and 120) because the portal venous collaterals or the engorged lymphatics at the hepatic hilum are not disturbed during hilar dissection, which consequently minimizes the risk of postoperative ascites. A vascular linear stapler is inserted and the left pedicle is transected. The intrahepatic glissonian approach reported by Machado et al.[98] is performed by small incisions on

two anatomic landmarks of the left glissonian pedicle. However, this technique is associated with a risk of injury of the middle hepatic vein or the glissonian pedicle because the vascular stapler is introduced intrahepatically without meticulous dissection. Also, the tip of the vascular stapler cannot be followed clearly because of limited vision and narrow space. Furthermore, the left glissonian pedicle is large and thick; it may not be successfully transected using a single vascular stapler.

Right Hepatectomy

Right hepatectomy is technically more challenging than left, and previous mastery of limited laparoscopic resections is a prerequisite. The patient is positioned supine on a split-leg table in a reverse Trendelenburg position. The ports sites are shown in Figure 127E.17. As previously detailed, the falciform and round ligaments are divided, and a tourniquet around the hepatoduodenal ligament is assembled. The cystic duct and artery are ligated and divided, and a replaced right hepatic artery is ligated and divided if present. A cholecystectomy is performed, but the gallbladder is left partially attached to liver so that it may be grasped and retracted for exposing the extrahepatic right glissonian pedicle. Gentle upper retraction of the cystic duct stump helps visualizing the right portal pedicle. The right branches of hepatic artery and portal vein are gently dissected and individually encircled with tapes to retract them for more secure division (Fig. 127E.18A). The right branch of the hepatic artery is divided between locking clips, and the right branch of the portal vein is divided with a linear stapler or between locking clips. Identification of the origin of the left branch of the portal vein should be assured before occluding the right portal branch (see Fig. 127E.18B). More distal visualization of the

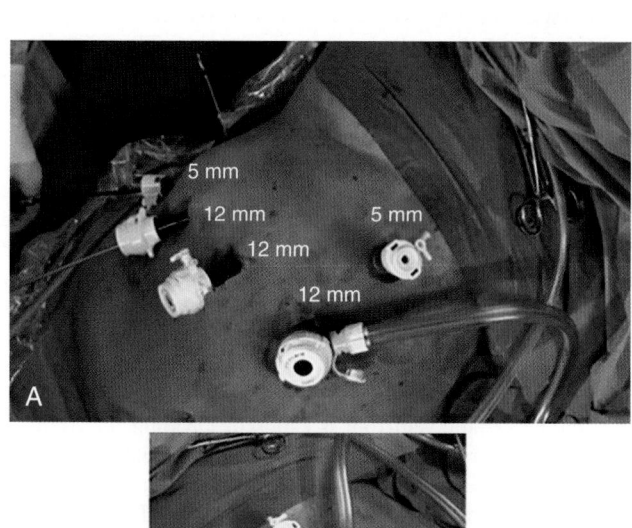
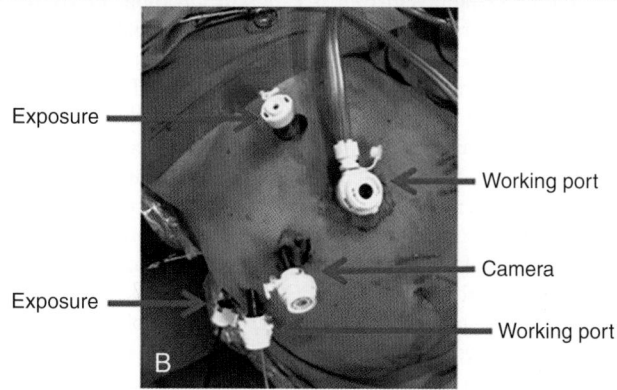

FIGURE 127E.17 **A–B,** Trocar placement in laparoscopic right hepatectomy

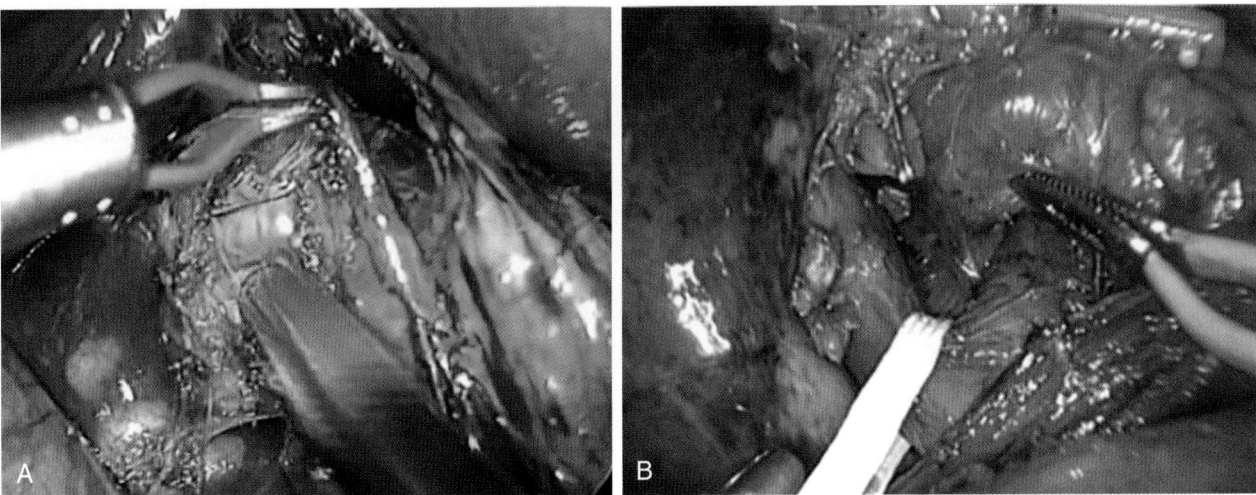

FIGURE 127E.18 Right hepatectomy: Hilar dissection. A, Dissection of right hepatic artery. **B,** Control of right portal vein. (Note: Portal vein bifurcation and left portal vein are well identified before right portal vein division; see Chapter 118A.)

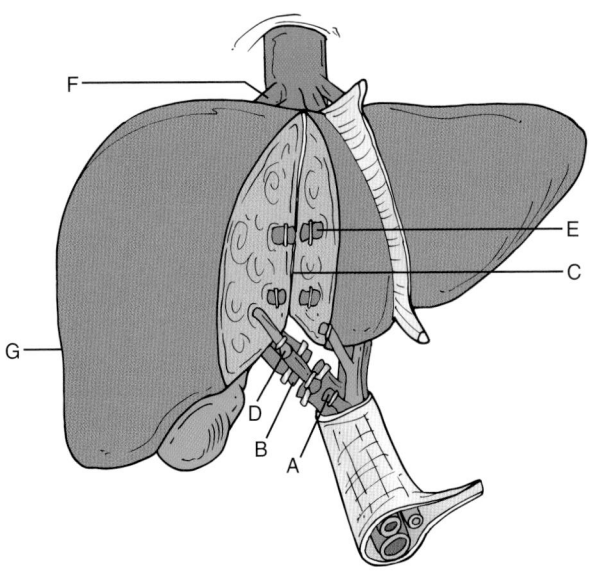

FIGURE 127E.19 Laparoscopic right hepatectomy by anterior approach, that is, without prior right liver mobilization. A, Division of right hepatic artery. **B,** Division of right portal vein. **C,** Transection. **D,** Intraparenchymal division of right bile duct. **E,** Division of middle vein tributary from segments V and VIII. **F,** Division of right hepatic vein using linear stapler after completion of parenchymal transection. **G,** Final mobilization of right liver. (See Chapter 118A.)

right glissonian pedicle to the bifurcation of anterior and posterior section is often possible laparoscopically and allows division of the branches at this level, thereby providing more safety in preserving hilar structures. The line of demarcation along the midplane of the liver is identified and marked, but the middle hepatic vein can be damaged because of deviation. Therefore it is crucial to determine the direction of the middle hepatic vein before transection. We should find the branch of the middle hepatic vein first and then look for the trunk along the branch. Laparoscopic ultrasonography ensures that the middle hepatic vein is completely avoided.[99] The parenchymal dissection can be done with or without initial mobilization of the right lobe; the latter is referred to as the anterior approach in open surgery and

is our preferred method (Fig. 127E.19). An advantage of the laparoscopic approach is the easier view of the infrahepatic and retrohepatic IVC, referred to as the caudal approach.[34] The absence of compression and manipulation of the tumor-bearing hemiliver before vascular control has several advantages. This approach avoids squeezing of tumor cells into the systemic circulation and avoids hepatic parenchymal tears especially for large and soft HCC. For the anterior approach, the right hepatic vein is not controlled before parenchymal transection. After ligation of the right hepatic artery and portal vein, parenchymal transection is started at the inferior edge of the liver in the anteroposterior direction along the line of demarcation. The previously described techniques are used. As progress is made cranially, the proximal hepatic veins branches draining segments V and VIII toward the middle hepatic vein are exposed on the transection area, which are clipped and divided (Fig. 127E.20). At the level of the hilar plate, the right bile duct's anterior and posterior branches are divided between clips or stapled. Division of the right bile ducts and the hilar plate allows the plane to be opened widely for easier parenchymal transection. The junction between the right liver and segment I is divided to allow exposure of the retrohepatic vena cava. The posterior Glisson capsule is now divided along the anterior surface of the vena cava, while systematically clipping and dividing or carefully treating by vessel sealant, the small bridging veins. The right hepatic vein is identified at its insertion into the vena cava and is transected with a linear stapler (Fig. 127E.21). The right lobe liver is now retracted laterally, as the hepatocaval ligament and the attachments of the right liver are freed from the diaphragm.

When parenchymal transection is to be performed after mobilization of the right liver, the right glissonian pedicle is dissected and divided as discussed for the anterior approach. A higher placed trocar very close to the patient's xiphoid process will help the mobilization between right liver and diaphragm. Next, the right triangular and coronary ligaments are divided. The liver is retracted to the left and anteriorly (Fig. 127E.22), and the short veins between the right liver and vena cava are clipped and divided. As progress is made cranially, the hepatocaval ligament is divided between clips, and the right hepatic vein is subsequently divided with a linear stapler. The liver is

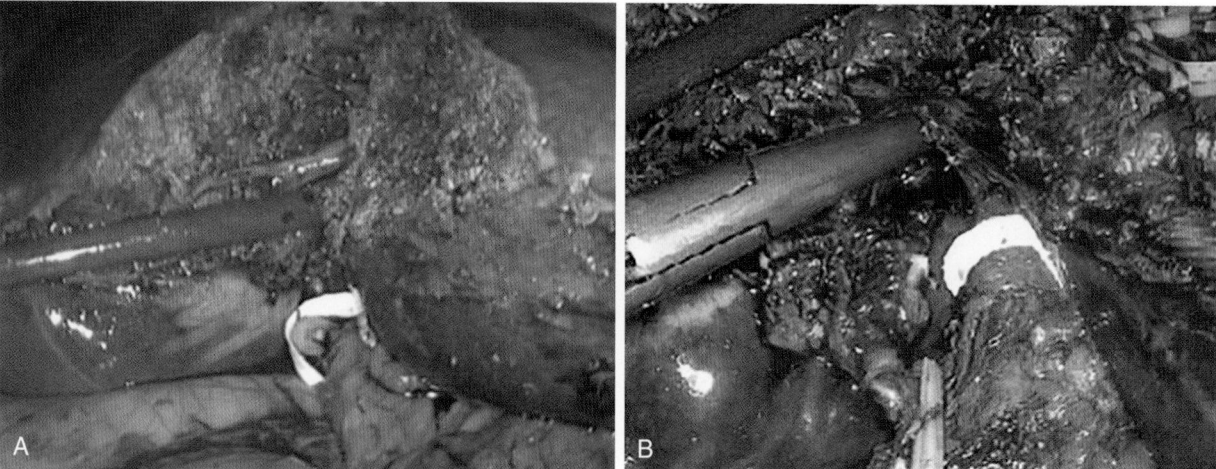

FIGURE 127E.20 Right hepatectomy: Transection and transparenchymal controls. **A,** Exposure of V5 during parenchymal transection. **B,** Right bile duct (see Chapter 118A).

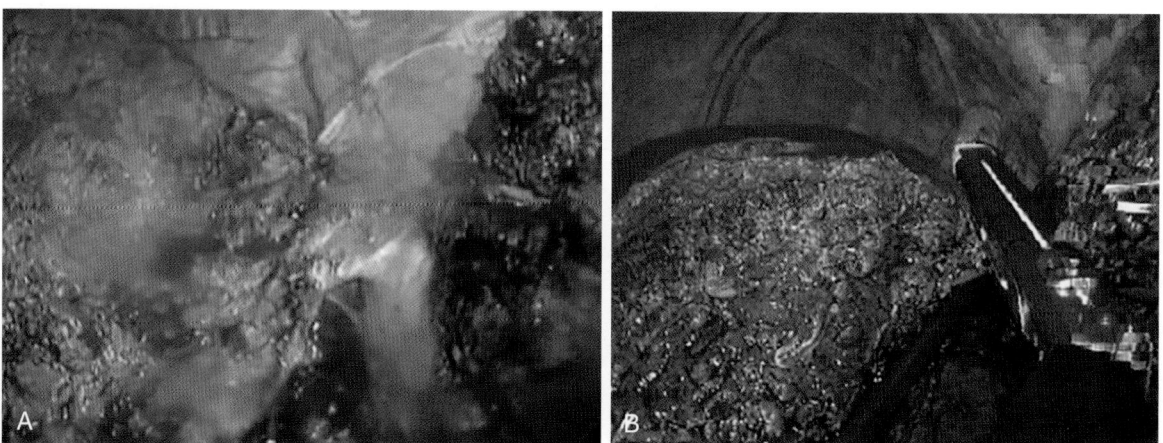

FIGURE 127E.21 Right hepatectomy: Right hepatic vein control after completion of transection. **A,** Exposure of right hepatic vein. **B,** Division of right hepatic vein by linear stapler (see Chapter 118A).

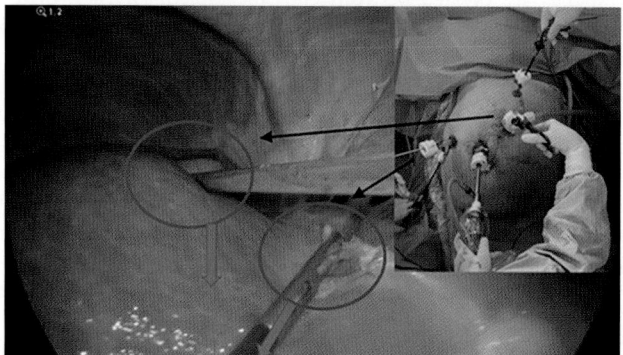

FIGURE 127E.22 Grasper to the falciform ligament that is pulling down and to the left, the liver.

now both completely mobilized and devascularized, and parenchymal transection is performed along the line of demarcation according to previously discussed principles. The remnant left liver is fixed in an orthotopic position by suturing falciform and round ligaments to the anterior peritoneum and diaphragm.

In the extrahepatic glissonian approach, the cystic artery and duct are divided and the gallbladder neck is dissected. The peritoneum of the hepatoduodenal ligament is dissected at the hepatic hilum. Retracting the round ligament and gallbladder allows a good surgical field of view. A Goldfinger is then meticulously extended between the hepatic parenchyma and the bifurcation of the right and left glissonian pedicles, so that the tip of the instrument is visualized. The right glissonian pedicle is encircled extrahepatically. Clamping the right glissonian pedicle allows the ischemic delineation of the right hemiliver. Hepatic parenchymal dissection along the Cantlie's line facilitates the insertion of an endoscopic stapler and division of the right glissonian pedicle.

Right Anterior Sectionectomy and Central Bisectionectomy

There are concerns that for the laparoscopic approach to be performed safely, surgeons would remove larger amounts of noncancerous liver parenchyma compared with open surgery.[86] Anatomic sectionectomy are often more difficult than major hepatectomy. For example, laparoscopic right hepatectomy for a tumor located in segment VIII would be technically easier

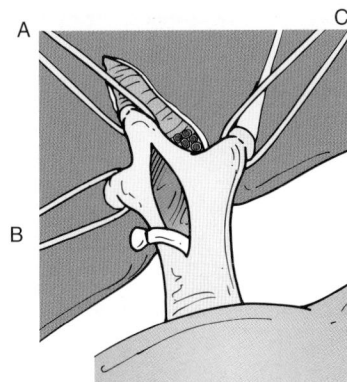

FIGURE 127E.23 Extrahepatic glissonian control of hepatic pedicles. **A,** Right anterior pedicle. **B,** Right posterior pedicle. **C,** Left pedicle (see Chapters 2 and 118A).

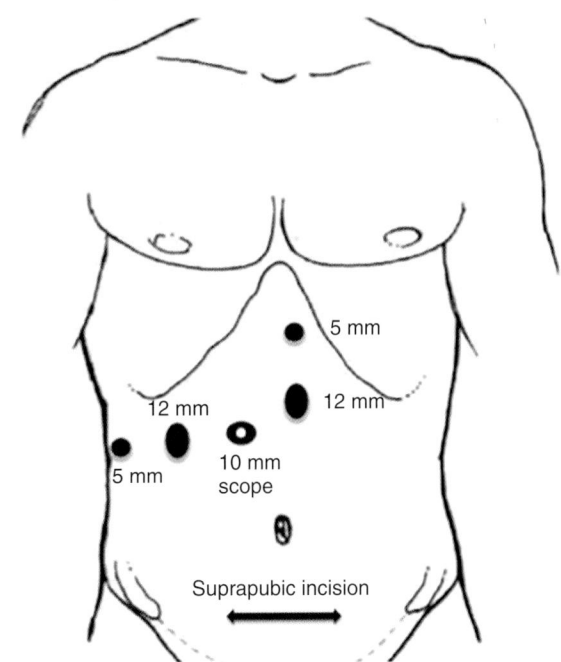

FIGURE 127E.24 Schema for trocar placement in laparoscopic right anterior sectionectomy.

than anterior sectionectomy or segmentectomy VIII. However, a more extensive resection by laparoscopic approach than would otherwise be necessary through an open approach should be avoided.

The anatomic parenchyma-preserving hepatectomy with glissonian pedicle transection is suggested for curative treatment of HCC (Fig. 127E.23).[100] The key of the glissonian pedicle approach[101] is dissecting and clamping the pedicle corresponding to the segment or section to be resected first, then confirming the ischemic territory, which includes the tumor, and finally dissecting the liver parenchyma along the anatomic segmental border. This procedure is designed to remove possible microvascular invasion of HCC, which spreads along the portal vein and improves disease-free survival. Because patients with HCC usually have concomitant hepatic dysfunction or liver cirrhosis, minimizing the volume of resection and leaving as much liver volume as possible are usually recommended. Therefore anatomic right anterior sectionectomy would be more appropriate surgical option than right hepatectomy if the tumor is limited to the right anterior section.

Laparoscopic right anterior sectionectomy has been first performed by Hwang et al.[102] It is one of the most challenging procedures because it involves transection of two hepatic parenchymal planes, in addition to controlling numerous branches coming from the right and middle hepatic veins and from the glissonian pedicles in the operative field. The risks of bleeding and/or bile leakage become higher with a larger plane of liver parenchymal transection. Cho et al.[19] showed that laparoscopic central hepatectomy and right anterior sectionectomy could be performed with comparable results to open liver resections.

The patient is put in a supine reverse-Trendelenburg position with legs splitting. Five ports are used as in right hepatectomy (Fig. 127E.24). An extrahepatic glissonian approach to dissect the right anterior pedicle is performed after cholecystectomy. After dissecting the anterior surface of hilar plate from the liver capsule, the right anterior glissonian pedicle can be recognized, and then it is dissected and looped (Fig. 127E.25A). After temporarily clamping the right anterior pedicle (see Fig. 127E.25B), the ischemic area shows the territory of segments V and VIII (see Fig. 127E.25C). In the cases of difficult clamping of the right anterior glissonian pedicle, the whole right glissonian pedicle is initially clamped to verify the margin of the plane between the right and left liver. Because the right glissonian pedicle is fully

exposed after division of this plane, the right anterior pedicle can be identified much easier. The positions of the middle and right hepatic veins are determined by intraoperative ultrasound (see Chapters 24 and 103). The parenchymal dissection is carried out along the demarcation line first on the Cantlie's line. Dissection is meticulously performed toward the cephalic direction along the right side of the middle hepatic vein until the insertion of the middle hepatic vein into the vena cava and toward the caudal direction until exposure of the hilar plate. In this manner, medial side dissection is completed. Transection on the lateral side is performed along the demarcation line between the right anterior and posterior sections. The small branches of the hepatic veins are controlled with Thunderbeat and the large branches of the right hepatic vein are controlled with clips. The middle and right hepatic veins are usually exposed at the cut surface and should be carefully preserved. Before complete division of the resected specimen, the right anterior glissonian pedicle is transected using a vascular stapler. During parenchymal transection, the use of an ICG fluorescence navigation system is also helpful for identifying the tumor margins and confirming the appropriate transection planes as reported previously.[103] The cut surfaces of the liver are checked. Bleeding and bile leakage are controlled meticulously (see Fig. 127E.25D).

If a more specific V or VIII single segmentectomy is planned, the tertiary branch of the glissonian pedicle corresponding to segment V or VIII can be identified during the parenchymal dissection at the cut surface (see Fig. 127E.25). After securing the segment V or VIII pedicle, the clamp at the right anterior pedicle is released, and the ischemic zone shows the territory of segment V or VIII.

Laparoscopic central bisectionectomy (anatomic resection of segments IV, V, and VIII) has been first performed by Gumbs et al.[104]; the first resection plane is along the right side of the umbilical fissure and the second resection plane is along the

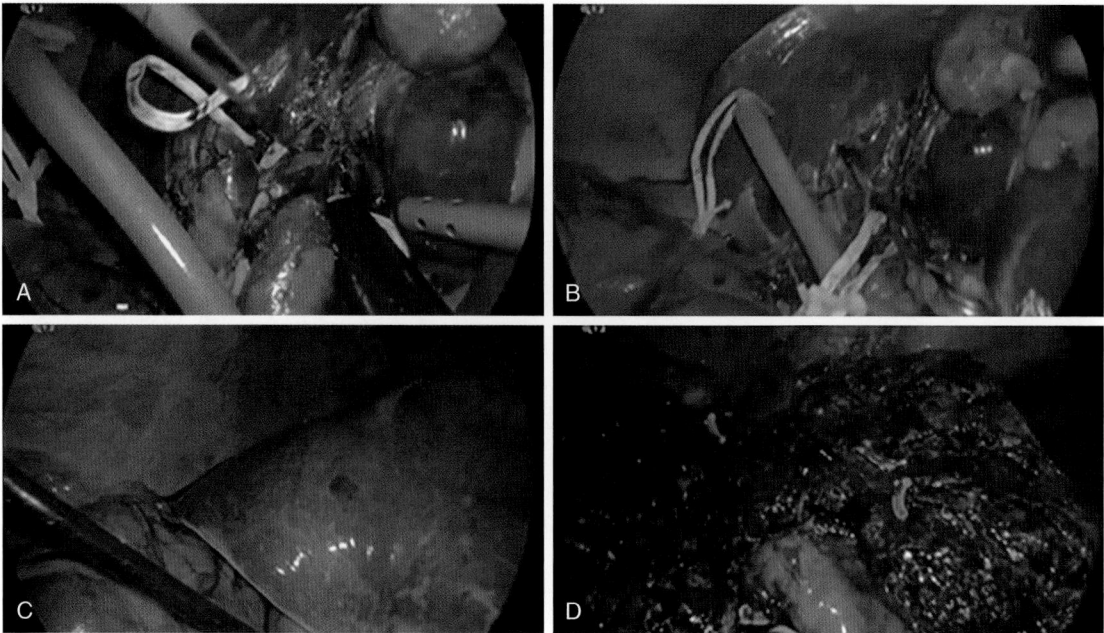

FIGURE 127E.25 A, Extrahepatic glissonian approach to right anterior pedicle. **B,** Temporary clamping of the right anterior pedicle. **C,** Delimitation of ischemic area of segments V and VIII. **D,** View of completed anterior sectionectomy (see Chapter 118B).

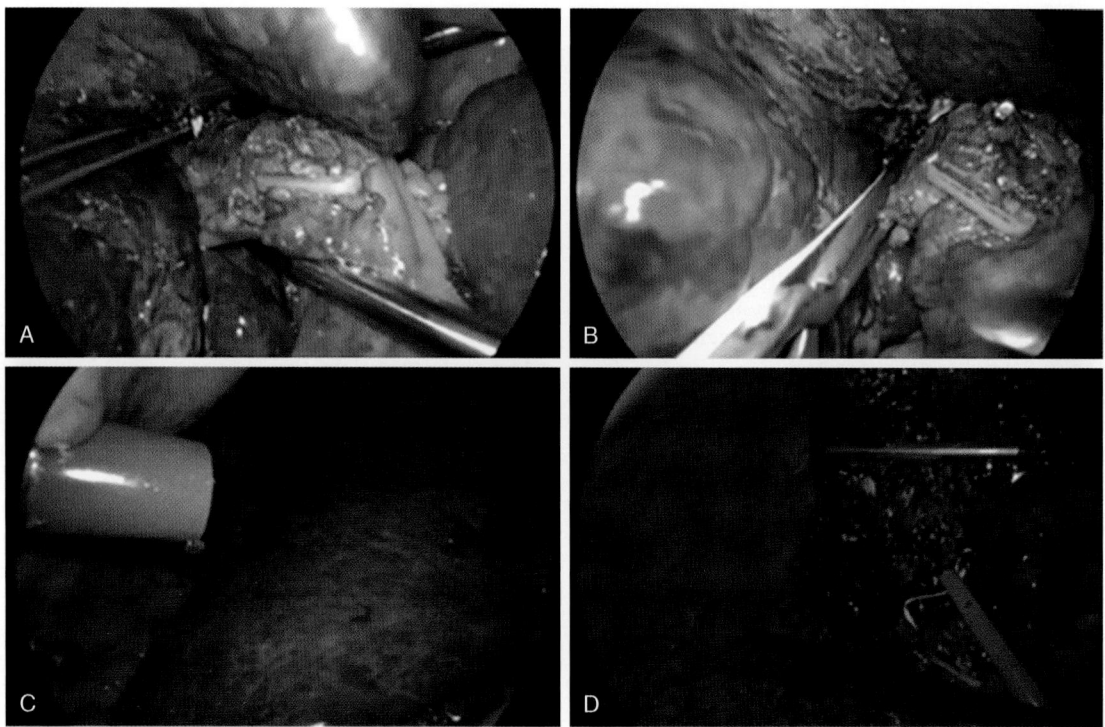

FIGURE 127E.26 A, Extrahepatic glissonian approach to right posterior pedicle. **B,** Temporary clamping of the right posterior pedicle. **C,** Delimitation of ischemic area of segments VI and VII. **D,** View of completed posterior sectionectomy.

right hepatic vein. The round ligament is retracted superiorly and to the patient's left for better exposure of the umbilical portion of left glissonian pedicle. The parenchymal dissection is then carried out along the patient's right side of the falciform ligament, which is the left border of segment IV. The portal pedicles of segment IV can be identified and controlled during

this step (Fig. 127E.26). Most of the branches only require double clipping. However, if a branch is thought to be large, a vascular stapler is used. The parenchymal transection is continued up to the junction of the middle hepatic vein and the left hepatic vein. The hilar plate is fully exposed after complete transection of the first resection plane, subsequently allowing for safe and easy isolation of the right anterior glissonian pedicle, which is looped and clamped using a laparoscopic bulldog clamp to verify the second resection plane, and the ischemic area of the right anterior sector is evaluated. The right anterior glissonian pedicle is divided using a vascular stapler after full exposure of the clamped pedicle during the second parenchymal transection. It is important to retract the right anterior glissonian pedicle with tape caudally and to the left and to apply the stapler as distally as possible to prevent stricture of the right posterior glissonian pedicle

In Hjortsjö's crook, as the liver parenchyma is divided, the specimen sides become redundant and the resection plane does not widen sideways but rather tilts forward and becomes poorly exposed. Therefore it is important to perform medial traction of the specimen at this time. The specimen is removed by dividing the middle hepatic vein using a vascular stapler and retrieved through a Pfannenstiel incision. The cut surfaces of the liver are checked. Bleeding and bile leakage are controlled meticulously.

Right Posterior Sectionectomy

Laparoscopic right posterior sectionectomy was first performed more than a decade ago.[105] However, because of its technical difficulty, it is classified as one of the most challenging procedures and thus not many studies regarding this procedure have been reported. Although there are studies[106,107] proposing that laparoscopic right posterior sectionectomy was feasible to perform compared with open right posterior sectionectomy, lesions located at posterior segments are still challenging compared with anterolateral segments.[108] For the right posterior section of liver, the patient is placed in the partial left lateral decubitus position with right arm elevated (see Fig. 127E.4). The right arm and shoulder are fixed to avoid plexus damage. A test is performed by changing the table position to a forced anti-Trendelenburg. Then, with a left tilt of the table, a forced left lateral position is also tested. Leg straps secure the thigh area and a lateral support pad placed in the left flank of the patient avoids lateral displacement while the patient position is adopted. With the table placed in a flat supine position, a tourniquet is placed around the portal pedicle and exteriorized at the left flank. The patient is then placed in a forced head-up position. By doing this, the liver literarily hangs from the diaphragm and vena cava. The dissection begins by division of the upper part of the falciform ligament, and then, from medial to lateral, the peritoneum is divided, thus exposing the anterior aspect of the middle and right hepatic veins. The division of the peritoneum is continued towards the right triangular ligament, which is now partially divided from above.

At this stage, a forced left lateral position is adopted by turning the table to a full left tilt. By doing this, the trocars on the right side become anterior. The surgeon, who remains between the patient's legs, now uses the three most external trocars. With this position, the liver tends by gravity to fall leftwards. Just by dividing the remaining triangular ligament and taking down the retroperitoneal attachments, it rotates anticlockwise until the lateral side of the vena cava is visible. The vena cava can be exposed by dividing the retrohepatic vessels with a bipolar sealing device or between clips. The cavo-caval ligament is divided, thus offering an excellent visualization and exposition of the right hepatic vein. The same procedures for extrahepatic glissonian approach previously described are performed to dissect the anterior surface of hilar plate. The advantage in laparoscopic right posterior sectionectomy is that the sulcus of Rouvière, apparent in 78% of patients,[109] serves as the easily identifiable anatomic landmark, because it contains the right posterior pedicle. Two hepatotomies are made, one above and one beneath Rouvière's sulcus. The right posterior glissonian pedicle can be identified and taped (see Fig. 127E.26A). After closure of the pedicle (see Fig. 127E.26B), the ischemic area shows the territory of the right posterior section of liver (see Fig. 127E.26C). The right hepatic vein is between the right anterior and posterior sections and is usually exposed on the cut surface during parenchymal dissection and should be carefully preserved (see Fig. 127E.26D).

CONCLUSION

Laparoscopic liver resection is a safe and feasible procedure for select patients when performed by appropriately trained surgeons. In well-selected patients, it offers considerable perioperative benefits compared with open hepatectomy. In addition, oncologic outcomes and survival for HCC and colorectal liver metastases are equivalent in nonrandomized trials. Although the indications for laparoscopic resection are somewhat rigid when it comes to lesion size and location, greater experience and newer technology are continually expanding its possibilities. Laparoscopic major and complex hepatectomies are now better standardized and are increasingly reported but require high levels of expertise.

Laparoscopic liver surgery is an expanding and exciting field and is likely to play an increasing role in the multidisciplinary approach to primary and secondary liver cancers.

The references for this chapter can be found online by accessing the accompanying Expert Consult website.

CHAPTER 127F

Robotic-assisted placement of hepatic arterial infusion pump

Benjamin D. Ferguson and T. Peter Kingham

INTRODUCTION

Hepatic arterial infusion was described nearly six decades ago as a regional treatment of hepatic tumors (see Chapters 50, 90, and 97). Robotic-assisted approaches to placement of hepatic arterial infusion pumps have become more prevalent following the rise of minimally invasive hepatobiliary techniques over the past 20 years.[1] The robotic-assisted approach to HAIP placement is associated with lower intraoperative blood loss compared with an open approach, and lower rate of conversion to open HAIP placement without a significant difference in operative time compared with a laparoscopic approach.[2] Sequential improvements in robotic surgery platforms have allowed for increasingly complex procedures involving minimally invasive liver resections and concomitant placement of hepatic arterial infusion pumps for patients with appropriate indications, most commonly for adjuvant or induction therapy in colorectal liver metastasis, though expanding uses for HAIP therapy and combinations with systemic therapies are the subject of several active trials. Robotic-assisted HAIP placement has a short learning curve for surgeons with robotic hepatobiliary experience,[3] and it can easily be combined with minimally invasive colorectal resection.

TECHNIQUE

The patient is positioned supine on a nonslip pad with a footboard in place. Monitoring lines are placed and a Foley catheter is inserted. The patient's arms are tucked and secured, and reverse Trendelenburg is tested to minimize patient movement once the operation has begun.

After prepping and draping the abdomen, an ideal pump pocket site is identified and marked, typically in the left hemiabdomen, with adequate space (2–3 fingerbreadths) inferior to the costal margin and superior to the anterior superior iliac spine. The subcutaneous pocket extends inferior to the incision. For obese patients, the pump pocket may need to be situated superior to the costal margin on the chest wall to minimize the risk of pump migration and optimize subsequent pump accessibility via palpation, as the subcutaneous fat layer is typically thinner in this region. Establishment of the ideal pump location before trocar placement ensures that port positions do not interfere with the eventual pump pocket.

The abdominal cavity is entered with open Hasson technique. A 12-mm balloon port is placed in the midline just inferior to the umbilicus. Diagnostic laparoscopy is performed using the robotic camera with careful inspection for evidence of extrahepatic disease, and any concerning lesions are biopsied and submitted for intraoperative frozen section analysis.

Additional 8-mm robotic trocars are inserted in the left upper quadrant superior to the planned pump pocket incision along the midclavicular line; right lower quadrant at the level of the umbilicus along the midclavicular line; and right hemiabdomen at the level of the umbilicus along the anterior axillary line (Fig. 127F.1). Care is taken to ensure a full handbreadth between port incisions. An additional 12-mm accessory port is placed in the left lower quadrant along the midclavicular line. The patient is placed into steep reverse Trendelenburg position (20°). A Nathanson liver retractor is placed in the subxiphoid area to retract the left lobe of the liver. The DaVinci Xi robot is docked on the right side of the patient. If the DaVinci Si robot is being used, it should be docked at the patient's head, with care taken to lower the bed sufficiently for the robotic boom and arms to clear the patient's face and endotracheal tube. A ProGrasp forceps is inserted in the right lateral trocar, a hook is inserted in the right lower quadrant trocar, and a bipolar cautery is inserted in the left upper quadrant trocar.

A cholecystectomy is routinely performed to avoid the risk of chemical cholecystitis.[4,5] Following this, dissection begins along the left side of the porta hepatis by incising the pars flaccida and gastrohepatic ligament. The right lobe of the liver is retracted cephalad with the ProGrasp forceps using the gallbladder or gentle pressure on the cystic plate if the patient has had a prior cholecystectomy. The common hepatic artery, proper hepatic artery, and right and left hepatic arteries are skeletonized circumferentially (Fig. 127F.2A). The common hepatic artery lymph node is excised. Dissection of the left hepatic artery is carried up 1 cm toward its first-order branches, and dissection of the right hepatic artery is carried distally for at least 2 cm or until the common bile duct is approached, as extrahepatic perfusion identified postoperatively frequently arises from its proximal small branches.[6] The right gastric artery is identified and divided between clips. The gastroduodenal artery is identified and dissected circumferentially. The supraduodenal artery and the superior posterior pancreaticoduodenal artery are identified and divided (see Fig. 127F.2A). A tie is placed along the gastroduodenal artery to minimize any barriers to placing the catheter into the artery, and clips are placed on the distal side of the vessel. Care is taken to identify and ligate all small collateral vessels and lymphatics in this space to prevent extrahepatic perfusion. Accessory or replaced right and/or left hepatic arteries, if present, are identified and dissected circumferentially. At the completion of the procedure, once the pump is successfully placed, the accessary or replaced arteries are ligated and divided between clips. The gastroduodenal artery is bathed in papaverine introduced percutaneously via a spinal needle (Fig. 127F.2B).

The pump is prepared at the back table by linkage of the catheters with a coupler, remote activation of the device, and flushing with heparinized saline to expunge gas bubbles and ensure a good seal at the linkage. The abdomen is desufflated.

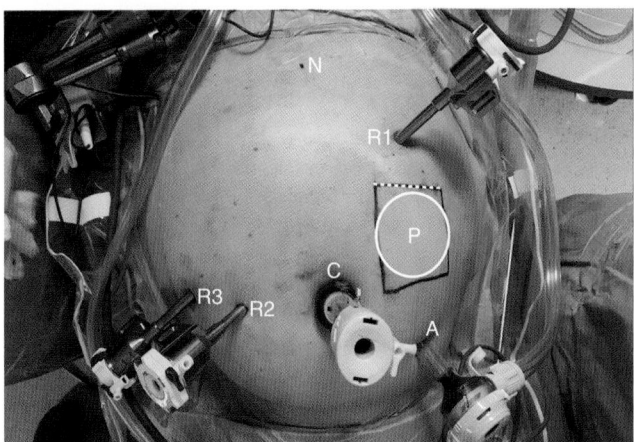

FIGURE 127F.1 Positioning of robotic and assistant ports. The *dotted line* indicates the incision created to develop the subcutaneous pocket and insert the hepatic arterial infusion pump. The *shaded circle* indicates the eventual position of the pump within the pocket. *A,* Assistant port; *C,* camera; *N,* Nathanson retractor; *P,* pump; *R,* robotic port.

A 7-cm incision is made at the site previously marked, and dissection is carried down to the anterior fascia overlying rectus abdominis and external oblique muscles. Fat is cleared caudally off the fascia to create a pocket large enough to comfortably accept the pump. A small fascial defect is created, and the pump catheter is introduced into the abdomen (Fig. 127F.2C). Excess extracorporeal catheter length is temporarily laid on the fascia under the pump. The pump is secured to the fascia at the floor of the pump pocket with 2-0 silk through its four suture loops, ensuring that the access port is positioned laterally and that the catheter is not kinked or entrapped by the sutures.

Insufflation is reestablished. The distal gastroduodenal artery is ligated with 2-0 silk at the level of the pancreatic head, and a metal clip is placed at the same level (Fig. 127F.2D). Accessory or replaced right and/or left hepatic arteries, if present, are temporarily occluded with a bulldog clamp (Fig. 127F.2E). A vascular bulldog clamp is placed across the proximal gastroduodenal artery at its origin from the common hepatic artery. Alternatively, two vascular bulldog clamps can be placed across the common and proper hepatic arteries to isolate the gastroduodenal artery

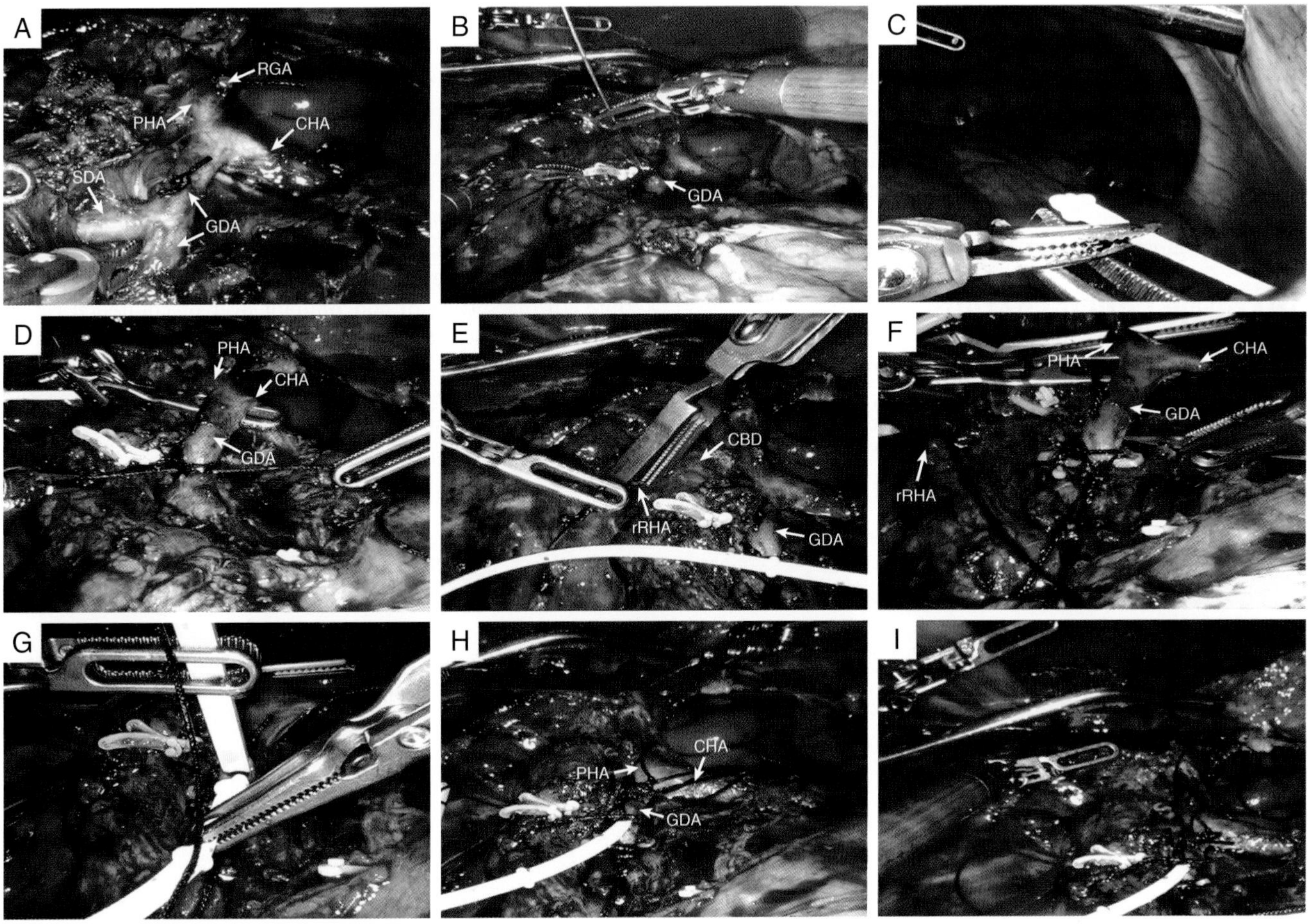

FIGURE 127F.2 Critical steps during robotic hepatic arterial infusion pump placement. **A,** Circumferential dissection of the hepatic artery and distal branches. **B,** Papaverine sprayed over the gastroduodenal artery. **C,** Introduction of the pump catheter into the abdomen. **D,** Ligation of the distal gastroduodenal artery at the level of the pancreas. **E,** Temporary occlusion of replaced or accessory right and/or left hepatic arteries, if present. These vessels are later ligated following confirmation of bilobar pump perfusion. **F,** Control of the hepatic artery proximal and distal to the gastroduodenal artery origin, and gastroduodenal arteriotomy. **G,** Retrograde insertion of the catheter into the gastroduodenal artery. **H,** The secured catheter with three silk ties. **I,** Confirmation of bilobar liver perfusion with absence of extrahepatic perfusion using methylene blue injection. *CBD,* Common bile duct; *CHA,* common hepatic artery; *GDA,* gastroduodenal artery; *PHA,* proper hepatic artery; *RGA,* right gastric artery; *rRHA,* replaced right hepatic artery; *SDA,* supraduodenal artery.

origin (Fig. 127F.2F). A loose 2-0 silk tie is laid behind the proximal gastroduodenal artery. Using a free #11 blade or robotic shears, an arteriotomy is sharply created in the distal gastroduodenal artery spanning one-third of the circumference of the vessel just proximal to the silk ligature (Fig. 127F.2F). The pump catheter is inserted retrograde into the gastroduodenal artery with its tip positioned at its origin from the common hepatic artery (Fig. 127F.2G). The vascular bulldog clamp is removed, and the loose silk tie is immediately tied adjacent to the catheter's distal bead with appropriate tension to appose the vessel wall around the catheter and affix its position, but not occlude the catheter lumen. An additional silk tie is placed adjacent to the catheter's second bead, and a third tie is placed equidistant between the two first ties (Fig. 127F.2H). The pump is flushed with heparinized saline after each tie is placed to confirm patency.

Methylene blue is infused through the pump, and the liver, stomach, duodenum, pancreas, and portal structures are examined to confirm bilobar hepatic perfusion and evaluate sites of extrahepatic perfusion, which, if present, are dissected further to identify and ligate sources of persistent collateral flow (Fig. 127F.2I). Redundant length of the pump catheter is pulled from the pump pocket into the abdomen, and the excess catheter is placed into the left upper quadrant.

The abdomen is again desufflated, and the robot is undocked. Trocars are removed under direct vision. After again confirming patency of the catheter by flushing heparinized saline, the pump pocket is closed in layers, with running 3-0 Vicryl for Scarpa fascia and deep dermal layers and running subcuticular 4-0 Monocryl for epidermis. The incision is dressed with Dermabond. Fascial defects at 12-mm port sites are closed with 0 Vicryl, and remaining skin incisions are closed with 4-0 Monocryl and dressed with Dermabond.

ANATOMIC CONSIDERATIONS

Aberrant anatomy of the hepatic artery may be identified in 30% to 50% of patients[7,8] (see Chapter 2). Hepatic artery variants can present challenges for intraoperative dissection as well as delivery of chemotherapy to the entire liver. Replaced or accessory arteries that are not ligated intraoperatively can continue to deliver native blood flow to liver segments, potentially limiting the intended effect of infusional therapy. Bilobar liver perfusion is routinely observed even with ligation of a replaced hepatic artery due to interlobar collateral perfusion. Furthermore, cannulation of vessels other than the gastroduodenal arteries in the setting of variant hepatic arterial anatomy is associated with more frequent postoperative and pump-related complications.[8] In patients with hepatic artery variants, we routinely cannulate the gastroduodenal artery and ligate replaced and accessory hepatic arteries. If the gastroduodenal artery is not amenable to a catheter, or a dissection occurs while placing the catheter, the catheter can be placed retrograde in either the left or right hepatic artery and cross perfusion within the liver usually leads to a functional pump.

SEQUENCING OF CONCOMITANT RESECTION

Any planned robotic hepatectomy is performed before pump placement, as technical complications that arise during placement of the pump could preclude subsequent resection, a low central venous pressure is only required for the resection portion, and resection after placement of the pump could result in dislodgement of the pump catheter or other pump malfunction. For combined colorectal resection and hepatic arterial infusion pump placement with or without hepatectomy, we perform the pump placement and hepatectomy portion first, because this often requires strict intraoperative volume restriction, followed by colorectal resection, which often includes creation of an enterostomy that would interfere with options for subsequent trocar placement. In addition, pump infection rates may be lower when the pump is placed and the pump pocket closed before the colon portion of the procedure. In the setting of concomitant liver or colorectal resection, the midline camera port is enlarged for use as a specimen extraction site.

The references for this chapter can be found online by accessing the accompanying Expert Consult website.

CHAPTER 128

Minimally invasive surgery techniques in transplantation

Choon Hyuck David Kwon, Kazunari Sasaki, and Amit Nair

The advent and refinement of minimally invasive surgery (MIS) techniques within the realm of oncologic hepatobiliary surgery[1] (see Chapter 127) has paved the way for the collateral development of this field in living donor liver transplantation (LDLT) (see Chapter 121). Further to the initial French report of laparoscopic donor left lateral segmentectomy two decades ago,[2] there has been a gradual accrual of literature in the arena of MIS living liver donation, with subsequent description of laparoscopic-assisted/hybrid or hand-assisted donor hepatectomy.[3,4] Indeed, the feasibility of pure laparoscopic liver donation has been recognized in more recent years,[5–8] with the predominant experience being reported from Far Eastern nations and Europe.[9,10] In addition, whereas the vast majority of these reports have focused on laparoscopic techniques, the impetus on robotic living liver donation has as yet been comparatively lacking in traction.[11,12]

The fundamental premise of living donation is one of donor safety,[13] as this procedure comes with no physiologic benefit to the donor (see Chapters 105, 109, and 121). As such, every effort should be made to minimize the risk of donor complications through the judicious selection of lobe laterality, leaving at least 30% functional liver remnant (FLR) (see Chapter 4) in the donor while permitting a minimum graft-recipient weight ratio (GRWR) of 0.8 or graft volume to standard liver volume (GV/SLV) of 35% to 40%.[14] Adequate experience of the surgical team is also crucial. Invariably, most described series of laparoscopic living donation have been undertaken by surgeons with proficiency in both laparoscopic oncologic hepatic resections (see Chapters 127D and 127E) and open liver donation (see Chapter 121), and this is of paramount importance in the safe undertaking of this procedure.[10,15] These facets notwithstanding, laparoscopic living donor hepatectomy serves to improve the recovery of the donors through the already known benefits related with MIS that include less intraoperative blood loss, shorter hospital stay, reduced postoperative analgesic requirements, and earlier return to normal activity.[16,17]

DONOR SELECTION

The candidacy of a prospective donor may vary across institutions and will not be discussed in detail in this chapter (see Chapters 105, 109, and 121). However, it is noteworthy to consider the difference in donor selection when the laparoscopic approach is considered. Considering the safety of the donor, with the addition to the complexity of the operation, it is recommended to start selecting donors with smaller livers, sufficient future remnant volume (see Chapter 4), and favorable anatomy before the learning curve of the program is accomplished. The presence of unfavorable hilar anatomy (see Chapter 2) as evidenced by early bifurcation of ipsilateral portal vein or bile duct is usually associated with wider Glissonian pedicles, and safe dissection and optimal division are more difficult, which may result in increased complications such as stricture or leakage of the bile duct.[18,19] With accumulation of experience, it is known that these obstacles can be overcome, but the application of a laparoscopic approach can yield increased frequency of multiple bile ducts of the graft, adversely affecting the recipient outcome. Therefore expansion of selection criteria for donors should be done with caution, weighing the advantages and the disadvantages of both the donor and the recipient outcome to have optimal results.[10,20–22]

We elaborate on our setup and technique for purely laparoscopic right, left with middle hepatic vein (MHV) and caudate lobe, left without MHV and caudate, and left lateral sectionectomy below.

OPERATING ROOM SETUP

Our preference for patient positioning is akin to the "French" system, where the donor is placed in a modified lithotomy position with legs abducted in stirrups to 20° to 30° (Fig. 128.1). For right hepatectomy, a degree of left tilting of the torso is beneficial for mobilization of the right lobe and facilitated by the placement of a cushion or rolled blanket behind the right scapular region. The patient should be firmly secured to the operating table to prevent sliding due to changes in table positioning during surgery.

The primary surgeon stands between the patient's legs while the camera operator is to the left of the patient's left leg. The first assistant is positioned to the left of the patient's torso, right of the camera operator (Fig. 128.2). The scrub nurse is to the left of and behind the primary operator and surgical instruments are placed in this area.

ANESTHETIC CONSIDERATIONS

The maintenance of low-volume anesthesia during liver parenchymal transection is key to curtail intraoperative blood loss (see Chapters 25 and 121). Good communication between the anesthesia and the surgical teams is key. The placement of a central venous catheter is not uniformly performed, and reliance on other indices of fluid status such as stroke volume variability can help further abrogate interventional risks to a living donor. To prevent kidney injury while maintaining a low-volume status during transection, the patient is kept dry throughout the operation until the parenchymal transection is complete, at which point the anesthesia team is informed to refill the depleted volume with intravenous (IV) bolus to reach euvolemic state before the surgery ends. If colloids are deemed to be necessary, they are given after the parenchymal transection is complete. Transversus abdominis plane (TAP) block with bupivacaine is routinely used for better postoperative pain control as part of our enhanced recovery after surgery (ERAS) protocol (see Chapter 27).

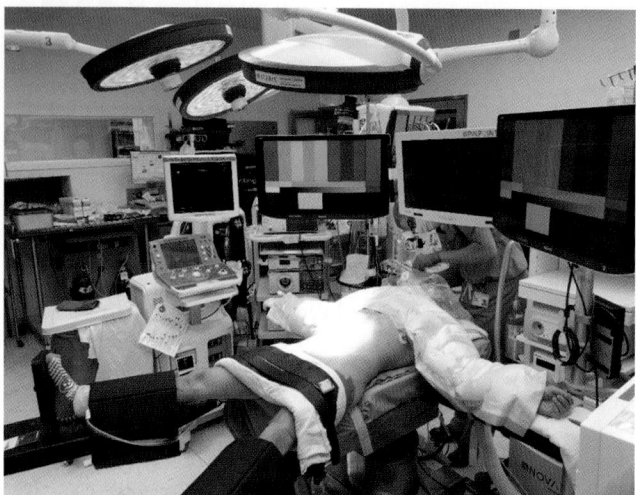

FIGURE 128.1   **The operating room setup.** Two large main screens are placed on both sides of the patient and a third monitor for ICG cholangiogram is placed at the center. Laparoscopic ultrasound can be seen on the far-right side.

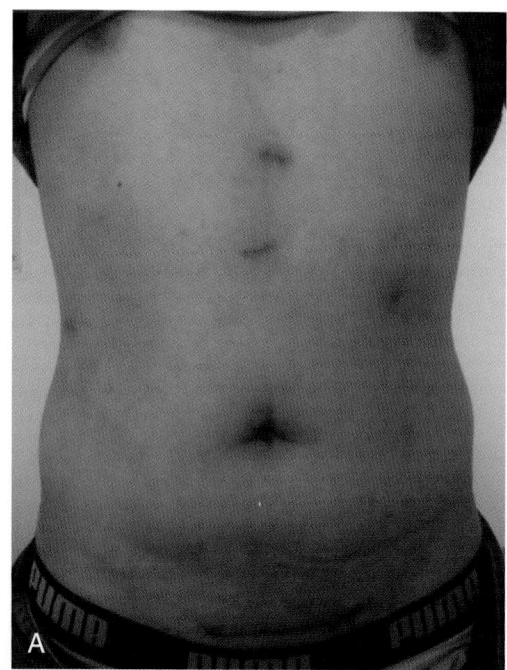

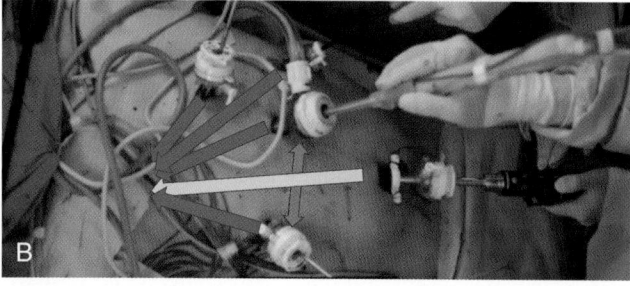

FIGURE 128.2   **A,** Port placement and the suprapubic incision used for a right liver and left with middle hepatic vein graft. **B,** The camera is approached between the right subcostal and epigastric midline ports *(yellow arrow),* which are used by the main surgeon. The subxiphoid and left subcostal ports are used by the first assistant standing on the left of the patient.

EQUIPMENT

The use of a three-dimensional (3D) flexible camera system (EndoEye Flex 3D, Olympus, Center Valle, PA) is our preference as it greatly facilitates depth perception and adequate visualization of tight corners,[10,23] thereby enabling safer dissection in the region of the root of the hepatic veins, posterosuperior right lobe, and short hepatic veins. In addition, spatial bimanual tasks such as intracorporeal suturing are eminently suited to and hastened by 3D visualization and this technology may indeed serve to reduce the learning curve for laparoscopic hepatectomy.[10] Two 3D monitors are placed beyond either shoulder of the patient angled inward toward the surgeon and should be positioned at eye level to prevent double vision (see Fig. 128.1).

We also place a third monitor positioned between both 3D monitors, which is used for indocyanine green (ICG) enabled endoscopic fluorescence imaging of the bile ducts (Pinpoint, Stryker, San Jose, CA). The ICG imaging technology allows real-time visualization of the bile ducts, which greatly facilitates and improves the accuracy of bile duct division compared with conventional cholangiogram (see Chapter 24).

With respect to laparoscopic insufflation, our inclination is toward the use of the AirSeal system (ConMed, Utica, NY) as this enables a stable degree of pneumoperitoneum despite the use of cavitron ultrasonic surgical aspirator (CUSA, Integra, Princeton, NJ) and the frequent requirement for suctioning. This helps promote operative flow and shorten times. However, the high-flow nature of the AirSeal system may cause increased CO_2 retention; therefore we keep it at a lower pressure level of 11 cm H_2O.

Ultrasonic shear device is deployed for dissection of the hepatic ligaments, some parts of hilar dissection, sealing vessels less than 2 mm in diameter, and for initial transection of the first 1 to 2 cm superficial layer of the liver as sizeable vascular structures are uncommon (Fig. 128.3) (see Chapters 121, 127D, and 127E). Battery powered cordless options afford more freedom with the instrument handling, but the counterparts with cords usually afford better energy delivery with improved bleeding control. New devices are constantly being developed, and the surgeon should be familiar with the advantages and disadvantages of each product line and choose the product best suited for one's preferences.

Precise dissection of the parenchyma is of vital importance in donor hepatectomy to keep the surgical field dry and have a clear vision in order to prevent any inadvertent injury to important structures or vessels (see Chapter 121). Crush clamp technique, either with or without coagulation function, ultrasonic shear device, and CUSA are the most commonly used methods for transection (see Fig. 128.3). Adding monopolar coagulator nosecone on the CUSA hand piece provides electrocautery without the need of instrumental change, which greatly improves hemostasis. Also, by turning off the laparoscopic mode, it can be used as a gentle suction device while transecting the liver. Notably, irrespective of instruments used, dissection should not be done blindly, especially in the deeper parenchyma, because this is where major bleeding events usually occur. Bipolar electrocautery has been our preferred instrument to safeguard bloodless parenchymal transection, and a second bipolar forcep in the tray allows rapid cycling of these instruments between cleaning of charred contact plates, which

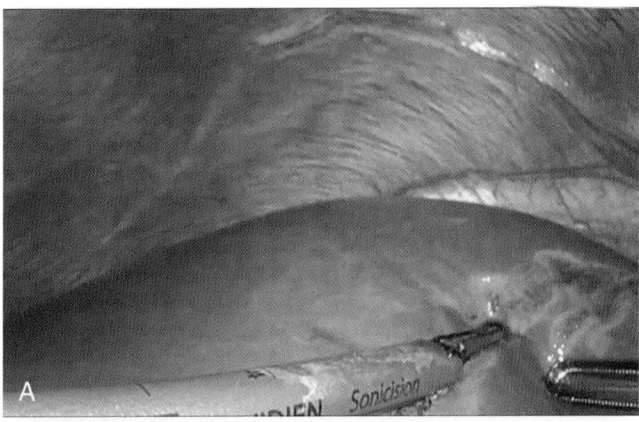

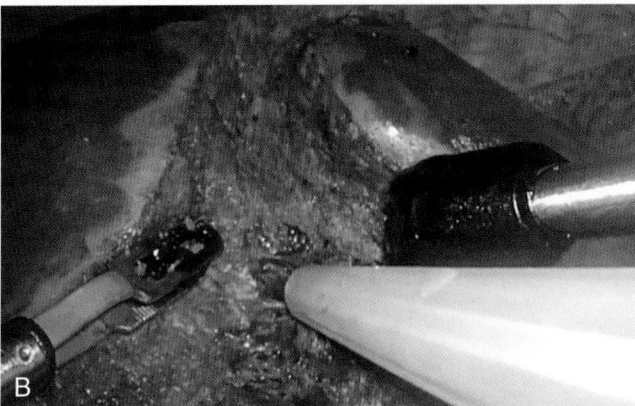

FIGURE 128.3 **A,** Parenchymal transection at the superficial layer up to 2 cm in depth can be done blindly using ultrasonic shear device. **B,** When deeper layers are dissected, CUSA and bipolar forceps with the aid of Aquamantys is used to finely dissect important structures and maintain a dry field.

allows parenchymal transection without interference of surgery. A supplemental soft coagulation instrument, handled by the assistant providing additional hemostasis, offers a smoother and more efficient transection.

MANAGEMENT OF PARENCHYMAL BLEEDING

The ability to control major bleeding is essential in ensuring the safety of the donor operation (see Chapters 25, 101, and 121); therefore a well-considered strategy is required before undertaking a laparoscopic program. Although blood loss is usually insignificant and patients do not require any transfusion, it is our preference to always have the suction device attached to the Cell Saver (Haemonetics, Boston, MA) in case significant bleeding occurs and autotransfusion becomes necessary. The use of bipolar electrocautery, energy-assisted coagulative devices, and/or vessel clips is typically the first step toward establishing hemostasis and is usually met with success. Temporary packing of the field with hemostatic agents (e.g., oxidized cellulose derivatives) or sponge and revisiting the area a few minutes later often proves beneficial.

In case of more brisk bleeding as will be seen with larger caliber vessels, bleeding control often only can be achieved through direct repair of the bleeding site either by clipping or suturing. In such circumstances, ensuring low central venous

pressure, including the use of 30% reverse-Trendelenburg positioning, with temporary increase of the insufflation pressure up to 15 mm Hg can help reduce the rate of bleed (see Chapters 25, 127D, and 127E). Temporary reduction of the tidal volume is proven to be effective as well. Regardless of the method used, reducing bleeding through counterbalance using pneumatic pressure should be done judiciously. CO_2 gas embolism[18] and hypercarbia inevitably occur, and although usually clinically insignificant when the duration is short, prolonged use may result in significant respiratory acidosis and hemodynamic instability. Finally, the application of the Pringle maneuver (see Chapters 101, 121, 127D, and 127E) can provide a summative effect to hemostatic control and can be resorted to without concern for graft outcomes in those recipients with projected good GRWR.[24]

Laparoscopic vascular clamps should always be prepared and be available in the operating room in case it becomes necessary for rapid bleeding control (Fig. 128.4) (see Chapters 127D and 127E). The threshold to convert to open (see Chapter 121) must remain low to ensure donor safety, but it is crucial that conversion is not rushed through because loss of the pneumoperitoneum will result in increased bleeding. Step-by-step strategy during conversion should be preplanned, and the whole team should be familiar with the process to prevent chaos.

LAPAROSCOPIC RIGHT HEPATECTOMY (ALSO SEE CHAPTER 127E)

Trocar Port Placement

Following establishment of pneumoperitoneum via the periumbilical 12 mm port, a 12 mm port is placed at the right subcostal region along the right anterior axillary line and a 5 mm (assistant) port is placed next in the left subcostal anterior axillary line (see Fig. 128.2). The round and falciform ligament is sectioned with an energy device in a caudocranial direction. At its inferior aspect, dissection is kept close to the abdominal wall so as to remove redundant fat with the ligament, and once anterior to the liver, this line is continued approximately 1 cm away from the liver surface. Dissection is thus carried out toward the diaphragm and base of the hepatic veins, exposing and dividing loose areolar tissue at the anterior apex of the bare area of the liver. The 12 mm epigastric (primary surgeon) midline port is now placed and another 12 mm (assistant) port is also inserted in the midline subxiphoid region, a few centimeters cranial to the aforementioned trocar. The right subcostal and the epigastric midline port are the main ports used by the primary surgeon, and the camera is positioned between these thus offering a good triangulation along the line of Cantlie (see Fig. 128.2).[15]

Right Lobe Mobilization

The mobilization of the right lobe may be done before or after the parenchymal division (see Chapter 127E). Mobilizing after, as in anterior approach, is easier because only the right lobe, and therefore a smaller liver mass, needs to be retracted and is the standard for all liver surgeries. However, with the living donors, mobilization is done first because in case of an urgent situation where the liver has to be retrieved during the course of transection, the graft can be quickly taken out (see also Chapter 118 on open hepatectomy).

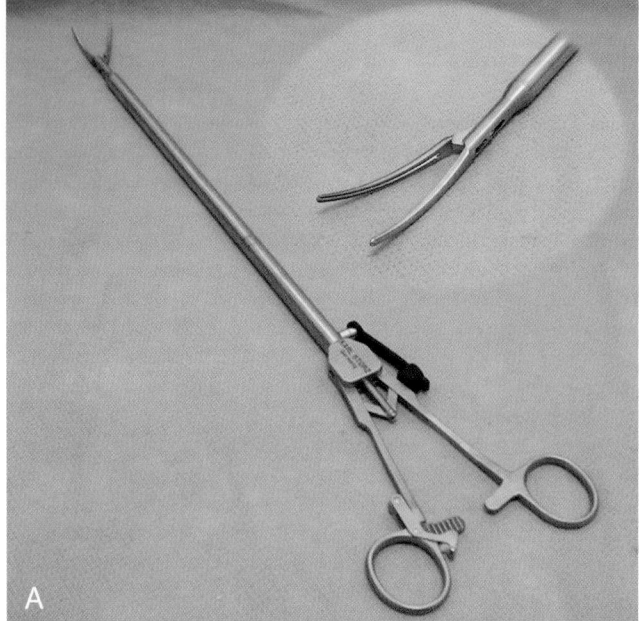

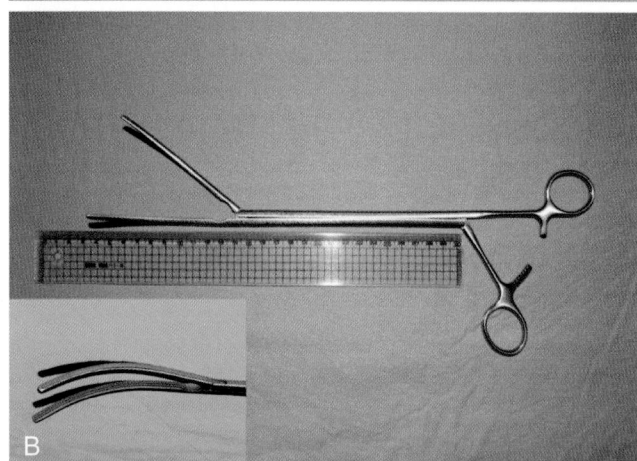

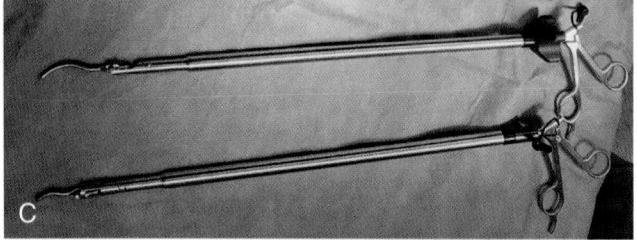

FIGURE 128.4 Vascular clamps should always be prepared and available in the operating room to manage major bleeding events. **A,** Laparoscopic vascular clamp. **B,** Chitwood deBakey clamp. **C,** Laparoscopic bulldog clamps.

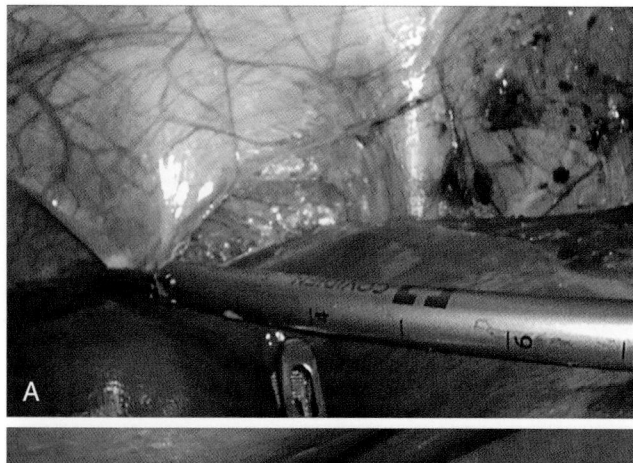

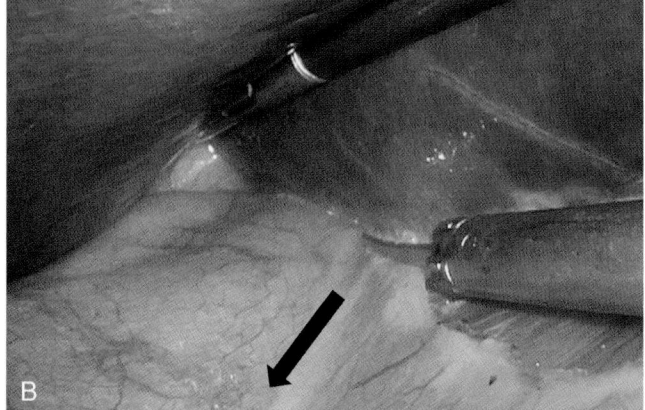

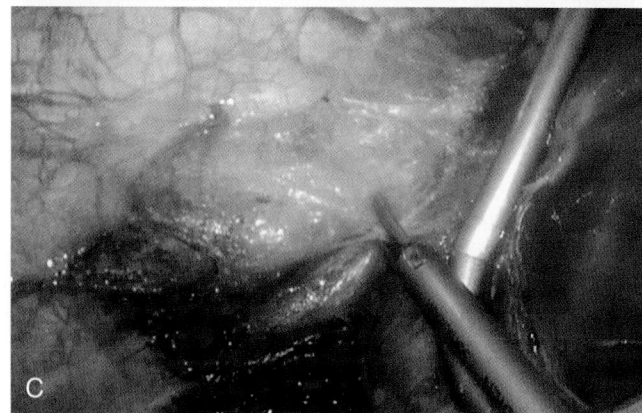

FIGURE 128.5 Mobilization of the right lobe. **A,** The coronary ligament is divided with ultrasonic shears. The subxiphoid port is used to have the best angle of approach. **B,** Right triangular ligament is divided. The assistant lifts the liver while the main surgeon pushes the kidney posteriorly to have a nice countertraction *(black arrow).* **C,** The lateral part of triangular ligament is taken last. The patient should be tilted left, and the dissection should be done using the right subcostal port until the vena cava become visible.

A systematic approach is vital in mobilization of the right lobe to not traumatize the liver (Fig. 128.5). First, the coronary ligament is divided. Caudal traction of the liver by the assistant using the round ligament improves visibility and provides countertraction. The dissection is best carried out through the subxiphoid port because it provides the safest angle of approach and may prevent injury to the diaphragm. Then the dissection of inferior aspect of triangular ligament follows. A snake retractor is placed underneath the right lobe to lift the liver in an anterior-cranial direction, and a posterior-caudal traction of the kidney facilitates the exposure to provide safe division of the ligament and prevent injury to the adrenal gland. The lateral aspect of the triangular ligament is dissected last. Tilting the patient to the left is essential to facilitate this phase of surgery and the gallbladder fundus may be used as a retraction tool in addition to the gentle traction using snake retractor. Dissection should be carried out using the right subcostal port because it provides the safest angle of approach. Mobilization of the lobe is carried out in a caudocranial and lateromedial direction concurrently, until the lateral aspect of the retrohepatic cava is exposed. Minor bleeding from the region of the cava is well addressed with bipolar electrocoagulation. The caval ligament, if present in a substantial form, is best left undisturbed at this juncture and can be divided from a medial side toward the conclusion of parenchymal transection.

Hilar Dissection

Cholecystectomy is now completed and the gallbladder will be retrieved later with the graft (see Chapters 36 and 127E). The cystic duct stump is retracted to the left-cranial direction by the assistant to open up the posterior-lateral aspect of the hilum to provide easy access to the right portal vein (RPV) and right hepatic artery (RHA). The use of hook electrocautery and the bipolar forceps is valuable at this stage (Fig. 128.6). It is important to proceed slowly, verifying every structure before coagulating with the hook electrocautery to prevent inadvertent injury of important structures. The artery is dissected out to an appropriate degree to allow placement of a silastic vessel loop around it, which is then fastened and retracted cranially to open up access to the RPV. The latter is now dissected proximally to positively identify its junction with the main portal vein and the takeoff of the left portal vein. The division of caudate tributaries is often necessary to permit better mobility and length to the right portal vein. The vein is similarly encircled with a vessel loop. The hilar plate is now lowered to expose the confluence of right and left bile duct and is marked using electrocautery. Bulldog clamps are then applied to the right portal vein and hepatic artery and 2.5 mg of ICG is given intravenously by the anesthesiologist. The line of demarcation is noted but a sharper image can be obtained using a near-infrared camera. After it is marked on the liver surface, the bulldog clamps are removed (Fig. 6, 11). Intraoperative ultrasound is performed to aid with the identification of the course of the middle hepatic vein (MHV) and the location of the segment 5 (V5) and segment 8 (V8) tributaries. The planned resection plane should lie at the right side of the MHV for conventional right hepatectomy, but in case MHV is included with the graft, the resection plane is planned to be on the left side of the MHV.

Parenchymal Transection and Bile Duct Division

Pringle maneuver is not routinely used in donors, but we recommend having it ready to be applied in case inflow control becomes necessary in the event of major bleeding (see Chapters 121, 127D, and 127E). Division of the hepatic parenchyma commences along the line of demarcation at the anterior border of the liver using the energy device, and working both in a cranial direction up to the groove between the right and middle hepatic vein and toward the initially made hilar plate demarcation point inferiorly (see Fig. 128.3). Leftward traction by the assistant using the falciform ligament or by gently grabbing the edge of the liver helps align the direction of the energy device parallel with the transection plane. Once the parenchyma is divided to a depth of 1 to 2 cm, our preference is to then start using the CUSA, as more delicate dissection of the parenchyma is necessary and sizeable venous vessels will be encountered in the field. Small vessels less than 2 mm can often be sealed and divided with monopolar electrocautery

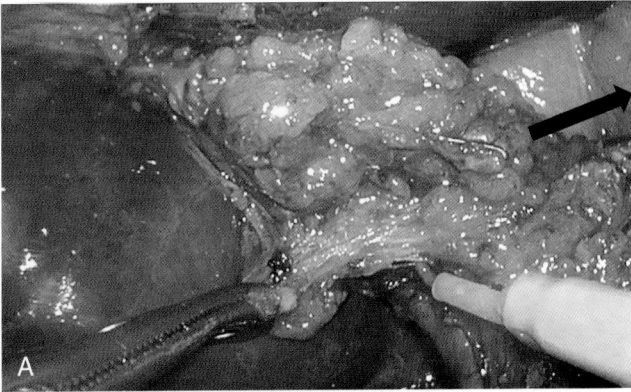
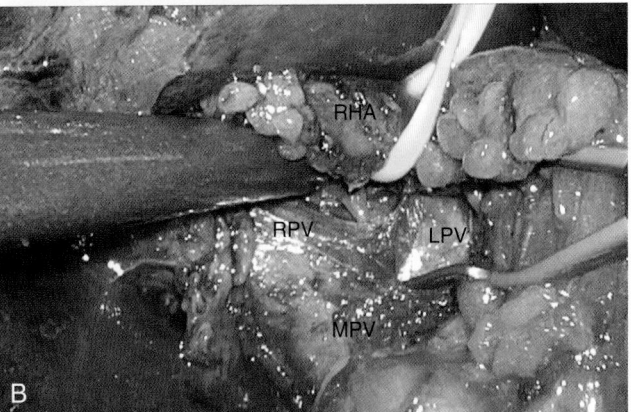
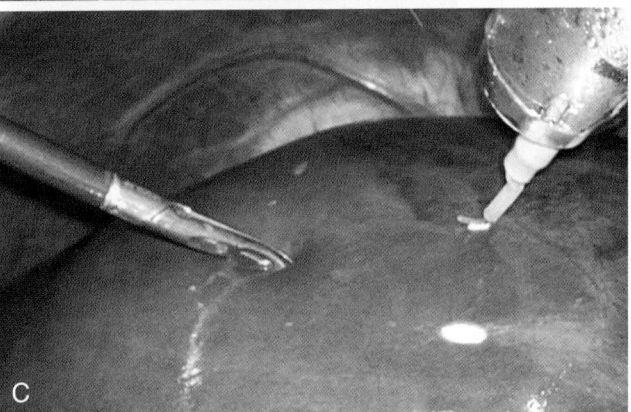

FIGURE 128.6 Hilar dissection. **A,** While the assistant is retracting the cyst duct in a left superior direction *(black arrow),* a hook monopolar electrocautery is used to dissect the soft tissues to skeletonize the right-side vessels. **B,** The portal vein is dissected using a gentle jaw opening movement with bipolar forceps. The right hepatic artery is encircled with vessel loop and retracted upward to have a good surgical field. **C,** Demarcation line between right and left liver can be observed and is marked using electrocautery.

or energy device, but larger branches are better controlled with metal or Hem-o-lok clips (Fig. 128.7). When clipping and dividing significant venous branches such as V5 or V8, two clips are usually applied on the patient side for safety reasons, whereas single Hem-o-lok may be used on the graft side for ease of clip removal on the back table for reconstruction of the outflow. Parenchymal transection is carried out until the hilar plate confluence becomes fully exposed. Then the caudate lobe is divided inferiorly. The gentle jaw opening movement of the forceps and sweeping allows safe dissection

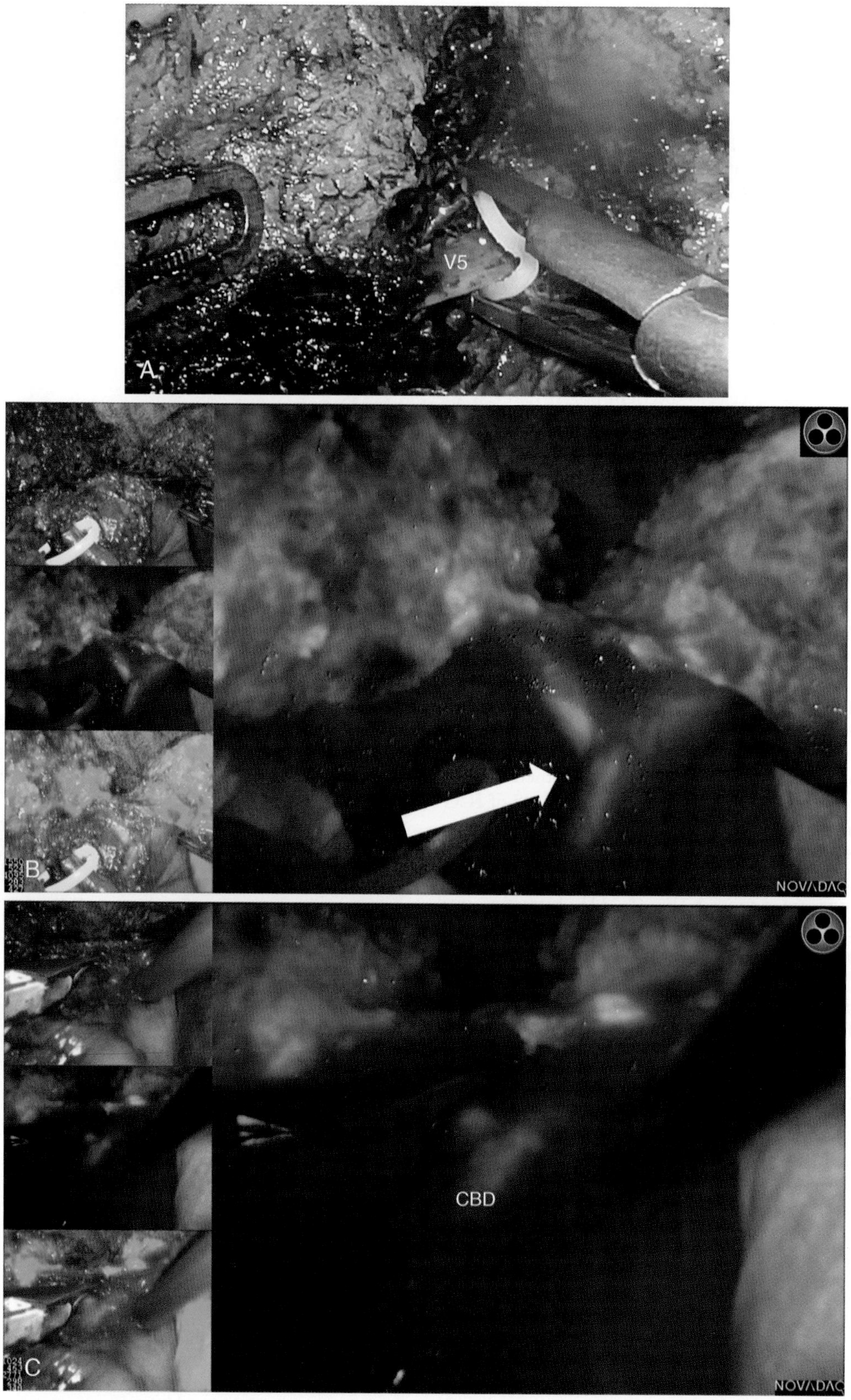

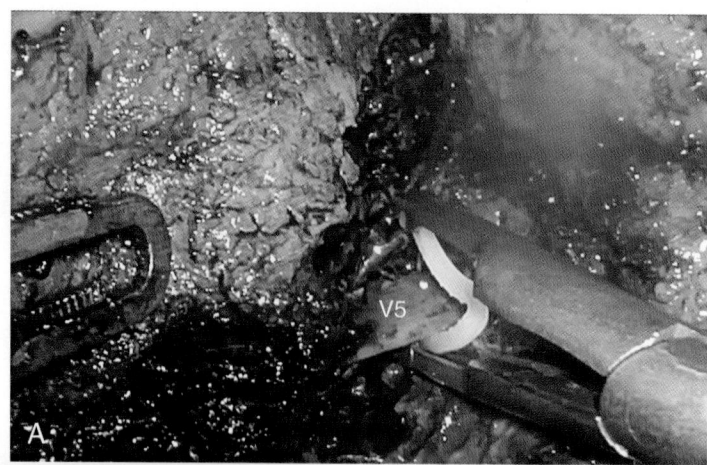

FIGURE 128.7 **Parenchymal transection and bile duct division. A,** V5 is dissected and clipped with a Hem-o-lok. **B,** Transection plane should be fully exposed when dividing the bile duct. The bifurcation of the right and left bile duct *(white arrow)* and the common bile duct (CBD) can be observed using indocyanine green (ICG) cholangiogram. **C,** The clip is applied in real time on the right bile duct, making sure the confluence and the left bile duct are not compromised.

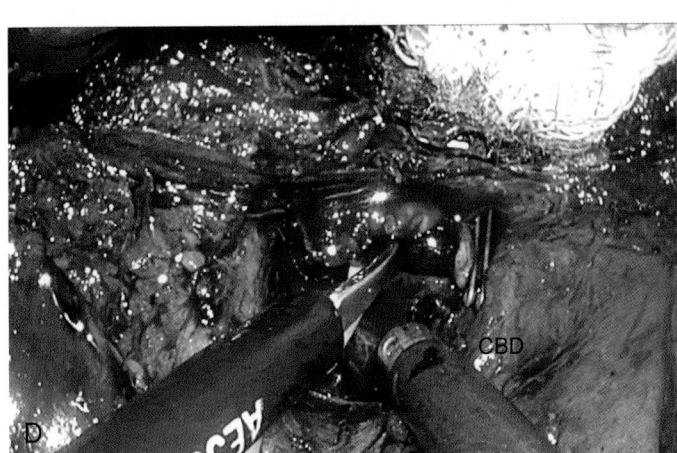
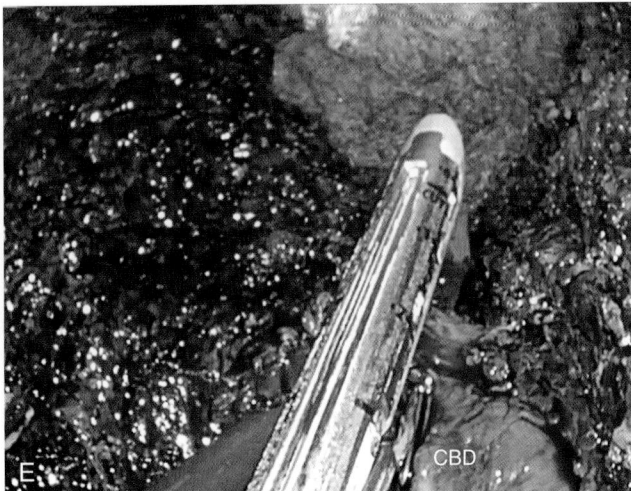

FIGURE 128.7 cont'd D, The right bile duct is divided after applying two secure clips on the remnant side. At least 1 to 2 mm length of left bile duct stump needs to remain, so the clips will not fall off. **E,** The remaining Glissonian sheath is divided using a stapler.

between the IVC and the caudate lobe, and any small short hepatic veins encountered along the way can be managed using small clips or energy device. Once the caudate lobe is transected past the right Glissonian pedicle, the right Glissonian sheath is encircled and exposed for bile duct division (see Chapter 127E).

The ICG cholangiogram allows real-time assessment of the biliary structure and provides a much more accurate division and management of the bile duct (see Chapters 20 and 121) (see Fig. 128.7). Because more than an hour has passed since the administration of ICG, a sufficient amount of ICG is excreted into the bile duct and provides good fluorescent imaging. Two metal clips are placed on the remnant side of the duct just beyond the site of proposed division of the right hepatic duct and is then divided sharply. The clip appliers may have to be approached through the umbilical port to provide the best angle. Brisk albeit small arterial bleeders may be encountered in the vicinity of the graft duct, which are controlled by temporarily applying a bulldog clamp. The use of any kind of energy devices or electrocautery is not recommended in this area to mitigate the risk of biliary ischemia and stricture. The remainder of the ipsilateral Glissonian sheath posterior to the divided bile duct is then sectioned with a stapler fire with a slimmer version cartilage to prevent biliary leaks from caudate branches that often lie within the sheath.

Final Steps and Organ Retrieval

Once the bile duct is divided, the transection plane, initially approached caudally, can be observed anteriorly, which can further be transected cranially along the retrohepatic cava (Fig. 128.8). The gentle sweeping and the use of jaw opening motion of the forceps allow safe dissection between the cava and the liver capsule providing a buffer space in between to allow safe use of the CUSA in this region. Multiple short hepatic veins are often found so care must be taken to prevent injury. Dissection is continued into the initially created groove between RHV and MHV. The remainder of the liver can be

dissected safely from the vena cava when approached medially. Accessory right inferior hepatic vein or the caval ligament is controlled with clips or with a stapler if considered to be large. If the surgical field is too narrow, making stapler application unsafe, stapling can be done at the final stage after the artery and portal veins have been divided. The RHV is encircled with umbilical tape. At this point the anesthesiologist is notified to initiate aggressive fluid resuscitation to return the patient back to euvolemic state (see Chapter 25).

A 10- to 13-cm Pfannenstiel incision is made in the suprapubic region and deepened. A small opening is made in the peritoneum to allow entry of a laparoscopic plastic bag and the right lobe is teased into it, along with the gallbladder. Additional muscle relaxant and 3000 IU of heparin is administered intravenously and allowed to circulate for 3 minutes before inflow vascular occlusion. The RHA is doubly clipped on the remnant aspect and the vessel then sharply divided. The RPV is stapled or clipped across at a safe distance from the bifurcation so as to avoid stricturing of the remaining vein. It is best to apply the stapler through the subxiphoid port to provide a perpendicular staple line to maximize the length of portal vein on the graft and prevent stricture of the remnant vein. Finally, the RHV is stapled, freeing the graft, which is then extracted via the Pfannenstiel incision after enlarging the peritoneal aperture appropriately, and taken to the back table for preparation toward implantation. The peritoneum is closed, and the abdomen is re-insufflated and closely monitored for any potential bile leak or bleeding (see Chapters 121, 127D, and 127E). Under adequate resuscitation, the cava is usually filled by now and any further bleeding from veins may be identified to be appropriately controlled. The resection surface is closely monitored for any potential bile leak. A closed suction drain is inserted via the left-sided 5 mm port site and placed across the resection bed of the liver. The remnant falx on the liver is sutured to the anterior abdominal wall to prevent postoperative torsion of the remnant. The 12 mm port sites and the extraction site are closed in layers.

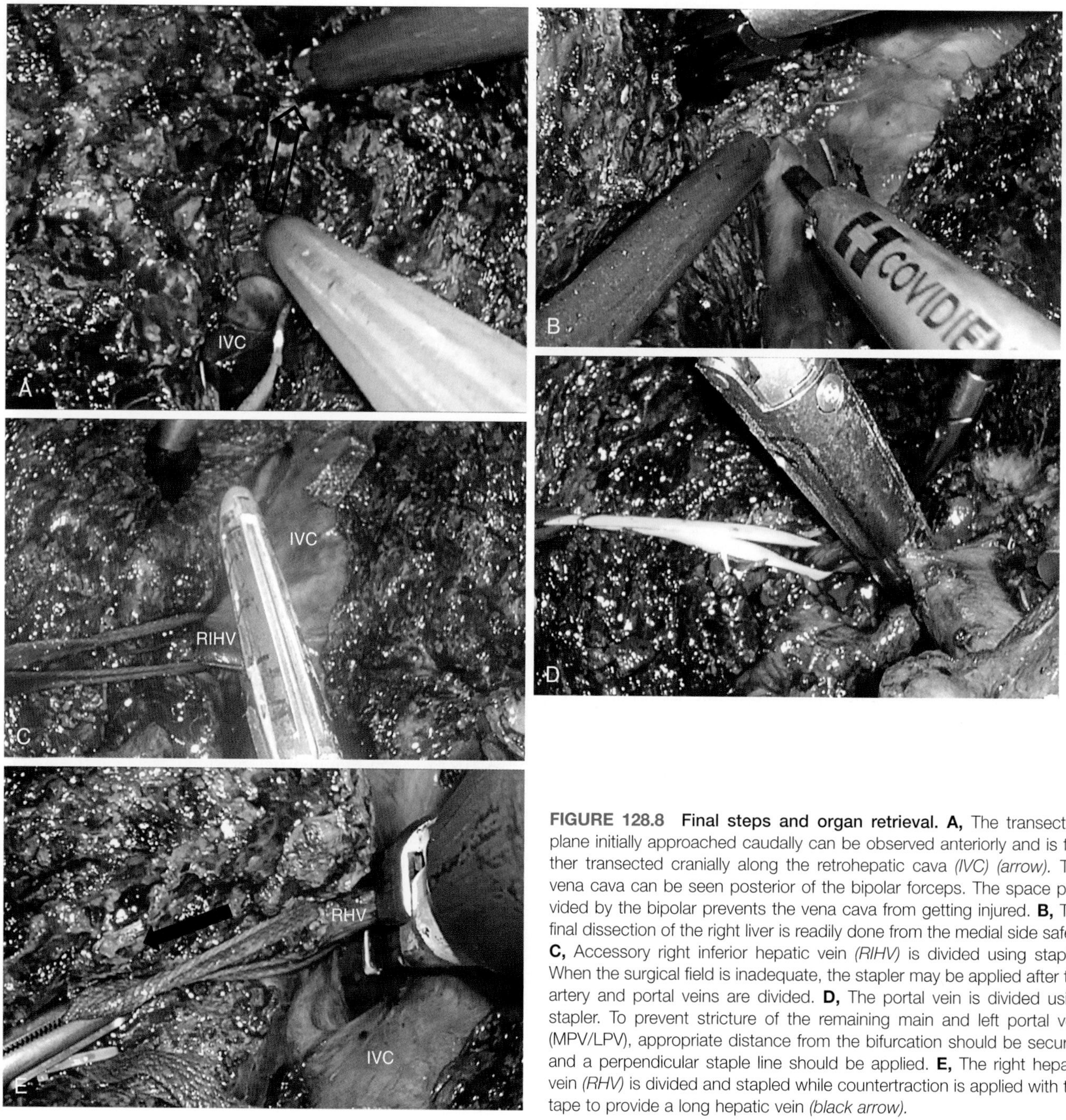

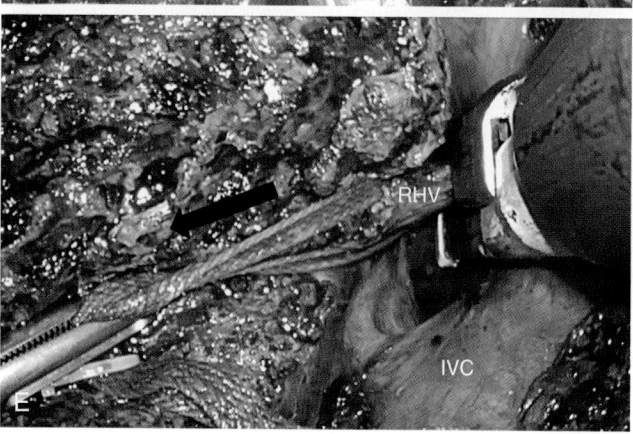

FIGURE 128.8 **Final steps and organ retrieval. A,** The transection plane initially approached caudally can be observed anteriorly and is further transected cranially along the retrohepatic cava *(IVC) (arrow).* The vena cava can be seen posterior of the bipolar forceps. The space provided by the bipolar prevents the vena cava from getting injured. **B,** The final dissection of the right liver is readily done from the medial side safely. **C,** Accessory right inferior hepatic vein *(RIHV)* is divided using stapler. When the surgical field is inadequate, the stapler may be applied after the artery and portal veins are divided. **D,** The portal vein is divided using stapler. To prevent stricture of the remaining main and left portal vein (MPV/LPV), appropriate distance from the bifurcation should be secured and a perpendicular staple line should be applied. **E,** The right hepatic vein *(RHV)* is divided and stapled while countertraction is applied with the tape to provide a long hepatic vein *(black arrow).*

LAPAROSCOPIC LEFT HEPATECTOMY WITH MHV AND THE CAUDATE LOBE (ALSO SEE CHAPTER 127E)

The right lobe is the most frequently used graft in adult LDLT, but our preference is always to resort to left lobe donation if recipient characteristics and GRWR permit its feasibility, as left-sided hepatectomy is associated with less risk to the donor. Besides leaving more FLR for the donor, the incidences of biliary and Clavien Grade II or above complications are shown to be less with left hepatectomy.[8,14]

Trocar Port Placement

The configuration of trocars is similar to that described for right hepatectomy, but because dissection along the Arantius ligament and the caudate lobe is necessary, the placement of the right subcostal and the main working ports is optimal when positioned 2 to 3 cm farther left as compared with right hepatectomy.

Mobilization of Left Lobe and Hilar Dissection

As the bare area of the liver is entered anteriorly, dissection is directed along the left triangular ligament thus freeing up the left lateral segment from the diaphragm (Fig. 128.9). Traction

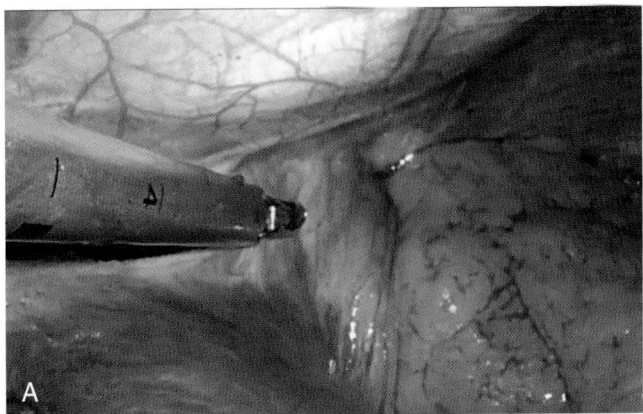

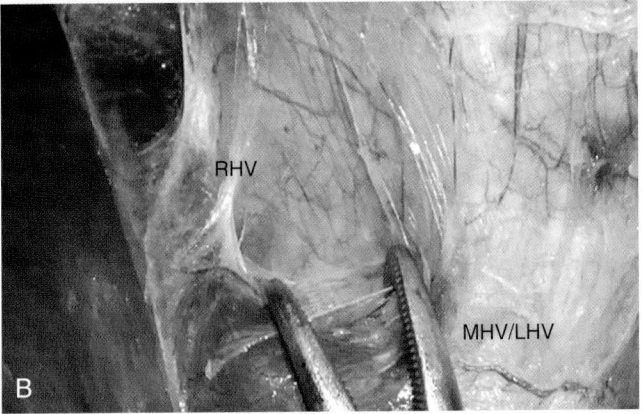

FIGURE 128.9 **Mobilization of the left lobe. A,** Left coronary ligament is divided. **B,** Loose areolar tissue is dissected to expose the base of the right, middle, and left hepatic veins *(RHV/MHV/LHV)*.

of the Falciform ligament toward the right iliac fossa by the assistant expedites this step. The base of the common stem of the middle and left hepatic veins is then delineated by further dissection of the loose areolar tissue over the bare area adjacent to the diaphragm (see also Chapter 118 on open hepatectomy).

Following cholecystectomy (see Chapters 36 and 127E), the peritoneal refection of the hepatoduodenal ligament and the left side of the hilum is skeletonized using a combination of hook electrocautery and bipolar forceps as previously described (Fig. 128.10). The left hepatic artery (LHA) is usually long redundant and easy to dissect, whereas the middle hepatic artery (MHA) to segment 4 is often small in caliber and close to the left hepatic duct and requires delicate dissection to prevent injury. The left portal vein lies behind the arteries and the arteries often have to be gently pulled away to obtain adequate space for dissection of the portal vein. Division of a caudate branch to the LPV can provide extra length and facilitate dissection of the portal vein, which is then encircled with vessel loops.

Bulldog clamps are applied to the inflow vessels, 2.5 mg of ICG is given, and near-infrared camera is used to identify the demarcation line (Fig. 128.11). The division plane is almost identical to that of right hepatectomy and likewise the transection plane should be on the right of the MHV in ultrasonogram evaluation. The inferior border should be heading toward the bifurcation of the left and right bile duct.

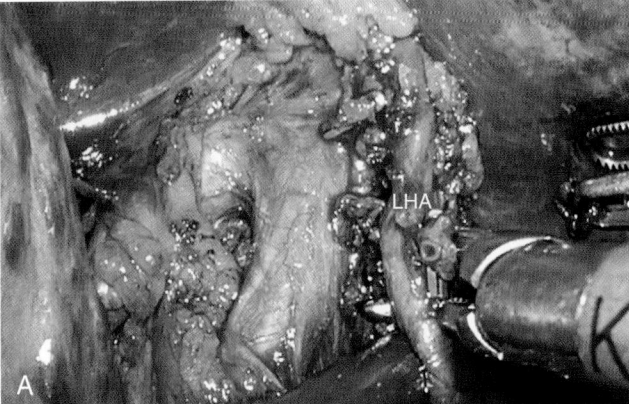

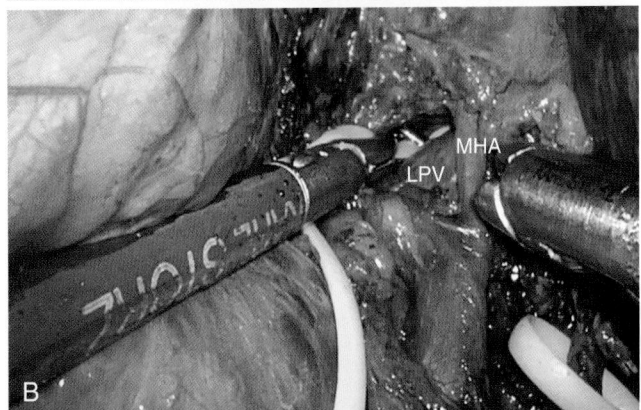

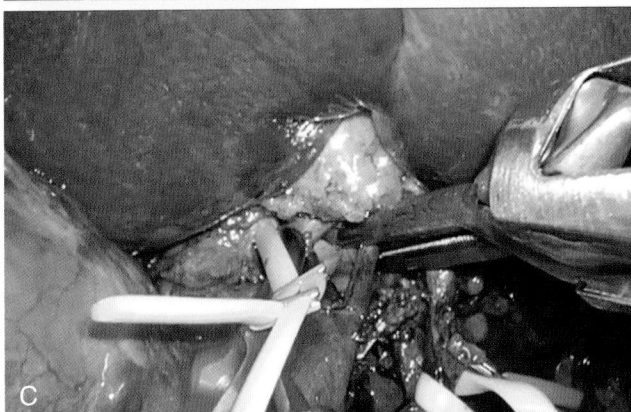

FIGURE 128.10 **Hilar dissection. A,** All the soft tissue surrounding the artery and portal vein is dissected with hook electrocautery and the left hepatic artery *(LHA)* is encircled. **B,** A vessel loop is placed around the left portal vein *(LPV)*. Portal vein behind the middle hepatic artery *(MHA)* can be observed. **C,** Bulldog clamp is temporarily applied to the left portal vein and the left and middle hepatic artery.

Caudate Lobe Mobilization

The lesser omentum is divided from the left side of the hilum up to the root of the left hepatic vein (LHV) to expose the caudate lobe (Fig. 128.12). This is facilitated by tilting the patient toward the right and with the use of a snake retractor to lift up the left lateral section (LLS). The presence of a replaced or accessory LHA would mandate dissecting out of this vessel toward its origin from the left gastric artery to garner extra length before its later division close to takeoff

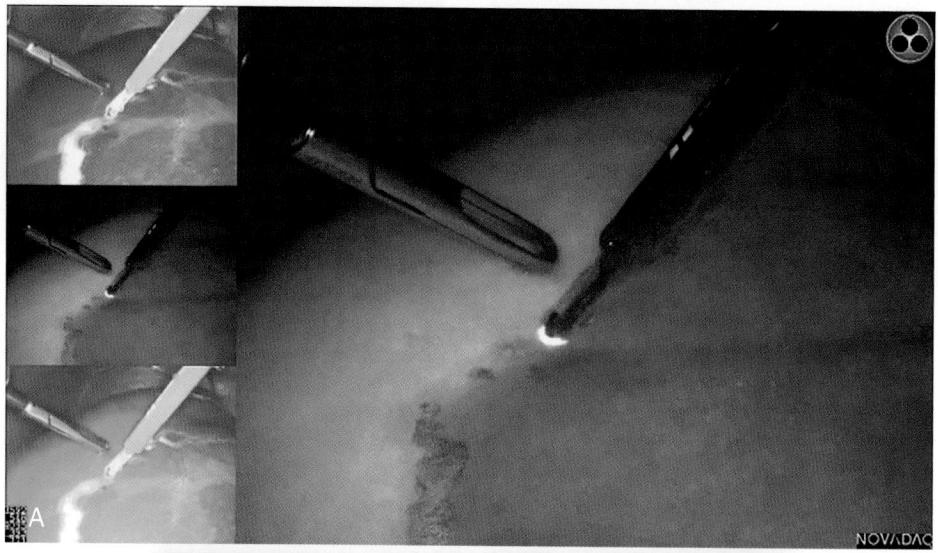

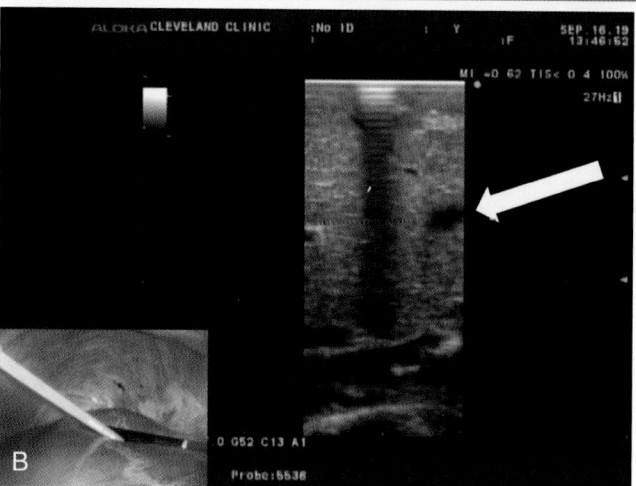

FIGURE 128.11 Identifying the correct resection plane. **A,** Indocyanine green 2.5 mg is given intravenously after the hepatic arteries and the portal vein are clamped. Good demarcation between the left and right lobe can be seen. **B,** Posterior shadowing *(white arrow)* of the marked area is shown on ultrasonography. The middle hepatic vein *(arrow)* on the left side of the shadowing is seen.

of the former. The terminal portion of the Arantius ligament is seen exiting the groove between the caudate and left lateral segments and is divided short of its termination on the LHV.

A gentle traction of the hepatoduodenal ligament to the right by the assistant exposes the lower part of Spiegel's lobe, which is lifted ventrally to expose the plane between the caudate lobe and the vena cava (see Fig. 128.12). Multiple short hepatic veins are usually present, which are carefully isolated and divided. This mobilization is continued as cranially as possible by gentle jaw opening movement with bipolar forceps, which can also efficiently control small bleedings. Use of monopolar electrocautery should be avoided in this area because it can aggravate injury and cause more bleeding. The caval ligament may be divided to provide additional exposure to allow further dissection cephalad, but excessive dissection, especially when the surgical exposure is inadequate, should not be done because bleeding from injuries to short hepatic veins may be difficult to control. Additionally, the deeper areas are often easier to approach anterior-medially at the

terminal stage of parenchymal transection, after the bile duct is divided.

Parenchymal Transection and Graft Removal

This is carried out as elaborated in the corresponding section in right donor hepatectomy (see Fig. 128.7). After the Glissonian pedicle is exposed, the caudate lobe is transected along the right side of Spiegel's lobe in the caudocephalad direction past the Glissonian pedicle. The Glissonian sheath, which includes the bile duct, is then encircled with a tape, and, using ICG cholangiogram to identify the biliary structure, the bile duct is clipped and divided at the exact desired location. The remaining Glisson is then divided using staplers (see Fig. 128.7). Now the previous caudally transected part of the caudate lobe becomes visible anteriorly and the remaining parenchymal division is done in a similar fashion as described for right hepatectomy until the base of the MHV and LHV on its medial side is reached (Fig. 128.13). Concurrently, any further tributaries from the left side of the caudate lobe are isolated and divided, thus freeing up the left hemigraft further. The MHV/

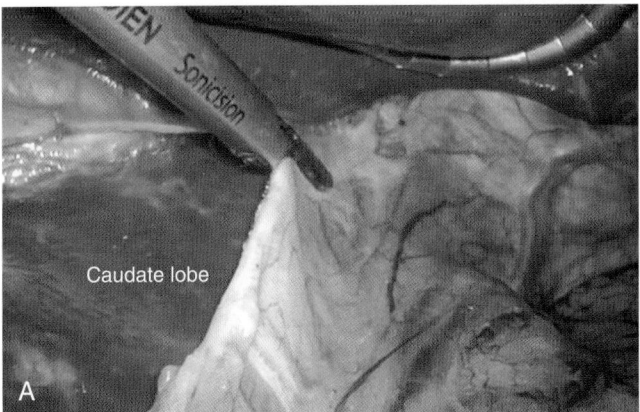

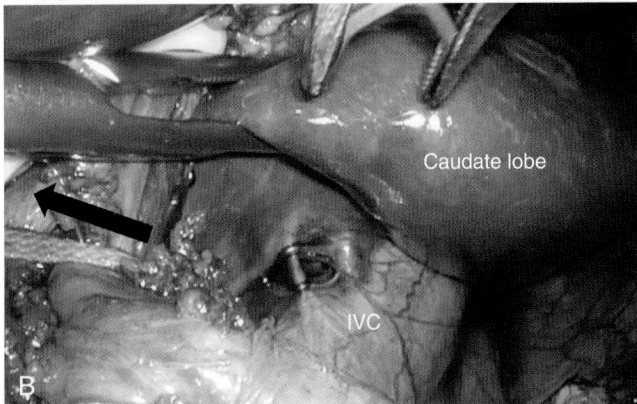

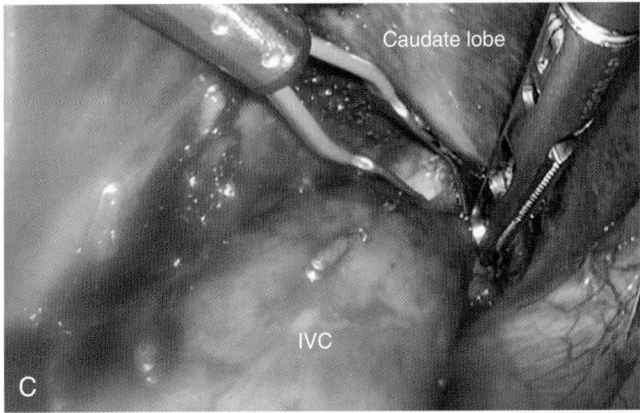

FIGURE 128.12 Caudate lobe mobilization. **A,** The lesser omentum is divided up to the root of the left hepatic vein to expose the caudate lobe. **B,** Gentle traction of the hepatoduodenal ligament to the right *(black arrow)* and anterior lift of the Spiegel's lobe exposes the plane between the caudate lobe and the vena cava. Short hepatic veins are often found, which are clipped and divided. **C,** Dissection is continued as cranially as possible by gentle jaw opening movement with the bipolar forceps. Small bleeding can easily be controlled with bipolar electrocautery.

LHV base is encircled with an umbilical tape to aid stapling. In case passing the tape around the veins is difficult, a Goldfinger may come handy.

A 9 to 11 cm Pfannenstiel incision is made, plastic bag is inserted, and the graft is placed inside it. After administration of IV heparin, inflow and outflow vessels are divided in succession and the graft is extracted via the Pfannenstiel incision.

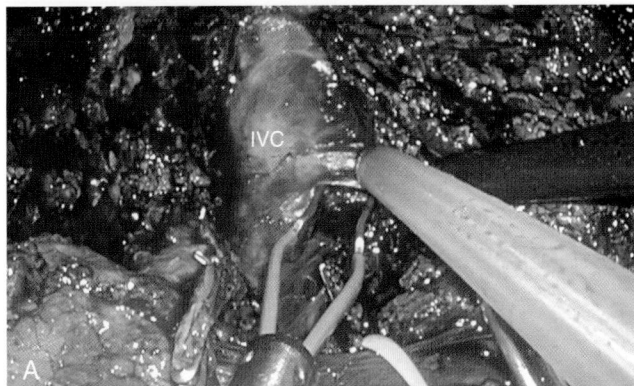

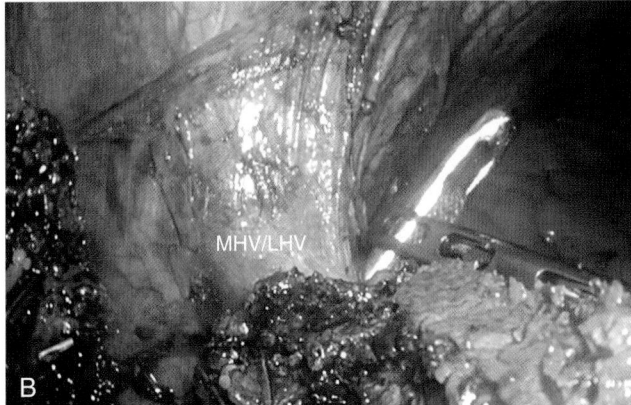

FIGURE 128.13 **A,** Tributaries from the caudate lobe are isolated and divided from the medical side up to the root of the hepatic veins to free the graft. **B,** A golden finger instrument is used to encircle a tape around the base of middle and left hepatic veins *(MHV/LHV)*.

LAPAROSCOPIC LEFT LATERAL SECTIONECTOMY (ALSO SEE CHAPTER 127D)

Left lateral section (LLS) grafts or left without the MHV are invariably used for pediatric recipients and smaller adults, in whom an acceptable GRWR can be realized despite the lower mean volume of these grafts. The preparatory steps are essentially the same as for left hepatectomy save a few key differences.

Transection Plane and Trocar Port Placement

Dependent on whether the plane of transection is along the Cantlie's line to include the segment 4 or through 0.5 to 1 cm right of the falciform ligament, an LLS graft (segments 2 and 3) or left graft without MHV is obtained, respectively. The resection plane should start superiorly from the groove between the MHV and LHV and end at the bifurcation of the main bile ducts inferiorly (Fig. 128.14).

Dependent on the location of the transection plane, the port site is shifted 2 to 5 cm left as necessary to maintain the optimal triangulation format as described previously. The right subcostal trocar port site is therefore placed somewhere between the anterior axillary and the midclavicular line and the main port between the midline and the left midclavicular line (see Fig. 128.2).

Parenchymal Resection and Hilar Dissection

The parenchyma is divided in the same fashion described previously. Large Glissonian branches feeding the segment 4a or

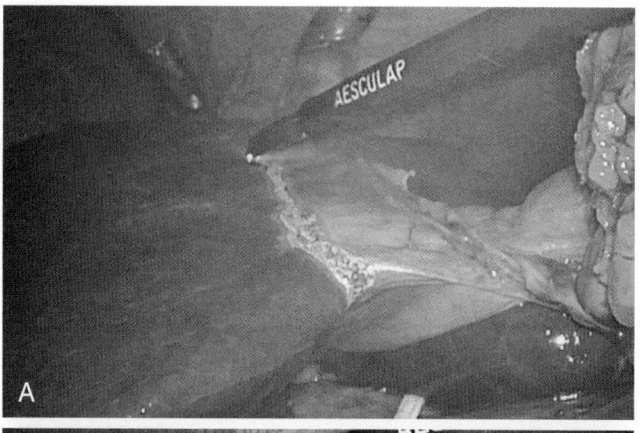

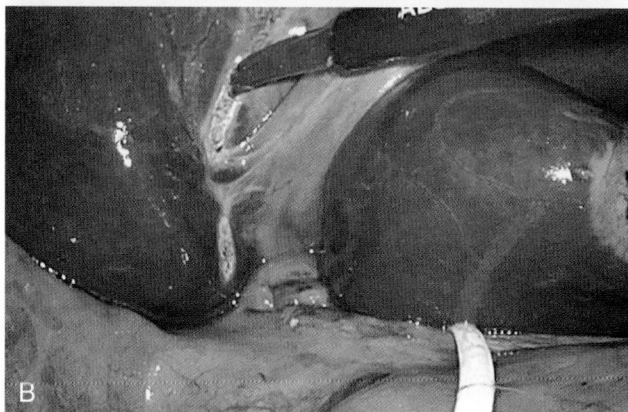

FIGURE 128.14   A, The plane of transection for left lateral sectionectomy is marked 0.5 to 1.0 cm to the right of falciform ligament superiorly and **(B)** the umbilical fissure inferiorly.

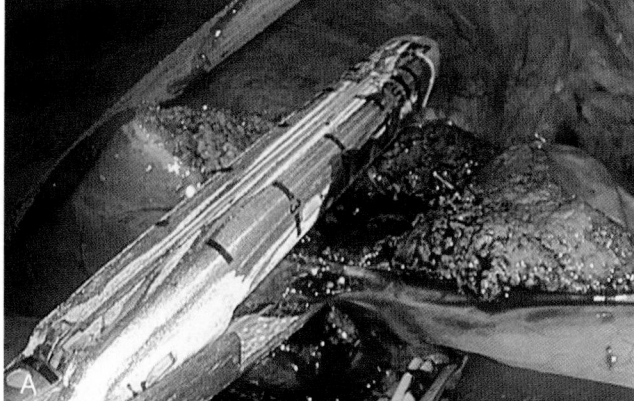

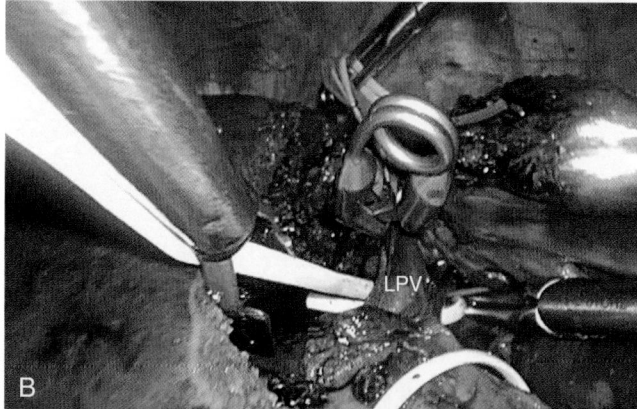

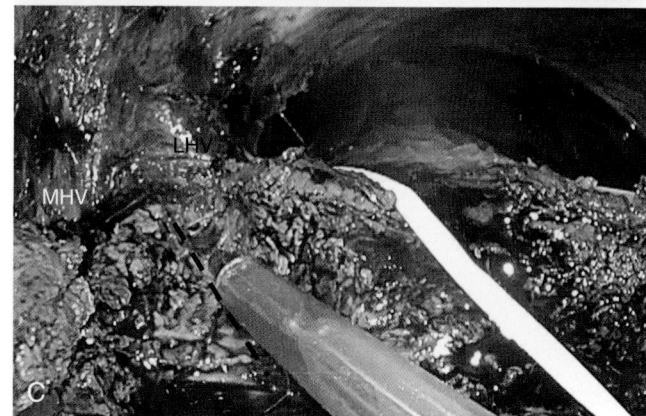

FIGURE 128.15   A, Large Glissonean branches feeding the segment 4a or 4b are usually present and often need to be stapled because of the size. **B,** After the left bile duct is divided, a tape is passed through toward the Arantius ligament to encircle the remaining Glissonean sheath. **C,** Parenchyma is divided until the LHV is isolated near its stalk intraparenchymally. Line of transection is shown in *broken line.*

4b are usually present and, depending on size, can either be clipped or stapled (Fig. 128.15). The transection plane should not head dorsally toward the IVC but should head toward the Arantius ligament, between the LLS and the caudate lobe. Once the parenchyma is transected enough to expose the hilar plate, the bile duct is divided using the ICG cholangiogram. A tunnel is made toward the Arantius ligament to encircle the remaining Glissonian sheath through which a stapler is applied to divide it. This opens up the plane between the anteriorly transected plane and the Arantius ligament, and the remaining parenchyma is transected cranially until the LHV is isolated near its stalk intraparenchymally and is encircled with an umbilical tape. Division of inflow and outflow vessels with subsequent graft extraction follows sequences as described earlier (see also Chapter 118 on open hepatectomy).

POSTOPERATIVE CONSIDERATIONS

The orogastric tube is routinely removed at the conclusion of surgery. Patients are commenced on clear fluids the following morning, and early ambulation is actively encouraged. As part of ERAS protocol (see Chapter 27), nonsteroidal antiinflammatory drugs (NSAIDs) and acetaminophen-based pain control are implemented with addition of patient-controlled analgesia (PCA) using opiates for breakthrough pain, but PCA is usually not necessary after the third postoperative day. Under most circumstances, patients have their urinary catheter removed the day after surgery and are able to resume a regular

diet by the third day, concurrent with cessation of PCA (see Chapter 26). Discharge from the hospital is usually achieved by postoperative day 5, at which point liver enzymes have stabilized. The surgical drain is removed before release from the hospital if there are no concerns with drainage.

TRANSITION FROM OPEN TO A LAPAROSCOPIC PROGRAM AND DISASTER PLANNING

The application of MIS in donor surgery has provided better quality of life and improved postsurgery recovery to donors, and is increasingly adopted, especially in established LDLT centers. It must be noted, however, that it is a surgery that requires double expertise, both in living donor hepatectomy and in advanced laparoscopic liver surgery, and it carries a very steep learning curve in a situation where utmost safety is needed. Therefore the surgical team must have ample experience in both the living donor hepatectomy (see Chapter 121) and advanced laparoscopic liver surgery (see Chapters 127D and 127E) before embarking on the program. Careful planning of the stepwise application should be well thought out beforehand for a safe and smooth transition from open to a laparoscopic program. It is preferable to have a transition period during which a hybrid approach is used with a gradual increase of the proportion done laparoscopically, instead of a sudden transition from open to a purely laparoscopic approach. This allows the surgical team to acquire the learning curve necessary during the transition period without jeopardizing the safety of the donor.

Last, disaster planning needs to be established both within the operating room and at the institutional level. A crisis management team should be readily available during surgery and the immediate postoperative period in order to prepare and protect the surgical team when a disaster occurs.

References are available at expertconsult.com.

Page number followed by *f* indicates figure, by *t* table, and by *b* box.

BLUMGART'S
Surgery *of the* Liver, Biliary Tract and Pancreas

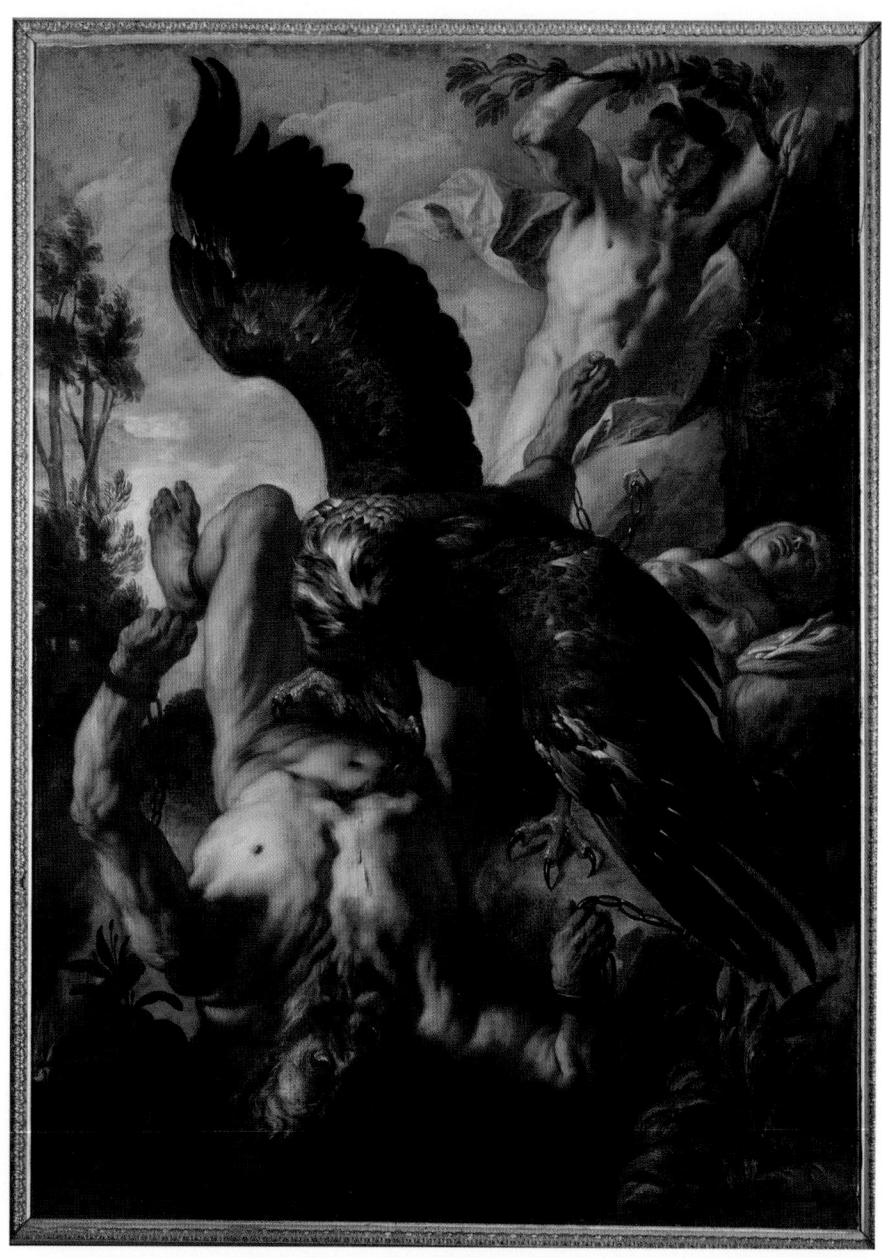

Prometheus, chained to the rocky Mount Caucasus, has his liver eaten by the eagle of Zeus.
Prometheus by Jacob Jordaens, 1640.
Walraff-Richartz Museum & Foundation Corboud, Cologne, Germany.
Photo: Rheinisches Bildarchiv Cologne, rba_c007696

BLUMGART'S
Surgery *of the* Liver, Biliary Tract and Pancreas

7th EDITION | VOLUME 1

EDITOR-IN-CHIEF

William R. Jarnagin, MD, FACS

ASSOCIATE EDITORS

Peter J. Allen, MD
William C. Chapman, MD, FACS
Michael I. D'Angelica, MD, FACS
Ronald P. DeMatteo, MD, FACS
Richard Kinh Gian Do, MD, PhD
Jean-Nicolas Vauthey, MD, FACS

EDITOR EMERITUS

Leslie H. Blumgart, BDS, MD, DSc(Hon),
    FACS, FRCS(Eng, Edin), FRCPS(Glas)

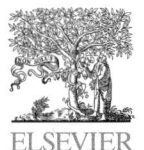

ELSEVIER

Elsevier
1600 John F. Kennedy Blvd.
Ste 1800
Philadelphia, PA 19103-2899

BLUMGART'S SURGERY OF THE LIVER, BILIARY TRACT, AND PANCREAS   ISBN: 9780323697842

Copyright © 2023 by Elsevier, Inc. All rights reserved.

Previous editions copyrighted 2017, 2012, 2007, 2000, 1994, and 1988 by Saunders, an imprint of Elsevier Inc.

Executive Content Strategist: Jessica McCool
Content Development Specialist: Casey Potter
Senior Content Development Manager: Laura Schmidt
Publishing services Manager: Deepthi Unni
Project Manager: Aparna Venkatachalam
Design Direction: Maggie Reid

Printed in India
Last digit is the print number: 9   8   7   6   5   4   3   2

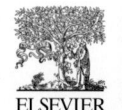
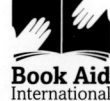
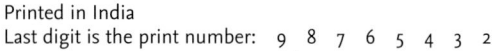

Working together
to grow libraries in
developing countries

www.elsevier.com • www.bookaid.org

This book is dedicated to Dr. Leslie H. Blumgart. Known as the "Professor," a term of respect and admiration, he is truly a giant in the field, one of the pioneering surgeons who helped establish and develop HPB surgery as a specialty in its own right. He served as a mentor and role model for a generation of surgeons, who strive to maintain the high standards that he established. For all that he has done for us and for the field of HPB surgery, we will be forever grateful.

EDITORS

EDITOR-IN-CHIEF

William R. Jarnagin, MD, FACS
Chief, Hepatopancreatobiliary Surgery
Benno C. Schmidt Professor of Surgical Oncology
Memorial Sloan Kettering Cancer Center;
Professor of Surgery
Weill Medical College of Cornell University
New York, New York

ASSOCIATE EDITORS

Peter J. Allen, MD
Professor of Surgery
Department of Surgery
Memorial Sloan Kettering Cancer Center
New York, New York

William C. Chapman, MD, FACS
Professor
Chief, Division of General Surgery
Chief, Abdominal Transplantation Section
Washington University School of Medicine
St. Louis, Missouri

Michael I. D'Angelica, MD, FACS
Attending Surgeon
Hepatopancreatobiliary Surgery
Enid A. Haupt Chair in Surgery
Memorial Sloan Kettering Cancer Center;
Associate Professor
Department of Surgery
Weill Medical College of Cornell University
New York, New York

Ronald P. DeMatteo, MD, FACS
Vice Chair, Department of Surgery
Chief, Division of General Surgical Oncology
Leslie H. Blumgart Chair in Surgery
Memorial Sloan Kettering Cancer Center
New York, New York

Richard Kinh Gian Do, MD, PhD
Associate Professor of Radiology
Weill Medical College of Cornell University;
Assistant Attending Physician
Department of Radiology
Memorial Sloan Kettering Cancer Center
New York, New York

Jean-Nicolas Vauthey, MD, FACS
Professor of Surgical Oncology
Chief, Hepato-Pancreato-Biliary Section
Bessie McGoldrick Professor in Clinical Cancer Research
Department of Surgical Oncology
University of Texas MD Anderson Cancer Center
Houston, Texas

EDITOR EMERITUS

Leslie H. Blumgart, BDS, MD, DSc(Hon), FACS, FRCS(Eng, Edin), FRCPS(Glas)
Member
Professor of Surgery and Attending Surgeon
Memorial Sloan Kettering Cancer Center;
Professor of Surgery
Weill Medical College of Cornell University
New York, New York

Ghassan K. Abou-Alfa, MD, MBA
Attending Physician
Medicine
Memorial Sloan Kettering Cancer Center
Professor
Medicine
Weill Medical College at Cornell University
New York, New York

Jad Abou-Khalil, MDCM MSc FRCSC
Assistant Professor of Surgery
Hepato-Biliary and Pancreatic Surgery
The Ottawa Hospital,
Clinician Investigator
Clinical Epidemiology
The Ottawa Hospital Research Institute,
Ottawa, Ontario, Canada

Alexandra W. Acher, MD
Department of General Surgery, Division of Surgical
    Oncology
University of Wisconsin,
Madison, Wisconsin

Rene Adam, MD, PhD
Professor of Surgery
Department of Hepato-Biliary Surgery
Paul Brousse Hospital,
Paris Saclay University,
Director of University Research Unit
"Chronotherapy, Cancers and Transplantation"
Paris-Saclay University,
Villejuif, French Guiana

Pietro Addeo, MD PhD
Attending Surgeon
Hepato-Pancreato-Biliary Surgery and Liver Transplantation
University of Strasbourg,
Strasbourg, France

Anil Kumar Agarwal, MS, MCh, FRCS, FACS
Director Professor & Head
GI Surgery & Liver Transplant
GB Pant Institute of Postgraduate Medical Education &
    Research & MAM College, Delhi University,
New Delhi, India

Davit L. Aghayan, MD, PhD
Postdoctoral Researcher
The Intervention Center
Oslo University Hospital,
Oslo, Norway
Visiting Professor
Department of Surgery N1
Yerevan State Medical University after M. Heratsi,
Yerevan, Armenia

Ola Ahmed, MD
Department of Abdominal Organ Transplantation
Washington University School of Medicine,
St Louis, Missouri

Matthew J. Aizpuru, MD
Resident Physician
Surgery
Mayo Clinic,
Rochester, Minnesota

Marc-Antoine Allard, MD, PhD
Centre Hépatobiliaire
Hôpital Paul Brousse,
Villejuif, France

Peter J. Allen, MD
Professor of Surgery
Chief of Surgical Oncology
Surgery
Duke University, School of Medicine
Durham, North Carolina

Thomas A. Aloia, MD, MHCM
Professor of Surgery
Surgical Oncology
UT MD Anderson Cancer Center,
Houston, Texas

Fernando A. Alvarez, MD
Chief
Division of HPB Surgery, Department of Surgery
Clínica Universitaria Reina Fabiola,
Córdoba, Argentina

Neda Amini, MD
Surgical resident
Surgery
Sinai hospital of Baltimore,
Baltimore, Maryland

Jesper B. Andersen, PhD
Associate Professor and group leader
University of Copenhagen,
Department of Health and Medical Sciences
Biotech Research and Innovation Centre,
Copenhagen, Denmark

Christopher D. Anderson, MD
James D. Hardy Chair
Department of Surgery
University of Mississippi Medical Center,
Jackson, Mississippi

Roi Anteby, MD MPH
Postdoctoral Research Fellow
Surgery
Massachusetts General Hospital,
Boston, Massachusetts
Resident
General Surgery
The Chaim Sheba Medical Center,
Tel Hashomer, Ramat Gan, Israel

Vittoria Arslan-Carlon, MD, FASA
Chief, Anesthesiology Service
Anesthesiology and CCM
Memorial Sloan Kettering Cancer Center,
New York, New York

Beatrice Aussilhou, MD
Department of HPB Surgery and Liver Transplantation
Hôpital Beaujon
Clichy, France

Joseph Awad, MD
Professor
Medicine-Gastroenterology and Hepatology
Vanderbilt University
Chief
Transplant Service
VA Tennessee Valley,
Nashville, Tennessee

Michele L. Babicky, MD
Hepatobiliary & Surgical Oncology
Center for Advanced Surgery
The Oregon Clinic,
Medical Director, Hepatobiliary & Pancreatic Cancer
Program Program
Providence Portland Medical Center,
Portland, Oregon

Philippe Bachellier, MD, PhD
Professor and Chairman
Hepato-Pancreato-Biliary Surgery and Liver transplant,
Pôle des Pathologies Digestives, Hépatiques et de la
Transplantation Hôpital de Hautepierre-Hôpitaux
Universitaires de Strasbourg
University of Strasbourg,
Strasbourg, France

Vinod P. Balachandran, MD
Assistant Attending
Department of Surgery
Assistant Member
Immuno-Oncology Service, Human Oncology and
Pathogenesis Program
Memorial Sloan Kettering Cancer Center
Member
Parker Institute for Cancer Immunotherapy
David M. Rubenstein Center for Pancreatic Cancer Research
Memorial Sloan Kettering Cancer Center,
New York, New York

Fiyinfolu Balogun, MD, PhD
Assistant Attending Physician
Gastrointestinal Oncology, Medicine
Memorial Sloan Kettering Cancer Center,
New York, New York

Andrew S. Barbas, MD
Surgery
Duke University,
Durham, North Carolina

Jeffrey Stewart Barkun, MD, MSc, FRSC (C)
Professor of Surgery, McGill University
Surgery
Hepatobiliary & Transplant Surgery
Surgery
McGill University Health Centre,
Montreal, Quebec, Canada

Claudio Bassi, FRCS, FACS, FEBS
Surgery
Pancreas Institute University of Verona,
Verona, Italy

Olca Basturk, MD
Associate Professor
Pathology
Memorial Sloan Kettering Cancer Center,
New York, New York

Maria del Pilar Bayona Molano, MD, DR-IR
Associate Professor
Interventional Radiology
UT Southwestern Medical Center,
Dallas, Texas

Rachel E. Beard, MD, FACS
Assistant Professor
Surgery
Rhode Island Hospital and Alpert Medical School of Brown
    University,
Providence, Rhode Island

Jacques Belghiti, MD
Emerite Professor
HPB Surgery & Liver Transplantation
Hospital Beaujon,
Clichy, France

Sean A. Bennett, MD, MSc, FRCSC
Assistant Professor
Surgery
Queen's University,
Kingston, Ontario, Canada

William Bernal, MD, FRCP, FFICM
Professor
Liver Intensive Therapy Unit
Institute of Liver Studies, Kings College Hospital,
London, England

Anton J. Bilchik, MD, PhD
Professor of Surgery, Chief of Medicine
Surgical Oncology
Saint John's Cancer Institute,
Santa Monica, California

Franz Edward Boas, MD, PhD
Associate professor
Interventional radiology
City of Hope Cancer Center,
Duarte, California

Morgan Bonds, MD
Assistant Professor of Surgery
Surgical Oncology
University of Oklahoma,
Norman, Oklahoma

Brooke C. Bredbeck, MD
House Officer
Surgery
University of Michigan,
Ann Arbor, Michigan

Lynn Brody, MD
Clinical Member
Radiology
Memorial Sloan Kettering Cancer Center,
New York, New York

Karen T. Brown, MD, FSIR
Professor
Department of Radiology
University of Utah Health Science Center,
Interventional Radiologist
Department of Radiology
University of Utah,
Salt Lake City, Utah

Jordi Bruix, MD, PhD
Senior Consultant
Bclc. Liver Unit
Hospital Clinic
Barcelona, Spain

Elizabeth M. Brunt, MD
Emeritus Professor (retired)
Pathology and Immunology
Washington University School of Medicine
St Louis, Missouri

Markus Büchler, Professor of Surgery, MD
Professor
Department of General,
Visceral and Transplantation Surgery
University of Heidelberg,
Heidelberg, Germany

Mark P. Callery, MD
William V. McDermott Professor of Surgery
Surgery
Harvard Medical School,
Chief, Division of General Surgery
Beth Israel Deaconess Medical Center,
Boston, Massachusetts

Juan C. Camacho, MD
Assistant Attending Radiologist
Interventional Radiology
Memorial Sloan Kettering Cancer Center,
New York, New York

Andre Campbell, MD
Professor of Surgery
UCSF, Department of Surgery
Zuckerberg San Francisco General Hospital and Trauma
    Center
San Francisco, California

Danielle H. Carpenter, MD
Associate Professor
Department of Pathology
Saint Louis University School of Medicine,
St Louis, Missouri

C. Ross Carter, MD, FRCS
West of Scotland Pancreatic Unit
Glasgow Royal Infirmary,
Glasgow, Scotland

Chung Yip Chan, MBBS, MMed(Surg), FRCS(Edin), MD
Department of Hepatopancreatobiliary and Transplant
    Surgery
Singapore General Hospital,
Singapore

See Ching Chan, MS, MD, PhD, FRCS
Honorary Clinical Professor
Surgery
University of Hong Kong,
Hong Kong, China

Rohit Chandwani, MD, PhD
Assistant Professor
Surgery/Cell & Developmental Biology
Weill Cornell Medicine,
New York, New York

William C. Chapman Sr., MD
Professor of Surgery
Surgery
Washington University in St Louis,
St Louis, Missouri

Harvey S. Chen, MD
General Surgeon
Department of Surgery
UCLA Medical Center,
Los Angeles, California

Daniel Cherqui, MD
Professor
HPB Surgery and Liver Transplantation
Paul Brousse Hospital - Paris Saclay University,
Villejuif, France

TT Cheung, MBBS, MS, MD, FRCS, FACS, FCSHK, FHKAM
Clinical Associate Professor
Chief of Division of Hepatobiliary and Pancreatic Surgery
The University of Hong Kong,
Hong Kong, China

Adrian Kah Heng Chiow, MBBS(Melb), FRCS(Ed), FAMS
Hepatopancreatobiliary Unit, Department of Surgery
Changi General Hospital,
Singapore

Clifford S. Cho, MD
C. Gardner Child Professor
Department of Surgery
University of Michigan Medical School,
Ann Arbor, Michigan

Yun Shin Chun, MD, FACS
Associate Professor
Surgical Oncology
The University of Texas MD Anderson Cancer Center,
Houston, Texas

Bryan M. Clary, MD, MBA
Professor and Chair
Department of Surgery
University of California at San Diego,
San Diego, California

Jordan M. Cloyd, MD
Surgical Oncologist
Surgery
The Ohio State University,
Columbus, Ohio

Maria V. Coats, PhD FRCS
Consultant HPB Surgeon
West of Scotland Pancreatic Unit
Glasgow Royal Infirmary,
Glasgow, United Kingdom

Joshua T. Cohen, MD
Resident
Department of General Surgery
Brown University,
Providence, Rhode Island

Kevin Christopher Conlon, MB, MCh, FRCSI, FRCSEd, FRCSGlas, FACS, MBA, MA, FTCD
Professor and Academic Head
Department of Surgery
Trinity College Dublin, Tallaght, Dublin 24
Consultant HPB Surgeon
Department of HPB Surgery
St Vincents University Hospital,
Consultant Surgeon
Tallaght University Hospital,
Dublin, Ireland

Louise C. Connell, MB Bch BAO, BSc, MRCPI
Medical Oncologist
Medicine, Gastrointestinal Oncology
Memorial Sloan Kettering Cancer Center,
New York, New York

Carlos Uriel Corvera, MD
Professor, Chief of Liver,
Biliary and Pancreatic Surgery
Surgery
UCSF, School of Medicine
Attending Surgeon
Surgery
VA Medical Center,
San Francisco, California

Anne M. Covey, MD
Attending Interventional Radiologist
Diagnostic Radiology
Memorial Sloan-Kettering Cancer Center,
Professor of Radiology
Diagnostic Radiology
Weill Medical College of Cornell University,
New York, New York

Christopher H. Crane, MD
Chief, Gastrointestinal Section
Radiation Oncology
Memorial Sloan Kettering Cancer Center,
New York, New York

John M. Creasy, MD
Fellow, Complex General Surgical Oncology
Department of Surgery
Duke University Medical Center,
Durham, North Carolina

Jeffrey S. Crippin, MD
Marilyn Bornefeld Chair in Gastrointestinal Research and
   Treatment
Internal Medicine
Washington University School of Medicine,
St Louis, Missouri

Nick Crispe
Professor
Pathology
Adjunct Professor
Immunology
University of Washington
Seattle, Washington

Michael I. D'Angelica, MD, FACS
Enid Haupt Chair in Surgery
Surgery
Memorial Sloan Kettering Cancer Center
Professor of Surgery
Surgery
Weil Cornell School of Medicine
New York, New York

Leonardo Gomes Da Fonseca, MD
Clinical Oncology
Instituto do Cancer do Estado de Sao Paulo,
University of Sao Paulo,
Sao Paulo, Brazil

Hany Dabbous
Professor
Tropical Medicine
Ain Shams University,
Cairo, Egypt

Christopher Danford
Gastroenterologist
Gastroenterology
Intermountain Medical Group,
Salt Lake City, Utah

Michael Darcy, MD
Professor, Interventional Radiology
Radiology
Washington University in St Louis,
St Louis, Missouri

Mark Davenport, ChM, FRCS (Eng), FRCS (Paeds)
Professor
Paediatric Surgery
Kings College Hospital,
London, United Kingdom

Yakira David, MBBS
Fellow
Gastroenterology
Icahn School of Medicine at Mount Sinai,
New York, New York

Ryan William Day, MD
Clinical Fellow
Division of Transplant Surgery
University of California, San Francisco,
San Francisco, California

Jeroen de Jonge, MD, PhD
Assistant Professor
Hepatobiliary and Transplant Surgery. Erasmus MC
Transplant Institute
Erasmus MC Rotterdam,
Rotterdam, Netherlands

Eduardo de Santibanes, MD, PhD
Professor
Surgery
University of Buenos Aires.,
Buenos Aires, Argentina

Martin de Santibañes, MD, PhD
Associate Professor of Surgery
Hepato-Biliary-Pancreatic unit and liver transplantation unit
Hospital Italiano,
Buenos Aires, Argentina

Roeland F. de Wilde, MD, PhD
Surgeon
HPB- & Transplant Surgery
Erasmus MC University Medical Center,
Rotterdam, Netherlands

Jean Robert Delpero,
Emeritus Professor
Department of Surgery
Institut Paoli Calmettes,
Marseille, France

Ronald P. DeMatteo, MD, FACS
The John Rhea Barton Professor and Chair
Department of Surgery
The University of Pennsylvania Health System,
Philadelphia, Pennsylvania

Danielle K. DePeralta, MD
Assistant Professor
Surgical Oncology
Northwell Health,
New York, New York

Niraj M. Desai, MD
Assistant Professor
Department of Surgery
Johns Hopkins University School of Medicine
Baltimore, Maryland

Shannan M. Dickinson, MBBS, FRANZCR
Assistant Attending
Department of Radiology
Memorial Sloan Kettering Cancer Center,
New York, New York

Euan J. Dickson, MBChB, MD, FRCS
Consultant Surgeon
West of Scotland Pancreatic Unit
Glasgow Royal Infirmary
Glasgow, United Kingdom

Christopher John DiMaio, MD
Director of Interventional Endoscopy,
Professor of Medicine
Division of Gastroenterology
Icahn School of Medicine at Mount Sinai
New York, New York

Richard Kinh Gian Do, MD, PhD
Associate Attending
Radiology
Memorial Sloan Kettering Cancer Center,
New York, New York
Associate Professor
Radiology
Weill Medical College of Cornell University,
New York, New York

Safi Dokmak, MD, PhD
HPB Surgery & Liver Transplantation
Hopital Beaujon,
Clichy, Hauts de seine, France

Majella Doyle, MD, MBA
Professor of Surgery
Department of Surgery
Washington University,
St Louis, Missouri

Jeffrey A. Drebin, MD, PhD
Chair
Department of Surgery
Memorial Sloan Kettering Cancer Center,
New York, New York
Professor
Department of Surgery
Weill Cornell Medical College,
New York, New York

Michael R. Driedger, MD
Surgical Oncology Specialist
Division of Hepatobiliary and Pancreatic Surgery
Mayo Clinic,
Rochester, Minnesota
General Surgery
Hepato-Pancreato-Biliary Surgery
Atrium Health,
Charlotte, North Carolina

Vikas Dudeja, MBBS, FACS
Associate Professor
Surgery
University of Alabama at Birmingham,
Birmingham, Alabama

Mark Dunphy, DO
Assistant Attending Physician
Radiology
Memorial Sloan Kettering Cancer Center,
New York, New York

Truman M. Earl, MD, MSCI
Professor of Surgery,
Chief Division of Transplant and Hepatobiliary Surgery
Department of Surgery,
Division of Transplant and Hepatobiliary Surgery
University of Mississippi Medical Center,
Jackson, Mississippi

Tomoki Ebata, MD, PhD
Professor and Chairman
Division of Surgical Oncology, Department of Surgery
Nagoya University Graduate School of Medicine,
Nagoya, Japan

Brett Logan Ecker, MD
Clinical Fellow
Department of Surgery
Memorial Sloan Kettering Cancer Center,
New York, New York

Bjorn Edwin, MD, PhD
Professor
The Intervention Centre
Oslo University Hospital,
Oslo, Norway
Professor
Department of HPB Surgery
Oslo University Hospital,
Oslo, Norway
Professor
Institute of Clinical Medicine
University of Oslo,
Oslo, Norway

Aslam Ejaz, MD, MPH
Assistant Professor
Department of Surgery
The Ohio State University,
Columbus, Ohio

Imane El Dika, MD
Assistant Attending
Department of Medicine
Memorial Sloan Kettering Cancer Center
New York, New York

Itaru Endo, MD, PhD
Professor
Department of Gastroenterological Surgery
Yokohama City University Graduate School of Medicine,
Yokohama, Japan

C. Kristian Enestvedt, MD, FACS
Associate Professor
Department of Surgery; Division of Abdominal Organ
Transplantation/Hepatobiliary Surgery; School of Medicine
Oregon Health & Science University,
Portland, Oregon

R. Eliot Fagley, MD
Section Head for Critical Care Medicine and Chief of Staff
Anesthesiology and Pain Medicine
Virginia Mason Medical Center
Seattle, Washington

Sheung Tat Fan, MD, PhD., D.Sc.
Emeritus Professor of Surgery
Department of Surgery
The University of Hong Kong
Hong Kong, China
Director
Liver Surgery and Transplant Centre
Hong Kong Sanatorium & Hospital,
Hong Kong, China

Olivier Farges, MD, PhD
Department of hepato-biliary and pancreatic surgery
Department of Surgery
Hôpital Beaujon, AP-HP, University Paris 7,
Clichy, France

Michael Steven Farrell, MD, MS
Acute Care Surgeon
Trauma
Lehigh Valley Health Network,
Allentown, Pennsylvania

Benjamin David Ferguson, MD, PhD
Assistant Professor
Department of Surgery
University of New Mexico
Albuquerque, New Mexico

Joana Ferrer-Fàbrega, MD, PhD
Associate Professor. Consultant
HepatoBilioPancreatic Surgery and Liver & Pancreatic
Transplantation Unit. ICMDiM.
Hospital Clínic. University of Barcelona,
Barcelona, Spain

Cristina R. Ferrone, MD
Professor of Surgery
Surgery
Massachusetts General Hospital,
Boston, Massachusetts

Ryan Fields, MD, FACS
Chief, Surgical Oncology; Professor of Surgery
Surgery
Barnes-Jewish Hospital & The Alvin J. Siteman
Comprehensive Cancer Center at Washington University
School of Medicine,
Kim & Tim Eberlein Distinguished Professor
Surgical Oncology
Washington University School of Medicine,
Co-Leader
Solid Tumor Therapeutics Program
Alvin J. Siteman Comprehensive Cancer Center
St Louis, Missouri

Mary Fischer, MD
Anesthesiology and Critical Care
Memorial Sloan Kettering Cancer Center,
New York, New York
Associate Professor
Anestesiology
New York Columbia Weill Medical College,
New York, New York

Yuman Fong, MD
Sangiacomo Chair and Chairman
Department of Surgery
City of Hope National Medical Center,
Duarte, California

Philippa Francis-West, PhD
Professor
Craniofacial
King's College London,
London, United Kingdom

Åsmund Avdem Fretland, MD, PhD
Attending Surgeon
The Intervention Centre
Oslo University Hospital
Attending Surgeon
Department of Hepato-Pancreato-Biliary Surgery
Oslo University Hospital
Oslo, Norway

Jonathan A. Fridell, MD
Chief, Abdominal Transplant Surgery
Surgery
Indiana University School of Medicine,
Indianapolis, Indiana

Scott L. Friedman, MD
Fishberg Professor of Medicine
Division of Liver Diseases
Icahn School of Medicine at Mount Sinai
Dean for Therapeutic Discovery
Icahn School of Medicine at Mount Sinai
New York, New York

Eva Galka, MD, FACS
Associate Professor of Surgery
Department of Surgery, Division of Hepatobiliary, Pancreatic,
& Gastrointestinal Surgery
University of Rochester,
Rochester, New York

David A. Geller, MD, FACS
Richard L. Simmons Professor of Surgery, Chief,
Division of Hepatobiliary and Pancreatic Surgery
Surgery
University of Pittsburgh,
Pittsburgh, Pennsylvania

Scott R. Gerst, MD
Attending Radiologist
Radiology
Memorial Sloan Kettering Cancer Center,
Director
Diagnostic Radiology, David H Koch Ctr for Cancer Care
Diagnostic Radiology
Memorial Sloan Kettering Cancer Center
New York, New York

Justin Theodore Gerstle, MD
Chief, Pediatric Surgery Service
Surgery
Memorial Sloan Kettering Cancer Center
New York, New York
Associate Professor
Surgery
Weill Cornell Medical College, Cornell University
New York, New York

Sepideh Gholami, MD
Assistant Professor
Surgery
University of California, Davis
Sacramento, California

Richard Gilroy, MBBS, FRACP
Medical Director of Hepatology and Liver Transplantation
Internal Medicine
Intermountain Medical Center
Murray, Utah

Brian K.P. Goh, MBBS, MMed, MSc, FRCSEd
Senior Consultant
Hepatopancreatobiliary and Transplant Surgery
Singapore General Hospital
Singapore
Clinical Professor
Duke-National University of Singapore Medical School
Singapore

Gregory J. Gores, MD
Executive Dean for Research, Professor of Medicine
Division of Gastroenterology and Hepatology
Mayo Clinic,
Rochester, Minnesota

John A. Goss, MD
Surgery
Baylor College of Medicine,
Houston, Texas

Brittany Dalia Greene, MD
Resident
Division of General Surgery, Department of Surgery
University of Toronto
Toronto, Ontario, Canada

Bas Groot Koerkamp, MD, MSc, PhD
Associate Professor of Surgery
Surgery,
Division of Hepatopancreatobiliary Surgery and Abdominal
Transplantation
Erasmus MC,
Rotterdam, Netherlands

Thilo Hackert, MD, MBA
Professor
Department of Surgery
University of Heidelberg
Heidelberg, Germany

Kate Anne Harrington, MB BCh BAO, FFR RCSI
Radiology
Memorial Sloan Kettering Cancer Center
New York, New York

Ewen M. Harrison, MB ChB, PhD, FRCS
Professor of Surgery and Data Science
Centre for Medical Informatics, Usher Institute
University of Edinburgh
Edinburgh, United Kingdom
Consultant HPB Surgeon
Clinical Surgery
Royal Infirmary of Edinburgh
Edinburgh, United Kingdom

Kiyoshi Hasegawa, MD, PhD
Professor
Hepato-Biliary-Pancreatic Surgery Division
Department of Surgery
Graduate School of Medicine, University of Tokyo
Tokyo, Japan

Haley Hauser, BA
Research Project Associate
Gastrointestinal Oncology Service, Department of Medicine
Memorial Sloan Kettering Cancer Center
New York, New York

Julie K. Heimbach, MD
Professor of Surgery
transplantation surgery
Mayo Clinic
Rochester, Minnesota

Alan W. Hemming, MD, MSc
Professor of Surgery
Surgery
University of Iowa
Iowa City, Iowa

Jonathan Hernandez, MD
Principal Investigator
Surgical Oncology
National Institute of Health
Bethesda, Maryland

Yuki Homma, MD, PhD
Department of Gastgroenterological Surgery
Yokohama City University
Yokohama, Japan

Christine A. Iacobuzio-Donahue, MD, PhD
Attending Pathologist
Pathology
Memorial Sloan Kettering Cancer Center
Affiliate Member
Human Oncology and Pathogenesis Program
Memorial Sloan Kettering Cancer Center
Director
David M. Rubenstein Center for Pancreatic Cancer Research
Memorial Sloan Kettering Cancer Center
New York, New York

Rami Imam, MD
Anatomic Pathologist
NYU Langone Hospitals
New York, New York

Oscar Cesar IMVENTARZA Sr., MD
Chief Liver Transplantation
Surgery & Transplantation
Hospital Garrahan,
Buenos Aires, Argentina
Chief Liver Transplantation
Surgery & Transplantation
Hospital Argerich
Buenos Aires, Argentina

Matthew Kalahasty Iyer, MD, PhD
Fellow
Department of Surgery
Duke University Hospital
Durham, North Carolina

William R. Jarnagin, MD, FACS
Chief, Hepatopancreatobiliary Service
Leslie H. Blumgart Chair in Surgical Oncology
Memorial Sloan-Kettering Cancer Center
New York, New York
Professor of Surgery
Weill Medical College of Cornell University
New York, New York

Shiva Jayaraman, MD, MESc, FRCSC, FACS
Associate Professor of Surgery
Surgery
University of Toronto
HPB and General Surgeon
Surgery
St. Joseph's Health Centre, Unity Health Toronto
Scientist
Li Ka Shing Knowledge Institute
Unity Health Toronto
Toronto, Ontario, Canada

Maria Jepperson
Radiologist
Radiology
Intermountain McKay-Dee Hospital
Murray, Utah

Michelle R. Ju, MD
Resident
Surgery
University of Texas Southwestern Medical Center
Dallas, Texas

Sean J. Judge, MD
Resident
Department of Surgery
University of California
Sacramento, California

Christoph Kahlert, MD
Universitätsklinikum Carl Gustav Carus Dresden
Klinik und Poliklinik für Viszeral-, Thorax- und Gefäßchirurgie
Universitätsklinkum Dresden
Dresden, Germany

Patryk Kambakamba, MD
Hepatobiliary Group
St. Vincent's University Hospital
Dublin, Ireland
MD
Department of Surgery
Cantonal Hospital of Winterthur
Winterthur, Switzerland

Ivan Kangrga, MD, PhD
Professor and Vice Chair for Health System Liaison
Department of Anesthesiology
Washington University in St. Louis, School of Medicine
St Louis, Missouri

S. Cheenu Kappadath, PhD
Professor
Department of Imaging Physics
UT MD Anderson Cancer Center
Houston, Texas

Paul J. Karanicolas, MD, PhD, FRCSC, FACS
Associate Professor
Surgery
University of Toronto
Toronto, Ontario, Canada

Seth S. Katz, MD, PhD
Assistant Clinical Member
Radiology
Memorial Sloan Kettering Cancer Center
New York, New York

Yoshikuni Kawaguchi, MD, MPH, PhD
Associate Professor/Lecturer
Hepato-Biliary-Pancreatic Surgery Division
Department of Surgery
The University of Tokyo
Tokyo, Japan

Kaitlyn J. Kelly, MD
Assistant Professor of Surgery
Division of Surgical Oncology
University of California San Diego
San Diego, California

Nancy E. Kemeny, MD
Professor of Medicine
Weill Medical College of Cornell University;
Attending Physician
Solid Tumor—GI Division
Memorial Sloan-Kettering Cancer Center
New York, New York

Adeel Khan, MD, MPH
Associate Professor of Surgery
Division of Abdominal Transplant, Department of Surgery
Washington University in St Louis
St Louis, Missouri

Tahsin M. Khan, MD
Surgical Oncology Research Fellow
Surgical Oncology Program
National Cancer Institute, National Institutes of Health,
Bethesda, Maryland

Heung Bae Kim, MD
Professor of Surgery
Department of Surgery
Harvard Medical School
Boston, Massachusetts
Director, Pediatric Transplant Center; Weitzman Family
Chair in Surgical Innovation
Boston Children's Hospital
Boston, Massachusetts

Woon Cho Kim, MD, MPH
Clinical Fellow
Surgery
University of California San Francisco
San Francisco, California

T. Peter Kingham, MD
Assistant Professor
Surgery
Memorial Sloan Kettering Cancer Center
New York, New York

Joseph Kingsbery, MD
Gastroenterologist
Medicine
Bay Ridge Gastroenterology
Brooklyn, New York
Clinical Instructor
Medicine
NYU Grossman School of Medicine
New York, New York
Clinical Instructor
Medicine
NYP Weill Cornell
Brooklyn, New York

Allan D. Kirk, MD, PhD
Professor and Chairman
Department of Surgery
Duke University
Durham, North Carolina

Russell C. Kirks Jr., MD
Hepatobiliary and Pancreatic Surgeon
St Joseph's/Candler
Savannah, Georgia

David Klimstra, MD
Chairman
Department of Pathology
Memorial Sloan-Kettering Cancer Center
New York, New York
Professor
Department of Pathology and Laboratory Medicine
Weill Medical College of Cornell University
New York, New York

Stuart Knechtle, MD, FACS
William R. Kenan, Jr. Professor of Surgery
Surgery
Duke University School of Medicine
Durham, North Carolina
Executive Director
Duke Transplant Center
Duke University School of Medicine
Durham, North Carolina

Jonathan B. Koea, MHB(Hons), MD
Professor
Department of Surgery
North Shore Hospital
Auckland, New Zealand
Professor
Department of Surgery
University of Auckland
Auckland, New Zealand

Norihiro Kokudo, MD, PhD
Professor
Surgery
National Center for Global Health and Medicine, 1-21-1
Toyama, Shinjuku-ku
Tokyo, Japan

Kevin M. Korenblat, MD
Professor of Medicine
Department of Internal Medicine
Washington University School of Medicine,
St Louis, Missouri
Medical Director, Liver Transplant
Barnes-Jewish Hospital
St Louis, Missouri

Lucy Zumwinkle Kornblith, MD
Assistant Professor of Surgery
Department of Surgery, Division of Trauma and Surgical
Critical Care
University of California San Francisco
San Francisco, California

Geoffrey Wayne Krampitz, MD, PhD
Assistant Professor
Surgery
Thomas Jefferson University
Philadelphia, Pennsylvania

Simone Krebs, MD
Assistant Attending
Department of Radiology
Molecular Imaging and Therapy Service
Memorial Sloan Kettering Cancer Center
New York, New York
Assistant Professor
Department of Radiology
Weill Cornell Medicine
New York, New York

Takafumi Kumamoto
Department of Gastroenterological Surgery
Graduate School of Medicine Yokohama City University
Yokohama, Japan

Choon Hyuck David Kwon, MD, PhD
Director of Laparoscopic Liver Surgery
General Surgery
Cleveland Clinic
Cleveland, Ohio
Professor of Surgery
General Surgery
Lerner College of Medicine of Case Western University,
Cleveland, Ohio
Section Head of HPB Surgery
General Surgery
Cleveland Clinic
Cleveland, Ohio

Kelly J. Lafaro, MD, MPH
Assistant Professor
Department of Surgery
Johns Hopkins University
Baltimore, Maryland

Hauke Lang, MA, MD, FACS
Professor
General, Visceral and Transplantation Surgery,
Unimedizin Mainz
Mainz, Germany

Michael J. LaQuaglia, MD
Clinical Fellow
Pediatric Surgery
Memorial Sloan Kettering Cancer Center
New York, New York

Michael P. LaQuaglia, MD
Joseph H. Burchenal Professor
Department of Surgery and Pediatrics
Memorial Sloan Kettering Cancer Center
New York, New York
Professor of Surgery
Department of Surgery
Weill Cornell Medical School
New York, New York

Nicholas F. LaRusso, MD
Charles H. Weinman Professor of Medicine
Molecular Biology and Biochemistry Internal Medicine
Mayo Clinic
Rochester, Minnesota

Rachel M. Lee, MD, MSPH
Resident Physician
Department of Surgery
Emory University
Atlanta, Georgia

**Ser Yee Lee, MBBS, MMed(Surgery), MSc, FAMS,
    FRCSEd, FACS**
Senior Consultant
Department of Hepatopancreatobiliary and Transplant
    Surgery
Singapore General Hospital
Singapore
Associate Professor
Duke - National University of Singapore (NUS) Graduate
Medical School
Singapore
Senior Consultant
Surgical Associates
Mount Elizabeth Medical Centre
Singapore

Riccardo Lencioni, MD
Professor
Department of Radiology
University of Pisa School of Medicine
Pisa, Italy
Director
Cancer Imaging Program
Pisa University Hospital
Pisa, Italy

Javier C. Lendoire, MD, PhD
Vice-Chairman
Liver & Transplant Unit
Hospital Dr Cosme Argerich
Buenos Aires, Argentina
Chairman
Liver Transplant Division
Instituto de Trasplantes y Alta Complejidad (ITAC)
Buenos Aires, Argentina

Galina Levin, MD
Associate Attending
Radiology
Memorial Sloan Kettering Cancer Center
New York, New York

Kewei Li, MD, PhD
Department of Pediatric Surgery
West China Hospital of Sichuan University
Chengdu, China

Michael E. Lidsky, MD
Assistant Professor
Surgery
Duke University
Durham, North Carolina

Jessica Lindemann, MD, PhD
General Surgery Resident
Department of Surgery
Washington University School of Medicine
St Louis, Missouri

David Linehan, MD
Professor, Chair
Surgery
University of Rochester
Rochester, New York

Roberto Carlos Lopez-Solis, MD, FACS
Associate Professor
General Surgery
West Virginia University School of Medicine
Morgantown, West Virginia

Patrick Daniel Lorimer, MD
General Surgeon
Surgical Oncology
Arizona Advanced Surgery, LLC
Scottsdale, Arizona

Ka Wing Ma
Orthopaedic surgeon
The University of Hong Kong
Pokfulam, Hong Kong

Shishir K. Maithel, MD, FACS
Professor of Surgery
Division of Surgical Oncology, Department of Surgery
Emory University, Winship Cancer Institute
Atlanta, Georgia

Giuseppe Malleo, MD, PhD
Associate Professor of surgery
Department of Surgery, Dentistry, Pediatrics and Gynecology
Unit of Pancreatic Surgery,
University of Verona Hospital Trust
Verona, Italy

Giovanni Marchegiani, MD, PhD
Dr Giovanni Marchegiani
Department of Surgery
Verona University Policlinico Borga Roma
Verona, Italy

James F. Markmann, MD, PhD
Chief, Division of Transplant Surgery
Surgery
Massachusetts General Hospital
Boston, Massachusetts
Claude E. Welch Professor of Surgery
Harvard Medical School
Boston, Massachusetts

J. Wallis Marsh, MD, MBA
Professor and Chairman
Surgery
West Virginia University School of Medicine
Morgantown, West Virginia

Robert CG Martin II, MD, PhD
Professor of Surgery
Sam and Loita Weakley Endowed Chair of Surgical Oncology
Surgery, Division of Surgical Oncology
University of Louisville
Louisville, Kentucky

Marco Massani, MD
Chief
Department of Surgery, Division of First General Surgery,
Hepato-Pancreato-Biliary Regional Referral Centre
Azienda ULSS 2 Marca Trevigiana, Ospedale Ca' Foncello,
Treviso, Italy

Ryusei Matsuyama, MD, PhD
Associate Professor
Gastroenterological Surgery
Yokohama City University School of Medicine
Yokohama, Japan

Aaron W.P. Maxwell, MD
Director of Interventional Oncology
Assistant Professor of Diagnostic Imaging
Department of Diagnostic Imaging
The Warren Alpert Medical School of Brown University,
Providence, Rhode Island

Oscar M. Mazza, MD
Professor of Surgery
Chief of Hepato-Biliary- Pancreatic Unit
Hospital Italiano
Buenos Aires, Argentina

Ian D. McGilvray, MD, PhD
Professor of Surgery
Surgery
University of Toronto
Toronto, Ontario, Canada
Head
Hepatopancreatic Biliary Surgical Oncology
University Health Network
Toronto, Ontario, Canada
Director
Toronto Video Atlas of Surgery
University Health Network
Toronto, Ontario, Canada

Caitlin A. McIntyre, MD
Fellow in Surgical Oncology
Department of Surgery
Memorial Sloan-Kettering Cancer Center
New York, New York

Sophia K. McKinley, MD, EdM
Resident physician
Surgery
Massachusetts General Hospital
Boston, Massachusetts

Jose Melendez
Vice President and Chief Medical Officer
HCA Healthcare
St. Mark's Hospital
Salt Lake City, Utah

Emmanuel Melloul, MD
Lausanne University Hospital
Visceral Surgery
Lausanne University Hospital
Lausanne, Switzerland

Robin B. Mendelsohn, MD
Associate Attending
Medicine, Gastroenterology, Hepatology and Nutrition
    Service
Memorial Sloan Kettering Cancer Center
New York, New York

Takashi Mizuno, MD., PhD.
Associate Professor
Division of Surgical Oncology, Department of Surgery
Nagoya University Graduate School of Medicine
Nagoya, Japan

Hunter Burroughs Moore, MD, PhD
Assistant Professor
Surgery-Transplant
University of Colorado
Denver, Colorado

Cristina Mosconi, MD
Department of Radiology
IRCCS Azienda Ospedaliero-Universitaria di Bologna,
Bologna, Italy

Santosh Nagaraju
Transplant Surgeon
Charleston Area Medical Center Health System
Charleston, West Virginia

Masato Nagino, MD, PhD
Professor and Chairman
Division of Surgical Oncology, Department of Surgery
Nagoya University Graduate School of Medicine
Nagoya, Japan

David M. Nagorney, MD, FACS
Professor of Surgery
Department of Surgery
Mayo Clinic
Rochester, Minnesota

Satish Nagula, MD
Associate Professor
Division of Gastroenterology, Department of Medicine
Icahn School of Medicine at Mount Sinai
New York, New York

Amit Nair, MD, FRCS
Assistant Professor
Division of Transplantation/Hepatobiliary Surgery
University of Rochester Medical Center
Rochester, New York

Navine Nasser-Ghodsi, MD
Fellow
Gastroenterology & Hepatology
Mayo CLinic
Rochester, Minnesota

Nadia Naz, MD, FAAP
Clinical Assistant Professor
Division of Gastroenterology, Hepatology, Pancreatology, and
    Nutrition
University of Iowa Health Care
Iowa city, Iowa

**John P. Neoptolemos, BA, MB, BChir, MA (Cambridge),
    MD, FRCS, FMedSci.**
Professor of Surgery
Department of General, Visceral and Transplantation Surgery
University of Heidelberg,
Heidelberg, Baden-Württemberg

James Neuberger, DM, FRCP
Hon Consultant Physician
Liver Unit
Queen Elizabeth Hospital
Birmingham, United Kingdom

Nicole M. Nevarez, MD
Surgical Resident
Department of Surgery
University of Texas Southwestern
Dallas, Texas

Timothy E. Newhook, MD
Assistant Professor
Surgical Oncology
The University of Texas MD Anderson Cancer Center,
Houston, Texas

Takehiro Noda, MD, PhD
Associate Professor
Department of Gastroenterological Surgery
Osaka University
Suita, Japan

Scott L. Nyberg, MD, PhD
Professor
Surgery
Consultant in Transplantation Surgery
Department of Transplantation Surgery
Mayo Clinic,
Rochester, Minnesota

Elisabeth O'Dwyer, MB BCh BAO
Molecular Imaging and Therapeutics Service
Memorial Sloan Kettering Cancer Center
New York, New York

Colm J. O'Rourke, BA(Hons.), PhD
Assistant Professor
BRIC, Department of Health & Medical Sciences
University of Copenhagen
Copenhagen, Denmark

Bruno C. Odisio, MD
Associate Professor
Interventional Radiology
The University of Texas MD Anderson Cancer Center,
Houston, Texas

RYOSUKE okamura, MD, PhD
Assistant Professor
Department of Surgery
Kyoto University Hospital
Kyoto, Japan

Karl Jürgen Oldhafer, Prof. Dr.
Department of Surgery
Asklepios Hospital Barmbek
Hamburg, Germany

Kim M. Olthoff, MD
Donald Guthrie Professor of Surgery
Division of Transplant Surgery, Department of Surgery
University of Pennsylvania
Associate Director
Penn Transplant Institute
Philadelphia, Pennsylvania

Franklin Olumba, MD
Research Fellow
Surgery
Washington University in St Louis School of Medicine
St Louis, Missouri

Susan Orloff, MD, FACS, FAASLD
Professor of Surgery and Chief, Division of Abdominal
Organ Transplantation/Hepatobiliary Surgery
Department of Surgery
Adjunct Professor
Department of Microbiology & Immunology
Oregon Health & Science University
Portland, Oregon

Christine E. Orr, MD, FRCPC
Assistant Professor
Department of Pathology and Molecular Medicine
Queen's University
Kingston, Ontario, Canada

Eileen M. O'Reilly, MD
Section Head, HPB/Neuroendocrine; Co-Director
Medical David M Rubenstein Center for Pancreas
Cancer Research
Medicine
Memorial Sloan Kettering Cancer Center
Professor of Medicine
Medicine
Weill Medical College of Cornell University
New York, New York

Chandrasekhar Padmanabhan, MD
Assistant Professor
Surgery
Vanderbilt Univeristy Medical Center
Nashville, Tennessee

Alessandro Paniccia, MD
Assistant Professor of Surgery
Department of Surgery
University of Pittsburgh
Pittsburgh, Pennsylvania

Theodore N. Pappas, MD
Professor
Surgery
Duke University
Durham, North Carolina

Valérie Paradis, MD, PhD
Professor
Pathology
Beaujon hospital,
Clichy, France

Rowan W. Parks, MD, FRCSI, FRCSEd
Professor
Clinical Surgery
University of Edinburgh
Edinburgh, United Kingdom

Timothy M. Pawlik, MD, MPH, MTS, PhD
Professor and Chair
Department of Surgery
The Ohio State University
Columbus, Ohio
The Urban Meyer III and Shelley Meyer Chair for Cancer
    Research
Wexner Medical Center at The Ohio State University
Columbus, Ohio

Cassandra D. Pierce-Raglione, MD
Director Emeritus
Surgical Oncology
Providence Portland Medical Center
Portland, Oregon

Venu G. Pillarisetty, MD
Professor
Surgery
University of Washington
Seattle, Washington

James Francis Pingpank Jr., MD
Associate Professor of Surgery
Department of Surgery
University of Pittsburgh
Surgical oncologist
UPMC Hillman Cancer Center
Pittsburgh, Pennsylvania

Henry A. Pitt, MD
Distinguished Professor of Surgery
Surgery
Rutgers RWJ Medical School
Chief of Oncologic Quality
Rutgers Cancer Institute of New Jersey
New Brunswick, New Jersey

Patricio M. Polanco, MD
Associate Professor
Surgery
University of Texas Southwestern Medical Center
Dallas, Texas

James J. Pomposelli, MD, PhD
Surgical Director of Liver Transplantation
Professor of Surgery
Department of Surgery
University of Colorado, Anschutz Medical Campus
Aurora, Colorado

John A. Powelson, MD
Associate Professor
Department of Surgery
Indiana University Medical School
Indianapolis, Indiana

Naveen Premnath, MD
Hematology and Oncology
University of Texas southwestern
Dallas, Texas

Motaz Qadan, MD, PhD
Associate Professor of Surgery; Gapontsev Family
Endowed Chair in Surgical Oncology
Surgery
Massachusetts General Hospital
Boston, Massachusetts

Nitya Raj, MD
Assistant Attending Physician
Department of Medicine,
Division of Gastrointestinal Medical Oncology
Memorial Sloan Kettering Cancer Center
New York, New York

Srinevas Reddy, MD
Faculty
Surgical Oncology
Ascension Columbia St. Mary's Hospital
Milwaukee, Wisconsin

Diane Reidy-Lagunes, MD, MS
Associate Attending
Medicine
MSKCC
Associate Professor of Clinical Medicine
Weill Cornell Medical College
New York, New York

Marsha Reyngold, MD, PhD
Assistant Attending
Department of Radiation Oncology
Memorial Sloan-Kettering Cancer Center
New York, New York

Teresa C. Rice, MD
Assistant Professor
Department of Surgery, Division of Transplant Surgery
Medical University of South Carolina
Charleston, South Carolina

Robert W. Rickert, Bachelor of Arts
Medical Student
Department of Surgical Oncology
University of Louisville
Louisville, Kentucky

John Paul Roberts, MD
Professor
Surgery
University of California San Francisco
San Francisco, California

Piera Marie Cote Robson, PhD, NP
Clinical Nurse Specialist
Departments of Nursing and Radiology
Memorial Sloan Kettering Cancer Center
New York, New York

Flavio G. Rocha, MD
Associate Professor of Surgery
Division of Surgical Oncology
Hedinger Chair and Division Head
Surgery, Division of Surgical Oncology
OHSU School of Medicine
Portland, Oregon

Garrett R. Roll, MD, FACS
Associate Professor
Department of Surgery, Division of Transplant
University of California San Francisco
San Francisco, California

Vineet Syan Rolston, MD
Assistant Professor
Gastroenterology
Memorial Sloan Kettering Cancer Center
New York, New York

Maxime Ronot, MD PhD
Professional
Radiology
Beaujon University Hospital
Clichy, France

Alexander S. Rosemurgy II, MD
Director of Hepatopancreaticobiliary Surgery
Surgery
Advent Health Tampa
Tampa, Florida

Charles B. Rosen, MD
Professor
Department of Surgery
Mayo Clinic
Rochester, Minnesota

Chady Salloum,
Doctor
Service de chirurgie hepatobiliopancreatique et transplantation
Hopital Paul Brousse Centre hepatobiliaire
Villejuif, France

Roberto Salvia, MD, PhD
Chief Executive of the Verona Pancreas Institute
Department of Surgery
Pancreas Institute
Verona, Italy

Hrishikesh Samant, MD FACG
Transplant Hepatologist
Hepatology
Ochsner Transplant Institute
New Orleans, Louisiana
Associate Professor
Gastroenterology and Hepatology
Lousiana State University Health
Shreveport, Louisiana
Director Hepatology
Gastroenterology and Hepatology
Ochsner-LSU
Shreveport, Louisiana

Kazunari Sasaki, MD
Clinical Associate Professor
General Surgery
Stanford University
Stanford, California

Mark A. Schattner, MD
Chief Attending
Department of Medicine
Division of Gastroenterology, Hepatology, and Nutrition,
Memorial Sloan Kettering Cancer Center
New York, New York

Gabriel T. Schnickel, MD, MPH
Professor of Surgery
Division of Transplant and Hepatobiliary Surgery, Department of Surgery
UC San Diego
San Diego, California

Richard D. Schulick, MD, MBA, FACS
Professor and Chair
Department of Surgery
Director
University of Colorado Cancer Center
University of Colorado School of Medicine
Aurora, Colorado

Max E. Seaton, MD
Surgical Oncology Fellow
Department of Surgery
Jackson Memorial Hospital / University of Miami
Miami, Florida

Yongwoo David Seo, MD
Resident Physician
General Surgery
University of Washington
Seattle, Washington

Jigesh A. Shah, D.O.
Assistant Professor
Surgery
UT Southwestern Medical Center
Dallas, Texas

Kevin N. Shah, MD
Assistant Professor
Surgery
Duke University Medical Center
Durham, North Carolina

Wong Hoi She, MBBS, FRCS, FCSHK, FHKAM
Consultant
Surgery
Queen Mary Hospital, The University of Hong Kong
Hong Kong, China

Junichi Shindoh, MD, PhD
Surgeon-in-chief
Hepatobiliary-pancreatic Surgery Division
Toranomon Hospital
Tokyo, Japan

Chaya Shwaartz, MD
Assistant Professor of Surgery
Abdominal Transplant & HPB Surgical Oncology
Department of General Surgery
University Health Network
Toronto, Ontario, Canada

Jason K. Sicklick, MD, FACS
Professor
Departments of Surgery and Pharmacology
Division of Surgical Oncology
University of California San Diego Cancer Center
University of California San Diego School of Medicine
UC San Diego Health
San Diego, California

Robert H. Siegelbaum, MD
Associate Attending Radiologist
Department of Radiology
Memorial Sloan Kettering Cancer Center
New York, New York

Martin Derrick Smith, MBBCh, FCS(SA), FEBS FRCS(Edin)
Professor
Surgery
University of the Witwatersrand, Johannesburg
Johannesburg, Gauteng

Kevin C. Soares, MD
Assistant Attending
Department of Surgery
Memorial Sloan Kettering Cancer Center
New York, New York
Assistant Professor
Department of Surgery
Weill-Cornell Medical College
New York, New York

Constantinos T. Sofocleous, MD, PhD, FSIR, FCIRSE
Interventional Oncologist/Radiologist
Department of Radiology
Memorial Sloan-Kettering Cancer Center
Professor Interventional Radiology
Weill-Cornell Medical College
New York, New York

Stephen B. Solomon, MD
Chief, Interventional Radiology Service
Director, Center for Image-Guided Intervention
Memorial Sloan-Kettering Cancer Center
New York, New York

Sanket Srinivasa, MBChB, PhD, FRACS
Consultant Surgeon
Waitematā District Health Board
North Shore Hospital
Auckland, New Zealand

Patrick Starlinger, MD, PhD
Associate Professor
Surgery
Mayo Clinic
Rochester, Minnesota

Tommaso Stecca, MD
Department of Surgery
Division of First General Surgery,
Hepato-Pancreato-Biliary Regional Referral Centre
Azienda ULSS 2 Marca Trevigiana, Ospedale Ca' Foncello,
Treviso, Italy

John A. Steinharter, MS
Hepatopancreatobiliary Service
Memorial Sloan Kettering Cancer Center
New York, New York
Medical Student
Robert Larner, MD College of Medicine UVM,
Burlington, Vermont

Camille Stewart, MD
Surgical Oncology Fellow
Surgery
City of Hope National Medical Center
Duarte, California

Lygia Stewart, MD
Professor of Surgery
Department of Surgery
University of California San Francisco and SF VAMC,
San Francisco, California
Chief General Surgery
Department of Surgery
San Francisco VA Medical Center
San Francisco, California

Janis Stoll, MD
Associate Professor of Pediatrics
Gastroenterology, Hepatology and Nutrition
Washington University School of Medicine
St Louis, Missouri

Iswanto Sucandy, MD FACS
Director
Hepatobiliary Surgery
Advent Health Tampa
Tampa, Florida
Associate Professor
Surgery
University of Central Florida
Florida

Paul V. Suhocki, MD
Associate Professor
Department of Radiology
Duke University Medical Center
Durham, North Carolina

James H. Tabibian, MD, PhD, FACP
Associate Professor
Vatche and Tamar Manoukian Division of Digestive Diseases
David Geffen School of Medicine at UCLA
Los Angeles, California
Director of Endoscopy
Department of Medicine, Division of Gastroenterology
Olive View-UCLA Medical Center
Sylmar, California

Nobuyuki Takemura, MD, PhD
Hepato-Biliary Pancreatic Surgery Division
Department of Surgery
National Center for Global Health and Medicine (NCGM),
Tokyo, Japan

Laura H. Tang, MD, PhD
Attending Pathologist
Pathology and Laboratory Medicine
Memorial Sloan-Kettering Cancer Center
New York, New York
Professor of Pathology
Department of Pathology and Laboratory Medicine
Weill Cornell Medical College
New York, New York

Cornelius A. Thiels, DO, MBA
Assistant Professor
Department of Surgery
Mayo Clinic
Rochester, Minnesota

Taner Timucin, MD, PhD
Associate Professor
Surgery & Immunology
Mayo Clinic
Chair
Division of Transplantation Surgery
Mayo Clinic
Rochester, Minnesota

Samer Tohme, MD
Assistant Professor of Surgery
Surgery
University of Pittsburgh
Pittsburgh, Pennsylvania

Guido Torzilli, MD, PhD, FESA, FACS, FAFC(Hon), FCBCD(Hon), FCHB(Hon)
Director
Division of Hepatobiliary and General surgery
Humanitas Research Hospital - IRCCS
Rozzano, Milano
Professor & Chairman
Director
General Surgery Residency Program
Humanitas University
Rozzano, Milano, Italy

Hop S. Tran Cao, MD, FACS
Associate Professor
Department of Surgical Oncology
The University of Texas MD Anderson Cancer Center
Houston, Texas

Simon Hing Yin Tsang, MB ChB, FCSHK, FHKAM
Honorary Clinical Associate Professor
Department of Surgery
The University of Hong Kong
Hong Kong, China
Consultant Surgeon
Department of Surgery
Queen Mary Hospital
Hong Kong, China

Simon Turcotte, MD, MSc
Associate Professor of Surgery
Hepatopancreatobiliary Surgery
Full Scientist
Cancer Axis
Centre de Recherche du Centre Hospitalier de l'Université de
    Montréal
Montréal, Quebec, Canada

Thomas van Gulik, MD, PhD
Professor
Department of Surgery
Amsterdam University Medical Centers, University of
    Amsterdam
Amsterdam, Netherlands

Andrea Vannucci, MD
Associate Professor of Anesthesiology
Department of Anesthesia and Critical Care
University of Chicago - Pritzker School of Medicine
Chicago, Illinois

Jean-Nicolas Vauthey, MD
Professor of Surgery
Surgical Oncology
MD Anderson Cancer Center
Houston, Texas
Fort Worth Living Legend Chair for Cancer Research
Chief of Hepatopancreatobiliary Surgery Section
Dallas Texas

Jack R. Wands, MD
Director
Gastroenterology/Liver Research Center
Rhode Island Hospital
Providence, Rhode Island

Julia Wattacheril, MD, MPH
Associate Professor of Medicine
Medicine
Columbia University College of Physicians and Surgeons,
New York, New York

Sharon Marie Weber, MD
Tim and MaryAnn McKenzie Chair of Surgical Oncology
Surgery
University of Wisconsin
Director for Surgical Oncology
UW Carbone Cancer Center
University of Wisconsin
Chair
Surgical Oncology
University of Wisconsin
Fellowship Director
Surgical Oncology
University of Wisconsin
Madison, Wisconsin

Alice C. Wei, MD MSc FRCSC FACS
Associate Attending Surgeon
Surgery
Memorial Sloan Kettering Cancer Center
New York, New York
Associate Professor
Surgery
Weill Medical College of Cornell University
New York, New York

Matthew Weiss, MD, MBA
Deputy Physician-in-Chief, Director of Surgical Oncology
Department of Surgery
Northwell Health Cancer Institute
Lake Success, New York

Jürgen Weitz, Professor, MD, MSc
Chair
Department of Gastrointestinal, Thoracic and Vascular
    Surgery
University Hospital Carl Gustav Carus,
Technische Universität Dresden
Managing Director
National Center for Tumor Diseases (NCT/UCC)
Dresden, Germany

Andrew David Wisneski, MD
Resident & Research Fellow
Surgery
University of California San Francisco
San Francisco, California

Christopher L. Wolfgang, MD, PhD
Chief, Surgical Oncology; Professor of Surgery,
Pathology and Oncology
Department of Surgery
The Johns Hopkins Hospital
Baltimore, Maryland

Dennis Yang, MD
Advanced Endoscopy Fellow
Gastroenterology
Advent Health
Director
Center for Interventional Endoscopy
Advent Health
Orlando, Florida
Professor
Medicine
Loma Linda University Health
Loma Linda, California

Hooman Yarmohammadi, MD
Associate Attending of Radiology
Radiology
Memorial Sloan-Kettering Cancer Center
New York, New York

Charles J. Yeo, MD, FACS
Samuel D. Gross Professor & Chair
Department of Surgery
Sidney Kimmel Medical College at Thomas Jefferson
    University
Philadelphia, Pennsylvania

**Theresa Pluth Yeo, PhD, MPH, AOCNP, ACNP-BC,
    FAANP**
Co-Director Jefferson Pancreas Tumor Registry
Department of Surgery
Professor
Jefferson College of Nursing
Acute Care Nurse Practitioner
Advanced Oncology Nurse Practitioner
Surgery
Thomas Jefferson University Hospital
Philadelphia, Pennsylvania

Adam Yopp, MD
Associate Professor
Surgery
UT Southwestern Medical Center
Dallas, Texas

Herbert Zeh, MD
Professor and Chair of Surgery
Surgery
UT Southwestern Medical Center
Dallas, Texas

Fangyu Zhou, MD
Postdoctoral Research Associate
Surgery
Washington University School of Medicine
St Louis, Missouri

Gazi B. Zibari, MD
Academic Chairman Dept of Surgery Program Director
Surgery Residency
Transplant
Willis Knighton Health System
Director, John C. McDonald Regional Transplant Center
Transplant
Willis Knighton Health System
Director, WK Advanced Surgery Center
Willis-Knighton Health System
Shreveport, Louisiana

George Zogopoulos, MD, PhD, FRCS(C), FACS
Associate Professor
Surgery and Oncology
McGill University
Attending Surgeon
Hepato-Pancreato-Biliary and Abdominal Organ Transplant
    Surgery
McGill University Health Centre
Montreal, Quebec, Canada

The seventh edition of *Blumgart's Surgery of the Liver, Biliary Tract, and Pancreas* was forged largely during the global COVID-19 pandemic, one of the most significant and devastating healthcare crises of the past century. As such, this has been among the most challenging editions to complete but is ultimately faithful to its long history and Dr. Leslie Blumgart's vision of embracing change to keep the book relevant to its readers. The COVID pandemic has profoundly impacted and disrupted all our lives, both professionally and personally, in ways none of us could ever have imagined. The completion of the seventh edition under such difficult circumstances thus represents a notable achievement and, on behalf of the section editors, I extend my sincere thanks to everyone who contributed.

The seventh edition once again relies heavily on associate editors to comprehensively cover the extraordinary advances over the past 5 years. As world-renowned experts in the field, the associate editors bring great insight to the book based on extensive personal experience. Dr. Jean-Nicolas Vauthey of the University of Texas MD Anderson Cancer Center once again joins Dr. William Chapman of Washington University in St. Louis in taking primary oversight of sections dealing largely with hepatic resection and transplantation, reflecting the substantial contributions they have made in these areas. Drs. Ronald DeMatteo, Michael D'Angelica, and Peter Allen bring their expertise to bear in the sections on basic science/ physiology, biliary tract, and pancreatic disease, respectively. Dr. Richard Kinh Gian Do's substantive improvements in the sections on liver, biliary, and pancreatic imaging include moving from modality-based to disease-based descriptions. Dr. T. Peter Kingham joins the editorship for this edition, taking charge of an expanded section on the technical aspects of liver, biliary, and pancreatic resection, including transplantation and minimally invasive approaches.

The current edition reflects advances in the molecular biology of benign and malignant HPB diseases, as well as significant improvements in imaging, therapeutics, and overall disease management. Indeed, since the last edition, great advances have been made in many areas, most notably in our understanding of the molecular underpinnings of malignant disease and the related explosion of treatment options, imaging technology, and minimally invasive/robotic surgery, and these are prominently featured in their respective sections.

As previously described, the organization of the book has been modified in that the sections on radiology are no longer separated by modality but rather by organ and disease type to provide a more rational view of imaging assessment. In addition, the technical aspects of HPB resectional surgery is now focused in a separate section. Furthermore, several new chapters have been added, while others have been expanded.

The general format has been maintained by covering all surgical aspects of the management of HPB disorders, whereas the radiologic, endoscopic, and other nonsurgical approaches are presented in detail and highlighted when they represent the preferred therapy. As with past editions, contributors were chosen largely based on their expertise and were asked to discuss specific topics based not only on the published literature but also on their own views and personal experience. Toward that end, overlap between chapters and discussion of controversy was encouraged to allow for conflicting points of view.

The initial section remains dedicated to general topics of HPB anatomy, physiology, and pathophysiology and thereby provides a solid foundation on which the remainder of the book is constructed. Chapter 2, "Surgical and Radiologic Anatomy of the Liver, Biliary Tract, and Pancreas," remains the cornerstone of this section; one of the most important chapters in the entire book, it provides the basis for understanding much of the material presented in subsequent chapters on physiology, molecular biology and immunology, imaging, and perioperative management.

In summary, the seventh edition attempts to include all aspects of the anatomy, pathology, diagnosis, and surgical and nonsurgical treatments related to HPB disorders, and all of the changes that have occurred since the last edition. We hope the work is of value to a wide range of readers, from seasoned HPB practitioners to surgical trainees and physicians in related disciplines. We have expanded our list of contributors to ensure the broadest and most contemporary viewpoints possible.

I would like to again express sincere thanks to the co-editors who have collaborated with me in this project, as well as all the contributors who generously gave their time to make this seventh edition possible. We hope that the readers find this text to be a valuable resource for many years to come.

W.R. Jarnagin, MD
New York, New York, 2022

ACKNOWLEDGMENTS

The Editors are indebted to our colleagues in surgery and other disciplines for their enthusiastic support and insightful contributions. We thank them for updating their areas of expertise, detailing recent advances, and highlighting areas of controversy and differing opinion – without them, this project would never have been possible. Special thanks to our respective staffs in New York, St. Louis, Houston, Durham (NC), and Philadelphia who have assisted in the preparation of this work. Finally, special thanks and appreciation are due to Erin Patterson, who provided much needed editorial support, and to Dee Simpson, Casey Potter, and all of the staff of our esteemed publisher, Elsevier, for their great support throughout the project.

CONTENTS

Hepatobiliary and pancreatic surgery: Historical perspective

Jacques Belghiti and Jean Robert Delpero

During the past decades, liver and pancreatic surgery have witnessed countless and tremendous changes, leading to disruptive innovations and continuous improvements regarding the safety, rapidity, precision, and overall efficiency of surgical procedures. The history of hepatobiliary and pancreatic surgery followed this dual path, and our goal was to unravel which innovations and, more importantly, which real progress marked the specialty. Because many innovations could not have happened outside a specific social environment and historical background, concomitant discoveries occurred frequently. In this context, while we report the work of various pioneers who are true heroes of our specialty, we also kept in mind that publication of the first series was probably the most relevant surrogate of innovation during the past 50 years.

HISTORY OF LIVER SURGERY

The history of liver surgery can be divided into three distinct periods: ancient times when concerns were focused on the liver's anatomy, from 1880 to World War II when surgical considerations were at the forefront, and over the last 50 years when good knowledge of anatomy and development of technology allowed safe liver resection.

The Ancient Period

Among all organs inspected in a sacrificial animal, the liver impressed the early observers as the most voluminous of the body and with its richness in blood. In Mesopotamia, the Assyrians and the Babylonians (2000–3000 BCE) believed that the liver was at the core of life, soul, emotions, and intelligence.[1] This belief continued through the ages, as confirmed by some literary passages from Greek tragedians referring to the liver as the seat of emotions. Even the Promethean myth may be interpreted in a way that the liver was chosen as the seat of the soul. In the following centuries in different cultures the link between the liver and the soul continued to persist. For example, in the Islamic world the prophet Mohammed used the term "moist liver" to refer to the soul, whereas among the modern Berber populations of North Africa, the depth of feelings is still used through the expression "You are my liver."[2] It is interesting to mention that we now know that liver disease affects brain functions.

Throughout antiquity, the most common fortune-telling method was the inspection of sacrificed animals. The liver was the single organ exploiting the custom of predicting the future among the Babylonians, Etruscans, Greeks, and Romans with the inspection of sacrificed animals.[3] Prediction of the future was based on specific findings obtained by observing the liver surface because two livers never looked the same. These priests developed sheep liver clay models that were used to instruct other priests. Models of sheep livers used by priests were found in Mesopotamia and in Italy during the Etruscan period (Fig. 0.1). These clay liver models are part of the history of liver anatomy along with several terms that were later incorporated into current anatomic terminology, including the right and left lobes, the gallbladder fossa, the umbilical fissure, and the caudate lobe and its processes described as papillary.[4] Pharaonic medicine did not pay much attention to the liver. However, the liver was considered important because it was the only organ to be preserved in the only canopic funerary jar with the human head called Amset (Fig. 0.2). In contrast, Greek academic achievements dominated the ancient period until 5th century BCE. Hippocrates (460–370 BCE) described the first rudiments of semiology and hepatic pathology. He described jaundice, edema, ascites, and palpation in search of hepatomegaly or splenomegaly and transmitted, through aphorisms, the first prognostic elements: "the prognosis is grim when in a yellow patient the liver is small and hard." Ancient Greeks described the treatment of abscess, puncture of ascitic fluid collection, and cauterization of war wounds. Both Prometheus and Tityus described two tragic mythical creatures that were punished by the fury of Zeus, and in both cases the carnivore birds devoured the liver; in the myth of Prometheus the eagle returned every day, but in the myth of Tityus the vultures appeared at every new moon. In these myths the liver was chosen as the immortal seat of the soul, but it remained impossible to determine whether Greek authors conceived the capacity of the liver parenchyma to regenerate.[1]

The Roman anatomist Gallien (130–201) was considered the father of modern medicine and pharmacology. Through the production of hundreds of books he named the liver as the main organ of the human body, arguing that it was the first of the organs to emerge in the formation of a fetus. For him "the liver is the source of the veins and the principal instrument of sanguification." Noticing the "cooked" aspect of food in the stomach and the central location of the liver in the venous system, he postulated that this digestive product resulted in chyme, which was transformed into blood in the liver, while the waste was eliminated in the bile and the excess water was carried by the urine. This arrangement, false in terms of blood circulation, remains accurate in terms of hepatic physiology.[5] Several centuries later Avicenna (980–1037), the father of early modern medicine, acknowledged the central role of the liver as "the seat of the nutritive or vegetative faculties." Throughout several centuries, many disorders were described as an alteration in the balance of humors produced by the liver, the gallbladder as the repository of fury, and the spleen as the receptacle of melancholy. Terms used to indicate the liver reflected the different interpretations of its role. In ancient Greek its name "hépar" might be related to pleasure, because this organ was looked on as the seat of the soul and of human feelings. In Romance languages the Latin

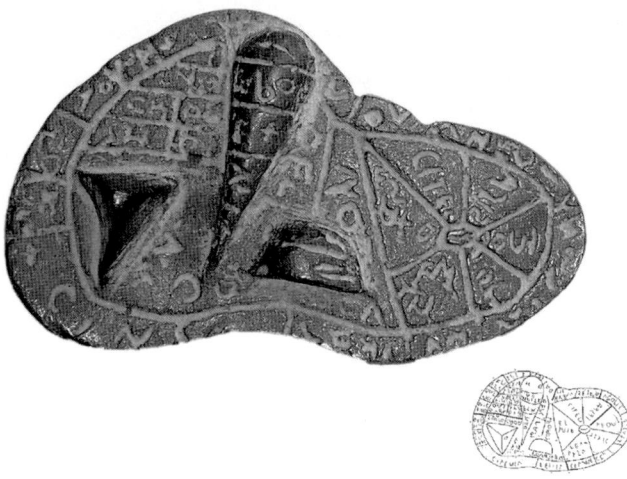

FIGURE 0.1 The liver of Piacenza. Etruscan Bronze with inscriptions dated to the late 2nd century BCE. (From the Municipal Museum of Piacenza, Italy.)

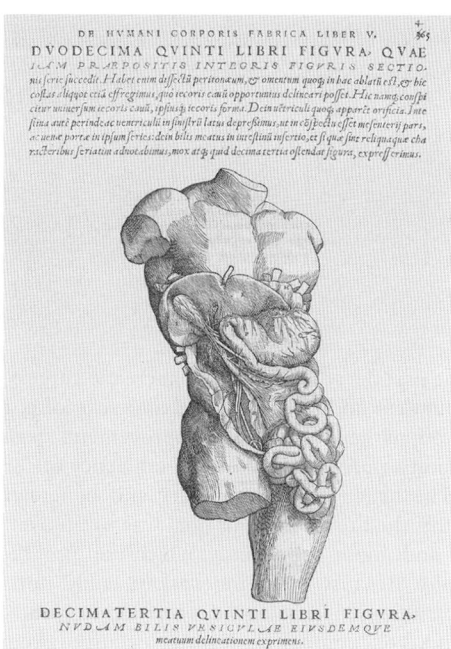

FIGURE 0.3 Andreas Vesalius (1514–1564). (From *De Humani Corporis Fabrica*, 1543.)

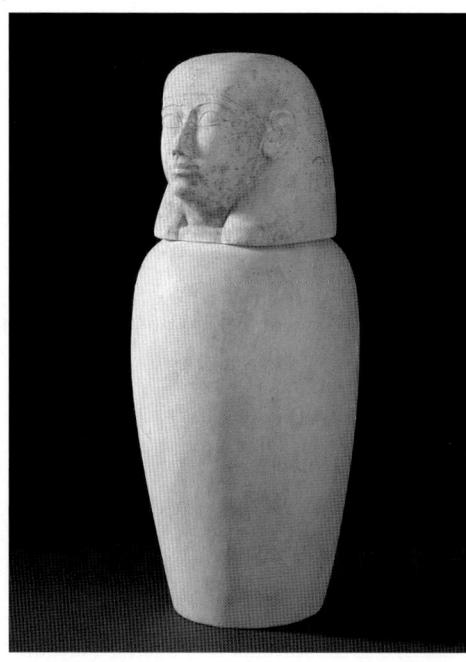

FIGURE 0.2 Egyptian funerary canopic jar with human head guardian of the liver. (Imsety [Amset], 600 BCE). (From the Science Museum of London.)

term *ficatum* was linked to the ancient practice of fattening geese with figs to make their livers more delicious. In the Early Modern Age, the liver became a recurring image used to indicate courage. The English term "liver" may derive from the Germanic term *lifere* connected to "life."[1]

The Renaissance

The writings of Greek physician Galen had dominated European medical thinking for over a millennium. Breakthrough knowledge concerning both liver anatomy and pathology emerged during the Renaissance in Italy. These improvements resulted from human autopsies performed by great artists and anatomists. The pioneer of these improvements was Antonio

Benivieni (1443–1502) in Florence who attempted to discover in his patients the etiology of biliary tract diseases. Most of the next phase of development of anatomic knowledge was centered around the University of Padua. In 1543 Andreas Vesalius (1514–1564) published innovative views of all organs arranged in three-dimensional (3D) space and interrelated. These anatomic drawings influenced the practice of operative techniques during the 16th and the 17th centuries (Fig. 0.3). Many of the eponyms that we now use in surgery were taken from famous anatomists of this school, including Johann Georg Wirsung (born in Augsburg Germany, 1589–1643), a German anatomist who was a long-time prosector in Padua. Years later, Giovanni Battista Morgagni (1682–1771) was promoted to the prestigious chair of anatomy and became the president of the University of Padua. In 1761 he published an outstanding analysis of biliary tract disease reporting the incidence of stones in male and female patients and describing the possible mechanisms by which calculi might be formed. He also considered the balance between conservative medical management and treatment by operation. Graduated from the University of Padua, the English physician William Harvey (1578–1657) is considered the greatest contributor to the study of anatomy and physiology. His description of the systemic circulation and the properties of blood pumped by the heart to the brain and the rest of the body ended the idea that the liver was the seat of blood formation. Harvey's student Francis Glisson (1597–1677) investigated the structure of the liver. His book *Anatomia Hepatis*, published in 1654, was the first major work devoted to the liver with the description of the hepatic capsule and of the investment of the hepatic artery, portal vein, and bile duct. Using casts and injection studies his description of hepatic anatomy appears close to images displayed today in 3D-computed tomography (CT) (Fig. 0.4). His name is given to the liver capsule, which is an important anatomic structure that continues to influence technical and oncologic approaches. Marcello Malpighi (1628–1694), regarded as the founder of microscopic anatomy, was the

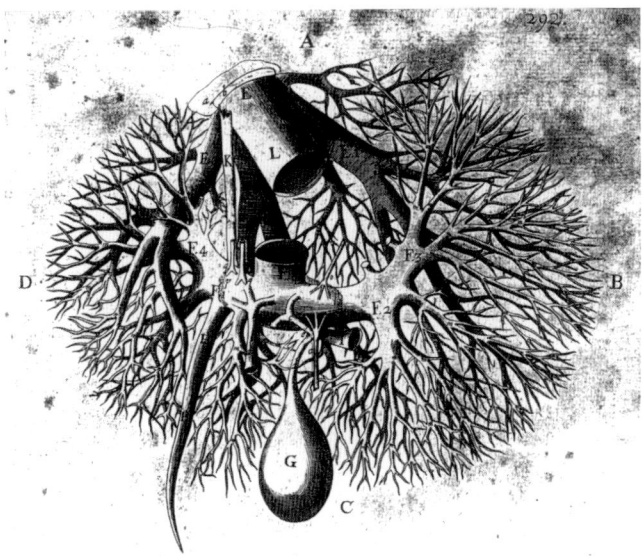

FIGURE 0.4   Francis Glisson (1597–1677). (From *Anatomia Hepatis*, 1654.)

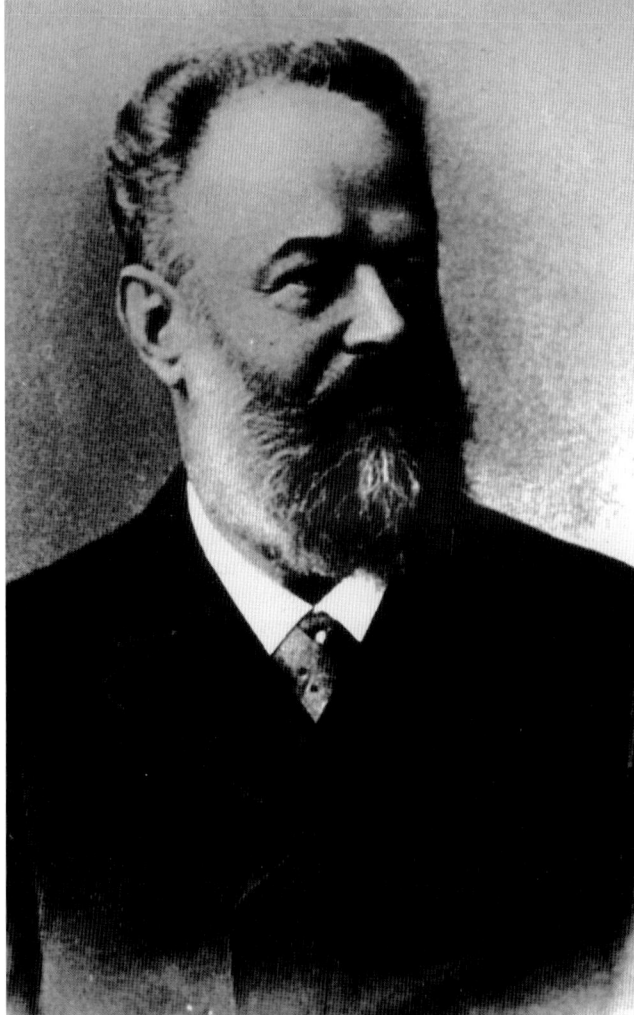

FIGURE 0.5   Carl Johann August Langenbuch (1846–1901), surgeon.

first to study liver glandular components. During the next century, scholars and anatomists focused on the formation of bile.

BILIARY SURGERY

The presence of gallstones in Egyptian mummies and the first description in the 6th century of human biliary concretions by Greek physician Alexander Trallianus had not been linked to a pathologic condition until the first description of obstructive jaundice in the beginning of the 17th century.[6] Until the publications of Giovanni Battista Morgagni, biliary symptoms were confused with multiple abdominal conditions and without attempted adequate therapy. Surgical therapy of the gallbladder started with Jean-Louis Petit (1674–1750), who was the first director of the French Royal Academy of Surgery created in 1731. He introduced the term biliary colic and identified gallbladder inflammation as different from liver abscesses. When the gallbladder adhered to the abdominal wall, he described a successful treatment of calculi removal through a small incision after a puncture. Nearly one century later, in 1853, Johann Ludwig Wilhelm Thudichum (1829–1901) from London, England, described a two-stage elective procedure, including the suture of the gallbladder to the abdominal wall, which served as a route for the removal of gallstone at a later date.[7] In 1867 in Indianapolis, Indiana, John Stough Bobbs (1809–1870) unknowingly performed the first cholecystostomy.[8] During surgery for an ovarian cyst, he found an inflamed sac and removed several gallstones in a large gallbladder. He closed the cholecystostomy incision and placed the gallbladder near the undersurface of the abdominal incision. The patient survived. This procedure was intentionally performed in 1878 by the American Marion Sims (1813–1883) and by the Swiss Theodor Kocher (1841–1917), who won the Nobel Peace Prize in medicine in 1909 for his work on the thyroid gland. His name is well known to surgeons who perform mobilization of the duodenum. While several surgeons were pursuing the construction of a gallbladder fistula and direct removal of stones, Carl Langenbuch (1846–1901) observed these measures as only

temporary relief. He was a brilliant surgeon who was appointed director of the Lazarus Hospital in Berlin at the age of 27 (Fig. 0.5). Concerned by clinical observations of patients suffering from biliary symptoms, on July 15, 1882, he performed the first cholecystectomy. He removed a chronically inflamed and thickened gallbladder containing two gallstones in a 43-year-old man who had been suffering from the disease for 16 years. The patient was discharged uneventfully from the hospital. This milestone procedure was performed after several years of investigations and accumulating results of animal experiments and numerous human cadaveric dissections showing that the gallbladder was not essential to life.[8] His innovation was received by the surgical community with skepticism, and, in some cases, with considerable disbelief. The debate between surgeons in favor of cholecystectomy versus those in favor of cholecystostomy was based on various pathophysiologic concepts and because of the technical difficulty of the procedure, at a time when anesthesia was not effective. In 1886 Justus Ohage (1843–1935) performed the first cholecystectomy in the United States in Minnesota, while a French surgeon named Jean-François Calot (1861–1944) described in 1890 the anatomic triangle of Calot, facilitating the technical aspect of cholecystectomy.[9] For the first time this debate was based on statistics comparing the mortality of the two approaches.[7] Initially considered as a risky procedure, William and Charles Mayo from the Mayo Clinic stated in 1899 that the cholecystectomy should be employed more frequently, and in 1903 William reported 65 cholecystectomies with only two deaths.[7] With a low risk rate, the long-term beneficial effect of cholecystectomy was solemnly established in 1917 by Charles Mayo in his address to the Clinical Congress of Surgeons of North America,[10] 35 years after Langenbuch's paper.

As soon as the cholecystectomy was feasible, there were several attempts to operate on the common bile duct (CBD), all of which resulted in the death of the patient.[11] Fatal issues resulted from the combination of jaundice, hemorrhage, infection, and technical difficulties.[6] Ludwig Georg Courvoisier (1843–1918), a surgeon from Basel, Switzerland, was the first to describe the successful removal of a stone from the CBD in 1889. The risk of postoperative peritoneal infiltration by bile after surgical exploration of the CBD limited the expansion of this approach. It began in 1897 when the German surgeon Johannes Otto Kehr (1862–1916) introduced the use of a T-tube for drainage and decompressing the biliary tree after exploration of the CBD. The T-tube is still used more than one century later. Kehr was one of the most outstanding biliary surgeons, opening the era of extensive biliary surgery, performing bilioenteric anastomosis, and describing resection of cancerous gallbladders, including hepatic resection.[12]

The first bilioenteric bypass was performed in 1880 by Alexander von Winiwarter (1848–1917), a surgeon from Vienna, who anastomosed the gallbladder with the colon for a patient with a malignant obstructive process.[13] A series of complications and re-operations ensued, but eventually after several months he was able to revise the original bypass to a cholecystojejunostomy. In 1887 two surgeons, Otto Kappeler in Switzerland and Dmitrievich Monastyrski in Saint Petersburg, almost simultaneously performed the first planned, one-stage cholecystojejunostomies in jaundiced patients with pancreatic cancer.[13] In 1889 the French surgeon Felix Terrier (1837–1908) performed the first successful cholecystoduodenostomy. The development of the cholecystectomy required the reconstruction of the biliary tract using the CBD, and Oskar Sprengel from Dresden, Germany, published the first report of a choledochoenterostomy[13] in 1891. The most innovative procedure was the use of a jejunal loop for relief of gastric obstruction, which was described in 1893 by César Roux (1857–1934) in Lausanne, Switzerland (Fig. 0.6), and adapted as a bilioenteric anastomosis with the gallbladder in 1904. This procedure was proposed at the French Congress of Surgery in 1908 with the CBD by Ambroise Monprofit, a surgeon from Angers, France.[12] The Roux-en-Y remains the most common bilioenteric anastomosis with the lowest incidence of reflux and cholangitis.

The approach of the ampulla to clear the CBD termination or to treat specific symptoms included papillotomy, sphincterotomy, and sphincteroplasty, which were gradually supplanted by the endoscopic approach.[12] In the 1960s various biliary-type symptoms and even pancreatitis were attributed to an abnormal pressure profile of the sphincter of Oddi, leading some surgeons, and, thereafter, endoscopists to develop various form of sphincterotomy and sphincteroplasty to treat these patients. After several decades of debate, the treatment of such sphincter dysfunction has fallen into disuse.[15] The development of biliary surgical procedures was associated with the occurrence of iatrogenic bile duct injury. The resulting biliary fistulas or strictures

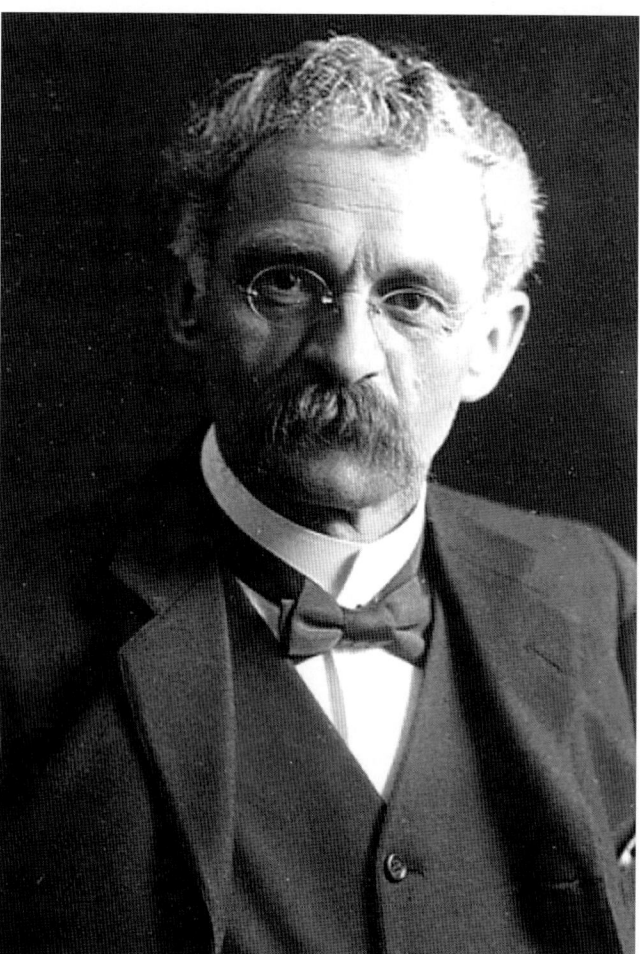

FIGURE 0.6 César Roux (1857–1934), surgeon.

necessitated the development of a new means of rerouting bile in the digestive tract. To treat a persistent biliary fistula after a cholecystostomy for a gallbladder empyema, Arthur Mayo-Robson (1853–1933), a surgeon from Leeds, England, performed an anastomosis between the gallbladder and the colon in 1889. The gradual practice of cholecystectomy and the increased risk of cholangitis and diarrhea using the colon led to establishing internal biliary drainage with the CBD. In 1905 William J. Mayo reported the first successful hepaticoduodenostomy reconstruction.[13] In 1909 Robert Dahl of Stockholm, Sweden, used a Roux-en-Y jejunal limb for the first time to manage a common hepatic duct fistula. Since its description, Dahl's approach remains widely used for the repair of various levels of damaged bile duct. In 1954 the description of a long extrahepatic course of the left hepatic duct in the hilar plate by Couinaud allowed several surgeons to perform hilar and intrahepatic biliary-enteric anastomoses in patients developing high biliary strictures.[16,17] However, the difficulty of these anastomoses with poor long-term results gave rise to the development of percutaneous and endoscopic methods for intubation and dilatation of the biliary tract, which are now the first-line treatment of biliary injuries. Direct reconstruction of the bile duct using various tissue substitutes, such as the gallbladder with gastric flaps, with or without stenting, was unsatisfactory, with numerous recurrent strictures due to the specific CBD arterial supply.[18]

Extensive surgery for biliary cancer was developed by Japanese surgeons starting at the end of the 1970s. Yuji Nimura (1943) from Nagoya was the pioneer of this approach, reporting the first large series of extended hepatobiliary and surrounding organ resection for locally advanced gallbladder and cholangiocarcinoma with a 3-year survival of 29%.[19] This aggressive approach was rapidly adopted by western surgeons, including Fortner in New York, Blumgart in the UK,[20] and Neuhaus in Berlin.[21] In the 21st century, factors contributing to preserve the leadership of Japanese surgeons for extensive surgery for hepatopancreatobiliary (HPB) cancer included technical meticulosity, progress in imaging, and preoperative management of the patients. Technical improvement using fine vascular surgical techniques and various vascular grafts have enabled surgeons to reconstruct portal, enous, and arterial flows. Progress in imaging diagnostics has enabled visualization of 3D anatomy, the extent of cancer progression, and hepatic segment volume. The most important innovation is preoperative management of the patient, including biliary drainage, which shifted from percutaneous transhepatic to endoscopic nasobiliary and portal vein embolization (PVE) for volume modulation.[22]

Good visualization of the biliary tree was quickly deemed essential for accurate diagnosis and treatment of biliary diseases. In 1924 Evarts Graham and Warren Cole discovered the diagnostic procedure of cholecystography. The first operative cholangiography was performed in 1931 by Argentinian Pablo Mirizzi (1893–1964). In 1968 one of the most innovative exploratory and therapeutic biliary procedures was published by William McCune (1909–1998) from George Washington University. He reported the first endoscopic cannulation of the ampulla in living patients to visualize both the CBD and the pancreatic duct.[23] In 1974 the first endoscopic treatment of choledocholithiasis with sphincterotomy of the ampulla was reported in Germany by Classen, with a first series of more than 200 patients published by Safrany in Munich.[24] Endoscopic retrograde cholangiopancreatography (ERCP) allowed physicians for the first time to obtain high-quality images of the common bile and pancreatic ducts. At present, magnetic resonance cholangiopancreatography (MRCP) is a quick, noninvasive method that can accurately evaluate the liver, gallbladder, bile ducts, pancreas, and pancreatic duct for disease. Percutaneous transhepatic biliary drainage and ERCP are now important tools for radiologic and endoscopic interventional procedures in patients with biliary obstacles or with postoperative complications.

Laparoscopic Cholecystectomy

The introduction of laparoscopic cholecystectomy was a surgical revolution with immediate acceptance by patients and surgeons based on clinical experience that became rapidly popular without randomized trials. Explorative abdominal laparoscopy was introduced in 1910 in Sweden by Hans Christian Jacobaeus (1879–1937). This procedure evolved as an effective diagnostic tool incorporating several technical improvements, including the Trendelenburg position, the use of carbon dioxide for insufflation, and the development of specific instruments. Since the 1970s, these instruments have also allowed gynecologists in Germany to use this approach for the exploration and treatment of gynecologic disorders. On September 12, 1985, Erich Muhe (1938–2005), from Erlangen, Germany, performed the first planned cholecystectomy using a local manufacturing laparoscope (Fig. 0.7). When he presented his

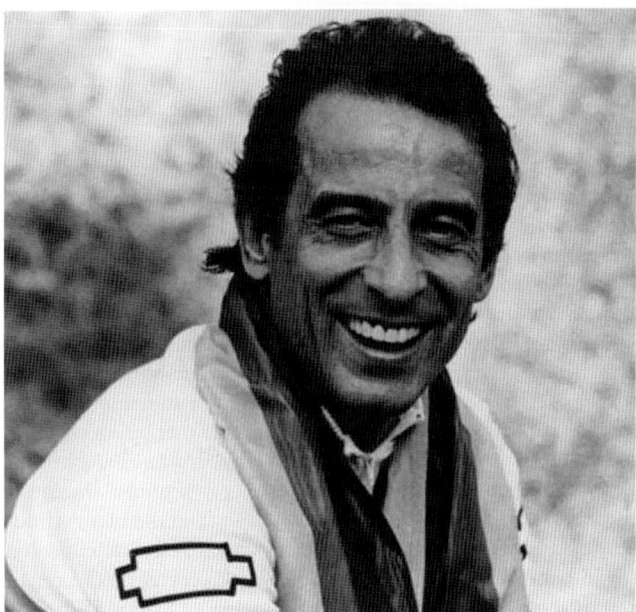
FIGURE 0.7 Erich Muhe (1938–2005), surgeon.

first series in front of his German colleagues in 1986, the technique was rejected and considered as dangerous with offending comments such as "Mickey Mouse surgery," while others remarked "small brain–small incision."[25] Reasons for rejection by the hierarchic German academic system included the predominant interest in transplantation and cancer treatments requiring large incisions. They had little interest in a gallbladder procedure with rapid medical dissolution and extracorporeal shock wave lithotripsy (presented by Gustave Paumgartner from Munich). Even though Muhe's technique was rejected, providentially the German Society of Surgery awarded him a top honor in 1992. Laparoscopic cholecystectomy has also been credited to French surgeons Philippe Mouret, François Dubois, and Jacques Perissat who were able to disseminate this innovation though video technology, publications in international scientific journals, and academic participation to a multinational congress. In 1989 Perissat presented his video at the American Gastrointestinal Endoscopic Surgeons (SAGES) meeting in Louisville, Kentucky. This presentation and Dubois' 1990 publication of a series of 36 cases of laparoscopic cholecystectomy found a large American audience.[26] This new technique was introduced in the United States in 1988 with the first large series published in 1991.[27] The advantages of laparoscopic cholecystectomy over open cholecystectomy were immediately accepted with a progressive disappearance of reluctance or contraindications, including pregnancy, obesity, severe cholecystitis, Mirizzi syndrome, acute pancreatitis, and the presence of CBD stones. CBD stones are usually extracted with ERCP, with laparoscopic cholecystectomy performed the following day after ductal clearance. Laparoscopic cholecystectomy provoked profound changes in the practice of biliary tract surgery with a 2-fold increase in the number of cholecystectomies performed worldwide. The beneficial effect of technical innovations such as single-incision laparoscopic surgery and robotic-assisted cholecystectomy has yet to be demonstrated in 2020.

PANCREAS SURGERY

For many years the pancreas remained off limits to anatomists because of its anatomic position and consistency. Considered as a "finger of the liver" in the Talmud, this organ was described around 300 BCE by Herophilus of Chalcedon and named by Rufus of Ephesus in Asia Minor (ca. CE 100) as the pancreas (etymologically: *pan* (πάγ), all; *kréas*, flesh).[27] This name was chosen in anticipation of a soft pancreas because it was considered as a gland in continuity with the omentum. In the Galenic framework the pancreas was considered as a conduit for the vasculature of vital organs and as a structural prop for the omentum. Its function was primarily to protect the retroperitoneal vessels. The anatomic reports of Galen remained uncontested until Vesalius' description of the mesenterico-portal circulation with a right venous trunk "*supported by a glandulous body.*" The view that the pancreas serves to "support" the intestines persisted when William Harvey described the blood circulation, considering that the pancreas was just a "pad" located behind the stomach to protect the great vessels of the retroperitoneum. When he was in Padua, Johann Georg Wirsung described in 1642 the ductal pancreatic system. He ignored the function of the duct, but he engraved his anatomic drawing on a copper plate (Fig. 0.8) and sent it to the main anatomists in Europe asking their opinion.[28] The authorship of this discovery was challenged by his trainee Moritz Hoffmann, and this controversy was complicated by the assassination of Wirsung in dubious circumstances in 1643, after which the name of the main pancreatic duct was referred to as "ductus Wirsungianus." Giovanni Domenico Santorini (1681–1737) studied a hundred

pancreatic dissections with the aid of magnifying glasses, and he is credited in 1724 with the discovery of an accessory pancreatic duct referred to as the Santorini duct. The first description of the tubercle or diverticulum that was later named the "ampulla of Vater" was attributed to Abraham Vater (1684–1751). The sphincteric muscle surrounding the CBD was described in 1654 by the anatomist Francis Glisson, and its function was rediscovered over two centuries later by Ruggero Oddi (1866–1913).[14]

Experimental studies contributed to the comprehension of the role of the pancreas in the digestive processes with the cannulation of pancreatic ducts in dogs by Regnier de Graaf (1641–1673) from Leyden. Herman Boerhaave (1668–1738), also from Leyden, described the pancreatic veins and arteries with precision. Giovanni Battista Morgagni, in 1761, described the pathologic aspect of this organ, including the description of what could be a pancreatic cancer. The depiction of the common channel of the pancreatic duct with the CBD by Sommering in 1796 reinforced the understanding of the excretory function, which was elucidated by the French physiologist Claude Bernard (1813–1878). In 1812 Johann Friedrich Meckel (1781–1833) described the embryologic development of the pancreas with the fusion of dorsal and ventral primordia, opening the comprehension of the pancreas divisum and the annular pancreas. In 1869 Paul Langerhans reported a microscopic description of the pancreatic tissue, including acinar cells as well as specific islets (referred to as islets of Langherans) with endocrine function.[29] In Europe, the ability to perform autopsies contributed to the further development of this knowledge, whereas in Japan the pancreas was not drawn in the book

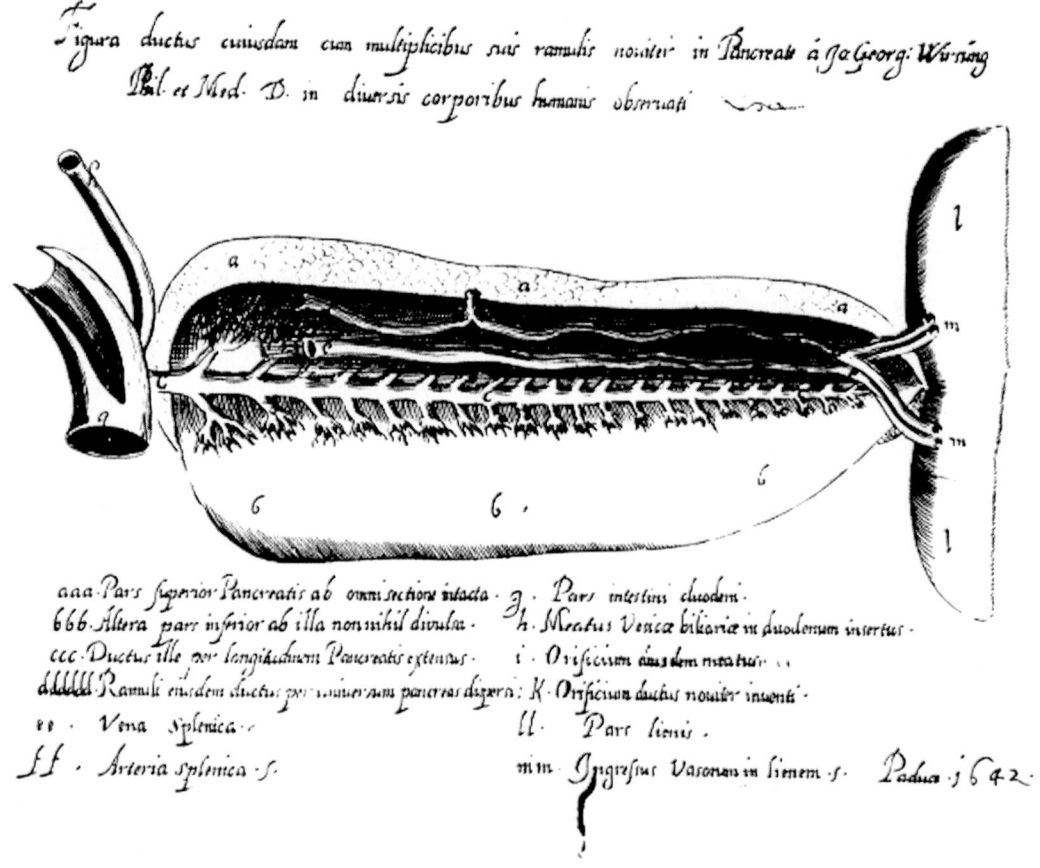

FIGURE 0.8 Imprint of the pancreatic ducts by Johann Georg Wirsung, 1642. (From Bo Palace, Padua, Italy.)

by anatomist Kouan Kuriyama in 1759, which illustrated the first recorded human dissection.[2] Nicholas Senn (1844–1908), who worked at the Rush Medical College of Chicago, observed how patients' skin was injured by the percutaneous drainage of pancreatic cysts. Diedrich Kulenkampff, a surgeon from Bremen, confirmed in 1881 that the fistula following the drainage of a traumatic cyst contained an alkaline juice capable of hydrolyzing starch, proteins, and fats in the absence of bile. The contribution of experimental surgery was important for discrimination between exocrine and endocrine function. In 1889 Joseph von Mering and Oskar Minkowski discovered the link between diabetes and the pancreas, reporting that removal of the pancreas induced diabetes in dogs and that subcutaneous pancreatic grafts prevented diabetes in these animals.[29] In 1909 Robert C. Coffey (1869–1933), from Portland, Oregon, published the first series of direct anastomosis of the pancreatic duct to the gastrointestinal tract. During the 19th century, experimental studies from Ivan Petrovich Pavlov (1849–1936) and his pupils from Russia added important contributions to the physiology of digestion, including the stimulation by the vagus nerve, the stimulation of pancreatic juice by a hormone called secretin, and the activation of this juice in the duodenal membrane by enterokinase.[29]

The beginning of pancreatic surgery in humans started with the treatment of cysts. In 1841 Friedrich Wilhelm Wandesleben (1800–1868) from Stromberg, Germany, reported the world's first operation on the human pancreas. In a 28-year-old man he drained pus and watery fluid from a pseudocyst secondary to a nonpenetrating abdominal trauma, but the patient died from respiratory failure 5 months later. In 1881 Carl Thiersch (1822–1895), from Munich, Germany, published a successful cyst drainage in a 38-year-old man with a persistent fistula from the pancreatic tail; the patient survived the operation. The chocolate-colored liquid of this cyst may be attributed to a complication of acute pancreatitis, suggesting that this procedure was one of the first surgical treatments of this disease. The first successful percutaneous drainage by marsupialization of the cyst on the abdominal wall was reported in 1882 by Karl Gussenbauer (1842–1903), who was a disciple of Theodor Billroth. This procedure triggered an increase in the number of operations performed on cysts with a dramatic 3% drop in mortality rate.[30] The differentiation between true pancreatic cysts from pseudocysts and cystic tumors was proposed in 1898 by Werner Körte (1853–1937) from Berlin. The first internal anastomosis of a pseudocyst with the duodenum was performed in 1911 by Louis Ombrédanne (1871–1956) from Paris, but the patient died 11 days after the procedure. In 1921 Rudolf Jedlička (1869–1926) in Prague, Czech Republic, performed what is considered to be the first pancreatic cystogastrostomy. The first cystojejunostomy was performed in 1923 by the German surgeon Adolf Henle (1864–1936). The first transgastric pancreatic cystogastrostomy was published in 1931 by Anton Jurasz (1882–1961), a professor of surgery at the University of Poznan (Poland). This innovative approach, known as the Jurasz procedure, became the standard approach for the treatment of mature pseudocysts in contact with the stomach.

Resection of pancreatic lesions started in 1867 with the removal of a pancreatic cyst by the German George Albert Lücke (1829–1884) in Bern. In 1882 in Berlin Friedrich Trendelenburg (1844–1924) performed the first distal pancreatectomy (DP) with splenectomy for a small solid tumor of the pancreatic tail in a 41-year-old female patient who died postoperatively from respiratory failure. The first central pancreatectomy for a

cystic lesion without closing the remaining pancreas was performed in 1885 by the Viennese surgeon Theodor Billroth (1829–1894). One year earlier, a successful total pancreatectomy (TP) was also attributed to Billroth.[30] In 1889 Giuseppe Ruggi (1844–1925) from Bologna, Italy, performed the first enucleation of a pancreatic mass.

Patients with obstructive jaundice due to pancreatic carcinoma were treated with various palliative operations (see "Biliary Surgery"). Until the beginning of the 20th century, pancreatic procedures in the head of the pancreas were scarce without touching the duodenum and without specific treatment of both the pancreatic remnant and the pancreatic duct. In 1904 Domenico Biondi (1855–1914) from Bologna, Italy, removed a pancreatic tumor with ligation of the pancreatic duct. At the Johns Hopkins Hospital in 1898 William Stewart Halsted (1852–1922) performed the first successful resection of an ampullary cancer through a transduodenal approach. After an en bloc resection of the ampulla, both pancreatic and bile ducts were re-anastomosed. The same year Alessandro Codivilla (1861–1912) performed the first pancreaticoduodenectomy (PD) in a patient with a pancreatic tumor adherent to the duodenum. The procedure consisted of resection of the pancreatic head, the duodenum, and part of the stomach followed by a cholecystojejunostomy and Roux-en-Y gastrojejunostomy without anastomosis or closure of the pancreatic stump. The patient died in the postoperative period. The breakthrough innovation of this surgery should be attributed to Walther Carl Eduard Kausch (1867–1928) who performed a safe two-stage resection of the pancreatic head in 1909 in Berlin. In a jaundiced 49-year-old male patient, he performed a cholecystojejunostomy followed 2 months later by pancreatic head resection with the pylorus and the first and second part of the duodenum. The posterolateral gastroenterostomy was associated with an anastomosis of the pancreatic stump with the third part of the duodenum. After a transitory pancreatic fistula, the patient died 9 months later after numerous episodes of cholangitis.[31] Anticipating the benefit of preoperative biliary drainage preventing postoperative complications due to the long-term preoperative jaundice, this procedure was a significant advance in pancreatic surgery, and some thought that the so-called Whipple procedure should be called the Kausch-Whipple procedure.

Two innovations before the publication of a PD described by Whipple in 1935 deserve consideration. The first innovation was a one-stage PD with a pancreatic anastomosis by Georg Hirschel from Heidelberg in 1914, and the second was the biliary-enteric anastomosis using the main bile duct, described in 1922 by Ottorini Tenani from Florence, Italy.[31] The two-stage procedure published in 1935 by Allen Oldfather Whipple (1881–1963) from the New York-Presbyterian Hospital (Fig. 0.9) was considered a surgical milestone, consisting of a complete resection of the head of the pancreas associated with a total duodenectomy, then suturing of the cut surface of the pancreas with nonabsorbable suture. This procedure resulted in a patient's 2-year survival after treatment for carcinoma of the ampulla of vater.[32] In Chicago in 1937 Alexander Brunschwig (1901–1969) introduced the concept of radical abdominal surgery with a dissection of the head of the pancreas on the right side of the superior mesenteric vein. Whipple modified this procedure, resulting in a single operative stage consisting of reconstruction with Roux en-Y jejunostomy and the end-to-side pancreatojejunostomy. This approach has become the standard technique for resection of the head of the pancreas.[32,33] This accurate utilization of his experience with modification based on the published experience

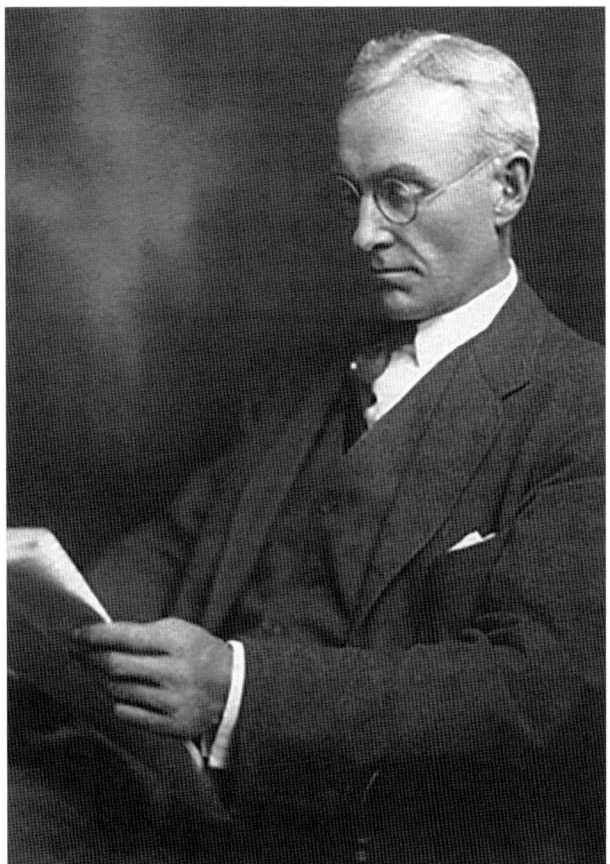

FIGURE 0.9   Allen Oldfather Whipple (1881–1963), surgeon.

of other surgeons warrants his designation as the father of pancreatic surgery. However, during subsequent decades, surgical resection of malignancies of the head of the pancreas was limited by a high rate of postoperative mortality (around 30%), a low rate of long-term survival (around 5% for pancreatic cancer), and several functional disorders. For several years palliative bypass alone resulted in better quality of life and similar survival. At the end of the 1980s, the trend of centralization at high-volume centers with surgeons specializing in pancreatic surgery resulted in a dramatic improvement of postoperative mortality rates at less than 5% in several institutions in the United States[34] and Germany.[35] John L. Cameron (1936) was a pioneer of the concentration of pancreatic surgery in specialized centers. This strategy is presently recommended more and more often and has improved the result of the procedure with better management of postoperative complications requiring interventional radiology.

The vast majority of immediate postresection complications are attributed to pancreatic leakage, and investigation into the best anastomotic technique raised considerable debate. Pancreaticojejunostomy was challenged by an anastomosis with the stomach aiming to inactivate pancreatic enzymes by the gastric acid, but this procedure did not show superiority.[36] Trends in the modification of the anastomotic method of the pancreatojejunostomy incorporated various methods of duct-to-mucosal anastomosis, with or without invagination or seromuscular jejunal anastomosis, and include the so-called Blumgart anastomosis using transpancreatic U-sutures with favorable outcome in some nonrandomized trials.[37] Another innovation was Peng's binding pancreaticojejunostomy technique with a near-zero fistula rate, which was not validated externally.[38] None of these

innovations resulted in significant progress except the external stenting of the main pancreatic published by R. Poon from Hong Kong, which can be recommended in patients with high risk of fistula.[39] Studies on this specific postoperative event were clarified by the international, uniformly accepted definition for pancreatic fistulae published in 2005 by the International Study Group on Pancreatic Fistulae (ISGPF).[40] Risk factors for postoperative pancreatic fistula (POPF) were dominated by the texture of the pancreatic gland and duct characteristics, such as the presence of a soft gland and/or a pancreatic duct less than 3 mm. The intraoperative tactile impression of the operative surgeon is currently surpassed by preoperative clinical and radiologic assessment,[41] but some scores, available online, have been recently developed for a better prediction of the risk of POPF. Medical and pharmacologic approaches preventing POPF remain controversial, including routine use of octreotide, perioperative nutrition, and decreasing the amount of intravenous fluids in the perioperative phase.[36]

Long-term survival after PD revealed functional disorders in more than half of patients, including delayed gastric emptying, dumping syndrome, exocrine insufficiency, diarrhea, long-term weight loss, and diabetes. The first innovative technical procedure aiming to preserve the gastrointestinal function was PD with pylorus preservation (PPPD), which was reported in 1944 by K. Watson from the UK and popularized in 1978 by Traverso and Longmire from Los Angeles.[31] In selected patients with localized tumors, this attractive procedure, which preserves both the entire stomach and pylorus function, gained worldwide popularity until the beginning of the 21st century, when multiple studies comparing classical PD with PPPD showed similar perioperative events and survival.[42] Delayed gastric emptying, which occurs in 25% of patients, was not significantly influenced by pylorus preservation or by the route of enteric reconstruction (antecolic vs. retrocolic). In 1993 the Johns Hopkins group, led by John Cameron, examined the medical approach of such complications with robust controlled trials demonstrating the beneficial effect of erythromycin on delayed gastric emptying.[43] The risk of postoperative diabetes observed in nearly one-third of patients after PD or DP is dramatically reduced in patients operated on for benign or low malignant potential tumors with pancreatic-sparing procedures.[44]

Recognition of hypersecreting endocrine tumors of the pancreas led to operations for these diseases. In 1926 at the Mayo Clinic in Rochester Russell M. Wilder (1885–1959) reported the first case of resection in the of pancreatic tumor with multiple intraabdominal metastases in which insulin was extracted.[1] The first successful enucleation of an insulinoma based solely on the patient's symptoms was reported in 1929 by Roscoe Graham in Toronto. Operating at the Mayo Clinic on a 49-year old woman with hyperinsulinism, James T. Priestley (1903–1979) performed the first TP in 1942, as he was unable to find the tumor during the laparotomy. The patient was cured by the operation, and the small tumor causing the syndrome was discovered by pathologic examination.[12] Accounting for less than 2% of all pancreatic neoplasms, neuroendocrine tumors of the pancreas include a wide range of heterogeneous neoplasms that are distinguished by symptoms related to the overproduction of the hormone from the cell of origin. The majority of these tumors are nonfunctional; however, they all may be identified with particular radiologic assessment, including nuclear medicine imaging. The scarcity of this disease and the complexity of the management of these patients with a favorable prognosis makes it necessary to centralize their management in high-volume centers.[44] Adenocarcinoma of the pancreas is a frequent tumor with a dreadful prognosis and the surgical approach remains the unique therapeutic option. During the 1960s and 1970s the lack of long-term survival motivated more radical resections, including TP with extensive lymph node dissection and vascular resection. This extensive approach was initiated by Joseph G. Fortner (1921–2007) from Memorial Hospital in New York, who proposed in 1973 a very unique extended technique of "regional pancreatectomy," including portal and arterial resection.[45] The high risk of this procedure contributed to its limited use.[12] The rationale for TP aiming to remove multicentric malignant foci with more complete lymphadenectomy was not sustained by any survival benefit compared with partial resection, whereas the morbidity of TP remains substantial. TP is presently considered as an exceptional oncologic option in patients with localized malignant tumor. Extensive dissection of nerve plexus and lymph nodes around the origin of the superior mesenteric artery was reported by O. Ishikawa from Osaka, Japan,[46] in 1988. However, several worldwide randomized controlled trials (RCTs), including one from Japan performed by Y. Nimura, showed that extended lymphadenectomy did not benefit from long-term survival; rather, it induced high morbidity and poor quality of life outcomes.[47]

Venous resection during PD was once considered in cases of tumor invasion, and initially in the 1950s restauration of the portal flow used a portocaval anastomosis with disastrous results. In the 1970s in Paris J.N. Maillard showed that a lateral venorrhaphy or a less than 3-cm resection was feasible after a complete mobilization of the mesentery. When larger resection is required to obtain cancer-free surgical margins, various types of autologous vein grafts are now used, including the left renal vein. The first approach using the artery during PD, which allowed early assessment of resectability,[48] was another technical innovation described in 1993 by Nakao from Japan. Except for the uncommon cases of successful en bloc resection with the celiac artery, first reported in 1997 by Y Nimura,[48] arterial involvement has remained a contraindication for resection. Improvement in imaging using high-resolution triphasic CT imaging with 3D reconstruction reduced the incidence of nontherapeutic laparotomies. In the beginning of the 21st century no more than 20% of patients were candidates for surgery, but gradually the use of chemotherapy resulted in two major advances, a higher rate of resection and an improved postoperative survival.[49] In 2020 surgery was not perceived as the unique treatment for patients with nonmetastatic pancreatic duct adenocarcinoma (PDAC). After pancreatic resection, adjuvant multiagent chemotherapy (gemcitabine plus capecitabine or modified FOLFIRINOX) become the standard of care.[50] The ability of neoadjuvant chemotherapy and radiotherapy to convert some patients from unresectable to resectable was an important advance. This strategy was effective in nearly two-thirds of patients with borderline resectable cancers characterized by tumor contact with either hepatic or mesenteric arteries or with the portal vein and mesenteric vein of greater than 180 degrees. Even in some patients initially considered as nonresectable for locally advanced tumors, this strategy allows a radiologic downstaging and more decisively a high rate of negative margins.[51] However, the morbidity of neoadjuvant treatment restricts the expansion of this strategy to patients whose cancer is resectable. In 2020 pancreatic cancer surgery was performed in high-volume centers with less than a 5% mortality rate and a 5-year survival rate of around 30% using adjuvant chemotherapy.[36] The trend to define a curative resection R0 with a free margin of 1 mm led to

dissection on the right side of the mesenteric artery with removal of the retroportal pancreatic parenchyma and lymphadenectomy of at least 15 lymph nodes.[52]

The concept of prophylactic surgery for benign precursors of pancreatic adenocarcinoma has changed the approach of pancreatic surgery over the last decade. The widespread use of high-quality imaging allowed the discovery of an increased number of asymptomatic cystic pancreatic lesions, including mainly intraductal papillary mucinous neoplasms (IPMNs). This cystic mucin-producing neoplasm with various grades of dysplasia has a risk of progression to adenocarcinoma with a dismal prognosis. The risk of pancreatic resection, including parenchyma-sparing procedures, was intended for select patients at risk for malignancy. The current consensus is to consider for resection patients with clinical symptoms and those in whom imaging detected a contrast-enhancing mural nodule (≥5 mm), a main pancreatic duct diameter greater than 10 mm, or a solid mass. The best approach to surveillance of patients not submitted to resection or at risk for cancer in the remnant pancreas remains controversial.[53]

The development of surgery in patients with chronic pancreatitis (CP) started in the beginning of the 20th century with the removal of pancreatic duct stones. This was first reported by Alfred Pearce Gould (1865–1922) in London.[29] The belief that pain of the pancreatitis is obstructive in nature led surgeons to try decompressing the parenchyma, with the first technical success reported by Merlin Du Val in 1954 in two patients operated on in the Bronx, New York. These patients underwent a transection of the pancreas at the junction of body and tail and a Roux-en-Y anastomosis with the pancreatic stump. In 1960 Partington and Rochell refined the decompression of the pancreas duct with a side-to-side longitudinal pancreaticojejunostomy after a complete opening of the pancreatic duct.[54] However, the inconstant efficacy of the drainage procedure on long-term pain relief led doctors to consider the use of pancreatic resection. In the 1970s resection procedures were undertaken in patients with severe painful PC, including pyloruspreserving pancreaticoduodenectomy, spleen-preserving DP, or even TP.[55] Considering the operative risk of these resections, procedures with a high rate of new-onset diabetes, and the intensification of exocrine pancreatic insufficiency, Hans Berger from Ulm University proposed an innovative partial resection of the head of the pancreas. Focusing on the inflammatory component of this disease, in 1980 he published a series of patients who underwent a partial resection of pancreatic head parenchyma preserving the duodenum and the CBD.[56] This approach, simplified by Charles F. Frey in 1987, reported a procedure combining a smaller amount of pancreatic resection and the absence of dissection of the portal system, and with a longitudinal pancreaticojejunostomy drainage was adopted during the next decades in Europe and in the United States.[57] A better knowledge of the natural history of patients with PC showing that pain can naturally disappear contributed to the decline of the surgical treatment of patients with PC. In 2020 the complications of PC, such as pseudocysts and the involvement of the biliary tree and duodenum, were challenged by endoscopic approach despite the poorer results of the latter.[58] By the end of the 19th century a correct clinical and pathologic description of acute pancreatitis was published by Reginald Fitz (1843–1913) from Harvard University.[59] In 1903 Von Mickulicz-Radecki (1850–1905), in Wroclau, Poland, advocated the drainage of pancreatic necrosis using gauze compresses, aiming to clean the necrosis and to prevent the false closure of the originating cavity. During the subsequent decades, despite a mortality rate over 50%, surgery was considered the best treatment. A more conservative approach was applied in the 1930s after the discovery of the value of blood amylase, which allowed early diagnosis of acute pancreatitis avoiding hazardous laparotomy in early stages of this disease. Conservative approaches, which prevailed until the early 1970s, remained associated with persistent high mortality despite advances in intensive care. CT diagnosis of necrosis and the characterization of pancreatic necrosis as infected versus sterile was a considerable advancement. The drainage of solely infected pancreatic necrosis proposed in 1991 by E.L. Bradley from Emory University in Atlanta was a disruptive approach associated with improvement of survival.[60] Open surgical necrosectomy was gradually substituted by less invasive interventions, including retroperitoneal surgical drainage, and percutaneous catheter drainage followed by endoscopic drainage when necessary, as demonstrated by several RCTs from the Netherlands.[61] The Atlanta classification of acute pancreatitis using prognosis scores of organ failures and the Balthazar radiologic CT scoring system of necrosis facilitated the evaluation of therapeutic procedures often altered by inherent selection bias.[62,63] The two main risks for acute pancreatitis, excessive alcohol intake and cholelithiasis, have long been recognized. In 1901 Eugene L. Opie (1873–1971) from Staunton, Virginia, observed the association of acute pancreatitis with gallstones impacted in the ampulla of Vater, causing him to propose a "common channel" hypothesis. Because the exact pathologic mechanism by which gallstones cause pancreatitis remains unclear, the role of ERCP also remains unclear except in patients with concurrent cholangitis or biliary obstruction.[64]

The history of pancreas transplantation started in 1893 when P. Watson Williams in Bristol, England, attempted to treat a 15-year-old boy developing diabetic ketoacidosis with subcutaneous xenotransplantation of a portion of a sheep's pancreas.[12] In 1921, at the University of Toronto, Frederick Grant Banting (1891–1941) reported the use of pancreatic extract and isolated insulin to treat diabetes mellitus in a man, for which he was awarded the Nobel Peace Prize in 1923. This discovery stimulated numerous animal studies with the first successful orthotopic transplantation in dogs in 1966 by Felix Largiarder in Zurich. In the same year, William Kelly (1922–2006) and Richard Lillehei (1928–1981) transplanted a segmental pancreas graft simultaneously with a kidney from a cadaver donor into a 28-year-old woman at the University of Minnesota. In 1967 Lillehei transplanted a whole pancreatic graft attached with the duodenum anastomosed to a Roux-Y jejunal host's segment.[65] Since the end of the 1970s, changes in surgical techniques involved venous drainage with a come-and-go from a recipient iliac vein to the mesenteric vein, and now drainage is done in the vena cava and pancreas. The benefit of combined kidney transplantation contributed to several technical changes. In 1983 Hans Sollinger from the University of Wisconsin described an innovative drainage of pancreatic secretion in the urinary bladder. In 1991 David Sutherland, from the University of Minnesota, showed the benefit of enteric drainage in a large series of transplanted patients.[66] In 1970 Sutherland and his team performed the first successful pancreas transplant from a living donor, and in 1999 he introduced laparoscopic DP harvesting.

The successful isolation of islet cells from the whole pancreas and their functional implantation in the spleen of dogs was a milestone.[67] The use of islet cells isolated from a cadaver in a diabetic patient with CP reported in 1977 by John S.

Najarian from the University of Minnesota raised a lot of hopes. Despite better separation of islet cells from a cadaveric pancreas, the facility used to infuse these cells into the recipient via the portal vein had several challenges that persisted into 2020, including the inconstant insulin independence of recipients who required adequate islet cells from multiple donors and lifelong immune suppression.

Laparoscopic procedures involving the pancreas started early in the 1990s for cancer staging, and within a few years both distal and proximal laparoscopic pancreatic resections were published. In 1994 Michel Gagner published the first case of laparoscopic PD in a patient with CP performed at the University of Montreal.[68] Two years later, the same group published a series of 12 patients with islet cell tumors, including 8 distal pancreatectomies and 4 enucleations.[69] The same year Alfred Cuschieri from the University of Dundee published a series of five patients who underwent DP with splenectomy for CP.[70] These two series of DP have initiated an extensive development of this approach for patients with benign or low malignant lesions of the distal pancreas. The gathering of pancreatic surgery in high-volume centers with rapid acquisition of technical skill and reducing operative time and conversion rates contributed to the adoption of this approach in all pancreatic centers. Laparoscopic DP become the standard procedure.[71] Unlike DP, the diffusion of laparoscopic PD in 2020 remains limited to experienced centers. The laparoscopic PD approach is a complex procedure, requiring three anastomoses with a high postoperative risk of fistula. In experienced hands, the robotic approach to DP, similar to the liver and the biliary tree, has the technical potential to compensate for the disadvantages of laparoscopy.

THE FORGOTTEN LIVER

Until the middle of the 19th century, there was little interest in the liver from a medical perspective because its main functions were unknown. The anatomic repositioning of the liver in the blood circulation, the description in 1651 by Jean Pecquet (1622–1674) of the real course of the lymphatic system from the mesentery to the thorax, and the extinction of the belief in the influence of liver humors led to a decline in the view of the supremacy of the liver. Liver surgery was restricted to the treatment of penetrating injuries, abscesses, and ascites. Since antiquity, puncturing the peritoneal cavity to sample fluid was an accepted treatment for ascites. The risk of brutal evacuation was reported by the Byzantine surgeon Pauï d'Aegina (625–690) who used a special pin called the "skolopion."

During antiquity, it was recognized that a wound with great effusion of blood under the right side of the hypochondra would not "permit life to continue even for a moment." In the medieval world, the question was who should proceed first: the surgeon and his attempts to stop such hemorrhage or the priest to hear confession from a subject likely soon to die.[72] However, when parenchyma evisceration was present through the wound without massive external bleeding, exceptional cases of successful treatment were reported, allowing the surgeon to address the bleeding and to excise a piece of the liver.[72] In 1816 the liver parenchymal compression was the most innovative approach described. It was described by Charles Bell (1774–1842), a surgeon in the British army at Waterloo. In 1888 Henry C. Dalton (1847–1917), a cardiac surgeon from Saint Louis University, reported successful control of bleeding in a patient suffering a laceration of the liver, using large and deep sutures. In a series of 69 cases of laparotomy for gunshot wounds, he recorded a survival rate of 5 survival among 10 liver wounds.[73] At the end of the 19th century, catgut suture and simple packing were procedures advocated in liver trauma.

The treatment of liver cysts and abscesses was only individualized during the 17th century without a significant development until the 19th century. This time line happened probably because such collections are often missed by physical examination and by the lack of accurate distinction between all types of purulent collections of the right hypochondra, including cholecystitis, subphrenic abscesses, and complications of perforated ulcers. It quickly became apparent that external drainage was an effective treatment in some patients. However, this maneuver was associated with several complications related to the etiology of the collection and to the skill of the operator. The puncture and simple incision of hydatid cysts advocated in 1825 by Joseph Recamier in Paris was promptly followed by some fatal outcomes. This changed in 1887 when a Russian surgeon names Nikolai Sklifosovsky reported three cases treated by a three-step procedure, including trocar aspiration of cyst contents, then marsupialization of the cyst wall to the abdominal cavity, and finally, washing the cyst lining with "corrosive sublimate."[72]

The Birth of Liver Surgery in the Middle of the 19th Century

Once the treatment of liver abscesses and the control of some penetrating injuries were recognized, some skillful surgeons tried to resect "abnormal liver tissue," as described by the founders of pathologic anatomy, including Carl Rokitansky (1804–1878) from the University of Vienna and Rudolf Virchow (1821–1902) in Berlin. Surgery became a science integrating anatomy, pathology, and physiology with the inclusion of the glycogenic function with the regulation of glucose in 1848 by Claude Bernard (1813–1878). In Boston, during the same period, John Collins Warren (1778–1856) of the Massachusetts General Hospital and founder of the *New England Journal of Medicine* performed the first public demonstration of a surgical procedure under ether anesthesia. Applying the revolutionary "germ theory" postulated by Louis Pasteur (1822–1895), the British surgeon Joseph Lister (1827–1912) developed the idea of sterile surgery (Fig. 0.10). This breakthrough innovation based on a new origin of infection and the changes in surgical practice were not easily accepted. Increasingly, however, the surgical community assimilated most of the familiar surgical accouterments and rituals of modern aseptic technique. The use of rubber gloves was promoted by William Steward Halsted (1852–1922) in 1890, and surgical masks were adopted in 1897 by Polish surgeon Johann von Mikulicz Radecki (1850–1905) from the University of Wroclaw. The use of anesthesia and the attention to asepsis contributed to shifting the act of surgery from a bloody act, when operations were done as rapidly as possible, to a meticulous procedure.

The German school of surgery was a dominant force for several decades. This was illustrated by the career of Theodor Billroth in Berlin, Zurich, and Vienna, where he pushed intestinal surgery to a higher level with successful removal of the esophagus, larynx, and rectum, including his most famous accomplishment, the first successful gastrectomy for gastric cancer. He introduced the concept of audits, publishing all results good and bad, and transmitted through his most brilliant student Theodor Kocher (1841–1907). These surgeons were characterized by their great attention to antisepsis, hemostasis, wound closure, and drainage.[74] This scrupulousness was influenced by

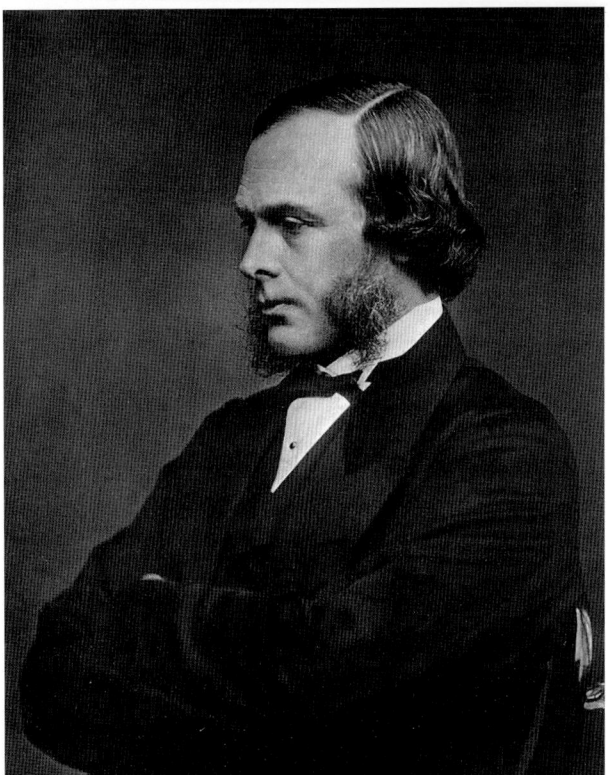

FIGURE 0.10 Joseph Lister (1827–1912).

laboratory attendance and experimental liver surgery on animals, which started in Berlin with Themistocles Gluck (1853–1942). It was further influenced by Bernhard von Langenbeck (1881–1887) who advocated that animal work must first be done, developing a series of experiments in the rabbit, cat, and dog in which, by manipulating the portal flow, he was able to successfully remove a large volume of the liver.[72] Carl Johann August Langenbuch performed the first cholecystectomy in 1882 (see Fig. 0.5). He performed the first elective hepatectomy on January 13, 1887, to remove a palpable mass in a 30-year-old woman. This mass, weighing 330 g, was apparently engorged liver parenchyma attached to the remaining liver by a bridge of fibrous tissue. The description of the resection did not mention any major vascular or biliary structures, and the abdominal incision was closed. Several hours later the patient was successfully operated on again for bleeding; after ligation of the bleeder vessel, evacuation of the blood, and closure of the abdomen the patient was discharged. After this, progressive technical improvements were popularized by Ernst von Bergmann (1836–1907). He was in favor of applying iodoform gauze on the raw surface of the liver with a partial closure of the abdomen so he could keep an eye on the impregnated gauze.[72] The first liver resection in the United States was performed in 1890 by Louis McLane Tiffany (1844–1916), a professor of surgery at the University of Maryland, who reported the successful removal of a portion of the left lobe of the liver.[72] Liver surgery in the United States was led by William Williams Keen (1837–1932) who worked in the US Army as a surgeon during the Civil War and spent 2 years studying in Paris and Berlin. As a professor of surgery in Jefferson Medical College in Philadelphia, he started his experience in liver resection on October 9, 1891, by operating on a young woman for a palpable tumor that had enlarged during her pregnancy and appeared attached to the edge of her liver. The depiction of the procedure included the use of the Paquelin cautery interposed by the ligation of large vessels, separating the liver substance from the tumor using his thumbnail, and approaching the two edges of the liver together with sutures.[72] In 1899 W. Keen published a compilation of 76 cases of liver resection, including 17 of his own patients with a mortality rate of 15%.[75] Before 1900, the restricted worldwide experience of liver resection reflected the rarity of palpable liver tumors, the reluctance to resect malignant tumors, and the difficulties of surgical extirpation while controlling bleeding. Thermocautery using heated vapor from a bottle filled with petroleum ether was an important technical innovation invented by the Frenchman Claude-André Paquelin (1836–1905). The control of vascular pedicles of tumors was advocated by the French surgeon Louis-Félix Terrier, who emphasized the benefit of "pediculization" of liver tissue from which a tumorous lesion seemed to arise. The resection of the strangulated pedunculated tumors were occasionally performed some days later. In fact, the control of hemorrhage from intraparenchymal vessels was dominated by manual tamponade often completed by the placement of iodoform gauze in the liver wound. In Berlin Ernst von Bergmann (1836–1907), concerned about the liver resection procedure, was in favor using gauze through the incision to watch for delayed hemorrhage and bile leak. Surprisingly, this latter complication was seldom mentioned. The management of digital compression during liver resection was extensively described in textbooks published around 1900 in Germany and France. In his textbook published in 1894, Langenbuch annunciated that liver surgery would be a new and adventurous specialty. This orientation was emphasized by the French surgeon Joseph-Antoine Pantaloni, who published a textbook titled *Chirurgie du foie et des voies biliaires* in 1899. Remarkably, he argued that as soon as the operation advanced from the edge to the central portions of the liver, before parenchymal transection, hemostasis should be controlled either by using the assistant's finger compression or by placement of broad parenchymal sutures. He showed that digital compression was also recommended to prevent air ingress into hepatic veins after observations of death from air embolism. Innovations concerning the suture of the liver were issued from ingenious procedures reinforcing the suture through very thin slices of decalcified and softened whalebone, similar to the pledgets used today.[72]

The Blossoming of Liver Surgery

Knowledge of liver anatomy allowed the development of liver surgery. Galen's concept of the liver as the place of manufacturing blood from ingested nutritive food described five lobes as five fingers enveloping the stomach to provide warmth for the digestion of food. This depiction of multiple lobes was issued from animal anatomy into human interpretation assuming one was similar to the other. Andreas Vesalius' representation of the liver in correct topographic position with two lobes separated by the falciform ligament (1555) was a turning point in the representation of this organ (see Fig. 0.3). In his book published in 1654, Francis Glisson depicted accurate liver anatomy with his specific triple vascular system structure (see Fig. 0.4). At the end of the 19th century the Scottish surgeon James Cantlie (1851–1926) and the Austrian anatomist Hugo Rex (1861–1936) debunked the classical division along the falciform ligament, showing instead that the boundary between the right and left livers is located on the line connecting the gallbladder bed to the inferior vena cava (IVC), which corresponds to the course of the middle hepatic vein. This simultaneous

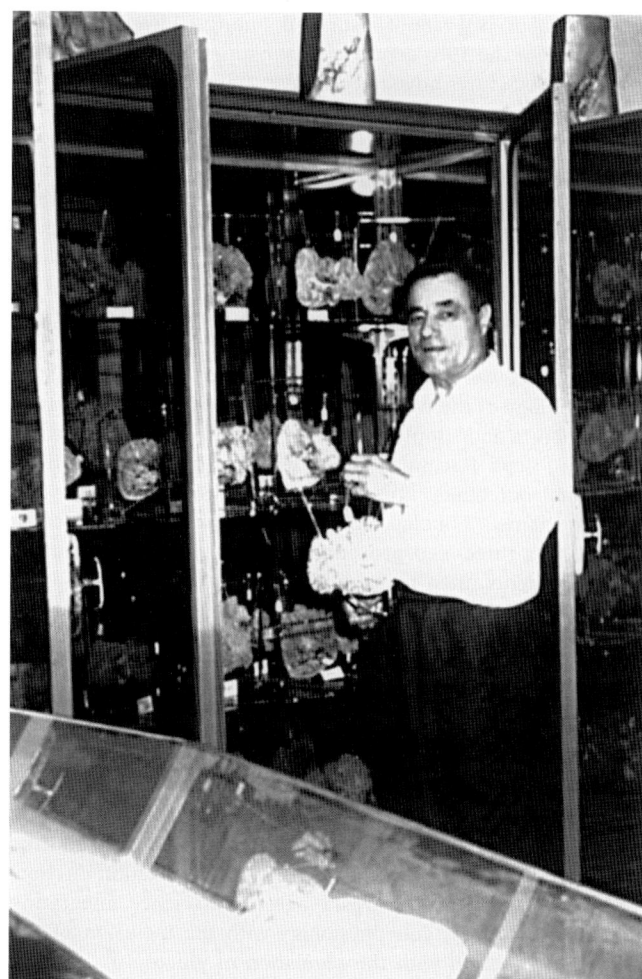

FIGURE 0.11 Claude Couinaud (1922–2008) working with his collection of liver casts.

anatomic discovery has been called the "Rex-Cantlie line." The major innovation of Claude Couinaud (1922–2008) (Fig. 0.11) was to confirm that right lobes and left lobes are not right and left livers and it was possible to divide the liver parenchyma into eight autonomous segments without intercommunication between the pedicles (blood vessels and bile ducts) of different segments.[76] This concept allowed surgeons to differentiate nonanatomic from anatomic resection. This latter type of resection is considered an oncologic resection, allowing transection along a well-defined line, avoiding necrosis, and preserving regeneration of the remnant liver. It is now well established that liver regeneration will occur not only if arterial and portal vascular inflow with biliary drainage are intact but also if there is complete venous drainage.[77] Before a liver resection, ensuring anatomic vascularization of the liver remnant is the main goal of radiologic investigations, confirmed by intraoperative exploration handled by the surgeon himself.

The possibility to obtain a pictorial view of the liver with penetrating imaging modalities was a breakthrough innovation allowing the location of nonpalpable tumors. In the middle of the 20th century, the first innovative imaging used was scintigraphy, which had the ability to clear colloidal particles from the blood into the Kupffer cells. The presence of a "cold" area due to the replacement of liver parenchyma by a malignant tumor, a benign lesion, a cyst, or an abscess was a considerable step forward for liver surgery.[72] Computerized axial tomography (CT scanning) resulted from an impressive collaboration between engineering and medicine involving an English electrical engineer, Sir Godfrey Hounsfield (1919–2004), and a physicist, Allan Cormack (1924–1998), culminating in them both winning the Nobel Peace Prize in 1979. Since its creation, this technology has gained impressive maneuverability with quick acquisition and accurate depiction of liver anatomy and its vascularization. Using 3D simulation, CT scanning allows visualization of intrahepatic blood vessels along with the calculation of the liver volume perfused by each pedicle. This technology initially developed in Germany at the end of the 20th century and was immediately adopted and developed in Japan and Korea for venous reconstruction in donor liver transplantations (LTs) and, subsequently, to prepare complex hepatectomies. The Nobel Peace Prize winning invention of magnetic resonance imaging (MRI) in 1977 by US physician and medical practitioner Raymond Vahan Damadian (1936) refined the exploration of the liver with better specification of both tumors and liver parenchyma analogous to a histologic approach.

The development of ultrasound for scanning the liver started around 1960 and rapidly became the first step in medical assessment of patients with liver disease. The quick adoption of ultrasound resulted because it was simple to use, there was no special preparation associated with it, and there was considerable improvement in the images provided. Studies in the United States detected gallstones and dilation of the biliary tree, liver abscesses, or tumors and their respective relationships with major vessels. Ultrasonic scanning facilitates liver biopsy and percutaneous cholangiography, and provides a sensitive means of detecting ascites. Introduced in biliary surgery by Bernard Sigel in the United States, intraoperative ultrasound (IOUS) was a revolution in liver surgery. In 1980 in Japan it was further developed with technical refinement allowing an accurate visualization of vascular structures and disclosure of small lesions.[78] IOUS made the liver transparent, allowing visualization of the complex layout of vessels impacting the surgical strategy. This innovation allowed identification of nonpalpable lesions and the development of oncologic resections according to the vascularization of the tumor. The introduction by Makuuchi of the concept of liver anatomic surgery using IOUS was a turning point in the practice of liver surgery (Fig. 0.13). This approach spread rapidly from Japan to France and Italy but appeared much later in the United States.

Technique of Liver Surgery

One of the greatest innovations in liver surgery was the temporary pedicular clamping proposed by James Hogarth Pringle (1863–1941), who was a surgeon of the Royal Infirmary in Glasgow with a passion for the treatment of trauma. In his paper published in *Annals of Surgery* in 1908, he reported reduction in liver bleeding by pinching of the portal vein and hepatic artery.[79] However, this maneuver was brutally attacked by European surgeons, predominantly the German school, who envisioned disastrous results from prolonged venous congestion of the splanchnic circulation.[72] Despite support in 1912 from John Mc Dill, who had a long and distinguished career in the US Army, the Pringle maneuver remained in the shadows for decades. The association of systematic control of the intrahepatic pedicle and resection was also a disruptive innovation. Initiated by Louis-Félix Terrier, this approach was perfected by the Vietnamese surgeon Tôn Thất Tùng (1912–1982), who was

trained in the French school of medicine in Hanoi. His outstanding knowledge of liver anatomy acquired by digital dissection of over 200 human livers, gave him a unique vision of regional anatomic demarcation for the 1930s. His comprehension of the segmental nature of liver substance allied with terrific dexterity allowed him to introduce intraparenchymal control of portal pedicles with finger fracture. By pressing liver tissue between the thumb and forefinger, until only vessels remained, this "digitoclasia" presaged the use of "hepatoclasia," which crushes the hepatic tissue with small Kelly clamps. His total commitment to his country during the colonial war between Vietnam and France and the latter against the United States have probably weakened his worldwide scientific reputation. He was one of the first exclusive liver surgeons who largely inspired French liver surgeons, inaugurating nearly 50 years in advance a true specialty. His intraparenchymal control of the first portal pedicles associated with hilar pedicle control remains the standard of liver surgery. The first publication in 1939 of the innovative approach by Tôn Thất Tùng included two successful cases of left lateral sectionectomies for patients with large hepatocellular carcinoma (HCC).[80] In 1948, after 220 published cases of liver resections, with the vast majority including left-side resection, it seemed that major resections were impossible. However, in 1949 Ichio Honjo in Japan, in 1951 J.L. Lortat-Jacob in France, and in 1952 J.K. Quattlebaum in the United states performed a right hepatectomy.[12,81] Although the French case was not the first, its report was the most renowned, with an accurate description of the procedure and a visionary consideration of the anatomic resection. In Paris in October 1951 Jean Louis Lortat-Jacob (1908–1992) (Fig. 0.12) operated on a 42-year-old man for a suspicious hydatid cyst; he discovered three tumors in the right lobe, corresponding to colorectal metastasis. His familiarity with esophageal surgery and with intrathoracic esophagogastric anastomosis led him to extend the incision to the right chest and, using this large approach, he completely mobilized the right liver toward the retrohepatic IVC. In contrast to contemporary surgeons, he did not start the section of the parenchyma immediately; instead, with his perfect knowledge of liver anatomy (learned from his friend Claude Couinaud), he controlled afferent and efferent vessels. The first step was hilar control of the right vessels and ducts followed by the division of minor hepatic veins to the IVC, and then he encircled and divided the right hepatic vein. Mostly, by finger fracture, the parenchyma was transected with ligature of the intraparenchymal vessels and ducts. He confessed to be surprised that there was no bleeding, but he was worried about the capacity of the remnant liver, which was "no bigger than a fist," to restore normal liver function. After an episode of jaundice and ascites, the patient was well 3 months later. During the report of this case on March 31, 1952, Lortat-Jacob imagined that the use of the right liver in transplantation could potentially solve some hepatic diseases once the problems of tolerance to tissue grafts and their rejection had been solved. Anticipating the use of a partial graft for LT, he was truly a visionary physician and surgeon who embodied the values of the modern liver surgeon.[82] Two years earlier, in March 1949, Ichio Honjo (1913–1987), a professor of surgery in Fukuoka, Japan, performed a right hepatic lobectomy for rectal metastasis in a 22-year-old man. This innovative procedure was performed through a large incision in the right and left quadrant associated with a long midline component. The liver was completely mobilized and the right branches of both the artery and the

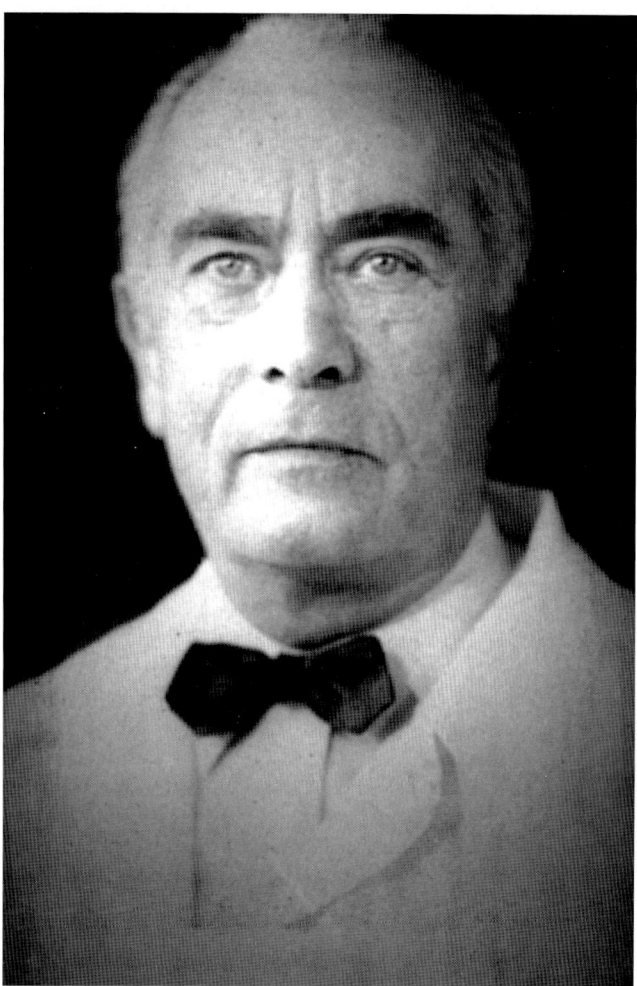

FIGURE 0.12 Jean-Louis Lortat-Jacob (1908–1992), surgeon.

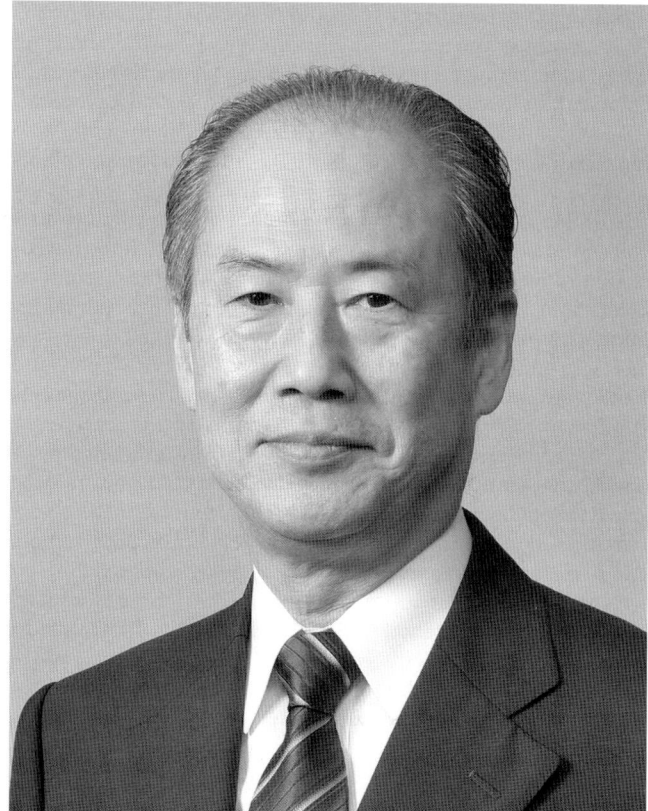

FIGURE 0.13 Masatochi Makuuchi (1946), surgeon.

portal vein were controlled. Once inflow was controlled, intra-parenchymal hemostasis was performed using silk sutures with the fear of compromising the vascularization of the remnant liver. The patient recovered uneventfully from this operation, which was reported in 1950 in a Japanese journal. This novel procedure escaped the attention of the Western surgical community until 1955 after its publication in an international journal. With this publication, Honjo inaugurated the next few decades of Japanese ascendency in liver surgery. In the 1980s the development of HCC in viral hepatitis was easier to detect radiologically and could be treated surgically. This situation was exploited by Japanese surgeons who were obsessed with minimal surgical risks. The establishment of the Liver Cancer Study Group of Japan in 1967 was focused on surgical mortality, which was approximately 1% in the 1990s.[77]

From this period, liver resection became a composite performance combining specific preoperative radiologic and biologic assessment, guided by IOUS, and including selective vascular clamping and sometimes preceded by PVE. The leadership of this school of thought was Masatoshi Makuuchi (1946), who can be considered one of the most innovative surgeons by the end of the 20th century (Fig. 0.13).

Makuuchi brought many innovations to liver surgery. A true Leonardo Da Vinci of our specialty, he established the safety limits for the extent of liver resection in injured livers using the indocyanine green (ICG) tolerance test, which is included in the so-called "Makuuchi criteria" for hepatic resection.[77] He described the extrahepatic division of the right hepatic vein in hepatectomy,[83] and introduced IOUS for the safety and quality of liver resections. He conceived preoperative PVE, which increases the volume of the future remnant liver and increases the tolerance of liver resection.[84] Makuuchi was the first in the world to perform surgery with an adult living donor, and further developed his interest in this field using venous drainage of partial grafts to define criteria for venous reconstruction.[85] He advocated hemihepatic vascular occlusion during liver resection in his first publication because it avoided splanchnic congestion and preserved vascularization of the remnant liver.[86]

Although the first Makuuchi maneuver did not have the same innovative success, his interest in the safety of vascular clamping led him to refine the procedure of the intermittent portal triad, and he was the first to demonstrate the safety of this type of clamping in harvesting a live liver graft.[87] Apprehension concerning the risk of ischemia induced by pedicle clamping outweighed its potential benefit to reduce bleeding. Several innovations aiming to reduce ischemia of the future remnant parenchyma were described. The first innovation was the refrigeration of the parenchyma. In 1963 Tong Ta Tung published an article in *The Lancet* about liver resection using portal clamping associated with refrigeration of the patient placed in a bathtub filled with ice to drop the body temperature to 30°C.[88] In 1974 Joseph Fortner (1921–2007) published a series of 29 patients with liver resection during vascular exclusion and hypothermic perfusion with only three postoperative deaths.[89] In the early 1990s Rudolf Pichlmayr (1932–1997), a transplant surgeon from Hannover, Germany, described a "bench procedure" with complete removal of a perfused liver allowing tumor resection in an organ free of blood. During this procedure, the patient remains anesthetized with a veno-venous bypass until the liver is reimplanted.[90] Daniel Azoulay from the Bismuth group, determined to push the limits of unresectability, clarified the indications of total vascular exclusion (TVE) associated with refrigeration.[91] However, the expansion of these major technical innovations remains limited with a decline due to the complexity of the procedure, the modest oncologic results, and the poor tolerance of diseased parenchyma with a high rate of postoperative liver failure.[92] The selective clamping of a hepatic lobe, a section, or even a liver segment promoted in the mid-1980s by Makuuchi limited the ischemia of the future remnant liver and facilitated the demarcation of the anatomic territories. For major hepatectomy, the division of the unilateral portal pedicle could be done by extensive hilar or suprahilar dissection as advocated by Bernard Launois.[12]

Although the selective control of pedicles becomes more complex for sectorial pedicles, selective vascular occlusion is still used by several western and Asian teams. The persistence of significant hemorrhage during the parenchymal transection, despite an effective portal pedicle clamping, revealed that the main source of bleeding originated from the hepatic veins and their tributaries. This was when anesthesiologists maintained high central venous pressure for liver surgery to keep ahead of the anticipated blood loss. Therefore the control of venous bleeding led many surgeons to exclude the liver from the splanchnic and systemic circulations by total inflow occlusion associated with clamping the IVC below and above the liver. TVE was described in 1966 a few years after the first LT by John Heaney from San Antonio.[72] At the end of the 1970s, Parisian Claude Huguet simplified and standardized this technique, which can be applied safely for as long as 60 minutes.[93] With an incredible talent for detecting and assuming innovations, Henri Bismuth and his team at the Hospital Paul Brousse published in 1989 their experiences with 51 patients that showed that the use of TVE allowed resection for some centrally located hepatic tumors associated in some cases with the reconstruction of vascular structures.[94] The routine use of TVE for major liver resection was doubted by a controlled study published in 1996, demonstrating that TVE is an invasive technique with nonnegligible morbidity and indicating that this procedure should be restricted.[95] One year later, a controlled study issued from the group of John Wong in Hong Kong showed that liver resections under vascular inflow control were safer than those performed without.[96] Although 1-hour continuous clamping is well tolerated in patients with normal underlying parenchyma, in 1992 K. Sugimachi from Fukuoka, Japan, introduced the concept of intermittent inflow occlusion in patients with chronic liver disease.[97] After years of debate concerning the respective durations of occlusions and reperfusion, the increased duration of surgery and blood loss from the transected surface during the perfusion controlled study demonstrated that intermittent clamping was better tolerated than continuous clamping.[98] The safety of a long duration of intermittent clamping, especially in patients with diseased parenchyma, was regularly reported in the early 2000s, rendering the attractive concept of ischemic preconditioning issued from cardiac surgery unnecessary in liver surgery. These debates on the safety of vascular clamping during liver resection were upended by R.M. Jones, a surgeon from Melbourne, Australia, who

demonstrated in 1998 that the reduction of the central venous pressure reduced intraoperative blood loss during liver surgery.[99] This breakthrough innovation requiring a new approach to anesthesiology allowed expert surgeons to perform routine liver resection with limited use of clamping.[100,101]

To minimize blood loss during hepatic resection many different methods have been used to cut the parenchyma, leaving vessels and biliary ducts that can be ligated or clipped. The finger fracture technique was subsequently improved through the use of surgical instruments such as a small Kelly clamp for blunt dissection (clamp crushing or "Kellyclasia"). In the 1990s ultrasonic dissectors, which were initially devoted to neurosurgery, were rapidly adopted in liver surgery and remain universally utilized because of their simplicity and the fascinating way they can selectively destroy and aspirate parenchyma cells leaving vascular structures almost intact. At the beginning of the 21st century several devices were developed, including the harmonic scalpel, LigaSure, TissueLink, and radiofrequency. None of these technical innovations have yet to emerge as a significant improvement with significant reduction of blood loss, biliary fistula, and duration of hospital stay. With a lower cost-effectiveness, Kellyclasia was not inferior to these technical innovations and remains widely used in open liver surgery, especially when associated with clamping a precise delimitation of the hepatic veins, which represents a true oncologic plan.[102,103]

A better definition of malignant liver lesions justifying resection was an important step in the 1980s. Leslie Blumgart (1931), especially after his move to Memorial Sloan Kettering Cancer Center in New York, developed an oncologic practice with great experience in resection for neoplasms. Advocating since the 1970s the resection of hilar cholangiocarcinoma and liver metastases, he built a surgical team with the highest expertise in various primary and secondary malignant liver tumors.[104] At the end of the 20th century, Blumgart contributed to the tremendous development of liver resection for colorectal liver metastasis in Western countries.[105] Whereas the surgical resection of benign liver lesions was declining,[106] the treatment of malignant tumors required a specific strategy, including anatomic resection for HCC and hilar cholangiocarcinoma and R0 resection in liver metastasis.[107] The anterior approach to major hepatectomy minimizing manipulation of the tumor-bearing liver was proposed by the Hong Kong group of John Wong,[108] and was facilitated by the "hanging maneuver" proposed by Belghiti and colleagues using a tape inserted between the anterior surface of the vena cava and the liver.[109] Since its introduction, this maneuver has gained worldwide popularity for large-sized liver tumors or tumor invading surrounding tissues and was subsequently applied to various anatomic resections with favorable oncologic results.[110] Although concomitant regional lymphadenectomy is not performed routinely, its prognostic value is important from the perspective of adjuvant treatment. The impact of postoperative morbidity on survival after resection of malignant tumors emphasizes the importance of measures such as preservation of venous drainage of the liver remnant and PVE.[107]

The unique regenerative abilities of the liver allow large liver resections and living donor LT (LDLT). The signals driving the process are complex but dominated by the portal flow. Enlargement of the left liver lobe was observed by Makuuchi in a patient with a hilar cholangiocarcinoma obstructing the right branch of the portal vein. This led him, in the 1980s, to develop an embolization of the right branch of the portal vein, which caused atrophy of the right liver balanced by the enlargement of the future remnant liver.[111] The introduction of this method was another disruptive innovation transforming the tolerance of patients after major resection of a diseased liver. In the 1990s PVE before major liver resection was widely adopted for several reasons, including its technical simplicity, its tolerance, and its efficiency.[112–114] The expansion of preoperative modulation of the liver volume using a vascular approach with the association of arterial embolization or hepatic vein occlusion was challenged by the two-step surgical procedure named "associating liver partition and portal vein ligation for staged hepatectomy" (ALPPS). This approach was proposed by Santibañez from Buenos Aires, Argentina, and Clavien from Zurich, Switzerland.[115] The high risk of this dual complex surgical procedure, which does not take into account the natural oncologic history and imposes a long hospital stay in a period aiming to enhance recovery after surgery (ERAS), explained why this innovation remains localized to certain centers only. In 2005 Guido Torzilli developed a conservative approach to multiple liver resections called parenchymal-sparing hepatectomy. This approach offered advantages over major hepatectomy in terms of tolerance without impairment of survival.[116] Since the beginning of the 21st century, the vast majority of patients operated on for malignant tumors had a diseased underlying liver parenchyma, including nonalcoholic steatohepatitis.[117] Parenchymal modifications decrease the tolerance of surgery emphasizing the need to use quantitative liver function tests. Measuring clearance of ICG, Makuuchi's group reported in 2003 a zero-mortality rate among more than 1000 hepatectomies.[118] However, during the last decade patients submitted to resection have been older and at higher risk with multiple illnesses, resulting in a liver resection stability of around 3%.[119] Therefore many liver surgeons put their hopes in the development of minimally invasive liver surgery.

Minimal Approach

The widespread use of laparoscopy in abdominal surgery, including biliary surgery, stimulated the development of laparoscopic liver resection (LLR). The first report in 1991 of LLR was from a gynecologic team who found incidentally superficial, small-sized benign tumors during laparoscopic surgery for gynecologic symptoms.[120] This innovative approach was exploited by multiple abdominal surgeons[12] until 1996 when Kaneko from Tokyo published the first series of 11 patients, including the first left lateral sectionectomy.[121] This Japanese team, still at the forefront of this procedure, used an innovative approach with accurate indications, including liver metastasis and HCC associated with cirrhosis. During the following years, LLR focused on lesions located in anterolateral segments that are more accessible laparoscopically and on anatomic resections with a small transection plane in a caudal-to-cranial direction.[122] In 1997 Huscher reported the first hemihepatectomy.[123] However, the expansion of this procedure was considerably slowed by the risk of major bleeding due to technical difficulties when mobilizing the right liver such as dissecting the IVC and controlling vascular and biliary pedicles in a large and deep area of transection.[122] Meanwhile advances in both instrumentations and technical skill caused the worldwide expansion of LLR, resulting in using this approach as a standard for left- and right-sided peripheral lesions as a routine procedure.[124] The advantages of LLR include better exposure with a magnified view through a minimal approach and decreasing postoperative pain, pulmonary complications, and ascites, resulting in a

shorter hospital stay. These advantages, however, were not sufficient to gradually replace conventional open liver resection. Even in experienced centers, right hepatectomy and resections of the posterior sector remains an exploratory procedure.[125]

To overcome the lack of 3D view and tactile sensation, which could impair oncologic value of LLR resection, intraoperative navigation using vascular and biliary reconstruction and an adjunct fluorescence camera for lesions not detectable with the naked eye have contributed to the improvement of LLR for resection of malignant tumors.[126] The laparoscopic surgical community is making efforts to organize consensus conferences and to promote prospective registries with scoring systems to grade the technical difficulty of this procedure.[127] In 2020, despite individual exploits such as living donor hepatectomies[128] or even total hepatectomies in the LT procedure,[129] the replacement of conventional open liver resection by LLR requires much more experience. The inexorable expansion of minimally invasive approaches has led the surgical community to explore robotic-assisted LLR. In 2003 Giulianotti published a series of abdominal procedures, including partial liver resection.[130] Despite the high cost of the robotic-assisted laparoscopic instrument, sold by a manufacturers that have monopolized the field, this innovation has been increasingly adopted by liver surgeons in the United States, Europe, China, South Korea, and Brazil. In 2008 S.B. Choi from Seoul reported the first series of a successful left lateral sectionnectomy.[131] The expansion of this procedure in the United States,[132] China,[133,134] and Korea was impressive.[135] The expansion of robotics in liver surgery are not only based on improved manipulation and instrumentation but also on the overall development of the digital artificial intelligence platform, facilitating the evaluation of the learning curve, integrating 3D reconstruction, and assessing surgical margins to achieve the standardization of surgical procedure.

Liver Transplantation

In the 1960s the success of kidney transplantation resulting from the use of effective immunosuppressive drugs opened the possibility to perform LT. This type of transplantation is forever attached to the name of Thomas Starzl (1926–2017) who initiated a procedure with multiple challenges.[135] Impressed during his residency by the consequences of the surgical treatment of portal hypertension, he started in 1958 with a National Institutes of Health (NIH) grant and an important experimental study on liver replacement in dogs. Francis Moore and Thomas Starzl published two important series of 30 and 80 cases of canine transplants, respectively, in 1960.[136] When Starzl moved to Denver in 1961, his activity was divided between kidney transplantation in humans and LT in dogs. His experience in animal models faced multiple problems, including anesthesia, organ preservation, reperfusion, hemodynamic tolerance of clamps, and bypass. The last key element highlighted by this work was "team construction," which is essential to the cohesion of a team.[135] With this background, in March 1963 he performed the first attempt at human LT in a 3-year-old who died intraoperatively. In 1964, after the failure of all attempts of LT by Starzl, Francis Moore in Boston, and Demirleau in Paris, a worldwide moratorium was imposed.[136] A few years later, a new enthusiasm for clinical LTs was generated by the advances in immunosuppression and the understanding that tissue matching was less important in liver grafting than in kidney transplantation. In 1967 the first successful LT was performed by Starzl in a pediatric recipient, and in 1968 it was performed by

Roy Calne (1930), the other pioneer of LT, in Cambridge, UK.[136] In 1968 the concept of brain death was accepted, which enabled a more controlled procurement procedure with improved graft quality. The first transplant unit outside of the United States was created by Roy Calne and associated with Roger Williams of Kings College Hospital in London. For nearly 20 years all immunologic and technical innovations were issued from Denver and Cambridge. In 1979 Roy Calne introduced the clinical use of cyclosporin, which improved graft tolerance with less toxicity.[137]

In June 1983, in Washington, DC, an NIH consensus conference evaluating the results of more than 500 cases in four centers worldwide with 1-year survival rates around 70% approved LT as a valid therapy for treatment of end-stage liver disease.[138] US centers were located in Denver and Pittsburgh, where Starzl moved in 1981 (Fig. 0.14); European centers were located in Cambridge–King's College, in Hannover headed by Pichlmayr, and in Groningen (the Netherlands) headed by Ruud Krom. In 1988 the use of University of Wisconsin (UW) solution extended the duration of organ preservation.[139] The growing experience in the United States and in European units in which Henri Bismuth established the European Liver Transplant Registry (ELTR) in 1985 contributed to select indications for LT, which have changed over the years. These changes were established during consensus conferences. Apart from the rational indications of irreversible toxic or viral parenchymal damages, malignancy was considered from the beginning of this procedure as an indication of LT. The firsts patients transplanted had unresectable tumors, but a low survival with a high rate of recurrence imposed a restrictive selection. In 1996 V. Mazzaferro defined the selection of cirrhotic patients who could benefit from LT in case of limited HCC.[140] The "Milan criteria" remains the focal point of the debates concerning this indication, and they represent nearly 20% of the worldwide indications of LT. This procedure treats the tumor and the underlying liver disease in patients with HCC, but many other primary and secondary liver tumors also can be cured by LT. The liver is the only organ whose transplantation can cure cancer. This characteristic can be partially attributed to the ability to administer more selective and less toxic immunosuppression regimens, because liver grafting stimulates less rejection compared with other transplanted organs.

For several decades, the LT procedure described by T. Starzl was well standardized and replicated worldwide after being exported by numerous surgeons trained in his center. After the resection of the native liver and enclosing the retrohepatic vena cava, the graft implantation procedure included vena cava anastomoses above and below the liver followed by reperfusion with the portal vein and then hepatic artery perfusion. The hemodynamic tolerance of total caval clamping was facilitated by the use of veno-venous bypass introduced in 1984. The preservation of the IVC described by Calne in 1968 was reintroduced 20 years later by Tzakis.[141] The "piggy-back" procedure requiring a single side-to-side caval anastomosis was rapidly widely used. In 1992 Jacques Belghiti from Beaujon Hospital in Paris described an LT procedure without the need for vena caval clamping.[142] The preservation of the vena caval flow permitted the preservation of the portal flow with a temporary portocaval shunt allowing hemodynamic stability, which is particularly important in patients with fulminant hepatitis who receive an LT.[143]

It was shown in a number of Asian centers that the involvement of liver surgeons in the world of transplantation was a strong factor stimulating technical innovations. In Europe, the

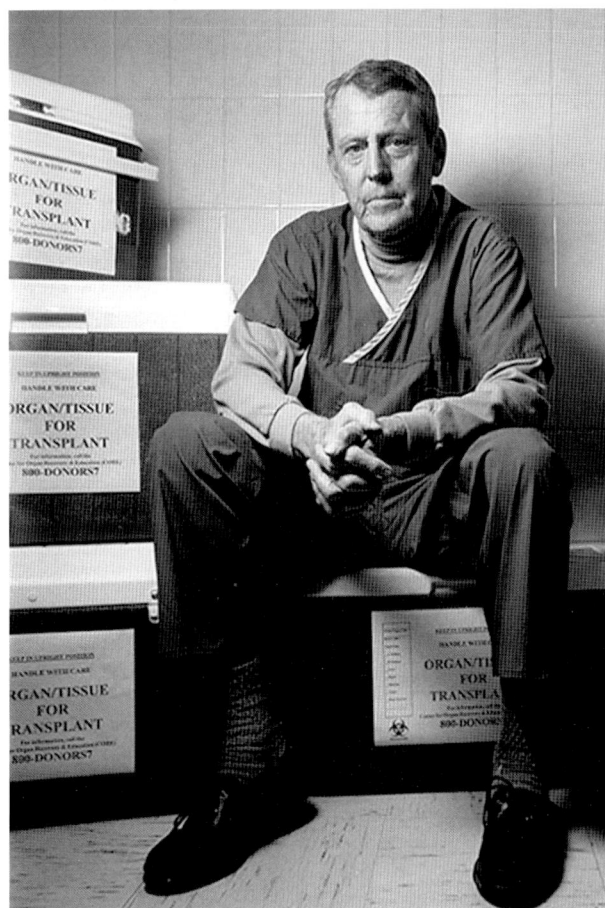

FIGURE 0.14 Thomas Starzl (1926–2017), surgeon.

LT community benefited from the connection of liver surgery with LT, particularly in Henri Bismuth's center. In 1984 Didier Houssin, also from this center, reported a reduced-size LT with ex vivo resection of an adult cadaveric liver to create an appropriately sized liver graft for an infant.[144] However, this technical innovation, which increased the number of pediatric LTs, had a negative impact on the adult population awaiting LT and is rarely used today. On the other hand, the ex vivo splitting of a cadaveric liver described in 1988 by Pichlmayer in Germany allowed transplantation to two recipients, usually a pediatric recipient for the left liver and an adult for the right side.[145] This procedure can increase the number of organs in the donor pool and is very attractive for that reason. It was later extended by Daniel Azoulay to include two adults.[146] However, the development of this technically demanding procedure had a limited expansion because it needed a good graft and a choice of two suitable recipients with an excellent organization. The concept of auxiliary liver transplantation (ALTx) was initially proposed to avoid a difficult native hepatectomy implanting a healthy liver graft placed heterotopically.[147] The high rate of vascular thrombosis, probably due to inadequate portal perfusion of the graft and inadequate drainage of hepatic blood flow, contributed to the abandonment of this approach. In 1991 G. Gubernatis from the Pichlmayer group published a successful case of fulminant hepatic failure using a new approach, in which a part of the native liver is resected and replaced by an auxiliary graft.[148] The use of an auxiliary graft, expectations of spontaneous regeneration of the native liver, and eventual withdrawal of immunosuppression drugs is based on the physiologic position of the hepatic graft.[149] The expansion of this innovation remains limited by the need of an excellent graft, the risk of vascular thrombosis, and the unpredictability of regeneration.[150]

The growth in indications and the improved results of LT has brought about the primary obstacle of it as an effective therapy, specifically, a wide discrepancy between candidates for the procedure and the number of available liver grafts. To overcome this situation, the transplant community attempted to establish a fair organ allocation, developed technical innovations, and extended the donor criteria. The organ allocation became rapidly crucial with several changes in prioritization of the candidates fluctuating from those who urgently need a graft and those who will get the most benefit. The medical and ethical debate concerning the allocation policy of cadaveric grafts remains focused on the Model for End-Stage Liver Disease (MELD) developed by Kamath and adopted in 2002 in the United States.[151] The MELD remains, after several adjustments, the best predictor of wait-list and post-transplant mortality.

The idea of removing part of the liver from a living donor was a strong motivation in pediatric transplantation. The unacceptability of a child dying while awaiting a graft stimulated the first attempt in 1988 by Raia in Brazil and the first success in 1989 by Strong in Australia, who transplanted a left lobe graft from mother to child.[136] The worldwide development of LDLT for children was accelerated by the possibility of obtaining an excellent small graft from a parent without major risk and few ethical issues. The first Western series of 20 cases was published in 1991 with an overall graft survival of 75% and patient survival of 85%.[152] LDLT was a true breakthrough innovation in Asian countries, allowing physicians to meet a need in countries where the availability of deceased donors was scarce. LDLT flourished in Japan where liver surgery was well developed but deceased donor graft donation was nonexistent. In 1989 Nagasue from Shimane performed the second successful pediatric case. In Kyoto University, Koichi Tanaka started a center in 1990 that concentrated a large number of cases and shortly became the world renowned for LDLT. He was the first to introduce microvascular surgery for hepatic artery reconstruction. During his time at Shinshu University, Makuuchi performed the world's first adult-to-adult LDLT, using a left liver graft in 1993.[153] However, it became quickly apparent that recipients with severe liver failure needed a large graft volume. In 1996 C.M. Lo performed the first right lobe harvesting at the University of Hong Kong.[154] This pivotal innovation, which facilitated and standardized worldwide adult LDLT, revealed that sufficient graft function and regeneration required complete venous drainage. This discovery, which prompted liver surgeons to revisit the anatomy of hepatic veins, was a subject of debate that ended with the rule to avoid graft congestion with venous reconstruction.[85]

Donor right hepatectomy is a major surgical procedure that exposes a donor with no illness or medical indication for surgery to an operation with significant morbidity and mortality and is the source of ethical concern. Because any undesirable event in the donor was unacceptable, the continuous attention to the postoperative course of the resected donor was one of the major advances that the surgeon community has benefited from with the LDLT experience. In this context S.Y. Lee in Seoul proposed the most intriguing technical innovations, using two left grafts from two donors in a single recipient.[155] Although this technique minimizes donor risk, the requirements of increased medical expertise and resources did not lead to wide acceptance.

However, the Asan Medical Center in Seoul headed by S.Y. Lee rapidly became the mecca of LDLT with hundreds of cases per year exploring all technical refinements, including vascular/biliary anastomosis, graft selection, countermeasures against small-for-size syndrome, and ABO-incompatible grafts.[156] Although ethical issues related to the use of unrelated living donors have been raised in some countries in Asia, in the Middle East and in Africa this procedure will continue to remain the predominant form of LT in countries where the combination of demographic, social, religious, economic, and political factors limits the use of a deceased donor. In the United States and Europe, LDLT stagnates to less than 2% of LT despite the persistent organ shortage and some innovative approaches minimizing donor trauma.[128] Proposed in 1995 by A. Casavilla in Spain and G. Kootstra in Maastrich, the use of donation after circulatory death (DCD) was put forth with considerable effort to expand the donor pool.[157] The initial use of these marginal grafts was associated with higher biliary complications, which dramatically decrease with appropriate donor and recipient selection and advances in cooling and pretransplant organ perfusion. DCD organs represented the fastest growing pool of organs for donation in the United States and Europe. The renewed interest in preservation technology was stimulated by the growing use of grafts with greater preoperative damage aiming to improve tolerance to ischemia but also to assess viability and function before transplantation. Oxygenated hypothermic and normothermic machine perfusion (NMP) have emerged as valid novel modalities for advanced organ preservation. The use of machine perfusion has several theoretical benefits, including organ repair, that may lead to improved organ quality, pretransplantation viability assessment of the donor organ, and extension of the amount of time between organ recovery and LT. Liver hypothermic machine perfusion (HMP) has been translated from the experimental state to clinical reality over the last decade. In 2010 Jean Emond and his group from Colombia University were the first to publish a series of patients who underwent LT of grafts preserved by nonoxygenated HMP with outcomes similar to a matched static cold storage (SCS) control group. Five years later the same group showed fewer biliary complications and shorter hospital stays by transplanting a series of 31 marginal grafts preserved under hypothermic dynamic conditions at 4°C to 8°C.[158] These results were confirmed by an international matched-case analysis, using a new machine perfusion called "*h*ypothermic *o*xygenated *p*erfusion" (HOPE).[159] Although HOPE become a widely used technology, in 2016 P.J. Friend from Birmingham, UK, published the first successful clinical application of an NMP functioning at 37°C.[160] The belief that cold storage is the best preservation procedure was cracked. In 2018 Friend published an RCT establishing the superiority of NMP regarding the utilization of liver grafts.[161] The "almost" physiologic effect of NMP can open ex situ clinical and experimental studies ranging from parenchymal remodeling, drug action, immunologic modification, and the generation of a chimeric organ.

In writing this historical description, we have drawn freely on the work of L. Blumgart[12] in his chapter from the previous edition and the recent book of T. Helling and D. Azoulay.[72] We are indebted to some excellent publications for allowing us to put into perspective several historical reviews, including S.A. Ahrendt,[13] F. Glenn,[6] T. Starzl,[135] and S. Navarro.[30] There will be some disputed claims concerning the "firsts," we mentioned, but we tried to relate a fascinating surgical story.

References are available at expertconsult.com.

PART 1

Liver, Biliary, and Pancreatic Anatomy and Physiology

CHAPTER 1

Embryologic development of the liver, biliary tract, and pancreas

Mark Davenport and Philippa Francis-West

INTRODUCTION

The liver's essential structure is one of layers of metabolically active hepatocytes arrayed along and around a vascular network carrying nutrient-rich blood derived from the products of intestinal absorption, otherwise semi-isolated from the systemic circulation. The biliary ducts are interleaved and intimate within this system and provide an excretory apparatus linking back with the intestinal tract.

The pancreas, by contrast, has two completely independent functional units. One is a relatively simple exocrine repository of initially inactive digestive enzymes; the other is a complex array of endocrine cells devoted to various homeostatic processes and feedback loops.

The first period of development is considered to extend from fertilization to form a single-celled zygote, or **ovum,** in the Fallopian tube to the implantation of the multicellular blastocyst into the wall of the uterus and lasts about seven days. Gastrulation in week three generates the three embryonic tissue layers: the ectoderm, mesoderm, and endoderm, which will contribute to various cell types within different organs. The first eight weeks post-fertilization are conventionally described as the **embryonic period**. They involve the formation of the major organs of the body and are followed by the **fetal period**, which involves further growth and maturation, extending to the time of birth and delivery.

Both the liver and pancreas start to develop during the embryonic period. Despite their very different functions and structures, the liver and pancreas initially arise from the same population of bipotent endodermal cells (Sox17, FoxA, Hhex, Gata-expressing), which can form either the liver or pancreas, depending on the growth factor signals from surrounding tissues. This region of endoderm also gives rise to the gallbladder and extrahepatic biliary system. Specification into the two different organs is dependent on the differential expression of the transcription factors PDX1 and PTF1A for the pancreas and HHEX, FOXA1/2, GATA4, HNF1β, and HNF4α for the liver. GATA4 and FOXA1/2 are known as "pioneer" transcription factors that are pre-assembled at liver-specific genes such as albumin, allowing a rapid induction of liver fate.

Gestational age is different from post-fertilization because it is measured from the last menstrual period, which effectively adds two weeks to the timeline described. Actually, this is a term seldom used by embryologists, but becomes more valid clinically by the end of the whole process.

Much of the work detailing the anatomy and timing of embryologic events was performed by Franklin Mall and later George Streeter in the Carnegie Institution in Baltimore, MD during the first part of the 20th century. From this ensued the widely-used classification of **Carnegie Staging** (stages 1–23).

DEVELOPMENT OF LIVER AND BILE DUCTS

Development of the liver can be divided into several phases (Fig. 1.1). During the early embryonic phase, there is induction of the liver diverticulum from the endoderm and growth with the formation of hepatoblasts to form the liver bud. The late embryonic period is defined by the onset of generation of hepatocytes, which will form the bulk of the liver, and of cholangiocytes, which will form the bile ducts. These two cell types arise from the bipotential hepatoblast that expresses markers of both hepatocytes and cholangiocytes. The fetal period is characterized by further differentiation of hepatocytes and cholangiocytes, which become organized into liver lobules and bile ducts, respectively. During this phase, there is maturation of the hepatocytes, together with further expansion of the liver and bile ducts at the periphery of the liver.[1]

This chapter provides an overview of key events and the growth factor signals and transcriptional factors required for liver development. More detailed information can be found in Gordillo et al.,[2] Ober and Lemaigre,[3] and Peruggoria et al.[4]

Weeks 4 to 5 Post-Fertilization (Carnegie Stages 10–15)

At the start of this period, the embryo measures about two to three mm, has implanted into the endometrial layer of the uterine wall, and externally is characterized by the formation of somites. The primitive endodermal intestinal tube has formed but is blind, occluded at either end by the buccopharyngeal and cloacal membranes and conventionally divided according to its three supplying arteries as foregut, midgut, and hindgut.

The liver and biliary tract arises initially as an endodermal bud from the distal foregut within the ventral mesogastrium, projecting into the mesenchyme of the **septum transversum**. This endodermal bud is formed from two endodermal origins: two lateral domains and the ventral midline of endoderm lip (VMEL), where the endoderm folds into the anterior intestinal portal.[5] The lateral and VMEL endodermal domains will generate the posterior and anterior parts of the liver, respectively. The liver primordia develops into a funnel-shaped structure with a lumen evident throughout, and from about 45 days the thicker-walled gallbladder also becomes evident.

Induction of the liver diverticulum is controlled by growth factors: bone morphogenetic proteins (BMPs) from the septum transversum and lateral plate mesoderm, together with fibroblast growth factors (FGFs) from precardiac mesoderm and signals from the surrounding endothelial cells (Table 1.1). Specifically, BMPs specify liver fate in the VMEL precursors, whereas FGFs induce liver formation in the lateral endodermal hepatic precursors. These growth factors induce or maintain the expression of the transcription factors FOXA1&2, HHEX,

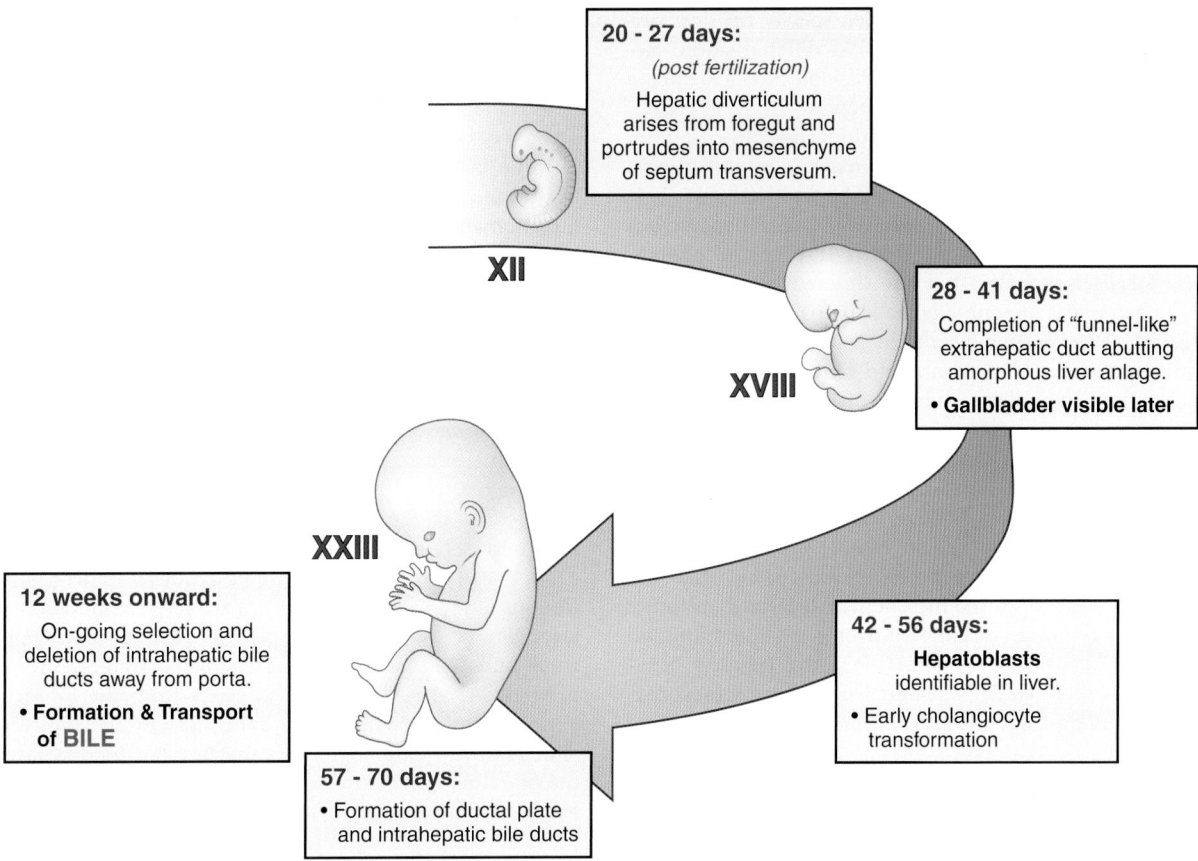

20 - 27 days:

(post fertilization)

Hepatic diverticulum arises from foregut and portrudes into mesenchyme of septum transversum.

XII

XVIII

28 - 41 days:

Completion of "funnel-like" extrahepatic duct abutting amorphous liver anlage.
- **Gallbladder visible later**

XXIII

12 weeks onward:

On-going selection and deletion of intrahepatic bile ducts away from porta.
- **Formation & Transport of BILE**

42 - 56 days:

Hepatoblasts identifiable in liver.
- Early cholangiocyte transformation

57 - 70 days:
- Formation of ductal plate and intrahepatic bile ducts

FIGURE 1.1 **Bile duct development timeline.** Roman numerals refer to Carnegie stages of embryo development.

TABLE 1.1	Genes Involved in Early Liver, Bile Duct, and Pancreas Development		
	DERIVATION	**POSSIBLE FUNCTION**	**CHROMOSOME**
BMP	Bone morphogenic protein	Growth factor family; multifunctional role.	Ch6 (Depends on member)
FGF	Fibroblast growth factor	Growth factor family; multifunctional role.	Ch10 (Depends on member)
VEGF	Vascular endothelial growth factor	The protein acts on endothelial cells, increasing permeability and inducing angiogenesis.	Ch6
PDX1	Pancreas/duodenum homeobox protein 1	Transcription factor; pancreas development	Ch13
HES-1	Hairy and enhancer of split 1 (*Drosophila*)	Transcription factor family; target of Notch signaling	Ch3
PROX-1	Prospero homeobox 1	Homeobox transcription factor; needed for hepatocyte formation.	Ch1
HNF-6 (*ONECUT-1*)	Hepatocyte nuclear factor	Transcription factor; needed for cholangiocyte formation.	Ch15
NOTCH 1-4	Mutation produced irregular ("notches") in wing tips of *Drosophila*.	Receptors for signaling network, which regulates interactions between physically adjacent cells.	Ch9
NEUROG3	Neurogenin 3	Basic Helix-loop-helix transcription factor; essential for endocrine lineage	Ch10
SOX-9	SRY (sex determining region Y)-box 9	Forms DNA-binding proteins; needed for cholangiocyte differentiation.	Ch17
WNT	Wg & Int standing for wingless-related integration (*Drosophila*)	Growth factor family; multifunctional roles. Canonical: cell proliferation & survival; Planar Cell Polarity: coordinated cell polarity and behavior	(Depends on member)
SHH	Sonic hedgehog	Early embryonic patterning, cell proliferation, and survival	Ch7
LGR-4	Leucine-rich repeat containing G protein-coupled receptor.	Gallbladder maturation	Ch11
PAX-6	Paired box - 6	Transcription factor; for endocrine cell lineage	Ch11
(C/EBP)	CCAAT/enhancer binding protein	Transcription factor; needed for hepatocyte formation.	N/A
PTF1A	Pancreas-specific transcription factor 1A	Transcription factor; pancreas development	Ch10

HNF1β, HNF4α, and GATA4&6, which specify the liver primordium and are needed for hepatoblast differentiation. Repression of the β-catenin (canonical Wnt) and Notch signaling pathways are also required for liver induction.

From the cranial aspect of the endodermal diverticulum emerge the primordial liver cells, known as the **hepatoblasts**. Hepatoblasts are the precursors of both hepatocytes and cholangiocytes and express markers of both lineages: hepatocytes (e.g., α-fetoprotein, albumin, HNF4α, HHEX) and cholangiocytes (HNF1β and CK19, a late differentiation marker). Initially hepatoblasts are cuboidal cells lining the invaginating diverticulum. Proliferation results in a "multilayered" pseudostratified endodermal structure and requires HHEX. Subsequently, the hepatoblasts reduce their cell–cell contacts, delaminate, and migrate into the septum transversum to become arranged in plates, initially three to four cells thick, which line the vascular sinusoids. This delamination phase requires the transcription factors PROX1, HNF6 (ONECUT1), and ONECUT2. The ingrowing columns of cells, known here as "cords" (sometimes "chords"), also have an intimate relationship with the mesenchymal-derived endothelial cells lining primitive vascular sinusoids. Proliferation and cell survival are controlled by paracrine Wnt, FGF, and hepatocyte growth factor (HGF) signaling from adjacent mesodermal cells, including from the closely opposed liver sinusoidal endothelial cells.

The embryonic liver is populated not only by the hepatoblasts but also by **hematopoietic cells,** originally derived from the yolk sac and then from the aorta-gonad-mesenchyme region and placenta. Hematopoietic cells will form the bulk of the liver, and hematopoietic maturation becomes the dominant feature during the second trimester. Hematopoietic cells produce Oncostatin M (OSM), which also increases hepatoblast proliferation, contributing to liver growth until late fetal development.

Weeks 6 to 8 Post-Fertilization (Carnegie 16–23)

The liver is by now a large, rounded mass of tissue called the *liver anlage* (German for "rudimentary organ or part") and the dominant organ by mass within the abdomen. Later, it will push the embryonic gut into the base of the umbilicus before it returns, and complete closure of the anterior abdominal wall occurs at around 12 weeks gestation. Failure of this return phase leads to an omphalocele (or exomphalos), of which the liver can form a major part.

Hepatoblasts are the parental cells for two key cellular progeny, **hepatocytes** and **cholangiocytes**, and differentiation occurs later at or around the seventh week (see Fig. 1.1). This common cellular origin has implications for malignant disease in adults. Notch signaling from the portal vein mesenchyme promotes cholangiocyte formation, and hence ductal development, whilst inhibiting hepatocyte development. Other growth factors needed for cholangiocyte cell fate include transforming growth factor (TGF)-β, BMPs, and FGFs. Cholangiocyte differentiation requires the HNF1β, HNF6, and SOX9 transcription factors. In contrast, hepatocyte induction requires FGF, HGF, and OSM signaling from the surrounding mesodermal cells, including the hematopoietic precursors and mesothelial cells that surround and line the liver lobes. Hepatocyte fate requires the transcription factors HNF4α and C/EBPα. The transcription factor PROX1 (and TBX3) determines which cell fate develops from the bipotential

hepatoblasts; in the absence of PROX1, fewer hepatocytes are formed, which is associated with an increase in cholangiocyte number.

Intrahepatic bile ducts only appear distinctly from about seven weeks gestation, and formation is organized by the portal vein.[6,7] At seven weeks, the portal venous network is infiltrating the liver anlage and becomes surrounded by a layer of mesenchyme. From this a cylindrical double cell layer of darkly staining cells adjacent to the portal vein emerges, which is termed the **ductal (or limiting) plate**. The bile ducts are generated from the dual-layer by a unique process of so-called *transient asymmetry*, whereby ductal plate cells resembling cholangiocytes (expressing SOX9 and CK19) on the side facing the portal tract are matched by ductal plate cells resembling hepatoblasts (expressing HNF4α) on the side facing the parenchyma.[8–11] After the formation of a lumen, the nascent bile duct becomes symmetrical, as hepatoblasts are replaced by cholangiocytes to form a double cell layer composed entirely of cholangiocytes, which will remodel to form a single-cell layer bile duct. Bile duct development is discontinuous along the portal vein, and selective remodeling of this layer generates an interconnected, single cell–lined network of small bile ducts within the mesenchymal architecture. Ductal progression and elongation proceeds from the hilum to the periphery and appears to be controlled by the noncanonical Wnt pathway. Cholangiocytes that are not incorporated into the bile ducts dedifferentiate into hepatocytes. At some point, extra- and intrahepatic systems coalesce at the interface of the porta hepatis, although the process is again imperfectly understood.[9,10] Hepatic arteries develop in association with the developing bile ducts and are thought to be induced by VEGF signals from the ductal plate.

The onset of hepatocyte polarity and generation of the polygonal shape characterizes the latter stages of this phase with structurally distinct apical, lateral, and basolateral domains. The basolateral surface abuts the blood-containing sinusoids, but is separated from them by the cell-free space of Disse. The apical aspect abuts onto adjacent hepatocytes, within which is the biliary canaliculus, the smallest component of the biliary network. These are delineated by tight junctions (desmosomes), with the remainder of this apical surface given over to gap junctions, which can be conduits between cells. The surface area of both the canaliculus and basolateral surfaces are multiplied by the presence of microvilli. This implies that the canaliculus is of hepatocyte origin, with later connections to the intrahepatic bile ducts emanating from the center. Nevertheless, the hepatocyte differentiation phase is most pronounced during the fetal stages and is linked to the reducing hematopoietic cell number as hematopoiesis shifts to the bone marrow.

The Ninth Week Onwards: The Fetal Phase

Bile acid synthesis starts at about six weeks, and bile is first observed in primitive cholangioles and then transported into the fetal gut from about 12 to 14 weeks gestation, implying completion of biliary continuity. The so-called "solid phase" of biliary development, formerly a widely held belief and an obvious corollary of biliary atresia, now appears erroneous.[12]

The other components of the mature liver parenchyma have different origins to the ones previously described. Kupffer cells are of a monocyte/macrophage lineage and appear at about five weeks gestation from fetal yolk sac precursors. Hepatic stellate cells are apparent by 10 weeks. These cells have molecular characteristics of all three germ layers and their origin is unclear, although some do appear to arise from the septum transversum. Mesodermal cells from the early liver anlage form the mesenchymal framework of the liver, including its perisinusoidal Ito cell population. Fetal liver stromal tissue consists of cells that express features of epithelium (Ck-8), mesenchyme (vimentin and osteopontin), and vascular smooth muscle actin (αSma).

The liver continues to develop throughout the fetal stage and after birth and is characterized by maturation, hepatocyte proliferation, and expansion of liver volume. Growth is controlled by OSM, glucocorticoids, HGF, and the canonical Wnt signaling pathway.[13] Hepatocyte maturation is more advanced in the center of the liver. Proliferation is highest at the periphery in response to paracrine signals from the overlying mesothelial cells. The bile ductal network also continues to develop at the periphery of the liver in response to Notch signaling. Until the late fetal stage, the bile ducts are all narrow. Then, there is remodeling and enlargement of the ducts at the center of the liver, potentially in response to the onset of bile flow.[1] Glycogen granules are present in fetal hepatocytes at about eight weeks, with the zenith of glycogen reserve achieved by the time of birth. Rapid onset of glycogenolysis over two to three days then depletes to about 10% of prenatal levels.

Vascular Events

The liver has a dual vascular supply, the portal venous system and the hepatic arterial system, which then drains by common hepatic venous channels into the vena cava and right atrium. The embryonic origins of the portal venous system are complex and involve two sets of paired venous structures: the vitelline and the umbilical veins together with posterior body wall venous structures such as the cardinal veins, which culminate in the inferior vena cava (IVC).

1. *Vitelline veins* (paired): These carry blood from the gut to an evolving sinusoidal plexus and are originally from the yolk sac—hence the name (*vitellus (Latin)*: color of yolk). Outside of the liver, they are interconnected to resemble a stepladder with the connections sometimes in front of and then behind the embryonic intestine. Remodeling and loss of some of these "steps" leads to the final arrangement of the S-shaped portal vein, which arises from the junction of the splenic vein and superior mesenteric veins anterior to the third part of the duodenum to then emerge from behind the junction of the first/second part of the duodenum to run in the free edge of the lesser omentum.

2. *Umbilical veins* (paired): These carry oxygenated blood passively back from the placenta to the right side of the developing heart at the *sinus venosus*. The right umbilical vein disappears early in gestation, leaving the other to be enveloped by the liver. This joins the left portal vein, which allows oxygenated blood into the sinusoids, although most continues into a low-pressure venous channel, the *ductus venosus* (or Duct of Arantius), which connects the left portal vein and the hepatic vein confluence. About 20% to 30% of this flow is shunted through this in the fetus, with progressive diminution as gestational age progresses. Oxygen saturation levels of about 80% can also be observed during the last trimester. By the time of birth and transition from the fetal circulation, the ductus closes functionally and later anatomically so the entire portal venous inflow is directed solely into the sinusoids. There is then a measurable increase in portal venous pressure after ductus closure. Commencement of enteral nutrition and consequent increases in intestinal perfusion also lead to increased sinusoidal liver perfusion and bile flow.

There are a number of different venous arrays within the posterior aspect of the abdominal cavity throughout embryonic and fetal life. The **posterior cardinal veins** are paired structures, which originally carry blood back from the lower half of the body. Their function declines during gestation, although they eventually will become the azygous[1] and hemiazygous veins.

The larger **IVC** is embryologically a much later structure and is formed from many different venous precursors, such as the **subcardinal veins** (to form the pre-renal portion) and **supracardinal veins** (to form the post-renal portion). The intrahepatic portion itself is an outgrowth from the **right subcardinal** vein subsumed in the evolving liver tissue (from about the sixth week) to anastomose with the hepatic vein confluence.

The ingrowth and indeed timing of the hepatic arterial network has been less intensively studied. Nonetheless, this is perceived as a relatively late event around about the time of the formation and expansion from the porta of the intrahepatic bile ducts. Thus there is a peribiliary arteriole plexus from the terminal branches of the hepatic artery at the periphery of the liver lobule, with arterial blood contributing to the sinusoidal network thereafter.

Clinical Correlates

Neonatal Cholestatic Syndromes

There are a large number of distinct cholestatic conditions that present during the neonatal period, with persistent jaundice and acholic stools. **Alagille's syndrome** is a multisystem genetic condition caused by loss of function mutations of the *JAG1* gene, a ligand for the Notch signaling pathway.[14] This leads to poor bile duct development (biliary hypoplasia), cardiac anomalies, vertebral anomalies ("butterfly" vertebrae), and an unusual "elfin-like" facies. **Biliary atresia** (see Chapter 40) encompasses a range of distinct variants, some of which may have their origins in embryonic life. Thus the **biliary atresia splenic malformation**[14] can be characterized as having an absent or poorly developed common bile duct and often an atrophic gallbladder in association with either polysplenia or asplenia and vascular anomalies, such as a pre-duodenal portal vein and an absent IVC. The pre-duodenal position of the portal vein is because of impaired development of the vitelline veins. Although this is not really thought of as pathologic in itself, it is clearly at risk of damage during dissection. Situs inversus is also present in about half of these infants – presumably reflecting randomness of the acquisition of visceral asymmetry. It is speculated that these key anomalies date the pathology to 20 to 40 days post-fertilization during the establishment of asymmetry in the embryo.[15]

It is not known when the pathology of the nonsyndromic forms of biliary atresia occurs, but presumably it must be either during or after organogenesis but independent of mechanisms that establish asymmetry. What appears clear is that in the vast

---

1 Azygous: From the Greek *azugos*, from a- "without" + zugon "yoke," the vein not being one of a pair.

majority, there is biliary obstruction biochemically evident by the time of birth.[16]

Congenital Portomesenteric Anomalies

The final functional result of the developed portomesenteric venous system is complete separation of it and the systemic venous system outside of the liver. Because of its complex heritage, this may not always be so, and as a result, there are a number of aberrant portosystemic connections described. The commonest is probably **persistence of the ductus venosus**. Normally there is fibrosis and anatomic closure beyond the first few weeks postnatally. This can be delayed and lead to a proportion of portomesenteric blood leaking into the circulation, not having gone through the sinusoidal network. Nevertheless, most close spontaneously within 2 years and rarely require surgical or endovascular closure.

The **Abernethy malformation**[17] is an interconnection of the portal vein and IVC, typically assuming an "H" shape at the inferior margin of the liver between the confluence of the left and right portal veins and the IVC. This is a permanent connection, and the degree of the functional venous bypass dictates its clinical consequences. Sometimes the entire portomesenteric venous flow bypasses the liver, with aplasia of the intrahepatic portal veins. This actually has no real consequence on liver "function" because its blood supply is then entirely derived from arterial sources. Nevertheless, presumably because of differing oxygen saturations within the sinusoids, there is a predisposition to the development of neoplasia, both benign with focal nodular hyperplasia and malignant with hepatoblastoma[18] (see Chapter 87). There are also potentially serious metabolic consequences with "unfiltered" blood entering the systemic venous system. Venous ammonia levels are usually high, and there is a predisposition to encephalopathy in later life and probably untoward effects on the developing brain, although this is poorly characterized. Surgical closure is certainly warranted and can reverse some of these histologic changes.[18]

PANCREAS

The pancreas is induced within the endoderm at Carnegie Stage (CS) 12. The pancreatic precursors arise within three locations: the ventral endodermal domain, the VMEL (both the ventral endodermal domain and the VMEL are common progenitors with the liver), and a dorsal domain to give rise to the dorsal and ventral pancreatic buds. Between CS13 and CS19, the multipotent pancreatic progenitors proliferate, and by CS19, cells of the exocrine lineage, the bipotential duct cells and acini cells, have started to differentiate. Generation of the endocrine lineage starts at CS21. At the end of the embryonic period, the ventral bud starts to rotate to unite with the dorsal pancreatic anlage. This chapter gives a brief overview of pancreatic development. For detailed reviews of pancreatic development, please see Jennings et al.[19] and Larsen & Botton.[20]

Development from Ventral and Dorsal Anlagen

The pancreas is derived from ventral and dorsal anlagen, which arise from the foregut diametrically opposite each other and are distinct from about day 26 to 32 (Fig. 1.2). The ventral duct is an off-shoot of the bile duct and maintains this bile duct connection throughout. The dorsal anlage will give rise to the head, body, and tail of the pancreas, whereas the ventral

bud gives rise to the uncinate (Latin – "shaped like a hook") process.

Actual fusion of pancreatic parenchyma occurs after a rotation of the ventral duct around the axis of the foregut at about 50 to 55 days. This differential heritage can still be evident histologically by staining for pancreatic polypeptide (PP). Thus, PP cells localize to the area derived from the ventral anlage, while the dorsal pancreas has larger lobules with PP-poor islets.

This process is also accompanied by a variable degree of interconnection of the ventral and dorsal ducts. Typically, the dominant flow of pancreatic secretions from body and tail and most of the head is preferentially directed through the ventral duct (of Wirsung). The entry of the smaller dorsal duct (of Santorini) is usually more proximal in the final duodenum and reputedly drains only the uncinate process.

The final phase of pancreatic development occurs later on during gestation. Initially, the junction of bile and pancreatic duct is outside of the wall of duodenum, but during the last trimester there is gradual absorption of this junction into the wall of the duodenum. The final arrangement is a common chamber (the ampulla of Vater), with each duct emptying in it but surrounded by its own sphincter to maintain bile and pancreatic juice separation.

Both pancreatic acinar tissue, ducts, and progenitor endocrine-active cells arise from the same multipotential precursor, with a process of layering and clustering of endodermal cells. Microlumens then form within the cluster and subsequently coalesce to form the lumen of a tubular gland. The first lineage decision is exocrine fate, with the generation of the bipotential ductal cells and the acini. Then endocrine cells are specified within the ducts to break away from the nascent glandular structure through the basal membrane into the surrounding mesenchyme. The endocrine cells aggregate and proliferate together as islet tissue. The first endocrine cells to form are the insulin-producing β-cells. Both insulin and glucagon can be detected in the fetal circulation by the fourth or fifth month of fetal development.

As in the developing liver, pancreatic development involves a series of steps: induction and proliferation of the early pancreatic progenitors followed by differentiation along various cell lineages. In contrast to induction of the liver, where BMP signaling is required, development of the pancreas requires an absence of BMP signaling. The absence of SHH signaling is also required for pancreatic fate: ectopic SHH promotes liver formation while inhibiting pancreatic induction. Although molecularly extremely similar, the ventral and dorsal pancreatic buds are also induced by different combinations of growth factor signals, reflecting their origin next to cardiac mesoderm/septum transversum/lateral plate mesoderm and notochord/dorsal aorta, respectively.

The developing pancreas is defined by PDX1, a member of the ParaHox group of homeodomain transcription factors, and SOX family genes are believed to be the key developmental genes required for normal human pancreas development[16,17]. PDX1 is an early marker for pancreatic progenitors that later "restricts" to the β-cells and is required for maintenance of β-cell fate and function (Gao et al., 2014). Pancreas-specific transcription factor 1A (PTF1a) is also an early marker of pancreatic progenitor cells, expressed slightly later than PDX1, and is needed to maintain PDX1 expression, providing a positive feedback loop.[21] SOX9 induces expression of FGFR3, a receptor

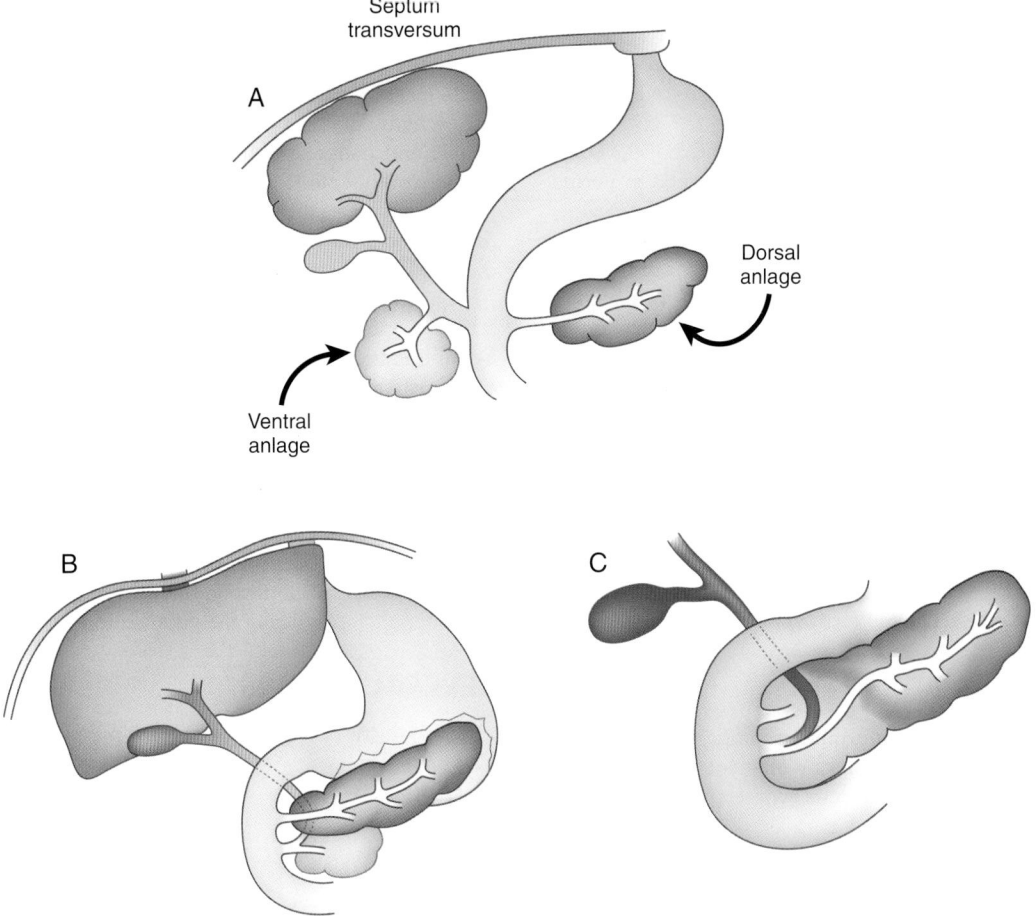

FIGURE 1.2 **Development of pancreas. A,** Initial separation with ventral anlage attached to developing biliary duct. **B,** Rotation of ventral anlage and bile duct behind duodenum. **C,** Fusion of the pancreatic anlagen with crossover of dorsal duct to now drain through the ventral orifice.

for FGFs which, together with Notch (and FGF10, BMP, retinoic acid and epidermal growth factor) signaling promotes proliferation of the pancreatic precursors. Mutations in PDX1, PTF1A, and SOX9 are all associated with pancreatic agenesis or hypoplasia. Mutations in GATA4 and 6 can also result in pancreatic agenesis. Because GATA4/6 normally repress Shh expression within the ventral pancreatic endoderm, this is because of ectopic Shh signaling and expansion of the hepatogenic domain.

A key step in pancreatic development is the lineage decision by pancreatic progenitor cells between the endocrine and exocrine lineage. Notch signaling has been identified as a master regulator of this fate decision switch.[22] Notch promotes ductal cell differentiation, while inhibiting endocrine cell differentiation. TGF-β signaling inhibits endocrine development. Specifically, the intracellular mediators of TGF-β signaling, Smad2 and Smad3, along with their inhibitor Smad7, have been found to play an intricate role in regulating pancreatic endocrine maturation and development. Genetic inactivation of Smad2 and Smad3 led to both a significant expansion of the embryonic endocrine compartment and a more robust islet proliferation in adult mouse pancreas after partial pancreatectomy. Genetic inactivation of Smad7 led to a significant decrease in the endocrine compartment with little β-cell proliferation after pancreatectomy in the adult mouse pancreas.[23,24] In contrast to

TGF-β, activin signaling promotes proliferation of the endocrine lineage. All the endocrine cells arise from a NeuroG3-expressing precursor cell, which is generated from the ductal tree and is present from weeks 7 to 35, with numbers peaking at week 12. The NeuroG3-expressing cells give rise to α- and γ-cells, which produce glucagon and pancreatic polypeptides, respectively, and β- and δ-cells, which secrete insulin and somatostatin, respectively. When NeuroG3 is deleted from cells, no pancreatic endocrine cells form,[25] whereas forced overexpression of NeuroG3 leads to cells prematurely committing to an endocrine lineage, which endocrine lineage is formed is dependent on the timing of NeuroG3 overexpression.[26] Thus NeuroG3 appears to be a critical and essential factor for endocrine differentiation.

Each endocrine cell type is characterized by a specific combination of transcription factors. Differentiation along the distinct lineages is also regulated by different signaling pathways. For example, TGF-β promotes β-cell development. Initially, pancreatic cells can co-express different endocrine factors, but eventually the majority will become restricted to one lineage via antagonistic feedback loops between these transcription factors. Therefore loss of one transcription factor will result in an increased number of cells of another lineage. This bipotentiality and the ability of specific transcription factors to direct fate may be exploited for therapies.

In vivo total ablation of β-cells (about 99%) can lead to α-cell conversion to β-cells via a bihormonal cell stage (glucagon positive/insulin positive).[27] Also, ectopic expression of PDX1 or PAX4 has been shown to induce α-cells or α-cell progenitors to convert to β-cells.[28,29]

In humans, loss of function mutations in *NEUROG3, GLIS3, PAX6, MNX1, NEUROD1,* and *NKX2.2* are linked to permanent neonatal diabetes myelitis (reviewed by Jennings et al.[19]). The essential role for NeuroG3 in specification of the endocrine lineage has been previously discussed, and the roles of the other transcription factors is being elucidated. These factors may influence development of specific lineages via specification of cell fate, survival, and/or proliferation. For example, Nkx2.2 is expressed as early and is co-expressed with PDX1, acting as a marker of multipotent pancreatic progenitor cells. Nkx2.2 expression eventually becomes restricted to NeuroG3-positive cells, persisting in all endocrine lineages except for δ-cells.[30,31] Nkx2.2-null mutant mice develop with no β-cells, reduced PP cells, an 80% reduction in α-cells, and no effect on δ-cells. Pax6 is also another marker of endocrine lineage, but unlike NeuroG3, it is not absolutely necessary for endocrine formation because null-mutant mice for Pax6 still form endocrine cells, albeit at a reduced rate.[32]

Clinical Correlates

See Chapter 53 for more information. Imperfect pancreatic fusion or persistence of an anterior element of the anlagen may lead to an **annular pancreas** where there is a ring of tissue surrounding the second part of the duodenum. Although of itself it is thought to be relatively benign, it can be associated with duodenal stenosis or even atresia. Some also seem to predispose to recurrent pancreatitis, presumably reflecting imperfect duct drainage.

Failure or imperfect fusion of dorsal and ventral pancreatic ducts leaves most of the parenchyma draining through the entire length of the dorsal duct and complete separation of bile and pancreatic ducts, and is then known as **pancreas divisum**. This mode of drainage seems to be less efficient and predisposes to recurrent or chronic pancreatitis, at least in children. Its relevance to clinical pancreatitis in adults has been disputed (see Chapters 55 and 57).

A **common channel** can be defined endoscopically in quite a high proportion of the population (~5%), most of whom are asymptomatic. Nevertheless, it does seem to predispose, again certainly in children, to recurrent pancreatitis and has been suggested as an etiologic factor for some choledochal malformations (see Chapter 46). Functionally, it allows free intermixing of bile and pancreatic secretions before they reach the duodenum. Such reflux into the biliary ducts can be quantified by measuring amylase in bile, and there is hypothetically a relationship that has been developed, particularly in Japan, with a predisposition to the development of neoplastic change in the bile duct and specifically the gallbladder.[33]

GENERAL READING

- Scoehnwolf GC, Bleyl SB, Brauer PR, Francis-West PH, eds. *Larsen's Human Embryology.* 5th ed. Churchill Livingstone, 2015.

The references for this chapter can be found online by accessing the accompanying Expert Consult website.

CHAPTER 2

Surgical and radiologic anatomy of the liver, biliary tract, and pancreas

Ronald P. DeMatteo*

ANATOMY OVERVIEW

Precise knowledge of the architecture of the liver, biliary tract, and pancreas and the related blood vessels and lymphatic drainage is essential for the successful performance of hepato-pancreaticobiliary surgical operations.

LIVER

The liver lies protected under the lower ribs, closely applied to the undersurface of the diaphragm and on top of the inferior vena cava (IVC) posteriorly (Fig. 2.1). Most of the liver bulk lies to the right of the midline, where the lower border lies near the right costal margin. The liver extends as a wedge to the left of the midline, between the anterior surface of the stomach and the left dome of the diaphragm. The upper surface is boldly convex and molded to the diaphragm, and the surface projection on the anterior body wall extends up to the fourth intercostal space on the right and to the fifth intercostal space on the left. The convexity of the upper surface slopes down to a posterior surface that is triangular in outline. The liver is invested with peritoneum except on the posterior surface, where the peritoneum reflects onto the diaphragm, forming the right and left triangular ligaments. The undersurface of the liver is concave and extends down to a sharp anterior border. The posterior surface of the liver is triangular in outline with its base to the right, and here the liver lying between the upper and lower "leaves" of the triangular ligaments is bare and devoid of peritoneum. The peritoneum reflects onto the right posterior liver from the medial aspect of Gerota's fascia, which is associated with the right kidney. The right adrenal gland lies beneath this reflection. The anterior border of the liver lies under cover of the right costal margin, lateral to the right rectus abdominis muscle, but it slopes upward to the left across the epigastrium. Anteriorly, the convex surface of the liver lies against the concavity of the diaphragm and is attached to it by the falciform ligament, left triangular ligament, and upper layer of the right triangular ligament.

Retrohepatic Inferior Vena Cava

The IVC runs to the right of the aorta on the bodies of the lumbar vertebrae, diverging from the aorta as it passes upward. Below the liver, the IVC lies behind the duodenum and head of the pancreas as a retroperitoneal structure passing upward behind the foramen of Winslow posterior to the right hilar structures of the liver. The renal veins lie in front of the arteries and join the IVC at almost a right angle on the left and obliquely on the right. The IVC is embraced in a groove on the posterior surface of the liver. The IVC comes to lie on the right crus of the diaphragm, behind the bare area of the liver; it extends to the central tendon of the diaphragm, which it pierces on a level with the body of T8, behind and higher than the beginning of the abdominal aorta. While the IVC courses upward, it is separated from the right crus of the diaphragm by the right celiac ganglion and, higher up, by the right phrenic artery. The right adrenal vein is a short vessel that enters the IVC behind the bare area. There may be a small accessory right adrenal vein on the right that enters into the confluence of the right renal vein and the IVC. Also, occasionally, a right adrenal vein drains directly into the posterior liver. The lumbar veins drain posterolaterally into the IVC below the level of the renal veins, but above this level, there are usually no vena caval tributaries posteriorly.

Hepatic Veins

The hepatic veins (Figs. 2.2–2.4) drain directly from the upper part of the posterior surface of the liver at an oblique angle directly into the vena cava. The right hepatic vein, which is larger than the left and middle hepatic veins, has a short extrahepatic course of approximately 1 to 2 cm. The left and middle hepatic veins may drain separately into the IVC but are usually joined, after a short extrahepatic course, to form a common venous channel approximately 2 cm in length that traverses to the left part of the anterior surface of the IVC below the diaphragm. In addition to the three major hepatic veins, there is the umbilical vein, which is single in most patients and runs beneath the falciform ligament between the middle and left hepatic veins; it empties into the terminal portion of the left hepatic vein, although, rarely, it drains into the middle hepatic vein or directly into the confluence of middle and left hepatic veins. This should not be confused for the umbilical vein from fetal circulation. In approximately 15% of patients, an accessory right hepatic vein is present inferiorly (see Fig. 2.3). Hepatic venous drainage of the caudate lobe is directly into the IVC, as described later.

   This classic description of the anatomy of the liver is sufficient for gross appreciation and for mobilization of the liver to allow access for repair of injuries, liver transplantation, or the placement of probes onto or into the liver substance. Hidden beneath this external gross appearance is a detailed internal anatomy, an understanding of which is essential to the performance of precise hepatectomy. This internal anatomy has been called the *functional* anatomy of the liver.

Functional Surgical Anatomy

The internal architecture of the liver is composed of a series of segments that combine to form sectors separated by scissurae

*The authors acknowledge Dr. Lucy E. Hann who coauthored this chapter in the fifth edition of this book. Much of her initial contribution is included here.

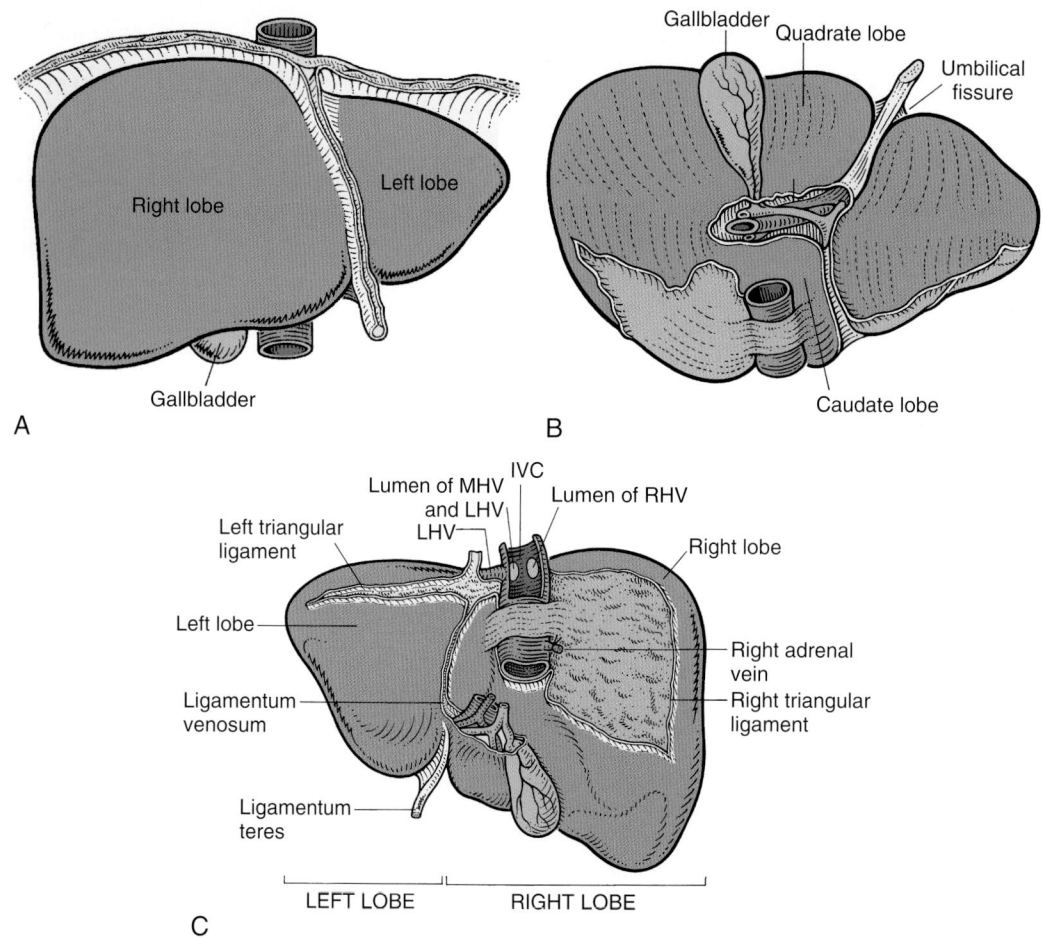

FIGURE 2.1 A, The liver as seen in situ has two main lobes, a large right and a smaller left, and conventional description places their line of fusion on the upper surface of the liver along the attachment of the falciform ligament at the inferior extent of which the ligamentum teres enters the umbilical fissure. **B,** With the liver flipped upward, the inferior surface of the right lobe is seen as the transverse hilar fissure, which constitutes the posterior limit of this lobe. The portion of the right lobe located anterior to the fissure is called the *quadrate lobe*, which is limited on the left by the *umbilical fissure* and on the right by the gallbladder fossa. Posterior to the hilar transverse fissure is a fourth lobe, the *caudate lobe*, which hugs the inferior vena cava (IVC) and extends upward on its left side. Thus the liver comprises two main lobes and two smaller lobes, separated by visible, well-defined fissures on the liver surface. **C,** The posterior aspect of the liver is shown. The IVC lies snugly in a deep groove within the bare area; the hepatic veins open directly into it. Within this bare area, the right suprarenal gland lies adjacent to the IVC, and the adrenal vein drains into the right of the IVC. The remainder of the bare area of liver is directly in contact with the diaphragm. To the left of the IVC, the caudate lobe slopes upward from the inferior to the posterior surface of the liver and is demarcated on the left by a fissure, within which lies the ligamentum venosum. The gastrohepatic omentum is attached to the ligamentum venosum, placing the caudate lobe within the lesser sac of the peritoneum. The left lobe of the liver is situated anteriorly in the supracolic compartment of the peritoneal cavity. The posterior surface of the left lobe is narrow; there is a very fine bare area on this side. While the vena cava traverses upward in the groove on the posterior surface of the liver, it is shielded on the right side by a layer of fibrous tissue that passes from the posterior edge of the liver backward toward the lumbar vertebrae and fans out posteriorly, especially in the upper part. Behind the IVC, a prolongation of this fibrous layer joins a less marked fibrous extension from the lateral edge of the caudate lobe. This layer of fibrous tissue, sometimes called the *ligament of the vena cava*, must be divided on the right, to allow surgical exposure of the IVC and the right hepatic vein, and on the left, to allow mobilization of the caudate lobe. Occasionally, the liver tissue embraces the vena cava completely, so that it runs within a tunnel of parenchyma. *LHV,* Left hepatic vein; *MHV,* middle hepatic vein; *RHV,* right hepatic vein.

that contain the hepatic veins (Fig. 2.5), as described by Couinaud (1957).[1] Together or separately, these constitute the visible lobes described previously. The internal structure has been clarified by the publications of McIndoe and Counseller (1927),[2] Ton That Tung (1939, 1979),[3,4] Hjörtsjö (1931),[5] Healey and Schroy (1953),[6] Goldsmith and Woodburne (1957),[7] Couinaud (1957),[1] and Bismuth and colleagues (1982).[8] Essentially, the three main hepatic veins within the scissurae divide the liver into four sectors, each of which receives a portal pedicle. The main portal scissura contains the middle hepatic vein and progresses from the middle of the gallbladder bed anteriorly to the left of

the vena cava posteriorly. The right and left parts of the liver, demarcated by the main portal scissura, are independent in terms of portal and arterial vascularization and biliary drainage (Fig. 2.6). These right and left livers are themselves divided into two by the remaining portal scissurae. These four subdivisions are referred to as *segments* in the description of Goldsmith and Woodburne (1957),[7] but in Couinaud's nomenclature (1957),[1] they are termed *sectors*.

The right portal scissura separates the right liver into two sectors: *anteromedial* (anterior) and *posterolateral* (posterior). With the body supine, this scissura is almost in the frontal

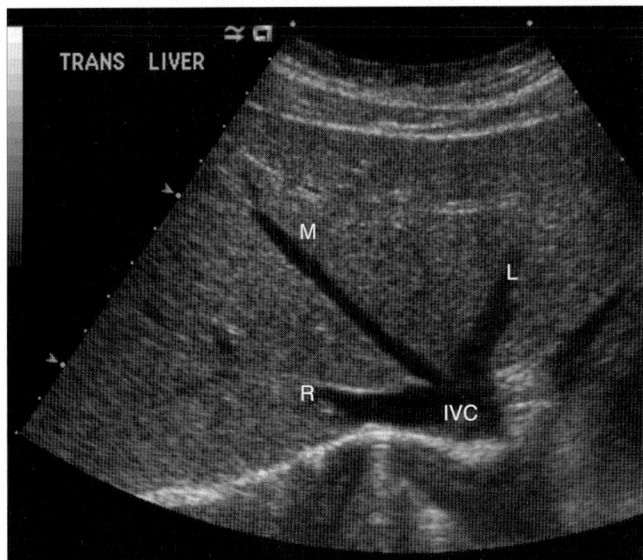

FIGURE 2.2 Transverse ultrasound image of the hepatic vein confluence shows the left *(L)*, middle *(M)*, and right *(R)* hepatic veins as they join the inferior vena cava *(IVC)*.

plane. The right hepatic vein runs within the right scissura. The left portal scissura divides the left liver into two sectors, but the left portal scissura is not within the umbilical fissure because this fissure is not a portal scissura, and instead it contains a portal pedicle. The left portal scissura is located posterior to the ligamentum teres and within the left liver, along the course of the left hepatic vein.

Although the description by Couinaud has been used widely, it is being replaced by an alternative terminology suggested by a committee of the International Hepato-Pancreatico-Biliary Association in 2000.[9] The main difference is that, in the alternative terminology, Couinaud's sectors are now referred to as *sections* (Table 2.1; see Chapter 103B for differences in the terminology of the various hepatic resections). Also, note that the left medial section, in the terminology of Strasberg (2005),[9] is composed of one segment (i.e., segment IV).

At the hilum of the liver, the right portal triad pursues a short course of approximately 1 to 1.5 cm before entering the substance of the right liver (Fig. 2.7). In some cases, the right anterior and posterior pedicles arise independently, and their origins may be separated by 2 cm. In some cases, it appears as if the left portal vein arises from the right anterior branch

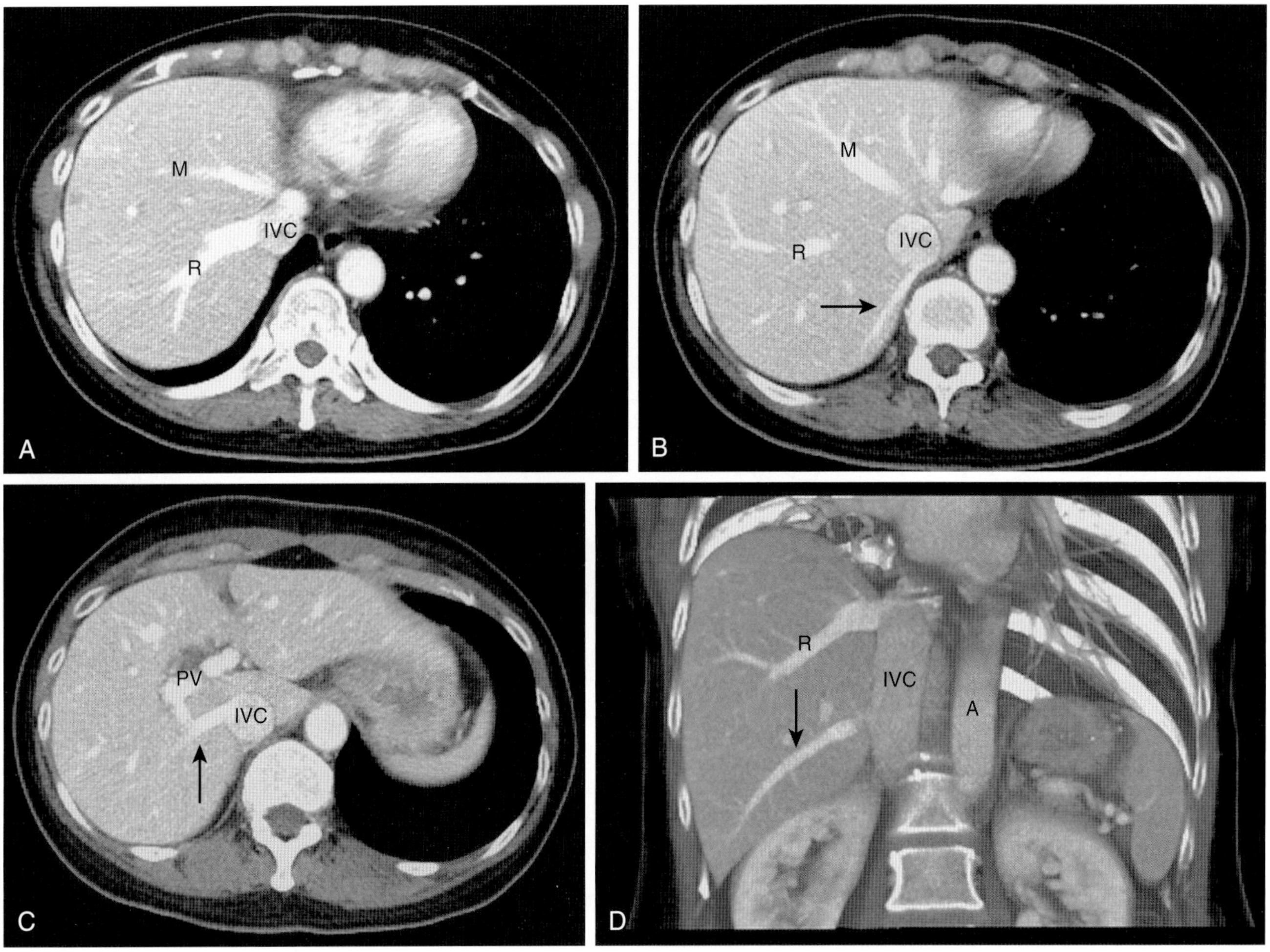

FIGURE 2.3 **Two inferior accessory right hepatic veins. A,** Contrast-enhanced computed tomographic (CT) image of the hepatic vein confluence. **B,** A small right inferior accessory vein *(arrow)* enters the IVC below the hepatic venous confluence. **C,** The second, larger right inferior accessory right hepatic vein *(arrow)* is seen more inferiorly. **D,** CT coronal reconstruction image shows the right hepatic vein *(R)* and one right inferior accessory vein *(arrow). A,* Aorta; *IVC,* inferior vena cava; *M,* middle hepatic vein; *PV,* portal vein; *R,* right hepatic vein.

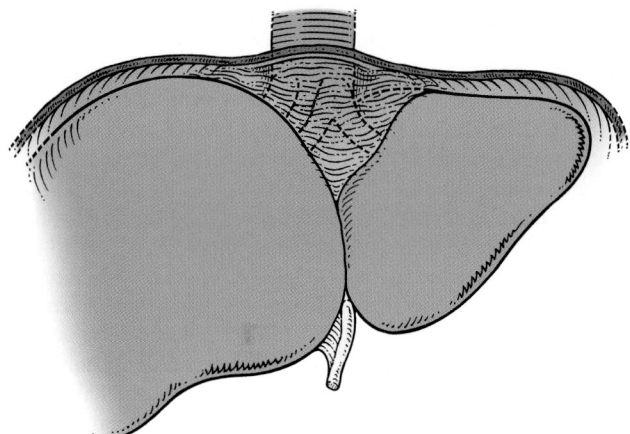

FIGURE 2.4 The anterior surfaces of the major extrahepatic veins and the inferior vena cava are retroperitoneal and masked behind the layers of the falciform ligament, while it splits and passes to the right and left triangular ligaments. The left and middle hepatic veins usually join within the liver and not outside the liver as depicted here for visual simplicity.

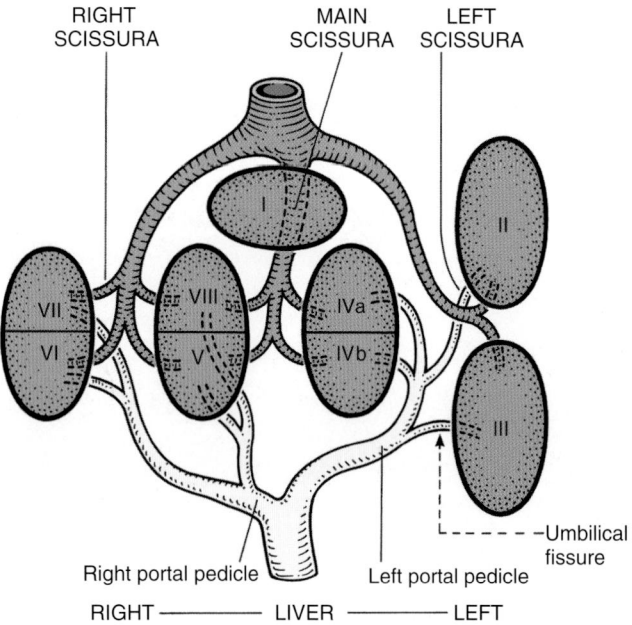

FIGURE 2.5 The portal vein, hepatic artery, and draining bile ducts are distributed within the liver in a beautifully symmetric pedicular pattern, which belies the asymmetric external appearance. Each segment (I to VIII) is supplied by a portal triad composed of a branch of the portal vein and hepatic artery and drained by a tributary of the right or left main hepatic ducts. The four sectors demarcated by the three main hepatic veins are called the *portal sectors* (now referred to as sections in the Brisbane terminology); these portions of parenchyma are supplied by independent portal pedicles. The hepatic veins run between the sectors in the portal scissurae; the scissurae containing portal pedicles are called the *hepatic scissurae*. The umbilical fissure corresponds to a hepatic scissura. The internal architecture of the liver consists of two hemilivers, the right and the left liver separated by the main portal scissura, also known as *Cantlie's line*. It is preferable to call them the *right* and *left liver* rather than the *right* and *left lobes* because the latter nomenclature is erroneous; there is no visible mark that permits identification of a true hemiliver.

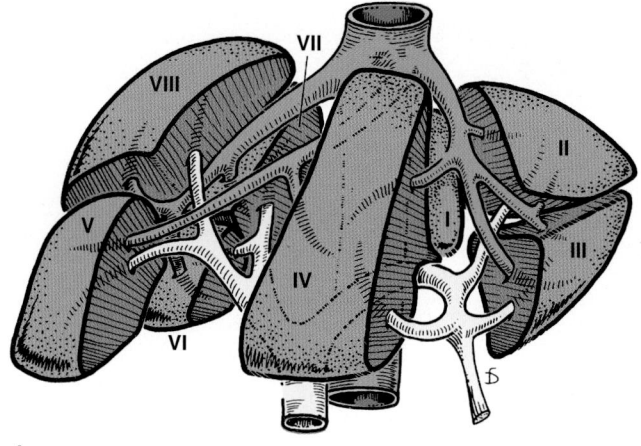

A

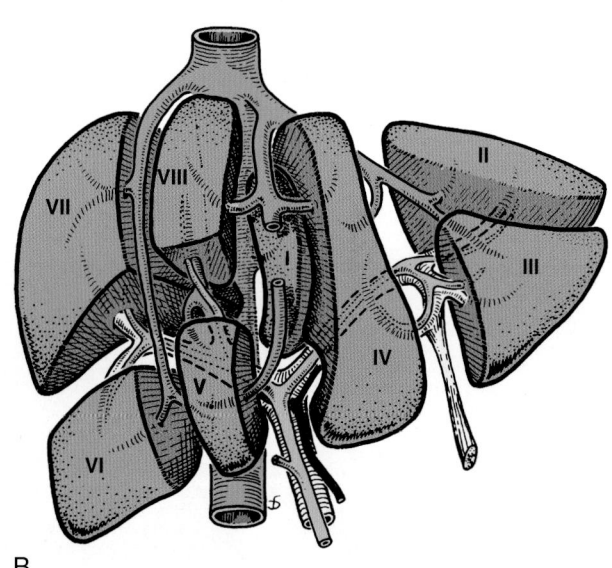

B

FIGURE 2.6 The functional division of the liver and its segments according to Couinaud's nomenclature. **A,** As seen in the patient. **B,** In the ex vivo position.

TABLE 2.1	Brisbane Terminology of Liver Anatomy and Resections	
ANATOMIC TERM	COUINAUD SEGMENTS	SURGICAL RESECTION
Right hemiliver/right liver	5–8	Right hepatectomy
Left hemiliver/left liver	2–4	Left hepatectomy
Right anterior section	5, 8	Right anterior sectionectomy
Right posterior section	6, 7	Right posterior sectionectomy
Left medial section	4	Left medial sectionectomy or Resection of segment 4
Left lateral section	2, 3	Left lateral sectionectomy or Bisectionectomy 2, 3
	4, 5, 6, 7, 8	Right trisectionectomy or Extended right hepatectomy
	2, 3, 4, 5, 8	Left trisectionectomy or Extended left hepatectomy

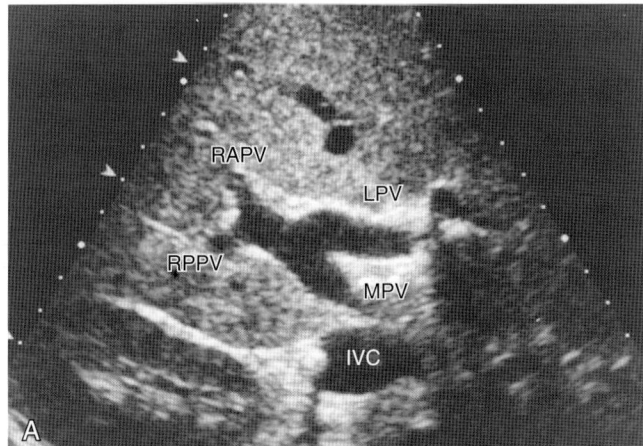

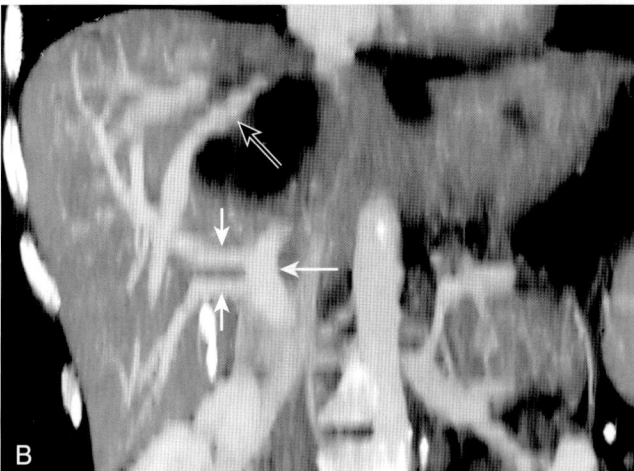

FIGURE 2.7 **A,** Transverse sonogram at the level of the portal vein bifurcation. The main portal vein *(MPV)* bifurcates into the left and right portal veins *(LPV and RPV)*. The RPV bifurcates shortly into the right anterior *(RAPV)* and right posterior *(RPPV)* branches, but the LPV has a longer horizontal course within the hilar plate. The inferior vena cava *(IVC)* is seen posteriorly. **B,** Coronal view of computed tomographic angioportography. Reconstruction shows the right hepatic vein *(open arrow)* and the portal vein *(large arrow)*; anterior and posterior sectional branches of the RPV *(small arrows)* are seen to arise directly and separately from the main portal trunk.

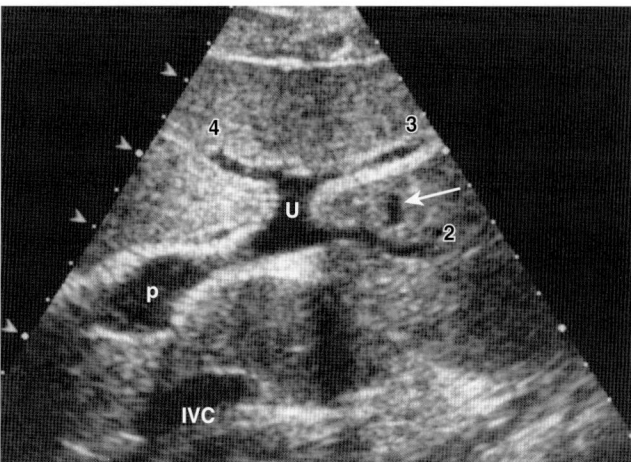

FIGURE 2.8 Transverse sonogram shows the branching pattern of the left portal vein *(P)*, which courses horizontally and into the umbilical fissure. The umbilical portion of the left portal vein *(U)* gives branches to the left hepatic segments (2 to 4). The left hepatic vein *(arrow)* and inferior vena cava *(IVC)* also are shown.

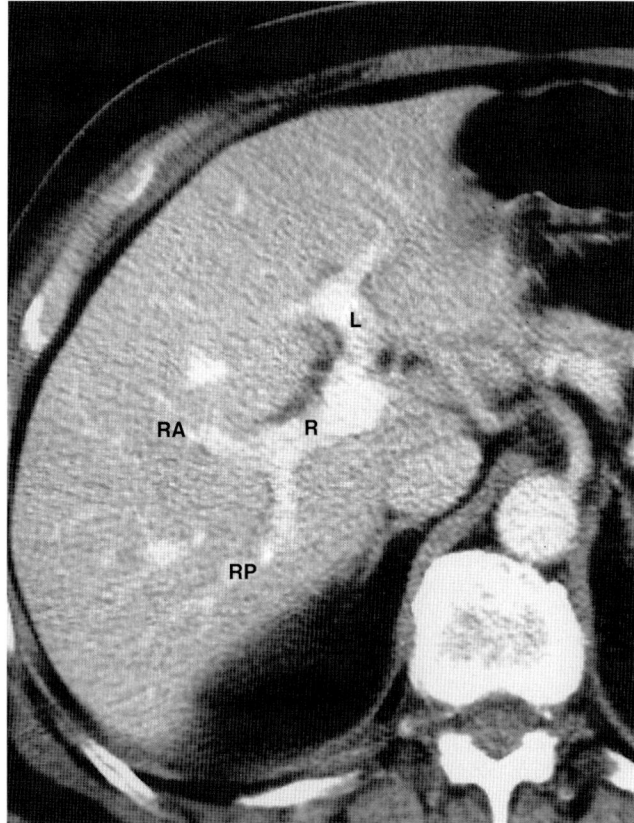

FIGURE 2.9 Contrast-enhanced computed tomographic image of the portal vein bifurcation. *L,* Left portal vein; *R,* right portal vein; *RA,* right anterior portal vein; *RP,* right posterior portal vein.

(see Fig. 2.40). On the left side, however, the portal triad crosses over approximately 3 to 4 cm beneath segment IV (formerly called the *quadrate lobe*), embraced in a peritoneal sheath at the upper end of the gastrohepatic ligament and separated from the undersurface of segment IV by connective tissue (hilar plate). This prolongation of the left portal pedicle turns anteriorly and caudally within the umbilical fissure, giving branches of supply to segment II first and then segment III and recurrent branches ("feedback vessels") to segment IV (Fig. 2.8; see Fig. 2.6). Beneath segment IV, the pedicle is composed of the left branch of the portal vein and the left hepatic duct, but it is joined at the base of the umbilical fissure by the left branch of the hepatic artery.

The branching of the portal pedicle at the hilum (Fig. 2.9), the distribution of the branches to the caudate lobe (segment I) on the right and left sides, and the distribution to the segments of the right (segments V through VIII) and left (segments II through IV) hemiliver follow a remarkably

symmetric pattern and, as described by Scheele (1994),[10] allow for the separation of segment IV into segment IVa superiorly and segment IVb inferiorly (see Fig. 2.6). This arrangement of subsegments mimics the distribution to segments V and VIII on the right side. The umbilical vein provides drainage of at least parts of segment IVb after

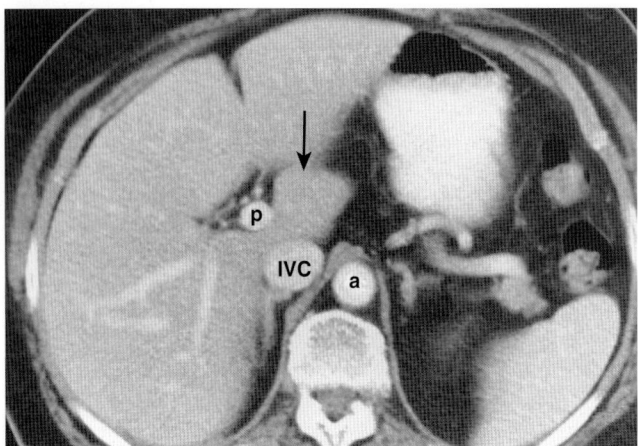

FIGURE 2.10 Contrast-enhanced computed tomographic scan of the liver shows the intimate relationship of the caudate lobe *(arrow)*, inferior vena cava *(IVC)*, portal vein *(p)*, and aorta *(a)*.

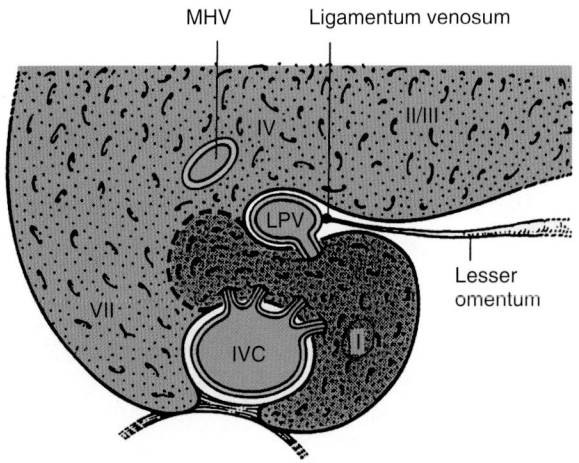

FIGURE 2.11 The main bulk of the caudate lobe (segment I; *dark area*) lies to the left of the inferior vena cava *(IVC)*; the left and inferior margins are free in the lesser omental bursa. The gastrohepatic (lesser) omentum separates the left portion of the caudate from segments II and III of the liver, while it passes between them to be attached to the ligamentum venosum. The left portion of the caudate lobe inferiorly traverses to the right between the left portal vein *(LPV)* and IVC as the caudate process, where it fuses with the right lobe of the liver. Note the position of the middle hepatic vein *(MHV)*.

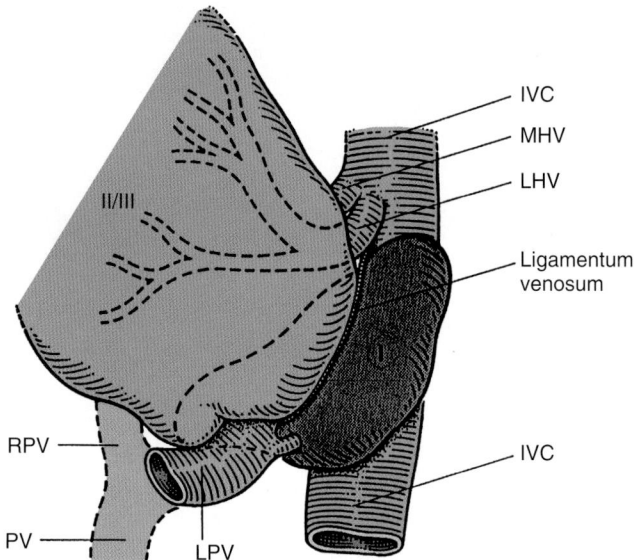

FIGURE 2.12 The caudate lobe *(shaded)* and segments II and III, rotated to the patient's right. Superiorly, the left portion of the caudate lobe is linked by a deep anterior portion, embedded in the parenchyma immediately under the middle hepatic vein *(MHV)*, reaching inferiorly to the posterior margin of the hilus of the liver and fusing anterolaterally to the inferior vena cava *(IVC)* on the right side to segments VI and VII of the right liver. The major blood supply arises from the left branch of the left portal vein *(LPV)* and the left hepatic artery, close to the base of the umbilical fissure of the liver. The hepatic veins *(MHV, LHV)* are short in course and drain from the caudate directly into the anterior and left aspect of the vena cava. *LHV,* Left hepatic vein; *PV,* main trunk of portal vein; *RPV,* right portal vein;

ligation of the middle hepatic vein, and it is important in the performance of segmental resections.

The caudate or segment I is the dorsal portion of the liver lying posteriorly; it embraces the retrohepatic IVC (Figs. 2.10 and 2.11). The caudate is intimately related to several major vascular structures. On the left, the caudate lies between the IVC posteriorly and the left portal triad inferiorly and the IVC and the middle and left hepatic veins superiorly (Fig. 2.12). The portion of the caudate on the right varies but is usually quite small. The anterior surface within the parenchyma is covered by the posterior surface of segment IV, the limit being an oblique plane slanting from the left portal vein to the left hepatic vein. Thus there is a caudate lobe with a constantly present left portion and a right portion of variable size. This portion of the caudate on the right is adjacent to the recently

described segment IX, which lies between it and segment XIII. The authors find segment IX of little practical clinical significance.

The caudate is supplied by blood vessels and drained by biliary tributaries from the right and left portal triad. Small vessels from the portal vein and tributaries joining the biliary ducts also are found. The right portion of the caudate, including the caudate process, predominantly receives portal venous blood from the right portal vein or from the bifurcation of the main portal vein, whereas on the left side, the portal supply arises from the left branch of the portal vein almost exclusively. Similarly, the arterial supply and biliary drainage of the right portion is most commonly associated with the right posterior sectional vessels and the left portion with the left main vessels. The hepatic venous drainage of the caudate is unique in that it is the only hepatic segment that drains directly into the IVC. These veins can sometimes drain into the posterior aspect of the vena cava if a significant retrocaval caudate component is present.

In the most common circumstance, the posterior edge of the caudate lobe on the left has a fibrous component, which fans out and attaches lightly to the crural area of the diaphragm, but it extends posteriorly, behind the vena cava, to link with a similar component of fibrous tissue (called the venal caval ligament) that protrudes from the posterior surface of segment VII and embraces the vena cava (see Figs. 2.1C and 2.11). In up to 50% of patients, this ligament is replaced by hepatic tissue, in whole or in part, and the caudate may completely encircle the IVC and may contact segment VII on the right side; a significant retrocaval component may prevent a left-sided approach to the caudate veins. The caudal margin of the caudate lobe can have a papillary projection that occasionally may attach to the rest of the lobe via a narrow connection. It is bulky in 27% of cases and can be mistaken for an enlarged lymph node on computed tomography (CT) scan (Fig. 2.13).

To summarize:

1. The liver is divided into two hemilivers by the main hepatic scissura, where the middle hepatic vein runs.

2. The left liver is divided into two sections. The Brisbane 2000 nomenclature describes the left lateral section (segments II and III) and the left medial section (segment IV).

3. The right liver is divided into an anterior section (segments V and VIII) and posterior section (segments VI and VII).

4. Segment I, the caudate lobe, lies posteriorly and embraces the IVC, its intraparenchymal anterior surface abutting the posterior surface of segment IV and merging with segments VI and VII on the right (Fig. 2.14; see Fig. 2.11).

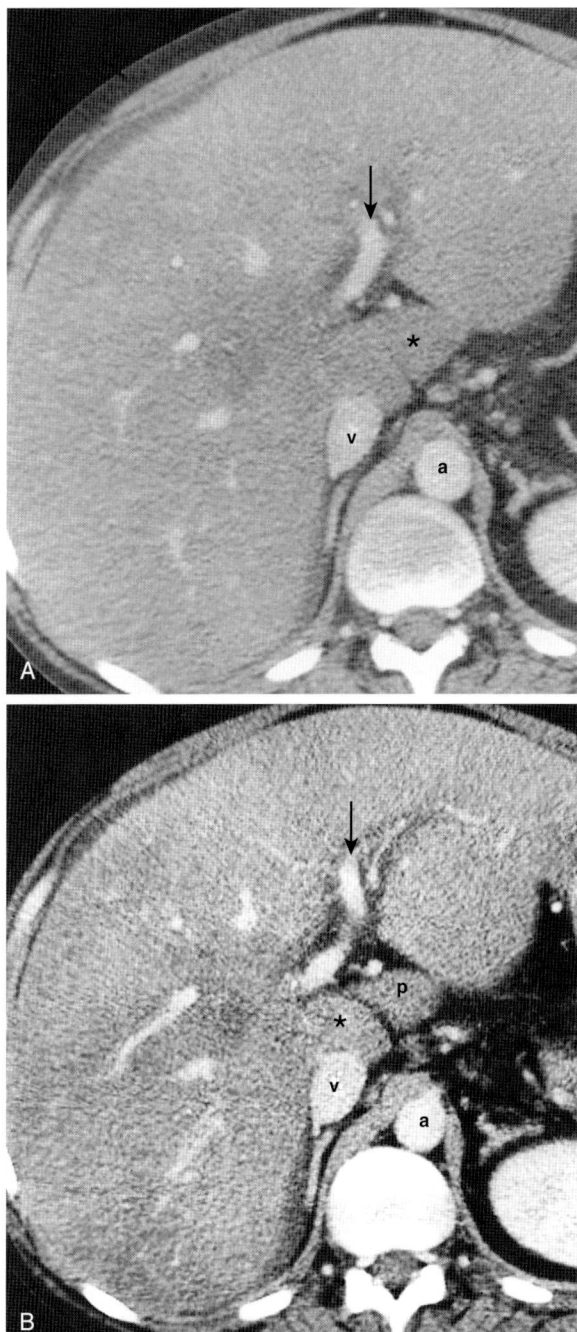

FIGURE 2.13 Computed tomographic image of the caudate lobe with papillary process. **A,** Caudate lobe *(asterisk)* positioned between the left portal vein *(arrow)* and inferior vena cava *(v)*. *a,* Aorta. **B,** Papillary process of the caudate *(p)* represents the lower medial extension of the caudate *(asterisk)* and may mimic a periportal lymph node *(Arrow)* indicates left portal vein.

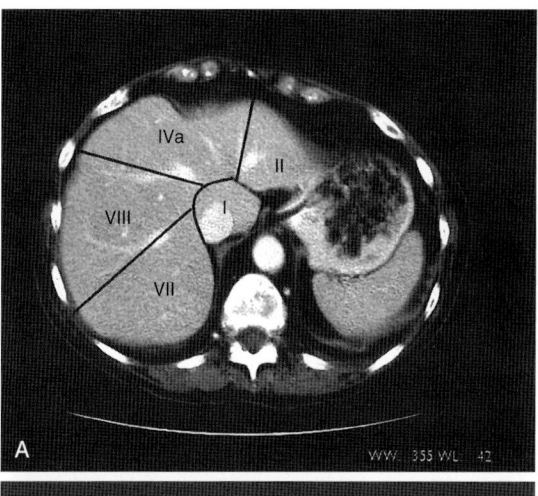

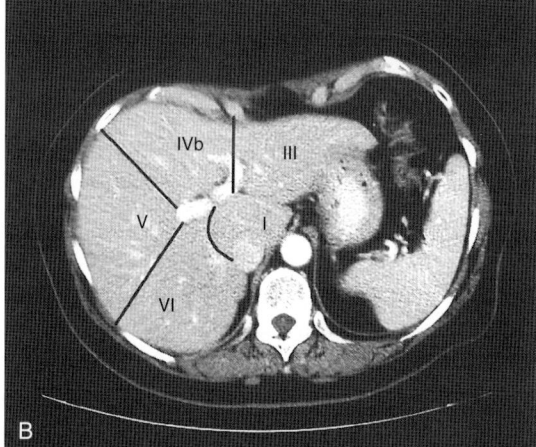

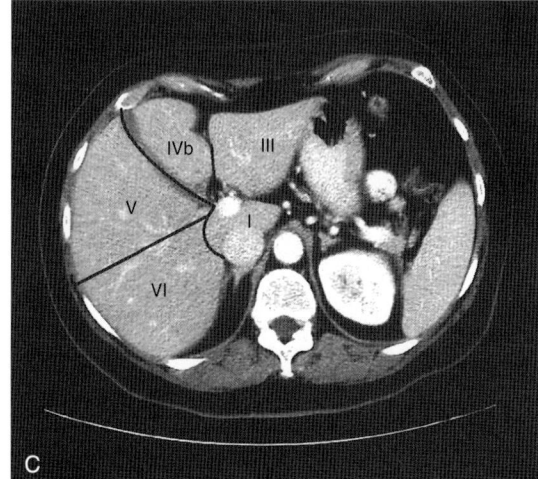

FIGURE 2.14 Hepatic segmental anatomy as shown by computed tomography at **A,** the level of the hepatic veins, **B,** at the portal vein bifurcation, and **C,** below the hepatic hilus.

Further details of segmental anatomy important in sectional or segmental resection are described in Chapters 101 and 102.

Surgical Implications and Exposure

All methods for precise partial hepatectomy depend on control of the inflow vasculature and draining bile ducts and the outflow hepatic veins of the portion of liver to be excised, which may be a segment, a subsegment, or an entire lobe. The remnant remaining after partial hepatectomy must be provided with an excellent portal venous inflow, hepatic arterial supply, and biliary drainage and unimpeded hepatic venous outflow. The classification of the various partial hepatic resection procedures, incisions and exposure, necessary mobilization of the liver, and the methods of control of the structures within the portal triads and of the hepatic veins are described in detail in Chapters 101 and 102.

BILIARY TRACT

Biliary exposure and precise dissection are the most important steps in any biliary operative procedure. A thorough understanding of biliary anatomy is necessary.

Intrahepatic Bile Duct Anatomy

The right and left livers are drained by the right and the left hepatic ducts, whereas the caudate lobe is drained by several ducts that join both the right and left hepatic ducts. The intrahepatic ducts are tributaries of the corresponding hepatic ducts, which form part of the major portal triads that penetrate the liver, invaginating Glisson capsule at the hilum. Bile ducts usually are located above the corresponding portal branches, whereas hepatic arterial branches are situated inferiorly to the veins. Each branch of the intrahepatic portal veins corresponds to bile duct tributaries that join to form the right and left hepatic ductal systems, converging at the liver hilum to constitute the common hepatic duct. The umbilical fissure divides the left liver, passing between segments III and IV, which may be bridged by a tongue of liver tissue. The ligamentum teres passes through the umbilical fissure to join the left branch of the portal vein.

The left hepatic duct drains the three segments—II, III, and IV—that constitute the left liver (Fig. 2.15). The duct that drains segment III is located slightly behind the left horn of the umbilical recess. It is joined by the tributary from segment IVb

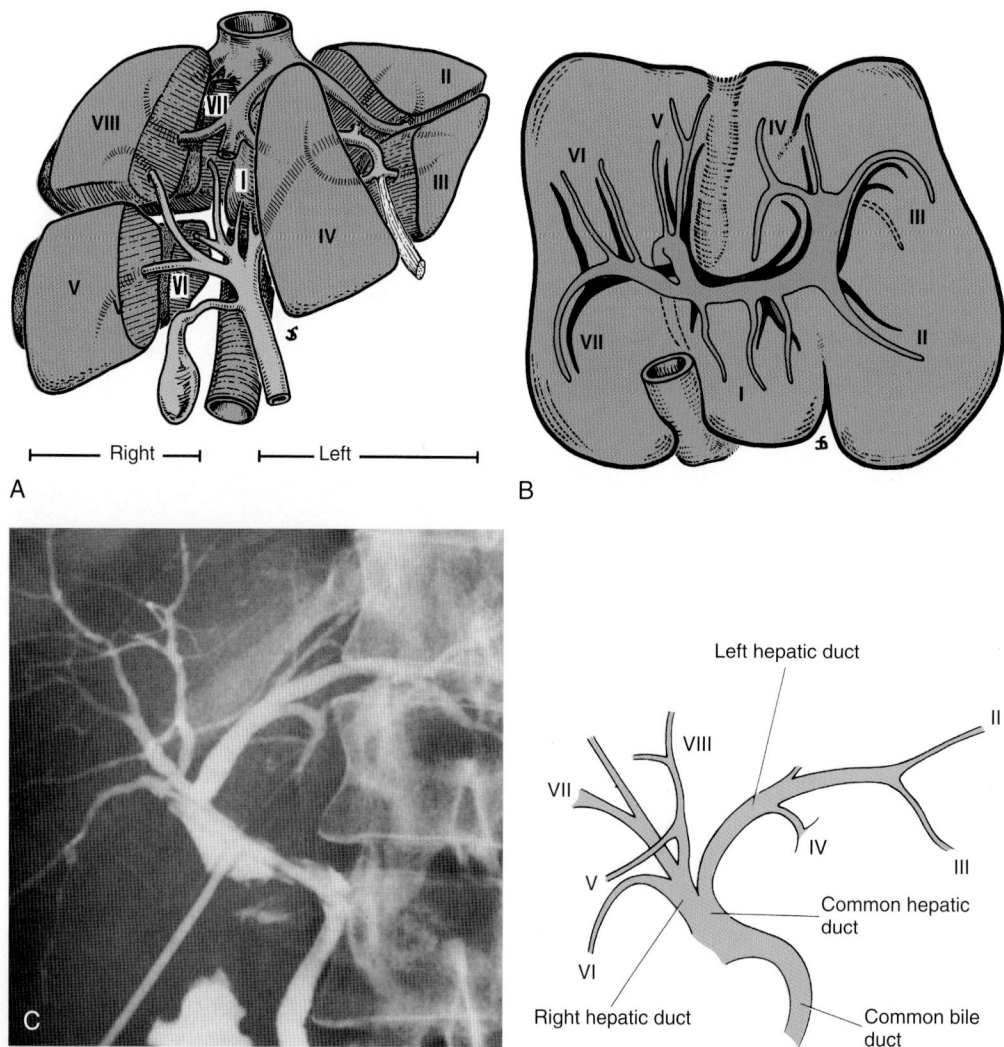

FIGURE 2.15   A, Biliary drainage of the two functional hemilivers. Note the position of the right anterior and right posterior sections. The caudate lobe drains into the right and left ductal system. **B,** Inferior aspect of the liver. The biliary tract is represented in black, and the portal branches are represented in white. Note the biliary drainage of segment IV (segment VIII is not represented because of its cephalad location). **C,** T-tube cholangiogram shows the most common arrangement of hepatic ducts.

to form the left duct, which is similarly joined by the duct of segment II and the duct of segment IVa, where the left branch of the portal vein turns forward and caudally. The left hepatic duct traverses beneath the left liver at the base of segment IV, just above and behind the left branch of the portal vein; it crosses the anterior edge of that vein and joins the right hepatic duct to constitute the hepatic ductal confluence. In its transverse portion, it receives a few small branches from segment IV.

The right hepatic duct drains segments V, VI, VII, and VIII and arises from the junction of two main sectional duct tributaries. The posterior or lateral duct and the anterior or medial duct are each accompanied by a corresponding vein and artery. The right posterior sectional duct has an almost horizontal course and constitutes the confluence of the ducts of segments VI and VII (Fig. 2.16). The duct then runs to join the right anterior sectional duct, as it descends in a vertical manner. The right anterior sectional duct is formed by the confluence of the ducts draining segments V and VIII. Its main trunk is located to the left of the right anterior sectional branch of the portal vein, which pursues an ascending course. The junction of these two main right biliary channels usually occurs above the right branch of the portal vein. The right hepatic duct is short and joins the left hepatic duct to constitute the confluence lying in front of the right portal vein and forming the common hepatic duct.

The caudate lobe (segment I) has its own biliary drainage.[6] The caudate lobe is divided into right and left portions and a caudate process. In 44% of individuals, three separate ducts drain these three parts of the lobe, whereas in another 26%, a common duct lies between the right portion of the caudate lobe proper and the caudate process and an independent duct that drains the left part of the caudate lobe. The site of drainage of these ducts varies. In 78% of cases, drainage of the caudate lobe is into the right and left hepatic ducts, but in 15%, drainage is by the left hepatic ductal system only. In about 7%, the drainage is into the right hepatic system.

Extrahepatic Biliary Anatomy and Vascular Anatomy of the Liver and Pancreas

The extrahepatic bile ducts are represented by the extrahepatic segments of the right and left hepatic ducts, joining to form the biliary confluence and the main biliary channel draining to the duodenum (Figs. 2.17 and 2.18). The confluence of the right and left hepatic ducts occurs at the right of the hilar fissure of the liver, anterior to the portal venous bifurcation and overlying the origin of the right branch of the portal vein. The extrahepatic segment of the right duct is short, but the left duct has a much longer extrahepatic course. The biliary confluence is separated from the posterior aspect of segment IVB of the liver by the hilar plate, which is the fusion of connective tissue enclosing the biliary and

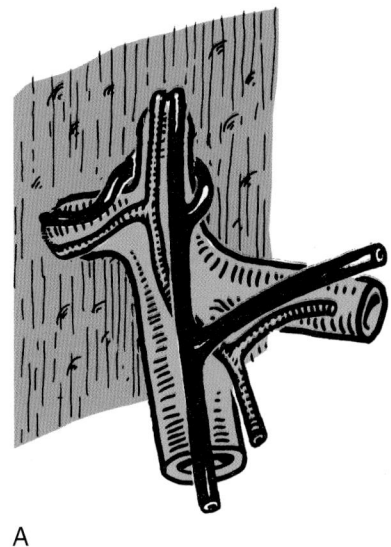

A

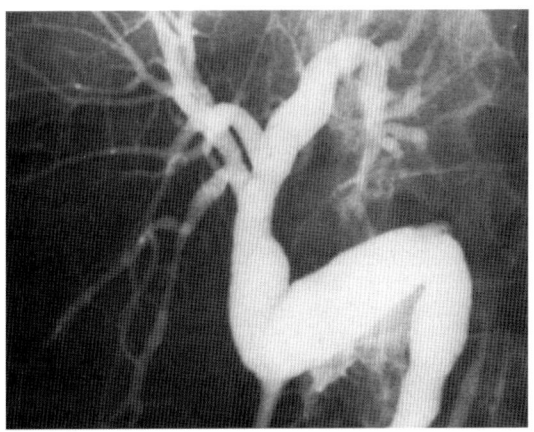

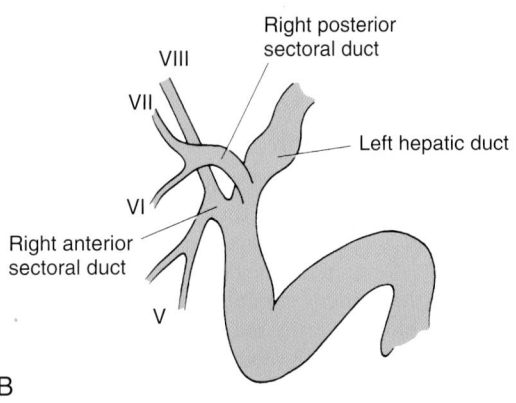

B

FIGURE 2.16 **A,** Biliary and vascular anatomy of the right liver. Note the horizontal course of the posterior sectional duct and the vertical course of the anterior sectional duct. **B,** Trans-tubal cholangiogram shows a common normal variant: the right posterior sectional duct drains into the left hepatic duct. In this case, the posterior duct is anterior to the posterior sectional duct. Frequently in this variant, the posterior duct passes posteriorly to the anterior sectional pedicle.

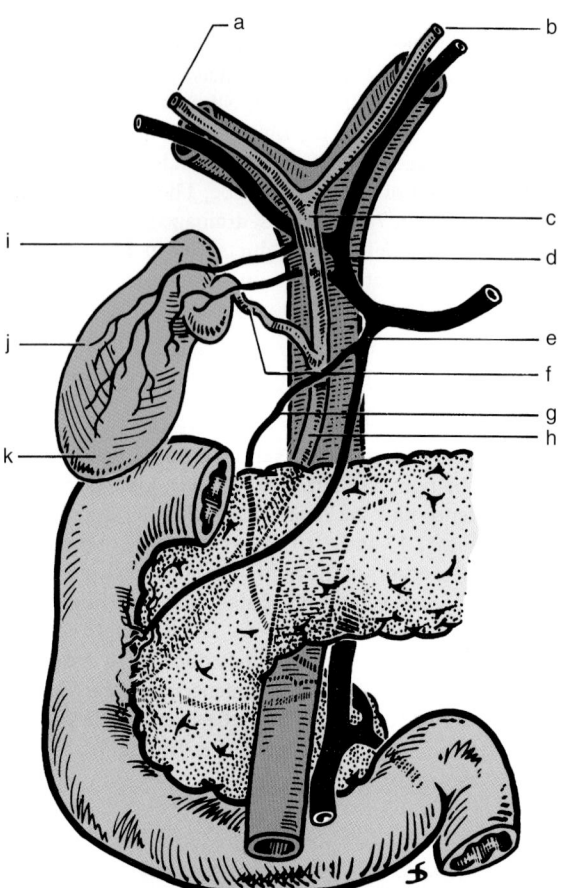

FIGURE 2.17 Anterior aspect of the biliary anatomy and of the head of the pancreas: right hepatic duct *(a)*, left hepatic duct *(b)*, common hepatic duct *(c)*, hepatic artery *(d)*, gastroduodenal artery *(e,* cystic duct *(f)*, retroduodenal artery *(g)*, common bile duct *(h)*, neck of the gallbladder *(i)*, body of the gallbladder *(j)*, fundus of the gallbladder *(k)*. Note particularly the position of the hepatic bile duct confluence anterior to the right branch of the portal vein, the posterior course of the cystic artery behind the common hepatic duct, and the relationship of the neck of the gallbladder to the right branch of the hepatic artery. Note also the relationship of the major vessels (portal vein, superior mesenteric vein, and superior mesenteric artery) to the head of the pancreas.

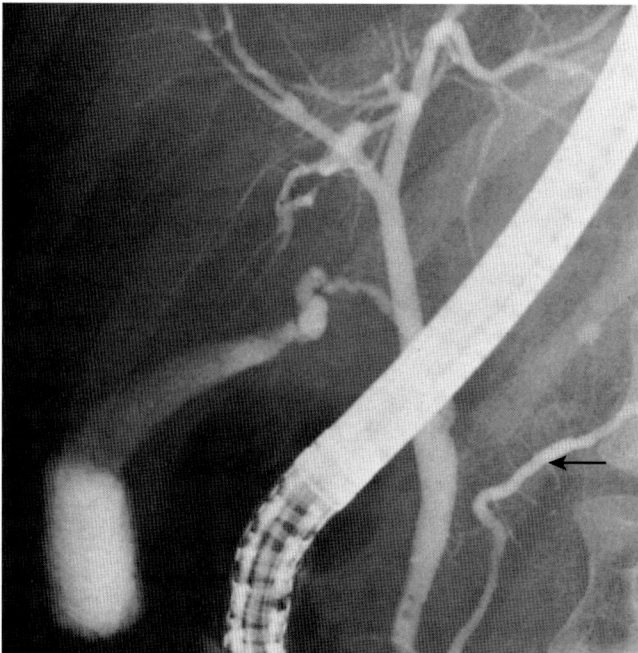

FIGURE 2.18 Endoscopic retrograde choledochopancreatogram showing the pancreatic duct *(arrow)*, gallbladder, and biliary tree.

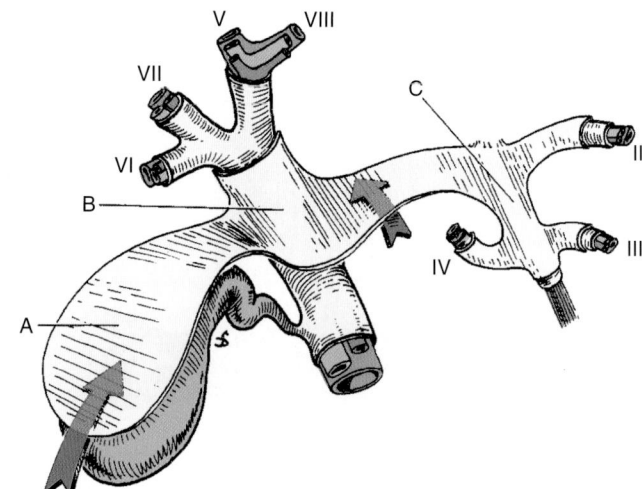

FIGURE 2.19 Anatomy of the plate system. A, Cystic plate, above the gallbladder. **B,** Hilar plate, above the biliary confluence and at the base of segment IV. **C,** Umbilical plate, above the umbilical portion of the portal vein. Large, *curving arrows* indicate the plane of dissection of the cystic plate during cholecystectomy and of the hilar plate during approaches to the left hepatic duct.

vascular elements with the Glisson capsule (Fig. 2.19). Because of the absence of any major vascular interposition, it is possible to open the connective tissue constituting the hilar plate at the inferior border of segment IV and, by elevating it, to display the biliary confluence and left hepatic duct (Fig. 2.20).

Main Bile Duct and Sphincter of Oddi

The main bile duct, the mean diameter of which is approximately 6 mm, is divided into two portions: the upper is called the *common hepatic duct* and is situated above the cystic duct, which joins it to form the lower portion, the common bile duct (CBD). Insertion of the cystic is variable and may be as low as the intrapancreatic portion of the bile duct. The common duct courses downward anterior to the portal vein, in the free edge of the lesser omentum; it is closely applied to the hepatic artery, which runs upward on its left, giving rise to the right branch of the hepatic artery, which crosses the main bile duct usually posteriorly, although in approximately 20% of cases, it crosses anteriorly. The cystic artery, arising from

the right branch of the hepatic artery, may cross the common hepatic duct posteriorly or anteriorly. The common hepatic duct constitutes the left border of the triangle of Calot, the other corners of which were originally described as the cystic duct below and the cystic artery above.[11] The commonly accepted working definition of the triangle of Calot recognizes, however, the inferior surface of the right lobe of the liver as the upper border and the cystic duct as the lower border.[12] Dissection of the triangle of Calot is of key significance during cholecystectomy because in this triangle runs the cystic artery,

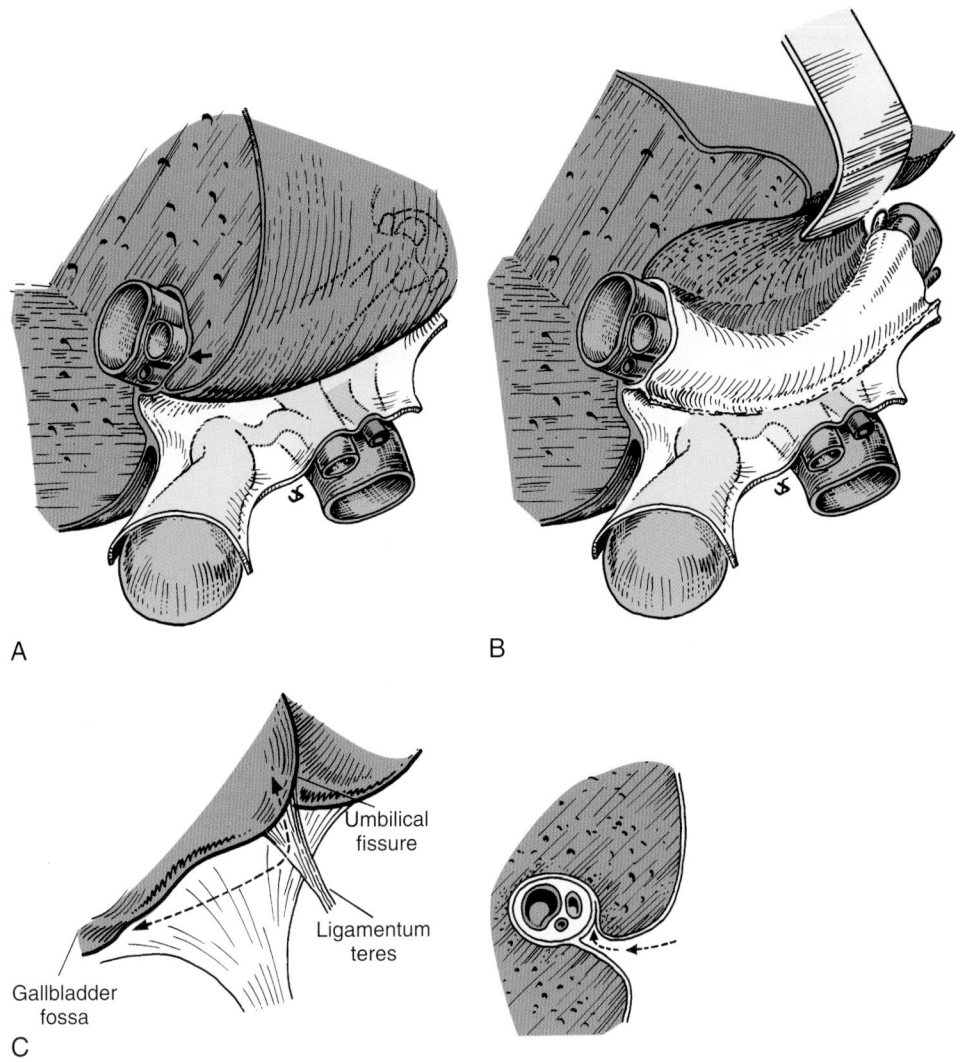

FIGURE 2.20   **A,** Relationship between the posterior aspect of segment IV and the biliary confluence. The hilar plate *(arrow)* is formed by the fusion of the connective tissue enclosing the biliary and vascular elements with the Glisson capsule. **B,** Biliary confluence and left hepatic duct exposed by lifting segment IV upward after incision of the Glisson capsule at its base. This technique, *lowering of the hilar plate,* generally is used to display a dilated bile duct above an iatrogenic stricture or hilar cholangiocarcinoma. **C,** Line of incision *(left)* to allow extensive mobilization of segment IV. This maneuver is of particular value for high bile duct strictures and in the presence of liver atrophy or hypertrophy. The procedure consists of lifting segment IV upward (**A** and **B**), then not only opening the umbilical fissure but also incising the deepest portion of the gallbladder fossa. *Right,* Incision of the Glisson capsule to gain access to the biliary system *(arrow)*. (**B,** From Hepp J, Couinaud C. L'abord et l'utilisation du canal hépatique gauche dans les reparations de la voie biliare principale. *Presse Med.* 1956;64:947–948.)

often the right branch of the hepatic artery, and occasionally a bile duct, which should be displayed before cholecystectomy (see Chapter 36). If there is a replaced or accessory common or right hepatic artery, it usually runs behind the cystic duct to enter the triangle of Calot (Fig. 2.21).

The common variations in the relationship of the hepatic artery and origin and course of the cystic artery to the biliary apparatus are shown in Fig. 2.22. Ignorance of these variations may provoke unexpected hemorrhage or biliary injury[13] during cholecystectomy and may result in bile duct injury during efforts to secure hemostasis (see Chapter 42). The union between the cystic duct and the common hepatic duct may be located at various levels. At its lower extrahepatic portion, the CBD traverses the posterior aspect of the pancreas, running in a groove or tunnel. The retropancreatic portion of the CBD approaches the second portion of the duodenum obliquely,

accompanied by the terminal part of the pancreatic duct of Wirsung.

Gallbladder and Cystic Duct

The gallbladder is a reservoir located on the undersurface of the right lobe of the liver, within the cystic fossa; it is separated from the hepatic parenchyma by the cystic plate, which is composed of connective tissue that extends to the left as the hilar plate (see Fig. 2.19). Sometimes the gallbladder is deeply embedded in the liver, but occasionally it occurs on a mesenteric attachment and may be susceptible to volvulus. The gallbladder varies in size and consists of a *fundus*, a *body*, and a *neck* (Fig. 2.23). The fundus usually, but not always, reaches the free edge of the liver and is closely applied to the cystic plate. The cystic fossa is a precise anterior landmark to the main liver incisura. The neck of the gallbladder makes an angle with the

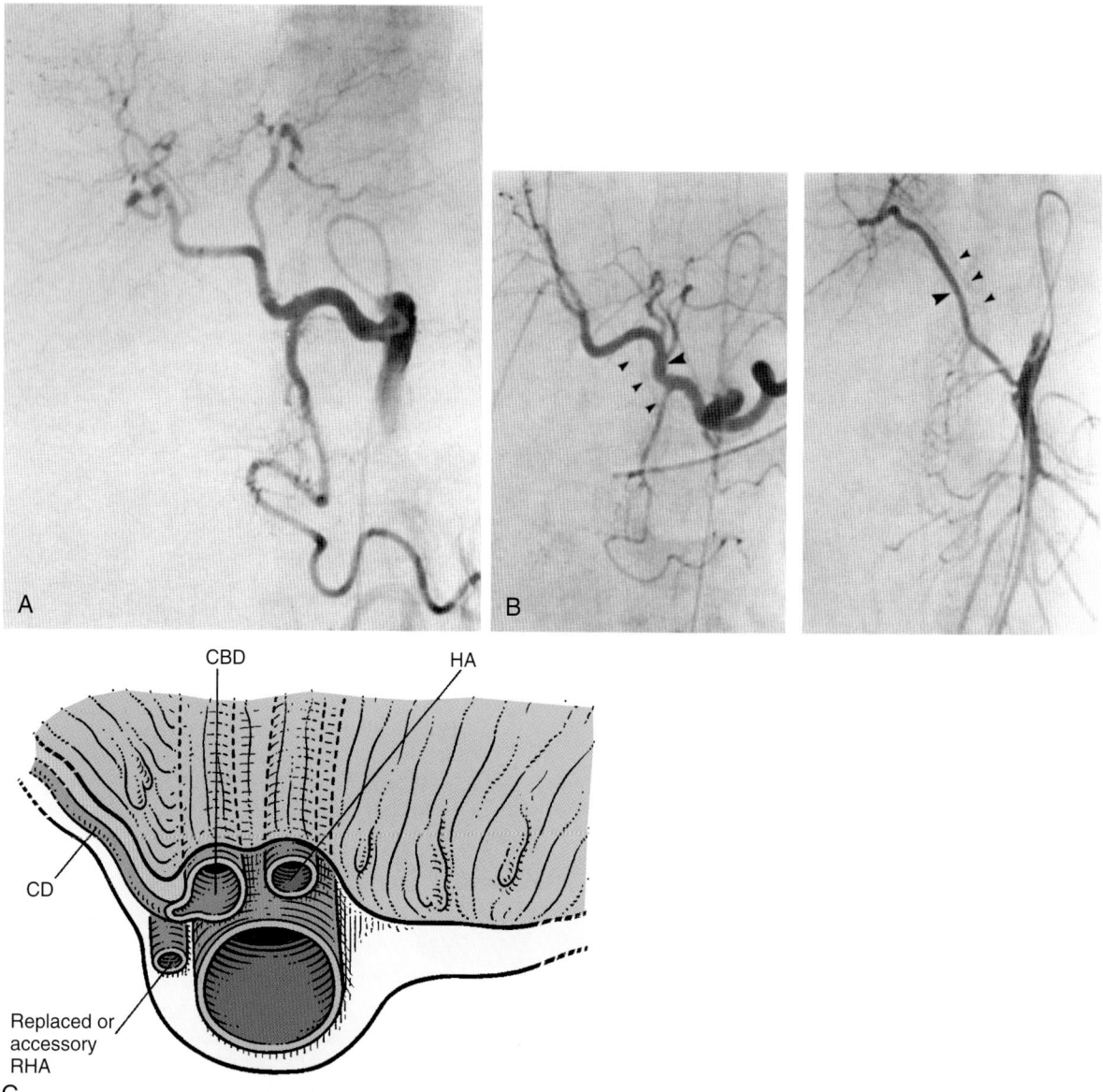

FIGURE 2.21 Hepatic artery variations shown by angiography. **A,** Replaced common hepatic artery arises from the superior mesenteric trunk. **B,** *Left,* The hepatic artery *(large arrowhead)* arises from the celiac axis. The small *arrowheads* indicate a drainage catheter in the bile duct. *Right,* An accessory right hepatic artery *(large arrowhead)* is arising from the superior mesenteric artery and lies lateral to the catheter *(small arrowheads)* in the common bile duct (CBD). **C,** The accessory right hepatic artery usually courses upward in the groove posterolateral to the *CBD,* appearing on the medial side of the triangle of Calot, usually running just behind the cystic duct *(CD).* This common variation occurs in about 25% of individuals. *HA,* Hepatic artery; *RHA,* right hepatic artery.

fundus and creates Hartmann's pouch, which may obscure the common hepatic duct and constitute a real danger point during cholecystectomy.

The cystic duct arises from the neck or infundibulum of the gallbladder and extends to join the common hepatic duct. Its lumen usually measures approximately 1 to 3 mm, and its length varies, depending on the type of union with the common hepatic duct. The mucosa of the cystic duct is arranged in spiral folds known as the *valves of Heister.*[12] Although the cystic duct joins the common hepatic duct in its supraduodenal segment in 80% of cases, it may extend downward to the retroduodenal or retropancreatic area. Rarely, the cystic duct may join the right hepatic duct or a right hepatic sectional duct (Fig. 2.24).

BILIARY DUCTAL ANOMALIES

Full knowledge of the frequent variations from the described normal biliary anatomy is required when any hepatobiliary procedure is performed (Fig. 2.25). The constitution of a normal biliary confluence by union of the right and left hepatic ducts, as described previously, is reported in only 72% of patients.[6] There is a triple confluence of the right anterior and posterior sectional ducts and the left hepatic duct in 12% of individuals,[1] and a right sectional duct joins the main bile duct directly in 20%. In 16% the right anterior sectional duct, and in 4% the right posterior sectional duct, may approach the main bile duct in this fashion. In 6%, a right sectional duct may join the left hepatic duct (the posterior duct in 5% and the

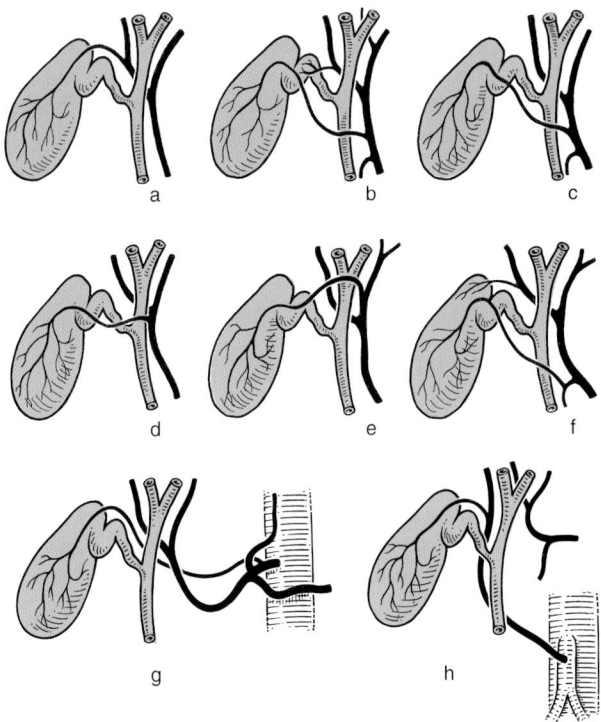

FIGURE 2.22 The main variations of the cystic artery: typical course *(a)*, double cystic artery *(b)*, cystic artery crossing anterior to main bile duct *(c)*, cystic artery originating from the right branch of the hepatic artery and crossing the common hepatic duct anteriorly *(d)*, cystic artery originating from the left branch of the hepatic artery *(e)*, cystic artery originating from the gastroduodenal artery *(f)*, cystic artery arising from the celiac axis *(g)*, and cystic artery originating from a replaced right hepatic artery *(h)*.

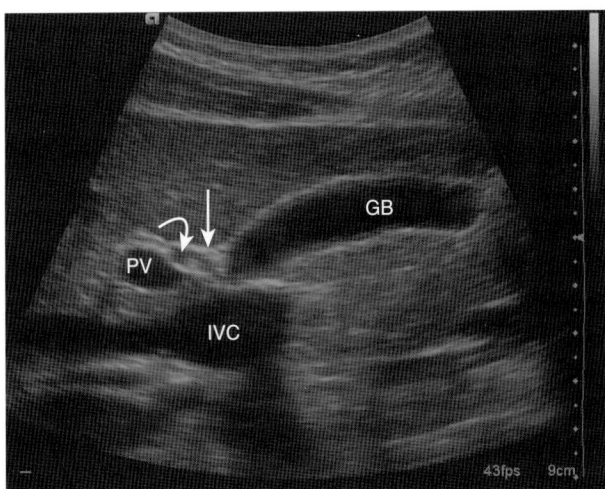

FIGURE 2.23 Longitudinal sonogram shows the relationship of the liver, gallbladder *(GB)*, portal vein *(PV)*, inferior vena cava *(IVC)*, hepatic artery *(curved arrow)*, and common bile duct *(straight arrow)*.

anterior duct in 1%). In 3%, there is an absence of the hepatic duct confluence, and the right posterior sectional duct may join the neck of the gallbladder, or it may be entered by the cystic duct in 2%.[1] In any event, these multiple biliary ductal variations at the hilus are important to recognize in resection and reconstructive surgery of the biliary tree at the hilus and during partial hepatectomy and cholecystectomy.

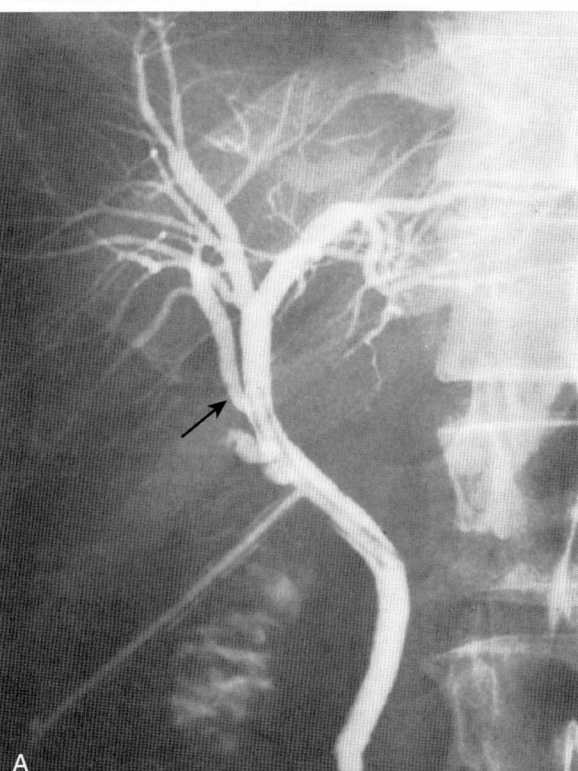

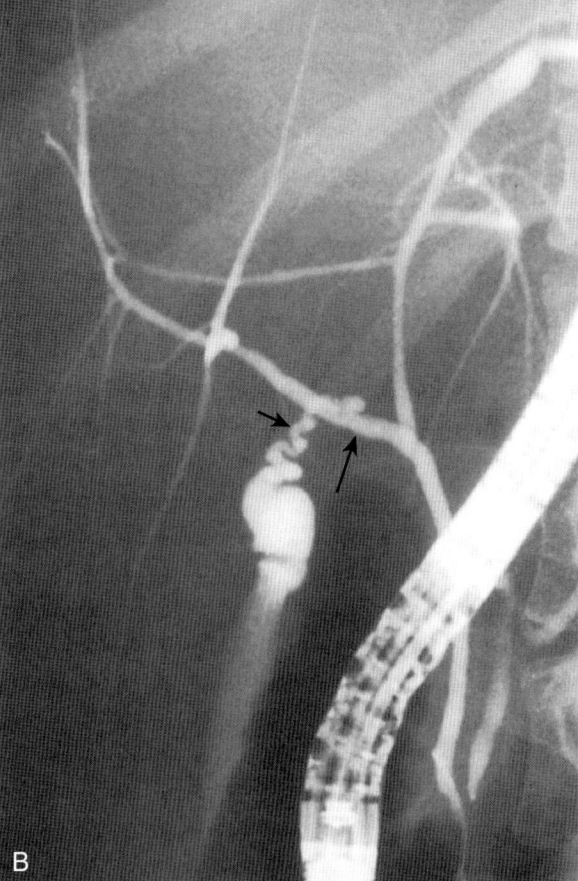

FIGURE 2.24 **A,** T-tube cholangiogram shows a very low insertion of a right sectional duct into the common hepatic duct *(arrow)*. **B,** Endoscopic retrograde choledochopancreatogram shows a low right sectional duct *(large arrow)* into which is draining the cystic duct *(small arrow)*, an uncommon but important normal variant.

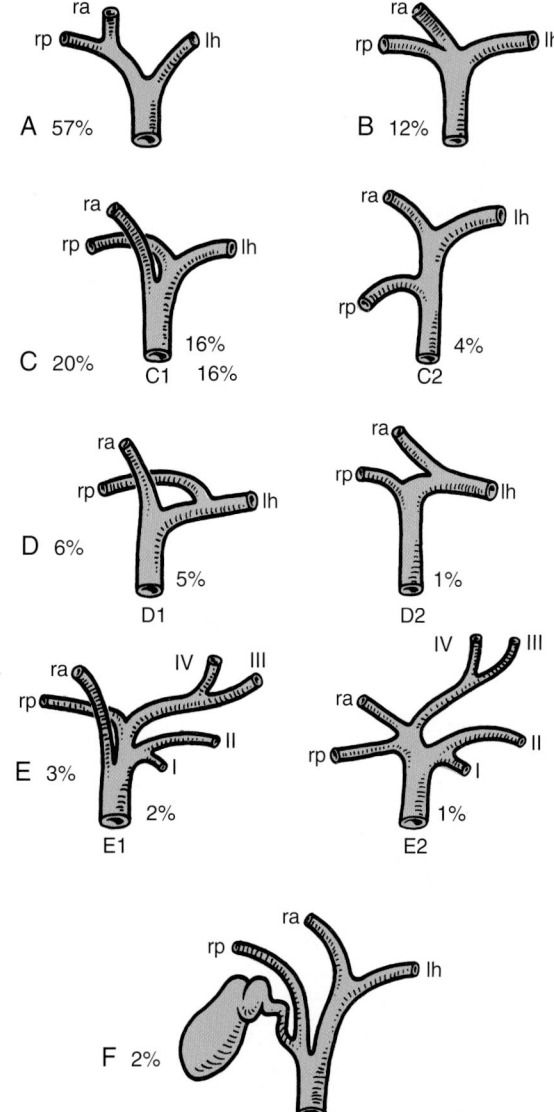

FIGURE 2.25 Main variations of the hepatic duct confluence. A, Typical anatomy of the confluence. **B,** Triple confluence. **C,** Ectopic drainage of a right sectional duct into the common hepatic duct. **D,** Ectopic drainage of a right sectional duct into the left hepatic ductal system. **E,** Absence of the hepatic duct confluence. **F,** Absence of right hepatic duct and ectopic drainage of the right posterior duct into the cystic duct. *C1,* Right anterior *(ra)* duct draining into the common hepatic duct; *C2,* right posterior *(rp)* duct draining into the common hepatic duct; *D1,* Right posterior sectional duct draining into the left hepatic *(lh)* ductal system; *D2,* right anterior sectional duct draining into the left hepatic ductal system. (From Couinaud C. *Le Foi: Études* Anatomiques *et Chirurgicales.* Masson; 1957.)

Intrahepatic bile duct variations also are common (Fig. 2.26).[6] The main right intrahepatic duct variations are represented by an ectopic drainage of segment V in 9%, of segment VI in 14%, and of segment VIII in 20%. In addition, a subvesical duct has been described in 20% to 50% of cases. This duct, sometimes deeply embedded in the cystic plate, joins either the common hepatic duct or the right hepatic duct. It does not drain any specific liver territory, never communicates with the gallbladder, and is not a satellite of an intrahepatic branch of the portal vein or hepatic artery. Although not of major anatomic significance, injury may

occur during cholecystectomy if the cystic plate is not preserved. This may lead to a postoperative biliary leak.

In 67% of patients,[6] a classic distribution of the main left intrahepatic biliary ductal system exists. The main variation in this region is represented by a common union between the ducts of segments III and IV in 25%, and in only 2% does the duct of segment IV join the common hepatic duct independently. Several anomalies of drainage of the intrahepatic ducts into the neck of the gallbladder or cystic duct have been reported (Fig. 2.27),[1,14] and these must be kept in mind during cholecystectomy (see Chapter 33).

ANOMALIES OF THE GALLBLADDER AND CYSTIC DUCT

Many anomalies of the accessory biliary apparatus have been described (Fig. 2.28).[15] Although rare, agenesis of the gallbladder,[16-18] bilobar gallbladders with a single cystic duct but two fundi,[19] and duplication of the gallbladder with two cystic ducts all have been described. A double cystic duct may drain a unilocular gallbladder,[20] and congenital diverticulum of the gallbladder with a muscular wall may also be found.[21] More frequently reported are anomalies of position of the gallbladder, which may be in an intrahepatic position, completely surrounded by normal liver tissue, or rarely may be found on the left of the liver.[22]

The mode of union of the cystic duct with the common hepatic duct may be angular, parallel, or spiral. An angular union is the most frequent and is found in 75% of patients.[23] The cystic duct may run a parallel course to the common hepatic duct in 20%, with connective tissue ensheathing both ducts. Finally, the cystic duct may approach the CBD in a spiral fashion. The absence of a cystic duct is probably an acquired anomaly, representing a cholecystocholedochal fistula.

BILE DUCT BLOOD SUPPLY

The bile duct may be divided into three segments: *hilar, supraduodenal,* and *retropancreatic.* The blood supply of the supraduodenal duct is essentially axial (Fig. 2.29).[24] Most vessels to the supraduodenal duct arise from the superior pancreaticoduodenal artery, right branch of the hepatic artery, cystic artery, gastroduodenal artery, and retroduodenal artery. On average, eight small arteries, each measuring approximately 0.3 mm in diameter, supply the supraduodenal duct. The most important of these vessels run along the lateral and medial borders of the duct and have been called the *3 o'clock* and *9 o'clock arteries.* Of the blood vessels vascularizing the supraduodenal duct, 60% run upward from the major inferior vessels, and only 38% of arteries run downward, originating from the right branch of the hepatic artery and other vessels. Only 2% of the arterial supply is nonaxial, arising directly from the main trunk of the hepatic artery as it courses up parallel to the main biliary channel. The hilar ducts receive a copious supply of arterial blood from surrounding vessels, forming a rich network on the surface of the ducts in continuity with the plexus around the supraduodenal duct. The source of blood supply to the retropancreatic CBD is from the retroduodenal artery, which provides multiple small vessels running around the duct to form a mural plexus.

The veins draining the bile ducts are satellites to the corresponding described arteries, draining into 3 o'clock and

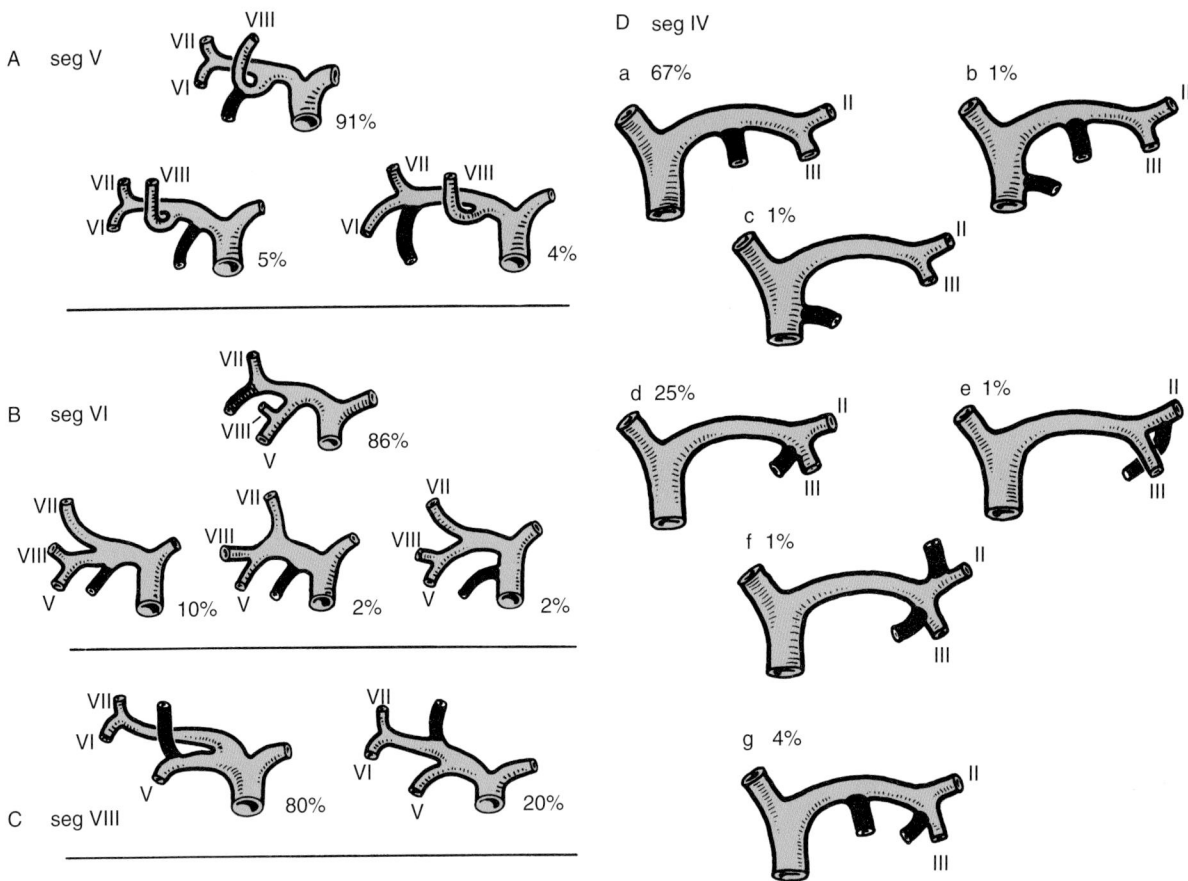

FIGURE 2.26 The main variations of the intrahepatic ductal system. **A,** Variations of segment V. **B,** Variations of segment VI. **C,** Variations of segment VIII. **D,** Variations of segment IV. There is no variation of drainage of segments II, III, and VII. *seg,* Segment.

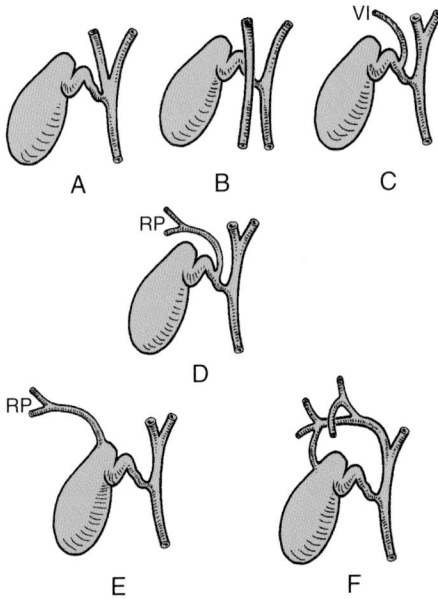

FIGURE 2.27 The main variations of ectopic drainage of the intrahepatic ducts into the gallbladder and cystic duct. **A,** Drainage of the cystic duct into the biliary confluence. **B,** Drainage of cystic duct into the left hepatic duct, associated with no biliary confluence. **C,** Drainage of segment VI duct into the cystic duct. **D,** Drainage of the right posterior *(RP)* sectional duct into the cystic duct. **E,** Drainage of the distal part of the right posterior sectional duct into the neck of the gallbladder. **F,** Drainage of the proximal part of the right posterior sectional duct into the body of the gallbladder.

9 o'clock veins along the borders of the common biliary channel. Veins draining the gallbladder empty into this venous system, not directly into the portal vein, and the biliary tree seems to have its own portal venous pathway to the liver.

ANATOMY OF BILIARY EXPOSURE

Biliary-Vascular Sheaths and Exposure of the Hepatic Bile Duct Confluence

Fusion of the Glisson capsule with the connective tissue sheaths surrounding the biliary and vascular elements at the inferior aspect of the liver constitute the plate system (see Figs. 2.19 and 2.20), which includes the hilar plate above the biliary confluence, the cystic plate related to the gallbladder, and the umbilical plate situated above the umbilical portion of the left portal vein.[1] Hepp and Couinaud[25] describe a technique whereby lifting segment IV upward and incising the Glisson capsule at its base offers good exposure of the hepatic hilar structures (see Fig. 2.20). This technique is referred to as *lowering of the hilar plate.* It can be carried out safely because only exceptionally (in 1% of cases) is there any major vascular interposition between the hilar plate and the inferior aspect of the liver, although tiny venules are common. This maneuver is of particular value in exposing the extrahepatic segment of the left hepatic duct because it has a long course beneath segment IV (see Chapter 42). It is not as effective in exposing the extrahepatic right duct or its secondary branches, which are short. The technique is of major

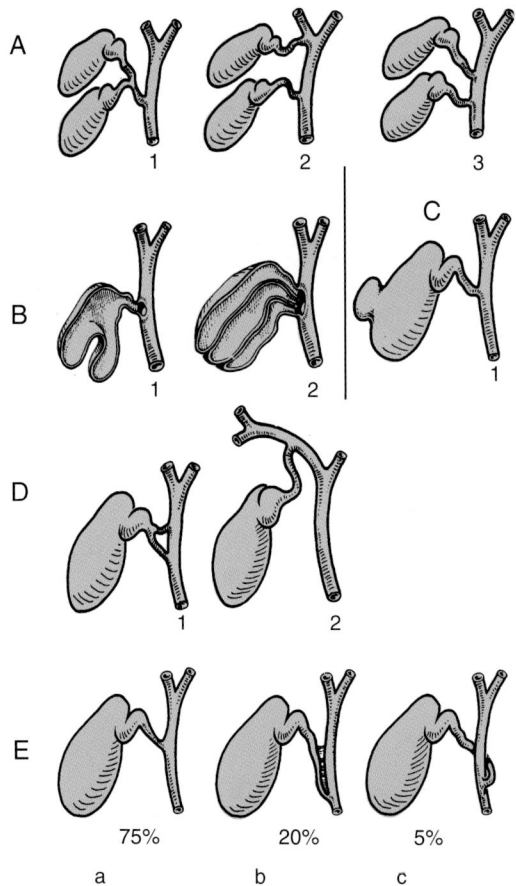

FIGURE 2.28 Main variations in gallbladder and cystic duct anatomy. **A,** Duplicated gallbladder. **B,** Septum of the gallbladder. **C,** Diverticulum of the gallbladder. **D,** Variations in cystic ductal anatomy. **E,** Different types of union of the cystic duct and common hepatic duct: angular union (a), parallel union (b), spiral union (c).

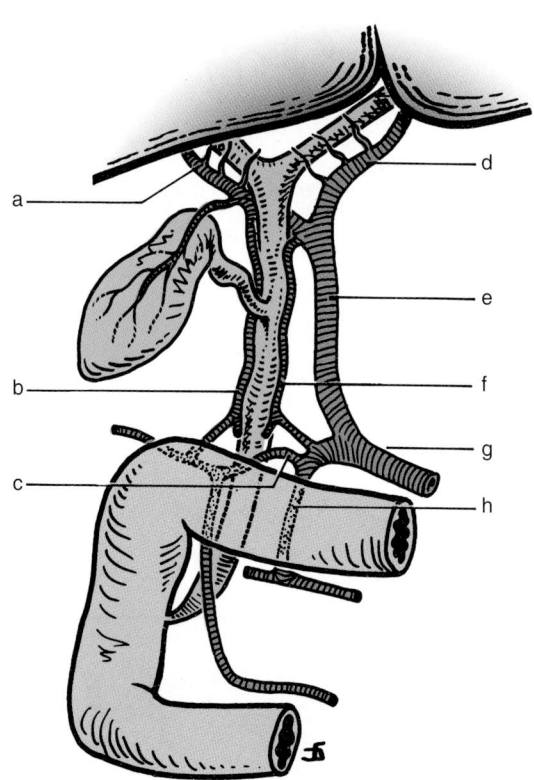

FIGURE 2.29 **The bile duct blood supply.** Note the axial arrangement of the vasculature of the supraduodenal portion of the main bile duct and the rich network enclosing the right and left hepatic ducts: right branch of the hepatic artery (a), 9 o'clock artery (b), retroduodenal artery (c), left branch of the hepatic artery (d), hepatic artery (e), 3 o'clock artery (f), common hepatic artery (g), and gastroduodenal artery (h).

importance for the identification of proximal biliary mucosa during bile duct repair after injury. Basically, an incision is made at the posterior edge of segment IV, where the Glisson capsule is attached to the hilar plate. The upper surface of the hilar plate can be separated from the hepatic parenchyma and, by lifting segment IV upward, display the hepatic duct convergence, which is always extrahepatic. Bile duct incision allows performance of a mucosa-to-mucosa anastomosis (see Chapters 32 and 42). Rarely, it may be hazardous to approach the biliary confluence in this manner, especially when anatomic deformity has been created by atrophy or hypertrophy of liver lobes and in patients in whom there appears to be a very deep hilum that is displaced upward and rotated laterally. Frequently, by a simultaneous opening of the deepest portion of the gallbladder fossa and the umbilical fissure (see Fig. 2.20C), good exposure of the biliary duct confluence, and especially the right hepatic duct, can be obtained without the necessity for full hepatotomy.

Umbilical Fissure and Segment III (Ligamentum Teres) Approach

The round ligament, which is the remnant of the obliterated umbilical vein, runs through the umbilical fissure to connect with the left branch of the portal vein. The round ligament is

sometimes deeply embedded in the umbilical fissure. At the junction of the round ligament and the termination of the left portal vein, elongations containing channels that are elements of the left portal system course into the liver. The bile ducts of the left lobe of the liver (Figs. 2.30 and 2.31A) are located above the left branch of the portal vein and lie behind these elongations, whereas the corresponding artery is situated below the vein. Dissection of the round ligament on its left side and division of one or two vascular elongations of segment III allow display of the pedicle or anterior branch of the duct of segment III (Fig. 2.32). In the event of biliary obstruction with intrahepatic biliary ductal dilation, a dilated segment III duct is generally easily located above the left branch of the portal vein. It is often preferable to split the normal liver tissue just to the left of the umbilical fissure to widen the fissure further, which allows access to the ductal system with no need to divide any elements of the portal blood supply to segment III (see Fig. 2.32; see also Chapters 32 and 42).

Surgical Approaches to the Right Hepatic Biliary Ductal System

Because of the lack of precise anatomic landmarks, exposure of the right intrahepatic ductal system is much more hazardous and imprecise than that of the left. In some cases of hilar cholangiocarcinoma, the planned surgical procedure—partial hepatectomy

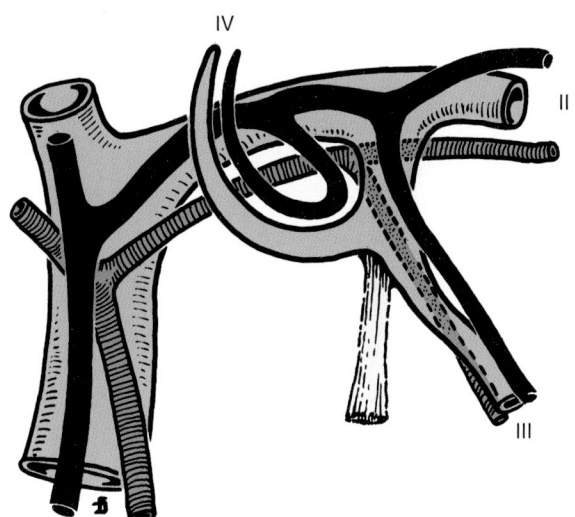

FIGURE 2.30 **Biliary and vascular anatomy of the left liver.** Note the location of the segment III duct above the corresponding vein. The anterior branch of the segment IV duct is not represented.

(see Chapters 51B, 101, 119B) or segment III duct bypass (see Chapters 32 and 42)—seems impossible at operation. In such a critical operative situation, intrahepatic right ductal system drainage is an option. Anatomically, the anterior sectional duct and its branches run on the left side of the corresponding portal vein. In essence, the end of the liver scissura, within which lies

the right branch of the portal vein, is opened through a short distance. The anterior sectional duct is displayed on the left aspect of the vein, and the dilated duct is opened longitudinally and sewn to a Roux-en-Y loop of jejunum (Fig. 2.33). Although this technique is rarely used, it may be valuable in selected cases. Preferably, the right-sided pedicles can be encircled and exposed by the technique used for pedicle exposure and control described for right-sided liver resection.

Exposure of the Bile Ducts by Liver Resection

This chapter does not detail exposure of the bile ducts by resection of liver substance. In essence, a segment of the left lobe may be amputated to expose the segment II or III ducts, or a similar procedure may be carried out after removal of the inferior tip of the right lobe. Finally, in some instances, removal of segment IV may be carried out to effect exposure of the biliary confluence. This procedure really represents a simple extension of the mobilization of segment IV after opening of the principal scissura and the umbilical fissure as described previously.

EXTRAHEPATIC VASCULATURE

Celiac Axis and Blood Supply of Liver, Biliary Tract, and Pancreas

The usual classic description of the arterial blood supply of the liver, biliary system, and pancreas is found in only approximately 60% of patients (Figs. 2.34–2.36). The right and the left hepatic arteries, the former in the right of the hilus of the liver

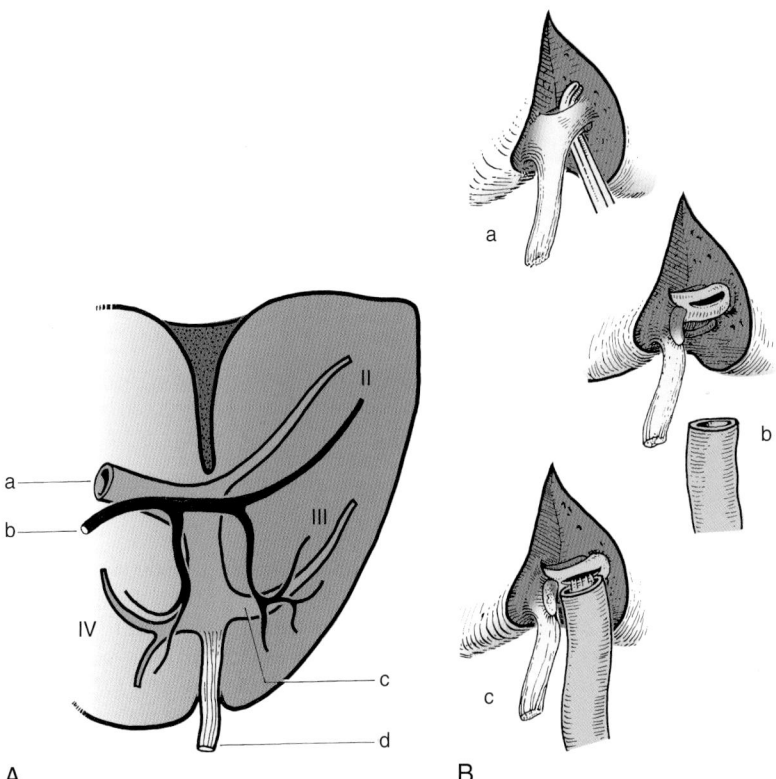

FIGURE 2.31 **A,** The biliary and vascular anatomy of the left liver. Note the relationship of the left horn of the umbilical recess with the segment III ductal system: left portal vein *(a)*, left hepatic duct *(b)*, segment III system—note that the duct *(black)* lies adjacent to the portal venous branch indicated *(c)*, ligamentum teres *(d)*. **B,** Segment III ductal approach: exposure of the left horn of the umbilical recess *(a)*, division of the left horn of the umbilical recess, including segment III portal vein branches *(b)*, exposure and opening of segment III duct: hepaticojejunostomy to the segment III ductal system *(c; see also Chapters 32 and 42).*

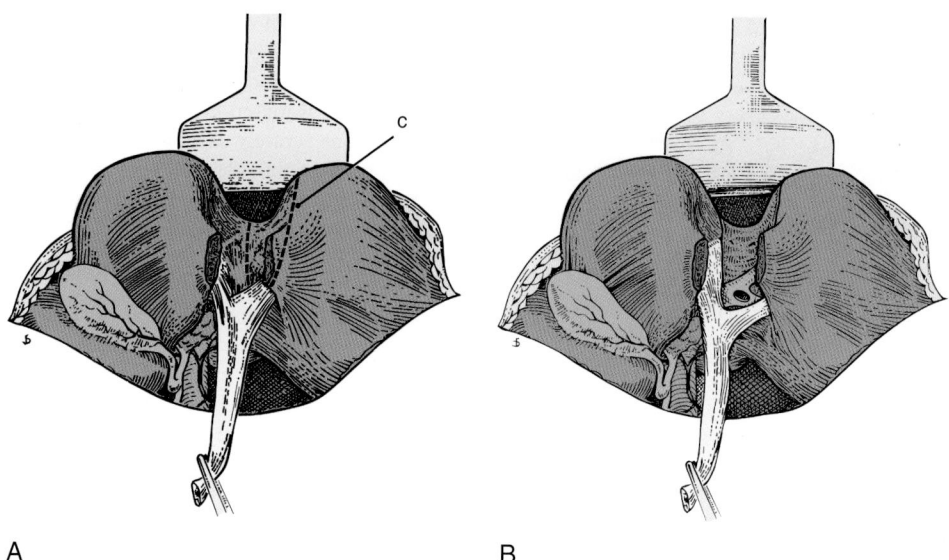

FIGURE 2.32 **A,** The liver is split to the left of the ligamentum teres in the umbilical fissure. It may be necessary to remove a small wedge of liver tissue *(c)*. **B,** Segment III duct is exposed at the base of the liver split, above and behind its accompanying vein, and is ready for anastomosis (see also Chapters 32 and 42).

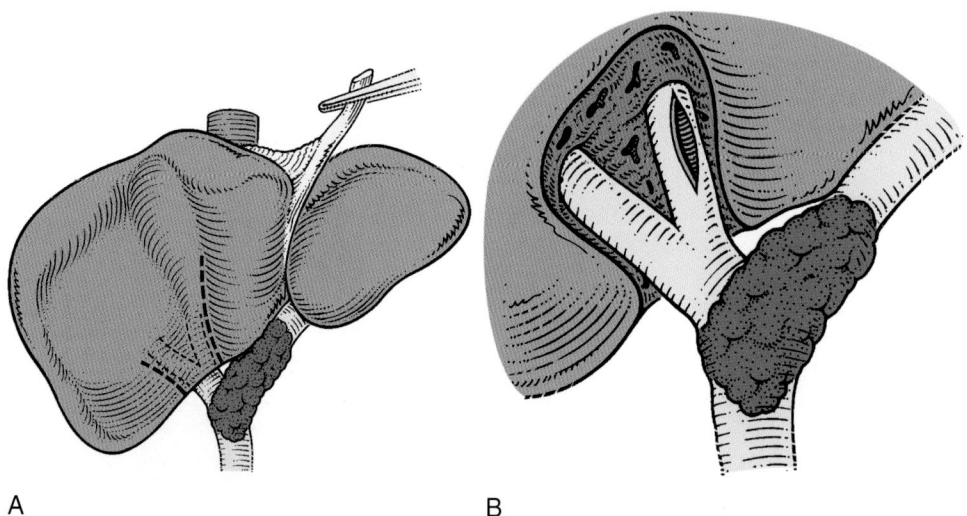

FIGURE 2.33 **A,** Anterior sectional approach. If necessary, the liver substance is opened through a short distance in the line of the right anterior sectional pedicle. **B,** The duct is displayed anterior and to the left side of the corresponding vein. This can be facilitated by using a posterior pedicular approach as described by Launois (see Chapter 101B).

and the latter in the left at the base of the umbilical fissure, become enclosed in the sheath of peritoneum, forming the right and left portal triads. In this sheath, further branching to the right anterior and posterior sections of the liver and on the left to segments II, III, and IV occurs within the respective pedicles, which also come to enclose the portal vein branches and the tributary bile ducts from these sections and segments. The arterial supply of the CBD was described earlier; it arises from branches of the hepatic artery, the gastroduodenal artery, and the pancreaticoduodenal arcades.

For practical surgical issues, the most important relationships in the anatomy of the pancreas concern the arterial blood supply and the venous drainage. The dorsal pancreatic artery is a major branch, usually arising from the splenic artery, but it can arise directly from the hepatic artery. When splenectomy is performed, it is important to establish the site of origin of the dorsal pancreatic artery to avoid distal pancreatic ischemia. The superior mesenteric artery (SMA) arises from the aorta posteriorly behind the pancreas and runs forward and upward to run first behind and then to the left of the superior mesenteric vein (SMV; see Fig. 2.35).

Variations in the Hepatic Artery

As a result of the complex embryologic development of the celiac axis and SMA, wide variations in the arterial supply of the liver are found (Fig. 2.37). These variations are important to

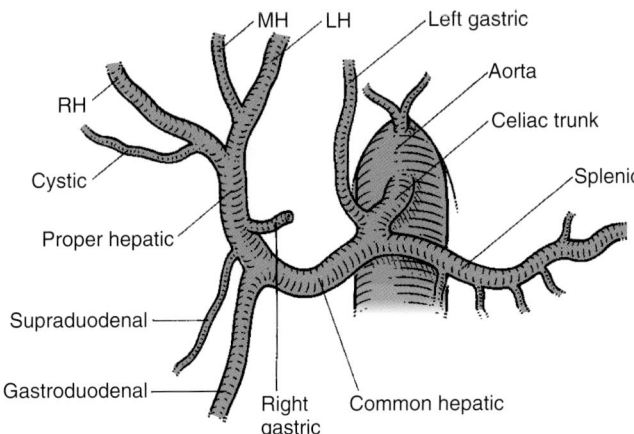

FIGURE 2.34 The celiac trunk is a short, thick artery originating from the aorta just below the aortic hiatus of the diaphragm and extending horizontally and forward above the pancreas, where it divides into the left gastric, common hepatic, and splenic arteries. An inferior phrenic artery, usually arising from the aorta or the splenic artery, occasionally arises from the celiac trunk. The left gastric artery curves toward the stomach and extends along its lesser curve, forming anastomoses with the right gastric artery. The splenic artery, the largest of the three celiac branches, takes a tortuous course to the left, behind and along the upper border of the pancreas and at the hilus of the spleen, where it splits into numerous terminal branches. The splenic artery usually approaches and runs superiorly to the splenic vein. An uncommon but dangerous abnormality can occur when the splenic artery runs inferiorly and behind the splenic vein, close to the splenic vein–mesenteric vein confluence. The left gastroepiploic artery and the short gastric arteries originate from one of these terminal branches. The common hepatic artery passes forward into the retroperitoneum, then curves to the right to enter the right margin of the lesser omentum, just above the pancreas, and ascends; it approaches the common bile duct (CBD) on its left side and runs usually anterior to the portal vein. While it turns upward just above the pancreas, it gives rise to the gastroduodenal artery, which also may originate from the right hepatic artery. This descends to supply the anterior, superior, and posterior surfaces of the first inch of the duodenum. The gastroduodenal artery can be duplicated and often has a small branch running with it toward the pylorus. The right gastric artery passes to the left along the lesser curve of the stomach, and anastomosis is to the left gastric artery. The continuation of the common hepatic artery, beyond the origin of the gastroduodenal artery and right gastric artery, is known as the *proper hepatic artery*, which usually soon divides into a right and a left branch. The left branch extends vertically, directly toward the base of the umbilical fissure, and usually gives off a branch known as the *middle hepatic artery (MH)*, which is directed toward the right of the umbilical fissure and is destined to supply segment IV of the liver. A further branch of the left hepatic artery *(LH)* courses to the left to supply the caudate lobe, and further smaller caudate branches arise from the left and right hepatic artery. The right hepatic artery *(RH)* usually passes behind the common hepatic duct and enters the cystic triangle of Calot; in some cases, it passes in front of the bile duct, which is important in surgical exposure of the CBD. The cystic artery usually arises from the right hepatic artery but has many variations.

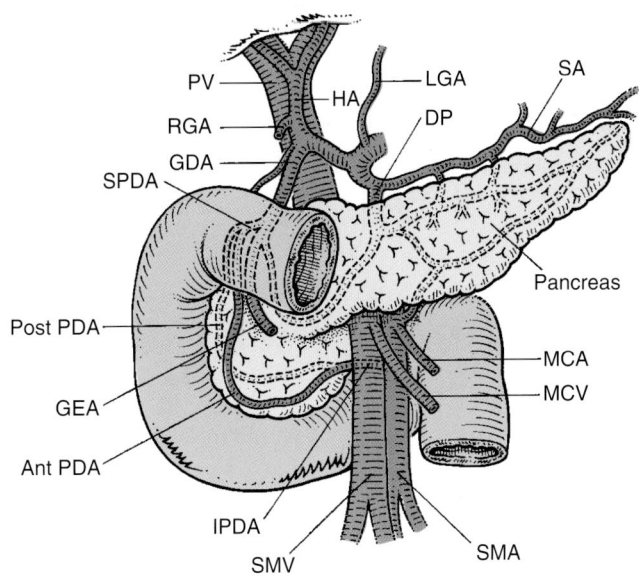

FIGURE 2.35 The primary arteries that supply the pancreas are the gastroduodenal artery *(GDA)*, which arises usually from the common hepatic artery *(HA)* as it crosses the portal vein *(PV)* above the pancreas proper, and the dorsal pancreatic artery *(DP)*, arising from the splenic artery *(SA)*. The superior pancreaticoduodenal arteries *(SPDAs)* arise from the GDA and join the inferior pancreaticoduodenal arteries *(IPDAs)* from the superior mesenteric artery *(SMA)*, forming two arcades along the anterior and posterior aspects of the head of the pancreas. The GDA, after giving rise to the pancreaticoduodenal artery *(PDA)*, passes forward and to the left as the right gastroepiploic artery *(GEA)*. The GDA is a good landmark for the identification of the portal vein above the pancreas, and surgical division of the GDA just at its origin from the common HA gives much greater access to the anterior surface of the portal vein at this site. The right gastric artery *(RGA)* also usually arises from the common HA just distal to the GDA, but it can arise from various sites. The GDA commonly divides into a larger right GEA and smaller SPDA. The right GEA runs forward between the first part of the duodenum and pancreas; the SPDA divides into anterior and posterior branches. The anterior superior PDA continues downward on the anterior surface of the head of the pancreas to anastomose with the IPDA, which arises from the SMA. The posterior superior PDA behaves similarly. *Ant,* Anterior; *LGA,* left gastric artery; *MCA,* middle colic artery; *MCV,* middle colic vein; *Post,* posterior; *SMV,* superior mesenteric vein.

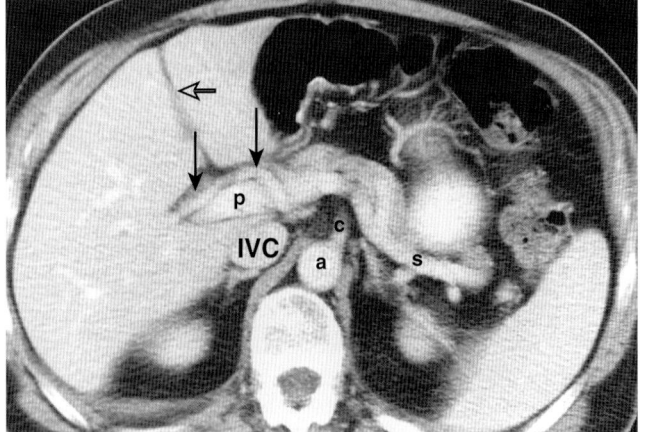

FIGURE 2.36 Computed tomographic image of the main portal vein shows the hepatic artery *(solid arrows)* coursing anterior to the portal vein *(p)*. The interlobar fissure *(open arrow)*, splenic vein *(s)*, celiac axis *(c)*, aorta *(a)*, and inferior vena cava *(IVC)* are also shown.

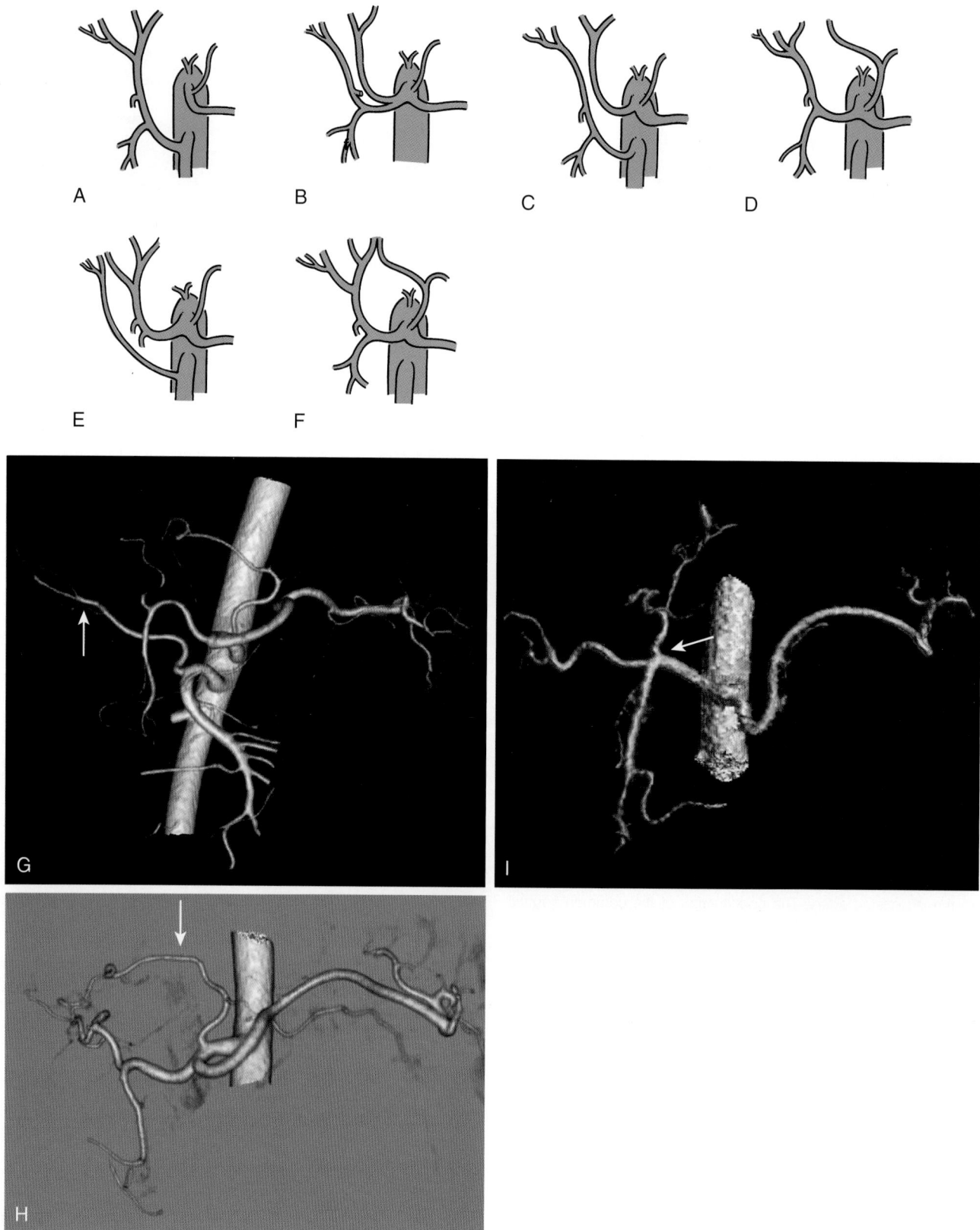

FIGURE 2.37   In approximately 25% of individuals, the right hepatic artery arises partially or completely from the superior mesenteric artery **(A, C, E)**; in a similar proportion of patients, the left hepatic artery may be partially or completely replaced by a branch arising from the left gastric artery, coursing through the gastrohepatic omentum to enter the liver at the base of the umbilical fissure **(D, F)**. Rarely, the right or left hepatic arteries originate independently from the celiac trunk or branch after a very short common hepatic artery origin, and the gastroduodenal artery may originate from the right hepatic artery **(B, C)**. Multidetector computed tomography (CT) angiogram demonstrating an accessory right hepatic artery *(arrow)* arising from the superior mesenteric artery **(G)**. Multidetector CT angiogram demonstrating a replaced left hepatic artery arising from the left gastric artery **(H)**. Another common arterial variant is the hepatic trifurcation **(I)**.

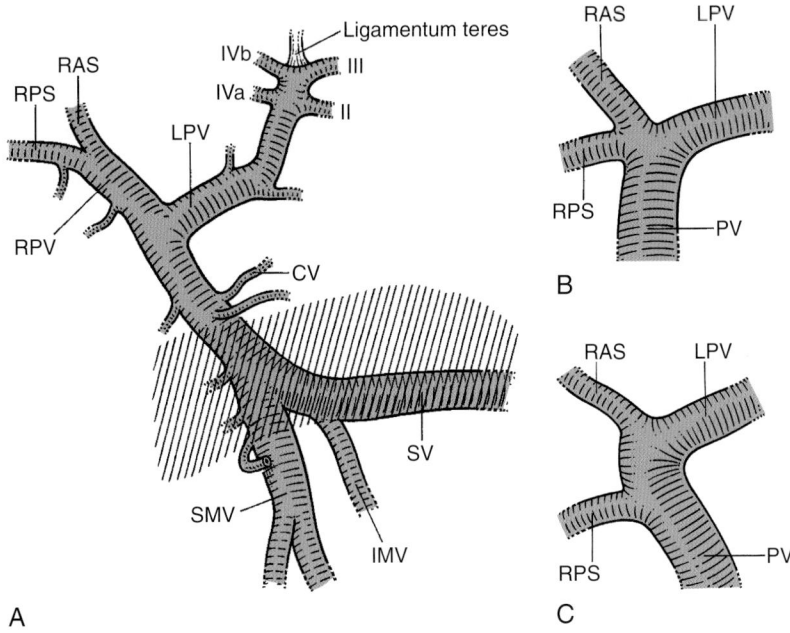

FIGURE 2.38 **A,** The superior mesenteric vein *(SMV)* at the root of the lesser omentum is usually a single trunk; two, or sometimes even three, branches may unite as the vessel enters the tunnel beneath the neck of the pancreas *(shaded)* to form a superior mesenteric trunk. This trunk ascends behind the neck of the pancreas and is joined by the splenic vein *(SV)*, which enters it from the left to form the portal vein *(PV)*, which emerges from the retroperitoneal upper border of the neck of the pancreas and ascends toward the liver within the free edge of the lesser omentum, lying behind the bile duct and the hepatic artery and surrounded by the lymphatics and nodes of the lesser omentum. During this course, it receives blood through the coronary vein *(CV)*, which communicates with esophageal venous collaterals, which connect with the gastric vein and the esophageal plexus. Sometimes a separate right gastric vein enters the PV in this area. A superior pancreaticoduodenal vein often enters the PV just above the level of the pancreas, and several smaller veins enter the SMV and PV from the right side beneath the neck of the pancreas. As the PV ascends behind the common bile duct and common hepatic duct, it approaches the hilus of the liver and bifurcates into two branches, a larger right *(RPV)* and a smaller left portal vein *(LPV)*. The branch on the left courses below the left hepatic duct to enter the umbilical fissure, in company with the left hepatic artery, and subsequently branches to supply the left liver segments (II-IV). Just before its entry into the umbilical fissure, it gives off a major caudate vein, segment I, which runs posteriorly and laterally to the left. Sometimes this vein consists of two or more branches; the right portal branch, which is much shorter in length before its entry into the liver, divides at the extremity of the hilus into the right anterior *(RAS)* and posterior *(RPS)* sectional branches and is accompanied by the respective arterial branches and biliary tributaries. **B,** The division of the portal vein may arise more proximally, however, and **C,** the right anterior and posterior sectional portal veins may arise independently from the portal venous trunk. *IMV,* Inferior mesenteric vein.

recognize. Failure to show all arteries feeding the liver at angiography may not only result in errors of diagnosis but also seriously mislead the surgeon or the interventional radiologist. In most cases, the hepatic artery arises from the celiac axis as described earlier, but it may be entirely replaced by a common hepatic artery that originates from the SMA. In this instance, the hepatic artery passes posterior and then lateral to the portal vein while it ascends and lies posterolateral to the CBD in the hepatoduodenal ligament, where it is susceptible to operative injury if not recognized. This applies to a right replaced or an accessory hepatic artery. Other variations in the origin of the common hepatic artery include its origin directly from the aorta and the persistence of a primitive embryologic link between the celiac and superior mesenteric systems. These variations are of considerable importance in controlling the arterial blood supply to the liver during hepatic resection, liver transplantation, devascularization of the liver, placement of intraarterial hepatic infusion devices, and in the resection of the head of the pancreas.

Portal Vein

The portal vein (Fig. 2.38) is formed behind the neck of the pancreas by confluence of the superior mesenteric and splenic

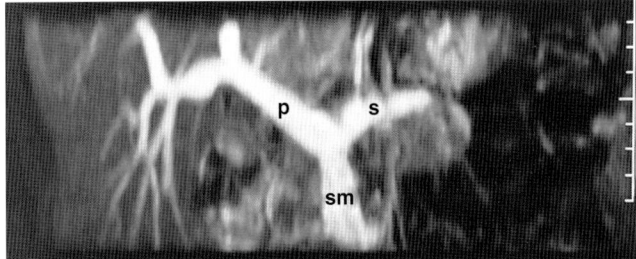

FIGURE 2.39 Magnetic resonance imaging of the splenoportal confluence: postcontrast, T1-weighted, three-dimensional gradient-echo coronal maximum intensity projection. Shown are the splenic vein *(s)*, portal vein *(p)*, and superior mesenteric vein *(sm)*.

veins (Fig. 2.39). The venous drainage of the pancreas usually runs parallel to the arterial supply. There are anterior and posterior and superior and inferior pancreaticoduodenal veins that drain to the portal vein and the SMV. The left gastric vein and the inferior mesenteric vein (IMV) usually drain into the splenic vein, but they can drain directly into the portal vein, whereas the various small splenic tributaries drain directly to the splenic vein.

The anatomic relationship of the pancreas to the SMV, the splenic vein, and the portal vein (see Fig. 2.38) is important in pancreatic resection (see Chapter 117). The uncinate process generally extends behind the SMV to a position adjacent to the SMA (see Fig. 2.35). Access to the portal vein behind the pancreas usually is obtained from below by elevating the pancreas from the surface of the SMV just before it joins the splenic vein. With the exception of the inferior pancreaticoduodenal veins, which enter the SMV at the inferior border of the pancreas, it is uncommon to see branches from the pancreas run directly posteriorly into the SMV. Fixation here is usually by an inflammatory or neoplastic process. Superiorly, the portal vein runs behind the pancreas and is identified first in the gap between the curvature of the splenic vein, splenic artery, common hepatic artery, and gastroduodenal artery. Division of the gastroduodenal artery provides much greater access to the superior surface of the portal vein, and this step is necessary to assess tumor involvement of the proximal portal vein. If difficulty is encountered in this area, division of the CBD, usually above the cystic duct, can provide excellent access to the right lateral aspect and anterior surface of the portal vein. The SMA can be approached behind the pancreas above the point at which it is embraced by the uncinate process at the origin from the aorta. This allows for dissection of the most proximal part of the SMA.

Occasionally, the middle colic artery and other vessels of supply to the colon can arise from the more proximal SMA, such that they pass through the pancreas; this abnormality should be searched for carefully. Division of the middle colic artery is usually not a problem, however, because the colon is well supplied with blood, and ischemia typically does not occur.

Of special importance to the surgeon is the direct relationship of the head of the pancreas to the duodenum and posteriorly to the right renal vein and the anterior surface of the IVC. The neck and body of the pancreas lie atop the SMA and the splenic vessels and their branches, the left renal vein, and, more laterally, the left kidney. The right gastroepiploic vein commonly drains into the anterior surface of the SMV just at the inferior border of the pancreas; this can often be involved by tumor, as can the anterior branch of the inferior pancreaticoduodenal vein; the middle colic vein may also join at this point. In mobilizing the SMV, these vessels are ligated so as to avoid bothersome hemorrhage. Abnormalities of the IVC are uncommon, with duplication of the vena cava and a left-sided vena cava seen rarely.

Several variations in anatomy and rare congenital anomalies of the portal vein are of surgical significance (Figs. 2.40–2.43). For example, performance of right hepatic resection, with division of what appears to be the right portal vein in a patient with absence of the left portal vein (see Figs. 2.42 and 2.43) can be fatal. Agenesis of the right branch of the portal vein is associated with agenesis of the right hemiliver and left liver hypertrophy. This may be associated with biliary and hepatic venous anatomic anomalies, which can compromise surgical approaches to the liver and to biliary repair.[26]

Portal venous blood is derived from the venous drainage of the stomach, small bowel, spleen, and pancreas, and this drainage is important when considering surgery of the pancreas and in patients with portal hypertension; it is described

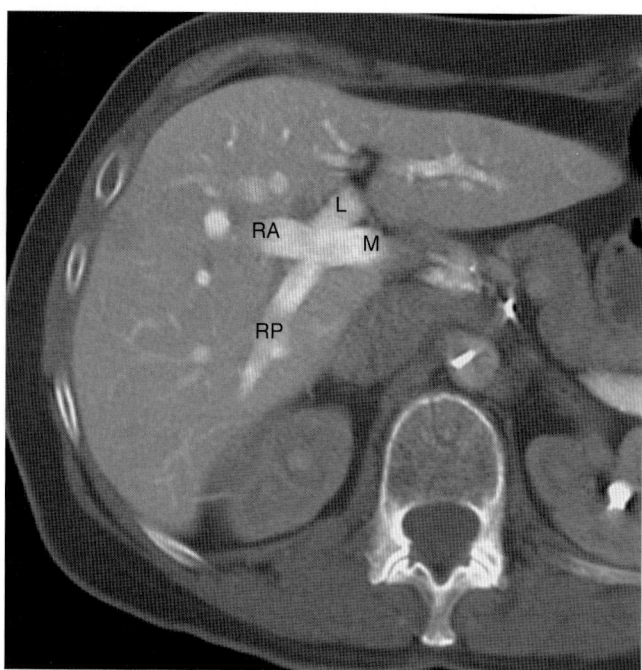

FIGURE 2.40   Contrast-enhanced computed tomographic scan of variant portal vein branching with trifurcation pattern. *L,* Left portal vein; *M,* main portal vein; *RA,* right anterior portal vein; *RP,* right posterior portal vein. (From Covey AM, Brody LA, Getrajdman GI, et al. Incidence, patterns, and clinical relevance of variant portal vein anatomy. *Am J Roentgenol.* 2004;183:1055–1064.)

in detail along with the description of the anatomy of the pancreas.

PANCREAS

The pancreas is a posteriorly situated retroperitoneal organ that lies transversely (Fig. 2.44). The organ is composed of a head, neck, body, and tail (see Chapter 1). The head is encompassed by the duodenum, whereas the tail rests in the splenic hilum (Figs. 2.45 and 2.46). A portion of the head inferiorly is termed the *uncinate process* and is intimately related to the SMV and SMA. Posteriorly, the pancreas is related to the IVC, aorta, left renal vein and kidney, and spleen. The portion lateral to the portal vein averages 56.4% of the total weight. The pancreatic capsule is loosely attached to the surface of the pancreas and is contiguous with the anterior layer of the mesocolon such that it can be dissected in continuity if necessary. The mesenteric attachments to the pancreas tend to be contiguous (see Fig. 2.46). The arterial blood supply and venous drainage and the relationships to the CBD are described and illustrated earlier (see Figs. 2.17, 2.29, 2.34, 2.35, and Fig. 2.38).

Pancreatic Duct

The duct of Wirsung, beginning in the distal tail as a confluence of small ductules, runs through the body to the head, where it usually passes downward and backward in close juxtaposition to the CBD (see Fig. 2.45). The sphincter of Oddi (Fig. 2.47) has been thoroughly studied[27,28] and consists of a unique

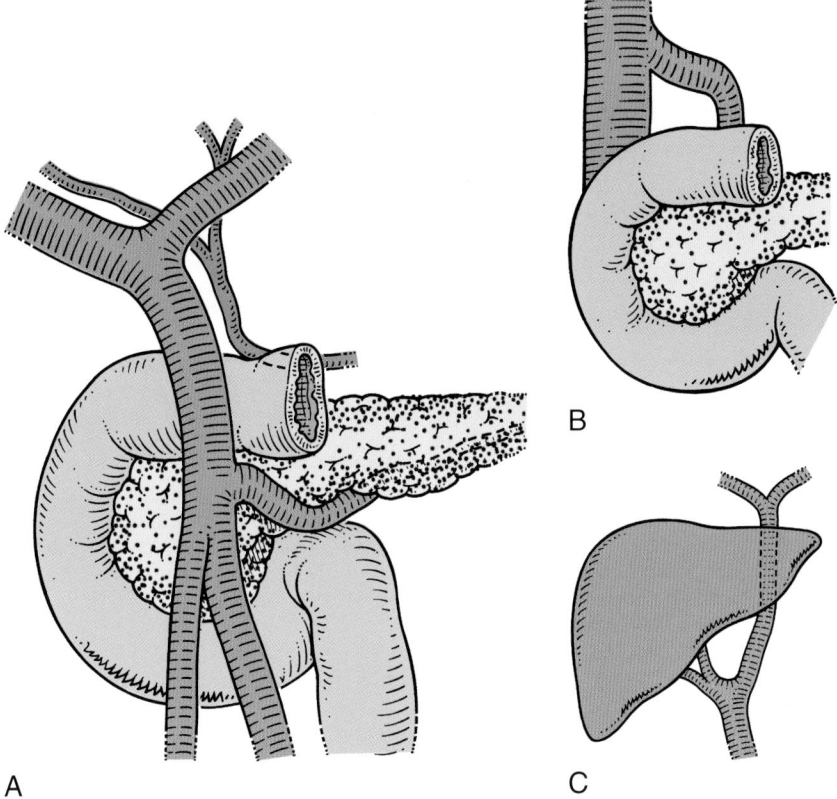

FIGURE 2.41 **A,** The portal vein anterior to the head of the pancreas and the duodenum may be in an abnormal position. **B,** Another rare but interesting anomaly is the entrance of the portal vein into the inferior vena cava. **C,** Very rare, the entrance of a pulmonary vein into the portal vein.

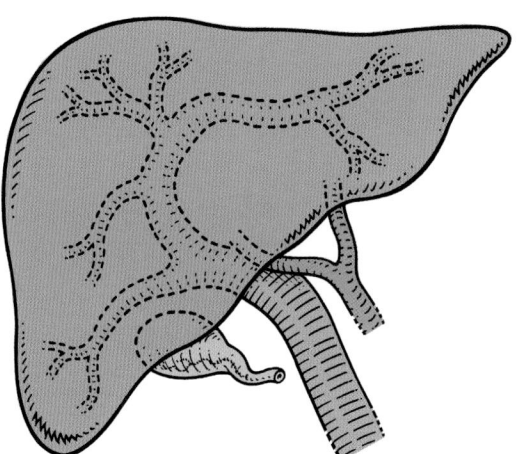

FIGURE 2.42 In a congenital absence of the left branch of the portal vein as described by Couinaud, the right branch courses through the right lobe of the liver, supplying it, and curves within the liver substance to supply the left lobe, which in such instances is usually smaller than normal.

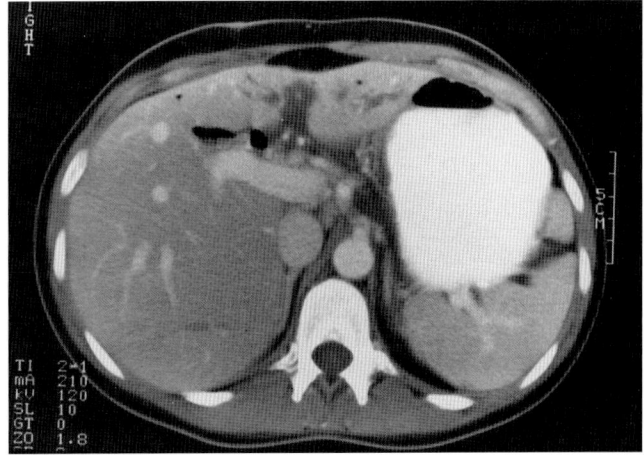

FIGURE 2.43 Computed tomographic scan in a patient with Caroli's disease shows a large right portal trunk. The left branch of the portal vein is absent, with findings confirmed at operation for left hepatic lobectomy.

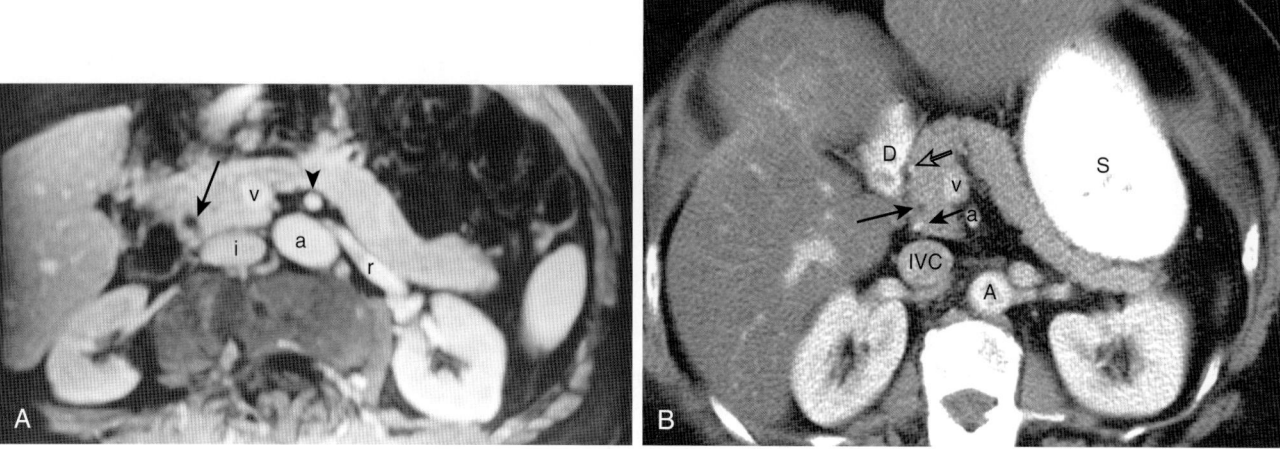

FIGURE 2.44 A, Magnetic resonance imaging of the pancreas, oblique axial reconstruction, T1-weighted three-dimensional gradient-echo technique. Aorta *(a)*, inferior vena cava *(i)*, common bile duct *(CBD; arrow)*, superior mesenteric vein at the splenoportal confluence *(v)*, superior mesenteric artery *(arrowhead)*, and left renal vein *(r)* are shown. **B,** Normal pancreatic anatomy. Postcontrast computed tomographic scan at the level of the pancreas. *A,* Aorta; *a,* superior mesenteric artery; *D,* duodenum; *IVC,* inferior vena cava; *S,* stomach; *v,* superior mesenteric vein; *long arrow,* CBD; *short arrow,* inferior pancreaticoduodenal artery; *open arrow,* gastroduodenal artery.

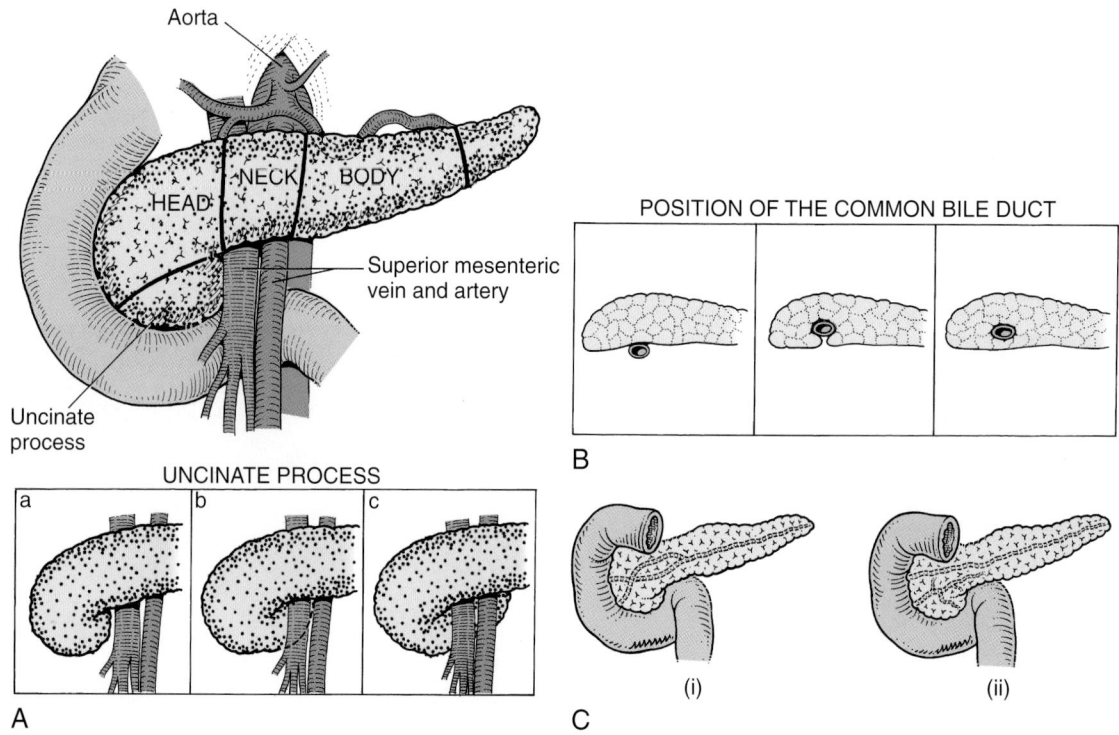

FIGURE 2.45 A, The head of the pancreas is globular with an extension, the *uncinate process,* which curves behind the superior mesenteric vessels and may end even before it embraces the superior mesenteric vein *(a),* or it may pass completely behind between the aorta and the left of the patient's superior mesenteric artery *(b, c).* All variations are commonly seen. Posteriorly, the head of the pancreas lies in juxtaposition to the inferior vena cava at the level of the entry of the left and right renal veins. The head of the pancreas forms a narrow *neck* in front of the superior mesenteric and splenic vein confluence. The neck joins to the *body* of the gland, which forms a narrow *tail.* **B,** The common bile duct (CBD) passes through the pancreas, either directly in the substance of the gland or initially with a posterior groove. **C,** The *duct of Wirsung* courses from left to right within the pancreas, curves downward approaching the CBD, and runs parallel with it, but separated from it, by the *transampullary septum* to enter the duodenum, 7 to 10 cm distal to the pylorus, at the *papilla of Vater* after traversing the *sphincter of Oddi.* An accessory duct, the *duct of Santorini,* runs more proximally in the head of the pancreas and usually terminates in the duodenum at an accessory papilla. Multiple variations of the ductal system occur, depending on the extent of development of the duct of Santorini, such that rarely the accessory duct can enter the duodenum inferior to the main duct. It can be in communication with the main duct directly *(i),* or it can occur in duplicate version known as *pancreas divisum (ii).* The duct of Santorini drains the body and tail of the organ, and the duct of Wirsung drains the head and the uncinate process.

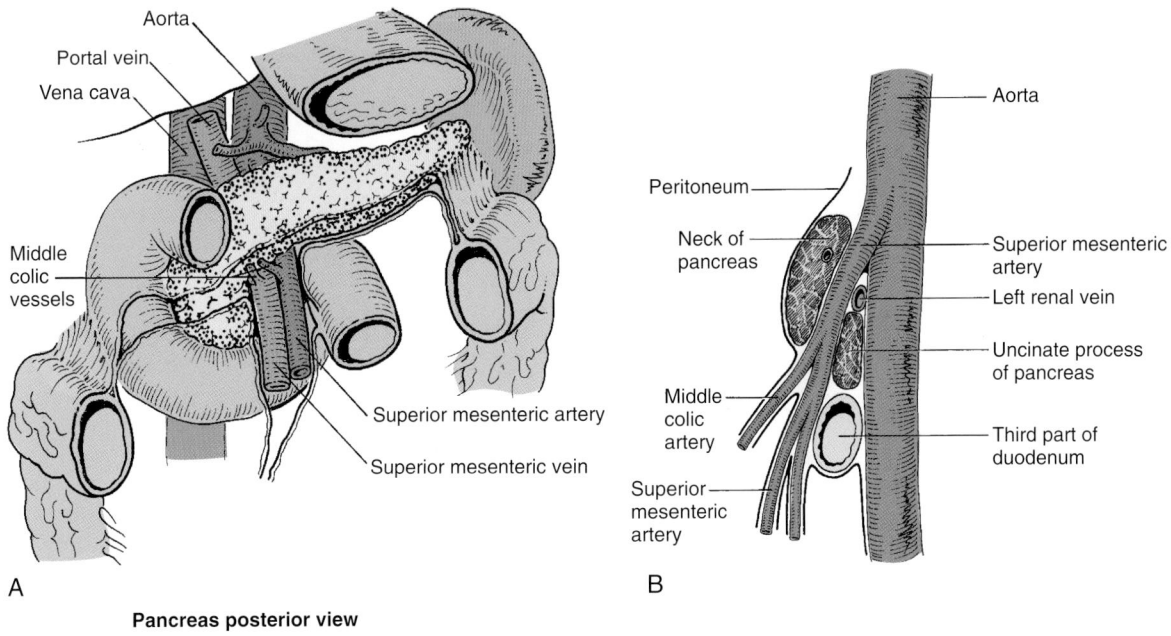

Pancreas posterior view

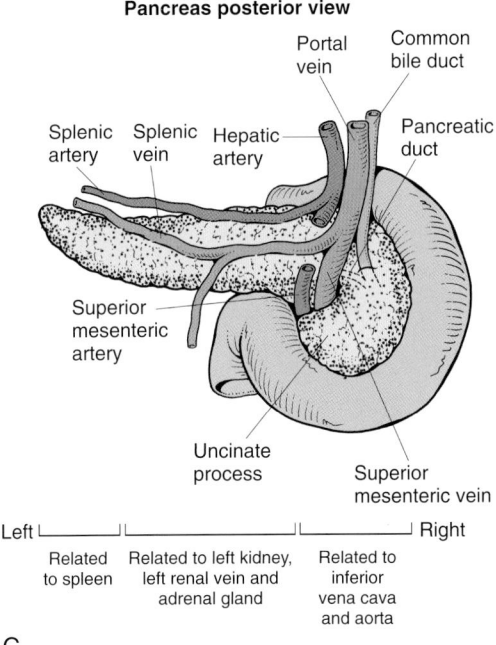

FIGURE 2.46 **A,** The anterior surface of the pancreas, covered by the posterior layer of the omental bursa or lesser peritoneal sac, can often be obliterated by adhesions. The transverse mesocolon arises from the lower border of the pancreas and envelops the middle colic vessels as they arise from the superior mesenteric vessels just beneath the pancreatic neck. **B,** The relationship of the pancreatic neck and uncinate process to the aorta and superior mesenteric artery. Note the position of the left renal vein and duodenum. **C,** The posterior relationships of the duodenal loop and pancreas. Note the relationship to the inferior vena cava, aorta, and hilum of the spleen.

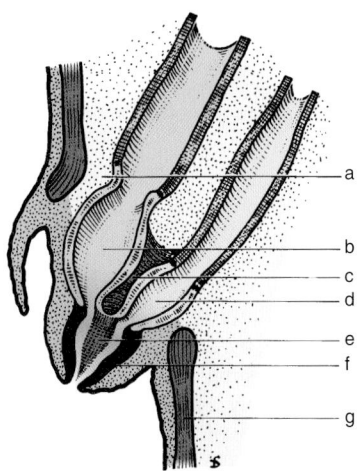

FIGURE 2.47 Schematic representation of the sphincter of Oddi: notch *(a)*, biliary sphincter *(b)*, transampullary septum *(c)*, pancreatic sphincter *(d)*, membranous septum of Boyden *(e)*, common sphincter *(f)*, smooth muscle of duodenal wall *(g)*.

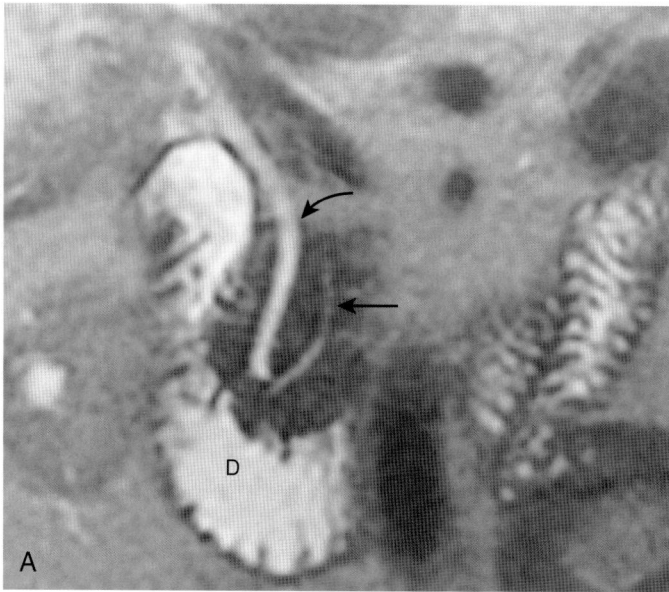

MRCP: PANCREAS DIVISUM

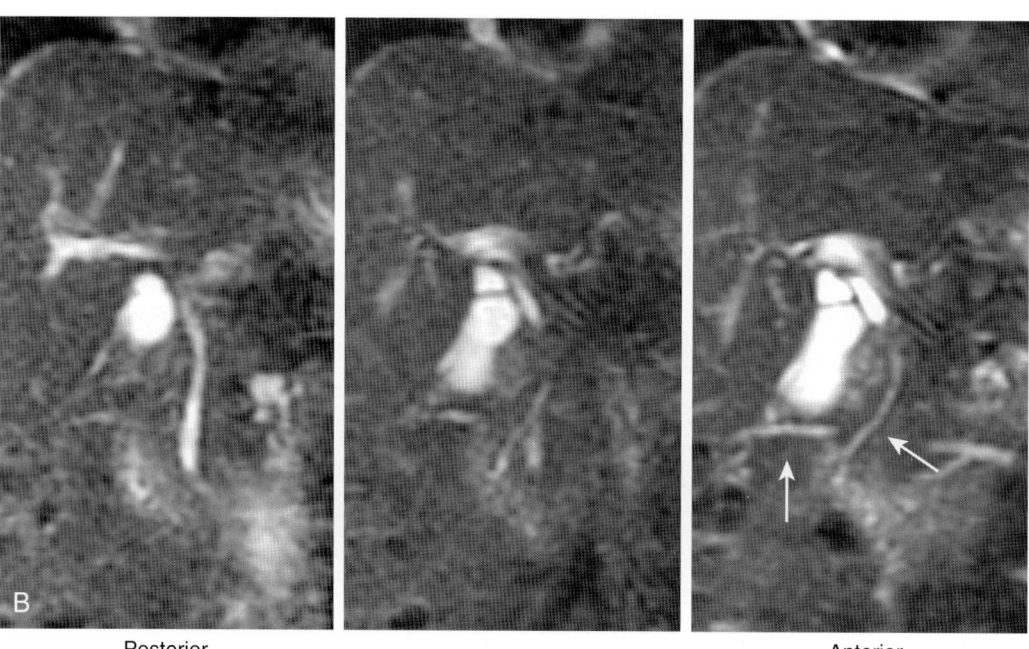

Posterior

Anterior

FIGURE 2.48   A, Magnetic resonance imaging cholangiography (MRCP), T2-weighted coronal image at the level of the ampulla, shows the duodenum *(D)* and the pancreatic head with common bile duct *(curved arrow)* and pancreatic duct *(straight arrow).* **B,** MRCP of pancreas divisum. Anterior projection shows variant anatomy with the duct of Santorini *(vertical arrow)* between the duodenum above the duct of Wirsung *(angled arrow).* The two ducts are separate; the duct of Santorini drains mainly the neck and body of the pancreas, and the duct of Wirsung drains mainly the uncinate process portion of the head of the pancreas.

cluster of smooth muscle fibers distinguishable from the adjacent smooth muscle of the duodenal wall. The papilla of Vater at the termination of the CBD is a small, nipple-like structure that protrudes into the duodenal lumen and is marked by a longitudinal fold of duodenal mucosa. The duct of Wirsung runs downward and parallel to the CBD for approximately 2 cm and joins it within the sphincter segment in 70% to 85% of patients; it enters the duodenum independently in 10% to 13% of patients and is replaced by the duct of Santorini in 2% of patients (Fig. 2.48; see Fig. 2.45). Rarely, the duct of Santorini

and the duct of Wirsung are separate, which is known as *pancreas divisum* (see Fig. 2.45Cii and Fig. 2.48B; see Chapters 1 and 53). The islets of Langerhans, which provide the endocrine component of the gland, are scattered throughout the pancreas.

Annular Pancreas

Annular pancreas is the development of a ring of pancreatic tissue that surrounds and often embraces the duodenum. This ring may contain a large duct and can be firmly affixed to the duodenal musculature. The duodenum beneath this annulus is

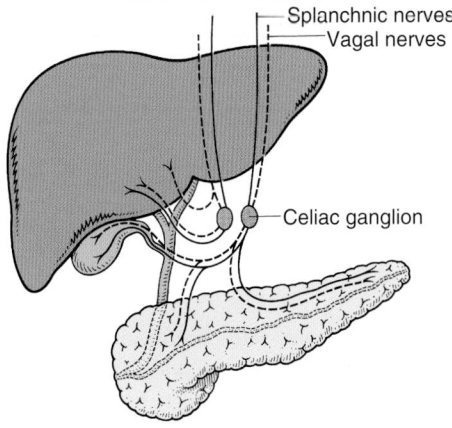

FIGURE 2.50 Note the distribution of sympathetic and parasympathetic nerves to the liver and pancreas from the celiac ganglion, mainly in association with major arteries.

often stenosed such that dividing this ring does not always relieve chronic duodenal obstruction. This accounts for the common process of applying duodenojejunostomy to relieve strictures caused by such an annulus (see Chapters 1 and 53)

LYMPHATIC DRAINAGE

Liver and Pancreas

The lymphatic drainage of the liver and gallbladder is mainly to nodes in the hepatoduodenal ligament and along the hepatic artery; this is shown in Fig. 2.49. The lymphatic drainage of the pancreas is predominantly to the nodes that lie in juxtaposition to the arteries and veins (Fig. 2.50B).

NERVE SUPPLY TO THE LIVER AND PANCREAS

The nerve supply to the liver and pancreas (see Fig. 2.50) is from branches of the celiac ganglion. It is composed of sympathetic and parasympathetic elements.

References are available at expertconsult.com.

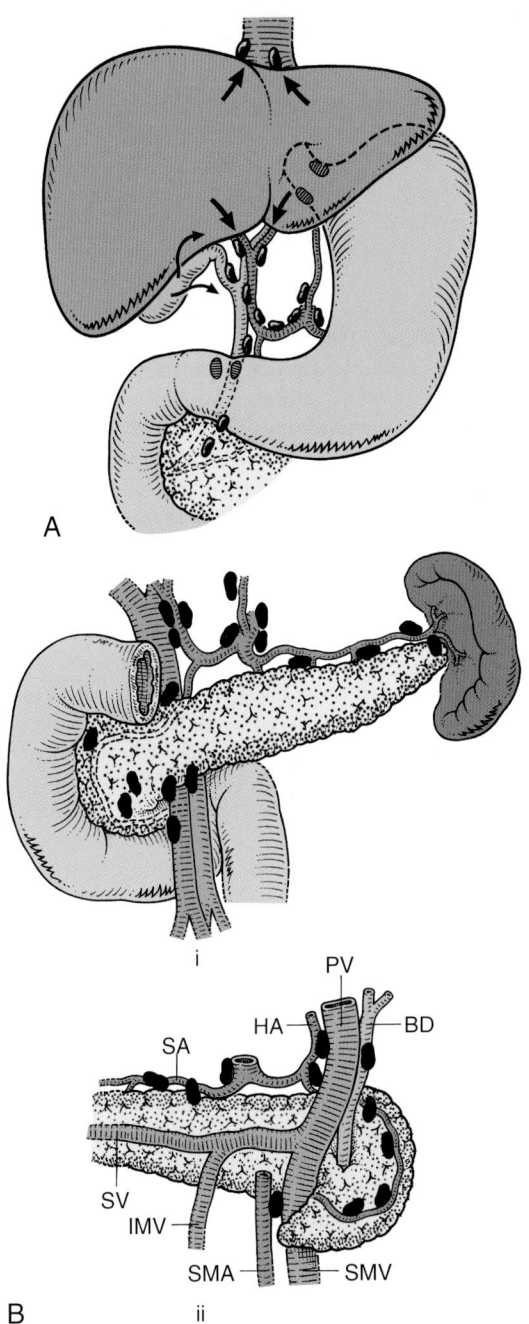

FIGURE 2.49 A, The liver drains principally to hepatoduodenal nodes at the hilus and along the hepatic artery and portal vein. The gallbladder drains partly to the liver, but it also drains via the cystic node to nodes of the hepatoduodenal ligament and to suprapancreatic nodes. **B,** Numerous nodes *(i)* lie along the superior mesenteric vein along the borders of the pancreas, draining back into the splenic hilar nodes; along the superior border of the pancreas to the superior pancreatic nodes; and to the celiac trunk and nodes at the base of the common hepatic artery. A large node commonly lodges in intimate association with the surface of the superior border of the pancreas and the right side of the common hepatic artery. This node often needs to be dissected and elevated to gain access to the anterior surface of the portal vein. Removal of this node often improves access, as does division of the gastroduodenal artery. Posterior pancreaticoduodenal nodes *(ii)* lie along the posterior pancreatic duodenal arterial arcade. *BD,* Bile duct; *HA,* hepatic artery; *IMV,* interior mesenteric vein; *PV,* portal vein; *SA,* splenic artery; *SMA,* superior mesenteric artery; *SMV,* superior mesenteric vein; *SV,* splenic vein.

CHAPTER 3

Pancreatic physiology and functional assessment

Alessandro Paniccia and Richard D. Schulick

The pancreas is a complex retroperitoneal gland with both endocrine (e.g., glucose homeostasis) and exocrine (e.g., nutrient digestion) functions. An adult human pancreas measures approximately 15 cm in length and weighs between 60 to 100 g; however, its size can vary because of aging or pathologic conditions (e.g., pancreatitis, neoplasia).[1,2] It is of endodermal origin and arises from two independent primordia: a ventral bud (derived from the hepatic diverticulum) and a dorsal bud (derived from the developing duodenum; see Chapter 1). Around the fifth week of gestation, the ventral bud rotates clockwise with the developing duodenum to fuse with the dorsal pancreatic bud.[3,4] Ultimately, the ventral bud will form the inferior pancreatic head and the uncinate process. The dorsal bud will constitute the majority of the pancreatic gland, representing the superior pancreatic head, the body, and the tail of the adult pancreas (see Chapters 1 and 2). During this process, the main ducts of the ventral and dorsal pancreatic buds fuse to form the main pancreatic duct (duct of Wirsung). The major pancreatic duct drains most of the organ's secretions through the major duodenal papilla (ampulla of Vater). A separate draining duct, arising from the dorsal pancreatic bud, usually persists and forms the minor pancreatic duct (duct of Santorini). The minor duct drains a portion of the pancreatic head secretions into the duodenum through the minor papilla, located 2 cm anterosuperior of the major papilla.[5]

The pancreas receives an abundant arterial vascular supply from branches of the celiac and superior mesenteric artery. The venous drainage follows the arterial supply, with venous effluents ultimately draining into the portal vein.[6] Furthermore, the pancreas is supplied by several neural sources, including sympathetic fibers from the splanchnic nerves, parasympathetic fibers from the vagus nerve, and peptidergic neurons (releasing amines and peptides; see Chapter 2).[7,8]

ENDOCRINE PANCREAS

The islets of Langerhans are the functional units of the endocrine pancreas and have a paramount role in maintaining glucose homeostasis. In light of their complex cytoarchitecture structure and regulatory system, they are de-facto *microorgan(s)* within the pancreas.[9] The pancreas of a healthy adult has approximately one million islets that are evenly distributed throughout the pancreatic gland and account for 1% to 2% of the organ's mass. Each islet ranges in size from 50 to 300 μm in diameter and contains a few hundred to a few thousand endocrine cells.[5]

Structure

There are at least five major cell types in each islet of Langerhans: α, β, δ, F, and ε cells. In humans, pancreatic α-cells, which principally secrete glucagon, represent approximately 35% of all islet cells. Pancreatic β-cells, which are responsible for the production and secretion of insulin and amylin, represent approximately 55% of islet cells. Pancreatic δ-cells, which principally secrete somatostatin, represent less than 10% of the islet cells, and pancreatic F cells, which secrete pancreatic polypeptide (PP), account for less than 5%. Finally, the ε cells, which secrete ghrelin, account for less than 1% of human islet cells.[10]

The distribution and cellular composition of the different cell types within the islet vary among species. Previous animal models with rabbits, rats, and mice demonstrated that β cells occupy the core of the islet of Langerhans and that non–β-cells are distributed toward the outside of the islet.[11] Recent studies in humans have demonstrated a different cytoarchitecture, where the majority of α-, β-, and δ-cells reside along the islet blood vessels without a specific order.[11] Furthermore, approximately 70% of human β-cells appear to be in contact with non–γ-islet cells, suggesting a predisposition for paracrine interaction.[9] The islet's regional location within the human pancreas is also essential to islet cytoarchitecture.[9] Islets located in the body and tail of the pancreas have a higher proportion of α cells and a lower proportion of F cells, whereas islets located in the uncinate process have a higher proportion of F cells and a lower proportion of α-cells. Notably, β-cells and δ-cells are present in nearly equal proportions throughout the pancreas.[5]

The islets are rich in axonal terminals and blood capillaries that participate in extensive neurohumoral and nonneuronal paracrine regulation. Studies using three-dimensional reconstruction of the axonal terminal field revealed that the autonomic innervation to the human islet of Langerhans is different from that previously identified in rodents.[8] Contrary to what was previously understood, human β cells receive minimal innervation from the parasympathetic cholinergic system.[8] Instead, sympathetic neural terminals penetrate the human islet of Langerhans to innervate the smooth muscle cells of the blood vessels, allowing fine regulation of islet blood flow. Consequently, sympathetic nerves indirectly influence downstream endocrine cells by regulating the local blood flow containing secreted endocrine hormone.[8]

The islets of Langerhans receive approximately 20% of the pancreatic arterial flow, with distribution significantly influenced by the different phases of digestion.[12] Furthermore, an insuloacinar portal system responsible for draining blood and secreted hormones from the islets of Langerhans to the pancreas' acinar element exists in several species, including humans.[13] Hormones secreted by the islet of Langerhans are directly transported to the acinar cells, where they can exert a local regulatory function. Besides, several neuropeptides, including neuropeptide-Y, gastrin-releasing peptide, and calcitonin gene-related peptide (CGRP), exert a local regulatory effect on endocrine and exocrine pancreatic function.

Synthesis and Storage of Insulin

In 1923 Banting and McLeod, two Canadian surgeons, were awarded the Nobel Prize in Physiology or Medicine for the discovery of insulin.[14] This 51–amino acid polypeptide is primarily responsible for maintaining serum glucose between 4 mM and 8 mM (70–140 mg/dL) during periods of feeding and fasting.[15] Moreover, insulin regulates lipid and protein metabolism. The gene responsible for encoding insulin is located on the short arm of chromosome 11 and leads to the translation of a preprohormone protein known as *preproinsulin* within the β-cell. Preproinsulin consists of a leading sequence of 24 amino acids, followed by three domains named "B," "C," and "A." Successive cleavage processes take place starting at the time of translation until the final secretion. First, cleavage of the leading sequence in the endoplasmic reticulum leads to the formation of proinsulin. As the proinsulin is arranged into secretory granules in the trans-Golgi, additional proteases cleave the central 31 amino acid C-peptide. This process leads to the formation of a mature insulin peptide composed of an A-chain and B-chain held together by two disulfide bonds, ready to be released in the secretory vesicle. Cleaved C-peptide and other intermediate products, such as proinsulin, remain present in the secretory granules and are eventually released with mature insulin.[5] The mature insulin peptide has a plasma half-life of 4 minutes. It is rapidly internalized by target organs expressing its receptor and degraded by the kidneys and liver.[16] Notably, C-peptide has a plasma half-life of 30 minutes and is excreted unchanged by the kidneys, making it a clinically meaningful marker of endogenous insulin secretion.[17]

Stimulus-Secretion Coupling for Insulin Secretion

The rise of islet cell transplantation has led to a renewed understanding of human β-cell regulation, building on earlier work completed in rodents (see Chapter 126). Insulin is released from β-cells through two mechanisms: unstimulated and stimulated secretion. Unstimulated secretion or basal insulin secretion occurs every 6 to 8 minutes.[18] Stimulated secretion of insulin occurs in response to several stimuli, including glucose, amino acids (e.g., arginine), acetylcholine (ACh), glutamate, and incretins such as gastric inhibitory peptide (GIP) and glucagon-like peptide-1 (GLP-1). The change in extracellular glucose concentration, however, is the dominant factor controlling β-cell function.

The primary glucose transporters on pancreatic β-cells are GLUT-2, highly expressed in rodents,[19] and GLUT-1 and GLUT-3, both expressed at high levels on human β-cells (Fig. 3.1).[20] The GLUT transporters allow equalization of the intracellular and extracellular glucose concentrations. If the glucose concentration exceeds 5 mmol/L, the intracellular β-cell glucokinase enzymes activate to allow fine regulation of insulin secretion.[21] Acting as a "glucose sensor," these enzymes are responsible for the phosphorylation of glucose to glucose-6-phosphate.[22,23] Glucose-6-phosphate accumulates in the β-cell, is metabolized, and contributes to an increase in cellular adenosine triphosphate (ATP). The β-cell membrane is rich in ATP-dependent potassium channels, which subsequently undergo closure in response to the surge in ATP, resulting in membrane depolarization.[24,25] Depolarization activates voltage-gated L-type calcium channels, leading to an influx of calcium into the cell.[15,26] The increased intracellular calcium concentration leads to margination of secretory granules, their fusion with the cell membrane, and exocytosis of their content,

including insulin and its intermediate products (e.g., C-peptide).[25] This process characterizes the "first phase" of insulin release, in which insulin is rapidly secreted within 3 to 5 minutes of glucose administration and terminates within 10 minutes. The loss of the first phase of insulin secretion is one of the earliest metabolic defects identified in type 2 diabetes mellitus (T2DM).[27] The "second phase" of insulin secretion is longer lasting (reaching a plateau in insulin secretion after 2–3 hours), and its regulation is not entirely understood.[28,29] Nevertheless, recent mathematic models suggest that the second phase is characterized by the recruitment and mobilization of intracellular granules containing insulin (as opposed to predocked granules as in the first phase) in a dose-dependent glucose response.[30]

The amino acid arginine (l-arginine) is another well-known insulin secretagogue. After uptake into the β-cells through a cationic amino-acid transporter (CAT), arginine leads to depolarization of cell membrane, which triggers calcium influx.[31] Furthermore, l-arginine can stimulate the release of GLP-1, which acts at its receptor (GLP-1R) to augment glucose-stimulated insulin secretion from pancreatic β-cells.[32,33]

The incretin effect further potentiates insulin secretion from pancreatic β-cells through the enteroinsular axis.[34,35] The incretin effect is the phenomenon whereby the presence of nutrients, especially carbohydrates, in the duodenal lumen stimulates cells in the gut mucosa to release potent insulin secretagogues.[36] The ingestion of nutrients stimulates duodenal and jejunal K cells to produce and release GIP, a well-studied incretin. Also, GLP-1 is produced and released by the L cells (also known as enteroglucagone cells), located in the distal small bowel, colon, and rectum. It has been shown that orally administered glucose can stimulate insulin secretion as much as 25% more than intravenously administered glucose, likely through the incretin effect.[37]

GIP and GLP-1 play significant roles in the enteroinsular axis, mainly through activation of adenylate cyclase and subsequent increase in intracellular cyclic adenosine monophosphate (cAMP). The increase in cAMP leads to the activation of protein kinase A, with subsequent phosphorylation and activation of exocytosis-related proteins. Furthermore, cAMP activates L-type calcium channels, culminating in insulin release (see earlier).

Acetylcholine (ACh) maintains a pivotal role in glucose homeostasis. In human islets, ACh acts primarily as a nonneuronal paracrine signal released from α-cells rather than as a neural signal, as previously described in rodent islets.[38] ACh stimulates the insulin-secreting β-cell via the muscarinic ACh receptors M3 and M5, causing insulin release.[39] The activation of the M3 receptor leads to calcium release from intracellular stores through a phospholipase C–mediated increase in inositol-1,4,5-triphosphate (IP3).[40] Additionally, ACh stimulates the somatostatin-secreting δ-cell via M1 receptors. Because somatostatin is known to inhibit insulin secretion, it appears that endogenous cholinergic signaling provides a direct stimulatory and indirect inhibitory input to β-cells, allowing further regulation of insulin secretion.[39]

Glucagon and Other Islet Hormones

The islets of Langerhans secrete many additional hormones, including glucagon (α-cells), somatostatin (δ-cells), pancreatic polypeptide (F cells), and ghrelin (ε-cells).[10] Furthermore, islets contain a variable, but small, number of cells responsible

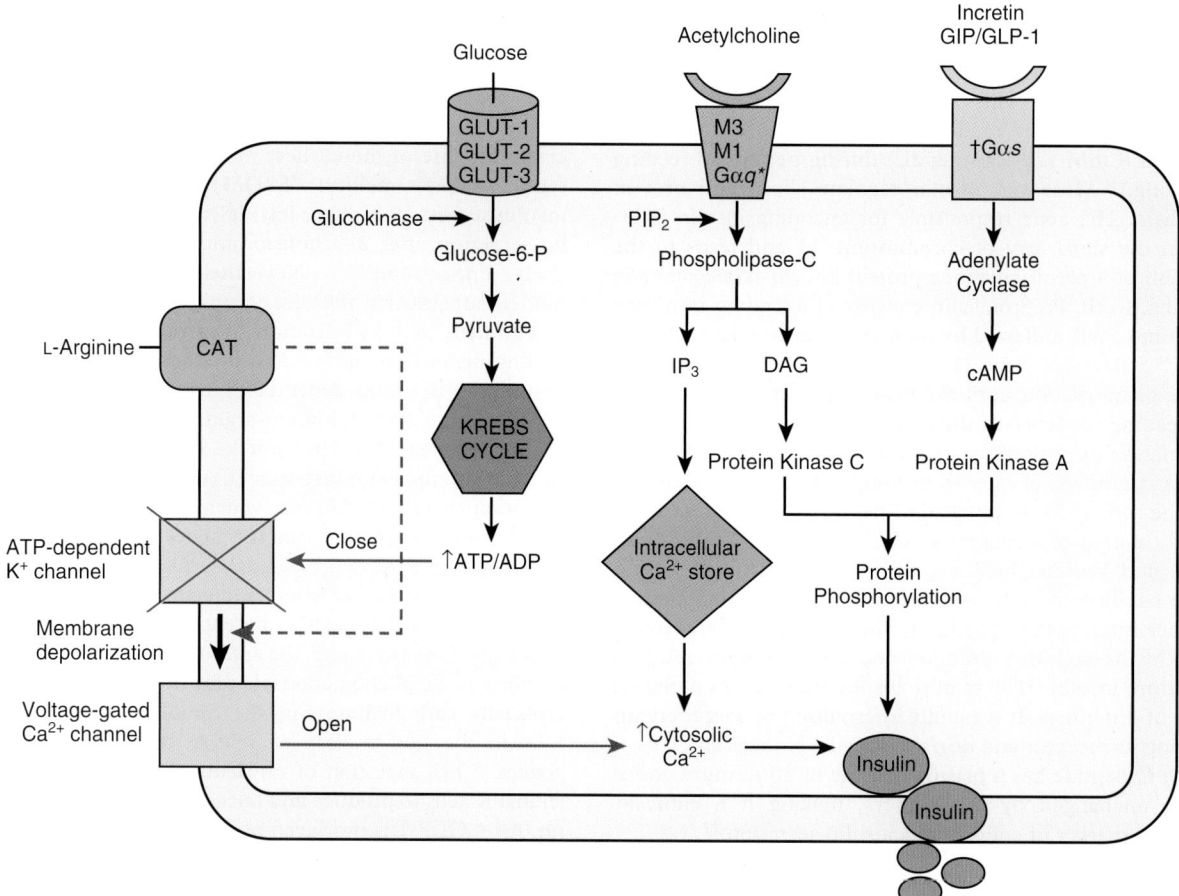

FIGURE 3.1　Stimulus-secretion coupling for insulin secretion. Insulin is secreted after food ingestion. Glucose, acetylcholine (ACh), incretins, and amino acids are the most important physiologic secretagogues. Glucose enters the human β-cell mainly via the glucose transporters GLUT-1 and GLUT-3 and, to a lesser extent, via GLUT-2. Once in the β-cell, glucose is phosphorylated to glucose-6-phosphate by an intracellular glucokinase (GCK) and eventually is metabolized to produce adenosine triphosphate (ATP), leading to an elevation of the cytosolic ATP/diphosphate (ADP) ratio. The increase in the intracellular ATP content is responsible for the closure of the ATP-dependent K^+ channel. The resulting increased membrane potential, caused by the closure of the ATP-dependent K^+ channel, prompts the opening of voltage-dependent Ca^{2+} channels, leading to an increase in intracellular Ca^{2+} levels. Arginine is a positively charged amino acid that depolarizes the β-cell after its uptake by a cationic amino-acid transporter (CAT); the membrane depolarization leads to the opening of voltage-dependent Ca^{2+} channels, allowing entry of Ca^{2+} into the cell. The increase in intracellular Ca^{2+} triggers exocytosis of insulin-containing secretory granules. ACh, released from vagal efferent and α-cell, binds to the muscarinic ACh receptor M3, which is coupled with a phospholipase C, resulting in the production of inositol-1,4,5-triphosphate (IP3) and diacylglycerol (DAG). Eventually, IP3 triggers the release of intracellular Ca^{2+}, and DAG causes activation of protein kinase C (PKC). The incretins (gastric inhibitory peptide [GIP] and glucagon-like peptide-1 [GLP-1]) bind to the extracellular domain of a G protein-coupled receptor to mediate signal transduction by activation of adenylate cyclase. The activated adenylate cyclase causes an increase of intracellular cyclic adenosine monophosphate (cAMP) concentrations leading to the activation of protein kinase A. Ultimately, the activation of protein kinase C and protein kinase A culminates with protein phosphorylation and secretion of insulin. *Gαq, Membrane-associated heterotrimeric G protein that activates *phospholipase C* (PLC); †Gαs, membrane-associated heterotrimeric G protein that activates the cAMP-dependent pathway by activating adenylate cyclase; *PIP2,* phosphatidylinositol-4,5-bisphosphate.

for secreting pancreastatin, serotonin, and vasointestinal polypeptide (VIP).[41–43] Glucagon, a 29–amino-acid peptide (molecular weight, 3.5 kDa), counteracts insulin's effect by increasing blood glucose concentration through stimulation of glycogenolysis, gluconeogenesis, and ketogenesis.[44] The secretion from islet α-cells directly into the portal system is mostly in response to protein ingestion. Glucagon at physiologic concentration exerts its function primarily in liver tissue through activation of cAMP pathways, where it promotes gluconeogenesis and, indirectly, ketogenesis.[45] Besides, glucagon indirectly stimulates fatty oxidation through the carnitine acylcarnitine translocase system (CAT). This process increases the ketone bodies β-hydroxybutyric acid and acetoacetic acid, which constitute metabolic fuel for other tissues. Glucagon inhibition is caused by increased

blood glucose concentration and by paracrine effects of insulin and somatostatin within the islet.[46]

Somatostatin, which acts primarily as an inhibitory hormone, is secreted by the islet δ-cell and by several other organs, including the hypothalamus and the D cells of the gastrointestinal (GI) tract. Among others, somatostatin inhibits insulin, glucagon, gastrin, and VIP. Its broad inhibition makes somatostatin and its pharmacologic analogs (e.g., octreotide) useful therapeutic agents in the medical management of secreting pancreatic neuroendocrine tumors (e.g., insulinoma; see Chapter 65) along with other medical diseases (e.g., Cushing's disease, acromegaly, carcinoid).[47] Furthermore, somatostatin analogs are used in the treatment of some surgical complications. For example, pasireotide, a multi-somatostatin receptor ligand, significantly decreased pancreatic leak complications after pancreatic surgery[48] (see Chapter 117).

Pancreatic polypeptide (PP) is produced and released by islet F cells; however, its physiologic role remains under investigation.[49] Some studies suggest that the absence of PP secretion, resulting from the removal of the uncinate process (rich in islet F cells) during pancreaticoduodenectomy, can lead to pancreatogenic diabetes (type 3c).[50]

Ghrelin, produced by the ϵ-cells, also known as the "hunger hormone," is a centrally active neuropeptide that participates in metabolic regulation, growth hormone release, and energy balance.[51,52] In particular, ϵ-cells participate in the regulation of various function of β-cells, including control of blood glucose levels as well as cellular growth. An increased understanding of ϵ-cells function and regulatory mechanism could lead to new therapeutic options for patients with diabetes mellitus.[53]

Pancreatitis Consequences on Endocrine Pancreas Function

Pancreatic endocrine insufficiency is a dreaded consequence of acute pancreatitis (AP). Recent studies suggest that after hospitalization for the first episode of AP, there is as much as a 40% risk of prediabetes or diabetes mellitus[54] (see Chapters 55 and 56).

Approximately 15% of newly diagnosed diabetes mellitus occurs within 12 months from the first episodes of AP, and the risk remains high, increasing significantly with time. It appears that the development of endocrine insufficiency is at least partially related to the severity of the episode of AP with an estimated 2-fold increase in the prevalence of endocrine pancreatic insufficiency after an episode of necrotizing pancreatitis.[55] The rate of insulin use within 5 years of the first episode of AP approaches 14%. Pancreatic necrosis and ethanol etiology represent strong risk factors for the development of pancreatic endocrine insufficiency.[55] Alternative mechanisms have been proposed and are currently under investigation, including both patients and disease-related factors, such as age, body mass index, family history, duration of pancreatic disease, presence of exocrine insufficiency, and pancreatic surgery. It is worth mentioning that the risk for diabetes mellitus can be as high as 80% in patients with chronic pancreatitis (CP; see Chapters 57 and 58).[56,57] Although pancreatogenic diabetes mellitus (type 3c) is most commonly the result of CP, it can also occur secondary to pancreatic cancer. In fact, the prevalence of diabetes mellitus in pancreatic ductal adenocarcinoma at the time of diagnosis is approximately 50%, and importantly, 75% of these patients are diagnosed with diabetes mellitus within 2 years before the diagnosis of cancer (see Chapter 62). Pancreatic polypeptide deficiency represents a distinctive feature of pancreatogenic diabetes and has been associated with reduced hepatic sensitivity to insulin.[58,59]

EXOCRINE PANCREAS

The exocrine pancreas constitutes 80% to 90% of the gland mass and secretes the majority of digestive enzymes, as well as approximately 2000 mL of colorless, odorless, and isosmotic alkaline protein-rich fluid (pH, 7.6–9.0) daily. It is mainly regulated by the neuroendocrine system, and it is integrated anatomically and physiologically with the endocrine pancreas, which helps modulate its function.[60]

Exocrine Pancreas Structure

The exocrine pancreas consists primarily of two distinct but integrated units: *the acinus* and *the ductal network*.

Acinus

The acinus is a functional unit mainly dedicated to digestive enzyme production and secretion (6 as much as 20 g daily). It is composed of 15 to 100 pyramidal-shaped cells (as much as 30 μm apical base height) known as *acinar cells*.[61] The acinar cells are polarized epithelial cells rich in rough endoplasmic reticulum and characterized by an abundance of secretory zymogen granules within the apex. The acinus is organized concentrically around a central lumen, which is in continuity with the proximal end of an *intercalated duct*, where it drains its secretions. Several acini form a pancreatic lobule, separated from other lobules by thin layers of connective tissue.

The Ductal Network

The ductal network serves two critical functions: transporting exocrine secretions from the acini to the duodenum and producing a solution rich in bicarbonate and electrolytes (Fig. 3.2). The bicarbonate and water released in the ductal network facilitate the transport and flushing of acinar secretions throughout the pancreatic ducts and, most importantly, optimize the pH of the solution in which pancreatic enzymes are secreted.[62]

The ductal network starts with small intercalated ducts originating from different acini, which then join to form an intralobular duct. This serves to drain an individual pancreatic lobule. Intralobular ducts then drain into larger interlobular ducts, which then empty into the main pancreatic duct, releasing the pancreatic secretions into the duodenum, through the ampulla of Vater.[63,64]

The ductal network is composed of highly specialized epithelial cells with varying morphologies and functions.[61] Cells of the intercalated duct are characterized by minimal cytoplasm and a squamous-shaped appearance. On the contrary, cells in the main pancreatic duct have an abundance of cytoplasm rich in mitochondria and are characterized by a cuboidal shape.

Ductal cells contain substantial levels of cytoplasmic carbonic anhydrase, an enzyme necessary for bicarbonate production.[65]

Centroacinar Cells

Cuboidal-shaped centroacinar cells are present at the junction between the acinus and the ductal cells of the intercalated duct. Recognized as morphologically distinct from acinar cells, centroacinar cells are smaller than acinar cells (~10 μm in diameter), have a high nuclear-to-cytoplasm ratio, and have long cytoplasmic processes that allow contact with other cells (i.e., centroacinar, acinar, and islet cells).[61,66,67] The role of centroacinar cells remains under investigation, but some authors suggest that centroacinar cells could represent multipotent progenitor pancreatic cells and potentially be involved in malignant transformation.[68,69]

Ductal Epithelial Compartment

Ductal epithelial compartments (also known as *pancreatic duct glands*) are distributed along the pancreatic ducts and resemble blind outpouchings or small branches originating from the pancreatic ducts. The cell lining of these outpouchings consists of columnar-shaped cells, characterized by abundant supranuclear

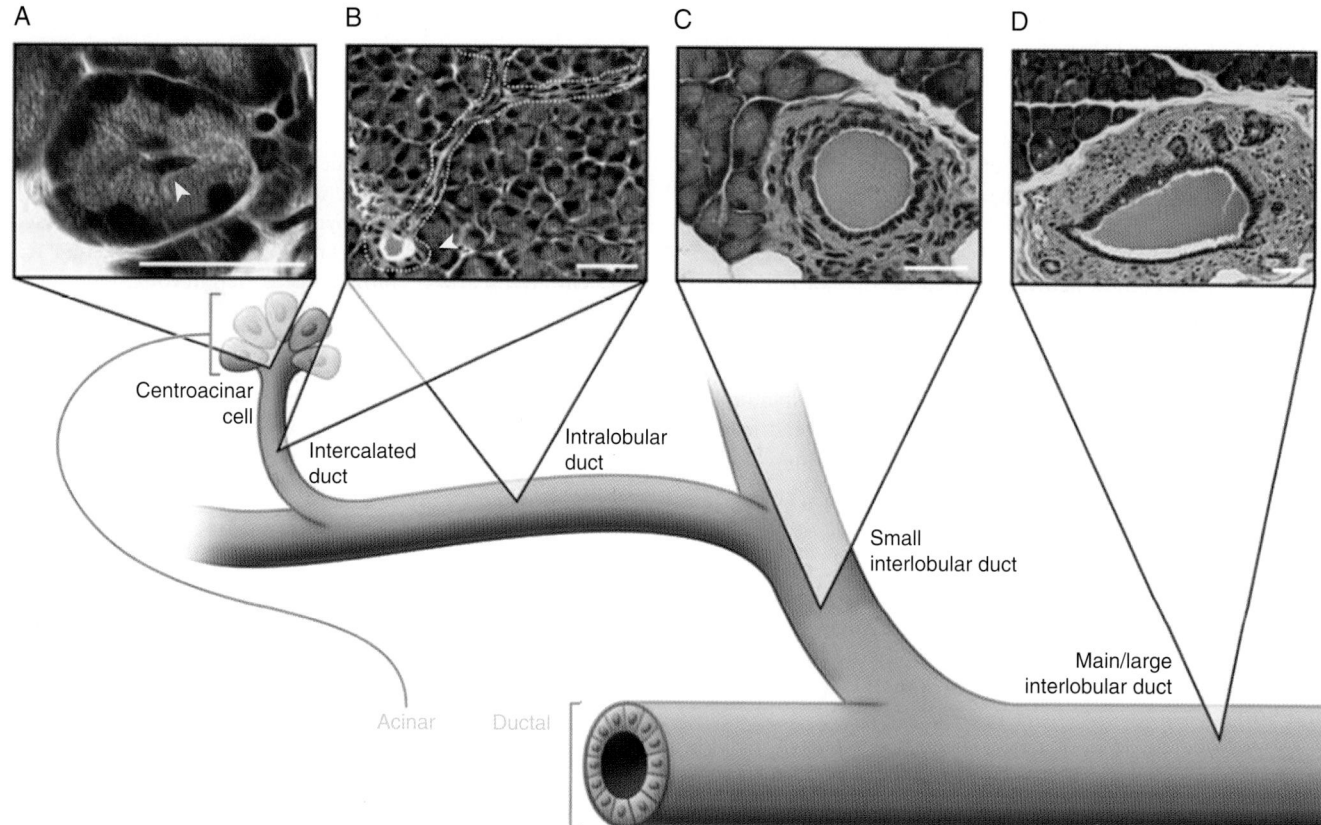

FIGURE 3.2 Anatomic organization of the pancreatic ductal network. **A,** Centroacinar cells are present at the junction between the intercalated duct and the acinar cell (*white arrowhead;* scale bar: 10 μm). **B,** Intercalated duct (also known as terminal duct) originates at the acini level and is composed of a cell characterized by minimal cytoplasm and a squamous-shaped appearance. The intercalated ducts merge into intralobular ducts (*white arrowhead*) that are lined by cuboidal epithelia and serve to drain an individual pancreatic lobule (*scale bar:* 10 μm). **C,** Intralobular ducts join to form small interlobular ducts that eventually merge into **(D)** larger interlobular ducts that are lined by cuboidal epithelium (scale bar: 10 μm). Exocrine pancreatic secretions ultimately reach the main pancreatic duct and are released in the duodenum through the ampulla of Vater (not shown). (Adapted from Reichert M, Rustgi AK. Pancreatic ductal cells in development, regeneration, and neoplasia. *J Clin Invest.* 2011;121:4572–4578.)

cytoplasm and basal-located nuclei.[61] Their physiologic function remains under investigation, although there is evidence to suggest that these cells undergo selective expansion during chronic epithelial injuries. Some authors have hypothesized that cells in the ductal epithelial compartment could contribute, at least in part, to the development of mucinous metaplasia and pancreatic intraepithelial neoplasia.[70]

Neurohormonal Regulation of Exocrine Pancreatic Function

Digestive and Interdigestive Periods of Pancreatic Secretion

Pancreatic exocrine secretion can be temporally categorized into an interdigestive and digestive secretion period. Between meals, the intestinal migrating myoelectric complex (MMC) is responsible for the cyclic stimulation of the exocrine pancreas (interdigestive period).[71] The cholinergic stimuli that regulate the MMC cause cyclic pancreatic secretion of a fluid rich in bicarbonate (every 60–120 minutes). These secretions appear to facilitate the removal of bacteria and food debris from the small intestine; however, definitive agreement on their function has not been reached.[72]

The digestive secretion period begins after the ingestion of a meal bolus and is characterized by three distinct phases:

cephalic, gastric, and intestinal. Each phase is determined by the location of the meal bolus in the GI tract, and it is regulated by different secretory signals.[72]

The cephalic phase, elicited by the anticipation of food, smell, taste, and chewing act, stimulates exocrine secretion via the vagus nerve.[73] In this initial phase, pancreatic secretions are mainly composed of digestive enzymes and low levels of bicarbonate, indicating an acinar-type secretion principally. ACh is the primary neurotransmitter, although acinar cells have been shown to express G protein-coupled receptors (GPCRs) for gastrin-releasing peptide (GRP) and VIP, suggesting a role for these peptides in the cephalic phase.[74,75]

The gastric phase is initiated once the meal reaches the stomach and is stimulated by gastric distention.[76] A low volume of enzyme-rich secretion characterizes this phase, and it is accompanied by minimal water and bicarbonate secretion.

The intestinal phase begins with the entry of chyme and gastric acid juice into the duodenum. In this phase, one of the main regulatory mechanisms is the vasovagal enteropancreatic reflex mediated through the dorsal vagus center. The presence of chyme in the duodenum activates efferent fibers of enteric neurons that stimulate intrapancreatic postganglionic neurons to release ACh. In addition, hydrogen ions (pH, ≤ 4.5) stimulate duodenal S cells to release secretin into the bloodstream.

Secretin acts primarily on ductal cells through its receptor GPCR, causing the release of fluid and bicarbonate and, to a lesser extent, acinar secretion.[77]

Water, Bicarbonate, and Ion Secretion from the Ductal Network

The role of the ductal network is of paramount importance for the optimal function of the exocrine pancreas. The ductal network cells are primarily under the control of secretin, which stimulates the centroacinar and ductal cells to release water and bicarbonate.[77] These secretions act as vehicles for the transport of inactive digestive zymogens from the acinar cells to the duodenum. Furthermore, their alkaline nature (pH, 7.6–9.0) helps neutralize the acidic chyme, in which nutrients are delivered from the stomach, resulting in an optimal neutral pH for the action of digestive enzymes. The concentration of sodium bicarbonate ($NaHCO_3$) in pancreatic secretions can reach up to 140 to 150 mM, and chloride secretion varies inversely to bicarbonate concentration, keeping $[HCO_3^-] + [Cl^-]$ constant at approximately 160 mM.[65]

Secretin promotes an increase of blood flow to the entire organ.[77] During a meal, the blood flow to the pancreas increases as much as 4 mL/min from a baseline of 0.2 or 0.3 mL/min.[72]

Regulation of Exocrine Secretion

Pancreatic secretions are tightly regulated through an intricate network of neural, humoral, and paracrine mediators. Many neurotransmitters, hormones, and growth factors have been reported to influence pancreatic exocrine function. These agents include but are not limited to, ACh and catecholamine, secretin (as earlier), nitric oxide (NO), VIP, GRP, neuropeptide Y, galanin, substance P, CGRP, gastrin/cholecystokinin (CCK), and enkephalins.[60,78,79]

Evidence suggests that muscarinic receptors (M1 and M3) are predominantly expressed on acinar cells and are involved in regulating exocrine function, making ACh the principal neurotransmitter.[80] This is supported by studies examining the mechanism of action of CCK. During the intestinal phase of pancreatic secretion, the I cell of the duodenum (also present in the jejunum) releases CCK primarily in response to products of the digestion of fat, protein, and, to a lesser extent, starch. CCK then causes the release of digestive enzymes and bile from the pancreas and gallbladder, respectively. Although only low levels of CCK receptor protein have been identified on human acinar cells, intrapancreatic vagal nerve terminals express CCK receptors.[81–83] These receptors bind CCK and release ACh in the proximity of acinar cells. This suggests that the cholinergic pathway regulates exocrine function. Additional studies support this hypothesis because the effect of CCK on pancreatic exocrine secretion can be prevented and almost abolished by atropine administration.[7,84–86]

Some ingested nutrients exert direct or indirect regulatory effects on pancreatic cells. Amino acids, especially phenylalanine, valine, methionine, and tryptophan, are potent stimulants of exocrine pancreatic secretion. Furthermore, intraluminal fatty acids, monoglycerides, and, to a lesser extent, glucose stimulate the secretion of digestive enzymes during the intestinal phase.[72]

Feedback Inhibitory Regulation

Feedback regulation to the exocrine pancreas is provided by signals originating in the proximal and distal intestine.

The main factors identified are monitor peptide, luminal CCK-releasing factor (LCRF), secretin-releasing factors (e.g., phospholipase A2), and peptide tyrosine tyrosine (PYY).[60,87–90] The action of these enzymes is dependent on the presence or the absence of intraluminal trypsin. Evidence suggests that trypsin inactivates monitor peptide and LCRF, therefore preventing augmentation of CCK release from the I cell. Once trypsin is occupied by the presence of meal chyme, monitor peptide and LCRF are not digested and can augment CCK release from the I cell. Eventually, the excess of digestive protease in the duodenal lumen leads to the digestion of both monitor peptide and LCRF, preventing further pancreatic enzyme secretion.[72]

Neuroendocrine L cells present in ileum and colon are stimulated by intraluminal oleic acid to release PYY. Oleic acid is a centrally active neuropeptide that exerts its action on the area postrema of the brain, decreasing vagal cholinergic mediation of CCK-stimulated pancreatic secretion.[7,91]

Digestive Enzymes

The exocrine pancreas releases proteolytic, amylolytic, lipolytic, and nuclease digestive enzymes. These enzymes are stored in zymogen granules either as proenzymes (i.e., trypsinogen, chymotrypsinogen, procarboxypeptidase, prophospholipase, proelastase, mesotrypsin) or as active enzyme (i.e., a-amylase, lipase, DNase, RNase).[92] In addition, the zymogen granules contain a trypsin inhibitor molecule known as *pancreatic secretory trypsin inhibitor* (PSTI).[93] PSTI forms a stable complex with trypsin near its catalytic site, preventing its undesired activation.[94]

After acinar stimulation, the zymogen granules fuse with the apical acinar cell membrane, releasing their contents in the pancreatic intercalated ducts that will eventually reach the intestinal lumen. A brush-border glycoprotein peptidase present on the duodenal lumen, known as *enterokinase*, activates trypsinogen by removing its N-terminal hexapeptide fragment. The active form of trypsin is responsible for the catalytic activation of the remaining pancreatic proenzymes.[92]

One characteristic of the acinar cell is its capacity to adapt the synthesis of digestive enzymes as a function of diet. Although the mechanisms by which acinar cells are capable of this adaptation remain under investigation, it is reasonable to believe that the regulation occurs at the level of gene transcription.

Stimulus-Secretion Coupling in Acinar Cell

An increase in the intracellular concentration of calcium is the major event that stimulates the acinar cells to release the secretory granules containing the digestive enzymes (Fig. 3.3).[95] Transmembrane heterotrimeric G proteins are the principal receptors for pancreatic acinar cell secretagogues and produce secondary messengers that ultimately act to release intracellular calcium.[96] Secretin and VIP bind to their specific GPCRs and cause activation of adenylate cyclase, generation of cAMP, and activation of protein kinase A.[77]

CCK, ACh, bombesin/GRP, PAR-2–activating protease, and substance P bind to their respective GPCRs, ultimately acting through the activation of phospholipase C and the production of IP3.[83,97] IP3 binds to its receptor in the endoplasmic reticulum and stimulates Ca^{2+} release. Ultimately, activated protein kinase A and protein kinase C phosphorylate specific intracellular proteins that lead to the secretion of pancreatic enzymes.

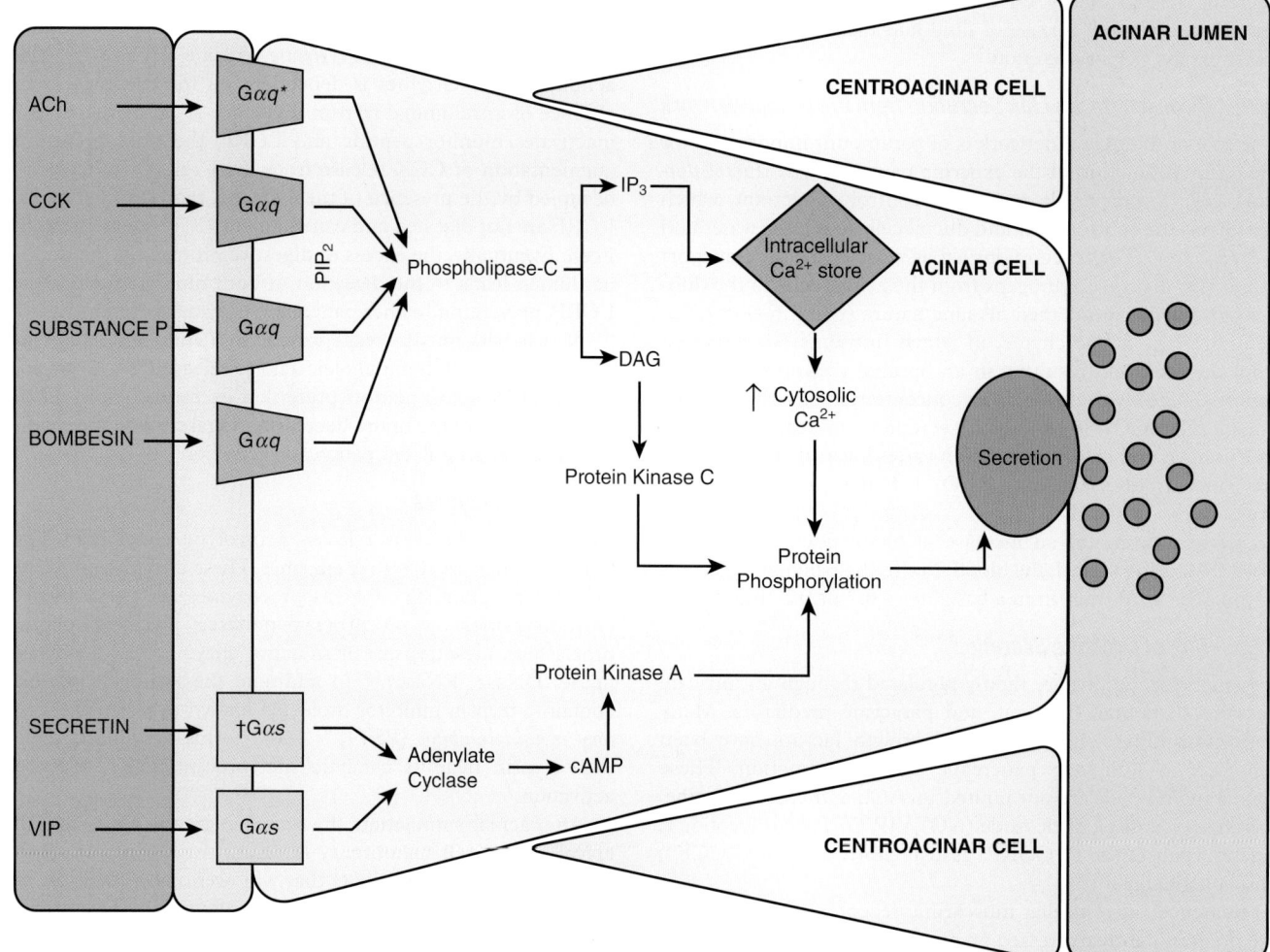

FIGURE 3.3 **Stimulus-secretion coupling in pancreatic acinar cell.** The primary secretagogues for acinar secretions bind to two types of cell surface heterotrimeric G protein receptors. Acetylcholine (ACh; the primary secretagogue for acinar secretion), cholecystokinin (CCK), substance P, and bombesin act through heterotrimeric G-protein–coupled receptors (GPCRs) associated with phospholipase C. This results in the production of two main messengers: inositol-1,4,5-triphosphate (IP3), which promotes the release of Ca^{2+} from intracellular stores; diacylglycerol (DAG), which prompts the activation of protein kinase C (PKC). The increase in cytoplasmic Ca^{2+} concentration and activated PKC leads to protein phosphorylation and digestive enzyme secretion. Secretin and vasoactive intestinal peptide (VIP) act through heterotrimeric GPCRs associated with adenylate cyclase. Elevation in cytoplasmic cyclic adenosine monophosphate (cAMP) levels causes the activation of protein kinase A (PKA), which ultimately leads to protein phosphorylation and digestive enzymes secretion. The centroacinar cells are terminal ductal cells in close contact with acinar cells and could represent progenitor multipotent pancreatic cells. *Gαq, Membrane-associated heterotrimeric G protein that activates phospholipase C (PLC); †Gαs, membrane-associated heterotrimeric G protein that activates the cAMP-dependent pathway by activating adenylate cyclase; PIP2, phosphatidylinositol-4,5-bisphosphate.

Stimulus-Secretion Coupling in the Ductal Cell

The apical and the basolateral portion of the ductal cells are involved in the stimulus-coupling secretion (Fig. 3.4). The apical membrane of ductal cells is equipped with cAMP-activated Cl^- channels (also known as the cystic fibrosis transmembrane conductance regulator), Cl^--HCO_3^- exchanger (SLC26A3/A6), and water channels aquaporin (AQP) 5. The basolateral membrane is rich in a Na^+-H^+ exchanger, N^+,K^+-ATPase, K^+ conductance channels, and AQP1 (localized in both apical and basolateral membrane). The interstitial portion of the ductal cells expresses receptors for the two major stimulants of ductal secretion: secretin and ACh.[65,98] Secretin binds to its cellular receptor, leading to the activation of adenylate cyclase and protein kinase A. ACh binds to the cellular receptor causing activation of protein kinase C and an increase in intracellular calcium concentration.

The result is the activation of cAMP-dependent Cl^- channel that releases intracellular Cl^- into the ductal space, increasing the amount of Cl^- available for the Cl^--HCO_3^- exchanger.

The high concentration of ductal Cl^- activates a Cl^--HCO_3^- antiport that results in an exchange of Cl^- for HCO_3^-. Furthermore, Na^+ and H_2O are released into the ductal space drowned by the ionic and osmotic gradient generated by the presence of bicarbonate in the duct lumen. Several K^+ channels are present in the ductal cell membrane and appear to have an essential role in generating and maintaining the electrochemical driving force for anion secretion. Ductal HCO_3^- secretion is not only regulated by GI hormones and cholinergic nerves but is also influenced by luminal factors: intraductal pressure, calcium concentration, and pathologic activation of protease and bile reflux.[65,98]

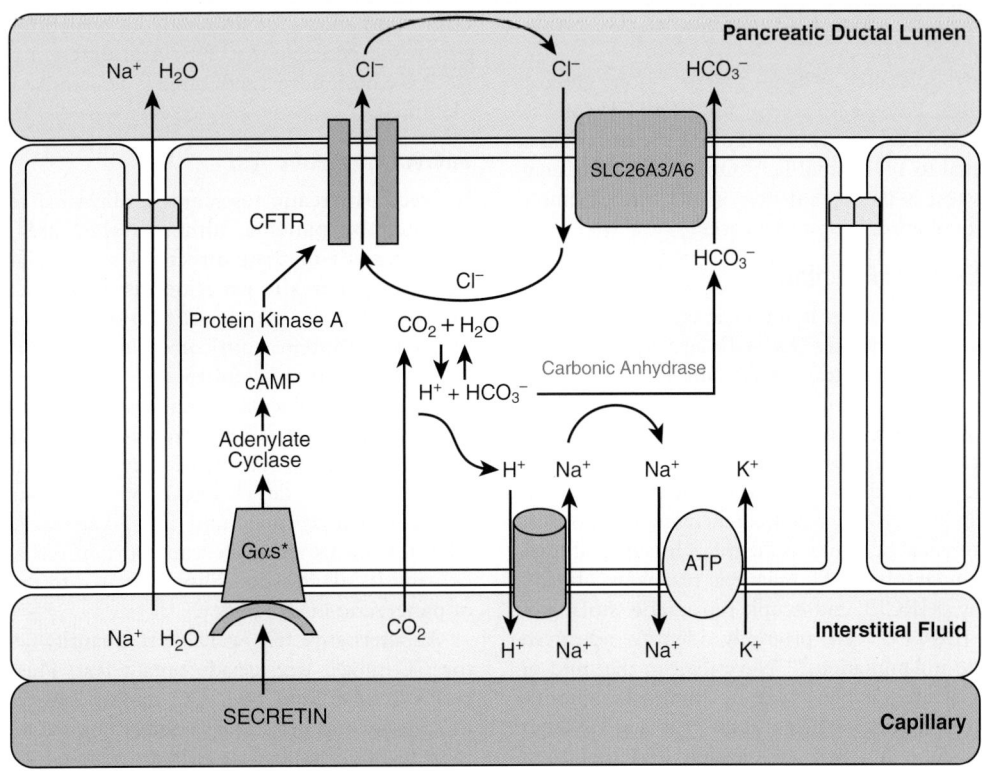

FIGURE 3.4 **Stimulus-secretion coupling in pancreatic ductal cells.** Carbon dioxide (CO_2) diffuses from the blood across the duct cell's basolateral membrane and is hydrated by carbonic anhydrase within the duct cell to form carbonic acid (H_2CO_3). Eventually, carbonic acid dissociates into H^+ and HCO_3^-. The extrusion of H^+ via Na^+-H^+ exchanger, located across the basolateral membrane, leads to the accumulation of bicarbonate (HCO_3^-) in the ductal cell. The intracellular bicarbonate (HCO_3^-) is then secreted into the ductal lumen by a chloride/bicarbonate (Cl^-/HCO_3^-) exchanger (SLC26A3/A6) in exchange for luminal Cl^-. The cystic fibrosis transmembrane conductance regulator (CFTR) channel recycles Cl^- back into the ductal lumen, making it available for a new exchange. Secretin, the most important ductal cell secretagogue, binds to its heterotrimeric G protein-coupled receptors, associated with adenylate cyclase located in the basolateral membrane. The resulting increase in cyclic adenosine monophosphate (cAMP) leads to the activation of protein kinase A (PKA), resulting in the activation of the CFTR channel. The activated CFTR channel accelerates the extrusion of Cl^- from the cell to the ductal lumen, causing the apical Cl^-/HCO_3^- to operate at a faster rate, leading to an increase in HCO_3^- secretion into the ductal lumen. The net passage of bicarbonate across the duct cell generates an ionic and osmotic gradient, which favors paracellular passage of sodium and water into the ductal space. *ATP,* Adenosine triphosphate; **Gαs,* membrane-associated heterotrimeric G protein that activates the cAMP-dependent pathway by activating adenylate cyclase.

FUNCTIONAL ASSESSMENT

Assessment of Endocrine Function

The evaluation of the endocrine pancreas revolves around the assessment of β-cell function. These assessments should consider the capacity of the β-cell to produce insulin, the response of the β-cells to secretagogue stimuli and the peripheral tissue resistance to insulin (characteristic of T2DM). Although each of these factors is important for accurate assessment of β-cell function, their evaluation under physiologic conditions can be cumbersome. Among the challenges is the nonlinear relationship between insulin secretion and insulin sensitivity, the nonconstant clearance of circulating insulin and hepatic extraction, and the dynamic insulin response to secretagogues stimuli. Several test "models" have been developed to account for the full range of factors that influence β-cell function; however, many are challenging to execute and lack standardization or accuracy.[99,100]

Methods for evaluation of β-cell function include basal measurement of plasma concentration of β-cell products, intravenous (IV) stimulation tests, and oral stimulation tests.

The simplest evaluation methods of β-cell function require basal measurement of plasma concentration of fasting insulin, fasting C-peptide, fasting proinsulin/insulin ratio, and the homeostatic model assessment test. However, these tests often lack standardization and are hindered by their wide range of sensitivity and specificity.[99]

The IV stimulation tests are mainly used for research purposes, and their clinical application is limited. These tests include the IV tolerance test, the hyperglycemic glucose clamp, the graded glucose infusion, and the arginine stimulation test.[99]

The oral stimulation tests are more commonly used in clinical practice and include the oral glucose tolerance test (OGTT) and the mixed meal tolerance test (MTT). The OGTT and the MTT provide a more physiologic stimulus to insulin secretion because these tests elicit the full incretin effect[101]; furthermore, both tests take advantage of mathematical models that normalize insulin secretion levels to varying plasma glucose concentrations.[99] The OGTT is widely used in clinical practice. After an overnight fast, subjects are administered an oral glucose load (approximately 75 g).[102] Blood samples are collected at baseline and at subsequent intervals to evaluate plasma concentration of insulin, glucose, C-peptide, and other parameters of interest.

Impaired glucose tolerance is defined by a 2-hour glucose value during an oral glucose tolerance test (OGTT) of 7.8 mmol/L to 11.0 mmol/L, whereas overt T2DM presents values greater than or equal to 11.1 mmol/L.[103] One of the significant limitations of this test is its dependency on the unpredictable and variable intestinal absorption of glucose.

Assessment of Exocrine Function

Exocrine pancreatic insufficiency in adults is often the result of pancreatic inflammatory processes (e.g., CP) and often a clinical problem after pancreatic or gastric surgery, and it leads to maldigestion of fat, protein, and carbohydrates[104] (see Chapters 58, 62, and 117). Ultimately, this will result in steatorrhea (>7 g of fecal fat in 24 hours), weight loss, and eventually malnutrition. The human pancreatic gland has a significant functional reserve; therefore more than 90% of pancreatic parenchyma must be lost before overt steatorrhea becomes evident.[105] Imaging studies (e.g., computed tomography [CT], magnetic resonance cholangiopancreatography [MRCP], endoscopic retrograde cholangiopancreatography [ERCP]) can promptly identify advanced stages of pancreatic inflammation.[106] Nevertheless, the mild or initial forms of CP are characterized by minimal anatomic changes and represent a diagnostic challenge.[107] It is in the latter scenario that pancreatic function tests would find their best application.

Pancreatic function tests (PFTs) can be grouped into two major categories: *indirect tests* and *direct tests* (Table 3.1).

Indirect PFTs are noninvasive tests that focus on evaluating the consequences resulting from diminished or absent digestive enzymes (e.g., steatorrhea).

Direct PFTs aim to quantify and characterize pancreatic secretory content (i.e., digestive enzyme, bicarbonate, and secretion volume); some tests require pancreatic stimulation by administering a meal or hormonal secretagogues (e.g., secretin, CCK). Direct PFTs are further divided into invasive, requiring GI instrumentation via a double-lumen gastroduodenal tube, and not invasive (often characterized by a lower sensitivity). Endoscopic versions of direct pancreatic tests have been developed (ePFT) in which pancreatic fluid secretions are collected directly from the second portion of the duodenum under direct visualization with an endoscope.[108,109] Besides, endoscopic

ultrasound allows for simultaneous structural evaluation of the pancreatic parenchyma.[110] Several different protocols for each test have been developed, but a gold standard test has not been identified.

Indirect Pancreatic Test

Indirect pancreatic tests are noninvasive tests that are well tolerated by patients, although they are characterized by lower sensitivity than direct tests, especially in the earlier stages of pancreatic exocrine insufficiency. One of the least invasive tests is the quantification of fecal fat. It can be qualitative (Sudan stain) or quantitative (72-hour stool collection) and often useful to evaluate the response to pancreatic enzyme replacement therapy.[111] In the most common form, patients are required to assume a diet of 100 g/day fat for 5 days and to collect the complete volume of feces for 3 days, starting on day 3. Fecal content greater than 7 g/day is considered abnormal, and it is diagnostic for steatorrhea. This test poses an unpleasant burden on laboratory personnel, and its diagnostic utility is limited to the advanced stages of pancreatic insufficiency.

An alternative test available to quantify fat malabsorption is the ^{13}C–mixed triglyceride breath test. This test requires the oral administration of a ^{13}C–market substrate and relies on the presence of intestinal pancreatic lipase activity. Ultimately, the ^{13}C–market substrate is hydrolyzed by the intestinal lipase, yielding $^{13}CO_2$ that is absorbed and eventually released across the pulmonary endothelium and quantified via mass spectrometry or infrared analysis. This test could represent a practical alternative to the fecal fat test, although it is subject to similar limitations of all indirect tests with limited accuracy for the early phases of pancreatic insufficiency.[112,113]

Direct Pancreatic Function Test

Noninvasive direct PFTs aim to quantify the fecal or serum levels of pancreas-derived enzymes (e.g., serum trypsinogen, fecal chymotrypsin, and fecal elastase). Although easy to perform and well tolerated by patients, noninvasive PFTs are hindered by their low sensitivity, often leading to inconclusive results, especially in the early phases of CP. Furthermore, fecal measurement of pancreatic enzyme can lead to false-positive results in the setting of nonpancreatic GI disturbances and diarrhea.

Serum trypsinogen is considered a sensitive and specific test for advanced pancreatic insufficiency, although its accuracy for earlier stages of pancreatic insufficiency is low. A serum trypsinogen concentration of less than 20 ng/mL is considered a reasonable cutoff for the diagnosis of pancreatic insufficiency.[114]

Fecal chymotrypsin concentration can be used for the evaluation of pancreatic insufficiency. Chymotrypsin is specifically synthesized and secreted by the acinar cells of the pancreas. This test is influenced by exogenous pancreatic enzyme administration and requires suspension of enzyme administration for at least 2 days before the test.[115] Furthermore, chymotrypsin is not an ideal marker because it is degraded during intestinal transit and can be diluted in the presence of diarrhea, leading to false-positive results.

Fecal elastase-1 appears to be a more reliable test compared with fecal chymotrypsin. Elastase-1 is not influenced by exogenous pancreatic enzyme administration, and it is more stable than chymotrypsin during intestinal transit. Evidence suggests

TABLE 3.1 Tests of Exocrine Pancreatic Function	
INDIRECT TESTS	**DIRECT TESTS**
Fecal fat quantification	**Noninvasive Tests**
Qualitative (Sudan stain)	Serum trypsinogen
Quantitative (72-hour stool collection)	Fecal chymotrypsin
	Fecal elastase-1
^{13}C-Mixed triglyceride breath test	
	Invasive Tests
	Lundh test
	Secretin test
	CCK test
	Secretin-CCK test
	Secretagogues and Imaging
	Secretin-enhanced MRI
	Secretin-enhanced MRCP

CCK, Cholecystokinin; *MRI,* magnetic resonance imaging; *MRCP,* magnetic resonance cholangiopancreatography.

that this study has a reasonably high sensitivity and specificity for pancreatic insufficiency.[116] Results obtained with the fecal elastase-1 test reliably correlate with the one obtained using imaging studies (ERCP, magnetic resonance neurography [MRN])[117] or the more sensitive direct invasive pancreatic tests (secretin test).[118,119] Level of fecal elastase-1 less than or equal to 15 μg/g of stool (enzyme-linked immunoabsorbent assay on spot fecal sample) are diagnostic for pancreatic insufficiencies in patients with CP.[120] Nevertheless, fecal elastase-1 tests are often unreliable after pancreatic resection, where pancreatic insufficiency results from a combination of factors not solely dependent on decreased pancreatic function (e.g., abnormal hormonal stimulation, abnormal mixing of food with digestive secretions, acidic intraluminal pH).[120] Furthermore, fecal elastase-1 levels are not influenced by the exogenous administration of pancreatic enzyme, and therefore this test cannot be used to evaluate the response to pancreatic enzyme replacement therapy.[116,121]

Invasive direct PFTs require the use of a double-lumen collection tube, with one lumen terminating in the duodenum to collect pancreatic secretions and one lumen resting in the gastric antrum to prevent gastric fluid from entering the duodenum. Correct tube placement is confirmed via fluoroscopy before administration of meal or secretagogues, and then pancreatic secretions are collected for 1 to 2 hours. Alternatively, an endoscope can be used, and pancreatic fluid can be collected directly through the cannulation of the pancreatic duct or through the suction channel of the endoscope under direct visualization from the duodenum. Of historic interest is the Lundh test,[122] where a physiologic stimulus to pancreatic secretion is obtained through the administration of a standardized meal (composed of 300 mL of solution containing 15% carbohydrate, 6% fat, and 5% protein). Endogenous secretin and CCK, released in response to the standardized meal, are necessary to stimulate pancreatic secretion, making the Lundh test dependent on normal duodenal mucosal function.[72,121] The hormone-stimulated tests are the cornerstone of the direct invasive pancreatic tests. These tests use the exogenous administration of secretin, CCK, or a combination of secretin-CCK as a more reliable method of pancreatic stimulation.[123,124]

The secretin test requires IV administration of a synthetic secretin bolus (0.2 μg/kg), followed by a continuous collection of duodenal fluid in four aliquots of 15-minute intervals each. The test measures bicarbonate concentration in each of the four aliquot samples. Exocrine insufficiency is evident when bicarbonate concentrations less than 80 mEq/L are recorded in each of the four aliquots, and severe exocrine insufficiency is diagnosed when bicarbonate concentration is less than 50 mEq/L.[125] Moreover, the test can quantify the total volume output as well as the total amount of bicarbonate secreted.

These measurements are employed as a secondary diagnostic test when bicarbonate concentrations are equivocal. Although theoretically useful, these tests are not commonly employed because they are hindered by the low accuracy caused by incomplete recovery of duodenal fluid.

Alternative approaches have been developed to overcome the challenges of gastroduodenal tube placement. One of these approaches is the purely endoscopic secretin test (ePFT). This test has been shown to have similar accuracy to the classic secretin test. Duodenal aspirates are obtained through an endoscope at 0, 15, 30, 45, and 60 minutes after secretin stimulation and analyzed for bicarbonate concentration.[109,126]

Another attempt made to overcome the limitations of duodenal fluid collection consists of the use of ERCP for the analysis of pure pancreatic secretion collected directly from the pancreatic duct, but the results obtained with this method have been unsatisfactory.[127] CCK tests using either CCK or a receptor agonist (e.g., cerulein) have been developed to measure pancreatic enzyme secretion. A simplified version of these tests measures lipase concentration from duodenal fluid collected over an 80-minute period and uses a cutoff lipase value of 780 IU/L.[128] Acinar and ductal pancreatic exocrine function can be evaluated simultaneously using the secretin-CCK test. This test requires continuous collection of duodenal fluid and measurement of total secretion output, bicarbonate concentration, and digestive enzyme concentration.[129] Some patients may have a more pronounced deficit of one specific enzyme; therefore measuring more than one digestive enzyme (i.e., amylase, lipase, and tryptase) in addition to bicarbonate can increase the sensitivity of this test. One pitfall of the secretin-CCK test is that the large amount of fluid released by the pancreas after secretin stimulation, combined with CCK-stimulated gallbladder contraction, ultimately results in dilution of the digestive enzymes. To avoid false positive results, some authors have advocated the use of perfusion markers, although no definitive agreement exists.

Of recent interest are tests combining secretagogues with imaging techniques. Examples of these tests are the secretin-enhanced MRI and the secretin-enhanced MRCP.[130–133] Secretin-enhanced MRI uses diffusion-weighted MRI imaging to evaluate increase in pancreatic capillary blood flow and pancreatic secretion after stimulation with secretin. In addition, secretin-enhanced MRCP allows evaluation of duodenal filling as a function of pancreatic secretion.[132,134] Although growing enthusiasm is developing around these tests, further studies are necessary to evaluate their performances with standard invasive tests.

The references for this chapter can be found online by accessing the accompanying Expert Consult website.

CHAPTER 4

Assessment of hepatic function: Implications for perioperative outcome and recovery

Sean Bennett and Paul J. Karanicolas

The limits of hepatic resectability are constantly expanding with our increased understanding of hepatic anatomy and refinements in surgical technique (see Chapters 2, 102, and 118B). In past years, partial hepatectomy was limited to anatomic resection and small-wedge resections, with a general consensus that two contiguous segments of hepatic parenchyma having adequate vascular inflow/outflow and biliary drainage was the minimum threshold for safe resection.[1,2] This conventional definition served the surgical community well but has required refinement for two reasons. First, a variety of techniques have been developed that allow more extensive resection than this definition suggests, including induced hypertrophy of the future liver remnant (FLR; e.g., two-stage hepatectomy, portal vein embolization [PVE], associating liver partition and portal vein ligation for staged hepatectomy [ALPPS]), and nonanatomic parenchymal-sparing resections (see Chapter 102). Indeed, through these and other techniques, it may be possible to safely resect tumors from all segments of the liver while maintaining adequate postoperative liver function. Second, patients selected for partial hepatectomy are increasingly treated with preoperative chemotherapy or have other risk factors for background liver injury; in these patients, the minimal requirement of two contiguous segments of liver is likely too liberal and puts patients at an unacceptable risk for posthepatectomy liver failure (see Chapters 69, 89, 90, 98, 101, and 102).

Given the trend toward more aggressive liver resections in patients at risk for background liver disease, thorough assessment of hepatic function is crucial. Liver function after hepatic resection is dependent on the quantity and quality of the FLR. Thus optimal assessment of fitness for liver resection would ideally incorporate some measure of FLR volume and function. This is particularly important in patients at risk for or documented evidence of background liver disease, including heavy alcohol consumption, hepatitis, cirrhosis, nonalcoholic steatohepatitis, and chemotherapy-associated liver injury, such as sinusoidal obstruction syndrome, steatosis, and chemotherapy-associated steatohepatitis (see Chapters 69 and 98). Surgeons contemplating major liver resection in patients with any of these risk factors should ensure that some measure of liver function, in addition to FLR volume, is considered. This chapter reviews these two critical components of FLR assessment in detail.

ASSESSMENT OF LIVER REMNANT VOLUME

Extent of liver resection (i.e., the number of segments resected) is strongly correlated with risk of postoperative liver insufficiency. Although this is intuitive and easily assessed, it is actually the volume of liver remaining (i.e., the FLR) that is more predictive of outcome and thus critical to accurately measure.

Furthermore, assessment of number of segments remaining is not sufficient because of substantial variability among patients in segmental anatomy and liver volume. In most patients, the right side of the liver represents more than half of the total liver volume (TLV); however, there is a broad range, from 49% to 82%, with the left side of the liver conversely ranging from 17% to 49%.[3] Thus formal radiologic assessment of volumetrics is required to accurately assess the FLR for anticipated major (i.e., >4 segments) liver resection (see Chapter 102).

Techniques of Volumetry

Formal measurement of liver volumes is most commonly accomplished by using computed tomography (CT) or magnetic resonance imaging (MRI).[4–7] Other imaging modalities may also be used, but CT and MRI are commonly obtained in patient care for characterization of lesions and operative planning, and therefore additional tests are typically not needed. Cross-sectional images obtained from either of these modalities are sequentially marked with the planned resection line, following which the surface area is derived and multiplied by the slice thickness (Fig. 4.1). Excellent correlation has been demonstrated between the planned FLR and the actual FLR radiologically,[8] as well as between the calculated resected liver volume and the surgical specimen.[9,10]

Because of the variability in total liver size based on patient body habitus, the FLR volume is typically expressed as a ratio of FLR to TLV. Although the measurement of the FLR is fairly standard, there are several variations to calculate the TLV. The simplest and most intuitive technique involves manually tracing the borders of the liver in a variety of planes and using software to calculate the total volume in the same manner as the FLR calculation. There are several limitations to this technique. Most notably, because resection is usually considered on the basis of hepatic tumors, the volume of the tumors is implicitly included in the measurement of the TLV. This is problematic because the tumor volume does not contribute to hepatic function and so provides a falsely elevated value of the TLV and hence a falsely diminished anticipated FLR ratio. Manually measuring the volume of each tumor and subtracting it from the TLV to yield the total functioning liver volume can correct this but can be labor intensive and prone to measurement error.[11] Some software packages can perform automated subtraction of the tumor volume. The direct measurement technique of TLV is further limited by the fact that the parenchyma beyond tumors may be abnormal because of biliary or vascular obstruction. These limitations typically do not apply to the assessment of the FLR, which usually does not contain tumors.

An alternative method referred to as the *total estimated liver volume* (TELV) was first proposed by Urata and colleagues in Japan for use in liver transplantation.[12] Rather than measuring

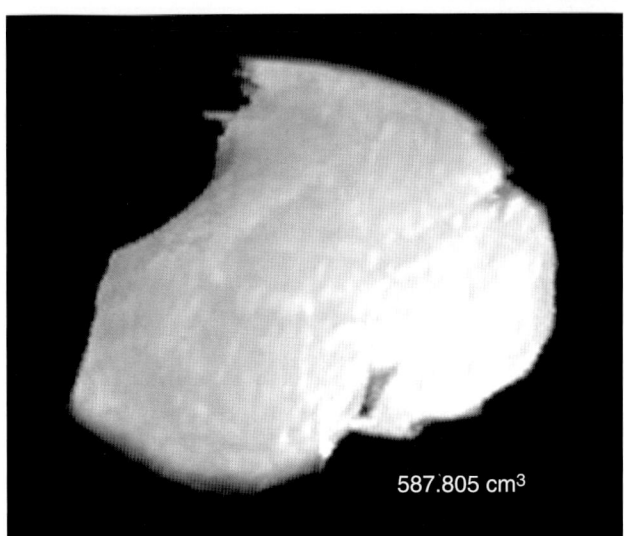

587.805 cm³

FIGURE 4.1 Volumetric assessment based on magnetic resonance imaging.

the TLV directly and subtracting the volume of liver tumors, this technique estimates the TLV based on body surface area (BSA). The formula was subsequently modified to apply to Western patients, based on the observation that Urata's formula underestimated TELV by an average of 323 cm³.[13,14] The resulting equation (TELV = −794 + 1267 × BSA) has been extensively studied and found to yield a precise estimate of TLV across institutions with different CT scanners and three-dimensional reconstruction techniques.[15] When the TELV is used as the denominator to calculate the FLR ratio (i.e., FLR/TELV), the resultant ratio is referred to as the *standardized FLR* (sFLR).

The measured TLV was compared with the TELV in a study of 243 patients who underwent major liver resection (three or more segments).[16] There was a strong correlation between the two measures across the population; however, in overweight patients (body mass index [BMI] > 25), TELV was significantly higher, yielding a lower sFLR in these patients. Based on the surgeons' thresholds, 47 patients were deemed to have insufficient liver volume for resection using TLV compared with 73 patients using TELV. According to institutional practices at the time, patients who had sufficient liver volume based on TLV underwent resection. The subset of patients who had insufficient volume based on TELV had significantly higher rates of post-hepatectomy liver failure (PHLF) and mortality than did the patients who had sufficient volume based on both calculations. Therefore the authors concluded that TELV (i.e., sFLR) is a better measure of postoperative hepatic insufficiency risk.

Increasingly sophisticated software packages are being developed that incorporate semi-automated and fully automated segmentation for both CT and MRI. A number of studies have shown these to be very accurate and time-efficient when compared with the gold standard of manual volumetry for TLV[5,17-19] and individual liver segment volumes.[20] These automated software packages have also been shown to be accurate and time-saving for living donor liver transplant patients[21] and for planning a standard right trisectionectomy.[22] Measuring the FLR for a resection not following a standard anatomic plane still requires manual volumetry.

Volumetric Thresholds

Despite the refinement in methods to measure the FLR, the clinical application of the information gathered remains controversial. It has long been clear that patients with lower FLR are at increased risk for hepatic dysfunction, but the exact threshold below which resection should not be performed is debated. Several studies have attempted to address this fundamental question, yielding different conclusions.[23-28] The variable results may be attributable to the heterogeneity of included patients (some having background liver disease and others healthy livers), methods used to calculate the FLR (TLV vs. TELV), indications for PVE, and definitions of hepatic dysfunction. Furthermore, only two studies analyzed their results using a formal receiving operator characteristic (ROC) curve to determine the optimal FLR threshold, and both studies were limited by small sample sizes.[23,27] Allowing for these admittedly crucial differences, the optimal cutoff for patients with a normal background liver appears to be between 20% and 30%. A 2006 expert consensus statement recommended a minimum of 20% FLR for major hepatic resection in a patient with a healthy liver and to consider PVE for any FLR less than that.[29]

Patients who have received preoperative chemotherapy are at risk for background liver injury that impairs regeneration after partial hepatectomy[30-32] (see Chapters 69, 98, and 102). There is general consensus that patients treated with extensive preoperative chemotherapy or who have evidence of background liver injury require a larger FLR to allow safe hepatectomy, although the exact threshold is again controversial. Two studies examined this question and performed formal ROC curve analyses, reporting optimal thresholds of 31% and 48.5%, respectively.[23,33] The largest study includes 194 patients undergoing extended hepatectomy on the right side, stratified by extent of preoperative chemotherapy, with long-duration chemotherapy defined as greater than 12 weeks (86 patients).[34] Using a minimum *P*-value approach, the authors concluded that the optimal cutoff value of FLR for preventing postoperative liver insufficiency in these patients was 30%. Patients who have received extensive chemotherapy and have an sFLR between 30% and 40% should be investigated closely for any suggestion of underlying liver dysfunction and could be considered for PVE.

The optimal FLR threshold in patients with documented underlying liver disease is even less certain, given the additional variability of defining the extent of background liver injury. Some authors advocate for PVE in all patients with chronic liver disease before right side hepatectomy, and others apply a conservative threshold as high as 40%.[35,36] Given the importance of background liver function, additional functional tests to assess the liver remnant should be considered before embarking on major hepatectomy in the setting of significant background liver disease.

Volumetry After Hypertrophy

In patients at increased risk for PHLF, hypertrophy of the FLR may be induced by preoperative ipsilateral PVE (see Chapter 102C).[37] Other techniques to achieve hypertrophy, such as the ALPPS procedure (see Chapter 102D) or radioembolization with yttrium-90 (see Chapter 94), are discussed in other chapters. Cross-sectional imaging is typically repeated 2 to 6 weeks after PVE, and the FLR (or sFLR) may be recalculated. The post-PVE FLR can be interpreted with the same thresholds previously discussed, although the degree of hypertrophy (DH), defined as absolute difference between FLR before and after PVE, appears to be more informative.[38] The authors of this study recommended that patients without cirrhosis undergoing PVE should have both an sFLR of at least 20% and a DH of at least 5% to undergo safe hepatectomy. In addition to its therapeutic intent, PVE functions as a diagnostic test analogous to a cardiac stress test; patients who do not experience substantial growth in the FLR after PVE should be suspected of harboring background liver disease and approached with caution.

Recognizing that the DH is contingent on the duration from PVE to reimaging, surgeons have proposed incorporating some measure of growth rate into consideration. The kinetic growth rate (KGR) may be calculated by dividing the DH by the number of weeks elapsed since PVE.[39] In one study of 107 patients who underwent liver resection for colorectal liver metastases with an sFLR volume of greater than 20%, KGR was a more accurate predictor of postoperative hepatic insufficiency than absolute sFLR or DH (area under the curve [AUC] 0.830).[39] In this study, patients with a KGR less than 2% per week suffered a 21.6% hepatic insufficiency rate and an 8.1% 90-day mortality rate compared with no hepatic insufficiency or 90-day mortality in patients with a KGR greater than 2% per week. In a similar study of 153 patients who underwent major hepatectomy after PVE, post-PVE absolute FLR correlated poorly with liver failure.[40] Both DH and KGR were good predictors of liver

failure (AUC 0.80 and 0.79, respectively). Notably, posthepatectomy liver failure did not develop in any patients with a KGR greater than 2.66% per week.

In summary, for patients with insufficient FLR (or sFLR) to safely undergo hepatectomy, response to PVE provides a good measure of the remnant liver's ability to hypertrophy. Post-PVE FLR should be interpreted in combination with some measure of extent of hypertrophy (either DH or KGR) to optimally predict a patient's risk for post-hepatectomy liver insufficiency.

ASSESSMENT OF LIVER REMNANT FUNCTION

Although a thorough assessment of the anticipated FLR volume is required before embarking on major hepatectomy, a complete assessment should ideally also account for the quality of the background liver that will be preserved. The optimal method to assess hepatic function would be accurate, noninvasive, inexpensive, specific to the remnant portion of the liver, and widely reproducible. Unfortunately, none of the techniques currently available fulfill all of these criteria, and therefore none are frequently used in routine assessment. Nevertheless, several newer techniques show promise and with further investigation may find a role in routine assessment of liver function (Table 4.1).

TABLE 4.1	Comparison of Tests Available for Assessment of Liver Function		
MODALITY	**RATIONALE**	**ADVANTAGES**	**LIMITATIONS**
Volume of liver remnant (MRI, CT)	Lower liver remnant volume is associated with worse outcomes	• Can be easily calculated with conventional imaging • Can be performed by surgeons • Incorporates planned resection	• Does not incorporate measure of underlying liver function • Threshold for safe resection in setting of background liver disease unclear
Response of liver remnant to portal vein embolization	Failure of liver to hypertrophy in response to portal vein embolization indicates underlying liver injury	• Can be easily calculated with conventional imaging • Can be performed by surgeons • Incorporates planned resection volume and underlying function	• Requires invasive procedure that may not be necessary in some patients
Clinical scoring systems (Child-Pugh, MELD, ALBI, etc.)	Scoring systems are associated with poor outcomes after other procedures	• Easy to calculate • Noninvasive	• Not sensitive enough for background liver dysfunction
ICG clearance	ICG is metabolized by the liver, and poor ICG clearance is indicative of underlying liver dysfunction	• Good measure of underlying liver function	• Time consuming • Measures total liver function, not specific to remnant • Altered based on environmental conditions
Hepatobiliary scintigraphy	^{99m}Tc- GSA binds to hepatocyte receptors; ^{99m}Tc- IDA derivatives are metabolized by the liver; poor uptake of either are indicative of liver dysfunction	• Provides anatomic and functional information • May be specific to remnant liver by combining with CT	• High inter-rater and inter-institution variability • Limited availability
Other measures of metabolic function (lidocaine-MEGX, galactose, etc.)	Metabolized almost exclusively by the liver (P450), and poor clearance indicates underlying liver dysfunction	• Correlated with other measures of total liver function	• Not widely available • Limited data related to clinical outcomes • High interrater variability • Time consuming • Measures total liver function, not specific to remnant • Altered based on environmental conditions
MRI with Gd-EOB-DTPA contrast	Taken up and cleared by hepatocytes, poor uptake indicates liver dysfunction	• Routinely available • Frequently used in preoperative assessment • May be specific to remnant liver • Provides other information	• Correlated with postresection clinical outcomes (PHLF and ICGR15) in only two small studies • Needs larger prospective trials
Transient elastography	Provides assessment of liver fibrosis	• Noninvasive • Fast	• User dependent • Not correlated with clinical outcomes • Poor PPV

ALBI, Albumin-bilirubin score; *CT,* computed tomography; *Gd-EOB-DTPA,* gadolinium ethoxybenzyl dimeglumine; *ICGR15,* indocyanine green retention (15 minutes); *MEGX,* monoethylglycinexylidide; *MRI,* magnetic resonance imaging; *PHLF,* post hepatectomy liver failure; *PPV,* positive predictive value; *SPECT,* single-photon emission computed tomography; ^{99m}*Tc-GSA,* technetium-99m–labeled galactosyl serum albumin; ^{99m}*Tc- IDA,* technetium-99m–labeled iminodiacetic acid.

Clinical Scoring Systems

The simplest, most widely available method to assess liver function relies on laboratory investigations either in isolation or combined into clinical scoring systems. Clinicians are familiar with conventional liver laboratory tests routinely used in clinical practice, including enzymatic measures of hepatocyte injury (alanine aminotransferase, aspartate aminotransferase, and alkaline phosphatase), and markers of hepatic metabolism bilirubin and synthetic function (albumin and international normalized ratio [INR]). Aberrations in any of these laboratory measures should prompt further investigation of background liver dysfunction, although none of them are sensitive or specific enough for surgeons to rely on exclusively.

The Child-Turcotte-Pugh scoring system was developed to predict the risk of death in patients undergoing surgical management of portal hypertension. The Child's score is easily calculated from three readily available laboratory tests (bilirubin, albumin, and INR) and two clinical findings (ascites and encephalopathy). The Child's score is a good marker of global liver function in a patient with cirrhosis and may help in the selection of patients appropriate for resection, particularly in the setting of hepatocellular carcinoma. In general, surgery is reasonable to consider in patients with class A cirrhosis, should be approached cautiously in patients with class B cirrhosis, and should be avoided in patients with class C cirrhosis. In patients without cirrhosis, the Child's score will almost always be normal even when there is substantial background liver dysfunction; in this setting, it does not predict postoperative liver dysfunction, and other tests are needed. Furthermore, it is important to recognize that significant portal hypertension may exist even in Child's A cirrhosis.

The Model for End-Stage Liver Disease (MELD) score is a mathematical equation frequently used in liver transplantation to allocate organs. The MELD score is similar to the Child-Pugh score in that it incorporates simple laboratory investigations, including serum bilirubin, creatinine, and INR, although it is more cumbersome to calculate. It was initially validated for the prediction of short-term survival in patients with cirrhosis and has subsequently been validated for long-term survival as well. In patients with cirrhosis undergoing partial hepatectomy, a MELD score greater than 8 is a strong predictor of perioperative mortality and decreased long-term survival.[41–43] In contrast, in patients without documented background liver injury, a MELD score is not strongly associated with inferior outcomes.[44–46]

First described in 2015, the albumin-bilirubin (ALBI) score categorizes patients into three risk groups based only on their serum albumin and bilirubin.[47] The calculation of the score requires a complex equation; however, a simple nomogram has been created to determine into which group a patient falls: A1, A2, or A3 (from best to worst). This model was developed from 1313 patients with hepatocellular carcinoma (HCC) in Japan and was validated in patients from other geographic regions, patients undergoing hepatectomy, and unresectable patients treated with sorafenib.[47] In patients undergoing resection, the ALBI was better able to predict survival than the Child-Pugh score and could better discriminate between Child-Pugh A patients. Further studies showed ALBI better able to predict both PHLF and survival after hepatectomy when compared with Child-Pugh[48] and MELD.[49]

Thus, in patients with cirrhosis being considered for partial hepatectomy, Child-Pugh and MELD scores provide good measures of global liver function. Surgeons should approach patients with Child-Pugh class B/C or MELD score greater than 8 with caution and consider alternative treatment approaches. Within the group of Child-Pugh A patients, use of the ALBI score can add further precision in predicting the risk for PHLF. Clinical scoring systems are not sensitive enough to detect background liver injury and subsequent risk of postoperative liver dysfunction in patients without cirrhosis; other methods of functional liver assessment are needed in these patients.

Measurement of Hepatic Uptake, Metabolism, and Elimination

Indocyanine Green Clearance

Indocyanine green (ICG) clearance is the quantitative measure of hepatic function most used worldwide. ICG is a water-soluble tricarbocyanine dye that binds to albumin and distributes rapidly and uniformly in the blood after intravenous (IV) injection. ICG is exclusively cleared from the bloodstream by the liver in a similar manner to bilirubin and toxins and then excreted unchanged into bile. Thus ICG clearance tests reflect blood flow–dependent clearance, hepatocyte uptake, and biliary excretion.

The conventional measurement of ICG clearance involves IV injection of ICG, followed by serial collection of venous blood at 5-minute intervals for 15 minutes. ICG clearance can also be measured noninvasively by pulse-spectrophotometry, which allows for real-time monitoring of liver function.[50,51] The results of ICG tests may be expressed as the percentage of ICG retained in the circulation 15 minutes after injection (ICG-R15), the plasma disappearance rate (ICG-PDR), and the elimination rate constant (ICG-k). Several studies have identified an association between elevated ICG-R15 and posthepatectomy complications, with proposed threshold values of ICG-R15 ranging from 14% to 20%.[52–54]

Despite the theoretical attractiveness of ICG clearance as a simple measure of hepatic function, several limitations have hampered enthusiasm for its widespread use. The results of ICG clearance tests are not reliable in patients with hyperbilirubinemia or in patients with intrahepatic shunting or sinusoidal capillarization. Further, ICG clearance testing is a measure of global liver function, so if there is heterogeneous uptake in the liver (e.g., the portion being resected does not function as well because of tumor, biliary obstruction, etc.), the results may be misleading. Finally, ICG testing does not incorporate the extent of resection, or conversely, the volume of the remnant that will remain. Researchers have attempted to mitigate some of these limitations by creating scoring systems and decision trees that incorporate ICG.[55–57] In one study of patients with cirrhosis, a combination of sFLR greater than 25% and an sFLR/ICG-R15 ratio greater than 1.9 predicted safety to undergo hepatectomy.[57]

Nuclear Imaging Techniques

Theoretically, nuclear imaging represents an attractive preoperative hepatic assessment, combining anatomic considerations (FLR volume) with both total and regional liver functional assessment. Several scintigraphic tests have been developed over the past few decades, but the most widely used radiopharmaceutical imaging methods for liver functional assessment are technetium-99m (^{99m}Tc)-labeled galactosyl serum albumin (GSA) scintigraphy and hepatobiliary scintigraphy (HBS) with

[99m]Tc-labeled iminodiacetic acid (IDA) derivatives. Both of these methods provide quantitative data on the total and regional hepatic function, although they are based on different principles and therefore interpretation varies.

^{99m}Tc-GSA is an analogue of a glycoprotein (ascites sialoglycoprotein) that binds to receptors on the hepatocyte cell membrane and is taken up by the hepatocytes. Chronic liver disease results in diminished hepatocyte glycoprotein receptors and subsequent accumulation of plasma glycoproteins. To perform dynamic scintigraphy, an IV bolus of ^{99m}Tc-GSA is administered, and images are obtained by using a gamma camera positioned over the heart and liver. Several parameters may be calculated to document the extent of hepatic ^{99m}Tc-GSA uptake, including the hepatic uptake ratio (LHL15 [receptor index: uptake ratio of the liver to the liver plus heart at 15 min]) and the blood clearance ratio (HH15 [blood clearance index: uptake ratio of the heart at 15 min to that at 3 min]). In patients with cirrhosis, ^{99m}Tc-GSA uptake corresponds well with other conventional liver function tests, including ICG clearance, and predicts histologic severity of disease better than ICG clearance in a substantial proportion of patients.[58,59] Several small studies have demonstrated an association between poor ^{99m}Tc-GSA uptake and postoperative complications after liver resection.[59-61]

^{99m}Tc-GSA uptake is limited by inter-operator and inter-institutional differences and does not provide a measure of regional liver function.[62] To address this limitation, ^{99m}Tc-GSA scintigraphy may be combined with static single-photon emission computed tomography–CT (SPECT-CT) to allow a three-dimensional measurement of ^{99m}Tc-GSA uptake. Results of dynamic SPECT-CT may help to predict postoperative liver failure; however, this method suffers from the same interobserver variability and environmental factors as dynamic ^{99m}Tc-GSA scintigraphy.[63-65] A single-arm prospective trial of 185 consecutive patients undergoing hepatectomy evaluated the predictive value of ^{99m}Tc-GSA SPECT-CT on PHLF and mortality.[66] SPECT-CT was used to calculate the ICG clearance specific to the predicted FLR and demonstrated very good correlation with postoperative bilirubin and INR levels, with a PHLF rate of 8% and 90-day mortality of 0.5%. Furthermore, 7 patients who would not have met their criteria for resection based on the overall ICG-R15 x FLR underwent hepatectomy without PHLF. This demonstrates the heterogeneity of liver function and the importance of measuring the function of the FLR rather than the TLV.

[99m]Tc-mebrofenin is an organic IDA derivative with similar properties to ICG: It has high hepatic uptake, low displacement by bilirubin, and low urinary excretion. The test is administered in an identical manner to ^{99m}Tc-GSA scintigraphy, using a gamma camera and calculating similar parameters and ratios. The uptake ratio, however, is divided by the patient's BSA to compensate for differences in metabolic requirements. ^{99m}Tc-mebrofenin HBS correlates well with ICG clearance and appears to be a good marker of post-resection liver function.[67-70] HBS may also be combined with SPECT-CT to allow for the calculation of both the function and volume of the FLR. An FLR function cutoff value of 2.7%/min/m[2] was shown to have a negative predictive value (NPV) of 97.6% and a positive predictive value (PPV) of 57.1% for PHLF.[68] The main limitation of HBS is, again, inter-observer and inter-institution variability. Although these techniques offer great advantages compared with more conventional methods, further research is needed to ensure that results are reproducible across different settings before wider application.

Other Measures of Metabolic Function

In addition to ICG, several other compounds are metabolized almost exclusively by the liver cytochrome P450 system and have been investigated as potential markers of hepatic function. For example, lidocaine is metabolized to monoethylglycinexylidide (MEGX) primarily in the liver. The MEGX test has been studied in transplantation and critical care medicine and appears to correlate with other measures of hepatic metabolism.[71,72] A small study demonstrated higher rates of postoperative liver insufficiency among Child-Pugh A patients who had a low MEGX value.[73] Unfortunately, the test is limited by poor reliability and the need for frequent monitoring; therefore its present application in preoperative assessment of liver function is investigational only. Galactose elimination capacity also accurately reflects metabolic function of the liver but is similarly limited by practical constraints and alterations due to environmental *conditions*.[74]

Magnetic Resonance Imaging Hepatic Agents

MRI with contrast enhancement offers high-resolution cross-sectional assessment of background liver anatomy and accurate characterization of hepatic tumors. MRI is more sensitive and specific than CT for the detection of primary and metastatic liver neoplasms and is used routinely at most centers before embarking on liver resection.[75] Gadolinium ethoxybenzyl dimeglumine (Gd-EOB-DTPA) is a liver-specific contrast agent that has as much as 50% hepatobiliary excretion in a normal liver.[76] Gd-EOB-DTPA improves the detection and characterization of focal liver lesions and diffuse liver disease. Given the hepatic uptake and elimination of Gd-EOB-DTPA, contrast-enhanced MRI may also provide functional assessment of the background liver (Fig. 4.2).

Several small studies have demonstrated correlation between Gd-EOB-DTPA uptake on MRI and conventional measures of liver function,[77-80] and with ^{99m}Tc-mebrofenin HBS.[81,82] Postoperative ICG-R15 can also be predicted well using pre-resection MRI.[83] There are several theoretical and practical advantages to using Gd-EOB-DTPA–enhanced MRI to assess liver function. First, MRI is routinely available and frequently used in the preoperative assessment of these patients, so no additional testing is required. Second, functional assessment may be focused on the planned FLR in cases of heterogeneous uptake, rather than calculating uptake for the whole liver as is the case in most other functional quantitative tests. Finally, MRI provides visual assessment of background liver injury, including steatosis and fibrosis, which may further assist in preoperative decision making.

MRI has been shown to be superior to sFLR volume and ICG-R15[84-86] at predicting PHLF. The most precise predictors for PHLF seem to use a combination of relative liver enhancement (RLE, difference in signal intensity between the unenhanced and hepatobiliary phases) or hepatocellular uptake index (HUI, difference in signal intensity between liver parenchyma and the spleen) specific to the FLR and patient weight. For example, Asenbaum et al. calculated an AUC of 0.9 for predicting PHLF for their outcome of functional FLR, which equals (FLR × remnant RLE)/weight.[86] Similar to using KGR as a measure of liver function after PVE, contrast-enhanced MRI can compare RLE and HUI before and after

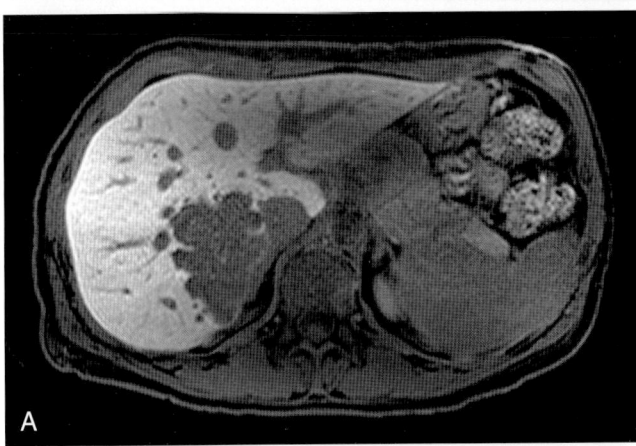

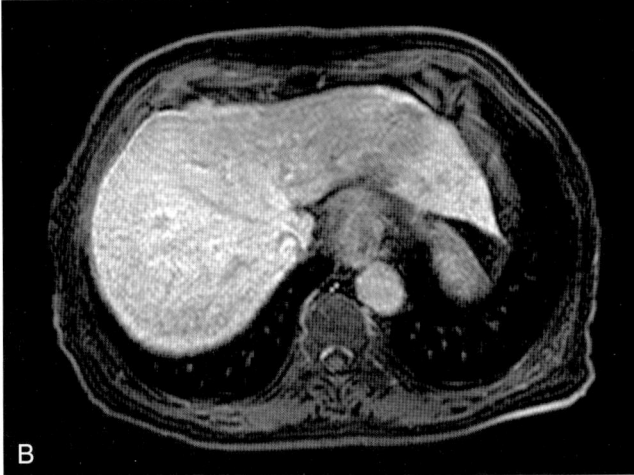

FIGURE 4.2 Magnetic resonance imaging with gadolinium ethoxybenzyl dimeglumine contrast on two patients demonstrating normal uptake **(A)** and diffusely decreased uptake **(B)**.

PVE. Studies performing MRI pre-PVE, post-PVE days 14 and 28, and 10 days post hepatectomy have shown that the increase in RLE from baseline to 14 days post-PVE is an excellent predictor of PHLF, and that beyond 14 days there is minimal improvements in FLR, KGR, and RLE.[87,88]

The availability and common use of MRI, combined with its ability to provide information on both the volume and the function of the FLR, give it the potential to be an extremely useful tool for the assessment of patients being considered for major hepatic resection. Early prospective studies demonstrate a relationship between Gd-EOB-DTPA uptake and clinical outcome postresection. Larger trials demonstrating its NPV and PPV for PHLF and mortality are needed.

Transient Elastography

Ultrasound transient elastography (TE) has been reported as a test to estimate the extent of liver fibrosis. Ultrasound TE has the clear advantages of being noninvasive and fast but is limited by significant inter-observer variability and anatomic variations.[89,90] Two studies of patients with HCC undergoing hepatectomy found ultrasound TE to have a high NPV of 98% but relatively poor PPV.[91,92] Therefore ultrasound TE may have a role in screening patients at low risk for PHLF, but a positive test should prompt further investigations and not necessarily preclude resection.

CT Texture Analysis

Texture analysis is an established technique that characterizes regions of interest in an image based on spatial variations in pixel intensity. On CT imaging, texture analysis can potentially quantify regional variations in enhancement that cannot be assessed by inspection. Several studies have shown potential utility of this technique for tumor diagnosis, characterization, and prognostication. Texture variables of preoperative CT scans show promise for predicting postoperative hepatic failure in single-institution[93] and multi-institution studies[94] and may represent a new means of preoperative risk stratification.

CONCLUSION

Hepatobiliary surgeons now have a variety of tools at their disposal to assist with preoperative assessment of hepatic function. The gold standard remains volumetric-based assessment of the FLR with cross-sectional imaging (CT or MRI). In patients in whom there is concern about insufficient liver volume or background liver injury, response to PVE provides a functional assessment of the FLR in addition to its therapeutic role. Quantitative measures of hepatic uptake, metabolism, and elimination, including ICG clearance, nuclear scintigraphy, and MRI hepatic-specific contrast agents, may have a role in assessment of patients with borderline FLR volume or background liver disease. MRI in particular seems poised to emerge as a complete package to diagnose occult metastases, assess FLR volumetry and FLR-specific function, and assess both the volumetric and functional response to PVE. Further refinement of these techniques may allow for the development of algorithms or decision aids that provide more precise prediction of postoperative hepatic insufficiency, ultimately decreasing postoperative morbidity and mortality.

The references for this chapter can be found online by accessing the accompanying Expert Consult website.

CHAPTER 5

Liver blood flow: Physiology, measurement, and clinical relevance

Edouard Girard and Simon Turcotte

Circulation in the liver is unique because of a dual afferent blood supply, derived from the hepatic artery (HA) and the portal vein (PV; see Chapter 2). The oxygen-rich arterial blood and the nutrient-rich PV blood merge in the hepatic parenchymal microcirculation to sustain the complex functions of the liver before returning to the heart through the hepatic veins (HVs). This chapter outlines how liver blood flow (LBF) is controlled to maintain the hepatic perfusion within an acceptable physiologic range, describes techniques used for LBF measurement, and explores clinical situations in which blood flow is altered.

PHYSIOLOGY

Liver Blood Supply

The peculiar double afferent blood supply to the liver (see Chapter 2) results in 75% to 80% of the entering blood being partially deoxygenated PV blood draining the stomach, intestine, spleen, and pancreas. The remainder is well-oxygenated blood from the aorta, carried by the HA. Mixing of arterial and portal blood occurs in terminal branches in the sinusoidal microcirculation around hepatocytes arranged into roughly polyhedral-shaped lobules, from their periphery toward their centrilobular venule (Fig. 5.1). The centrilobular venules drain into the HVs and into the inferior vena cava (IVC). Although the liver mass constitutes approximately 2.5% of the total body weight, the liver receives nearly 25% of the cardiac output. The total LBF ranges between 800 to 1200 mL/min, which is equivalent to approximately 100 mL/min per 100 g liver wet weight. The liver blood volume is estimated to range from 25 to 30 mL per 100 g of liver wet weight, which accounts for 10% to 15% of the total body blood volume. The sinusoids hold 60% of the blood volume, whereas the remaining 40% lies in large vessels (HA, PV, and HV).[1,2] Of note is the high compliance of the liver, calculated as the change in its blood volume per unit change in venous pressure. The liver thus acts as an important blood reservoir because its blood volume can expand considerably in cardiac failure or, in case of bleeding episodes, can compensate as much as 25% of the hemorrhage by rapid expulsion of blood into the circulation.[3,4]

Hepatic Artery

The HA normally supplies approximately 25% of the total blood flow to the liver (25 to 30 mL/min per 100 g of liver tissue) in a high-pressure/high-resistance system. The mean pressure in the HA is similar to that in the aorta. The HA provides as much as 50% of the liver's oxygen requirement because of the greater oxygen content found in arterial blood. In addition, the HA provides the exclusive blood supply to the intrahepatic bile ducts through the peribiliary plexus (Fig. 5.2). In the hepatic lobules, the hepatic arterioles empty directly or via peribiliary plexi into the sinusoids. Direct artery-to-HV connections do not usually exist but may arise in liver disease.

Within the liver parenchyma, the pressure in the arterial system is reduced toward that existing in the portal circulation and sinusoids. This is suggested to be achieved mainly by (1) the presinusoidal arteriolar resistance in the peribiliary plexus and (2) the intermittent closure of the arterioles, which protect the portal bloodstream from arterial pressure.[5] In the event of HA occlusion, numerous intrahepatic collaterals can provide a source of arterial blood. Additionally, extrahepatic collateral supply can develop after HA ligation and depends on the site of occlusion. If the common HA is interrupted, revascularization occurs through extrahepatic collaterals arising from (1) the inferior phrenic arteries and (2) from the gastroduodenal arteries, which derive blood flow from the superior mesenteric artery.[6] Ligation of the proper HAs leads to revascularization mainly via a hypertrophied inferior phrenic circulation, which can develop connections with HAs within the liver.[7] If only the right or left HA is interrupted, intrahepatic translobar anastomoses reestablish arterial flow in the ligated system.[8] Thus complete long-term dearterialization of the liver by any form of arterial vascular occlusion is difficult to achieve.

Portal Vein

The PV normally carries approximately 75% of the total blood flow to the liver (90 mL/min per 100 g of liver weight) in a valveless, low-pressure/low-resistance venous system. The inferior and superior mesenteric veins join with the splenic vein to form the PV, and jointly they collect the venous outflow from the entire prehepatic splanchnic vascular bed (the intestinal tract from the lower esophagus to the rectum plus the pancreas and spleen). The PV pressure ranges between 6 and 10 mm Hg in humans when measured by direct cannulation.[9] PV pressure depends primarily on the degree of constriction of mesenteric and splanchnic arterioles, coupled with the intrahepatic vascular resistance. Because portal blood is derived from postcapillary beds, it is partly deoxygenated. However, because of its large volume flow rate, it may supply 50% to 70% of the liver's normal oxygen requirement. During fasting states, the oxygen saturation in the portal blood approaches 85%, which is greater than other systemic veins. Hepatic oxygen supply is diminished if portal blood flow is significantly reduced, but the effect is minimized by an increase in oxygen extraction from the HA blood and not by increasing flow.[10]

Hepatic Veins

The HV system is the systemic drainage tract of the entire splanchnic circulation. A total LBF of 1.5 L/min is considered the normal value in the average male, but the range can be quite wide (1–2 L/min). In normal conditions, the free pressure in

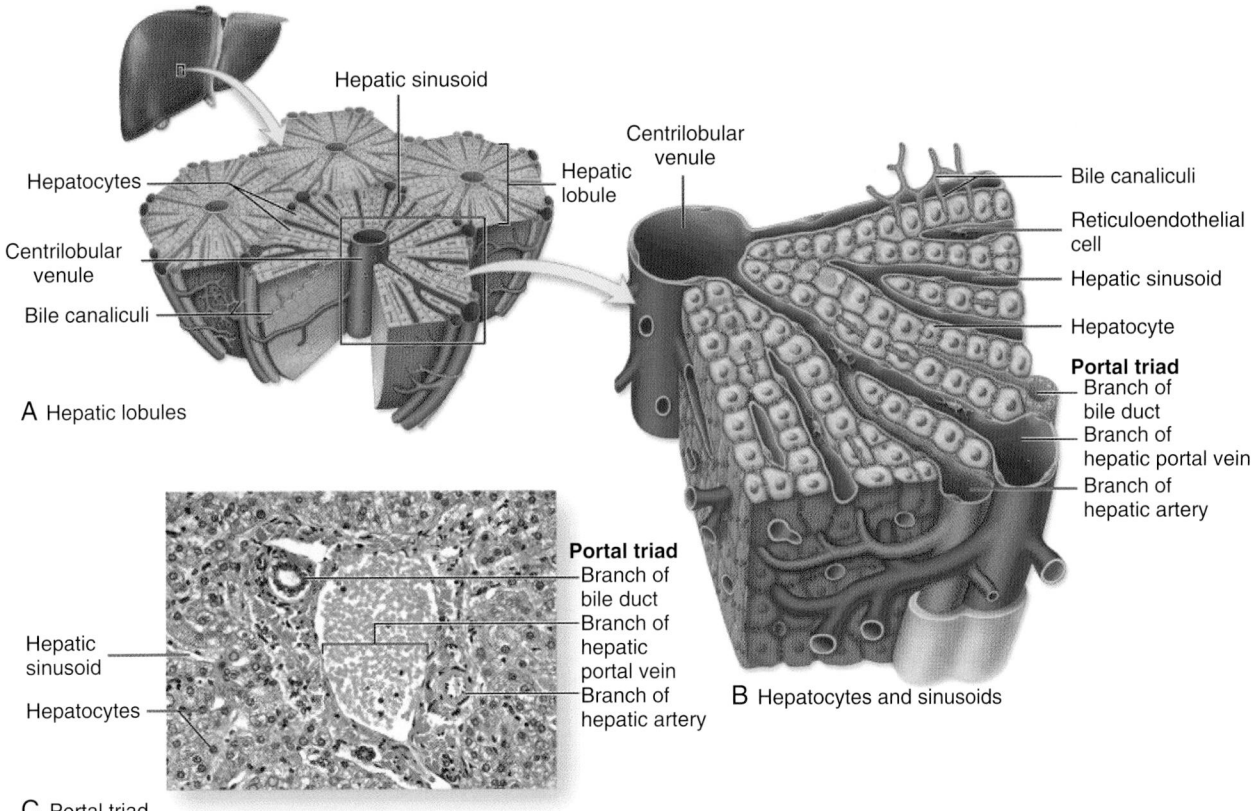

FIGURE 5.1 **The liver microcirculation.** The liver is composed of thousands of roughly polyhedral structures called *hepatic lobules*, which are the basic functional units of the organ. Hepatic lobules of some mammals, such as the pig, are delimited on all sides by connective tissue but have much less connective tissue and their boundaries are more difficult to distinguish in humans. **A,** A small central vein projecting through the center of each hepatic lobule and several sets of blood vessels defining the periphery. The peripheral vessels are grouped primarily in connective tissue involving the portal tracts in the space of Mall, which include a branch of the portal vein, the hepatic artery, and the bile duct. These make up the portal triad. **B,** Both blood vessels to each lobule give off sinusoids, which run between plates of hepatocytes and drain into the central vein. **C,** Micrograph showing components of the portal triad within the space of Mall (hematoxylin and eosin; ×220). (From Mescher AL. *Junqueira's Basic Histology: Text and Atlas*. 12th ed. McGraw-Hill; 2009.)

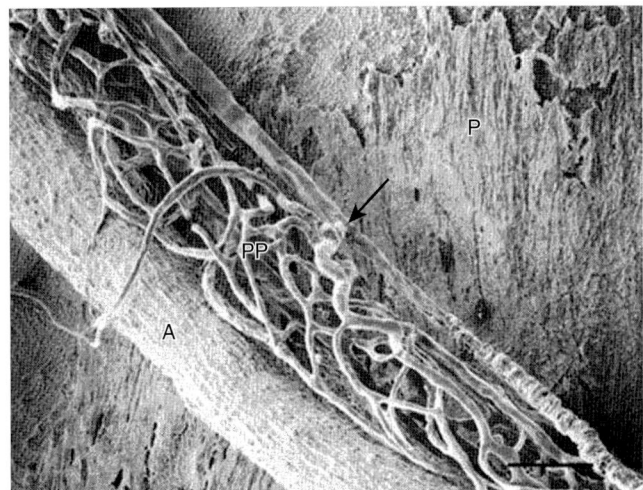

FIGURE 5.2 **Arterial peribiliary plexus.** A cast of the portal vein *(P)*, hepatic artery *(A)*, and peribiliary arterial plexus *(PP)* of a rat, showing a connection between a small artery and the plexus *(arrow)*. The peribiliary plexus forms a dense sheath around the bile duct. Bar = 100 μm. (From Grisham JW, Nopanitaya W. Scanning electron microscopy of casts of hepatic microvessels: Review of methods and results. In Laut W, ed. *Hepatic Circulation in Health and Disease*. Raven Press; 1981:98.)

the HVs and IVC is 1 to 2 mm Hg and is 1 to 5 mm Hg lower than the pressure measured in the sinusoids and PV. The portal pressure gradient, defined as the difference in pressure between the PV and the IVC, has been a useful clinical indicator of the perfusion pressure of the liver with portal blood.[11] The pressure gradient in the liver is thus extremely low, in the range of 5 mm Hg compared with all other organs, where it is in the range of 115 mm Hg.[12] Hepatic venous blood is normally approximately two-thirds saturated with oxygen, but this may be markedly reduced during periods of low delivery of oxygen to the liver, when oxygen is extracted by hepatocytes. In resting states, the liver accounts for approximately 20% of the total oxygen consumption of the body.

Hepatic Microcirculation

Although the organization of the liver into morphologic and functional units has been a matter of debate, the hexagonal polyhedral-shaped hepatic lobule, encompassing hepatic microvascular subunits consisting of a portal triad of terminal branches of the HA, PV, and bile duct; a network of sinusoids; and an efferent centrilobular venule is a widely accepted framework[13,14] (see Fig. 5.1). The portal triads, surrounded by lymphatics and autonomous nerves, all travel together in

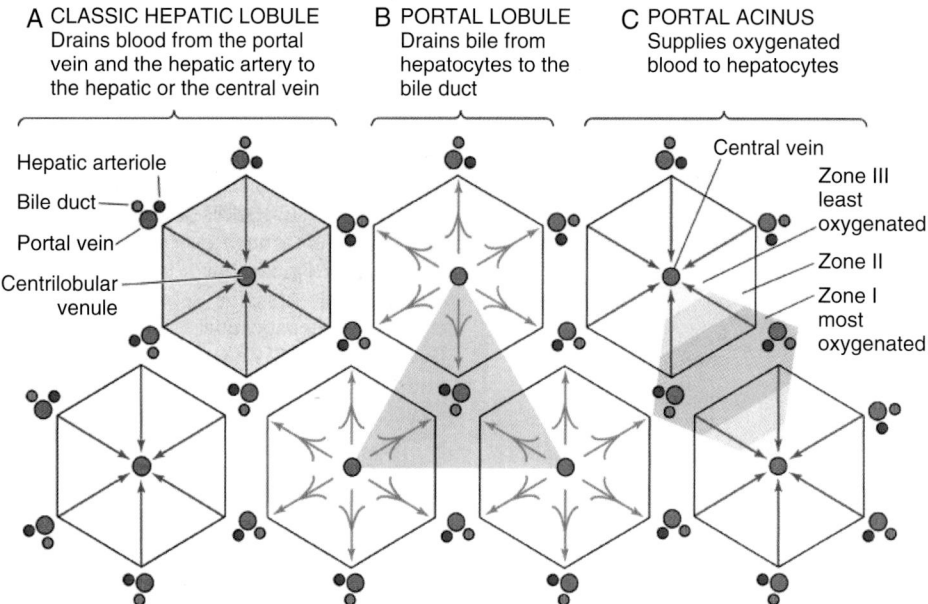

A CLASSIC HEPATIC LOBULE
Drains blood from the portal vein and the hepatic artery to the hepatic or the central vein

B PORTAL LOBULE
Drains bile from hepatocytes to the bile duct

C PORTAL ACINUS
Supplies oxygenated blood to hepatocytes

Hepatic arteriole
Bile duct
Portal vein
Centrilobular venule

Central vein
Zone III least oxygenated
Zone II
Zone I most oxygenated

FIGURE 5.3 **Structure-function conceptual liver units.** To this day, there is no complete consensus on whether the microvascular unit of the liver should be referred to as a lobule, centering on a hepatic vein, or an acinus, centering on a "portal triad" consisting of a terminal branch of the hepatic artery, portal vein, and bile duct, encased within a limiting plate of cells defining the space of Mall. Three related conceptual units emphasizing different aspects of hepatocyte activity have been proposed. **A,** The *classic lobule* emphasizes the endocrine function of hepatocytes as blood flows past them toward the centrilobular venule. **B,** The *portal lobule* emphasizes the hepatocytes' exocrine function and the flow of bile from regions of three classic lobules toward the bile duct in the portal triad at the center. The area drained by each bile duct is roughly triangular. **C,** The *liver acinus* concept proposed by Rappaport emphasizes the different oxygen and nutrient contents of blood at different distances along the sinusoids, with blood from each portal area supplying cells in two or more classic lobules. Each hepatocyte's major activity is determined by its location along the oxygen/nutrient gradient: periportal cells of zone I get the most oxygen and nutrients and show metabolic activity generally different from the pericentral hepatocytes of zone III, exposed to the lowest oxygen and nutrient concentrations. (From Boron WF, Boulpaep EL, eds. *Medical Physiology: A Cellular and Molecular Approach.* Saunders Elsevier; 2005.)

parallel in the space of Mall, through the liver parenchyma, and form portal tracts. Lymphatics transport proteins and other macromolecules that are trapped extravascularly because of hindrance of hepatocellular uptake, as in the case of cirrhosis, which will, in turn, contribute to ascites formation (see Chapters 74 and 79). The hepatic sinusoids correspond to the capillary bed of the liver and represent the segment of the microcirculation in which supply of nutrients and removal of metabolic products by hepatocytes takes place. Bile canaliculi closely assemble around hepatocytes and collect bile flowing in an opposite direction from blood in the sinusoids. As depicted in Figure 5.3, histologic and physiologic studies of the liver have given rise to three related ways to view the liver's microcirculation, emphasizing different functional aspects useful for the classification of various pathologic processes.

Apart from the absence of a basement membrane, the structural peculiarity of hepatic sinusoids is their unique lining, consisting of endothelial cells with flattened processes perforated by small fenestrae. These open fenestrations are arranged in clusters of 10 to 50 pores, forming so-called "sieve plates" with a diameter of 150 to 175 nm (Fig. 5.4). The sieve plates occupy as much as 8% of the endothelial surface and are not uniform in size or distribution throughout the length of the sinusoids. There is a decrease in diameter but an increase of frequency from periportal to centrilobular zones, which results in higher centrilobular porosity.[15,16] The fenestrae are dynamic structures that contract and dilate in response to alterations of sinusoidal blood flow and perfusion pressure.[17] Red blood cells

(RBCs) remain restricted within the sinusoids, whereas molecules as large as albumin can pass through the fenestrations and enter the small space of Disse before making contact with the microvilli of the hepatocytes.[12]

As represented in Figure 5.5, other unique cellular components, such as the hepatic stellate cell (HSC)[18] and the Kupffer cell (KC), are found in the hepatic sinusoids and may regulate the sinusoidal microcirculation in response to various mediators.[19] External to the endothelium cell lining, HSCs (also known as fat-storing cells, Ito cells, or hepatic perisinusoidal lipocytes) are contractile cells distributed homogeneously around the exterior of the endothelial cells in the space of Disse, which is the space between the basal microvilli-rich surfaces of the hepatocytes and the sinusoidal lining cells. In addition to their well-known importance in retinol metabolism and as key actors in the hepatic fibrogenic response to injury (see Chapters 7 and 74), HSCs are capable of compressing the sinusoidal diameter by squeezing the endothelial cells and therefore play a central role in the regulation of blood flow through hepatic sinusoids.[20,21] KCs are liver-specific macrophages, and, in contrast to HSCs, are anchored to the luminal side of the sinusoids. They account for approximately 15% of the liver-cell population and constitute approximately 80% of the total population of macrophages in the body.[12] By their large bodies, with cytoplasmic process that sometimes reach the opposite wall of a sinusoid, KCs represent a flow hindrance and can secrete large amounts of the vasodilator nitric oxide, but their direct regulation role of the sinusoidal microcirculation is debated.[12,22]

Control of Liver Blood Flow

The hepatic blood flow required to meet the physiologic function of the liver is mainly controlled by intrinsic physiologic mechanisms that are independent of extrinsic innervation and vasoactive agents. Instead, the interrelationship of arterial and portal inflow circuits is the major contributor to hepatic perfusion.

Liver-Intrinsic Blood Flow Regulation

THE HEPATIC ARTERIAL BUFFER RESPONSE. Adequate and homogeneous blood flow to the liver is necessary to sustain hepatic

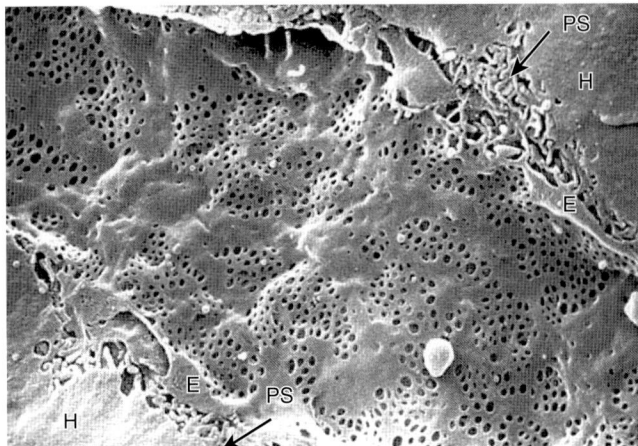

FIGURE 5.4 Fenestrations in endothelial sinusoid lining. Electron microscopy of the luminal surface of the endothelium lining a sinusoid in the liver shows grouped fenestrations. At the border are seen cut edges of the endothelial cell *(E)* in this discontinuous sinusoid and hepatocytes *(H)*. Between these two cells is the thin perisinusoidal space *(PS)*, into which project microvilli from the hepatocytes surface. Blood plasma passes freely through the fenestrations into the perisinusoidal space, where the voluminous membrane of hepatocytes acts to remove many high- and low-molecular-weight blood components and nutrients for storage and processing. Proteins synthesized and secreted from hepatocytes, such as albumin, fibrinogen, and other blood proteins, are released into the perisinusoidal space (×6500). (From Mescher AL. *Junqueira's Basic Histology: Text and Atlas*, 12th ed. McGraw-Hill; 2009; and Eddie Wisse, Electron Microscopy Unit, Department of Pathology, University of Maastricht, The Netherlands.)

functions and clearance of metabolites. Because the liver does not control portal blood flow, which is simply the outflow of the extrahepatic splanchnic organs, the main mechanism by which hepatic blood flow can remain constant relies on modulation of the hepatic arterial flow (Fig. 5.6). Although this phenomenon was observed in the late 19th and early 20th centuries,[23,24] it was characterized and coined as the hepatic arterial buffer response (HABR) by Lautt in 1981.[25]

HABR represents the ability of the HA to produce compensatory flow changes at the presinusoidal level in response to changes in PV flow (see Fig. 5.6): If portal blood flow is reduced, the HA dilates and increases its flow into the sinusoids, and the HA constricts when the portal flow is increased.[26,27] In patients undergoing abdominal surgery, a temporary occlusion of the PV resulted in a sharp increase in HA flow of about 30%, whereas temporary occlusion of the HA did not have significant effect on PV flow. The HABR seems to operate under various physiologic and pathologic conditions and has even been suggested to operate prenatally.[28] The HABR appears mainly regulated by the washout of adenosine, a potent vasodilator. Although adenosine is produced at a constant rate and secreted into the space of Mall (see Fig. 5.1), its concentration depends on the rate of washout from the space of Mall into the sinusoids. When portal blood flow decreases, less adenosine is washed away, and the elevated adenosine concentration leads to dilation of the HA. Of importance, the source of the extracellular adenosine found in the space of Mall remains to be elucidated. If portal blood flow is severely reduced, the buffer response results in the HA dilating maximally, as demonstrated by the inability to produce additional dilation in response to intraarterial infusion of adenosine. Conversely, when portal flow is doubled, the HA constricts to a maximal extent, as demonstrated by the inability of intraarterial norepinephrine to produce further constriction.[27] Although the HABR is sufficiently powerful to regulate the vascular tone in the HA over the full range from maximal vasodilation to maximal vasoconstriction, this mechanism is capable of buffering 25% to 60% of the decreased portal flow.[29]

Although adenosine appears to be the main mediator of the HABR, a possible contribution of the afferent sensory nerves and neuropeptides is suggested by studies in fully denervated animal livers[30] and in transplanted human livers,[31,32] in which

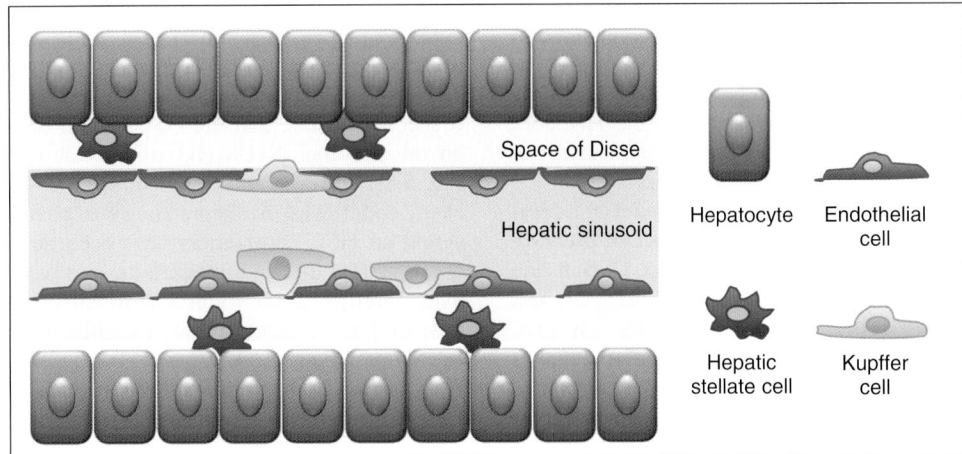

FIGURE 5.5 Hepatic stellate and Kupffer cells relation to the liver microcirculation. Contractile hepatic stellate cells are distributed homogeneously around the exterior of the endothelial cells in the space of Disse, the space between the basal microvilli-rich surfaces of the hepatocytes and the sinusoidal lining cells. Kupffer cells, which are liver-specific macrophages, are anchored to the luminal side of the sinusoids. They can secrete vasoactive mediators, and their large bodies may represent sinusoidal flow hindrance.

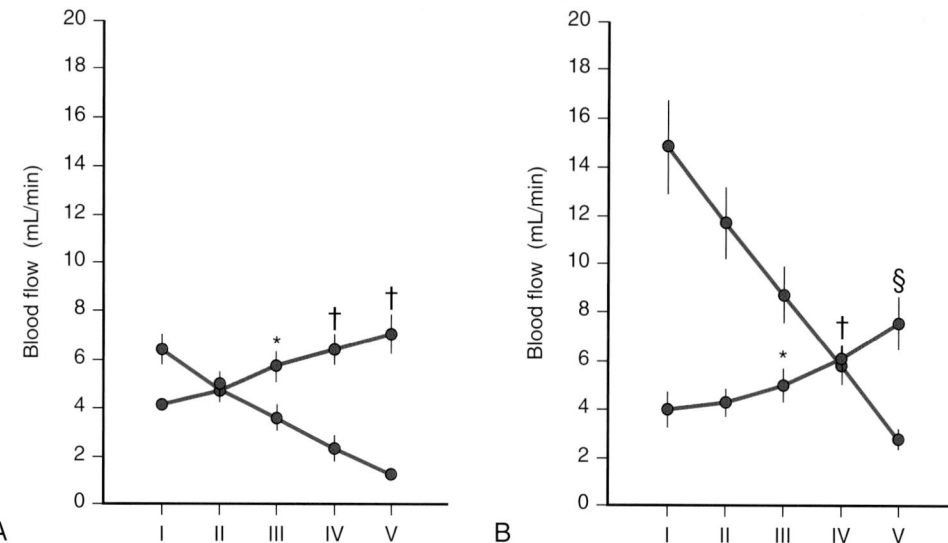

FIGURE 5.6 Hepatic arterial buffer response in cirrhotic **(A)** and control livers **(B).** Upon reduction of portal venous blood flow *(red),* there is a constant increase of hepatic arterial blood flow *(blue).* The portal flow is markedly diminished in cirrhotic liver, but the buffer response is preserved. Values are means ± standard error of triplicate measurements per animal (*n* = 6). *$P < .05$ vs. I and II; †$P < .05$ vs. I, II, and III. §$P < .05$ vs. I, II, II, and IV. (From Richter S, Mücke I, Menger MD, Vollmar B. Impact of intrinsic blood flow regulation in cirrhosis: Maintenance of hepatic arterial buffer response. *Am J Physiol Gastrointest Liver Physiol.* 2000;279(2):G454–G462.)

the HABR upon partial PV occlusion is partially impaired.[33,34] It has also been shown that hydrogen sulfide (H_2S), a vasoactive gaseous mediator produced within the liver, appears to almost double the HABR by increasing the HA conductance, and, in turn, its inhibition has the opposite effect.[35]

THE HEPATIC INFLOW IS NOT CONTROLLED BY LIVER-INTRINSIC METABOLIC NEEDS.
Until the mid-1970s, the HA flow was believed to be under metabolic control of the liver. As for most organs, the liver metabolism, estimated by its oxygen requirements, was postulated to participate in vascular inflow control. It has, however, been established that the liver normally receives more oxygen than it requires and can extract more oxygen to compensate for reduced delivery.[3,36,37] Additionally, the unique one-way sinusoidal flow arrangement precludes substances diffusing back from the hepatic parenchyma or venous blood into the HA resistance vessels. Among other studies, this concept has been exemplified by isovolemic hemodilution or upregulation of hepatic enzymes, leading to oxygen deprivation to the liver parenchyma, which does not result in HA dilation.[10,38] Therefore the hepatic metabolic demands do not control the HA flow, even if the liver parenchymal cells can release large quantities of potent vasoactive molecules during metabolic stress.

The term autoregulation refers to the tendency for local arterial blood flow to remain constant in the face of pressure changes in the arteries that perfuse a given organ. Overall, the degree of autoregulation is considered small in the liver, and mixed results have been reported in animal models.[39] In fact, the adenosine washout may well account for HA autoregulation because endogenous adenosine produced by the HA tributaries can contribute to high presinusoidal adenosine concentration in situations where hepatic clearance is impaired by a reduction in the portal flow, leading to HA vasodilation.[40]

REGULATION OF INTRAHEPATIC RESISTANCE AT THE SINUSOIDAL LEVEL.
Sinusoidal blood pressure and vascular resistance are so

low that a pressure gradient across the liver from the PV inflow to the HV outflow is only approximately 5 mm Hg. The low-pressure gradient is remarkable, considering that 30% of the inflow to the liver sinusoids is provided by the HA under arterial pressure. How the hepatic pressure gradient is maintained has been studied in multiple animal models. About 60 years ago, Knisley suggested the presence of sphincter-like structures at the entrance and exit of sinusoids that maintain the PV pressure gradients, but these proved to be species dependent.[12,22,41] In humans, although smooth muscle cells are found throughout all segments of the hepatic microvascular subunits, no such sphincter-like structures have been described for controlling intrahepatic blood flow.

In contrast, there is a growing body of evidence that contracting cells associated with the sinusoids, such as the HSCs and the sinusoidal endothelial cells, through a complex interplay with vasoactive mediators, may dynamically regulate the hepatic microvascular blood flow. With such a low sinusoidal perfusion pressure, local regulators at a single-cell level may actively control the flow within the sinusoids toward the HVs. It seems plausible that the HSCs could dilate to pull outward on the endothelial cells and enlarge the sinusoidal space (see Fig. 5.5); however, this does not seem to have been shown.[22] Many endothelial mediators known to control vascular tone by acting on HSC contractility have been described (Table 5.1), notably: (1) the endothelium-derived relaxing factor nitric oxide (NO),[42] (2) the endothelium-constricting factor endothelin-1 (ET-1),[43,44] and (3) two vasodilatory gaseous molecules: carbon monoxide (CO)[45,46] and H_2S.[47,48] With the exception of H_2S, a direct contribution of these vasoactive agents to the HABR is not well established.[39]

Liver-Extrinsic Factors Affecting Liver Inflow

ENDOGENOUS FACTORS
Blood Gas Tensions. Hypercarbia (partial pressure of carbon dioxide in arterial blood [$PaCO_2$] > 70 mm Hg) increases PV

TABLE 5.1 Liver-Intrinsic Vasoactive Molecules and Pathways Regulating the Microcirculation

VASOACTIVE AGENT	FUNCTION	ENZYME SYSTEM	CELLULAR SOURCE AND DISTRIBUTION	TARGET CELL	PATHWAYS
Thromboxane A_2	Vasoconstriction, platelet activation and aggregation, leukocyte adhesion	COX-1, COX-2	SEC, KC	SEC, platelet, leukocyte	TxA_2R
Prostaglandin I_2	Vasodilation, inhibition of platelet aggregation	COX-1, COX-2	SEC	SEC, HSC	PGI_2R
Angiotensin II	Vasoconstriction	ACE	HSC	HSC	AT_1
Nitric oxide	Vasodilation	eNOS	SEC	VSMC, HSC	sGC
Nitric oxide	Vasodilation	iNOS	SEC, KC, VSMC, HSC, HC	VSMC, HSC	sGC
Endothelin-1	Vasoconstriction		SEC, HSC, KC	VSMC, HSC, SEC, KC	ET_AR, $ET_{B2}R$
Endothelin-1	Vasodilation		SEC, HSC, KC	SEC	$ET_{B1}R$
Carbon monoxide	Vasodilation	HO-1	SEC, KC, VSMC, HSC, HC	VSMC, HSC	sGC
	Vasodilation	HO-2	HC	VSMC, HSC	sGC
Hydrogen sulfide	Vasodilation	CSE (CBS)	HSC, HC	VSMC	K_{ATP} channels

ACE, Angiotensin-converting enzyme; *AT₁,* type 1 of angiotensin II; *CBS,* cystathionine-synthase; *COX-1, COX-2, cyclooxygenase*-1 and 2, respectively; *CSE,* cystathionine-lyase; *eNOS,* endothelial constitutive nitric oxide synthase (type III); *ETₐR,* endothelin type A receptor; *ET_{B1}R,* endothelin type B1 receptor; *HC,* hepatocytes; *HO-1,* inducible heme oxygenase; *HO-2,* constitutive heme oxygenase; *HSC,* hepatic stellate cells; *iNOS,* inducible nitric oxide synthase (type II); *K_{ATP},* adenosine triphosphate (ATP)-sensitive potassium channel; *KC,* Kupffer cells; *PGI₂R,* prostaglandin I₂ receptor; *SEC,* sinusoidal endothelial cells; *sGC,* soluble guanylate cyclase; *TxA₂R,* thromboxane A₂ receptor; *VSMC,* vascular smooth muscle cells.

From Vollmar B, Menger MD. The hepatic microcirculation: Mechanistic contributions and therapeutic targets in liver injury and repair. *Physiol Rev.* 2009;89:1269–1339.

flow and decreases HA flow in dogs,[49] whereas hypocarbia ($PaCO_2$ < 30 mm Hg) decreases both.[50] Systemic hypoxia (partial pressure of oxygen in arterial blood [PaO_2] < 70 mm Hg) causes a decrease in arterial flow but has no effect on the contribution from the PV.[51] The response to metabolic acidosis is similar to that induced by hypercarbia, whereas metabolic alkalosis has essentially no significant effect.[52] The sympathetic nervous system is thought to be responsible for the HA vasoconstriction observed in hypercarbia and hypoxia.[53]

Sympathetic Nervous System. The liver is a significant blood reservoir, and 50% of its blood volume may be mobilized by nerve stimulation.[54] Denervation experiments have shown that the sympathetic nervous system is not involved in basal arterial tone in the liver.[53] Hepatic sympathetic nervous stimulation causes HA vasoconstriction and reduced blood flow, which appears secondary to an autoregulatory response.[1] Sensory denervated rats and pigs have a diminished arterial buffer response on partial occlusion of the PV.[34] Portal pressure increases as a result of an increase in PV resistance, but portal flow does not decrease unless there is a decrease in intestinal or splenic blood flow caused by simultaneous sympathetic stimulation of these vascular beds. Although the HA contains both α-adrenergic and β-adrenergic receptors, the PV system is believed to contain only α-receptors.[55] At low doses, epinephrine causes hepatic and mesenteric arterial vasodilation, whereas at high doses, vasoconstriction occurs in the HA and PV vascular beds and in the mesenteric circulation.[1,55]

Other Endogenous Vasoactive Agents. Intraportal administration of exogenous vasoactive agents affects HA resistance.[56] The mechanisms underlying this intrahepatic transvascular effect are not understood, but it is likely that the close anatomic association between arterioles and venules could permit this and may be a means by which HA blood flow is finely controlled by endogenous agents, such as gut hormones. Gastrin, secretin, cholecystokinin, and vasoactive intestinal peptide

cause vasodilation of the HA. Hepatic blood flow is profoundly increased by glucagon as a consequence of its strong vasodilatory action on the mesenteric vasculature, but insulin has little hemodynamic effect on the hepatic circulation. In addition, antagonists of calcitonin gene–related peptide and neurokinin significantly reduce HA blood flow, suggesting the presence of their receptors on the arterial vasculature.[33] Histamine causes HA dilation and, in the dog only, HV constriction. Bradykinin is a potent HA vasodilator that has little effect on the PV system. The HA vascular bed is dilated by most prostaglandins; however, prostacyclin does not affect HA flow but increases portal blood flow through a vasodilator effect on the prehepatic vascular bed. Vasopressin decreases portal flow and pressure by mesenteric arterial vasoconstriction but has variable effects on the HA. Serotonin is believed to mediate vasoconstriction of portal radicles.

Liver-extrinsic NO causes vasodilation in the HA and mesenteric vascular beds. Endothelin molecules can exert a powerful and prolonged generalized systemic constriction[21,57] that also has a direct effect on the hepatic blood flow. Endothelins reduce hepatic perfusion,[58] increase portal pressure,[59-62] and reduce sinusoidal diameter.[21,59,63] Angiotensin decreases HA and portal blood flow and is one of the few substances to produce a significant vasoconstrictor effect on the HA. In contrast, H_2S, either endogenously or exogenously, can reverse the norepinephrine-induced vasoconstriction in an NO-independent fashion.[64]

PHYSIOLOGIC STATES AND EXOGENOUS FACTORS

Age. Liver size and blood flow decrease with age in humans. Similarly, apparent liver blood flow per unit volume of liver (liver perfusion) falls with age.[65] Age does not seem to affect sinusoidal dimensions or sinusoidal density, but rather the geometry and the complexity of the sinusoidal network changes. These small age-related changes in the architecture of the liver sinusoidal network may influence hepatic function and reflect broader aging changes in the microcirculation.[66] The reduced elimination of both capacity-limited and flow-limited drugs, which is seen in the elderly, predisposed to adverse drug reactions, is likely because of these morphologic combined with physiologic changes.[67] Reduction in the activity of drug-metabolizing enzymes are probably of less significance in the healthy aged population.

Food Intake. Postprandial hemodynamic changes have been studied extensively in animals and humans. A meal induces a marked vasodilatation of the mesenteric artery with a consequent increase in PV flow, and compensatory vasoconstriction of the HA. The intrahepatic hemodynamic changes are greater in the right lobe of the liver, with a more significant increase of portal flow velocities on that side, in association with a bilateral reciprocal HA response that may be maximal on both sides.[68] The meal composition did not influence the magnitude of the hemodynamic changes but rather the timing of the response.[69,70]

Anesthesia. The effect of anesthetic agents on the LBF has been mainly studied in animal models some 30 years ago. HA and PV blood flow decreases passively in parallel with cardiac output during halothane inhalation, with little change in vascular resistance.[71,72] Enflurane has been found to have similar effects as those of halothane, although there is a decrease in HA vascular resistance as part of a generalized decrease in peripheral vascular resistance.[71] NO concentrations of 30% to 70% reduce HA and PV flow, possibly as a result of a generalized stimulatory action on α-adrenergic receptors.[73] Isoflurane seems to have minimal effects on HA and PV flows, and the intravenous (IV) agent fentanyl may have little effect on prehepatic splanchnic blood flow.[74] Thiopentone in low doses vasoconstricts the HA and mesenteric vascular beds.[75]

The effect of regional anesthesia on the LBF is poorly characterized. Sympathetic block might logically improve flow by reducing splanchnic vascular resistance, whereas reductions in systemic vascular resistance and cardiac output might offset this beneficial effect.[76] Thoracic epidural anesthesia caused a reduction in blood flow in mesenteric arteries that was associated with a decrease in systemic mean arterial pressure.[77]

Intermittent positive pressure ventilation predictably reduced splanchnic perfusion via a reduction in preload with a fall in cardiac output. The splanchnic circulation is also susceptible to more direct effects of positive pressure ventilation. The use of very large tidal volumes, high levels of positive end expiratory pressure (PEEP), and high inspiratory pressures have been shown to reduce splanchnic perfusion. These effects appear to be because of increased HV pressures and mesenteric vascular resistance, with reduced portal blood flow.[76]

MEASUREMENT OF LIVER BLOOD FLOW AND LIVER PERFUSION

The earliest methods of measuring LBF involved direct invasive techniques, such as intravascular devices or venous outflow collection.[23,78,79] Currently, measurement of hepatic venous pressure gradient (HVPG) remains the gold standard technique to assess portal hypertension[11] (see Chapters 74 and 85). Indirect determination of blood flow by the use of a variety of indicator-clearance techniques were subsequently developed, often confounded by the presence of liver disease. Some of these techniques remain useful to estimate liver function when planning major hepatectomies. By far today, Doppler ultrasound (D-US)

BOX 5.1 Summary of Methods Commonly Used for Measuring Liver Blood Flow

Flow in Single Vessels
Transjugular hepatic veins and wedge pressure measurement
Doppler ultrasound
Four-dimensional flow magnetic resonance imaging (MRI)

Total Liver Blood Flow
Hepatocyte clearance of Indocyanine green (ICG)

Hepatic Tissue Perfusion
Contrast-enhanced ultrasound
Contrast-enhanced computed tomography (CT)
Contrast-enhanced MRI
Isotopic imaging Scintigraphy (technetium 99m pertechnetate, albumin or sulfur-based colloids)

---

is the most common first-line noninvasive technique used to assess liver vascularization and guide clinical management. The available methods are discussed under three broad headings: (1) flow in single blood vessels, (2) total LBF, and (3) hepatic tissue perfusion. The techniques most commonly used for clinical use are listed in Box 5.1.

Flow in Single Vessels and Assessment of Portal Hypertension

Invasive Techniques

ELECTROMAGNETIC FLOWMETER PROBES. The direct and continuous measurement of HA and PV blood flow with electromagnetic flowmeter probes remains the best available means of assessing individual vessel flow. The technique has found widespread application in experiments using large animals, but not in clinical situations because of the vascular dissection required for placement of the probes. It is with this technique that total LBF in anesthetized subjects was determined to be approximately 1 L/min, of which approximately 25% was supplied by the HA.[80] Electromagnetic flowmeter probes have been used in the investigational setting intraoperatively to assess the hemodynamic status of the cirrhotic liver[81] and for intraoperative and postoperative measurement of PV and HA blood flow in liver resection and transplantation.[31,32,82] A typical experimental preparation using electromagnetic flowmeter probes is illustrated in Figure 5.7.

TRANSJUGULAR HEPATIC VENOUS PRESSURE MEASUREMENT. Because portal hypertension is responsible for most clinical consequences of cirrhosis, measurement of PV pressure is critical to guide the clinical management of patients with chronic liver diseases. Currently, the accuracy of invasive techniques has not been surpassed by noninvasive measurement. Direct measurements of portal pressure can be performed through transhepatic or transvenous catheterization of the PV, but are rarely used because of the risk of intraperitoneal bleeding and visceral perforation. Instead, measurement of HV direct pressure and wedge pressure by a transjugular approach has been developed as a safe and reproducible technique to assess portal hypertension (Fig. 5.8). As mentioned earlier, the pressure gradient between the PV and the IVC represents the liver portal perfusion pressure, and its normal value is as high as 5 mm Hg.

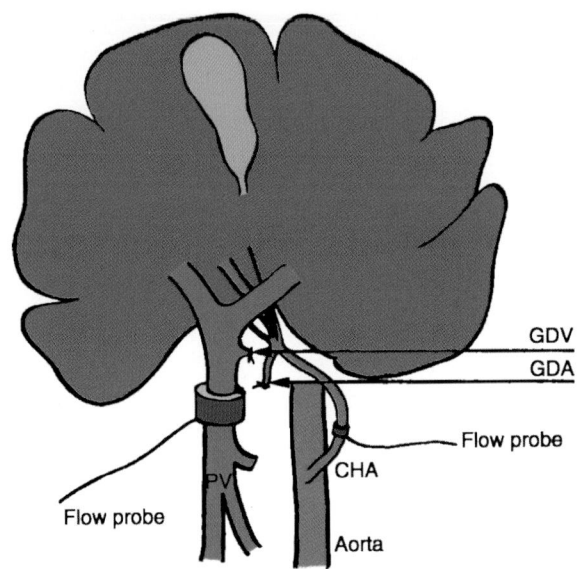

FIGURE 5.7 Experimental arrangement for measuring liver blood flow in the dog with electromagnetic flow probes. Probes are placed around the portal vein *(PV)* and common hepatic artery *(CHA)*. The gastroduodenal vein *(GDV)* and gastroduodenal artery *(GDA)* are ligated as illustrated to ensure that the flows measured by the probes are those that actually perfuse the liver.

The HVPG is calculated with the difference between wedged hepatic venous pressure (WHVP) and free hepatic venous pressure (FHVP; see Chapter 85). It is based on the concept that when the blood flow in a HV is blocked by a wedged catheter, the static column of blood transmits the pressure from the preceding communicated vascular territory, in this case, the hepatic sinusoids. Thus the WHVP is a measurement of the hepatic sinusoidal pressure and not of the portal pressure itself. In cirrhosis, even if the intersinusoidal communications are lost because of fibrosis and nodule formation, it has been well demonstrated that WHVP adequately reflects portal pressure.[83,84] The use of balloon-tipped catheters is recommended to measure HVPG[85] because the volume of the liver circulation that is measured is larger than that obtained by wedging the catheter tip, which enhances the reliability and accuracy of the measurement.[86]

Noninvasive Techniques

DOPPLER ULTRASOUND. Named after Christian Doppler for the phenomenon he described, the principle of flow estimation by Doppler is simple: flow is a product of the average velocity of the blood measured in the vessel of interest and the cross-sectional area of the vessel. Two forms of D-US devices exist. The first consists of a flowmeter with a US probe that is placed directly on the vessel; measurement with such a device is invasive. The second consists of a combined image scanner and flowmeter (duplex) by which flow in a vessel can be measured transcutaneously and noninvasively. In experiments performed on anesthetized dogs, good correlation was found between PV flow measured by a transcutaneous D-US and electromagnetic flowmeter probes fitted to the PV.[87] Because the development of color Doppler and better probe resolution with high-frequency transducers has improved accuracy, and because the technique provides morphologic assessment of the liver, is cheap, and can be performed at the bedside, D-US has become a widespread

first-line technique. In patients with known cirrhosis, D-US has greater than 80% specificity diagnosing clinically significant portal hypertension, but the sensitivity may not exceed 70%, particularly in compensated patients.[11] Inversion of flow within the PV is 100% specific for clinically significant portal hypertension. D-US is very accurate for detecting PV, HV, and HA thrombosis.[88] Additionally, D-US is useful in the noninvasive follow-up of transjugular intrahepatic portosystemic shunt (TIPS; see Chapter 85).[89]

FOUR-DIMENSIONAL FLOW MAGNETIC RESONANCE IMAGING. Since its original description in the 1980s,[90] phase contrast-enhanced magnetic resonance imaging (MRI) has seen broad clinical acceptance for the visualization and quantitative evaluation of blood flow in the heart and large vessels.[91] Further developments have led to time-resolved, three-dimensional (3D) phase-contrast MRI with 3D velocity encoding, which is often referred to as "four-dimensional (4D) flow MRI." Although standard two-dimensional (2D) MRI allows for the evaluation of blood flow in a single 2D slice, 4D flow MRI can provide information on the temporal and spatial evolution of 3D blood flow, with full volumetric coverage of any vascular region of interest.[92] This method can be used to monitor hepatic blood flow in patients with portal hypertension, in particular for noninvasive longitudinal hemodynamic monitoring before and after TIPS placement (Fig. 5.9).[93]

Total Blood Flow

Clearance Techniques

Substances reaching the liver via the HA or PV are equally well extracted,[56] and the rate of disappearance from the bloodstream of an indicator substance exclusively cleared by the liver is proportional to LBF. First applied to humans by Bradley and colleagues in 1945,[94] indirect clearance methods of LBF measurement rely on the Fick equation.

The Bradley's group originally used IV-injected bromosulfophthalein, removed from the bloodstream and excreted into the bile entirely by hepatocytes. The total hepatic blood flow was calculated by deriving a value for the rate of hepatic bromosulfophthalein removal using the rate of IV infusion of dye that maintained the arterial concentration at a constant level and the arteriovenous concentration difference of bromosulfophthalein. The mean value obtained in healthy individuals was 1.5 L/min. Other hepatic clearance techniques have been investigated in the past, such as colloidal clearance by the hepatic KC[95] and hepatocyte removal of galactose,[96] sorbitol,[97] rose bengal,[98] or propranolol.[99] The more complete hepatic extraction of these substances overcomes the need to cannulate an HV in patients with normal liver function. A modification of the colloid extraction method developed in the 1980s allows the derivation of the ratio of HA to total LBF, termed the "hepatic perfusion index." The basis of the technique is the ability to determine by dynamic scintigraphy the temporal separation of accumulating hepatic activity after reticuloendothelial uptake from the arterial and portal supplies after the IV administration of a bolus of technetium-99m–sulfur colloid.[100]

Indocyanine green (ICG) is now the most commonly used substance dependent on hepatocyte extraction into the bile. It was initially devised for the measurement of blood flow and later used for the assessment of liver function by measuring functional hepatocyte mass (see Chapter 3). HV cannulation

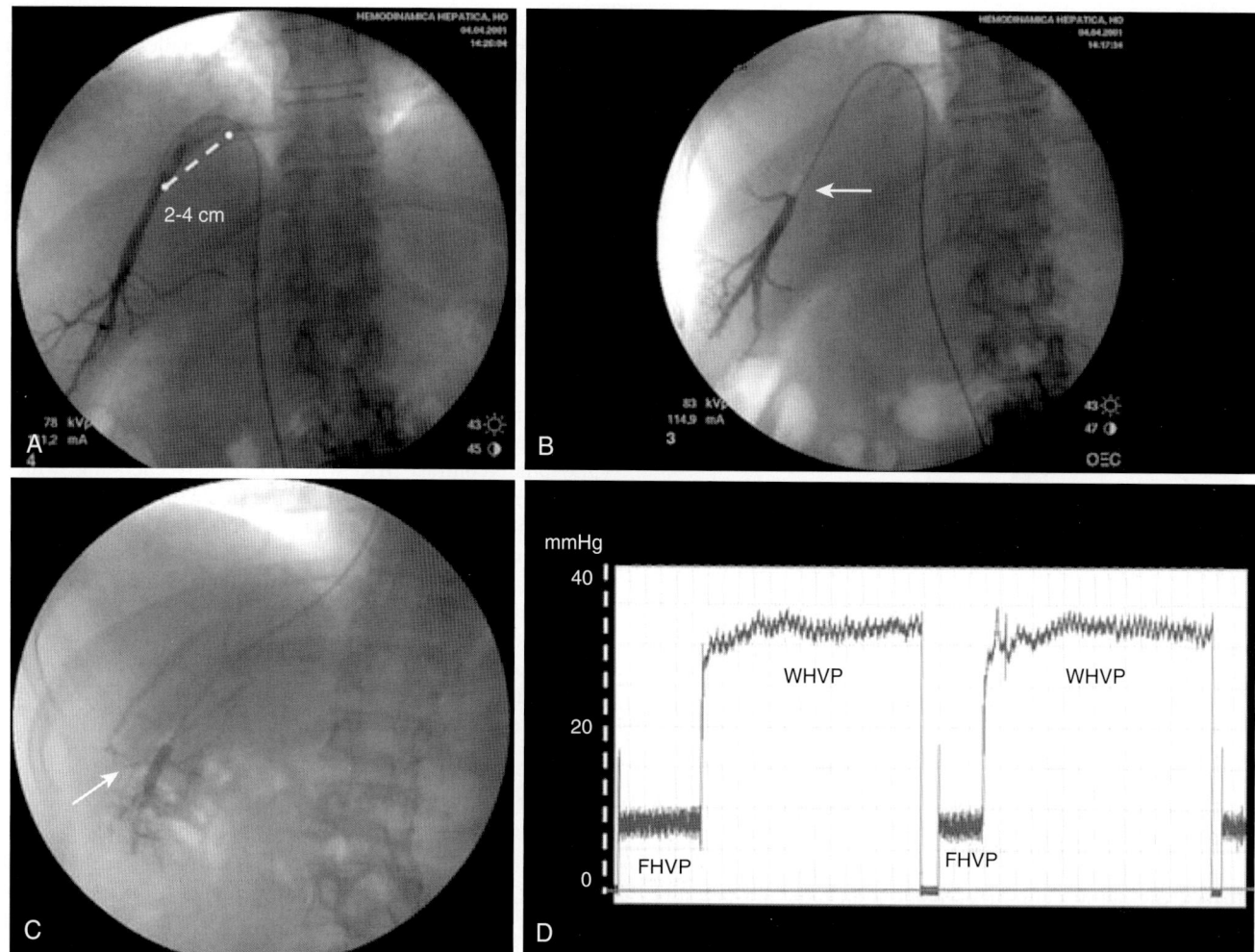

FIGURE 5.8 **Measurement of hepatic venous pressure. A,** Free hepatic venous pressure *(FHVP)* is measured by maintaining the tip of the catheter free in the hepatic vein at 2 to 4 cm from its opening into the inferior vena cava. **B,** Wedged hepatic venous pressure *(WHVP)* is measured by occluding the hepatic vein by inflating the angiographic balloon *(arrow)* at the tip of the catheter. Adequate occlusion of the hepatic vein is confirmed by slowly injecting 5 mL of contrast dye into the vein with the balloon inflated. Please note the typical wedged pattern distal to the balloon. **C,** A washout of contrast dye through communications with other hepatic veins *(arrow)* prevents a correct measurement of the hepatic venous pressure. **D,** Typical tracing of pressures measured in the hepatic vein obtained using a multichannel recorder and adequately calibrated transducers. (From Berzigotti A, Seijo S, Reverter E, Bosch J. Assessing portal hypertension in liver diseases. *Expert Rev Gastroenterol Hepatol.* 2013;7[2]:141–155.)

was initially performed to calculate the true extraction efficiency of ICG because of its incomplete hepatic removal.[101] Many investigators now use a simplified version of the original method, in which ICG is administered as a single IV bolus instead of as an infusion, and hepatic extraction efficiency is determined from an analysis of the clearance curve derived from peripheral blood sampling or pulse dye densitometry, by using an optical sensor placed on the finger.[102,103] ICG plasma disappearance rate is the most commonly used parameter, with a normal range between 16% and 25% per minute and near-complete disappearance at 20 minutes.[104] It is now the most widely used quantitative liver function test in the clinical setting.[105] Limitations of this technique include variations in hepatic blood flow caused by intrahepatic and extrahepatic shunting, or portal thrombosis, which is common in liver disease.

Other Techniques of Physiologic Interest

INDICATOR DILUTION. The indicator dilution method relies on the application of the Stewart-Hamilton principle, also derived

from the Fick equation.[106] In principle, the hepatic blood flow is proportional to the amount of hepatic blood that has diluted an introduced indicator. This method involves the injection into the HA and PV of a labeled substance that is not removed by the liver; changes in HV concentration are measured by blood sampling or by monitoring the hepatic isotope activity with an external detector. Such a method is therefore independent of hepatocellular function and reliable, provided the indicator remains in the vascular space and is not excreted before sampling. A modified thermal dilution technique has been used to measure portal blood flow in humans.[107] Indicator dilution methods overestimate true blood flow to hepatic tissue when intrahepatic or extrahepatic shunts are present, although it is possible to measure azygos blood flow by thermal dilution in patients with cirrhosis.[108]

INDICATOR FRACTIONATION. The measurement of regional blood flow by fractional distribution of cardiac output was first described by Sapirstein in 1956.[109] Briefly, a known amount of

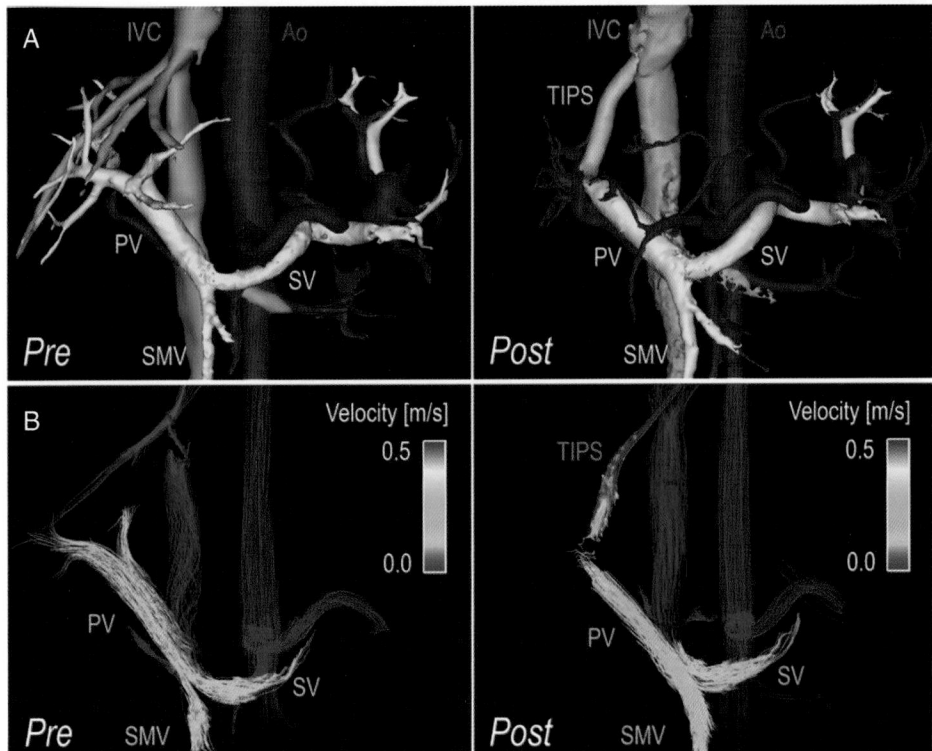

FIGURE 5.9 Four-dimensional flow magnetic resonance imaging *(MRI)*-based visualization and quantification of hemodynamics in the portal system before and after transjugular intrahepatic portosystemic shunt *(TIPS)* for portal hypertension. **A,** Segmentation of four-dimensional *(4D)*-flow angiograms obtained before (pre) and two weeks after (post) TIPS placement show arteries *(red)*, veins *(blue)*, portal vasculature *(yellow)*, and TIPS *(gray)*. **B,** Velocity-coded 4D-flow MRIs obtained before (pre) and 2 weeks after (post) TIPS placement show velocity distribution in the portal circulation. Color-coded streamlines show increased blood flow in the superior mesenteric vein *(SMV)*, splenic vein *(SV)*, and portal vein *(PV)* in response to TIPS placement. Note the high velocity in the TIPS, with a signal dropout at the proximal end of the TIPS are because of disordered flow. *Ao,* Aorta, *IVC,* inferior vena cava. (From Bannas P, Roldán-Alzate A, Johnson KM, et al. Longitudinal monitoring of hepatic blood flow before and after TIPS by using 4D-flow MR imaging. Radiology. 2016;281[2]:574–582.)

radioactive microspheres is injected into the left ventricle, and a reference sample is withdrawn from a peripheral artery at a known rate. The microspheres are then extracted from the various vascular beds, where they have lodged in proportion to the cardiac output. The HA blood flow can be determined directly by this method, but the portal flow contribution is found indirectly by addition of the flow values in the prehepatic splanchnic organs. Examination of the intrahepatic distribution of microspheres has provided a means of assessing the pattern of arterial flow in different liver regions.[110] Because the microsphere method requires the postmortem removal of the organs of interest for radioactivity or colorimetric measurement, the additional determination of tissue weight enables flow per gram (i.e., tissue perfusion) to be calculated. Microspheres may be used to determine the extent of portosystemic shunts. The fractional distribution in the liver may be measured with respect to systemic (lung) activity after PV injection, or it may be estimated by injecting a second radioactive microsphere directly into the splenic or mesenteric venous system.[111]

Hepatic Tissue Perfusion

Contrast-Enhanced Ultrasound

If D-US allows to quantify flow in single vessels, contrast-enhanced US with microbubble contrast agents allows to quantify hepatic tissue perfusion. Advantages over other imaging

techniques are the use of purely endovascular agents, which circumvent the issue of extravascular leakage, the equipment lightweight and readiness, and the avoidance of exposure to x-rays or radionuclide tracers.[112] Dynamic image sequences are obtained after contrast injection, which then varies in local concentration over time. The change in intensity over time can then be modeled to obtain parameters describing the microcirculation. A software program is used to estimate liver perfusion along three main types of analysis: organ transit time of the contrast, tissue reperfusion kinetics, and enhancement intensity curves.[113]

Computed Tomography

A concentrated iodinated contrast medium is used as tracer in computed tomography (CT), and it is injected at high flow. This technique is inexpensive, readily accessible, quick, highly reproducible, and provides morphologic information.[112] It offers good spatial and temporal resolution, and quantification of the tracer is straightforward because the density concentration relationship is linear (Fig. 5.10). It is most commonly used to delineate acute liver parenchymal injuries and the precise localization and vascularization pattern of suspected liver lesions. The information gained by CT scan to guide clinical decision making outweighs risks related to radiation and the potential nephrotoxicity of iodinated contrast, which can also be reduced by optimizing the acquisition settings, improving detectors, and using reconstruction algorithms.[114]

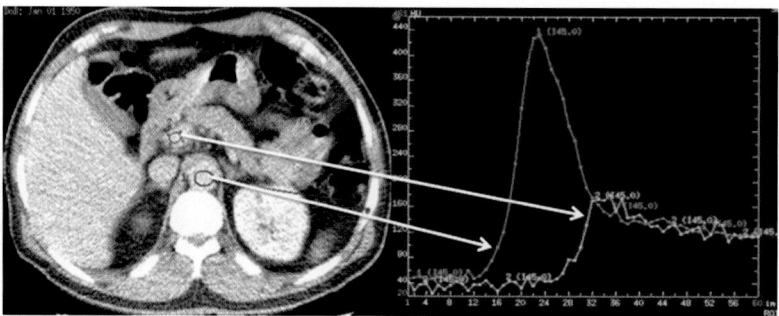

FIGURE 5.10 Example of signal to time curve obtained on computed tomography (**CT**). The signal to time curve (image on the right) is obtained after positioning the regions of interest in the afferent vessels (aorta and portal vein). The change in tracer concentration over time is obtained by rapid signal sampling (in this case density). The perfusion parameters are extracted from an analysis of these curves. (From Ronot M, Lambert S, Daire JL, et al. Can we justify not doing liver perfusion imaging in 2013? *Diagn Interv Imaging.* 2013;94[12]:1323–1336.)

Magnetic Resonance Imaging

Significant correlation between MRI and thermal dilution probe flow measurements using 1.0T T1-weighted sequences in pigs was first described in 1999.[115] This technique does not necessitate radiation, with good spatial and temporal resolution. The main technique used for MRI perfusion measurement is dynamic contrast-enhanced MRI (DCE-MRI) after injection of a gadolinium chelate.[92,116] Unlike CT, in which the tracer concentration curve over time is proportional to changes in attenuation measured in Hounsfield units, the curve is more difficult to obtain in MRI because the relationship between signal intensity and tracer concentration is not linear. Concentration is related to the relaxivity of the medium and requires measurement of T1, which can be performed using samples of increasing gadolinium concentration.[112] Of note, MRI sequences that are affected by molecular diffusion (diffusion MRI) are influenced by the microperfusion. The diffusion MRI signal depends on the speed of the circulating blood and the microvascular architecture. The restriction in diffusion seen in cirrhotic liver may be because of changes in microperfusion components rather than reduction in pure hepatic diffusion.[117] Ongoing research is evaluating specific use of MRI to assess liver perfusion.

Isotopic Imaging

Scintigraphic methods to calculate liver perfusion parameters were first described in the 1970s. Images are generally acquired after IV injection of a radiopharmaceutical (technetium 99m pertechnetate, albumin, or sulfur-based colloids).[112] Liver enhancement is analyzed by regions of interest and the arterial and portal components are separated; the renal enhancement peak represents the beginning of portal enhancement of hepatic parenchyma.[118] Scintigraphic studies based on positron emission tomography have assessed the feasibility of studying hepatic perfusion.[119] Isotopic imaging, however, is often hindered by poor spatial and temporal resolution.[112]

Other Techniques

INERT GAS CLEARANCE. By exploiting the fact that radioactive gases such as krypton (^{85}Kr) and xenon (^{133}Xe) distribute equally between tissue and blood according to a specific partition coefficient, the rate of clearance of such gases can be measured after their injection into the hepatic blood supply. After injection and rapid diffusion throughout the liver, the gas

clears from the tissue into the blood and is almost completely eliminated from the body after a single passage through the lungs. The clearance rate is proportional to hepatic tissue perfusion, which may be calculated by using a standard formula.[120] The first to use the inert gas method in the hepatic circulation were Aronsen and colleagues (1968a),[121] who recorded the γ-emissions of ^{133}Xe after the injection of a saline solution of the isotope into the PV. β-Emissions of ^{85}Kr are recorded by a Geiger-Müller tube or semiconductor (silicon) detector placed on or immediately above the exposed liver surface, whereas the γ-emissions of ^{133}Xe are monitored transcutaneously by a single scintillation crystal or a γ-camera; the latter device allows simultaneous measurement of hepatic tissue perfusion in many regions of interest. Inert gas techniques involve minimal trauma to the patient, and their accuracy is not markedly affected by the presence of hepatic cellular disease or nonperfusion shunts. Reproducibility of the results, even within the same subject, has been a concern.

LASER DOPPLER FLOWMETRY. Laser Doppler flowmetry (LDF) is a technique for the real-time measurement of microvascular RBC perfusion in the liver. By illuminating the tissue with low-power laser light and capturing the backscattered light with independent photodetectors, the Doppler shift of moving cells can be transmitted as an electrical signal. Linearity of the LDF signal from the liver with total organ perfusion has been shown,[122] and the technique has been shown to be sensitive to rapid changes in organ flow.[123] The technique has been applied successfully to measure LBF during liver transplantation in humans.[124] A major drawback of the technique is that, because of the small volume of tissue interrogated by the laser, the LDF signal can only be used to measure arbitrary, instead of absolute, blood perfusion in a single area.

IN VIVO FLUORESCENT MICROSCOPY. Intravital microscopy was first described in the microvessels of the frog tongue by Waller in 1846.[125] Using this technique, individual sinusoids and terminal venules can be visualized, and changes in their diameters and the velocities with which erythrocytes pass through them can be seen.[126] The introduction of fluorescent dyes has broadened the spectrum of in vivo microscopy in the liver from morphologic analysis to the study of pathologic events. From a hemodynamic point of view, however, intravital fluorescent microscopy has problems of interpretation.[127] In perfused liver, a 2.5-fold increase in PV blood flow has been found to be associated with only a 22% increase in sinusoidal RBC velocity, suggesting that changes in PV blood flow have only a minor effect on the capillary transit time.[128]

NEAR-INFRARED SPECTROSCOPY. Near-infrared spectroscopy is a noninvasive technique that uses light transmission and absorption to measure hemoglobin and mitochondrial oxygenation. In contrast to visible light, which can only penetrate a few millimeters, near-infrared light (700–1000 nm) can be detected through as much as 80 mm of tissue. The application of this technology to monitor liver oxygenation has been validated in models of endotoxic shock in pigs[129] and by intraoperative quantification of congestion and mitochondrial redox during HV occlusion in living-donor transplantation.[130]

CLINICAL RELEVANCE

Hemorrhagic Shock, Hypoperfusion, and Ischemia-Reperfusion Injury

Total LBF decreases approximately in relation to the degree of the hemorrhage, and PV blood flow decreases in parallel to cardiac output; but similar to the coronary, pulmonary, and cerebral circulations, HA flow does not decrease until extremely low blood pressures are reached. As a result, the hepatic oxygen supply tends to be maintained, although oxygen extraction greatly increases to preserve normal total oxygen consumption.[131] Hepatic blood volume can increase significantly in cardiac failure and can compensate as much as 25% of hemorrhage from its large-capacitance vessels.[132]

The clinical entity known as shock liver has long been recognized, typically related to cardiogenic or hemorrhagic shock.[133] Hepatic dysfunction caused by hypoperfusion is manifested pathologically by centrilobular necrosis and clinically by abdominal pain, cholestatic jaundice, and marked elevation of serum aminotransferases. Three phases of liver injury attributed to ischemia were proposed by Champion and colleagues (1976),[134] whereby the initial hepatic dysfunction would resolve as long as no additional insults (e.g., sepsis) were incurred. Gottlieb and colleagues (1983)[135] showed that hepatic dysfunction in humans after trauma was related to a reduced hepatic blood flow rate as much as 70% of resting levels. Hepatic blood flow was markedly reduced after injury, and although total splanchnic oxygen delivery was decreased, oxygen consumption remained normal as a result of increased hepatic extraction.

In the ischemic state, upregulation of acute-phase proteins (C-reactive protein, fibrinogen, ceruloplasmin, haptoglobin) is prioritized versus production of other hepatic proteins, such as albumin and transferrin.[136] More recently, hemorrhagic shock has been recognized to result in generalized vascular endothelial dysfunction and impaired endothelial biosynthesis of NO. Endothelial NO that continues to be expressed by the liver during ischemia is believed to protect against the initial hepatic injury arising from severe hemorrhage. By contrast, more prolonged hemorrhagic shock (>6 hours duration) induces greatly increased production of NO because of activation of an inducible NO synthase enzyme in hepatocytes and KCs.[137]

In the transplantation era, the consequences of ischemia and reperfusion for the liver have been increasingly investigated and understood. The damage to the hepatic endothelium and parenchyma that results from postischemic reperfusion is caused by numerous interrelated phenomena, including the action of locally liberated oxygen-derived free radicals and excess formation of vasoconstrictor agents.[138] Endogenous NO tends to protect the liver in the early reperfusion period after hepatic ischemia.[139] Ischemia is also the primary signal for heat-shock protein production in liver tissue. Experimental studies of heat-shock protein preconditioning through intermittent portal clamping demonstrated attenuated aminotransferase elevations and improved bile production after ischemia[140].

Liver Atrophy

Liver atrophy results from a significant reduction of LBF containing hepatotrophic substances (see Chapter 6). The degree of atrophy depends on the degree of blood flow deprivation and may be distributed according to the source of deprivation, including PV or HA blood flow or their combination. Atrophy and fatty degeneration of the canine liver after total portal diversion through an Eck fistula initially was reported more than a century ago.[141] Partial or complete diversion of PV blood flow from the liver results in atrophy. Complete PV flow diversion with interruption of all PV collaterals results in more profound liver atrophy than the partial deviation of PV flow resulting from side-to-side portacaval anastomoses.[142]

Liver atrophy after portal diversion is not believed to be the result of a decrease in absolute volume flow, but instead it is because of the effective loss of hepatotrophic substances in the portal blood. Rats subjected to portal flow diversion with portacaval transposition had a decrease in relative liver weight[143] despite the effective preservation of portal perfusion from the IVC.[144] Dogs with "partial portacaval transposition"[145] or "splanchnic flow division"[146] with diversion of pancreaticogastroduodenosplenic blood had atrophy in liver lobes, although normal tissue perfusion was shown in all regions of the liver.[147]

Histologically, arterial obstruction results in ischemic changes, such as mitochondrial swelling, cell membrane disruption, platelet aggregation, and widening of the spaces of Disse.[148] The fate of the liver after ligation of the HA depends largely on the extent of a functional collateral arterial circulation.[6] If limited collaterals are present, liver infarction and necrosis may occur after HA ligation, resulting in death. Nevertheless, HA ligation results only in transient ischemic changes in the periphery of the hepatic acinus (zone III, see Fig. 5.3) in the presence of adequate collaterals. Atrophy after HA ligation can occur in liver segments that have compensatory collateral supply to prevent necrosis. The effects of HA flow absence are magnified by the presence of low PV blood flow, limited oxygen saturation, and superimposed infection.[6]

Impact of Acute and Chronic Bile Duct Obstruction on Liver Blood Flow

Bile duct obstruction can affect hepatic hemodynamics significantly. In general, LBF is reduced in the presence of chronic biliary obstruction, leading to hepatic dysfunction. Conversely, acute increases in bile duct pressure from early obstruction result in a reflexive increase in LBF, which attempts to maintain adequate flow in the face of an increased pressure gradient opposing secretion and excretion of bile (see Chapter 8). Most evidence suggests that the hemodynamic response of the liver to biliary obstruction is related, directly or indirectly, to changes in bile duct pressure. Given the limited space of Mall in the portal triad (see Fig. 5.1), it is conceivable that increased biliary pressures may compress the portal capacitance vessels, leading to increased arterial flow.[149] Acute serial increases in bile duct pressure in dogs with complete bile duct obstruction increased HA blood flow by 250% but did not affect PV blood flow. Although increased portal vascular resistance is the accepted underlying cause, the primary site of this resistance change has been considered to be presinusoidal,[150] sinusoidal,[151] or postsinusoidal.[152] The precise mechanism for reduction in LBF after chronic bile duct obstruction thus remains to be fully elucidated. It should be noted that the combination of biliary and PV obstruction greatly accelerates atrophic changes, which has important implications for resection of hilar cholangiocarcinoma (see Chapters 51 and 119B).

Relief of long-term obstruction does not result in the return of normal hemodynamics, suggesting irreversible intrahepatic vascular damage.[153] Furthermore, a 23% reduction in effective LBF persisted for one to five years after operative decompression in patients with choledocholithiasis and jaundice for more than two weeks preoperatively.[154] Hunt (1979)[155] serially measured LBF daily for one week after bile duct ligation in rats, using the ^{133}Xe clearance technique to document the early hemodynamic response. Total LBF decreased steadily after the first postoperative day to a plateau level of approximately 50% of the preoperative value five days after operation. Mathie and colleagues (1988)[156] confirmed the decrease in total LBF after bile duct ligation by measuring the individual PV and HA components of LBF. Using electromagnetic flowmeters in dogs with complete bile duct ligation, HA and PV blood flow were observed to decrease by 36% and 44%, respectively; they also showed a 200% increase in intrahepatic portal resistance but a lesser increase in HA resistance. Similarly, dogs with chronic bile duct ligation had decreased PV flow and had developed sinusoidal portal hypertension and extensive portosystemic shunting.[151]

Chronic biliary obstruction can thus result in two hemodynamic consequences: portal hypertension associated with secondary biliary fibrosis (see Chapter 74) and shock after biliary tract decompression. Approximately 20% of patients with prolonged biliary obstruction experience clinically significant portal hypertension.[157,158] The operative risk of biliary decompression in these patients is significant. Technical difficulties of stricture repair—dense fibrous adhesions, hilar ductal involvement, and infection—are complicated by the risk of hemorrhage from subhepatic and periductal varices and potential postoperative liver failure. In addition to the hemodynamic consequences of chronic bile duct obstruction, sudden decompression of the obstructed biliary tree also causes an abrupt decrease in wedged HV pressure, PV pressure, and arterial pressure within 30 minutes of decompression in jaundiced dogs, leading to hypotension and shock.[152] Similarly, Steer and colleagues (1968)[159] reported that rapid needle decompression of an obstructed biliary tree in jaundiced dogs induced a decreased arterial pressure, central venous pressure, and PV pressure within one hour. They concluded that sudden decompression of chronic biliary obstruction leads to sequestration of fluid within the liver, resulting in a decrease in the effective circulating plasma volume and subsequent hypotension.

Liver Resection and Regeneration

The adult liver exhibits a remarkable potential to restore its cellular mass in response to injury through hepatocyte hyperplasia. Hepatic regeneration of the normal liver remnant proceeds rapidly after partial hepatic resection[160,161] (see Chapters 6). Partial liver resection without devascularization normally produces little change in total blood flow to the liver. This occurs because the major contributor to total flow, the PV, is affected less by events occurring within the liver than by control mechanisms in the arterial resistance vessels of the prehepatic splanchnic bed. On the other hand, the failure of the liver to directly control its PV flow may result in portal hyperperfusion of a reduced parenchymal mass. Because essentially the same total blood flow is redistributed to a smaller mass of liver tissue, a corresponding increase in tissue perfusion (mL/min per unit tissue weight) would be anticipated in the in situ remnant. Experimental studies support these expectations; an increase in hepatic tissue perfusion was observed in rats immediately after two-thirds hepatectomy.[162–164] This increase in hepatic perfusion is primarily because of PV inflow, because HA blood flow is low, and because HA resistance is high even 24 hours after partial hepatectomy in rats.

In humans, an immediate increase in tissue perfusion of approximately 120% occurs in the liver remnant.[165] A 60% partial hepatectomy results in a doubling of the portal flow in the 40% of remnant liver tissue.[166] Experimental evidence has suggested that intrahepatic shear stress from increased portal flow is a regulator of liver regeneration.[167,168] The significance of blood flow in relation to liver regeneration, however, continues to be debated since Mann (1944)[169] suggested that regenerative hyperplasia of the liver after partial resection was a function of portal blood flow and that the process could be prevented by portal flow diversion. However, regenerative hyperplasia normally occurs after partial liver resection in portacavally transposed animals, in which there is no direct supply of portal blood nor the usual posthepatectomy increase in hepatic tissue perfusion.[170]

Liver Blood Flow and Hemodynamic Studies in Liver Transplantation

The HA buffer response is conserved after orthotopic liver transplantation (OLT) despite denervation.[31,39] In a series of experiments by Payen and colleagues (1990),[32] serial clamping of the PV every 12 hours for seven days after OLT resulted in reciprocal increases in HA flow. OLT of a normal donor organ does not normalize the splanchnic and systemic hemodynamic alterations of end-stage liver disease.[171] In fact, total hepatic blood flow remains elevated six months after OLT[172,173] mainly because of PV blood flow.[31,174] This suggests that baseline LBF may be under direct sympathetic control, which is lost after OLT, leading to an unopposed rise. Azygos flow also remains elevated, and other portosystemic shunts have been documented up to four years after OLT.[173] Ligation of these portosystemic collateral pathways has been shown to increase PV blood flow.[175]

The hemodynamic consequences of OLT in human patients are difficult to interpret for several reasons: (1) the causes of liver failure in end-stage transplant candidates are diverse; (2) immunosuppressive drugs are used, such as cyclosporine, which causes arterial hypertension; and (3) to control systemic hypertension after OLT, patients may also be given vasodilators, which can cause persistently increased cardiac output. Cardiac output data have been conflicting, with one group reporting persistently elevated values[172] and others showing decreases two weeks and two months after OLT.[173] Gadano and colleagues (1995)[176] emphasized that factors such as anemia and sepsis may account for the deranged hemodynamics after OLT. In a retrospective series of 970 patients, new-onset heart failure developed in as many as 10% of patients after OLT after a median follow-up of 5.3 years, the majority of which were of nonischemic etiology.[177]

Small-for-Size Syndrome

The advent of living-donor partial liver transplantation and the enlargement of the resectable limit has introduced the phenomenon of small-for-size syndrome, whereby the pressure of the full portal flow traveling through a small liver remnant leads to a marked decreased arterial inflow, hypothesized to result from an intact HABR.[178] In a porcine model, portal flow to split grafts with a graft-to-recipient liver volume ratio of 2:3 and 1:3 was inversely correlated to graft size.[179] In patients with right lobe living-donor transplantation, the grafts are subjected to more than double increases of portal blood flow, whereas the arterial flow is strikingly decreased, likely to maintain total blood flow within an acceptable physiologic range.[180,181] The consequences of inadequate HA flow range from mild cholestasis and delayed synthetic function to ischemic cholangitis and parenchymal infarct[182] (see Chapter 111).

Although arterial flow impairment appears to result from an active HABR, it has repeatedly been ascribed to the splenic artery steal syndrome in the past.[183,184] This phenomenon describes the impaired HA flow by shifting the main blood flow to the splenic or gastroduodenal artery in patients with hypersplenism. In whole-organ liver recipients analyzed by D-US, HA vasoconstriction in response to portal hyperperfusion and exaggerated HABR produces a high resistive index with poor arterial perfusion.[185] In a retrospective analysis of 650 OLTs, a 5.1% incidence of splenic artery syndrome has been reported, and prophylactic treatment with ligation of the splenic artery for patients at risk for development of splenic artery syndrome has been advocated.[186] A prospective study has suggested that preoperative embolization of the splenic artery leads to improved postoperative living-donor graft function.[187] Because splenic artery occlusion reduces the resistance to distal HA flow by reducing flow in the splenic circulation, and consequently PV flow, it has been suggested to revise the name of splenic artery steal syndrome to splenic artery syndrome, thereby underlining that the cause is portal hyperperfusion and not arterial siphoning.[185]

Portal Hypertension

Portal hypertension is a state of sustained increase in the intraluminal pressure of the PV and its collaterals, associated with the most severe complications of cirrhosis, including ascites, hepatic encephalopathy, and bleeding from gastroesophageal varices[188] (see Chapters 74, 79, and 80). A mean HVPG greater than 12 mm Hg has classically been used to define portal hypertension because variceal bleeding does not occur at lower pressures than this.[189] Measurement of HVPG is now considered one of the best surrogates of clinical events, using different thresholds to guide the management of cirrhotic patients, and a value of 10 mm Hg and greater is predictive of varices formation and liver decompensation (Table 5.2).[11]

Hemodynamics of Portal Hypertension

Hemodynamic factors that influence portal hypertension are best understood by the flow-resistance principle that applies to the PV system. Portal pressure depends on two basic components: portal blood *flow* and hepatic portal vascular *resistance*. Portal hypertension may result from a significant increase in hepatic portal inflow from the prehepatic splanchnic vasculature, an increase in intrahepatic portal resistance, or both. Although simple in concept, multiple factors may influence both the components of the system and the pathophysiology of portal hypertension.

Increased portal pressure, diminished hepatic portal blood flow, and an extensive extrahepatic collateral venous network supplied by a hyperdynamic splanchnic and systemic circulation characterize the hemodynamics of portal hypertension in cirrhotic patients. Extrahepatic shunts may account for at least 50% of the portal flow, whereas 80% of portal flow actually reaching hepatocytes has been observed to bypass the sinusoidal vascular bed via intrahepatic shunts.[206] The magnitude of extrahepatic shunt flow in patients with cirrhosis was measured directly by thermal dilution assessment of azygos blood flow; a value 300 mL/min greater than in patients without portal hypertension was noted.[108] The HA probably provides a greater relative contribution to the total LBF in patients with cirrhosis than in healthy individuals, although it also was shown that 33% of the arterial blood may flow through intrahepatic shunts to the systemic venous circulation.[207] Vallance and Moncada proposed the hypothesis that the low peripheral vascular resistance in portal hypertension may be caused by the stimulated

TABLE 5.2 Prognostic Significance of Hepatic Venous Pressure Gradient Thresholds According to the Compensated or Decompensated Stage of Cirrhosis

CLINICAL SETTING	HVPG (mm Hg)	INCREASED RISK OF THRESHOLD
Compensated cirrhosis	10	Presence[189] and development of gastroesophageal varices[190] First clinical decompensation in patients without varices[191] Development of HCC[192] Decompensation after surgery for HCC[193,194]
	12	Variceal bleeding[189,195–198]
	16	First clinical decompensation in patients with varices[199] and mortality[200]
Decompensated cirrhosis	16	Variceal rebleeding and mortality[201]
	20	Failure to control variceal bleeding in patients actively bleeding from varices[202,203]
	22	Mortality in patients with alcoholic cirrhosis and acute alcoholic hepatitis[204]
	30	Spontaneous bacterial peritonitis[205]

HCC, Hepatocellular carcinoma.

From Berzigotti A, Seijo S, Reverter E, Bosch J. Assessing portal hypertension in liver diseases. *Expert Rev Gastroenterol Hepatol.* 2013;7(2):141–155.

production of NO induced by endotoxemia in 1991. The initial experimental evidence was provided by Pizcueta and others,[208] who showed an increase in systemic and splanchnic vascular resistance in cirrhotic rats after the administration of an NO inhibitor. Although endotoxemia is likely responsible for the decompensation in end-stage cirrhosis, the hemodynamic alterations are because of NO in animal models.[209,210] Constitutive NO synthase seems to be upregulated in discrete anatomic locations, such as in the endothelium of the mesenteric artery and in the esophageal, gastric, and jejunal mucosa.[211]

The direction of portal blood flow has been proposed as a contributor to the pathophysiology of portal hypertension. The progression of intrahepatic disease and increasing sinusoidal pressure has been postulated as contributing to reversal of flow in the PV, which further aggravates the injury by depriving the liver of nutrients.[212] Gaiani and colleagues[213] reported an incidence of 3.1% reversed, or *hepatofugal*, PV flow in 228 patients assessed. Intrahepatic portal flow reversal has been described in as many as 9% of patients and seen almost exclusively in those with Child's C cirrhosis.[214]

In portal hypertension, the increased mesenteric blood flow in the hyperdynamic stage may be relatively less important than the elevated intrahepatic portal resistance caused by the interplay of local regulatory mechanisms affecting sinusoidal hemodynamics.[215] The traditional view of the source of increased portal pressure is fibrotic encroachment around portal radicles, leading to increased resistance. The pathogenesis of cirrhosis involves initial hepatocyte necrosis and inflammation with subsequent transformation of HSCs into myofibroblasts. HSC activation results in the collagenization of the space of Disse[216] (see Chapter 7). Several factors have been implicated in HSC activation, such as inflammatory mediators, cytokines, growth factors, and endothelin[217] (see Chapter 10). Capillarization of sinusoidal endothelial cells occurs by defenestration or loss of endothelial cell pores and the appearance of a basement membrane.[218] In the cirrhotic liver, the sites of vascular resistance are still unclear. However, because portal and hepatic venules can be found within fibrous septa, constriction or distortion of portal venules, hepatic venules, or both may be involved.[219] Disruption of hepatic architecture, with the development of fibrous septa and abnormal nodules and circulation, leads to a sustained intrahepatic portal resistance and portal pressure. Although PV blood flow progressively decreases in cirrhosis, arterial resistance decreases and arterial flow increases, suggesting an intact buffer response. Studies in cirrhotic rats have demonstrated higher HA flows compared with normal control rats under baseline conditions.[220] This finding was confirmed by using intraoperative measurements in patients with end-stage cirrhosis undergoing living-donor liver transplantation.[221] Clinically, the vasodilation of the splanchnic circulation likely serves to increase flow in the extrahepatic collateral circulation, leading to variceal hemorrhage.

Treatment of Portal Hypertension

Medical and surgical management strategies for portal hypertension strive to improve patient survival by the reduction of pressure and flow in extrahepatic variceal vessels, mainly esophageal and gastric vessels, while preserving adequate portal flow to the liver (see Chapters 79–85). Portosystemic shunting and pharmacologic reduction of portal flow can provide effective decompression, but both deprive the liver of portal flow.

Multiple pharmacologic agents have been investigated to reduce portal hypertension by diminishing hepatic portal inflow from the mesenteric vascular bed. At a dose that decreases the heart rate by 25%, the β-blocker propranolol significantly reduced the risk of rebleeding in cirrhotic patients who were otherwise in good condition[222] (see Chapter 80). Propranolol exerts its action by two mechanisms: decreased cardiac output as a result of β_1-adrenergic cardiac receptor blockade and antagonism of β_2-adrenoceptors in the splanchnic vasculature, which leaves the vasoconstrictive influence of α-adrenergic receptors unopposed, resulting in a decreased portal flow and pressure. Vasopressin causes generalized peripheral vasoconstriction,[223] whereas the effect of somatostatin is specific to the splanchnic vascular bed[224] and results from glucagon-release inhibition and direct vasoconstriction. Serotonin may play a significant role in maintaining increased portal pressure, and smooth muscle serotonin-receptor antagonists have been shown to lower the pressure in cirrhosis.[225,226]

Although it was originally thought that intrahepatic portal resistance in cirrhosis was irreversible, evidence has supported that it can be reduced pharmacologically.[227] The nitrovasodilators isosorbide dinitrate and isosorbide mononitrate were observed to lower the portal pressure in portal hypertensive animals[228] and to increase hepatic (but not azygos) blood flow in patients with cirrhosis,[229] suggesting that they may act by reducing intrahepatic PV resistance. Application of nitroglycerin by transdermal tape to patients with cirrhosis resulted in a reduction in portal pressure without affecting hepatic blood flow,[230] and IV nitroglycerin caused a 24% decrease in intrahepatic portal resistance in patients with cirrhosis.[215] In animal models, intrahepatic portal resistance can be reduced by prostaglandin E_2, the endothelin receptor antagonist isoprenaline, nitroprusside, papaverine, and verapamil.[227,231–233]

The use of TIPS, first reported by Rössle and colleagues (1989),[234] now largely replaces shunt surgery. TIPS is currently the treatment of choice for recurrent variceal bleeding in patients who are refractory to conservative medical management[235] (see Chapter 85).

Surgical treatment of portal hypertension may be performed by one of the many portosystemic shunt procedures; the initial clinical application of the portacaval shunt was reported 50 years after its description by Eck[236] (see Chapters 83 and 84). The hemodynamic consequences of shunt surgery depend on the particular shunt performed, the nature and severity of the disease, and the hemodynamic condition of the patient. End-to-side portacaval shunts divert all portal blood flow away from the liver, whereas less complete diversions reduce portal flow in proportion to the degree to which the shunt reduces portal pressure. The HA flow may increase by 100%, but even a maximal flow increase can usually only partly compensate for loss of portal flow.[237] Hepatic oxygen consumption tends to be maintained by increased oxygen extraction from the available arterial supply. Total portacaval shunts are very effective in reducing portal pressure and preventing bleeding from esophageal varices. However, because of bypass of the hepatic circulation, liver failure and encephalopathy are common complications of the operation. Therefore partial shunts, such as the side-to-side, mesocaval, and proximal or distal splenorenal shunts, are preferred when technically feasible. Selective shunts, such as the distal splenorenal (Warren) shunt, in which the gastrosplenic collaterals are decompressed via the splenic vein into the left renal vein, leaving the PV intact, are effective but usually too time consuming for use in emergency operations.

Current consensus on treatment approaches are here summarized for prevention and treatment of variceal bleeding in patients with cirrhosis.[188,238]

PREVENTION OF VARICEAL BLEEDING. All patients with cirrhosis should be screened by endoscopy for varices at diagnosis. The treatment of underlying liver disease, when possible, may reduce portal hypertension and prevent its clinical complications. There is no pharmaceutical agent proven effective to prevent the formation of varices. Patients with small varices with red marks or Child-Turcotte-Pugh C cirrhosis have an increased risk of bleeding and should thus be treated with nonselective β-blockers. Patients with medium to large varices also can benefit from endoscopic band ligation for the prevention of the first variceal bleeding episode (primary prophylaxis; see Chapter 80). In centers where adequate resources and expertise are available, HVPG measurements can routinely be used for prognostic and therapeutic indications (see Table 5.2). A decrease in HVPG of at least 20% from baseline or to 12 mm Hg or less after chronic treatment with a nonselective β-blocker has been demonstrated to be clinically relevant in the setting of primary prophylaxis of variceal bleeding.

TREATMENT OF ACUTE BLEEDING (SEE CHAPTER 81). Critical initial steps include airway protection, particularly in patients with altered mental status or those with hemodynamic instability, resuscitation with fluid and blood products, and correction of coagulopathy and thrombocytopenia. Patients with variceal hemorrhage are often bacteremic as a result of a concomitant infectious process (spontaneous bacterial peritonitis, urinary tract infection, or pneumonia), and clinical trials have shown better outcomes when empiric antibiotic therapy is initiated early. Vasoconstrictive drugs that reduce portal pressure (somatostatin and vasopressin analogues) and endoscopic variceal ablation (ligation and sclerotherapy) are the mainstay of initial management (see Chapters 80 and 81). As shown in single trials and by meta-analysis, this initial strategy controls 80% to 85% of bleeding episodes.[239] Early assessment of prognosis is important to guide further management because patients at high risk for treatment failure benefit from early TIPS placement (within 72 hours; see Chapter 85).[240] An HVPG of 20 mm Hg or higher, Child-Turcotte-Pugh class C, and active bleeding at endoscopy are the variables most consistently found to predict five-day rebleeding treatment failure.[241] TIPS may not be an option in some cases, such as in face of portal thrombosis, in which case a surgical shunt or a devascularization procedure[242] is indicated (see Chapters 82–84). Emergency portacaval shunt has a success rate of 95% in stopping bleeding in this context. The death rate of the operation is, however, not insignificant, but generally related to the status of the patient's liver function. Approximately 40% of patients experience encephalopathy after portacaval surgical shunting. Hepatic insufficiency is accelerated, and liver failure is the cause of death in approximately two-thirds of those who die after an emergency portacaval shunt. Balloon tamponade should only be used in massive bleeding as a temporary measure until definitive treatment is instituted.[238]

Blood Flow in Hepatic Tumors

It has been demonstrated that tumors of the liver, whether primary or secondary, are generally perfused with arterial blood.[243]

Hepatocellular carcinoma and liver metastases from neuroendocrine tumors are, however, more arterialized and less necrotic than most other liver tumors. The arterial uptake of hepatic solid lesions thus provides important differential diagnosis information when assessed by CT scan and MRI performed with IV contrast, provided that images are acquired at time of arterial enhancement in addition to venous enhancement[244] (see Chapters 14, 15, 89, and 91). The neovasculature of tumor tissue lacks smooth muscle and therefore does not respond to vasoconstrictor agents, enabling increased delivery and retention of chemotherapeutic drugs.

A variety of transarterial techniques have been used to selectively embolize and deliver chemotherapy to liver tumors, taking advantage of the fact that they derive disproportionately greater blood supply from the HA circulation compared with the surrounding liver (see Chapter 94). Embolization is often performed with Gelfoam, which dissolves after a few weeks, but other inert agents are also used and are probably more effective for occluding vessels. Some centers use inert particles without chemotherapy (i.e., bland embolization), but most combine the procedure with chemotherapy (i.e., transarterial chemoembolization [TACE]). Doxorubicin, mitomycin, and cisplatin in various combinations are the drugs most often given. The embolized material causes temporary blood flow interruption and potentially improves the uptake of chemotherapeutic agents in tumor tissue and, consequently, reduces systemic toxicity.[245] Lipiodol and drug-eluting beads, which lodge in the tumor, have also been used as a carrier for chemotherapy. More recently, radioactive microspheres emitting Yttrium-90 have been used (see Chapter 94B). These procedures are mainly performed in the palliative setting for patients with liver confined malignancies not amenable to liver resection or transplantation. It remains unclear if the addition of chemotherapeutic agents provides much benefit beyond the necrosis produced by occlusion of the HA supply alone.[246–252]

Increasing evidence supports that HA infusion of chemotherapy delivered by catheters connected to subcutaneously placed ports or pumps can also be effectively used to deliver high doses of chemotherapy directly to the liver for the treatment of patients with colorectal cancer liver metastasis and unresectable intrahepatic cholangiocarcinoma[253–257] (see Chapter 97).

Effect of Laparoscopy on Liver Blood Flow

The use of a CO_2 pneumoperitoneum in laparoscopic surgery has been demonstrated to substantially reduce PV in parallel with the rise of the intraperitoneal pressure.[258,259] The reduction in hepatic blood flow is because of a number of factors, including mechanical compression of the mesenteric veins, humoral vasoconstriction of the mesenteric bed and increased portal venous pressure caused by hypercapnia, local absorption of CO_2, and increased release of vasopressin.[260] Conflicting data exist in support of the maintenance of the HABR effect in high-pressure pneumoperitoneum. Rat models using fluorescent microspheres supported preserved HA flow during decreased PV flow,[261] but this was not supported by others[262] who saw a parallel decrease in arterial and portal venous flows during laparoscopy. Most surgical teams use a 10 to 15 mm Hg pneumoperitoneum during laparoscopic liver resection, which allows good control of bleeding[263] (see Chapter 127). A case-matched analysis suggested that the positive pressure of pneumoperitoneum was probably the main factor explaining the decreased blood loss during laparoscopy when compared with open liver surgery.[264] Some groups have suggested the avoidance of head-up positioning and pressures greater than 15 mm Hg during laparoscopy to preserve LBF.[265,266] So far, no major accident related to the use of a CO_2 pneumoperitoneum during laparoscopic liver resection has been reported in approximately 6,000 cases.[267] Furthermore, a swine model has been used to prospectively demonstrate that multiple gas embolisms frequently occur during laparaoscopic liver resection without significant modification of hemodynamics.[268,269] Although PEEP may increase central venous pressure, there is no strong published evidence that this or other lung protective ventilation strategies are significantly associated with increased bleeding during open or laparoscopic hepatectomy.[270]

Acknowledgments

Thank you to Drs. Blumgart, Wheatley, Mathie, and Rocha for their previous contributions to this chapter.

References are available at expertconsult.com.

CHAPTER 6

Liver regeneration: Mechanisms and clinical relevance

Jeroen de Jonge and Kim M. Olthoff

INTRODUCTION TO LIVER REGENERATION

The ability of the liver to regenerate was recognized by the Greeks in the ancient myth of Prometheus, the Titan god of forethought, who gave fire to the mortals and angered Zeus. Prometheus was chained to the Caucasus mountains and each day he would be tormented by Zeus' eagle Ethon as it devoured his liver. Each night, the damaged liver would be restored so the eagle could begin anew, illustrating the liver's unique power to regenerate. This regenerative capacity is what allows transplant surgeons to successfully remove or transplant portions of a liver, with the remnant portion then rapidly growing to the original volume, and also allows for restoration of function after hepatocyte mass loss from toxic injury or inflammation.

The terms *regeneration*, *hyperplasia*, and *hypertrophy* are used synonymously in literature, but hyperplasia is the most precise from a cellular standpoint. The damaged or resected hepatic lobes do not grow back in the same way that a lizard's tail regrows, but rather there is a hyperplastic response (defined as increasing in cell number) in the remnant liver, leading to its hypertrophic appearance (defined as enlarging liver size). This process is highly regulated and involves multiple cell types, extrahepatic signals, complex molecular pathways, and cellular interactions. A delicate balance is required for initiation of regeneration, exerting a growth response, and maintaining normal metabolic function. The inability to maintain this process leads to poor liver function and ultimately liver failure after surgery, whereas a successfully orchestrated response results in restoration of normal liver function.

CLINICAL RELEVANCE OF LIVER REGENERATION

Hepatobiliary surgery is now routinely and safely accomplished for malignant and benign disease. This technical success in both resection and transplantation relies on the remarkable ability of the liver to regain most of its functional mass within a matter of weeks[1] (see Chapters 101 and 109). Factors that limit the achievement of curative tumor resection and small-for-size (SFS) transplantations make up the high morbidity and mortality rates associated with insufficient volume of the liver remnant or transplanted graft. As hepatobiliary and transplant surgeons continue to expand the magnitude and complexity of liver resection and explore the limits of living donor liver transplantation (LDLT), understanding the mechanisms behind liver regeneration is essential for clinical practice. Many tumors that were previously considered to be unresectable are now amenable to complete resection through induction chemotherapy and innovative treatment strategies to increase liver remnant volume.[2] There are several techniques, including portal vein embolization (PVE) or portal vein ligation (PVL), additional hepatic vein embolization, and (the most extreme) associating liver partition and PVL for staged hepatectomy (ALPPS; see Chapter 102D). They cause atrophy of the ipsilateral hemiliver and hypertrophy

of the contralateral side and are particularly valuable in patients who have underlying liver disease. Many patients with underlying liver disease are now considered suitable candidates for liver resection, even with Child-Pugh grade A cirrhosis and minimal portal hypertension.[3-5]

Regeneration also is crucial in liver transplantation. In deceased donor transplantation, hepatocyte loss occurs in the form of ischemia/reperfusion (I/R) injury because of the necessary preservation period from procurement to implantation and damage that may have occurred in the donor (see Chapters 105 and 111). Because of the scarcity of organs, more "marginal" organs are accepted for transplantation, which have increased need for regeneration and recovery in the environment of I/R injury (see Chapter 109). One of the landmark advances in liver transplantation is the ability to use segmental liver grafts obtained from either a deceased donor or a living donor. In the latter situation, success of the procedure relies on relatively rapid hepatic regeneration in both donor and recipient. The minimal amount of functional liver necessary for successful transplantation or for safe recovery in the donor is a major concern. Donor graft size, recipient weight, portal hypertension, I/R injury, and the recipient's disease severity all contribute to the amount of post-transplant regeneration and recovery needed.[6] Efforts to decrease the amount of liver removed from the donor to minimize donor risk results in smaller grafts for the recipients and real challenges in postoperative recovery.

BASIC CHARACTERISTICS OF LIVER REGENERATION

Models of Liver Regeneration

Liver regeneration is most clearly shown in the experimental model that was pioneered in 1931 by Higgins and Anderson.[7] In this model, a simple two-thirds partial hepatectomy (PHx) is performed, without damage to the lobes left behind. This leads to enlargement of the residual lobes to make up for the mass of the removed lobes in five to seven days. Other well-known models of liver regeneration are associated with extensive tissue injury and inflammation and include the use of hepatic toxins, such as ethanol (EtOH),[8] carbon tetrachloride (CCl_4),[9] and galactosamine (GalN)[10]; bile duct ligation[11] or PVL[12]; and I/R injury.[13] Newer models include transgenic albumin promoter urokinase-type plasminogen activator (u-PA) fusion constructs,[14] Fah/Rag2 knock-out mice,[15,16] and PHx in zebrafish.[17] In each model, the different toxic agents injure specific liver cell subpopulations. Therefore, PHx is the preferred in vivo model to study the regenerative response. Debonera demonstrated that regenerative signaling observed in a rat liver transplant model of I/R injury is similar to that observed after PHx.[18] The most recent instrument to study liver regeneration, when proliferation is impaired, is lineage tracings using cyclization recombinase

(Cre) recombinase–mediated cell labeling.[19] In its classical setting, a traced cell population harbors two transgenes. The first expresses Cre under the control of cell-specific regulatory elements. The Cre activity is modulated by fusing a mutated ligand-binding domain of the estrogen receptor (ER), which is sensitive to tamoxifen but insensitive to estrogen. Upon addition of tamoxifen, CreER eliminates a locus of X-over P1 (loxP)–flanked stop cassette and induces transcription of the second transgene, coding for a reporter protein. Although this represents the gold standard for defining cell fate, this strategy is not without pitfalls, which may explain the sometimes-controversial results.[20]

General Features of Liver Regeneration

It is well established that liver regeneration after surgical resection is carried out by growth and proliferation of existing mature hepatocyte populations. These include hepatocytes, biliary and fenestrated endothelial cells, Kupffer cells, platelets, and Ito cells (stellate cells; Fig. 6.1). The kinetics of cell proliferation and the growth factors produced by proliferating hepatocytes suggest that hepatocytes provide the mitogenic stimuli leading to proliferation of the other cells. The degree of hepatocyte proliferation is directly proportional to the degree of injury.[21,22] Immediately after liver resection, the rate of DNA synthesis in hepatocytes begins to increase as they exit the resting state of the cell cycle (G_0) and enter G_1, traverse to DNA synthesis (S phase), and

ultimately undergo mitosis (M phase). The first peak of DNA synthesis occurs at 40 hours after resection in rodents and at seven to 10 days in primates. In small animals, the regenerative response returns the liver to the pre-resection mass in one week to 10 days. Clinical studies from living donor transplantation suggest that a significant amount of regeneration occurs in human within two weeks after resection and is nearly complete at three months after resection.[23–25]

After resection, hepatocyte proliferation starts in the periportal areas of the lobules and then proceeds to the pericentral areas by 36 to 48 hours. Liver histology at day three to four after PHx is characterized by clumps of small hepatocytes surrounding capillaries, which change into true hepatic sinusoids. The hepatic matrix composition also changes from high laminin content to primarily containing fibronectin and collagen types IV and I. After a 70% hepatectomy, restoration of the original number of hepatocytes theoretically requires 1.66 proliferative cycles per residual hepatocyte. In fact, most of the hepatocytes (95% in young and 75% in very old rats) in the residual lobes participate in one or two proliferative events.[26] Hepatocytes have an almost unlimited capacity to regenerate as transplantation of several hundreds of healthy hepatocytes can repopulate a whole damaged liver in a calculated minimum of 69 doublings.[27] Interestingly, the mechanisms associated with how a liver knows when to stop regenerating are much less clear than the starting mechanisms.

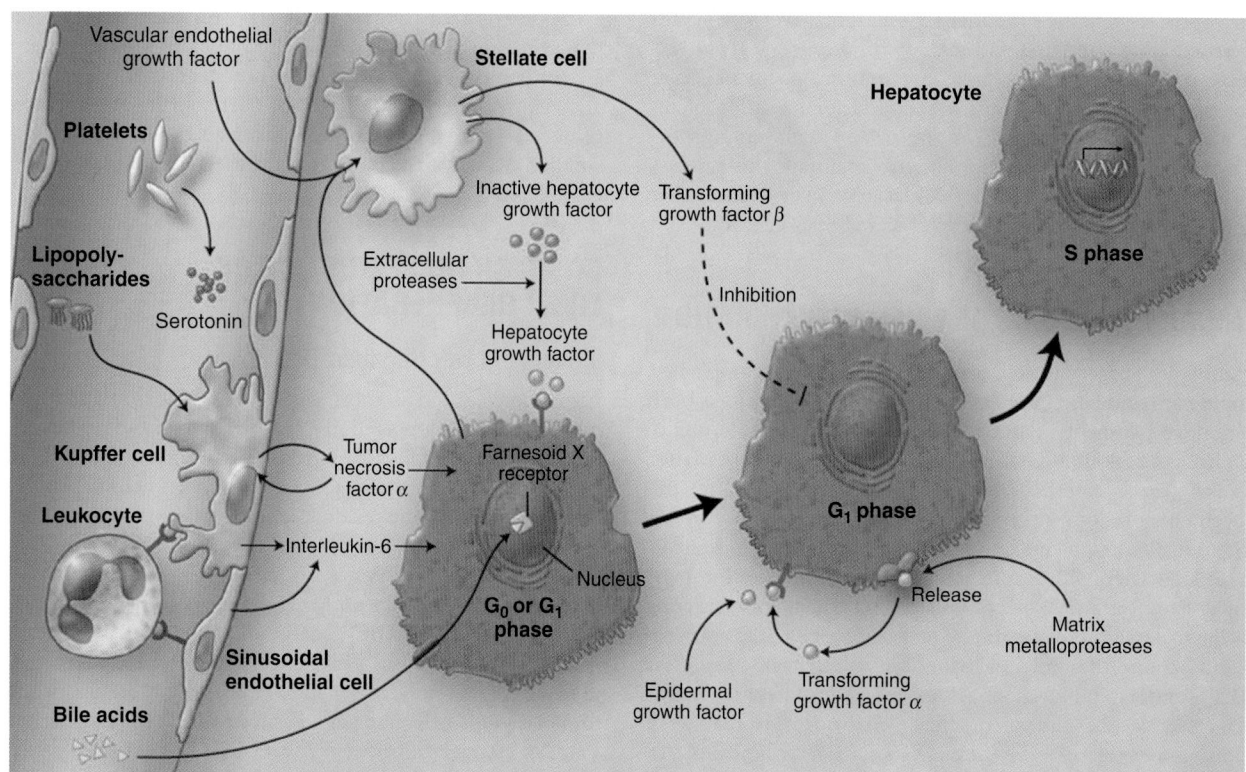

FIGURE 6.1   Pathways of liver regeneration initiated by major hepatectomy. After hepatectomy, nonparenchymal cells, such as stellate cells, Kupffer cells, leukocytes, and platelets, are activated by soluble factors. As a result, Kupffer cells release tumor necrosis factor-α and interleukin-6. The cytokines cause a priming of the remnant hepatocytes, and concurrently, extracellular proteases such as urokinase-type plasminogen activator convert inactive hepatocyte growth factor to its active form. The cytokines and the growth factors act in concert to initiate the reentry of quiescent hepatocytes (in the G_0 phase) into the cell cycle from the G_1 phase to the S phase, resulting in DNA synthesis and hepatocyte proliferation. The metabolic burden is indicated by the accumulation of bile acids in the blood, which enter the hepatocytes and drive increased protein and DNA synthesis. To signal the end of proliferation, transforming growth factor-β blocks further replication. (Original from Clavien P-A, Petrowsky H, DeOliveira ML, Graf R. Strategies for safer liver surgery and partial liver transplantation. *N Engl J Med* 2007;356:1545–1559. Reprinted with permission.)

Contribution of Liver Stem Cells to Regeneration

In contrast to other regenerating tissues (bone marrow, skin), primary liver regeneration after surgical trauma is not dependent on a small group of progenitor cells (stem cells). However, in response to toxic liver damage inflicted by agents such as galactosamine, hepatocytes are unable to replicate. In this situation a population of cells known as "oval cells" proliferates to replace the hepatic parenchyma.[28] In distinct approaches to determine whether cells other than hepatocytes themselves could be the source of new hepatocytes in oval cell injury, two groups found no evidence of such liver stem/progenitor cells.[29,30]

In the human situation, hepatic progenitor cells (HPCs) were presumed to participate in repopulation of the liver after acute massive necrosis and have also been identified in chronic liver disease.[31] The human HPCs originate from the canals of Hering[32–34] and play an important role in acetaminophen-induced injury.[35] Huch et al. described conditions allowing for the long-term expansion of these adult bile duct–derived bipotent progenitor cells from human liver,[36] which enables disease modeling, toxicology studies, and regenerative medicine. More recent studies have shown the contribution of HPC is very much context dependent, with hepatocyte senescence after injury being a major driver for HPC expansion and their hepatocytic differentiation. The rapidity of regeneration after PHx suggests a minimal involvement of stem cells in this response, but new stem/progenitor hepatocytes have been located either randomly throughout the lobule or at opposite ends of the portal vein-hepatic vein axis. It was reported that different regeneration stimuli trigger different regenerative responses; after toxic liver damage, stem cell–dependent proliferation is seen along the central vein,[37,38] whereas homeostatic proliferation is present throughout the whole liver.[39] The presence of regenerative stem cells at the portal rim has refueled the streaming liver debate.[40–42]

Altogether, there remains considerable disagreement of the exact role of stem/progenitor cells in liver regeneration and homeostasis.[19,43]

Induction of Proliferation: Priming and Cell-Cycle Progression

Within minutes after PHx, specific immediate early genes are activated in remnant hepatocytes.[44,45] These 70 to 100 genes include proto-oncogenes, which play an important role in normal cell-cycle progression, such as c-jun, c-fos, c-myc, and K-Ras,[46–48] and the transcriptional factors nuclear factor (NF)-κB, signal transducer and activator of transcription 3 (STAT3), activator protein-1 (AP-1), and CCAAT enhancer binding protein beta (C/EBPβ).[49,50]

Historically, the onset of liver regeneration has been attributed to a flow-dependent response by which increased relative flow after PHx resulted in hepatocyte proliferation and hyperplasia.[51] A more recent experimental partial liver transplant model demonstrates that increased portal flow is essential for liver regeneration. Nevertheless, portal hyperperfusion (flow that exceeds 250 mL/100 g/min) completely abolishes the process[52] (see "Portal Inflow and Hepatic Outflow").

Very early experiments in parasymbiotic rats demonstrated the existence of humoral factors in the induction of liver growth after PHx.[53] Interleukin (IL)-6 and tumor necrosis factor (TNF)-α have since been identified as the earliest factors triggering activation of several transcription factors during regeneration[54,55] (Fig. 6.2). In IL-6 deficient or TNF-α receptor

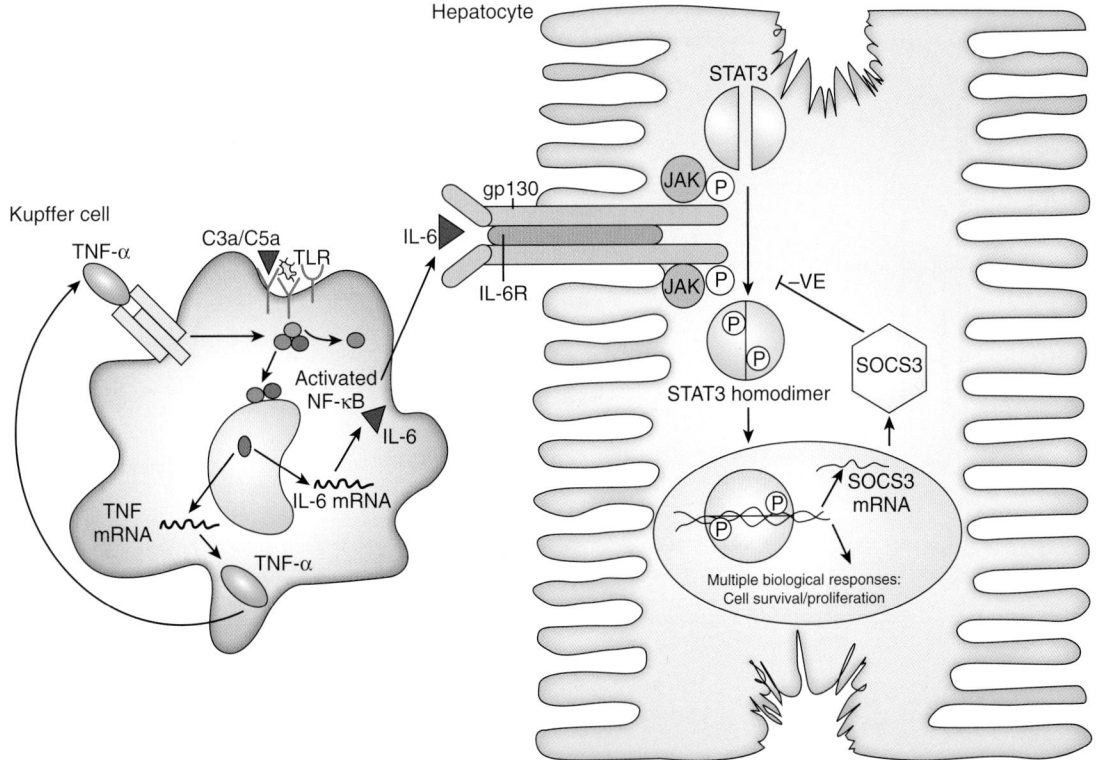

FIGURE 6.2 Stimulated by components of the innate immune system, Kupffer cells produce and secrete interleukin (IL)-6 and tumor necrosis factor (TNF)-α to kick-start the regenerative response. IL-6 helps stimulate hepatocyte proliferation via signal transducer and activator of transcription 3 (STAT3) activation; in turn, this response is negatively regulated by suppression of cytokine signaling-3 (SOCS3). (Original from Alison MR, Islam S, Lim S. Stem cells in liver regeneration, fibrosis and cancer: The good, the bad and the ugly. *J Pathol.* 2009; 217:282–298. Reprinted with permission.)

deficient mice, liver regeneration after hepatectomy is delayed[56] but not completely abolished.[57,58] Therefore other blood-derived mitogens, such as hepatocyte growth factor (HGF), were identified as putative hepatic growth factor during liver regeneration.[59] Hepatocytes in normal liver are not ready to respond to mitogenic signals without a set of "priming" events that switch them into a responsive state. This has been described by Fausto, who identified the *priming factors* involved in initiating and triggering the hepatic response to injury and concomitant *growth factors* and their receptors, which allow for competent hepatocytes to progress through the cell cycle.[60] Priming is accomplished by the release of preformed cytokines that subsequently activate transcription factor complexes and allow the cell to exit G_0 into G_1 of the cell cycle. This group includes TNF-α and IL-6.[61]

TNF signaling through TNF receptor (TNFR)-I initiates liver regeneration after PHx with IL-6 as the key target. Knockout mice that lack TNFR-I showed an almost complete inhibition of NF-κB binding and a severe defect in hepatocyte replication after PHx. IL-6 reverses the deficiency in hepatocyte replication imposed by the lack of TNFR-I and corrects the defects in STAT3 and AP-1 binding but does not reverse the inhibition of NF-κB binding.[55] This solved a long-standing riddle in the understanding of liver regeneration by identifying TNF as the initiator of IL-6.

IL-6 activates the Janus kinase (JAK)/STAT3 and MAPK signaling pathways via the gp130/IL-6R complex. This leads to activation of an array of immediate and delayed early genes required for normal liver-specific metabolic functions, repair, and hepatoprotection from injury.[62–64] STAT3 is crucial for cells to progress from G_1 to S phase and for activating the c-myc gene, a gene required for cell-cycle progression.

Other intracellular signaling pathways that involve the receptor tyrosine kinases p38 mitogen-activated protein kinase (MAPK), protein kinase R-like ER kinase (pERK), and c-jun-NH2-terminal (JNK) are also rapidly activated. Progression through the cell cycle is regulated by cyclins and cyclin-dependent kinases (CDKs). Various combinations bind to form kinase complexes that are active at distinct points within the cell cycle and tightly controlled by several mechanisms, including binding by CDK–inhibitory proteins, such as p21. Feedback signals to this process are provided by suppression of cytokine signaling-3 (SOCS3) and transforming growth factor (TGF)-β, also regulated by IL-6. Other studies confirmed the importance of NF-κB[65–67] and showed immediate upregulation of apoptotic genes (Fas and caspases) in livers that failed because of excessive resection[68] (Fig. 6.3).

So far, a few factors have been identified to be possibly responsible for the release of these priming cytokines and growth factors in the onset of liver regeneration. The first is endotoxin lipopolysaccharide (LPS), produced in the gut by Gram-negative bacteria. Circulating LPS is an extremely strong signal for Kupffer cells to produce TNF and start the cascade, resulting in hepatocyte replication. Rats treated

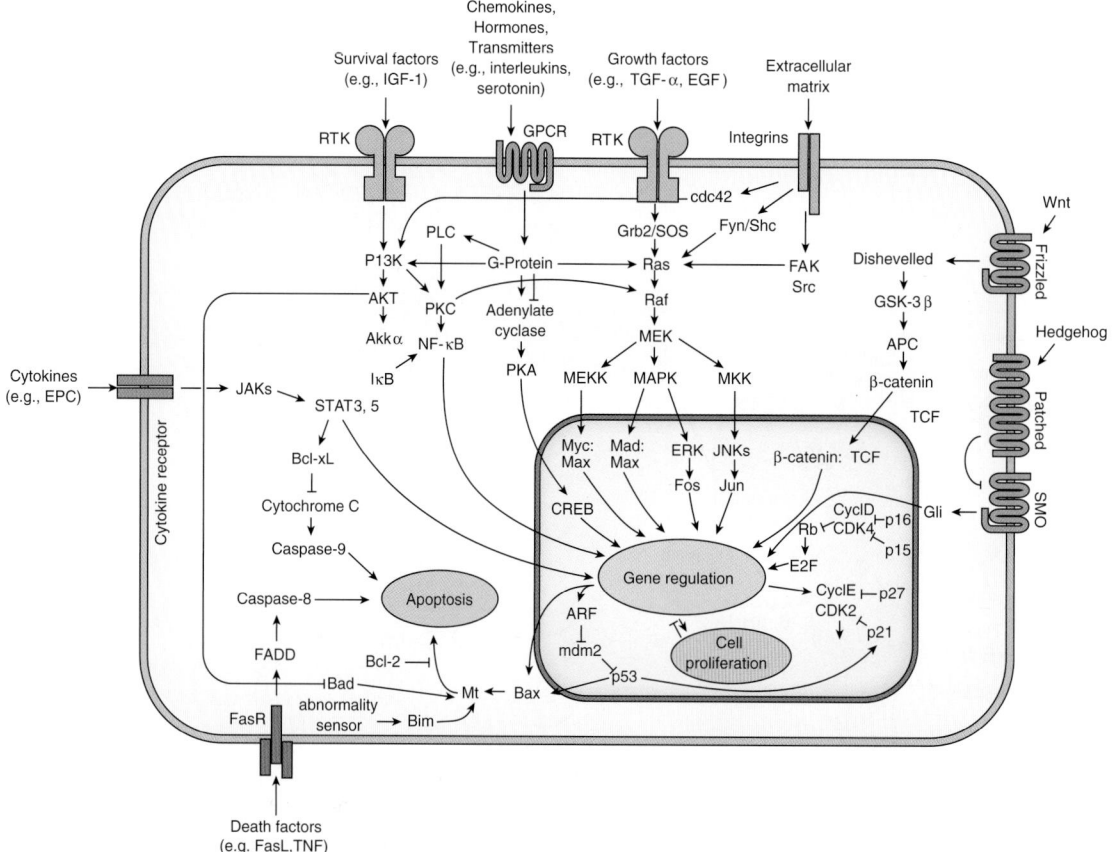

FIGURE 6.3   Intracellular pathways of liver regeneration. Multiple intracellular signaling pathways are rapidly activated. Progression through the cell cycle is regulated by cyclins and cyclin-dependent kinases (cdks), tightly controlled by several mechanisms, including binding by cdk–inhibitory proteins, such as p21. Modification of https://foundation.wikimedia.org/wiki/File:Signal_transduction_v1.png, uploaded by Roadnottaken, adapted from figure 23-12 in Molecular cell biology. Lodish, Harvey 5 ed: New York : W. H. Freeman and Co., 2003, p949. ISBN: 0-7167-4366-3

with antibiotics and germ-free rodents have a delayed peak of DNA replication after PHx, confirming the importance of LPS.[69]

Another major finding is the demonstration that cytokine activation and DNA replication are severely impaired in mice lacking the complement components C3a and C5a.[70] In particular, mice lacking both C3a and C5a have impaired production of TNF and IL-6 after PHx and poor activation of NF-κB and STAT3.

Distinct Intracellular Pathways in Maintaining Liver Regeneration

After the priming phase, concomitant growth factors are essential to progress hepatocytes into cell division. Growth factors include the potent hepatocyte mitogens HGF, TGF-α, and heparin-binding epidermal growth factor (HB-EGF). This process is further controlled by co-mitogens, such as insulin, glucagon, steroid and thyroid hormone, and epinephrine, which facilitate activity of the mitogens, and by downregulation of growth factor inhibitors, such as activin A and TGF-β.

The HGF/c-Met pathway is important for sustaining DNA synthesis after injury and activates various downstream pathways that involve PI3K, ERK, and AKT.[71] This pathway cross-talks with the Wnt/β-catenin signaling pathway, which has come to the forefront in liver biology over the last several years.[72] Increased levels of HGF result in β-catenin dissociation along with nuclear translocation[73] and upregulation of downstream targets of this pathway such as cyclin D1, c-myc, uPAR, matrix metalloproteinases (MMPs), and epidermal growth factor receptor.[74] Vascular endothelial growth factor (VEGF) interacts with endothelial cells in the liver to increase HGF production from nonparenchymal cells.[75]

In the initiation of HGF, urokinase-type plasminogen activator (uPA) appears to play an important role. uPA and its downstream effector, plasminogen, increase within one to five minutes after PHx and rapidly cleave the HGF precursor, pro-HGF. Blocking uPA delays the appearance of HGF, and thereby delays liver regeneration, whereas blocking plasminogen-activator inhibitor (PAI) accelerates the release of HGF and liver regeneration.[76]

Another humoral factor that triggers the concerted regenerative response in hepatocytes has been discovered; extracellular adenosine triphosphate (ATP) has emerged as a rapidly acting signaling molecule that after PHx leads to rapid and transient activation of JNK signaling, induction of immediate early genes c-Fos and c-Jun, and activator protein-1 (AP-1) DNA-binding activity.[77] Recent studies directly link mitochondrial bioenergetics to several markers of postoperative liver function after resection; early lactate clearance and postoperative alanine aminotransferase (ALT) strongly correlated with mitochondrial energy state,[78] as well as with enhanced growth of the future liver remnant (FLR).

The control of inflammatory signals is also necessary to allow for the progression of the regenerative pathways. The NF-κB inhibitory and ubiquitin-editing A20 protein (tnfaip3) plays a key role in the liver's protective response to injury, particularly its antiinflammatory effects.[79] A20 is significantly upregulated in the liver after PHx and protects hepatocytes from apoptosis and ongoing inflammation by inhibiting NF-κB.[80,81] A20 also allows for proliferation and optimizes metabolic control and energy production after liver regeneration, as demonstrated by increased enzymatic activity of cytochrome c oxidase or

mitochondrial complex IV.[82] A20-based therapies could be beneficial in future prevention and treatment of hepatic failure after liver resection. The cytokine induced form of nitric oxide synthase (iNOS) also seems to play an important role in scavenging oxygen radicals and protecting from apoptosis, caused by an uncontrolled inflammatory reaction mediated through IL-6 and TNF-β.[83]

The mechanisms of regeneration were also studied in the transplant setting, where microarray analysis of SFS rat liver grafts showed upregulation of vasoconstrictive and adhesion molecule genes at early time points after reperfusion, with later increases in genes associated with inflammation and cell death and downregulation of genes related to energy metabolism.[84] These pathways have been confirmed in the situation of clinical deceased donor and LDLT.[85,86]

Remodeling of the Liver

Remodeling of the newly regenerated liver tissue begins with the repopulation and maturation of nonparenchymal cells, such as endothelial, stellate, and biliary epithelial cells (see Chapter 1).

Newly formed hepatocytes form clusters into which replicating endothelial cells invade to form new sinusoids. To restore normal architecture, stellate cells, which are located between endothelial cells and hepatocytes, synthesize extracellular matrix (ECM) proteins and TGF-γ1, which can regulate the production of hepatic ECM. VEGF, angiopoietins 1 and 2, TGF-α, fibroblast growth factor (FGF)-1 and FGF-2, and HGF all are likely involved in the angiogenic process. Angiostatin, an inhibitor of angiogenesis, causes delayed and suppressed liver regeneration in mice.[87,88] Remodeling of the ECM is associated with the activation of the urokinase/plasminogen pathway and the MMP pathway. MMPs not only remodel the ECM but also regulate immune responses[89] and participate in modulation of vascular integrity at the endothelial cell–cell junctions in steatotic livers after I/R injury.[90] MMPs, in combination with HGF, EGF, and TGF-β1, act to remodel the ECM, changing the levels of several ECM proteins, such as collagen, fibronectin, laminin, and entactin. The maturation and thickening of the ECM seems to have an inhibitory effect on proliferating hepatocytes, potentially signaling the end of rapid regeneration.[91]

The role of the ECM has been increasingly studied and plays an important role in regeneration, influencing proliferation, differentiation, and termination signals that regulate the regenerated liver size. The ECM was regarded as "that stuff between cells" but now is considered to be the dictator of metabolic liver zonation and is a hepatic growth/size rheostat during development, homeostasis, and regeneration. The interaction between LGR4/5 receptors and their cognate RSPO ligands potentiate Wnt/β-catenin signaling and promote proliferation and tissue homeostasis.[92] Also, the role of mechanical forces and mechanosensing in regulating liver regeneration is being increasingly studied. Increased shear stress after liver resection is picked up by the cells through mechanosensors on their membranes, which include glycocalyx, primary cilia, caveolae, ion channels, receptor tyrosine kinases, and G proteins and G protein-coupled receptors.[93] These mechanosensing mechanisms either generate molecular signals that further activate downstream signaling pathways, such as Yes-associated protein (YAP), or directly transduce mechanical signals by regulating the actomyosin cytoskeleton. α-Catenin is now considered a key mechanosensor for direct cell–cell tension and pressure, leading to proliferation. Additionally, the ECM maintains the differentiation state of hepatocytes. Increased rigidity favors hepatocyte proliferation,[94] with hepatocytes remaining differentiated on softer support of fibrillar collagen meshwork and committing into dedifferentiation on stiffer support of monomeric collagen-coated dish.[95] On rigid surfaces, hepatocytes exhibit epithelial to mesenchymal transition and switch into fibroblast-like morphology.[96] In this context, it is interesting that temporary fibrosis is seen during normal liver regeneration and resolves over time.[97,98]

Maintaining Liver Function During Regeneration

After volume loss, hepatocytes must adapt rapidly and seek a compromise between maintenance of continued differentiated function and cellular replication to permit survival. After toxic injury, resection, or transplantation, the balance is dramatically shifted to the crucial tasks of recovery and regeneration at the expense of normal hepatic metabolism. The success of restoring lost liver mass, repairing tissue injury, and resolving inflammation determines the ability of the liver to support normal metabolic function and determines the ability of the liver to recover. (Fig. 6.4). Several of the expressed immediate early genes encode enzymes and proteins that are involved in regulating gluconeogenesis, a very important process after PHx to compensate for the lost glycogen content and to produce sufficient glucose for the whole organism.[99,100] There is rapid increased expression of genes involved in glucose homeostasis after PHx. Most notably, these include phosphoenolpyruvate carboxykinase (PEPCK), glucose-6-phosphatase (G6Pase), and hepatic insulin–like growth factor binding protein 1 (IGFBP-1), controlled at the level of transcription by insulin (downregulation), glucagon/adenosine 3',5'-cyclic monophosphate (cAMP;

upregulation), and glucocorticoids (upregulation).[44,101] Insulin itself can be a potent growth factor mediated through the insulin receptor, and insulin and glucagon have long been established as important "gut-derived" growth factors.[102] Liver-specific transcription factors (hepatocyte nuclear factors [HNFs]) have an important role in determining the level of glucose production, fatty acid metabolism, and liver-specific secreted proteins. C/EPBα regulates expression of genes involved in hepatic glucose and lipid homeostasis, has antiproliferative properties, and is downregulated during liver regeneration after hepatectomy.[103,104]

During early regeneration, the liver accumulates fat before the major wave of parenchymal growth. Suppression of hepatocellular fat accumulation is associated with impaired hepatocellular proliferation after PHx, indicating that hepatocellular fat accumulation is specifically regulated during, and may be essential for, normal liver regeneration.[105] Unlike pathologic steatosis, this transient regeneration-associated steatosis in hepatocytes is a physiologic process observed in every regenerating liver. Acute energy deprivation provokes hypoglycemia, mobilization of peripheral fats, and a switch to lipid usage.[106] In mice, indirect calorimetry revealed that lipid oxidation is the primary energy source early after hepatectomy.[107] This was regulated by downregulation of phosphatase and tensin homolog (PTEN), a key inhibitor of the phosphoinositide 3-kinase (PI3K)/protein kinase B (AKT)/mammalian target of rapamycin (mTOR) axis that regulates growth and metabolic adaptations after hepatectomy.

Some data show that decreasing lipid peroxidation levels by vitamin treatment after PHx produces an attenuation of cellular apoptosis and a marked increase in the proliferation process,

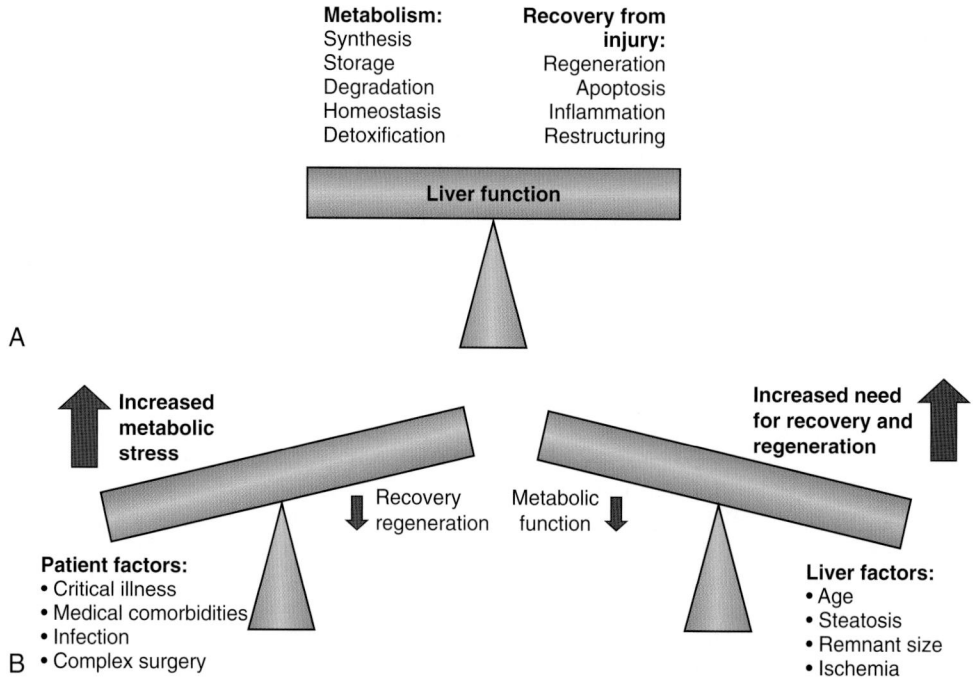

FIGURE 6.4 Metabolic balance between regeneration and maintaining liver function. **A,** In times of relative quiescence, there is a balance within the liver of metabolic function and continuous liver cell replacement or restructuring as needed. **B,** In times of stress or after injury or resection, there is an increased need for metabolic function or regeneration and recovery. If metabolic need is great as a result of conditions within the patient, there may not be sufficient energy balance within the liver to regenerate sufficiently, and the liver may not recover. If the requirements for regeneration and repair are overwhelming, there may be decreased metabolic function, affecting patient outcome.

suggesting that the modulation of lipid peroxidation also has a role in the liver regeneration process.[108] Hepatocytes in the periportal regions that divide and replicate after PHx require mitochondrial fatty acid beta oxidation. Peroxisome proliferator–activated receptor (PPAR)-α may be a crucial modulator controlling energy flux important for repair of liver damage and regeneration.[109,110] Data from experimental models of liver transection, combined with PVL to promote liver regeneration, showed an overwhelming inflammatory response that interfered with the peroxisome proliferator-activated receptor-γ coactivator (PGC-1α) mitochondrial biogenesis pathway. This resulted in the accumulation of immature and malfunctioning mitochondria in hepatocytes during the early phase of liver regeneration[111] and showed close association with growth of the FLR.[78] Also, increased expression of augmenter of liver regeneration (ALR), a potent hepatotrophic factor with important regulatory functions in cellular respiration, was shown. ALR is one of the strongest hepatic cell mitogens and also modulates mitochondrial biogenesis and ATP synthesis.[112]

In a microarray analysis of gene expression profiles after LDLT, it was demonstrated that C/EBPα was downregulated, as was HNF-4α and PPAR-α.[85] Expression of many other liver-specific genes, such as IGFBP1 and G6Pase, is regulated in the basal state by HNF1. The transcriptional activity of HNF1 is upregulated during liver regeneration by binding of HNF1 to the growth-induced transcription factors STAT3 and AP-1.[113]

New insights into how the liver fulfills the adaptive response to metabolic needs during regeneration may come from the tight regulation of lipid, glucose, and bile acid (BA) metabolism through the class III NAD1-dependent histone deacetylase SIRT1 114. The role of SIRT1 as a key regulator of the regenerative response of the liver, controlling BA homeostasis, protein synthesis, and cell proliferation through deacetylation of farnesoid X receptor (FXR) and histones, and regulation of mTOR was established.[115] SIRT1 is activated in situations of low energy availability and links nutritional status with metabolic homeostasis. It regulates adenosine monophosphate–activated protein kinase (AMPK). Contrary to SIRT1, mTOR is activated in high-energy conditions and controls cell growth and proliferation.[116] mTORC1 promotes protein synthesis, and this axis is essential to regulate the cell cycle during liver regeneration after PHx. BA is also essential for the regeneration of the liver after PHx,[117] although, when present in excess, BA can be toxic and promote hepatocyte death. Therefore a fine regulation of BA metabolism is essential to preserve liver homeostasis and a proper response to injury. FXR (NR1H4) is the master regulator of BA, lipid, and glucose metabolism. Through the activation of FXR, BAs regulate their hepatic metabolism and also promote hepatocellular proliferation. FXR is also expressed in enterocytes, where BAs stimulate the expression of FGF15/19, which is released to the portal blood. Through the activation of FGFR4 on hepatocytes, FGF15/19 regulates BA synthesis and finely tunes liver regeneration as part of the "hepatostat."[118,119]

Termination of Proliferation

The size of the liver is highly regulated and is controlled by the functional needs of the organism. This observation implies the existence of a master regulator of the liver/body mass ratio (i.e., a "hepatostat").

From LDLT we know that differences are present between donors and recipients in the percentage reconstitution of the standard liver volume (80 vs. 93% at 3 months), which is probably caused by the need for functional liver mass to compensate for long-standing liver disease.[23]

The most well-known antiproliferative factors within the liver are TGF-β and related family members such as activin.[120] TGF-β is produced mainly by hepatic stellate cells, but in the early phase it forms inhibitory complexes with SKI proto-oncogene (SKI) and SKI-like proto-oncogene (SnoN),[121] rendering hepatocytes initially resistant to TGF-β.[122] The downregulation of miR23b may further contribute to activation of the TGF-β1/Smad3 signaling pathway during the termination stage.[123] Upon activation, Smad2, Smad3, and Smad4 assemble in a common complex, translocate into the nucleus, and activate target genes that negatively regulate the cell cycle.[124] Reactive oxygen species (ROS) enhance synthesis and activation of TGF-β,[125] which may account for the reduced regeneration after ischemia and reperfusion. Interacting with the TGF-β/Smad signaling could restore regeneration in a model of SFS liver grafts.[126]

Similarly, activin A blocks hepatocyte mitogenesis and shows diminished signaling during liver regeneration when its cellular-receptor level is reduced. Its receptor level is restored once liver regeneration is terminated.[127] The level of activin receptor mRNA expression was shown to be an important determinant in the magnitude of regeneration in PVL and PHx.[128,129] Suppressors of cytokine signaling (SOCS) are important negative regulators of cytokine signaling that prevent the tyrosine phosphorylation of STAT proteins.

Of the cytokines, both IL-1 and IL-6 are involved in the termination of proliferation.[130] The administration of exogenous IL-1β suppressed DNA synthesis post-PHx,[131] and increased expression of IL-1β has also been observed in a shrinking liver lobe of a rat PVL model, indicating that IL-1β is involved in the process of cellular atrophy.[132] The suppression of IL-1β was shown to promote liver regeneration in rat models of classic 70% PHx and 90% extended hepatectomy.[133]

The IL-1 is secreted by Kupffer cells, regulated by prostaglandin E2 (PGE2), and suppressed by heparin and PGE1 after PHx.[134] The effect is mediated through the IL-1 receptor as its antagonist (IL-1Ra), a competitive inhibitor of IL-1α and IL-1β and antiinflammatory protein, inhibits facilitated liver regeneration.[135] IL-1 appears to contribute to the cessation of liver regeneration in a reduced-size liver transplantation model by reducing HGF and promoting TGF-β release.[136] Another study showed that IL-1β inhibits the FGF19 signaling pathway, which regulates cell growth and metabolism of hepatocytes in liver regeneration.[137]

IL-6 signaling in the liver causes the rapid upregulation of SOCS3, which correlates with a feedback loop and the subsequent downregulation of phosphorylated STAT3, thereby terminating the IL-6 signal.[138] Also the role of C/EBPα, a key regulator of liver proliferation, in the termination of regeneration has been demonstrated. Complex formation of C/EBPα and chromatin remodeling protein HDAC1 represses other key regulators of liver proliferation: C/EBPα, p53, FXR, SIRT1, PGC1α, and TERT. The C/EBPβ-HDAC1 complexes also repress promoters of enzymes of glucose synthesis PEPCK and G6Pase. Proper cooperation of C/EBP and chromatin remodeling proteins seems essential for the termination of liver regeneration after surgery and for maintenance of liver functions.[139] Additional work strongly implicates the detection of blood BA levels by nuclear receptors as a regulator of liver growth.[117]

The Hippo signaling pathway and its downstream effectors, YAP and transcriptional coactivator with PDZ-binding motif (TAZ), have also been identified as key regulators of cell proliferation and organ size.[140] Overexpression of YAP in a transgenic mouse model leads to massive liver hyperplasia, reaching 25% of body weight. The core component of the mammalian Hippo pathway is a kinase cascade in which mammalian Ste20-like kinases 1/2 (MST1/2) phosphorylates and activates large tumor suppressor 1/2 (LATS1/2). LATS1/2 then phosphorylates the transcriptional coactivators, YAP and TAZ, downregulating their function and increasing their degradation by the proteasome.[141] During regeneration in a rat model, YAP was activated one day after PHx through decreased activation of core kinases MST1/2, as well as LATS1/2 by three days after PHx. At day seven, reaching normal liver size, YAP nuclear levels and target gene expression returned to baseline.[142]

In aged mice, it was shown that MST1 and LATS1 activity was increased, leading to anomalous Hippo signaling and nonregenerating livers.[143] It is therefore suggestive that the Hippo kinase pathway has a decisive role in determining overall liver size.[144–147]

LIVER ATROPHY

Classically, atrophy is triggered by an obstruction of portal venous blood flow and/or results from chronic obstruction of the bile duct. When atrophy occurs unilaterally, the opposite lobe of the liver responds with a hypertrophic response. This response has been capitalized on by hepatobiliary surgeons and interventional radiologists, who perform selective PVE to induce hypertrophy of potentially small remnant lobes before resection, or ligate the portal vein intra-operatively in the two-staged ALPPS procedure (see Chapters 102C and 102D). In slow-onset atrophy, the liver frequently is significantly distorted, and anatomic landmarks can be markedly changed, most commonly seen accompanied by a rotation of the liver and portal triad structures (Fig. 6.5).

Mechanisms of Liver Atrophy

The death of liver cells in atrophy generally is divided into necrosis and apoptosis. The distinction is important because necrosis is a nonregulated traumatic disruption of a cell that occurs when it encounters overwhelming injury, whereas apoptosis is an inducible, highly orchestrated cascade of events that

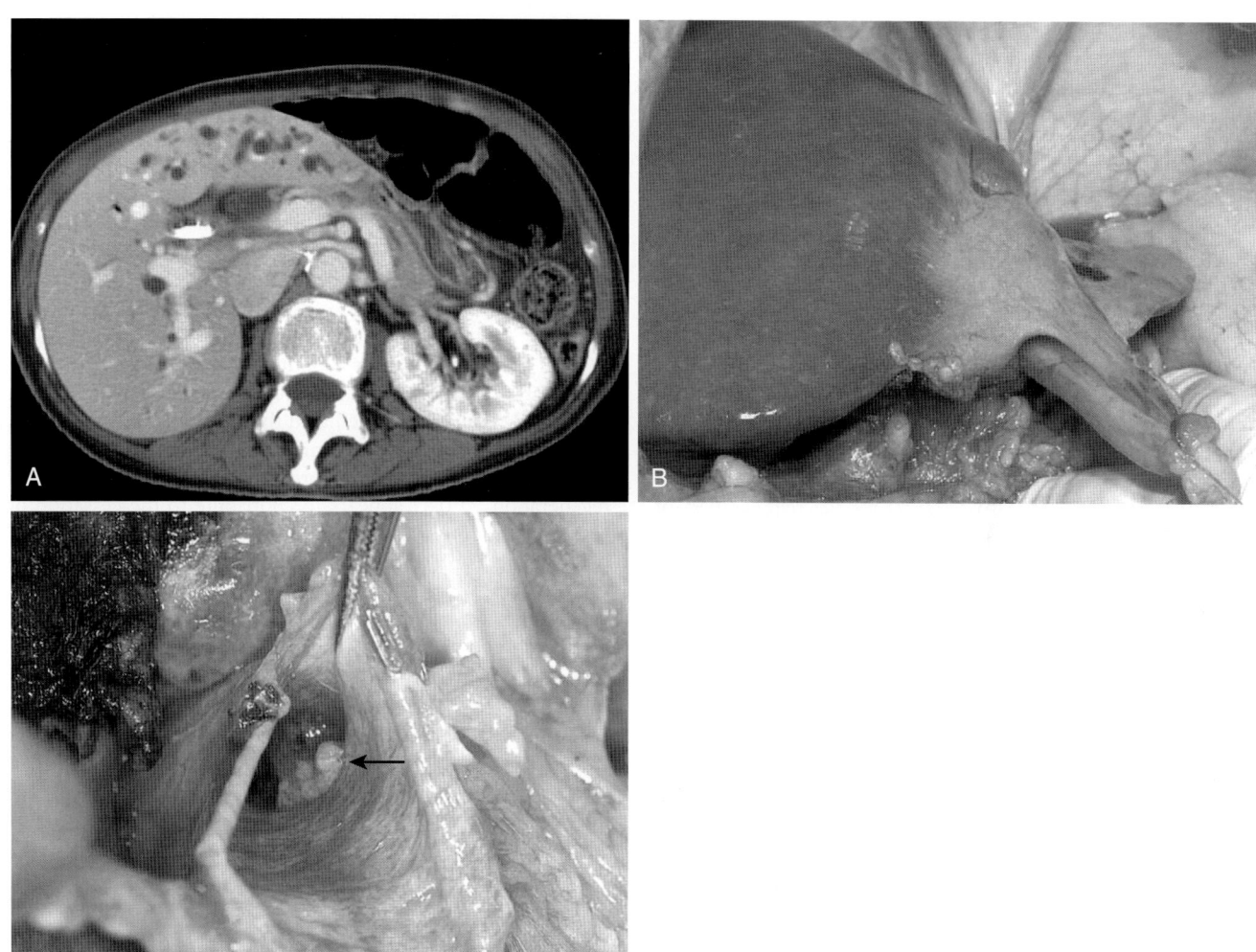

FIGURE 6.5 **Hepatic atrophy. A,** Computed tomography (CT) appearance of the liver in a patient with papillary hilar cholangiocarcinoma involving the left hepatic duct. Note the atrophic left lobe and intrahepatic ductal dilation predominantly on the left. **B,** Gross appearance of the liver in the same patient. Inset shows intraluminal view of the common bile duct, with tumor extruding from the left hepatic duct *(arrow).*

is physiologic. Necrotic cells lose membrane integrity, leak lysosomal enzymes, and induce a large inflammatory response. Apoptosis is energy dependent and allows cells to shrink and die without inducing inflammation.

Portal Vein Embolization/Ligation–Induced Hepatic Atrophy

For more information, see Chapter 102C.

The liver has the remarkable potential to maintain its total volume by adjusting lobes differently in response to extrahepatic stimuli; atrophy of the ligated lobe is the result of apoptosis, whereas increased portal flow in the nonembolized lobe induces proliferation and activates several cytoplasmic growth–promoting signal transduction pathways.[148,149] Ischemic necrosis of centrilobular areas of the liver predominates in the first three days of cell death. Areas peripheral to the necrotic liver cells predominantly undergo apoptotic cell death, and apoptosis persists long after necrosis subsides. Oxygen levels and mitochondrial function help determine which cells will undergo necrosis or apoptosis.[150] Models of portal vein ischemia in rats have confirmed a caspase-dependent apoptosis and have indicated that Kupffer cells are involved in generating reactive oxygen substrates and other acute-phase reactants, culminating in mitochondrial dysfunction and apoptosis.[151,152]

Interestingly, in a research environment when the contralateral lobes are resected after PVL, the regenerative stimulus of a 70% hepatectomy can counteract the atrophy of the ipsilateral liver, leading to a low but prolonged regenerative response of the portally deprived liver lobe.[153]

Biliary-Induced Hepatic Atrophy

The molecular mechanisms involved in biliary obstruction leading to hepatic atrophy are much more centered on apoptosis, with little or no involvement of acute necrosis. Cholestasis results in the accumulation of toxic bile salts, which induce apoptosis through the Fas-mediated pathway. In this case, TNF-α and Fas ligand bind to the Fas death receptors, leading to a cascade of intracellular events, including cytochrome c release from mitochondria and activation of apoptosis-mediating caspases. In Fas-deficient mice, bile duct ligation resulted in impaired apoptosis and less injury and fibrosis compared with wild-type mice.[154–156] More recent data, however, suggest a nonischemic model of necrosis/oncosis as the predominant process leading to cell death after common bile duct ligation, with cell swelling and without apoptotic caspase 3 activation.[157]

Clinical Causes of Atrophy

In addition to the purposeful ligation of the portal vein to induce hypertrophy, there are rare situations of portal vein thrombosis in noncirrhotic patients. If occurring acutely, this can be associated with bowel inflammation, pancreatitis, and hypercoagulable states. After umbilical vein catheterization in the newborn, liver volumes were shown to be 25% smaller than the expected standard liver volume. Creating a meso-portal surgical shunt between the superior mesenteric vein and the umbilical portion of the left portal vein achieved significant liver regeneration with a 28% increase in the liver volume.[158]

Perihilar cholangiocarcinoma is a frequent cause of biliary atrophy, induced by progressive occlusion of a major bile duct (see Chapter 51B). Biliary occlusion, often accompanied by portal vein compromise and leading to atrophy of the liver, occurs approximately 20% of the time with this disease and has significant

surgical implications. Benign post-cholecystectomy bile duct strictures can also lead to hepatic atrophy 10% to 15% of the time.[159,160] Choledocholithiasis and hepatolithiasis are infrequent causes of atrophy, as are benign tumors, such as papillomas, cystadenomas, and granular cell tumors (see Chapters 37A, 39, and 48).

Strictures caused by parasitic biliary infections, such as *Clonorchis sinensis* and *Ascaris lumbricoides*, also have been known to cause biliary obstruction and associated atrophy of the liver (see Chapter 45). Occlusion of the hepatic artery alone would not induce atrophy, although arterial radio-embolization techniques are currently used to treat hepatocellular carcinomas and increase resectability. Lobar radioembolization with Yttrium-90 or Holmium-166 can cause atrophy of a lobe through β emission, causing necrosis. This way, "radiohepatectomy" allows for growth of the contralateral lobe with a median increase of 24% after three months,[161,162] which may enable resection.

CLINICAL FACTORS INFLUENCING LIVER REGENERATION

Patient-Related Factors

Age and Cellular Senescence

Liver age is a significant factor in hepatocellular regeneration. Older livers do not regenerate as quickly as younger livers and show delayed regeneration after acute injury and impaired function after liver transplantation.[163,164] Rodent models have shown reduced and delayed thymidine kinase uptake in older animals after PHx, and there is a striking difference in the magnitude of DNA synthesis and timing of hepatocyte replication between young and old livers.[165]

This aging effect was attributed to cellular senescence by Hayflick in 1961. First introduced to describe the limited proliferative ability of human fibroblasts in cell culture, senescence has been discovered in vivo in many types of tissues, and the number of senescent cells increases with age.[166] In senescence, the p53 and Rb signaling pathways become activated, leading to activation of p21Cip1 (CDKN1A). p21Cip1 is the inhibitor of cyclin E/ CDK2 complex and promotes cell cycle arrest at the G1/S phase of the cell cycle. In old mouse livers, the CDK inhibitor p21 is expressed at high levels, as is cyclin B1, a regulator of G2/M phase of the cell cycle.[167] Also, aging switches the C/EBPα pathway of growth arrest in liver from CDK inhibition to repression of E2F transcription. This blocks the activation of the c-myc promoter in old livers after PHx and in tissue culture models.[168,169]

Once it becomes senescent, the cell stops dividing permanently but remains metabolically active. When cells in an organ become senescent, the entire organism can be affected through the senescence-associated secretory phenotype (SASP). Senescence is generally considered beneficial as a tumor suppressive or anticancer process because the senescent cells cannot divide. On the other hand, cellular senescence may cause loss of regenerative capability of the liver.[170] Any repetitive wave of insult that can cause damage to hepatocytes, such as alcohol intake, hepatitis viral infection, immune disorder, or autophagy deficiency, promotes senescence in hepatocytes and may compromise liver regeneration. The normal liver contains a basal level of senescent hepatocytes (3%–7%), but in chronic hepatitis and cirrhosis the liver may exhibit 50% to 100% of hepatocytes in senescence.[166]

Senescent hepatocytes secrete SASP factors with an abnormal level of proinflammatory cytokine/chemokines, such as CCL2, stimulating the production of TGF-β from hepatic macrophages, which can promote the conversion of nonsenescent cells to senescent cells in a paracrine manner. The inhibition of TGF-β–TGFβ-R1 interaction by specific inhibitors or the depletion of macrophages reduced senescence progress and enhanced liver regeneration.[171]

Aging has been also shown to be associated with a progressive decline in growth hormone secretion and Foxm1B expression.[172] Treatment of old mice with growth hormone can restore hepatocyte proliferation with increased Foxm1B and cyclin B1 expression and significant reduction in p27 protein levels.[173] Recently, a critical role of the glycogen synthase kinase 3β- cyclin D3 pathway in the loss of the regenerative capacity in old livers was shown, which could be overcome by exogenous growth hormone substitution.[174]

Biliary Obstruction or Diversion

Cholestasis results in the accumulation of toxic bile salts, which induce apoptosis through the Fas-mediated pathway. In this pathway, TNF-α and Fas ligand bind to the Fas death receptors, leading to cytochrome c release from mitochondria and activation of apoptosis-mediating caspases. In Fas-deficient mice, bile duct ligation resulted in impaired apoptosis and less injury and fibrosis compared with wild-type mice.[154–156] Other molecular mechanisms involved in reduced regenerative capacity with biliary obstruction are suppressed expression of c-myc,[175] C/EBP, and cyclin E.[176] Production of HGF,[177] EGF,[178] and IL-6 [179] is also altered. Finally, biliary obstruction also impairs enterohepatic circulation, thus negatively affecting the regenerative capacity. Clinically relevant is that external biliary drainage for obstructive jaundice markedly suppresses liver regeneration after PHx,[180] whereas internal biliary drainage preserves this capacity.[181] The mechanism was demonstrated in a rat model in which oral bile acids were given before PHx. Liver regeneration was significantly increased through activation of the farnesoid X receptor signaling pathway.[182]

Diabetes Mellitus

Insulin is one of the most important hepatotrophic factors in portal venous blood.[102] The binding protein of IGF, a molecule similar to insulin, also rises substantially after PHx.[183,184] Thus impaired secretion of insulin and IGF in diabetic patients prevents liver regeneration after PHx, as reflected by decreased synthesis of RNA, DNA, and protein on the first postoperative day.[185] Enhancement of mitochondrial phosphorylate activity in the remnant liver after PHx is inhibited in proportion to the severity of impaired insulin secretion. Insulin gene transfer via the spleen enhances liver regeneration without causing liver damage and improves nutritional status after hepatectomy in diabetic rats.[186] Multiple regression analysis in clinical PVE has shown that diabetes mellitus is a risk factor for reduced hypertrophy in the nonembolized lobe[187] (see Chapter 102C). These results demonstrate the importance of insulin in hepatic regeneration, and strict glucose control should be aimed for in liver surgery and PVE.[188]

Nutritional Status

The literature on the effect of nutritional status on liver regeneration is contradictory. Hepatic regeneration is metabolically intensive and requires a large amount of energy. Liver regeneration after hepatectomy is associated with a derangement in energy metabolism, measured by a decrease in the ratio of ATP to its hydrolysis product inorganic phosphate. This depleted energy status is mirrored in biochemical indices of liver function, and restitution parallels the course of restoration of hepatic cell mass.[189] Nutritional support is undoubtedly the most physiologic manner to enhance liver regeneration, but there still is little, if any, clear information regarding the effect of specific nutrients on liver regeneration in humans.[190,191]

From animal models, we know that malnutrition is associated with higher postoperative mortality and reduced regeneration after PHx.[192] When improving nutritional status, enteral feeding should be preferred because rats given enteral nutrition showed much better weight gain after 70% hepatectomy than those given isocaloric nutrition parenterally.[193]

Recently, a small trial with supplementation with branched chain amino acids-enriched nutrients showed improved nutritional state in LDLT recipients in the early post-transplant period and shortened the post-transplant catabolic phase.[194] Supplementation of glutamine, one of the sources of DNA and protein synthesis, has been shown to promote liver regeneration.[195] Essential fatty acids, components of the cell membrane and precursors of several functional mediators, also play an important role in hepatic regeneration. Interestingly, dextrose supplementation has an inhibitory effect on liver regeneration, associated with increased expression of C/EBPα, p21, and p27,[196] although this effect was not found in a previous study.[197]

On the other hand, the most recent preclinical studies investigated the effect of short-term starvation (12–23 hours) and showed beneficial results in protecting against apoptosis and necrosis, associated with I/R. Mechanisms involved higher levels of betahydroxybutyric acid and consequently an increase of heme oxygenase-1 and autophagy activity and inhibition of high-mobility group box 1 (HMBG1) release, NF-κB activation, and NLRP3 inflammasome activity.[198] In this light, an interesting concept is the mathematical "network of interaction prediction model,"[22] which indicates that halving the metabolic load for 48 hours after a 85% liver resection could rescue the regenerative process.

Gender

Sex steroids are known to induce transient hepatocellular proliferation and to improve fatty acid metabolism.[199] Estrogen receptors are found on hepatocytes and serum estradiol is increased substantially after PHx in rodents and humans.[200] Pretreatment of rats with 17β-estradiol induces hepatocyte DNA synthesis in vitro and accelerates liver regeneration in vivo; administration of tamoxifen, a mixed estrogen agonist/antagonist, slows regeneration when given soon after PHx.[201] In contrast, testosterone levels decline in men and in male rats after PHx. Nevertheless, there is no clinical evidence that shows significant differences between the sexes in man after liver resection. In murine models, gender may also have a positive effect on regeneration of transplanted partial grafts.[202] In humans, the latency of bilirubin level reduction was shorter in women than in men, suggesting that a female factor promotes bilirubin recovery after liver transplantation. Estrogen was shown to significantly promote Cytochrome P450 (CYP) 2A6, a bilirubin oxidase, facilitating bilirubin metabolism in regenerating liver.[203] Generally, estrogen may be responsible for the better tolerance to various stresses because of a reduced inflammatory response and a reduced oxygen radical production, leading to improved hepatic regeneration.[204]

Intrinsic Liver Disease

Steatohepatitis

The regenerative response of the liver can be seriously affected by preexisting intrinsic liver conditions, such as steatohepatitis, fibrosis, and cirrhosis (see Chapters 7, 69, and 74). Steatohepatitis is a condition met more frequently in the general population, and nonalcoholic fatty liver disease (NAFLD) and steatohepatitis (NASH) have become an epidemic[205] that poses significant challenges in the management of patients undergoing liver resection. Hepatic steatosis affects regeneration on several molecular levels.[206] Lipid accumulation has been associated with hepatocyte mitochondrial damage caused by free radical injury. Steatotic livers in rats show delayed mitosis and increased mortality after PHx, which may be because of abnormal TNF and IL-6 signaling.[207] The coordinated induction of Jnks and Erks is disrupted after PHx in fatty livers of ob/ob mice (a model for steatohepatitis), with enhanced AKT and inhibition of PEPCK.[208] Cyclin D1 induction is abolished along with STAT3 and reduced ATP levels, which may arrest cell-cycle progression. Hepatocyte mitochondrial damage associated with lipid accumulation is caused by free radical injury from fatty acid oxidation. Abnormalities in induction of CYP450 may be one mechanism in the pathophysiology of these findings in fatty livers and may contribute to poor regeneration.[209–211] The presence of underlying steatosis has a considerable impact on operative morbidity and mortality after major hepatic resection,[212–214] with a significantly higher rate of complications if marked steatosis ($\geq$30%) is present.[215] Interestingly, in a clinical setting of major hepatectomies, BMI did not impact liver regeneration during the first two months, but the kinetic growth rate per week between two and seven months postoperatively was less among overweight and obese patients. Also in this series, risk of a major complication was greatest among obese patients.[216] Steatohepatitis, or acute inflammation in the setting of fatty infiltration, carries an even higher risk and eventually results in fibrosis and cirrhosis.[217]

Inflammation: Viral Hepatitis and Bacterial Infections

Inflammation in general and some viral infections, such as hepatitis B and C and murine cytomegalovirus specifically,[218–220] have been reported to inhibit hepatic regeneration (see Chapter 68).

A factor that links inflammation directly to regeneration is mitochondrial calcium uptake 1 (MICU1), the gatekeeper of the mitochondrial calcium uniporter (MCU). Loss of MICU1 leads to an enhanced and sustained proinflammatory response post PHx with a failure of hepatocytes to enter the cell cycle and large-scale hepatic necrosis through Ca^{2+} overload-induced mitochondrial permeability transition pore (PTP) opening.[221] Prevention of mitochondrial Ca^{2+} overload rescued liver regeneration in MICU1 knock-down mice.

The precise mechanism responsible for viral infection–related suppression is unclear, although it may be partly mediated by the inhibition of cell cycle–dependent molecules. In hepatitis B virus (HBV) infection, it was shown that liver regeneration is delayed through a reduced activation of the insulin receptor. HBV induces expression of the insulin receptor via activation of the NF-E2-related factor 2, leading to increased

intracellular amounts of insulin receptor in the hepatocytes. However, intracellular retention of the receptor simultaneously reduces the amount of functional insulin receptors on the cell surface and thereby attenuates insulin binding. Consequently, hepatocytes are less sensitive to insulin stimulation leading to delayed liver regeneration.[222]

Concomitant bacterial infections also alter liver regeneration. Earlier reports showed enhanced liver regeneration in rats after inflammation before hepatic resection because of stimulation of lipopolysaccharide, upregulation of proinflammatory cytokines, such as IL-6 and TNF-α and HGF,[223,224] all of which are chief mediators of hepatic regeneration. More consistent with clinical observations, a recent study showed significantly delayed regeneration kinetics in a rat model of combined liver resection and intraperitoneal sepsis, with hyperinflammation and increased liberation of pro-inflammatory cytokines.[225] The relation between inflammation and poor liver regeneration was confirmed in patients with early allograft dysfunction (EAD) occurring in the first week after liver transplantation. EAD was associated with an inflammatory response in the perioperative period, and a specific pattern of 25 cytokines, chemokines, and immunoreceptors. Patients with EAD showed higher MCP-1 (CCL2), IL-8 (CXCL8), and RANTES (CCL5) chemokine levels in the early postoperative period, suggesting upregulation of the NF-kB pathway, in addition to higher levels of chemokines and cytokines associated with T-cell immunity, including MIG (CXCL9), IP-10 (CXCL10), and IL-2R.[226]

Pharmacologic Therapy

Many exogenous agents can affect liver regeneration, including frequently prescribed drugs and neoadjuvant chemotherapy. Numerous medications associated with induction of steatosis may interfere with liver regeneration and include certain antiarrhythmic agents, antibiotics, antiviral agents, anticonvulsants, steroids, calcium channel blockers, statins, and antiglycemic medications. β-Blockers and nonsteroidal anti-inflammatory drugs (NSAIDs) may exert a direct negative influence on liver regeneration. β-Blockers decrease portal blood flow to the liver and, blocking the trophic effects of epinephrine and NSAIDs, directly inhibit cyclooxygenase, part of the CEBPβ-mediated liver regenerative pathway, but there is no clinical evidence reflecting increased morbidity or mortality. Nonetheless, any potential harmful effect of any medication must be considered before resection.

There are an increasing number of patients having liver surgery after neoadjuvant or induction chemotherapy. Major drawbacks of hepatotoxic chemotherapy are the sinusoidal obstruction syndrome (SOS), associated with oxaliplatin (Eloxatin, Sanofi Aventis)[227] and the chemotherapy associated steatohepatitis (CASH),[228] which is associated with irinotecan (Campto, Pfizer). This chemotherapy-associated steatohepatitis increases postoperative mortality and specifically deaths from postoperative liver failure.[229] Sinusoidal obstruction also impairs liver regeneration after extensive liver resections and increases postoperative morbidity, but may be prevented by administering concomitant Bevacizumab (Avastin, Hoffmann–LaRoche).[230,231] Bevacizumab, a monoclonal antibody targeting VEGF, is given in combination with cytotoxic chemotherapy, to improve resectability[232] and survival in patients with metastatic colorectal cancer.[233] Well-designed preclinical studies have demonstrated that inhibition of angiogenesis can inhibit wound healing.[234] Bevacizumab does not appear to adversely affect the results of PHx in humans.[235] Animal studies have demonstrated that liver regeneration depends on VEGF and angiogenesis.[87] In a murine model, anti-VEGF receptor therapy slightly impaired liver regeneration and cell proliferation after PHx compared with control.[236] Clinically, no differences in postoperative liver insufficiency were seen if stopped at least six to eight weeks before hepatic resection.[237,238]

Regarding the effect of Sorafenib (Nexavar, Bayer), a multikinase inhibitor used for treatment of hepatocellular carcinoma, conflicting results have been reported in experimental research. Sorafenib did not impact on liver regeneration when ceased before surgery; however, administration during and after hepatectomy affected liver regeneration in rodent models.[239,240] Reduced phospho-ERK levels and wound-healing complications were observed. In another rat experiment however, no significant change in liver regeneration related to Sorafenib exposure was found.[241]

Liver Transplantation

Regeneration also is crucial in liver transplantation (see Chapters 105 and 111). In deceased donor transplantation, hepatocyte loss occurs in the form of I/R injury because of the necessary preservation period from procurement to implantation and damage that may have occurred in the donor. Regenerative mechanisms are actively engaged after transplantation, depending on the length and degree of preservation injury.[18,242] Similarly, hepatocytes lost to the alloimmune response require replacement. Regeneration also is necessary in the setting of transplanting an SFS graft into a larger recipient. This is the case in the setting of adult-to-adult living donor transplantation (AALDLT).[6] Ischemic injury is minimized in AALDLT, in that the preservation period is short; however, this technique supplies a graft that is by definition too small, requiring vigorous immediate hepatocyte proliferation. By transplanting only 50% to 60% of what is the expected liver volume in adults, recipients (and donors) must rely on the rapid regeneration of a partial liver in addition to maintaining the basic metabolic functions required of the liver. The National Institutes of Health (NIH)-sponsored study in adult-to-adult living donor transplantation (A2ALL) has investigated the role of numerous donor and recipient factors in regeneration. The size of the remnant liver or graft had the greatest impact on rate and quantity of regeneration.[23]

In a pilot study investigating molecular mechanisms associated with human liver regeneration, differences in hepatic gene expression were noted between donors with complete regeneration compared with those with less successful regeneration. Genes mainly related to cell proliferation, inflammation and metabolism, metabolic pathways (aminoacyl tRNA synthesis), and stress pathways (acute phase response) were among the most significantly regulated pathways. In contrast, the poor regeneration group demonstrated very little change in expression before and after resection. The lack of significant change in genomic profile in the poorly regenerating livers suggests a possible inhibition or delay in initiation of recovery and regeneration molecular pathways.[243]

Ischemic Injury

Warm and cold ischemic injury is an unavoidable component of transplantation. After prolonged cold ischemia of whole liver grafts, there is initiation of the cell-cycle pathways with upregulation of markers of liver regeneration as previously described. When ischemic injury is significant, there is a greater expression and activation of cytokines, transcription factors, and immediate early genes and a greater magnitude of hepatocellular replication up to a certain "point of no return," after which the damage is too extensive and the liver or allograft is unable to maintain functional homeostasis and regenerative capabilities, which results in liver dysfunction and graft failure.[98,244,245]

Other studies have demonstrated that lack of blood flow occurring during cold preservation for transplantation markedly deteriorates the protective phenotype of liver sinusoidal endothelial cells (LSEC) by downregulating the expression of the transcription factor Kruppel-like Factor 2 (KLF2), which orchestrates the transcription of a variety of protective genes, including the endothelial synthase of NO (eNOS), the antithrombotic molecule thrombomodulin, and the antioxidant transcription factor Nrf2.[246–248]

Minimal Transplanted Liver Mass

The amount of liver mass transplanted has been shown to be an important factor after transplantation. Early experimental studies addressing regeneration after transplantation showed that an SFS graft adapts to its environment and achieves a size equal to the original native liver.[249] It became apparent that graft size-to-recipient ratio was crucial when it became clear that grafts that were too small had decreased survival.[250] These findings correlated with early clinical experience in living donor transplantation, in that some SFS segmental grafts developed a "small-for-size syndrome" that was associated with significant functional impairment, shown by prolonged cholestasis and histologic changes consistent with ischemic injury and associated with poor outcome. Liver grafts with a graft volume of less than 40% of calculated standard liver volume were associated with poor graft survival and prolonged hyperbilirubinemia.[251–254] The development of segmental graft dysfunction in the A2ALL study was also associated with worse patient outcome.[23] Animal models of partial liver graft transplantation have studied the interplay between the regenerative response and ischemic injury in the setting of 50% and 30% size grafts. The partial grafts showed a robust regenerative response if the ischemic injury was minimal. It became apparent, however, that when these partial grafts were subjected to ischemic injury of moderate to prolonged time periods, there was a significant effect on survival, with extensive hepatic necrosis, the inability to initiate or maintain the regenerative response, and decreased survival. These findings show the diminished tolerance of SFS grafts for additional injury beyond transplantation itself.[245,255]

Although ischemic injury in AALDLT is minimized, the amount of critical liver mass required for transplantation in living donation remains in question. Most centers have defined liver mass as graft-to-recipient body weight ratio or as a percentage of the standard liver volume. No uniform method of measuring or reporting graft volume in relation to the recipient has been established. Clinical experience with living donor and split grafts has led to an accepted lower limit of 0.8% graft-to-recipient body weight ratio, or 40% of the standard liver volume, although significantly smaller liver segmental grafts up to 0.47% to 0.49% have been used successfully.[256,257] Donor and recipient characteristics and graft factors significantly influence these minimal accepted standard volumes. Patients with fulminant hepatic failure, severe portal hypertension, and significant disease severity as manifested by a high Model for End-Stage Liver Disease (MELD) score (see Chapter 4) and patients with significant metabolic stress may require more liver volume than stable patients transplanted under elective conditions. The accumulation of additional stressful stimuli, such as sepsis or renal failure, may push a relatively small graft into failure.

Effect of Immunosuppression

Within the graft environment, the host immune response needs to be inhibited to avoid acute allograft rejection, and inhibition of this response may interfere with the recovery of liver grafts, requiring active regeneration of hepatocytes. Glucocorticoids, routinely used in immunosuppression protocols, have been shown to inhibit cell cycle progression markedly in PHx models and in transplant models with ischemic injury.[258–260] Cyclosporine and tacrolimus may have differential effects on regeneration in a dose-dependent fashion.[261] Sirolimus, with its antiproliferative action, interferes with hepatocyte replication.[262,263] The rapid hepatocyte replication and smaller liver mass also may interfere with metabolism and pharmacokinetics of certain drugs. Preliminary studies have shown that AALDLT recipients require lower doses of tacrolimus in the early postoperative period than patients receiving whole grafts.[264] The ability to measure functional recovery of these recipients would help in the assessment of hepatocellular function and metabolic demands in these regenerating partial liver grafts.

Donor Age

As with liver regeneration in the nontransplant setting, old grafts do not regenerate as quickly as young livers. A clinical study of living donors showed a greater graft/standard liver volume in the young donor livers post-transplant compared with middle-aged and old donor grafts. The old livers also had a higher prothrombin time in the early period postoperatively.[265] Statistics from the United Network for Organ Sharing database show that the graft survival of older living donor grafts is inferior to younger grafts,[266] and increasing donor and recipient age affected both short-term and long-term survival in the NIH A2ALL study.[23,267] In the deceased donor transplant setting, grafts older than 55 to 60 years of age have poorer long-term survival combined with longer cold ischemic times.[268] Age may affect the regeneration and recovery of the living donor and the recipient. Many groups limit the upper age limit of the donor into the 50 to 60 year range, although no definite age has been specified.

Portal Inflow and Hepatic Outflow

In both liver resection and partial liver graft transplantation, in addition to the reduced cell mass, portal blood flow dynamics are altered, leading to increased portal blood flow and pressure. Hepatic regeneration is triggered by shear stress on the sinusoidal endothelium and is implicated in more rapid regeneration[269,270] and increased recovery, if portal flow is increased to about two times baseline level.[271,272] Ultimately, this is shown in a model of PVL, where the mere ligation of the portal vein branch is responsible for overwhelming alterations of both hepatic structure and physiology.[273] In the ligated lobe, the total blood flow halves, with increased fraction of arterial blood flow and development of extensive necroapoptotic lesions and loss of higher liver functions. Meanwhile, a hyperperfusion (~230%) of mainly (>97%) portal blood flow with reverse hepatic artery

buffer response takes place in the nonligated lobe, with intensive rise in mitotic activity and increased functionality after 14 days.

Significant portal hyperperfusion, on the other hand, is regarded as central to the problem in SFS grafts, leading to decreased regeneration and increased mortality.[52,175,274,275]

Significant and persistent portal hyperperfusion caused a loss of hepatic arterial buffer response with hypoxia and significantly increased anaerobic metabolism, hepatocellular injury, and loss of function.[276] In a pig model of 20% inflow reduction to the left portal vein, a robust regenerative response and increase in total liver volume and function was seen on the right side mediated through TNF-α, IL-6, and NOS2 in the early phase, without causing atrophy or loss of liver function on the left side.[277]

In addition to portal venous inflow alteration, the hepatic venous outflow may be altered during surgery, even causing outflow obstruction of areas of the liver remnant or liver graft. Postoperative liver hypertrophy ratios and even function parameters were shown to be significantly impaired in living donor liver grafts with the large-outflow-obstruction areas, compared with small-outflow-obstruction areas.[278] Segments with poor venous drainage become atrophied with time.[279]

Microbiome

The intestinal content is rich in microorganisms and in metabolites generated from both the host and colonizing bacteria. Via the gut-liver axis, the microbiome exerts an immense impact on liver integrity and function, and research has emerged to support that the gut microbiota may promote liver regeneration.[191,280]

LPS are the major components of the outer membrane of gram-negative bacteria. Although it was initially thought that bacteria negatively influence liver regeneration, evidence indicates that endotoxin is necessary for liver regeneration. Gut-derived endotoxin administered both before and after PHx induced hepatic DNA synthesis and release of several hepatotrophic factors such as insulin.[281] Conversely, hepatic DNA synthesis in mice was impaired when gut-derived endotoxin was prevented from reaching the liver.[282] In addition, conditions that eliminate bacteria or reduce endotoxin (gut sterilization using neomycin and cefazolin, reduction of endotoxin and BAs using cholestyramine, and neutralization of the lipid A portion of circulating endotoxin by polymyxin B) could inhibit DNA synthesis following 2/3 hepatectomy. The observed LPS-induced hepatocyte proliferation results from HGF activity. Treatment of rats with a combination of LPS and HGF increased JNK and AP-1 DNA binding, through c-JUN and STAT3 upregulation.[283] LPS-HGF modulation of hepatocyte proliferation indicates potential contribution from the gut microbiota to the liver regeneration program. It is important to note, however, that not all endotoxin-releasing bacteria are beneficial for liver regeneration. In mice, orthotopic liver transplantation was associated with increased hepatic inflammation and increased portal endotoxin levels after surgery, often leading to liver injury and rejection.[284] When *Bifidobacterium*, *Lactobacillus*, *Bacteroides*, and *Eubacterium* were increased and *Enterobacteriaceae* was reduced, portal LPS levels and Kupffer cell activation decreased, which was beneficial for preventing liver injury found in rats after orthotopic liver transplantation. These findings suggest differential effects of specific bacteria on liver regeneration. Interestingly, PHx caused fluctuating changes in the gut microbiome, which paralleled the biological processes of regeneration.[285]

Besides the direct role of bacteria, microbial enzymes are responsible for the synthesis of various BAs, which play an important role as "hepatostat," balancing the need for liver regeneration through activation of the FXR receptor (see earlier). In humans, cholic acid (CA) and chenodeoxycholic acid (CDCA) are primary BAs entering the intestinal lumen that undergo deconjugation, dehydroxylation, epimerization, and oxidation using bacterial enzymes. Conjugation increases the aqueous solubility of BAs and renders them largely impermeable to the intestinal epithelium, thus preventing them from exiting the intestinal lumen. The conversion from their primary form to the secondary BAs deoxycholic acid (DCA) and lithocholic acid (LCA) is also mediated via bacterial enzyme 7α-dehydroxylase. Therefore the composition of BAs depends on the bacterial composition.[286]

EXPERIMENTAL STRATEGIES TO PROMOTE LIVER REGENERATION

Although there has yet to be developed any reliable intervention to improve liver regeneration in the clinical realm, numerous approaches have been successful in the experimental setting.[287]

Because fat metabolism has been shown to be of major importance, several experimental strategies have been developed to improve liver regeneration. In a model of high-fat-diet induced steatosis, supplementation of omega-3 fatty acids revealed improvements in I/R injury and regenerative capacity, interestingly in both lean and fat mice.[288] In the situation of an SFS fatty liver remnant, the expression of ApoA-1 was decreased in hepatocytes with steatosis and was inversely associated with the concentration of oleic acid. Exogenous ApoA-1 administration effectively attenuated hepatocyte steatosis and promoted liver regeneration at day two after major hepatectomy. Because ApoA-1 treatment increased the expressions of PGC1α and its target genes, ApoA-1 may accelerate regeneration of SFS fatty liver grafts through regulating mitochondrial function.[289] This mechanism was supported by another study that supplemented nicotinamide to promote liver regeneration and restore liver function after PHx in mice. Nicotinamide significantly upregulated the NAD–dependent protein deacetylase sirtuin1 (SIRT1), which also targets PGC1α and mitochondrial biogenesis.[290]

A third study supplementing fish oil during and after PHx in mice showed faster restoration of ALT and total bilirubin levels through AMPK activation.[291]

Another strategy that may be useful in an SFS situation is blockage of specific receptors or peptides. The blockage of the receptor for advanced glycation end-products (RAGE) showed improved survival in a rat hepatectomy model.[292] TGF-β1, a potent growth inhibitory polypeptide, was found to rise after SFS transplantation, forming a heteromeric receptor complex. Phosphorylation of this complex activates Smad2 and Smad3, which leads to regulatory proteins that exert their inhibitory effect on hepatocyte proliferation.[293] Inhibiting TGF-β dependent cell cycle arrest may hold future promise.[126] Recently, preclinical evidence showed that silencing the Hippo core kinases MST1 and MST2 with small interfering RNA provokes hepatocyte proliferation in quiescent livers and rescues liver regeneration in aged mice after PH. This has

therapeutic potential to improve regeneration in nonregenerative disorders.[143]

Finally, the FXR, as the key mediator of proliferative bile salt signaling, was targeted by the potent obeticholic acid (OCA) in a model of PVE and in partial resection, showing accelerated liver regeneration through induction of intestinal FGF15.[294,295] In the situation of cholestasis, however, it exacerbates biliary injury by forced pumping of BAs into an obstructed biliary tree.

CLINICAL IMPLICATIONS

When to Stimulate Liver Regeneration Preoperatively?

The assessment of hepatic function before resection is difficult (see Chapter 4), but we do know that the risk for perioperative complications increases when the remnant liver volume is too small, particularly in diseased or biliary compromised livers[296,297] (see Chapters 101 and 102A). Hepatic function seems to recover quickly after resection but is difficult to measure. Conventional clinical blood tests and liver biopsy do not give the full picture of hepatic function. Child's classification and MELD scores apply primarily to cirrhotics and can provide a good clinical assessment, but they are only rough estimates of functional reserve. Bilirubin, albumin, international normalized ratio, and platelet count become abnormal only in advanced cirrhosis. Magnetic resonance (MR) imaging or computed tomography (CT) can measure residual liver volume (LV) accurately, but quantitative functional testing is not as precise. Traditional techniques to measure the LV to be resected before hepatectomy can lead to inaccurate estimates of functional residual liver (FRL) volumes because of the presence of dilated bile ducts, multiple tumors, undetected lesions, compromised liver volume caused by cholestasis or previous chemotherapy, cholangitis, vascular obstruction, steatosis or cirrhosis, or segmental atrophy and/or hypertrophy from tumor growth (see Chapter 4). Accurate preoperative assessment by CT or MR volumetry is important because significant interpatient variation exists in hepatic volumes. In LDLT, total liver volume (TLV) and FRL can generally be relied on to predict postresection function because the donor liver is normal. However, the TLV of the recipient's diseased liver is not a useful index of function. Values calculated from graft weight-to-recipient body weight ratio (GRBWR) or standardized liver volume (SLV) based on recipient BSA are used to predict minimum adequate graft volume.[298,299] In segmental graft liver transplantation, a GRBWR greater than 0.8% or a graft weight ratio (graft weight divided by standard liver weight of recipient) greater than 40% have been generally recommended to achieve graft and patient survival greater than 90%[253]; however, these parameters can be stretched somewhat if the graft is younger and of excellent quality. In comparison, extended resection of 80% of functional parenchyma can be performed in the absence of chronic liver disease for hepatobiliary malignancies.[300] Recommended minimal functional remnant LV after extended hepatectomy is greater than 25% in a normal liver and greater than 40% in an "injured" liver, with moderate to severe steatosis, cholestasis, fibrosis, or after chemotherapy.[301]

Quantitative liver function tests measure the liver's ability to metabolize or extract test compounds and can identify patients with impaired function at earlier stages of disease but have limited application in predicting a liver's ability to regenerate after major resection. Indocyanine green clearance (IGC) is regarded as an accurate assessment of functional reserve and can help predict mortality,[302] but more is being learned about measuring hepatic function in diseased livers using quantitative functional testing, such as methionine breath tests, cholate clearance, liver single-photon emission CT scans, and liver scintigraphy and phosphorus 31 MR spectroscopy.[303] When compared with ICG and CT volumetric data, hepatobiliary scintigraphy is a reproducible accurate tool to assess functional liver uptake and excretion, preoperative liver function reserve, and remnant liver function and allows for monitoring of postoperative liver function regeneration.[304] One of the drawbacks of hepatobiliary scintigraphy is that it does not give reliable information about liver function in patients with biliary obstruction, such as cholangiocarcinoma patients. In this case, the maximum liver function capacity (LiMAx) test has been proposed as a breath test for the perioperative assessment of liver function.[305] This test is based on the metabolization of 13C-methacetin in the liver acinus by liver-specific enzyme CYP1A2 into acetaminophen and carbon dioxide ($13CO_2$). The latter can then be determined in the exhaled air, and a ratio of $13CO_2/12CO_2$ is built to eventually calculate the maximum liver function capacity. In the last years, several studies have been published regarding the use of the LiMAx test to predict mortality and perioperative liver function.[306]

Assessment of future remnant volume/function distinguishes those who will most likely benefit from preoperative liver enhancement techniques with PVE and additional hepatic vein embolization.

The Use of Portal Vein Embolization to Promote Regeneration

The selective embolization technique increases tolerance to major hepatic resection by reducing the liver volume that requires resection and inducing hypertrophy of the FLR to approximate target limits in patients with large tumors or abnormal liver function (see Chapter 102C). Criteria for selection of patients for PVE before major hepatectomy are FLR size; factors compromising liver function, including previous chemotherapy, hepatitis, and cholestasis; and the planned complexity of the procedure.[296,307] It is recommended when predicted FLR is less than 20% to 25% in a normal liver and less than 40% in a liver with compromised function.[297,308] Stimulation by PVE increases circulating IL-6 and TNF-α,[309,310] with activation of the mitogenic cascade, similar to PHx. In fact, marginal contralateral regeneration of less than 5% after PVE is a strong predictor of liver failure after subsequent liver resection.[311] A significant increase in DNA synthesis and mRNA expression of HGF has been observed in the nonembolized or ligated lobe,[132] whereas HGF expression is only slightly elevated and negative regulators of hepatocyte proliferation, such as TGF-β and IL-1β, are strongly expressed in the shrinking ligated lobe. It is important to keep in mind that these factors also may promote tumor outgrowth in the FLR, and continuation of chemotherapy during PVE for malignant conditions should be considered.[312,313]

Associating Liver Partition With Portal Vein Ligation for Staged Hepatectomy

In 2012 a radical new surgical procedure was introduced to stimulate liver regeneration in patients with a small FLR[314]

(see Chapter 102D). In this two-step approach, the liver parenchyma is transected between segments 2/3 and 4, with concomitant ligation of the right portal vein. Between one week and ten days later, impressive hypertrophy of the left lateral segments has occurred, with a median volume increase of 74% (range 21%–192%)[315] and, in a second stage, an extended right hemihepatectomy can be performed. The procedure was initially hampered by high mortality (11%–19%) and high morbidity (up to 40%),[316,317] but with increasing experience and better patient selection, better results are gained without perioperative mortality.[318] In an experimental model comparing ALPSS with PVL and PHx, the gene expression profile after ALPPS showed a more similar expression pattern to PHx than PVL at the early phase of the regeneration. Early transcriptomic changes and predicted upstream regulators, however, showed many overlapping molecular mechanisms and pathways,[319] but unique differences were found in the IGF1R, ILK, and IL-10 pathways, whereas the activity of the interferon pathway was reduced.[320]

Although ALPPS is a unique technique to boost regeneration in selected patients, many recommend considering alternative approaches, such as adequate portal and hepatic vein embolization, before an all-operative approach is attempted.[321,322]

Ischemic Preconditioning to Stimulate Regeneration

Liver resection, transplantation, and trauma can result in prolonged deprivation of tissue oxygen, converting cellular metabolism to anaerobic pathways. Reperfusion, and consequently the restoration of oxygen delivery, lead to liver injury. This phenomenon is known as I/R injury, which impairs liver regeneration.[323] The first clinical attempt to minimize ischemic injury during liver resection was performed by interrupting long ischemic intervals with multiple short periods of reperfusion.[324] The protective effect of ischemic preconditioning (IPC) involves many different mechanisms, including inhibition of apoptosis and preservation of cellular ATP content in patients undergoing major liver resection.[325,326] A recent cDNA microarray study in humans demonstrated that IPC triggers the overexpression of IL-1Ra, iNOS, and *Bcl-2*, which counteracts the ischemia-induced proinflammatory and proapoptotic activation.[327] IPC has also been described as promoting liver regeneration via the upregulation of cytokines, such as TNF-α, IL-6, and various heat shock proteins (HSPs), and the downregulation of TGF-β.[328] IPC by 10 minutes of portal triad inflow occlusion and 10 minutes of reperfusion was shown to be effective both in liver resection, particularly in patients with mild to moderate steatosis,[325] and liver transplantation.[329,330] There was no difference in protecting potential between intermittent clamping (15 minutes ischemia and five reperfusion) or IPC with subsequent inflow occlusion for a maximum of 75 minutes, except for patients over 65 years of age, who benefited more from intermittent clamping to attenuate liver injury. Pharmacologic induction of HSPs could play a beneficial role in the recovery of liver function after hepatectomy, but clinical trials have not yet been conducted.

Regenerative Potential of the Liver After Chemotherapy

As previously discussed, an increasing number of patients with tumors undergo extensive chemotherapy with multiple drugs before surgery (see Chapters 69 and 98). The complication rate and mortality after major liver resection is increased in those patients compared with patients who are not receiving these drugs.[228,229] The deleterious effect of chemotherapy on regeneration seems to increase with the total number of cycles given and shows a sharp rise after five courses.[331] Therefore we advocate no more than six cycles of FOLFOX/FOLFIRI (5-FU, Leukovorin, Oxaliplatin/Irinotecan) containing chemotherapy before liver resection with three weeks in between. The anti-VEGF monoclonal bevacizumab has a long half-life and theoretically should be stopped six to eight weeks before surgery, necessitating close collaboration with the medical oncologist in the timing of surgery. Results from PVE before major liver resection under continuous bevacizumab, however, showed no deterioration in increase in FLR volume four weeks after PVE.[238] Recently significantly impaired hypertrophy was reported in the same situation,[332] but this may also be attributed to extensive concomitant chemotherapy.[333] Thus the optimal window between the completion of bevacizumab and surgery remains uncertain.[2]

Regeneration and Harnessing Inflammation

Liver regeneration involves an intricate play between many factors, especially ECM components and inflammatory chemokines, also involved in liver damage. Continuous enhancement of ECM and inflammatory chemokines (e.g., in cholestasis) negatively regulate liver regeneration.[334] Upon tissue injury, danger signals (danger-associated molecular patterns [DAMPs]) are released from necrotic hepatocytes, such as high-motility group box 1 (HMGB-1), HSPs, and DNA fragments, and recognized via TLR receptors in resident macrophages (Kupffer cells). Attracted by the release of chemokines and inflammatory cytokines (TNF-α, IL-1β, and IL-6), neutrophils are the first cells to reach inflamed tissues. Armed with a plethora of enzymes, they invade the liver, facilitated by the lack of the common basal lamina and tight junctions of liver sinusoidal endothelial cells (LSECs), and find easy passage to the Disse space.[335] During normal liver regeneration, neutrophils have crucial functions in liver repair by promoting the phenotypic conversion of proinflammatory monocytes/macrophages to proresolving macrophages, involving ROS, granulocyte colony-stimulating factor, and NADPH oxidase 2 (Nox2).[336]

Balancing the positive and negative effects of the inflammatory reaction is key for the outcome of liver regeneration in inflammatory environments, such as combined I/R injury, cholestasis or postoperative (bacterial) infection in liver resection, and transplantation. The advantages of inflammation in the regenerative process need to be weighed against the disadvantage of uncontrolled inflammation in which friendly inflammatory fire causes more harm than good. The key question is: Which of the known regenerative cytokines or signaling molecules can be harnessed without compromising regeneration? This complex balance becomes clear from evidence that the single perioperative administration of glucocorticoids reduced systemic inflammatory cytokine release (TNF-α and IL-6) and showed benefits in postoperative bilirubin levels and reduced postoperative complications.[337,338] Apparently, the positive effect of steroids to prevent a systemic inflammatory response syndrome (SIRS) outweighed the risk of abolishing the onset of liver regeneration.[339]

NEW HORIZONS AND FUTURE PERSPECTIVES

Therapeutic Use of Stem Cells

In addition to hepatocyte proliferation and hepatic progenitor cells in liver regeneration, bone marrow (BM)–derived cells have the ability to engraft as hepatocytes.[340–342] In the discussion of the mechanism whereby the hematopoietic stem cells acquire a hepatocyte phenotype, both fusion of stem cells and hepatocytes[343,344] and transdifferentiation of stem cells into hepatocytes have been proven.[345,346] Evidence for BM-to-hepatocyte transition has been demonstrated by analyzing liver samples after male-to-female BM transplantation in rodents and humans.[347–349] Estimates of repopulation by hematopoietic stem cells vary from 0.01% up to 40% but are often overestimated.[350]

The highest levels of BM-derived hepatocytes were found in humans with severe liver disease, suggesting that tissue damage may promote engraftment as hepatocytes. The major fraction of mobilized BM stem cells expresses the chemokine receptor CXCR4. At the same time, the mRNA level of its ligand (SDF-1) is increased in the damaged liver tissue. These results provide a clue that CXCR4/SDF-1 interaction may be important for the mobilization of progenitor stem cells from BM to the damaged liver.[351]

Clinically, the release of adult stem cells from BM was demonstrated after partial liver resection for benign and malignant conditions[352,353] and BM-derived stem cells increased the regeneration of contralateral liver after clinical PVE 2.5-fold.[354] Additional studies report that mesenchymal stem cells (MSCs) also promote liver repair in cases of liver damage.[341] MSCs, isolated from human umbilical cords,[355] adipose tissue,[356], BM,[357] or rat BM[358] improved the liver function of rodents undergoing acute liver damage (e.g., carbon tetrachloride injections).

The therapeutic effects of MSCs or MSC-derived hepatocytes in liver injury can be explained by three primary mechanisms. First, MSCs generate cells that function as normal hepatocytes after fusing with metabolically defective hepatocytes.[343,348,359] The second mechanism is soluble factors secreted by MSCs in response to acute damage. Infusion of human MSC–conditioned medium into rats treated with D-galactosamine (i.e., acute liver damage) improved liver function after 24 hours,[360,361] with a 90% decrease in apoptosis and a threefold increase in the number of proliferating hepatocytes. The same was shown after 70% hepatectomy, with upregulated hepatic gene expression of cytokines and growth factors relevant for cell proliferation, angiogenesis, and antiinflammatory responses.[362,363]

Finally, the paracrine effects of MSCs may be exerted by sharing of shed microvesicles (MVs).[364] Intercellular exchange of protein and RNA-containing microparticles is an increasingly important mode of cell–cell communication and MSCs may redirect the behavior of differentiated hepatic cells by horizontal transfer of mRNA shuttled by MVs.[365,366]

In the context of disease, infusion of (BM) MSC has shown some beneficial effects in patients with liver failure.[367] In chronic liver failure, some Phase I trials involving the injection of autologous BM cells to cirrhotic patients have reported modest improvements in clinical scores.[368,369] The latest publications in this field indicate that the use of MSCs is safe and has a beneficial effect on liver fibrosis.[370–375]

Future studies should address the number of cells needed to obtain therapeutic effect and the frequency of administration in liver regeneration after liver surgery or transplantation.

Decellularized Hepatic Matrix and Hepatic Tissue Engineering

Because of the shortage of organs for transplant, research on alternate modalities, such as hepatic tissue engineering, has gained momentum. The applications of such engineered organs could be seen not only in the setting of transplantation but also as support for failing liver function after large resections.

An innovative advance in this field has been the realization of an important role of ECM in the maintenance of differentiated hepatocyte phenotype. Recently, strategies were developed to derive intact ECM from a liver using a decellularization process (Fig. 6.6).

This strategy is based on removal of cells from an organ, leaving a complex mixture of structural and functional proteins that constitute the ECM,[376] which is then re-seeded with an appropriate population of cells[377,378] and connected to the blood stream and biliary system. Using the whole organ acellular matrix as a three-dimensional scaffold for seeding hepatocyte-like cells, a fully functional transplantable bioengineered liver graft may become a reality.

One of the major remaining obstacles toward clinical application is now to choose a cell source for liver repopulation. So far, adult primary hepatocytes have been the primary choice, but scarcity of high-quality human hepatocytes limits tissue-engineering applications.

With the advent of technologies enabling reprogramming of adult somatic cells to a pluripotent state (induced pluripotent stem cell [iPS]), it may now become possible to generate the large numbers of inducible human hepatocytes (iHeps) needed to recellularize a liver bioscaffold.[379–385] There is, however, concern about the plasticity of these cells to form bile ducts, a main

hurdle to usefulness in clinically transplantable liver matrix engineering. A solution to this problem may come from recently discovered bipotential liver organoids.[36] These cells are positive for *Lgr5*, the receptor for the Wnt agonist R-spondin. They are able to differentiate into both hepatocytes and cholangiocytes, as precursors of bile ducts, depending on culture media composition. Recently these organoids were shown to be able to activate the regenerative program through the transcriptional regulation of stem-cell genes and regenerative pathways, including the YAP-Hippo signaling pathway.[386]

The intricate spatiotemporal environment of a decellularized liver matrix, with additional use of nonparenchymal cells of the liver, may provide the ideal niche for functional differentiation of such organoids. This is truly an evolving and timely field with much ongoing research in which knowledge of liver regeneration is crucial, and partnership between clinical scientists and bioengineers is essential.

The Role of miRNA in Liver Regeneration

A family of tiny regulatory RNAs, known as microRNAs (miRNAs), was found to have profound roles in the control of diverse aspects of hepatic function and dysfunction, including hepatocyte growth, stress response, metabolism, viral infection and proliferation, gene expression, and maintenance of hepatic phenotype.[387,388] miRNAs are small endogenous noncoding RNAs that post-transcriptionally repress the expression of protein-coding genes by base-pairing with the 39 untranslated regions (UTRs) of the target messenger RNAs.[389,390]

In 2002, miR-122 was identified as an abundant miRNA in the liver[391] and characterized as the most frequent miRNA isolated in the adult liver.[392] Using distinct protocols to silence miR-122, evidence for the overall importance of miR-122 in the regulation of liver metabolism was found.[393,394] Silencing miR-122 in high-fat fed mice resulted in a significant reduction of hepatic steatosis, which was associated with reduced cholesterol synthesis rates and stimulation of hepatic fatty-acid oxidation. The clinical relevance of miRNAs was shown in differences in spontaneous recovery from acute liver failure. Patients with spontaneous recovery from acute liver failure showed significantly higher serum levels of miR-122 and liver tissue levels compared with nonrecovered patients, with strong downregulation of miRNA target genes that impair liver regeneration, including heme oxygenase-1, programmed cell death 4, and the cyclin-dependent kinase inhibitors p21, p27, and p57.[395]

After partial liver resection, miR-122 and miR-21 are upregulated, but other miRs are downregulated: miR-22a, miR-26a, miR-30b, miR378, Let-7f, and Let-7g. Inhibition of miR33 improves liver regeneration after PHx in mice, indicating that miRNAs are critical regulators of hepatocyte proliferation during liver regeneration.[396–399] Also in liver transplantation, distinct patterns of successful and failed regeneration could be discerned, with inhibition of miRNA 150, 663, and 503 being associated with successful regeneration.[400]

SUMMARY

In the last century, knowledge about liver regeneration has rapidly evolved from a truly mythical black box event into a growing understanding of the pathways involved in this amazingly complex multistep process. Much has been learned

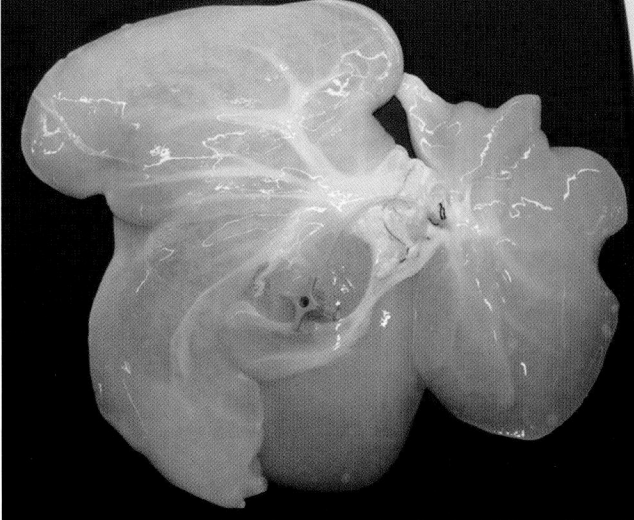

FIGURE 6.6 Decellularized liver scaffold. A pig liver was treated with 4% Triton X-100 and 0.1% NH$_3$ for approximately 16 hours at a low flow rate of 60 mL/min. Vascular structures such as the vena cava retain their strength, whereas the liver extracellular matrix is totally disposed of all cell types.

about the dynamics and redundant intracellular signaling pathways of liver regeneration, but less is still known about the exact signals that initiate and stop liver regeneration. Our advanced knowledge on liver regeneration and prevention of liver failure have led to safer extreme liver resections for benign and malignant diseases and the use of living liver donors in liver transplantation.

Despite our better understanding, there has been little structured advance in therapeutic options in cases of liver failure caused by insufficient liver regeneration. New challenges lie ahead in the use of therapeutic strategies to enhance liver regeneration in patients in whom normal regeneration fails. This will push the possibilities of liver resection to the next level. Furthermore, while promoting liver cell proliferation, we must be very cautious not to stimulate tumor growth in patients with primary or metastatic liver tumors as a consequence of our therapy.

The references for this chapter can be found online by accessing the accompanying Expert Consult website.

CHAPTER 7

Liver fibrogenesis: Mechanisms and clinical relevance

Scott L. Friedman

Liver fibrosis represents a scarring response to either acute or chronic liver injury. After acute liver injury, parenchymal cells regenerate to successfully preserve hepatocellular mass and function. This acute process is associated with an inflammatory and fibrogenic response but with limited deposition of extracellular matrix (ECM). In contrast, prolonged liver injury leads to sustained production of growth factors, proteolytic enzymes, angiogenic factors, and fibrogenic cytokines. These events culminate in the accumulation of ECM, forming septa that coalesce into broad bands of scar tissue encircling nodules of hepatocytes and leading to altered microvascular structure[1,2] (Fig. 7.1). This late stage of fibrosis, termed *cirrhosis*, ultimately impairs liver function and leads to portal hypertension and its complications, including ascites, encephalopathy, and hepatocellular carcinoma, or primary liver cancer (see Chapters 74 and 79).

Typically, progression of fibrosis to cirrhosis evolves for decades before clinical events ensue, but disease may progress more rapidly after repeated episodes of severe acute alcoholic hepatitis and subfulminant hepatitis (especially because of drug toxicity). In addition, there have been reports of rapidly progressive acute hepatitis C virus (HCV) with fibrosis in men coinfected with human immunodeficiency virus (HIV),[3] a syndrome that has become much rarer, with good control of HIV using highly active antiretroviral therapies.[4]

Genetic and environmental factors also influence the course of liver diseases. For example, in HCV infection, polymorphisms in a number of candidate genes involving the inflammatory (e.g., Toll-like receptor 4 [TLR4])[5] or the immune[6] responses may influence the progression of liver fibrosis in humans. Although genetic polymorphisms in these and other pathways have been linked to progression risk in HCV, they have become far less relevant with the development of direct-acting antiviral drugs that cure the infection in more than 95% of patients, regardless of the disease stage or risk factors.[7] Unfortunately, the development of a similar genetic risk score for nonalcoholic fatty liver disease (NAFLD) has been elusive, possibly because the disease is more heterogeneous. Nonetheless, genetic determinants have been identified that influence the risk and severity of NAFLD[8] (see Chapter 69).

The main etiologies of liver fibrosis in Western countries are chronic HCV and hepatitis B virus (HBV) infection, alcohol abuse, and nonalcoholic steatohepatitis (NASH; see Chapters 68 and 69). As a generalized tissue response to chronic injury, fibrosis also occurs in many other organs (heart, lung, kidneys) and typically represents the result of an ongoing inflammation. Remarkably, as many as 45% of all deaths are related to some kind of fibrosis,[9] which underscores the importance of this response and explains the growing interest in this field of research. For decades, fibrosis was considered an irreversible disease that progresses to cirrhosis with a greater risk for hepatocellular carcinoma and with development of liver failure. This meant that the only potential treatment for liver fibrosis was liver transplantation once cirrhosis was present.

Research during the past 35 years has yielded increasing insight into the cellular and molecular mechanisms of this disease, uncovering an orchestrated pathophysiology, identifying the hepatic stellate cell (HSC) as the central cell type in fibrogenesis,[10] and, most importantly, revealing the potential reversibility of the disease and the hope for effective antifibrotic drugs.

MOLECULAR AND CELLULAR MECHANISMS OF FIBROSIS

The anatomic arrangement of the parenchymal and nonparenchymal cells of the liver contributes to its unique role as an immune organ and helps explain how the liver responds to an insult. The liver is composed primarily of epithelial cells (hepatocytes and cholangiocytes), as well as resident nonparenchymal cells that include resident hepatic macrophages (Kupffer cells), sinusoidal endothelium, and HSCs. In addition to Kupffer cells, several specialized immune cells have been characterized, including dendritic cells, natural killer (NK) cells, and natural killer T (NKT) cells, which reveal that the liver represents a key organ in the regulation of innate immunity[11,12] (see Chapter 10).

The liver capsule extends as septae into the liver, delineating hepatic lobules that form the structural units of the liver. The lobule forms a hexagonal structure with portal triads (including branches of the hepatic portal vein, the hepatic artery, and the bile duct) localized in the periphery of the lobule and with a portal vein branch in the center (see Fig. 7.1; see Chapter 5). Hepatocyte plates radiate outward from the central vein and are separated from each other by sinusoids. The latter form the connecting element between the branches of the hepatic portal veins and hepatic arteries with the central vein. Kupffer cells, NK cells, NKT cells, and dendritic cells, all of which are important components of the innate immune system, reside in the hepatic sinusoids. The subendothelial space between the sinusoidal endothelium and hepatocytes is also termed the *space of Disse*. Thus the HSCs, which lie in the space of Disse, have direct contact with endothelial cells and hepatocytes. Sinusoidal endothelial cells are highly fenestrated, which allows for unimpeded flow of plasma from sinusoidal blood into the space of Disse. Through this arrangement, hepatocytes and HSCs are exposed directly to plasma derived largely from venous blood draining the intestine.

Common Triggers of Hepatic Fibrogenesis

Ongoing insult to the liver will lead to an increased inflammatory state with activation of HSCs, which ultimately tilts the profibrotic and antifibrotic balance toward fibrosis. Viral infection, reactive oxygen species (ROS), endoplasmic reticulum stress with protein misfolding,[13] damage associated molecular patterns (DAMPs), pathogen-associated molecular patterns,[14] and bile acids are among the most common stress signals for the

Normal liver

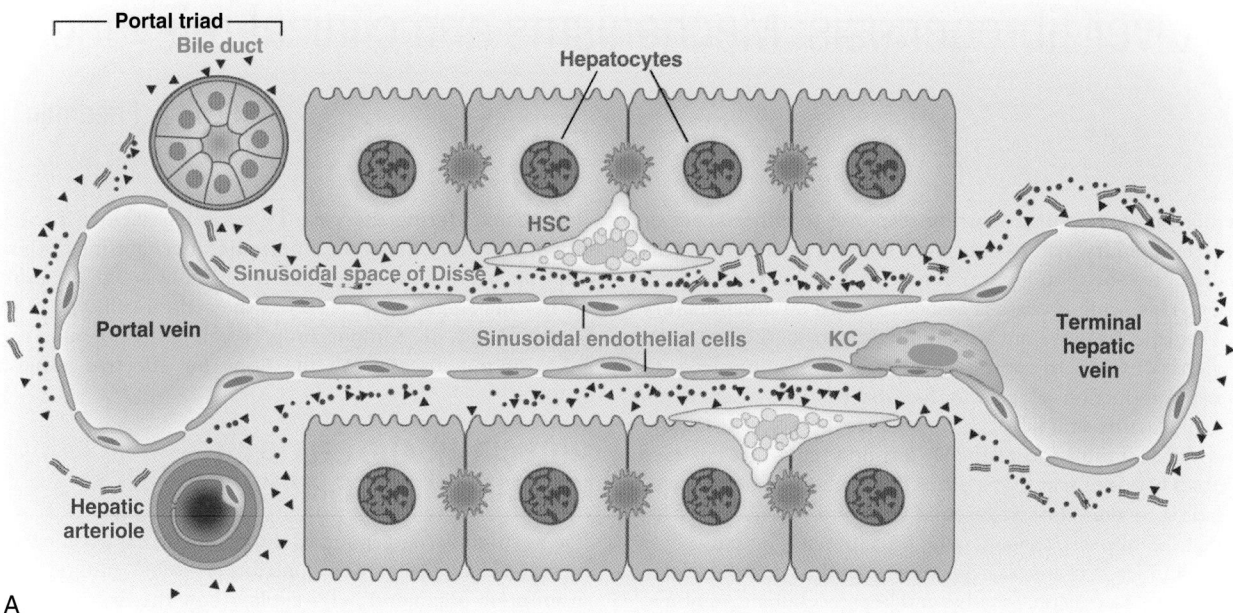

A

Fibrotic liver

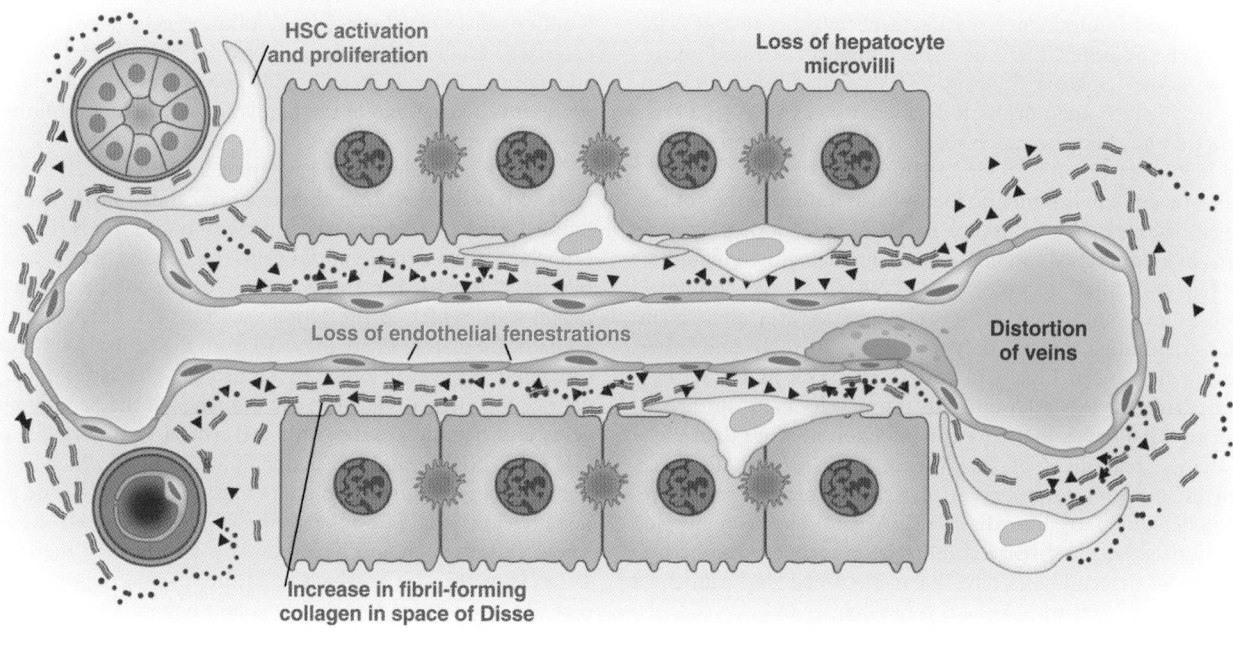

B

⸺ ⸺ ⸺ Fibril-forming collagens (types I, III,V)

∴∵∷ Basement membrane collagens (types IV,VI)

▼▶◀▲ Glycoconjugates (laminin, fibronectin, glycosaminoglycans, tenascin)

FIGURE 7.1 **Matrix and cellular alteration in hepatic fibrosis.** Normal liver parenchyma contains epithelial cells (hepatocytes) and nonparenchymal cells: fenestrated sinusoidal endothelium, hepatic stellate cells (HSCs), and Kupffer cells (KCs). **A,** Sinusoids are separated from hepatocytes by a low-density basement membrane–like matrix confined to the space of Disse, which ensures metabolic exchange. Upon injury, the HSCs become activated and secrete large amounts of extracellular matrix (ECM), resulting in progressive thickening of the septa. **B,** Deposition of ECM in the space of Disse leads to the loss of both endothelial fenestrations and hepatocyte microvilli, which results in both the impairment of normal bidirectional metabolic exchange between portal venous flow and hepatocytes and the development of portal hypertension. (From Hernandez-Gea V, Friedman SL. Pathogenesis of liver fibrosis, *Annu Rev Pathol* 2011;6:425–456.)

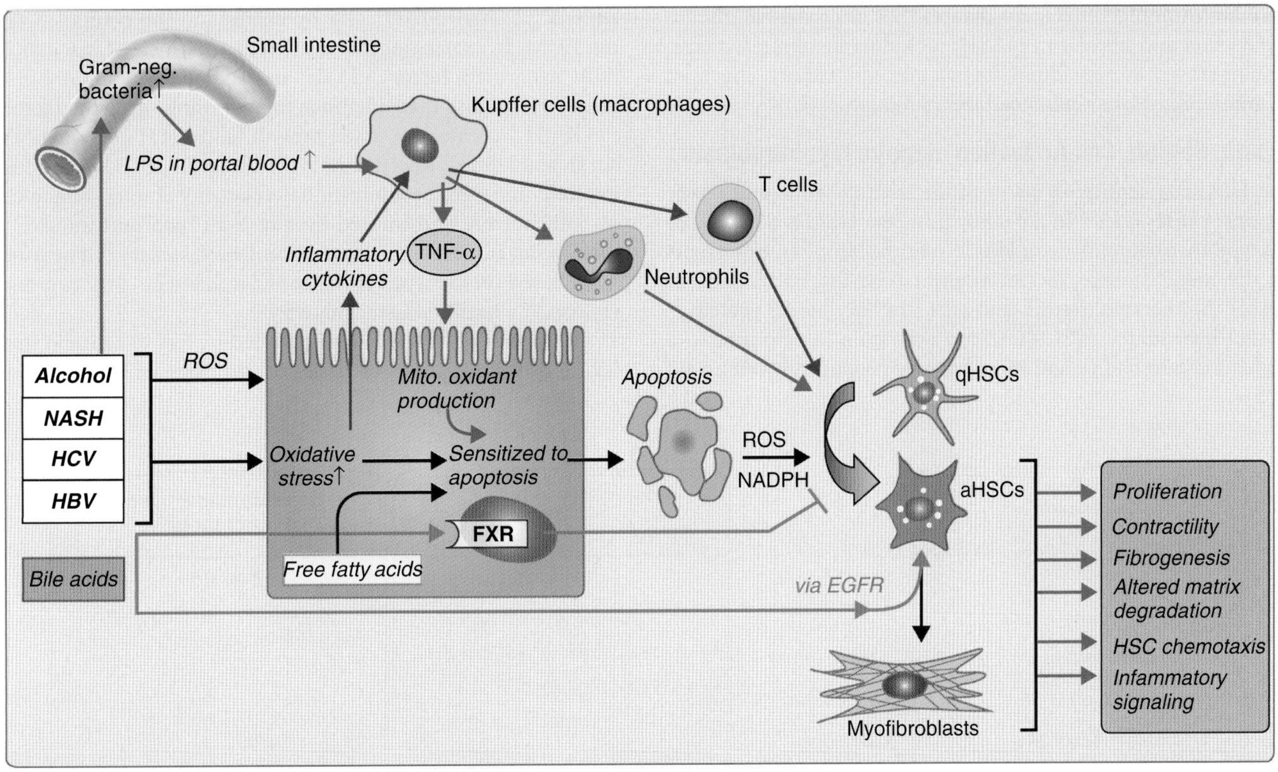

FIGURE 7.2 **Pathways of cellular injury and fibrosis.** This diagram depicts the key pathways of cellular injury and fibrosis. The main causes of chronic liver injury are alcohol, nonalcoholic steatohepatitis (NASH), viral infection, and injury from bile acids in cholestatic conditions. All factors activate hepatic stellate cells (HSCs), which is a key event in liver fibrogenesis. Alcohol can promote gram-negative bacterial overgrowth of the small intestine and/or reduced gut integrity, thereby increasing lipopolysaccharide (LPS) in the portal blood. LPS activates Kupffer cells (hepatic macrophages), which increase the mitochondrial oxidant production in hepatocytes by way of tumor necrosis factor-α (TNF-α), thereby sensitizing them to apoptosis. Kupffer cells also promote local accumulation of T cells and neutrophils, which, along with apoptotic hepatocytes, stimulate the activation of HSCs. Damage to hepatocytes by NASH or infection with hepatitis B or C viruses (HBV, HCV) promotes oxidative stress, further sensitizing hepatocytes to apoptosis. Free fatty acids also increase the intracellular oxidative stress of hepatocytes. Bile acids inhibit activation of HSCs via a farnesoid X receptor (FXR) pathway. *aHSCs,* Activated HSCs; *EGFR,* endothelial growth factor receptor; *ERK-1,* extracellular signal-regulated kinase-1; *mito.,* mitochondrial; *NADPH,* reduced nicotinamide adenine dinucleotide phosphate; *qHSCs,* quiescent HSCs; *ROS,* reactive oxygen species; *TNF-α,* tumor necrosis factor-α.

liver (Fig. 7.2). Additionally, free cholesterol promotes fibrogenesis by indirect activation of HSCs,[15] which may be relevant to the pathogenesis of NAFLD (see Chapter 69).

In alcoholic liver disease, ethanol decreases gut motility, increases epithelial permeability, and promotes overgrowth of gram-negative bacteria. Consequently, lipopolysaccharide (LPS) concentration is elevated in portal blood, through the TLR4 signaling complex, to generate ROS via reduced nicotinamide adenine dinucleotide phosphate (NADPH) oxidase.[16-19] Oxidants then upregulate nuclear factor kappa B (NF-κB) in Kupffer cells, which leads to increased tumor necrosis factor-α (TNF-α) production (see Fig. 7.2). In turn, TNF-α induces neutrophil infiltration and stimulates mitochondrial oxidant production in hepatocytes, which are then sensitized to undergo apoptosis. Furthermore, ROS and acetaldehyde, the main degradation product of alcohol, both activate HSCs and stimulate inflammatory signals. Interestingly, many of the same gut defects in alcoholic liver disease are now also implicated in NASH, with additional focus on the nature of the microbiome as well as the integrity of the gut mucosa as determinants of this disease.[8,20-22]

Bile acids are hepatotoxic agents and typically target hepatocytes but may also injure biliary epithelium.[23] In addition to their potential role in provoking damage, bile acids are also ligands for nuclear receptors, in particular the farnesoid X receptor (FXR), which drives an entire cellular program that can alter hepatocellular metabolism and bile secretion and composition.[24] Remarkably, the therapeutic benefit of vertical sleeve gastrectomy has also been ascribed to FXR signaling in an animal model, raising the possibility that intestinal FXR alone may be sufficient to drive weight loss and improve metabolic parameters in NASH.[25,26]

Oxidant stress, mediated by ROS, is a common mediator of injury in many liver diseases in which damaged hepatocytes become apoptotic or necrotic, thereby releasing ROS[27] and NADPH oxidase, which both activate HSCs.[28] Injured hepatocytes also release inflammatory cytokines and soluble factors that activate Kupffer cells and stimulate the recruitment of activated T cells. This inflammatory milieu further stimulates the activation of resident HSCs.

NAFLD is increasingly prevalent because of increased rates of childhood and adult obesity in the United States and Western Europe[29] (see Chapter 69). In fact, the percentage of liver transplantations performed for this indication is rapidly rising and is overtaking viral hepatitis not only because of curative antiviral therapy for HCV but also because of the rising prevalence of metabolic syndrome, which predisposes to NAFLD.[30] NAFLD can progress to NASH, with consequent fibrosis and cirrhosis.[22] Although a hierarchy of disease causality is still lacking, there are multiple convergent defects that clearly drive disease progression and fibrosis in NASH, including insulin resistance, oxidant stress, altered adipokine balance, lipotoxicity, effects of the microbiome, and enhanced inflammation.[21,22,31,32]

Hepatic Stellate Cell Activation: Hepatic Myofibroblasts

The HSC is a central regulator of the liver's fibrotic and repair responses (Fig. 7.3).[10] In a healthy liver, the HSC is a quiescent cell type that contains cytoplasmic retinoid droplets, representing the major storage site for vitamin A in the body, and expresses the markers desmin and glial fibrillary acidic protein.[33] During liver injury, HSCs undergo activation in response to a range of inflammatory and injury signals produced by damaged hepatocytes and biliary cells, by changes in the composition of the ECM, by proangiogenic growth factors such as vascular endothelial growth factor (VEGF) and angiopoietin, and by fibrogenic cytokines that include transforming growth factor-β (TGF-β1), connective tissue growth factor (CTGF), angiotensin II, and leptin.[1] Recent studies using single cell RNA sequencing have uncovered significant heterogeneity among stellate cells in both normal and injured liver in both man and mouse,[34–36] reinforcing earlier studies that documented stellate cell heterogeneity based on the types of intracellular filaments they express as assessed by immunohistochemistry.[37]

Activation of HSCs is accompanied by loss of retinoid droplets and accumulation of α-smooth muscle actin, a myogenic

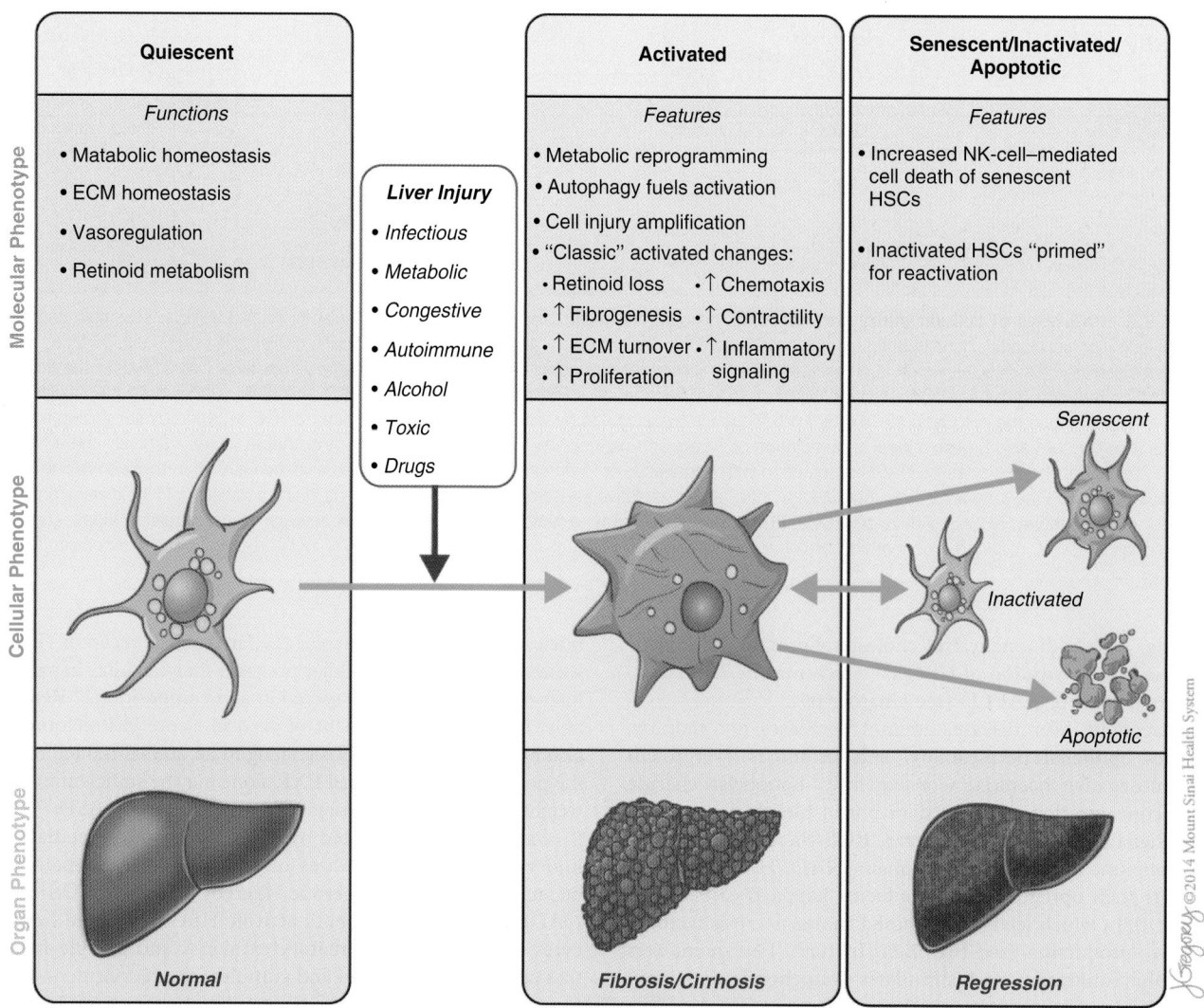

FIGURE 7.3 Functions, features, and phenotypes of hepatic stellate cells in normal and diseased liver. Hepatic stellate cells may exist as several different phenotypes with distinct molecular and cellular functions and features, each of which contributes significantly to liver homeostasis and disease. Quiescent stellate cells are critical to the normal metabolic functioning of the liver. Liver injury provokes transdifferentiation of quiescent stellate cells to their activated phenotype, leading to metabolic reprogramming, increased autophagy to fuel the metabolic demands, amplification of parenchymal injury, and the development of "classic" phenotypic features of activated hepatic stellate cells/myofibroblasts. Through these changes, activated stellate cells drive the fibrotic response to injury and the development of cirrhosis. As liver injury subsides, activated stellate cells can be eliminated by one of three pathways: apoptosis, senescence, or reversion to an inactivated phenotype. Senescent stellate cells are more likely to be cleared by natural killer (NK)-cell–mediated cell death, whereas inactivated stellate cells remain "primed" to respond to further liver injury. This reduction in the number of activated stellate cells contributes to the regression of fibrosis or cirrhosis and repair of the liver in most, but not all, patients. The relative contribution of these three pathways of stellate cell clearance to fibrosis regression is not yet clear. *ECM,* Extracellular matrix; *HSCs,* hepatic stellate cells. (From Lee YM, et al. Pathobiology of liver fibrosis—a translational success story. *Gut* 2015;64:830–841.)

filament that confers increased cellular contractility. Activated HSCs are characteristically positive for α–smooth muscle actin and desmin and are called *hepatic myofibroblasts* (MFB),[33] a cell type that is also characteristic of wound healing in a range of tissues, including the skin, kidney, lung, bone marrow, and pancreas.[9,38–41] The relative importance of each fibrogenic cell type in liver fibrogenesis may depend on the origin of the liver injury. Fate-tracing studies using genetically engineered reporter mice implicate stellate cells as the dominant source of MFBs in parenchymal liver disease[42]; however, a contribution from biliary portal fibroblasts is important in cholestatic liver disease.[43,44]

HSC activation can be divided conceptually into two phases. First there is *initiation*, with early changes in gene expression and phenotype, resulting from paracrine stimulation, primarily because of changes in surrounding ECM, as well as exposure to lipid peroxides and products of damaged hepatocytes. Next there is *perpetuation*, which results from the effects of these stimuli on maintaining the activated phenotype and generating fibrosis. Within the nucleus, a growing number of transcription factors regulate HSC activation, including peroxisome proliferator–activated receptors (PPARs), retinoid receptors, liver X receptor, REV-ERBα, NF-κB, FXR, GATA4, vitamin D receptor, JunD, Kruppel-like factor 6, and FOXF1.[45,46] A number of general and cell type–specific membrane receptors and signaling pathways also control HSC biology, including receptor tyrosine kinases, chemokine receptors, and integrins.[45,47] Not only is HSC activation under transcriptional control, but a growing range of epigenetic changes further regulates this HSC transdifferentiation into myofibroblasts.[48–50]

As previously noted, portal fibroblasts and bone marrow–derived MFBs[51–53] have also been identified as collagen-producing cells in the injured liver, although their overall contribution is minor. Earlier studies implicated epithelial-mesenchymal transition as a source of fibrogenic cells, but more recent findings strongly refute its importance in liver.[54]

Functions of Hepatic Myofibroblasts

Hepatic MFBs have functions that are distinct from their quiescent cells of origin. They are profibrogenic and promitotic, they have a chemotactic and vasoregulatory role, and they control the degradation of ECM. They also have important immune and phagocytic functions.[55–58] The regulation of ECM accumulation and degradation by HSCs is reviewed in the next section.

Fibrogenesis

The major profibrogenic signal in liver is the cytokine TGF-β1. TGF-β1 is secreted mainly by MFBs[59] but also by platelets cells[60] and liver macrophages.[61] It functions by activating the type II TGF-β receptor, which recruits the type I TGF-β receptor. SMAD2 and SMAD3 then associate with the TGF-β1 receptor, are phosphorylated, and recruit SMAD4. This triheteromeric complex then translocates to the nucleus, where it activates profibrogenic transcription factors.[62] TGF-β also activates the mitogen-activated protein kinase (MAPK) p38 pathway, which stimulates additional SMAD-independent collagen type 1 synthesis[62] and, in contrast to the SMAD-dependent collagen type 1 synthesis, also leads to a post-transcriptionally regulated stabilization of the collagen type 1 messenger RNA (mRNA).[63] Local activation of TGF-β1 at the cell surface by integrins has led to the prospect of antagonizing integrins as an antifibrotic therapy.[64] In addition to TGF-β1, CTGF[65] and

Hedgehog signaling have also been implicated as important fibrogenic mediators in liver injury and repair.[66,67]

Proliferation

The predominant stimulus to MFB proliferation is the mitogen platelet-derived growth factor (PDGF)[68] in addition to other mitogens, including epidermal growth factor, VEGF, and fibroblast growth factor.[47] All pathways downstream of the β-PDGF receptor, the key receptor isoform in HSCs, promote proliferation. First, c-Jun N-terminal kinase is stimulated through MAPK; second, PDGF receptor stimulates the RAS/RAF complex, followed by mitogen-induced extracellular kinase and extracellular signal-regulated kinase engagement; and third, the PI3K pathway is activated, leading to AKT (protein kinase B) activation and phosphorylation of the 70S6 kinase.[68]

Immunoregulation

The liver is a microenvironment of diminished immunogenicity, which is necessary to cope with the high exposure of antigens from the portal vein[69,70] (see Chapter 10). This feature also accounts for the tolerance of liver transplantation across ABO barriers and may contribute to the chronic nature of HBV or HCV, in which the virus persists despite the development of an immune response. Upon entry of the antigen to the sinusoid, classic antigen-presenting cells (Kupffer cells, dendritic cells) are first encountered. Subsequently, HSCs in the space of Disse may contact antigens.[58] Indeed, HSCs display a wide range of immunoregulatory functions and are an essential part of the liver's immune response.[56,57]

Hepatic MFBs produce a range of proinflammatory and antiinflammatory cytokines (see Chapter 10) and recruit lymphocytes through secretion of chemokines (monocyte chemoattractant protein-1, interleukin-8 [IL-8], C-C chemokine 21 [CCL21], regulated on activation, normal T-cell expressed and secreted [RANTES], C-C chemokine receptor 5 [CCR5]),[71–73] thus amplifying the inflammatory response. Nevertheless, upon activation, they exert a profound immunosuppressive activity by inducing T-cell apoptosis.[74] In the setting of liver transplantation, MFB can induce T-cell apoptosis via programmed death ligand-1[74] and may foster local immunotolerance of the liver. In liver fibrosis, MFBs may further regulate the contribution of lymphocytes to the course of hepatic fibrosis by ingesting disease-associated lymphocytes[75] or by activating in response to engulfment of apoptotic bodies.[76]

The interaction between HSCs and immune cells is bidirectional. T cells activate HSCs by interferon-γ (IFN-γ), which upregulates both stimulatory (CD80, CD86, CD54) and inhibitory (B7-H1) surface molecules and enhances both inflammatory and suppressive cytokines. The inhibitory molecules, however, are thought to override the stimulatory counterparts, resulting in immunosuppression. Lymphocytes can also mediate hepatic fibrosis by activating HSCs. CD8-positive T lymphocytes are more fibrogenic toward stellate cells than CD4 T lymphocytes.[55] This may explain, in part, why patients co-infected with untreated HIV and HCV have accelerated fibrosis because their CD4:CD8 cell ratios are reduced. Of the CD4-positive T lymphocytes, previously called T-helper cells, the humoral immunity mediated by T-helper 2 cells (Th2) is profibrogenic in liver injury, whereas the cell-mediated immunity by the Th1 cells via IFN-γ, TNF-α, and IL-2 is antifibrogenic.[77]

HSCs can also function as antigen-presenting cells.[58] They can interact with bacterial LPS directly via TLR4, which amplifies their activation. TLR4 signaling leads to downregulation of a TGF-β pseudoreceptor, BMP (bone morphogenic protein), and activin membrane-bound inhibitor, which thereby amplifies fibrogenic activity of MFBs.[78] Signaling through TLR4 may be elicited not only by exogenous ligands, including LPS, but also by endogenous ligands, including high-mobility group box 1 protein.[79] The discovery of endogenous ligands for TLR4 has been part of a larger recognition that many cells, including HSCs, possess an intracellular complex known as the *inflammasome*, which transduces signals arising from cellular damage.[80-82] The inflammasome is especially pertinent to understanding the pathogenesis of inflammation and fibrosis in NAFLD and NASH.

Vasoregulation

MFBs play an important role in the regulation of sinusoidal blood flow and may contribute to portal hypertension that is characteristic of advanced liver disease (see Chapter 74). The release of endothelin-1 (ET-1) can stimulate their contraction through the endothelin type A (ETA) receptor,[83] thereby promoting tissue contraction, increasing portal resistance, and generating portal hypertension. On the other hand, MFBs and endothelial cells also secrete nitric oxide (NO), which is the physiologic antagonist of ET-1.[84]

Structural Features of Hepatic Fibrogenesis

In hepatic fibrosis, the total amount of collagen is increased up to sixfold, whereas the parenchymal mass (e.g., hepatocytes) is progressively diminished (see Chapter 74). The composition of the ECM changes with progression of disease (see Fig. 7.1). Collagen type IV in the space of Disse is replaced by interstitial, or fibrillar, collagens, primarily types I and III. Additionally, the discontinuous basal membrane beneath the sinusoidal endothelial cells is replaced by a continuous basement membrane, and sinusoidal fenestrations are reduced. This decreased porosity (also known as *capillarization*), combined with perisinusoidal fibrosis, scar contraction, and formation of intrahepatic shunts, contribute to increased hepatic venous pressure and portal hypertension. Fibrillar collagens that are produced by MFBs also interact with MFBs via discoidin domain receptors and integrins,[85] thereby inhibiting apoptosis and increasing MFB proliferation.

With the maturation of the fibrotic scar, not only is the amount of collagen increased, but the scar also becomes increasingly insoluble through chemical cross-linking by lysyl oxidase 2 (LOXL2), tissue transglutaminase, and a disintegrin and metalloproteinase with thrombospondin-type repeats metalloproteinase with thrombosponin type I motif (ADAMTS2).[86] Indeed, HSCs are an important source of these cross-linking enzymes.[87] Cross-linking makes the fibrous septa progressively resistant to proteolysis by matrix metalloproteinases (MMPs). The longstanding clinical dogma that the slower the pace of injury, the less reversible the scar, is supported by animal studies in which even advanced fibrosis of short duration is reversible. Thus the reversibility of a scar may be limited primarily by the extent of collagen cross-linking. Clinically, increased septal thickness and smaller nodule size as assessed by liver biopsy, both of which reflect more advanced stages of fibrosis, are significant predictors of worse clinical outcomes.[88] Efforts to therapeutically increase the solubility of collagen have tested an antibody to LOXL2, which has marked antifibrotic effects in animal models of fibrosis in liver and other organs.[89] These findings led to its evaluation in clinical trials to treat fibrosis and cancer, which unfortunately showed no efficacy. These negative

results may indicate a lack of sufficient penetration of the antibody to sites of cross-linking rather than disproving the role of LOXL2 in matrix homeostasis, however.

Regulation of Collagen Deposition and Degradation

The deposition and degradation of collagen are tightly regulated. MMPs are the key enzymes that degrade fibrillar collagens (collagen types I and III) and noncollagenous ECM substrates.[90] The tissue inhibitor metalloproteinases (TIMPs) are their major antagonists by inactivating proteases and by inhibiting MFB apoptosis.[91]

Both altered levels of interstitial collagenases and increased levels of MMP inhibitors in liver injury create an imbalance that favors reduced degradation of fibrillar collagens in hepatic fibrosis. The interstitial collagenases MMP-1, MT1-MMP, MMP-8, and MMP-13 in humans and MMP-13 in rodents unwind the triple-helical collagen type I, which is the principal collagen in the fibrotic liver, so that each α-chain is presented to the active site of the enzyme that cleaves the collagen.[90] Other MMPs (e.g., MMP-2) cannot unwind the triple-helical collagen and thus cannot degrade intact collagen type I alone. In early liver injury, MMP-2 degrades the low-density basement membrane present in the subendothelial space.[92] Its replacement with fibril-forming matrix impairs hepatocyte differentiation and function. During progressive fibrosis, expression of MMP-1 (humans) or MMP-13 (rodents) is decreased, and MMP-2 expression increases.[64] In parallel, the expression of TIMP-1 and TIMP-2, which inhibit the collagen-degrading MMPs, is increased.[93,94] Matrix type 1 metalloproteinase (MT1-MMP) is another interstitial collagenase whose contribution to overall matrix degradation in liver has not been established.[95]

Hepatic macrophages are key cellular determinants of matrix degradation, with some contribution by dendritic and other inflammatory cells.[96] In mouse models, macrophages augment fibrogenesis during progression of liver fibrosis, whereas during resolution, they hasten matrix degradation through increased production of MMP-13.[97] More importantly, there is substantial heterogeneity of macrophages in liver injury and resolution to account for these divergent activities, with a subset known as Ly6C[lo] cells implicated in degrading matrix during fibrosis regression.[82,98,99] Despite these major advances in identifying the key fibrolytic cell in liver fibrosis regression, it is not clear which is the major interstitial collagenase in fibrosis regression because MMP-1 is only expressed at low levels in liver. As noted, other interstitial collagenases may be more important in ECM degradation.

DIAGNOSIS AND CLINICAL MONITORING OF HEPATIC FIBROSIS

Many patients with chronic liver disease may initially present with late-stage fibrosis because earlier stages are often asymptomatic. Thus clinicians must have a high index of suspicion for occult fibrosis, especially in patients with unexplained elevations of liver enzymes, splenic enlargement, stigmata of liver disease, and/or laboratory or imaging findings suggestive of portal hypertension (see Chapter 77).

When chronic liver disease is suspected, the liver biopsy remains the gold standard for diagnosing and staging liver fibrosis. However, it is an invasive procedure with risk of adverse events and, equally important, a high likelihood of sampling variability,[100,101] as well as inter- and intra-pathologist variability.[100]

At least one third of biopsies may differ by one fibrosis stage between the right and left hepatic lobes in HCV[102] and NAFLD.[101] Smaller biopsy specimens are associated with an increase in reported diagnoses of mild and moderate fibrosis at the cost of more severe fibrosis, representing an understaging of fibrosis.[100]

There are several commonly used histologic staging systems for fibrosis (see Chapter 74). The Histology Activity Index score reported by Knodell includes three stages,[103] whereas the Ishak score differentiates six stages, including two stages of cirrhosis ("incomplete" and "complete" cirrhosis).[104] The METAVIR score (an acronym derived from a French Investigator group) is a simple, widely applied five-stage scoring system[105] that is the most commonly used worldwide for staging HCV infection. It incorporates the fibrosis scores F0 to F4, and the activity scores A0 to A3, which assess the amount of necroinflammation.

For NAFLD, a separate scoring system for grading inflammation and staging fibrosis has been widely adopted,[106] which captures key histologic features of disease progression that are distinct from viral liver disease (see Chapter 69). Specifically, NAFLD and NASH, as well as alcoholic liver disease, are primarily centrilobular in distribution rather than periportal like viral liver diseases. The NAFLD Brunt/Kleiner stages are stage 0 = no fibrosis, stage 1 = perisinusoidal or periportal fibrosis (1a: mild, zone 3; 1b: moderate, zone 3; 1c: portal/periportal), stage 2 = periportal and perisinusoidal fibrosis, stage 3 = bridging fibrosis, and stage 4 = cirrhosis.

For fibrosis staging, there is increasing reliance on absolute quantification of collagen in liver biopsy samples as assessed by computerized morphometry, instead of using a discontinuous scoring system composed of separate stages. Indeed, collagen proportionate area assessment is far more predictive of clinical outcomes, even in NASH, and therefore its use is rapidly gaining popularity because it is objective and quantitative.[107–109]

There is a great need for reliable, quantitative noninvasive diagnostics for fibrosis, and recent studies indicate progress. Cross-sectional imaging studies such as computed tomography (CT) and magnetic resonance (MR) imaging can demonstrate features of advanced liver disease, such as nodularity and signs of portal hypertension (splenomegaly, enlarged caudate lobe, esophageal varices). Advances in MR methods include MR elastography,[110] MR fat fraction, and other related technologies.[111] There are also efforts to develop newer MR probes that may enable quantification of total liver collagen or elastin content.[112,113]

Biochemical parameters associated with hepatocyte injury (aspartate aminotransferase [AST], alanine aminotransferase [ALT]), cholestatic liver injury (bilirubin, alkaline phosphatase), impaired liver synthetic function (apolipoproteins, cholesterol, coagulation factors, α2-macroglobulin, hyaluronic acid, albumin, globulins), or impaired hepatic clearance of endogenous or exogenous substances from the circulation (bilirubin, bile acid, caffeine, lidocaine metabolites, bromsulphalein, methacetin, indocyanine green, cholate, or ammonia)[114] can provide information on the presence and cause of the disease. These tests all assess impaired liver function in fibrosis and may prove to be more quantitative and sensitive than tests of liver injury or morphology. Indeed, pulmonary function tests (e.g., spirometry) have been a mainstay of clinical assessment in lung disease rather than tissue analysis of lung for decades. Continued progress in using functional rather than structural assessment of liver disease is expected but not yet widely adopted in clinical trials or clinical practice.

Biochemical Tests

A more direct approach incorporates serum molecules associated with fibrosis, including those involved in deposition or degradation of ECM, as well as specific fibrogenic cytokines associated with fibrosis. A number of combination serum tests have been evaluated for predicting fibrosis stage and outcomes, with improving sensitivity and specificity. To date, no single molecule, but rather combinations of different components, demonstrate the best sensitivity and negative predictive values to exclude significant fibrosis.

The most studied combination serum tests are the AST-to-platelet ratio index,[115] the Fibrosis-4 (FIB-4) index,[116] the enhanced liver fibrosis (ELF) test,[117,118] and the FibroTest (FT; Biopredictiv, Paris).[119] Newer biomarker scores include the HepaScore[120] and measurement of collagen propeptides.[111,121] All these biochemical tests range from sufficient to excellent in ruling out significant fibrosis (F3 to F4) when the proper cutoff value is chosen,[118] but they are less useful in distinguishing mild from moderate fibrosis. Ongoing efforts are seeking to combine blood tests with other modalities (e.g., liver stiffness) to enhance their diagnostic accuracy.[122] The sensitivities of the tests vary based on the etiology of the liver disease. A further difficulty of these tests is the absence of an ideal gold standard, in view of the liver biopsy's significant sampling variability and interlaboratory differences. The lack of a true gold standard means that the utility of serum tests can never be fairly evaluated when compared with biopsy.[123]

Overall, the performance of serum markers is approximately comparable.[122] Although it is unlikely that these markers alone will suffice in assessing short-term disease progression in clinical trials of antifibrotic drugs or in management of chronic liver diseases, they do predict long-term outcomes and therefore remain of great interest.[124,125]

Cytokines and Chemokines Associated With Hepatic Fibrosis

Of the cytokines and chemokines that are associated with hepatic fibrosis, TGF-β1 is the dominant stimulus for the production of ECM by HSCs. Hepatic mRNA levels of TGF-β1 are increased in chronic liver disease in association with increases in mRNA levels of type I collagen.[126] TGF-β serum levels not only correlate with fibrosis scores but also may indicate necroinflammation, although their measurement is not sufficiently predictive to be used as a clinical biomarker.

Stiffness Assessments

An alternative approach to fibrosis assessment is the measurement of liver stiffness using a number of devices, the first of which, Fibroscan (FS), uses vibration-controlled transient elastography; other devices that use either vibration controlled– or shear wave elastography[127] are now widely available but have less clinical validation than FS. As noted previously, stiffness can also be assessed by MR elastography, which has the advantage of assessing the entire liver[128] and can be combined with other MR-based methods to assess liver fat content or other imaging characteristics.[129,130]

For FS, the stiffer the liver tissue, the faster a wave propagates. Results are expressed in kilopascals (kPa). With the Fibroscan, the virtual cylinder of tissue that is assessed is at least 200 times larger than a biopsy sample and therefore is far more representative of the hepatic parenchyma. Thus FS may provide a more accurate and reproducible picture of cirrhosis than liver biopsy. There is also potential value to FS in early stages of disease, where fibrosis may be unevenly distributed and thus underestimated by liver biopsy. Furthermore, FS has very low interobserver variability. However, its accuracy is limited in patients with obesity, ascites, or acute hepatitis. FS has been evaluated extensively.[122,131]

It is important to remember that stiffness can arise from edema or inflammation, not only fibrosis, and thus interpretation of the results in the proper clinical context is essential because acute hepatitis can yield stiffness values comparable to cirrhosis. Also, the ability to perform the test and the accuracy of data may be reduced in obese patients, although newer probes can better overcome this problem. When FS has been combined with FT in HCV patients, both tests agreed in 70% to 80% of subjects, with increasing concordance in higher stages of liver fibrosis. Compared with the liver biopsy, results were confirmed in 84% to 94% of cases, with a tendency of FS/FT to underestimate fibrosis.[132] To assist in this effort, an additional technology has been added to FS, called controlled attenuation parameter (CAP score), which can estimate liver fat content and therefore is especially useful in assessing patients with NAFLD or NASH[133] (see Chapter 69).

In patients with more advanced disease, assessment of vascular changes can predict outcomes. Specifically, the measure of the pressure gradient across the liver, or hepatic venous pressure gradient (HVPG), is highly predictive of clinical deterioration.[134] Because the technique cannot be widely replicated in large clinical trials, however, efforts are underway to develop noninvasive imaging approaches that can capture the same information as HVPG without the need for hepatic catheterization.[135]

In aggregate, all these noninvasive approaches can accurately distinguish between patients with little or no fibrosis and those with advanced disease, but they are less reliable at discriminating intermediate stages of fibrosis. They show a high level of variability because of interlaboratory differences, but on the other hand, the patients at risk for false-positive results are well defined. Although the combination of FT, FS, or the ELF panel in NAFLD patients are potential alternatives to liver biopsy, their value in individual patient management still needs to be validated and standardized.[136]

Despite its limitations, to date no single test can match the overall information from liver biopsy histology (inflammation, fibrosis, steatosis, architecture), and thus phase 3 clinical trials testing drugs for fibrosis or NASH still require liver biopsy as an endpoint (see later), although phase 2 proof-of-concept trials may rely on noninvasive markers instead of biopsy. The role of noninvasive alternatives so far lies first in improving the fibrosis staging and grading made from liver biopsies and, second, in reducing the number of liver biopsies by screening patients with abnormal liver tests to identify patients with a higher probability of liver fibrosis who need further evaluation or therapy. There is great interest in establishing the value of noninvasive tests in predicting disease progression or response to therapy by combining serum markers with noninvasive tests of liver function and hepatic blood flow. To date, however, this goal has not fully materialized.

THERAPEUTIC STRATEGIES

The elucidation of pathways of hepatic fibrogenesis has provided a rational framework for developing antifibrotic therapies in chronic liver disease (Fig. 7.4). Methods to attack several points are under development, and it may ultimately be advantageous to combine more than one therapy for maximal efficacy. To date, no antifibrotic therapy has been approved for clinical use, but dozens are currently in clinical trials, primarily for NASH with fibrosis.

Reversibility of Fibrosis: "Point of No Return"

Fibrosis is no longer considered as an irreversible and progressive state in all patients. Liver fibrosis of different etiologies is usually reversible by removing the causative agent.[137] For example, a decrease in the viral load of HBV patients,[138] clearance of HCV with pegylated IFN and ribavirin or direct-acting antivirals,[139] cessation of ethanol intake, weight loss or bariatric surgery in patients with NASH,[140] decreased iron or copper in hemochromatosis or Wilson disease, or immunosuppressive therapy in autoimmune diseases can limit fibrosis progression experimentally and clinically. Even cirrhosis can regress in some patients. In fact, removing the causative agent is still the most effective antifibrotic therapy. As previously noted, efforts to treat fibrosis are focused almost exclusively on NASH because this represents a growing fraction of patients with advanced liver disease, and there are no approved therapies.[22,141]

Although fibrosis, inflammation, and bile duct proliferation decrease when the damaging stimulus is withdrawn, regenerative nodules may become autonomous and grow progressively. This raises a key question of whether there is a "point of no return" for advanced fibrosis, wherein even complete clearance of the underlying disease will no longer yield an improvement. Increased cross-linking of the collagen fibrils over years makes the fibrous septa progressively resistant to proteolysis by metalloproteinases, and hypoxia stimulates secretion of proangiogenic factors by HSCs, such as VEGF and angiopoietin-1, which induce proliferation and motility.[142] However, antagonism of VEGF in particular may be deleterious because it also plays a role in restoration of liver architecture after cessation of experimental liver injury.[143] Overall, as many as 70% of patients with cirrhosis will have regression of fibrosis once the primary etiology is mitigated, but in those in whom the disease still progresses, there may be a positive feedback loop between angiogenesis and fibrogenesis, which persists even when the primary etiology is cleared, leading to sustained abnormalities of the intrahepatic vasculature. The tremendous efficacy of direct-acting antivirals in curing HCV in even advanced patients with cirrhosis provides an opportunity to better refine the "point of no return," but is limited by the fact that biopsies are not routinely performed in patients with a sustained virologic response (i.e., cure of HCV) from these medications.[144] Nonetheless, as we learn more about regression of fibrosis after cure of HCV, it is likely that antifibrotic treatments will be considered for those with HCV cirrhosis who do not show reversibility well after virologic cure (e.g., > 3–5 years).

Prevention of Hepatocyte Apoptosis in Liver Injury

Apoptosis of hepatocytes during liver injury is a proinflammatory event associated with Kupffer cell and HSC activation.[145] In the surgical setting, reduced hepatocyte damage is pursued by decreasing the time of vascular occlusion (Pringle maneuver) during resection or shortening the ischemia-reperfusion time in transplant surgery. Experimental approaches to reduce ischemia-reperfusion injury, (e.g., intermittent clamping or drugs) merit continued development to preserve hepatocyte integrity.

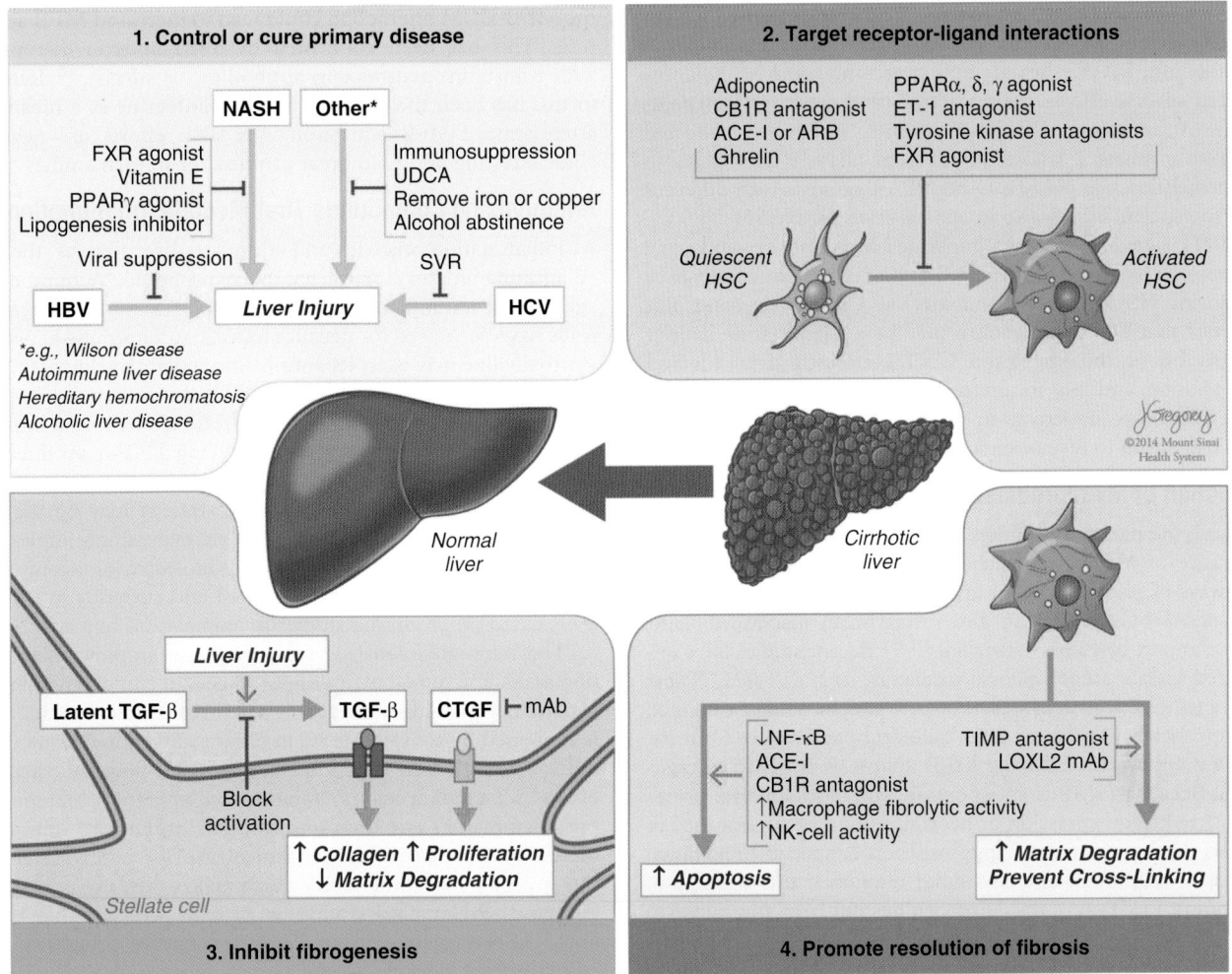

FIGURE 7.4 Mechanisms by which antifibrotic therapies may lead to fibrosis regression. 1. Disease-specific therapies that control or cure the underlying disease are still the most effective antifibrotic approach. **2.** Targeting receptor-ligand interactions with either established or experimental drugs to reduce hepatic stellate cell (HSC) activation will attenuate fibrosis development, with multiple potential strategies under development. **3.** Inhibition of the most potent of the profibrogenic pathways, for example, preventing activation of latent TGF-β, or blocking the activity of CTGF, are among the more promising antifibrotic strategies. **4.** Resolution of fibrosis can be promoted by enhancing the apoptosis of activated hepatic stellate cells either with drugs or through the activity of either NK cells or fibrolytic macrophages, and by increasing degradation of extracellular matrix, or by preventing its cross-linking with antagonists to LOXL2. *ACE-I,* Angiotensin converting enzyme-I inhibitor; *CB1R,* cannabinoid receptor type 1; *CTGF,* connective tissue growth factor; *ET-1,* endothelin 1; *FXR,* farnesoid X receptor; *HBV, HCV,* hepatitis B and C virus, respectively; *LOXL2,* lysyl oxidase 2; *mAb,* monoclonal antibody; *NASH,* nonalcoholic steatohepatitis ; *NF-κB,* nuclear factor kappa B; *NK,* natural killer; *PPAR,* peroxisome proliferator–activated receptor; *SVR,* sustained virologic response; *TGF-β,* transforming growth factor-β; *TIMP,* tissue inhibitor of metalloproteinase; *UDCA,* ursodeoxycholic acid. (From Lee YM, Wallace MC, and Friedman SL. Pathobiology of liver fibrosis—a translational success story, *Gut* 2015;64:830–841.)

Caspase Inhibitors

Apoptosis is a functional antagonist to mitosis. Together they regulate homeostatic cell turnover. The two main pathways of apoptosis are the extrinsic pathway, which is death ligand–death receptor–mediated and is dependent on caspase-8, and the intrinsic pathway, which is regulated by BCL2-induced mitochondrial dysfunction and downstream activation of caspase-9 and its effector caspases: 3, 6, and 7. Caspase inhibitors were developed to minimize apoptotic death of hepatocytes in chronic liver injury by inhibiting the caspases that contribute to the apoptotic cascade, with the lingering concern that such an approach could promote the survival of preneoplastic hepatocytes. Nonetheless, caspase inhibitors have been well tolerated in clinical trials to date but with no clear evidence of efficacy in patients with inflammatory liver diseases or acute-on-chronic liver failure.

Inhibition of Hepatic Stellate Cell Activation or Inactivation of Myofibroblasts

Oxidant stress in the form of ROS released by injured hepatocytes through the action of NADPH oxidase is a potent fibrogenic stimulus. Thus antioxidants, including vitamin E,[146] silymarin, cysteamine,[147] or *S*-adenosyl-l-methionine,[148] may benefit fibrosis, particularly in patients with alcohol-induced liver disease and NASH, in which oxidant stress plays an especially important role. In principle, antioxidants should be efficacious in all inflammatory liver diseases; however, efforts to establish the activity of antioxidants are confounded by the uneven quality of commercially available products, especially as these compounds are typically available over-the-counter and their potency is not monitored.

Given their widespread use in diabetes, PPARγ agonists have been tested in clinical trials both in NASH and HCV, but their activity is modest and is associated with unwanted weight gain, especially in patients with NASH.[146] With an improved formulation, PPARγ ligands may overcome some of their unwanted adverse effects in clinical trials and merit further evaluation. A combined PPARα,δ agonist, elafibranor, showed promise in phase 2 trials,[149] but recent phase 3 data failed to confirm efficacy in NASH. Other PPAR agonists with different subtype specificity are also in clinical trials for NASH.

WNT signaling has been implicated in pulmonary and renal fibrosis and has also been reported to promote hepatic fibrosis by enhancing HSC activation and survival. On the one hand, this suggests that WNT antagonism may be a useful target in liver fibrosis, but on the other hand, WNT is a critical signal for liver regeneration, and thus its antagonism could be deleterious.[150] In fact, efforts are underway to explore the value of therapeutic WNT agonism to reverse cirrhosis and advanced liver disease.

Induction of Myofibroblast Apoptosis

Because the natural resolution of fibrosis leads to apoptosis and clearance of MFBs, approaches that exploit these endogenous pathways of resolution merit attention. In addition to apoptosis, activated HSCs/MFBs can also revert to an inactivated state, driven in part by PPARγ signaling.[151,152] Recent studies have uncovered specific transcriptional regulators, such as Tcf21,[153] that promotes deactivation of stellate cells,[154] which could be exploited therapeutically to promote HSC quiescence and reduce fibrosis.

One approach to driving MFB apoptosis is TIMP antagonism. Because TIMP is antiapoptotic and blocks matrix proteases,[91] reduced expression or neutralization favors clearance of MFBs through increased apoptosis and enhanced breakdown of scar.[155] Although animal studies reinforced this strategy of inhibiting TIMP-1,[156] this approach has not been translated to humans yet.

Delivery to stellate cells of an shRNA to block heat shock protein 47 (hsp47), which is required for proper collagen folding, has been reported in an animal model.[157] Hsp47 inhibition leads to accumulation of misfolded collagen, which promotes HSC apoptosis to reduce the number of fibrogenic cells.[95] A phase 2 trial using this formulation in patients post–HCV SVR is underway, with improvement in histology as the primary endpoint.

There are also receptor-ligand–mediated pathways of MFB apoptosis that are potential therapeutic targets. For example, activation of the cannabinoid 1 (CB1) receptor leads to increased collagen deposition and protects MFB from apoptosis, whereas the CB2 receptor is proapoptotic via induction of intracellular oxidative stress. Correspondingly, CB1 knockout mice or CB1 antagonist–treated mice,[158] as well as CB2 receptor–stimulated mice,[159] display less fibrosis and more MFB apoptosis than control mice after CCl_4 or thioacetamide (TAA) treatment or bile duct ligation (BDL). Also, CB2 knockout mice developed increased fibrosis in a CCl_4 model.[160] Whereas trials of a systemic CB1 receptor antagonist for obesity and NASH were discontinued because of central nervous system (CNS) effects, newer peripheral CB1 antagonists that do not enter the CNS are under development.

Blocking Myofibroblast–Extracellular Matrix Interactions

The ECM and MFBs interact in a positive feedback mechanism that could be amenable to therapeutic antagonism. MFBs interact with ECM via α/β-integrins,[161] thereby decreasing apoptosis and increasing proliferation of MFBs. Thus blocking

the MFB-ECM interaction could lead to increased MFB apoptosis. This has been confirmed by α3β2-integrin disruption with echistatin, neutralizing antibodies, or siRNA.[162] Related to this has been the proposal to block integrins as a means of attenuating TGF-β activation[64,163]; such efforts are nearing clinical testing and hold great promise for human studies.

Antagonizing Compounds That Mediate Inflammation

As inflammation precedes and stimulates liver fibrosis, the use of antiinflammatory drugs has been proposed. A number of agents have antiinflammatory activity. For example, corticosteroids have been used for decades to treat autoimmune hepatitis. Pentoxifylline may exert its antifibrotic activity by downregulating TGF-β1 and CTGF signaling,[164] but it can upregulate TIMP-1, thereby reducing its antifibrotic effect. It also inhibits NF-κB in Kupffer cells, thereby reducing TNF-α production, the impact of which is uncertain.

A more rational antiinflammatory strategy may be the antagonism of chemokines because they are increasingly implicated in human liver disease.[72,73,165] Small-molecule antagonists of chemokine receptors are well tolerated and currently in clinical trials based on promising studies in animals and humans.[166]

The renin-angiotensin system may also amplify inflammation and has assumed major importance in the understanding of hepatic fibrosis. Angiotensin II is a vasoconstrictive peptide that is expressed by activated HSC in chronically injured livers.[167] It induces hepatic inflammation and stimulates fibrogenic actions of HSCs, including cell proliferation, cell migration, secretion of proinflammatory cytokines, and collagen synthesis.[168] Inhibitors of this system have been in clinical use for antihypertensive therapy for a substantial time, which makes their use in humans attractive. Preliminary studies in patients with chronic HCV and NASH suggest a positive effect on fibrosis progression by administering blocking agents, but definitive trials are lacking.

Ursodeoxycholic acid (UDCA) has a beneficial effect on fibrosis in primary biliary cirrhosis. Similarly, a modified derivative of UDCA, nor-UDCA, reduces inflammation, fibrosis, and portal pressure in an animal model.[169] Interestingly, UDCA also activates the pregnane X receptor, which has antifibrotic properties.[170]

More recently, ligands for FXR, another nuclear receptor, have been developed, which are also antifibrotic in animal models and in a Phase 3 clinical trial in NASH[171]; however, these promising results did not yet earn US Food and Drug Administration (FDA) approval.

Selectively Antagonizing Pathways of Hepatic Stellate Cell Activation

Fibrogenic, proliferative, proangiogenic, vasoconstrictive, and proinflammatory mediators work synergistically toward hepatic fibrogenesis in the setting of chronic liver injury. Thus efforts are underway to antagonize the specific mediators driving these pathways.

Multiple approaches have been directed toward blocking the profibrogenic TGF-β signaling pathway. However, systemically blocking the TGF pathway has theoretical limitations, because apart from stimulating wound healing and fibrosis, TGF-β is also a central inhibitor of uncontrolled inflammation and essential in inducing epithelial differentiation and in triggering apoptosis. This raises safety concerns for the general and long-term use of TGF-β inhibition, especially in patients with chronic hepatic inflammation. The use of integrin antagonists that inactivate TGF-β only at the stellate cell surface (see earlier) may mitigate this concern, but clinical data are still awaited.

To antagonize PDGF, imatinib mesylate (Gleevec), a clinically approved tyrosine kinase inhibitor, attenuates proliferation and migration and fibrosis in animal models,[172,173] and newer related drugs such as nilotinib, show promise as well.[174] Sorafenib, a multi-kinase inhibitor approved for treatment of liver cancer, also shows antifibrotic activity in animal models,[175] attesting to the contribution of receptor tyrosine kinases such as PGDFR in fibrosis as well as cancer. However, sorafenib has adverse effects (e.g., rash, diarrhea, hand-foot syndrome), which may be acceptable to patients with cancer but would not be acceptable to asymptomatic patients with fibrotic liver disease. Thus better-tolerated kinase inhibitors are an appealing class of antifibrotic compounds.

Apart from blocking HSC-stimulating factors, activating HSC inhibitory factors is yet another possibility. Hepatocyte growth factor (HGF) inhibits HSC activation.[176] However, potential procarcinogenic effects are probable and would limit its therapeutic use.

In rodents, the blockade of the ETA receptor, which leads to vasoconstriction or scar-contraction upon binding of ET-1, and the administration of vasodilators (prostaglandin E_2 and NO donors) have antifibrotic qualities.[83,84] At one point, ET receptor blockade was highly attractive; however, clinical trials of these drugs for other indications demonstrated unacceptable liver toxicity,[177] and thus their development was halted until safety concerns can be more thoroughly addressed.

Bone marrow–derived mesenchymal stem cells have an antifibrotic effect, and multiple clinical trials have been conducted. A key problem with autologous and stem cell and bone marrow therapies to date has been their incomplete characterization, such that the exact composition of cells being transplanted is not standardized.[178] Recent human trials reinforce the safety of stem cell therapies,[179,180] but evidence of clinical efficacy is still awaited. A key goal of future studies is to understand and fully control the cellular composition of stem cell therapies to reliably demonstrate efficacy and reproducibility.

Enhancing Extracellular Matrix Degradation

Although no antifibrotic drug is approved for clinical use in patients with liver fibrosis, the broad and rational development of a range of promising compounds means that success is likely in the near future. The challenge ahead is to further refine therapeutic targets and to establish efficacy of these new drugs in vivo in animal models and in clinical trials. Equally challenging is the need to define clear and robust endpoints for clinical trials to ensure that a therapeutic benefit is apparent, based on improvement in noninvasive markers, improvement in biopsy, and, most importantly, by improving clinical outcomes.

References are available at expertconsult.com.

CHAPTER 8

Bile secretion and pathophysiology of biliary tract obstruction

Henry A. Pitt and Attila Nakeeb

OVERVIEW

Bile secretion is one of the major functions of the liver, which serves two major purposes: (1) the excretion of hepatic metabolites—including bilirubin, cholesterol, drugs, and toxins—and (2) the facilitation of intestinal absorption of lipids and fat-soluble vitamins. More recently, through their interaction with the gut microbiome, bile acids also have been found to have important signaling functions. Through receptor activation, bile acids regulate lipid, glucose, and energy metabolism. Alterations in bile secretion also may contribute to cholelithiasis (see Chapter 33) and its potential complications, such as cholecystitis (see Chapter 34) and choledocholithiasis (see Chapters 37 and 38). On the other hand, obstruction of bile flow results in alterations of coagulation, the immune system, and all organ functions. This chapter will discuss the physiology of bile secretion, the pathophysiology of bile obstruction, and the management of obstructive jaundice.

BILE SECRETION

Bile Formation

The two primary roles of bile in normal physiology are the excretion of organic compounds, such as bilirubin and cholesterol, and the intestinal absorption of lipids. Bile secretion results from the active transport of solutes into the canaliculus, followed by the passive flow of water. Water constitutes approximately 85% of the volume of bile. The major organic solutes in bile are bilirubin, bile salts, phospholipids, and cholesterol. Bilirubin, the breakdown product of spent red blood cells, is conjugated with glucuronic acid by the hepatic enzyme glucuronyl transferase and is excreted actively into the adjacent canaliculus. Normally, a large enzyme reserve exists to handle excess bilirubin production, which might exist in hemolytic states.

Bile salts are steroid molecules synthesized by hepatocytes. Bile salts account for approximately 72% of the biliary lipids. The primary bile salts in humans, cholic and chenodeoxycholic acid, account for approximately 80% of those produced. The primary bile salts, which are then conjugated with either taurine or glycine, can undergo bacterial alteration in the intestine to form the secondary bile salts, deoxycholate and lithocholate. The purpose of bile salts is to solubilize lipids and facilitate their absorption. Phospholipids are synthesized in the liver in conjunction with bile salt synthesis and account for approximately 24% of biliary lipids. Lecithin is the primary phospholipid in human bile, constituting more than 95% of its total. The final major solute of bile is cholesterol, which accounts for 4% of the lipids. Cholesterol also is produced primarily by the liver with a small contribution from dietary sources.

The normal volume of bile secreted daily by the liver is 750 to 1000 mL. Bile flow depends on neurogenic, humoral, and chemical control. Vagal stimulation increases bile secretion, whereas splanchnic stimulation causes vasoconstriction with decreased hepatic blood flow and thus results in diminished bile secretion. Gastrointestinal hormones—secretin, cholecystokinin, gastrin, and glucagon—all increase bile flow, primarily by increasing water and electrolyte secretion. This action probably occurs at a site distal to the hepatocyte. Finally, the most important factor in regulating the volume of bile flow is the rate of bile salt synthesis by hepatocytes. This rate is regulated by the return of bile salts to the liver by the enterohepatic circulation.

Bile Composition

The components of hepatic and gallbladder bile are essentially the same, but the concentration varies considerably because of the ability of the gallbladder to absorb water (Table 8.1). The gallbladder absorbs water both actively via sodium-hydrogen (Na^+/H^+) pumps and passively through aquaporin channels. Both chloride (Cl^-) and bicarbonate (HCO_3^-) are absorbed by the gallbladder epithelium via the cystic fibrosis transmembrane regulator (CFTR).[1] The secretion of hydrogen ions and the absorption of bicarbonate by the gallbladder alter the acid-base balance from basic in hepatic bile to acidic in gallbladder bile.

The gallbladder mucosa also absorbs calcium (Ca^{+2}) and magnesium (Mg^{+2}). Nevertheless, calcium absorption is not as efficient as the absorption of sodium and water, which leads to a significantly greater relative increase in the concentration of calcium in the gallbladder. Similarly, the concentration of bilirubin, which is not actively absorbed by the gallbladder, may be as high as 10-fold. Thus precipitation of calcium bilirubinate crystals, the major component of pigment gallstones, is much more likely to occur within the gallbladder. In addition, the biliary lipids, bile salts, phospholipids, and cholesterol all become more concentrated in the gallbladder. While gallbladder bile becomes concentrated, several changes occur in the capacity of bile to solubilize cholesterol. The solubility in the micellar fraction is increased, but the stability of the phospholipid-cholesterol vesicles is greatly decreased. Because cholesterol crystal precipitation occurs preferentially by vesicular, rather than micellar, mechanisms, the net effect of concentrating bile is an increased tendency to form cholesterol crystals.[2]

Bile Salt Secretion

Bile is secreted from the hepatocyte into canaliculi, which drain their contents into small bile ducts. Secretion of bile salts is the major osmotic force for the generation of bile flow. Bile acids are formed at a rate of 500 to 600 mg per day. The bulk of the bile salt pool is maintained in the gallbladder, followed by the liver, the small intestine, and the extrahepatic bile ducts.

TABLE 8.1	Composition of Hepatic and Gallbladder Bile	
CHARACTERISTICS*	HEPATIC BILE	GALLBLADDER BILE
Sodium	160	270
Potassium	5	10
Chloride	90	15
Bicarbonate	45	10
Calcium	4	25
Magnesium	2	4
Bilirubin	1.5	15
Proteins	150	200
Bile acids	50	150
Phospholipids	8	40
Cholesterol	4	18
Total solids	—	125
pH	7.8	7.2
Significant ranges may be seen.		

*All determinations are milliequivalents per liter, except for pH.

Bile acids are synthesized from cholesterol via two main pathways: a classic pathway leads to the formation of cholic acid, and an alternative pathway results in the synthesis of chenodeoxycholic acid. The classic pathway is the predominant mode of bile acid synthesis in humans. As a result, 60% to 70% of the bile acid pool consists of cholic acid and its metabolite deoxycholic acid, with chenodeoxycholic acid occurring less commonly in human bile.[3,4]

In plasma, bile acids circulate bound to either albumin or lipoproteins. In the space of Disse within the liver, bile salt uptake into the hepatocytes is very efficient. This process is mediated by sodium-dependent and sodium-independent mechanisms. The sodium-dependent pathway accounts for more than 80% of taurocholate uptake but less than 50% of cholate uptake.[5] In recent years, a number of transport proteins have been identified that play a key role in this process (Fig. 8.1). The bile salt transporter is termed the *sodium-taurocholate cotransporting polypeptide* (NTCP) and is exclusively expressed in the liver and located in the basolateral membrane of the hepatocyte. Sodium-independent hepatic uptake of bile acids is mediated primarily by a family of transporters termed the *organic anion transporting polypeptides* (OATPs). In contrast to NTCP, these transporters have a broader substrate affinity and transport a variety of organic anions, including the bile salts. OATP-C is the major sodium-independent bile salt uptake system, but OATP-A also takes up bile acids, and OATP-8 mediates taurocholate uptake.

Intracellular bile acid transport occurs within a matter of seconds. Two mechanisms may be responsible for bile acid transcellular movement: One involves transfer of bile acids from the basolateral membrane to the canalicular membrane via bile acid–binding proteins[6]; the other moves cellular bile salts through vesicular transport. In contrast, the transport of bile salts across the canalicular membrane of hepatocytes represents the rate-limiting step in the overall secretion of bile salts from the blood into bile.

Bile salt concentrations are 1,000-fold greater within the canaliculi than in the hepatocytes. This gradient necessitates an active transport mechanism, which is an adenosine triphosphate (ATP)-dependent process. The ATP-binding cassette transporter ABCB 11 (formerly known as the *bile salt export pump* [BSEP])

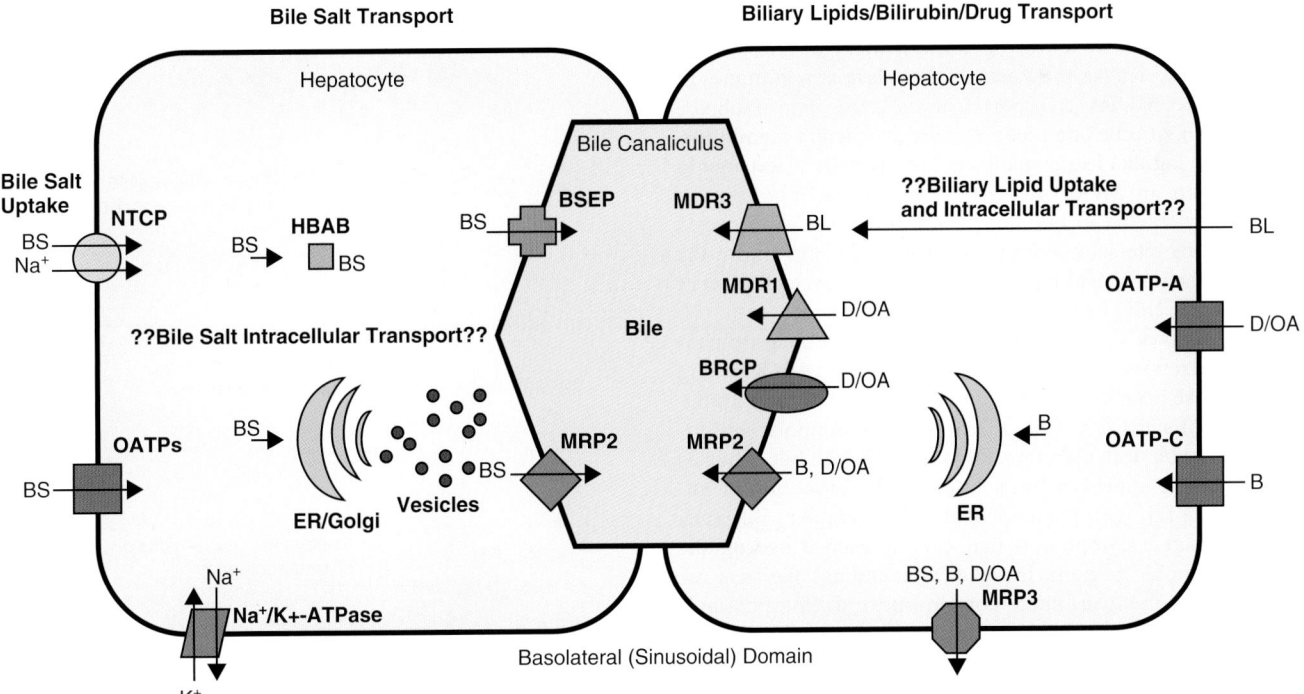

FIGURE 8.1 Bile formation in human liver. *ATP,* Adenosine triphosphate; *B,* bilirubin; *BL,* biliary lipids; *BRCP,* breast cancer–related protein; *BS,* bile salts; *BSEP,* bile salt export pump; *D/OA,* drugs/organic anions; *ER,* endoplasmic reticulum; *HBAB,* hepatic bile acid–binding protein; *MDR1* and *MDR3,* multidrug-resistance proteins 1 and 3, respectively; *MRP3,* MDR-related protein-3; *NTCP,* Na⁺-taurocholate cotransporting polypeptide; *OATPs (A, C, 8),* organic anion transporting polypeptides.

plays a key role in this process.[7] The ABC transporters mediate the transport of metabolites, peptides, fatty acids, cholesterol, and lipids in the liver, intestines, pancreas, lungs, kidneys, brain, and in macrophages. Although ABCB 11 is the major transporter for monovalent bile salts into the canaliculus, MDR-related protein-2 (MRP2), a member of the multidrug-resistant protein family, also transports sulfated and glucuronidated bile salts into the canaliculus. MRP2 also mediates the export of multiple other organic anions, including conjugated bilirubin, leukotrienes, glutathione disulfide, chemotherapeutic agents, uricosurics, antibiotics, toxins, and heavy metals.[8]

Recent studies suggest that bile acids are signaling molecules that regulate lipid, glucose, and energy metabolism.[9] This function of bile acids is mediated primarily by the nuclear receptor farnesoid X receptor (FXR) and the G-protein–coupled receptor TGR5. Bile acids in the small and large intestine regulate the gut microbiome, incretin secretion, and the production of fibroblast growth factors 15 and 19 (FGF15/FGF19).[10] These FGFs, in turn, modulate lipid, glucose, and energy metabolism and may play a role in the rapid improvement in glycemic control after gastric bypass surgery. In addition, FXR and TGR5 receptors exist in other tissues, such as the heart and the kidneys, and, therefore, may help to explain the dysfunction that occurs in these organs with biliary obstruction.[11]

Biliary Lipid Secretion

Compared with bile salts, the biliary lipids, phospholipids and cholesterol play a secondary role in the formation of bile. Phospholipids and cholesterol are formed primarily from low-density lipoproteins circulating in plasma and from de novo synthesis by hepatocytes. Less is known about the secretion of biliary lipids compared with bile salt secretion; however, biliary lipid secretion is crucial for cholesterol disposal, intestinal absorption of dietary lipids, and cytoprotection against bile acid–induced hepatocyte and cholangiocyte injury.[12]

Phospholipid secretion involves the delivery of phospholipids to the inner leaflet of the canalicular plasma membrane. In humans, the MDR3 transporter translocates phospholipids from the inner to the outer leaflet of the canalicular membrane. Progressive familial intrahepatic cholestatis type 3 develops in humans with an MDR3 deficiency.[3] These patients have no phosphatidylcholine in bile and therefore do not form mixed micelles with bile salts. As a result, toxic bile salts injure the biliary epithelium, resulting in neonatal cholestasis, cholestasis of pregnancy, and cirrhosis in adults.

Less is known about the role of transporter proteins in cholesterol secretion, but the ABC transporters ABCG5 and ABCG8 have been demonstrated to be involved in the elimination of plant steroids.[13] Cholesterol is highly nonpolar and insoluble in water and, therefore, also is insoluble in bile. The key to maintaining cholesterol in solution is the formation of micelles, a bile salt–phospholipid–cholesterol complex. Bile salts are amphipathic compounds that contain both a hydrophilic and hydrophobic portion. In aqueous solutions, bile salts are oriented with the hydrophilic portion outward. Phospholipids are incorporated into the micellar structure, allowing cholesterol to be added to the hydrophobic central portion of the micelle. In this way, cholesterol can be maintained in solution in an aqueous medium.

The concept of mixed micelles as the only cholesterol carrier has been challenged by the demonstration that much of the biliary cholesterol exists in a vesicular form. Structurally, these vesicles are made up of lipid bilayers of cholesterol and phospholipids. In their simplest and smallest form, the vesicles are unilamellar, but an aggregation may take place, leading to multilamellar vesicles. Present theory suggests that in states of excess cholesterol production, these large vesicles also may exceed their capability to transport cholesterol, and crystal precipitation may occur (Fig. 8.2).

Bilirubin Secretion

Heme is released at the time of degradation of senescent erythrocytes by the reticuloendothelial system. Heme is the source of approximately 80% to 85% of the bilirubin that is produced daily. The remaining 15% to 20% is derived largely from the breakdown of hepatic hemoproteins. Both enzymatic and nonenzymatic pathways for the formation of bilirubin have been proposed. Although both may be important physiologically, the microsomal enzyme heme oxygenase—found in high concentration throughout the liver, spleen, and bone marrow—plays a major role in the initial conversion of heme to biliverdin, which is then reduced to bilirubin by the cytosolic enzyme biliverdin reductase before being released into the circulation. In this "unconjugated" form, bilirubin has a very low solubility and is bound avidly to plasma proteins, primarily albumin, before

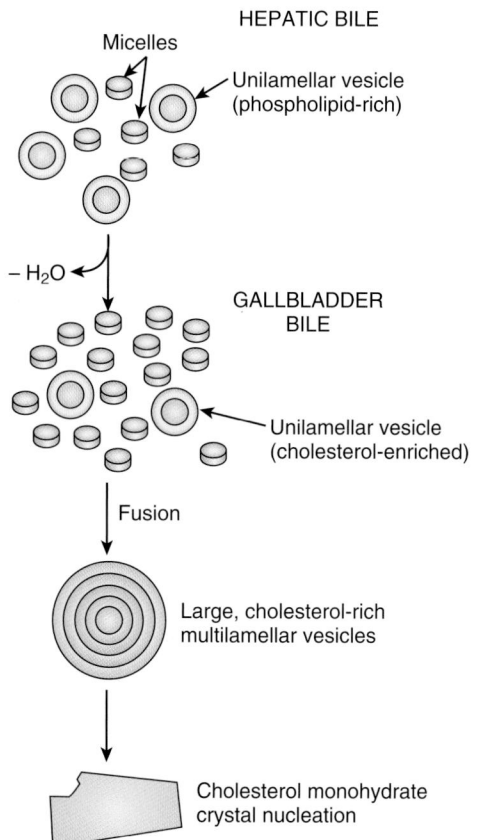

FIGURE 8.2 Concentration of bile leads to net transfer of phospholipids and cholesterol from vesicles to micelles. Phospholipids are transferred more efficiently than cholesterol, leading to cholesterol enrichment of the remaining (remodeled) vesicles. Aggregation of these cholesterol-rich vesicles forms multilamellar liquid crystals of cholesterol monohydrate. (From Vessey DA. Metabolism of drugs and toxins by the human liver. In Zakin D, Boyer TD, eds. *Hepatology: A Textbook of Liver Disease.* 2nd ed. WB Saunders 1990:1492.)

uptake and further processing by the liver. The liver is the sole organ capable of removing the albumin-bilirubin complex from the circulation and esterifying the potentially toxic bilirubin to water-soluble, nontoxic, monoconjugated and deconjugated derivatives.

In the sinusoidal membrane of the hepatocyte, bilirubin is taken up by OATP-C, a membrane transporter belonging to the OATP family.[14] OATP-C is involved with the uptake of both conjugated and unconjugated bilirubin, but unconjugated bilirubin also can cross hepatic sinusoidal membranes by a diffusion process. In the hepatocyte, bilirubin binds to a driver of glutathione-*S*-transferase and is catalyzed by bilirubin uridine-5′-diphosphate glycosyltransferase to form bilirubin glucuronides. Mutations in the gene encoding bilirubin UDP-glycosyltransferase are associated with the unconjugated hyperbilirubin syndromes, Crigler-Najjar and Gilbert syndromes.[15]

Bilirubin glucuronides are excreted into the bile canaliculus primarily via MRP2, which also plays a role in the transport of glucuroniductal bile salts and a wide spectrum of organic anions, including the antibiotic ceftriaxone. MRP3, which is expressed in the basolateral membrane of hepatocytes and cholangiocytes, also participates in the transport of bilirubin monoglucuronide. In addition, MRP3 may prevent intracellular accumulation of conjugated bilirubin, bile salts, and other organic anions in cholestatic situations.

Bile Flow

The bile ducts, gallbladder, and sphincter of Oddi act in concert to modify, store, and regulate the flow of bile. Bile flow is primarily driven by bile salt secretion. During its passage through the bile ductules, canalicular bile is modified by the absorption and secretion of electrolytes and water. Bicarbonate secretion by the bile ducts plays an important role in bile salt–independent bile flow. The gastrointestinal hormone secretin increases bile flow primarily by increasing the active secretion of chloride-rich fluid by the bile ducts. Bile duct secretion also is stimulated by other hormones, such as cholecystokinin and gastrin. The bile duct epithelium is capable of water and electrolyte absorption, which may be of primary importance in the storage of bile during fasting in patients who have previously undergone cholecystectomy. The main functions of the gallbladder are to concentrate and store hepatic bile during the fasting state and deliver bile into the duodenum in response to a meal. The usual capacity of the human gallbladder is about 40 to 50 mL. Only a small fraction of the bile produced each day would be stored, were it not for the gallbladder's remarkable absorptive capacity.

The enterohepatic circulation provides an important negative feedback system on bile salt synthesis. Should the recirculation be interrupted by resection of the terminal ileum or by primary ileal disease, abnormally large losses of bile salts occur. This situation increases bile salt production to maintain a normal bile salt pool. Similarly, if bile salts are lost through an external biliary fistula, increased bile salt synthesis is necessary. Except for those unusual circumstances in which excessive losses occur, however, bile salt synthesis matches losses, maintaining a constant bile salt pool size. During fasting, approximately 90% of the bile acid pool is sequestered in the gallbladder.

Enterohepatic Circulation

Bile salts are synthesized and conjugated in the liver; secreted into bile; stored temporarily in the gallbladder; passed from the

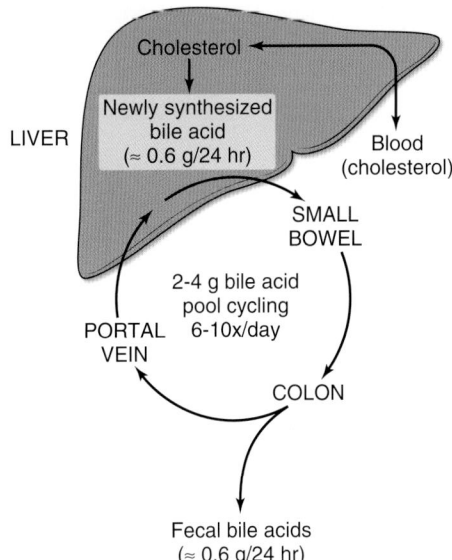

FIGURE 8.3 **Enterohepatic circulation of bile salts.** Cholesterol is taken up from plasma by the liver. Bile acids are synthesized at a rate of 0.6 g/24 hr and are excreted through the biliary system into the small bowel. Most of the bile salts are reabsorbed in the terminal ileum and are returned to the liver to be extracted and reextracted. (Modified from Dietschy JM. The biology of bile acids. *Arch Intern Med.* 1972;130:482–474.)

gallbladder into the duodenum; absorbed throughout the small intestine, especially in the ileum; and returned to the liver via the portal vein. This cycling of bile acids between the liver and the intestine is referred to as the *enterohepatic circulation* (Fig. 8.3). The total amount of bile acids in the enterohepatic circulation is defined as the *circulating bile pool*. In this highly efficient system, nearly 95% of bile salts are reabsorbed. Thus, of the total bile salt pool of 2 to 4 g, which recycles through the enterohepatic cycle 6 to 10 times daily, only about 600 mg is actually excreted into the colon. Bacterial action in the colon on the two primary bile salts, cholate and chenodeoxycholate, results in the formation of the secondary bile salts, deoxycholate and lithocholate. In fact, the bile acid signature of an individual is very dependent on gut microbial modification.[10,11] Bacterial enzymes modify primary bile acids through deconjugation, dehydrogenation, dehydroxylation, and sulfation reactions. In turn, bile acids restrict bacterial proliferation and overgrowth. However, the physiology of bile salts, biliary lipids, bilirubin, bile flow, and the enterohepatic circulation is dramatically altered when the bile ducts become obstructed.

BILIARY OBSTRUCTION

The evaluation and management of the patient with biliary obstruction is a common problem facing the general surgeon. Over the past 40 years, significant advances have been made in our understanding of the pathophysiology, diagnosis, and management of the jaundiced patient. Similarly, advances have been made in perioperative and operative management that have resulted in improved survival of the jaundiced patient. Obstructive jaundice affects multiple organ systems, including hepatic, renal, cardiovascular, hematologic, and immune systems. This section will review the causes, pathophysiology, and management of biliary obstruction.

TABLE 8.2 Classification of Jaundice

DEFECT IN BILIRUBIN METABOLISM	PREDOMINANT HYPERBILIRUBINEMIA	EXAMPLES
Increased production	Unconjugated	Congenital hemoglobinopathies, hemolysis, multiple transfusions, sepsis, burns
Impaired hepatocyte uptake	Unconjugated	Gilbert disease, drug induced
Reduced conjugation	Unconjugated	Neonatal jaundice, Crigler-Najjar syndrome
Altered transport and excretion	Conjugated	Hepatitis, cirrhosis, Dubin-Johnson syndrome, Rotor syndrome
Biliary obstruction	Conjugated	Choledocholithiasis, benign strictures, chronic pancreatitis, sclerosing cholangitis, periampullary cancer, biliary malignancies

Causes of Jaundice

Jaundice may result from (1) increased production of bilirubin, (2) impaired hepatocyte uptake of bilirubin, (3) reduced conjugation of bilirubin, (4) altered transport or excretion of bilirubin into the bile canaliculus, or (5) obstruction of the intrahepatic or extrahepatic biliary tree (Table 8.2). Overproduction, impaired uptake, and reduced conjugation of bilirubin all lead to a predominantly unconjugated hyperbilirubinemia. Altered transport and excretion and biliary ductal obstruction result in hyperbilirubinemia that is primarily conjugated. Some patients have multiple defects in normal metabolism. For example, secondary hepatocellular dysfunction may develop in a patient with biliary obstruction from a tumor. Therefore these classification systems may be simplifications of more complex disease processes.

Diseases that cause bile duct obstruction may be further divided into conditions that cause (1) complete obstruction, (2) intermittent obstruction, (3) chronic incomplete obstruction, or (4) segmental duct obstruction (Box 8.1). Patients with complete biliary obstruction will have clinical jaundice, and those with intermittent obstruction may experience symptoms (pain, pruritus, fevers) and biochemical changes without necessarily experiencing clinical jaundice. Hepatic fibrosis can eventually develop in patients with chronic incomplete obstruction (see Chapter 7) and biliary cirrhosis (see Chapters 7 and 74).

Pathophysiology

Biliary obstruction produces local effects on the bile ducts, which lead to derangements of hepatic function and, ultimately, to widespread systemic effects. Jaundiced patients are at increased risk for hepatic dysfunction, renal failure, cardiovascular impairments, nutritional deficiencies, bleeding problems, infections, and wound complications. Importantly, perioperative mortality and morbidity are increased in patients with biliary obstruction.

Hepatobiliary

Hepatocytes are arranged in plates along which blood flows from portal to central veins. Within these plates, the small apical domains of adjacent hepatocytes form a tubular lumen, the canaliculus, which is the site of primary bile formation. From the canalicular network, bile flows to the small ductules and subsequently to the larger ducts. With biliary obstruction, the bile canaliculi become dilated, and the microvilli are distorted and swollen. In patients with long-standing obstruction, intrahepatic bile ductule proliferation occurs with an increase in the length and tortuosity of the canaliculi.

The biliary system normally has a low pressure (5–10 cm H_2O); however, in the setting of complete or partial biliary obstruction, biliary pressure can approach 30 cm H_2O. While

BOX 8.1 Lesions Commonly Associated With Biliary Tract Obstruction

Type I: Complete Obstruction
Tumors of the head of the pancreas
 Common bile duct ligation
 Cholangiocarcinoma
 Gallbladder cancer
 Parenchymal liver tumors (primary or secondary)

Type II: Intermittent Obstruction
Choledocholithiasis
 Periampullary tumors
 Duodenal diverticula
 Choledochal cyst
 Polycystic liver disease
 Biliary parasites
 Hemobilia

Type III: Chronic Incomplete Obstruction
Strictures of the common bile duct
 Congenital biliary atresia
 Traumatic (iatrogenic)
 Sclerosing cholangitis
 Post radiotherapy
 Stenosis of biliary-enteric anastomosis
 Chronic pancreatitis
 Cystic fibrosis
 Sphincter of Oddi stenosis

Type IV: Segmental Obstruction
Traumatic
 Intrahepatic stones
 Sclerosing cholangitis
 Cholangiocarcinoma

biliary pressure increases, the tight junctions between hepatocytes and bile duct cells are disrupted, resulting in an increase in bile duct and canalicular permeability. Bile contents can freely reflux into liver sinusoids, causing a marked polymorphonuclear leukocyte infiltration into the portal triads. This inflammatory response is followed by increased fibrinogenesis with deposition of reticulin fibers, which undergo conversion to type I collagen (see Chapter 7). The extrahepatic bile ducts exhibit mucosal atrophy and squamous metaplasia, followed by inflammatory infiltration and fibrosis in the subepithelial layers of the bile duct.[16]

In addition to the structural effects of biliary obstruction on the bile ducts, elevated biliary pressure can alter bile production by hepatocytes. In the setting of biliary obstruction and elevated biliary pressure, bile becomes less lithogenic because of a relative decrease in cholesterol and phospholipid secretion compared with bile acid secretion. With the relief of biliary obstruction and the normalization of biliary pressures, the recovery of cholesterol and phospholipid secretion is more rapid than bile acid secretion; therefore bile is more lithogenic in this setting. This phenomenon may lead to premature occlusion of decompressive biliary stents placed for the management of obstructive jaundice.

Several authors have reported impairment of both macrovascular and microvascular perfusion of the liver in obstructive jaundice (see Chapter 5). Intravital fluorescence microscopy has shown a significant increase in the number of nonperfused sinusoids after three days of extrahepatic obstruction. This alteration in hepatic perfusion may help explain the increased risk for hepatocellular dysfunction when performing liver resections in patients with obstructive jaundice (see Chapter 101). Extrahepatic biliary obstruction and jaundice also can alter important secretory, metabolic, and synthetic functions of the liver. When biliary pressure rises higher than 20 cm H_2O, hepatic bile secretion is diminished, and hepatocytes cannot excrete efficiently against the high pressure. As a result, excretory products of the hepatocytes reflux directly into the vascular system, leading to systemic toxicity (see Chapters 10 and 43).

Patients with jaundice have a decreased capacity to excrete drugs, such as antibiotics, that are normally secreted into bile.[17] The increased concentration of bile acids associated with obstructive jaundice results in inhibition of the hepatic cytochrome P450 enzymes and, therefore, a decrease in the rate of oxidative metabolism in the liver. In addition, bile acids in abnormally high concentrations can induce apoptosis (programmed cell death) in hepatocytes. The synthetic function of the hepatocyte also is decreased with obstructive jaundice, as evidenced by decreased plasma levels of albumin, clotting factors, and secretory immunoglobulins (IgA).[16]

Kupffer cells are tissue macrophages that are the predominant cell type of the hepatic reticuloendothelial system (see Chapters 10 and 11). Normally, infectious agents, damaged blood cells, cellular debris, fibrin degradation products, and endotoxin absorbed or formed in the portal circulation are effectively filtered by Kupffer cells and removed from the systemic circulation. Kupffer cells also play an interactive role with hepatocytes, modulating synthesis of hepatic proteins. Obstructive jaundice has been shown to have profound effects on Kupffer cells, including decreased endocytosis, phagocytosis, clearance of bacteria and endotoxin, and expression of the major histocompatibility complex class II antigen, with a consequent diminished ability to process antigen.[18,19] Biliary obstruction also has been shown to increase levels of proinflammatory cytokines, including tumor necrosis factor (TNF)-α and interleukin (IL)-6 (see Chapters 10 and 11).

Cardiovascular

In addition to hepatic dysfunction, obstructive jaundice may cause severe hemodynamic and cardiac disturbances. Experimental animals with obstructive jaundice tend to be hypotensive and exhibit an exaggerated hypotensive response to hemorrhage. Studies in experimental animals have demonstrated that bile duct ligation (1) decreases cardiac contractility; (2) reduces left ventricular pressures; (3) impairs response to β-agonist drugs, such as isoproterenol and norepinephrine; and (4) decreases peripheral vascular resistance. Padillo and others[20] have shown in

13 patients a negative correlation between serum bilirubin and left ventricular systolic work. Successful internal biliary drainage in these patients was associated with a significant increase in cardiac output, compliance, and contractility. The combination of depressed cardiac function and decreased total peripheral resistance most likely makes the jaundiced patient more susceptible to the development of postoperative shock than nonjaundiced patients.

Renal

The association between jaundice and postoperative renal failure has been known for many years. The reported incidence of postoperative acute kidney injury has been reported to be as high as 10% but varies depending on the nature of the procedure. Moreover, the mortality rate in patients with jaundice in whom renal failure developed has been reported to be as high as 70%.[21] Important factors that may play a role in the development of renal failure in obstructive jaundice include (1) depressed cardiac function, (2) hypovolemia, (3) bile salt–mediated effects on renal FXR and TGR5 receptors, and (4) endotoxemia.

The decreased cardiac function associated with obstructive jaundice leads to a decrease in renal perfusion. Decreased cardiac output also may result in stretching of the atrium and increased production of atrial natriuretic peptide (ANP). This hormone is known to cause natriuresis, to counter the action of water- and sodium-retaining hormones, to inhibit the thirst mechanism, and to produce peripheral vasodilation. Plasma levels of ANP have been shown to be increased in both experimental animals and in patients with extrahepatic biliary obstruction.[20]

In addition to the direct effects of jaundice on the heart and peripheral vasculature, the increased serum levels of bile acids associated with obstructive jaundice have a direct diuretic and natriuretic effect on the kidney that results in significant extracellular volume depletion and hypovolemia. The infusion of bile into the renal artery of dogs results in increased urine flow, natriuresis, and kaliuresis. This diuretic effect may be mediated by increased prostaglandin E_2 production by the kidney[22] and/or by their effect on FXR and TGR5 receptors.

Another significant factor in the development of renal failure is endotoxemia (Fig. 8.4). Approximately 50% of patients with obstructive jaundice have endotoxin in their peripheral blood.[23] This phenomenon may be the result of decreased hepatic clearance of endotoxin by Kupffer cells and a lack of bile salts in the gut lumen that normally prevent absorption of endotoxins and inhibit anaerobic bacterial growth. Endotoxin also causes renal vasoconstriction and redistribution of renal blood flow away from the cortex and disturbances in coagulation that include the activation of complement, macrophages, leukocytes, and platelets. As a result, glomerular and peritubular fibrin is deposited. This factor, in combination with reduced renal cortical blood flow, results in the tubular and cortical necrosis observed in jaundiced patients with renal failure (see Chapter 10).

Coagulation

Disturbances of blood coagulation are commonly present in jaundiced patients. The most frequently observed abnormality is prolongation of the prothrombin time. This problem results from impaired vitamin K absorption from the gut, secondary to a lack of intestinal bile. This coagulopathy is usually reversible with parenteral administration of vitamin K. Decreased bile

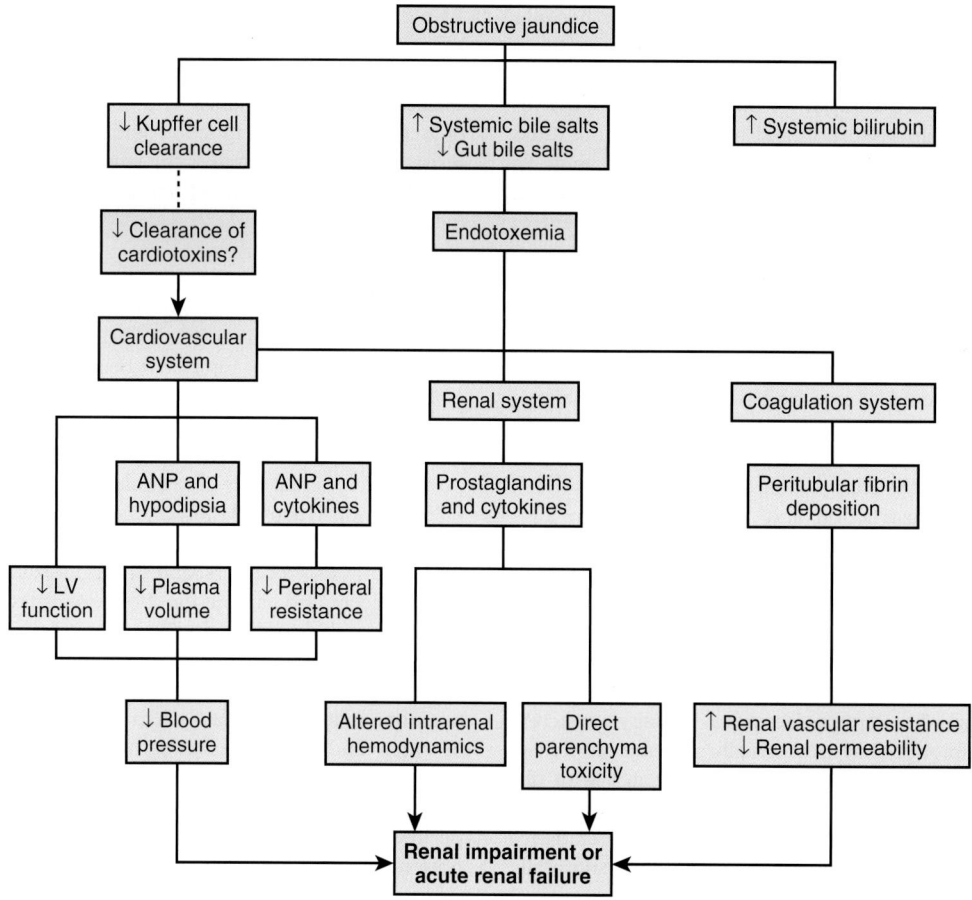

FIGURE 8.4   Obstructive jaundice leads to renal impairment or acute kidney injury. *ANP,* Atrial natriuretic peptide; *LV,* left ventricular.

levels in the small intestine may result in diminished absorption of other fat-soluble vitamins and fats, which results in weight loss and loss of calcium. This latter factor, as well as the earlier-mentioned increase in circulating endotoxin, may further contribute to clotting abnormalities.

In experimental animals, endotoxin affects metabolism of factors XI and XII and causes platelet and direct endothelial damage.[23] Moreover, endotoxin release in patients with jaundice results in a low-grade, disseminated intravascular coagulation, with increased fibrin degradation products. Hunt and colleagues have shown that patients with jaundice with circulating endotoxin or increased fibrin degradation product levels before surgery are at increased risk for hemorrhagic complications. In addition to problems with endotoxemia, patients with coexisting cirrhosis often have additional problems related to thrombocytopenia from hypersplenism and fibrinolysis. Portal hypertension in patients with cirrhosis also exacerbates these coagulation disorders.

Immune System

Surgery in patients with jaundice is associated with a higher rate of postoperative septic complications compared with those without jaundice, due in large measure to defects in cellular immunity that make them more prone to infection (see Chapters 10 and 11). Cainzos and colleagues[24] have demonstrated an association between jaundice and altered delayed-type hypersensitivity. Only 16% of 118 patients with jaundice

were immunocompetent, compared with 76% of 59 healthy controls, when tested with a panel of seven skin antigens. As mentioned earlier, the ability of the reticuloendothelial system, specifically Kupffer cells, to clear bacteria and endotoxin from the circulation also is reduced in obstructive jaundice. Studies in humans also have demonstrated decreased T-lymphocyte proliferation,[25] decreased expression of adhesion molecules,[26] and altered monocyte functions.[27] Septic manifestations in jaundiced patients result from cellular immune insufficiency (T-lymphocytes) induced by release of cytokines (TNF-α, IL-1, IL-6, interferon-γ), prostaglandins, and other inflammatory mediators.[16]

The absence of bile from the intestinal tract also plays a role in the infectious complications seen in patients with obstructive jaundice. Bacterial translocation from the gut is increased in the setting of bile duct obstruction.[28] Obstruction causes a disruption of the enterohepatic circulation and results in loss of the emulsifying antiendotoxin effect of bile acids; therefore a larger pool of endotoxin is available within the intestine for absorption into the portal circulation. The combination of reduced or absent bile in the intestine and impaired cellular immunity and reticuloendothelial cell function appears to be a major factor contributing to more frequent infective complications in the jaundiced patient.

Acute cholangitis is a bacterial infection of the biliary ductal system, which varies in severity from mild and self-limited to severe and life threatening (see Chapter 43). The clinical triad associated with cholangitis—fever, jaundice, and pain—was first described in 1877 by Charcot. Cholangitis results from a combination of two factors: significant bacterial concentrations in the bile and biliary obstruction. Although bile from the gallbladder and bile ducts is usually sterile, in the presence of common bile duct stones or other obstructing pathology, the incidence of positive cultures increases. Likewise, instrumentation of the biliary tree also greatly increases rates of bile colonization. The most common organisms recovered from the bile in patients with cholangitis include *Escherichia coli*, *Klebsiella pneumonia*, the enterococci, and *Bacteroides fragilis*.[29] Even in the presence of high biliary bacterial concentrations, however, clinical cholangitis and bacteremia will not develop unless obstruction causes elevated intraductal pressures.[30]

Normal biliary pressures range from 7 to 14 cm H_2O. In the presence of bacteribilia and normal biliary pressures, hepatic venous blood and perihepatic lymph are sterile. With partial or complete biliary obstruction, however, intrabiliary pressures rise to 20 to 30 cm H_2O, and organisms rapidly appear in both the blood and lymph. The fever and chills associated with cholangitis are the result of systemic bacteremia caused by cholangiovenous and cholangiolymphatic reflux.

The most common causes of biliary obstruction are choledocholithiasis (see Chapter 37), benign strictures (see Chapter 42), biliary-enteric anastomotic strictures (see Chapter 32), and periampullary or proximal biliary cancers (see Chapters 49, 50 and 59). Before 1980, choledocholithiasis was the cause of approximately 80% of the reported cases of cholangitis. In recent years, however, malignant strictures have become a frequent cause, especially after the placement of biliary stents. Endoscopic cholangiography, percutaneous transhepatic cholangiography, and stent placement via either the endoscopic or percutaneous route are all known to cause bacteremia, and these procedures are frequently performed in patients with a presumptive diagnosis of malignant obstruction.[31]

Wound Healing

Delayed wound healing and a high incidence of wound dehiscence and incisional hernia have been observed in patients with jaundice undergoing surgery. Patients with obstructive jaundice have decreased activity of the enzyme propyl hydroxylase in their skin. Propyl hydroxylase is necessary for the incorporation of the amino acid proline into collagen, and its activity has been used as a measure of collagen synthesis. Grande and colleagues[32] measured skin propyl hydroxylase activity in 95 patients with extrahepatic bile duct obstruction and 123 nonjaundiced control patients undergoing cholecystectomy. The patients with jaundice had only 11% of the skin propyl hydroxylase activity of the controls. In the subgroup of patients with jaundice secondary to malignancy, propyl hydroxylase activity was less than 7% of controls. With relief of obstruction, the activity increased to 22% of controls. Interestingly, in patients with jaundice secondary to benign obstruction, the activity increased to 100% of controls.

Other Factors

Other problems that face patients with jaundice are anorexia, weight loss, and malnutrition. Appetite is adversely influenced by the lack of bile salts in the intestinal tract. In addition, patients with pancreatic or periampullary malignant lesions may have partial duodenal obstruction or abnormal gastric emptying, in some cases secondary to tumor infiltration of the celiac

nerve plexus. Patients with pancreatic or ampullary tumors also may have pancreatic endocrine and exocrine insufficiency. This latter problem may further compound other nutritional defects that, in turn, may exacerbate the immune deficits of the patient with jaundice.

Several recent observations suggest that the many physiologic derangements induced by obstructive jaundice take a long time to reverse. For example, Koyama and colleagues[33] have shown that hepatic mitochondrial function does not return to normal even seven weeks after relief of obstruction. This same prolonged effect of obstructive jaundice has been noted with lymphocyte, polymorphonuclear, and Kupffer cell function. Therefore, even patients who have had temporary relief of biliary obstruction via percutaneous or endoscopic stents are likely to remain at risk for significant complications after surgery because derangements in hepatic function are likely still present at the time of operation. Moreover, an analysis by Strasberg and colleagues[34] suggests that preoperative jaundice may adversely affect long-term survival in patients with resected pancreatic cancer.

Management

Historically, the only option for the relief of obstructive jaundice was operative intervention. With the development of therapeutic techniques such as percutaneous (see Chapters 31 and 52) and endoscopic stenting (see Chapters 20 and 30), balloon dilation, and endoscopic sphincterotomy, however, many nonoperative options for the relief of obstructive jaundice are now available. The surgeon must determine the safest and most effective therapy for each individual patient and must adequately prepare each patient for surgery or nonoperative therapeutic intervention.

Patients with obstructive jaundice and those with hepatocellular disease severe enough to cause jaundice are prone to many secondary problems. Patients with jaundice are at increased risk for the development of kidney injury, gastrointestinal bleeding, infections, and wound complications (see earlier section on *Pathophysiology*). Cardiac, pulmonary, and renal function must be considered in every patient undergoing major abdominal surgery. In addition, special attention must be focused on the patient with jaundice's nutritional status, coagulability, immune function, and presence or absence of biliary sepsis. Complications related to portal hypertension, such as ascites, varices, and encephalopathy, also may develop in patients with chronic liver disease and cirrhosis, and these abnormalities may require specific treatment (see Chapters 74 and 77–85).

Cardiopulmonary

In assessing cardiopulmonary status, the patient's age, history of recent myocardial infarction, and the presence of congestive heart failure, significant valvular heart disease, or a disturbance of normal cardiac rhythm all have been correlated with increased operative risk.[35] In addition, patients with severe pulmonary disease may not be candidates for extensive abdominal surgery (see Chapter 26).

Renal

Patients with jaundice, especially those with cirrhosis and cholangitis, are at increased risk for renal insufficiency. The maintenance of adequate blood volume and the correction of dehydration are extremely important if renal complications are to be avoided. Fluid management can be quite complex in patients with jaundice because both excess and insufficient fluids may be problematic. Therefore selected patients may benefit from invasive hemodynamic monitoring to assist with goal-directed fluid management.

Certain oral bile salts have been shown to be efficacious in preventing the development of postoperative kidney injury. In a study by Cahill,[36] 54% of 24 patients with jaundice not given oral bile salts before surgery were found to have systemic endotoxemia, which was associated with renal impairment in two-thirds of the cases. In comparison, none of the eight patients with jaundice given 500 mg of sodium deoxycholate every eight hours for 48 hours before surgery had portal or systemic endotoxemia. Moreover, none of these eight patients had evidence of renal impairment (see Chapter 26).

Nutrition

Malnutrition is a significant risk factor for surgery in the setting of obstructive jaundice (see Chapter 26). Halliday and colleagues[37] noted that patients who died in the postoperative period after surgery for obstructive jaundice had a significant reduction in body weight, midarm circumference, total body potassium, and reactivity to skin test antigens preoperatively. In a study from Italy,[38] enteral hyperalimentation was found to significantly decrease operative morbidity and mortality in a group of patients treated with 20 days of preoperative percutaneous biliary drainage. Although most patients with benign biliary problems are adequately nourished, various degrees of malnutrition are frequently present in patients with malignant obstruction. Therefore patients with malignant obstructive jaundice should be evaluated for evidence of malnutrition and have nutritional support instituted if necessary.

Coagulation

Patients with obstructive jaundice, cholangitis, or cirrhosis all are prone to excessive intraoperative bleeding. The most common clotting defect in patients with obstructive jaundice is prolongation of the prothrombin time (PT), which is usually reversible by the administration of parenteral vitamin K. Patients with severe jaundice and/or cholangitis also may develop disseminated intravascular coagulation (DIC), which may require infusion of platelets and fresh frozen plasma. Reversal of DIC also requires control of the underlying sepsis, which should include biliary drainage in patients with cholangitis in addition to systemic antibiotics.

In cirrhotic patients, clotting abnormalities are often multifactorial and include thrombocytopenia secondary to hypersplenism, prolongation of PT and partial thromboplastin time (PTT), and fibrinolysis. Vitamin K should be administered if the PT is prolonged. If no effect is seen and/or if the PTT is also prolonged, fresh frozen plasma should be given. Thrombocytopenia usually can be managed by intraoperative platelet infusions. If the patient has a shortened clot lysis time and hypofibrinogenemia, ε-aminocaproic acid may be indicated (see Chapter 26).

Pruritus

Pruritus is often a distressing problem in the jaundiced patient. The exact cause of pruritus remains obscure, but increased circulating levels of bile salts, histamines, and central nervous system opiate receptors have been implicated. In some patients, relief from itching can be obtained by bile salt–binding agents, such as cholestyramine. Various sedatives and antihistamines also can provide relief of itching in jaundiced patients. However, relief of biliary obstruction remains the most effective method for managing pruritus, and improvement can occur rapidly after stent placement, although occasionally it can take a week or so.

Cholangitis

Biliary sepsis also has been identified as a major risk in jaundiced patients (see Chapter 43). Cholangitis occurs when partial or complete obstruction of the bile duct exists, resulting in increased intraluminal pressure and infected bile proximal to the obstruction. Patients with cholangitis may present with right upper quadrant abdominal pain, fever, and/or jaundice (Charcot's triad). Patients with "toxic" cholangitis—Charcot's triad plus shock and mental confusion (Reynold's pentad)—have significant mortality with appropriate antibiotic therapy alone and therefore require emergent biliary decompression.

Gigot and associates[39] identified seven prognostic factors that are indications for urgent biliary decompression: (1) acute kidney injury, (2) liver abscess, (3) cirrhosis, (4) high malignant stricture, (5) percutaneous transhepatic cholangiography, (6) female gender, and (7) advanced age. However, emergent surgical treatment is associated with significant morbidity and mortality; therefore both percutaneous and endoscopic biliary drainage have been proposed as effective therapy for the 5% to 10% of patients with cholangitis who are unresponsive to conservative therapy. Lai and colleagues[40] have shown, in a series of 82 patients with severe acute cholangitis, that endoscopic drainage is associated with a lower morbidity (34% vs. 66%) and mortality (10% vs. 32%) than operative drainage. Current concepts in the initial management and treatment of cholangitis have been summarized in the Tokyo Guidelines.[41,42]

Preoperative Drainage

The preoperative relief of jaundice and the reversal of its systemic effects by either endoscopic or transhepatic biliary decompression has been proposed as a method to decrease the risk of surgery in jaundiced patients. However, several prospective randomized studies have shown that the routine use of preoperative biliary drainage (PBD) does not reduce operative morbidity or mortality in patients with obstructive jaundice (see Table 8.3).[43–48] In addition, meta-analyses also concluded that preoperative biliary drainage increased ($P < .001$), rather than decreased, overall complications from surgery and the drainage procedure provided no benefit in terms of reduced mortality or decreased hospital stay.[49–51] In addition, insufficient evidence exists to determine whether endoscopic plastic or metal stents or percutaneous transhepatic drains are better than no drainage.[49] However, endoscopic ultrasound (EUS)-guided biliary drainage may have an advantage over percutaneous drainage when ERCP fails.[52] Moreover, several retrospective studies have documented a higher incidence of infectious complications (wound infection, pancreatic fistula) and even mortality in patients undergoing pancreatic or biliary tract resection after preoperative biliary decompression.[51,53]

A criticism of some of the prospective studies is that the duration of preoperative drainage (10–18 days) may have been inadequate to reverse the multiple metabolic and immunologic abnormalities associated with severe obstructive jaundice. Both animal and human studies demonstrate that the recovery of various metabolic and immune functions requires at least

TABLE 8.3 Prospective Randomized Trials of Preoperative Biliary Drainage (PBD)

FIRST AUTHOR	TYPE OF DRAINAGE	MORTALITY, PBD	MORTALITY, NO PBD	MORBIDITY, PBD	MORBIDITY, NO PBD
Hatfield[43]	Percutaneous	4/29	4/28	7/29	4/28
McPherson[45]	Percutaneous	11/34	6/31	17/34	13/31
Pitt[46]	Percutaneous	3/37	2/38	30/37	20/38
Lai[44]	Endoscopic	6/43	6/44	28/43	18/44
Wig[48]	Percutaneous	1/20	4/20	12/20	10/20
van der Gaag[47]	Endoscopic	15/102	12/94	75/102	37/94
Total (%)		40/265 (15.1)	34/255 (13.3)	169/265 (63.8)*	104/255 (40.0)

*$P < .001$ vs. no PBD.

six weeks to pass after the relief of biliary obstruction.[54] Similarly, animal studies strongly suggest that return of bile to the intestinal tract has significant advantages over external biliary drainage.[55]

Although the data suggest that routine PBD may be of limited benefit, PBD may have some value in selected patients with advanced malnutrition, biliary sepsis, and hilar malignancies that require liver resection.[56] Regarding the latter, most of the published data regarding PBD focus on patients with periampullary malignancy. Patients with proximal biliary obstruction undergoing major hepatic resection represent an entirely different subgroup, but a multicenter European study suggests that those requiring right hepatectomy benefit from preoperative drainage of the future liver remnant (see Chapters 51, 52, and 101). In patients with perihilar cholangiocarcinoma, percutaneous drainage is associated with less cholangitis and pancreatitis compared with endoscopic drainage.[57,58] Preoperatively placed transhepatic catheters also may be of value in the operating room during difficult biliary dissections in patients with proximal biliary tumors or strictures, and they may aid in the placement of long-term transhepatic stents. Finally, preoperative drainage is required in patients receiving neoadjuvant therapy. In these patients, metal stents have fewer problems with cholangitis at no additional cost, although plastic stents are preferable for patients with hilar cholangiocarcinoma in whom surgery is planned.[59]

SUMMARY

Over the past few decades, tremendous strides have been made in our understanding of bile secretion and our ability to care for the jaundiced patient. Clinicians now have a better understanding of normal bile salt, biliary lipid, and bilirubin physiology and can classify the diseases that cause jaundice as defects in normal metabolism. Similarly, investigators have elucidated the multiple pathophysiologic effects of jaundice that explain why jaundiced patients are at risk for increased perioperative morbidity and mortality.

The references for this chapter can be found online by accessing the accompanying Expert Consult website.

Molecular and cell biology of hepatopancreatobiliary disease: Introduction and basic principles

Caitlin A. McIntyre and Rohit Chandwani

INTRODUCTION

In recent years, there has been an increased understanding of the molecular and cellular processes that govern hepatopancreatobiliary (HPB) diseases. These processes, which include those that are immune-mediated, involve chronic inflammation or processes of neoplastic transformation and are driven by factors such as genomic alterations, epigenetic modification, and dysregulated cell signaling pathways. These principles are integrally intertwined, as evidenced by crosstalk between genetic and epigenetic regulation, post-translational modifications, and cell signaling pathways. The primary goal of this section is to provide a foundation outlining the biologic principles that govern benign and malignant HPB diseases and bring light to the complex interactions between such principles. Each of these themes will be explored in depth in Chapters 9B to 9E.

SIGNALING PATHWAYS

For further information, see Chapters 9B to 9E.

Cell signaling pathways play an integral role in the mechanisms of numerous cellular processes. There is significant crosstalk between pathways, and the same signaling pathway may serve multiple functions within the same cell or organ, which is dependent on the stage of development, surrounding microenvironment, or other selective pressure. A number of cell signaling pathways are important for normal pancreatic and liver development. Differentiation and proliferation of both hepatocytes and cholangiocytes are components of normal liver development (see Chapter 1). These processes involve multiple pathways at various stages of development and include Notch, Hedgehog, Wnt/β-catenin, PI3K (phosphatidylinositol-3 kinase)/PTEN, mTOR, nuclear factor (NF)-κB, and transforming growth factor (TGF)–β signaling.[1] In malignancy, these signaling pathways are often hijacked, and *RAS* and p53 signaling are also commonly altered in HPB malignancies.

Notch Signaling

The Notch pathway plays a significant role in cell fate determination and homeostasis of several adult tissues. Notch receptors and ligands are transmembrane proteins, with four Notch receptors (Notch1–4) and five Notch ligands (Dll1, Dll3, Fll4, Jagged1, and Jagged2) found in mammals.[2] Interactions between receptor and ligand on adjacent cells results in several proteolytic cleavages of the Notch receptor at three distinct sites (S1, S2, and S3), releasing the Notch intracellular domain (NICD). NICD translocates to the nucleus, where it binds CBF1/RBPj, displacing co-repressor complexes, and recruits coactivator molecules, including Mastermind-like (Maml).[3] In the liver, Notch signaling is critical to the development of the intrahepatic biliary system (see Chapter 1) and is also crucial in liver regeneration (see Chapter 6). This pathway is activated during liver repair and has a clear role in biliary regeneration, although its utility in hepatocyte regeneration is less clear.[4] Notch1 and Jagged1 are both induced by hepatectomy and injury, directing the formation of biliary cells. Alagille syndrome, which is characterized by an autosomal dominant mutation in Notch2 or Jagged2 (encodes a ligand in the Notch pathway), results in malformation of the intrahepatic biliary tree as well as other abnormalities.[5–7] In liver malignancies, the role of Notch signaling is ambiguous. Notch1 knockout mice develop proliferation and dedifferentiation of endothelial cells with eventual spontaneous development of hepatic angiosarcoma, suggesting a tumor suppressive role.[8] By contrast, constitutive expression of both activated Notch1 and the intracellular domain of Notch2 lead to spontaneous hepatocellular carcinoma (HCC) at 12 months.[9,10]

In the pancreas, Notch signaling is similarly critical to tissue homeostasis. Activation in pancreatic progenitors prevents specification into either endocrine or exocrine lineages, whereas inhibition of the pathway results in premature differentiation to neurogenin-3 (*Ngn3*+) expressing endocrine cells. As in the liver, injury to the adult tissue unveils developmental Notch signaling to permit regeneration following pancreatitis.[11]

Hedgehog

Sonic hedgehog (SHH) is an essential pathway involved in cell growth and tissue patterning. Canonical SHH signal transduction consists of multiple Hedgehog (Hh) ligands, two transmembrane receptors (Patched [PTCH1, PTCH2] and Smoothened [SMO]), and the glioma-associated oncogene homolog (GLI) family of transcription factors (GLI1, GLI2, GLI3). When Hh ligands bind to the receptor Patched, it blocks the inhibitory effect of Patched on the co-receptor Smoothened. Active SMO leads to GLI protein activation with nuclear translocation and activation of target genes. Hedgehog signaling is involved in normal pancreatic and liver development, with mouse models indicating the need for Shh for appropriate organogenesis.

Hh ligands are largely absent in the adult liver but are reactivated in response to liver injury and at times of liver regeneration. In injury, epithelial cells produce Hh ligands that act in a paracrine fashion on mesenchymal-type cells. The pathway is critical to crosstalk among multiple cell types and specifically promotes viability of progenitor cells and activates hepatic stellate cells. Hedgehog signaling plays a role in chronic liver disease with upregulation of PTCH and GLI factors in nonalcoholic fatty liver disease (NAFLD), biliary cirrhosis, and hepatitis B (HBV) and C (HCV).[12–14] Hedgehog signaling has also been identified in the development of HCC, with correlative data suggesting poorer outcomes in patients with increased SMO.[15–17] Similarly, in the pancreas, Hedgehog signaling is enhanced early in tumorigenesis and in stromal fibroblasts, with conflicting data suggesting either supportive or restraining roles for enhanced Hedgehog signaling.[18,19]

Wnt/β-Catenin

The Wnt/β-catenin pathway is critical for both pancreatic and liver development and for regeneration. β-Catenin, a cytoplasmic protein, is typically maintained in a phosphorylated state and targeted for degradation by adenomatous polyposis coli (APC) product, casein kinase 1 (CK1), and glycogen synthase kinase-3 (GSK3)-β. Nevertheless, when Wnt proteins, typically glycosylated and acylated moieties, engage the Frizzled (Fz) receptor in the context of a ternary complex, hypophosphorylated β-catenin is released where it can translocate to the nucleus and induce target gene expression.[20]

Similar to Notch, fibroblast growth factor (FGF), and bone morphogenetic protein (BMP) signaling, Wnt signaling is central in the determination of endodermal patterning. Wnt is initially suppressed in early liver development and then activated later, and this pathway is critical to metabolic zonation in the liver. In both hepatectomy and injury models, β-catenin is important for regeneration and the hepatocyte proliferation that occurs. In the pancreas, the absence of β-catenin in animal models leads to disrupted development of the exocrine pancreas.[21] Similarly, gain-of-function experiments show that Wnt pathway activation also results in a hypoplastic pancreas after abnormal acquisition of intestinal features.[22]

Wnt/β-catenin pathways are commonly altered in benign and malignant tumors of the liver. Mutations or deletions of the β-catenin gene, *CTNNB1*, or mutations in other genes or aberrant expression of proteins in the pathway, result in cytoplasmic stabilization and nuclear translocation of β-catenin and ultimately dysregulated transcription of cell cycle regulatory proteins. β-Catenin mutated hepatic adenomas account for approximately 10% to 15% of hepatic adenomas and are associated with an increased risk for transformation into HCC[23] (see Chapters 87–89). Additionally, abnormal expression of β-catenin is noted in 17% to 40% of HCC and 50% to 75% of hepatoblastoma.[24–28] In pancreatic cancer, β-catenin stabilization results in the formation of pancreatic tumors, affirming an oncogenic role across the spectrum of HPB disease.

Innate Immune Response Pathways

Many signaling pathways are involved in normal immune function and in dysregulation of immune mechanisms and chronic inflammation. Toll-like receptors (TLR) are cell surface receptors found on dendritic cells and macrophages and play a key role in the innate immune system.[29] They recognize pathogen-associated molecular patterns (PAMPs; specific microbial components that are conserved between species) or damage-associated molecular patterns (DAMPs; components of dying cells) and activate multiple signaling pathways in immune cells, including the myeloid differentiation primary response (MyD88) and TIR-domain-containing-adapter-inducing interferon-β (TRIF) pathways, resulting in activation of NF-κB and, ultimately, an inflammatory response. TLRs (specifically TLR2, TLR4, and TLR9 expressed on Kupffer cells) have been shown to play a role in the development of alcoholic liver disease, nonalcoholic steatohepatitis (NASH), and HCC, likely through interactions with host intestinal flora, which subsequently

results in activation of multiple proinflammatory pathways[30] (see Chapters 69, 74, and 89). Cytokines are small peptide molecules secreted by both immune and nonimmune cells that act through cell surface receptors. Examples include interferons (IFNs), interleukins (ILs), and tumor necrosis factors (TNF). IFNs have been shown to play a role in host defenses against viruses, and IFN-α has been used to treat HCV infection (see Chapter 10).

Key Metabolic Pathways

A number of signaling pathways are imperative for normal metabolism of glucose and fatty acids in the liver. These include the PI3K/Akt/mTOR, AMP-activated protein kinase, and protein-kinase A (PKA) pathways. Transcription factors such as FOXO1, liver X receptor (LXR), farnesoid X receptor (FXR), SRE-binding protein 1 (SREBP1), and peroxisome proliferator-activated receptors (PPAR) are key regulators of metabolism in the liver.

Many of these pathways are dysregulated in liver disease, including NAFLD and HCC (see Chapters 69 and 89). Recent emphasis has been placed on the mechanisms behind the development of NAFLD and NASH, given that this spectrum of disease is increasing in incidence worldwide and accounts for a subset of HCC cases annually. Interestingly, previous data have demonstrated that approximately 50% of HCC cases associated with NAFLD are in patients who are not cirrhotic,[31] further highlighting the importance of better understanding the mechanisms behind NAFLD. The development of NAFLD is multifactorial in origin and is a complex interaction between insulin resistance, dysregulation of fatty acid metabolism, the microbiome, activation of the innate immune system, and increased inflammation through cytokine signaling. Insulin and glucagon signaling through the PI3K/Akt/mTOR and PKA pathways, respectively, regulate gluconeogenesis and fatty acid metabolism in the liver; dysregulation of these pathways contributes to insulin resistance.[32] Additionally, TLRs have been shown to contribute to insulin resistance through fatty acid activation of TLR4 in mouse models.[33] PPARs are essential transcription factors for fatty acid β-oxidation, and dysregulation of these factors is believed to contribute to the development of NAFLD. For example, prior data have demonstrated that PPAR-α expression was decreased in patients who had NASH, steatosis, ballooning of hepatocytes, and fibrosis on liver biopsy compared with those who did not.[34]

Signaling Pathways in Cancer

Dysregulated cellular signaling is a hallmark of cancer, and certain pathways are frequently altered in HPB cancers. Many of these signaling pathways do not play a significant role in normal development or response to injury, but instead, when mutated, lead to aberrant cell growth. Two commonly altered signaling pathways in HPB cancers are the p53 and RAS pathways because *TP53* and *KRAS* are among the most frequently mutated genes in pancreatic and biliary cancers.[35,36] *TP53* encodes a tumor suppressor protein, which is present in normal cells and has a diverse role in many cellular functions including DNA repair, cell cycle regulation, and apoptosis. *TP53* alterations can result in either gain-of-function or loss-of-function mutations of p53, ultimately resulting in uncontrolled cell proliferation and tumor development. Although *KRAS* is one of the most commonly altered genes, additional mutations occur in other members of the RAS pathway, including *NRAS* and

BRAF. Mutations in this pathway result in constitutive activation of RAS/RAF and increased signaling through MEK/ERK, resulting in uncontrolled cell proliferation.

A number of additional signaling pathways are dysregulated in HPB cancers, including MYC, vascular endothelial growth factor (VEGF), and platelet-derived growth factor (PDGF). Unlike the frequently altered p53 and RAS pathways, these additional pathways can be targeted with small molecule inhibitors, and recent studies have supported the use of these agents in hepatobiliary cancers. For example, sorafenib, which targets the Raf/VEGF/PDGF pathways, has been shown to improve overall survival (OS) in patients with advanced HCC (see Chapter 89) and is US Food and Drug Administration (FDA)-approved for first-line therapy in these patients.[37] Similarly, regorafenib, which targets VEGF2, is approved as a second-line agent in patients with HCC.[38] Pemigatinib, a small molecule inhibitor of FGFR2, has recently demonstrated a survival benefit in patients with intrahepatic cholangiocarcinoma (CC; see Chapter 50).[39]

EMERGING THEMES

For more information, see Chapters 9B to 9E.

Oncogenic Viruses

Chronic primary infections of the liver and the biliary tree have been shown to have an association with the development of cancer; the most common of these infections are HBV and HCV (see Chapter 68). HBV and HCV are strongly associated with the development of HCC; approximately 44% of worldwide cases of HCC are attributed to HBV, whereas 21% are attributed to HCV.[40] The mechanism of carcinogenesis differs between the two viruses. Genomic instability from HBV viral DNA integration into the host cell genome is the primary mechanism of carcinogenesis in HBV infection; however, this is coupled with the effects of viral proteins, epigenetic regulation, and aberrant cell signaling.[41] On the contrary, HCV infection results in persistent inflammation leading to cirrhosis, which is believed to be a mechanism of carcinogenesis in HCV. Nevertheless, given that not all patients with HCC arising in the setting of HCV infection have cirrhosis, virus-specific proteins and immune-mediated mechanisms also play a significant role in carcinogenesis.[42]

Chronic Inflammation

Chronic inflammation results from dysregulation of the immune system and can ultimately lead to fibrosis and cancer development. Foreign antigens or self-antigens produced by damaged hepatocytes lead to recruitment of immune cells and release of proinflammatory cytokines and chemokines, such as IL-1β, IL-6, and TNF-α. Specifically, neutrophils and macrophages are directed to the site of injury, and subsequently, natural killer (NK) cells, dendritic cells, and T-cells are recruited. In response to release of inflammatory mediators released by immune cells, quiescent hepatic stellate cells (HSCs) are activated and differentiate into myofibroblast-like cells (see Chapter 7). Studies in mice have demonstrated that HSCs are the primary source of myofibroblasts in cholestatic, toxin-induced, and fatty liver diseases.[43] These myofibroblast-like HSCs deposit extracellular matrix (ECM), a process that is promoted by matrix metalloproteinases (MMPs). Persistent liver inflammation results in further hepatocyte damage, and continued release of proinflammatory cytokines from hepatocytes, lymphocytes, and even the ECM itself. Withdrawal of the inciting agent can halt progression of this process; however, persistent inflammation results in continued deposition of collagen and liver fibrosis.

Examples of inflammation in the liver and carcinogenesis are seen in both CC (see Chapter 50) and HCC (see Chapter 89). Liver fibrosis and cirrhosis are associated with the development of HCC, which can result from multiple benign processes including steatosis, viral infection, or alcohol-induced liver disease. Although the cause of the underlying liver cirrhosis may differ, the pathophysiology of the development of cirrhosis and subsequent carcinogenesis are parallel. Similarly, long-standing primary sclerosing cholangitis (PSC) and chronic biliary stasis are associated with the development of CC, although immune activation in this case is less well understood. Analogous associations between chronic inflammation and malignancy are also seen in pancreatic cancer because chronic pancreatitis is associated with an increased risk for pancreatic adenocarcinoma.[44,45]

Cellular Plasticity

Cellular plasticity refers to changes to lineage specification and cell fate that occur with physiologic stress and are most commonly epigenetic or transcriptional in origin. Plasticity in cell fate is a hallmark of multiple inflammatory and neoplastic pathologies in HPB disease. Importantly, both the liver and pancreas do not display significant evidence of stem cell compartments, such that plasticity of terminally differentiated cells is critical to responses to injury. In the pancreas, acinar-to-ductal metaplasia (ADM) is the transition of acinar cells to ductal cells and occurs in the setting of chronic inflammation or pancreatitis (see Chapters 57 and 58). ADM is a precursor to pancreatic intraepithelial neoplasia (PanIN) and, ultimately, pancreatic ductal adenocarcinoma (PDAC; see Chapter 59) and represents a complex transdifferentiation event (i.e., direct conversion from acinar-to-ductal) that is also accompanied by features suggestive of a dedifferentiated phenotype (i.e., reversion within the pancreatic lineage). Notch and β-catenin pathways are reactivated, and several progenitor markers are expressed. Acinar cells readily acquire features of both ductal and progenitor cells in response to pancreatic injury, a cellular plasticity that is critical to tissue homeostasis.[46] Loss of acinar cell identity after injury is reversible with regeneration, such that the pancreas can regain its normal architecture and function. Regeneration of the acinar compartment is dependent on the reactivation of several aforementioned developmental pathways, including β-catenin signaling, Hedgehog signaling, and the Notch pathway. In tumorigenesis, the reprogramming of acinar cells is enforced by oncogenic *KRAS*, such that the acinar compartment cannot undergo this process of redifferentiation.

In the liver, hepatocytes can differentiate into cholangiocytes at times of injury or chronic inflammation, leading to the development of CC. In chronic liver disease, ductular proliferations containing cells that simultaneously express markers of hepatocytes and bile ducts are found. Interestingly, data have demonstrated that CCs that microscopically appear similar to HCC or combined HCC-CC are not necessarily derived from biliary epithelium (see Chapter 50). Evidence for biliary epithelial cell conversion into hepatocytes exists in rodent models of liver injury with either iethoxycarbonyl-1,

4-dihydrocollidine (DDC) or thioacetamide (TAA), wherein lineage-tracing makes clear that the hepatocyte compartment can be reconstituted in part by bile duct epithelial cells.[47]

Epithelial-mesenchymal transition (EMT) occurs in both normal development and pathologic processes such as cancer progression. EMT is a process during which epithelial cells undergo a series of transitions (e.g., loss of cell-to-cell adhesion, changes in morphology) to gain increased mobility.[48] This is important in the escape of tumor cells from the primary site and the development of distant metastases. In hepatobiliary disease, this accounts for metastatic disease to the liver, which is more common than primary liver tumors. EMT is well understood to reflect another outcome of cellular plasticity, whereby a mesenchymal cell fate is acquired by either internalization or downregulation of epithelial transcripts such as E-cadherin, along with concomitant increases in intermediate filament proteins, such as vimentin.[49]

Immune Cell Engagement

The liver is a lymphoid organ in many respects and plays an important role in immune tolerance. Given first-pass metabolism from the portal vein, there is significant antigen exposure to cells in the liver. A subset of cells within the liver are resident immune cells, including lymphocytes and Kupffer cells (macrophages). Many cell types in the liver have the potential to act as antigen presenting cells (APCs). These include the resident immune cells, such as Kupffer cells, hepatic dendritic cells, and sinusoidal endothelial cells, yet even hepatocytes and biliary epithelial cells can act as APCs during chronic inflammation and express class II major histocompatibility complexes (MHCs; see Chapters 5 and 7).[50]

Immune-mediated diseases are common in the liver and biliary tract. Immune-mediated cholangiopathies include primary biliary cirrhosis (PBC), PSC, and autoimmune cholangitis (see Chapters 41, 43, and 74). These are diseases of the intrahepatic biliary tree of which the underlying causes are largely unknown but believed to be immune in origin and ultimately result in biliary stasis. PBC is an autoimmune disorder characterized by disappearance of the intrahepatic bile ducts, and patients are characteristically antimitochondrial antibody–positive, whereas PSC is characterized by progressive inflammation and fibrosis of the intra- and extrahepatic bile ducts. Inflammatory-mediated destruction of the biliary tree can result in fibrosis, and ultimately cirrhosis, in many patients with PBC and PSC, given the persistent chronic inflammation. Similarly, we see immune cell engagement in primary liver pathophysiology. Autoimmune hepatitis involves antibody-mediated destruction of hepatocytes thought to be precipitated by environmental triggers, which results in activation of both the innate and adaptive immune systems; however, the mechanisms of it are not well understood. Viral hepatitis infection involves various components of the immune system. HBV and HCV infections both involve activation of the innate immune system, and immune evasion results in a chronic infection, which is more common in HCV.

Another important area to address regarding immune cell engagement is the use of immunotherapy in hepatobiliary malignancies. Immunotherapy has been largely ineffective in most HPB cancers. For example, recent trials evaluating pembrolizumab (KEYNOTE-240) and nivolumab (CheckMate 459) in HCC did not demonstrate a meaningful survival benefit compared with best supportive care and sorafenib, respectively[51,52] (see Chapter 99).

Tumor mutational burden (TMB) is defined as the number of mutations per coding area of tumor genome and has been shown to correlate with neoantigen expression. Neoantigen expression, and ultimately TMB, is related to response to immunotherapeutic agents.[53,54] There are additional biomarkers that can inform of the response to immunotherapy, including PD-L1 expression, but these have been shown to be poorly correlated with TMB.[55] HPB cancers are thought to be poorly responsive to immunotherapy secondary to the dearth of neoantigen expression resulting in a lack of immune cell engagement.[56]

A subset of HPB tumors have an increased TMB, including microsatellite stable PDAC (see Chapters 9D, 61, and 62) and CC (see Chapters 9C, 9E, 50, and 51), viral-induced HCC (see Chapters 9B, 68, and 89), and liver-fluke associated CC (see Chapters 9C, 9E, and 50). Immunotherapy has been shown to be more effective in this subset of patients. For example, KEYNOTE-158 evaluated pembrolizumab in patients with non-colorectal cancers with high microsatellite instability (MSI[hi]), including PDAC and CC, and demonstrated an overall response rate of 18.2% and 40.9%, respectively[57] (see Chapters 50, 66, 67, and 99).

Complex Genomic Alterations

The genomic landscape of HPB cancers has been well characterized over the last decade, and there has been an increased understanding of the driver genes that underlie carcinogenesis in these malignancies. In PDAC, the four well-established driver genes are *KRAS*, *TP53*, *CDKN2A*, and *SMAD4*[35] (see Chapters 9D and 59). Similar drivers, such as *KRAS* and *TP53*, are noted in biliary tract cancers, as well as additional, commonly altered genes such as *IDH1*, *IDH2*, and *PIK3CA*[36] (see Chapters 9C and 9E). Alterations in *KRAS* and *TP53* have been shown to be associated with decreased overall survival in PDAC and CC.[36,58] In addition to single nucleotide variants, copy number alterations (CNA) and large-scale chromosomal aberrations, including chromothripsis, are noted in CC, gallbladder cancer, and PDAC (see Chapters 9C–9E, 49, 50, and 59).

Although there are distinguishing mutations in the genomic drivers, HPB cancers are overall characterized by a paucity of mutational events. Previous studies have demonstrated a lower rate of somatic point mutations in pancreatic and hepatobiliary cancers compared with other cancer types.[59] As mentioned previously, a lower TMB is associated with fewer neoantigens and a decreased response to immunotherapeutic agents. By contrast, HCC in particular is noteworthy for profound structural variants and depression of transposable elements, which can also be found in the regenerative nodules of cirrhotic patients, long before the development of apparent malignancy.[60]

Unlike other tumor types such as non–small cell lung cancer and colorectal cancer, HPB cancers are also characterized by very few actionable genomic alterations, although recent studies have demonstrated some promise. For example, ivosidenib is a targeted inhibitor of mutated *IDH1* and has recently been shown to improve progression-free survival compared with placebo in patients with *IDH1*-mutated intrahepatic CC[61] (see Chapters 9C, 9E, and 50). Additionally, data suggest that patients diagnosed with PDAC who have germline

BRCA1 and *BRCA2* mutations treated with platinum-based chemotherapy and poly-adenosine diphosphate (ADP) ribose polymerase (PARP) inhibitors have improved outcomes[62–64] (see Chapters 9D, 61, and 62). Additional drivers of tumorigenesis have been identified and successfully targeted in a subset of KRAS-wildtype PDAC. These include *ALK* alterations that can be targeted with tyrosine kinase inhibitors,[65,66] *NRG1* rearrangements that have been treated with ERBB inhibitors,[67] and *NTRK* fusions.[68]

Epigenetic Mechanisms

Epigenetic alterations involve those exclusive of changes to the DNA sequence itself and include chromatin modification and post-transcriptional regulation. Recent studies have provided increasing evidence that epigenetic regulation plays a role in the development of many cancers, and, in particular, emerging evidence has supported this finding in HPB cancers. In PDAC, mutations have been found in the genes that encode *MLL2 (KMT2D)*, *MLL3 (KMT2C)*, and *KDM6A*, which encode proteins responsible for post-translational modifications, and *ARID1A*, which encodes a protein subunit of the SWI/SNF complex that is integral for chromatin remodeling[69,70] (see Chapter 9D). Among these, *ARID1A* and *KDM6A* appear to confer a basal or squamous transcriptional phenotype to PDAC, which is associated with poorer outcomes and with chemoresistance. Epigenetic mechanisms are also critical to defining organotropism and metabolic rewiring in metastatic disease.[71] Chromatin-based enhancer reprogramming also occurs in the absence of a genetic event and permits metastasis of established tumors.[72] Together, these data suggest that epigenetic regulators and chromatin plasticity drive aggressive behavior in this cancer.

In CC, mutations to the isocitrate dehydrogenase enzymes *IDH1* and *IDH2* are common resulting in the abnormal production of the oncometabolite 2-hydroxyglutarate (2-HG).

α-Ketoglutarate (α-KG), a key intermediate in the tricarboxylic acid (TCA) cycle, is diminished, and histone and DNA demethylases that require α-KG are affected so that there are resultant increases in DNA hypermethylation and altered gene expression (see Chapters 9C and 9E). Recently, it has been shown that p53 also preserves α-KG levels such that mutations to this tumor suppressor represent an alternate means by which cancers appear to hijack chromatin-modifying enzymes to alter transcriptional landscapes.[73] In HCC, chromatin regulators also appear central across the spectrum of malignancy, with elegant studies indicating that clonal mutations to these regulators first appear in cirrhosis and accumulate in full-blown HCC.[60] The key chromatin regulators mutated include *ARID1A*, *BAP1*, and *ARID2*, with *ARID1A* notably displaying distinct oncogenic and tumor suppressive roles in initiation and progression of HCC[74] (see Chapters 9B and 9C).

CONCLUSION

In conclusion, the molecular and cellular basis of HPB disease is a complex interaction between genetic alterations, epigenetic modifications, and immune dysregulations that alter several key conserved signaling pathways. The confluence of these mechanisms serves broadly to disrupt epithelial cell fate and homeostasis of the organ. Much progress has been made in understanding these processes in the last decade, allowing for improved therapeutic intervention for some disease. Subsequent chapters in this section will explore these principles in more depth to provide a greater understanding of molecular and cellular mediators that define benign and malignant HPB diseases.

The references for this chapter can be found online by accessing the accompanying Expert Consult website.

Molecular and cell biology of liver carcinogenesis and hepatitis

Takehiro Noda and Jack R. Wands

OVERVIEW OF MOLECULAR ETIOLOGY

Recent advances in molecular genetics have emphasized the multistep process of tumorigenesis. It is evident that cancer is a genetic disease involving aberrant chromosome rearrangements, genetic mutations, and epigenetic silencing of tumor suppressor genes.[1] Independent of the etiology, hepatocellular carcinoma (HCC) generally develops where sustained hepatocyte turnover occurs in the setting of injury-inflammation-regeneration, which leads to the accumulation of chromosomal aberrations (see Chapters 68 and 89). The monoclonal populations of hepatocytes become preneoplastic and, after additional genomic alterations, change into dysplastic cells and eventually HCC.[2] Accumulated genetic alterations in preneoplastic lesions and HCC result in the activation, as well as inactivation, of many growth factor signal transduction pathways involved in hepatic transformation. It is believed that increased hepatocyte turnover associated with chronic liver injury may be a major feature of hepatic oncogenesis. However, another central question is whether hepatitis viruses, the leading cause of HCC worldwide, directly contribute to the development of this disease. Accumulating evidence suggests that chronic hepatitis B virus (HBV) and hepatitis C virus (HCV) infection play a direct role in the molecular pathogenesis of HCC through specific viral–cellular protein interactions[3] (see Chapter 68). In this chapter, we discuss the molecular mechanisms of liver carcinogenesis and focus on the role of HBV and HCV.

EPIDEMIOLOGY

Primary liver cancer was the fourth leading cause of cancer death in 2015 after lung, colorectal, and stomach cancer.[4] It is estimated that 782,000 new patients with the disease were diagnosed in 2012.[5] The 5-year survival rate is less than 15% in developed countries, and the United States has a survival rate of 20.3%, making liver cancer the second most fatal tumor after pancreatic cancer.[6] Presumably because of its poor prognosis, liver cancer is the second leading cause of cancer death in men and the sixth among women in the world. It is estimated that about 745,000 individuals worldwide died from this disease in 2012.[5] It is one of the few neoplasms with a steadily increasing incidence and mortality in the United States.[7]

Primary liver cancer comprises a heterogeneous group of malignant tumors with different histologic features. The unfavorable prognosis varies from hepatocellular carcinoma (HCC) and intrahepatic cholangiocarcinoma (iCCA) to mixed hepatocellular cholangiocarcinoma (HCC-CCA), fibrolamellar HCC, and the pediatric neoplasm hepatoblastoma[8] (see Chapters 50, 87, and 89). The most common is HCC, which accounts for 70% to 85% of all hepatic tumors.[9] Approximately 80% of HCC is caused by chronic infection with HBV or HCV (see Chapter 68). The HCC burden is unevenly distributed worldwide; areas where tumors are most prevalent include West and Central Africa and East and Southeast Asia, with China alone accounting for more than 50% of the world cases.[5] The incidence of HCC varies with both geographic location and ethnicity. For example, HCV is the leading etiology of HCC in the United States, Europe, Japan, and South America, whereas HBV is the major cause in the majority of Asian and African countries.[10]

Trends in HCC incidence are likely to be different in regions of high and low persistence of HBV and HCV infection.[11] Comparative studies performed between 1977 and 1982 and between 1993 and 1997 show that the incidence of HCC in Hong Kong, Shanghai, Singapore, and Japan has begun to decrease.[12] The fall in incidence is apparently because of vaccination against HBV, which has been accomplished in greater than 80% of newborns,[13] because chronic HBV infection in those countries is usually acquired through mother-to-newborn or sibling-to-sibling transmission at a young age. Although HBV vaccination reduces the incidence of HCC, many unvaccinated persons are still infected with HBV (257 million in 2015), mostly in Asia and sub-Saharan Africa.[14]

The incidence of HCC has increased in some countries, such as Australia, the United States, and the United Kingdom, probably as the result of chronic HCV infection and nonalcoholic steatohepatitis (NASH; see Chapter 69). The annual incidence of liver cancer increased from 2.6 per 100,000 population for the years 1978 to 1980 to 8 per 100,000 in 2010, of which at least 3 of 4 cases are because of HCC.[15] Reasons for this increased incidence are not entirely clear but may reflect a greater prevalence of NASH and role of persistent HCV infection.[16] Recent advances in direct-acting antiviral (DAA) agents for HCV will cure most individuals with chronic HCV infection, and it has been estimated that reducing the frequency of chronic HCV infection by 90% would eliminate 15% of HCC in the United States.[17] However, there is debate over the effects of DAA agents on tumor progression.[18]

The age of onset of HCC varies in different parts of the world. HCC tends to occur later in life in Japan, North America, and European countries, where the median age of onset is above 60 years. In contrast, in parts of Asia and most African countries, HCC is commonly diagnosed in the age range of 30 to 60 years.[19] In the United States, however, recent trends have revealed a peak incidence shifting toward a relatively younger age group.[15]

Significant gender and ethnic variation in incidence, as well as mortality from HCC, has also been found; male rates are nearly triple that of females.[5] The most likely explanation for gender variation is that men have more risk factors, such as exposure to hepatitis virus infection, excessive alcohol intake, smoking, and increased iron stores in the liver.[11] In addition, androgen levels may accelerate the progression of HCC through interaction with the HBV genome.[20,21] The incidence of HCC also varies with race and ethnicity in the same area. In the United States, the incidence and subsequent mortality rates are two times greater in Asians than African Americans, which are two times greater than those found in Caucasians.[11] These variations are explained, in part, by the accumulation of major risk factors in each ethnic group.

RISK FACTORS

Unlike most malignancies, HCC has well-established extrinsic risk factors that account for at least 80% of tumors (namely chronic infection with HBV or HCV; see Chapter 68). Key epidemiologic aspects of HBV- and HCV-induced HCC are summarized in Table 9B.1. Chronic HBV infection is the leading cause of HCC, and it has been estimated that there are 350 to 400 million HBV carriers, which account for 5% of the global population. About 59% of HCC patients in developing countries and 23% of HCC patients in developed countries are chronically infected with HBV.[22] Risk factors for HBV-related HCC include demographic features such as male sex, older age, Asian or African ancestry, family history of HCC, viral properties (higher levels of HBV replication; HBV genotype; longer duration of infection; co-infection with HCV, human immunodeficiency virus [HIV], or hepatitis delta virus), clinical factors (cirrhosis), and environmental factors (exposure to aflatoxin, heavy intake of alcohol or tobacco).[23] The 5-year cumulative incidence rates of HCC from HBV-related cirrhosis are 17% in highly endemic areas and 10% in Europe and the United States.[24] HBV can cause HCC in the absence of cirrhosis, although approximately 70% to 90% of HBV-related HCC cases develop in patients with this disease.[25] Nucleoside/nucleotide analogues that suppress viral replication are associated with risk reduction of HCC in patients with chronic hepatitis B.[26] Aflatoxin B1 (AFB1) is produced by *Aspergillus flavus* and related fungi that contaminate corn, rice, and peanuts in China and sub-Saharan Africa. High rates of dietary exposure to AFB1 increase the risk for HCC 4-fold. When people with chronic HBV infections are exposed to AFB1, the relative risk for HCC dramatically increases to about 60-fold.[27] This synergistic effect between AFB1 exposure and chronic HBV infection is an important observation because in some regions of the world, AFB1 exposure and chronic HBV infection rates are high.

Chronic HCV infection is the second leading cause of HCC. The estimated number of HCV carriers worldwide is 180 million, which accounts for 2% of the global population. Approximately 33% of HCC tumors in developing countries and 20% of HCC in developed countries are attributable to persistent HCV infection.[22] According to cross-sectional and case-control studies, HCC risk is increased 15- to 20-fold in HCV-infected people compared with the HCV-negative population.[28] Patients with HCV-induced cirrhosis are at particularly high risk for the development of HCC, with an annual incidence of HCC ranging from 0.5% to 10%. Sustained virologic response (SVR) with DAA agents has emerged as the most dominant modifier of HCC in patients with HCV.[23] Although DAA is likely to change the epidemiology of HCV-related HCC in those who are treated, most HCV-infected populations remain untreated. The DAAs offer a chance for

TABLE 9B.1	Comparison of Epidemiologic Features between HBV- and HCV-Induced HCC	
	HBV*	**HCV**
Virus carriers (% of global population)	350-400 million (5%)	180 million (2%)
Highly prevalent areas	Asia, sub-Saharan Africa, Melanesia, Micronesia	Africa, South and East Asia, South America
Relative risk of HCC	5- to 100-fold*	15- to 20-fold
5-year cumulative incidence rates of HCC from cirrhosis	10% (Europe and United States) 17% (East Asia)	17% (Europe and United States) 30% (Japan)

HBV, Hepatitis B virus; HCC, hepatocellular carcinoma; HCV, hepatitis C virus.

*Depends on multiple factors, including HBV load, presence of cirrhosis, and exposure to aflatoxin B1.

From El-Serag HB, Kanwal F. Epidemiology of hepatocellular carcinoma in the United States: Where are we? Where do we go? *Hepatology.* 2014;60:1767–1775, and El-Serag HB. Epidemiology of viral hepatitis and hepatocellular carcinoma. *Gastroenterology.* 2012;142:1264–1273.

cure of patients with advanced cirrhosis, older age, and alcohol use. These patients had a poor response to interferon (IFN)-based therapies. However, there was no evidence for differential occurrence of HCC or recurrence risk after SVR attributable to DAA or IFN-based therapy.[29]

Excessive ethanol consumption (>50–70 g/day) is another well-defined risk factor for HCC. Alcoholic cirrhosis is the second most common risk factor for HCC in the United States and Europe.[19,30] There was a linear increase of a relative risk for HCC by 5-fold when 60 to 140 g/day alcohol was consumed. The 5-year cumulative HCC incidence in alcoholic cirrhosis without HBV and HCV infection is 8%[31]; however, it is unlikely that ethanol itself has a direct carcinogenic effect. Rather, excessive ethanol ingestion indirectly affects hepatocarcinogenesis through the promotion of cirrhosis. Indeed, greater than 80% of HCC tumors found in alcoholics develop in the background of a cirrhotic liver. A synergistic effect between heavy alcohol consumption and hepatitis virus infection has been observed in several studies. The relative risk for HCC attributable to heavy alcohol consumption alone was only 2.4-fold, whereas in combination with chronic HCV infection, it increased to 50-fold.[32] Others have reported that concomitant HCV infection in alcoholics increases the risk for HCC 2-fold, whereas HBV infection moderately increases this risk 1.2- to 1.5-fold.[30,33]

Growing evidence now suggests that metabolic dysfunction, including obesity, diabetes, and nonalcoholic fatty liver disease (NAFLD), are important risk factors for HCC, especially in developed countries[34] (see Chapter 69). Several large cohort studies revealed that obesity is a definitive risk factor for HCC, with the 1.5- to 4-fold increased risk. Men are more susceptible to obesity-associated HCC than women. NAFLD-associated HCC also occurs frequently in the absence of cirrhosis.[35] Diabetes mellitus has also been established as a moderately strong risk factor for HCC, with a two- to four-times higher risk.[11,36] The use of metformin is associated with decreased risk, and the use of insulin or sulfonylureas may increase HCC risk. Longer duration of diabetes may be associated with an incremental increase in risk.[37–39] More recently,

NASH, the more aggressive form of NAFLD, is considered to be a cause of a large proportion of cryptogenic cirrhosis, which is risk for HCC development. However, the overall incidence of HCC in patients with NAFLD is lower than in patients with other well-established etiologies, such as chronic viral infection.[36]

Cigarette smoking is one risk factor for HCC. The HCC risk of current and former smoking was 1.55 and 1.39 times, respectively.[40] Cirrhosis of any cause increases the risk for HCC, with an annual incidence between 2% and 4%.

GENETIC AND EPIGENETIC ALTERATIONS

Chronic inflammation accompanied by sustained cycles of injury and regeneration of hepatocytes over 20 to 40 years promotes the development of liver fibrosis, cirrhosis, and eventually HCC (Fig. 9B.1A; see Chapter 7). Pathologically, HCC occurs early within cirrhotic nodules, which can form in areas of adenomatous hyperplasia or dysplasia. These cells eventually become more atypical, and the malignant transformation process is completed.[41] HCC is like other malignancies and represents a DNA disease with accumulation of many alterations in oncogenes and tumor suppressor genes. The accumulation of genetic aberrations that induces cellular transformation may take 20 to 40 years, suggesting that liver carcinogenesis involves a multistep process.

Cirrhosis may represent end-stage liver disease as a result of persistent HBV or HCV infection. Because about 80% of HCC tumors originate from cirrhotic liver, it is evident that continuous rounds of cellular injury, followed by regeneration fundamentally contributes to the oncogenic processes. The sustained cycles of injury and repair increase the chance of genomic alteration. Furthermore, the host inflammatory response to viral infection, including activation of stellate cells, causes the release of proinflammatory cytokines, which accelerate hepatic carcinogenesis by augmenting oxidative stress and DNA damage.[42–44] Continuous rounds of this process in the presence of inflammation not only increase the chance of genomic alterations but also produce chromosome instability. For example, hyperploidy has been observed in 43% of dysplastic peritumoral regions and in about 50% of HCC tumors.[45] The molecular mechanisms underlying such genomic instability include telomerase dysfunction, defective segregation of chromosomes, and an impaired DNA damage response (see Fig. 9B.1B).

Recent advances in genome-wide analysis, including whole-genome sequencing and DNA array technologies, have provided more detailed information on the alterations of oncogenic or tumor suppressive genes.[46–48] Accordingly, development of molecularly targeted therapy for HCC will be challenging. Nevertheless, several frequently mutated genes, such telomerase reverse transcriptase (TERT), the tumor suppressor gene (TP53), the β-catenin gene (CTNNB1), the axis inhibition protein 1 gene (AXIN1), the AT-rich interactive domain 1A [SWI-like] gene (ARID1A), tuberous sclerosis complex 1/2 (TSC1/TSC2), and the nuclear factor (erythroid derived 2)-like 2 (NFE2L2), are found in HCC. The key genes of major signaling pathways are involved by genetic alterations; TP53 in p53-Rb and CTNNB1 and AXIN1 of WNT (wingless type)/β-catenin pathways, as well as ARID1A in chromatin remodeling, TSC1/TSC2 in phosphatidylinositol-3-kinase (PI3K)/mechanistic target of rapamycin (mTOR) pathway, NFE2L2 in nuclear factor

(erythroid-2 like) factor 2(NRF2)-KEAP1 pathway.[49] Newly identified alterations in these genes can suggest potential therapeutic and diagnostic opportunities.

Telomerase is a key enzyme for cell survival that prevents telomere shortening and the subsequent cellular senescence that is observed after many rounds of cell division. Absence of telomerase activity and shortening of telomeres have been implicated in hepatocyte senescence and the development of cirrhosis, a chronic liver disease that can progress to HCC.[50] In human HCC, telomere shortening has been shown to have a positive correlation with increased chromosome instability—chromosomal gains, losses, and translocations—by promoting chromosomal fusions.[51] In some HBV-induced HCC tumors, the viral genome is integrated into the TERT locus, which results in increased expression of telomerase.[48,52] Direct sequencing of the TERT promoter region has revealed that 59% of HCCs have recurrent somatic mutations, which may result in the activation of TERT, and TERT promoter mutation are frequently associated with CTNNB1 mutations.[53] Other findings related to telomerase biology indicate amplification of telomerase RNA component gene (TERC) mRNA and allelic loss of chromosome 10p, where a putative telomerase inhibitor resides.[54,55] Re-activated telomerase enzyme maintains the shortened telomere length in these tumor cells and prevents them from undergoing apoptosis.

DNA damage-response pathways are safeguards that regulate cell-cycle checkpoints and prevent DNA-damaged cells from further proliferation. Several studies report that the functions of key regulatory molecules, including p53, mouse double-minute 2 (MDM2), retinoblastoma 1 (RB1), and p16INK4a (also known as CDKN2A [cyclin-dependent kinase inhibitor 2A]) were impaired in human HCC. The p53 protein, encoded by the TP53 gene, is a master molecule that maintains genome integrity by inducing cell-cycle arrest, followed by activation of DNA repair systems. Moreover, TP53 is one of the most mutated genes in HCC, and the mutations often result in loss of function. The frequency ranges between 11% and 35%, depending on the regions of the world. The regional difference in the frequency is attributable to a specific mutation caused by AFB1 exposure. TP53 missense mutations in codon 249 (R249S) were found in more than 50% of AFB1-related HCC and appeared to be the main cause of AFB1-induced liver cancer.[56,57] Therefore TP53 mutations in HCC can be frequently found in Africa and Asia where people are exposed to a high level of AFB1. Other mutations of TP53 are found in 20% to 40% of HCC without molecular evidence of AFB1 exposure.[11] The aberration of the p53 pathway can be caused by molecules that inappropriately regulate p53 functions. The MDM2 is an E3 ubiquitin ligase targeting tumor suppressor proteins, including p53 and RB1. Strikingly, gankyrin (encoded by Proteasome 26S Subunit, Non-ATPase 10[PSMD10]), which promotes such protein degradation by MDM2, was highly overexpressed in human HCC.[58,59] More recently, genome-wide copy number variation analysis identified IFN regulatory factor 2 (IRF2) as a novel tumor suppressor gene in HCC that activates the p53 pathway and revealed that IRF2 loss-of-function mutations were frequently and exclusively found in HBV-related HCC.[46] The CDKN2A gene encodes for two splice-variant products, including p16INK4a and p14ARF, which positively regulate the p53 and RB1 signaling pathways. The expression of the CDKN2A gene was suppressed in 30% to 70% of human HCC as a result of methylation of the

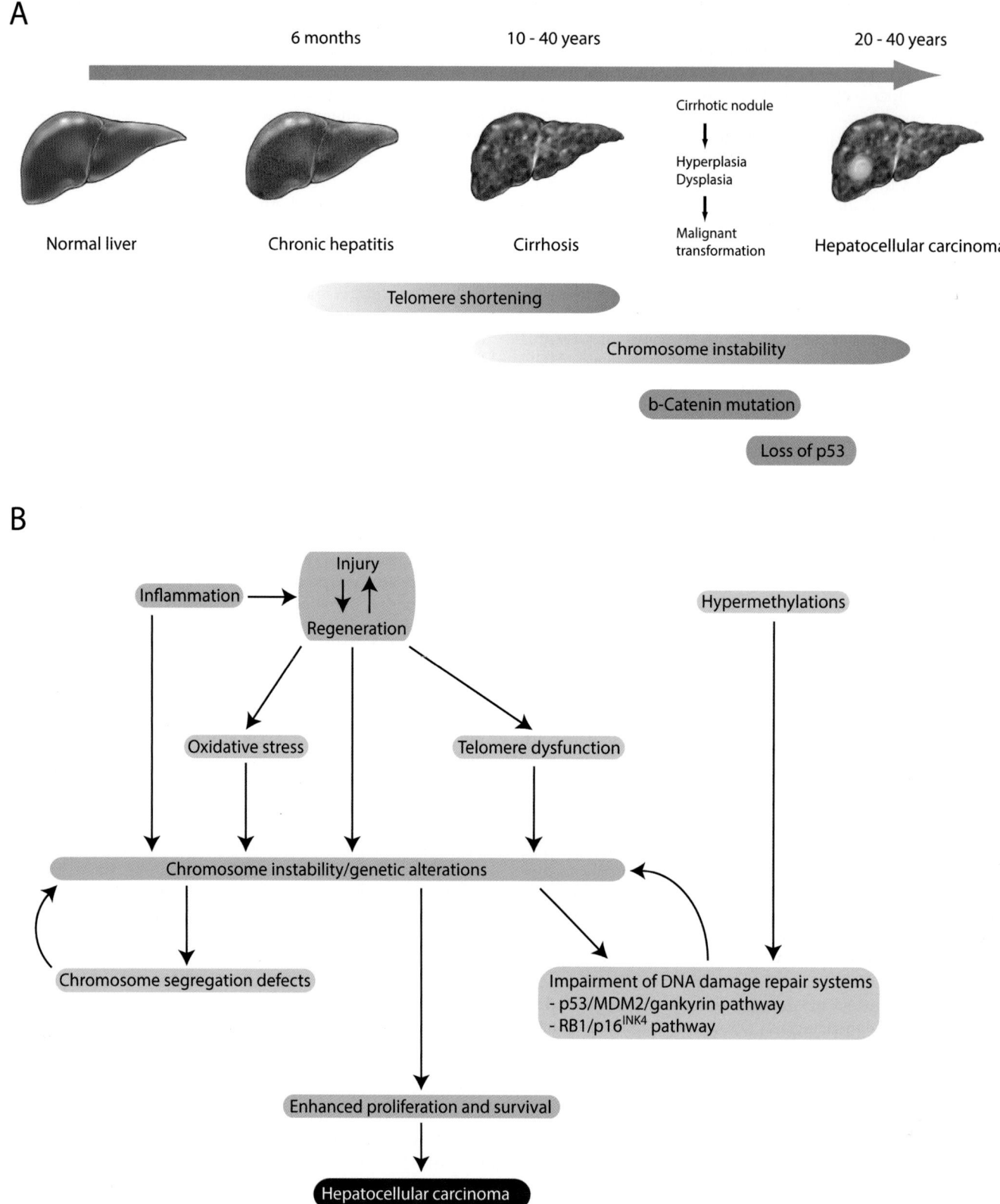

FIGURE 9B.1   A, Diagram showing progression of liver disease and genetic events accompanied by chronic inflammation. **B,** Common mechanisms underlying hepatocarcinogenesis. A number of factors contribute to chromosome instability and other genetic alterations, which lead to the formation of hepatocellular carcinoma.

promoter region.[60–63] Loss of heterogeneity of chromosome 9p, where *CDKN2A* is located, was found in 15% to 20% of tumors.[64–66] Interestingly, *CDKN2A* deletion rarely occurs in HCC when *TP53* is also mutated.[67] Taken together, impairment of the p53 and RB1 pathways is a common genetic feature of HCC development, growth, and progression.

The canonical WNT pathway plays a central role in the development of many tumor types and is a key regulator of β-catenin, which is encoded by the *CTNNB1* gene. *CTNNB1* is one of the most frequently mutated genes in HCC, ranging from 20% to 40%.[57,68] The activating mutations frequently occur in exon 3, which result in the nuclear accumulation of β-catenin, thereby inducing WNT-responsive gene expression. Indeed, nuclear accumulation of β-catenin is associated with a more aggressive phenotype and with poor prognosis in HCC patients.[69] Another frequently mutated gene in the canonical WNT pathway is *AXIN1*, a gene encoding a cytoplasmic protein that negatively regulates WNT signaling. *AXIN1* mutations are found in about 10% of HCC.[46,70] Loss-of-function mutations of *AXIN1* lead to a decrease in degradation of β-catenin and to nuclear localization of this protein.

Epigenetic regulation of the genome is a fundamental determinant of global gene expression. Epigenetic regulators have come to be recognized as tumor suppressors because next-generation sequencing of cancer genomes has defined frequent mutations in epigenetic regulators, including chromatin remodeling proteins and histone-modification proteins. In HCC, the AT-rich interactive domain *ARID* family, including *ARID1A*, *ARID1B*, and *ARID2*, was found to be mutated in 6% to 17% of HCC genomes.[46,48,71] Through the interaction with the switch/sucrose nonfermentable (SWI/SNF) chromatin-remodeling complex, ARID family proteins bind transcription factors and recruit the remodeling activity to a specific gene. Mechanisms underlying tumor development by loss-of-function mutations of *ARID* family genes are not known in detail, but it is highly likely that *ARID* mutations are associated with tumor proliferation, dedifferentiation, and inhibition of apoptosis.[72] MLL and MLL3 are histone methyltransferases that positively regulate gene transcription. The *MLL* gene translocations are frequently found in infant leukemia, but the significance of loss-of-function mutations of *MLL* family in HCC remains to be determined.[73]

TSC1/*TSC2* are both negative modulators of mTOR cascade, and their inactivation promotes mTOR signaling.[74] The mutations of *TSC1* or *TSC2* are described in 2% to 5% of HCC.[49,75] *TSC1*/*TSC2* mutations are closely associated with the scirrhous HCC subtype, defined by marked stromal fibrosis.[76]

NRF2 encoded by *NFE2L2* is centrally involved in counteracting such oxidative stress by enhancing adaptive oxidative stress and hence survival. NRF2 is negatively regulated and targeted to proteasomal degradation by Kelch-like ECH-associated protein 1 (KEAP1). The activating *NFE2L2* mutation is identified in 6% to 7% of adult HCC.[46] The dysregulation of the KEAP1-NRF2 molecular pathway is observed in human HCC. The protein NRF2 is frequently mutated and activated at early steps of the tumorigenic process.[77] These key genetic alterations in HCC are summarized in Table 9B.2.

It is evident that the expression and function of oncogenes and tumor suppressor genes are affected by copy number because of chromosomal gains and losses and by point mutations

TABLE 9B.2	Genetic Alterations Frequently Found in HCC	
GENE SYMBOL	**GENETIC ALTERATION**	**FREQUENCY (%)**
Telomere Maintenance		
TERT	Promoter activation	20-60
WNT/β-Catenin		
CTNNB1	Gain-of-function mutation	20-40
AXIN1	Loss-of-function mutation	3-16
Cell Cycle		
TP53	Loss-of-function mutation	11-35
CDKN2A	Loss of heterozygosity	
Promoter inactivation	15-20	
30-70		
Proliferation		
IRF2	Loss-of-function mutation	5
IGF2R	Allelic loss	0-13
Epigenetic Modifier		
ARID1A/1B	Loss-of-function mutation	7-17
ARID2	Loss-of-function mutation	6-16
PI3K-mTOR Pathway		
TSC1	mTOR signaling	2
TSC2	mTOR signaling	5
Nrf2-Keap1 Pathway		
NFE2L2	Oxidative stress	5

HCC, Hepatocellular carcinoma.

From Ding J, Wang H. Multiple interactive factors in hepatocarcinogenesis. *Cancer Lett.* 2014;346:17–23; and Marquardt JU, Thorgeirsson SS. SnapShot: Hepatocellular carcinoma, *Cancer Cell.* 2014;25:550; and Totoki Y, Tatsuno K., Covington K. R., et al. Trans-ancestry mutational landscape of hepatocellular carcinoma genomes. *Nat Genet.* 2014;46:1267–1273.

in the genes. However, recent studies have revealed that epigenetic mechanisms—such as DNA methylation and short, noncoding RNA (21–23 nucleotides) species, or microRNA (miRNA)—also contribute to aberrant expression of oncogenes and tumor suppressor genes. In human HCC, aberrant DNA methylation patterns have been detected.[2,78,79] More importantly, hypermethylation has been observed at the earliest stages of HCC development, and the extent of hypermethylation tends to increase with tumor progression.[80] Specific gene targets for hypermethylation include *CDKN2A*, prostaglandin-endoperoxide synthase 2 *(PTGS2)*, *CDH1*, *PYCARD*, *GADD45B*, and *DLC1*. Among these genetic elements, it has been shown that *CDKN2A*, *GADD45B*, and *PTGS2* expression were directly affected by methylation, using human HCC cell lines.[61,62,81,82]

In addition, miRNA contributes to mRNA instability by hybridizing with its complementary target sequence, followed by degradation, so that a protein cannot be generated. Several studies reveal aberrant expression of some miRNAs in human HCCs compared with the adjacent, non-tumorous counterparts. Many miRNAs perform tumor suppressor function by downregulating oncogene expression. Nevertheless, other miRNAs are oncogenic functions by downregulating tumor suppressor genes or upregulating oncogene expression levels to promote liver cancer development. For example, miR-21 is expressed in human HCC; it targets the phosphatase and tensin (PTEN) tumor suppressor gene.[83] Also, miR-21 promotes hepatic lipid accumulation and hepatocarcinogenesis by interacting with the HBP1-p53-SREBP1C pathway.[84] MicroRNA-122, which targets the cyclin G_1 cell-cycle regulator, is abundant in normal hepatocytes and is essential for homeostasis of hepatocytes. Its implication in hepatocarcinogenesis was revealed using knockout mice and clinical samples.[85,86] The MicroRNA 193a-5p appears to prevent liver tumorigenesis by reducing levels of nucleolar and spindle-associated protein 1 (NUSAP1).[87] The expression of miR-26a is diminished in murine and human tumors, resulting in enhanced activity of cyclin D2 and E2 to promote cell proliferation. Moreover, when exogenous miR-26a is overexpressed in mice prone to form multiple HCCs, substantial protection from disease progression is observed, indicating a possible therapeutic approach for this disease.[88] These findings indicate that epigenetic and posttranscriptional regulation of gene expression plays an important role in hepatic oncogenesis.

SIGNAL TRANSDUCTION PATHWAYS

Genetic alterations of oncogenes and tumor suppressor genes impinge on a wide variety of signal transduction pathways involved in proliferation and tumor cell viability. Although the spectrum of affected signal transduction pathways in HCC cells is more heterogeneous compared with that of affected signals in other tumor types, key pathways are commonly dysregulated in human HCC, such as the WNT/β-catenin, erythroblastosis (ERB)-B receptor tyrosine kinase (ERBB)/extracellular signal-regulated protein kinase (ERK)/PI3K, and insulin-like growth factor (IGF)/insulin receptor substrate (IRS)/ERK/PI3K cascades (Fig. 9B.2).

The WNT/β-catenin pathway has a role in physiologic embryogenesis and regulates cell proliferation, motility, and differentiation. WNT proteins are ligands that bind to Frizzled (FZD) cell-surface receptors to stabilize β-catenin in the cytoplasm, followed by translocation to the nucleus, where it upregulates WNT-responsive genes.[89] In the absence of WNT signaling, the amount of cytosolic β-catenin is low as a result of proteolytic degradation produced by the action of glycogen synthetase kinase-3β (GSK-3β)/adenomatosis polyposis coli (APC)/AXIN kinase destruction complex. However, when WNT ligands bind to the FZD/low-density-lipoprotein receptor-related protein-5/6 (LRP-5/6)/Disheveled (DVL) receptor complex, phosphorylation of β-catenin by GSK-3β is inhibited to allow its accumulation in the cytoplasm. The β-catenin molecules are then transported into the nucleus and bind to T-cell factor (TCF)/leukocyte enhancer factor (LEF) transcription factors; this complex acts as transcriptional regulators. Finally, the TCF/LEF/β-catenin complex promotes activation of target genes, including cyclin D1 (CCND1), myelocytomatosis viral oncogene (MYC), PTGS2, and JUN, which leads to proliferation of HCC cells.[90] The frequency of β-catenin nuclear accumulation varies between 17% and 75%, as determined by immunohistochemical staining.[69,91,92] Nuclear accumulation of β-catenin is an excellent biomarker for activation of WNT signaling in HCC. The activation of β-catenin occurs at an earlier stage of the oncogenic process in dysplastic cells, suggesting that the WNT/β-catenin cascade is directly involved in tumor formation.[2,93–95]

The major cell-surface molecules in WNT/β-catenin signaling are FZD receptors. There are 10 FZD receptors (FZD1 to FZD10) in humans. Indeed, studies reveal that 23% to 59% of HBV-related HCCs overexpress the FZD7. Through the interaction with a FZD-ligand WNT3, overexpressed FZD7 leads to the activation of this pathway in human tumors and HCC cell lines.[96,97] The functional consequences of FZD7 overexpression are enhanced cell motility and invasion. In murine HCC models, overexpression of FZD7 occurs in dysplastic nodules and HCC tissue but not in normal liver.[95,98] The FZD7 overexpression is a common event during hepatic oncogenesis in that it promotes tumor cell motility and invasion.

Receptor tyrosine kinases (RTKs) and subsequent signal transduction, including the mitogen-activated protein kinase (MAPK) pathway and the PI3K/AKT pathway, play a central role in tumor cell proliferation and survival. The ERBB family (especially ERBB1), MET proto-oncogene, and IGF-1 receptor (IGF-1R) are the RTKs frequently activated in HCC cells. The ERBB family consists of four RTKs, including ERBB1/EGFR/HER1, ERBB2/HER2/NEU, ERBB3/HER3, and ERBB4/HER4.[99] When ligands bind to the ERBB1 receptor, autophosphorylation occurs that leads to an association with the growth factor receptor–bound protein 2 (GRB2) adaptor molecule and PI3K. When phosphorylated ERBB1 binds to GRB2, the complex activates the rat sarcoma (RAS) oncoprotein, resulting in enhancement of RAF serine/threonine kinase activity. Activated RAF kinase triggers MEK/ERK kinases, as well as ERK, which translocates to the nucleus and upregulates the transcription of oncogenes such as FBJ murine osteosarcoma viral oncogene homolog, JUN, and MYC. When phosphorylated ERBB1 binds to PI3K, ERBB1 activates PI3K and the downstream AKT kinase. AKT phosphorylates a number of important molecules, including mTOR, GSK-3β, and inhibitor of kappa B kinase (IKK) to promote proliferation and viability of tumor cells. TSC1/TSC2 are both negative modulators of AKT/mTOR cascade.

ERBB1 and ERBB3 were overexpressed in 68% and 84% of HCC, respectively, which correlates with an aggressive phenotype.[100] Ligands for ERBB include epidermal growth factor (EGF), transforming growth factor (TGF)-α, heparin-binding EGF (HB-EGF), amphiregulin, β-cellurin, and epiregulin. In this regard, TGF-α and HB-EGF proteins may play a role in the pathogenesis of HCC. TGF-α was frequently upregulated at an earlier stage of tumor formation.[101,102] The upregulation of TGF-α was linked to the oncogenic process.[103] The HB-EGF protein was a potent mitogen for hepatocytes, detected in about 60% of HCC cases.[104] Moreover, overexpression of HB-EGF was found at an earlier stage of HCC with moderately or well-differentiated features,[105] suggesting that HB-EGF is an important ligand in initiation of this disease. As a consequence, MAPK activity is increased in HCC, compared with adjacent non-tumorous tissues.[106,107]

The IGF signaling cascade regulates energy metabolism and cell growth. It consists of ligands, receptors, adaptors, and subsequent MAPK and PI3K/AKT pathways. The ligands IGF-1, IGF-2, and insulin bind to receptors of IGF-1R homodimers and heterodimers consisting of IGF-1R and insulin receptors and activate their kinase domain. Activated receptors phosphorylate adaptor proteins such as IRS-1 and IRS-2, which are able to trigger the MAPK and PI3K/AKT signaling cascades. Negative regulators are IGF-2R and IGF-binding proteins (IGFBPs). IGF-2R is a decoy receptor to which IGF-2 exclusively binds, but no

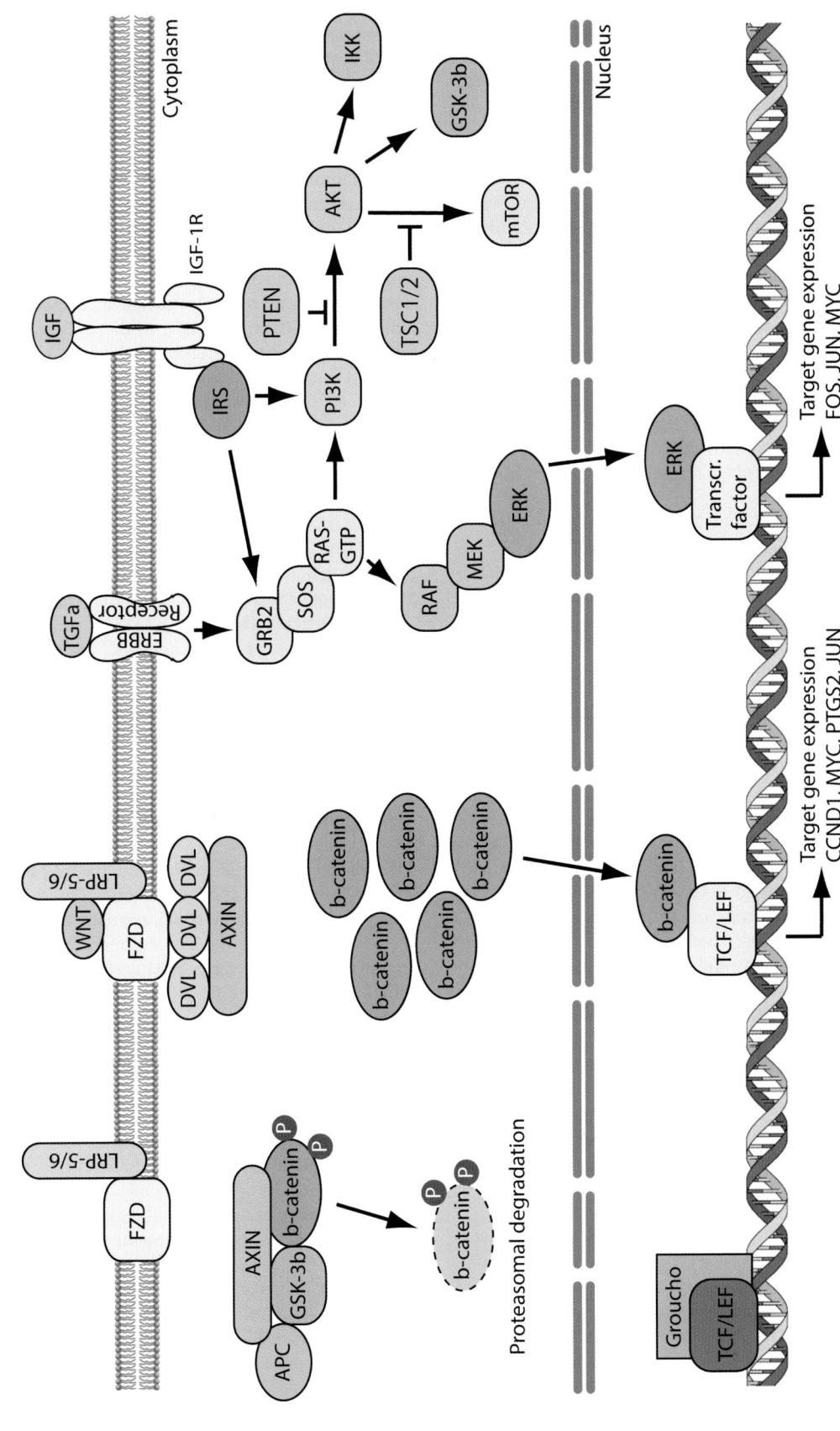

FIGURE 9B.2 Schematic diagram showing the major components of three signal-transduction pathways involved in hepatic oncogenesis. In the WNT/β-catenin cascade, accumulation of β-catenin is regulated by WNT ligands. The ERBB and IGF/IRS pathways both use downstream activation of several kinases, including the RAS/RAF/MEK/ERK and PI3K/AKT cascades. *AKT,* v-Akt murine thymoma viral oncogene homolog; *APC,* antigen-presenting cell; *AXIN,* ***; *ERK,* extracellular signal-regulated protein kinase; *DVL,* Disheveled (receptor); *ERBB,* erythroblastosis (ERB)-B receptor tyrosine kinase; *FZD,* Frizzled (receptor); *GRB2,* growth factor receptor–bound protein 2; *GSK,* glycogen synthetase kinase; *GTP,* guanosine triphosphate; *IGF-1R,* insulin-like growth factor-1 receptor; *IKK,* inhibitor of κB kinase; *I/R,* ischemia/reperfusion; *IRS,* insulin receptor substrate; *LEF,* leukocyte enhancer factor; *MEK,* mitogen-activated protein kinase; *mTOR,* mammalian target of rapamycin; *SOS,* son of sevenless homolog; *TCF,* T-cell factor; *TGF,* transforming growth factor; *transcr.,* transcription; *WNT,* wingless type.

activation of downstream molecules occurs. IGFBP-3, a predominant form of IGFBPs, is a neutralizing peptide that binds to circulating IGF-1 and IGF-2.[108]

Many lines of evidence have established that dysregulation of IGF pathway is involved in the malignant transformation, cancer development, and even resistance to anticancer agents. The same is true for HCC. Comprehensive analysis of 104 HCC cases revealed that IGF pathway activation, namely the presence of phosphorylated IGF-1R, was found in 21% of the cases.[109] Overexpression of IGF-2, downregulation of IGFBP-3, or allelic losses of *IGF2R*, which all lead to the activation of the pathway, was found in 25% of the cases. Another report revealed that the IGF-2 ligand was overexpressed in 16% to 40% of tumors, as well as in dysplastic tissue, suggesting that IGF-2 may act by autocrine and/or paracrine mechanisms.[110] IRS adaptor molecules are also important in HCC development. IRS-1 is overexpressed in the majority of human HCCs.[111,112] Constitutive MEK/ERK pathway activation may also occur via downregulation of a RAF kinase inhibitor protein (RKIP); this event promotes HCC cell proliferation and migration.[113] Indeed, downregulation of RKIP was found in 90% of human HCC and suggests that it plays a role as a tumor suppressor protein.

The PI3K/AKT/mTOR and RAS/RAF/mitogen-activated protein kinase pathways are activated in around 5% to 10% of HCC by amplification of the FGF19/CCND1 locus. Also, inactivating mutations of *TSC1* or *TSC2* (2%–5%) lead to activation of mTOR signaling in a subset of HCC.[49,114] Homozygous deletion of *PTEN*, an inhibitor of the PI3K kinase, has been identified in approximately 1% to 3% of HCC.

The angiogenic pathway is the most important molecular target in HCC because HCC is usually a highly vascular tumor.[115] Angiogenesis is a complex process regulated by many factors, such as vascular endothelial growth factor (VEGF), platelet-derived growth factor (PDGF), and basic fibroblast growth factor (bFGF). VEGF and its receptors VEGF-R1, -2, and -3 are overexpressed in HCC, and overexpression of VEGF is associated with poor prognosis.[116,117] PDGF recruits pericytes and smooth muscle cells around new vessels. bFGF is involved in endothelial cell migration, capillary branching, and the activity of proteases, which are essential for angiogenesis. These growth factors bind and stimulate their corresponding receptors on angiogenic cells and activate the subsequent signal pathways, including MAPK, PI3K/AKT, SRC, and phospholipase C (PLC)-γ pathways. Sorafenib is a small-molecule multikinase inhibitor that inactivates VEGF receptors, PDGF receptors, v-Kit Hardy-Zuckerman 4 feline sarcoma viral oncogene homolog (KIT), and B-Raf proto-oncogene (BRAF).[118] It is the first drug proven to be effective in advanced HCC[119] (see Chapter 99). The antiangiogenic approach may become a mainstream of the systemic treatment of HCC, and in fact, many clinical trials for use of such agents are currently underway.[120]

Oxidative stress is a process whereby the body receives stimulation from harmful endogenous or exogenous factors. Free radicals, including reactive oxygen species (ROS) and reactive nitrogen species, which are common metabolic products of several oxidation-reduction (redox) reactions in the cells, are increased when oxidative stress occurs. A transcription factor, NRF2, was found to play a key role in promoting HCC pathogenesis.[121] The oxidative stress pathway is altered by activating mutations of NRF2 (coded by *NFE2L2*) or inactivating KEAP1 in 5% to 15% of the cases, preventing proteasome degradation of NRF2 physiologically induced by KEAP1/CUL3 complex ubiquitinylation.[46]

LIVER CANCER STEM CELLS

There exists a hierarchy in a tumor in terms of the potential to divide and of cell-specific functions that differentiated cells exert. A small population of tumor cells with the highest potential and an undifferentiated state gives rise to a bulk tumor population. Such undifferentiated tumor cells, called cancer stem cells (CSCs) or tumor-initiating cells, are able to self-renew and produce differentiated cells by asymmetric division.[122,123] The clinical importance of CSC theory is that CSCs are generally resistant to conventional anticancer agents and radiotherapy, and when CSCs are brought to distant organs, they can form metastatic lesions. Therefore eradication of cancer cells is so difficult that we should target a few therapeutic-resistant CSCs, as well as the more differentiated bulky tumor cell population sensitive to conventional treatment. In HCC, identification of surface markers has moved toward a deeper understanding of liver CSCs. Liver CSC surface markers include CD133, CD90, epithelial cell adhesion molecule (EpCAM), CD13, CD24, OV6, and CD44.[124] They are necessary for the effective targeting of liver CSCs to find specific pathways for the expansion and maintenance of stem cell properties. The pathways of TGF-β, Janus-activating kinase (JAK)/signal-transducer and activator of transcription 3 (STAT3), NOTCH, and PI3K/AKT/mTOR are identified as regulatory networks essential for the activation and functions of liver CSCs.[125–127] Taken together, analysis of the cancer cells in HCC supports the presence of cells with stem cell properties. However, definitive specific markers for these putative CSCs have not yet been found and a liver CSC has not been isolated and characterized.

HEPATITIS B VIRUS (SEE CHAPTER 68)

HBV is the prototype member of the *Hepadnaviridae* family. Viral members of this group also infect ducks, ground squirrels, and woodchucks. These small, partially double-stranded DNA viruses contain four overlapping open reading frames (ORFs), including preC/core, preS/S, P, and X, except for the duck, in which X is missing (Fig. 9B.3A and B). PreC/core ORF encodes the precore protein, a precursor of hepatitis B early antigen (HBeAg), and core protein (HBcAg), a component of the nucleocapsid. PreS/S ORF encodes for three proteins, including large (L), middle (M), and small (S; HBsAg) proteins. The S accounts for approximately 90% of all protein produced from preS/S transcripts. The P gene encodes for a DNA-dependent DNA polymerase, which also has reverse transcriptase and RNase H activities. The partially double-stranded HBV genome (approximately 3.2 kb in length) exists within a nucleocapsid. The X region encodes for a multifunctional protein, HBx. Although HBx is not a component of HBV particles, it is believed to play a crucial role in viral replication. Acute and chronic infection of the liver with HBV appears not to produce cytopathic effects on hepatocytes; however, several components of the viral particles activate the host's immune response, and cytotoxic T cells (CTLs) eliminate HBV-infected hepatocytes.[128,129] Such immune responses induce sustained cycles of hepatocyte injury and regeneration that contribute to cirrhosis and HCC tumor formation.

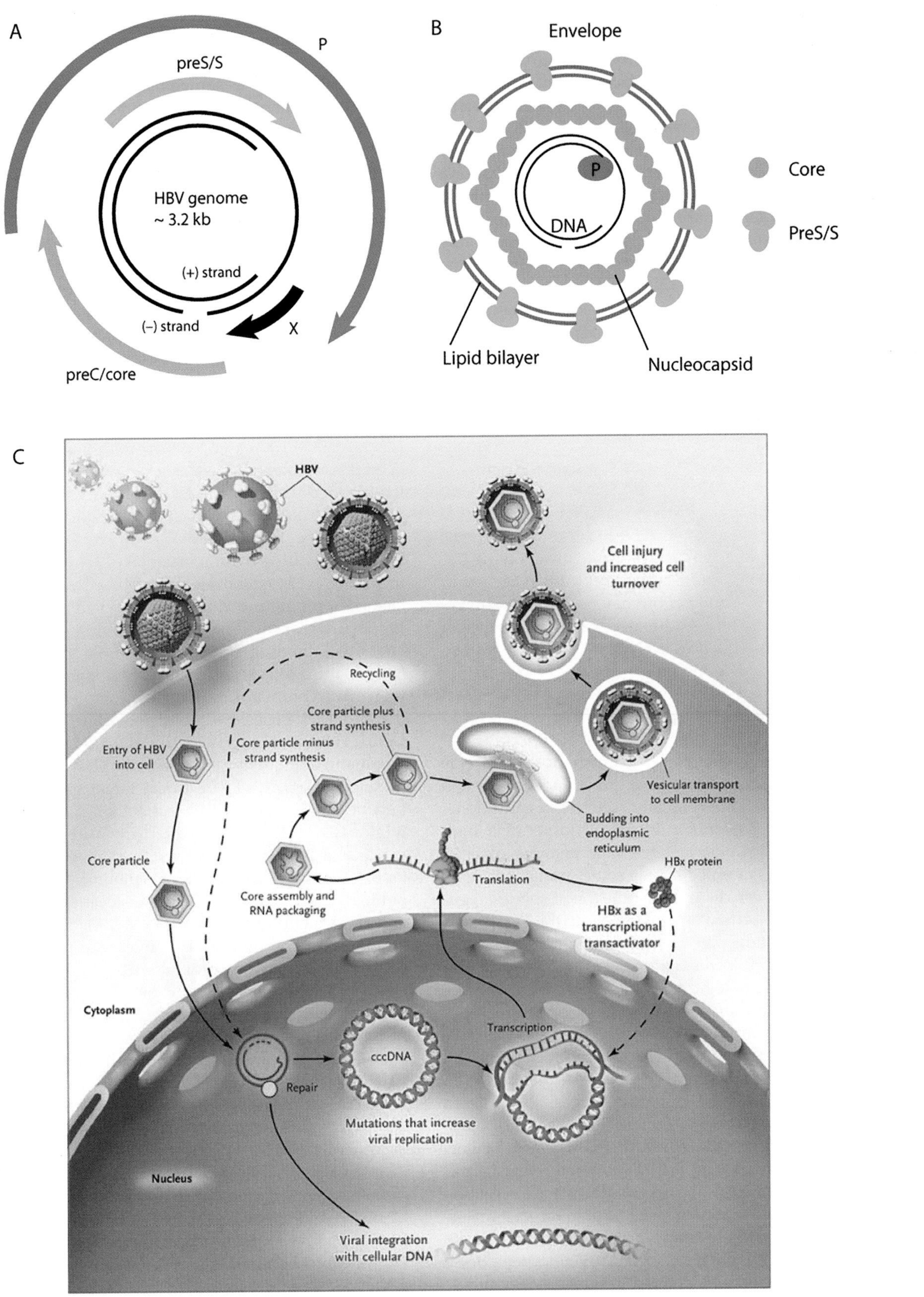

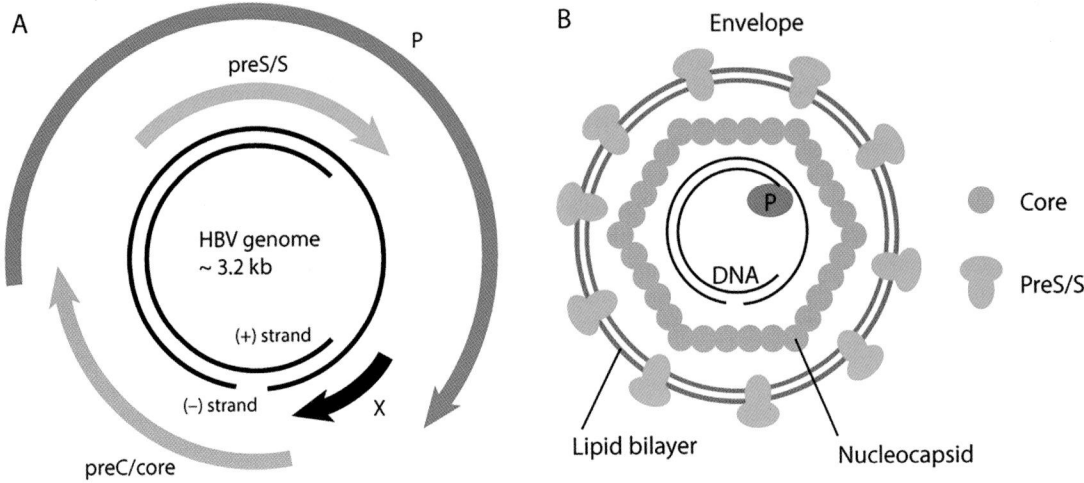

FIGURE 9B.3 **A,** Structure of the hepatitis B virus (HBV) DNA genome, showing the four open reading frames involved in generation of preC/core, preS/S, P, and X proteins. **B,** Structure of infectious HBV particle, showing the nucleocapsid containing an HBV genome and polymerase (P) and an envelope derived from the lipid bilayer, where preS/S proteins are embedded. **C,** Life cycle of HBV, showing viral entry through receptors, followed by uncoating and translocation of HBV DNA to the nucleus, where it is repaired to generate a covalently closed circular DNA (cccDNA) form that serves as the template for transcription of the pregenomic and other viral mRNA necessary for replication. (Used with permission from Wands JR. Prevention of hepatocellular carcinoma. *N Engl J Med* 2004;351:1567–1570. All rights reserved.)

A liver bile acids transporter, sodium taurocholate cotransporting polypeptide (NTCP, encoded by *SLC10A1*) was identified as a functional host cell receptor for HBV entry.[130–132] EGF receptor (EGFR) plays a role as a cofactor of NCTP for HBV internalization.[133] After internalization of HBV, the envelope glycoprotein is subsequently removed (see Fig. 9B.3C). The partially double-stranded DNA is repaired to form a covalently closed circular DNA (cccDNA) moiety in the nucleus to serve as a stable template for transcription of the pregenomic mRNA and other species required for productive viral replication. This cccDNA template remains in the nucleus during chronic viral infection and may persist in the liver for the lifetime of the individual.[134]

HBV can promote carcinogenesis by three different mechanisms: (1) a classic retrovirus-like insertional mutagenesis with the integration of viral DNA into host cancer genes like *TERT*; (2) the promotion of genomic instability as the result of both the integration of viral DNA into the host genome and the activity of viral proteins; and (3) the ability of wild-type and mutated/truncated viral proteins (HBx, HBc, and preS) to affect cell functions, activate oncogenic pathways, and sensitize liver cells to mutagens.[135]

The DNA of the HBV integrates randomly into hepatocyte chromosomes and acts as a nonselective insertional mutagenic agent. Secondary chromosomal rearrangements involving duplications, translocations, and deletions reveal that the major oncogenic effect of HBV integration may be increased by genomic instability of the host's cellular DNA. The presence of integrated HBV DNA sequences in cellular DNA from human HCCs was initially reported in the early 1980s.[136] Integration of HBV DNA into the host genome occurs at early steps of clonal tumor expansion. In about 80% of patients with HBV-related HCC, fragments of viral DNA have been found integrated into the host genome.[137] HBV integration at specific genomic sites is thought to provide a growth advantage to a clonal cell population that eventually accumulates additional mutations. Most HCCs contain integrated forms of a high molecular weight. However, a large-scale analysis of HBV DNA integration sites revealed that, in some special instances, the integration event can disrupt the function of specific regulatory genes.[138] The insertion of viral DNA into the *TERT* locus is observed in HBV-induced HCC and then telomerase reactivation is found. The HBV integration event into the *TERT* locus is an important pathologic event in these tumors. Another gene family recurrently affected by HBV integration includes those involved in calcium signaling. Studies indicate that HBV DNA had inserted into the gene encoding for SERCA (sarco/endoplasmic reticulum calcium adenosine triphosphatase), which plays a pivotal role in regulating intracellular calcium levels and shows as a second messenger involved in cell proliferation and programmed cell-death pathways.[139] Collectively, cellular genes involved in chromosomal integrity and in growth factor–mediated signaling pathways are occasionally targeted by HBV integration events, but in the vast majority of tumors, the viral integration is random throughout the host genome.[138,140] Thus integration of HBV into hepatocyte DNA produces specific and nonspecific genetic alterations that contribute to hepatocarcinogenesis. Recently, next-generation sequencing of 399 HBV integration breakpoints from 81 HBV-induced HCCs has shown that recurrent HBV integration points are near coding genes, including *TERT*, *MLL4* coding mixed lineage leukemia protein 4, and *CCNE1* coding

cyclin 1.[141] The expression of integrated genes is upregulated in tumors compared with the normal tissue.

Studies on murine models expressing HBV-related transgenes such as *HBx*, as shown in Fig. 9B.4, as well as truncated preS/S regions, provide evidence for their role in hepatic tumor development.[142,143] HBx is a multifunctional regulatory protein that is both required for HBV cDNA transcription/viral replication and thought to contribute to HBV oncogenicity. HBx is a 154–amino-acid molecule highly conserved among mammalian hepadnaviruses, and it has multifunctional and pleiotropic properties that modulate cellular functions, including transcription, signaling cascades, DNA repair, protein degradation, and cell-cycle control.[144] During viral replication, HBx is localized in the cytosol with a minor fraction present in the nucleus. Cytosolic HBx activates the RAS/RAF/MEK/ERK, PI3K/AKT pathway, SRC kinase, and JAK/STAT cascades, leading to increased cell proliferation.[145] Constitutive expression of HBx also promotes hepatocarcinogenesis, in combination with activation of the insulin/IGF-1/IRS-1/MEK/ERK cascade.[146] In addition, nuclear HBx has been reported to act as a transcriptional coactivator, although it does not directly bind to DNA. The mechanism of chromatin remodeling of HBx can be either transcriptional activation or repression of transcription by different mechanisms. HBx binds many nuclear proteins and regulates the transcription, including cyclic adenosine monophosphate (cAMP) response element–binding protein (CREB), activating transcription factor 2 (ATF2), activating enhancer binding protein 2 (AP-2), and CREB-binding protein/p300.[145] Suppressor of zeste 12 homolog (SUZ12) is an essential component of the polycomb repressive chromatin remodeling complex 2 (PRC2) that silences target genes by repressive trimethylation of H3 on Lys27, H3K27me3.[147] HBx induces the downregulation of the chromatin remodeling components SUZ12 and the overexpression of SUZ12/PRC2 direct target genes, including the hepatic CSC markers BMP and activin membrane-bound inhibitor (BAMBI) and EpCAM.[148] EpCAM and DLK1 overexpression is also mediated by HBx demethylation of CpG islands involving a complex containing enhancer of zeste homolog 2 (EZH2), ten-eleven translocation 2 (TET2) enzyme, and DNA methyltransferase (DNMT3L).[149,150]

Several reports indicate an interaction between HBx and p53 tumor suppressor protein. HBx binds to p53 in the nucleus and inhibits expression of p53-responsive genes. Nuclear HBx also alters the association of p53 with transcription factors, such as excision repair cross-complementation group 3 (ERCC3) and transcription factor IIH (TFIIH), which are involved in nucleotide excision repair.[151–153] Moreover, HBx expression has been shown to block p53-mediated apoptosis, and it provides a clonal selective advantage to HBV-infected hepatocytes.[153–155]

Interestingly, HBx can trigger the release of calcium ion from mitochondria, leading to the enhanced replication of HBV DNA through interaction with a proline-rich tyrosine kinase 2 (PYK2) and SRC kinase.[156] Calcium release and localization of HBx in mitochondrial membranes cause oxidative stress, in which ROS are produced.[157,158] ROS directly damage DNA, leading to aberrant DNA replication. HBx also influences the androgen signaling pathway, which may explain, in part, the known male predominance of HBV-induced HCC.[159] Taken together, these findings indicate that HBx plays a complex and pleiotropic role in the multistep process of tumor development.

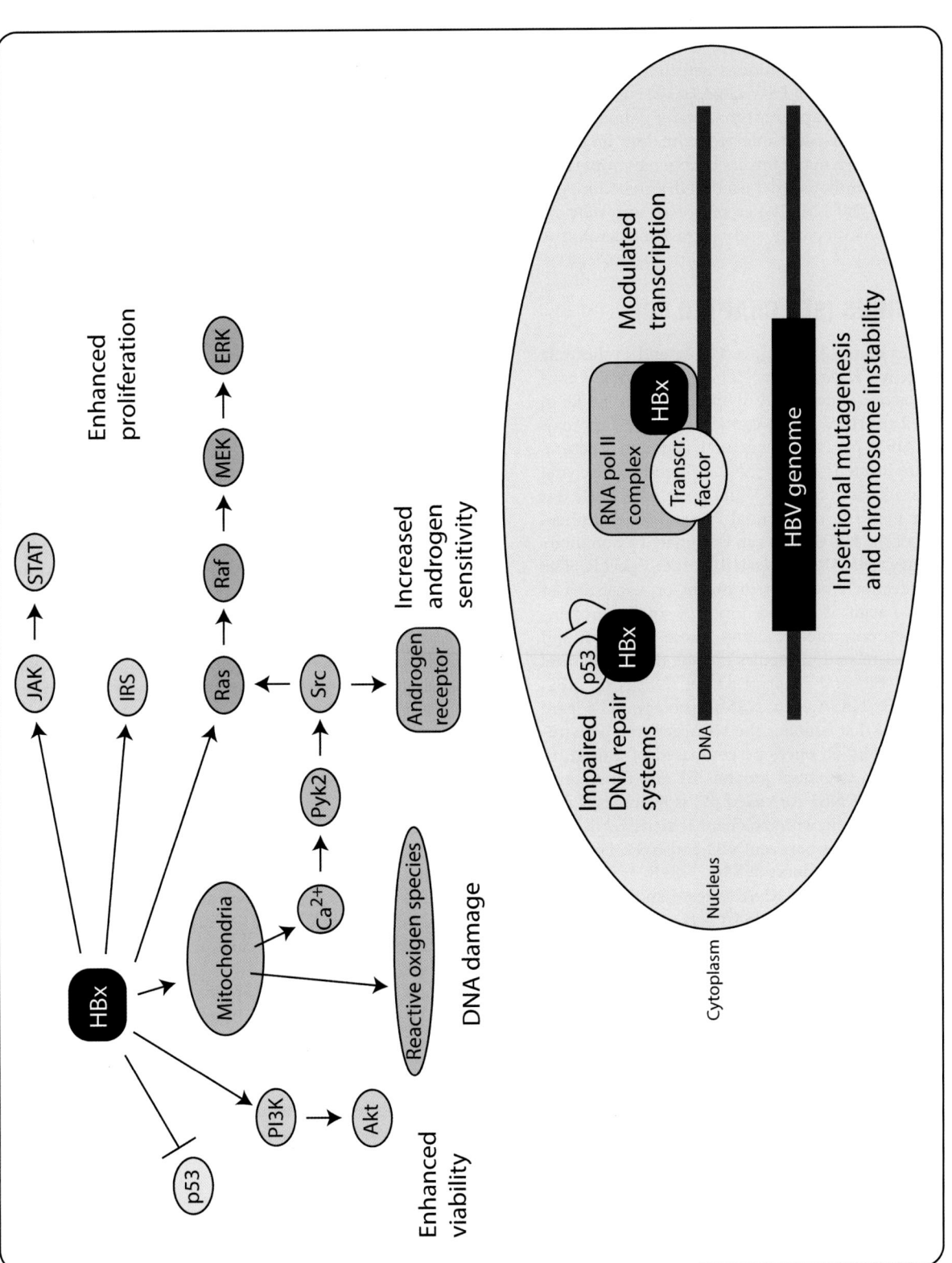

FIGURE 9B.4   Characteristics of the HBx protein and its involvement in tumor formation. HBx plays a crucial role in hepatitis B virus (HBV)-induced carcinogenesis. HBx is located in the cytoplasm and activates cellular signaling cascades. This viral nonstructural protein also inhibits p53-mediated apoptosis. Nuclear HBx modulates a set of transcription factors through interaction with a RNA polymerase complex. The HBV genome integrates into the host genome during persistent viral infection and promotes chromosome instability. *AKT,* v-Akt murine thymoma viral oncogene homolog; *ERK,* extracellular signal-regulated protein kinase; *HBx,* hepatitis B virus X protein; *IRS,* insulin receptor substrate; *JAK,* Janus-activating kinase; *MEK,* mitogen-activated protein kinase; *PI3K,* phosphatidylinositol-3-kinase; *PYK,* proline-rich tyrosine kinase; *RAF,* Raf-1 proto-oncogene; *RAS,* rat sarcoma (oncoprotein); *SRC,* sarcoma; *STAT,* signal-transducer and activator of transcription; *transcr,* transcription.

Evidence has been accumulating that the risk for HCC is substantially increased by viral factors, such as the level of HBV replication produced by naturally occurring mutations in the core and precore promoter regions.[160–162] A high viral replication phenotype places the infected liver at greater risk for transformation, as shown in Fig. 9B.3C. Finally, with the development of diagnostic techniques sensitive enough to detect very low levels of serum HBV DNA (<100 copies/mL), it has become increasingly apparent that many patients with chronic HCV infection also are infected with low levels of HBV. In this setting, HBV maintains its oncogenic properties, and evidence has accumulated that occult HBV infection, defined as less than 10,000 virions per mL of serum, may be associated with chronic hepatitis and cirrhosis of heretofore unknown origin.[134]

HEPATITIS C VIRUS (SEE CHAPTER 68)

HCV is a member of the *Flaviviridae* family and is the only member of the genus *Hepacivirus*.[163] The HCV genome consists of a single positive-strand RNA of approximately 9.6 kb in length (Fig. 9B.5A). HCV RNA contains a large (approximately 9.0 kb) ORF in which structural and nonstructural coding regions are located near the 5′ and 3′ ends of the viral genome, respectively. Both 5′ and 3′ untranslated (UTR) domains have been found to be essential for viral RNA replication. Translation of the HCV RNA can be initiated by an internal ribosome entry site (IRES) located in the 5′ UTR. The single ORF encodes for a polyprotein precursor, consisting of about 3,000 amino acids; it is cleaved into 10 smaller proteins by the action of several proteases derived from both host and virus. These 10 viral-related molecules include three structural (core [C], E1, and E2) and 7 nonstructural (NS; NS1, NS2, NS3, NS4A, NS4B, NS5A, and NS5B) proteins. The core forms a nucleocapsid that contains the HCV genome. The nucleocapsid is covered by an envelope composed of a lipid bilayer, in which the two structural proteins E1 and E2 are embedded. The function of NS1 (or called p7) is hypothesized to be a transmembrane protein with ion channel activity. NS2 is a metalloprotease that cleaves between NS2 and NS3. The NS3 is a serine protease that produces NS4A, NS4B, NS5A, and NS5B viral proteins; it also has RNA helicase and nucleoside triphosphatase (NTPase) activity. NS4A acts as a cofactor for NS3 activity, and NS4B is an integral membrane protein located on the cytoplasmic side of endoplasmic reticulum (ER); it has been implicated in the assembly of replicase complex. The NS5A protein is believed to act as a component of RNA replicase complex, and it plays a role in evasion of the host's cellular immune response. The NS5B is an RNA-dependent RNA polymerase essential for the replication of the HCV genome.

The life cycle of HCV consists of at least six different stages: *attachment/entry, translation, processing, genome replication, assembly,* and *release* into the circulation (see Fig. 9B.5B). HCV particles attach to the hepatocyte cell-surface membrane and enter the cell via key proteins such as CD81, SR-BI, claudin-1, and occludin. After entry into the hepatocyte, the nucleocapsid is delivered to the cytoplasm, and the HCV RNA is released and immediately translated. The large polyprotein is processed on the cytoplasmic side of the ER, and nonstructural proteins form a complex and initiate replication of the RNA genome in collaboration with some host proteins. Viral particles are assembled from the structural proteins, and the RNA genome becomes encased between membranes derived from lipid droplets and the ER. Assembled particles are delivered to the plasma membrane and released into the blood by exocytosis. Importantly, the entire process related to HCV replication is restricted to the cytoplasm; unlike HBV, the viral RNA does not form a DNA intermediate, and thus the HCV genome does not integrate into the host's cellular DNA.

HCV is an RNA virus with a predominantly cytoplasmic life cycle.[164] All potentially pro-oncogenic events are therefore likely to be restricted to the cytoplasm, suggesting indirect mechanisms of hepatocarcinogenesis. Although HCV infection leads to chronic inflammation, steatosis, fibrosis, and oxidative DNA damage, several HCV proteins, including core protein, have been shown to have direct oncogenic effects and to upregulate mitogenesis.[165] The accumulation of oxidative stress and DNA damage in a setting of restricted cell-cycle checkpoint control and/or accelerated cell division is thought to compromise gene and chromosome stability and to form the genetic basis for malignant transformation.[166] These mechanisms promote chronicity of HCV infection, which promotes hepatic inflammation, cirrhosis, and HCC (Fig. 9B.6).

At least four HCV proteins, including core, NS3, NS5A, and NS5B, have been proposed to have cellular transforming potential when transiently or stably expressed in cultured cells or in transgenic mice expressing the different viral proteins or the intact HCV polyprotein as depicted in Fig. 9B.6. The HCV core protein has been shown to have transforming potential in vitro.[167] The core protein is also localized at the cytoplasmic surface of the ER and on lipid droplets and relates to the induction of liver steatosis and is localized to the outer membrane of mitochondria, leading to alterations of apoptosis and lipid metabolism.[168,169] In addition, HCV core binds numerous cellular proteins and modulates the RAF/MEK/ERK signal transduction pathway.[135] The core protein also augments the TGF-β pathway by upregulating TGF-β expression in hepatic stellate cells to promote fibrosis.[170] Enhanced proliferation of HCC cells has been demonstrated by overexpression of the HCV core protein in vitro. This phenomenon was because of upregulation of WNT1 expression, suggesting a functional link between HCV core expression during active viral replication and subsequent activation of the WNT/β-catenin signaling cascade.[171] The core has been shown to induce ROS production via interaction with heat shock protein Hsp60.[172]

NS3 has been shown to complex with the wild-type p53 protein.[173] By modulating the activity of p53, NS3 inhibits transcription of the leucine carboxyl methyltransferase 2 (*LCMT2*) gene, which encodes a cell-cycle regulator, p21WAF1/CIP1. In addition, it has been found to repress *LCMT2* promoter activity in a dose-dependent manner and stimulates cell growth.[174] The NS3 protein binds and co-localizes with the mitochondrial antiviral signaling protein, MAVS, that activates NF-κB and IFN regulatory factor 3.[175]

The NS5A protein may act as a transcriptional modulator through interactions with other cellular proteins, such as GRB2, p53, p21WAF1/CIP1, and CDK2. The functional consequences have been inhibition of hepatocyte apoptosis, leading to persistent HCV infection.[176] One potential mechanism by which NS5A may be able to exert an effect on gene expression and cellular growth is through functional associations with p53 and TATA box–binding proteins (TBPs). The overexpression

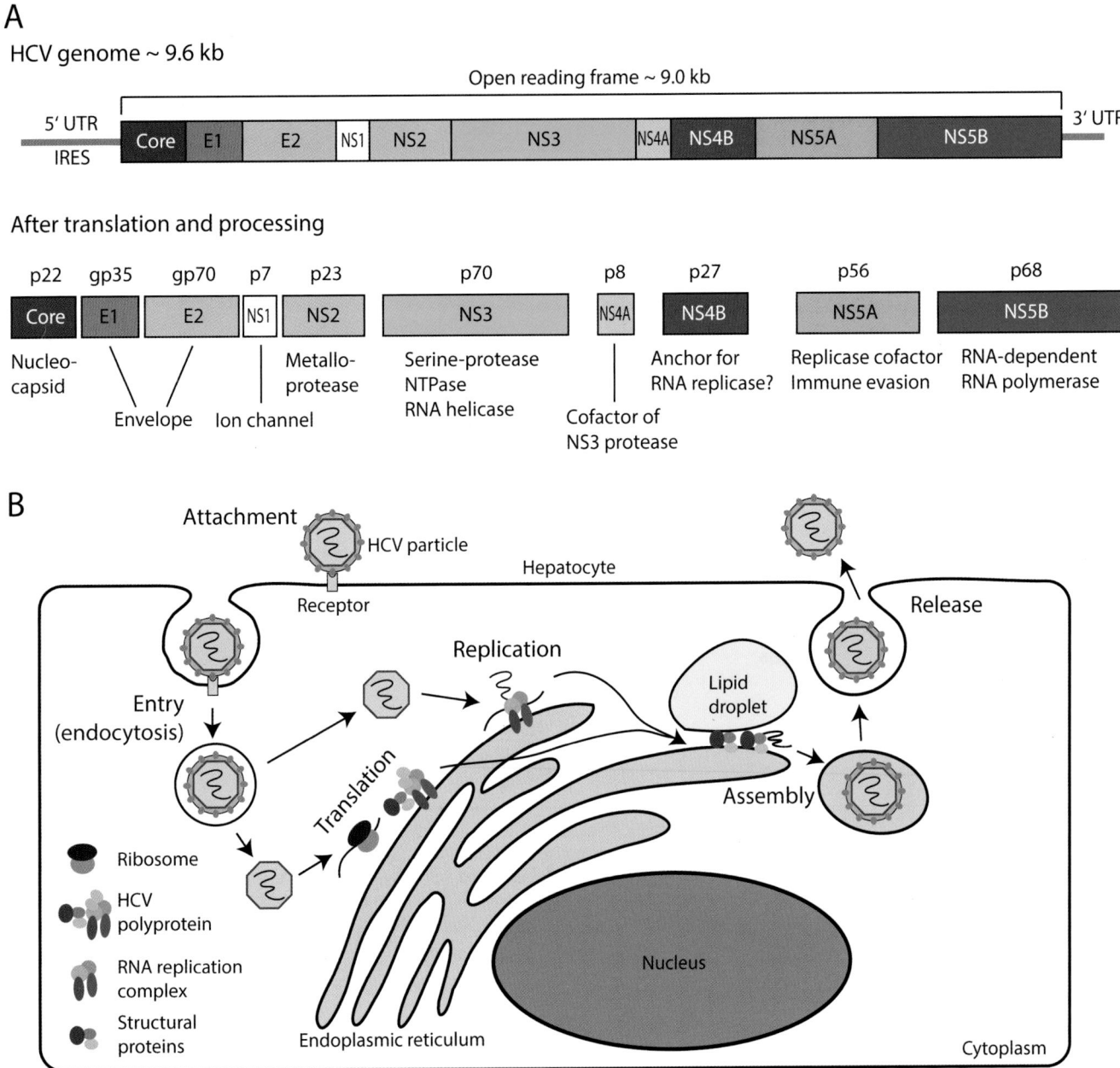

FIGURE 9B.5 Diagram of hepatitis C virus (HCV) and the replication process. **A,** Components of the HCV genome showing the structure of HCV RNA. HCV proteins, including their role in HCV replication, are presented. **B,** Life cycle of HCV showing the known steps of viral replication, including attachment/entry, translation, replication, processing, assembly, and release of virus into the blood. *IRES,* Internal ribosome entry site; *NS,* nonstructural; *NTPase,* nucleoside triphosphatase; *UTR,* untranslated region.

of NS5A also induces oxidative stress and activates the signaling pathways such as STAT3, PI3K, and NF-κB, resulting in the stabilization and accumulation of β-catenin in the cytoplasm and nucleus through inactivation of GSK-3β.[177–180]

Another possible pathway activated in HCV-induced HCC involves oxidative stress generated by increased production of ROS during persistent viral infection. Indeed, ROS production in the liver has been found to be increased in HCV core transgenic mice.[181] Moreover, iron loading in transgenic mice expressing the full-length HCV genome promotes HCC formation, again implicating chronic oxidative stress in the pathogenesis of HCV-mediated HCC.[182] The mechanisms underlying oxidative

stress–induced hepatocarcinogenesis involve increased chromosome instability and mutations in the host cellular DNA produced by the action of ROS.[183,184] Moreover, HCV directly induces lipid accumulation in hepatocytes as a result of ER stress because viral replication occurs on the ER membranes, where the core impedes ER functions.[185] Hepatic steatosis induced by HCV infection promotes oxidative stress and ROS production.[186] Collectively, many of the HCV proteins are believed to contribute to hepatocyte transformation during persistent viral infection through stimulation of cell proliferation, increased cell survival, induction of genomic instability, and promotion of immune evasion.

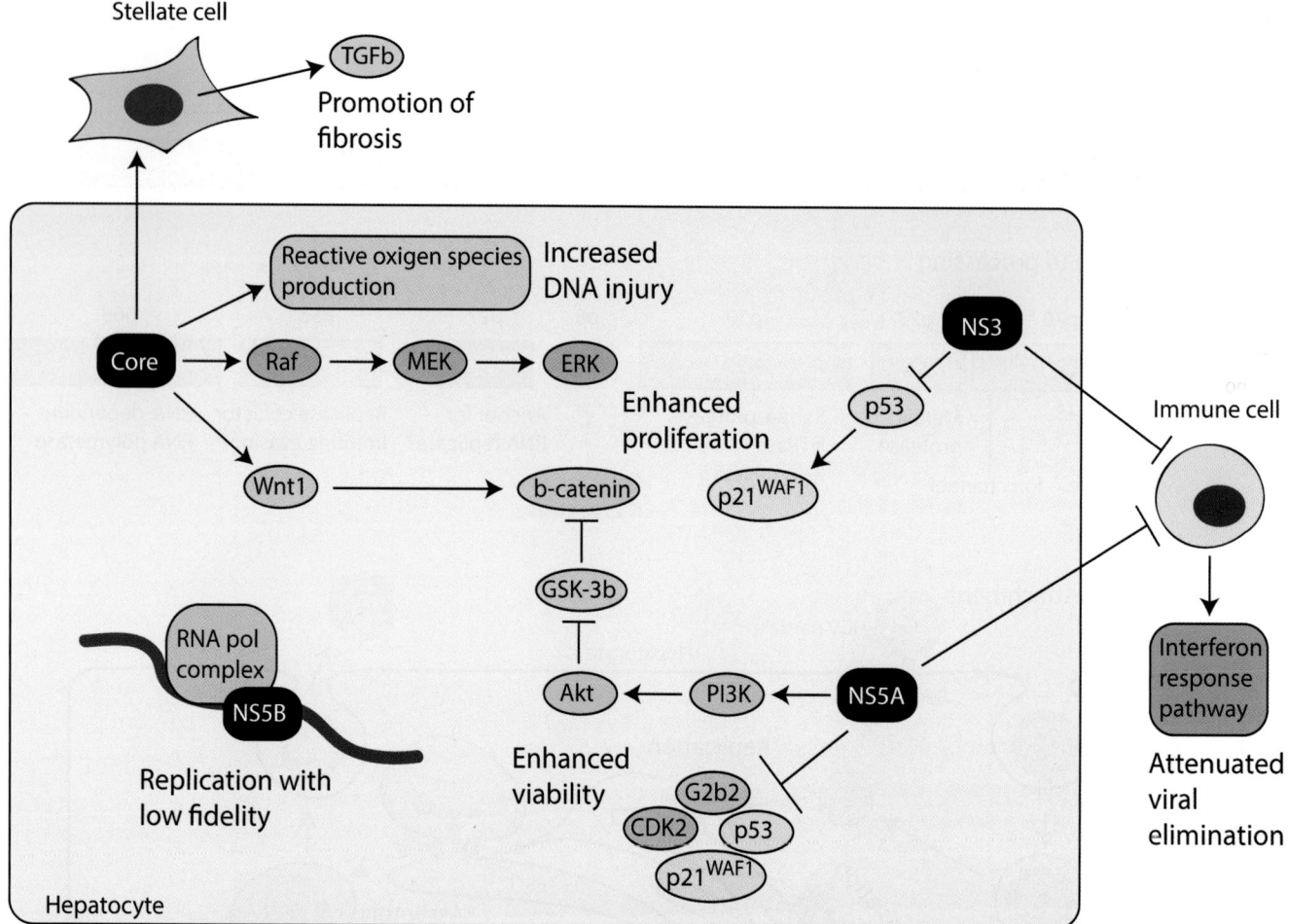

FIGURE 9B.6   Pathogenic role of hepatitis C virus (HCV) proteins. This diagram illustrates how HCV proteins, including core, NS3, NS5A, and NS5B, may modulate cellular function. Such proteins promote hepatocarcinogenesis in diverse ways via activation of signaling pathways and stellate cells, and they suppress immune responses to the virus and generate oxidative stress in the liver. *AKT*, v-Akt murine thymoma viral oncogene homolog; *CDK2*, cyclin-dependent kinase 2; *ERK*, extracellular signal-regulated protein kinase; *GRB2*, growth factor receptor-bound protein 2; *GSK-3β*, glycogen synthetase kinase-3β; *MEK*, mitogen-activated protein kinase; *NS*, nonstructural; *PI3K*, phosphatidylinositol-3-kinase; *pol*, polymerase; *TGF-β*, transforming growth factor-β; *WNT*, wingless type.

FUTURE DIRECTIONS

In the postgenomic era, comprehensive examination of tumors via next-generation sequencing and microarray technologies makes it highly likely that molecular genetic changes evolving from normal liver to dysplasia to HCC will be more precisely defined. Over the past few decades, significant progress has been made in epigenetic analysis, miRNA function, and genomic profiling of HCC, which will greatly enhance our understanding of the molecular oncogenesis of HCC. Some novel driver mutations of HCC have been identified and tremendous effort has been applied to the development of drugs that target these key genetic mutations. Furthermore, the benefit of immunotherapy for HCC has been highlighted and the development of immune checkpoint inhibitors are under intense investigation. Clinical trials exploring the efficacy and safety of molecular-targeted agents or immune checkpoint inhibitors are now ongoing. The characterization of the molecular biology of liver carcinogenesis and hepatitis may lead to the development of preventive approaches and the establishment of new treatment strategies for HCC. These investigations emphasize the importance of unraveling the molecular mechanisms of liver carcinogenesis, which may ultimately result in "personalized" medical approaches for this devastating disease.

References are available at expertconsult.com.

Advances in the molecular characterization of liver tumors

Colm J. O'Rourke and Jesper B. Andersen

OVERVIEW

Tumors of the hepatobiliary (HB) system are among the most challenging tumors to effectively manage in the clinic. At time of diagnosis, only approximately 25% of gallbladder carcinoma (GBC) patients,[1] 30% of cholangiocarcinoma (CCA) patients,[2] and 30% of hepatocellular carcinoma (HCC) patients[3] are eligible for curative therapy through surgical resection (see Chapters 49–51 and 89). The direct result of this is overall 5-year survival rates of less than 5% in GBC,[4] 7% to 20% in CCA,[2] and less than 18% in HCC.[5] Tumors spanning the HB system are unified by late diagnosis, innate aggressive behavior, rapid chemoresistance, and dismal prognosis.[6] These cancers display ominous epidemiologic trends,[7,8] are highly resistant to most systemic therapies,[9] and are projected to increase in global health burden over upcoming decades.[2,5,10] To mitigate such adverse projections, robust molecular characterization of HB cancers is fundamental. In this chapter, we discuss the diverse molecular characterization strategies that have been pursued to elucidate the molecular basis of these diseases. In particular, we focus on the contribution of mutations, structural alterations, and epigenome remodeling in HB cancers. Finally, we evaluate the impact of integrative -omics approaches to stratify these heterogeneous cancers into homogenous, clinically impactful subtypes.

Mutational Burden and Signatures

To understand the molecular origins of the intrinsically aggressive disease trajectories of HB malignancies, increased mutational burden and/or rates may be suggested as a plausible mechanism. Surprisingly, comparative mutational profiling across cancers indicates these subsets of tumors are exceptionally unremarkable in this regard, falling approximately midway between leukemias (toward the lower end) and melanomas (at the upper end of the spectrum).[11] On average, whole-exome sequencing (WES) studies have detected nonsynonymous mutation frequencies of 39 per tumor (median) in intrahepatic CCA (iCCA; see Chapter 50),[12] 35 per tumor (median) in extrahepatic CCA (eCCA; see Chapter 51),[12] 64 per tumor (median) in GBC[12] (see Chapter 49), and 64 per tumor (median) in HCC[13] (see Chapter 89). Although it is clear that there is significant variation in mutational burden between HB cancers, significant heterogeneity also exists within HB cancer subtypes. Certain etiologic backgrounds have been confirmed to correlate with higher mutational loads, such as liver fluke-associated CCA versus noninfected CCA.[14] The mutation loads of HB tumors are of particular interest, given that tumor mutation burden (TMB) is positively correlated with increased likelihood of neoantigen production, potentially resulting in beneficial response to checkpoint inhibitor therapies.

Beyond the exome, whole-genome sequencing (WGS) studies remain somewhat underevaluated in HB cancers, with some notable exceptions,[15–17] but this approach holds significant potential to inform on important features of cancer biology. Such areas include the pro-tumorigenic impact of retrotransposon reanimation,[18] viral integration with insertional mutagenesis,[19] enhancer function,[20] and intergenic long ncRNAs (lncRNAs).[21] WGS analysis has also been applied to successfully discern multicentric HCC from HCC with intrahepatic metastasis,[15] a distinction that is important in determining patient eligibility for surgical resection.

Diverse exogenous and endogenous mutagenic processes are active in individual HB patients, collectively contributing to the total mutation burden of a given tumor. Analysis of mutational signature patterns in whole-exome and whole-genome sequencing data enable such mutagenic processes to be extrapolated, providing insight into the evolutionary processes that shaped the cancer genome. In total, 81 mutational signatures have been identified,[22] although the causative mutagenic process is only known for some of these signatures. General signatures found across HB cancers include those associated with nucleotide excision repair deficiency, 5-methylcytosine deamination, and aging.[17,23,24] Examples of mutation signatures found to be enriched in specific HB cancers include an aflatoxin-associated signature in HCC[23,25] and an APOBEC-associated signature in eCCA and GBC.[12] Further, a liver cancer–specific signature has also been identified, associating with alcohol exposure, transcription-coupled damage, and beta-catenin (CTNNB1) mutations.[26] The existence of such a liver-specific signature is perhaps unsurprising, given the associated hepatic exposure to diverse mutagens when carrying out its physiologic function in detoxification.

Structural Rearrangements

Although less prevalent than single nucleotide variants (SNVs), structural variants (SVs) occur frequently in cancer genomes and are more likely to affect endogenous gene expression and function. Recurrent structural alteration signatures have been identified in HCC and are associated with diverse clinicopathologic and molecular features, including alcohol consumption, tumor protein P53 (TP53) mutation status, and size of genomic alterations.[26] Copy number alterations (CNAs) typically affect genes also observed to be recurrently mutated. Specifically, recurrent amplification of oncogenes has been reported, including cyclin D1 (CCND1) and MYC proto-oncogene, BHLH transcription factor (MYC) in HCC,[23] and CCND1 (11q13.3) in CCA.[24] Telomerase reverse transcriptase (TERT) amplification occurs in approximately 10% of HCC patients.[23] Conversely, tumor suppressor genes frequently undergo copy number loss, most commonly in cyclin dependent kinase inhibitor 2A (CDKN2A) in HCC[23] and CCA.[24] Consistent with such overlap of gene targets shared by mutation and structural processes, an inverse correlation between mutation (M-class) and structural copy number (C-class) was observed in iCCA, indicative of different perturbation mechanisms driving the same disease phenotype.[27] Such findings highlight the importance of applying multiple genomic readouts (mutation and copy number analysis) to HB tumors when considering allocation of patients to targeted therapy trials.

Additional pathogenetic mechanisms have also been reported to induce genomic insults with a single event. Chromothripsis involves the localized catastrophic shattering of a chromosomal arm followed by random re-ligation of the sections by the endogenous DNA damage and replication system.[28] Such wanton repair yields a multitude of structural variants, with current criteria for chromothripsis calling invoking more than 30 rearrangements and more than 10 translocations on a single arm.[29] Although chromothripsis is estimated to occur in 2% to 3% of cancer genomes, a WGS study of 88 HCC specimens detected enrichment of these events in 6% of tumors.[30] Specifically, chromothripsis was found to affect chromosome arm 1q, 8q, and 5p. Interestingly, such regions are the recurrent targets of non–shattering-associated chromosomal anomalies also, indicating convergent perturbation of resident genes by these two independent phenomena as important in hepatocarcinogenesis. Biliary tumors have also been reported to exhibit chromothripsis, linked in particular to whole-genome duplications.[31] Indeed, genome duplication has been shown to be frequent and highly clonal in iCCA.[32] Additionally, *TP53* mutations have been linked with localized chromosome shattering in liver[30] and other cancers.[33]

Recurrently mutated genes are diverse and heterogeneous across HB malignancies, exhibiting low-to-intermediate mutation frequencies. Furthermore, the exact mechanism of genomic perturbation appears to be redundant to some extent, with common targets such as *TP53* altered by SNVs and SVs. However, neither mutational loads nor mutational mechanisms appear to alone govern the aggressive behavior of these tumors, exemplified by the apparently unremarkable clinical trajectory of hypermutated patients and patients harboring chromothriptic events. Therefore the molecular basis for the overall aggressive behavior of HB cancers compared with other cancers, as well as the heterogeneous disease trajectories between HB patients, appears to lie in the specific genes and networks affected.

Mutational Landscapes in Hepatobiliary Cancers

Statistical modeling predicts that three driver gene mutations are sufficient to induce advanced cancer,[34] and pan-cancer analysis of tumors suggests that cancer genomes contain four to five mutations on average, 57% of which are clinically actionable.[35] However, with two recent notable exceptions (fibroblast growth factor receptor 2 *[FGFR2]* fusions[36] and isocitrate dehydrogenase 1 *[IDH1]* mutations[37] in iCCA), genomic alteration-guided targeted therapies have not drastically impacted treatment of HB malignancies (see Chapter 9E). One reason is that many of the most recurrently altered genes remain undruggable. These include undruggable hotspot mutations in the notorious oncogene, KRAS proto-oncogene, GTPase *(KRAS)*, which are detected in approximately 5% of biliary tract cancers (BTCs)[17] and 1% of HCCs.[35] Diverse mutations also arise in the tumor suppressor gene, *TP53*, in 31% of HCCs[35] and 16% of BTCs,[17] with these alterations being similarly undruggable (see Chapters 9B, 9C, and 9E). Additionally, recurrent alterations are found in genes whose pathobiologic roles in HB malignancies remain poorly characterized. Prime examples of

these include recurrent alterations in chromatin remodeler complex members,[23,24] with emerging evidence supporting a tumor suppressor-like role for these genes in HB transformation, including AT-rich interaction domain 1A *(ARID1A)*[38] and BRCA1-associated protein 1 *(BAP1)*.[39]

Another issue is the relatively low recurrence frequencies of candidate driver alterations between patients, making design of sufficiently powered trials difficult, especially for BTCs, which are considered rare diseases. In fact, genomic evidence highlights that BTCs are highly distinct based on tumor location within the biliary tract. *IDH1/2* mutations and *FGFR2* fusions exclusively occur in iCCA,[12] whereas protein kinase CAMP-activated catalytic subunit alpha *(PRKACA)* and protein kinase CAMP-activated catalytic subunit beta *(PRKACB)* fusions preferentially occur in eCCA[12] and erb-B2 receptor tyrosine kinase 2/3 *(ERBB2/3)* mutations preferentially occur in GBC.[12,40] These data suggest that BTC patients should potentially be stratified by anatomic location before trial development, further challenging statistical power in these rare patient demographics.

Remarkably, a minority of HB patients appear to lack any single known driver alteration.[31] A logical explanation for this is that rare variant genes with extremely low alteration frequencies have driver-like capabilities in their altered forms. Successfully identifying such instances will require careful functional validation using gene editing technologies, such as CRISPR. However, formally testing such rare variants may be complicated further if some variants only exert driver-like function in combination with other specific genomic insults. Even among the most commonly mutated genes, tendencies towards mutual exclusivity have been reported in HB cancers, such as between *IDH1* and *TP53* in iCCA[41] (see Chapters 9E and 50). Therefore contextualizing specific genetic insults among the wider oncogenic programs will be paramount to successfully modeling HB tumors, and this importantly includes consideration of genetic and nongenetic mechanisms (Fig. 9C.1).

Epigenome Reprogramming in Hepatobiliary Cancers

Epigenome reprogramming is pervasive throughout HB transformation.[42] This involves coordinated biochemical modification of DNA, RNA, and proteins, triggering alterations in gene expression programs that are entirely reversible, unlike mutations. The importance of epigenome remodeling to HB carcinogenesis is highlighted by detection of recurrent mutations in epigenetic genes in HB cancers, such as *ARID1A, ARID2, BAP1*, lysine methyltransferase 2D *(KMT2D)*, lysine methyltransferase 2C *(KMT2C)*, and polybromo1 *(PBRM1)*.[43] Such mutants globally affect epigenome homeostasis, contributing to tumor development. However, cancer-associated epigenome reprogramming also occurs in the absence of mutations in epigenome regulators, in which instance the tumor microenvironment plays an important role. Genetic insult-bearing hepatocytes undergo transformation into HCC in the presence of an apoptotic microenvironment in mice, but transform into iCCA in a necroptotic microenvironment[44] (see Chapter 9E). These data highlight the potential for microenvironment-triggered epigenome reprogramming, in particular emphasizing the potential of epigenome alterations to dynamically adapt to challenges such as chemotherapy.

DNA methylation, the addition of a methyl group to cytosine to generate 5'-methylcytosine (5mC), is by far the best characterized epigenetic modification in HB cancers. Although

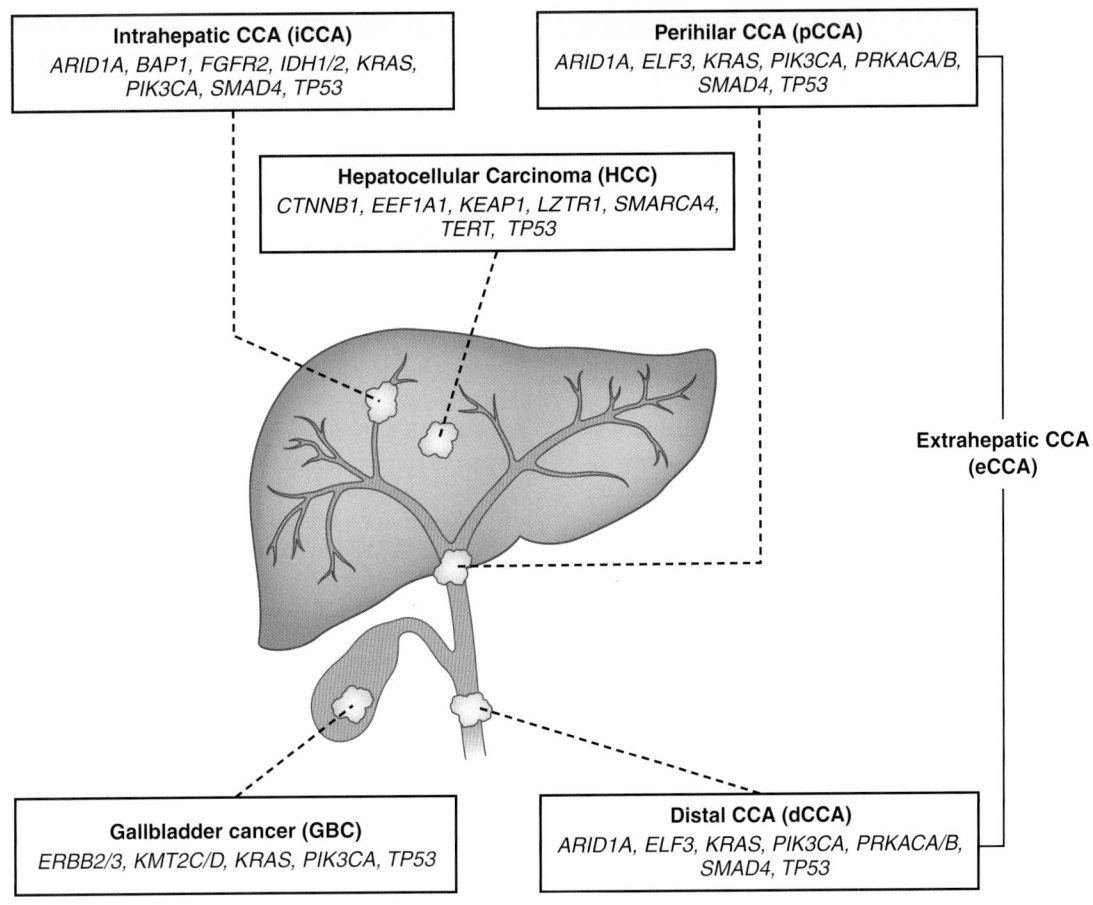

Intrahepatic CCA (iCCA)
ARID1A, BAP1, FGFR2, IDH1/2, KRAS, PIK3CA, SMAD4, TP53

Perihilar CCA (pCCA)
ARID1A, ELF3, KRAS, PIK3CA, PRKACA/B, SMAD4, TP53

Hepatocellular Carcinoma (HCC)
CTNNB1, EEF1A1, KEAP1, LZTR1, SMARCA4, TERT, TP53

Extrahepatic CCA (eCCA)

Gallbladder cancer (GBC)
ERBB2/3, KMT2C/D, KRAS, PIK3CA, TP53

Distal CCA (dCCA)
ARID1A, ELF3, KRAS, PIK3CA, PRKACA/B, SMAD4, TP53

FIGURE 9C.1 Overview of hepatobiliary (HB) cancers and the most frequently genetically altered genes. *ARID1A/B*, AT-rich interaction domain 1A/B; *BAP1*, BRCA1-associated protein 1; *CTNNB1*, catenin beta 1; *EEF1A1*, eukaryotic translation elongation factor 1 alpha 1; *ELF3*, E74-like ETS transcription factor 3; *ERBB2/3*, erb-b2 receptor tyrosine kinase 2/3; *FGFR2*, fibroblast growth factor receptor 2; *IDH1/2*, isocitrate dehydrogenase 1/2; *KEAP1*, kelch-like ECH associated protein 1; *KMT2C/D*, lysine methyltransferase 2C/D; *KRAS*, KRAS proto-oncogene, GTPase; *LZTR1*, leucine zipper-like transcription regulator 1; *PIK3CA*, phosphatidylinositol-4,5-bisphosphate 3-kinase catalytic subunit alpha; *PRKACA/B*, protein kinase cAMP-activated catalytic subunit alpha/beta; *SMAD4*, SMAD family member 4; *SMARCA4*, SWI/SNF related, matrix associated, actin dependent regulator of chromatin; *TERT*, telomerase reverse transcriptase; *TP53*, tumor protein p53.

global loss of 5mC is a hallmark of cancers, including HCC, CCA appears to be the exception to the rule and retains 5mC levels comparable to normal cells.[45] This is likely in part contributed to by *IDH1* and *IDH2* mutations (enzymes which function as rate-limiting competitors for Ten-Eleven-Twelve [TET] deoxygenases involved in the DNA demethylation pathway) that are prevalent in approximately 10% to 25% of iCCAs[42] and 1% of HCCs.[23] *IDH* mutations result in production of the oncometabolite, 2-hydroxyglutarate (2-HG), in place of α–ketoglutarate (α-KG). α-KG is required as a cofactor by multiple enzymes, including TET demethylases, so 2-HG production compromises DNA demethylation leading to DNA hypermethylation. At the cellular level, mutant IDH can inhibit differentiation of hepatic progenitors which, in conjunction with mutated *KRAS*, prompts stem cell pool expansion and neoplastic transformation into iCCA in vivo.[46] Most notably, the phase III ClarIDHy trial evaluated the mutant IDH1 inhibitor, ivosidenib, in *IDH1* mutant iCCA patients and found treatment to significantly increase progression-free survival from median 1.4 months (placebo group) to 2.7 months[37] (see Chapters 9E and 50). However, it remains difficult to extrapolate the extent to which this therapeutic benefit arises from

epigenetic effects as distinct from other α-KG-dependent processes, especially metabolism.

DNA methylation alterations occur during the earliest stages of transformation and can still be detected in advanced stage tumors, including signatures associated with hepatitis B, hepatitis C, alcohol consumption,[47] and nonalcoholic steatohepatitis (NASH; see Chapter 69).[48] Later in HB tumor evolution, de novo DNA methylation reprogramming has been reported to contribute to postsurgical HCC recurrence.[49] Like mutations, patterns of aberrant methylation are recurrent across HB tumors, suggesting that altered functionality of these affected loci are pro-oncogenic. In general, aberrant DNA methylation primarily targets developmental pathways, reactivating HOX,[50] WNT,[51] and SOX17[52] signaling; however, excluding IDH mutants, which represent a minority of HB tumors, the exact mechanisms promoting characteristic epigenome remodeling in wild-type tumors remain unclear. One example of such a mechanism involves ubiquitin like with PHD and ring finger domains 1 (UHRF1), which is overexpressed in a subset of aggressive HCC, causing DNA methyltransferase 1 (DNMT1) destabilization and DNA hypomethylation.[53] Further, although the existence of "epi-drivers" has been suggested, such as ephrin B2

(EFNB2) and septin 9 (SEPT9),[54] functionally confirming their existence remains elusive because of technical challenges in precisely editing the epigenetic landscape of narrow genomic windows.

Beyond DNA methylation, other epigenetic modalities remain less well described. Mutations in chromatin remodeling complex members are among the most common alterations detected in CCA and HCC, presumably leading to altered chromatin accessibility profiles. Integrative genomic analysis previously highlighted the histone modification profiles of HCC to be grossly altered compared with normal liver, with remodeling most drastic at enhancer regions.[55] Altered epigenetic landscapes at such loci were associated with altered transcription of candidate epi-drivers catechol-o-methyltransferase (COMT) and flavin containing dimethylaniline monooxygenase 3 (FMO3), genes which are influential in HCC prognosis. Multiple studies have also highlighted important roles for micro-RNA (miRs) in HB cancers. These approximately 22 nucleotide noncoding transcripts bind to their target mRNA(s), causing sequestration and degradation of the mRNA, thereby functioning as posttranscriptional regulators. These small miRs have a large impact on diverse features of HB cancers, including miR-21-mediated resistance of CCA to heat shock protein inhibitors through regulation of dnak heat shock protein family (HSP40) member (DNAJB5)[56] and miR-1249-mediated resistance to gemcitabine and cisplatin through the regulation of the clonal expansion of CD133+ BTC cells.[57] Clearly, many diverse and recurrent perturbation mechanisms are active and exert clinically impactful consequences in HB cancers, emphasizing the need for integrated molecular profiling.

Molecular Subtyping of Hepatobiliary Cancers

Although iCCA is the least prevalent anatomic subtype among BTCs, it has received the greatest attention regarding molecular subtyping (see Chapters 9E and 50). Single gene mutation–based stratification of these tumors into IDH1/2-gr, KRAS-gr, TP53-gr, and the remainder (referred to as "undetermined" [Udt-gr]) demonstrated unique oncogenic programs associated with each subtype that translated into distinct therapeutic vulnerabilities in vitro.[58] Specifically, IDH-gr tumors were hypersensitive to RNA synthesis inhibitors, KRAS-gr to topoisomerase inhibitors, TP53-gr to polo-like kinase 1 (PLK1) inhibitors, and Udt-gr to mammalian target of rapamycin (mTOR) inhibitors. Transcriptomic approaches have suggested survival subclasses based on KRAS mutations and EGFR-HER2 signaling,[59] as well as "proliferation" and "immune" subtypes.[60] DNA methylation-based approaches argue for iCCA stratification into four subgroups based on IDH1/2 status and DNA methylation profiles classified as low, intermediate, or high,[61] as well as highlighting DNA hypermethylation-associated CpG>TpG mutation events.[16] An immune-based subclassification approach has also been suggested for iCCA. In this scheme, tumors can be stratified into lymphoid, myeloid, mesenchymal, and immune-desert phenotypes.[62] The validity of this approach is further supported by single cell RNA-sequencing (scRNAseq) studies, which have identified fundamental cross-talk networks between iCCA-associated immune cells, tumor cells, and microenvironment cells.[63,64]

Although GBC has not been molecularly stratified to date, four molecular subclasses of eCCA have recently been identified.[65] These include a metabolic subclass associated with bile acid metabolism signatures, a proliferation subclass associated with MTOR signaling, a mesenchymal subclass associated with transforming growth factor-beta (TGF-β) signaling, and an immune subclass associated with high lymphocyte infiltration.

Compared with BTC, molecular stratification of HCC is much more formalized and can be split into six biological subtypes: AKT/mTOR, P53/cell cycle regulation, epigenetic modifiers, MAP kinase, oxidative stress, telomere maintenance, and Wnt/β-catenin.[66] Significant mutual inclusivity (CTNNB1 and TERT) and exclusivity (CTNNB1 and TP53) of key drivers has been consistently highlighted.[66] In addition, approximately 25% of HCCs exhibit an inflammatory phenotype, which was further stratified into adaptive T cell response and exhaustion subtypes.[67] Such immune diversity has also been emphasized in scRNAseq studies, especially the role of tumor-associated macrophages (TAMs) in the inflammatory response and patient outcome[68] (see Chapter 9B).

Independent of diagnosis, molecular subtypes that span iCCA and HCC have also been reported in the Asian population.[69] The TIGER-LC consortium integrated genomics, transcriptomics, and metabolomics, unveiling two clusters of tumors independent of classification as iCCA or HCC. One subtype was associated with mitotic checkpoint anomalies and mutations in epithelial cell transforming sequence 2 oncogene (ECT2) and PLK1. In contrast, the other subtype was characterized by obesity, bile acid metabolism, and T cell infiltration. These findings emphasize the potentially over-constraining implications of umbrella diagnostic terms, such as HCC and BTC, and may support molecularly guided basket trial approaches in HB cancers as a whole.

Future Perspectives

In 2020 the clinical impact of molecular characterization of HB tumors was epitomized by the US Food and Drug Administration (FDA) approval of pemigatinib as a second-line treatment for FGFR2 fusion-positive advanced iCCA and ivosidenib as a second-line treatment for IDH1 mutant advanced iCCA after successful phase III trials[36,37] (see Chapter 50). Although the clinical management of these patients has been historically changed, these cases represent only a small minority of the HB cancer demographic. Significant additional work is required to apply molecular characterization into tangible therapeutic strategies for the majority of HB patients. Although molecular characterization has largely focused on inter-patient differences, these same approaches must now be applied to characterize intra-patient differences over time because HB cancers are dynamic diseases. This will necessitate molecular profiling of precursor lesions to understand primary tumor induction, metastatic lesions to understand tumor dissemination, and pre- and post-treatment samples to decipher the molecular basis of treatment response and chemoresistance.

The references for this chapter can be found online by accessing the accompanying Expert Consult website.

Advances in the molecular characterization of pancreatic cancer and pre-malignant lesions

Rami Iman and Christine Iacobuzio-Donahue

PANCREATIC CANCER OVERVIEW

Pancreatic ductal adenocarcinoma (PDA), commonly referred to as "pancreatic cancer" is the fourth most common cause of cancer in both men and women. PDA remains a devastating diagnosis, with an overall survival rate of no greater than 10%.[1,2] In 2020 approximately 57,600 Americans will be diagnosed with PDA, and approximately 47,050 will die of it[1] (see Chapters 61 and 62).

The past two decades have seen an exponential increase in our understanding of the molecular basis and etiology behind PDA.[3–6] Still, the clinical management of this disease, including primary prevention, early detection, and better targeted treatment options, has not changed significantly during the past decade. Currently, the only cure for this disease is surgical resection. Unfortunately, only approximately 20% of the patient population is seen with resectable disease.[7] This chapter aims (1) to show that even though every tumor has a number of common molecular events, it is the differences among tumors that have clinical implications and (2) to set the stage for the future, which will include a discussion of successful early detection and treatment strategies for this deadly disease.

Progression Model of Pancreatic Ductal Adenocarcinoma

In the first era of pancreatic cancer research (Figs. 9D.1 and 9D.2), the fields of molecular biology and pathology combined to establish a paradigm that PDA culminates from a multistep progression model.[3] The second era of pancreatic research (see Figs. 9D.1 and 9D.2) led to the identification of targetable recurrent alterations in PDA and possible targets for therapy (Fig. 9D.3). This slow, sequential process may be the reason PDA is primarily a disease of people in their sixth and seventh decades of life. Definable pathologic markers on this stepwise progression, which follows a similar model first developed in colon carcinogenesis, are lesions referred to as *pancreatic intraepithelial neoplasia* (PanIN)[3] (Fig. 9D.4A–C). These lesions are believed to be precursor lesions to pancreatic cancer. PanIN lesions are thought to develop years before the emergence of PDA and are pathologically graded as low-grade PanIN lesions without cytologic dysplasia (PanIN-1) (see Fig. 9D.4A) to intermediate lesions (PanIN-2) with cytologic abnormalities such as pseudostratification, crowding, or nuclear enlargement (see Fig. 9D.4B) to high-grade lesions (PanIN-3) that consist of full-thickness dysplasia/carcinoma in situ (see Fig. 9D.4C). Although low-grade PanIN lesions are common incidental findings, high-grade PanIN lesions are more common in the pancreata of patients with PDA (see Chapter 59).

Key evidence supporting that PanIN lesions are precursors to PDA is that similar hallmark molecular defects are found in PanIN lesions adjacent to invasive cancers.[8–12] Kirsten rat sarcoma oncogene *(KRAS)* mutations are frequently found in early PanIN lesions, including PanIN-1,[13] whereas genes involved in DNA repair mechanisms or transforming growth factor-β (TGF-β) signaling, such as for tumor protein 53 (TP53) and SMAD4, respectively, are altered in the latter stages of this progression model.[14] It has also been shown that a higher frequency of PanIN lesions may be found in pancreata of patients with an inherited risk of PDA, again supporting the hypothesis that PanINs are true precursors to PDA.[13]

Once a PDA has formed, additional genetic changes continue to occur with time, thereby creating subclones (intratumoral heterogeneity) that seed metastases (e.g., peritoneal or distant).[15] It has been estimated that it takes an average of 6.8 years for a parental pancreatic ductal adenocarcinoma (PDAC) clone to give rise to a given metastatic lesion.[15]

Intraductal Papillary Mucinous Neoplasm

The intraductal papillary mucinous neoplasm (IPMN) is a well-accepted clinical and pathologic entity (see Fig. 9D.4D; see Chapters 59 and 60).[16] IPMNs typically produce radiographically identifiable pancreatic ductal dilation, which may predominantly involve the main pancreatic ducts (main duct type IPMN), the secondary ducts (branch duct type IPMN), or both types of ducts (mixed type) (see Chapter 17). The distinction between the branch duct type and main duct type IPMNs is important, because the former are more likely to involve the head and uncinate process of the pancreas and are associated with lower-grade dysplasia and fewer invasive carcinomas.[17] Approximately 30% to 40% of resected IPMNs harbor an invasive adenocarcinoma, and adenocarcinoma is most strongly associated with main duct IPMNs. Approximately half of invasive carcinomas arising within IPMNs are so-called *colloid* (mucinous) carcinomas, and most of the remainder are tubular adenocarcinomas; the latter is histologically indistinguishable from invasive ductal adenocarcinomas that arise in the setting of PanINs.[18] Colloid carcinomas associated with IPMNs have a relatively good prognosis compared with other pancreatic carcinomas of the ductal type and have a 5-year survival of 60%[19] (see Chapters 61 and 62).

PanINs and IPMNs show some overlapping features (see Chapter 59). For example, both are inherently intraductal lesions composed predominantly of columnar, mucin-producing cells that may grow in a flat configuration or may produce papillae; these lesions show a range of cytologic and architectural atypia and can give rise to invasive adenocarcinomas of the pancreas (see Fig. 9D.4E). An important feature that distinguishes the two lesions is that PanINs are microscopic lesions and IPMNs are macroscopic. Nevertheless, recognition of an IPMN and its distinction from a PanIN lesion is important for two reasons: (1) IPMN-associated colloid carcinomas have a significantly better prognosis than either PanIN- or IPMN-associated tubular adenocarcinomas[20] and (2) IPMNs have a propensity to

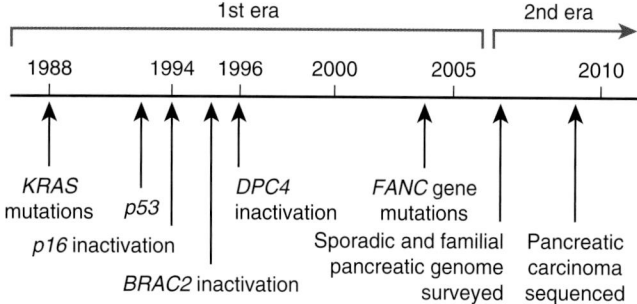

FIGURE 9D.1 Genetic landmark discoveries in pancreatic cancer research. The first era is highlighted by the discovery of tumor suppressor genes such as *DPC4* and loss of p16. The second era is highlighted by genomic profiling of discovery and validating sets of isolated and purified tumors from pancreatic cancer patients.

be multifocal lesions, therefore, patients who undergo partial pancreatectomy and are left with a remnant pancreas need to be followed for life, even when the lesion originally resected was a noninvasive IPMN.[21]

Genetic analyses of IPMNs have disclosed abnormalities in many of the same genes altered in conventional ductal adenocarcinoma, including mutations in the *KRAS2*, *TP53*, and *CDKN2A* genes, although the frequency and stage of neoplastic progression at which these alterations occur in IPMNs differ from PanINs.[16,22] For example, in contrast to PanINs, IPMNs harbor *KRAS* mutations in only half of analyzed cases.[23] Moreover, abnormalities in *SMAD4*, which are

present in 30% of PanIN-3 and 55% of PDA, are rare in IPMNs.[24] IPMNs may also contain genetic alterations of genes that are specific to this form of neoplasia. Activating mutations in *GNAS* have been found in more than 70% of IPMNs, and a subset shows genetic inactivation of *RNF43*.[23] Interestingly, correlations between phenotypic differentiation of IPMNs (described later) and mutations have been identified: *GNAS* mutations are more common in gastric and intestinal type IPMNs than in pancreaticobiliary type IPMNs, whereas *KRAS* mutations are more common in gastric and pancreaticobiliary type IPMNs.[23] Molecular testing of pancreatic cyst fluid for *GNAS* and *KRAS* mutations may help support a diagnosis of IPMN and distinguish it from other cystic lesions, including neuroendocrine tumors with cystic degeneration, benign pseudocysts, and solid and cystic pseudopapillary neoplasms. However, a negative result does not rule out a mucinous cystic neoplasm.[25]

Another distinction between PanINs and IPMNs relates to the expression of the caudal differentiation factor CDX2, a marker of intestinal differentiation. Most IPMNs express CDX2, in particular IPMNs associated with an invasive colloid carcinoma, whereas this is uncommon both in PanINs and in the subset of IPMNs that give rise to invasive cancers resembling ductal adenocarcinomas.[26] CDX2 expression in IPMNs is generally associated with expression of MUC2, an intestinal epithelial apomucin, whereas the absence of CDX2 expression usually is associated with expression of MUC1, a biliary apomucin, and concomitant lack of expression of MUC2. These findings have suggested that there may be two divergent pathways of carcinogenesis within the pancreatic ducts.[18] The first is a

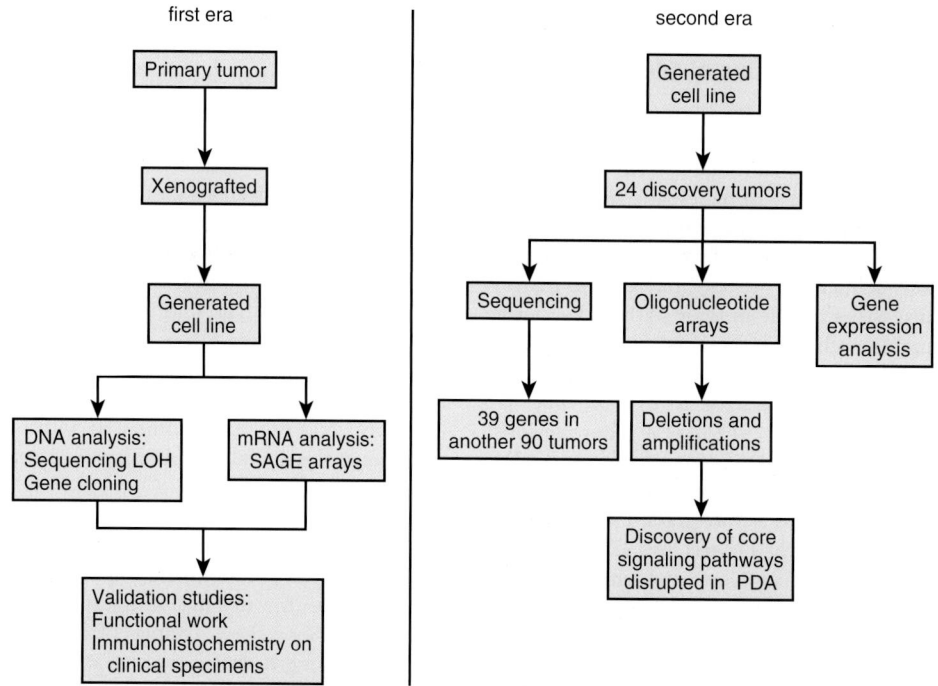

FIGURE 9D.2 Simplified flowchart of genetic discoveries performed in the two eras of genetic research. In the first era *(left)*, resected pancreatic cancers were xenografted, and genomic DNA was isolated for genetic analysis of a region or putative tumor suppressor or oncogene. In the second era *(right)*, combining advances in equipment and techniques and high-throughput sequencing allowed a genomic survey of the pancreatic cancer genome. *LOH*, Loss of heterozygosity; *mRNA*, messenger RNA; *PDA*, pancreatic ductal carcinoma; *SAGE*, serial analysis of gene expression. Data from Ding J, Wang H: Multiple interactive factors in hepatocarcinogenesis, Cancer Lett 346: 17–23, 2014; and Marquardt JU, Thorgeirsson SS: SnapShot: hepatocellular carcinoma, Cancer Cell 25: 550, 2014; and Totoki Y, et al. Trans-ancestry mutational landscape of hepatocellular carcinoma genomes, Nat Genet. 46: 1267–73, 2014.

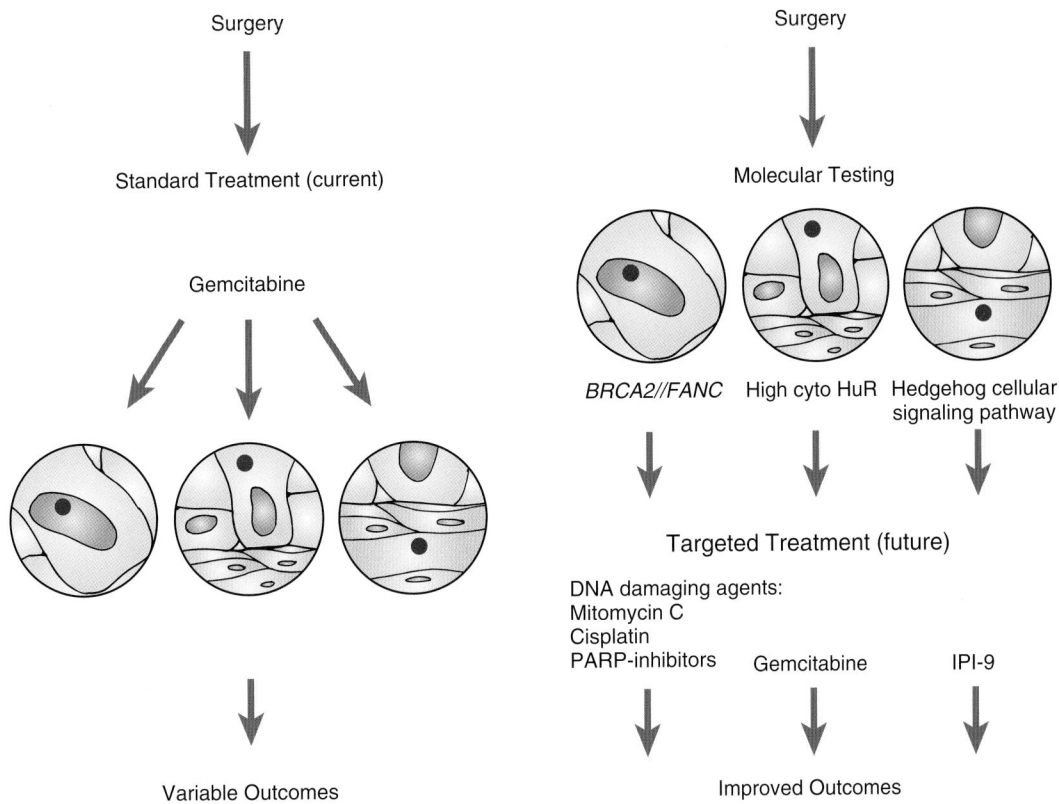

FIGURE 9D.3 **Targeted treatment strategy of PDA.** *Left,* The current strategy. *Right,* The future. IPI-9 is the abbreviation for IPI-926, an agent that inhibits the Hedgehog cellular signaling pathway (the stromal component of PDA). *cyto,* Cytoplasmic; *HuR,* human antigen R; *PDA,* pancreatic ductal adenocarcinoma; *PARP,* poly (ADP-ribose) polymerase. (Courtesy Jennifer Brumbaugh, Thomas Jefferson University, Philadelphia.)

so-called *intestinal pathway* that gives rise to CDX2- and MUC2-expressing IPMNs that progress to colloid carcinomas, which have a better prognosis. The second is a pancreatobiliary pathway that gives rise to *CDX2*-negative, MUC2-negative, and MUC1-expressing PanINs and a subset of IPMNs, both of which can progress to conventional ductal adenocarcinomas, which have a poorer prognosis.

MUC5AC, a gastric foveolar mucin, is a secretory product normally expressed by surface mucus cells in the stomach and bronchial tract. MUC5AC expression is typically absent in the normal pancreas and hyperplastic lesions, whereas MUC5AC has consistently been shown to be aberrantly expressed in PDAC and its associated premalignant lesions, including all subtypes of IPMNs.[27] It has been suggested that MUC5AC expression in pancreatic tumors may play a role in the tumor cells evading the host immune response, as well as contributing to the invasive motility of pancreatic cancer cells.[28] Overexpression of MUC5AC relays a poorer prognosis in PDAC.[29]

Intraductal Tubulopapillary Neoplasm

Intraductal tubulopapillary neoplasm (ITPN) is an intraductal neoplasm of the pancreas with distinct genetic and immunophenotypic features that are different from IPMNs and conventional ductal adenocarcinoma (see Chapter 59). ITPNs were first described in 2009 and included as a distinct diagnostic entity in the 2010 World Health Organization (WHO) classification of tumors of the gastrointestinal tract.[30] ITPNs account for 3% of intraductal neoplasms of the pancreas.[30] They have a slight female predominance and typically present with nonspecific abdominal symptoms.[31] Histologically, ITPNs are composed of nodules with back-to-back tubular glands lined by cuboidal cells with eosinophilic to amphophilic cytoplasm. Rare papillae may be seen, although the predominant architectural pattern is tubular.[30] The glandular crowding results in the formation of large circumscribed cribriform structures with central comedo type necrosis. Intracellular mucin is typically minimal. An invasive carcinoma is identified in up to 70% of cases.[32] The prognosis of ITPNs with an invasive carcinoma is regarded as better overall than that of ductal adenocarcinoma, with a 5-year overall survival rate of 71% in ITPN in contrast to a 5-year overall survival rate of 21% in PDAC.[31]

The immunophenotype of ITPNs shares some overlap with pancreaticobiliary type IPMNs. Expression of MUC1 and MUC6 is commonly seen in both ITPNs and pancreaticobiliary type IPMNs, whereas MUC5AC expression, which is highly expressed in all subtypes of IPMNs, is rarely reported in ITPNs.[27] MUC2 labeling, which is observed in the intestinal type IPMNs, is consistently not seen in ITPNs.[30]

Genetic alterations characteristic of PDAC and IPMNs are typically absent in ITPNs. Mutations in *KRAS,* for example, are seen in 7.1% of ITPNs, whereas they are observed in 80% of IPMNs.[33] *GNAS* mutations, which are found in more than 70% of IPMNs, have not been reported in ITPNs.[33] Somatic mutations in *PIK3CA* have also been described in 27% of ITPNs, whereas these alterations are typically absent in IPMNs.[34] Although both intraductal pancreatic neoplasms share morphologic and immunophenotypic characteristics,

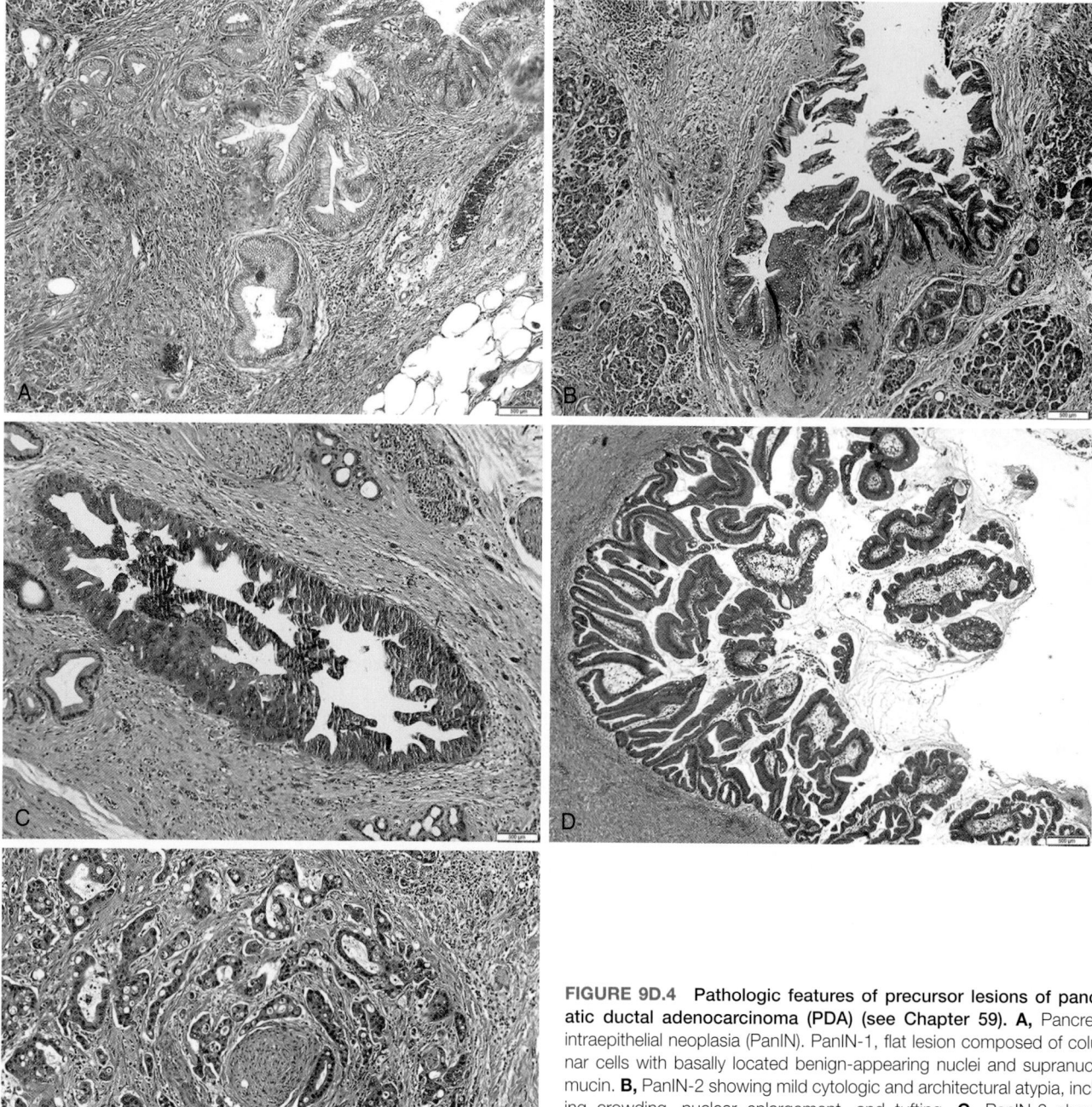

FIGURE 9D.4 Pathologic features of precursor lesions of pancreatic ductal adenocarcinoma (PDA) (see Chapter 59). **A,** Pancreatic intraepithelial neoplasia (PanIN). PanIN-1, flat lesion composed of columnar cells with basally located benign-appearing nuclei and supranuclear mucin. **B,** PanIN-2 showing mild cytologic and architectural atypia, including crowding, nuclear enlargement, and tufting. **C,** PanIN-3 showing complex papillary architecture with budding of epithelial cells into lumen and severe cytologic atypia of lining cells. **D,** Intraductal papillary mucinous neoplasm (IPMN) with low-grade dysplasia showing well-formed papillae lined by mucin-containing cells. **D,** IPMN with high-grade dysplasia with complex branching papillae and cells showing marked cytologic atypia. **E,** Invasive, moderately differentiated PDA forming angular abortive glands and invading perineural spaces.

both are recognized as distinct intraductal entities based on the differences in their genetic alterations.

Intraductal Oncocytic Papillary Neoplasm

Intraductal oncocytic papillary neoplasm (IOPNs) were formally considered as a variant of IPMNs; however, advancements in the understanding of the molecular and immunophenotypic features of IOPNs have led to the reclassification of these lesions as a distinct diagnostic entity in the 2018 WHO

classification of tumors of the gastrointestinal tract (see Chapters 59 and 60). IOPNs account for 4.5% of all intraductal neoplasms of the pancreas.[35] They typically present in female patients most commonly either as an incidental finding or with symptoms associated with tumoral mass effect. IOPNs have a unique histologic appearance characterized by complex arborizing papillae with delicate fibrovascular cores lined by cuboidal to columnar cells with granular, eosinophilic cytoplasm and a round, centrally located nucleus with a prominent eccentric nucleolus. Architecturally, the cells form cribriform spaces with intraluminal mucin. IOPNs are essentially regarded to exhibit high-grade dysplasia due to the degree of architectural and cellular complexity commonly seen.[35]

Although there are overlapping clinicopathologic characteristics between IOPNs and IPMNs, IOPNs exhibit distinct molecular alterations. IOPNs are reported to harbor recurrent mutations in *ARHGP26*, *ASXL1*, *EPHA8*, and *ERBB4*, although none occur at a high enough frequency to be considered entity-defining genomic alterations.[36–38] Mutations in *KRAS* and *GNAS*, by contrast, have rarely been reported.[36] The recently described novel *DNAJB1-PRKACA* oncogenic fusion has been found to be a mutated subset of intraductal pancreatic neoplasms with oncocytic morphology.[39] The novel fusion was first described in the fibrolamellar variant of hepatocellular carcinoma and had previously been considered to be diagnostic of this entity.[40]

Immunohistochemically, IOPNs exhibit diffuse labeling for MUC1 and MUC6 in 50% and 29% of cases, respectively. Interestingly, 61% of IOPNs label for HepPar-1, a marker of hepatocellular differentiation. In situ hybridization for albumin, a more specific marker for hepatocellular differentiation, is consistently negative in these cases.[37]

The distinction between IOPNs and IPMNs is critical as IOPNs are regarded to have a better overall prognosis. Invasive carcinoma is associated with IOPNs in about 30% of cases.[41] The predominant morphology of invasive tumors is that of a tubular adenocarcinoma composed of oncocytic tumor cells similar to the preneoplastic lesion.[41] Invasive carcinoma associated with IOPNs has a relatively good prognosis with a 5-year survival approaching 100%.[41]

GENETICS OF PANCREATIC DUCTAL ADENOCARCINOMA (SEE CHAPTER 9A)

Genomic (DNA) Alterations in Pancreatic Cancer

The multitude of genetic abnormalities in pancreatic cancer have many characteristics similar to other solid tumors; thus they include point mutations in critical genes, chromosomal (copy number) aberrations, mitochondrial DNA mutations, telomeric abnormalities, and epigenetic silencing by methylation of defined promoter DNA sequences. An individual pancreatic tumor contains on average 63 genetic alterations, primarily point mutations. Only a small subset of these mutations is required for tumorigenesis.[4]

The field of analyzing the genetics of pancreatic cancer can be broken down chronologically (see Fig. 9D.1). First, landmark studies starting in the late 1980s and spanning nearly two decades are highlighted by the discovery of *KRAS* activation, *SMAD4* and *BRCA2* mutations, and *CDKN2A* silencing (see Figs. 9D.1 and 9D.2, left). Some of these discoveries spurred new lines of investigation in the field of pancreatic cancer as well as specific classification of PDA subtypes.[42] More recently, with the help of advanced DNA sequencing technology, investigators have been able to sequence the entire genomes of various pancreatic cancer subtypes (see Figs. 9D.1 and 9D.2, right).

Copy Number Aberrations

Although now considered primitive, valuable cytogenetic analysis performed more than a decade ago found that chromosomal aberrations occur in virtually every pancreatic cancer. Cytogenetic analyses of pancreatic cancers have shown multiple, nonrandom numeric, and structural changes.[43,44] The most common numeric abnormalities include losses of chromosomes 6, 12, 13, and 18 and gains of chromosomes 7 and 20. Structural abnormalities (intrachromosomal break points) frequently involve 1p and 1q, 3p, 4q, 6q, 7q, 17p, 11p, 11q, 15q, 16q, and 19q.[45] The technical limitations of conventional cytogenetics have presented challenges for identifying genes that are affected by chromosomal breaks. Allelotyping identifies areas of gross chromosomal loss by using polymorphic microsatellite markers to determine regions of genomic loss compared with matched healthy tissues, also known as *loss of heterozygosity* (LOH) analysis. Allelotyping operates on the basic principle of the two-hit hypothesis, which postulates that tumor suppressor genes require biallelic inactivation. This most commonly happens by intragenic mutation in one allele, followed by loss of genetic material in the other allele. Identifying regions of single or biallelic loss or mutation holds the potential to understand the role of neighboring novel and well-known tumor suppressor genes. A landmark allelotype analysis of pancreatic cancers was performed using approximately 80 pancreatic cancer xenografts and 386 microsatellite markers.[46] This work discovered allelic losses in chromosome regions in proximity to tumor suppressor genes *CDKN2A*, *TP53*, and *SMAD4*. Allelotype analysis of PanIN lesions also has been performed using microdissected samples, and as expected, LOH is seen in many of the same chromosomal regions as invasive cancer, including 9p, 17p, and 18q.[47,48] Although the changes are conserved in most synchronous precursor lesions (i.e., the same allele is lost in PanIN and associated cancers), there is occasional clonal divergence between high-grade PanIN lesions harboring genetically distinct changes from the synchronous invasive cancer.[48] These findings may have important clinical implications in regard to tumor heterogeneity and clonal cancer cell drug resistance.

Comparative genome hybridization (CGH) identifies genomic amplifications and deletions and differentially labels normal and tumor genomic sequences with different dyes. The relative ratio of the two dyes indicates regions of cancer-associated losses or gains, with a ratio of 1:1 consistent with no change in copy number compared with healthy DNA. Conventional CGH is performed on metaphase spreads and suffers from both low resolution and the inability to precisely map the various regions of amplifications and deletions.[49] The resolution of array CGH is significantly better than the conventional technique, ranging from 500 to 30 kb, permitting the precise mapping of deletion and amplicon boundaries and genes targeted therein. Array technology also provides the ability to use probes more efficiently to study amplification of a larger number of genes. Array CGH analysis of pancreatic cancers has identified numerous recurrent copy number aberrations, including amplifications of the myelocytomatosis oncogene (c-*MYC*) (8q), epidermal growth factor receptor gene (*EGFR*) (7p), *KRAS* (12p), *AKT2* (19q), and *NCOA3* (20q) and deletions of *SMAD4* (18q), *CDKN2A* (9p), *FHIT* (3p), and *MAP2K4* (17p).[50–52]

Utilizing high-density single-nucleotide polymorphism arrays, Calhoun and colleagues[51] surveyed all the commercially available pancreatic cancer cell lines. In brief, this study provided high-resolution and detailed break-point mapping of these cell lines and found two subclasses of cancer cell lines, original chromosomal instability (CIN) and holey CIN genotypes.[51]

Perhaps global classification of tumor cells with high-density arrays will become part of a prognostic or predictive molecular signature panel in the future.

Specific Gene Mutations

Allelotyping provides insight into areas harboring tumor suppressor genes, but it cannot qualify areas of enhanced genomic expression, as happens with oncogene activation. Simplistically, wild-type tumor suppressor genes can "put the brakes" on the speeding vehicle (the cell), but if mutated, these "brakes" become defective, and the vehicle cannot stop. Using a similar automobile analogy, protooncogenes, in a mutated form known as *oncogenes,* become the "accelerators," and these "go signals" are often critical in transforming normal cells to a malignant phenotype.

Much like other solid tumors, genes altered in pancreatic cancer include three functional classes: *oncogenes, tumor suppressor genes,* and *caretaker genes.* A family of caretaker genes recognized as disrupted in pancreatic cancer are genes of the Fanconi anemia complementation group, which are involved in homologous recombination-based DNA damage repair.[53] Patients with Fanconi anemia present with a wide variety of clinical issues, including aplastic anemia and a high risk of developing cancer. *BRCA2* is a member of this DNA repair pathway and is mutated in a subset of familial pancreatic cancers.[54] This has led to the search for mutations in other Fanconi anemia genes in pancreatic cancer. Somatic mutations of two genes in the core complex, *FANCC* and *FANCG,* were discovered but are rare in sporadic pancreatic cancers.[55] Through other modern techniques, Jones and colleagues[5] discovered *FANCN (PALB2)* as another mutated gene found in familial pancreatic cancers.

Mutations in this core complex and in this DNA repair mechanism have major therapeutic implications (Fig. 9D.5 and Table 9D.1; see "Familial Pancreatic Cancer").[56] Unlike most in vivo experiments, xenografted mice with isogenic cell lines (*FANCC* deficient and proficient) experienced regression of tumor after a single dose of the available mitomycin C intra-strand cross-linking drug.[57] Although other than *FANN, FANCC,* and *FANCG,* mutations in the Fanconi complementation group have not yet been described, and the frequency of these mutations in PDA appear to be low, it is likely that defects in other *FANC* genes yet to be thoroughly investigated (i.e., *FANCA*) are the direct cause of some familial and sporadic PDAs.

Oncogenes

Perhaps the best evidence that *KRAS* activation is an early and important event in tumorigenesis comes from decades of research on pancreatic cancer. The *KRAS* oncogene on chromosome 12p is the most commonly altered oncogene, with as many as 90% of pancreatic cancers containing mutations on codons 12, 13, and 61.[58] Activating mutations impair the intrinsic guanosine triphosphate (GTP)ase activity of the *KRAS* gene product, resulting in a protein that is constitutively active in intracellular signal transduction. *KRAS* mutation happens early in the pathway to oncogenesis, with approximately 30% of PanIN-1 lesions harboring *KRAS* mutations.[59,60] The first mouse model of pancreatic cancer was generated by constitutive overexpression of mutant *KRAS2* in murine pancreatic ductal epithelium, underscoring its importance in pancreatic oncogenesis.[61] This model

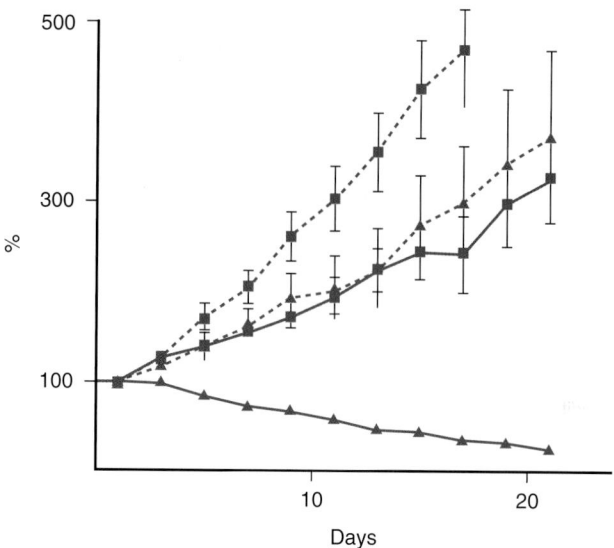

FIGURE 9D.5 Preclinical model shows an example of a successful targeted treatment strategy against a Fanconi-deficient tumor. A single-dose treatment with mitomycin C (5 mg/kg) of pancreatic cancer cell lines xenografted into nude mice. Note the hypersensitivity and tumor regression in the *FANCC*-deficient PL11 cells *(squares)* compared with the retrovirally corrected *FANC*-proficient PL11 cells *(triangles).* *Solid lines* indicate treated mice; *gray lines* indicate no-treatment controls. Similar sensitivity was seen in the *BRCA2*-deficient CAPAN1 xenografted cells. (From van der Heijden MS, et al. In vivo therapeutic responses contingent on Fanconi anemia/BRCA2 status of the tumor. *Clin Cancer Res.* 2005;11[20]:7508–7515.)

was further developed into a powerful and useful preclinical model for PDA progression.[62] Several good sources on mouse modeling and pancreatic cancer have been published.[63–66]

Rarely, pancreatic cancers with wild-type *KRAS* genes harbor point mutations of *BRAF,* another gene in the RAS/RAF/mitogen-activated protein kinase (MAPK) signaling pathway, thereby explaining why mutations of these genes occur in mutually exclusive patterns in pancreatic cancer.[67] This highlights the importance of identifying different molecular targets that lead to similar pathways in pancreatic cancer development and of finding a drug that can target one pathway, not one gene. Studies have shown that targeting *KRAS* may have potential in modulating angiogenesis in tumorigenesis. Matsuo and colleagues[68] showed that oncogenic overexpression of *KRAS* increases production of angiogenesis, promoting CXC chemokines and vascular endothelial growth factor (VEGF) from human pancreatic duct epithelial cells. This upregulation acts through the MAPK pathway and c-JUN signaling.[68] *KRAS* mutation has been shown to be associated with increased *VEGFA* expression and poorer prognosis in pancreatic carcinoma.[69] Yet, targeting *KRAS* activation in PDA patients has shown no success. Perhaps *KRAS* activation is a critical early event in pancreatic tumorigenesis, but once cells become malignant, there is no need for constitutive *KRAS* activation, or for oncogenic addiction, for that matter.

Other oncogenes implicated in pancreatic cancers include *MYC* and *EGFR,* which can be mutated *(GNAS)* or amplified *(MYC)* in various subsets of cancers. Overexpression of *MYC* transcripts occurs in approximately 50% to 60% of pancreatic

TABLE 9D.1 Genetic Syndromes With Inherited Predisposition to Pancreatic Cancer

SYNDROME/DISEASE	GENE(S)	GENETIC TESTING CONSIDERATIONS	RISK OF PANCREATIC ADENOCARCINOMA	AVAILABLE TARGETED THERAPY/ CLINICAL CORRELATES
Hereditary breast/ ovarian cancer syndrome (HBOCS)	BRCA1 BRCA2	NCCN test criteria require personal or family history of breast and ovarian cancer	BRCA1: 2.26-fold[*] BRCA2: 3- to 9-fold[†]	Cross-linking chemotherapeutics (mitomycin C, cisplatin, chlorambucil, melphalan) PARP inhibitors
Peutz-Jeghers syndrome (PJS)	STK11 (LKB1)	Diagnosis of index case is generally based on clinical findings/ working definition[‡]	132-fold; lifetime risk ~36%[§]	Reports of a PJS-associated cancer with loss of the wild-type STK11 allele, together with a germline mutation in the other allele. Some sporadic PDAs exhibit somatic mutations of STK11[ǁ]
Hereditary pancreatitis	PRSS1, SPINK1, CFTR, CTRC	Testing guidelines are based on symptoms with or without family history of pancreatitis[¶]	50- to 67-fold; lifetime risk 44%[a,b]	Tumor susceptibility is presumably due to mitogenic stimulation and clonal outgrowth of PDA cells as part of the normal healing responses that occur subsequent to repeated rounds of tissue destruction[b]
FAMM melanoma syndrome	CDKN2A	Documented patients/families with multiple melanomas	13- to 39-fold[†]	Somatic p16 alterations were identified in 80% of PDAs[c]
HNPCC-Lynch syndrome	MLH1, MSH2, MSH6, PMS2	Bethesda Guidelines[†] (tumor MSI/ IHC) and Amsterdam Clinical Criteria II (germline studies)		MSI-H pancreatic cancer may have a better prognosis after resection, possibly because of intensive immunoreaction to the tumor[d]
Familial adenomatous polyposis (FAP)	APC	APC is considered in individuals with ≥20 colon adenomas	Relative risk 4.46[e] Lifetime risk ~2%[f]	Some theorize that pancreaticobiliary secretions affect the development of adenomas and cancer in this area[g]
Cystic fibrosis (CF)	CFTR	Genotyping identifies patients with class IV and V mutations, which are likely to represent those with a functioning pancreas[h]	Relative risk 5.3[i]	Modifier genes or environmental factors may also be important in stratifying risk (e.g., mucin genes are found in both CF and PDA)[j]

[*]From Thompson D, et al. Cancer incidence in BRCA1 mutation carriers. *J Natl Cancer Inst.* 2002;94(18):1358–1365.

[†]From Brand RE, et al. Advances in counseling and surveillance of patients at risk for pancreatic cancer. *Gut.* 2007;56(10):1460–1469.

[‡]From Giardiello FM, et al. Increased risk of cancer in the Peutz-Jeghers syndrome. *N Engl J Med.* 1987;316(24):1511–1514.

[§]From Giardiello FM, et al. Very high risk of cancer in familial Peutz-Jeghers syndrome. *Gastroenterology.* 2000;119(6):1447–1453.

[ǁ]From Su GH, et al. Germline and somatic mutations of the STK11/LKB1 Peutz-Jeghers gene in pancreatic and biliary cancers. *Am J Pathol.* 199;154(6):1835–1840.

[¶]From Ellis et al. Genetic testing for hereditary pancreatitis: guidelines for indications, counseling, consent, and privacy issues. *Pancreatology.* 2001;1(5):405–415.

[a]From Lowenfels AB, et al. Hereditary pancreatitis and the risk of pancreatic cancer: International Hereditary Pancreatitis Study Group. *J Natl Cancer Inst.* 1997;89(6):442–446.

[b]From Howes N, et al. Clinical and genetic characteristics of hereditary pancreatitis in Europe. *Clin Gastroenterol Hepatol.* 2004;2(3):252–261.

[c]From Rozenblum E, et al. Tumor-suppressive pathways in pancreatic carcinoma. *Cancer Res.* 1997;57(9):1731–1734.

[d]From Nakata B, et al. Prognostic value of microsatellite instability in resectable pancreatic cancer. *Clin Cancer Res.* 2002;8(8):2536–2540.

[e]From Giardiello FM, et al. Increased risk of thyroid and pancreatic carcinoma in familial adenomatous polyposis. *Gut.* 1993;34(10):1394–1396.

[f]From Burt RW. Colon cancer screening. *Gastroenterology.* 2000;119(3):837–853.

[g]From Wallace MH, et al. Upper gastrointestinal disease in patients with familial adenomatous polyposis. *Br J Sur.* 1998;85(6):742–750.

[h]From Krysa J, et al. Pancreas and cystic fibrosis: the implications of increased survival in cystic fibrosis. *Pancreatology.* 2007;7(5–6):447–450.

[i]From Maisonneuve P, et al. Risk of pancreatic cancer in patients with cystic fibrosis. *Gut.* 2007;56(9):1327–1378.

[j]From Singh AP, et al. MUC4 expression is regulated by cystic fibrosis transmembrane conductance regulator in pancreatic adenocarcinoma cells via transcriptional and post-transcriptional mechanisms. *Oncogene.* 2007;26(1):30–41.

FAMM, Familial multiple mole; *HNPCC,* hereditary nonpolyposis colorectal cancer; *IHC,* immunohistochemical; *MIS-H,* microsatellite instability, high frequency; *MSI,* microsatellite instability; *NCCN,* National Comprehensive Cancer Network; *PARP,* poly (ADP-ribose) polymerase; *PDA,* pancreatic ductal adenocarcinoma.

Modified from Showalter SI, et al. Identifying pancreatic cancer patients for targeted treatment: the challenges and limitations of the current selection process and vision for the future. *Expert Opin Drug Deliv.* 2010;7(3):1–12.

cancers and has been shown to cooperate with *KRAS*.[50,70,71] NTRK gene fusions have also been detected in less than 1% of pancreatic adenocarcinomas.[72] First-generation TRK inhibitors appear to be well tolerated in patients with NTRK fusion-positive pancreatic cancer, although acquired resistance through both kinase domain mutation in NTRK genes and downstream mutations in the MAPK pathway remains a therapeutic challenge.[72,73]

Tumor Suppressor Genes

CDKN2A, on chromosome 9p, is the most commonly inactivated gene in pancreatic cancers, occurring in 90% of patients.[74,75]

CDKN2A belongs to the cyclin-dependent kinase inhibitor family and inhibits cell cycle progression through the G_1-S checkpoint mediated by cyclin-dependent kinases such as CDK4 and CDK6. Homozygous deletions (40%), intragenic mutation with loss of the second allele (40%), and epigenetic silencing by promoter methylation (10% to 15%) all contribute to gene inactivation. Loss of *CDKN2A* function occurs throughout the process of oncogenesis, with lesions appearing in different PanINs: 30% of PanIN-1A and PanIN-1B, 55% of PanIN-2, and 71% of PanIN-3 lesions show loss of nuclear p16 protein expression.[76] The *CDKN2A* homozygous deletions encompass the methylthioadenosine phosphorylase *(MTAP)* gene in approximately 30% of pancreatic cancers, which offers potential therapeutic benefit because targeted therapies have been developed that specifically inhibit the growth of *MTAP*-deficient cells.[77]

As many as 80% of pancreatic cancers contain an inactivation of the *TP53* gene on chromosome 17p. Such inactivation most often occurs via intragenic mutation combined with loss of the second allele, although homozygous deletions also occur in some PDAs. The TP53 *(p53)* protein leads to cell cycle arrest and activates apoptosis in the presence of DNA damage. It is believed that loss of TP53 function allows cells to survive and divide, despite the presence of damaged DNA, leading to accumulation of additional genetic abnormalities and, eventually, to neoplasia. Nuclear overexpression of the TP53 protein does not correlate well with mutation status. By immunohistochemistry, TP53 accumulation is seen only in the advanced PanIN-3 lesions, consistent with TP53 being a "late" genetic event in pancreatic cancer progression.[78] PDA cells with a mutant *TP53* have been shown to have a greater propensity for metastases.[79] Of note, in an experimental model, the *BRCA2* gene could not be artificially disrupted in cancer cells with intact wild-type *TP53* status.[80,81]

Inactivation of the *SMAD4* gene on chromosome 18q21 occurs in 55% of pancreatic cancers by homozygous deletions (30%) or by intragenic mutations and loss of the second allele (25%). Loss of *SMAD4* function interferes with intracellular signaling cascades downstream of the TGF family of cell surface receptors, leading to decreased growth inhibition and uncontrolled proliferation. Although *SMAD4* alterations are most common in PDA, they are also frequently seen in other carcinomas, occurring in approximately 15% of colorectal carcinoma and 10% of gastric carcinoma.[82] Similar to *TP53*, loss of *SMAD4* function is a late genetic event in pancreatic carcinoma progression, with loss of *SMAD4* seen only in a few PanIN-3 lesions.[78] Examination of resected tumor specimens found that *SMAD4* inactivation portends a poorer prognosis and greater potential to metastasize.[42,83] Moreover, in a study of PDA patients who underwent autopsy, loss of *SMAD4* was highly correlated with extensive metastatic burden. Identification of downstream targets might allow restoration of SMAD4-dependent signaling in pancreatic cancer, yielding an improved prognosis.[84]

Several tumor suppressor genes are inactivated in smaller numbers (5% to 10%) of pancreatic cancers, including *STK11* (chromosome 19p),[85] *TGFBR1* (chromosome 9q), *TGFBR2* (chromosome 3p), *RB1* (chromosome 13q),[86] and *MAP2K4* (chromosome 17p).[87] *MAP2K4* function has been explored in a number of models, yet the main reason for its loss in pancreatic cancer is still unknown.[88]

Separately, DNA-level abnormalities in the switch/sucrose nonfermentable (SWI/SNF) complex gene member AT-rich interaction domain 1A *(ARID1A)* have been reported in approximately 14% of PDAs in provisional TCGA data, mostly gene deletions and truncating mutations, whereas another 6% of PDA have decreased messenger RNA (mRNA) *ARID1A* levels without corresponding DNA abnormality, suggesting an epigenetic aberration.[82,89] *ARID1A* and other SWI/SNF members remodel chromatin, thus controlling the transcription and expression of various genes. Abnormalities in *ARID1A* have been associated with upregulation of the phosphoinositide-3-kinase (PI3K) pathway as well as sensitivity to PI3K and AKT inhibition.[90]

Mixed-lineage leukemia 3 *(MLL3* or *KMT2C)* is a gene involved in histone methylation and transcriptional coactivation. It functions as a tumor suppressor and is recurrently mutated in approximately 18% of pancreatic carcinoma, with the most common mutation type being truncating mutations (frameshift and nonsense mutations).[82,89]

Other Caretaker Genes

In addition to classic oncogenes or tumor suppressor genes, caretaker genes (beyond Fanconi anemia–related genes) have been shown to play a role in oncogenesis. In theory, caretaker genes do not influence cell growth and proliferation directly but rather prevent the accumulation of DNA damage and cumulative mutations within key exonic sequences that make up the human genome. Loss of function of the DNA damage repair genes *(MLH1, hMSH2)* occurs in a small subset of pancreatic cancers in the familial setting but has been reported to occur in approximately 17% of sporadic, nonfamilial cases.[91–93] Histologically, these microsatellite instability (MSI) cancers comprise poorly differentiated cancers with a syncytial growth pattern, expanding tumor margins, extensive necrosis, and intratumoral lymphocytic infiltrates. This uncommon variant has been termed *medullary cancer* to distinguish it from the more common PDAC.[94] Although findings in colon cancer have attempted to correlate MSI status with response to 5-fluorouracil, other studies have questioned these claims.[95]

Telomere Length Abnormalities

Telomeres are hexameric repeats of the sequence TTAGGG at the ends of chromosome arms that confer stability to chromosomes during cell division and prevent the ends from becoming "promiscuous."[96] In other words, intact telomere structure guards against chromosomal fusion and thus may prevent CIN.[97,98] In fact, telomeric dysfunction has been hypothesized to be one of the more important gateways of CIN, a signature of most solid cancers characterized by aneuploidy and extensive chromosomal rearrangements. The development of direct visualization of in situ telomere length was a breakthrough for understanding telomere length abnormalities and cancer development.[99] A study by van Heek and colleagues[11] showed that telomere length abnormalities are one of the earliest demonstrable genetic aberrations in pancreatic cancer, with greater than 90% of the lowest grade PanIN lesions showing marked shortening of telomeres, compared with normal duct epithelium.[11] It has been hypothesized that intact telomeres may serve as "caretakers" in the pancreatic ducts and that the loss of telomeres in PanIN lesions sets the stage for progressive accumulation of chromosomal abnormalities, eventually culminating in neoplasia.

Alternative Genetic Silencing: Epigenetic Abnormalities

Although the classic two-hit hypothesis postulated that tumor suppressor gene silencing occurs by a combination of intragenic mutations and allelic loss, it has become apparent since the

1990s that epigenetic mechanisms of silencing are probably as important in terms of frequency and prevalence in many cancers.[100] Epigenetic silencing occurs predominantly through hypermethylation of so-called *CpG islands* in the promoter region of tumor suppressor genes, leading to transcriptional abrogation. In cancers, preferential hypermethylation of the promoter occurs in the neoplastic cells with consequent downregulation of gene expression, but this does not occur in the corresponding normal counterpart. Epigenetic silencing is seen frequently in pancreatic cancers and tends to involve genes that function in tumor suppression or in critical homeostatic pathways (e.g., *CDKN2A*, E-cadherin, retinoic acid β, osteonectin, *SOCS1*) or in both.[101,102]

Aberrant methylation of genes is also found in precursor lesions of pancreatic cancers and tends to occur in intermediate- or late-stage lesions (PanIN-2 and PanIN-3).[103] Although there has been extensive work on the role of promoter hypermethylation in the pathogenesis of cancers, more recent data suggest that promoter hypomethylation in candidate genes also may be important in cancer development and progression. Genes showing preferential hypomethylation in pancreatic cancers (*SERPINB5, S100P, MSLN, PSCA,* and *CLDN4*) are usually overexpressed in the cancers compared with healthy pancreas, suggesting that epigenetic mechanisms can affect gene expression in either direction.[104]

Aberrant epigenetic silencing by promoter methylation also has been reported in IPMNs, including methylation of the *SOCS1* and *CDKN2A* genes.[105] Global analyses of gene expression in IPMNs have revealed the overexpression of *LCN2, LGALS3, CTSE, CLDN4,* and three members of the trefoil factor family, *TFF1, TFF2,* and *TFF3*.[106,107] These global analyses also have shown that CLDN4, CXCR4, S100A4, and MSLN all are expressed at significantly higher levels in invasive IPMNs than in noninvasive IPMNs, suggesting that these proteins may contribute to the process of invasion.[108]

Core Signaling Pathways Disrupted in Pancreatic Cancer

The modern era of molecular biology has progressed to allow high-throughput surveying of the pancreatic cancer genome (see Figs. 9D.1 and 9D.2, right), bringing some clarity to our understanding of the interactions of molecular pathways in tumorigenesis. This high-throughput analysis revealed that pancreatic cancers contain an average of 63 genes that are genetically altered.[4] In this work, Jones and colleagues used a combination of modern molecular techniques to report that 67% to 100% of all pancreatic cancer genomes surveyed had a genetic abnormality in 12 core signaling pathways and processes. These pathways, confirmed by later studies as well, include apoptosis, DNA damage control, regulation of G_1-to-S phase transition, Hedgehog signaling, hemophilic cell adhesion, integrin signaling, c-JUN N-terminal kinase signaling, KRAS signaling, regulation of invasion, small GTPase-dependent signaling (other than KRAS), TGFB signaling, and WNT/NOTCH signaling.[4,89]

Recently, genetic aberrations in the axon guidance pathway genes have been identified in genes in the SLIT/ROBO pathway (mutations and deletions in *SLIT, ROBO1,* and *ROBO2*), ephrins *(EPHA5* and *EPHA7),* and class 3 semaphorins (amplifications and mutations in *SEMA3A* and *SEMA3E*).[89] These genes have been implicated in cell growth, metastasis, and invasion,[109] overlapping with some of the pathways listed in the previous paragraph.

Unlike certain subtypes of leukemia that are driven by single "targetable" oncogenes, we have learned that pancreatic cancers

result from genetic alterations of large numbers of genes that function through a distinct number of pathways. The study by Jones and colleagues[4] suggested that it may be beneficial to target the physiologic effects of disrupted pathways rather than individual target genes. In fact, targeting multiple pathways or multiple points in the pathway may be in line with the early preclinical and clinical success stories of the concept of "synthetic lethality."[110]

FAMILIAL PANCREATIC CANCER

Approximately 10% of pancreatic cancers show familial aggregation[111] (see Chapter 61). The presence of two first-degree family members with pancreatic cancer confers a 6- to 18-fold increased risk of the disease in other first-degree relatives. This risk is increased 32- to 57-fold in families with three or more first-degree relatives with pancreatic cancer.[112,113] Only a minority of these familial cancers is caused by a recognized cancer syndrome associated with germline mutations in known genes. Included in Table 9D.1 are possible "targeted therapies" for the genes and disorders germane to pancreatic cancer. Thus this table underscores the significance for understanding the inherited lesion that may have contributed to the pancreatic cancers found in these families.

For example, as mentioned earlier in this chapter, Fanconi anemia is characterized as a rare, autosomally recessive cancer syndrome that results initially from a mutation in one of the multiple *FANC/BRCA* complementation groups in the *FANC/BRCA* pathway.[114] One gene in this pathway, *BRCA2*, is associated with a greatly increased risk of cancer when deleted via a biallelic mutation. The *BRCA* genes play a critical role in DNA repair via RAD51 repair pathways.[115] Loss of functional *BRCA1* and *BRCA2* conveys CIN to cells by impairing the critical function of DNA double-stranded break repair.[110] It has been well established that DNA damaging agents such as mitomycin C or cisplatin effectively kill cells with loss of *BRCA2* or related genes (see Fig. 9D.5).[116]

Currently, poly (adenosine diphosphate-ribose) polymerase (PARP) inhibitors have similar promising results as intrastrand cross-linking agents in early-phase trials in other cancer types (ovarian, breast).[117] Certainly, pancreatic cancer is a logical tumor system in which to test novel PARP inhibitors in combination with other DNA-damaging agents. Targeting the *FANC-BRCA* pathway with PARP inhibitors similarly has been shown to lead to synthetic lethality, creating a convenient and fortuitous therapeutic window.[110] The makeup of this therapeutic window relies on the fact that healthy cells will have an intact DNA repair mechanism and thus will be capable of managing and repairing the damage put forth by a DNA-damaging agent. In contrast, the tumor will be unable to repair such damage due to loss of a key aspect of this repair mechanism (i.e., *BRCA2;* see Fig. 9D.5).

Identification of mutations in the *FANC-BRCA* pathway in familial cancers has the potential to shed light on the treatment of sporadic cancers as well. It has been suggested that perhaps as many as 25% of sporadic breast and ovarian cancers manifest a *BRCA*-like phenotype.[118] The data have been derived from *BRCA1, FANCC, FANCG,* and *FANCF* methylation studies.[118] Further studies are warranted, but future banking of sporadic pancreatic cancers to study all of the tumor characteristics, such as posttranscriptional modification, polymorphisms, and CGH analysis, along with thorough analysis of family history may reveal a "*BRCA*ness" among certain sporadic pancreatic tumors, aiding in the personalization of therapy.[119] Focused DNA-repair microarray analysis may also shed light on other cancer susceptibility genes.

Of note, a recent report demonstrated that *PALB2*, formerly known as *FANCN*, is a gene inherited in a mutant form that produces a stop codon in a small percentage of familial PDAs. This gene was discovered to be mutated in 3 of 96 familial pancreatic cancers, each producing a different stop codon.[5] Truncating mutations in *PALB2* were not found in any of the 1084 patients of similar ethnicity used as a control cohort in a similar study, thus ruling out a polymorphic sequence variant. This information suggests that next to *BRCA2*, *PALB2* is the second most commonly mutated gene in hereditary pancreatic cancer.[5] Thus most familial pancreatic cancers have no known genetic bases at this time, although many believe an autosomal dominant inheritance of a rare mutant allele is the most likely cause of these cancers. Of apparently "sporadic" (nonfamilial) pancreatic cancer patients, 7% harbor germline mutations in the *BRCA2* gene, and this low-penetrance pattern is peculiar to cancers arising in the Ashkenazi Jewish population.[120] Perhaps no single gene is responsible for the other familial forms of PDA, the carcinogenesis of which may be the best example that core pathways collaborate with the environment[121]; thus no single gene from one pathway will prove to be disrupted in the complex process of tumorigenesis in this familial form of pancreatic cancer.

Several other known genetic syndromes associated with PDA exist, including familial atypical mole and multiple melanoma syndrome (FAMM) and Peutz-Jeghers syndrome (PJS). FAMM results from the microdeletion of *CDKN2* on chromosome 9p21.3, particularly *p16INK4a*[122,123] (see Chapter 61). As a result, CDK4/6 function is uninhibited. FAMM kindred have also been reported to harbor *CDK4* mutations that prevent CDKN2 binding, as opposed to *CDKN2* microdeletions, in some cases.[124] Patients with FAMM have an approximately 80% lifetime risk of melanoma and a 20% lifetime risk of PDA.[125] PJS is an autosomal dominant syndrome caused by mutations of the tumor suppressor *STK11 (LKB1)*. This syndrome is best known for polyps throughout the small and large intestine with an arborizing pattern of musculature, and these patients develop various types of carcinoma, including PDA. PDA develops in approximately one-fourth of patients with PJS by age 75 years.[126]

Another condition that may progress to PDA is hereditary pancreatitis (see Chapters 54, 55, and 57). These patients carry germline mutations in the *PRSS1* gene, which encodes cationic trypsinogen. Multiple mutations have been described; the original was R117H, which resulted in the elimination of a hydrolysis site in trypsin and an inability to inactivate trypsin.[127] Patients with hereditary pancreatitis are at a 35-fold relative risk for PDA by age 75 years. Diet modification, including lowering triglyceride intake, as well as abstaining from smoking or drinking, are advised to decrease the risk of progression to chronic pancreatitis.

TRANSCRIPTOMIC (RNA) ABNORMALITIES IN PANCREATIC CANCER (SEE CHAPTER 9A)

Several studies have analyzed pancreatic cancers and compared their gene expression profile with healthy pancreas tissue to identify differentially overexpressed and underexpressed genes.[128–135] A comprehensive analysis of pancreatic cancer using high-density oligonucleotide microarrays identified 217 genes as overexpressed 3-fold or greater in cancers versus healthy tissue.[132] Six genes (keratin 19, retinoic acid–induced 3, secretory leukocyte protease inhibitor, stratifin, tetraspan 1, and transglutaminase 2) were found to be overexpressed in pancreatic cancer by three platforms: oligonucleotide, cDNA microarrays, and serial analysis of gene expression (SAGE). The future role of one or all of these six genes in early detection or therapy remains to be elucidated.

The identification of differentially expressed genes not only serves the further understanding of the basic biology of pancreatic cancers, it also provides a fertile ground to identify markers for early diagnosis, imaging, and novel therapeutic strategies. Mesothelin *(MSLN)* was identified by SAGE as a gene overexpressed in pancreatic cancers, and it was confirmed by immunohistochemistry to be restricted to the neoplastic epithelium.[136] This identification led to the development of a pancreatic cancer vaccine targeted to the mesothelin antigen and the development of antimesothelin antibody-conjugated immunotoxins.[137] Phase 1 clinical trials showed that investigated antimesothelin drugs are well tolerated, and patients with advanced cancers often achieve stable disease on antimesothelin therapy.[138,139] In 2013, the US Food and Drug Administration (FDA) granted the antimesothelin drug CRS-207 approval for use in combination therapy with GVAX, a drug that stimulates the granulocyte-macrophage colony-stimulating factor.[140]

Posttranscriptional Regulation (see Chapter 9A)

In recent years, strong evidence has shown that posttranscriptional regulation of genes can directly affect both the tumorigenesis process[141,142] and cancer cell susceptibility to chemotherapy.[95,143,144] Posttranscriptional gene regulation can have the same effect on gene expression as a genetic mutation or methylation of a promoter. One potent mechanism of posttranscriptional regulation involves RNA-binding proteins. One such RNA-binding protein that has been shown to be important in a number of tumor systems is Hu antigen R (HuR), a ubiquitously expressed member of the *HU* family that mediates cellular response to stress and DNA damage by posttranscriptional regulation.[145] Elevated HuR cytoplasmic expression is detected in tumors with poor pathologic features and poor predicted outcomes.[142] It is has been shown that during times of certain cellular stressors, brought on by agents such as ultraviolet C (UVC) irradiation, heat shock, hypoxia, tamoxifen,[146] and actinomycin D, HuR can bind to certain apoptotic or survival mRNA transcripts by binding to AU-rich elements in the 3′ untranslated region (UTR) of these mRNAs. In regard to tumorigenesis, HuR has been shown to bind to and stabilize proteins such as p21, p53, and cyclin A.[144] For instance, Gorospe and colleagues[144] showed that HuR can enhance translation of proteins such as p53 under stress from UVC irradiation. Thus the role of HuR in cellular stress and damage gives it a likely pivotal role in both the tumorigenesis process and in the acute cellular response to chemotherapy in pancreatic cancer cells.

In vitro and in vivo studies have shown that PDAs with HuR overexpression were dramatically sensitive to gemcitabine, the standard chemotherapeutic treatment for pancreatic cancer, when compared with a control group.[143,147] Patients who had low cytoplasmic HuR levels had a 7-fold increase in mortality compared with patients who had elevated cytoplasmic HuR levels (Fig. 9D.6).[143]

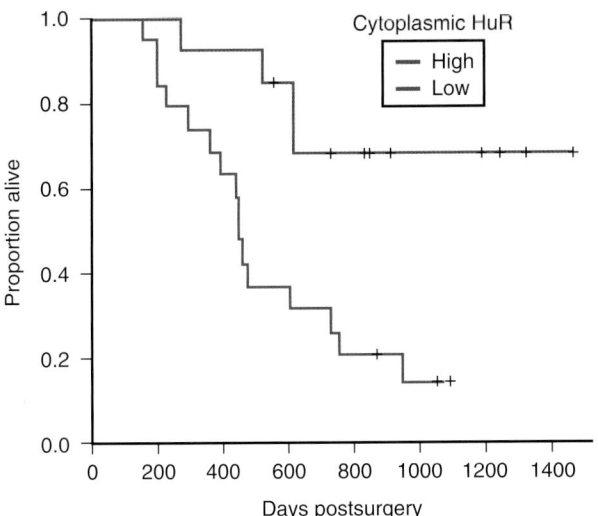

FIGURE 9D.6 Tumor human antigen R (HuR) cytoplasmic status can stratify pancreatic cancer patients treated with standard-of-care chemotherapy (gemcitabine) into two groups: responders (high cytoplasmic HuR) versus nonresponders (low cytoplasmic HuR). (From Costantino CL, et al. The role of HuR in gemcitabine efficacy in pancreatic cancer: HuR up-regulates the expression of the gemcitabine metabolizing enzyme deoxycytidine kinase. *Cancer Res.* 2009;69[11]:4567–4572.)

MicroRNAs

MicroRNAs (miRNAs) are defined as short, noncoding regions of RNA sequences (22 nucleotides) that can potently regulate gene expression patterns; miRNAs have been shown to regulate a number of disease- and developmental-related genes, and they are tissue specific in expression.[148] These miRNA-specific attributes make them putative, powerful, and unique candidate biomarkers.[149] Discovering the presence of miRNAs in pancreatic cancer may be extremely valuable, although understanding the significance of these miRNAs may be more difficult and tedious, as miRNAs have been shown to distinguish between various disease states and tissues, including pancreatitis, PDA, IPMN, and healthy specimens.[149] Further, it has been shown that a miRNA molecular signature can stratify long- and short-term survivors.[150]

MOLECULAR GENETICS OF OTHER PANCREATIC NEOPLASMS

Acinar Cell Carcinoma (see Chapter 59)

Unlike PDA, acinar cell carcinomas (ACCs) activating mutations in *KRAS* are uncommon.[151] Whole-exome sequencing of

17 ACCs revealed hot spot–activating mutations, including *GNAS* p.R201C in two tumors and *BRAF* p.V600E in one tumor, as well as mutations in tumor suppressors, including *SMAD4*, *TP53*, retinoblastoma 1 *(RB1)*, phosphatase and tensin homolog *(PTEN)*, and *ARID1A*.[152] In addition to point mutations and indels, *SND1-BRAF* fusions were identified in 6 of 44 (14%) either pure or mixed differentiation ACCs. Transfectants expressing this fusion have shown increased MAPK pathway activity as well as sensitivity to the MAP/extracellular signal-regulated protein kinase (ERK) kinase (MEK) inhibitor trametinib.[151] Epigenetic changes have also been identified, including MSI in 10% to 20% of ACCs.[152,153]

Pancreatic Neuroendocrine Tumors (see Chapters 59 and 65)

Pancreatic neuroendocrine tumors (PanNETs) also have different molecular profiles than either PDAs or ACCs. PanNETs lack *KRAS*, *SMAD4*, and *CDKN2A* mutations, and only very rarely (approximately 3%) harbor *TP53* mutations. Instead, the sporadic forms of this tumor frequently harbor death domain–associated protein/gene *(DAXX)*/alpha-thalassemia X-linked mental retardation protein/gene *(ATRX)* mutations (43%) or multiple endocrine neoplasia type 1 *(MEN1)* mutations (44%).[154]

In addition to sporadic forms, PanNETs are also seen as a component of various inherited tumor syndromes associated with germline mutations, including *MEN1*, due to mutations that cause loss of function of the *MEN1* and *VHL* genes in MEN and von Hippel Lindau syndromes, respectively.[155,156] PanNETs occurring in association with these syndromes are thought to follow a less aggressive course more often.

FINAL THOUGHTS AND PERSPECTIVES

We are currently at an interesting and critical time in studying the molecular aspects of pancreatic cancer. The research community has incredible resources at its disposal, ranging from patient databases to complex sequencing equipment. This coming of age of pancreatic cancer research must include surgeons, pathologists, molecular biologists, and medical oncologists collaborating toward ultimately better and more personalized patient care. Current research will also need to provide better early detection markers so that physicians can have more opportunities to prevent cancer from forming, instead of attempting to cure it before it is too late.

References are available at expertconsult.com.

Advances in the molecular characterization of biliary tract and gallbladder cancer

Ryosuke Okamura and Jason K. Sicklick

BILIARY TRACT CANCERS

First described by Durand-Fardel in 1840,[1] biliary tract tumors arise from cholangiocytes residing in the biliary tree. The biliary tract cancers include intrahepatic cholangiocarcinoma (IHCC, within the liver; see Chapter 50), extrahepatic cholangiocarcinoma (EHCC, within the extrahepatic biliary tree; see Chapter 51), and gallbladder cancer (GBCA, within the gallbladder; see Chapter 49). Recently, it has been recognized that some subtypes of IHCC can arise from hepatic progenitor cells or have stem cell features[2] (see Chapter 9C). Thus combined or mixed hepatocellular cholangiocarcinoma (C-HCC), which has cells with a phenotype that is intermediate between hepatocellular carcinoma (HCC) and cholangiocarcinoma (CCA), is occasionally seen and considered to be a subtype of IHCC (see Chapters 47, 50, and 89). These biliary tract cancers constitute a rare set of malignancies and mostly present as locally advanced or metastatic disease. Because of their rarity, as well as their common cell of origin, systemic treatment for all these tumor types has been identical, but chemotherapeutic regimens lack significant response rates. In patients with advanced disease, goals of systemic chemotherapy are still palliative in nature (see Chapters 47 and 49–51). With fairly recent developments in next-generation sequencing (NGS) and other molecular techniques; however, comprehensive molecular profiling now enables the identification of unique genetic signatures among these cancers and is important in clinical trial design using drugs to target specific pathways.

CLASSIFICATION

The vast majority of biliary tract tumors are adenocarcinomas,[3] and they most often arise at or near the biliary confluence. The latter fall under the general category of EHCCs (see Chapter 51), which are further subcategorized into *hilar CCA* (also known as *Klatskin tumor*) and *distal CCA,* with the transition occurring proximal to the cystic duct in the current American Joint Committee on Cancer TNM Classification and National Comprehensive Cancer Network (NCCN) guidelines.[4,5] These are further categorized as perihilar CCA by their precise location with reference to the biliary bifurcation and the hepatic lobar ducts. This classification is most useful for descriptive purposes and for operative planning. In contrast to the perihilar tumors, the distal CCAs account for a relatively small fraction of all bile duct tumors. Mid-bile duct tumors are even less common and often turn out to represent tumors of the gallbladder or cystic duct. Diffuse involvement of the entire biliary tree is a very rare condition, affecting a very small fraction of patients with biliary tract cancer. CCA may also arise from the intrahepatic bile ducts, giving rise to the subgroup known as IHCC (or peripheral CCA; see Chapter 50). IHCCs can also be subcategorized by their growth characteristics into three groups: *mass-forming*, *periductal-infiltrating*, or *intraductal growing* types.[6] Until recently, International Classification of Disease (ICD) codes combined IHCC with HCC under the code for primary liver tumor,[7,8] but these are clearly different entities, and the second and third editions of the ICD for Oncology (ICD-O-2/3) have attempted to correct for this issue. In ICD-O-2, hilar tumors were assigned a unique histology code, but this was cross-referenced to the topography code for intrahepatic rather than extrahepatic tumors. Under the third ICD-O-3 edition, hilar tumors are cross-referenced to either location.[9] In addition to the aforementioned coding issues, many tumors previously referred to as liver adenocarcinoma of unknown primary site were likely unrecognized IHCCs. Together, these changes in ICD classification have influenced observed changes in the incidence rates of IHCC and EHCC.

EPIDEMIOLOGY

Although rare, biliary tract cancer has a distinctly higher incidence in certain demographic groups and geographic regions (see Chapters 49, 50, and 51). GBCA has a higher incidence among females and in South America, whereas IHCC is more common in Asia.[10] The peak incidence of the biliary tract cancers is the seventh decade of life, with a slightly higher male predilection.[1] In the United States, an estimated 6,300 new IHCC cases were diagnosed, whereas 12,360 new EHCC or GBCA cases were diagnosed in 2019.[11–13] Outside of the United States, the incidence rates vary globally, presumably reflecting differences in infectious causes, environmental risk factors (i.e., sedentary lifestyles, alcohol, smoking, and diet), exposure to toxic chemicals, and genomics. The highest incidence rate is in Northeast Thailand (age-standardized incidence rate [ASIR]: 85/100,000 population), where it occurs approximately 100 times more often than in the West.[14] High prevalence of carcinogenic liver flukes is associated with the high incidence rates of biliary tract cancers. Nevertheless, in the United States, IHCC and EHCC incidence rates have steadily increased from 1999 to 2013 across sex and racial/ethnic groups (estimated annual percent change [eAPC]: 3.2% for IHCC and 1.8% for EHCC). Also, in other countries (e.g., Japan, Australia, and many European countries), increased rates for IHCC are widely reported.[14] In contrast, the overall GBCA incidence rate has been stable or declining, although it increased among African Americans (eAPC: 1.8%) and people aged less than 45 years (eAPC: 1.8%).[10,15] The increased incidence of IHCC and EHCC may be attributable, in part, to the fact that several risk factors (e.g., cirrhosis and obesity) have increased globally over recent decades.[14] The increased detection of early stage or smaller tumors may also be considered a reason, as would be expected if the increase were only because of an improvement in diagnostic modalities, such as magnetic resonance imaging (MRI) and computed tomography (CT).[7,16,17]

Epidemiologic data over the last few decades have also shown that the mortality rate of IHCC is rising globally, whereas the mortality rates of EHCC and GBCA have decreased in most countries.[18,19] The GBCA mortality rates declined after the increase of cholecystectomy. Despite recent imaging modality developments, most patients presenting with unresectable or metastatic disease still typically die within 12 months of diagnosis. In addition to a lack of highly efficacious systemic therapies, sepsis from cholangitis, frequently related to interventions performed for biliary obstruction and progressive liver failure, contribute to the high mortality.[16] Although biliary tract tumors remain relatively rare, there has been increased interest in studying the biology of these diseases in recent years.

CHRONIC BILIARY INFLAMMATION AND CHOLESTASIS

Clinical Risk Factors

There are multiple risk factors for biliary tract cancers. The heterogeneous tumor phenotypes and molecular findings can be explained by a complicated interaction between the unique genetic background of a patient and their exposure to the risk factors.[14] Reported risk factors for these tumors are a diverse group of conditions that include infectious causes, congenital conditions, inflammatory diseases, drugs, environmental exposures, and toxins.[14,20,21] Congenital biliary duct cysts (including Caroli disease; see Chapter 46) and cholangitis (including primary sclerosing cholangitis [PSC]; see Chapter 41) are established as well-known risk factors. The high prevalence of these diseases affects the high incidence rates in the female population of Asian countries (e.g., China and Japan). In addition, previous studies found that biliary cirrhosis, cholelithiasis, hepatolithiasis, alcoholic liver disease, nonalcoholic fatty liver disease/steatohepatitis (NAFLD/NASH), nonspecific cirrhosis, diabetes type II, thyrotoxicosis and chronic pancreatitis, obesity, chronic hepatitis B virus infection (HBV), hepatitis C virus (HCV) infection, human immunodeficiency virus (HIV) infection, and smoking were associated with the development of biliary tract cancers[21,22] (see Chapters 49–51). A recent systematic review suggests that the rising global incidence of IHCC may be associated with increases in diabetes type II, alcoholic liver diseases, and cholelithiasis.[23] Liver flukes (*Opisthorchis viverrini* and *Clonorchis sinensis*) are also major causes in East Asia, especially in Thailand and Laos. Thorotrast, which was previously used as an intravascular contrast agent, is also carcinogenic and associated with a 64-fold increased odds ratio of developing CCA.[24] Occupational exposures to 1,2-dichloropropane or asbestos have become well-known as strong risk factors in recent years. Some studies using nationwide databases support that inflammatory bowel disease is associated with the increased risk for these cancers as well.[25,26] Based on the aforementioned predisposing factors, a common theme of chronic biliary epithelial inflammation appears to be a predisposing factor for the development of biliary tract cancers. PSC is the most common condition predisposing to CCA, with incidence rates of 0.5 to 1.5 per 100 person-years reported in patients with PSC (400-fold the risk in the general population).[27,28] Although the incidence of CCA in pediatric PSC patients is very rare, CCA in adult PSC patients is seen most commonly less than 1 year after the diagnosis of PSC.[29,30] Congenital abnormalities of the biliary tree, congenital hepatic fibrosis, and choledochal cysts (cystic dilatations of the bile ducts) also carry a 15% risk of malignant change.[31,32] Furthermore, with untreated choledochal cysts, the risk of biliary tract cancers increases to 28%.[33,34] Biliary stasis, reflux of pancreatic juice, activation of bile acids, and deconjugation of carcinogens are speculated as mechanistic drivers of carcinogenesis related to the theme of chronic inflammation.[35]

Biology of Clinical Risk Factors

Several underlying mechanisms play a role in the induction of chronic biliary inflammation and cholestasis.

Bile Content and Deconjugation of Xenobiotics

Polymorphisms in bile salt transporter proteins (i.e., BSEP, ATP8B1, and ABCB4) can lead to unstable bile content and deconjugation of environmental toxins (i.e., xenobiotics) previously conjugated in the liver.[36,37] In the background of congenital bile duct abnormalities, this process increases the risk of CCA.[38] Individuals who are heterozygous for bile salt transporter polymorphisms are thought to have an increased predisposition to cancer as adults, following exposure to cofactors that result in chronic inflammation in the biliary tree.[38]

DNA Mutagens

Promutagenic DNA adducts have been identified in biliary tract cancer tissue, indicating exposure to DNA-damaging agents.[39] Although the mechanisms have not been fully elucidated, Thorotrast has a very long half-life and induces biliary tract cancers, possibly because of the release of alpha particles with high linear energy transfer, inducing mutations in various oncogenes and tumor suppressor genes, which leads to their activation.[40] Inflammatory conditions, such as chronic viral infections (e.g., HBV and HCV) or alcoholic/nonalcoholic hepatitis, promote carcinogenesis by producing reactive oxygen and nitrogen species from inflammatory and epithelial cells, activating reparative tissue proliferation, and creating a local environment rich in cytokines and other growth factors, ultimately resulting in DNA damage.[41,42] Exposures to 1,2-dichloropropane and asbestos fibers also increase DNA double-strand breaks.[43,44]

Inherited Syndrome

Lynch syndrome, an autosomal dominant predisposition for DNA mismatch repair, is associated with a high incidence of colorectal, endometrial, stomach, ovary, pancreas, ureter and renal pelvis, bile duct, and brain tumors. The associated lifetime risk for bile duct cancer in patients with Lynch syndrome is 1% to 4% (Cancer.Net, https://www.cancer.net/cancer-types/lynch-syndrome). Although hereditary and not environmental, deficiency of DNA repair is a recurrent theme in the development of biliary tract cancers.

MOLECULAR PATHOGENESIS

The molecular pathogenesis of biliary tract tumors has recently become an area of vigorous investigation (see Chapters 9A and 9C). In the era of advanced molecular analyses, including NGS, rapid progress is being made in our understanding of the genomic basis of these malignancies. Tumor profiling of biliary tract cancers has revealed that molecular profiles differentiate

IHCC, EHCC, and GBCA and that every tumor has both biologically complex and individually unique molecular alterations, suggesting individualized therapeutic options. It is beyond the scope of this chapter to document every known molecular alteration reported or associated with biliary tract cancers. Instead, we focus on recurrent themes in altered signaling pathways that together result in the pathogenic phenotypes and potential drug targets (Fig. 9E.1).

Biology of Biliary Epithelial Injury and Repair

Similar to the development of other tumors, biliary tract carcinogenesis is thought to be a multistep process dependent on the interaction between environmental factors and host genetic factors. Most of the putative environmental risk factors for

CCA result in chronic biliary inflammation, leading to tissue-repair mechanisms and, ultimately, carcinogenesis.

Conceptually, exposure to an inflammatory stimulus would not have the same effect on each cell because of changes in perfusion (e.g., centrilobular versus periportal), as well as differential levels of cytochrome P450 (CYP) expression, exposure to bile salt concentrations, and exposure to inflammatory components (e.g., cytokines and immune surveillance cellular components, such as Kupffer cells and hepatic stellate cells; see Chapters 7 and 10). Based on this, the concept of heterogeneity can be inferred where distinct clonal populations may arise based on differential response to stimuli. In this section, we review the underlying host factors associated with bile tract cancers.

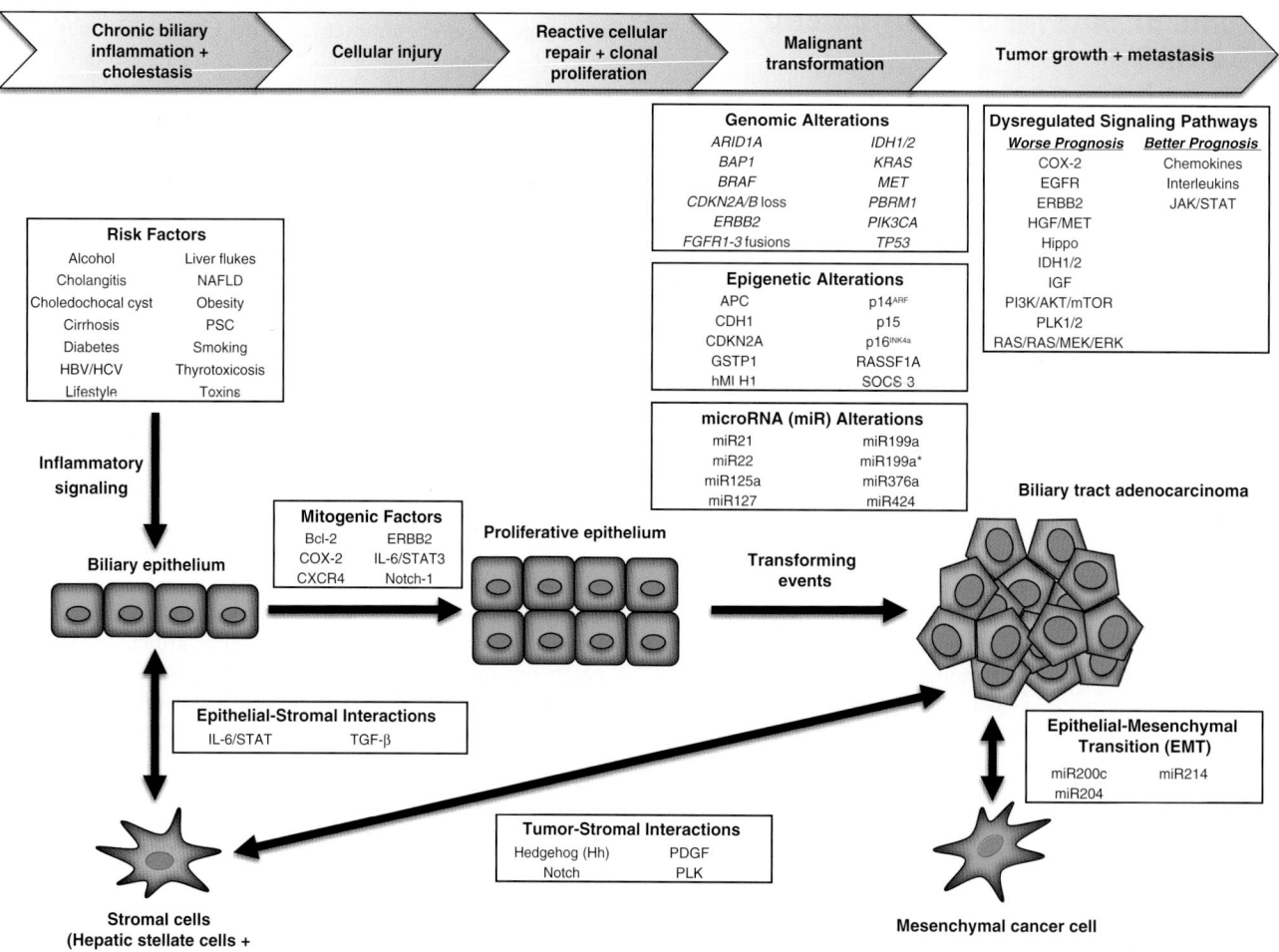

FIGURE 9E.1 Vogelgram of biliary carcinogensis. The progression from benign biliary epithelium to biliary tract adenocarcinoma occurs through a series of stages, including chronic biliary inflammation and cholestasis caused by several risk factors, followed by cellular injury, reactive cellular repair, clonal proliferation, malignant transformation, tumor growth, and metastasis. Each one of these steps is regulated by many factors, including epithelial-stromal interactions, mitogens, genomic alterations, epigenetic alterations, microRNAs, dysregulated signaling pathways, epithelial-tomesenchymal transitions, and tumor-stromal interactions. *APC,* Adenomatosis polyposis coli; *ARID1A,* AT-rich interaction domain 1A; *BAP1,* BRCA1-associated protein 1; *Bcl-2,* B-cell chronic lymphocytic leukemia/lymphoma; *BRAF,* B-Raf protooncogene; *CDH1,* cadherin 1; *CDKN,* cyclin-dependent kinase inhibitor; *COX-2,* cyclooxygenase-2; *EGFR,* epidermal growth factor receptor; *ERBB2,* ERB-B2 receptor tyrosine kinase 2; *FGFR1-3,* fibroblast growth factor receptor 1–3; *GSTP1,* glutathione-S-transferase pi 1; *HBV,* hepatitis B virus; *HCV,* hepatitis C virus; *HGF,* hepatocyte growth factor; *hMLH1,* human mutL homolog 1; *IDH1/2,* isocitrate dehydrogenase 1/2; *IGF,* insulin-like growth factor; *IL-6,* interleukin-6; *JAK,* Janus-activating kinase; *KRAS,* Kirsten rat sarcoma; *mTOR,* mechanistic target of rapamycin; *NAFLD,* nonalcoholic liver disease; *PBRM1,* polybromo 1; *PDGF,* platelet-derived growth factor; *PI3K,* phosphatidylinositol-3-kinase; *PIK3CA,* phosphatidylinositol-4,5-bisphosphate-3-kinase catalytic subunit alpha; *PLK,* polo-like kinase; *PSC,* primary sclerosing cholangitis; *SOC-3,* general sugar transporter; *STAT,* signal-transducer and activator of transcription; *TGF-b,* transforming growth factor-β; *TP53,* tumor protein 53.

Genetic Polymorphism at Cytochrome P450

Genetic polymorphisms exist in the CYP450 enzyme complex, a large family of constitutive and inducible enzymes that play a central role in the oxidative metabolism of both environmental toxins and endogenous compounds. These polymorphisms play a critical role in how endogenous and exogenous toxins are biotransformed by the liver. Similar to many other cancers, which rely on a sequence of chronic injury and repair, the development of CCA may be partially regulated by the host ability to respond toxic to insults.

Several CYPs are involved in the metabolism of oxysterols, that are cholesterol oxidation products with expression that may be dysregulated in inflammation-related diseases, including cancer. For instance, 1,2-dichloropropane, a DNA mutagen as previously mentioned, influences the proliferation and apoptosis of cholangiocytes via CYP450.[45] CYP39A1, which can metabolize 24-hydroxycholesterol, is downregulated in 70% of CCA and plays an important role in the inflammatory response and oxidative stress.[46] Low expression of CYP39A1 correlates with disease metastasis. Also, CYP2A6 and CYP2E1 are upregulated in *Opisthorchis*-associated CCA and indicate that enhanced CYP2A6 activity and diminished CYP2E1 activity are involved in the progression of CCA.[47] Finally, molecular profiling of EHCC specimens demonstrated significant enrichment of CYP-metabolic pathways, including transcription factors such as glutathione-S-transferase α1 (GSTA1) and GSTA3, which may cause abnormal gene expression and tumorigenesis through CYP450-metabolic pathways.[48] Differential CYP activity may be involved in the initiation and/or progression of disease via modulation of chronic inflammation, metabolism of exogenous compounds (e.g., drugs, tobacco, and nitrosamines), viral hepatitis, parasitic infestation, and recurrent cholangitis.[14]

MRP2/ABCC2

Multidrug resistance–associated protein 2 (MRP2/ABCC2) is one of the adenosine triphosphate-binding cassette (ABC) transporters expressed on the apical membrane of hepatocytes and cholangiocytes. ABCC2 plays an important role in the biliary clearance of endogenous and exogenous toxic compounds. The ABCC2 variant c.3972C>T in exon 28 has been shown to be associated with the risk of carcinogenesis.[49]

MUTYH and NEIL1

It was recently found that the human mutY DNA glycosylase (h-MUTYH) and Nei-like DNA glycosylase (NEIL) 1 genes encode DNA glycosylases involved in repair of oxidative base damage, and mutations in these genes are associated with CCA.[50] NEIL1 G83D was identified in PSC and CCA.[51]

Activation-Induced Cytidine Deaminase

Other work has also suggested that chronic inflammation can play a critical role leading up to CCA. The proinflammatory cytokine-induced aberrant production of activation-induced cytidine deaminase (AID), a member of the DNA/RNA-editing enzyme family, links bile duct inflammation to an enhanced genetic susceptibility to mutagenesis that leads to CCA.[52] Ectopic AID production is induced in response to tumor necrosis factor-α (TNF-α) stimulation via a nuclear factor kappa B (NF-κB)–dependent pathway. Aberrant expression of AID in biliary cells results in the generation of somatic mutations in tumor-related genes, including tumor protein 53 (TP53), c–myelocytomatosis viral oncogene (c-MYC), and the promoter region of the cyclin-dependent kinase inhibitor A (CDKN2A) sequences. In human tissue specimens, reverse transcription polymerase chain reaction analyses revealed that AID was significantly increased in 28 of 30 (93%) CCA tissues, whereas only trace amounts of AID were detected in the normal liver. Immunohistochemistry showed that all of the CCA tissue samples examined showed overproduction of endogenous AID protein in cancer cells. Moreover, immunostaining for AID was detectable in 16 of 20 biliary epithelia in PSC.

Human CYP1A2 and Arylamine N-Acetyltransferases (NAT1 and NAT2)

The *CYP1A2*, *NAT1*, and *NAT2* genes have been shown to be potential modifiers of an individual's susceptibility to certain types of cancers. In a previous study evaluating the relationship between *CYP1A2*, *NAT1*, and *NAT2* polymorphisms in Thai CCA patients, a total of 216 CCA patients and 233 control subjects were genotyped using PCR.[53] Two *CYP1A2* alleles (CYP1A2*1A wild type and *1F), six *NAT1* alleles (NAT1*4 wild type, *3, *10, *11, *14A, and *14B), and seven *NAT2* alleles (NAT2*4 wild type, *5, *6A, *6B, *7A, *7B, and *13), were analyzed. The *CYP1A2*1A/*1A* genotype conferred a decreased risk of the cancer (adjusted odds ratio [OR], 0.28; 95% confidence interval [CI], 0.08 to 0.94) compared with *CYP1A2*1F/1*F*. Frequency distributions of rapid *NAT2*13* and two slow alleles, *6B and *7A, were associated with lower risk of CCA. This study suggests that the *NAT2* polymorphism might be a modifier of individual risk of CCA.

Trefoil Factor Family

Trefoil factor family 1 (TFF1) is critical for mucosal protection and tumor suppression in the stomach. To examine its role in CCA, specimens with varying degrees of dysplasia were examined. These included IHCC as a result of hepatolithiasis, biliary epithelial dysplasia with hepatolithiasis, hepatolithiasis without dysplasia or carcinoma, IHCC without hepatolithiasis, and control normal livers.[54] TFF1 expression in the biliary epithelium was increased in hepatolithiasis compared with control livers ($P < .01$). In biliary epithelial dysplasia and noninvasive IHCC with hepatolithiasis, TFF1 was extensively expressed, and MUC5AC gastric mucin was usually colocalized with TFF1. However, TFF1 expression was significantly decreased in invasive IHCC, despite preserved expression of MUC5AC. A total of four missense mutations were detected: three were found in two noninvasive IHCC with hepatolithiasis (29%) and one in invasive IHCC (11%). Loss of heterozygosity of the TFF1 gene was not detectable. The decreased expression of TFF1 in invasive IHCC may be explained by the methylation of the TFF1 promoter region. Upregulation of TFF1 coupled with MUC5AC in biliary epithelium in hepatolithiasis, biliary epithelial dysplasia, and noninvasive IHCC may reflect gastric metaplasia and early neoplastic lesion. Under such conditions, decreased TFF1 expression is critical for the maintenance of the epithelial barrier and mucosal protection and can lead to increased cell proliferation and then to the invasive character of IHCC.

Biliary Epithelial Proliferation

Ultimately, the underlying chronic biliary inflammation, which may be modified by toxin exposure, along with modulation by endogenous host factors or inherited gene polymorphisms, may lead to an exaggerated repair response that results in cholangiocyte proliferation.

Mitogenic Factors

Identification of several mitogenic stimuli with resultant increases in DNA, RNA, protein synthesis, and immune modulation have been implicated in the carcinogenesis of biliary tract tumors. The liver fluke *Opisthorchis viverrini* can generate mitogenic substances, such as glutathione-S-transferases (GSTs), which act as a secretory product that may play an important role in promoting the genesis of CCA. GST has a proliferative function on NIH-3T3 murine fibroblasts and MMNK1 nontumorigenic human bile duct epithelial cells in a dose-dependent manner, with subsequent in vitro activation of both phospho-AKT (v-akt murine thymoma viral oncogene homolog 1; pAKT) and phospho-ERK (extracellular signal regulated kinase; pERK).[55] Other mitogens can activate these pathways. Recombinant human TFF2 can stimulate proliferation and trigger phosphorylation of epidermal growth factor receptor (EGFR) with downstream ERK activation, displaying potential mitogenic impact in CCA via EGFR/mitogen-activated protein kinase (MAPK) activation.[56] Moreover, TFF family members have been assessed as potential biomarkers in CCA. Gene copy number, messenger ribonucleic acid (mRNA) levels, and protein expression were evaluated in bile duct epithelium biopsies collected from individuals with CCA, precancerous bile duct dysplasia, and from disease-free control participants. The TFF1, TFF2, and TFF3 mRNA levels were significantly increased in CCA tissue.

In healthy tissues, cellular senescence results in irreversible growth arrest. This is prevented, however, in malignant cells by maintenance of chromosomal length via telomerase activity. This is observed in CCA cells but not in normal cholangiocytes. Interleukin-6 (IL-6) is partially responsible for this because it acts as an autocrine promoter of the cell growth of CCA. IL-6 stimulation leads to enhanced telomerase, decreased cellular senescence, and thereby increased CCA growth.[57] Moreover, in conjunction with hepatocyte growth factor (HGF), IL-6 increases CCA cell growth in vitro and induces a rapid release of prostaglandin synthesis, followed by downstream signal transduction via MAPKs, protein kinase C, and calmodulin.[58] Taken together, these, and probably other mitogens, drive the proliferation of CCA.

Malignant Transformation

Gene Expression Analysis

In 2009 Miller and colleagues investigated the molecular alterations in carcinomas of the biliary tree, including IHCC, EHCC, and GBCA, using frozen specimens from patients who underwent surgical resection.[59] Unsupervised hierarchical clustering analysis revealed that cancers from these different sites did not cluster separately, implying that there was no difference in the global gene expression patterns between the biliary cancer subgroups. However, as NGS techniques have advanced, unique molecular patterns across the subtypes of biliary tract cancer have been revealed. The molecular spectrum of biliary tract cancers is depicted in Fig. 9E.2.[60] *IDH1/2* and *BAP1* mutations, as well as *FGFR2* fusions, are more common in IHCC, whereas *KRAS* (23%–38%), *TP53* (14%–49%), and *SMAD4* mutations are more frequent in EHCC. Finally, activating *ERBB2/ERBB3* and PIK3CA mutations, as well as inactivating *PTEN* and *TSC1* mutations, are more commonly observed in GBCA[61] (see Chapter 9C).

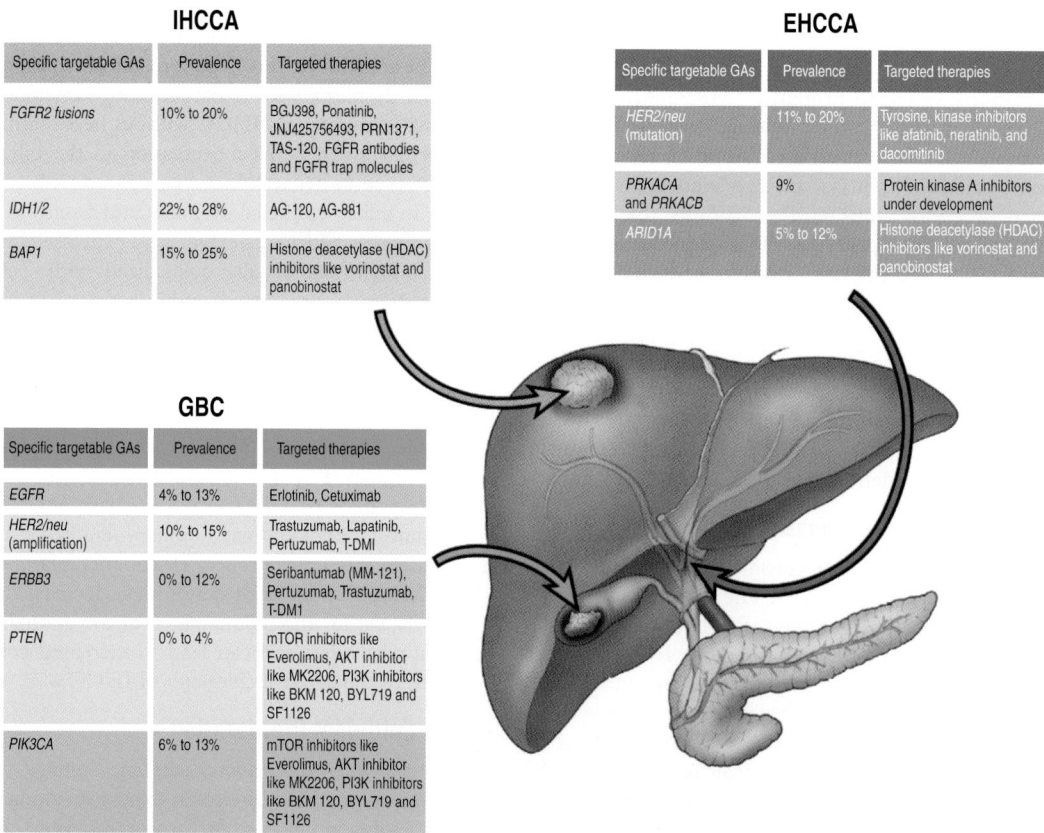

IHCCA

Specific targetable GAs	Prevalence	Targeted therapies
FGFR2 fusions	10% to 20%	BGJ398, Ponatinib, JNJ425756493, PRN1371, TAS-120, FGFR antibodies and FGFR trap molecules
IDH1/2	22% to 28%	AG-120, AG-881
BAP1	15% to 25%	Histone deacetylase (HDAC) inhibitors like vorinostat and panobinostat

EHCCA

Specific targetable GAs	Prevalence	Targeted therapies
HER2/neu (mutation)	11% to 20%	Tyrosine, kinase inhibitors like afatinib, neratinib, and dacomitinib
PRKACA and *PRKACB*	9%	Protein kinase A inhibitors under development
ARID1A	5% to 12%	Histone deacetylase (HDAC) inhibitors like vorinostat and panobinostat

GBC

Specific targetable GAs	Prevalence	Targeted therapies
EGFR	4% to 13%	Erlotinib, Cetuximab
HER2/neu (amplification)	10% to 15%	Trastuzumab, Lapatinib, Pertuzumab, T-DMI
ERBB3	0% to 12%	Seribantumab (MM-121), Pertuzumab, Trastuzumab, T-DM1
PTEN	0% to 4%	mTOR inhibitors like Everolimus, AKT inhibitor like MK2206, PI3K inhibitors like BKM 120, BYL719 and SF1126
PIK3CA	6% to 13%	mTOR inhibitors like Everolimus, AKT inhibitor like MK2206, PI3K inhibitors like BKM 120, BYL719 and SF1126

FIGURE 9E.2 **Molecular patterns of biliary tract cancers.** From Jain A, Javle M. Molecular profiling of biliary tract cancer: A target rich disease. *J Gastrointest Oncol.* 2016;7(5):797–803.

Pre–Next-Generation Sequencing

With the revolutionary changes that are occurring in genomics, the cost, sequencing time, and analysis time of NGS has significantly decreased during the past decade. Whole-exome sequencing (WES) and targeted sequencing of several hundred cancer-specific genes have provided significant insight and a deeper understanding of the oncogenes and tumor-suppressor genes involved in biliary tract carcinogenesis. In the era preceding NGS, several studies showed abnormal expression of the Kirsten rat sarcoma (KRAS) oncogene in 21% to 100% of cases, as well as alteration in the TP53 tumor suppressor gene in up to 37% of archival CCA specimens.[62] These genetic alterations were associated with a more aggressive phenotype in biliary tract tumors.[62] KRAS and TP53 mutations were also been identified in bile and pancreatic juice of affected patients,[62,63] but neither KRAS nor TP53 mutational analysis was shown to be superior to conventional cytopathology in the diagnosis of pancreaticobiliary tumors. However, combined pathologic analysis and mutation analysis increased diagnostic sensitivity.[62–64]

Next-Generation Sequencing in Biliary Tract Cancers

Compared with older studies, which relied on sequencing one gene a time, more recent studies have capitalized on NGS to narrowly or broadly characterize tumors. Although the biliary tract cancers were frequently grouped together by biologic, histologic, and clinical trial assignment, their somatic genomic landscapes are distinct from each other, suggesting that different treatment strategies are necessary for clinical trial design in each individual cancer. The first study to begin delineating these differences was reported by Borger and colleagues in 2012.[65] They studied 287 tumors from gastrointestinal cancer patients, including biliary tract, colorectal, gastroesophageal, hepatic, pancreatic, and small intestine carcinomas, and evaluated 15 known cancer genes for 130 site-specific gene mutations (Table 9E.1). Since this publication in 2012, several additional studies have been reported using WES analysis in biliary tract cancers. Study differences in alteration frequencies of each gene can be attributable to tissue sources (primary tumor or metastatic sites), sample size, depth of sequencing, and other factors. The most common genomic alterations are listed in Table 9E.2.

IDH1 and IDH2 Mutations

Combining several cohorts of biliary tract cancers, mutations in IDH1 and IDH2 were found in 15% to 29% and 3% to 6% of IHCC cases, respectively, whereas none or few were identified in EHCC or GBCA cases (see Chapters 9C and 50). Therefore IDH1 mutations were defined as a molecular feature of IHCC and also suggested as a potential therapeutic target specific to IHCC. IDH1 and IDH2 play roles in normal cellular metabolism and in conferring cellular protection against oxidative damage.[66] Mutant IDH blocks hepatocyte differentiation and promotes IHCC by cooperating with KRAS mutations.[67] In a multicenter randomized controlled study, the ClarIDHy study, a small molecule IDH inhibitor, ivosidenib, improved progression-free survival in CCA patients with mutant IDH1.[68] Also, preclinical studies have suggested that IDH1 mutations in other types of cancer confer sensitivity to PARP inhibitors[69–71] (see Chapter 9C).

FGFR2 Fusions

FGFR2 is a receptor tyrosine kinase (RTK), which plays an important role in cell differentiation, growth, and angiogenesis.[72] FGFR genomic alterations occur more frequently in IHCC

TABLE 9E.1 Most Common Somatic Mutations by Biliary Tract Tumor Subtype

	IHCC (N = 40)	EHCC (N = 22)	GBCA (N = 25)
AKT1	3%	0%	0%
APC	0%	0%	4%
BRAF	3%	0%	0%
CTNNB1	0%	0%	4%
IDH1	20%	0%	0%
IDH2	3%	0%	0%
KRAS	5%	23%	4%
NRAS	5%	0%	4%
PIK3CA	0%	0%	12%
PTEN	3%	0%	0%
TP53	5%	14%	4%

AKT1, v-AKT murine thymoma viral oncogene homolog 1; APC, adenomatosis polyposis coli; BRAF, B-Raf protooncogene; CTNNB1, β1-catenin; EHCC, extrahepatic cholangiocarcinoma; GBCA, gallbladder cancer; IDH1/2, isocitrate dehydrogenase 1/2; IHCC, intrahepatic cholangiocarcinoma; KRAS, Kirsten rat sarcoma; NRAS, neuroblastoma RAS viral (v-ras) oncogene homolog; PIK3CA, phosphatidylinositol-4,5-bisphosphate-3-kinase catalytic subunit alpha; PTEN, phosphatase and tensin; TP53, tumor protein 53.

From Borger DR, Tanabe KK, Fan KC, et al. Frequent mutation of isocitrate dehydrogenase (IDH)1 and IDH2 in cholangiocarcinoma identified through broad-based tumor genotyping. *Oncologist*. 2012;17:72–79.

TABLE 9E.2 Common Somatic Alterations by Biliary Tract Tumor Subtype

	IHCC	EHCC	GBCA
BAP1	10%-20%	0%-5%	2%
BRAF	3%-7%	0%	0%-6%
ERBB2	0%-4%	4%-7%	4%-16%
FGFR2	5%-50%	0%	
IDH1	15%-29%	0%-5%	0%
IDH2	3%-6%	0%	0%
KRAS	6%-25%	23%-38%	4%-13%
PIK3CA	0%-6%	0%	6%-12%
TP53	5%-18%	14%-49%	4%-47%

EHCC, Extrahepatic cholangiocarcinoma; GBCA, gallbladder cancer; IHCC, intrahepatic cholangiocarcinoma.

patients of younger age (≤40 years), earlier cancer stage presentation (TNM stage I/II), and Caucasian race.[73] FGFR2 alterations, mostly fusions, are seen in 5% to 50% of IHCC and these FGFR2 activating alterations confer sensitivity to FGFR inhibitors (e.g., erdafitinib and pemigatinib).[74] Clinical trials have demonstrated the meaningful antitumor activity and better overall survival time of FGFR inhibitors in IHCC harboring fusions[75–77] (see Chapters 9C and 50).

ERBB Family

ERBB2 (as also known as HER2/neu) is a member of the ERBB family in the same capacity as EGFR and has been already well-established in many types of cancer. Amplification or overexpression of ERBB2 leads to tumor proliferation and oncogenesis of CCA cells. Amplification and mutation of ERBB2 more frequently occurs in GBCA and EHCC than IHCC.[78] *ERBB2* amplification and activating mutations may confer sensitivity to ERRB2-targeted drugs, which are now being evaluated in ERBB2-altered biliary tract cancers. According to data from the pre-NGS era, overexpression of EGFR can be seen in 11% to 27% of IHCC cases and 5% to 19% of EHCC cases.[79,80] A subgroup analysis of the randomized controlled study evaluating the additional efficacy of an anti-EGFR small molecule inhibitor to chemotherapy indicated a longer progression-free survival in patients with CCA.[81]

Other Targetable Genomic Alterations

Alterations in DNA repair or homologous recombinant gene are targetable with drugs that are associated with DNA repair mechanisms. For instance, the *BAP1* (BRCA1 associated protein-1) gene encodes an enzyme regulating the ubiquitin-proteasome protein degradation pathway and acts as a tumor suppressor gene. Inactivation of this gene leads to carcinogenesis, whereas germline *BAP1* inactivation increases susceptibility to several malignancies, including CCA.[82] *BAP1* mutations are seen in 10% to 20% of IHCC cases and 0% to 5% of EHCC/GBCA cases. Clinical and preclinical studies suggest that *BAP1*-mutation can be a target from EZH2 inhibitors, PARP inhibitors, and HDAC inhibitors.

NTRK fusions are also known drivers of oncogenesis by activating the downstream effectors, including the MAPK and PI3K/AKT pathways.[83] Although this alteration is exceedingly rare in biliary tract cancers, the antitumor activity of NTRK inhibitors is remarkable. Clinical trials demonstrating the efficacy of NTRK inhibitors (i.e., larotrectinib and entrectinib) for patients with *NTRK* fusions included a few patients with CCA, who all responded, and their responses were often long-lasting.[84,85] A nonrandomized study demonstrated that molecularly matched therapeutic regimens based on NGS genomic profiling was significantly associated with longer progression-free survival and higher disease control rate than regimens unmatched to genomic alterations (mostly gemcitabine-based regimens) in advanced biliary tract cancers (Okamura R, Kurzrock R, Mallory RJ, et al. Comprehensive genomic landscape and precision therapeutic approach in biliary tract cancers. *Int J Cancer.* 2021;148(3):702-712. doi:10.1002/ijc.33230).

Epigenetic Alterations

Many human cancers have aberrant epigenetic alterations. Epigenetic mechanisms involved in gene regulation include DNA methylation, histone modification, and noncoding RNAs. Studies defining the role of these epigenetic alterations in the tumorigenesis of biliary tract cancers have emerged. Aberrant promoter hypermethylation of specific genes, such as cell-cycle associated and DNA repair genes, is associated with tumor progression and metastasis in CCA. Point mutation in CpG islands of the cell-cycle regulator, P16INK4A, result in inactivation of the gene and lead to the proliferation or vascular invasion of CCA cell.[86] Inactivation of the *MLH1* gene, a DNA mismatch repair gene, contributes to the tumorigenesis of CCA.[87] The DNA mismatch repair deficiency is a major molecular pathway of genetic instability in cancer. High microsatellite instability (MSI-High) is one of the most predictive biomarkers of responsiveness toward immune checkpoint blockade. Furthermore, promoter hypermethylation of SOCS-3 (regulator of glucose transport), which is implicated in IL-6/signal-transducer and

activator of transcription 3 (STAT3) activation, has been noted in 27% of CCA cells. Other relevant aberrantly methylated genes include runt-related transcription factor 3 *(RUNX3)*, which is altered in 42% of IHCC tumors, and p14ARF, which prevents *TP53* degradation and hence cell-cycle arrest, has been reported as altered in 18% of tumors.[20] Histone methylation can also result in transcriptional activation, although it depends on the type of amino acid and its position in the histone tail.[88] Histone deacetylase (HDAC) regulates cell cycle progression and differentiation, and its overexpression in CCA is associated with the malignant behavior and poorer disease-free survival in CCA.[89] The inhibition of HDAC suppresses the tumor growth in CCA cells.[90] Noncoding RNAs also regulate the tumorigenesis in CCA and may be important targets for cancer therapy. A long, noncoding RNA (lncRNA), actin filament associated protein 1 antisense RNA1 (AFAP1-AS1), is reported to promote the tumor growth and metastasis of CCA cells in vivo.[91] The BRCA-1 associated protein-1 (BAP1) is a chromatin modulator, and BAP1-dependent expression of lncRNA, nuclear paraspeckle assembly transcript 1 (NEAT-1), modulates sensitivity to gemcitabine in CCA.[92] Targeting these epigenetic alterations by specific inhibitors may be a promising treatment option in CCA.

microRNA Alterations

Emerging evidence has recently suggested that the expression of noncoding RNAs, such as microRNAs (miRs), is important in carcinogenesis because they can modulate the expression of many genes that regulate critical properties, such as cell survival, autophagy, stemness, and response to therapy. As a result, miRs have been linked to tumor heterogeneity, as well as significant determinants of genomics-based patient stratification. Several miRs are reported to promote the tumorigenesis of cholangiocarcinoma (e.g., miR-21, miR-155) and to suppress the tumor development. For instance, the increased expression of miR-21 is associated with the tumor growth and metastasis of CCA and modulates chemotherapy-induced apoptosis by regulating PTEN-dependent activation of phosphatidylinositol-3-kinase (PI3K) signaling pathway.[93] MiR-1249 expression is increased in biliary tract cancers and mediates chemotherapy resistant, by regulating the clonal expansion of CD133+ cells.[94] Also, the expression of miR-24 leads to the decrease of a tumor suppressor gene *MEN1*, and miR-24 inhibition possibly attenuates the tumor progression of CCA.[95] miRs are promising as biomarkers for predicting survival and treatment response.

Tumor Growth and Metastasis
Dysregulated Signaling Pathways

The progression and metastasis of biliary tract tumors appear to be driven by a variety of cellular signaling pathways involved in responses to embryonic/stem cell signaling pathways (e.g., Hh, WNT, NOTCH, HIPPO), growth factors (e.g., EGF, FGF, HGF/ mesenchymal-to-epithelial transitions [MET], VEGF), intracellular signal transduction (e.g., KRAS/RAF/MEK/ERK), cytokine signaling (e.g., IL-6/STAT), and cell-cycle progression (e.g., polo-like kinases [PLKs]).[2]

Embryonic Signaling

It is increasingly recognized that embryonic signaling pathways are important in the carcinogenesis of numerous types of cancer. The Hedgehog (Hh), Wnt/β-catenin, NOTCH, and HIPPO signaling pathways are important regulators of proliferation, survival, self-renewal, and development in embryos and cancers in adults (see Chapter 1). The Hh pathway was initially reported be overexpressed in CCA.[96] Hh has been also shown to regulate tumor-stromal interactions in the liver that stimulate the proliferation, migration, and invasion of CCA cells.[97] Hh also directly regulates the viability of CCA.[98] Similarly, the NOTCH pathway has been shown to regulate cell proliferation, apoptosis, migration, invasion, and epithelial-mesenchymal transition (EMT) while working in concert with TP53 to regulate cell viability.[99] Aberrant expression of NOTCH receptors 1 and 3 play a role during cancer progression, and the NOTCH pathway protein DLL4 correlates with poor survival in EHCC and GBCA.[100] Multiple studies have suggested that the Wnt/β-catenin pathway also plays the key role in progression of CCA cells, although genomic mutations in genes, including adenomatosis polyposis coli (APC), are rare. Finally, the HIPPO signaling pathway regulates proliferation and apoptosis of cholangiocarcinoma cells via the yes-associated protein 1 (YAP1) and also promotes angiogenesis by regulating the expression of secreted pro-angiogenic proteins.[101,102] Nuclear YAP expression was shown to represent a biomarker of response to FGFR-directed therapy.[103] Overall, these developmental signaling pathways appear to be important in disease progression, whereas cross talk between these pathways needs further investigation.

Growth Factor Receptor

FGFR2 gene fusions are found in 9% to 25% of IHCC and promote cell proliferation, survival, and apoptosis of cancer cells. FGFR inhibitors for CCA with *FGFR* fusions have already been approved by the US Food and Drug Administration (FDA; see Chapters 9C and 50). Overexpression of EGFR occurs in 10% to 32% of CCAs, although somatic mutations in EGFR family members are rare. Furthermore, aberrant phosphorylation of EGFR activates MAPK, and p38 signaling can increase cyclooxygenase-2 (COX-2). In turn, this can inhibit apoptosis while enhancing tumor growth. However, although in vitro EGFR inhibition with erlotinib has shown cell proliferation of CCA cells, in vivo dual blockage of EGFR and ERBB1/ERBB2 with lapatinib is necessary. The hepatocyte growth factor (HGF)/MET pathway is rarely mutated in biliary tract tumors, but amplification of MET, the HGF receptor, has been reported in IHCC. In turn, HGF/MET can activate many pathways, including MAPK, PI3K, and STAT, and can stimulate migration and invasion in CCA cells. VEGF is a signal protein produced by cells that stimulates angiogenesis. Alterations occur in almost half of IHCCs and correlate with a poor prognosis. Although the application of targeted therapies such as sorafenib, which targets wild-type BRAF and vascular endothelial growth factor receptor (VEGFR), has been studied, the preclinical data have been disappointing in CCA models.

IL-6/JAK/STAT Cytokine Signaling

IL-6 is an inflammatory cytokine and mediates JAK/STAT activation, which modulates cell growth and survival of CCA cells.[104] The overexpression of IL-6 may result from epigenetic silencing of SOCS-3 in CCA cells.[105] Binding of IL-6 to its receptor (gp130) results in heterodimerization with the Janus kinases (JAK1, JAK2, or TYK2). In turn, this drives activation of STAT3 (i.e., the JAK/STAT pathway) and/or the MAPK pathway. NOTCH and JAK-STAT signaling cross-talk during RAS-induced CCA. A preclinical study suggested that combined

inhibition of the two pathways can prevent RAS-induced lineage conversion from hepatocytes to CCA.[106]

Polo-Like Kinases

The Polo-like kinases (PLKs) are a family of serine/threonine kinases involved in key regulatory processes, including cell-cycle progression (G2/M transition) and cytokinesis. Targeting PLK-1 has been shown to increase the efficacy of 5-fluorouracil,[107] whereas PLK-2 is a mediator of Hh signaling in CCA.[108] A preclinical study showed that inhibition of PLK can sensitize CCA cells to cisplatin-induced apoptosis with proteasomal Bcl-2 degradation.[109]

Epithelial-to-Mesenchymal Transition

EMT, MET, and, epithelial-mesenchymal interactions (EMI) are often lumped together under the term EMT.[110] In the former phenomenon, however, epithelial cells lose their polarity and cell-cell adhesion while gaining migratory and invasive properties to become mesenchymal. This is thought to be involved in the initiation of metastasis. TGF-β1, an EMT-related protein, is highly expressed in CCA. A previous study indicates that the high TGF-β1 levels correlate with cancer metastasis and survival in patients with CCA.[111] Also, Snail and β-catenin regulate EMT in CCA, and overexpression is found in about 50% of IHCCs.[112]

Tumor-Stromal Interactions

Hepatic stellate cells (HSCs) are stromal cells in benign hepatic parenchyma that possess both neural and myofibroblastic features (see Chapter 7). HSCs are the major cell type involved in hepatic fibrosis and cirrhosis. In addition, portal myofibroblasts can contribute to hepatic fibrosis. The tumor-stromal microenvironment is a key component of the development and progression of CCA. Several pathways appear to regulate this process. For instance, the Hh pathway regulates HSC.[113] In turn, HSCs stimulate the proliferation, migration, and invasion of CCA cells and also promote angiogenesis through Hh pathway activation. This renders CCA cells more susceptible to necrosis by Hh inhibition.[97] Moreover, myofibroblast-derived platelet-derived growth factor-BB protects CCA cells from TRAIL (TNF-α–related apoptosis-inducing ligand) cytotoxicity by a Hh-dependent process.[114] Finally, expression of the Hh target gene osteopontin is an independent predictor of survival in IHCC patients.[115] In addition, other mechanisms activate tumor-associated angiogenesis and lymphangiogenesis. CCA cells have an interaction with vascular endothelial cells via VEGFR2-VEGFA, which leads to tumor angiogenesis via upregulation of the PI3K/AKT pathway.[116,117] Cancer-associated fibroblasts upregulate the ERK/JNK pathway and stimulate lymphatic endothelial cells via VEGFR3 engagement. That promotes lymphangiogenesis and tumor cell intravasation in CCA.[118]

SUMMARY

In the last decade, we have gained significant insight into the environmental risk factors, genomic alterations, tumor heterogeneity, and epithelial-mesenchymal interaction/transitions associated with the development of biliary tract adenocarcinomas. We are gaining a more comprehensive understanding of the molecular pathogenesis of CCA, which relies on the underlying themes of chronic inflammation to the biliary epithelium, host-mediated response, and subsequent development of the malignant phenotype. Many new candidates for targeted therapy based on molecular profiling have emerged, including the MET, EGFR, ERBB2, FGFR, JAK/STAT, RAS/RAF/MAPK, PI3K/AKT/mTOR, Wnt/Hh/Notch/Hippo, and IDH pathways. Data have also emerged on the role of epigenetics and miRs, providing the potential for further studies in these areas. Identifying and cataloging somatic alterations and associating these alterations with clinical outcomes may assist in the development of novel therapeutic interventions, enhance early diagnosis, identify at-risk individuals, and ultimately improve survival.

The references for this chapter can be found online by accessing the accompanying Expert Consult website.

CHAPTER 10

Fundamentals of liver and pancreas immunology

Yongwoo David Seo, Ian Nicholas Crispe, and Venu G. Pillarisetty

INTRODUCTION

The immune system manifests two strategies of host defense termed *innate* and *adaptive* immunity (Fig. 10.1).[1] Innate immunity refers to the nonspecific first line of defense against danger signals from pathogens or tumor cells. The repertoire of innate immune cells includes natural killer (NK) cells, macrophages, and dendritic cells (DCs). Innate immune cells sense both tissue injury and pathogens through pattern recognition receptors (PRRs) that trigger a rapid response. PRRs bind to well-conserved molecules from microbes, including lipopolysaccharide, other bacterial cell wall moieties, and pathogen nucleic acids. PRR signaling and the ensuing response may lead to destruction of the invading pathogen or tumor via phagocytosis or release of various cytotoxic or inflammatory agents. Innate immunity may also activate antigen-presenting cells (APCs), leading to the activation of T and B cells and leading to adaptive immunity, and such crosstalk bridges the nonspecific initial response to a highly specialized system capable of long-lasting immunologic memory.

Adaptive immunity involves antigen-specific responses, which occur de novo during an initial immune response or rapidly upon repeat exposure to a particular pathogen. The adaptive immune system comprises T and B lymphocytes that circulate within the blood, lymphatic tissues, and nonlymphoid organs, including the liver. T and B cells express specific cell-surface receptors capable of recognizing particular antigens. T-cell activation requires presentation of antigen by APCs such as DCs. APCs mediate antigen presentation to T cells within the context of major histocompatibility complex molecules (MHC I or MHC II). In addition, APCs provide a critical "second signal" through co-stimulatory molecules, and the response is further modulated by secreted cytokines (Fig. 10.2). Classically, CD4+ helper T cells recognize antigen in the context of MHC II, whereas CD8+ cytotoxic T cells engage antigen loaded onto MHC I molecules. Several subsets of CD4+ cells (T helper, or Th cells) orchestrate and polarize the immune response to address particular challenges.

Although activation of innate and adaptive immunity is essential for combating pathogens and malignant cells, overly exuberant immune responses can result in severe tissue damage. The immune system is normally able to distinguish self from nonself and is controlled by numerous regulatory mechanisms. During T-cell development, autoreactive cells are deleted through negative selection in the thymus. Regulatory T cells (Tregs) and myeloid-derived suppressor cells (MDSCs) regulate immune responses in the periphery and prevent autoimmunity. Immunoinhibitory receptors, including programmed death-1 (PD-1) and cytotoxic T-lymphocyte–associated protein 4 (CTLA-4), modulate T-cell function, working in concert with suppressor cells to regulate immune responses. As will be discussed later, Tregs, MDSCs, and immunoinhibitory pathways in the liver cooperate to create a highly tolerogenic milieu. Intrahepatic tolerance is a fundamental aspect of liver immunology that reflects its position at the interface between ingested exogenous antigens and the systemic circulation.

The balance between tolerance and immunity in the liver is tightly regulated by intrahepatic immune cells and associated signaling pathways. Several features of liver immunology point to the skewing of this balance toward tolerance under normal physiologic conditions. First, the fact that the liver is one of the most common sites for metastatic disease suggests that malignant cells are able to exploit intrahepatic immunosuppression. Second, compared with other solid organ transplants, liver allografts do not require immunosuppression in certain strains of mice and require less immunosuppression in humans. Third, the immune system is often unable to clear chronic hepatitis B and C viral infections. Additionally, oral ingestion or portal vein injection of foreign proteins can lead to tolerance in animal models. Conversely, the liver is the site of several autoimmune processes, including primary sclerosing cholangitis and primary biliary cirrhosis. Despite the prominent role that the intrahepatic immune system plays in disease, the study of liver immunology remains underdeveloped.

On the other hand, in a normal physiologic state, the pancreas does not appear to have a major impact on the overall immune response. However, malignancies of the pancreas such as ductal adenocarcinoma demonstrate significant immune evasion, which pose unique therapeutic challenges. Here, we review our current understanding of liver and pancreatic immunology and the complex interplay of cells and cytokines therein.

Anatomic Considerations in Liver Immunology

Because the vascular supply of the liver derives principally from the portal venous system draining the gut, a heavy antigen load is delivered to the liver. Portal venous blood flows slowly through the vast network of hepatic sinusoids, which are discontinuously lined by fenestrated endothelium lacking a basement membrane (Fig. 10.3; see Chapters 2 and 5). The sluggish flow of blood allows for the efficient capture of antigens by leukocytes traveling in the blood within the sinusoids and by the endothelial cells lining the sinusoids. The liver reticuloendothelial system, comprising liver sinusoidal endothelial cells (LSECs) and Kupffer cells (KCs), is very efficient at extracting antigens from portal blood. LSECs capture and process antigen at levels comparable to professional APCs, such as DCs.[2] The microscopic anatomy of the liver also favors the ability of bloodborne leukocytes to interact with hepatic parenchymal cells and resident immune cells of the liver. The microanatomic and rheologic features of the hepatic sinusoids facilitate highly efficient antigen presentation and interactions among immune cells.

Tolerance and Immunosuppression

From a teleologic perspective, tolerance to oral antigens is clearly advantageous. In experimental animal models and clinical liver transplantation studies, a greater propensity for graft acceptance

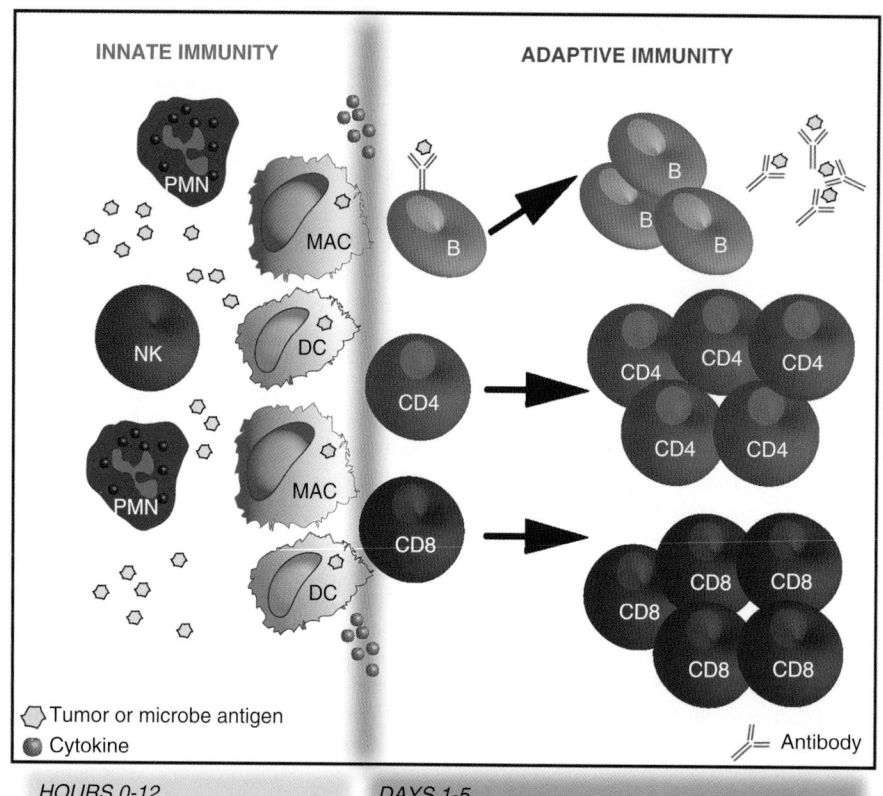

FIGURE 10.1   Innate and adaptive immunity. A, *Innate immunity* includes the body's initial defenses against infection. It includes certain complement proteins, epithelial barriers, natural killer *(NK)* cells, neutrophils (polymorphonuclear *[PMN]*), phagocytes such as macrophages *(MACs)*, and antigen-presenting cells such as dendritic cells *(DCs)*. Innate immune cells may directly kill tumor or infected cells, and then present antigen to adaptive immune cells. **B,** In contrast, *adaptive immunity* refers to the precisely targeted immune mechanisms that occur later in the immune response. The adaptive immune system has B-cell–mediated humoral (dissolved) and T-cell–mediated cellular components. The innate and adaptive immune systems overlap extensively, communicating by direct cellular contact or cytokine secretion. B-cell secretion of antibodies functions to block infections and trigger the destruction of pathogenic organisms. T-cell–mediated immunity occurs after antigen presentation and leads to direct cellular lysis by CD8 T cells with support from the CD4 arm.

has been noted compared with transplantation of other solid organs. A liver transplant protects a kidney allograft transplanted simultaneously from the same donor.[3] Unfortunately, primary and metastatic tumors in the liver exploit intrahepatic immunosuppression to evade destruction by the immune system. A deeper understanding of liver tolerance may support therapeutic interventions to stimulate immunity for cancer or control liver immune cell function for inflammatory conditions.

LIVER IMMUNE CELLS

Among the liver's nonparenchymal cells (NPCs), one quarter are leukocytes. The composition of the intrahepatic leukocyte population is markedly different from that seen in other organs. The liver contains most of the cellular components of innate and adaptive immunity. Importantly, liver immune cells demonstrate unique functional properties that tend to promote a tolerogenic milieu.

Antigen-Presenting Cells

Experimental and clinical observations that antigens passing through the liver can lead to tolerance make the understanding of intrahepatic antigen presentation particularly relevant.[4] APCs play a crucial role in driving adaptive immune responses

and bridging innate to adaptive immunity. DCs, LSECs, KCs, and B cells all play a role in antigen presentation within the liver. The context in which an APC presents an antigen can dramatically alter the response of antigen-specific T cells. Specifically, when antigen presentation occurs in conjunction with the appropriate co-stimulatory molecules, T cells proliferate and develop an immunogenic phenotypic and functional profile (Fig. 10.4). In contrast, antigens presented in the absence of co-stimulation or presence of immunoinhibitory signals lead to anergy or activation-induced T-cell death, two of the mechanisms of peripheral tolerance induction and maintenance.

Dendritic Cells

DCs are a heterogeneous population of leukocytes primarily responsible for the capture of antigens in the periphery and subsequent presentation to immune effector cells. DCs are the most potent APCs of the immune system. Immature DCs are specialized to capture antigens and then migrate to lymph nodes, where they can interact with T cells. After an encounter with a pathogenic stimulus, such as bacterial lipopolysaccharide, DCs undergo phenotypic and functional changes, whereby their ability to capture antigens is diminished, but they increase their expression of class II and T-cell co-stimulatory molecules. Co-stimulatory molecule expression is essential in facilitating

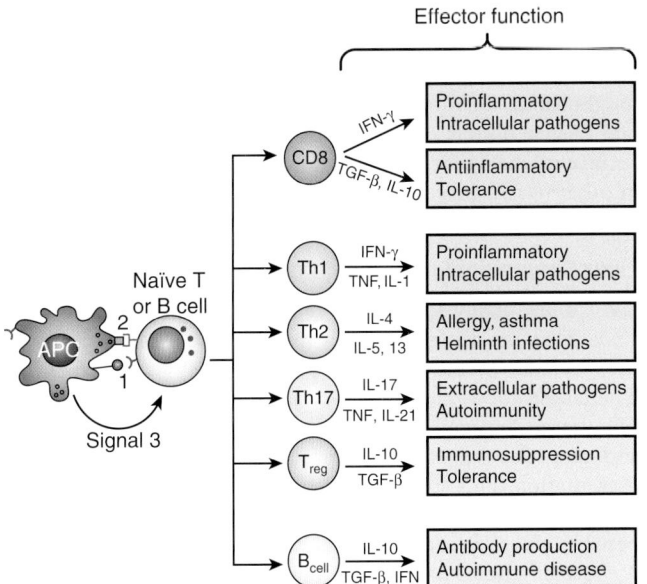

FIGURE 10.2 **Antigen-presenting cell (APC) instruction of T and B cells.** Signals 1 (antigen presentation), 2 (co-stimulation), and 3 (cytokine production) between APCs and naïve T or B cells govern the subsequent adaptive immune response. Naïve CD4[+] T cells can differentiate into four types of T cells—Th1, Th2, Th17, and Treg—each with a distinct cytokine profile and specific effector function. In turn, programmed CD4[+] T cells modulate CD8[+] T cells that can differentiate into either cytotoxic or regulatory cells capable of killing foreign pathogens or suppressing immune responses, respectively. B cells can also differentiate into cytokine and antibody-producing cells, which play a role in responses against tumors, pathogens, and autoimmune diseases. *APCs,* Antigen-presenting cells; *IFN-γ,* interferon-γ; *IL,* interleukin; *TGF-β,* transforming growth factor-β; *TNF,* tumor necrosis factor.

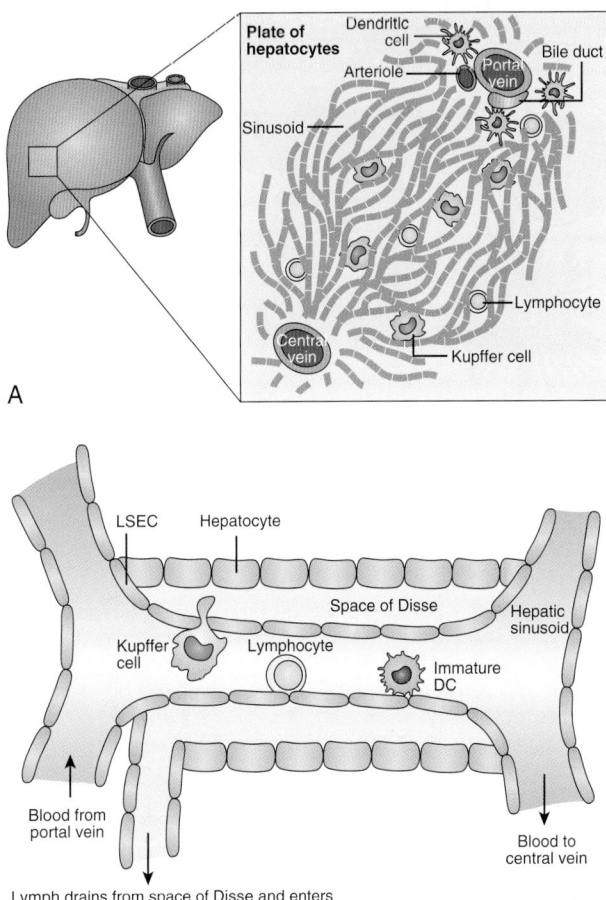

A

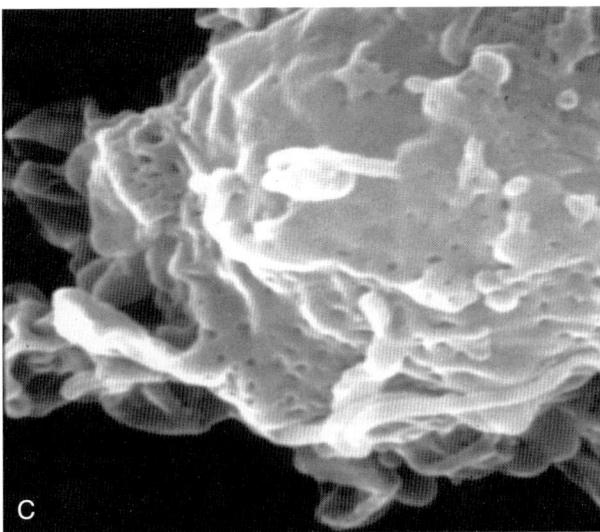

B

Lymph drains from space of Disse and enters lymphatic capillaries in the portal area

antigen presentation and efficient T-cell activation. Inflammatory conditions often promote a process of maturation, whereby DCs increase expression of MHC and co-stimulatory molecules, enabling efficient antigen presentation and T-cell activation. However, liver DC phenotype and function is somewhat unique, as we discuss later.

When compared with DCs from the spleen, CD11c[+] liver DCs were immature and only weakly immunostimulatory.[5] In contrast to spleen DCs, liver DCs were heterogeneous in their expression of MHC class II and co-stimulatory molecules. Myeloid (CD11b[+]) and lymphoid (CD8α[+]) liver DCs, which each comprise approximately 10% of the total population of DCs in the liver, were as able to activate T cells as their splenic counterparts were. The bulk of the remaining cells, which had low-to-no expression of CD11b and CD8α, were poor T-cell stimulators. The presence of these atypical DCs accounted for the weakly activating nature of liver DCs on the whole. More recently, using a transgenic mouse in which CD11c[hi] DCs can be depleted selectively, we found that activation of antigen-specific CD8[+] T cells in the liver only occurred in the presence of CD11c[hi] DCs.[6]

As in the mouse, freshly isolated DCs from human liver exhibit tolerogenic properties when compared with autologous blood DCs. Human liver DCs are weaker stimulators of T cells and produce the antiinflammatory cytokine interleukin-10 (IL-10), which induces the differentiation of naïve CD4[+] T cells into regulatory T cells with suppressive function.[7]

C

FIGURE 10.3 **Microvascular hepatic anatomy.** **A,** The liver is organized as lobules defined by their relation to portal vascular bundles and central veins. **B,** Liver sinusoidal endothelial cells (LSECs) line the hepatic sinusoids and have fenestrated membranes. A variety of immune cells exist within the sinusoids and are able to traverse the sinusoidal membrane to enter and exit the space of Disse, which is in contact with hepatocytes (From Crispe IN. Hepatic T cells and liver tolerance, *Nat Rev Immunol.* 2003;3:51–62.) **C,** Scanning electron micrograph of LSEC (×20,000) demonstrated the classic fenestrated cell membrane. (From Katz SC. Liver sinusoidal endothelial cells are insufficient to activate T cells. *J Immunol.* 2004;173:230–235.)

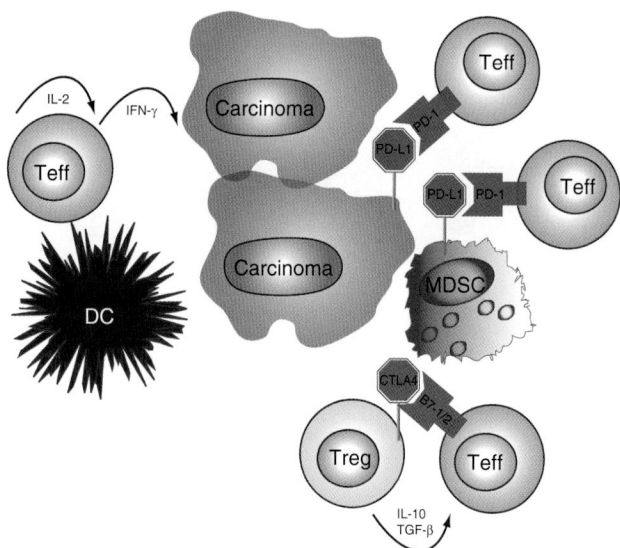

FIGURE 10.4   Context of antigen presentation determines T-cell activation status. The three main APCs are dendritic cells (DCs), macrophages, and B cells. The immune response depends on the context in which antigens are presented to T cells. The type of APC and the presence or absence of co-stimulatory molecules are important in determining whether a T cell has no response (anergy) or is activated. Presentation of antigen by an APC to a T cell typically result in triggering of an adaptive immune response *(left)*, unless suppressor cells or immunoinhibitory signals intervene *(right)*. *APC,* Antigen-presenting cell; *IFN,* interferon; *IL,* interleukin; *MDSC,* myeloid-derived suppressor cells; *PD-L1,* programmed death ligand-1; *Teff,* effector T cell; *TGF-β,* transforming growth factor-β; *Treg,* regulatory T cells. (From Khan H, et al: The prognostic value of liver tumor T cell infiltrates, *J Surg Res* 191:189–195, 2014.)

Kupffer Cells

Liver macrophages, referred to as *Kupffer cells,* are the primary phagocytic cells of the liver (see Chapter 7). KCs represent the largest pool of macrophages in the body, derived in part from monocytic precursors in the blood and partly from fetal precursors that seed the liver early and maintain themselves by cell division in situ. They are typically found in the hepatic sinusoids; however, they also can migrate through the space of Disse to interact with hepatocytes (see Fig. 10.3). KCs play a major role in antigen presentation and have been implicated in portal venous tolerance, possibly by regulating T-cell responses to antigens in the context of immune tolerance to liver allografts.[8] On the other hand, more recent murine model work has demonstrated the ability of KCs within the sinusoids to effect CD8 T-cell activation to antigens in an intercellular adhesion molecule-1 dependent manner.[9]

Multiple lines of evidence from flow cytometry, lineage-tracing, and single-cell RNA sequencing suggest that KCs consist of two subsets. In the mouse, there is clear evidence that one subset derives from precursors in the yolk sac and/or the fetal liver and maintains itself locally for the life of the animal. These cells express more molecules linked to endocytosis and to immune tolerance, which the alternative subset of KCs derives from blood monocytes, and are increased in abundance during emergency repopulation of the liver. Recent evidence has shown that embryo-derived KCs remain resistant to irradiation via upregulation of a kinase inhibitor Cdkn1a, which may have implications in understanding radiation-induced liver

diseases.[10] In humans, lineage-tracing experiments are not possible, but genes expressed by two clusters of macrophage-like cells identified on the basis of differential gene expression argue for the same dichotomy. The distinction between KC subsets and DCs in human liver is complicated by the concern that cell surface markers that clearly distinguish macrophages from DCs in other tissues may not be absolute among liver myeloid cells, and this remains an active area of investigation.

Liver Sinusoidal Endothelial Cells

LSECs are highly specialized cells that line the hepatic sinusoids. They are distinguished by the presence of fenestrations in their cellular membranes (see Fig 10.3; see also Chapter 7). The fenestrations are believed to facilitate the selective passage of antigens between the sinusoid and the hepatic parenchyma and may also increase the surface area available for antigen presentation. This strategic placement puts LSECs in the ideal position to interact with antigens and immune cells passing between the liver and the portal venous system.

Several studies have shown that, in addition to serving as a structural component of the hepatic sinusoids, LSECs are immune cells with the ability to capture and present antigen to T cells.[11] As with KCs, considerable controversy surrounds the immunologic function of LSECs. In contrast to earlier work, we have shown that although LSECs are highly capable of capturing various antigens in vivo and in vitro, they lack the ability to activate T cells in the absence of exogenous co-stimulation.[2] The differences in results may derive from the use of more specific methods of cell isolation in the latter study. The finding that LSECs are not independently capable of triggering a T-cell–mediated immune response does not, however, exclude the possibility that LSECs, in concert with DCs or KCs, play an important role in antigen presentation in the liver.

Effector Cells

T Cells

Like other liver immune cell populations, intrahepatic T cells have unique properties enabling them to contribute to maintenance of a tolerogenic milieu. T cells are a heterogeneous population of adaptive immune cells with both effector and suppressor subtypes. CD4+ helper T cells orchestrate immune responses, CD8+ cytotoxic T cells destroy infected host or malignant cells, and Tregs play an immunomodulatory role. The liver also contains multiple nonclassical T-cell subsets, including NKT cells and γδ T cells. The nature of the interactions between APCs and T cells polarizes T-cell differentiation and thus determines the outcome of a particular immune response.

The liver contains a full complement of T-cell subsets, although the relative proportions of each population are different when compared with lymphoid organs. Conventional or classical T cells express the αβ T-cell receptor in association with either CD4 or CD8. These are the most prevalent T cells in the body and account for about one third of the murine liver T-cell population. In contrast, unconventional T cells expressing NK markers or the γδ T-cell receptor comprise a greater proportion of liver T cells, approximately 50% and 10%, respectively. Immunosuppressive Tregs expressing FOXP3 are heavily represented in the liver. Among the classical T cells, the liver also contains *Th17 cells,* which are capable of producing the highly inflammatory cytokine IL-17. Th17 cells play an important role in the promotion of inflammatory and fibrotic disorders affecting the liver.

The diversity of conventional T cells is based on their recognition of specific peptide antigen motifs within the context of MHC class I or II molecules expressed by APCs. The αβ T-cell receptor is highly variable, and numerous T cells, each recognizing a different antigen presented by APCs, are present in the immune system. CD8$^+$ T cells respond to peptides presented on MHC class I molecules, which are expressed by nearly every cell in the body, excluding erythrocytes. Activated CD8$^+$ T cells become cytotoxic T lymphocytes. CD4$^+$ helper T cells recognize antigens presented on MHC class II molecules on the surface of professional APCs. CD4$^+$ T-cell subsets, Th1 and Th2 cells, then regulate and amplify the immune response by secreting cytokines, which affect nearby effector cells.

γδ T Cells

The γδ T-cell receptor is relatively invariant and can recognize multiple nonpeptide antigens without the need for MHC presentation. γδ T cells represent 10% of liver T cells, whereas they comprise only a small proportion (<5%) of T cells in the blood or lymphoid organs. γδ T cells also are abundant at other environmental interfaces, including the skin and mucosal surfaces. Through secretion of activating and modulatory cytokines, γδ T cells help orchestrate early responses to atypical bacterial and viral pathogens. γδ T cells can also promote antitumor immunity through their early secretion of interferon-γ (IFN-γ).[12] Conversely this cell type has immunosuppressive properties as well.[13] The high proportion of γδ T cells in the liver suggests that they have an important immunologic role, but further investigation is required. As with most lymphocyte populations, heterogeneity among liver γδ T cells precludes simple generalizations concerning their functions.

Natural Killer T Cells

NKT cells share characteristics of conventional T cells and NK cells and are defined by the presence of several T cell and NK cell surface markers. Most NKT cells react against glycolipid antigens in the context of CD1d, which is an MHC class I–like glycoprotein. CD1d is expressed on APCs and hepatocytes. NKTs express invariant T-cell receptor chains that are conserved across species, suggesting an important role for NKT cells in the innate immune response to pathogens. Activated NKT cells are capable of producing IFN-γ and IL-4, which are the prototypical Th1 and Th2 cytokines, respectively.

NKT cells constitute a relatively large proportion of T cells found in the liver compared with other organs. In addition, a local expansion of NKT cells is seen in several models of liver injury, such as partial hepatectomy. NKT cells play a role in inflammatory diseases and in clearance of infection from the liver. Depletion of NKT cells abrogated the effects of experimentally induced hepatitis in a mouse model, and mice lacking NKT cells are susceptible to viral and bacterial infections. NKT cells also play a part in tumor surveillance in the liver. In murine primary and metastatic tumor models, NKT cells can mediate tumor rejection, in part because of their ability to secrete IFN-γ.[14] Work in other murine models suggests that liver NKTs have the capacity to suppress T-cell proliferation and hence contribute to immunosuppression in the liver.[13]

Natural Killer Cells

NK cells are innate responders and, unlike T cells, do not possess receptors for specific peptide antigens. By expressing a variety of activating and inhibitory receptors, NK cells can bind ligands on their target cells. The resulting activation of NK cells causes the release of lytic granules, or cytokines such as IFN-γ, which kill the infected host or tumor cell in an MHC-unrestricted fashion. NK cells are a major component of murine and human liver lymphocytes and mediate inflammatory reactions seen in viral and autoimmune hepatitis. Bulk human liver NK cells possess weaker lytic capabilities when compared with autologous blood NK cells[15] because the liver has a greater proportion of NK cell subtypes with weaker cytolytic function when compared with blood NK cells.

B Cells

B cells mediate adaptive immune responses, delivering humoral immunity through antibody production. B cells may also function as APCs. Although hepatic B cells have received very little attention, they make up a significant proportion of liver lymphocytes. They play prominent roles in viral and autoimmune disease affecting the liver.[16] MDSCs in the liver suppress hepatic B cells through downregulation of CD80, which is a co-stimulatory molecule involved in T-cell activation.[17] This may be a mechanism through which hepatic B-cell function is altered to contribute toward intrahepatic tolerance.

OVERVIEW OF PANCREATIC IMMUNOLOGY

The immune milieu of the exocrine pancreas is less exhaustively studied than that of the liver, and there is a less conspicuous immune cell compartment in the absence of disease. Besides lacking the richness of antigen-presenting cells and specialized cell types, such as the sinusoidal endothelial cells, many conditions such as pancreatic adenocarcinoma have been characterized by a dense stromal fibrosis, which was initially thought to exclude components of the effector cells from the peritumoral area.[18] However, more recent work has highlighted a nuanced view of the balance of T-cell activation and immunosuppressive elements within the pancreas, which will be highlighted in subsequent sections.

Immunoinhibitory Pathways of the Liver and Pancreas

Suppressive or co-inhibitory signaling pathways are important mediators of tolerance and immune evasion within both the liver and pancreas. The immunoinhibitory receptors receiving the most attention in laboratories and clinical trials are the checkpoint molecules CTLA-4 and PD-1.[19,20] The PD-1 and CTLA-4 axes are pivotal regulators of T-cell activity that can be usurped by tumors to induce T-cell suppression (see Fig. 10.4). CTLA-4 is expressed on activated T cells and constitutively on Tregs, and blocking the activity of CTLA-4 enables T-cell functional rescue. Like CTLA-4, PD-1 is a co-inhibitory receptor but with distinct biologic properties. PD-1 has two known ligands: programmed death ligand-1 (PD-L1) and PD-L2. Many tumors and suppressive immune cells express PD-L1, and PD-1 engagement by PD-L1 results in T-cell functional exhaustion.[21] Exhausted T cells have a markedly diminished capacity for cytokine production, proliferation, and tumor lysis.

Tregs are a subset of CD4$^+$ T cells that mediate tolerance by suppressing antigen-specific T cells.[22] Differentiation of Tregs is programmed by the FOXP3 transcription factor, which is also useful for identifying Tregs experimentally. Immunosuppression by Tregs is mediated through numerous mechanisms, including secretion of tolerogenic cytokines and expression of PD-L1. MDSCs work in concert with Tregs to promote an immunosuppressive environment. MDSCs are a heterogeneous group of cells derived from a myeloid lineage pathway. Phenotypically, MDSCs have features of immature neutrophils, monocytes, or NK cells. MDSCs express PD-L1 and promote T-cell suppression through production of suppressive cytokines such as IL-10. Tregs and MDSCs are likely both important contributors to baseline liver tolerance, as well as suppression of immune responses to cancer in the liver and pancreas.

CYTOKINES

Cytokines are small proteins that play a primary role in the human response to a variety of stimuli. These nonstructural proteins participate in the communication between cells. Pleiotropic in nature, many cytokines can produce both proinflammatory and antiinflammatory effects, depending on the timing, levels, and context in which they are secreted. Cytokines are crucial mediators in the development of hepatic diseases, as well as regeneration and repair, so it is reasonable to suppose they play a similar role in pancreatic pathophysiology. Elucidation of the mechanisms of these mediators will allow an enhanced understanding of the natural history of liver, biliary, and pancreatic surgical diseases. Although produced by all nucleated cells, constitutive production of most cytokines is low in the absence of noxious stimuli. This section reviews these stimuli, as well as the specific mediators involved, in the pathophysiology of liver, biliary, and pancreatic disease.

Immune Recognition and Toll-Like Receptors

Immune response to microbial pathogens and biologic insults requires quick identification of the threat to minimize damage to the host. The innate immune system is a first-line defense against microbial pathogens, providing the ability to distinguish self from non-self via cell-surface receptors expressed in many cell types. Additionally, central to this defense mechanism is the ability to recognize cellular damage.

The liver, biliary system, and pancreas play a vital role in development of immunologic responses because of their close physiologic relationship with the gut. Portal blood entering the liver contains a diverse load of antigens and microbial products, which functions to shape immunologic tolerance, as well as an organized response of inflammatory mediators.[23] Recognition of cellular damage and microbial products is accomplished via intracellular and cell-surface–expressed pattern recognition receptors (PRRs).[24]

An example of essential PRRs in the liver is the family of Toll-like receptors (TLRs). TLRs are a family of at least 10 transmembrane receptors found in cells throughout the human body. Although essential for protective immunity in the normal state, aberrant or prolonged responses can produce catastrophic effects on the host. Accordingly, TLRs have been demonstrated to be essential in the development of multiple hepatic diseases and continue to be investigated as potential therapeutic targets.

Endotoxins and the Immune Response

Exclusive to gram-negative bacteria, lipopolysaccharide (LPS) is one of the most studied pathogen-associated activators of inflammation. An activator of proinflammatory cytokines, LPS plays a large role in tissue damage and development of septic shock, classifying it as an endotoxin.[25] Although the exact mechanism of LPS pathogenesis in human disease remains undefined, its role in activation of the host innate immune response

TABLE 10.1 Host Defense Responses to Lipopolysaccharide and Endotoxemia

ACUTE-PHASE RESPONSE	HOST DEFENSE
Thermoregulation	Elevated core temperature Antimicrobial response
Immunologic	Complement activation Leukocytosis (neutrophilia) Proinflammatory response (IL-1α, IL-1B, TNF-α, IL-1R, TGF-β, protease inhibitors) B-cell stimulation, antibody production
Coagulation	Decreased protein C Decreased antithrombin III Increased cell adhesion Activation of coagulation cascade Increased tissue factor production Prostaglandin production Platelet aggregation, platelet-activating factor Fibrinogen
Metabolic	Lipolysis Mobilized amino acids Altered glucose metabolism Increased corticosteroid production

IL, Interleukin; *IL-1R,* interleukin-1 receptor; *TGF-β,* transforming growth factor-β; *TNF-α,* tumor necrosis factor-α.

is well understood (Table 10.1). Increasing insight into the downstream effects of the LPS response is likely to open up potential areas for targeted treatment.

The host innate immune recognition and response to LPS is highly ordered and is crucial to preventing overwhelming infection and resultant sepsis. Although it is crucial that the high sensitivity of the system allows rapid mobilization of host protective mechanisms, self-limitation of this response is just as vital, preventing irreversible tissue damage and allowing return to homeostasis. Extensive study has recognized a strictly ordered sequence of interactions with multiple extracellular and cell-surface host proteins, including LPS-binding protein (LBP), CD14, myeloid differentiation protein-2 (MD-2), and TLR4.[26,27]

Initiation of the host innate immune response to LPS is binding of it to LBP to form the LPS-LBP complex.[28] The importance of LBP in beginning this inflammatory cascade is noted by the rise in LBP ribonucleic acid (RNA) and protein synthesis during the initial acute phase of endotoxic shock.[29] LBP, a 58 kDa glycoprotein secreted by hepatocytes into the bloodstream, binds the lipid A portion of LPS with high affinity and facilitates transfer to, and the subsequent effects of, CD14+ cells.

The initial signal-transducing component of this pathway is TLR4. Although expressed at low levels in healthy hepatic cells, increasing evidence points to altered LPS-TLR4 complex signaling in the pathogenesis of chronic liver disease. This complex, with the addition of the extracellular protein MD-2, functions to catalyze the intracellular signaling cascade.[30]

This system of signaling and enhanced response to LPS to activate the innate immune response is advantageous to the host in that it can provide enhanced protection from gram-negative induced infection. However, an unregulated response can cause an extremely damaging host response, as is seen with overwhelming sepsis. Specific regulatory mechanisms are needed to prevent the potential shock, multisystem organ failure, or possible death that can result without modulation of the previously described signaling pathways.

Macrophages previously exposed to LPS demonstrate reduced responses to repeat stimulation; this LPS tolerance is important for the negative regulation of the systemic inflammatory response.[31] At the cell-surface level, RP 105 (radioprotective 105), a homolog of TLR4, can function to competitively inhibit the interaction between LPS and TLR4.[32] At the TIR domain of TLR4, overexpression of TRIAD3A, an E3 ubiquitin-protein ligase inhibitor, functions to promote degradation of TLR4 and downregulation of NF-κB.[33] These examples, along with multiple additional proteins that function to regulate TLR4 signaling, can prove to be potential targets to counteract destructive inflammatory responses.

Tumor Necrosis Superfamily

The tumor necrosis factor (TNF) superfamily is composed of more than 20 primarily type II transmembrane proteins with more than 30 receptors. This family of ligands acts on the immune response, cell proliferation, and apoptosis.[34,35] Induction of the inflammatory response by TNF-α acts on vascular endothelial cells, producing vasodilation and capillary permeability that increase trans-endothelial passage of fluid via alterations of adhesion molecules, increased production of nitric oxide, and cyclooxygenase (COX). Further cellular damage and deleterious inflammatory effects are produced by the triggering effect of TNF-α on secondary mediators, such as IL-1, IL-6, IL-10, IFN-γ, platelet-activating factor, epinephrine, cortisol, and growth hormone. This activation contributes to the wide range of physiologic effects seen with overwhelming septic shock.[36]

TNF-α has long been investigated as a potential chemotherapeutic agent because of its antiproliferation properties and effects on vascular permeability.[37] Systemic use has been limited, however, by its significant side effects. Low-dose TNF-α administration in healthy volunteers produced an acute activation of neutrophils, accompanied by a rapid increase in plasma concentrations of IL-6, IL-8, and acute-phase proteins. Additionally, participants demonstrated a sustained decrease in lymphocytes, basophils, and eosinophils.[38] Because of the increased doses of TNF-α needed in chemotherapeutic regimens, such as with isolated limb perfusions, continuous monitoring of systemic leakage and infusion rate adjustment is necessary.[39]

Interleukin-1

IL-1 is a potent factor in activation of the innate immune system and inflammatory response. Because the cytoplasmic domain of the IL-1 receptor type I is homologous to those of TLRs, similar activation of proinflammatory immune responses would be expected.[40] Unlike most other cytokine families, however, the IL-1 family includes members that actively function in suppression of the innate immune response.[41]

IL-1 primarily produces an immune response via gene expression of multiple inflammatory mediators. This is observed with the IL-1–mediated production of COX-2 and inducible nitric oxide synthase, as well as increased expression of intercellular adhesion molecule-1 and vascular cell adhesion molecule-1.[42] These products, as well as interaction with and potentiation of other cytokines, result in the symptoms of inflammation, vasodilation, and movement of activated inflammatory cells to tissues, which are seen with activation of the innate immune response. Stimulation of IL-1 can occur via LPS, as is seen with other cytokine families. However, other factors, such as TNF-α, complement C5a, hypoxia, or IL-1 ligands per se, can induce increased IL-1 messenger RNA transcription.

Interleukin-6

IL-6 is involved in inflammation through effects on cell differentiation, proliferation, and apoptosis, and is active in other functions, including immune regulation and oncogenesis.[43] IL-6 belongs to a nine-member superfamily of cytokines, which includes leukemia inhibitory factor, oncostatin M, cardiotrophin-1, neurotrophic factor, and IL-11. Signal transduction for all members of this family uses the signal-transducing receptor glycoprotein 130 kDa (gp130), making this a potential target for future therapies. Upon formation of gp130 homodimers by ligand binding, signaling is carried forward primarily by the Janus activating kinase/signal transducer and activator of transcription pathway.

IL-6 has a wide range of effects, both in the hematopoietic system and in the innate immune response, including a substantial role in the balance between IL-17–producing T cells and regulatory T cells. IL-6 overproduction and upregulation of Th17 cells is thought to be a critical factor in development of multiple autoimmune disorders.[43] IL-6 and IL-11, with known effects on cell proliferation, are felt to play a crucial role in the development of hepatocellular carcinoma (Fig. 10.5). Current studies are underway investigating inhibition of these cytokines in solid tumors.

Transforming Growth Factor-β

Transforming growth factor-β (TGF-β) is another pleiotropic cytokine involved in many aspects of cellular function, including differentiation, migration, angiogenesis, and apoptosis.[44] It is stored as an intracellular latent form until it is activated by several factors, including MMPs, integrins, and thrombospondin 1.[46] The downstream effects of this cytokine are quite context- and cell-dependent. The primary signaling mechanism is through the phosphorylation of SMAD2 and SMAD3, allowing

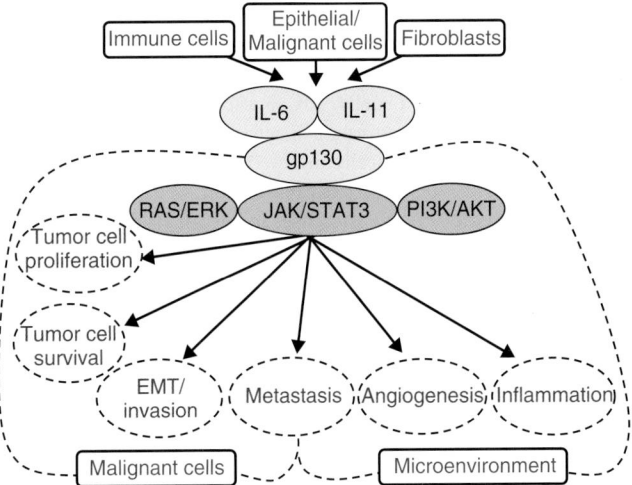

FIGURE 10.5 Interleukin *(IL)*-6 and IL-11 signaling in cancer. IL-6 and IL-11, produced by immune cells, fibroblasts, and epithelial and malignant cells, activate the JAK/STAT3, SHP-2-RAS-ERK, and PI3K-AKT pathways, through which they induce cell proliferation, survival, EMT/invasion, metastasis, angiogenesis, and inflammation. *AKT,* Protein kinase B; *EMT,* epithelial-to-mesenchymal transition; *ERK,* extracellular signal-regulated kinase; *gp130,* glycoprotein 130; *JAK,* Janus activating kinase; *PI3K,* phosphatidylinositol-3-kinase; *RAS,* rat sarcoma (protein); *STAT,* signal transducer and activator of transcription. (From Taniguchi K, Karin M. IL-6 and related cytokines as the critical lynchpins between inflammation and cancer. *Semin Immunol.* 26:54–74, 2014.)

translocation into the nucleus and resultant gene activation.[47] Additionally, activation can occur via SMAD-independent pathways, primarily through MAPKs.

Paradoxically, TGF-β can function to arrest growth, as well as act as a tumor promoter. The functional switch can occur at many points in the signaling pathway. In the SMAD-dependent pathway, location of formation of the active complex appears to play a role in conversion to oncogenic properties because increased phosphorylation of the linker region of SMAD3, in preference to the C-terminal region, is seen in many advanced tumors.[48] Although less common, mutations can also play a role in tumor development, which is seen with increased SMAD4 inactivation in pancreatic carcinoma.[49] Additionally, aberrant TGF-β signaling has been implicated in the progression of hepatic fibrosis through the increased production of connective tissue growth factor by hepatic progenitor cells[50] (see Chapter 7).

Type I Interferons (Interferon-α and Interferon-β)

Type I IFNs refers to a family of structurally similar cytokines that are crucial in the immune response to viral infection. IFN-α is secreted by immune cells, whereas IFN-β is secreted by multiple cell types, such as fibroblasts, in response to viral infection. Type I IFNs have direct antiviral action by triggering virally infected cells to produce enzymes that interfere with viral RNA or DNA replication. They also lead to the increased expression of MHC class I molecules on the surface of virally infected cells, increasing their likelihood of being killed by cytolytic CD8+ T cells. Additionally, type I IFNs inhibit cellular proliferation. IFN-α has been used clinically in the treatment of viral hepatitis and as an adjuvant therapy for melanoma.

Type II Interferons (Interferon-γ)

IFN-γ, a type II IFN, is the archetypal proinflammatory cytokine associated with antitumor immune responses. IFN-γ activates macrophages and plays a crucial role in bridging innate and adaptive immunity by increasing antigen presentation through the MHC class I and II pathways.[51] It is produced by T cells, B cells, NKT cells, DCs, and macrophages. IFN-γ promotes Th1-driven cytotoxic T-cell responses, which are essential for clearance of virally infected cells or tumors. In addition, IFN-γ promotes MHC expression on APCs and enhances NK cell cytotoxic activity. Increases in serum IFN-γ levels have been correlated with favorable clinical responses to immunotherapy treatments.

However, IFN-γ is a double-edged sword. In addition to promoting APC activation and antiviral immunity, it participates in adaptive resistance, a phenomenon whereby the activation of T cells leads to IFN-γ secretion and the activation of genes encoding co-inhibitory molecules, in particular PD-L1.[52,53]

Cytokine Regulation in the Liver and Pancreas

Hepatic response to inflammation and parenchymal injury produce a variety of effects in the host, both locally and systemically. Although cytokine expression in the liver is low at baseline, as a nonspecific first line of defense from bacterial products from the hepatic circulation, a rapid, orchestrated response is needed for host protection.

Hepatic cytokine contribution has been demonstrated in human studies, where cannulation of the hepatic vein after intravenous endotoxin administration revealed that large amounts of both TNF-α and IL-6 in the systemic circulation were derived from the splanchnic bed.[54] Increasing evidence has also defined the role of hepatic stellate cells in recruitment and induction of infiltrating leukocytes, amplifying the inflammatory response. Infiltration of T cells and NK cells can enhance production of TNF-α, FASL, and TGF-β in virally induced hepatic injury.[55] Increasing levels of these cytokines are found in both hepatic injury and regeneration.

Cytokines and the Pancreas

Defining the effects of specific cytokines in pancreatic dysfunction is complicated by the pleiotropic effect of these molecules. Pancreatic islet cells produce multiple cytokines in the healthy state, regulating β-cell function and replication. Increasing IL-1 levels stimulates β-cell proliferation to respond to exogenous stressors. Nevertheless, prolonged stress has been implicated in islet cell dysfunction and destruction. Mouse models have demonstrated the role of TGF-β in the progression of type 1 diabetes, and elevated concentrations of this cytokine have been implicated in increased microvascular complications in children with diabetes.[56]

TGF-β has also been studied as a contributing factor in the development of chronic pancreatic inflammation (see Chapters 57 and 58) and pancreatic adenocarcinoma (see Chapter 59). Elevated levels are found in patients with chronic pancreatitis, correlating with progression of fibrosis and insulin resistance. It has been postulated that insensitivity to TGF-β stimulation, with resultant elevated levels, results in a switch from inhibitory effects to increased proliferation of pancreatic adenocarcinomas, in concert with additional cytokine influence. Accordingly, elevated TGF-β1 and TGF-β2 receptor levels have been associated with advanced cancers, with a trend toward worse overall survival.[57]

Nitric Oxide

Altered redox states and oxidative stress have been extensively studied in a multitude of disease states because of their participation in inflammation and apoptosis.[58] Oxidative stress implies an imbalance between oxidant and antioxidant agents; when the capacity of the antioxidant system is overwhelmed, a harmful level of redox state is achieved and the potential for cellular damage arises.

Central to the balance of redox states in hepatocytes is nitric oxide (NO). NO is a small, hydrophobic molecule with a short half-life. Created by nitric oxide synthase (NOS), NO can be greatly increased via production by inducible NO synthase (iNOS). iNOS is expressed in all hepatic cells, and its production can be induced by IL-1, TNF-α, and LPS.[59] NO plays a complicated role in hepatocyte cellular function. In steady-state low-redox conditions, NO plays a protective role in the liver, having been demonstrated to inhibit apoptosis and abate mitochondrial dysfunction.[60,61] NO also functions as a cytoprotective molecule by acting as an electron acceptor for S-nitrosylation, causing inhibition of caspase activity.[62] Upregulation of iNOS is also an important factor in the propagation of the inflammatory response, which can play a protective role. NO induces the expression of heat-shock protein 70.[63] These proteins may function by refolding damaged proteins in the liver, modulating caspase activation, and regulating expression of heme oxygenase-1, conferring a protective mechanism from apoptosis. NO also can bind soluble guanyl cyclase, which can increase intracellular cyclic guanosine monophosphate, suppressing apoptosis and caspase activity.[64]

TABLE 10.2 Roles of iNOS in Hepatic Injury

CONDITION/INDUCERS	NO EFFECT	MECHANISM
In Vivo		
Endotoxemia	Protective Toxic	Inhibition of apoptosis Oxidative stress Circulatory failure
TNF-α	Protective	Inhibits apoptosis
CCl₄	Protective	Decreases oxidative stress
Liver Regeneration	Protective	Inhibits apoptosis
Ischemia/reperfusion	Toxic	Oxidative damage
Hemorrhagic shock	Toxic	Direct toxicity, activates inflammation
Alcoholic liver injury	Protective	Unclear
In Vitro		
TNF-α, FAS antibody	Protective	Inhibits caspase/apoptosis HSP70 upregulation
H_2O_2	Protective	Heme oxygenase-1 upregulation
Acetaminophen	Protective	Modulates GSH levels

CCl_4, Carbon tetrachloride; *GSH*, reduced glutathione; H_2O_2, peroxide; *HSP70*, 70-kDa heat-shock protein, *iNOS*, inducible nitric oxide synthase; *NO*, nitric oxide; *TNF-α*, tumor necrosis factor-α.

Modified from Li J, Billiar TR. Nitric oxide. IV. Determinants of nitric oxide protection and toxicity in the liver. *Am J Physiol.* 1999;276:G1069–G1073.

In conditions of oxidative stress and altered redox states, upregulation of iNOS has been associated with deleterious effects because of continued oxidative damage and propagation of inflammation. Studies in mice have demonstrated reduced hepatic damage with inhibition of NO synthesis, and iNOS has been implicated in ethanol-induced hepatic injury.[65] Viral hepatitis has also been associated with increased iNOS expression, with several studies suggesting an association between levels of iNOS induction and disease severity.[66] Thus it appears that the NO functioning in either a protective or destructive role can vary depending on cellular levels and redox conditions (Table 10.2).

IMMUNE SYSTEM IN NONMALIGNANT LIVER DISEASES

Intrahepatic immune cells play prominent roles in myriad inflammatory, infectious, and neoplastic diseases affecting the liver. Our understanding of liver immune cell biology and crosstalk among intrahepatic immune cell subsets has greatly informed our appreciation of liver disease pathogenesis. The following sections highlight the role of the hepatic immune system in a variety of diseases affecting the liver.

Transplantation

Transplant immunology has shed significant light on the unique properties of the liver as an immunologic organ (see Chapter 104). Unlike other organs, the liver can be accepted across MHC barriers in animal models of transplantation.[67] In addition, systemic donor-specific tolerance often develops in liver allograft recipients.[68] In humans, liver transplants confer protection for other organs from the same donor,[69] and recipients can often be weaned off immunosuppression altogether.[70]

BOX 10.1 Factors Contributing to Hepatic Tolerance

- Immunosuppression via release of soluble MHC class I antigens
- Distinct lymphocyte population with distinct functions (KCs, DCs, NK, and NKT cells, LSECs)
- Constant antigen load from the portal circulation
- Induction of activated T-cell apoptosis
- Microchimerism
- Immature phenotype and tolerogenic function of resident liver APCs (DCs, KCs, LSECs)
- Altered Th1 versus Th2 profile within the liver (favoring Th2)
- Presence of suppressor cells (Tregs and MDSCs)
- Immunoinhibitory pathways (CTLA-4, PD-1)

APCs, Antigen-presenting cells; *CTLA-4*, cytotoxic T-lymphocyte–associated antigen-4; *DCs*, dendritic cells; *KCs*, Kupffer cells; *LSECs*, liver sinusoidal endothelial cells; *MDSC*, myeloid-derived suppressor cells; *MHC*, major histocompatibility complex; *NK*, natural killer; *NKT*, natural killer T cell; *PD-1*, programmed death-1; *Treg*, regulatory T cells.
Modified from Gershwin ME, Vierling JM, Manns MP, eds. *Liver Immunology.* Hanley and Belfus; 2003.

The unique ability of allografts to resist rejection and promote extrahepatic tolerance speaks to the immunosuppressive properties of hepatic immune cells.

The development of mouse models of orthotopic liver transplantation has provided an opportunity to gain mechanistic insight into the regulation of immune responses in the liver.[71] Factors that contribute to hepatic tolerance (Box 10.1) include microchimerism and induction of activated T-cell apoptosis. Defined as the persistence of donor cells in allograft recipients, microchimerism has been postulated to be a prerequisite for organ allograft acceptance.[72,73] The high antigenic load derived from the donor liver coupled with persistence of donor APCs within lymphoid tissues of the recipient may provide a continuing source of allostimulation.[74,75] The persistent activation of alloreactive recipient T cells is thought to result in exhaustive deletion and induction of systemic tolerance. The role of specific donor-derived liver APCs, such as DCs and KCs, in contributing to chimerism-induced tolerance remains unclear. Although freshly isolated liver DCs have been shown to exhibit tolerogenic potential via the production of IL-10,[7] others have shown that donor-derived liver DCs prime recipient T cells to differentiate into proinflammatory subtypes that promote rejection.[76]

The immunoregulatory role of KCs has also been extensively investigated. KCs have been implicated in the induction of oral tolerance and in lymphocyte apoptosis, which has been a proposed mechanism of immunosuppression in liver transplantation.[77] More recently, KCs have been shown to play a crucial role in induction of antigen-specific T-cell tolerance[78] and are thought to suppress T-cell response via the production of prostaglandins.[79] Despite evidence of the tolerogenic potential of KCs, the use of gadolinium chloride to suppress KC function has not been shown to impact survival of liver allografts in mouse models of liver transplantation. The disparate findings concerning the role of KCs in liver transplantation may reflect the opposing effects of tolerogenic MDSCs and proinflammatory macrophages, both of which share considerable phenotypic overlap with KCs.

The overall bias of intrahepatic T-cell responses toward tolerance and apoptosis might account for the survival of liver allografts.[80] Activated T cells and their subsequent apoptosis within the liver are thought to be another critical component in the induction of hepatic tolerance and the acceptance of liver allografts. Recently, hepatic stellate cells (HSCs) have been found to mediate liver T-cell apoptosis via the PD-L1/PD-1 axis.[81] HSCs may also induce expansion of Tregs as another mechanism of influencing T-cell tolerance.[82]

Although the hepatic immune system has been shown to clearly play an important role in liver and systemic tolerance, definitive mechanisms in humans remain elusive. It is likely that multiple suppressive cell types and several overlapping immunoinhibitory pathways interact to form a network of tolerance within the intrahepatic space. Understanding the mechanisms controlling the tolerogenic propensity of the liver is of great significance in transplantation because it will permit the design of novel approaches to reduce immunosuppressive-related morbidity and mortality.

Hepatitis

Hepatitis B virus (HBV) and hepatitis C virus (HCV) are noncytopathic and hepatotropic and cause acute and chronic liver disease (see Chapter 68). The worldwide burden of disease is immense, with an estimated 500 million people infected with either of these two viruses. The cost to society is magnified when the increased risk for cirrhosis and liver cancer in those infected with HBV and HCV are taken into account. Immune-mediated or inflammatory destruction of liver parenchyma is a common final pathway in viral hepatitis. The presence of large numbers of KCs and DCs in the liver, which produce TNF-α in response to viral antigens, leads to high local levels of inflammatory cytokines and untoward host cell damage. Similarly, T cells, NKT cells, and NK cells in the liver produce IFN-γ, which also serves to amplify the local immune response by activating KCs and DCs. Consistent with this, chronic active hepatitis is morphologically identified by piecemeal necrosis and a predominantly mononuclear cell infiltrate.[83]

Despite immune cell activation and inflammatory cytokine production, the host is frequently unable to clear HBV or HCV. Therefore, to achieve successful viral control and limit collateral damage, a sustained, antigen-specific immune response is necessary.[84,85] Recognition of multiple viral epitopes by the host is also advantageous because it offers some protection against the emergence of mutants that escape the immune system. Unfortunately, effective T-cell responses against HBV and HCV are susceptible to suppression by the PD-1/PD-L1 immunoinhibitory access and Treg.[86] The tolerogenic predisposition of the liver may suppress adaptive immunity to HBC and HCV, accounting in part for the persistence of these infections.

Emerging research tools that will undoubtedly shed more light on the immune mechanisms underlying viral persistence and resistance to treatment include the development of chimeric mice that are reconstituted with human hepatocytes and immune cells.[87] The transplantation of human hepatocytes into immunodeficient mice will allow for large-scale screening of therapeutics against human hepatitis viruses, and an immunocompetent humanized murine HCV infection model has also been developed.[88] Chimeric murine models will enable researchers to study the in vivo effects of human hepatotropic viruses on human immune responses to infection for the first time.

Autoimmune Hepatitis

Autoimmune hepatitis (AIH) is an idiopathic disorder that leads to cirrhosis as a manifestation of an overactive hepatic immune system (see Chapter 105). AIH likely reflects an imbalance between proinflammatory immune responses and immunosuppressive factors, the latter including PD-1/PD-L1, Treg, and

MDSC. It has a female predominance and is characterized by elevated levels of immunoglobulin G (IgG) autoantibodies.[89] An experimental model of autoimmune hepatitis is based on the treatment of mice with concanavalin A (ConA), a plant lectin known to activate T cells in vitro. A single intravenous injection of ConA leads to severe liver damage and is associated with the activation of CD4$^+$ T cells and the production of TNF-α and IFN-γ. Further studies showed that NKT cells are the most important subset of CD4$^+$ T cells involved in mediating ConA hepatitis. The importance of NKT cells in mediating autoimmune liver damage is also supported by the observation that injection of α-galactosylceramide, an activator of NKT cells through CD1d binding, leads to a similar form of injury as that seen in ConA hepatitis. AIH has also been linked with dysfunction of Tregs, leading to a hyperfunctional Th17 compartment and excessive inflammation.[90] The pathogenesis of AIH highlights the critical importance of balance between proinflammatory and antiinflammatory immune processes within the liver.

Primary Biliary Cirrhosis

Primary biliary cirrhosis (PBC) is an autoimmune liver disease that leads to the destruction of intrahepatic bile ducts and subsequent cholestasis and cirrhosis[91,92] (see Chapter 105). Most cases of PBC are associated with antimitochondrial (95%) and antinuclear (50%) antibodies directed against self-antigens. Dysregulated CD4$^+$ helper T cells and CD8$^+$ cytotoxic T lymphocytes are thought to be important in the pathogenesis of PBC. This is supported by the findings of lymphoid infiltration of the portal tracts and aberrant expression of MHC class II on biliary epithelial cells. Because biliary epithelial cells are the primary target of injury in PBC, their expression of MHC molecules and cytokines likely plays an important role in the pathogenesis of this disease. The degree of Th17 activity within the liver of PBC patients has been associated with severity of disease, and IL-17 promotes excessive fibrosis.[93] In addition to pathogenic T-cell function, biliary epithelial cells from patients with primary biliary cirrhosis attract mononuclear cells via the chemokine CX3CL1 and overexpress the inflammatory cytokines IL-6 and TNF-α.[94]

Primary Sclerosing Cholangitis

Primary sclerosing cholangitis (PSC) results from fibrosis of the intrahepatic and extrahepatic bile ducts[95] (see Chapters 41 and 105). The pathogenesis is thought to result from immune activation within the liver after bacteria gain access to the portal circulation via a diseased intestinal epithelium. The disease is associated with T cells infiltrating the portal tracts. In addition, an increase in production of circulating proinflammatory cytokines has been shown to correlate with disease progression. Pathologic Th17 cell activation in response to bacteria and PRR activity contributes to inflammation in PSC patients.[96] The end result is biliary cirrhosis and a markedly elevated risk for cholangiocarcinoma (CCA). Most cases of PSC are associated with underlying inflammatory bowel disease, specifically ulcerative colitis.

Ischemia/Reperfusion Injury

Liver ischemia/reperfusion (I/R) injury is a well-recognized consequence of trauma, circulatory shock, partial hepatectomy, and liver transplantation (see Chapters 106 and 113). It contributes to the shortage of organs available for transplantation and is a major determinant of postoperative allograft dysfunction and morbidity.[97] During liver I/R, the release of endogenous molecules signal danger to the host by activating innate immune cells through their interaction with TLRs.[98] Such "danger signals," or *danger-associated molecular patterns* (DAMPs), can be classified as intracellular proteins, nucleic acids, or components of the extracellular matrix that are released after host cell injury. The ensuing host innate immune response results in untoward collateral tissue damage that culminates in hepatocyte death and a systemic inflammatory response. The injury stems from the inability of TLRs on innate immune cells to distinguish infectious ligands from DAMPs released by autologous tissue. The need for effective approaches to manage patients with I/R-induced organ damage is highlighted by the fact that current treatment is merely supportive care.

In a murine model of segmental liver I/R, hepatic DCs and TLR9 played critical roles in modulating the host immune response.[7] Hepatocyte DNA released during ischemia binds TLR9 in a variety of liver immune cells that then cause liver damage. In contrast, DCs respond to host DNA by curtailing injury via production of antiinflammatory IL-10, which confers protection by suppressing the function of inflammatory monocytes that migrate to the liver from the bone marrow. Human liver DCs also have a propensity to secrete large amounts of IL-10 at baseline and after TLR activation.[7] T cells also play a role in I/R tissue injury, with Th17 cells promoting influx of neutrophils.[99] Improved understanding of the complex interactions between DAMPs and PRRs on immune cells will promote the development of rational, more effective approaches to limit liver I/R injury.

TNF-α also appears to play a central role in I/R injury. Murine models have demonstrated a significant increase in TNF-α levels after 90 minutes of ischemia, followed by 60 minutes of reperfusion.[100] Although the exact mechanism stimulating TNF-α release is not yet defined, it appears that production is significantly influenced by KC activation. In rats, KCs isolated from the liver after I/R demonstrated a several hundred-fold increase in TNF-α production compared with controls. Treatment with anti–TNF-α antibodies significantly decreased both TNF-α and IL-6 production.[101] Mediation of the effects of TNF-α occurs primarily through activation of NF-κB. Translocation to the nucleus and binding activity of NF-κB increased as much as 66% after 5 minutes of ischemia.[102] Additionally, inhibition of NF-κB activation has demonstrated significantly decreased hepatic apoptosis and caspase-3 activity.[103] This is similar to findings with induction of heme oxygenase-1, which functions to suppress TNF-α/TNFR1-directed hepatic apoptosis.[104]

NOS also appears to be a factor in hepatic ischemia-reperfusion injury. The endothelial isoform of NOS (eNOS) has most clearly been defined as a protective molecule during reperfusion. eNOS knockout mice demonstrated increased severity of hepatic injury after ischemia compared with their wild-type counterparts. Additionally, TNF-α expression was upregulated to a level five times that in the wild-type mice,[105] suggesting a protective effect from cytokine injury. This protection has demonstrated effects beyond the liver because NO has also been shown to reduce the incidence of onset of hepatopulmonary syndrome in transplanted rats.[106]

IMMUNE SYSTEM IN MALIGNANT LIVER DISEASES

Evidence on the importance of the hepatic immune system in malignancy comes from data, which reveal that (1) when compared with autologous blood, human liver specimens from patients with malignancy contain a disproportionately higher percentage of NK cells with reduced antitumor function[15] and (2) the hepatic T-cell infiltrate predicts survival after surgery in patients with metastatic colorectal liver cancer.[107] Tumor-infiltrating lymphocytes (TILs) indicate a specific host response to tumor antigens. TILs may be used with therapeutic intent or studied for prognostic information.[108] TILs have been demonstrated to predict outcomes in a wide variety of solid tumors, with the magnitude of this effect being dependent on tumor site and disease stage.[109] An increasing number of studies have focused on TILs as predictors of outcome for primary and metastatic liver tumors. Our evolving understanding of intrahepatic antitumor immunity promises to enable development of novel therapeutic approaches using immunomodulatory agents and adoptive cell therapy.

Immune Response to Primary Liver Cancer

Hepatocellular carcinoma (HCC) is one of the most common malignant tumors worldwide (see Chapter 89). The immune response to neoplastic cells has been shown to be a potential determinant of survival in HCC patients.[110–112] High densities of DCs, T-cell subsets, and tumor-associated macrophages have all been reported to be favorable prognostic factors in HCC.[113] TIL responses to HCC occur in a more complex biologic context than metastatic tumors, given the underlying inflammatory processes that drive HCC carcinogenesis and progression.

HCC TILs have been compared with T cells in adjacent normal liver tissue, and HCC TILs reflect a more immunosuppressed state. HCC TIL populations have been shown to contain a higher number of Tregs compared with normal surrounding liver.[114] Increased ratios of Tregs (FOXP3+) to total T cells (CD3+) were independently associated with poorer differentiation. Furthermore, high FOXP3+ to CD8+ TIL ratios were associated with shorter overall and disease-free survival times in HCC patients on both univariate and multivariate analysis.[114] Immune suppression within HCC may also be attributed to increased expression of PD-1 on TILs. As noted earlier, PD-1 is an immunoinhibitory receptor that suppresses T-cell division and cytokine production.[115] PD-1 is engaged by PD-L1, which has been detected on HCC tumor cells. The presence of Tregs and PD-1+ TILs reflect an immunosuppressive milieu but may represent a therapeutic opportunity because anti–PD-1 antibodies are now in clinical use for a variety of solid tumors.

TIL responses have also been studied in patients with biliary tract cancers. CCA is the second most common primary intrahepatic malignancy, and most patients are not candidates for potentially curative surgical intervention (see Chapter 50). A study of 123 patients with intrahepatic CCA who underwent curative surgical resection revealed that IL-17+ (Th17) and FOXP3+ (Treg) TILs were enriched predominantly within CCA tumors, whereas CD8+ TILs were most abundant at the tumor margin. IL-17+ TIL counts were an independent predictor of decreased patient survival, reflecting the importance of the Th17/Treg balance in liver diseases.[116] Similar to HCC, tumor expression of PD-L1 was correlated with CCA stage and tumor differentiation.[117] Improving our understanding of CCA immune responses and tumor-driven immunosuppression may offer insights into novel therapeutic options and improve risk stratification.

Immune Response to Metastatic Cancer in the Liver

The high prevalence of metastatic disease to the liver is likely because of multiple factors, including the unique characteristics of the liver immune system. As delineated earlier, the primary mediators of innate and adaptive immunity found in the liver (DCs and T cells) are unique in their distribution of subtypes and skew toward tolerogenic function.[5,13] In addition, the liver contains suppressive cells, such as Tregs and MDSCs, that may also promote the establishment of metastatic colonies within the intrahepatic space.

Several studies suggest that intrahepatic adaptive immune responses to colorectal cancer liver metastases (CRCLM) are predictive of recurrence and death after resection (see Chapter 90). Both CD4[+] and CD8[+] T cells are activated within CRCLM, and activated CD4[+] T helper cells may promote tumor-selective activity of cytotoxic CD8[+] T lymphocytes.[118] After hepatic resection, patients with high numbers of CD8[+] intratumoral T cells were more likely to survive 10 years or longer. Among patients who survived for 10 years or more, 31% had high levels of CD8[+] T cells. In contrast, only 8% of those who survived less than 2 years had a high level of CD8[+] TIL.[107] Ratios of TIL subsets have been studied as well and may provide more biologic insight than individual TIL counts. In patients with CRCLM, high CD8[+] to CD4[+] TIL ratios were an independent predictor of long-term survival after resection, after adjusting for multiple variables, including clinical risk score. In a more recent study, high CD4[+] to CD3[+] and CD8[+] to CD3[+] TIL ratios were a significant correlate of improved and recurrence-free survival.[119]

As reported in the setting of primary liver cancer, TIL ratios, including FOXP3[+] Treg, are predictive of outcome after CRCLM resection. High FOXP3[+] to CD4[+] and FOXP3[+] to CD8[+] TIL ratios were independent predictors of shorter overall survival. Overall survival at 5 years for patients with a high FOXP3[+] to CD4[+] TIL ratio was 34% compared with 51% for patients with a low ratio (odds ratio [OR] = 1.6; P = .03). Similarly, 5-year survival was 35% in those with a high FOXP3[+] to CD8[+] ratio compared with 46% in those with a low FOXP3[+] to CD8[+] TIL ratio (hazard ratio [HR] = 1.5; P = .05)[119]. FOXP3[+] TIL counts were also found to be predictors of outcome after resection of neuroendocrine tumor liver metastases.[120] Tumor MHC I expression has also been correlated to immune infiltrates and outcome.[121]

A critical finding from studies of CRCLM is that although patients with favorable TIL profiles are more likely to have a good outcome, the majority of individuals do not demonstrate an effective intratumoral immune response. We speculate that immunosuppressive intrahepatic immune cells and immunoinhibitory pathways limit the function of effector T cells. This presents a therapeutic opportunity to deliver effective adoptive cellular immunotherapy in conjunction with suppressive pathway inhibition to overcome the factors curtailing endogenous antitumor immunity.

Immune Response to Pancreatic Adenocarcinoma

Pancreatic ductal adenocarcinoma (PDA) is the fourth most common cause of cancer death in the United States and has a rising incidence[122] (see Chapters 61 and 62). It has been recognized in murine models and human tissue that PDA is surrounded by dense stromal fibrosis; however, although there is a dearth of effector cells within mouse models, in human PDA there appears to still be significant populations of T cells into the tumor milieu.[123] Early evidence demonstrated improved survival with higher densities of CD8[+] T cells and DCs[124]; conversely, myeloid cell types, including MDSCs, and Tregs were enriched in poorly differentiated PDA.[125] Immunosuppressive

M2 phenotype macrophages also appear to suppress tumor killing activity by effector T cells via secretion of cytokines such as IL-10 and TGF-β; DCs in the circulation and within the microenvironment also appear to be suppressed by IL10 and TGF-β secretion from MDSCs and tumor cells.[126] Increased Treg within the tumor microenvironment and in peripheral blood has been associated with decreased survival[127]; higher expression of leukocyte adhesion molecules, such as CD166, produced by endothelial cells in the stroma appear to enhance Treg migration into the PDA microenvironment.[128]

PDA cells also appear to evade the immune response using checkpoint molecules, including by expressing PD-L1[129]; similar mechanisms modulating CTLA-4 have also been described.[130] The immunosuppressive milieu also tends to shift CTL phenotypes away from the effector Th1 to the more suppressive Th2 subtype via IL-10[131,132]; higher ratios of the Th2 to Th1 ratio seen in PDA has been associated with worse outcomes.[133] Despite this, there is recent evidence that demonstrates the presence of clonally expanded effector T cells, further lending credence to the idea that the adaptive immune response against PDA exists but is kept at bay by the immunosuppressive microenvironment.[134] This complex interplay between activation and suppression, modulated by both cellular and soluble components of the adaptive response (Table 10.3), has likely contributed to the difficulty in medical therapy against the disease.

Current Advances in Immunotherapy Against Liver and Pancreatic Malignancies (see Chapters. 66, 6,7 and 99)

Although many investigators have attempted to manipulate the immune system for the treatment of cancer,[135] few attempts have been made to directly target intrahepatic immune cells. The primary goal of cancer immunotherapy, particularly for liver tumors, is to deliver or induce potent antitumor immunity while reversing intrahepatic suppression. Reversal of intrahepatic tolerance has been accomplished in animal models by activating liver immune cells, depleting suppressor cells, or blocking immunoinhibitory pathways, such as the PD-1/PD-L1 axis. IL-12 production by DCs activates NK cells toward protection against tumor in a mouse melanoma liver metastasis model.[136] Despite having less lytic potential than blood NK cells, human liver NK cells have the capacity to become potent antitumor cells when activated in the presence of KCs and TLR3 ligands.[15]

In addition to DCs, recent work on the role of peritumoral monocytes in patients with HCC has garnered much attention among immunologists and hepatologists alike. Activated monocytes in the peritumoral stroma of HCC have been shown to foster a state of tolerance and promote tumor progression via the expression of an immunosuppressive molecule, PD-L1.[137] Furthermore, tumor expression of PD-L1 was recently shown to serve as a predictor of recurrence in patients with resected HCC.[138]

Recent trials have finally put into clinical practice the promises of immunotherapy that have been shown mechanistically (see Chapter 99). Before these trials, the tyrosine kinase inhibitor sorafenib had been the one and only data-driven choice for systemic therapy for advanced HCC.[139,140] Although there was the introduction of levatinib (a vascular endothelial growth factor [VEGF] receptor kinase inhibitor) as a noninferior alternative to sorafenib,[141,142] there has been a rapid increase in the number of immunotherapeutics approved for both second-line

TABLE 10.3	Factors Involved in Modulating T Cell Programming in Pancreatic Adenocarcinoma	
	FUNCTION IN T-CELL PROGRAMMING	**RELEVANCE TO PDA IMMUNE MICROENVIRONMENT**
Cytokines		
IL-2	• Promotes differentiation, survival, and function of Treg	• IL-2 mediates increased proliferation and expansion of Treg within the tumor microenvironment to decrease tumor targeting
IL-4	• Shifts macrophages from activated M1 subtype to immunosuppressive M2 subtype	• May play a role in enhanced activity of the M2 subtype within the tumor milieu
IL-10	• Inhibits expression of IL-12, thereby downregulating T-cell activation	• Immunosuppressive M2 macrophages produce IL-10 to reduce T-cell activation in and around the tumor
IL-12	• Induces Th1 differentiation • Increases IFN-γ production, thereby enhancing cytotoxic activity	• Administration of IL-12 in vitro modulated T cells from PDA patients toward Th1 subtype
Soluble Factors		
IFN-γ	• Induces Th1 differentiation • Increases antigen processing and presentation to T cells • Upregulates expression of class I and II MHC molecules	• Cytotoxic cells targeting the tumor kill malignant cells in part via release of IFN-γ
TGF-β	• Inhibits T-cell activation and proliferation • Induces differentiation of Treg and Th17 • Inhibits macrophage activation	• PDA tumor cells release TGF-β, thereby directly reducing T-cell activation
TNF-α	• Causes systemic inflammation and fever	• Monoclonal antibodies against TNF-α have demonstrated decreased infiltration of Treg into PDA
Cell Surface Receptors		
CTLA-4	• Competes with the binding of activating co-stimulatory molecules on T cells, leading to decreased activation • Serves as an immune checkpoint via increased expression in T cells after activation	• A phase II trial involving ipilimumab, a CTLA-4 inhibitor, did not demonstrate any benefit in survival or outcomes in patients with advanced PDA
PD-1	• Binds to ligands present on APCs to downregulate T-cell activity • Terminates peripheral effector cell activity	• PDA expresses higher levels of PD-L1, the ligand for PD-1, which leads to decreased T-cell activation
• CCR2	• Important in monocyte chemotaxis	• CCR2 appears to mediate recruitment of M2 macrophages into the PDA microenvironment, thereby decreasing immune activation
• CXCR4	• Important in homing to bone marrow niche, as well as T-cell co-signaling	• CXCR4 and PD-1 combination blockade with chemotherapy showed enhanced disease control rate in a phase II trial • CXCR4 blockade leads to increased trafficking of T cells to PDA

CCR, Chemokine receptor type; *CTLA-4*, cytotoxic T-lymphocyte-associated protein 4; *CXCR*, C-X-C chemokine receptor type; *GM-CSF*, granulocyte-macrophage colony stimulating factor; *IFN-γ*, interferon gamma; *IL*, interleukin; *M-CSF*, macrophage colony stimulating factor; *PD-1*, programmed cell death protein 1; *TGF-β*, transforming growth factor beta, *Th*, T helper; *TNF-α*, tumor necrosis factor alpha.

Modified from Seo YD, Pillarisetty VG. T cell programming in pancreatic adenocarcinoma: A review. *Cancer Gene Therapy*. 2017;24(3): 106–113.

and now first-line treatments. Pembrolizumab, a PD-1 inhibitor, was one of the first to gain US Food and Drug Administration (FDA) approval for treatment of advanced HCC not responsive to sorafenib[143]; nivolumab (another PD-1 inhibitor) and combination nivolumab plus ipilimumab (a CTLA-4 inhibitor) have since been added to this list of second-line therapies.[144,145] Most recently, combination atezolizumab (a PD-L1 inhibitor) and bevacizumab (a direct VEGF inhibitor) demonstrated improved overall and disease-free survival rates compared with sorafenib in unresectable HCC as first-line therapy.[146]

Although the immunosuppressive nature of the intrahepatic space has long been thought to be the cause of ineffective antitumor immunity, it seems this suppressive milieu can be overcome with combination immunotherapy as noted previously.

Another rapidly expanding indication for immunotherapy is the treatment of deficient mismatch repair and microsatellite instability-high (dMMR/MSI-H) tumors in the liver, most notably CRCLM. dMMR tumors were early on shown to respond to immune checkpoint inhibition across tumor types, likely as a result of higher mutation burden, leading to more immunogenicity[147]; this has led to the first FDA approval of a drug agnostic of disease site, namely pembrolizumab for dMMR/MSI-H tumors.[148] Although hepatobiliary tumors have a low prevalence of MSI-H phenotypes, colorectal cancer has one of the highest rates at 6% to 20%.[149] Nivolumab and nivolumab plus ipilimumab have demonstrated durable response rates in MSI-H tumors, particularly in the setting of previous systemic therapy failures.[150] Most notably, pembrolizumab has recently shown superior progression-free survival compared with conventional systemic chemotherapy (16.5 months vs. 8.2 months) as first-line therapy for MSI-H metastatic CRC, further cementing the role of immunotherapy as a mainstay of treatment of unresectable CRCLM.[151]

Still in transition from concept to bedside, genetically modified chimeric antigen receptor T cells (CAR-Ts) offer another potential avenue to providing effective antitumor immunity for CRCLM. CAR-Ts are produced from patient autologous T cells, using a retroviral system to engineer expression of an immune receptor that is activated upon engagement of tumor antigens such as carcinoembryonic antigen (CEA). A phase I Hepatic Immunotherapy for Metastases (HITM) trial demonstrated the safety and encouraging signals of clinical efficacy of hepatic artery anti-CEA CAR-T infusions in patients with CRCLM.[152]

Within pancreatic adenocarcinoma, initial trials evaluating efficacy of PD-1 and PD-L1 blockade did not demonstrate any meaningful improvement in clinical outcomes[18]; multiple subsequent trials using different combinations of immunotherapy have failed to show any benefit. However, there has been recent work that aims to activate the effector component while simultaneously breaking the immunosuppressive elements. Mouse model work initially demonstrated that combination blockade of PD-1 and CXCR4 (a chemokine receptor for CXCL12, thought to be immunosuppressive and produced by cancer-associated fibroblasts) yielded tumor killing in a synergistic way.[153] This was confirmed by our work using an organotypic slice culture model of PDA, in which ex vivo treatment of combination PD-1 monoclonal antibody and AMD3100 (an FDA-approved CXCR4 inhibitor) released T cells from the stroma, allowing them to get adjacent to tumor cells and then achieve tumor kill.[134,154] The recent phase II COMBAT trial in metastatic PDA using combination CXCR4 and PD-1 blockade confirmed the increase in CD8 T-cell infiltration while decreasing MDSC and Treg populations; furthermore, it demonstrated a disease control rate of 77% out to 2 years when combined with chemotherapy.[155]

FUTURE DIRECTIONS

The examples listed above encapsulate our ability to translate understanding of the nuanced immune microenvironment of complex diseases of the liver and pancreas and to turn these concepts into targetable therapies that confirm our hypotheses in treatment settings. Much more work needs to be performed to elucidate the complex interplay between the adaptive immune response, immune tolerance, immune evasion, and suppression within morbid diseases such as HCC and PDA. However, recent advances give hope that the paradigm-shifting era of immunotherapies will soon make headway into decreasing the mortality of advanced liver and pancreatic malignancies.

The references for this chapter can be found online by accessing the accompanying Expert Consult website.

CHAPTER 11

Infections in hepatic, biliary, and pancreatic surgery

Sanket Srinivasa and Ryan C. Fields

Infections cause significant morbidity and mortality in patients undergoing hepatopancreatobiliary (HPB) surgery. In the era of more extensive resections in elderly comorbid patients with the greater use of perioperative chemoradiotherapy and biliary instrumentation, surgical-site infection (SSI) rates after HPB procedures can be as high as 20% to 40% with an added substantial risk of intraabdominal infections.[1] Infection is associated with increased hospital stay, operative times, transfusions, blood loss, intensive care unit use, and readmission rates.[2] In addition to these short-term sequelae, long-term sequelae include worse oncologic outcomes.[3] This chapter will outline the range of infectious complications that may accompany resections of the liver, biliary tree, and pancreas with important surgery-specific risk factors discussed. Potential strategies for mitigating infection risk in the perioperative period are also discussed.

RISK FACTORS FOR SURGICAL-SITE INFECTION

There are inherent protective host mechanisms within the liver and pancreas (Table 11.1; see Chapter 10). Some of these are altered in the perioperative phase or from the pathology mandating intervention, such as bacterial colonization of bile from preoperative stenting or instrumentation of the hepatic inflow.[4,5] There are two important sources of risk regarding the development of a postoperative SSI. Both *patient*-specific factors and *surgery*-related factors combine to yield varying degrees of risk. Surgery-related risk factors are discussed specifically as they pertain to hepatic, pancreatic, and biliary operations.

Patient-Related Risk Factors

Patient-related risk factors may not always be modifiable at the time of operation, but it is important to be aware of them while the patient receives care. They include age, nutritional status, diabetes, smoking, obesity, coexisting infections at a remote body site, colonization with microorganisms, altered immune response, and length of preoperative stay.[6] Interventions to modify these risk factors can be employed throughout the perioperative period from initial consultation until long-term follow-up (Tables 11.2 to 11.4).

SURGERY-SPECIFIC RISK FACTORS

Hepatic Resection (See Chapters 101 and 102)

Preoperative Risk Mitigation

Hepatic resection removes Kupffer cell mass, which is the liver's principal mechanism for clearing the portal inflow of enteric microorganisms and their associated toxins. Hepatic resection also decreases bile production with a consequent impairment of the chemical and immunologic effects of bile salts. Resection with biliary reconstruction or biliary stenting also bypasses the sphincter of Oddi and predisposes patients to bilioenteric reflux and cholangitis.[4] Depending on the extent of resection, a normal healthy liver in a reasonable surgical candidate may be able to compensate for these changes. However, this may not be the case for the patient with diseased liver parenchyma. The preoperative mitigation of the risk of postoperative infectious complications after hepatic resection therefore begins with a full appreciation of the preexisting condition of the patient's liver. Adjunctive assessments such as liver biopsy and measurement of portal venous pressures may be necessary when there is uncertainty concerning the health of the liver.

Yang and colleagues (2014)[32] found cirrhosis and hepatolithiasis to be independent preoperative risk factors for the development of postoperative SSIs. Garwood and colleagues (2004)[33] showed that the extent of hepatic resection, age, and comorbidity is associated with postoperative infectious complications. Schindl and colleagues (2005)[34] established a relationship among the extent of resection, residual liver volume, and the development of infection. Although a precise residual liver volume to predict postoperative infection could not be found, there was a significant relationship linking severe hepatic dysfunction and postoperative infection (see Chapter 102). Furthermore, severe hepatic dysfunction could be predicted by small residual liver volume and high body mass index (BMI). Nanashima and colleagues (2014)[35] similarly demonstrated that liver failure was significantly associated with deep SSIs. A recent study has similarly proposed that the future liver remnant (FLR) should be more than 45% in patients older than 69 to minimize postoperative complications including sepsis.[36]

If the risk of postoperative hepatic dysfunction is deemed too high for formal resection, then other treatment modalities may be needed. For example, parenchymal-sparing techniques, such as segmental hepatectomy (see Chapter 102B), ablation (see Chapters 95 and 96), or arterial-based modalities (see Chapters 94, 97, and 100) may be required. Preoperative portal vein embolization can be considered in certain patients in whom the FLR volume is too low and/or of poor quality. There is also increasing enthusiasm in facilitating resection by using hepatic vein embolization or ALPPS (see Chapters 102C and 102D). When the risk of postoperative complications is prohibitive, then *not* operating or ablating may be the prudent course of action. It should, however, be noted that nonoperative strategies such as yttrium-90 radioembolization are also associated with infectious complications,[5] and efficacy for many of these modalities has yet to be established.

The use of systemic chemotherapy is increasingly common in the overall treatment plan for patients undergoing hepatic resection, especially in patients with colorectal liver metastases (see Chapters 50 and 97–99). Neoadjuvant chemotherapy may increase the risk of infection due to its negative effects on the

TABLE 11.1   Normal Host Defense Mechanisms in the Hepatobiliary System and Pancreas

	HEPATOBILIARY	PANCREAS
Physical	Biliary sphincter	Pancreatic sphincter
	Hepatic tight junctions	Pancreatic tight junctions
	Bile flow	Pancreatic juice flow
	Mucus	Mucus
	Cilia	Cilia
Chemical	Bile salts	Pancreatic fluid
Immunologic	Kupffer cells	—
	Immunoglobulin A	Immunoglobulin A
	Fibronectin	Complement
	Complement	

liver, including steatosis, steatohepatitis, and sinusoidal obstruction syndrome (see Chapter 69). It is, however, an important part of multimodal management of hepatic tumors, especially colorectal liver metastases, and confers superior oncologic outcome.[37] Scilletta and colleagues (2014)[38] suggested that neoadjuvant chemotherapy was *not* a significant risk factor for SSIs in patients undergoing liver resection for colorectal hepatic metastases.

Nordlinger and colleagues (2008)[39] conducted a randomized controlled trial comparing liver resection for resectable colorectal liver metastases in patients with and without perioperative chemotherapy. Perioperative chemotherapy was defined as six cycles of 5-fluororuracil plus leucovorin and oxaliplatin (FOLFOX4) before and after surgery. There were 182 patients within each arm of the study. Infectious complications that were analyzed included wound, intraabdominal, and urinary infections. There was a trend toward higher rates of these complications in the perioperative chemotherapy group, but it was not statistically significant. In the setting of resectable colorectal cancer liver metastasis, chemotherapy before hepatectomy is safe from a postoperative infectious standpoint and remains indicated overall to achieve optimal oncologic outcomes. Liver-directed chemotherapy via hepatic artery infusion pumps also does not seem to increase the risk of infectious complications[40] (see Chapters 69, 97, and 98).

Preoperative nutrition also requires careful consideration. A recent review by Walcott-Sapp et al. (2018)[41] has expanded on the importance of recognizing malnutrition before hospital admission and considering oral supplementation with high-calorie, high-protein drinks and avoiding unnecessary preoperative fasting in the immediate preoperative phase. A recent trial by Russell et al. (2019)[42] also evaluated the value of immunonutrition in patients undergoing elective hepatectomy, but the majority of patients did not have malnutrition and there were no differences in outcome between the two groups (see Chapters 26 and 27).

Other preoperative contributors to postoperative infectious complications after hepatic resection include advanced age, presence of diabetes mellitus, obesity, presence of an open wound, hypernatremia, hypoalbuminemia, elevated serum bilirubin, dialysis, comorbid conditions, repeat hepatectomy, and hepatic steatosis.[33,42–47] Because many of these preexisting conditions may not be modifiable before the time of operation, any resection must be considered in light of the general condition of the patient.

Operative Risk Mitigation

There are several operative risk factors that are associated with postoperative infectious complications. These include bile leaks, surgery duration, increased blood loss, and iatrogenic bowel perforation.[35,44,45,48–50] It is thus important to mitigate these factors; one deliberate strategy can be intraoperative identification and treatment of bile leaks. Numerous strategies have been proposed for this including the use of indocyanine green, methylene blue, hydrogen peroxide, or air[51] (see Chapters 24 and 25).

An intraoperative air leak test has been shown to be effective in the detection of bile leaks, thus, decreasing the rate of postoperative biliary complications.[52] This maneuver involves the placement of a transcystic catheter that is used to inject air into the biliary tree after the upper abdomen is submerged in saline and the distal common bile duct is occluded. Bile leaks are identified at the site of streaming air bubbles and are directly repaired. The authors compared the rates of postoperative biliary complications among 103 patients who underwent air-leak testing and 120 matched patients who underwent hepatic resection before air-leak testing was used. None of the hepatic resections in either group were accompanied by biliary reconstruction. The authors noted a significantly lower rate of postoperative bile leaks in the air leak–tested group (1.9% vs. 10.8%, $P = .001$).

Minimally invasive approaches (laparoscopic/robotic) have also reported lower rates of wound infections and lower rates of pulmonary complications with comparable rates of bile leak and noninferior oncologic outcomes.[53,54] Although laparoscopic liver resections are commonly used for minor hepatectomy, major hepatectomy is also increasingly performed using minimally invasive techniques.[55]

Regarding parenchymal transection techniques, no one method or combination of methods has been shown to be convincingly superior, although a recent network meta-analysis has suggested (with significant caveats) that energy devices may be best in reducing overall complications[56] (see Chapter 118). It is thus recommended that the surgeon use the technique that is most familiar, while limiting the amount of necrotic liver parenchyma left behind.[57] It is also important to suction any pooled blood and bile at the end of the operation.

Perioperative Antibiotics

A reasonable approach to the prevention of SSI in the setting of hepatic resection would be to administer antimicrobial prophylaxis for all elective hepatic resections regardless of anticipated bilioenteric reconstruction. The recommended antimicrobial agent for biliary tract procedures from the Clinical Practice Guidelines for Antimicrobial Prophylaxis (https://www.ashp.org) is cefazolin. This online resource is frequently updated and can be used to guide antibiotic choice in line with institutional considerations. Other options include cefoxitin because it is a single agent with broad coverage. Whatever agent is used, it should be given within 60 minutes of skin incision and re-administered appropriately intraoperatively to maintain adequate tissue levels. There is no evidence to support routine use of postoperative antibiotics.

Drains

The rationale for leaving an intraabdominal drain is to detect and prevent biloma formation in the event of bile leakage after hepatic resection (see Chapters 28 and 118). Bile leakage and

TABLE 11.2 General Preoperative Interventions to Prevent Surgical-Site Infection

INTERVENTION	EVIDENCE	REFERENCES
Reduce hemoglobin A1c levels to <7% before operation	Class II data	Mangram et al. (1999)[7]
Smoking cessation 30 days before operation	Class II data	Mangram et al. (1999)[7]
Administer specialized nutritional supplements or enteral nutrition to patients at severe nutritional risk for 7-14 days preoperatively; preoperative parenteral nutrition should not be routinely used, except selectively in patients with severe underlying malnutrition	Class I and class II data with significant heterogeneity	Anonymous (1991)[8]; Mangram et al. (1999)[7]; Weimann et al. (2006)[9]
Adequately treat preoperative infections, such as urinary tract infections	Class II data	Mangram et al. (1999)[7]

Modified from Horan TC, Gaynes RP, Martone WJ, Jarvis W, Emori TG. CDC definitions of nosocomial surgical site infections: a modification of CDC definitions of surgical wound infections. *Infect Control Hosp Epidemiol.* 1992;13:606–608.

TABLE 11.3 General Perioperative Interventions to Prevent Surgical-Site Infection

INTERVENTION	EVIDENCE	REFERENCES
Remove hair only if it will interfere with the operation; hair removal by clipping immediately before the operation or with depilatories; no preoperative or perioperative shaving of surgical site	Class I data	Anderson et al. (2008)[10]; Bratzler (2006)[11]; Kjønniksen et al. (2002)[12]; Mangram et al. (1999)[7]; Springer (2007)[13]
Use an antiseptic surgical scrub or alcohol-based hand antiseptic for preoperative cleansing of the operative team members' hands and forearms	Class II data	Anderson et al. (2008)[10]; Mangram et al. (1999)[7]
Prepare the skin around the operative site with an appropriate antiseptic agent, including preparations based on alcohol, chlorhexidine, or iodine/iodophors	Class II data	Anderson et al. (2008)[10]; Digison (2007)[14]; Mangram et al. (1999)[7]
Administer prophylactic antibiotics for most clean-contaminated and contaminated procedures, and selected clean procedures; use antibiotics appropriate for the potential pathogens	Strong class I data	Anonymous (1999)[15]; Bratzler (2006)[11]; Classen et al. (1992)[16]; Mangram et al. (1999)[7]; Springer (2007)[13]
Administer prophylactic antibiotics within 1 hr before incision (2 hr for vancomycin and fluoroquinolones)	Strong class II data	Anonymous (1999)[15]; Bratzler (2006)[11]; Classen et al. (1992)[16]; Mangram et al. (1999)[7]; Springer (2007)[13]
Use higher dosages of prophylactic antibiotics for morbidly obese patients	Limited class II data	Forse et al. (1989)[17]; Mangram et al. (1999)[7]
Use vancomycin as a prophylactic agent only when there is a significant risk of MRSA infection	Class I data	Anderson et al. (2008)[10]; Anonymous (1999)[15]; Bolon et al. (2004)[18]; Finkelstein et al. (2002)[19]; Mangram et al. (1999)[7]
Provide adequate ventilation, minimize operating room traffic, and clean instruments and surfaces with approved disinfectants	Class II and class III data	Anderson et al. (2008)[10]; Mangram et al. (1999)[7]
Avoid "flash" sterilization	Class II data	Anderson et al. (2008)[10]; Mangram et al. (1999)[7]
Carefully handle tissue, eradicate dead space, and adhere to standard principles of asepsis	Class III data	Anderson et al. (2008)[10]; Mangram et al. (1999)[7]
Leave contaminated or dirty infected wounds open, with the possible exception of wounds following operations for perforated appendicitis	Limited class I, class II data	Brasel et al. (1997)[20]; Cohn et al. (2001)[21]; Mangram et al. (1999)[7]
Redose prophylactic antibiotics with short half-lives intraoperatively if operation is prolonged (for cefazolin if operation >3 hr) or if there is extensive blood loss	Limited class I, class II data	Mangram et al. (1999)[7]; Scher (1997)[22]; Swoboda et al. (1996)[23]
Maintain intraoperative normothermia	Class I data, some contradictory class II data	Anderson et al. (2008)[10]; Barone et al. (1999)[24]; Bratzler (2006)[11]; Mangram et al. (1999)[7]; Sessler & Akca (2002)[25]; Springer (2007)[13]; Walz et al. (2006)[26]

MRSA, Methicillin-resistant *Staphylococcus aureus.*

Modified from Kirby JP, Mazuski JE. Prevention of SSI. *Surg Clin North Am.* 2009;89(2):365–389, viii.

TABLE 11.4	General Postoperative Interventions to Prevent Surgical-Site Infection		
INTERVENTION		**EVIDENCE**	**REFERENCES**
Discontinue prophylactic antibiotics within 24 hours after the procedure (48 hr for cardiac surgery and liver transplant procedures); preferably, discontinue prophylactic antibiotics after skin closure		Class I data	Anonymous (1999)[15]; Bratzler (2006)[11]; DiPiro et al. (1986)[27]; Mangram et al. (1999)[7]; Springer (2007)[13]
Maintain serum glucose levels <200 mg/dL on postoperative days 1 and 2		Class II data	Anderson et al. (2008)[10]; Bratzler (2006)[11]; Carr et al. (2005)[28]; Furnary et al. (1999)[29]; Lazar et al. (2004)[30]; Springer (2007)[13]; Zerr et al. (1997)[31]
Monitor wound for the development of surgical-site infection		Class III data	Anderson et al. (2008)[10]; Mangram et al. (1999)[7]

Modified from Kirby JP, Mazuski JE. Prevention of SSI. *Surg Clin North Am.* 2009;89(2):365–389, viii.

subsequent biloma formation is an important contributor to infectious complications after hepatic resection. However, the overall trend reflected in the literature does not support the routine use of drains in elective hepatic surgery. Foregoing prophylactic drainage after elective hepatic surgery is consistent with the general notion that drainage may be unnecessary in most gastrointestinal (GI) operations. Petrowsky and colleagues (2004)[58] studied the value of prophylactic drainage in GI surgery in a systematic review and meta-analysis, concluding that many GI operations can be safely performed without the use of drains. Regarding liver surgery specifically, this article suggests that surgical drains do not necessarily prevent biloma formation and do not always prevent the need for percutaneous drainage. A grade A recommendation was given against prophylactic drainage in elective hepatic resection. This is supported by several randomized studies[59–61] and a systematic review.[62] A more recent multicenter international prospective study also concluded that intraoperatively placed surgical drains do not prevent the need for additional percutaneous drainage.[63] Another study evaluating hepatectomy within the United States showed that routine drain placement did not prevent nor diagnose bile leaks and was associated with more interventions, a higher rate of readmissions, and longer length of stay.[64] However, practical considerations such as urgent access to image-guided drain insertion postoperatively if required often affect clinical decision making and individual high-risk cases (e.g., central resections, complex nonanatomical resections, and high bilioenteric anastomosis) may warrant prophylactic drain placement. A reasonable strategy may be to avoid routine drain placement unless specific concerns exist and remove drains as early as possible postoperatively.

Postoperative Risk Mitigation (see Chapter 27)
Nasogastric Decompression

Pessaux and colleagues (2007)[65] conducted a randomized clinical trial examining the utility of postoperative nasogastric decompression after elective hepatectomy. The authors randomized 200 patients to nasogastric tube use versus no nasogastric tube. The use of a nasogastric tube was significantly associated with an increased rate of pneumonia and atelectasis but did not reduce overall surgical complications, medical morbidity, in-hospital mortality, duration of ileus, or length of hospital stay. The authors concluded that routine nasogastric decompression offers no benefit. A recent randomized trial confirmed this finding.[66] There is no role for routine nasogastric tube placement in elective hepatectomy.

Early Enteral Nutrition and Enhanced Recovery Pathways

The concept of early enteral nutrition has been studied in patients undergoing liver resection. Richter and colleagues (2006)[67]

conducted a systematic review of early enteral nutrition following open liver resection, concluding that it is safe and that it decreases the incidence of postoperative complications compared with parenteral nutrition. The authors noted a statistically significant lower rate of wound infections and catheter-related infections with early enteral feeding versus parenteral nutrition. However, pneumonias and intraabdominal abscesses were not significantly decreased. It should be noted that enteral nutrition in this review was, in general, started on the second postoperative day via an operative jejunal tube. Placement of jejunal feeding catheters in the otherwise healthy liver resection patient is not to be encouraged. In general, resumption of oral intake with caloric supplementation as soon as practical is recommended unless contraindicated, in which case enteral nutrition is preferable to parenteral nutrition.

Enhanced recovery after surgery (ERAS) pathways have shown promise in improving postoperative outcomes in patients undergoing liver surgery[68] (see Chapter 27). Important components of ERAS pathways include continuing nutrition as long as 2 hours before hepatic resection, avoidance of a nasogastric tube, and early postoperative diet resumption. A recent randomized trial has shown decreased overall complications, although there was no statistically significant differences in infectious complications likely due to a small sample size.[69] An updated systematic review similarly shows decreased overall complications in two of four trials.[70] ERAS pathways should therefore be considered for those patients undergoing routine hepatectomy.

Blood Glucose Control

Dysglycemia has been studied in patients undergoing hepatectomy specifically. Huo and colleagues (2003)[71] demonstrated increased hepatic decompensation in diabetic patients undergoing hepatic resection for hepatocellular carcinoma. Little and colleagues (2002)[72] showed an association with increased mortality in diabetic patients undergoing hepatectomy for colorectal cancer metastasis. Ambiru and colleagues (2008)[73] and Li and associates (2017)[74] demonstrated an increase in SSI in HPB surgery patients with poor postoperative blood glucose control. Therefore tight glycemic control is paramount after hepatectomy and can be achieved using sliding scales and continuous insulin infusions.

Preoperative Biliary Drainage in the Hilar Cholangiocarcinoma Patient (see Chapter 51B)

Preoperative biliary drainage before hepatic resection for extrahepatic hilar cholangiocarcinoma requires careful consideration. Postoperative outcomes after liver resection tend to be worse in patients with obstructive jaundice.[75] However, preoperative instrumentation of the biliary system is associated with cholangitis and increased infectious complications.[76,77] Liu and colleagues (2011)[78] concluded that preoperative drainage should not be routinely performed if it can be avoided. However, there are data to suggest that there is a role for preoperative biliary decompression in certain scenarios, including very small FLR patients[79] and perhaps for right-sided resections.[80] It is thus reasonable to consider biliary drainage via endoscopic retrograde cholangiography or percutaneous transhepatic cholangiography and portal vein embolization in patients with a very small FLR.

Pancreatic Resection

The most commonly performed resections include pancreaticoduodenectomy and distal pancreatectomy (typically with splenectomy when performed for cancer). These may also be accompanied by major vascular resection and multivisceral resection when resecting borderline resectable or locally advanced disease. Hence the studies of infectious complications after pancreatectomy focus on these two procedures. Enucleation and central pancreatectomy are less common procedures (see Chapter 117).

Infectious complications after pancreatic resection may include SSI or organ/deep space infection. The latter can be further categorized by the contributing anastomosis: intraabdominal abscesses, or infected fluid collections can be related to an infected bile, pancreatic, or enteric leak, or a combination of these. Organ/space infection after distal pancreatectomy is typically related to pancreatic leak and less commonly due to iatrogenic injury to surrounding structures (colon, stomach) (see Chapter 28). Patients are also at risk for the development of abscesses not related to anastomotic leakage or secondary to an infected hematoma. Furthermore, these patients can develop infections in remote sites, including bloodstream infections, cholangitis, respiratory tract infections, urinary tract infections, and *Clostridium difficile* infections.

General risk factors for SSI discussed earlier apply to patients undergoing pancreatic resection; however, there are risk factors specific to pancreatic resection that warrant discussion including potential strategies to decrease incidence or limit consequences by prompt diagnosis and initiation of treatment.

Preoperative Risk Mitigation
Age

Elderly patients undergoing pancreatic resection may not necessarily be at higher risk of infectious complications but are more likely to experience a greater decline in function and higher mortality if they have a complication that is suggestive of diminished physiologic reserve.[81] It is thus worth considering overall frailty and patient comorbidity should be considered alongside the potential for oncologic gain rather than age alone.

Body Mass Index and Nutritional Status

Elevated BMI is a risk factor for infectious complications following pancreatic cancer. House and colleagues (2008)[82] studied postoperative complications in 356 patients who underwent pancreaticoduodenectomy for pancreatic adenocarcinoma with the goal of identifying preoperative patient and radiographic factors associated with postoperative morbidity. Complications developed in 38% of this patient population; the most common pancreatic complications were fistula/abscess, wound infection, and delayed gastric emptying. Wound infection rates were significantly higher in those patients with a BMI greater than or equal to 30 ($P = .03$). The authors also determined that the degree of visceral fat as seen on preoperative axial imaging correlated with higher rates of overall complications and pancreatic fistula. This may also be related to the quality of the pancreas, as a soft, fat-replaced pancreas is likely to be at increased risk of postoperative pancreatic fistula.[83]

Greenblatt and colleagues (2011)[84] used the ACS-NSQIP database in an attempt to formulate a prediction tool for patients undergoing pancreaticoduodenectomy. The authors examined preoperative factors that might predict perioperative morbidity and mortality. Although this study was not designed to predict who would incur an infectious complication specifically, the authors found that the most frequent complications after pancreaticoduodenectomy included sepsis (15.3%), SSI (13.1%), and respiratory complications (9.5%). The overall complication rate in 1342 patients was 27.1%. Elevated BMI was a significant predictor of morbidity (after adjusting for confounding variables), and morbidity increased incrementally with BMI. Other predictors included older age, male gender, dependent functional status, chronic obstructive pulmonary disease, steroid use, bleeding disorder, leukocytosis, elevated serum creatinine, and hypoalbuminemia.

Kelly and colleagues (2011)[85] attempted to identify preoperative and operative risk factors for the development of complications after distal pancreatectomy. The authors also used the multi-institutional prospective ACS-NSQIP database. Their efforts concerned the development of a risk score for patients undergoing distal pancreatectomy. The study population included 2322 patients. The overall 30-day complication and mortality rates were 28.1% and 1.2%, respectively. Similar to the analysis conducted by Greenblatt and colleagues (2011),[84] this study was not designed to specifically address infectious complications. However, the most common complications were sepsis, SSI, and pneumonia. Multivariate analysis determined that high BMI was a preoperative predictor of postoperative morbidity. The other preoperative variables associated with postoperative complications included male gender, smoking, steroid use, neurologic disease, preoperative systemic inflammatory response syndrome/sepsis, hypoalbuminemia, elevated creatinine, and abnormal platelet count.

Poor preoperative nutritional status is another important risk factor for SSI and other postoperative morbidity in patients undergoing pancreatic resection. La Torre and colleagues (2013)[86] noticed a relationship between malnutrition and morbidity after pancreatic surgery in their retrospective evaluation of data collected from 143 patients undergoing pancreatic resection for cancer. Malnutrition was defined by using several different validated screening tools and was an independent risk factor for overall morbidity, which included SSI. Shinkawa and colleagues (2013)[87] confirmed these findings in an examination of 64 patients with pancreaticoduodenectomy with regard to potential perioperative risk factors for SSI. Using multivariate logistic regression analysis on perioperative factors, the authors identified pancreatic fistula and a nutritional risk index (NRI) of 97.5 or less as independent risk factors for SSI.

As noted previously, modification of preoperative risk factors may be difficult or even impossible before pancreatectomy. This is particularly true if the indication for resection is cancer or suspicion of cancer, which is common. In these instances, proceeding to the operating room expeditiously may be the prudent course of action, especially in the clearly resectable and otherwise healthy operative candidate. However, more than one-third of patients about to undergo pancreaticoduodenectomy can be considered borderline candidates from a medical standpoint.[88] These patients are at significant risk for postoperative morbidity (including infectious complications) as well as mortality. Therefore, as suggested by Tzeng and colleagues,[99] surgeons should strongly consider improving the condition of the patient to mitigate infectious/overall morbidity and mortality in these "borderline resectable type C" patients before surgery. Those patients receiving neoadjuvant therapy should take advantage of this time and use it as a "window of opportunity" to modify BMI, improve nutritional/functional status, control hypertension, and/or quit smoking. For patients seen with surgically resectable tumors but significant reversible functional deficits, it may be worthwhile to administer neoadjuvant therapy while the patient is medically optimized. Regardless of whether neoadjuvant therapy consists of chemoradiation or chemotherapy alone, either type of preoperative therapy is considered safe with regard to postoperative complications.[89–92]

Preoperative Biliary Drainage (see Chapters 30 and 117)

Preoperative biliary drainage in the setting of an obstructing pancreatic head mass continues to be debated. Earlier studies suggested that perioperative mortality is higher when pancreaticoduodenectomy is performed in the presence of hyperbilirubinemia.[93–95] More recent work has also shown preoperative jaundice to be a poor prognostic factor with regard to overall survival for patients undergoing resection of the head of the pancreas for adenocarcinoma.[96] However, routine preoperative biliary drainage in this setting may not be ideal.

Healthy patients with an intact sphincter of Oddi and a normal biliary system have sterile bile. However, obstructive jaundice in the setting of a mass in the head of the pancreas results in bile stasis. This in turn promotes colonization of the biliary system, especially after the bile ducts are interrogated and drained via stents.[97] The presence of bacteria in the biliary system is known as *bacterobilia*. When normal host defense mechanisms present in the liver and biliary tree are overwhelmed by a critical level of bacterobilia and the biliary tree is not adequately drained, then pathogenic enteric organisms may reach the systemic circulation through the liver, causing sepsis (i.e., cholangitis).[4]

It is rare for a patient with pancreatic cancer to be seen with cholangitis without having undergone attempts at biliary decompression. However, should this happen, the required treatment is antibiotics with biliary drainage as described in the Tokyo Guidelines.[98,99] In the United States, typical drainage procedures include decompression via the percutaneous transhepatic approach or via endoscopic retrograde cholangiography. More commonly, cholangitis develops during or soon after attempted biliary decompression in the patient who is undergoing elective preoperative biliary drainage. Unfortunately, these patients who develop cholangitis preoperatively are at increased risk for postoperative complications, especially those related to infection and pancreatic fistula.[100,101]

The mere presence of bacterobilia, often related to preoperative biliary drainage, increases the risk of infectious complications in the postoperative setting.[97,102–108] Therefore preoperative biliary drainage in a patient with resectable disease should be given thoughtful consideration, especially in light of a multicenter, randomized trial that showed routine preoperative biliary drainage increases the rate of postoperative complications in general.[109]

There are patients who routinely undergo preoperative biliary drainage. One group includes those patients with borderline resectable pancreatic head cancers who receive several months of neoadjuvant therapy before surgery. Although these patients may experience an increase in postoperative infectious complications with prolonged preoperative biliary drainage, the procedure appears to be relatively safe, and its associated risks are not prohibitive.[110,111] With the increasing use of neoadjuvant chemotherapy and the requirement for tissue diagnosis via endoscopic ultrasound, it is likely that most patients will undergo preoperative stenting.

Another group of patients in whom preoperative biliary drainage may be routinely indicated includes symptomatic patients with significant jaundice who are expected to wait more than 1 week for surgical referral. Preoperative biliary drainage in this cohort also appears to be relatively safe, as demonstrated by Howard and colleagues (2006).[4] The authors of this study examined the relationship between bacterobilia (based on intraoperative bile cultures) and infectious complications in 138 patients undergoing an operation (including a biliary enteric anastomosis) for obstructive jaundice. Eighty-six (62%) patients had preoperative biliary stenting, whereas 52 (38%) did not. Ninety-one patients had bacterobilia, 69 from the stented group and 22 from the other group. Overall infectious complications occurred in 31 patients (22.4%), with the majority occurring in the stented group (23 vs. 8). However, this difference was not statistically significant. Stented patients did have a significantly higher rate of wound infection ($P = .03$) and bacteremia ($P = .04$) on subset analysis. The authors concluded that preoperative stenting increases the number of patients with positive intraoperative bile cultures, bacteremia, and wound infection. However, they also noted that preoperative stenting does not increase overall infectious morbidity, noninfectious morbidity, mortality, or hospital length of stay. The authors ultimately state that preoperative biliary drainage is not unreasonable in the jaundiced patient awaiting referral to an appropriate surgical center.

Operative Risk Mitigation (see Chapter 117)
Preoperative Antibiotics

The current Clinical Practice Guidelines for Antimicrobial Prophylaxis recommend a single preoperative dose of cefazolin. The guidelines do not recommend continuing antimicrobial coverage beyond 24 hours postoperatively. Despite these guidelines, antimicrobial prophylaxis specifically for pancreatic resections has not been well evaluated in terms of the specific agent to use and its duration. Donald and colleagues (2013)[112] suggested that guideline-recommended antimicrobial prophylaxis may not be appropriate for patients undergoing pancreaticoduodenectomy. They presented an argument for broadening perioperative antibiotic coverage with the use of piperacillin-tazobactam. Other authors have advocated for the selection of perioperative antimicrobial prophylaxis that is based on preoperative bile cultures obtained at the time of preoperative biliary drainage.[113,114] An option is to administer cefoxitin preoperatively for reasons previously mentioned in the section "Hepatic Resection."

Wound Protectors

Dual-ring wound protectors are increasingly used in open abdominal surgery as they provide retraction and decrease the incidence of SSIs.[115] In two trials evaluating their use in pancreaticoduodenectomy, conflicting results have been obtained.

The study by Bressan et al. (2018)[116] showed a significant decrease in SSI (21% vs. 44%) in patients randomized to receiving wound retractors. All patients in this study had preoperative biliary stents. The trial by De Pastena et al. (2020),[117] however, did not demonstrate any improvement in SSI in patients who were randomized to receiving wound protectors (7% in both groups, $P = .59$), even when the groups were stratified by whether preoperative biliary stenting was required (9% vs. 8%, $P = .54$). The difference in outcomes may be explained by the low baseline incidence of SSI in the study by De Pastena et al. A pragmatic approach may thus be to consider the use of wound protectors depending on the patient's individual risk of SSI (e.g., whether they have had preoperative stents, etc.), the additional exposure provided in terms of retraction, and the institutional incidence of SSI to determine whether a clinically significant improvement is likely to be seen.

Other Operative Risk Factors

Pancreatic fistula is one of the most important risk factors determining postoperative morbidity following pancreatic resection.[87,118,119] Behrman and colleagues (2008)[118] retrospectively studied 196 pancreatectomy patients with an aim to identify risk factors for intraabdominal sepsis. Approximately 16% of these patients developed an infected intraabdominal fluid collection, and overt pancreatic fistula as well as soft pancreatic remnants, were found to be statistically significant factors associated with its development. The authors also observed that infected fluid collections may occur relatively early in the postoperative course, and surgeons should have a low threshold to image and drain these collections.

Sugiura and colleagues (2012)[119] retrospectively examined risk factors for SSI in 408 patients who underwent pancreaticoduodenectomy. An incisional SSI developed in 61 patients, whereas an organ/space infection developed in 195 patients. The following were identified as significant risk factors for incisional SSI on multivariate analysis: length of operation greater than 480 minutes (odds ratio [OR], 3.22), main pancreatic diameter less than or equal to 3 mm (OR, 2.18), and abdominal wall thickness greater than 10 mm (OR, 2.16). Also, the following were significant risk factors for the development of organ/space SSI: pancreatic fistula (OR, 7.56), use of semi-closed drainage system (OR, 3.68), BMI greater than 23.5 (OR, 3.04), main pancreatic duct diameter less than or equal to 3 mm (OR, 2.21), and operation longer than 480 minutes (OR, 1.78).

Schmidt and colleagues (2009)[120] studied preoperative and perioperative risk factors for the development of a pancreatic fistula in pancreaticoduodenectomy patients. Their multivariate analysis showed that an invaginated pancreatic anastomosis and closed suction intraperitoneal drainage were predictive of a pancreatic fistula, whereas chronic pancreatitis and preoperative biliary stenting were protective of a pancreatic fistula. Schoellhammer and associates (2014)[121] have suggested that no one pancreatic anastomosis is superior and that more studies are needed to identify the best anastomotic technique. Recent work has suggested that externalized pancreatic duct stents may decrease pancreatic fistulae in high-risk anastomoses.[122]

A recent randomized trial studied pasireotide as a possible adjunct to prevent postoperative pancreatic fistula.[123] Pasireotide is a somatostatin analogue with a longer half-life than octreotide. The authors randomly assigned 300 patients undergoing either pancreaticoduodenectomy or distal pancreatectomy to either perioperative pasireotide or placebo. The primary end point was the occurrence of pancreatic fistula, leak, or abscess of grade 3 or higher. This end point was significantly lower in those patients treated with pasireotide (9% vs. 21%, $P = .006$). The authors concluded that this perioperative medication decreases the rate of clinically significant postoperative fistula, leak, or abscess in patients undergoing pancreatic resection. These findings, however, have not been widely replicated in other institutions in nonrandomized studies.[124]

Pancreatic fistula remains a clinically relevant problem in distal pancreatectomy also. Hamilton and colleagues (2012)[125] conducted a randomized controlled trial examining the efficacy of mesh-reinforced stapled closure of the distal pancreas. The authors randomly assigned 54 patients to mesh reinforcement and 46 patients to non-mesh reinforcement, in which the primary outcome was clinically significant pancreatic leak. International Study Group of Pancreatic Fistula (ISGPF) grade B and C leaks occurred more frequently in the patients without mesh reinforcement (20% vs. 1.9%, $P = .0007$).

Other operative risk factors contributing to postoperative infectious morbidity after pancreatic resection include longer operative times[114,119,126–128] and need for perioperative blood transfusion.[126] Procter and colleagues (2010)[127] performed a retrospective analysis of 299,359 general surgical procedures (including pancreatectomy), identified through the ACS-NSQIP database, looking for risk factors associated with infectious complications. Their multivariate analysis suggested that increased operative duration is an independent risk factor for infectious complications and hospital length of stay. This was confirmed by Ball and colleagues (2010),[126] who conducted a retrospective analysis on only pancreaticoduodenectomy patients identified via the ACS-NSQIP database. Their study involved 4817 patients and determined that longer operative times were associated with both morbidity and mortality. Also, there was a linear relationship between preoperative RBC transfusion and 30-day morbidity. This led the authors to suggest blood transfusion and operative time as quality indicators for pancreaticoduodenectomy.

The use of intraperitoneal drains remains contentious among pancreatic surgeons. Despite a large amount of literature within the recent past suggesting that intraperitoneal drainage may be unnecessary and even harmful,[129–136] a randomized prospective multicenter trial concluded that "elimination of intraperitoneal drainage in all cases of pancreaticoduodenectomy increases the frequency and severity of complications."[137] This most recent study randomized 137 patients undergoing pancreaticoduodenectomy. Half of the patients had an intraperitoneal drain left in place, whereas the other half did not. These patients were followed prospectively for a range of complications. The study was stopped early because there was a substantial difference in mortality between the two groups. The drained patients had a mortality of 3%, whereas the undrained group experienced a 12% mortality rate. Beyond this, pancreaticoduodenectomy without intraperitoneal drainage was significantly associated with an increase in the number of complications per patient, an increase in the number of patients who had at least one complication rated at grade 2 or higher, and a higher average complications severity. From an infectious standpoint, pancreaticoduodenectomy without intraperitoneal drainage was associated with a higher rate of intraabdominal abscess (25% vs. 10%, $P = .027$). This study therefore provides strong evidence supporting the placement of intraperitoneal drains at the time of pancreaticoduodenectomy. Taken in the context of other contemporary literature on this subject, the best approach to peritoneal drainage remains unclear and should be individualized to the specific patient. Also, placing a drain intraoperatively does not always obviate the need for a percutaneous drainage procedure in the early postoperative period.[131] If placed at the time of pancreaticoduodenectomy, the timing of drain removal is also controversial. Recent prospective studies, including a randomized trial, have suggested that early drain removal based on drain amylase levels can lower the rate of postoperative complications, including infectious ones.[138,139] A reasonable strategy would be to leave a non-suction drain posterior to the pancreaticojejunostomy and measure daily drain amylase for the first 3 postoperative days and remove the drain on day 3 if drain amylase is less than 30 and outputs are acceptable in quantity and character in an otherwise well patient.

Minimally invasive pancreatic resections, either laparoscopic or robotic, have begun to be implemented worldwide and are discussed separately in a dedicated chapter (see Chapter 127). Laparoscopic distal pancreatectomy has been shown to be associated with improved short-term outcomes, decreased blood loss, and decreased infectious complications.[140] Minimally invasive pancreaticoduodenectomy has a steep learning curve and may be regarded as in the evaluation stage outside of high-volume expert centers. In one study evaluating the last decade of outcomes across the United States, laparoscopic pancreaticoduodenectomy was associated with decreased pulmonary complications although no formal data on infectious complications were reported.[141]

To summarize, risk mitigation at the operative level for a pancreaticoduodenectomy or distal pancreatectomy consists of the efficient performance of the operation using careful operative technique in an effort to avoid unnecessary blood loss. There are no universally agreed on techniques to reduce pancreatic fistula during the performance of pancreaticoduodenectomy. The pancreaticoenteric anastomosis during pancreaticoduodenectomy is still performed according to surgeon preference but must be done meticulously. With regard to distal pancreatectomy, stapled closure of the pancreas with bioabsorbable mesh buttress appears promising in the prevention of pancreatic fistula. Perioperative administration of pasireotide has demonstrated efficacy in reducing pancreatic fistula after pancreaticoduodenectomy and distal pancreatectomy in one study but is not otherwise widely used. The use of intraperitoneal drains and the timing of their removal remain controversial, but most surgeons use drains especially after pancreaticoduodenectomy. Minimally invasive techniques confer benefit in distal pancreatectomy and remain under evaluation for pancreaticoduodenectomy.

Postoperative Risk Mitigation (see Chapter 27)

Two hundred and sixty-five HPB surgery patients were studied by Ambiru and colleagues (2008)[73] and were prospectively evaluated for the development of SSI. Multivariate analysis showed that poor postoperative blood glucose was an independent risk factor for SSI. The rate of SSI was 20% in those patients with blood glucose levels below 200 versus 52% in those without insulin infusion therapy ($P < .01$). Therefore blood glucose control in the postoperative setting is of particular concern in the post-pancreatectomy patient, especially because some patients who were not previously diabetic may eventually require insulin therapy.

A high proportion of patients undergoing pancreatic resection experience some sort of complication with infectious complications being relatively common. It is not unreasonable therefore to *expect* a complication and remain vigilant to avoid "failure-to-rescue" scenarios. Early detection of deviation from the normal postoperative course must be recognized with prompt diagnosis and treatment of complications.

Infectious Complications and Oncologic Outcome

The oncologic outcomes from HPB malignancy remain poor with a few notable exceptions (e.g., colorectal liver metastases). An increasing body of evidence shows that postoperative complications not only delay immediate recovery but also worsen long-term oncologic outcome.[3,142] This may be partly due to an inability to receive adjuvant therapy but also has to do with postoperative immune modulation adversely impacting tumor biology. Decreasing the burden of infectious complications is thus paramount from both a perioperative and oncologic standpoint.

SUMMARY

HPB surgery is increasingly carried out in elderly patients often with advanced malignancy. Infectious complications are a major contributor to morbidity and mortality but can be addressed throughout the perioperative period using patient-specific and institutional interventions to mitigate risk and improve perioperative and oncologic outcomes.

References are available at expertconsult.com.

PART 2

Diagnostic Techniques

CHAPTER 12

Clinical investigation of hepatopancreatobiliary and pancreatic disease

Marco Massani and Tommaso Stecca

INTRODUCTION

The clinical approach to the patient diagnosed with hepatopancreatobiliary (HPB) disease must be systematic without neglecting clinical elements that could prove illuminating in the diagnostic process. The correct interpretation of symptoms and signs could be challenging, demanding great judgment, because even subtle clinical manifestations may forecast unattended events. A meticulous, detailed history and physical examination, followed by a few laboratory tests, are of great value. The clinical history should focus on the symptoms of HPB disease and their nature and pattern of onset and progression as well as potential risk factors. The modern and almost ubiquitous availability of second-level radiologic or endoscopic investigations must not subtract the physician from the analytical approach to the patient; "scan first, clinic later" must be avoided.

This chapter describes the common symptoms and signs of HPB disease, the value of basic investigations, and how this initial assessment guides further management. Clinical presentations and investigations of specific HPB diseases are also detailed.

LIVER DISEASE

The liver is an organ with a broad set of critical biologic functions, a unique dual vascular supply, and several distinct cell types that contribute to its physiologic functions and its potential pathology. Liver disease encompasses infectious, malignant, and chronic disease processes arising from a wide range of etiologies, which generally present with a few clinical patterns classified as hepatocellular, cholestatic, or mixed.[1] In hepatocellular diseases (e.g., steatosis, alcoholic liver disease [ALD], and viral hepatitis), the clinical and biochemical scenario is dominated by liver damage, inflammation, and necrosis. In cholestatic diseases (e.g., bile duct—gallstones or malignant—obstruction, biliary cirrhosis), bile flow obstruction predominates. In the mixed form, both characteristics are present.

The results from the last Global Burden of Diseases, Injuries, and Risk Factors Study (GBD) on the burden of chronic liver disease (CLD) revealed that globally in 2017, cirrhosis caused more than 1.32 million deaths (66.6% in males) compared with less than 899,000 deaths in 1990. These deaths constituted 2.4% of all deaths, with an age-standardized death rate of 16.5 per 100,000 population, which was at its lowest in the high-income countries and at its highest in sub-Saharan Africa. Globally, 31.5% of cirrhosis deaths in males were caused by hepatitis B, followed by alcohol-related liver disease (27.3%), hepatitis C (25.5%), nonalcoholic steatohepatitis (NASH; 7.7%), and other causes (8.0%). In females, hepatitis C (26.7%) was the leading cause, followed by hepatitis B (24.0%), alcohol-related liver disease (20.6%), NASH (11.3%),

and other causes (17.3%).[2] However, the scenario of CLDs in the United States has changed over the past 30 years. Hepatitis C is decreasing, whereas hepatitis B and alcohol-related liver disease remain stable. In contrast, the prevalence of nonalcoholic fatty liver disease (NAFLD) is increasing alongside the epidemic of obesity and type-2 diabetes mellitus (T2DM).[3] In 2014, in the United States, the average yearly healthcare expenses in patients with CLD was $19,390 dollars, with nationwide healthcare expenses estimated at $29.9 billion (2.6% of the total nationwide for adults; see Chapters 68, 69, and 74).[4]

Many patients come to the clinician's attention not because of complaints of symptoms but because of the alteration of biochemical liver enzyme (aminotransferases) or function test results (prothrombin time/INR [PT/INR], bilirubin, and albumin) as part of routine physical examination or screening blood tests.[5] Almost 10% to 17% of patients with unexplained liver enzyme elevation have previously unsuspected CLD.[6] Clinicians should be able to accurately and efficiently recognize CLD given the high prevalence of morbidity associated with the liver tests and their significant costs and the consequences associated with cirrhosis. The patient evaluation path should lead to the determination of the etiologic diagnosis, severity (grading), and stage of disease.

CLINICAL HISTORY

The physician should begin the history by focusing on the symptoms of liver disease (the nature, pattern of onset and progression) and on potential risk factors to provide clues toward the underlying etiology of liver injury, which may help to differentiate acute injury from CLD. The duration of liver injury, particularly in the absence of symptoms, is not always certain. The clinical history should then proceed with a systematic inquiry into family history, drug history, social circumstances, employment, and travel. Commonly, it is the set of symptoms and the way in which they have arisen, rather than a specific symptom, that directs the determination of etiology.[7]

Presenting symptoms may include abdominal discomfort, anorexia, nausea, vomiting, fatigue, malaise, fever, rash, itching, or jaundice.

Fatigue (described as lethargy, weakness, malaise, an increased need for sleep, or a loss of energy) is the most common and characteristic symptom. Typically, fatigue arises after exertion and is often intermittent and variable in severity. Abdominal pain is a common presenting symptom to be investigated for site, severity, radiation, and the rapidity of onset. Localization in the right upper quadrant, because of the distention or irritation of the richly innervated Glisson capsule, is usually marked by tenderness over the liver area. Severe pain may also indicate gallbladder disease, liver abscess, veno-occlusive disease, or acute hepatitis. A history of weight loss may point to a malignant process. Nausea and vomiting should be recorded along with a history of itching, jaundice, and the color of urine and stools. Jaundice is the hallmark symptom of liver disease and is best detected by the examination of the sclera or the mucous membranes below the tongue. The loss of functioning hepatocellular mass leads to hypoalbuminemia, which can manifest as a shortness of breath, ankle swelling, abdominal distension, and ascites, all of which can occur in many acute and chronic HPB disorders. Gastroesophageal varices and splenomegaly are consequences of portal hypertension and can clinically manifest as hematemesis or melena, thus requiring urgent endoscopic investigation. The increased peripheral conversion to estrogen resulting from the decreased hepatic metabolism and catabolism of androstenedione results in palmar erythema, spider nevi, gynecomastia, decreased body hair, and testicular atrophy. Terry nails (white nails) are characterized by a silver-white pallor that can range from the proximal to the entire nail bed, obscuring the nail lunula.

Accurate recording of alcohol intake is important in assessing the cause of liver disease, focusing on whether alcohol abuse or dependence is present (the CAGE questionnaire is recommended)[8] and on planning management and treatment because heavy alcohol use impacts CLD outcomes.

A past medical history should be obtained and include any major illnesses and any abdominal surgery. A record of comorbidities and exercise tolerance should be made because this will guide the surgeon in assessing fitness for future intervention if required.

PHYSICAL EXAMINATION

A physical examination is a fundamental complement to, rather than a substitute for, diagnostic investigations. Indeed, physical signs need to be used with additional clinical criteria to augment the probability of identifying patients with CLD. Physical signs are generally of low sensitivity for the diagnosis, and signs with higher specificity are associated with clinically decompensated disease.[9] Typical findings in CLD are: jaundice (Fig. 12.1), hepatomegaly (Fig. 12.2), liver tenderness, splenomegaly, spider nevi, palmar erythema (Fig. 12.3), and scratching injuries. Ascites, edema, sarcopenia, collateral circulation, hepatic *fetor*, and encephalopathy are signs of advanced disease. Signs related to

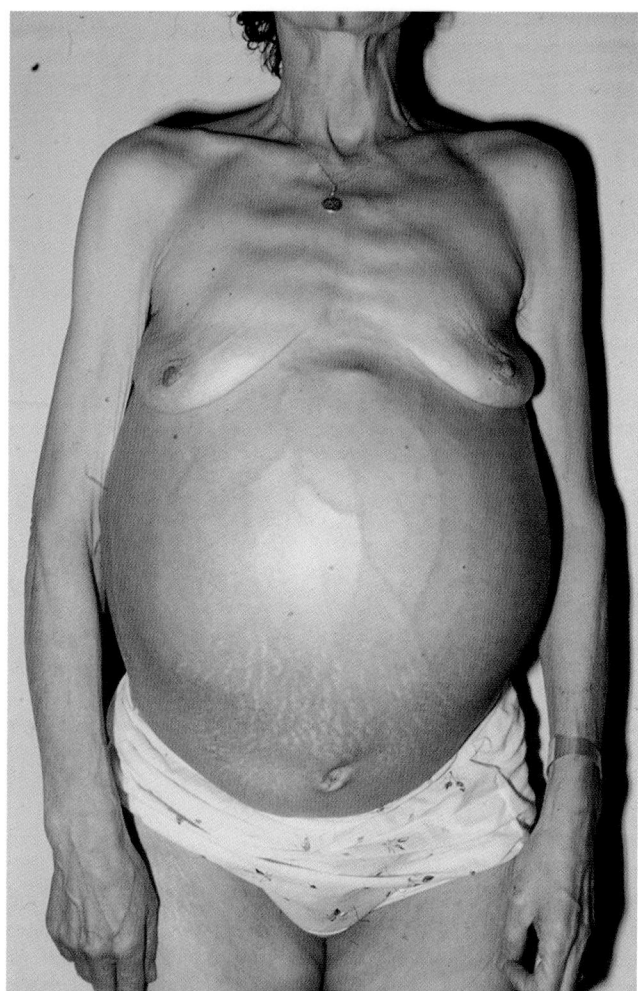

FIGURE 12.2 Massive hepatomegaly.

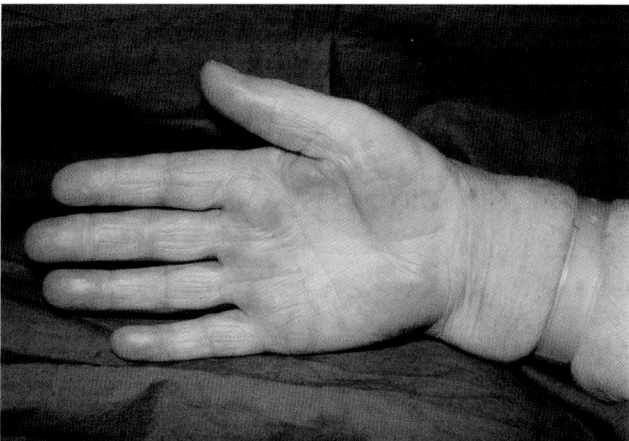

FIGURE 12.3 Palmar erythema.

alcohol abuse are gynecomastia (Fig. 12.4), parotidomegaly, facial telangiectasia, Dupuytren contracture, and testicular atrophy (see Chapters 74, 76, and 77).

When inspected under natural light, jaundice can be noted within the sclera or the mucous membranes below the tongue. Jaundice can usually be observed when the bilirubin level is above 43 μmol/L (2.5 mg/dL). Hyperpigmentation is typical of

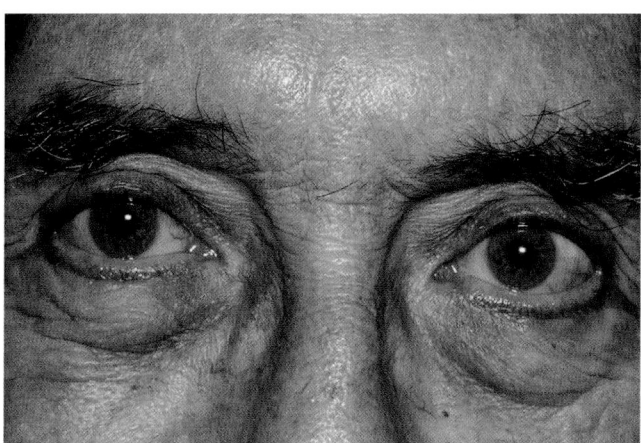

FIGURE 12.1 Jaundice.

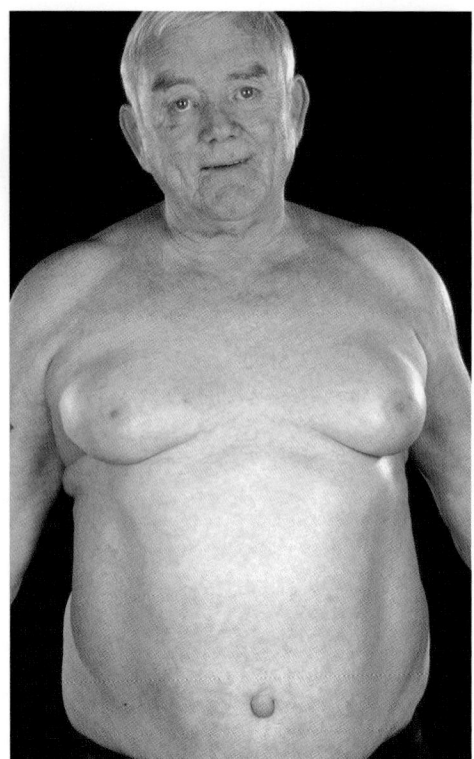

FIGURE 12.4 Bilateral gynecomastia.

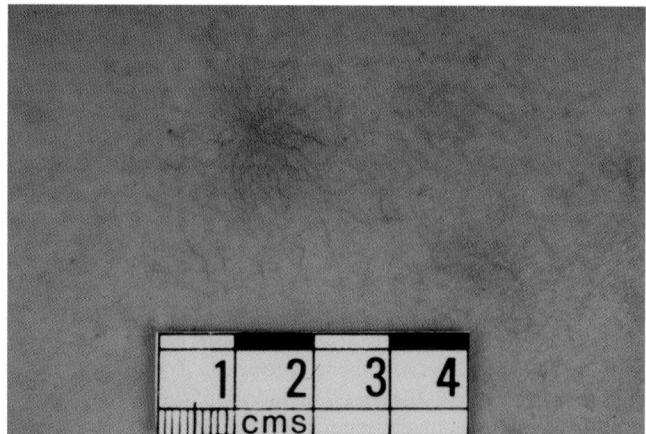

FIGURE 12.5 Spider nevus in a patient with cirrhosis.

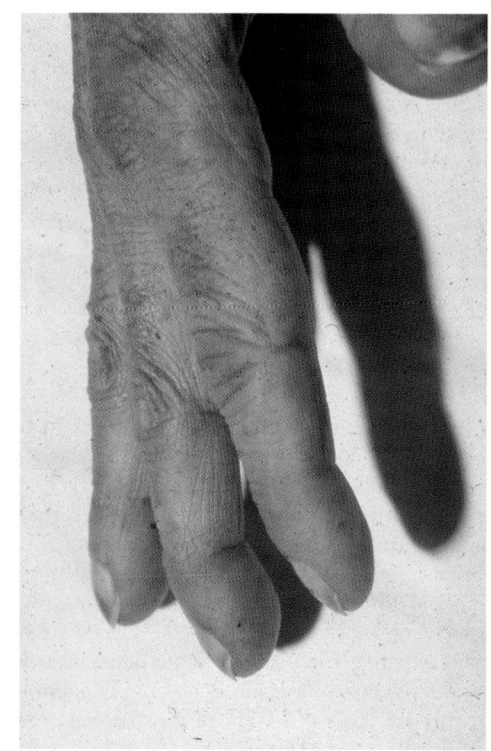

FIGURE 12.6 Clubbing of fingernails.

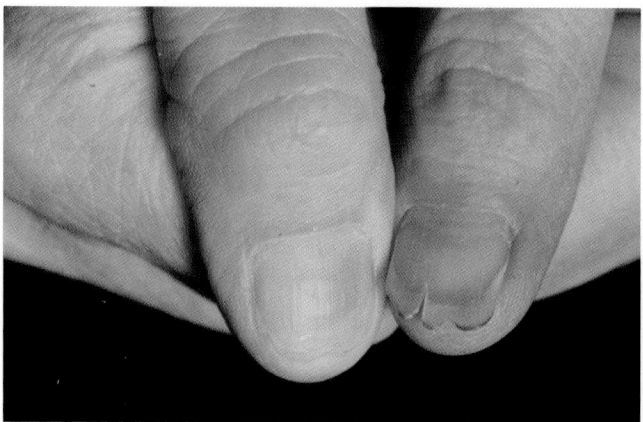

FIGURE 12.7 Koilonychia.

advanced CLD, such as primary biliary cirrhosis and sclerosing cholangitis, whereas in hemochromatosis, pigmentation is slate-gray. Spider nevi are superficial, tortuous, arterial skin lesions with a central arteriole and numerous small radiating vessels (Fig. 12.5). Usually found in the vascular territory of the superior vena cava (arms, face, and upper torso), more than two or three is likely to be abnormal. Palmar erythema may also develop in healthy individuals and is frequently found during pregnancy. Hippocratic fingers (clubbing; Fig. 12.6), white nails (Terry nails), koilonychia (Fig. 12.7), and asterixis are all features of CLD. During eye examination attention should be paid to the pallor, scleral icterus, xanthelasma, and Kayser-Fleischer rings. Physical findings of hepatic encephalopathy include asterixis and flapping tremors of the body and tongue. When there is a portal-venous shunt, a characteristic fruity, ammoniacal, odor—called *fetor hepaticus*—occurs because of exhaled thiols. During abdominal examination, particular attention should be paid to any scars from previous abdominal surgery, abdominal distension, and areas of discoloration. Ascites (Fig. 12.8) is appreciated by detecting shifting dullness by careful percussion. Portal hypertension may present with cutaneous manifestations such as visible collateral veins radiating from the umbilicus called *caput medusae* (Fig. 12.9).

Palpation of the abdomen should begin with a general light palpation, looking for obvious masses and areas of tenderness. The healthy liver is usually impalpable. Reduction in liver size is also important because this may occur in cirrhosis and certain types of hepatitis. A lobe may undergo hypertrophy and become palpable, and this may occur in the presence of hemiliver atrophy or after liver resection. Marked hepatomegaly is typical of cirrhosis, veno-occlusive disease, infiltrative disorders such as amyloidosis, metastatic or primary cancers of the liver,

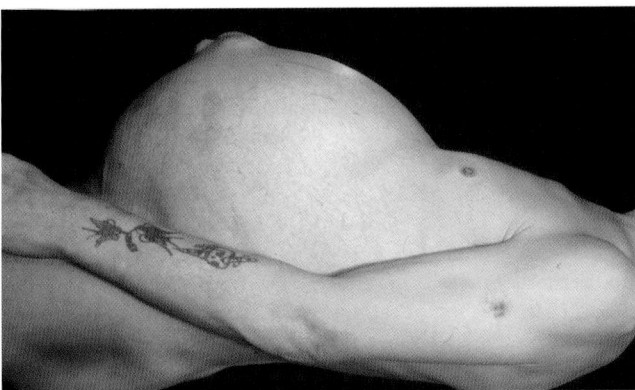

FIGURE 12.8 Ascites with an everted umbilicus and venous distension in a patient with cirrhosis.

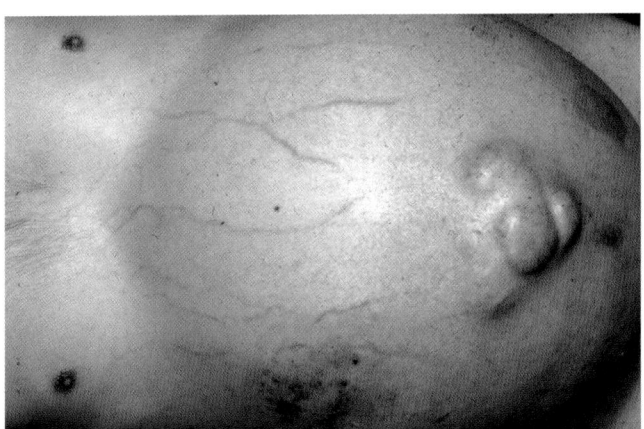

FIGURE 12.9 Caput medusae.

BOX 12.1 Causes of Hepatomegaly
Variant Anatomy Riedel lobe Low-lying diaphragm **Inflammatory** Hepatitis Abscesses, amebic and pyogenic Schistosomiasis Cirrhosis, early Sarcoid Biliary obstruction, especially extrahepatic **Metabolic** Amyloid Steatohepatitis Glycogen storage disease **Hematologic** Leukemias Lymphomas Myeloproliferative disorders Sickle cell disease Porphyrias **Tumors** Primary, benign and malignant Secondary **Cardiovascular** Cardiac failure Hepatic vein obstruction

and alcoholic hepatitis. Careful assessment of the liver edge may also reveal unusual firmness, the irregularity of the surface, or frank nodules. A hard, knobby liver often indicates the presence of metastases, whereas smooth enlargement may be because of cirrhosis.

Causes of hepatomegaly are listed in Box 12.1.

Splenomegaly may occur in many medical conditions. Splenomegaly can be difficult to find but is significant in liver disease. Percussion may be useful, and if ascites is present, the spleen may be ballotable. If the spleen is sufficiently enlarged, the notch on its anterior border may become palpable (Fig. 12.10).

Causes of splenomegaly are listed in Box 12.2.

CLINICAL FEATURES OF LIVER DISEASE

Portal Hypertension

Portal vein pressure normally ranges from 7 to 12 mm Hg. Portal hypertension is characterized by an abnormal increase in pressure within the portal venous system and is defined as a hepatic venous pressure gradient (HVPG) higher than 5 mm Hg[10] (see Chapter 74). It becomes clinically significant at values ≥10 mm Hg. According to the hydraulic analogy of Ohm's law, the main determinants of portal pressure are blood flow and vascular resistance. The primary factor is a marked increase in the intrahepatic vascular resistance to portal blood flow because of both

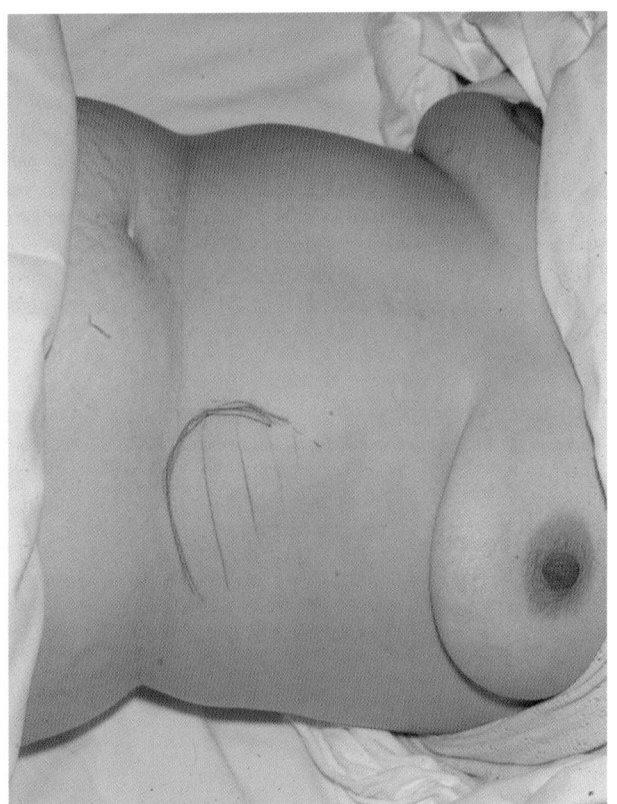

FIGURE 12.10 Splenomegaly.

BOX 12.2 Causes of Splenomegaly

Infection
Acute: viral, bacterial
Chronic: tuberculosis, brucellosis
Parasitic: malaria, schistosomiasis

Hematologic
Leukemias
Hemolytic anemias
Hemoglobinopathies
Portal hypertension, especially extrahepatic

Neoplastic
Lymphomas
Myeloproliferative disorders
Secondary deposits

Inflammatory
Rheumatoid
Systemic lupus
Amyloidosis

mechanical obstruction from fibrosis and the contraction of the portohepatic bed. Second, arteriolar splanchnic dilation and hyperdynamic circulation aggravate and perpetuate portal hypertension syndrome.[11] Any condition that interferes with portal venous blood flow or vascular resistance can lead to portal hypertension. The causes are listed in Table 12.1 and can be classified according to the anatomic location in prehepatic, hepatic, and posthepatic cases.[12] The definitive diagnosis requires the use of invasive interventional radiology methods to measure the HVPG by hepatic vein catheterization. Serum surrogate markers for cirrhosis include the aspartate aminotransferase-to-platelet ratio index, the Forns index, and the FibroTest. Ultrasound (US) allows us to assess the hepatic parenchyma and the surrounding structures (splenomegaly is the most sensitive sign of portal hypertension). Doppler US can be used to assess hepatic vein flow patterns and waveforms. Tissue elastography is a noninvasive method of measuring liver stiffness and predicting liver fibrosis. The results are expressed in kPa, but they should be interpreted with caution in the setting of acute liver damage in CLD because of the effect of edema and inflammation. Liver biopsy is still the gold standard for the diagnosis of CLD even though it is an

invasive procedure, and concerns about serious complications and sampling variations may limit its use[11] (see Chapter 23).

An accurate diagnosis can be made relying on the presence of portal-hypertension-related complications, namely esophageal and gastric varices, variceal bleeding, ascites, spontaneous bacterial peritonitis, splenomegaly, and hepatic encephalopathy (see Chapters 74 and 76).

The increased flow through portosystemic collaterals remodels the esophageal and gastric vessels (more common in noncirrhotic portal hypertension). Variceal bleeding may be a life-threatening complication and is seen when the pressure gradient reaches 12 mm Hg with continuous bleeding when greater than 20 mm Hg (see Chapters 80 and 81). Arterial vasodilatation, sodium and water retention, and increased sinusoidal pressure are determinants of ascites progression (see Chapter 79). The net positive balance of ammonia induced by intrahepatic portosystemic shunts, decreased urea and glutamine synthesis, and shortened muscle mass are responsible for hepatic encephalopathy. Ammonia reaches cerebral astrocytes through hepatic portosystemic shunts and is metabolized into glutamine, thus providing an osmotic pull toward cerebral edema (see Chapter 77).

Alcoholic Liver Disease

ALD covers a wide range of hepatic injuries related to the amount of alcohol consumed and to the duration of drinking, including simple steatosis, fatty liver, alcoholic hepatitis, fibrosis, and cirrhosis.[13] ALD is a chronic, relapsing disease affecting approximately 10% of the general population in Western countries, and it is one of the 30 most frequent causes of death in the world. Diagnosis can be made based on clinical and laboratory features alone in patients with a history of prolonged alcohol abuse for which no other causes can be found.[14] The 2014 World Health Organization (WHO) report on alcohol stated that Eastern European countries have the highest annual per capita alcohol consumption (11–13 L per person), and North Africa and the Middle East have the lowest (0–2 L per person). The estimated annual per capita consumption in the United States is 10 L per person.[15] A recent study by the Global Burden of Disease 2016 Alcohol Collaborators reported that the safest level of drinking is none.[16] An alcohol intake of 60 g per day is associated with hepatic steatosis in 60% to 90% of individuals; less than half of those individuals who continue to drink will develop fibrosis, and only 10% to 20% will eventually

TABLE 12.1 Etiologies of Portal Hypertension

| PREHEPATIC | HEPATIC | | | POSTHEPATIC |
	PRESINUSOIDAL	SINUSOIDAL	POSTSINUSOIDAL	
Portal vein thrombosis	Schistosomiasis	Cirrhosis	Veno-occlusive disease	Budd-Chiari syndrome
Splenic-arteriovenous fistula	Nodular regenerative hyperplasia	Acute hepatitis	Sinuoidal obstruction syndrome	Congestive heart failure
	Cholangiopathy	Acute fatty liver of pregnancy		
	Liver metastases	Amyloidosis		
	Sarcoidosis	Mastocytosis		
	Amyloidosis	Gaucher disease		
	Polycystic liver disease			
	Congenital hepatic fibrosis			

develop cirrhosis. Alcoholic liver damage can be found in otherwise asymptomatic people. Clinical features of more severe, symptomatic ALD are jaundice, ascites, or encephalopathy, but many have nonspecific symptoms, especially anorexia, nausea, vomiting, abdominal discomfort, or diarrhea. Some patients present with infections such as pneumonia or are found to have injuries such as rib fractures. Patients also present because of damage to other organs such as the pancreas, brain, heart, or peripheral nerves. Typical laboratory findings include transaminase levels with aspartate aminotransferase levels more than twice that of alanine aminotransferase levels; an increased mean corpuscular volume, gamma-glutamyltranspeptidase, and IgA to IgG ratio; a prolonged prothrombin time; a low albumin level; and a decreased platelet count.[13] According to the European Association for the Study of Liver Diseases (EASL),[17] the American Association for the Study of Liver Diseases (AASLD),[18] and the American College of Gastroenterology (ACG)[19] guidelines, liver biopsy is not routinely recommended for all suspected ALD cases, but it is useful in cases of aggressive forms. Histologic features are hepatic steatosis, inflammation, and Mallory-Denk bodies. US, computerized tomography (CT), and magnetic resonance imaging (MRI) detect liver steatosis, cirrhosis, and portal hypertension with different levels of sensitivity and specificity according to the stage of fibrosis. Transient elastography has excellent diagnostic accuracy for the diagnosis of advanced fibrosis and cirrhosis. The Child-Turcotte-Pugh (CTP) score and Model for End-Stage Liver Disease (MELD) assess the severity and prognosis of liver disease. Severe forms of ALD are defined as a MELD score ≥ 18, with mortality ranging between 30% and 60% without therapy.[14]

Autoimmune Liver Disease

The term autoimmune liver diseases encompasses a group of chronic immune-mediated disorders that are distinct in the target of liver injury, the pattern of serologic tests, and their clinical findings (see Chapter 105). The diagnosis is obtained from the characteristic phenotype of each disorder and the exclusion of secondary liver diseases (e.g., viral, alcoholic, or drug-induced hepatitis). The most important autoimmune liver diseases are as follows:
- *Autoimmune hepatitis (AIH):* AIH is characterized by hepatocellular injury and typical interface hepatitis at histology. AIH is about four times more common in females than males. Serologic findings include increased levels of transaminases, marked polyclonal hypergammaglobulinemia, and typical non–organ-specific autoantibodies.[20]
- *Primary biliary cholangitis (PBC;* formerly known as primary biliary cirrhosis): PBC is characterized by autoimmune injury of small bile ducts that leads to chronic nonsuppurative cholangitis and subsequent fibrosis. PBC is the most common chronic cholestatic liver disease in women. Biochemical signs of cholestasis and the presence of anti-mitochondrial antibodies (AMAs) are the main serologic findings.[21]
- *Primary sclerosing cholangitis (PSC):* PSC is a chronic immune-mediated disease affecting intra- and extrahepatic bile ducts, leading to cholestasis, liver fibrosis, multifocal biliary strictures, liver cirrhosis, and, ultimately, liver failure (see Chapter 41). PSC has a male predominance (more than 60%) and diagnosis is confirmed through magnetic resonance cholangiopancreatography (MRCP) or endoscopic retrograde cholangiopancreatography (ERCP). PSC is characterized by the absence of any disease-specific autoantibodies and poor response to immunosuppression. It must also

be taken into account that in approximately 70% of PSC patients, inflammatory bowel disease (IBD) is diagnosed (e.g., mainly ulcerative colitis)[22].

Such diseases, characterized either by hepatocellular injury (i.e., AIH) or by predominant cholestatic features (i.e., PBC and PSC), have a progressive course that may cause liver failure and may even require transplantation.

Budd-Chiari Syndrome

Budd-Chiari syndrome is the eponym used for referring to a heterogeneous group of conditions characterized by partial or complete hepatic venous outflow obstruction (see Chapter 86). It is a rare and potentially life-threatening condition, and the estimated incidence in Western countries is one in 2.5 million cases per person per year. The obstruction can be located at any level, from the small hepatic veins to the junction of the inferior vena cava. The increase in hepatic sinusoidal pressure leads to portal hypertension and liver congestion, which may ultimately progress to hepatic fibrosis and cirrhosis. The most common causes are, for example, an underlying hypercoagulable or a prothrombotic state because of congenital diseases or myeloproliferative disorders, malignancy, and pregnancy. Secondary causes are direct compression from primary or secondary liver masses or abscesses and the extension of a thrombus from renal cell carcinoma. The clinical presentation ranges from acute failure to asymptomatic (up to 20% of cases), and it depends on the rapidity and extent of obstruction and the presence of collateral veins. The classic triad comprises abdominal pain, ascites, and hepatomegaly. Laboratory analyses provide little help in the diagnosis but are useful in understanding the etiology and predicting the severity of disease, the likelihood of mortality, and the possible response to therapy. Imaging techniques (US, MRI, and CT) play an important role in the diagnosis, classification, and severity assessment of the disease, documenting intrahepatic collaterals and areas of reduced perfusion and necrosis as well as providing appropriate images for therapeutic planning.[23,24]

Hemochromatosis

Hemochromatosis is defined as a systemic iron overload most commonly caused by the autosomal-recessive inheritance of a C282Y substitution in the HFE gene (hereditary hemochromatosis [HH] type 1). It can also be caused by mutations in other genes (non-HFE-related: HAMP, HJV, TFR2, SLC40A1) or by acquired iron overload (hematologic disorders, excessive iron supplementation, metabolic syndrome, and chronic alcoholism).[25] Type 1 HH is the most common mutation associated with a clinical disease, with the frequency of a homozygous C282Y mutation reported to be 0.4% in European countries. Diagnosis involves a strategy that combines clinical, imaging, and biologic data. Patients are asymptomatic for many years and develop symptoms at approximately 30 to 40 years of age in men and 40 to 50 years of age in women. The disease is frequently first recognized by elevated iron indices (transferrin saturation and serum ferritin) or by parameters that indicate organ-specific iron overload (mild hypertransaminasemia and hyperglycemia). Common presenting symptoms that may lead to clinical diagnosis of HH include fatigue, arthralgia, and a loss of libido. Chronic iron overload organ damage results in clinical HH including hepatic cirrhosis and hepatocellular carcinoma, dilated cardiomyopathy or cardiac rhythm disorders, diabetes mellitus, hypogonadism, chronic fatigue, lethargy, joint pain, and skin bronzing. Liver biopsy has been replaced by the combined evaluation of biochemical and imaging findings, but it still has a role in assessing hepatic complications such as fibrosis. Transient elastography is a useful noninvasive test for detecting significant liver fibrosis, and liver MRI can be used to assess the presence of elevated hepatic iron in a quantitative fashion.[26,27]

Polycystic Liver Disease

Adult polycystic liver disease (PLD) is a rare inherited autosomal dominant condition characterized by more than 20 fluid-filled biliary epithelial-lined cysts in the liver (see Chapter 73). Three PLD entities are recognized in adults. PLD can occur in the setting of two distinct hereditary disorders: as the primary presentation of autosomal-dominant PLD or associated with polycystic kidneys in autosomal-dominant polycystic kidney disease (ADPKD). Microhamartomas (Von Meyenburg complexes) may occur in isolation or in the context of PLD and ADPKD, are usually asymptomatic, and require no management or follow-up examination. Genetic mechanisms or signaling defects are the root cause of ductal structures becoming separated from the biliary tree, finally resulting in cyst formation. The proteins affected in ADPKD are located at the cilium, which has led to its classification it as a ciliopathy. On the other hand, hepatic cysts in ADPLD are lined by cholangiocytes; therefore this form is defined as a cholangiopathy.[28,29] Although PLD is most often asymptomatic, one in five patients experience symptoms, with the most common symptoms being abdominal pain or distention, early satiety, nausea, dyspnea, and lower back pain. In rare cases, cyst compression may lead to ascites, biliary obstruction, and portal thrombosis. Patients can experience acute liver cyst complications, including infection, rupture, torsion, and hemorrhage. Cross-sectional imaging (CT or MRI) characterizes liver cyst burden and determines appropriate treatment. In symptomatic patients, surgical therapy is the mainstay of treatment tailored to the extent of disease for each patient. Management options include cyst aspiration and sclerosis, open or laparoscopic fenestration, liver resection with fenestration, and liver transplantation.[30,31]

Liver Disease in Pregnancy

Pregnancy-associated liver diseases occur in 3% to 5% of pregnant women. There are many potential causes of liver disease in pregnancy, including non-pregnancy related pre-existing liver disease (viral, cirrhosis and portal hypertension, autoimmune) or those that are coincidental with pregnancy (autoimmune, viral, vascular, and drug-induced hepatotoxicity). Pregnancy-related liver disease can be classified according to the time of onset (early or late pregnancy): hyperemesis gravidarum in the first trimester; intrahepatic cholestasis in the second half; and acute fatty liver of pregnancy, preeclampsia with hepatic involvement including hemolysis, elevated liver enzymes and low platelet (HELLP) syndrome and liver rupture/infarction in the third trimester. Pregnancy-associated diseases can carry a high mortality rate for both mothers and babies and require rapid diagnosis and urgent delivery if at the severe end of the spectrum. In cirrhotic women who become pregnant, hepatic decompensation occurs in 10% and this can be predicted by the MELD score. Many physiologic changes occur in a pregnant woman, some of which can mimic those seen in CLD, including hyperdynamic circulation, a procoagulation state, palmar erythema, spider nevi, gallstones, and an increase in alkaline phosphatase and alpha fetoprotein. Elevations in transaminases, bilirubin, or

prothrombin time require further assessment, indicating a pathologic state. Acute fatty liver of pregnancy may present to the surgeon with liver subcapsular hematoma or rupture with massive intraabdominal bleeding. Laparotomy for clot evacuation and hemostasis may be required. The management is supportive, and mortality is high.[32,33]

Acute Liver Failure

Acute liver failure (ALF) is the clinical manifestation of sudden and severe hepatic injury, and it has an incidence of fewer than 10 cases per million persons per year in the developed world (see Chapters 77 and 78). In the developing world, viral causes predominate (see Chapter 68), with hepatitis E infection recognized as a common cause; other rare viral causes of acute liver failure include hepatitis B virus, herpes simplex virus, cytomegalovirus, Epstein–Barr virus, and parvoviruses. In the United States and western Europe, most cases arise from drug-induced liver injury, mostly commonly because of acetaminophen. Other causes of ALF are neoplastic infiltration, Budd-Chiari syndrome, heatstroke, mushroom ingestion, metabolic diseases such as Wilson's disease, acute ischemic hepatocellular injury, or hypoxic hepatitis. Nevertheless, a large proportion of cases are still of unknown origin. The clinical presentation usually includes hepatic dysfunction, abnormal liver biochemical values, and coagulopathy; encephalopathy may develop, with multiorgan failure and death occurring in up to half the cases.[34,35] Diagnostic liver biopsy is not routinely recommended. Various prognostic evaluation systems are in use worldwide, of which the Model for End-Stage Liver Disease (MELD) and the King's College Hospital criteria are the best known. A MELD score of 30.5 (fixed cutoff value) should be used for prognosis, and higher scores predict a need for liver transplantation.[36] When symptoms seriously progress under continuous supportive medical care, deceased-donor liver transplantation (DDLT) becomes the only therapeutic option. In countries where cadaveric donors are scarce, living-donor liver transplantation (LDLT) is another option.

Benign Liver Masses[37,38] (see Chapter 88)
Hepatic Hemangioma

Hepatic hemangioma is the most frequent benign liver lesion with a prevalence of 5% in the population, and it is more frequent in women between 30 and 50 years of age. It consists of "cavernous" vascular spaces lined by endothelial cells, varying in dimension (capillary hemangiomas, giant or cavernous hemangiomas), while remaining asymptomatic. Radiologic investigations such as CT and MRI are extremely reliable in the diagnosis because of the unique centripetal vascularization (see Chapter 14). Spontaneous bleeding is rare. For smaller lesions that may have an uncertain diagnosis, radiologic follow-up is preferable, but it is not required after a diagnosis of classical hemangioma. Surgery must be considered and is reserved in cases of lesions that have grown beyond 10 cm or in patients symptomatic for compression or recurrent pain (generally after thrombotic/hemorrhagic phenomena).

Focal Nodular Hyperplasia

Focal nodular hyperplasia (FNH) is the second most common benign liver lesion, with a prevalence of 3%. Up to 90% of cases of FNH are diagnosed in women between 35 and 50 years of age. Generally, FNHs are small, solitary lesions of less than 5 cm, but they can be larger and multiple in 20% to 30% of cases. FNH originates from the hepatic stellate cell response to an irritative stimulus such as increased blood flow, which produces the typical central radial scar. In most cases, the size is stable over time, the lesions are asymptomatic, and complications (rupture and malignant degeneration) are extremely rare. Biopsy is not indicated to confirm the diagnosis of typical FNH. Surgical treatment is reserved for cases of symptomatic, exophytic lesions or those with increases in size. Patients with definitive radiologic diagnosis do not need follow-up.

Hepatocellular Adenoma

Hepatocellular adenoma (HA) is a rare benign liver lesion affecting less than 0.012% of the population that is commonly diagnosed in women between 35 and 40 years of age. HAs can be solitary or multiple, ranging in dimension from a few millimeters up to 30 cm. HAs are characterized by specific radiologic peculiarities but also by a significant risk for complications such as rupture, bleeding, and malignant degeneration (in lesions greater than 5 cm). Numerous studies have shown a causative role of sex hormones (oral contraceptives or hormone-releasing intrauterine devices and anabolic hormones in men) in their development. The recent increase in incidence is closely related to the increased prevalence of obesity and metabolic syndrome. MRI has the greatest sensitivity in identifying HA but also in diagnosing the different variants of adenoma. Liver biopsy can help identify HA subtypes and the specific underlying genetic alterations. Surgical treatment is always expected in men because of the non-negligible risk for malignant degeneration. In women, however, surgery must be considered in the case of adenomas greater than 5 cm in size, in lesions that are exophytic, and in those with an increase in size of more than 20% during radiologic follow-up (see Chapters 88 and 89).

Simple Hepatic Cysts

The vast majority of simple hepatic cysts are benign and derive from a congenital failure of a bile duct to communicate with the bile tree. These cysts are generally less than one centimeter in diameter, but they can grow up to 30 cm. These cysts are often asymptomatic, but patients with larger lesions can manifest with abdominal pain and epigastric and postprandial fullness. The presence of multiple cysts (more than 20); cysts larger than 5 cm; or cysts with internal septa, calcifications, fenestrations, internal loculations, alterations of the wall, or "daughter" cysts must lead to further investigations because of their malignant potential (cystadenoma or cystadenocarcinoma) or the potential for congenital diseases (polycystic liver disease) or parasitic infections (hydatid cysts). Simple liver cysts, asymptomatic and without signs of suspicion, do not require treatment or radiologic follow-up. Symptomatic simple liver cysts, on the other hand, can be treated surgically by laparoscopic "fenestration" (see Chapter 73).

GALLBLADDER AND BILIARY TRACT DISEASE

Gallbladder

The most common form of gallbladder disease is cholelithiasis, which affects more than 20 million Americans, with an annual direct cost of more than 6.3 billion dollars (see Chapter 33). The usual presentation of uncomplicated gallstones is biliary colic (see Chapter 34). The pain is characteristically steady, is moderate to severe in intensity, and is epigastric or in the right quadrant postprandially; the pain lasts several hours and then gradually subsides. The pain often radiates to the back and to the right shoulder. If pain persists with the onset of fever or leukocytosis, it should raise suspicion for complications such as acute cholecystitis (AC), gallstone pancreatitis, or ascending cholangitis. Upper right quadrant tenderness and guarding exacerbated by inspiration (Murphy's sign) suggest AC. A palpable, distended gallbladder—"Courvoisier's gallbladder"[39]—in the presence of obstructive jaundice may suggest malignant obstruction of the biliary tree mainly because of pancreatic head lesions. Nevertheless, a nonpalpable gallbladder does not exclude a malignant process and is the rule in hilar obstruction. On the other hand, an intermittently palpable gallbladder may suggest the presence of a periampullary carcinoma.[40] Acute cholecystitis in the presence of bacteria-containing bile may progress to suppurative infection in which the gallbladder fills with purulent material, a condition referred to as empyema of the gallbladder.

Gallstones and Biliary Colic

The prevalence of gallstone disease varies significantly among ethnicities and its incidence increases with age and is higher in women. In developed countries, gallbladder stones are present in 10% to 20% of the adult population. As stated by the third National Health and Nutrition Examination Survey, in the United States 6.3 million men and 14.2 million women aged 20 to 74 had gallbladder disease.[41] In Europe, according to the Multicenter Italian Study on Cholelithiasis (MICOL), the overall incidence of gallstone disease was 18.8% in women and 9.5% in men.[42] Symptoms (biliary colic) occur in 1% to 4% of patients annually, and 20% become symptomatic within 20 years of diagnosis. Nearly 35% to 50% of symptomatic patients do not experience further biliary pain, even if no definitive predictive factor for biliary recurrence has been clearly identified in symptomatic patients. After the first episode of colic, 1% to 3% of patients per year will manifest a complication (AC, acute cholangitis, acute biliary pancreatitis, obstructive jaundice), whereas in asymptomatic patients, the rate is 0.1% to 0.3% annually.[43]

Major risk factors for cholesterol gallstones (the most common type in Western countries) include advancing age, sex, race, family history, pregnancy, and parity. Additional risk factors include high-calorie and low-fiber diets, low physical activity, rapid weight loss, metabolic syndrome, hormonal therapy, and obesity.

Biliary colic, radiating pain, and the use of analgesics are symptoms that are significantly associated with the presence of gallstones.[44] The pain is usually severe in intensity with an abrupt beginning or with a progressive crescendo that is thought to relate to the distention of the gallbladder after acute and usually transient obstruction of the cystic duct. The symptoms are often present shortly after a meal and last from 30 minutes to a few hours and then resolve. A duration longer than 5 hours most often indicates AC. The patient is afebrile with tenderness in the epigastrium but no peritonism.[45] Even though dyspepsia, heartburn, bloating, and flatulence are often present in these patients, they are not characteristic of gallstone disease, and they usually persist after cholecystectomy. Laboratory tests are usually normal and do not contribute to the diagnosis of uncomplicated colic. With an accuracy for detecting gallstones reaching 95%, abdominal US is the imaging technique of choice. In the case of a normal US finding, MRI is recommended, while in patients with unexplained acute and/or recurrent pancreatitis endoscopic US (EUS) is helpful[43] (see Chapters 16, 20, 22, and 30).

Several risk factors for cholesterol, pigment, and mixed gallstones exist and general preventive measures are plausible. A healthy lifestyle and diet, regular physical activity, and an ideal body weight might prevent gallstones and biliary colic. The administration of ursodeoxycholic acid (UDCA) to the general population as a preventive drug has no indication, and conflicting results are available on the protective effect of statins or ezetimibe.

There have been no randomized clinical trials, clinical observations, or prospective studies assessing the benefit of cholecystectomy in asymptomatic patients. Approximately 0.7% to 2.5% of this group of patients will develop symptoms related to gallstones with an annual incidence of complications of 0.1% to 0.3%. The overall morbidity and mortality risk of surgery outweighs the probability of complications, thus giving no recommendation for routine surgical treatment.

On the other hand, cholecystectomy should be performed in symptomatic patients. Half of them will have recurring colic within 1 year, but surgical treatment may not be necessary if symptoms have not occurred within the last 5 years or after one isolated episode.[43]

Gallstones in the Bariatric Population

The prevalence of obesity among adults in the United States has increased dramatically during recent decades among all race/sex groups but also worldwide with a greater surge of obesity prevalence in lower- and middle-income developing countries than in higher-income countries. In the United States, according to the third National Health and Nutrition Examination Survey, 58 million people are at least 20% overweight, with a greater prevalence in black and Hispanic females, where obesity approaches 50%.[46,47] Increased BMI and female sex are decisive risk factors for the development of gallstones, acting together with diabetes mellitus and insulin resistance. Additionally, increasing BMI, waist circumference, and serum triglycerides increase the risk for symptomatic gallstones. The pathogenic mechanisms involved in the formation of gallstones are the supersaturation of bile with cholesterol, increased propensity to cholesterol crystallization, stone aggregation, and defective gallbladder emptying. Additional factors are insulin resistance, dyslipidemia, sedentary lifestyle, hormone replacement therapy, and fast-food consumption.

Gallbladder stasis and increased cholesterol saturation in bile have been implicated as major predisposing factors in the development of sludge and gallstones if weight loss, either with very-low-calorie diets or with bariatric surgery without cholecystectomy, is too rapid (more than 1.5 kg/week). The lithogenic effect is seen after 4 weeks, although it generally appears within 7 to 18 months. Approximately one-third of patients may develop gallstones after bariatric surgery, with a greater risk after a gastric bypass procedure with 28% to 71% of these patients becoming symptomatic and up to one-third of patients eventually requiring urgent cholecystectomy by 3 years.[47,48] Lytholytic hydrophilic UDCA has become the standard prophylactic treatment for gallstone formation after rapid weight reduction. Nevertheless, the adoption of prophylactic cholecystectomy is still controversial. Some centers routinely perform it; however, this may be associated with an increase in the overall operative time, the length of stay (LOS), and related complications.[43,48]

Acute Cholecystitis

Cholecystitis may be acute or chronic. Four different forms of AC are described: acalculous, xanthogranulomatous, emphysematous, and torsion of the gallbladder (see Chapter 34). Acalculous cholecystitis is typical of critically ill patients; xanthogranulomatous cholecystitis is because of an impacted stone and is characterized by wall thickening and increased intraluminal pressure; emphysematous cholecystitis is caused by gas-forming anaerobes; and torsion of the gallbladder results in compromised vascular supply.[45] AC is the most common complication of gallstone disease and occurs in 10% to 20% of untreated patients. Chronic cholecystitis is the result of repeated episodes of AC and is characterized by thickened gallbladder walls, mucosal atrophy, and fibrosis. In patients discharged home without operation after an episode of AC, the probability of gallstone-related events is 14%, 19%, and 29% at 6 weeks, 12 weeks, and 1 year, respectively.[49] According to the 2016 European Association for the Study of Liver Disease guidelines, the 2016 World Society of Emergency Surgery guidelines, and the 2018 Tokyo Guidelines, the diagnosis of AC is based on clinical findings, laboratory data, and imaging. The Tokyo Guidelines for the diagnosis and management of AC were originally published in 2007 and have recently been updated. These are summarized in Box 12.3. Patients with AC have severe and worsening right upper quadrant pain lasting for several hours, radiating to the interscapular area or right shoulder. It is usually associated with tenderness on palpation (Murphy's sign). Nausea and vomiting are often present. Systemic signs of inflammation are fever and elevated C-reactive protein and white blood cell (WBC) count. Blood urea nitrogen, creatinine, albumin, and arterial blood gas analysis may be required to further assess the severity of AC. US is the first-choice imaging method for the morphologic diagnosis of AC because of its low invasiveness, ease of use, cost-effectiveness, and widespread use.[43,49,50]

Biliary Obstruction

Biliary obstruction can occur anywhere along the extrahepatic biliary system and can have various benign and malignant etiologies. These include choledocholithiasis, choledochal cysts, Mirizzi's syndrome, infectious diseases (parasitic cholangiopathy), inflammatory and autoimmune disease (AIDS cholangiopathy, autoimmune cholangiopathy), and neoplastic strictures (cholangiocarcinoma, pancreatic head cancer, ampullary carcinoma).[51]

Malignant biliary tract obstruction is often asymptomatic until the disease is significantly advanced. Jaundice is usually the presenting symptom in up to 90% of pancreatic head cancer

---

BOX 12.3 The 2018 Tokyo Guidelines Diagnostic Criteria for Acute Cholecystitis

A. Local signs of inflammation
   1. Murphy's sign
   2. Right upper quadrant mass/pain/tenderness
B. Systemic signs of inflammation
   1. Fever
   2. Elevated C-reactive protein
   3. Elevated white blood cells count
C. Imaging findings
   Imaging findings characteristic of acute cholecystitis

Suspected diagnosis: one item in A + one item in B
Definite diagnosis: one item in A + one item in B + C

and distal cholangiocarcinoma (dCCA) patients and may also be seen with gallbladder carcinoma (see Chapters 49, 51, and 62). Accompanying symptoms are pale stools, dark urine, itching, right upper quadrant discomfort, nausea, weight loss, anorexia, and night sweats. Symptoms suggestive of pancreatic carcinoma include dull epigastric pain radiating to the back, Courvoisier's gallbladder, dyspepsia, new-onset diabetes, or acute pancreatitis (AP). Hilar cholangiocarcinoma (hCCA) is a rare malignancy that affects hepatic duct confluence (see Chapter 51B). Patients typically present with jaundice because of a proximal biliary stricture, which in a significant proportion of patients (up to 15% of resected patients) can have benign pathology (inflammatory strictures, sclerosing cholangitis, or IgG4-related cholangiopathy).[52]

Laboratory tests depict a cholestatic process, and direct serum bilirubin, alkaline phosphatase, and gamma-glutamyl transpeptidase are elevated. Tumor markers are usually nonspecific. CA 19-9 is elevated not only in pancreatic cancer but also in other gastrointestinal (GI) cancers (cholangiocarcinoma, gastric cancer, colorectal cancer, esophageal cancer, and hepatocellular cancer) and benign processes (AC or AP) as well as biliary obstruction per se, thus limiting its specificity.[51]

Diagnostic modalities include transabdominal US, CT scan, and MRI/MRCP (see Chapter 13). MRCP has excellent sensitivity and specificity for demonstrating the level and presence of biliary obstruction. Additional modalities that are both diagnostic and allow therapeutic interventions include EUS with EUS-BD or without guided biliary drainage, ERCP, and percutaneous transhepatic cholangiopancreatography (PTC)[52,53] (see Chapters 20, 22, 30, 31, 37C, and 51B).

Asymptomatic Bile Duct Dilatation

An incidentally found asymptomatic dilated common bile duct (CBD) is a common finding because of the widespread use of abdominal imaging. The mean diameter of a normal CBD ranges from 4 to 8 mm, but in most studies, a CBD diameter greater than 7 mm is considered abnormal. Patient presentation can be asymptomatic or symptomatic, with normal or abnormal liver function tests. A recent systematic review documented that in 9% to 73% of patients a diagnosis can be found and is most commonly benign. The most common causes are: CBD stones, chronic pancreatitis (CP), periampullary diverticulum, and cholecystectomy. Malignancy is identified in 12% of patients. Potential predictors of malignancy include jaundice, age, and coexisting CBD and intrahepatic duct dilation. There are no definitive recommendations on the approach, imaging modalities, or follow-up. However, the symptomatic patient and/or patients with abnormal liver function tests need further investigation. The truly asymptomatic patient should be followed closely with clinical and laboratory follow-up to help decide whether any additional imaging would be appropriate. Even though these patients often undergo further evaluation with different radiologic techniques, EUS is the primary imaging modality of choice.[54]

Choledocholithiasis

Choledocholithiasis, commonly from gallbladder stones, is the main etiology of nonmalignant biliary obstruction (see Chapter 37). It is estimated that up to 10% of patients concomitantly have a stone or multiple stones in the CBD after cholecystectomy. In 1987 Taylor and Armstrong demonstrated that stones migrated in only 3% of patients with a normal cystic duct diameter of less

than 4 mm versus in 32.5% of patients with a duct diameter of greater than 4 mm.[55] Stones found in the CBD may be primary, secondary, residual, or recurrent. Primary stones may arise intrahepatically or within the CBD and occur more often in the Asian population (see Chapters 39 and 44). These stones are thought to originate as a consequence of bacteriobilia and are often attributed to biliary stasis (bile duct stricture, papillary stenosis, periampullary diverticulum, the reflux of the duodenal contents into the bile duct) and abnormalities of the sphincter of Oddi. Secondary stones are the most common stone type in the United States. These stones migrate from the gallbladder to the CBD through the cystic duct.[56] Secondary CBD stones may recur after cholecystectomy or after endoscopic sphincterotomy with a wide range of incidences from 4% to 24%. Risk factors for recurrence are periampullary diverticulum type I or II, angulation along the course of the CBD, multiple CBD stones, bile duct dilation, and muddy stones. Residual stones are missed at the time of cholecystectomy but present within 2 years, whereas recurrent stones develop more than 2 years after surgery.[45,57]

Many patients are asymptomatic and are incidentally found to have choledocholithiasis during an abdominal US for cholelithiasis or abnormal liver function tests. Symptomatic patients complain of right upper quadrant or epigastric pain, nausea, vomiting, intermittent or persistent jaundice, colorless stools, dark urine, and AP. Transabdominal US is the most appropriate initial imaging study in most patients even though its sensitivity ranges from 13% to 89%. CT scans may be performed after US, particularly when malignancy is suspected. Endoscopic US and MRCP have better sensitivity for detecting CBD stones than transabdominal US or conventional CT and are less invasive than ERCP.[57,58]

Cholangitis

Acute cholangitis is characterized by biliary infection and concomitant obstruction with various benign and malignant causes (see Chapter 43). The bacteriobilia and the elevated intraductal pressure allow bacterial and endotoxin translocation into the vascular and lymphatic system. Cholangitis is a potentially life-threatening condition if not treated with antibiotic therapy and if biliary obstruction is not resolved. The diagnosis is based on clinical presentation, laboratory results, and diagnostic imaging. Acute cholangitis has long been diagnosed on the basis of Charcot's triad of fever, jaundice, and abdominal pain. Patients with more severe forms may also have hypotension and altered mental status, a constellation called Reynold's pentad. US and CT scan with contrast help to identify the underlying cause and to exclude other diagnoses. Other imaging modalities include MRCP, MRI, EUS, and ERCP. Poor prognostic predictive factors include a WBC count greater than 20,000 cells/mm^3, total bilirubin greater than 10 mg/dL, temperature greater than 39°C, serum albumin less than 3.0 g/dL, and age greater than 75.[43,45,59,60] The diagnostic criteria for acute cholangitis are based on the Tokyo Guidelines, relying on the three items of systemic inflammation, cholestasis, and imaging, with moderate diagnostic accuracy (sensitivity 91.8%, specificity 77.7%). The Tokyo Guidelines for the diagnosis and management of acute cholangitis were originally published in 2007 and have recently been updated.[61] These are summarized in Box 12.4.

Acalculous ("Functional") Biliary Pain

Patients may complain of symptoms typical of biliary pain without detectable gallstones. When no structural abnormalities exist or pain continues after cholecystectomy, biliary pain is

---

BOX 12.4   The 2018 Tokyo Guidelines for the Diagnosis and Management of Acute Cholangitis

A. Systemic inflammation
  1. Fever and/or shaking chills
  2. Laboratory data: evidence of inflammatory response
B. Cholestasis
  1. Jaundice
  2. Laboratory data: abnormal liver function tests
C. Imaging
  1. Biliary dilatation
  2. Evidence of the etiology on imaging (stricture, stone, stent etc.)
Suspected diagnosis: one item in A + one item in either B or C
Definite diagnosis: one item in A, one item in B and one item in C

Note:

A-2: Abnormal white blood cell counts, increase of serum C-reactive protein levels, and other changes indicating inflammation
B-2: Increased serum ALP, GGT, AST, and ALT levels
Other factors that are helpful in diagnosis of acute cholangitis include abdominal pain (right upper quadrant or upper abdominal) *and a* history of biliary disease, such as gallstones, previous biliary procedures, and placement of a biliary stent.
In acute hepatitis, marked systematic inflammatory response is observed infrequently. Virologic and serologic tests are required when differential diagnosis is difficult.

Thresholds:

A-1. Fever > 38°C
A-2. Evidence of inflammatory response
WBC (×1000 microliters) < 4 or > 10
CRP (mg/dL) ≥ 1
B-1. Jaundice T-Bil ≥2 (mg/dL)
B-2. Abnormal liver function tests
ALP (IU) > 1.5 × STD
GGT (IU) > 1.5 × STD
AST (IU) > 1.5 × STD
ALT (IU) > 1.5 × STD
(STD is upper limit of normal value.)

ALP, Alkaline phosphatase; *ALT,* alanine aminotransferase; *AST,* aspartate aminotransferase; *CRP,* C-reactive protein; *GGT,* gamma glutamyl transpeptidase; *T-Bil,* total bilirubin; *WBC,* white blood cells.

BOX 12.5   Rome III Criteria for Functional Gallbladder Disorder

Diagnostic Criteria
Must include *all* of the following:
1. Criteria for functional gallbladder and sphincter of Oddi disorder
2. Gallbladder is present
3. Normal liver enzymes, conjugated bilirubin, and amylase/lipase

Diagnostic Criteria for Functional Gallbladder and Sphincter of Oddi Disorders
Must include episodes of pain located in the epigastrium and/or right upper quadrant and *all* of the following:
1. Episodes lasting 30 minutes or longer
2. Recurrent symptoms occurring at different intervals (not daily)
3. The pain builds up to a steady level
4. The pain is moderate to severe enough to interrupt the patient's daily activities or lead to an emergency department visit
5. The pain is not relieved by bowel movements
6. The pain is not relieved by postural change
7. The pain is not relieved by antacids
8. Exclusion of other structural disease that would explain the symptoms

Supportive Criteria
The pain may present with one or more of the following:
1. Pain is associated with nausea and vomiting
2. Pain radiates to the back and/or right infrasubscapular region
3. Pain awakens from sleep in the middle of the night

BOX 12.6   Rome III Criteria for Functional Biliary Sphincter of Oddi Disorders

Must include *both* of the following:
1. Criteria for functional gallbladder and sphincter of Oddi disorder (see Box 12.5)
2. Normal amylase/lipase

Supportive criterion
Elevated serum transaminases, alkaline phosphatase, or conjugated bilirubin temporally related to at least two pain episodes

---

considered "functional." In these patients, the symptoms may be caused by an alternative diagnosis or may originate in a dysfunctional biliary system.[62,63] Box 12.5 includes the Rome III criteria for the diagnosis of functional gallbladder disorder.[64]

These patients have normal laboratory tests and upper endoscopy findings and a scrupulous search for gallstone disease is negative. Furthermore, in an attempt to identify the gallbladder as the culprit in acalculous biliary pain, several studies have used cholecystokinin infusion to reproduce the pain; however, this test has no validity. Thus functional biliary pain is a diagnosis of exclusion. Laparoscopic cholecystectomy results in only 50% of patients obtaining symptom relief compared with 81% in gallstone disease.[63] Surgery should not be offered on the basis of a symptomatic diagnosis, and patients should be counseled regarding the uncertainty of its outcome.

Sphincter of Oddi Dysfunction

The sphincter of Oddi is composed of three sphincters of smooth muscle fibers that surround the distal CBD, main pancreatic duct, and the ampulla of Vater. Its contractility regulates antegrade and retrograde flow through the pancreatobiliary tree. A

dyskinetic or stenotic sphincter results in the clinical syndrome called "sphincter of Oddi dysfunction" (SOD), formerly called "papillitis" (Box 12.6).[64,65] The most adopted classification system is the Milwaukee classification scheme proposed by Hogan and Geenen in 1988.[66] SOD is classified into biliary types I, II, and III based on upper abdominal symptoms and biochemical and imaging findings. The classification was then broadened to include patients with pancreatic-type pain and relapsing pancreatitis. The diagnosis, however, is still controversial and the classification system has been questioned. Some authors believe that the symptoms could be a consequence of sludge/gravel passage with papillary stenosis (type I), stone passage without stenosis (type II), or a functional disorder (type III).[67] The Evaluating Predictors and Interventions of SOD (EPISOD) trial and the EPISOD2 observational study demonstrated that SOD type III patients with a presumed hypertensive and/or dyskinetic sphincter of Oddi did not benefit from endoscopic sphincterotomy even after 5 years of follow-up, as recently demonstrated by Cotton et al. Thus SOD type III should now be termed functional pain.[68–70] The diagnosis is typically made after cholecystectomy. Biliary SOD can present as episodic, postprandial right upper quadrant pain with or without cholestasis. Pancreatic SOD is characterized by more prolonged pain, radiating to the back, and can be associated with pancreatitis. It is important to point out that clinicians must ensure that a diagnosis of occult malignancy is not being missed in patients with ductal dilation and abnormal pancreatic or liver function tests. There is no gold-standard technique for the diagnosis of SOD. Manometry is not widely available and requires expertise; measurements vary according to catheter equipment, sphincter lumen size and spasm, and probe position.[67,71]

PANCREAS

Pancreatic diseases, including CP, pancreatic cancer, and diabetes mellitus occur in more than 10% of the world population. However, there is a lack of robust estimates of the worldwide incidence and mortality of pancreatic disease in the general population. According to the 2018 update of the burden and cost of GI, liver, and pancreatic diseases in the United States in 2014, there were more than 3.0 million hospital admissions in the United States for a GI disease at a cost of $30.6 billion dollars. Pancreatitis was one of three most common discharge diagnoses overall. The combined cost of pancreatitis, GI hemorrhage, and gallbladder disease was nearly $12 billion dollars.[72]

The clinical manifestations of pancreatic diseases vary. Patients with AP or CP may present with hypertriglyceridemia, vitamin B12 malabsorption, hypercalcemia, hypocalcemia, hyperglycemia, ascites, pleural effusions, and chronic abdominal pain with or without an increase in blood pancreatic enzymes (see Chapters 54–58). Weight loss, jaundice, itching, abdominal pain radiating to the back, early satiety, and anemia may indicate a malignant pancreatic process. The relative inaccessibility of the pancreas to direct clinical examination and the nonspecificity of the abdominal pain associated with pancreatic disease may make the diagnosis difficult. The number of observations of hyperamylasemia and hyperlipasemia in the general population are increased because general practitioners tend to include amylase and lipase more frequently in routine blood tests and because of the constant evaluation of this biochemical alteration in the emergency departments. With neither amylase nor lipase being specific for pancreatitis, it is important for the clinician to be aware of different causes of hyperamylasemia and hyperlipasemia, especially when the clinical diagnosis of pancreatitis is unclear; these causes include benign pancreatic hyperenzymemia (also known as Gullo's syndrome), diabetic ketoacidosis, head injury, trauma, acute liver failure, chronic renal failure, severe burns, shock, abdominal and cardiac surgery, toxic epidermal necrolysis, and Stevens-Johnson syndrome.[73,74] Pancreatic disease may also occur in patients with IBD because of the disease itself (Crohn disease) or because of side effects of medications used in the treatment (azathioprine, 6-mercaptopourine, 5-aminosalicylate, and corticosteroid treatment).[75] Imaging technologies have given clinicians an unprecedented toolbox to aid in clinical decision making. Currently, endoscopy, CT, and MRI are the core imaging methodologies for pancreatic diseases. Depending on the imaging modality used, the resulting images can reflect the anatomy, metabolism, or molecular aspects of the tissue of interest.[76]

Acute Pancreatitis

AP is the most common disease of the exocrine pancreas and is one of the most common reasons for hospitalization with a GI disease (see Chapters 55 and 56). Estimates of AP incidence and mortality in the general population vary greatly in the published literature and the epidemiology of pancreatitis has changed over time for many reasons, including population growth and migration, changes in patterns of alcohol consumption and tobacco smoking, rising rates of obesity and the recognition of metabolic causes of pancreatitis, and the increasing use and improving quality of imaging modalities. A recent systematic review and meta-analysis by Xiao et al. reported a global pooled incidence of AP of 34 cases per 100,000 individuals in the general population per year, with no statistically significant difference between the sexes. The disease predominantly affects those who are middle-aged or older. North America and West Pacific regions have a high incidence of disease (more than 34 cases per 100,000 individuals in the general population per year), whereas Europe is a low-incidence region (29 cases per 100,000 individuals in the general population per year). After the first episode of AP, recurrence will develop in 21% of patients and CP will develop in 36% of patients after recurrent AP. Xiao reported a pooled mortality from an episode of AP of 1.16 per 100,000 individuals in the general population per year, with persistent organ failure and infected pancreatic necrosis being the major determinants.[77,78] Although the case fatality rate for AP has decreased over time, the overall population mortality rate for AP has remained unchanged.[79]

The most common causes of AP are gallstone disease and alcohol abuse, which account for almost 75% of recognized cases. Numerous drugs have been involved in AP pathogenesis, the most strongly associated of which are azathioprine, 6-mercaptopurine, didanosine, valproic acid, angiotensin-converting enzyme (ACE) inhibitors, and mesalamine. AP has been associated with genetic mutations in the genes encoding cationic trypsinogen (PRSS1), serine protease inhibitor Kazal type 1 (SPINK1), cystic fibrosis transmembrane conductance regulator (CFTR), chymotrypsin C, calcium-sensing receptor, and claudin-2. Other causes of AP are hypertriglyceridemia, ERCP, trauma, surgery, viral infection, exposure to smoking and other environmental toxins, or effects of coexisting diseases such as obesity and diabetes, autoimmune pancreatitis as part of the multiorgan disorder called IgG4-related disease, and "nonalcoholic duct destructive pancreatitis" (also called idiopathic duct-centric CP).[80,81]

The clinical presentation of AP is characterized by constant, usually severe, upper abdominal pain, constant in intensity and persistent for several hours. The pain is mostly epigastric, occasionally generalized and radiating to the back or to the chest or flanks. Patients experience pain relief when sitting forward or worsening when lying flat. Symptoms may mimic the acute presentation of almost any acute abdominal pain but also myocardial infarction, pneumonia, and pleurisy. However, an acute episode may also be painless. Nausea and vomiting are also common, and sequestered fluid in the small bowel may lead to rapid and severe dehydration. Hiccoughs can also occur because of diaphragmatic irritation secondary to the extension of the inflammatory process tracking up via the retroperitoneum. The presentation of the patient can also be critical and dominated by a clinical picture of profound shock with tachycardia, tachypnea, hypotension, anuria, and mental status alteration. On the other hand, patients may be have a paucity of symptoms, with few physical signs. The patient may be afebrile on admission, but the progression of the inflammatory process leads to fever, facial flushing, and mild jaundice. Pancreatic ascites and pleural effusion may be present. Abdominal examination reveals epigastric tenderness and guarding. Abdominal

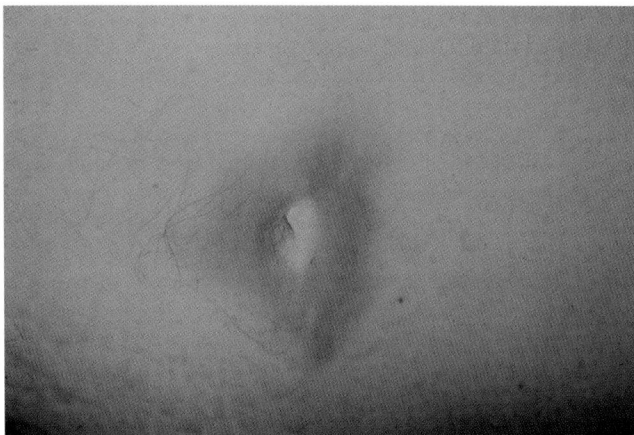

FIGURE 12.11 Cullen sign (periumbilical bruising).

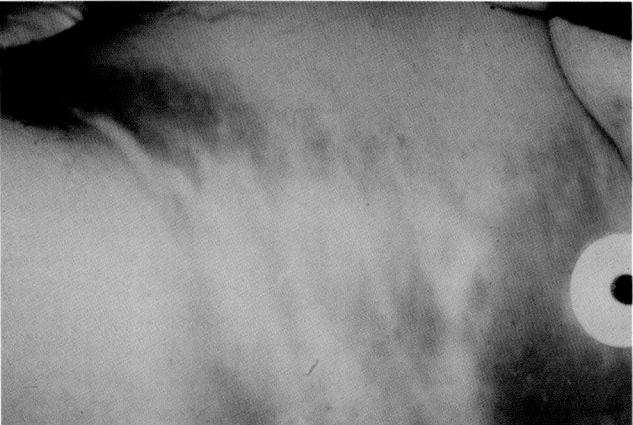

FIGURE 12.12 Grey-Turner sign (flank bruising).

distension with diminished peristalsis is a sign of the presence of a paralytic ileus. Later features may include mottled skin or livedo reticularis and lace-like purplish discoloration of the skin, which may appear up to 3 days from the clinical onset. Abdominal periumbilical ecchymosis, Cullen sign (Fig. 12.11), ecchymosis of the flank, and Grey-Turner sign (Fig. 12.12) result from the diffusion of fat necrosis and inflammation associated with retroperitoneal or intraabdominal bleeding. Although not specific, these signs are associated with a severe course and high mortality.[79,80]

Diagnosis and Severity Scoring

According to the 2012 revision of the Atlanta classification, the diagnosis of AP is established by the presence of at least two of the following criteria: abdominal pain consistent with the disease, serum lipase or amylase levels that are at least three times the upper limit of the normal range, and characteristic findings from abdominal imaging.[82] AP is divided into two phases. The first "early phase" occurs in the first week after onset (coinciding with the first day of pain), and the clinical scenario is dominated by the systemic inflammatory response. In this setting, the presence and degree of organ failure determine the severity and treatment. After the second week, the "late phase" starts, which can last for several weeks and is characterized by local complications and persistent organ failure.[80] Most episodes of AP are

mild and self-limiting. The last version of the classification system updated the definitions of severity in AP: Mild AP consists of no organ failure and no local or systemic complications.[83] Moderately severe AP is defined as local or other systemic complications and/or transient organ failure lasting less than 48 hours. Severe AP is defined as persistent organ failure lasting more than 48 hours. The determinant-based classification in 2012 introduced a fourth group with higher mortality, termed "critical," characterized by persistent organ failure and infected pancreatic necrosis.[84]

The ability to understand which patient will have a severe course of disease allows the clinician to triage the patient to an intensive care unit (ICU) and start an effective treatment early. The degree of the elevation of the serum amylase or lipase level has no prognostic value.[80] The prediction of severity is based on clinical, biochemical, and imaging findings (Box 12.7).[79] Several scoring systems have been validated to incorporate those findings in various combinations, including the Acute Physiology and Chronic Health Evaluation II (APACHE II), the APACHE combined with scoring for obesity (APACHE-O), the Glasgow scoring system, the Harmless Acute Pancreatitis Score (HAPS), PANC 3, the Japanese Severity Score (JSS), Pancreatitis Outcome Prediction (POP), and the Bedside Index for Severity in Acute Pancreatitis (BISAP). All of these methods have a high false-positive rate, are complex, and are not routinely used.[80] Pancreatic imaging is performed to determine the etiology of AP when the clinical situation is uncertain, to determine the severity, to evaluate complications, and to guide intervention. According to the American College of Gastroenterology Guidelines, a transabdominal US is recommended in all patients with suspected AP.[79] Because the majority of patients will have a mild, self-limited disease, CT scans are not routinely advocated. A CT scan is not required at the timepoint of admission unless the diagnosis is equivocal, clinical predictors suggest a severe course, conservative treatment is not followed by clinical improvement, or the patient is deteriorating. Moreover,

---

BOX 12.7 Acute Pancreatitis: Predictors of Severity

Clinical Findings:
Age >55 years
Obesity (BMI > 30 Kg/m²)
Altered mental status
Comorbid disease
Systemic inflammatory response syndrome (defined by the presence of > 2 of the following: pulse > 90 beats/min, respirations > 20/min or PaCO₂ >32 mm Hg, temperature >38°C or <36°C, WBC count >12,000 or <4000 cells/mm³ or >10% immature cells).

Laboratory Findings
BUN > 20 mg/dL
Rising BUN
HCT > 44%
rising HCT
Elevated creatinine

Radiologic Findings
Pleural effusion
Pulmonary infiltrates
Multiple or extensive extrapancreatic collections

BMI, Body mass index; *BUN,* blood urea nitrogen; *HCT,* hematocrit; *WBC,* white blood cell.

contrast-enhanced CT (CECT) is relatively contraindicated in patients with iodinated contrast agent allergies or impaired renal function. The initial CT assessment should be performed 72 to 96 hours after the onset of symptoms.[76] In the diagnostic process, EUS, MRCP, and ERCP are indicated to evaluate the biliary duct system (see Chapters 16, 17, 20, 22, 30, and 37C). ERCP should be performed early (<24 hours) in patients with acute cholangitis. MRCP is an accurate modality and its selective use reduces the need for ERCP.[85] Nevertheless, negative findings on MRCP do not exclude the presence of small CBD stones (<5 mm), for which EUS is superior.[86] Contrast-enhanced US (CEUS) has been used in some centers for the diagnostic evaluation of patients with pancreatitis. One study found CEUS to be equivalent to CECT and clinical scoring, with a sensitivity and specificity in detecting severe AP of 91% and 100%, respectively, compared with CT.[87]

Chronic Pancreatitis

Before 2016, CP was defined by relying on clinicopathologic features that were the expression of signs and symptoms of defined pathology (chronic inflammation, irreversible fibrosis without infection; see Chapters 57 and 58). This definition led to years of delay between symptom onset and diagnosis, failing to identify the etiology and to predict the clinical course. In 2016 an International Working Group defined CP as "a continuing inflammatory disease of the pancreas, characterized by irreversible morphologic change, and typically causing pain and/or permanent loss of function." The new definition addresses the disease mechanism as a "pathologic fibro-inflammatory syndrome of the pancreas in individuals with genetic, environmental, and/or other risk factors who develop persistent pathologic responses to parenchymal injury or stress." In addition, it defines the end-stage disease as "pancreatic atrophy, fibrosis, pain syndromes, duct distortion and strictures, calcifications, pancreatic exocrine dysfunction, pancreatic endocrine dysfunction, and dysplasia."[88]

The evaluation of the patient should start with a thorough history and a review of all risk factors, the characteristics of the pain, related conditions (e.g., steatorrhea and/or vitamin deficiency), and physical examination. Patients usually suffer from debilitating abdominal pain, malnutrition, osteoporosis, fat-soluble vitamin deficiency, and pancreatic endocrine failure (type 3c diabetes mellitus).[89]

A systemic review by Sankaran et al. in 2015 of high-quality cohort studies quantified the frequency of transition from the first episode of AP to recurrent acute pancreatitis (RAP) and CP. After the first episode of AP, RAP developed in 21% of patients; and after RAP, CP developed in 36% of patients. Transition was higher in patients with alcohol-induced versus biliary pancreatitis.[90] According to the systematic review by Xiao et al., the global pooled incidence of CP is 10 cases per 100,000 individuals in the general population per year.[77]

The diagnosis relies on exposure risk, underlying predisposition, and imaging and pancreatic function tests. The M-ANNHEIM multiple risk factor classification, published in 2007,[91] and the TIGAR-O (Toxic-Metabolic, Idiopathic, Genetic, Autoimmune, Recurrent and Severe Acute Pancreatitis and Obstructive) Pancreatitis Risk/Etiology Checklist version 2.0, updated in 2019,[92] are used to categorize the etiology and evaluate the impact and interaction of various risk factors on the course of the disease. Cross-sectional imaging is recommended for the first-line diagnosis. In 2017 a systematic review and meta-analysis of 43 studies compared the performances of

CT, MRI, and EUS, demonstrating that the sensitivity and specificity did not differ significantly among these modalities[93] (see Chapters 16, 17, and 22). However, EUS should be used if there is uncertainty after cross-sectional imaging.[94] Secretin-enhanced MRCP should be used if the former modalities are not diagnostic, thus identifying subtle ductal abnormalities that may provide morphologic clues for the diagnosis.[89] The prevalence of exocrine pancreatic insufficiency (EPI) ranges from 40% to 75% in patients with CP, and the risk is highest in those with alcohol and/or tobacco use or fibrocalcific pancreatitis. EPI is investigated with direct and indirect pancreatic function tests, including hormonal (CCK stimulation test and secretin stimulation test) and nonhormonal (fecal elastace-1 test, 13C-mixed triglyceride test, serum trypsinogen/trypsin test) tests. Because of the low sensitivity, these tests should be used only to support the diagnosis.[95] Genetic testing is recommended in patients in whom the etiology of CP is unclear; the primary goal is to identify pancreatitis-associated disorders that promote the pathogenic process, provide prognostic information, and identify possible targets for therapy. Patients should be evaluated for cationic trypsinogen (PRSS1), anionic trypsinogen (PRSS2), serine protease inhibitor Kazal-type 1 (SPINK1), and cystic fibrosis transmembrane conductance receptor (CFTR) gene mutations.[89]

Pancreatic Cancer

Clinical manifestations of pancreatic cancer are heterogeneous and may be absent until the lesion is unresectable (see Chapter 62). Typical symptoms include epigastric or mid-back pain, anorexia, early satiety, weight loss, diabetes mellitus, and obstructive jaundice. The clinical manifestations also include appetite loss, pale stools, dark urine, unusual bloating, unusual belching, constipation, and diarrhea. These symptoms may help the clinician suspect the diagnosis; however, approximately 50% of patients are more likely to have had three or more consultations for cancer symptoms before referring to the HPB surgeon.[96,97] Up to 80% of patients lose glycemic control over 3 years before the diagnosis of pancreatic cancer. New-onset diabetes is an early manifestation and a unique phenomenon of pancreatic cancer.[98,99] Abdominal pain is the most common presenting complaint, insidious in nature, and frequently has been present for 1 or 2 months at the time of diagnosis. This abdominal pain has a visceral gnawing quality and is generally epigastric but may radiate to the flanks and/or to the back.[100] The pain frequently exacerbates at night, is sleep disturbing, and may worsen in the postprandial period and in the supine position.[101] The compromise of the body and tail of the pancreas usually gives rise to severe back pain that is the result of splanchnic nerve and/or celiac plexus infiltration. Perineural invasion is a characteristic of pancreatic cancer and has a high prevalence of approximately 80% to 100%. It is related to a poor prognosis and is strongly associated with local recurrence after curative resection.[102,103] Postprandial pain may be secondary to an increase in secretory ductal pressure because of neoplastic obstruction of the duct of Wirsung. Because of CBD obstruction, on physical examination, the gallbladder may be distended and palpable (Courvoisier's gallbladder). An abdominal mass, fixed and hard, accompanied by ascites is a late sign and usually heralds inoperability. The Trousseau sign of malignancy or Trousseau's syndrome (*thrombophlebitis migrans*) is a systemic sign of neoplastic disease, but it is uncommon and nonspecific. Together with pain, jaundice and weight loss are generally later clinical features. Weight loss may be the only presenting symptom until pain indicates peripancreatic tissue invasion. Lesions of the pancreatic head usually manifest as jaundice and severe pruritus; when jaundice occurs with tumors of the body or tail of the pancreas, it usually signifies hilar liver or nodal metastases.

CT, MRI, and EUS are the imaging technologies usually involved in the detection of solid or cystic pancreatic lesions (see Chapters 16, 17, and 22). CT is required for full staging of the disease. Multiphasic CECT is the most ubiquitous imaging test with a sensitivity of 89% to 97% compared with histopathology.[104,105] Its sensitivity reaches 100% for tumors larger than 2 cm, but it falls to 77% for smaller tumors.[106] Tumors less than 1 cm can be isoattenuating on CT, thus making their detection challenging.[76] MRCP and MRI have a better sensitivity for small, isoattenuating lesions that subtly narrow the pancreatic duct. EUS combined with endoscopic-guided fine-needle aspiration has a sensitivity of 90% for detecting pancreatic cancer, but it is not widely available.[107]

Numerous novel studies about the molecular imaging of pancreatic cancer have been published so far, although these imaging techniques are early in clinical development. A promising agent would be one with high specificity (>90%) and sensitivity for cancer over benign disease.[76] Vascular endothelial growth factor receptor 2 (VEGFR2) is overexpressed during the neoangiogenic neoplastic process and has been detected in mouse adenocarcinoma vasculature using CEUS with a contrast agent of VEGFR2-targeted microbubble.[108] The same approach has been adopted using Thy1-targeted microbubble (a membrane glycoprotein), which was able to reliably detect pancreatic cancer as small as 3 mm in mouse models.[109] Other potential targets have been found in the tumoral stroma (IGF-1[110] and SPARC[111]), in the cytoskeleton (plectin[112]), and in the abnormal glycosylation of carbohydrate antigen 19-9 (CA19-9, the sialyl Lewis antigen).[113]

ASSESSMENT OF FITNESS FOR MAJOR HEPATOPANCREATOBILIARY SURGERY (SEE CHAPTERS 26 AND 27)

The median age for HPB cancer diagnosis is 66 years[114] and the number of patients will continue to rise in the future, thus making surgical resections high risk because of age, frailty, and multiple comorbidities. Preoperative care needs special attention to decrease morbidity and mortality.[115] Elderly patients' health status requires an accurate assessment, which can be achieved by a multidimensional diagnostic tool, the comprehensive geriatric assessment (CGA), which evaluates the medical, functional, and psychosocial status of these patients[116] and helps to identify vulnerable patients at increased risk for poor surgical outcomes. The functional status and the resulting risk of postoperative complications can be assessed by various screening tools, such as the Activities of Daily Living (ADL), the Instrumental Activities of Daily Living (IADL),[117] the Time Get-Up-and-Go (TUG) test,[118] the Six-Minute Walk Test (6MWT),[119] and the Cardiopulmonary Exercise Test (CPET).[120] Frailty is a clinically relevant domain defined by the presence of three or more of the following criteria: unintentional weight loss of more than 10 lbs in the previous year, self-reported exhaustion, weakness measured by grip strength, slow walking speed, and low levels of physical activity.[121] Frail patients are at increased risk for postoperative complications, increased LOS, and discharge to nursing facilities.[122] Several tools assess frailty, including the Groningen Frailty Index (GFI), the Vulnerable Elders Survey-13 (VES-13), and Fried's

frailty criteria assessment. Sarcopenia is a term describing morphometric data indicating a loss of skeletal mass and can be preoperatively assessed by CT-based measurements, and its presence has been associated with poorer surgical outcomes.[123] Malnutrition has been shown to correlate with increased morbidity, the severity of postoperative complications, and the LOS. Some of the more common parameters are weight loss, serum protein levels, immunocompetence, and anthropometric indicators.[124] Various tools exist for clinical use, including the Mini Nutritional Assessment examination (MNA), the Short Nutritional Assessment Questionnaire (SNAQ) Nutritional Risk Screening-2002 (NRS-2002), and the Geriatric 8 (G8). Postoperative delirium is associated with poorer surgical outcomes including morbidity, mortality, and discharge to nursing facilities. Patients at risk can be assessed by the Mini-Mental Status Examination (MMSE), the Mini-Cog assessment, and the Montreal Cognitive Assessment (MoCA).[125] As of yet, there is no consensus on the screening tool that should be used to adequately identify vulnerable oncogeriatric HPB patients. In 2013, Badgwell et al. identified the following CGA variables associated with a poorer outcome: weight loss greater than 10% within 6 months, American Society of Anesthesiologist (ASA) risk assessment score ≥2, Eastern Cooperative Oncology Group (ECOG) performance score ≥2, polypharmacy, and distant metastatic disease.[126] In 2014 Huisman et al. demonstrated that a TUG score greater than 20 identified twice as many surgical oncogeriatric patients as an ASA score ≥3 at risk for postoperative complications (50% vs. 24.8%).[118]

Other tools and scoring systems have been devised over time to assist in quantifying the surgical risk. The American College of Surgeons National Surgical Quality Improvement Program (ACS NSQIP) surgical risk calculator (http://riskcalculator.facs.org) collects high-quality standardized clinical data on preoperative risk factors and postoperative complications. It offers surgeons the ability to estimate patient-specific postoperative risk in a patient-friendly format, helping to decide which operation to perform and offering insights about the morbidity and mortality risk.[127] The Physiologic and Operative Severity Score for the Enumeration of Mortality and Morbidity (POSSUM), developed in 1991 by Copeland et al., has been evaluated extensively in both general surgery and HPB surgery. When used correctly, POSSUM can usefully predict morbidity and mortality in the surgical treatment of HPB patients.[128–131]

During the preoperative evaluation of HPB patients, other factors must be assessed to determine the postoperative risk. Postresection liver failure (PLF) remains the most important factor associated with postoperative mortality after major liver resections.[132–134] Liver function can be determined by combined analysis of results from volumetric liver assessments, liver functional MRI, and the indocyanine green clearance retention test (see Chapters 4 and 102). Total liver volume (TLV), future remnant liver volume (FRLV), and remnant liver volume percentage (RLV%) can be calculated by CT- or MRI-based volumetric liver analysis. In healthy livers, approximately 25% of the liver parenchyma needs to be preserved to prevent PLF. In damaged, postchemotherapy or cirrhotic livers, up to 50% of the liver parenchyma needs to be spared.[135–138] MRI-based T1 relaxometry with the liver-specific contrast agent gadolinium-ethoxybenzyl diethylene-triaminepentaacetic acid (Gd-EOB-DTPA) is an emerging method for assessing overall and segmental liver function.[139] Functioning areas of the liver exhibit shortening of the T1 relaxation time, and reduced liver function correlates with decreased Gd-EOB-DTPA accumulation in hepatocytes during the hepatobiliary phase. The indocyanine green retention rate at 15 minutes (ICG-R15) has been widely used as a routine guideline in Eastern countries for making appropriate surgical decisions in hepatocellular carcinoma patients and is considered the most predictive test of operative mortality after hepatectomy compared with other tests such as the aminoacidic clearance test or the aminopyrine breath test.[140] The ICG retention value at 15 minutes (ICG R15) describes the percentage of circulatory retention of indocyanine green during the first 15 minutes after bolus injection. In healthy patients, it is between 8% and 15% and the cutoff indicative of the need for a major hepatectomy is between 14% and 17%.[141,142] Minor resections may be performed for values that reach 22%, and limited hepatectomies may be performed for values up to 40%.

The references for this chapter can be found online by accessing the accompanying Expert Consult website.

CHAPTER 13

Cross-sectional imaging of liver, biliary, and pancreatic disease: Introduction and basic principles

Richard Kinh Gian Do

INTRODUCTION

Cross-sectional imaging of the liver, biliary tree, and pancreas can be performed with ultrasound, computed tomography (CT), or magnetic resonance imaging (MRI). Positron emission tomography (PET) is most often performed in combination with CT (PET-CT) and has more recently been performed in conjunction with MRI (PET-MRI). This chapter will emphasize basic principles of ultrasound, CT, and MRI that highlight the strengths and limitations of each technique for the ordering clinicians.

ULTRASOUND

Ultrasound as an imaging modality has tremendous versatility, is low-cost, and has real-time capability and portability. Ultrasound is considered safe at clinical, diagnostic levels, with no confirmed harmful biologic effects on the operator or patient. Use of Doppler ultrasound also allows for the assessment of blood flow dynamics (see Chapter 5). Despite these advantages, certain limitations influence the applicability of ultrasound. Ultrasound waves are unable to penetrate bone or air, which can obscure lesions and limit the field of view. The quality of ultrasound imaging and its interpretation are also operator dependent, which means they are influenced by skill and experience.

Different ultrasound transducers are optimized for specific frequencies. Lower-frequency transducers have poorer resolution with greater depth of penetration and thus are used to image deeper structures such as abdominopelvic tissues. Higher-frequency transducers have better spatial resolution, but higher-frequency sound attenuates rapidly and has poorer tissue penetration. Higher frequency ultrasound is best used for superficial soft tissues, such as the thyroid, and it can also be used to assess liver surface nodularity.

Echogenicity of tissue refers to the reflection or transmission of ultrasound waves relative to surrounding tissues. Based on gray scale imaging, a structure on the image display can be characterized as anechoic (uniformly black), hypoechoic (dark gray), or hyperechoic (light gray) (Fig. 13.1). Acoustic artifacts often occur, many of which are clinically useful. For example, acoustic enhancement is described when there is increased through-transmission of sound waves in fluid-containing structures, making tissue behind the fluid appear artificially bright, a characteristic of cystic structures (see Fig. 13.1). Certain artifacts are useful to hepatobiliary imaging in particular. Acoustic shadowing occurs when a structure attenuates sound more rapidly than surrounding tissues and casts a dark acoustic shadow beyond the object. This occurs with strong reflectors, such as calcifications, or strong attenuators, such as dense tumors. Acoustic shadowing is a feature of gallstones and, in

conjunction with mobility, aids in distinction between gallstones and gallbladder polyps (see Chapter 33). Comet tail artifact is a type of reverberation that occurs when two reflective interfaces are closely spaced, such as within a punctate crystal, producing posterior echoes that are parallel, evenly spaced echogenic bands with a triangular tapered shape. Comet tail artifact allows for the identification of surgical clips and is also a feature of gallbladder adenomyomatosis. Twinkle artifact is a color Doppler artifact that helps to detect and verify crystals and calcifications, particularly if a calculus does not demonstrate acoustic shadowing. Twinkle artifact occurs posterior to strong reflectors and appears as turbulent color Doppler flow with a mix of red and blue pixels; however, spectral Doppler tracing demonstrates noise. Additional artifacts have been described and are outside the scope of this chapter; the reader is referred to specialized texts.[1–3]

Liver Ultrasound

A normal liver is smooth in contour and uniform in echogenicity. Hepatic parenchyma is hypoechoic to the spleen and either isoechoic or minimally hyperechoic to renal parenchyma (see Fig. 13.1C). Liver size is most commonly determined sonographically by a longitudinal image of the right lobe. Treece et al. found that when the liver measures 15.5 cm or greater in the midhepatic line, hepatomegaly is present in 75% of patients.[4] In the right midclavicular line, the normal mean length is 10 cm, with a standard deviation of 1.5 cm.[5] In most patients the measurement of liver length suffices, but hepatic shape can be variable, and thus three-dimensional ultrasound volumetric analysis can aid evaluation.[6,7] Ultrasound images are obtained through available acoustic windows, avoiding bone and air, which will vary the appearance of the liver compared with the standard transverse planes of CT and MRI.

Doppler ultrasound is used to identify and evaluate blood flow in vessels based on the backscatter of blood cells (see Fig. 13.1D). Doppler imaging allows for the assessment of vessel patency, direction of blood flow, flow velocity, and spectral waveforms.[8] Three different Doppler displays are available: color, power, and spectral Doppler. Color Doppler provides information about the direction of motion and differences in flow velocity. Limitations of color Doppler imaging include dependence on angle of insonation, inability to display the entire Doppler spectrum in the image, and artifacts caused by aliasing and noise. Power (or amplitude) Doppler is a complementary technique that displays total amplitude of the echo signal but not flow direction. Power Doppler signal is more sensitive for flow detection than color Doppler and is less dependent on the angle of insonation. It is not subject to aliasing and is less sensitive to noise. Power Doppler is most useful in showing areas of low flow, depicting slow flow in an area of subtotal occlusion and demonstrating intralesional vascular patterns. In spectral

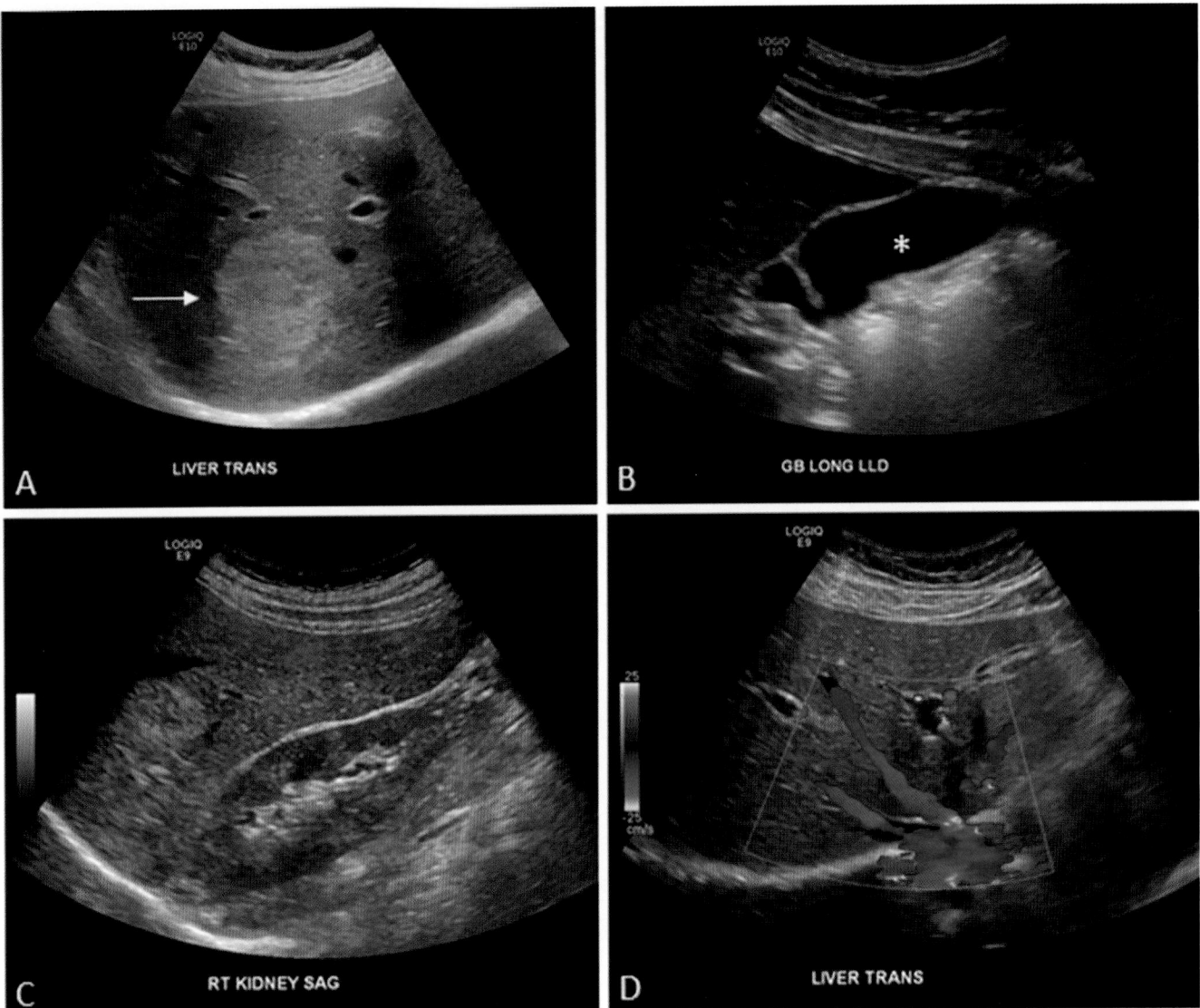

FIGURE 13.1   Liver ultrasound. A, A liver mass in the right hepatic lobe is hyperechoic, or brighter, than the liver parenchyma. **B**, The gallbladder (*) is anechoic (black) and as a fluid-containing structure, shows through transmission of sound waves, making posterior soft tissues brighter. **C**, The liver is usually isoechoic or slightly hyperechoic to renal parenchyma. **D**, Doppler images demonstrate blood flow in the hepatic veins.

Doppler, a sample volume cursor is placed within the target vessel and displays a waveform of the entire range of velocities during time, rather than the mean velocity as in a color Doppler image. Arterial waveforms are characterized as *high resistance* by limited flow during diastole or *low resistance* by continuous flow during diastole. At sites of stenosis, flow is not laminar; instead, flow becomes turbulent, and the spectral Doppler waveform reflects the red blood cells moving at varying velocities.

COMPUTED TOMOGRAPHY

CT excels as a cross-sectional imaging tool for hepatopancreatobiliary disease and provides high-resolution anatomic imaging that relies on differences in the ability of various tissues to attenuate x-ray beams. Relative to MRI, CT remains superior at in-plane and z-axis (interslice) resolution. Since its inception in the 1970s, the usage of CT has increased exponentially with key innovations such as helical scanning in the late 1980s and

multi-detector (MD) CT beginning in the late 1990s,[9] both contributing to the speed of CT image acquisition. The reduction in scanning times (several seconds for the entire study) greatly decreased motion artifacts and allowed multiphasic evaluation (hepatic arterial, portal venous, and delayed phases) of the liver and pancreas (Fig. 13.2). Current CT scanners can obtain images with resolution below 1 mm in all planes (i.e., isotropic submillimeter voxels), yielding smoother images when the data acquired in the axial plane are reformatted in the coronal, sagittal, and oblique planes.

With higher resolution data, many types of postprocessing[10] aided by voxel isotropy and digital display, include maximum intensity projection (MIP), where processed images depict only the brightest structures within the specified data volume.[10–15] Using portal venous phase source images, MIP images produce a more robust depiction of portal venous and hepatic venous anatomy (see Fig. 13.2; see also Chapter 5). Volume-rendered reconstructions provide a lifelike three-dimensional (3D) model of complex anatomy that can be rotated in any direction,[11,12,14,15]

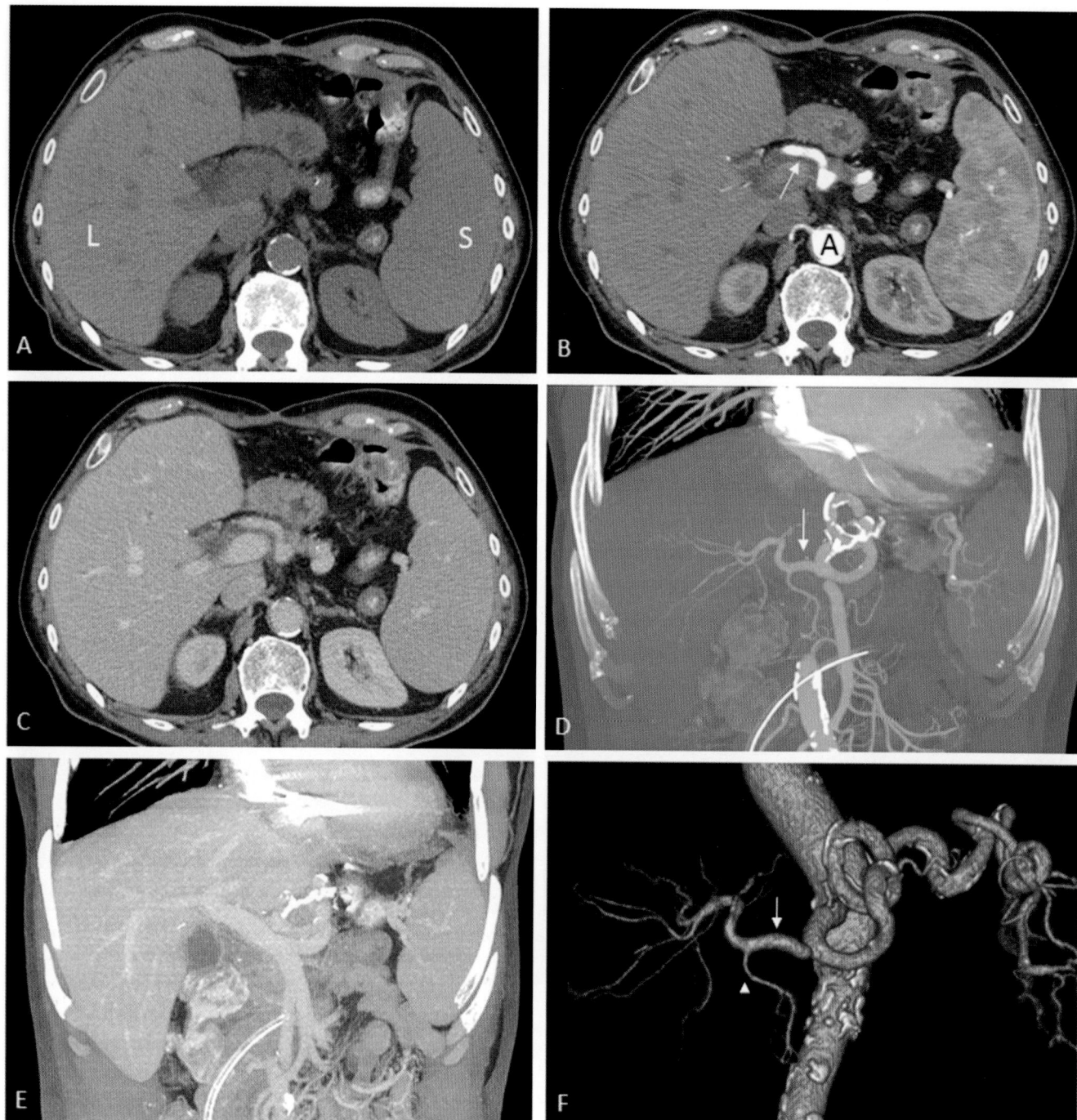

FIGURE 13.2 Multiphasic computed tomography imaging. A, Noncontrast computed tomography (CT) images of the upper abdomen, showing the unenhanced liver *(L)* and spleen *(S)*. **B,** Early arterial phase image shows enhancement of the aorta *(A)* and common hepatic artery *(arrow)*. **C,** Portal venous phase image shows enhancement of the portal and hepatic veins. **D,** Maximum intensity projection (MIP) image depicting visceral arteries. **E,** MIP image of abdomen in the portal venous phase image. **F,** 3D reconstruction of the celiac, splenic, and hepatic arterial anatomy, including the gastroduodenal artery *(arrowhead)*. Calcified plaques on the abdominal aorta appear brighter than the contrast within the arteries.

transforming the numerous axial images into an interactive 3D model that may be more intuitive to the surgeon. Hepatic arterial anatomy can be similarly displayed (see Fig. 13.2), and the relationship of tortuous vessels to the hepatic parenchyma and lobar anatomy can be depicted clearly. It is also possible to view a rotating model that depicts the relationship of a mass to the adjacent vessels from any angle to help the surgeon conceptualize

preoperatively what would be encountered at surgery (see Chapters 2 and 118–122).

Although MRI offers superior tissue contrast and capability for functional imaging (and thus superior lesion characterization), the superior spatial resolution, ease of interpretation, greater availability, and lower cost of CT maintain it as the most frequently requested modality in evaluating the liver and pancreas. A major drawback remains usage of ionizing radiation, with a trend in past decades toward decreasing exposure of the patient population. Dose reduction in multiphasic CT studies of the liver and pancreas CT have been a priority.[16] With a lower dose, however, CT images become noisier, requiring new reconstruction algorithms to "smooth out" the images, such as adaptive statistical iterative reconstruction (ASIR) and model-based iterative reconstruction.[17–19] Lower-dose and new reconstruction algorithms are not without limitations because they may reduce the conspicuity of liver metastases.[20]

Dual-energy CT (DECT) is another recent development using either a single radiation source that alternates beam energies ("rapid switching" or rsDECT) or two radiation sources of differing energies ("dual source" or dsDECT) to produce CT images. For the liver, biliary system, and pancreas, applications include "material-specific imaging" and "virtual monochromatic imaging."[21] In the liver, "virtual iron images" may be used for quantitation of hepatic iron deposition without interference from coexisting steatosis,[22] whereas "virtual non-iron images" can be created for fat quantitation independent of concomitant siderosis[23] (see Chapter 69). "Virtual iodine mapping" may also aid in identifying tumor thrombus and distinguishing it from bland thrombus in the setting of hepatocellular carcinoma (HCC; see Chapter 89).[24] In the pancreas, lower kilovolt peak images from "virtual monochromatic" dsDECT[25] and lower kiloelectron volt images from virtual monochromatic rsDECT[26] have been shown to improve conspicuity of hypovascular tumors, such as typical ductal adenocarcinoma. Lower-energy virtual monochromatic images may also provide more robust surface-rendered 3D arterial images, whereas virtual higher-energy images have less apparent metallic artifact around biliary stents and clips.[21]

Computed Tomography in Liver Imaging

State-of-the-art CT evaluation of the liver may include any combination of the following: precontrast, contrast-enhanced early arterial phase (CT angiography), late arterial phase, portal venous phase, and/or delayed phase. Routine CT is usually performed only in the portal venous phase because common liver metastases, such as those from colon cancer, are commonly hypovascular relative to adjacent normal liver parenchyma (see Chapter 90). On the other hand, hypervascular neoplasms such as hepatocellular adenomas and HCC and certain metastases (see Chapters 88, 89, and 91), including neuroendocrine tumors, renal cell carcinoma, melanoma, and thyroid cancer, are generally evaluated using a multiphasic protocol that includes precontrast, late arterial phase, and portal venous images, with the addition of delayed phase images for HCC.[27,28]

Early arterial phase high-resolution images (CT angiography) are obtained to assess tumor involvement of arteries and evaluate variant celiac axis anatomy.[29] Identification of variant anatomy (see Chapter 2) is crucial to decisions regarding hepatic arterial embolization (see Chapter 94) and placement of hepatic arterial chemoinfusion pumps (see Chapter 97); gains in image resolution during the MDCT era have allowed CT angiography to largely supplant invasive direct catheter angiography for planning placement of intraarterial chemoinfusion pumps[30] (see Chapter 21). Vascular mapping may now also be performed with CT.

In planning for surgery and other locoregional therapy, portal and hepatic veins can be identified as anatomic landmarks to localize tumors to specific hepatic segments (see Chapter 2) and to assess the proximity of lesions to the inflow and outflow vessels. This information determines the extent of potential hepatic resection required to achieve clear surgical margins. If a proposed operation will be extensive, postprocessing of CT images with 3D volume rendering can also identify segmental or lobar hepatic atrophy and compensatory hypertrophy.

Computed Tomography in Pancreatic Imaging

CT imaging of the pancreas relies on the differential intravenous (IV) contrast enhancement between tumor tissue and normal pancreatic parenchyma. The use of IV contrast agent is mandatory for accurate diagnosis, and timing of the contrast injection and accurate delivery of the appropriate volume requires the use of a dedicated CT power injector.[31] The precontrast scan permits evaluation of pancreatic calcifications and allows for localization of the gland and pertinent arteries in the z-axis for subsequent acquisition of contrast-enhanced phases. IV contrast medium is injected at a high flow rate of 4 to 6 mL per second. The late arterial or pancreatic parenchymal phase, acquired roughly 30 to 40 seconds after initiating contrast injection, is designed to maximize differences in contrast enhancement between pancreatic neoplasms and adjacent normal pancreatic tissue and is also useful in evaluating hypervascular liver metastases seen in patients with pancreatic endocrine neoplasms (see Chapter 91). Last, the portal venous phase acquired approximately 70 to 90 seconds from the start of IV contrast injection provides the best evaluation of hepatic metastases from pancreatic ductal adenocarcinoma[32,32] (see Chapter 62) and, in some cases, offers the best contrast to identify the primary pancreatic lesions themselves. The dedicated pancreas protocol uses oral water as a negative contrast agent administered before the examination to aid distinction of enhanced vessels from the gastrointestinal tract[33–35] and to facilitate identification of tumor invasion into the adjacent bowel.

MAGNETIC RESONANCE IMAGING

MRI is a cross-sectional multiplanar imaging technique. MRI uses magnetic fields and radiofrequency pulses to generate images with outstanding tissue contrast and excellent spatial resolution. The principles of nuclear magnetic resonance were first described in the 1940s by Bloch et al.[36] and Purcell et al.[37] as a method for in vitro chemical analysis; these principles were later used by Damadian[38] and Lauterbur[39] to design MRI for in vivo imaging. Today, MRI is used extensively as a medical imaging tool throughout the body to visualize and distinguish normal and pathologic tissue.

Principles of Magnetic Resonance Imaging

Liver MRI used in clinical practice consists of a combination of T1- and T2-weighted images (T1w and T2w), as well as diffusion-weighted imaging (DWI), obtained before or after IV contrast administration (Fig. 13.3). The variety of contrast available to MRI is a result of the signal available from the magnetic moment (or spin) present in hydrogen atoms (H^1) because of its abundance in the human body in the form of water and fat. Other nuclei that may be imaged by MRI include phosphorus (P^{31}), sodium (Na^{23}), and carbon (C^{13}), but these are used mostly in the research setting. A measurable signal is generated from the magnetic moment after excitation by a radiofrequency (RF) pulse; signal is generated as the excited

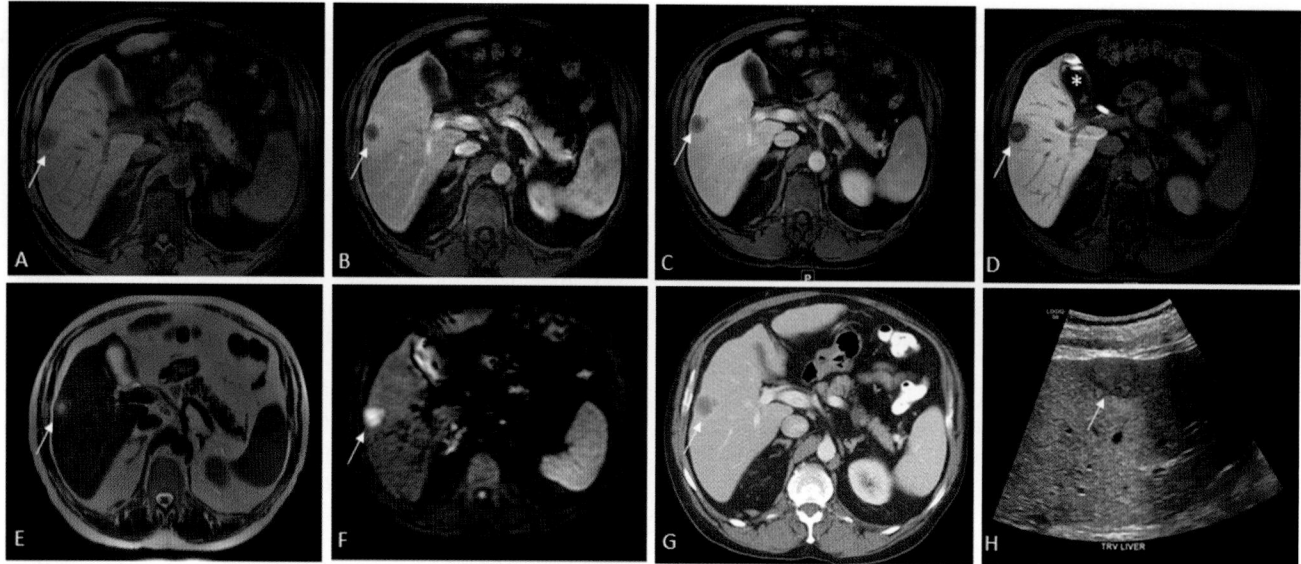

FIGURE 13.3 Magnetic resonance imaging of liver metastasis. **A**, Precontrast T1-weighted image with fat suppression shows a hypointense (dark) right hepatic metastasis *(arrow)*. **B**, Perilesional hyperenhancement is seen on T1-weighted imaging in the arterial phase. **C**, The liver metastasis is hypovascular in the portal venous phase. **D**, Postcontrast delayed hepatobiliary phase shows a hypointense liver metastasis. Hyperintense hepatobiliary contrast (Gd-EOB-DTPA) is seen excreted into the gallbladder (*) and common hepatic duct. **E**, The right hepatic metastasis is hyperintense (bright) on T2-weighted imaging. **F**, Diffusion-weighted imaging shows hyperintense signal (or diffusion restriction) in the right hepatic metastasis. **G**, Contrast-enhanced CT image in the portal venous phase shows the same hypovascular right hepatic metastasis. **H**, Ultrasound image of the liver metastasis shows the expected hypoechoic appearance.

nuclei return to equilibrium, releasing energy in the form of an electromagnetic field that is captured by a receiver coil. The strength of this emitted signal determines the signal intensity (SI) of a tissue. The precise tissue SI depends on several factors, including its intrinsic longitudinal relaxation (T1), transverse relaxation (T2), proton density (the number of nuclei present), flow, and the coil itself. T1w and T2w images are created by manipulating the RF pulse and various electromagnetic fields during imaging.

Differences in T1 and T2 relaxation times intrinsic to various soft tissues (e.g., fat, muscles, water) can be exploited to improve image contrast and diagnostic accuracy. For example, free water is low signal on standard T1w imaging and markedly high signal on T2w imaging. Thus so-called heavily T2w imaging sequences (e.g., used in magnetic resonance [MR] cholangiopancreatography) highlight high water content structures, such as bile and pancreatic ducts, while reducing the signals of other organs. DWI is used to highlight differences in water diffusion. The higher proportion of cell membranes in rapidly dividing cells contributes to restricted diffusion of cancer cells. DWI of the liver is thus used to help detect hepatic metastases and may also be used to assess changes in the liver parenchyma, such as liver fibrosis.[40]

Magnetic Resonance Imaging of the Liver

MRI is routinely used to evaluate diffuse and focal liver abnormalities. Normal hepatic parenchyma is brighter (hyperintense) than the spleen on T1w images, whereas on T2w images, the spleen is relatively brighter than the liver (see Fig. 13.3). Although most hepatic lesions are low in signal intensity on T1w images, they have more variable intensity on T2w images, with cysts (see Chapter 73) and hemangiomas (see Chapter 88) having the highest T2 signal intensity in general. Precontrast and

postcontrast T1w imaging is also performed to assess enhancement patterns of the liver parenchyma and liver lesions, similar to a multiphasic CT. If a hepatobiliary contrast agent is used, additional transitional phase and delayed hepatobiliary phase images are acquired.

MRI contrast agents for hepatobiliary imaging are divided into two categories: *extracellular* fluid (ECF) and hepatobiliary contrast agents. After IV injection, ECF agents, such as gadopentetate dimeglumine (gadolinium diethylenetriaminepentaacetic acid [Gd-DTPA]), distribute within the intravascular compartment and rapidly diffuse through the extravascular space, similar to the action of iodinated contrast agents in CT imaging. Hepatobiliary-specific contrast agents behave similar to traditional ECF contrast agents when first injected, but they are taken up to varying degrees by functioning hepatocellular tissue and are excreted in bile over time. Hepatobiliary specific agents include mangafodipir trisodium, gadobenate dimeglumine, and gadoxetic acid disodium (Gd-EOB-DTPA). Both gadobenate dimeglumine (MultiHance; Bracco Imaging, Cranbury Township, NJ) and gadolinium-ethoxybenzyl-diethylenetriamine pentaacetic acid (Eovist/Primovist; Bayer Healthcare, Wayne, NJ) have been approved in the United States. Gd-EOB-DTPA has become the preferred hepatobiliary contrast agent given its rapid uptake by normal liver parenchyma that allows for hepatobiliary phase imaging at approximately 20 minutes after IV injection. These agents provide comprehensive information about the hepatic parenchyma, bile ducts, and liver vasculature.[41,42]

Magnetic Resonance Imaging Cholangiopancreatography

MR cholangiopancreatography (MRCP) is an imaging technique used to evaluate the bile and pancreatic ducts and plays an important role in imaging benign disorders, as well as in comprehensive evaluation of malignancies of the biliary system.[43-45] Heavily T2w images are used to provide an overview of biliary and pancreatic ductal anatomy, by reducing the signal of surrounding nonfluid structures. Cross-sectional images and maximum intensity projection images (see Fig. 13.2) are produced with current MRCP techniques, and projection images are similar to direct contrast-enhanced cholangiograms obtained with either endoscopic retrograde cholangiopancreatography (ERCP) or percutaneous transhepatic cholangiography. MRCP is a noninvasive imaging tool, eliminating the potential morbidity associated with ERCP or PTC.[46]

The basic principle of MRCP is to use T2w imaging to highlight stationary or slowly moving fluid, including bile, as high in signal intensity; surrounding tissues, including retroperitoneal fat and the solid visceral organs, with shorter T2 values, are markedly reduced in signal. In addition to heavily T2-weighted sequences, MRCP protocols also include routine T1w, T2w, and DWI sequences obtained during a liver MRI.

MAGNETIC RESONANCE IMAGING SAFETY CONSIDERATIONS

MRI is an attractive alternative to CT imaging because of the lack of ionizing radiation and the higher safety profile of MR gadolinium contrast agents. However, physicians should be aware of some important considerations, including MR contrast deposition and the risk of interactions between the patient (including their implants) with the MR scanner. In a worst-case scenario, patients can die if placed in an MRI without proper implant screening, as some have after torsion of brain aneurysm clips.[47] MRI facilities should all have screening programs in place to address contraindicated devices, under new MRI safety guidelines proposed by the American College of Radiology.[48] However, referring physicians should become familiar with their local imaging centers' approach to MRI safety, and specifically their ability to scan patients with MR-conditional or MR-unsafe pacemakers and defibrillators.

Unlike iodinated contrast used for CT imaging, MRI gadolinium-based contrast agents (GBCAs) have no association with contrast-induced nephropathy, and contrast-enhanced (CE) MRI is an alternative for patients with moderate to severe renal failure. Administration of GBCAs in patients with severe or end-stage renal insufficiency carries a small risk of nephrogenic systemic fibrosis (NSF). NSF is a serious and potentially fatal complication related to free gadolinium deposition within soft tissues and organs, with resulting scleroderma-like fibrosis. The exact causal mechanism of NSF remains unknown, but the risk of NSF increases in patients with an estimated glomerular filtration rate (eGFR) less than 30 mL/min, and particularly in patients with end-stage disease (eGFR < 15 mL/min). Gadolinium contrast usage in these patients should only be performed if essential, after careful evaluation of risks versus benefits, and with consultation with a nephrologist, if available. Since NSF was initially described, the rapid international investigation, dissemination of information, and swift adjustment to policy have led to a precipitous drop in reported NSF cases. In multiple countries, NSF has essentially disappeared since 2009.[49-51] In recent years, macrocyclic GBCAs have emerged as preferred contrast agents for patients undergoing MRI because of the lower risk of NSF and gadolinium deposition.[52]

The references for this chapter can be found online by accessing the accompanying Expert Consult website.

CHAPTER 14

Imaging features of benign and malignant liver tumors and cysts

Kate Anne Harrington

INTRODUCTION

The increased frequency of cross-sectional imaging with improved imaging techniques has resulted in the increased detection of liver lesions. The majority of incidentally discovered liver lesions are benign, even in the oncologic population.[1,2] Although ultrasound (US) can be useful in screening for and detecting liver lesions, lesion characterization is mostly performed using computed tomography (CT) or magnetic resonance imaging (MRI). Contrast-enhanced ultrasound (CEUS) provides real-time dynamic assessment capability, with high spatial and temporal resolution, making it a valuable component of multimodality imaging. This method is more widely used in Europe and Asia, with US Food and Drug Administration (FDA) approval of microbubble contrast agents for noncardiac use only granted since 2015.

MRI has more advantages than CT in the evaluation of liver lesions, notwithstanding the avoidance of patient exposure to ionizing radiation that occurs with CT. The numerous sequences that are at the radiologist's disposal with MRI means that many lesions can be accurately diagnosed on imaging.

BENIGN LIVER TUMORS

For more information on benign liver tumors, see Chapter 88.

Hemangioma

Hepatic hemangiomas are benign vascular tumors of the liver and have an estimated incidence of anywhere between 4% and 20%.[3,4] Most hemangiomas are found incidentally on imaging studies such as ultrasound and CT. The most typical forms of hemangioma are cavernous and flash-filling hemangiomas.

On US, hemangiomas are characteristically homogeneously hyperechoic, well-circumscribed masses with subtle posterior acoustic enhancement (Fig. 14.1A). A hyperechoic rim may also be seen in a portion of hemangiomas, particularly if the hemangioma was predominantly isoechoic to liver. Increased echogenicity is because of multiple vascular interfaces within hemangiomas. Although hemangiomas are vascular, flow is extremely slow, and usually no Doppler signal is evident.[5] If a US shows a classic appearance of hemangioma and the patient has no risk factors, history of underlying liver disease (hepatitis, alcohol abuse, fatty liver, etc.), or malignancy, then no follow-up imaging needs to be performed.[6,7] It should be noted that those with a history of malignancy and at an increased risk for hepatocellular carcinoma (HCC) should be further evaluated upon the identification of an echogenic liver lesion. In a study of 1,982 patients with cirrhosis, US depicted hemangioma-like lesions in 44 patients; on follow-up, half of these proved to be HCCs, and half were hemangiomas.[8]

Larger hemangiomas often lack characteristic features because of central fibrosis, necrosis, and myxomatous degeneration

and can appear heterogeneously hyperechoic (see Fig. 14.1B). When the background liver itself becomes hyperechoic as a result of steatosis, hemangiomas may appear hypoechoic to liver parenchyma.[5,9]

On CT, hemangiomas are typically hypoattenuating to surrounding liver on noncontrast imaging. In patients with hepatic steatosis, the liver is typically diffusely decreased in attenuation, thereby decreasing the conspicuity of hypoattenuating hemangiomas. However, fatty sparing around the rim of the hemangioma can occur, resulting in the presence of a hyperattenuating rim on noncontrast CT.[10]

MRI is ideal for characterizing hemangiomas and is the preferred modality for characterization with a high sensitivity and specificity.[11] On T2-weighted imaging, hemangiomas are T2 bright, nearly similar in intensity to cerebrospinal fluid (CSF).[3] On diffusion-weighted imaging (DWI), hemangiomas appear hyperintense on low b-values and remain hyperintense at higher b-values, similar to malignant lesions. Nevertheless, they will also have high apparent diffusion coefficient (ADC) values, a phenomenon known as T2 shine-through. This can be useful when differentiating from metastases, which have lower ADC values.[12]

The classical enhancement pattern of cavernous hemangiomas seen on multiphase contrast-enhanced imaging done on US, CT, and MRI is typically peripheral, nodular, discontinuous enhancement on arterial phase, with centripetal fill-in on portal venous phase and persistent homogenous enhancement on later postcontrast phases (Fig. 14.2). The peripheral areas of enhancement follow the same attenuation or signal intensity of blood vessels (such as the hepatic artery or portal vein).[13–15]

Caution must be used when assessing enhancement on MRI using a hepatocyte specific contrast agent such as gadoxetate disodium (Gd-EOB-DTPA). The overlapping extracellular phase and hepatobiliary excretion of this contrast may confound the typical hemangioma enhancement pattern and lead to the appearance of "pseudowashout" in the late dynamic phase.[16] Because hemangiomas do not contain hepatocytes, they become gradually hypointense on the transitional and hepatobiliary phase. For this reason, we prefer not to use gadoxetate disodium as the contrast agent for initial liver lesion characterization and use a traditional extracellular fluid contrast (ECF) agent instead, such as one of the macrocyclic gadolinium agents (e.g., gadobenate dimeglumine, gadoterate meglumine, gadoteridol).

Flash-filling hemangiomas are often small lesions (under 1 cm in diameter) and appear as diffusely hypervascular, homogenous lesions. Homogenous enhancement is seen in the arterial phase, and enhancement density/intensity follows that of the aorta in subsequent phases.[15]

Larger hemangiomas tend to follow the cavernous type enhancement pattern criteria, although giant hemangiomas

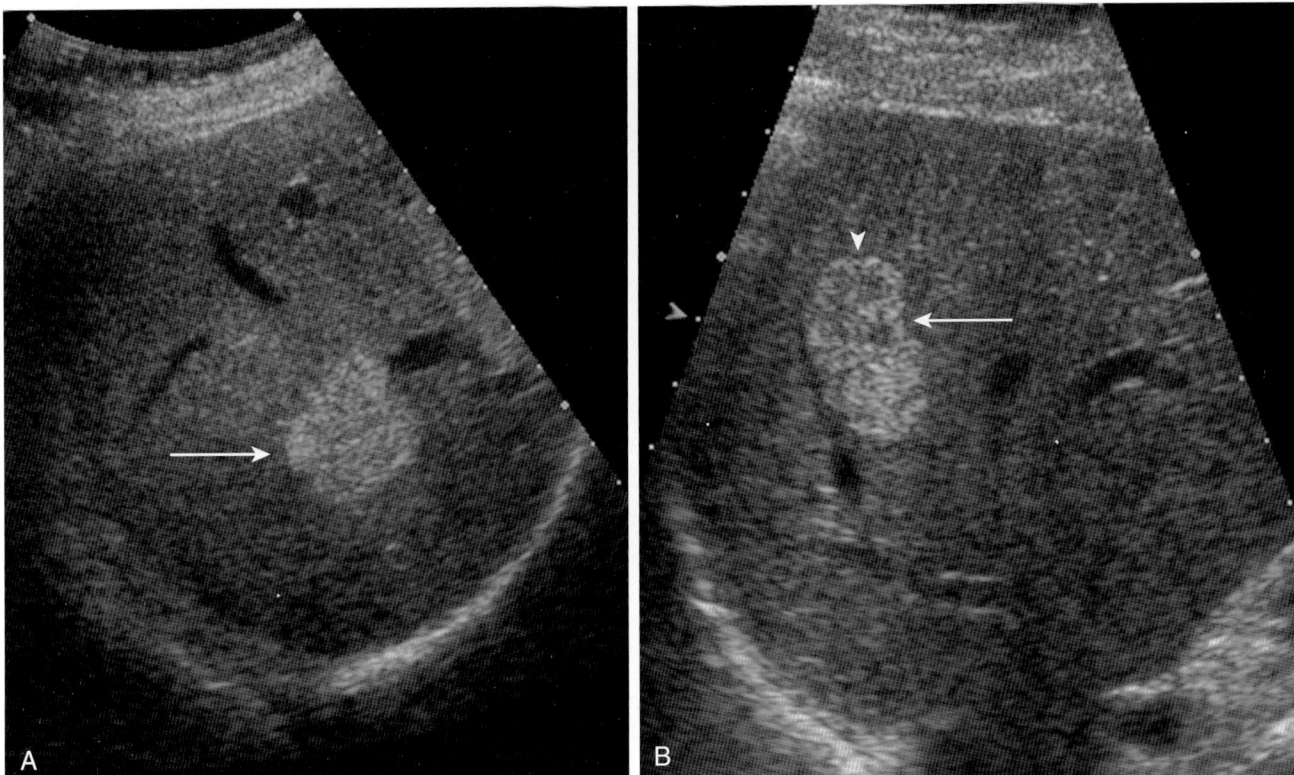

FIGURE 14.1   Hemangiomas. A, Longitudinal sonogram of the right lobe shows a brightly echogenic hemangioma *(arrow)* with a circumscribed border. **B,** Atypical hemangioma *(arrow)* with areas of internal heterogeneity, a result of fibrosis or myxomatous degeneration, and a thin echogenic rim *(arrowhead).*

(>6–10 cm) may also have variable signal intensity and a central scar.[17] Giant hemangiomas often do not completely fill in with contrast on delayed phases.

Calcification in hemangiomas is rare and is reported in 10% to 20% of cases,[18] although our own experience is much lower than 10%. Calcifications may correspond to phleboliths and are most easily detected on CT.

Sclerosed and sclerosing hemangiomas are a rare type of hemangioma where degeneration and intralesional fibrosis and hyalinization occurs (Fig. 14.3). These hemangiomas do not exhibit typical appearances on MRI because of loss of normal vascular channels. Markedly sclerosed hemangiomas lack the classic T2 hyperintense signal on MRI and may even become isointense to the liver parenchyma. Commonly, they demonstrate little or minimal arterial-phase enhancement and show variable progressive enhancement in portal venous and delayed phases.[19] Some sclerosed hemangiomas may not achieve any enhancement on any phase, particularly if the lesion shows marked sclerosis on histopathologic evaluation.[19] Additional features that may be seen in sclerosed hemangiomas include capsular retraction and peritumoral arterial enhancement.[20] Thus, sclerosed hemangioma are easily mistaken for metastatic disease in the liver and may require biopsy for definitive diagnosis.

Focal Nodular Hyperplasia

Focal nodular hyperplasia (FNH) is the second most common solid benign liver lesion after hemangioma. Pathologically, FNH contains all the elements of normal liver, may have a central fibrous scar, and is surrounded by hepatocytes and small bile ducts. FNH has been associated with oral contraceptive use, as well as chemotherapy in the pediatric age group, although the former association is not definitive.[21]

On US, FNH has a smooth lobulated contour and variable echogenicity. A key to US diagnosis of FNH is the characteristic Doppler appearance of a central feeding artery with tortuous spoke-wheel vascularity.[22] A recognized feature of FNH is the presence of a central scar, yet this is usually better depicted on CT, MRI, or CEUS.[14]

On CT, FNH is isoattenuating or slightly hypoattenuating to adjacent liver on noncontrast imaging. If a central scar is present, it is hypointense on precontrast phase.[23] Although described as a typical feature, a scar is usually only seen on CT in approximately 20% to 50% of cases.[24,25]

On MRI, most FNH are isointense to normal liver parenchyma and nearly invisible on T1- and T2-weighted images (Fig. 14.4). Occasionally, some lesions may be mildly T1 hypointense or minimally T2 hyperintense. When discussing relative T1 and T2 signal, a normal background liver parenchyma is assumed. In a liver with iron deposition, which diffusely lowers the signal intensity of the liver parenchyma, T1 and T2 relative hyperintensity can be expected.[21] A central scar can be seen more frequently on MRI and is hypointense on T1-weighted images and hyperintense on T2-weighted images (see Fig. 14.4).[24]

After intravenous (IV) contrast administration, the typical enhancement pattern of FNH is diffuse homogenous hyperenhancement in the arterial phase, followed by fading to background hepatic attenuation/intensity by the portal venous phase (see Fig. 14.4).[26–28] Fading to background hepatic parenchyma signal should be distinguished from "washout," where a lesion becomes darker than background liver. When a central scar is

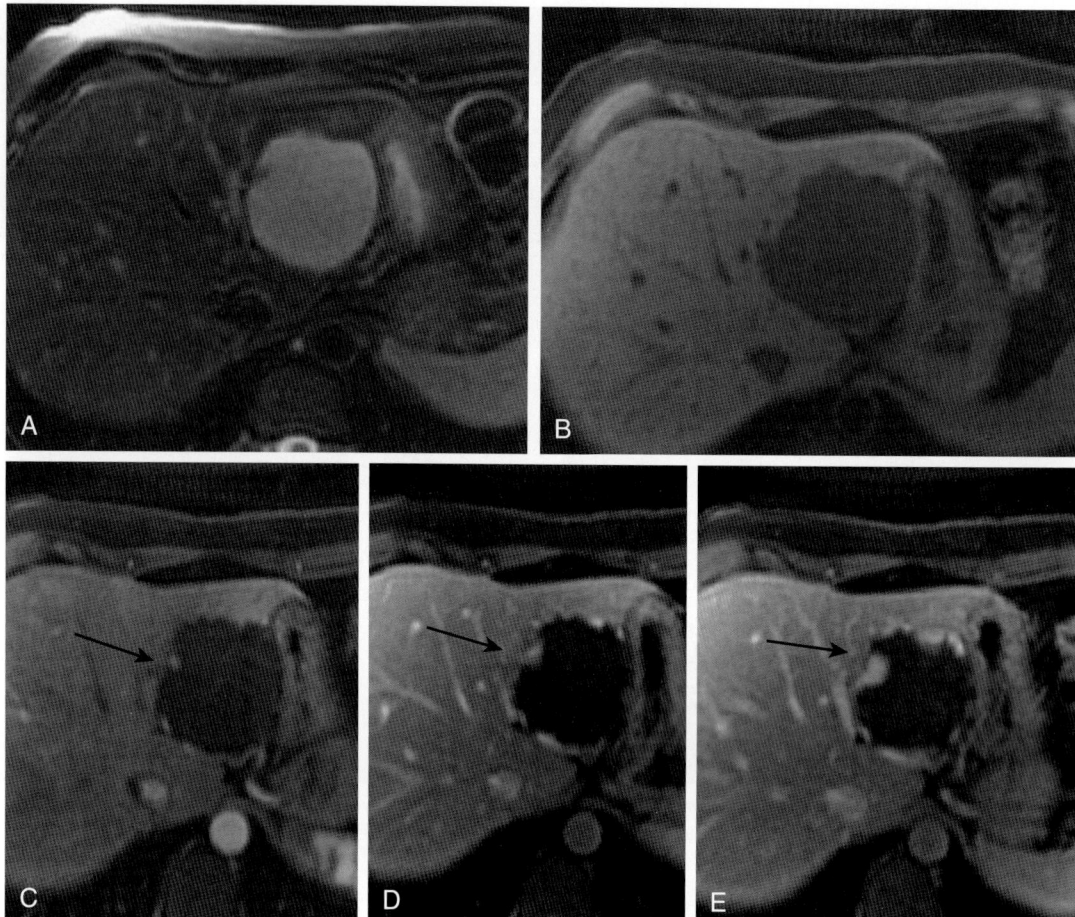

FIGURE 14.2 Cavernous hemangioma. A, Fat-saturated T2-weighted image shows a mass that is hyperintense to hepatic parenchyma, with well-defined margins. **B,** Precontrast T1-weighted fat saturation image at the same level shows the mass to be low in signal compared with background parenchyma. **C–E,** Multiphase T1-weighted postcontrast image in arterial, portal venous and equilibrium phases respectively shows progressive, peripheral nodular enhancement within this mass *(arrows).*

present, it enhances on delayed phases, beginning at approximately 3 minutes when using ECF contrast agents.[29] When a hepatocyte-specific contrast agent is used, lesional enhancement similar to or higher-than-normal to background hepatic parenchyma during the delayed hepatobiliary phase is expected in the majority of FNHs (Fig. 14.5). Of note, with the use of a hepatobiliary-specific agent such as gadoxetate disodium, a central stellate scar, if present, does not progressively enhance on later dynamic phases and will appear relatively hypointense, reflecting the absence of hepatocytes and the presence of fibrous tissue within the scar.[29]

Hepatocellular Adenoma

Hepatocellular adenoma (HCA) is a benign hepatocellular tumor; however, unlike FNH, it is a true neoplastic lesion with associated complications, such as abdominal pain, bleeding, and, rarely, malignant degeneration. HCAs have been traditionally associated with oral contraceptive use in women of childbearing age or anabolic steroid use in men. More recently, metabolic syndrome associations such as diabetes mellitus and obesity have also been recognized as risk factors.[30] Adenomas are usually solitary, with multiple lesions seen in less than 30% of cases.[31] Adenomatosis has been a term typically reserved for the presence of greater than 10 adenomas, first described in

1985.[32] However, adenomatosis does not refer to a particular type of adenoma, and it has become apparent that clinical features and histologic subtype are more important than the number of adenomas present.[31]

Over the past decade, HCAs have been further characterized and subtyped by their specific morphologic and immunohistochemical phenotype, with the most recent classification in 2017 describing eight subtypes.[33] Four additional subtypes were added to the already described hepatocyte nuclear factor (HNF)1α-inactivated HCA (H-HCA), inflammatory HCA (IHCA), β-catenin-activated HCA (β-HCA) and "unclassified" subtypes. The newly added subtypes were β-HCA exon 7/8, β-IHCA exon 3, β-IHCA exon 7/8, and sonic-hedgehog HCA (sh-HCA), some of which were previously lumped together in the "unclassified" section. When considering HCA diagnosis for a liver lesion on imaging, correlation with patient demographics is important because men with metabolic syndrome or anabolic steroid use and adenomas with β-catenin-activated mutations are at a much higher risk for malignant degeneration.

On US, HCAs have variable echogenicity but are often hyperechoic because of intratumoral fat content. Internal hemorrhage within adenomas may produce cystic areas.[23] Vascular flow is usually detected on Doppler imaging; however, the pattern of flow is nonspecific and may be seen as exclusively intralesional

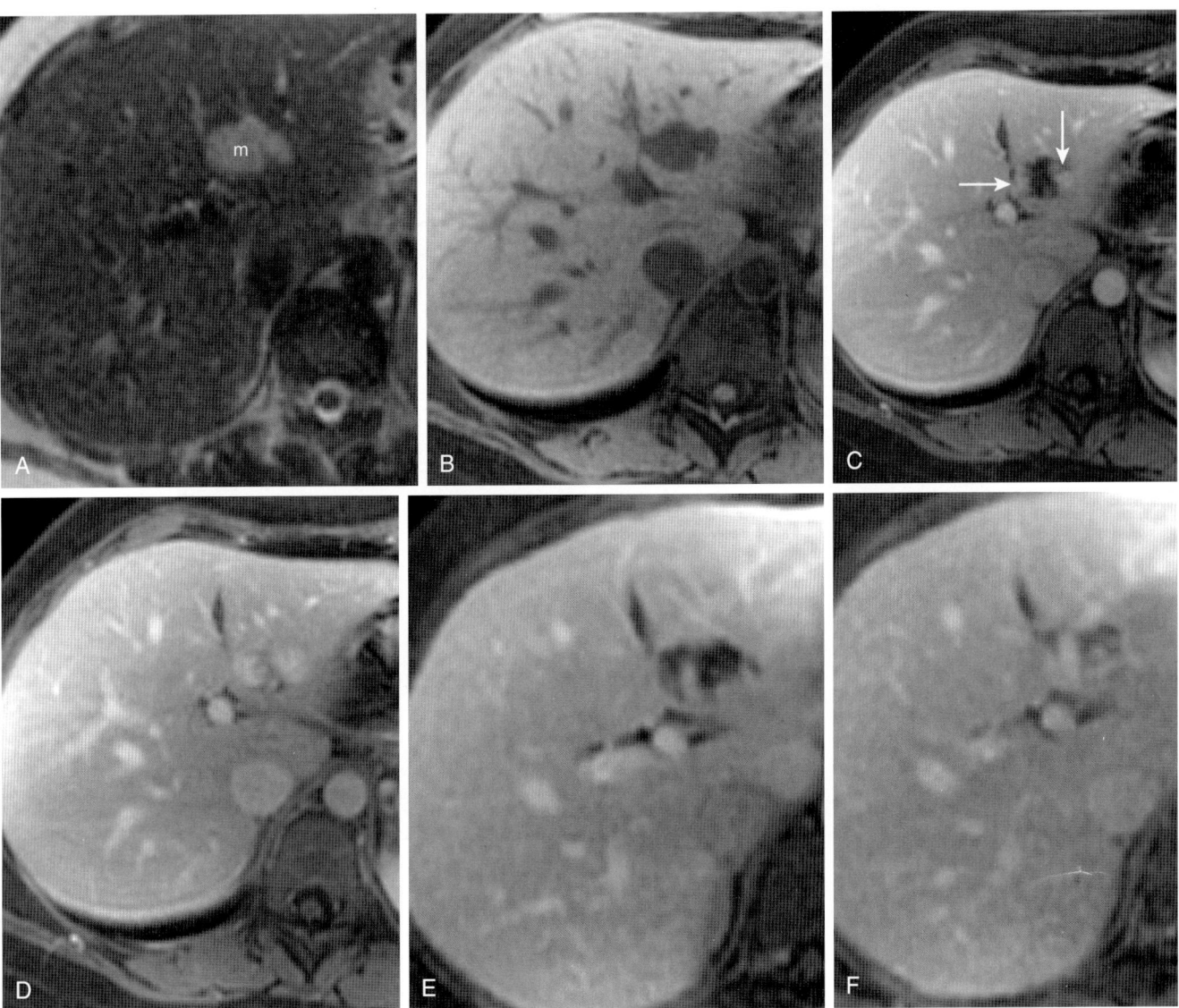

FIGURE 14.3 Hepatic hemangioma undergoing sclerosis. A, Heavily T2-weighted image (echo time [TE] 150) shows a mass (m) that is hyperintense to hepatic parenchyma with well-defined margins. **B**, Precontrast T1-weighted fat saturation image at the same level shows the mass to be low signal compared with background parenchyma. **C**, T1-weighted postcontrast image in early portal venous phase shows peripheral nodular enhancement within this mass *(arrows)*. Portions of the lesion fail to show enhancement during this phase. **D**, Equilibrium phase T1-weighted image postcontrast shows the lesion has partially filled in toward the central portion. This constellation of findings is typical for hepatic hemangioma. **E–F**, The same lesion 5 years later on T1-weighted postcontrast scans in portal venous and equilibrium phase imaging shows less avid enhancement and has shown slight size decrease, consistent with developing sclerosis. Sclerosing hemangiomas may show size decrease with less avid enhancement, associated capsular retraction, and lower T2 signal than nonsclerosed hemangiomas.

or perilesional or both perilesional and intralesional flow.[34] On CEUS, HCAs demonstrate homogenous arterial hyperenhancement, with rapid and complete, usually centripetal, filling. On later phases of imaging contrast enhancement, characteristics are heterogenous, with some lesions demonstrating washout and others remaining iso- or hyperenhanced. It should be noted that washout in portal or later phases on postcontrast imaging on CT or MRI is not a typical feature of adenoma. It has been postulated that washout demonstrated on CEUS is because the microbubbles remain intravascular compared with the ECF contrast agents, which may see diffusion across the vascular endothelium into the tumor interstitium.[34]

The CT appearance of adenomas often overlaps with FNH and HCC. Adenomas tend to have similar attenuation to normal liver on unenhanced images. Larger adenomas, however, are more heterogenous in appearance than smaller lesions, depending on their predilection to hemorrhage and/or the presence of fat. The characteristic pattern of contrast enhancement is variable degrees of arterial hyperenhancement and fading or persistent enhancement in later phases, depending on the HCA subtype. For example, strong arterial hyperenhancement with persistent enhancement in portal venous and subsequent delayed sequences is more typical for inflammatory HCA (Fig. 14.6).[34]

MRI is preferred to CT for identification of intracellular fat and for better characterization of HCA. Furthermore, certain imaging features on MRI have been shown to be associated with different subtypes to date.[35–38]

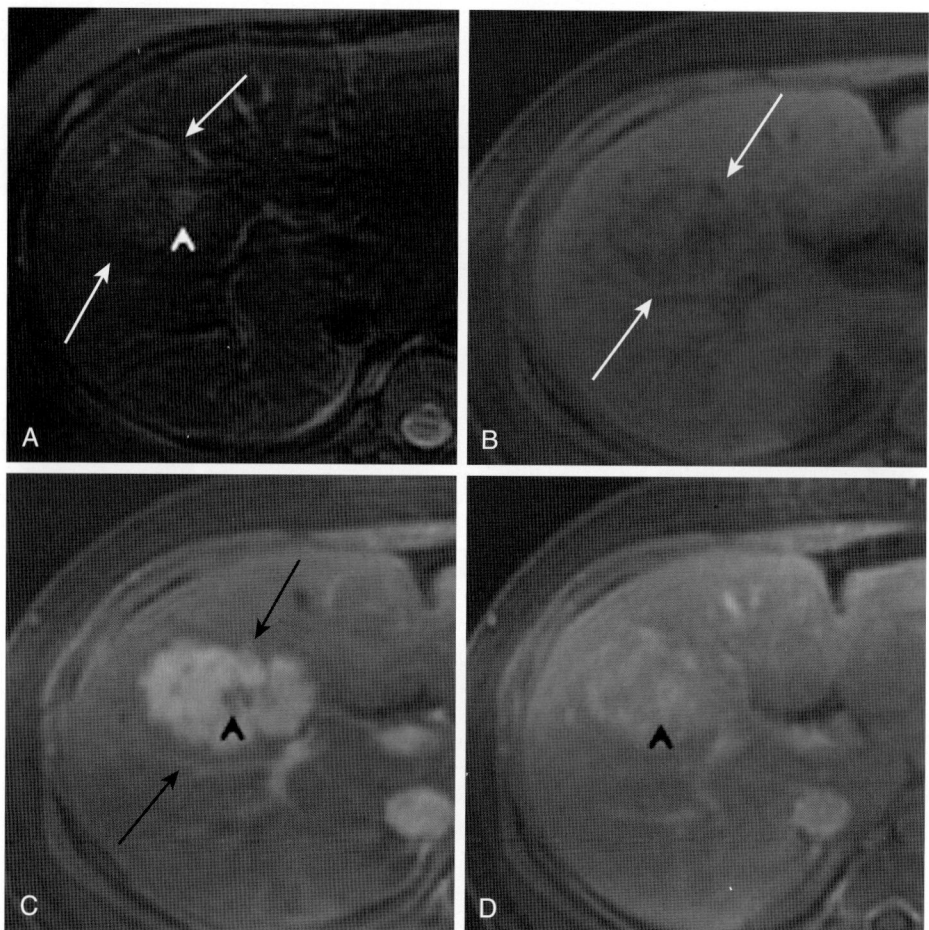

FIGURE 14.4   Focal nodular hyperplasia (FNH). A, T2-weighted image shows a mass that is isointense to hepatic parenchyma *(arrows)*. Centrally, within this mass is a hyperintense focus *(arrowhead)*. **B**, A precontrast, T1-weighted gradient-echo image shows the mass *(arrows)* to be almost isointense to liver. **C**, Arterial dominant phase T1-weighted gradient-echo sequence shows that the mass enhances intensely with respect to hepatic parenchyma *(arrows)*. The central focus, which was bright on the T2-weighted images, does not show enhancement on this phase of the injection *(arrowhead)*. **D**, Postcontrast equilibrium phase image shows the mass to be isointense to background hepatic parenchyma. The central portion of scar shows delayed enhancement *(arrowhead)* characteristic of FNH.

H-HCAs are more likely to have diffuse, homogenous intratumoral fat deposition compared with other subtypes (Fig. 14.7). This can be demonstrated by diffuse signal drop-out on out-of-phase compared with in-phase T1-weighted imaging. They also typically enhance less avidly in the arterial phase and are heterogeneously low in signal in the delayed hepatobiliary phase.

A specific feature of I-HCAs is the presence of marked sinusoidal dilatation, which manifests as moderate diffuse intralesional hyperintensity or a rim of hyperintensity (known as the "atoll sign") on T2-weighted images and corresponding arterial hyperenhancement with persistent delayed enhancement on postcontrast imaging. A "crescent sign" has also been recently proposed, which is similar to the atoll sign, but the rim of T2 hyperintensity and hyperenhancement is incomplete or crescent-shaped.[36] Some I-HCAs may show focal or heterogenous fat deposition.[37] I-HCAs also have a propensity for internal hemorrhage, which can manifest as T1 hyperintensity or hemosiderin deposition, as seen by signal drop-out on in-phase imaging.[36] Intralesional hemorrhagic changes, however, are non-specific, with such changes also seen in other subtypes. For example sh-HCAs, which account for approximately 4% of HCAs, have also been noted to have a predilection to hemorrhage.[39] β-HCAs

have no specific differentiating characteristics. They tend to show moderate, often heterogenous arterial-phase enhancement, which may persist but is variable in the late dynamic and delayed phases. These lesions show diffuse glutamine synthetase expression from upregulation, although they may be heterogenous. This is in contradistinction to FNH, which show map-like glutamine synthetase expression distribution adjacent to hepatic veins.[38] Unclassified HCAs have no specific genetic or histopathologic abnormalities. Similarly, no specific imaging features have been identified for these lesions.

Traditionally, HCAs are expected to be hypointense on the hepatobiliary phase when using hepatocyte-specific contrast agent, in contrast to FNHs, which retain the same contrast agent and appear iso- to hyperintense.[40] Iso/hyperintense uptake by FNH has been shown to correlate to expression of hepatocyte proteins such as OATPB1/B3.[41] Nevertheless, increasing studies have noted the retention of hepatocyte-specific contrast in a small proportion of adenomas, particularly the β-HCA subtype.[42] This is thought to be explained by the expression of hepatocyte transport proteins such as OATPB1/B3 that can be seen in β-HCAs.[41] The majority of adenomas do not display OATPB1/B3 expression, however, and the evaluation of

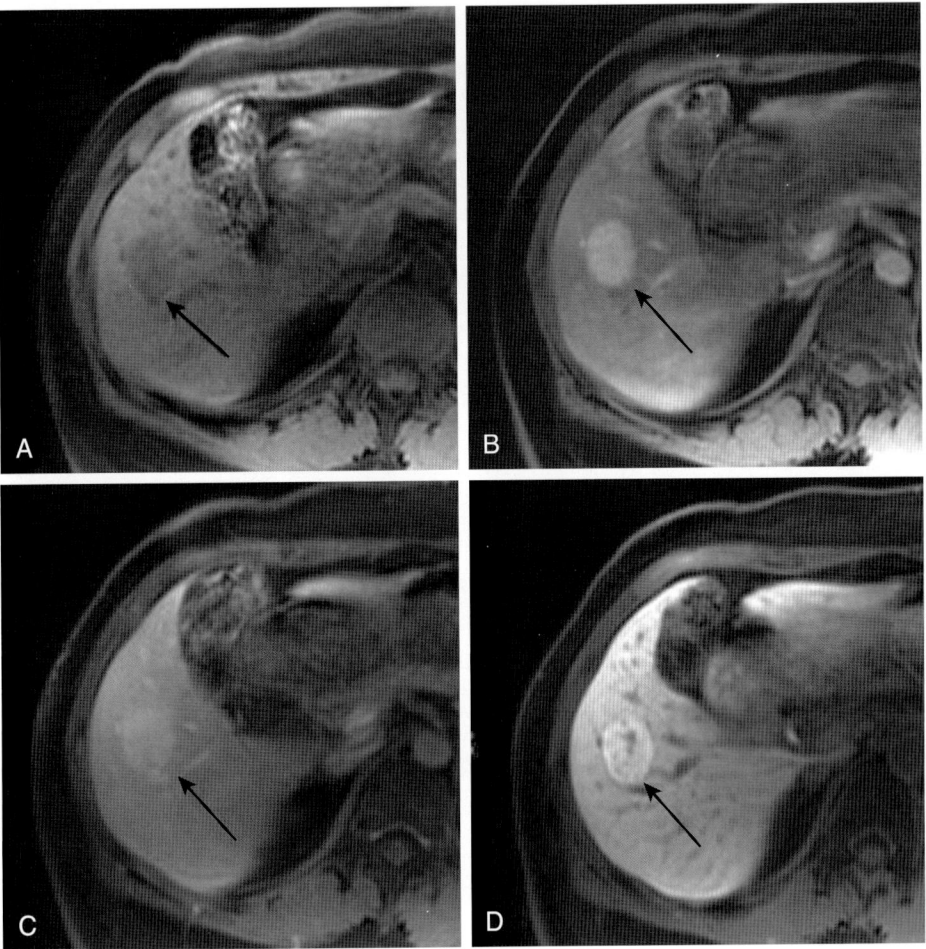

FIGURE 14.5 **Focal nodular hyperplasia (FNH). A**, Precontrast T1-weighted image demonstrates a mildly T1 hypointense lesion in the right lobe of liver *(arrow)*. **B**, Arterial-phase T1-weighted sequence shows that the mass is diffusely hyperenhancing *(arrow)*. **C**, Portal venous phase demonstrates mild persisting hyperenhancement of the FNH *(arrow)*. **D**, Postcontrast hepatobiliary phase imaging shows retention of hepatocyte specific contrast, with mild hyperintensity of the FNH relative to the liver *(arrow)*.

hepatocyte-specific contrast uptake in a lesion remains helpful in the differentiation of FNH from adenoma, when an HCA has low signal in the delayed hepatobiliary phase.[40] Care should also be taken in the interpretation of perceived retention of hepatocyte-specific contrast in some lesions, which may instead be explained by inherent hyperintensity on precontrast T1 imaging because of the presence of blood products or relative to underlying hepatic parenchymal steatosis.[42]

Angiomyolipoma and Other Benign Fat-Containing Hepatic Tumors

Angiomyolipoma

Hepatic angiomyolipoma (HAML) is an uncommon tumor and is seen more frequently in women. HAML is generally considered a benign, solitary tumor made up of three elements: smooth muscle, thick-walled blood vessels, and mature adipose tissue.[43] HAML imaging features may vary based on the relative proportions of the three elements within a lesion, which makes this lesion often challenging to diagnose on imaging.[43] Although intralesional fat is typical in HAMLs, they can often show brisk, avidly enhancing soft tissue components with washout, which can overlap with other liver malignancies, such as HCC (see Chapter 89), and some lesions may present without

detectable fat (Fig. 14.8).[44] Tortuous vessels and enlarged early draining veins to either portal veins or hepatic veins are features that have been associated with HAML.[43-46] Intralesional hemorrhage may be seen in a small proportion of cases.[44]

At US, HAMLs are typically well-demarcated, echogenic lesions, similar in appearance to hemangiomas. On CT, intralesional fat is evidenced by fat density tissue (< -20 HU). On MRI, the signal characteristics of macroscopic lipid follow that of subcutaneous fat and demonstrate signal drop out on T1-weighted and T2-weighted fat-saturated sequences. Microscopic fat can also be seen in HAML, seen as signal drop-out on out-of-phase compared with in-phase T1-weighted images.[46]

Enhancement on multiphase CT and MRI is typically a heterogeneous pattern of hyperenhancement on arterial phase with washout on portal venous or delayed phase; however, gradual and prolonged enhancement may also be observed.[43] Peripheral rim enhancement caused by peripheral tumor vessels may also be seen, a feature which the reader must be careful not to misdiagnose as a tumor capsule typically seen in a HCC.[43,44] On contrast-enhanced images using gadoxetic acid, HAMLs typically appear hypointense on delayed hepatobiliary phase.[46] In summary, if a well-demarcated, hypervascular, macroscopic fat-containing tumor is seen with peripheral enhancement, if it has no tumor capsule, and if there are early draining

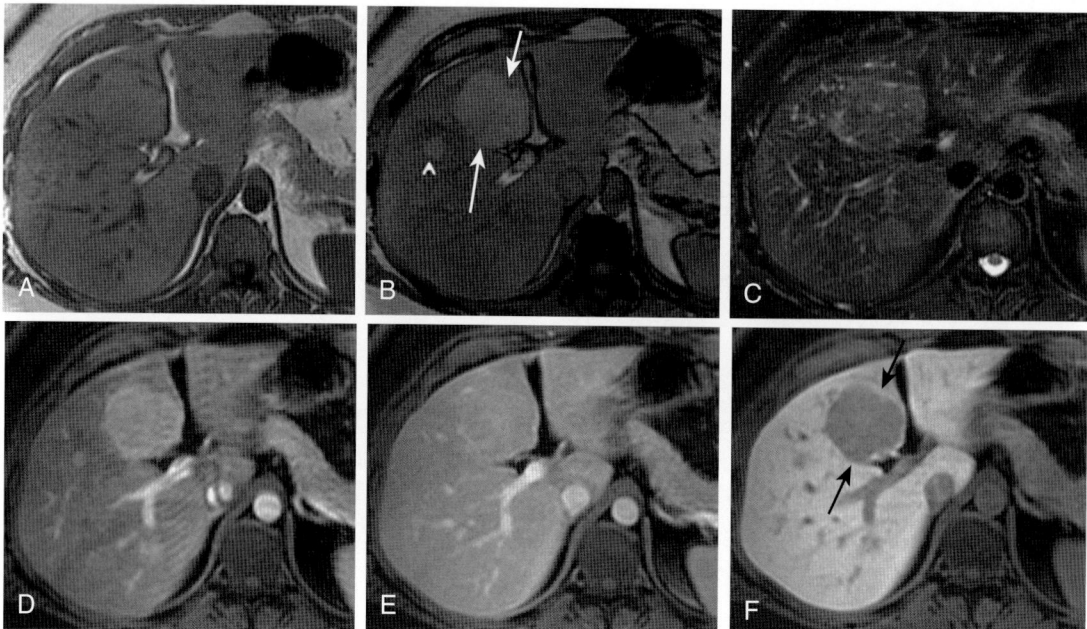

FIGURE 14.6   **Adenoma. A–B,** In- and out-of-phase T1-weighted imaging shows background hepatic steatosis with diffusely decreased signal intensity of the hepatic parenchyma on out of phase imaging. A mass in segment 4 is isointense to liver parenchyma on in phase imaging and relatively hyperintense on out of phase because of background steatosis *(arrows).* An adjacent smaller adenoma is also visualized *(arrowhead).* **C,** The mass is minimally hyperintense to hepatic parenchyma on fat saturated T2-weighted. **D,** Arterial-phase T1-weighted sequence demonstrates diffuse hyperenhancement. **E,** Portal venous phase image shows the mass fades to isointensity to background liver. **F,** Delayed-phase image using hepatobiliary contrast demonstrates the lesions do not retain contrast *(arrows).*

veins, an angiomyolipoma should be considered, particularly in patients without cirrhosis.

Myelolipoma

Hepatic myelolipoma is a rare benign tumor containing mature adipose and myeloid tissue in varying degrees, with only a handful of published case reports in the medical literature.[47] Imaging features reflect the tumor composition with heterogenous enhancement of myelogenous components and regions of macroscopic fat appearing as low attenuating fat density tissue on CT and signal intensity identical to subcutaneous fat on T1-weighted and T2-weighted sequences.

Lipoma

Hepatic lipomas are composed entirely of mature adipose tissue with expected imaging features, including echogenic lesions on US, density values consistent with fat on CT, and following the signal intensity of subcutaneous fat on all sequences on MRI. Lipomas show minimal to no enhancement on CT or MRI, distinguishing them from other fat-containing lesions in the liver.[48]

Hepatic Peliosis

Hepatic peliosis (also called *peliosis hepatis*) is a rare benign vascular disorder characterized by sinusoidal dilatation and numerous blood-filled spaces within the liver. The size of the lesions typically vary from 1 mm to several centimeters.[49] Numerous etiologies have been associated with hepatic peliosis, such as drugs (ocular cicatricial pemphigoid [OCP], corticosteroids, chemotherapy), infection (leprosy, tuberculosis [TB]), underlying systemic disease (diabetes mellitus, hematologic disorders), immunocompromised status (acquired immunodeficiency syndrome [AIDS], post-transplant) and toxins (arsenic, thorium oxide).

Nevertheless, up to 50% of cases are idiopathic.[49] US imaging may demonstrate hyperechoic lesions on a background of normal liver parenchyma or hypoechoic lesions in a steatotic liver. Posterior acoustic enhancement may be seen.[50] On CEUS, a transient "fast surge" of central enhancement has been described.[50] On nonenhanced CT, lesions are usually hypodense to liver and rarely hyperdense secondary to hemorrhage. Calcifications within peliotic lesions have also been described.[49] On MRI, lesions are typically iso- or mildly hypointense on T1-weighted and hyperintense on T2-weighted imaging.[51] T1-weighted hyperintense foci may also be seen, representing hemorrhage. Postcontrast multiphase imaging on CT and MRI typically shows arterial hyperenhancement with globular central enhancement, termed the "target sign," and corresponds to the "fast surge" of central enhancement seen at CEUS.[49,52] Enhancing lesions tend to demonstrate a centrifugal enhancement pattern on successive phases of postcontrast imaging, with persistent hyperenhancement.[49] Some lesions may become isoattenuating or isointense on later phases of imaging, and small lesions may not be detected at all by CT because of their size.[53] Other lesions may not show any enhancement because of the presence of thrombosis. On the hepatobiliary phase of imaging, lesions may have ill-defined margins and demonstrate low signal intensity.[51] Lesions of hepatic peliosis typically do not demonstrate mass effect on adjacent hepatic vessels, unlike other liver tumors.[53]

Cystic Liver Lesions (see Chapters 72 and 73)
Hepatic Cysts

Simple hepatic or biliary cysts are common benign liver lesions and have no malignant potential. They are usually diagnosed incidentally and are almost always asymptomatic. Simple cysts

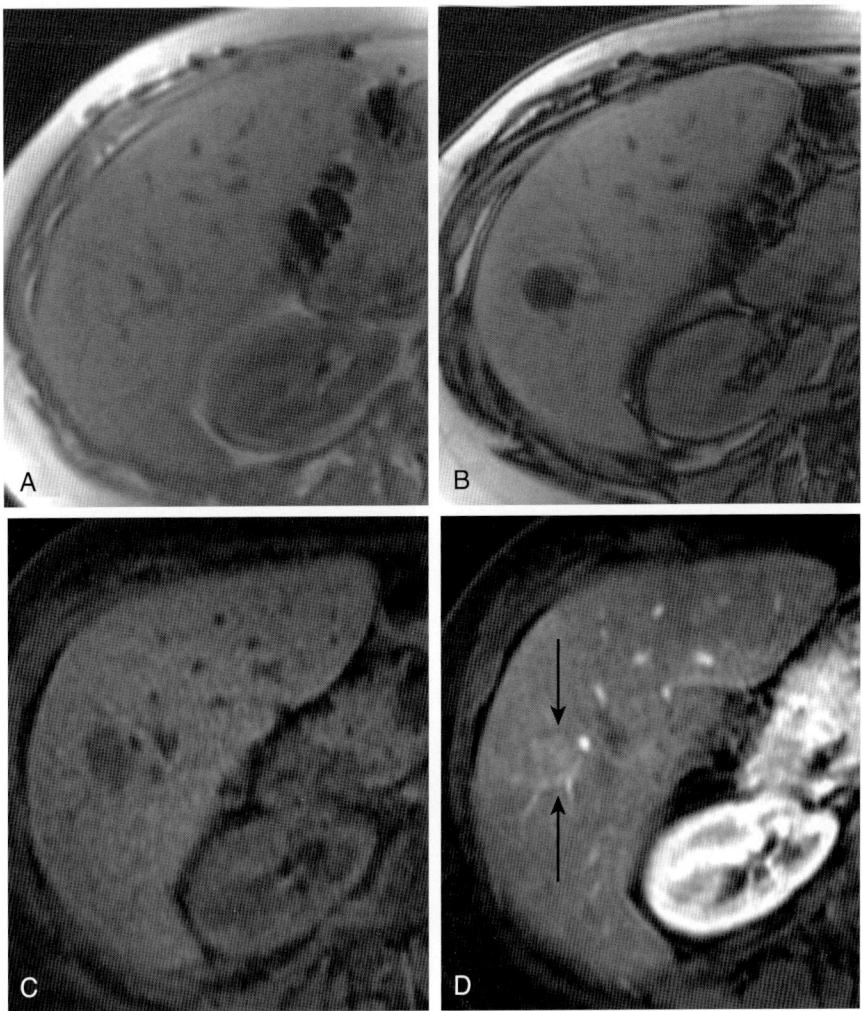

FIGURE 14.7 **Adenoma. A–B,** In- and out-of-phase imaging shows a mass that is isointense on in-phase imaging, which demonstrates diffuse loss of signal on out-of-phase imaging consistent with intratumoral fat content. **C,** Precontrast fat-saturated T1-weighted imaging shows the lesion to be hypointense relative to liver parenchyma because of fat content. **D,** Arterial-phase T1-weighted imaging demonstrates faint arterial enhancement *(arrows)*.

increase in prevalence with age, with the majority of incidental cysts seen in those greater than 60 years of age.[4] Certain diseases are associated with the presence of numerous hepatic cysts, such as autosomal dominant polycystic kidney disease, polycystic liver disease, and von Hippel-Lindau (Fig. 14.9).[54] Simple cysts typically demonstrate imaging characteristics of an uncomplicated fluid-filled structure across all imaging modalities. On ultrasound, the cyst is typically anechoic and well-circumscribed, with either a round or slightly lobular contour, and has no perceptible wall.[55] Cysts typically demonstrate posterior acoustic enhancement, which describes increased echoes of the structures seen distal to the cyst because of easier transmission of US waves through the fluid-filled cyst relative to adjacent organ tissue. Occasionally, thin internal septa may be seen. On CT, a cyst is homogenously hypoattenuating relative to background liver. At MRI, cysts are homogenously T1 hypointense and markedly T2 hyperintense, similar to CSF. Cysts do not enhance on postcontrast imaging.[54] Complications such as cyst rupture, intracystic hemorrhage, or biliary obstruction are rare but may occur in large cysts.[56] Intracystic hemorrhage is manifest by internal echoes and/or thickened septa on US, density higher than that of simple fluid on CT (>20 HU), and hyperintense signal on T1-weighted MR sequences.

Polycystic Liver Disease

Polycystic liver disease (PLD) is characterized by the presence of multiple fluid-filled liver cysts, arbitrarily defined as greater than 20 cysts.[57] Ultrasound is recommended in the initial evaluation and in the diagnosis of PLD, and the lesions will appear as simple or minimally complex cysts as previously described (see "Hepatic Cysts"). Cysts can vary in size from 1 mm to more than 12 cm. The role of CT or MRI is mostly to enable classification of disease severity or to evaluate for intracystic or volume-related complications. Volumetric studies can be performed using semi-automated software that allows for postprocessing and liver segmentation of acquired CT or MRI to estimate height-adjusted total liver volume (htTLV). The greater the htTLV, the greater the disease severity.[58]

Biliary Hamartoma

Biliary hamartomas, also known as *von Meyenburg complex*, are benign tumors composed of small, dilated biliary structures lined by bland biliary epithelium and often containing inspissated bile. Tumors are usually small, measuring less than 1 cm in size.[59] On US, hamartomas may be hyperechoic, hypoechoic, or mixed echogenicity, and a comet-tail artifact (linear, tapering

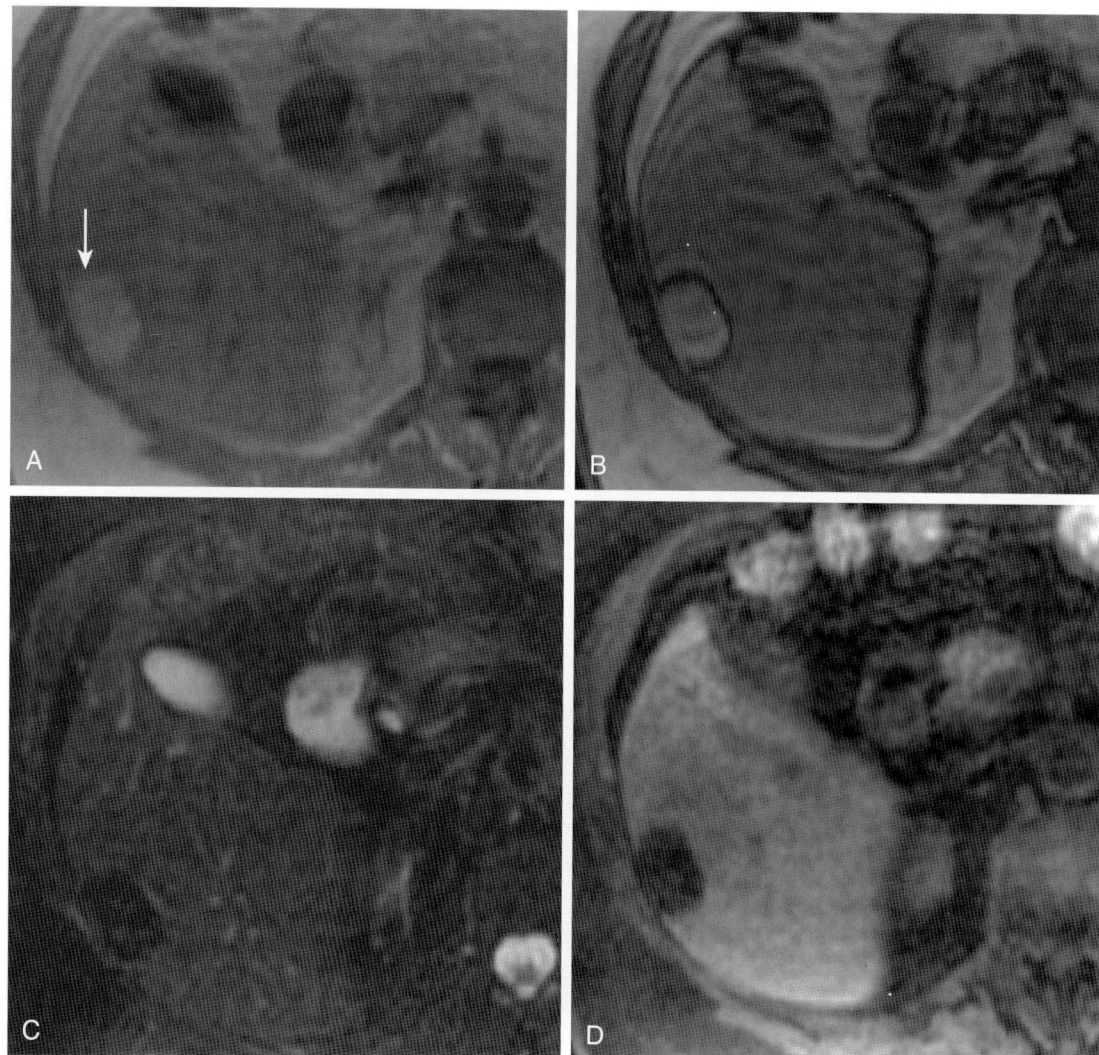

FIGURE 14.8 **Angiomyolipoma. A,** T1-weighted in-phase image shows a high-signal right hepatic mass *(arrow)*. **B,** T1-weighted out-of-phase image shows low signal at its margin because of chemical shift artifact between the mass and surrounding liver, confirming the presence of bulk fat. **C,** Axial T2-weighted image with fat saturation shows the mass is dark, similar to subcutaneous fat. **D,** Axial T1-weighted fat saturation image shows the mass is dark as well.

trail of echoes just distal to a strongly reflective surface) may be seen. On CT, multiple, small, hypoattenuating nodules are usually seen diffusely throughout the liver. These lesions typically have a more ill-defined margin, compared with simple liver cysts, which are well defined. These lesions typically do not demonstrate enhancement on CT,[60] but they can be hard to distinguish from metastatic disease when small. On MRI, lesions are hypointense on T1-weighted imaging and markedly hyperintense on T2-weighted imaging. The appearance of these numerous lesions on heavily T2-weighted imaging, such as MR cholangiopancreatography (MRCP), has been likened to a "starry sky" (Fig. 14.10). Communication with the bile ducts is typically not seen.[61] Endocystic mural nodules are also a feature, better seen on MRI than on CT, and are isointense on T1-weighted and intermediate signal on T2-weighted imaging, giving an irregular lesion contour.[62] These nodules demonstrate enhancement on contrast-enhanced MRI.[63] Thin, peripheral enhancement has also been described, although it was attributed to enhancement of adjacent, compressed liver parenchyma.[63] Differential diagnoses for the presence of numerous

tiny cystic-appearing lesions include hepatic microabscesses, metastases, peribiliary cysts, and Caroli disease. The lack of communication with the biliary system helps differentiate biliary hamartomas from Caroli disease.

Caroli Disease

Caroli disease is a congenital autosomal recessive disease that results in multifocal, saccular, or fusiform dilatation of large intrahepatic bile ducts, which may be diffuse or segmental. Caroli syndrome is the term used when Caroli disease and congenital hepatic fibrosis coexist. In the Todani classification of biliary cysts, Caroli disease is classified as Type V (see Chapter 46).[64] The dilated ducts may measure up 5 cm in size and contain sludge or calculi.[65] The lesions appear cystic on US, CT, and MRI. On contrast-enhanced imaging, Caroli disease often shows fibrovascular bundles with strong enhancement within focally dilated biliary ducts. This appearance has been termed the "central dot sign" and corresponds to a portal vein branch or portal radicle that protrudes into the lumen of the dilated duct.[66] MRCP can demonstrate saccular or fusiform cystic foci

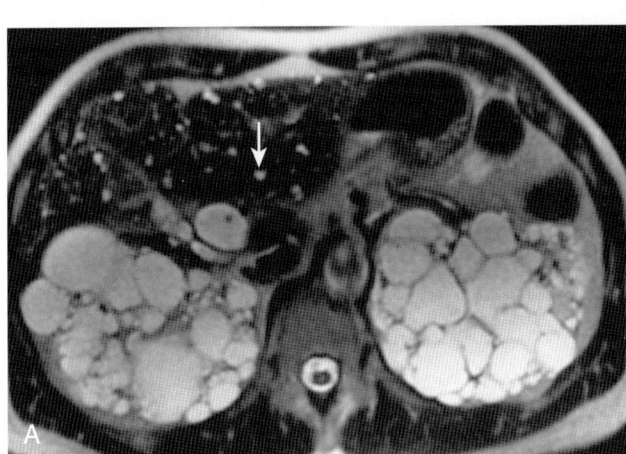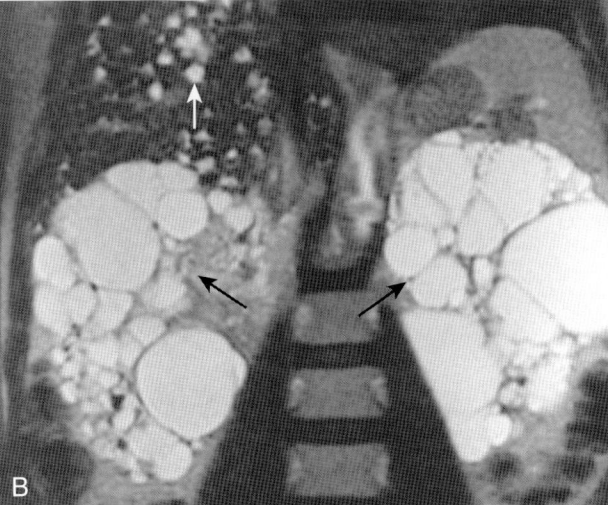

FIGURE 14.9 **Hepatic cysts associated with polycystic kidney disease. A,** Axial T2-weighted image at the level of the kidneys shows bilaterally enlarged kidneys with multiple hyperintense cysts. Little normal renal parenchyma is present at this level, and multiple small hepatic cysts *(arrow)* are seen. **B,** Coronal T2-weighted images through the kidneys show similar findings of enlarged kidneys containing multiple cysts *(black arrows),* and small hepatic cysts are identified *(white arrow).*

that are in communication with the biliary tree. Occasionally, filling defects may be seen that represent intraluminal calculi. Hepatocyte-specific MRI contrast agents can also be used to demonstrate communication with the biliary tree.[55]

Biliary Cystadenoma

Biliary cyst adenoma (BCA) is a rare, slow-growing neoplasm arising from the bile ducts, with a strong predilection to occur in middle-aged women (see Chapter 88B).[67] BCA was reclassified

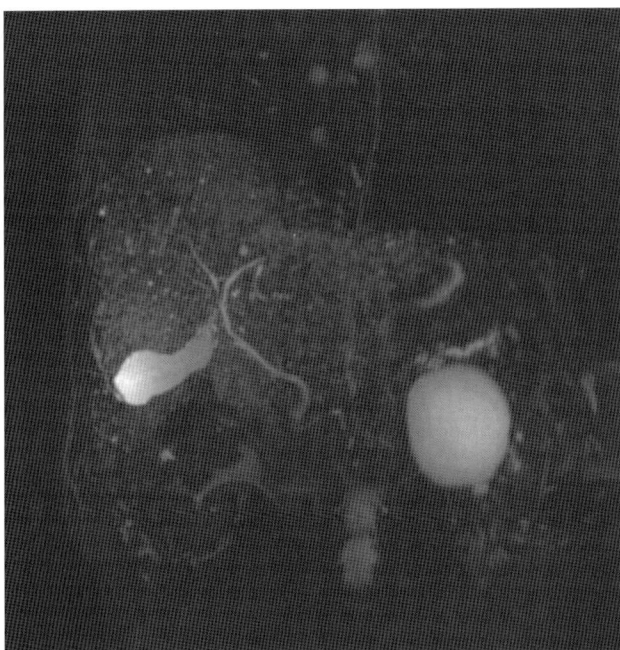

FIGURE 14.10 **Biliary hamartoma.** Coronal magnetic resonance cholangiopancreatography (MRCP) maximum intensity projection (MIP) of the liver demonstrates numerous tiny T2 hyperintense bile duct hamartomas scattered throughout the hepatic parenchyma, resembling a "starry sky."

as a mucinous cystic neoplasm (MCN) of the liver according to the 2010 World Health Organization (WHO) classification, but for the purposes of this chapter, it will be referred to as BCA because this term is still mostly in use. Although generally benign, these lesions are considered to be premalignant and have the potential to develop into biliary cystadenocarcinoma (BCAC) in up to 20% to 30% of cases.[67] BCAs are more often solitary cystic lesions and seen within the left hepatic lobe.[67] Sonographically, BCA may be multilocular, with cystic locules demonstrating different echogenicities, depending on cyst fluid content. They may have mural nodularity, nodular thickened septations, papillary excrescences, and mural or septal calcifications.[67–69] CEUS typically demonstrates a honeycomb pattern of enhancement of the cyst septations and mural nodules, with hyperenhancement more likely to be seen in the arterial phase.[70] Although CEUS is useful to demonstrate intratumoral vascularity, there are no significant differences in enhancement patterns between BCA and BCAC.[71] US is more sensitive than CT in the detection of intracystic septations; however, CT offers a more accurate depiction of cyst size and anatomic location.[69] On CT, BCAs are predominantly low attenuating, with density values measuring that of fluid (<20 HU) and tend to be multiloculated with internal septations or mural nodules. The density of loculated cyst fluid can vary, depending on its content, and may be hemorrhagic, mucinous, proteinaceous, or bilious. Rarely, they may be unilocular, and minimally complex lesions on CT may be difficult to differentiate from simple hepatic cysts. Occasionally, upstream or downstream biliary ductal dilatation may be seen in BCA, a feature that is rare in simple hepatic cysts.[72] Mural calcification can occur rarely.[73]

On MRI, the lesions may be of low, intermediate, or increased signal on T1-weighted images, again depending on cyst fluid content. Proteinaceous or hemorrhagic material are typically hyperintense in signal on T1-weighted imaging and fluid-fluid levels may be seen in the presence of internal hemorrhage.[74] BCAs are usually hyperintense on T2-weighted sequences (Fig. 14.11).

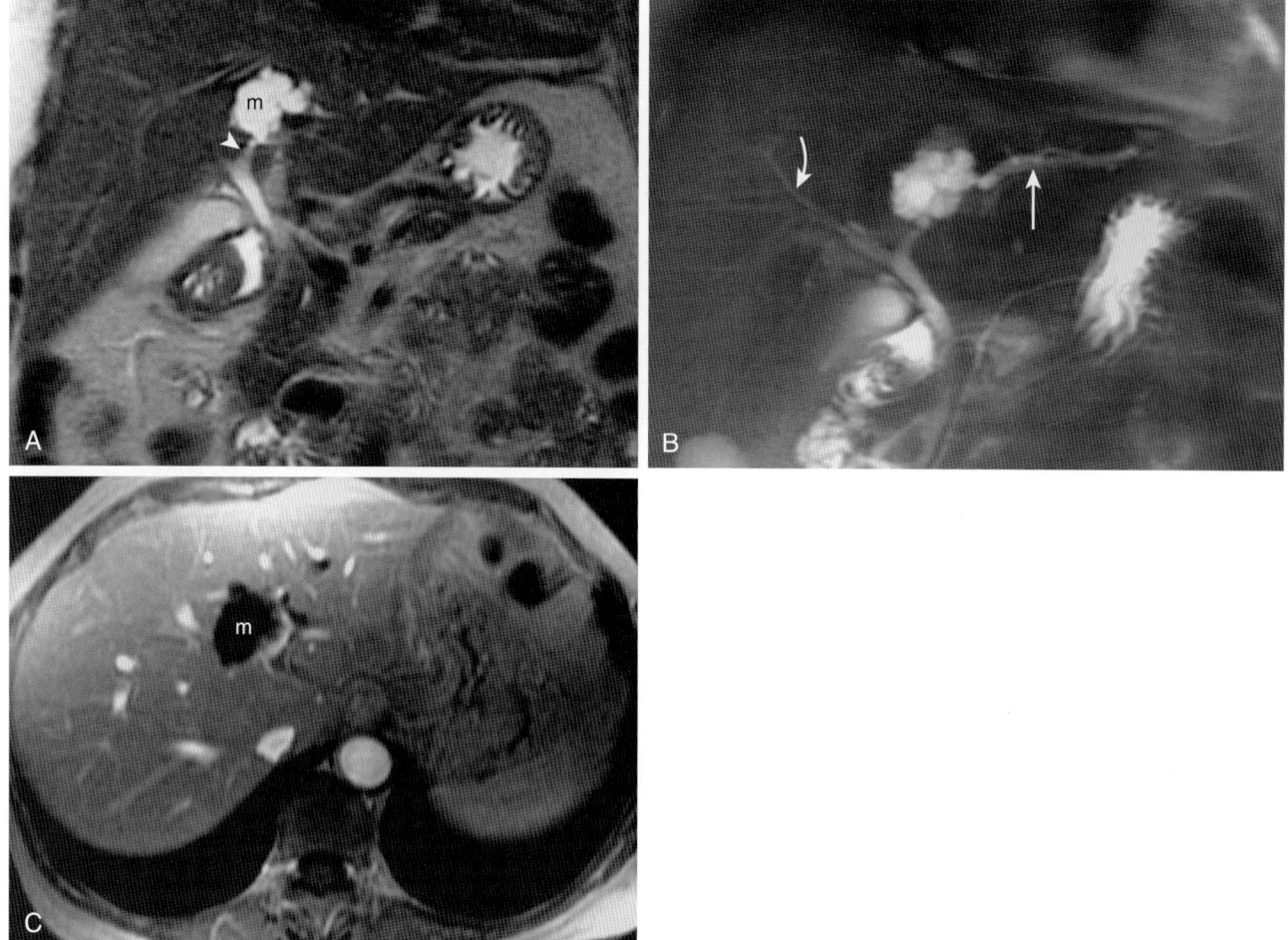

FIGURE 14.11 **Biliary cystadenoma. A,** Coronal T2-weighted image shows a lobulated mass (m) in close proximity to the left hepatic duct *(arrowhead)*. **B,** Projection image in the coronal oblique plane shows the well-defined hyperintense mass to be in continuity with a mildly dilated left-sided biliary radicle *(straight arrow)*. The normal right-sided biliary radicle *(curved arrow)* is easily seen with this technique. **C,** Postcontrast, T1-weighted gradient-echo image shows no enhancement within this mass (m).

Contrast-enhanced imaging typically demonstrates enhancement of septa and mural nodules. Intracystic debris in a hemorrhagic cyst can mimic mural nodules, and care should be taken to ensure true nodule enhancement has occurred by examining precontrast and postcontrast series.[72] Communication with the biliary ductal system on delayed hepatobiliary phase imaging with hepatocyte-specific contrast agents has been reported, helping to differentiate these tumors from non-neoplastic, simple hepatic cysts.[75] Infectious cysts may also communicate with the biliary tree, however.

Hepatic Abscess and Infection (see Chapters 11, 70, 71)

A hepatic abscess is an inflammatory collection in the liver from a bacterial (pyogenic), parasitic, or fungal infection.

CT is generally the modality of choice in recent postoperative or at-risk patients in whom there is a clinical suspicion of a hepatic pyogenic abscess. Patients with more atypical symptoms may present a diagnostic dilemma. Although some patients show symptoms suggesting abscesses, others do not. Abscesses are found more frequently in the right lobe of liver.[76] On US, pyogenic abscesses can vary in appearance and may even appear solid, particularly if infected with *Klebsiella pneumoniae*. More

often, they appear cystic, with debris and thickened septations. There is typically absence of internal Doppler signal, but the abscess wall is usually vascular.[77]

The CT appearances of pyogenic abscesses can vary widely. They may appear as small, low-attenuating, well-defined masses and may be widely scattered or clustered with a tendency to coalesce (Fig. 14.12). The appearance of coalesced smaller abscesses into a larger multiloculated abscess has been called the "cluster sign."[78] Larger abscesses may range in appearance from unilocular cystic cavities with smooth outer margins to highly complex and septated structures with internal debris and irregular conforms. The attenuation value of the abscess cavity depends on the age of the abscess; it becomes lower as the abscess matures. Intralesional gas may be present, either in the form of gas bubbles or an air-fluid level, and can be a feature of up to 20% of abscesses.[77] Other associated features include pneumobilia and thrombophlebitis.[55]

On MRI, pyogenic abscesses are hyperintense on T2-weighted images. A peripheral rim of signal hyperintensity indicating perilesional edema may also be seen surrounding the abscess wall. Pyogenic abscesses are generally hypointense on T1-weighted images, unless they have hemorrhagic or proteinaceous debris

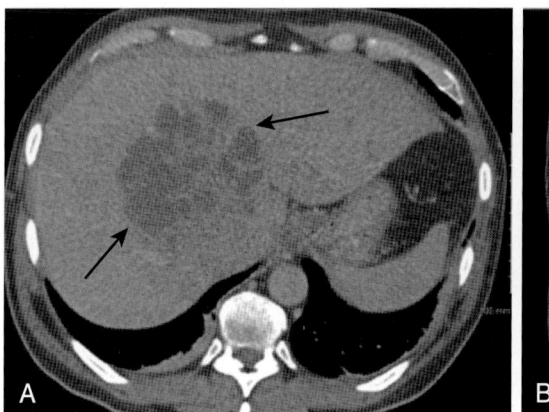
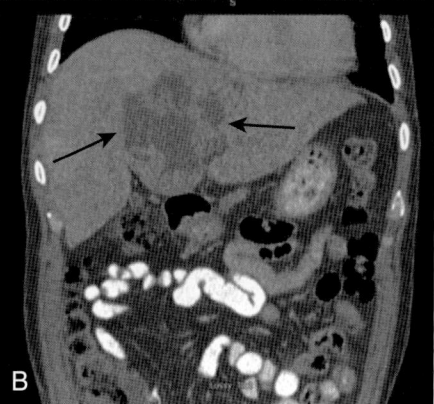

FIGURE 14.12 Hepatic abscess. **A–B**, Postcontrast axial and coronal computed tomography (CT) demonstrating low attenuating, irregularly lobulated mass in the central right hepatic lobe *(arrows)*. Smaller, discrete cystic lesions are seen within this region, which are tending to coalesce into adjacent larger lesions, a feature that can be seen in some hepatic abscesses called the "cluster sign."

within them, in which case they will appear hyper- or isointense. If gas is present, it typically manifests as signal voids on all sequences, which is more pronounced on T1-weighted in-phase gradient echo sequences because of greater magnetic susceptibility.[77] In the case of *K. pneumoniae* infection, the "turquoise sign" has been described, which refers to the presence of hypointense, thin, septal bands on T2-weighted images that resemble the turquoise mineral.[77]

Abscesses typically have thick walls that enhance after administration of contrast material on either CT or MRI. The central, pus-filled portion does not enhance. A "double target" sign may be seen, which describes the presence of hepatic parenchymal enhancement peripheral to the enhancing wall, secondary to increased capillary permeability.[55] The imaging findings of abscesses can overlap with malignancies, although some features on postcontrast imaging can suggest abscess over tumor. On multiphase imaging, arterial rim enhancement that persists into portal venous or transitional phase is typical for abscesses, compared with arterially rim-enhancing malignant lesions that fade or wash out by the portal venous or transitional phase.[79,80] Perilesional hyperemia and patchy liver parenchymal enhancement may also be frequently seen in abscesses.[80] On the delayed hepatobiliary phase using hepatocyte-specific contrast, the periphery of the abscess is low in signal, corresponding to damaged hepatocytes.[81] A significant size discrepancy between the measurable lesion on precontrast T1-weighted images and hepatobiliary phase images is therefore more frequently observed in abscesses than in tumors.[79] DWI may be a valuable tool in differentiating hepatic abscesses from malignancy. The abscess periphery typically shows "T2-shine through" (i.e., high *b*-value on DWI and ADC) compared with malignant tumors, which typically demonstrate peripheral diffusion restriction.[81] Conversely, central abscess pus-filled cavities demonstrate diffusion restriction.[82]

Hydatid or echinococcal cysts (EC) occur because of infection with a parasite called *Echinococcus granulosus* ingested through contaminated food (see Chapter 72). EC is most commonly seen in the right hepatic lobe and imaging appearances vary depending on the stage of the cyst.[83] EC have a variable appearance on ultrasound and may appear as simple fluid-filled cysts. However, the cyst wall usually has a hypoechoic layer bordered by an echogenic line on each side, representing the

layers of the cyst membrane; inner germinal and acellular laminated layers (the endocyst) and outer, fibrous layer (the pericyst). Multiple floating, internal echoes may also be seen, especially on repositioning the patient, which are termed "hydatid sand" and represent parasite larva called *protoscolices*. Detachment of the endocyst from the pericyst can result in characteristic imaging appearances on US, CT, and MRI. A localized split resembles "floating membranes" within the cyst, and a complete membrane detachment has been called the "water lily" sign.[84] The membrane is hyperattenuating relative to mother cyst fluid on CT and hypointense on T2-weighted imaging. Some cysts are multivesicular in appearance, containing daughter cysts or cysts-within-a-cyst. These clustered daughter cysts can also produce a "spoke-wheel" pattern. Numerous daughter cysts, along with detached membranes and hydatid sand, can make the cyst appear as a solid mass on US.[83] On CT, daughter cysts are seen as small hypodense, peripheral foci within the mother cyst because they are usually lower in density than the mother cyst fluid.[55] A proportion of EC may have partial or complete pericystic rim calcification and/or calcification of internal septa (Fig. 14.13).[85] As healing progresses, all components within the cyst generally become more densely calcified. Partial calcification does not always indicate parasite death; however, it is implied when complete calcification occurs.[85]

Superinfection may complicate hydatid cysts, particularly if there has been membrane disruption and/or intrabiliary cyst rupture. The cysts appear less well-defined and may demonstrate air-fluid levels. Postcontrast imaging typically shows cyst rim-enhancement and perilesional hypervascularity.[84] Other complications of EC include mass effect on adjacent structures and cyst rupture into the biliary tree or into adjacent viscera.[84]

Fungal microabscesses generally manifest in immunocompromised patients as numerous tiny abscesses disseminated throughout the liver. The classical imaging finding on US describes the "bull's eye" appearance of a round hyperechoic lesion with a hypoechoic rim. An additional hypoechoic central focus can occasionally be present and give a "wheels-within-wheels" appearance.[86] Most commonly, however, abscesses appear as small, nonspecific, hypoechoic nodules.[77] On contrast-enhanced CT, fungal abscesses are small, hypodense lesions, ranging from several millimeters to 1.5 cm in size. The "bulls-eye" appearance

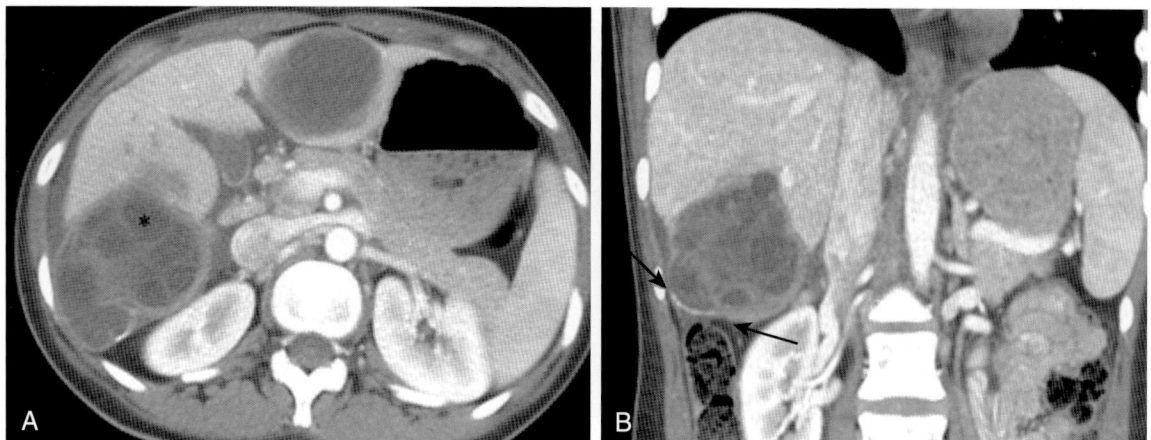

FIGURE 14.13 **Echinococcal cyst. A,** Postcontrast portal venous phase axial computed tomography (CT) demonstrating two complex cystic liver masses in the left and right lobes. The right lobe mass contains small daughter cysts, resulting in a cyst within a cyst appearance *(asterisk)*. **B,** Postcontrast portal venous phase coronal CT of the same cyst demonstrating thin, partial rim calcification of the pericyst.

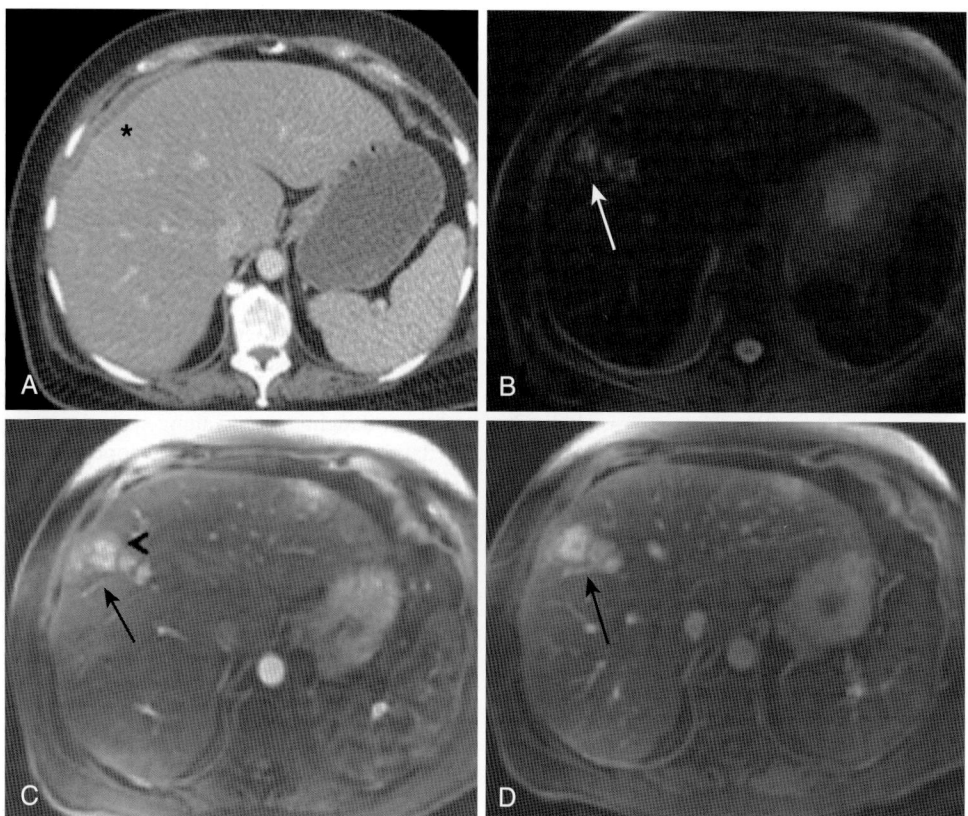

FIGURE 14.14 **Fungal abscesses. A,** Postcontrast portal venous phase axial computed tomography (CT) demonstrating only subtle hyperenhancement in the peripheral right lobe of liver *(asterisk)*. No obvious lesion is discernable. **B,** Axial fat-saturated T2-weighted magnetic resonance imaging (MRI) at the same level reveals clustered, ill-defined T2 hyperintense lesions consistent with microabscesses with surrounding parenchymal edema *(arrow)*. Also note the diffusely decreased signal of the hepatic and splenic parenchyma, consistent with transfusional hemosiderosis in this patient with a history of leukemia. **C,** Axial postcontrast T1-weighted images in the arterial phase demonstrating peri-abscess hyperemic change *(arrowhead)*. **D,** Axial postcontrast T1-weighted images in portal venous phase shows persistent abscess and peri-abscess parenchymal enhancement *(arrow)*.

on CT appears as a small, high-attenuation focus centrally surrounded by a low-attenuating zone. Authors have reported significant increase in sensitivity and lesion conspicuity using arterial-phase CT, compared with portal venous phase CT, when evaluating liver lesions in immunocompromised patients suspected to have hepatosplenic fungal infections (Fig. 14.14).

The addition of an arterial phase may also yield additional imaging findings that would support an infective etiology, such as transient hepatic parenchymal hyperemia.[87] On MRI, the lesions are most conspicuous on T2-weighted sequences and are seen as hyperintense foci (see Fig. 14.14). Ring enhancement may be seen on early postcontrast phases, and the abscesses may also

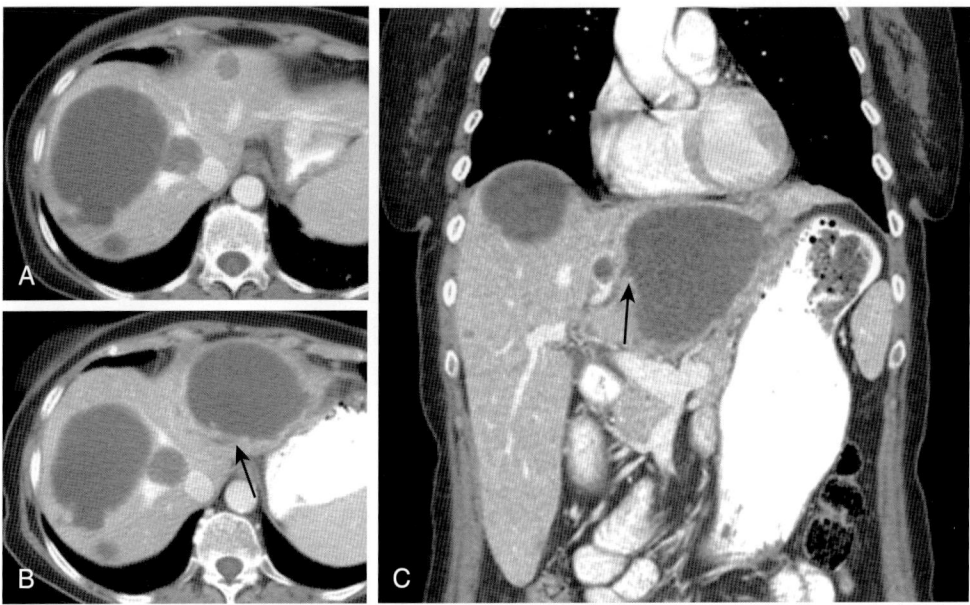

FIGURE 14.15   Biloma. A, Postcontrast portal venous phase axial computed tomography (CT) in a patient with metastatic liver disease. In the right lobe, the patient has already undergone embolization, and a low attenuating fluid filled structure consistent with biloma is seen *(asterisk)*. In the left lobe, an untreated low attenuating metastasis is also visualized *(arrow)*. **B,** Postcontrast portal venous phase axial CT after left hepatic lobe emboliza-tion with a new fluid density lesion now seen at the site of the left lobe liver metastasis *(arrow)*. **C,** Postcontrast portal venous phase coronal CT demonstrates communication of the cystic lesion with a mildly prominent bile duct *(arrow)* and is consistent with a biloma. Previously embolized right lobe metastasis is again seen on this image *(asterisk)*.

show diffusion restriction.[77] The MRI appearances of fungal abscesses varies as the infection evolves and with treatment. For example, in the early stages of infection and in the presence of neutropenia, the disease may be occult on MRI. The "dark ring" sign describes the emergence of susceptibility artifact (signal drop-out) at T1-weighted gradient echo imaging, such as in-phase images, and corresponds to iron accumulation in macro-phages at the periphery of the abscess in patients on antifungal treatment.[55,88]

Ciliated Hepatic Foregut Duplication Cyst

A ciliated hepatic foregut duplication cyst (CHFC) is a rare congenital hepatic cystic lesion that develops secondary to em-bryonic foregut cell migration, and although it is considered a benign entity, it carries a risk for transformation into squamous cell carcinoma. CHFC is typically solitary, most commonly located in the subcapsular segment 4, and typically measures less than 3 cm in size.[89,90] Imaging appearances are nonspecific. CHFC is typically hypoechoic or anechoic on US. It is usually hyperdense on CT because of its thick mucoid content. On MRI, hyperintensity on T2-weighted images is typical; however, T1-weighted signal intensity can vary depending on cyst fluid content. It does not demonstrate enhancement on contrast administration.[90,91]

Biloma

A biloma is an encapsulated collection of bile outside of the biliary tree. It may occur secondary to trauma, spontaneously, or represent an iatrogenic complication after an interventional procedure or liver surgery (see Chapter 11; Fig. 14.15). Bilious fluid has the same density as water on imaging and both US and CT can reliably demonstrate the presence of loculated fluid within or around the liver. Post-traumatic bile duct injuries may

be subtle in the acute setting, manifest by nonspecific small peri- or intrahepatic fluid collections or ascites. Follow-up imag-ing demonstrating an enlarging cystic fluid collection should increase suspicion for a biliary leak.[92] In the postsurgical setting, distinguishing between a biliary leak and other postprocedural collections is not reliable by these modalities. Hepatobiliary scintigraphy using technetium-99m-labeled iminodiacetic acid demonstrates physiologic biliary excretion and, although it can be used to demonstrate the presence of an active biliary leak, its inherent poor spatial resolution limits the precise identification of the bile leak location. Although ERCP can be performed to identify the exact location of the biliary leak, it is nonetheless an invasive procedure with significant potential complications and is therefore usually reserved for nonsurgical therapeutic management (see Chapter 12). MRCP performed without con-trast is useful in the diagnosis of bile leaks, and the addition of hepatobiliary-specific contrast material results in a reliable diagnostic technique that provides functional information on the biliary tree.[92,93] The diagnosis of a biliary leak is achieved by demonstrating the presence of biliary contrast extravasation on delayed hepatobiliary phase postcontrast imaging.[94]

MALIGNANT TUMORS

Hepatocellular Carcinoma (see Chapter 89)

HCC is the most common primary hepatic malignancy world-wide. The most significant risk factors include the presence of cirrhosis and infection with hepatitis B and C viruses. Approxi-mately 80% of HCC tumors develop in cirrhotic livers. The diffusely heterogenous, multinodular parenchyma in cirrhotic livers can increase the difficulty in distinguishing focal hepatic lesions on imaging (Fig. 14.16).[95,96] These nodules represent a

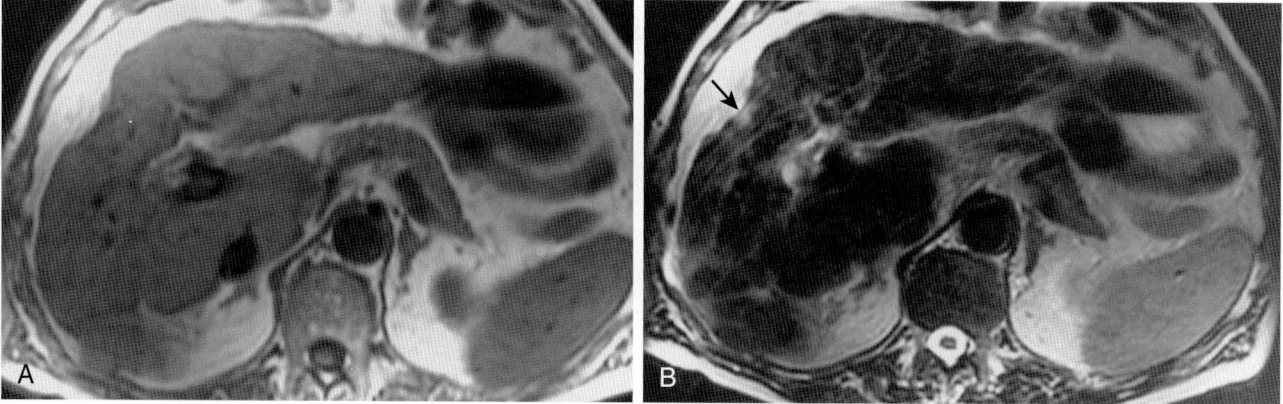

FIGURE 14.16 **Liver with cirrhotic configuration. A,** T1-weighted spin-echo image at the level of the portal vein shows hypertrophy of the left lobe and caudate with atrophy of the right lobe of the liver. **B,** T2-weighted image of the liver at the same level shows mildly heterogeneous signal in the atrophied right lobe. Note also the focal hepatic scarring *(arrow).*

spectrum, from regenerative or dysplastic nodules to HCC. The American Association for the Study of Liver Diseases (AASLD) issued revised recommendations in 2018, recommending US imaging every 6 months, with or without serum α-fetoprotein (AFP), as the recommended modality used to screen for HCC in at-risk patients.[97] When used as a surveillance test, US has a sensitivity of around 63%.[98]

On US, HCC tumors are often nonspecific in appearance and may be hypo- or hyperechoic.[99] CEUS has been shown to be useful in the diagnosis of HCC, particularly in small HCCs less than 2 cm in size, where it has a sensitivity and specificity of 0.81 and 0.86, respectively.[100] However, current AASLD guidelines do not recommend CEUS as a diagnostic tool.

Subsequent diagnostic evaluation should be performed with multiphase CT or MRI, both demonstrating similar diagnostic cabilities.[97,101] The additional advantage of MRI compared with CT in the evaluation of HCC is that malignancies show differences in signal intensity, diffusion, blood pool, and functional hepatocyte enhancement and growth, compared with regenerative or dysplastic nodules or background cirrhotic parenchyma. MRI also has an advantage over other modalities in assessing vascular invasion.

The enhancement patterns at multiphasic CT and MRI using extracellular agents are essentially the same, and the hallmark pattern is that of arterial-phase hyperenhancement with washout appearance in the portal venous or delayed phase (Fig. 14.17). Washout refers to the reduction in enhancement of the tumor relative to background liver parenchyma.[102] In addition to washout, peritumoral capsules, which are low in signal intensity on the arterial dominant phase and enhance later, are an important feature and their absence has been associated with microvascular invasion.[103] If using hepatocyte-specific contrast agents, assessment of washout is confined to the portal venous phase and should not be characterized in the transitional or hepatobiliary phases.[104] When using hepatocyte-specific contrast agents, HCC tumors generally show hypointensity in the delayed hepatobiliary phase of imaging compared with surrounding liver in the majority of cases. Hepatocyte-specific contrast agents have been shown to be more sensitive in the detection of small HCCs or premalignant lesions than extracellular agents.[105,106]

On other MRI sequences, HCC is generally hypointense on T1-weighted and mild to moderately hyperintense on T2-weighted imaging.[107] HCC with intracellular fat can be detected by signal loss on out-of-phase imaging (Fig. 14.18). Fat is associated with early HCC and can also be seen in dysplastic nodules.[108] Intracellular lipid may be an important clue to small HCCs, especially those without typical enhancement patterns, because early HCC are sometimes hypovascular in the arterial phase.[109,110] Larger lesions may be heterogenous because of areas of necrosis. An infiltrative appearance has been associated with more aggressive subtypes, as does the presence of macrovascular invasion.[111]

Because of the complexity of imaging features and overlap, as well as multimodality availability, there have been organized efforts to improve report standardization and communication regarding imaging findings in patients at risk for HCC. The Liver Imaging Reporting and Data System (LI-RADS), an initiative supported by the American College of Radiology, and the Liver and Intestinal Organ Transplant Committee (OPTN) have also issued guidelines regarding HCC classification. LI-RADS was revised in 2018 to facilitate integration of the diagnostic algorithm into the AASLD 2018 HCC clinical practice guidelines. The 2018 diagnostic algorithm describes a four-step approach to the assessment of liver lesions at multiphase CT or MRI in the untreated high-risk population for HCC.[102] The algorithm is intended for use only in patients who are considered high risk for HCC and are without histologic diagnosis or have undergone previous treatment. As a result LI-RADS categories are designed to have high specificity but at the expense of sensitivity.[112] Major features that are seen in HCC include non-rim arterial-phase hyperenhancement (the presence of this feature is mandatory for LR-5 categorization), non-peripheral "washout," enhancing "capsule," and threshold growth. Ancillary features favoring HCC include nodule-in-nodule or mosaic appearance, intralesional fat or blood products, and are also incorporated into the LI-RADS imaging interpretation algorithm (https://www.acr.org/Clinical-Resources/Reporting-and-Data-Systems/LI-RADS/CT-MRI-LI-RADS-v2018; Fig. 14.19). A separate category of LR-TIV (tumor in vein) is assigned for observations that are definitely malignant, with unequivocal enhancing soft tissue in vein. Although tumor in vein is most frequently associated with HCC, it is not exclusive to HCC, with macrovascular invasion also seen in other non-HCC liver tumors, such as intrahepatic cholangiocarcinoma (Fig. 14.20).[113] Although continued revisions are inevitable,

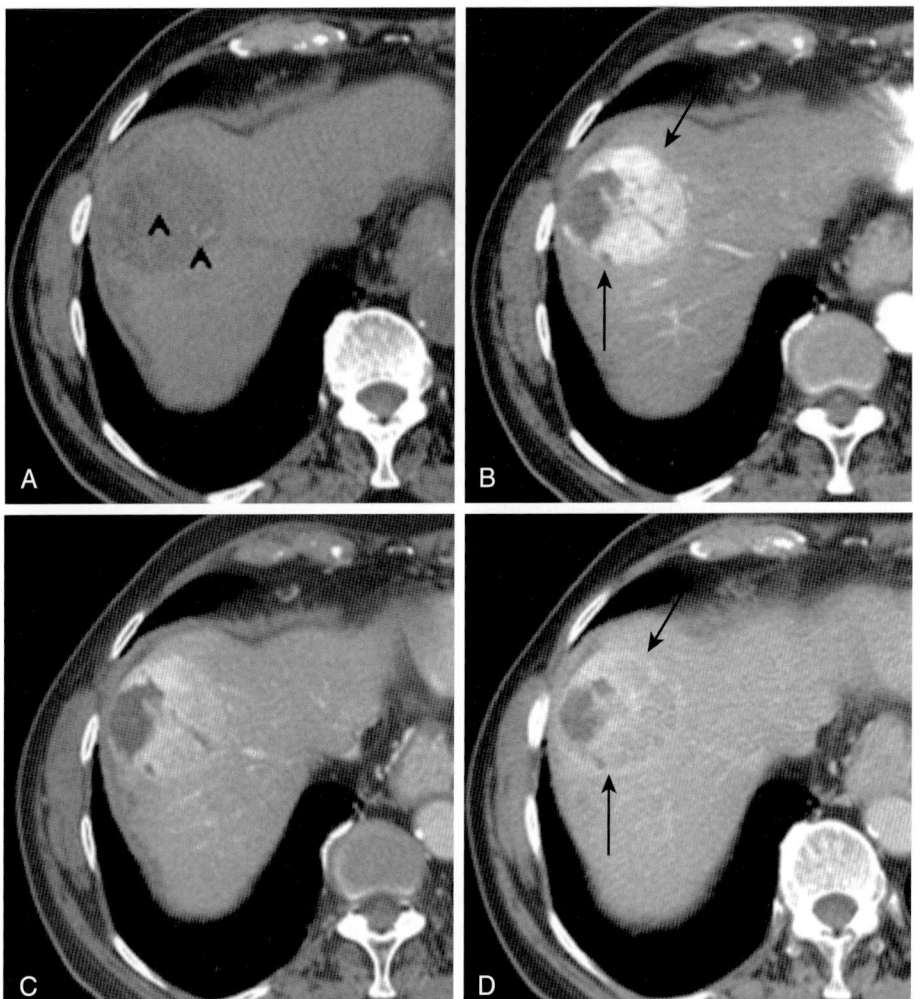

FIGURE 14.17 Hepatocellular carcinoma. A, Precontrast axial computed tomography (CT) image demonstrating a lesion that is mildly hypointense to background liver containing scattered areas of hyperattenuation suggestive of blood products *(arrowheads)*. **B,** Late arterial-phase enhancement demonstrates heterogenous non-rim arterial enhancement of the mass *(arrows)*. **C–D,** Portal venous and delayed phase imaging respectively demonstrating progressive washout appearance with capsule, best appreciated on delayed phase *(arrows)*.

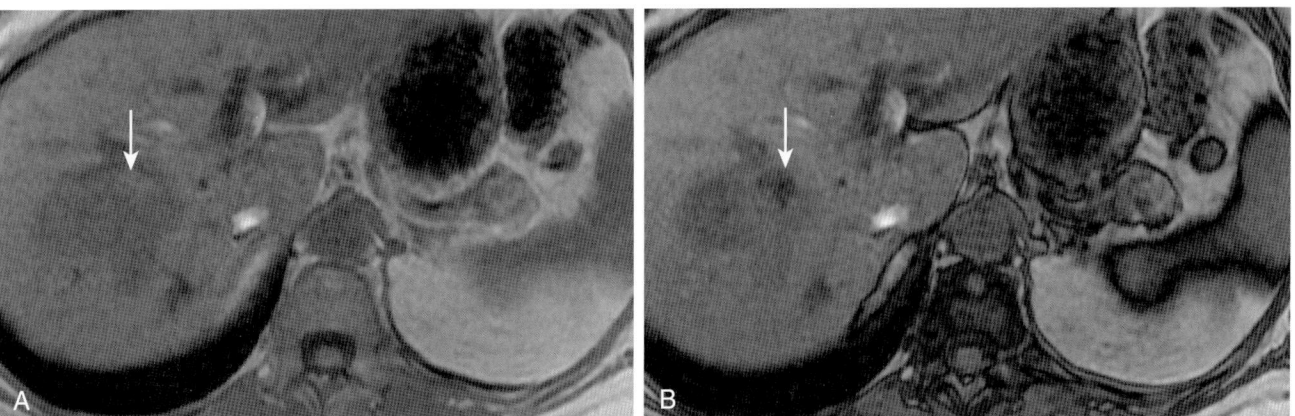

FIGURE 14.18 Hepatocellular carcinoma containing intracellular lipid. A, T1-weighted in-phase gradient-echo image shows a mass in the liver that is darker than normal parenchyma, with a small internal area of brighter signal *(arrow)*. **B,** T1-weighted out-of-phase gradient-echo image shows the same area *(arrow)* has lost signal, which is consistent with an admixture of fat and water-containing tissue.

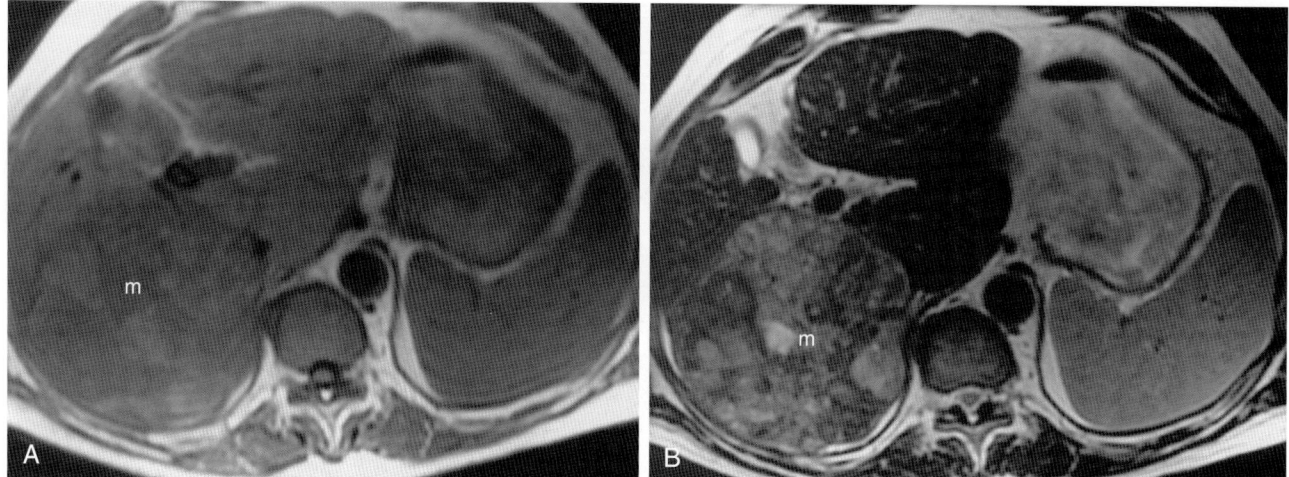

FIGURE 14.19 **Large hepatocellular carcinoma showing a mosaic pattern. A**, T1-weighted image shows a large heterogeneous mass (m) in the liver. Note the hypertrophied left hepatic lobe and caudate. **B**, T2-weighted image also shows the mass (m) to be heterogeneous, with islands of tissue that are hyperintense with respect to other portions of the same mass. This pattern is known as the mosaic pattern, and it can be seen in hepatocellular carcinoma, especially when the lesion is large.

consensus guidelines will encourage report standardization, improve communication, and ultimately improve decision making. Agreement among readers using newer algorithms tends to be moderate to substantial for expert readers but lower among novices, suggesting implementation of these criteria may require a learning curve.[113–115]

Intrahepatic Cholangiocarcinoma (see Chapter 50)

Intrahepatic cholangiocarcinomas (IHCCs) account for approximately 10% of biliary duct cancers, and the majority of these are of the peripheral, mass-forming subtype.[116] A less common intrahepatic subtype is the periductal-infiltrating type, which appears as thickened bile duct walls and longitudinal tumor extension along the bile ducts. Intrahepatic intraductal-growth types are rare and usually present as a small intraluminal papillary tumor within a dilated bile duct.[117] Increasingly, mass-forming IHCCs are seen to arise on a background of cirrhosis, making distinguishing these lesions from HCC difficult on imaging.[118]

On US, IHCC may present as a focal hepatic mass, which may be solitary or with satellite lesions, and may appear hypo- or hyperechoic. The number of tumors present has been shown to be a significant prognostic indicator, with multiple lesions associated with a poorer outcome.[119]

Diagnostic workup and staging generally involves modalities such as CT and MRI. CT angiography with multiphase imaging offers improved spatial resolution and similar accuracy to MRI to assess vascular involvement and exceeds MRI accuracy when assessing for nodal and distant metastases.[120] On CT, IHCC is usually low-attenuating on noncontrast imaging. The precontrast phase is useful for the detection of intraductal stones and differentiating stones from tumor.[121] Capsular retraction and peripheral biliary ductal dilatation have also been described as features, but are not seen in every case.[117]

On MRI, IHCC generally have low T1-signal intensity, high heterogenous T2 signal, and lobulated margins. Enhancement patterns are similar on both multiphase contrast-enhanced CT and MRI using extracellular contrast agents, with tumors often showing peripheral enhancement in the arterial phase and gradual centripetal fill-in on delayed phases because of the central abundant fibrous stroma.[121,122] The initial rim of arterial enhancement, representing viable tumor cells histologically, is typically continuous and can demonstrate washout on later phases of imaging (Fig. 14.21).[123] Non-rim arterial enhancement may be seen in smaller lesions, particularly in cirrhotic livers, and can therefore appear similar to small HCCs, making imaging diagnosis difficult.[118] Caution should be used in the interpretation of images using hepatocyte-specific contrast, such as gadoxetic acid, since a "pseudo-washout" appearance can be seen on the later transitional phase of imaging because of the progressive enhancement of background liver, which can also mimic the appearance of HCC.[124] The presence of washout should therefore be assessed only on the portal venous phase of hepatocyte-specific contrast agents to avoid misidentification of this feature. On hepatobiliary phase, a target appearance has also been described, which is represented by a rim of hypointensity and central "cloud-like" hyperintensity.[121]

The presence of a target sign on DWI has also been described in IHCC, which refers to a rim of hyperintensity and central low intensity on high *b*-value images and a rim of hypointensity on the corresponding ADC map, again reflecting peripheral hypercellular tumor cells and central fibrous stroma.[125] A targetoid appearance of a liver lesion on DWI or postcontrast imaging in a patient at risk for HCC is sufficient to classify that lesion as LI-RADS M.

Combined hepatocellular cholangiocarcinoma (cHCC-CC) is a rare primary hepatic malignancy with both HCC and IHCC components and, accordingly, can mimic either HCC or IHCC, with imaging features more frequently overlapping with IHCC.[126] One study showed that 6.5% of cHCC-CC can be misclassified as HCC, even when using LI-RADS criteria,[127] and diagnosis is more challenging in smaller lesions.[113]

Fibrolamellar Carcinoma (see Chapter 89)

Originally considered within the HCC spectrum and formerly termed "fibrolamellar HCC," this malignant hepatocellular tumor's distinct clinical, pathologic, and imaging features have led to the newer nomenclature. Fibrolamellar carcinoma (FLC)

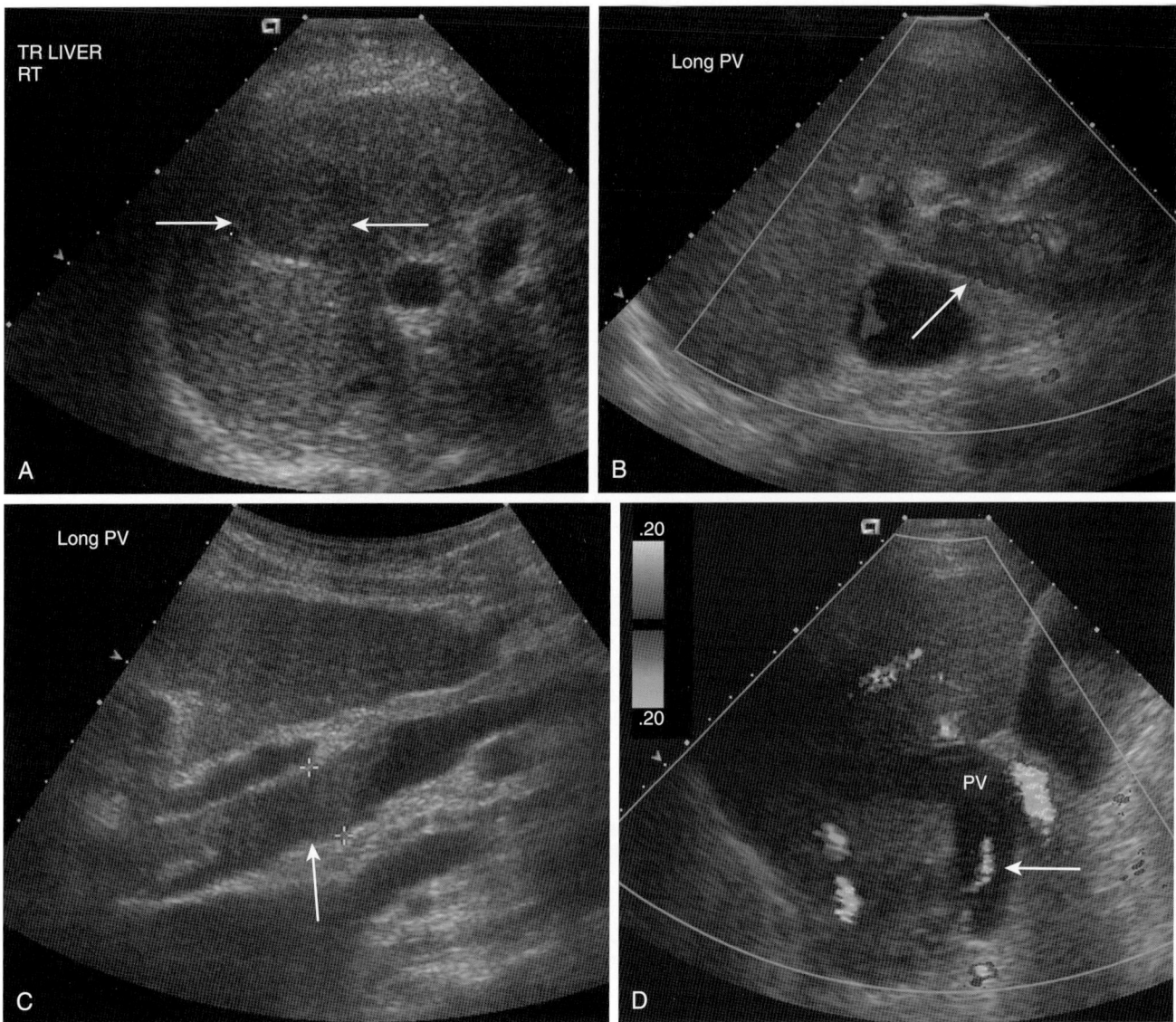

FIGURE 14.20 **Hepatocellular carcinoma (HCC) with portal vein thrombosis. A,** Transverse image shows a hypoechoic HCC in the right hepatic lobe *(arrows).* **B,** Transverse image of the main portal vein reveals only a trickle of blood flow *(arrow).* The lumen is nearly filled with echogenic thrombus. **C,** Longitudinal image of the main portal vein shows the extent of thrombus *(arrow).* **D,** Color Doppler image of the main portal vein confirms arterial flow *(arrow)* within the hypoechoic thrombus; this is pathognomonic for tumor thrombus. *PV,* Portal vein.

occurs in young adults, average age of presentation is 25 years, and it occurs in the absence of cirrhosis or risk factors for liver disease.[128,129] It frequently presents as a large, well-demarcated, solitary mass with a mean diameter of greater than 11 cm, and a central scar can be seen in 46% to 73% of cases.[130,131] A common diagnostic dilemma for radiologists is to distinguish FLC from either FNH or conventional HCC, both of which can present as a large solitary mass with a central scar. Metastatic disease is common at presentation in FLC, both in the abdomen and chest, with adenopathy being prominent in a majority of cases.[129,130]

On US, appearances are variable and nonspecific, occasionally showing calcifications and a central hyperechoic scar.[132] There is little literature published on its appearance at CEUS.

On unenhanced CT, FLH usually appears as a large, hypoattenuating, solitary mass with well-defined lobular margins and a central low-attenuating scar. Calcification, a finding that is used to help differentiate this lesion from FNH, can be seen

in 43% to 64% of cases, and when seen is typically associated with a central scar.[129–131] On MRI, FLC is frequently low on T1-weighted and high on T2-weighted imaging.[130,133] The central scar, if present, tends to be low in signal on T1-weighted and T2-weighted images because of fibrous changes. This is a distinguishing characteristic from FNH, in which if a central scar is present, it is typically increased in T2 signal. However, some FLC central scars can also show increased T2 signal. Therefore, the presence of increased T2 signal is not a reliable discriminator.[130] A scar that is low in T2 signal, on the other hand, is seldom seen in FNH and should raise the suspicion for FLC (Fig. 14.22).

FLCs usually show more heterogenous enhancement on arterial phase on either CT or MRI, compared with FNH. Imaging findings are more variable on later phases, with regions of washout sometimes demonstrated.[131,133] The central scar tends not to enhance on portal venous and later phases of postcontrast imaging, in contrast to FNH scars, which typically do.

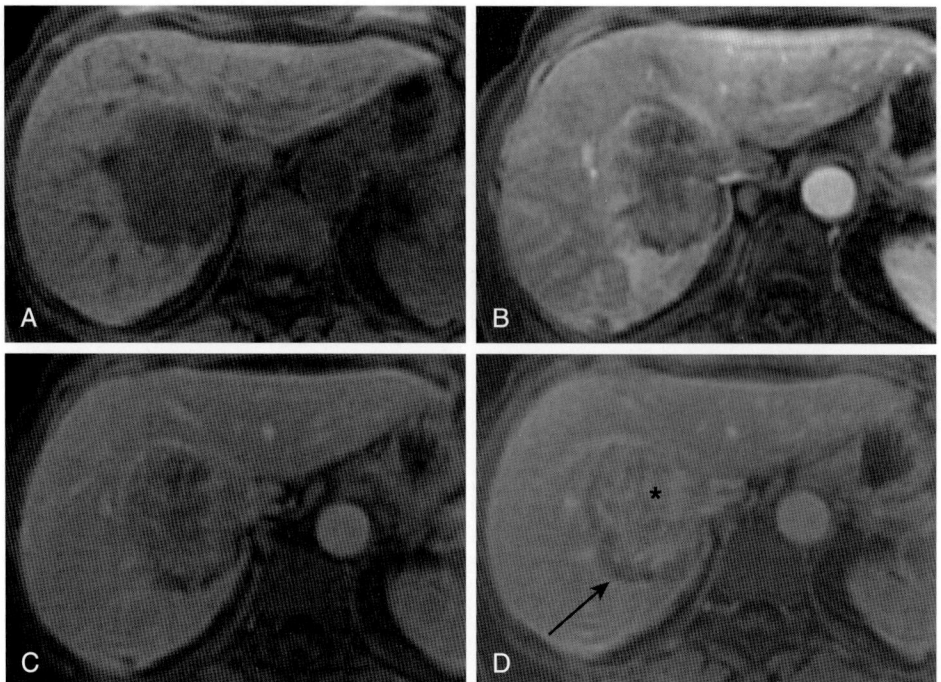

FIGURE 14.21 **Mass forming intrahepatic cholangiocarcinoma. A**, T1-weighted in-phase gradient-echo image shows a peripheral hypointense mass. **B**, T1-weighted fat saturation postcontrast-enhanced image in late arterial phase shows peripheral enhancement. **C**, T1-weighted postcontrast-enhanced image in portal venous phase shows only partial filling of the mass. **D**, T1-weighted postcontrast-enhanced image in equilibrium phase shows progressive central filling of the mass representing central fibrous stroma *(asterisk)* and washout of the peripheral rim of viable tumor cells *(arrow)*.

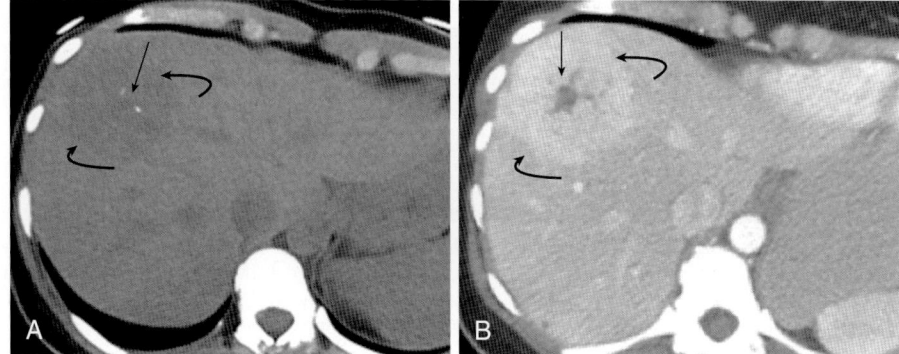

FIGURE 14.22 **Fibrolamellar carcinoma. A**, Precontrast axial CT image demonstrates a solitary mass in the right lobe of the liver *(curved arrows)*. Clustered punctate foci of calcification is noted centrally *(arrow)*. **B**, Portal venous phase postcontrast imaging demonstrates an enhancing mass *(curved arrows)*. A central low attenuating scar *(arrow)* is visible and corresponds to the region of central punctate calcification, more easily apparent on precontrast imaging.

However, FLC scar enhancement on delayed phase has been described in a small proportion of cases.[130,131] Partial uptake may be seen on hepatobiliary phase of imaging using hepatocyte-specific contrast agents; FLC nonetheless typically remains hypointense relative to background liver.[133]

Epithelioid Hemangioendothelioma

Hepatic epithelioid hemangioendothelioma (HEH) is a rare tumor of vascular origin and is considered to be a low-to-intermediate grade malignancy with variable clinical behavior (see Chapter 87).

HEH tumors are typically multifocal and located in the peripheral, subcapsular regions of the liver.[134] As the disease progresses, these nodules tend to coalesce to appear as a large infiltrative, peripheral liver mass. Capsular retraction is also frequently observed in HEH.[134,135] On US, discrete nodules of variable echogenicity may be seen or the liver may have a diffusely heterogenous echotexture in regions of coalesced tumor involvement.[136]

On noncontrast CT, central low density change and capsular retraction are frequently seen, with occasional central calcification also reported.[137] Postcontrast features seen on both CT and MRI include arterial ring-like enhancement and target-like enhancement on portal venous phase.[134,135,137] The target sign typically refers to the target appearance of the lesion on T2-weighted imaging, with a central core of high

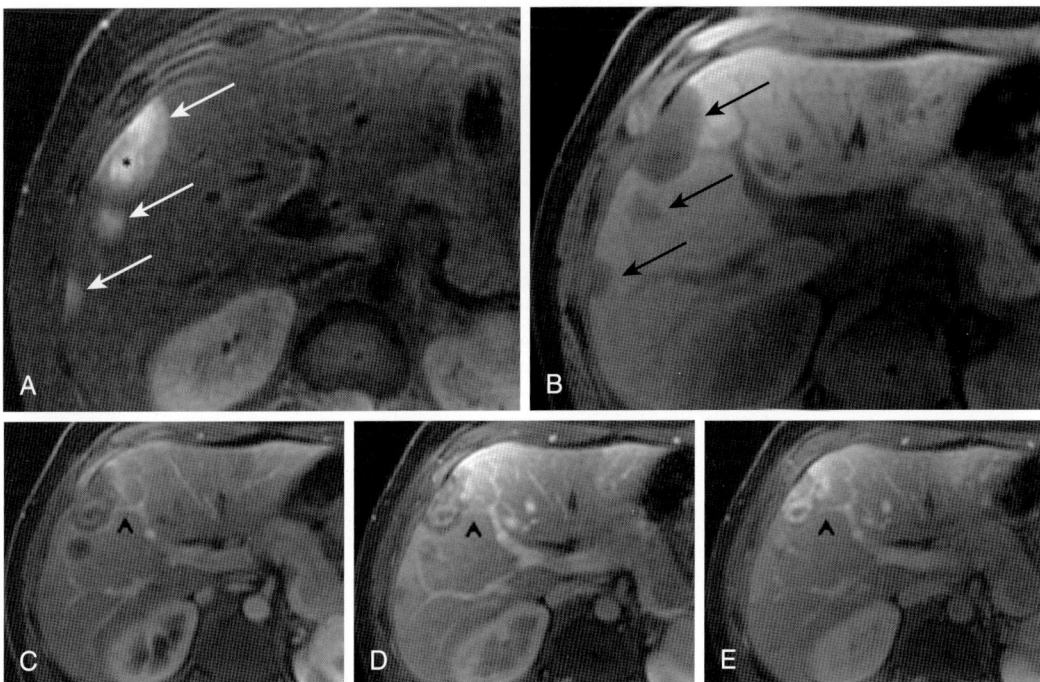

FIGURE 14.23 **Epithelioid hemangioendothelioma. A,** Fat saturated T2-weighted axial image demonstrating multiple liver lesions in a peripheral, subcapsular distribution *(arrows)*. The lesions are centrally T2 hyperintense *(asterisk)* with a surrounding halo of lower signal intensity, likened to a "target" appearance. **B,** Fat saturated T1-weighted axial image demonstrates a corresponding low T1 signal intensity *(arrows)*. The surrounding halo is very slightly higher in intensity on T1-weighted imaging. **C–E,** Postcontrast images in the late arterial, portal venous, and equilibrium phases demonstrate arterial ring-like enhancement with more of a target-like enhancement pattern on later phases of imaging. A portal vein branch is seen extending towards the tumor with abrupt termination at the tumor margin, which has been likened to a "lollipop" in appearance. The vessel represents the lollipop stick *(arrowhead)*.

signal, representing fibrosis stroma, surrounded by a rim of low-signal intensity, reflecting proliferating tumor cells. A mildly hyperintense halo may also be seen in the presence of an avascular rim because of invasion of hepatic sinusoids and small vessels by tumor cells. This target-like appearance may also be seen on DWI, on nonenhanced T1-weighted images, and on postcontrast hepatobiliary phase using hepatocyte-specific contrast.[134,135,138] Although usually diffusely low in signal on nonenhanced T1-weighted imaging, a small proportion of HEH lesions demonstrate low central signal intensity surrounded by a thin hyperintense ring and a peripheral low signal halo, which has also been called the "T1-weighted-dark-bright-dark ring sign."[135] In the case of postcontrast hepatobiliary phase imaging, HEH may have a central hypointense core surrounded by a rim of mild signal intensity, also described as a "core pattern."[139] The "lollipop" sign refers to the presence of a hepatic vein or portal vein branch (the stick) extending towards the tumor (the candy of the lollipop) and then terminating at the margin or just within the lesion rim because of the vessel branch occlusion.[140] It can be seen in up to half of cases of HEH and, when seen, is considered a characteristic finding (Fig. 14.23).[137]

Hepatic Angiosarcoma and Other Mesenchymal Tumors

Primary hepatic angiosarcoma (HAS) is a rare but aggressive hepatic malignancy, with a median survival reported as less than 6 months. It has been associated with a variety of environmental exposures, most notably, thorium dioxide (Thorotrast), arsenic, and radiation exposure.[45] When arising in the setting of thorium dioxide exposure, thorium deposition can be seen

as high-attenuating foci within the liver, perihepatic lymph nodes, and spleen. Underlying cirrhosis is often present (see Chapter 87).[141]

On US, HAS is usually heterogeneously hyperechoic, reflecting its vascular origin.[141] On nonenhanced CT, HAS most commonly presents as either multiple, bilobar masses, one of which is usually dominant, or as a solitary mass.[141,142] Because of the tumor's vascular nature, tumor heterogeneity with multiple regions of mixed attenuation or foci with fluid-fluid levels may be seen, representing intratumoral hemorrhage.[45,143] On MRI, HAS is typically high in T2 signal and low in T1 signal. Hemorrhagic foci within the lesion will demonstrate increased T1-weighted signal.

On postcontrast imaging on either CT or MRI, HAS enhancement on multiphase imaging tends to follow that of blood pool, although the pattern of enhancement can be highly variable, including nodular, rim, branching, or diffuse patterns. Heterogenous arterial enhancement is typically seen, although regions of hyperenhancement are typically small relative to tumor size.[141] Washout is typically not seen, and its absence can be a helpful factor in distinguishing HAS from HCC.[141] In a proportion of cases, enhancement patterns resemble that of hemangiomas to a varying degree, such as the presence of centripetal fill-in (Fig 14.24).[142,144] "Reverse hemangioma" centrifugal pattern has also been described in a number of cases.[141] Splenic metastases are common and, if present, offer a clue to the diagnosis of HAS. A proportion of cases may present with capsular rupture and subcapsular hematoma and hemoperitoneum.

Other rarer tumors of mesenchymal origin include leiomyosarcoma, fibrosarcoma, Kaposi sarcoma, and solitary fibrous

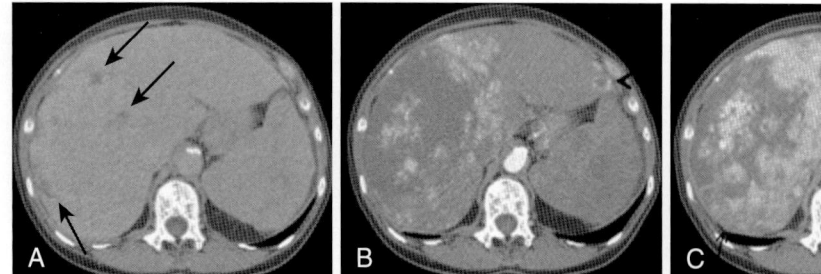

FIGURE 14.24 **Hepatic angiosarcoma. A**, Precontrast axial computed tomography (CT) image demonstrates scattered areas of vague liver heterogeneity *(arrows)*. **B–C**, Postcontrast imaging in the arterial and portal venous phase respectively demonstrates the full extent of a dominant, heterogeneously enhancing mass replacing most the right the hepatic lobe *(arrows)*. The irregular tumoral enhancement is similar to that of blood pool with progressive, centripetal enhancement on the later portal venous phase. A smaller mass is also seen in the left lobe of liver *(arrowhead)*.

tumor (previous called "hemangiopericytoma"). The imaging features of these tumors are nonspecific on US, CT, and MRI. On MRI they are generally of low signal intensity on T1-weighted images and hyperintense on T2-weighted images, with heterogenous enhancement.[145,146]

Undifferentiated embryonal sarcoma (UES) is usually seen in the pediatric population; however, cases have been reported in the adult population. These tumors tend to have extensive cystic and necrotic change and may be mistaken for hepatic abscesses or other cystic liver masses.[147] Discrepancy between a predominantly solid appearance on US, and cystic appearance on CT has been described as a classical feature of UES.[145]

Primary Hepatic Lymphoma

Primary hepatic lymphoma (PHL) is a rare hepatic tumor and refers to liver-confined lymphoma without involvement of lymph nodes, bone marrow, spleen, or other lymphomatous structures.

In order of frequency, PHL may present as a solitary mass, multiple lesions, or a diffuse infiltrative process, with the most common imaging manifestation of a solitary mass seen in about 60% of cases.[148,149] When multiple lesions are present, typically one of these lesions is dominant.[150] In contrast, multiple lesions without a dominant mass or an infiltrative pattern are the main

imaging appearances seen in lymphoma with secondary involvement of the liver (SHL).[150] SHL is relatively easier to diagnose because of concomitant involvement of other organs, especially spleen and generalized lymphadenopathy.

On US, lesions are typically hypoechoic with case reports of lesions appearing anechoic and mimicking cysts. Nevertheless, absence of posterior acoustic enhancement should hint as to the presence of a solid lesion.[149,151] PHL is typically hypoattenuating on CT.[149] On MRI, an "insinuative" growth pattern has been described, which is shown by tumor growth without displacement of hepatic vessels or biliary ducts.[148] This appearance has also been described as the "vessel penetration sign."[151] Lesions are typically homogenously T1 hypointense and T2 hyperintense; however, signal intensity may be heterogenous in the presence of blood products or necrosis.[149] Postcontrast imaging on both CT and MRI demonstrate variable, nonspecific appearances, typically heterogeneously enhancing, but hypoattenuating or hypointense relative to background liver on multiphase imaging (Fig. 14.25). Arterial and portal venous rim enhancement can be seen in a proportion of cases.[148,149]

Restricted diffusion is typically seen, with one study noting that ADC values were significantly lower in PHL when compared with both benign liver lesions and other primary hepatic lesions.[148]

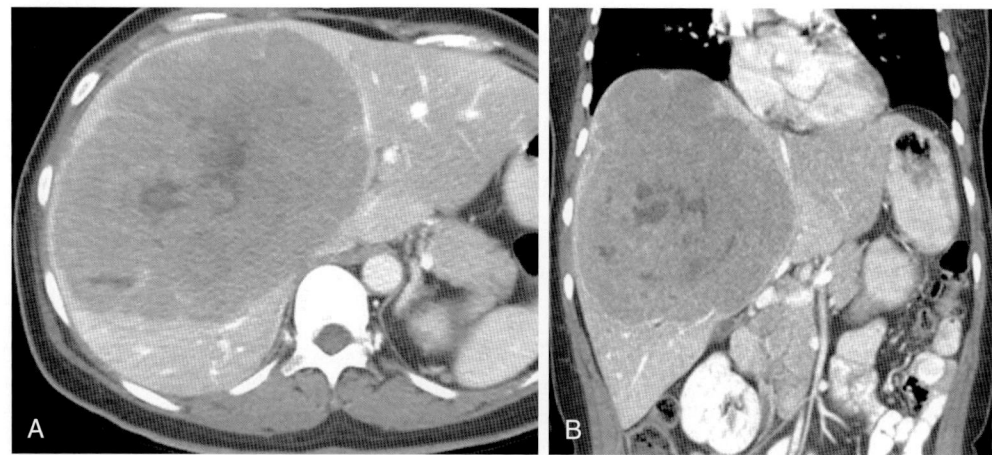

FIGURE 14.25 **Primary hepatic lymphoma. A–B**, Computed tomography (CT) axial and coronal contrast-enhanced images in the portal venous phase shows a large, solitary mass in the liver, with rather nonspecific features and demonstrating heterogeneous enhancement, hypoattenuating relative to background liver.

Imaging characteristics of lymphoma, however, are nonspecific and overlap with other malignant hepatic lesions.

Biliary Cystadenocarcinoma

Biliary cystadenocarcinoma (BCAC) is a rare neoplasm arising from the bile ducts. BCAC is usually a result of malignant transformation of BCA; however, it can also arise de novo (see Chapter 88B).[55] Imaging features of BCAC overlap with BCA and although the presence of "high-risk" features such as mural nodularity, solid components, septations, and papillary excrescences have a high negative predictive value of 91%, the positive predictive value is low at 11%. Tumor size is also a poor discriminator of BCAC from BCA.[67] Mural nodules greater than 1 cm in size are more likely to occur in BCAC, however.[71]

The references for this chapter can be found online by accessing the accompanying Expert Consult website.

CHAPTER 15

Imaging features of metastatic liver cancer

Galina Levin and Richard Kinh Gian Do

OVERVIEW

Imaging plays a central role in the characterization of liver lesions and detection of liver metastases in patients at risk. As treatment options for patients with metastatic liver disease have proliferated over the past decade (see Chapters 90–92), timely and accurate characterization of liver lesions is increasingly important.

Several imaging modalities, such as ultrasonography (US), computed tomography (CT), and magnetic resonance imaging (MRI), can be used in the detection of hepatic metastases. The choice of imaging tests may vary greatly between different institutions based on availability, expertise, preferences of the referring physicians and radiologists, and unique patient factors (for example, MRI-unsafe implanted devices, claustrophobia, impaired renal function, and contrast allergies). Conventional US is the most widely available technique, but its sensitivity is significantly affected by patient factors, such as obesity, bowel interposition between the liver and abdominal wall, and shadowing artifact from excessive bowel gas. Although new US contrast agents have significantly increased the sensitivity of hepatic lesion detection,[1,2] contrast-enhanced US (CEUS) is not yet widely available in the United States.

According to the current National Comprehensive Cancer Network guidelines, PET/CT (positron-emission tomography/CT) is recommended for the initial staging of only some newly diagnosed tumors, such as lung, esophageal, head and neck, cervical cancers and lymphoma. In tumors that frequently metastasize to the liver such as colorectal, pancreatic, and gastric cancers, PET/CT is not routinely recommended for the initial staging in most cases (see Chapter 18).[3] According to the American College of Radiology (ACR) Appropriateness Criteria for presurgical assessment of suspected hepatic metastases, traditional US carries a rating of 3 (on a scale of 1 to 9 with 1, 2, and 3 denoting "usually not appropriate" and 7, 8, and 9 denoting "usually appropriate"). In comparison, MRI, CT, and PET/CT carry ratings of 9, 8, and 6, respectively. CT and MRI are currently the most widely used modalities for the initial detection and surveillance of metastatic liver lesions and for presurgical planning.[4]

The goal of this chapter is to review the imaging characteristics of hepatic metastases, to compare the strengths and weaknesses of various imaging modalities, and to highlight important pearls and pitfalls of image interpretation.

ULTRASOUND

Background

US has been used since the 1970s, and conventional US has unique advantages, such as low cost, lack of radiation, and widespread availability. However, US is less sensitive than other imaging modalities for liver metastases. Experience and technique of the doctor or technician acquiring US images may also vary significantly. Some studies report sensitivity of US in detection of liver metastases to be as low as 38%.[1] Although US contrast agents were introduced and used worldwide since the 1990s, United States Food and Drug Administration (FDA) approval of the first contrast agent for liver lesions in children and adults took place in 2015.[5] CEUS uses microbubbles that enable the demonstration of tissue perfusion similar to contrast enhancement in CT and MRI, but with subtle differences. Numerous studies demonstrate increased sensitivity and specificity of CEUS compared with conventional US, with sensitivities ranging between 72% and 96% and specificities between 93% and 98%.[2] For example, in a prospective study that evaluated detection of hepatic metastases with US, CEUS, and contrast-enhanced CT (CECT) in 253 patients with suspected hepatic metastases from various primary malignancies, CEUS improved sensitivity from approximately 40% to 83% and specificity from 63% to 84%. The sensitivity and specificity of CECT in the same study was demonstrated to be 89% and 89%, respectively.[6]

According to the latest guidelines and good clinical practice recommendations for CEUS in the liver from 2012 that involved collaboration of multiple leading ultrasound societies worldwide, the indications for liver CEUS are the following[7]:

- Incidental findings on conventional US
- Lesion(s) or suspected lesion(s) detected with US in patients with a known history of a cancer, as an alternative to CT or MRI
- Patients with contraindications to CT and MRI contrast administration
- Inconclusive MRI/CT findings
- Inconclusive biopsy results

US contrast agents are not nephrotoxic and are safe for use in patients with renal failure and even dialysis. These contrast agents are also safe in patients with iodine contrast allergies. The overall rate of severe allergic reactions is lower compared with iodinated CT contrast and is comparable to magnetic resonance (MR) contrast agents.[5,8]

Imaging Findings

Although most metastases are hypoechoic (darker) with respect to the underlying liver parenchyma (Fig. 15.1A–B), some metastases can also be isoechoic (similar to) and hyperechoic (brighter) to adjacent liver (Fig. 15.2A–B). Echogenicity of liver metastases can vary, based on primary tumor and based on the composition of underlying liver parenchyma that can be affected by hepatic steatosis, prior chemotherapy treatments, and other forms of liver disease. Thus primary (benign or malignant neoplasms) and metastatic liver lesions may have

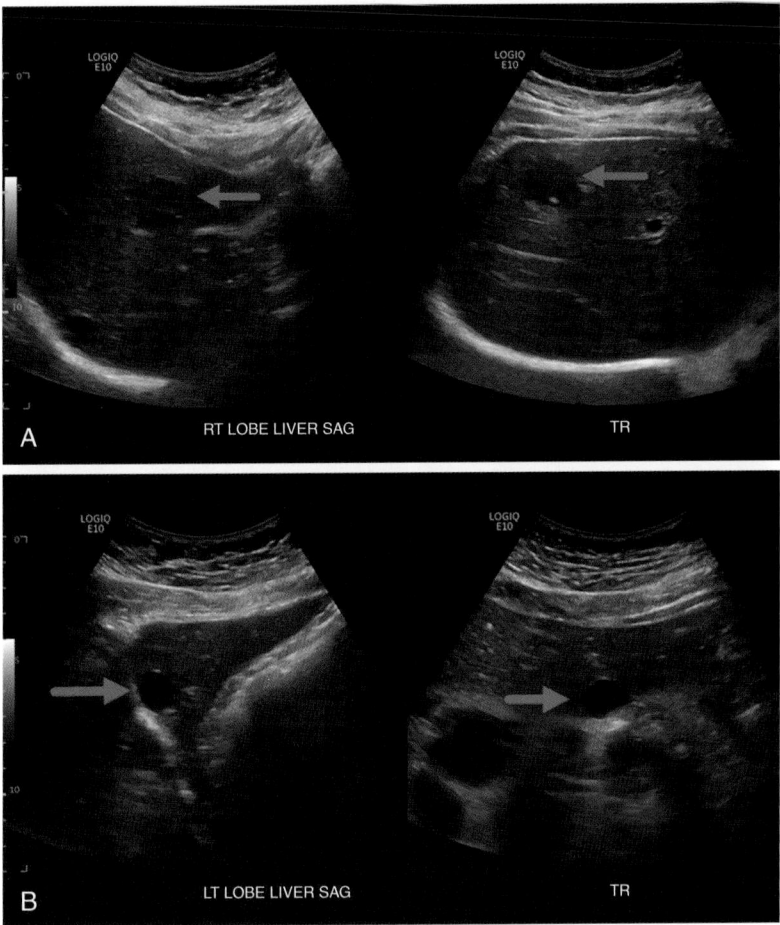

FIGURE 15.1   Hypoechoic hepatic metastasis and a cyst in the same patient with breast cancer. **A,** Sagittal and transverse grey scale ultrasound images demonstrate a hypoechoic lesion *(arrow)* with a poorly defined, slightly irregular wall. **B,** Sagittal and transverse ultrasound images in the same patient demonstrate a simple cyst *(arrow)*. Note the difference in echogenicity when compared with the metastasis. The cyst is anechoic *(completely black)* and has a thin, sharp wall.

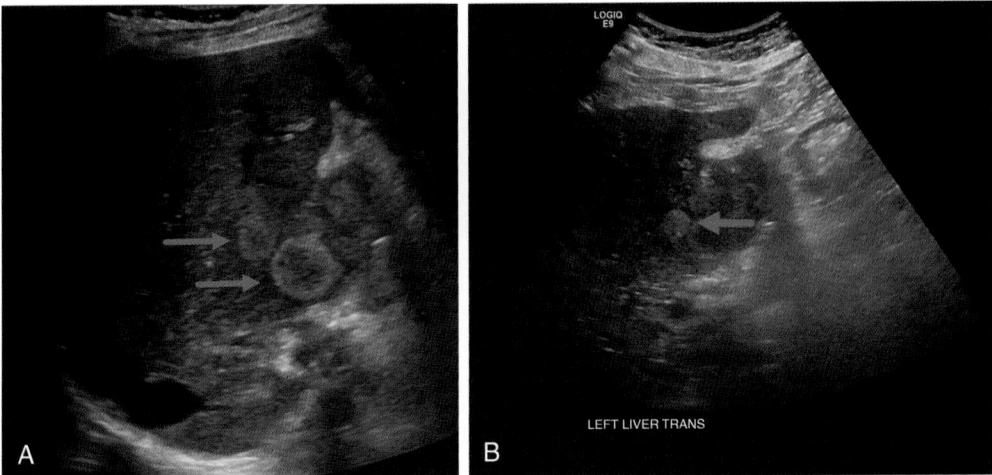

FIGURE 15.2   Hyperechoic metastases in a patient with metastatic neuroendocrine tumor. **A,** Grey-scale ultrasound image demonstrates two adjacent metastases *(arrows)* with markedly echogenic periphery and relatively hypoechoic center. **B,** Another metastasis in the same patient *(arrow)* is completely hyperechoic.

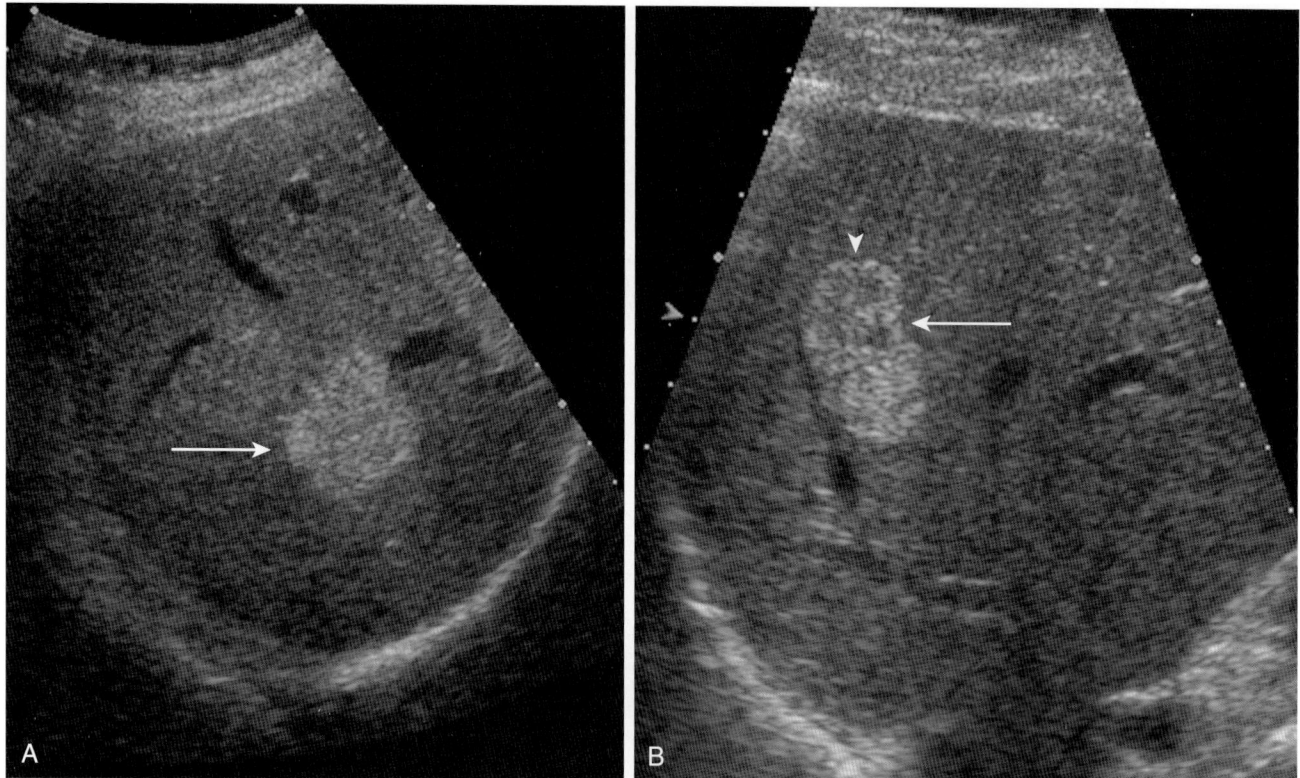

FIGURE 15.3.   Hemangiomas. A, Longitudinal sonogram of the right lobe shows a brightly echogenic hemangioma *(arrow)* with a circumscribed border. **B,** Atypical hemangioma *(arrow)* with areas of internal heterogeneity, a result of fibrosis or myxomatous degeneration, and a thin echogenic rim *(arrowhead)*.

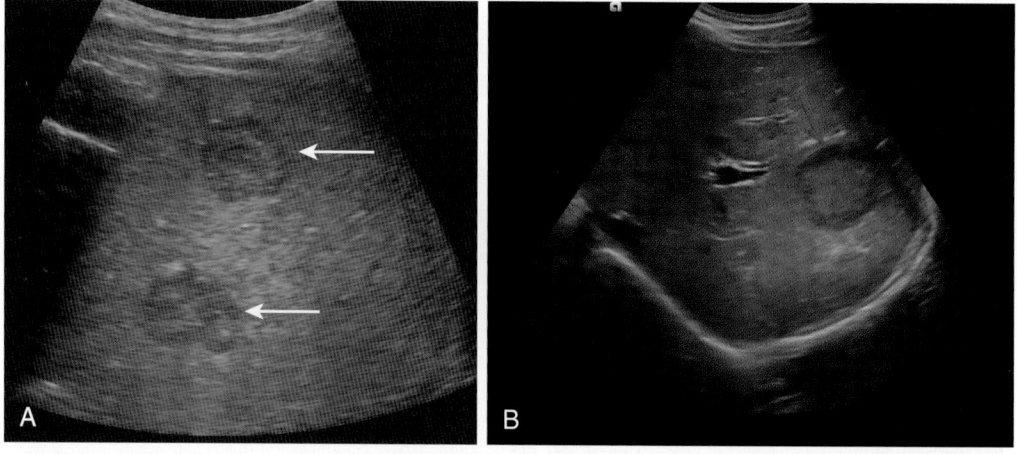

FIGURE 15.4   Hypoechoic halo sign. A, Ultrasound image demonstrates metastatic neuroendocrine tumor in the liver with a subtle peripheral hypoechoic halo **B,** Ultrasound image demonstrates focal lymphomatous involvement of the liver with a prominent hypoechoic halo *(arrow)*.

similar US characteristics (Compare Fig. 15.2B with Fig. 15.3); for example, metastases and hemangiomas (see Chapter 88A) may both demonstrate hyperechoic appearance with respect to adjacent liver.

A hypoechoic halo sign (bull's eye sign) is a helpful way to distinguish benign from malignant lesions. This is a sign of difference in acoustic impedance along the periphery compared with the center of the lesion, which reflects parenchymal compression and active growth on pathologic correlation. Therefore the halo sign is usually indicative of an expansile, malignant mass, such as a metastasis or a primary hepatic neoplasm (Fig. 15.4).[9]

Liver metastases demonstrate variable enhancement when evaluated with the CEUS technique. The arterial phase imaging characteristics vary between no enhancement, rim enhancement, and diffuse hyperenhancement. There is rapid, complete washout on the portal venous phase (Fig. 15.5). In contrast, hepatocellular carcinoma (HCC) demonstrates a later washout, and benign lesions demonstrate minimal or absent washout. Cholangiocarcinoma (see Chapter 50) demonstrates rapid washout on CEUS (unlike on CT and MRI where it demonstrates progressive delayed enhancement) and, therefore, cannot be reliably distinguished from a metastasis.[10]

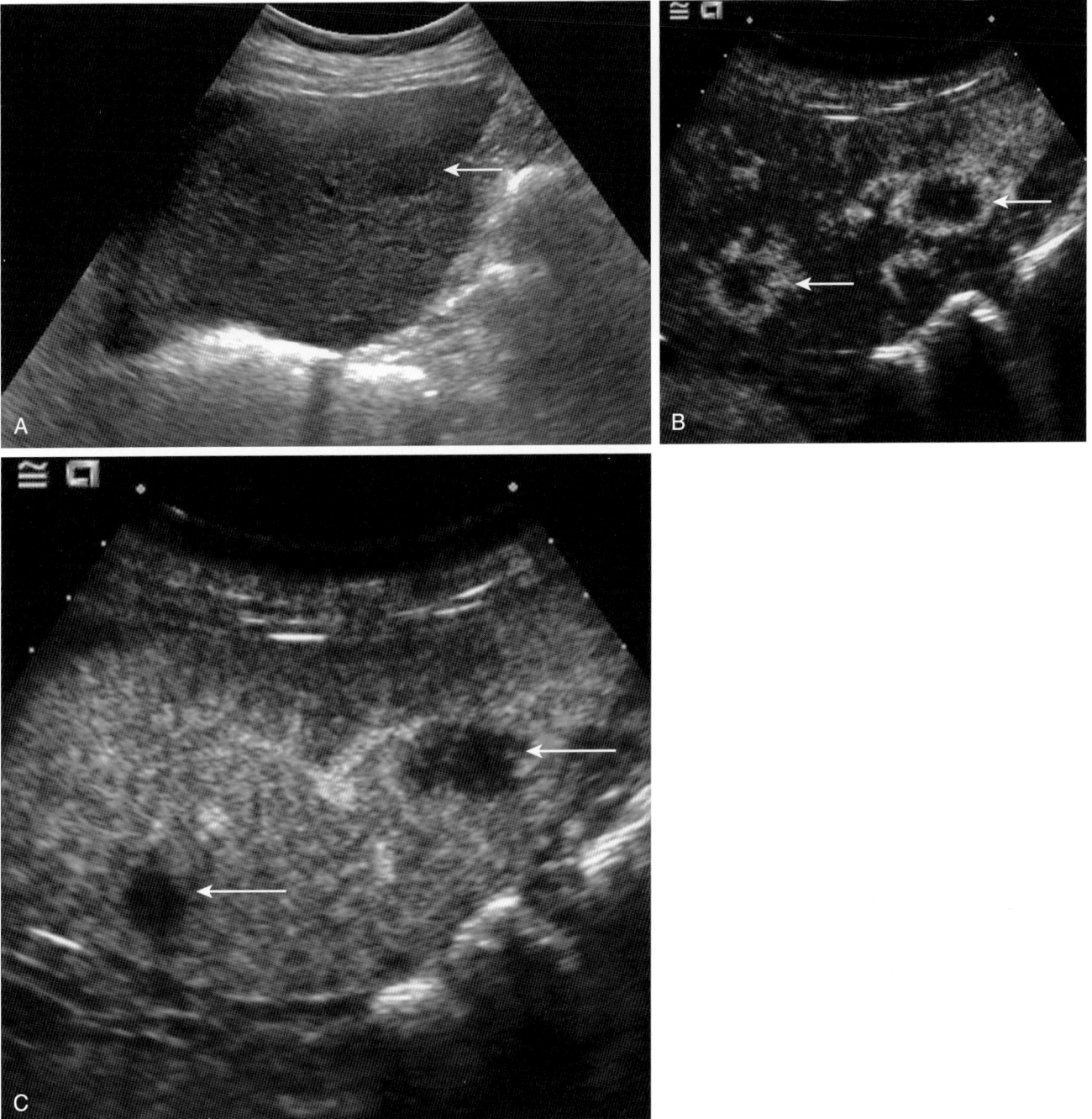

FIGURE 15.5   **Hepatic metastases evaluated with contrast-enhanced ultrasound. A,** Gray-scale image reveals a hypoechoic mass *(arrow)* representing a metastasis. **B,** In the arterial portal phase after contrast injection, the liver metastases *(arrows)* have peripheral rim enhancement, and an additional lesion is now evident. **C,** The metastases *(arrows)* show complete washout of contrast in less than a minute; image taken at 54 seconds. (Courtesy Stephanie R. Wilson.)

Limitations and Pitfalls

The quality of images is highly dependent on the operator's skill and patient's body habitus, with both traditional US and CEUS. Small lesions, particularly less than 0.5 cm, are usually not adequately visualized and characterized. Liver lesions subjacent to interposed bowel may be completely obscured by the shadowing artifact from air contained within bowel loops. Specific anatomic location also plays a role. For example, lesions adjacent to the diaphragm (particularly in segments VII and VIII) or near the heart are technically challenging to image

because of motion and may be missed. Deep lesions in a setting of fatty liver are poorly visualized secondary to decreased acoustic penetration.[5]

Peribiliary metastases are particularly challenging to diagnose, even with CEUS. One study demonstrated that in a group of 35 patients with proven peribiliary metastases, only one was visualized with CEUS. In the same study, all peribiliary lesions were detected on MRI.[11]

Occasionally benign entities can mimic metastases on traditional US and CEUS. In the setting of hepatic steatosis, benign lesions, such as focal nodular hyperplasia (FNH), which is

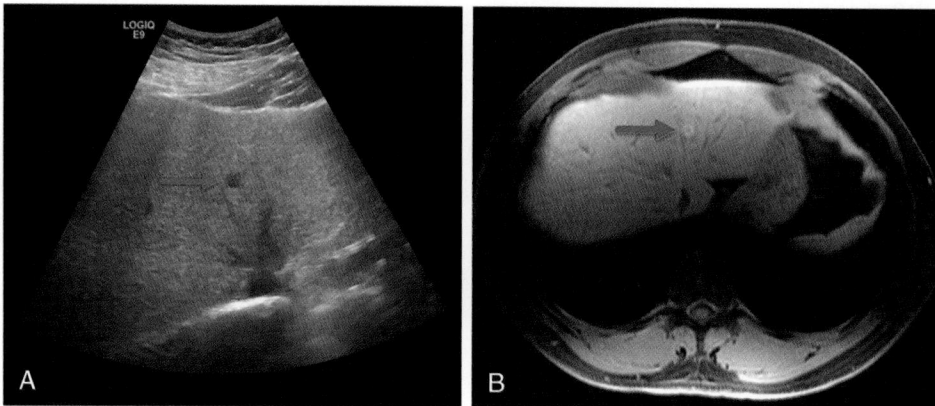

FIGURE 15.6   Focal lesion in a patient with colon cancer. **A,** Ultrasound image demonstrates a small hypoechoic lesion seen on the background of hepatic steatosis. This raised a concern for metastatic disease. **B,** Magnetic resonance imaging (MRI) with Gd-EOB-DTPA obtained for further evaluation. Axial T1 postcontrast MRI image obtained during a hepatobiliary phase revealed peripheral hyperenhancement, consistent with focal nodular hyperplasia (FNH).

usually isoechoic to normal liver parenchyma, will appear hypoechoic (dark) relative to the liver (see Chapter 88A). A hypoechoic lesion is often interpreted as metastatic disease (Fig. 15.6). Focal fatty sparing or focal fat can mimic a mass lesion, particularly if it demonstrates an unusual shape or occurs in an atypical location. One study that looked at detection of metastases occult on conventional US with CEUS and MRI in cancer patients with hepatic steatosis demonstrated that in 1 out of 37 patients, CEUS misinterpreted geographic hepatic steatosis as metastases, which was correctly diagnosed with MRI.[12]

Abscesses can be isoechoic, hypoechoic, or hyperechoic relative to the hepatic parenchyma and can present as a solid, partially cystic, or a predominantly cystic lesion (see Chapter 70).[13] Acoustic through transmission and lack of internal flow on Doppler interrogation favors an abscess rather than a neoplastic process. However, necrotic or cystic metastases may contain substantial cystic components and may not demonstrate appreciable internal vascularity, which makes it difficult to differentiate them from an abscess. Other benign entities, such as tuberculosis (TB), sarcoidosis, and inflammatory pseudotumors, may present as mass lesions and can mimic metastatic disease.[14,15]

COMPUTED TOMOGRAPHY

Background

CT is the most commonly used technique in the United States for the initial staging and surveillance for metastatic disease because this modality allows for assessment of the liver as well as other potential sites of metastatic disease in the lungs and pelvis. According to several meta-analyses performed between 2010 and 2019, the sensitivity of CECT in detection of hepatic metastases ranges between 74% and 83%.[16–19] The sensitivity of CT is dependent on image acquisition technique and parameters, particularly slice thickness and phase of enhancement. Lower slice thickness improves the detection and characterization of liver metastases. For example, use of 2.5-mm slice thickness resulted in a 46% increase in lesion detection rate in one study when compared with 10-mm slice thickness and an 18% increase when compared with 5-mm slice thickness images.[20]

Use of intravenous (IV) iodinated contrast is necessary to optimize the sensitivity and specificity of CT. Noncontrast CT

images have limited utility in the evaluation of liver lesions with certain exceptions, such as hemorrhagic and calcified lesions that have higher density than underlying liver parenchyma. Previously embolized or ablated lesions are also frequently higher in density because of either postprocedural changes or embolization material, so the noncontrast phase is helpful in the post-treatment setting to accurately assess for the presence of enhancement.

Imaging Findings

Metastases can be hypovascular, hypervascular, or isovascular (i.e., enhance less, similar, or greater) with respect to the background liver parenchyma. Most metastases (e.g., colorectal, pancreatic adenocarcinoma, and lung) are hypovascular relative to the liver and are best visualized on the portal venous phase of enhancement, which is acquired approximately 60 to 80 seconds after the injection of contrast (Fig. 15.7). The portal venous phase is usually sufficient for detection of most hypovascular metastases. However, 88% of hypovascular metastases demonstrate some degree of arterial hyperenhancement, most commonly either partial or complete peripheral ring hyperenhancement on the arterial phase of CT. This pattern of enhancement has been suggested to have a high positive predictive value for malignancy, near 98%.[21] Utilization of the arterial phase for detection of hypovascular metastases remains controversial. Some studies report no added value with the addition of the arterial phase.[22,23] However, there are studies that report improved sensitivity for lesion detection in the range of 8% to 13%. The most significant increase in the detection of metastases is observed with lesions less than 1 cm.[24,25] The delayed phase is usually not helpful because both hypervascular and hypovascular metastases become less conspicuous a few minutes after the injection of contrast.

Hypervascular liver metastases are less common and are most commonly observed with primary tumors, such as melanoma, neuroendocrine neoplasms, renal cell carcinoma, and thyroid cancer (see Chapters 91 and 92). Numerous studies have demonstrated advantages of multiphasic imaging in evaluation of hypervascular liver metastases (Fig. 15.8). For example, 14% of melanoma metastases are not seen on the portal venous phase images when the arterial phase of enhancement is not provided.[26] Ten percent of hepatic metastases from renal cell carcinoma are missed if only the portal venous phase is used.[27]

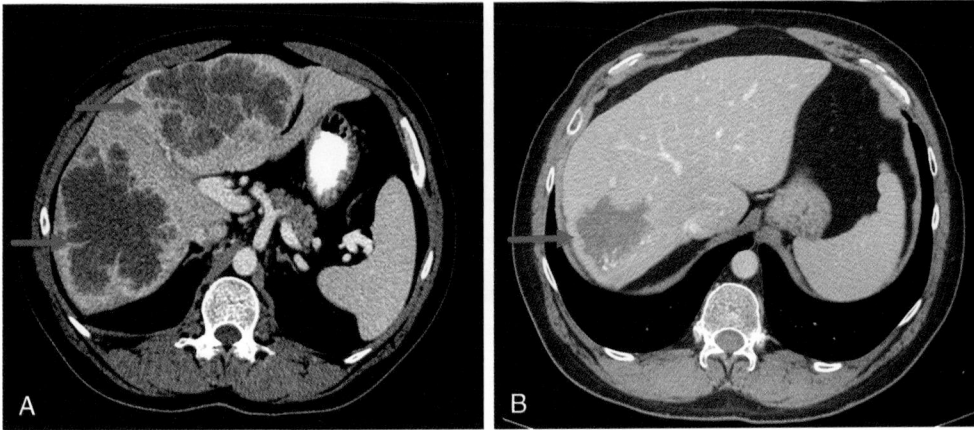

FIGURE 15.7 **A,** Axial computed tomography (CT) image in a patient with colorectal cancer obtained during the portal venous phase. Hypovascular metastases with faint rim of peripheral hyperenhancement *(arrows).* **B,** Axial CT image in the same patient obtained a few months after initiation of chemotherapy demonstrates decreased metastases and new tiny calcifications along the posterior border of the residual metastasis.

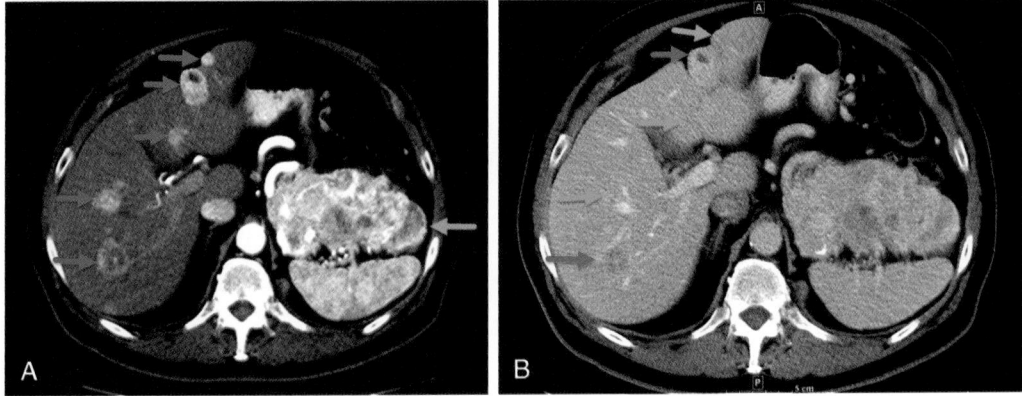

FIGURE 15.8 **Hypervascular metastases in a patient with a pancreatic neuroendocrine tumor best seen on the arterial phase. A.** Axial computed tomography (CT) image obtained during an arterial phase demonstrates five hypervascular metastases *(red arrows).* Note primary pancreatic tumor in the left abdomen *(green arrow)* **B.** Axial CT images in the same patient obtained during the portal venous phase shows that only some metastases are visible *(red arrows).* Three additional metastases *(green arrows)* blend into background parenchyma.

Noncontrast images have been shown to add value in evaluation of a subset of lesions that are isodense on the portal venous and arterial phases. For example, a study of patients with primary hypervascular malignances other than HCC demonstrated maximum sensitivity of 96% in detection of liver metastases when a combination of noncontrast and portal venous phases was used. Use of portal venous and arterial phases without the noncontrast phase resulted in sensitivity of 78%.[28] Therefore multiphasic imaging that includes noncontrast, arterial, and portal venous phases is usually recommended for the evaluation of hypervascular liver metastases (Fig. 15.9).

Liver metastases can also appear cystic with primary malignancies that are cystic in appearance, such as ovarian and mucinous cancers. Additionally, rapidly growing hypervascular tumors can produce cystic-appearing lesions because of central necrosis. Necrotic metastases usually retain irregular peripheral rim of hyperenhancing tissue while the center of the lesion shows absence or minimal enhancement (Fig. 15.10). "Peripheral washout sign," a "targetoid" pattern of enhancement, can be seen in some metastases. This sign has a high specificity for malignancy. However, it is not specific for metastasis and may

be seen with primary liver malignancies as well (Fig. 15.11; see Chapter 14).[8]

Some metastases may demonstrate calcifications both at presentation and after chemotherapy treatment (see Fig. 15.7B). Mucinous gastrointestinal (GI) and ovarian tumors are considered common primaries to develop calcified liver metastases and calcifications within metastatic lymph nodes. A study from 2010 that evaluated for the presence of calcifications within liver metastases in different subtypes of colon cancer did not reveal any correlation between calcifications and the histologic subtype and differentiation degree of the primary malignancy (see Chapter 90).[29]

The appearance of hepatic metastases varies not only with the primary tumor type but also with changes in the underlying liver parenchyma and with treatment (see Chapters 69, 97, and 98). Hypovascular metastases may appear hyperdense or hypervascular on the background of hepatic steatosis or may become isodense on portal venous phase, limiting sensitivity of CT (Fig. 15.12). Colorectal liver metastases in patients with biopsy-proven hepatic steatosis were detected on CT only 65% of the time in one study, and only 11% of lesions measuring up

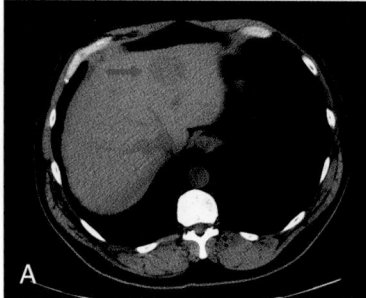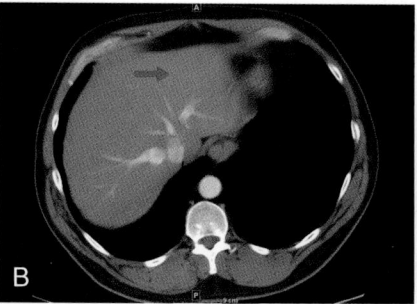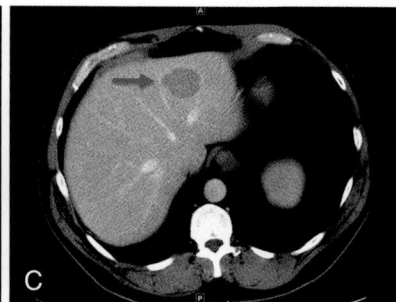

FIGURE 15.9 Neuroendocrine metastasis that is isodense on the arterial phase. **A,** Axial noncontrast computed tomography (CT) image demonstrates good visualization of the metastasis (red arrow). **B,** Axial arterial phase CT image. The same metastasis blends into the hepatic parenchyma. **C,** Axial CT image obtained during the portal venous phase shows washout of the lesion.

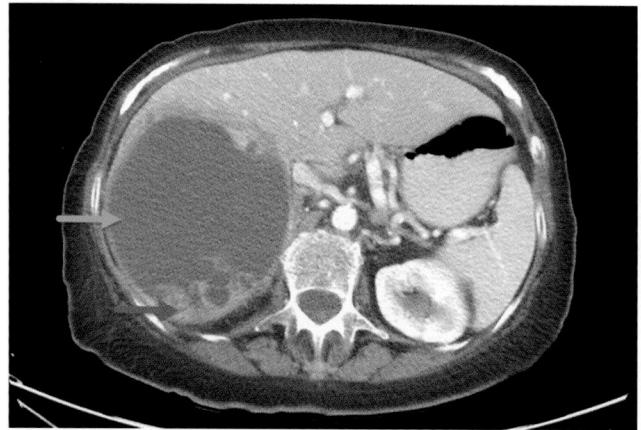

FIGURE 15.10 Cystic metastasis in a patient with endometrial sarcoma, initial presentation before treatment. Axial computed tomography (CT) image obtained during the portal venous phase demonstrates a large metastasis with a substantial low density/cystic central component reflecting necrosis (green arrow). A thick irregular peripheral rind represents remaining vascular tumor (red arrow).

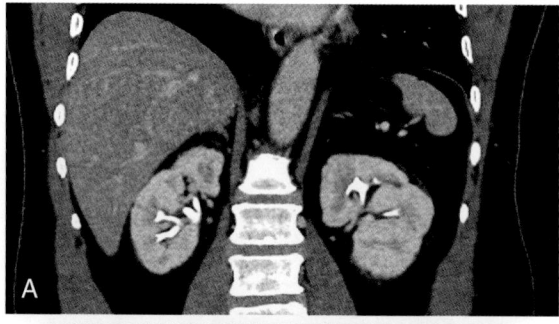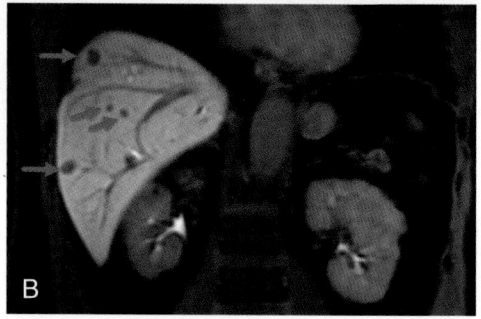

FIGURE 15.12 Hepatic metastases in a patient with hepatic steatosis and metastatic appendiceal neuroendocrine tumor. **A,** Coronal computed tomography (CT) image obtained during portal venous phase does not demonstrate metastases. **B,** Coronal magnetic resonance (MR) image obtained during a hepatobiliary phase with Gd-EOB-DTPA reveals several small metastases (arrows).

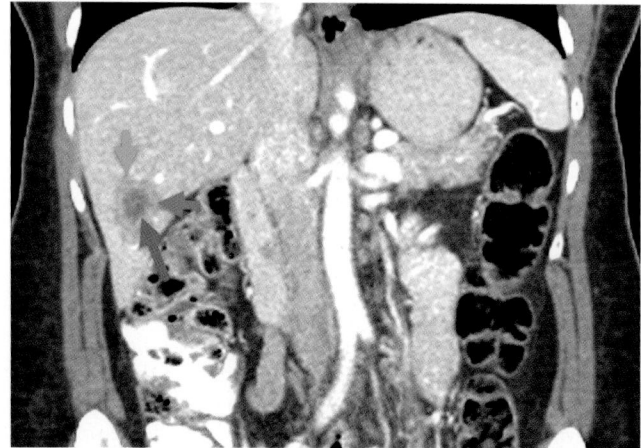

FIGURE 15.11 Liver metastasis with a "peripheral washout sign" in a patient with breast cancer. Postcontrast coronal computed tomography (CT) image demonstrates a faint dark rim around the lesion (green arrow). Note low density center probably related to necrosis (red arrow) and a grey rim of intervening viable tumor (blue arrow).

to 1.0 cm were detected.[30] Chemotherapy and liver-targeted therapies may change the morphology of metastases or the overall degree and pattern of enhancement or calcifications or may lead to the development of cystic components (Fig. 15.13; see Chapters 69, 97, and 98). For example, marked change in enhancement is seen for GI tumor metastases treated with imatinib.[31] Occasionally, treated metastases may mimic cysts and hemangiomas. Therefore, careful review of prior imaging studies is critical for assessment of change in lesion size and enhancement characteristics before and after the initiation of treatment.

Limitations and Pitfalls

Multiple factors can affect lesion detection on CT, including patient imaging characteristics, imaging technique, and specific locations in the liver. Although CT modality offers superior

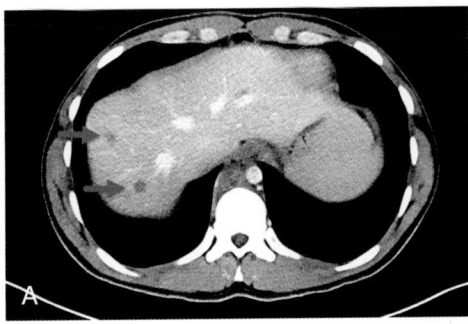
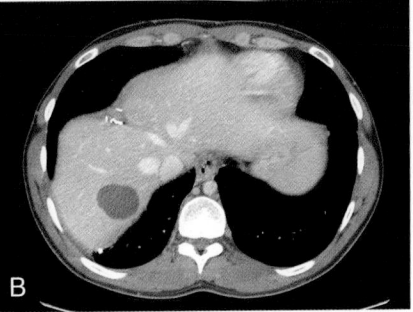

FIGURE 15.13 **Change in density of metastases after chemotherapy. A,** Hypovascular solid metastases in a patient with testicular germ cell tumor at presentation before treatment. **B,** Residual metastasis in segment 7 after chemotherapy demonstrates low density similar to a cyst.

resolution (with potential for submillimeter voxel resolution) compared with MRI, it has lower contrast resolution. Liver lesions that are smaller than 1.0 cm are not as accurately characterized by CT.[32–35]

A disadvantage associated with CT is the risk for ionizing radiation, which is proportional to the radiation dose. Although significant dose reduction for some protocols, such as lung cancer screening or renal colic, may provide sufficient diagnostic information, reducing dose in liver imaging results in decreased diagnostic accuracy. One prospective study that looked at accuracy of regular-dose CT and reduced-dose CT (approximately 60%–70% dose reduction) in the same patients with nonliver primary malignancies demonstrated a drop in sensitivity from 91% to 79%.[36] Thus low contrast technique is not recommended for dedicated liver imaging.

Liver metastases may be missed on CT for various reasons. A study that looked at characteristics of liver metastases from various primary tumors missed on CT noted that hepatic steatosis (see Chapter 69) and subcapsular location contributed to the highest fraction of missed lesions. For instance, 36 of 53 (67%) subcapsular lesions were missed, whereas 11 of 14 (78.6%) lesions in a setting of hepatic steatosis were missed.[37] Decreased detection of subcapsular lesions when compared with more centrally located lesions is probably in part related to the fact that perceptual errors on imaging in general are more common with peripheral ("corner of film" phenomenon) rather than central locations of interest. Subcapsular lesions may also be mistaken for structures outside of the liver, for example, focal lobulation of the diaphragm. Detection of peribiliary lesions can also be challenging on CT. In a study evaluating detection of peribiliary metastases by different modalities, CT correctly identified only 22.8% of such metastases, whereas all peribiliary lesions were detected on MRI.[11] Although most cases of high hepatic tumor burden are detected on CT, CT-occult extensive infiltrative pattern of tumor spread leading to liver failure has been described in the literature, most commonly with breast carcinoma.[38]

Effective chemotherapy can lead to complete resolution of metastases on CT images, a phenomenon referred to as radiologically disappearing liver metastases (DLM; see Chapters 90, 97, and 98). However, this does not always correlate with complete pathologic response. For example, radiologic-pathologic correlation of colorectal DLM demonstrated that only 66% that were subsequently resected represented a true complete response.[39] This emphasizes the importance of evaluating prechemotherapy imaging in preoperative surgical planning.

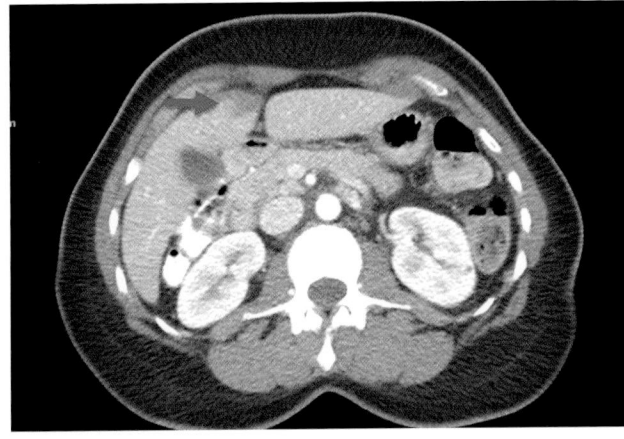

FIGURE 15.14 Hepatic pseudolesion around the falciform ligament. Axial computed tomography (CT) image with intravenous contrast demonstrates a triangular area of hypoenhancement (*arrow*) abutting the falciform ligament that is related to either focal fat or perfusional anomaly and should not be misinterpreted as a metastasis.

Occasionally, benign processes can mimic metastatic disease. One of the most common pseudolesions in the liver is focal hypoenhancement around the falciform ligament, which may result either from focal fat deposition or anomalous venous supply (Fig. 15.14). It usually occurs in the left hepatic lobe, either along one side or both sides of the falciform ligament. Geographic shape and typical location are two of the most important key findings that help to distinguish this pseudolesion from a neoplastic process. Focal hepatic steatosis and areas of fatty sparing of an ovoid shape or in unusual locations can mimic metastases. If this is suspected, then further evaluation may be performed with liver MRI, which includes in- and opposed-phase T1-weighted imaging to confirm the presence of lipid (Fig. 15.15A–C).

Other benign entities, such as sarcoidosis, TB, fibrosis, and infection, may have imaging characteristics that are similar to those of metastatic disease. Atypical hemangiomas can mimic metastases on both CT and MRI modalities. Atypical hemangiomas can demonstrate calcifications, central necrosis, adjacent capsular retraction, and hyalinization/fibrosis. Either all or some of the classic enhancement characteristic that include peripheral, discontinuous, nodular, and centripetal contrast pooling may be absent and preclude a definitive diagnosis on imaging. Therefore a biopsy is sometimes warranted in equivocal cases (see Chapter 88A).

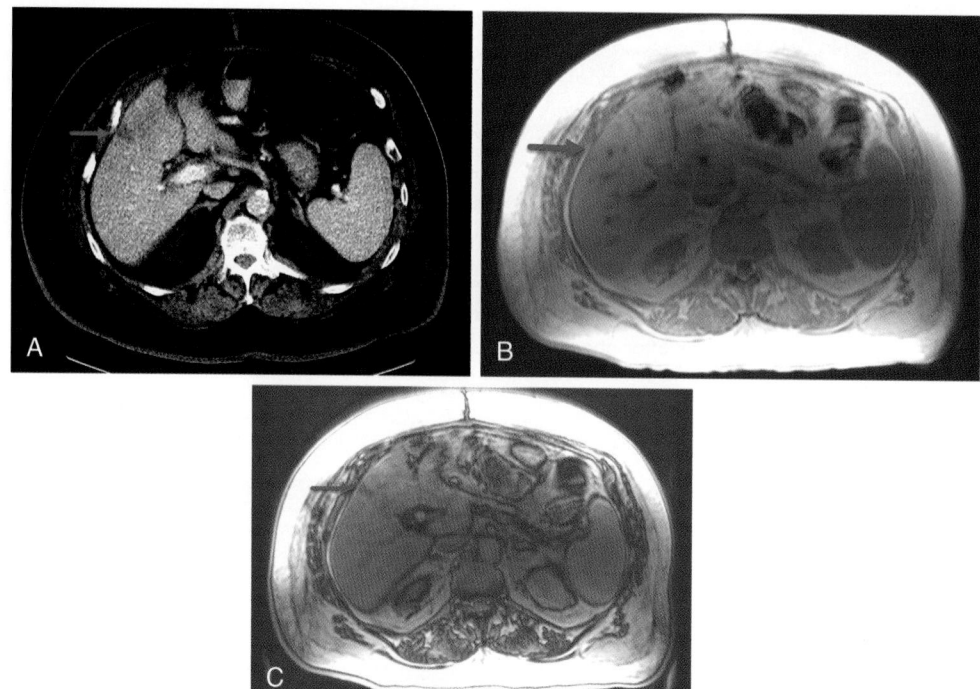

FIGURE 15.15 Hepatic steatosis in a patient with pancreatic cancer after chemotherapy. **A,** Axial postcontrast computed tomography (CT) image obtained during restaging examination demonstrates a new hypodense lesion *(arrow)*. **B,** Axial in-phase magnetic resonance (MR) image does not reveal a focal abnormality in the region of interest *(arrow)*. **C,** Axial out-of-phase MR image shows an area of signal loss *(darker focus)* compared with in-phase reflect presence of microscopic fat *(arrow)*. There is also mildly decreased signal throughout the entire right hepatic lobe as well. These findings are consistent with diffuse hepatic steatosis and more focal fat deposition.

PET/CT AND PET/MRI

Background

Fluorine-18-2-fluoro-2 deoxy-D-glucose (FDG) PET/CT is widely used in the evaluation of metastatic disease and provides both anatomic and metabolic information on the liver (see Chapter 18). According to the ACR Appropriateness Criteria for suspected liver metastases, PET/CT is not recommended as a first-line imaging modality.[4] Early meta-analyses performed between 2002 and 2005 suggested that PET/CT is superior to other modalities in the detection of liver metastases,[40,41] but more recent studies performed since 2010 in patients with colorectal and other primary tumors have highlighted superior sensitivity of MRI over PET/CT on a per patient as well as per lesion basis.[42–45]

One of the major strengths of PET/CT is its ability to diagnose extrahepatic metastatic disease, such as in nonenlarged lymph nodes or peritoneal disease. This can lead to change in management in 8% to 25% of patients with colorectal and other primary tumors.[46–48] Another use of PET/CT is to assess treatment effect by demonstrating decreased FDG uptake within treated metastases.

PET/MRI is a new hybrid technology that was approved by the FDA in 2011. Evaluation for hepatic metastases is the most common indication for PET/MRI of the liver. This test offers the advantages of high tissue contrast and physiologic information combined in one test. In a patient with hepatic metastases, a multiphasic contrast-enhanced MRI of the liver combined with PET images offers a comprehensive assessment of the presence and viability of hepatic and distant metastases. Because PET/MRI is a relatively new imaging technology, the research

data regarding specificity and sensitivity are more limited. Nevertheless, a recent meta-analysis from 2019 indicates increased sensitivity and specificity of PET/MRI compared with PET/CT with sensitivity and specificity of these modalities of 95.4%/99.3% and 68%/95.8%, respectively.[49] Several studies have demonstrated superiority of PET/MRI over CECT and PET/CT. However, there are no data at this time to suggest that PET/MRI is advantageous over hepatocyte-specific agent MRI for the detection of hepatic metastases. A retrospective study by Donati et al. that evaluated hepatic metastases from various malignancies with and without prior chemotherapy demonstrated the sensitivities of PET/MRI, gadoxetate disodium MRI, and PET/CT to be 93%, 91%, and 76%, respectively. For lesions up to 1 cm, the sensitivities of the same modalities were 70%, 80%, and 30%, respectively.[50] Another retrospective study that looked at detection of colorectal cancer metastases in patients with PET/MRI, gadoxetate disodium MRI, CECT, and PET/CT also demonstrated superior sensitivity of PET/MRI compared with CECT and PET/CT but no significant difference between PET/MRI and MRI alone.[51]

In addition to F-18, other radiopharmaceutical agents that target specific tumors have emerged in recent years. For example, 68Ga-DOTA-TATE is used in the evaluation of neuroendocrine tumors and 68Ga-prostate specific membrane antigen (PSMA) is used for the evaluation of prostate cancer metastases. These agents can be used with either PET/CT or PET/MRI (see Chapter 18).

Imaging Findings

Evaluation of PET images is usually performed qualitatively by assessing the tumor to background contrast ratio (Fig. 15.16A–B).

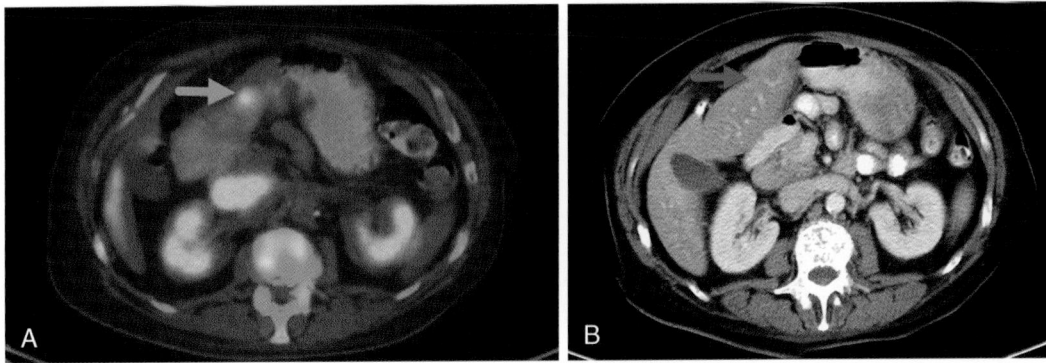

FIGURE 15.16 Hepatic metastasis in a patient with adenocarcinoma of unknown primary. **A,** Axial fused positron emission tomography (PET)/computed tomography (CT) image demonstrates a hypermetabolic lesion in the left hepatic lobe *(arrow)*. **B,** CT in the same patient does not a reveal a metastasis in the expected location *(arrow)*. Moderate hepatic steatosis is present that probably limits visualization of that metastasis.

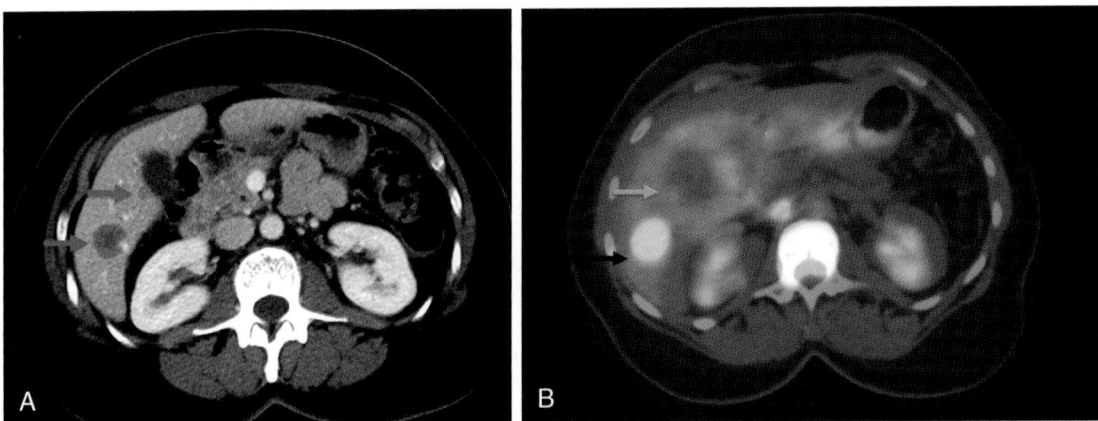

FIGURE 15.17 Hepatic metastases in a breast cancer patient. **A,** Axial contrast-enhanced computed tomography (CT) image demonstrates two metastases in the right hepatic lobe. **B,** Positron emission tomography (PET)/CT obtained on the same day demonstrates hypermetabolism within the larger lesion. However, the subcentimeter lesion adjacent to the gallbladder is not visualized.

Normal liver parenchyma demonstrates a relatively high baseline metabolic activity when compared with lung or muscle. Most hepatic metastases demonstrate hypermetabolism on PET/CT and typically have a standardized uptake value (SUV) of greater than 3.

Limitations and Pitfalls

PET/CT has a limited role in the detection of subcentimeter lesions (Fig. 15.17A–B).[52,53] False negatives may occur with tumors demonstrating low level metabolic activity, such as mucinous tumors.[54] A retrospective study that looked at FDG-PET/CT in the assessment of colorectal cancer metastases showed a significantly lower sensitivity with mucinous tumors. Sensitivity for mucinous cancers was 58%, and it was 92% for nonmucinous metastases.[55]

Sensitivity of FDG-PET/CT is significantly lower in patients with colorectal cancer after neoadjuvant chemotherapy.[56] A prospective study that looked at accuracy of FDG-PET and triphasic CT in colorectal liver metastases demonstrated a drop in sensitivity of FDG-PET from 93.3% to 49% after neoadjuvant chemotherapy. For lesions less than 1 cm, sensitivity before and after chemotherapy was 33% and 17%, respectively. Thus lack of hypermetabolism within liver lesions in the setting of recent chemotherapy does not exclude the presence of viable metastases.[57]

False positives may occur with inflammatory and infectious processes, such as abscesses and postradiation changes. Although benign liver lesions usually demonstrate uptake similar to that of background liver parenchyma (see Chapter 88), focally increased uptake within hemangiomas, FNH, and hepatocellular adenomas has been reported.[58,59] False positive uptake within either benign liver lesions or primary liver tumors have been described in the literature with 68Ga-DOTA-TATE and 68 Ga-PSMA as well (Fig. 15.18).[60-62]

MAGNETIC RESONANCE IMAGING

Background

Continuous improvements in MRI scanner hardware and software, in diffusion-weighted imaging (DWI), and increased use of hepatobiliary contrast agents have led to marked improvement in image quality and accuracy of MRI for liver imaging. MRI is considered superior to CT in hepatic lesion detection and characterization. Based on ACR Appropriateness Criteria for the initial staging of disease and surveillance after treatment of the primary malignancy, CT carries a higher rating than MRI because of its ability to evaluate the lungs and other sites of extrahepatic disease. However, MRI has a higher rating than CT when it comes to presurgical assessment of liver metastases.[4]

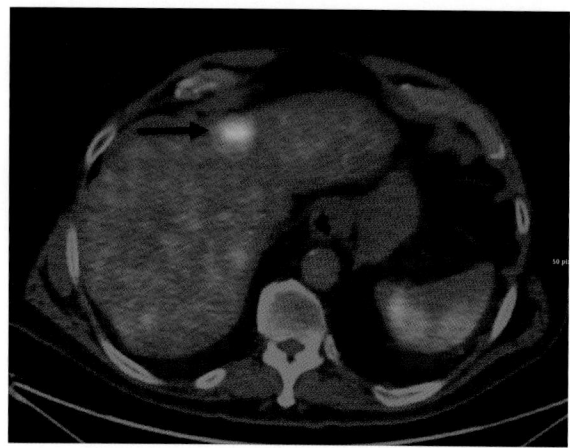

FIGURE 15.18 False positive with 68 Ga-PSMA positron emission tomography (PET). Axial fused images from a 68 Ga-PSMA PET in a patient with prostate cancer shows focal uptake in the liver *(arrow)*. A metastasis was suspected. However, biopsy revealed a cholangiocarcinoma. This lesion was subsequently resected.

As hepatocyte-specific contrast agents (e.g., gadoxetate disodium, Gd-EOB-DTPA) have been increasingly used, meta-analyses published after 2010 have demonstrated the superiority of MRI in its sensitivity when compared with CT and PET/CT with colorectal and other metastases, particularly with respect to subcentimeter liver lesions.[16,35,63] For example, a prospective cohort study by Asato et al. from 2017 reports the overall sensitivity of MRI with DWI versus CT as 91.4% versus 80.9%. For lesions less than 1 cm, sensitivities for MRI with DWI versus CT were 73.3% and 56%, respectively.[63] A meta-analysis by Choi et al. from 2018 that included patients with colorectal and other primary malignancies reports sensitivities for hepatocyte-specific MRI, CT, and PET as 93.1%, 82.1%, and 74.1%, respectively.[19] A prospective study published by Sivesgaard et al. from 2018 evaluated diagnostic accuracy of CT, hepatocyte-specific MR, and PET/CT in 76 colon cancer patients with and without prior chemotherapy and/or ablative treatments. It demonstrated the highest per lesion sensitivity for MRI (85.9%–83.8%), followed by PET/CT (72.0%–72.1%) and CT (62.3%–69.1%). Sensitivities for lesions up to 1 cm sensitivities were as follows: MRI (91.5%–95.1%), PET/CT (86.5%–89.3%), and CT (79.2%–82.40%). MRI detected additional metastases in 18 patients compared with CT and 17 patients compared with PET/CT. Of note is that PET/CT was interpreted in combination with CECT in this study, which may account for the higher sensitivity of PET/CT compared with other studies. No significant per lesion specificity was found between modalities.[64]

A meta-analysis by Vilgrain et al. looked at sensitivities of DWI alone versus gadoxetic-enhanced (hepatocyte specific agent) MRI in 3,854 metastases from various primary tumors in 1,989 patients. Although a relatively small difference in sensitivities was found between DWI-MR and gadoxetic acid-enhanced MR (87.1% vs. 90.6%), the combination of two techniques was shown to have the highest sensitivity of 95.5%. Similar results were noted when limiting the analysis to colorectal liver metastases and metastases smaller than 1 cm.[65] Although delayed hepatobiliary-phase imaging produces very high contrast between the tumor and the normal liver parenchyma, hypointense (dark) lesions on delayed phase could either be benign or malignant

(e.g., metastasis or a cyst). Thus it is importance to use all MR sequences to optimize lesion detection and characterization.

Additional data have recently emerged with regard to cost-effectiveness and improved mortality of patients imaged with hepatocyte-specific agents. A randomized multicenter trial (the VALUE study group) by Zech et al. published in 2014 reported a decreased need for additional imaging, higher diagnostic confidence, and a lower rate of intraoperative change of plans in patients with colorectal cancer who underwent initial imaging with hepatobiliary agent MRI compared with extracellular-contrast agent MRI and CECT.[66] A study by Kim at al. in 2018 demonstrated increased 5-year survival rate in patients with colon cancer who underwent gadoxetic acid enhanced-MRI in addition to CT when compared with patients who underwent only CT (70.8% vs. 48.1%). In this study, MRI detected 39 additional synchronous liver metastases initially missed on CT in 26 patients.[67]

Imaging Findings

Most liver metastases are hypovascular and hypervascular on multiphasic contrast-enhanced MRI, similar to CECT, but the superior contrast resolution of MRI enhances its sensitivity for liver metastases (see Chapters 90–92). In addition, the use of T1-weighted imaging, T2-weighted imaging, and DWI provides additional signal characteristics for liver lesions that improve the accuracy of MRI compared with other imaging modalities. Most metastases are hypointense (darker than liver parenchyma) on T1-weighted images and mildly hyperintense (slightly brighter than liver) on T2-weighted images (Fig. 15.19A–E). Notable exceptions to this rule are hemorrhagic and melanoma liver metastases because blood products and melanin both demonstrate high signal on T1-weighted images (Fig. 15.20). Other types of malignancies can also occasionally produce T1 hyperintense liver metastases because of high protein content.

Most metastases are not as bright on T2-weighted images as hemangiomas and cysts, except when there is extensive necrosis or cystic components. Occasionally a target sign can be seen on T2-weighted images, where there is a markedly hyperintense center of the lesion (liquefactive necrosis) that is surrounded by a rim of more solid tissue. On T1-weighted images, there is usually a corresponding donut sign, a low signal intensity rim, and an even more hypointense (darker) center.[68]

DWI is a sequence that is wonderfully suited for detection of liver metastases. The signal in DWI is affected by the movement of water molecules in the tissues of interest. The signal intensity of liver lesions on DWI remains high in lesions with higher cellularity, such as liver metastases, compared with benign lesions. Numerous studies have demonstrated that DWI is more sensitive for the detection of liver lesions compared with CT.[35] DWI, however, suffers from relatively low special resolution and is more susceptible to artifacts because of motion or field inhomogeneities (Fig. 15.21). T1-weighted imaging, T2-weighted imaging, and DWI sequences should be used in combination with contrast-enhanced sequences for a comprehensive evaluation of patients with liver metastases.

Limitations and Pitfalls

Although MRI does not carry the risk associated with ionizing radiation or the risk of contrast-induced nephropathy, liver MRIs are lengthy examinations compared with CT (around 20–30 minutes compared with <5 minutes) and is poorly

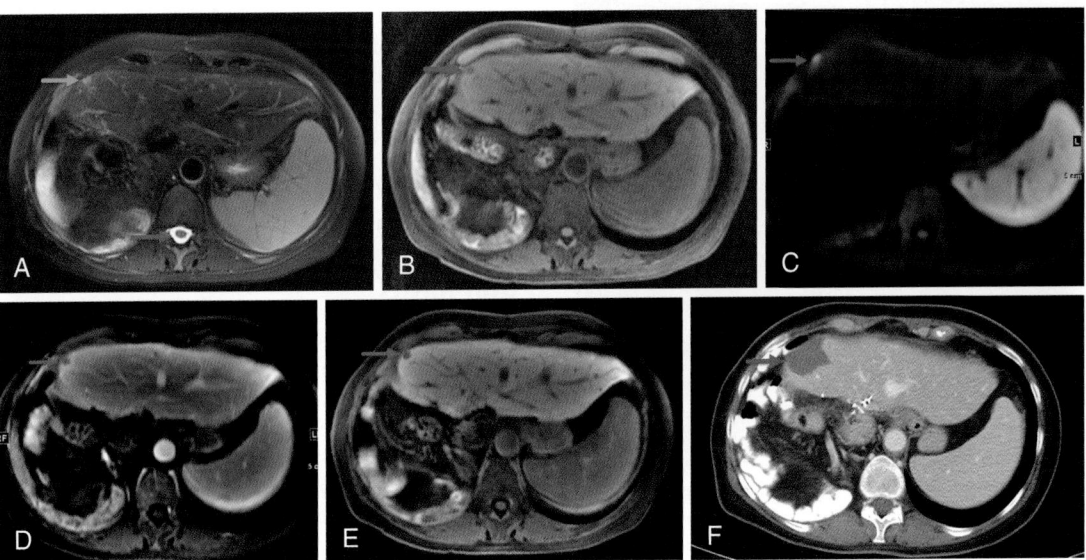

FIGURE 15.19 **Usual magnetic resonance imaging (MRI) characteristic of hepatic metastases.** Axial MRI images in a patient with colon cancer and prior right hepatectomy. **A.** T2-weighted image shows a subcentimeter lesion that is brighter than adjacent liver parenchyma *(green arrow)* but not as bright as cerebrospinal fluid in the spinal canal *(red arrow)*. **B,** T1-weighted image with fat suppression. The lesion is slightly darker than the liver *(arrow)*. **C,** Diffusion-weighted imaging (DWI). The lesion is markedly hyperintense *(arrow)*. **D.** Postcontrast portal venous phase. The lesion is hypoenhancing with respect to adjacent liver *(arrow)*. **E.** Delayed/ hepatobiliary phase. The metastasis is hypointense, but is more conspicuous because of increased contrast between the lesion and the enhancing hepatic parenchyma *(arrow)*. **F.** Axial CT image from a follow-up examination showing subsequent ablation of the metastasis.

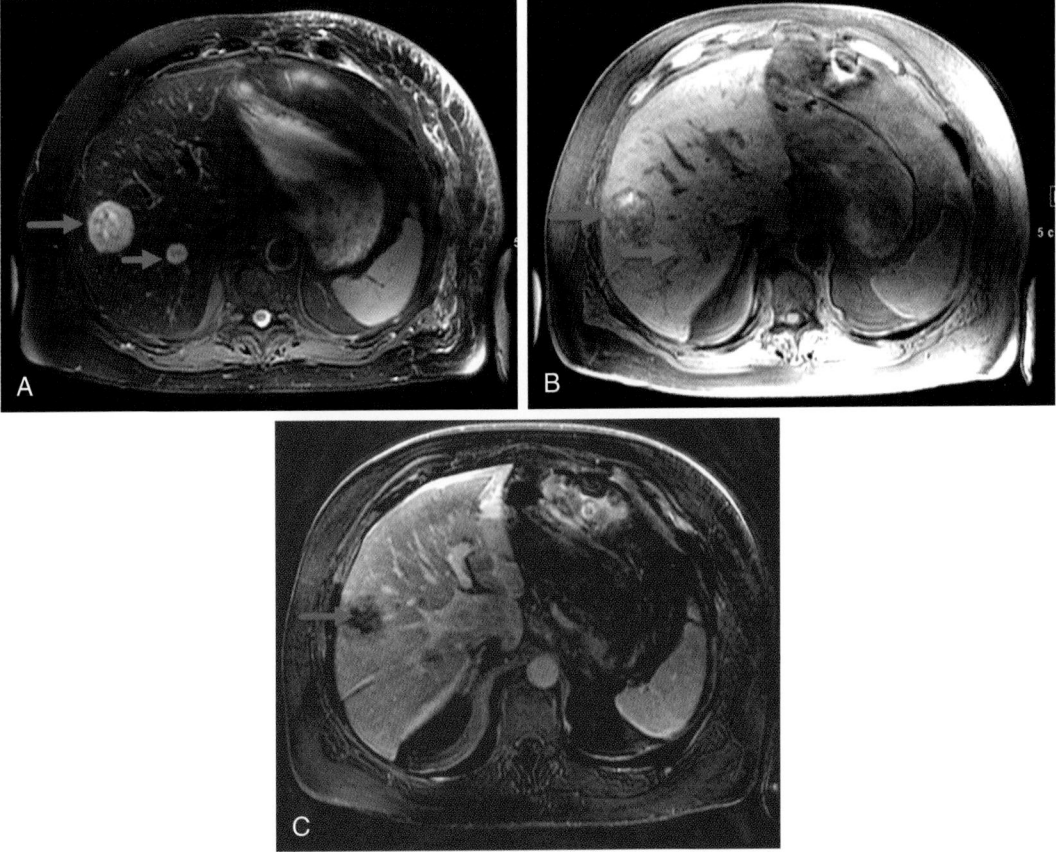

FIGURE 15.20 **Melanoma metastases. A.** Axial two-weighted images demonstrates two adjacent metastases that are moderately brighter than adjacent liver *(arrows)*. **B.** Axial T1-precontrast image shows that the larger metastasis is partially hyperintense, probably because of the presence of melanin *(arrow)*. However, the second smaller metastasis is isointense and is not well seen. **C.** Axial subtraction image demonstrates a doughnut sign *(arrow)*. Peripheral rim of enhancing viable tissue and central hypoenhancement probably due to necrosis.

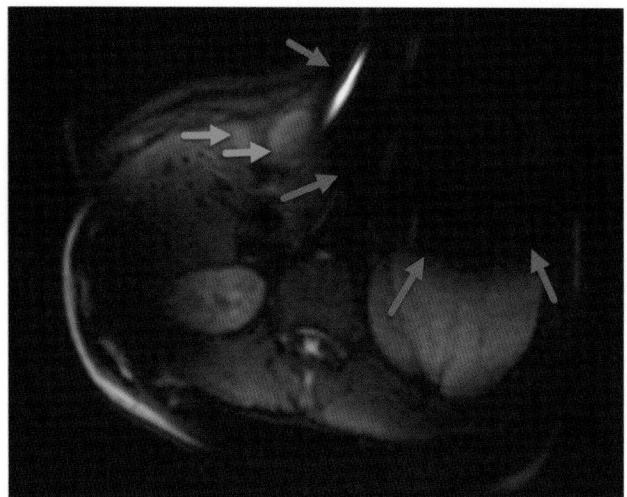

FIGURE 15.21 Axial magnetic resonance (MR) diffusion-weighted imaging (DWI) demonstrates an artifact from a hepatic arterial infusion pump *(red arrows)* that partially obscures the hepatic metastases *(green arrows)*.

tolerated in a minority of patients. MRIs are susceptible to motion and other artifacts and, therefore, may not be ideal in patients who are unable to follow breath-holding instructions or who are unable to remain supine and still in the MRI scanner. Liver lesions in the left hepatic lobe, in proximity to the stomach and heart, may be obscured because of peristalsis or susceptibility artifact from intraluminal gas. Because of lower spatial resolution and susceptibility to motion, MRI technique may be less desirable than CT for the delineation of complex variant vascular anatomy in the upper abdomen.

Imaging of disappearing colorectal metastases remains a challenge even when using hepatocyte-specific contrast agents (see Chapter 90). A retrospective review of resected colorectal liver metastases that were imaged with preoperative gadoxetate-MRI revealed that 38.5% of lesions demonstrated "disappearance" on MRI. Fifty-five percent of those lesions demonstrated viability on pathology.[69]

SUMMARY

Multiple modalities can be used to image hepatic metastases. Traditional US is the least sensitive, least specific, most operator-depended modality and is most frequently affected by patient factors. CEUS is a rapidly evolving technique that shows much higher sensitivity and specificity than conventional US and approaches accuracy that is comparable to that of CT and MRI in some studies.[2] However, CEUS is not yet widely available in the United States. Therefore the most frequently used modalities in the initial detection and surveillance of hepatic metastases in the United States are CECT and MRI, with PET/CT reserved for detection of extrahepatic disease. MRI shows superior sensitivity for presurgical assessment of liver metastases.[4] PET-CT may play a complementary role in specific situations, such as in response assessment, or for specific tumors, such as neuroendocrine liver metastases with new radiotracers. PET-MRI is emerging as a technique for liver metastases detection that may play a larger role in the near future.

References are available at expertconsult.com

CHAPTER 16

Imaging features of gallbladder and biliary tract disease

Scott R. Gerst and Richard K. Do

In the past decade, the combination of increased computing processing power and technologic improvements in acquisition across all modalities have imparted significant advances in medical imaging, including imaging of the biliary tract and gallbladder. This chapter will review current methods of evaluating the most common abnormalities of the biliary system.

As the gallbladder resides in a somewhat anterior right upper quadrant location, ultrasound is ideal for initial imaging (Fig. 16.1), with computed tomography (CT) and magnetic resonance imaging (MRI) utilized for more complex cases. The intrahepatic bile ducts closely follow the portal venous system, merging from the left and right hepatic lobe into the right and left hepatic ducts. The confluence of the right and left hepatic ducts forms the main bile duct, which is called the common hepatic duct superiorly, and becomes the common bile duct (CBD) once the cystic duct inserts. The CBD becomes retroperitoneal at the level of the pancreatic head, typically joining the pancreatic duct just before entering the ampulla of Vater (see Chapter 2).

On axial CT, the CBD is a circular structure of fluid attenuation (0–20 Hounsfield units [HUs]) within the posterolateral aspect of the pancreatic head on a contrast-enhanced scan. It is normally less than or equal to a 9-mm caliber, although a diameter up to 10 mm may be observed in elderly patients or in patients post-cholecystectomy. Measurement of the extrahepatic duct is usually performed near the crossing of the hepatic artery, with measurement of the lumen from inner wall to inner wall.

Intrahepatic bile ducts are best evaluated by MRI due to its superior tissue contrast, particularly on T2-weighted images. Contrast-enhanced CT also demonstrates intrahepatic bile ducts in normal subjects. Delineation of variant biliary anatomy is possible on CT or MRI, particularly if the biliary tree is dilated (Fig. 16.2; see Chapter 2). Dilated intrahepatic ducts should measure greater than 2 mm, or greater than 40% of the adjacent portal vein. The "double-track" sign, traditionally described on ultrasound, is caused by dilated bile ducts running parallel to portal vein branches (Fig. 16.3). The pattern of bile duct dilatation should be assessed to determine whether it is symmetric or localized to a portion of the liver. Imaging can usually differentiate intrahepatic from extrahepatic, as well as the etiology, of obstruction (Fig. 16.4).

When evaluating biliary and gallbladder disorders, MRI with MR cholangiopancreatography (MRCP) is an excellent method.[1,2] A combination of heavily T2-weighted images for ductal anatomy, intermediate T2-weighted and T1-weighted images for surrounding structures, and diffusion-weighted imaging (DWI) provide a comprehensive evaluation of benign and malignant biliary abnormalities. Hepatic lesions, diffuse liver disease, adenopathy, or other visceral abnormalities are also evaluated with the addition of dynamic T1-weighted sequences acquired with intravenous gadolinium

contrast. MRCP offers high sensitivity and specificity in evaluating ductal dilatation, strictures, and intraductal abnormalities.[3–7] MRCP is noninvasive, or minimally invasive with the addition of intravenous contrast, eliminating the added morbidity associated with endoscopic retrograde cholangiopancreatography (ERCP) or percutaneous transhepatic cholangiography (PTC).[7,8]

BENIGN DISEASES OF THE BILIARY TRACT

Biliary Hamartoma

Bile duct hamartomas are common benign tumors composed of disorganized bile ducts and ductules surrounded by a fibrocollagenous stroma. The tumors are generally multiple, range from 1 to 15 mm, rarely communicate with the biliary tree, and are scattered throughout the liver.[9] They are most often confused with cysts, although they may also be mistaken for metastases or microabscesses with delayed marginal enhancement on CT or MRI.[10,11] On MRI, they appear cystic (Fig. 16.5), and may show a small internal mural nodule related to the fibrocollagenous component (see Chapters 47, 48, and 88).

Bile Duct Adenoma

Bile duct adenomas are rare benign epithelial neoplasms, usually incidentally detected and asymptomatic. They are usually solitary and without specific imaging findings, although hyperenhancement has been reported in some series.[12] Definitive diagnosis can be made only at histologic analysis. Internal heterogeneous enhancement has been reported on MRI, with reported hypointensity on delayed hepatobiliary phase imaging using hepatocyte contrast agents[13] (see Chapters 47 and 48).

Cholelithiasis

Ultrasound is usually the modality of choice in the evaluation of uncomplicated cholelithiasis or cholecystitis due to its high sensitivity and lower cost, but choledocholithiasis is more effectively imaged by MRI.[14] On MRI, gallstones are well-circumscribed, low-signal filling defects within a fluid-filled gallbladder or common duct on T2-weighted and MRCP images (Fig. 16.6). Coronal T2-weighted imaging, performed routinely with MRI, readily identifies common duct stones. MRCP can also be obtained to evaluate whether retained stones are present after cholecystectomy, although surgical clip artifact may limit visualization of the adjacent portion of the main bile duct. A negative MRCP may obviate the need for ERCP (see Chapters 33 and 34).

Given that most gallstones in Western countries are mixed cholesterol stones and noncalcified, CT is limited for stone detection, but it may reveal unsuspected gallstones during studies performed for other reasons. On CT, gallstones are visible when either calcified or containing material of substantially lower attenuation than the surrounding bile (such as trapped

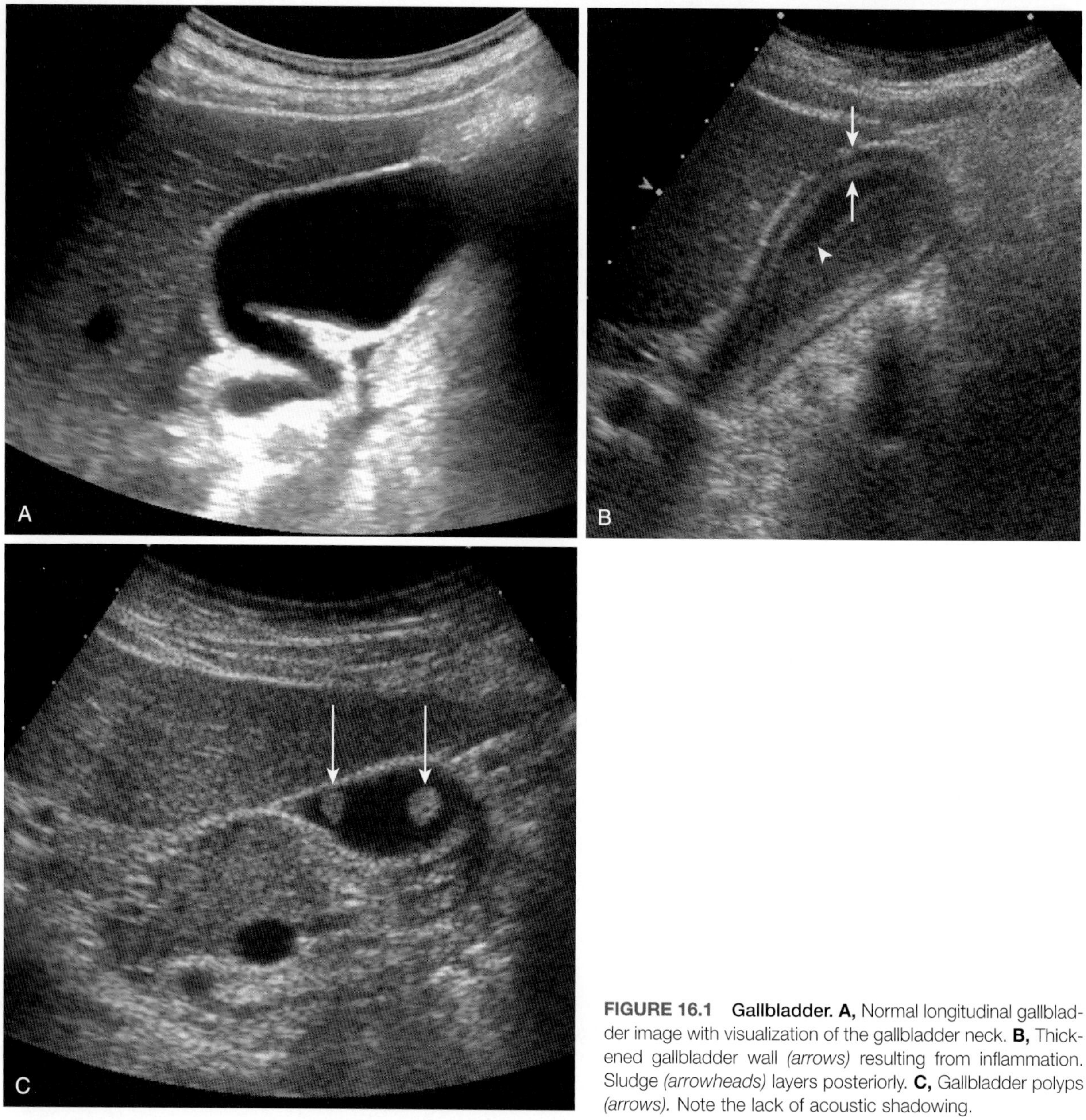

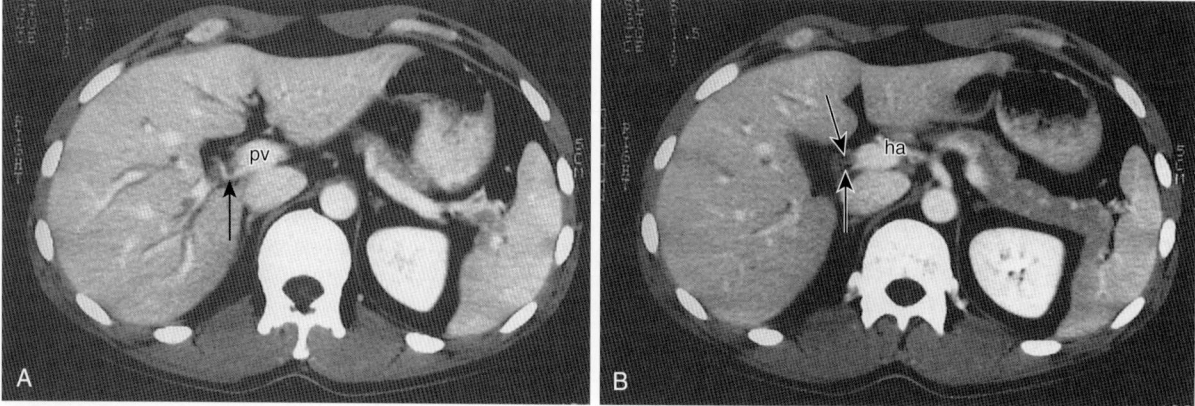

FIGURE 16.1   Gallbladder. A, Normal longitudinal gallbladder image with visualization of the gallbladder neck. **B,** Thickened gallbladder wall *(arrows)* resulting from inflammation. Sludge *(arrowheads)* layers posteriorly. **C,** Gallbladder polyps *(arrows).* Note the lack of acoustic shadowing.

FIGURE 16.2   Contrast-enhanced computed tomography in a patient with a minimally dilated biliary system. A, The intrahepatic bile ducts are seen as branching, low-attenuation structures adjacent to the portal veins. At the porta hepatis, the hepatic artery *(arrow)* is seen to pass between the main portal vein *(pv)* and the common hepatic duct. **B,** Scan caudal to the porta hepatis shows the common hepatic duct and the cystic duct running adjacent to each other in the hepatoduodenal ligament *(arrows).* The hepatic artery *(ha)* is in a more medial position.

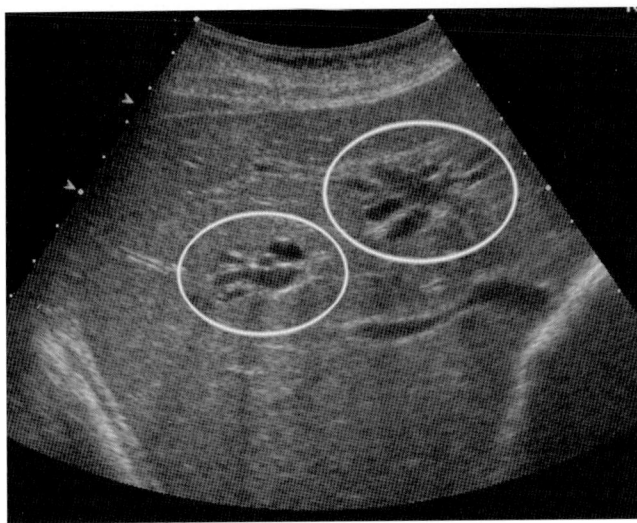

FIGURE 16.3 Biliary obstruction from choledocholithiasis. **A,** Transverse sonogram of the liver reveals the "double-track" sign *(circled areas)*, consistent with intrahepatic biliary dilatation.

nitrogen gas or high cholesterol content). Newer dual energy CT techniques have shown promise in detecting noncalcified cholesterol stones and acute cholecystitis.[15,16]

On ultrasound, gallstones are echogenic, mobile, and demonstrate posterior acoustic shadowing when imaging is optimized and when 3 mm or greater in size (Fig. 16.7). Ultrasound is technique and operator dependent. It is important to scan patients in different positions to differentiate gallstones from polyps, as polyps are fixed. Optimized Doppler analysis may also help, as stones are associated with "twinkle artifact" and polyps often show vascularity. Stones fixed in the gallbladder neck are frequently associated with cholecystitis. If large stones or multiple stones fill the entire gallbladder lumen, there may be little surrounding bile, limiting ultrasound evaluation due to acoustic shadowing. Identification of the "wall echo shadow" sign, produced by echoes from the anterior gallbladder wall, echogenic stones, and posterior acoustic shadowing produced by the stones, is helpful (Fig. 16.8). A porcelain gallbladder has echogenic calcification in the gallbladder wall. Gallbladder sludge is echogenic nonshadowing bile that sometimes takes on a rounded shape called "tumefactive" sludge. Sludge can

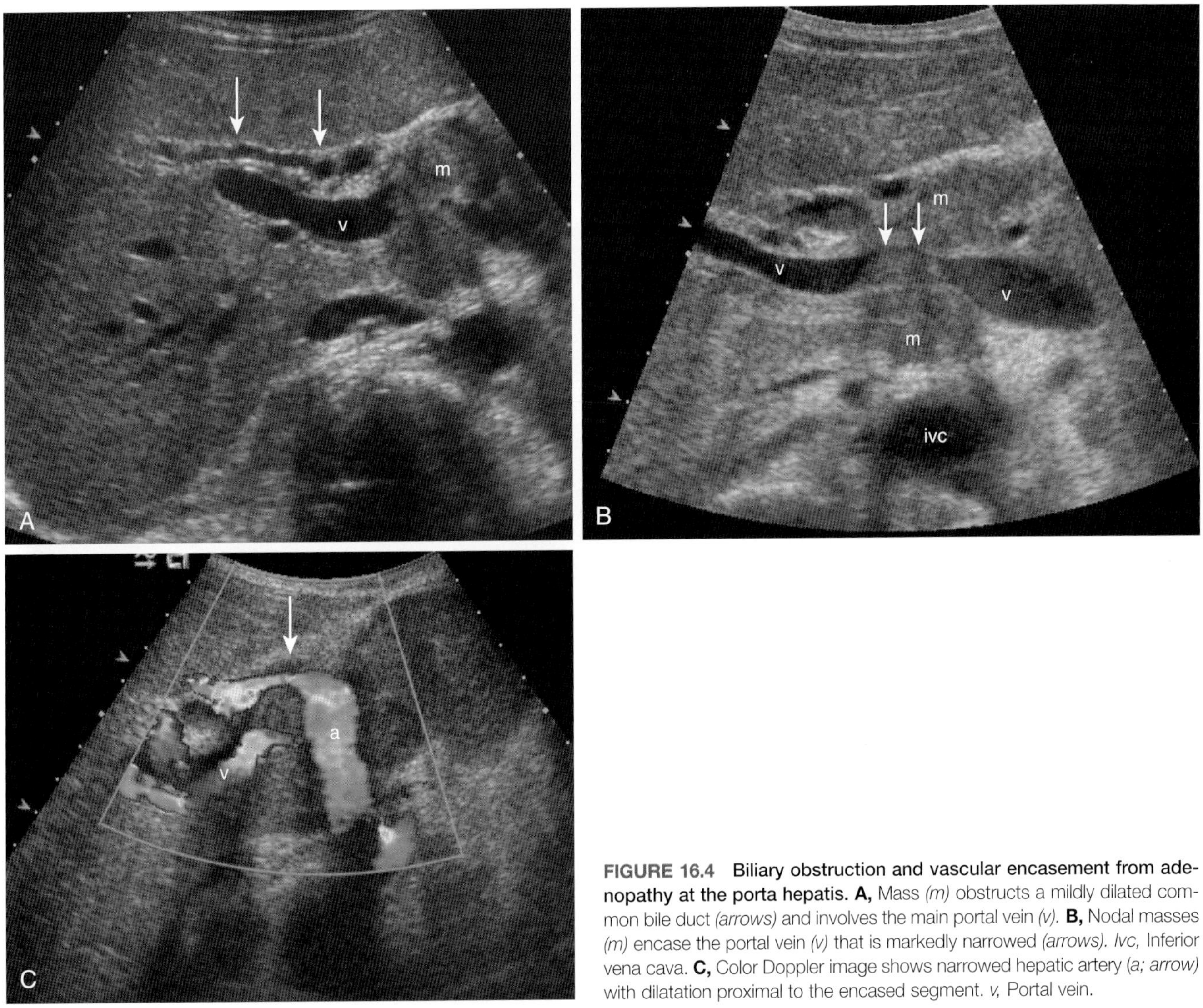

FIGURE 16.4 Biliary obstruction and vascular encasement from adenopathy at the porta hepatis. **A,** Mass *(m)* obstructs a mildly dilated common bile duct *(arrows)* and involves the main portal vein *(v)*. **B,** Nodal masses *(m)* encase the portal vein *(v)* that is markedly narrowed *(arrows)*. *Ivc,* Inferior vena cava. **C,** Color Doppler image shows narrowed hepatic artery *(a; arrow)* with dilatation proximal to the encased segment. *v,* Portal vein.

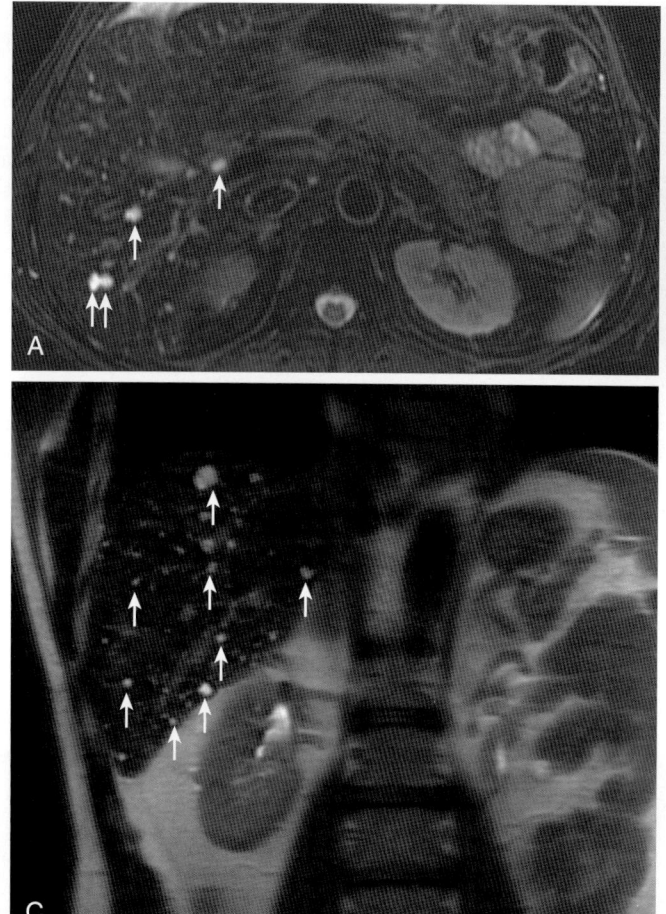

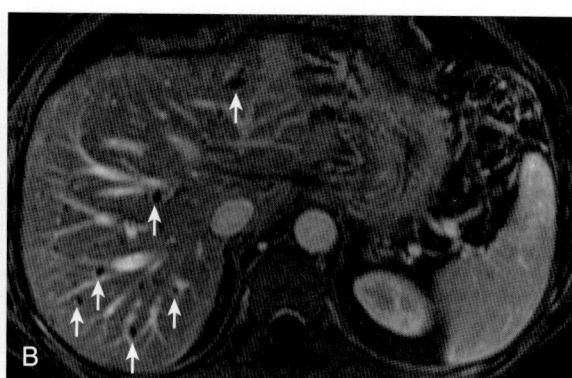

FIGURE 16.5 **Adult male with multiple biliary hamartomas. A,** T2-weighted axial magnetic resonance imaging (MRI) with fat saturation shows multiple *(arrows)* high-signal cystic-appearing foci. **B,** Axial T1-weighted fat saturation image acquired in portal venous phase post intravenous gadolinium, with subtraction of precontract image, shows lack of significant enhancement within the structures *(arrows),* and no abnormal surrounding parenchymal enhancement. **C,** Coronal T2-weighted MRI again demonstrates multiple high T2 cystic-appearing lesions *(arrows).*

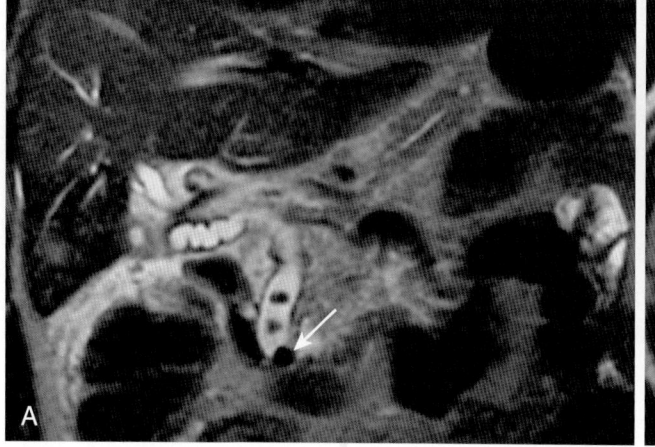

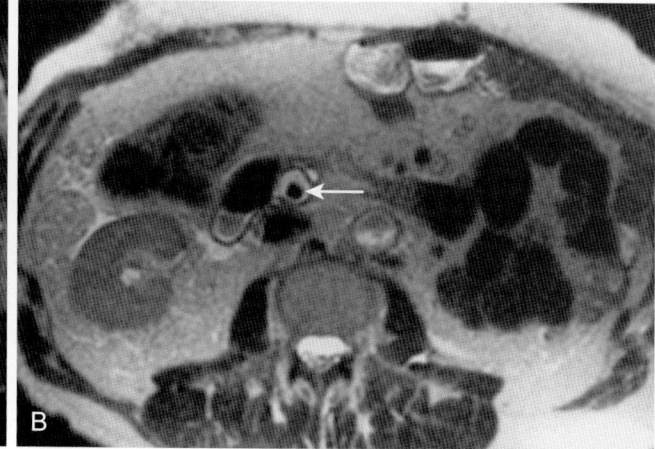

FIGURE 16.6 **Choledocholithiasis. A,** Coronal T2-weighted single-shot fast spin-echo image through the common duct in a patient after cholecystectomy shows multiple stones within the common bile duct. Note the distal stone impacted at the level of the ampulla *(arrow).* **B,** Axial T2-weighted image with the same technique also shows a stone, surrounded by bile, in the distal common bile duct *(arrow).*

obscure the interfaces of small stones. Sludge is avascular, and it usually changes with positional variation, albeit slowly.

Choledocholithiasis and Biliary Obstruction

MRCP is the imaging modality of choice for choledocholithiasis, as it has the highest sensitivity and specificity.[8,16] Intrahepatic calculi are rare in Western countries, but they most frequently occur in association with iatrogenic bile duct strictures

(Fig. 16.9). Bile duct calculi appear as intraluminal filling defects on MRCP, or echogenic foci on ultrasound (Fig. 16.10). Calculi may form or reflux into intrahepatic ducts, and small calculi can be mistaken for air. Because there is little bile surrounding intraductal calculi, and because the stones may be small, acoustic shadowing may not always be elicited on ultrasound, which has poor sensitivity in detecting choledocholithiasis. On CT, dense intraluminal calcification or a *target sign*

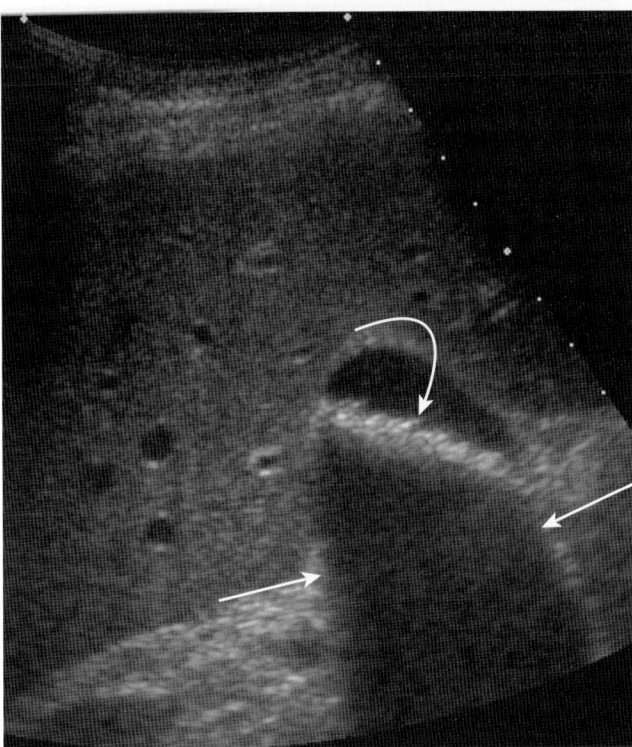

FIGURE 16.7 Gallstones *(curved arrow)* layering in the gallbladder produce an acoustic shadow *(straight arrows)*.

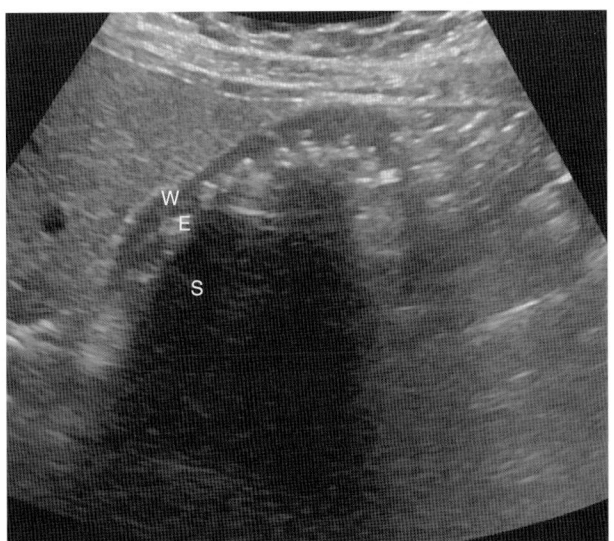

FIGURE 16.8 **Gallstones.** Gallstones fill the gallbladder lumen, producing a wall-echo-shadow *(WES)* sign from the anterior gallbladder wall, the echogenic anterior surface of gallstones, and posterior acoustic shadowing by the gallstones.

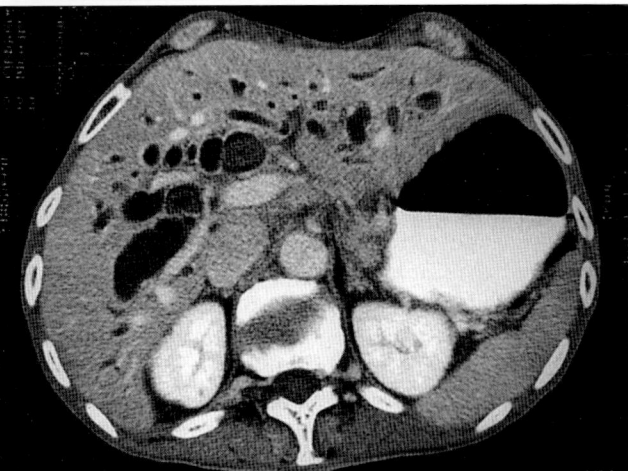

FIGURE 16.9 **Intrahepatic cholelithiasis.** Intrahepatic duct dilation is seen after recurrent anastomotic stricture formation at a hepaticojejunostomy. Several laminated, noncalcified calculi can be seen within the dilated ductal system.

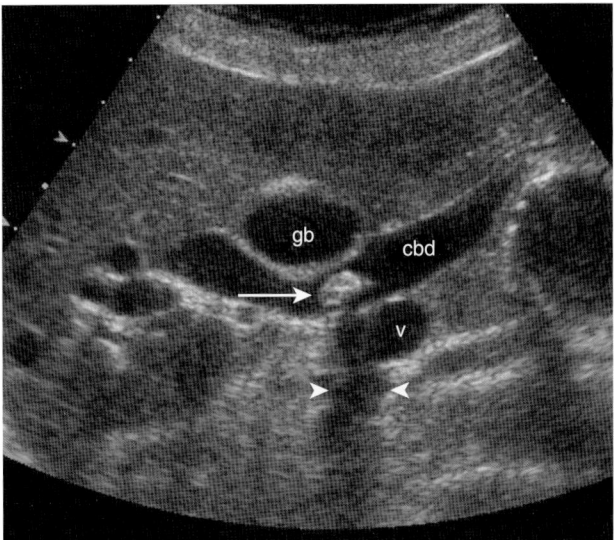

FIGURE 16.10 **Choledocholithiasis.** Longitudinal view of the common bile duct *(cbd)* shows an echogenic stone *(arrow)* that produces acoustic shadowing *(arrowheads)*. *gb,* Gallbladder; *v,* portal vein.

representing a halo of bile surrounding a higher attenuation stone are reliable indicators of intraductal calculi. Cholesterol stones may blend imperceptibly with surrounding bile, although dual-energy CT may have value in demonstrating these stones as either hypoattenuating or hyperattenuating relative to bile, depending on the energy level.[16] In addition, a minority of patients with choledocholithiasis have no biliary ductal dilatation (see Chapters 37–39 and 44).

On ultrasound, debris or thick bile within the ducts may cause internal echoes within ducts or fluid levels, but they do not shadow and will shift with positional variation. Adherent intraductal clot as well as intraductal tumors often show no associated acoustic shadowing and will not shift with position.[17,18] Obstruction as a result of biliary ascariasis is associated with tubular structures within the bile duct, and movement of the worms is pathognomonic[19] (see Chapter 45). MRI and MRCP are superior to CT, which is of less value when stones are small and noncalcified and bile duct dilation is minimal or absent. Intrahepatic choledocholithiasis may have an unusual appearance, with segmental or subsegmental biliary radicles filled with calculi (see Chapter 44). In Asian patients with recurrent pyogenic cholangitis who subsequently form bile pigment stones, the debris filling the biliary system generally has higher attenuation than normal bile on CT. Marked bile duct dilation is present, and often the larger intrahepatic ducts are dilated without side-branch dilation. Eccentric and diffuse extrahepatic bile duct wall thickening is usually seen.[20]

In biliary obstruction, both the pattern of obstruction and appearance of the duct wall are useful for diagnosis. A spectrum of chronic progressive, cholestatic disorders exists, with etiologies varying from recurrent infection to autoimmune disorders, and unknown. Recurrent pyogenic cholangitis is related to repeated bacterial infections and is evidenced by dilated ducts with intraductal calculi and segmental dilatation (Fig. 16.11) (see Chapter 44). Lobar atrophy may also be present. Of note, intraductal papillary mucinous tumor of the bile ducts may be confused with recurrent pyogenic cholangitis on imaging, because both diseases involve repeated episodes of incomplete

biliary obstruction and evident intraluminal masses or filling defects (see Chapters 47 and 51).[21]

Sclerosing cholangitis may be primary and of unknown etiology, or secondary and due, for example, to autoimmune disorders, infection, or ischemia (see Chapter 41). It causes a beaded appearance of the ducts with wall thickening and enhancement, strictures, and discontinuous areas of dilatation (Fig. 16.12); dilated ducts contain debris such as pus, sludge, or sloughed epithelium. Primary sclerosing cholangitis (PSC) carries an increased risk of cholangiocarcinoma, and MRCP remains the most sensitive and specific noninvasive imaging modality to assess these patients and to detect concomitant cholangiocarcinoma.[22,23] Mural thickening of the ducts also is seen with HIV-associated cholangiopathy; however, HIV-associated cholangiopathy often shows added papillary stenosis, a finding not typically seen in PSC.[24]

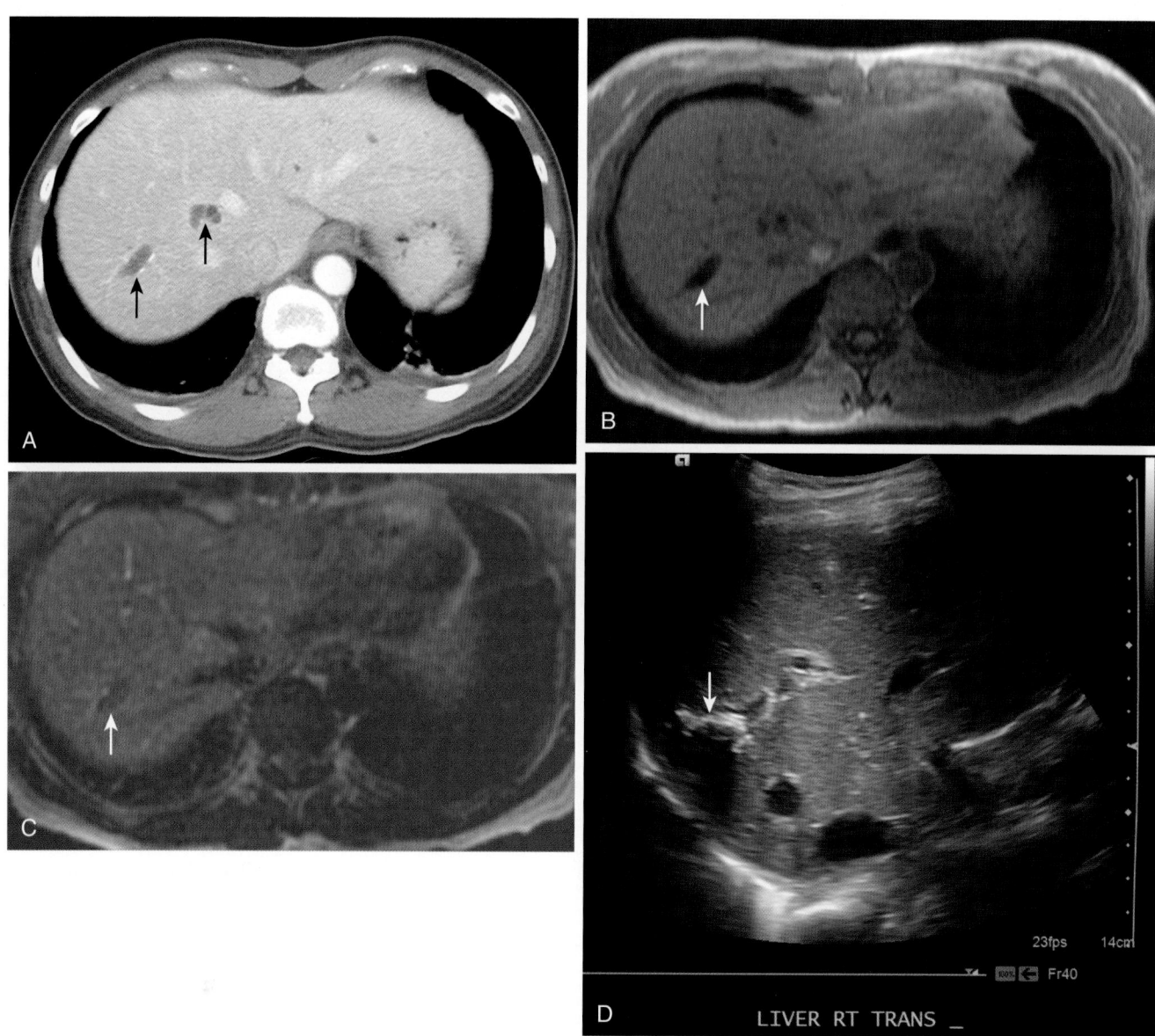

FIGURE 16.11 Recurrent pyogenic cholangitis. **A,** Axial computed tomography (CT) image post intravenous contrast shows dilated low attenuation intrahepatic ducts *(arrows)*. **B,** Axial T1 weighted in phase magnetic resonating imaging (MRI) shows lower signal than expected for bile *(arrow)*. **C,** Axial T2-weighted fat saturation image confirms there is no high signal bile corresponding to the area of dilatation. **D,** Ultrasound confirms echogenic calculus *(arrow)* with acoustic shadowing *(arrowheads)* in this location.

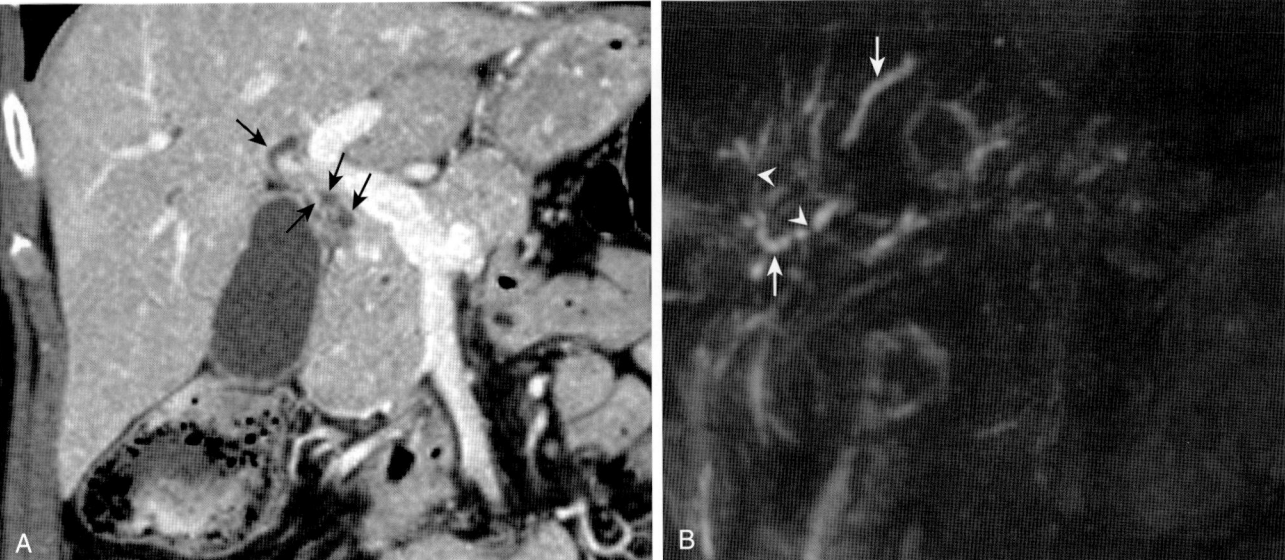

FIGURE 16.12   Primary sclerosing cholangitis in a patient with ulcerative colitis. A, Coronal reconstructed computed tomography (CT) image post intravenous contrast shows periductal high attenuation enhancement *(arrows)* consistent with inflamed, thickened duct walls, with scattered bilobar dilated ducts *(*)*. **B,** Coronal T2-weighted three-dimensional magnetic resonance cholangiopancreatography (3D MRCP) shows intrahepatic duct beaded appearance with dilatation *(arrows),* and multiple strictures *(arrowheads).*

In patients with biliary obstruction who are being considered for surgical resection or palliative biliary drainage, the distribution of ductal dilatation should be carefully evaluated to determine management. Any isolated biliary ductal segments that do not communicate with the main ducts should be noted, because isolated segments may alter surgical approach, and biliary drainage may require placement of multiple catheters.[25]

Hyperplastic Cholecystoses and Gallbladder Polyps

Hyperplastic cholecystoses, such as cholesterolosis and adenomyomatosis (ADM), can cause focal or polypoid gallbladder wall thickening. Cholesterolosis results from abnormal cholesterol deposits in the gallbladder wall creating wall irregularities or polypoid intraluminal masses. Cholesterolosis usually presents as multiple small (1–10 mm) nonshadowing polyps arising from the nondependent wall with echogenic speckles and lobular contour on ultrasound. Cholesterol polyps are benign with no malignant potential.[26,27] ADM is a benign hyperplastic cholecystosis with no known inherent malignant potential that results from hyperplasia of both the mucosa and muscularis propria of the gallbladder wall (see Chapter 49). ADM has an association with chronic inflammation and calculi, as does gallbladder carcinoma, and may confound the diagnosis of an underlaying carcinoma on imaging, particularly when segmental.[28] Intramural diverticula are called *Rokitansky-Aschoff sinuses*; they trap bile that accumulates cholesterol crystals appearing as cystic spaces in a thickened gallbladder wall with a characteristic comet tail artifact on ultrasound in ADM[27] (Fig. 16.13).

On MRI, the normally low T2 signal gallbladder wall may appear focally and diffusely thickened, with multiple punctate intramural high T2 signal foci throughout. Focal wall thickening is most common in the fundus; when it occurs in the gallbladder body, there may be annular constriction producing an hourglass-shaped gallbladder.

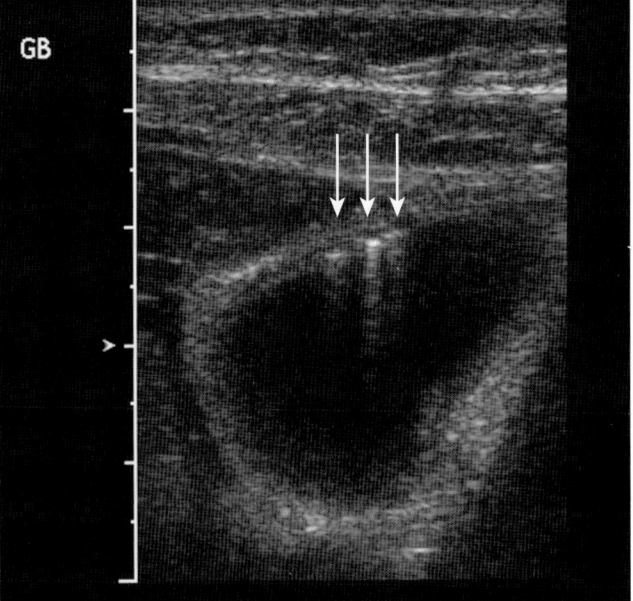

FIGURE 16.13   Gallbladder adenomyomatosis with bright reflectors in the gallbladder wall *(arrows)* producing comet tail artifact secondary to sound reverberation.

The majority of incidentally detected polypoid gallbladder lesions are nonneoplastic and represent cholesterol polyps or inflammatory polyps.[29] Rarely, these may be neoplastic, such as adenomatous polyps, and malignant transformation to adenocarcinoma is a concern (see Chapter 49). Adenomatous polyps tend to be solitary and uniformly hyperechoic, yet they become more heterogeneous as they increase in size; they may either be pedunculated or sessile. Thickening or irregularity of the gallbladder wall adjacent to a polyp may represent malignancy.

In patients with polypoid gallbladder lesions, risk factors for malignancy include patient age (>60 years), coexistence of gallstones, and size of the polypoid lesion (>10 mm in diameter).[30] Surgical consultation for asymptomatic polyps greater than 10 mm and for symptomatic gallbladder polyps irrespective of size has been proposed.[31] Often, asymptomatic gallbladder polyps smaller than 10 mm are followed sonographically; those smaller than 6 mm may be followed at extended intervals.[32]

Cholecystitis

For the diagnosis of cholecystitis, ultrasound has moderate to high sensitivity and specificity.[33] Ultrasound findings of acute calculous cholecystitis include gallstones, gallbladder wall thickening greater than 3 mm, pericholecystic fluid, and a positive sonographic Murphy sign. Gallstones, wall thickening, and Murphy sign together have a positive predictive value of 92% to 95%[33] (Fig. 16.14). Of note, gallbladder wall thickening is nonspecific, and diffuse thickening without primary gallbladder disease occurs in systemic processes such as hypoalbuminemia, congestive heart failure, ascites, hepatitis, and pancreatitis.[34] CT and MRI are generally not used for initial detection of acute cholecystitis. Occasionally, patients with cholecystitis display a confusing clinical picture and may undergo CT examination before the precise nature of the disease is clear, with MRI used as a problem-solving alternative, to further evaluate for choledocholithiasis or complicated cholecystitis (see Chapter 34).

In emphysematous cholecystitis, echogenic air within the gallbladder wall produces reverberation artifact on ultrasound. In this entity, there is the possibility of gallbladder necrosis, gangrene, and perforation. Gangrenous cholecystitis occurs more often in patients with diabetes mellitus or a white blood cell count greater than 15,000 cells/mL.[35] Ultrasound features of gangrenous cholecystitis include floating intraluminal membranes from sloughed mucosa, shadowing foci from air in the gallbladder wall, disrupted gallbladder wall, and pericholecystic abscess formation.[36] CT is preferable when evaluating for complications such as pericholecystic abscess, emphysematous cholecystitis, or gallbladder perforation, and can identify patients in need of emergency surgery. CT findings most specific for acute gangrenous cholecystitis are gas in the gallbladder wall or lumen, intraluminal membranes, irregular gallbladder wall enhancement, and pericholecystic abscess.[37]

Although gallbladder distension, wall thickening, and gallstones are often present in acute cholecystitis, these are nonspecific signs that occur in most patients with chronic cholecystitis as well. Ill-defined pericholecystic lucency on CT, or heterogeneous increased T2 signal on MRI within the hepatic parenchyma adjacent to the gallbladder, suggests gallbladder inflammation (Fig. 16.15).

Mirizzi Syndrome

Mirizzi syndrome is an uncommon condition in which the common hepatic duct is obstructed extrinsically by calculi impacted in or extruded from a Hartmann pouch or adjacent cystic duct. Cholecystobiliary and cholecystoenteric fistulae are common complications, and there is an increased risk of malignancy of the gallbladder (see Chapter 49). It is clinically important to recognize the diagnosis preoperatively to address the cause of obstruction. The typical CT features of Mirizzi syndrome are an impacted gallstone (eccentrically located relative to the bile duct) and associated dilation of the proximal biliary system with a normal-caliber downstream system. An irregular cavity with surrounding edema and inflammation may be seen adjacent to the gallbladder neck (Fig. 16.16). Although all typical findings may not be present on CT, direct cholangiography or MRCP can be obtained to further evaluate the nature of the obstruction and to search for the presence of a biliary fistula.

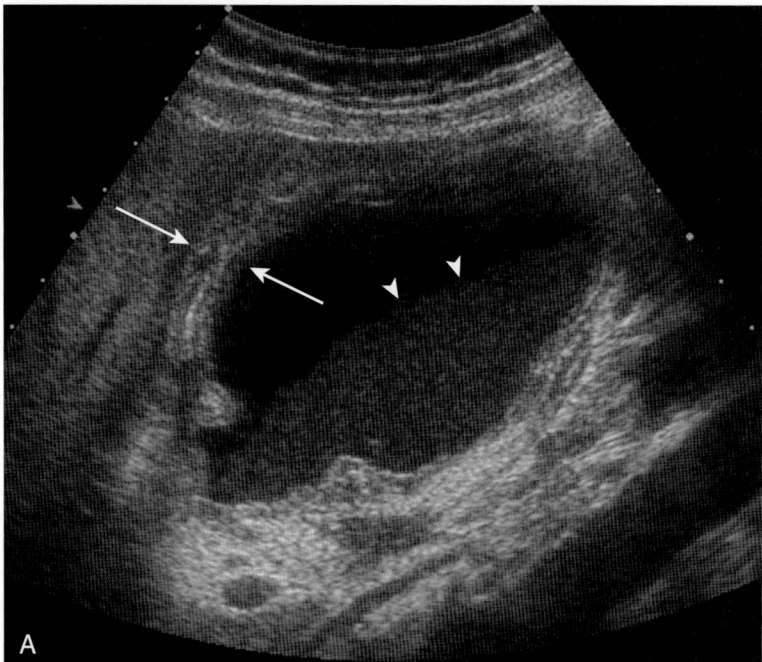
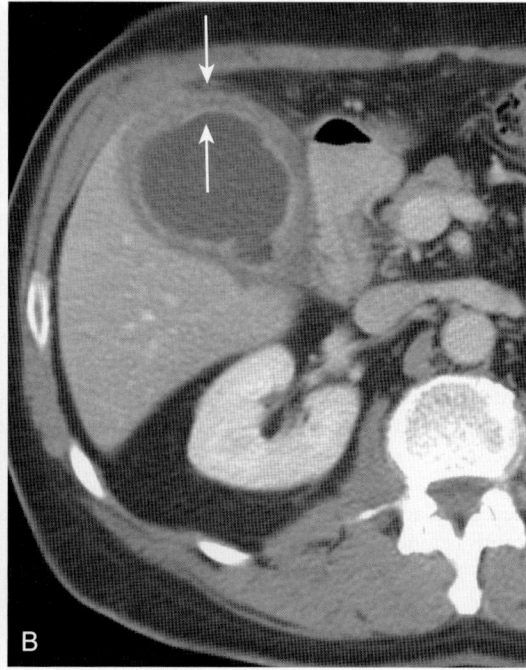

FIGURE 16.14 Acute cholecystitis. A, Longitudinal sonogram shows a distended gallbladder with thickened irregular wall *(arrows)* and layering sludge *(arrowheads).* **B,** Computed tomographic scan shows gallbladder wall thickening *(arrows).*

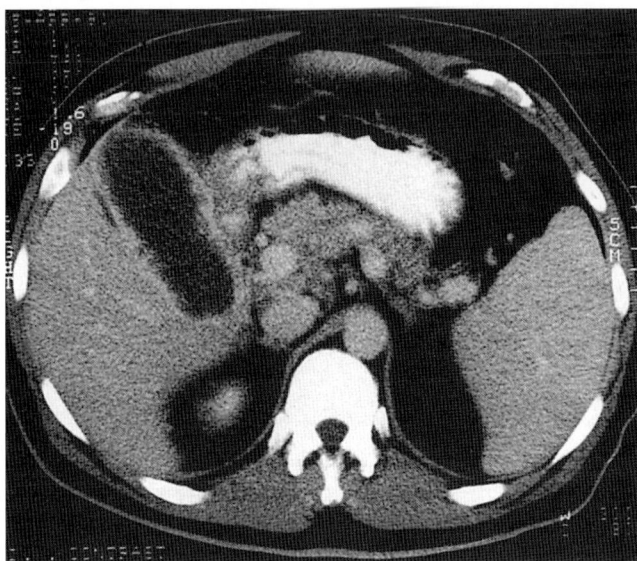

FIGURE 16.15 **Acute cholecystitis.** Computed tomography shows a distended, thick-walled gallbladder with pericholecystic fluid. No gallstones are seen.

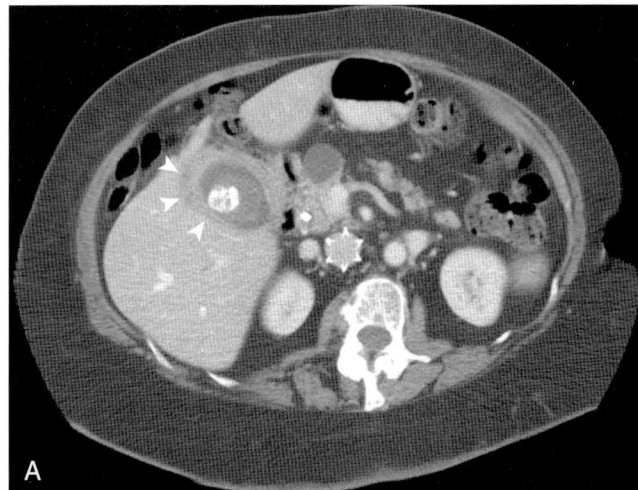

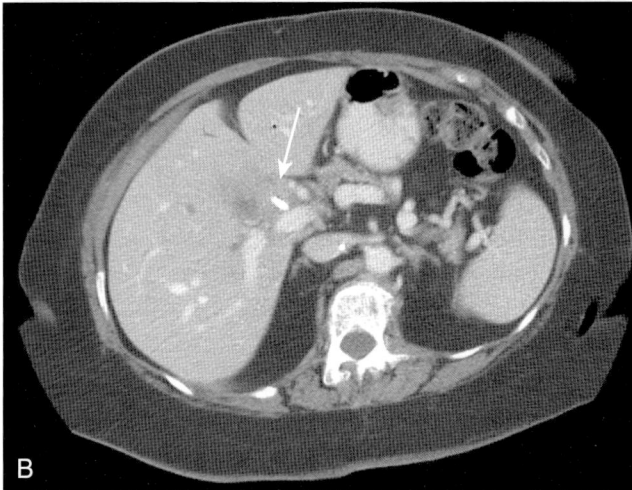

FIGURE 16.16 **Mirizzi syndrome. A,** Contrast-enhanced computed tomography reveals a large calcified gallstone associated with gallbladder wall thickening and extensive pericholecystic inflammatory change *(arrowheads)*. **B,** Extensive inflammatory change surrounds the internal biliary stent *(arrow)*.

Choledochal Cysts

Choledochal cysts, a rare congenital anomaly that usually presents before 10 years of age, manifest as dilatation of the extrahepatic bile ducts with possible associated intrahepatic duct dilatation (see Chapter 46). The presenting classic triad includes a palpable mass, abdominal pain, and jaundice (need ref). Cysts may be associated with chronic inflammation and increased risk for cholangiocarcinoma. Five types of cysts have been described[38-40]: *type I* fusiform extrahepatic duct dilatation (Fig. 16.17), *type II* extrahepatic duct diverticulum, *type III* choledochocele from a dilated terminal CBD, *type IV* multifocal dilatation, and *type V* cystic dilatation of the intrahepatic bile ducts that is synonymous with Caroli disease. Caroli disease belongs to a group of hepatic fibropolycystic diseases and is a hepatic manifestation of autosomal recessive polycystic kidney disease (ARPKD).[41] The cysts may be large, and the connection with the bile duct is not always evident on ultrasound. On imaging, it is important to demonstrate the connection with the bile ducts to differentiate this condition from multiple cysts or biliary hamartomas. Arterial flow from the fibrovascular bundle at the margin of the saccules and central enhancing portal venous branch or "central dot sign" may also aid in diagnosis on CT or MRI. Types I and IV have been further subdivided, and recently, there have been advocates for dropping the numeric classification system for more descriptive, clinically meaningful nomenclature.[42] MRI is well suited to diagnose and classify these cysts. Not only can three-dimensional (3D) MR cholangiograms depict the normal and abnormal anatomy, but direct coronal imaging and delayed scans post hepatocyte-specific gadolinium-based contrast agents can be obtained for further evaluation.[9]

MALIGNANT BILIARY TUMORS

Gallbladder Carcinoma

In 2020 there will be nearly 12,000 new cases of gallbladder carcinoma within the United States, with risk factors including female gender, age, and gallstones[43,44] (see Chapter 49). *Porcelain gallbladder,* a term used to describe calcification within the gallbladder wall, places a patient at some increased risk for gallbladder carcinoma. Older studies suggested that 10% to 25% of patients with a porcelain gallbladder develop gallbladder carcinoma, but more recent reports indicate that the risk may be lower, probably less than 10%, and related to the type of calcification (lower risk with complete calcification of the entire wall compared with selective calcification).[45-47] Many patients with gallbladder carcinoma are diagnosed with advanced disease, but the majority have earlier stage gallbladder carcinoma detected incidentally after elective cholecystectomy for symptomatic gallstone disease.

The CT imaging appearances of gallbladder carcinoma include a mass replacing the gallbladder (seen in 40%–65% of patients), focal or diffuse gallbladder wall thickening (seen in 20%–30%) (Figs. 16.18 and 16.19), and an intraluminal polypoid mass (seen in 15%–25%) (Fig. 16.20).[48,49] When the mass occupies the gallbladder lumen, it can result in a displaced or "trapped" stone that is fixed in position due to intraluminal tumor. Additional imaging findings associated with gallbladder carcinoma reflect the pattern of disease spread. The most common mode by which gallbladder carcinoma spreads is direct invasion into the adjacent organs. The liver is the organ most

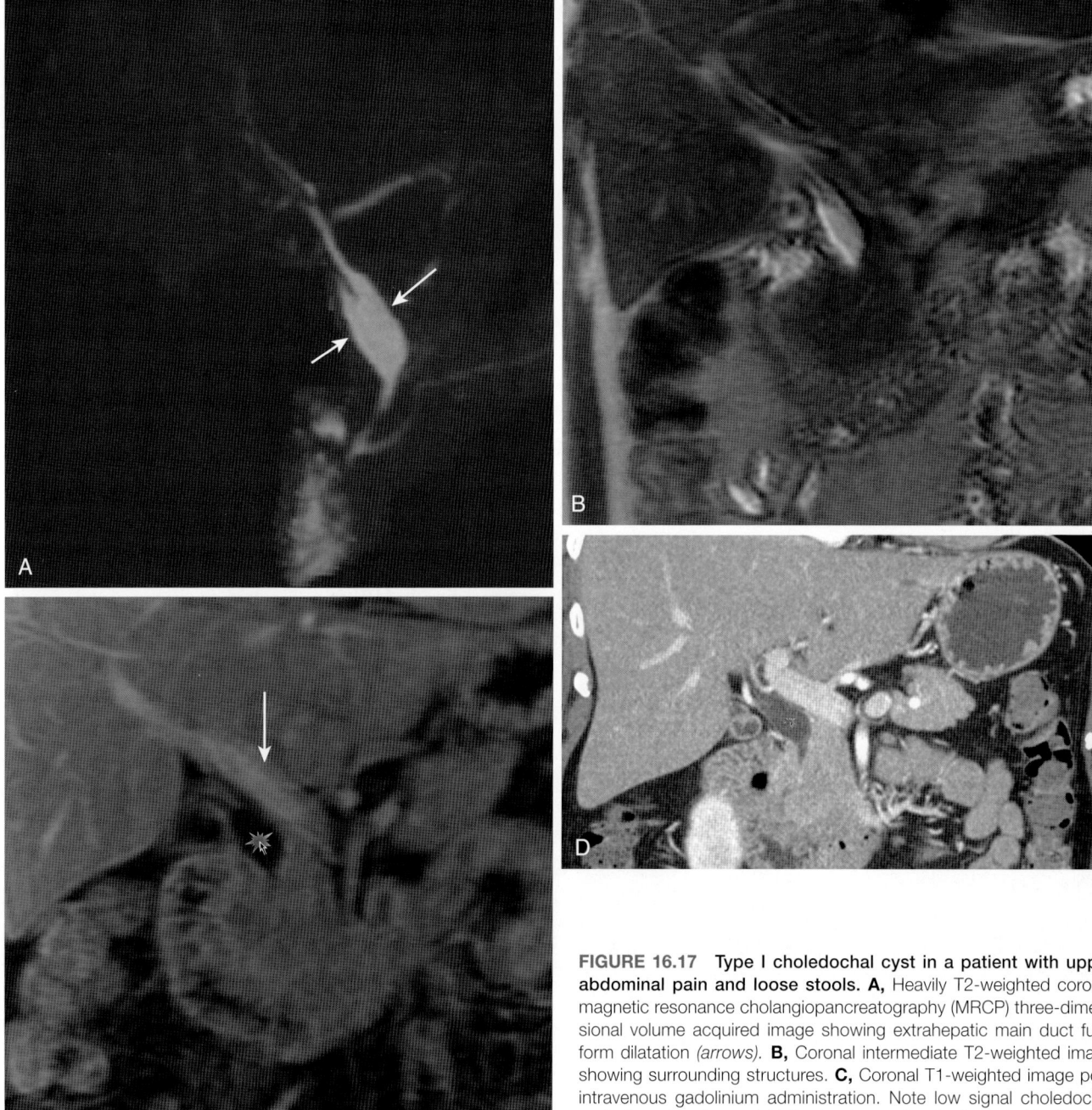

FIGURE 16.17 Type I choledochal cyst in a patient with upper abdominal pain and loose stools. **A,** Heavily T2-weighted coronal magnetic resonance cholangiopancreatography (MRCP) three-dimensional volume acquired image showing extrahepatic main duct fusiform dilatation *(arrows)*. **B,** Coronal intermediate T2-weighted image showing surrounding structures. **C,** Coronal T1-weighted image post intravenous gadolinium administration. Note low signal choledochal cyst (*) and enhanced high signal portal vein *(arrow)*. **D,** Coronal contrast-enhanced computed tomography (CT), showing low attenuation dilated main bile duct (*) consistent with type I choledochal cyst.

frequently invaded, followed by the bile duct, adjacent bowel, or pancreas. Air may be seen within the gallbladder lumen if tumor results in an enteric fistula. Tumors involving the infundibulum or cystic duct may invade directly and obstruct the CBD or portal vein, precluding surgical resection.

MRI offers improved characterization of gallbladder cancer compared with other modalities. However, differentiation from concurrent inflammatory conditions may be difficult with any modality. As opposed to inflammation-associated wall thickening with maintained mucosal and submucosal layers, gallbladder cancer typically shows irregular intermediate to high T2

signal thickening of the gallbladder wall, with early and prolonged heterogeneous enhancement, often in patients with multiple gallstones.[50] Cholelithiasis is a predisposing condition. On ultrasound, in addition to a mass involving the gallbladder wall or replacing the gallbladder, secondary signs of gallbladder cancer include discontinuity of the echogenic mucosal lining, absence of echogenic specks seen in cholesterol crystals, and high-velocity arterial flow greater than 60 cm/s (Fig. 16.21).

Gallbladder carcinoma often contiguously extends into hepatic segments IVB and V, or into the hepatic hilum, possibly directly involving the main bile duct with secondary biliary obstruction. Adjacent adenopathy may also be present. CT or MRI are the preferred modalities to accurately determine tumor resectability (see Chapter 119A) and distant disease spread, including peritoneal metastases.[51,52] Although CT remains the standard for initial imaging for gallbladder carcinomas, with reported overall accuracy of 85%, MRI offers similar accuracy for evaluating the primary tumor or hepatic metastases, with improved soft tissue contrast.[53,54]

DWI offers added sensitivity and specificity for extent of the primary tumor, and simultaneous ability to better assess for regional nodal or hepatic metastatic disease.[50] Fluorodeoxyglucose (FDG) positron emission tomography (PET) imaging may also provide improved sensitivity and specificity for nodal or distant metastatic disease.[55]

In the era of laparoscopic surgery for gallstone disease, it is important to assess the gallbladder carefully on preoperative ultrasound to exclude occult gallbladder cancer and to plan an appropriate surgical approach. Approximately 47% of gallbladder carcinomas are detected incidentally at laparoscopic cholecystectomy.[56] A serious potential complication of laparoscopic cholecystectomy is the inadvertent dissemination of unsuspected gallbladder carcinoma including involvement along the port tracts and abdominal wall (Fig. 16.22).[57] For patients with incidental discovery of carcinoma on laparoscopic cholecystectomy, re-exploration with definitive resection and re-excision of laparoscopic port sites is recommended.[56,58]

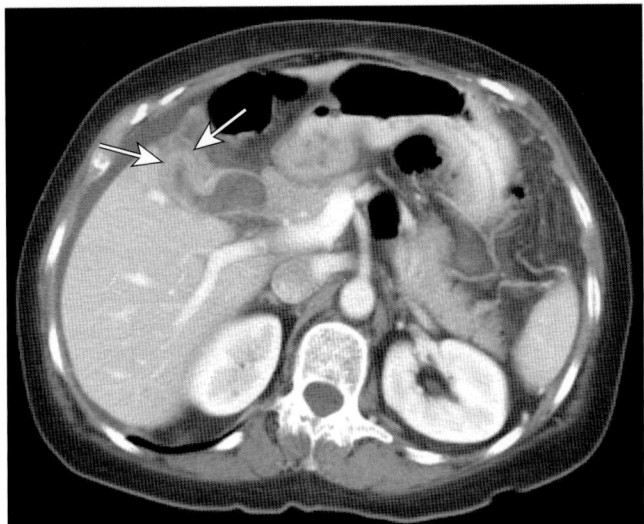

FIGURE 16.18 Contrast-enhanced computed tomography reveals focal gallbladder wall thickening *(arrows)* in a patient with gallbladder cancer.

Extrahepatic Cholangiocarcinoma

Cholangiocarcinoma is a relatively rare adenocarcinoma of the bile duct epithelium presenting mostly after the sixth decade of life (see Chapter 51). Although most patients have no known risk factors, conditions conferring increased risk include liver fluke infestation (see Chapter 45), PSC (see Chapter 41), choledochal cyst (including Caroli disease; see Chapter 46), hepatolithiasis (see Chapters 39 and 44), bile stasis, abnormal choledochopancreatic junction, hepatitis C viral infection, cirrhosis, alcoholic liver disease, ulcerative colitis, type 2 diabetes, thyrotoxicosis, and pancreatitis.[59]

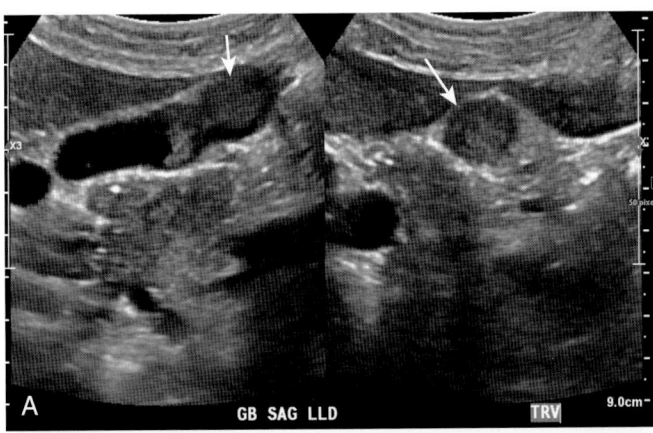

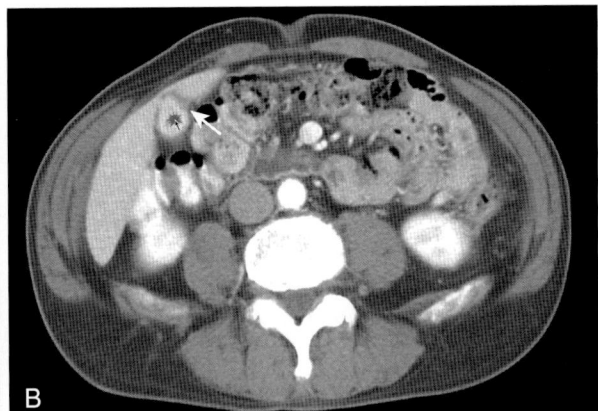

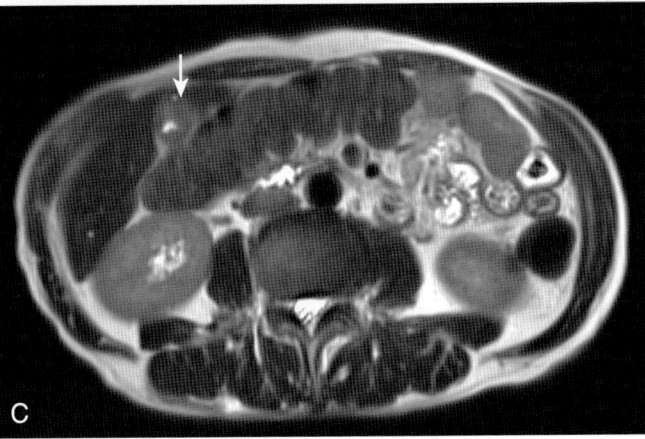

FIGURE 16.19 Gallbladder carcinoma. **A,** Patient with fatty liver. Screening ultrasound revealed irregular nodular soft tissue involving the gallbladder fundus with poor delineation of surrounding wall *(arrows)*. **B,** Axial computed tomography (CT) shows enhancement of the soft tissue *(*)* with infiltrated fat plane between gallbladder fundal wall and liver *(arrow)*. **C,** Axial T2-weighted magnetic resonance imaging (MRI) also shows poor delineation of the wall and obliteration of fat plane between gallbladder wall and liver *(arrow)*. Pathology showed adenocarcinoma, with tumor invasion of the perimuscular connective tissue adjacent to liver.

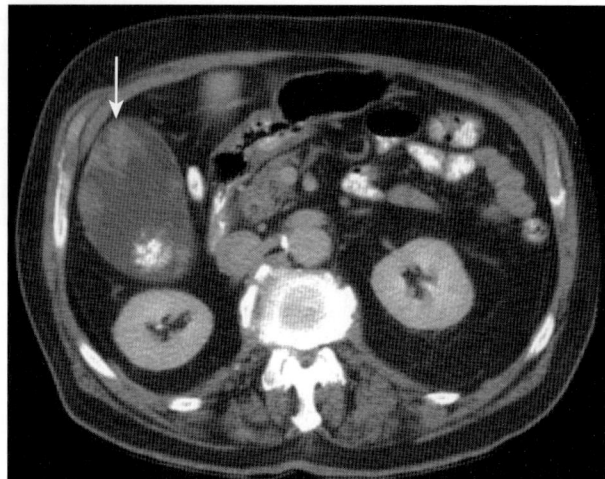

FIGURE 16.20   **Gallbladder carcinoma.** The gallbladder is distended and contains calcified stones. Nodular soft tissue emanates from the gallbladder wall into the lumen *(arrow)*.

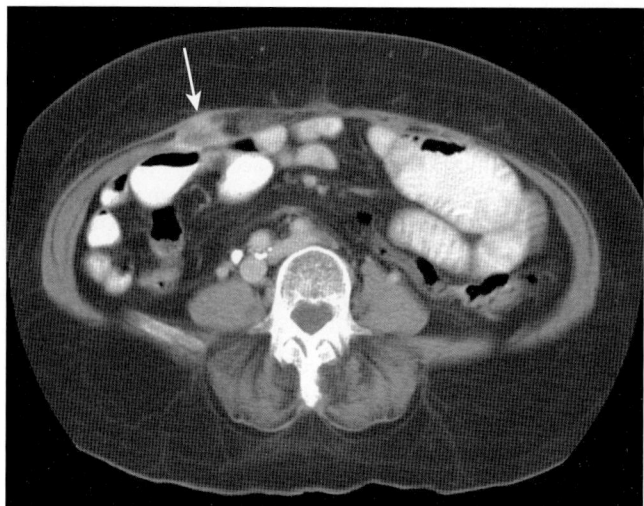

FIGURE 16.22   Contrast-enhanced computed tomography in a patient who had previously undergone laparoscopic cholecystectomy. The enhancing mass *(arrow)* within the anterior abdominal wall reflects recurrent gallbladder carcinoma within a laparoscopic port tract.

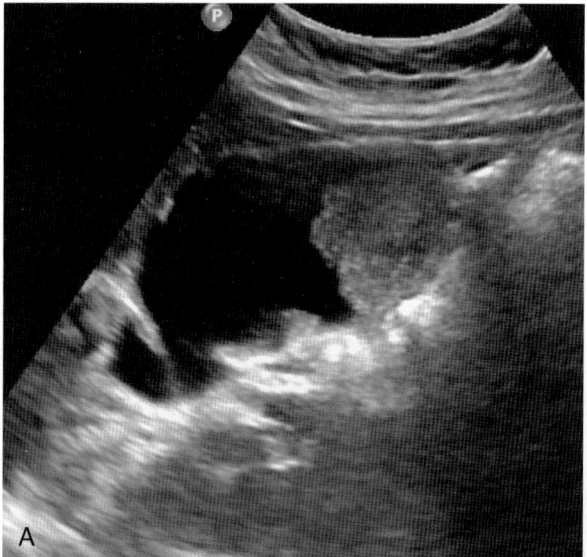

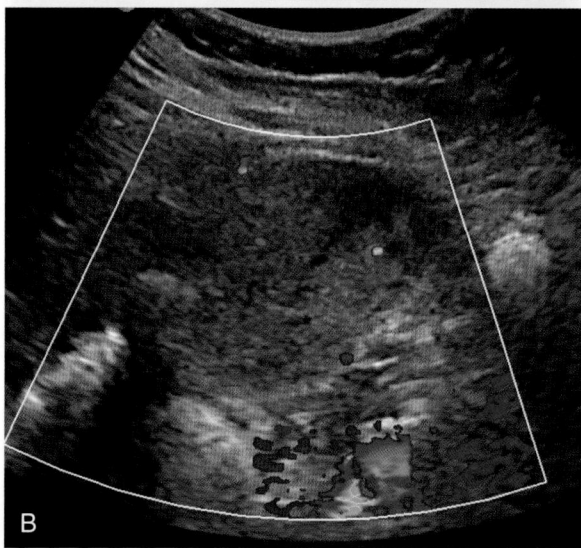

FIGURE 16.21   **Gallbladder carcinoma. A,** Gray scale longitudinal image of the gallbladder shows a solid irregular mass in the fundus. **B,** Transverse color Doppler image of this lesion demonstrates internal vascularity, suspicious for tumor. Pathology demonstrated gallbladder adenocarcinoma.

In 1997 the Liver Cancer Study Group of Japan categorized cholangiocarcinoma into three subtypes based on macroscopic appearance (*mass forming*, *periductal infiltrating*, and *intraductal growing*), corresponding in older literature to the terms "nodular," "sclerosing/infiltrating," and either "exophytic" or "papillary," respectively (see Chapter 47). A combination of periductal infiltrating and mass-forming types is also common. Cholangiocarcinoma has also been divided by the seventh edition of the American Joint Committee on Cancer Staging Manual[60] into perihilar, distal, and intrahepatic types, which are distinct clinical and radiologic entities[61] (see Chapter 51).

The perihilar location is most common at 60% to 70% and is generally associated with a component of biliary obstruction, whereas distal sites are less common at 20% to 30%, and intrahepatic is the least common at 5% to 15%.[62,63]

Preoperative high-resolution CT or MRI with MRC are typically used to address the following factors that determine resectability per the staging system for hilar cholangiocarcinoma developed by Jarnagin and colleagues[25]: level and extent of tumor, vascular invasion, hepatic lobar atrophy, and distant metastatic disease (Fig. 16.23) (see Chapters 51B and 119B).

On MRI, bile duct tumors typically show intermediate, mildly increased T2 signal that is less bright than fluid in the dilated bile ducts. The level of obstruction and continuity of the tumor with the vasculature are well evaluated with MRI.[64] CT angiography with multiphasic imaging offers improved spatial resolution to MRI, with similar accuracy to assess vascular involvement. Tumor extent along the portal veins and hepatic arteries can also be identified with multiphase CT angiography. CT is the preferred modality to assess for distant metastases.[65]

Focused assessment of ductal, portal venous, and hepatic arterial involvement is performed in staging and preoperative imaging. The portal vein and hepatic artery status and extent of ductal spread help determine surgical approach, because long-term survival is possible only with en bloc resection of the liver and the extrahepatic biliary ducts.[66]

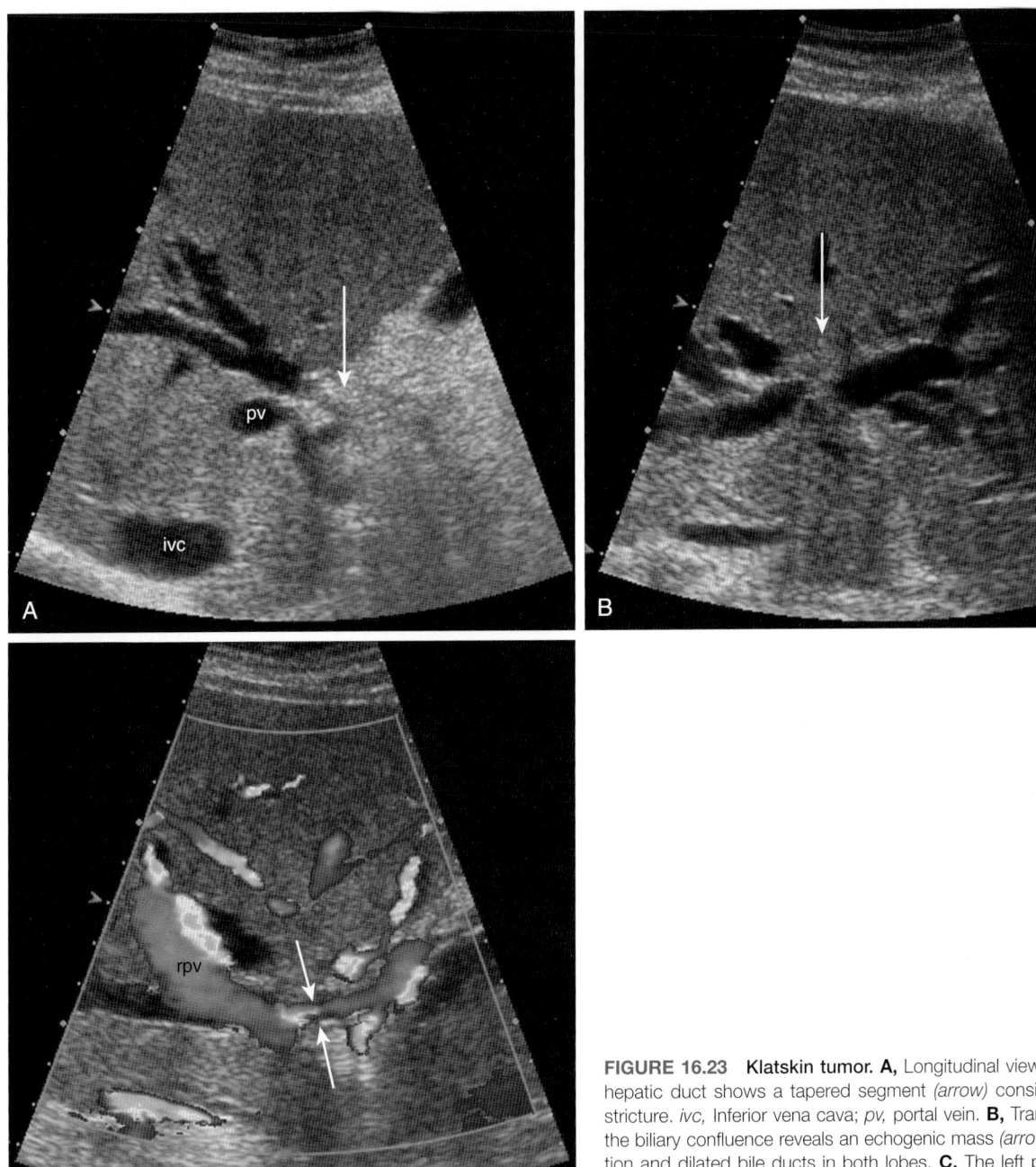

FIGURE 16.23   Klatskin tumor. A, Longitudinal view of the common hepatic duct shows a tapered segment *(arrow)* consistent with tumor stricture. *ivc,* Inferior vena cava; *pv,* portal vein. **B,** Transverse image at the biliary confluence reveals an echogenic mass *(arrow)* at the bifurcation and dilated bile ducts in both lobes. **C,** The left portal vein is narrowed and encased *(arrows),* as shown on color Doppler transverse image. *rpv,* Right portal vein.

On CT, individual dilated bile ducts can be traced to the point(s) of obstruction (Fig. 16.24), and to evaluate the cause of biliary obstruction. On meta-analysis,[67] multidetector row CT (MDCT) has a sensitivity and specificity of 89% and 92%, respectively, for portal venous involvement, and 84% and 93%, respectively, for hepatic arterial involvement (and 86% accuracy in assessing extent of ductal involvement). Moderate lobar atrophy is typically caused by long-standing obstruction of the ipsilateral bile duct; however, associated portal venous obstruction causes rapid and marked atrophy of the affected lobe (Fig. 16.25).[66,68] Atrophy should also be recognized and reported when biliary decompression is under consideration, because drainage of an atrophic lobe does not relieve jaundice and is only indicated to relieve biliary sepsis.[66]

Perihilar tumors of the periductal infiltrating morphologic subtype often appear as focal duct wall thickening with obliteration of the lumen,[61] but may only manifest as ductal enhancement or merely narrowing. Although most biliary strictures are malignant, correlation with serum IgG4 levels may better assess for possible IgG4 sclerosing cholangitis (see Chapter 42). Malignant strictures tend to be longer (≥18–22 mm) and have a thicker wall (≥2 mm) than benign strictures, and they may show bile duct hyperenhancement.[69] Mass-forming perihilar tumors, like their intrahepatic counterparts, are heterogeneous hypovascular masses with peripheral rim enhancement in the arterial and portal phase and central enhancement in delayed phases. In perihilar malignancies, hypoenhancing soft tissue infiltration of adjacent periductal fat may also be visible with delayed-phase

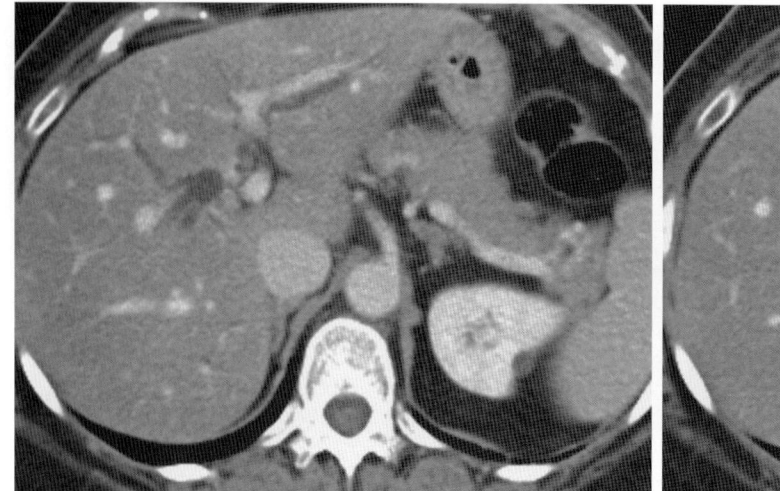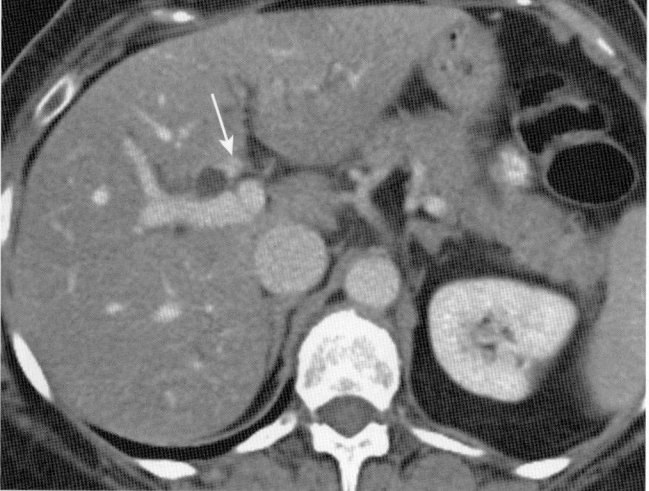

FIGURE 16.24 Cholangiocarcinoma. Contrast-enhanced computed tomography at two levels through the liver (*left* and *right*) reveals bilobar central intrahepatic biliary duct dilation as a result of an obstructing enhancing mass at the hepatic hilum (*arrow*).

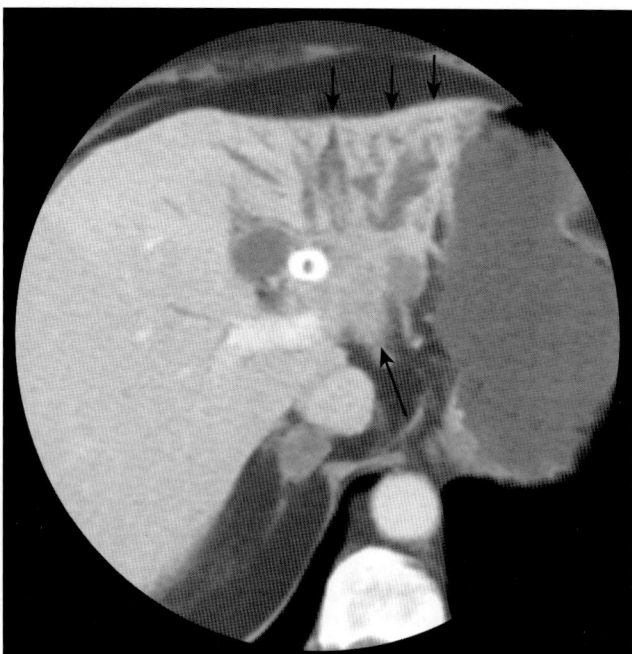

FIGURE 16.25 Infiltrative hilar cholangiocarcinoma. Reformatted oblique axial image. The infiltrative mass (*long arrow*) in the left hepatic lobe causes left intrahepatic biliary ductal dilation (*short arrows*). Tumor extends along the central portion of the right portal vein with mild atrophy of the left lobe.

hyperenhancement, although this infiltration may sometimes be hypervascular (Fig. 16.26).[59]

Although operator dependent, ultrasound in expert hands may be helpful in the preoperative imaging evaluation of local tumor extent for hilar tumors but should be performed before intervention or stent placement to avoid pneumobilia and artifact, which may obscure both tumor and level of obstruction after biliary decompression. The majority of hilar cholangiocarcinomas are isoechoic, which renders their delineation challenging on ultrasound as well.

On ultrasound, extrahepatic cholangiocarcinoma may show infiltrative tumor spread along the duct walls, nodular mural thickening, or appear papillary. Intraductal papillary neoplasms of the bile duct (IPNBs) (see Chapter 60), including mucinous cystic neoplasm of the bile duct, may be intrahepatic or extrahepatic, typically manifest as a polypoid expansile intraductal mass, and have a better prognosis and surgical outcome (Fig. 16.27).[70,71]

Contrast-enhanced ultrasound (CEUS) in experienced hands may also aid the diagnosis and staging of cholangiocarcinoma.[72,73] Ultrasound and CEUS are focused on local tumor extent and are preferably performed before any intervention. CT and MRI remain essential for evaluation of regional and distant disease, even if the tumor is visible on ultrasound.

The least common intraductal-growing tumor subtype (8%–18%) predominantly shows multiple lesions along various segments of the bile ducts with papillary histologic features differentiating them from the other types of cholangiocarcinoma.[74] The World Health Organization endorses the term "intraductal papillary neoplasm of the bile ducts" to encompass all variants of biliary intraductal neoplasia, which has been recognized as a biliary counterpart of pancreatic intraductal papillary mucinous neoplasm. These tumors, particularly the mucin-secreting subtype, are more often resectable with a more favorable prognosis.[75] On CT, asymmetric biliary dilation is usually noted with enhancing, expansile, and well-defined intraductal soft tissue mass in the most dilated ducts. Unlike mass-forming or periductal-infiltrating subtypes, there is no invasion of adjacent liver parenchyma.[59,61]

DISTAL CHOLANGIOCARCINOMA

The periductal infiltrating subtype is also the most common form involving the CBD. The radiologic and pathologic features are identical to those perihilar in location. The assessment and treatment of distal bile duct cancers is similar to that of pancreatic head carcinoma[76] (see Chapters 59 and 117A).

The less common intraductal subtype of cholangiocarcinoma is most often found involving the CBD. Imaging features are identical to its appearance in the perihilar region. Enhancement

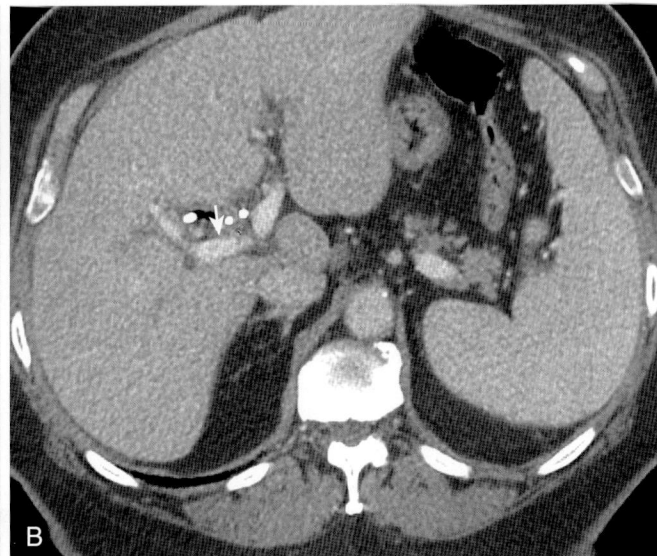

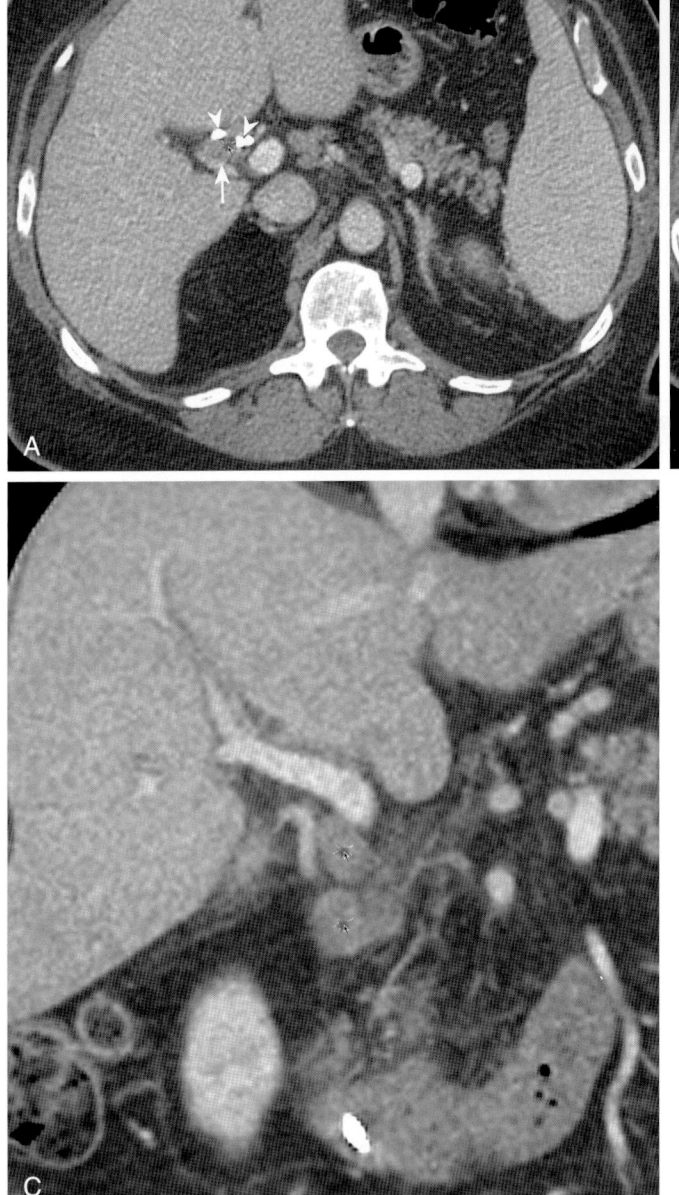

FIGURE 16.26 Hilar cholangiocarcinoma in a patient with painless jaundice. **A,** Axial contrast-enhanced computed tomography (CT) shows hilar hypoenhancing biopsy–proven cholangiocarcinoma *(*)* inseparable from right hepatic artery *(arrow)*. Note hyperattenuating biliary stent *(arrowheads)*. **B,** Axial CT image at another level confirms tumor *(*)* abutting the portal vein at its bifurcation, with greater abutment of the right portal vein *(arrow)*. **C,** Coronal reconstructed CT image shows periportal lymphadenopathy *(*)* suspicious for metastatic disease.

of the mass is generally noted where tumor remains fixed along the duct wall, and there may be segmental asymmetric thickening and enhancement of the duct wall. The subset of intraductal mucinous tumors, considered a precursor to cholangiocarcinoma, may cause marked extra or intrahepatic duct dilatation, with low attenuation mucin on CT, high T2 signal on MRI, and hypoechoic or anechoic findings on ultrasound. The tumors may be small and not visible on imaging, or larger and fungating, with some tumors friable with sloughing resulting in intermittent or partial biliary obstruction.[21,77]

Biliary Cystic Tumors (Cystadenoma and Cystadenocarcinoma)

Biliary cystadenomas (BCAs) are uncommon benign cystic lesions that occur predominantly (90%) in women between 42

and 55 years of age and are more common within the left lobe (see Chapters 47 and 88B). Although benign, these lesions may recur after excision and have the potential to develop into biliary cystadenocarcinomas (BCACs). BCACs at presentation are more evenly distributed between men and women and generally occur a decade later.[78] BCAs are most often intrahepatic (83%), but they may also occur within the extrahepatic bile ducts (13%) or gallbladder (0.02%).

On CT, biliary cystic tumors (BCTs) tend to be multiloculated cystic lesions with internal septations; only rarely are they unilocular (Fig. 16.28). The attenuation of the cyst fluid depends on its content, which may be hemorrhagic, mucinous, proteinaceous, or bilious. Calcifications may be present within the wall of the cyst or within septa, and septa may enhance with intravenous contrast (Fig. 16.29). Although ultrasound and

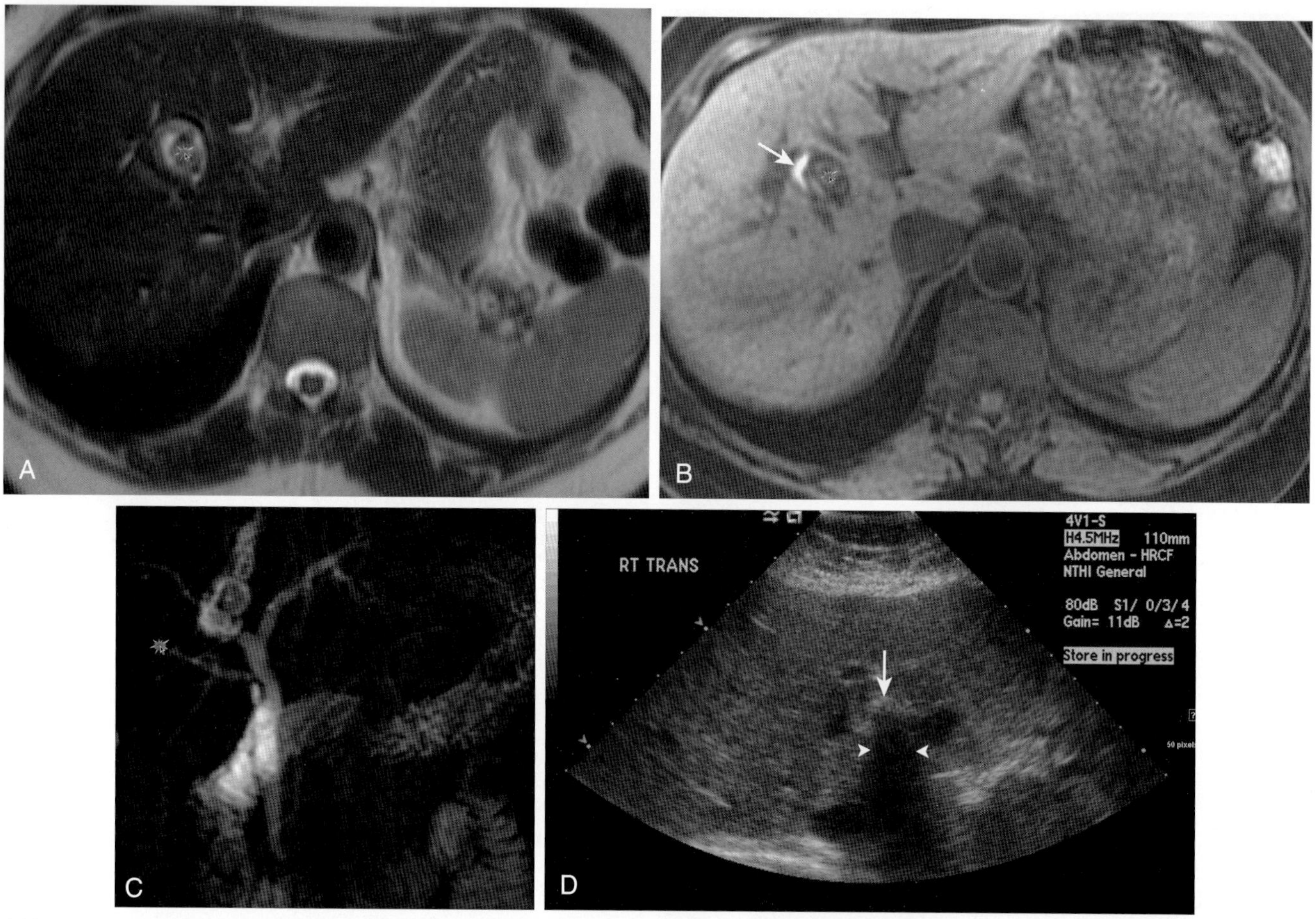

FIGURE 16.27 **Intraductal papillary carcinoma. A,** Axial T2-weighted magnetic resonance (MR) image shows expanded right intrahepatic bile duct (*arrows*) with heterogeneous filling defect *(*)*. **B,** Axial T1-weighted fat saturated MR image shows marginal high T1 signal (*arrow*) along the filling defect *(*)*. **C,** Coronal three-dimensional (3D) MR cholangiopancreatography volume acquired image also shows the expanded duct and intraductal mass *(*)*. **D,** Axial ultrasound image in the region of interest shows marginal echogenic apparent calculus *(arrow)* with acoustic shadowing *(arrowheads)*. Pathology revealed 1-cm intraductal papillary carcinoma, with marginal pigment stones accounting for the high T1 signal in **(B).**

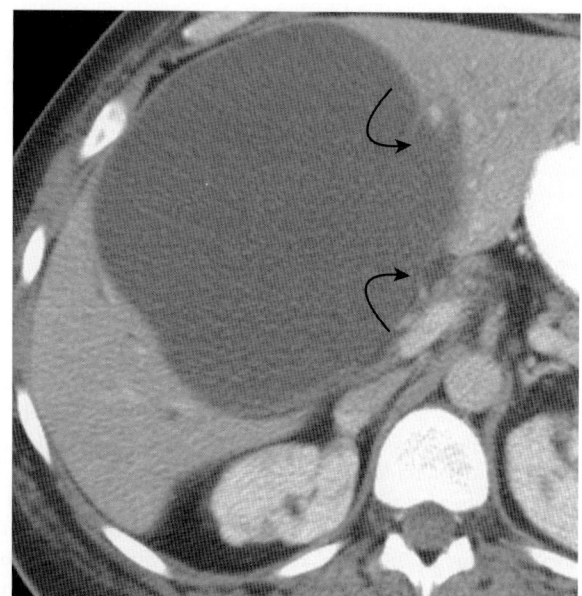

FIGURE 16.28 **Biliary cystadenoma.** Contrast-enhanced computed tomography reveals a large cystic mass with a very subtle internal septation *(curved arrows)*.

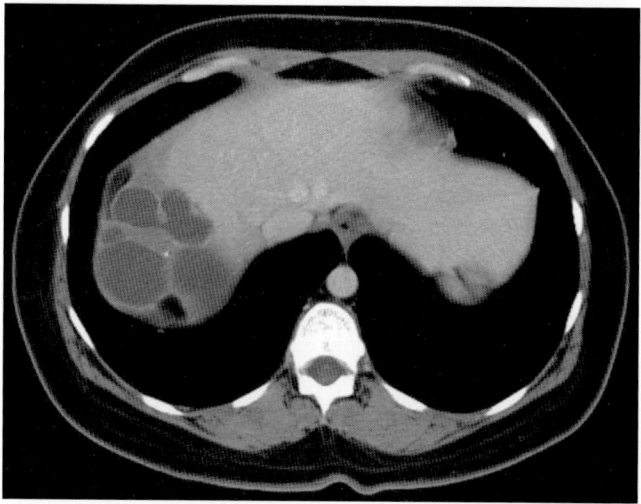

FIGURE 16.29 **Recurrent biliary cystadenoma after resection.** Multiloculated cystic lesion is seen at the resection margin containing enhancing septa and calcification.

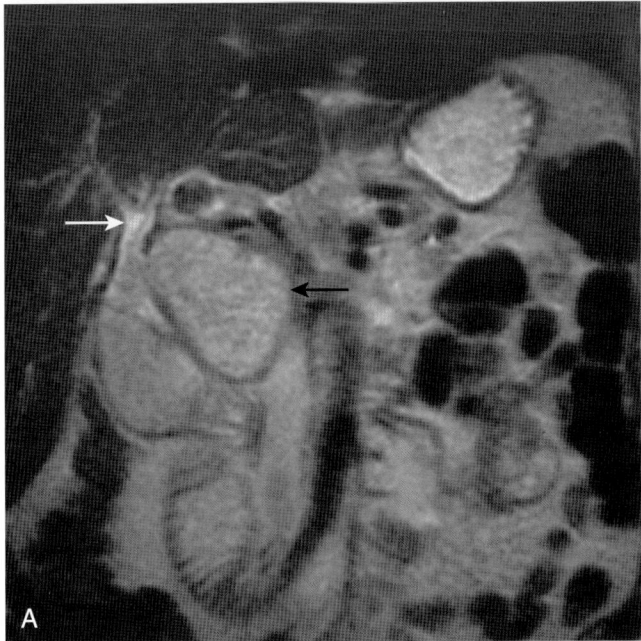
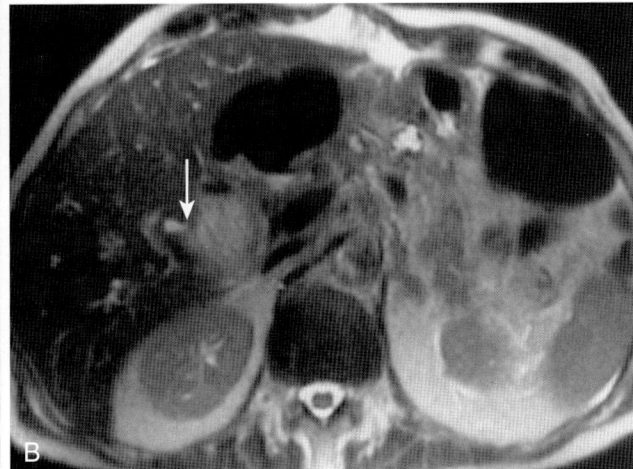

FIGURE 16.30   Afferent loop syndrome. A, Coronal T2-weighted sequence in a patient after pancreaticoduodenectomy for pancreatic carcinoma. The patient has a hepaticojejunostomy with a patent anastomosis *(white arrow)*. The afferent loop is markedly dilated *(black arrow)* compared with other loops of bowel. No mechanical obstruction was noted. **B,** Axial T2-weighted image through the level of the anastomosis *(arrow)* shows the site to be patent without evidence of a stricture. The afferent loop is dilated.

MRI are considered more sensitive than CT for detection of septa and complexity, the accuracy of imaging in distinguishing the different types of complex and simple hepatic cystic lesions from BCA remains low.[78,79] Multiple studies have also shown no reliable imaging features to predict BCAC over BCA in the absence of gross tumor.[80,81]

(MR) Postoperative Biliary Complications

Complications from surgical procedures include bile leaks, abscess formation, and biliary strictures (see Chapters 28, 117A, 188, and 119). MRCP is uniquely suited for the assessment of the postoperative biliary tract, including the assessment of bile leaks and abscesses. Bile duct injuries after surgery can be multifactorial, but the result is commonly a stricture at the anastomotic site (see Chapters 42 and 52). Surgical clips near the anastomosis may create streak artifacts during CT scanning, but contemporary clips are less problematic for MRI. MRI has multiplanar capabilities and superior tissue contrast, and MRCP sequences can minimize susceptibility to artifacts to allow improved visualization of the region of the anastomosis and improved diagnostic confidence (Fig. 16.30). More recently, hepatocyte contrast agents also allow delayed hepatobiliary phase scans by opacifying the biliary tree, which may improve diagnostic confidence to evaluate for active biliary leak, anatomic variants, and choledocholithiasis.[9,82]

The references for this chapter can be found online by accessing the accompanying Expert Consult website.

CHAPTER 17

Imaging features of benign and malignant pancreatic disease

Shannan M. Dickinson and Seth S. Katz

INTRODUCTION TO PANCREATIC IMAGING

Transabdominal ultrasound (US) is a noninvasive, inexpensive, and rapid method of evaluating morphologic changes in the pancreas and may be used as an initial investigation in the setting of abdominal pain or suspected obstructive jaundice. However, considerable limitations reduce its diagnostic utility; these include overlying bowel gas obscuring the pancreas and limitations related to the patient's body habitus.[1] If a pancreatic mass or parenchymal abnormality is found at US, further assessment with contrast-enhanced computed tomography (CT) or magnetic resonance imaging (MRI) should be performed. If CT is performed in the workup of a pancreatic mass, particularly in suspected pancreatic ductal adenocarcinoma (PDAC), it should be performed as a multiphase pancreatic protocol study, with imaging in the pancreatic parenchymal/late arterial phase and the portal venous phase. MRI with Magnetic resonance cholangiopancreatography (MRCP) is also a mainstay of pancreatic imaging and can provide detailed assessment of the pancreatic and bile ducts. Secretin-enhanced MRCP is an advanced imaging technique, with limited availability. The technique can be used to improve visualization and assessment of the pancreatic ductal system and to assess exocrine gland function.[2]

CONGENITAL CONDITIONS, VARIANTS, AND BENIGN ALTERATIONS

Pancreatic Divisum

Pancreatic divisum is the most common congenital pancreatic ductal anatomic variant, resulting from failure of fusion of the ventral and dorsal pancreatic anlages (Fig. 17.1; see Chapters 1 and 53). This results in the majority of pancreatic parenchyma draining via the dorsal duct into the minor papilla.[3] The ventral duct, which generally does not communicate with the dorsal duct,[3] joins the common bile duct to empty into the major papilla. Pancreas divisum may be seen on high-spatial-resolution and thin-section multidetector CT[4]; however, MRI is generally superior in visualizing the pancreatic duct, with T2 sequences offering similar visualization to dedicated MRCP sequences.[5] MRI will demonstrate the dominant dorsal duct emptying into the minor papilla, superior to the level of the bile duct, with the ventral duct sometimes too small to discretely visualize on MRI[6] or even absent.[3]

Annular Pancreas

Annular pancreas is present when a complete or incomplete ring of pancreatic tissue encircles the second portion of the duodenum (D2; Fig. 17.2; see Chapters 1 and 53).[7] MRI will demonstrate the encircling, or partially encircling pancreatic tissue, and sometimes the small associated annular duct that drains the annular portion.[6] An incomplete ring is demonstrated by pancreatic tissue extending in both a posterolateral and anterolateral direction around the D2 or, in some cases, only in the posterolateral direction.[7] Pancreatic tissue extending only in an anterolateral direction around the D2 is less specific for incomplete annular pancreas.[7]

Fatty Infiltration

Fatty replacement of pancreatic tissue may be focal or diffuse and can occur in diabetic, obese, or elderly patients.[6,8] Complete fatty replacement of the pancreas is seen most commonly in patients with cystic fibrosis or Schwachman-Diamond syndrome.[6,8] In severe cases, the pancreas will be clearly visible and will have the same density (CT) or signal (MRI) to the mesenteric fat (Fig. 17.3).[8] In this setting, the presence of the ductal system differentiates fatty replacement from agenesis.[8] Fatty replacement may not be homogeneous, with the anterior pancreatic head more severely affected, compared with the posterior pancreatic head peribiliary tissue, which can be spared.[8,9] This nonhomogeneous fatty replacement may mimic a mass or neoplasm on CT (Fig. 17.4); however, MRI can usually differentiate fatty replacement changes from neoplasm.[6]

PANCREATITIS

Acute Pancreatitis

The 2012 revised Atlanta classification provides standardized clinical and radiologic nomenclature for acute pancreatitis and associated complications.[10] The classification defines two distinct types of acute pancreatitis: interstitial edematous pancreatitis (IEP) and necrotizing pancreatitis (NP), depending on the absence or presence of necrosis, respectively (see Chapters 55 and 56).[10,11]

Imaging of the pancreas is not necessarily required in the setting of mild cases of acute pancreatitis because the diagnosis can be based on clinical symptoms and serology.[10,11] Nevertheless, imaging may be required to make the diagnosis if one of the aforementioned factors is negative or to assess for a causative factor, the most common being gallstones (see Chapter 33).[11,12] Early US can be performed with a limited purpose of identifying gallstones or to demonstrate bile duct dilatation; however, stones in the distal duct may not be identified.[13] Standard contrast-enhanced CT (CECT) abdomen is the most common modality used, and a multiphase pancreatic protocol is typically unnecessary.[12] MRI/MRCP may also be used, particularly in the setting of iodinated contrast allergy, renal failure, or suspicion of choledocholithiasis.[11,12] Nevertheless, MRI scan time is long compared with CT, and the availability of MRI should be

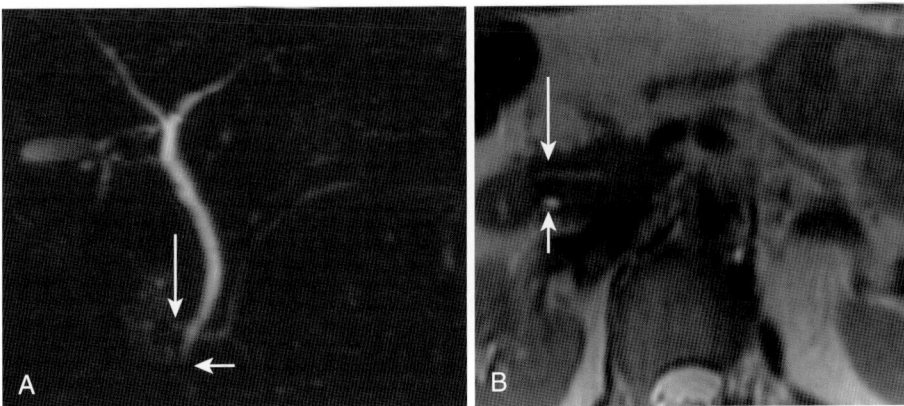

FIGURE 17.1   Pancreatic divisum. Three-dimensional (3D) Magnetic resonance cholangiopancreatography (MRCP) reconstruction **(A)** and an axial T2-weighted magnetic resonance image (MRI) **(B)** demonstrating the main pancreatic duct *(long arrow)* separately entering into the duodenum, superior to the common bile duct *(short arrow)*. In image **(A)** the ducts cross, rather than coalesce to both empty into the duodenum at the ampulla.

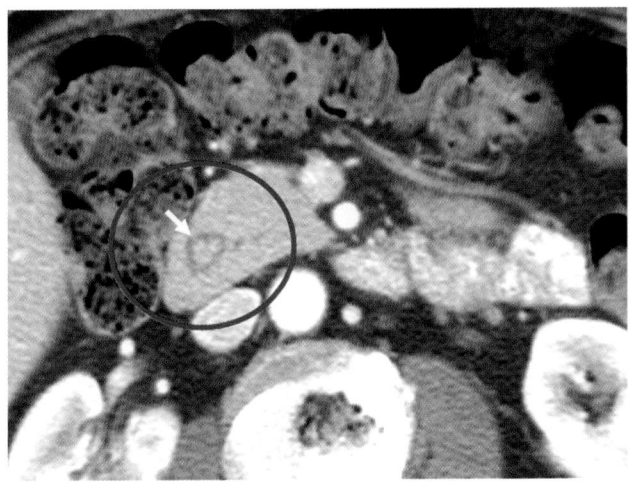

FIGURE 17.2   Annular pancreas. Axial computed tomography (CT) in portal venous phase demonstrating annular pancreas *(red circle)* with pancreatic parenchyma completely encircling the proximal duodenum *(arrow)*.

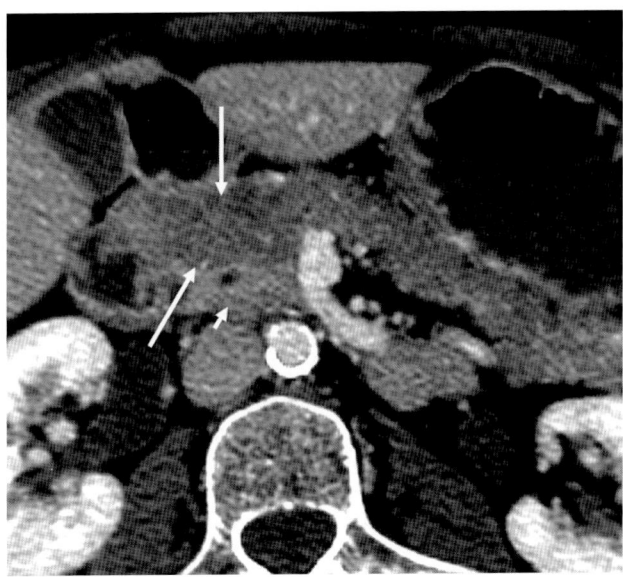

FIGURE 17.4   Fatty infiltration with pseudomass. Axial computed tomography (CT) in portal venous phase. Diffuse fatty infiltration of the pancreas, most marked at the anterior pancreatic head *(long arrows)*, mimicking a hypoenhancing pancreatic mass. This is demarcated by a region of fatty sparing at the posterior peribiliary pancreatic head *(short arrow)*.

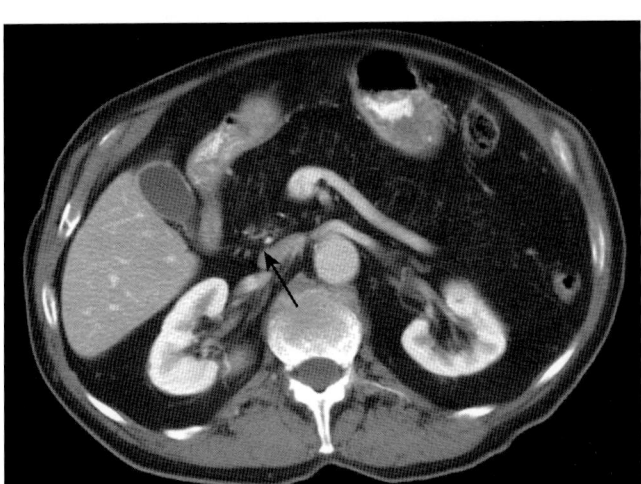

FIGURE 17.3 Axial computed tomography (CT) in portal venous phase demonstrating extensive fatty replacement of the pancreas, appearing isodense to the mesenteric fat. Minimal pancreatic acinar tissue is visible in the posterior aspect of the pancreatic head *(arrow)*, where there can be peribiliary sparing.

considered.[12] Imaging in pancreatitis should ideally be performed five to seven days after pain onset, when necrosis is clearly definable and local complications have developed.[10] Earlier imaging within the first few days after pain onset may miss or be equivocal for necrosis and correlates poorly with clinical severity.[10,14]

The CT Severity Index (CTSI)[14] and later modified CT Severity Index (mCTSI)[15] both define specific radiologic criteria for grading the severity of acute pancreatitis and complications. The CTSI score is based on pancreatic changes, the presence and amount of necrosis (none, ≤30%, 30%–50%, and >50%), and peripancreatic fluid collections.[14] The mCTSI includes similar criteria, with a simplified definition of the amount of necrosis (none, ≤30%, and >30%), and includes extrapancreatic findings, such as pleural effusions and ascites.[13,15] A study involving almost 400 patients demonstrated no significant difference between CTSI and mCTSI in evaluating the severity of acute pancreatitis.[16]

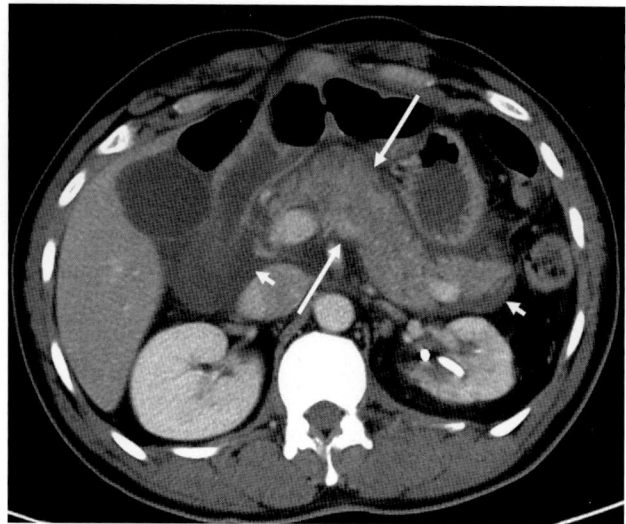

FIGURE 17.5 Axial computed tomography (CT) in portal venous phase demonstrating acute interstitial edematous pancreatitis with diffuse edematous enlargement of the pancreas with mild hypoenhancement *(long arrows)*; note there are no nonenhancing parenchymal regions. Small amount of reactive fluid surrounding and adjacent to the pancreas *(short arrows)*.

Interstitial Edematous Pancreatitis

IEP is the more common form of acute pancreatitis and, at imaging, usually appears as diffuse or focal pancreatic enlargement with a small amount of peripancreatic fluid (Fig. 17.5).[11] The pancreatic parenchyma will generally enhance less than a normal pancreas because of the presence of interstitial edema.[11] However, there should be no nonenhancing parenchymal regions or peripancreatic necrotic collections; if these are present, the diagnosis of NP should be made.[11]

According to the 2012 revised Atlanta criteria, any peripancreatic fluid collection occurring within the first 4 weeks of IEP is classified as an "acute peripancreatic fluid collection" (APFC; see Chapter 54). Because there is no necrosis in IEP, the APFC will contain only fluid and appear as homogeneous fluid attenuation (0–20 HU) at CT and fluid signal intensity on T2-weighted MRI imaging, conforming to the retroperitoneal structures, and without a well-defined wall.[10,11] These usually resolve spontaneously without intervention and most APFC will remain sterile. In 10% of cases, the peripancreatic collections persist for more than four weeks,[17] and these are termed pancreatic pseudocysts (see Chapter 54).[10] Like APFC, pseudocysts should not include any solid components or debris. Pseudocysts will appear as homogeneous fluid attenuation CT and hyperintense on T2, with a well-defined enhancing capsule.[11] A connection between the pseudocyst and the main pancreatic duct may be present, best visualized on MRI/MRCP (Fig. 17.6). On transabdominal US, pseudocysts typically appear as a circumscribed, smooth-walled spherical anechoic lesion with posterior acoustic enhancement.

Necrotizing Pancreatitis

Necrotizing pancreatitis (NP) is defined by necrosis involving the pancreatic parenchyma and/or the peripancreatic soft tissues. Involvement of both parenchyma and peripancreatic soft tissues is the most common form, occurring in 75% of cases.[10] Involvement of the peripancreatic tissues alone without

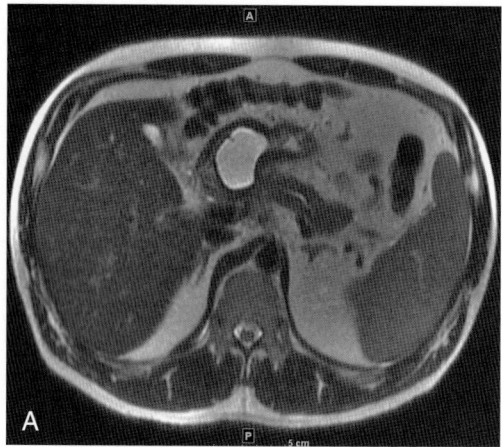

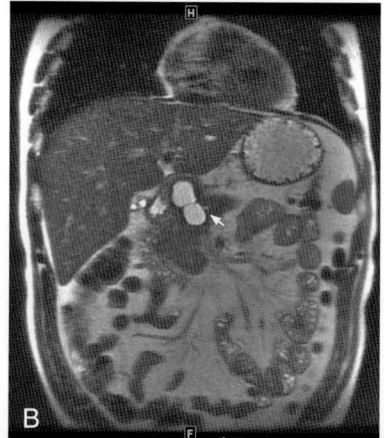

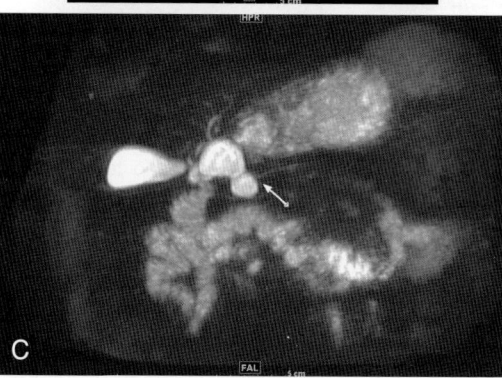

FIGURE 17.6 **Pseudocyst communication with main duct.** Axial T2-weighted magnetic resonance imaging (MRI) **(A)** demonstrates a pseudocyst adjacent to the pancreatic head. Coronal T2-weighted images **(B)** and maximum intensity projection (MIP) T2-weighted images **(C)** demonstrate communication between the pseudocyst and the main pancreatic duct *(arrows)*.

parenchymal necrosis occurs in 25%, and pancreatic necrosis alone without peripancreatic collections is the least common, occurring in 5%.[10]

At early imaging within the first few days of pain onset, NP will appear as patchy enhancement, potentially indistinguishable from IEP, and with potential underestimation of the eventual extent of necrosis.[10] At around five to seven days, the necrotic, nonenhancing parenchyma will become demarcated, and peripancreatic necrotic collections may develop (Fig. 17.7).[10] If parenchymal necrosis is present, the amount of necrosis should be estimated according to either the CTSI or mCTSI

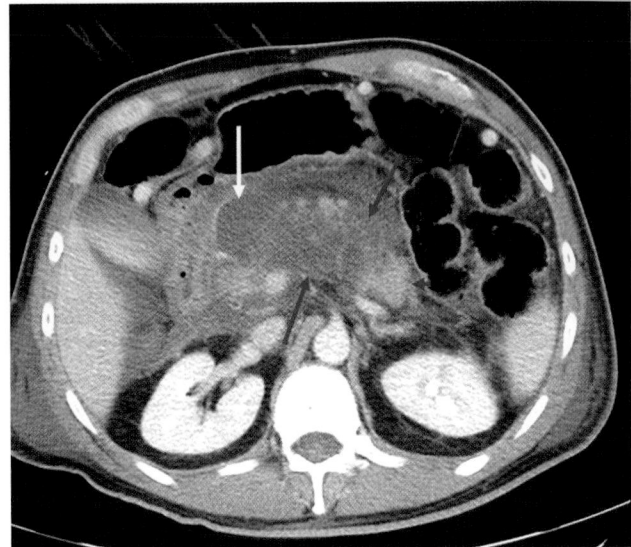

FIGURE 17.7 Axial computed tomography (CT) in the portal venous phase. Necrotizing pancreatitis with regions of nonenhancing pancreatic parenchyma at the pancreatic neck and body *(long red arrows)*, with sparing of the pancreatic tail, with preserved normal enhancement *(short red arrow)*. An acute necrotic collection *(long white arrow)* is present anterior to the pancreatic head.

systems.[14,18] Parenchymal necrosis predominantly affects the neck and body, and the head and tail may be spared. If there is confluent necrosis extending over 2 cm at the head, neck, or body, the pancreatic duct may be disrupted and pancreatic fluid from the isolated non-necrotic distal body or tail will leak into soft tissues, causing fistulas and collections.[19] The disrupted

duct may be best identified with ERCP or secretin MRCP. The isolated duct may not be dilated.[19]

Pancreatic and peripancreatic fluid collections occur in NP, and these have different and specific terms to the fluid collections found in IEP. A collection present within the first four weeks of NP is termed an "acute necrotic collection" (ANC). These can occur within the pancreas or peripancreatic tissue, are often multiple, loculated, and can extend into the pelvis.[11] ANC contain a variable amount of fluid, debris, and necrotic tissue.[10] At imaging, the debris and necrotic tissue will appear as nonenhancing solid components or fat globules.[11] The term ANC is still used in NP to describe any fluid collection, even if the collection lacks debris.[10] After four weeks, the collections will become encapsulated with a well-defined, thick enhancing wall, termed "walled off necrosis" (WON).[10] These can occur in both the pancreatic parenchyma and peripancreatic tissues and may form coalescent collections.[11] MRI is superior to CT in demonstrating the internal debris present with WON.[20] The internal debris usually appears as dependant, nonenhancing T2 hypointense material on MRI,[21] and as soft tissue or high attention on CT (Fig. 17.8). Infected necrosis does not have specific imaging findings; air within the necrotic areas can indicate infection but may also be secondary to fistula.

Leaked pancreatic proteolytic enzymes can cause weakening of vessel walls and the formation of pseudoaneurysms, most commonly involving the splenic, gastroduodenal, and pancreaticoduodenal arteries, and may lead to life-threatening hemorrhage (see Chapter 115). If hemorrhage is clinically suspected, a multiphase CT with both arterial and portal venous phases should be performed.[12] On imaging, pseudoaneurysms will show a connection to an adjacent vessel and enhance similar to arteries.[22] Other local complications that may be evident on imaging include splenic or

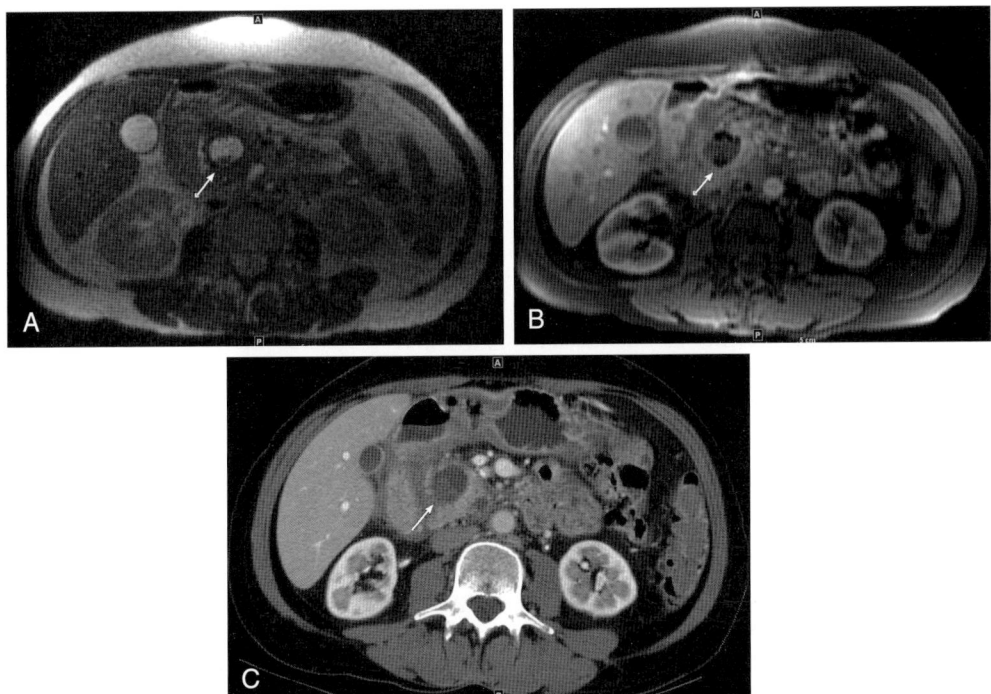

FIGURE 17.8 Walled off necrosis. A, Magnetic resonance imaging (MRI) demonstrates a T2 hyperintense focus at the pancreatic head with hypointense debris *(arrow)* exhibiting blooming artifact on **(B)** fat-saturated T1-weighted contrast images. **C,** Contrast-enhanced computed tomography (CT) 1 week later shows the fluid-attenuation and nonenhancing debris within the walled-off necrosis.

portal vein thrombosis, gastric outlet obstruction, and colonic necrosis.[10]

Chronic Pancreatitis

Although transabdominal US may be the initial modality used in the assessment of chronic abdominal pain, a frequent symptom of chronic pancreatitis (CP), it has the lowest accuracy and is not recommended for initial assessment.[1,23] CT and MRI/MRCP are ideal first choices because they have comparable diagnostic performance and are noninvasive.[23] CT is best for visualization of pancreatic calcification, whereas ductal and early parenchymal changes are better evaluated on MRI.[1] The role of ERCP and EUS is discussed in Chapters 20 and 22, respectively (also see Chapters 57–58).

Pancreatic calcification is commonly seen in CP and is the most specific CT imaging feature.[24] Chronic alcoholic pancreatitis is the most common cause of pancreatic calcification in the United States, although CP related to other causes such as hyperparathyroidism and tropical pancreatitis may also cause calcifications.[25] Importantly, pancreatic calcification is characteristically seen in other causes of pancreatitis, such as gallstones, drugs, viruses, and trauma.[25] The calcifications are always present within the ductal system; however, this may be difficult to discern on imaging.[24] The calcifications can vary widely in size, ranging from punctate to large coarse foci.[24] The distribution may also vary from focal to diffuse involvement, with the pancreatic head usually more prominently affected than the tail.[24,25] Coarse calcifications are a definite sign of CP,[26] and innumerable punctate calcifications strongly suggest CP.[27] The number and size of calculi are independent of disease duration and the degree of gland atrophy.[28] Although calcifications are more frequently detected with increasing CP severity, the degree of calcification is not indicative of clinical severity or vice versa.[28,29] Many patients with severe exocrine dysfunction may have a normal-appearing pancreas on CT.[1]

Although MRI/MRCP may be normal in early CP,[1] it is an excellent modality to assess the pancreatic duct with strong correlation to ERCP findings.[30] Dilatation of the main duct (>3.5 mm) is commonly seen and the duct may have a variable smooth, beaded, or irregular appearance with strictures.[1,24] The dilatation of the main duct with alternating strictures and stenoses causes a classic "chain of lakes" appearance.[31] Side branch dilatation can be seen predominantly in advanced cases on MRCP but may be missed in early disease.[32] Intraductal calculi will be seen as filing defects in high signal pancreatic fluid.[32] Features that favor ductal dilatation because of CP over PDAC-related ductal obstruction include the presence of intraductal or parenchymal calcifications, irregular ductal dilatation, relative limited gland atrophy, and, of course, the lack of a discrete mass.[1] Secretin MRI can help in the diagnosis of early CP by assessing the exocrine parenchyma and ductal response to secretin.[1]

MRI is also very sensitive to detect parenchymal abnormalities associated with CP, and these may precede ductal abnormalities.[1,33] Fat-suppressed T1 is best for evaluating the pancreatic parenchymal atrophy and fibrosis seen with CP. Early on, this will appear as subtle areas of decreased T1 signal within the pancreas[1] and later as more diffuse parenchymal fibrosis and atrophy. On dynamic postcontrast MRI, the fibrotic parenchyma in CP will demonstrate delayed and reduced enhancement compared with a normal pancreas.[1] The fibrotic parenchyma in CP can demonstrate restricted diffusion with low ADC compared with normal pancreas.[1]

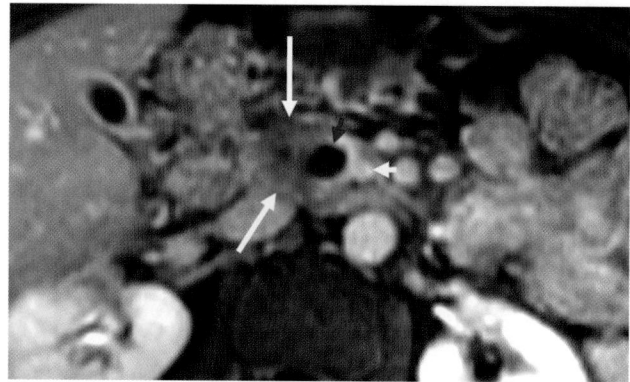

FIGURE 17.9 Axial postcontrast T1 fat-saturated magnetic resonance imaging (MRI), chronic pancreatitis with an ill-defined hypoenhancing inflammatory mass at the pancreatic head *(long arrows)*. Note normal enhancing parenchyma at the medial pancreatic head *(short arrow)*. The common bile duct *(short red arrow)* is markedly hypointense because of pneumobilia.

Pseudocysts can be observed in CP without any clinical or biochemical evidence of acute pancreatitis.[24] Some CP patients can experience superimposed episodes of acute pancreatitis, and therefore imaging features, such as fluid collections, peripancreatic stranding, and abscesses, may be present.[24]

Pseudotumors or focal benign inflammatory masses may occur in CP, with a small series reporting the presence in nearly 30% of patients.[24] The masses most commonly occur in the pancreatic head and are often indistinguishable from PDAC; additionally patients with chronic pancreatitis are at increased risk for PDAC.[34,35] On CT, calcification in the mass favors an inflammatory mass over PDAC.[24] On MRI, ductal structures and the duct penetrating sign in the mass are indicative of an inflammatory mass, whereas these findings are absent in PDAC.[36] On postcontrast T1 sequences, inflammatory masses are usually ill-defined and poorly demarcated, whereas PDAC will show relative demarcation to normal pancreas (Fig. 17.9).[37] Both inflammatory masses and PDAC will usually have lower ADC values compared with normal pancreas, and PDAC has been demonstrated to have significant lower ADC values compared with inflammatory masses[38]; however, the ADC values in PDAC can be variable (as discussed later).

Groove Pancreatitis

Groove pancreatitis is an inflammatory plate-like mass involving the groove between the pancreatic head, duodenum, and the common bile duct that may be partially cystic. The cystic change may be associated with duodenal stenosis and wall thickening, which may lead to abdominal pain and vomiting.[39,40]

Classic imaging features include loss of fat planes between the pancreatic head and the duodenum. Associated ill-defined sheet-like soft tissue will demonstrate arterial phase hypoenhancement and progressive patchy delayed enhancement because of fibrosis, often with small cysts or even a multilocular cystic mass.[41] Coarse calcifications may be visible at CT (Fig. 17.10). At MRI, groove pancreatitis is typically hypointense to pancreatic parenchyma on T1-weighted images and is of variable signal intensity on T2-weighted images, depending on the acuity of the process, decreasing in signal with chronicity and increasing fibrosis.[42] Decreased T1 signal can also be seen in the pancreatic head or diffusely. There is often narrowing of both the lower common

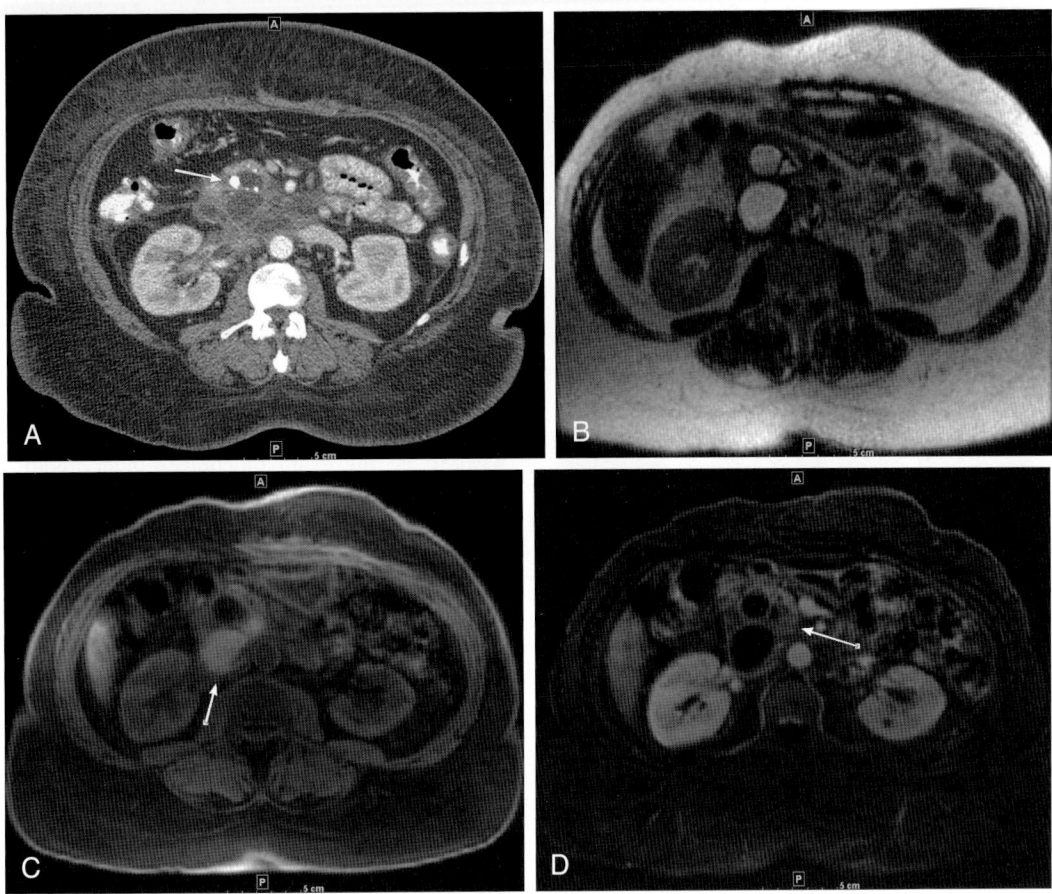

FIGURE 17.10   **Groove pancreatitis in a 60-year-old woman with history of pancreatitis, alcohol, and tobacco use. A,** Contrast-enhanced computed tomography (CT) demonstrates a multicystic lesion at the region of the pancreaticoduodenal groove, with several coarse calcifications *(arrow)* and sheet-like soft tissue effacing fat planes. **B,** Axial T2 hyperintense magnetic resonance imaging (MRI) demonstrates cystic components and hypointense surrounding tissue. **C,** Fat-saturated T1-weighted precontrast MRI demonstrates hemorrhage or proteinaceous material within some of the cystic components *(arrow).* **D,** T1 postcontrast subtraction imaging reveals no enhancement of the cystic foci, but some enhancement of surrounding tissue *(arrow)* in the portal venous phase.

bile duct and main pancreatic duct, with upstream ductal dilatation (more often of the bile duct) and widening of the space between the two. Cystic components of mixed size and complexity are often best seen on T2-weighted images along the thickened duodenal wall, a sign that carries some specificity.[41] Because the entity can be extremely difficult to distinguish from necrotic PDAC, groove pancreatitis is often a diagnosis of exclusion.

Autoimmune Pancreatitis

Two types of autoimmune pancreatitis (AIP) are recognized; type 1 is the most recognized type, which is a multi-organ disease that is associated with elevated immunoglobulin G4 (IgG4) levels.[43,44] Type 2 AIP is a pancreatic specific disease not associated with an elevated IgG4.[43,44]

Both type 1 and type 2 AIP will appear similar on imaging; however, type 2 is more frequently focal (85% of cases) and will lack extrapancreatic disease (see Chapter 54).[43] AIP causes enlargement of the pancreas in a focal, multifocal, or diffuse pattern.[45] Focal AIP most commonly affects the pancreatic head.[46] Diffuse AIP is characterized by sausage-shaped enlargement of the pancreas with loss of normal pancreatic contour lobulations and clefts (Fig. 17.11). A capsule-like rim or "halo"

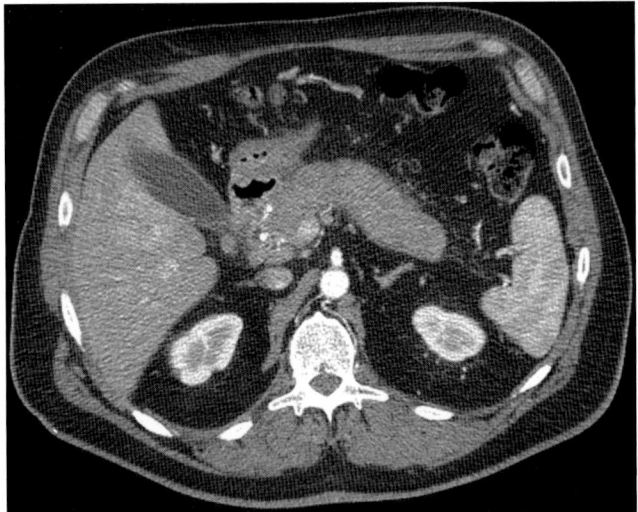

FIGURE 17.11   **Axial computed tomography (CT) in pancreatic parenchymal/late arterial phase.** Diffuse autoimmune pancreatitis as evidence of diffuse enlargement of the pancreas with hypoenhancement. Note the lack of surrounding fluid.

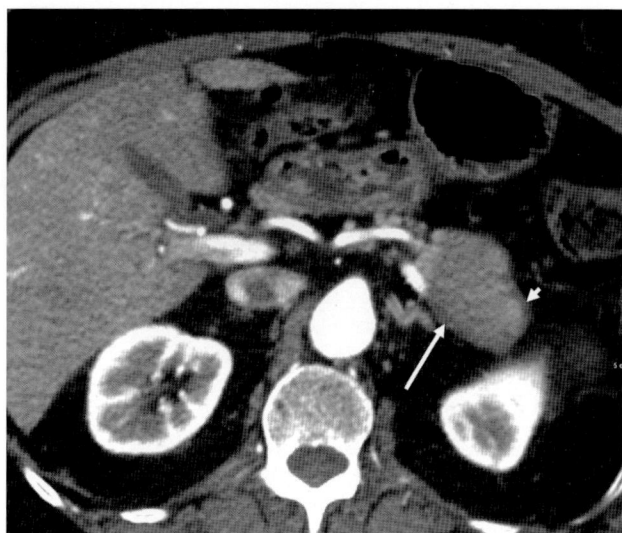

FIGURE 17.12 Focal autoimmune pancreatitis. Axial computed tomography (CT) in pancreatic parenchymal/late arterial phase with focal mass-like enlargement and hypoenhancement of the pancreatic tail *(long arrow)*, with a small hypoenhancing halo *(short arrow)* partially surrounding the mass.

in the peripancreatic tissue is common and characteristic of AIP and is thought to correspond to inflammatory soft tissue (Fig. 17.12).[47,48]

On CT, the affected regions of the pancreas will demonstrate progressive enhancement, hypodense to normal pancreas in the pancreatic parenchymal phase, iso/hypodense in the portal venous phase, and hyperdense in the delayed phase.[47–49] This is in contrast to PDAC, a frequent differential diagnosis in the case of focal disease, which is more commonly hypodense in both pancreatic parenchymal and portal venous phases.[49] The characteristic capsule-like rim or "halo" will appear hypodense on CT, hypointense on T1 and T2 MRI, and demonstrate delayed postcontrast enhancement.[47,50]

On MRI, the affected area will appear hypointense on precontrast T1 and heterogeneously hyperintense on T2.[47,50] On MRCP there is generally diffuse multifocal irregular narrowing of the pancreatic duct.[51] The pancreatic duct may not be visualized at all in the affected regions.[48,52] Upstream pancreatic duct dilatation and parenchymal atrophy is rare but has been reported.[48] Tapered narrowing and enhancement of the distal common bile duct is commonly seen, and multiple biliary strictures may be evident.[51,53] AIP will demonstrate restricted diffusion with low ADC; this generally normalizes with corticosteroid treatment.[54]

Extrapancreatic lesions are common in type 1 AIP, reported in 45% to 92% of patients.[45,48,55,56] The lesions can involve numerous organs throughout the body. Common manifestations include hilar, peripancreatic, and para-aortic lymphadenopathy; biliary duct wall thickening; soft tissue masses in the kidneys, ureters, orbits, and retroperitoneum with retroperitoneal fibrosis; and swelling of the salivary and lachrymal glands.[55] Renal involvement, demonstrated in up to 35% of patients, most commonly involves the renal cortex. These lesions are hypoenhancing and may manifest as diffuse patchy involvement, round or wedge-shaped lesions, or as small peripheral cortical nodules.[57] Lesions will decrease with corticosteroid treatment.[57]

CYSTIC PANCREATIC LESIONS

Cystic pancreatic lesions as a group include a large number of benign, premalignant, and malignant entities (see Chapter 60).[58] The five most common constituents that include the vast majority of cases are: complications of pancreatitis, including pseudocyst (described previously), the mucinous entities of intraductal papillary mucinous neoplasm (IPMN) and mucinous cystic neoplasm (MCN), and serous cystic neoplasms like serous cystadenoma (SCA). Pancreatic neuroendocrine tumors can also appear as predominately cystic lesions and are described later in this chapter.

MRI and CT are the preferred modalities for the noninvasive characterization of cystic lesions.[59,60] Both imaging modalities have similar utility with dedicated protocols,[61–63] although a consensus of radiologists had traditionally deemed MRI to be the exam of choice—older iterations of current guidelines cite MRI's superior contrast resolution facilitating recognition of septa, nodules, and duct communication, and the benefit of avoiding radiation exposure.[64,65]

Cystic lesions may also be detected by transabdominal US, but at a lower rate than MRI or CT[66] and with limited ability to distinguish between cystic neoplasms and pseudocysts (40%–50% specificity).[67] Therefore the role of US in the evaluation of cystic pancreatic lesions remains limited, in sharp contradistinction with EUS, which plays a major role in the diagnostic workup of these lesions (see Chapter 22).

Cystic Pancreatic Tumors

Intraductal Papillary Mucinous Neoplasm

IPMNs are mucin-producing neoplasms that arise from the main pancreatic duct or its branches and exhibit a spectrum of dysplasia from low-grade to high-grade to invasive carcinoma (see Chapter 60–62).[68] They are the most common cystic neoplasms and may represent up to 30% of all cystic pancreatic lesions. As cross-sectional imaging, and particularly MRI, have become more common, IPMNs are now being discovered frequently as incidental small pancreatic cystic lesions on scans obtained for other indications.[58,69]

IPMNs can be classified into main duct, branch duct, and mixed type varieties, based either on imaging appearance or histopathology.[70–75] The importance of this distinction is highlighted in an analysis of a group of studies from 2003 to 2010 demonstrating that, among main duct and mixed-type IPMN, prevalence of invasive carcinoma was 44% to 45% versus only 16.6% in the branch duct type (overall 30.8% prevalence in 3568 specimens).[65] Among IPMNs without invasive carcinoma, actuarial risk of future carcinoma development is also much higher among main and mixed types.[76]

On CT or MRI, it is largely the mucin produced by the tumor that is identified rather than the neoplastic epithelium itself. When present, however, visible enhancing mural solid nodules may actually represent the cellular elements. Such nodules and main duct dilatation are associated with the presence of invasive cancer and high-grade dysplasia (Fig. 17.13)[77–80]; therefore they are given considerable import in the revised 2017 international consensus Fukuoka guidelines (discussed later).

Main duct IPMN is characterized on CT or MRI by diffuse or segmental dilatation of the main pancreatic duct to more than 5 mm caliber, without another identifiable cause of obstruction (Fig. 17.14). At MRI, this is best seen on

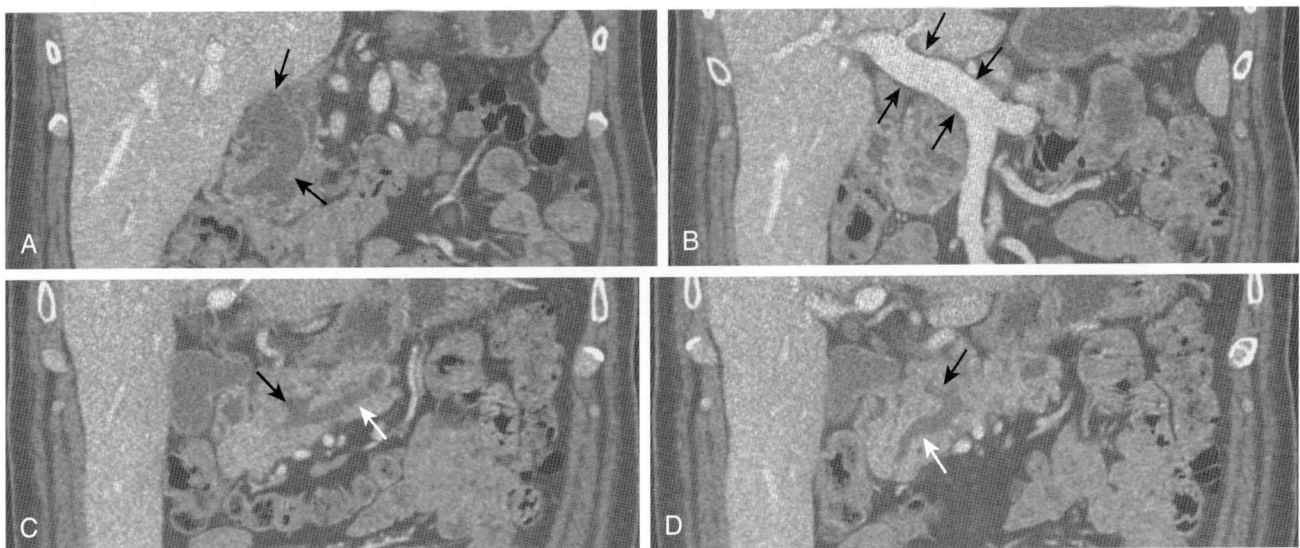

FIGURE 17.13 Coronal computed tomography (CT) in the portal venous phase demonstrates an intraductal papillary mucinous neoplasm (IPMN)-associated tumor. A, C, D, These show dilatation/expansion of the main *(white arrows)* and branch *(black arrows)* pancreatic ducts by invasive adenocarcinoma. **B,** Normal appearing portal vein *(black arrows)* with no evidence of tumor vascular encasement (no tumor vascular involvement was found at surgery or at pathologic examination).

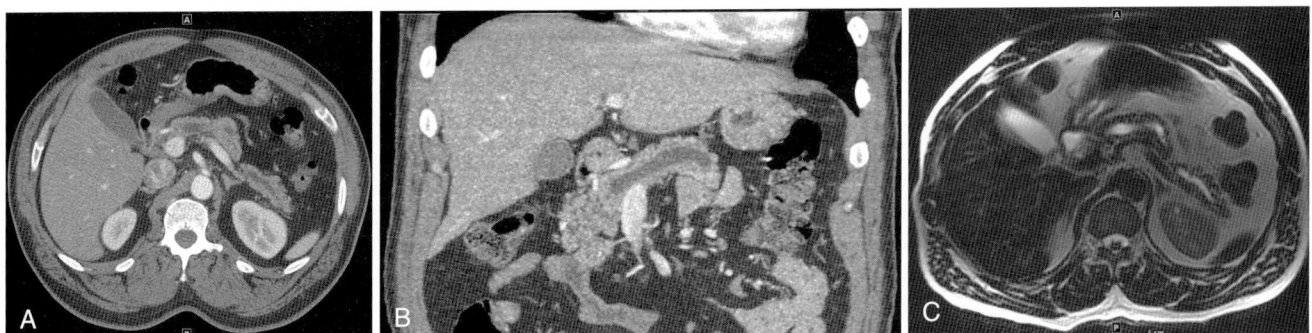

FIGURE 17.14 Main duct intraductal papillary mucinous neoplasm (IPMN). A, Axial and **(B)** coronal contrast-enhanced computed tomography (CT) and **(C)** axial T2-weighted magnetic resonance imaging (MRI) demonstrates dilation of the main pancreatic duct to 9 mm caliber.

T2-weighted images where fluid in the duct has markedly hyperintense signal. Mural nodules, mucin globules, or a dilated major or minor papilla bulging into the duodenal lumen may be seen.[81]

Branch duct IPMN can occur anywhere in the gland, most commonly in the pancreatic head, and may be multifocal in approximately 30% of cases.[82] They appear as a cluster of round or tubular lesions or a single lesion with fluid attenuation (0–20 HU) on CT or T2 hyperintense fluid signal on MRI with no or few septa (Fig. 17.15). A microcystic pattern has also been described, in which multiple thin septa separate numerous fluid-filled spaces.[81,83] Communication with a nondilated main pancreatic duct is often seen, particularly at thin-section three-dimensional (3D) MRCP images.[84] The presence of the lesion in the pancreatic head may compress the common bile duct, resulting in dilation of the intrahepatic bile ducts. As with the main duct type, mural nodules may be present. A mixed-type IPMN is designated when features of both branch and main duct types are present.

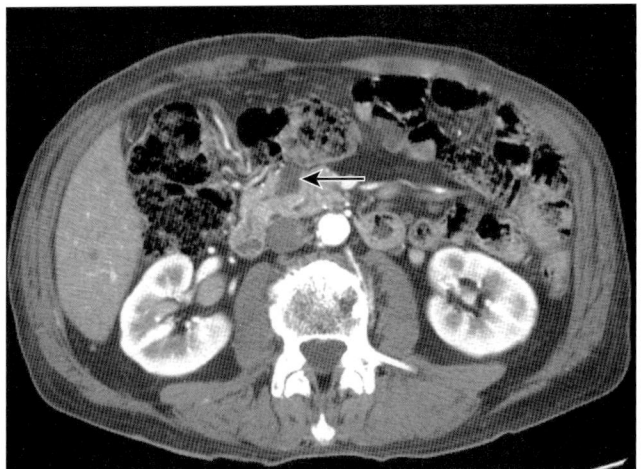

FIGURE 17.15 Axial computed tomography (CT) in the arterial phase of contrast enhancement shows a fluid-attenuation intraductal papillary mucinous neoplasm (IPMN) in the pancreatic head *(arrow).*

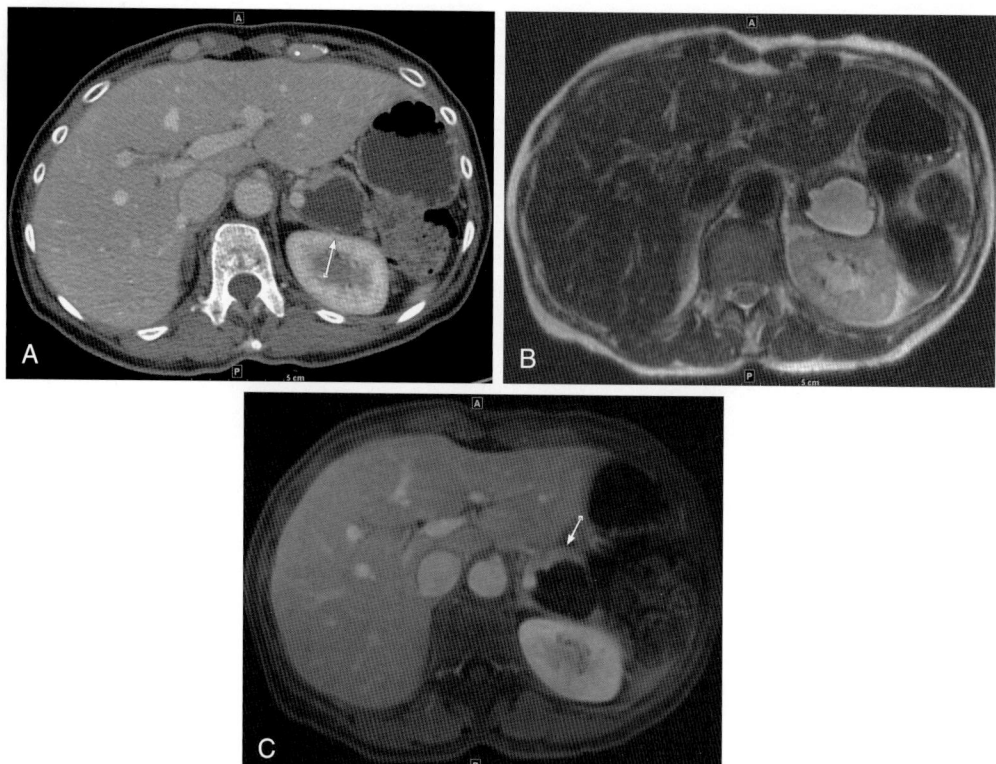

FIGURE 17.16 **Mucinous cystic neoplasm in a 55-year-old woman. A**, Computed tomography (CT) demonstrates an ovoid cystic lesion with a punctate mural calcification *(arrow)* in the pancreatic tail. The lesion is hyperintense on axial T2 hyperintense magnetic resonance imaging MRI **(B)**. **C**, Post contrast fat-saturated T1-weighted MRI demonstrates a thickened pseudocapsule and a barely perceptible thin septation.

Mucinous Cystic Neoplasms

Characterized histologically by the presence of progesterone and estrogen receptor-positive ovarian-type stroma, mucinous cystic neoplasms (MCNs) have been considered nearly exclusively tumors of perimenopausal women (see Chapter 60).[58] Although there is a growing body of case reports of tumors considered by pathology to be MCN in males,[85] a pathology review continues to describe the entity as nearly exclusively a lesion of women.[86] MCNs are a pathologically heterogeneous group, including benign mucin-producing epithelium, dysplasia, carcinoma in situ, and invasive tumor (mucinous cyst adenocarcinoma).

The typical appearance of MCN is a loculated cystic lesion occurring most commonly in the pancreatic body or tail (90%–95%). Morphologically, they appear as round or ovoid—"orange-like," rather than the more "grape-like" clustered appearance of IPMN, with locules or pauciseptate individual cystic components, which are larger than the typical cystic components seen with serous cystadenoma (Fig. 17.16). Unlike IPMN, the lesions tend to be solitary and only rarely demonstrate communication with the main pancreatic duct if there is associated fistula formation. Mildly thickened, enhancing septa are common in MCN, and a delayed enhancing pseudocapsule may be seen.[82] Peripheral calcification may be demonstrated on CT. On MRI, the lesions appear as simple fluid with T2 hyperintensity and usually T1 hypointensity, despite the mucinous contents, although occasionally lesions may have a more variable T1-weighted signal.[87] Features that can be associated with malignancy (mucinous cystadenocarcinomas) are a thick wall (>2 mm), thick septations, and calcification within the wall or

septa (Fig. 17.17).[88] In any case, the presence of internal enhancing soft tissue elements is indicative of carcinoma.

Serous Cystadenoma

Pancreatic serous cystic neoplasms represent about 20% of all cystic pancreatic lesions and approximately 30% of cystic neoplasms (see Chapter 60).[58] They are largely benign serous cystadenoma (SCA) with extremely rare instances of malignant serous cystadenocarcinoma,[89] which can only be diagnosed on imaging in the presence of metastases.[86] SCAs are indolent tumors with a slight female predilection, usually presenting in the 5th to 7th decades of life, often as an incidental radiographic finding in asymptomatic patients. Previously, these tumors had been called microcystic adenomas, a term that has fallen out of favor because of reported macrocystic and oligocystic variants.[90]

SCA tumors most commonly occur in the pancreatic body and tail and may vary in size from 1 mm to several centimeters; they may be large at the time of discovery because of their slow-growing and potential asymptomatic nature. The lesions are generally lobulated and surrounded by a fibrous capsule. SCA tumors are typically comprised of numerous tiny cysts, which appear fluid-attenuation on CT and hyperintense on T2-weighted MRI. The individual cysts may be variable in size, but are typically less than 1 cm.[87] The cysts are sometimes so small that the cystic nature of the lesion becomes difficult to appreciate, with the appearance dominated by highly vascularized fibrous septa arranged in a honeycomb configuration radiating from a central nidus (Fig. 17.18). In this case, MRI is often superior to CT in demonstrating the tiny cystic regions.[91–93] At

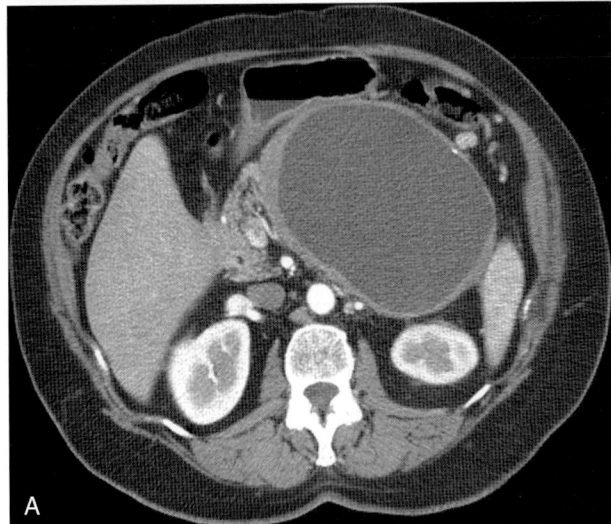

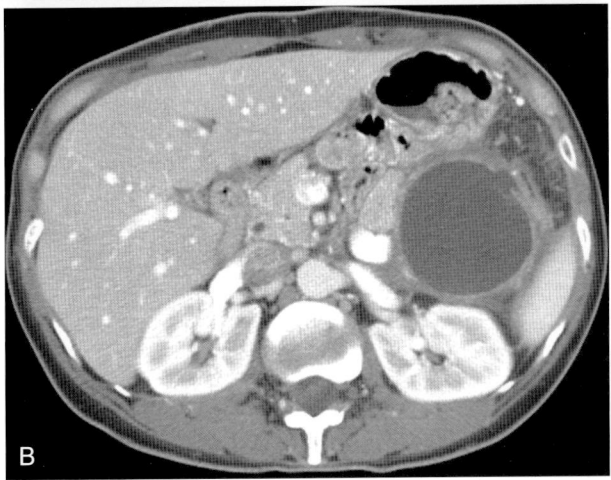

FIGURE 17.17 **Arterial phase axial computed tomography (CT) shows mucinous cystadenocarcinoma. A,** Thick-walled cystic lesion with punctate mural calcification in the pancreatic body and tail. **B,** A different patient with mural ulceration in the anterolateral aspect of the thick-walled mucinous adenocarcinoma at the pancreatic tail.

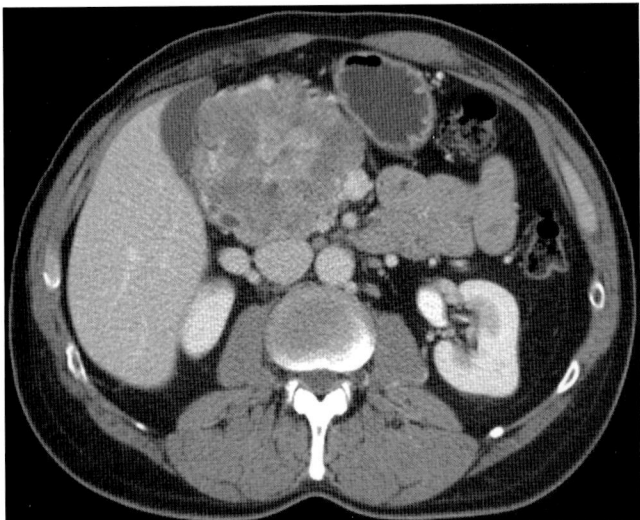

FIGURE 17.18 Portal venous phase axial computed tomography (CT) shows a typical lobulated serous cystadenoma (SCA) with enhancing radiating septa in the pancreatic head.

MRI, hemorrhage may be seen as higher T1-weighted signal, and the central nidus may enhance on delayed postcontrast imaging (Fig. 17.19). Stellate calcification of the central nidus strongly suggests the diagnosis of SCA; however, it is only seen in approximately 30% of cases.[81] This feature may also be identified at US.[94,95] Transabdominal US is otherwise not well suited as a characterization tool because numerous tiny cystic spaces may create multiple interfaces and not be resolved individually, causing the cystic component to appear echogenic or solid appearing. Nevertheless, internal architecture with honeycomb or spongy appearance can sometimes be delineated at higher frequency magnified US imaging (Fig. 17.20).

In contrast to IPMN, SCA do not communicate with the pancreatic duct.[86] In the absence of classic features suggesting SCA, such as multicystic morphology with a central nidus, differentiation from mucinous entities (particularly IPMN) may be challenging,[96–99] and many cases are still diagnosed only upon resection.[100]

Differentiating Cystic Pancreatic Tumors

One of the chief imaging challenges is distinguishing the mucinous lesions of IPMN and MCN, which have malignant potential, from other benign pancreatic cystic lesions (pseudocyst and SCA).[63] To address this issue, several guidelines have been proposed within the past decade for imaging work-up and management of cystic lesions. The aforementioned revised 2017 international consensus Fukuoka guidelines,[59] and a section of the white paper produced by the incidental findings committee of the American College of Radiology (ACR), also updated in 2017,[60] are two of the more influential papers. Although there are differences in focus and recommendations, both guidelines support under certain circumstances a role for imaging surveillance that had been suggested by previous work.[91,93]

The 2017 ACR white paper proposes an algorithmic approach to all incidentally detected cystic lesions lacking solid elements in asymptomatic patients. The paper stratifies the approach with five separate algorithms based on patient age, lesion size, and presence of discernible communication with the main duct, with roles for imaging surveillance of varying frequency and length and further characterization by EUS.[60]

The 2017 international consensus Fukuoka guidelines, being aimed at already-suspected mucinous lesions (not restricted to asymptomatic patients), puts more emphasis on two groups of features: "high-risk stigmata," including main duct caliber greater than 9 mm and enhancing mural nodule greater than 5 mm, and "worrisome features," including main duct 5 to 9 mm caliber, abrupt caliber transition (more dilated upstream) with distal gland atrophy, nonenhancing mural nodules, size greater than 3 cm, associated lymphadenopathy, and change in size greater than 5 mm over two years. Imaging-only surveillance is recommended only for lesions without any of these imaging features in patients also without any of three specified clinical features (obstructive jaundice, elevated carbohydrate antigen [CA] 19-9, and pancreatitis).[59] One potential problem in applying this approach has been that agreement on the presence of certain imaging features may not be repeatable among radiologists.[101] Although the two guidelines have made a strong contribution to the management approach of these lesions, neither has gained universal acceptance as yet, and they may evolve with time. Challenging cases may be discussed at tumor boards using a combination of clinical judgment and imaging data to guide management decisions.

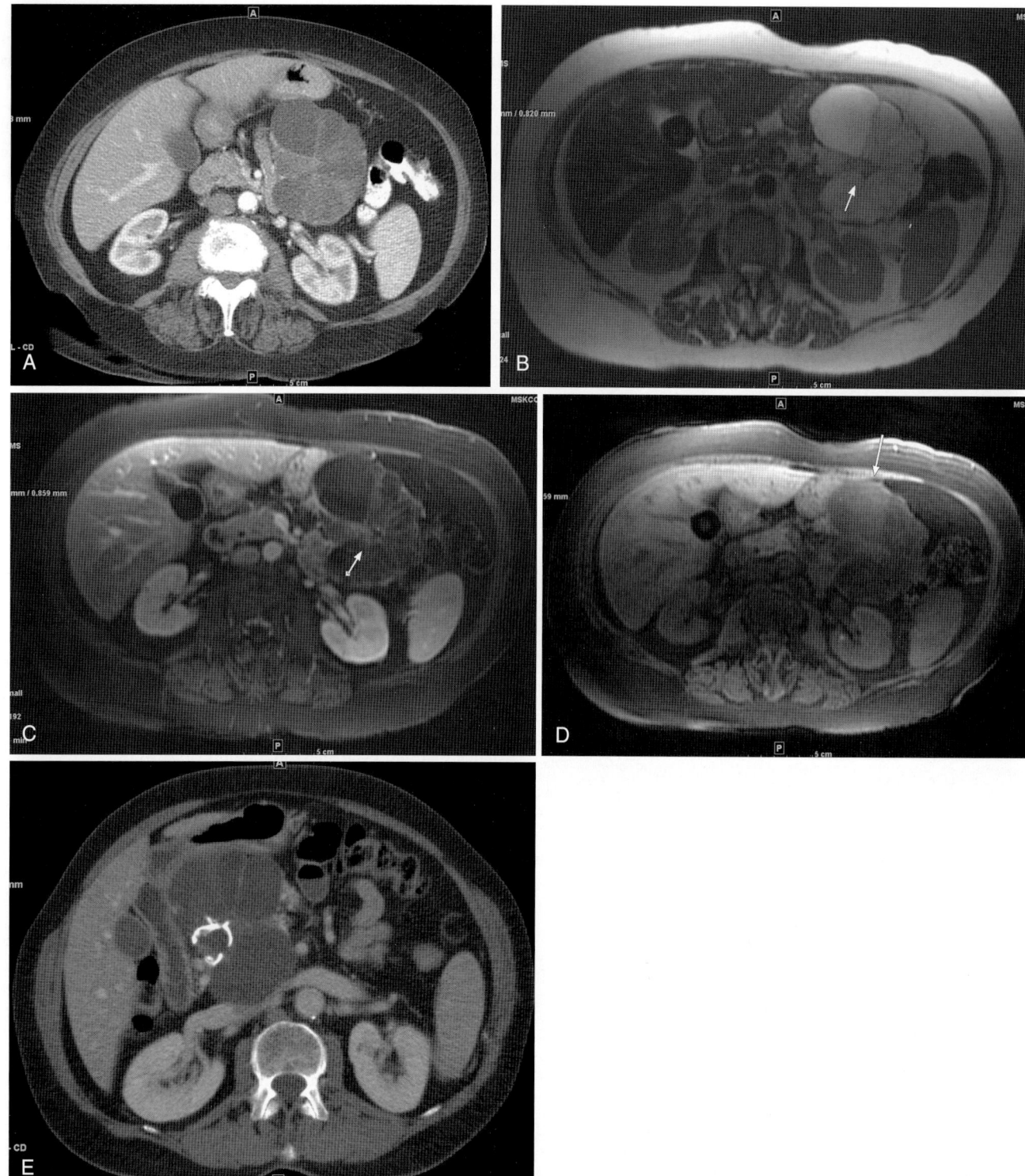

FIGURE 17.19   Serous cystadenoma (SCA). A, Contrast-enhanced computed tomography (CT) demonstrates a lobulated cystic lesion radiating around a central nidus. **B**, Axial T2-weighted magnetic resonance imaging (MRI) demonstrates the T2 hypointense central nidus *(arrow)* that enhances on postcontrast fat-saturated T1-weighted MRI **(C)** *(arrow)*. **D**, Precontrast fat-saturated T1-weighted MRI demonstrates hemorrhage or protein-aceous material in an anterior cystic component *(arrow)* that developed in the year after the CT image in **A**. **E**, CT of another patient demonstrates a SCA in the pancreatic head with calcification of the central nidus.

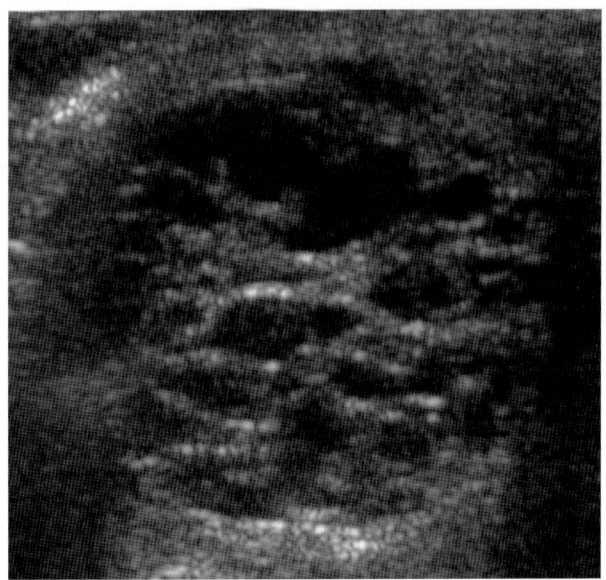

FIGURE 17.20 Serous cystadenoma of the pancreas. Magnified transverse intraoperative ultrasound images of the pancreatic tail demonstrate the typical honeycomb architecture of the lesion with anechoic areas bounded by echogenic septa.

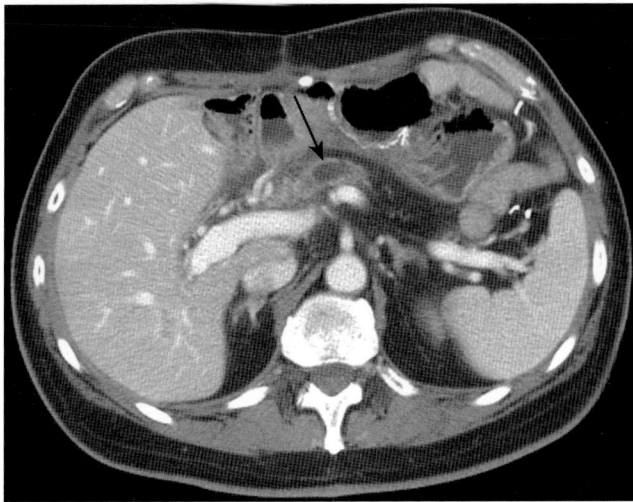

FIGURE 17.21 Axial computed tomography (CT) in portal venous phase shows abrupt cut off of the pancreatic duct with upstream dilatation *(arrow)* secondary to a small hypoenhancing pancreatic head/neck ductal adenocarcinoma.

Other Cystic Pancreatic Lesions

Lymphangiomas are congenital malformations of the lymphatic system, which result from obstruction of the lymph flow and formation of multiloculated serous, serosanguineous, or chylous cystic lesions. They are indolent, often incidentally discovered, and tend to occur more commonly in women. They can be seen as peripancreatic or pancreatic lesions[58] and may reach a large size up to 25 cm (average 12 cm).[102] On CT, they appear as well-circumscribed, often multilocular fluid attenuation lesions with an enhancing capsule, thin septa, and, rarely, calcification. At MRI, they have the typical T2 hyperintense signal of fluid with T2 hypointense fibrous septa.[103,104] On US, they appear complex because of internal septa and also may have internal echoes if they are secondarily infected. Rare calcifications can produce acoustic shadowing.

SOLID PANCREATIC LESIONS

Pancreatic Ductal Adenocarcinoma

Imaging is used in PDAC for initial diagnosis, assessment of resectability, and detection of metastatic disease (see Chapters 61 and 62). The National Comprehensive Cancer Network (NCCN) recommends that any patient with a clinical suspicion of PDAC and evidence of a dilated pancreatic or bile duct or stricture should undergo initial evaluation with a pancreatic protocol CT.[105] NCCN endorses a dual-phase pancreatic protocol with imaging obtained in the pancreatic parenchymal and portal venous phases.[106] The NCCN recommends CT as the preferred modality for preoperative assessment because it is widely available and can be extended to include both the chest and pelvis for staging purposes. MRI can be used if a CECT is contraindicated, or as a problem-solving tool, particularly if a suspected tumor is not visible on CT or for the characterization of indeterminate liver lesions.[105] A 2016 meta-analysis found that CT and MRI were comparable in diagnosis and assessment

of vascular involvement.[107] Nevertheless, MRI is more sensitive in detecting hepatic metastases[108] (see Chapter 15).

In the setting of a known pancreatic tumor, high-quality imaging of the pancreas should be performed, even if standard portal venous phase CT imaging is available. This should be performed within four weeks of surgery, after the completion of neoadjuvant therapy (if applicable), and before stenting whenever possible.[105]

In addition, the NCCN recommends the use of the PDAC radiology reporting template,[106] which is a consensus statement from the American Pancreatic Association and Society of Abdominal Radiology.[105] This template facilitates a comprehensive and standardized approach in the reporting of PDAC to optimize treatment recommendations.[106] In particular, the template standardizes terminology for tumor vascular involvement, with an at least 180-degree degree tumor vascular contact classified as abutment and a greater than 180-degree tumor vascular contact classified as encasement.[106]

On CT, PDAC typically appears as an ill-defined solid mass, hypoattenuating to normal pancreatic parenchyma in both the pancreatic parenchymal and portal venous phases.[109] Tumors are often accompanied by secondary signs of abrupt pancreatic duct cut-off (Fig. 17.21), pancreatic or bile duct obstruction, upstream pancreatic atrophy, and/or contour abnormality.[110] These secondary signs are important clues to the presence of PDAC and may be present on CT many months before patients becoming symptomatic with disease.[111]

Tumors located in the pancreatic head may cause dilatation of both the pancreatic and bile ducts, which is called the "double-duct sign."[112] Pancreatic tail tumors generally present later, are larger, and are more infiltrative at the time of diagnosis.[113]

Approximately 5% of PDACs are isoattenuating to normal pancreas on both phases of dual-phase pancreatic protocol CT, and these have been shown to have increased survival compared with hypoattenuating tumors.[114] Additionally small tumors (≤20 mm) are more likely to be isoattenuating and difficult to discretely visualize; however, they are often accompanied by secondary signs.[110] In the case of suspected PDAC

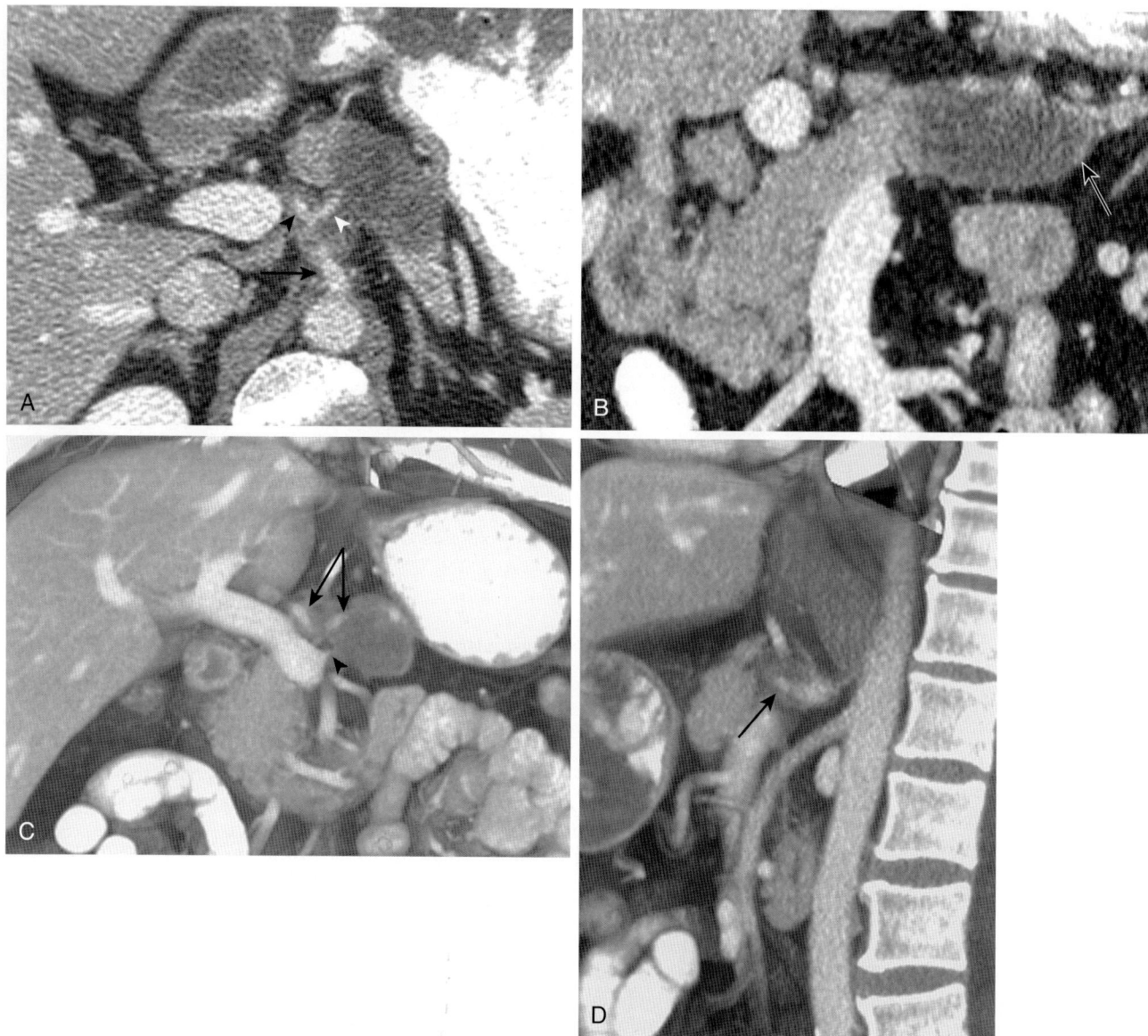

FIGURE 17.22 **Pancreatic ductal adenocarcinoma with vascular encasement. A,** Hypoenhancing tumor in the body and tail of the pancreas tracks posteriorly to encase the celiac axis, the proximal hepatic artery *(black arrowhead),* and the splenic artery *(white arrowhead).* **B,** Curved multiplanar reconstruction showing the tumor *(arrow)* in the body and tail of the pancreas. **C,** Coronal volume-rendered image shows the tumor occluding the splenic vein *(arrowhead)* and encasing celiac axis branches *(arrows).* **D,** Sagittal volume-rendered image shows tumor encasing the celiac axis *(arrow).*

without visible tumor on pancreatic protocol CT, further assessment should be considered with endoscopic US (EUS), MRI, or positron emission tomography (PET)/CT.[105,110]

Detailed assessment of tumor vascular involvement is required to ultimately determine the resectability of the tumor and should be described using the previously described standardized terms of abutment (≤180 degrees) and encasement (>180 degrees).[106] Vessel deformity, narrowing, or occlusion are specific signs of vascular invasion (Fig. 17.22).[115–118] PDAC tumors are associated with peritumoral dense fibrotic reaction, which can abut or encase vessels.[119] It is often impossible to differentiate between benign fibrous soft tissue or tumoral vascular involvement, a common scenario after neoadjuvant therapy where differentiation between active tumor, treated tumor, tumor fibrosis, and treatment-related fibrosis is challenging.[120–123]

On MRI, PDAC generally appears hypointense to normal pancreatic parenchyma on precontrast T1 imaging and remains predominantly hypointense in the arterial/parenchymal phases.[112] The T2 signal is variable.[124] The conspicuity of tumors may be affected by pancreatic parenchymal changes related to upstream obstructive pancreatitis, or CP, which causes decreased T1 and increased T2 parenchymal signal changes.[110] Both the pancreatic and bile ducts are well visualised on MRCP, and tumor-related duct obstruction may be abrupt or gradual, with a smooth or beaded appearance of the dilated duct.[112] Tumors can have variable restricted diffusion because this depends on both tumor differentiation and density of fibrosis.[125]

Pancreatic Neuroendocrine Neoplasms

Pancreatic neuroendocrine neoplasms are a diverse group of tumors with varying clinical, functional, and histopathologic features (see Chapter 65).[126] They may be well-differentiated tumors (PNETs) or poorly differentiated carcinomas (PNECs). The 2017 revised World Health Organization (WHO) grading system[127] further classifies PNETs into grades according to number of mitoses and Ki-67 index. Grade 1 (<2 mitoses/10 HPF, <3% Ki-67) and grade 2 (2–20 mitoses/10 HPF, 3%–20% Ki-67) PNETs are considered low-grade tumors. Grade 3 PNETs are well-differentiated tumors, but have a higher mitotic rate (>20/10 HPF) or Ki-67 index (>20%) and have a worse prognosis compared with low-grade (grade 1 and grade 2) PNETs.[128] Poorly differentiated neoplasms are classified as carcinomas (PNECs), with high mitotic rates (>20/10 HPF) and Ki-67 indices (>20%), and they demonstrate aggressive behavior.[128]

Well-differentiated neoplasm (PNETs) are usually solitary, except in the setting of familial syndromes, such as multiple endocrine neoplasia syndrome type 1 (MEN1), von Hippel-Lindau disease (VHL), neurofibromatosis type 1 (NF-1), and tuberous sclerosis (TSC).[129] PNETs are considered functional or nonfunctional, depending on whether hormones secreted by the tumor cause systemic symptoms. Functional PNET manifest early because of clinical symptoms related to pathologic hormone secretion, with the most common being insulinoma. Functioning tumors tend to be small homogeneous masses without local invasion or distant metastases.[129,130]

Nonfunctional tumors are usually larger and present later with symptoms related to mass effect.[129,131] These larger tumors demonstrate heterogeneous enhancement because of areas of cystic degeneration and necrosis.[129] Local soft-tissue invasion, vascular invasion, and metastases are more commonly demonstrated in larger, nonfunctioning, clinically silent tumors.[130] Calcification can occur in larger lesions and is more commonly associated with lymph node and liver metastases, compared with noncalcified tumors.[130,132]

CT is regarded as first-line imaging for PNET, and triphasic CT imaging protocol should be used; this not only aids in detection of the primary tumor but also helps to improve visualization of metastatic disease.[133] A noncontrast scan before the multiphase CT is useful in demonstrating tumoral calcification; the tumor is typical isodense to normal pancreas on noncontrast CT.[133]

On MRI, PNETs will generally demonstrate nonspecific signal hypointensity on precontrast T1 and moderate hyperintensity on fat-suppressed T2 compared with normal pancreas, with smaller tumors appearing more homogenous and larger tumors appearing heterogeneous.[134,135] PNET will generally demonstrate restricted diffusion because of high cellularity, and this feature may aid in the detection of nonhypervascular tumors.[136] Additionally, lower ADC values were more commonly demonstrated in PNETs, with more aggressive behavior compared with PNETs that had benign features.[137]

Smaller tumors generally show homogeneous enhancement on both CT and MRI and are hypervascular to normal pancreas on arterial and pancreatic parenchymal phases (Fig. 17.23). Larger tumors usually demonstrate heterogeneous hypoenhancement on arterial phases and may be hypo or iso-enhancing to normal pancreas on portal venous and delayed phases.[138] Obstruction of the pancreatic duct can occur in PNET, a feature that is often indicative of more aggressive behavior.[137] The appearance of metastases is dependent on the vascularity of the primary PNET; hypervascular primary tumors will generally have hypervascular metastases.[133,134] Well-differentiated PNETs

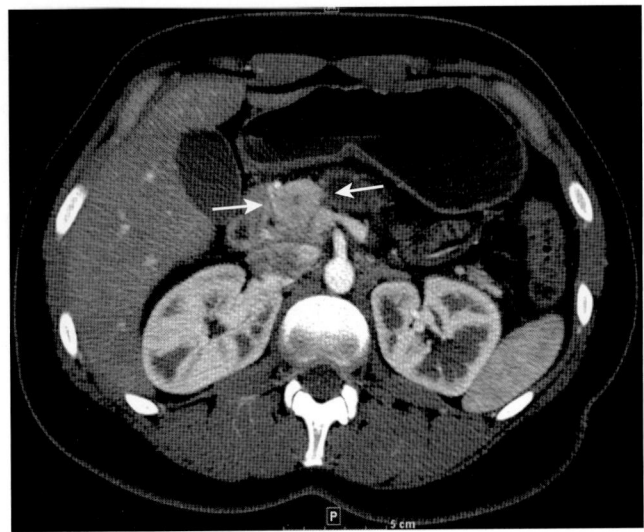

FIGURE 17.23 Axial computed tomography (CT) in pancreatic parenchymal/late arterial phase. A well-differentiated pancreatic neuroendocrine tumor (PNET) appearing as a hypervascular mass in the pancreatic head (*arrows*).

are usually avid on somatostatin receptor (SSTR) imaging (e.g., ^{68}Ga-DOTATATE PET and ^{111}In-octreotide), and these scans can be useful in demonstrating the extent of disease (see Chapter 18).[131]

A PNET may also appear as cystic neoplasm in 10% to 17% of cases,[86] usually in nonfunctioning tumors, and these most commonly appear in the pancreatic body and tail. These appear as well-circumscribed unilocular or multilocular cystic lesions with an arterially enhancing, often slightly nodular rim.[81,139] The rim may be somatostatin-receptor avid on SSTR imaging but will not typically be avid in the cystic component (Fig. 17.24).[81,129] Patients with cystic PNET are 3.5 times more likely to have MEN1,[139] and PNET should be a differential for a cystic pancreatic lesion in the setting of known MEN1.[140]

With regard to specific tumor types, almost all insulinomas arise in the pancreas, with no site predilection.[129] Approximately half of somatostatinomas occur in the pancreas, most commonly in the pancreatic head with an average size of 5 to 6 cm.[129,141,142] It is reported that up to half of patients have metastatic disease at the time of presentation, typically involving lymph nodes or liver.[129,141] Most glucagonomas originate in the pancreatic body and tail and are often large tumors (5–6 cm) because of delayed presentation.[129] Vasoactive intestinal peptide tumors (VIPomas) most frequently occur in the pancreatic tail, with a 5-cm average size at diagnosis.[143] Most VIPomas are aggressive, with metastases present in 60% to 80% of cases at presentation.[129] Gastrinoma tumors are more commonly extrapancreatic and multiple, occurring in the gastrinoma triangle; however, if they occur in the pancreas, they usually average 3 to 4 cm in size[141] and can demonstrate rim enhancement.[135]

Poorly differentiated carcinomas (PNECs) occur most frequently in the pancreatic head and typically appear as ill-defined, heterogeneous masses with rim enhancement (Fig. 17.25). They are commonly associated with biliary obstruction, invasion of adjacent soft tissue, and nodal or hepatic metastatic disease.[129] PNECs can demonstrate more restricted diffusion compared with well-differentiated PNETs.[144] PNECs

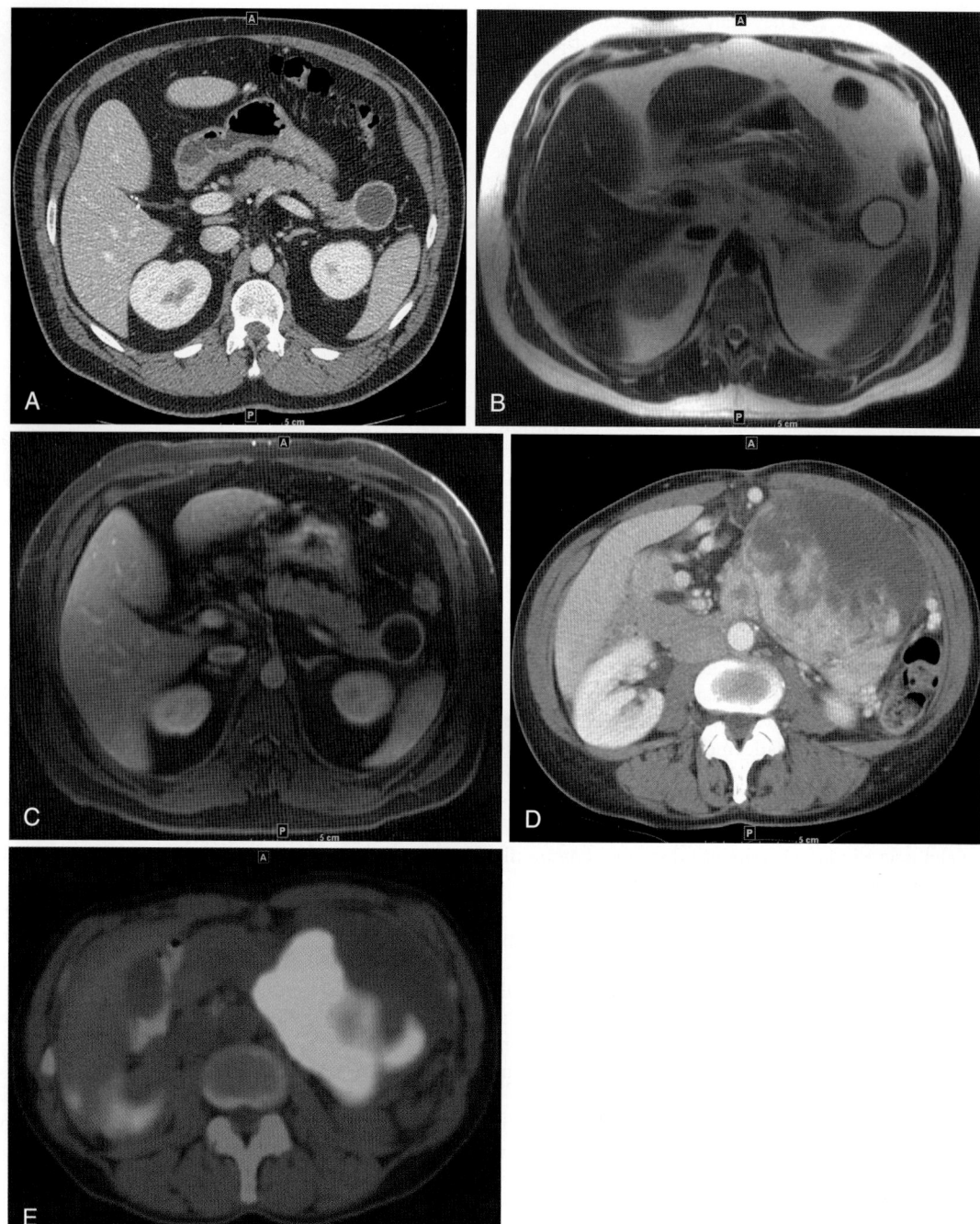

FIGURE 17.24 **Cystic pancreatic neuroendocrine tumor (PNET). A**, Contrast-enhanced computed tomography (CT) in the portal venous phase demonstrates a rounded pancreatic tail cystic lesion with slightly thick hyperenhancing rim. **B**, Magnetic resonance imaging (MRI) shows the T2 hyperintense cyst with hypointense rim. **C**, Postcontrast fat-saturated T1-weighted MRI in the arterial phase again demonstrates the hyperenhancing rim. **D**, CT in another patient with a larger PNET with cystic and solid components. **E**, Fusion imaging from a somatostatin receptor (⁶⁸Ga-DOTATATE) positron emission tomography (PET)/CT demonstrates tracer uptake in the solid elements and physiologic uptake in the liver and right kidney.

are more typically FDG avid and usually demonstrate little or no uptake on SSTR imaging (see Chapter 18).

Pancreatic Lymphoma

Lymphoma can occur in the pancreas in both primary and, more commonly, secondary forms. It may appear as solitary nodular, multinodular, or diffuse disease.[50,145,146]

On CT, the affected region will appear hypodense to normal pancreas, without cystic or necrotic areas.[147,148] On MRI,

lymphoma is typically T1 hypointense and T2 hyperintense to normal pancreas.[50,145] On postcontrast imaging, lymphomatous regions demonstrate homogenous hypoenhancement to pancreas in both arterial and delayed phase.[50,145]

Diffuse lymphomatous involvement of the pancreas is less common and may mimic acute pancreatitis.[145] Features of acute pancreatitis, such as peripancreatic stranding, peripancreatic fluid collections, and fat necrosis are usually absent in pancreatic lymphoma.[145] Vascular encasement can occur but

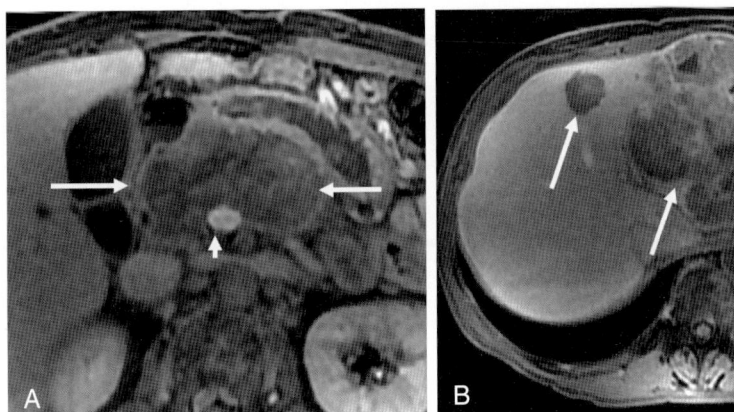

FIGURE 17.25   Pancreatic neuroendocrine carcinoma with liver metastases. A, Axial T1 postcontrast T1-weighted fat-saturated magnetic resonance imaging (MRI) in portal venous phase at the level of the pancreas demonstrating a hypovascular mass *(long arrows)* encasing the superior mesenteric vein *(short arrow)*. **B,** Axial postcontrast T1-weighted fat-saturated MRI demonstrating multiple hypovascular liver metastases *(long arrows)* and a hypovascular peritoneal metastasis in the left upper quadrant *(short arrow)* abutting the left hepatic lobe.

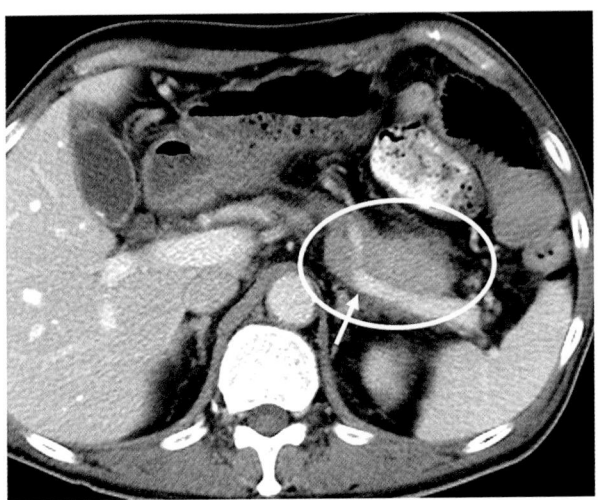

FIGURE 17.26   Focal pancreatic lymphoma. Axial computed tomography (CT) in portal venous phase demonstrates a slight hypoenhancing mass in the pancreatic tail *(white oval)* encasing, but not occluding, the splenic vein *(white arrow)*.

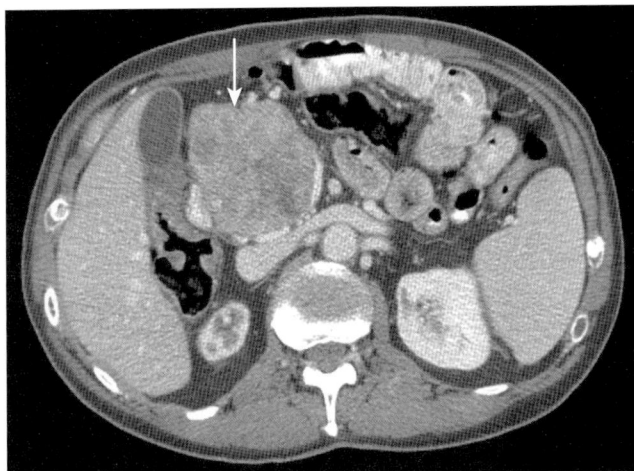

FIGURE 17.27   Acinar cell carcinoma. Axial computed tomography (CT) in portal venous phase demonstrating an encapsulated, partially exophytic heterogeneous pancreatic head mass *(arrow)*.

will generally lack features of vascular infiltration, such as vessel deformity (Fig. 17.26).[145,147]

Pancreatic duct obstruction can occur, but this is generally because of ductal displacement or compression rather than invasion. This is in contrast to PDAC where duct obstruction is more common and occurs because of tumoral invasion of the duct.[147,148] Evaluation of the pancreatic duct with secretin MRI may be useful to distinguish between a patent but compressed duct (duct-penetrating sign) or an infiltrated duct; the latter suggests PDAC.[149] Bile duct dilatation can reportedly occur in 42% of patients with primary pancreatic non-Hodgkin lymphoma.[147,148]

Lymph node involvement below the level of the renal veins can be seen with lymphoma, but is rare in PDAC cases.[148] Differentiating pancreatic lymphoma and autoimmune pancreatitis can also be difficult because both have overlapping imaging appearances; however, lymphoma is more often bulky in appearance. Challenging with corticosteroid treatment is not recommended because enlargement in both pancreatic lymphoma and autoimmune pancreatitis can decrease with treatment.[145]

Acinar Cell Carcinoma

Acinar cell carcinoma (ACC) generally appears as a large, oval pancreatic mass, without site predilection, in older men.[150–153] The tumors are typically well marginated, encapsulated, and partially or completely exophytic (Fig. 17.27).[153,154]

Intratumoral necrotic regions are common, particularly in larger tumors and may be because of local necrosis secondary to the release of pancreatic enzymes and impairment of blood supply.[153,155] These cystic/necrotic regions are seen as heterogeneously hypodense areas on CT and T1-hypointense, T2-hyperintense areas on MRI.[154,155] On MRI, the tumor has nonspecific signal hypointensity on precontrast T1 and iso/hypointensity on T2, relative to normal pancreas.[151,155] Tumors commonly have an enhancing capsule and demonstrate hypoenhancement to pancreas on both arterial and portal venous phases.[150,152,156] Intratumoral hemorrhage (T1-hyperintense areas on MRI) and calcification (best seen on CT) are less common reported features.[151,153,155] Restricted diffusion may also be present.[150]

ACC rarely show biliary or pancreatic duct dilatation, which is thought to be because ACC originates in acinar cells of the

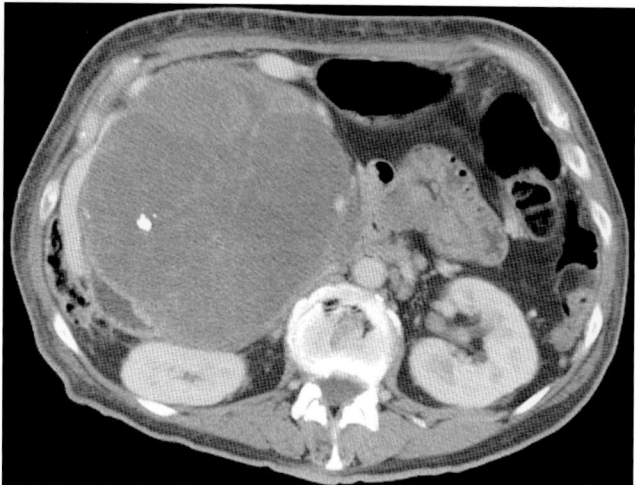

FIGURE 17.28   Solid pseudopapillary neoplasm (SPN). Axial computed tomography (CT) in portal venous phase demonstrating a large, heterogeneous but predominately hypoenhancing pancreatic head mass with some internal calcification.

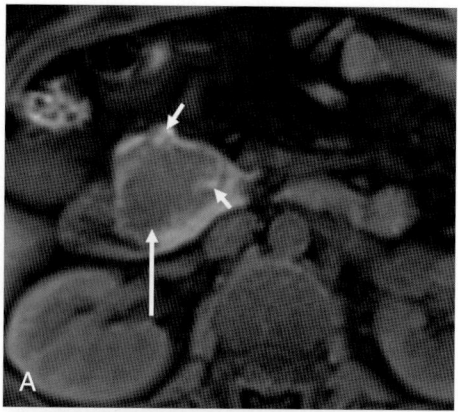

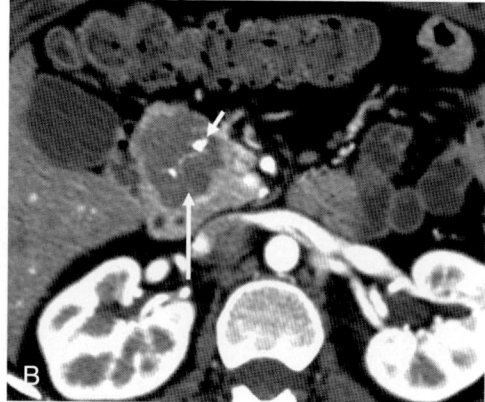

FIGURE 17.29   Solid pseudopapillary neoplasm (SPN). Axial precontrast T1 fat-saturated magnetic resonance imaging MRI (**A**) demonstrating a hypointense mass at the pancreatic head (*long arrow*) with internal T1 hyperintense foci (*short arrows*), which represent internal hemorrhagic or calcified components. Axial CT in pancreatic parenchymal/late arterial phase (**B**) showing the hypoenhancing mass (*long arrow*) with internal calcifications (*short arrow*).

pancreas rather than the ductal epithelium.[151,155,156] ACC can be metastatic, with metastatic disease most commonly involving regional lymph nodes and the liver.[155]

Features helpful in differentiating ACC from PDAC include presence of necrotic regions, well-defined margins, exophytic mass, large size, presence of enhancing capsule, and lack of biliary or pancreatic duct obstruction.[154,156] Hypovascular PNET and solid pseudopapillary tumor may appear similar as large, well-marginated masses with internal calcification and cystic regions; however, solid pseudopapillary tumor almost exclusively occurs in young females and more commonly demonstrates intratumoral hemorrhage.[157,158]

Solid Pseudopapillary Neoplasm

Solid pseudopapillary neoplasms (SPNs) are typical large solid tumors with cystic areas related to hemorrhage and necrosis; however, small tumors tend to be completely solid (Fig. 17.28).[159] Tumors located in the pancreatic body and tail are generally larger, and pancreatic tail lesions may invade the spleen.[159] The lesions typically appear sharply demarcated from pancreatic parenchyma and encapsulated,[157,159] in contrast to PDAC. However, the tumor capsule can frequently show discontinuous areas[160,161] and may not be seen at all in some lesions, particularly larger lesions.[159,162] A common tumor feature is amorphous or scattered calcification,[159,162] which is rare in PDAC.[160] Pancreatic duct obstruction can occur with SPN,[160] but this feature is inconsistently shown across small case series to be associated with malignant SPN over benign SPN.[161,163] Vascular invasion can be seen in malignant SPN.[163]

On MRI, tumors frequently demonstrate internal hyperintensity on precontrast T1 imaging related to hemorrhagic necrosis (Fig. 17.29).[157] Cystic or fluid regions with layering T1 hyperintense hemorrhagic debris may be seen.[162] On multiphase postcontrast imaging, the tumor will typically show early peripheral heterogeneous enhancement of the solid portions, with progressive fill-in on the delayed phase.[164] The fibrous tumor capsule may be evident as a T1/T2-hypointense rim, with some discontinuous regions, and commonly demonstrates early and more hyperintense enhancement compared with the tumor.[164]

Pancreatic Metastases

In a Japanese autopsy series involving patients with malignant tumors, 15% had pancreatic metastases (excluding primary pancreatic cancer metastases), and approximately half of these were solitary (see Chapter 64).[165] The most common tumors metastasizing to the pancreas vary across autopsy studies but are commonly from the kidney, gastrointestinal tract, lung, lymphoma, and breast.[165–168]

Pancreatic metastases may be solitary, multiple, or demonstrate diffuse involvement,[169,170] with no known site predilection.[171,172] Metastases are generally round or ovoid, with discrete margins.[168,171] The imaging features of the pancreatic metastases are dependent on the imaging characteristics of the primary tumor. Metastases from renal cell carcinoma, hepatocellular carcinoma, and thyroid carcinomas are typically hypervascular, whereas those from the lung, breast, and gastrointestinal tract are generally hypovascular.[170,173] Hypervascular metastases show avid enhancement in the arterial or pancreatic parenchymal phase, with wash-out on portal and delayed phase imaging (Fig. 17.30).[171] Because of this feature, such metastases may not be appreciated unless arterial phase imaging is performed as part of a multiphase pancreatic protocol.[174,175] Small hypervascular metastases more often show homogenous enhancement, whereas larger lesions may demonstrate heterogeneous or peripheral enhancement because of the presence of central necrosis.[168,171,176]

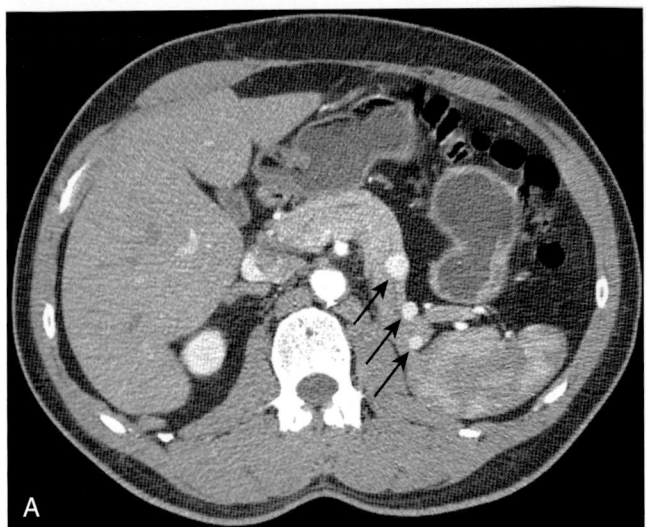
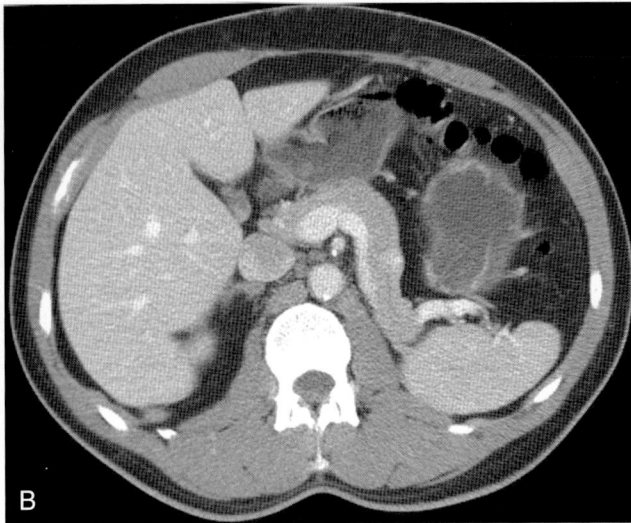

FIGURE 17.30   **Renal cell carcinoma metastatic to pancreas. A,** Computed tomography (CT) in pancreatic parenchymal/late arterial phase shows hypervascular pancreatic metastases *(arrows).* The metastases become more inconspicuous/ isodense to pancreas on the portal venous phase **(B).**

On MRI, both hypo- and hypervascular metastases will typically demonstrate nonspecific hypointensity to pancreas on precontrast T1 imaging, show moderate or heterogeneous T2 hyperintensity, and may show restricted diffusion.[171,175]

Pancreatic metastases are usually found in the setting of widely metastatic disease. Nevertheless, pancreatic metastases from renal cell carcinoma (RCC) are commonly isolated or oligometastatic and may occur several years after the initial RCC diagnosis.[170–172,177,178] Differentiating solitary RCC metastases from PNET is challenging because both could have an identical appearance on multiphase CT.[170,171] Additionally, uptake on SSTR imaging is not pathognomonic of PNET because a number of case studies show somatostatin expression in RCC metastases.[179–182] Ultimately biopsy may be required to differentiate between the two tumors.

Solitary hypovascular metastases may be particularly difficult to differentiate from PDAC. Although metastases may obstruct the pancreatic duct,[168,183,184] they may compress, rather than invade, the duct (as opposed to PDAC), and this is seen as a "duct-penetrating sign" on MRI.[173] Metastases may be considered in the setting of a large pancreatic head tumor without biliary/pancreatic duct obstruction or infiltration of retropancreatic fat.[185] An additional differentiating imaging feature favoring metastases is a lack of vascular invasion.[186,187]

Intrapancreatic Accessory Spleen

Intrapancreatic accessory spleen (IPAS) is ectopic spleen tissue within the pancreas, which appears as a mass-like entity, and is reported to occur in 7% to 10% at an autopsy series.[188,189] IPAS is generally small (1–3 cm) and commonly found in the pancreatic tail.[190,191] This may occur by two mechanisms: via congenital presence of accessory spleen or via splenosis after splenectomy or splenic trauma.[192]

IPAS should be hyperattenuating (CT) and hyperintense (MRI) to normal pancreatic parenchyma on all postcontrast phases (Fig. 17.31).[193,194] Further, IPAS should demonstrate identical precontrast T1 and T2 signal to normal spleen on MRI, which is hypointense and hyperintense to pancreas parenchyma, respectively.[194] Rarely the IPAS T2 signal may be hyperintense to normal spleen because of the presence of a higher white to red pulp ratio.[194]

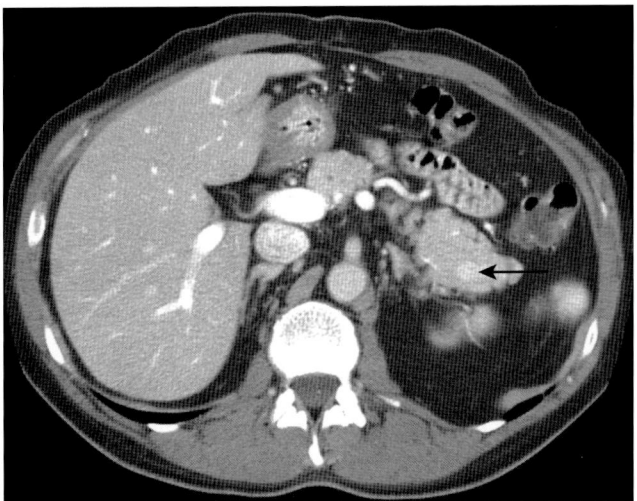

FIGURE 17.31   **Intrapancreatic accessory spleen (IPAS).** Axial computed tomography (CT) in pancreatic parenchymal/late arterial phase demonstrates a rounded hypervascular mass in the pancreatic tail *(arrow).*

On both CT and MRI, the enhancement pattern of IPAS will be similar, if not identical, to normal spleen.[195] When large, the mass will show typical splenic heterogeneous arterial phase enhancement because of the different blood flow rates between splenic red and white pulp.[195] When small, however, IPAS will be homogeneously enhancing. Thus the appearance of IPAS can be similar to other pancreatic tumors on multiphase CT and MRI, particularly hypervascular PNETs and metastases. Additionally, a small increase in the size of IPAS can occur because splenic size can be variable over time, affected by physiologic factors.[196]

If conventional CT or MRI are not definitive in the diagnosis of IPAS, then further confirmation is possible with either technetium-99m (^{99m}Tc) sulphur colloid or ^{99m}Tc heat damaged red blood cell scintigraphy (see Chapter 18).

The references for this chapter can be found online by accessing the accompanying Expert Consult website.

The role of nuclear medicine in diagnosis and management of hepatopancreatobiliary diseases

Simone Krebs, Elisabeth O'Dwyer, and Mark Dunphy

Nuclear medicine uses radioactive pharmaceuticals, or *radiopharmaceuticals*, for diagnostic imaging and internal radiotherapy of a variety of diseases. This chapter discusses clinical applications of diagnostic nuclear medicine imaging for the care of patients with hepatic, pancreatic, and biliary (hepatopancreatobiliary [HPB]) diseases. Radioembolization of liver tumors with radiolabeled microspheres is discussed more extensively in Chapter 94B.

In general, the role of diagnostic nuclear medicine imaging (NMI), or *scintigraphy*, including *positron emission tomography* (PET), is to provide HPB clinicians with a noninvasive method to aid in detecting and localizing certain types of HPB disease and to evaluate HPB organ function and the effects of treatment. In general, NMI can be considered a clinical assay of cellular biology in the tissues of patients; the in vivo tissue accumulation, or uptake, of *most* radiopharmaceuticals depends on the biomolecular composition of living cells in body tissues, as well as tissue perfusion.

The diagnostic accuracy of scintigraphy varies according to the specific scintigraphic study (including the specific radiopharmaceutical used and how it is assayed) and the specific disease or condition being studied. The HPB specialist must integrate diagnostic data from any scintigraphic study of a particular patient with signs, symptoms, and data from other relevant assays for optimal diagnostic accuracy and therapeutic decision making. NMI has a major positive impact on patient care, improving therapeutic strategy.

This chapter discusses the published clinical evidence regarding the impact of nuclear medicine in HPB diseases and focuses on state-of-the-art nuclear medicine. As such, it concentrates predominantly on published medical literature from the past 15 years. In our experience, most clinical nuclear medicine research publications before then often employ methodology and technology that is no longer reflective of current state-of-the-art clinical practice in nuclear medicine. The state-of-the-art in nuclear medicine, in its diagnostic and therapeutic procedures, has improved rapidly in the past 15 years and continues to evolve and innovate, including major improvements in commercially available nuclear imaging camera systems (particularly the advent of hybrid "fusion imaging" camera systems), image data processing, new types of instrumentation, and clinical introduction of new radiopharmaceuticals, both for diagnostic imaging and nuclear therapy.

Therefore we strongly advise the reader to note the dates of nuclear medicine references cited in HPB bibliographies and other guidelines, especially when these make judgments on the diagnostic accuracy or clinical impact of nuclear medicine; sometimes guidelines cite outdated nuclear medicine research from decades past. Such guidelines might be designed in recognition that nuclear medicine clinical practice varies worldwide, as reflected in the often widely varying diagnostic sensitivities and specificities reported by different medical centers performing a particular NMI procedure and the variation of hardware (e.g., scanners) and techniques (e.g., administered tracer doses, software-based data-processing algorithms) employed in different centers.

After an introduction to the pharmacology and technology of diagnostic imaging and therapy in radiopharmaceuticals and the general role of nuclear medicine in HPB diseases, we discuss current nuclear medicine procedures for specific HPB clinical indications. For diagnostic imaging procedures, discussion focuses on how well a particular clinical NMI study performs for a specific HPB indication, in terms of its diagnostic accuracy (sensitivity, specificity) and potential pitfalls, including necessary patient preparation, when applicable. The chapter also includes a concise look at select new, currently investigational radiopharmaceuticals relevant to HPB disease.

RADIOPHARMACEUTICALS

Nuclear medicine specialists prescribe radiopharmaceuticals for diagnostic imaging and internal radiotherapy of a variety of diseases. Radiopharmaceuticals can be placed into three major categories of applications in HPB disease: detection and evaluation of cancerous HPB tumors, treatment of HPB cancers, and evaluation of HPB organ function (and indirectly for detection of disease entities causing HPB organ dysfunction).

A radiopharmaceutical is a radioactive compound containing a *radionuclide,* also referred to as a "radioisotope" (radioactive isotope). A radioisotope is an energetically unstable atom that will achieve a stable or more stable, lower-energy state (transitioning from a *parent* to a *daughter* state) by releasing (radiating) energy (radiation) in some form (e.g., emitting a gamma ray, positron particle, or beta particle, as discussed later). The release of energy by the (parent) radioisotope atom may be called a *physical decay, disintegration,* or *transition.* The energy decay makes the elemental atom either become a different isotope of the same element (e.g., the radioisotope technetium 99m [^{99m}Tc] decays to the stable isotope technetium 99 [^{99}Tc]) or become a different element by *transmutation* (e.g., the radioisotope ^{18}F decays to become a stable form of the element oxygen, ^{18}O). Other forms of nuclear decay are possible (e.g., transitions from a higher-energy unstable radioisotope to a lower-energy, but still unstable, daughter radioisotope). A radiopharmaceutical is administered in a trace amount (with no detectable radiobiologic effects) or therapeutic amount for use as a diagnostic imaging agent or therapeutic agent. A radiopharmaceutical also contains other active and inactive ingredients in the compound formulation. In the radiopharmaceutical, the elemental radioisotope atom typically is incorporated within a molecule by chemical bonding. The molecule is said to be *radiolabeled.*

As with any pharmaceutical, each type of radiopharmaceutical has in vivo *pharmacokinetic* (PK) properties specific to and determined by its molecular structure and associated physicochemical properties. PK properties include the radiopharmaceutical's distribution in tissues throughout the body *(biodistribution)*, metabolism, and bodily elimination (by hepatobiliary and urinary excretion for all relevant radiopharmaceuticals). The in vivo PK properties are also determined, to some degree, by the physicochemical properties of excipients (vehicles) in the radiopharmaceutical formulation (e.g., formulation of an orally administered radiopharmaceutical compound may affect its bioavailability and biodistribution), as well as by the route of administration (e.g., peripheral intravenous [IV] injection, hepatic arterial catheter infusion).

The mass-amount of radioactive molecules in any prescribed radiopharmaceutical formulation is only a *trace* amount, typically in the picogram (pg) range. This tiny mass-dose of radioactive molecule is incapable of exerting detectable *pharmacologic* effects on body tissues in vivo, but the typical pg amounts of radioactive molecules emit radioactivity sufficient for diagnostic imaging and therapeutic applications. With exceptions, the nonradioactive constituents of radiopharmaceutical compounds typically used only for clinical diagnostic imaging are present in somewhat higher mass-amounts but are still scant, typically less than 100 micrograms (µg), and allergic reactions, other side effects, or pharmacodynamic effects are rarely reported. Nuclear medicine specialists may prescribe the radiopharmaceutical compound to be administered in conjunction with a relatively high and biologically effective mass-amount of a nonradioactive, or *unlabeled*, version of the same compound or a related compound, with *therapeutic* intent (relevant compounds are discussed later).

The terms "radiotracer," "tracer dose," and "radiotracer dose" commonly refer to the use of trace amounts of a radiolabeled molecule to study molecular biology. The trace amount of radioactivity and the trace mass of the administered radiotracer are unable to affect (and therefore unable to interfere with measurements of) the biomolecular system or target being assayed. Following this common convention, in this chapter we use *radiotracer* to refer to radiopharmaceutical administered for diagnostic imaging. We use *therapeutic radionuclide* to refer to administration of a relatively high amount of radioactivity with the intent of inducing therapeutic radiobiologic effects in vivo, as discussed later. The radioactivity emitted by a therapeutic radiopharmaceutical may be useful for diagnostic imaging, as well as radiotherapy. The approach of combining diagnostic imaging and therapy using a same molecule or at least very similar molecules, which are either radiolabeled differently or given in different dosages, is known as theranostics.

Fluorodeoxyglucose Positron Emission Tomography

In the past 25 years, fluorodeoxyglucose (FDG) PET has rapidly emerged as a revolutionary imaging modality in clinical oncology, demonstrating diagnostic efficacy in tumor staging and tumor-response evaluation for histologies across a variety of cancers. FDG, or 2-deoxy-2-(^{18}F)fluoro-d-glucose, is an analogue of glucose; fluorine-18 occupies the molecular $2'$ position in which a hydroxyl group is found in glucose. The substitution affects the metabolism of FDG compared with glucose. In vivo, IV FDG extravasates into tissues, followed by its uptake into tissue cells by glucose transporter proteins. Once FDG enters the cell, hexokinase converts FDG to FDG-6-phosphate, which cannot be metabolized further, thus trapping the tracer intracellularly. Blood FDG concentrations decrease to relatively low levels 45 to 90 minutes after injection; at this point, further FDG uptake in most tissues is relatively minor, and after that time, FDG concentrations in most tissues and tumors remain relatively stable. Acquiring a single FDG PET scan, beginning 45 to 90 minutes after injection, has become the standard clinical approach. Usually, as for HPB cancer imaging, the scan spans from "eyes to thighs," including the entire head or extremities only if there is a patient-specific clinical reason.

The basic rationale for using FDG PET for tumor detection is the observation that neoplastic cells typically accumulate FDG more than the non-neoplastic cells of origin and that the difference in FDG concentration between the tumor and surrounding normal tissues in an organ is detectable by PET. This *avidity* of tumors for FDG manifests on PET images as a "hot spot," or a *focus*, of FDG accumulation that is of abnormally high concentration relative to other, healthy tissues.

Why are some tumors FDG avid and other are not very avid? The physician-scientist and Nobel laureate Otto Warburg long ago observed in multiple tumor cell lines that he studied an abnormally high rate of glycolysis in cancer cells compared with their normal cellular counterparts, even in the presence of normal levels of oxygen. In normal cells with adequate environmental oxygen, glucose metabolism is typically directed into the mitochondrial tricarboxylic acid (TCA) cycle; glucose–TCA cycle metabolism yields the maximal amount of energy substrate (adenosine triphosphate [ATP]) from each glucose molecule metabolized for meeting the bioenergetic needs of the cell. The TCA cycle depends on oxygen to function; in normal cells, if environmental oxygen is low, glucose metabolism instead occurs in the cytosol by an oxygen-independent glycolytic process that yields much less ATP per glucose molecule. In cancer cells, however, Warburg observed that glucose metabolism occurred predominantly by glycolysis in the cytosol, regardless of whether or not the tumor cells were well oxygenated. This preference of tumor cells is the *Warburg effect*. According to the Warburg hypothesis, cancer cell metabolism of glucose was inefficient because it yielded fewer ATP molecules per glucose cell, and this inefficiency was caused by a defect in the mitochondrial metabolism of cancer cells. The Warburg effect remains a valid observation, although not a universal phenomenon among all cancer cell lines and types (i.e., glucose metabolism of some cancer cell lines is essentially the same as the glucose metabolism of normal cell counterparts). The Warburg hypothesis, however, is outdated; the shift of glucose metabolism from the mitochondrial TCA cycle to cytosolic glycolysis is not an inefficient use of glucose. Rather, it is a "repurposing" of glucose. In multiple cell lines, abnormal cytosolic glycolysis has become understood as advantageous to cancer cell proliferation. Cytosolic glycolysis yields fewer ATP molecules, but it yields glucose-derived metabolites during the multiple intermediate steps of glycolysis that the cell can use in other anabolic pathways as components for synthesizing macromolecules necessary for building cellular biomass before cell division and tumor growth. To meet the bioenergetic needs of these cells, instead of predominantly relying on glucose, these cells depend on other nutrient molecules, notably glutamine, to fuel the TCA cycle.[1]

The Warburg effect explains the avidity of tumors for FDG, the glucose analogue, when visualized by PET, but only in part. PET visualizes the FDG avidity of tumors at the macroscopic tissue level (again, with spatial resolution of ~2 mm). The "FDG-avid tumor" visualized by PET and described in PET/computed tomography (CT) reports represents a complex composite of FDG avidities of tumor cells and nonneoplastic cell constituents within the tumor internal microenvironment under the influence of complex biomolecular and other processes. Detected FDG avidity in a particular tumor often does primarily represent tumor cell FDG avidity (i.e., the sum of FDG uptake from all tumor cells within the tumor) more than the FDG avidity of other cells in the same tumor. However, the FDG avidity of other constituents of the tumor microenvironment sometimes contributes to a clinically significant degree, particularly in the posttreatment setting, potentially causing diagnostic confusion, as discussed. In certain cases, overall *tumor* FDG avidity can be caused, in relatively large part or even primarily, by tumor cellular constituents other than the neoplastic cells, such as infiltrating inflammatory cells, especially when the tumor cells do not have intrinsically high FDG avidity and when inflammatory cells are present in relatively high tissue concentrations. For example, inflammatory cells can accumulate around the necrotic cores of tumors before treatment and can infiltrate heavily throughout tumors after treatment. Standard FDG PET guidelines often advise that posttreatment PET be deferred for 6 to 8 weeks after chemotherapy and 2 to 3 months after radiotherapy. It was empirically observed in clinical PET trials that successfully treated tumors often demonstrate apparently suspicious residual FDG avidity in the first few weeks after treatment because of inflammatory cells infiltrating the treated tumors, presumably to clear the necrotic/apoptotic debris associated with successful treatment.

Whenever using PET to characterize or localize tumors, the oncologist (and imaging specialist) should be aware of key factors that affect the apparent FDG avidity of a tumor and the diagnostic *sensitivity* of FDG PET: tumor size; cancer treatment(s); and background organ FDG avidity. As the Nyquist principle indicates, the apparent FDG avidity of subcentimeter tumors will be underestimated because such small lesions fall below the spatial resolution of PET technology. It is still possible for PET to detect a subcentimeter tumor if the tumor is so FDG avid that the FDG accumulation in tumor is detectably higher than that in background tissues of the organ involved, but many subcentimeter tumors lack apparent FDG avidity and may be reported as "too small to characterize by FDG PET." Additionally, the *specificity* of FDG can vary in the setting of coexisting benign pathologies, leading to false-positive results. For example, specificity of FDG PET is lower for patients who live in areas where tuberculosis (TB) is endemic. Furthermore, TB lesions absorb FDG and can mimic tumors on FDG PET.

Cancer treatments, depending on action and efficacy, also affect apparent tumor FDG avidity.[2] Tumor FDG avidity represents the sum of the FDG avidity of constituent tumor cells. Various studies indicate FDG PET is unable to detect *microscopic* residual disease; for example, a partially treated tumor containing FDG-avid cells may be of macroscopic size on CT or magnetic resonance imaging (MRI) but may contain a depleted cell population with a sum FDG avidity that appears minimal to nil on PET imagery. For staging, FDG PET is expected to be less accurate after therapy than before therapy.[2] FDG PET can also be false positive, detecting FDG uptake at a former tumor site in the absence of residual disease. With systemic therapy, residual FDG uptake may indicate inflammatory cells (extremely FDG

avid, when active) infiltrating tissues to remove the debris of treated disease. Radiotherapy and surgery, for tumor treatment or resection, both evoke local tissue inflammation that can be greatly FDG avid, mimicking local residual or recurrent neoplastic disease on PET imagery. FDG PET is usually deferred for several weeks after surgery or radiotherapy, when evaluation for local disease is desired.

Certain organs and organ systems have marked FDG avidity consistently or variably that may exceed that of primary tumors and metastases, obscuring tumor detection. For example, the brain is consistently FDG avid because it normally depends on glucose metabolism; FDG PET has limited sensitivity for detection of brain metastases. FDG is excreted through the urinary tract; the radioactive signal from excreted FDG in the collecting systems typically obscures PET evaluation of the kidneys and urinary bladder. The liver, lungs, and other tissues have lesser degrees of background FDG avidity that usually do not obscure tumor detection significantly.

Besides tumor detection, for disease (re)staging, FDG PET may be used to evaluate tumor response to cancer therapy. Frequently, FDG PET is performed twice, before and after therapy, for comparison, using *changes* in tumor FDG avidity as an index of changes in tumor cell population size (i.e., tumor response). Marked *decreases* in tumor FDG avidity during therapy have frequently predicted favorable clinical outcomes, whereas stable or increasing FDG avidity portend worse outcomes across a variety of cancers. Evaluation of tumor FDG avidity after cytotoxic therapy without a pretreatment PET study for comparison can be performed but can yield potentially confusing findings; for example, reactive lymph nodes and partially treated metastatic adenopathy can have similar appearances on PET. Tumors may have marked residual FDG avidity after treatment, which may provoke concerns about tumor resistance. If a pretreatment FDG PET had been obtained, however, the residual FDG avidity might have been observed as a marked decrease from baseline tumor FDG avidity, suggesting a favorable tumor response. In other words, the *change* in tumor FDG avidity before versus after treatment can be more predictive of tumor response than merely the posttreatment FDG avidity alone. As mentioned, certain tumor histologies seem frequently to lack FDG avidity, despite the presence of viable, macroscopic neoplastic disease. A lack of tumor FDG avidity on a posttreatment PET scan can be potentially misleading as an indicator of tumor response, unless a pretreatment PET scan has demonstrated the tumor being treated was originally FDG avid.

DIAGNOSTIC IMAGING IN NUCLEAR MEDICINE

In general, diagnostic NMI is a noninvasive procedure that uses scanning hardware to examine the distribution of a radiopharmaceutical within the internal environment of the body. As discussed, imaging the in vivo distribution of a radiopharmaceutical can be considered as an in vivo assay of radiopharmaceutical pharmacokinetics, not just in blood but also in tissues/organs throughout the body. No radiopharmaceutical compound yet designed has been found to bind exclusively to one particular biologic molecule. Some compounds, however, such as radiolabeled antibodies, radiolabeled "small molecules," and other types of agents, do bind with very high selectivity and affinity to relatively few biologic molecules and not at all to other types of molecules and are called "targeted agents." Still, the biophysiologic processes and biologic molecules targeted by such agents for diagnostic imaging (or "targeted therapy") of a particular condition of interest can almost invariably be found in other physiologic or pathologic conditions, again precluding 100% specificity. For example, the biologic molecule prostate-specific membrane antigen (PSMA, now more properly referred to as glutamate carboxypeptidase II), once thought to be uniquely expressed by prostate tissues and thus a good biomarker for prostate cancer (e.g., for imaging by PSMA-targeted radiolabeled antibody), was later found to be expressed by certain other tissues in the body and in the neovasculature of most tumors. However, PSMA is highly expressed in only a few types of nonprostatic tissues and therefore still possesses high selectivity for prostatic tissues. Therefore "perfect" specificity should not be expected for diagnostic imaging agents, even radiolabeled antibodies, considering the underlying imperfect pharmacologic and biologic specificity, as well as potentially misleading imaging artifacts.

In diagnostic NMI, the image is produced by the radiopharmaceutical administered to the patient. Once administered, the radioisotope physically decays with a characteristic radioactive emission pattern, producing energy or *photons*. These photons are detected by nuclear scanner (e.g., PET scanner or gamma camera) and an image is created.

Does the biodistribution of the radioisotope atoms visualized by the nuclear scan represent the biodistribution of the administered radiopharmaceutical (molecules)? If the radiopharmaceutical does not undergo in vivo chemical transformation to another form (e.g., catabolite or metabolite) before imaging of the patient, the answer is yes. Otherwise, the *radioisotope* biodistribution imagery may represent a composite of biodistributions, including those of the (unmodified) administered *radiopharmaceutical* and the radioactive products of in vivo chemical reactions (i.e., reaction products that still incorporate the radioisotopic atom). Usually, in vivo *metabolism* of the radiopharmaceutical causes in vivo production of metabolites, one or more of which include the radioisotope; these are *radiometabolites*. Such metabolism may be the diagnostic imaging target of the nuclear scan (e.g., PET imaging with F-18 FDG to detect tumor concentrations of the FDG metabolite). Some radiometabolites may be radiolabeled molecules, or in vivo metabolism may yield radioisotope in free, unattached elemental form. These radiometabolites often have different in vivo PK properties from the intact parent radiopharmaceutical. Thus the radiotracer biodistribution visualized by nuclear imagery will represent a combination of biodistributions: that of the intact radiopharmaceutical and that of one or more radiometabolites. In vivo metabolism occurs but typically does not interfere with diagnostic interpretation. On the contrary, metabolism may yield a radiometabolite "trapped" in a tissue of interest, such as enzymatic trapping of the PET imaging FDG in tumor cells; the cytoplasmic enzyme hexokinase yields the radiometabolite FDG-6-phosphate, which is trapped intracellularly. This chapter discusses the meaning of each radiopharmaceutical scintigraphic biomarker scan relevant in HPB diseases. Once administered to a patient, the radioisotope used for diagnostic imaging emits radiation that can be detected by a nuclear scanner.

Diagnostic imaging with radiopharmaceuticals, in standard clinical practice, may be referred to in various ways, including (1) using general terms such as nuclear imaging or *scintigraphy,* (2) referring to one of two general types of scintigraphic camera technology (PET, single-photon emission computed tomography [SPECT]/single-photon emission tomography [SPET]), and (3) using the procedure involved (e.g., theranostic imaging). The term *scintigraphy* (Latin *scintilla,* "spark") in medicine refers to the light produced by crystalline detectors in clinical scintigraphic cameras when those crystals are struck by gamma rays emitted from radiopharmaceuticals (e.g., as emitted from within a patient scanned after receiving a radiopharmaceutical injection). These scintillations produced in the crystalline detectors are recognized and processed by the camera system to yield nuclear imagery.

Of the basic types of scans found in a radiology department (e.g., plain radiography, CT, MRI, ultrasound [US]), *diagnostic NMI* scans are typically of the longest duration, in terms of both the time the patient must physically spend with the scanner and the time required for the entire study (start to finish), often with necessary delays before scanning or between scanning (i.e., if the patient is scanned more than once after a single radiopharmaceutical administration) to allow the radiopharmaceutical time to undergo desired in vivo physiologic processes. The total duration of a diagnostic NMI study thus depends on a variety of technical, biologic, and typical clinical logistical variables. Most frequently, a radiopharmaceutical is administered intravenously by bolus injection. After the injection, a standard time-delay may be necessary before the patient undergoes scanning to allow the radiopharmaceutical to spread throughout the body and achieve a biodistribution considered optimal for imaging. To acquire data for a single image, the time that a patient spends "in front of the camera" must be of sufficient duration for the scanner to collect a statistically robust number of radioactive signals, or *counts,* to ensure that the derived imagery will be satisfactory for visual analysis. Low-count images are visually "noisy." How long it takes for the camera to collect enough photons for a sufficient-quality diagnostic image depends primarily on the intrinsic properties of the radioisotope involved, how much radiopharmaceutical is administered, how well the radiopharmaceutical concentrates in tissues of interest (e.g., tumors) compared with surrounding tissues in vivo, how well the camera system detects photons, and how the photon data are constructed into imagery. Depending on the type of nuclear imaging study, before imaging even starts, there may be a standardized delay after the radiopharmaceutical administration to allow the radiopharmaceutical time to achieve an in vivo biodistribution considered optimal (i.e., one hour after FDG injection before PET scan acquisition). Lastly, the imaging specialist decides whether to have the patient undergo scanning at additional time points or using special techniques, if it is thought necessary to increase the diagnostic accuracy of the study. The referring clinician's staff can help prepare patients mentally by advising them of the prolonged duration typical of diagnostic NMI.

Nuclear scanners may be categorized into two general types: PET scanners and standard *gamma cameras*. Their designs are tailored to image two fundamentally different types of radiopharmaceuticals (radioisotopes): those that emit positrons (for PET cameras) and those that emit gamma rays (for standard gamma cameras). As mentioned previously, images are created from photons produced by decaying radioisotopes administered to the patient, which are detected by nuclear scanners. The scanner system processes the photon data and reconstructs it into an image that can be presented as a two-dimensional (2D), or *planar*, image or as a (virtual) three-dimensional (3D) image (e.g., allowing display of sections of data in conventional axial, coronal, and sagittal views, similar to CT). Images may represent biodistribution at one or a few time points or can display time-dependent changes in biodistribution in cinematic fashion.

Planar images of radiotracer biodistribution in the anterior-posterior plane will result in an image in which in vivo tracer accumulations in two or more organs or other tissues may overlap (in the 2D plane) and thus potentially obscure detection or evaluation of the radiotracer uptake of interest (e.g., tumor detection). Tomographic (SPECT and PET) nuclear imaging can help avoid this potential issue by permitting tracer biodistribution to be evaluated in three dimensions. However, the limited spatial resolution of scintigraphic imaging may make it difficult to localize a particular tracer accumulation in a small tissue structure (e.g., tracer uptake in a small tumor may be hidden if the tumor is located within or immediately adjacent to a normal organ that also accumulates tracer). Additionally, for single-photon imaging agents, SPECT often requires a significantly longer duration scan than a 2D planar scan using standard SPECT camera systems, and often 2D imaging may be sufficient for the clinical data desired. The necessity for SPECT imaging is guided by the reason for a particular examination, available clinical research, and the particular patient context. For PET, by definition, tomography (3D imaging) is always used, involving ring-type dedicated PET camera systems with sophisticated signal analysis algorithms.

The advantage of PET imaging versus single-photon gamma imaging is that the PET permits a more precise determination of where the radiation originated, when using the coincidence-detection method. Thus the scan imagery reconstructed from PET data has a much better spatial resolution (typically 4–5 mm, vs. <1 mm on CT) than that reconstructed from single-photon gamma data (typically 12–15 mm). According to the Nyquist principle, this superior resolution results in PET-acquired data providing superior *quantification* of radioactivity concentrations in imaging data analyses compared with single-photon imaging. As one potential advantage versus PET imaging, single-photon imaging can simultaneously detect and distinguish two or more different gamma-emitting radiopharmaceuticals in a single patient in vivo, whereas PET imaging cannot distinguish between different PET isotopes. Gamma rays emitted by non-PET isotopes for single-photon imaging can have a variety of signature energy levels, which can distinguish it and be separated by signal processing.

Fusion Imaging

Scintigraphic imaging of PET and single-photon emission radiopharmaceuticals are often combined with CT imaging for fusion imaging: PET/CT and SPECT/CT, respectively. In *fusion imaging,* the 3D imagery of PET or SPECT is combined with CT data so that tracer biodistribution/localization is visualized within the internal anatomy. Clinical studies have, overall, demonstrated that fusion imaging can have a *synergistic* effect on the accuracy of scintigraphy and CT image analyses for various clinical applications. A notable general example is improved accuracy for detection of radiotracer-avid tumors; often, on fusion imagery, scintigraphy (PET or SPECT) highlights findings poorly detected or easily overlooked on CT, or vice versa. The CT information also serves as data for an important technical function, called *attenuation correction,* which improves the quantitative accuracy of measurements derived from PET or SPECT analyses. Fusion imaging has done much to rescue diagnostic nuclear medicine from its former moniker (deserved or not) of "unclear medicine."

One important caveat remains regarding the CT scans involved in fusion PET/CT and SPECT/CT imaging: the *companion* CT scan. The quality of the companion CT image can vary considerably; it can be of standard diagnostic quality (i.e., exactly the same technical-quality CT scan as obtained from a separate, stand-alone, state-of-the-art CT scanner), or it can be of inferior diagnostic quality (e.g., if acquired with a lower current [mA], yielding relatively noisier images, with less detail and greater susceptibility to certain artifacts, such as beam hardening). Chest imaging may be acquired at pulmonary end expiration rather than the standard maximal pulmonary inspiration, limiting evaluation. The CT might be acquired with the patient's upper extremities positioned along the torso if the patient cannot tolerate having the arms raised (the standard chest CT position) for the 15 to 25 minutes of a standard torso FDG PET/CT, often creating a beam hardening artifact. Additionally, oral and IV iodinated contrast material more routinely used in standard CT protocol are not always used. Nevertheless, a noncontrast low-dose companion CT performed typically is sufficient for the basic needs of the PET or SPECT scan, providing sufficient anatomic detail to identify what tissues are involved in radiotracer uptake within an organ and providing attenuation correction, a modification of the scintigraphic data based on tissue densities and depth measured by CT that improves scintigraphic image quality, especially for quantification (e.g., for PET quantitative measurements known as the standardized uptake value [SUV]). Decay photons emitted from within deeper or denser body tissues will lose more energy from tissue interactions than photons from superficial or less dense tissues. The attenuation correction attempts to account for that artifact to provide more accurate measurement of tissue tracer concentrations.

Beyond CT, clinical PET/MRI systems are already available at a few major medical centers with increasing use in the setting of certain pathologies (e.g., prostate cancer and neuroimaging). The advantages of PET/MRI include simultaneous acquisition to improve registration of fusion images, lower radiation dose, superior soft-tissue contrast, and availability of multiparametric imaging. To date, the clinical use of PET/MRI has been limited by availability of accurate attenuation correction algorithms and problem of motion artifacts, including respiratory motion. With the advent of machine learning programs, however, these problems are being overcome and its use in clinical practice is expected to grow accordingly.

"Can I Order Two Nuclear Medicine Scans on the Same Day?"

The distinction between positron-emitting (PET) and solely gamma photon–emitting (non-PET) isotopes is relevant for referring specialists primarily because of this question. Unlike positron-emitting radioisotopes, the gamma ray–emitting isotopes of radiopharmaceuticals used for single-photon imaging come in a variety of energy levels. Gamma cameras can distinguish and potentially use these energy levels to separate the biodistributions of one radioisotope from another if a patient were to receive two radiopharmaceuticals with different radioisotopes simultaneously (i.e.,, by having the camera only accept detected photons of the energy level characteristic of the particular radioisotope of interest, then doing the same for the other radioisotopes). However, the energy emissions of different single-photon imaging radioisotopes can overlap, particularly if one of the radioisotopes emits relatively high-energy emissions, because some emitted rays will lose energy and fall into the energy (keV) range of the other radioisotope. The 511 keV coincidence gamma rays of PET radiopharmaceuticals are relatively high energy and will interfere with imaging of single-photon radiopharmaceuticals (whether to a significant degree depends on other technical factors). Thus, after a PET scan, some period of delay is necessary, to allow the PET radiopharmaceutical to undergo physical decay and biologic clearance from the patient, before performing another imaging study with a single-photon radiopharmaceutical or another PET radiopharmaceutical.

Practically, if a patient receives ^{18}F-FDG for FDG PET, the patient should wait more than 20 hours before a subsequent nuclear study is performed, based on the known half-life of ^{18}F (~1.9 hours), the amount of tracer we administer to a patient (maximal tracer dose of 12 mCi), and a common rule of thumb of waiting 10 half-lives for a radioisotope to decay sufficiently before allowing imaging with another radiopharmaceutical. In general single-photon radiopharmaceutical imaging, however, studies can be performed immediately before PET scan as the photons of non-PET radioisotopes typically are relatively low energy and thus cannot interfere with detection of the relatively high-energy 511 keV photons of PET radiopharmaceuticals. A few non-PET radioisotopes do emit high-energy photons at or above the 511 keV range, but even the presence of these high-energy photons from a prior non-PET radiopharmaceutical injection do not necessarily preclude immediately performing a PET study. Because the high-energy photons of the non-PET radioisotope are not produced as pairs, these photons will strike PET detectors in random directions. The PET scanner, however, will ignore photons that are not detected in the coincidence pattern typical of annihilation photon pairs. As such, the PET scanner often can detect the desired PET radiopharmaceutical signal without significant interference from any residual non-PET radiopharmaceutical in the patient's system.

Radiation Dose in Nuclear Medicine

When administered solely for diagnostic imaging, conventional radiopharmaceuticals expose the receiving patient to a low radiation dose, typically one or more orders of magnitude below the level of radiation exposure conventionally accepted as being associated with an increased risk for harmful radiation effects, based on decades of dosimetric research. Certain radiopharmaceuticals are administered at relatively high doses of radioactivity with therapeutic intent; the administered radioactivity is sufficiently high (and concentrates in body tissues at levels sufficient) to induce acute radiobiologic effects on diseased tissues and other organs within a patient, with potential therapeutic benefit as well as adverse side effects. The radiation dose absorbed by the patient from the radiopharmaceutical is determined by the specific type of radioactive isotope involved, the administered activity (amount) of radiopharmaceutical (quantified in becquerels, typically megabecquerels [MBq], or curies, typically millicuries [mCi]), and the pharmacokinetics and distribution of radiopharmaceutical throughout the body (biodistribution), which is again determined by the physicochemical characteristics of the radiopharmaceutical molecule (or element).

NUCLEAR MEDICINE AND LIVER CANCER

Hepatocellular Carcinoma

For more information on hepatocellular carcinoma (HCC), see Chapter 89.

Detection and Staging

HCC is detected and characterized by CT and MRI (see Chapter 14). Both 2020 National Comprehensive Cancer Network (NCCN) guidelines[3] and 2018 European Association for the Study of the Liver (EASL) guidelines[4] do not recommend PET/CT for detection of HCC because of its limited sensitivity.

HCC is FDG avid in less than 40% of HCC cases, with the majority of well-differentiated HCC tumors not avid or demonstrating avidity close to background liver on 18F-FDG PET, thus limiting sensitivity of detection (Fig. 18.1). Inherently low FDG avidity is because of the (1) HCC lower levels of glucose transporter-1 expression and (2) overexpression of the enzyme glucose-6-phosphatase, which hydrolyzes FDG-6-phosphate to FDG, which can be transported out of the cell.[5] However, increased glucose transporter expression has been demonstrated in poorly differentiated HCC, with increased FDG avidity on PET (Fig. 18.2); thus non-avid HCC appears to be associated with a less aggressive tumor and a more favorable patient prognosis.[6]

Tumor-to-liver uptake ratio (TLR) has been shown to correlate more closely with HCC doubling time and represents metabolic activity of HCC more precisely than SUV, with one study performed in 116 patients showing that a higher TLR (>1.62) was associated with poorer prognosis and presence of extrahepatic metastases.[7,8] Additionally, FDG-avid portal vein thrombosis has been shown to be an independent predictor for progression-free survival (PFS) and overall survival (OS), irrespective of avidity of primary HCC.[9] Thus PET/CT may be of potential prognostic value before surgical resection, liver transplantation, or locoregional therapy.

Extrahepatic metastasis (most commonly lung, abdominal nodes, and bone) have been found in 37% of patients during staging with poorly differentiated HCC more frequently likely to metastasize.[10] A positive statistical correlation between FDG avidity of primary HCCs and tendency of extrahepatic metastasis has been shown, suggesting that metastatic HCC lesions would also have increased FDG uptake. FDG PET has demonstrated high sensitivities of 77% to 100% for detecting extrahepatic metastasis, notably bone metastasis, with one study demonstrating superior diagnostic detection compared with bone scintigraphy.[11–13] Thus PET may have a role in detecting extrahepatic disease, but current NCCN and EASL guidelines do not support routine use. NCCN recommends continued use of bone scintigraphy with ^{99m}Tc–radiolabeled bisphonates, such as methylenediphosphate (MDP), for staging of HCC patients with bone lesions.

Additional PET tracers have been studied in HCC with Carbon 11 (^{11}C) acetate[14] and ^{11}C choline[15] and perform better than FDG PET for detection of well-differentiated HCC but are inferior compared with CT/MRI. Also, ^{11}C has a physical half-life of 20 minutes, requiring an onsite cyclotron or nearby producer for manufacturing of tracer, thus further limiting its widespread routine clinical use. ^{68}Ga-PSMA has recently been proposed as a potential tracer in HCC. PSMA plays a major role in regulating angiogenesis and endothelial cell recruitment, which occurs early in HCC and throughout hepatic tumorigenesis. Nearly 95% of HCCs stain positive for PSMA in the tumor vasculature and early prospective trials have shown that ^{68}Ga-PSMA PET has outperformed ^{18}F-FDG PET in the detection of HCC and extrahepatic disease.[16]

Tumor-Response Evaluation

FDG PET/CT has become a *tumor-response radiologic biomarker* with a major clinical impact on the management of a growing

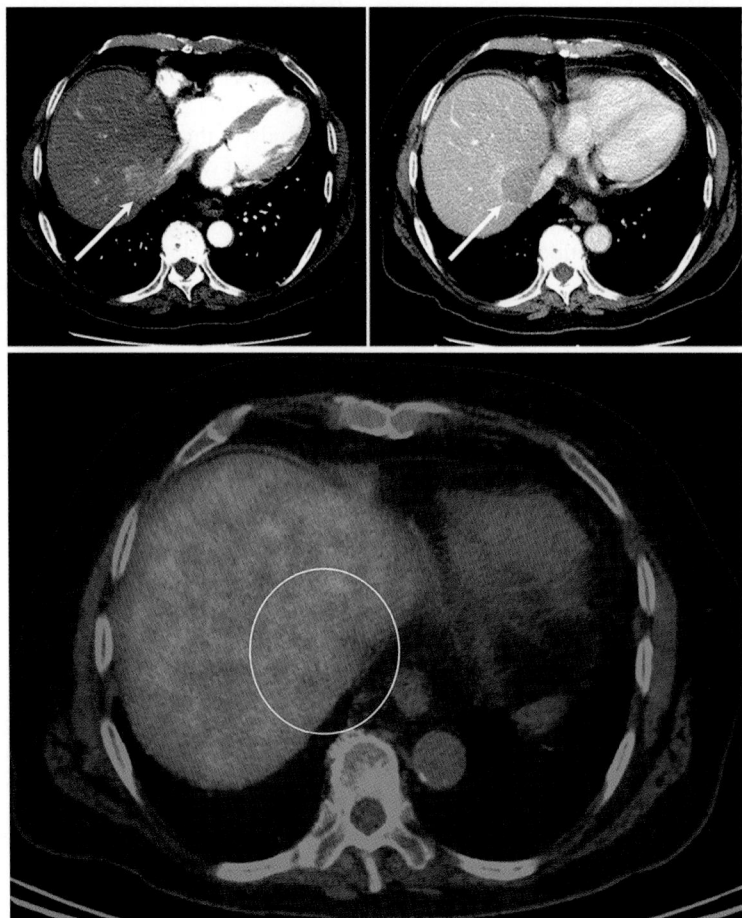

FIGURE 18.1 Well-differentiated hepatocellular carcinoma (HCC) on fluorodeoxyglucose (FDG) positron emission tomography (PET)/ computed tomography (CT). Multiphasic, contrast-enhanced CT of segment 8 lesion *(arrow, top left image)* contiguous with the inferior vena cava (IVC), which demonstrates with arterial phase hyperenhancement, washout, and enhancing capsule on delayed-phase imaging *(arrow, top right image)*, diagnosed as HCC based on imaging characteristics. Corresponding fused axial 18F-FDG PET/CT *(circle, bottom image)* does not show uptake in lesion above background liver, suggestive of well-differentiated HCC.

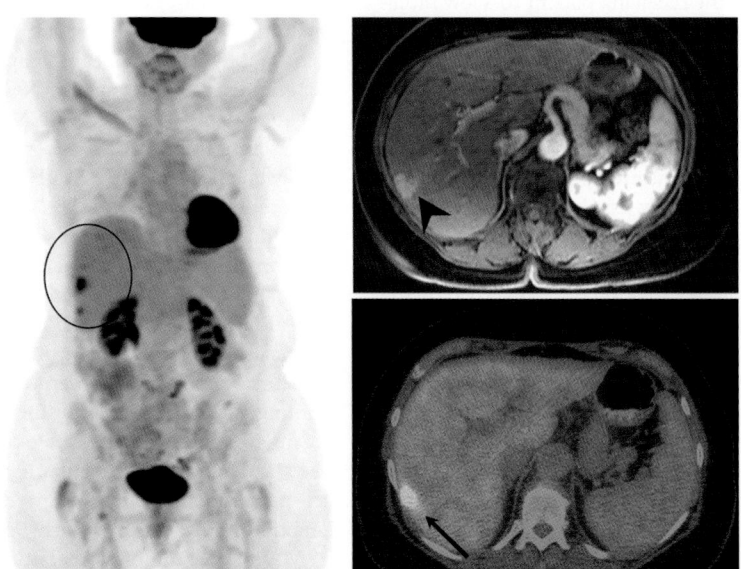

FIGURE 18.2 Poorly differentiated hepatocellular carcinoma (HCC) on fluorodeoxyglucose (FDG) positron emission tomography (PET)/ computed tomography (CT). Maximum intensity projection (MIP) image from 18F-FDG PET/CT *(left)* shows multiple right hepatic lobe FDG-avid lesions *(circled)* in a patient with known multifocal HCC. Arterial phase MRI *(top right image)* shows dominant segment 7 lesion with arterial phase hyperenhancement *(arrowhead)*, which demonstrates avidity above background liver on corresponding fused 18F-FDG PET/CT *(arrow, bottom right image)*, typical of poorly differentiated HCC. Poorly differentiated HCCs are more frequently likely to metastasize, with metastatic lesions also more likely to demonstrate increased FDG uptake.

number of other cancers (e.g., it is standard of care in breast cancer, lymphoma, esophageal cancer, and gastric cancer). In these types of cancer, overall robust clinical literature demonstrates that a therapy-induced decrease in tumor FDG avidity, as a biomarker of a decrease in tumor metabolism and tumor cell mass, correlates with histopathologic response and is often prognostically powerful, especially when conventional changes in tumor volume (e.g., anatomic criteria such as RECIST) measured by CT or MRI failed to predict either pathologic response or prognosis.[17] Nevertheless, unlike cancers such as invasive ductal breast cancer or high-grade lymphoma, which are frequently FDG avid, HCC frequently demonstrates minimal to no FDG avidity, therefore limiting the role of PET-response evaluation. As such, PET is not currently routinely recommended for HCC tumor response to therapy.

Still, the role of PET/CT has been shown to be potentially useful in certain post-treatment scenarios. In previous studies of HCC patients who underwent curative surgical resection or liver transplantation, high FDG uptake in an HCC showed a significant association with tumor recurrence, especially early recurrence.[18–20] Furthermore, retrospective studies have shown that when PET/CT is used in combination with Milan criteria (a solitary tumor ≤5 cm in diameter or 2 to 3 tumors ≤ 3 cm in diameter) with or without serum alpha fetal protein (AFP) for selecting candidates for liver transplantation, patients who are beyond the Milan criteria but have a negative PET/CT had clinical outcomes comparable with those within Milan criteria.[21] Furthermore, in candidates who met Milan criteria but had an FDG-avid HCC, higher rates of recurrence were seen than in those who had low FDG-avid HCC.[22,23] Thus a FDG PET finding has been found to be an independent predictive factor for tumor recurrence. Along with Milan criteria and serum AFP and FDG PET, it could provide additional information for making decisions regarding liver transplantation for HCC patients.

Locoregional therapy (e.g., ablation or transarterial chemoembolization [TACE]) is a preferred treatment option for patients with unresectable or nonoperable liver-confined disease (see Chapters 94 and 96). The prognostic value of FDG PET has been assessed in HCC patients treated with locoregional therapy, which suggests longer PFS and OS in patients with low FDG uptake of HCCs, again suggesting significant associations between FDG avidity of HCCs and clinical outcomes.[24]

Recurrence

HCC recurrence typically manifests as tumor regrowth at a prior site of treatment (e.g., ablation) or as tumor appearing at a new site in the liver. PET/CT is not routinely recommended for surveillance in the post-treatment HCC patient. However, Hayakawa et al. evaluated FDG PET/CT for detecting recurrent HCC postoperatively in patients with either suspected recurrence on CT or MRI (group 1) or suspected recurrence because of abnormal serum tumor markers but with no disease evident on CT or MRI (group 2). FDG PET/CT had a 53% and 41% sensitivity and 100% specificity for recurrent tumor in both groups 1 and 2, respectively. The data from group 1 support the idea that FDG PET/CT cannot replace CT or MRI as the first-line imaging modality for detection of recurrence; the data from group 2 support the hypothesis that FDG PET/CT may be of value as second-line imaging if CT or MRI fails to detect recurrence.[25] Wang et al. reported a remarkably high sensitivity of FDG PET/CT for HCC detection of 97%,

with a specificity of 83% ($n = 32$).[26] FDG PET/CT has reported sensitivity no greater than 90% (usually much lower) for HCC in the pretreatment setting.[12]

Colorectal Cancer Metastasis to Liver

For more information on colorectal cancer (CRC) metastasis to liver, see Chapter 90.

The most recent guidelines from the NCCN (2020),[27] European Society of Medical Oncology (ESMO),[28] and European Registration of Cancer Care (EURECCA)[29] agree on the potential roles and limitations of FDG PET/CT in clinical management of CRC and only recommend PET/CT in certain clinical circumstances (e.g., potentially surgically curable metastatic disease). As such, this discussion focuses on the CRC patient with potentially resectable liver metastases.

In CRC patients with liver metastases, but no extrahepatic metastases, complete resection of liver metastases improves long-term survival better than other treatments currently available. (see Chapters 90, 97, and 98). Before surgery, it is essential to confirm that liver metastases are likely resectable (based on CT and/or MRI imaging) and that no extrahepatic metastatic disease is present. CRC metastases occur most commonly in the liver, followed by the lungs, with metastases in the central nervous system, bones, adrenal glands, and spleen occurring in less than 10% of CRC patients.[30]

FDG PET/CT is extremely sensitive in detection of liver and lung metastases,[31] the two most common viscera to be involved by metastatic disease at initial presentation.[32] FDG PET/CT has long been recognized as superior to conventional CT for detecting hepatic metastases,[33–35] with decreasing sensitivity for both modalities in characterizing subcentimeter hepatic lesions.[36,37] FDG PET/CT and MRI are equivalent in diagnostic sensitivity for liver metastases, but MRI is more sensitive in identifying subcentimeter liver lesions than FDG PET/CT (i.e., with greater sensitivity). As such, PET/CT is not routinely indicated in primary staging of CRC in current NCCN guidelines. ESMO 2014 colorectal cancer guidelines agree with current NCCN guidelines regarding the role of FDG PET-CT.[28]

However, FDG PET/CT is considered a diagnostic adjunct to staging in patients with an equivocal finding on CT/MRI or in patients with potentially surgically curable metastatic disease (M1), as demonstrated on CT/MRI, but require evaluation for unrecognized metastatic disease that would preclude the possibility of surgical management. Patients planning to undergo hepatic resection based on conventional imaging will be found to have extrahepatic disease by FDG PET in 18% to 32% of cases (Fig. 18.3),[37–39] changing management in 20% to 40% of cases in early clinical PET trials[36,37] and changing management in curative-intent surgery in as many as 25% of patients in a later trial.[40] Fernandez et al. found that patients with hepatic metastases who underwent FDG PET for preoperative staging had a much higher 5-year survival rate than historic controls.[41] A randomized, controlled trial (RCT) of patients with resectable metachronous metastases assessed the role of PET/CT in the workup of potential curable disease.[42] This study showed that while PET/CT did not impact survival, surgical management was changed in 8% of patients after PET/CT, with additional sites of metastatic disease detected in 2.7% of patients (bone, peritoneum/omentum, abdominal nodes), thus precluding surgical resection. In addition, 1.5% of patients had more extensive hepatic resections and 3.4% had additional organ surgery. However, 8.4% of patients in the PET/CT arm had

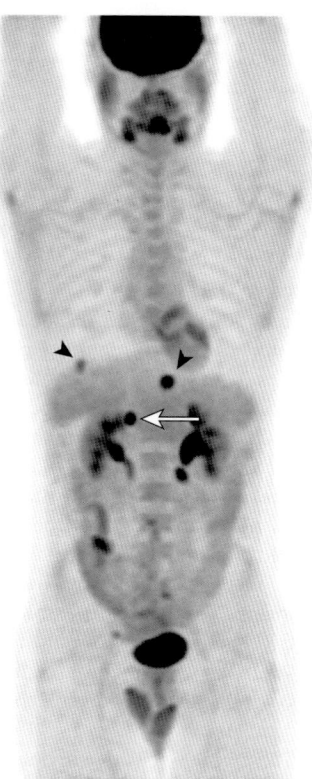

FIGURE 18.3 Role of fluorodeoxyglucose (FDG) positron emission tomography (PET)/computed tomography (CT) in colon cancer. Maximum intensity projection (MIP) image from FDG PET/CT of a colon cancer patient on chemotherapy being considered for locoregional therapy of known liver metastases. The MIP image demonstrates FDG-avid liver metastases *(arrowheads)* and FDG-avid extrahepatic disease, a subcentimeter right adrenal metastases with intense hypermetabolic activity *(arrow)*, new compared with a previous FDG PET scan and not appreciated on CT.

false-positive results, many of which required additional imaging with biopsies or other imaging modalities.

Additionally, current NCCN guidelines for CRC do not advocate routine use of FDG PET/CT for post-treatment follow-up imaging of patients with no evidence of distant metastatic disease by contrast-enhanced CT/MRI because of the potential risk for false-negative (e.g., non-avid necrotic liver lesions after chemotherapy) or false-positive findings (e.g., post treatment or surgery tissue inflammation). NCCN guidelines also do not recommend PET/CT in long-term monitoring: a small RCT reported earlier detection of recurrences with PET and suggested improved clinical outcomes compared with conventional CE imaging,[43] but larger trials are required to further investigate its utility.

The utility of FDG PET/MRI in the follow-up of treated CRC patients has been investigated, with initial studies showing promising results. When compared with current standard-of-care imaging, PET/MRI changed clinical management in 35.7% of cases: 21.5% upstaging cases and 14.2% downstaging cases ($P < .001$).[44] However, larger multicenter prospective studies with larger patient numbers are required to confirm these preliminary results.

NCCN guidelines also suggest clinicians consider FDG PET/CT for evaluation of patients with serial elevations of serum carcinoembryonic antigen (CEA) levels without an identifiable

source after standard IV contrast CT or colonoscopy. A systematic review and meta-analysis of 11 trials (510 patients) reported pooled estimates of sensitivity and specificity for FDG PET/CT for detection of occult tumor recurrence (after conventional CT workup) of 94% (95% confidence interval [CI], 89%–97%) and 77% (95% CI, 66%–86%), respectively.[45]

THE ROLE OF NUCLEAR MEDICINE IN LOCOREGIONAL LIVER THERAPY

Although surgical resection often provides the best patient outcomes for patients with HCC or metastatic liver lesion, some patients are not surgical candidates (e.g., because of the extent of tumor, underlying liver disease, or comorbid conditions). In these patients, locoregional therapies (e.g., ablation, transarterial chemoembolization, or radioembolization) can be offered typically as a palliative therapy, although it can offer curative extent in certain cases. Locoregional therapies will be discussed in more detail in Chapters 94 and 96, but we will briefly touch on the role of nuclear medicine in workup, therapy, and surveillance in this setting.

THE ROLE OF NUCLEAR MEDICINE IN HEPATIC ARTERIAL INFUSION THERAPY

Hepatic arterial infusion therapy (HAIT) is direct infusion of a therapeutic compound (e.g., chemotherapeutic, embolic, or radioembolic agents) to treat malignant liver tumors (primary or secondary; see Chapters 94, 97, and 100). Clinical studies demonstrate that arterial infusion improves tumor uptake of certain chemotherapeutic agents compared with portal venous or systemic venous infusion.[46] Cancerous liver tumors derive/stimulate a nutrient blood supply from the arterial system by tumor neoangiogenesis as opposed to normal hepatic parenchyma, which receives blood supply mostly from the portal venous system.

Hepatic arterial infusion scintigraphy (HAIS), also called hepatic arterial perfusion scintigraphy, is the imaging of the biodistribution of a radionuclide delivered directly into liver through an arterial catheter, typically in the (proper) hepatic artery, for delivery of chemotherapy, or potentially into hepatic lobar or segmental arterial branches, when HAIS is conducted associated with HAIT radioembolization (e.g., treatment with ^{90}Y-radiolabeled resin or glass microspheres or ^{131}I-radiolabeled lipiodol).

The role of HAIS is to:
(1) predict that infused macroaggregated albumin (MAA) is properly distributed throughout the downstream liver or targeted hepatic subregion before HAIT,
(2) ensure that no extrahepatic infusion caused by variant anatomy is present before HAIT,
(3) calculate lung shunt volumes before *radioembolic* HAIT is performed,
(4) predict or measure hepatic radiation dosimetry, before or after HAIT, and
(5) ensure the integrity and function of an infusion system before administration of medication (e.g., post placement of a hepatic intraarterial pump reservoir-catheter system, which is used to deliver local chemotherapy).

Placement of the arterial catheter used for HAIT and HAIS involves different possible techniques, most commonly placed intermittently into the hepatic artery during an interventional radiology (IR) procedure. In certain institutions, catheters may connect to a subcutaneously implanted port or an infusion pump system to allow slow, continuous drug infusion of hepatic arterial chemotherapy (more commonly performed in the United States). The tracer used for HAIS for treatment planning is ^{99m}Tc MAA, a radiolabeled particulate, 25 to 50 μm in mean diameter, which physically occludes the first microvascular lumen it encounters. The infusate tracer, several hundred thousand MAA particles, labeled with a trace amount of radioactivity, are suspended in a small volume of saline (e.g., 2 cc) and injected into a transiently placed hepatic artery catheter or hepatic pump (see Chapter 97) by a trained operator (e.g., physician or nurse) and remain intact in vivo for several hours, allowing imaging of the distribution of tracer. Injection of an infusate can be slow (e.g., <1 cc/min), which mimics somewhat the slow rate typical of pump-infusions in HAI chemotherapy. Fast injection of infusate (e.g., ≥1 cc/sec; bolus) allows rapid introduction of infusate into the hepatic artery, creating turbulence in the bloodstream that mixes infusate and blood more homogeneously and more rapidly and, as a result, bolus infusions of tracer infusate are typically not advised for HAIS because the bolus pressure may cause retrograde flow of tracer into other celiac branches and artifactual extrahepatic tracer accumulations.[47] Extrahepatic tracer accumulations, when tracer is infused slowly, are usually because of variant hepatic arterial anatomy, such as branches supplying extrahepatic viscera (e.g., stomach, pancreas, gastrointestinal [GI] tract) and could lead to complications (e.g., GI ulceration) if not identified before HAIT. True aberrant arterial branches typically must be embolized before HAIT to avoid extrahepatic organ toxicity.

SPECT/CT provides excellent anatomic localization of infused ^{99m}Tc MAA. Alternatively, ^{99m}Tc-labeled SC scintigraphy can immediately precede HAIS, to provide a gross outline of hepatic (and splenic) anatomic contours (Fig. 18.4). Because ^{99m}Tc-MAA HAIS and ^{99m}Tc-SC scintigraphy use the same ^{99m}Tc isotope, a larger amount (activity, MBq) of ^{99m}Tc MAA is administered than ^{99m}Tc sulphur colloid (SC), so that the

signal on the subsequent HAIS scan *predominantly* represents ^{99m}Tc MAA. However, confusion can arise regarding overlap between ^{99m}Tc-SC and ^{99m}Tc-MAA signals, as in evaluation of the homogeneity of ^{99m}Tc-MAA hepatic distribution. Additionally, if any delay occurs after ^{99m}Tc SC is injected, before ^{99m}Tc-MAA scintigraphy is performed, ^{99m}Tc-SC catabolic breakdown and release of free pertechnetate can yield gastric tracer-uptake, potentially mimicking extrahepatic infusion of the stomach on ^{99m}Tc-MAA scintigraphy. Obtaining dynamic images of ^{99m}Tc-MAA uptake as it is infused slowly for two minutes or more permits detection of increases in hepatic or extrahepatic tracer uptake indicative of true ^{99m}Tc-MAA signal, whereas any residual ^{99m}Tc-SC or free-pertechnetate signal will remain unchanged during dynamic imaging of the ^{99m}Tc-MAA infusion (Fig. 18.5). ^{99m}Tc-MAA SPECT/CT without ^{99m}Tc SC has the advantage of having SPECT imagery that solely represents ^{99m}Tc-MAA biodistribution, although CT typically is associated with a higher radiation dose to the patient than ^{99m}Tc-SC scintigraphy.

Abnormal HAIS findings include subtotal hepatic infusion (in nonselective angiography cases), extrahepatic organ infusion, catheter obstruction, and catheter leakage (Fig. 18.6) and typically require additional investigation (e.g., fluoroscopy or CT hepatic angiography) to guide subsequent management. In a clinical study of patients with implanted hepatic arterial pump-catheter systems, HAIS studies revealed abnormalities in 9% of patients after pump implantation; the abnormalities were predominantly extrahepatic infusion (63% of abnormal studies), but 12% demonstrated abnormal subtotal intrahepatic infusion (i.e., infusion distributed to only a portion of the liver, when infusion of the entire liver was expected). Abnormal subtotal intrahepatic infusion (i.e., regions of devoid of infusate

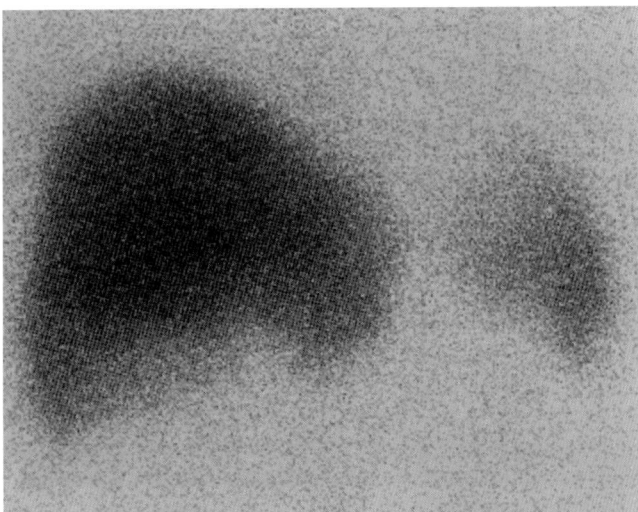

FIGURE 18.4 Normal appearance of technetium 99m (^{99m}Tc)–labeled sulfur colloid scintigraphy. An anterior projection of the abdomen is shown. The larger mass at left is the liver. The smaller mass is the spleen. Sulfur colloid tracer accumulation in vertebral marrow is sometimes faintly detectable, although not in this patient.

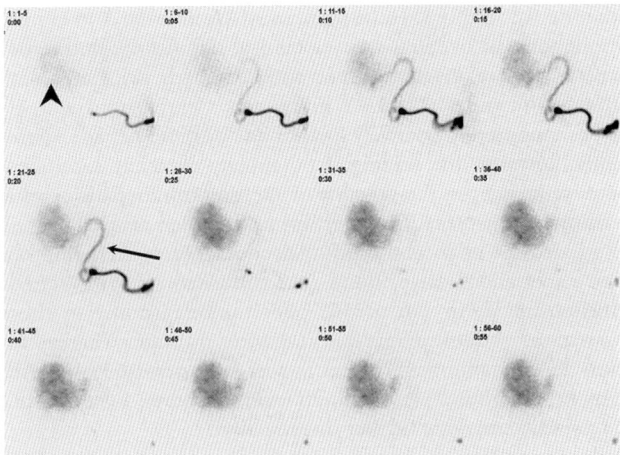

FIGURE 18.5 Normal appearance of hepatic arterial infusion scintigraphy. Serial anterior projection planar images were obtained during slow bolus injection of technetium 99m (^{99m}Tc) macroaggregated albumin (MAA) into the common hepatic artery via an implanted hepatic pump-catheter system at rate of five seconds/frame. On the first image, before the ^{99m}Tc MAA has reached the liver, faint activity is detectable in the liver *(arrowhead)*; this faint activity is from ^{99m}Tc-labeled sulfur colloid tracer, used immediately before to obtain a gross anatomic outline. The ^{99m}Tc MAA is visualized transiting through the pump catheter as it is slowly infused *(arrow)*. Progressive accumulation of the ^{99m}Tc-MAA infusate throughout the liver is visualized as the infusion is completed. No abnormal extrahepatic accumulation of ^{99m}Tc-MAA infusate is evident.

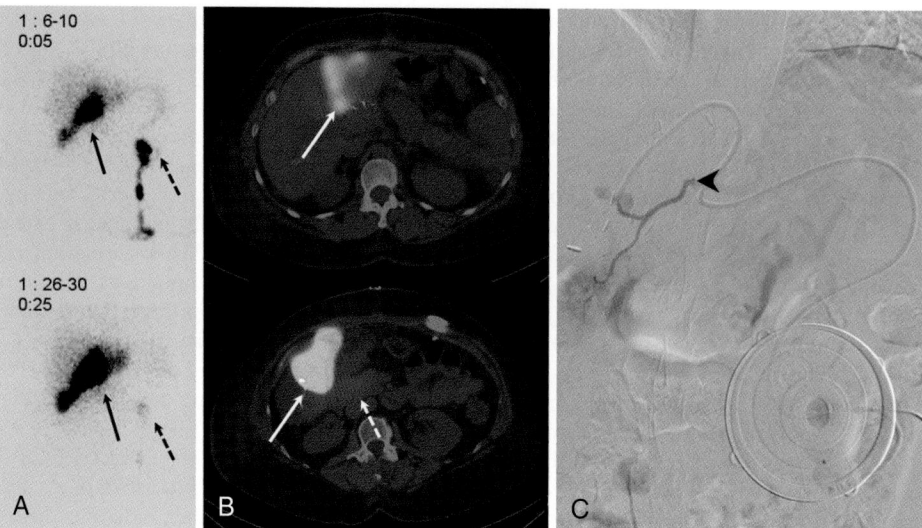

FIGURE 18.6 Abnormal hepatic arterial infusion scintigraphy (HAIS). A 67-year-old woman with colon cancer with liver metastases after a recent hepatic arterial pump placement for intraarterial chemotherapy and HAIS performed to ensure patency of system before chemotherapy infusion. **A,** Two selected anterior abdominal images are shown from a series of five-second-per-frame images acquired during a one-minute infusion of technetium 99m (^{99m}Tc) macroaggregated albumin (MAA) into the common hepatic artery via a hepatic pump-catheter system. The *top image* was obtained at five seconds and the *bottom image* at 25 seconds into the infusion show abnormal progressive accumulation of ^{99m}Tc MAA only into the left lobe of liver *(solid arrow)* and in the gastropancreatic region *(dashed arrow)*. **B,** Corresponding single-photon emission computed tomography (SPECT)/computed tomography (CT) images from HAIS showing accumulation of ^{99m}Tc-MAA into the left lobe of liver *(solid arrow)* and in the gastropancreatic region *(dashed arrow)*. **C,** Spot fluoroscopic image from angiography identifying celiac origin stenosis *(arrowhead)* with resultant reversal of arterial blood flow to the left hepatic artery. Additionally, the right hepatic artery was replaced to the superior mesenteric artery (not shown). These findings accounted for abnormal HAIS.

uptake) should be distinguished from heterogenous intrahepatic distribution of MAA infusate, which occurs probably in part because of laminar flow phenomenon. The laminar flow phenomenon can occur in the presence of a large hepatic tumor mass, which appears to draw hepatic arterial flow away from other hepatic regions. Heterogenous MAA infusate distribution throughout the liver has no *clear* clinical significance and in our experience is relatively common and not clearly associated with adverse outcomes. If MAA infusate is clearly, unexpectedly *absent* (not merely relatively low) in one or more hepatic subregions, however, the finding is potentially clinically significant because it suggests the possibly of aberrant intrahepatic arterial anatomy, a misplaced catheter, or an occluded arterial branch (e.g., stenotic or thrombosed). Anecdotal cases, including our own experiences, have found that abnormal subtotal hepatic infusion on HAIS can predict poor tumor response in those subregions without detectable receipt of infusate, whereas tumors in the same patient that appear well perfused on HAIS respond favorably.[48] As such, abnormal subtotal hepatic infusion always warrants further investigation.

In the setting of *hepatic pump* HAIS abnormalities, pump fluoroscopy evaluation fails to find corresponding abnormalities in approximately 25% of cases.[49] In those cases, HAIS was repeated, and the previously identified HAIS abnormality was no longer evident scintigraphically in almost all cases. In the few cases in which the HAIS abnormality persisted, fluoroscopic or CT studies were again repeated, and a corresponding aberrant vessel was successfully identified. This study recommended evaluating abnormal HAIS findings by fluoroscopic correlative imaging initially; if radiographic correlation is found, HAIS is repeated in two to three weeks, seeking spontaneous normalization of HAIS.

Radioembolization therapy with yttrium 90 (^{90}Y)–labeled glass or resin microspheres delivered by hepatic intraarterial catheter infusion is used for treatment of colorectal metastases or HCC (see Chapter 94B). Patients before therapy undergo HAIS to delineate hepatic perfusion and extrahepatic supply, as previously mentioned, but also dosimetry to calculate dose to tumor, and lung shunt fraction (LSF) needs to be calculated on ^{99m}Tc-MAA imaging before treatment because radiation-induced pneumonitis and sclerosis can occur because of hepatopulmonary shunting of radioembolic microspheres and is a potential major toxicity concern. Significant shunting is estimated at LSF greater than 15%, which requires treatment modification before HAIT to reduce complications or not treating if LSF is greater than 20%.[50] Immediately after therapy, typically SPECT/CT is performed to evaluate technical success, although in certain centers, ^{90}Y-PET/CT is used instead.

After radioembolization dosimetry, SPECT or PET/CT, performed within 24 hours of treatment, has been employed in certain institutions because it enables rapid and precise prediction of efficacy on a per-lesion basis and allows for early treatment adaptation in case of undertreatment of the lesions. One study showed that in chemo-refractory mCRC, patients treated with radioembolization that absorbed dose determined on post radioembolization ^{90}Y-PET/CT correlated with metabolic response, and higher lesion mean absorbed doses were associated with prolonged OS.[51]

There is no standard protocol for pre- and postradioembolization imaging, with CT being the most commonly used modality. The role of FDG PET/CT has been suggested as a promising radiologic assay for detecting a favorable liver tumor response to ^{90}Y microsphere radioembolization.[52] One study showed that increased metabolic activity of the lesion pretherapy was associated with decreased liver PFS postradioembolization with authors recommending use of FDG PET/CT as part of work-up before therapy.[53] Furthermore, the current data are heterogenous with regards to FDG PET/CT in the setting of evaluating postembolization treatment response of liver metastasis versus HCC because well-differentiated HCC does not typically accumulate FDG as previously discussed. As such, current guidelines do not recommend use of PET/CT routinely in pre- and postradioembolization imaging.

THE ROLE OF POSITRON EMISSION TOMOGRAPHY IN PERCUTANEOUS LIVER ABLATION

Percutaneous ablation of hepatic malignancies, HCC or liver metastases, can be considered in patients who are not surgical candidates or as a bridging strategy before curative therapy (e.g., resection or transplantation[27]; see Chapter 96). As discussed previously, FDG PET/CT has been shown to be superior to CT or MRI alone in staging patients with hepatic metastases and can often lead to a change in the treatment plan in patients being considered for percutaneous ablation. In one study, pre-ablation PET/CT led to a change in clinical management in 26% of patients in whom extrahepatic disease was identified and ablation was not performed.[54] Another study found that PET/CT altered the clinical management in 25% of potential radiofrequency ablation (RFA) candidates with colorectal hepatic metastases in whom extrahepatic disease was missed by conventional imaging, and systemic chemotherapy was offered instead of performing ablation.[55] PET/CT imaging can be used within the IR suite to guide ablation in PET-avid CT occult lesions. Additionally, periprocedural PET/CT can be used to determine technical success and permits immediate repeat tumor ablation as needed.[56]

Recurrence after percutaneous ablation of hepatic malignancy is, unfortunately, not uncommon. After ablation of HCC, local recurrence rates of 11% to 36% have been reported, with more frequent recurrence occurring after treatment of larger lesions and lesions close to large vessels. Metastatic colorectal cancer recurs even more frequently after ablation than in HCC, with reported rates over 50%. High quality post-ablation surveillance imaging is required to identify residual or recurrent tumor to allow early identification of recurrent or residual disease and retreatment. However, it can be challenging to distinguish recurrent or residual disease from normal treatment response. Immediately after thermal ablation of the liver, the central area of post-ablation necrosis is surrounded by a zone of hyperemia and a peripheral rim of mild reactive change, which appears as a central nonenhancing area of necrosis, with a rim of increased enhancement compared with normal liver tissue in the hyperemic zone on contrast enhanced CT or MRI (see Chapters 14 and 15). The rim of increased enhancement may mask residual viable tumor in the early post-ablation period. Cells destroyed by thermal ablation lose their ability to concentrate glucose within the cell; thus, on FDG PET/CT, there is a corresponding photopenic area.[57] Glucose metabolism within the zone of hyperemia, however, is unaltered and normal FDG uptake or a rim of uniform, low-grade FDG uptake surrounding the ablation site may be present. If focal areas of increased FDG uptake are seen adjacent to the photopenic area of necrosis within 48 hours of ablation, residual macroscopic tumor is suspected. From 72 hours to 6 months after

ablation, a band of regenerative tissue containing neutrophils and fibroblasts develops surrounding the ablation zone that demonstrates variable degrees of both peripheral enhancement and also increased FDG uptake surrounding the ablation site because of inflammatory changes; however, FDG PET/CT seems more sensitive for determining the treatment effect and detecting local recurrence because of combined functional and anatomic information. Chen et al. retrospectively reviewed 33 lesions treated with RFA in 28 patients and reported that PET/CT demonstrated superior sensitivity and accuracy (94.1% and 87.9%, respectively) compared with MRI (66.7% and 75%, respectively) and multiphase contrast-enhanced CT (66.7% and 64.3%, respectively).[58] To date, however, there are no established guidelines for when to perform post-ablation PET/CT, with some centers proposing intervals of 3 to 6 months for the first year after ablation, and over 95% of local recurrences identified within 1 year of treatment.[59]

NUCLEAR MEDICINE AND BILIARY TRACT CANCERS

Intrahepatic and Extrahepatic Cholangiocarcinoma

For more information on intrahepatic and extrahepatic cholangiocarcinoma, see Chapters 50 and 51.

Cholangiocarcinomas include all tumors originating in the epithelium of the bile duct, with intrahepatic cholangiocarcinoma being more common than extrahepatic and the second most common primary hepatic tumor. Cholangiocarcinomas are typically FDG avid. A recent meta-analysis of 47 studies found that FDG PET/CT had an overall sensitivity of 91.7% and specificity of 51.3% for detection of cholangiocarcinoma with sensitivity of 88.4% and specificity of 69.1% for lymph node invasion.[60] PET/CT performed better for the detection of distant metastases and local recurrence, with a sensitivity and specificity of 85.4% and 89.7% and 90.1% and 83.5%, respectively.

A previous meta-analysis found PET/CT had higher diagnostic sensitivity for intrahepatic tumors than for perihilar and other extrahepatic tumors.[61] As such, there is growing evidence that [18]FDG-PET should be incorporated into the current standard of care for the staging (lymph node and distant metastases) and identification of relapse to guide treatment selection, especially if standard of care imaging MRI/CT are equivocal. Although the role of PET/CT for diagnosis of the primary tumor is not currently recommended by NCCN because of low sensitivity,[3] emerging evidence indicates that it may be useful for the detection of regional lymph node metastases and distant metastatic disease in patients with otherwise potentially resectable disease.[62,63] However, FDG-avid inflammation along the biliary tree (i.e., cholangitis) can mimic or obscure detection of FDG-avid biliary tumor.

Gallbladder Cancer

For more information on gallbladder cancer, see Chapter 49.

Gallbladder cancer is often diagnosed at an advanced stage because of the aggressive nature of the tumor; often its symptoms mimic benign conditions, including biliary colic or chronic cholecystitis. The role of PET has not been established in the evaluation of patients with gallbladder cancer, but evidence from retrospective studies indicates that it may be useful for the detection of radiologically occult regional lymph node and distant metastatic disease in patients with otherwise potentially resectable disease.[63,64] No prospective trials, however, have been performed to date to confirm the role of PET/CT. Additionally, false positives related to an inflamed gallbladder can make interpretation troublesome.

Pancreatic Adenocarcinoma

For more information on pancreatic adenocarcinoma, see Chapters 61 and 62.

Detection and Staging

The standard diagnostic workup for pancreatic cancer is high-quality contrast-enhanced CT with pancreatic protocol.[65] The role of PET/CT remains unclear, and current guidelines only recommend the role of PET/CT in certain circumstances (e.g., borderline resectable disease, markedly elevated CA 19-9, large primary tumors, or large regional lymph nodes) to detect extra-pancreatic metastases.

PET/CT has long been reported to be a highly sensitive method for detecting pancreatic cancer, with reported sensitivity of 85% to 97%; however, PET/CT lacks specificity with reported rates of 61% to 94%.[66–68] A 2012 meta-analysis of 16 studies with 804 patients found FDG PET/CT offered a diagnostic sensitivity of 87% and specificity of 83%.[69] A 2014 meta-analysis (including much of the same data as the 2012 analysis) obtained similar results: FDG PET/CT for evaluation of suspected pancreatic cancer was calculated to offer pooled sensitivity of 90% and specificity of 76%.[70] Typically pancreatic adenocarcinoma presents as a focally hypermetabolic focus; however, benign conditions, such as focal acute pancreatitis and mass forming chronic pancreatitis can also present as hypermetabolic foci.[62]

One possible reason for the relatively low specificity of PET/CT may be because of misdiagnosis of a benign condition, such as mass-forming pancreatitis, as a pancreatic adenocarcinoma. This is a challenging diagnosis on multiple imaging modalities because chronic inflammation in mass-forming pancreatitis leads to fibrosis of pancreatic parenchyma and thus demonstrates similar imaging characteristics to pancreatic adenocarcinoma on CT (a hypodense mass with mild or no enhancement; see Chapter 17). The reported sensitivity and specificity of CT for differentiating chronic pancreatitis from cancer were 82% to 94% and 83% to 90%, respectively,[71] with similar results in MRI (sensitivity of 93% and specificity of 87%). Early studies suggested that FDG PET could reliably differentiate between mass-forming pancreatitis and pancreatic adenocarcinoma because overexpression of the glucose transporter 1 is increased in pancreatic cancer but not in chronic pancreatitis, which revealed the possibility of diagnosing pancreatic cancer from mass-forming pancreatitis.[66,72] However, the value of FDG-PET/CT in differentiating pancreatic cancer from chronic pancreatitis remains controversial because high FDG uptake caused by increased glycolytic activity in inflammatory cells such as neutrophils and activated macrophages has been seen in pancreatitis, including mass-forming pancreatitis,[73] and its utility remains unclear in diagnosis.

Another potential cause of low sensitivity of PET/CT in detection of pancreatic adenocarcinoma may be because of characteristics of the tumor. If the lesion is predominantly cystic then the lesion is typically FDG PET–negative, regardless of whether it is benign or malignant. However, some benign or low-grade malignant solid pancreatic lesions (e.g., solid pseudopapillary tumors) can be as FDG avid as malignant solid pancreatic adenocarcinomas.[74] In fact, if a solid tumor has activity close to blood pool activity (i.e., minimal FDG avidity), it is more likely to be a pancreatic adenocarcinoma or neuroendocrine tumor than a solid pseudopapillary tumor (which usually demonstrate FDG avid significantly above blood pool).[75]

The main potential utility of FDG PET/CT in pancreatic cancer is as an *adjunct in staging*. One study showed that sensitivity of detecting metastatic disease for PET/CT alone, standard CT alone, and the combination of PET/CT and standard CT were 61%, 57%, and 87%, respectively. Studies have shown that clinical management of 11% of patients with invasive pancreatic cancer and resectability status in at least 20% to 30% of patients were changed based on PET/CT findings because PET/CT detected metastatic lesions that were not identified by the standard staging protocol in these patients.[76,77]

Because of the low-dose noncontrast companion CT, however, PET/CT is limited in tumor(T) staging. Nonenhanced companion CT often fails to detect vascular invasion.[78,79] Studies have shown that FDG PET/CT combined with contrast-enhanced CT offers superior diagnostic accuracy compared with standard PET/CT (performed with a noncontrast, low-dose CT) with diagnostic sensitivity of 91% (95% CI, 86%–96%) versus 88% (95% CI, 78%–100%), and specificity of 88% (95% CI, 73%–100%) versus 81% (95% CI, 69%–94%), respectively, although these were not statistically significant differences ($P > .05$).[69] Also, contrast-enhanced PET/CT is not commonly performed in routine clinical practice because it does not replace the multiphase contrast-enhanced CT (pancreatic protocol) required for accurate diagnosis and staging (see Chapter 17). PET/CT utility in detecting nodal(N) metastasis is limited, with a reported sensitivity of 0% to 57%,[26] perhaps because lymph node size is not a reliable parameter for the evaluation of metastatic involvement in pancreatic adenocarcinoma, and small nodes (<5 mm) are difficult to detect because of spatial resolution.

Conversely, for detection of distant metastases, FDG PET/CT appears to have relatively high specificity of 91% to 100%,[26] especially for lung and bone metastases.[78] However, detection of liver metastases with FDG PET/CT has a reported sensitivity of 22% to 88%; this wide variance is probably accounted for by the reduced sensitivity of PET in detection of subcentimeter lesions because of the partial volume averaging effect. Despite the variability in reported percentages, clinical studies predominantly report that FDG PET/CT seems to perform better than conventional CT for detection of liver metastases, although most studies were underpowered.[26] MRI offers superior diagnostic sensitivity for liver metastases compared with FDG PET/CT on a per-lesion basis, particularly for detection of subcentimeter liver metastases. The sensitivity of FDG PET/CT for detection of bone metastases is superior to standard CT because bone metastases may only be associated with subtle osteolytic changes on CT or may be CT occult because they are predominantly bone marrow–based. MRI is at least as diagnostically accurate as FDG PET/CT for detection of osseous metastases. Other common metastatic sites include lungs and peritoneum, with the diagnostic accuracy of FDG PET/CT appearing similar to that of standard CT; a dedicated contrast-enhanced CT scan improves PET/CT detection of peritoneal metastases significantly compared with PET with a nondiagnostic companion CT.

PET/MRI has been shown to be equivalent to PET/CT for determination of resectability and staging tumors.[80] The combination of diffusion-weighted imaging (DWI) and metabolic markers (metabolic tumor volume) appears to predict advanced stage tumor and is correlated with progression-free survival.[81]

Pancreatic Tumor Response and Recurrence

FDG PET/CT for detecting pancreatic cancer response is superior in general to conventional CT or MRI for predicting favorable histopathologic response and for predicting patient outcomes.[82] Multiple clinical trials have shown that changes in pancreatic tumor hypermetabolic activity, measured by comparing a pretreatment PET scan with a post-treatment or on-treatment PET scan, correlated with (predicted) histologic response, radiologic (CT or MRI) response, or patient response (e.g., overall survival or progression-free survival).[26] Topkan et al. demonstrated that in patients with locally advanced *unresectable* pancreatic carcinoma treated with chemoradiotherapy (5-fluorouracil [5-FU] and gemcitabine), patients who demonstrated above-average decreases in tumor hypermetabolic activity demonstrated superior median overall survival (17.0 vs. 9.8 months; $P = .001$), progression-free survival (8.4 vs. 3.8 months; $P = .005$), and locoregional progression-free survival (12.3 vs. 6.9 months; $P = 0.02$) compared with poor responders.[83] The predictive value of a favorable "metabolic response" on FDG PET/CT remained statistically significant for each of these three outcomes on multivariate analysis. Others have reported statistically significant correlations between favorable FDG PET/CT tumor metabolic response to chemoradiotherapy and favorable survival outcome in unresectable, locally advanced pancreatic cancer as well.[76,77,84] One study showed similar predictive power of FDG PET/CT for treating unresectable disease treated with chemotherapy alone[85] (see Chapter 66).

For resectable pancreatic cancer, studies have shown FDG PET/CT can predict histologic response to neoadjuvant chemotherapy. Heinrich et al. initially showed in patients treated with neoadjuvant gemcitabine and cisplatin that although both PET responders and nonresponders had microscopic disease after surgery, the responders had less microscopic disease,[86] and neither PET nor histologic response correlated with survival outcomes. Later studies compared metabolic response on PET/CT of other neoadjuvant regimes (namely, nab-paclitaxel plus gemcitabine vs. gemcitabine alone because the MAPCT trial proved that nab-paclitaxel and gemcitabine demonstrated superior efficacy versus gemcitabine alone for patients with metastatic pancreatic cancer). The nab-paclitaxel plus gemcitabine arm demonstrated an increased metabolic response compared with gemcitabine alone and its metabolic response by PET (best response at any time during study) was associated with longer overall survival (OS; median 11.3 vs. 6.9 months). Also in both arms more patients experienced a metabolic response than a RECIST-defined size response.[87] As a result of this study, the NCCN now recognizes the role of PET/CT in tumor response in the neoadjuvant chemotherapy setting.

FDG PET/CT also has a role in detection of recurrence in pancreatic adenocarcinoma, although it is not recommended by guidelines currently. Pancreatic cancer recurrence can be detected by elevation of serum levels of the tumor marker with high diagnostic sensitivity, but serum assays do not distinguish the anatomic location of the disease recurrence (e.g., in a tumor resection bed or as new metastases). Small studies indicate that FDG PET/CT after conventional CT in the setting of suspected recurrence will change therapeutic management in as many as 44% of patients,[88] and FDG PET/CT identifies local pancreatic cancer recurrence in the surgical bed better than standard CT or MRI.[88] FDG PET/CT detected local recurrence with 67% to 96% sensitivity versus 39% to 50% sensitivity for CT and/or MRI.[26,89] FDG PET/CT appears superior to conventional CT for detection of recurrence in lymph nodes, peritoneal implants, and bones. Diagnostic sensitivity and specificity for FDG PET/CT are typically greater than 90% for suspicious FDG-avid lymph nodes, peritoneal lesions, and bone lesions compared with CT, which has a sensitivity of approximately 60% for nodal metastases, 50% for peritoneal recurrence, and less than 5% for recurrence as bone metastatic disease.[89] As mentioned previously, MRI has superior sensitivity to FDG PET/CT for detection of liver lesions and thus detection of recurrent liver metastases.

Gastroenteropancreatic Neuroendocrine Tumors

For more information on gastroenteropancreatic (GEP) neuroendocrine tumors (NETs), see Chapters 65, 87, and 91.

NETs are epithelial neoplasms with predominant neuroendocrine differentiation, which are classified according to their embryonic origin: foregut (bronchial, gastric, duodenal, pancreatic); midgut (ileal, jejunal, cecal); or hindgut (distal colonic, rectal). NET tumors are classified according to grade or Ki-67 expression: low grade (G1) indicates less than 3%, intermediate grade (G2) is 3% to 20%, and high grade (G3) is greater than 20%. NETs are variable in their presentation depending on whether the tumor is functioning or nonfunctioning. Although generally considered rare because of low incidence of 2.5 to 5 per 100,000 in the United States, NETs have a higher prevalence than more aggressive and common malignancies, such as pancreatic or gastric adenocarcinoma.[90] For the purpose of this discussion, we will concentrate on GEP-NETs.

Imaging

The somatostatin receptor (SSTR) family consists of different subtypes and belongs to the group of G-protein–coupled receptors. Approximately 70% to 90% of GEP-NETs express different SSTRs, predominantly subtype 2 and, to a lesser degree, subtypes 1 and 5 receptors.[91,92] There have been major developments in diagnostic options available to patients in the last 5 years in the United States, thus allowing for the development of "personalized" therapeutic options. In June 2016, the Food and Drug Administration (FDA) approved the use of PET tracer ^{68}Ga-radiolabeled SSTR analogue ^{68}Ga-DOTATATE for the diagnosis of NET. Before this, there was a disparity in standards of practice for the diagnostic workup of NETs in the United States compared with Europe and the rest of world. In the United States, the FDA-approved radiotracers for NET imaging were planar and SPECT/CT imaging with the Indium-111 (^{111}In) radiolabeled analogue of the SSTR-binding octapeptide, octreotide (^{111}In pentetreotide). In Europe and elsewhere, however, PET tracers with ^{68}Ga-SSTR analogues, notably ^{68}Ga-DOTATOC, ^{68}Ga-DOTANOC, and ^{68}Ga-DOTATATE, were approved for workup of NETs.[93]

Octreotide was the first somatostatin analogue (SSA) introduced into clinical practice. In 1994, ^{111}In–diethylenetriamine pentaacetic acid (DTPA)–octreotide (Octreoscan, Mallinckrodt, St. Louis, MO) was approved by the FDA as a clinical imaging agent because it demonstrates high affinity for SSTR2 with sensitivity of greater than 80% for diagnosis of well-differentiated (grades 1 and 2) tumors.[94,95] Typically, planar and SPECT images are obtained 24 and 48 hours after tracer injection with SPECT/CT imaging, allowing for both functional and anatomic localization simultaneously. ^{68}Ga-SSTR PET/CT tracers have been repeatedly shown to offer significantly superior diagnostic sensitivity for SSTR-overexpressing NETs in multiple clinical trials, compared with ^{111}In pentetreotide scintigraphy on a per-lesion and per-patient basis, and allow for earlier imaging time points (1–3 hours after tracer injection) for increased patient convenience.[95]

SSTR-targeted scintigraphy is often used to predict tumor response to SSTR-targeted therapy (e.g., with octreotide or other SSAs). Studies have showed that ^{68}Ga-DOTATATE PET/CT changed treatment in 36% of patients compared with ^{111}In pentetreotide[96] and 41% of patients compared with conventional diagnostic imaging,[97] mainly because of the detection of additional findings. [68]Ga -DOTATATE PET/CT is also associated with no significant toxicity and lower radiation exposure compared with ^{111}In pentetreotide scintigraphy, and thus [68]Ga -DOTATATE PET/CT should preferentially be used when available.

Physiologic uptake of SSAs is seen in pituitary, thyroid, kidney, liver, and spleen. [68]Ga -DOTATATE PET/CT tracers are most sensitive for low-grade NETs (low Ki-67 index). High-grade NETs (high Ki-67 index) indicate a loss of SSTR expression and dedifferentiation and, therefore, FDG PET/CT should be considered for characterization instead of ^{68}Ga-SSTR PET/CT in these cases. Insulinomas, which predominantly express SSTR2 and SSTR5,[98] are typically avid on ^{68}Ga-SSTR PET/CT imaging, with reported sensitivity up to 90%.[99,100] As with other types of NET, higher-grade or poorly differentiated tumors are better assessed with FDG-PET/CT. ^{68}Ga-SSTR-PET/MRI has been used in imaging of NET and has been shown to improve the detection of liver metastases, particularly when hepatobiliary phase imaging is used.[101] However, detection of bone and lung metastasis may be slightly limited compared with PET/CT.[102]

Although ^{68}Ga-SSTR PET/CT has been shown to be both sensitive and specific for NET, false positives have been reported. Skoura et al. found 1.1% (14/1258) of false positives in ^{68}Ga-DOTATATE PET/CT performed in 728 patients with confirmed or suspected neuroendocrine tumors, with the majority of cases stemming from inflammatory causes (e.g., reactive nodes) or physiologic uptake in organs, which normally express SSTR2 (e.g., uncinate process of pancreas and adrenal glands).[97] Additionally, osteoblasts have been shown to express SSTR2; thus osteoblastic processes, including degenerative change, fractures, or hemangiomas can be SSTR avid.[103] There have also been case reports of non-neuroendocrine tumors, which are SSTR avid on ^{68}Ga-SSTR PET/CT (e.g., medullary thyroid cancer).

Peptide Receptor Radionuclide Therapy

If GEP-NETS are resectable, surgery is the primary approach (see Chapters 65 and 91). In patients with unresectable metastatic disease, however, multiple lines of therapy are used, including SSA therapy, targeted therapy (e.g., mTOR inhibitor everolimus or tyrosine kinase inhibitor sunitinib), or chemotherapy agents (e.g., capecitabine-temozolomide). In patients with metastatic SSTR expressing G1 and G2 NETs, who have failed first-line somatostatin treatment, peptide receptor radionuclide therapy (PRRT) is also an established treatment option.

PRRT exploits the molecular profile of NETs, which frequently overexpress SSTRs, allowing for the use of SSTR as a target for therapy (so-called theranostics). PRRT relies on the combination of the SSTR ligand and the selected radioisotope, preferentially a medium- to high-energy β emitter, which generates radiation-induced DNA damage, with ^{111}In, ^{90}Y, and lutetium 177 (^{177}Lu) being the most commonly studied radionuclides.[94,104] When combining the SSTR ligand and radioisotopes other than ^{111}In, however, a universal chelator molecule needs to be developed, which results in the introduction of 1,4,7,10-tetraazacyclodecane-1,4,7,10-tetraacetic acid (DOTA).[105] Development of different ligands with higher affinity and preferential targeting of selected somatostatin subtypes can lead to the introduction of agents such as ^{177}Lu and ^{90}Y DOTA-TOC, DOTA-TATE, and DOTA-NOC. [90]Y is a β emitter with a half-life of 2.7 days and maximal tissue penetration of 12 mm; ^{177}Lu is a medium-energy β emitter with a half-life of 6.7 days and maximal tissue penetration of 2 mm, but which also emits low-energy gamma rays, which enables scintigraphy and subsequent dosimetry with the same therapeutic compound and thus is the current preferred radionuclide for clinical practice.

^{177}Lu-DOTATATE received FDA approval for treatment of metastatic, SSTR-positive, well-differentiated GEP-NET in January 2018 after the results of the Neuroendocrine Tumors Therapy (NETTER-1) and ERASMUS trials. The NETTER-1 trial was the first RCT to evaluate the efficacy and safety of ^{177}Lu-DOTATATE in patients with advanced, progressive, SSTR-positive, grade 1 GEP NETs, demonstrating that patients that received PRRT with long-acting SSA had improved PFS compared with patients receiving long-acting SSA alone (at 20 months: 65.2% vs. 10.8%). The ^{177}Lu-DOTATATE group also demonstrated an increased response rate of 18% versus 3% in the control group, and patients in the ^{177}Lu-DOTATATE arm reported an increased quality of life (Fig. 18.7). Nevertheless, OS has not yet been demonstrated in the ^{177}Lu-DOTATATE arm, but preliminary data suggest a survival benefit.[106] In the United States, ^{177}Lu-DOTATATE (Luthathera, Advanced Accelerator Applications SA, Saint-Genis-Pouilly, France) is administered in four cycles of 7.4 GBq (200 mCi) every 8 weeks. Long-term serious side effects of PRRT include renal failure and myelodysplastic syndrome (MDS)/leukemia, with the ERASMUS trial reporting rates of 2% and 3%, respectively, after more than four years of follow-up. Kidney protection using co-infusion of positively charged amino acids is mandatory in PRRT,[107] as is vigilant monitoring of blood counts and renal function.

Currently, the NETTER-2 trial is ongoing and looking at whether combination ^{177}Lu-DOTATATE and long-acting SSA therapy prolongs PFS in patients with grade 2 and 3 GEP-NET when given as a first-line therapy compared with long-acting SSA alone (NCT03972488).[108] Additional approaches to improve antitumoral efficacy include combination therapies (e.g., PRRT) and radio-sensitizing chemotherapeutic agents (e.g., capecitabine),[109–111] PRRT and targeted therapy (e.g., everolimus)[112] and combined radionuclide PRRT, including ^{177}Lu combined with α-emitters radionuclides.

Applications of PRRT in the neoadjuvant setting to achieve tumor size reduction and thus allow curative surgery are also under investigation. Another approach in targeting somatostatin relies on the implementation of a binding-receptor antagonist instead of a receptor agonist, which may be of particular benefit

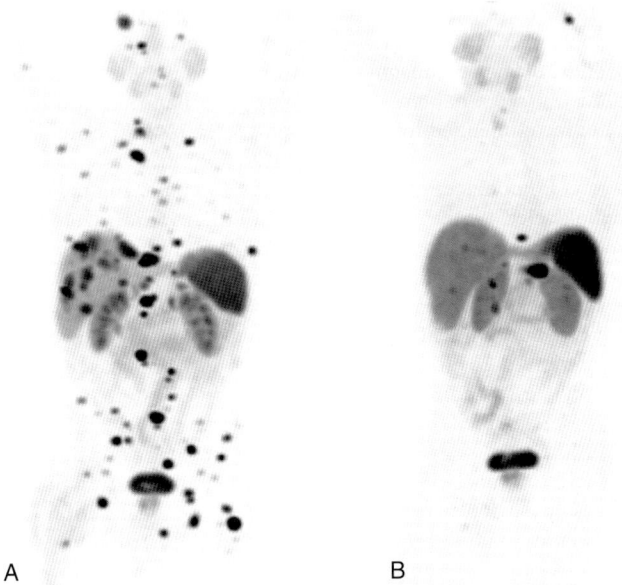

FIGURE 18.7 ^{177}Lu-DOTATATE peptide receptor radionuclide therapy (PRRT). **A,** Maximum intensity projection (MIP) image from ^{68}Ga-DOTATATE positron emission tomography (PET)/computed tomography (CT) in 75-year-old man with symptomatic well-differentiated insulin secreting neuroendocrine tumor with liver and bone metastases. Patient had been previously treated with octreotide therapy and hepatic arterial embolization but had increasing episodes of symptomatic hypoglycemia. Patient was referred for consideration of ^{177}Lu-DOTATATE with pre-PRRT ^{68}Ga-DOTATATE PET/CT showing widespread somatostatin receptor expressing bone, nodal and liver metastases. **B,** MIP image from ^{68}Ga-DOTATATE PET/CT after four cycles of ^{177}Lu-DOTATATE PRRT in the same patient showing significant reduction in volume of somatostatin receptor expressing bone, nodal, and liver metastases, and the patient reported significant improvement in volume of hypoglycemia episodes.

in the setting of heavily pretreated NET patients. Whereas binding of SSTR agonists leads to receptor-mediated internalization, degradation, and intracellular trapping, the somatostatin antagonist is not internalized, offering the possibility to bind to more receptor sites and have a longer retention time.[113–115] Radiolabeled SSTR antagonists, initially ^{111}In-DOTA-BASS and more recently ^{177}Lu-satoreotide tetraxetan (also known as ^{177}Lu-DOTA-JR11,[177]Lu-IPN01072, and ^{177}Lu-OPS201), have been investigated with early promising results.[116–121]

THE ROLE OF NUCLEAR MEDICINE IN NON-ONCOLOGIC HEPATOBILIARY PATHOLOGIES

Hepatobiliary Scintigraphy

Hepatobiliary scintigraphy (or cholescintigraphy) refers to diagnostic imaging of radiotracers that assess hepatic perfusion, hepatocellular function, and hepatobiliary drainage. The most common clinical application of hepatobiliary scintigraphy is for detection of cholecystitis, including *acute* cholecystitis, typically induced by cystic duct obstruction, and *chronic* cholecystitis, typically associated with impaired gallbladder ability to contract normally (see Chapter 34). State-of-the-art hepatobiliary scintigraphy has high diagnostic sensitivity and specificity for detection of both acute and chronic cholecystitis, typically greater than 95%, when an optimal approach is used. Other notable but less common clinical indications for hepatobiliary scintigraphy are listed in Box 18.1; the diagnostic accuracy varies for each.

Because information regarding hepatic function and biliary drainage can usually be diagnosed with clinical examination and

---

BOX 18.1 Clinical Indications for Hepatobiliary Scintigraphy

1. Functional biliary pain syndromes in adults
2. Functional biliary pain syndromes in pediatric patients
3. Acute cholecystitis
4. Right upper quadrant pain variants
5. Biliary system patency
6. Bile leak
7. Neonatal hyperbilirubinemia (biliary atresia versus neonatal hepatitis "syndrome")
8. Assessment of biliary enteric bypass (e.g., Kasai procedure)
9. Assessment of liver transplant
10. Afferent loop syndrome
11. Assessment of biliary dilation (e.g., choledochal cyst)
12. Calculation of gallbladder ejection fraction
13. Functional assessment of the liver before partial hepatectomy
14. Demonstration of anomalous liver lobulation
15. Enterogastric (duodenogastric) reflux assessment
16. Esophageal bile reflux after gastrectomy
17. Sphincter of Oddi dysfunction
18. Differentiation of focal nodular hyperplasia from other hepatic neoplasms

From Tulchinsky M, Ciak BR, Delbeke D, et al: SNM practice guideline for hepatobiliary scintigraphy 4.0. *J Nucl Med Technol* 38:210-218, 2010; and American College of Radiology, Society for Pediatric Radiology: ACR-SPR practice parameter for the performance of hepatobiliary scintigraphy. Amended 2017 (Resolution 40). www.acr.org.

---

blood tests, in general, most hepatobiliary medical society guidelines recommend diagnostic hepatobiliary scintigraphy in only a very few specific clinical indications and typically only as a second-line imaging modality. EASL Guidelines (2016) recommend abdominal US as the primary noninvasive imaging procedure to distinguish intrahepatic from extrahepatic cholestasis, with MR cholangiopancreatography (MRCP) and endoscopic ultrasound (EUS) as potential next diagnostic imaging investigations for unexplained cholestasis[122] (see Chapters 16 and 22). Hepatobiliary scintigraphy is not recommended for the investigation of cholestasis.

Hepatobiliary scintigraphy uses an iminodiacetic acid (IDA)–derivative pharmaceutical radiolabeled with [99m]Tc. This has been colloquially known as "HIDA scan" because HIDA (or ^{99m}Tc-radiolabeled IDA compound, lidofenin) was the preeminent radiopharmaceutical in use at the time that hepatobiliary scintigraphy was introduced into clinical practice. Nevertheless, lidofenin is not commonly used in clinical practice because it has been replaced by ^{99m}Tc-radiolabeled disofenin or mebrofenin, which offer more favorable in vivo pharmacokinetics.

The radiolabeled IDA compounds share common PK properties, differing predominantly in degrees or particular characteristics. All are injected intravenously and bind loosely to plasma proteins, mainly albumin; exiting the bloodstream, the IDA tracers dissociate from plasma proteins in the space of Disse and then undergo hepatic uptake by hepatocytes, followed by hepatic excretion into the intrahepatic biliary tree and subsequent clearance by biliary flow into the intestines via the sphincter of Oddi.

These compounds also share PK properties with bilirubin. Bilirubin, the end-product of heme catabolism, is taken up from the blood circulation into hepatocytes by a high-affinity, sodium-independent, organic anion transport protein shared with IDA radiotracers. Inside hepatocytes, bilirubin is metabolized to a more water-soluble conjugated form; the IDA radiotracers, however, do not change form. Conjugated bilirubin and the IDA radiotracers both exit hepatocytes by energy-dependent *active transport* (particularly transporter ABCC2),[123] then are excreted into the biliary tree, along with other components of bile (e.g., cholesterol, bile acids).

In marked hyperbilirubinemia, the hepatic uptake of IDA radiotracers can be inhibited by competition in carrier-mediated transport of IDA radiotracers because of the high circulating levels of bilirubin, which uses the same transporters. In severe hyperbilirubinemia, a higher activity (MBq) of IDA radiotracer may be injected but not in hopes of reducing competitive inhibition by "mass effect," because the higher radiotracer dose still involves only nanogram (trace) amounts of IDA compound. Rather, the liver will likely absorb the same percentage of the radiotracer dose, regardless of the activity. It is hoped, however, that this absorbed percentage, by using a higher administered activity (MBq), will yield more photons and more signal from the liver and biliary tree for better-quality scintigraphic image. In moderate to severe hyperbilirubinemia, ^{99m}Tc-radiolabeled mebrofenin is probably preferable to disofenin because mebrofenin has higher hepatic extraction.[124]

Hepatobiliary scintigraphy is first an assay of hepatic parenchymal function (see Chapter 4). Hepatic excretion of the radiolabeled IDA compounds is an energy-dependent, active transport process, dependent on intact hepatocellular function. An absent or abnormally low hepatic uptake of IDA radiotracer is indicative of hepatic parenchymal dysfunction, often a diffuse hepatic pathology (e.g., hepatitis). One proposed definition of "poor hepatic uptake" is hepatic tracer

uptake that is visually equivalent, in scintigraphic intensity, to that of tracer present in the cardiac blood pool 5 minutes after injection. Normally, hepatic tracer concentration should be greater than that of circulating tracer in the cardiac blood pool tracer by 5 minutes after injection.[125] However, uptake of IDA radiotracers can remain relatively intact in the acute phase of hepatic injury, noting again that hepatocellular uptake of IDA radiotracers is not ATP dependent. In the early acute phase of hepatic injury, the cessation of ATP-mediated hepatocellular excretion of IDA radiotracers may precede any significant (i.e., scintigraphically detectable) decrease in overall hepatic uptake of IDA radiotracer. The differential analysis and clinical scenarios where this may be encountered are discussed later. Essentially, however, a marked decrease in IDA radiotracer and bile excretion and an associated lack of bile (tracer) flow through the biliary tree are signs of a severe hepatic dysfunction, which may be caused by a primary hepatic dysfunction (e.g., severe hepatitis) rather than a mechanical obstruction of biliary tree drainage (and thereby secondary hepatic dysfunction).

Bile production depends on normal hepatocellular function (see Chapter 8). If hepatic parenchymal dysfunction is severe, bile production and bile flow will slow down, perhaps even stop, until hepatocellular recovery. Similarly, with severe hepatic parenchymal dysfunction and associated scant hepatic IDA radiotracer uptake, hepatic excretion of the IDA radiotracer and its drainage through the biliary tree will also be scant or undetectable on scintigraphy.

Normal Hepatobiliary IDA Radiotracer Scan

This section discusses hepatobiliary scintigraphy with the commonly used ^{99m}Tc-labeled IDA tracers mebrofenin and disofenin, unless otherwise specified. Again, although colloquially called a "HIDA scan," this, in fact, refers to imaging with lidofenin, which is not used in common routine practice. Scintigraphy with mebrofenin and disofenin yields similar findings in healthy individuals after standard preparation. Patient preparation varies, depending on the specific clinical indication, but usually includes fasting (unless the patient has no gallbladder; e.g., after cholecystectomy) and avoiding or counteracting recent use of opioids (Box 18.2).[124]

Current guidelines advise a fasting period of at least two hours, but preferably six hours, for adults, likely based on the normal gastric (and duodenal) clearance times after a typical solid meal. For infants, a fasting period of only two hours is typical, likely because the infant diet is liquid, and gastroduodenal

---

BOX 18.2 Hepatobiliary Scintigraphy: Key Points

A "normal" hepatobiliary scan appearance is defined by the amount of tracer present in the blood pool, liver, biliary tree, and bowels, at different times after injection.

Normal Patient Preparation
Fasting (only if gallbladder present):
- 2 hours for infants
- 2–4 hours
- ≥2–6 hours for adults
- But not >24 hours fasting
Opioids: wait ≥4 half-lives or use opioid antagonist (e.g., naloxone).

clearance of liquid meals is faster than that of solid meals. Physiologically during feeding, the gallbladder contracts, moving bile from gallbladder lumen out the cystic duct into the common bile duct (CBD) and the duodenum to aid digestion of food entering from the stomach. The duodenum, receiving a bolus of nutrients from the stomach, releases the hormone cholecystokinin (CCK); CCK causes contraction of the gallbladder and relaxes the sphincter of Oddi, allowing concentrated bile from the gallbladder stores to be pumped into the duodenal lumen. Thus, in the recently fed patient with relatively high levels of circulating CCK, the gallbladder often will be contracting, and excreted tracer may not enter the gallbladder lumen, potentially mimicking the appearance of a pathologic cystic duct obstruction and being misdiagnosed as consistent with acute cholecystitis on scintigraphy. In the fasting state, neural and hormonal impulses cause the sphincter of Oddi to be predominantly closed and the cystic duct of the gallbladder to remain predominantly open. This halts bile flow into the intestines (via sphincter of Oddi) and creates a pressure gradient directing bile (and IDA tracer) into the gallbladder. During fasting, some phasic contractions of gallbladder and relaxation of the sphincter of Oddi still occur, possibly to churn the bile and avoid precipitation of some bile constituents. Therefore a normal variability (i.e., range of normal values) occurs in the time required to observe excreted tracer in the gallbladder and bowels in well-prepared, healthy individuals.

Prolonged fasting for longer than 24 hours (including during hyperalimentation) is also associated with excreted IDA tracer failing to enter the gallbladder lumen, creating a potentially misleading appearance scintigraphically. This is likely attributable to accumulation of biliary sludge in the gallbladder lumen, obstructing the cystic duct in a nonpathologic manner. Clinical research demonstrates that for patients who have undergone prolonged fasting, it is beneficial to administer a synthetic CCK octapeptide (sincalide) to "clean out" the gallbladder as part of patient preparation for hepatobiliary scintigraphy. Pretreatment with sincalide is typically 0.02 μg/kg intravenously during 30 to 60 minutes by slow infusion. One guideline suggests that hepatobiliary tracer injection can occur 15 to 30 minutes after slow sincalide infusion pretreatment.[124] However, sincalide administration is associated with increased side effects, particularly crampy abdominal pain. Furthermore, sincalide can induce a contractile spasm of the gallbladder neck, especially if given as a bolus, creating a cystic duct obstruction lasting approximately one hour.[126]

Opioid medications (e.g., morphine) acutely induce strong, prolonged contraction of the sphincter of Oddi. If a patient has recently received opioid medications, passage of excreted radiotracer from the biliary tree into the duodenum can be delayed as a side effect. If biliary-to-bowel transit is delayed beyond three to four hours after injection from lingering opioid effects, this can mimic the appearance of CBD obstruction. To avoid this potential diagnostic pitfall, patients should avoid opioid medications before hepatobiliary scintigraphy; one guideline suggests waiting for four times the half-life of the particular opioid drug.[124] Alternatively, naloxone may be administered to attempt to reverse the opioid effects.[127] Additional forms of patient preparation for less common indications of hepatobiliary scintigraphy are discussed later.

The in vivo hepatobiliary parameters typically assessed on scintigraphy are hepatic uptake and excretion of the administered IDA tracer and subsequent biliary drainage of the excreted

radiotracer through the biliary tree into the small bowel (Fig. 18.8). Typically, hepatobiliary scintigraphy begins with a series of consecutive planar images of the liver region (1 frame/minute) for total acquisition of 60 minutes, starting at the time of radiotracer-injection. ^{99m}Tc-labeled IDA tracers clear rapidly from the bloodstream with elimination predominantly by hepatobiliary excretion. The tracers achieve maximal hepatic concentration approximately 10 minutes after injection and are detectable in the extrahepatic biliary tree within 30 to 60 minutes after injection. Excreted tracer passes from the biliary tree into the duodenum via the sphincter of Oddi and is detectable in the intestines in 80% of healthy people within one hour after injection. Biliary-to-bowel transit can take longer in some healthy individuals, especially if sincalide was administered before investigation (a paradoxical phenomenon).[128] Excreted tracer that enters the intestines remains in the intestines, with no significant intestinal tracer reabsorption or enterohepatic recycling of radiotracer.

Lastly, the gallbladder should be visualized within 30 to 60 minutes after injection, typically the endpoint of the study. Gallbladder nonvisualization after one hour in the proper clinical setting is highly suggestive of cystic duct obstruction, most commonly associated with acute cholecystitis. In these patients, additional imaging for 30 minutes after IV morphine administration or delayed imaging can be performed to confirm the diagnosis. As mentioned previously, the radiotracer ^{99m}Tc-lidofenin is now rarely used compared with current agents such as ^{99m}Tc-radiolabeled disofenin and mebrofenin, which have more favorable pharmaceutics with increased hepatic clearance (both with half-times of ~15–20 minutes vs, ~40 minutes with ^{99m}Tc-lidofenin). However, older literature and certain guidelines often suggest obtaining delayed imaging at three to four hours after radiotracer injection, based on original ^{99m}Tc-lidofenin imaging. With increased hepatic clearance of ^{99m}Tc-disofenin and ^{99m}Tc-mebrofenin, however, delayed gallbladder imaging (>1 hours) is not typically possible because the liver is often essentially "empty" of radiotracer by two to four hours after injection. Nevertheless, with a severely ill patient, such as a patient with severe hepatocellular dysfunction, suspected CBD obstruction, or suspected biliary atresia, uptake and secretion of biliary tracer by dysfunctional hepatocytes may be abnormally delayed or biliary flow through the biliary tree may be greatly slowed, thus allowing for delayed imaging with ^{99m}Tc-disofenin and ^{99m}Tc-mebrofenin up to 24 hours after injection.[129]

Analysis of hepatobiliary scintigraphy is typically based on visual detection of tracer in expected locations at expected time points as previously discussed, with semiquantitative visual estimation of whether the amount of tracer present in the blood pool, liver, biliary tree, and bowels is appropriate for the time point after injection also employed. Quantitative analysis may be performed with region of interest (ROI) analysis, although it is not routinely performed in clinical practice. Nuclear medicine societies provide detailed guidance documents with technical protocols for image acquisition protocols.[44]

Pathology in hepatobiliary scintigraphy is thus indicated by one or more of the following:

- An abnormally low amount of hepatic tracer uptake
- An abnormally prolonged hepatic retention of tracer
- An abnormally delayed appearance of excreted tracer in the biliary tree
- An abnormally delayed appearance of excreted tracer in the intestines

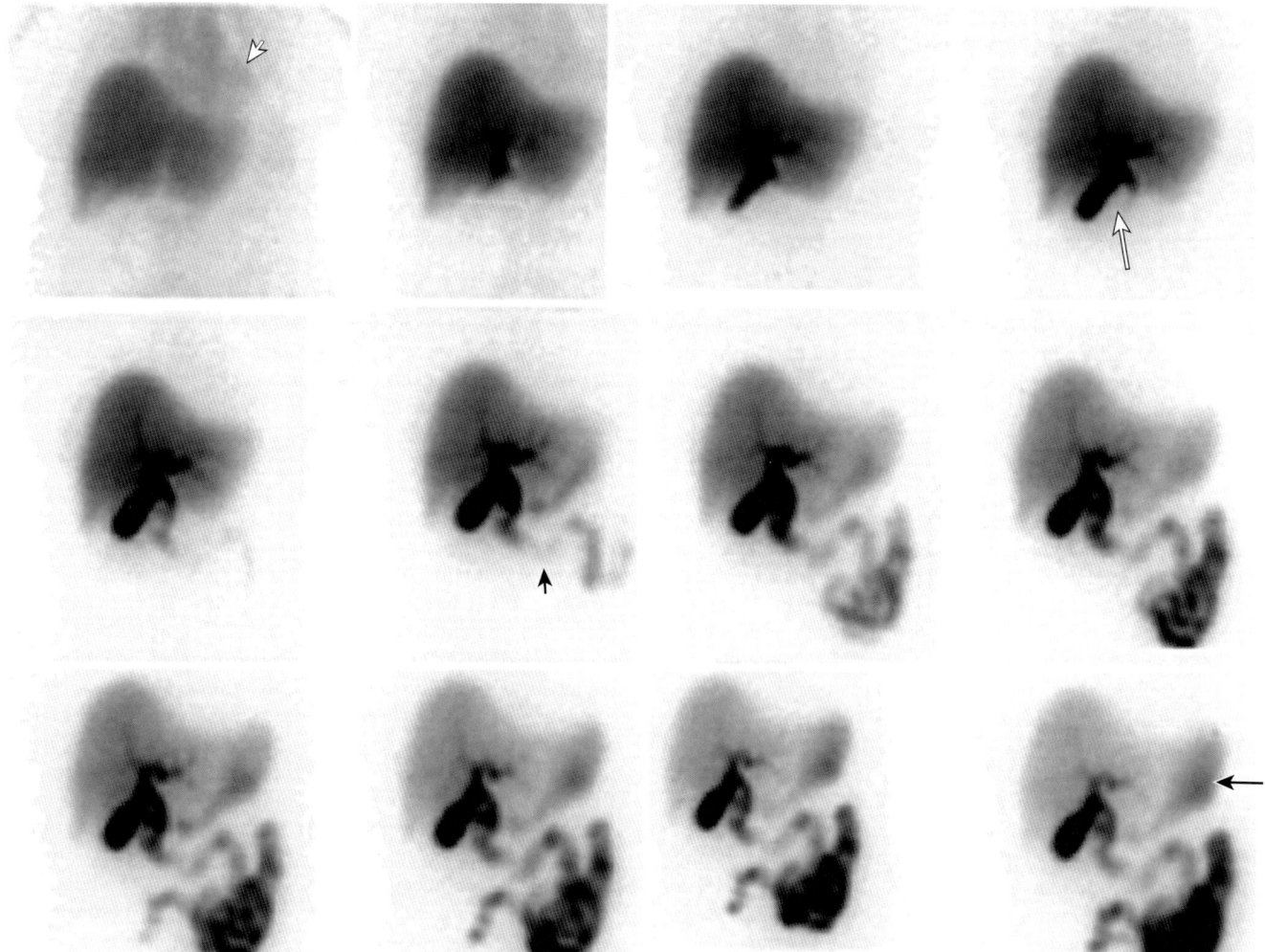

FIGURE 18.8 Normal hepatobiliary iminodiacetic acid study. Serial images of the liver, in anterior projection, acquired beginning immediately after tracer injection; each image is five minutes in duration. The serial images show prompt systemic clearance of radiotracer (e.g., disappearing cardiac blood pool, *gray arrowhead*) via hepatic uptake, followed by prompt hepatobiliary excretion of tracer. Excreted tracer flows promptly through the extrahepatic biliary tree, including into the gallbladder lumen *(large arrow)*. Excreted tracer passes from biliary tree into the duodenum, carried away into distal bowel loops by peristalsis *(black arrowhead)*. One atypical incidental finding is enterogastric reflux of the biliary tracer *(small arrow)*.

Augmented Hepatobiliary Scintigraphy

Hepatobiliary scintigraphy can employ pharmacologic interventions, most notably with phenobarbital, morphine, and sincalide.

Phenobarbital is used in cholescintigraphic evaluation of neonatal jaundice (see Chapters 1 and 40). Patient pretreatment with phenobarbital will stimulate bile production and biliary flow and increase the likelihood of visualizing hepatobiliary radiotracer excretion, if biliary atresia is absent. It reduces the likelihood of false-positive scintigraphic appearance of biliary flow obstruction.

Morphine is used in cholescintigraphic evaluation of gallbladder cystic duct obstruction (see Chapter 34). If accumulation of excreted biliary tracer in gallbladder lumen is not observed in the expected time frame, morphine administration normally contracts the sphincter of Oddi and relaxes any physiologic gallbladder contraction; this increases the likelihood that biliary radiotracer can accumulate within the gallbladder, if no pathologic obstruction of the gallbladder cystic duct (e.g., associated with calculous or acalculous cholecystitis)

is present. It reduces the likelihood of false-positive scintigraphic appearance of gallbladder cystic duct obstruction. Because morphine contracts the sphincter of Oddi, scintigraphically, entry of biliary tracer into small intestines is typically confirmed visually before use of morphine, first to exclude CBD obstruction before attempting to exclude a cystic duct obstruction. If the decision to use morphine is made based on nonvisualization of the gallbladder but the injected biliary tracer has already essentially cleared from the liver and biliary tree into the bowels, it is often necessary for patients to receive a "booster" injection of biliary tracer before administration of morphine to renew a flow of radiotracer through the biliary tree.

Sincalide is used in cholescintigraphy for evaluation of gallbladder cystic duct or CBD obstruction or gallbladder dyskinesia (see Chapters 34 and 37). Patient treatment with sincalide causes contraction of the gallbladder and relaxation of the sphincter of Oddi. Sincalide can be given before radiotracer to evacuate the gallbladder lumen if gallbladder accumulation of a biliary sludge is possible (e.g., from patient hyperalimentation or prolonged fasting) or evident sonographically; such sludge can impede gallbladder accumulation of biliary tracer, creating a scintigraphic appearance mimicking a cystic duct obstruction (false positive). If the gallbladder lumen accumulates biliary tracer (i.e., there is no cystic duct obstruction) but gallbladder dyskinesia is suspected, sincalide can then be administered 30 to 60 minutes after tracer administration to assess gallbladder ejection fraction (normal >38%).

Gallbladder Ejection Fraction

The scintigraphic hallmark of cholecystitis is *gallbladder dyskinesia,* defined as gallbladder ejection fraction (GBEF) less than 38%, on sincalide-stimulated cholescintigraphy.[124,129] Gallbladder dyskinesia can be seen in both acute and chronic cholecystitis because both cause dysfunction of inflamed gallbladder smooth musculature. The GBEF study begins after the expected tracer accumulation in the gallbladder lumen has been visualized (see Chapter 34).

Medications can interfere with interpretation of GBEF, most notably morphine. If morphine augmentation has been used, sincalide GBEF testing can still be performed with normal GBEF reliably excluding gallbladder dyskinesia; however, low GBEF results are nondiagnostic. Other medications associated with low GBEF include atropine, calcium channel blockers, octreotide, progesterone, indomethacin, theophylline, benzodiazepines, and histamine-2 receptor antagonists. As such, patient medications should be reviewed at the time of the study. Additionally, a variety of conditions other than cholecystitis have been associated with low GBEF results, including obesity, diabetes mellitus, celiac disease, cirrhosis, and myotonic dystrophy.

Clinical Uses of Hepatobiliary Scintigraphy

ACUTE CHOLECYSTITIS. Acute cholecystitis is the most common clinical indication for cholescintigraphy, although abdominal US remains the first-line imaging modality (see Chapters 16 and 34). The reported sensitivity and specificity of cholescintigraphy for suspected acute calculous cholecystitis ranges from 87% to 98% and 81% to 100%, respectively.[129] Kaoutzanis et al. retrospectively reviewed patients presenting to the emergency department with acute upper abdominal pain ($n = 406$) who underwent investigation for acute cholecystitis, using abdominal US ($n = 132$), scintigraphy ($n = 46$), or both ($n = 228$), as per the referrer wishes.[130] The sensitivity for acute cholecystitis was 73% for US alone, 92% for scintigraphy alone, and 98% for both. Although this study is limited because of its retrospective nature and nonrandomization of imaging investigation performed, the findings indicate that hepatobiliary scintigraphy (1) continues to have a standard role in the evaluation of the patient with acute abdominal pain, especially if combined with abdominal US, and (2) offers high sensitivity for preoperative diagnosis of acute cholecystitis, alone or combined with US, in the correct clinical context.

Acute cholecystitis in adults is almost always associated with a pathologic obstruction of the cystic duct, whether secondary to cholelithiasis impacted in the cystic duct or acalculous cholecystitis (i.e., inflammation and edema in the walls of the gallbladder neck, occluding the duct). Nonvisualization of the gallbladder at 60 minutes is suggestive of cystic duct obstruction and thus acute cholecystitis.

As previously discussed, however, in a minority of healthy patients without pathologic obstruction of the cystic duct, the gallbladder lumen does not accumulate excreted tracer within 1 hour because of a physiologic obstruction of inward biliary flow associated with physiologic contractions of the gallbladder. These contractions are typically stopped by adequate fasting; however, in a small percentage of patients, they persist. To increase the diagnostic specificity of gallbladder nonvisualization as a scintigraphic biomarker of cystic duct obstruction, guidelines suggest obtaining either delayed imaging 3 to 4 hours after injection or morphine administration to stimulate the sphincter of Oddi.[42] If the gallbladder remains nonvisualized after these strategies, cystic duct obstruction can be diagnosed with greater specificity.

The "cystic duct sign" is a nonelongated, spot-like focus of tracer accumulation in the expected location of the cystic duct along the common hepatic and bile duct course and can mimic gallbladder tracer accumulation. However, the cystic duct sign represents a focal accumulation of biliary radiotracer within the proximal cystic duct (closest to and communicating with the common duct), which can occur in cystic duct obstruction when cholelithiasis obstructing bile passage from the gallbladder is lodged more distally within the cystic duct. The cystic duct sign should be suspected when biliary tracer accumulation in the gallbladder region is not elongated but rather is more spot-like and smaller than usual. In cases of diagnostic uncertainty, a suspected cystic duct sign can be evaluated further by SPECT/CT to confirm an absence of excreted tracer in the gallbladder lumen.

The "rim sign," seen in 25% to 35% of patients with acute cholecystitis, describes an abnormal "blush" of activity around the gallbladder fossa, which can occur in flow phase imaging because of inflammation of the surrounding hepatic parenchyma. The rim sign has been associated with an increased risk for complicated cholecystitis, specifically gangrene and gallbladder perforation, and is sensitive but not specific for acute cholecystitis.[129]

Acalculous acute cholecystitis occurs in less than 10% of adult patients with acute cholecystitis but is associated with a high morbidity and mortality (see Chapter 34). Most patients with acute acalculous cholecystitis have cystic duct obstruction caused by multiple different etiologies, including fibrosis, anomalous vessels, and tumor, but most commonly because of inspissated bile, debris, and local edema. In most patients, the diagnosis can be made with cholescintigraphy; however, cholescintigraphy appears to have less diagnostic sensitivity for *acalculous* acute cholecystitis compared with *calculous* acute cholecystitis (70%–80% vs. 95%).[124,129] Additionally, approximately 25% of patients with acute acalculous cholecystitis do not have cystic duct obstruction but rather direct inflammation of the gallbladder wall secondary to ischemia.[129] Thus, gallbladder tracer accumulation can occur, a false-negative finding. In patients with gallbladder tracer accumulation, however, the presence of the rim sign or abnormally low GBEF can increase diagnostic sensitivity, although poor gallbladder contraction can also be seen in chronic cholecystitis.[129] As mentioned previously, acalculous cholecystitis is relatively uncommon in adults; in pediatric patients, however, acute cholecystitis is more frequently acalculous. Cholescintigraphy remains the imaging examination of choice when acalculous cholecystitis is suspected.

CHRONIC CHOLECYSTITIS. Patients with chronic cholecystitis typically present with recurrent biliary colic (typically chronic calculous cholelithiasis; see Chapter 34). If cholelithiasis is seen on US, then the patient is referred for cholecystectomy. As such, cholescintigraphy is rarely indicated as part of a work-up, unless patients present with atypical symptoms, which the physician suspects are not attributed to chronic calculous cholecystitis, or chronic acalculous cholecystitis is suspected.

Cholelithiasis is commonly seen, but one study showed that only 15% of patients developed biliary colic after 20-year follow-up.[131] The cystic duct is typically patent in chronic cholecystitis; therefore, if tracer accumulates in the gallbladder during cholescintigraphy and a normal GBEF is seen, then symptomatic chronic cholecystitis is unlikely.[132] Acalculous chronic cholecystitis is reported to occur in approximately 5% to 25% of patients, attributed to gallbladder lymphocyte infiltration and fibrosis similar to gallbladders with the calculous form of the disease but without stones and thus is associated with low GBEF and gallbladder dyskinesia.

EXTRAHEPATIC BILE DUCT OBSTRUCTION. In cholescintigraphy performed in normal healthy volunteers, tracers undergo hepatobiliary drainage with detectable passage of excreted tracer into the duodenum within one hour after injection in a majority of cases, but can take up to two hours in approximately one-third

of people, probably because of transient/phasic physiologic contraction of the sphincter of Oddi. In healthy volunteers, with relatively delayed passage of tracer into the small bowel, excreted tracer is visible in the extrahepatic biliary tree, awaiting passage into the bowel once the sphincter of Oddi relaxes. Additionally, patients pretreated with sincalide before cholescintigraphy paradoxically seem to be more likely to demonstrate a nonpathologic delay in biliary transit into the bowel, especially if sincalide is infused relatively rapidly.[128]

Pathologic obstruction of the common hepatic duct or CBD can be diagnosed by cholescintigraphy (Fig. 18.9). Extrahepatic bile duct obstruction can be caused by cholelithiasis (choledocholithiasis or, rarely, Mirizzi syndrome; see Chapters 34 and 37) or tumor (e.g., pancreatic head mass compressing adjacent duct; see Chapters 49, 51, 62, 63, and 67). Tumor-associated biliary obstruction is usually identifiable by structural imaging (CT, US, or MRI) because biliary duct dilation is often already present at diagnosis. Obstructive choledocholithiasis, in contrast, often presents clinically as an acute biliary-type pain; in the first 24 to 72 hours after bile duct obstruction by choledocholithiasis, bile duct distension may not yet be marked enough to be

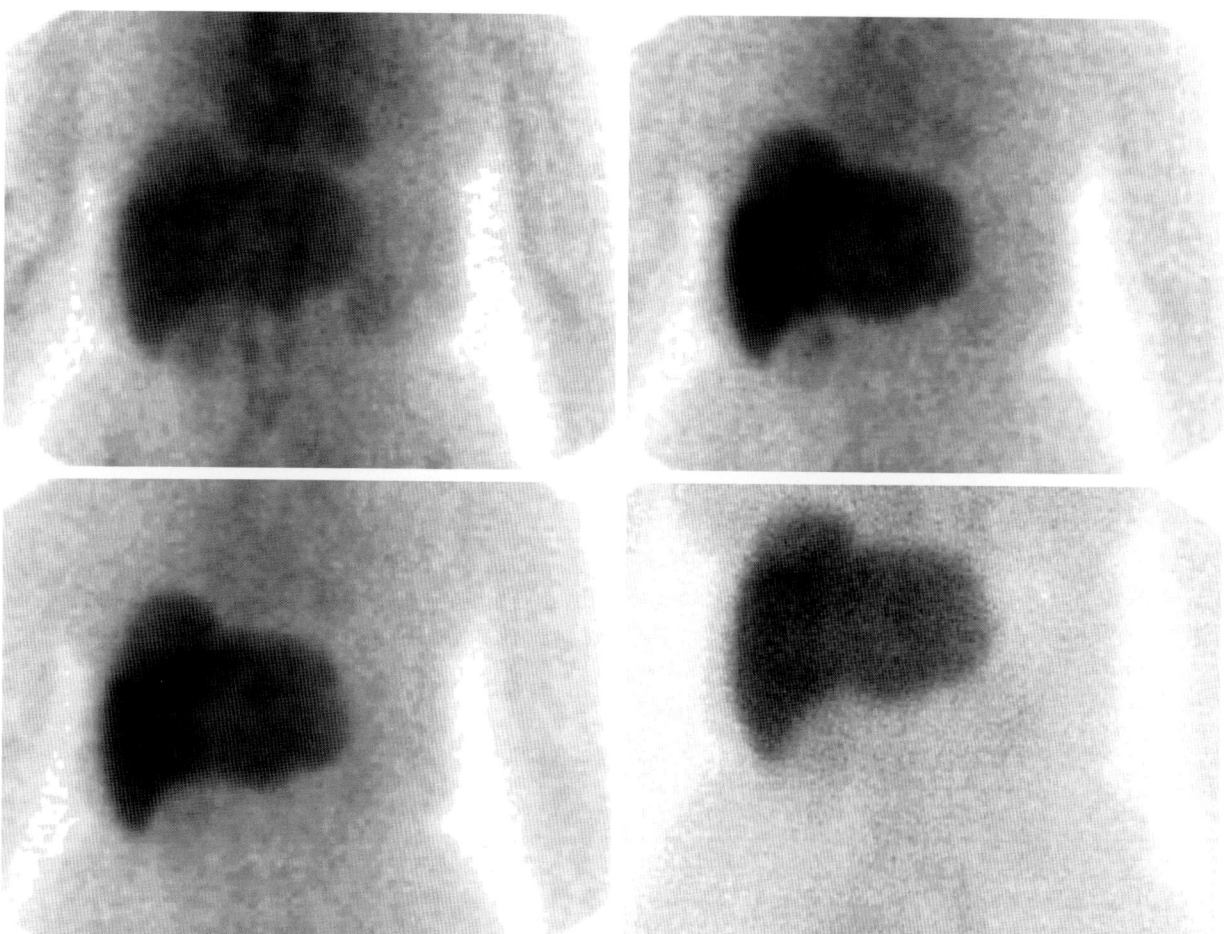

FIGURE 18.9 Complete biliary obstruction. Images were obtained immediately after injection and at 30 minutes, 60 minutes, and three hours. No severe hepatocellular dysfunction is evident; systemic tracer clearance is somewhat delayed (cardiac blood pool still detectable at 30 minutes), but the liver demonstrates prompt, visually distinct tracer uptake. No excreted tracer is detectable in the extrahepatic biliary tree at one hour after tracer injection. This constellation of scintigraphic findings is suspicious for an acute high-grade extrahepatic bile duct obstruction, in the proper clinical setting. If hepatocellular function is impaired, continued absence of detectable excreted extrahepatic tracer at three to four hours after injection increases diagnostic confidence.

suspicious on structural imaging. Cholescintigraphy can confirm a clinical suspicion of acute extrahepatic bile duct obstruction in patients with negative structural imaging. Additionally, patients with previously treated bile duct obstruction can have persistent bile duct dilation after treatment; if these patients return to the clinic with suspicious biliary colic, structural imaging may demonstrate a chronically distended bile duct of uncertain significance. Cholescintigraphy can confirm a clinical suspicion of acute recurrent extrahepatic bile duct obstruction in such patients. Acute extrahepatic bile duct obstruction has been described as having cholescintigraphic appearances that favor either a "high-grade" or a lesser, "partial" degree of biliary obstruction.[129] An acute high-grade obstruction of the extrahepatic biliary tree can be diagnosed if the following findings are present:

- The patient has good hepatic function, as indicated by blood tests and on cholescintigraphy by rapid hepatic tracer-uptake and rapid tracer clearance from the blood pool.
- Excreted biliary tracer is not detectable or scantly present in the extrahepatic biliary tree by one hour after injection.

If these two findings are present, extrahepatic bile duct obstruction is the likely diagnosis, and other etiologies are relatively rare.[133] If hepatic function is poor, however, passage of excreted tracer into the extrahepatic bile ducts can be *delayed* because hepatic bile production is slow (Fig. 18.10). Hepatic function may be poor because of a true bile duct obstruction (in which case it was more likely chronic than acute) or because of a separate nonobstructive etiology (e.g., hepatitis or cirrhosis). If hepatic function is poor, delayed imaging will improve test specificity (i.e., help avoid false diagnosis of bile duct obstruction).[133]

A partial obstruction of the extrahepatic bile ducts is associated with the following cholescintigraphic appearance:
- Hepatic uptake is normally prompt (unless the patient also has hepatic dysfunction unrelated to biliary obstruction).
- Excreted tracer appears promptly within the extrahepatic biliary tree.
- Clearance of excreted tracer from the extrahepatic biliary tree is absent or scant during the first hour after injection.
- Further clearance of excreted tracer from the extrahepatic biliary tree into the small bowel, after sincalide administration or at delayed time points, is less than expected.

Normally, approximately half of biliary tracer has passed from the hepatobiliary tree into the small bowel by one hour after tracer injection, and a progressive decline in the net amount of tracer in the extrahepatic biliary tree is usually visibly evident

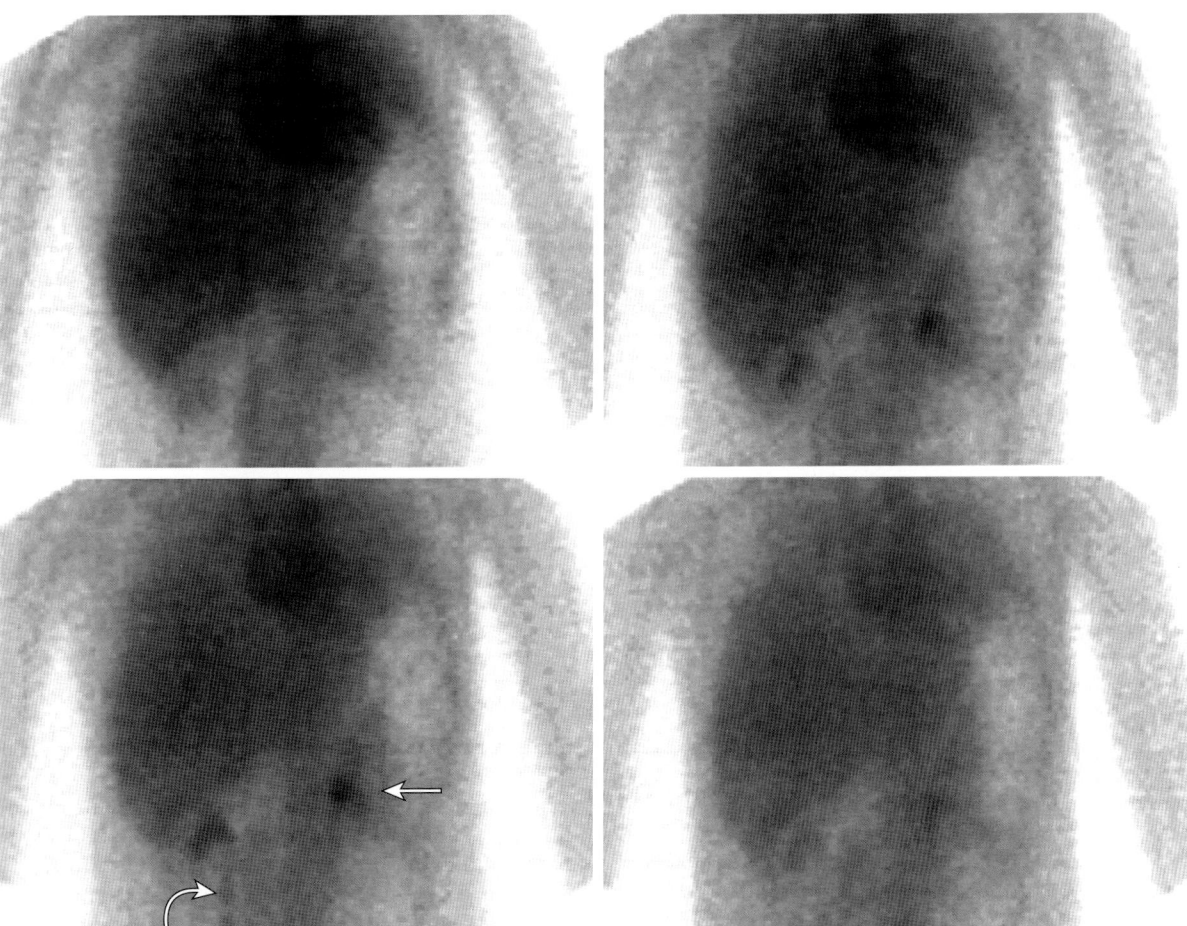

FIGURE 18.10   This study shows severe hepatocellular dysfunction, with the kidneys exhibiting increased clearance of the tracer. Note the parallel reduction in activity in the cardiac blood pool and the liver. The two bright foci beneath the liver are caused by activity in the pelvis of the right and left kidneys. The *straight arrow* points to the left renal pelvis; the *curved arrow* points to the right ureter. Images were acquired at two, 15, 25, and 60 minutes after injection.

scintigraphically within the first hour.[134] However, an absence of bowel activity at one hour after tracer injection is sensitive for partial obstruction (~98%), but is not highly specific because of the normal variation in drainage of bile into bowel associated with phasic physiologic contractions of the sphincter of Oddi.[135] Delayed imaging can be obtained to allow for detection of biliary passage into the bowel, allowing for the possibility of a physiologic contraction of the sphincter of Oddi. Alternatively, relaxation of the sphincter of Oddi can be induced by sincalide treatment to avoid delay and can be used in the setting of cholelithiasis. The gallbladder, if present, must accumulate excreted tracer normally, before use of sincalide, to exclude cystic duct obstruction. If clearance of excreted tracer from the extrahepatic biliary tree into the bowel remains less than expected after sincalide administration or at delayed time points, a partial bile duct obstruction can be diagnosed with a specificity of approximately 85%.[129]

POSTCHOLECYSTECTOMY SYNDROME AND SPHINCTER OF ODDI DYSFUNCTION. *Postcholecystectomy syndrome* refers to the recurrence of abdominal pain after cholecystectomy, which occurs in 10% to 40% of patients who have had cholecystectomy for symptomatic chronic cholecystitis and more commonly occurs in women[136] (see Chapters 34 and 36). Onset of symptoms can occur from two days up to 25 years after surgery. Hepatobiliary causes for the recurrent pain include retained and recurrent stones, biliary stricture, tumors, a cystic duct remnant, and obstruction of the sphincter of Oddi. The explanation for presentation after cholecystectomy is that the biliary system no longer has a pressure-release mechanism, formerly served by the gallbladder, which increased pressure, producing the pain. In the majority of patients, however, other extrahepatic disorders (e.g., reflux esophagitis, gastritis, irritable bowel syndrome, chronic pancreatitis) are responsible for the postcholecystectomy pain syndrome.[137]

Sphincter of Oddi dysfunction is a poorly understood clinical entity that occurs weeks, months, or years after cholecystectomy in 1% to 14% of patients,[138,139] presenting as either recurrent episodic biliary colic pain (stage I), recurrent pain associated with elevated liver enzymes or dilated ducts (stage II), or episodic pain with elevated liver enzymes and dilated biliary ducts (stage III).[140] The dysfunction can be caused by true stenosis or secondary to spasm of the sphincter. The establishment of a diagnosis and treatment approaches is challenging. Sphincterotomy, advocated as effective therapy, can be associated with bleeding and pancreatitis. Cholescintigraphy and sphincter of Oddi manometry have been explored as assays to confirm diagnosis in support of therapeutic intervention. All biliary causes for the postcholecystectomy pain syndrome have a similar scintigraphic pattern on cholescintigraphy, that of a partial biliary obstruction. Various protocols assessing qualitative image analysis based on cholescintigraphy have been published recommending an infusion of sincalide during three to 10 minutes, completed 15 minutes before radiotracer injection.[141] Another study, however, indicated that sphincter of Oddi manometry is superior to scintigraphy.[142] Subsequently, another report indicated that although the sensitivity of scintigraphy is less compared with superior manometry, the higher accuracy in predicting treatment success compares favorably.[143] Furthermore, manometry is rarely used anymore because of the frequent occurrence of serious side effects, particularly pancreatitis.

BILIARY TRACT COMPLICATIONS AFTER SURGERY. Cholescintigraphy can positively impact diagnostic evaluation of patients for biliary tract complications associated with a variety of procedures, such as laparoscopic cholecystectomy, partial hepatic resections, or liver transplantation (see Chapters 28, 32, and 42). Bile duct injuries may lead either to biliary duct obstruction or bile leakage but are generally rare, with a reported rate of 0.39% after laparoscopic cholecystectomy.[144] CT and US are first-line imaging modalities to evaluate for suspected complications; nonspecific findings include fluid collection in the gallbladder fossa or peritoneal cavity. Cholescintigraphy allows for the noninvasive evaluation of the biliary tree for obstruction and leakage and can be used to characterize fluid collections detected by US or CT, particularly benefiting from the use of SPECT/CT to visualize both the fluid collection (on CT) and the abnormal tracer accumulation within the collection on fusion SPECT/CT. Most leaks are observed at the cystic duct stump, and characteristic scintigraphy findings include tracer accumulation at the gallbladder fossa, near the porta hepatis or in the subphrenic space. SPECT/CT is also advantageous for patients with complicated postsurgical hepatobiliary anatomy (e.g., status after hepaticojejunostomy), to help clarify biliary flow patterns.

LIVER TRANSPLANTATION. A biliary stricture is one of the most common biliary complications after liver transplantation, with incidence varying depending on the type of biliary reconstruction and with a higher incidence in patients undergoing duct-to-duct anastomosis[145] (see Chapter 111). Endoscopic retrograde cholangiopancreatography (ERCP), MRCP, and US are typically used for diagnosis of stricture; although the role of hepatobiliary scintigraphy has been studied in post-transplantation, it is not currently recommended in guidelines. Hepatobiliary scintigraphy with IDA-type tracers has been shown to provide accurate diagnosis of biliary complications in adult and pediatric patients.[145–147] Nevertheless, hepatobiliary scintigraphy cannot reliably distinguish between cholestasis and rejection, which is typically diagnosed by liver biopsy.[145,148] Hepatobiliary scintigraphy can have a role in diagnosis of biliary leaks after transplantation, especially Roux-en-Y choledochojejunostomy bile leaks, which can be difficult to diagnose on ERCP because of alternation of anatomy.

The Role of Hepatobiliary Scintigraphy in Pediatric Imaging

NEONATAL JAUNDICE. The incidence of neonatal jaundice in the United States has been increasing, currently affecting approximately two-thirds of newborns[149] (see Chapter 1). In most infants, the etiology of jaundice is physiologic; however, high concentrations of unconjugated bilirubin may cause permanent neurologic damage, known as chronic bilirubin encephalopathy or kernicterus. Even moderately elevated levels of bilirubin may induce permanent neurodevelopmental impairment (NDI) or bilirubin-induced neurologic dysfunction (BIND). The various etiologies include infections, isoimmunization, inherited disorders of bilirubin conjugation and transport, and biliary malformation. Biliary atresia, inspissated bile syndrome, and choledochal malformation are associated with a relatively good clinical outcome after surgery. Early establishment of the underlying cause is a key factor to improve associated morbidity and mortality rates. In pathologic jaundice, neonatal hepatitis and biliary atresia account for 70% to 80% of cases. Alagille syndrome and α_1-antitrypsin deficiency account for 10% to

15%.[150] The clinical dilemma is that the diseases have similar clinical presentations and blood test findings, but biliary atresia, if present, requires urgent surgical intervention for optimal pediatric outcomes. ^{99m}Tc-IDA cholescintigraphy plays a valuable role in the evaluation of neonatal jaundice. Hepatobiliary scintigraphy is performed with ^{99m}Tc-labeled mebrofenin as the preferred agent because of its high hepatic extraction.

BILIARY ATRESIA. Biliary atresia is a common cause of neonatal cholestasis jaundice and occurs in one in 10,000 to 15,000 newborns[151] (see Chapters 1 and 40). Biliary atresia develops either during embryogenesis or the perinatal period, with progressive inflammatory sclerosis of the intrahepatic and extrahepatic biliary ducts. The cause of biliary atresia is unknown, although several mechanisms have been postulated, including viral etiologies.[152,153] Early diagnosis within the first two months after birth is crucial to prevent irreversible liver damage. Treatment is based on palliative hepatoportoenterostomy (Kasai procedure) and often, ultimately, liver transplantation.

Biliary atresia shows high-grade biliary obstruction with a persistent hepatogram and no biliary-to-bowel transit over 24 hours. The negative predictive value of the study is high (approximately 100%) and thus cholescintigraphy is typically used to exclude biliary atresia because the detection of excreted biliary tracer in the gallbladder or bowels effectively excludes biliary atresia.[129] However, false-positive studies can be seen in biliary atresia or severe hepatocellular dysfunction (e.g., from hepatitis). Thus patient preparation for cholescintigraphy should include administration of phenobarbital (5 mg/kg/day) for up to five days before the test to activate liver excretory enzymes and increase bile flow, and cholescintigraphy imaging should continue at multiple time points up to 24 hours after tracer injection to allow for possible markedly slow biliary flow. A 2013 meta-analysis reported a pooled sensitivity and specificity of 98.7% (range, 98.1%–99.2%) and 70.4% (68.5%–72.2%), respectively, for diagnosis of biliary atresia. Its near-perfect sensitivity for biliary atresia makes cholescintigraphy an effective assay for excluding biliary atresia. Its limited specificity demonstrates that a lack of biliary tracer transit into gallbladder or bowel, as a scintigraphic biomarker, has insufficient specificity to positively diagnose atresia and guide decision making on whether surgical intervention is necessary.[154] If there is equivocal gallbladder filling on planar imaging, SPECT/CT imaging can be used to help diagnosis.[155] Thus cholescintigraphy is diagnostically useful as a means to "rule out" biliary atresia.

Hepatobiliary Sulfur Colloid Imaging

In the past, scintigraphy with radiolabeled SC provided a useful means for gross structural evaluation of liver and spleen; however, with the increased availability of CT and MRI, which provide far superior structural/anatomic delineation of organs, SC imaging has been almost entirely replaced for hepatobiliary imaging, except in a few very specific indications, most commonly as a diagnostic adjunct for hepatic arterial perfusion scintigraphy (as discussed previously), for detection of splenosis, and, rarely, for characterization of suspected focal nodular hyperplasia (FNH).

Colloid scintigraphy is an umbrella term, because a variety of radiolabeled colloid particulates have been developed for human studies. In the United States, ^{99m}Tc-labeled SC is the only radiocolloid in common use for clinical hepatic scintigraphy. ^{99m}Tc-labeled SC is a particulate compound. ^{99m}Tc-labeled

SC particulates administered to humans range from 0.1 to 1.0 μm in size. After IV injection, ^{99m}Tc-labeled SC normally localizes at its highest concentration in the liver, followed by lesser uptake in the spleen and relatively low uptake in bone marrow (see Fig. 18.4). This liver-spleen-marrow biodistribution reflects the removal of ^{99m}Tc-labeled SC particulates from the bloodstream by phagocytes in the reticuloendothelial system (including hepatic Kupffer cells). Blood clearance is normally rapid (two to three minute half-life), allowing scintigraphy to begin 20 to 30 minutes after injection. In a few hours, catabolism of ^{99m}Tc-labeled SC can become evident by scintigraphic signs of catabolic production of free ^{99m}Tc pertechnetate; signs of ^{99m}Tc pertechnetate include (delayed–time point) accumulation of radioisotope in stomach and thyroid and urinary radioisotope excretion. Splenic concentration of ^{99m}Tc-labeled SC normally is less than the scintigraphic intensity of hepatic concentration. *Colloid shift* is an abnormality in colloid biodistribution that occurs when hepatic ^{99m}Tc-labeled SC concentration is visually less than splenic concentration because of abnormally low hepatic uptake or abnormally high splenic uptake of ^{99m}Tc-labeled SC (e.g., in diffuse hepatic diseases such as advanced cirrhosis and severe hepatitis or causes of hypersplenism).[156] It was hypothesized that hepatic colloid uptake could be a semiquantitative biomarker of hepatic function; however, this has not been shown to be true, with one study showing no correlation between scintigraphic semiquantitative uptake measurements and Child-Pugh classification.[157]

Hepatic lesions can be colloid tracer "cold" or "hot" lesions; however, because of limited resolution of the planar and SPECT scans, only hepatic lesions greater than 1.5 to 2 cm can be reliably detected. The differential of cold or photopenic lesion, foci of absent or relatively low hepatic colloid uptake, is broad, but includes HCC, liver metastases, adenoma, and hepatic abscess.[158] However, the only reported "hot" hepatic lesion is focal nodular hyperplasia because SC is taken up by Kupffer cells in the reticuloendothelial system, which are found in abundance in FNH. Intense focal uptake is thought to be quite specific for FNH but has relatively poor sensitivity of 60% to 70% for detection of FNH.[159,160] The finding of diminished colloid uptake in the right and left liver lobes, with sparing of the caudate lobe, has been associated with Budd-Chiari syndrome (hepatic vein thrombosis).

Splenosis, or ectopic splenic tissue, is an acquired condition (typically after trauma or splenectomy) where foci of splenic tissue is autoimplanted in various compartments of the body, which then recruits local blood supply and, as a result, can grow over time and present serious diagnostic problems because they can mimic malignant lesions (e.g., peritoneal metastases in pancreatic cancer). Although splenosis typically demonstrates similar imaging characteristics to the spleen on CT and MRI, it can be diagnostically challenging, especially in the postsplenectomy oncology patient. The diagnosis of splenosis can be confirmed with ^{99m}Tc-labeled SC scan, which will demonstrate increased uptake in lesions greater than 1.5 to 2.0 cm with sensitivity increased with SPECT imaging. If ^{99m}Tc-labeled SC scan fails to confirm the presence of splenic tissue, [99m]Tc- tagged heat-damaged red blood cell (RBC) scan with autologous erythrocytes is the gold standard of imaging, being capable of specifically proving splenic tissue. Intrapancreatic accessory spleen (IPAS), a normal variant, can be a mimic of malignancy (e.g., pancreatic neuroendocrine tumors [PNET]). If conventional CT or MRI are not definitive in the diagnosis of IPAS, then further confirmation is possible with 99mTc-labeled SC +/− ^{99m}Tc- tagged heat-damaged RBC scan. These scans are both highly specific and best differentiate IPAS from PNET because the PNET will not show uptake.[161,162] 68Ga-SSR PET/CT and octreotide scans are not reliable to differentiate between IPAS and PNET because false-positive IPAS tracer uptake has been reported.[163–165]

Incidental Liver Lesions

The differential diagnosis of an incidental liver lesion is broad and includes benign lesions, such as hemangioma, FNH, hepatic adenoma, and regenerative nodules, and malignant lesions, including HCC or metastases (see Chapters 14, 15, and 87). Characterization and detection of liver lesions usually begins with US, CT, or MRI, which can be sufficient for diagnosis.[166,167] The role of scintigraphy in characterizing liver lesions is typically limited and confined to second-line imaging, but it can be helpful in select cases when the differential diagnosis has been narrowed by initial evaluation of the liver lesion by CT/US/MRI, clinical history, and blood test findings. The American College of Radiology suggests a limited role for nuclear scintigraphy in characterization of incidentally discovered lesions, with CT or MRI always the preferred initial imaging modality.[141] If a patient has a *known* extrahepatic malignancy and CT/MRI characterization is indeterminate, PET/CT, typically FDG, is potentially helpful for further characterization, especially if the patient had previously tracer-avid extrahepatic disease. Also, nuclear imaging may have a role in characterization of certain benign lesions if conventional imaging remains uncertain, as discussed later.

Focal Nodular Hyperplasia

FNH is a regenerative mass lesion of the liver and the second most common benign liver lesion (see Chapters 14 and 88). It is commonly asymptomatic and requires no treatment. ^{99m}Tc SC imaging may be useful in characterizing FNH, especially when combined with SPECT imaging, if findings are equivocal on conventional imaging. SC is taken up by Kupffer cells in the reticuloendothelial system, which are found in abundance in FNH, thus appearing as a hot lesion. When present, intense focal uptake is thought to be quite specific for FNH but has quite poor sensitivity of approximately 60% to 70% for the detection of FNH.[159,160,168] This, in part, may be because of the size of the lesion: SPECT sensitivity for detection is decreased in lesions less than 1.5 cm because of spatial resolution of SPECT camera and increased risk for partial volume–averaging effects that diminish the detectability of tracer uptake by colloid-avid FNH lesions and background hepatic uptake or because of the paucity of Kupffer cells in certain FNH, which then appear photopenic or with uptake similar to background liver. Additionally, hepatic adenomas may rarely contain Kupffer cells and be associated with uptake similar or slightly greater than background liver.

Cholescintigraphy, using biliary tracers such as ^{99m}Tc-radiolabeled disofenin or mebrofenin, have been used in characterization of FNH. Hepatocytes in the FNH lesion produce bile; however, biliary canaliculi within the FNH are often characterized by disordered drainage connections with the remainder of the intrahepatic biliary tree and therefore, on cholescintigraphy, demonstrate abnormal focal accumulation and prolonged focal retention of a biliary radiotracer. Early studies suggest cholescintigraphy had promising diagnostic sensitivity (e.g., 92%)[169]; however, with the advent of hepatobiliary contrast agents used in MRI, this technique is not used in modern clinical practice. Additionally, well-differentiated HCC are reported to demonstrate a similar cholescintigraphic phenotype, as an abnormal focal, prolonged retention of biliary tracer.

The FDG PET appearance of FNH is variable, ranging from mild hypermetabolic, isointense to mild hypometabolic avidity compared with surrounding hepatic FDG uptake, but is rarely, if ever, intensely FDG avid.[170]

Hemangioma

Hepatic hemangioma is the most common benign liver lesion (see Chapters 14 and 88). It is typically characterized on US or contrast-enhanced CT or MRI and is only incidentally seen on nuclear studies performed for other indications. On ^{99m}Tc-labeled SC scintigraphy, hemangiomas appear as a photopenic or "cold" lesions, and on FDG PET, they typically demonstrate avidity equivalent or less than cardiac blood pool activity and also generally less than surrounding liver FDG uptake. There have been reported cases of hemangiomas that demonstrate intense avidity on ^{68}Ga-PSMA PET/CT, used in prostate cancer imaging, probably because PSMA plays a major role in regulating angiogenesis and endothelial cell recruitment, and thus is expressed in hemangiomas.

Hemangioma also demonstrates a scintigraphic hot-spot appearance on radiolabeled RBC) studies, with increased sensitivity in lesions at least 1.0 to 1.5 cm because smaller lesions tend to blend into surrounding hepatic tracer uptake because of partial volume averaging associated with the limited spatial resolutions of SPECT. The liver hot-spot appearance on ^{99m}Tc-labeled RBC scintigraphy has been described as pathognomonic for a hemangioma; however, there have been case reports with other pathologic entities (e.g., inflammatory adenoma demonstrating a liver hot-spot appearance).

Assessment of Pancreatic Function

For more information, see Chapter 3.

Clinical research into development of tracer-based PET assays of endocrine and exocrine pancreatic functional mass is ongoing. Diabetes mellitus (both type 1 and type 2) is associated with loss of insulin producing tissue or β-cell mass. Preservation of β-cell mass is being investigated to prevent diabetes progression, and thus a reliable noninvasive biomarker of β-cell mass would be an important aid to diabetes research. A candidate radiotracer of β-cell mass that has been studied includes dihydrotetrabenazine (DTBZ), a novel PET imaging agent,[171] which appears promising, but further validation studies are needed before it can be considered for routine clinical practice. Pancreatic exocrine function, which can be impaired postoperatively or with certain diseases (e.g., chronic pancreatitis) is currently measured with invasive direct or noninvasive but lengthy indirect tests (e.g., requiring patient stool collection). Researchers have evaluated pancreatic uptake of the PET radiotracers, such as ^{11}C methionine and ^{11}C acetate, as noninvasive, real-time biomarkers of exocrine pancreatic function.[172] These PET assays remain investigational, although preliminary data is encouraging.

References are available at expertconsult.com.

CHAPTER 19

Emerging techniques in diagnostic imaging

Richard Kinh Gian Do

The field of radiology has undergone tremendous growth over recent decades, with continuous advances in diagnostic imaging that include innovations in medical devices, such as the creation of dual energy–source multidetector computed tomography (CT); innovations in imaging agents, such as new hepatocyte-specific gadolinium (Gd)-binding contrast agents for magnetic resonance imaging (MRI); increases in use of functional imaging, such as for magnetic resonance (MR) diffusion-weighted imaging, and innovations in image analysis tools, such as texture analysis, as well as the application of deep learning/artificial intelligence. In this chapter, we will review a few emerging techniques in diagnostic imaging with relevance to hepatopancreatobiliary tumors.

DUAL-ENERGY COMPUTED TOMOGRAPHY

Medical imaging with CT has benefited from the development of multidetector technology, leading to faster scanning of the abdomen with higher-resolution images, resulting in submillimeter isotropic image voxels that allow for multiplanar reformatting and three-dimensional volume rendering (see Chapter 13). New dose modulation techniques have also reduced the radiation dose exposure for patients. An exciting innovative technique in CT imaging relevant to hepatopancreatobiliary tumors is dual-energy CT (DECT).[1,2] To understand the utility of DECT, a few physical principles underlying CT imaging are worth reviewing.

CT is based on the application of x-rays, which represent electromagnetic waves (photons) of very high energy and very short wavelengths that can pass through most objects, allowing us to "see" through the body. The degree of x-ray attenuation by different elements in our body is proportional to the number of electrons present. The higher the atomic number of an element, the greater the number of electrons present that can interact with x-rays. Put simply, x-rays will be more frequently scattered or absorbed by the photoelectric effect when they travel through bones, which are high in calcium atoms (Ca^{20}), than when traveling through other soft tissues made predominantly of hydrogen (H^1), carbon (C^6), nitrogen (N^7), and oxygen (O^8), which are lower in atomic number. The density of atoms present is another factor contributing to x-ray attenuation; lungs are radiolucent (dark) on plain film and CT because of the much lower density of atoms (and electrons) present in the air within the lungs. On the other hand, the use of iodinated contrast agents in contrast-enhanced CT (CECT) is partly based on the high attenuation of iodine (I^{53}), which can more easily scatter and absorb x-rays because of the higher number of electrons, thereby making vessels and enhancing organs brighter than surrounding tissues.

With single energy (or routine) CT, the x-rays are generated from accelerating electrons in a x-ray tube subject to a peak voltage, kVp, with a predictable energy spectrum of the emitted x-rays. The addition of a second x-ray beam with a different kVp allows us to create CT images based not only on electron density but also on the concentration of distinct elements present in the body. DECT thus takes advantage of the "signature" x-ray interaction profile of distinct elements, such as calcium (Ca^{20}) and iodine (I^{53}).

The potential applications of DECT are numerous but are primarily separated into two functions. The first is in changing the image contrast, such as by increasing the conspicuity of tumors that enhance using iodinated contrast. At lower x-ray energy, the attenuation of iodinated contrast is magnified compared with other elements in soft tissue, which can alter the conspicuity of subtle enhancing lesions. Potential applications include improving hepatocellular carcinoma (HCC) detection[3] (see Chapter 89), liver metastasis detection[4] (see Chapters 90–92), and pancreatic cancer or pancreatitis detection[5,6] (Fig. 19.1; see Chapters 55–59, 62). A second application of DECT relies on the quantification of specific elements, such as calcium or iodine. Quantifying iodine can improve our ability to measure treatment response, such as in therapies in which tumor vascularization (and enhancement) is affected and changes in tumor attenuation are informative.[7] Fat quantification, in patients at risk for hepatic steatosis, for example, is also another potential application of this technique.[8] Although DECT is gaining in popularity as the applications multiply, a number of obstacles remain, including standardization and differences in hardware and software between vendors.[9] Nevertheless, the potential quantification of certain elements by DECT, including iodine uptake, is attractive to radiologists who are increasingly exploring quantitative tools in medical imaging.

FUNCTIONAL IMAGING WITH MAGNETIC RESONANCE IMAGING

The similarities between MRI and CT are evident: cross-sectional high-resolution imaging of abdominal organs, using intravenous (IV) contrast to highlight differences in enhancement. Analogous to advances in CT, progress in MRI technology has benefited from hardware upgrades generating more rapid and higher-resolution images. The added value for MRI over CT, however, comes from the ability to image patients without the risk of ionizing radiation and from exploiting new soft tissue contrast mechanisms (see Chapters 13–17).

MRI is based on the principles of nuclear magnetic resonance (NMR), which harnesses the inherent magnetic properties of protons (H^1) and their electromagnetic interactions. For example, tissue contrast can be generated from differences in chemical environment that affect tissue relaxivity (e.g., T1- vs. T2-weighted imaging), differences in microscopic and macroscopic motion (e.g., diffusion-weighted imaging [DWI] and vascular flow-sensitive imaging), electromagnetic environment (e.g., susceptibility imaging), and many others. The soft tissue contrast mechanisms generated by MRI are numerous and growing, with new sequences exploiting different biologic states

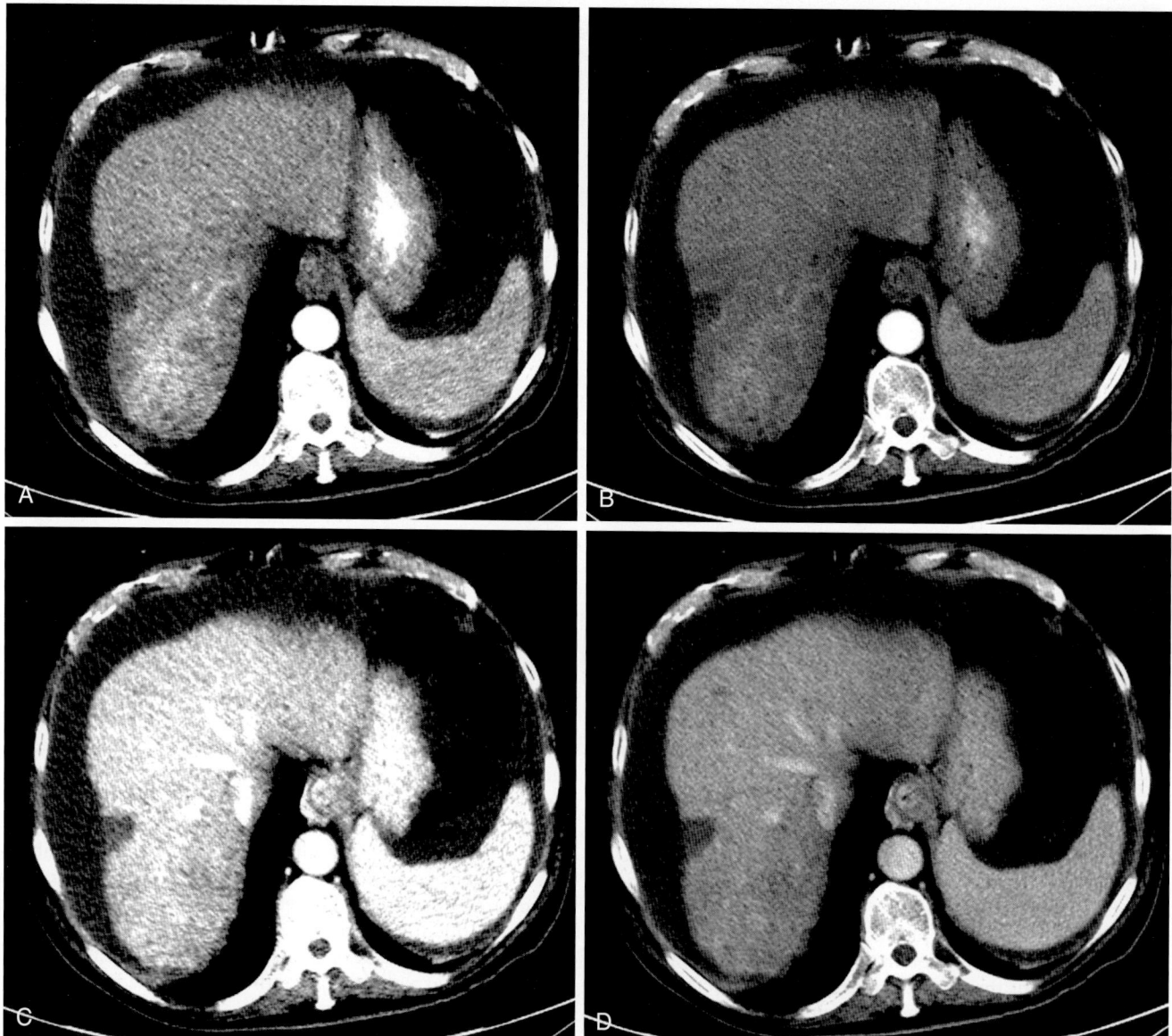

FIGURE 19.1 Computed tomography (CT) images of a patient with infiltrative hepatocellular carcinoma obtained by dual-source dual-energy CT. Arterial phase **(A and B)** and portal venous phase images **(C and D)** on liver windows demonstrate an ill-defined right posterior hepatic mass with arterial phase hyper enhancement, better appreciated on the arterial phase of lower (60) KEV images **(A)** than traditional higher (77) KEV images **(B)**. At a lower KEV **(A and C),** image noise is increased compared with higher KEV images **(C and D).**

(e.g., oxygenation of hemoglobin) being developed continuously. Two applications of MRI that emphasize function (and not just form) are dynamic contrast-enhanced MRI (DCE-MRI) and diffusion-weighted MR imaging (DWI or DW-MRI).

DCE-MRI is a technique that noninvasively characterizes the vasculature of organs and tumors and has the potential to provide predictive or prognostic response biomarkers in multiple cancers.[10] Tumor response to chemotherapy has traditionally been assessed by measurements of tumor size, such as through guidelines from the Response Assessment Criteria in Solid Tumors. With cytotoxic therapies, response is measured by the magnitude of tumor reduction in size. Because new targeted therapies may inhibit vascularization or act as cytostatic agents, however, traditional response criteria based on tumor shrinkage may underestimate therapeutic effectiveness. With DCE-MRI,

calculations of tumor vascularity are used to better predict tumor response to antiangiogenic or targeted therapy. DCE-MRI is based on the repeated imaging of an organ or body part during several minutes, during which the initial uptake and subsequent distribution of IV administered contrast are recorded (Fig. 19.2). Although DCE-CT is also technically feasible, the increased ionizing radiation associated with obtaining multiple CT images has limited its development. With MRI, the arrival and distribution of Gd contrast throughout the vasculature and interstitial space is continuously imaged, and through pharmacokinetic modeling, the changes in signal intensity of an organ (or tumor) of interest are converted into perfusion parameters.[11]

Quantitative perfusion parameters obtained from DCE-MRI reflect the rate of exchange of Gd from vessels to the interstitial space and include K^{trans}, a volume transfer constant

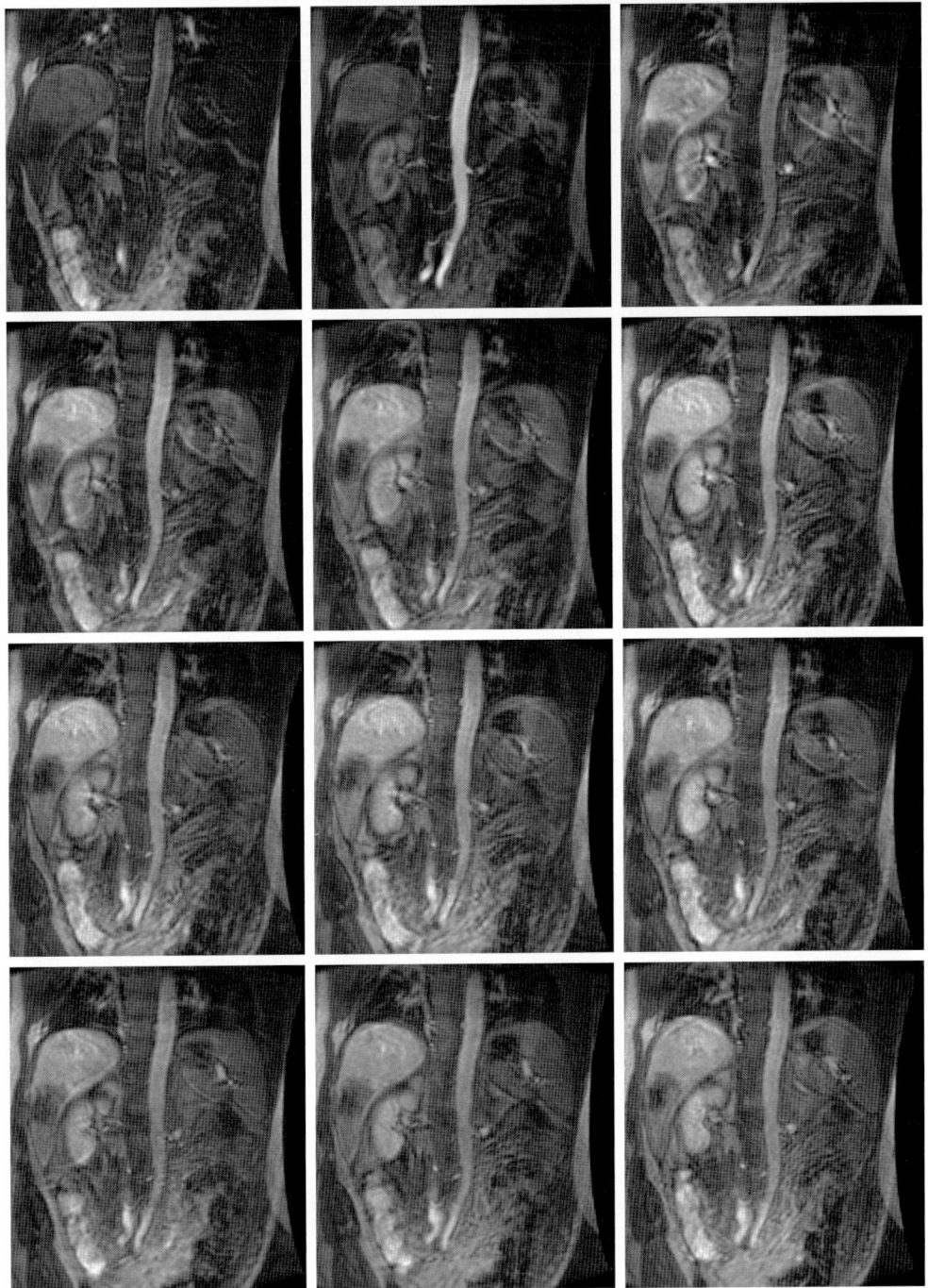

FIGURE 19.2 Consecutive oblique coronal magnetic resonance images (MRI) were obtained of the abdomen every 5 seconds, before *(first panel, top left)* and immediately after intravenous contrast administration. Contrast can be seen arriving in the abdominal aorta *(middle panel, top row),* before enhancing the periphery of the right hepatic lobe peripheral cholangiocarcinoma, on subsequent frames. The entire tumor was imaged during this dynamic contrast-enhanced MRI sequence, with only a single representative slice through the middle of the tumor shown at various time points.

between blood plasma or vascular space (VS) and extracellular extravascular space (EES); *kep*, the rate constant between EES and VS; and *ve*, the fractional vascular volume. These perfusion parameters were initially applied for evaluation of antiangiogenic therapy, but their use has expanded to other targeted chemotherapy agents. Although there has been an increasing number of studies evaluating the utility of DCE-MRI in hepatobiliary tumors,[12,13] the imaging protocols for DCE-MRI have differed among medical centers, limiting comparison of studies

and clinical adoption of this technique. Efforts are ongoing to reduce the variability and improve standardization of imaging parameters by the Quantitative Imaging Biomarker Alliance, formed by the Radiological Society of North America.

An extension of DCE-MRI that is unique to liver imaging is the use of hepatobiliary contrast agents to simultaneously assess vascular supply (through both the hepatic artery and portal vein) as well as hepatic function.[14] Although the majority of MR contrast agents containing Gd are excreted through the kidneys and are predominantly limited to the vascular and extracellular space in distribution, gadoxetate disodium (Gd-EOB-DTPA) also undergoes uptake by hepatocytes and gets excreted through the biliary tree. Thus it is often referred to as a *dual-function contrast agent*, allowing the evaluation of both tumor and liver parenchymal enhancement in the same study.[15]

DWI is an alternative and complementary functional imaging technique to DCE-MRI that can help predict and monitor tumor response to therapy.[16–18] With DWI, one can measure the apparent diffusion coefficients (ADCs), which provide an estimate of the magnitude of water diffusion in biologic tissues. When ADC is measured in tumors, it provides an indirect measure of tumor cellularity at baseline and necrosis after treatment. There is an inverse relationship between ADC and tumor cellularity, which is explained by the presence of cell membranes in proliferating tumors, which act as barriers to water motion. Thus rapidly growing tumors with smaller diving cells will be lower in ADC. Most treatments will lead to disruptions of cell membrane integrity, resulting in greater water diffusion and subsequent increases in ADC. In HCC[19] and colorectal liver metastases,[20,21] ADC can be used to assess response to chemoembolization and chemotherapy, respectively. A study using DWI to monitor HCC response to sorafenib is also promising.[22] As an indirect measure of tumor cellularity and necrosis, DWI is ideally suited as a biomarker to assess therapy response. Similar to DCE-MRI, clinical adoption of DWI for hepatopancreatobiliary tumors will depend on further standardization of ADC measurements, a challenge that is not trivial because of field inhomogeneity and motion inherent to the upper abdomen, given its proximity to the lungs and heart, as well as from interspersed small and large bowel containing gas.

DIAGNOSTIC CRITERIA

Although functional imaging techniques such as DCE-MRI and DWI are quantitative methods to measure tumor properties, the majority of diagnostic radiology still relies on the subjective interpretations of images. For example, CT and MRI have a critical role in the initial assessment of hepatobiliary lesions, such as in the characterization of a solitary liver mass that is incidentally discovered. A hypervascular solitary tumor may represent a benign neoplasm (e.g., focal nodular hyperplasia), a tumor with malignant potential (e.g., hepatocellular adenoma), or a primary malignancy, such as HCC. The temporal pattern of tumor enhancement, the heterogenous appearance of the tumor, and the conspicuity of the tumor with respect to the adjacent liver parenchyma on different MRI sequences are a few of the imaging features used by interpreting radiologists as diagnostic clues. Although CT and MRI techniques may be standardized across different medical centers, the variability in imaging interpretation between different radiologists can remain substantial. Thus an emerging body of research has focused on the diagnostic performance of radiologists. One of the criticisms of early retrospective studies that report on the accuracy of imaging modalities for different clinical questions has been the use of consensus interpretation among expert readers.[23] Individual interpretation, rather than consensus interpretation, is the norm in routine clinical practice. The referring clinician is thus dependent on the training and expertise of the diagnostic radiologist who is assigned to interpret their patient's imaging study at a particular point in time.

A method to reduce the potential variability among diagnostic radiologists is the establishment of diagnostic imaging criteria. For example, multiple criteria for the diagnosis of HCC have been published by various societies in different countries.[24] The role of imaging diagnosis for HCC is unique in its potential impact in patient care, guiding the choice of treatment and even affecting the allocation of liver transplants. The American College of Radiology (ACR) first released a set of guidelines for the diagnosis of HCC termed the *Liver Imaging Reporting and Data System* (LI-RADS) in 2013[25] (see Chapter 89). LI-RADS has been regularly updated to incorporate new literature over time (http://www.acr.org/quality-safety/resources/LIRADS), and in 2018, LI-RADS was adopted into the American Association from the Study of Liver Diseases (AASLD) clinical practice guidance for HCC.[26] At the core of the LI-RADS diagnostic criteria are the definitions of major imaging features, such as arterial phase hyperenhancement, washout appearance, and capsule, which are used to make a definitive diagnosis of HCC.

The concept of washout on CT and MRI is straightforward, described as decreased enhancement in a lesion when compared with the liver parenchyma after initial enhancement on the arterial phase. With LI-RADS, the suggestion is to recognize this finding only when it is unequivocally present. The possibility that different radiologists may interpret "washout appearance" with some variability was well known.[27] In fact, a large interobserver variability study since the first release of LI-RADS demonstrated that there was only moderate agreement between radiologists for the detection of "washout appearance."[28] The agreement for the definitive diagnosis of HCC based on imaging criteria for LI-RADS, AASLD, and Organ Procurement and Transplantation Network (OPTN) guidelines was also moderate to substantial at best. Thus, despite efforts at standardization with the development of diagnostic guidelines, variability in the performance of diagnostic radiologists can remain substantial in specific clinical scenarios and a source of uncertainty for clinical management. Further efforts to reduce this variability may come in the form of accreditation programs, similar to that required for breast imagers through the ACR Mammography Accreditation Program and the federal Mammography Quality Standards Act. These studies are important acknowledgments of the variability inherent in diagnostic imaging that extend beyond the imaging techniques themselves.

RADIOMICS

Variability in the interpretation of medical imaging partly stems from the inherent subjectivity of visual assessments performed by diagnostic radiologists. One method to reduce this variability will come from the use of computer software to aid in the interpretation of medical images and the quantification of imaging features. Radiomics is a growing field of study, with a focus on improving image analysis through the extraction of large amounts of advanced quantitative features of medical images, through automatic or semiautomatic software that can provide more and better information than a physician.[29] The quantification of imaging features can include the description of tumor enhancement at the individual pixel level on CT or MRI, the measurement of tumor heterogeneity by texture analysis, the description of tumor border with respect to the surrounding organ, and many others. The features that are reproducible and most informative are then analyzed for their relationship with treatment outcomes or gene expression (i.e., radiogenomics). An underlying hypothesis for radiomics is that

FIGURE 19.3 Example of textural differences in liver parenchyma on computed tomography images from two patients **(A and B).** Sample with magnified rectangular regions of interest demonstrate greater heterogeneity in the second patient **(B)** than the first patient **(A),** which can be quantified by texture parameters.

genomic and proteomic data from malignancies can be represented in macroscopic image-based features and is correlated to tumor heterogeneity on medical images.

Until recently, the heterogeneity of tumors on imaging was commonly observed but seldom assessed qualitatively by diagnostic radiologists or quantitatively by computer software. Tumor heterogeneity observed on imaging has the potential to reflect molecular and cellular dynamics that may be specific to individual patients and may be predictive of response to targeted therapies that are increasingly in use.[30] Gatenby and colleagues propose that heterogeneity in tumor enhancement is based on perfusion deficits, which can generate significant microenvironmental selection pressures, and that adaptive response to heterogeneity can lead to the emergence of genetic variations within tumors. Quantifying tumor heterogeneity on imaging, to uncover differences in genetic background of individual tumors, can thus form the basis for patient-specific therapies in cancer treatment.

Tumor heterogeneity in medical images can be investigated by texture analysis, defined as the measurement of variations in pixel intensity levels (i.e., gray-scale level) as a function of space. Thus, rather than subjective visual assessment of tumor heterogeneity, one can provide quantitative measures of heterogeneity based on accepted texture parameters, such as contrast, entropy, and other higher-order statistics (Fig. 19.3). Radiomics studies in multiple cancers and hepatopancreatobiliary tumors in particular have increased in recent years.[31] In pancreas cancer, for example, tumor radiomics on CT images are associated with genotype and stromal content, which may help select patients for upfront surgery versus neoadjuvant therapy.[32] Preoperative evaluation of HCC radiomics also shows potential in identifying microvascular invasion.[33]

Texture analysis is not limited to the analysis of tumors. During the development of liver cirrhosis, the liver acquires a characteristic nodular contour, and the liver parenchyma also develops a heterogeneous appearance with an increasingly reticular enhancement pattern. A number of studies have investigated the potential of texture analysis to quantify liver fibrosis by MRI.[34,35] Texture analysis of liver parenchyma also has the potential to predict liver failure after major hepatic resection and predict recurrence of liver metastases.[36,37]

A criticism of radiomics and texture analysis is the potential lack of reproducibility in texture features generated from computer algorithms.[38,39] An alternative approach to analyzing medical imaging without relying on texture analysis is the use of machine learning (ML) techniques. This approach usually requires very large data sets of images, and early studies show potential applications in multiple settings, such as in the diagnosis of liver tumors[40] or the application of LI-RADS categories for patients at risk for HCC.[41] Further multi-institutional studies are needed to generate sufficiently large validation studies before clinical use.

SUMMARY

The field of radiology has undergone tremendous progress in recent decades, with continual investments in imaging technologies to produce more rapid and higher-resolution scanning. Novel imaging devices, contrast agents, and functional techniques continue to emerge and provide improvements in biologic insight for medical decision making. Nevertheless, the variability inherent to imaging technique and diagnostic radiologists themselves can affect the diagnostic performance of an imaging study and is increasingly the subject of investigation. This acknowledgment is leading to the emergence of standardization in radiologic reports and image acquisition parameters, as well as greater interest in the use of computer-based image analyses.

References are available at expertconsult.com

CHAPTER 20

Direct cholangiography: Approaches, techniques, and current role

Robert H. Siegelbaum and Robin B. Mendelsohn

DIRECT CHOLANGIOGRAPHY OVERVIEW

Direct cholangiography, the introduction of contrast medium into the biliary system, can be performed under fluoroscopic guidance percutaneously, endoscopically, or intraoperatively via surgically placed catheters. The nonoperative techniques are percutaneous transhepatic cholangiography (PTC) and endoscopic retrograde cholangiopancreatography (ERCP). Magnetic resonance imaging (MRI) and contrast-enhanced computed tomography (CECT), however, have virtually eliminated the need for direct cholangiography (see Chapters 13 and 16).[1–3] Currently, ERCP and PTC are typically performed only as part of a planned outpatient or inpatient interventional procedure, such as stone extraction, stent placement, biliary drainage, or stricture dilation (see Chapters 30, 31, and 37c).

Magnetic resonance cholangiopancreatography (MRCP) and CECT are noninvasive imaging tests that do not require sedation and are generally considered to be safe. Imaging protocols with multiplanar reconstruction are standard and allow a large field of view, enabling visualization of the entire biliary tree and pancreatic duct (Fig. 20.1). Reconstructed three-dimensional data sets can be displayed in multiple projections, allowing for excellent visualization of the biliary tree and pancreatic duct. Injection of contrast dye under fluoroscopic guidance, on the other hand, is limited to visualization of structures in direct continuity with the opacified, nonisolated segments of the biliary tree (Fig. 20.2). While performing direct cholangiography with PTC, simultaneous cross-sectional imaging may be required to ensure that the entire biliary tree has been opacified, even with multiple percutaneous puncture sites and injections. Cross-sectional imaging of the liver can be performed in a fluoroscopy room with rotational angiography or by direct CT imaging if available. Furthermore, MRCP and CECT provide superior diagnostic accuracy when compared with PTC or ERCP, allowing visualization of the bile duct wall, structures contiguous to the biliary tree (such as cysts and neoplasms), and structures adjacent to the liver.

PERCUTANEOUS TRANSHEPATIC CHOLANGIOGRAPHY

History

Fluoroscopic imaging of the biliary tree was first reported by Burckhardt and Müller in 1921,[4] who performed cholecystocholangiography via percutaneous puncture of the gallbladder. The first report of PTC was by Huard and Do-Xuan-Hop in 1937,[5] who performed cholangiography with Lipiodol, a suboptimal contrast agent. Transhepatic cholangiography as a diagnostic tool gained popularity 15 years later, after Carter and Saypol's (1952)[6] discussion of PTC with the use of a water-soluble contrast agent. In the ensuing years, many investigators[7–12] described a variety of different techniques, including the use of sheathed or unsheathed needles of various sizes and different puncture sites. These procedures were associated with a significant risk of bile peritonitis, especially in obstructed biliary systems, and less frequently, bleeding. Fine-needle transhepatic access to the biliary tree was first developed at Chiba University and was presented by Ohto and Tsuchiya (1969),[13] and later by Tsuchiya (1969).[14] Numerous additional reports have also described decreased complications with fine-needle transhepatic access, and this technique has generally been accepted as the standard[15–22] (see Chapter 31).

Evaluation of the biliary tree by noninvasive imaging techniques have largely replaced transhepatic cholangiography (see Chapters 13 and 16). In 1985 Kadir[23] reported that less than 5% of patients referred for evaluation of biliary disease required concomitant drainage procedures. With continued advancement of cross-sectional imaging techniques, in particular MRCP (see Chapters 13, 16 and 19),[24–28] percutaneous fluoroscopic imaging of the biliary tree with contrast injection is typically performed only as part of a planned interventional procedure.

Imaging evaluation of the biliary tree with MRCP or CECT is noninvasive, does not require sedation, and is generally regarded as safe (see Chapters 13 and 16). With direct needle puncture and contrast injection in the biliary tree, only bile ducts in continuity with the punctured duct are visualized. In the presence of bile duct isolation, multiple percutaneous needle punctures may be required to visualize the entire biliary tree (see Fig. 20.2). Even with multiple transhepatic bile duct needle punctures, CT imaging performed at the time of the procedure can be helpful to ensure that the biliary tree has been fully imaged. Alternatively, MRI and CECT can image the entire biliary system and can demonstrate the presence and severity of bile duct isolation (see Fig. 20.1). MRI or CECT can visualize the bile duct wall, liver, and surrounding structures, often providing more clinical information that could be relevant to patient care.

Preprocedural Preparation

Patients should undergo cross-sectional imaging (CECT or MRI) before fluoroscopic imaging of the biliary tree. This is particularly so in patients who have undergone prior liver surgery or liver resection. MRI or CECT are the imaging modalities of choice because these studies depict the level of bile duct obstruction, patency of the portal venous system, the relationship of the liver and bile ducts to other structures, and the presence of tumors or lobar atrophy. Knowledge of this information could improve the chance of successful and safe bile duct puncture (see Chapter 31).

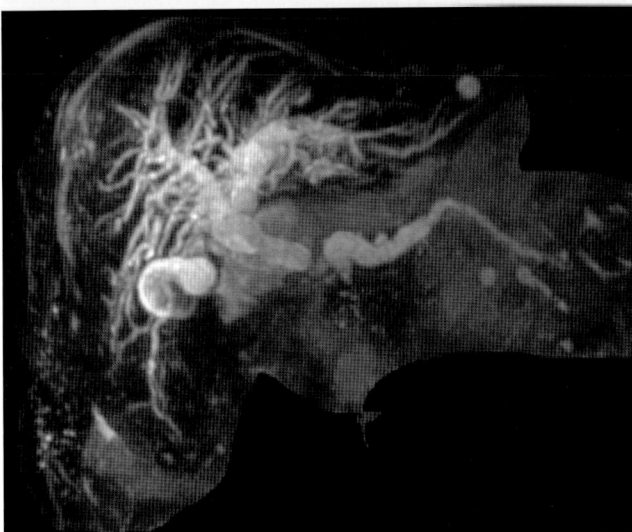

FIGURE 20.1 Magnetic resonance cholangiopancreatography. Three-dimensional maximum intensity projection image showing marked dilatation of the intrahepatic and extrahepatic biliary tree, as well as the pancreatic duct, in a patient with a head of pancreas mass (see Chapters 16 and 17).

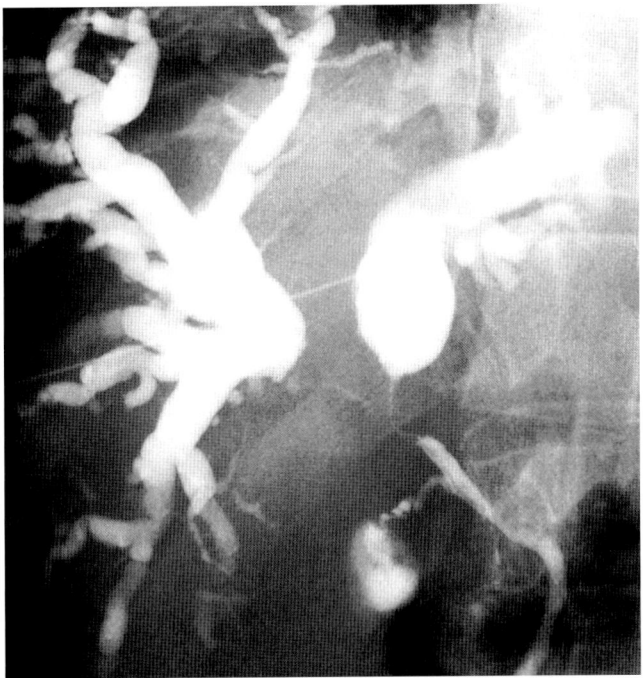

FIGURE 20.2 Hilar cholangiocarcinoma involving first-order right and left hepatic ducts. Separate needle punctures were required to fill the right and left ducts.

Coagulation parameters and platelet count should be checked before the procedure and corrected if necessary. Informed consent is obtained in accordance with institutional policy, specifically including a discussion of the risks, benefits, and alternatives of the procedure. Patients generally receive moderate sedation or monitored anesthesia care. All patients should receive broad-spectrum intravenous (IV) antibiotic coverage according to institutional guidelines or preferences.

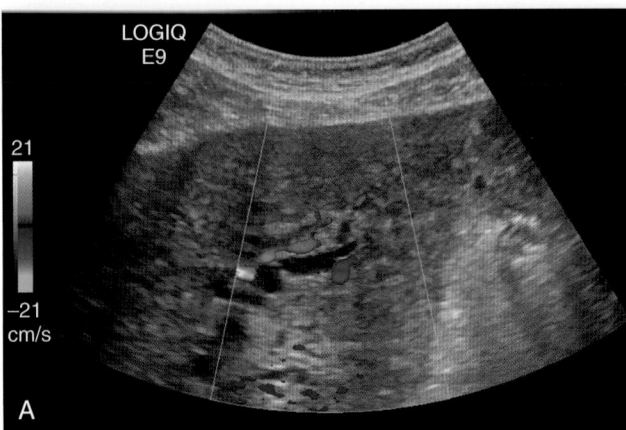

A

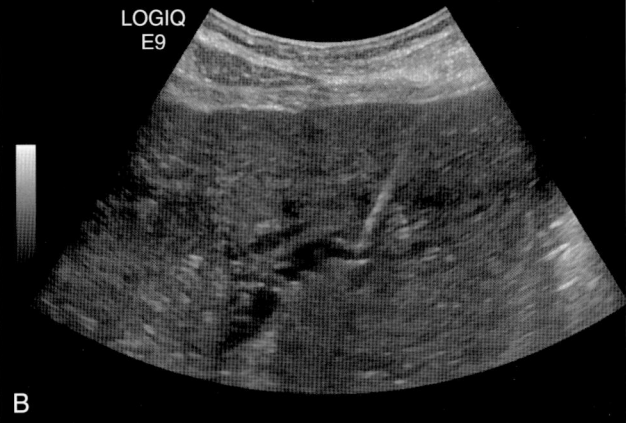

B

FIGURE 20.3 Real-time ultrasound guidance can be helpful for the initial puncture in the presence of bile duct dilatation. **A,** Color Doppler image of the left liver revealing a dilated segment III bile duct. **B,** Static grayscale ultrasound image taken during puncture of the dilated bile duct with an echogenic 21-gauge needle.

Procedure

Although typically not present in modern fluoroscopy suites, PTC is ideally performed on a tilting fluoroscopic table—another reason why these techniques have been largely supplanted by CECT and MRI. Because the specific gravity of contrast material is greater than that of bile, less contrast dye is typically required to fully delineate the biliary tree when the table is tilted.

Right-Sided Puncture

When performing a puncture of a right-sided bile duct, a site is selected in the right midaxillary line, typically one or two interspaces below the costophrenic angle. Needle puncture sites are ideally below the ninth intercostal space to avoid inadvertent crossing of the pleural space. The skin is prepped and draped using standard techniques and a subcutaneous anesthetic agent such as lidocaine is infused. A small dermatotomy is made with a No. 11 blade scalpel. A 21- or 22-gauge, 15- to 20-cm Chiba-style needle is advanced under fluoroscopic guidance superior to the closest rib to the target puncture site to avoid injury to an intercostal vessel or nerve. Real-time ultrasound guidance can be helpful for the initial puncture in the presence of bile duct dilatation.[29] The puncture site and direction of puncture are chosen based on evaluation of the patient's cross-sectional imaging studies (Fig. 20.3A–B). A small amount of water-soluble contrast agent is injected while slowly withdrawing the needle until a bile duct is identified. Injection of contrast agent into a bile duct has the appearance of oil being dropped in water. Inadvertent opacification of a vascular structure is recognized by the rapid clearance of the contrast agent. If a bile duct is not entered during withdrawal of the needle, the needle is reintroduced in a slightly different direction. It is generally considered best practice not to withdraw the needle completely from the liver to minimize the number of punctures through the liver capsule. When opacification of the biliary tree is challenging, particularly in the case of a nondilated biliary tree, the same puncture site may be used multiple times before selecting a new percutaneous access site. If successful puncture of a bile duct is unlikely from that site after multiple attempts, a new site should be chosen. In patients with biliary obstruction, gentle injection of 10 mL of iodinated contrast is typically sufficient for bile duct opacification. A larger volume of contrast material is typically required in nonobstructed systems. When the bile ducts are visualized, fluoroscopic images should be acquired and stored in multiple projections to identify specific portions of the biliary tree and to completely delineate abnormal findings, if present. Of note, care should be taken to avoid puncture of the gallbladder or an extrahepatic bile duct.

Left-Sided Puncture

Considerable variation is present in size and anatomic position of the left lateral segments of the liver. Careful review of preprocedural cross-sectional imaging is recommended to select an optimal puncture site. Although left-sided punctures can be performed through the right liver via an anterior axillary line approach to the segment IV bile ducts, a subxiphoid approach to a bile duct in segment II or segment III is generally preferred. As in punctures of right-sided bile ducts, percutaneous access to the biliary tree can be simplified by using real-time ultrasound guidance in the presence of dilated bile ducts.[29]

Success Rate and Accuracy

Percutaneous opacification of the biliary tree is successful in 95% to 100% of patients with biliary obstruction.[19,21,30] A success rate of 60% to 95% is reported for nondilated biliary systems. The likelihood of success in a nondilated system is increased by the number of needle passes performed.[31] No current radiologic descriptions of obstructed bile ducts are pathognomonic for differentiation of benign and malignant disease.[32,33] Bile cytology and review of cross-sectional imaging can be helpful in conjunction with fluoroscopic images in diagnosing the cause of the obstruction.

Pitfalls in Interpretation

Lack of Opacification

Failure to inject an adequate volume of contrast agent can result in incorrect interpretation of the level of obstruction. This pitfall can occur in the setting of complete obstruction and can be identified by the presence of a hazy margin at the level of the apparent (false) obstruction (Fig. 20.4).[34] In high bile duct obstruction, especially when associated with variant anatomy, isolated segments of the biliary tree can be visualized only by direct puncture. If an incorrect bile duct is selected or if puncture of an additional bile duct is needed but not performed, the diagnosis of bile duct injuries and bile leaks can be missed. This is a clear limitation of direct cholangiography versus noninvasive imaging techniques.

Ductal Dilatation

The absence of bile duct dilatation does not exclude the presence of clinically significant obstruction. Disorders such as sclerosing cholangitis, acquired immunodeficiency syndrome (AIDS), and chemotherapy-induced biliary sclerosis can present with bile duct fibrosis, impeding the ability of the bile ducts to become dilated. Conversely, bile duct dilatation does not always imply the presence of an obstructed biliary system. For

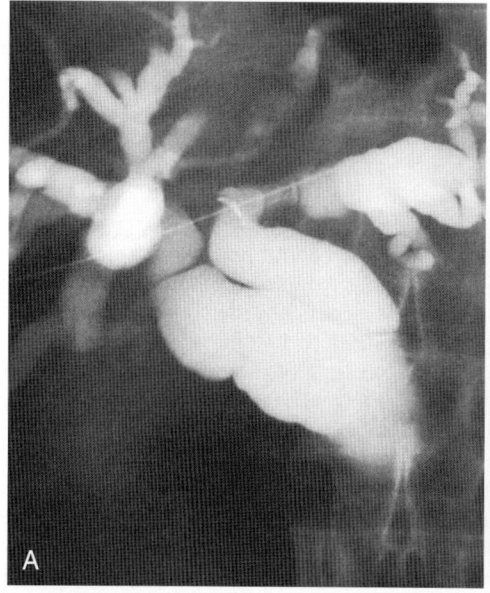
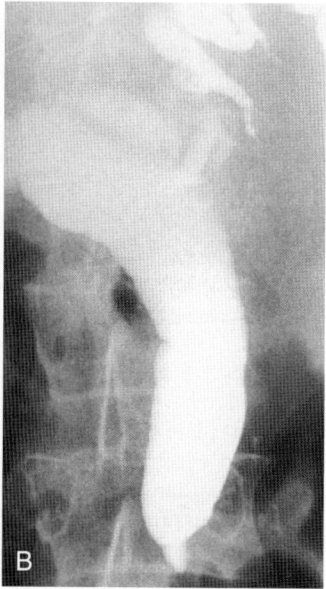

FIGURE 20.4   **Ampullary carcinoma. A,** With the patient supine, contrast pools proximally, giving a false impression of a high bile duct obstruction. The spurious nature of the level is suggested by the hazy inferior margin to the contrast column. **B,** With the patient sitting semierect, the contrast pools at the true point of obstruction, which is sharply defined.

example, dilatation that may be seen in patients with Caroli disease, or choledochal cysts, can have the radiographic appearance of bile duct dilation without the presence of obstruction.

Complications

Significant complications of PTC are rare and occur in approximately 3% of patients.[19] The most common major complications are bile leak (1%–2%), sepsis (2%–3%), and bleeding (0.2%–0.4%). Other rare complications include pneumothorax, biliothorax, injury to the colon, and abscess formation. Puncture below the ninth intercostal space should decrease the incidence of chest complications. The risk for infectious complications, such as sepsis and abscess formation, can typically be decreased with proper antibiotic coverage. Care should be taken to not over-distend the bile ducts with contrast media because opacification and incomplete drainage of the biliary tree can be a source of cholangitis,[29] particularly in the presence of bile duct isolation.

ENDOSCOPIC RETROGRADE CHOLANGIOPANCREATOGRAPHY

History

ERCP (see Chapter 30) was first described in 1968[35] and rapidly became accepted as an important diagnostic modality for patients with hepatobiliary and pancreatic diseases.[36–39] Advances in technology and training over the last 50 years have enhanced and expanded the scope of ERCP. The addition of an elevator to the side-viewing duodenoscope helped facilitate cannulation of the papilla of Vater.[40–42] The development of therapeutic applications through ERCP, including sphincterotomy[43–45] and stenting,[46,47] has transformed ERCP from a diagnostic into a therapeutic procedure. ERCP is considered to be an advanced procedure, requiring skills more difficult to learn than routine endoscopic procedures, and is offered as an additional year of training beyond the standard gastroenterology fellowship.

Indications

Diagnostic ERCP has largely been replaced by noninvasive imaging techniques and is rarely performed without a therapeutic component. In 2002 the National Institutes of Health sponsored a consensus conference on ERCP and issued a statement proposing the indications for ERCP.[48] They concluded that ERCP, MRCP, and endoscopic ultrasound have comparable sensitivity and specificity in the diagnosis of common bile duct (CBD) stones. They stated that avoidance of unnecessary ERCPs is the best way to reduce the number of complications and that endoscopists performing ERCPs should have appropriate training and expertise. In 2005 the American Society of Gastrointestinal Endoscopy published guidelines stating that, based on expert opinion, ERCP is primarily a therapeutic procedure for the management of pancreaticobiliary disorders.[49] ERCP is currently rarely performed without a therapeutic component.

Technique

Most ERCPs are performed as outpatient procedures in a hospital setting, although they can also be performed in ambulatory centers. Given that ERCP is a complex procedure, requiring special equipment and training, the risks and benefits of the procedure must be heavily considered before proceeding (see Chapter 30). Patients should be alert, oriented, and able to give informed consent. The next of kin can provide consent in the rare cases where patients are unable to give informed consent. Patient age and clinical picture are important. Older age is not a risk factor for ERCP. Elderly patients have the same risks of bleeding and perforation as younger patients and actually have a lower risk of pancreatitis.[50]

After consent is obtained, the patient is brought into a room with a C-arm for availability of fluoroscopy during the procedure. IV sedation is given under monitored control. In the past, drug combinations of narcotics, such as meperidine and droperidol, and benzodiazepines, such as midazolam or diazepam, were used. More recently, this has been replaced by propofol, a short-acting sedative and amnestic with a rapid recovery profile. Studies have shown that propofol is more effective than sedation with midazolam, is safe, and is associated with a faster postprocedure recovery.[51,52] In some centers, general anesthesia may be used if the endoscopic procedure is expected to be difficult, the patient has significant comorbid medical conditions, or there are any signs of functional or mechanical intestinal obstruction. Oxygen is administered by nasal cannula to avoid hypoxemia, which has been described in 40% of patients undergoing ERCP.[53] The patient's electrocardiogram, blood pressure, oxygen saturation, and overall condition are continually monitored throughout the procedure by a dedicated nurse. Antibiotics are not given routinely for diagnostic procedures. All endoscopic equipment used for this procedure, including the endoscopes, is either chemically disinfected or gas sterilized.

The patient is usually placed in a semiprone position with special positioning of the arms to help optimize access to the ampulla of Vater. A side-viewing duodenoscope is used to afford excellent visualization of the ampulla of Vater. In patients with postoperative anatomy, a standard forward-viewing upper endoscope, pediatric colonoscope, or single balloon enteroscope may be needed to successfully approach the ampulla. An initial endoscopic evaluation of the stomach and duodenum is performed before cannulation of the ampulla. The ampulla is usually located in the second portion of the duodenum but, in rare instances, may be found more proximal or distal (see Chapter 2). It is usually easily identified, although in some cases, it may be distorted because of malignancy or edema from pancreatitis, hidden behind a fold, or within a diverticulum. The orifice of the CBD is usually located on the left upper corner of the ampulla. In most patients, the CBD and main pancreatic duct share a common channel. In a minority of patients, the orifices are separate. The minor papilla is located about 1 to 2 cm above the major papilla. The CBD is selectively cannulated with either a cannula or sphincterotome. Studies have shown that access to the biliary tree is easier and faster with a sphincterotome, compared with a cannula.[54–56] Some endoscopists have been using guidewire-assisted cannulation. Whether insertion of a guidewire, as opposed to the more conventional technique of contrast injection, should be the preferred technique to access the bile ducts remains controversial. A guidewire does not produce the hydrostatic pressure associated with contrast injection and decreases the risk for trauma to the pancreatic duct, thereby theoretically decreasing the risk for post-ERCP pancreatitis. The data, however, are mixed. A meta-analysis looking at 12 randomized controlled trials (RCTs) with 3,450 patients concluded that wire-guided technique had a higher cannulation success rate (84% vs. 77%) and a lower risk of post-ERCP pancreatitis (3.5% vs. 6.7%).[57] Nevertheless, a prospective trial with 1,249 patients showed no significant difference in post-ERCP pancreatitis in the guidewire group (5.2%) compared with the contrast injection group (4.4%).[58]

There are techniques to help facilitate access to the bile duct in difficult cannulations (see Chapter 30). Excess duodenal motility can be controlled by bolus injections of 0.25 to 1 mg of IV glucagon. If the pancreatic duct is inadvertently cannulated, placement of a pancreatic duct stent may help cannulation by both blocking the pancreatic duct orifice and providing more information to the endoscopist about the angle of the bile duct, especially in cases of distorted anatomy (Fig. 20.5).[59] Another technique involves placing a guidewire into the pancreatic duct, which adds more information about the optimal

angle to approach cannulation (Fig. 20.6). The studies are limited, but a recent review concluded that the sole use of pancreatic guidewire does appear to be associated with an increased risk of pancreatitis.[60] Other more invasive maneuvers, including precut sphincterotomy with or without pancreatic duct stent placement, may also improve success rate but are associated with an increased risk of complications, including bleeding, perforation, and pancreatitis, even in experienced hands.[61]

Duodenal diverticula are common and almost always are located near the papilla in the descending duodenum. Although

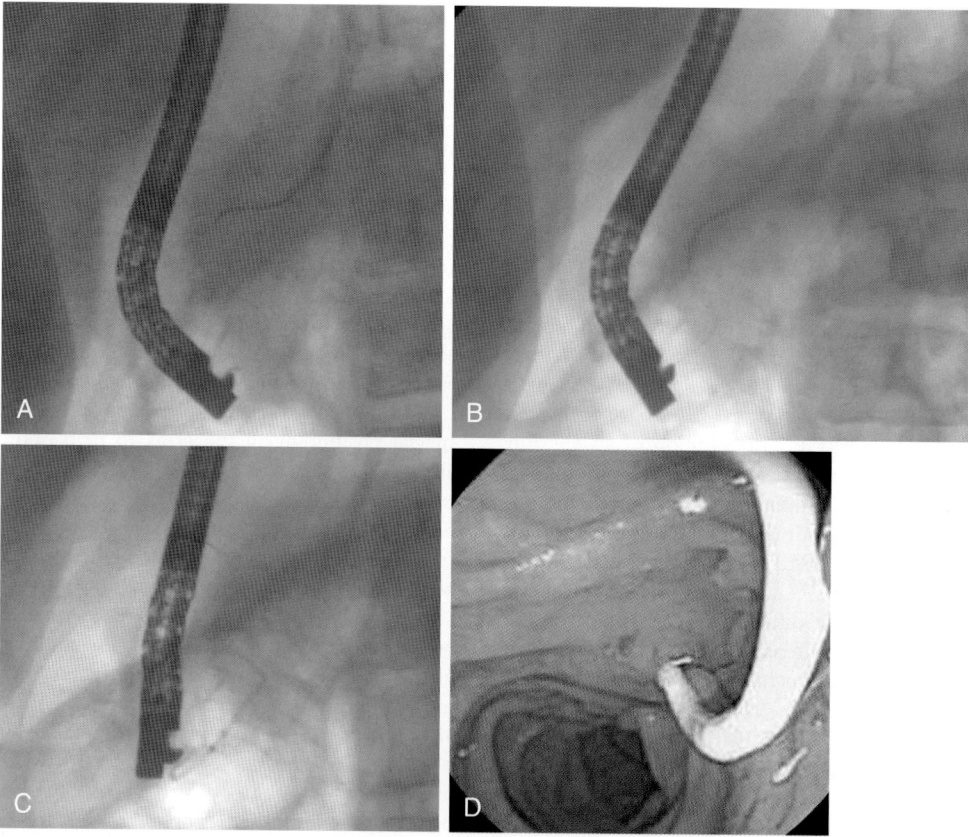

FIGURE 20.5 Pancreatic duct stent placement. **A,** Wire placement into the pancreatic duct. **B,** Contrast injection to confirm position in pancreatic duct. **C,** Placement of a 5 French (F) × 5-cm pancreatic duct stent with a full external pigtail and a single internal flap. **D,** Endoscopic view of 5F pancreatic duct stent.

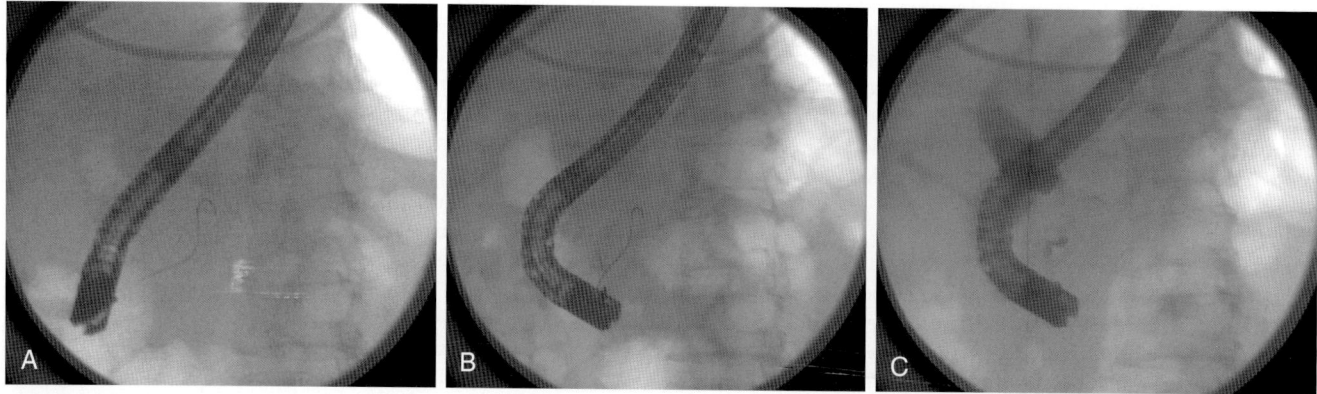

FIGURE 20.6 Guidewire placement in pancreatic duct to facilitate bile duct cannulation. **A,** Wire placement into pancreatic duct. **B,** This provided more information to the endoscopist about the angle of the bile duct, and the CannulaTome was adjusted under fluoroscopic guidance. **C,** Contrast injection confirmed position in common bile duct.

usually asymptomatic, diverticula have been shown to be associated with choledocholithiasis. Periampullary diverticula may make cannulation more difficult, but the data are mixed[62,63] (see Chapter 30).

In patients with surgically altered anatomy, ERCP may be quite challenging. In patients with a Billroth II gastrojejunostomy, success rates for bile duct cannulation are much lower.[64] The papilla is found in the afferent limb, which may be difficult to traverse. In addition, the orientation of the ampulla is upside down compared with standard ERCP. In patients with Roux-en-Y gastrectomies, it is often difficult even to reach the papilla, given the long Roux limb. If the papilla is identified, cannulation may still be extremely difficult because of the location and position of the ampulla.[65] Single balloon enteroscopy has been reported to have high procedural success rates and should be considered first-line intervention when biliary access is required after Roux-en-Y gastric bypass, Billroth II gastrojejunostomy, or hepaticojejunostomy[66] (see Chapter 30). This is mostly only offered in tertiary care centers.

Once the bile duct is selectively cannulated, a contrast agent is injected under fluoroscopic control, with subsequent radiographic images obtained of the duct anatomy. Choice of contrast agent differs among endoscopists. Many choose to use half strength contrast when looking for stones. Material for pathologic and cytologic evaluation can be obtained from either the biliary or pancreatic duct system, with a variety of dedicated endoscopic biopsy forceps and cytology brushes. Pathologic and cytologic material may be obtained from the ampulla of Vater, duodenum, and stomach for diagnostic purposes during the procedure as well.

Pancreatography

Imaging the pancreatic duct can be an important adjunct to cholangiography during ERCP. Strictures, stones, and other obstructing lesions can be identified. Most recommend guidewire cannulation of the pancreatic duct over contrast injection because this produces less hydrostatic pressure in the duct, possibly decreasing the risk for post-ERCP pancreatitis. In general, the pancreatic duct is about 20 cm in length and variable in caliber. With increasing age comes progressive atrophy and fibrosis of the pancreas. The diameter of the main pancreatic duct also increases with age, although one study found no difference in pancreatic duct length among patients younger than 40 years compared with older patients. Duct diameter throughout the pancreas was significantly greater, however, in patients older than 40 years.[67]

Anatomic variations, such as pancreas divisum (Fig. 20.7), also may be identified on a pancreatogram (see Chapter 2). This abnormality has been described in 7.5% of ERCP procedures and can be confirmed by cannulation of the main pancreatic duct through the orifice in the minor papilla.[68]

Cholangioscopy and Pancreatoscopy

Cholangioscopy and pancreatoscopy involve using miniature endoscopes through the channel of the duodenoscope, allowing for direct visualization of the bile and pancreatic ducts, respectively (see Chapters 30). A new skill set is necessary to perform these procedures, given that this technique uses two different endoscopes. Diagnostic cholangioscopy may be used to evaluate indeterminate biliary strictures and filling defects. Similarly, diagnostic pancreatoscopy may be used to evaluate pancreatic strictures and intraductal papillary mucinous neoplasms. Studies

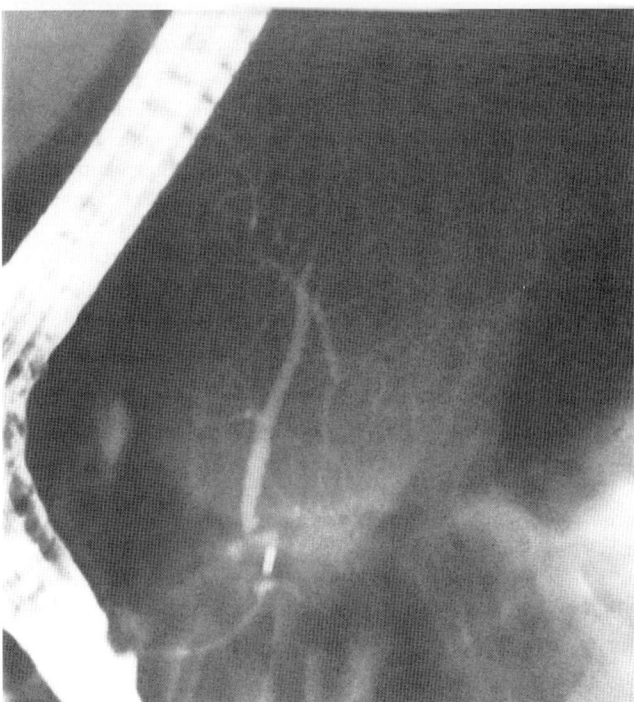

FIGURE 20.7 **Pancreas divisum.** The cannula is in the major papillary orifice, and contrast injection opacifies the proximal portion of the major pancreatic duct (Wirsung). Injection through the minor papillae allows opacification of the duct of Santorini and the distal duct of Wirsung (see Chapter 53).

have shown that it is an accurate diagnostic tool for patients with pancreaticobiliary disorders.[69-71] One prospective multicenter study of 87 patients reported that endoscopists were able to distinguish benign from malignant indeterminate biliary lesions 92.1% of the time with cholangioscopy with visualization alone.[72] A recent systematic review and meta-analysis looking at 13 original articles concluded that cholangioscopy has very high diagnostic capability to diagnose malignant biliary obstruction.[73] Complications of cholangiopancreatoscopy include bacteremia, bleeding, and pancreatitis. One retrospective study reported that complications of cholangiopancreatoscopy are increased compared with ERCP alone and are associated with a much higher risk of cholangitis.[74]

Complications

Complications of ERCP include those associated with endoscopic procedures in general, as well as those specific to ERCP. Incidence rates of complications vary in the literature. A systematic survey of prospective studies reviewed 21 studies with 16,855 patients and reported a specific complication rate of 6.9% and a mortality rate of 0.33%.[75] The experience of the endoscopist and case volume also has an impact on the complication rate. In a study conducted in Austria, endoscopists performing more that 50 ERCP procedures per year were compared with those performing fewer than 50 per year. Those in the higher case-volume group had a significantly higher success rate (86.9% vs. 80.3%; $P < .001$) and a lower overall complication rate (10.2% vs. 13.6%; $P = .007$).[76]

Pancreatitis

The most common complication of ERCP is pancreatitis, with reported incidences ranging from 1% to 40% but most frequently reported around 3% to 5%.[75,77–80] The incidence of post-ERCP pancreatitis in children is quite low, about 2.5% in one study.[81] The consensus classification defined post-ERCP pancreatitis as the clinical picture of new or worsened abdominal pain with amylase at least three times normal at 24 hours after the procedure and requiring hospitalization.[82] They further defined it as mild if hospitalization is two to three days, moderate if hospitalization is four to 10 days, and severe if hospitalization is more than 10 days, if there is a pseudocyst or hemorrhagic pancreatitis, or if an intervention is required. Post-ERCP pancreatitis should be distinguished from transient asymptomatic hyperamylasemia, which occurs in 40% to 75% of cases and disappears within one to two days.[43,83] Most cases of post-ERCP pancreatitis are mild and usually resolve in a few days with conservative measures of bowel rest and IV fluids. The management is the same as for pancreatitis from other causes.

Multiple potential mechanisms have been proposed to explain the pathogenesis of post-ERCP pancreatitis. Mechanical injury to the pancreatic duct from manipulation of the papilla, instrumentation of the pancreatic duct, or injection of the pancreatic duct likely play a role.[84] Similarly, thermal injury from electrocautery leading to edema and possible obstruction of the duct has been invoked.[85] Hydrostatic pressure from contrast injection leading to injury is also likely a component. The contrast itself theoretically may cause a chemical or allergic injury. However, the use of nonionic contrast medium of low osmolarity has shown no advantage over the less expensive ionic contrast medium in preventing ERCP-related pancreatitis,[86] and a meta-analysis showed no significant difference in post-ERCP pancreatitis among different contrast media.[87]

Although it remains unclear whether these mechanisms work independently or in conjunction, recent data have helped to elucidate both patient- and procedure-related risk factors that are independently associated with post-ERCP pancreatitis. These risk factors are additive.[88] Patient-related factors include younger age, female sex, normal serum bilirubin, recurrent pancreatitis, history of post-ERCP pancreatitis, and sphincter of Oddi dysfunction. Procedure-related factors include difficult cannulation, pancreatic duct injection, precut sphincterotomy, pancreatic sphincterotomy, minor papilla sphincterotomy, balloon sphincteroplasty, ampullectomy, and sphincter of Oddi manometry. One study showed that trainee participation was an independent risk factor.[77] Most studies, however, have not shown a correlation between case volume and rates of pancreatitis.[80,88,89]

Specific techniques and measures to decrease the risk of pancreatitis have been evaluated. The risk of pancreatitis is reduced by minimizing the number of attempts of cannulation, avoiding pancreatic duct cannulation if not necessary, and minimizing the volume of contrast injected into the pancreatic duct to avoid overdistension or "acinarization" of the pancreatic duct.

Placement of a temporary pancreatic duct stent may also reduce the risk. One meta-analysis demonstrated that the use of pancreatic duct stents in high-risk patients decreased the rate of post-ERCP pancreatitis by about two-thirds.[90] Their use is not routinely recommended but is reserved for high-risk patients. Studies have shown a benefit of pancreatic duct stents in biliary sphincterotomy for sphincter of Oddi dysfunction, precut sphincterotomy, balloon sphincteroplasty, endoscopic ampullectomy, and difficult cannulation.[90–92]

Many pharmacologic agents have been studied. A recent systematic review included 85 RCTs and 28 meta-analyses evaluating pharmacologic prevention of post-ERCP pancreatitis. They concluded that rectal nonsteroidal antiinflammatory drugs (NSAIDs) were beneficial, especially in high-risk patients. Data on bolus-administered somatostatin, sublingual nitroglycerin, and some protease inhibitors were considered promising, but confirmatory studies are necessary.[93]

NSAIDs inhibit prostaglandin synthesis, phospholipase A_2 activity, and neutrophil/endothelial cell attachment, which are all thought to play a major role in the pathogenesis of pancreatitis and thus may have a role in post-ERCP pancreatitis prevention. A meta-analysis that included 10 RCTs with a total of 2,269 patients concluded that NSAID use decreased the risk for post-ERCP pancreatitis (risk ratio [RR] 0.57; 95% confidence interval [CI], 0.38–0.86; $P = .007$).[94] Nevertheless, these studies were extremely heterogeneous in regard to type of NSAID and to route and timing of administration. A placebo-controlled, double-blind RCT of high-risk patients showed that patients who received rectal indomethacin immediately after the procedure were less likely to develop post-ERCP pancreatitis than the control group (9.2% vs. 16.9%; $P = .0005$) and were less likely to develop moderate to severe pancreatitis (4.4% vs. 8.8%; $P = .03$).[95] A meta-analysis that specifically looked at studies of rectal indomethacin and included four studies with 1,470 patients showed that the rate of pancreatitis was significantly lower using indomethacin compared with placebo (odds ratio [OR], 0.49; CI, 0.34–0.71; $P = .0002$).[96] A network meta-analysis compared rectal indomethacin to pancreatic duct stenting and concluded that rectal indomethacin alone was superior to pancreatic duct stenting in post-ERCP prevention (OR, 0.48; 95% CI, 0.26–0.87).[97] The European Society of Gastrointestinal Endoscopy guidelines recommend routine prophylactic use of rectal NSAIDs immediately before or after ERCP in all patients without a contraindication.[98]

Somatostatin and its analogue octreotide inhibit pancreatic secretions, decrease sphincter of Oddi pressure, modulate cytokines, and lead to apoptosis of pancreatic acinar cells, and therefore may be protective against post-ERCP pancreatitis. They have been studied extensively, with conflicting results. One meta-analysis included seven homogeneous high-quality studies involving 3,130 patients and concluded that somatostatin administered as a bolus was effective in prevention of post-ERCP pancreatitis.[99] A different meta-analysis looked at 17 studies with a total of 3,818 patients and found that somatostatin and high-dose octreotide prevented post-ERCP pancreatitis if given over 12 hours or in bolus form.[100] Subsequent RCTs have yielded mixed results. One double-blinded, placebo-controlled RCT involved 391 patients in three hospitals. Patients were randomized to receive 3 mg of somatostatin in 500 mL normal saline (NS) infused for 12 hours, starting 30 minutes before the ERCP or 500 mL NS infused for 12 hours, starting 30 minutes before the ERCP. They found a significantly lower risk for pancreatitis in the somatostatin group (3.6% vs. 9.6% in the placebo group; $P = .02$).[101] Another study involved 133 patients who were randomized to a bolus of somatostatin infusion before ERCP, followed by continuous infusion for 12 hours, a bolus of somatostatin before ERCP only, and placebo alone; no significant differences were found among the three groups.[102] A recent RCT of 510 patients randomized to an IV bolus of 250 µg of somatostatin before cannulation, followed by a four-hour continuous infusion of the drug at 250 µg/hr, or placebo with NS, showed no significant difference in rates of post-ERCP pancreatitis.[103] Future research is necessary to elucidate the role of somatostatin in prevention of post-ERCP pancreatitis.

Nitroglycerin acts as a smooth muscle relaxant and subsequently may decrease sphincter of Oddi pressures, thereby decreasing the risk of post-ERCP pancreatitis. Only three out of seven RCTs showed that nitroglycerin was effective, but two of the three positive studies used sublingual nitroglycerin.[93] One compared 2 mg sublingual nitroglycerin given five minutes before endoscopy with placebo in 186 patients and found a lower incidence of pancreatitis in the nitroglycerin group (7/90 vs. 17/96; $P < .05$).[104] The second one enrolled 74 patients and randomly assigned them to 5 mg sublingual glyceryl trinitrate versus 100 mg vitamin C, five minutes before the ERCP. They found a significant difference in post-ERCP pancreatitis in the study group (7.9%) compared with placebo (25%; $P = .012$).[105] In both studies, however, the consensus definition for pancreatitis was not used, which may account for the high rates of pancreatitis in the control groups. One RCT of 300 patients showed that the combination of rectal indomethacin and sublingual nitroglycerin was superior to rectal indomethacin alone at prevention of post-ERCP pancreatitis (6.7% vs. 15.3%; $P = .016$).[106] More studies are needed to further clarify the benefit of nitroglycerin in post-ERCP pancreatitis.

Protease inhibitors, such as gabexate mesylate, nafamostat mesylate, and ulinastatin, have been investigated, given that activation of proteolytic enzymes likely contributes to the pathogenesis of pancreatitis. A meta-analysis of 18 studies with a total of 4,966 patients showed a significant, yet small, risk reduction in post-ERCP pancreatitis with the protease inhibitors.[107] They stated there was no solid evidence to support their use at this time.

A pilot study investigated whether aggressive periprocedural hydration reduced the risk of post-ERCP pancreatitis and found that none of the patients in the aggressive hydration group developed pancreatitis compared with 17% of patients in the standard hydration group.[108] A subsequent prospective multicenter RCT looked at 385 patients randomized to aggressive IV hydration (3 mL/kg/h during ERCP, a 20 mL/kg bolus and 3 mL/kg/h for eight hours after ERCP) with either lactated Ringer's or NS or standard IV hydration with lactated Ringer's (1.5 mL/kg/h during and hours after ERCP) and found that the rate of post-ERCP pancreatitis was significantly lower for the aggressive lactated Ringer's group.[109] A recent systematic review and meta-analysis reviewing 10 RCTs with 2,200 patients concluded that aggressive hydration with lactated Ringer's during the perioperative ERCP period can prevent pancreatitis.[110]

Many other agents have been investigated, including secretin, corticosteroids, allopurinol, and topical epinephrine, with conflicting results, and are not recommended at this time.

Infection

A serious complication of ERCP is the development of postprocedure infectious complications, most commonly cholangitis (see Chapter 43) and cholecystitis (see Chapter 34). In a systematic survey of 21 prospective studies with 16,855 patients, the incidence of infectious complications was 1.4%.[75]

Cholangitis most commonly occurs when there is failed or incomplete biliary drainage. The risk is increased in patients with hilar obstruction and sclerosing cholangitis, given the increased risk of incomplete drainage.[80,111,112] Other risk factors include jaundice, small endoscopy center, and delay in performing ERCP.[80,113] Treatment involves supportive care with antibiotics and decompression of the obstruction. Studies have shown that prophylactic antibiotics significantly reduce the frequency of procedure-related bacteremia but have not shown

a difference in rates of cholangitis.[114] Two meta-analyses failed to demonstrate a benefit of giving routine prophylactic antibiotics.[115,116] Antibiotics added to the injected radiographic contrast medium are also of no benefit.[117]

It has also been found that endoscopic instruments used in ERCP can be the source of serious infections In 2015 the US Food & Drug Administration (FDA) published a safety communication stating that the design of the duodenoscope may impede effective cleaning and lead to the transfer of multi-drug resistant organisms and subsequent infections, leading to outbreaks and deaths (https://www.fda.gov/medical-devices/medical-device-safety). A recent meta-analysis estimated the contamination rate of 15.25% in reprocessed duodenoscopes.[118] Multiple societies released guidelines focusing on reprocessing techniques.[119] In 2019 the FDA reported that the rate of transmitted infections decreased significantly. They recommended to transition to duodenoscopes with innovative designs to enhance safety (https://www.fda.gov/medical-devices/safety-communications/fda-recommending-transition-duodenoscopes-innovative-designs-enhance-safety-fda-safety-communication#disposable). There are currently ongoing studies with multiple disposable devices.

Bleeding

Bleeding is a rare complication of diagnostic ERCP and is most commonly seen with sphincterotomy. Risk factors for post-sphincterotomy bleeding include bleeding during the procedure, concomitant thrombocytopenia or coagulopathy, anticoagulation started within three days of the sphincterotomy, and low case volume of the endoscopist.[79]

Rarely, there may be a Mallory-Weiss tear from scope trauma or submucosal hemorrhage from manipulation of the papilla.[80] There have been case reports of intraperitoneal hemorrhage from injury to abdominal vessels, liver, and spleen.[120,121]

Perforation

The most common type of perforation associated with ERCP is retroperitoneal perforation, which is usually associated with sphincterotomy, with an incidence ranging from 0.5% to 2.1%.[82] In their systematic survey of 21 prospective studies with 16,855 patients, Loperfido and colleagues (1998)[80] reported 101 perforations (0.6%) and 10 deaths from perforation (0.06%). Free bowel wall perforation is quite rare and is usually associated with a structural abnormality, such as a stricture or Billroth II gastrectomy.[122]

The management of the perforation depends on the size, location, and clinical picture. Free bowel wall perforations usually require surgery. Use of endoscopic clips for the treatment of duodenal perforations has also been reported.[123,124]

DIRECT CHOLANGIOGRAPHY AND PANCREATOGRAPHY BY PERCUTANEOUS TRANSHEPATIC CHOLANGIOGRAPHY OR ENDOSCOPIC RETROGRADE CHOLANGIOPANCREATOGRAPHY

The anatomy of the bile ducts is discussed in Chapter 2. Knowledge of the common variations of ductal branching is essential for accurate interpretations of cholangiograms, and these are shown in Figs. 20.8 and 20.9; segmental nomenclature is summarized in

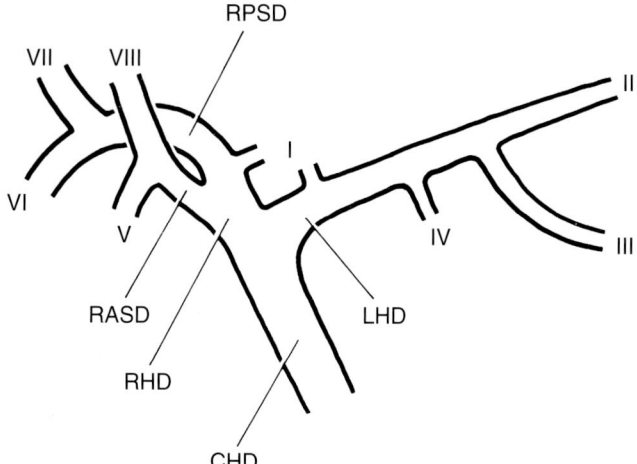

FIGURE 20.8   **Standard intrahepatic ductal anatomy.** The segments are numbered according to Couinaud's description (see Table 20.1). *CHD,* Common hepatic duct; *LHD,* left hepatic duct; *RASD,* right anterior sectoral duct; *RHD,* right hepatic duct; *RPSD,* right posterior sectoral duct. (See Chapter 2.)

Table 20.1. In the right lobe, the posterior segments lie more laterally than the anterior segments, so that the most lateral ducts on a cholangiogram are usually segments VI inferiorly and VII superiorly. The posterior sectoral duct is often recognizable by an arched course near the confluence (Figs. 20.10 and 20.11B). A right sectoral duct crosses to the left to join the left hepatic duct in 28% of cases, according to Healey and Schroy (1953)[125]; in 22%, this is the posterior sectoral duct (see Figs. 20.9B and 20.11B), and in 6%, this is the anterior duct (see Figs. 20.9C and 20.11D). Occasionally, a right sectoral or segmental duct, posterior more often than anterior, courses inferiorly and enters the common hepatic duct directly (Fig. 20.12). The confluence of the right and left ducts takes the form of a trifurcation rather than a bifurcation in 12% of cases according to Couinaud (1957; see Fig. 20.9A).[126]

In the left lobe, the superior and inferior lateral segment ducts, segments II and III, unite in the line of, or to the right of, the umbilical fissure in 92% of cases. In the latter instance, the quadrate lobe, segment IV, may drain wholly or partially into the segment II duct. Rarely, segment II and III ducts join at or close to the confluence (see Figs. 20.9E and 20.11C), and

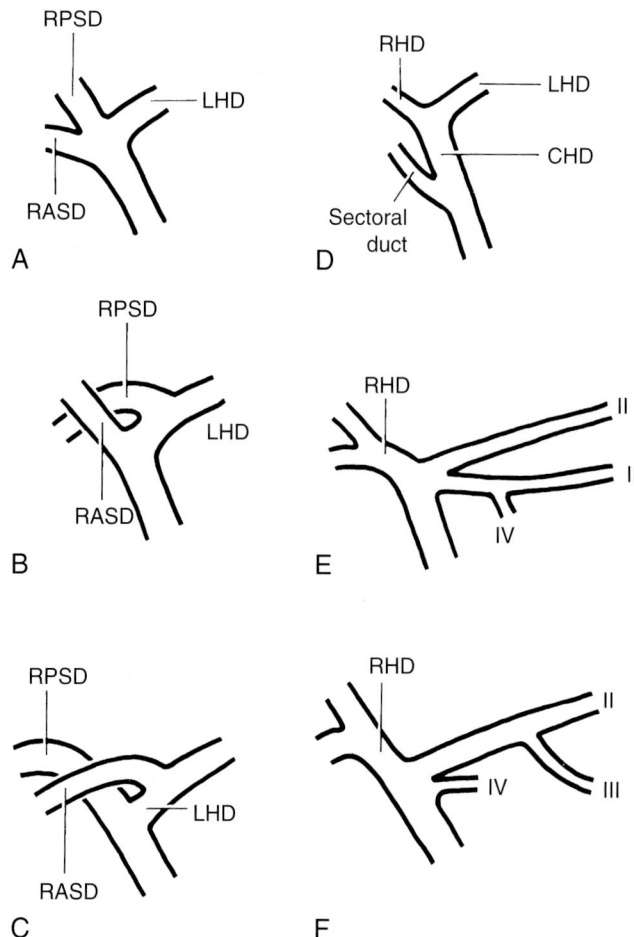

FIGURE 20.9   **Variations of perihilar ductal anatomy.** *CHD,* Common hepatic duct; *LHD,* left hepatic duct; *RASD,* right anterior sectoral duct; *RHD,* right hepatic duct; *RPSD,* right posterior sectoral duct. (See Chapter 2.)

TABLE 20.1	Segmental Nomenclature
I	Caudate lobe
II	Left lateral superior segment
III	Left lateral inferior segment
IV	Left medial segment or quadrate lobe
V	Right anterior inferior segment
VI	Right posterior inferior segment
VII	Right posterior superior segment
VIII	Right anterior superior segment

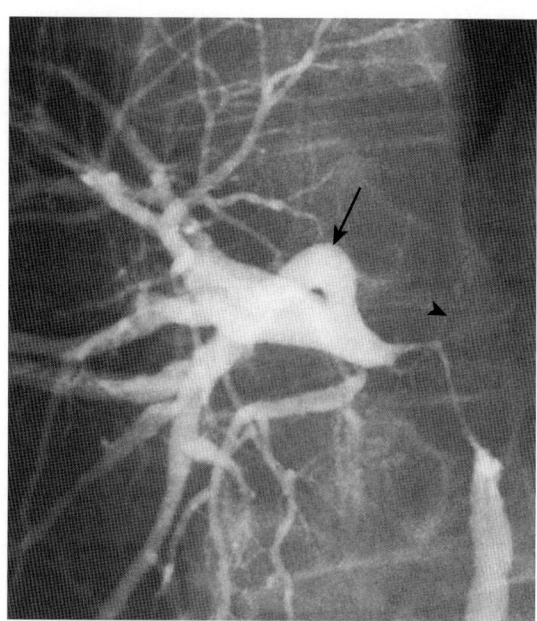

FIGURE 20.10   Hilar cholangiocarcinoma involving first-order right hepatic duct, proximal common hepatic duct, and faintly opacified left hepatic duct *(arrowhead).* Note the characteristic arched course of the right posterior sectoral duct *(arrow).* (See Chapter 2.)

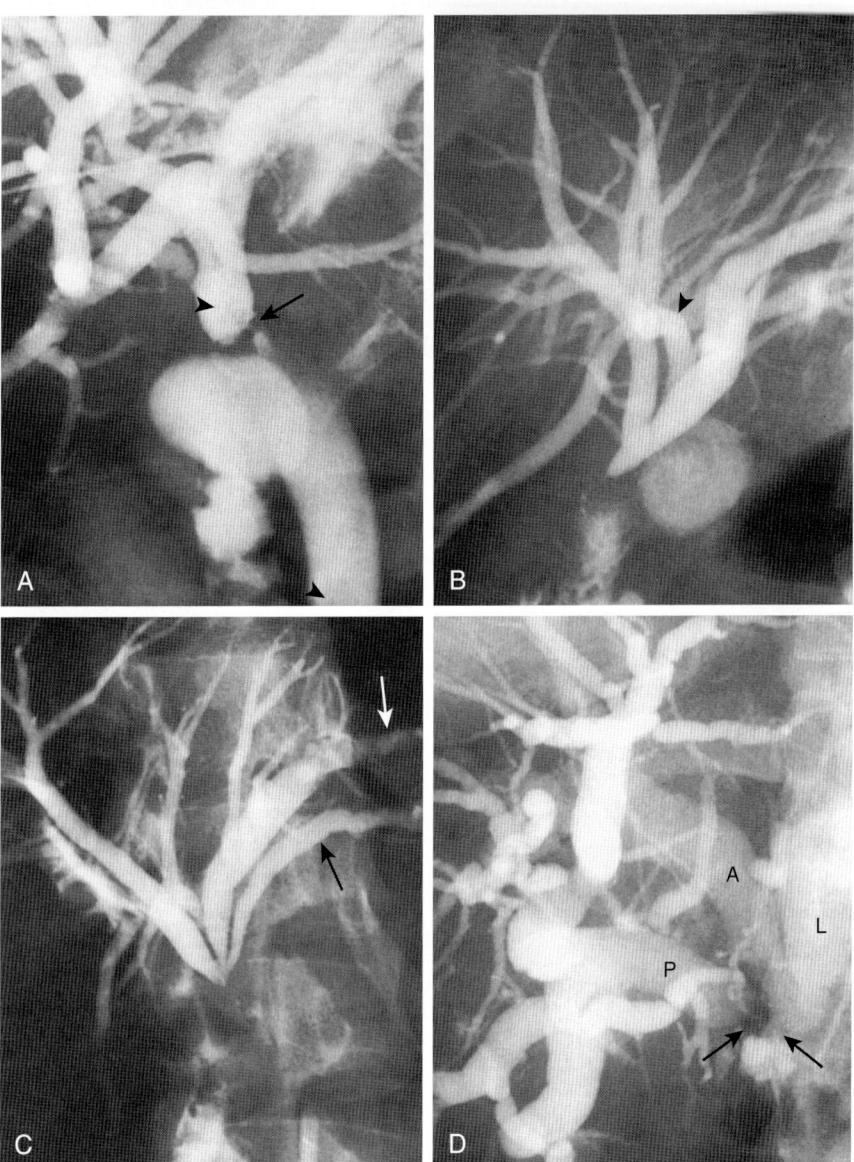

FIGURE 20.11 Postcholecystectomy strictures graded according to Bismuth. **A,** Grade I (>2 cm from the confluence of the right and left hepatic ducts; *arrowheads*): Calculi lie above and below the stricture *(arrow)*. **B,** Grade II (<2 cm from the confluence): There has been a previous hepatojejunostomy; the right posterior sectoral duct *(arrowhead)* has an exaggerated arched course and enters the left hepatic duct as a normal variant. **C,** Grade III (the confluence is involved by stricture, but the right and left hepatic ducts are not completely separated): Ducts of segment II *(white arrow)* and segment III *(black arrow)* join the confluence independently as a normal variant. **D,** Grade IV (the right and left ducts are separated by the stricture): The right anterior sectoral duct *(A)* is draining into the left hepatic duct *(L)*, which is separated from the right posterior sectoral duct *(P)* by the stricture *(arrows)*. (See Chapter 42.)

segment IV drains directly into the common hepatic duct in 1% of cases (see Fig. 20.9F).[125]

The caudate ducts are often difficult to identify. Usually two or three ducts drain most commonly into the right posterior sectoral duct, right hepatic duct, or left hepatic duct.[125] The recognizable caudate ducts are usually a few centimeters long and drain downward or to the right.

The left hepatic duct (average length, 17 mm) is considerably longer than the right hepatic duct (average length, 9 mm) and has a longer extrahepatic course. The normal diameters of the main bile ducts as measured at PTC are shown in Table 20.2. These figures are greater than the true duct dimensions because of some distension produced by direct cholangiography,

together with considerable magnification occurring on any fluoroscopic "spot film." The magnification is of the order of 40%[127] and affects all structures in the image, including calculi, tubes, and strictures.

The upper limits of normal for the diameter of the extrahepatic bile ducts as measured by ERCP vary between 9 and 14 mm.[128] Combined radiologic and manometric studies[129] have shown that even in the absence of extrahepatic cholestasis, the diameter of the bile ducts and the pressure difference therein increases with advancing age. The diameter of the bile ducts as measured by ultrasonography is less than those measurements obtained during ERCP.[128] Anatomic abnormalities of the hepatobiliary system include cystic dilations (Fig. 20.13) of the bile duct or

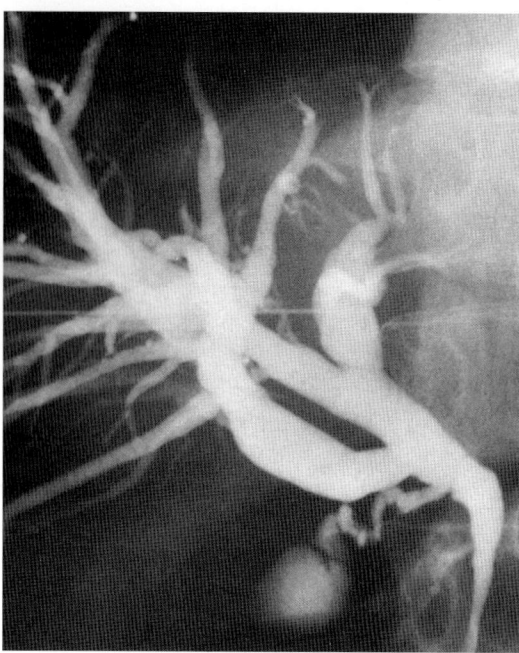

FIGURE 20.12 Pancreatitis producing a typical, incomplete long stricture of the common bile duct. The right posterior sectoral duct has a low entrance into the common hepatic duct, an uncommon but important normal variant. (See Chapter 2.)

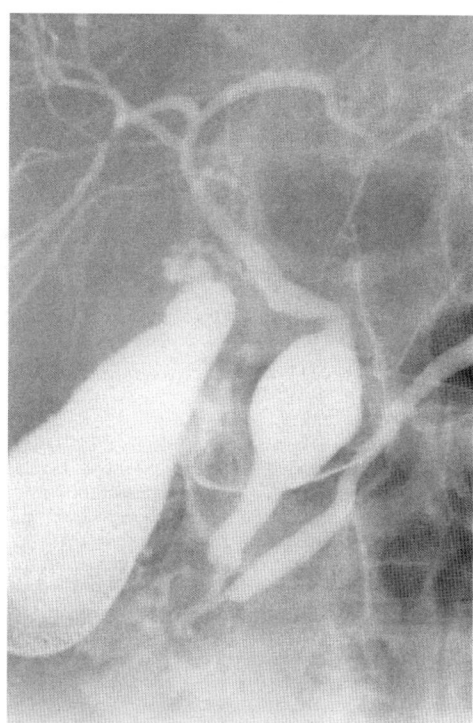

FIGURE 20.13 Choledochal cyst. (See Chapter 46.)

TABLE 20.2 Average Duct Diameters Measured Directly From 50 Normal Percutaneous Transhepatic Cholangiography Examinations
DUCT DIAMETER (mm)
Right hepatic = 4.7
Left hepatic = 5.2
Common hepatic = 6.5
Common bile = 7.6

From Okuda K, Musha H, Nakajima Y, et al. Frequency of intrahepatic arteriovenous fistula as a sequela to percutaneous needle puncture of the liver. *Gastroenterology.* 1978;74:1204–1207.

of the intrahepatic bile ducts (Caroli disease; see Chapter 46). There is a wide variation in where the cystic duct joins the common hepatic duct. A low junction with a correspondingly long cystic duct (Fig. 20.14) may result in difficulties if not recognized. This is especially true when a cholecystojejunostomy is performed as a palliative biliary bypass for carcinoma of the head of the pancreas, and the jaundice either is not relieved or recurs rapidly in the postoperative period.

Interpretations

Because of its inherent weakness of only allowing visualization of the bile duct lumen, the main problem with the use of direct cholangiography is its lack of specificity. There are few, if any, pathognomonic radiologic findings. Many disease entities, from benign to malignant, overlap greatly in their cholangiographic appearances. The combination of history, blood markers, associated radiologic findings, and clinical scenario can often significantly narrow the differential diagnosis. However, it must be stressed strongly that because the cholangiographic appearance of many biliary diseases may be indistinguishable, biopsy is often required to rule out malignancy or to confirm suspected diagnosis.

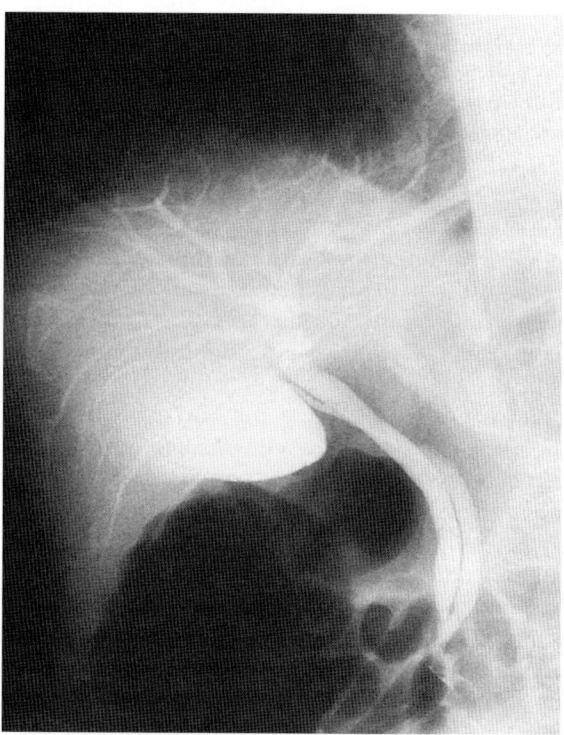

FIGURE 20.14 Long cystic duct.

Bile Leaks

Bile leaks are seen as sites of free extravasation of contrast agent at a site of bile duct injury. Injury may be secondary to trauma, but most commonly it is iatrogenic in nature. Associated bilomas may be seen at the point of bile leak. Diagnosis of bile leak can usually be made by noninvasive imaging techniques, such as ultrasound, CT or MRI, but because the intrahepatic bile ducts are usually not dilated, a bile leak may not be evident on imaging. Cholescintography with technetium 99m–hepatic iminodiacetic acid (hepatobiliary iminodiacetic acid [HIDA] scan) may be useful for diagnosis when the other imaging modalities are inconclusive. ERCP can diagnose bile duct leaks effectively but is usually reserved for cases when a therapeutic intervention is anticipated.

Filling Defects

Air Bubbles, Blood Clots, Calculi, Primary and Secondary Bile Duct Cancers, and Parasitic Diseases

Air bubbles, although confusing, most commonly declare themselves by their perfectly circular shape and their distribution to nondependent structures. Blood clots in the bile duct are seen more frequently with PTC than with ERCP. Hemobilia can sometimes take more than 48 hours to resolve, and when it is more severe, it can be cast-like and may mask other filling defects (see Chapter 116).

Calculous disease (see Chapter 37A, B and C) remains the most common filling defect in the biliary system. Distinguishing characteristics of gallstones and primary bile duct calculi include a faceted appearance and disposition to move to gravity-dependent positions. Calculi may be seen as discrete filling defects (Figs. 20.15 and 20.16) or cast-like structures filling entire ducts, as occurs in recurrent pyogenic cholangitis, cystic diseases of the bile ducts, or even proximal to strictures of any etiology. Impacted calculi may be difficult to differentiate from strictures or tumors.

Primary bile duct cancer (see Chapter 51A and B), specifically papillary cholangiocarcinomas, can also present as cholangiographic filling defects (Fig. 20.17). T-shaped filling defects may also be detected (Fig. 20.18),[130] and papillary bile duct cancers may cause filling defects as a result of mucin

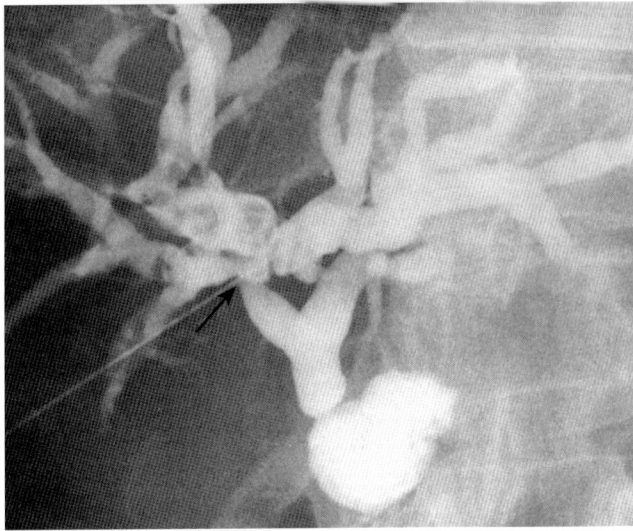

FIGURE 20.16 Benign stricture of the right hepatic duct *(arrow)* with multiple ductal calculi proximal to it. The hepatojejunostomy is partially strictured.

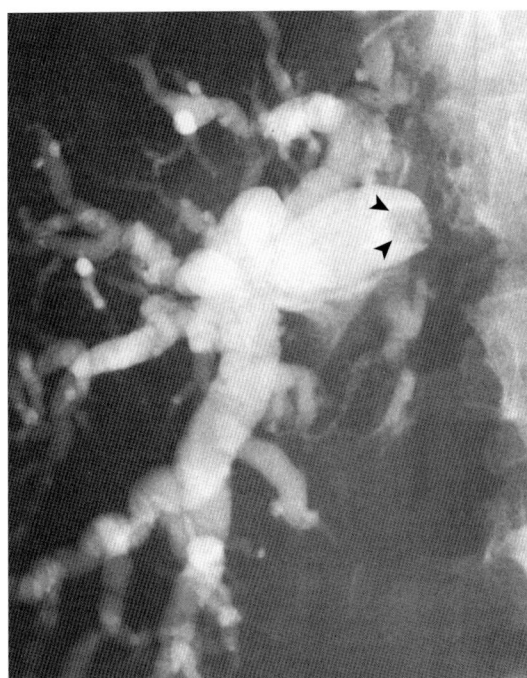

FIGURE 20.17 Papillary hilar cholangiocarcinoma *(arrowheads)*. Only the right ducts are opacified. (See Chapter 51A and B.)

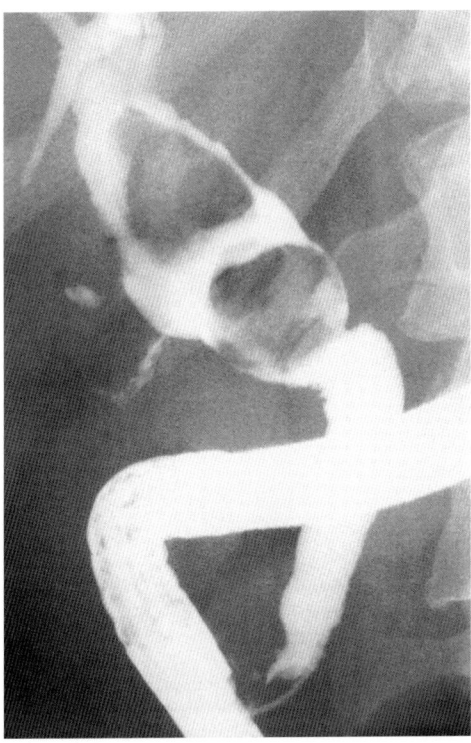

FIGURE 20.15 Choledocholithiasis.

production (Fig. 20.19). Other malignancies, including melanoma and intraductal metastases, such as colon cancer, are also more unusual causes of cholangiographic filling defects.[131]

Parasitic infections, such as hydatid disease (see Chapter 72) and infections with *Ascaris lumbricoides* or *Clonorchis sinensis* (see Chapter 45), are diseases with worldwide distribution that can also present cholangiographically as intraductal filling defects. A proportion of hepatic hydatid cysts (5%–10%) rupture into the bile ducts and may simulate choledocholithiasis. Calcified cysts are easy to recognize on radiographs, and daughter cysts can cause biliary obstruction. When the calcified cyst is not obvious,

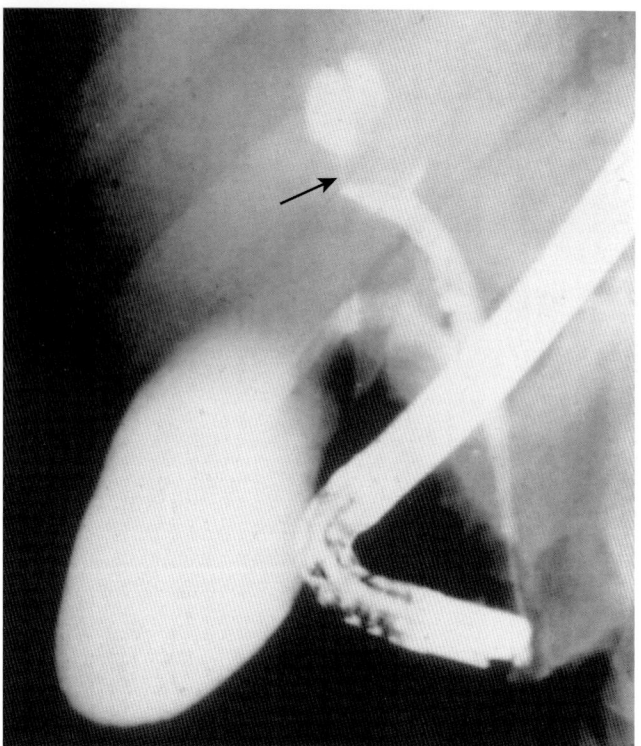

FIGURE 20.18 "Golf tee" appearance of a papillary bile duct cancer *(arrow)* involving the common hepatic duct. (See Chapter 51A and B.)

biliary strictures with obstruction may be noted on cholangiogram. The biliary ducts can show considerable irregularities in caliber and extensive displacement of the intrahepatic branches secondary to the mass effect of a large hydatid cyst.[132–134]

A. lumbricoides is a commonly seen helminth with a prevalence of 90% in some parts of Africa and Asia (see Chapter 45). If the worm passes through the sphincter of Oddi, it may cause acute pancreatitis or a cholestasis syndrome.[135] In the acute stage, the worm occasionally may be found and extracted from the ampulla, and it can be detected in the biliary tract by cholangiography.

Eating raw meat has been associated with *C. sinensis* infestation. The prevalence of this disease has been estimated to be 60% of the general population of Hong Kong, based on stool ova examinations. This worm can penetrate through the papilla into the bile ducts. In an ERCP study of 31 consecutive patients, the typical filamentous, wavy, or elliptic appearance of the worm in the bile ducts was believed to be pathognomonic. Other common cholangiographic findings include widely dilated extrahepatic bile ducts, which are filled with biliary sludge and stones, and intrahepatic duct strictures, which are predominantly found in the branches of the left hepatic duct.[136] The eggs of *C. sinensis* act as a nucleus for the development of the bile duct stones.[137] Naval and colleagues (1984)[138] reported successful endoscopic biliary lavage to eliminate the eggs.

Invasion of *Fasciola hepatica* into the biliary tract also may cause serious lesions (see Chapter 45). In the chronic stage, *F. hepatica* infection can resemble sclerosing cholangitis.[139] The appearance on ERCP is that of dilated bile ducts with unexplained sludge in the distal bile duct (Figs. 20.20 and 20.21).

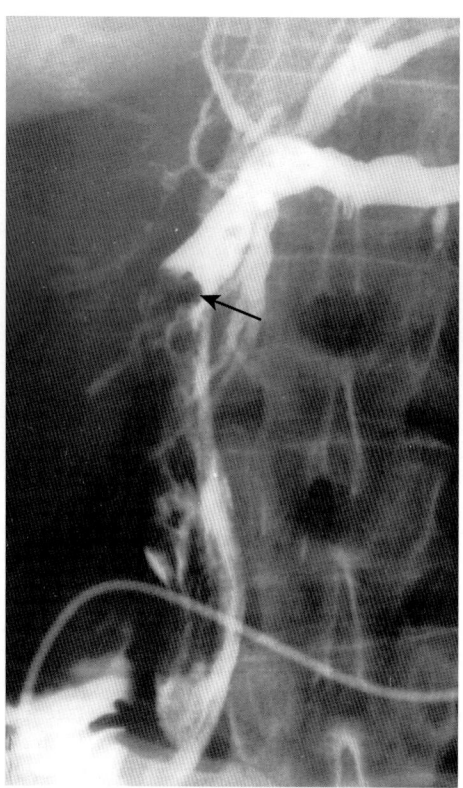

FIGURE 20.19 Nasobiliary cholangiogram opacifying left hepatic ducts. Main left hepatic duct contains a small mucin-secreting papillary cholangiocarcinoma *(arrow)*. The mucin results in expansion of the common bile duct below the tumor and appears as strand-like filling defects. (Courtesy Dr. A. Speer.)

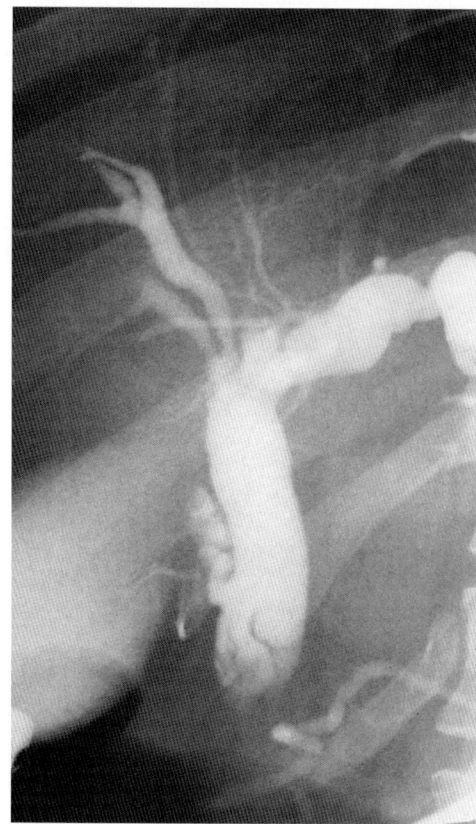

FIGURE 20.20 Liver flukes in the distal bile duct presenting as "biliary sludge." (See Chapter 45.)

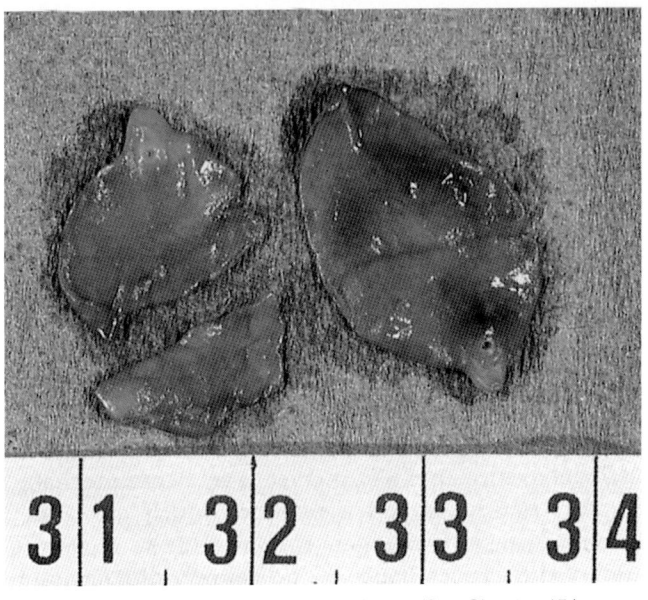

FIGURE 20.21 Extracted liver flukes. (See Chapter 45.)

CONCLUSION

The role of direct cholangiography in the diagnosis of biliary disease has been largely supplanted by less invasive imaging modalities, such as MR cholangiography and CT with contrast. The ability to visualize the entire biliary tree, the bile duct wall, and other structures other than the bile duct lumen increases the diagnostic accuracy and clinical utility of these noninvasive techniques, which have become the gold standard for cholangiography. Direct cholangiography is generally reserved for clinical scenarios involving concomitantly planned therapeutic interventions.

References are available at expertconsult.com.

CHAPTER 21

Diagnostic angiography in hepatobiliary and pancreatic disease: Indications

Aaron W.P. Maxwell and Hooman Yarmohammadi

OVERVIEW

Once a mainstay of diagnosis in hepatobiliary and pancreatic diseases, indications for catheter angiography have changed significantly in the past three decades. This is mainly because of the widespread adoption of noninvasive imaging modalities such as multidetector computed tomography (MDCT) and magnetic resonance imaging (MRI). These imaging techniques can accurately demonstrate both vascular and nonvascular structures associated with the hepatobiliary and pancreatic systems without the risks of conventional diagnostic angiography (see Chapters 16 and 17).

Historically, indications for catheter angiography have included the identification and characterization of focal liver lesions, the delineation of hepatic arterial anatomy before liver resection or transplantation, the assessment of vascular invasion by pancreatic cancer or cholangiocarcinoma, and the ascertainment of the organ of origin of an abdominal mass. Because of their improved sensitivity and specificity, however, computed tomography (CT) angiography and magnetic resonance angiography (MRA) have together all but replaced catheter angiography for these indications. Presently, catheter angiography is principally reserved for anatomic delineation before contemporaneous catheter-based interventions, including embolization of gastrointestinal (GI) bleeding (see Chapter 28), hepatic artery embolization (see Chapter 31), chemoembolization (see Chapter 94A), radioembolization (see Chapter 94B), and chemoperfusion (see Chapters 97 and 100).

Contemporaneous with advances in CT and MRI, recent developments in imaging technology have enabled greater visualization of vascular anatomy during conventional catheter angiography. Cone beam CT (CBCT) is one such example, which allows the user to perform a three-dimensional (3D) rotational acquisition using the fluoroscope to generate a volumetric data set akin to helical CT within a smaller field of view. CBCT images can undergo multiplanar reformatting for improved visualization of vascular anatomy, as may be associated with a target lesion such as a liver tumor. In addition, many vendors offer software packages for automated vessel tracking, which serve to highlight tumor-feeding vessels to improve outcomes for embolization or infusion procedures. Hybrid imaging, or image fusion, techniques have further advanced the field of modern catheter angiography. Such techniques allow the operator to superimpose angiographic and cross-sectional imaging data in real-time to help facilitate improved visualization and targeting of lesions during therapeutic interventions. Data from both MDCT and MRI examinations obtained before the procedure can be used. The images can be post-processed and rendered in a 3D format to provide an anatomic depiction that would not be available by either technique alone.

In this chapter, we will discuss angiographic anatomy relevant to hepatobiliary and pancreatic surgery and discuss current indications for performing catheter angiography relevant to the hepatobiliary and pancreatic systems. Additionally, we will discuss localization of occult neuroendocrine tumors of the pancreas. Our discussion on splanchnic veins will include venographic anatomy, venous sampling, techniques of catheter-based venous imaging, and venous imaging before surgical or percutaneous venous interventions.

Angiography Technique

In recent years, technologic advances have resulted in significant improvements in angiographic imaging. Cut-film angiography has been replaced with digital flat-panel detectors and biplane angiography units. Biplane angiography is capable of producing high-quality images in 3D views. These advances in technology allow for less contrast while minimizing radiation exposure to both patients and interventionalists.

Depending on the procedure, catheter angiography may be performed under conscious sedation or general anesthesia. Most angiographic procedures are performed on an outpatient basis; however, some patients may require overnight stay primarily for pain control after embolization-based interventions or for symptoms related to recovery from anesthesia. All patients are seen in the clinic before the diagnostic or interventional catheter angiography procedure. During this visit, indications for performing the procedure are reviewed. Additionally, patients are assessed for any history of cardiopulmonary or renal disease. Prior history of angiography or other surgical interventions are also assessed. A thorough physical examination, which includes a detailed pulse examination and an assessment of the airway, lungs, and heart, is performed. Finally, patients' performance status is evaluated. Most institutions either use Eastern Cooperation Oncology Group (ECOG) performance status or Karnofsky performance status. The procedure is explained to the patient in detail and after a discussion of the risks and benefits of the procedure, written informed consent is obtained.

Relevant laboratory parameters reviewed before catheter angiography include serum creatinine and estimated glomerular filtration rate, hemoglobin and hematocrit levels, platelet count, and prothrombin time and international normalized ratio (INR). For liver-directed interventions such as embolization, serum bilirubin is also assessed. Additionally, a baseline 12-lead electrocardiogram (ECG) may be considered in patients with known or suspected cardiac disease. In patients with significant comorbidities, cardiology or geriatric consultation should be considered before the procedure to ensure the safety of conscious sedation or general anesthesia.

In patients with a history of preexisting renal impairment, prophylactic measures may be considered to lower the risk of further reductions in glomerular filtration rate related to the injection of iodinated contrast media during catheter angiography. Although multiple agents, including sodium bicarbonate and N-acetyl cysteine infusion, have been evaluated in randomized clinical trials (RCTs), intravenous (IV) hydration with normal saline (NS) solution before and/or subsequent to catheter angiography is the only measure currently recommended for this purpose.

The risk of bleeding from the puncture site is low, and hematomas complicate 1% of femoral punctures and 3% of nonradial upper extremity punctures. An abnormal bleeding profile related to thrombocytopenia or an elevated INR increases the risk of hemorrhage, but there is only weak association between magnitude of INR elevation and procedure-related hemorrhage. The need to correct an underlying coagulopathy is dependent on the specific procedure to be performed and the preference of the angiographer. Based on the current recommendations from the Society of Interventional Radiology (SIR) consensus guideline, diagnostic catheter angiography (arterial intervention with access size up to 6 French [F]) is classified as a procedure with a low risk of bleeding. For this procedure, SIR recommends platelet count above $20,000 \times 10^6$ per liter and an INR of less than or equal to 1.8 for femoral access and 2.2 for radial access.[1] Patients are advised to stop eating 6 hours before the procedure. IV hydration is recommended before, during, and after the arteriogram to diminish adverse effects of contrast media on renal function. The patient should also be encouraged to take ample fluids by mouth after the procedure.

The right common femoral artery is the most common access site. The left common femoral artery, axillary artery, brachial artery, or radial artery may be used as alternatives when clinically appropriate. In the past few years, there has been growing interest and expertise with radial artery access, particularly with interventional cardiology procedures. With appropriate technique, including ultrasonographic guidance at the time of arterial puncture, the trans-radial approach is associated with low risk of bleeding or vessel injury and affords patients the advantage of immediate ambulation after catheter angiography. Additionally, recent studies have demonstrated comparable procedural and clinical outcomes with the trans-radial approach when compared with the trans-femoral approach.[2]

For all arterial access procedures, the desired puncture area is cleansed, and the patient is draped in a sterile fashion. In most centers, arterial entry is performed under real-time ultrasound guidance using a 21-gauge micropuncture set. The use of ultrasonography allows for assessment of the quality of the common femoral artery, depicts the position of the profunda femoris, and detects the presence of aberrant veins extending ventral to the puncture site. After entry into the vessel, the appropriate catheter is inserted for catheterization of the target vessel. After diagnostically adequate images are obtained, the catheter is removed, and one of a variety of closure devices is deployed to seal the arteriotomy; manual pressure may also be applied for 15 to 20 minutes, or until hemostasis is achieved. Patients are observed in a postprocedural area until they have recovered from sedation, and most can be discharged home 2 to 4 hours later.

HEPATOBILIARY AND PANCREATIC ARTERIAL ANATOMY

Arterial Anatomy

Arterial anatomy has been discussed elsewhere (see Chapter 2) and will only be briefly reviewed here. The most frequently

encountered anatomy (Fig. 21.1) is the left gastric artery, splenic artery, and common hepatic artery (CHA) taking origin from the celiac axis. The CHA divides into the gastroduodenal artery (GDA) and proper hepatic artery, with the latter dividing into the right and left hepatic arteries (RHA and LHA, respectively). The right gastric artery most often originates from the base of the left hepatic artery, and the cystic artery most often originates from the right hepatic artery, but considerable variations in the origins of these arteries exist.[3] Moreover, accessory duodenal arteries, either representing a supraduodenal or a retroduodenal artery, are frequently encountered; this is critical to recognize when planning embolization, chemoembolization, and radioembolization.

The normal arterial supply to the liver is shown in Fig. 21.2, which shows the commonly recognized variations of the LHA,

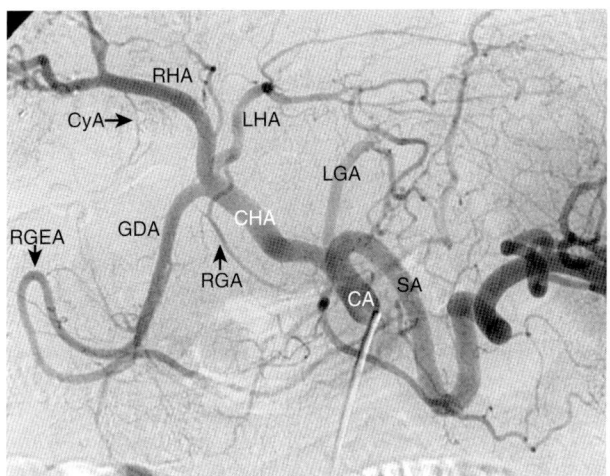

FIGURE 21.1 Conventional celiac artery anatomy. *CA,* Celiac axis; *CHA,* common hepatic artery; *CHA,* cystic artery; *GDA,* gastroduodenal artery; *LGA,* left gastric artery; *LHA,* left hepatic artery; *RGA,* right gastric artery; *RGEA,* right gastroepiploic artery; *RHA,* right hepatic artery; *SA,* splenic artery. (See Chapter 2.)

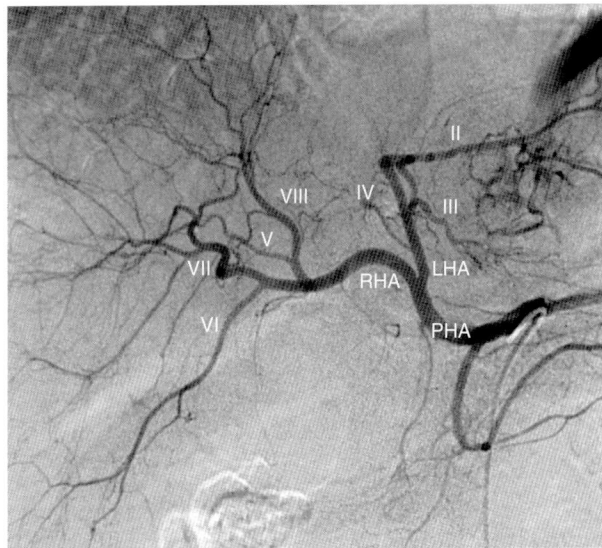

FIGURE 21.2 Arterial anatomy of the liver. *LHA,* Left hepatic artery; *PHA,* proper hepatic artery; *RHA,* right hepatic artery. Additional vessels are labeled in accordance to the Couinaud segment they supply. (See Chapter 2.)

taking origin from the left gastric artery, and the RHA taking origin from the superior mesenteric artery (SMA). It is important to recognize that either a part or the entirety of the RHAs and LHAs may have these variant origins. When the entire vessel has a variant origin, it is termed *replaced*. If the entire trunk does not take a variant origin, the vessel is termed *accessory*. For example, if the right lobe is supplied by an RHA originating from the CHA, as well as an RHA taking origin from the SMA, the latter would be termed an *accessory RHA*. If the entire right lobe was supplied by an artery taking origin from the SMA, it would be called a *replaced RHA* (see Chapter 2).

In most patients, the arteries to Couinaud segments I, II, III, and IV are branches of the LHA, and arteries to segments V, VI, VII, and VIII are branches of the RHA. The most variable segmental branch is to segment IV. Although most frequently arising as a branch vessel from the LHA, the segment IV artery may also take origin from the RHA, assuming the misnomer of a "middle hepatic artery" in older works. Separate origins of segment IVa, usually from the LHA, and segment IVb from the RHA are frequently identified. Also, a branch from the segment IV artery is often seen extending outside of the liver toward the abdominal wall along the midline, supplying the falciform ligament (Fig. 21.3). Recognition of this vessel is important when conducting embolization, chemoembolization, or radioembolization to avoid nontarget embolization, which may result in ischemia or radiation dermatitis to the periumbilical region.

The RHA conventionally divides into an anterior (ventral) and a posterior (dorsal) branch. The anterior branch usually is more vertically oriented and supplies segments V and VIII. The posterior branch is usually more horizontally oriented and supplies segments VI and VII. More than one projection is usually required to ascertain with certainty which is the anterior branch

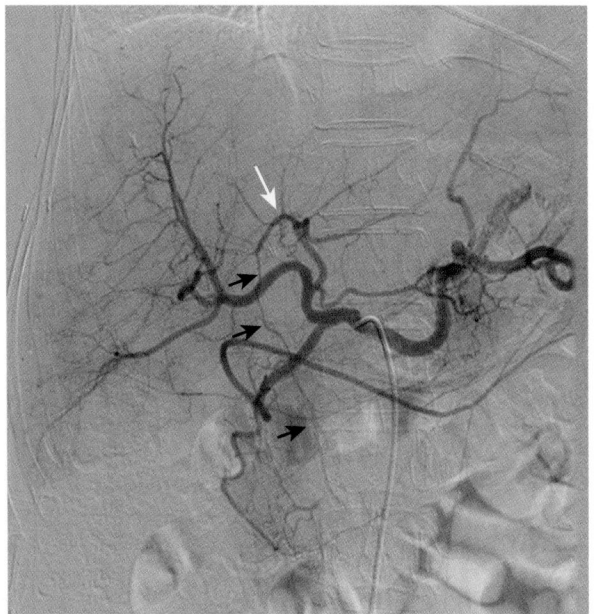

FIGURE 21.3 Subtracted angiography from celiac artery demonstrating the falciform artery *(black arrow)* arising from segment 4 hepatic artery branch *(white arrow)*. This artery courses inferiorly with an inverted V-shaped distal branches and supplies the anterior abdominal wall, superior to the umbilicus.

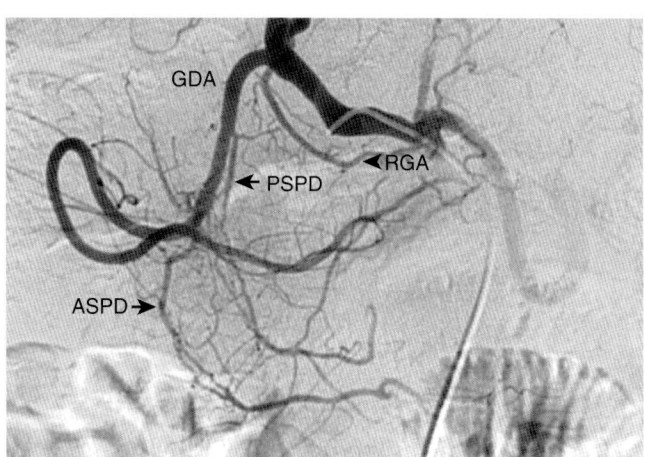

FIGURE 21.4 Arterial anatomy of the pancreas. *ASPD,* Anterior superior pancreaticoduodenal artery; *GDA,* gastroduodenal artery; *PSPD,* posterior-superior pancreaticoduodenal artery; *RGA,* right gastric artery. (See Chapter 2.)

and which the posterior branch. In the right anterior oblique projection, the anterior branch moves medially, and the posterior branch moves laterally when compared with the posteroanterior (PA) projection. The entire segmental arterial supply to the liver should be accounted for before hepatic arterial therapy, major hepatic resection, partial hepatectomy (see Chapters 101 and 118), or living donor liver transplantation (LDLT, see Chapters 109 and 125). Adjunctive techniques such as CBCT may be used, as necessary, to achieve optimal delineation of hepatic vascular anatomy.

The arterial supply to the pancreas is somewhat variable. The most consistent supply is to the pancreatic head, formed by a rich anastomotic arcade between the superior pancreaticoduodenal (SPD) artery arising from the GDA and the inferior pancreaticoduodenal (IPD) artery arising from the SMA (Fig. 21.4). There, variable arteries give rise to both anterior and posterior divisional branches. Additional pancreatic arterial supply includes the transverse pancreatic artery, which runs along the middle portion of the long axis of the pancreas and may take origin from the arterial arcade in the head of the pancreas, directly from the GDA, or as a branch of the dorsal pancreatic artery, which variably originates from the CHA or the splenic artery (Fig. 21.5). The transverse pancreatic artery may anastomose distal with the pancreatica magna artery, which typically arises from the splenic artery. A number of small branches from the splenic artery supply the pancreatic body and tail, but the number and location of these arteries vary and must be identified in each individual patient when clinically relevant (see Chapter 2).

Venous Anatomy

The splenic vein and superior mesenteric vein (SMV) join to form the main portal vein (see Chapter 2). The inferior mesenteric vein (IMV) usually enters the splenic adjacent to the confluence, but it may also enter the SMV either at or just caudal to the confluence. The coronary vein most often drains into the cephalic aspect of the main portal vein just beyond the confluence of the SMV and splenic vein. The number and location of veins draining the pancreas is variable. Multiple small, unnamed veins drain directly into the splenic vein. Typically,

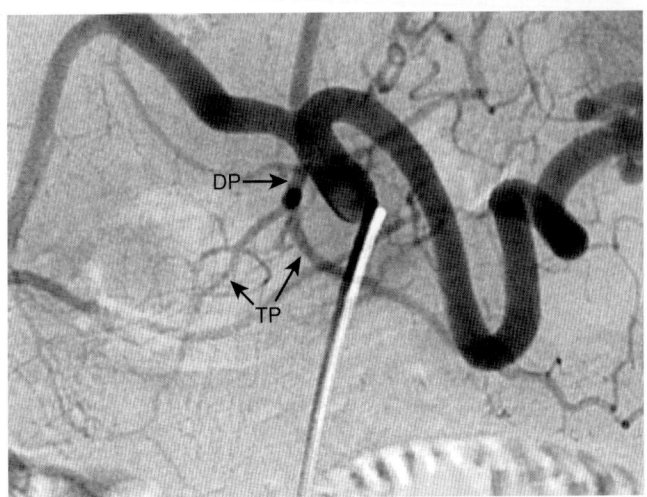

FIGURE 21.5 Arterial anatomy of the pancreas. *DP,* Dorsal pancreatic artery; *TP,* transverse pancreatic artery. (See Chapter 2.)

the anterior SPD vein drains directly into the portal vein, and the posterior SPD vein drains into the SMV. The IPD veins drain into the SMV at the caudal margin of the pancreas, and the portal vein courses obliquely cephalad from near the midline toward the liver, where it divides to supply the right and left lobes. This division, as well as the division into segmental branches, is variable and must be delineated when clinically relevant for each individual patient.

ANGIOGRAPHY INDICATIONS

As mentioned earlier in this chapter, historical indications for performing diagnostic catheter angiography, including assessments of vascular invasion before potential pancreatic or biliary surgery, characterization of focal liver lesions, and preoperative arterial mapping before major hepatic resection, have been replaced by multidetector computed tomography angiography (MDCTA). MDCTA provides higher sensitivity and diagnostic accuracy for these indications. On rare occasion, there is a specific piece of critical anatomic information that cannot be ascertained with certainty by MDCTA, such as the origin and course of the artery to segment IV before a living donor partial hepatectomy. In these circumstances, catheter angiography can be a useful adjunctive technique.

On extremely rare occasions, large tumors are identified on cross-sectional imaging, but the organ of origin cannot be determined. The majority of these are large sarcomas of the retroperitoneum but excluding a pancreatic source may be difficult. A similar situation can occur with large right adrenal or renal tumors blending with the hepatic parenchyma. In these highly selected cases, catheter angiography can be useful in delineating the organ of origin by demonstrating the primary arterial supply.

Currently, the most common indication for arteriography is planning an arterial-based intervention such as embolization (see Chapter 94A), chemoembolization (see Chapter 94A), radioembolization (see Chapter 9B), or chemo-perfusion (see Chapters 97 and 100) to treat a primary or metastatic hepatic malignancy. These specific interventions will be discussed elsewhere in this book. Inadvertent administration of embolic particles, radiation particles, or chemotherapeutic agents into arteries supplying the stomach or duodenum can lead to significant adverse outcomes, including death.[4] Small anastomotic connections between intrahepatic branches to the lower esophagus, stomach, and diaphragm are of equal importance.[5]

As previously described, most modern angiography suites are equipped with CBCT imaging technology. This technology uses a fixed C-arm system equipped with a flat-panel detector and requires 3D CT volumetric images.[6] CBCT has improved feasibility, effectiveness, and safety of many image-guided procedures by allowing the interventionalist to identify extrahepatic perfusion from aberrant hepatic arterial branches (Fig. 21.6).

Other current indications of performing catheter angiography in the hepatobiliary and pancreatic system are as follows:
1. Treatment of bleeding/hemorrhage from liver, spleen and pancreas (see Chapters 113, 114, and 116)
2. Diagnosis of arterial occlusive diseases
3. Diagnosis and treatment of arterial stenosis
4. Treatment of visceral arterial aneurysms (see Chapter 115)
5. Diagnosis of vasculitis
6. Diagnosis of other visceral vascular disease
7. Localization of functional pancreatic neuroendocrine tumors (see Chapter 65)

These indications will be discussed in the following sections.

Treatment of Bleeding/Hemorrhage

Bleeding from the liver, spleen, or pancreas is most often secondary to iatrogenic or noniatrogenic trauma, but it may occur spontaneously in patients with mycotic aneurysms, pancreatitis, or collagen vascular diseases. Angiography is usually not used to ascertain whether arterial hemorrhage is present but rather to precisely localize and treat the offending vessel. Embolization of arterial bleeding will be discussed elsewhere in this book (see Chapters 28, 115, and 116), but salient features will be reviewed in this chapter.

Splenic Bleeding

The most common cause of bleeding from the spleen is blunt trauma, and nonoperative management is currently the standard of practice. Splenic artery embolization has been established as a method to increase the success rate of nonoperative management of traumatic splenic injuries.[7] A comparative study between two cohorts consisting of 625 patients over a 15-year period revealed an improved success rate of nonoperative management from 77% to 96% with the advent of splenic embolization.[8] The indications for splenic arteriography and splenic arterial embolization are based on CT findings and include active contrast blush beyond or within the splenic parenchyma, pseudoaneurysm, an associated large hemoperitoneum, and a high-grade splenic injury.[7] Moreover, the American Association for the Surgery of Trauma recommends angiography for grade III, IV, and V splenic injuries.[9]

Two techniques are used to perform splenic embolization. The first is occlusion of the proximal splenic artery with coils or Amplatzer plugs (AGA Medical, Plymouth, MN), and the second is selective small intrasplenic arterial embolization with a gelatin sponge or coils. Distal super-selective particle embolization has also been described. Collaterals through the short gastric arteries and the gastroepiploic arcade usually maintain splenic viability after proximal splenic artery occlusion, whereas distal intrasplenic embolization generally results in a variable degree of splenic infarction, depending on the size of the artery

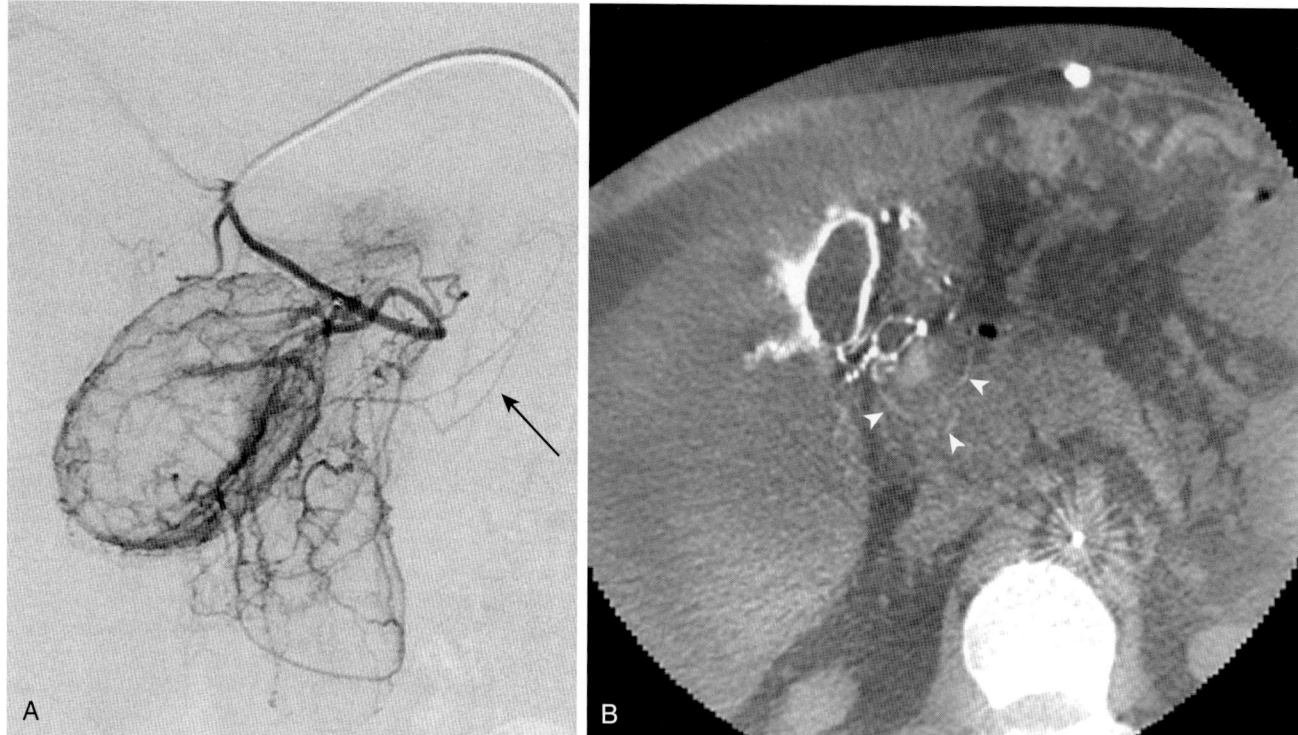

FIGURE 21.6 Extrahepatic perfusion detected with C-arm computed tomography (CCT). **A,** Selective cystic arteriogram shows the gallbladder and several branches extending medially *(arrow).* **B,** CCT performed during contrast injection of the cystic artery confirms aberrant perfusion of the duodenum *(arrowheads).* (Courtesy Daniel Sze, Stanford University.)

occluded because intrasplenic arteries have no significant collateral routes. Both techniques have equivalent rates of major infarctions and infections requiring splenectomy.[10] Distal splenic embolization is associated with higher rates of infarction; however, these infarctions are limited to the segments just distal to the site of embolization and are often of no clinical relevance.

In summary, the current literature is inconclusive regarding whether the proximal or distal embolization should be used, although results from a recent systematic review and meta-analysis suggested proximal embolization may reduce the risk for postprocedure complications.[11] Minor complications, including fever, pleural effusion, and partial splenic infarction, have been reported in up to 34% of patients using both techniques. Major complications, including splenic abscesses, splenic infarction, splenic atrophy, and postprocedure bleeding, have been observed in 14% of patients.[10]

Hepatic Bleeding

Arterial hemorrhage from the liver may be encountered from blunt or penetrating trauma (see Chapter 113) but is most commonly because of an iatrogenic injury related to biopsy (see Chapter 23) or percutaneous transhepatic biliary drainage (PTBD; see Chapters 31 and 52). Arteriographic findings indicating a source of hemorrhage include extravasation, pseudoaneurysm formation, and arteriovenous fistula (see Chapter 115). In contrast to the spleen, a rich collateral network exists in the hepatic arterial bed, making proximal occlusion of the offending artery ineffective in many cases. Therefore super-selective catheterization using coaxial microcatheters to deposit coil-spring emboli both distal and proximal to the area of injury is

the preferred technique for embolization when a discrete bleeding site can be identified (Fig. 21.7). The use of liquid embolic agents such as n-cyanoacrylate glue may also be considered since these agents may achieve rapid and focal hemostasis even in the setting of diminished thrombus formation because of coagulopathy or thrombocytopenia. For more diffuse injuries with multiple bleeding sites secondary to blunt trauma, using particulate embolization with a gelatin sponge may be a useful adjunct.

As with blunt splenic injuries, nonoperative management has become the preferred method of management in hemodynamically stable patients. The success rate of this management exceeds 90%.[12] Two main indications for hepatic angiography and embolization are primary hemostatic control in a hemodynamically stable patient that has radiographic evidence of active arterial hemorrhage and adjunctive hemostatic control after surgical exploration and packing of a hepatic parenchymal injury with evidence of continued bleeding or hemodynamic instability. Additionally, patients who present with hemodynamic instability can be successfully resuscitated with embolization.[13] The yield of arteriography in identifying an arterial injury amenable to embolization is higher when the CT scan suggests a vascular injury.

Complications after embolization of a hepatic arterial injury secondary to blunt trauma are relatively frequent.[14] In a retrospective study, Letoublon et al. reported a 70% liver complication rate.[14] These complications include hepatic ischemia, infarction, hepatic failure, gallbladder ischemia, bile leak, and abscess formation. The relative contribution of the embolization to these complications may be difficult to distinguish from sequelae of the underlying traumatic injury.

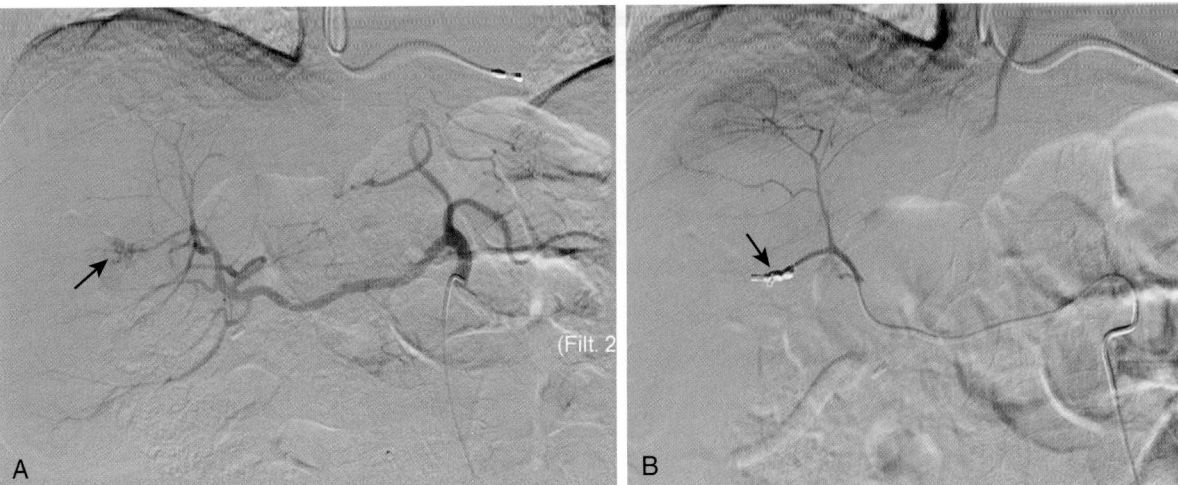

FIGURE 21.7 A, Digital subtracted angiography from celiac axis demonstrates active extravasation of contrast *(black arrow)* from the corresponding location of a liver biopsy consistent with post-liver biopsy bleeding. **B,** The injured/bleeding artery was embolized by coil embolization *(black arrow)*. No further extravasation of contrast is detected on post-coil angiography.

Procedure-related iatrogenic injury to the hepatic artery may be suspected when a patient develops intracatheter or pericatheter hemorrhage after PTBD or when melena develops secondary to hemobilia after an intervention through the hepatic parenchyma. CT in these patients may or may not reveal an abnormality, and patients should undergo hepatic arteriography when a clinical suspicion of a hepatic arterial injury exists even in the absence of negative cross-sectional imaging. Patients with iatrogenic injuries usually have a single, discrete bleeding source that can be addressed with super-selective embolization techniques. Identification of a bleeding source may require provocation maneuvers, such as biliary catheter removal during the angiography. Complications related to the embolization procedure tend to be lower when compared with patients who have had blunt trauma because the traumatic injury to the liver is less extensive.

Pancreas Bleeding

Bleeding from the pancreas is uncommon and usually encountered in patients with pancreatitis (see Chapters 56 and 58) or pancreatic surgery (see Chapters 28, 62, and 117). Post-traumatic bleeding from the pancreas is not frequently encountered in clinical practice. Pancreatic hemorrhage typically localizes to the retroperitoneum but may extend from the retroperitoneum into the peritoneal cavity or into the GI tract via communication with the pancreatic duct, a condition termed "hemosuccus pancreaticus."

Vascular complications are seen in 25% of patients suffering from pancreatitis and are usually arterial in origin. Proteolytic enzymes combined with intense inflammation can erode small arterial branches and create foci of extravasation or small pseudoaneurysms. Although this complication is encountered in only 2% to 5% of cases, it may be life threatening. Pseudocysts may erode into small arterial branches, leading to hemorrhage within the pseudocyst, or may erode into larger arterial branches and create a large pseudoaneurysm (Fig. 21.8; see Chapter 115). These pseudoaneurysms are most frequently identified in the splenic artery or its branches (60%–65%), followed by the GDA (20%–25%),

pancreaticoduodenal arteries (10%–15%), hepatic artery (5%–10%), and left gastric artery (2%–5%).[15,16]

The sensitivity of MDCT for the identification of pseudoaneurysms in patients with acute pancreatitis has been reported as high as 90%, obviating the need for angiography in most instances. However, small pseudoaneurysms arising from one or more intrapancreatic or peripancreatic arteries may not be visible using cross-sectional imaging.[17] As with hepatic bleeding, conventional catheter angiography may be warranted in patients with clinical and/or laboratory evidence of significant active or recurrent hemorrhage of a pancreatic source despite unrevealing CT imaging. When the bleeding site is identified angiographically, it can be controlled with embolotherapy in up to 88% of patients.[18]

Angiography and embolization is also feasible and safe in treatment of hemorrhagic complications after pancreatic surgery[19,20] (see Chapters 28, 62, and 117). Yekebas et al. reported significant hemorrhage in 5.7% of 1669 consecutive patients after partial or total pancreatectomy.[19] In a more recent study, Casadei et al. reported significant hemorrhage in 9.8% of 182 patients after pancreatic resection for pancreatic and periampullary diseases.[20] Bleeding may manifest clinically as GI hemorrhage, retroperitoneal or intraperitoneal hematoma, or bleeding through percutaneous or surgically placed drains. When a pancreaticojejunal anastomosis has been created, disruption of the anastomosis may lead to false localization of the bleeding site. Specifically, an extraluminal bleeding site may drain into the bowel through the dehisced anastomosis, or bleeding from the bowel at the anastomosis may extend outside the lumen to cause an intraperitoneal hematoma or hemorrhage through a drain. Angiography can be extremely useful in the diagnosis and treatment of these patients. In 25 of 43 patients undergoing angiography to diagnose and treat post-pancreatectomy hemorrhage, a bleeding site was located and embolized with an 80% success rate in controlling the hemorrhage.[19] The relatively low rate of positive angiograms may be explained by the high incidence of venous bleeding encountered in the post-pancreatectomy patient. Many of these patients develop regional portal hypertension as a result of splenic, portal, or

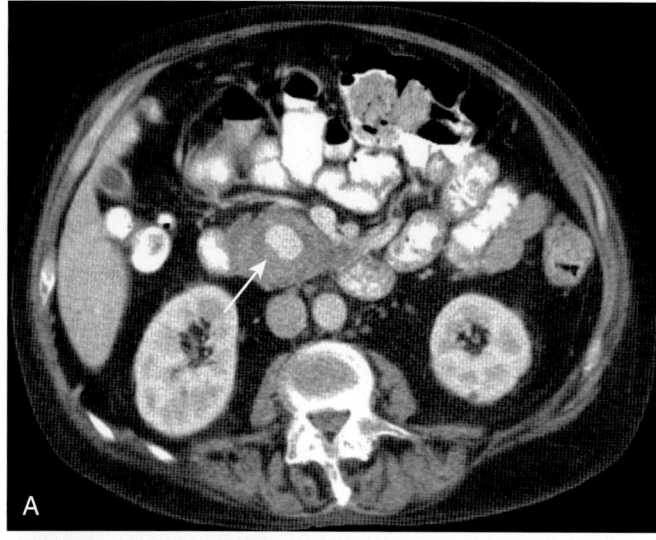

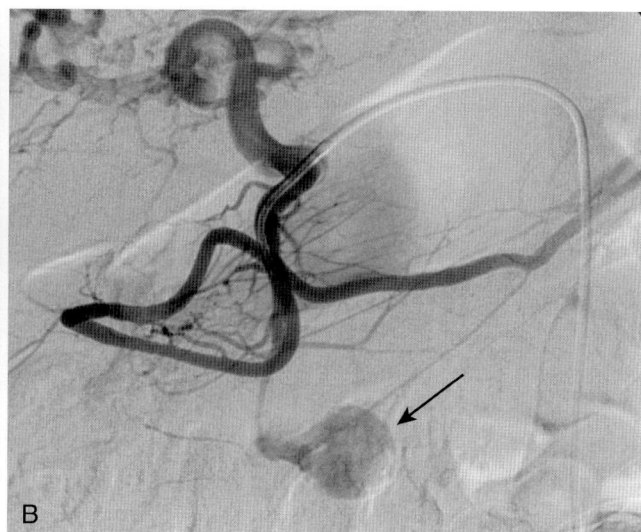

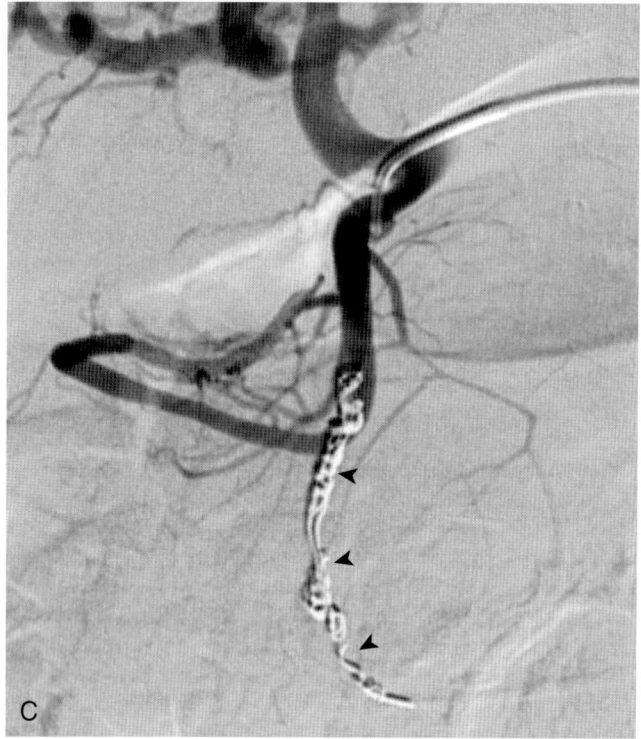

FIGURE 21.8 Pseudoaneurysm secondary to pancreatitis treated with coil embolization. **A,** Contrast-enhanced computed tomography reveals a pseudoaneurysm in the pancreatic head *(arrow)*. **B,** Selective gastroduodenal arteriogram reveals the pseudoaneurysm *(arrow)* taking origin from a branch of the anterior-superior pancreaticoduodenal artery. **C,** The pseudoaneurysm is occluded with coils *(arrowheads)*. (See Chapter 115.)

SMV compression or occlusion secondary either to the underlying pathology or a surgical complication. Venous extravasation is rarely identified by arteriography but may be suggested by CT. If the underlying etiology is compression of the splenic or portal veins, percutaneous transvenous stenting may be potentially useful.

Diagnosis of Arterial Occlusive Disease

Many arterial disorders that involve the primary branches of the celiac trunk, as well as the SMA, can be assessed adequately with MDCT or MRA. However, delineation of pathology in smaller branches, such as with vasculitis, may require the increased morphologic detail afforded by catheter angiography.

Arterial occlusive disease as a result of atherosclerosis and compression of the celiac axis by a median arcuate ligament are common diseases that do not generally influence the conduct of hepatobiliary or pancreatic surgery. The principal exception

is in the performance of orthotopic liver transplantation (OLT), when preservation of brisk hepatic arterial flow is essential (see Chapter 111). In that circumstance, the inflow must be corrected either by surgical or endovascular interventions. Another potential area of concern is pancreaticoduodenectomy, particularly in jaundiced patients. In this situation, sacrifice of the GDA is required, which interrupts the retrograde arterial flow from the SMA to the liver and may uncommonly result in hepatic ischemia and necrosis. Likewise, fibromuscular dysplasia may rarely involve the SMA, but associated clinical sequelae are extremely uncommon. The SMA may also be compromised in very rare circumstances by a median arcuate ligament.

Diagnosis and Treatment of Arterial Stenosis

Hepatic arterial anastomotic stenoses are observed in up to 11% to 12% of patients after OLT (see Chapter 11).[21,22]

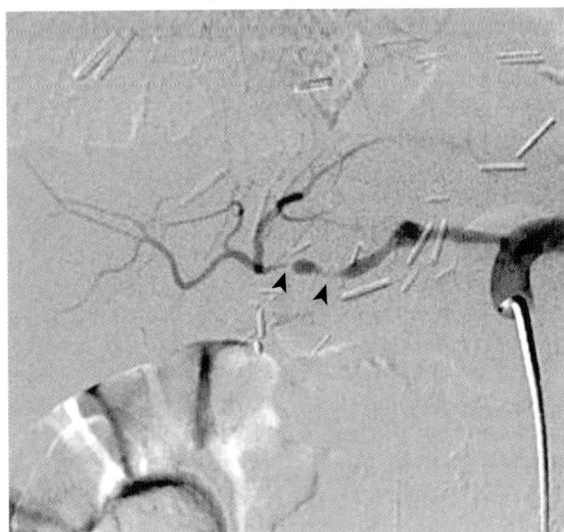

FIGURE 21.9 Hepatic artery stenosis after orthotopic liver transplantation. Celiac arteriogram shows mild diffuse narrowing of the hepatic artery with two areas of critical stenosis *(arrowheads).* (See Chapter 111.)

Although these stenoses are usually detected by surveillance duplex ultrasound and confirmed with MDCTA, catheter angiography is often performed to improve morphologic delineation and assess the degree of stenosis in preparation for endovascular treatment.[23] Stenoses of the hepatic artery may also be more diffuse than suggested on noninvasive imaging studies such as ultrasound or CT (Fig. 21.9). Anastomotic stenoses of the hepatic artery anastomosis may lead to allograft dysfunction and biliary ischemia with the potential for diffuse biliary infarction if untreated. Severe stenosis may lead to hepatic artery thrombosis, which may yield irreversible allograft damage and necessitate re-transplantation. When a hepatic arterial stenosis is identified, endovascular therapy, including balloon angioplasty with or without stent placement, is warranted, with high published rates of technical success and few major complications.[24]

Treatment of Visceral Arterial Aneurysms

Visceral artery aneurysms are rare entities that involve the celiac, splenic, superior mesenteric, or inferior mesenteric arteries and their branches (see Chapter 115). The prevalence of visceral artery aneurysm is 0.1% to 2%.[25,26] True aneurysms involve all three vessel walls and are usually atherosclerotic or developmental in origin and differ from those encountered in pancreatic inflammatory disease, which are typically pseudoaneurysms. Depending on the size and location of the aneurysm, mortality from rupture ranges from 25% to 100%.[27]

The splenic artery is the most commonly affected artery (60%), followed by the hepatic artery (20%–50%). Splenic artery aneurysms in women of childbearing age are of particular concern because of their propensity to rupture during childbirth. Most splenic aneurysms are saccular and located in the mid to distal segment of the artery.[28] The rate of rupture ranges from 3% to 20%.[29] Size is the primary variable when considering intervention, with most societies and providers recommending definitive therapy for aneurysms greater than or equal to 2.0 cm in size. The endovascular treatment approach for splenic artery aneurysms depends on the tortuosity

and location of the aneurysm. Covered stent placement may be used to exclude the aneurysm sac from the parent vessel, resulting in aneurysm thrombosis, and coil embolization may be used in patients with large or tortuous vessels where stenting is not feasible.[25] As with aneurysms elsewhere in the body, both proximal and distal coil embolization across the aneurysm neck is advised to prevent retrograde aneurysm sac perfusion, potentially resulting in postembolization aneurysm enlargement and rupture.

Traditionally, surgical resection or ligation of visceral artery aneurysms was considered the standard of care; however, endovascular treatments have largely supplanted open resection. Large studies have reported technical success rates ranging from 89% to 98%.[25,26,30] Endovascular treatments are associated with shorter hospital stay compared with surgical repair (3.8 vs. 12 days). Operative mortality and morbidity are both elevated relative to endovascular therapies for visceral aneurysms, particularly those that arise secondary to infection or inflammation (e.g., pancreatitis) or in the setting of prior surgical intervention.

Diagnosis of Vasculitis

Vasculitis

Vasculitides involving the hepatic arterial system may require catheter angiography for definitive diagnosis because of the technique's increased spatial and temporal resolution since the characteristic microaneurysms and areas of arterial narrowing or irregularity may not be apparent by MDCT. The most common vasculitis with hepatic and pancreatic involvement is polyarteritis nodosa, which may not lead to symptoms despite involvement of the visceral arteries, although pancreatitis, cholecystitis, and hepatic dysfunction may be observed.

Arterial abnormalities in the liver and pancreas have also been identified in patients with systemic lupus erythematosus and Wegener granulomatosus. In most patients, the underlying diagnosis is apparent, and the angiographic findings do not represent a diagnostic dilemma.

Diagnosis of Other Visceral Vascular Disease

Segmental Arterial Mediolysis

Segmental arterial mediolysis (SAM) is a rare arteriopathy affecting vascular smooth muscle, resulting in the development of aneurysms, dissections, thrombosis, and, uncommonly, vessel rupture. SAM is most commonly seen in older adults and the cause remains unknown. Clinical manifestation are often nonspecific, and cross-sectional imaging may fail to identify or adequately delineate the true extent of the pathology, necessitating catheter angiography for reliable characterization of the relevant findings. Multifocal lesions with skip areas involving the superior mesenteric, hepatic, renal, and middle colic arteries in patients in their fourth to sixth decades are typical (Fig. 21.10). Medical treatment with immunosuppressants is not effective in patients with SAM, and endovascular interventions, including angioplasty, embolization, and stenting, represent the primary approach to therapy.[31]

Hereditary Hemorrhagic Telangiectasia

Hereditary hemorrhagic telangiectasia (HHT), also known as *Osler-Weber-Rendu syndrome,* is an autosomal dominant vascular dysplasia characterized by telangiectasias of the skin and mucous

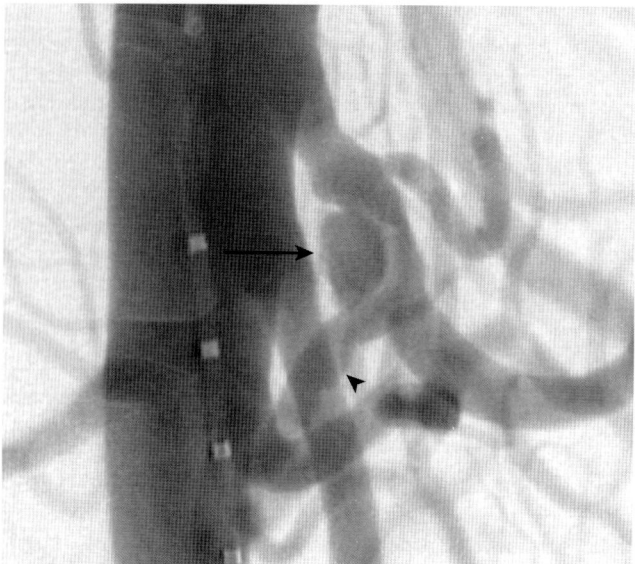

FIGURE 21.10 Segmental arterial mediolysis (SAM). Abdominal aortogram reveals a dissection with a small aneurysm in the celiac artery *(arrow)* as well as undulating irregularity of the common hepatic artery *(arrowhead)* typical of SAM.

membranes. HHT is also associated with arteriovenous malformations (AVMs) in the pulmonary and hepatic circulation, which may be life-threatening. Diagnosis is primarily clinical based on the Curacao criteria, which incorporates epistaxis, mucosal telangiectasia, visceral AVMS, and family history. Cross-sectional imaging, including ultrasound, CT, or MRI, plays a fundamental role in detecting visceral involvement in HHT. The hepatic arterial malformations that shunt blood into the hepatic venous system may be initially noted on a cross-sectional imaging study, but the findings may be nonspecific. Catheter angiography can be diagnostic by depicting arteriovenous or arterioportal shunting (Fig. 21.11).[32] Although HHT

has previously been treated with transcatheter techniques, embolotherapy has currently fallen out of vogue because of the risk of precipitating hepatic failure. OLT is curative if the patient develops high-output cardiac failure.

Peliosis Hepatis

Peliosis is a rare abnormality of the reticuloendothelial system that is most commonly encountered in the liver (peliosis hepatis). The name is derived from the Greek word "pelios," which means "lead-colored," referring to extravasated blood. Pathologically it is characterized by blood-filled cystic spaces that range in size from a few millimeters to multiple centimeters, distributed randomly in the liver. This abnormality has been associated with HIV infection and with the use of certain drugs, including immunosuppressives, antimetabolites, and oral contraceptives. Although usually benign, it has been associated with spontaneous massive hemorrhage and therefore may be encountered angiographically during the investigation of hepatic bleeding.[33] Angiographically (Fig. 21.12), the lesions are easily visible as a disorganized collection of amorphous channels not dissimilar to those observed in HHT or hepatic hemangioma; however, the lack of shunting to the hepatic venous system distinguishes it from HHT, and the absence of sharp definition with persistence into the late venous phase distinguishes it from hemangioma. Peliosis hepatis should be among the differential diagnosis of multiple hypervascular lesions in a patient with long-standing history of oral contraceptive drug use and with no prior history of cancer.[34]

Localization of Functional Pancreatic Neuroendocrine Tumors

Calcium stimulation arteriography for the detection of pancreatic endocrine tumors was developed and described in 1991.[35] Although unnecessary when imaging can confidently detect the offending pancreatic lesion, it is an extremely useful adjunct when the location of the lesion cannot be defined with confidence using noninvasive techniques (Fig. 21.13; see Chapter 65). To perform the localization, 1 mL of 10% calcium

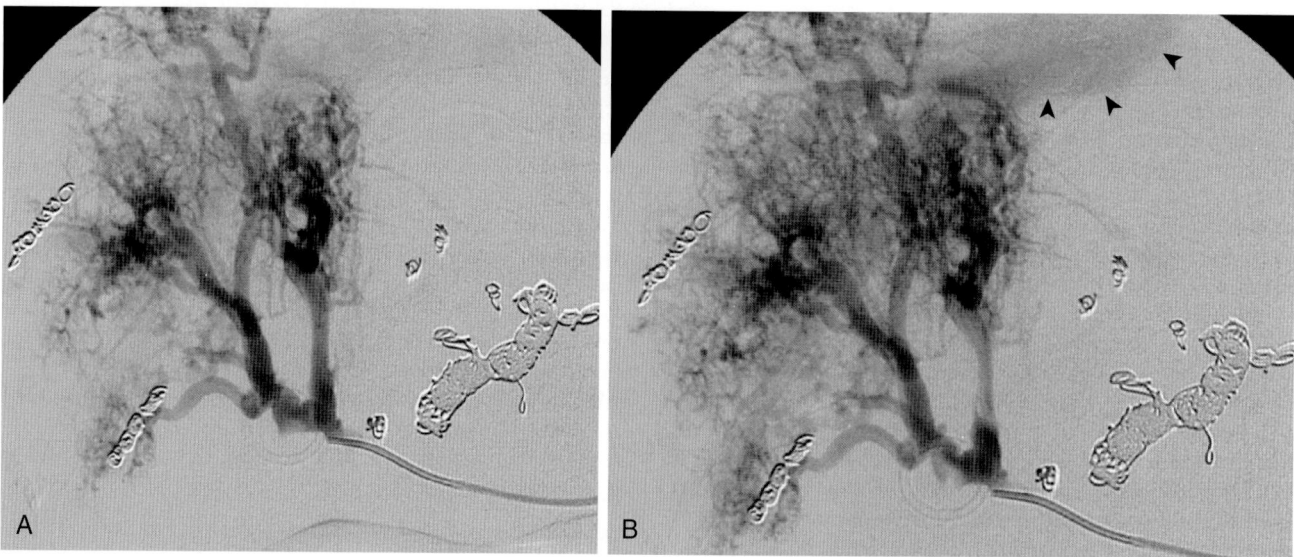

FIGURE 21.11 Hereditary hemorrhagic telangiectasia (HHT). **A,** Selective hepatic arteriogram shows disorganized and dilated intrahepatic vessels typical of HHT. Coils are being placed preoperatively for impending liver transplantation. **B,** Slightly later in the sequence, early opacification of the hepatic vein is visible *(arrowheads)*.

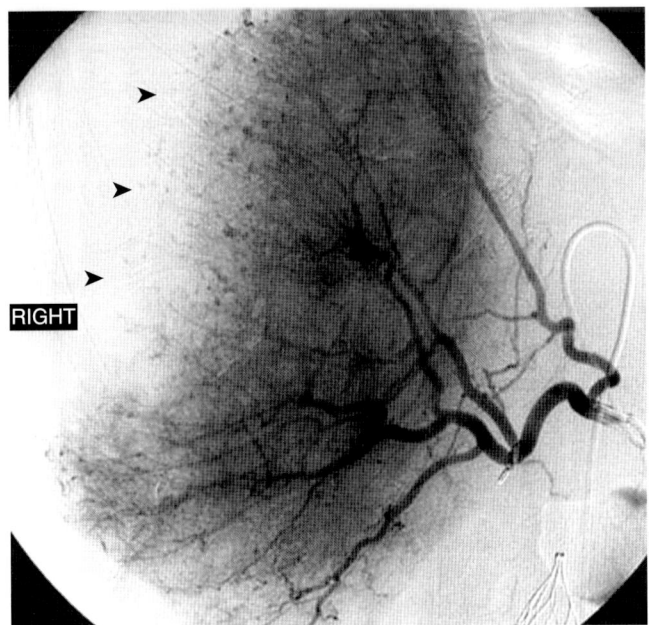

FIGURE 21.12 **Peliosis hepatitis.** Multiple small contrast collections can be seen within the hepatic parenchyma. This patient had spontaneous hemorrhage that created displacement of the hepatic parenchyma *(arrowheads).*

gluconate solution is selectively and sequentially injected via a microcatheter into small arteries supplying differing anatomic regions of the pancreatic parenchyma to provoke degranulation of hormone into the portal venous circulation. Serial blood samples taken from the hepatic vein and hormone level measurements are made. These measurements can then be

correlated with the anatomic location of injection, allowing for confident tumor localization.

Given the heterogeneity of arterial supply to the pancreas, the operator must interrogate branches arising from the GDA, the SMA, and the splenic artery to ensure complete coverage of the pancreatic head, uncinate process, body, and tail. The origin of small branches supplying the pancreas from the splenic artery and CHA are important to note in determining the approximate areas of pancreatic arterial supply. In the aforementioned article by Guettier et al., calcium stimulation arteriography was the most sensitive technique for localizing surgically proven insulinomas with an accuracy of 84%, a false-negative rate of 11%, and a false-positive rate of 4%.[36]

Percutaneous transhepatic sampling of the splenic, superior, and portal venous system can also be performed to diagnose occult hormonally-active neuroendocrine tumors (NET) of the pancreas. This may be done in conjunction with calcium stimulation, as described, or it may be performed without stimulation because of the higher concentration of the hormone when obtained directly or adjacent to the venous tributary.

Insulinomas

Insulinoma originates from β cells and is the most frequently hormonally active pancreatic NET. More than 90% of insulinomas are solitary, benign tumors for which surgical resection is curative. These tumors are the most common tumors originating from the islets of Langerhans (see Chapter 65). The most effective method of diagnosing insulinoma is a combination of dual-phase thin-section CT scan and endoscopic ultrasound (EUS; see Chapters 17 and 22).[37] In a series of 75 surgically-proven insulinomas, the sensitivities of CT and MRI were 28% and 35%, respectively.[36] This series incorporated cross-sectional imaging dating back to the late 1980s that likely reduced the

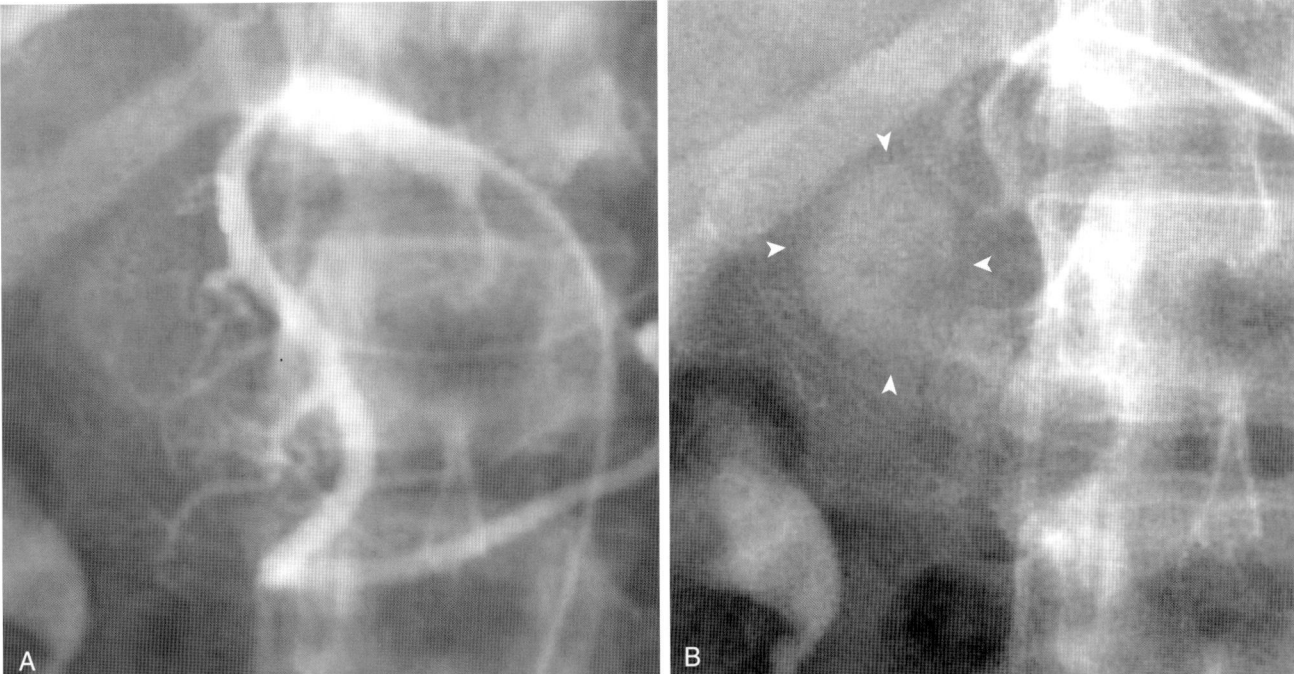

FIGURE 21.13 **Insulinoma. A,** Selective gastroduodenal arteriogram shows no definite abnormality during the arterial phase. **B,** A subtle area of hypervascularity is identified during the capillary phase, possibly representing an insulinoma *(arrowheads).* This was confirmed as the region of tumor by calcium stimulation with venous sampling. (See Chapter 65.)

overall sensitivity. When cross-sectional imaging techniques were examined after 1994, the sensitivity of CT and MRI improved to 80% and 70%, respectively, because of improved imaging technology.[38] More recent literature has shown even more favorable results, with 22 of 23 (96%) insulinomas identified before surgery using dual-energy CT technology.[39] The sensitivity of EUS in detecting and localizing insulinomas ranges from 82% to 94%.[40]

Gastrinomas

Gastrin-secreting NET are the cause of Zollinger-Ellison syndrome, and in approximately one third of the cases are accosiated with multiple endocrine neoplasia (MEN) type 1. Fifty percent of gastrinomas occur in the pancreas, with the duodenum being the most common extrapancreatic location. Approximately 60% to 90% of gastrinomas are malignant. When a sporadic gastrinoma is identified, surgical resection is indicated. The role of surgery in patients with MEN type 1 is more controversial because of multiplicity of tumors and lack of an established survival benefit (see Chapter 65).

The diagnosis and location of a gastrinoma can be established with a combination of somatostatin receptor scintigraphy (see Chapter 18) and EUS (see Chapter 22) in approximately 90% of patients. When an occult gastrinoma is encountered, angiography has been used for localization. The principles are identical to the localization of insulinomas; however, secretin has been used in addition to calcium gluconate as the stimulating agent. Sensitivities of arterial stimulation venous sampling (ASVS) in the detection of gastrinomas have ranged from 70% to 100%.[41,42]

Angiographically, gastrinomas are less hypervascular and more difficult to detect compared with insulinomas. Sensitivity of angiography alone without ASVS is less than 50%. Moreover, the 50% extrapancreatic location makes detection more difficult, often requiring superselective catheterization to evaluate the duodenum.

Glucagonoma

Glucagonomas may occur sporadically or may be associated with MEN type 1. They originate from α cells of the pancreatic islets. These tumors are usually larger than gastrinomas or insulinomas at presentation, therefore localization can generally be achieved with cross-sectional imaging or EUS. Equchi et al. reported 8 patients with pancreatic hypervascular tumor and elevated serum glucagon level wherein glucagonomas were successfully localized using the ASVS technique.[43]

VENOGRAPHIC TECHNIQUES

MDCT, magnetic resonance venography, and ultrasound are usually sufficient for depiction of the major visceral venous trunks and their primary branches in the vast majority of patients. Cross-sectional imaging can accurately depict the relationship of a mass in the pancreas to both the splenic veins and SMVs. It also has the advantage of simultaneous opacification of all of the venous structures. However, in certain clinical situations, it is desirable to visualize the venous structures with a higher level of clarity. These situations include planning for percutaneous venous interventions in situations where occlusions are suspected or occasionally to plan a surgical portosystemic shunt.

The most common technique to visualize the splanchnic vein is transarterial portography, in which selective splenic and

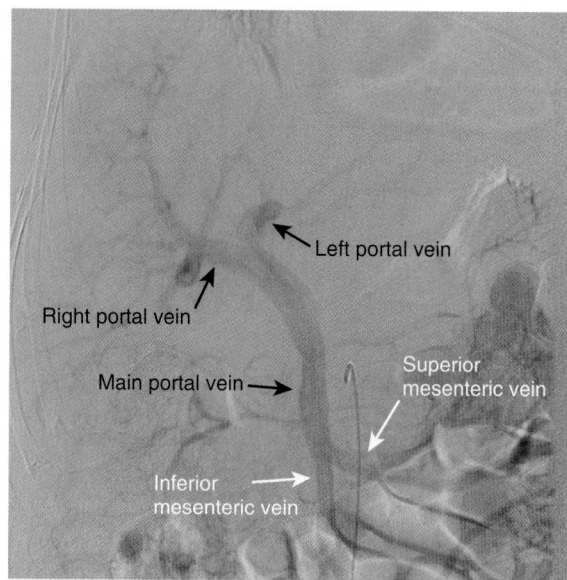

FIGURE 21.14 Arterial portography in a patient with hepatocellular carcinoma. During the venous phase of superior mesenteric arterial injection the inferior and superior mesenteric veins are opacified and join to form the main portal vein. The main then branches into left and right portal veins.

superior mesenteric arteriograms are performed with delayed imaging into the venous phase, depicting the splenic veins and SMVs, respectively (Fig. 21.14). When detailed visualization of the venous anatomy is required, a higher dose of contrast media can be used for the arterial injection, increasing the clarity of the venous opacification.

When an extremely detailed evaluation is required, a combination of transarterial portography and MDCT can be performed (Fig. 21.15). The improved spatial and soft tissue contrast resolution of MDCT coupled with multiplanar and 3D reconstruction allows for visualization of venous anatomy that cannot be an-otherwise achieved by any other single technique. This is particularly useful in the presence of portal vein occlusion, when a complex venous reconstruction or bypass is being considered. Fig. 21.16 demonstrates a portovenography performed using a transsplenic access. The patient with unresectable pancreatic cancer presented with portal hypertension and ascites. Area of narrowing was treated with stent placement (see Fig. 21.16B).

Direct venography of the splanchnic veins can be achieved by three routes: *transjugular, transhepatic,* and *transsplenic.* In the transjugular approach, a catheter is placed into the jugular vein and advanced into a hepatic vein. Free and wedged hepatic pressures can be obtained through this catheter to calculate corrected sinusoidal pressure in patients being assessed for portal hypertension. A biopsy of the hepatic parenchyma (transjugular liver biopsy) may also be performed during this procedure, when indicated. Injection of carbon dioxide through a catheter wedged in a hepatic vein or through a balloon catheter will often yield an image of the portal vein. If direct portography is warranted, one of several specially designed needles can be inserted to puncture the portal vein through the intervening hepatic parenchyma. A catheter is then advanced into the portal, splenic, or superior mesenteric venous system. This procedure is performed almost exclusively in patients

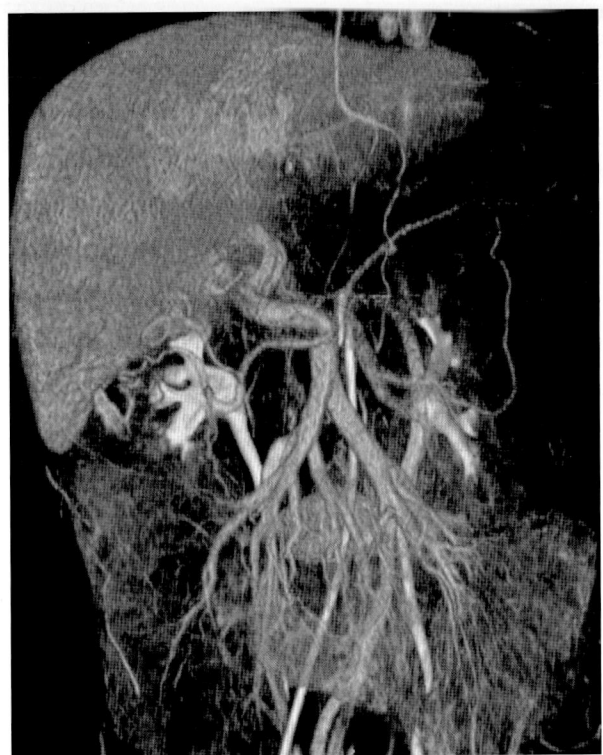

FIGURE 21.15 Multidetector computed tomography with three-dimensional reconstruction after superior mesenteric arterial injection. The superior mesenteric vein and cavernous transformation are easily visualized.

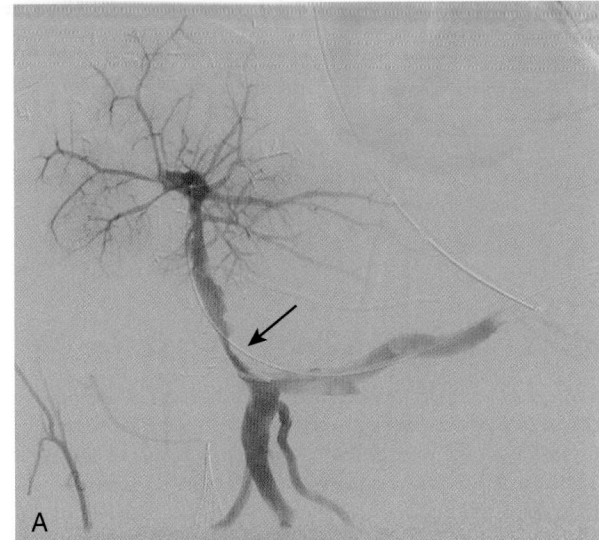

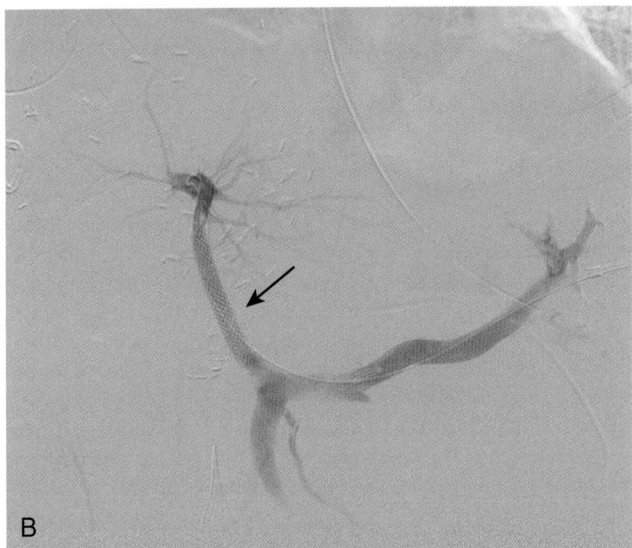

FIGURE 21.16 **A,** Trans-splenic portovenography in a patient with unresectable pancreatic cancer causing narrowing in the main portal vein *(black arrow).* **B,** The area of narrowing was treated with stent placement *(black arrow).* The final run demonstrates free flow of contrast through the treated area consistent with successful treatment.

undergoing a transjugular intrahepatic portosystemic shunt (TIPS), but it is also used to manage selected patients with portal and SMV thrombosis.[44]

The portal venous system may also be accessed by a percutaneous transhepatic approach.[45] After sterile preparation of the right upper quadrant, an intrahepatic portal venous radicle is punctured under real-time ultrasonographic guidance, permitting a vascular access sheath to be placed using a Seldinger technique. Standard guidewire and catheter manipulations are then used through the sheath for selectively catheterizing the splenic vein and the SMV or its branches. Once diagnostic images have been acquired or venous interventions have been performed, the catheter is removed. The transhepatic tract is then occluded by a variety of techniques including insertion of Gelfoam pledgets, deployment of coils, or injection of fibrin glue. The transhepatic venographic procedure is usually performed as part of a direct pancreatic venous sampling, lobar portal venous embolization to stimulate contralateral hypertrophy before major hepatic resection, assessment and management of an anastomotic portal venous stenosis after OLT, pharmacomechanical lysis of a splanchnic vein thrombosis, or rarely to control bleeding from a splanchnic vein.

Percutaneous injection of the splenic parenchyma can also be used to delineate the anatomy of the splenic and portal veins and the draining tributaries. This examination is somewhat antiquated and has been generally replaced by MDCT or magnetic resonance venography. In infants, cross-sectional imaging may be inconclusive, and transarterial portography is risky because of the diminutive size of the femoral arteries; however, it remains an alternative in planning a portosystemic shunt procedure.

Percutaneous catheterization of the splanchnic veins is also possible from a transsplenic approach using a technique identical to that described for transhepatic catheterization.[46] This procedure is usually done in conjunction with a percutaneous procedure to assess a portal vein stenosis or occlusion after OLT, but it may also be used in conjunction with the assessment and treatment of a splenorenal venous bypass, when access cannot be achieved from the systemic venous circulation.

The references for this chapter can be found online by accessing the accompanying Expert Consult website.

CHAPTER 22

Endoscopic ultrasound of the biliary tract and pancreas

Vineet Syan Rolston, Joseph Patrick Kingsbery, and Mark Andrew Schattner

IMAGING AND DIAGNOSIS

The diagnosis of benign and malignant diseases of the pancreas and biliary tree historically have relied on a detailed history and complete physical examination, with correlation of the results of clinical chemistries. Imaging of the hepatic and pancreatic parenchyma and ductal anatomy has, however, evolved as critical for accurate diagnosis and for guiding therapy. Ultrasonography (US), computed tomography (CT), and magnetic resonance imaging (MRI) have become important noninvasive modalities in the routine investigation of pathologic conditions of the biliary tree or pancreas (see Chapters 12 and 13).

Invasive procedures for imaging the biliary and pancreatic ductal systems, primarily percutaneous cholangiography (PTC) (see Chapter 20) or endoscopic retrograde cholangiopancreatography (ERCP) (see Chapter 31) remain important therapeutically, but diagnostically, these have been almost entirely replaced by less invasive modalities. Endoscopic ultrasonography (EUS) has become an essential tool for the diagnosis and treatment of pancreatic and biliary pathology. Its high-resolution images complement the more general findings of cross-sectional imaging and result in a higher sensitivity for diagnosis of early-stage disease and detection of smaller lesions. Linear array echoendoscopes permit guided passage of needles and devices through the endoscope, allowing biopsies to be obtained and permitting therapeutic interventions. This chapter discusses the techniques of endosonography in the diagnosis, staging, and treatment of benign and malignant disease of the pancreas and biliary tree.

Endoscopic Ultrasound Technique

The pancreas is located posterior to the stomach and is readily seen by EUS imaging through the wall of the stomach and duodenum. With the transducer in the duodenum, the pancreatic head and uncinate process, ampulla of Vater, pancreatic ducts, common bile duct (CBD), and the surrounding vascular and nodal structures can be visualized. With the transducer in the stomach, the pancreatic body and tail, gallbladder, and left lobe of the liver are seen. Additionally, the celiac, splenic, hepatic, and superior mesenteric arteries, as well as the splenic, superior mesenteric, and portal veins are all seen in detail (see Chapter 2).

The normal pancreatic parenchyma has a homogeneous echogenic appearance (Fig. 22.1), and tumors usually appear hypoechoic, often with irregular borders, in sharp distinction from healthy tissue (Fig. 22.2). Small tumors of the pancreas that are often missed by CT or MRI are readily imaged by EUS. For example, islet cell tumors, which are often encapsulated and small, are more readily detected on EUS than cross-sectional imaging and appear as well-demarcated hypoechoic lesions (see Chapter 65). Other neuroendocrine tumors, such as gastrinomas, may be isoechoic within the pancreatic parenchyma and

difficult to identify without careful, tedious, real-time imaging (Fig. 22.3). Ampullary tumors are also often seen and staged on EUS because of their proximity to the duodenal wall, CBD, and pancreatic duct (Fig. 22.4) (see Chapter 59). Extrahepatic bile duct tumors can also be detected and described in detail with EUS imaging (Fig. 22.5).

Cysts of the pancreas are generally anechoic and well demarcated and thus easily identified even when small (see Chapter 60). Some cysts may have internal echoes or solid nodules, which raise concern for a mucinous lesion or associated tumor (Figs. 22.6 and 22.7). Cysts can easily be distinguished from vascular structures using Doppler flow. Serous cystadenomas may also appear isoechoic with the pancreas and require careful imaging for proper identification (Fig. 22.8).

Endoscopic Ultrasound–Guided Fine-Needle Aspiration and Biopsy

The development of linear array echoendoscopes, which scan an area orthogonally in line with the endoscope (thus in line with the biopsy channel), has allowed the development of EUS-guided fine-needle aspiration (EUS-FNA) and fine-needle biopsy (EUS-FNB). The indications for EUS-guided aspiration or biopsy include pathologic confirmation of a suspected pancreatic or periampullary cancer, evaluation of pancreatic masses, bile duct lesions or abnormal lymph nodes, and aspiration of pancreatic cysts. EUS-guided needle puncture has also provided the platform for therapeutic EUS-guided techniques (see Chapter 30).

Endoscopic Ultrasound Fine-Needle Aspiration Technique

Within the duodenum or stomach, the EUS probe is positioned near the target lesion, typically less than 3 cm away. The area is then interrogated with Doppler flow to ensure the absence of significant vascular structures in the needle path. A 25-gauge, 22-gauge, or 19-gauge needle can then be directed into the target lesion. The tip and shaft of the needles used for FNA produce a bright, hyperechoic image. This allows the needle to be followed in real time to ensure precise positioning within the target lesion (Fig. 22.9). Ideally, a cytopathologist or cytotechnologist should be present at the time of the FNA to determine the cellular adequacy of the specimen, improve diagnostic yield, and reduce the need for additional pass of the biopsy needle.[1] (Khoury et al, 2019). Alternatively, multiple punctures (six to seven) should be performed to ensure an adequate cytologic specimen.[2] Cyst fluid can also be aspirated and sent for cytology, tumor markers, and chemical analysis (Fig. 22.10). More recently, the development of needles that can obtain core samples (FNB) allows tissue with preserved architecture to be acquired, as opposed to purely cytologic specimens.[3] Several maneuvers have been described to improve diagnostic yield, including the use of a "fanning" technique, whereby multiple

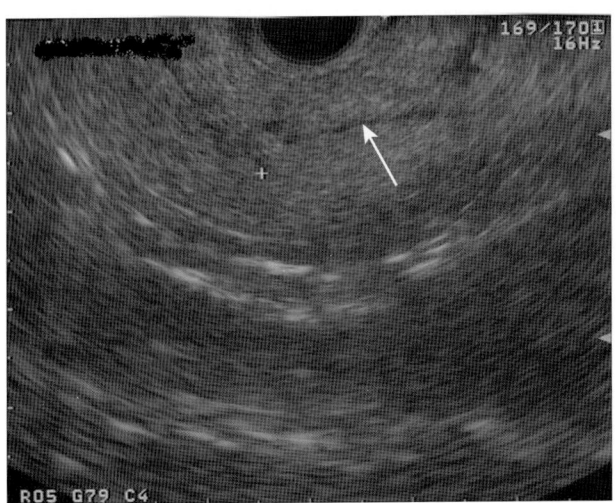

FIGURE 22.1 Normal endoscopic ultrasound image of the body of the pancreas with thin main pancreatic duct *(arrow)*.

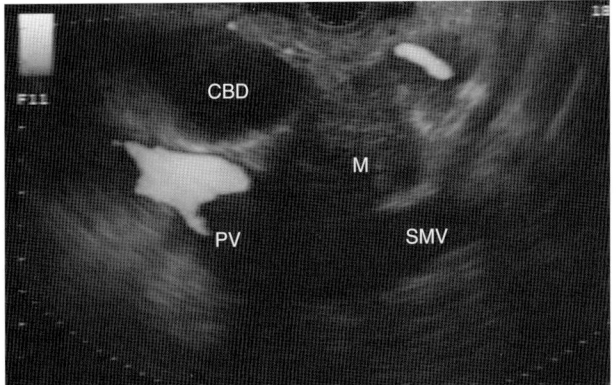

FIGURE 22.2 Solid, irregular, hypoechoic mass *(M)* in the pancreatic head seen with abrupt termination of a dilated common bile duct *(CBD)* and contact with the portal confluence (portal vein *[PV]* and superior mesenteric vein *[SMV]*). Cytology obtained by endoscopic ultrasound–guided fine-needle aspiration proved to be adenocarcinoma.

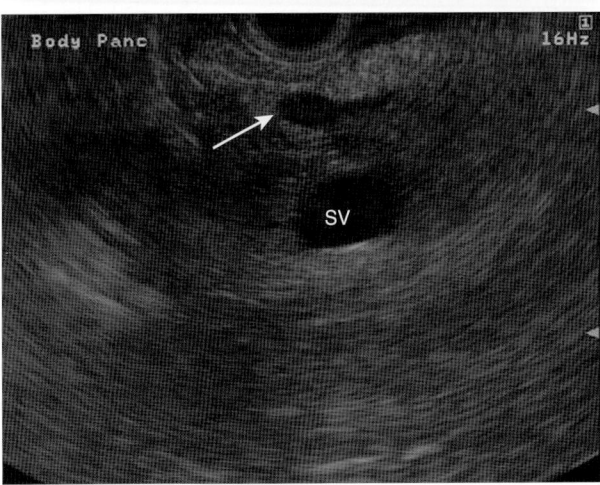

FIGURE 22.3 Small, well-circumscribed, hypoechoic appearance of an insulinoma *(arrow)* in the body of the pancreas with splenic vein *(SV)* below.

areas are sampled within a lesion, particularly the peripheral area of lesion to improve yield and reduce the number of passes required for diagnosis.[4] The use of suction for FNA of lymph nodes or solid masses has been suggested to have improved cellularity; however, it may yield more bloody samples.[5,6] The reinsertion of a stylet within the fine needle does not appear to increase yield, may increase the bloodiness of the sample, and can increase procedural time.[7] However, the use of a stylet slow-pull technique may confer some advantage for diagnostic yield.[8]

DIAGNOSIS OF PANCREATIC CANCER

Endoscopic Ultrasound Fine-Needle Aspiration and Biopsy of Solid Pancreatic Lesions

Solid masses of the pancreas may represent a primary pancreatic cancer (see Chapter 62), neuroendocrine tumor (see Chapter 65), metastatic lesion (see Chapter 64), or focal pancreatitis (see Chapter 55). These masses may be difficult to visualize on

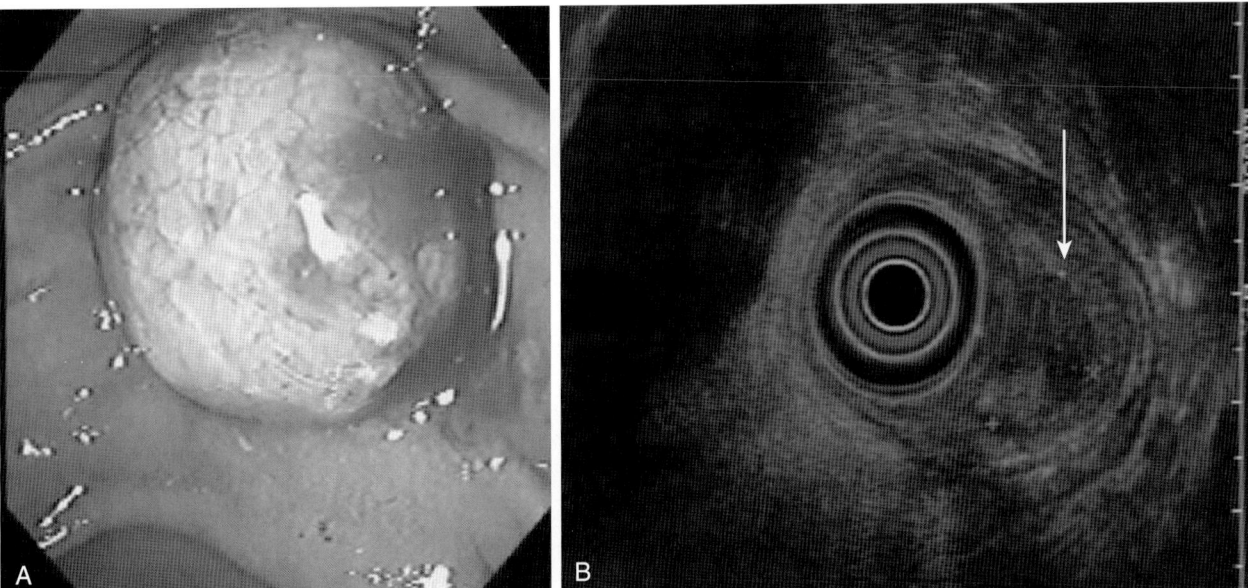

FIGURE 22.4 Endoscopic **(A)** and endoscopic ultrasound **(B)** imaging of an ampullary tumor *(arrow)*.

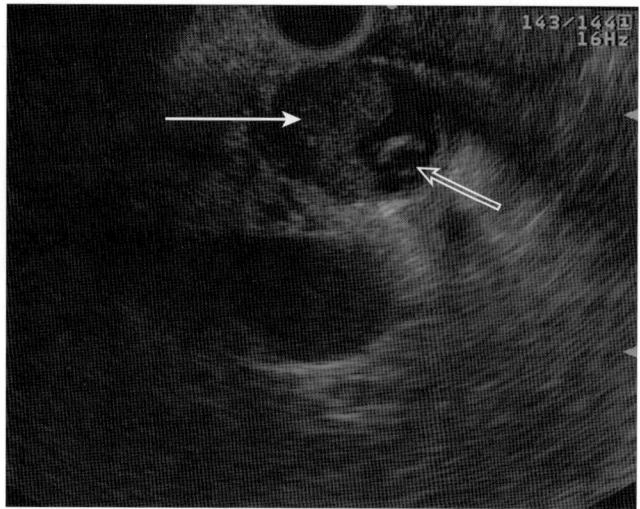

FIGURE 22.5 Hypoechoic mass appearance of cholangiocarcinoma of the common bile duct *(solid arrow)* with biliary stent visible *(open arrow).*

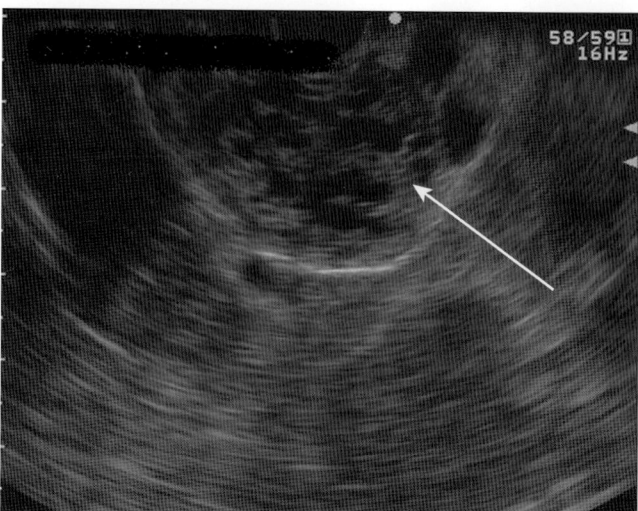

FIGURE 22.8 Typical microcystic appearance of a serous cystadenoma in the head of the pancreas *(arrow).*

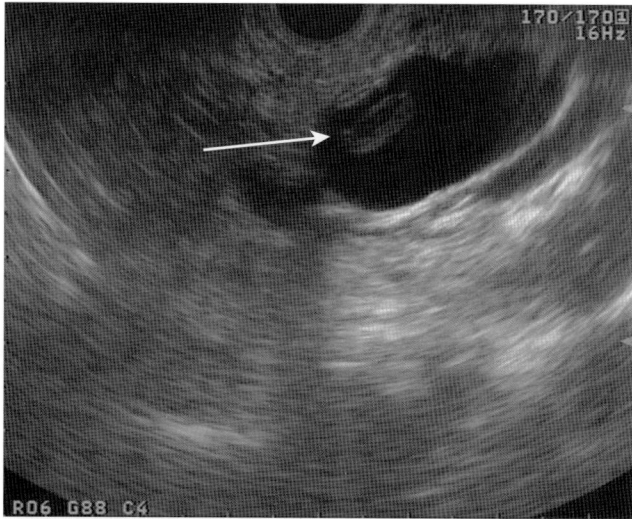

FIGURE 22.6 Mucinous cystic lesion in the head of the pancreas with mural nodule *(arrow).*

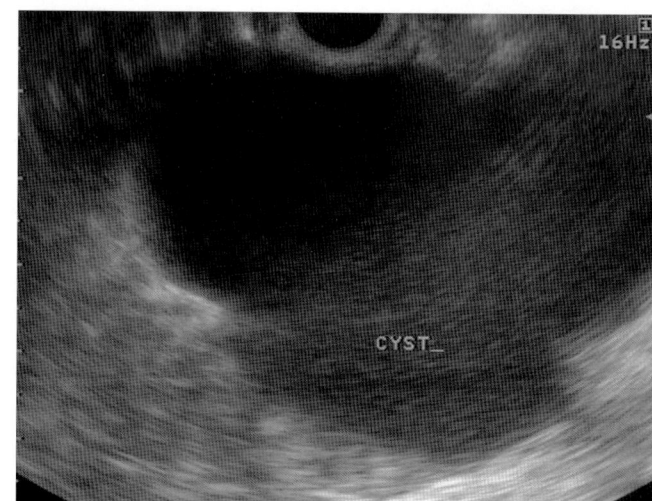

FIGURE 22.9 Bright appearance of fine-needle aspiration of a solid mass in the head of the pancreas.

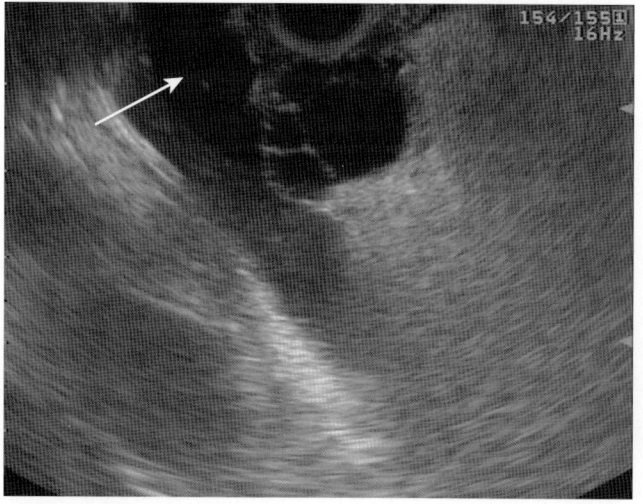

FIGURE 22.7 Multiseptated mucinous cystic lesion in the head of the pancreas *(arrow).*

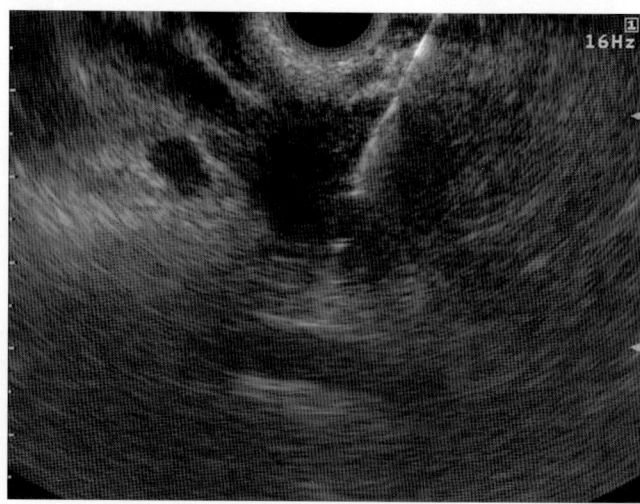

FIGURE 22.10 Fine-needle aspiration of cyst fluid.

TABLE 22.1 Imaging Characteristics and Fluid Analysis of Pancreatic Cystic Lesions

	EUS MORPHOLOGY	COMMUNICATION WITH PANCREATIC DUCT	FLUID AMYLASE	FLUID CEA	FLUID CYTOLOGY
Retention cysts	Unilocular, thin walled	No	Variable	Low	Normal duct or centroacinar cells
Pseudocyst	Unilocular, thick-walled with debris	Yes	Very high	Low	Inflammatory cells, no epithelial cells
Serous cystadenoma	Microcystic with central calcification	No	Low	Low	Small cuboidal cells, positive glycogen stain
Mucinous cystadenoma	Macrocystic with thick septations	Occasionally	Low	High	Atypical ductal cells, positive mucin stain
IPMN	Dilated, tortuous pancreatic duct and/or side branches	Yes	High	High	Atypical ductal cells, positive mucin stain

CEA, Carcinoembryonic antigen; *EUS,* endoscopic ultrasound; *IPMN,* intraductal papillary mucinous neoplasm.

noninvasive imaging when small. EUS allows high-resolution imaging of the pancreas as well as facilitating guidance of FNA and FNB.

Some solid lesions in the pancreas may not need preoperative biopsy if the result of biopsy would not change the decision to resect the lesion. Current surgical guidelines recommend proceeding to surgery for resectable pancreatic lesions for which surgery is indicated without first obtaining a diagnostic biopsy.[9] However, patients with locally advanced pancreatic lesions require histologic diagnosis before initiating chemotherapy or radiation. Biopsy is also indicated before surgical resection for those patients in whom there is suspicion for autoimmune pancreatitis (see Chapter 54).

EUS-FNA has been shown to have superior diagnostic accuracy for pancreatic malignancy than percutaneous CT-guided and US-guided approaches, especially for small lesions.[10] EUS-FNB has a diagnostic accuracy similar to EUS-FNA; therefore either EUS-FNA or FNB is the preferred modality for diagnostic sampling of pancreatic lesions.

Recent randomized controlled trials assessing EUS-FNA and FNB tissue acquisition reported diagnostic accuracies of 81% to 100% and 85% to 94% for FNA and FNB, respectively.[6,11–14] In these studies, there was an equivalent complication rate of between 0% and 3% for both FNA and FNB, with bleeding, abdominal pain, and pancreatitis the most common complications cited.

There is some suggestion that FNB produces a superior specimen with preserved tissue architecture over FNA samples. A retrospective study looking at EUS sampling of pancreatic lesions using a 22-gauge FNA needle and 25-gauge FNB needle in 76 patients found no difference in safety or technical success; however, the 25-gauge FNB needle produced a higher amount of diagnostic material and superior preservation of tissue architecture despite the smaller caliber needle.[15] Additionally, a large retrospective study found that EUS-FNB was superior to EUS-FNA in obtaining tissue for genomic testing compared with FNA samples (90.9% vs. 66.6%, respectively). More research is needed in this area, as molecular testing is becoming more common and more directed therapies are becoming available.[16]

Endoscopic Ultrasound Fine-Needle Aspiration of Pancreatic Cystic Lesions

Cystic lesions of the pancreas remain a diagnostic and therapeutic challenge (see Chapter 60). The differential diagnosis

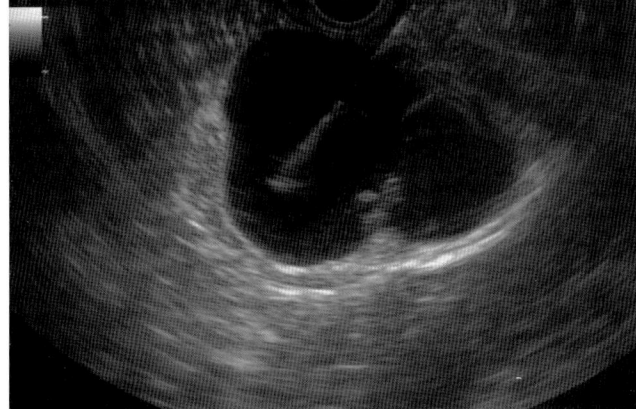

FIGURE 22.11 Large debris-filled pseudocyst adjacent to the tail of the pancreas.

includes retention/simple cysts, pseudocysts, cystic neoplasms, and cystic degeneration of solid masses (Table 22.1). EUS provides detailed imaging of the entire pancreas, including location and number of cysts; size; ductal dilatation or communication; signs of chronic pancreatitis; cyst wall thickness; mural nodules; papillary projections; and intracystic structures such as septations, debris, and mass components.

Retention cysts are benign dilated segments of the pancreatic duct secondary to focal duct disruption. Under EUS they are generally small, thin-walled, and unilocular; they carry no malignant potential and can be left untreated

Pseudocysts develop as a result of acute inflammation (see Chapters 55 and 56). On EUS, they are thick walled as they become chronic and may have debris within the cyst cavity (see Fig. 22.11). They can be seen in or adjacent to the pancreas and often communicate with the pancreatic duct. FNA will yield thick fluid with inflammatory cells, but there is an absence of epithelial cells. Tumor marker levels (carcinoembryonic antigen [CEA]) in the cyst fluid are low or undetectable; in contrast, fluid amylase is usually markedly elevated.

Regarding cystic neoplasms, it is important to distinguish mucinous and papillary tumors from serous lesions (see Chapter 60). Serous tumors have no malignant potential and do not require resection unless symptoms occur or they encroach on vascular structures, specifically the portal and superior mesenteric and splenic veins. Typically, serous cystadenomas are composed of a honeycomb of microcysts with no communication with the pancreatic duct (see Fig. 22.8). They can be large and exhibit central stellate calcification on imaging studies. Papillary lesions and solid pseudopapillary tumors carry the risk of malignant transformation and should be referred for resection. Mucinous lesions (mucinous cystic neoplasm [MCN] and intraductal papillary mucinous neoplasm [IPMN]) also harbor malignant potential. Mucinous cysts are generally composed of one or more large cystic spaces with thickened walls or septa (see Fig. 22.7). Features that may indicate malignant potential of MCNs include size ≥3 cm in size, rapid increase in cyst size during surveillance, mural nodules, mass-forming lesions, and peripheral egg-shell calcifications.[17] In the case of IPMNs, distinguishing main-duct from side-branch types is important clinically because the former is associated with malignancy in as many as 62% of patients.[18] Although cross-sectional imaging may help in this regard by demonstrating a dilated pancreatic duct characteristic of main-duct IPMN, communication with the main pancreatic duct can also be demonstrated on EUS.

Although these anatomic characteristics are helpful, EUS cyst morphology alone is insufficient to characterize the lesion.[18-20] Aspiration of cyst fluid via EUS-FNA can further aid in the diagnosis. Cyst fluid can be analyzed for tumor markers, amylase, and molecular markers, and it provides material for cytopathologic assessment. Cyst fluid tends to be paucicellular; thus the sensitivity and negative predictive value of cytology is low.[21,22] The presence of thick, viscous fluid and a positive mucin stain is suggestive of a mucinous lesion. The concentration of several tumor markers in pancreatic cyst fluid has been examined, and CEA has been found to be the most useful. Higher concentrations of CEA most accurately predict mucinous lesions, although the optimal cutoff is not universally agreed on, a cyst-fluid CEA concentration of more than 192 ng/mL predicts a mucinous lesion with a sensitivity of 73%, specificity of 84%, and an accuracy of 79%.[19,23]

Although helpful for diagnosing mucinous lesions, cyst-fluid CEA levels do not correlate with the presence of malignancy.[24] Another limitation of cyst-fluid CEA analysis is that it requires aspiration of at least 1 mL of fluid, which can be difficult if the cavity is small or the fluid is very viscous, making it difficult to pull through a fine needle. More recently, cyst-fluid DNA analysis has shown promise in differentiating mucinous from nonmucinous cysts. This analysis can be done on as little as 200 μL of fluid. The presence of a *KRAS* mutation, high DNA content, and loss of polymorphic alleles are indicators of mucinous cysts. In a large validation study, early *KRAS* mutation followed by allelic loss was 96% specific and 37% sensitive for a malignant cyst.[25] Interleukin-1β (IL-1β) has recently been identified as a potential biomarker for high-grade dysplasia or malignancy.[26] Cyst fluid aspirated ahead of surgical resection was found to contain higher concentrations of IL-1β in specimens with evidence of high-grade dysplasia or carcinoma. Nonetheless, a reliable and sufficiently sensitive biomarker for malignancy is still lacking.

The use of a EUS-guided through-the-needle biopsy forceps device has had promising results for further evaluation of cysts. A disposable needle is introduced through a standard 19-guage EUS-FNA needle to allow sampling of the cyst wall, mural nodules, or septae, and may provide greater sensitivity and specificity for both identification of cyst type and risk-stratification of mucinous cysts.[27]

Complications of Endoscopic Ultrasound Fine-Needle Aspiration and Biopsy

EUS-FNA of the pancreas is a safe procedure. The reported rate of pancreatitis is 0% to 2%.[28-31] (see Chapter 55) In a multicenter analysis of almost 5000 EUS-FNAs of solid pancreatic masses, the incidence of pancreatitis was 0.3%, and most cases were clinically mild.[28] EUS-guided aspiration of pancreatic cysts is similarly safe, with a pancreatitis rate of less than 1% and an overall complication rate of about 2%.[32] Bacteremia is uncommon following EUS-FNA of solid lesions, with a rate similar to that for diagnostic upper endoscopy; thus prophylactic antibiotic administration is unwarranted.[33,34] However, early data evaluating EUS-guided cyst aspiration showed increased infectious complications leading to the recommendation of routine antibiotic prophylaxis for all patients undergoing this procedure.[35] Major extraluminal hemorrhage is a rare complication and occurs at a rate of less than 1%.[36]

STAGING OF PANCREATIC CANCER

The method of staging generally practiced in the United States is that published by the American Joint Committee on Cancer (see Chapter 62). It follows the tumor-node-metastasis (TNM) staging system and is outlined in Table 22.2.

TABLE 22.2	AJCC Staging of Pancreatic Cancer
	TNM DEFINITIONS
Primary Tumor (T)	
TX	Cannot be assessed
T0	No evidence of primary tumor
Tis	Carcinoma in situ
T1	Tumor confined to pancreas, ≤2 cm in diameter
T2	Tumor confined to pancreas, >2 cm in diameter
T3	Extrapancreatic extension, no celiac axis or SMA involvement
T4	Involvement of celiac axis or SMA
Regional Lymph Nodes (N)	
NX	Cannot be assessed
N0	Regional lymph node metastases absent
N1	Regional lymph node metastases present
Distant Metastases (M)	
MX	Cannot be assessed
M0	Distant metastases absent
M1	Distant metastases present
AJCC TNM	
Stage 0	Tis, N0, M0
Stage I	
IA	T1, N0, M0
IB	T2, N0, M0
Stage II	
IIA	T3, N0, M0
IIB	T1-T3, N1, M0
Stage III	T4, N0-N1, M0
Stage IV	T1-T4, N0-N1, M1

AJCC, American Joint Committee on Cancer; *SMA,* superior mesenteric artery; *TNM,* tumor-node-metastasis.

From Edge SB, Byrd DR, Compton CC, eds. *AJCC Cancer Staging Manual.* 7th ed. New York, NY: Springer, 2010.

Endoscopic Ultrasound Tumor-Node-Metastasis Staging

Some of the first reports of EUS imaging of the pancreas described its ability to detect and diagnose pancreatic and periampullary tumors.[37,38] However, subsequent studies evaluated the ability of EUS to stage tumors and assess appropriateness of resection.[39,40] Although the general approach to the preoperative evaluation of pancreatic cancer has focused on the TNM stage, the usefulness of such staging is questionable, particularly because the T stage does not necessarily correlate with resectability. The role of EUS and CT scan for staging of pancreatic lesions is complementary in nature. EUS may offer a superior sensitivity for evaluating tumor invasion of the portal vein; however, it is lower than CT for tumor invasion in the celiac artery, superior mesenteric artery, and superior mesenteric vein.[41-43]

Perhaps the most useful application of EUS is the diagnosis of small pancreatic tumors (<3 cm) in patients with equivocal radiologic imaging. Several studies have demonstrated that EUS is superior to CT scanning for evaluation of pancreatic lesions smaller than 3 cm.[44,45] In addition, EUS far exceeds CT and MRI in the diagnosis and staging of tumors of the ampulla of Vater to determine whether local or radical resection may be appropriate.[46,47] EUS has also demonstrated greater sensitivity for detecting small pancreatic neuroendocrine tumors <2 cm and insulinomas[48] (see Chapter 65). Other reports, as well as our own experience, have shown the usefulness of EUS in evaluating patients with dilated pancreatic and/or bile ducts but no demonstrable cause. EUS in this setting has been useful in the identification of small tumors of the ampulla, pancreas, or bile duct and nonneoplastic causes, such as stone disease, chronic pancreatitis, or abnormal anatomy.[49] Therefore, when a pancreatic mass is suspected but cannot be identified by standard imaging modalities, EUS should be considered if further clarification is clinically warranted. A large retrospective series reported a high specificity for EUS in predicting the absence of pancreatic cancer, with a negative predictive value of 100%, when the results of EUS showed a normal pancreas.[49]

Preoperative Reassessment After Neoadjuvant Chemoradiotherapy

Studies on the treatment of pancreatic cancer have recently focused on neoadjuvant treatment with chemotherapy and radiation therapy, followed by attempted radical resection (see Chapter 66). Several studies have investigated the ability of EUS to reassess patients who have completed neoadjuvant therapy, with most suggesting that EUS is no better than CT for determining resectability. In one report, EUS correctly assessed residual tumor stage in 40% of patients and node status in 90%, but it incorrectly suggested venous invasion in 43%.[50] These results suggest that inflammatory changes in the tumor bed, pancreas, and lymph nodes alter the anatomy and blur the distinction between normal tissue planes and between tumor and normal tissue.

DIAGNOSIS AND STAGING OF CHOLANGIOCARCINOMA

Primary bile duct cancers (see Chapters 51 and 59) usually present with painless jaundice. Although transcutaneous US and CT scanning reliably show biliary dilatation, they are less accurate for delineating tumors, especially if tumors are smaller than 2 cm. ERCP is the dominant invasive modality used to evaluate extrahepatic bile duct strictures. Diagnostic specimens can be obtained by deployment of a cytology brush against the stricture, but the sensitivity is low, with a yield of only 40% to 50%.[51-53] EUS has now emerged as a useful diagnostic and staging technique in this regard using linear and radial echoendoscopes. If a biliary stricture is visualized, malignancy is suggested by the presence of an irregular, thickened (>3 mm) bile duct wall (see Fig. 22.5). Hypoechoic infiltration invading through the biliary wall layers or an adjacent pancreatic mass can also be seen. The accuracy of EUS-FNA in the diagnosis of bile duct strictures has a reported sensitivity ranging from 43% to 86%[54-56] (Table 22.3). The results of a large single-center experience suggest that EUS can be very useful in the assessment of extrahepatic cholangiocarcinoma.[57] Tumor detection was superior with EUS compared with triphasic CT scan and MRI. EUS-FNA added significant diagnostic yield, particularly with distal bile duct tumors, with an overall sensitivity of 73%. In addition, EUS determined resectability with a sensitivity and specificity of 53% and 97%, respectively. The disadvantage of EUS-FNA is the potential for transperitoneal seeding and is generally not recommended if the patient is a candidate for curative liver transplantation.[58] The more recent development and use of per-oral cholangioscopy is a useful tool, allowing direct visualization of the biliary tree and targeted biopsies, with a reported sensitivity of 60% and specificity of 98% for diagnosis malignant biliary strictures.[59]

Endoscopic Ultrasound–Guided Intervention

Tumor Localization

Radiotherapy is increasingly important in the management of pancreatic cancer, but stereotactic radiation is limited by respiratory motion and accurate assessment of tumor size and location in real time. A role for EUS-guided intratumoral placement of gold fiducials in localizing pancreatic tumors for targeted radiation therapy has also been demonstrated, which limits radiotherapy toxicity to the surrounding.[60-62] Gold fiducial markers can be backloaded into a 19-gauge or 22-gauge delivery system.[63] Alternatively, multifiducial delivery systems have been developed to allow for placement of multiple markers, with

TABLE 22.3 Performance Characteristics for EUS in the Diagnosis and Staging of Pancreatic, Ampullary, and Extrahepatic Biliary Tumors

	SENSITIVITY	SPECIFICITY	ACCURACY
Pancreatic Tumors			
Diagnosis[a]			
Tumor >3 cm	86%–95%	94%–99%	86%–94%
Tumor <3 cm	85%–95%	87%–100%	93%–100%
Tumor staging	–	–	72%–98%
Nodal staging	–	–	44%–66%
Ampullary Tumors	–	–	
Diagnosis	–	–	93%–100%
Resectability	–	–	61%–88%
Bile Duct Tumors	–	–	
Diagnosis[a]	–	–	43%–86%
TN staging	–	–	60%–80%

[a]Includes the use of fine-needle aspiration to obtain cytology.
EUS, Endoscopic ultrasound; *TN*, tumor node.

technical success of delivering at least three fiducials into the target area of 92%[64] (see Chapter 67).

Celiac Plexus Neurolysis

In patients with pain as a result of pancreatic cancer, EUS-guided celiac plexus neurolysis (CPN) has been shown to be a safe and effective alternative to surgical or percutaneous approaches (see Chapters 62 and 67). The celiac axis is easily identified using a linear-array echoendoscope positioned in the stomach (Fig. 22.12), and it provides a quick method of palliating cancer-related pain in patients undergoing staging and diagnosis of pancreas cancer. Two large meta-analyses demonstrated improved sustained pain relief in 72% to 80% of patients at a follow-up range of 1 to 6 months.[65,66] In addition, decreased analgesic requirements and fewer opioid-induced side effects can be expected after EUS-guided neurolysis.

However, there is significant variation in the literature with regards to technique as well as assessments of pain score. Multiple iterations of the procedure (bilateral celiac trunk injection, 10 cc vs. 20 cc of ethanol, broad injection to include the superior mesenteric artery, direct injection into celiac ganglion) have been studied to optimize palliation.[67–70]

More recently, there has been interest in celiac ganglion radiofrequency ablation (RFA) for pancreatic cancer pain palliation. In a recent prospective randomized controlled trial, 26 patients with pain related to pancreatic cancer underwent EUS-CPN (12) or EUS-RFA (14). The authors found that EUS-RFA provided more pain relief and improved the quality of life for patients with pancreatic cancer at 2- and 4-weeks post-treatment more than EUS-CPN. This is a relatively new technique and deserves more investigation.[71]

Drainage of Pseudocysts and Peripancreatic Collections

Pancreatic and peripancreatic fluid collections are common after pancreatic injury (see Chapter 56) The revised Atlanta Classification of acute pancreatitis updates the definitions of these fluid collections and makes an important distinction between fluid collections due to interstitial edematous pancreatitis and those due to necrotizing pancreatitis.[72]

Fluid collections related to interstitial edematous pancreatitis are classified by the timing of their formation: acute peripancreatic fluid collections occur within the first 4 weeks of pancreatic injury and are characterized by nonencapsulated fluid-filled collections. Fluid collections that develop after the first 4 weeks of injury are referred to as pseudocysts and typically have a well-defined capsule surrounding them.

Fluid collections that form as the result of necrotizing pancreatitis are similarly classified by their timing of formation: acute necrotic collections form in the first 4 weeks and are nonencapsulated, heterogeneous, nonliquefied material. Those that form after 4 weeks are referred to as walled-off necrosis and are made of encapsulated heterogeneous nonliquefied material.

Although many pancreatic and peripancreatic fluid collections will resolve spontaneously over time, drainage is indicated in the setting of infection or if persistently symptomatic.[73]

The role for EUS is as a minimally invasive and effective technique for guiding drainage of pancreatic pseudocysts and walled-off necrosis[74,75] (see Chapters 28, 30, and 56) or after pancreatic resection has been established. A fine needle is used to puncture the fluid collection, and a guidewire is used for transluminal stenting. Using real-time imaging and Doppler flow, intervening organs and vascular structures can be avoided. Thus there are fewer complications, such as bleeding and perforation, compared with the percutaneous approach.

A randomized trial comparing surgical and endoscopic drainage showed equal efficacy of the surgical and endoscopic approach, but with a shorter length of hospital stay for endoscopic drainage. Currently, endoscopic drainage is generally considered the first-line of care for pancreatic and peripancreatic fluid collection management.[75]

Early experience with transluminal endoscopic drainage involved creating a fistula between the fluid collection and the luminal gastrointestinal (GI) tract with placement of plastic stents through the fistula to maintain patency. More recently, self-expanding metal stents and lumen-apposing metal stents have been used for this purpose, with a larger lumen allowing passage of semisolid and necrotic debris. A meta-analysis comparing metal and plastic stents for drainage of pancreatic fluid collections identified 7 studies with 681 patients (340 metal, 341 plastic) with metal stents superior in both clinical success (93.8% vs. 86.2%). Additionally, metal stents were associated with fewer adverse events compared with plastic (10.2% vs. 25%). Adverse events for transluminal drainage of pancreatic and peripancreatic fluid collections include bleeding, stent migration, infection, and perforation.[76]

EUS-Guided Biliary Drainage

In patients with advanced abdominal malignancies, simultaneous duodenal and biliary obstruction can occur. Traditionally, these patients have required percutaneous or surgical biliary drainage because transpapillary decompression via ERCP is often not possible. EUS-guided transduodenal or transgastric biliary drainage is a novel approach that allows internal drainage.[77–79] Like pseudocyst drainage, the dilated CBD or left hepatic duct is localized with EUS and punctured with an FNA needle. A cholangiogram is performed (Fig. 22.13A), followed by guidewire insertion, dilation of the tract, and deployment of a self-expandable metal stent across

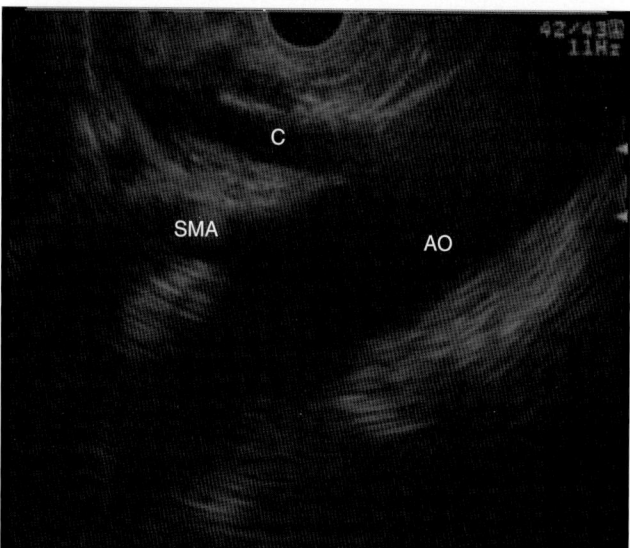

FIGURE 22.12 Endoscopic ultrasound appearance of the longitudinal course of the aorta (AO) with celiac (C) and superior mesenteric artery (SMA) origins.

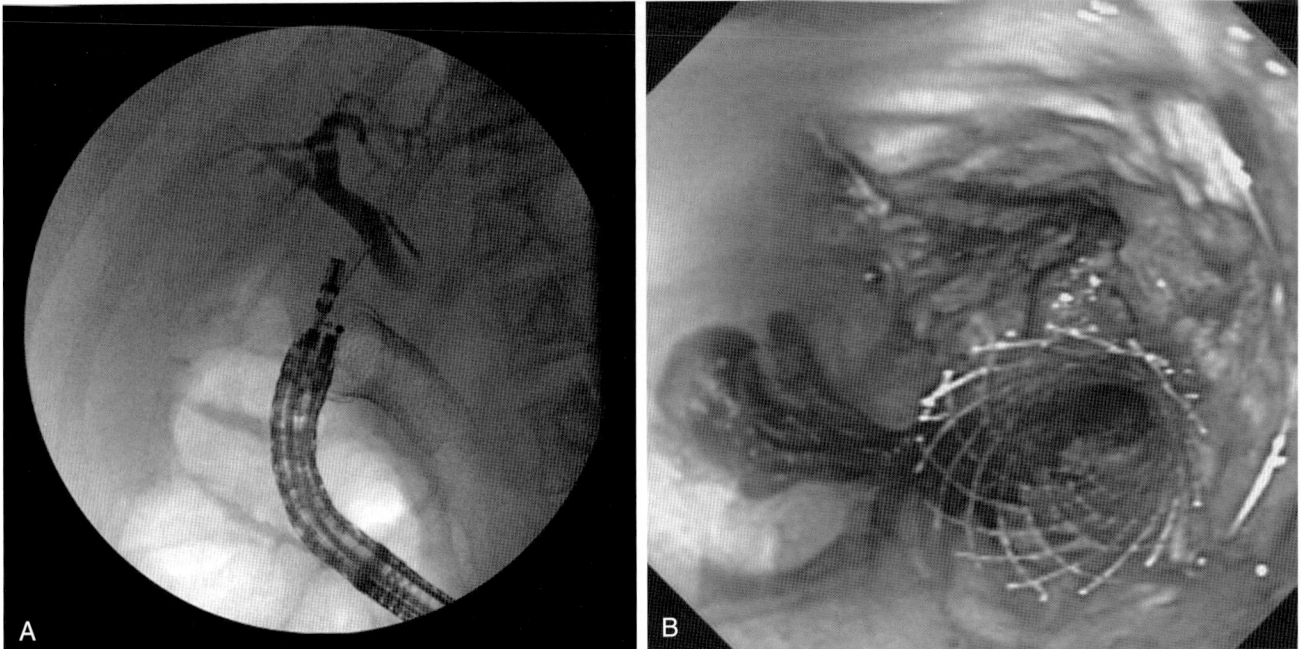

FIGURE 22.13 **A,** Cholangiogram obtained by endoscopic ultrasound (EUS)-guided puncture of the common bile duct by fine-needle aspiration in preparation for EUS-guided biliary drainage. **B,** EUS image after deployment of self-expanding metal stent.

the choledochoduodenostomy or hepaticogastrostomy tract (see Fig. 22.13B). EUS-guided biliary drainage was compared with percutaneous drainage in patients who failed ERCP[80] (see Chapter 30). EUS-guided biliary drainage was equally effective, with fewer adverse events, reduced need for reinterventions, and reduced cost (see Chapter 30).

More recent studies have shown superiority of EUS-BD to ERCP in patients with duodenal stenosis, patients with altered anatomy, and in patients with indwelling duodenal stents.[81–83]

Novel Therapeutics

EUS-guided ethanol ablation of cysts has been previously reported.[84,85] Patients with asymptomatic, unilocular pancreatic cysts were treated by injection and lavage of the cyst with ethanol through an FNA needle, with complete cyst resolution documented in 30% to 35% of patients. More recently, ethanol has been combined with paclitaxel, with complete resolution achieved in 62% to 78% of patients.[86] RFA of pancreatic cysts has also been described recently in a small series of patients.[87] Despite these advances, concerns remain about residual epithelium, which could remain after ablation. In addition, evidence that ablation reduces the risk of malignancy, the need for resection, or continued surveillance is lacking.

The use of lumen-apposing metal stents has allowed for the creation of EUS-guided gastroenterostomy (EUS-GE) for treatment of gastric outlet obstruction. By utilizing EUS to identify duodenum or jejunal loops adjacent to the gastric wall, and typically with the aid of a water-filling technique to distend the distal bowel, the electrocautery system of a lumen-apposing stent can be deployed. Khashab and colleagues demonstrated that while technical success for EUS-GE is lower than that of surgical gastrojejunostomy, EUS-GE has a similar clinical success rate and adverse event rate, offering a noninferior and less invasive option for treatment of gastric outlet obstruction.[88]

Mendelsohn and associates demonstrated good technical and clinical success in the presence of peritoneal carcinomatosis, encouraging the use of this therapy for palliative purposes.[89]

The use of a EUS-guided fine-needle injection (EUS-FNI) confers the ability to provide treatment to a targeted lesion. Therapies include the use of fiducial markers directly into malignant tissue as well as interstitial brachytherapy to general gamma rays and damaged local tissue.[90] Other uses of FNI include direct delivery of antitumor agents to a lesion, including lymphocytic cultures to induce cytokine release, immature dendritic cells to generate T-cell immune responses, and viral vectors.[91–93]

Ongoing work for targeting the mutant KRAS oncogene in pancreatic cancer includes the use of loading platforms to deliver siRNA targeted against KRAS mutations for antitumor effects. Animal models have yielded promising results by impeding growth of pancreatic tumor cells and prolonged mouse survival.[94] Clinical trials are underway to determine efficacy in humans.

SUMMARY

EUS is an essential tool in the evaluation of patients with abnormalities that involve the pancreas and the biliary tree. It provides detailed images of the pancreas and bile ducts and complements the findings of noninvasive radiographic imaging. For patients seen initially with suspected pancreatic or bile duct cancer, multidetector CT scanning assists in identifying those with obvious masses, metastatic disease, and vascular involvement. The usefulness of EUS in this setting is limited, except to provide tissue diagnosis using EUS-guided FNA, in localizing lesions, or in management of the complications of metastatic disease. For patients with small tumors, ampullary lesions, or equivocal findings detected by CT or MRI, the high sensitivity of EUS helps provide a diagnosis, with a high accuracy for tumor staging and determining resectability. Because EUS has poor sensitivity for identifying distant metastatic disease, CT scanning and laparoscopy will remain important tools in the evaluation of patients with pancreatic and bile duct cancer who are being considered for surgery. EUS-FNA and EUS-FNB are safe and valuable tools in the evaluation of patients with a suspected solid or cystic mass of the pancreas or extrahepatic bile ducts. It has a higher diagnostic sensitivity and specificity than noninvasive imaging and allows tissue sampling and molecular testing as part of the same procedure. Similarly, EUS-FNA has evolved from a diagnostic to a therapeutic procedure in the management of biliary and pancreatic disease.

References are available at expertconsult.com.

CHAPTER 23

Image-guided liver biopsy

Juan Camacho, Lynn A Brody, and Anne M Covey

INTRODUCTION

Percutaneous image-guided needle biopsy (PNB) is the cornerstone for diagnosis and treatment of many diseases involving the liver. Minimally invasive, PNB is an effective outpatient procedure with a low complication rate. The success of PNB requires proper patient selection, optimal procedural technique, and optimal postprocedure management.

Interventional radiology (IR, which also stands for interventional radiologists) plays a central role in patient management because of the need for image-guided tissue sampling procedures. Several oncology trials have demonstrated that molecular and biomarker targeted therapies have a higher chance of clinical success,[1] and such studies require tissue for analysis. PNB may also prevent unnecessary surgery for lesions with benign pathology.[1] Finally, tissue obtained at PNB can allow for histologic grading that has both prognostic and treatment implications.[2]

The role of PNB has increased beyond simply obtaining a diagnosis, and tissue obtained from PNB can now predict disease susceptibility to treatment and provide prognostic information. In addition, tissue-based biomarkers can be used to prescribe a tumor-specific treatment regimen because they can predict response to targeted therapies and/or immunotherapy.[3] As a result, an increased volume of tissue per biopsy and repeated sampling from the same target are often required.

Because the results of PNB are so impactful for optimal care of patients with a liver mass or at risk for cirrhosis, obtaining adequate specimens is critically important. This also holds true for clinical trials in which inadequate specimens have been shown to be a cause of ineligibility for oncology patients.[4] For example, in the National Cancer Institute–Molecular Analysis for Therapy Choice (NCI-MATCH) trial, almost 15% of biopsy samples were inadequate for molecular analysis; this proved to be a major impediment in the treatment of patients for whom a trial was the last resort.[5] Therefore, with PNB, IR can help improve patient outcomes through the study of biomarkers and optimization of specimen acquisition techniques. This chapter will explore the equipment and modalities used to perform PNB, the preprocedural and postprocedural patient care, sample adequacy concepts, and quality metrics, as well as future perspectives in the era of personalized medicine.

NEEDLE BIOPSY MODALITIES AND EQUIPMENT

PNB involves advancing a needle under imaging guidance into a target to obtain tissue or cells for diagnosis. PNB can be performed using aspiration techniques with a thin hollow needle (18–25 gauge) for cytologic evaluation or by using a cutting tool (core needle biopsy [CNB]), which uses a larger needle (9–20 gauge) that has a capturing mechanism to allow for the extraction of a piece of tissue. Of the two, only CNB allows for gross histologic evaluation[6] (Fig. 23.1). Both techniques can provide material for immunohistochemistry and molecular characterization.

Aspiration techniques include fine needle aspiration (FNA), fine needle capillary sampling (FNCS), and large needle aspiration (LNA). These techniques are generally considered safer and potentially less traumatic compared with CNB. During FNA, samples are acquired by using suction from a syringe until tissue/cells are collected. FNCS consists of placing a fine needle into the target, followed by rotating the tip within the target without aspiration until the sample ascends the needle by capillary action. An LNA is similar to an FNA but performed with a larger bore needle, is often useful to aspirate fluid for cytology, and may be preferred for thicker fluids/secretions. Ideally, an on-site cytopathologist or cytotechnologist can provide an immediate evaluation of the sample quality; this has been shown to increase the sensitivity of the biopsy, shorten the procedure time, and minimize the number of passes required to obtain a diagnostic specimen.[7,8]

A CNB is most commonly performed with 16- to 21-gauge needles that have an automated cutting mechanism and a variable throw or length of tissue sampled (5–30 mm). The specific needles are selected based on target size and presence of vascular structures or other organs in the path of or beyond the margins of the targeted lesion. The needle length is chosen after determining the depth of the target, based on the preprocedural imaging. Although FNA can provide excellent diagnostic information for metastatic disease, infection, and lymphoma, CNB samples are more likely to render definitive diagnosis for most primary liver tumors. To confirm adequacy of the specimen, a touch preparation can be prepared on a glass slide for immediate evaluation by a cytopathologist or cytotechnologist. Before placement in formalin or saline, the core of tissue is placed on a glass slide and gently moved over the slide to allow some cells to collect on the surface. Care should be taken to avoid excessive vigorous touch preparations because this has been shown to deplete the cellularity and DNA content of the specimen.[9]

Core samples are commonly placed in formalin. Occasionally, specimens may be sent "fresh" to pathology in saline or on saline-soaked gauze for special studies. Because cells placed in saline eventually undergo cell lysis related to osmotic shifts of saline into the cell, a specimen in saline needs to be fixed or frozen within a few hours to avoid deterioration of the tissue sample. Tissue also may be snap frozen for future studies. The preferred method for processing tissue may vary from institution to institution, and the preference of the pathologists reviewing the material should be ascertained before initiating a biopsy. For core biopsies obtained to evaluate organ parenchyma, end-cut rather than side-notch needles may yield more diagnostic samples in terms of number of portal triads.[10] In the setting of organ dysfunction or failure, no touch preparation is required; specimens are sent in formalin or saline, depending on the indication and the preference of the pathologist.

Many authors advocate performing both FNA and CNB to maximize the diagnostic yield of every biopsy.[11–13] CNB is particularly useful in most solid primary liver lesions, such as

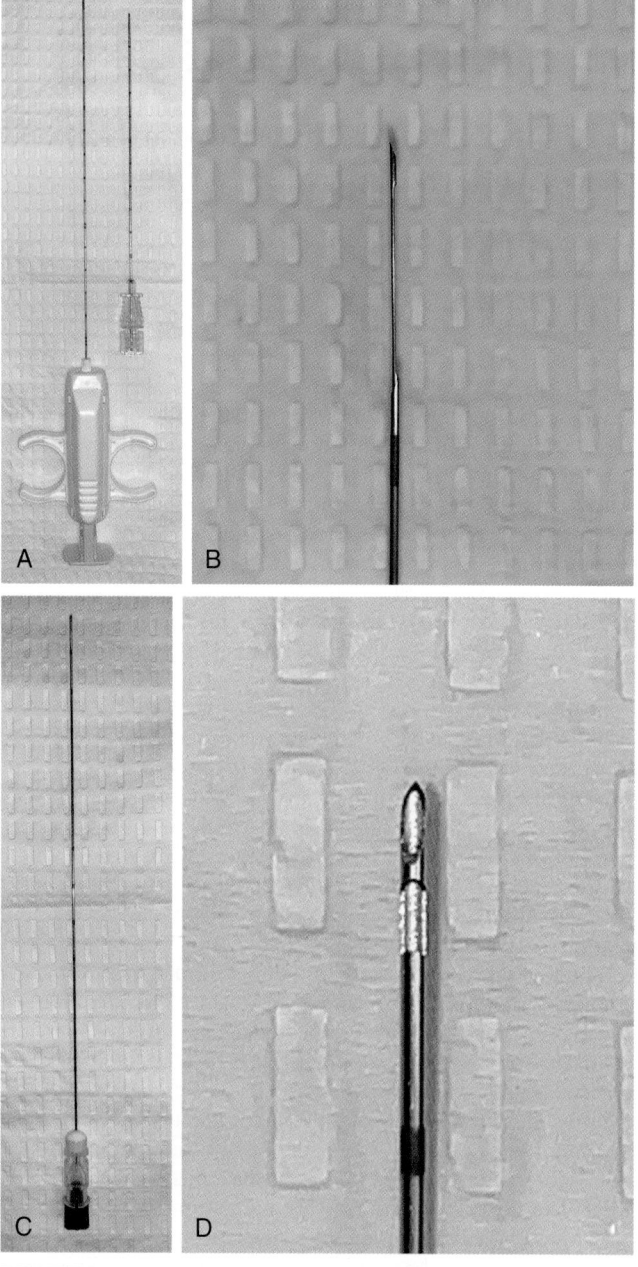

FIGURE 23.1 **Fine and core biopsy needles. A,** Panoramic view of a semi-automatic core needle biopsy gun, demonstrating the finger notches and, in this case, a retracted plunger that conceals the specimen notch. **B,** Magnified lateral view of the tip of a semi-automatic core needle biopsy gun exposing the specimen notch when the plunger is deployed. **C,** Panoramic view of a fine needle for biopsy (in this case, a Westcott-style needle with the stylet in place). **D,** Magnified anterior view of the Westcott-style needle without the inner stylet, demonstrating the beveled tip and the notch in the sidewall of the needle just proximal to the tip, which facilitates the operator's ability to choose more precisely the location from which the cells will be aspirated.

well-differentiated hepatocellular carcinoma (HCC) or nodular hyperplasia in the setting of cirrhosis and in confirmation of benign diagnoses, including hemangioma, adenoma, or focal nodular hyperplasia (FNH; see Chapter 87).[14,15]

IMAGE GUIDANCE MODALITIES

For more information, see Chapter 13–17.

Preprocedural target evaluation is crucial to adequately select the best imaging modality for a specific target lesion. Multiple imaging modalities are available. For a summary of advantages and disadvantages of each imaging modality, please refer to Table 23.1.

For many lesions that can be seen with ultrasonography (US), ultrasound is ideal for PNB. Because it is located just under the diaphragm, the liver is susceptible to respiratory motion. Smaller lesions and lesions in proximity to critical structures benefit the most from US because of the ability to visualize the needle in real-time as it is advanced from the skin into the target. Another advantage of US is the ability to image in virtually any plane, which allows the operator to plan trajectories that might be impossible using computed tomography (CT) or magnetic resonance (MR) guidance. The fact that US does not use ionizing radiation is also relevant, especially for children and pregnant patients. US has been shown to result in a shorter procedure time and a lower cost when compared with CT-guided interventions.[16] The ability to successfully and safely place a biopsy needle in a lesion is unfortunately operator-dependent and has a relatively steep learning curve. Further, US imaging is limited or impossible in air-filled/gas-filled structures, such as the lung or bowel, and the sound waves cannot penetrate bone.

CT is a common modality for guiding PNBs because it provides superb anatomic detail. IRs are very familiar with cross-sectional imaging, making it the modality of choice for deep intra-abdominal structures or for those that cannot be adequately imaged with US (i.e., lung, pancreas, adrenal glands, retroperitoneal lymph nodes, bone). Many manufacturers offer CT fluoroscopy as an option on diagnostic scanners. This produces CT images in near real time. CT fluoroscopy can expose the operator to ionizing radiation, but some physicians prefer it because of the near immediacy between needle manipulation and image availability.

Cone-beam CT (CBCT), also sometimes referred to as *C-arm CT*, uses a flat-panel x-ray detector that rotates around the patient; the x-rays are divergent, forming a cone. Images can be reconstructed in multiple planes, and three-dimensional reconstructions can be performed. The soft tissue resolution is not nearly as good as with conventional CT, but the resolution for lung and bone is adequate for biopsy guidance. Further, available biopsy path–planning and needle-navigation software may assist the operator with needle placement.[17]

MR imaging (MRI)–guided biopsy has been made possible by the advent of open-bore MRI systems that provide access to patients during imaging and the availability of nonferrous biopsy needles and monitoring equipment. The superior contrast resolution of MRI allows for the targeting of lesions that are difficult to visualize with US and noncontrast CT, and the ability of MRI to image in any plane enhances the safe targeting of lesions where access in the axial plane would be more dangerous or more difficult.[18] However, there is a limited selection of MRI-safe biopsy needles and there is considerable artifact on the MRI images; this makes biopsy of small lesions challenging.

Fluoroscopy is useful in the abdomen for guiding bile duct biopsies. Benign and malignant biliary strictures often have similar cholangiographic appearances and rarely can be distinguished based on imaging alone[19,20] (see Chapter 16 and 20).

TABLE 23.1	Commonly Used Imaging Modalities for Image-Guided Biopsy			
MODALITY	REAL TIME	COMMON TARGETS	LIMITATIONS	ADVANTAGES
Ultrasound	Yes	• Soft tissue lesions • Solid visceral organs • Omental and peritoneal lesions	• Operator dependent • Susceptible to artifacts • Unable to use in deeper lesions, some bone lesions, or gas-filled organs • Dense calcifications may obscure needle	• Multiplanar • Nonionizing radiation • Real time allows accurate targeting of mobile structures
CT	Nearly (CT fluoroscopy)	• Thoracic • Pelvic • Musculoskeletal • Retroperitoneal • Deep abdominal viscera-liver, adrenal, pancreas, omentum	• Ionizing radiation • Metal artifacts • Positioning and patient motion • Targets can only be accessed in one plane and gantry angulation is not widely available	• Requires less operator skill than ultrasound • Allows in-plane visualization of the entire path to the lesion • Allows multiplanar reconstructions (not in real time) • High resolution and contrast
Fluoroscopy	Yes	• Endoluminal biopsies, commonly brush biopsies – bile ducts, ureter • Transjugular liver, renal biopsies • Selected bone lesions	• Ionizing radiation • Not cross sectional • Two-dimensional	• Widely available • Multiplanar
X-Ray	No	Stereotactic – breast	Ionizing radiation	Visualize and sample calcifications
MR	Nearly (MR Fluoroscopy)	• Breast • Prostate • Abdominal lesions	• High cost/infrastructure required • Requires special equipment	• Nonionizing • Multiplanar • Excellent contrast and spatial resolution • Ideal for "occult" lesions not well seen using other modalities
PET-CT	No, although often used in combination with CT	• Any FDG avid target	• Susceptible to miss-registration, particular in areas with significant respiratory motion • High cost • Additional radiation exposure	• Useful for lesions that may have different components (necrosis) • Very sensitive – can show malignant changes before morphologic changes on CT

Lesions originating within the duct may be sampled by either an endoluminal or a direct percutaneous approach. Percutaneous transhepatic biliary drainage allows direct access to the biliary tract for endoluminal biopsy (see Chapter 31). Biopsy forceps or brush-biopsy catheters can be used through the existing tract to obtain tissue samples of suspicious areas. The sensitivity of forceps biopsy is in the range of 40% to 80%, higher than that of brush biopsy, which is in the range of 30% to 60%. Specificity for each approaches 98%.[12,21,22] Combining forceps and brush biopsy of the bile duct may provide superior results to either alone. Studies have noted the sensitivity of brushing alone of 49%, forceps alone of 69%, and combined of 80%; with specificity for malignancy of 100%.[23] However, a new percutaneous forceps biopsy technique cites sensitivity of 93.3%, specificity of 100%, positive predictive value of 100%, and negative predictive value of 70%, with overall accuracy of 94.2%.[24] Alternatively, after the biliary tree is opacified, a direct PNB of a bile duct lesion may be targeted with fluoroscopy, using a transhepatic approach.[25,26] After contrast injection into the indwelling biliary drainage catheter to delineate the targeted bile duct abnormality, a fine needle is advanced through the abdomen to the target and a specimen is obtained. Confirmation of accurate needle position is made by obtaining oblique fluoroscopic images and by real-time fluoroscopy, when the needle is seen to move the duct or the indwelling catheter or both. Fluoroscopy can also be used to guide nontargeted transvenous biopsies of the liver.

Occasionally, a lesion is only well demonstrated by ^{18}F-fluorodeoxyglucose (FDG) positron emission tomography (PET) imaging (see Chapter 18). In these cases, it is possible to use the combination of PET and CT to guide accurate needle placement. Certain lesions may also have varying FDG avidity; PET guidance allows the most hypermetabolic portion of a lesion to be targeted. Operators should be mindful of the patient as a source of radiation; the major source of radiation to the operator during PET-guided interventions was found to be the time spent in close proximity to the patient.[27]

New technology that requires further development into clinical practice allows for the fusion of multiple modalities. For example, CT and MRI scans can be overlaid with real-time US images to achieve the clarity of the CT or MR and the real-time visualization capabilities of US. PET images can also be fused. Additionally, robotic guidance systems have entered the market in an effort to optimize speed and accuracy for needle placement (Fig. 23.2).

PREPROCEDURE EVALUATION

With the exception of nontarget liver biopsy, all patients undergoing PNB should have preprocedural imaging. Careful evaluation of the images by an IR is mandatory for the procedure to be successful because adequate imaging will determine the proper imaging modality for guidance, patient positioning, and

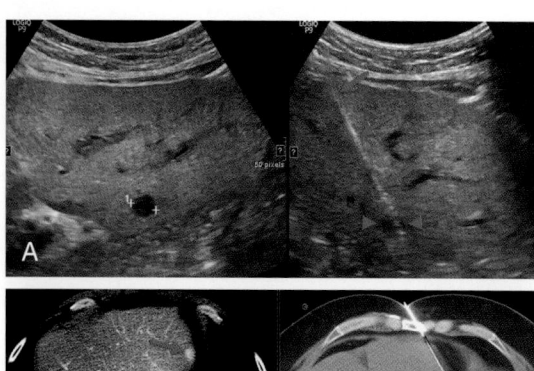

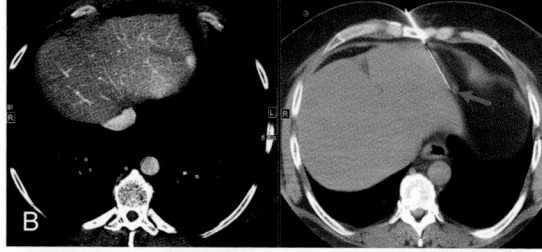

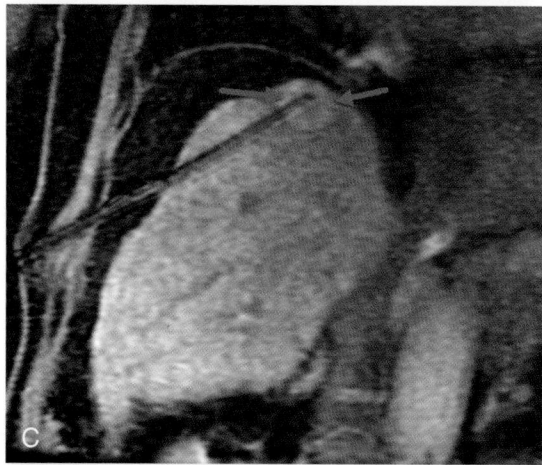

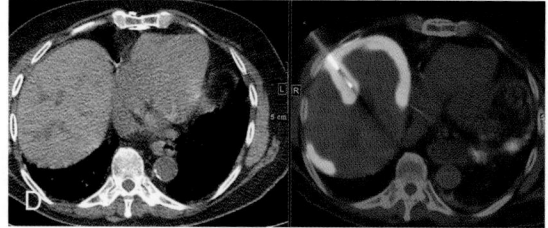

FIGURE 23.2 **Image-guided liver biopsy. A,** An 82-year-old male with a history of lymphoma was found to have a hypoechoic liver lesion not seen on computed tomography (CT; *arrowheads*). Ultrasound-guided biopsy was performed. Real-time ultrasound guidance allowed for placement of the needle *(arrows)* in a relatively avascular trajectory. **B,** A 27-year-old male with sarcoma and a solitary liver lesion *(arrow)*. CT is useful for lesions high in the liver where ultrasound is limited by interposed air or bone. **C,** A 77-year-old man with cirrhosis, hepatopulmonary syndrome, and liver lesion suggestive of hepatocellular carcinoma. Magnetic resonance (MR) guidance allows for multiplanar planning of needle paths, as in this case in which coronal imaging was used. **D,** A 74-year-old with a remote history of lymphoma and smoldering myeloma. Areas of positron emission tomography (PET) avidity in the liver were seen without CT or ultrasound correlate. PET guidance was used to perform the biopsy and confirm the diagnosis of recurrent lymphoma.

preferred access/sampling technique.[6] Main objectives for PNB may include diagnosis of the etiology of diffuse parenchymal diseases, microbiology diagnosis in infectious diseases, histologic diagnosis of a focal lesion, histologic classification of a malignancy, pathologic staging of a malignancy, or molecular diagnostic testing.

Absolute contraindications for a PNB are rare and are basically limited to lack of safe access. Relative contraindications are related to conditions that increase the risk for complications and include coagulopathy (depending on target location), inability to sedate or provide general anesthesia, and significant comorbidities.[6] Table 23.2 lists the general approach to common medication classes that should be considered before any biopsy procedure.

Liver-Specific Considerations

The indication for liver biopsy can be broadly grouped into two categories: (1) Random (nontarget) liver biopsy for diagnosis of hepatocellular disease, and (2) targeted liver biopsy for tissue diagnosis of a liver mass. With refinements in abdominal imaging, benign diseases are often confidently diagnosed on imaging alone, obviating the need for a biopsy; this is particularly helpful in cases of suspected adenomas and hemangiomas because these highly vascular lesions have a higher risk for procedural complications.

Certain locations in the liver can be more technically difficult in terms of visualizing and accessing the lesion, particularly with masses that are closer to the dome and/or more anterior. In these instances, patient cooperation with deep inspiration and/or decubitus or semirecumbent positioning can be helpful, although the need for deep inspiration in particular limits the ability to sedate the patient for the procedure, because sedated patients are typically not able to cooperate with breathing instructions. When multiple liver lesions with similar diagnostic imaging characteristics are present, the choice of which lesion to biopsy is made based on lesion visibility and location. A needle trajectory that passes through normal parenchyma before accessing the lesion is preferred to minimize the risk for hemorrhage and tract seeding.[29–31]

Focal Liver Lesions

Focal liver lesions may be solitary or multiple. For a solitary lesion, several benign conditions—cyst, hemangioma, FNH, and adenoma—often can be diagnosed confidently by high-quality cross-sectional imaging, obviating the need for biopsy[32–34] (see Chapter 14). These diagnoses should be considered in all solitary liver lesions, unless they are known to be new in the setting of a known cancer or in patients at risk for primary HCC.

HCC may also be diagnosed based on imaging and clinical criteria (see Chapter 14 and 89). According to the integrated Liver Imaging Reporting and Data System (LI-RADS) and the American Association for the Study of Liver Diseases (AASLD) and National Comprehensive Cancer Network (NCCN) guidelines, liver lesions identified on screening US that are larger than 1 cm in patients with cirrhosis or chronic hepatitis can be diagnosed as HCC based on a single CT or MRI study demonstrating classic findings of arterial enhancement and portal venous or delayed-phase washout[35,36] (see Chapter 14). When the diagnosis of HCC is considered and these criteria are not met or if patients are to be treated with systemic therapy, biopsy may be required. Smaller, encapsulated tumors are more likely to be well differentiated, and tissue cores are required to distinguish a well-differentiated tumor from normal or cirrhotic liver. Because of the risk for tumor seeding,[30,31,37] when a curative treatment is possible, biopsy for HCC should be performed only after surgical consultation and after referencing the most

TABLE 23.2 General Approach to Medications Addressed Before Percutaneous Image-Guided Needle Biopsy[28]

MEDICATION CLASS	LOW PROCEDURAL RISK	HIGH PROCEDURAL RISK	MEDICATION RESUME
Glycoprotein IIb/IIIa inhibitor	Withhold 24 hours before procedure		24 hours
Direct thrombin inhibitors	Continue	Withhold 2–4 hours before procedure and check activated partial thromboplastin time (aPTT)	4–6 hours after procedure
Direct factor Xa inhibitors	Continue	eGFR ≥30 mL/min: withhold 4 doses eGFR <30 mL/min: withhold 6 doses Emergent: Use reversal agents as appropriate (i.e., andexanet alfa).	24 hours
Nonsteroidal antiinflammatory drugs (NSAIDs)	Continue	Hold for five days if possible, minimum three days	24 hours after procedure
Parenteral direct P2Y$_{12}$ inhibitors	Defer until patient is off medication. If emergent, withhold 1 hour before procedure, discuss with cardiology	Defer until patient is off medication. If emergent, withhold one hour before procedure, discuss with cardiology	4–6 hours after procedure
Intermediate-acting NSAID	Continue	Hold morning of procedure	24 hours after procedure
Reversible phosphodiesterase II inhibitor	Continue	Continue	4–6 hours after procedure
Thienopyridines (P2Y$_{12}$ platelet inhibitors)	Continue	Withhold for five days before procedure	4–6 hours after procedure
Low molecular weight heparin	Continue	Prophylactic dose: withhold one dose Therapeutic dose: last dose 24 hours before the procedure Check anti-Xa level if renal function is impaired	12 hours after procedure
Heparin	Continue	Stop 4–6 hours before procedure.	6–8 hours after procedure
Phosphodiesterase (PDE) inhibitor	Continue	Hold morning of procedure	Resume day after procedure
Reversible adenosine diphosphate (ADP) receptor antagonist	Continue	Withhold five days before procedure	Day after procedure
Vitamin K antagonist	Do not withhold if preprocedure international normalized ratio (INR) <3. For INR >3 (mechanical heart valves), consider bridging for cases that are high risk for thrombosis	Withhold for five days. Confirm INR <1.8 preprocedure. Consider bridging for high thrombosis risk patients. If stat or emergent, use reversal agent.	Bridged patients: same day High risk for bleeding patients: resume day after procedure. High thrombosis risk cases may benefit from bridging

Adapted from Patel IJ, Rahim S, Davidson JC, et al. Society of Interventional Radiology Consensus Guidelines for the periprocedural management of thrombotic and bleeding risk in patients undergoing percutaneous image-guided interventions-part II: Recommendations: Endorsed by the Canadian Association for Interventional Radiology and the Cardiovascular and Interventional Radiological Society of Europe. *J Vasc Interv Radiol.* 2019;30(8):1168–1184.e1

current imaging and clinical criteria. The AASLD position paper on liver biopsy reinforces caution based on concern for needle-track seeding, sampling error, and possible increased rate of recurrence post-transplant in Child B or C cirrhotic patients with stage I to III tumors greater than 3 cm and α-fetoprotein greater than 200 ng/mL.[38] However, an accurate diagnosis of HCC is extremely important because confirmation of diagnosis alters the priority for liver transplantation.[39]

Multifocal solid liver lesions most commonly represent metastatic disease. In such cases, biopsy may be requested to (1) confirm the presence of metastatic disease in a patient with a known primary, (2) establish tumor type and stage simultaneously at initial presentation, (3) acquire tissue for genetic analysis, and (4) obtain required samples for patients undergoing experimental therapies.

Liver Parenchymal Biopsy

Core liver biopsy is used to grade and stage liver disease in patients with abnormal liver function studies, chronic hepatitis,

and known or suspected cirrhosis (see Chapters 68, 69, and 74). Gastroenterologists have historically performed most liver biopsies without imaging guidance; however, unusual anatomy, obesity, and other exigencies occasionally make imaging-guided biopsy advisable. Adequate tissue cores can be obtained with needles that are 20 gauge and larger, although needles 18 gauge and larger provide a more generous specimen for analysis.[40,41] It has been suggested that specimens of at least 1 cm in length are preferred.[42] Biopsy may also be performed in transplanted livers and in living donors before transplant. Indications for this last group are controversial, and it is recommended to follow the recommendations of the Vancouver Forum[43] in performing biopsy in potential donors who have a clinical or imaging-based reason to do so, but not as a matter of routine.[44]

Transvenous Liver Biopsy

Transjugular liver biopsy is a useful alternative to PNB in patients with coagulopathy or significant ascites or when hepatic venous pressure measurements are required.[45] Although transvenous

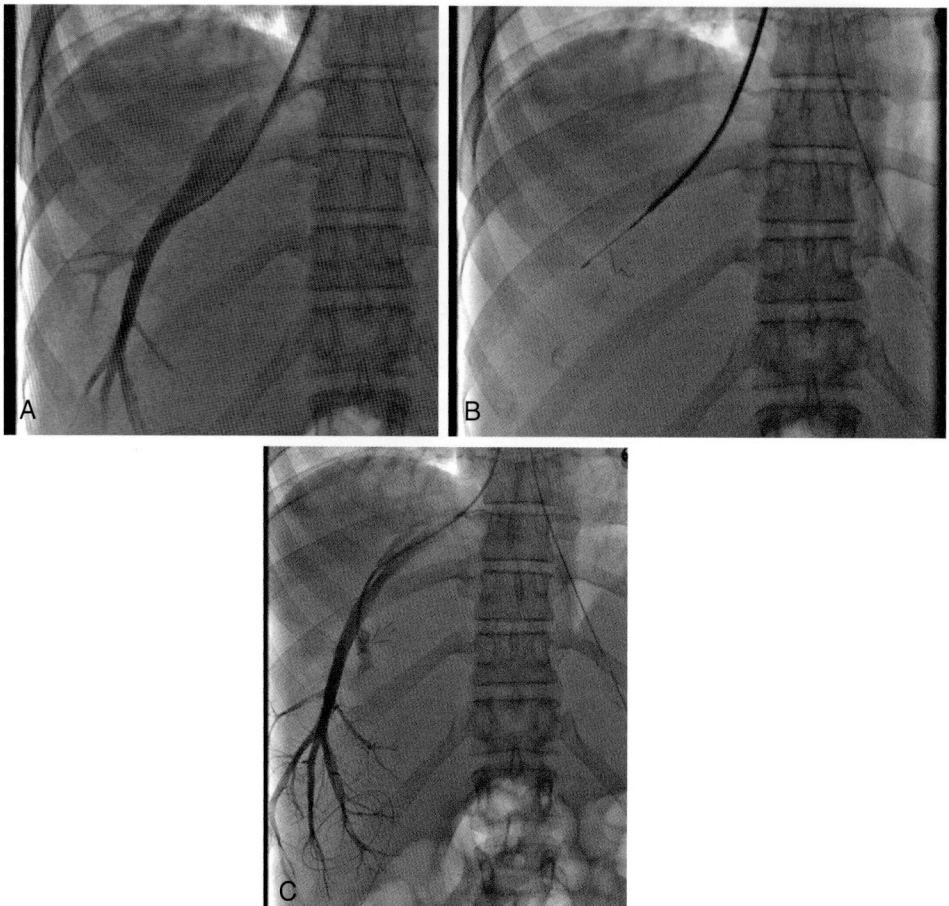

FIGURE 23.3 **Transjugular liver biopsy. A,** A right hepatic venogram is shown via a catheter placed in the right internal jugular vein in a 29-year-old female with aplastic anemia and liver failure. **B,** The trough of an 18-gauge core biopsy needle is advanced into the liver parenchyma *(arrow)*. **C,** Right hepatic venogram after biopsy shows contrast in the biopsy tract *(arrow)* and no evidence of extracapsular hemorrhage.

biopsy is seemingly more invasive than PNB, the risk for significant bleeding in patients with coagulopathy is minimized using a transvenous approach because bleeding from the biopsy site tracks back into the venous circulation and not into the abdominal cavity. Proper technique to avoid puncture of the liver capsule is crucial to optimize safety.

In this technique, a venous sheath is introduced into a hepatic vein (most commonly the right hepatic vein from a right internal jugular approach; Fig. 23.3). Pressure measurements may be obtained to evaluate the source (presinusoidal, sinusoidal, or postsinusoidal) and degree of portal hypertension. A biopsy needle is introduced through the sheath into the liver parenchyma to obtain histologic samples. Care must be taken to avoid performing the biopsy too peripherally because this increases the risk for capsular puncture and secondary intraperitoneal hemorrhage.

Transvenous biopsy is useful for nontargeted parenchymal biopsy and, in rare circumstances, for biopsy of focal lesions with or without the aid of additional imaging techniques like US.[46,47]

ASCITES. Historically, ascites has been considered a relative contraindication to liver biopsy. Some studies have suggested a higher complication rate in the presence of ascites, although

the validity of their results can be questioned because of the lack of image guidance and other co-existing confounding variables, such as coagulopathy or thrombocytopenia. Other studies have demonstrated that the presence of ascites did not result in a significant difference in the major complication rate.[48,49]

Many have advocated for ascites drainage before visceral interventions. The theoretical advantage of this approach is to allow a potential tamponade effect of the abdominal wall against the needle entry site in the liver. If a therapeutic paracentesis is being performed with a drain, some also advocate leaving the drain in place because this may help to identify a hemoperitoneum earlier, which may facilitate a prompt treatment. The utility of preprocedural drainage has not been demonstrated in the literature.

PROCEDURAL OUTCOMES AND COMPLICATIONS

Diagnostic yield for percutaneous liver biopsy ranges from 83% to 100%.[50,51] Outcomes are also influenced by size of the lesion, pathology, and the use of FNA or CNB. For example, accuracy for diagnosis of HCC has been reported to be greater than 86%, although nondiagnostic samples are more frequent in lesions smaller than 2 cm.[52,53]

Complications

Death after PNB is rare. Mortality in large series is under 0.01%, and it is more frequent in patients with cirrhosis or in those with underlying malignancy.[54] Major hemorrhage requiring transfusion or intervention ranges from 0% to 3.4%[48,55] (Fig. 23.4). Some authors advocate placing absorbable gelatin sponge (Gelfoam) pledgets in the biopsy tract, but this has not been shown definitively to decrease the risk of major bleeding.[56]

Additional risks include bleeding, pneumothorax, infection, bile leak, and needle-tract seeding of tumor. To minimize the risk of bleeding, patients should have relevant laboratory work before biopsy, including a complete blood count and coagulation profile. Although criteria differ from institution to institution and from physician to physician, a platelet count of greater than 50,000 μL and an international normalized ratio (INR) less than 1.5 are acceptable in most cases. Biopsy in thrombocytopenic patients can be performed with platelet coverage, although the decision to proceed with biopsy should be considered carefully. For patients with an elevated INR, transfusion of plasma or supplementation with vitamin K should be considered. One additional consideration is that patients with cirrhosis may have altered coagulation not accurately reflected by the INR. In these patients, measuring thromboelastography may more accurately predict the risk of bleeding and therefore inform judicious use of prophylactic blood products before biopsy. Elevated partial thromboplastin time (PTT) in patients not on heparin is usually because of circulating antiphospholipid cardiolipins and is not typically clinically significant. A test of bleeding time may be performed to evaluate the significance of an elevated PTT in select patients. It is advisable to have patients stop antiplatelet medications, if possible, to minimize the risk of bleeding; however, the risk of stopping antiplatelet therapy must be weighed against the risk of bleeding from the biopsy. Occasionally, the balance favors performing the biopsy while the patient remains on regular medication(s).

Pain out of proportion to imaging findings after liver biopsy may be because of bile peritonitis.[57,58] Care should be taken to minimize needle passes through the gallbladder, cystic duct, or dilated bile ducts. If the gallbladder is inadvertently punctured, it should be aspirated as completely as possible before removing the needle. Bile leaks resulting in discernible collections are rare after liver biopsy in the absence of downstream biliary obstruction.

Lesions in the dome of the liver sometimes require an approach for biopsy that crosses the lung base, putting patients at risk for pneumothorax. Pneumothorax occurs in approximately 30% of transthoracic procedures and requires placement of a chest tube in approximately 6% to 12% of cases. The risk of pneumothorax is typically related more to patient than technical factors, although depth of the target lesion, number of pleural surfaces transgressed, and patient positioning (e.g., prone positioning decreases the risk of pneumothorax) have been shown to affect the likelihood. Elderly patients and patients with underlying chronic obstructive pulmonary disease are more prone to pneumothorax that requires treatment.[59-61]

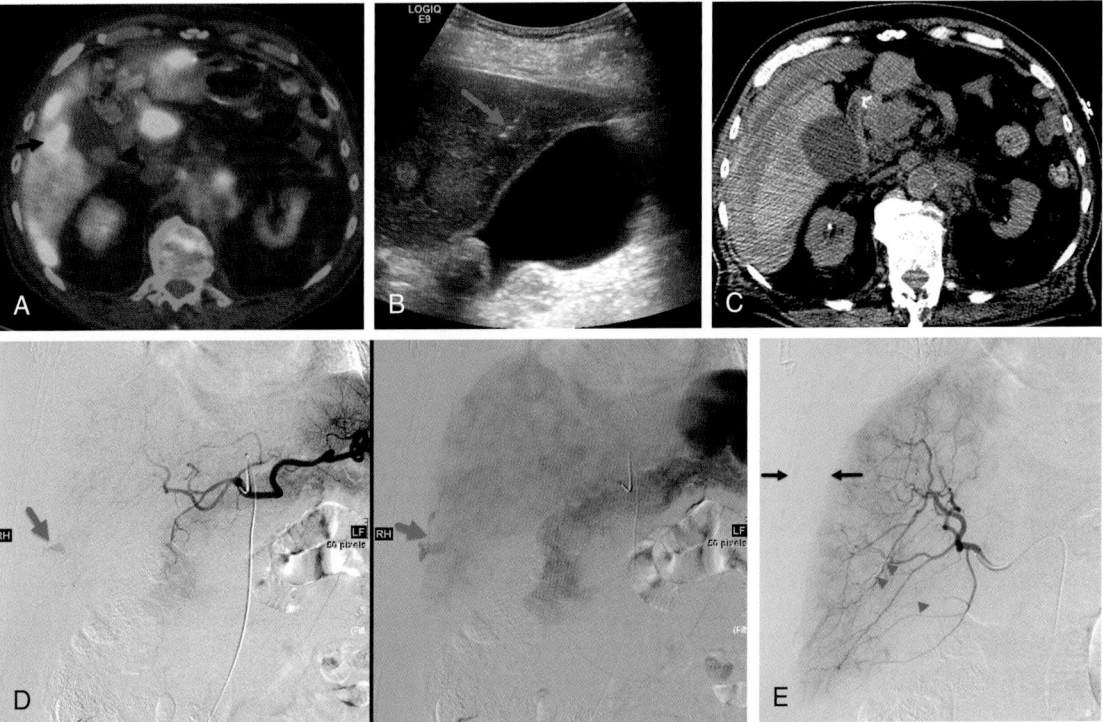

FIGURE 23.4 **Liver biopsy complicated by hemorrhage. A,** Positron emission tomography (PET) shows multiple ¹⁸F-fluorodeoxyglucose (FDG) avid liver lesions *(arrow)* in a 78-year-old male with gastric cancer. **B,** A 22-gauge FNA *(arrow)* was performed to confirm the presence of metastatic disease. The patient developed hypotension, pain, and tachycardia in the recovery room after the procedure, and **C,** a noncontrast computed tomography (CT) was performed showing acute hemoperitoneum. **D,** Celiac angiography was performed showing active extravasation from a right hepatic artery branch *(arrows).* **E,** The bleeding right hepatic artery branch was selectively catheterized and embolized with coils *(arrowheads).* Notice the gap between the liver edge and the abdominal wall because of hemoperitoneum.

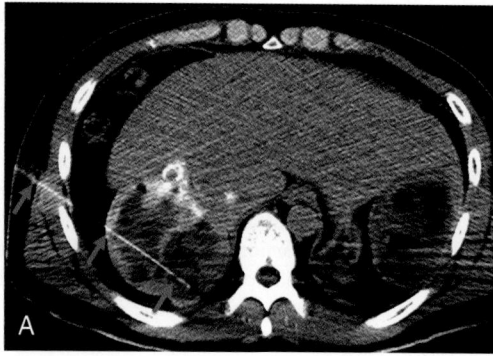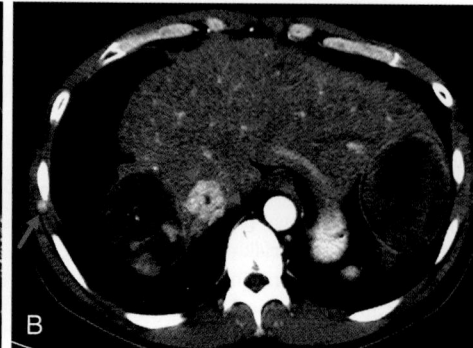

FIGURE 23.5 **Track seeding. A,** Combination embolization and ethanol ablation was performed to treat an area of residual viable tumor in a 47-year-old male with hepatocellular carcinoma (HCC). Note the path of the 20-gauge needle *(arrows)* used for ethanol ablation. **B,** 20 months later, in addition to an intrahepatic recurrence *(arrowheads)* there is evidence of track seeding in the abdominal wall *(arrow)* that was not evident on 4 interval scans.

Another feared complication is tract seeding (Fig. 23.5). Multiple studies have found an incidence of seeding ranging from 0% to 6%. Two large meta-analyses demonstrated an incidence of 2.7% and median risk of 2.29%.[29,30] High rates of tract seeding have also been suggested after liver biopsy in colorectal metastases.[62] In other large surveys of percutaneous biopsy from all sites and malignancy types published in the literature, however, the reported overall seeding rate was 0.005% to 0.009%.[63]

SAMPLE ADEQUACY AND CLINICAL IMPLICATIONS

The evaluation of sample adequacy in the setting of parenchymal liver disease is considered when the total core sample measures 20 to 25 mm long and/or allows evaluation of more than 11 complete portal tracts. The specimen adequacy in oncologic samples refers to the availability of obtaining tissue for both histopathologic and biomarker analysis.[64–67] For example, at least 50 viable cells per tissue section are needed for fluorescent *in situ* hybridization (FISH) testing, and a minimum of 200 ng of DNA (about 500 cells) is needed for genotyping. These numbers are changing rapidly because of improved sensitivity of multiple diagnostic platforms and current techniques allowing genotyping with less than 10 ng of DNA.[68] Mutational analysis requires at least 10% malignancy cell content.[68] From a practical standpoint, a 21-gauge needle aspirate can yield 100 cells and a CNB sample 500 cells.[59,69]

These pathologic biomarkers can have significant impact in diagnosis, prediction of response, and overall prognosis, allowing treatment monitoring and potentially screening of relatives. Most common pathologic biomarkers predictive of a potential response to a given intervention are further detailed in Table 23.3.

QUALITY ASSURANCE, BIOPSY LIMITATIONS, AND FUTURE DIRECTIONS

IRs are the gatekeepers tasked with evaluating relative risks and potential rewards by selecting adequate targets for biopsy. This evaluation requires expertise in assessing safety, optimal sampling technique, potential complications, and image guidance to obtain the necessary specimens for pathologic analysis. To this end, the National Institutes of Health (NIH) has issued

TABLE 23.3 Common Mutations Found in Frequent Primary and Metastatic Malignancies to the Liver and Therapeutic Implication

MALIGNANCY	MUTATIONS	TARGETED MEDICATION
Melanoma	BRAFV600E	Vemurafenib
	BRAFV600E or V600K	Dabrafenib, Trametinib, Cobimetinib
	BRAF V600X	Nivolumab
	PD-L1	Pembrolizumab
Lung cancer	EGFR	Afatinib, Erlotinib, Gefitinib
	EGFR T790M	Osimertinib
	EML4—ALK	Ceritinib, Crizotinib, Alectinib
	KRAS	Erlotinib, Gefitinib
	ROS1	Crizotinib
	PD-L1	Pembrolizumab
Breast	ESR1 and HER2-HER2	Everolimus Lapatinib Pertuzumab, Trastuzumab, Trastuzumab-emtansine
	ESR1 and PGR	Tamoxifen, Anastrozole, Exemestane, Letrozole
Gastric	HER2	Trastuzumab
GIST	c-KIT	Imatinib, Sunitinib
Pancreatic	EGFR and KRAS	Erlotinib
Colorectal	EGFR and KRAS-ESR1 and PGR and HER2-	Cetuximab, Panitumumab Palbociclib Fulvestrant
Renal	ESR1 and HER2-BRAF V600X	Everolimus Nivolumab
Ovarian	BRCA	Olaparib

several recommendations that can help improve the quality of the samples obtained for clinical trial purposes and that can be summarized under the following five premises[70]:
1. Include IR on any research proposal requiring tissue sampling.
2. Communicate with IR to establish the biopsy needs, including number of cores required, preferred tumor region to be sampled, and designated time points when sampling should be performed.
3. If safe and feasible, recommend collecting up to five cores per biopsy to allow molecular diagnostic testing.

4. Standardize the biopsy procedure as much as possible.
5. Review each case with an IR to ensure preprocedural successful planning.

Biopsy Limitations

Although biopsy is the standard of care for many pathologies, innate limitations include sampling error, the subjective nature of the interpretation, the cost of the procedure in standard of care facilities, and the associated potential complications previously described.

A biopsy is only able to evaluate a very small piece of parenchyma, which may or may not represent a diffuse process, leading to sampling error because it is well known that pathology may not affect the parenchyma uniformly.[71,72] In addition, diagnostic accuracy and disease staging is directly related to specimen size, and small biopsy samples may be nondiagnostic or may not reveal cirrhosis, even when cirrhosis is present.[73]

Biopsy interpretation is subjective. Although pathologists have well-established criteria for diagnosis and staging of multiple liver diseases, there is interobserver and intraobserver variability. For example, in one study of pathologic staging of fibrosis, interobserver and intraobserver variability was approximately 80%; however, concordance for inflammatory activity and fat content was under 50%.[74]

Cost associated with percutaneous image-guided procedures should not and cannot be ignored. Every biopsy involves an expert IR and a pathologist in addition to technologists, nurses, and, in some cases, an anesthesiologist. The average direct costs of a percutaneous liver biopsy are $1,558 (in 2016 U.S. dollars),[75,76] and this can be significantly higher for a transvenous procedure.

Future Directions

Advances in diagnostic imaging and pathology will revolutionize PNBs in the near future. Radiogenomics is a field that studies the relationship between imaging phenotypes and the underlying genetic characteristics of a tumor. Radiogenomics has the potential of determining the ideal site to biopsy or even obviate the need for tissue diagnosis[68] (see Chapters 13 and 19).

Another field that is growing at an accelerated pace within diagnostic radiology is quantitative radiology, which measures the structural and biologic parameters of medical images to obtain metrics that can provide a "virtual biopsy." These measurements can potentially determine not only disease status but also severity, treatment response, and future outcomes.[77]

Optical molecular imaging is also an emerging imaging modality that allows for characterization of tissue in real time. By using a molecular tracer in tissues, suspicious areas of any body part can potentially be biopsied or resected.[68] These tracers include the development of theranostics, such as nanoparticles, which combine both therapeutics and diagnostics in one package for image-guided therapy. This strategy has been explored in tumors, such as colorectal cancer, in which CEA, the folate receptor alpha (FRα), and the epidermal growth factor receptor (EGFR) present in tumor cells are actively being used as targets.[78]

The additional potential development of smart needles that can identify molecular characteristics of lesions confirming the ideal site for sampling is a revolutionary concept.[68] Efforts are also underway to design steerable needles that allow for greater control and maneuverability to make the path to a lesion safer.[68] All of these concepts align with the development of robotically assisted guided intervention programs.[68]

A parallel field to tissue sampling that has grown at an accelerated rate is the field of "liquid biopsy." Liquid biopsy platforms can detect circulating tumor cells (CTCs), circulating tumor DNA (ct-DNA), and microvesicles containing RNA within a peripheral venous blood sample. Obtaining a peripheral blood sample is significantly safer than even a minimally invasive biopsy. Liquid biopsy may offer an alternative evaluation of tumor burden, as well as new biomarkers that can be followed over time at a potentially lower cost. More importantly, liquid biopsy may better reflect the spectrum of heterogeneity present in any given tumor.[79,80]

CONCLUSION

PNB is a well-established and safe diagnostic tool, and it is an important instrument in the diagnosis of tumors, for determining the cause of organ dysfunction/staging, and for documenting recurrent or metastatic disease. Increasingly, needle biopsy is required to provide material for genetic analysis. Complications are infrequent, and most are easily treated or self-limiting. Tract seeding has been reported but occurs infrequently. It is important to remember that there is no such thing as a "negative" biopsy.[81] If a diagnosis of malignancy is not made, a specific benign diagnosis needs to be confirmed. If nonspecific findings are evident on cytology, including inflammatory or reactive changes, fibrous tissue, or normal site tissue, or, if atypical cells are present, either another biopsy can be performed, or the lesion should be closely followed up with imaging depending on the pretest probability of disease. The role of biopsy in patient management is evolving in tandem with the development of associated fields, including functional and molecular imaging. Until biopsies are no longer necessary, every effort should be made to keep morbidity low and diagnostic rates high.

The references for this chapter can be found online by accessing the accompanying Expert Consult website.

CHAPTER 24

Intraoperative diagnostic techniques

Ola Ahmed and M. B. Majella Doyle

OVERVIEW

The management of hepatobiliary and pancreatic disease has evolved greatly since the 1990s. Today's operative surgeon has several valuable adjuncts to aid in accurate preoperative evaluation and planning for benign and malignant disease. Advances in contrast-enhanced computed tomography (CT), endoscopic ultrasound (EUS), magnetic resonance imaging (MRI; see Chapters 13–17), and endoscopic retrograde cholangiopancreatography (ERCP; see Chapters 20 and 30) have revolutionized the treatment of benign and malignant hepatobiliary and pancreatic disease. Despite these advances in the modern era, present-day management of these conditions relies on the appropriate use of intraoperative diagnostic modalities, particularly when confronted with challenging and unanticipated findings during surgical exploration. This chapter will review the intraoperative utility of ultrasound (US), cholangiography, and laparoscopy in hepatobiliary and pancreatic surgery.

INTRAOPERATIVE ULTRASONOGRAPHY

Intraoperative US (IOUS) is commonly used during both open and laparoscopic procedures to provide accurate real-time imaging. It can be a valuable tool in the assessment of hepatic and biliary anatomy, evaluation of biliary calculi, localization of tumors, determination of the extent of and/or resectability of disease, and determination of the extent of mesenteric vascular involvement in the case of pancreatic tumors.[1]

Hepatic Disease

Evaluation of the Liver

IOUS of the liver was first introduced into clinical practice in the early 1980s and rapidly became routine practice for the management of malignant liver disease.[2–4] Early reports demonstrated the advantages of IOUS, which in some cases altered the operative management of hepatic malignancy not only by delineating the proximity major vascular and biliary structures but also by detecting hepatic tumors not revealed on preoperative imaging (Fig. 24.1). In a study of 100 consecutive patients undergoing preoperative imaging for colorectal liver metastases, contrast-enhanced and unenhanced IOUS identified an additional 47 liver nodules that were not viewed using MRI, and these new findings resulted in the modification of a previously planned procedure.[5] In a similar study of 102 patients with colorectal liver metastases, contrast-enhanced IOUS altered 22% of planned surgical procedures because of the additional diagnosis of nodules or more accurate visualization of vascular invasion.[6] The yield of IOUS is highly dependent on the type and quality of preoperative imaging obtained and although additional intraoperative findings may not influence all planned resections, it remains an integral adjunct to parenchymal assessment and operative planning.

When evaluating the liver parenchyma, the sonographer must first evaluate the extent of intrahepatic disease and then assess for vascular occlusion or invasion. Sonographic features of liver tumors vary. The surgeon should anticipate the need for assistance in the case of ambiguous or challenging lesions and communicate with radiologists preoperatively so that personnel and equipment are readily available.

The sonographer should be familiar with the characteristics of common parenchymal lesions (see Chapters 13–15). Hemangiomas are typically soft when palpated and either lack any visible flow or demonstrate minimal flow compared with the adjacent liver parenchyma. They typically appear hyperechoic with well-demarcated margins and may demonstrate posterior echo enhancement.[7] In contrast, colorectal liver metastases are usually hyperechoic or isoechoic with adjacent liver parenchyma and are frequently surrounded by an ill-defined hypoechoic rim that may give the lesion a bull's-eye or target appearance. Mucinous variant colorectal cancer metastases may contain calcification that produces acoustic shadowing. Hepatocellular carcinoma (HCC) frequently invades major vascular structures and may be associated with portal lymphadenopathy.[8]

Technical Considerations

Examination of the liver should always start with inspection of the organ and the entire peritoneal cavity followed by palpation. IOUS is then applied with increasing pressure to accurately delineate the spatial relationship of hepatic tumors to major vascular and biliary structures. Intraoperative transducers appropriate for liver surgery include high-frequency (6–10 MHz) T-shaped linear- or curvilinear-array transducers. These probes provide excellent high-resolution images and can identify lesions as small as approximately 1 to 2 mm in size at depths of penetration of approximately 10 to 12 cm. Transducers with color-flow Doppler imaging enable further discrimination of tumors and normal hepatic vasculature.

Techniques for IOUS continue to evolve, with some units now routinely performing laparoscopic IOUS. Particular attention must be given to port placement in this scenario.[9] Typically, no coupling gel is required because of the natural surface moisture of the liver. The transducer is initially held in a transverse position, and the survey of the liver begins by first identifying the confluence of the right and left portal pedicles. Next, all segmental pedicles on the right are visualized, followed by those on the left. Each hepatic vein is visualized by scanning peripherally and then by traversing toward the vena cava. Identifying the hepatic veins can be achieved by placing the transducer cranially in a midline position and angling towards the heart. The confluence of the left and middle vein has a characteristic appearance and should be observed in all sonographic examinations. Only light pressure should be applied to the liver. If the entire liver is to be scanned (e.g., to search for metastases), sequential overlapping sagittal strokes are made sweeping

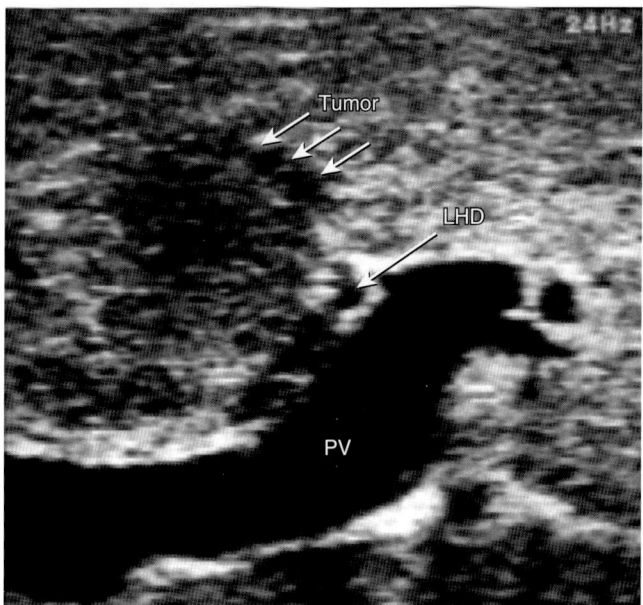

FIGURE 24.1 Intraoperative ultrasound view of a tumor *(arrows)* at the base of segment IV. The confluence of the right and left portal venous branches is shown *(PV)*. Dilation of the left hepatic duct *(LHD)* is indicated and suggests possible involvement by tumor.

from superior to inferior, beginning at the most lateral margin of segment II and traveling toward the right. More focal scanning can be used to localize impalpable lesions situated deep within the liver parenchyma. Special care must be taken when imaging the superior portion of the right liver, the posterior subdiaphragmatic bare area, and surface lesions, such as hamartomas, because these areas are particularly challenging to completely visualize. Once the lesion has been delineated and measured, photographic documentation should be obtained and saved.

The planned surgical margin of the lesion may be outlined using electrocauterization of the liver capsule because it will produce acoustic shadowing. The depth of the lesion can be estimated using its relationship to other structures or direct measurement.

Biliary Disease

Evaluation of the Biliary Tree

As laparoscopic cholecystectomy has become the standard of care for gallbladder disease, the use of laparoscopic US (LUS) during this procedure has emerged as an alternative to cholangiography (see Chapters 37 and 38). In this scenario, IOUS has a reported sensitivity and specificity over 90% for detecting choledocholithiasis and is recommended as the primary screening modality for evaluating bile duct calculi because of its safety, efficiency, and overall cost-effectiveness.[10] IOUS is at least as good as cholangiography, if not better, at detecting stones during laparoscopic cholecystectomy.[11] LUS in particular has the added advantage of reducing the risk for biliary and vascular injury. A recent systematic review compared LUS with intraoperative cholangiography (IOC) during laparoscopic cholecystectomy and found that routine LUS reduced bile duct injuries to almost 0% and resulted in a reduced procedure time when compared with IOC.[12] However, proficiency with IOUS requires

some time to develop and has a longer learning curve, which may explain why it is not used more liberally for biliary disease.

LUS is a useful adjunct for staging gallbladder carcinoma and cholangiocarcinoma (see Chapters 49–51). Sonographic findings not only reveal subtle liver metastases but also may help to define the local extent of these tumors and their relationship to the ductal system.[13,14] Doppler and color flow images may help distinguish biliary sludge from polyps and other intraluminal tumors. Other applications of LUS include evaluating biliary strictures and malignant biliary obstructions in the planning of surgical reconstructions, such as biliary bypass procedures.

Technical Considerations

The biliary tree and gallbladder are imaged best from a right subcostal port or from the periumbilical port. Sonographic examination of the gallbladder is approached through the liver by using a 5- or 7-MHz transducer. A nasogastric or orogastric tube should be placed for decompression. The bile ducts can be visualized through a compressed duodenum or gastric antrum using a 7-MHz transducer, but placing the transducer directly on the ducts should be avoided because reverberation artifact limits its sensitivity. Color flow images are helpful for distinguishing the common bile duct (CBD) from the portal vein, for identifying the insertion of cystic duct into the CBD, and for identifying any aberrant biliary anatomy during surgery.

Pancreatic Disease

Evaluation of the Pancreas

The principal application of IOUS for pancreatic disease is during staging laparoscopy (SL) in patients with pancreatic malignancy. In such cases, it can be used to further evaluate pancreatic lesions and their proximity to or invasion into vascular structures, concurrent liver metastases, and potential resectability. Approximately 20% to 35% of patients deemed initially resectable on preoperative imaging demonstrate occult metastases and/or locally invasive disease, which preclude curative resection (see Chapter 62).

Other applications for US in pancreatic surgery include localizing islet cell tumors (see Chapter 65). These particularly small lesions may be difficult to visualize or palpate in the body or tail, and sonographic images may help delineate these and other malignant or premalignant tumors in the distal portions of the pancreas.[15] In addition, US can help identify and characterize pancreatic ductal abnormalities and areas of necrosis in pancreatitis and may be useful during drainage procedures, such as cystogastrostomy (see Chapters 56 and 58).

Technical Considerations

When IOUS is performed laparoscopically, a right upper or left upper quadrant port is used to orient the probe transversely along the long axis of the pancreas. Frequently, a periumbilical port is required to image the head, neck, and uncinate process. A range of probes, most commonly "I" or "T" shaped and convex, with different forms and frequencies can be used, ranging from 7.5 MHz to 10 MHz.[16] The standard approach requires access into the retrocavity and direct contact between the probe and the pancreas. When this is difficult to achieve, the IOUS can be performed through the acoustic window of the left lobe of the liver or by pushing onto the gastric wall or overlying omentum.[16]

INTRAOPERATIVE CHOLANGIOGRAPHY

IOC is most used during elective cholecystectomy to define biliary anatomy and to assess for choledocholithiasis. It is rarely necessary or helpful in assessing the extent of biliary tumors or during hepatic resection.

Choledocholithiasis

In terms of diagnosing choledocholithiasis, IOC has a sensitivity ranging from 59% to 100% and specificity of 93% to 100%.[17] The procedure itself is highly operator dependent, and there is ongoing debate regarding its routine use during laparoscopic cholecystectomy. Most cases of choledocholithiasis are suspected on clinical grounds with elevated liver enzymes and are often visualized during preoperative US, ERCP, or magnetic resonance cholangiopancreatography (MRCP; see Chapter 16). The incidence of clinically silent choledocholithiasis is low, occurring in roughly 1 in 25 cases of biliary colic.[18,19] Even when missed during cholecystectomy, these residual stones rarely, if ever, cause symptoms or become clinically relevant. As a result, routine application of IOC for the evaluation of unsuspected choledocholithiasis may subject patients to unnecessary bile duct explorations or ERCP studies, with considerable cost to both patients and providers.[20]

Biliary Injuries

Proponents of routine IOC argue that its use can help identify and prevent bile duct injuries, a rare but major complication during laparoscopic cholecystectomy (see Chapter 36). Iatrogenic injuries are typically because of either a technical error, in which the CBD is inadvertently transected or occluded with a surgical clip, or misidentification of the duct.

The Stewart-Way classification categorizes bile duct and vascular injuries into four classes based on the mechanisms of injury.[21] Class I injuries involve an incision (i.e., an incomplete transection) of the CBD without duct loss and typically occur when the CBD is mistaken for a cystic duct but the injury is recognized before complete transection. Class II injuries represent lateral injury to the common hepatic duct. Class III injuries are the most common and represent a CBD mistaken for a cystic duct, transected and partially excised before immediate intraoperative recognition. Finally, class IV injuries occur when a right hepatic duct is mistaken for a cystic duct.

Ideally, if IOC is performed, it should be before dividing the presumed cystic duct. If cannulation of the CBD, rather than the cystic duct, occurs, the cholangiocatheter can be removed, and the ductotomy can be addressed by primary repair or by placing a T-tube, without the need for formal biliary reconstruction. A T-tube for large defects would allow the CBD to heal without stricture formation, and the tube can be removed nonoperatively several weeks after the cholecystectomy following cholangiography. The alternative scenario is complete transection of the CBD, a class III injury. In the absence of cholangiography, this transection is seldom recognized intraoperatively, typically presents postoperatively, and results in significant patient morbidity. Management requires an open bilioenteric anastomosis for repair; thus IOC has the potential to not only prevent bile duct injury but also mitigate its impact if injury does occur.

Controversies

Critics of routine cholangiography suggest that such an approach increases the risk of ductal complications (i.e., stricture) and pancreatitis, wastes time and money, and is seldom indicated if the critical view of safety is achieved (see Chapters 36 and 37). Proponents argue that routine cholangiography is a safe, accurate, quick, and cost-effective method for evaluating the bile duct.[22,23] Although we favor a selective approach, we recognize that the success of either approach is highly variable and likely to depend on each surgeon's familiarity with cholecystectomy and cholangiography. Whether selective or routine cholangiography is adopted, it is critical that surgeons develop a familiarity with the interpretation of the cholangiogram. Way et al. reported that out of 252 laparoscopic bile duct injuries, only 25% were recognized at the index operation.[21]

Technical Considerations

The critical view of safety during laparoscopic cholecystectomy is an important first step before performing IOC.[24] The gallbladder is retracted laterally, and the cystic duct and artery are dissected free and cleared of the fat and overlying peritoneum in Calot's triangle. A clip can be applied to the infundibular junction to stop the flow of contrast into the gallbladder or bile from the gallbladder during the procedure. A small incision (<50% of the duct circumference) is made in the cystic duct adjacent to the gallbladder neck. Laparoscopically, the cystic duct is best approached from a right subcostal port or from the periumbilical port (we prefer the former). A 60-cm, tapered 5-Fr cholangiocatheter is then advanced directly into the cystic duct through the ductotomy. A specialized cholangiogram clamp, often termed an *Olsen cholangiogram clamp,* or clip secures the catheter in place. In the open setting, the cholangiocatheter can be secured using a silk ligature. Alternatively, a percutaneous method may be used, where access to the cystic duct is achieved via a separate puncture in the abdominal wall by using at least a 2-inch, 14-gauge needle. A 5-Fr cholangiocatheter is guided through this needle and directly into the cystic duct. Regardless of approach, the catheter is first flushed with saline to confirm its patency, then radiographic contrast is infused, and fluoroscopic images are obtained. A complete study demonstrates flow of contrast into the duodenum and shows opacification of both the right and left hepatic ducts.

STAGING LAPAROSCOPY

Hepatobiliary and pancreatic malignancies are often very aggressive, and despite refinements in several preoperative diagnostic modalities, occult disease missed on imaging is discovered at the time of operative intervention in 20% to 25% of patients. In this setting, SL can clarify resectability, identify metastatic disease, and help specialty surgeons tailor curative and palliative operations for patients with hepatobiliary and pancreatic malignancies (Box 24.1). Controversy still exists,

---

BOX 24.1 Benefits of Laparoscopic Staging

Avoids unnecessary exploratory laparotomy
Excludes unnecessary chemotherapy/chemoradiation in patients with imaging occult metastatic disease
Shorter time to initiation of adjuvant therapy
Allows appropriate patient selection of those with locally advanced disease
Decreased procedure-related morbidity
Reduced hospital cost

however, and some critics may argue the procedure is of limited benefit in an era of more effective and high-quality preoperative imaging. The benefits of SL include shorter recovery, decreased hospital stay, decreased morbidity, improved quality of life, shorter time to initiation of adjuvant therapy, and reduced hospital costs. Disadvantages include increased potential morbidity, increased operating room times and costs, and potential port-site seeding (Box 24.2).

Surgical Technique

Technical Considerations

SL is typically performed under general anesthesia. The patient is placed supine on the operating table and fully prepared as for laparotomy. The abdomen is marked for the intended open incision, which is traditionally a bilateral subcostal incision two to three fingerbreadths below the costal margin. In the case of pancreatic disease, access to the peritoneum is made through a 1-cm subumbilical incision; for hepatobiliary cases, a 1-cm incision is made along the midclavicular line. For both, the fascia and peritoneum are incised under direct vision, a blunt 5- or 10-mm port is placed, and insufflation is begun with the initial flow rate set at 2 L/min and gradually increased to 15 L/min to achieve an intra-abdominal pressure of 10 to 14 mm Hg.

We use a 5- or 10-mm, 30-degree angled telescope to inspect the abdomen. Although we prefer a multiport technique to facilitate obtaining biopsy specimens and LUS, a single-port approach is also described. Two more ports are placed under direct vision, in the left and right upper quadrants. For pancreatic cases, another 5-mm port is inserted along the incision line to the right of the midline (Fig. 24.2). The peritoneal cavity is systematically assessed and adhesions are divided to facilitate adequate inspection of the abdominal viscera and peritoneum. All four quadrants are examined for evidence of peritoneal deposits; biopsies are taken of any suspicious lesions using standard biopsy forceps, and samples are sent for histologic examination (Fig. 24.3). If clinically indicated, peritoneal cytology can be sampled at this time by instilling 200 mL of warm normal saline into the peritoneal cavity followed by gentle agitation. The irrigant is aspirated from the right and left subhepatic spaces and from the pelvis, and a sample is sent for cytologic examination.

Once the peritoneum is inspected, attention is turned to the anterior and posterior surfaces of the left lateral segment of the liver and the anterior and inferior surfaces of the right lobe (Fig. 24.4). Next, the hepatoduodenal ligament, the foramen of Winslow, and hilum of the liver are examined for lymphadenopathy (Fig. 24.5). Any suspicious nodes are excised and sent for pathology analysis. The patient is then placed in the 10-degree Trendelenburg position, and the omentum is retracted into the left upper quadrant. The ligament of Treitz and inferior surface of the transverse mesocolon are inspected for metastatic deposits and lymphadenopathy (Fig. 24.6).

The operating table is then leveled and the left lateral segment of the liver is elevated superiorly with a retractor via the

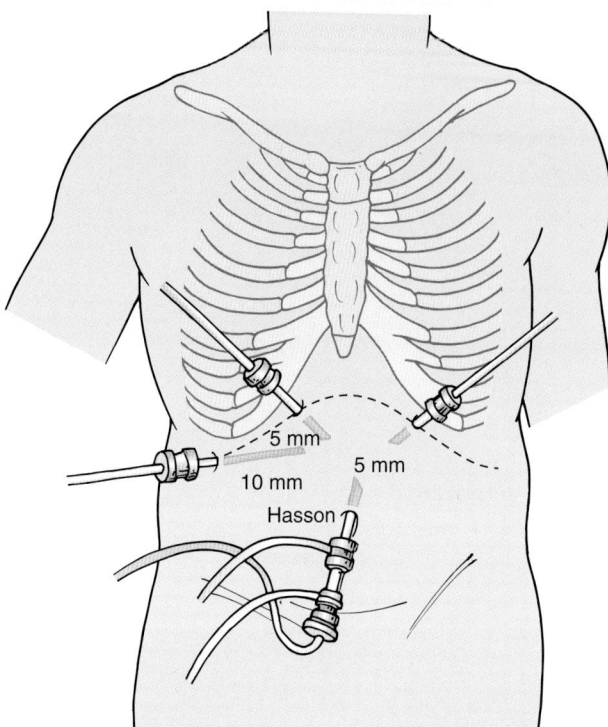

FIGURE 24.2 Port placement for laparoscopic staging. For patients undergoing staging for hepatobiliary diseases, the camera may be placed along the line of a subcostal incision.

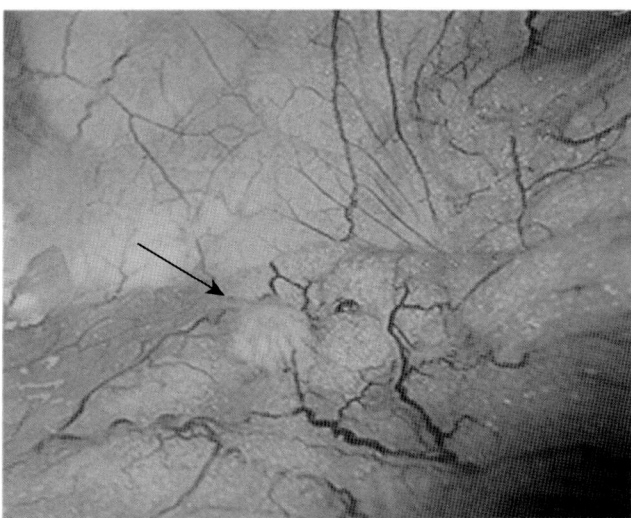

FIGURE 24.3 Peritoneal nodule. *Arrow* indicates a metastatic deposit, which can be sampled easily using a cup forceps to obtain a biopsy.

left upper quadrant port. The lesser omentum is opened to visualize the caudate lobe of the liver and the vena cava. Care should be taken to evaluate for, and avoid damage to, aberrant left hepatic arterial anatomy. From this vantage point, the anterior aspect of the head of the pancreas, posterior wall of the stomach, and "gastric pillar," which contains the left gastric artery and vein, can be seen (Fig. 24.7). The left gastric artery can be followed to its origin to allow inspection of the celiac axis (Box 24.3).

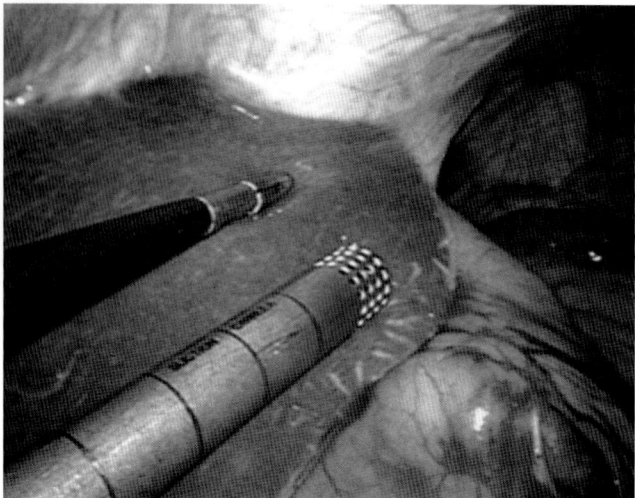

FIGURE 24.4 Examination of the liver. A blunt 10-mm instrument is used in conjunction with a 5-mm grasper.

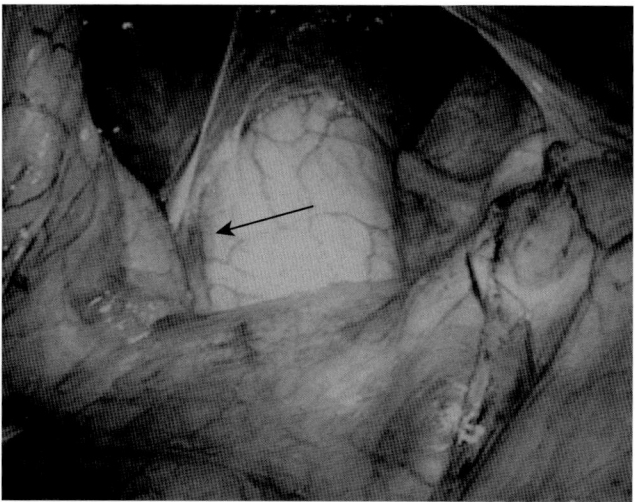

FIGURE 24.5 The hepatoduodenal ligament can be examined from the left (shown) or right side. Periportal adenopathy *(arrow)* is shown.

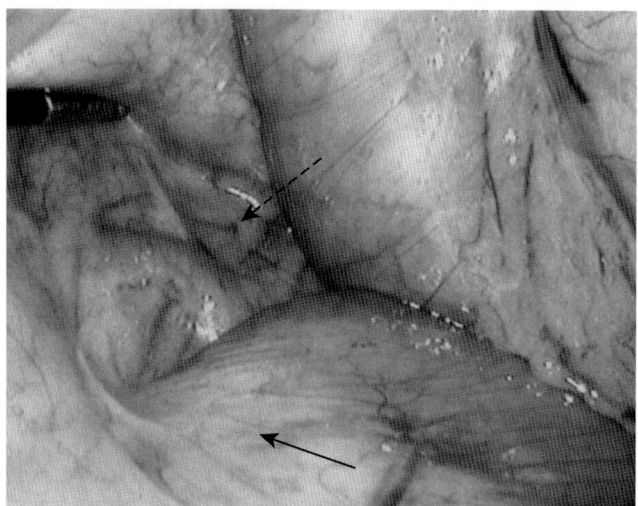

FIGURE 24.6 Examination of the ligament of Treitz. Proximal jejunum *(solid arrow)* and inferior mesenteric vein *(dashed arrow)* are shown.

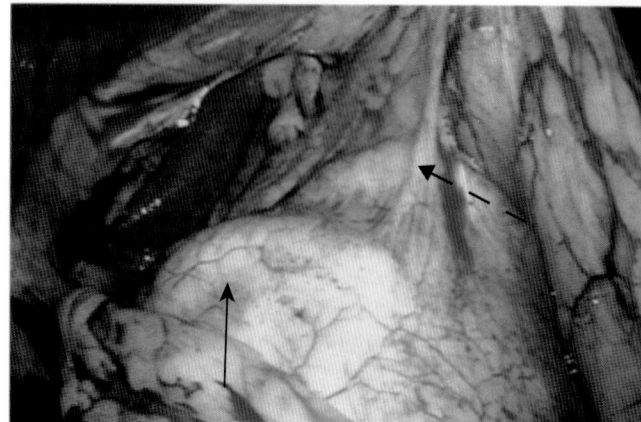

FIGURE 24.7 Lesser sac. The "gastric pillar" *(dashed arrow)* and hepatic artery *(solid arrow)* are shown.

BOX 24.3 Steps for Staging Laparoscopy

Examination of peritoneal cavity
Placement of laparoscopic trocars
Instillation of 200 mL of normal saline and aspiration of cytologic specimens
Assessment of primary tumor
Examination of the liver and porta hepatis
Division of gastrohepatic omentum and examination of caudate lobe, vena cava, celiac axis, and lesser sac
Identification of the ligament of Treitz and inspection of the mesocolon, duodenum, and jejunum
Laparoscopic ultrasound

From Conlon KC, Brennan MF. *Laparoscopy for staging abdominal malignancies.* Mosby: 2000.[25]

LAPAROSCOPIC ULTRASOUND

US can be used as an adjunct in diagnostic laparoscopy. A systematic examination of the liver, biliary tree, and pancreas takes place as previously described. A 6- to 10-MHz T-shaped linear- or curvilinear-array transducer is placed over the left lateral segment to assess segments I, II, and III. The probe is moved to the right liver and placed on the dome of the liver. The vena cava is visualized posteriorly, and the hepatic and portal veins are seen as the probe is moved anteriorly.

Placement of the probe in the transverse direction over the hepatoduodenal ligament allows the common hepatic duct, CBD, hepatic arteries, and portal vein to be visualized (Fig. 24.8). Similarly, at the confluence of the portal vein, the splenic and superior mesenteric veins can be identified. Finally, the superior mesenteric artery is delineated, and its relationship to any pancreatic tumor is assessed. The probe is placed on the gastrocolic omentum and advanced first caudally and then through the window in the gastrohepatic omentum. LUS can help facilitate pathology biopsies and needle aspirations of any suspicious lesions (Fig. 24.9; Box 24.4).

Complications

Morbidity associated with SL is uncommon, occurring in only 1% to 2% of cases. Major complications are similar to those for other laparoscopic procedures and include hemorrhage, visceral perforation, and infection. A misconception is that

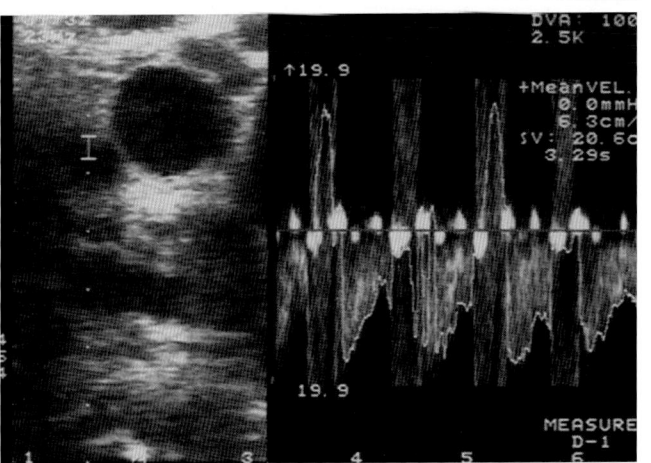

FIGURE 24.8 Laparoscopic ultrasound of the hepatoduodenal ligament. Doppler capability facilitates identification of the hepatic artery.

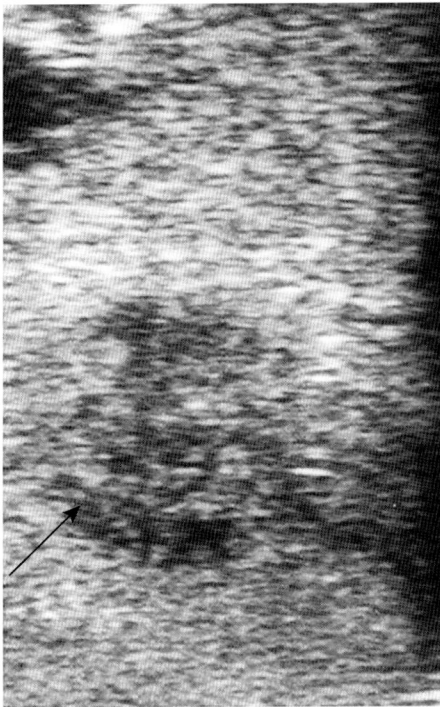

FIGURE 24.9 Hepatic metastasis *(arrow)* in a patient with pancreatic adenocarcinoma.

BOX 24.4   Steps for Laparoscopic Ultrasound
Insertion of laparoscopic ultrasound probe
Examination of liver: left lateral segment, right lobe
Transverse scan of hepatoduodenal ligament
Identification of superior mesenteric artery, portal vein, splenic vein
Examination of pancreas
Assessment of tumor

From Minnard EA, Conlon KC, Hoos A, et al. Laparoscopic ultrasound enhances standard laparoscopy in the staging of pancreatic cancer. *Ann Surg.* 1998;228:182–187.[26]

suspected malignancy precludes SL examination. An additional concern of laparoscopic intervention is port site tumor implantation. In an early study of 1650 laparoscopies for upper gastrointestinal malignancy, port site implantation occurred in 0.79%

of patients at a median 8.2 months postoperatively.[27] The findings of this study further suggested that recurrence is a marker of more advanced disease rather than being an event resulting from the laparoscopy. Overall, Shoup et al. concluded that SL can be performed safely in the setting of presumed malignancy and others have demonstrated that the incidence of port-site recurrence (3%) is equivalent to that of open wound recurrence in patients who had an exploratory laparotomy alone (3.9%).[28,29]

STAGING LAPAROSCOPY FOR POTENTIALLY RESECTABLE DISEASE

Hepatobiliary Malignancy

Determining the resectability of hepatobiliary malignancy begins with CT or MRI; however, laparoscopy can play an effective role in detecting occult disease and spare open curative resections in the presence of advanced metastatic disease. In addition to the quality of preoperative imaging, the yield of laparoscopy depends on the underlying disease and can range from 16% to 57%.[30] For example, hilar cholangiocarcinoma infrequently gives rise to peritoneal disease; however, it is often unresectable because of local tumor extension and/or vascular involvement, which is difficult to determine laparoscopically. The yield of laparoscopy is therefore lower than for other diagnoses, such as gallbladder cancer, which frequently results in peritoneal disease (see Chapter 51).

In patients with HCC, laparoscopy can be used to evaluate for cirrhosis and aid in determining resectability (see Chapter 89). In a study of 60 patients with HCC who underwent SL, approximately 30% of patients were spared nontherapeutic laparotomy.[31] In a prospective analysis of 401 patients with potentially resectable hepatobiliary malignancy, unresectable disease was discovered at the time of laparoscopy in 84 cases and 69 patients had unresectable disease identified during open exploration, for an overall false-negative rate of 22%.[32] In total, SL spared 1 in 5 patients a laparotomy while also reducing hospital stay and morbidity.

Laparoscopy is most accurate for identifying peritoneal deposits (80% accuracy) and hepatic disease (63% accuracy) and is least accurate for identifying nodal metastases (7% accuracy) and vascular invasion (18% accuracy).[32] Factors that can improve the yield of laparoscopy include the surgeon's preoperative judgment regarding the likelihood of resectability, the completeness of laparoscopic staging examinations, the addition of LUS, and the primary diagnosis. The yield was highest with gallbladder adenocarcinoma and cholangiocarcinoma and lowest with colorectal metastases.

Laparoscopic staging can be used in the evaluation of colorectal metastases (see Chapter 90). Approximately one half of all patients with new diagnoses of colorectal cancer will subsequently develop liver metastases, yet only 20% are candidates for curative hepatic resection. Most authors agree that hepatic cirrhosis, extrahepatic tumor spread, and significant bilobar disease are relative contraindications for hepatic resection. However, in patients with known colorectal cancer and liver metastases, evidence for its routine use has not been conclusively established and is reported to add limited additional value.[33,34] In a large series of 274 patients with colorectal metastases undergoing open hepatectomy, unresectable disease was found in 12 patients (4.4%) patients at the time of surgery. The authors suggest that unresectability could have been determined in

5 patients with laparoscopy; however, route SL is still not encouraged.[35]

In an effort to improve the yield of SL for hepatic colorectal metastases, a study used a clinical risk score (CRS) to try to determine which patients are more likely to have disease that is occult on preoperative imaging. The CRS uses five clinical parameters; each is shown as an independent predictor of outcome after resection and each criterion is assigned 1 point. Forty-two percent of patients with a CRS greater than 2 had unresectable disease detected at laparoscopy versus none of the patients with CRSs of 0 to 1 (Box 24.5).[36] The score was later validated in a study of 200 patients with colorectal metastases who underwent SL and had the benefit of predicting the likelihood of finding incurable disease ($P < .001$) and determining curability ($P < .001$).[37] Laparoscopy did not change the management of any patient with a CRS of 0 or 1; however, it did alter the course of patients with a score of 2 to 3 (18/129 patients affected) and a score of 4 to 5 (21/40 patients affected). Using such a risk scoring system to help guide the addition of laparoscopy to higher-risk patients could improve the overall yield from laparoscopy.

Pancreatic and Periampullary Malignancy

Our approach for staging pancreatic adenocarcinoma is illustrated in Fig. 24.10. A minority of patients with pancreatic and periampullary malignancies (see Chapter 62) are suitable candidates for curative resection. Similar to the management of other hepatobiliary malignancies, initial diagnostic evaluation begins with high-resolution contrast-enhanced CT. Imaging studies can predict resectability in 57% to 88% of cases.[38] Other useful imaging modalities that may augment CT evaluations include MRI, ERCP, EUS, and positron-emission tomography (PET). However, sub-centimeter metastases on the surface of the liver or peritoneal cavity are not always evident on CT, MRI, or PET scanning and may be picked up laparoscopically.

The Society of Surgical Oncology guidelines from the 2009 consensus statement regarding the pretreatment assessment of pancreatic cancer state the following regarding the use of laparoscopy:

1. For apparent resectable pancreatic cancer, SL should be used selectively on the basis of clinical parameters that optimize yield. These include pancreas head tumors of greater than 3 cm, tumors of the pancreas body and tail, equivocal findings on a CT scan, and high cancer antigen 19-9 levels (>100 U/mL).
2. For locally advanced unresectable pancreatic cancer without radiographic evidence of distant metastasis, SL may be used to rule out subclinical metastatic disease to optimize treatment selection.

A recent Cochrane review included 16 studies and a total of 1146 patients in a meta-analysis to determine the role of SL after CT in pancreatic and periampullary cancers.[39] The study concluded that laparoscopy may decrease the rate of unnecessary laparotomies in patients with resectable disease on CT scanning by avoiding 21 unnecessary laparotomies in 100 people for which a curative resection was planned. These findings demonstrate that, despite refinements in imaging techniques, peritoneal disease is not easily revealed on CT.

As imaging has improved, the yield of laparoscopy has been challenged. In 1996, Conlon et al. reported the Memorial Sloan Kettering experience. In a review of 115 patients between the

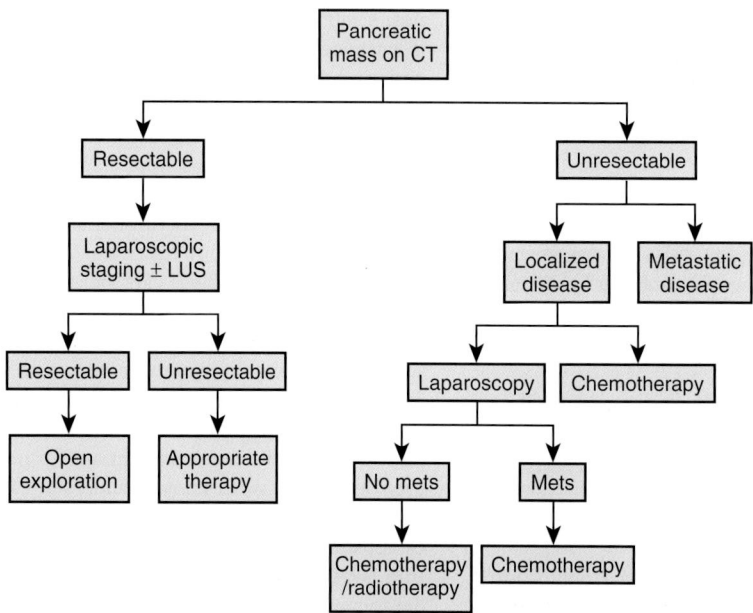

FIGURE 24.10 Use of laparoscopic staging in the management of adenocarcinoma of the pancreas. *CT,* Computed tomography; *mets,* metastases; *LUS,* laparoscopic ultrasound.

BOX 24.6 Criteria for Unresectability in Pancreatic Cancer

Histologically confirmed hepatic, serosal, peritoneal, or omental
metastases
Tumor extension outside pancreas
Celiac or high portal node involvement confirmed by frozen section
Extensive portal vein involvement by tumor or invasion/encasement
of celiac axis, hepatic artery, or superior mesenteric artery

Data from Conlon KC, Brennan MF. *Laparoscopy for staging abdominal malignancies.*
Mosby: 2000; and Conlon KC, Minnard EA. The value of laparoscopic staging in upper gastrointestinal malignancy. *Oncologist* 1997;2:10–17.

---

years of 1992 and 1994 deemed resectable based on imaging, 38% had findings at the time of SL that precluded resection (Box 24.6).[40] However, in an updated review of their experience, the yield of the procedure has decreased. In a review of 1045 patients with imaging-determined pancreatic and peripancreatic tumors, 12% of patients with pancreatic tumors had findings on diagnostic laparoscopy that precluded resection. The yield was greater for patients diagnosed with pancreatic adenocarcinoma and less for patients with tumors of the ampulla, distal bile duct, duodenum, and neuroendocrine tumors. The decrease in sensitivity between the time periods is likely in part because of the improvement in preoperative imaging with the addition of MDCT scanners and thin-slice imaging.[41]

In addition to the benefits related to recovery from laparoscopy, several authors have found that the laparoscopic approach to staging may be superior to open exploration for the detection of occult metastases. Contreras et al. determined that within a 4-year period, occult metastases among 52 patients with potentially resectable pancreatic tumors were more likely to be detected during SL when compared with open explorations (32% vs. 18%).[42] Other centers have reported similar results, as detailed in Table 24.1.

LUS may further increase the sensitivity of SL; however, it can be technically demanding, and it is unclear if many centers routinely use this adjunct. In an early study of pancreatic tumor staging with laparoscopy and LUS, John and colleagues demonstrated that additional staging information and a change to the initial decision of resectability was provided when LUS was utilized.[49] A study of 50 patients similarly reported 96% specificity and 92% sensitivity when laparoscopic US was combined with SL.[50] Vollmer et al. studied 72 patients with pancreatic head cancers and found that 22 patients had metastatic disease that precluded resection; laparoscopy alone identified 14 of these 22 patients; the remaining 8 patients had major vessel encasement or liver metastases revealed by LUS.[45] Similarly, in a prospective study of 90 patients, LUS altered the planned surgical treatment in 14% of patients, whose SL procedures were equivocal.[26] Sonography was particularly useful in identifying venous (42%) and arterial (38%) involvement, which precludes curative resection.

TABLE 24.1 Reviews on Staging Laparoscopy for Pancreatic Cancer

REFERENCE	N	NO. RESECTABLE ON CT	NO. RESECTABLE ON CT BUT UNRESECTABLE AT LAPAROSCOPY	LAPAROSCOPY CHANGED OPERATIVE PLAN (%)
Reddy et al., 1999[43]	109	99	29	29
Jimenez et al., 2000[44]	125	70	39	31
Conlon & Brennan, 2000[25]	577	577	211	36
Vollmer et al., 2002[a45]	72	72	22	31
Doran et al., 2004[46]	305	190	28	15
Contreras et al., 2009[42b]	58	58	18	31
Mayo et al., 2009[47b]	86	86	24	28
White et al., 2008[48]	1045	1045	145	14

[a]Excluding ampullary malignancies.
[b]Pancreatic adenocarcinoma only (including head and body/tail).
CT, Computed tomography.

Controversies

Some critics of routine SL believe that unresectable disease caused by vascular involvement or local extension can only be confirmed during open explorations.[51] Others suggest that the role for laparoscopy is limited only to those patients who do not require some form of palliation, either biliary or gastric bypass.[52] This is determined in part by the type of malignancy.[45] SL has not been shown to be useful among patients with ampullary or duodenal tumors because these cancers tend to present earlier and are less likely to have metastatic disease at the time of presentation. The relative yield of diagnostic laparoscopy may be lower at centers that have an aggressive palliative surgical approach, whereas even if a disease is unresectable, laparotomy is performed regardless for palliative intervention with bypass. Finally, some argue that SL is costly, time consuming, and of decreasing diagnostic yield because of improvements in radiologic imaging techniques.[53,54]

The references for this chapter can be found online by accessing the accompanying Expert Consult website.

PART 3

Anesthetic Management, Pre- and Postoperative Care

CHAPTER 25

Liver and pancreatic surgery: Intraoperative management

Mary Fischer, Vittoria Arslan-Carlon, and Jose Melendez

OVERVIEW

Improvements in patient selection criteria, advances in hepatopancreatobiliary (HPB) surgical techniques, and perioperative care have enabled increasing numbers of older and previously deemed inoperable patients to undergo HPB surgery. Despite this increase in comorbidities, recent studies have documented the progressive safety of liver[1-4] and pancreas surgery[5-7]; nonetheless, morbidity remains significant even at tertiary care centers.[4,5,8-12] This chapter addresses the unique perioperative anesthetic considerations of patients undergoing HPB operations, with emphasis on the role of the anesthesia care provider (ACP) to improve morbidity.

PREOPERATIVE EVALUATION

Risk and Outcome Improvement

Components for the ACP to consider that influence postoperative morbidity include, but are not limited to, comorbid medical conditions, perioperative care to modify risk, and the ability to rescue should an adverse event occur. Identifying patients at increased risk of a poor outcome before surgery remains challenging, and what the anesthesiologist can do to improve perioperative outcome is not always obvious (see Chapter 27).

There are several scoring systems to assist clinical risk assessment. By entering data into a multivariable prediction model, an individualized patient risk score for certain morbidities and mortality can be included to guide surgical planning and informed consent.[13] Surgical risk prediction models, such as the Physiological and Severity Score for the Enumeration of Mortality and Morbidity (POSSUM), are not always based solely on preoperative data, nor are they procedure specific, and they are complex to use.[14] Anesthesiologists prefer a less complicated risk score, such as the American Society of Anesthesiologists' Physical Status Score (Table 25.1),[15] which scores a patient on a scale that other patients may be compared, not the individualized risk prediction of an adverse outcome.[16] However, even if the anesthesiologist knows the risk prediction or risk score, it may not be apparent which anesthesia management factors are independent risk factors for perioperative morbidity and amenable to preventive measures to improve outcome. Another option is to use a biomarker, such as plasma B-type natriuretic peptide concentrations, to predict complications; however, there is no biomarker specific to HPB surgery.[17] No scoring system provides a clear identification of which elective surgery should proceed safely, and risk scores must be viewed in their clinical context.

Anesthetic management can be a Sophie's choice: modifying one component to prevent a complication that leads to increasing risk by a different pathway. Anesthetic care, like all of life, has risk, and this risk is determined by the preoperative presence of one or more comorbidities that significantly augment the incidence of postoperative adverse events. A key component of complications after surgery is the failure to recognize the patients at risk so that appropriate assessments occur before surgery.[18] Because anesthesia care is facilitative rather than therapeutic, the main outcome of anesthesia care has been traditionally measured in terms of absence of "complications." Today it is rare for a patient to develop complications due directly to the act of anesthesia, yet anesthesia clinical decisions may impact the perioperative outcome. Given that anesthetic drugs are short-acting, it is not obvious that consequences of anesthetic management could last more than hours or days after surgery. There is arguably a shift toward avoiding anesthesia-related harm after surgery, such as the maintenance of normothermia, antibiotic dosing and glucose control (prevention of surgical site infection), thromboprophylaxis and β-blockade or prescribing target-controlled fluid management, opioid-sparing analgesia, or up-to-date intraoperative ventilation. The choices we make in the operating room may have an impact not only during the case, or in the immediate postoperative time, but long after the patient is discharged from the postanesthesia care unit (PACU).[19]

The occurrence of a 30-day postoperative complication is more important than the preoperative patient risk and intraoperative factors in determining the survival after surgery.[20] Postoperative morbidity has been shown to adversely affect long-term outcome after HPB surgery; therefore efforts aimed at reducing perioperative morbidity will not only reduce usage of resources but will likely further enhance the therapeutic benefit of resection.[21-24] Given the impact of anesthesia intervention on long-term postoperative outcomes and costs, a natural evolution of the Michigan Surgical Quality Collaborative has been to expand the data collection and collaboration efforts to include the anesthesiology provider and process. The Multicenter Perioperative Outcomes Group (MPOG) has built a comprehensive perioperative patient registry based on electronic healthcare data. Preoperative and intraoperative data are collected and used to identify variations in anesthetic care and optimal care patterns.[25] The data collected are used as a foundation of collaboration between surgeons and anesthesiologists to establish process of care and outcome measures to recommend best practice clinical standards where prospective effectiveness trials may be absent.

Although it is not possible to alter all risk factors, such as age, or avoid every potential consequence, such as pain, there are modifiable risk factors. Detailed evaluation and correction of all modifiable risk factors combined with best practice guidelines are our best choices to help avoid the most preventable

TABLE 25.1 American Society of Anesthesiologists' Physical Status Score (ASA-PS)

ASA CLASSIFICATION		EXAMPLES
ASA I	A normal healthy patient	Healthy; no smoking; no or very minimal drinking
ASA II	A patient with mild systemic disease	Smoker; more than minimal drinking; pregnancy; obesity; well-controlled diabetes; well-controlled hypertension; mild lung disease
ASA III	A patient with severe systemic disease, not incapacitating	Diabetes, poorly controlled hypertension; distant history of MI, CVA, TIA, cardiac stent; COPD; ESRD; dialysis; active hepatitis; implanted pacemaker; ejection fraction below 40%; congenital metabolic abnormalities
ASA IV	A patient with severe systemic disease that is a constant threat to life	Recent history of MI, CVA, TIA, cardiac stent; ongoing cardiac ischemia or severe valve dysfunction; implanted ICD; ejection fraction below 25%
ASA V	A moribund patient who is not expected to survive without the operation	Ruptured abdominal or thoracic aneurysm; intracranial bleed with mass effect; ischemic bowel in the face of significant cardiac pathology
ASA VI	A patient who has already been declared brain-dead and whose organs are being removed for transplant	

Note: The addition of an "E" indicates emergency surgery.

COPD, Chronic obstructive pulmonary disease; *CVA,* cerebrovascular accident; *ESRD,* end-stage renal disease; *ICD,* internal cardiac defibrillator; *MI,* myocardial infarction; *TIA,* transient ischemic attack.

complications. Before undergoing surgery, optimization of chronic medical conditions is of critical importance. Hyperglycemia should prompt evaluation of glycemic control including fasting glucose and HgbA1c levels. Uncontrolled diabetes has been associated with adverse postoperative outcomes including wound infections or organ space infection.[26] Chronic cardiopulmonary comorbidities may require preoperative intervention and even modification of intraoperative approach. Functional status workup may identify correctable deficits that can be addressed preoperatively with physical conditioning, nutritional counseling, blood glucose control, and smoking cessation. To decrease patient anxiety, any complete preoperative evaluation of a patient undergoing HPB surgery should include extensive, preoperative education including education material and the opportunity to ask questions of the multidisciplinary team. Medical guidelines have rapid turnover, with medical reversal a reality, and staying current to apply evidence-based practice is recognizing that the correct "scientific answer" may shift over time.[27,28] Not only is the patient population becoming older with ever-expanding comorbidities, but improvements in the medical management of some chronic illnesses mean that the implications of such illnesses may be quite different today than years past. Select patients might be better served having HPB surgery at a major medical center where the multidisciplinary care team provides optimum preparation of patients as well as the ability and availability to minimize the impact on patients when adverse events occur.[29,30]

Cardiac Evaluation

Although the perioperative event rate has declined because of better anesthetic and surgical techniques, perioperative cardiac complications remain a significant problem. The first step in preoperative care is an adequate identification of patients at risk for perioperative cardiac events. Clinical history, physical examination, and review of a baseline electrocardiogram usually provide enough data to estimate cardiac risk. Estimation of a stable patient's cardiac risk can be derived from the Lee Revised

Cardiac Risk Index (LRCRI), a simple index that identifies six independent risk factors to provide the risk of a cardiac complication in percentages.[31] The risk of a perioperative major cardiac event (PMCE), defined as cardiac death, myocardial infarction (MI), or pulmonary edema within 30 days postoperatively, is the summation of an individual patient's risk and functional capacity and the cardiac stress related to the surgery.

There are active cardiac conditions that may lead to cancellation of the procedure, unless the surgery is emergent, but most PMCE risk is silent, and the LRCRI has shown only moderate predictive performance.[32] The absence of coronary computed tomographic angiography findings of coronary artery disease confers low PMCE risk regardless of clinical risk, and some have suggested adding this noninvasive test to the LRCRI.[33] The 2014 American College of Cardiology/American Heart Association (ACC/AHA) guidelines on perioperative cardiovascular evaluation and care for noncardiac surgery are an excellent framework for evaluating cardiac risk in the perioperative period for patients with clinical risk factors.[34]

Cardiac functional status or capacity, as determined by doctors assessing patients with a brief set of questions, can be expressed in metabolic equivalents or simply the inability to perform various activities such as climbing two flights of stairs or walking four blocks.[35,36] A patient's cardiac functional status has been thought to be positively associated with postoperative outcomes.[35,36] The Measurement of Exercise Tolerance before Surgery (METS) prospective cohort study concluded that subjectively assessed preoperative functional capacity did not accurately identify patients with poor cardiopulmonary fitness or predict morbidity or mortality.[37] How this will affect the ACP's choice for additional cardiac evaluation is unclear. Over the years, perioperative management has shifted from treating coronary obstruction with coronary revascularization toward medical therapy aiming at prevention of myocardial oxygen supply and demanding mismatch and coronary plaque stabilization. Today preoperative cardiac testing, cardiac stenting, and coronary revascularization are only performed for the same indications as the nonoperative setting.[38,39]

The risks and benefits of continuing perioperative medical management are complex. Perioperative β-blockade (PBB) has been shown to reduce the incidence of perioperative ischemic events and MI in patients with coronary artery disease but confers questionable benefit and possible harm in patients without coronary artery disease.[40,41] The PeriOperative Ischemic Study Evaluation (POISE) trial completely transformed the premise of PBB, finding PBB stroke morbidity outweighed any PMCE prevention.[42] POISE confirmed what clinical anesthesiologists had experienced: increased intraoperative hypotension and bradycardia in low-risk patients with newly initiated PBB. PBB guideline revisions followed rapidly in 2009. The guidelines recommended continuation of β-blockers for patients who are already on them and the initiation of PBB for high-risk patients, but not to initiate PBB in low-risk patients in the perioperative period. β-Blockers should still be used to manage acute hypertension and tachycardia perioperatively in patients at risk for myocardial supply and demand imbalance. Similarly, balancing the risk-to-benefit ratio of dual antiplatelet therapy (APT) or aspirin interruption and the risk of stent thrombosis versus continuation and the risk of bleeding is challenging. The POISE-2 trial showed that perioperative aspirin did not reduce PCME at 30 days but did increase perioperative bleeding.[43] Only a small number of patients in this trial had coronary stenting, and patients with a bare-metal stent (BMS) for less than 6 weeks or a drug-eluting stent (DES) for less than 1 year were excluded.

Contemporary data suggest that approximately one in five patients with coronary stent implantation will require noncardiac surgery within 2 years of their coronary intervention.[44] Patients with freshly placed coronary stents presenting for liver surgery pose a significant challenge to anesthesiologists. It is no surprise that anesthesiologists must consistently stay current with rapidly evolving guidelines for the perioperative management of these patients. Some of the clinical questions that arise include the following: How soon can a stented patient undergo surgery? Should a patient continue APT during the perioperative period? What is the risk for surgical bleeding versus coronary thrombosis in this population? In 2016 the ACC/AHA guidelines recommended delaying noncardiac surgery 30 days after BMS implantation and 6 months after DES implantation. However, if the risk for delay for 6 months was greater that the risk for ischemia, elective surgery could be considered at 3 months.[45]

Communication among the patient's cardiologist, surgeon, and anesthesiologist is essential for the management of patients with active or quiescent coronary artery disease. At the authors' institution, the medical consult takes into account both the ACC/AHA patient's number of clinical factors (does the patient have an active cardiac condition; planned surgery, low or high risk; good functional capacity; further testing required) and the LRCRI (high-risk type of surgery; history of ischemic heart disease; history of congestive heart failure; history of cerebrovascular disease; diabetes mellitus [insulin dependent]; renal insufficiency [creatinine > 2]), to determine whether the patient is at acceptable risk to proceed to the planned surgery or if there is the need for further testing before surgery or pharmacologic intervention perioperatively.[38]

In HPB patients with a history of alcohol abuse, cardiac assessment needs to stress the evaluation of myocontractile function. Two basic patterns of alcohol-induced cardiomyopathy have been shown: left ventricular dilation with impaired systolic function and left ventricular hypertrophy with diminished compliance and normal or increased contractile performance.

Geriatric Evaluation

Elderly patients with impaired functional status have been shown to have increased morbidity and mortality when undergoing HPB surgery.[46,47] More than 80% of pancreatic cancers are diagnosed in patients older than 65 years old. Although age should not preclude surgery, at-risk elderly patients should have a comprehensive geriatric assessment and a multidimensional diagnostic tool used to test functional performance and mental status. Frailty has emerged as an important perioperative risk factor. Diagnosis of frailty is especially important in managing geriatric patients. It is a clinical syndrome in which three or more of the following criteria are met: unintentional weight loss of greater than 10 pounds within the previous year, self-reported exhaustion, weakness measured by grip strength, slow walking speed, and low levels of physical activity. Over 300 different types of frailty assessments have been created and used, but there is really no gold standard. Evidence of sarcopenia, which clinically manifests itself as a loss of skeletal mass, strength, and decreased physical performance, is often used to assess frailty. The most commonly used Fried phenotype looks at frailty as a syndrome, something with signs and symptoms that can be measured. In this case, 1 point is assigned to things like walking speed and weight loss, for a final score between 0 and 5.[48] The frailty index is defined as the ratio of the number of deficits present in an individual to the total number of age-related health variables considered. The key here is that the deficits are measured across multiple domains. One compares the number of deficits with the total number measured and ends up with a score between 0 and 1. The clinical frailty score uses a scale of 1 to 9 where each number is associated with a short vignette and an image. The electronic rapid fitness assessment (eRFA) is a questionnaire developed at our institution and used by all the doctors of the geriatrics service to gauge and understand an older patent's level of fitness.[49] At the authors' institution, all patients over 65 deemed at increased risk are referred to a geriatric specialist. This service also advises on medications to be used with caution and nonpharmacologic strategies to reduce delirium and analgesics while the patient is in the hospital.

Delirium (temporary inability to focus attention and think clearly) occurs in one of five older patients who undergo major surgery. Delirium is associated with a slower recovery and a poorer outcome, and a vicious circle may be initiated (delirium, physical restraint, and medication to treat delirium; postoperative complications; then more delirium). Korc-Grodzicki used comprehensive geriatric assessment components to predict the development of postoperative delirium and other comorbidities in patients undergoing varying abdominal surgeries. The study population included 416 patients, of which 20% of patients underwent HBP surgeries. Charleston comorbidity index score greater than 3, patients with a history of falls 6 months before surgery, instrumental activities of daily living scores of less than 8, and abnormal mini-cog test results were all predictive of postoperative delirium. In this study, patients who developed postoperative delirium had longer median length of hospital stays and greater likelihood of discharge to a skilled nursing facility.[50] Randomized studies have shown that multicomponent interventions can reduce the incidence of delirium and/or related complications.[51] We advocate a daily protection and intervention program based on early-start and supporting treatment, with increased monitoring, better pain relief, avoidance of polypharmacy, and good nutrition, but from a prevention or therapeutic point of view, there is no one target for decreasing the incidence after surgery. It has been suggested by some studies that the routine use of perioperative medications, such as dexmedetomidine[52] or ketamine[53] can prevent postoperative delirium; however, available evidence does not support this. Gabapentin may reduce postoperative delirium, perhaps by reducing pain and opioid administration.

Pulmonary Evaluation

Despite steady advances in care, patients with respiratory disease are still at increased risk for postoperative pulmonary complications (PPCs). PPCs continue to rival cardiovascular complications in frequency and severity after hepatic surgery.[4]

There are many limitations of studies that examine risk factors for PPCs, but there are some consistent patterns. Important risk factors for PPCs are the presence of pulmonary disease, cigarette smoking, low preoperative arterial oxygen saturation, acute respiratory infection during the previous month, age, preoperative anemia, site of surgery (with upper abdominal, especially near the diaphragm, or intrathoracic surgery being the highest risk), surgery duration of at least 2 hours, and emergency surgery.[54,55] Despite the increased risk of PPCs in patients with preexisting pulmonary disease, no prohibitive level of pulmonary function has been established for which surgery is contraindicated. Neither abnormal pulmonary function testing nor arterial blood gas analysis are useful in predicting risk. Thus these tests are only justified as part of an effort to optimize preoperative pulmonary status, either with an immediate perioperative course of systemic corticosteroids or antibiotics, or to advise if surgery should be delayed.[56] Poor functional capacity and especially low anaerobic threshold have been associated with a high risk of postoperative complications and death. Submaximal cardiopulmonary exercise testing is a noninvasive objective test that measures a patient's anaerobic threshold and patients with low subjective functional capacity or dyspnea may benefit from this test of cardiopulmonary reserve to determine complication risk.[57] Although it seems reasonable to assume that fitter patients will have better outcome, a recent study suggested that cardiopulmonary exercise testing should not be used as a barrier to patients undergoing liver surgery.[58] Potential interventions to reduce PPCs include smoking cessation, preoperative exercise training, early mobilization, postoperative parental nutrition, and optimal treatment of pain.[59]

Although obesity presents the anesthesiologist with significant challenges, obesity per se is not a significant risk factor for PPCs and should not be used to deny a patient HPB surgery. There are two subsets of obese patients: one group is "the metabolically healthy but obese" and the other group is the "metabolically unhealthy but obese."[60] When an obese patient has three or more of the following criteria, abdominal obesity, increased triglycerides, decreased high-density lipoprotein, elevated cholesterol, hypertension, and glucose intolerance, the patient has a 2.5 increased incidence of PPCs.[61] Obese patients are at risk of suffering from several respiratory derangements, including obstructive sleep apnea (OSA), obesity-hypoventilation syndrome, and restrictive impairment. The increase in body mass also results in increased oxygen consumption and carbon dioxide production. With these issues in mind, it is not surprising that acute PPCs are twice as likely in OSA patients.[62] Many patients with OSA are undiagnosed,

but there is a strong relationship between obesity and OSA. The American Society of Anesthesiologists (ASA) addressed this issue with practice guidelines, including assessment of patients for possible OSA before surgery and careful postoperative monitoring for those suspected to be at risk.[63] It is unclear whether screening for OSA will affect surgical morbidity, but it is reasonable to question obese patients about symptoms that may suggest sleep apnea before HPB surgery. At Memorial Sloan Kettering Cancer Center (MSKCC), all obese patients are given the STOP (Snoring, Tiredness, Observed apnea, high blood Pressure)-Bang (Body mass index, Age, Neck circumference, and gender) questionnaire.[64] Given the association of obesity and OSA with multiple medical conditions (increased risk of venous stasis, pulmonary embolism, hypertension, cerebral vascular accidents, cardiomyopathy, arrythmias, and ischemic heart disease) the anesthesiologist is in a position to have an informed discussion with the patient about the increased risk of morbidity and mortality and work with other members of the patient's care team to determine whether any interventions should be initiated before surgery in an effort to minimize the risk of complications.[65] Polysomnography is the gold standard for diagnosis of OSA, but it is expensive and a limited resource. The most reasonable approach is to check room air-pulse oximetry. If the patient has an oxygen saturation level less than 96%, further evaluation is warranted. A 2-week period of continuous positive airway pressure (CPAP) therapy has been shown to be effective in correcting abnormal ventilatory drive and improving cardiac function.[66]

Venous Thromboembolism Prophylaxis

In patients undergoing general surgery, the risk of venous thromboembolism (VTE) varies depending on both patient and procedure-specific factors.[67] Patients having cancer surgery have a moderate risk for VTE.[68-70] Guidelines recommend low-molecular-weight heparin (LWMH) for patients undergoing general surgery procedures with at least moderate (3%) risk of VTE, if the risk of bleeding does not negate the risk of VTE.[67] After HPB surgery, the risk of VTE (deep vein thrombosis, pulmonary embolus) is not insignificant and is higher in the obese patient. After major hepatectomy, the concern for postoperative bleeding, combined with an erroneous presumption of protection because of the coagulopathy, often preclude the use of routine prophylaxis despite evidence to the contrary.[71] In a recent retrospective review at our institution, postoperative VTE occurred in 2.6% of patients and was independently associated with higher postoperative international normalized ratio (INR) and LWMH had no relationship to VTE incidence or bleeding complications.[72] Patients with more extensive liver resections and higher operative blood loss had a higher incidence of VTE. Despite an elevated INR and lower platelet count, a patient having major liver cancer surgery is in a normocoagulable or even a hypercoagulable state and at risk for VTE; yet there is no consensus of opinion for pharmacologic prophylaxis.[73] The ACP and the surgeon should discuss risk versus benefit.

Pancreatic cancer is among the most common malignancies associated with thrombosis, as it occurs in 50% of patients[74] (see Chapter 62). Prophylaxis against postoperative VTE should be tailored to the patient's level of risk. The Caprini score, which can be potentially used for such purposes, estimates VTE risk by adding various points for VTE risk factors.[75] Current recommendations strongly advise effective and preventive strategies for all hospitalized patients who are defined as moderate to high risk for VTE and are awaiting pancreatic surgery. LMWHs appear to be effective and are potentially associated with a lower risk of bleeding when the first dose is administered 12 hours preoperatively.[67,76]

Hepatic Evaluation

Risk factors and symptoms of liver disease are not as well defined as in other organ systems. There is no single biomarker for liver dysfunction; instead, the diagnosis of liver disease requires a high degree of suspicion, with a careful probing of the clinical history to identify specific risk factors for liver disease, such as previous blood transfusions, jaundice, travel, tattoos, high-risk sexual behavior, illicit drug use, excessive alcohol intake, or chemotherapy[77] (see Chapter 4).

The goal of preoperative screening is to determine the presence of preexisting liver disease without the need for extensive or invasive monitoring. Liver function tests can measure different aspects of hepatic function, but as a group of tests, they lack specificity and are often affected by nonhepatic function. These biochemical markers cannot quantify hepatic cellular dysfunction. In contrast, anesthesiologists are often confronted with abnormal hepatic function tests in asymptomatic patients. In general, for asymptomatic patients with mildly elevated alanine and aspartate aminotransferase levels and a normal bilirubin concentration, cancellation of surgery is rarely indicated

Most hepatic resections are performed for metastatic cancer. In these patients the quantity of hepatocyte dysfunction, whether induced by preoperative alcohol, chemotherapy, or metabolic syndrome, is more elusive to identify. In patients with significant abnormalities, additional investigation is warranted, given the higher risk to patients having HPB surgery to evaluate whether there is underlying cirrhosis or steatosis. Serologic testing to exclude viral hepatitis and human immunodeficiency virus should always be performed.

The etiology of hyperbilirubinemia may have an obstructive or nonobstructive cause. No matter the root cause, jaundice adversely affects outcome. Unlike elevated bilirubin associated with hepatocyte disturbance, obstructive jaundice is typically seen in patients with bile duct obstruction and is not a contraindication for HPB surgery, if it is being performed to remove the cause of the obstruction. Biliary sepsis may contribute to the exacerbation of perioperative hemodynamic instability. In situations where there is clinical concern for the development of acute cholangitis, rapid biliary decompression and intravenous (IV) antibiotics should be administered preoperatively, and surgery should be delayed until the infection resolves. Patients with hyperbilirubinemia are a subset of patients with an increased risk of renal compromise after low central venous pressure (LCVP)-assisted hepatectomy.[78] The surgeon and anesthesiologist must have a detailed discussion of risk versus benefit.

Alcohol Use Disorder

Patients with unhealthy alcohol use face increased perioperative risks from the medical consequences associated with alcohol consumption as well as from physiologic dependence and withdrawal. Up to 50% of patients presenting for gastrointestinal (GI) cancer surgery have alcohol use disorder. Studies have found that many surgical patients have not had been appropriately assessed for alcohol use in the preoperative evaluation.[79] Abstinence from drinking, as imposed by a hospital admission, places patients at risk for alcohol withdrawal syndrome (AWS). The preoperative evaluation of patients with unhealthy alcohol

use should include effective screening strategies to identify the presence of heavy alcohol use, detect end-organ damage secondary to alcohol consumption, and prompt intervention to address alcohol use before surgery. There are several screening tools to identify alcohol use disorder. The authors' preference is to use the CAGE (cut down, annoyed, guilty, eye opener) questionnaire. AWS prophylaxis should begin on admission to the hospital. Evidence supports the use of benzodiazepines as first-line treatment.[80] Two strategies are recommended: either a fixed-dosage or an as-needed regimen triggered by symptoms. These patients may have increased or decreased anesthesia requirements during induction and maintenance. The most common 90-day postoperative complications are infections, bleeding, and cardiopulmonary insufficiency; however, these complications are only increased if the patient has alcohol abuse at the time of surgery.[81] For those patients with alcohol abuse at the time of surgery, the development of AWS is associated with a longer hospital stay and increased mortality.[79]

Blood Conservation

Patient blood management is based on the three pillars: detecting and treating preoperative anemia, reducing the loss of red blood cells (RBCs) perioperatively, and optimizing the treatment of anemia.[82] Thorough preoperative planning is essential to avoid perioperative allogeneic transfusion. Any history of bleeding disorders and management of anticoagulation must be evaluated, including discontinuation of drugs that adversely affect clotting (e.g., acetylsalicylic acid, nonsteroidal antiinflammatory drugs [NSAIDs], and anticoagulants). In patients with anemia, iron therapy may help optimize the starting operative hemoglobin. Preoperative autologous donation (PAD) also has been used to reduce the need for allogeneic RBC products.[83] However, PAD may not avoid allogeneic blood because almost half of the patients who donate blood before surgery are anemic on the day of surgery, and preoperative strategies to augment the RBC mass require more time than is generally reasonable for optimal efficacy. Patients with low hemoglobin levels at the start of surgery are at an increased risk of receiving allogeneic blood.[84] In addition, PAD is costly, it can be associated with clerical errors, and for every two units donated, usually only one unit gets transfused.[85] If the patient is optimized and surgery is bloodless, the autologous units are discarded. Other blood conservation strategies, such as intraoperative blood salvage (cell saver) and acute normovolemic hemodilution (ANH), have been used successfully for patients having major liver resections and for Jehovah's Witnesses.[86] ANH has been shown in two prospective studies to reduce the number of RBCs transfused per patient in major liver resections.[87,88] A score with good discriminatory ability to predict the necessity of RBC transfusion during liver resection was developed,[89] and, subsequently, this score was incorporated into a nomogram to predict which patients would benefit from ANH to decrease transfusion during hepatic resection.[90] At our institution a randomized controlled trial (RCT) of ANH in patients undergoing major pancreatic surgery showed no reduction in RBC transfusion.[91]

INTRAOPERATIVE STRATEGIES FOR HEPATOPANCREATOBILIARY SURGERY

At tertiary care centers HPB surgery has evolved into a discrete specialty in which HPB surgeons manage the complexity of both liver and pancreas surgery. Like HPB surgeons, anesthesiologists must master the intraoperative management of liver and pancreas surgery. Although many elements are similar between liver and pancreas anesthetic care for preoperative preparedness, i.e., "ready for surgery," some intraoperative elements are procedure specific.

Fluid Management for Hepatopancreatobiliary Surgery: Pancreas

One of the most common interventions made by ACPs is the administration of IV fluid. Many questions have arisen, and much controversy has emerged regarding how much fluid should be given perioperatively, which fluids should be given, when they should be given, and whether outcomes can be influenced. Because preoperative fluid status and perioperative fluid shifts are difficult to measure, and correct therapy remains uncertain, the assessment of intravascular volume status, the maintenance of hemodynamics, and the need for transfusion for patients undergoing HPB surgery remain an important clinical decision in the perioperative setting. Past research to identify the perfect recipe of fluid administration during abdominal surgery suffered from standardization of regimens and the goals chosen to influence the amount of fluid prescribed. Although liberal, standard, conservative or restrictive has been and still remains in the eye of the beholder, contemporary fluid therapists emphasize that administering more fluid (typically crystalloid) than is needed to patients undergoing surgery has been associated with harm.[92] Preoperative volume loading and routine replacement of insensible and third space losses should be abandoned in favor of rational fluid therapy, zero-based fluid therapy or demand-related fluid protocols to avoid any collateral damage that may be caused by interstitial edema. There is evidence-based medicine to support this contemporary approach to fluid therapy. Mechanical bowel preparation and overnight fasting are less common and are no longer recommended before HPB surgeries.[92] Intraoperative evaporated fluid losses during surgery are at most 1cc/kg/hr.[93] Modern tracer studies do not support the existence of a third space.[94] Therefore filling of this theoretical space is moot and the term should be abandoned; fluid is either intravascular or shifted into the interstitium.

Focusing on intraoperative fluid management, the key question is whether administration of fluids will result in a clinically relevant increase in cardiac output, thereby enhancing tissue perfusion and oxygen delivery.[95] Furthermore, a strategy that does not require an empiric fluid challenge to determine whether fluid administration would increase cardiac output has the obvious benefit of preventing fluid administration and volume overload–induced complications in patients who are fluid nonresponsive.[96] Unfortunately, methods that have been used in the past to assess volume status and volume responsiveness are unreliable.

There are many opinions regarding fluid management in the operating room; nonetheless, as a whole, fluid administration is based on textbook guidelines for surgery-specific replacement of blood loss and maintenance fluid requirements. The standard approach used to deliver these goals uses maintenance background fluid therapy that replenishes fluid lost by urinary output and perspiration then adding additional fluid boluses for blood loss or fluid shifts. It is accepted practice to adjust the dose of fluid in response to some form of end point. Conventional end points include urine output, blood pressure, and heart rate. For the higher risk patient or surgery, basic invasive

monitoring such as arterial pressure of CVP may be added. This traditional fluid management strategy is unreliable because the traditional static end point parameters, such as blood pressure, heart rate, urine output, and CVP, used to diagnose hypovolemia and the response to a fluid challenge are unreliable.

Goal-directed individual fluid therapy (GDT) based on the optimization of cardiac output or using dynamic indices of blood flow and arterial pressure to guide fluid requirement has appeal and has become more common.[96] The availability of minimally invasive hemodynamic monitoring techniques (esophageal Doppler, arterial waveform analysis) and the use of dynamic parameters of fluid responsiveness allow the use of protocolized GDT strategies. Functional hemodynamics parameters provide a numeric representation of the patient's fluid responsiveness and are more reliable than using standard static parameters, such as blood pressure, heart rate, urine output, or even CVP.[97] A recent meta-analysis supports GDT for patients having abdominal surgery to improve postoperative recovery and decrease complication rates, yet liver and pancreas surgeries were excluded.[98]

HPB surgery exposes patients to periods of cardiovascular insufficiency, either because of anesthesia-induced loss of vasomotor tone and baroreceptor responsiveness or because of blood loss and mechanical obstruction to blood flow. In all cases, stroke volume will fall as well as global oxygen delivery to the tissues. GDT is targeted to detect hypovolemia and hypoperfusion early (at or before anesthetic induction) to be proactive to avoid hypoperfusion.[99] Because surgery also creates a cytokine storm, the combination of relative hypoperfusion and immune modulation will alter the microcirculation, causing subclinical damage. Whether GDT for HPB surgery can rescue patients from this insult is unknown.

Based on the growing evidence supporting GDT, clinical societies have published guidelines for operative fluid management recommending that all ACPs should have a perioperative fluid plan using an algorithm guided by the most appropriate and accurate monitor. While acknowledging that the benefits of perioperative GDT have yet to be proven, experts believe the bulk of clinical research supports the implementation of a two-step GDT plan containing colloid and balanced solutions for major abdominal surgery. All ACPs should implement a two-step GDT plan, which begins immediately after induction of anesthesia. First, determine whether the patient requires hemodynamic support of augmentation of cardiovascular function. Second, if the need is apparent and the patient is fluid responsive, fluid bolus therapy should be considered and guided by appropriate changes in stroke volume.[100]

Pancreatic Anastomotic Leak

The Whipple procedure, or pancreaticoduodenectomy (see Chapters 62 and 117) is an extensive and relatively long procedure with the potential for large fluid losses. Whether intraoperative fluid management influences outcome after pancreatic surgery is a controversial topic. Postoperative GI dysfunction is a frequent complication in these surgical patients. Although the pathogenesis of GI complications is multifactorial, gut hypoperfusion, secondary to hypovolemia or cardiac dysfunction, plays a key role.[101] Although healthy patients may tolerate a 25% to 30% decrease in blood volume without changes in systemic arterial pressure or heart rate, splanchnic perfusion is compromised after 10% to 15%reduction in intravascular volume.[102] Selective vasoconstriction of mesenteric arterioles, mediated primarily by the renin-angiotensin system, contributes to the maintenance of systemic arterial pressure and the perfusion of nonmesenteric organs.[103] This response occurs at the expense of splanchnic hypoperfusion that often outlasts the period of the hypovolemic insult or low-flow state, promoting abdominal damage.

GI dysfunction presents with clinical signs and symptoms ranging from impaired motility[101] and inability to tolerate enteral diet to ischemic injury.[104] The type of surgery is important; for example, in abdominal surgery, poor oxygen delivery is significantly associated with anastomotic leak,[102] especially in GI segments highly dependent on oxidative phosphorylation.[105] Pancreaticoduodenectomy has a unique set of conditions, including three different anastomoses, giving rise to complications such as ileus, anastomotic leak, and pancreatic fistula formation. One of the postoperative GI complications of interest for pancreatic surgery, anastomotic leak, would seem to be the one most affected by excessive fluid administration. Hypervolemia (typically too much crystalloid) can damage the glycocalyx, a layer of membrane-bound proteoglycans and glycoproteins that coats healthy vascular endothelium and plays an important role in managing vascular permeability by acting as a second barrier to extravasation.[106] The most common manifestation of hypervolemia is edema of the gut wall and prolonged ileus. A study in rats undergoing a bowel resection and anastomosis showed that excessive crystalloid results in submucosal intestinal edema, lower anastomotic bursting pressure, and a decrease in the structural stability of intestinal anastomosis in the early postoperative period.[107]

Retrospective single-center studies for pancreatectomies examining an association of anastomotic leak and higher amounts of perioperative fluid therapy report contradictory results.[108–113] Two prospective RCT at MSKCC may be bringing us closer to identifying a safe range of intraoperative fluids that does not affect morbidity for patients undergoing pancreatectomy at high-volume centers. An RCT of hemodilution for patients undergoing pancreatectomy in which the hemodilution cohort received two more liters of intraoperative fluid than the liberal arm of our RCT of liberal versus restrictive fluid therapy[114] showed an increased incidence of pancreaticoduodenectomy anastomotic leak (ANH 21% vs. standard deviation [STD] 7.7%).[91] Both RCTs had fluid therapy guided by empiric end points. GDT has been advocated as the strategy to best maintain oxygen delivery and minimize splanchnic hypoperfusion, and a meta-analysis of major surgeries has shown it decreases major and minor GI complications in the perioperative period.[115] The authors know of no trial that has looked at GDT and its effect on anastomotic leak for pancreatic surgery.

Fluid Management: Liver Surgery

For hepatic resection, a relationship between extent of intraoperative blood loss and mortality and morbidity has been consistently shown. To minimize blood loss, it is common anesthesia practice to perform liver resections with the CVP less than 5 mm Hg. The blood loss resulting from a vascular injury is directly proportional to the pressure gradient across the vessel wall and the fourth power of the radius of the injury. If the CVP is lowered from 15 to 3 mm Hg, the blood loss through a vena caval injury consequently falls by a factor greater than 5. LCVP not only lessens the pressure component of the equation but also minimizes the radial component of flow by reducing vessel distention (Fig. 25.1). LCVP anesthesia is designed

to preclude vena caval and hepatic venous distention, facilitate mobilization of the liver and dissection of retrohepatic vena cava, minimize hepatic venous back bleeding during parenchymal transection, and facilitate control of inadvertent venous injury[78] (see Chapter 118).

LCVP anesthesia is often performed in combination with surgical inflow and outflow vascular control (Pringle technique) before parenchymal transection.[116]

In 1996 the authors developed and reported a simple, effective, and reproducible technique for decreasing the intraoperative blood loss in patients undergoing liver resection based on fluid restriction and the vasodilatory effects of anesthetic agents.[78] Around the same time, a complex LCVP management technique was described[117] that used epidural blockade and IV nitroglycerin. These patients often required intraoperative dopamine for systemic pressure support. The technique seemed cumbersome, adding an unnecessary level of complexity to an already challenging situation. Despite this, both approaches contributed to improved outcomes and continue to be practiced at major institutions.[118–120]

Over time several other techniques of LCVP have been advocated: administration of diuretics, low tidal volume (TV) ventilation with positive end-expiratory pressure (PEEP) reduction, hypovolemic hemodilution, and so forth. Recent comparison of fluid restriction or vasodilation to lower CVP concluded that either seemed equally effective.[121] To reduce intraoperative blood loss the current practice of liver surgery in high-volume centers restricts the intraoperative fluid infusion to reduce CVP during parenchymal resection.[122]

Low Central Venous Pressure Technique: General Anesthesia

LCVP-assisted hepatic resection at the authors' institution has evolved over the years but is still true to the two original pillars: fluid restriction and pharmacologic vasodilation. This anesthetic technique was historically dependent on the presence of a central venous catheter to provide hemodynamic information and expeditious and reliable access in case rapid resuscitation

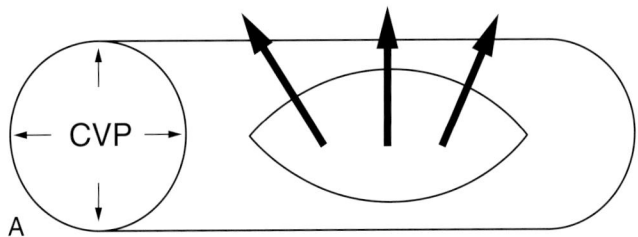

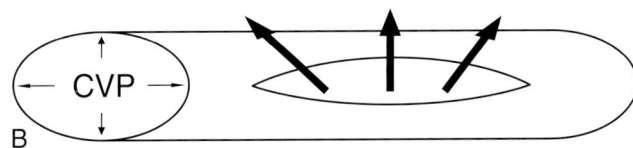

FIGURE 25.1 Vena caval injury profile under various central venous pressure (CVP) conditions. **A,** High CVP. **B,** Low CVP. Increased CVP leads to distention of the vena cava, with ensuing enlargement in diameter of injury and increase in the bleeding driving pressure.

was required.[78] However, in the modern era of bloodless hepatic resection, to avoid the morbidity associated with central vein cannulation, our clinical practice has abandoned the routine use of central venous lines. The authors have not adopted surrogate measures of CVP: external jugular venous pressure, peripheral venous pressure, inferior vena cava diameter using transesophageal echocardiography, inferior vena cava collapsibility using hand-carried ultrasound devices, or stroke-volume variation.[119] Instead, the success of our LCVP is currently based on surgical visual inspection of the vena cava or the amount of venous back bleeding as reported by the surgeon.[123] Patients should still be prepared for large-volume transfusion, although this is infrequently needed. Close cooperation between the anesthesiologist and the surgeon continues so that likely difficulties can be anticipated, and appropriate measures can be taken. Fluid management is an important aspect of the LCVP anesthesia. Intraoperative fluid management is divided into the following two phases.

Phase 1: Prehepatic

Prehepatic resection starts at anesthesia induction and ends at the completion of parenchymal transection and hemostasis. During this phase, inflow control of the portal vein and hepatic artery are achieved, and the vena cava and hepatic veins are dissected. Sixty percent of the time hepatic parenchymal transection is performed with intermittent inflow occlusion (Pringle technique) applied.[4]

This phase avoids fluid excess and takes advantage of the vasodilatory effects of anesthetic drugs. Preoperative overnight fluid replacement is withheld, and maintenance fluid requirement at 1 mL/kg/hr of balanced crystalloid solution is infused until the liver resection is completed. Intermittently, small fluid boluses or vasoactive drugs may be given to maintain hemodynamic stability. Some extent of permissive oliguria caused by decreases in antidiuretic hormone or permissive relative hypotension while peripheral tone is decreased will allow for continued minimal fluid infusion until the specimen is delivered.

Anesthesia is maintained with a combination of isoflurane or sevoflurane in oxygen and fentanyl. Isoflurane provides vasodilation with minimal myocardial depression.[124] Consistent with its minimal effect on cardiac output and systemic pressure, fentanyl has no effect on liver blood flow and oxygen delivery and, given its lack of toxic metabolites, can be administered like any abdominal surgery without any dosing reduction.[125] As tolerated, a background infusion of dexmedetomidine or ketamine may be added to minimize narcotic dosage. Shortly before transection of the liver, sublingual nitroglycerin is applied. This combination of inhalational agent, fentanyl, and sublingual nitroglycerin readily provides the favorable LCVP environment for hepatic resection.

Postresection: Phase 2

Posthepatic resection, the second phase, begins once the specimen has been delivered and hemostasis secured. During this phase, the goal of fluid prescription is to leave the operating room with a normovolemic patient. Early proactive GDT may compromise the effectiveness of LCVP on decreased blood loss. Although most liver surgery does not result in profound tissue hypoperfusion, some degree of hypoperfusion does occur with the Pringle technique, adding tissue perfusion injury before resuscitation. There is presently no approved treatment for

ischemia reperfusion injury (IRI), which is the inflammation that occurs when blood flow is returned to healthy liver tissue after diseased tissue has been surgically removed. IRI can harm the vascular barrier and the endothelial glycocalyx and results in part from the deposition of complement, a protein that kills liver cells and impairs regeneration.[99] GDT has been shown to be effective when combined in an enhanced recovery after liver surgery (ERAS) program.[120,126] (see Chapter 27). A recent randomized trial for hepatic surgery at our institution showed intraoperative GDT was a safe technique and allowed for less intraoperative fluid, but it did not influence overall 30-day morbidity.[131] The optimal perioperative fluid resuscitation strategy for liver surgery remains undefined.

Renal Dysfunction

The common assumption is that urine output must be maintained above a certain level to prevent acute kidney injury (AKI); therefore low urine output should be treated with crystalloid boluses.[127,128] Yet, in the intraoperative period, oliguria defined as urine output less than 0.5mL/kg/hr is extremely common and often occurs as a neurohormonal response to surgical stress, rendering it an unreliable marker of volume status. In a large retrospective analysis, it was reported that 85% of postoperative patients not developing AKI had a urine output less than 0.5mL/kg/hr, surprisingly significantly more patients than those who developed AKI (75%).[129] Recently, using a large national database, procedure-specific risk of perioperative AKI for patients undergoing intraabdominal surgery was evaluated.[130] The results demonstrated that among patients undergoing intraabdominal surgery, the risk of severe AKI varies considerably, depending on the specific procedure. HPB procedures (liver and pancreas, elective and emergent) had a 1.8 % incidence of acute renal failure with an adjusted risk of 1%. The authors hypothesized that AKI may be a spectrum of diseases with different causes and consequences that depend on the clinical context in which it occurs. A retrospective review in a similar time period, as in the report by Kim and colleagues, evaluated severe clinical AKI following LCVP-assisted liver resection.[130] Clinically relevant AKI was rare (<1%) and resolved in half of these patients during a short follow-up period.[118] These results are mirrored by analysis of postoperative morbidity after liver resections.[132] Whereas Kim only had severe end points (creatinine >2, dialysis) to analyze, and may have underestimated the incidence of clinically significant AKI defined by the RIFLE (Risk, Injury, Failure, Loss of kidney function, and End-stage kidney disease) criteria, this review analyzed laboratory data and was able to apply the RIFLE criteria to the incidence of biochemical AKI[118]. Although biochemically defined renal dysfunction was a relatively common event (16%) in patients undergoing LCVP-assisted liver resection, it was a transient phenomenon, and its clinical significance was limited.

The incidence of biochemical acute renal failure is not in and of itself an argument against the use of LCVP anesthesia for liver resections. Some permissive, clinically nonrelevant renal dysfunction is a very common event in this patient population, and it is consistent with published literature regarding other types of major operations.[133] The evidence does not support LCVP-assisted liver surgery increasing the incidence of significant AKI. A retrospective review of a series of 1153 liver resections found that epidural anesthesia (EDA) and/or EDA

LCVP-assisted liver surgery significantly increases the incidence of AKI (defined by the Acute Kidney Injury Network [AKIN] criteria) following major resections but not minor liver resections.[134]

Blood Conservation, Transfusion

The ACP not only has a pivotal role in reducing blood loss during hepatic surgery but also contributes to intraoperative blood conservation and controls transfusion protocol for all HPB surgery. Transfusion-free surgery, better known to the public as bloodless surgery, can only be achieved by the application of blood management techniques to decrease allogeneic transfusion. The three pillars of blood conservation are (1) build up the patient's own blood volume, (2) reduce blood loss, and (3) recycle the patient's own blood.[82] The ACP should be familiar with recycling techniques, such as intraoperative RBC salvage and hemodilution, which are maneuvers that may contribute to reduced allogeneic RBC transfusion in major liver surgery. Autologous RBC salvage (intraoperative autotransfusion) involves recovery of the patient's shed blood from a surgical wound, washing or filtering, and reinfusion of the blood into the patient. HPB operations often are performed for cancer. Cell salvage had been excluded in oncologic surgery because of the concern for potential dissemination of cancer cells, but the availability of leukocyte-depleting filters allows its use during cancer surgery. Another transfusion-sparing technique is ANH. This is a recycling technique that can be performed intraoperatively by the anesthesiologist. Blood is removed from the patient after induction and replaced with crystalloid or colloid fluid. The removed blood is stored at room temperature in the operating room and is returned to the patient at the conclusion of the operation. Two randomized studies of ANH in major hepatic resection showed a significant reduction in the percentage of patients requiring allogeneic RBC transfusion.[87,88] An important factor in selection of patients who may benefit from ANH is predictably the likely operative blood loss. Studies have shown that the threshold for utilizing ANH is a predicted blood loss of 0.2 of the patient's estimated total blood volume. Therefore utilizing ANH must be selective and reserved for those cases in which substantial blood losses are expected. In a randomized trial of 114 patients undergoing major liver resection and allocation of intraoperative management using a transfusion nomogram, low blood loss cases were more effectively identified with reduced ANH use in patients least likely to benefit.[90] A similar trial showed no benefit of ANH in patients undergoing pancreatectomy.[91]

Tolerance of normovolemic anemia is important, and care must be taken not to confuse the momentary helpful effect of RBC transfusion on hypotension and hypovolemia with an outcome benefit. A restrictive approach to blood transfusion with a threshold of 7 g/dL has been shown to reduce blood use and not cause harm in critically ill patients,[136] as well as in liver resection patients.[137]

In a recent review, Kingham and colleagues[4] reported that transfusions have decreased by 50% over two decades, but perioperative blood loss and transfusion remain associated with morbidity. Cannon and colleagues[138] specifically showed that transfusion with packed RBCs was associated with postoperative complications in patients undergoing hepatectomy. The correlation of transfusion with complications should not be interpreted as a direct cause-and-effect relationship; instead, what is important is that patients undergoing liver surgery and receiving very few units of blood transfusion nevertheless have higher complication rates.[139] There are increased infectious complications in those transfused: the more transfusions that are done, the higher the rate of total complications and infectious complications. The cause is not known, but one possible mechanism proposed is "transfusion-related immunomodulation."[140] In addition, patients who have received blood stored 29 days or more have twice the rate of infection. It has been suggested that the reason for this observation is that as stored RBCs break down they release cytokines that can lower immune function.[141] One could hypothesize that by reducing transfusion, complications would also be reduced. A prospective trial of ANH reduced RBC transfusion but did not reduce morbidity.[87]

Most HPB surgery is performed for cancer, and studies have examined the association of cancer progression and RBC transfusion for primary and metastatic cancer. Because it was reported in the journal *Anesthesiology* that blood transfusion in rats promoted cancer progression,[142] there has been a perception that an anesthesiologist's choice to transfuse RBCs can influence long-term survival. Human studies have not supported animal data, however. A retrospective review of 1300 hepatectomy patients with metastatic colorectal cancer reported the major effect on survival is in the immediate postoperative period, but transfusion did not predict long-term survival.[139] Patients receiving only autologous blood or spared-blood transfusion from ANH also did not have better disease-free survival.[131,139] Postoperative complications, especially infectious and other tumor-related factors, such as tumor-infiltrating lymphocytes, are more dominant determinants of long-term cancer survival.[143] The magnitude of operative blood loss during resection of hepatocellular carcinoma was found to be a predictor of recurrence and survival rates; however, the blood loss was found to be related to tumor characteristics and extent of surgery.[144] RBC transfusions are indisputably associated with an increase in mortality and morbidity in liver surgery; however, transfusion may be a surrogate marker of one or more other variables that is more directly related to the complication. Abdominal infections are the most common complication of modern HPB surgery.[4] Postoperative complications in cancer patients have been shown to reduce disease-free survival and disease-specific survival.[22,118] The mechanism is unknown, but perioperative inflammation and infection are a current theory.

CHOICE OF ANESTHESIA AND HEMODYNAMICS

The impact of anesthesia and surgery on hepatic blood flow (HBF) has important implications for intraoperative management. The liver is unique in that it receives a dual afferent blood supply equivalent to about 20% of the cardiac output. The majority of HPF (70%) is via the portal vein and flows through the hepatic sinusoids, hepatic veins, vena cava, and back to the right atrium, and the remainder is derived from the hepatic artery. It is a low-resistance reservoir that can store blood during hypervolemia and a source of blood during times of hypovolemia. Although hepatic outflow may vary, hepatic inflow is constant by the reciprocal relationship of portal vein flow and hepatic artery flow.[145] When portal venous flow increases, hepatic arterial flow decreases, and when portal vein flow decreases, hepatic arterial flow increases. This is the hepatic arterial buffer response because the hepatic artery adjusts its tone to keep HBF at a steady state. The reverse is not true; hepatic arterial tone does not affect portal venous flow (see Chapter 5).

Veins, particularly splanchnic veins, are much more compliant than arteries,[146] and with a higher density of α-adrenergic receptors, are more sensitive to sympathetic activation than arteries.[147] HBF is directly proportional to perfusion pressure (mean arterial or portal vein pressure minus hepatic vein pressure) across the liver and inversely related to splanchnic vascular resistance. Autoregulation of HPB is not prominent; therefore total HBF (arterial plus portal) can be modified by "surgery-related" factors, such as stimulation, retraction, or manipulation, and several "anesthesia-related" factors, such as positive pressure ventilation, anesthetic technique, or drug effect on perfusion pressure or splanchnic vascular resistance.

Oxygen delivery to the liver may already be marginal because most of the blood flow is with desaturated hemoglobin delivered via the portal vein. A well-planned anesthetic maximizes the relationship between oxygen supply and demand, with the premise that reductions in systemic pressure will reduce HBF. A good rule of thumb is anything that could result in significant reductions of systemic pressure and/or blood flow (cardiac output–induced hypotension, hypovolemia, anesthetic overdoses) should be avoided.

Volatile anesthetics reduce HBF in a dose-dependent fashion by affecting cardiac output and systemic pressure. Isoflurane has been considered the agent of choice in cases in which preservation of splanchnic blood flow is required. Liver blood flow and the hepatic artery buffer response are maintained better in the presence of isoflurane than with any other volatile anesthetic agent.[148] In addition, isoflurane attenuates the increases in hepatic oxygen consumption associated with surgery and liver manipulation. Desflurane is shown to have no deleterious effects on liver function and hepatocyte integrity. Desflurane anesthesia is associated with significantly greater gut blood flow than equipotent isoflurane. This difference cannot be explained by systemic hemodynamics alone. There is no difference in total hepatic flow between isoflurane and desflurane groups, however, implying that an intact hepatic arterial supply buffers response with desflurane.[149] Sevoflurane seems to be like isoflurane and desflurane with a few exceptions. Indocyanine green clearance is better preserved during sevoflurane anesthesia. Sevoflurane seems like isoflurane in its effect on regional HBF.[150] Nitrous oxide is used extensively in patients with hepatic disease. It is not shown to contribute to hepatic disease exacerbation.[151] The sympathomimetic effects of nitrous oxide decrease HBF.

Intravenous Anesthetics and Muscle Relaxants

Inhaled anesthetics supply all the aspects needed for anesthesia in one package, but today most anesthesiologists choose multiple drugs to reach their goals: immobility, amnesia, suppression of autonomic reflexes, muscle relaxation, and analgesia. Over the last several decades, dramatic advances have been made in IV anesthesia, with the result that total IV anesthesia is now a workable alternative to the traditional inhalation anesthetic. Anesthesiologists using multiple drugs take advantage of the interactions of drugs with different mechanisms of action but similar therapeutic effects. The therapeutic goal of the anesthetic can often be achieved with less toxicity and faster recovery than when the individual drugs are used alone in higher doses.

The liver plays a major role in biotransformation, the process through which drugs are broken down into metabolites that can be more easily eliminated. The main mechanisms that affect hepatic elimination of a drug are changes in HBF and changes in the ability of the liver cells to biotransform a drug for excretion. These two mechanisms, hepatocyte function and HBF, have an important role in the choice of anesthetics for patients undergoing hepatobiliary surgery because even small changes in liver function or blood flow can change the concentrations of drugs and their metabolites. High-extraction drugs (ketamine, flumazenil, morphine, fentanyl, sufentanil, lidocaine) are directly related to liver blood flow and essentially cleared as they pass through the liver. Protein binding, enzymatic induction, intrahepatic shunting, and the effect of anesthetics on liver blood flow may affect the elimination of drugs with a high-extraction rate. Reductions in metabolic clearance result in increases of peak drug level with minimal change in the elimination half-life. Low-extraction drugs are those whose concentration is little changed after passage through the liver and depend on the intrinsic clearance (liver size, total enzyme capacity) of the liver. The elimination of drugs with a low-extraction rate (benzodiazepines) depends more on the metabolic capacity of the liver and less on the HBF. In patients with impaired liver function, such drugs experience a prolonged length of activity with no increase in peak levels.

The safety of IV anesthetic agents and muscle relaxants is uncontested, yet, increasingly, anesthesiologists prefer agents that are not influenced by liver function or using multiple drugs for the same effect despite liver dysfunction. Although the use of opioids is appropriate during HPB surgery and the management is like other abdominal surgery, remifentanil, a short rapidly acting opioid, given by continual infusion and metabolized by plasma esterases, is gaining in popularity over fentanyl. The muscle relaxants atracurium and cisatracurium both undergo Hoffman degradation and ester hydrolysis, neither of which is dependent on liver function. Dexmedetomidine, an α2-agonist, and ketamine do depend on hepatic function; however, perioperatively, their weak analgesic effects decrease the minimum alveolar concentration of volatile vapors and the postoperative opioid requirements.[152,153]

Analgesia Strategies

Effective analgesia in HPB surgery is important for postoperative respiratory function, compliance with physiotherapy, mobilization, and prevention of complications. Different analgesic strategies are needed for open and laparoscopic surgery. There is evidence supporting the use of wound catheters or transversus abdominis plane blocks. The POP-UP study demonstrated that continuous wound infiltration is noninferior to epidural analgesia in HPB surgery.[154] Medial open transversus abdominis plane catheter analgesia conferred superior analgesia versus IV patient-controlled analgesia (PCA) following liver resection.[155] Single-shot spinal opioid administration may provide adequate analgesia for both laparoscopic and open pancreatic surgery. Intrathecal morphine and PCA have been shown to provide acceptable postoperative outcomes in patients undergoing open liver resection.[156] In a recent survey of HPB surgeons in Canada, IV PCA and epidural analgesia were used in similar proportions, with very few surgeons reporting routine use of regional nerve blocks such as transversus abdominis plane catheters.[157]

Epidural Anesthesia and Analgesia

In recent years HPB surgery, performed under general anesthesia and a thoracic epidural block, that may be used intraoperatively or solely to provide postoperative analgesia, has increased as providers have taken a growing interest in ERAS protocols (see Chapter 27). Guidelines for ERAS almost unanimously include the use of regional analgesia when appropriate. Level 1 evidence for the use of epidurals in open abdominal surgery stems from their ability to reduce PPCs[158] and provide multimodal analgesia, thereby reducing opioid-related adverse effects.

In contrast to pancreatic surgery, there remains an unclear role for EDA or analgesia in the setting of liver surgery. The most commonly used incisions are subcostal or midline, with significant cephalic retraction of the chest wall. Therefore the patient's pain is more like a postthoracotomy patient's pain. Although thoracic extrapleural analgesia (EPA) provides superior pain relief for thoracoabdominal operations[159] and reduces PPCs,[158] the risk versus benefit of an indwelling catheter with EDA for liver operations is controversial due to the role the liver plays in the postoperative coagulation cascade[135] and the possibility that EDA may drive increased fluid therapy and transfusion[160] or AKI.[134] In addition, the number one complication following hepatectomy is abdominal infections, with PPCs, less common than thoracic surgery and resulting more from the act of surgery (pleural effusion or bile leak) than the patient's comorbidity. The decision to consider the use of epidurals in liver surgery is further complicated by potential for perioperative hypotension, which may be exacerbated by management of patients using LCVP technique. EDA may be used to provide LCVP conditions during hepatic surgery.[120,161] Despite many animal and human studies, the effects of thoracic EDA on HBF are not entirely clear. EDA can interfere with the numerous factors affecting HBF: hemodynamics, autonomic nervous system, circulating neurohumoral agents, and local metabolites (adenosine) either by sympathetic blockade, systemic hemodynamics, or even the circulating effects of local anesthetics.[162] Splanchnic veins, with their higher density of α-adrenergic receptors, play the main role in maintaining a ratio between stressed (Vs) and unstressed blood volume (Vu).[146] Vu is hemodynamically inactive, but when venoconstriction changes it, this is equivalent to a transfusion of a significant amount of blood. Controlled ventilation and EDA both decrease venous return (VR) and must be associated with an increase in Vs to maintain hemodynamics. Decreased Vs and VR can be restored by fluid infusion to fill up the increased venous capacity or by an α-agonist to increase sympathetic tone of the compliant veins, which robs from Vu to give to Vs. If fluid is infused to counteract the hemodynamic effects of EPA, this may lead to excessive hydration and increased packed RBC transfusion after hepatectomy. The clinical advantage of using a vasopressor is that it maintains tissue blood flow but avoids fluid infusion. However, a clinician who practices LCVP should realize that this approach might decrease the margin of safety. Low Vu per se is not harmful and up to 1000 mL of blood may be lost without change in standard hemodynamic parameters. However, beyond this point, when the mobilization of blood

from Vu to Vs is approximately complete, even minor reduced VR, whether by the Pringle technique, vena caval compression, or blood loss, can quickly lead to hemodynamic deterioration. Vasopressors during LCVP-assisted liver surgery are certainly justified; however, it may delay recognizing dangerous hypovolemia.

Nonetheless, enthusiasts point out that there may be several other advantages to regional anesthesia, especially when combined with postoperative EPA: better pain control, attenuation of the stress response, decreased requirement of volatile anesthetics, and a reduction in the need for perioperative opioids. The avoidance of the need for perioperative opioid-based analgesia cannot be overstated. Aside from well-established immediate adverse effects attributed to opioids, perioperative opioids may have longer-lasting implications. The Centers for Disease Control and Prevention recently rated prescription opioid abuse among the top five health threats, and the so-called opioid crisis in the United States has been linked to the over prescription of opioids by well-intentioned providers.

Perhaps the strongest arguments for the use of thoracic EDA for liver surgery is its possible modulation of the immune response and its possible effect on tissue microperfusion.[162] Preclinical data, animal studies, and retrospective reviews demonstrate the potential for a decreased recurrence rate in some cancer types. Animal studies have shown that EDA could have an important role in modifying tissue microperfusion and protecting tissue from ischemic damage, regardless of the effects on hemodynamics. The notion that anesthesiologists may be able to impact the short-term and long-term outcome for a cancer patient simply by incorporating regional anesthesia is appealing, although unproven in human studies and more prospective randomized research is needed. Recently, basic science and retrospective reviews have suggested that the anesthetic management during cancer surgery may influence the patient's long-term survival. There are several multicenter prospective trials underway to examine whether the use of regional anesthesia can truly decrease cancer recurrence. What is perhaps the most intriguing and an immediate hypothesis for HPB surgery is whether EDA can improve immune function and increase resistance to postoperative infection.

Surgical stress and pain may induce lymphocyte depletion, which may be associated with the risk of postoperative infectious complications. Although circulating cytokines related to monocyte activation and phenotype alterations are not influenced by postoperative pain reduction compared with systemic opioid treatment, there has been evidence in animals that EPA influences lymphocyte distribution, increases the postoperative CD4/CD8 ratio and B cells, and decreases natural killer cells. This preservation of immunity has not been shown in human studies.[163] EDA combined with EPA has been shown to significantly reduce the amount of postoperative inflammatory response in patients by altering the circulating leukocyte surface molecules CD11b and CD62L (L-selectin), which are known to be more sensitive markers of the early detection of postoperative stress response inflammatory markers.[164] If there is an attenuated neutrophil adhesive capability by EDA/EPA, and if this improves patient resistance to infection, this may be more important for HPB surgery than for other types of surgery because of the role that the liver plays in the immune and inflammatory process.

An elevated INR or decreased platelet count can influence the timing of the removal of the catheter because of a theoretical risk of spinal hematoma.[162] In recent years, bloodless hepatic surgery, the known hypercoagulable state despite elevated INR and decreased platelet counts, and the safety of an indwelling catheter in other surgeries in patients who undergo anticoagulation postoperatively allows for re-evaluation of the modern age risk versus benefit in patients undergoing liver resection. There are no clinical guidelines as to the safety of epidural use solely for the patient undergoing liver surgery. The guidelines for the placement and removal of neuraxial analgesia in patients with coagulation defects outlined by the American Society of Regional Anesthesia (ASRA) apply to hepatic resection as well.[165]

Today, most ACPs believe that epidural use is safe in liver surgery. The vasodilatory effect of volatile anesthetics may safely be treated with vasopressor support and is expected to terminate at the end of surgery. The sympathetic blockage of epidural analgesic results in relative hypotension, which can be treated with temporary vasopressor support and does not require aggressive fluid resuscitation, but this treatment approach may need to be continued in the immediate postoperative time. At tertiary care centers, where an acute pain anesthesia service and ACP work closely with the surgeon to evaluate epidural function, volume status and potential complications, its benefits may outweigh its risks. There is a paucity of randomized trials examining this controversy, however.

The ASA postoperative evidenced-based pain management guidelines are generalized and can be confusing when adapted to liver surgery. The web-based PROSPECT (Procedure-Specific Postoperative Pain Management) is a collaborative group of anesthesiologists, surgeons, and surgical scientists that recommend optimal postoperative pain management that is specific for different surgical procedures, as well as arguments for and against the invasiveness of the analgesic technique and the consequences of pain on outcome. Hepatic surgery is not represented, and what operation is transferable is unclear. Recent 2016 guidelines by the ERAS society specifically outline current evidence and recommendations for optimal postoperative pain management in liver surgery that support use of intrathecal or wound infusion catheters.[166] Despite recognizing improved pain control, ERAS society recommendations are less enthusiastic regarding patient-controlled epidural anesthetic given potential delay in removal with elevated INR/prothrombin time and reported increased risk of kidney failure secondary to hypotension.[167]

After HPB surgery, most patients are extubated in the operating room. Until recently, it was tacitly assumed that postoperative pain was essentially the pain of inflammation plus, perhaps, some direct pain from cutting nerves. Subsequently, it has been demonstrated that there are important differences between pain from surgery and pain from inflammation.[168] More important from a clinical perspective, some drugs are effective to treat either surgery pain or inflammation, such as opioids, whereas others are unique to the setting. A better understanding of the pain pathways and the concerted effort by ERAS to shorten and uncomplicate hospital stay, especially in the older patient, has drawn attention to the success of multimodality analgesia. Postoperative pain management has evolved considerably from the use of parental or neuraxial opioid monotherapy to multimodal opioid-sparing analgesia. The options include NSAIDs/cyclo-oxygenase-2 inhibitors, local anesthetics, N-methyl-d-aspartate antagonists, α_2-antagonists, thoracic epidural catheters, single-dose intrathecal, transverse abdominis plane blocks, IV PCA, and local analgesia including local wound injection catheters for the incisional wound.[169] Although opioids have stood the test of

time to anchor postoperative pain, these drugs, whether infused epidurally or parentally, are not without adverse effects; consequently, targeted multimodality opioid-sparing analgesic algorithms are ubiquitous. These algorithms may not be safe for patients having hepatic surgery; instead, choices must be based on an individual basis, given the liver's role in drug biotransformation and coagulation.

CARDIOPULMONARY

Cardiopulmonary complications are no longer the major postoperative morbidity for HPB patients. This improvement parallels decreased blood loss, decreased transfusion rate, and improved perioperative fluid and hemodynamic management.

Cardiac Dysfunction

The incidence of postoperative MI may be explained by better patient selection and optimization; however, the absence of benefit of preoperative revascularization in the face of known coronary artery disease may be explained, first, by the overall skill with which ACPs manage perioperative stressors, and second by the nature of perioperative MI. Ischemia can occur due to excess demand versus supply (type 2 MI)[170] as triggered by hypertension, tachycardia, hypoxia, anemia, or hypotension. ACPs can and do manage these conditions both intraoperatively and postoperatively. Ischemia can also occur with acute plaque rupture and thrombosis formation.[170] These events occur more often in the operative setting due to increased hypertension, tachycardia (shear forces), hypercoagulability, and surgery-associated inflammatory response. The perioperative period is particularly risky for patients with coronary stents who may already have a disrupted coronary endothelial lining and are predisposed to stent thrombosis. Fearful of the risk for surgical bleeding, well-meaning surgeons may inappropriately advise patients to discontinue their dual APT which not only reverses the antiplatelet effect but also leads to an exaggerated rebound thrombogenic effect. The POISE trials give credibility to a calculated strategy of decreasing heart rate while avoiding perioperative hypotension (avoid MI and stroke). The ACP should be able to manage these hemodynamic issues that can precipitate an MI, but the triggers to inflammation and hypercoagulation are poorly understood and not yet modifiable by an anesthetic method. The ACPs involved in nonpreventable events may have their clinical vigilance and ability to rescue the patient questioned, or they may feel as personally responsible as those involved in preventable events.[171]

Myocardial injury after noncardiac surgery is common and not necessarily revealed by ischemic features (symptoms or electrocardiographic findings). A large international study reported that an elevated troponin T, irrespective of ischemic features, independently predicted 30-day mortality.[172]

Pulmonary Dysfunction

PPCs include pneumonia, respiratory failure, bronchospasm, pleural effusions, atelectasis, hypoxemia, and exacerbation of underlying chronic lung disease. Atelectasis and pleural effusion are common consequences of anesthesia and surgery after HPB surgery. With aggressive postoperative pulmonary toilet and early mobilization, these minor problems resolve without the need for further intervention.

At least three mechanisms contribute to impaired pulmonary function in the postoperative period. First, respiratory muscles disrupted by surgical transection (abdominal muscles) will not function normally. Second, patients may limit motion of respiratory muscles to minimize postoperative pain. Finally, stimulation of the visceral afferent nerves markedly changes the activation of respiratory muscles. For example, removal of the gallbladder activates vagal efferent, which produces a reflex inhibition of diaphragmatic activity. Of note, laparoscopic surgery may ameliorate the first two mechanisms but not the third, and significant decrements in pulmonary function may still be observed after laparoscopic surgery.

ACPs play a key role in the prevention of PPCs. Preoperative preparation, intraoperative management, and immediate postoperative care can have a major impact on the occurrence of this morbidity. It has long been known that the induction of general anesthesia, both total IV anesthesia and inhaled anesthesia, decreases lung volume and promotes dependent zone atelectasis.[173,174] To improve oxygenation, ACPs apply a high TV and high fraction of inspired oxygen (FiO_2). High FiO_2 via absorption atelectasis has also been linked to the development of atelectasis during the postoperative period.[175] After HPB surgery, like all abdominal surgery, this impaired oxygenation caused by intraoperative atelectasis persists for days after the surgical procedure.[176] An association, but not a causal effect, of atelectasis and PPC has been reported.[177] There is experimental work that links atelectatic areas of the lung to translocation and increased bacterial growth, providing an optimal nidus for infection.[178] Regardless of the etiology, PPCs increase 30-day mortality.[54]

The use of high TV (10–15 mL/kg) ventilation, encouraged to prevent atelectasis, results in high peak ventilatory airway pressure, which has been shown to be associated with acute lung injury.[179] Low TV ventilation (TV 6–8 mL/kg ideal body weight) with PEEP (6–8 mm H_2O) and recruitment maneuvers every 30 minutes (lung protective ventilation) has demonstrated reduced mortality in patients with acute respiratory distress syndrome and decreased PPCs in patients at risk of PPCs after abdominal surgery.[180] Yet, most anesthesiologists decrease TVs without the addition of PEEP or respiratory maneuvers (likely because of their effects on hemodynamics), which in a large retrospective cohort may have led to increased mortality.[181] The authors speculated that this resulted from increased atelectasis from lower intraoperative TV ventilation. Lung protective ventilation is being proposed as a standard of care to be bundled into ERAS or perioptimal care to further decrease the incidence of PPCs and serve as a measure of the quality and safety of care. Effective strategy during pancreatic surgery should involve the application of a protective ventilation strategy (lower TVs <8 mL/kg, PEEP = 6–12 mm Hg and recruitment maneuvers) to improve respiratory function during the postoperative period and to reduce the clinical signs of pulmonary infection.[182] On the other hand, during liver surgery, the ACP must weigh the evidence for lung protective ventilation and the effect of high PEEP and respiratory maneuvers on decreased VR or liver congestion on a patient-by-patient basis.

Postoperative respiratory failure is most commonly defined as the need for mechanical ventilation for more than 48 hours or unplanned postoperative reintubation. The nature and magnitude of the preexisting respiratory conditions determine the effect of a given standard anesthetic on respiratory function. The ACP plays a key role in the prevention of respiratory muscle-related PPCs. In patients with obstructive lung disease,

high airway resistance favors deep slow respiration, which may not be possible in patients with large abdominal incisions. The treatment of this pain with opioids will reduce minute ventilation and respiratory drive. A meta-analysis of patients undergoing thoracic and abdominal surgery showed that the odds of developing postoperative pneumonia was reduced nearly 50% in patients receiving epidural versus IV analgesia, fueling the controversy of this choice in patients after HPB resection.[158]

Particular attention must be paid to anesthetic elimination and residual drug effect, especially sedative, analgesic, and neuromuscular blockers, in posthepatectomy patients who have altered drug pharmacodynamics and pharmacokinetics. In a recent prospective cohort study, the use of intermediate-acting neuromuscular blocking agents was associated with postoperative desaturation (90%) and reintubation, regardless of train-of-four monitoring and use of reversal agents.[183] In a cohort of 33,769 surgical cases, planned reintubation within the first 3 days after surgery was associated with a 72-fold increased risk of in-hospital mortality.[184]

The findings of a recent systematic review and meta-analysis suggest that the use of early CPAP for the prevention of hypoxemia after abdominal surgery may reduce the incidence of PPCs compared with just supplemental oxygen.[185]

Anticipated respiratory compromise after HPB surgery in patients without an epidural may preclude early extubation, especially in combination with any baseline abnormality in gas exchange. If a patient must be placed on mechanical ventilation, diaphragmatic weakness, atrophy, and respiratory muscle fatigue can occur within hours. Like all muscles, complete rest can lead to diaphragm atrophy, and modes that allow patient triggering, such as assist-control ventilation, are necessary to maintain diaphragm muscle function.[186]

SPECIAL CONSIDERATION LIVER SURGERY: AIR EMBOLUS

The goal of keeping a low central pressure to minimize back bleeding from the liver sinusoids during transection must be counterbalanced by a central pressure that minimizes the risk of air entrainment. The risk of intraoperative air emboli is likely to increase under LCVP anesthesia. Elimination of nitrogen from the anesthetic gas mixture is necessary to permit expiratory nitrogen monitoring for air emboli. Restriction of nitrous oxide in the gas mixture prevents the diffusion-mediated increase in the size of circulating air. Transesophageal echocardiography can be used to monitor air emboli, but this technology is sensitive and overdiagnoses clinically insignificant events. At our institution, during open hepatectomy, surgical and anesthesia vigilance and communication are the keys to detect and treat air emboli. With surgical watchfulness and rapid occlusion of open venous channels, and our monitoring of end-tidal carbon dioxide and hemodynamics, LCVP anesthesia results in a low incidence of clinically significant air emboli.

Minimally Invasive Liver Resection

Anesthesiologists continually adjust strategies as innovative surgical techniques evolve. The benefits of laparoscopic liver resection (LLR) have been associated with less blood loss and earlier postoperative recovery,[22] although all the comparisons reported are retrospective and therefore associated with a huge selection bias. Pneumoperitoneum induces predictable pulmonary and renal responses as well as phasic hemodynamic changes. Intraperitoneal insufflation and head-up tilt result in impairment of HBF secondary to decreases in cardiac output.[187,188] In well-selected patients, the consequences of these changes are not relevant. However, the challenges of the pneumoperitoneum, positioning, and mechanical ventilation on cardiopulmonary function in addition to longer surgical time may not be the correct choice for every patient. Before positioning, the patient should be prepared the same as for an open case, including the ability to do large-volume transfusion in case inadvertent major vessel bleeding occurs. A protocol should be in place as well as a fully open instrument tray and equipment available in case the robot must be undocked emergently to convert to open surgery. It is important that the anesthesiologist and surgeon have a discussion before the start of the laparoscopic or robotic liver case because the risk versus benefit of LCVP-assisted hepatic resection is less clear.

The pneumoperitoneum compresses the portal vein, reduces portal blood flow, and seems to reduce hepatic back bleeding during transection. Decreasing blood loss for open resection is based on keeping the radius of an inadvertent venous injury small and the pressure head low so that less blood will be lost through the opening. However, retractions can distort vessels and stent them open during LLR. Fluid management is complicated by compromised hemodynamics resulting from positioning and decreased lung compliance. Renal parenchyma and venous compressions during pneumoperitoneum are the etiology of oliguria during LLR. The effects are reversible and usually cause no harm. Yet, many anesthesiologists prefer to optimize intravascular volume to minimize the effects of intraabdominal pressure (IAP) on renal and cardiac function. The issue of gas embolism (GE) during LLR is still debated. Some authors consider it little or no problem, and some consider it a real threat to patient safety.[189] The debate centers on the theory that GE occurs when the IAP exceeds CVP.[190] The opposite situation, when CVP exceeds IAP, does not prevent GE because it can occur irrespective of whether CVP is greater or less than IAP.[191] Positive pressure ventilation causes rhythmic variations in VR for both pressure and flow. With an open vein because of entrainment during the phase with higher flow, gas from the abdomen might reach the venous circulation. Both carbon dioxide and the argon beam coagulation (ABC) during liver surgery have been associated with GE.[192]

Ablation

Major hepatectomies have decreased, whereas hepatectomy with concurrent surgery and repeat hepatectomies with or without simultaneous ablation have increased. The development of ablative techniques for tumor ablation has been one of the major advances for liver cancer (see Chapter 96). Ablation therapy for benign or malignant liver tumors is often used as an alternative to surgery, the principal aim being to ablate the undesirable areas without damaging the surrounding healthy tissue. At our institution, ablation is mostly used for parenchymal-sparing procedures during a concurrent major hepatectomy or when comorbid conditions preclude major liver surgery. The treatments currently available, such as low-temperature cryosurgery, nonselective chemical ablation, focused ultrasound, radiofrequency ablation (RFA), microwave ablation (MWA), or electroporation, have their own specific advantages, disadvantages, and applications. At our institution, the ACP may care for patients undergoing an ablative procedure during open or laparoscopic surgery or percutaneous ablation in the interventional suite. Experience and rapidly changing technology have overcome many of the issues that challenged the ACP in the early years of RFA or cryotherapy and replaced them with newer concerns. RFA is by far the most frequently used procedure; however, for technical reasons, MWA and irreversible electroporation (IRE) are becoming common. MWA is faster and can be used for larger tumors, creating greater cell lysis.[193] IRE requires the use of an electrocardiogram synchronizer to protect the patient from arrhythmias and dense muscle relaxation to prevent upper muscle body contraction.[194] Despite synchronization, intraoperative cardiac events (hypertension; arrhythmias) as well as an increase in potassium levels are common during IRE but rarely impair completion of the procedure.[167]

References are available at expertconsult.com.

CHAPTER 26

Nutrition and perioperative critical care in the hepatopancreatobiliary surgery patient

Russell C. Kirks Jr, R. Eliot Fagley, and Flavio G. Rocha

Assessment of patient nutritional status and functional reserve allows surgeons to identify malnourishment and potential recovery before major abdominal surgery. Evolving nutritional and fluid management strategies, along with improving anesthesia, pain management, and hemodynamic monitoring, seek to minimize homeostatic alterations. Although specific surgical procedures, modalities, and disease states may each present specific challenges to perioperative management, these two efforts are now being understood to play a synergistic and cooperative role in patients' physiology and recovery.

NUTRITIONAL AND FUNCTIONAL ASSESSMENT

Gauging nutritional and functional status along with medical comorbidity portends a patient's functional reserve. The ideal preoperative assessment should quantify the severity of malnutrition and depletion of lean body mass, estimate a patient's physiologic reserve, and juxtapose these with the magnitude of metabolic stress induced by a surgical intervention.[1] The idea that aspects of a patient's nutritional status and functional reserve can be improved before a scheduled procedure is known as *prehabilitation*.

A thorough nutritional assessment (NA) should include: (1) a clinical gastrointestinal (GI) and dietary history; (2) a physical and/or radiographic assessment of muscle mass; (3) a strength and functional assessment; (4) an evaluation of serum nutritional markers; and (4) a determination of nutrient requirements. Historical questions should identify the degree and rate of weight loss over the previous month and 6 months, use of alcohol, duration of jaundice, and altered stool pattern. Clinical or radiographic evidence of gastric emptying abnormality, severe gastroesophageal reflux disease, or intestinal obstruction may alter the method by which nutritional supplementation is delivered.

Anthropometric tests incorporated into NA have the benefits of objectivity, rapidity, and reproducibility. A variety of anthropometric measurements, such as hand grip strength, may be used not only as a surrogate of muscle wasting but also to assess protein-energy malnutrition.[2] Used in combination with assessment of objective clinical and laboratory parameters and patient-reported assessment of eating and nutrient intake, these assessments can be used to provide a more complete clinical picture of nutrition and as part of an estimation of immediate postoperative complications.[3-5]

SERUM BIOCHEMICAL MARKERS

Although no single laboratory value is by itself indicative of nutritional sufficiency, many have the benefit of being easily obtainable through simple blood tests. Serum albumin has been extensively studied as a marker for nutritional status, and low levels have been shown to be a sensitive predictor of adverse surgical outcomes.[6-9] In the setting of liver disease, serum albumin may be more difficult to interpret as a nutritional marker because of its correlation with intrinsic liver function.[10] Serum albumin should not be used as a sole prognosticator of nutritional status given its relationship as an acute phase reactant. Unlike albumin, prealbumin is thought to be a better indicator of nutritional status given its half-life of 48 hours. As such, short-term fluctuations in nutritional standing can be more accurately assessed using serum prealbumin.[11] Unfortunately, like albumin, prealbumin levels can vary with chronic disease states.

Given the limitations of anthropometric and biochemical assays, more accurate methods of NA have incorporated key features of both to create predictive nutritional scoring systems. A number of different schemas exist, including the Nutritional Risk Index (NRI), Nutritional Risk Score (NRS), Subjective Global Assessment (SGA), and Malnutrition Universal Screening Tool (MUST).

Sarcopenia

Body mass index (BMI) is widely used in patient risk models but fails to account for the diversity of body composition. A relative dearth of lean muscle mass, called sarcopenia, is associated with functional impairments, physical disability, perioperative complications, prolonged hospital length of stay, and poorer long-term outcomes in cancer patients.[12-16] Unlike cachexia, sarcopenia develops over a long period of time and is not necessarily associated with weight loss.[17] Thus many patients who fall into a normal range for weight and BMI may have unrecognized sarcopenia. Patients who are both obese by BMI calculation and sarcopenic are categorized as having "sarcopenic obesity." Sarcopenic obesity has been reported as one of the most powerful independent predictors of poor survival for patients with cancer and is associated with impaired functional status and decreased ability to tolerate chemotherapy, surgery, and other invasive therapies.[18,19]

The most clinically applicable method used to identify sarcopenia uses computed tomography (CT) imaging to estimate lean muscle mass of the psoas muscle of a single CT image at the L3 level normalized for height (total psoas area in mm^2/ height in m^2).[12,20] Patients are sarcopenic if these values are less than $385 \ mm^2/m^2$ in women or less than $545 \ mm^2/m^2$ in men. In retrospective studies, sarcopenic patients who underwent liver transplantation, liver resection, and pancreatic resection had increased perioperative complications, increased postoperative mortality, and worse overall and recurrence-free survival.[14,15,21-25]

The pathophysiology of sarcopenia is not well understood but poor nutrition, alterations in hormonal and other signaling pathways, and inflammatory factors and cytokines are thought to be

TABLE 26.1 Comparison of Comorbidity Factors Assessed in Modified Frailty Indices

MODIFIED 11-ITEM FRAILTY INDEX (mFI-11)	MODIFIED 5-ITEM FRAILTY INDEX (mFI-5)
History of diabetes mellitus	Diabetes mellitus (insulin- or noninsulin-dependent)
History of congestive heart failure	Congestive heart failure (within 30 days of surgery)
History of either COPD or pneumonia	COPD or pneumonia
Functional status 2 (not independent)	Dependent functional health status (total or partial) at time of surgery
Hypertension requiring medication	Hypertension requiring medication
History of either transient ischemia attach or cerebrovascular accident	
History of myocardial infarction	
History of either peripheral vascular disease or rest pain	
History of cerebrovascular accident with neurologic deficit	
History of either PCI, PCS, or angina	
History of impaired sensorium	

Scores calculated by assigning a 1 (for presence of comorbidity) or 0 (for absence of comorbidity). Higher scores suggest higher frailty and less physiologic reserve.
COPD, Chronic obstructive pulmonary disease; *PCI,* percutaneous coronary intervention; *PCS,* prior cardiac surgery.

the principal mechanisms behind the development of sarcopenia in the chronically ill.[26,27] Investigations seeking to mitigate the effects of sarcopenia have reported that exercise combined with supplemental protein or amino acids can reverse sarcopenia in the elderly.[28,29] These observations support the practice of prescribing exercise and supplemental protein to sarcopenic patients before hepatopancreatobiliary (HPB) surgery.[28]

Frailty

Whereas sarcopenia describes a specific and quantifiable finding, frailty comprises a more global assessment of physiology and resilience. Initially considered to be synonymous with age, frailty describes a depletion of physiologic reserves culminating in both a higher degree of vulnerability to physiologic stressors and a simultaneous decrement in the ability to recover from these physiologic challenges.[30] Considering the physiologic challenges of HPB diseases and major abdominal surgery, the assessment of frailty and incorporation into perioperative planning and patient selection is gaining interest. With an aging population,[31] a surgeon can expect to encounter more elderly and potentially more frail patients.

Frailty is a risk factor for multiple adverse outcomes such as surgical complications, mortality, and loss of functional independence.[32–34] In regards to postsurgical complications, the idea of diminished physiologic resilience contributes to increases in failure-to-rescue events, suggesting that these patients are less likely to recover from postsurgical complications even if they are managed appropriately.[35,36] With increased postoperative complications, length of stay, disposition care requirements, and healthcare-associated costs due to frailty, modifying frailty could potentially alter costs associated with healthcare.[37–39]

Assessment and quantification of frailty is based on comorbidity and functional capability. Tools such as the 11-variable modified Frailty Index (mFI) are used to identify patients at higher risk for postoperative complications, disposition to facilities rather than home, and longer lengths of stay in oncologic surgical.[40–42] A 5-factor modified frailty index has also been derived from American College of Surgeons National Quality Improvement Project (ACS-NSQIP) data. Comparing the 5- and 11-factor frailty indices across surgical subspecialties supports the predictive ability of the shorter 5-factor frailty

index for the prediction of mortality, postoperative complications, and 30-day readmission in general surgery procedures. This study did not specifically parse out HPB or surgical oncology patients[43] (Table 26.1).

Identifying frail patients allows for their enrollment in programs designed to improve modifiable risk factors when a surgery is planned or a period of observation, such as during or following neoadjuvant therapy, is included in a treatment plan. Degree of medical optimization, nutritional goals, and exercise prescription would be tailored to a patient's specific needs.[44,45] Prehabilitation of frail patients has not been studied extensively in a HPB surgery population. Prehabilitation efforts performed in non-HPB abdominal surgery population focus on smoking cessation, improving exercise tolerance, stress elimination, and nutritional improvement.[46–48]

NUTRITIONAL FOCUS: LIVER AND BILIARY DISEASE

Patients with liver disease, biliary obstruction, bacterial or viral infection, or malnutrition have impaired antioxidant defenses coupled with increased oxidant stresses.[49] Additional factors that deplete hepatic antioxidants include smoking, alcohol ingestion, general anesthesia, and surgery.[50] Chronic liver disease further alters bile salt pools and enterohepatic circulation of bile salts, leading to impaired micelle formation and consequently malabsorption of fat and fat-soluble vitamins.

Obstructive Jaundice

Approximately 45% to 70% of patients with obstructive jaundice present with malnutrition because of anorexia resulting in diminished oral intake.[51] The primary nutritional deficit resulting from obstructive jaundice is malabsorption of fat and fat-soluble vitamins in addition to trace minerals. Biliary sepsis in patients with obstructive jaundice contributes to malnutrition by shifting protein synthesis from anabolic protein synthesis to acute-phase protein synthesis.[52] Although some authors have advocated preoperative biliary drainage (PBD) in patients undergoing HPB surgery, multicenter trials and Cochrane analysis have demonstrated no evidence to support or refute routine biliary drainage and stenting in patients with malignant HPB diseases awaiting surgery.[53,54] Conversely, PBD should probably be performed in patients undergoing extended hepatectomy to improve the health of the planned remnant. To reverse the catabolic effects of chronic endotoxemia and restore hepatic protein synthesis, patients with cholangitis should be treated with biliary decompression for at least 4 weeks before major HPB surgery (see Chapter 43).

For patients with pancreatic disease presenting with recent-onset obstructive jaundice, PBD may not be required in the absence of profound malnourishment or deconditioning. Although routine PBD is discouraged in such patients because of substantial increases in the incidence of postoperative infectious complications,[55] patients with long-standing obstructive jaundice, cholangitis, and those who are planned to receive neoadjuvant therapy before resection benefit from biliary decompression during this period.

Such patients are best managed with internal biliary drainage as part of a comprehensive nutritional repletion program. Internal drainage can be accomplished by endoscopic drainage, percutaneous biliary access with internal stenting, or rendezvous procedure (see Chapters 30 and 31). For patients managed with external biliary drainage, bile refeeding may be a consideration: prolonged external drainage and discarding of bile occurring in the setting of biliary obstruction or disconnection culminates in dehydration, metabolic acidosis, progressive loss of biliary protein, and nutrient malabsorption. Most patients can tolerate bolus infusion of bile into their small bowel of 150 mL or less every 4 hours. If a patient has percutaneous jejunal feeding access, it is preferable to provide bile refeeding in a continuous manner. An alternative to enteric bile refeeding is to provide oral bile salts (ursodeoxycholic acid, 300 mg QID) to form micelles for fat absorption.[56]

Hepatic Steatosis

The presence, degree, and evolution of hepatic steatosis may all be considerations in the operative assessment and planning for patients undergoing hepatic resection (see Chapter 69). Classically defined by the presence of 5% or greater of triglycerides in hepatic parenchyma based on biopsy, many studies characterize the degree of steatosis based on severity.[57-60] Although the most common etiology of steatosis is because of nonalcoholic fatty liver disease (NAFLD), chemotherapy-associated steatosis (CAS) describes a change in intrahepatic fat (IHF) composition over time during chemotherapy administration. The degree of steatosis and presence of inflammation may alter the detection and tracking of hepatic lesions and size of the planned remnant when hepatectomy is planned.

Cytotoxic chemotherapy administered in the treatment of colorectal liver metastases (CRCLM) may also contribute to hepatic steatosis or steatohepatitis. CAS has been described as a result of many current regimens used in the treatment of colorectal cancer and CRCLM including irinotecan and fluorouracil.[61-63] An additional description of etiologic factors of steatosis and chemotherapy-associated changes is provided in Chapter 69.

The degree of steatosis can contribute to the development of postoperative complications. Retrospective studies have found that patients undergoing hepatic resection were at significantly higher risk for infectious, wound-related, GI, and hepatobiliary complications when the background liver was characterized by at least 30% steatosis.[64-66] Severe steatosis can also increase operative time and increase transfusion requirements.[65] The degree of steatosis, with potential correlation to remnant function, also correlates with increasing overall postoperative morbidity,[67] post-hepatectomy liver failure (PHLF),[68] increased intensive care unit (ICU) stay, and increased hospital length of stay.[69]

Liver parenchymal modification has been described in bariatric literature via low-calorie diets (800–1000 kCal/day for 4 weeks).[70,71] Further dietary studies focusing on intrahepatic fat burden demonstrate that drastic changes in intrahepatic fat can be achieved in short periods of time.[72,73] Pharmacologic interventions have also been investigated as measures to decrease intrahepatic fact and mitigate the inflammatory changes of steatohepatitis,[74,75] but the duration of medication use in these studies may limit their practical use in the prior liver resection.

Cirrhosis and Liver Failure

Cirrhosis causes multiple hormonal and metabolic alterations, yielding loss of fat and muscle mass, glucose intolerance, insulin resistance,[76] increased plasma glucagon and catecholamines,[77] elevated serum free fatty acids,[78] hypoproteinemia, and hyperammonemia.[79] These metabolic aberrations eventually lead to increased skeletal muscle proteolysis with muscle wasting and increased peripheral lipolysis, leading to hyperglycemia and hyperlipidemia.[80] Added risk factors for malnutrition include protein-restricted diets used in an effort to prevent encephalopathy. The practice of routine protein restriction should be abandoned in an already malnourished patient because it exacerbates the problems inherently associated with malnutrition (see Chapters 77 and 78).

NUTRITIONAL FOCUS: PANCREATIC DISEASE

Many factors contribute to perioperative nutritional deficits and malnutrition in patients with benign or malignant pancreatic disease. Patients with abdominal pain related to pancreatic disease may have profound malnutrition because of food avoidance, dietary restriction, exocrine or endocrine insufficiency, pancreatic and/or biliary duct obstruction, and chronic malabsorption. Patients with severe acute pancreatitis and particularly those with acute superimposed on chronic pancreatitis are at risk for profound malnutrition and metabolic derangement because of the catabolic effects of critical illness and sepsis.

Pancreatic Cancer

Pancreatic cancer (PC) is associated with a severe metabolic derangement referred to as "cancer anorexia-cachexia syndrome"[81,82] (see Chapter 62). This syndrome is associated with anorexia, tissue wasting, malnutrition, weight loss, and a loss of compensatory increase in feeding. The pathogenesis is dependent on disorders of carbohydrate, protein, lipid, and energy metabolism mediated by proinflammatory cytokine elaboration and an overall increase in leptin.[83,84] PC patients have the highest incidence of cachexia among patients with cancer; up to 80% of such patients have cachexia at the time of initial diagnosis. Increasing severity of anorexia-cachexia in PC patients interferes with therapy and correlates with short survival.[19,85] For this reason, patients with PC are perhaps the most likely of all patients undergoing HPB surgery to benefit from nutritional support strategies.

Pancreatic Exocrine Insufficiency

Benign and malignant conditions of the pancreas can produce biliary and/or pancreatic duct obstruction resulting in maldigestion and malabsorption. The majority of patients with PC present with malnutrition and weight loss, with 75% found to have pancreatic exocrine insufficiency (PEI) at presentation.[86] The etiology of PEI in patients with PC is incompletely understood but likely related to main pancreatic duct obstruction, glandular atrophy, age- or cancer-related pancreatic exocrine senescence, and potentially reduced exocrine function because of previous pancreatitis. Because PEI is so common in patients with pancreatic cancer, an argument can be made to provide pancreatic enzymes to all symptomatic patients at the time of diagnosis. Asymptomatic patients, on the other hand, should be evaluated for PEI by fecal elastase 1 assay. The nutritional consequences of untreated or unrecognized steatorrhea can lead to significant weight loss, malnutrition, vitamin deficiencies, poor quality of life, and delays in therapy.[87,88]

NUTRITION SUPPORT OF HPB SURGERY PATIENTS

The primary goal for nutritional support (NS) in patients before and after HPB surgery is to restore health and function as quickly as possible; this is facilitated by the support of normal digestion and intestinal absorption. Although no data support the routine use of NS in well-nourished patients undergoing HPB surgery, patients who are profoundly malnourished or deficient in specific vitamins probably benefit from NS.[28,89,90]

The majority of patients with HPB disease who are malnourished do not require specialized NS to correct their nutritional deficits because in most circumstances, their malnutrition is the consequence of inadequate caloric intake over prolonged periods of time. There are no consensus guidelines on a specific duration of nutritional repletion required to achieve a certain level of risk reduction of operative complications. Experts recommend at least 7 days and preferably 2 to 3 weeks of oral nutritional repletion in patients who have profound malnutrition or until such time that the serum prealbumin rises into a normal range.[28,91]

Routes of Feeding

The most common and physiologic manner of NS is an oral diet tailored to the patient's needs. If the patient is unable to consume an oral diet or meet their estimated caloric needs orally, enteral tube feeding access should be considered. Although nasoenteral feeding may be suitable for a short duration of feeding, jejunal, gastric, or gastrojejunostomy tubes should be considered for a longer duration of feeding. Supplementation with pancreatic enzymes, bile salts, and/or bile refeeding may enhance absorption in instances of PEI or biliary diversion, respectively. There is no clinical evidence to support the administration of supraphysiologic amounts of substrate (e.g., more than 5 mg/kg/min of glucose or more than 2 g protein/kg/day).[89,92]

If a patient fails to meet their total nutritional needs by combined oral and enteral routes, the addition of parenteral nutrition (PN) is appropriate. The increased infectious complications and costs associated with PN mandate that it is used only in patients with anatomic abnormalities of the GI tract in whom EN is not feasible or fails.[93–97] The physiologic benefits of enteral nutrition (EN) over PN are maintenance of intestinal immunity and gut integrity, prevention of intestinal microbial translocation, reduced postoperative infections and sepsis, and lesser expense.[98–100] Routine PN has not been found to

convey benefit to patients undergoing HPB operations in the first 2 weeks postoperatively.[101] Prolonged PN can cause hepatocellular steatosis and cholestasis.[102] It is important that, when PN is used, patients are not given excess calories (e.g., they should receive less than 30 kCal/kg/day) and glycemic control (serum glucose 100–150) is maintained with insulin.

Nutrition Support As Part of Enhanced Recovery After Surgery Programs

Perioperative care regimens have changed substantially over the last decade with the advent of Enhanced Recovery After Surgery (ERAS) protocols[103] (see Chapter 27). ERAS is a multimodal and multidisciplinary management pathway that's goal is to maintain and more quickly restore health and function to patients by mitigating the catabolic stress response to operation. A central tenet of ERAS is to limit preoperative fasting and restore oral intake as soon as possible postoperatively. Current ERAS guidelines for pancreatic resection recommend the use of preoperative oral carbohydrate supplementation 2 to 3 hours before anesthesia.[104–106] This practice has been shown to reduce psychological and physiologic stress, improve glycemic control during and after surgery, reduce skeletal muscle proteolysis and weakness, restore bowel motility, and reduce delayed gastric emptying after pancreaticoduodenectomy (PD).[105,107] The feasibility, safety, and utility of ERAS in patients undergoing HPB operations has recently been established and leads to reduced morbidity and shorter hospital length of stay.[104,108,109]

The majority of patients treated within an ERAS protocol who do not experience a major complication have rapid return of bowel function and tolerate ingestion of a normal regular diet within 24 to 48 hours of surgery independent of the type of operation.[110,111] Conversely, patients who deviate from postoperative recovery expectations usually have an underlying complication such as intraabdominal collection, fistula, or systemic infection. In a systematic review of the literature, Kagedan reported on 10 ERAS studies in patients undergoing PD. In the majority of studies, patients were allowed access to and tolerated solid food on the first or second postoperative day.[110] A systematic review of five feeding routes after PD concluded that an oral diet is the preferred route of feeding and that there is no evidence to support routine EN or PN after PD.[112] Current ERAS guidelines suggest most patients after hepatectomy can begin eating on day 1 after surgery,[113] and a post-PD diet is resumed based on patient tolerance.[106] Prolonged routine nasogastric decompression in patients undergoing PD and hepatectomy is not needed.[111,114]

PERIOPERATIVE CRITICAL CARE IN HEPATOBILIARY AND PANCREATIC SURGERY

Intraoperative and perioperative management of patients undergoing HPB surgical procedures is affected by malnutrition, frailty, treatment-related physiologic changes, and disease-related physiologic disturbances related to chronic liver disease. Nutrition- and disease-related factors can predispose to postoperative complications or physiology, requiring postoperative management in an ICU setting. In addition to optimizing a patient's nutrition and potentially improving stress tolerance before surgery, careful preoperative assessment, planning, and intraoperative monitoring may reduce the perioperative risks of morbidity and mortality of HPB surgery.

PREOPERATIVE ASSESSMENT AND CARE OF PATIENTS WITH LIVER DISEASE

Patients with cirrhosis and portal hypertension have higher morbidity and mortality rates, not only after HPB surgical and nonsurgical procedures but also after major nonhepatic interventions[115,116] (see Chapters 75, 101, and 102). When evaluating perioperative risks for patients with chronic liver diseases, three main factors should be considered: hepatic reserve, comorbid conditions, and the complexity of the planned surgical procedure. The development of splenomegaly and thrombocytopenia without documented portal hypertension has been noted in patients undergoing systemic chemotherapy, including those receiving chemotherapy before planned liver resection for metastatic disease.[117–119] In the absence of cirrhosis as a causal agent, this may reflect underlying sinusoidal injury in the liver parenchyma.[118,119] Mindfulness of potential portal hypertensive physiology should be considered in these patients with similar consideration given to the extent and timing of hepatectomy. Ascites, upper GI bleeding, poor nutritional state, anemia, thrombocytopenia, electrolyte disorders with or without acute kidney injury (AKI), and preoperative infection are additional risk factors for perioperative complications and mortality among cirrhotic patients undergoing surgery.[120]

Assessing Liver Function

Several tools are available to assess hepatic reserve (see Chapter 4). The most frequently used are the Child-Turcotte-Pugh (CTP) and the Model for End-Stage Liver Disease (MELD) scores.[121] The CTP score describes the degree of hepatic synthetic dysfunction and is based on the presence of hepatic encephalopathy, degree of ascites, prothrombin time, and serum levels of albumin and bilirubin. The score allows for categorization of cirrhosis into three classes: Class A (5–6 points) refers to well-compensated cirrhosis; class B (7–9 points) and class C (10–15 points) describe cases of cirrhosis that are in a state of mild and severe decompensation, respectively. The mortality rates for elective or emergent extrahepatic surgery range from 0% to 7.1% for class A, 50% for class B, and 84% to 100% for class C cirrhosis.[122] Practical limitations of the CTP scoring system include variability and interobserver subjectivity in the estimation and detection of both ascites and encephalopathy.[123] An additional limitation in surgical series is that many patients found to have hepatic encephalopathy would not be considered for hepatectomy; this has led certain groups to propose changes in the calculation of CTP scoring in which hepatic encephalopathy is replaced with platelet count to provide a more objective assessment of severity of portal hypertension.[124]

In 2000 the MELD score was developed as a prognostic index for 3-month mortality after a transjugular intrahepatic portosystemic shunt (TIPS) procedure.[125] The MELD score is based on the international normalized ratio (INR), serum bilirubin, and creatinine levels. Because the calculation uses a natural logarithmic function, several application-based and internet calculators are available for ease of use. In 2016 the MELD score was updated by the incorporation of serum sodium level to yield the sodium-modified MELD, or MELD-Na, based on accumulating evidence that hyponatremia was an additional powerful predictor of mortality in cirrhotic patients.[126–128]

The MELD score ranges from 6 to 40. Moderate MELD scores (>9) correspond to poor outcomes after hepatic resection for HCC.[129] The MELD score correlates well with the CTP score and is an accurate predictor of postoperative mortality in cirrhotic patients undergoing elective and emergent surgery.[130,131] The predictive utility of the MELD-Na score has been studied in cirrhotic populations undergoing non-HPB surgical procedures with findings that support the idea that worsening liver function (as assessed by MELD-Na) increases the chances of postoperative complications, loss of independence, and mortality.[132–134] In the setting of changing demographics related to the etiology of end-stage liver disease from hepatitis C virus to fatty liver disease, subtle changes in the predictive validity of the MELD score has are being explored.[135,136]

Portal Hypertension

Portal hypertension confers a higher risk of in-hospital mortality.[115] Ascites and varices related to portal hypertension are associated with increased risks for postoperative morbidity and complication, hospital mortality, and loss of independence at discharge in cirrhotic patients undergoing various surgical procedures.[115,132,137] Although invasive measures such as hepatic venous gradient can predict clinical decompensation in patients with cirrhosis,[138] incorporating predictive scales such as MELD-Na, noninvasive tools such as elastography, and simple factors such as platelet count[124] may relegate invasive portal pressure measurements to equivocal cases in which diagnostic dilemma arises (see Chapters 77, 79, and 80).

Cirrhotic patients undergoing preoperative multidisciplinary evaluation benefit from hepatology assessment and management to assess for the presence and degree of portal hypertension; this allows for diagnosis of esophageal varices as well as treatment, if needed, to control or minimize ascites. Although medical therapy such as octreotide or diuretics can lead to improvement in portal and systemic hemodynamics,[139] this improvement may not extend to tolerance of liver resection. TIPS is indicated for patients with ascites refractory or intolerant to diuretics, but patients who undergo TIPS should be closely monitored for hepatic encephalopathy.[140] β-Blockers are contraindicated in cirrhotic patients with refractory ascites, and these patients should avoid abdominal surgery because of the high rates of postoperative morbidity and death.[141]

Coagulopathy

Coagulation abnormalities are frequent in cirrhotic patients and are the result of many causes, including decreased hepatic synthetic function, malnutrition, vitamin K deficiency, thrombocytopenia, and dysfibrinogenemia.[142] There is no clear correlation between an increased risk for hemorrhage and a prolonged PT or activated partial thromboplastin time (aPTT).[143] In the absence of bleeding, routine fresh frozen plasma (FFP) transfusions to correct prolonged PT-INR and aPTT are no longer advocated.[144] Excessive FFP transfusions can lead to volume overload and may exacerbate ascites. Administration of cryoprecipitate is advocated when serum fibrinogen levels are less than 100 mg/dL in the presence of bleeding.[145] Data on the benefits of fibrinogen concentrates are limited to trauma and massive hemorrhage.[146] Transfusion of platelets is recommended before invasive procedures for moderate thrombocytopenia of less than 50,000/μL.[147] Adjunctive desmopressin may be considered as rescue therapy for refractory hemorrhage, particularly when AKI is present, but conflicting results persist about its benefits in chronic liver disease.[148]

Cardiovascular and Respiratory Parameters

Respiratory alkalosis tends to develop in patients with chronic liver disease. Increased abdominal girth in the setting of tense ascites can lead to a restrictive ventilatory defect with reduced functional residual capacity (FRC); therapeutic paracentesis may lead to improvement in respiratory parameters.[149] Cirrhotic patients typically have a hyperdynamic hemodynamic profile because of low systemic vascular resistance, high cardiac output, and vasodilatation of the pulmonary, splanchnic, and peripheral beds.[150,151] Patients with alcoholic liver disease and iron overload are predisposed to cardiomyopathy and cardiac arrhythmias.[151]

Hepatopulmonary syndrome (HPS) is relatively common in advanced cirrhosis and is often associated with portopulmonary hypertension. Signs and symptoms of HPS include hypoxemia, platypnea, orthodeoxia, clubbing, and spider angiomata.[152] Transthoracic echocardiography with agitated saline or bubble contrast allows for the identification of intrapulmonary and right-to-left intracardiac shunts indicative of HPS.[153] HPS signals an overall worse prognosis in patients with cirrhosis.[154] General anesthesia in patients with HPS is associated with increased perioperative risk.[155] Preoperative partial pressure of oxygen in arterial blood (PaO_2) of 50 mm Hg or a macroaggregated albumin scan shunt fraction of 20% or higher are associated with prohibitive mortality rates from cardiorespiratory complications.[156,157]

Infection

Patients with cirrhosis are at increased risk for infection, particularly spontaneous bacterial peritonitis (SBP).[158] In patients with cirrhosis, infections increase mortality 4-fold with a median mortality rate of 38%,[159] which can be accentuated by additional comorbidities.[160] Risk factors for SBP include GI hemorrhage, metabolic alkalosis, dehydration, hyponatremia, and a high MELD score.[161] SBP can be confirmed by a diagnostic paracentesis. If SBP is present, elective surgery should be deferred until the infection has been adequately controlled.

Assessment for Pancreatobiliary Surgery

Nutritional and functional assessments play a role in patient selection before pancreatobiliary surgery, but other scoring systems seek to predict overall major complications or procedure-specific complications. The Preoperative Pancreatic Resection (PREPARE) score is based on several variables, including vital signs, laboratory values, comorbidity assessment via American Society of Anesthesiologists (ASA) category, and etiology of disease. The PREPARE score is accurate in identifying low- and high-risk patients for pancreatic surgery based on the projected occurrence of morbidity classified as grade III or above by the Clavien-Dindo classification.[162,163] Additional perioperative risk calculators intended to enrich preoperative discussion and planning, such as those based on NSQIP data, may require additional disease-specific input to fully capture and describe potential risk associated with PD.[164,165] Other predictors of PD-specific postoperative morbidity include pathology, texture of the pancreas, pancreatic duct diameter, and operative blood loss.[166] Ongoing efforts seek to determine the most sensitive and specific data points to be used to produce highly predictive tools to predict PD-specific postoperative complications in open and minimally invasive PD populations.[167,168]

Additional Perioperative Considerations in HPB Surgical Patients

Anemia

Anemia is a common complication of chronic liver disease even in the absence of decompensation or esophageal varices.[142] Anemia is caused by many factors, including bleeding, hemolysis, splenic sequestration, hepatic dysfunction, and malnutrition. Iron supplementation should be administered only in the presence of documented deficiency. Autologous blood transfusion and administration of erythropoietin have been used successfully to mitigate the need for red blood cell transfusions.[169,170]

The presence of chemotherapy-related anemia is identified in up to 75% of patients.[171] The etiology of this anemia is multifactorial and includes treatment-associated myelosuppression and, in the HPB patient, potential nutritional, appetite-related, and disease-related contributions. Comparisons of parenteral iron administration alone[172] and erythropoietin, along with parenteral iron,[173] have not focused on HPB patients or on the recuperation of hemoglobin before surgical resection.

Electrolytes

Hyponatremia in the setting of chronic liver disease is attributed to an impaired ability to excrete free water and can be found concurrently with other sequelae if it occurs in the setting of cirrhosis with portal hypertension.[174] The causes of hyponatremia should be elucidated and addressed through various strategies, such as correction of fluid deficit or fluid restriction, and cautious and transient use of vasopressin-2 (V2)-receptor antagonists.[175] Hypokalemia and hypomagnesemia can result from the use of loop diuretics, chronic respiratory alkalosis, or malnutrition in various HPB diseases and should be addressed before surgery to limit cardiac arrhythmias.

Acute hypocalcemia can occur during hepatectomy or liver transplantation because of the massive citrate load associated with blood transfusion.[176] Administration of intravenous (IV) calcium should be considered in the setting of intraoperative hemorrhage and hypotension because it helps maintain vascular muscle tone and may enhance hemostasis. Intraoperative and postoperative serum levels of potassium, calcium, magnesium, and phosphorus should be monitored, and abnormalities should be promptly corrected.[177]

INTRAOPERATIVE MANAGEMENT

The core components of the intraoperative care of HPB surgical patients include careful selection of anesthetic, narcotic, and sedative agents; management of mechanical ventilation; maintenance of intravascular volume in the setting of hemorrhage and fluid shift/loss; glucose control and correction of electrolyte disorders; avoidance of hypothermia; and adjustment to blood losses in the setting of relative anemia and coagulopathy (see Chapter 25).

Selection of Anesthetic, Narcotic, and Sedative Agents

The choices and doses of anesthetics, muscle relaxants, analgesics, and sedatives should account for the degree of impairment in hepatic synthetic function and clearance.[178] Endotracheal intubation and induction are achieved in patients with liver disease similar to that in the general population. Presuming normal airway anatomy, atracurium, and cisatracurium are the preferred neuromuscular blocking agents to facilitate intubation because they are not metabolized through the hepatic or renal system.[178] If a rapid-sequence induction is required, the anesthesiologist is safe to use succinylcholine, a depolarizing neuromuscular blocking agent, or rocuronium, a steroid-based nondepolarizing neuromuscular blocking agent. Rocuronium has a reversal agent, sugammadex, which introduces an additional layer of safety, and makes poor hepatic clearance less problematic. Isoflurane, sevoflurane, and desflurane remain the preferred inhalational anesthetic agents in patients with liver disease because they undergo less hepatic metabolism.[179] Of the three agents, isoflurane is more frequently selected because of its minimal effects on hepatic blood flow, although the clinical applicability of this selection is somewhat theoretical. Enflurane and halothane are no longer used in clinical practice (see Chapter 25).

Most narcotic, sedative, and analgesic agents are extensively metabolized in the liver, and their half-life is often altered in patients with chronic liver disease.[180] Cirrhosis delays the elimination of alfentanil, whereas the metabolism of fentanyl, sufentanil, and remifentanil does not seem to be affected.[181] Decreased protein binding and increased volumes of distribution hinder the clearance of midazolam in cirrhotic patients.[182] Remifentanil is sometimes favored for induction because of rapid onset and elimination. Propofol is also preferred versus midazolam for sedation during surgical or endoscopic procedures because of shorter recovery time, more favorable pharmacokinetics, and less propensity to exacerbate subclinical encephalopathy.[183]

Management of Mechanical Ventilation

From a ventilatory perspective, low to moderate tidal volume (Vt) is essential to mitigate effects of higher Vt including abdominal hypertension, respiratory alkalosis, potential barotrauma, and reduced ventricular preload.[184] Patients with chronic liver disease are at increased risk for hypoxemia because of increased shunt fraction, diffusion abnormalities, ventilation-perfusion mismatch, and decreased FRC.[185]

Ventilatory changes during minimally invasive liver resection can be affected by institution of pneumoperitoneum, patient positioning, and strategies used to temper bleeding while operative control is obtained. Changes in mechanical ventilation rate and tidal volume may be requested during episodes of bleeding to decrease thoracic and resulting hepatic venous pressure while laparoscopic control of bleeding is obtained. Decreased respiratory rate or periods of apnea can contribute to respiratory acidosis. Therefore minute ventilation should be closely monitored, and consideration should be given to regular intraoperative arterial blood gas monitoring.

Fluid/Blood Loss and Hemodynamic Parameters

Careful patient selection, attention to the volume of hepatic tissue resected, and reduction in intraoperative blood loss contribute to improved perioperative morbidity and mortality (see Chapters 25, 101, and 102). Decreased effective circulatory volume is frequently present in cirrhotic patients despite total body fluid overload.[150] The initial periods of surgery are often associated with abdominal and thoracic pressure changes and fluid shifts resulting from the evacuation of ascites or when pneumoperitoneum is established. HPB surgery may also be marked by intraoperative hemorrhage, which is exacerbated by portal hypertension and coagulopathy.

The importance of minimization of intraoperative blood loss is highlighted in both hepatic and pancreatic surgery. Although blood loss can be an indicator of case complexity, intraoperative blood transfusion is a harbinger of morbidity and mortality in patients undergoing hepatic resections[186] and is also associated with increased morbidity, mortality, and worsened oncologic outcomes in PD.[187–189] Anesthetic techniques aimed at maintaining a low central venous pressure (CVP) during hepatic resection are associated with a reduction in blood loss, renal failure, and mortality.[190] Strategies combining low CVP with pneumoperitoneum of 10 to 14 mm Hg are commonly used perioperative practices for minimally invasive hepatectomy[191,192] (see Chapter 25).

The physiologic challenges of maintaining low CVP under anesthesia include hemodynamic monitoring in the setting of low CVP, the contribution of pneumoperitoneum, and the technique chosen for maintenance of low CVP. Administering IV fluids in the immediate preoperative period may reduce hemodynamic alterations and prevent complications related to hypovolemia, such as postoperative AKI. Although a low CVP is a generally agreed-upon target, large volumes of blood products or IV fluids are sometimes necessary to maintain cerebral and cardiac perfusion. Once hepatic transection has been completed and bleeding is controlled, many protocols allow for a more liberal fluid or colloid administration to restore intravascular volume when low CVP anesthesia is used for liver resection (see Chapter 25).

With technology allowing for indirect CVP assessment and calculation of stroke volume variation, routine central venous access for guidance of intraoperative resuscitation is being re-evaluated. Stroke volume variation is a useful indicator of intraoperative blood loss and response to resuscitation and can safely guide the administration of IV fluid during hepatic resection.[193,194] Studies comparing the use of stroke volume variation (SVV) monitoring against direct CVP monitoring show that SVV-based resuscitation allows for similar control of CVP and minimization of bleeding.[193,195] Monitoring strategy does not seem to affect postoperative length of stay or postoperative morbidity.[196] Intraoperative transesophageal echocardiography may also be employed in high-risk patient populations, although special expertise is required in employing this modality.

POSTOPERATIVE MANAGEMENT

Despite careful planning, cautious patient selection, and judicious intraoperative monitoring and management, some patients experience AKI, infectious complications, ICU admission, postoperative hepatic insufficiency, and postoperative mortality. Cirrhosis increases the risk for AKI, sepsis, ICU admission, and postoperative mortality, particularly when associated with alcohol dependence, hepatic encephalopathy, and GI hemorrhage.[197] High MELD score, admission to the ICU, and need for organ replacement therapy (pulmonary and/or renal) are predictors of increased length of stay and both short- and long-term mortality.[198,199]

Postoperative Hepatic Failure

Hepatic failure, often manifested as encephalopathy, hyperbilirubinemia, development of ascites, and coagulopathy, can lead to acute respiratory failure, renal failure with/without hepatorenal syndrome, and bleeding complications. Whereas decompensation of cirrhosis can occur after abdominal procedures or

TABLE 26.2 Clinical Findings and Potential Additional Therapies Described by Grade of Posthepatectomy Liver Failure

	PHLF GRADE A	PHLF GRADE B	PHLF GRADE C
Definition	Abnormal INR and bilirubin on POD 5 but no deviation in clinical management	Deviation in regular postoperative care but without invasive intervention	Deviation from postoperative care, requiring invasive intervention
Location of Patient Care	Surgical ward	Intermediate level or ICU	ICU
Additional Investigations that May Be Required	None	Liver/abdominal ultrasound with hepatic vascular evaluation; CXR; Blood, sputum, urine, potentially ascites cultures	As grade B, but needs neurologic evaluation (CT head) to exclude stroke or structural disease
Liver Function	INR <1.5; No symptoms of hyperammonemia	INR ≥1.5 but <2; potentially some somnolence or confusion	INR ≥2; Hepatic encephalopathy
Pulmonary	SpO2 >90%, nasal cannula or simple face mask allowed	SpO2 <90% despite use of nasal cannula or simple face mask	Severe hypoxemia, SpO2 ≤85% despite high FiO2
Renal Function	Adequate UOP BUN <150 mg/dL No symptoms of uremia	UOP ≤0.5 mg/kg/h BUN <150 mg/dL No symptoms of uremia	Nonoliguric renal failure despite diuretics BUN ≥150 mg/dL Clinical uremia
Potential Additional Therapies	Routine care	Albumin, FFP, diuretics, non-invasive ventilation	Intubation and mechanical ventilation, hemodialysis, extracorporeal liver support, liver transplantation

BUN, Blood urea nitrogen; *CT,* computed tomography; *CXR,* chest x-ray; *FFP,* fresh frozen plasma; *FiO2,* fraction of inspired oxygen; *ICU,* intensive care unit; *INR,* international normalized ratio; *PHLF,* posthepatectomy liver failure; *POD,* postoperative day; *SpO2,* arterial oxygen saturation; *UOP,* urine output.

illness, PHLF specifically describes a decrement in liver function after liver resection (see Chapter 77).

The development of PHLF depends on the size and health of the liver remnant remaining after hepatectomy. Several postoperative criteria have been used in predicting PHLF and mortality. The 50-50 criteria, a combination of prothrombin time of less than 50% (or PT-INR > 1.7) and serum bilirubin greater than 50 μmol/L (or > 2.9 mg/dL), has been validated as an excellent predictor of death on days 3 and 5 for patients admitted to the ICU for PHLF.[200,201] The Mullen criteria (bilirubin peak > 7 mg/dL on postoperative days 1–7) were found to be more accurate than the 50-50 criteria in predicting death from hepatic failure after liver resection.[202]

Although various methods exist to diagnose PHLF based on laboratory values, additional work has devised a classification system to describe the clinical impact of PHLF so that degree of morbidity can be described universally and independent of the differing systems used to diagnose PHLF. In this consensus statement, PHLF is determined by increased INR and hyperbilirubinemia on or after postoperative day 5; in cases of elevated values before surgery, the definition includes rising levels after surgery. The classification system bases its gradation of liver failure not on specific symptoms but on the impact on postoperative care, including location of care and additional measures used to treat symptoms (Table 26.2):[203]

Acute Renal Failure and Hepatorenal Syndrome

AKI occurs in approximately 15% of patients who undergo liver resection and correlates to preexisting cardiovascular disease, preoperative serum alanine aminotransferase elevation, underlying renal disease, and diabetes mellitus[204] (see Chapter 25). Postoperative AKI in patients with chronic liver disease may be caused by the administration of nephrotoxic drugs, intraoperative hypotension or hemorrhage, hypovolemia, intrinsic renal disease, and hepatorenal syndrome (HRS).[205] Initial management of mild increase of serum

creatinine may be treated with volume expansion, withdrawal of diuretic therapy if it is being used, and search for nephrotoxic drugs. Further progression of renal dysfunction or failure to respond may require further assessment and exclusion of postoperative complications.[206]

HRS, an alarming postoperative renal complication in patients with advanced-stage liver disease, represents a functional renal failure caused by intrarenal vasoconstriction combined with splanchnic vasodilation; this may be precipitated by infection or intravascular volume depletion.[207] There are two types of HRS: type 1 HRS is often associated with a rapid deterioration of renal function concomitant with deterioration in liver function. Type 2 HRS is characterized by a more gradual and less severe form of renal impairment often associated with refractory ascites[174] (see Chapter 77).

Vasoconstrictor agents, either alone or in combination with albumin or TIPS, are the main therapies for HRS[208,209] (see Chapter 85). Continuous or intermittent renal replacement therapies should be offered to patients who do not respond to vasoconstrictors or TIPS and to prospective candidates for liver transplantation; recovery of renal function can be achieved in as many as 50% of patients.[210] Terlipressin may be more effective for HRS related to sepsis or systemic inflammatory conditions.[211,212] Its United States Food and Drug Administration (FDA) approval is pending (early 2020) for use in type 1 HRS. Noradrenaline has been compared with terlipressin without findings of significant outcome difference in randomized trials.[206]

Anemia and Hemorrhage

Among patients with cirrhosis, postoperative anemia may warrant transfusion of red blood cells, particularly in the setting of surgical or GI hemorrhage. Hematocrit should be kept between 21% and 24% because excessive blood transfusions can lead to increased variceal rebleeding.[213] In cirrhotic patients, the risk of postoperative variceal rupture and bleeding is increased by excessive blood transfusion, large-volume ascites, increased portal pressure, and infection, particularly when coagulopathy and thrombocytopenia coexist.[214] For patients with acute variceal hemorrhage, a MELD score greater than or equal to 18, transfusion requirement greater than or equal to 4 U of red blood cells within the first 24 hours of admission, and active bleeding at endoscopy are independent predictors of 6-week mortality and variceal rebleeding within the first 5 days.[215] Variceal hemorrhage warrants transfusion of blood products and treatment aimed at modulating portal pressure[216,217] (see Chapter 81).

The traditional strategy of FFP transfusion to correct coagulopathy in patients who are not bleeding has been abandoned because of the absence of correlation between an increased risk for hemorrhage and a prolonged PT or aPTT. Moreover, FFP transfusion may lead to volume overload and does not decrease the risk for bleeding.[143,218] Data on the successful use of four-factor prothrombin and fibrinogen complex in patients with liver cirrhosis and postoperative hemorrhage are lacking. Algorithms may include prothrombin concentrate in treatment of life-threatening hemorrhage in decompensated cirrhotic patients, but this may increase the risk for thromboembolic events.[219–221]

Sedative and Pain Management

In patients with cirrhosis, sedative and narcotic agents undergo increased volume of distribution, slow hepatic metabolism, and prolonged elimination.[181] Associated renal dysfunction should prompt adjustment of the doses of sedative and analgesic medications to prevent an exacerbation of hepatic encephalopathy and other complications.[182]

Narcotics can have unpredictable effects because of variable metabolism. In general, hydromorphone and fentanyl have cleaner side effect profiles, and so are often used judiciously, often in reduced doses, in patients with liver disease. Nonsteroidal antiinflammatory agents (NSAIDs) should be used sparingly because of the potential for peptic ulceration, fluid retention from inhibition of renal prostaglandin synthesis, precipitation of hepatorenal syndrome, and bleeding caused by antiplatelet activity, GI irritation, and renal failure.[180]

Optimal postsurgical analgesia is chosen based on several factors, including level of comfort provided, limitation of postoperative mobility, safety of use and potential complications, and patient satisfaction. Postoperative pain control strategies include intravenous patient-controlled analgesia (PCA), epidural catheters, and regional therapies, including wound/abdominal wall catheters or nerve blocks (see Chapter 25).

Although epidural anesthesia has been used for decades, postoperative hypotension from alteration of sympathetic tone may limit return to mobilization and can raise concerns for other causes of hypotension (i.e., intraabdominal hemorrhage) after major HPB surgery. Theorized limitations in the use of epidural analgesia include concern for coagulopathy at the time of catheter removal, leading to a longer indwelling catheter time. A retrospective view of patients undergoing liver resection containing 15% cirrhotic (CPT A) patients found an 8% rate of postponement of catheter removal due to coagulopathy at the time when epidural would have been removed by clinical indication.[222] Additional retrospective studies have found up to 32% of patients receiving FFP or vitamin K before epidural replacement to obtain a goal INR ≤1.3.[223] Perioperative conditions may portend post-hepatectomy, such as cirrhosis, preoperative INR ≥1.3, preoperative platelet count ≤150,

major hepatectomy, and intraoperative estimated blood loss ≥1000 mL.[224] Prediction of more severe postoperative coagulopathy could serve to influence the pain control strategy.

Local anesthetic instillation in the transversus abdominis preperitoneal (TAP) and paravertebral locations may also be used to treat pain from abdominal incisions for HPB surgery. A randomized study comparing epidural against bilateral paravertebral block measuring visual pain scoring, incentive spirometry use, and use of opioid PCA (in both groups) found improved pain scores at 24 hours postoperatively in the epidural group, whereas incentive spirometer use and PCA use did not differ.[225] Other regional blocks or infusion catheters are being explored as an alternative to epidural analgesia, both with and without concurrent use of PCA.[226,227] Current ERAS Society guidelines for patients undergoing open hepatectomy as part of an ERAS protocol suggest consideration of wound catheters or intrathecal opiates rather than thoracic epidural analgesia[113] (see Chapter 25).

Phosphate Metabolism After Hepatectomy

Hypophosphatemia is a frequent occurrence in the early days after hepatectomy and should be corrected.[228] Failure to develop hypophosphatemia is a marker of postoperative hepatic insufficiency and mortality and may be evident in the early postoperative period before the traditional markers defining PHLF become evident.[229,230] In patients who develop PHLF, the later development of hypophosphatemia may signal the beginning of recovery.[231]

Postoperative Care after Pancreaticoduodenectomy

Postoperative complications of PD, such as anastomotic leak, fistula, and abdominal collections, vary with the type of pancreatoenteric anastomosis, pancreatic texture, size of the main pancreatic duct, and intraoperative blood transfusion.[168] As many as 18% of patients may require ICU admission for postoperative complications of PD. Delayed admission to the ICU for septic shock carries a mortality rate of close to 20%.[232] Protocol-driven elimination of variation in perioperative care based on evidence from clinical trials has led to the development of ERAS recommendations for routine postoperative and perioperative management of patients undergoing PD[106]; these recommendations and their supporting evidence are further discussed elsewhere in this volume (see Chapters 27 and 117).

In conclusion, evolutions in preoperative patient assessment including evaluation of sarcopenia, frailty, and comorbidity are allowing surgeons to identify and potentially intervene on patients at higher risk for perioperative morbidity and functional decline. Nutritional optimization, perioperative physiologic homeostasis, and consideration of disease-specific challenges are being increasingly employed in a cooperative manner in the care of HPB surgery patients with guidance from evidence-based multidisciplinary groups such as the ERAS Society. Although ongoing work explores the best ways to identify at-risk HPB surgery patients and the strategies most effective in preoperative physiologic and functional improvement, collaborative effort between surgeons, anesthesia staff, intensivists, rehabilitation or prehabilitation providers, and nursing embodies a global approach to perioperative care of this patient population.

The references for this chapter can be found online by accessing the accompanying Expert Consult website.

CHAPTER 27

Enhanced recovery programs in hepatobiliary surgery

Timothy E. Newhook and Thomas A. Aloia

INTRODUCTION

In the 1990s, initial reports of fast-track surgical principles detailed their application to cardiac surgery patients with the goal of reducing intensive care unit (ICU) stay.[1] Afterward, a novel multimodal approach to perioperative care was described by Kehlet and Mogensen, resulting in a dramatic reduction in length of hospital stay (LOS) after colectomy.[2,3] After overcoming much skepticism and scrutiny, the ensuing paradigm shift in perioperative care of the surgical patient has resulted in their principles being applied across disciplines and in the formation of the Enhanced Recovery After Surgery (ERAS) Society (https://www.erassociety.org), which aims to disseminate and implement enhanced recovery best practices globally.[4] Since the introduction of these practices, enhanced recovery program (ERP) principles have been successfully applied across the surgical spectrum and have now been adopted in other procedural (e.g., stem cell transplantation) and non-procedural (e.g., medical hospitalist) care.

Principles of enhanced recovery have been increasingly incorporated into the care of hepatobiliary (HB) surgery patients, with clinical trials and individual reports documenting improved outcomes with these programs.[5,6] Perhaps the earliest description of experience with ERPs and HB surgery came from Scotland, when Mackay and O'Dwyer published their small series of early discharge "fast-track" liver resection patients.[7] In the same year, van Dam et al. described their initial experience with 61 patients who underwent hepatectomy under an ERP and compared outcomes with 100 consecutive hepatectomies before initiation of the protocol.[8] Hepatectomy patients resumed oral intake earlier and had a decreased LOS compared with traditional pathway patients, along with similar rates of morbidity and mortality.[8] Since that time, there has been an explosion of literature involving enhanced recovery after HB surgery, evaluating proposed pathways and operative strategies within an ERP framework.

HB surgery is unique from other fields in gastrointestinal (GI) surgery because of differing patient comorbidities and underlying chronic diseases that may require intervention, and thus the perioperative care plans must be different. Recent advances in surgical planning, perioperative care, and operative techniques have resulted in decreased morbidity and mortality after HB surgery.[9,10] Despite this, HB surgery remains difficult, with recognized rates of major complications as high as 30%, and mortality of up to 5% even at high-volume centers.[11,12] Of particular concern are high rates of digestive and pulmonary complications associated with HB surgery. Therefore a shift toward perioperative care aimed at a reduction in these adverse outcomes via early intervention allows for a faster, more efficient recovery. Lastly, it is important to note that ERPs are management strategies predicated on safe, effective, and meticulous surgical technique to deliver optimal outcomes and

derive maximal benefit from these programs. In other words, an ERP cannot make up for substandard surgery.

HB surgery remains complex, with perioperative variables not found in other surgical disciplines; it also requires significant contributions from many members of the HB surgery care team. These major operations can be incredibly complex, requiring a large multidisciplinary effort that may function more effectively with a standardized plan. Therefore implementation of such a protocol for patients undergoing HB surgery requires commitment from surgeons, trainees, anesthesiologists, nursing staff, and patients themselves to adhere to the common core principles discussed below.

THE "4 PILLARS" OF ENHANCED RECOVERY PROGRAMS

Fundamental surgical principles, such as thromboembolic prophylaxis, prophylactic antibiosis, appropriate application of minimally-invasive approaches, and minimization of drains/lines/tubes are critical to ERPs. In addition, modern ERP approaches consist of effective patient education and engagement, upon which stand "4 pillars" of enhanced recovery: early postoperative feeding, goal-directed fluid therapy, opioid-sparing analgesia, and early ambulation (Fig. 27.1).[13,14] These core components occur at different phases of the ERP along the spectrum of care of an HB surgical patient and will be discussed later in this chapter.

The foundation of all ERPs, patient engagement and education, is of critical importance. Much of enhanced recovery requires the participation of the patient (i.e., early ambulation) and thus all efforts within the pathway rest on a solid foundation of patient engagement. Effective education of both the patient and caregiver(s) in advance of and during recovery allows for a "team approach" that will lead to improved and enhanced outcomes.

Along with the "4 pillars," other critical aspects of a comprehensive ERP are detailed later along the phases of care for HB surgical patients (Table 27.1). Other aspects or program-specific elements exist; however, the following subjects remain most concordant with major published guidelines.

PREOPERATIVE PHASE

Preoperative Patient Evaluation

A thorough preoperative evaluation is imperative for any patient being considered for HB surgery. A complete history and physical examination should include a review of all comorbidities, surgical history, medications, and detailed oncologic history. Determination and quantification of receipt of any prior cytotoxic/targeted/immunologic therapies is paramount. Specific to HB surgery, any risk factors for hepatic dysfunction,

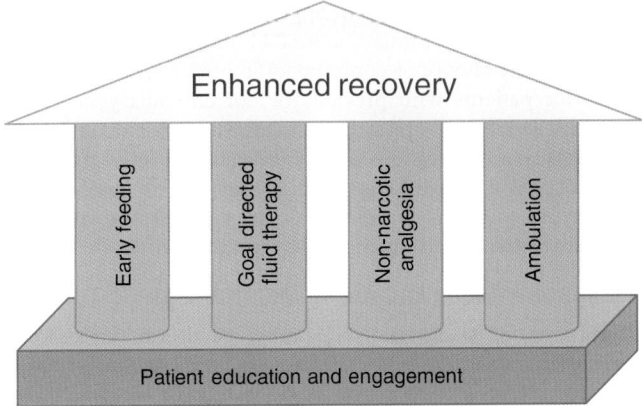

FIGURE 27.1 The "4 pillars" and foundation of enhanced recovery programs (ERPs). (From Kim BJ, Aloia TA. What is "enhanced recovery," and how can I do it? *J Gastrointest Surg*. 2018;22[1]:164–171.)

TABLE 27.1 Essential Elements of Enhanced Recovery Programs by Preoperative, Perioperative, and Postoperative Phases of Care for the HB Surgery Patient

PREOPERATIVE PHASE	PERIOPERATIVE PHASE	POSTOPERATIVE PHASE
Patient Evaluation	Clear Liquids up to 2 hours pre-procedure	**Early Mobilization**
Medical Optimization	VTE prophylaxis	**Goal-Directed Fluid Therapy**
Prehabilitation	Antimicrobial prophylaxis	Prevention of PONV
Nutritional Assessment	Avoidance or early discontinuation of NGT or abdominal drains	**Early Nutrition**
Education and Engagement	**Goal-Directed Fluid Therapy**	**Opioid-Sparing Analgesia**
	Neuraxial and Regional Anesthesia	Educate on Discharge Criteria
	Opioid-Sparing Analgesia	
	Minimally-invasive Surgical Approaches, if possible	

portal hypertension, or cirrhosis should be ascertained by inquiring about prior HB surgical history, including endoscopic procedures and detailed social history. Physical examination should include detection of any signs of hepatic dysfunction, including jaundice, ascites, or prior surgical scars.

Optimization of chronic comorbidities, both medically and with intervention, is critical to the quality of recovery after HB surgery (see Chapters 25 and 26). Borderline operability from a medical perspective must be uncovered because these patients (age >75 years, dependent function, lung disease, ascites/varices, myocardial infarction, stroke, steroids, weight loss >10%, and/or sepsis) have a threefold higher mortality after hepatectomy.[15] Moreover, patients with more comorbidities are more likely to be discharged to a skilled nursing facility or nonroutine discharge after hepatopancreatic surgery.[16] Optimization of

comorbidities before planned hepatectomy may greatly influence outcome and allow for adherence to ERP principles.

Patient functional status must be evaluated thoroughly and potentially improved before planned HB surgery. Evaluation of functional status may be performed using reported grading tools (i.e., Eastern Cooperative Oncology Group Performance Status, Karnofsky Score, MD Anderson Symptom Inventory, Timed Up And Go).[17–22] The concept of frailty as it applies to HB surgery is in evolution; however, objective tools such as these may identify patients that may be best suited for a coordinated "prehabilitation" program before surgical intervention. This allows for an improved "starting point" before physiologically stressful, complicated HB surgery. As it pertains to cardiopulmonary fitness, structured exercise programs have been shown to improve quality of life scores and exercise capacity before planned hepatectomy for colorectal liver metastases.[23] Moreover, prehabilitation may be used as an opportunity to institute dietary and exercise programs aimed at reducing hepatic steatosis for patients deemed high risk and undergoing planned hepatectomy.[24] Clearly, there are prime opportunities to potentially improve perioperative outcomes via preoperative optimization of HB surgical patients in the context of a comprehensive ERP (see Chapter 26).

Determining a patient's baseline use of pain medications, primarily opioids, can be critical to the success of an enhanced recovery approach. Preoperative opioid use has been reported in almost 25% of patients reporting for surgery, and preoperative opioid prescriptions are associated with higher postoperative opioid requirements and increased readmissions.[25–27] Moreover, opioid tolerance is associated with decreased compliance with ERPs, particularly in the postoperative period.[28] Therefore this information is imperative because it may inform regional anesthesia strategies and postoperative multimodal therapy.

Preoperative Education and Patient Engagement

Patients being cared for along an ERP for HB surgery must be engaged and educated thoroughly on the goals of the program and the reasons behind care decisions. Educational materials on operative approaches and expectations for day-to-day care while in the hospital, including pain control, diet, and ambulation, should be provided in a format that is easy to comprehend. Patients will require detailed information regarding opioid-sparing analgesia, including the use of multimodal agents and the efficacy of initial and repeated regional anesthetic nerve blocks. Although no studies have evaluated education, there is a shared recognition that these educational efforts create excitement in patients about the potential for decreased LOS after their HB surgery and increase their willingness to work toward this enhanced recovery. Beyond allowing for understanding of expectations, these efforts reduce patient anxiety and lead to increased compliance.[29] The ERAS Society recommendations for liver surgery are that "routine and dedicated preoperative counseling and education" be provided to patients before undergoing liver surgery.[4]

Preoperative Nutrition

As with any elective surgical procedure, consideration of a patient's baseline nutritional status and evaluation of potential nutritional deficits is critical during preparation for HB surgery (see Chapter 26). Important factors to consider include recent weight loss and obesity, body mass index (BMI), and laboratory evaluation of nutritional indices, such as albumin, prealbumin, ferritin, and relevant vitamins and micronutrients.[14,30] Beyond incorporation within the history and physical, several screening instruments are available, which may augment evaluation and have been shown to be useful in clinical practice.[31,32]

When possible, every attempt should be made to remediate nutritional deficiencies. The ERAS Society recommendations for liver surgery suggest that patients found to be "at risk" receive 7 days of oral nutritional supplementation before elective liver surgery. At-risk patients are defined as having greater than 10% to 15% weight loss within 6 months, BMI less than 18.5 kg/m², and serum albumin less than 30 g/L without any signs of liver or renal dysfunction.[4]

PERIOPERATIVE PHASE

Perioperative Nutrition and Carbohydrate Loading

An integral aspect of ERPs is maintaining homeostasis and limiting the surgical stress response, as well as avoiding catabolism. Despite dogmatic guidelines of prolonged fasting before general anesthesia (nil per os after midnight), modern recommendations include the allowance of clear liquids up to 2 hours and solid food 6 hours before general anesthesia, as long as there are no concerns for gastroduodenal functional impairment.[33,34] The role of preoperative carbohydrate loading is established for patients undergoing colorectal operations and is likely also applicable to HB surgical patients.[4,35,36] Patients receiving preoperative carbohydrate loading before other interventions have been shown to have less anxiety, malaise, nausea, and perioperative insulin resistance in clinical trials.[37] Although more evidence is required before strong recommendation for carbohydrate loading before HB surgery, data on the adverse effects of starvation are compelling enough that they should be considered.

Venous Thromboembolism Prophylaxis

Perioperative venous thromboembolism (VTE) results in significant morbidity and mortality, and patients with malignancy are at higher risk for development of these complications. Concerns for bleeding after HB surgery has traditionally resulted in resistance to at least preoperative VTE chemoprophylaxis; however, a large percentage of patients undergoing hepatopancreatobiliary surgery have been shown to be hypercoagulable.[38] Major hepatectomy itself is an independent risk factor for the development of VTE.[39] Moreover, VTE rates increase with extent of hepatectomy and this risk exceeds that of major bleeding, strongly supporting the use of preoperative and early postoperative VTE chemoprophylaxis.[40] Graded compression stockings and intermittent pneumatic compression/sequential compression devices (SCDs) can be placed before anesthesia induction and continued until ambulation, and this can further decrease the risk for VTE after HB surgery.[36] Indeed, guidelines for liver surgery recommend administration of low-molecular-weight heparin (LMWH) or unfractionated heparin 2 to 12 hours preoperatively and the use of SCDs.[4]

Antimicrobial Prophylaxis and Surgical Site Infection Prevention

Routine use of antimicrobial prophylaxis for liver surgery remains inconsistent; however, national guidelines aimed at reducing complications after surgery recommend prophylaxis within 1 hour before incision, appropriate re-dosing based on case duration, and continuation for 24 hours after surgery.[13,41,42] Surgeons may choose to continue antibiotics for more than 24 hours for patients with previous or current biliary drainage; however, evidence supporting this practice is inconclusive. Similarly, skin preparations that include alcohol (e.g., chlorhexidine-alcohol 2%) are recognized as superior to povidone-iodine alone solutions in prevention of surgical site infection (SSI) for patients undergoing HB surgery.[4,43]

Nasogastric Tubes and Abdominal Drainage

Routine use of nasogastric (NG) drainage after major abdominal surgery is largely being abandoned, and some major studies have revealed their prophylactic use to be detrimental.[44] Specific to HB surgery, a randomized trial of 210 patients undergoing hepatectomy failed to reveal any difference in overall morbidity, pulmonary complications, frequency of postoperative emesis, or time to oral intake between patients with or without prophylactic NG tubes until flatus or bowel function.[45] Moreover, a NG tube has been identified as independently associated with postoperative pulmonary complications after hepatectomy.[46]

Data for prophylactic abdominal drainage after HB surgery are mixed; however, supporters use them as potential indicators for biliary complications, such as bile leak and prevention of subdiaphragmatic abscesses. However, these drains may serve to impair patient mobilization postoperatively and may also result in increased pain and need for opioid medications. Therefore abdominal drains should be omitted if possible, particularly when intraoperative identification of bile leak tests (e.g., air-leak test) are performed and results are negative.[30,47–49]

Intraoperative Fluid Management

Reduction in the volume of fluid administered after major abdominal surgeries has resulted in significantly decreased morbidity[50] (see Chapter 25). Intraoperative fluid management for patients undergoing HB surgery within an ERP is unique compared with other major abdominal operations. This starts with avoidance of bowel preparations and prolonged preoperative fasting for HB operations, thus avoiding dehydration.[30] Intraoperative fluid management should be goal-directed, focusing on maintaining euvolemia and avoiding excess crystalloid fluids. Goal-directed fluid therapy (GDFT) aims to optimize end-organ perfusion by monitoring various dynamic markers of resuscitation status, including central venous pressure (CVP), cardiac output/index (CO/CI), and noninvasive stroke volume variation (SVV) as examples. In place of invasive CVP monitoring, the SVV can guide GDFT and results in improved intraoperative fluid administration and decreased postoperative morbidity.[51] However, this is more complex for HB operations because maintenance of a low CVP during hepatic transection results in reduced blood loss and lower rates of blood transfusion.[52] This highlights the critical importance of establishing an individualized plan for fluid management with all team members to realize improved outcomes.

Neuraxial and Peripheral Regional Anesthesia Techniques

The goal of a pain control regimen with ERPs is to limit the postoperative neuroendocrine stress response, allow for early ambulation, and maintain homeostasis. These goals are achieved by limiting opioid use as much as possible, while ensuring pain control that facilitates full patient function and activity. To achieve this balance, liberal use of opioid-sparing analgesia and neuraxial blocks is advised. Opioid-sparing analgesia begins before the operating room and continues through a patient's recovery, and regional anesthesia techniques augment pain control and thus reduce the need for opioids postoperatively. Neuraxial and peripheral regional anesthesia techniques (i.e., transversus abdominal plane [TAP], blocks, epidural catheters) are indispensable components of standardized multimodal analgesia strategies to limit opioid consumption while ensuring adequate acute pain control (see Chapter 25).

Neuraxial blockade to cover the incisional area for HB surgery typically includes thoracic epidural anesthesia (TEA), which has been shown to be superior to analgesia and result in earlier return of GI tract function.[53,54] Epidurals should be performed by experienced practitioners to cover the incisional area and are most beneficial for open surgery. TEA has resulted in superior pain control, patient experience, and decreased opioid consumption without increased length of stay as compared with intravenous (IV) patient-controlled analgesia (PCA) after HB surgery in randomized trials.[55,56] Moreover, there may be oncologic benefit compared with IV analgesia, with TEA being associated with improved recurrence-free survival after resection of colorectal liver metastases.[57] Use of TEA for HB surgery is the most supported by high-level evidence; however, trials comparing TEA with regional anesthesia techniques are ongoing.

As alternatives to neuraxial blockade, peripheral techniques are emerging, such as the TAP and quadratus lumborum (QL) block. These approaches may result in decreased perioperative hypotension and urinary retention that may result from TEA, thus potentially allowing for more efficient return to homeostasis. In studies comparing these approaches with TEA, with some revealing similar pain control, there are conflicting data on opioid consumption being higher or lower than epidural.[58,59] For example, epidural analgesia was associated with the lowest inpatient opioid use after pancreatectomy, likely because all patients with TAP blocks may get concomitant IV-PCA.[27] Studies comparing peripheral and neuraxial analgesia techniques as they pertain to ERPs for HB surgery are clearly needed.

Operative Approach

Most complex HB surgery is performed with an open approach; however, experienced centers have reported improved short-term and similar long-term outcomes with minimally invasive surgery (MIS) approaches[60–62] (see Chapter 127). Application of MIS approaches to various aspects of HB surgery, particularly minor hepatectomy and left lateral sectionectomy, have become standard practice and recommended by international consensus guidelines.[63,64] Despite this, few studies have evaluated the integration and impact of MIS into ERPs for HB surgery. A randomized trial resulted in decreased LOS for MIS liver surgery patients cared for under an ERP compared with traditional care; however, MIS compared with open HB surgery has not been shown to result in faster recovery within ERPs.[65,66] Regardless, MIS HB surgical approaches dovetail with many of the core pillars of enhanced recovery, including resulting in decreased postoperative complications, lower intraoperative blood loss, faster time to oral intake, and decreased need for opioid pain medications.[4,60,67–69] Application of MIS HB surgical techniques must be selected for patients with respect to safety and efficiency within the context of an ERP and be performed by surgeons experienced in these approaches.

POSTOPERATIVE PHASE

Early Mobilization

Enhanced recovery principles center on rapid return to homeostasis, and early postoperative mobilization and ambulation is critical to completing an ERP.[70] As one of the four pillars of ERPs, it is imperative that patients and team members embrace this intervention. Early ambulation may have tremendous positive impacts on pulmonary function, VTE prevention, and resumption of GI function and is also associated with successful completion of an ERP.[70] As previously mentioned, limiting abdominal drains, urinary catheters, invasive lines, and enteric tubes allows for more efficient mobility and prevents further barriers to this critical, simple intervention. Select patient populations will benefit from involvement of physical and occupational therapists.

Postoperative Fluid Resuscitation

Once out of the operating room, GDFT remains important for HB surgical patients. Not only does over or under-resuscitation result in potential cardiopulmonary and renal complications, but it also overall impedes return to homeostasis. Postoperative trends in hemodynamics and urine output should guide fluid therapy. Moreover, certain serum laboratory values can help with assessment of intravascular volume, such as serum brain natriuretic peptide (BNP). According to a BNP-guided fluid management protocol, management of bolus fluids, diuresis, and fluid rate adjustments resulted in a fourfold reduction in cardiopulmonary and renal complications after hepatectomy.[71] When integrated within ERPs, interventions such as this allow for more refined fluid management during recovery from HB surgery (see Chapters 25 and 26).

Postoperative Nausea and Vomiting Prophylaxis

Nausea and emesis can be common after surgery, and efforts should be made to limit or prevent these debilitating symptoms. Team members must evaluate patients for known risk factors for postoperative nausea and vomiting (PONV), and a multimodal prevention approach is also recommended. The use of two antiemetic medications is advocated for by ERAS Society guidelines.[4]

Diet and Nutrition

Rapid return to homeostasis and prevention of catabolism are facilitated by optimizing and maintaining cellular metabolism. Early postoperative nutrition, such as clear liquids on postoperative day 0 and regular diet on postoperative day 1, can shorten the interruption in cellular metabolism and is well-tolerated within an ERP for HB surgery.[13] It is our preference to avoid a full-liquid diet if possible because many patients may be lactose intolerant.[30] Avoidance of NG tubes, encouragement of early ambulation, oral laxatives, and limitation of IV fluid replacement are all part of the multimodal approach to allow for early diet resumption after HB surgery (see Chapter 26).

Pain Control and Opioid-Sparing Analgesia

Opioid-sparing analgesia is absolutely imperative to the success of ERPs and a pillar of these strategies. Opioids are helpful for treating acute pain after HB surgery; however, their adverse effects are counterproductive to recovery. These medications can decrease gastric emptying and increase pyloric sphincter tone, thus potentiating or inducing PONV and can also cause paralytic ileus. Inability to initiate oral intake ensues, leading to a chain reaction that collapses the enhanced recovery effort. Therefore narcotic limitation, and sometimes omission, can exponentially hasten return of homeostasis. A multimodal approach to pain control supports the opioid-sparing theme, and this is a true perioperative approach. Many non-narcotic adjuncts can be started preoperatively, such as gabapentin, pregabalin, nonsteroidal antiinflammatory drugs (NSAIDs; i.e., Celecoxib), and acetaminophen. These medications form the basis of night of surgery analgesia, obviating the need for high-dose parenteral narcotics. Preoperative education, support, and continual discussion regarding the ability to avoid opioids with adequate analgesia will ensure the success of this approach (see Chapter 25).

Benefits of neuraxial blockades initiated in the intraoperative setting continue postoperatively. For example, TEA has been shown to result in significant decrease in opioid use and improved patient reported outcomes, as compared with IV-PCA in a randomized controlled trial of HB surgery patients.[55] Moreover, regional anesthesia can be helpful as a "rescue" strategy within ERPs after HB surgery for patients struggling with acute pain control. For patients who did not receive neuraxial blockade or block preoperatively, these may be used in the postoperative setting to augment the opioid-sparing approach. Each institution may have particular aptitude in placing a particular type of block, so local preference is acceptable provided blocks are offered and widely applied.

The benefits of opioid-sparing analgesia within ERPs can be seen across the entire patient surgical experience, from accelerating functional recovery to decreasing opioid need after discharge. After implementation of an HB-specific ERP at MD Anderson Cancer Center, patients were much less likely to require a prescription for traditional opioids at discharge or require opioids at their initial postoperative clinic visit.[72] Although pain scores were similar between patients on ERP versus traditional care pathways, traditional care pathways were a predictor of requiring opioids at first follow-up.[72] The efficacy of ERP management clearly extends beyond the traditional perioperative period.

FUTURE OF ENHANCED RECOVERY FOR HB SURGERY

The field has made considerable progress since the initial introduction of ERP principles in surgery, particularly as applied to HB surgery patients. But what does the future hold as we move forward? Clearly, the future likely involves more minimally invasive approaches to HB surgical patients, including anesthesia techniques. Moreover, the application of ERP principles themselves are being increasingly applied before and longer after the initial perioperative period.

With an aging population, more advanced tumors presenting for surgery, and more patients undergoing preoperative therapy, a multidisciplinary approach to preoperative optimization of patients is becoming critical. Prehabilitation programs and other medical optimization approaches have been garnering increasing attention in recent times because it is recognized that poor exercise capacity is strongly associated with worse outcomes after HB surgery.[73–75] Therefore patients who are deconditioned by their underlying disease, physical condition, or treatment strategy should be advised to participate in a preoperative multidisciplinary conditioning program to optimize outcomes. Evaluation of these programs, including what interventions lead to improved outcomes, synergy within ERPs, and compliance are an important area of future research within enhanced recovery. Moreover, an organized enhanced recovery approach to HB surgery patients is important, and implementation, audit of consistent variables, and measured compliance are paramount to the program's success and sustainability.[76,77] Adherence to implementation science principles will help to push ERPs across practices. Since the explosion of literature early in the ERP journey, most studies have focused on individual program elements and outcomes, and the language of these variables is not consistent. Moreover, few studies include data on compliance of their program variables when communicating their results.[77] Moving towards consistent language with consistent variables will allow cross-program comparisons and, ultimately, better outcomes for HB patients.

CONCLUSION

Since the initial reports on enhanced recovery for patients after major abdominal surgery, great progress has been made to expand these principles to complex disciplines, such as HB surgery. By focusing on perioperative strategies for maintaining homeostasis and a rapid return to baseline, patients and members of their multidisciplinary care team have made tremendous improvements in short-term and long-term outcomes. Because HB surgery patients may have unique disease and management characteristics, this makes their ERPs distinct from other complex abdominal surgeries. Going forward, with technique refinements and the expansion of principles across the phases of HB surgical patient care, the multidisciplinary ERP approach will likely evolve to become the standard of care.

The references for this chapter can be found online by accessing the accompanying Expert Consult website.

CHAPTER 28

Postoperative complications requiring intervention: Diagnosis and management

Franz Edward Boas and Stephen B. Solomon

IMAGING AND IMAGE-GUIDED THERAPY OF COMPLICATIONS AFTER PANCREATECTOMY

Imaging After Pancreatectomy

Computed tomography (CT) is the most common imaging modality for evaluation of the pancreas after surgery. Complications that can be detected on CT include anastomotic leak, abscess, fistula, and bleeding (see Chapters 62 and 117).

Fluid collections, such as seromas, abscesses, and pancreatic pseudocysts, can be identified on CT (Fig. 28.1). Rim enhancement suggests abscess or pseudocyst. Gas within a collection suggests infection or enteric leak. Enteric leaks can have a thin tract containing gas and fluid, extending from an enteric anastomosis to an abscess. Oral contrast given before the CT can leak into the abscess, which is diagnostic of an enteric leak.

Postoperative bleeding can be evaluated using a CT angiogram, which should include noncontrast and arterial phases. Hematomas are visible on noncontrast CT as high density (greater than 20 Hounsfield units) collections. Active arterial bleeding is seen as extravasation of contrast on arterial phase contrast-enhanced CT (CECT) scans. On delayed phase images (if obtained), the extravasated contrast continues to spread if there is active bleeding. On the other hand, a pseudoaneurysm (which can bleed intermittently) is an enhancing structure next to an artery, which maintains its shape on delayed CT images (Figs. 28.2 and 28.3).

Magnetic resonance cholangiopancreatography (MRCP) is a fluid-sensitive magnetic resonance imaging (MRI) sequence that clearly shows the pancreatic duct, bile ducts, fistulas, and fluid collections. The MRCP is typically reconstructed into axial and coronal slices, as well as a three-dimensional (3D) images. The site of a pancreatic fistula can be identified in 75% of patients on CT, compared with 93% on MRCP.[1]

Interventional Radiology Procedures Postpancreatectomy

Many postpancreatectomy complications are managed using image-guided percutaneous interventions, reducing the need for reoperation. After pancreaticoduodenectomy, 12% to 22% of patients require percutaneous intervention,[2,3] including intra-abdominal abscess drainage (72%), percutaneous biliary drainage (PBD; 18%), and angiography with or without embolization (10%).[4]

Image-Guided Abdominal Drainage

Postoperative abscesses can be drained percutaneously, using ultrasound or CT guidance (see Fig. 28.1). Small abscesses (<3 cm) can usually be treated with antibiotics alone, but larger collections require both antibiotics and drainage. Complications of image-guided drainage of fluid collections are infrequent but include bleeding, sepsis, and peritonitis.

Abscesses are typically drained using the Seldinger technique. A needle is advanced into the collection under ultrasound or CT guidance. After aspirating fluid, a stiff guide wire is placed through the needle into the collection. The needle is then removed, and a drain is placed over the wire into the collection. Typically, 8 to 10 French (Fr) drains are placed in thin, serous collections, and 10 to 12 Fr drains are placed in thick bloody or purulent collections.[5] Larger drains are available for very thick collections, up to 20 Fr for locking loop drains and 36 Fr for straight drains. Biliary-type drains (which have additional side holes) may be helpful for long, multiloculated collections.

After catheter placement, the abscess is emptied, and specimens are sent for gram stain and culture. The fluid can also be sent for amylase (to evaluate for pancreatic leak) and bilirubin (to evaluate for bile leak). Drain fluid to serum bilirubin ratio greater than five indicates a bile leak,[6] and drain amylase to serum ratio greater than five indicates a pancreatic leak.[7]

Drain Management

The drain should be flushed with normal saline two to three times per day to prevent clogging. Drainage from loculated collections can be improved by injecting tissue plasminogen activator (tPA) into the tube. One report showed an 89% success rate using tPA to drain abscesses refractory to simple catheter drainage.[8] In a postsurgical patient, the benefit of tPA should be weighed against the risk of bleeding.

If the drain output remains high, this suggests an ongoing pancreatic or enteric leak. The drain should be positioned adjacent to the leak for optimal drainage. When output from the drain decreases, the locking loop drain can be exchanged for a straight drain to collapse the abscess cavity adjacent to the leak. The straight drain can be slowly pulled back over days or weeks in an attempt to close the fistula. Occasionally, a persistent fistula is seen on abscessogram, even after the patient is doing well clinically, with no residual abscess cavity and no output from the drain. This is a one-way fistula, and the drain can usually be safely removed. Management of persistent pancreatic leaks is discussed later (see "Interventional Management of Pancreaticocutaneous Fistulas").

Minimal output from the drain indicates that the drainage is complete or that the drain is clogged or malpositioned. Pus leaking around a drain suggests that the drain is clogged and should be assessed with cross-sectional imaging or a tube study. Clogged drains can be exchanged over a guidewire.

An abscess drain can typically be removed when the output is less than 20 mL a day, the patient has no fever or pericatheter leakage, and the drain flushes easily. An abscessogram or CT

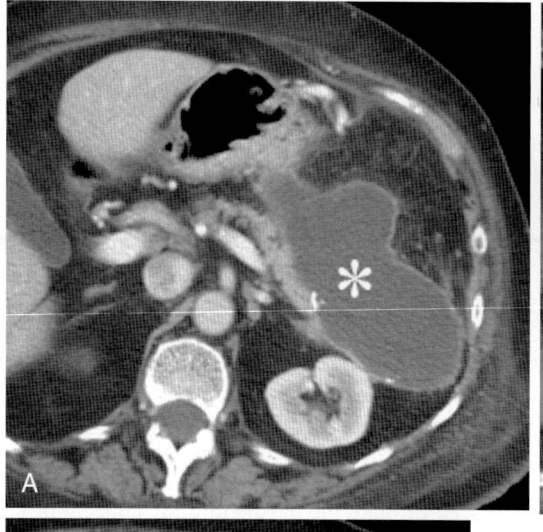
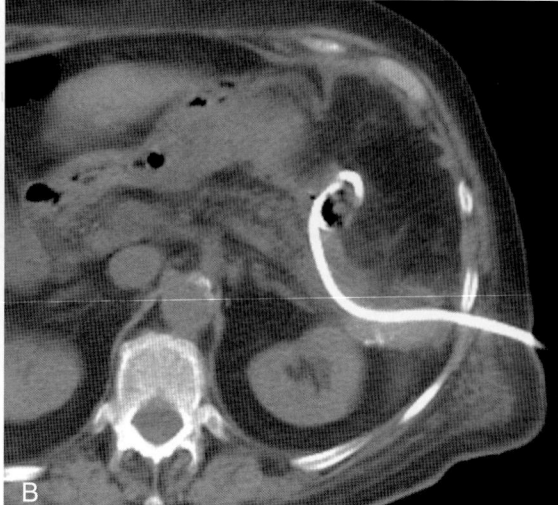
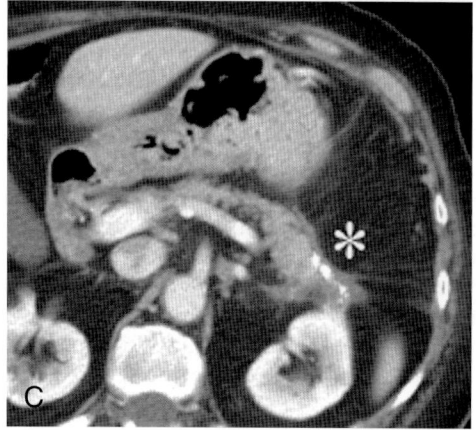

FIGURE 28.1 **A 77-year-old female patient after distal pancreatectomy for neuroendocrine tumor. A,** Postoperative development of a large rim-enhancing fluid collection in the operative bed, suspicious for abscess or pseudocyst *(asterisk).* **B,** Computed tomography (CT)-guided drainage of the fluid collection with a 10-French (Fr) drainage catheter. Rust-colored fluid was aspirated and sent for analysis, which showed elevated amylase and negative culture, consistent with a pancreatic leak. The catheter was removed after the output had diminished. **C,** CT follow-up 10 months after drain removal showed resolution of the fluid collection *(asterisk).*

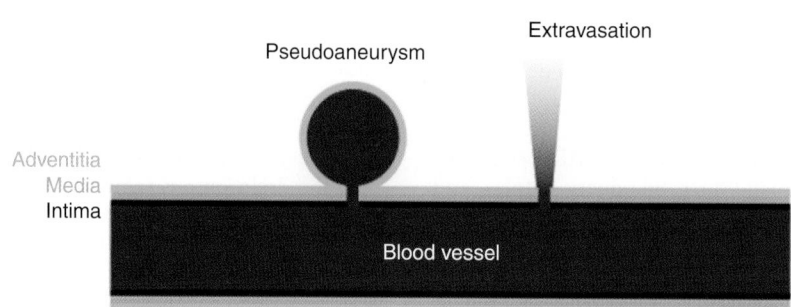

FIGURE 28.2 A pseudoaneurysm is a contained arterial rupture, which can bleed intermittently. On angiogram or computed tomography (CT) angiogram, it looks like a round enhancing structure. On the other hand, active extravasation of contrast looks like a jet of contrast on angiography, which continues to spread on delayed images.

scan can be performed before drain removal to ensure resolution of the cavity. An abscessogram shows if the tube is clogged or malpositioned, as well as the size of the residual collection and any fistulas. A CT scan shows the position of the tube and any undrained collections. On CT, a residual collection around an abscess drain indicates a clogged or poorly functioning drain.

The median drainage time is 11 days for sterile fluid collections, 29 days for abscesses, and 30 days when there is a pancreatic leak.[2]

Interventional Management of Pancreaticocutaneous Fistulas

Pancreatic leaks with pancreaticocutaneous fistulas can develop after pancreatic surgery. Most fistulas resolve after one month of conservative therapy, including jejunal feedings, somatostatin analogues, pseudocyst drains, and endoscopic stent placement in the pancreatic duct.[9,10] The fistula is likely to persist if there is complete transection of the pancreatic duct, if there is a downstream ductal stricture, or if it is a high-output fistula.[9]

Several percutaneous approaches have been described for reconnecting the pancreas to the gastrointestinal (GI) tract to

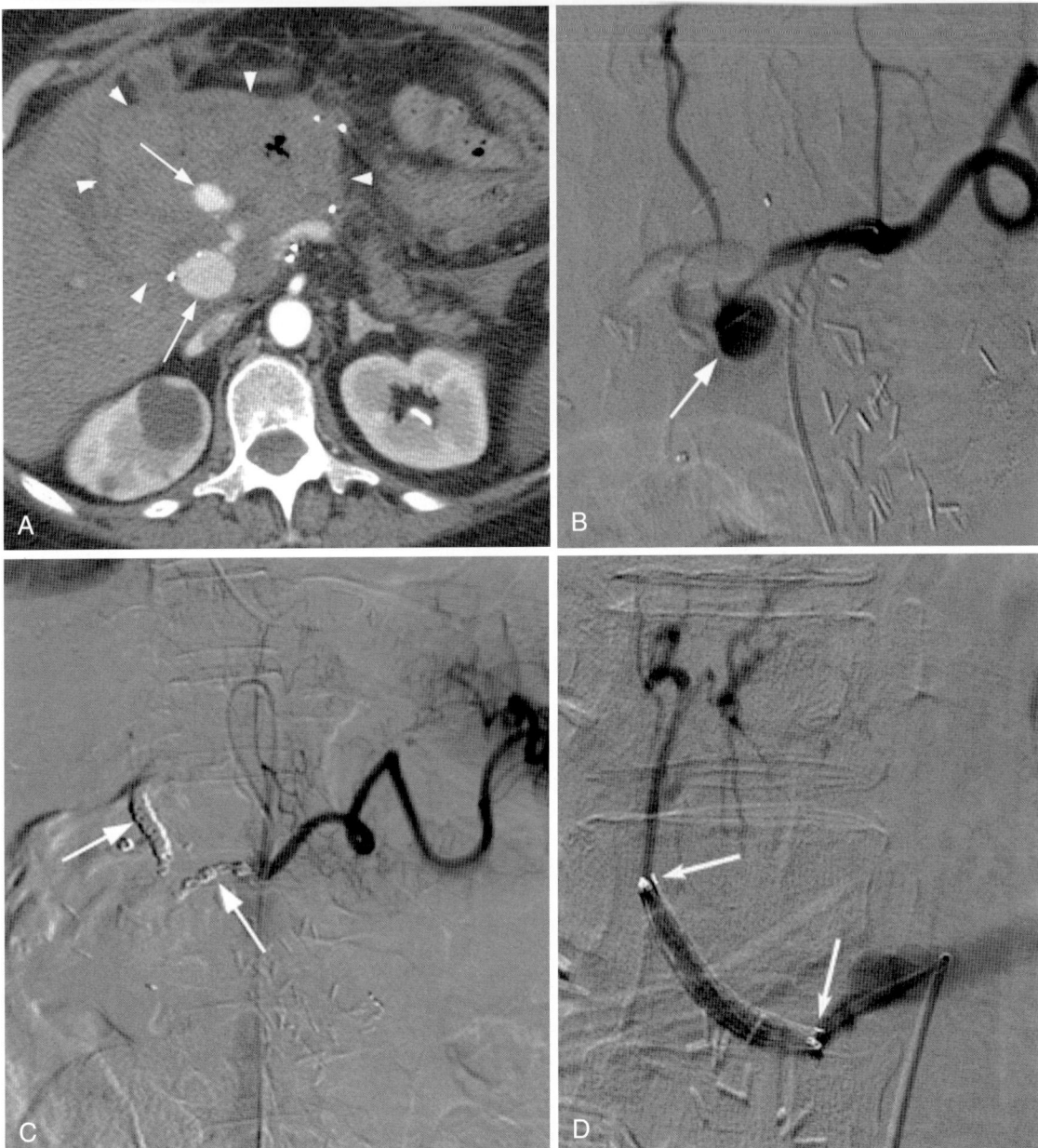

FIGURE 28.3 **A 63-year-old female patient had clinical evidence of bleeding 3 weeks after pancreaticoduodenectomy for pancreatic adenocarcinoma. A,** Computed tomography (CT) angiogram showed a large hematoma *(arrowheads)* in the subhepatic space, with highly enhancing components within this hematoma, consistent with a pseudoaneurysm *(arrows)* at the origin of the gastroduodenal artery. **B,** Catheter angiography confirmed a pseudoaneurysm *(arrow)* of the gastroduodenal artery, which was treated by occluding both the proper hepatic (outflow) and common hepatic arteries (inflow) with stainless steel coils. **C,** Postembolization angiogram showed coils in the hepatic arteries *(arrows)*, with no enhancement of the hepatic arteries or the pseudoaneurysm of the gastroduodenal artery. **D,** A 46-year-old male had gastroduodenal artery stump bleeding after pancreaticoduodenectomy, which was treated by placement of a covered stent *(between arrows)* into the hepatic artery. Covered stent placement preserves hepatic arterial flow.

divert pancreatic fluid away from the fistula and allow it to heal. Cystogastrostomy (surgical, endoscopic, or percutaneous) can be performed if there is a pseudocyst associated with the fistula. If the pancreatic duct is dilated (>4 mm), then it can be punctured percutaneously, allowing for placement of a drain from the pancreatic duct to the stomach or bowel.[11] However, the pancreatic duct is frequently nondilated because it is decompressed into the cutaneous tract. If the pancreatic duct is not dilated, then a snare can be placed into the duct via the cutaneous

fistula, providing a target for percutaneous puncture and drainage of the duct into the stomach.[12]

Management of Hemorrhage: Angiography, Embolization, and Covered Stent Placement (see Chapters 21, 31, and 115)

Hemorrhage is seen in less than 10% of patients after pancreatectomy but is associated with high mortality.[13] Major bleeding is seen on average 19 days after surgery and is usually preceded by a smaller sentinel bleed.[14] Therefore even a small amount of

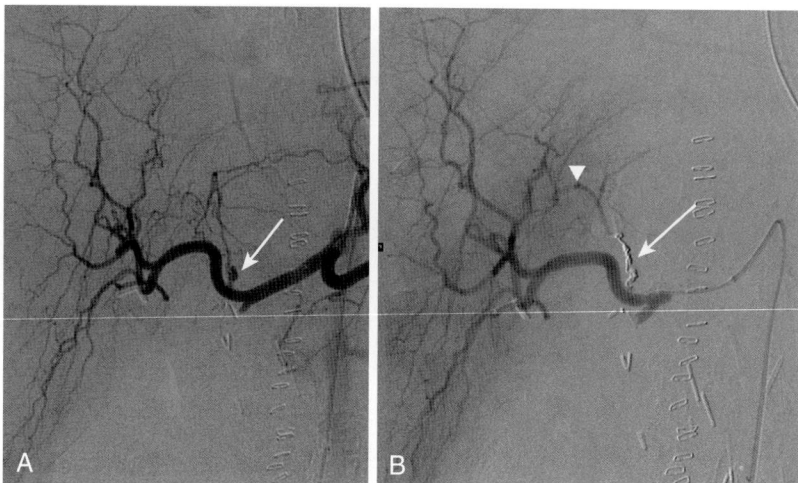

FIGURE 28.4   A 72-year-old female patient developed hemoperitoneum after pancreaticoduodenectomy. A, Angiogram showed a small pseudoaneurysm of the left hepatic artery *(arrow)*. **B,** After coil embolization *(arrow)*, the left hepatic artery is now supplied by the right hepatic artery, via intrahepatic collaterals *(arrowhead)*.

increased bleeding from surgical drains or GI bleeding more than three days after pancreatic surgery should be evaluated immediately. Bleeding can be because of vessel injury during surgery or because of pancreatic fluid eroding the vessel wall.

In hemodynamically stable patients, CT angiography can identify the bleeding vessel. CT angiogram is most likely to be positive if performed when the patient is actively bleeding. Hemodynamically unstable patients should proceed directly to catheter angiography and intervention or to the operating room.

Pseudoaneurysms and arterial extravasation after pancreatic surgery occur in the gastroduodenal artery (GDA) most commonly, followed by the hepatic artery, superior mesenteric artery (SMA), and splenic artery[15] (see Chapter 115). Selective coil embolization across the pseudoaneurysm is successful in approximately 85% of patients.[16] In an otherwise normal liver, the right or left hepatic arteries can be safely coil embolized (Fig. 28.4) because the embolized lobe of the liver will be supplied by the portal vein and intrahepatic arterial collaterals.[17] The proximal splenic artery can also be safely coil embolized without complete splenic infarction, because of collateral arterial supply to the spleen.[18]

Pseudoaneurysms and arterial extravasation can also be treated using a covered stent to exclude the pseudoaneurysm while preserving distal flow.[19,20] Covered stents are particularly helpful for GDA stump blowouts (where coil embolization might not be technically possible), distal splenic artery pseudoaneurysms (where embolization has a higher risk of splenic infarction), common and proper hepatic artery pseudoaneurysms (to preserve arterial flow to the liver), and SMA pseudoaneurysms (to preserve flow to bowel).

Examples of embolization and covered stent placement for bleeding after pancreatic surgery are shown in Figs. 28.3 and 28.4.

IMAGING AND IMAGE-GUIDED THERAPY OF COMPLICATIONS AFTER HEPATECTOMY

Imaging After Hepatectomy

Ultrasound, CT, hepatobiliary iminodiacetic acid (HIDA) scan, and MRI/MRCP can be used to evaluate the liver and biliary system. Postoperative bilomas, hematomas, and abscesses can be detected with these imaging modalities.

The typical appearance of a biloma on imaging is that of an encapsulated fluid collection adjacent to the liver resection plane. Rim enhancement of a fluid collection suggests infection, but this is not a specific finding. In some cases, aspiration may be required to distinguish between infected and noninfected collections. A postoperative biloma, hematoma, or seroma might initially be sterile but can progress to become an abscess. Gas within a collection suggests infection or enteric leak.

A HIDA scan, also known as hepatobiliary scintigraphy, is a nuclear medicine scan that can show biliary leaks.[21] Although ^{99}Tc-HIDA has largely been replaced by other radiotracers (which have improved liver uptake), the term "HIDA scan" remains in common use. A normal HIDA scan initially shows radiotracer uptake in liver, followed by excretion of radiotracer into the bile ducts, gallbladder, and small bowel. Pooling of tracer elsewhere indicates a bile leak. HIDA scans are typically two-dimensional (2D) images acquired with a gamma camera, but fused 3D images can also be obtained, using a single photon emission computed tomography (SPECT)/CT scan. The 3D images can be helpful for more precise anatomic localization (see Chapter 18).

MRCP is an MRI protocol optimized for seeing the bile ducts. It can show the anatomy of the biliary tree and any associated bilomas. MRCP can also show a biliary leak, when it is performed using an intravenous (IV) contrast agent that is excreted into the bile ducts, such as gadoxetate (Eovist).[22] (Typically, MRCP is performed without IV contrast.) MRCP has higher resolution than a HIDA scan and can show the biliary tree more clearly than CT (see Chapter 16).

Acute and subacute hematomas appear as high density collections on CT. In addition, active bleeding can be demonstrated by contrast media extravasation on CECT.

Interventional Radiology Procedures Posthepatectomy
Intrahepatic Abscess Drainage

Small pyogenic liver abscesses can be successfully treated with antibiotics alone. Large (>3 cm) unilocular abscesses can be treated with percutaneous drainage and antibiotics. Large multiloculated abscesses have a lower success rate with percutaneous drainage and might require surgery.[23] Intracavitary tPA can help drain multiloculated collections that are refractory to simple percutaneous drainage.[8] When biliary obstruction is present, relief of the obstructed biliary tree is mandatory for successful abscess treatment. Abscesses located near the dome of the liver may be technically more difficult to drain without transgressing the pleura. Transpleural abscess drains carry a risk of empyema.

Interventional Management of Bilomas and Bile Leaks

After liver resection, bile can leak from a bile duct injury, bilioenteric anastomosis, or the cut surface of the liver. Bile leakage can cause bile peritonitis and bilious fluid collections that can become infected. These fluid collections can be drained percutaneously, under CT, or using ultrasound guidance. When an infected biloma is drained, the fluid can initially appear purulent, then may turn bilious if there is a continued bile leak after the infection clears. Ideally, the drain should be placed near the bile leak to provide optimal drainage.

The amount of drain output allows for monitoring of the amount of bile leak over time. Small bile leaks can resolve spontaneously.[24] Persistent drainage greater than 100 mL a day (at 10 days posthepatectomy) should be treated with ERCP and placement of a plastic biliary stent or PBD placement, which decompresses the biliary system and diverts bile flow away from the defect in the bile ducts, allowing the leak to heal (Fig. 28.5). Complete transection of a bile duct at the hilum typically requires surgical repair.

PBD is the preferred treatment for high bile duct injuries (at or above the bifurcation) and bilioenteric anastomotic leaks, both of which are difficult to access endoscopically. ERCP is less invasive than PBD and is the preferred treatment for leaks from the cut surface of the liver and for accessible common duct leaks (see Chapters 20, 30, and 31).

PBD healed 88% to 100% of postoperative bile leaks, after an average of one to three months of drainage.[25,26] Retrievable covered stents can be placed for common duct leaks.[27] Intractable bile leaks can be managed with surgery, portal vein embolization,[28] or bile duct embolization with N-butyl cyanoacrylate glue.[29]

Interventional Management of Biliary Strictures

Postoperative biliary strictures can occur after hepatectomy, cholecystectomy, choledochojejunostomy, liver transplant, and other procedures. These strictures can be caused by direct biliary injury from surgery, ischemia, or recurrent tumor. Benign and malignant strictures can be difficult to distinguish on imaging, and biopsy may be required. Biliary strictures can cause jaundice, cholangitis, and pruritis (see Chapters 31 and 42).

Low bile duct obstruction (common bile duct or common hepatic duct not involving the bifurcation) can be relieved via ERCP and placement of a plastic or metal biliary stent across the obstruction. High bile duct obstruction and bilioenteric anastomotic strictures (both of which are difficult to access endoscopically) can be treated with PBD or metal stent placement. Metal stents are typically only used for malignant obstruction because they have a limited patency rate (30 months on average when used for benign disease).[30] However, retrievable covered stents can be used to treat benign biliary strictures[31,32] (see Chapter 30).

If the biliary stricture cannot be crossed percutaneously, an external biliary drain can be placed. If the biliary stricture can be crossed, an internal/external biliary drain is placed, which has side holes both above and below the obstruction. An internal/external biliary drain can be capped if there is no leak, infection, or significant blood in the bile and should be flushed daily with 10 mL normal saline to maintain patency.

Biliary drains are typically exchanged every three months to prevent clogging, but are exchanged more frequently if cholangioplasty or other interventions are planned. An over-the-wire cholangiogram can be performed through a sheath that does not cross the bile duct injury to evaluate for persistent leak or stenosis. If the bile duct injury has resolved on the cholangiogram, then an external biliary drain can be placed to maintain access to the bile ducts. This external drain should be capped for two weeks without flushing. If the patient passes the capping trial (no fever, no significant leakage around the tube, no rise in bilirubin), then the drain can be safely removed.

Benign biliary strictures are typically managed with endoscopic placement of a plastic biliary stent or percutaneous internal/external biliary drainage. Cholangioplasty can be performed

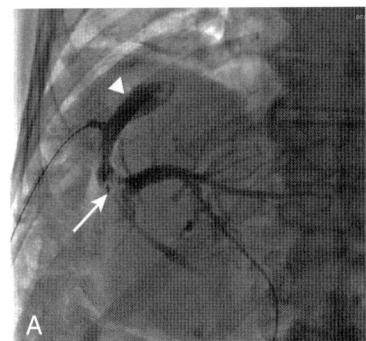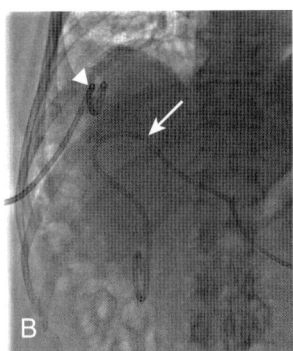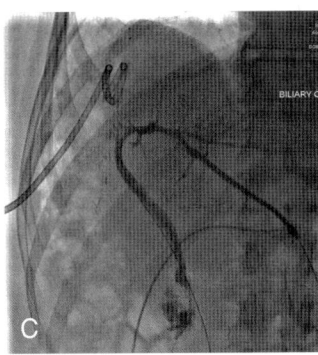

FIGURE 28.5 **A 57-year-old male patient with metastatic colon cancer developed a bile leak after extended right hepatectomy.** A biloma drain was placed, which was draining 700 mL of bile per day. **A,** Percutaneous cholangiogram shows a bile leak *(arrow)* into the biloma cavity *(arrowhead)*. **B,** A left internal/external biliary drain *(arrow)* was placed to divert bile away from the biloma drain *(arrowhead)*. **C,** After two months of biliary drainage, biloma drain output decreased to 15 mL per day. Follow-up cholangiogram shows resolution of the bile leak. The internal/external biliary drain was converted to an external biliary drain for a two-week capping trial before removal.

using a high pressure balloon during biliary drain placement or exchange. High pressures and prolonged cholangioplasty (up to 15 minutes) are typically required to overcome the dense fibrous tissue around biliary strictures. An 8-mm balloon can be used for intrahepatic strictures, and a 10- to 12-mm balloon for common duct strictures. Cholangioplasty can be repeated at two to 14 day intervals.[33] For benign biliary strictures, cholangioplasty and internal/external biliary drainage have a long-term (25 years) primary success rate of 59% and a secondary success rate of 80%[33] (see Chapter 31).

Malignant biliary obstruction can be relieved with a biliary drainage catheter to treat cholangitis or pruritis, or to lower bilirubin for chemotherapy. A metal biliary stent can be placed (percutaneously or endoscopically) for palliation of unresectable symptomatic biliary obstruction in patients with limited life expectancy. Metal biliary stents placed for malignant obstruction remain patent for an average of 11 months.[34]

The references for this chapter can be found online by accessing the accompanying Expert Consult website.

CHAPTER 29

The impact of hepatobiliary interventions on health and quality of life and health

Piera Marie Cote Robson

THE CONCEPTS OF HEALTH AND QUALITY OF LIFE

Promotion of health and restoration of quality of life is central to the delivery of healthcare. There is limited value in engaging in a medical intervention if there is no anticipated impact on health or improvement in quality of life. This chapter will explore the concepts and tools used to measure health and quality of life and will summarize current research on how hepatobiliary interventions impact patients' perceptions of their health and quality of life.

Health

The Constitution of the World Health Organization (WHO) defines health as a "state of complete physical, mental, and social well-being, not merely the absence of disease."[1] This definition integrates three components of well-being (physical, mental and social) into a holistic view of health. Physical health reflects the physiologic and biologic components of health and the maintenance of homeostasis.[2] Mental health is the aspect of health that relates to a person's mental status or their psychological and emotional state.[2] Social health is the ability of a person to engage in the social aspects of life and fill roles within society.[2]

The WHO takes the position that the measurement of health is as important as evaluating the severity of disease. Over time, the perception of disease has evolved from the biomedical concept of disease to the broader biopsychosocial model of disease. The biomedical concept restricts the focus of disease to one of "organic malfunction."[3] This narrow view was broadened in the biopsychological model, which was first proposed by George Engel in 1977.

"To provide a basis for understanding the determinants of disease and arriving at rational treatments and patterns of healthcare, a medical model must also take into account the patient, the social context in which he [sic] lives, and the complementary system devised by society to deal with the disruptive effects of illness, that is, the physician role and the health care system."[4]

The biopsychological model encourages healthcare professionals to incorporate all aspects of health into their clinical care and decision making, weighing various aspects of health, as needed, to optimally address the patient's clinical presentation.[3]

The attention to the effect of a person's social situation on health has gained increased attention in this century, particularly with regard to how societal differences impact health and health equality.[5] Social determinants of health (SDH) are the "conditions in the environments in which people are born, live, learn, work, play, worship, and age that affect a wide range of health, functioning, and quality-of-life outcomes and risks."[6]

The key areas of SDH are "economic stability, education, social and community context, health and health care, neighborhood and built environment."[6] To achieve population health, the WHO has called for the evaluation of SDH in clinical care and the incorporation of SDH into research so that the effect of SDH on a person's health can be recognized, addressed, and measured.

As the biopsychological model has gained acceptance, the question turns from whether health should be assessed to how best evaluate it. The evaluation of health necessarily includes the biomedical aspects provided by objective clinical data. Incorporated into this evaluation are assessments of psychological health including depression, delirium, and suicide screening.[7–9] Social aspects of health are incorporated into patient assessment by exploring social determinants of health such as by assessing financial toxicity and food and housing insecurity.[10] A patient's well-being is evaluated using a measure of quality of life (QOL).[11]

Quality of Life

QOL has been frequently defined as the "individual's perception of their position in life in the context of their culture and value systems in which they live and in relation to their goals, expectations, standards, and concerns."[11] The concept of QOL reflects the experience of an individual and is an evaluation of their own life.[12] It is built on culture, experience, values, goals, expectations, and standards.[11] In the very broadest of terms, QOL is multidimensional and influenced by many factors outside the realm of health/disease, including self-esteem, spirituality, financial security, job satisfaction, and personal freedom.[13] The WHO Quality of Life Group (1998) offered a succinct definition of QOL as "a subjective evaluation that is embedded in a cultural, social and environmental context."[13]

QOL was first discussed in the literature in the 1960s when it was realized that the extension of life through a medical intervention did not always result in the improvement of QOL.[14] It was also recognized that medical interventions, at times, resulted in a cost to QOL.[14,15] The term "health-related quality of life" (HRQOL) is often use to describe QOL related to healthcare experiences. HRQOL does not consider factors that affect QOL that are outside of the purview of the healthcare system including cultural, economic, and political factors.[16] Excluding factors that are not managed by clinicians offers an incomplete view of the person by excluding social well-being from assessment, and it devalues the impact of SDH on the health of individuals. It undermines the holistic approach of the biopsychosocial model and takes a narrow view of QOL similar to the narrow view of the biomedical model of disease.[17]

The assessment of QOL is an assessment of a patient-reported outcome (PRO) measure. PRO is "used as an umbrella term for different concepts for measuring subjectively perceived health status."[18] PRO includes any direct report by a patient of their health condition that has not been interpreted by a clinician or anyone else.[19] PRO measures can assess a single value at one point in time or measure change in that value over time.[18] The psychometrical approach to PRO measures is used most commonly in healthcare. This approach refers to the individual reporting of the presence and quality of perceived symptoms, the functional state, QOL, health behaviors, satisfaction, and emotional and mental status.[18] How the individual reports these measures is their prerogative; however, consensus has not been achieved regarding the definition of concepts measured by PROs. As such, there is an opportunity for additional research in this field.[18]

The interrelationships between different PROs have not been clearly defined. Wilson and Cleary developed a conceptual framework to describe the relationships between five different measures of health.[16] The five measures of health are physiologic and biologic factors, symptoms, functioning, general health perceptions, and overall QOL. This linear model depicts the relationships on a continuum from biologic and physiologic processes to symptoms to function followed by health perceptions, which result in QOL. The framework depicts characteristics of the individual and environment as moderators of health measures. This is a parsimonious model that describes and explains health and can be used to evaluate health outcomes and their relationships with QOL.

Patient report is the key feature of PRO measures. For practical reasons, initial investigations of QOL and other PRO measures used the external judgment of observers, typically nurses or clinicians, to evaluate treatment impact. Examples of this are the commonly used measures of performance such as the Karnofsky Performance Scale (KPS) Index[20] and the Eastern Cooperative Oncology Group (ECOG) Performance Index.[21] These are measures of function and performance, but they are not PROs because they provide the clinician's perception of the patient's status, not the patient's report of their function and performance. This method of evaluating patient outcomes is inherently biased by the observer's own internal standards. Multiple studies evaluating the degree of agreement between the proxy ratings of QOL by observers to patient assessments have consistently found very little correlation between the two measures.[22–27] In clinical trial research, up to 76% of cases with severe symptoms are underreported by providers.[28–30]

The validity of QOL instruments and rigor of results is contingent on patients' reporting. Unfortunately, this requisite self-reporting can become an issue when patients are followed over time because disease status and symptoms worsen, making completion more challenging. With time, patients are less likely to fill out instruments, leading to nonrandom missing data, which is a significant challenge in QOL research.[31,32] Feinstein[33] coined the term "sensibility" of QOL instruments to denote the practical issues related to implementation of QOL measurements. All PRO measures must be evaluated before use from the perspective of the patient. The number of items in a measure, the thought required to complete the measure, and the time required to complete a measure can lead to "questionnaire burn-out" and subsequent patient noncompletion. Other issues, such as literacy and preferred language, may prohibit patients from completing instruments independently.

Measurement of Quality of Life

Essential to the assessment of QOL are instruments developed specifically to measure the construct of QOL. As with the conceptual evolution, assessment of QOL in the clinical setting has been progressive. In the field of oncology, there was a need to assess the "quality of survival" since early chemotherapeutic treatments were severely toxic and there were few options to mitigate the adverse effects.[34] In 1982 the Eastern Cooperative Oncology Group published criteria to measure the toxicity from treatment. All included measures were objective clinical parameters except for their novel performance status scale.[21] In the absence of specific measures of QOL, some researchers reported the ECOG scale and the KPS as surrogates for QOL despite being single unidimensional parameters of performance. With time, the void of valid and reliable instruments for QOL assessment has been filled with multidimensional instruments of QOL with well-established psychometric properties.

The availability of QOL instruments has led to increasing acceptance of their importance as a necessary outcome measure in oncology and surgery. The WHO lists benefits of QOL assessment in clinical practice, including improved decision making, enhanced physician and patient relationship, and better evaluation of treatments.[35] Through the assessment of QOL, a physician learns which patient's domains are most impacted, and this understanding can drive clinical decisions.[36] The assessment of QOL improves the physician and patient relationship by increasing the physician's understanding of the patient's experience.[36] Lastly, QOL assessment allows the physician to evaluate the relative merits and effectiveness of treatment options from a patient's perspective.[35,36]

The acceptance of QOL as an important parameter to assess does not overcome the challenges of implementing assessment into routine clinical practice. There are inherent limitations in the assessment and measurement of QOL. As a subjective measurement, individual benefit may go unrecognized within the results of the entire sample.[37] In many cases, specific detected numeric differences in two assessments (e.g., presurgery to postsurgery) have not been correlated with the clinical implication of the findings.[38] Finally, patients may not be able to adequately reflect their experience within the context of an instrument.[39] These limitations need to be acknowledged and present opportunities for additional research and instrument development.

QUALITY OF LIFE AS AN OUTCOME MEASURE IN SURGERY: WHY AND WHEN?

Surgery, as a specialty, is unique in the immediateness of the intervention and its largely irreversible effects. The goal of the surgeon is to repair, remove, or revise pathologic processes and initiate healing. The ultimate goal is evaluation of the impact of surgery on QOL with preoperative and postoperative assessment of QOL. Presurgical QOL information should be integrated into the informed consent process and postsurgical QOL information should guide clinical decision making and be used as a marker of surgical success. A recent review of 33 randomized surgical oncology trials, in which QOL data were collected, indicated that in two-thirds of trials, the QOL information influenced clinical decision making and/or facilitated the surgical consent process.[40] Integration of the QOL data was more common among later trials included in the systematic review, reflecting the progressively increased value attached to these outcomes by surgeons.[10] On a similar note, it has been shown that communicating both technical procedural–related information and QoL information to the patient and their family facilitates an improved physician-patient relationship, reconciles patient expectations, and improves patient satisfaction.[41–45] Furthermore, although QOL measurement tools have evolved from generic to disease/site specific, and subsequently have become more sensitive, focus on QOL as a predictive/prognostic variable of outcomes such as morbidity, mortality, and survival has increased. Meta-analysis of 30 randomized clinical trials with QOL data from the European Organization for the Research and Treatment of Cancer (EORTC) Quality-of-Life Questionnaire (QLQ)-C30 (core 30 items; Fig. 29.1) revealed

ENGLISH

EORTC QLQ-C30 (version 3)

We are interested in some things about you and your health. Please answer all of the questions yourself by circling the number that best applies to you. There are no "right" or "wrong" answers. The information that you provide will remain strictly confidential.

Please fill in your initials:

Your birthdate (Day, Month, Year):

Today's date (Day, Month, Year):   31

	Not at All	A Little	Quite a Bit	Very Much
1. Do you have any trouble doing strenuous activities, like carrying a heavy shopping bag or a suitcase?	1	2	3	4
2. Do you have any trouble taking a <u>long</u> walk?	1	2	3	4
3. Do you have any trouble taking a <u>short</u> walk outside of the house?	1	2	3	4
4. Do you need to stay in bed or a chair during the day?	1	2	3	4
5. Do you need help with eating, dressing, washing yourself or using the toilet?	1	2	3	4

During the past week:	Not at All	A Little	Quite a Bit	Very Much
6. Were you limited in doing either your work or other daily activities?	1	2	3	4
7. Were you limited in pursuing your hobbies or other leisure time activities?	1	2	3	4
8. Were you short of breath?	1	2	3	4
9. Have you had pain?	1	2	3	4
10. Did you need to rest?	1	2	3	4
11. Have you had trouble sleeping?	1	2	3	4
12. Have you felt weak?	1	2	3	4
13. Have you lacked appetite?	1	2	3	4
14. Have you felt nauseated?	1	2	3	4
15. Have you vomited?	1	2	3	4
16. Have you been constipated?	1	2	3	4

<u>Please go on to the next page</u>

FIGURE 29.1 European Organization for the Research and Treatment of Cancer Quality-of-Life Questionnaire (EORTC QLQ-C30). A user's agreement is required to use this scale and can be accessed through the website at: https://qol.eortc.org/questionnaire/eortc-qlq-c30/

Continued

ENGLISH

During the past week:	Not at All	A Little	Quite a Bit	Very Much
17. Have you had diarrhea?	1	2	3	4
18. Were you tired?	1	2	3	4
19. Did pain interfere with your daily activities?	1	2	3	4
20. Have you had difficulty in concentrating on things, like reading a newspaper or watching television?	1	2	3	4
21. Did you feel tense?	1	2	3	4
22. Did you worry?	1	2	3	4
23. Did you feel irritable?	1	2	3	4
24. Did you feel depressed?	1	2	3	4
25. Have you had difficulty remembering things?	1	2	3	4
26. Has your physical condition or medical treatment interfered with your <u>family</u> life?	1	2	3	4
27. Has your physical condition or medical treatment interfered with your <u>social</u> activities?	1	2	3	4
28. Has your physical condition or medical treatment caused you financial difficulties?	1	2	3	4

For the following questions please circle the number between 1 and 7 that best applies to you

29. How would you rate your overall <u>health</u> during the past week?

    1   2   3   4   5   6   7

Very poor   Excellent

30. How would you rate your overall <u>quality of life</u> during the past week?

    1   2   3   4   5   6   7

Very poor   Excellent

FIGURE 29.1 cont'd

that the addition of QOL parameters (physical functioning, pain, anorexia) to sociodemographic and clinical variables provides prognostic value and significantly improves the predictive accuracy of models of survival.[46] Moreover, patient scores within the physical functioning domain have been shown to be an independent predictor of survival for multiple different cancers.[47–49]

More specific to hepatobiliary surgery, global QOL, social well-being, and physical functioning have all been shown to independently predict survival outcomes in patients with colorectal liver metastases (CRLMs) and to add to the prognostic value

of survival models, including standard biomedical data.[50–52] Similar findings have been observed among patients with hepatocellular carcinoma (HCC).[53] Whether QOL simply reflects a highly sensitive instrument of patients' overall health status not evaluated elsewhere, or whether QOL impacts other important areas, such as self-care/treatment adherence and thus survival, is unknown. What is clear is that measurement of QOL to aid informed consent and clinical decision making, to facilitate physician-patient relationship and manage expectations, and to help improve prognostication is requisite to optimize care of surgical patients.

As with any outcome measure, it is essential to identify the clinical scenarios in which assessment is appropriate. Consequently, it is incumbent on surgeons to define these relevant settings where QOL endpoints will result in clinically meaningful/actionable outcomes. It is suggested that the most pertinent scenarios for surgical patients include evaluation of palliative interventions or procedures in which survival outcomes are thought to be equivocal and/or survival outcomes similar, but morbidity/side-effect profiles differ significantly.[40,54–58] In fact, the intention of palliative surgery is to mitigate physical symptoms in patients with noncurable disease, with the primary goal of improving or maintaining QOL.[59] Inclusion of QOL measurements in studies in which these specific scenarios are encountered will maximize the clinical applicability of the QOL outcomes observed.

Psychometric Properties of Quality of Life Instruments

Before using an instrument for clinical or research purposes, the psychometric properties of the instrument must be evaluated and understood. These properties should guide the selection of the instrument. For QOL results to be respected on the same level as other measured clinical variables, established rigor of measurement tool is essential and depends on three primary concepts: reliability, validity, and responsiveness/sensitivity, which are described in this section.

Reliability is the degree to which a method of measurement consistently assigns scores to individuals or measures the attribute of interest.[60] A measure's reliability reflects the ability to identify the true score as opposed to measurement error. Therefore a measure that has perfect reliability would only identify the true score; however, perfect measures do not exist.[60,61] There are two key types of reliability: stability reliability and equivalence reliability.[61] Stability reliability is evaluated when the attributes are expected to be stable. Equivalence reliability evaluates whether all items consistently measure the attributes of the tool and whether individuals obtain similar scores on similar measures.[61] Within these two types of reliability are the different ways reliability can be measured. Test-retest reliability, which is a type of stability reliability, is the evaluation of score when the same test is given to the same group of individuals at different times. The degree to which the two overall scores, as well as individual items, are correlated is an indicator of stability reliability. A reliability coefficient of the comparison is generated.[62] Internal consistency reliability is an indicator of equivalence reliability and is an indicator of the degree to which the items of a measure covary, or hang together, conceptually. Internal consistency often uses the Cronbach alpha statistic (ranging from 0.00 to 1.00), which can be generated after only one administration of the test (an advantage of this method of assessing reliability). Nevertheless, this means it is specific to the population using the instrument and should be repeated with each test administration. Alternate forms (or parallel forms) reliability is a means of demonstrating equivalence reliability by using different versions of an instrument to determine whether the scores remain constant. Questions are pulled from a question bank and should test the same concept. The means, variances, and Cronbach alphas of both tests should be approximately equivalent. The researcher makes a decision regarding the approach to establish reliability based on the concept or attribute being measured.[60,61,63,64]

Validity is the degree to which an instrument successfully measures the attribute/construct that it is intended to measure. There are multiple types of validity.

- Content validity is the degree or extent to which the content of the measure encompasses the domain or concept that is being addressed in the measure. Content validity exists if, out of all possible items that might be used to identify the domain/construct, the items selected are representative of the concept or domain.[60,61,63,64]
- Criterion validity is the degree to which a measure's scores correlate with another measure's scores. Criterion validity is the correlation between the measure and the "gold standard" for assessment of that attribute.[60,61,63,64] There are two types of criterion validity: predictive and concurrent.
  - Predictive validity provides a predictive indicator of the extent to which future performance on a criterion can be predicted based on performance on a prior measure.[60]
  - Concurrent validity is the degree to which a measure can be used to determine an individual's current position or standing on the criterion being measured.[60]
- Construct validity is the degree to which an instrument measures the attribute/construct under investigation.[60]
- Convergent validity is the degree to which two measures that measure the same construct/attribute are related to each other.[60]
- Discriminant validity is the degree to which two measures that measure different constructs/attributes should not be related to each other.[60]

A key aspect of validity is that it is not a property of the measure. Validity is a property of the scores obtained from a population with a purpose for the measurement.[61,64] Therefore the evidence for validity must be provided each time a measure or an instrument is used. This means that different sources of evidence must be woven into the argument that the use of the specific measure was appropriate to evaluate the construct/attribute in the designated population. Additionally, the interpretation of scores must be supported using evidence from the current study and past studies, and the evidence gathered during the current study can inform future use of the measure/instrument.

Responsiveness is the ability of an instrument to detect and measure changes during time and treatments. A good instrument is stable when nothing has changed and capable of detecting even small changes when they occur. Responsiveness is dependent on the number of items in a questionnaire as well as the number of potential responses. From a practical standpoint, the number of items and associated responses must be optimized to ensure sufficient responsiveness without creating overly cumbersome questionnaires in which respondents experience "question fatigue," leading to increased rates of nonresponse and missing data.

The content of QOL instruments typically includes multiple domains containing information on a specific area of health/disease, such as physical, social, emotional, role, and global functioning. In turn, each domain contains a number of items (questions or statements) for which respondents must provide an answer, either on a Likert scale or in visual analogue form. Each item is individually scored, and scores from all items in a given domain are summed to give each domain a specific score.[65]

QUALITY OF LIFE INSTRUMENTS AND INTERPRETATION

Early in the history of QOL assessment in cancer clinical trials, no standard instrument was used, and the default was simply ad hoc trial-specific questionnaires that prohibited comparison across trials and often even among patients with the same disease.[66] These findings prompted a new era in QOL research heralded by the development of multiple standardized tools/instruments to measure QOL. There are now more than 600 QOL PRO measures, of varying quality, and the sheer number of measures highlights the expansion of the QOL field.[67] There is a need to carefully select measures of QOL for strong psychometric properties and established use in similar populations. The former ensures that the instrument will accurately measure the concept of QOL and the latter supports comparability of the findings.

To date, no "gold-standard" instrument exists for the evaluation of QOL. Generic instruments are used in many surgical trials such as the Medical Outcomes Survey 36-Item Short Form (SF-36). Although these instruments provide a broad overview

of the patient's QOL, care must be taken to choose an instrument that is intended to measure QOL and is not simply a PRO measure of another related construct. The advantage of a generic instrument is that it permits comparison across disease states and treatment types. Patient burden must also be considered since these surveys can be time consuming to complete and, in the end, the effort invested may not result in data with adequate sensitivity to identify changes in QOL specifically related to different diseases and/or treatments. Two commonly used generic instruments used in the oncologic setting are the EORTC, presented in Table 28.1A, and the Functional Assessment of Cancer Therapy-General (FACT-G). These types of instruments focus more on expected changes specifically related to cancer and its treatment. Consequently, they are more sensitive to QOL changes and are good for comparisons across different cancer diagnoses but are not generalizable to other disease states.

Disease-specific tools focus on a single disease state. There are only six validated and reliable instruments that were designed for disease specific assessment of hepatobiliary or pancreatic cancers.[80] Three are disease-specific instruments of the EORTC,[77–79,81–83] two are disease specific scales of the

TABLE 29.1A Generic and Disease-Specific Health-Related Quality-of Life-Measurement Instruments

INSTRUMENT	AUTHOR, YEAR, COUNTRY	TYPE OF INSTRUMENT	DESCRIPTION OF QUALITY-OF-LIFE MEASURES	INTERPRETATION	HPB-SPECIFIC MODULES	COMMENTS
Medical Outcomes Study 36-Item Short Form (SF-36)	Ware, 1992, US[68]	Generic profile based	36 items 8 health-status scales: General health perceptions Physical functioning Role limitations due to physical problems Role limitations due to emotional problems Social functioning Bodily pain Vitality (energy/fatigue) General mental health	8 health-status scale scores Items in each scale are summed and averaged to give a single score (0-100) for each health status *Higher scores = better quality of life (QOL)*	No	Comparison across broad range of disease states and treatments Less sensitive to changes in disease/health status
EuroQoL EQ 5D-5L	EuroQoL Group, 1990, UK[69]	Generic value/preference based	EQ-5D-5L (descriptive system): 5 dimensions, 5 levels of severity: Mobility, self-care, usual activities, pain/discomfort, anxiety/depression	Each dimension given a 1-digit number expressing the level selected Numbers from each dimension are combined to give 5-digit number corresponding to a specific health state; preference value is then assigned based on empirically derived valuations (0-1)	No	Self-administered with minimal responder bias Revision of EQ-5D-3L, increased levels of severity from 3-5 to improve sensitivity and reduce ceiling effect
Spitzer Quality-of-Life Index (QLI)	Spitzer, 1981, Australia[70]	Generic index	EQ-VAS (visual analogue scale) 5 items: Activity Daily living Health Support Outlook	VAS: quantitative measure of overall health perceived by respondent (self-rated) *Higher score = better QOL*	No	3 types of data produced: 1. Profile indicating extent of the problems in each domain 2. Population-weighted health index 3. Self-rated assessment of health status

TABLE 29.1A   Generic and Disease-Specific Health-Related Quality-of-Life-Measurement Instruments—cont'd

INSTRUMENT	AUTHOR, YEAR, COUNTRY	TYPE OF INSTRUMENT	DESCRIPTION OF QUALITY-OF-LIFE MEASURES	INTERPRETATION	HPB-SPECIFIC MODULES	COMMENTS
FACT-G (Functional Assessment of Cancer Treatment–General)	Cella, 1993, US[71]	Disease specific: cancer	27 items, 4 domains: Physical (7) Social/family (7) Emotional (6) Functional (7)	Each item scored 0-4 on Likert scale; items in given domain are summed to give overall score for each domain Scores for each domain summed to give overall score *Higher score = worse QOL*	Yes	Comparable across different cancers Moderate sensitivity to changes over time Published data exists regarding clinically important changes over time, allowing improved interpretation
EORTC QLQ-C30 (European Organization for Research and Treatment of Cancer-Core Quality-of-Life Questionnaire)	Aaronson, 1993, Netherlands[72]	Disease specific: cancer	30 items; 9 multiitem scales + 6 single items: *5 functional scales:* Physical Role Social Cognitive Emotional *1 Global Health/QOL Scale* *3 symptom scales:* Pain Fatigue Nausea/vomiting	Each item in a scale is scored, and an overall scale score from 0-100 is reported *Higher-score functional/ global scales = better QOL*	Yes	Comparable across different cancers Sensitive to cancer-related changes overtime Published data exists regarding clinically important changes during time, allowing for improved interpretation
Gastrointestinal Quality-of-Life Index (GQLI)	Eypasch, 1995, Germany and Canada[73]	Disease specific: any GI disease	36 items, 5 response categories (recall over 2 wk): Core symptoms items Physical items Psychological items Social items Disease-specific items	Scores from all questions are summed and a single score is reported *Higher score = better QOL* Scores from all items are summed, and a single score is reported *Higher score = better QOL*	No	Assesses QOL pertaining to a variety of diseases of the liver, pancreas, and biliary system Single score lacks sensitivity to change

TABLE 29.1B   Disease Specific Health Related Quality of Life Measurement Instruments

CORE QUESTIONNAIRE	MODULE	AUTHOR, YEAR, COUNTRY	DESCRIPTION OF QUALITY-OF-LIFE MEASUREMENT	COMMENTS
Functional Assessment of Cancer Therapy (FACT)	Hepatobiliary subscale (HS) FACT + HS = FACT-Hep	Heffernan et al, 2002, US[74]	Specific disease: Metastatic or primary liver cancer, pancreatic cancer, CCA, GBCA FACT-G + 18-item subscale, including HPB-specific concerns related to: Jaundice GI obstruction Fatigue/energy Each item scored (0-4) and summed to give overall subscale score	HS can be combined with physical and functional domain scores of FACT-G to give Trial Outcome Index (TOI) 7 additional questions (nonscored) at end of HS, addressing HAIP and biliary drainage
	FACT Hepatobiliary Symptom Index-8 (FHSI-8)	Yount et al, 2002, US[75]	Specific disease: Metastatic or primary liver cancer, pancreatic cancer, CCA, GBCA 8 key symptoms from 18-item HS scale including: Pain Nausea Fatigue (× 2 items) Jaundice Weight loss Back Pain Stomach Pain/discomfort *Developed in response to clinician concern regarding the time and resources required to complete and interpret multidimensional QOL assessments*	Brief index with good correlation with scores on FACT-G and FACT-Hep Capacity to discriminate patients based on performance status/ treatment; status adequate but not as good as FACT-G subscales or HS Developed primarily based on pancreatic cancer

Continued

TABLE 29.1B   Disease Specific Health Related Quality of Life Measurement Instruments—cont'd

CORE QUESTIONNAIRE	MODULE	AUTHOR, YEAR, COUNTRY	DESCRIPTION OF QUALITY-OF-LIFE MEASUREMENT	COMMENTS
European Organization for Research and Treatment of Cancer–Quality-of-Life Questionnaire–Core 30 (EORTC QLQ-C30)	Pancreatic carcinoma (QLQ-PAN26)	Fitzsimmons et al, 1998, UK[76]	Specific disease: Diseases of the pancreas, not oncology specific 26-item subscale, including items concerning pancreas: Symptoms Treatments Emotional issues	Commonly used although no information on psychometric properties in oncology population Examples: Pain (abdominal, back, positional, night) Dietary restrictions GI symptoms Cachexia Weight loss Jaundice Pruritus Ascites
	Colorectal liver metastases (QLQ-LMC21)	Kavadas et al,[77] 2003, UK	Specific disease: CRLM 21-item subscale. including items concerning CRLM-specific: Symptoms Treatment Emotional issues	Examples: Pain (abdominal, back) Eating problems (early satiety) Fatigue Lethargy Jaundice Taste Tingling hands/feet Stress Loss of enjoyment
	Hepatocellular carcinoma (QLQ-HCC18)	Blazeby et al, 2004, UK[78]	Specific disease: HCC 18-item subscale, including items concerning HCC-specific: Symptoms Treatments Emotional Issues	Examples: Fatigue Body image Jaundice Nutrition Pain Fevers
	Cholangiocarcinoma, Gallbladder Carcinoma (QLQ-BIL21)	Friend et al, 2011, UK[79]	Specific disease: CCA and GBCA 21-item subscale, including items concerning CCA/GBCA-specific: Symptoms Treatments Emotional issues	Examples: Eating Satiety Jaundice Fatigue Anxiety Pain Stress Worry

CCA, Cholangiocarcinoma; *CRLM*, colorectal liver metastases; *GBCA*, gallbladder carcinoma; *GI*, gastrointestinal; *HAIP,* hepatic arterial infusion pump; *HCC*, hepatocellular carcinoma; *HPB*, hepatopancreatobiliary; *QOL*, health-related quality of life; *UK*, United Kingdom; *US*, United States.

FACT,[74,75] and one is the QOL for patients with Liver Cancer Treatment (QOL-LC).[84] These instruments use the modular approach, which is specific to patients with cancer. It refers to the use of a core cancer questionnaire in conjunction with validated modules for specific disease sites (i.e., pancreas, liver, biliary modules).[56] This approach is based on the premise that, although there are similar effects of disease/treatment across cancers, each primary tumor site is also associated with a unique set of QOL concerns. Use of a modular approach increases the sensitivity to detect small, yet clinically relevant, changes in QOL. This method has been popularized by the EORTC, in which the core EORTC QLQ-C30 questionnaire is paired/supplemented with a site- and/or symptom-specific instrument. The FACT hepatobiliary subscale (FACT-Hep) is an example of a modular instrument (Fig. 28.2). The comprehensive nature of these tools provides increased sensitivity; however, practicality, in terms of time

and resources required to complete, may be prohibitive in some settings. Based on this, attempts to develop brief scales that adequately correlate with the more extensive evaluations have been attempted. Yount et al.[75] developed and tested an eight-item symptom scale from the FACT-Hep that correlated well with overall FACT-G scores; however, the ability to discriminate patients based on performance status/treatment status was limited. Overall, these simplified indices are not as sensitive or reliable as longer multidimensional evaluations of QOL; however, their practicality makes them attractive alternatives.

QOL is more than the sum of its parts, and it is likely that a global assessment in the form of an index is complementary to, rather than an alternative to, individual domain evaluation. It is generally accepted that a single assessment of patients' perceptions of overall QOL is improved over aggregation of individual domain scores, where each domain is given equal importance and a "mean" QoL is estimated.[85,86] Ideally, optimal QOL assessment strategies should include both global- and domain-specific measurements.

The vast array and potential combinations of available measurement tools can be overwhelming and make interpretation/evaluation of QOL literature difficult. To critically appraise QOL literature, it is essential to understand the psychometric properties so that judgment as to the robustness of the results can be made. Table 28.2 outlines QOL levels of evidence based on the psychometric properties of the measurement tool(s) used.[44] Guyatt et al.[87] and Wu et al.[88] have published review articles that present a standardized approach to critical appraisal and provide a means by which QOL can be integrated into evidence-based medicine.

FACT-Hep (Version 4)

Below is a list of statements that other people with your illness have said are important. **Please circle or mark one number per line to indicate your response as it applies to the <u>past 7 days.</u>**

	PHYSICAL WELL-BEING	**Not at all**	**A little bit**	**Some-what**	**Quite a bit**	**Very much**
GP1	I have a lack of energy.....................................	0	1	2	3	4
GP2	I have nausea..	0	1	2	3	4
GP3	Because of my physical condition, I have trouble meeting the needs of my family......................	0	1	2	3	4
GP4	I have pain...	0	1	2	3	4
GP5	I am bothered by side effects of treatment....................	0	1	2	3	4
GP6	I feel ill..	0	1	2	3	4
GP7	I am forced to spend time in bed..................................	0	1	2	3	4

	SOCIAL/FAMILY WELL-BEING	**Not at all**	**A little bit**	**Some-what**	**Quite a bit**	**Very much**
GS1	I feel close to my friends...............................	0	1	2	3	4
GS2	I get emotional support from my family........................	0	1	2	3	4
GS3	I get support from my friends.........................	0	1	2	3	4
GS4	My family has accepted my illness.................................	0	1	2	3	4
GS5	I am satisfied with family communication about my illness...	0	1	2	3	4
GS6	I feel close to my partner (or the person who is my main support)	0	1	2	3	4
Q1	*Regardless of your current level of sexual activity, please answer the following question. If you prefer not to answer it, please mark this box ☐ and go to the next section.*					
GS7	I am satisfied with my sex life..	0	1	2	3	4

English (Universal)
Copyright 1987, 1997

16 November 2007
Page 1 of 3

FIGURE 29.2   Functional assessment of cancer treatment–hepatobiliary questionnaire (FACT-Hep). (Courtesy Dr. David Cella copyright 1987, 1997. Permission for use must be obtained by contacting Dr. David Cella at www.FACIT.org or d-cella@northwestern.edu.)

Continued

FACT-Hep (Version 4)

Please circle or mark one number per line to indicate your response as it applies to the <u>past 7 days</u>.

	EMOTIONAL WELL-BEING	Not at all	A little bit	Some-what	Quite a bit	Very much
GE1	I feel sad..	0	1	2	3	4
GE2	I am satisfied with how I am coping with my illness.........	0	1	2	3	4
GE3	I am losing hope in the fight against my illness...............	0	1	2	3	4
GE4	I feel nervous...	0	1	2	3	4
GE5	I worry about dying...	0	1	2	3	4
GE6	I worry that my condition will get worse...........................	0	1	2	3	4

	FUNCTIONAL WELL-BEING	Not at all	A little bit	Some-what	Quite a bit	Very much
GF1	I am able to work (include work at home)........................	0	1	2	3	4
GF2	My work (include work at home) is fulfilling.....................	0	1	2	3	4
GF3	I am able to enjoy life...	0	1	2	3	4
GF4	I have accepted my illness..	0	1	2	3	4
GF5	I am sleeping well...	0	1	2	3	4
GF6	I am enjoying the things I usually do for fun....................	0	1	2	3	4
GF7	I am content with the quality of my life right now..............	0	1	2	3	4

English (Universal)
Copyright 1987, 1997

16 November 2007
Page 2 of 3

FIGURE 29.2 cont'd

TABLE 29.2	Levels of Evidence in Health-Related Quality-of-Life Evaluation	
LEVEL OF EVIDENCE	**METHODOLOGY/APPROACH**	**EXPLANATION**
Low	Single items (symptoms/performance/VAS)	Often developed for a single study Typically not psychometrically validated
Middle (A)	Conversion of preexisting tools	Adaptation of tools from traditional psychology and psychiatry Assumes measures are reliable and valid in cancer patients (example: Beck Depression Inventory)
Middle (B)	Assessment of a single QOL domain	Measurement of multiple single items within a single domain of QOL Typically focused on physical well-being and/or measurement of treatment toxicities/side effects (example: performance scores)
High	Multidimensional assessments	Highest level of QOL evidence Multiple subscales evaluating multiple domains (physical, social, emotional, role, spiritual, etc.) Disease specific (example: FACT, EORTC QLQ-C30, FLIC)

EORTC-QLQ-C30, European Organization for the Research and Treatment of Cancer Quality-of-Life Questionnaire–Core 30; *FACT,* Functional Assessment of Cancer Therapy; *FLIC,* Functional Living Index-Cancer; *QOL,* health-related quality of life; *VAS,* visual analogue scale.
From Table 1 in Passik SD, Kirsh KL. The importance of quality-of-life endpoints in clinical trials to the practicing oncologist. *Hematol Oncol Clin North Am.* 2000;14(4):877–886.

FACT-Hep (Version 4)

Please circle or mark one number per line to indicate your response as it applies to the <u>past 7 days.</u>

	ADDITIONAL CONCERNS	Not at all	A little bit	Some-what	Quite a bit	Very much
C1	I have swelling or cramps in my stomach area	0	1	2	3	4
C2	I am losing weight	0	1	2	3	4
C3	I have control of my bowels	0	1	2	3	4
C4	I can digest my food well	0	1	2	3	4
C5	I have diarrhea (diarrhoea)	0	1	2	3	4
C6	I have a good appetite	0	1	2	3	4
Hep 1	I am unhappy about a change in my appearance	0	1	2	3	4
CNS 7	I have pain in my back	0	1	2	3	4
Cx6	I am bothered by constipation	0	1	2	3	4
H17	I feel fatigued	0	1	2	3	4
An7	I am able to do my usual activities	0	1	2	3	4
Hep 2	I am bothered by jaundice or yellow color to my skin	0	1	2	3	4
Hep 3	I have had fevers (episodes of high body temperature)	0	1	2	3	4
Hep 4	I have had itching	0	1	2	3	4
Hep 5	I have had a change in the way food tastes	0	1	2	3	4
Hep 6	I have had chills	0	1	2	3	4
HN 2	My mouth is dry	0	1	2	3	4
Hep 8	I have discomfort or pain in my stomach area	0	1	2	3	4

English (Universal)
Copyright 1987, 1997

16 November 2007
Page 3 of 3

FIGURE 29.2 cont'd

QUALITY OF LIFE STUDIES IN HEPATOBILIARY CANCER

The development of reliable, valid, and sensitive measurement tools for use in cancer patients and, more specifically, in patients with hepatobiliary malignancy, has led to an increase in the number and quality of studies assessing QOL in patients with hepatopancreatobiliary (HPB)-related malignancy.

The following sections highlight the current status of QOL as it pertains to definitive surgical management as well as palliative interventions in patients with advanced HPB malignancies.

Tables 28.3 to 28.7 summarize the most recent reports in the literature as well as landmark studies on QOL in the setting of HPB malignancy.

Pancreatic Resection

Despite advances in surgical technique and perioperative care after pancreatic resection, morbidity remains common (20%–30%; see Chapters 27, 62, and 66). Furthermore, in the setting of pancreatic cancer, even with complete resection, long-term survival is rare. It is therefore not surprising that with high morbidity and less than optimal survival outcomes, the impetus

TABLE 29.3 Studies of Pancreatic Surgery and Health-Related Quality of Life

FIRST AUTHOR, JOURNAL, YEAR	POPULATION (PATIENT WITH)	STUDY PURPOSE/QUALITY-OF-LIFE ENDPOINT	STUDY DESIGN, N, AND QOL ASSESSMENT TIME POINTS	QUALITY-OF-LIFE INSTRUMENT	QUALITY-OF-LIFE RESULTS	COMMENTS
Pancreatic Resection						
Nguyen, Journal of Gastrointestinal Surgery, 2003[89]	Periampullary cancer randomized to PD or a RPD (PD + retroperitoneal lymph node dissection)	Primary outcome: postoperative QOL	Cross-sectional, N = 105 (55 PD and 50 RPD); QOL assessed at a single, nonstandard postoperative time point	FACT-Hep	Assessments were completed at mean 2.1 yr after surgery. No differences at long-term follow-up in QOL and GI functional status between PD and RPD. RPD patients had a statistically significantly higher postoperative complication rates (43% to 29%, $P = .01$)	
Van Heek, Annals of Surgery, 2003[90]	Unresectable periampullary cancer randomized to undergo a double bypass (HJ + GJ) or a single bypass (HJ)	Primary outcome: development of GOO Secondary end point: QOL	Prospective randomized trial, N = 65 (36 HJ + GJ, 29 HJ alone) QOL assessed preoperatively, at discharge, and q1mo for 6 mo	EORTC QLQ-C30 + PAN26 module	2/36 HJ + GJ and 12/29 HJ patients developed GOO ($P < .01$). After an initial decline with surgery, QOL returned to baseline by 4 mo postoperatively and was not different between groups	Completion rates were >90% in both groups for the first 4 mo postoperatively and 75% in the last 2 mo
Billings, J Gastrointestinal Surgery, 2005[91]	Periampullary disease (benign and malignant) requiring TP	Primary outcome: longitudinal QOL	Cross-sectional matched design, N = 27 TP; TP cohort age/gender matched 1:1 with IDDM cohort; QOL assessed at a single, nonstandard, postoperative time point	SF-36 Health Survey, Audit of Diabetes-Dependent QOL (ADD QOL), EORTC Pan26, nonvalidated institutional survey	Mean follow-up time: 7.5 yrs postoperatively. TP cohort had lower SF-36 role, and physical and general health scores ($P < .05$). ADD QOL scores were decreased but not different from IDDM controls	Only evaluated TP patients alive with no disease at time of survey administration (mean, 7.5 yr), "healthy-survivor" bias
Nieveen van Dijkum, British Journal of Surgery, 2005[92]	Resectable pancreatic tumors (benign and malignant) undergoing PD compared with unresectable pancreatic tumors undergoing double bypass (HJ + GJ)	Primary outcome: longitudinal QOL	Prospective longitudinal, N = 114 (PD = 72, HJ + GJ = 42); assessed preoperatively, postoperatively, and at 1.5-, 3-, 6-, 9-, and 12-mo follow-up	Medical outcomes study (MSO-24), gastrointestinal QOL index (GIQLI)	After an initial decline, QOL scores returned to baseline at 3 mo postoperatively in both groups. Rapid decline in QOL was observed in both groups in the 8th wk before death	
Schmidt, Annals of Surgical Oncology, 2006[93]	Pancreatic tumors (benign and malignant) undergoing PD with PG or PJ reconstruction	Primary outcome: QOL and long-term morbidity	Cross-sectional, N = 104 (PG = 63, PJ = 41); QOL assessed at a single, nonstandardized, postoperative time point	EORTC QLQ-C30 + PAN26 module, nonvalidated institutional evaluation of GI symptoms	104/133 surviving patients responded to questionnaires (mean assessment time, 6.4 yr postoperatively). Global QOL was the same between PJ and PG groups. PG group had significant decrease in multiple GI symptoms but increase in steatorrhea, early satiety, and food aversion. PJ patients had no change in GI symptoms but did report reduced jaundice-related symptoms	Only evaluated subset of patients alive at the time of survey administration (mean, 6.5 yr), "healthy-survivor" bias

Study	Population	Outcome	Study Design	QOL Instrument	Results	Completion Rates
Shaw, Hepaticogastroenterology, 2005[94]	Pancreatic tumors (benign and malignant) undergoing PD	Primary outcome: longitudinal QOL	Cross-sectional matched design, N = 49 PD; PD cohort age/gender matched 1:1 with patients undergoing open cholecystectomy for benign disease; QOL assessed at a single, nonstandardized postoperative time point	EORTC QLQ-C30 + PAN26 module	Mean assessment at 42 mo postprocedure. Global health status was similar between PD and matched controls. Patients with malignant indication for PD had decreased physical and role functioning as well as more symptoms of fatigue, muscle weakness, and failure to gain weight compared with patients undergoing PD for benign disease	Completion rates: preoperative 100%, 4 wk 100%, 12 wk 16/19 (84%)
Wehrmann, European Journal of Gastroenterology and Hepatology, 2005[95]	Unresectable pancreatic head cancer with pancreatic duct obstruction and postprandial epigastric pain undergoing endoscopic pancreatic duct stenting	Primary outcome: QOL and pain control	Prospective longitudinal, N = 20; QOL assessed preprocedure and 4 and 12 wk postprocedure	Spitzer QLI	Successful procedure in 19/20 patients. Patients reported a significant improvement in pain and QOL at 4 wk (P < .01) but decreased again at 12 wk to preprocedure values	
Muller-Nordhorn, Digestion, 2006[96]	Consecutive patients admitted to hospital with various stages of pancreatic cancer	Primary outcome: QOL in patients with pancreatic cancer; Secondary outcome: relation of symptoms to QOL	Cross sectional matched design, N = 45 (44% stage 4) QOL assessed at a single time point following admission to hospital	EORTC QLQ-C30 and EuroQol (EQ-5D-3L)	Global QOL as well as all subscale measures were decreased among patients with pancreatic cancer. Fatigue and pain were significantly associated with worse QOL	
Schniewind, British Journal of Surgery, 2006[97]	Pancreatic head cancer undergoing PD or PPPD	Primary outcome: longitudinal QOL	Prospective longitudinal, N = 91 (PPD = 34, PPPD = 57); QOL assessed preoperatively and at 3, 6, 12, and 24 mo postoperatively	EORTC QLQ-C30 + PAN26 module	QOL, global as well as all subscales, declined postoperative but returned to baseline by 3-6 mo in both groups. Among survivors, no differences were observed in QOL	Completion rates: precperative 56%, 3 mo, 72% of survivors; 24 mo, 56% of survivors
Han, Hepatogastroenterology, 2007[98]	Pancreatic mass (benign and malignant) treated with PD or PPPD and alive without at ≥3 yr	Primary outcome: long-term gastrointestinal functional outcomes and QOL	Cross-sectional, N = 67 (23 PD and 44 PPPD); QOL assessed at a single, nonstandardized postoperative time point	EORTC QLQ-C30	PD patients reported less steatorrhea and diabetic symptoms but reported more flatus, diarrhea, and fatigue compared with PPPD patients. Mean scores on global QOL subscales were higher in the PPPD group than the PD group (P > .05).	
You, Surgery, 2007[99]	Patients with MEN-1 undergoing PD for pancreaticoduodenal neoplasm	Primary outcome: perioperative outcomes and survival; Secondary outcome: QOL	Cross-sectional, N = 28; QOL assessed at a single, nonstandard postoperative time point	EORTC QLQ-C30 and a unique symptom index	Assessed QOL at mean 5.4 yr postoperatively. Global measures of QOL among the treated group were no different than those of the general population; however, symptoms of nausea/vomiting, diarrhea, and appetite loss were greater (P ≤ .02). Compared with asymptomatic patients, symptomatic patients reported a significantly lower QOL (P = .05)	

Continued

TABLE 29.3 Studies of Pancreatic Surgery and Health-Related Quality of Life—cont'd

FIRST AUTHOR, JOURNAL, YEAR	POPULATION (PATIENT WITH)	STUDY PURPOSE/ QUALITY-OF-LIFE ENDPOINT	STUDY DESIGN, N, AND QOL ASSESSMENT TIME POINTS	QUALITY-OF-LIFE INSTRUMENT	QUALITY-OF-LIFE RESULTS	COMMENTS
Crippa, *Journal of Gastrointestinal Surgery,* 2008[100]	Various stages of newly diagnosed pancreatic cancer (treatment course at enrollment unknown)	Primary outcome: QOL and survival by stage/treatment	Prospective longitudinal, N = 92 divided into 3 groups: Group 1: localized disease treated surgically (28, 30.5%) Group 2: locally advanced disease (34, 37%) Group 3: metastatic disease (30, 32.5%) QOL assessed at enrollment, then 3- and 6-mo follow-up	FACT-Hep	Median OS for the entire cohort, 9.8 mo. In group 1 (resected), QOL was significantly improved (P = .03). Group 2 (locally advanced, various treatments) experienced no change, and group 3 (metastatic disease, various treatments) experienced a persistent decline over time	Survival poor overall, but QOL improved with surgery
Kostro, *Acta Chirugica Belgica,* 2008[101]	Potentially resectable pancreatic cancer, subsequently undergoing curative PD or palliative double bypass (HJ + GJ) or laparotomy alone	Primary outcome: longitudinal QOL	Prospective longitudinal, N = 54 (26 PD, 17 DBP, 11 laparotomy); QOL assessed preoperatively and at 1, 2, 3, and 6 mo postoperatively	EORTC QLQ-C30 + PAN26	No differences in global QOL between the patient groups. Palliative HJ + GJ was associated with increased symptoms immediately postoperatively but acceptable QOL. Eight wks before death, all subscales and global QOL declined rapidly	Completion rates: preoperatively 100%, 1 mo 46/54 (85%), 2 mo 42/54 (78%), 3 mo 31/54 (57%), 6 mo 22/54 (41%)
Halloran, *Pancreatology,* 2011[102]	Patients undergoing partial pancreatectomy for pancreatic cancer	Primary outcome: pancreatic exocrine insufficiency Secondary outcome: QOL, nutrition, symptoms	Prospective longitudinal, N = 40; QOL assessed only postoperatively at 1.5, 3, 6, and 12 mo	EORTC QLQ-C30	Overall, QOL increased at 6 (P = .03) and 12 mo (P < .01) Physical and role functioning were increased at 3 mo (P = .03); social functioning was improved at 6 and 12 mo (P = .03 and P < .01, respectively) Trend toward worse QOL in patients who experienced exocrine insufficiency	QOL was not measured preoperatively; baseline = postoperative (6 wk); improvements in QOL may be inflated
Ljungman, *World Journal of Surgery,* 2011[103]	Resectable periampullary cancer	Primary outcome: cost utility of curative treatment for pancreatic cancer Secondary outcome: QOL	Retrospective cohort, N = 119; QOL assessed preoperatively, early postoperatively (<1 yr), or late postoperatively (1-5 yr), compared with age-matched healthy controls	SF-36 Health Survey and Utility Index (SF-36-6D preference-based utility index, scored 0 = death to 1 = perfect health)	QOL index lower in study patients compared with controls at all time points (P < .05) QOL index (0.69) at long-term follow-up was not different from index scores preoperatively (0.65) or early postoperatively (0.63) in the treated group	QOL data available for only 58 patients (37 early and 27 late); late data subject to "healthy-survivor bias"
Walter, *European Journal of Surgical Oncology,* 2011[104]	Advanced pancreatic cancer undergoing palliative resection (PR) or double bypass (HJ + GJ)	Primary outcome: longitudinal QOL between PR and HJ + GJ	Prospective longitudinal, N = 86 (61 HJ + GJ, 25 PR); QOL assessed preoperatively, at discharge, and 3 and 6 mo postoperatively	EORTC QLQ-C30	Outside of worse scores on physical functioning subscales at 6 mo, the HJ + GJ group had significantly better QOL and improved symptoms compared with PR group	Completion rates: baseline 100%, discharge 78/86 (91%), 3 mo 58/86 (67%), 6 mo 41/86 (48%)

Study	Population	Outcome	Study design	Instrument	Results	Notes
Chan, *Journal of Gastrointestinal Surgery*, 2012[105]	Periampullary cancer undergoing PD	Primary outcome: longitudinal QOL	Prospective longitudinal, N = 37; QOL assessed preoperatively, 1, 3, 6, and 12 mo postoperatively	SF-36 Health Survey	One mo postprocedure, significant decline in physical function (P < .01) and emotional role (P < .03). At 3 mo, mental health increased significantly (P = .02); 6 mo, physical role (P < .01), physical pain (P = .01), social function (P = .01) improved significantly. At 12 mo, these changes were sustained as well as significant improvement in vitality (P = .02) and emotional role (P < .01)	Completion rates: preoperative 100%, 1 mo 29/37 (78%), 3 mo 26/37 (70%), 6 mo 28/34 survivors (82%), 12 mo 28/28 survivors (100%)
Mbah, *Journal of the Pancreas*, 2012[106]	Pancreatic cancer undergoing pancreatectomy	Primary outcome: QOL following pancreatectomy in patients with and without complication	Prospective longitudinal, N = 34 QOL assessed preoperatively and at 2-3 wk, 6 wk, 3, and 6 mo postoperatively	EORTC QLQ-C30 and FACT-Anemia	After an initial postoperative decline, QOL returned to baseline at 6 wk. Overall, complication rate was 21%, with no difference in QOL scores among those who did and did not have complications (P = .11). At 6 mo, scores on cognitive functioning significantly declined (P = .02).	QOL data collected as part of a prospective trial examining the safety of intraoperative autotransfusion during oncologic resections; QOL stratified by anemia at discharge was also evaluated
Belyaev, *Langenbecks Archives of Surgery*, 2013[107]	Pancreatic disease (benign and malignant) undergoing pancreatic resection	Primary outcome: longitudinal QOL comparison by procedure and diagnosis	Retrospective cohort, N = 174 (105 malignant, 69 benign); QOL assessed preoperatively and at 3 and 24 mo postoperatively; included comparison to age-matched population norms	SF-36 Health Survey	QOL was worse compared with population norms at all time points, P = .03. Early postoperative QOL was best in patients undergoing distal pancreatectomy and worst with TP. Patients with cancer, as opposed to benign diagnosis, had lower postoperative QOL and persistent decline to 24 mo. Patients with benign tumors/pancreatitis had initial drop, followed by slow trend toward recovery at 24 months.	Completion rates: preoperatively 100%, 3 mo 133/174 (76%), 24 mo 83/174 (48%)
Roberts, *HPB (Oxford)*, 2014[108]	Pancreatic tumors (benign or malignant) treated with TP	Primary outcome: overall QOL and diabetes-specific problems between TP and matched IDDM	Cross sectional matched design, N = 28 TP; TP cohort age/gender matched to IDDM group; QOL assessed at a single, nonstandardized postoperative time point	EORTC QLQ-C30 +PAN26 module and Problem Areas in Diabetes Scale	Physical (P < .01), cognitive (P < .01), and social functioning (P = .02), as well as working ability (P = .01), were worse in TP compared with IDDM groups. Symptoms of fatigue, nausea/vomiting, and insomnia were also worse (P ≤ .01); however, no differences in diabetes-specific problems were observed	88/123 TP were dead at time of survey administration; 28 of the remaining 33 returned surveys
Epelboym, *Journal of Surgical Research*, 2014[109]	Pancreatic tumors treated with TP	Primary outcome: morbidity/mortality post-TP Secondary outcome: overall, pancreas-specific and diabetes-specific QOL following TP	Cross sectional matched design, N = 17 TP; TP cohort matched on age/gender/operative indication to patients who underwent PD and had or developed diabetes postoperatively (PD + DM); QOL assessed at a single, nonstandardized postoperative time point	EORTC QLQ-C30 + PAN26 module and Audit of Diabetes-Dependent Quality of Life (ADD-QOL)	QOL assessed at median 45 mo postoperatively. Overall and pancreas-specific measures of QOL were not different between TP and PD + DM groups. Diabetes negatively impacted QOL and was not different between TP and PD + DM groups.	TP patients had more hypoglycemic events (2 requiring hospitalization), but given small numbers, this was not statistically significant

Continued

TABLE 29.3 Studies of Pancreatic Surgery and Health-Related Quality of Life—cont'd

FIRST AUTHOR, JOURNAL, YEAR	POPULATION (PATIENT WITH)	STUDY PURPOSE/ QUALITY-OF-LIFE ENDPOINT	STUDY DESIGN, N, AND QOL ASSESSMENT TIME POINTS	QUALITY-OF-LIFE INSTRUMENT	QUALITY-OF-LIFE RESULTS	COMMENTS
Serrano, *International Journal of Radiation Oncology Biology Physics*, 2014[110]	Resectable or borderline resectable pancreatic cancer undergoing neoadjuvant chemoradiation	Primary outcome: QOL during and after chemoradiation and surgery	Prospective multi-institutional Phase II clinical trial, N = 55; QOL assessed at baseline, after 2 cycles of neoadjuvant therapy, after surgery, at 6 mo from initiation of therapy, and 6-mo intervals for 2 yr	EORTC QLQ-C30 + PAN26 module and FACT-Hep	After 2 cycles of chemoradiation, QOL was not different from baseline. Global QOL was not statistically (EORTC QLQ-C30) or clinically (FACT-G) different from baseline at the conclusion of chemoradiation; however, pancreatic pain was improved, scores of physical function declined, and diarrhea symptoms increased significantly. Among patients who underwent resection global, QoL and most subscales returned to baseline measures by 6 mo	QOL assessed as part of a Phase II clinical trial of neoadjuvant chemoradiation (gemcitabine + oxaliplatin + radiation) in patients with resectable or borderline resectable pancreatic cancer; compliance in nonoperated group poor and not included in longer-term analysis
Eshuis, *British Journal of Surgery*, 2015[111]	Scheduled for PD for oncologically indicated disease	Primary outcome: Compare QOL between retrocolic and antecolic gastroenteric reconstruction after PD and correlate findings with DGE	Single institution RCT, N = 73 (38 retrocolic, 35 antecolic), QOL assessed at baseline, 2, 4, and 12 weeks postoperatively	EORTC QLQ-C30 and PAN 26; GIQLI	Statistically significant differences for any QOL outcomes between study groups were not found. QOL declined for both groups at 2 and 4 weeks and improved by 12 weeks. QOL outcomes in were statistically significantly worse in DGE group in QLQ-C30 global health status and all functional scales except cognitive (Cohen's d = 0.53-0.96, $P < .0450$) at two weeks postoperatively. In GIQLI scores were statistically significantly worse in DGE group in total score, physical well-being, and mental well-being (Cohen's d =0.65-0.98, $P < .023$) at 2 weeks postoperatively. The group differences resolved by 12 weeks.	Response rate 88% across time points
Hartwig, *Annals of Surgery*, 2015[112]	Locally advanced or centrally located pancreatic tumors undergoing TP	Primary outcome: perioperative morbidity/mortality and survival Secondary outcome: longitudinal QOL overall and compared with healthy controls	Prospective longitudinal, N = 81 (25 benign disease, 56 malignant disease), TP cohort age/gender matched to healthy controls; QOL assessed preoperatively and 1, 2, 3, 4, and 5 yr	EORTC QLQ-C30 + PAN26	No difference in global QOL scores between TP patients and matched controls; however, all functional scale scores (physical, emotional, social, role, cognitive) were significantly lower at all time points in the TP group. Global QOL and functional scales were not different based on indication for operation (benign vs. malignant), but symptoms were greater among patients undergoing TP for malignant disease at yr 1 and 2 ($P < .01$)	596 TP or completion pancreatectomy were included in primary analysis; QOL assessment was available in only 81 patients who had follow-up at study center

Reference	Population	Aim	Study design	Instrument	Results	Comments
Heerkens, British Journal of Surgery, 2015[113]	Pancreatic resection for pancreatic or periampullary malignancy or premalignancy	Primary outcome: Describe QOL after pancreatic resection	Prospective longitudinal quasi experimental single institution study, N = 68, assessed QOL at baseline, 1, 3, 6, 12 months except if hospitalized at time of assessment.	EORTC-QLQ-C30; SF-36	QLQ-C30 Global Health had a clinically relevant worsening at 1 month in 50% of subjects ($P = .010$). Scores were equal to or improved from baseline levels at 6 months in 88% and 79%, respectively. At 12 months, 87% and 97% returned to baseline or better, respectively. Similar trends were seen in the physical and social scales.	Follow-up instrument completion 57%–94% across assessments. Study limited to those well enough to be outpatients at time of assessment. Mean scores were not evaluated; instead clinical relevance, defined as a greater than 10% change from baseline, were used.
Williamsson et al., British Journal of Surgery, 2015	PD for malignant and benign disease	Evaluate safety, outcomes, and patient experience after PD before and after implementation of fast-track recovery program.	Retrospective study of control group (retrospective chart review) and fast-track group (prospectively entered database); N = 100 (50 fast-track, 50 control); QOL assessed 2 weeks before and 4 weeks after PD	EORTC QLQ-C30 and EORTC QLQ-PAN26	70% completion rate of instruments. In both groups, QOL deteriorated in most aspects after surgery. There were no group differences noted.	
De Rooij et al., Annals of Surgery, 2018[115]	Left-sided, confined (Yonsei criteria[116]) pancreatic tumors (benign, pre-malignant, malignant) undergoing MIDP or ODP	Primary outcome: compare time to functional recovery between MIDP ODP. Secondary outcome: compare QOL	Patient-blinded, multicenter RCT, N = 108 (51 MIDP, 57 ODP), assessed QOL at 14, 30, 90 days postoperatively.	EORTC-QLQ-C30	Overall global health score was higher for MIDP than ODP mean difference 4.97 (95% CI -1.22 to 11.16, $P = .12$, corrected for baseline scores). MIDP had higher rate of grade B and C postoperative fistulas (RR 1.72 (95% CI 0.96-3.09, $P = .07$), whereas ODP had higher rate of DGE (RR 0.30 (95% CI 0.09-1.03, $P = .04$).	
Shin et al., HPB, 2019[117]	PD with duct to mucosa PJ	Describe outcome differences in those with and without external and internal pancreatic stents	Prospective, single institution longitudinal study, N = 185 (97 external stenting, 88 internal stenting), QOL assessed at 1-2 weeks and 1 year.	EORTC QLQ-C30 and EORTC QLQ-PAN26	There was no statistically significant differences between groups at 1-2 week and 1 year in the global health status, functional scales, or the pancreatic cancer-specific scales (all $P > .170$).	
Van Hilst, British Journal of Surgery, 2019[18]	Pancreatic tumors (benign, pre-malignant, malignant) undergoing MIDP or ODP	Describe cost-effectiveness and QOL after distal pancreatectomy	Patient-blinded, multicenter RCT, N = 104 (48 MIDP, 56 ODP), QOL assessed at baseline and 365 days post resection (first 90 days reported by de Rooij et al.[115])	EORTC QLQ-C30	Completion rates of 65% of the 97 patients who were alive at 1 year. The global health score and seven categories of the PAN-26 were comparable at 1 year between groups (all $P > .153$)	

DBP, Double bypass; DGE, delayed gastric emptying; DM, diabetes mellitus; DP, distal pancreatectomy; EORTC QLQ-C30, European Organization for the Research and Treatment of Cancer Quality-of-Life Questionnaire–Core 30; FACT, Functional Assessment of Cancer Therapy; GI, gastrointestinal; GJ, gastrojejunostomy; GOO, gastric outlet obstruction; HJ, hepaticojejunostomy; IDDM, insulin-dependent diabetes mellitus; MEN-1, multiple endocrine neoplasia-1; MIDP, minimally invasive ductal pancreatectomy; MSO, Medical Outcomes Study; ODP, open distal pancreatectomy; OS, overall survival; QOL, quality of life; PAN26, pancreatic cancer module; PD, pancreaticoduodenectomy; PG, pancreaticogastrostomy; PJ, pancreaticojejunostomy; PPD, pylorus-preserving pancreaticoduodenectomy; QLI, Quality-of-Life Index; RCT, randomized controlled trial; RPD, radical pancreaticoduodenectomy; RR Relative risk SF-36, 36-item Short Form; TP, total pancreatectomy.

TABLE 29.4 Studies of Hepatic Resection and Health-Related Quality of Life

FIRST AUTHOR, JOURNAL, YEAR	POPULATION (PATIENT WITH:)	STUDY PURPOSE/ QUALITY-OF-LIFE ENDPOINT	STUDY DESIGN, N, AND ASSESSMENT TIME POINTS	QUALITY-OF-LIFE INSTRUMENT	QUALITY-OF-LIFE RESULTS	COMMENTS
Hepatic Resection						
Poon, *Archives of Surgery*, 2001[119]	HCC undergoing HR	Primary outcome: longitudinal QOL	Prospective longitudinal, N = 76 (66 HR, 10 controls—unresectable HCC treated with TACE); QOL assessed every 3 months for 2 years	FACT-G, translated into Chinese	At 3 mo, global QOL, PWB, EWB, and SWB significantly improved over baseline and were maintained out to 2 yr among the HR group; no changes were observed in QOL measures among unresected controls at 3 mo, and decline was observed starting at 9 mo. Disease recurrence was associated with a significant decline in mean QOL ($P < .001$)	Disease recurrence was treated with TACE, systemic chemotherapy, and/or BSC
Chen, *Hepatobiliary and Pancreatic Disease International*, 2004[120]	Primary hepatic cancer undergoing HR	Primary outcome: short-term and longitudinal QOL	Prospective longitudinal, N = 36; QOL assessed preoperatively; at 2, 5, and 10 wk; 4, 6, and 9 mo; and 1, 1.5, and 2 yr postoperatively	Gastrointestinal QOL Index (GQLI)	Mean GQLI was decreased at 2-10 wk postoperatively, followed by a gradual return to baseline by 4 mo, and at 9 mo. Mean GQLI scores were increased above baseline measures. Disease recurrence was associated with a steady decline in QOL.	47% (17/36) patients died by 9-mo follow-up
Langenhoff, *British Journal of Surgery*, 2006[121]	Hepatic malignancy undergoing HR (CRLM, CCA, HCC, and other hepatic metastases)	Primary outcome: short-term and longitudinal QOL	Prospective cohort, N = 97 (group 1 = HR [n = 60], group 2 = unresectable at laparotomy [n = 19], group 3 = unresectable at presentation [n = 20]); QOL assessed at baseline and 0.5-, 3-, 6-, and 12-mo follow-up	EORTC QLQ-C30 and EQ-5D-3L + EQ-VAS	Group 1: decrease in global and functional QOL domains; decrease in EQ-VAS and symptoms at 2 wk, with return to baseline at 3 mo; stable or improved out to 12 mo. Group 2: decrease in global and functional QOL domains; decrease in EQ-VAS and increased symptoms at 2 wk, with continued decline and ongoing symptoms. Group 3: no change in global, functional, or symptoms, QOL domains, or EQ-VAS at 2 wk or 3 mo, decrease in global and functional domain-specific QOL at 6 mo	
Eid, *Cancer*, 2006[122]	Hepatic malignancy undergoing HR or surgical RFA (CRLM, CCA, HCC, other metastases)	Primary outcome: comparison of QOL based on type of surgical intervention	Prospective longitudinal, N = 40 (24 major hepatectomy, 8 minor hepatectomy, 8 surgical RFA); QOL assessed at baseline, discharge, first postoperative visit, 6 wk, 3 mo, and 6 mo	FACT-Hep, FHSI-8, POMS, EORTC QLQ-C30 + PAN26 module; global rating of change scales (6 domains, scales −7 to +7)	Major hepatectomy associated with decrease in physical and functional domain scores on FACT-Hep at 6 wk compared with minor resection or RFA. No differences in QOL measures at 3 and 6 mo were observed between interventions. A similar trend was observed for all QOL measures (POMS, EORTC QLQ-C30/PAN36, FHSI-8, global rating scales)	

Study	Population	Primary outcome	Design	Instrument	Findings	Notes
Lee, *Journal of Surgical Oncology*, 2007[123]	HCC	Primary outcome: QOL in HCC compared with population norms and between treatment type	Cross-sectional cohort, N = 161 (121 HR, 31 TACE, 8 PEI, 1 BSC) QOL assessed at single time point	WHOQOL-BREF and EORTC QLQ-C30 (Taiwanese translation)	Compared with population norms, HCC was associated with decrease in social and psychological domains and improved environment domains; HR was associated with improved QOL compared with TACE/PEI/BSC	70% Hepatitis B
Martin, *Surgery*, 2007[124]	CRLM, CCA, or HCC undergoing HR	Primary outcome: time to return to baseline QOL	Prospective longitudinal N = 32 (24 major hepatectomy, 8 minor hepatectomy); QOL assessed at consent, discharge, first postoperative visit, 6 wk, then 3, 6, and 12 mo	FACT-HEP, FHSI-8, EORTC QLQ-C30 + PAN26 module, POMS; global rating scale (6 domains, scales −7 to +7)	Major hepatectomy associated with decline in all measures of QOL postoperatively; QOL nadir scores observed at 6 wk, with return to baseline values by 3 mo. Minor resection was associated with decrements in all measures at discharge; nadir QOL scores observed at initial postoperative visit and returned to baseline by 6 wk postoperatively	Major hepatectomy = ≥3 Couinaud segments
Dasgupta, *British Journal of Surgery*, 2008[125]	Hepatic malignancy undergoing HR (CRLM, CCA, HCC, other metastases)	Primary outcome: longitudinal QOL	Prospective longitudinal, N = 103 (74 CRLM, 9 CCA, 8 HCC, 12 other); QOL assessed at baseline, 6, 12, and 36-48 mo	EORTC QLQ-C30	Decrease from baseline to 6 mo in physical functioning domain and increase in dyspnea/fatigue. At 12 mo, physical function and fatigue return to baseline but dyspnea persistent. Survivors with no recurrence at 36-48 mo had improved global QOL over patients with disease recurrence	44/103 (43%) alive at last follow-up
Banz, *World Journal of Surgery*, 2009[126]	HR for benign or malignant disease at least 6 mo before analysis	Primary outcome: impact of postoperative diagnosis (benign/malignant) on QOL	Cross-sectional cohort, N = 135 (89 malignant disease, 46 benign disease); QOL assessed at a single, nonstandardized postoperative time point	EORTC QLQ-C30 + LM21 module	Patients who underwent hepatic resection for malignant disease had similar general, global, and self-assessed QOL relative to those with benign diagnoses. However, physical function scores and pain, fatigue, and social function scores were worse in the malignant group	QOL assessment at a mean of 27 mo postoperatively
Bruns, *World Journal of Gastroenterology*, 2010[127]	HR for benign or malignant disease at least 3 mo before analysis	Primary outcome: QOL and identification of variables associated with/predictive of decrease QOL	Cross-sectional cohort, N = 96 (76 malignant [21 primary, 55 metastases], 20 benign); QOL assessed at a single, nonstandardized postoperative time point	SF-12 (mental component scale [MCS] + physical component scale [PCS]), ad hoc symptom and pain scale	MCS significantly lower among patients with benign vs. malignant diagnosis as well as primary vs. metastatic cancers ($P < .05$). No difference in QOL based on sex, age, or postoperative complications. Increase in symptoms/pain and decreases in daily activities were associated with worse PCS/MCS	QOL assessed once between 3-36 mo postoperatively

Continued

TABLE 29.4 Studies of Hepatic Resection and Health-Related Quality of Life—cont'd

FIRST AUTHOR, JOURNAL, YEAR	POPULATION (PATIENT WITH:)	STUDY PURPOSE/ QUALITY-OF-LIFE ENDPOINT	STUDY DESIGN, N, AND ASSESSMENT TIME POINTS	QUALITY-OF-LIFE INSTRUMENT	QUALITY-OF-LIFE RESULTS	COMMENTS
Wiering, *British Journal of Surgery*, 2011[128]	≤4 CRLM with no EHD undergoing HR	Primary outcome: short-term and longitudinal QOL	Prospective longitudinal, N = 138 (117 curative HR, 19 unresectable at laparotomy); QOL assessed at baseline, then 3 wk, 6 wk, and every 3 months for 3 yr	EQ-5D-3L + EQ-VAS	Overall, decline in global QOL at 3 and 6 wk postoperatively. Curative HR was associated with return of global QOL to baseline at 3 mo and stabilization to 3 yr. Patients found to be unresectable at laparotomy had persistent decline in QOL during the study period. Disease recurrence associated with decline in QOL during time. Patients with recurrence amenable to re-resection had global QOL scores similar to patients never experiencing recurrence	
Rees, *Journal of Clinical Oncology*, 2012[129]	CRLM undergoing HR	Primary outcome: longitudinal QOL	Prospective longitudinal, N = 232; QOL assessed preoperatively and at 3, 6, and 12 mo postoperatively	EORTC QLQ-C30 + LM21 module	Twenty percent of patients had severe symptoms at baseline. At 3 mo postoperatively, all functional scales decreased, proportion with severe symptoms increased, and functional scales returned to baseline at 6 mo and stabilized thereafter. Ten percent of patients continued to have severe problems with pain and sexual function 1 yr postoperatively	
Miller, *American Journal of Surgery*, 2013[130]	Hepatic malignancy undergoing HR of > 2 segments (CRLM, CCA, HCC, other metastases)	Primary outcome: impact of anemia and postoperative complications on short term QOL	Prospective longitudinal, N = 41 (16 CRLM, 9 HCC, 4 CCA, 12 other); QOL assessed preoperatively, at first postoperative visit, then 1.5, 3, and 6 mo postoperatively	EORTC QLQ-C30, FACT-Anemia, global change rating scale (−7 to +7)	Social and functional domains scores lower in anemic group at all time points. Major complications associated with increased pain at 6 wk and 6 mo but no difference in any domain-specific QOL scales	Anemia defined at discharge as <10 g/dL; 34% overall complication rate, 25% major complication rate
Mise, *World Journal of Surgery*, 2014[131]	HCC undergoing HR	Primary outcome: longitudinal QOL Secondary outcome: identification of perioperative predictors of QOL	Prospective longitudinal, N = 69; QOL assessed preoperatively and every 3 months for a year.	SF-36 Health Survey	PCS did not change after surgery. At 9 mo, MCS were significantly improved versus baseline and population norms; female sex, age > 70 yr, thoracoabdominal incisions, tumors > 5 cm, and ICGR-15 < 10% were associated with worse PCS at 3 mo; no clinical variables were predictive of MCS at 3 mo	

Study	Population	Primary outcome/purpose	Study design	Instrument	Results	Comments
Rees, *British Journal of Surgery*, 2014[132]	CRLM treated with HR ≥ 5 yr before assessment	Primary outcome: long-term QOL	Long-term follow-up of prospective cohort, $N = 68$; QOL assessed at single, nonstandardized time point ≥ 5 yr postoperatively	EORTC QLQ-C30 + LM21 module	Overall, scores in all domains excellent at long-term follow-up and were significantly improved from baseline; <5% of patients reported severe symptoms; persistent symptoms included peripheral neuropathy, sexual dysfunction, constipation, and diarrhea	QOL assessment at median of 8 (6.9–9.2) yr postoperatively
Studer et al., *British Journal of Surgery*, 2018[133]	Malignant and benign tumors requiring liver resection	Evaluate long-term QOL after liver resection	Prospective, single institution, longitudinal study, $N = 188$ (130 malignant, 58 benign), QOL assessed at baseline, 1, 3, 6 and 12 months.	EORTC QLQ-C30, LMC21	There was no difference in global health status between baseline and 1 month assessment. At 3, 6, 12 months, global health status improved, with benign tumors having a statistically significantly better score than malignant tumors ($P \leq 0.006$ at all time points).	Data on instrument completion rates not provided, limited data on scores provided.
Wang et al., *Medicine*, 2019[134]	HCC undergoing resection	Compare effect of intervention on depression, anxiety, QOL, and survival	Single-institution RCT, $N = 136$ (68 comprehensive education and care program group, 68 control group); QOL assessed at baseline, 3, 6, 9 and 12 months after resection.	EORTC QLQ-C30	The intervention group had statistically significantly higher global health status scores at 12 months compared with the control group ($P < .05$). Still, there was no statistically significant difference in global health status at time points before 12 months ($P > .05$). There was no statistically significant group differences in symptom scores at any time point ($P > .05$).	

BSC, Best supportive care; CCA, cholangiocarcinoma; CRLM, colorectal liver metastases; EHD, extrahepatic disease; EORTC QLQ-C30, European Organization for the Research and Treatment of Cancer Quality-of-Life Questionnaire–Core 30; EWB, emotional well-being; FACT-G, Functional Assessment of Cancer Therapy–General; FHSI-8, FACT-Hepatobiliary Symptom Index-8; HCC, hepatocellular carcinoma; HR, hepatic resection; QOL, health-related quality of life; ICGR-15, indocyanine green retention rate at 15 minutes; LM21, colorectal liver metastases module; PAN26, pancreatic cancer module; PEI, percutaneous ethanol injection; POMS, profile of mood states; PWB, physical well-being; RFA, radiofrequency ablation; SF-12, 12-item Short Form; SWB, social well-being; TACE, transarterial chemoembolization; VAS, visual analogue scale; WHOQoL-BREF, World Health Organization Quality-of-Life–BREF (abbreviated) assessment.

TABLE 29.5   Studies of Locoregional Therapy for Hepatic Tumors and Health-Related Quality of Life

FIRST AUTHOR, JOURNAL, YEAR	POPULATION (PATIENT WITH)	STUDY PURPOSE/ QUALITY-OF-LIFE END POINT	STUDY DESIGN, N, AND QOL ASSESSMENT TIME POINTS	QUALITY-OF-LIFE INSTRUMENT	QUALITY-OF-LIFE RESULTS	COMMENTS
Locoregional Treatments						
Steel, *Psychooncology,* 2004[135]	HCC treated with TACE (cisplatin) or ⁹⁰Y radioembolization	Primary outcome: QOL and survival	Prospective cohort, N = 28; QOL assessed preprocedure and 3, 6, and 12 mo postprocedure	FACT-Hep	Overall, QOL and scores on all subscales declined from baseline to 6 mo for both groups. At 3 mo, FWB and overall QOL scores are higher in ⁹⁰Y group (P < .01). At 6 mo, FWB remains significantly improved over TACE, but overall QOL was not different	Overall, survival at 6 mo not different between groups; only 14 patients evaluable at 6 mo
Ruers, *Annals of Surgical Oncology,* 2006[136]	Nonresectable CRLM treated with surgical ablation ± resection vs. systemic chemotherapy (CTX)	Primary outcome: comparison of longitudinal QOL and survival	Prospective longitudinal, N = 201 (117 HR, 45 surgical ablation, 39 CTX) survival data; QOL assessed preprocedure and at 3, 6, 9, and 12 mo for randomly selected members of the cohort; N = 109 (53 HR, 29 surgical ablation, 27 CTX)	EuroQoL-5D-3L and EORTC QLQ-C30	Baseline QOL similar between groups. All groups experienced an initial decline in QOL and physical function at 3 wk postprocedure. Ablation and HR groups return to baseline at 3 mo, whereas CTX did not. HR was associated with higher QOL than both ablation and CTX; however, QOL in ablation group was significantly higher than CTX group from 3-12 mo	All patients underwent initial laparotomy; no difference in median OS between ablation and CTX groups (31 and 26 mo, respectively)
Wang, *Quality of Life Research,* 2007[137]	HCC treated with TACE or TACE+ percutaneous RFA	Primary outcome: short-term postprocedure QOL	Prospective longitudinal, N = 83 (43 TACE, 40 TACE + RFA); QOL assessed preprocedure and 3 mo postprocedure	FACT-G (Chinese translation)	TACE + RFA group higher overall FACT-G, SWB, and FWB scores at 3 mo postprocedure (P < .01). Predictors of QOL were Child-Pugh class and tumor recurrence	
Bonnetain, *Quality of Life Research,* 2008[138]	Advanced HCC treated with tamoxifen, TACE, or BSC in the palliative setting (primarily alcohol-related cirrhosis)	Primary outcome: determine the value of baseline QOL scores in predicting overall survival	Retrospective evaluation of 2 randomized clinical trials, N = 489; QOL assessed at baseline only	Spitzer QLI	Higher Spitzer QLI at baseline associated with increased median OS (P < .01). In addition to common variables used in classification systems (Okuda/CLIP/BCLC), QOL was the single best prognostic factor for survival	Combined QOL data from 2 RCTs of palliative treatment for HCC: (1) tamoxifen to best supportive care (N = 416), (2) TACE to tamoxifen only (N = 122)
Kalinowski, *Digestion,* 2009[139]	Unresectable liver; only neuroendocrine tumor metastases treated with ⁹⁰Y	Primary outcome: safety and efficacy of ⁹⁰Y Secondary outcome: longitudinal QOL	Prospective longitudinal, N = 9; QOL assessed preprocedure, and 3, 6, 9, 12 mo postprocedure	EORTC QLQ-C30 + LMC21 module	Overall, an initial decrease in mean QOL scores occurred after ⁹⁰Y. At 6 mo, the majority of patients had improvement in QOL scores, followed by a trend toward decline QOL at 12 mo.	Late decline in QOL was associated with tumor recurrence/disease progression
Kuroda, *Journal of Gastroenterology and Hepatology,* 2010[140]	HCC treated with percutaneous RFA with and without postprocedure BCAA supplementation	Primary outcome: comparison of hepatic function and nutritional status following RFA with and without BCAA supplementation Secondary outcome: QOL	Prospective cohort, N = 49; QOL assessed preprocedure and 1 yr	SF-36 Health Survey	BCAA group experienced improvement in overall health as well as physical and social functioning (P < .05 for all subsets); QOL did not change in no-BCAA group following RFA	Hepatitis C patients only

Study	Population	Design	Outcomes	Instrument	Findings	
Wible, *Journal of Vascular and Interventional Radiology*, 2010[141]	Previously untreated HCC undergoing TACE	Prospective longitudinal, N = 73 (≥3 TACE N = 23); QOL assessed preprocedure and 4, 8, and 12 mo postprocedure	Primary outcome: QOL Secondary outcome: QOL in patients treated with ≥3 TACE procedures	SF-36 Health Survey	Baseline QOL significantly lower compared with population norms. Mental health score at 4 mo postprocedure, but not at 8 or 12 mo, was improved ($P = .05$). No other changes in QOL were observed in study cohort over time. The subset of patients undergoing ≥3 TACE procedures with improved mental health after first and second procedures, whereas bodily pain improved ($P < .01$, $P = .05$, respectively), and vitality scores declined ($P = .04$) after first procedure only	Completion rates: 4 mo 48/73 (66%), 8 mo 38/73 (52%), 12 mo 28/73 (38%)
Eltawil, *HPB (Oxford)*, 2012[142]	Unresectable, nonablatable primary hepatic tumors (HCC and ICC) undergoing TACE	Prospective longitudinal, N = 48 patients; QOL assessed before first TACE and before each subsequent procedure (3-4 mo)	Primary outcome: QOL and treatment efficacy	WHOQoL-BREF	Overall QOL did not decline in the 12 mo after TACE. After third TACE procedure (~1 yr), a trend toward a decline in the physical health domain was observed ($P = .08$) and coincided with increasing AFP and tumor size.	
Shun, *Oncologist*, 2012[143]	HCC treated with TACE	Prospective cohort, N = 89; QOL assessed within 3 days before discharge, and 4 and 8 wk	Primary outcome: short-term QOL following single TACE procedure Secondary outcome: variables associated with changes in postprocedure QOL	SF-12 Health Survey, Symptom distress Scale (SDS), Hospital Anxiety and Depression Scale (HADS)	Mean QOL was improved from discharge to 8 wk postprocedure. At all timepoints, physical component scores were lower than mental component scores. Factors associated with lower physical component scores: age, new diagnosis, higher levels of symptom distress, and depression. Factors associated with lower mental component scores: male sex, recurrent disease, higher levels of anxiety, and depression	
Toro, *Surgical Oncology*, 2012[144]	HCC undergoing HR, TACE, percutaneous RFA, or NT	Prospective longitudinal, N = 51 (14 HR, 15 TACE, 9 RFA, 13 NT); QOL assessed preprocedure and 3, 6, 12, and 24 mo postprocedure	Primary outcome: QOL in all patients with HCC regardless of treatment	FACT-Hep (Italian translation)	Postoperatively, all domains of QOL significantly improved in the HR group and were significantly higher compared with all other treatments. Mean PWB and EWB after RFA was improved compared with TACE and NT	Percentage change in QOL from baseline was calculated at each time point. The average percentage change in each group was used for comparison
Salem, *Clinical Gastroenterology and Hepatology*, 2013[145]	HCC treated with TACE or ⁹⁰Y	Prospective cohort, N = 56 (27 TACE, 29 ⁹⁰Y); assessed preprocedure and 2 and 4 wk postprocedure	Primary outcome: short-term postprocedure QOL	FACT-Hep	No difference in overall QOL between treatment groups. At 4 wk, ⁹⁰Y had a greater improvement in SWB, FWB, embolotherapy-specific score (ESS), and a trend toward better overall QOL and TOI compared with TACE group	⁹⁰Y patients had greater tumor burden and more advanced disease; ESS consists of the following items: pain, bothered by treatment side effects, ability to work, diarrhea, and appetite

Continued

TABLE 29.5 Studies of Locoregional Therapy for Hepatic Tumors and Health-Related Quality of Life—cont'd

FIRST AUTHOR, JOURNAL, YEAR	POPULATION (PATIENT WITH)	STUDY PURPOSE/ QUALITY-OF-LIFE END POINT	STUDY DESIGN, N, AND QOL ASSESSMENT TIME POINTS	QUALITY-OF-LIFE INSTRUMENT	QUALITY-OF-LIFE RESULTS	COMMENTS
Hamdy, Journal of the Egyptian Society of Parasitology, 2013[146]	HCC treated with percutaneous RFA or TACE	Primary outcome: short-term postprocedural QOL	Prospective cohort design, N = 120 (40 TACE, 40 RFA, 40 HCV without HCC [controls]); QOL assessed preprocedure and 1 mo postprocedure	SF-36 Health Survey	At baseline, RFA and TACE groups had significantly worse physical function, energy/fatigue, pain, and general health compared with controls. Significant improvements in all QOL domains were observed at 1 mo in the RFA group (P < .05) but not the TACE group	Hepatitis C patients only
Huang, British Journal of Surgery, 2014[147]	Small HCC (<3 cm) treated with HR or percutaneous RFA	Primary outcome: longitudinal QOL and survival	Prospective longitudinal, N = 389 (HR, RFA); QOL assessed preprocedure, and 3, 6, 12, 24, and 36 mo postprocedure	FACT-Hep	Baseline QOL was similar between groups. For both groups, following an initial postprocedural decline, QOL consistently improved and exceeded baseline values at 6–12 mo. Compared with HR, RFA group had significantly higher overall QOL scores at all time points. On multivariate analysis, HR was independently associated with worse QOL	Hepatitis B patients only; no difference in DFS and OS between groups; survey completion rates >95% at all time points
Kolligs et al, Liver International, 2015[148]	Unresectable liver: only HCC, with preserved hepatic function treated with SIRT or TACE	Primary outcome: safety and short-term postprocedure QOL	Pilot randomized controlled trial, N = 18 (8 SIRT, 10 TACE) QOL assesses preprocedure and 1, 6, and 12 wk postprocedure	FACT-Hep	Efficacy of treatment for local tumor control was similar between groups (73% disease control TACE vs. 77% disease control SIRT). At baseline, SIRT patients had significantly worse PWB scores; however, no differences were observed between groups in overall QOL or subscales at 6 or 12 wk postprocedure	SIRTACE was an open-label multicenter randomized control pilot study; TACE at 6-wk intervals until fully treated or disease progression (gold standard) vs. single session SIRT
Anota et al., BMJ Open, 2016[149]	HCC ineligible for curative treatments	Explore associations between QOL and Phase I dose in Phase I trial of idarubicin-loaded TACE beads by evaluating time to deterioration in at least one QOL domain	Prospective, three group design; N = 21; Groups: 5 mg, 10 mg, 15 mg; QOL assessed at baseline, 15, 30, 60 days post TACE	EORTC QLQ-C30	Completion rates 81%–100% across time points. 90% of patients developed a deterioration in one or more QOL score. Patients at 10 mg dose had longer times to deterioration for global scores and physical and pain domains.	Design highlights novel method of incorporating QOL assessment into phase I clinical trials.
Xu et al., Integrative Cancer Therapies, 2016[150]	HCC undergoing TACE	Evaluate effect of decoction treatment on post-embolization syndrome	Double blind, placebo controlled RCT, N = 140 (50 neither placebo or decoction, 40 placebo, 50 Jian Pi Li Qi decoction administered day of procedure and for 3 days after). QOL assessed at baseline and daily for 3 days after the procedure.	MDASI-GI	The Jian Pi Li Qi decoction group demonstrated a statistically significant improvement on day 2 in the following symptoms of pain, fatigue lack of appetite, drowsiness dry mouth and constipation (p < .005).	Excluded patients who could not tolerate placebo or decoction (n = 5)

Study	Population	Purpose	Study design	QOL instrument	Results
Rostas et al, *The American Journal of Surgery,* 2017[151]	Unresectable hepatic metastases from ocular melanoma treated with DEB loaded with doxorubicin	Describe QOL following treatment with DEB loaded with doxorubicin	Prospective, longitudinal, multi-center trial; N = 20 receiving 3 treatments; baseline, 3-7 days after each treatment	FACT-Hep	Completion rates were 90%. No statistically significant differences were found between baseline and 3rd treatment in SWB, EWB, FWB, or FACT-G score (p> .127). PWB and FACT-Hep total scores were statistically significantly different between baseline and the 2nd treatment assessment (p < .025). There was a statistically significant decrease in FACT-Hep TOI after each treatment in pairwise analysis (P = .003).
Vilgrain et al., *The Lancet,* 2017[152]	Locally advanced, inoperable HCC	Compare efficacy and safety of sorafenib treatment with SIRT with ^{90}Y	Multi-institution, open-label, phase 3 RTC, N = 459 (237 SIRT, 222 sorafenib), QOL assessed at baseline and every 3 months.	EORTC-C30, EORTC QLQ-HCC18	QOLf global health status subscore was statistically significantly better in the SIRT group than the sorafenib group (group effect P = .005, time effect P < .001).
Prince et al., *The Journal of Nuclear Medicine,* 2018[153]	Inoperable liver metastases refractory to systemic treatment undergoing embolization	Evaluate efficacy of ^{166}Ho-microspheres. Demonstration of change in QOL after the procedure was a secondary outcome.	Prospective, single institution, longitudinal study, N = 37, QOL assessed at baseline, 1 and 6 weeks, and every 3 months.	EORTC	Global QOL declined from baseline to 1 week (83 (IQR 67-83) to 42 ([IQR 56-86]) and recovered at 6 weeks to 67 (IQR 56-83). The worst symptoms peaked at 1 week post-procedure (fatigue, eating, pain, and emotional problems).
Xing et al., *BMC Cancer,* 2018[154]	Advanced unresectable HCC with infiltrative characteristics and portal vein thrombosis treated with ^{90}Y radioembolization	Evaluate effect of ^{90}Y radioembolization on QOL and survival	Prospective, single institution, longitudinal study, N = 30, QOL assessed at baseline, 1, 3, 6 months post procedure	SF-36	Completion rates declined with time (1 month 100%, 3 months 87%, 6 months 67%). No statistically significant change in 8 domains of SF-36 at any time point compared with baseline.

AFP, α-Fetoprotein; *BCAA,* branched-chain amino acids; *BCLC,* Barcelona Clinic Liver Cancer Classification; *BSC,* best supportive care; *CLIP,* Cancer of the Liver Italian Program HCC (hepatocellular carcinoma) classification system; *CRLM,* colorectal liver metastases; *CTX,* systemic chemotherapy; *DEB,* drug-eluting beads; *DFS,* disease-free survival; *EORTC QLQ-C30,* European Organization for the Research and Treatment of Cancer Quality-of-Life Questionnaire–Core 30; *EWB,* emotional well-being; *FACT,* Functional Assessment of Cancer Therapy; *FACT-G,* FACT-General; *FWB,* functional well-being; *HAE,* hepatic artery embolization; *HCC,* hepatocellular carcinoma; *HCV,* hepatitis C virus; *Hep,* hepatobiliary; *HR,* hepatic resection; *QOL,* health-related quality of life; *ICC,* intrahepatic cholangiocarcinoma; *MDASI-GI,* MD Anderson Symptom Inventory-Gastrointestinal Module; *NT,* no treatment; *Okuda,* Okuda Prognostic Classification; *OS,* overall survival; *PWB,* physical well-being (FACT); *QLI,* Quality-of-Life Index; *RCTs,* randomized controlled trials; *RFA,* radiofrequency ablation; *SF-36,* 36-item Short Form; *SIRT,* selective internal radiotherapy; *SWB,* social well-being (FACT); *TACE,* transarterial chemoembolization; *TOI,* Trial Outcome Index; *WHOQoL-BREF,* World Health Organization Quality-of-Life project (short form of WHOQoL-100); ^{90}Y, yttrium-90 radioembolization.

TABLE 29.6 Studies of Palliative Intervention for Malignant Gastric Outlet Obstruction (GOO) and Health-Related Quality of Life

FIRST AUTHOR, JOURNAL, YEAR	POPULATION (PATIENT WITH)	STUDY PURPOSE/ QUALITY-OF-LIFE END POINT	STUDY DESIGN, N, AND QOL ASSESSMENT TIME POINTS	QUALITY-OF-LIFE INSTRUMENT	QUALITY-OF-LIFE RESULTS	COMMENTS
Gastric Outlet Obstruction						
Mehta, *Surgical Endoscopy*, 2006[155]	Malignant GOO randomly assigned to DS or LGJ (56% pancreatic cancer)	Primary outcome: morbidity, pain and short-term QOL	Randomized clinical trial, N = 27 (14 LGJ, 13 DS); QOL assessed preprocedure and 1 mo postprocedure	SF-36 Health Survey	13/14 successful LGJ vs. 10/13 successful DS. LGJ had more postprocedure complications and longer LOS. Mean physical health score in the DS group was improved at 1 mo ($P < .01$), whereas no changes in QOL were observed in the LGJ group	In-hospital mortality, rates high for both groups: 23% (3/13) LGJ and 17% (2/12) DS
Schmidt, *American Journal of Surgery*, 2009[156]	Malignant GOO undergoing palliative intervention: surgical bypass, PEG, PEJ, or ES	Primary outcome: short-term QOL	Prospective cohort, N = 47 (16 surgical bypass, 7 PEJ/PEG, 24 ES); QOL assessed preprocedure and 1 and 3 mo postprocedure	EORTC QLQ-C30 + STO22 module	At 3 mo, both ES and surgery groups had improved global QOL, physical and role functioning, with decreased GOO symptoms compared with baseline (statistically significant only in ES group). In the surgical group, there was a significant decline in physical functioning at 1 mo; however, this rebounded by 3 mo. No changes were observed in the PEG/PEJ group	Median OS = 64 days; only 10 patients completed QOL questionnaires at all time points (5 ES and 5 surgery); initial procedural success rates: 70% ES vs. 100% surgical bypass
Van Hooft, *Gastrointestinal Endoscopy*, 2009[157]	Malignant GOO undergoing palliative ES	Primary outcome: symptom palliation (GOO-SS) Secondary outcome: safety, efficacy, and global QOL	Multicenter single-arm prospective trial, N = 51; QOL assessed preprocedure, at 4 wk, and bimonthly	EORTC QLQ-C30, EQ-5D-3L+VAS	GOO symptoms (GOO-SS) consistently improved postprocedure, whereas global QOL (QL2 subscale and EQ-VAS) was unchanged following ES	Median OS = 62 days; technical success ES 98%. Clinically, stent dysfunction occurred in 7 patients (14%), migration in 1 patient (2%)
Van Hooft, *Scandinavian Journal of Gastroenterology*, 2010[158]	Malignant GOO undergoing palliative ES	Primary outcome: identify predictors of survival from baseline evaluation	Combined data from 2 multicenter single-arm prospective trials, N = 101; baseline QOL assessment only	EORTC QLQ-C30, EQ-5D-3L + EQ-VAS	WHO performance status (HR, 2.63; 95% CI, 1.68 to 4.12, $P < .01$); prescription narcotic use (HR, 2.42; 95% CI, 1.38 to 4.25, $P < .01$), and pain score of the EORTC (HR, 1.01; 95% CI, 1.00 to 1.01, $P = .04$) independently associated with worse OS	Median OS = 82 days, although statistically significant the HR for EORTC pain score = 1.01, clinical relevance questionable
Dolz, *Gastroenterology Hepatology*, 2011[159]	Malignant GOO undergoing palliative ES	Primary outcome: procedural technical success, clinical efficacy, and short-term QOL	Multicenter, single-arm prospective trial N = 71 (38 duodenal tumors, 15 recurrent tumors localized to GJ anastomosis, 18 antral tumors); QOL assessed preprocedure and 1 mo postprocedure	EuroQol - 5D-3L	Symptoms of GOO were significantly improved postprocedure, whereas no change in QOL was observed. Stent efficacy was dependent on tumor location (GJ anastomosis [87%] > duodenal [70%] > antral [29%])	Median OS = 91 days, 29/71 (40%) completed both preprocedure and postprocedure assessments
Van den Berg, *Endoscopy*, 2013[160]	Malignant GOO undergoing palliative ES (54% pancreatic cancer)	Primary outcome: procedural technical success and clinical efficacy Secondary outcome: QOL	Multicenter, single-arm, prospective trial, N = 46; QOL assessed preprocedure and bimonthly until death	EORTC QLQ-C30 and EQ-5D-3L + EQ-VAS	Global QoL reflected by health status (QL2) and EQ-VAS demonstrated significant improvement between baseline and the mean scores during total follow-up. Data from EORTC scales not presented	Median OS = 87 days, technical success = 89%, clinical success = 72%, periprocedural complication = 57% (one or more complications)

CI, Confidence interval; DS, Duodenal stent; EORTC QLQ-C30, European Organization for the Research and Treatment of Cancer Quality-of-Life Questionnaire–Core 30; EQ-VAS, EuroQol Visual Analogue Scale; ES, endoscopic stent; GOO-SS, gastric outlet obstruction symptom scale; HR, hazard ratio; LGJ, laparoscopic gastrojejunostomy; LOS, length of stay; OS, overall survival; PEJ, percutaneous endoscopic jejunostomy; QL, quality of life; QOL, health-related quality of life; SF-36, 36-item Short Form; STO22, EORTC gastric specific QoL Module.

TABLE 29.7 Studies of Malignant Biliary Obstruction and Health-Related Quality of Life

FIRST AUTHOR, JOURNAL, YEAR	POPULATION (PATIENT WITH)	STUDY PURPOSE/ QUALITY-OF-LIFE END POINT	STUDY DESIGN, N, AND QOL ASSESSMENT TIME POINTS	QUALITY-OF-LIFE INSTRUMENT	QUALITY-OF-LIFE RESULTS	COMMENTS
Malignant Biliary Obstruction						
Abraham, *Gastrointestinal Endoscopy*, 2002[161]	MBO undergoing palliative intent ES (66% distal obstruction, 12.5% mid-CBD obstruction, 21.5% hilar or intrahepatic obstruction)	Primary outcome: short-term QOL	Prospective cohort, $N = 50$; QOL assessed preprocedure and at 1 mo postprocedure	SF-36 Health Survey	Overall, decrease in T-bili from baseline to 1 mo postprocedure was associated with significant improvements in social function and mental health; however, if baseline T-bili was very high (≥ 14 mg/dL), no improvement in social function was observed	84% of patients experienced at least a 33% reduction in T-bili postprocedure; 25% mortality at 1 mo
Chan, *Journal of Gastrointestinal Surgery*, 2005[162]	MBO undergoing ES as initial drainage procedure	Primary outcome: stent patency Secondary outcome: morbidity, mortality, and short-term QOL	Randomized double-blinded controlled trial of ciprofloxacin vs. placebo before ES for MBO, $N = 94$ (50 placebo, 44 ciprofloxacin); QOL assessed preprocedure and 1 mo postprocedure	SF-36 Health Survey	Baseline QOL was similar between groups. Compared with baseline, at 1-mo follow-up, social functioning scores improved in the ciprofloxacin group and were significantly different from placebo ($P = .05$). All other subscales and summative QOL measures were not different between groups	Median OS and stent patency were not different between groups; however, cholangitis was less common in the ciprofloxacin group
Artifon, *American Journal of Gastroenterology*, 2006[163]	Metastatic pancreatic cancer with MBO undergoing surgical bypass (choledochojejunostomy or cholecystojejunostomy) or ES	Primary outcome: cost of care Secondary outcome: short-term QOL	Prospective randomized trial, $N = 30$ (15 surgery, 15 ES); QOL assessed preprocedure and 30, 60, and 120 days postprocedure	SF-36 Health Survey	For the entire cohort, QOL scores improved at 30 and 60 days postprocedure, followed by decline to preprocedure levels at 120 days. ES was associated with significantly higher QOL than surgery at 30 days ($P = .04$) and 60 days ($P = .05$)	Median OS and postprocedural morbidity were not different between groups; overall cost of care from treatment to death was significantly reduced with ES ($4270 USD) vs. HJ ($8320 USD)
Saluja, *Clinical Gastroenterology and Hepatology*, 2008[164]	Unresectable gallbladder carcinoma with hilar obstruction undergoing ES or PTBD with plastic stent	Primary outcome: short-term QOL and clinical effectiveness of biliary drainage	Prospective randomized trial, $N = 54$ (27 ES, 27 PTBD); QOL assessed preprocedure and 1 and 3 mo postprocedure	WHOQoL–BREF-26 and EORTC QLQ-C30	At 1 mo postprocedure, no change was observed in global QOL for either group; however, symptom scale scores were improved in both PTBD and ES. At 3 mo, both groups showed a trend toward improvement in all domains of QOL assessed. PTBD was associated with improved physical and psychological scores compared with ES ($P = .02$) as well as greater improvement in symptom scores at 3 mo	Median OS was not different between groups. Clinical procedural success was higher in the PTBD group (89%) vs. ES (41%), and cholangitis was less common with PTBD (11%) compared with ES (48%)
Robson, *Annals of Surgical Oncology*, 2010[165]	MBO undergoing PTBD	Primary outcome: short-term QOL, symptom control, morbidity/mortality and procedural efficacy	Prospective cohort, $N = 109$; QOL assessed preprocedure and 1 and 4 wk postprocedure	FACT-Hep and VASP	VASP scores (pruritus symptoms) significantly improved during time; however, overall QOL as measured by mean FACT-Hep scores were significantly decreased at 1 and 4 wk postprocedure	Median OS = 4.7 mo, mortality 10% at 1 wk, 28% by 8 wk; 100% technical procedural success but 50% major complications

Continued

TABLE 29.7 Studies of Malignant Biliary Obstruction and Health-Related Quality of Life—cont'd

FIRST AUTHOR, JOURNAL, YEAR	POPULATION (PATIENT WITH)	STUDY PURPOSE/ QUALITY-OF-LIFE END POINT	STUDY DESIGN, N, AND QOL ASSESSMENT TIME POINTS	QUALITY-OF-LIFE INSTRUMENT	QUALITY-OF-LIFE RESULTS	COMMENTS
Larssen, *Surgical Endoscopy*, 2011[166]	Malignant GI obstruction undergoing ES SEMS	Primary outcome: short-term QOL. Secondary outcome: comparison of physician- and patient-rated treatment effect	Prospective cohort, N = 162 (40 [25%] biliary); QOL assessed preprocedure and 2 wk postprocedure	EORTC QLQ-C30 ± STO22 ± PAN26	Global QOL as well as nausea/vomiting, and appetite loss, and pruritus symptoms were significantly improved in patients with biliary obstruction treated with SEMS. Both patients and physicians reported symptom improvement; however, degree of improvement reported by physicians was higher than that of patients.	In addition to biliary obstruction, study cohort included patients undergoing esophageal, duodenal, and colonic SEMS
Artifon, *Journal of Clinical Gastroenterology*, 2012[167]	MBO with history of a failed ERCP undergoing PTBD or EUS-CD	Primary outcome: clinical and technical procedural success. Secondary outcome: cost, morbidity, and QOL	Prospective randomized trial, N = 25 (13 EUS-CD, 12 PTBD); QOL assessed preprocedure and 7 and 30 days postprocedure	SF-36 Health Survey	No difference in QOL measured at 7 or 30 days postprocedure for either group	One hundred percent clinical and technical success in both groups; complication rates and procedural costs not different between groups. Median OS = 8.7 mo
Aggarwal, *Brachytherapy*, 2013[168]	MBO undergoing palliative ILBT with access via PTBD	Primary outcome: symptom control, QOL, and survival	Prospective longitudinal, N = 18; QOL assessed pre-PTBD, post-PTBD, pre-ILBT, post-ILBT, and follow-up	EORTC QLQ-C30	Significant improvement in overall QOL post-PTBD, post-ILBT, and at last follow-up. Physical and social functioning scores were improved at all time points, as was insomnia symptom scale. The percentage of patients who reported pruritus and icterus declined at each time point	
Barkay, *Journal of Clinical Gastroenterology*, 2013[168]	MBO undergoing ES	Primary outcome: longitudinal QOL	Prospective longitudinal, N = 164; QOL assessed preprocedure, at 30 and 180 days postprocedure	FACT-G	Significant improvement in global QOL and PWB, EWB, and FWB subscales at 30 and 180 days. Weight loss, appetite, pruritus, and pain improved significantly at both time points	
Moses, *World Journal of Gastroenterology*, 2013[169]	Infrahilar MBO undergoing ES randomly assigned to pcSEMS or PS	Primary outcome: time to stent failure. Secondary outcome: morbidity, mortality, KPS, QOL	Multicentered prospective randomized trial, N = 85 enrolled; 74 with QOL data (36 PS, 38 pcSEMS); QOL assessed preprocedure at baseline and 1, 3, 6, 9, 12, and 15 mo	SF-36 Health Survey	At baseline, SEMS group had significantly worse physical functioning scores; no differences were observed between groups thereafter. At 1 mo, vitality was improved, and at 6 mo physical functioning was improved in the pcSEMS group. PS was associated with significant improvement in subscales of bodily pain, social functioning, and mental health at 1 mo	Time to stent failure significantly longer among the pcSEMS group, and cholangitis was less common; no difference in OS
Castiglione et al., *Abdominal Radiology*, 2020[170]	Malignant obstructive jaundice undergoing PTBD	Compare QOL between right and left drainage approaches to PTBD	Prospective, single institution RCT, N = 64 (31 right access, 33 left access), QOL assessed daily postoperatively for 7 days	EORTC QLQ-BIL21	Jaundice, tiredness, anxiety, and pain scales was worse in right sided drainage group (p < .03). There was no difference between groups in treatment and weight loss scales (P > .38)	The ability to randomize to right or left suggests there was clinical equivalence to the two approaches.

BMS, Bare metal stent; *CBD*, common bile duct; *EWB*, emotional well-being; *EORTC QLQ-C30*, European Organization for the Research and Treatment of Cancer Quality-of-Life Questionnaire-Core 30; *EORTC QLQ-BIL21*, European Organization for the Research and Treatment of Cancer Quality-of-Life Questionnaire-Biliary 21; *ERCP*, endoscopic retrograde cholangiopancreatography; *ES*, endoscopic stenting; *EUS-CD*, endoscopic ultrasound-guided cyst drainage; *FACT*, Functional Assessment of Cancer Therapy; *FWB*, functional well-being; *GI*, gastrointestinal; *ILBT*, intraluminal brachytherapy; *KPS*, Karnofsky Performance Score; *MBO*, malignant biliary obstruction; *OS*, overall survival; *pcSEMS*, partially covered self-expanding metallic stent; *PAN26*, pancreatic cancer module-26; *PTBD*, percutaneous transhepatic biliary drainage; *PS*, performance score; *PWB*, physical well-being; *QOL*, health-related quality of life; *SEMS*, self-expanding metallic stent; *SF-36*, 36-item Short Form; *STO22*, EORTC gastric specific QoL Module; *T-bili*, total bilirubin; *WHOQoL–BREF-22*, World Health Organization Quality-of-Life assessment (abbreviated version, 22 items); *VASP*, visual analogue scale for pruritus assessment.

for robust QOL evaluation among patients undergoing pancreatic resection has gained significant momentum. As a consequence of this increased interest, study design and methodology have improved greatly and appreciably enhanced the quality of this expanding body of knowledge (see Table 28.3).

Patients with pancreatic cancer often experience considerable symptoms and are at increased risk for impaired QOL compared with population norms.[103,105,107] Results of QOL evaluation after pancreatic surgery are divergent and heavily dependent on the cohort studied and the timing of evaluation relative to surgery. Among well-selected patients with localized, resectable disease, QOL at 3 months after surgery was reportedly improved.[100,171] Unfortunately, the beneficial findings reported in these studies appear to be the exception, with the great majority of investigations reporting stability and/or a decline in QOL scores after pancreatic resection.[92,96,97,100,103,105–107,118,172] The heterogeneity observed in these studies is likely multifactorial and related, but not limited, to differences in disease stage, the QOL instrument used, timing/frequency of measurement, and length of follow-up.

Early postoperative evaluation of QOL typically represents a transient state, primarily reflective of a patient's recovery from the acute effects of surgery. These findings certainly allow surgeons to better inform patients, improve the consent process, and help tailor expectations. However, longer-term follow-up post-pancreatectomy is requisite to unveil the true clinical impact of surgical resection on QOL outcomes. In a recent prospective longitudinal study, QOL 12 months after pancreaticoduodenectomy (PD) for periampullary malignancies was evaluated using the SF-36 survey. Despite the heterogeneity in cancer subtypes included, and initial decrements, significant improvements were observed in the majority of subscales when measured at 12 months.[105] Similarly, significant improvements in QOL domains assessed with the EORTC QLQ-C30 were observed among a group of patients undergoing partial pancreatectomies for pancreatic adenocarcinoma at 6 and 12 months postoperatively. Although baseline measurements were obtained postoperatively, and absolute QOL improvement is most certainly overestimated in this later study, the overall conclusions remain the same.[102] After pancreatectomy, patients tend to experience surgery-related decline in QOL, although the overwhelming majority of data support a gradual improvement/return to baseline within the first postoperative year.

To date, several studies have compared QOL of patients undergoing different types of partial pancreatomy—classic PD versus radical pancreaticoduodenectomy (RPD) versus pylorus-preserving pancreaticoduodenectomy (PPPD) versus parenchyma-preservation/-sparing pancreatectomy (PSP), with different reconstruction techniques—pancreaticogastrostomy (PG) versus pancreaticojejunostomy (PJ), for a mix of benign and malignant indications.[89,94,98,99,102,109,115,117,118,173] In general, patients undergoing partial pancreatectomy for benign disease, regardless of the type (PD, RPD, PPPD, and PSP) had similar long-term global ratings of QOL as well as comparable social, functional, and role scores on the EORTC QLQ-C30. Furthermore, studies of long-term QOL among patients with completely resected malignant tumors also suggest that QOL trends follow the same postoperative trajectory independent of the type of resection and/or reconstruction.

Total pancreatectomy (TP) is a procedure associated with substantial and irreversible long-term consequences related to pancreatic insufficiency. Patients undergoing TP are dependent on orally administered exogenous pancreatic enzymes to prevent malabsorptive syndromes/chronic diarrhea as well as strict insulin administration regimens to balance blood sugars and mitigate long-term diabetic complications. Not surprisingly, TP has the potential to substantially influence many QOL domains. In a longitudinal study of 32 patients undergoing TP for locally advanced central tumors (benign and malignant), QOL was assessed postoperatively and annually for 4 years thereafter. Interestingly, no difference in the mean global QOL scores between healthy norms and the entire TP population was observed; however, physical functioning among the TP group was significantly lower. Compared with benign counterparts, patients undergoing TP for malignant disease had higher symptom scale scores, suggesting a greater negative impact on QOL among this group. The number of patients evaluable at each time point in this study was low, and longer-term outcomes are subject to the "health survivor" bias.[112]

Billings and colleagues[91] compared QOL outcomes of 27 long-term survivors (mean, 7.5 years) treated with TP for malignancy with age- and gender-matched controls. TP patients experienced a negative impact on their QOL and health status compared with the general population; however, compared with patients with insulin-dependent diabetes mellitus (IDDM) from other causes, the differences were no longer observed. Similarly, Epelboym and colleagues[109] compared QOL between patients treated with TP versus PD with IDDM. Patients in the TP group had a slightly higher number of hypoglycemic events, but no significant differences were observed in global QOL scores. A subsequent study matched TP patients to IDDM patients and compared global QOL scores using the EORTC-QLQ-C30 plus the PAN26 module and diabetes-specific QOL scores. Overall, TP patients reported worse global QOL compared with matched IDDM patients; however, when using the diabetes-specific measurement tool, there were no significant differences.[174] These findings suggest that although TP impacts QOL, the changes observed are comparable to those seen in patients with IDDM alone and/or other types of pancreatic resection. This suggests that if TP is indicated, concerns regarding the impact of pancreatic insufficiency on QOL should not obviate intervention in well-selected patients.

Many patients with pancreatic cancer are seen late with disease that is not amenable to curative resection. Although less common in the era of percutaneous and endoscopic interventions, some patients may require or may be best served with surgical palliation of gastric and/or biliary obstructions (see Chapter 69). In a randomized study, Van Heek et al. compared QOL after prophylactic double bypass with hepaticojejunostomy (HJ) plus gastrojejunostomy (GJ) to single biliary bypass (HJ) alone. In terms of QOL measures, no differences were observed between groups. However, an 18% reduction in the risk of gastric outlet obstruction and need for repeat intervention was observed in the HJ-plus-GJ group. QOL was not reassessed or compared among those who did and did not develop obstructive symptoms requiring secondary intervention. This is unfortunate because this may have influenced longer-term QOL.[90] Palliative resection for advanced carcinoma of the pancreatic head has been suggested as an alternative to prophylactic surgical bypass (HJ plus GJ), with the potential added benefit of reducing pain associated with advanced pancreatic malignancy. When directly compared, no differences have been shown in terms of operative morbidity/mortality and/or overall survival between palliative resection and bypass. Furthermore, despite the idea that resection improves pain control, and potentially QOL, it has been observed that patients treated with palliative resection actually experience significantly greater declines in emotional, cognitive, and social-functioning scales as assessed by the EORTC QLQ-C30 compared with surgical bypass alone.[104] In combination, these findings suggest that resection provides no advantage in terms of survival or QOL. Consequently, use of resection as a means of palliation for advanced pancreatic head tumors should be used sparingly.

To reiterate, the primary goal of palliative care is symptom management and maintenance of QOL. To this end, pancreatic stenting for the relief of intractable malignant pain has been evaluated. Wehrmann et al. assessed overall QOL using the Spitzer Quality-of-life Index (QLI), as well as pain control and opioid analgesic use, at baseline and every 4 weeks after intervention in patients with unresectable pancreatic carcinoma. Stenting was associated with significantly improved pain control at 4 weeks, which persisted out to 12 weeks. QLI scores paralleled pain scores and were improved versus baseline at the 4-week time point, with return to baseline levels at 12 weeks.[95] Stenting of the pancreatic duct in select patients with advanced pancreatic malignancy and significant pain transiently improves pain control and QOL and is most certainly a reasonable option for palliation of these patients (see Chapter 69).

Hepatic Resection

In the early eras of hepatic surgery, mortality ranged from 30% to 60%, and elective intervention was rare. Similar to pancreatic resection, however, improvement in surgical technique, perioperative care, and multidisciplinary team management has led to significant decreases in morbidity and mortality (from >50% down to 2%–3%) associated with hepatic resection (Jarnagin et al. 2002; see Chapter 103).[175] As a consequence, hepatic resection has become the standard of care for definitive management of many hepatic tumors. The increased use of hepatectomy for both primary and metastatic hepatic cancers has undoubtedly improved survival outcomes; however, questions regarding the impact of hepatic resection on QOL remain. At present, there are a number of studies that address QOL as it pertains to hepatic resection and treatment of hepatic tumors (see Table 28.4).

QOL in the early postoperative period primarily reflects procedure-related factors (e.g., incisional pain, mobility limitations, complications). To date, multiple studies have evaluated the short-term impact of hepatic resection on QOL.[120–122,124,128,130] Among patients undergoing hepatectomy for primary hepatic cancer (HCC/intrahepatic cholangiocarcinoma [ICC]), a significant decline in mean scores on the Gastrointestinal QOL Index (GQLI) was observed 2 to 10 weeks postoperatively.[120] The initial decline was followed by a gradual return to baseline by 4 months, and in patients without recurrence, mean GQLI was greater than baseline assessment by 9 months. This postoperative trend in QOL after hepatic resection has been observed in multiple studies[121,122,124,128,130,133] and appears similar regardless of underlying tumor type (primary/metastatic) or QOL measurement tool used (e.g., EORTC QLQ-C30, FACT-G, FACT-Hep, GQLI). Although the extent of resection may alter the degree/duration of QOL decline postoperatively, in the absence of disease recurrence, the overall trend remains the same.[120,122,124,126] In direct contrast to patients undergoing curative resection, patients found to have unresectable disease at the time of laparotomy experience a steady decline in global QOL and all functional subscales, with persistence of symptoms throughout follow-up.[121,136] Laparotomy for hepatic malignancy, without resection of disease, negatively impacts both early and longer-term QOL outcomes. As such, meticulous preoperative evaluation is essential to avoid subjecting patients to futile intervention.

Compared with short-term postoperative QOL, longitudinal evaluation (≥3 to 6 months) after hepatic resection is less reflective of the technical procedure and more likely related to patient- and disease-specific factors.[126,127,133] Overall, patients with HCC have worse psychological and social functioning compared with population norms,[123] and not surprisingly, patients amenable to complete resection have improved QOL compared with HCC treated with transarterial chemoembolization (TACE), percutaneous ethanol injection, and/or best supportive care[144] (see Chapters 91, 96, and 98). In a long-term evaluation of hepatic resection for HCC in patients with persevered hepatic function, significant improvements in mean QOL and subscale scores were observed at 3 months and persisted out to 2 years follow-up.[119] Similar improvement was not observed in a control group with HCC undergoing TACE. Chen and colleagues[120] also observed similar long-term trends in patients undergoing hepatic resection for HCC. However, findings from these studies contrast with those of Mise and colleagues,[131] in which no change in the physical component scale on SF-36 and minimal change on the mental component scale were observed after hepatectomy for HCC. The measurement tools used in these studies differed (disease-specific FACT-G vs. generic SF-36) in terms of sensitivity to change and may account for the observed differences. It is likely that longer-term QOL assessment in patients with HCC is heavily dependent on the type and severity of underlying hepatic disease as well as other associated comorbidities. Future studies stratifying for these potential confounders are necessary.

CRLMs are the most common indication for hepatic resection, and multiple studies have assessed longer-term QOL outcomes among these patients[50,121,126,127,132,176] (see Chapter 92). Based on the literature, there is general consensus that after an initial postoperative decline, global QOL tends to return to baseline and at times exceeds baseline scores during longer-term follow-up. Likewise, disease-specific symptoms and symptom scales tend to follow a similar trajectory after hepatectomy for CRLMs. However, a recent study by Rees and colleagues[177] using the EORTC QLQ-C30 in conjunction with the liver-specific module found that as many as 10% of patients had persistent severe symptoms of pain and decrements in sexual function at 1 year after resection of CRLMs. Longer-term follow-up of this study cohort suggests that, even at a median of 8 years follow-up, 5% of patients still have significant symptoms.[132] This study did not account for the use of preoperative or postoperative chemotherapy or further treatments. Consequently, it is difficult to discern if the reported persistent symptoms are related to CRLMs, hepatic resection, previous surgery for primary tumor, or ongoing oncologic therapy.

Overall survival is increased among patients with resectable CRLMs. Unfortunately, disease recurrence requiring further oncologic therapy is the norm and may influence QOL. In a well-designed prospective study by Wiering and colleagues,[128] patients undergoing hepatic resection and having less than or equal to four CRLMs were followed for 3 years, and QOL was assessed at predefined time points. Overall, disease recurrence was associated with a decline in QOL as measured by the

EQ-5D-3L plus EQ-VAS (visual analogue scale). This decline in QOL, however, was mitigated by the ability to undergo repeat curative resection of recurrent disease. QOL scores of patients who underwent complete re-resection were similar to those of patients who never experienced a recurrence. Dasgupta and colleagues[125] also report a decrement in global QOL on the EORTC QLQ-C30 in the setting of recurrence. Similar decrements in QOL have been observed after recurrence of HCC[119,120] and after repeat resection of recurrent HCC, QOL trends parallel to what is seen with CRLMs.[178] At present, it is reasonable to suggest that recurrence of disease after hepatic resection for malignancy portends worse QOL; however, this decrement may be transient if complete surgical re-excision can be achieved.

Locoregional Treatment of Hepatic Tumors

Locoregional therapy (LRT), including hepatic arterial embolization, selective internal radiotherapy (SIRT), and ablation, may be used with curative and/or palliative intent for both primary and metastatic tumors of the liver (see Chapters 96–98). These therapies treat disease/symptoms using percutaneous methods, thereby avoiding the morbidity of an open or laparoscopic surgical procedure. In addition to bland hepatic artery embolization (embolization with particles alone), chemotherapy and radiotherapy may be delivered to the liver locally via TACE and yttrium-90 (^{90}Y) microsphere radioembolization (see Chapter 96). Ablative therapies vary by the agent/energy source used to induce cell damage/death and include thermal (radiofrequency, microwave, or cryotherapy; see Chapters 98B and 98C), electrical (irreversible electroporation; see Chapter 98C), and chemical (alcohol injection; see Chapter 98D) techniques. The use of LRT to treat hepatic tumors has increased substantially, and the impact on morbidity/mortality and survival has been well documented. In general, these types of "hard" clinical outcomes are similar across LRTs; as such, studies evaluating QOL and LRT for primary and metastatic hepatic tumors are rapidly emerging (see Table 28.5).

HCC is the most common primary hepatic tumor (see Chapter 91). Because HCC typically arises in the setting of underlying cirrhosis, treatment decisions are dependent on tumor characteristics/disease burden, hepatic function, and performance status. Transplant and hepatic resection are the primary curative therapies; however, these are limited to a minority of patients (see Chapters 103 and 115). As a consequence, LRT has emerged as the mainstay of treatment for many patients with HCC. Although some patients may be rendered disease free, LRT in the setting of HCC is typically noncurative and offered to provide local disease control and ameliorate symptoms. As a consequence, interest in QOL associated with LRT has focused primarily on this population of patients. Although LRT is used in the treatment of hepatic metastases from neuroendocrine tumors (NET) and CRLMs, limited data are available regarding the impact of LRT on QOL in these populations.[136,139]

Compared with published population norms, patients with HCC have lower overall QOL.[146,154] Multiple studies have evaluated short-term (0–3 months) postprocedural QOL among patients with HCC treated with LRT.[137,143,145,146,148–150] In general, regardless of modality (TACE/^{90}Y radioembolization/radiofrequency ablation [RFA]) and/or QOL instrument used, most patients experience a transient decrement in overall QOL very early (1–3 weeks) after intervention. This is typically

followed by an improvement in most subscales/domains (physical, emotional, social, mental/psychological), global QOL, and symptoms.

The impact of LRT on longer-term QOL has also been extensively evaluated.[135,140–142,144,147,152,154] Similar to short-term evaluations, most longitudinal studies report an initial early decline in QOL regardless of LRT modality. Nevertheless, because the natural history of HCC differs based on the etiology of underlying hepatic disease (i.e., hepatitis C virus cirrhosis vs. hepatitis B virus cirrhosis), it is not surprising that reported longitudinal QOL outcomes with LRT treatment of HCC vary (see Chapters 70 and 76). Steel and colleagues[135] found a persistent decrease in global QOL and all subscales from baseline to 6 months after TACE (cisplatin) or ^{90}Y radioembolization. Interestingly, in this study, despite having greater disease burden and lower reported QOL at treatment initiation, patients undergoing ^{90}Y radioembolization had better functional well-being at 3- and 6-month follow-up when compared with those treated with TACE. Vilgrain et al.[152] reported statistically significant differences in the two randomized treatments (sorafenib arm vs. SIRT arm). The QOL global health status subscore of the EORTC was statistically significantly better in the SIRT group than the sorafenib group. Other studies of TACE[141,142] and RFA[140] for unresectable HCC have reported no significant changes in QOL parameters during longer-term follow-up. Toro and colleagues[144] evaluated longitudinal QOL among patients undergoing hepatic resection, RFA, TACE, or no treatment (NT). With the exception of the NT group, all patients (resection, RFA, TACE) reported persistent improvements in QOL from 3 to 24 months. In this study, compared with TACE and NT groups, patients treated with RFA had significantly better physical and emotional well-being. Improved longer-term QOL after LRT was also observed in a recent study comparing hepatic resection with RFA in patients with small (<3 cm) HCC.[147] QOL is not only important as a clinical outcome, but correlational studies have also shown that among patients undergoing transarterial embolic therapy for HCC, baseline QOL is actually one of the strongest predictors of overall survival.[138]

The studies are nonrandomized and thus subject to inherent disease- and patient-related selection bias. Apart from the earlier discussed RCT comparing chemotherapy regimen with SIRT,[152] the only other known RCT evaluating QOL explored the impact of a herbal extract on reducing postembolization syndrome.[150] The Jian Pi Li Qi decoction arm demonstrated statistically significant improvement on day 2 postembolization in the following symptoms of pain, fatigue, lack of appetite, drowsiness, dry mouth, and constipation ($P < .005$).

To date, no single LRT modality has consistently been shown to be superior to others in terms of QOL outcomes. Review of the literature suggests that, in general, ^{90}Y radioembolization and RFA are associated with better QOL compared with TACE[135,137,144–146] and TACE in combination with RFA yields better outcomes than TACE alone.[137] TACE and ^{90}Y radioembolization are typically used to treat multifocal unilobar/segmental disease, whereas RFA is indicated for small solitary lesions or low-volume multifocal disease; as such, comparison between treatments without randomization or matching for extent of disease/hepatic function is limited. A single, small, randomized pilot study of TACE versus selective internal radiotherapy was recently completed. QOL was a secondary endpoint of the trial, and when using the FACT-Hep scale, no significant differences were observed between the treatments arms at 6 or 12 weeks of follow-up.

Despite the limitations of the available literature, small sample sizes, heterogenous patient populations, and lack of randomization, it is reasonable to conclude that QOL after LRT for HCC is improved in the short term, whereas longer-term outcomes vary and are likely strongly influenced by patient- and disease-specific variables. Furthermore, the clinical indications and patient populations amenable to TACE versus RFA versus ^{90}Y radioembolization are inherently different. At present, no one form of LRT has consistently been associated with superior QOL. Overall, in patients with unresectable, non-transplantable liver, only HCC treatment with LRT provides local disease control and likely improves the overall QOL for patients during the first 6 to 12 months after intervention.

Palliative Treatments

Surgery for tumors of the pancreas, liver, and bile ducts has improved over time; however, as many as 85% of patients with HPB malignancies are seen late with advanced-stage disease that is not amenable to surgical intervention. In this setting, significant complications related to the precarious location of these tumors are common and often require intervention to ameliorate associated symptoms. The goal of treatment in this setting is palliative. It is therefore critical that interventions minimize morbidity and improve symptoms to maintain or improve QOL.

Gastric Outlet Obstruction

Malignant gastric outlet obstruction (GOO) occurs when the pyloric channel or duodenum is externally compressed by tumor and/or internally obstructed because of local tumor invasion (see Chapter 69). It is a debilitating complication of advanced malignancies, occurring in 10% to 20% of periampullary cancers.[90,179] The predominant symptoms associated with GOO include early satiety, bloating, nausea, vomiting, reflux, and abdominal pain, often leading to anorexia, weight loss, and cachexia. Treatment of GOO is essential not only to improve symptoms but also to allow suitable candidates to return to or initiate other oncologic therapy. Before the development of endoscopic and minimally invasive techniques, treatment of GOO required laparotomy and open surgical bypass (GJ). More recently, advancements in both laparoscopic and endoscopic techniques have led to the development of less invasive means of treating GOO, including laparoscopic GJ (LGJ), percutaneous endoscopic gastrostomy/jejunostomy (PEG/PEJ), or endoscopic/radiologic duodenal stenting (DS). At present, determining which intervention to use requires a balanced assessment of life expectancy, risks and benefits of each intervention, the potential need for repeat intervention, and the overall impact on QOL. In the context of palliative interventions for GOO, QOL has only been assessed as the primary outcome in one study; however, it has been assessed extensively as a secondary outcome (see Table 28.6). It should be noted that many studies of QOL related to treatment of GOO have used a tool designed specifically for this patient population called the Gastric Outlet Obstruction Scoring Scale (GOO-SS).[157,159,160] Although the scale only evaluates a single domain (physical), it is often reported as a surrogate for QOL.

There remains a paucity of research on QOL in this population. There is a single randomized trial of 27 patients with malignant GOO (56% pancreatic cancer) treated with DS ($n = 13$) versus LGJ ($n = 14$) that has been completed.[155] The underlying fragility of this group of patients is highlighted by the high rate of hospital mortality (DS at 17% and LGJ at 23%). Not surprisingly, LGJ was associated with longer hospital stay (LOS) and greater postprocedural complications compared with DS. However, the procedural success rate in the DS group (77%) was lower than in the LGJ group (100%). Physical and mental QOL scores on the SF-36 at baseline were similar between groups. Among evaluable patients at 1 month follow-up ($n = 13$, 6 LGJ and 7 DS), patients treated with DS had improved physical QOL scores, whereas no changes in QOL were observed in the LGJ group. The authors concluded that DS provided improved palliation versus LGJ based on decreased LOS, morbidity, and increased physical QOL at 1 month; however, this must be viewed in light of the decreased procedural success rates of DS and need for potential repeat intervention. Similarly, Schmidt et al.[156] observed improvements in global QOL, physical and role functioning, and a decrease in symptoms after palliative intervention (endoscopic stenting [ES] and surgical bypass) among 50 patients with malignant GOO at 3 months post-procedure.

DS is the most recent addition to the armamentarium of procedures available to palliate GOO, and prospective trials evaluating safety and efficacy have also included an evaluation of QOL outcomes and/or symptom relief.[157,159,160] In terms of symptom relief, evaluated with GOO-SS, placement of ES was consistently associated with symptom improvement and increased oral intake across studies. In two of three studies reporting QOL outcomes, no changes in global measures of QOL were observed at 1 month follow-up.[157,159] Although no untreated GOO control group was included, and the QOL in this population was not documented, it is likely that QOL would decline with progressive/untreated GOO and that stability of global measures represents a positive QOL outcome. Conversely, the most recent study by van den Berg and colleagues[160] reported significant improvements in global QOL after ES. This study compared preprocedural QOL measure with the mean QOL for the entire follow-up period (not standardized post-procedure time point); as such, the conclusions regarding QOL outcomes are difficult to interpret.

Overall, studies reporting on QOL after palliative procedures for GOO are limited in size, follow-up, and, most importantly, response rates.[179] Reported median overall survival of patients with advanced/end-stage malignancy and GOO ranges from 3 to 4 months; therefore even short-term follow-up can be difficult, and results are inherently biased in that patients returning questionnaires/surveys represent a "healthy survivor" subgroup.[179,180,181] Furthermore, QOL is most commonly reported as a secondary outcome of safety and efficacy trials; as such, established QOL instruments were not used and full data are not reported (e.g., single global measures reported as means, little evaluation of subscales), and the robustness of analysis and methodology is suboptimal. Despite this, available literature would suggest that relief of obstruction obviates the main symptoms associated with GOO, leading to a stabilization of QOL. The palliative nature of intervention for GOO demands assessment of QOL. At present, additional prospective studies with QOL as a primary outcome measure are necessary to define the true relationship between treatment of malignant GOO and QOL.

Malignant Biliary Obstruction

Malignant biliary obstruction (MBO) is common in the setting of pancreaticobiliary cancers (see Chapters 49, 51, and 65). In fact, jaundice is often the initial clinical presentation of these tumors. Hyperbilirubinemia is associated with increased perioperative risk in certain situations and is a contraindication to many chemotherapy regimens. Furthermore, biliary obstruction may be associated with symptoms of anorexia, weight loss, pruritus, and malabsorption, leading to significant functional impairment. As such, intervention to alleviate MBO is undertaken for two primary reasons: to allow initiation of definitive oncologic therapy (surgery and/or chemotherapy) and/or to palliate associated symptoms. In the past, surgical bypass with HJ was the mainstay of treatment for MBO. In the current era, however, ES and image-guided percutaneous transhepatic biliary drainage (PTBD) are the most common procedures used to relieve jaundice (see Chapters 29 and 30).[167,182-185] Intraluminal brachytherapy (ILBT) has also been proposed as a mechanism to treat MBO. Initial reports regarding ILBT for MBO suggest an improvement in QOL; however, research in this area is limited.[168] Decisions regarding the type of intervention for MBO are complex and must take into account not only anatomic location but also life expectancy, intended future oncologic therapy, safety/efficacy, and QOL. To date, multiple studies have evaluated management strategies for MBO, which have included analysis of QOL outcomes (see Table 28.7).

Several studies have assessed different methods of achieving decompression of the biliary tree and compared subsequent impact on QOL. Surgical bypass for MBO is uncommon in developed countries and data pertaining to its impact on QOL are limited. In a study from Brazil, where surgical bypass remains common, a comparison was made between ES and surgical bypass (choledochojejunostomy or cholecystojejunostomy) in patients with metastatic pancreatic cancer.[163] Regardless of treatment type, global QOL improved from baseline at the 30- and 60-day follow-up, respectively, but returned to preprocedure values by 120 days. However, global QOL scores in patient treated with ES were significantly higher at all time points compared with the surgery group. No differences in procedural complications or survival were observed between groups. The equivalence in morbidity and mortality between procedures with improved QOL suggests ES may be superior to surgical bypass in select patients.

Techniques of ES and PTBD for MBO continue to evolve. Similarly, studies evaluating not only safety/efficacy of these interventions, but also QOL, continue to increase. ES for MBO is associated with reasonable clinical and technical success. Reduction in total bilirubin levels by at least one-third of preprocedural values with ES has been associated with improved social and mental functioning as measured by SF-36; however, these QOL improvements appear to be mitigated by the absolute preprocedure bilirubin (preprocedure total bilirubin $\geq$ 14 mg/dL; no change in QOL parameters).[161] Furthermore, in an assessment of 40 patients undergoing ES with self-expanding metal stents (SEMS), global QOL on the EORTC QLQ-C30 was improved, as were symptoms of nausea/vomiting, appetite, and pruritus at 2 weeks after the procedure.[166] Using the FACT-G questionnaire, Barkay et al.[186] also evaluated ES for MBO and found improvement in global QOL and physical, emotional, and functional well-being at both 1 and 6 months follow-up. Likewise, a recent study comparing partially covered self-expandable metal stents with plastic stents revealed no difference between treatments in terms of QOL but a general trend in both arms toward an improvement in global QOL and subscales.[169] Taken in concert, these findings suggest that ES

for MBO improves short-term QOL and symptoms; however, conclusions regarding longer-term QOL outcomes are limited by the substantial decrements in survey completion with prolonged follow-up.

In a prospective evaluation of 109 patients with MBO presenting for PTBD, significant improvements in pruritus symptoms were observed, but overall QOL, as assessed by FACT-Hep, significantly declined during the 4-week period after PBD.[165] The mortality rate was extremely high (28% at 8 weeks post-PBD), highlighting the degree of illness and frailty among this patient population.[165] A recent study randomized patients to either the right or left access approach before PTBD and assessed QOL in the 7 days after the procedure.[170] Although the study found the right access group had worse scores in jaundice, tiredness, drain care, and anxiety scales, the study was limited by duration of follow-up and assumption of equivalence in drainage approaches.[170] PTBD followed by ILBT has recently been touted to reduce localized tumor burden and result in improved biliary drainage and symptom relief. In a study of high-dose ILBT, 18 patients with advanced pancreaticobiliary or metastatic cancer underwent PTBD, followed by two ILBT sessions 1 week apart.[168] In conjunction with significant improvement in symptoms (100% resolution of pruritus), global QOL, as well as physical and social functional scores, were improved at all assessment points.[168] It appears that PTBD alone significantly improves biliary obstructive symptoms; however, in the absence of further treatments, QOL seems to decline in a fashion expected of end-stage pancreaticobiliary cancers.

ES was initially preferred to PTBD because drainage was internal and thought to be more readily achievable. However, advances in image-guided interventions and the development of internal stents for percutaneous delivery mean adequate internal drainage can be achieved with both PTBD and ES. The growing number of techniques and methods for ES and PTBD has led to multiple comparative evaluations of the two procedures. Saluja et al.[164] randomly assigned patients with unresectable gallbladder carcinoma and hilar obstruction to undergo either PTBD or ES. At the 1-month follow-up, no significant change in overall QOL was observed between the groups; however, at 3 months, a trend toward improvement was noted in both. Compared with ES, PTBD was associated with significantly greater improvement in the physical and psychological domains of QOL. Both groups experienced improvement in symptoms, but PBD was associated with significantly greater improvements in fatigue compared with ES. Conversely, evaluation of patients randomly assigned to PBD or endoscopic ultrasound-guided choledochoduodenostomy (EUS-CD) revealed no significant change in QOL in the 30 days after intervention.[167] Furthermore, there were no significant differences between the PBD and EUS-CD groups. It appears that, regardless of procedure performed, relief of obstruction per se provides symptom relief and at best stabilizes QOL, which among this fragile cohort likely represents a positive outcome.

CHALLENGES IN HEALTH-RELATED QUALITY-OF-LIFE RESEARCH AND FUTURE DIRECTIONS

Despite the widespread implementation of QOL assessment, interpretation of findings and implementation at the clinical practice level is a significant challenge. Merely stating a *P* value, indicating a statistical difference, is the standard; however, determining how this is to be interpreted clinically is a challenge and is one of the major criticisms of QOL research. To date, this has significantly limited the clinical applicability of QOL research outcomes. As of 2005, only 25% of QOL studies reported on the clinical significance, and thus applicability, of their findings.[187] Several methods have been suggested to rectify this issue, including establishment of a minimal important difference (MID)—the smallest difference in a score in the domain of interest that a patient perceived as beneficial and that would mandate a change in patient management.[188] Two primary methods for determining a MID for QOL outcomes exist: distribution based (estimate based on observed scores in a sample) and anchor based (compare, or anchor, QOL differences/changes to other clinical variables or patient's subjective assessment). Although imperfect, a MID provides a means by which to place QOL into a clinical context. Proponents for both forms of measurement of MID exist; however, a combination of both methods, where feasible, likely yields the most clinically useful and accurate information.[189]

Longitudinal studies of QOL are essential in the current era, where disease treatments are becoming more and more complex and survival "with" disease is common. However, this assessment is subject to several biases, including "response shift," whereby patients recalibrate their internal standards regarding QOL during the course of treatment/follow-up and "healthy survivor"; as time passes, sicker patients are less likely to complete surveys, and therefore longer-term results are heavily biased toward patients who are faring the best. Although methods exist to attempt combating these issues, their use is rare and the approaches lack validation. Furthermore, long-term studies are often limited by the logistics of survey administration and practicality.

Missing data is a common and critical concern when interpreting QOL data. The consequences of missing QOL information depends on both the amount and the cause of missing data. It is to be expected that some information will be missing at random; the real concern comes when "missingness" is not a random event. There are multiple mechanisms by which to assess the importance of missing data, including comparison of statistical means from patients with complete follow-up to those with incomplete follow-up, to see if there is a difference between groups in QOL indices. If this is indeed the fact, data are nonignorable missing data and must be accounted for or explained. Given the significant impact of missing data in QOL assessment, especially in studies during time, the best method to deal with it is, in fact, preventive. Trials assessing QOL should be designed in a fashion such that implementation strategies and rigorous follow-up are in place at the outset.

Future directions in QOL are based on item response theory and include computerized adaptive testing in which patients' responses to a given question will prompt the subsequent line of questions, thus individualizing surveys. Furthermore, the use of electronic surveys is increasingly become part of standard clinical care such that questionnaires are completed before each clinic visit, immediate feedback is generated for the patient and treating physician, and important patient-centered concerns may be addressed and decisions made. Likewise, in response to increasing fervor surrounding personalized medicine, QOL researchers have developed GENEQoL, an initiative assessing potential links between QOL outcomes and genetics. Given that QOL may be predictive of clinical outcomes, the ultimate goal of such investigations would be the development of a QOL genetic signature to be used as a predictor of patient outcomes.[190,191]

QOL research in surgery is in its infancy and, as such, faces many challenges, from study design and implementation to clinical application. However, it is encouraging that enthusiasm surrounding development of this field continues to rise among surgeons and institutions alike. In the future, collaboration between surgeons, statisticians, qualitative researchers, and most importantly, patients will be essential to further the development and clinical application of QOL outcomes in surgery. Furthermore, as the landscape of medicine continues to evolve, become more complex, and offer more life-saving/prolonging treatments, there is no doubt that QOL measurement and understanding will become increasingly valuable and essential for optimal patient care.

Acknowledgments

This chapter was fully reviewed and revised for this edition. The foundation was laid by past authors of the 4th and 5th editions, Michael D'Angelica, Sofija Pitka, Steven D. Passik, and Julie Leal. There is grateful acknowledgement for their past contribution.

References are available at expertconsult.com.

PART 4

Techniques of Biliary Tract Intervention: Radiologic, Endoscopic, and Surgical

CHAPTER 30

Interventional endoscopy for biliary tract disease: Technical aspects

Yakira David, Dennis Yang, and Christopher DiMaio

EQUIPMENT NEEDED FOR STANDARD ENDOSCOPIC RETROGRADE CHOLANGIOPAN-CREATOGRAPHY CANNULATION

Before attempting cannulation of the biliary tree for standard endoscopic retrograde cholangiopancreatography (ERCP), the appropriate equipment must be assembled (see Chapter 20). At baseline that equipment should include[1]:

- Side-viewing duodenoscope with biopsy channel of at least 3.2 mm to 4.2 mm
- Guidewire[2,3]:
  - Hydrophilic or Hydrophilic tipped
  - Diameter: 0.018, 0.025, and 0.035 inches. The 0.035 inch is most commonly used, but the 0.025 size can be useful in smaller papillae and the 0.018 inch in the pancreatic duct. Although these have the advantage of being able to access narrower orifices, their smaller size makes them more pliable and more difficult to control.
  - Tip: angled or straight-tipped
  - Length:
  - Long-wire (420–480 cm) – This allows for universal exchange capabilities across all devices and brands and is also needed for complex rendezvous endoscopic ultrasound (EUS)–assisted cholangiopancreatography and single-operator cholangioscopy. It, however, does not allow for control by the endoscopist and instead relies heavily on excellent coordination with communication with a trained endoscopy assistant.
    - Short-wire system (184–270 cm) – Allows exclusive control of the guidewire by the endoscopist because it can be locked in place both at the level of the elevator and externally at the biopsy port to allow for easy exchange of devices over the wire.
- Standard cannulation catheters (typically have two to three lumens to facilitate concurrent passage of a guidewire and contrast injection)
  OR:
- Sphincterotome – This includes an electrosurgical cutting wire at the distal end of the catheter. This is used primarily to perform a sphincterotomy. Additionally, applying tension on the cutting wire results in bowing of the sphincterotome which aligns its axis to facilitate cannulation.
- Access (pre-cut) papillotomy catheters – These are used for precut sphincterotomies or biliary fistulotomies. The most commonly used of these catheters is the *needle-knife* (NK), which has a retractable electrosurgical cutting wire.

ENDOSCOPIC RETROGRADE CHOLANGIOPAN-CREATOGRAPHY STANDARD CANNULATION TECHNIQUE

There are two main techniques that can be used to cannulate the biliary system: traditional contrast-assisted biliary cannulation and guidewire-assisted biliary cannulation.[4]

Traditional Contrast-Assisted Biliary Cannulation

In traditional contrast-assisted biliary cannulation, the catheter is engaged with the papillary orifice and contrast is injected to delineate the trajectory and pathway of the bile duct. Afterwards, the catheter and/or a guidewire can be inserted directly into the bile duct. One of the main risks of this is inadvertent injection of contrast into the pancreatic duct, which increases the risk for post-ERCP pancreatitis (PEP; see Chapter 55).

Guidewire-Assisted Biliary Cannulation

This involves confirmed cannulation of the bile duct with a guidewire before the injection of any contrast. There are two methods to achieve this:

- *Touch guidewire technique:* The tip of the catheter can be engaged with the biliary orifice and then the guidewire can be advanced into the common bile duct under fluoroscopic guidance. This technique may be associated with higher cannulation rates.[5]
- *No-touch technique:* Alternatively, the guidewire can be advanced one to two mm beyond the tip of the catheter and then advanced directly through the papillary orifice oriented towards the bile duct under fluoroscopy.

Guidewire-assisted biliary cannulation has been found to be superior to the contrast-assisted biliary cannulation technique because it results in higher rates of primary biliary cannulation, less need for precut sphincterotomy, and a lower risk of PEP.[6]

DIFFICULT BILIARY CANNULATION

Difficult biliary access is defined as the inability to achieve selective biliary cannulation by standard ERCP techniques within 10 minutes or five cannulation attempts or failure of access to the major papilla.[7] Repeated attempts at biliary cannulation are independently associated with an increased risk of PEP. There are a few strategies that have been established to facilitate biliary cannulation in such instances.

Pancreatic Duct Wire or Stent Placement to Facilitate Biliary Access

In the "double-wire technique," a guidewire is deliberately placed in the pancreatic duct while the biliary cannulation device is preloaded with a second guidewire to reattempt biliary cannulation. Theoretically, the pancreatic guidewire assists by straightening the common channel and common bile duct (CBD), thus facilitating biliary cannulation. Furthermore, the direction of the pancreatic wire exiting the papilla on endoscopy may provide anatomic cues regarding the optimal axis for biliary cannulation. Although this technique has been associated with high rates of cannulation in difficult situations, it has not been conclusively shown to be superior to standard cannulation and may be associated with an increased risk of PEP.[8,9] Placement of a pancreatic duct stent facilitates biliary duct cannulation and also reduces the risk of PEP by ensuring pancreatic duct drainage and by minimizing further inadvertent entry into the pancreatic duct on repeated attempts at biliary cannulation.[8,9]

Access "Precut" Sphincterotomy for Biliary Access

Access "precut" sphincterotomy refers to the technique of incising the papilla before obtaining biliary access. Precutting can be a useful technique to achieve selective bile duct cannulation when standard approaches fail. The needle-knife (NK) catheter is typically used for this procedure. The NK catheters have a retractable bare electrosurgical cutting wire that extends from the tip of the catheter. The exposed needle can then be inserted into the papillary orifice, and the cut is directed upward in the axis of the bile duct, generally in the 11 to 12 o'clock position. Another variation of this technique involves using the NK to begin an incision above the ampullary orifice to directly access the CBD by creating a biliary fistula ("fistulotomy").

Precut sphincterotomy has been associated with biliary cannulation rates exceeding 90%.[10,11] Nevertheless, precutting is not without risk because the incision is performed without the guidance of a wire within the duct. Earlier experience with precut sphincterotomy demonstrated an increased risk of complications such as PEP, bleeding, and perforation.[12,13] Nevertheless, given that precut sphincterotomy has traditionally been used as a second option or last resort during difficult cannulation, it has been suggested that precut sphincterotomy may be a surrogate marker of difficult cannulation and not an independent predictor of PEP.[14,15] More recent data have indicated no overall increased risk of complications when compared with persistent attempts at cannulation and may even be associated with a lower risk of PEP compared with repeated attempts at cannulation.[10,11,16,17,18] Some centers have modified this technique and perform a "shallow" precut sphincterotomy, which uses only three mm of the NK, which has demonstrated overall lower complication rates.[19] These centers have even advocated for this to be used as the first-line approach for all ERCPs.[20]

Overall, there is good evidence to recommend early precut sphincterotomy in cases of challenging biliary cannulation but not enough to recommend this universally as the first-line approach for all ERCPs. It is important to emphasize that this approach should be performed by an experienced biliary endoscopist familiar with the nuances and technical aspects of this approach.[4]

Transpancreatic Precut Sphincterotomy

Transpancreatic precut (transeptal) sphincterotomy (TPS) for biliary access was first described by Goff and is thus sometimes known as the Goff technique.[21] In this technique, after selective cannulation of the pancreatic duct, precut sphincterotomy is performed by cutting the septum between the pancreatic and bile duct with the standard sphincterotome directed cephalad toward the bile duct. Since its introduction, several studies have demonstrated high rates of bile duct cannulation without increased complication rates compared with other precut techniques used for difficult biliary cannulation, when used in expert hands.[22,23] To reduce the risk of PEP after TPS, it is further recommended that a pancreatic stent be left in situ.[4]

The decision on the type of precut technique used can be determined based on papilla morphology (e.g., for protuberant papilla where NK fistulotomy may be preferential) or based on the presence of inadvertent pancreatic duct cannulation (where transpancreatic precut sphincterotomy may be preferred).[24] It is again crucial that any of these precut techniques be performed by an expert endoscopist.[4]

TECHNIQUES FOR BILIARY ACCESS IN PATIENTS WITH SURGICALLY ALTERED ANATOMY

ERCP in patients with surgically altered anatomy can be technically difficult. There are two main challenges that need to be overcome to successfully complete the procedure. The first challenge is to reach the papilla or bilioenteric anastomosis in altered luminal anatomy. The second challenge is to be able to cannulate and perform the intended intervention from an altered position with the available endoscopes and accessories.

Endoscopic Retrograde Cholangiopancreatography in Patients With a Bilroth II Gastrojejunostomy

In Bilroth II anatomy, the distal stomach is resected and an end-to-side gastrojejunostomy has been created. From the gastrojejunal anastomosis, an afferent limb leads toward the proximal duodenum, whereas the efferent limb leads to the distal small bowel. In the Braun variation, there is additionally a side-to-side jejuno-jejunostomy between the afferent and efferent limbs. ERCP is performed by intubating the afferent limb and cannulating the papilla from a caudal angle. Although the afferent limb may be short, identification of the limb and navigating through the sharp angulation of this limb can be challenging with the conventional side-viewing duodenoscope, and even more so with the Braun variation. An alternative is to perform the entire procedure with a forward-viewing gastroscope or pediatric colonoscope. This can be further aided by placing a transparent cap on the tip of the endoscope, which facilitates navigation through the tortuous afferent limb and stabilizes the scope position for selective biliary cannulation. Other options for afferent limb intubation and biliary cannulation include use of balloon-assisted enteroscopy, spiral enteroscopy, or use of an anterior oblique-viewing endoscope.[25,26] There are limitations, however, to using these endoscopes because they lack elevators, which aid with biliary cannulation, and there are less ERCP-directed accessories available.

When using a duodenoscope, the papilla is usually visible en face upon reaching the second portion of the duodenum. From this position, the papilla appears rotated by 180 degrees, and as such biliary cannulation generally proceeds toward the five o'clock position instead of the 11 o'clock position used for standard ERCP. Hence standard straight cannulas may be preferable for selective bile duct cannulation compared with the upward-curved papillotomes. Alternative devices that have been explored to facilitate bile duct access in these patients include the Bilroth II sphincterotome with a downward "reversed bow" curved wire, rotatable sphincterotomes, pull-type sphincterotomes, or triple-lumen needle-knives. In expert hands these have success rates of over 90%.[27,28,29]

Despite the inherent challenges of Bilroth II anatomy, the success rates for ERCP are similar amongst the different techniques used. In a large single-center series of 713 patients, the success rate for afferent limb intubation and biliary or pancreatic duct cannulation using the duodenoscope was 87% and 94%, respectively.[30] Similarly, ERCP success rates with over-tube-assisted enteroscopy (single-balloon [SBE], double- balloon [DBE], spiral enteroscopy) exceeded 90% in patients with Bilroth II anatomy.[25,31] A systematic review comparing the different techniques has reported rates of access and selective biliary cannulation exceeding 95% for both side-viewing and forward-viewing endoscopy.[32]

In additional to the potential risks associated with conventional ERCP, Bilroth II anatomy increases the risk of adverse events, including perforations at the gastrojejunal anastomosis or within the afferent limb itself.[30] The risk of this has been noted to be marginally higher with side-viewing endoscopy.[32,33]

At this time, some society guidelines recommend the side-viewing endoscope as a first option with forward-viewing endoscopes (gastroscope, pediatric colonoscope, and balloon enteroscope) as the second choice in cases of failure.[4] Given that there are pros and cons to both side-viewing conventional endoscopes and forward-viewing scopes, the endoscopist should be familiar with multiple techniques and be prepared to change strategies on a case-by-case basis, depending on the intraprocedural findings.

Transoral Endoscopic Retrograde Cholangiopancreatography in Patients with a Roux-en-Y Anatomy

Roux-en-Y reconstruction has been used in bariatric gastric bypass, gastric resections, pancreaticoduodenectomy (Whipple procedure), resection of biliary malignancies, reconstruction of benign biliary strictures, and in some cases of liver transplant (see Chapters 42, 117A, and 119A).

Briefly, in patients with Roux-en-Y anatomy, the jejunum is divided into two segments close to the ligament of Treitz. The distal segment of this is anastomosed to the stomach or gastric remnant and forms the "Roux" limb. A jejunojejunal anastomosis is then formed by anastomosing the proximal segment further down on the distal segment. Proximally, this connects to the duodenum and the biliary system and forms the "biliopancreatic" limb.

Before attempting ERCP, a comprehensive review of the patient's operative reports, imaging, and prior procedures are necessary, and a discussion with their surgeon would be ideal to develop a strategic approach.[34] Emphasis should be placed on the type of resection and anastomosis, length of both limbs, and whether there is a native papilla or other type of bilioenteric anastomosis.

Roux-en-Y anatomy poses a major challenge for ERCP, given the length of bowel that must be traversed to reach the papilla or bilioenteric anastomosis. This is often prohibitive for duodenoscopes, and again the altered orientation makes cannulation difficult. To improve success rates, various combinations and adaptations of forward-viewing and side-viewing scopes have been employed.

Push enteroscopy (using a forward-viewing enteroscope or push colonoscope) can be an alternative when the biliopancreatic limb cannot be reached with the duodenoscope.[35,34] Deep enteroscopy platforms, including SBE, DBE, and spiral enteroscopy, were developed to allow access to the distal small bowel and have quoted success rates of reaching the papilla of up to 86%.[25,31,36–39] Although the longer enteroscopes may facilitate navigation through the surgically altered anatomy compared with the duodenoscope, this advantage comes with several limitations. First, the lack of a side-viewing perspective and an elevator can potentially make cannulation more difficult. Second, there are limited accessories specifically designed to use with the longer endoscopes to perform diagnostic and therapeutic interventions. The use of larger-diameter biliary stents can be limited by the size of the working channel of the endoscope, and even smaller-caliber accessories may be difficult to advance through the channel when the longer endoscope is torqued or looped in the surgically altered bowel. Lastly, these procedures can be long (median ranging from one to three hours), with the increased risk of prolonged general anesthesia.[25] Success rates of device-assisted enteroscopy range from 70% to 86% across multiple studies, with the main limiting factor being the enteroscopy, as cannulation rates are upwards of 85% once the papilla or bilioenteric anastomosis is reached.[36–40]

Alternatives to Transoral Access for ERCP in Surgically Altered Anatomy

Transoral ERCP in patients with Roux-en-Y gastric bypass (RYGB) can be challenging given the relatively longer Roux and biliopancreatic limbs that must be traversed. Hence, alternative access routes through the remnant stomach directly to the native papilla have been explored.

Percutaneous Transgastric ERCP – This involves creation of a gastrostomy to the excluded stomach and can be done via open surgery or via a percutaneous gastrostomy placed by interventional radiology, but is most commonly performed laparoscopically.[41] In laparoscopic-assisted transgastric ERCP, a 15-mm trocar is inserted into the excluded stomach is used to pull it adjacent to the abdominal wall, and is secured with a purse-string suture. The duodenoscope can then be inserted through the trocar into the excluded stomach and advanced in an anterograde manner to the papilla. If subsequent ERCPs are anticipated, a gastrostomy tube may be inserted to maintain and allow for maturity of the gastrostomy tract over two to four weeks.[34] This technique has quoted success rates of up to 100% and low rates of severe adverse events, even in lower volume community hospitals.[41–48] It has the advantage of facilitating use of standard side-viewing duodenoscopes and ERCP accessories, which improves success rates of cannulation and interventions when compared with enteroscopy-assisted ERCP.[49,50] Additionally, laparoscopy allows for diagnosis and management of internal hernias, adhesions, and cholecystectomy if indicated in the same setting (see Chapter 24). Coordination between gastroenterology and surgical teams and maintenance of a sterile field are the main challenges with this approach.[42]

As an alternative to this multidisciplinary approach, a technique using percutaneous- assisted transprosthetic endoscopic therapy has been described.[51,52] In this technique, an enteroscope is advanced transorally into the excluded stomach, followed by the creation of a percutaneous endoscopic gastrostomy. The gastrostomy tract is then dilated to allow for the placement of a fully covered esophageal self-expanding metal stent (SEMS). A duodenoscope can then be advanced through the stent to perform antegrade ERCP. This has just been described in a single-center case series, however, and has not been widely adopted.[52]

EUS-Directed Transgastric ERCP (EDGE) – This is another option for patients with RYGB (see Chapter 22). It involves the creation of a fistula between the gastric pouch or proximal Roux limb and the excluded stomach under EUS guidance, using a lumen-apposing metal stent (LAMS). A duodenoscope is then inserted orally and advanced through this fistula to the excluded stomach, and the ERCP is completed in the standard manner. There is a risk of acute stent migration when attempting ERCP in the same session that the LAMS is placed, which can lead to a free perforation of both the gastric pouch/roux limb or the excluded stomach. Because of this risk, some centers perform a "staged EDGE" whereby the ERCP is performed in a separate session after placement of the LAMS.[53,54] However, if a single-stage EDGE is desired, such as in cases of acute cholangitis, some investigators have reported success with anchoring the LAMS in place using either an over-the-scope clip (OTSC) or with endoscopic suturing.[55,56] This procedure has technical and clinical success rates ranging from 91% to 100%, with main adverse events being related to bleeding, perforation, and stent dislodgement.[53,57-60] There is also concern for weight regain because of the creation of the gastro-gastric fistula, although weight loss has actually been more common in the short term.[58,61] The fistula often closes spontaneously after removal of the LAMS or can be closed by endosuturing or by using an OVESCO if necessary[53,54]. The EDGE procedure has higher clinical and technical success when compared with enteroscopy-assisted ERCP but does have more adverse events.[62] When compared with the laparoscopic transgastric approach, the EDGE procedure has similar success and adverse event rates but has shortened procedure times and shorter hospital stays.[54,61]

EUS-Directed Transenteric ERCP (EDEE) – This technique has been recently described and involves the creation of an enteroenteric anastomosis to facilitate ERCP in non–RYGB surgical anatomy (e.g., Whipple, hepaticojejunostomy, Bilroth II, and duodenal switch).[63] The pancreaticobiliary limb is first identified either by enteroscopy or via direct EUS puncture from the stomach, duodenum, or jejunum and filled with a solution of contrast, saline, and methylene blue. A target is then identified where the distance between the two luminal walls is less than 1 cm and there are no intervening vascular structures on Doppler. EDEE is then performed using either a 15 mm or 20 mm LAMS. A standard duodenoscope can then be passed through the LAMS to facilitate completion of the ERCP. In

this study, 22% of ERCPs were done in the same session as the LAMS placement but did not demonstrate any increased risk of adverse events compared with those that were done in a separate session. Additionally, despite no stent fixation being done for any of the procedures, there were no occurrences of stent migration. This procedure has technical and clinical success rates of up to 100% and 94.4%, respectively, with an adverse event rate of 5.6%. This procedure provides an additional option to access the pancreaticobiliary region in patients with complicated surgically anatomy in institutions where this expertise is available.

In summary, selection of the appropriate technique for biliary access in patients with surgically altered anatomy should be individualized and would likely involve a combination of methods and endoscopic tools based on patient factors and operator's expertise.

EUS-GUIDED BILIARY ACCESS/DRAINAGE

ERCP success rates for biliary and pancreatic duct decompression can be anywhere from 76% to 98% depending on operator expertise, alterations in anatomy, and the etiology of biliary obstruction (see Chapter 20).[64] Alternative methods of biliary decompression have traditionally included percutaneous transhepatic drainage or surgery (see Chapters 20, 31, 42, and 52). With the advancement of curvilinear-array echoendoscopes and peripheral devices, EUS-guided biliary drainage (EUS-BD) has become increasingly reported either via an intrahepatic (hepaticogastrostomy) or extrahepatic (choledocho-duodenostomy) approach (Fig 30.1A). This approach has been found to have better clinical success outcomes and less adverse events when compared with percutaneous drainage.[65]

EUS-BD has conventionally been used as a second-line therapy when ERCP is unsuccessful.[4,66] Nevertheless, there are increasing reports, including two randomized controlled trials (RCTs), of EUS-BD being used as the primary procedure for biliary decompression with comparable success rates and decreased adverse event rates compared with ERCP.[67,68] In cases of malignant biliary obstruction, these techniques have a pooled technical and clinical success rate of 95% and 97%, respectively, and adverse event rates (mainly biliary peritonitis and cholangitis) of 19%.[69] At this time, given inter-institution variations in access to EUS, it cannot be universally recommended as the initial procedure for biliary decompression.

There are three main EUS-guided techniques: rendezvous, anterograde stenting, and direct transluminal drainage, which are described in detail in the following sections.

Rendezvous Technique

The EUS rendezvous technique was first described by Mallery et al. in 2004 and involves EUS-guided wire placement into the bile duct in an antegrade fashion to facilitate subsequent retrograde biliary cannulation (see Chapter 20).[70] The point of biliary duct entry (intrahepatic vs. extrahepatic) depends on accessibility and which route facilitates wire manipulation. Nevertheless, accessing the extrahepatic bile ducts from the second portion of the duodenum has been associated with a higher success rate.[71] Whether it is through an intrahepatic or extrahepatic approach, a therapeutic linear echoendoscope is used to visualize the bile duct from the stomach or small intestine. Once an avascular plane has been identified using

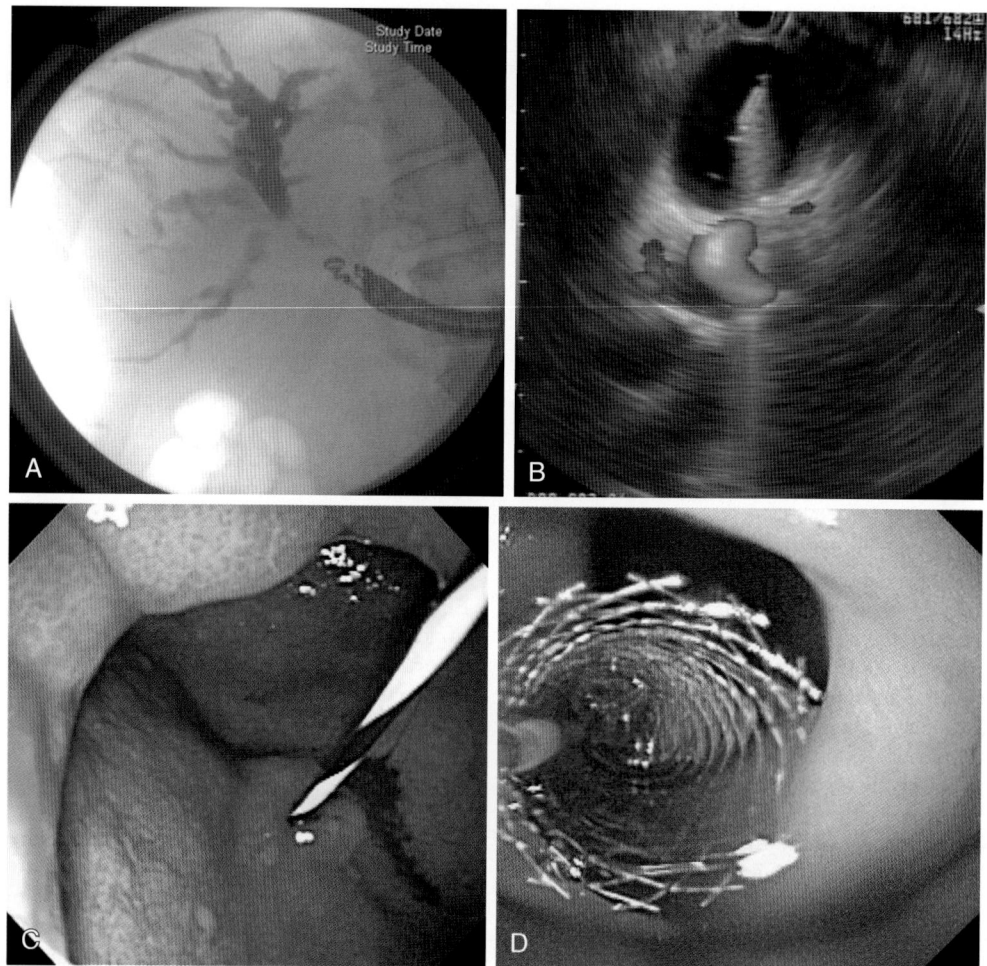

FIGURE 30.1 Endoscopic ultrasound (EUS)–guided biliary drainage. **A,** Cholangiogram showing complete distal bile duct obstruction with diffuse upstream dilation. **B,** The common bile duct is accessed by using an EUS needle. **C,** A guidewire is left across the choledochoduodenostomy. **D,** After dilating the tract, a stent is successfully deployed.

Doppler ultrasonography, an EUS needle is advanced into the bile duct (see Fig 30.1B). Bile is aspirated, and contrast is injected to confirm position inside the bile system. A hydrophilic guidewire is then advanced antegrade through the EUS needle and into the bile duct and manipulated across the papilla. The needle is first exchanged out over the wire, followed by an exchange of the echoendoscope over the wire. The duodenoscope is then inserted transorally adjacent to the indwelling wire and advanced to the duodenum, with visualization of the wire traversing the papilla. The distal end of the indwelling guidewire can be grasped with forceps or snare and withdrawn through the accessory channel, and a cannulation catheter can be backloaded over the guidewire and re-advanced to the papilla. Alternatively, biliary cannulation can be accomplished in the standard retrograde fashion adjacent to the indwelling wire. Overall success and complication rates of the EUS-guided rendezvous technique are quoted as 80% to 86% and 10% to 15%, respectively.[72,73]

Antegrade Biliary Drainage

This technique is useful in cases where conventional or even rendezvous ERCP cannot be performed because of inaccessibility of the papilla (e.g., because of proximal luminal obstruction or altered surgical anatomy, such as in RYGB). Similar to

the previously detailed rendezvous technique, the bile duct is identified and accessed from the stomach or small intestine. The transmural tract is then dilated over the guidewire with either a balloon catheter or bougie to allow anterograde advancement of a stent into the bile system with subsequent deployment across the biliary obstruction and through the papilla. Success rates from various case series range from 57% to 100%, and complication rates range from 0% to 6%.[74,75]

Transluminal Biliary Drainage

In cases where anterograde or rendezvous techniques for transpapillary drainage cannot be accomplished (e.g., impacted biliary calculi, papillary stenosis, and tumor infiltration), an EUS-guided transluminal approach can facilitate biliary decompression.

In the original variations of this procedure, the bile duct was accessed under EUS guidance, with placement of a guidewire similar to described above. The fistula tract was then dilated, and a stent was deployed over the guidewire (see Fig 30.1C and D). This technique was initially performed with plastic stents.[76] It was subsequently performed with SEMS[77] and then LAMS,[78] in an attempt to improve patency and reduce leakage and migration. More recently, with the introduction of electrocautery-enhanced LAMS (ECE-LAMS), this procedure can be reduced to a single step wherein the biliary duct is punctured with the ECE-LAMS system and the stent is deployed without the need for guidewire placement or fistula tract dilation. This procedure has been associated with technical and clinical success rates of 88% to 93% and 97% to 100%, respectively, with overall adverse event rates (mostly mild) of up to 36%.[79-81]

TECHNIQUES FOR THE MANAGEMENT OF CHOLEDOCHOLITHIASIS

Complications of cholelithiasis accounts for over 300,000 hospital admissions annually at a cost of over four billion dollars.[82] Choledocholithiasis is present in 10% to 15% of patients with symptomatic gallstones and can result in significant morbidity and mortality related to biliary obstruction, ascending cholangitis, and pancreatitis.[83] Up to one-third of CBD stones may pass spontaneously, but for those that do not, ERCP with biliary sphincterotomy and stone extraction is considered the first-line management (Fig 30.2A; see Chapter 37).[83-85]

Biliary Sphincterotomy

Endoscopic sphincterotomy (EST) aims at opening the terminal part of the CBD by cutting the papilla and sphincter muscles. The basic technique of sphincterotomy has not changed significantly since its initial description. The standard sphincterotome, the Erlangen "pull-type" model, consists of a catheter containing an electrosurgical cutting wire exposed 20 to 25 mm near the tip of the sphincterotome. The leading tip distal to the wire, the "nose," is five to ten mm in diameter. Once deep biliary cannulation has been achieved, the sphincterotome is retracted slowly, until one-fourth to one-half of the wire length is exposed outside the papilla. The sphincterotome is slightly bowed so the cutting wire is in contact with the roof of the papilla.

The incision is made by upward lifting of the sphincterotome with pressure against the papillary roof, but not excessively, to avoid a rapid large incision ("zipper"; see Fig 30.2B). It is recommended that a current mode with alternating cutting and coagulating phases (e.g., Endocut) be used because this reduces the rates of uncontrolled cutting ("zipper"), PEP, and postsphincterotomy bleeding.[4,86] The size of the sphincterotomy varies on a case-by-case basis and can be limited by the length of the intraduodenal portion of the CBD. In general, the sphincterotomy should be of adequate size to allow the passage of the stone in the CBD. The size of sphincterotomy can be

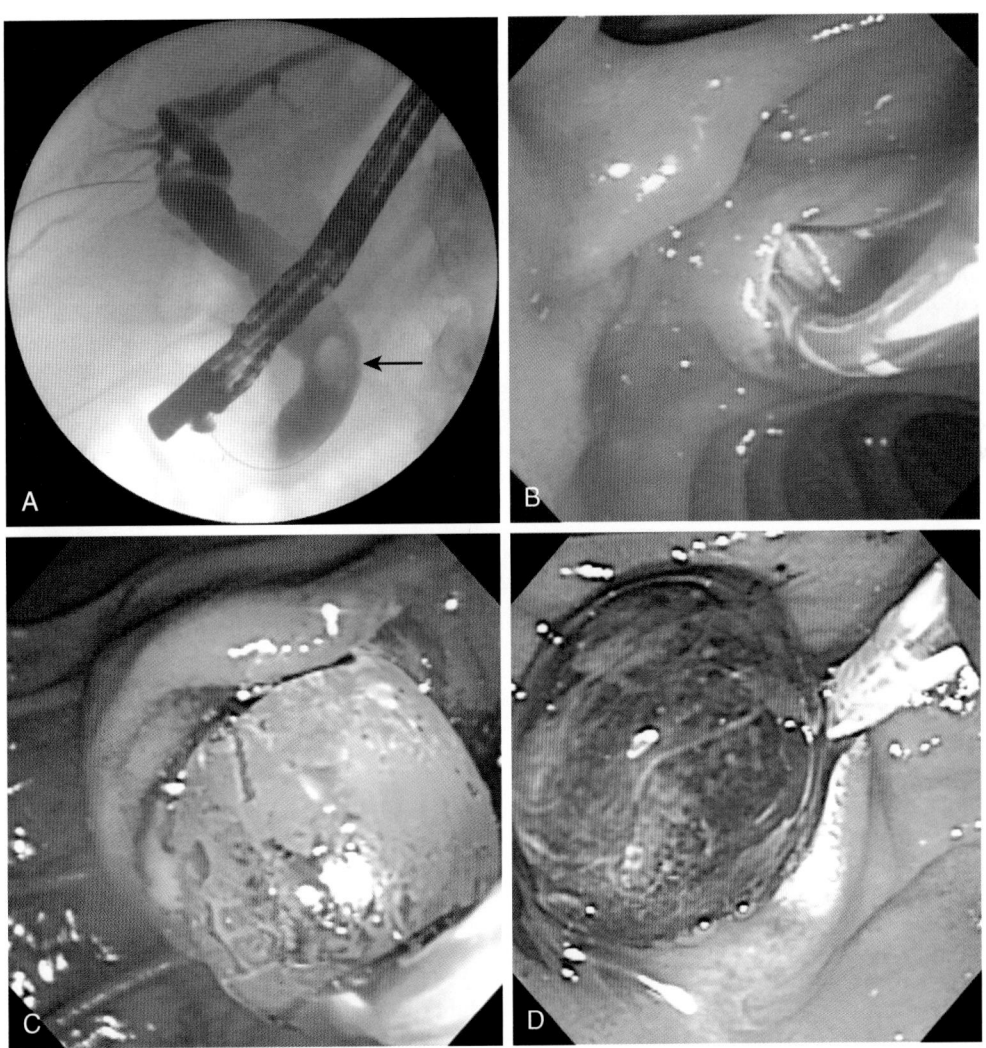

FIGURE 30.2 Endoscopic management of choledocholithiasis. **A,** Cholangiogram showing diffusely dilated biliary system with stone in the common bile duct *(arrow)*. Biliary sphincterotomy **(B),** followed by sphincteroplasty **(C)**. **D,** Extraction of large stone.

gauged by the ability to move the bowed sphincterotome across the opening, by passing an inflated balloon catheter through the site, and/or by eliminating the tapering or "pinch" of the intra-ampullary bile duct seen on fluoroscopy.

Endoscopic Balloon Papillary Dilation

Endoscopic balloon dilation (EBPD; also known as sphinctero-plasty) of the biliary sphincter muscle can be used as an alternative or adjunct to sphincterotomy. The main advantage of sphincteroplasty is that it results in transient widening of the biliary sphincter such that it remains intact and functional after the procedure. This reduces duodenobiliary reflux, which, in turn, reduces cholangitis and stone recurrence. Additionally, because there is no cutting involved, there is a lower risk of procedure-related bleeding. Thus, use of this technique may be preferred to sphincterotomy in patients who are at increased risk of bleeding because of medications or underlying coagulopathy. It can also be helpful in facilitating biliary cannulation in patients with surgically altered anatomy in whom standard sphincterotomy cannot be performed safely or is technically difficult.

Standard EBPD can be used for calculi less than 8 mm in size and involves the dilation of the papilla with a balloon diameter up to 10 mm.[4,87] In this procedure, after selective biliary cannulation and placement of a guidewire in the bile duct, a balloon-tipped catheter (i.e., CRE balloon or Hurricane RX dilation balloon; Boston Scientific, MA) is advanced over the guidewire. The deflated balloon is positioned across the papilla and inflated with radiopaque contrast medium under both endoscopic and fluoroscopic visualization (see Fig. 30.2C). The inflated balloon is maintained until the "waist" corresponding with the biliary sphincter disappears. The optimum time for balloon inflation has not been defined, but longer inflation times (five minutes vs. 1 min) have been associated with increased rates of stone clearance and a decreased risk of PEP.[88,89] It is recommended that this technique be performed with an 8 mm balloon irrespective of the size of the CBD.[4] Earlier approaches to this technique selected balloon sizes that were less than the size of the CBD because of concern for bile duct injury[90]; however, it has been demonstrated that using a standard 8 mm balloon size irrespective of the size of the CBD did not result in any increased risk of perforation. Additionally, use of smaller size balloons has been associated with increased risk of PEP, compared with either larger balloons or ESR.[4]

Endoscopic papillary large balloon dilation (EPLBD) is a modification of this technique for removal of large bile duct stones in which the papilla is dilated with a balloon greater than 10 mm with or without EST.[91,92] For this technique, it is recommended that the balloon size not exceed the size of the distal bile duct because of the risk of perforation.[93] Overall EPLBD has been associated with comparable and even higher rates of stone clearance, with less additional interventions for stone clearance and comparable rates of adverse events compared with EST.[87,94–97] It is recommended that, for large stones, EPLBD should be done after EST because this has been found to have higher rates of complete stone clearance compared with EST alone.[83,85,98,99] Additionally, ELBD has been found to be an effective alternative to and reduces the need for mechanical lithotripsy for large bile duct stone removal.[96,99]

Stone Extraction

Bile duct stone extraction after sphincterotomy or sphinctero-plasty can be performed using either extraction balloon catheters or wire baskets, which are equally effective (>80%–92.3% clinical success rates) and safe (6.6%–11.8% adverse event rates; see Fig. 30.2D).[100–102]

Extraction balloon catheters are available in different sizes (8.5–20 mm) and in most centers are the standard first-line approach for stone extraction, given their ease of use and lack of risk of becoming entrapped within the duct. The extraction balloon is inflated (to the diameter of the bile duct) above the stone and pulled back gently to the level of the papilla. In the setting of multiple stones, it is important to remove the stones individually, starting with the most distal one, to avoid stone impaction.

Similarly, there are also a variety of wire baskets in different sizes and configurations. The stone is entrapped between the wires when the basket is closed, and subsequent removal is achieved by traction removal of the basket in the axis of the bile duct. The effective traction of the wire basket often allows for effective removal of medium to large stones within the CBD or stones that are "floating" within a dilated bile duct and thus easily slip around a balloon.[103] Conversely, the extraction balloon may be more suitable for the removal of small stones/fragments that are difficult to entrap between the wires or when opening of the basket is constrained by duct caliber and has been found to be more efficacious than wire baskets in achieving complete clearance if there are more than four bile duct stones or if they are less than 6 mm.[101,102]

Biliary Stenting

In difficult cases of choledocholithiasis in which the bile duct cannot be completely cleared with the previous techniques, plastic or fully covered SEMS should be placed as a temporizing measure.[83,100] This strategy maintains biliary drainage and is found to reduce the stone burden at subsequent ERCP. This is thought to be because of direct mechanical friction between the stent and the stones, which results in their disintegration, and papillary dilation, which results in their passage.[83,100] It is recommended that these stents be removed or exchanged after two to six months to reduce the risk of cholangitis. These stents inevitably become occluded and as such should not be used as destination therapy for management of bile duct stones.[83,100]

Lithotripsy

Standard stone extraction techniques may fail when a stone is large, impacted, or proximal to a stricture or when stones are multiple. A variety of modalities are currently available to fragment these difficult stones before extraction, including mechanical lithotripsy, endoscopic intraductal lithotripsy, and extracorporeal shock-wave lithotripsy.

Mechanical Lithotripsy

Mechanical lithotripsy has been the most frequently used lithotripsy approach, given its ease of use and availability. It is recommended for difficult stones that have not been able to be cleared with sphincterotomy and EPLBD.[100] Success rates range from 63% to over 90%, depending on CBD size relative to the size of the stone.[97] More than one procedure may be necessary to achieve complete duct clearance.

There are two variations to the technique of mechanical lithotripsy: an external-type lithotripter/out-of-the-scope (OTS) method and an integrated through-the-scope (TTS) method.

The TTS method is recommended for elective cases.[100] Here, a special lithotripsy basket contained within a metal sheath is inserted through the accessory channel of the endoscope. Once the stone is captured within the basket, forceful traction on the wires against the metal sheath results in stone fragmentation.[104]

The OTS method is used as a "salvage" method when a standard basket engages a large stone and becomes lodged at the papilla.[100] In this method, the stone is captured within a standard Dormia basket, the basket handle is cut off, and the endoscope is removed. A coiled metal sheath is inserted over the wire until its tip is in contact with the stone, and mechanical lithotripsy is performed by turning the crank handle, crushing the stone between the basket wires and the metal tip of the sheath.[104]

The most common adverse events include PEP, hemorrhage, basket entrapment, basket wire rupture, traction wire fracture, or a broken handle and can occur in up to 13% of cases.[105] Other types of lithotripsy, sphincterotomy extension, or stenting are options for management of these complications. The most common reason for failure is large stones exceeding 3 cm in size.[105]

Endoscopic Intraductal Lithotripsy

Intraductal shock-wave lithotripsy is an alternative modality for the fragmentation of refractory calculi. It can be performed with fluoroscopic guidance only but is preferably performed under direct visualization via cholangioscopy. The two methods used to accomplish this are electrohydraulic lithotripsy (EHL) and laser lithotripsy (LL). They both involve irrigation of the bile duct with a saline solution and the generation of shock waves through this fluid medium, which shatter the calculi. The fragments are then removed by standard methods.[104]

In **electrohydraulic lithotripsy (EHL),** a bipolar electrode probe is positioned about one to two mm from the stone. A charge is transmitted across the electrodes, which creates a spark. This, in turn, causes expansion of the surrounding fluid, which generates a shock wave, which shatters the intraductal stones.[104]

Laser lithotripsy (LL) is based on the principle of transforming optical energy into mechanical energy. In LL, focusing the high-power density laser light on the surface of the calculi results in the transformation of matter into a plasma state, which is a gaseous collection of ions and free electrons. Subsequently, the plasma expands, inducing an oscillation wave with tensile/compressive forces that create cavitation of the stone surface and ultimately shatter the stone.[104]

Intraductal lithotripsy is associated with better rates of duct clearance compared with conventional therapies, including mechanical lithotripsy, with success rates upwards of 90%.[105–110] Although both modalities are efficacious and head-to-head RCTs are lacking, LL may be more successful at duct clearance than EHL.[108] Adverse events occurred in up to 11.3% of cases and were mainly because of cholangitis, pancreatitis, and hemorrhage and may be higher in EHL than LL.[105,107–109]

Extracorporeal Shock-Wave Lithotripsy

Extracorporeal shock-wave lithotripsy (ESWL) can be considered when conventional techniques have failed and intraductal lithotripsy is not feasible.[100] It involves initial placement of a nasobiliary tube by interventional radiology to aid with stone visualization. Under ultrasound or fluoroscopic guidance, high pressure electrohydraulic or electromagnetic energy is delivered to the liquid medium in the bile duct, which generate shock waves and results in stone fragmentation.[84,104] Multiple ESWL sessions are generally required and final duct clearance rates range from 60% to 90%.[84,111] ERCP may have to be performed after ESWL for stone fragment removal. Adverse events, including hemobilia, cholangitis, pancreatitis, and cardiac arrhythmias, have been reported in 9% to 35% of cases.[100] Additionally, recurrence of bile duct stones have occurred in up to 20% of patients.[112] The need for ESWL has decreased as the effectiveness of intraductal lithotripsy has improved, with several studies suggesting superior ductal clearance and fewer treatment sessions with LL compared with ESWL.[100,108]

TECHNIQUES FOR THE MANAGEMENT OF BILIARY STRICTURES

ERCP with stenting is a well-standardized technique commonly used to relieve biliary obstruction secondary to both benign and malignant disease. The goal is to relieve the biliary obstruction that can potentially lead to complications, such as jaundice, pruritus, cholangitis, chronic liver disease, and liver failure. Biliary stricture characterization can be a diagnostic challenge that requires a multidisciplinary approach with the integration of laboratory testing, noninvasive, and invasive imaging, and tissue sampling methods. This section focuses on the technical aspects and outcomes associated with endoscopic management of benign and malignant biliary strictures. Advances in endoscopic imaging and tissue sampling for the diagnosis of biliary strictures will be covered later in this chapter.

Types of Biliary Stents

Plastic Stents

Plastic biliary stents are composed of polyethylene, polyurethane, or Teflon. Stent diameter and length range from 5Fr to 12Fr and 5 to 18 cm, respectively.[113] Plastic stents are available in a variety of configurations: straight, angled, curved, with flaps (flanged), or coiled at one or both ends (single or double pigtail) for anchorage. All plastic stents are radiopaque, some with additional markers at the proximal and distal end of the stents to facilitate visualization under fluoroscopy. Insertion is via a push catheter over a guidewire. Duration of stent patency is largely dependent on the size of the inner diameter, with 10Fr and larger stents remaining patent, on average, for approximately three months, and stent occlusion developing secondary to bacterial colonization, sludge, tissue debris, or bilioduodenal reflux.[114] Shorter patency times may be observed in patients undergoing chemotherapy for pancreatic adenocarcinoma.[114]

Self-Expandable Metal Stents

SEMS are composed of stainless steel or a variety of metal alloys, such as nitinol (nickel and titanium combination) or platinol (platinum core with nitinol encasement). This material is malleable, which allows the SEMS to adapt to many configurations without compromising radial expansile force. SEMS are configured into a cylinder by interwoven wires and are deployed from a constrained position within a delivery catheter. Stent diameter and length vary from 6 mm to 10 mm and 4 to 12 cm, respectively.[113] The larger stent diameter compared with plastic stents results in increased duration of stent patency (on average, six–12 months). SEMS can be covered, partially covered, or uncovered. The covering consists of a silicone, polycaprolactone, polyether polyurethane, polyurethane,

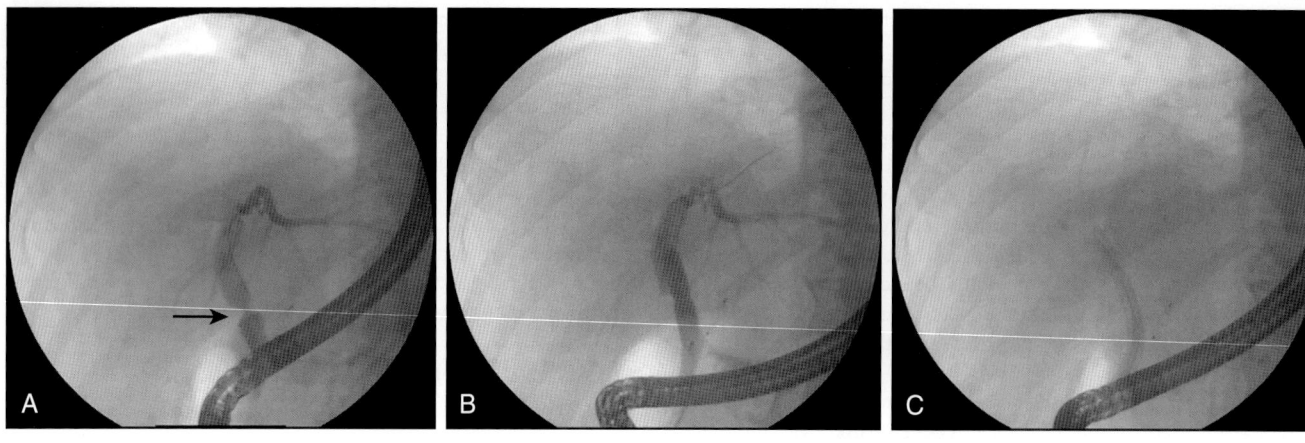

FIGURE 30.3   A, Cholangiogram showing a benign biliary anastomotic stricture *(arrow)* after orthotopic liver transplantation. Balloon dilation across the stricture **(B),** followed by placement of three plastic biliary stents **(C).**

TABLE 30.1 Etiologies of Biliary Strictures	
BENIGN ETIOLOGIES	**MALIGNANT ETIOLOGIES**
Iatrogenic (postoperative)	Pancreas carcinoma
Cholecystectomy	Cholangiocarcinoma
Biliary anastomosis	Ampullary carcinoma
Chronic pancreatitis	Gallbladder carcinoma
Autoimmune pancreatitis	Hepatocellular carcinoma
Primary sclerosing cholangitis	Metastasis
Autoimmune sclerosing cholangiopathy	
Ischemic	
Vasculitis	
Infectious (viral, parasitic, HIV cholangiopathy, tuberculosis)	
Radiation therapy	
Postsphincterotomy	
Portal biliopathy	
Abdominal trauma	

HIV, Human immunodeficiency virus.

or expanded polytetra-fluoroethylene fluorinated ethylene propylene lining.[113] Covering reduces tumor or hyperplastic tissue ingrowth but is associated with a higher migration rate compared with uncovered metal stents because of decreased tissue anchoring.[114] Partial or fully covered SEMS can typically be removed or repositioned, whereas uncovered stents are difficult to remove because of tumor ingrowth or benign tissue hyperplasia.[113]

Endoscopic Management of Benign Biliary Strictures

There are numerous etiologies of benign biliary strictures. Many cases of benign biliary strictures are secondary to postoperative iatrogenic injury, after cholecystectomy or at the site of a biliary anastomosis after biliary surgery or liver transplantation (Fig 30.3A). Benign biliary strictures may also result from ischemic injury and/or inflammatory processes such as primary sclerosing cholangitis or chronic pancreatitis (Table 30.1; see Chapter 42). Comprehensive evaluation of a biliary stricture and its etiology should always be sought before any therapeutic endoscopic intervention so as to rule out any underlying malignant etiology. Magnetic resonance cholangiopancreatography (MRCP) is a noninvasive imaging modality that can accurately delineate the biliary anatomy, site, and length of the

biliary stricture and thus provide useful information for ERCP planning[115] (see Chapter 16).

Endoscopic Technique

ERCP with stricture dilation and biliary stenting is currently recommended as the first-line intervention for the management of biliary strictures[116,117] (see Chapter 39B). It is performed after a detailed assessment of the type and site of the biliary stricture. The key technical step is to negotiate the stricture and achieve biliary access with the use of a guidewire. This process can be challenging, and the use of different sizes and types of hydrophilic guidewires in addition to guidewire manipulation with steerable catheters or sphincterotomes is often necessary. Although not required in all cases, biliary sphincterotomy may need to be performed to facilitate subsequent therapy, including stricture dilation and stent placement.

Stricture Dilation

Stricture dilation can be performed using push-type dilation catheters (bougies) or hydrostatic balloons (range, 4–10 mm in diameter) when the stricture is not amenable to mechanical dilation. The balloon is inflated with diluted contrast material to the maximum atmospheric pressure allowable and is kept inflated until the stricture "waist" is obliterated, generally after 30 to 60 seconds (see Fig. 30.3B). Dilation can be safely performed to a diameter 1 to 2 mm larger than the downstream bile duct diameter, but caution must be exercised in anastomotic strictures that are less than four weeks old.[117] Depending on the etiology, stricture dilation alone is associated with high restricturing rates, and thus stent placement is often pivotal in maintaining patency.[117,118] One exception is for primary sclerosing cholangitis (PSC), where serial dilation alone may provide adequate therapeutic benefit.[119,120]

Biliary Stenting

Two types of stents can be used: plastic and covered SEMS (cSEMS). For plastic stents, placement of a single plastic stent has poor outcomes for resolving benign biliary strictures. Instead, it is recommended that multiple side-by-side plastic stents be placed during the index ERCP (number and caliber of stents limited by size of the bile duct and stricture; see Fig. 30.3C).[121] These can be sequentially exchanged with additional stents placed each time, usually at three month intervals for up to 12 months.

Alternatively, a single cSEMS can be placed and exchanged periodically until stricture resolution is achieved (see Fig. 30.2C).[116] It is important to highlight that placement of a fully covered SEMS (FCSEMS) may potentially block drainage of a neighboring duct (including the cystic duct); thus these stents are preferably restricted to distal bile duct strictures and must be used cautiously in patients with an in situ gallbladder because mechanical obstruction of the cystic duct and resultant cholecystitis may ensue.[122–124] It must be noted, however, that concomitant obstruction of the cystic duct by tumor or the presence of gallstones may be stronger predictors of cholecystitis than stent type alone.[122,125]

Both stents have demonstrated similar efficacy with stricture resolution rates of up to 95% in plastic and 100% for cSEMS and recurrence rates of up to 20% across multiple etiologies of benign strictures.[56,126–133] Nevertheless, cSEMS have the ability to exert greater radial force, which results in more sustained stricture dilation, and require fewer stent exchanges when compared with plastic stents.[56,127,128,134] Recurrence rates may be higher in chronic pancreatitis than in anastomosis or surgical strictures.[135] Adverse events occurred in up to 23% and were mainly because of stent migration or occlusion. The importance of compliance with stent exchanges must be emphasized to patients to reduce the risk of stent occlusion and resulting cholangitis.[121]

To date, the ideal number of stents, the type of stent, and the duration of stent placement for benign stricture resolution remain highly debated and often vary on a case-by-case basis.

Endoscopic Management of Malignant Biliary Strictures

Malignant biliary obstruction is most frequently seen in the setting of pancreaticobiliary malignancy, but it can also be because of many other etiologies (see Table 30.1). When indicated, endoscopic therapy is considered the mainstay therapy for biliary decompression. A careful multidisciplinary review of the indication and appropriateness of any endoscopic intervention should be sought before any procedure.

Preoperative Biliary Drainage

The routine need for preoperative biliary decompression in patients with resectable pancreaticobiliary disease remains controversial (see Chapters 50–51B and 62). From a technical standpoint, the placement of a short plastic or metal biliary stent does not appear to interfere with subsequent pancreaticoduodenectomy.[136,137] However, meta-analyses of the current literature indicate that routine preoperative biliary drainage may be associated with increased postoperative complications (in particular, wound infection) when compared with patients who proceed directly to surgery.[138,139] As such, routine preoperative biliary drainage in patients with resectable malignant obstruction is not recommended and should be reserved for cholangitis, severe symptomatic jaundice, and pre-neoadjuvant chemotherapy and in cases of delayed surgery.[140–143] If stenting is required for these reasons, the shortest-length FCSEMS has been recommended because these were associated with better patency rates and lower infection rates and did not interfere with subsequent pancreaticoduodenectomy if indicated.[136,141,144] A more recent prospective multicenter RCT, however, suggests that uncovered SEMS (UCSEMS) and FCSEMS have similar success rates despite prior concerns of tumor in growth in UCSEMS. Stent lengths of 6 and 8 cm were found to have longer patency times than 4 cm.[143] Additional multicenter trials are

needed to further validate these findings. It must be noted that if the definitive diagnosis and/or staging of the biliary stricture is not certain, an UCSEMS should not be placed because it has poor long-term patency and removal is difficult.[140] Plastic biliary stents or a FCSEMS can be placed for biliary decompression while workup is completed.

Palliative Biliary Drainage of Distal Bile Duct Obstruction

Distal malignant biliary obstructions are typically defined as those distal to the cystic duct insertion, although this definition is suboptimal, given the substantial anatomic variability of the cystic duct insertion site. Therapeutic options include surgical bypass, percutaneous decompression, and endoscopic stenting. A large meta-analysis of 2,436 patients demonstrated that endoscopic stenting was associated with a lower risk of procedural complications than traditional surgical bypass.[145] A large meta-analysis of 20 RCTs, which included 1,713 patients, demonstrated improved stent patency for distal biliary obstruction with SEMS versus plastic stents.[146] In light of this, SEMS are recommended over plastic stents for the treatment of distal malignant bile duct obstruction.[140] In terms of what type of SEMS is superior, a meta-analysis of 11 RCTs demonstrated no difference in stent failure or mortality between cSEMS and UCSEMS. There was a higher rate of migration and sludge with cSEMS, whereas tumor ingrowth was more likely with UCSEMS.[147] Ultimately, the optimal stent choice depends on various factors, including establishment of diagnosis, need for reinterventions, operator's expertise, cost analysis, and the patient's life expectancy.[143]

Palliative Biliary Drainage of Proximal Bile Duct Obstruction (Hilar)

Malignant biliary obstructions at the biliary confluence can be technically challenging (see Chapter 51B). The extent of the biliary obstruction is commonly classified based on the modified Bismuth-Corlette classification and can be summarized as follows: Bismuth type I strictures involve the proximal common hepatic duct (CHD) but not the confluence of the left and right ductal systems, type II involves the confluence but spares the segmental hepatic ducts, type IIIa and IIIb involve either the right or left segmental hepatic ducts, respectively, whereas both segmental hepatic ducts are involved in type IV.[148] Biliary drainage with stent placement can be particularly difficult in those with advanced complex strictures (Bismuth type II and above). Evaluation with noninvasive imaging (i.e., MRCP) to delineate the anatomy is mandatory for preprocedural planning and helps limit contrast injection during the ERCP and the risk of contaminating undrainable segments. Furthermore, evaluation of the side of the liver (i.e., lack of atrophy, patent portal vein branch, and lack of extensive segmental biliary involvement) that will provide biliary drainage to the most functional parenchyma is critical. It is of utmost importance that the best approach (including percutaneous approaches) be evaluated in a multidisciplinary review.

In patients with strictures that do not involve the confluence of the right and left hepatic ducts (Bismuth type I), adequate biliary drainage is often achieved by placing a single biliary stent. Controversy exists as to whether both lobes of the liver need to be drained when a bifurcation lesion obstructs both lobes. The main determining factor associated with effective drainage is the liver volume to be drained. Drainage of 50% of the liver volume has been found to represent effective biliary drainage and is associated with improved median survival.[149–151] Thus the goal of endoscopic therapy should be directed at achieving drainage volume greater than 50%, irrespective of whether unilateral or multisegmental stenting is performed.[140]

Both unilateral and bilateral stents may have similar technical success rates, although bilateral metal stent placement has been found to have decreased need for reintervention and improved symptom-free stent patency.[152–154] However, a recent multicenter retrospective study found a higher rate of adverse events (PEP, bleeding, perforation, and cholangitis) and death with bilateral compared with unilateral stent placement.[155] Given these potential benefits and risks, it is important to individualize the decision on stent placement based on the patient's anatomy and clinical scenario.

Several studies have suggested that an SEMS is preferable to a plastic stent, based on higher rates of successful drainage, prolonged patency, and prolonged survival and lower rates of complications.[156,157] The use of UCSEMS is preferred for proximal malignant biliary strictures because placement of a covered stent can potentially obstruct drainage of adjacent ducts.[140] For stent implantation, a guidewire is advanced across the malignant stricture into the duct preselected for drainage (Fig 30.4A). After wire placement, if necessary, dilation of a tight stricture can be performed with a balloon catheter or bougie (see Fig 30.4B). A sphincterotomy is not necessary when the distal ends of the stents are positioned within the duct, which may reduce the risk of poststenting cholangitis. On the other hand, stent revision is technically less demanding and more accessible when the distal end of the stents protrude out of the papilla (see Fig 30.4C). Regardless of stent positioning, all patients who undergo endoscopic therapy for these complex strictures should receive prophylactic antibiotics.

In summary, endoscopic stenting of proximal biliary obstruction is challenging. Preprocedural cross-sectional imaging and multidisciplinary review is essential in the selection of the target parenchyma for drainage and the optimal approach (percutaneous vs. endoscopic). If endoscopic approaches are favored, this planning will, in turn, help maximize biliary drainage by targeting the dominant biliary systems, limit the use of contrast during the procedure, and avoid intubating atrophic segments or areas that cannot be effectively drained.

Adjunctive Therapies for Biliary Strictures

In addition to stenting, a few adjunctive therapies are available to remodel and treat the stricture, which can have implications on stent patency, quality of life, and survival.

Photodynamic Therapy

Photodynamic therapy (PDT) is based on the ability of photosensitizers to generate cytotoxic oxygen species in the target tissue upon exposure to light of an appropriate wavelength. Photosensitizing agents (sodium porfimer or aminolaevulinic acid) are injected intravenously preprocedurally, and ERCP is subsequently performed two to four days thereafter. A catheter with a quartz fiber coupled with a diode laser emitting a wavelength of 630 nm is inserted into the bile duct through the accessory channel of the endoscope. The catheter is directed against the photosensitized malignant cells, causing tumor cell death by the generation of oxygen-free radicals. This procedure can also be done under direct visualization via cholangioscopy.[158]

A meta-analysis of six studies, which included 170 patients, as well as subsequent retrospective studies have demonstrated improved survival (Weighted mean difference [WMD] 265 days; 95% confidence interval [CI]: 154–376; $P = .01$; $I(2) = 65\%$) and improved quality of life as measured by Karnofsky scores (WMD 7.74; 95% CI: 3.73–11.76; $P = .01$; $I(2) = 14\%$) with PDT with stenting compared with stenting alone.[159,160] The main adverse effects of PDT are cholangitis, which can be seen in up to 50% of patients, and photosensitivity.[159,160]

Radiofrequency Ablation

Radiofrequency ablation (RFA) relies on the generation of high-frequency alternating electromagnetic energy resulting in thermal injury to the target tissue. A variety of RFA probes designed to be used with an ERCP scope are commercially available. The probe is inserted into the working channel of the duodenoscope and advanced into the bile duct over a guidewire. Unlike PDT, ERCP-guided RFA requires direct contact of the probe with the malignant stricture. Upon correct positioning of the probe under fluoroscopy, the probe is activated and the ablative energy is delivered directly to the target tissue, resulting in local coagulative necrosis.[161]

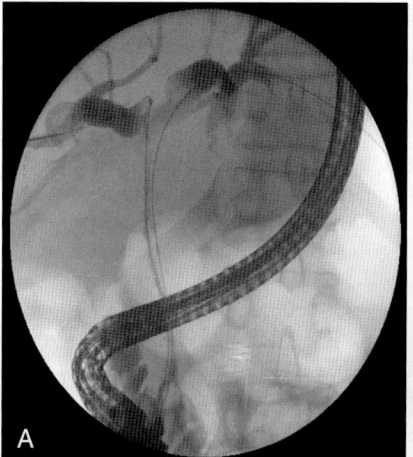 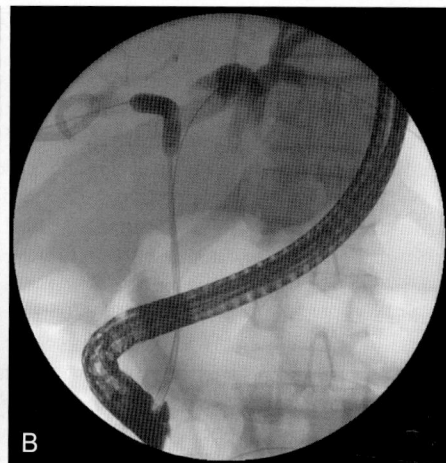 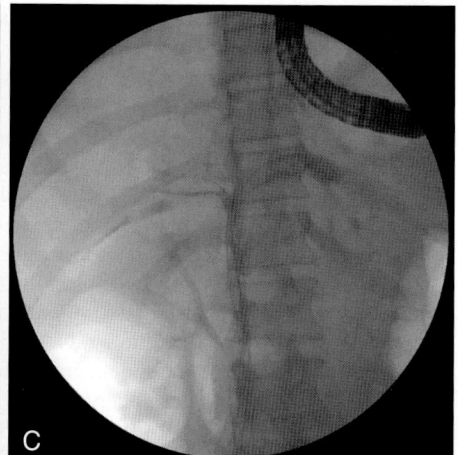

FIGURE 30.4 A, Cholangiogram showing a type IIIb malignant hilar obstruction with upstream dilation of the right and left hepatic ducts. Balloon dilation across the stricture **(B)** and placement of bilateral uncovered metal biliary stents to drain both lobes of the liver **(C)**.

Recent studies have confirmed the safety and efficacy of RFA as an adjunct to SEMS in patients with a malignant biliary stricture. A meta-analysis of nine observational studies, including 505 patients, demonstrated that the addition of RFA to biliary stenting was safe and resulted in longer stent patency times with pooled WMD in stent patency of 50.6 days (95% CI, 32.83–68.48) favoring patients receiving RFA and improved survival (hazard ratio [HR] 1.395; 95% CI, 1.145–1.7; $P < .001$).[162] RFA was also found to have similar survival to patients treated with PDT with a median survival of 9.6 versus 7.5 months, respectively ($P = .799$).[163] Further studies, including RCTs, over a longer period are needed to validate these preliminary findings.

TECHNIQUES FOR THE MANAGEMENT OF BILE LEAKS

Bile leak is a well-known complication from injury to the biliary tree, either secondary to trauma or iatrogenic after laparoscopic cholecystectomy, liver resection, or transplantation (see Chapter 28). Bile leaks can be classified as either high grade or low grade. High-grade leaks demonstrate rapid extravasation of contrast during cholangiogram, whereas low-grade leaks exhibit contrast extravasation only after near complete intraductal filling has occurred (Fig 30.5A). The aim of endoscopic therapy is to decrease the transpapillary pressure gradient, thus favoring transpapillary bile flow rather than extravasation at the site of the leak.

This can be achieved by performing a biliary sphincterotomy, placing a transpapillary biliary stent, or both. In most instances, placement of a plastic biliary stent (7Fr or 10Fr) is sufficient without the need of a sphincterotomy and its potential associated risks[164] (see Fig. 30.5B). Nevertheless, both stenting alone and stenting with sphincterotomy demonstrated superior outcomes when compared with sphincterotomy alone.[165,166] It is not necessary to place the proximal end of the stent beyond the site of the leak because reduction of the pressure inside the duct alone is generally sufficient. Typically, the stent is left in place for approximately four to six weeks. Various studies have reported endoscopic success rates for the management of bile leaks between 70% to 100%, with high-grade leaks being associated with lower success rates.[167,168] In the minority of cases in which the bile leak is refractory to endoscopic therapy with plastic stent placement and/or sphincterotomy, upsizing the stent or placing multiple plastic stents (MPS) can be performed in subsequent sessions until resolution is documented.[167] An alternative to this is to temporarily place a single FCSEMS, which has been shown to be an effective rescue therapy for refractory bile leaks and may be superior to MPS.[140,169,170]

It should be noted that, in the presence of a perihepatic bile collection, endoscopic stenting alone does not result in the reabsorption of the established biloma. Thus symptomatic bilomas will need to be drained percutaneously. An output of less than 10 mL per day through a percutaneous drain is associated with bile leak resolution and can be used as a surrogate indicator for stent removal. Successful EUS-guided transenteric/transgastric drainage of bilomas with SEMS has been described, but additional prospective studies are required for validation.[171]

ENDOSCOPIC MANAGEMENT OF AMPULLARY ADENOMAS

Ampullary adenomas are dysplastic glandular lesions that arise from either the major or minor duodenal papilla (see Chapter 63). These lesions can occur sporadically or arise in the context of genetic syndromes, such as familial adenomatous polyposis (FAP). If not removed, ampullary adenomas can undergo malignant transformation to ampullary cancer, with a reported incidence from 25% to 85%.[172] With advances in therapeutic endoscopy, endoscopic ampullectomy/papillectomy has become an acceptable alternative therapy to surgery for ampullary adenomas.[173]

Diagnosis and Local Staging

Before endoscopic ampullectomy, preoperative assessment with both a forward- and side-viewing endoscope is routinely performed to further characterize the lesion. Endoscopic findings, including spontaneous bleeding, friability, ulceration, and induration, are often associated with malignant lesions. Biopsies obtained during endoscopy can assess for dysplasia or unsuspected

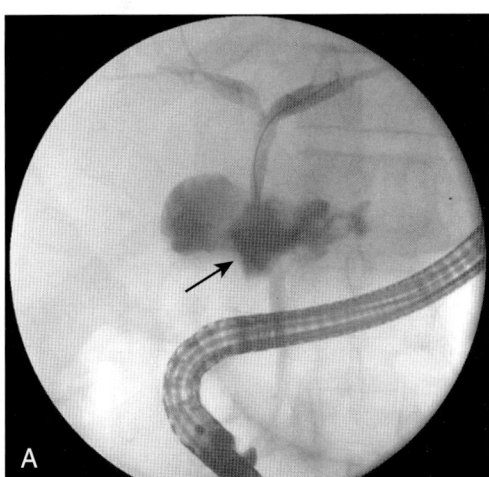
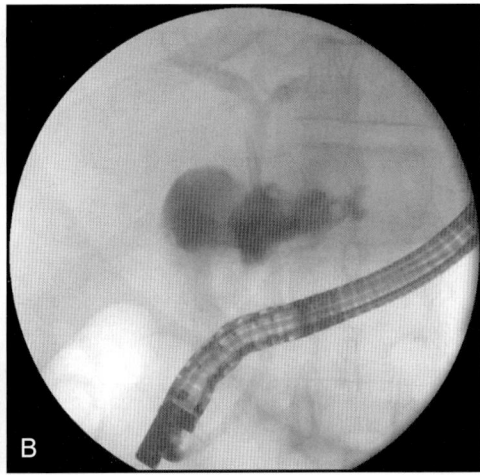

FIGURE 30.5 A, Cholangiogram showing contrast extravasation *(arrow)* at the biliary anastomosis in a patient after liver transplantation, consistent with bile leak. **B,** Bile leak treated by placing a plastic stent across the biliary anastomosis.

carcinoma, although malignancy may be missed in up to 30% of tumors when forceps biopsy specimens are obtained.[174,175] Hence, other advanced imaging modalities, including narrow-band imaging, confocal laser endomicroscopy, and high-definition white light endoscopy, have been proposed as complementary techniques to help predict histologic characteristics of ampullary lesions, but further multicenter trials are needed to validate these techniques.[176]

EUS has been shown to be superior to computed tomography (CT), angiography, and magnetic resonance imaging (MRI) for local tumor staging, including assessment of the size of lesion and involvement/infiltration of the periampullary wall layers, the CBD, and the pancreatic duct, in addition to identification of malignant periampullary lymph nodes.[177] When performed, EUS can help stratify which lesions are amenable to endoscopic ampullectomy. ERCP with both biliary and pancreatic duct evaluation, and intraductal ultrasound (IDUS) can also aid in the detection of tumor extension into either ductal system. Many experts agree that smaller lesions (<1 cm) without suspicious signs of malignancy (ulceration, spontaneous bleeding, biopsies positive for high-grade dysplasia or carcinoma) may not require EUS evaluation before endoscopic resection.[177]

Endoscopic Therapy

Endoscopic ampullectomy (papillectomy) can be considered once malignancy has been reasonably excluded. This procedure is performed with the standard monopolar diathermic snare used for colon polypectomy. The aim of endoscopic excision is to obtain complete removal of the ampullary lesion, preferably en bloc (Fig. 30.6A and B). When performing this technique, it is common for the intra-ampullary portions of the CBD and pancreatic duct to be removed as well. Submucosal injection is not routinely recommended because the center of the ampullary lesion is generally tethered down by the bile and pancreatic duct. Thus submucosal injection may actually raise the surrounding mucosa, create a depressed center ("valley effect"), and interfere with en bloc excision and subsequent attempts at bile and pancreatic duct access.[177]

For most ampullary lesions, the tip of the snare is positioned against the wall of the duodenum at the superior aspect of the mass. The snare is then slowly opened, and the snare catheter advanced slowly to allow the open snare to drape downward over the lesion encircling it. Once achieved, the snare is slowly closed while simultaneously advancing the snare catheter toward the base of the lesion, followed by polypectomy. Thermal therapy (i.e., argon plasma coagulation, monopolar and bipolar coagulation, neodymium:yttrium-aluminum-garnet laser) can be used to fulgurate any residual tissue after piecemeal or incomplete resection, with caution to avoid excessive tissue destruction around the biliary and pancreatic duct orifices.[177] Additionally, in cases where there is intraductal extension, intraductal RFA or ablation with a cystotome has demonstrated high therapeutic success rates, even in malignant neoplasms.[178,179]

A meta-analysis of 29 studies including 1,751 patients demonstrated a pooled complete resection rate of 94.2%. Adverse events occurred in 24.9% of them, with the majority being because of PEP (11.9%). Follow-up ranged from 9.6 to 84.5 months and demonstrated recurrence in 11.8% of patients.[180]

Prophylactic pancreatic stenting is recommended after an ampullectomy because it has been found to reduce the risk of PEP.[177,180] Whether ERCP with pancreatic and biliary sphincterotomy/stent placement is performed preresection or postresection often depends on the endoscopist's preference (see Fig 30.6C). Because identification of the pancreatic orifice after ampullectomy can be challenging, some endoscopists favor performing pancreatography with iodinated contrast diluted with methylene blue or indigo carmine before resection. The blue-stained pancreatic orifice can theoretically be more readily identified adjacent to the bile-stained biliary orifice, and thus facilitate postresection cannulation.[177] Prophylactic biliary sphincterotomy and/or stenting is neither widely performed nor uniformly recommended unless there is concern for inadequate biliary drainage after ampullectomy.[177]

Patients who have undergone endoscopic ampullectomy should undergo routine surveillance, given the risk of recurrence.[177] Endoscopic surveillance should be performed with a side-viewing duodenoscope; the timing interval and duration of surveillance is dependent on several factors, including histology and margin status of resected specimen, history of FAP, and the patient's age and comorbidities. Furthermore, any specimen with unexpected malignancy should be referred for surgical consultation.

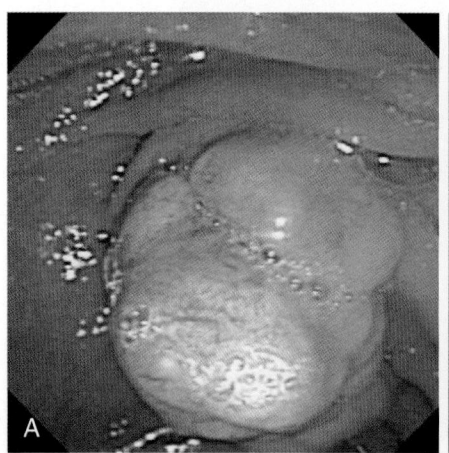 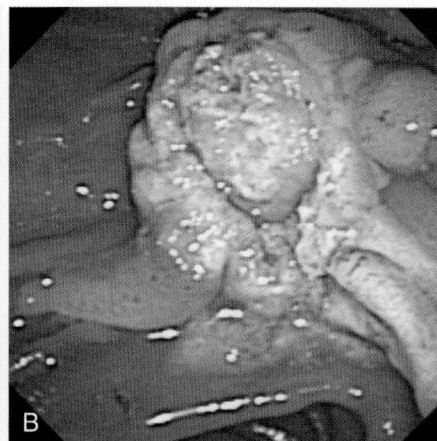 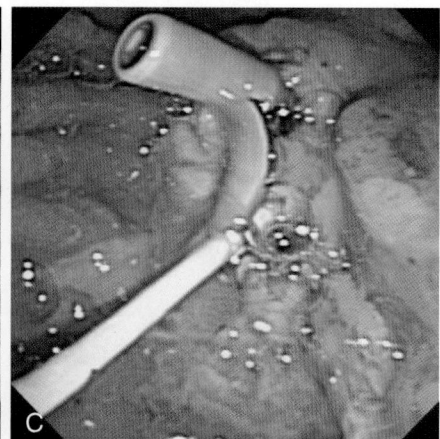

FIGURE 30.6 Endoscopic ampullectomy. **A,** Ampullary adenoma. Ampullectomy with en bloc resection **(B),** followed by biliary and pancreatic duct stenting **(C).**

Endoscopic Biliary Tissue Acquisition and Advanced Imaging Techniques

The role of ERCP as a diagnostic tool has significantly diminished with the advent of multiple noninvasive imaging tests of the biliary system, including high-resolution CT and MRCP. One notable exception to this trend is the need for ERCP with tissue sampling in suspected malignant biliary obstruction.

Biliary Tissue Acquisition and Analysis

Intraductal Brushings

Intraductal brushing during ERCP is the standard first-line approach for tissue acquisition of biliary strictures, primarily because of wide availability and technical feasibility. The technique involves advancing the sheathed cytology brush over a guidewire into the bile duct to the proximal end of the stricture. The brush is then advanced out the catheter, and multiple to and fro movements are performed with the brush across the stricture for approximately 10 passes. The brush is then withdrawn into the catheter and removed as a unit, which has been shown to improve diagnosis.[173] Repeated brushing with consecutive brushes may increase diagnostic yield.[181]

The diagnostic yield of brush cytology for biliary strictures is low, with a meta-analysis of 16 studies demonstrating sensitivities ranging from 6% to 64%.[173] The poor sensitivity of brush cytology has often been attributed to sampling error and low cellular yield because of the scirrhous nature of cholangiocarcinoma and because pancreatic adenocarcinomas frequently cause only extrinsic compression of the distal bile duct, rather than frank invasion.

Biliary Intraductal Biopsies

Endobiliary forceps biopsy during ERCP is an alternate technique routinely used for tissue sampling of biliary strictures. A variety of flexible forceps are available in adult (7Fr) and pediatric (5Fr to 6Fr) calibers. Similar to other accessories, the forceps can be advanced into the bile duct. A prior sphincterotomy may facilitate this process but is not essential in the presence of an indwelling guidewire in the biliary system.[182,183] Although previous studies have suggested that tissue sampling with forceps provided the highest yield for detection of malignancy, a recent meta-analysis indicates that both brushings and biopsy are comparable and have limited sensitivity (pooled sensitivity of 45% and 48%, respectively).[184] A combination of both of these techniques leads to only a moderate improvement in sensitivity of 59.4%.[184]

A major advancement in the ability to evaluate and sample biliary strictures is the development of digital cholangioscopy devices that allow for direct visualization of the stricture and targeted cholangioscopy-guided tissue biopsies. This modality is currently the most high yield in the evaluation of indeterminate biliary strictures. A detailed discussion is included in the following section of this chapter.

Molecular Analysis of Tissue Samples

Chromosomal abnormalities are typically seen in malignant biliary strictures, and there are various techniques to assess this, with the goal of improving diagnostic sensitivity when compared with conventional histocytopathology.

Flow cytometry has been commonly used to identify aneuploidy in tissue specimens. Older data have shown that flow cytometry for DNA evaluation yields improved sensitivity (42%) but at the expense of lower specificity of 70% and 77% for the diagnosis of malignant biliary strictures.[185] Furthermore, flow cytometric analysis requires large cellular samples, which can be challenging with current endoscopic tissue sampling techniques. As a result of these limitations, flow cytometry is less frequently used in the analysis of biliary specimens.[186]

Digital image analysis (DIA) is another technique that had been investigated to increase the diagnostic yield of routine cytology. DIA uses a computer assessment to quantify DNA content, chromatin distribution, and nuclear morphology to assess for aneuploidy. In a single-center prospective study, DIA had a higher sensitivity (39%) compared with routine cytology (18%), albeit with a significantly lower specificity (77% vs. 98%, respectively).[187] For patients with negative cytology and histology who were later proven to have malignancy, however, DIA identifies the diagnosis of malignancy in only 14% of cases.[188] With these shortcomings in diagnosis and improvements in other techniques such as FISH (fluorescent in-situ hybridization), DIA is used less commonly.[186]

FISH is a cytogenetic technique that uses fluorescent probes that selectively bind to specific portions of selected chromosomes, allowing assessment of polysomy via fluoroscopic microscopy. The presence of multifocal polysomy in particular is a strong predictor of cholangiocarcinoma.[189] A potential advantage of FISH is that it requires fewer cells for analysis compared with routine cytology or flow cytometry. A meta-analysis of six studies on 828 patients with PSC demonstrated a sensitivity and specificity for the diagnosis of cholangiocarcinoma of 68% and 70%, respectively.[190] Another study of biliary strictures of varying etiologies noted that, compared with brush cytology alone, FISH resulted in an increase in sensitivity from 39.5% to 63.9% with a similar specificity of 94.3%.[191] Sensitivity can be further improved by using a combination of FISH probes 1q21, 7p12, 8q24, and 9p21, which, in a single center study, was found to have a sensitivity of 93% and a specificity of 100%.[192] Because of the improved sensitivity of FISH when cytology is negative for malignancy, it is currently recommended for the diagnosis of cholangiocarcinoma in PSC patients (see Chapter 41).[193]

Next-generation sequencing has been recently applied to biliary strictures and has resulted in an increased sensitivity of diagnosis of cholangiocarcinoma of 77% in brushing and 83% in biopsy specimens.[194]

Overall, ERCP with brush cytology and/or intraductal biopsies should be performed in the initial evaluation of indeterminate biliary strictures. Advanced cytologic methods, such as FISH and next-generation sequencing, can potentially improve sensitivity, especially in the setting of negative cytology and histology. It should be stressed that a multidisciplinary review of the indication for biliary tissue sampling is of critical importance. Some strictures do not require biopsy if surgery is indicated on clinical and radiologic grounds, and other biopsy approaches may be more appropriate.

Advanced Endoscopic Biliary Imaging

Peroral Cholangioscopy

Peroral cholangioscopy is a technique that permits direct endoscopic visualization of the bile ducts by using miniature endoscopes and catheters inserted through the accessory port of a duodenoscope. In the endoscope-based ("mother-daughter") system, a small, thin endoscope (daughter) is inserted through the accessory channel of the duodenoscope (mother). The main limitation of this system is the requirement of two separate endoscopists to operate each scope during the procedure.

Single-operator cholangioscopy has also been developed and involves advancement of the digital cholangioscope over a guidewire through the working channel of a therapeutic duodenoscope. These initially consisted of fiberoptic probes but have since evolved to use high-resolution digital technology. The digital SpyGlass system (Boston Scientific Corp) has been available since 2015. It has two dedicated irrigation channels and four-way tip deflection. A biliary sphincterotomy is often required to allow passage of the catheter into the duct. In addition to the channel for the optical probe, the catheter includes a 1.2-mm accessory channel and two 0.6-mm irrigation channels.[195]

Alternatively, direct cholangioscopy can also be performed using ultraslim endoscopes originally designed for pediatric or transnasal esophagogastroduodenoscopy. This requires a previous ERCP with a large sphincterotomy or sphincteroplasty. Direct cholangioscopy can be performed with the tandem technique, which involves placing a guidewire into the bile duct via a duodenoscope, which is then withdrawn, and then advancing the ultraslim endoscope over the guidewire. The alternative is the freehand intubation technique in which the ultraslim endoscope is advanced independently to the papilla. The bile duct is then cannulated with a guidewire over which the endoscope is advanced. Although this has the advantage of needing a single operator and having a larger working channel (2 mm), which permits use of a wider range of accessories, it does carry a risk of air embolism. To reduce this risk, it is recommended to use only carbon dioxide insufflation or water irrigation to clear the bile duct.[195]

Peroral cholangioscopy has been primarily used for the management of refractory choledocholithiasis (discussed earlier in this chapter) and for the evaluation of indeterminate biliary strictures. Cholangioscopy allows direct visualization and inspection of mucosal abnormalities of the biliary epithelium (Fig 30.7A–C). Various classification systems that include

features such as vessel and pit pattern, papillary projections, and ulceration have been found to improve diagnostic accuracy and interobserver agreement for diagnosis of cholangiocarcinoma in indeterminate biliary strictures.[98,196] Despite a definitive consensus on criteria for diagnosis of cholangiocarcinoma, a meta-analysis of six studies demonstrated that direct single-operator cholangioscopy had a pooled sensitivity and specificity of 94% and 95%, respectively, for diagnosing malignancy among indeterminate strictures by visual interpretation alone.[197]

Furthermore, direct visualization during cholangioscopy also permits selective targeted tissue sampling and results in adequate biopsies in more than 90% of cases.[198] A meta-analysis of 10 studies demonstrated a sensitivity of 60.1% for cholangioscopy-guided biopsies in the diagnosis of malignant biliary strictures.[199] In a prospective randomized study, it was found that three biopsies resulted in a sensitivity of 76.9%.[200] When combined with visualization assessment, the overall sensitivity of digital single-operator cholangioscopy (DSOC) guided biopsies can increase to 87%.[197] In a recent international multicenter prospective RCT, first-pass sensitivity of DSOC-guided biopsy samples was significantly higher than ERCP-guided brushing (68.2% vs. 21.4%; $P < .01$). The overall accuracy of DSOC was also significantly better that ERCP-guided brushings (87.1% vs. 65.5%; $P = .05$).[201] Overall, there was no difference in adverse events with DSOC compared with ERCP intraductal biopsies or brushings.[201]

Overall, cholangioscopy represents an evolving novel technology for the evaluation of indeterminate biliary strictures, exclusion of occult malignancy, and management of biliary stones.

Endoscopic Ultrasound

Transduodenal endoscopic ultrasound with fine-needle aspiration (FNA) has also been used for the evaluation and tissue diagnosis of extrahepatic biliary strictures (see Chapter 22). A meta-analysis of 20 studies including 957 patients demonstrated a specificity of 100% for both proximal and distal biliary strictures. Nevertheless, the sensitivity for distal strictures was

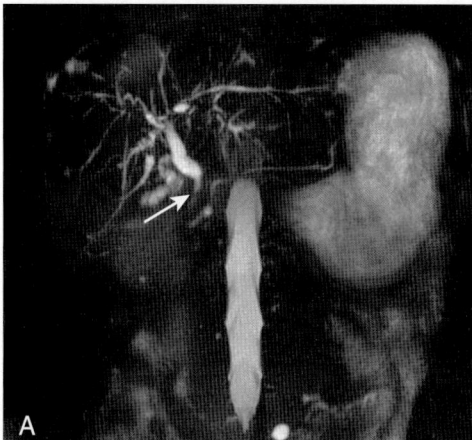
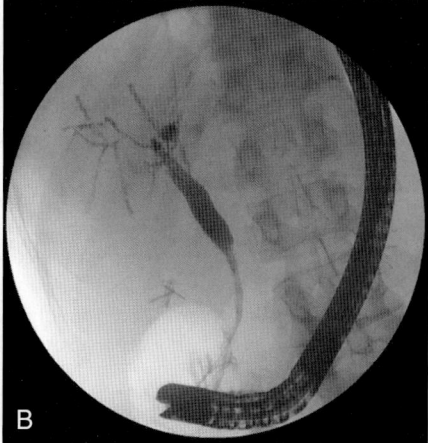
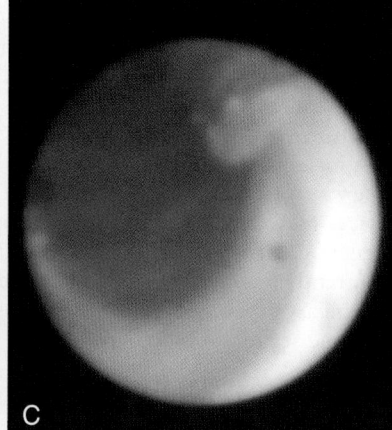

FIGURE 30.7   Evaluation of a dominant common bile duct stricture (CBD) in primary sclerosing cholangitis (PSC). **A,** Magnetic resonance cholangiopancreatography revealing a long-segment distal CBD stricture *(arrow)* with upstream biliary dilation. **B,** Cholangiogram showing long CBD stricture, upstream extrahepatic dilation, and intrahepatic ducts with beading consistent with PSC. **C,** Direct visualization of the bile duct with peroral cholangioscopy reveals a smooth, scarred stricture.

83% compared with 76% for proximal strictures.[202] This is likely because of the proximity of the distal segment of the CBD to the duodenal wall rather than the proximal perihilar segments, which impacts visualization and tissue acquisition. The pooled adverse event rate was 1%, with the main event being self-controlled bleeding. When combined with ERCP, diagnostic sensitivity increases to 85.8%, with a specificity of 87.1%.[203] There is a theoretical risk of tumor seeding with EUS-FNA. One study of 191 patients who were planned for liver transplantation for cholangiocarcinoma reported rates of seeding of up to 83% in patients who had undergone transperitoneal FNA (either percutaneously or via EUS) of hilar strictures compared with 8% in those who did not undergo FNA.[204] This study, however, only had three out of 16 FNAs that were performed via EUS as opposed to percutaneously, and separate analysis of tumor seeding in each group was not performed. Additionally, more recent studies seem to temper this concern and have not demonstrated any difference in overall (HR 1.36; 95% CI, 0.93, 1.99, $P = .112$) or progression-free survival (HR 0.98, 95% CI 0.63–1.53, $P = .944$) or the development of tumor seeding in patients who underwent EUS FNA compared with those who did not.[205,206] Because of potential risk of tumor seeding, however, EUS-FNA can disqualify patients from liver transplantation for perihilar cholangiocarcinoma in some centers and as such should be performed cautiously and after multidisciplinary discussion on patients who are otherwise potential transplant candidates.[207–209]

Endoscopic Intraductal Ultrasound

The evolution of EUS has led to the development of small-caliber ultrasound probes (2.9 mm or less in diameter) for biliary endosonography. These IDUS mini probes are introduced through the accessory channel of the duodenoscope over a guidewire and advanced into the bile duct. IDUS operates at higher frequencies (12–30 Mhz), with penetration of 2 cm at higher image resolution (0.07–0.18 mm) compared with standard EUS.[210] The bile duct appears as three layers on IDUS. The innermost hyperechoic layer corresponds to the mucosa and bile interface. The middle hypoechoic layer corresponds to the discontinuous fibromuscular layer, whereas the outermost hyperechoic layer represents the subserosal fat plane.[210] IDUS has been used for the evaluation of suspected choledocholithiasis. It has been found to have a sensitivity for detecting choledocholithiasis of 95%, which is superior to either MRCP (80%) or ERCP (90%).[211] IDUS was additionally more sensitive at detecting stones less than 8 mm in size in the setting of CBD greater than 12 mm compared with ERCP. As such, it has been suggested that IDUS may be most useful in patients who have a high likelihood of choledocholithiasis but a negative ERCP.[212] With the high diagnostic accuracy of EUS (sensitivity of 89% and specificity of 94%) for detecting choledocholithiasis in patients with suspected choledocholithiasis, however, the role of IDUS in the diagnostic algorithm of biliary stone disease remains to be determined.[83,210]

Several studies have reported IDUS findings in strictures concerning for biliary malignancy. These criteria include the presence of localized wall thickening, polypoid lesions, sessile lesions, intraductal infiltrating lesions, and size greater than 10 mm.[213–215] The sensitivity of predicting malignancy in bile duct strictures has been found to be greater than 90%

and can be more sensitive than EUS, especially in more proximal strictures.[210,214,216] Furthermore, IDUS has been shown to improve local tumor staging for cholangiocarcinomas in various studies, even compared with standard EUS.[217] Conversely, the restricted depth of penetration with IDUS and the inability to perform FNA significantly limits its utility for assessing advanced tumor extension and nodal and metastatic staging.

IDUS is a promising advanced endoscopic imaging modality that permits high-resolution images of the bile system. This advantage is hindered by the limited depth of penetration and ability to examine more distal sites. Further studies are needed to validate its place as an adjunct imaging tool to ERCP and EUS.[195]

Confocal Laser Endomicroscopy

Confocal endomicroscopy (CLE) allows real-time high-resolution evaluation of gastrointestinal mucosal histology in vivo. Imaging is achieved by the projection of a low-power laser light passed through a confocal aperture. The focused beam targeted on a specific layer of tissue is then captured by a photodetection device and transformed into electrical signals processed into grayscale images.[218] Because CLE relies on tissue fluorescence, intravenous fluorescein dye (5–10 mL of 10% fluorescein) is administered to highlight tissue structures (individual cell structures, vasculature) before imaging. The lack of contrast uptake by neoplastic tissue results in a contrasted dark appearance compared with adjacent normal structures.[195]

There are two currently available CLE systems: endoscope-based CLE (eCLE) and probe-based CLE (pCLE). The former is too large because the CLE is integrated in the tip of the endoscope, and thus biliary examination is generally performed with pCLE probes that can be inserted through the accessory channel of the duodenoscope. The laser (488 nm, blue light) is transmitted through thousands of optimal fibers within the probe (the cholangioflex probe is 9 mm in diameter), and subsequent confocal image data is collected at a frame rate of 12 frames/ second, with a limited field of vision of 325 μm. pCLE can be challenging because optimal imaging requires significant probe and patient stability.

The indications for pCLE in biliary disease have not been established, but studies have suggested a potential role in the evaluation of biliary strictures suspicious for malignancy. CLE has been found to have a pooled sensitivity of 90% and specificity of 72% to decipher between benign and malignant strictures in the evaluation of indeterminate biliary stenosis in a meta-analysis of eight prospective studies.[219] The Miami criteria has been developed to identify malignant strictures and include findings of thick white (>20 μm) and dark bands (>40 μm), epithelial structures, and dark clumps. A combination of two of these findings was found to have a sensitivity of 97% and specificity of 33% for diagnosing malignancy.[220] Additionally, the Paris criteria was developed and validated for identification of inflammatory strictures. The criteria for this includes multiple thin white bands, dark granular pattern with scales, increased space between scales, and thickened reticular structures. When the Paris criteria was retrospectively applied to videos of the same strictures used to previously validate the Miami criteria, it was found to have a sensitivity of 81% and specificity of 83.3% for diagnosing malignant strictures, thereby reducing false positives.[221] A more recent randomized prospective trial found that when using a combined Miami and Paris classification, real-time pCLE had a sensitivity of 89% and specificity of 71% when compared with ERCP alone. When combined with tissue sampling, the sensitivity of pCLE was 89% with a specificity of 88%.[222]

Despite these promising preliminary results, there have been discrepancies in the interpretation of pCLE findings between endoscopists for both benign and malignant pancreaticobiliary lesions, which indicates the need for dedicated training.[223]

Overall, pCLE is a promising technique for evaluating indeterminate biliary strictures, but further studies are needed to improve accuracy and interobserver agreement.

The references for this chapter can be found online by accessing the accompanying Expert Consult website.

CHAPTER 31

Radiologic hepatobiliary interventions

Karen T. Brown and Anne M. Covey

RADIOLOGIC HEPATOBILIARY INTERVENTIONS

Minimally invasive hepatic intervention is indicated in a wide range of pathologic conditions and can be generally divided into vascular, biliary, and hepatic parenchymal procedures. The objective of this chapter is to provide a broad overview of the spectrum of interventions that can be performed percutaneously using imaging guidance. Greater detail will be found in individual chapters devoted to each topic.

Vascular Procedures

The liver is an extremely vascular organ with nutrient supply from both the portal vein and hepatic artery and drainage via the hepatic veins. These vessels are common targets for the interventional radiologist.

Portal Vein

The majority of the nutrient blood flow to the liver is via the portal vein, which drains the splanchnic circulation and spleen. The most common abnormality involving the portal vein is portal hypertension, typically as a sequela of cirrhosis (see Chapters 74, 79, 81, and 85). Clinical manifestations of portal hypertension include splenomegaly, thrombocytopenia, varices, ascites, and liver failure. In 1969 Rosch and colleagues[1] reported the first case of transjugular intrahepatic portosystemic shunt (TIPSS) in dogs (see Chapter 85). Thirteen year later, Colapinto and colleagues (1982)[2] reported the first human application of TIPSS. In this procedure, a path is created from the hepatic vein to the portal vein through the liver parenchyma, thereby decreasing portal pressure and relieving patients from intractable ascites or acute variceal bleeding. Initially the tract was formed with serial dilators or balloon dilation, with limited success. When the Palmaz metallic balloon expandable stents became available in the mid-1980s,[3] procedural success improved, and the technique gained widespread acceptance. Further refinement using covered self-expanding stents has improved long-term patency, making this a viable option not only for patients with life-threatening hemorrhage but also as a means to control intractable ascites.[4,5]

The most significant complication of TIPSS is hepatic encephalopathy because of the volume of blood shunted past the liver parenchyma (see Chapter 77). As a result, the presence of hepatic encephalopathy is a relative contraindication to the procedure. Other contraindications include right heart failure, hepatic vein occlusion, and sepsis. The risk of cardiac decompensation after TIPSS can be predicted noninvasively.[6]

In patients with hepatic encephalopathy and portal hypertension or patients with "left-sided (sinistral) portal hypertension" (gastric varices because of splenic vein occlusion), balloon-occluded retrograde transvenous obliteration (BRTO) or balloon-occluded antegrade transvenous obliteration (BATO) may be preferable to TIPSS. BRTO and BATO refer to procedures in which a high-risk or bleeding gastric varix is catheterized and

sclerosed, typically with a mixture of Ethiodol, Sotradechol, and air agitated through a three-way stopcock.[7] In patients with isolated sinistral portal hypertension because of occlusion of the splenic vein, recanalization of the occluded splenic vein or embolization of the splenic artery may be considered.[8]

In some cases, portal vein narrowing or occlusion because of extrinsic compression by tumor may cause symptoms similar to those seen in cirrhotic portal hypertension. In such cases, placement of a self-expanding stent can relieve varices and ascites. This is most commonly seen in patients with locally advanced pancreaticobiliary cancer, where portal vein stenting may also improve thrombocytopenia, broadening chemotherapy options.

Another procedure that has gained widespread acceptance is portal vein embolization (PVE) as an adjunctive procedure before hepatic resection (see Chapter 102C). Patients with a suboptimal future liver remnant (FLR), which can be assessed volumetrically (i.e., with computed tomography [CT] or magnetic resonance imaging [MRI]) or functionally (e.g., indocyanine green clearance), may undergo contralateral PVE to induce preoperative hypertrophy of the FLR[9] (see Chapter 102C). In patients with cirrhosis, most surgeons believe that a FLR of greater than 40% of the total liver volume (TLV) is optimal. For patients without underlying liver disease, a FLR of greater than 25% is thought to be acceptable. Other risk factors for impaired liver function include diabetes, prior chemotherapy, and steatosis, and therefore the desired volume of the FLR is best assessed on a case-by-case basis.

PVE to improve the safety of hepatic resection was first proposed by Makuuchi and colleagues in 1990.[10] Initially, this procedure was performed via a transileocolic approach that required laparotomy and general anesthesia. Although ligation of a portal vein branch can be carried out during a laparotomy, today this procedure is most commonly performed percutaneously, typically as an outpatient procedure. A wide range of agents have been used to perform the procedure, including ethanol, Gelfoam, thrombin, polyvinyl alcohol, glue, spherical embolic agents, coils, and sclerosing agents. No agent has proven superior; each is expected to increase the absolute FLR/TLV in the range of 8% to 10%. Complications are uncommon, the most significant being nontarget embolization to the main portal vein or portal vein supplying the FLR, which could preclude operation. This occurs in less than 1% of patients.[11]

Liver hepatic venous deprivation is another technique to improve contralateral hepatic hypertrophy before major hepatic resection. In this procedure, both the portal and hepatic veins in the hemiliver to be resected are embolized to maximize growth of the FLR and allow major hepatic resection.[12]

Hepatic Artery

Unlike portal vein interventions, which are most commonly undertaken to treat the sequela of portal hypertension or, in the case of PVE, as adjunct to hepatic resection, most transarterial interventions in the liver are done to effect treatment of unresectable malignancy or for control of bleeding in the setting of trauma (see Chapters 21, 94, 113, 115, and 116).

Both primary and metastatic liver tumors derive the majority of trophic blood supply from the hepatic artery, unlike the non–tumor-bearing parenchyma, which receives the majority of nutrient flow from the portal vein (see chapter 5). Therefore administering a treatment to the artery can affect tumor regression while minimizing collateral damage to the underlying parenchyma.

In the mid-1970s, it was recognized that the unusual dual vascular supply to the liver might allow effective transarterial treatment for hypervascular metastases from neuroendocrine tumors, as well as primary hepatocellular carcinoma (HCC). Subsequently, transarterial treatments have been applied to a wide variety of hypervascular tumors, including sarcoma and breast cancers, as well as some tumors that are not particularly hypervascular by imaging, such as colon cancer or cholangiocarcinoma (see Chapter 94).

Different forms of treatment have been administered via the hepatic artery to treat such tumors, including chemotherapy infusion, bland (particle) embolization (transcatheter arterial embolization [TAE]), transarterial chemoembolization with lipiodol (TACE), embolization with drug-eluting beads (DEB-TACE), and radioembolization (RAE; see Chapter 94). Two randomized trials have demonstrated improvement in overall survival in patients with HCC treated with TACE compared with patients who received best supportive care.[13,14] To date, there has been no study demonstrating a significant difference in overall survival among any method of embolization, including TACE, DEB-TACE, TAE, or RAE.[15,16]

Indications for arterially directed therapy include control of symptoms (e.g., pain or hormonal-related symptoms because of neuroendocrine liver metastases; see Chapter 91), control of tumor in the liver to prolong survival, progression of disease after systemic treatment, and local tumor control to maintain eligibility for liver transplant in select patients with HCC (see Chapter 89). Transarterial therapies are rarely, if ever, curative and instead are intended to be repeated upon disease progression. In cases of minimal disease burden, ablation may be performed in conjunction with embolization as a potentially curative therapy (see Chapter 96). In this instance, performing the embolization immediately before ablation has the advantage of depositing contrast-laden particles within the tumor to assist in targeting with the ablation device and also decreasing the "heat sink" effect, whereby flowing blood continues to "cool" the tumor margin, potentially increasing the risk of local recurrence. Occluding arterial blood flow may increase the zone of ablation.[17] In some cases, the angiogram may identify additional sites of disease undetected on preprocedure imaging, changing the treatment plan.

Selection criteria differ slightly with each treatment option. Broadly speaking, patients with unresectable disease involving less than 50% of the liver without underlying liver disease or with well-compensated (Childs-Pugh score A–B7) cirrhosis may be candidates. In the past, portal vein occlusion was considered an absolute contraindication because of the reported higher complication rate and risk of death. More recently, series of patients with portal vein occlusion treated with TAE, TACE, and RAE have been shown to respond to treatment without a significant increase in complications, thus supporting its use in this group of patients with limited treatment options.[18-22]

The complication profiles differ slightly between the various transarterial therapies. TACE is infrequently associated with bone marrow suppression and alopecia. Radiation-induced liver failure occurs in 1% to 2% of patients who undergo RAE; however, radiologic findings of cirrhosis and portal hypertension are seen in greater than 50% of patients with neuroendocrine tumor treated with whole liver RAE at a mean of 4.1 years after treatment.[23] With varying frequency, intra-arterial therapy is associated with arterial sclerosis and arterial occlusion, which can make future intervention more difficult.[24] This is more commonly seen with TACE and DEB-TACE than with TAE.[25,26] The clinical relevance of this angiographic finding is that over time tumors can derive arterial supply from nonhepatic collateral vessels, making treatment more challenging and creating a higher risk of nontarget embolization. Branches that commonly give rise to extrahepatic tumor supply include the right phrenic, internal mammary, gastroduodenal, intercostal, and renal capsular arteries.

Complications include nontarget embolization, liver failure, vessel injury, and postembolization syndrome. Postembolization syndrome occurs in the majority of patients, other than those treated with RAE, and consists of some degree of pain, fever, and/or nausea that can last for several days. Prolonged pain may suggest nontarget embolization to the pancreas, resulting in pancreatitis, or to the gallbladder or upper gastrointestinal (GI) tract, resulting in cholecystitis or gastric or duodenal ulceration.

The hepatic artery is also a vessel that may require intervention after liver transplant. After primary graft malfunction, hepatic artery thrombosis (HAT) is the second leading cause of graft failure after liver transplant and is a major cause of transplant-related mortality (see Chapter 111). This complication can result from technical issues with the anastomosis, including disparate diameters of donor and recipient vessels, and tension on, or kinking of, the anastomosis. In most cases, HAT occurs within the first 100 days and manifests as fulminant hepatic necrosis and/or biliary tract ischemia and necrosis, resulting in sepsis. Because these patients are immunosuppressed to prevent graft rejection, the gram-negative sepsis resulting from biliary necrosis can be very difficult to treat (see Chapter 111).

Early posttransplant screening Doppler ultrasound (US) can be used to detect abnormal flow in the hepatic artery. If this test is abnormal, a contrast study (US, CT, or angiography) should be considered. To salvage the organ, a precious resource, revascularization is often attempted after documentation of abnormal flow, even in asymptomatic patients.[27]

Other hepatic artery complications may develop post-transplant, including stenosis and pseudoaneurysm. As with occlusion, revascularization with catheter-directed thrombolysis, angioplasty, and/or stent placement is effective in the majority of cases with hepatic artery stenosis. Pseudoaneurysm is a rare but potentially fatal complication that may be treated with a covered stent graft (see Chapters 111 and 115).

After blunt abdominal trauma, the liver is the second most commonly injured abdominal organ after the spleen (see Chapter 113). The American Association for the Surgery of Trauma Injury Scoring Scale was developed to help guide management of these patients.[28] Injuries to the hepatic artery include pseudoaneurysms, which can be unifocal or multiple, resulting in a "starry sky" appearance of multiple sites of extravasation/injury on angiography. Focal extravasation or pseudoaneurysm is usually treated with coil embolization of the affected vessel distal and proximal to the injury, or with a covered stent. In the case of multifocal injury, particle embolization of the hepatic artery may be performed. Because of the dual blood supply to the liver discussed earlier, embolization of the hepatic artery in the presence of a patent portal vein is rarely of clinical consequence. Hepatic artery injury may occur after iatrogenic hepatic interventions, either surgical or percutaneous, such as biliary drainage or TIPSS, and is treated similarly with coil embolization or covered stent placement.

Hepatic Vein

The least common vascular target of endovascular intervention in the liver is the hepatic vein. Budd-Chiari is a potentially life-threatening disease of heterogeneous etiology, resulting in obstruction of hepatic venous outflow that occurs in less than one per million persons (see Chapter 86). Acutely, patients are symptomatic with abdominal pain and ascites, and over time, centrilobular fibrosis and cirrhosis may develop. Initial therapy includes systemic anticoagulation, but the benefit of anticoagulation alone is debatable. Patients with ongoing symptoms may benefit from thrombolysis, venoplasty, and/or stent placement and, in some cases, TIPSS[29] (see Chapter 85).

Stenosis of the intrahepatic or suprahepatic inferior vena cava may occur as a complication after orthotopic liver transplantation, and symptomatology mimicking Budd-Chiari may ensue. Elevated velocities by Doppler US suggest the diagnosis, and a pressure gradient of greater than 6 mm Hg across the stenosis at venography is diagnostic.[30] Venoplasty or, in select cases, stent placement can alleviate symptoms and preserve graft function.

Biliary Intervention

Noninvasive imaging of the biliary tree with contrast-enhanced CT (CECT) and MRI have virtually eliminated the need for invasive percutaneous transhepatic cholangiography to diagnose biliary tract disorders (see Chapters 16 and 20). As a result, percutaneous transhepatic cholangiography is rarely performed for diagnostic purposes alone but rather at the time of planned biliary intervention. Percutaneous transhepatic biliary drainage or stent placement can be performed to relieve symptoms caused by obstructive jaundice, including pruritus, anorexia, and cholangitis. Biliary drainage can also be performed to lower the bilirubin preoperatively, to allow for chemotherapy or, in the setting of bile leak, to divert bile.[31] Less common indications include access to treat biliary stone disease or to facilitate intraductal therapies, such as brachytherapy.

In general, bile duct obstruction below the common hepatic duct (i.e., "low" bile duct obstruction)[32] is best treated endoscopically because placement of a plastic or self-expanding metal stent (SEMS) can drain the entire biliary tree through the normal orifice of the sphincter of Oddi. In cases of high bile duct obstruction, (at or above the cystic duct insertion) percutaneous drainage is preferred because this allows a specific duct to be targeted for drainage without contamination of potentially isolated, undrained ducts (see Chapters 20 and 52).

Ideally, the need for drainage and optimal plan for a given patient is made by multidisciplinary consensus involving hepatobiliary surgeons, gastroenterologists, and interventional radiologists. Preprocedure planning must include high-quality imaging of the liver and biliary tree. CECT and MRI are extremely useful to show biliary anatomy and pathology (see

Chapter 16). In some cases, US may add additional information about the level of obstruction and patency of portal vein branches, but US alone is not sufficient for preprocedure planning. A dose of prophylactic broad-spectrum antibiotic to cover enterococci, streptococci, and aerobic and anaerobic gram-negative bacilli is recommended before biliary intervention. This is particularly important when there has been bile duct reconstruction or biliary instrumentation because, in this setting, the incidence of colonized bile is high.

With malignant biliary obstruction in the absence of signs or symptoms of cholangitis, placement of a primary SEMS may be performed. Compared with plastic stents, metal stents have a longer median patency (3–9.1 months vs. 1.8–5.5 months), but there is no difference in overall patient survival.[33] When feasible, primary stent placement is preferred because it does not require an exteriorized device. Additionally, if there are incompletely drained ducts, having a catheter may put patients at risk for developing cholangitis because bile colonization occurs within 48 hours, and when a primary stent is placed, there is less opportunity for contaminating incompletely drained ducts. Finally, in high bile duct obstruction, stents can often be placed above the papilla. Without reflux of bowel contents or an exteriorized device, the sterility of the biliary tree is maintained so that if or when patients present with occluded stents, the likelihood of presenting with cholangitis is diminished.

Metal stents also may be covered with polyurethane, with the goal of preventing tumor ingrowth, resulting in improved patency. Unfortunately, this has not been shown to be the case, and increased complications of acute cholecystitis[34] and stent migration have been seen.[35] Covered stents are not generally indicated in high bile duct obstruction because of the risk of occluding undrained segmental bile ducts. Further studies are needed to establish the indications for covered versus bare metal stents.

Bile Duct Biopsy

In some cases, the etiology of biliary obstruction may not be evident at the time of drainage. Bile obtained at the time of drainage may be sent for cytology, but diagnostic sensitivity is relatively low. Bile duct biopsy may be helpful in establishing a diagnosis of intraductal pathology (e.g., cholangiocarcinoma) and in differentiating recurrent tumor from ischemic/postoperative stricture (see Chapters 22 and 51). At the time of biliary drainage, endoluminal brush or forceps biopsy of the stricture depicted by cholangiography can be used to obtain a sample. These techniques are most useful for intraductal pathology (e.g., cholangiocarcinoma) in contradistinction to extrinsic masses that may cause biliary obstruction (e.g., hilar adenopathy or parenchymal liver mass). In cases in which establishing a diagnosis is difficult, the biliary tree can be opacified through an indwelling drainage catheter, and the stricture targeted with a percutaneous fine needle.[36] Cholangiographic-guided needle biopsy can be used to diagnose both intraductal and extraductal causes of obstruction.

Percutaneous Cholecystostomy

Percutaneous cholecystostomy is most commonly indicated for the treatment of acute acalculous cholecystitis in severely ill hospitalized patients but may also be used to treat calculous cholecystitis in patients who are too sick for, or in whom comorbidities preclude, definitive cholecystectomy (see Chapters 34 and 35). It may also be performed to provide access to the gallbladder or biliary tree for stone removal or, in rare instances, to provide biliary drainage in patients with common bile duct (CBD) obstruction distal to the insertion of the cystic duct. When performed in the setting of gallstones, it is often used as a temporizing measure to allow the resolution of sepsis and optimization of the patient's medical conditions for subsequent cholecystectomy.

In cancer patients with bile duct obstruction, it is not uncommon to see cholecystitis complicating SEMS placement when gallstones are present and the stent covers the cystic duct orifice, particularly when contrast is seen within the cystic duct or gallbladder. Some of these patients undergo subsequent cholecystectomy but, in palliative situations, the patients may live with a cholecystostomy catheter. Cholecystostomy has been reported effective as definitive therapy in very-high-risk patients with calculous cholecystitis who have remained asymptomatic after catheter placement.[37] After cholecystostomy, clinical resolution of infection occurs within 24 to 48 hours in the vast majority of cases. When performed for acalculous cholecystitis, the catheter can be capped once it begins to drain bile, a clear sign that the cystic duct is patent, but the catheter should not be removed until tract maturation has occurred. In general, this occurs within two to three weeks.[38] Tract maturation may happen earlier when a transhepatic rather than transperitoneal route to the gallbladder has been employed. If stone removal from the gallbladder is to be undertaken, this should also be performed after tract maturation.

Biliary Stone Disease

Stones can be removed from the gallbladder or biliary tree using a variety of approaches and methods (see Chapters 30, 36, and 37). When there is a retained CBD stone after cholecystectomy and a T-tube has been left in place, this is accomplished via the T-tube tract following tract maturation. When choledocholithiasis occurs in a patient with remote cholecystectomy, it can be performed through a transhepatic approach if endoscopy is unsuccessful. Choledocholithiasis may present with cholangitis or be asymptomatic. The first step in stone removal is placement of a percutaneous biliary drainage catheter. After a period of two to three weeks of drainage, during which a mature tract forms, the biliary catheter is exchanged for a large diameter sheath. The first order of business then is balloon sphincterotomy, followed by pushing smaller calculi into the duodenum using a balloon. If the stones are too large to pass through the dilated ampulla, they can be broken up using baskets, snares, or even lithotripsy. Once the duct is thought to be clear, the internal external drainage catheter is replaced. The patient returns in one to two weeks, and sheath cholangiography is performed to look for retained stones. If the ducts are clear, the internal external catheter is replaced with an external drain above the ampulla and then capped. If the patient does well with the catheter capped, it can be removed without further imaging.

Bile Duct Injury

The bile duct can be injured from blunt or penetrating trauma but is probably most commonly injured at the time of surgery (see Chapters 28, 32, 42, and 113). There was a fairly high rate of bile duct injury when laparoscopic cholecystectomy was initially introduced, at least in part related to lack of operator experience, now mostly related to unrecognized bile duct anomalies (see Chapters 2 and 36). When the bile duct is clipped or transected, there is little that can be done percutaneously other than draining the obstructed duct or diverting the transected one. When postoperative strictures occur, patients may present with cholangitis, pruritus, or jaundice. Percutaneous access to the biliary tree is established first, and then the stricture is crossed. An internal external catheter is left across the stricture for a couple of weeks as tract maturation occurs. The patient returns, and the stricture is dilated with a balloon.[39] When applied to bilioenteric anastomoses, success is likely in the majority of patients, with stricture recurrence in as few as 5% of patients on long-term follow-up.[40] Dilation of the CBD is not likely to be successful using a balloon of less than 10 mm. If an acceptable result is not seen when the patient returns for a repeat study after their first dilation, the stricture can be redilated, sometimes with a larger balloon. Strictures particularly resistant to dilation have been treated by some operators by using cutting balloons with good, durable results.[41]

Hepatic Cysts

Liver cysts occur in up to 5% of the population and are incidentally seen on cross-sectional imaging (see Chapters 73 and 88B). They can enlarge slowly and rarely become symptomatic, although symptoms from mass effect may develop if they impinge on adjacent structures. In addition, bleeding may occur into the cyst, causing pain. A simple liver cyst should be differentiated from a cystic tumor. The most common mimic of the simple cyst is a cystadenoma that has the potential to become a cystadenocarcinoma (see Chapter 88B). Unfortunately, cross-sectional imaging studies do not reliably distinguish between these two entities. Metastases that become necrotic can also appear cystic; however, history and previous imaging will usually make the distinction.

Treatment of simple liver cysts is not typically indicated unless the patient is symptomatic and the symptoms are clearly related to the cyst. Simple aspiration can provide temporary relief, and, when the symptoms are relieved, serves as proof of association, but recurrence after aspiration is very high. Drainage and sclerosis have been reported, but have generally been replaced by laparoscopic unroofing of the cyst, which is typically well tolerated by the patient and avoids problems associated with an indwelling catheter (see Chapter 73). Cystadenomas, because of the risk of malignancy, require surgical resection.

Hepatic Abscess

Most liver abscesses in the United States are pyogenic, caused by bacteria (see Chapter 70). Amebic abscesses caused by *Entamoeba histolytica* and fungal abscesses each account for about 10% of liver abscesses (see Chapter 71). Pyogenic liver abscesses are usually polymicrobial, and an etiology can often be discovered. Ascending hematogenous infection from the GI tract is a common etiology, and patients with diverticulitis or appendicitis may present with a liver abscess. Appearance on cross-sectional imaging is usually that of a complex collection with many internal septa, resembling a cauliflower. Despite this appearance, these can be successfully treated percutaneously in combination with antibiotics, although catheter drainage may be prolonged.[42] Imaging should include the pelvis, with careful evaluation for a potential source.

Patients who develop bile duct obstruction, particularly in the setting of bactibilia related to previous biliary-enteric bypass, transampullary stent placement, or a preexisting percutaneous drain, also may present with a liver abscess, although in this situation it is often better classified as an infected biloma and is usually less complex in appearance. Causes of infected biloma include stent obstruction, recurrent tumor, or anastomotic stricture, and a catheter placed into a biloma for drainage will continue to drain bile until the causative obstruction is eliminated.

Liver abscess can also occur as a complication after embolization of liver tumors in the patient group with compromised sphincter of Oddi and bactibilia[43] (see Chapter 94). This should always be considered in the preprocedure evaluation of patients undergoing hepatic artery embolization that have had a previous pancreatoduodenectomy or colonized bile for any reason. True liver abscesses should be distinguished from "perihepatic" collections that occur postoperatively, are not in the parenchyma of the liver, and are usually much easier to treat (see Chapters 28 and 101).

Amebic Abscess

Unlike pyogenic hepatic abscess, amebic abscesses are typically associated with travel history to an endemic region (see Chapter 71). At presentation, patients almost universally have fever and abdominal pain. Hepatomegaly occurs often, particularly with large cysts. When cysts are small, aspiration may be necessary to differentiate amebic from pyogenic abscess because amebic antibodies may not be detected at presentation, although they typically appear later. Symptoms resolve quickly with administration of metronidazole, and intervention beyond that is rarely needed unless there has been rupture. A randomized trial of 57 patients with abscesses 5 to 10 cm in size found that although fever and pain resolved sooner in the group treated with aspiration and metronidazole, compared with metronidazole alone, the difference was not statistically significant, and there was no difference in morbidity, mortality, treatment failure, days to normalization of leukocytosis, or duration of hospital stay between the two groups.[44]

Echinococcal Cysts

Hydatid cystic disease is a parasitic disease caused by *Echinococcus granulosa* (see Chapter 72). The larvae of this parasite cause the disease, which is endemic in Mediterranean, Middle Eastern, and South American countries and in New Zealand and Turkey, where people are in close contact with sheep and dogs. The most common site of disease is in the liver (50%–80%), followed by the lung (5%–30%). Surgery is the primary method of treatment; however, percutaneous approaches have been investigated in recent years. In 2005 Paksoy and colleagues[45] reported on 59 patients with 109 hydatid cysts that were treated percutaneously, injecting either hypertonic saline or albendazole sodium as the scolicidal agent. All patients were given 10 mg/kg/day of albendazole, beginning 48 hours before their procedure, and this was continued for two months after the procedure. Directly before the procedure, they received diphenhydramine and hydrocortisone to prevent anaphylactic reactions. Treatment was safe and effective in both groups, with only one recurrence in the group treated with hypertonic saline. This compares well with a reported 4% incidence of recurrence after surgery. Although all cysts returned to their initial size directly after aspiration and injection, successful treatment was associated with decrease in size over time.

Hepatic Ablation

Tumors

Small primary and metastatic tumors in the liver may be completely eradicated by chemical or thermal ablation (see Chapter 96). The most common tumors treated with ablation include HCC and colorectal liver metastases. Improved screening of patients with risk factors for HCC has resulted in detection of small tumors amenable to curative resection or ablation. Colorectal cancer is the third most common malignancy in the United States, and most disease-related deaths are secondary to metastatic disease. Up to 50% of patients with colorectal cancer will develop liver metastases during the course of their disease (see Chapter 90). In almost half of these patients, disease is limited to the liver, and up to 25% of these patients have resectable disease. More effective systemic chemotherapy (see Chapters 97 and 98) and advances in techniques of hepatic resection (see Chapter 101) have combined to improve survival and increase rates of hepatic resection. Concomitantly, there have been advances in interventional radiologic techniques of percutaneous thermal ablation, including radiofrequency, microwave, laser, and cryoablation, as well as irreversible electroporation (see Chapter 96). All of these techniques are less costly, safer, and result in shorter hospital stays than hepatic resection and can be applied in place of surgical resection in well-selected cases, although the risk of local recurrence is higher.[46–51] There are other tumors that might be treated with ablation, assuming they meet number, size, and location criteria for successful treatment.

Criteria for Treatment

Even the most advanced ablative techniques are limited with regard to the tumor size that can be successfully treated. It has recently been shown that an ablative margin is critical to a successful ablation, with a margin of at least 5 and ideally 10 mm on CT four to eight weeks after ablation associated with the best local tumor control.[52] Most commercially available ablation systems result in an elliptic volume of coagulative necrosis, with a maximum long axis of 5 cm, limited by properties of the local tumor/tissue environment. For this reason, successful ablation, with a low rate of local tumor recurrence is seen most often in tumors less than 3 cm in size, and the best results are obtained in tumors 2.5 cm or smaller. Larger tumors, or those with complex geometry, are unlikely to be effectively treated by attempting to extend the thermal effect by using multiple overlapping applications. The location of the tumor may also limit effectiveness of ablation or ability to use the technique safely. Tumors that are adjacent to high-flow blood vessels (portal vein, hepatic vein, inferior vena cava) will be cooled where they are in contact with the blood vessel so that the application of heat will be less effective at that margin and the risk of recurrence higher. Subcapsular tumors can be difficult to treat effectively. Structures that may be injured by heat or cold, such as bile ducts and other adjacent organs, might preclude safe treatment, although irreversible electroporation has been developed, in part, to address that issue. Ideal patients for percutaneous ablation should have oligometastatic disease with three or fewer tumors, all less than 3 cm in size, that are not adjacent to a major bile duct or bile duct branch or in contact with any high-flow vessel, especially one greater than 5 mm in size. Local tumor recurrence and survival rates are both related to the number of tumors treated, and the best outcome is found in patients with a solitary tumor.

Size criteria can be extended in HCC or other vascular tumors that can be embolized first. In this instance, addition of ablation to embolization provides several theoretical advantages. In the first instance, it provides a method of "double kill," whereby the tumor is exposed to two tumoricidal events: ischemia and lethal temperature.[53] Because embolization results in cessation of flowing arterial blood, the primary blood supply to hepatic tumors, heat resulting from ablation does not need to overcome the cooling effects of flowing blood in the tumor or immediate environment, theoretically increasing efficiency of the process, resulting in more effective heating of the tissue. Second, when ablation is performed directly after embolization, it becomes much easier to radiologically target small tumors in the 1- to 2-cm range because they retain dense contrast. Finally, it is possible to target areas within the tumor that may show less deposition of embolic material and in which recurrence is likely.[54]

The following chapters will provide a more detailed discussion of these techniques, as well as more in-depth consideration of indications, outcomes, and potential complications of radiologic hepatic interventions.

References are available at expertconsult.com.

CHAPTER 32

Bile duct exploration and biliary-enteric anastomosis

Brooke C. Bredbeck and Clifford S. Cho

OVERVIEW

Minimally invasive techniques to manage biliary pathology have reduced the need for open operative intervention. Although open exploration for biliary disease has become less common, specific situations like obstructive common duct stones not amenable to endoscopic therapy or restoration of biliary-enteric continuity following resection of bile duct tumors remain indications for surgical approaches. It is important to have a thorough understanding of biliary anatomy (see Chapter 2) and a familiarity with various options for operative exposure and management (see Chapter 42). Operative techniques encompassing bile duct exploration and biliary-enteric bypass will be the focus of this chapter.

ANATOMY

Knowledge of extrahepatic biliary anatomy and an appreciation of anatomic variants are essential for safe operative conduct (see Chapter 2). The intrahepatic bile ducts draining the various sections ultimately coalesce into the right hepatic duct draining the right hemiliver and the left hepatic duct draining the left hemiliver. These converge at the liver hilum to form the common hepatic duct, which is generally the most anterior structure and lies along the right border of the porta hepatis at this location. In approximately 80% to 90% of cases, the right hepatic artery courses posterior to the common hepatic duct toward the right liver; however, in a minority of cases, it can be found anterior to the duct. The right hepatic duct has a short extrahepatic segment (approximately 1.5–2 cm) in contrast to the left hepatic duct, which traverses beneath segment IVB for approximately 3 to 4 cm after exiting the liver parenchyma. When segment IVB is broad, the left hepatic duct assumes a longer extrahepatic course with a transverse orientation, as opposed to a shorter and more oblique orientation when segment IVB is narrow (Fig. 32.1). The left hepatic duct and left portal vein travel within a peritoneal reflection of the gastrohepatic ligament; exposure of these structures is facilitated by lowering the hilar plate at the base of segment IVB (Fig. 32.2). As the left hepatic duct and left portal vein enter the umbilical fissure, they are joined by the left hepatic artery, and vascular branches to segments II, III, and IV travel with biliary drainage from these segments. To maximize access to these structures, a bridge of hepatic tissue at the base of the umbilical fissure (bridging segments III and IV) must often be divided (Fig. 32.3). The ligamentum teres (obliterated umbilical vein) at the base of the falciform ligament runs across the umbilical fissure, separating segment IV from segments II and III. Segment I hepatic ducts flow into both the right and left biliary systems, with the majority of drainage entering the left hepatic duct just proximal to common hepatic duct.

Safe operative conduct requires a close familiarity with anatomic variations of biliary drainage, as they occur in up to 25% of patients.[1] There are a number of ductal anomalies related to the convergence of the left and right hepatic ducts and the insertion of the cystic duct. Although the left biliary system is fairly consistent, the right biliary system is prone to anatomic variation; the most common variants include the right anterior or posterior section ducts traversing a longer extrahepatic course before joining the left biliary system[2] (see Chapters 2 and 42).

BILE DUCT EXPLORATION

Overview

It is estimated that approximately 10% of the US adult population is affected by cholelithiasis, with nearly one-third of these patients requiring cholecystectomy over their lifetime (see Chapter 33). Approximately 10% to 15% of patients undergoing cholecystectomy have choledocholithiasis, and common bile duct stones remain the most common indication for biliary exploration[3] (see Chapters 32 and 37). There are a number of techniques available for evaluation and clearance of the common bile duct, including percutaneous, endoscopic, laparoscopic, and open methods (see Chapters 30, 31, and 37). Although open common bile duct exploration (CBDE) is only necessary in a small subset of patients, it is performed at a similar rate to the laparoscopic approach: a review of the NSQIP database between 2008 and 2013 revealed that just over half of 2,635 CBDEs were performed in an open manner.[4] This subset includes patients undergoing an open cholecystectomy (or a laparoscopic cholecystectomy converted to open) in which choledocholithiasis is suspected, patients with large or multiple stones, and patients requiring transduodenal sphincteroplasty (see Chapter 117D). Because percutaneous, endoscopic, and laparoscopic modalities are discussed in alternate chapters, OBDE will be the focus of the following section.

Incision and Exposure

A right subcostal incision affords satisfactory exposure of the gallbladder, portal structures, and duodenum. Division of the lateral peritoneal attachments of the right colon, followed by mobilization of transverse colon mesentery off of the duodenum, provides visualization of the duodenum (see Chapters 37 and 117). A generous Kocher maneuver facilitates access to the common bile duct located in the lateral border of the hepatoduodenal ligament. Cephalad retraction of the undersurface of the liver at the base of segment IVB will optimize visualization of the extrahepatic biliary system (Fig. 32.4) (see Chapter 119). Additionally, cholecystectomy can enhance exposure of the hepatoduodenal ligament and facilitate intraoperative transcystic cholangiography, which can help to delineate biliary anatomy. Dissection of the gallbladder and cystic duct also identifies the confluence of the cystic duct and common bile duct. Once the common bile duct has been successfully identified,

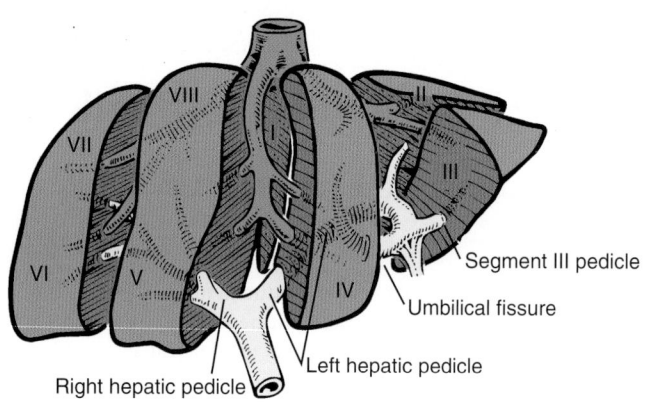

FIGURE 32.1 Diagrammatic expanded view of the liver showing its segmental structure (see Chapter 2). Elements of the portal triad are distributed to the right and left liver on a segmental basis. The left hepatic duct always pursues an extrahepatic course beneath the base of segment IV in the groove separating segment IV from the caudate lobe (segment I; see Fig. 32.2). The ligamentum teres marks the umbilical fissure and runs to join the umbilical portion of the left branch of the portal vein. Each portal triad is composed of the hepatic artery, portal vein, and biliary duct. Note the distribution of the left portal triad in the umbilical fissure; major branches recur to segment IV medially, and two major branches pursue a lateral course to segments II and III of the left lobe.

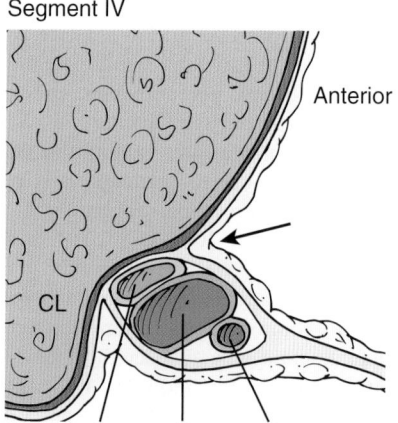

FIGURE 32.2 Sagittal section showing the relationship of segment IV and caudate lobe to the left portal triad, which is encased within a reflection of the lesser omentum that fuses with the Glisson capsule at the base of segment IV. The *arrow* indicates the point of incision for the dissection to lower the hilar plate (see also Fig. 32.5). *A,* Left hepatic duct. *B,* Left branch, portal vein. Note the left hepatic artery *(C)* joins the left duct and left branch of the portal vein at the umbilical fissure (see Chapter 2).

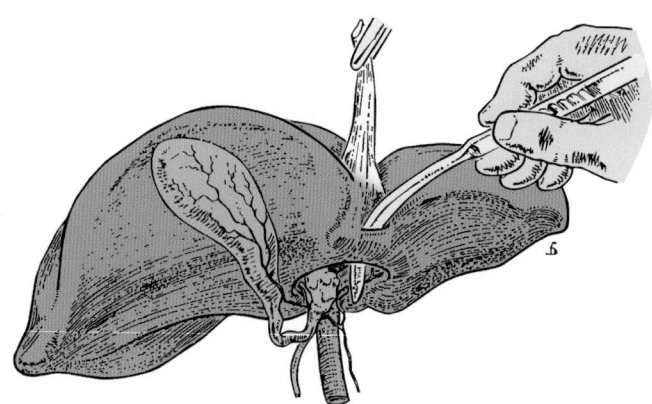

FIGURE 32.3 The bridge of liver tissue frequently present between the base of segment IV and the left lobe of the liver can be divided (see Chapter 2), as illustrated in this approach to a patient with hilar cholangiocarcinoma. This is conveniently done by passing a curved director beneath it and cutting it with diathermy. Such division can be useful in aiding an approach to the left hepatic duct, particularly if the course of the duct is vertical and the base of segment IV is short. If the bridge of tissue is present, the maneuver is always necessary to allow dissection of the segment III duct (see Fig. 32.8).

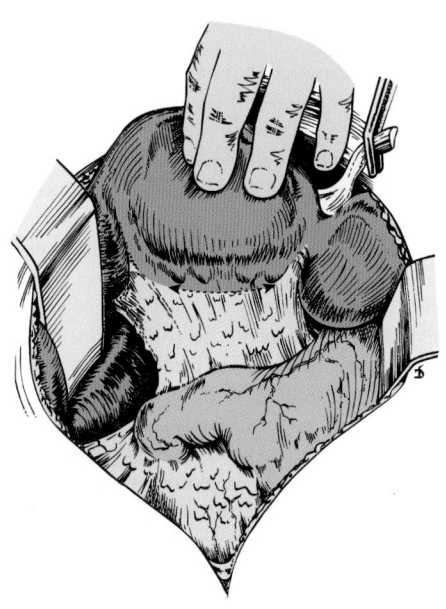

FIGURE 32.4 To optimize exposure of the extrahepatic biliary system, the undersurface of the liver at segment IVB is retracted cephalad. Also depicted here is the initial line of incision for an approach to the left hepatic duct by lowering of the hilar plate. The incision is made at precisely the point at which the Glisson capsule reflects to the lesser omentum (see Fig. 32.2).

the overlying peritoneal tissue can be dissected free to allow access to the anterior portion of the duct (see Chapters 37, 42, and 117D).

Supraduodenal Exploration

The anterior aspect of the common bile duct is exposed, and two stay sutures are placed on either side of the midpoint of the planned longitudinal incision (see Chapter 37). The choledochotomy should be located anteriorly to avoid compromising

blood vessels that typically run along the medial and lateral aspects of the common bile duct and common hepatic duct. To avoid injury to the cystic duct, the site of cystic duct insertion should be identified, as this may occur in a medial or posterior location. During the incision, caution should be taken to avoid injuring the posterior wall of the duct. The length of the choledochotomy will depend on the diameter of the duct and size of stones present with the lumen, but is generally 1 to 2 cm. Another consideration regarding the location of this incision is proximity to the duodenum; in the event that a choledocho-duodenostomy may be required for appropriate drainage, every effort should be made to position the incision distally enough to permit a tension-free anastomosis to the proximal duodenum.

After choledochotomy, flushing of the duct (distally toward ampulla) with saline irrigation can result in expulsion of stones. Following this, a deflated Fogarty balloon catheter is passed distally through the ampulla into the duodenum. Once the tip of the catheter is palpated within the duodenal lumen, the balloon is inflated, and the catheter is withdrawn until resistance is encountered, indicating that the balloon is positioned against the sphincter of Oddi. The balloon is slowly and partially deflated while applying continuous tension, allowing passage into the distal common bile duct. At this point, the balloon is carefully reinflated, and the catheter is swept proximally, sweeping retained stones up toward the cholodochotomy. This process is repeated until no stones return. The catheter is then passed proximally to retrieve any stones within the common hepatic duct and intrahepatic biliary tree. Rigid instruments such as clamps or stone forceps can cause injury to the bile duct and should therefore be used with caution. A choledochoscope can be utilized to visualize remnant stones, which can be captured with basket retrieval in which the basket is passed beyond the stone, opened, and pulled back to ensnare the stone. The choledochoscope and associated basket with stone are then withdrawn. At the conclusion of duct exploration, confirmation of proximal and distal duct clearance is performed either by choledochoscopy or completion cholangiography.[5]

Transduodenal Exploration

When an impacted stone at the distal common bile duct cannot be cleared via choledochotomy, a transduodenal approach can be employed. A 2- to 4-cm longitudinal incision on the lateral aspect of the second portion of the duodenum allows visualization of the ampulla. Stay sutures are placed on either side of the incision to maximize exposure (see Chapters 37 and 117D). If there is difficulty visualizing the ampulla, a small catheter can be passed through the choledochotomy into the duodenum. A sphincterotomy is performed at the 11 o'clock position to follow the direction of the bile duct, and the sphincter is incised to the level of the impacted stone or probe. This location minimizes the chance of pancreatic duct injury, which is generally located opposite the planned sphincterotomy site. The stone is then extracted, and the common bile duct mucosa is approximated to the duodenal mucosa with absorbable sutures (sphincteroplasty) to avoid postoperative papillary stenosis. Once again, a catheter is passed to ensure resolution of obstruction, and choledochoscopy or cholangiography is used to confirm the absence of residual stones. The duodenotomy is typically closed in one layer.[5] If sphincteroplasty is not successful, the obstruction can be bypassed with a choledochoduodenostomy (discussed later).

T-Tubes

T-tube insertion for choledochotomy closure has historically been used to drain bile in the setting of common bile duct or papillary edema and to facilitate postoperative duct access. Disadvantages include tube migration, obstruction, and bile leak. A meta-analysis of open CBDEs found that primary closure is equivalent in morbidity and mortality and decreases both operative time and hospital stay compared with T-tube

closure.[6] Another meta-analysis found primary closure superior to T-tube closure in laparoscopic CBDE when comparing rates of postoperative biliary peritonitis, operative time, length of hospital stay, and hospital expenses.[7] If a T-tube is employed, use of a 14-French (Fr) or larger size will permit cholangiography and choledochoscopy. The T-tube is prepared by cutting two limbs at lengths that will not traverse into the left or right hepatic duct proximally or into the duodenum distally, and excising the back wall of the horizontal portion of the T (to minimize the risk of tube occlusion and to facilitate eventual tube removal). The tube is inserted through the choledochotomy, and the remainder of the duct is closed with fine absorbable sutures around the tube. Care should be taken to leave enough redundancy in the intraperitoneal portion of the tube to avoid tension (and possible tube dislodgement) in the event of significant postoperative abdominal distension. Postoperatively, the T-tube is placed to dependent drainage until resolution of postoperative papillary edema allows physiologic flow of bile into the duodenum. If persistently elevated output or drainage around the tube occurs, investigation via cholangiography can identify malfunction, dislodgement, or distal obstruction secondary to retained stone. If the results of a repeat cholangiogram at approximately 2 to 3 weeks are normal, the T-tube may be removed. If choledocholithiasis persists, the T-tube can be clamped to promote stone passage. If signs or symptoms of cholangitis occur, the tube can be unclamped and repeat imaging is obtained. Residual obstruction may be amenable to stone extraction via T-tube or endoscopic or percutaneous access (see Chapter 37A).

Outcomes

Open CBDE is safe and effective, although endoscopic and laparoscopic modalities may now have more favorable risk profiles as these techniques have matured (see Chapters 30, 37B, and 37C). The most recent Cochrane review primarily reflects outcomes from the early endoscopic and laparoscopic era, with 10 of 16 trials published before 2000. Within this analysis, open CBDE and endoscopic retrograde cholangiopancreatography (ERCP) had similar rates of mortality (1% vs. 3%) and morbidity (20% vs. 19%), respectively.[8] A recent prospective randomized trial demonstrated lower morbidity and shorter length of stay for laparoscopic versus open CBDE.[9] Compared with laparoscopic CBDE, a recent meta-analysis found that endoscopic retrograde cholangiogram and sphincterotomy was associated with a higher common bile duct stone clearance rate and lower postoperative bile leakage rate, but a higher rate of pancreatitis.[10] Although it may incur greater morbidity compared with less invasive techniques, open CBDE overall remains a highly effective and safe way to clear common bile duct stones, especially when other modalities are not an option (see Chapter 38).

BILIARY-ENTERIC ANASTOMOSIS

Overview

There are three key aspects to consider when planning a biliary-enteric anastomosis: identification of a healthy segment of bile duct tissue proximal to the site of obstruction; preparation of a segment of alimentary tract such as duodenum or, more commonly, Roux-en-Y jejunal limb; and construction of a mucosa-to-mucosa anastomosis (see Chapter 42). It is important to use preoperative imaging to clearly delineate the biliary anatomy before undertaking operative intervention for biliary decompression, but invasive cholangiography is no longer necessary to delineate biliary anatomy in the great majority of cases. Cross-sectional imaging with magnetic resonance imaging (MRI)/magnetic resonance cholangiopancreatography (MRCP) (or high-resolution computed tomography [CT]) can accurately characterize the anatomy of the biliary tree and underlying pathology (see Chapter 16). Instrumentation of the biliary tree introduces bacterial contamination that, in a setting of biliary stasis, can result in cholangitis, periductal inflammation, and a higher risk of postoperative infections. Likewise, insertion of a percutaneous drain into an excluded biliary segment will result in bacterial colonization of static bile. If that hepatic segment cannot be decompressed by a subsequent operative intervention, it will not be possible to remove the external drain without risking refractory cholangitis. These complexities underscore the critical importance of an experienced multidisciplinary team reviewing and treating complex biliary obstruction, particularly at the biliary confluence.

Depending on the underlying pathology, there are a number of options for restoring biliary continuity with the alimentary tract. For instance, benign etiologies such as iatrogenic bile duct injury, strictures from previous biliary-enteric operations, choledochal cysts, or inflammatory strictures may require restoration with Roux-en-Y choledochojejunostomy or hepaticojejunostomy. Additionally, benign proximal biliary strictures as well as malignancy (cholangiocarcinoma) may require anastomosis between intrahepatic ducts and jejunum (see Chapters 42, 51, and 119B). Choledocholithiasis refractory to local exploration may require choledochoduodenostomy. Benign ampullary adenomas and papillary stenosis that fail endoscopic management may be treated with transduodenal surgical ampullectomy. Finally, the gallbladder may also be utilized to facilitate drainage (cholecystoduodenostomy and cholecystojejunostomy). Although nonoperative measures can be utilized in most situations, familiarity with the various surgical techniques enables appropriate restoration of biliary-enteric continuity when the situation demands.

Incision and Exposure

A right subcostal incision with or without an upper midline extension or a left subcostal extension followed by upward elevation and cephalad retraction of the costal margin provides adequate exposure for construction of any biliary-enteric anastomosis (see Chapters 37 and 42). The ligamentum teres is ligated and divided, and the falciform ligament is divided to its most cephalad extent on the diaphragm. Retraction of the ligamentum teres is helpful for optimal visualization of the vascular inflow and biliary drainage of segments II, III, and IV. If direct decompression of the gallbladder is not to be undertaken, cholecystectomy can be advantageous for identification of the cystic duct, which can be dissected to its point of insertion onto the common hepatic duct. Cholecystectomy will also expose the cystic plate, which runs in continuity with the hilar plate. By lowering the hilar plate, the left hepatic duct may be exposed as it runs against the base of segment IVB.[11] Mobilization of the right colon with caudal retraction, followed by a generous Kocher maneuver, will further enhance exposure for biliary-enteric bypass.

Caution must be exercised in the setting of long-standing biliary obstruction or conditions associated with ipsilateral hepatic atrophy and contralateral hypertrophy. In the scenario of marked right hemiliver atrophy, the liver hilum and portal structures will become rotated in a counterclockwise manner. Consequently, the portal vein will assume a more anterior location and the common bile duct or common hepatic duct will be posteriorly displaced. Hypertrophy of segment IV protrudes over the porta hepatis and may provide additional complexity for access to the hilum and left biliary system.[12]

Hepaticojejunostomy

Roux-en-Y hepaticojejunostomy is used to create a large tension-free anastomosis to healthy hepatic ducts that drain all biliary segments. The proximal jejunum should reach easily to the hepatic duct confluence in the right upper quadrant, where the biliary anastomosis will take place. If this approach is not feasible due to tumor infiltration or a high stricture, drainage can be obtained via the right hepatic duct or left hepatic duct (discussed later). Moreover, ducts draining segments II and III can be utilized when the left hepatic duct is not accessible.[2] Disadvantages include the necessity for two anastomoses and exclusion of bile from the duodenum (see Chapters 37 and 42).

Approach to Right Hepatic Duct

As the portal pedicles enter the liver parenchyma, they remain enclosed within a fibrous sheath derived from Glisson capsule (see Chapter 2). Access to the right portal pedicle containing the right hepatic duct can be achieved by isolating the pedicle in an extrahepatic location or by exposing the pedicle via intrahepatic dissection (see Chapter 42). The extrahepatic approach begins by lowering the hilar plate; the peritoneum along the posterior aspect of segment IV is divided, allowing separation of Glisson capsule from the peritoneal reflection enveloping the porta hepatis. By reflecting the base of segment IV in a cephalad direction, this dissection effectively exposes the confluence of the right and left hepatic duct. By continuing this plane of dissection to the right (onto the cystic plate), the right hepatic duct may be exposed.[13] If the extrahepatic portion of the right hepatic duct is too short to be visualized in this way (as is often the case), the intrahepatic approach may be used. This requires hepatotomies in the caudate process just posterior to the porta hepatis and along the base of the gallbladder fossa. A blunt right angle clamp may be passed between these hepatotomies to encircle the right pedicle, which can then be delivered for further dissection to identify the right hepatic duct, or the anterior or posterior sectional ducts (Fig. 32.5).[14]

Approach to Left Hepatic Duct

The left hepatic duct traverses an extrahepatic course below segment IVB from the umbilical fissure to the porta hepatis. After ligation of the ligamentum teres with a firm tie, retraction is applied to elevate the left hemiliver. The bridge of tissue at the base of the umbilical fissure contains no large vessels and can be divided to provide mobility of the base of segment IVB, and to enhance exposure of the left portal pedicle (see Fig. 32.3). The left hepatic duct runs with the left portal vein and is exposed by lowering the hilar plate (Fig. 32.6). Dissection toward the hepatic confluence to expose an adequate segment of the left hepatic duct is facilitated by retracting segment IVB anteriorly[2] (see Chapter 42).

Approach to Segment III Duct

The presence of a bulky unresectable tumor at the hepatic hilus may require construction of a more proximal anastomosis. This can be achieved by exposing the biliary drainage of the left

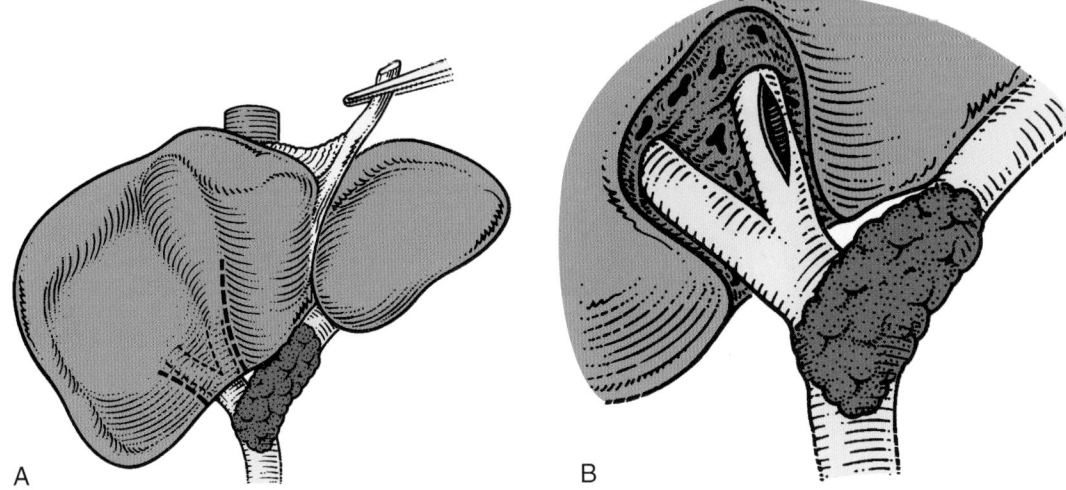

FIGURE 32.5 **A,** Exposure of the right hepatic pedicle in the setting of a cholangiocarcinoma extending into the left hepatic duct. Intrahepatic exposure of the right hepatic duct is accomplished initially by controlling the right portal pedicle. After performing hepatotomies in the caudate process just posterior to the porta hepatis and along the base of the gallbladder fossa, a blunt right angle can be used to facilitate encircling and delivery of the right pedicle. The overlying hepatic parenchyma is further dissected, which allows identification of the right hepatic duct and the anterior or posterior sectional ducts. **B,** The relevant duct, usually the anterior sectoral duct, is opened, and anastomosis is carried out.

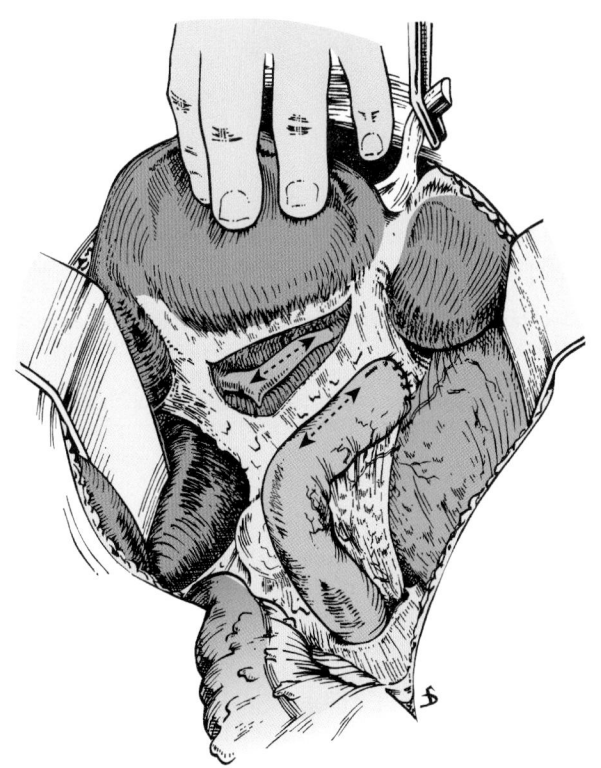

FIGURE 32.6 The hilar plate is lowered, and the left hepatic duct is exposed for dissection. The exposure is carried medially and to the right to expose the confluence and the right hepatic duct.

hemiliver within the umbilical fissure.[11,15,16] If the left hemiliver has not atrophied from long-standing biliary obstruction, unilateral left-sided biliary decompression will effectively relieve obstructive jaundice and restore hepatic function, even when the biliary drainage of the excluded right hemiliver remains obstructed. In a series evaluating segment III bypass for malignant

biliary obstruction, patients experienced durable relief of jaundice and pruritis, with an 80% patency rate at one year.[15]

After ligation and retraction of the ligamentum teres, the band of liver parenchyma at the base of the ligamentum teres joining segment III and IVB (if present) is divided to enhance exposure of the segment III duct (which, if dilated, may be more readily apparent). This exposure can be facilitated by fashioning a superficial hepatotomy along the left of the ligamentum teres, through which the segment III duct may be exposed and opened without risk of injury to the vascular pedicle to segment III (Fig. 32.7). In circumstances in which identification is difficult, localization can be confirmed by aspiration with a small gauge needle. On occasion, a wedge resection of a portion of segment III can also be performed to provide exposure of the segment III duct (Fig. 32.8).[11] To prepare for biliary-enteric anastomosis, the duct should be dissected free for 1.5 cm but should not be cleared circumferentially (to minimize devascularization injury). A defunctionalized jejunal loop is then brought up in a retrocolic fashion and prepared for anastomosis (see Chapter 42).

Construction of Anastomosis

For the purposes of Roux-en-Y reconstruction, the most proximal loop of jejunum that can be brought to lie against the planned site of anastomosis without tension is selected. The jejunum is transected and a Roux limb of 50 to 70 cm is passed in a retrocolic fashion through the avascular portion of the transverse mesocolon to the right of the middle colic artery. The jejunojejunostomy may be fashioned in a sutured or stapled manner. We do not typically employ a transanastomotic stent; however, if a stent is to be used, it is preferable to pass the stent through the cut hepatic duct before construction of the anastomosis. The stent may be affixed against the duct wall with a single 4-0 or 5-0 absorbable catgut suture, which is tied on the outside of the duct wall (Fig. 32.9); this maneuver helps to avoid inadvertent dislodgment of the tube during placement of the anastomotic sutures. When more than one biliary duct

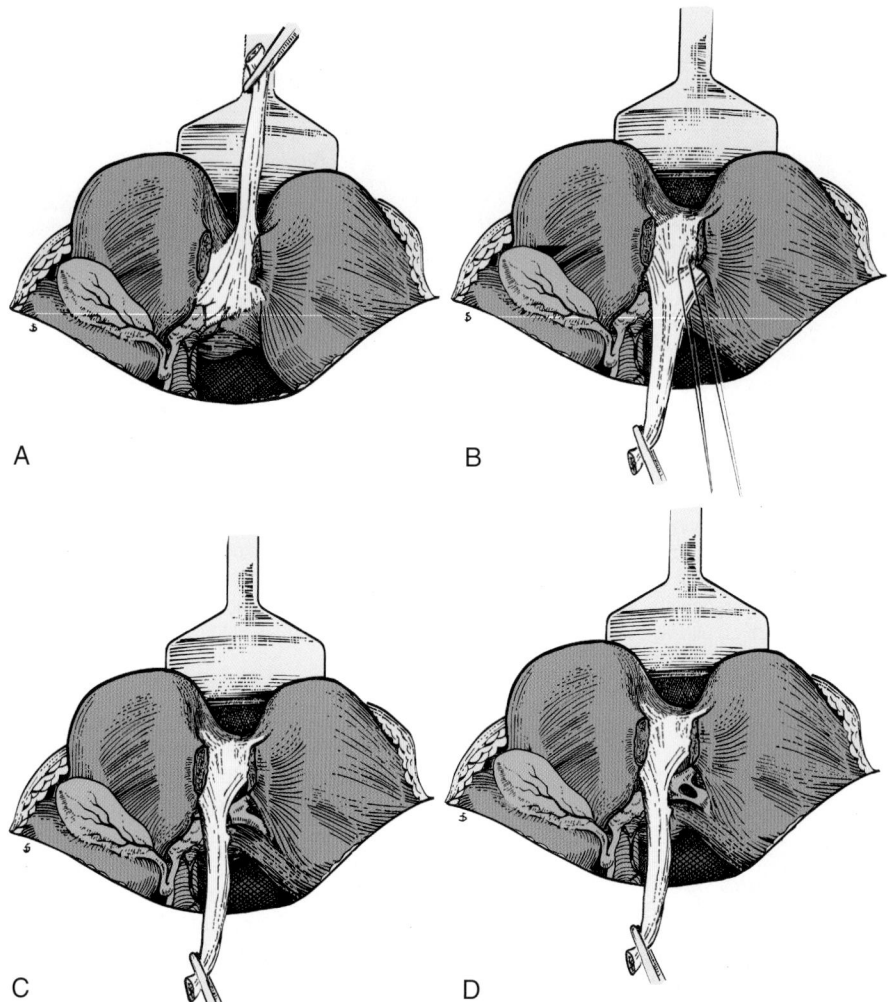

A

B

C

D

FIGURE 32.7   **A,** The liver is held up so that its inferior surface is seen. The bridge of liver between segment IV and the left lobe of the liver has been divided. The base of the ligamentum teres is seen. **B,** The ligamentum teres is then pulled downward. The peritoneum of its upper surface on the left side is incised, and the extensions passing into the liver are exposed. The left sides of these extensions are divided between ligatures, which must be passed carefully using aneurysm needles. This part of the dissection is tedious and should be carried out meticulously because hemorrhage within the recess adjacent to the segment III duct can be difficult to control. **C,** The segment III duct is exposed. **D,** The duct is opened longitudinally for anastomosis, which is carried out by the technique illustrated in Fig. 32.13.

orifice is present, it is preferable to create a single duct orifice by approximating the two ducts with a single row of 4-0 or 5-0 absorbable sutures (Fig. 32.10).

The hepaticojejunostomy may be performed using an end-to-side or side-to-side anastomosis. Side-to-side anastomosis usually requires less dissection (preserving vascular supply) and allows for a wider anastomosis, which may decrease risk of stricture.[17] A study examining the two anastomoses in a series of 125 type 1a choledochal cysts found that about 10% of the end-to-side group experienced stricture after two years follow-up, compared with none in the end-to-side group.[18]

A side-to-side anastomosis is especially useful in the setting of left hepatic duct or segment III duct hepaticojejunostomy (see Fig. 32.6). Additionally, benign strictures (e.g., iatrogenic) can be approached in this fashion. When decompression is undertaken at the level of the proximal hepatic duct, increased length may be achieved by extending the incision onto the left hepatic duct. A longitudinal ductotomy of approximately 2.5 to 3.0 cm is performed, with a corresponding jejunotomy on the

antimesenteric border, 2 cm from the staple line. An anterior row of full-thickness, single interrupted 4-0 or 5-0 absorbable sutures passed from outside to inside are retracted to allow exposure for placement of the posterior row. Full-thickness, single interrupted 4-0 or 5-0 absorbable sutures approximate the inferior edge of the duct to the superior edge of jejunum. Following placement, the posterior row of sutures is tied. Subsequently, the preplaced anterior row of sutures is used to complete the anastomosis; they are passed from inside to outside on the jejunum, and the knots are tied.[17]

For an end-to-side hepaticojejunostomy, the bile duct segment is transected, and an adjacent jejunotomy is fashioned at a safe distance from the mesenteric margin of the bowel approximately 2 cm from the staple line. The jejunotomy length should be shorter than the ductotomy, as the bowel is more pliable than the duct. An anterior row of full-thickness, single interrupted 4-0 or 5-0 absorbable sutures is placed in the bile duct passed from inside to outside and working from the patient's left to right. This row of sutures, with needles intact, is

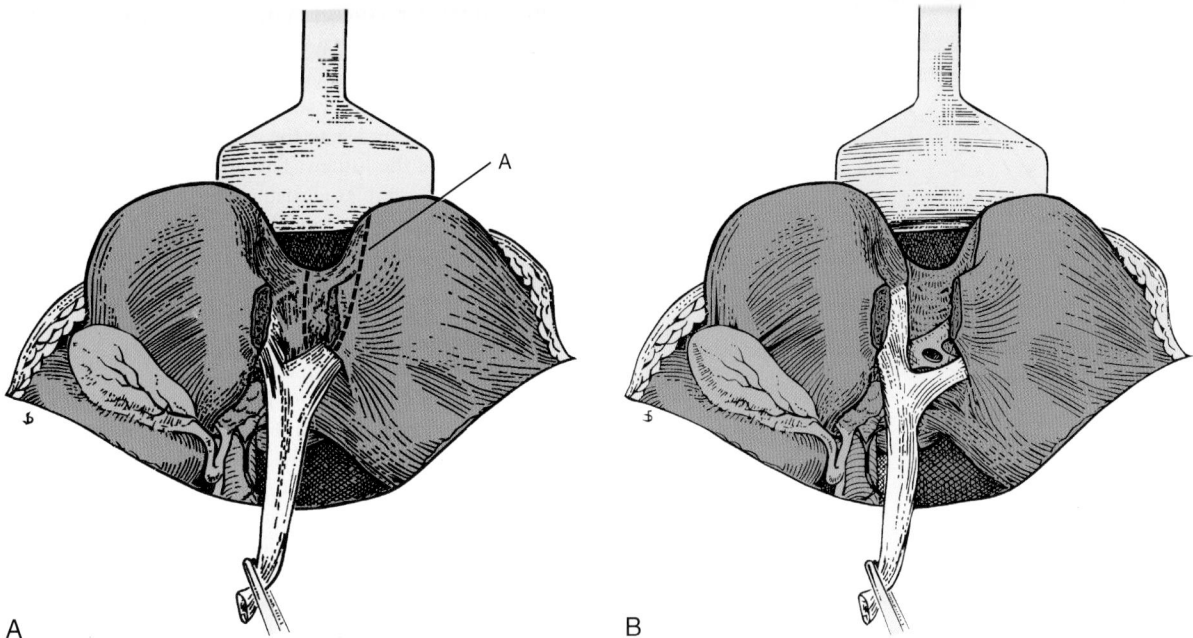

FIGURE 32.8 **A,** The liver is split to the left of the ligamentum teres in the umbilical fissure, and it may be necessary to remove a small wedge of liver tissue. **B,** The segment III duct is exposed at the base of the liver split above and behind its accompanying vein and is ready for anastomosis.

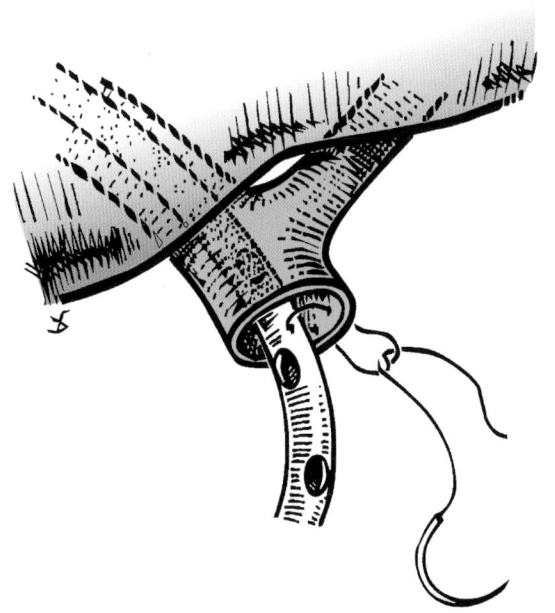

FIGURE 32.9 Manner of fixation of transanastomotic tubes. Note the introduction of the absorbable suture in a mattress fashion across the ductal wall, proximal to the future site of anastomosis. This secures the tube conveniently during anastomosis.

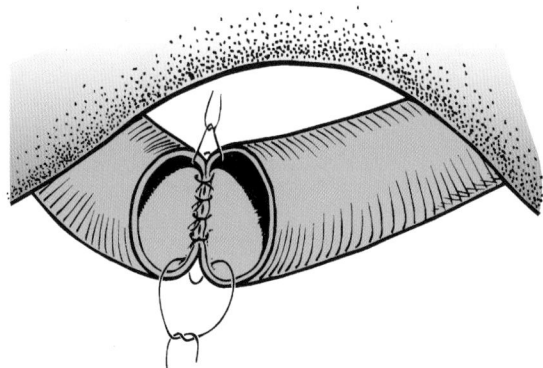

FIGURE 32.10 Adjacent ductal orifices may be approximated before anastomosis.

The previously placed row of anterior sutures is then used to complete the anastomosis. Each needle is passed through the jejunum, tied, and cut short; the corner stay sutures are then cut (see Chapters 42 and 119B).

Choledochojejunostomy

In cases of distal obstruction, a choledochojejunostomy decompresses the biliary tree, using the common hepatic or common bile duct. Causes of distal obstruction include ampullary stone(s), iatrogenic injuries, benign strictures not amenable to endoscopic management, and unresectable periampullary tumors in which biliary stenting is not effective. Advantages of a surgical approach versus nonoperative decompressive modalities are long-term patency and durability without the need for repeat stent placement or revision.

Choledochojejunostomy can be performed as an end-to-side or side-to-side anastomosis. For the end-to-side technique, a cholecystectomy with cystic duct ligation is performed followed

retracted and elevated; this maneuver effectively pulls the anterior aspect of the duct away, facilitating exposure and placement of the posterior row of sutures (Fig. 32.11). A single, full-thickness posterior row of interrupted 4-0 or 5-0 absorbable sutures is used to approximate the inferior edge of the biliary duct to the superior edge of jejunum, also working from patient's left to right. These sutures are tied and cut short except for the two corner sutures, which are secured with clamps.

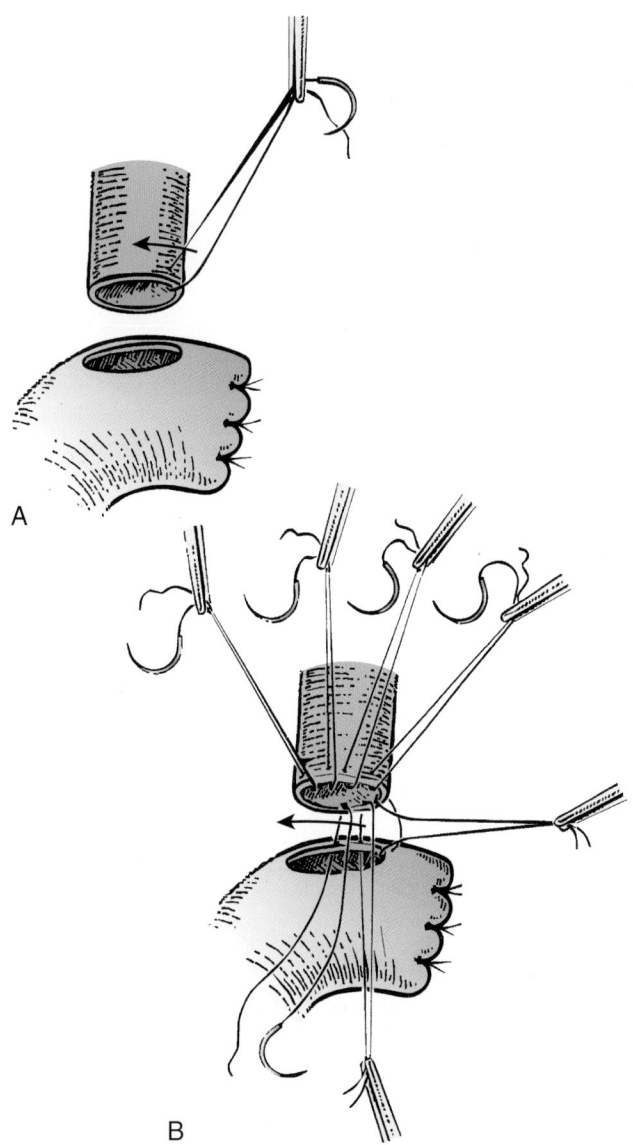

FIGURE 32.11 **A,** The initial step in the creation of hepaticojejunostomy Roux-en-Y. The anterior layer of suture (3-0 Vicryl) on the bile duct is inserted first, and the sutures are passed from the inside out, starting from the patient's left and working toward the right. The needles are retained, and the sutures are kept in order. **B,** The anterior layer of sutures is elevated. This displays the posterior ductal wall, and the posterior row of sutures is now placed, again from left to right.

by ligation of the common bile duct or common hepatic duct (hepaticojejunostomy) at the level of planned transection. The duct is opened at the level of the planned anastomosis, and the endobiliary stent (if present) is removed. If desired, bile cultures may also be collected at this time. The remainder of the common bile duct is transected, and the distal stump is oversewn with 3-0 absorbable suture. It is important to identify a healthy, well-vascularized duct proximal to the level of injury or pathology to avoid ischemic stricture. Similarly, care should be taken to avoid excessive circumferential dissection of the duct, as this can compromise its blood supply. A 50- to 70-cm Roux-en-Y limb of jejunum is passed in a retrocolic position to the right of the middle colic vessels, and positioned to reside adjacent to the proximal bile duct in a tension-free manner. The posterior

wall of the duct is sutured to the jejunum with a running 3-0 or 4-0 absorbable suture. The tail of the suture and needle are left intact. A jejunotomy is fashioned along the duct, and single interrupted 3-0 or 4-0 absorbable sutures are used to approximate the jejunal mucosa to the duct mucosa, with the knots tied on the inside of the lumen. The anterior portion of the anastomosis is then completed using the running suture used to construct the posterior row (Fig. 32.12). Because of the small lumen, the anastomosis is generally completed with a single layer to avoid narrowing. Placement of a sponge circumferentially around the anastomosis allows for an intraoperative test to confirm absence of a large bile leak.

The alternative approach of constructing a side-to-side anastomosis offers the advantages of less devascularization with the use of a nontransected duct, and preservation of biliary-duodenal continuity (in case future ERCP should be desirable).[17] To perform this anastomosis, the anterior surface of the duct is exposed and opened longitudinally for a distance of 2.5 to 3.0 cm, avoiding the medial and lateral locations of periductal vasculature. The biliary-enteric anastomosis can then be completed in a similar manner as described for side-to-side hepaticojejunostomy (see previous discussion). A single, interrupted anterior (or right) row of sutures allows exposure for placement of the posterior (or left) row approximating duct to jejunum, followed by completion of the anterior row[17] (see Chapters 42 and 119B).

Choledochoduodenostomy

While choledochoduodenostomy has the physiologic advantage of enabling bile flow into the duodenum, this procedure is effective only for distal strictures or impacted stone(s) in the distal common bile duct. After mobilization of the hepatic flexure of the colon, a generous Kocher maneuver is performed to allow sufficient mobility of the duodenum to enable construction of a tension-free anastomosis. The gallbladder is removed and the cystic duct is ligated. A 2.5- to 3.0-cm longitudinal incision is made on the anterior surface of the supraduodenal common bile duct. Correspondingly, the duodenum adjacent to the common bile duct is incised longitudinally along its superolateral border (Fig. 32.13). This produces incisions that are perpendicular to one another (unlike the parallel configuration used during hepaticojejunostomy). As with the hepaticojejunostomy, the duodenotomy is generally shorter in length than the ductotomy. The anastomosis is then constructed in a manner that anastomoses the bile duct transversely to the longitudinally oriented duodenotomy. Three corner 4-0 or 5-0 absorbable sutures are placed: the first two are positioned between the midpoints of the ductotomy and proximal and distal aspects of the duodenotomy, and the third is placed between the distal aspect of the common bile duct incision and midpoint of the superior lip of the duodenotomy. Traction on the three corner sutures reorients the distal portion of the ductotomy transversely, facilitating placement of the posterior row of absorbable sutures between the superior edge of the duodenotomy and the distal half of the common bile duct. Full-thickness sutures are used to approximate the ductal mucosa to duodenal mucosa. A fourth corner suture can then be placed between the proximal end of the ductotomy and the midpoint of the anterior duodenal wall. Retraction of this fourth corner suture tents the remaining anterior wall of the anastomosis forward, facilitating placement of the remaining anterior row of sutures (Fig. 32.14). As before, use of a single row of sutures minimizes the risk of anastomotic narrowing (see Chapter 42).

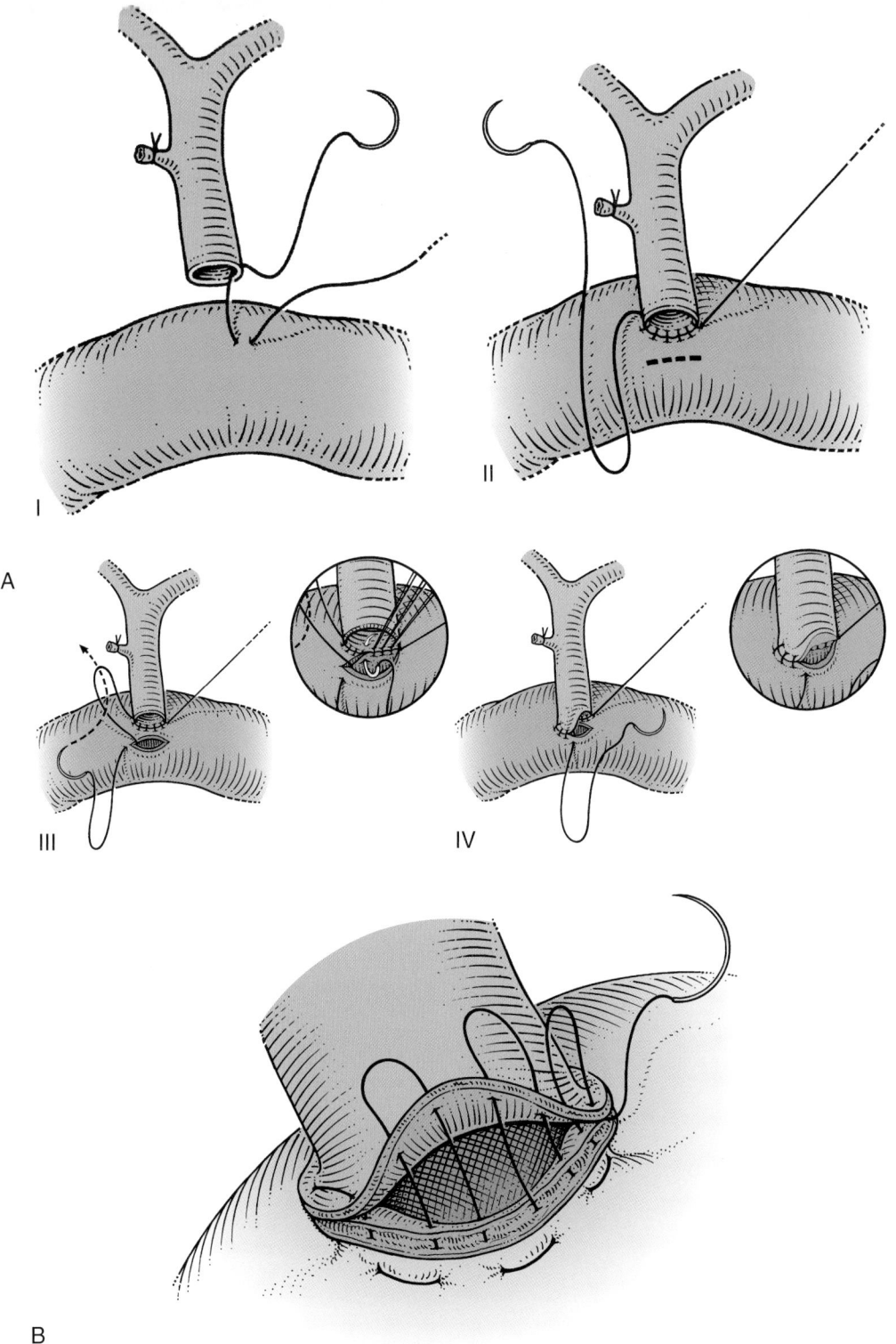

FIGURE 32.12 **A,** Technique for end-to-side anastomosis of the bile duct below the hilus to jejunum. *I,* A 3-0 Vicryl suture is used, and the serosa of the jejunum is sutured to the full thickness of the bile duct. *II,* This suture is developed as the posterior wall of the bile duct is attached to the jejunal serosa. The *dotted line* marks the point of incision in the jejunum, which is made after the posterior layer is attached. *III,* The suture is now developed either as a continuous or an interrupted suture on the anterior layer. The posterior layer of the jejunal mucosa is not sutured directly to the bile duct mucosa. Several interrupted sutures may be inserted before completing the anterior layer, however, to approximate the mucosa *(inset).* *IV,* The anastomosis is completed. The *inset* shows the posterior layer with mucosal apposition. **B,** Alternatively, the jejunum may be opened, and a mucosa-to-mucosa anastomosis may be performed with a continuous polydioxanone suture as illustrated.

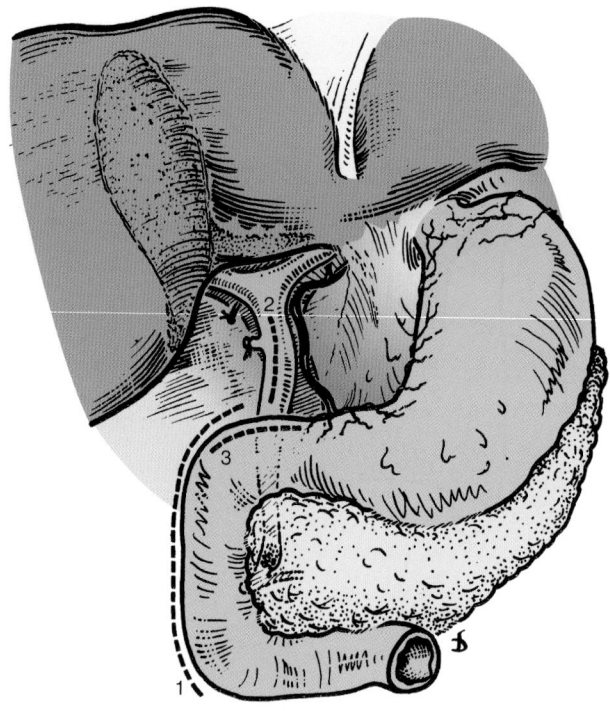

FIGURE 32.13   **After the gallbladder is removed, the common bile duct is removed through a conventional longitudinal incision following a Kocher incision** *(1)* **freeing the lateral duodenum around the common duct.** Routine common duct exploration is carried out. If indications for a choledochoduodenostomy exist, the anastomosis is performed. The incision in the common duct *(2)* is extended to 2.5 cm by direct measurement. In almost all instances, the incision in the duct carries into the common hepatic duct. The incision in the postbulbar duodenum *(3)* is slightly smaller because the stoma in the duodenum stretches to approximate the choledochal incision.

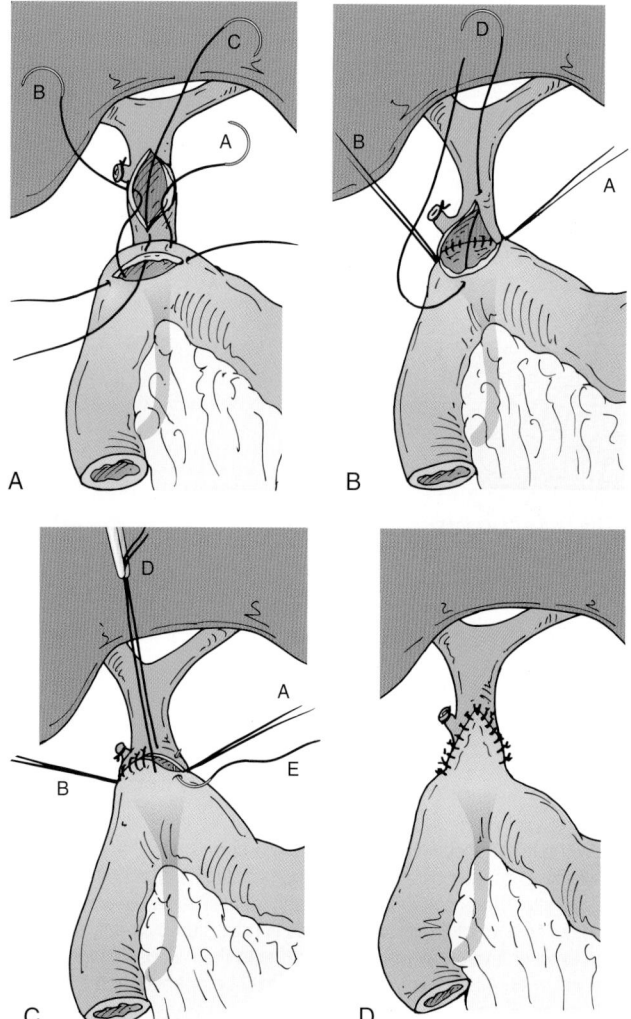

FIGURE 32.14   **A,** Each side of the choledochoduodenostomy is bisected by suture *(A* and *B)* of absorbable material (Vicryl or PDS) that passes from the end of the duodenal incision through the midpoint of the choledochal incision. Likewise, the duodenal incision is bisected by a suture through the posterior wall of the duodenal incision and the lower apex of the choledochal incision *(C)*. These stitches convert part of the longitudinal choledochotomy incision into a transverse ostium. The lax approximation of the duodenal and choledochal incisions occurs, with the duodenum mobilized, by placing tension on a lateral stay suture *(A* or *B)* and the middle stay suture *(C)*. **B,** Sutures may be placed to complete the posterior suture line approximating the common bile duct to the posterior duodenal incision. After placement of the sutures, they are tied so that the knots are within the lumen. The anterior wall is similarly approximated using a suture bisecting the anterior duodenal incision *(D)* and through the original apex of the bile duct incision. **C,** With this bisecting suture *(D)* tented forward, each of the segments between the tied lateral stay suture and this anterior suture is similarly approximated using interrupted sutures with the knots tied on the outside. The anastomosis is completed by completing the third segment of this triangle with sutures placed between the remaining lateral stay suture and the bisecting, anterior suture *(D)*. It is important in the placement of these last sutures that they do not catch the posterior suture line. The benefit of placing all the sutures in one line of the triangular closure and tying them all after placement is that it allows an internal inspection before the lumen of the choledochoduodenostomy is obscured. A single row of sutures is all that is used. A second row does nothing but decrease the choledochoduodenostomy orifice size and should be avoided. The sutures should be placed close enough for a bile-tight approximation. Digital pressure on the duodenum or the common duct should give no evidence of leakage. **D,** The completed anastomosis allows a thumb-sized defect to be palpated through the duodenal tongue that has been brought on to the common bile duct and common hepatic duct. The anastomosis may be drained or not, according to preference (the leak rate is 1%). The presence of a closed-suction drain (Jackson-Pratt type) obviates the need for a subsequent percutaneous drainage catheter if this uncommon complication occurs.

Transduodenal ampullectomy

Transduodenal ampullectomy is used for benign ampullary tumors and strictures not amenable to endoscopic therapy, as well as symptomatic pancreas divisum. It is substantially less morbid than the alternative of pancreaticoduodenectomy and generally well tolerated, with success rates of over 80%.[19] After adequate exposure, a longitudinal duodenotomy on the anterior surface of D2 is made to gain access to the ampulla. It can be helpful to place stay sutures of 3-0 PDS along the duodenal mucosa circumferentially around the ampullary mass, as retraction of these sutures can help to visualize the area surrounding the ampulla. As the ampullary mass is excised, stay sutures of 4-0 or 5-0 PDS can be placed along the cut edges of the biliary and pancreatic ducts to facilitate their identification. After excision of the ampulla, the biliary and pancreatic ducts are joined with sutures to create a common ostium. Reinsertion of the duct is accomplished with interrupted duct-to-mucosa sutures of 4-0 or 5-0 PDS, and the duodenotomy is closed in one layer (Fig. 32.15) (see Chapter 117D).

Cholecystoduodenostomy and Cholecystojejunostomy

Less common approaches to biliary bypass are cholecystoduodenostomy or cholecystojejunostomy. The cholecystoenteric bypass is relatively easy to construct, but long-term patency rates are suboptimal compared with maneuvers that directly decompress the extrahepatic biliary ducts. As a result, use of cholecystoduodenostomy or cholecystojejunostomy is limited to circumstances of advanced malignancy that require simple operative interventions and only short-term palliation.[20] Cholecystoenterostomy may be suitable in situations where major tumoral obstruction obscures access to the porta hepatis; however, the obstruction must not extend to the level of the cystic duct insertion. The presence of cholelithiasis is another consideration, as significant stone burden within the gallbladder makes this operative strategy less attractive.

Operatively, the gallbladder and cystic duct are evaluated to ensure their suitability for biliary decompression. To construct a cholecystoduodenostomy, a Kocher maneuver is used to provide enough duodenal mobility for a tension-free anastomosis. If cholecystojejunostomy is performed, the most proximal loop of jejunum that will easily lie adjacent to the gallbladder is selected; a Roux-en-Y is not routinely performed. The gallbladder fundus is secured to the antimesenteric border of duodenum or jejunum with interrupted 3-0 absorbable sutures. A cholecystotomy is performed and the gallbladder evacuated of stones and bile; a bile specimen can be sent for analysis. Continuity with the common hepatic duct is confirmed, and a corresponding enterotomy mirroring the cholecystotomy is fashioned. An anterior row of sutures is then placed to complete the anastomosis (Fig. 32.16) (see Chapter 37).

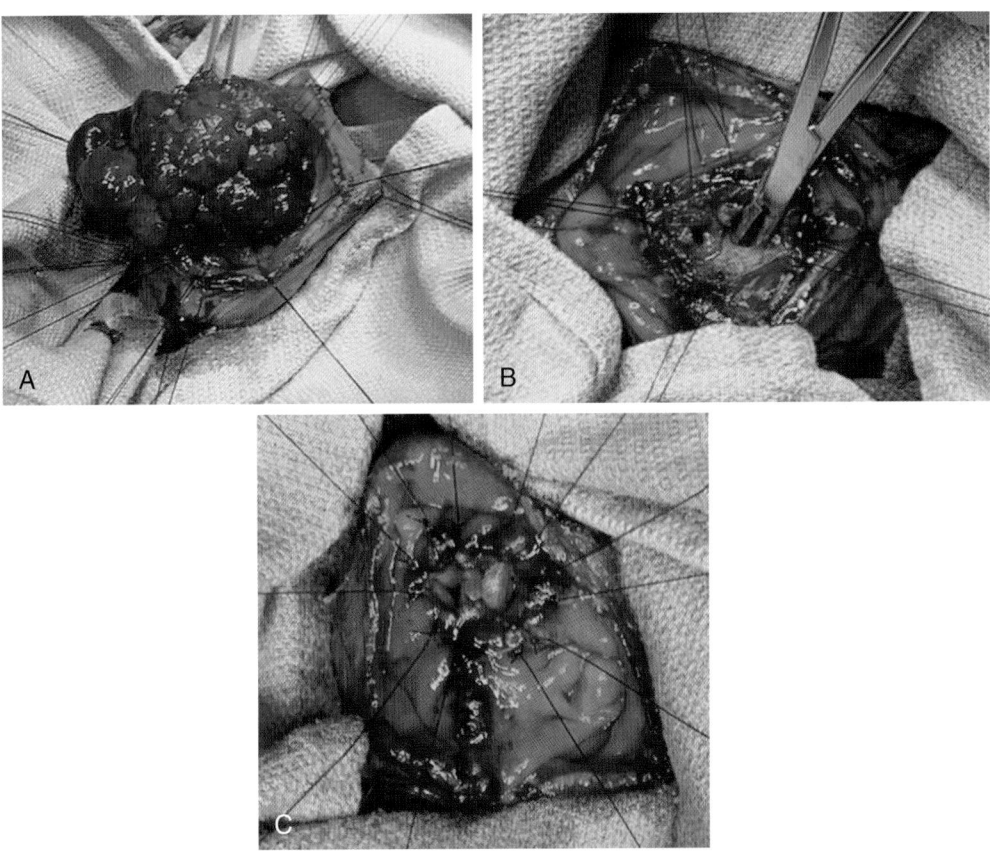

FIGURE 32.15 Technique of transduodenal ampullectomy. A, Stay sutures of 3-0 PDS are placed along the duodenal mucosa circumferentially about the ampullary mass to facilitate exposure of the periampullary space. **B,** On removal of the ampullary mass, the luminal openings of the distal common bile duct and pancreatic duct are visible (the instrument is indicating the pancreatic duct orifice). **C,** The anastomosis is completed with a series of interrupted 4-0 PDS sutures between the common bile duct and pancreatic duct wall and the surrounding duodenal mucosa (see Chapter 117D).

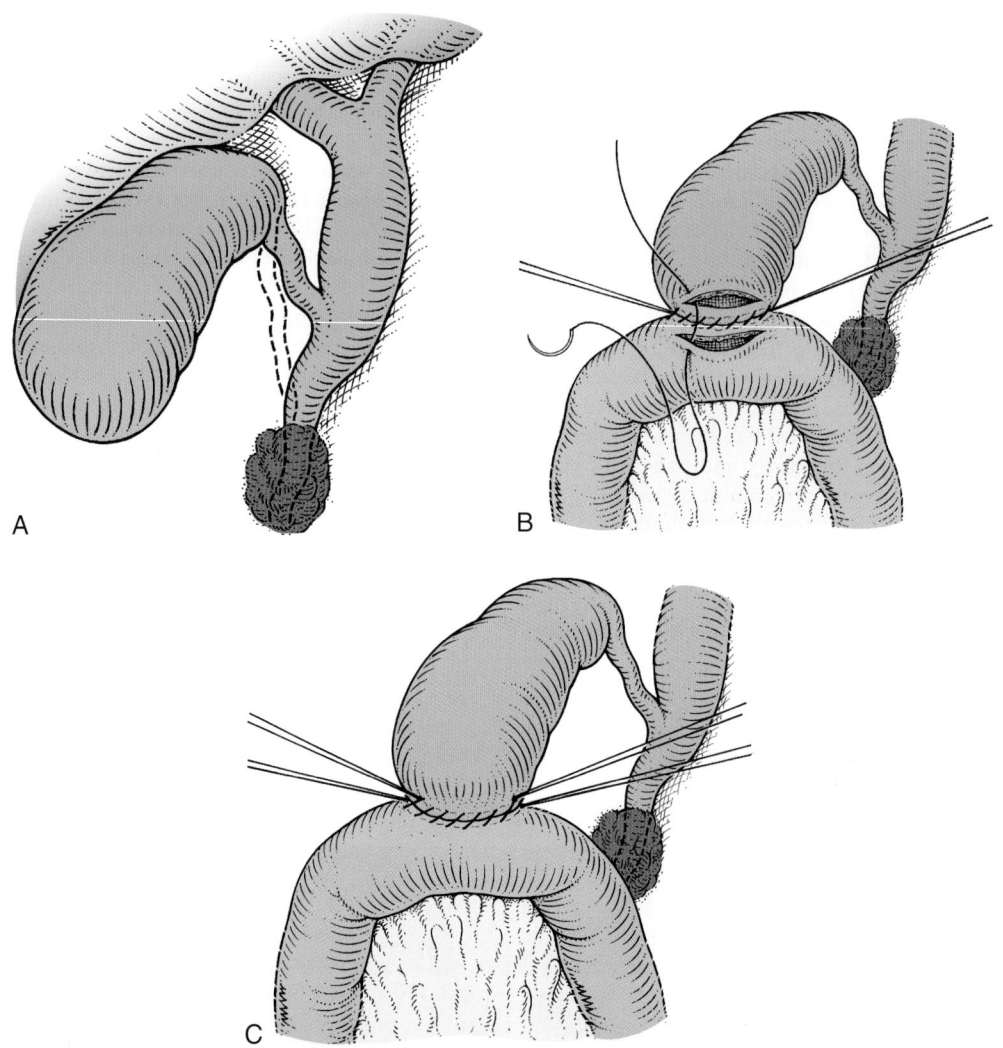

FIGURE 32.16 Technique of cholecystojejunostomy. A, The cystic duct should join the common bile duct above the tumor. If it enters at the level of the tumor *(dashed line)*, the procedure is contraindicated. **B,** The posterior layer of the anastomosis is performed with a running suture between the openings at the fundus of the gallbladder and the jejunum. **C,** The anterior layer of the side-to-side anastomosis is completed.

Outcomes

A recent single institution retrospective analysis of 45 patients undergoing reconstruction after biliary injury measured a postoperative biliary fistula rate of 3%, and a biliary stricture rate of less than 5% over four years.[17] Other analyses have also confirmed the safety and longevity of biliary decompression, with low rates of fistula and stricture formation necessitating subsequent operative intervention.[15,21–23] Although the limited number of patients requiring biliary-enteric bypass prohibits comparative analysis of the various techniques, the larger series demonstrate low perioperative morbidity and mortality and adequate long-term patency.

In patients undergoing bypass for benign disease, consideration should be given to prolonged clinical monitoring, as there appears to be both a risk of delayed stricture and an elevated risk of cholangiocarcinoma. In a review of 1,003 patients undergoing biliary decompression, cholangiocarcinoma developed in 5.8% of patients after transduodenal sphincteroplasty, 7.6% of patients after choledochoduodenostomy, and 1.9% of patients after hepaticojejunostomy after an interval of 132 to 218 months.[24]

The references for this chapter can be found online by accessing the accompanying Expert Consult website.

Biliary Tract Disease

C. Malignant Tumors

SECTION I. Inflammatory, Infective, and Congenital

A. Gallstones and Gallbladder

CHAPTER 33

The natural history of symptomatic and asymptomatic gallstones

Sean J. Judge and Sepideh Gholami

INTRODUCTION

The aim of this chapter is to describe established and novel findings on the natural history of gallstones. Gallstones have been a scourge of humankind for millennia. Each year surgeons perform over 700,000 cholecystectomies in the United States alone, with an estimated annual cost of approximately $6.2 billion USD.[1,2] The annual rate of hospital admissions for acute cholecystitis and the associated hospital charges continue to increase,[3] highlighting the great burden gallstone disease places on the American healthcare system. Despite these increasing trends, a substantial proportion of the population have asymptomatic gallstones that will likely never come to the attention of the individual or medical provider. In this chapter we focus on the epidemiology and natural history of symptomatic and asymptomatic gallstones and the evolving understanding of the many factors that may influence development of complications. The implications of these findings for the diagnosis and treatment of gallstones disease and directions for future research are also discussed.

HISTORICAL PERSPECTIVE

Humans have recorded gallstone disease since the beginning of written medical communication. Indeed, it is documented that ancient Greeks and Egyptians suffered from the disease.[4] In that time and for the following years, treatment consisted of various herbal remedies. The first recorded operation for gallstone disease was performed by Jean-Louis Petit in 1743. When exploring a patient with abdominal pain and an erythematous abdomen, Petit lanced the abdominal wall, opened the gallbladder, and removed the stones. He then allowed the gallbladder to fistulize, thus performing the first cholecystostomy[5] (see Chapter 35). Over a century later, the American surgeon John Stough Bobbs performed the first deliberate cholecystostomy after identifying an inflamed and stone-filled gallbladder in a young woman undergoing laparotomy. He proceeded to incise the gallbladder, remove the stones, and close the organ without extirpation or drainage.[6] It was Carl Langenbuch, a pioneering German surgeon, who

ushered in the modern era of gallbladder surgery by proposing removing the gallbladder as opposed to removing stones alone.[7] An additional century passed before another pioneering German surgeon, Erich Mühe, performed the first laparoscopic cholecystectomy in 1985[8] and set the stage for the minimally invasive approach to gallbladder disease (see Chapter 36).

Dr. Mühe presented his work to the Congress of the German Surgical Society in 1986.[9] The lecture was not the success he had hoped and was only published as a brief abstract in the proceedings.[9] At the 1990 meeting of the Society of American Gastrointestinal Surgeons (SAGES), several French surgeons were recognized for their early work in laparoscopic cholecystectomy, but Dr. Mühe was not acknowledged. It was not until 1999 when he was recognized by SAGES for performing the first laparoscopic cholecystectomy.[10]

CLASSIFICATION AND NOMENCLATURE

Gallstones are firm masses formed within the biliary tract as precipitations of cholesterol or bilirubin and have distinct etiologies (see Chapter 8). Gallstones are categorized by their color or primary chemical component, notably cholesterol (yellow), black pigment, or brown pigment stones. The location of the mass dictates the terminology used (i.e., cholelithiasis is within the gallbladder, choledocholithiasis is within an extrahepatic bile duct, and hepatolithiasis is within an intrahepatic bile duct; Fig. 33.1).[11] In the United States, the most common form of gallstones is cholesterol stones formed within the gallbladder, and as such, this will be the major focus of this chapter. Further clarification should be made regarding the term "gallstone disease," which represents the manifestation of gallstones and ensuing signs or symptoms. Therefore patients with gallstones may be asymptomatic (stones discovered incidentally) or symptomatic (presence of gallstone disease). Gallstone disease can be separated into uncomplicated disease (biliary colic, chronic cholecystitis) or complicated disease (acute cholecystitis, obstructive jaundice, gallstone ileus, acute gallstone pancreatitis) based on the manifestation (see Chapters 37 and 38).

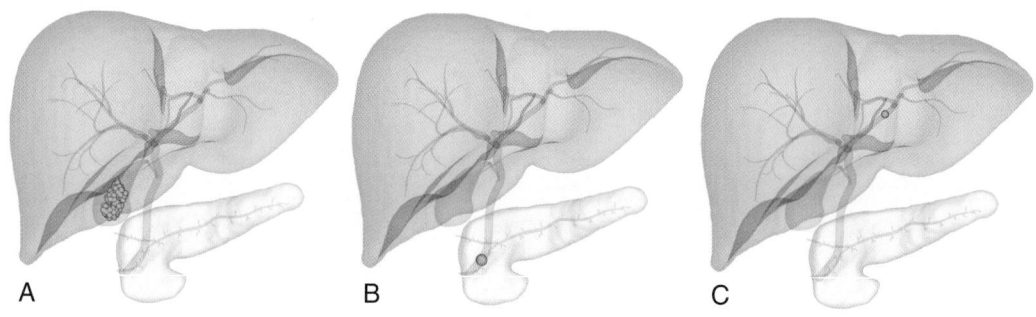

FIGURE 33.1 Common sites for stone formation and obstruction within the biliary system. **A**, Cholelithiasis, **B**, choledocholithiasis, and **C**, hepatolithiasis determined by stones *(green spheres)* located in the gallbladder, common bile duct, and intrahepatic bile duct, respectively. (Images courtesy Dr. Thomas W. Loehfelm, Department of Radiology, University of California, Davis.)

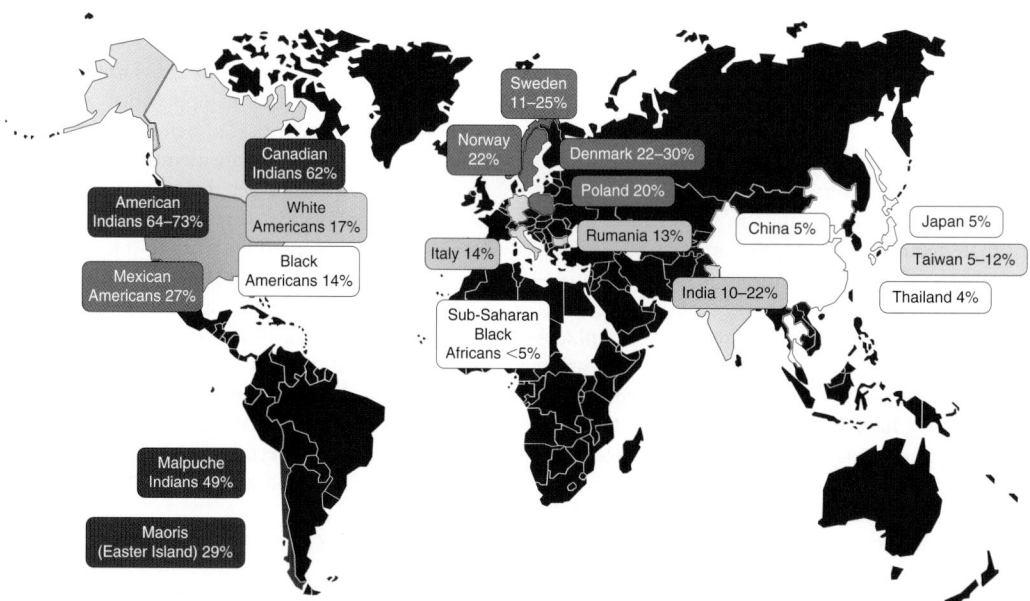

FIGURE 33.2 Worldwide prevalence of gallstones in women based on ultrasonographic studies. (With permission from Stinton LM, Shaffer EA. Epidemiology of gallbladder disease: Cholelithiasis and cancer. *Gut and Liver*. 2012;6[2]:172–187.)

PREVALENCE AND EPIDEMIOLOGY OF GALLSTONES

The prevalence of gallstones in a given population is multifactorial and primarily driven by gender, age, diet, ethnicity, and genetics. In 1993 the NIH estimated that approximately 10% to 15% of the US adult population had gallstones.[12] Since that time, expanded data on the global prevalence of gallstones have revealed the broad ranges of gallstone prevalence observed across various countries and ethnicities, including the United States,[13–15] South America,[16–20] Europe,[21–30] Asia,[31–35] and Africa.[36–38] The estimated global prevalence of gallstones in women is shown in Fig. 33.2. Research from the National Institute of Diabetes and Digestive and Kidney Diseases (NIDDK) has provided some of the best insight into the prevalence of gallstones within US populations. Implemented through the National Health and Nutrition Examination Survey (NHANES) III by the US Centers for Disease Control and Prevention (CDC) from 1988 until 1994, 14,294 people aged 20 to 74 years underwent screening and completed ultrasound examinations of the gallbladder for detection of stones.[14] The overall prevalence of gallstones was 5.5% in men and 8.6% in women. Gallstone prevalence increased with age, with reported 17.2% in men and 16.4% in women by age 60 to 74 years. The NHANES III study revealed substantial variation in gallstone prevalence according to race and ethnicity with the lowest prevalence in non-Hispanic Black men (3.9%) and highest in Mexican-American women (12.8%).

American Indians are estimated to have the highest rates of gallstones and gallbladder disease in the world.[39] Prevalence of gallstones in separate American Indian communities in four states—Arizona, Oklahoma, North Dakota, and South Dakota—were 18% in women and 17% in men.[13] When using a composite score of the presence of stones and prior cholecystectomy, the overall prevalence in this population was 64% in women and 30% in men.[13]

NATURAL HISTORY OF SYMPTOMATIC GALLSTONES

For uncomplicated disease, most typically biliary colic, current treatment recommendations include elective cholecystectomy in patients fit for surgery. This is based on results from older studies showing a high prevalence of continued symptoms, an eventual need for cholecystectomy, and a significant rate of complications (Table 33.1). Thistle et al. published a report evaluating patients from the National Cooperative Gallstone Study, which investigated the efficacy of chenodeoxycholic acid in patients with gallstones.[40] Using the placebo group to determine the natural history of gallstones in symptomatic patients over 2 years, the authors detected a 69% cumulative incidence of biliary symptoms. This was corroborated in a larger study following 556 symptomatic patients in the Health Insurance Plan of Greater New York where nearly 65% of patients described either unchanged or increased symptoms.[41] During a median follow-up of 5.7 years, 44% of symptomatic patients underwent cholecystectomy and 8% of the symptomatic patients developed complications from their gallstone disease, including acute cholecystitis and obstructive jaundice. Friedman et al. followed 298 mildly symptomatic patients over 25 years within the Kaiser Northern California System.[42] In this extensive follow-up period, 9% experienced severe (acute cholecystitis, obstructive jaundice, biliary pancreatitis) gallstone disease, 25% experienced nonsevere (biliary colic) gallstone disease, and 31% of patients underwent cholecystectomy.

Results from a more recent Italian study showed a relatively benign natural history for symptomatic gallstones by following 213 patients for nearly 10 years.[43] The authors reported that 64% of individuals experienced decreased symptoms, 25% reported unchanged symptoms, and only 11% reported an increase in symptoms. Even for those individuals initially reporting severe symptoms, complete resolution was obtained in 52%.[43] Despite this high rate of resolution, the authors reported a 9% complication rate, similar to prior publications. With the likelihood of persistent or worsening symptoms (~30%–70%) and risk of complications (~6%–9%), cholecystectomy for symptomatic patients remains the appropriate treatment given the relatively low risk of the operation in patients fit for surgery. Additional large studies on this topic appear unlikely because there is uniform consensus among clinicians.

NATURAL HISTORY OF ASYMPTOMATIC GALLSTONES

In contrast to symptomatic gallstones, the debate over the natural history and treatment of asymptomatic gallstones is rooted within the medical and surgical giants of America. Sir William Osler wrote, "The gall-bladder will tolerate the presence of large numbers [of stones] for an indefinite period of time" and concluded that the presence of gallstones in asymptomatic patients is not an indication for surgery.[44] Concurrently, in 1911 William Mayo stated that the "innocent" gallstone is a myth and early cholecystectomy decreased the mortality and morbidity associated with prolonged gallbladder disease.[45] As larger cohorts with more diverse patients were published, the consensus has become a watchful waiting strategy for most patients with asymptomatic gallstones because the cumulative rate of symptom development appears to be around 10% to 30%, with an even lower rate of complications (0%–8%; Table 33.2).

The earliest evaluation of the natural history comes from Comfort et al. who published their experience with incidental gallstones at the Mayo Clinic in 1948.[46] The authors identified 112 patients with incidental gallstones found during abdominal surgery, and over 10 to 20 years, biliary colic developed in 19% of these patients.[46] Nearly 40 years later, Gracie and Ransohoff published one of the most cited articles describing the natural history of stones in asymptomatic male and female faculty members from the University of Michigan.[47] During the follow-up period of approximately 24 years, biliary symptoms developed in 13% of patients and 40% of the total cohort underwent cholecystectomy (cholecystectomy rate of 88% in those who developed symptoms). With a reported complication rate of 2%, they concluded that the "the innocent gallstone is not a myth."

In the last twenty years, further comprehensive studies have set out to gain a better understanding of these rates and elucidate risk factors for the development of symptoms or complications. Halldestam et al. prospectively identified Swedish citizens

---

TABLE 33.1 Reports and Details on the Natural History of Symptomatic Gallstones

| STUDY | NO. OF SYMPTOMATIC PATIENTS | YEARS OF FOLLOW-UP | INCIDENCE RATE | | |
			BILIARY SYMPTOMS (%)	CHOLECYSTECTOMY (%)	COMPLICATIONS (%)
Thistle et al. (1984)[40]	112	2	69	6	—
McSherry et al. (1985)[41]	556	5.7, median	36 decreased 39 unchanged 25 increased	44[a]	8
Friedman et al. (1989)[42]	298	25	9 severe 25 non-severe	31 overall 85 for severe 95 for non-severe	9
Attili et al. (1995)[21]	38	10	6 acute cholecystitis	45	6
Festi et al. (2010)[43]	213	9, mean	64 were decreased 25 were unchanged 11 were increased	—	9

[a]Includes six choledochoduodenostomies and two cholecystostomies.

TABLE 33.2 Reports and Details on the Natural History of Asymptomatic Patients

STUDY	NO. OF ASYMPTOMATIC PATIENTS	YEARS OF FOLLOW-UP	BILIARY SYMPTOMS (%)	INCIDENCE RATE CHOLECYSTECTOMY (%)	COMPLICATIONS (%)	COMMENTS
Comfort et al. (1948)[46]	112	10–20	19	21	—	51 patients developed symptoms. Dyspepsia, n = 30 (27%) Biliary colic, n = 21 (19%)
Gracie and Ransohoff (1982)[47]	123	24	13	40	2	Cholecystectomy rates: Remained asymptomatic, 39% Developed symptoms, 88%
Thistle et al. (1984)[40]	193	2	31	3	—	—
McSherry et al. (1985)[41]	135	4	10	7	2	An additional 5 patients had incidental cholecystectomies
Friedman et al. (1989)[42]	123	25	19 overall 6 severe 13 non-severe	16 71 for severe 94 for non-severe	6	Cumulative probability of any event after diagnosis: 0.18, 5 yr 0.30, 10 yr 0.34, 15 yr 0.41, 20 yr
Cucchiaro et al. (1990)[48]	139	5	11	6	1	9 cholecystectomies Incidental, n = 3 Elective, n = 4 Emergency, n = 2
Wada et al.[a] (1990)[49]	680	13, median	20	—	—	—
Juhasz et al. (1994)[50]	110	6, median	15	18	5	8-yr median follow-up on subset of cohort shows 27% developed symptoms and 33% underwent cholecystectomy
Attili et al. (1995)[21]	118	10	12, 2 yr 16, 4 yr 26, 10 yr	24	3	1 death from gallbladder adenocarcinoma
Angelico et al. (1997)[51]	47	10	15, 10 yr	23	0	—
Halldestam et al. (2004)[52]	120[b]	7, median	12	8[c]	4	1 death from gallbladder adenocarcinoma
Festi et al. (2010)[43]	580	9, mean	22	14	<1	—
Sood et al. (2015)[53]	213	4, mean	11, 4 years 14, 10 years	Not reported	—	—
Shabanzadeh et al. (2016)[54]	664	17, median	20	7 in patients without complications	8	Noted increased rates of biliary colic in patients who were aware of gallstones

[a]Abstract only. Article in Japanese

[b]Includes gallstones, sludge, and cholesterolosis

[c]10 of 14 patients with symptoms underwent cholecystectomy. Study does not report prophylactic cholecystectomy rate in patients who remained asymptomatic.

aged 35 to 85 years for the presence of asymptomatic gallstones.[52] During a median follow-up of 7 years, 12% of the cohort developed biliary symptoms, 8% underwent cholecystectomy, and 4% experienced gallstone-related complications (acute cholecystitis, obstructive jaundice, and gallstone pancreatitis). The authors only identified younger age as a risk factor for the development of gallstone-related events.[52] The most current and comprehensive analysis on this topic was published by Shabanzadeh et al. in 2016[54] and determined prediction rules for risk stratification in asymptomatic individuals. The authors followed 664 people with asymptomatic gallstones from the general population of urban Copenhagen, Denmark and during a median follow-up of 17 years, 20% of individuals developed symptoms of gallstone disease, and 8% experienced gallstone-related complications.[54] A unique component of this study involved nondisclosure of ultrasound results creating cohorts of patients who were either aware or unaware of their asymptomatic gallstones. Interestingly, the most significant predictor of gallstone-related events was awareness of gallstones, but as the authors note, this may be secondary to the protopathic bias or may reflect a confounding variable in which those who were aware of their stones before enrollment likely had symptoms that prompted evaluation and may not have been truly asymptomatic.[54]

Extensive studies over the course of nearly 80 years have provided significant evidence for the relatively benign natural history of asymptomatic gallstones. In contrast to symptomatic stones, most patients with asymptomatic gallstones (~70%–90%) will never experience gallstone-related symptoms, and even more (90%–99%) will never experience complications of their gallstones. As such, prophylactic cholecystectomy is not appropriate in asymptomatic patients within the general population.

RISK FACTORS FOR GALLSTONE DISEASE (SEE CHAPTER 8)

As identified in the recent work from Shabanzadeh[54] and Sood,[53] there appear to be factors that increase the risk of gallstone-related events in patients with asymptomatic stones. Ignoring the confounding factor of gallstone awareness, the authors identified large stones greater than 10 mm, female gender, and two or more stones as independent predictors of all gallstone-related events. Female gender was determined as a risk factor for gallstone disease in asymptomatic Malaysian citizens.[53] Apart from these observations in the general public, specific populations and clinical scenarios require further discussion because of increased rates of either stone formation or complications.

Bariatric and Metabolic Surgery Patients

Obesity[55,56] and rapid weight loss[57–59] are both considered risk factors for gallstone formation, but the magnitude of the risk of developing gallstone disease in these populations remains controversial. Specifically, in patients undergoing weight loss surgery (sleeve gastrectomy or Roux-en-Y gastric bypass), practice has changed from a concurrent prophylactic cholecystectomy to intervening only in patients with preoperative biliary symptoms. A prior report in patients undergoing gastric exclusion surgery showed nearly 30% of patients developed gallstone disease after bariatric surgery, with most occurring in the first 24 months postoperative.[60] These results were followed by work from Swartz et al. evaluating 692 patients undergoing

Roux-en-Y gastric bypass (96% laparoscopic) from 2003 to 2004 at a single center using a protocol of postoperative ursodeoxycholic acid therapy. Approximately 15% of patients required subsequent cholecystectomy during a mean follow-up of 7.5 months.[61] Authors also discovered an indirect relationship between the duration of ursodeoxycholic acid therapy and the rate of cholecystectomy; specifically, patients who did not use therapy had a 25% rate of cholecystectomy compared with 10% in those that were adherent to therapy for 6 months.[61] The authors concluded that bariatric surgery patients can be managed like the general population, with significant benefit from ursodeoxycholic acid therapy.[61] These results support the Choosing Wisely guidelines, which states that during weight loss surgery the gallbladder should not be routinely removed unless clinically indicated because of the associated risk of surgery without clear evidence showing benefit of removing a normal or asymptomatic gallbladder.[62]

Hemolytic Disorders

Hematologic disorders resulting in increased red blood cell (RBC) hemolysis are associated with increased rates of pigment gallstones because of elevated efflux of bilirubin. Most commonly, these disorders include sickle cell anemia (SS) and hereditary spherocytosis (HS). The rates of gallstones and gallstone disease in SS were investigated through The Jamaican Cohort Study evaluating 100,000 consecutive infants from 1973 until 1981.[63] Three hundred fifteen infants with homozygous SS were identified, and gallstones developed in 31% of patients and were present in almost 10% of SS patients by the time of their first ultrasound (5 patients were < 6 years of age); 7 individuals underwent cholecystectomy for gallstone-related events (~2%).[63] This study suggests that gallstones are a common manifestation of SS, but rates of complications necessitating surgery are low.

Incidence and complication rates for adults with SS were investigated by researchers at King's College Hospital tracking all SS patients between 2003 and 2013.[64] Gallstones were identified in 44% of patients and gallstone-related complications occurred in 26% during the 11-year follow-up period. Authors identified a perioperative complication rate of approximately 10% in SS patients undergoing cholecystectomy.[64] Given the increased risk for surgical complications, there is a limited role for prophylactic cholecystectomy in this population.

Similar to SS disease, patients with HS show high rates of pigment gallstones. In a retrospective study from the Johns Hopkins Hospital analyzing 58 patients who underwent splenectomy for HS between 1960 and 1979,[65] gallstones were present in 21% of all patients. Since many of these patients eventually undergo splenectomy to remove the site of RBC hemolysis, there has been controversy regarding performing concomitant cholecystectomy. After splenectomy, the risk of pigment stone formation is markedly reduced and some surgeons have performed cholecystolithotomy at the time of splenectomy to remove the stones and preserve the gallbladder.[66] Current guidelines from the British Society of Hematology support cholecystectomy only in patients with symptomatic gallstone disease undergoing splenectomy.[67]

Transplant Patients

Solid organ transplant patients may be at increased risk for gallstone formation and increased complications from gallstone disease (see Chapter 111). Kilic et al. evaluated the Nationwide

Inpatient Sample (NIS) database to identify heart transplant recipients who underwent cholecystectomy between 1998 and 2008.[68] The authors identified 1,687 patients (75% laparoscopic) who underwent post-transplant cholecystectomy and found increased mortality in open cases compared with laparoscopic, as well as in urgent or emergent cases compared with elective cases. On multivariate analysis, urgent or emergent admission, open operation, and complicated gallstone disease were independent predictors of inpatient mortality, supporting the use of prophylactic cholecystectomy in heart transplant patients with asymptomatic gallstones or mildly symptomatic gallstone disease.[68] Kao et al. arrived at a similar conclusion through use of a decision analysis algorithm based on the option for pre-transplant cholecystectomy, post-transplant cholecystectomy, or expectant management.[69] For heart transplantation, the authors determined post-transplant prophylactic cholecystectomy to have the lowest mortality, whereas the preferred strategy in kidney/pancreas transplant patients was expectant management.[69] Although there are no guidelines mandating prophylactic cholecystectomy in heart transplant candidates or recipients, patients may benefit from elective operations for asymptomatic gallstones.

Immunotherapy Patients

Immune checkpoint inhibition (ICI) and other systemic immunotherapies (e.g., interleukin [IL]-2, IL-15) have been associated with extensive side effects and toxicities,[70–72] but to date, there does not appear to be a correlation with increased gallstone formation or gallstone disease. Notably, both IL-2[73] and ICI[74] have been associated with acalculous gallbladder pathology mimicking acute cholecystitis, and differentiating the etiologies is critical to avoid inappropriate surgical management in patients often requiring cessation of immunotherapy and initiation of systemic steroids.

GALLSTONES AND THE MICROBIOME

The influence of the gut microbiome on health and disease has been extensively explored in the last few decades. There have been recent advances in the understanding of the impact of intestinal microbiome on bile acids and subsequent role in both gallstone formation[75] and other gastrointestinal (GI) diseases.[76] Recently, this was explored further in a study evaluating the microbiome profile of feces, bile, and gallstones in patients undergoing cholecystectomy that compared this profile with the feces of healthy individuals.[77] The authors found significant differences in feces microbiome diversity between gallstone patients and healthy individuals and noted higher microbiome diversity in the bile compared with the feces in patients with gallstones.[77] These observations have been investigated in animal models, using a diet-induced cholesterol gallstone mouse model.[78] Notably, germ-free mice had increased cholesterol gallstone formation, which normalized after fecal microbiota transfer with known commensal organisms.[78] As this field continues to expand, further details regarding the interconnectedness of the gut-microbiome-liver axis will be elucidated with potential for predictive biomarkers, preventive measures, and therapeutics.

The references for this chapter can be found online by accessing the accompanying Expert Consult website.

CHAPTER 34

Cholecystitis

Alexandra W. Acher, Kaitlyn J. Kelly, and Sharon M. Weber

OVERVIEW

Cholecystitis, a common condition usually resulting from complications of cholelithiasis, occurs in two forms: acute and chronic. Acute cholecystitis requires urgent intervention, typically with antibiotics and cholecystectomy. In the setting of acute cholecystitis, cholecystectomy is optimally performed within 72 hours of symptom onset. If urgent cholecystectomy is not feasible, cholecystectomy can be performed electively, provided symptoms have resolved with medical management. Chronic cholecystitis is the manifestation of ongoing, intermittent inflammation and biliary colic. Patients with this condition benefit from elective cholecystectomy. A less common version of cholecystitis is acute acalculous cholecystitis, which occurs most often in critically ill patients. Although gallstones are, by definition, absent in this condition, cholecystectomy specimens in patients with acute acalculous cholecystitis often reveal biliary sludge (see Chapter 33).

ACUTE CHOLECYSTITIS

Pathogenesis

The cause of acute calculous cholecystitis is an impacted gallstone in the outlet of the gallbladder, either in the infundibulum or in the cystic duct.[1] The impacted gallstone results in gallbladder distension and edema with acute inflammation, which eventually can result in venous stasis and obstruction, followed by thrombosis of the cystic artery. Ultimately, ischemia and necrosis of the gallbladder can occur. Because the fundus of the gallbladder is the greatest distance from the cystic arterial blood supply, it is more sensitive to ischemia and is the most common location for necrosis of the gallbladder. The acute inflammation of cholecystitis may be complicated by secondary biliary infection. Positive bile cultures are found in approximately 20% of patients with acute cholecystitis,[2] the most common of which are gram-negative bacteria of gastrointestinal origin, such as *Klebsiella* spp. and *Escherichia coli*. The incidence of bactobilia has been reported to be as high as 60% in patients who have had endoscopic sphincterotomy or other biliary instrumentation[3] (see Chapters 30 and 31).

Clinical Manifestations

Most patients with acute cholecystitis are seen with severe, constant, right upper quadrant abdominal or epigastric pain, sometimes with radiation to the subscapular area. This pain may be preceded by intermittent, self-limited bouts of abdominal pain from episodes of biliary colic. Acute cholecystitis is frequently associated with fever and leukocytosis, findings that are not present in cases of uncomplicated biliary colic. Patients also may have a Murphy's sign (inspiratory arrest on palpation of the right upper quadrant of the abdomen). Other presenting symptoms include nausea, vomiting, and anorexia.

Differential Diagnosis

Several disease processes can present similarly to cholecystitis and should be considered in the differential diagnosis. These include peptic ulcer disease, gastritis and gastroenteritis, irritable bowel syndrome, inflammatory bowel disease, right lower lobe pneumonia, and biliary dyskinesia. An initial chest radiograph is generally sufficient to assess for a right lower lobe infiltrate. The other diagnoses should be entertained and worked up appropriately in symptomatic patients without gallstones on ultrasound (US).

The Tokyo Guidelines are also a useful tool to assess the likelihood of acute cholecystitis and can be used to assist in diagnosis.[4] These guidelines are based on three clinical and diagnostic categories: local signs of inflammation (Murphy's sign or right upper quadrant mass or right upper quadrant tenderness), systemic signs of inflammation (fever, elevated C-reactive protein, elevated white blood cell [WBC] count), and imaging findings suggestive of cholecystitis (pericholecystic fluid, gallbladder wall edema, luminal debris and stone impaction). For patients who present with one item from each category, validation studies demonstrate a guideline sensitivity and specificity of 91% and 97%, respectively.[5] Additionally, the Tokyo Guidelines stratify presentations of acute cholecystitis according to risk of 30-day mortality: 1.1% for mild acute cholecystitis (Grade I), 0.8% for moderate acute cholecystitis (Grade II), and 5.4% for severe acute cholecystitis (Grade III; $P < .0001$).[4] Online calculators allow for easy access and use of this tool.

Diagnostic Evaluation and Imaging

Abdominal US (see Chapter 16) is useful for assessing patients suspected to have acute cholecystitis. Typical findings include gallstones, gallbladder wall thickening (>4 mm), and pericholecystic fluid (Fig. 34.1). In addition, the sonographer can assess for pain and inspiratory arrest when the gallbladder is directly compressed by the US probe (sonographic Murphy's sign). Typically, conventional grayscale imaging is used, which, together with clinical picture and sonographic Murphy's sign, is sensitive and specific for diagnosing acute cholecystitis, with an overall accuracy of greater than 90% (Pinto et al., 2013). Other ultrasound techniques that assess blood flow, such as Doppler and color velocity imaging, may improve accuracy in selected cases.

Hepatobiliary scintigraphy (see Chapter 18) is a useful study in selected patients when the diagnosis is uncertain. This nuclear medicine study is performed with derivatives of aminodiacetic acid (hepatoiminodiacetic acid, isopropylacetanilido iminodiacetic acid, or diisopropylacetanilido iminodiacetic acid), which are taken up by hepatocytes and secreted in bile. When the tracer is labeled with technetium, scintigraphy allows for visualization of the extrahepatic biliary system. A normal scan delineates the biliary tree, including the gallbladder, and shows prompt emptying of the agent into the duodenum. Nonvisualization of the gallbladder on scintigraphy implies obstruction of the cystic duct and is

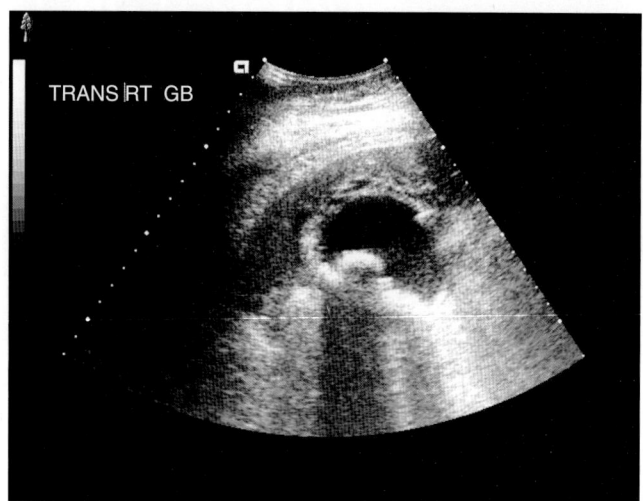

FIGURE 34.1 Transverse view of the gallbladder on ultrasound in a patient with calculous cholecystitis, revealing gallstones and gallbladder wall thickening.

consistent with acute cholecystitis (Fig. 34.2). Hepatobiliary scintigraphy is not useful in patients with reduced hepatic function because it depends on hepatic excretion of bile, but it is accurate in approximately 90% of patients with acute cholecystitis and may be more accurate than US alone in some presentations.[6]

An added utility of scintigraphy is that in addition to gallbladder filling or nonfilling, it can also be used to quantify gallbladder emptying. Abnormal emptying is defined as an ejection fraction (EF) of 35% or less on scintigraphy, although cutoff values of between 35% and 40% have been reported.[6] The evaluation of EF is potentially useful for patients with symptoms suggestive of biliary dyskinesia or chronic acalculous cholecystitis but usually unnecessary in cases of acute cholecystitis because 90% of acute cholecystitis is secondary to cholelithiasis obstruction of the cystic duct.[6] Consensus on the utility of scintigraphy EF in diagnosing biliary dyskinesia or chronic cholecystitis remains debated. This is in part because of reliance on retrospective data limited by selection bias and because

of inconsistent indications and variability in EF cutoff values.[6] In a study of 141 symptomatic patients with normal US and scintigraphy demonstrating normal gallbladder filling and an EF of 35% or less who underwent cholecystectomy, 95% had symptom relief and 41% had cholecystitis on histologic evaluation of the gallbladder.[7] A recent meta-analysis of studies from 1980 to 2016 ($n = 29$ studies) examining the use of scintigraphy EF in the diagnosis of biliary dyskinesia or cholecystitis found only two randomized controlled trials (RCTs) and 27 observational studies.[8] This meta-analysis demonstrated that of the patients who underwent cholecystectomy, the chance of symptom improvement was similar in patients with a low EF versus those with a normal EF (risk ratio [RR] 1.09, $P = .07$). However, they also found that in patients managed medically, symptom improvement was more likely in patients with normal EF than those with a low EF (RR 2.37, $P < .0005$). Because of the heterogeneity of studies and bias inherent in retrospective data, no definitive conclusions could be drawn regarding how to interpret a normal EF in the setting of biliary symptoms and unclear imaging findings.[8] In the setting of biliary pain with unclear US findings, however, a low EF is considered a reliable indicator of a biliary etiology.[6,8]

Hepatobiliary scintigraphy is more involved, more expensive, and requires a longer time than US; however, it should be considered in certain cases.[9–11] Guidelines have suggested a diagnostic approach that starts with US for patients with biliary symptoms. If no gallstones are definitively identified, this should be followed by esophagogastroduodenoscopy to exclude alternative causes of symptoms, such as peptic ulcer disease or gastritis. If the endoscopy is negative, hepatobiliary scintigraphy should follow.

Computed tomography (CT; see Chapter 16) can also help diagnose acute cholecystitis and provides more detailed anatomic information than US. CT is particularly useful in patients whose symptoms suggest a complication such as pericholecystic abscess or an alternative diagnosis. The CT findings of acute cholecystitis are the same as those seen on US and include wall thickening, pericholecystic stranding or fluid, distension of the gallbladder, high-attenuation bile, and subserosal edema. CT is generally less sensitive than US for diagnosing

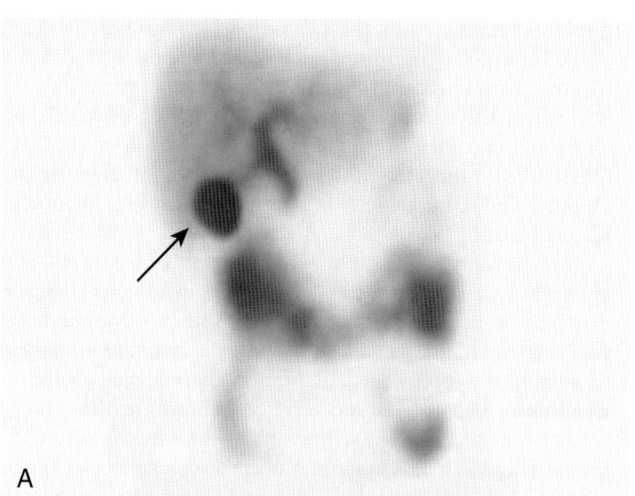
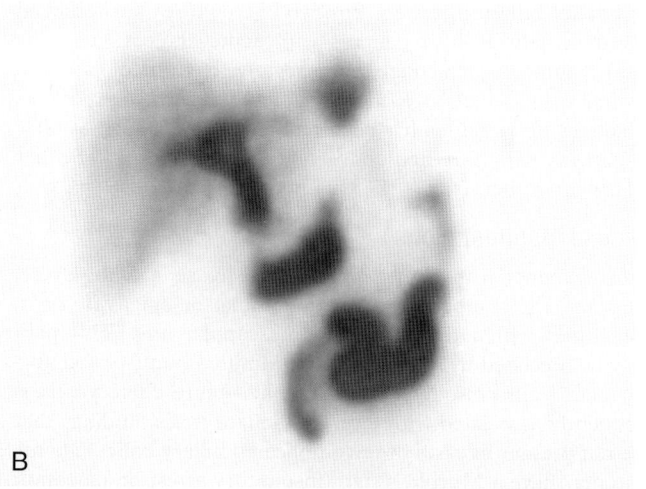

FIGURE 34.2 A, Normal hepatoiminodiacetic acid (HIDA) scan demonstrating contrast-filled gallbladder *(arrow).* **B,** Abnormal HIDA scan demonstrating nonfilling of the gallbladder consistent with cystic duct obstruction. (Courtesy Dr. Scott Perlman, University of Wisconsin Hospital and Clinics)

acute cholecystitis, particularly early in the course, when the imaging findings may be subtle.[12,13]

Treatment

Initial treatment with antibiotics active against enteric bacteria should begin as soon as the patient is diagnosed with acute cholecystitis. Additionally, oral intake should be held, and appropriate intravenous (IV) fluid resuscitation should be started in preparation for surgery. Parenteral analgesics should be administered as needed.

The definitive treatment for acute cholecystitis is cholecystectomy (see Chapter 36). From the time this operation was first performed in 1882 by Langenbuch, open cholecystectomy has been the standard of care for patients with acute cholecystitis. With the advent of laparoscopic cholecystectomy in the 1980s, the standard approach has changed such that cholecystectomy is now routinely performed laparoscopically. The benefits of laparoscopic cholecystectomy are discussed in Chapter 36, but they include a shorter postoperative stay and decreased analgesia requirements.[14] Although the laparoscopic approach is now standard for most cases, it is interesting to note that two prospective randomized studies suggested little or no difference in intraoperative or postoperative complications or length of stay between laparoscopic versus small-incision open cholecystectomy[15,16]; however, most of these patients underwent elective rather than urgent cholecystectomy.

Early analysis of the results of laparoscopic cholecystectomy in patients with acute versus chronic cholecystitis showed increased morbidity and mortality rates for patients with simple or complicated acute cholecystitis. Because of the increased morbidity and mortality, acute cholecystitis initially was considered a relative contraindication to laparoscopic cholecystectomy.[17] Subsequent reports, however, have shown improved safety of this technique in the acute setting.[18–21] The conversion rate to an open procedure is higher for patients with acute cholecystitis compared with patients undergoing elective cholecystectomy,[22]

but most patients with acute cholecystitis (>80%) can undergo successful laparoscopic cholecystectomy.[23] Retrospective series have reported that risk factors for conversion to open cholecystectomy include obesity,[24] elevated WBC count and elevated bilirubin,[25,26] previous surgery,[26] and male gender.[26]

Other novel surgical approaches to cholecystectomy have been proposed to treat patients with symptomatic gallstones, including *mini-laparoscopic cholecystectomy* (see Chapter 36), which uses 2- to 3-mm ports[27]; mini-cholecystectomy,[28] in which a small (mean, 5.5 cm) incision is used to remove the gallbladder; single-incision laparoscopic cholecystectomy; and natural orifice transluminal endoscopic (NOTES) cholecystectomy with transvaginal extraction. Prospective randomized studies evaluating the safety of these techniques are lacking, but existing data suggest decreased postoperative pain and improved cosmesis at the expense of slightly longer operating times with these techniques.

Laparoscopic subtotal cholecystectomy (LSC) has also been evaluated as a means of decreasing the conversion rate to open procedure in patients with acute cholecystitis[29,30] (see Chapter 36). Subtotal cholecystectomy can be of two types: fenestrating or reconstituting[31] (see Figs. 34.3 and 34.4). A subtotal fenestrating cholecystectomy involves excising the peritonealized gallbladder (anterior surface) and leaving the posterior wall of the gallbladder in situ. The remnant mucosa may be cauterized, any stone burden is evacuated, and the cut edge of the gallbladder can then be oversewn or cauterized. The cystic duct can also be sutured closed from the luminal/ mucosal side to avoid injury to the common bile duct[31] (see Chapter 36). In contrast, a reconstituting subtotal cholecystectomy involves excising the peritonealized gallbladder, extracting any stones, and closing (sewing or stapling) the inferior gallbladder in a way that *preserves a small lumen and patent biliary drainage* through the cystic duct.[31] Drains are typically left after either approach.

Each subtotal cholecystectomy technique has different advantages and disadvantages, and their feasibility depends on

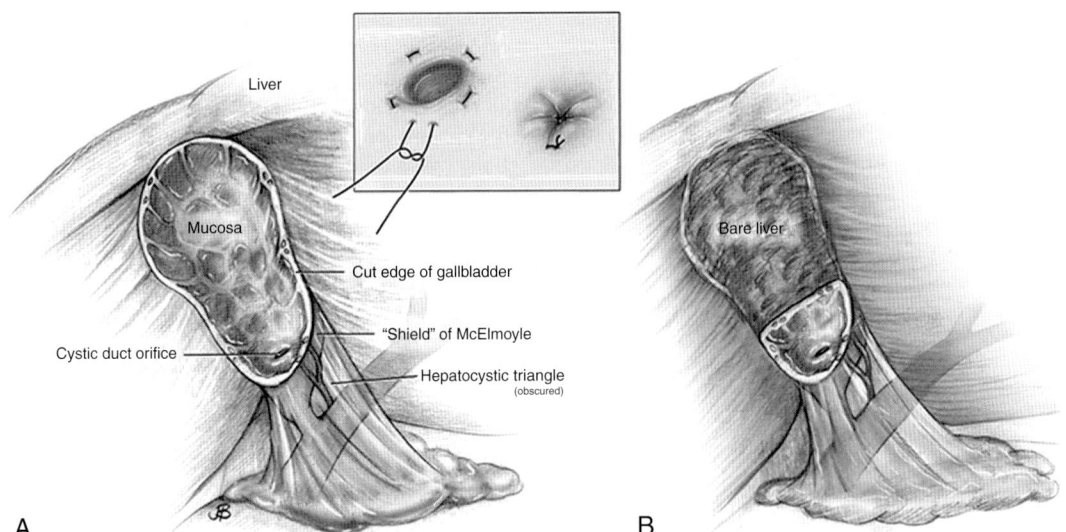

FIGURE 34.3   Schematic of a subtotal fenestrating cholecystectomy. (From Strasberg SM, Pucci MJ, Brunt LM, Deziel DJ. Subtotal cholecystectomy-"fenestrating" vs "reconstituting" subtypes and the prevention of bile duct injury: Definition of the optimal procedure in difficult operative conditions. *J Am Coll Surg.* 2016;222:89–96.)

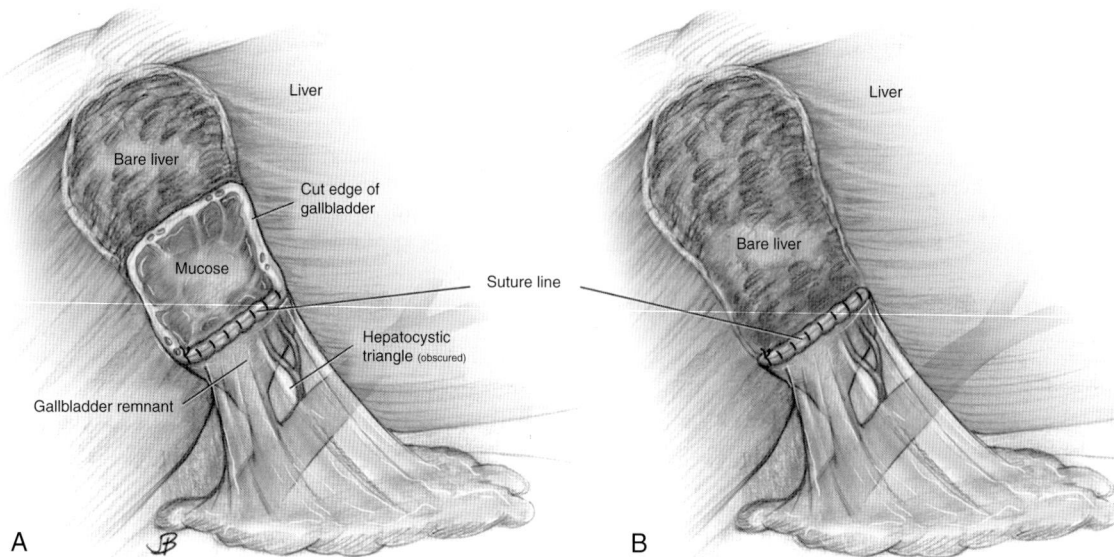

FIGURE 34.4 Schematic of a subtotal reconstituting cholecystectomy. (From Strasberg SM, Pucci MJ, Brunt LM, Deziel DJ. Subtotal cholecystectomy-"fenestrating" vs "reconstituting" subtypes and the prevention of bile duct injury: Definition of the optimal procedure in difficult operative conditions. *J Am Coll Surg.* 2016;222:89–96.)

patient presentation and anatomy. In a retrospective multi-institutional study[32] comparing outcomes after subtotal fenestration versus reconstituting cholecystectomy (median follow-up of six years, interquartile range [IQR] 5–10 years), fenestration was associated with a higher risk of bile leak (18% vs. 7%, $P < .02$), wound infection (11% vs. 3%, $P < .02$) and longer hospitalization (median 5 days, IQR 3–17 days vs. three days, IQR 2–6 days, $P = .005$). However, reconstitution was associated with an increased risk of recurrent biliary pathology (18% vs. 9%, $P < .02$). Interestingly, in this study patients who underwent subtotal fenestrating cholecystectomy had an increased risk of subsequent completion cholecystectomy (9% vs. 4%, $P < .02$) despite a lower risk of recurrent cholecystitis. This may be reflective of the fact that patients underwent completion cholecystectomy for various indications such as choledocholithiasis and biliary colic, in addition to recurrent cholecystitis. There was, however, no difference in reintervention rate (endoscopic retrograde cholangiopancreatography [ERCP] or completion cholecystectomy) between those patients who underwent subtotal fenestrating versus reconstituting cholecystectomy (32% vs. 26%, $P = .21$). Laparoscopic cholecystectomy remains the standard therapy for definitive treatment of patients with acute cholecystitis. Conversion to an open approach or performing either type of subtotal cholecystectomy is appropriate for high-risk cases where a laparoscopic approach may be unsafe.

In patients with a high perioperative risk related to sepsis, duration of presenting symptoms, or underlying medical comorbidities, initial treatment of acute cholecystitis with percutaneous cholecystostomy tube placement is preferred (see Chapter 35). The standard of care for this high-risk patient cohort is percutaneous cholecystostomy tube followed by interval cholecystectomy, which is typically performed at least six to eight weeks after tube placement. Percutaneous cholecystostomy is placed under US or CT guidance[33] and decompresses the gallbladder by evacuating the infected bile and relieving the pain associated with gallbladder distension from outlet obstruction.

Most patients (>80%) have immediate clinical improvement after biliary decompression.[33–35]

The incidence and severity of complications after percutaneous cholecystostomy tube placement is low and relatively benign.[34,36–38] Approximately 33% of patients who undergo cholecystostomy tube for acute cholecystitis will experience tube-related complications.[39] The most common complications include tube displacement, tube site skin infection, and tube site pain.[39,40]

After resolution of the acute inflammatory process, the standard of care includes interval cholecystectomy in patients without contraindications to surgery. Laparoscopic cholecystectomy can often be performed successfully,[37] but the conversion from a laparoscopic to open approach is relatively increased in this population. In patients with previous percutaneous cholecystostomy, the rate of conversion from a laparoscopic to open approach ranges from 14% to 32%.[37,41] This is in contrast to the relatively low conversion rates for elective cholecystectomy (5%)[42] and emergent cholecystectomy performed for acute cholecystitis (6%).[43] Overall, compared with patients who were treated with antibiotics and delayed cholecystectomy, patients who underwent percutaneous cholecystostomy tube followed by interval cholecystectomy had shorter overall hospital stay and decreased cost,[36] although there is clearly selection bias, which can make these differences difficult to evaluate.

There is a subset of patients who are unable to undergo interval cholecystectomy, either because of prohibitive anticipated surgical morbidity and mortality or because of other considerations (i.e., noncurative cancer). These patients have two options for tube management: tube removal or indefinite tube continuation (sometimes referred to as a destination tube). The criteria for cholecystostomy tube removal include resolution of the obstructive inflammatory process and patency of the cystic and common bile ducts. Biliary patency can be assessed via a clamp trial where the cholecystostomy tube is clamped and the patient self-monitors for any recurrent symptoms or via cholecystography to confirm tube position and duct patency.

The most concerning complication after cholecystostomy tube removal in nonsurgical patients is recurrent cholecystitis. Recurrent cholecystitis after cholecystostomy tube removal is reported to be between 10% to 21%, although these numbers are skewed by the selection bias of retrospective research and the high mortality (43%) of nonsurgical patients.[39,44] Risk factors for recurrent cholecystitis after cholecystostomy tube removal include tube removal within 44 days of percutaneous placement (OR 5.6; 95% confidence interval [CI]: 1.25–23.2; $P = .02$) and history of choledocholithiasis (OR 24.4; 95% CI: 2.7–220.7; $P = .005$). Patients who underwent a successful clamping trial before tube removal had lower rates of recurrent cholecystitis (OR 0.10; 95% CI 0.01–0.8; $P = .03$).[44]

Advancements in endoscopic technologies and techniques have led to expanded options for definitive nonoperative management of acute cholecystitis. Lumen-apposing self-expandable metallic stents (LASEMS) have historically been used for transgastric drainage of pancreatic pseudocyst or walled off necrosis[45] (see Chapter 56). They have more recently, however, been adapted to offer transduodenal or transgastric gallbladder drainage in patients unfit for cholecystectomy. One such stent is the AXIOS stent (AXIOS; Xlumena Inc, Mountain View, CA), a fully covered self-expandable nitinol-based stent with anchoring flanges on opposing ends that inhibit post-placement migration. Its use in cholecystitis as a means of achieving biliary decompression has only been described in case reports of anywhere from one to 30 patients. A systematic review[45] of 11 studies (78 patients total) found that AXIOS/LASEMS placement from duodenum or stomach to the gallbladder was successfully achieved in 97% of patients and relieved symptoms in 99.6% of patients. Minor procedure-associated complications included transient fever ($n = 1$), hematochezia ($n = 1$), and pain ($n = 1$). There were no procedure-associated major complications and no reports of stent migration. Stents were removed within one to two weeks in 10 out of the 11 studies, after establishment of a fistulous tract between the gallbladder and either duodenum or stomach. Only one study ($n = 27$ patients) examined long-term outcomes (three months): three patients developed mucosal ingrowth and two patients developed recurrent cholecystitis from an obstructed stent.[45] Any consideration of LASEMS should occur at initial diagnosis and treatment planning as LASEMS are not compatible with other biliary drainage approaches (i.e., percutaneous cholecystostomy tube). LASEMS could offer a nonoperative management strategy for acute cholecystitis in patients unfit for surgery; however, multiinstitutional RCTs are needed to definitively understand the short- and long-term risks and benefits of this approach and the most appropriate population for its application.

Timing of Surgery

The optimal interval of time between the diagnosis of acute cholecystitis and definitive treatment with cholecystectomy has been the subject of many prospective randomized trials, with nine evaluating open cholecystectomy and five evaluating laparoscopic cholecystectomy.[23,46] The concern in operating on patients with early cholecystitis (typically defined as <72 hours) is the fear of increased operative complications, including common bile duct injury (see Chapter 36). The downside of performing delayed cholecystectomy (weeks after the diagnosis of cholecystitis) is that a subset of patients will develop recurrence

cholecystitis before cholecystectomy, leading to readmission and urgent surgery.[23] In multiple randomized prospective trials evaluating the timing of open cholecystectomy, patients undergoing early operation did not experience any increase in perioperative morbidity or mortality and had a shorter total length of hospital stay compared with patients undergoing delayed operation.[47,48] In addition, a meta-analysis of these trials demonstrated that more than 20% of patients did not respond to medical management while awaiting definitive treatment, and approximately half of these patients required urgent surgical treatment as a result.[23] Additionally, no increase in morbidity was seen in patients undergoing early (<72 hours from symptom onset) versus late (>72 hours from symptom onset) cholecystectomy with either laparoscopic ($P = .6$) or open ($P = .2$) approach. However, patients undergoing delayed cholecystectomy had significantly prolonged total hospitalization and higher cost of care compared with patients who underwent early cholecystectomy.[23]

Injury to the common bile duct (see Chapters 36 and 42) is a feared complication of any cholecystectomy but particularly for those performed in the setting of acute cholecystitis. Acute severe inflammation can obscure biliary anatomy and predispose to biliary injuries and complications. Multiple prospective randomized trials have demonstrated (Table 34.1) that although early cholecystectomy is associated with a significant increase in operation time compared with delayed cholecystectomy ($P = .002$), there is no significant difference in postoperative morbidity or mortality, including the incidence of common bile duct injury.[46]

No significant difference has been found in the conversion rate (laparoscopic to open approach) in early versus delayed cholecystectomy. Nevertheless, conversion to open surgery was higher (20%–30%) in patients with acute cholecystitis compared with patients undergoing elective laparoscopic cholecystectomy in the nonacute setting. Perhaps the most important finding was that in all but one study, patients randomly assigned to delayed cholecystectomy did not respond to medical management (supportive care and antibiotics) in 15% to 30% of cases. Although patients in the early surgery group generally experienced a longer postoperative hospital stay ($P = .004$), most of these trials demonstrated a decrease in overall length of hospital stay (surgical admission plus readmission) in the early compared with the delayed group (cumulative $P < .001$).[18-21,53] Early cholecystectomy has also been demonstrated to be more cost effective than delayed cholecystectomy. This was illustrated in a meta-analysis of studies of various designs performed by Lau and colleagues,[54] which concluded that early surgery was more cost effective because of its associated reduced overall length of hospital stay and avoidance of readmissions for recurrent symptoms. Early laparoscopic cholecystectomy is therefore the preferred surgical technique for patients with acute cholecystitis.

Catena and colleagues[55] have proposed the use of a harmonic scalpel for improved hemostasis and biliostasis in laparoscopic cholecystectomy, and preliminary data suggested it may decrease the conversion rate to open procedure in patients undergoing laparoscopic cholecystectomy for acute cholecystitis. A prospective RCT subsequently confirmed these findings.[55]

The majority of trials examining early versus delayed laparoscopic cholecystectomy define "early" as within 72 hours of symptom onset, but the impact of the time from symptom

TABLE 34.1 Results of Prospective Randomized Trials Comparing Early Versus Delayed Laparoscopic Cholecystectomy for Acute Cholecystitis

REFERENCE	N	DEFINITION	MORBIDITY RATE	LENGTH OF STAY (DAYS)	CONVERSION TO OPEN CHOLECYSTECTOMY
Ozkardes et al., 2014[49]	60	Early: <24 hours Late: 6–8 weeks	27% 0	5 8	13% 0%
Saber & Hokkam, 2014[50]	120	Early: <72 hours Late: 6–8 weeks	NR NR	2 6	5% 2%
Gutt et al., 2013[51]	618	Early: <24 hours Late: 7–45 days	12% 34%	5 10	10% 12%
Macafee et al., 2009[52]	72	Early: <72 hours Late: 3 months	22% 11%	6 6	3% 3%
Kolla et al., 2004[53]	40	Early: <4 days Late: 6–12 weeks	20% 15%	4 10	25% 25%
Johansson et al., 2003[19]	145	Early: <7 days Late: 6–8 weeks	18% 10%	5 8	31% 21%
Lai et al., 1998[20]	104	Early: <24 hours Late: 6–8 weeks	9% 8%	8 12	24% 8%
Lo et al., 1998[21]	99	Early: <3 days Late: 6–8 weeks	29% 13%	6 11	11% 23%

NR, Not recorded.

onset to cholecystectomy on outcomes has also been examined in more detail. A nonrandomized prospective study by Tzovaras and colleagues[56] assessed 129 patients undergoing laparoscopic cholecystectomy for acute cholecystitis. Patients were divided into three groups according to the time from symptom onset to cholecystectomy: less than three days, between four and seven days, and greater than seven days. This study found no significant difference in conversion rate (laparoscopic to open), morbidity, or postoperative hospital stay among these groups and suggested that cholecystectomy may be safe even if performed up to or after seven days from symptom onset. The results of this study, however, should be interpreted in the context of its inherent selection bias because the timing of surgery was determined by surgeon discretion rather than randomization of clinically similar groups.

CHRONIC CHOLECYSTITIS

Pathogenesis and Clinical Manifestations

Chronic cholecystitis may result after one or more episodes of acute cholecystitis, or it may evolve, initially without symptoms, merely from the presence of gallstones. In most cases, patients describe at least one episode of abdominal pain that is clinically consistent with biliary colic. The term *colic* is a misnomer because the pain from chronic cholecystitis is usually constant in nature and is similar to that seen initially with acute cholecystitis, although it is self-limited and often less severe. The pain associated with chronic cholecystitis seems to be the result of intermittent obstruction of the gallbladder outflow.

There are numerous well-described risk factors for the development of gallstones and subsequent chronic cholecystitis. Patients at particularly high risk include obese women, in whom pathologic changes of chronic inflammation are found even in the absence of gallstones[57,58]; this may be because of an increase in the cholesterol saturation of bile in obese patients[59] (see Chapter 8). These patients are often asymptomatic.

Xanthogranulomatous cholecystitis is a subtype of chronic cholecystitis that can appear similar to gallbladder cancer on imaging studies[60] (see Chapter 49). It is characterized by the presence of destructive inflammation of the gallbladder wall, often accompanied by proliferative fibrosis. The histologic appearance is that of foamy histiocytes in a background of acute and chronic inflammatory cells. This process can result in the appearance of asymmetric gallbladder wall thickening and/or mass formation in the gallbladder wall and can be difficult or impossible to distinguish from gallbladder cancer (Fig. 34.5). Further confusing this picture, serum cancer antigen 19-9 levels can be elevated in xanthogranulomatous cholecystitis.[61]

Diagnostic Imaging

US examination of the gallbladder most often reveals circumferential thickening of the gallbladder wall with cholelithiasis (see Chapter 16). In advanced cases, a small, shrunken gallbladder with a thickened wall and multiple gallstones are seen. Discomfort may be reproduced with direct pressure on the gallbladder with the US probe. Commonly, particularly in obese patients and in those with mild symptoms, the US examination shows no particular gallbladder wall abnormalities.[57]

Treatment

Elective cholecystectomy is the treatment of choice for patients with symptoms of chronic cholecystitis (see Chapter 36). In most (≥90%) cases, cholecystectomy can be accomplished laparoscopically. Patients occasionally are seen with atypical pain (left hypochondrium) or with minimal or no pain but, rather, intermittent nausea or bloating. In such cases, evaluation for other possible causes of symptoms should be undertaken, particularly if the US shows gallstones but no sequelae of chronic cholecystitis. In cases where there is asymmetric gallbladder wall thickening or mass formation concerning for malignancy, a laparoscopic exploration is reasonable, but with a low threshold for conversion to an open operation. The surgeon should be prepared to perform a definitive gallbladder cancer operation, including liver resection

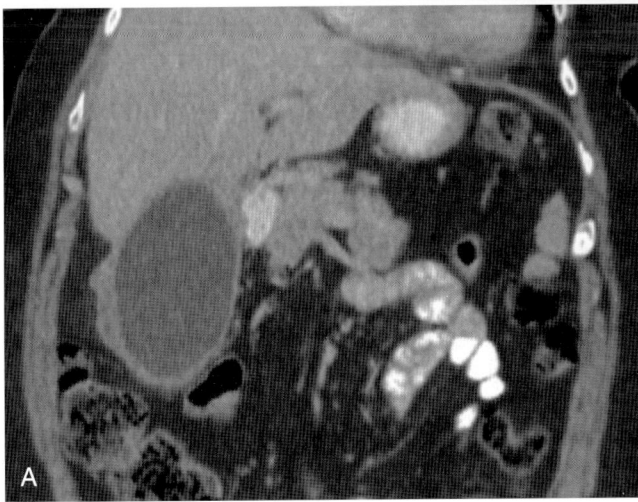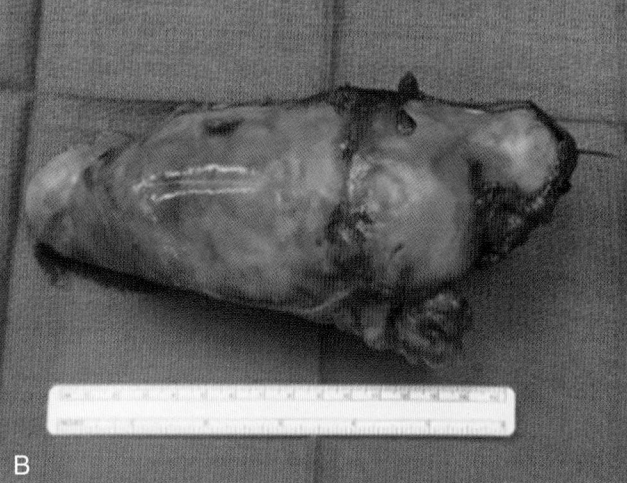

FIGURE 34.5   **A,** Coronal image of a patient seen with chronic right upper quadrant pain and a distended gallbladder with asymmetric wall thickening concerning for malignancy. **B,** Gross image of the resected gallbladder, which was firm and markedly abnormal. Final pathology demonstrated xanthogranulomatous cholecystitis.

and regional lymphadenectomy. In these cases, it is critical to avoid gallbladder perforation or spillage intraoperatively. Frozen-section analysis of any grossly abnormal tissue can be considered, but it is often appropriate to proceed with a cancer operation if gross findings are suspicious for malignancy (see Chapter 49).

ACUTE ACALCULOUS CHOLECYSTITIS

Pathogenesis

Acalculous cholecystitis usually occurs in patients with coexisting acute major illnesses, such as generalized sepsis, major trauma, or burns, or in those undergoing a prolonged recovery from major operations who are unable to tolerate oral intake.[62] It has been speculated that in such situations, there is no stimulus for gallbladder contraction, the bile becomes inspissated, and biliary sludge forms. The exact pathogenesis is unknown but likely involves some combination of ischemia, biliary stasis, and sepsis.[63,64] Inspissated bile and sludge seem to play some causative role as well. Although this condition traditionally has been described in the patient groups mentioned earlier, several reports suggest an increase in the de novo presentation of acalculous cholecystitis in the outpatient population, including patients with atherosclerotic vascular disease, as is seen in hypertension and diabetes.[65–67] Overall, acalculous cholecystitis represents approximately 5% to 15% of all cases of acute cholecystitis. A male predominance is seen in cases of acalculous cholecystitis, in contrast to acute calculous cholecystitis, which occurs more commonly in women.[66,68,69]

A prospective study evaluating trauma patients with serial US examinations found that the incidence of acalculous cholecystitis in severely injured patients (injury severity score $\geq$ 12, requiring intensive care for > four days) was 11%,[70] which is similar to other reports.[71] In addition, three factors were correlated with an increased risk for acalculous cholecystitis in this high-risk population: (1) high injury-severity score, (2) increased heart rate, and (3) transfusion requirement at the time of admission. This study suggests that more acutely injured patients, who are

expected to require prolonged ventilatory and nutritional support, are at higher risk for acalculous cholecystitis.[70]

Clinical Manifestations

Part of the difficulty in making the diagnosis of acalculous cholecystitis is that many patients seen with this condition are critically ill and require ventilatory support and sedation. The symptoms and signs are often masked by the patient's underlying condition or the interventions used to treat it.[68] In the outpatient population seen with acalculous cholecystitis, the diagnosis is more straightforward, mimicking the signs and symptoms of acute calculous cholecystitis.[66]

The most frequent physical and laboratory findings are fever, right upper quadrant pain, leukocytosis, and hyperbilirubinemia. These findings are often nonspecific, however, in the setting of sepsis and critical illness.[68] The incidence of gangrene and perforation seems to be increased in patients with acalculous cholecystitis compared with acute calculous cholecystitis, likely because of the delay in diagnosis that is common with this disease. Severe gallbladder complications such as gangrene, perforation, and empyema occur more commonly in older patients with elevated WBC counts.[66,69] In many series, the risk of severe gallbladder complications was found to be 50% to 60%.[68,69,72] This high risk may be the result of the disturbance in capillary microcirculation, which has been shown in pathologic studies on gallbladder specimens after cholecystectomy for acalculous cholecystitis.[63,64] In addition, partly as a result of the severity of the patient's underlying condition, the mortality rates are as high as 15% in some series.[69]

Diagnostic Evaluation and Imaging

Imaging algorithms for patients with suspected acalculous cholecystitis are similar to algorithms for patients with acute cholecystitis. The initial imaging test is usually US, which classically reveals gallbladder distension, a thickened gallbladder wall, and biliary sludge without stones[69] (Fig. 34.6; see Chapter 16). The difficulty with interpreting these findings is that many critically ill, parenteral nutrition–dependent patients have these findings.

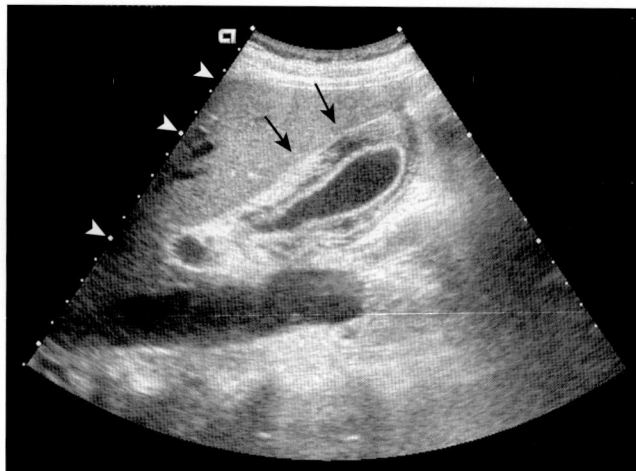

FIGURE 34.6 Ultrasound of a patient with acalculous cholecystitis reveals marked thickening of the gallbladder wall *(arrows)*.

Partly because of this difficulty, the accuracy of US to diagnose acalculous cholecystitis has been highly institution dependent, with some series showing it to be highly sensitive and specific[70] and others showing it to be less accurate.[68] US is widely available and easy to use, even in critically ill patients, because it can be performed at the bedside, and it is inexpensive. US should be performed as the initial imaging modality for suspected acalculous cholecystitis.

The natural history of abnormalities visualized on US in critically ill patients is unclear; a prospective trial assessed 255 critically ill trauma patients with serial US examinations. In this trial, all patients with US findings consistent with acalculous cholecystitis also had significant clinical symptoms of abdominal pain and/or distension, hemodynamic instability, or organ failure. All patients with US findings suggestive of acalculous cholecystitis underwent cholecystectomy and all had acalculous cholecystitis on final pathology. A subset of patients had positive US findings without significant clinical symptoms and within this subset, US findings normalized within three weeks. In addition, 15% of patients experienced hydrops of the gallbladder without clinical symptoms with eventual normalization of US findings observed in all.[70] These findings suggest that although many critically ill patients may develop US abnormalities consistent with acalculous cholecystitis, the combination of clinical symptoms and positive imaging findings is crucial in distinguishing patients who may benefit from intervention.

Because of the difficulty establishing a diagnosis in these critically ill patients, CT has been used as an additional diagnostic adjunct. The advantage of CT is that imaging of the entire chest, abdomen, and pelvis can be obtained; this is particularly important in this patient cohort, in whom clinical signs and symptoms may be misleading or may result from other causes. CT may be more sensitive and specific than US,[73,74] but it has the disadvantage of requiring transport of the patient outside of the intensive care unit.

When a patient's diagnosis is questionable based on physical findings or US evaluation or both, hepatobiliary scintigraphy may also be employed (see Chapter 18). In past reports, a high rate of false-positive scintigraphy results were seen in patients with acalculous cholecystitis[74], but more recent evaluation

of this modality has shown improved accuracy in diagnosing acalculous cholecystitis.[66,68] In some series, scintigraphy has been found to be more sensitive than CT or US in diagnosing acalculous cholecystitis.[66,68,75,76] The specificity of hepatobiliary scintigraphy can be improved by administering morphine to cause constriction of the sphincter of Oddi and improve gallbladder filling (see Chapter 16). This maneuver decreases the incidence of false-positive studies and improves specificity, but it does not result in improvements in sensitivity compared with conventional scintigraphy.[68,77,78] As discussed previously, evaluation of gallbladder EF with scintigraphy can aid in diagnosis of acalculous cholecystitis and chronic cholecystitis. However, caution should be exhibited in interpreting a normal EF in the setting of clinical symptoms, as various studies have reported symptom relief with either surgery or medical management in this population[6,8].

Treatment

The definitive treatment for acalculous cholecystitis is cholecystectomy, which can be performed laparoscopically in most cases. In patients who are critically ill, placement of a percutaneous cholecystostomy tube allows decompression of the gallbladder and drainage of contained, infected bile (see Chapter 35); this allows time for the patient to recover from the acute illness before considering proceeding with cholecystectomy.[36,79] Percutaneous cholecystostomy may be the definitive treatment for acalculous cholecystitis because there is no chronic obstruction of the gallbladder outlet as in acute cholecystitis.[35,80]

COMPLICATIONS OF CHOLECYSTITIS

Gangrenous Cholecystitis

Gangrenous cholecystitis is a more common finding in diabetic patients with acute cholecystitis who present with a leukocytosis.[81] In addition, the risk of gangrenous cholecystitis is higher in patients with acalculous cholecystitis, likely owing to the delay in diagnosis that commonly occurs in this disease.[68,69,72] As previously mentioned, the most common site for necrosis to occur is in the fundus. Full-thickness necrosis is by definition always present in patients with gangrenous cholecystitis, but this condition may or may not result in free perforation of the gallbladder. In patients with free perforation, bile-stained abdominal fluid is present.

Because these patients are generally ill, imaging with CT scan is often performed. Findings most specific for acute gangrenous cholecystitis on CT scan include air in the wall or lumen, intraluminal membranes, an irregular wall, or pericholecystic abscess. As expected, a contrast-enhanced CT scan may show a lack of mural enhancement in patients with gangrenous cholecystitis.[82]

Empyema

In cases of empyema, the gallbladder is filled with purulent bile. This condition usually is associated with acute cholecystitis and occurs in the setting of infected bile and an obstructed cystic duct. Most patients with empyema have calculous cholecystitis, but empyema also can occur in patients with acalculous disease.[83] The clinical course can mimic that of an intra-abdominal abscess from other causes, and patients are often seen initially with clinical manifestations of sepsis. Patients with gallbladder empyema require urgent cholecystectomy or percutaneous cholecystostomy, depending on the severity of illness at the time of presentation.[83] Critically ill patients may be best served by a temporary cholecystostomy tube followed by elective cholecystectomy.

Emphysematous Cholecystitis

Emphysematous cholecystitis is a rare entity that results from the presence of gas-forming bacteria in the bile. Emphysematous cholecystitis may be seen in association with acute or gangrenous cholecystitis, and it is more common in men and patients with diabetes.[84] The diagnosis occasionally can be made by simple abdominal radiographs, but more often it is diagnosed on US (Fig. 34.7) or CT scan[82,85,86] (Fig. 34.8). Patients should receive IV antibiotics to include coverage for *Clostridium* species, followed by emergent cholecystectomy.

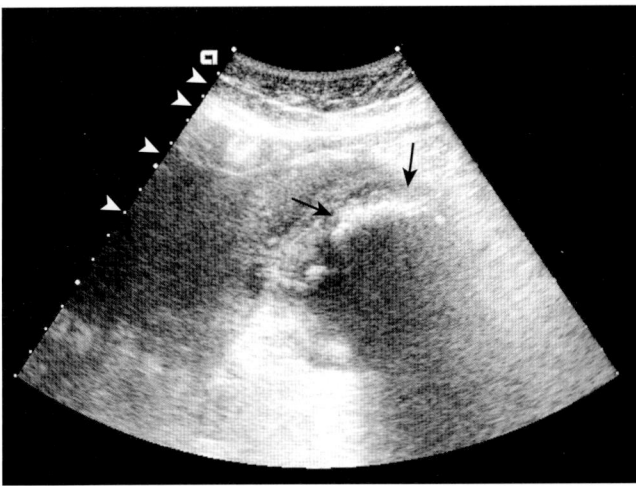

FIGURE 34.7 Ultrasound of the gallbladder revealing air within the gallbladder wall *(arrows)* consistent with emphysematous cholecystitis.

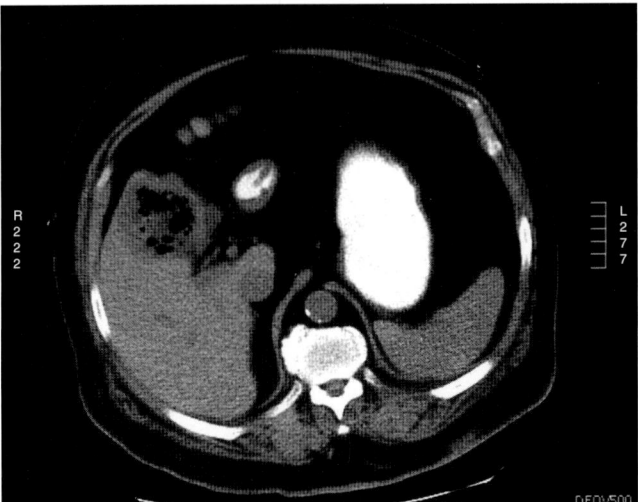

FIGURE 34.8 Computed tomography scan (noncontrast) in a patient with emphysematous cholecystitis showing gallbladder filled with air.

Mirizzi Syndrome

Mirizzi syndrome is defined as biliary obstruction secondary to cholecystitis related to large gallstones. It occurs in 0.3% to 3% of patients undergoing cholecystectomy[87] (see Chapter 37–38). An impacted stone in the gallbladder infundibulum or cystic duct can compress the bile duct, usually at the level of the common hepatic duct (type I), or a stone can erode from the gallbladder or cystic duct into the common hepatic duct, resulting in a cholecystocholedochal fistula (type II). Patients are seen with symptoms of acute cholecystitis but with the additional finding of hyperbilirubinemia and elevated alkaline phosphatase. A laparoscopic approach to this condition has been shown to result in high conversion and complication rates and is generally not recommended.[87,88] Open cholecystectomy is the gold standard for treatment when this condition is identified preoperatively. If inflammation has obliterated the triangle of Calot, a partial cholecystectomy with removal of any stones may be all that is possible and usually resolves the condition. In the acute setting, the biliary obstruction often resolves after cholecystectomy and resolution of the inflammatory process. In some cases, however, the chronic inflammation leads to fistulation from the gallbladder to the bile duct, or a biliary stricture results, both of which will complicate the operative procedure and may require biliary reconstruction (see Chapter 42).

Cholecystoenteric Fistula

Cholecystoenteric fistula, or perforation of the gallbladder into an adjacent hollow organ, is a rare complication of acute cholecystitis. The duodenum and the transverse colon are the most common sites of fistulation, which results in decompression of the gallbladder and may result in brief symptomatic improvement. This complication occurs most frequently in women in their sixth to seventh decades and has been shown to be associated with Mirizzi syndrome or an additional hepatobiliary abnormality such as gallbladder cancer[89–91] (see Chapters 37-38, 42, 49). Contamination of the biliary tree by enteric organisms may result, and patients may be seen with cholangitis and pneumobilia. Approximately 10% to 15% of patients with cholecystoenteric fistulae will pass gallstones into the small intestine and be seen with small bowel obstruction, termed *gallstone ileus*. In patients with cholecystocolonic fistula, chronic diarrhea is the most common presenting symptom in nonemergent cases.[91]

Patients with cholecystoenteric fistula require cholecystectomy with takedown and closure of the fistula. When cholecystoenteric fistula is encountered at the time of surgery, concomitant Mirizzi syndrome should be considered. Patients with gallstone ileus require removal of the obstructing stone via enterotomy,[90] and it is important to perform a thorough examination of the bowel for any other stones. Fistula takedown and cholecystectomy can be performed at the same procedure or at a second, delayed procedure if the patient is too unstable to tolerate a prolonged initial operation, or if the pericholecystic inflammation is so severe as to make initial cholecystectomy unsafe.

Bouveret Syndrome

Bouveret syndrome is defined as gastric outlet obstruction secondary to gallstone impaction facilitated by a bilioenteric fistula[92] (Fig. 34.9). Gallstone ileus is estimated to occur in less than 0.5% of patients with clinically relevant cholelithiasis.[92] Bouveret syndrome represents only 1% to 3% of all cases of

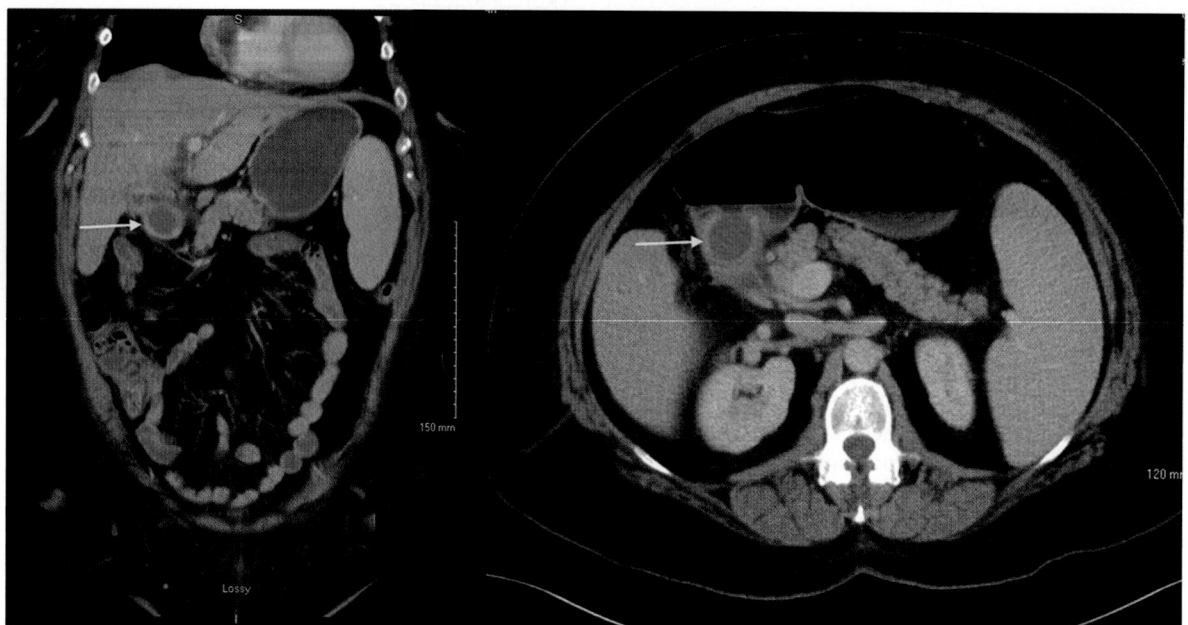

FIGURE 34.9 Coronal and axial cuts from a computed tomography scan in a patient presenting with Bouveret syndrome, demonstrating a large hyperlucent stone *(arrows)* obstructing the first portion of the duodenum with associated gastric distension and outlet obstruction.

gallstone ileus. It is hypothesized to occur secondary to inflammatory remodeling and stone-associated pressure necrosis after acute cholecystitis. Risk factors include female gender, older age, and stones greater than 2.5 cm in diameter. The presenting symptoms can range from nonspecific (nausea, abdominal pain) to complete foregut outlet obstruction. Because of its rarity and potential for vague presenting symptoms, its inclusion on the differential for foregut symptoms is often overlooked.

Diagnosis is facilitated by abdominal imaging. The pathopneumonic findings on abdominal plain films are Rigler's triad (dilated stomach, pneumobilia, and a radio-opaque duodenal shadow), but abdominal films are only diagnostic in about 30% of presentations. US offers more anatomic detail of the bilioenteric fistula and can also characterize the gallbladder; however, sensitivity is variable and user-dependent. A more sensitive modality is contrast-enhanced multi-detector CT, which allows for simultaneous evaluation of the bilioenteric fistula, the gallbladder, and the anatomic relationship between inflammatory change and surrounding structures (i.e., porta hepatis, pancreas). Esophagoduodenoscopy is the most sensitive diagnostic modality and is potentially therapeutic.[92]

Treatment can be facilitated from either endoscopic or surgical approaches. Endoscopic removal can be achieved through direct mechanical removal, mechanical lithotripsy, laser lithotripsy, extracorporeal shockwave lithotripsy, or intracorporeal electrohydraulic lithotripsy. A described complication from lithotripsy is distal enteric obstruction from stone fragmentation. Unfortunately, endoscopic stone extraction is only successful in about 10% of cases. However, because of its less invasive nature, it is generally recommended before any surgical approach. Surgical approach must consider both patient comorbidity and the anatomy of the bilioenteric fistula as it relates to surrounding structures. Surgery can include enterolithotomy with or without closure of the bilioenteric fistula and cholecystectomy (usually done in a multi-stage operation) but depending on the degree of inflammation and location of the impacted stone can also include more invasive approaches. Although the optimal surgical approach is a topic of continued debate, many argue for enterolithotomy alone because it minimizes risk in a typically older population. Although difficult to study because of its rarity, the risk of recurrent biliary symptoms or enteric obstruction after enterolithotomy alone is estimated to be less than 10%.[92]

The references for this chapter can be found online by accessing the accompanying Expert Consult website.

CHAPTER 35

Percutaneous treatment of gallbladder disease

Jad Abou Khalil, George Zogopoulos, and Jeffrey S. Barkun

OVERVIEW

The first reports of an operative cholecystostomy are attributable to Johannes Fabricius (1618) and Stalpert Von Der Wiel (1667) who described the procedure as occurring almost by happenstance upon the incision of an abdominal wall abcess.[1] The following two centuries revealed further sporadic reports, until Marion Sims, an American surgeon in Paris, performed a clearly intentional cholecystostomy in 1878. Kocher and Tait[2] formalized the procedure in 1878, many months after and independently of Sims' efforts.

At a time when cholecystectomy had become the gold standard for the management of most acute gallbladder diseases, operative cholecystostomy remained an attractive alternative in situations of significant patient comorbidity or intraoperative risk, often as a bridge to cholecystectomy[3,4] (see Chapters 33 and 36).

The first description of an ultrasound-guided percutaneous cholecystostomy (PC) for acute cholecystitis followed the development of percutaneous biliary drainage for the management of obstructive jaundice and dates back to 1980.[5,6] Early case series showed encouraging results in patients who were not candidates for cholecystectomy,[7] and ensuing cohort studies popularized its use in circumstances in which cholecystectomy was not feasible (see Chapter 36). The popularity of this procedure has persisted into the laparoscopic era. In the absence of comparative data, PC has supplanted open and laparoscopic alternatives to cholecystostomy and become widely accepted as a treatment for cholecystitis in situations in which surgical intervention is not feasible or deemed too risky. A review of nationwide medical administrative data confirms that the number of PCs performed in the United States for all indications increased 6-fold between 1994 and 2004. The vast majority of PCs, 97% in that time period, have been performed by interventional radiologists.[8] An examination of the National Inpatient Sample database demonstrated that between 1998 and 2010, 1.5% of calculus and 7.5% of acalculous cholecystitis cases in the United States were treated with PC.[9]

In addition to its use for the management of acute cholecystitis, PC also provided its early practitioners with the opportunity to investigate the management of gallstone disease nonsurgically by chemical dissolution, mechanical extraction, or lithotripsy of gallbladder calculi.[6,10] However, these approaches are not curative and have largely been abandoned because of the high rates of recurrence of cholelithiasis and cholecystitis. Furthermore, the logistical hurdles required for their safe administration and the superiority of laparoscopic cholecystectomy (LC; see later) have made these treatments impractical. In this chapter, we will examine the indications and contraindications for PC and illustrate some of its technical aspects and potential complications. We will place a particular emphasis on the quality of the evidence available in the literature and propose guidelines for the management of patients considered for PC.

INDICATIONS AND CONTRAINDICATIONS FOR PERCUTANEOUS CHOLECYSTECTOMY

Acute Calculous Cholecystitis in High-Risk Patients

Despite the dearth of high-quality data, the use of PC in patients with acute calculous cholecystitis (ACC) at high risk for surgery has become commonplace. In reviews of surgical databases, patients who receive PC are demonstrably older and have greater medical comorbidity than those receiving LC.[9,11]

A systematic review of cohort studies examining PC for ACC identified 53 studies examining the question; however, differences in outcome reporting, biases in control selection, and the significant heterogeneity of study populations made it impossible to draw conclusive recommendations on clear indications in high-risk surgical patients.[12] The review confirmed that mortality rates after PC are high (15.4% vs. 4.5% with cholecystectomy), likely indicating selection biases favoring the use of PC in patients with higher comorbidity. Although the high mortality rate is likely inflated by the higher mortality in early cohorts, it remains elevated in contemporary cohorts, reflecting the high-risk population in whom PC is performed.

Only three randomized studies examining the use of PC in acute cholecystitis have been published; however, they ask different questions, and have significant methodologic limitations. Hatzidakis and colleagues[13] randomly assigned 123 high-risk patients (Acute Physiology and Chronic Health Evaluation [APACHE] score > 12) with ultrasound-proven ACC or acute acalculous cholecystitis (AAC) to ultrasound-guided PC versus conservative medical therapy (63 and 60 patients, respectively; see Chapter 34). In this trial, ultrasound-guided PC was unsuccessful in 5% of patients who had to undergo computed tomography (CT)-guided PC. The authors were unable to demonstrate a difference in symptom resolution after 3 days or in 30-day mortality and concluded that PC was indicated if symptoms failed to resolve after 3 days of conservative medical management. The study, however, had significant methodologic flaws. There was no pre-planned power analysis, no measures taken to conceal allocation, and no attempt to blind the investigators, the patients, or the care providers. Moreover, an evolving procedural learning curve within the study period made PC appear more morbid than it likely is in more experienced hands. The conclusion of this trial (i.e., that PC should be delayed until more conservative measures have failed to improve symptoms within 3 days) is counter to the current thinking, which promotes the use of early PC if it is to be used at all. This early use of PC is supported by observational cohorts where delayed PC is associated with more bleeding complications and an increased length of stay.[14]

The second randomized trial by Akyürek et al.[15] randomly assigned 70 patients with ultrasound-proven AAC to PC followed by early LC 3 to 4 days later or to conservative management with delayed LC 8 weeks after recovery (33 patients).

In this study, PC followed by early LC decreased hospital length of stay and costs compared with conservative management with delayed LC. There was no difference in the proportions of conversion to open cholecystectomy at operation. The authors did not define inclusion or exclusion criteria, and no definition was provided for "a high-risk" surgical patient. The study was also not adequately powered to detect meaningful differences in the outcomes it compared. Furthermore, the trial did not state how randomization was performed and lacked blinding or allocation concealment. Of note, the analysis was performed strictly per-protocol and there was a notable 13% drop-out rate. Such methodologic shortcomings make it difficult to make recommendations based on this study.

A Cochrane Collaboration Systematic Review[16] on the use of PC in high-risk patients with ACC identified the aforementioned two randomized trials,[13,15] grading their quality as very low and their risk of bias as very high. The group was unable to generate any recommendation on the usefulness of PC compared with conservative therapy, calling for higher-quality randomized trials.

The largest multicenter randomized trial to date, the CHOCOLATE (Acute Cholecystitis in High-Risk Surgical Patients: Percutaneous Cholecystostomy Versus Laparoscopic Cholecystectomy) trial provides us with the highest-level evidence.[17] It randomized high-risk patients with ACC, defined as patients with an APACHE II score between 7 and 15, to PC versus LC. The trial excluded critically ill patients (APACHE II score > 15), those not considered to be surgical candidates, and patients with delayed presentations (>7 days from symptom onset). In this population, as in the literature at large, patients undergoing PC had a rapid improvement in their symptoms, but the incidence of major complications was greater in the PC group at an interim analysis (12% vs. 65%, respectively; $P < .001$). Healthcare utilization and cost were also greater in the PC group. The major morbidity increase in the PC group was driven by reinterventions. Importantly, the 65% morbidity rate far exceeds what would be considered standard for PC. Nevertheless, it is clear from this study that patients who are physiologically able to tolerate a cholecystectomy should be offered surgery rather than PC. As a result of this trial and other data, the 2018 Tokyo Guidelines on the management of cholecystitis now recommends a cholecystectomy even in patients with a Tokyo grade II or III acute cholecystitis if they have a Charlson Comorbidity Index less than 6 , American Society of Anesthesiologists (ASA) class of 2 or less, good functional status, favorable organ system failure (defined as cardiovascular or renal organ system failure rapidly reversible during admission and before laparoscopic cholecystectomy for acute cholecystitis), and no negative predictive factors. This is in contrast to the 2013 guidelines, which recommended PC more liberally for acute cholecystitis grades II and III.[18]

In conclusion, despite the absence of convincing high-level evidence, and based mainly on retrospective unmatched cohorts, PC is frequently performed in patients with ACC who do not respond to medical therapy and who are deemed unfit for surgery because of age or medical comorbidity. The evidence suggests that LC should be offered to patients with acute cholecystitis who can tolerate surgery.

Acute Calculous Cholecystitis With Delayed Presentation

PC, followed by interval LC, has been used in the specific context of ACC late in the course of the disease, hoping that conversion to open cholecystectomy would be less than during LC at the index presentation. This was the subject of a retrospective cohort study of patients with an ASA score of 1 or 2 presenting with ACC after more than 72 hours of symptoms who did not respond to nonoperative treatment for 48 hours. It compared early PC with PC and delayed LC 4 weeks later (48 patients) to LC (43 patients). The authors found a lower frequency of conversion to open surgery, shorter hospital stay, and fewer total complications with PC and delayed LC (40% vs. 19%; $P = .029$ in the early LC vs. early PC and delayed LC group).[19] The main methodologic limitation of the study was selection bias: It is unclear how patients in the early cholecystectomy group were selected, and no attempt was made to adjust for baseline differences between the groups. Zehetner and colleagues[20] analyzed patients with ultrasound-confirmed ACC presenting more than 72 hours after symptom onset. They compared 23 patients treated with PC with those treated by LC. The authors pair-matched patients for age, sex, race, body mass index, diabetes, and sepsis. Contrary to the previous study, the authors demonstrated increased length of hospital stay (LOS) with PC and no difference in major morbidity; however, there was a significant proportion of conversion to open surgery in the non-PC group (17%) and a trend toward higher 30-day mortality in the PC group (13%). The deaths in the PC group were because of advanced cancer, illustrating the significant selection bias that went into treatment attribution, a bias that was not accounted for by matching on basic demographic characteristics in a very small sample.

Acute Acalculous Cholecystitis

The use of PC in high-risk patients with AAC is supported by many cohort studies demonstrating decreased morbidity and mortality when compared with LC or open cholecystectomy[21,22] (Fig. 35.1). However, when compared with conservative medical therapy, different studies reach different conclusions, with some large studies showing no benefit attributable to PC. An examination of 43,341 patients with AAC and severe sepsis or shock within the California Office of Statewide Health Planning and Development Patient Discharge Database (1995–2009) demonstrated that patients undergoing PC had the greatest number of comorbidities and were the sickest. No difference in survival, however, was found between PC and medical management after extensive multivariate adjustment.[23] This remained true in the subgroup of patients with severe sepsis or shock and those dependent on mechanical ventilation. In fact, patients seemed to fare best when they could undergo cholecystectomy alone or were treated with PC followed by cholecystectomy. The study did not consider short-term outcomes, LOS, symptom control, and quality-of-life measures. This large study of medico-administrative data is the strongest evidence that PC might not offer a mortality benefit over medical management in patients with AAC who are deemed unfit for surgery, but this conclusion is clouded by significant residual confounders that cannot be adjusted for in a medico-administrative database. An analysis of 58,518 patients with AAC from another medico-administrative database, the National Inpatient Sample,[9] demonstrated that, after multivariate adjustment (for sex, age, race, Charlson index, and hospital teaching status), PC remained associated with increased odds of death, increased LOS, and decreased odds of gallbladder-specific and total complications compared with surgery, indicating that in both ACC and AAC, its use was reserved for select sicker patients. The study did not compare PC with nonoperative management, and there is no doubt that residual

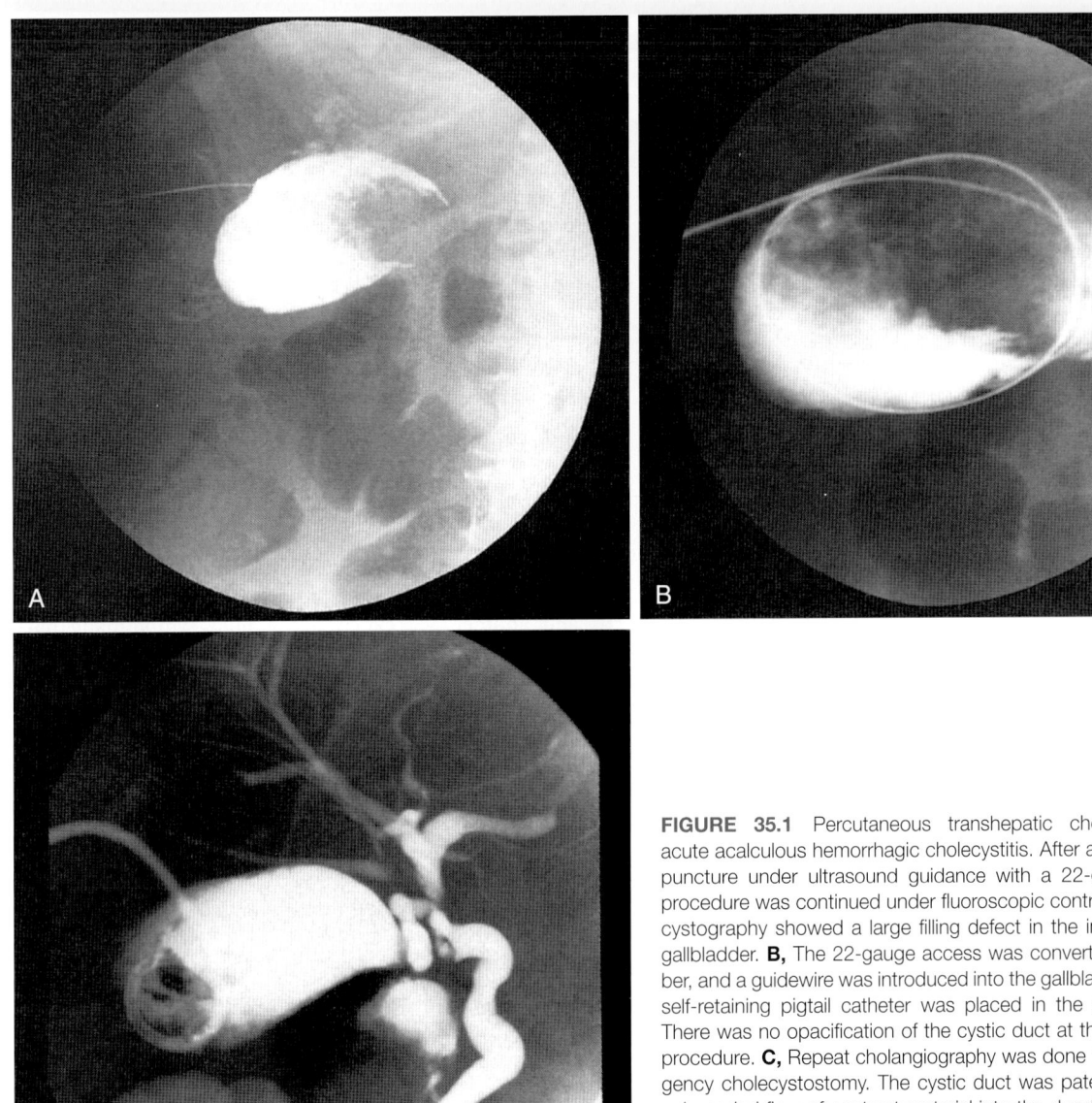

FIGURE 35.1 Percutaneous transhepatic cholecystostomy for acute acalculous hemorrhagic cholecystitis. After an initial gallbladder puncture under ultrasound guidance with a 22-gauge needle, the procedure was continued under fluoroscopic control. **A,** Direct cholecystography showed a large filling defect in the infundibulum of the gallbladder. **B,** The 22-gauge access was converted to a larger caliber, and a guidewire was introduced into the gallbladder. A 6.5-French self-retaining pigtail catheter was placed in the gallbladder lumen. There was no opacification of the cystic duct at the time of the initial procedure. **C,** Repeat cholangiography was done 1 week after emergency cholecystostomy. The cystic duct was patent, and there was unimpeded flow of contrast material into the duodenum. Most of the debris within the gallbladder had disappeared. The cholecystostomy catheter was removed 1 week after cholecystostomy; elective cholecystectomy was not required.

statistical confounding is a concern in such large retrospective databases.

Therefore whether or not PC in critically ill patients with AAC offers a survival advantage over medical treatment alone remains unclear because our knowledge is derived from retrospective cohort studies with varying degrees of risk adjustment and significant residual confounding.[24]

Some data exist that indicate that in patients with AAC, a PC can constitute a definitive treatment without the need for a delayed cholecystectomy. Calculous etiology and presence of pus in the gallbladder are independent predictors of recurrence of cholecystitis after PC.[25] Most patients with AAC treated with PC will not experience a recurrence of the cholecystitis[26] (in one series of PC for AAC, 21% of patients died in hospital, and 18% of patients treated with PC died from unrelated causes in the months after discharge).[27]

Special Populations

Pregnancy

Although the safety of LC is well established in the second trimester of pregnancy,[28,29] most surgeons are reluctant to operate in the first and third trimesters out of fear of spontaneous abortion and preterm labor. PC may thus provide a safe temporizing measure for pregnant patients seen with severe biliary colic or cholecystitis in the first and third trimester who fail conservative medical therapy. The evidence to support this approach is scarce, and no large cohort or controlled trial has examined this question. Two small studies have reported the feasibility and safety of PC in pregnancy for acute cholecystitis and biliary colic in a limited number of patients. Allmendinger et al.[30] published a case report of two pregnant patients who underwent PC for cholecystitis at 30 and 32 weeks of gestation, respectively, followed by elective cholecystectomy in the postpartum phase. Chiappetta Porras et al.[31] described a cohort of 122 patients treated for symptomatic cholelithiasis in the first trimester, among which four cholecystostomies in the first trimester for cholecystitis and four gallbladder aspirations in the third trimester (three for biliary colic and one for cholecystitis) are described. These case reports and case series suggest that PC is feasible during pregnancy and may be used as a safe alternative to operative intervention after failure of medical management, but its use should be limited when a safe laparoscopic cholecystectomy can be performed.

Sepsis of Unknown Origin in the Intensive Care

In the critically ill patient with persistent sepsis of unknown origin, PC affords a safe and rapid therapeutic intervention in the event of suspected AAC or ACC, and it can be used to exclude the gallbladder as the septic focus. Two case series describe such an approach: In 24[32] and 82 patients,[33] PC resulted in resolution of sepsis in 58% and 51% of patients, respectively. These case series were, however, not followed by controlled trials. Moreover, it is possible that the incidence of AAC was higher compared with contemporary practice because of different intensive care practices, such as prolonged enteric starvation. We postulate that "diagnostic PC" has less utility in the modern intensive care setting.

Conclusion

PC should be reserved for patients who are not medically fit to undergo open cholecystectomy or LC.[34] It may be used as a bridge to cholecystectomy in patients failing medical therapy for ACC who are not fit for surgery at the time of presentation, and it could be used as definitive therapy in patients with AAC.

TECHNICAL ASPECTS AND COMPLICATIONS

Insertion Technique

1. Drainage versus aspiration: Drainage has been demonstrated to be superior to simple aspiration of the acutely inflamed gallbladder in a single randomized trial[35] and is currently the most widely used approach.
2. Operator: Most commonly, PC is performed by radiologists[8] (see Chapter 30) under ultrasonographic guidance, but a single publication reports on a series performed by surgeons,[36] with acceptable results and improved access times, although this experience may not be generalizable to most institutions. Regardless of who performs the procedure, it is advisable that only individuals highly facile with ultrasonographic or CT-guided interventional techniques perform PC and that there be regular institutional quality monitoring, according to proposed procedure-specific quality-control benchmarks.[37]
3. Approach: Patient preparation consists of skin disinfection and standard sterile precautions, procedural sedation, and either prophylactic administration or ready availability of atropine because vagal reactions have been documented.[38] PC is performed under direct ultrasound or computed tomography (CT) guidance, with equivalent success and complication rates.[39] After the planned anatomic course is identified, the gallbladder is entered using a finder needle, and a guidewire is inserted into it, with a size 7- to 10-French

pigtail catheter inserted over the guidewire using a Seldinger technique. Other catheters, such as a central venous catheter, can be used in lieu of a pigtail catheter and may be of use in certain institutional settings, but data on catheter displacement and patency times with these other options are limited.[40] A catheter placed by transhepatic access is preferred to the transperitoneal route. The transhepatic tract matures faster than the transperitoneal tract (2 weeks vs. 3 weeks, respectively), allowing faster removal of the catheter as well as less bile leaks and bile peritonitis.[41] The transhepatic approach is safer because it avoids the peritoneum in patients with significant ascites or bowel interposition.[42] However, it is associated with the potential for pneumothorax, bleeding, and hemobilia.[10]

Complications

In experienced hands, PC has both a high technical success rate (>98.9%)[12] and a low complication rate. Documented complications include hemorrhage (2.5%), pneumothorax (0.5%), and postprocedural catheter dislodgement (<1%).[37] After catheter withdrawal, 3% of patients experience severe bile peritonitis and another 3% experience a mild symptomatic biliary leak.[43] Bile leaks are associated with transperitoneal access[44] and may require operative therapy or repeat PC. In a systematic review of 35 papers, displacement of the PC catheter was reported in 8.6%; however, this may be an underestimation in an outpatient population.[12] In a cohort described by Smith et al.,[11] catheter-related complications occurred in 14.5% of patients, including tube dislodgement in 10 of 143 (7%), extra-abdominal peritube bile leak in 7 of 143 (5%), pain in 4 of 143 (3%), and occlusion in 4 of 143 (3%). These complications were managed mostly with tube repositioning or upsizing, and none required operation.

Management of the Percutaneous Cholecystectomy Catheter and the Gallbladder

As already stated, the catheter tract usually matures after 2 weeks for transhepatic catheters and after 3 weeks for transperitoneal drains. A cholecystogram can be obtained before removal of the catheter 3 to 6 weeks after insertion, but imaging is not necessary in cases where a small-bore catheter was placed and where the cystic duct was patent at insertion. In AAC, assuming the resolution of precipitating factors, PC is considered curative, and LC is not mandatory because 70% of patients may not experience a recurrence.[26] There remains a debate as to whether PC can be considered curative after ACC.[45] Recurrence rates of cholecystitis after PC in ACC without interval cholecystectomy vary between studies: from 4.1% at 1 year in one study[46] to 11.7% at 38 months in another.[47] A cohort from the United Kingdom shows a recurrence rate as high as 22% at 1 year but also a 1-year mortality of 37% after index admission, mainly from medical causes unrelated to gallstone disease.[44] Although cholecystectomy may be desirable after PC for ACC, a review of a large medico-administrative database demonstrates that PC is, in fact, only followed by elective cholecystectomy in 40% of patients at 1 year, whereas an additional 18% die without undergoing cholecystectomy.[48] It is therefore prudent to weigh the risk of interval LC with the patient's concurrent medical comorbidities, evolving surgical risks, and life expectancy against the risk of recurrence and ensuing morbidity and mortality.

PERCUTANEOUS TREATMENT OF GALLSTONES: TECHNIQUES OF HISTORIC INTEREST

Many techniques have been developed in an attempt to avoid the need for elective cholecystectomy. The 1980s saw the rise in popularity of extracorporeal shock-wave lithotripsy (ESWL), which in association with oral bile salt therapy, promised to clear the gallbladder of gallstones without resorting to surgery. Its use, however, was limited to patients with less than three cholesterol stones of 2 cm or less in size, and it required multiple treatments over months. The proportion of patients with recurrent cholelithiasis at 6 years was 69%, making ESWL an unacceptable option for most patients.[49] Moreover, it has been proven to not be a cost-effective approach,[50] and its use has been largely abandoned.

Methyl tert-butyl ether (MTBE), a cholesterol solvent, has been used to dissolve gallbladder calculi after the placement of a PC. Its use, however, is cumbersome, requires specialized equipment and tubing that will not be destroyed by MTBE, and involves bothersome, prolonged administration over many days.[51] Its use is mainly of historic interest.

A publication has suggested the use of PC as an adjunct to cystic duct stenting in patients deemed unfit for LC.[52] Only four patients were described in this study, and no information on long-term patency of this technique was described. A small series has described the feasibility of endoscopic ultrasound-guided transduodenal drainage of the gallbladder; however, this experience has not been reproduced to date.[53]

The references for this chapter can be found online by accessing the accompanying Expert Consult website.

CHAPTER 36

Cholecystectomy techniques and postoperative problems

Morgan Bonds and Flavio Rocha

OVERVIEW

Cholecystectomy is one of the most frequently performed general surgery procedures in the United States (US) with over 500,000 being performed annually.[1] There are many reasons for this, including the frequency of gallbladder disease and indications for intervention in the US population. The advent of laparoscopic cholecystectomy in the 1980s also resulted in a rapid rise in the number of cholecystectomies because of the reduced postoperative recovery, reduced pain, and ability to complete the procedure in the outpatient setting.[2,3] As familiarity with laparoscopy has increased, the incidence of open cholecystectomy has steadily decreased. This chapter will address techniques of open cholecystectomy because this approach is still used when laparoscopy is contraindicated or technically impossible. Appropriate laparoscopic cholecystectomy techniques will also be discussed, including strategies to prevent common bile duct injuries (CBDI), which are an avoidable source of severe morbidity with this procedure. Alternative minimally invasive approaches and common complications will also be addressed.

INDICATIONS

Symptomatic gallstones are the primary reason a patient requires cholecystectomy (see Chapters 33 and 34). In the US, approximately 5% to 22% of the population has cholelithiasis.[4] Cholelithiasis can lead to several pathologic conditions including biliary colic, acute cholecystitis, gallstone pancreatitis, or choledocholithiasis, but the majority of patients with cholelithiasis will remain asymptomatic (see Chapter 33). As such, prophylactic cholecystectomy in asymptomatic patients is typically not warranted. Nevertheless, cholecystectomy may be indicated for certain populations with asymptomatic cholelithiasis. An example is sickle cell anemia where hepatic and vaso-occlusive disease can be indistinguishable from acute cholecystitis.[5]

Gallbladder polyps without cholelithiasis can be an indication for cholecystectomy (see Chapter 49). Resection is recommended for gallbladder polyps greater than or equal to 10 mm and in patients with biliary symptoms in the setting of gallbladder polyps of any size.[6] Cholecystectomy is also often performed concomitantly with other procedures. Examples include pancreaticoduodenectomy and major anatomic liver resections. Cholecystectomy at the time of bariatric surgery is controversial. It is thought that biliary symptoms increase after extreme weight loss. Nevertheless, a systematic review and meta-analysis reported that concomitant cholecystectomy increases postoperative morbidity and operative time[7] (see Chapter 34).

Timing of cholecystectomy can vary by indication. Acute cholecystitis cases should proceed to the operating room as early as possible. A recent study using a Swedish registry found that adverse events, mortality, and CBDIs were higher in patients who underwent cholecystectomy more than 4 days after admission.[8] These data suggest the optimal timing for cholecystectomy is within 48 hours of admission for acute cholecystitis.

LAPAROSCOPIC CHOLECYSTECTOMY TECHNIQUES

Laparoscopy has become the standard access for removing the gallbladder. Multiple studies have shown a decrease in postoperative pain, an earlier return to normal activity, a decrease in hospital length of stay (LOS), and a reduction in incisional hernia development for laparoscopic cholecystectomy when compared with open cholecystectomy.[9–12] Familiarity with the anatomy of the porta hepatis, including common biliary and vascular variations, can reduce complication rates for both laparoscopic and open cholecystectomy, particularly for challenging cases presenting with significant inflammation.

Operating Room Setup

Before beginning any procedure, the surgeon must ensure that all equipment is present and functional, which includes equipment for potentially necessary procedures such as cholangiography or need for conversion to laparotomy (Box 36.1).

Port Placement and Exposure

Once pneumoperitoneum is obtained, a 5- or 10-mm port is placed in the periumbilical region. A 30-degree laparoscope is inserted, and the abdominal cavity is inspected. One 5-mm trocar is placed along the right anterior axillary line 2 centimeters below the costal margin. The other 5-mm port is placed at the midclavicular line on the right at the edge of the liver. A fourth port (5- or 10-mm) is placed in the subxiphoid region and should be placed 2 to 4 centimeters below the xiphoid depending on the location of the gallbladder and falciform ligament (Fig. 36.1). A fifth port can be placed in the location deemed most appropriate for additional retraction, if necessary.

Dissection and Critical View of Safety

An atraumatic grasper is placed through the most lateral port and grasps the fundus of the gallbladder to retract it cephalad and laterally. This raises the liver edge and exposes the neck of the gallbladder and the porta. With the gallbladder retracted cephalad, a second atraumatic grasper is placed through the midclavicular port to manipulate the infundibulum of the gallbladder. Adhesions should be taken down until the gallbladder infundibulum can be seen. Retraction of the infundibulum caudally and to the right exposes the triangle of Calot. A cautery instrument placed through the xiphoid port opens the peritoneum in the triangle of Calot (Fig. 36.2). This should be started at the edge of the gallbladder neck to avoid iatrogenic injury to aberrant hepatic vasculature or bile ducts. Dissection of the peritoneum is continued on both sides of the gallbladder 1 to 2 mm from the liver edge.

Attention is next turned to obtaining the critical view of safety (CVS).[13] This technique has been shown to reduce the rates of iatrogenic bile duct injuries[14] (see Chapters 32 and 42). In fact, a recent multisociety consensus statement recommended CVS for identification of the cystic duct and cystic artery during laparoscopic cholecystectomy, and when CVS was not attainable, a subtotal cholecystectomy should be performed rather than attempting a fundus-first approach[15] (see Chapter 34).

Attachments at the neck of the gallbladder are dissected using a combination of blunt and cautery assisted dissection. It is useful to serially retract the infundibulum medially and laterally to fully dissect the triangle of Calot. Carrying dissection to the level of the common bile duct (CBD) is not indicated because this only increases the risk for iatrogenic injury. Blunt dissection with a Maryland grasper or right-angle grasper can help create a window behind the cystic duct by spreading in the avascular tissue. The gallbladder is dissected off the liver edge, exposing the cystic plate. The criteria for CVS have been met when (1) there are only two structures seen entering the gallbladder, the cystic duct and cystic artery; (2) the lower third of the cystic plate is exposed; and (3) tissue has been cleared from the hepatocystic triangle so that all structures can be clearly identified anteriorly and posteriorly (Box 36.2).[16] These views are demonstrated in Fig. 36.3. If any question or doubt about the anatomy is encountered, a cholangiogram should be performed to reorient the surgeon (see Chapter 24).

Most surgeons attempt the CVS during laparoscopic cholecystectomy, but in practice it is rarely achieved. An evaluation of 160 online videos of laparoscopic cholecystectomy found only one video accomplished a passing CVS score.[17] The safe cholecystectomy curriculum can be found free of charge at the

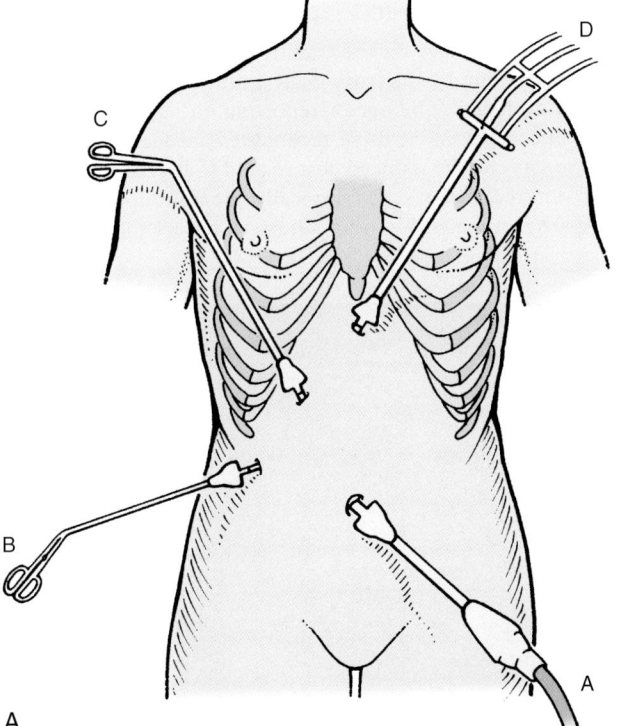

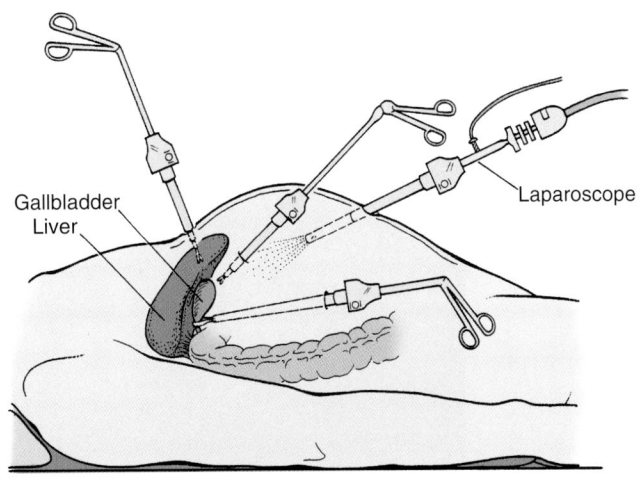

FIGURE 36.1 Positions for insertion of trocars during laparoscopic cholecystectomy. The laparoscope **(A)** is positioned in the periumbilical region, the graspers for gallbladder retraction **(B)** and manipulation **(C)** are positioned in the right upper quadrant (RUQ) along the subcostal region, and the subxyphoid region **(D)** is used for the dissector, diathermy, and clip appliers.

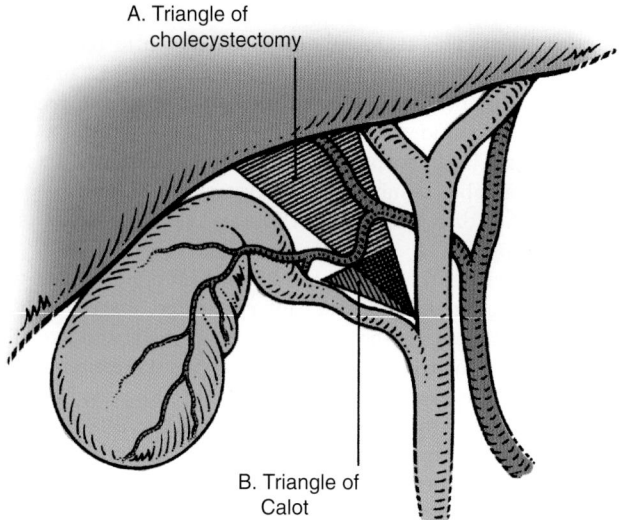

A. Triangle of
cholecystectomy

B. Triangle of
Calot

FIGURE 36.2 **A,** Triangle of cholecystectomy limited by the common hepatic duct, right hepatic duct, cystic duct, and inferior liver edge. **B,** The triangle of Calot limited by the common hepatic duct, cystic duct, and cystic artery.

BOX 36.2   Doublet Scoring for Critical View of Safety

Criteria for Achieving Critical View of Safety
Two structures connected to gallbladder:
• Only two structures clearly seen entering the gallbladder.
Cystic plate:
• Approximately 1/3 of cystic plate is clearly visible.
Clearance of hepatocystic triangle:
• Hepatocystic triangle is cleared of tissue so visibility of cystic structures and plate is unimpeded and the surgeon is certain no other structures are in the hepatocystic triangle.

Society of American Gastrointestinal and Endoscopic Surgeons (SAGES) website.[18]

Completion of Cholecystectomy

Once all critical anatomy is confirmed, the cystic artery and duct are clipped and divided. Care should be taken to avoid tenting the CBD with clips placed too distally on the cystic duct. The tips of the clip should be directly visualized to be free before closing to avoid inadvertent injury to other structures and ensure the clip completely occludes the artery or duct. If it is not possible to secure a clip completely across a structure, an Endoloop device can be used to ligate it. Scissors are used to divide the cystic artery and duct. In rare cases with a large inflamed cystic duct that cannot accommodate clips, endovascular staplers can be used to divide and secure the duct. These situations, however, should raise the level of concern regarding possible injury to the CBD, and the surgeon should consider intraoperative cholangiography if there is any concern whatsoever regarding the anatomy. Cautery is avoided for division because of the increased risk for necrosis resulting in clip slippage. The gallbladder is dissected off the cystic plate from the infundibulum to the fundus with electrocautery. Blindly placing clips, clamps, or cauterizing at this time risks causing hemorrhage or inadvertent injury to the hepatic blood supply, superficial biliary pedicles, or middle hepatic vein branches and should be avoided (Fig. 36.4). Before completely freeing the gallbladder from the liver, the gallbladder is used for retraction to inspect the cystic plate for hemostasis and inspect that clips are still securely placed on the cystic duct and artery.

Specimen removal is performed through the periumbilical incision because it is easy to enlarge this incision to extract large gallstones. Bag extraction is performed with videoscopic visualization to ensure the bag does not rip and specimen contents are not lost. Spilled bile or debris should be completely irrigated and cleared with suction to prevent subsequent migration or abscess formation. The fascia of port sites greater than 10 mm are closed to prevent development of incisional hernias although some surgeons elect not to close the epigastric site because herniation is unlikely in that location.

Three-Port and Two-Port Techniques

Attempts to improve on the traditional four-port laparoscopic cholecystectomy by decreasing the number of port sites have been introduced. The series reporting these techniques are small but suggest that these techniques are feasible and safe. Proponents cite the reduced cost related to fewer trocars, fewer scars, and reduced cost.[19,20] Typically, the right upper quadrant ports are eliminated by using suture to retract the gallbladder

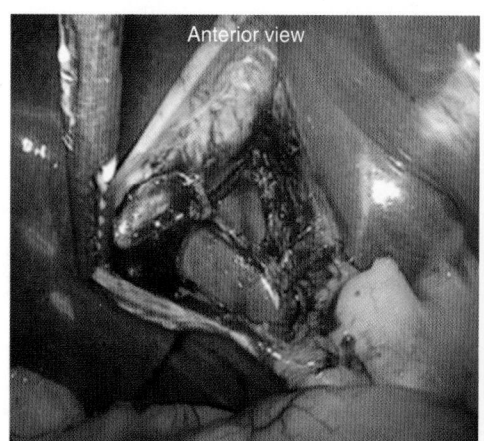
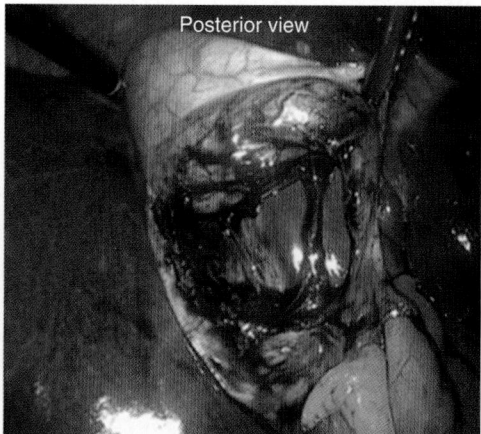

Anterior view   Posterior view

FIGURE 36.3 **A,** Critical view. Hepatocystic triangle is dissected free of all tissue except for the cystic duct and artery, and one-third of the cystic plate on the liver bed is exposed. When this view is achieved, the two structures entering the gallbladder can only be the cystic duct and artery. **B,** Critical view of safety during laparoscopic cholecystectomy.

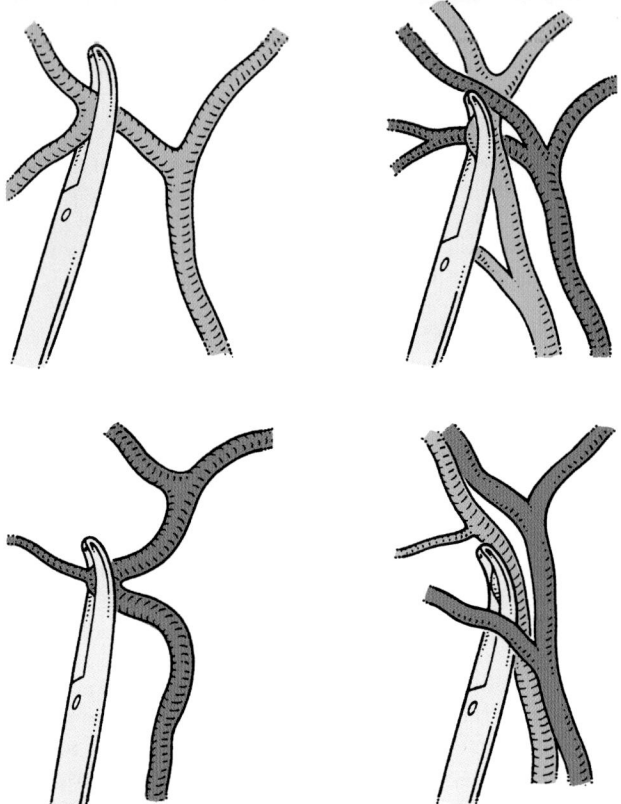

FIGURE 36.4   Blind placement of clips or clamps for hemostasis can result in injury to the hepatic artery or bile duct.

in their stead.[21] A small randomized controlled trial (RCT) with 217 patients compared four-port with three-port cholecystectomy and found no difference in length of operation or morbidity, including iatrogenic bile duct injuries; however, there was also no difference in pain medication required between groups.[22] Currently, there are no obvious advantages that these techniques offer over the four-port technique.

Single-Incision Laparoscopic Cholecystectomy

Single-incision laparoscopic cholecystectomy (SILC) is the extreme attempt at reducing the number of ports for laparoscopic cholecystectomy. SILC is performed through a single transabdominal incision, usually at the umbilicus. There are specifically designed single-port systems and instruments available that have been approved by the US Food and Drug Administration (FDA).

Several RCTs comparing SILC with standard laparoscopic cholecystectomy have been performed, although most are hampered by low accrual. A 2017 trial from Egypt enrolled 187 patients. SILC had a statistically significant longer operating time and conversion rate compared with three-port laparoscopic cholecystectomy; the only advantage to SILC in this study was the aesthetic score.[23] In addition to the absence of benefit to the patient, SILC induces significantly more stress on the surgeon. A double-blind RCT measured surgeon heart rate and salivary cortisol before being randomized to either SILC or traditional laparoscopic cholecystectomy, after clipping the cystic duct and while closing skin. SILC was associated with higher heart rates and cortisol levels. Surgeons also reported the surgical workload was more demanding with

SILC.[24] Careful patient selection is necessary to optimize the use of this technique. It is critical to understand that the CVS should be obtained regardless of the number of laparoscopic ports used to reduce the risk of vasculobiliary injury during minimally invasive cholecystectomy.

Robotic-Assisted Laparoscopic Cholecystectomy

The use of robotic assisted laparoscopic surgery has significantly increased in recent years. This upswing in robotic surgery is because of a combination of aggressive marketing resulting in patient demand. This platform is attractive to surgeons as well because it offers the benefits of 3-dimensional (3D) visualization, improved ergonomics, and an easier learning curve compared with laparoscopy. Robotic laparoscopic cholecystectomy has been proposed as an ideal tool to improve skill and confidence using the robotic platform[25] (see Chapter 127A).

Despite similar outcomes, robotic surgery is associated with significantly higher costs than laparoscopy. The upfront cost of purchasing a robotic console is approximately 2 million dollars. In addition, there is the cost of maintenance and replacement of disposable instruments. A single institution analysis reported lower readmission rates with robotic cholecystectomy in propensity matched patients, but the overall hospital costs and operative time were significantly larger.[26] These cost discrepancies must be considered when deciding on the optimal minimally invasive approach to cholecystectomy.

CONTRAINDICATIONS

Contraindications to this procedure are divided into two categories: (1) contraindications to cholecystectomy and (2) contraindications to laparoscopy. Absolute contraindications to operative cholecystectomy include refractory coagulopathy and intolerance of general anesthesia (see Chapter 35). The 2018 Tokyo Guidelines do not discourage cholecystectomy for patients with severe sepsis and end-organ failure (Grade III cholecystitis) if supportive care is available and the operating surgeon feels the patient can withstand the procedure.[27]

Relative contraindications include severe cardiopulmonary disease, pregnancy, and cirrhosis with portal hypertension, but ultimately the decision is made based on clinical judgment (see Chapter 75). The presence of cirrhosis can complicate many abdominal surgical interventions. Laparoscopic cholecystectomy in cirrhotic patients is especially challenging because it can be difficult to retract the stiff, friable liver and avoid the potential for bleeding from the associated coagulopathy. Outcomes between Childs-Pugh A/B cirrhotic patients undergoing laparoscopic cholecystectomy and those with normal liver function are similar with the exception that operative times are longer and there is a trend towards increased rates of conversion to open cholecystectomy[28] in the former. Laparoscopic cholecystectomy is also feasible in cirrhotics with portal hypertension.[29] When performing laparoscopic cholecystectomy in a cirrhotic patient, the surgeon must be aware of aberrant portosystemic venous collateralization in the liver bed, porta hepatis, and abdominal wall. It is recommended that an energy-sealing device be available to limit blood loss during dissection. Hemostatic agents and argon beam should be readily available to assist with hemostasis. The procedure should be converted to an open procedure for significant bleeding.

CONVERSION TO OPEN

Although laparoscopy is the preferred approach for cholecystectomy, there are many situations that may necessitate conversion to open procedure. The decision and timing of intraoperative conversion to laparotomy depends on the surgeon's experience, comfort with laparoscopic and open techniques, and patient factors (anatomy and pathology). There is no consensus on when conversion is necessary as long as patient safety is the ultimate priority. Contemporary conversion rates are reported to be between 5% to 15%.[30,31]

Reasons to consider conversion include unclear anatomy despite cholangiography, intraoperative complication, failure to progress, and pathology not amenable to laparoscopic or postoperative endoscopic techniques. Independent factors associated with conversion to open cholecystectomy include prior upper abdominal surgery, pericholecystic fluid, acute cholecystitis, and emergent cholecystectomy.[32] Conversion has been described as a "complication" of laparoscopy by some; however, this view is untenable and conversion should be regarded as mature judgment because it can prevent disastrous complications in challenging cases.

OPEN TECHNIQUE

Incision

The traditional incision used for an open cholecystectomy is a right subcostal or Kocher incision. This incision is created 2 centimeters below the right costal margin and extends from the midline to the lateral edge of the right rectus muscle. This incision can be extended superiorly along the midline if further exposure is needed.

Dissection

Retrograde Cholecystectomy

When performing a retrograde cholecystectomy, the critical view of safety must be identified before removing the gallbladder from the liver. Although this is the usual approach during laparoscopic cholecystectomy, it can be more difficult for an unexperienced surgeon without the magnification of laparoscopy and difference in exposure. The same principles must be maintained to prevent inadvertent biliary injury.

The fundus of the gallbladder is grasped with a Kelly or similar clamp. Peritoneum overlying the infundibulum is incised. The incision is extended along the anterior and posterior gallbladder, being careful to stay close to the edge of the gallbladder. Once the cystic duct is identified, a suture ligature is passed around it and used to place tension on the duct for better exposure and to prevent stone migration into the CBD. The CVS has been achieved once all fibroadipose tissue is cleared from the hepatocystic triangle, only two structures are seen clearly entering the gallbladder, and a third of the cystic plate is seen (see Box 36.2). Any stones palpated within the cystic duct are "milked" back into the gallbladder. The cystic artery can be ligated with either clips or sutures then divided. If cholangiography is indicated, it is performed at this time. Ligation and division of the cystic duct occurs next.

To complete the retrograde cholecystectomy, the gallbladder is dissected off the cystic plate using cautery. The dissection plane is kept close to the gallbladder to avoid entering the cystic

plate and deeper liver parenchyma. Brisk bleeding from liver parenchyma lacerations tend to be venous in nature because distal branches of the middle hepatic vein can be located immediately deep to the cystic plate (see Chapter 2). These can usually be treated by holding constant pressure over the area for 5 to 10 minutes. Hemostatic agents may be beneficial in these instances as well. If these techniques fail, deep hemostatic sutures can be placed. Nevertheless, one must be aware of the location of the right portal pedicle and its anterior branch, which can be close to the base of the gallbladder fossa.

Antegrade, or Fundus-Down Cholecystectomy

Antegrade cholecystectomy is an alternate technique for cholecystectomy, but this technique should not be used in the presence of severe inflammation that obstructs visualization of the cystic duct. As with the fundus-down laparoscopic technique, there is still significant risk of biliary injury in these cases without proper visualization of the cystic duct and artery.

A clamp is used to grasp the fundus of the gallbladder; another clamp is used to grasp the peritoneum on the liver edge to provide countertraction. An incision is made in the gallbladder serosa approximately 5 millimeters from the liver edge with cautery. A dissection plane is developed between the superior gallbladder wall and the cystic plate. Again, care is taken to avoid entering the cystic plate and lacerating the liver parenchyma. This plane is continued medially and laterally toward the gallbladder neck. An energy-sealing device can be used on edematous or vascularized peritoneum. Dissection is performed posterior and lateral to fully free the gallbladder from the cystic plate. This best exposes the cystic artery and duct. The cystic artery is ligated and transected as it enters the gallbladder wall. The infundibulum is dissected free to expose the cystic duct. One should not dissect more than 1 centimeter of the cystic duct because this increases risk of CBDI. Once the cystic duct is visualized, it can be ligated with suture or clips and divided. The gallbladder is removed, and the abdomen is closed.

PARTIAL OR SUBTOTAL CHOLECYSTECTOMY

Subtotal cholecystectomy is the recommended technique for treating severely inflamed gallbladders when the CVS cannot be safely obtained[16] (see Chapter 34). Fibrosis and inflammation can cause the cystic duct to shorten and fuse with the CBD; this can lead to the surgeon mistaking the CBD for the cystic duct (Fig. 36.5). In these cases, it is best to err on the side of caution and avoid dissecting in the hepatocystic triangle. Cholecystitis can be managed safely until inflammation has subsided, but CBDIs have significant long-term morbidity. In these cases, a partial or subtotal cholecystectomy, in which a portion of the gallbladder is removed and gallstones are extracted while leaving the posterior wall of the gallbladder in place, is the procedure of choice for source control and surgical management.

This technique can be used either open or laparoscopically, and the technique is similar for both. To perform a safe subtotal cholecystectomy, all dissection should be performed above the "the line of safety," which runs between the sulcus of Rouviere.[33] These landmarks are seen in Fig. 36.6. The gallbladder is drained and opened with cautery at the fundus. Bile, stones, and debris are suctioned or set aside for future extraction in a specimen bag in a laparoscopic approach. This incision is

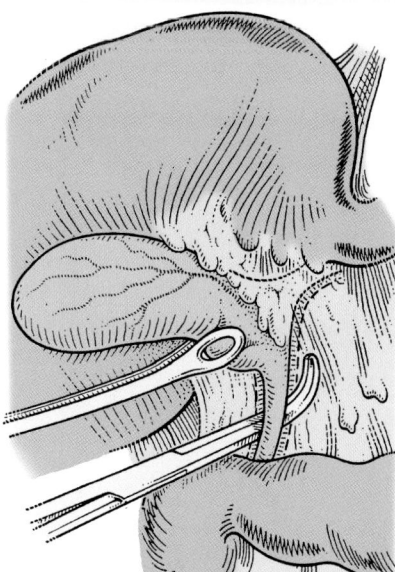

FIGURE 36.5 The common hepatic duct can be mistaken for the cystic duct when the region of the infundibulum cannot be delineated because of fibrosis and inflammation.

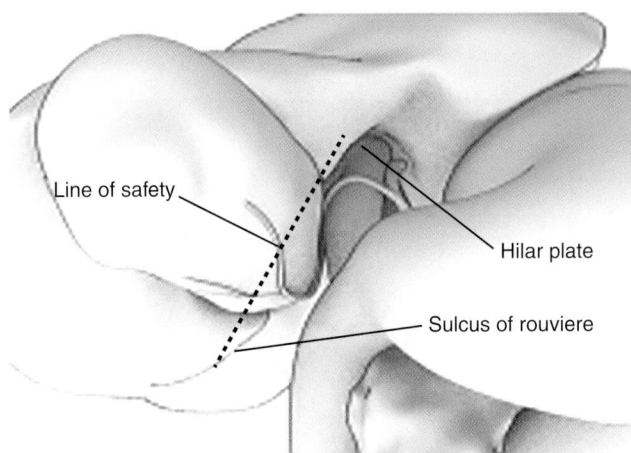

FIGURE 36.6 The limit of proximal dissection for subtotal cholecystectomy is the "line of safety" between the sulcus of Rouviere and hilar plate. The ensures dissection occurs away from the common bile duct in the setting of severe inflammation. (From Purzner RH, Ho KB, Al-Sukhni E, Jayaraman S. Safe laparoscopic subtotal cholecystectomy in the face of severe inflammation in the cystohepatic triangle: A retrospective review and proposed management strategy for the difficult gallbladder. *J Can Chir*. 2019;62:402–411.)

extended to the gallbladder neck without dissecting the cystic duct or artery. The anterior wall of the gallbladder is then completely removed, and the posterior wall is left on the cystic plate (Fig. 36.7). The remnant mucosa is then coagulated with either cautery or argon beam. A drain should be placed near the gallbladder stump to drain potential bile collection.

Subtotal cholecystectomies, both open and laparoscopic, are being performed more frequently, and conversion to open procedure is becoming less common.[34] As one may expect, there is a higher risk of bile leaks and subphrenic collection with subtotal cholecystectomy compared with standard cholecystectomy.

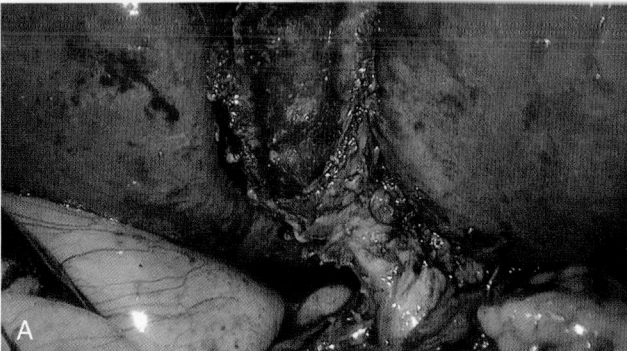

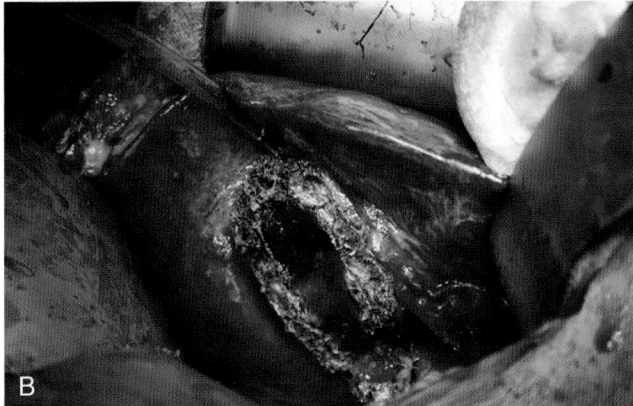

FIGURE 36.7 A–B, Laparoscopic subtotal cholecystectomy and open subtotal cholecystectomy demonstrating the anterior wall excised and a small strip of the posterior wall left attached to the liver. The remnant mucosa can then be either removed or coagulated with cautery or argon laser.

One study found the relative risk of bile leak after subtotal cholecystectomy was as high as 3-fold; these were more common if the gallbladder remnant was left open.[33]

ANATOMIC VARIATIONS

An intimate knowledge of gallbladder and biliary anatomy, as well as common variations, is essential to perform a safe cholecystectomy (see Chapter 2). Variations in gallbladder anatomy such as duplicated, left-sided, bilobed, or congenitally absent gallbladder are rare, and they are typically identified preoperatively. As such, this section will focus on relevant biliary anatomy and variations that can potentially lead to inadvertent injury (see Chapter 42).

Significant variations of the cystic duct and hepatic duct junction exist (Fig. 36.8; see Chapter 2). The common hepatic duct can range in length from 1 to 7.5 centimeters. A large series of magnetic resonance cholangiopancreatographies demonstrated that 40.7% of patients had some variant in biliary tree anatomy. In this study, 5% of subjects had medial cystic duct insertion.[35] Anomalous extrahepatic bile ducts occur in up to 12% of patients, with the most common being an anomalous right sectoral duct that empties into either the common hepatic or cystic duct.[36] Fig. 36.9 demonstrates common anatomic biliary variation of the right sectoral ducts. When these variations occur, they often represent the only biliary drainage for the corresponding segment(s) of the liver. Thus injury or obstruction of these ducts results in liver atrophy or obstructive cholangitis in that segment. It should be noted that true duplication of the

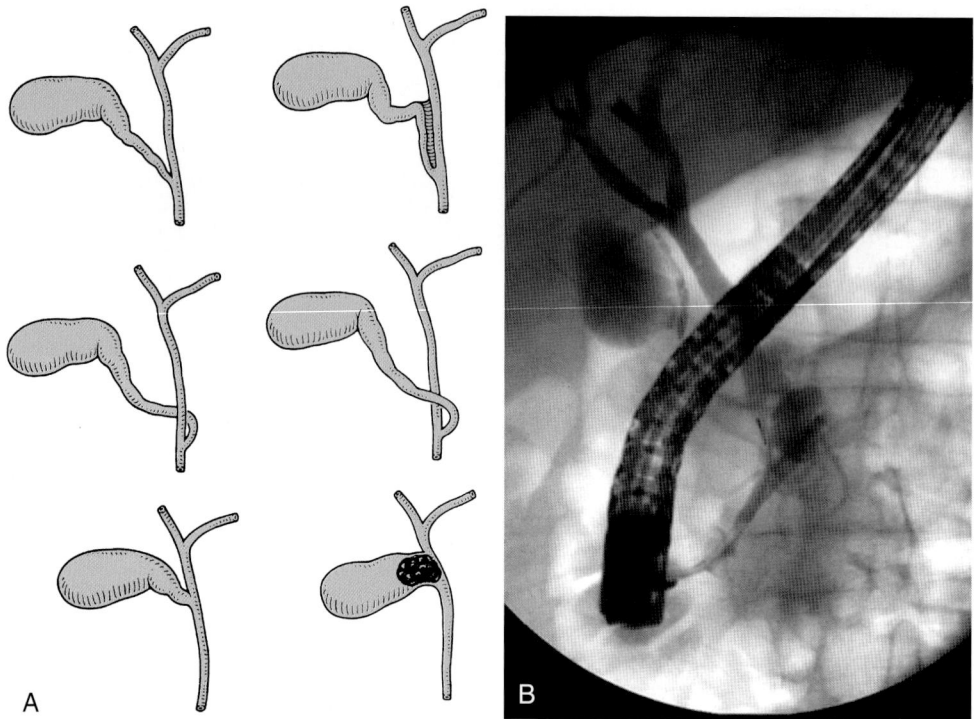

FIGURE 36.8 **A**, Variations in the confluence of the cystic duct and common hepatic duct. **B**, High insertion of the cystic duct demonstrated on endoscopic retrograde cholangiopancreatography.

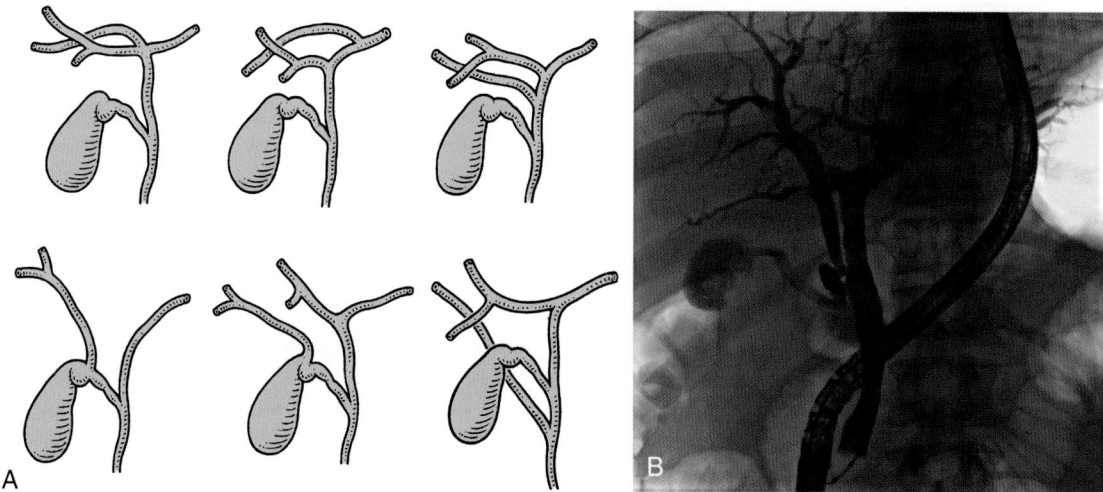

FIGURE 36.9 **A**, Variations in the confluence of the extrahepatic bile ducts and cystic duct. **B**, Cholangiogram demonstrating a cystic duct inserting into the right anterior section bile duct.

cystic duct is exceedingly rare, and cholangiography should be performed if the surgeon believes such an anomaly has been encountered (see Chapter 24).

Arterial anatomic variations are also common and can contribute to morbidity after cholecystectomy (see Chapter 2). Typically, the cystic artery originates from the right hepatic artery (76%) but may also branch off the left, common, or proper hepatic arteries.[37] Arterial injury may accompany a bile duct injury resulting in a combined vasculobiliary injury. The right hepatic artery is involved in 92% of these injuries because of its proximity to the CBD and can significantly add to the difficulty of bile duct repair[38] (see Chapter 42).

POSTOPERATIVE MANAGEMENT

Most patients undergoing elective laparoscopic cholecystectomy are discharged the same day because of the decreased pain profile associated with this minimally invasive technique. A patient admitted with acute cholecystitis is often observed in the hospital overnight postoperatively because of infectious concerns. Elderly patients, comorbid patients, patients requiring significant analgesia postoperatively, and patients with complicated procedures may also benefit from postoperative admission. The patient is allowed a diet shortly after surgery. Oral narcotics for postoperative incisional pain can be prescribed for pain control, but many patients recover with only over-the-counter pain medications, including nonsteroidal antiinflammatories and acetaminophen. Routine follow-up by the surgeon in clinic can occur between 1 and 4 weeks after surgery.

IMMEDIATE POSTOPERATIVE COMPLICATIONS

Biliary Injury

Biliary injury remains the most feared complication of cholecystectomy (see Chapters 28 and 34). It has been shown that bile duct injuries have a 30-day mortality rate of 2% in a large database study.[39] Another prospective cohort of 800 patients with CBDI referred to a single center reported the mean survival after iatrogenic biliary injury was 17.6 years, and patients also had a worse physical quality of life and loss of productivity; at long-term follow-up, 34.9% were receiving disability benefits.[40] Although these injuries are rare, occurring at a rate of 0.08% and 0.25%, the impact on patients is significant.

Intraoperative cholangiography has been proposed to reduce iatrogenic bile duct injury during laparoscopic cholecystectomy[41] (see Chapter 24). Nevertheless, recent retrospective studies show a higher incidence of CBDI when intraoperative cholangiogram is performed (0.25% vs. 0.12%). This is likely because cholangiography is used more frequently during challenging cases.[42] Proper biliary anatomy identification and interpretation of the cholangiography images are required for it to aid in prevention of CBDI. The CVS, as described earlier, remains the current standard technique to reduce the incidence of CBDI during cholecystectomy.

Inflammation of the gallbladder increases the risk of CBDI. As the grade of cholecystitis severity increases, the risk of CBDI rises.[43] The "classic injury" occurs when the CBD is mistaken for the cystic duct and ligated. This is thought to occur when the gallbladder is retracted too aggressively to the right, causing the cystic duct to lie parallel and adjacent to the CBD. Dissection is then continued along the CBD superiorly until an "aberrant" or "duplicated" duct is encountered. If this duct is subsequently divided, a more proximal bile duct injury will occur (Fig. 36.10).

If a CBDI is identified at the time of surgery, the surgeon must assess the extent of the injury, their own experience repairing these injuries, the patient's condition, and the hospital resources. A hepatobiliary surgeon should be called to assess the situation if one is available. When a specialist is not available, the best course of action is to place a drain near the porta hepatis, close the patient, and initiate transfer to a center with hepatobiliary expertise. Proceeding with gallbladder extraction after identifying a biliary injury is not recommended because it risks amplifying the injury[38] (see Chapter 42).

CBDIs are often not discovered during the index procedure. Patients with ongoing abdominal pain, fevers, or ileus should alert the surgeon to a potential complication. The initial diagnostic test should start with abdominal ultrasound followed by computed tomography (CT) of the abdomen if a complication is suspected. If excessive peritoneal fluid is present, percutaneous drainage should be performed. The type of injury should be determined next and this can be done with magnetic resonance cholangiopancreatography (MRCP), percutaneous transhepatic cholangiography, and/or endoscopic retrograde cholangiopancreatography (ERCP). Simple postoperative leaks can be managed with drainage alone or drainage and ERCP placement of

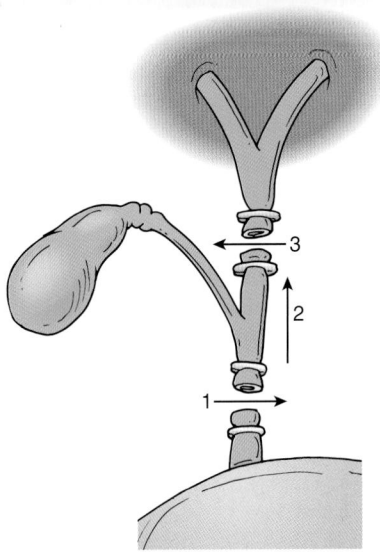

FIGURE 36.10 Pathogenesis of the "classic" injury. *1.* The common bile duct is mistaken as the cystic duct and is clipped and divided. *2.* The dissection is carried up along the left side of the common hepatic duct in the belief that this is the underside of the gallbladder. *3.* The common hepatic duct is transected while the surgeon tries to dissect what they believe is the gallbladder from the liver bed. If the structure is recognized as a bile duct at this point, it is often thought to be a second cystic duct or an accessory duct. While the common hepatic duct is divided, the right hepatic artery is often injured. (From Strasberg SM, Helton WS. An analytical review of vasculobiliary injury in laparoscopic and open cholecystectomy. *HPB (Oxford).* 2011;13:1–14.)

biliary stents.[44] Several centers with advanced gastroenterologists are beginning to manage selected patients with complex injuries with percutaneous-endoscopic rendezvous procedures with promising long-term results.[45] Further details regarding repair of biliary injuries are discussed elsewhere in this textbook (see Chapter 42).

Bleeding

Clinically significant bleeding occurs in 0.1% to 1.9% of laparoscopic cholecystectomies. Bleeding can arise from (1) the liver, (2) an abdominal arterial source, or (3) port sites. Significant bleeding from the liver bed tends to be from the terminal branches of the middle hepatic vein. Bleeding from the gallbladder fossa that appears venous in nature can be controlled laparoscopically with hemostatic agents and applied pressure. Visualization can be improved by lifting the liver and increasing the pressure of pneumoperitoneum. Clips or sutures can be placed in the cystic plate for hemostasis if all landmarks are identified to avoid injury to underlying portal structures. If visualization is lost, pressure should be applied to the area with sponge and grasper while converting to laparotomy. During laparotomy, one should keep pressure on the venous injury because air embolus is possible and can be severe. Acute hemodynamic decline in the postoperative period should raise concern for significant bleeding, which is likely because of a dislodged clip. As with any laparoscopic procedure, bleeding can occur from trocar insertion.

Retained Common Bile Duct Stones

Common bile duct stones are present in approximately 5% to 15% of patients presenting for cholecystectomy.[46–48] Those suspected of having choledocholithiasis should undergo preoperative diagnostic MRCP or ERCP, especially if the surgeon is not comfortable exploring the CBD laparoscopically. Choledocholithiasis is not an indication for laparotomy in the modern era. Laparoscopic bile duct exploration at the time of cholecystectomy has been shown to reduce hospital LOS and overall cost compared with endoscopic treatment followed by cholecystectomy[49] (see Chapter 37).

Retained common duct stones after cholecystectomy are rare. In one single center study, the incidence of postoperative ERCP for suspected retained stones was 1.8%.[50] As with patients with presumed choledocholithiasis, those suspected of having a retained CBD stone should be studied with either MRCP or ERCP depending on facility capabilities. Endoscopic sphincteroplasty with stone extraction is the most widely accepted treatment for this condition in the current era. The details of CBD stone management are discussed in other chapters (see Chapters 37 and 38).

Gallbladder Perforation

Entering the gallbladder during cholecystectomy is a common event, particularly during the learning phase of the procedure. Careful retraction is essential because spillage of bile and stones can result in serious complications. Intraperitoneal spillage of stones can lead to abscess and fistula formation.[51] In patients with incidental gallbladder carcinoma, bile spillage at the time of cholecystectomy resulted in higher rates of carcinomatosis (24% vs. 4%) compared with those without spillage, as well as poorer disease-free survival[52] (see Chapter 49).

DELAYED COMPLICATIONS OF CHOLECYSTECTOMY

Remnant Gallbladder and Cystic Duct Stones

Recurrent stone formation in a remnant gallbladder or cystic duct is rare. Most patients present with pain similar to their precholecystectomy symptoms, and it can occur at any time from 4 months to 25 years after surgery. Remnant gallbladder stones are usually associated with subtotal cholecystectomy. Diagnosis requires a study that delineates the biliary anatomy, such as MRCP or ERCP. Endoscopic ultrasound, intraoperative cholangiogram, and percutaneous transhepatic cholangiogram can also be useful in obtaining a diagnosis of retained stones.[53]

Treatment of cystic duct stones can be managed in a variety of ways. Some stones are amendable to endoscopic retrieval or lithotripsy, whereas others require a surgical intervention to extract the stone and ligate the cystic duct closer to the common duct.[54] Treatment of a remnant gallbladder typically requires resection to prevent further stone formation. Depending on the situation and surgeon skill set, completion cholecystectomy can be performed either open or laparoscopically with low morbidity.[55–57]

Biliary Strictures

Benign strictures of the CBD occur in up to 2.7% of laparoscopic cholecystectomies and 0.5% of open cholecystectomies.[58,59]

These strictures arise from an injury to the bile duct that was unidentified in the immediate postoperative period. Causes include incomplete transection, clipping or ligation, thermal injury, or ischemic devascularization of the bile duct. Commonly, patients with benign biliary strictures present with symptoms consistent with obstructive jaundice (see Chapter 42).

Options for management of biliary strictures are varied. Endoscopic treatment is typically the first approach, with surgery reserved for those who do not respond to endoscopic therapy.[60] Endoscopic stenting has been shown to result in 67% of patients being symptom-free for 28 months, and having a normal ERCP after stenting was predictive of not reforming a stricture.[61] Nevertheless, surgery remains the mainstay of therapy for benign biliary strictures after cholecystectomy. A recent meta-analysis showed that a surgical approach had an 84% long-term patency rate.[62] Further description of the management of benign and malignant biliary strictures will be addressed elsewhere in the book (see Chapters 30 and 31).

Postcholecystecomy Diarrhea

Postcholecystecomy diarrhea is defined as three or more loose stools per day after removal of the gallbladder. It is difficult to assess the prevalence of this disorder. Etiology is likely multifactorial in nature. One factor may be the increased number of bile salts in the colon because of continuous bile flow into the gut, which leads to secretory diarrhea.[63] Recent evidence showed that the gut microbiome of patients with postcholecystectomy diarrhea is altered. Compared with healthy patients, patients with diarrhea after cholecystectomy had significantly higher levels of *Proteobacteria,* which may be pathogenic in this process.[64] Currently, the recommended therapy is the administration of bile-acid binding agents and antidiarrheals; however, these have variable results.[63]

CONCLUSION

Cholecystectomy remains the gold standard for the management of gallbladder disease in the developed world, with the vast majority now performed minimally invasively with excellent results. Most patients now undergo this operation in an ambulatory setting. Attempts at improving outcomes from laparoscopic cholecystectomy will continue to drive the development of novel surgical tools and techniques. Although relatively safe, there is room to reduce the number of CBDIs because these have a significant impact on patient quality of life and overall survival. These gains will be achieved with improved outreach and education regarding the CVS and when to pursue alternative procedures instead of forging ahead with total cholecystectomy. As new technology arises, surgeons must always keep in mind the safety of the patient alongside the development of new techniques.

The references for this chapter can be found online by accessing the accompanying Expert Consult website.

Stones in the bile duct: Clinical features and open surgical approaches and techniques

Bryan Clary and Gabriel T. Schnickel

OVERVIEW

The first successful common bile duct exploration (CBDE) by Thornton in 1889 and the introduction of catheter-based biliary decompression by Courvoisier and Kehr marked the initial efforts in treating choledocholithiasis. Open cholecystectomy and bile duct exploration were performed commonly as the standard treatment for patients with choledocholithiasis for many years with good success and low rates of morbidity and mortality (Table 37A.1). During this era of open operative interventions, the percentage of retained stones was only 1% to 3%, and long-term follow-up revealed that revisional surgery was necessary in about 10% of the patients.[1–4]

In the last several decades, however, there has been a shift away from open cholecystectomy and CBDE with improvements in noninvasive imaging and increasing sophistication of percutaneous and endoscopic interventions (see Chapters 19, 29, 30, and 36C). Beyond the widespread availability of endoscopic retrograde cholangiopancreatography (ERCP), the increased use of laparoscopy and minimally invasive techniques has made open CBDE an infrequently used tool. The significant trend toward laparoscopic surgery including cholecystectomy, intraoperative cholangiogram (IOC), and CBDE over the last several decades has impacted the experience of surgical trainees. This has resulted in limited experience in open biliary surgery, specifically open cholecystectomy and open CBDE. Chief residents complete training with an average of a single CBDE, open or laparoscopic.[5]

Although the majority of cholecystectomies are now performed laparoscopically (see Chapter 35), laparoscopic CBDE (LCBDE; see Chapter 36B) has not been similarly embraced. This is in part because of the wide availability of ERCP but also in part because the technical demands of LCBDE do not lend themselves to routine use by most general surgeons. Surveys of general surgeons practicing in a rural area of the United States demonstrated that the preferred approach to choledocholithiasis was ERCP (75%), followed by laparoscopic (21%) or open (4%) exploration.[6] Analysis of practice patterns in large hospital systems more than a decade later found a similar underutilization of LCBDE with less than 30% of patients undergoing a single-stage laparoscopic cholecystectomy with LCBDE.[7] There is also broad variability in terms of evaluation and treatment of choledocholithiasis across geographic regions. A multicenter trial found that when choledocholithiasis was suspected, laparoscopic cholecystectomy with IOC was the most common initial procedure in seven institutions followed by ERCP in four and magnetic resonance cholangiopancreatography (MRCP) in one.[8]

Despite these considerations, there remain indications for open CBDE. This chapter presents a review of the clinical features of choledocholithiasis with an emphasis on the technical aspects of open CBDE.

ORIGIN OF CHOLEDOCHOLITHIASIS

CBD stones are broadly classified by their location of origin (see Chapter 32). Secondary stones, those that originate in the gallbladder and migrate into the bile duct, are the most common. Chemically, these stones tend to be cholesterol or black-pigment stones. Primary CBD stones, in contrast, originate within the CBD and are predominantly brown-pigment (calcium bilirubin) stones. Primary stones occur in patients with congenital absence of the gallbladder and in those whose CBD had been cleared at the time of prior cholecystectomy. CBD stones that occur in the immediate postcholecystectomy period should be assumed to be secondary stones that are the result of an incompletely cleared CBD. Secondary stones are the most commonly observed CBD stones, particularly in Europe and North America. Primary stones are encountered more commonly in Asia and are associated with a high incidence of intrahepatic bile duct stones seen in Southeast Asian countries such as Taiwan, Hong Kong, and Singapore[9] (see Chapter 39). The relative prevalence of intrahepatic bile duct stones in all gallstone cases in Taiwan is extremely high (>50%) and coexisting intrahepatic and extrahepatic bile duct stones are found in approximately 70% of these patients.

Typical presentations for inflammatory, infective, and congenital choledocholithiasis include biliary colic, jaundice, cholangitis (see Chapter 43), and pancreatitis (see Chapter 55). Of these, pain from biliary colic tends to be the most common symptomatic manifestation of CBD stones. In many cases, the intermittent obstruction and passage of CBD stones will result in fluctuating elevation of bilirubin and hepatocellular enzymes. If untreated for a long period of time, these recurrent episodes may lead to secondary biliary cirrhosis. In contrast to the intermittent obstruction that results in biliary colic, persistent CBD obstruction can result in cholangitis, which may display the Charcot's classic triad (fever/rigors, jaundice, and right upper quadrant pain) or the Reynold's pentad (Charcot's triad plus hypotension and altered mental status) (see Chapter 43). Pancreatitis is the second most frequent symptomatic presentation of CBD stones (see Chapter 55), and depending on the timing of cholangiography, CBD stones can be identified in up to 50% of these patients. Patients who have symptomatic bile duct stones are at risk of experiencing further symptoms or complications if left untreated. More than one-half of patients who had retained bile duct stones experienced recurrent symptoms during a follow-up period of 6 months to 13 years,[10] and 25% developed serious complications.[11] The potential for serious sequelae related to CBD stones makes the identification and

TABLE 37A.1 Mortality Rates of Biliary Reoperation for Retained or Recurrent Bile Duct Stones

REFERENCE	NUMBER OF OPERATIONS	NUMBER OF DEATHS (%)
Saharia et al. (1977)[76]	30	0
Jones (1978)[96]	22	0
McSherry & Glenn (1980)[18]	341	7 (2%)
Allen et al. (1981)[78]	47	1 (2%)
De Almeida et al. (1982)	22	1 (5%)
DenBesten & Berci (1986)[13]	86	2 (2.3%)
Girard (2000)	88	0
TOTAL	920	15 (1.6%)

definitive treatment of patients with CBD stones of great importance.

The potential long-term sequelae of untreated clinically significant stones have led some to advocate for routine intra-operative cholangiography at the time of cholecystectomy so that clearance of the duct at the time of surgery can be ensured. The clinical significance and natural history of asymptomatic CBD stones, however, is unpredictable, as many small stones will pass spontaneously without incident. During the era of open cholecystectomy, the practice of routine cholangiography was common, and studies from this period demonstrated an incidence of choledocholithiasis approaching 10% to 15% in patients without any clinically evident common duct involvement.[12–18] Proponents of a more selective approach to cholangiography, however, note that the percentage of clinically significant stones is far lower than the 10% to 15% of patients who will have cholangiographic findings of CBD stones when routine cholangiography is used.

The use of selective intraoperative cholangiography in laparoscopic cholecystectomy series demonstrates similar findings.[19] Collins and colleagues identified filling defects consistent with stones in 4.6% of patients on IOC.[20] In these patients, access was maintained for the performance of postoperative cholangiograms. At 48 hours, 26% of patients had a normal cholangiogram, and an additional 26% had evidence for passage of the stones by 6 weeks. Only 22 patients (2.2%) had persistent CBD stones at 6 weeks after laparoscopic cholecystectomy and underwent ERCP for retrieval.[20]

PREOPERATIVE DIAGNOSIS

In the absence of clinical signs such as cholangitis or pancreatitis, preoperative identification of choledocholithiasis typically relies on serum liver function tests (LFTs) and imaging studies. The utility of LFTs in predicting the presence of CBD stones has been demonstrated by a number of groups.[21,22] Serum bilirubin and alkaline phosphatase are typically the most commonly used laboratory values; however, a raised γ-glutamyltransferase (GGT) level has been suggested to be the most sensitive and specific laboratory indicator of CBD stones. A GGT value greater than 90 U/L has been proposed to indicate a high risk of choledocholithiasis, with sensitivity and specificity of 86% and 75%, respectively.[21]

Transabdominal ultrasound (TUS) alone has a low sensitivity (25%–60%) for detection of CBD stones and is highly operator dependent.[23,24] When used in conjunction, clinical examination, laboratory studies, and ultrasonography (typically the first-line imaging modality) (see Chapter 15) are sensitive in 96% to 98% and specific in 40% to 75% for identification of patients with choledocholithiasis.[25–28] Liu and colleagues stratified precholecystectomy patients into four groups of descending risk of choledocholithiasis based on guidelines incorporating clinical evaluation, serum chemistry analysis, and TUS. The occurrence of choledocholithiasis in these groups (group 1, extremely high risk; group 2, high risk; group 3, moderate risk; group 4, low risk) was 92.6%, 32.4%, 3.8%, and 0.9%, respectively. Triaging patients in this manner resulted in preoperative identification of choledocholithiasis by ERCP in 92.3% of the patients who were subsequently referred for endoscopic clearance.[28] Similarly, the American Society of Gastrointestinal Endoscopy (ASGE) identified several predictors of choledocholithiasis in their guidelines for the use of endoscopy in the evaluation of CBD stones.[29] CBD stones seen on TUS or cross-sectional imaging, clinical evidence of ascending cholangitis, and bilirubin greater than 4 mg/dL were identified as high-risk criteria for choledocholithiasis and patients should move directly to ERCP. They suggest that any other risk factors, such as those mentioned previously, should prompt additional investigation with MRCP, endoscopic ultrasonography (EUS), or IOC at the time of cholecystectomy. ERCP requires cannulation of the papilla and is associated with a significant risk of adverse events in up to 15% of patients and severe adverse events including death or prolonged hospital stay in approximately 2%. For this reason, ERCP should be reserved for individuals in the high-risk category or with CBD stones confirmed by MRCP or EUS. When taken in sum, these data suggest that the ERCP is best reserved as a therapeutic measure for patients with a high probability of CBD stones, rather than as an initial diagnostic test.

Like TUS, standard computed tomography (CT) scanning has a low sensitivity for the detection of bile duct stones and is most useful in documenting biliary dilation or excluding mass lesions as a cause of biliary obstruction (see Chapter 18). Newer techniques of CT cholangiography use contrast agents excreted in the biliary tree, which when combined with high-resolution helical scans and three-dimensional reconstructions can give accurate and detailed information about the biliary tree.[30,31] The sensitivity of this technique can be as high as 97%, and the specificity is 75% to 96%.[30–38] Although these data suggest accuracy comparable to MRCP (see Chapter 19), helical CT cholangiography is limited by several issues: (1) possible allergic reactions to the contrast agents (as high as 15% in one series using intravenous iotroxate),[33] (2) suboptimal ductal contrast opacification in the presence of significant jaundice,[36,37] and (3) limited visualization of intrahepatic duct branches.[33,39]

MRCP has become the gold standard for noninvasive biliary imaging since its introduction in 1991 and has been recommended by some as the preoperative noninvasive modality of choice for the detection of CBD stones[40–44] (see Chapter 17). MRCP provides precise anatomic detail of the biliary tract and has a sensitivity of 81% to 100% and a specificity of 92% to 100% in detecting choledocholithiasis.[41,45] The accuracy of MRCP in diagnosing CBD stones is comparable with that of ERCP (see Chapters 19 and 20) and IOC (see Chapter 23).[41,46]

As a diagnostic test, MRCP has largely replaced ERCP, once considered the gold standard of preoperative bile duct imaging, because the nonselective use of ERCP in all patients with suspected choledocholithiasis detects CBD stones in less than 50%.[47,48] Although both MRCP and ERCP are effective at detecting choledocholithiasis, a randomized trial looking at an MRCP first versus ERCP first approach to patients with suspected CBD stone disease found equivalent patient outcomes. Importantly, those in the MRCP arm were 50% less likely to have a subsequent ERCP.[49]

Indiscriminate use of ERCP exposes over half of patients to unnecessary procedure-related morbidity and mortality[50]; thus ERCP is better used as therapeutic intervention rather than a diagnostic one. Although MRCP is currently the most accurate noninvasive imaging modality for choledocholithiasis, it may miss stones smaller than 5 mm in diameter and can underestimate the number of stones detected.[46] Furthermore, it is expensive when compared with TUS or CT, not readily available at smaller facilities, and may not be technically feasible in obese patients or those with significant claustrophobia.

EUS has also emerged as an alternative to ERCP and MRCP for preoperative assessment of bile duct stones and was initially described in 1990[51,52] (see Chapter 16). EUS and MRCP are both highly accurate in detecting choledocholithiasis, with EUS having a slight edge because of its increased sensitivity at detecting small stones (97% vs. 90%).[53] EUS may be particularly useful in patients in which MRCP may be limited such as patients with obesity, claustrophobia, metal clips, cardiac pacemaker, or inability for breath holding. EUS also provides the advantage of immediate transition to therapeutic ERCP if diagnostic findings warrant. A systematic Cochrane review of the literature, including 18 studies involving 2532 participants, found both EUS and MRCP to be highly accurate at diagnosing CBD stones and found no difference in sensitivity or specificity between the two modalities.[54] Randomized controlled trials (RCTs) have also demonstrated that EUS-guided ERCP can avoid unnecessary ERCP in up to two-thirds of patients when compared with using ERCP alone for diagnosis of choledocholithiasis.[55] Furthermore, selective use of ERCP based on EUS findings resulted in reduced risk of overall complications and post-ERCP pancreatitis (PEP).

TIMING AND SEQUENCE OF INTERVENTIONS

Suspected Choledocholithiasis Before Cholecystectomy

In patients with suspected choledocholithiasis, selecting and sequencing the laparoscopic, open, and endoscopic therapeutic modalities can be challenging. Before the popularization of therapeutic laparoscopy, precholecystectomy endoscopic clearance of the CBD was uncommon. Several studies did not reveal any morbidity or mortality advantage with preoperative endoscopic sphincterotomy (ES)[56–58] and one actually showed an increased rate of morbidity in patients who underwent preoperative ERCP, followed by open cholecystectomy, compared with the group that was treated with single-stage open cholecystectomy and CBDE.[58] A systematic review of the literature, including eight trials with 737 participants, comparing open CBDE versus ERCP for clearance of CBD stones found no significant difference in morbidity or mortality. However, open CBDE was more effective at clearing CBD stones than ERCP.[59]

The expansion of therapeutic laparoscopy saw a rise in the popularity of preoperative ERCP CBD clearance for patients with suspected choledocholithiasis, in part because laparoscopic CBDE is more technically challenging than laparoscopic cholecystectomy alone (see Chapters 36B and 36C). For surgeons who are comfortable with LCBDE, the data support single-stage laparoscopic management (laparoscopic cholecystectomy and IOC with CBDE in those with CBD stones) over preoperative ERCP, followed by laparoscopic cholecystectomy. Several prospective RCTs compared these two treatment strategies (Cuschieri et al., 1999; Rogers et al., 2010; Sgourakis et al., 2005) and found that the two groups had equivalent success rates of duct clearance and patient morbidity, but a significantly shorter hospital stay was reported with the single-stage laparoscopic treatment.[22,60,61] Single-stage laparoscopic cholecystectomy with LC + CBDE results in fewer procedures, the shortest length of stay and most cost-effective treatment for patients with CBD stones. Despite these findings it continues to be underutilized in measures of current practice patterns with less than one-third of patients received single-stage LC + LCCBDE versus laparoscopic cholecystectomy with preoperative or postoperative ERCP.[7]

When LCBDE is not part of the surgeon's armamentarium, the decision to perform a precholecystectomy ERCP should be weighed carefully because it is not without complications. Although most post-ERCP complications are mild to moderate in severity,[62] the risk of severe complications, such as pancreatitis, bleeding, infection, and perforation, need to be weighed against the likelihood that ERCP will find clinically relevant CBD stones. ERCP has an overall complication rate of 10% and a mortality rate less than 0.5%.[63–66] In a systematic review of 108 RCTs with 13,296 participants the incidence of PEP was 9.7% and up to 14.7% in the high-risk population. Most cases are mild to moderate and the mortality rate associated with PEP was 0.7%. Despite advances in equipment and techniques the rate of PEP has not decreased in the modern experience with a rate of 10% in studies since 2000.[67] Additionally, the increased financial cost of preoperative ERCP should be considered when evaluating its role in the treatment of suspected stones.

Accurately predicting which patients will have clinically relevant choledocholithiasis can be challenging. Several studies have shown that a "negative" ERCP is performed in 40% to 70% of patients because most of these biochemical and radiographic abnormalities were the result of transient biliary obstruction secondary to stones that passed preprocedurally into the duodenum.[58,63,65,66,68] As mentioned earlier in this chapter, the 2019 ASGE guidelines suggest immediate ERCP for patients in the high-risk category: (1) CBD stone on ultrasound or cross-sectional imaging, (2) total bilirubin >4 mg/dL and dilated CBD, and (3) ascending cholangitis. EUS or MRCP are recommended for intermediate-risk patients, whereas low-risk patients may proceed to cholecystectomy. Treatment strategies for patients stratified to the low- and high-likelihood groups are generally agreed on. Patients who are in the low risk for choledocholithiasis group should go directly to laparoscopic cholecystectomy (with or without IOC) because CBD clearance is unlikely to be necessary.

For patients in the high-risk group, particularly those needing biliary decompression for treatment of acute cholangitis and in patients with severe gallstone pancreatitis and evidence of persistent choledocholithiasis, precholecystectomy ERCP is warranted. Patients with multiple medical comorbidities, limited life expectancy, or other issues that would make them poor surgical candidates, ERCP with ES and biliary decompression can sometimes be used as the definitive management without cholecystectomy[60,69] (see Chapter 29). This strategy is not ideal for patients who are acceptable surgical candidates, however, because there is a risk of recurrent biliary symptoms if cholecystectomy is not performed. In a prospective randomized trial published in 1995 by Hammarström and colleagues, an expectant policy after ES was compared with open cholecystectomy combined with CBDE. It was reported that 20% of the patients after ES alone needed cholecystectomy during follow-up.[2] A prospective randomized trial of high-risk patients performed by Targarona and colleagues (1996) comparing ES and subsequent open cholecystectomy to ES alone resulted in similar findings.[4] They noted patients who underwent elective open cholecystectomy had significantly fewer recurrent biliary symptoms (6% vs. 21%) and needed fewer readmissions (4% vs. 23%) than patients who did not undergo surgery after ES.

In contrast to the general consensus of how to treat high- and low-likelihood patients, the question of how to treat intermediate-risk patients has been the subject of some debate. A recent RCT examined an up-front cholecystectomy and IOC strategy against preoperative ERCP and subsequent cholecystectomy for intermediate-risk patients.[70] Fifty patients were randomized to each group, and differences in length of stay, number of subsequent CBD interventions, morbidity, mortality, and quality of life were analyzed. No significant difference was found in morbidity or quality of life; however, patients who underwent cholecystectomy as the initial procedure had a significantly shorter length of stay (median, 5 days vs. 8 days; $P < .001$) and fewer common duct investigations. A systematic review of seven trials including 746 participants compared single-stage LC + LCBDE versus two-stage preoperative ERCP + LC or LC + postoperative ERCP.[71] The authors found no difference in morbidity or mortality but a lower rate of retained stones in the single-stage group. Together a single-stage LC + CBDE provides the best clearance of the bile duct, the shortest length of stay, and is more cost-effective with equivalent morbidity and mortality.

Common Bile Duct Exploration at Time of Open Cholecystectomy

Therapeutic laparoscopy has become routine in much of the world, and as laparoscopic experience has grown, surgeons have become increasingly more comfortable using LCBDE when choledocholithiasis is noted intraoperatively. In areas of the developing world, however, where access to endoscopic, radiologic, and laparoscopic expertise is limited, open cholecystectomy and bile duct exploration remains a mainstay of treatment. Even in settings where laparoscopy and endoscopy are readily available, however, there will still be some patients in whom an open approach to CBDE may be required (see Chapters 36B and 36C). Principal among these include patients with (1) large or impacted CBD stones and who have failed previous endoscopic interventions; (2) a need for biliary enteric drainage; (3) anatomic considerations that preclude endoscopic treatment, such as prior gastric resection, gastric bypass or duodenal diverticula; and (4) complex situations requiring an open approach for cholecystectomy, including those with Mirizzi syndrome, biliary-enteric fistula, severe cholecystitis, or a high index of suspicion for cancer.

Postcholecystectomy Choledocholithiasis (See Chapter 38)

Incidence

The majority of initial operations for gallstone disease, with or without demonstrated choledocholithiasis, are curative, but some patients will develop sequelae of choledocholithiasis postcholecystectomy. Approximately 1% to 2% of all patients who undergo cholecystectomy have stones left in the CBD that require further intervention.[72] Retained calculi occur rarely after open cholecystectomy without CBDE (Bergdahl & Holmlund, 1976), whereas the incidence in those who undergo open cholecystectomy with concomitant CBDE is slightly higher but still reported to be less than 5%.[73–75] Retained CBD stones occur with higher frequency after positive CBDE than after a negative one. The rate of recurrence increases to approximately 20% after a second operation on the biliary tract for choledocholithiasis,[76,77] and this rate increases after subsequent reoperation.[78]

Treatment

Endoscopic and percutaneous methods remain the preferred modalities when managing recurrent or retained CBD stones (see Chapters 30 and 36C). The open surgical approach is reserved for patients who have failed nonoperative treatments. Decision making is further influenced by clinical presentation, condition of the patient, institutional expertise, and presence or absence of a T-tube.

RETAINED STONES IN THE PRESENCE OF A T-TUBE. Along with the rise in popularity of laparoscopic biliary surgery decreasing use of T-tube biliary drainage has also occurred. When LCBDE is performed, primary closure has been shown to be safe, and routine use of postexploration T-tubes is no longer common[79–81] (see Chapters 31 and 42). If a T-tube is present, it provides nonsurgical options for accessing the biliary tree postoperatively. In the presence of a T-tube, retained CBD stones in the immediate postoperative period can be managed with observation, mechanical extraction, or ES.

In the initial weeks after CBDE, 10% to 25% of retained stones found on postoperative cholangiography will pass spontaneously into the duodenum, and as such interventions are not undertaken, assuming there is no evidence of obstruction or cholangitis. If calculi persist after 4 to 6 weeks, treatment options include radiologic approach through the T-tube tract (see Chapter 30) or ERCP (see Chapter 29). Because of its high success rate and low morbidity and mortality, nonoperative mechanical extraction through the T-tube tract is an attractive treatment choice. A success rate of 95% has been reported with a morbidity rate of only 4%,[82] Burhenne reported no deaths in a series of 661 consecutive patients.[83] When complications do occur, they can be treated medically in most instances, and only 0.2% of cases have required surgery.[82]

ES also has been shown to be effective in the management of retained stones in the early postoperative period after exploration of the CBD with a T-tube still in place.[2,84] Although ES has the considerable advantage that it can be carried out as soon as retained stones are discovered, treatment may be unnecessary in some patients because stones may pass spontaneously. Some authors have suggested that mechanical stone extraction through the T-tube tract is superior to ES because of its high success rate and lower morbidity profile, although modern endoscopic equipment may mitigate some of the post-ERCP hemorrhagic complications seen in earlier series.[85,86] Regardless, the safety and efficacy of percutaneous intervention through the T-tube makes it an ideal choice for initial postoperative interventions, and ES is best used in the early postoperative period before a T-tube tract is well formed, if the patient is clinically unstable, the T-tube is inappropriate in size and position, or mechanical extraction through the T-tube has failed. If these techniques fail, operative management can be undertaken with the expectation of a high success rate and acceptable morbidity and mortality.[16,87]

RETAINED OR RECURRENT STONES IN THE ABSENCE OF A T-TUBE.
ES is the procedure of choice and should be attempted first in patients without a T-tube in place[87,88] (see Chapters 29 and 36C). Most reports of ES indicate a success rate in achieving overall clearance of stones from the CBD of more than 85%.[63,71,89] Although early complication rates for ES range from 5% to 15%, emergency surgery is uncommonly required and most complications can be managed conservatively. Hemorrhage, pancreatitis, cholangitis, and perforation are the most frequent complications, and mortality usually is reported at 0.5% to 2%.[85,88] Long-term complication rates, mainly from stenosis or new stones or both, are low (<10%), and most complications can be managed endoscopically.[2,63,88,89]

Although initial ES has a success rate of 80% to 90% stents may be placed when the duct cannot be completely cleared of stones for biliary drainage and subsequent attempts at clearance. The success rate of subsequent attempts varies widely in the literature from 44% to 96% and success depends on size, shape, and number of residual stones. The 2019 ASGE guidelines recommend ES with large balloon dilation in patients with difficult or large CBD stones. A meta-analysis of nine RCTs found ES + large balloon dilation more effective at stone clearance than ES alone (odds ratio [OR] 2.8). Lithotripsy, either mechanical or cholangioscopy assisted, is an effective technique to address difficult or refractory stone disease. Success rates also vary widely in the literature and frequently require multiple attempts with a complication rate up to 25%. The most common complication being cholangitis.[53] Additionally, percutaneous transhepatic rendezvous techniques can sometimes aid in duct clearance, particularly if there is difficulty cannulating the ampulla. Often, however, failures of endoscopic management will be the result of large impacted stones or anatomic issues that are not ameliorated by a percutaneous approach. Definitive stenting with metal stents in uncleared ducts carries a high rate of morbidity and mortality and should be approached with caution. In such settings, operative management is the most reasonable alternative.[87] Reoperation for retained stones can be performed safely, with operative mortality less than 2%.[16] Miller and colleagues reported 237 patients with CBD stones treated by CBDE or ES.[90] Success was higher and mortality was lower for the operatively managed group. The complication rate was similar, but the complications tended to be more serious and more apt to require surgery in the ES group.[90] A systematic review performed by Dasari and colleagues found that duct clearance in patients undergoing open bile duct exploration was superior to ES, but it should be noted that most series that compare open cholecystectomy/CBDE to ES are from the era of open surgery, which also corresponds to the early days of ERCP and ES.[71] Therefore caution should be used in extrapolating these data to the modern endoscopic

experience. Nevertheless, these findings reinforce that surgery can be a valuable, effective, and safe tool in the treatment of recurrent/retained CBD stones, even if confined to the subset of patients who fail ES.

In patients with anatomy that is unfavorable for conventional ERCP and ES such as those with history of gastric resection or gastric bypass, laparoscopic-assisted ERCP provides an alternative approach for CBD clearance. Laparoscopic-assisted ERCP utilizes a laparoscopic approach to the remnant stomach, which is accessed via trocar for introduction of the duodenoscope for conventional ERCP. A multicenter study of 579 patients looking at laparoscopic-assisted ERCP in patients with previous Roux-en-Y gastric bypass found a procedure success rate of 98% with an adverse event rate of 18%.[91] Adverse events were related to laparoscopy in 10% and ERCP in 7% and both in 1%. The gastrostomy can be closed surgically at the end of the procedure or a G-tube left in place for subsequent access if indicated. Together this is a viable alternative for certain patients, although it carries a higher complication profile than conventional ERCP + ES alone.

When reoperation is required for retained CBD stones, the optimal procedure is complete removal of all stones via choledocholithotomy, choledochoscopy, placement of a T-tube (in many cases), and completion cholangiography. This procedure is adequate for most patients, and the overall failure rate has been reported as low as 3%.[16] Others, however, have reported significantly higher failure rates,[76,78] which has prompted some authors to recommend biliary-enteric drainage in all patients with previous choledocholithotomy.[78,92] Tompkins and Pitt (1982) and Cameron (1989) emphasized, however, that concomitant biliary drainage should not be regarded as mandatory procedure in all patients with retained or recurrent stones.[87,93] In general, biliary-enteric drainage at reoperation is appropriate in the following scenarios: (1) stricture or stenosis of the distal bile duct or sphincter of Oddi, (2) marked dilation of the duct of 2 cm or more, (3) multiple or primary bile duct stones, (4) inability to remove all stones from the duct, and (5) a third operation.

Transduodenal sphincteroplasty, choledochoduodenostomy, and choledochojejunostomy are effective methods of biliary enteric drainage[94–96] (see Chapter 31). With the wide availability of ERCP, operative sphincteroplasty is rarely required because ES is sufficient in most cases. In the presence of a long distal CBD stricture, ES is not an appropriate choice because it does not address the primary obstructive issue. For ducts smaller than 1 to 1.5 cm in diameter, sphincteroplasty is the preferred operative approach as this avoids possible anastomotic stricture formation, but it does carry a greater risk of postoperative pancreatitis. Occasionally, recurrent or primary stones will be seen in patients with dilated ducts and a widely patent sphincter after sphincteroplasty or sphincterotomy. In such cases, choledochoduodenostomy or Roux-en-Y choledochojejunostomy is necessary. Side-to-side or end-to-side choledochoduodenostomy and end-to-side Roux-en-Y choledochojejunostomy are excellent drainage options for CBDs larger than 1.5 cm and offer better decompression of an extremely large duct. CDD can be performed end to side or side to side depending on the situation. Although side to side has been reported to have a higher rate of sump syndrome more recent reviews have not found this to be the case.[97] In the context of previous biliary pancreatitis, patients who present for reoperation with multiple stones and an incompletely cleared proximal biliary system may be better served with an end-to-side choledochoduodenostomy as opposed to a side-to-side technique because it minimizes the chance of stones dropping distally and causing recurrent pancreatitis. Sump syndrome, the development of cholangitis, hepatic abscess, or pancreatitis caused by stones, sludge, or debris or food lodged in the CBD obstructing normal biliary drainage, is an uncommonly observed complication of choledochoduodenostomy and should be managed initially by endoscopic modalities. If ERCP fails to improve symptoms, the choledochoduodenostomy can be converted to a Roux-en-Y choledochojejunostomy. Laparoscopic or open approaches to choledochoduodenostomy are options with a low complication rate that allow easier subsequent endoscopic access to the biliary tree and more physiologic biliary drainage and do not require an entero-enteric anastomosis.[98]

Clinical Experience With Reoperation

Girard reviewed all patients who underwent reoperation for retained or recurrent choledocholithiasis at the Maisonneuve-Rosemont Hospital between 1969 and 1990. Eighty-five patients with preoperatively confirmed choledocholithiasis underwent a total of 88 operations. Eighty-five of these operations were second procedures, and three patients required a third operation. Three types of bile duct reoperation were performed: choledocholithotomy with T-tube drainage (64 patients), choledocholithotomy with side-to-side choledochoduodenostomy (15 patients), and choledocholithotomy with transduodenal sphincteroplasty (6 patients). Choledocholithotomy with T-tube drainage in one patient and choledocholithotomy with side-to-side choledochoduodenostomy in two patients were performed at a third operation. The average hospital stay was 9.3 days. There were no deaths in the series despite the fact that 43 of 85 patients were older than 60 years and 44 patients had associated risk factors. Six minor complications were observed, none of which necessitated urgent surgery. Two patients (3%) of the 64 who had choledocholithotomy with T-tube drainage developed recurrent bile duct stones 4 and 5 years after a second operation, and side-to-side choledochoduodenostomy was performed.[99]

To summarize, ES has become the first-line therapy for retained or recurrent bile duct stones, but surgery can be performed safely with low mortality and morbidity when required. Surgery remains a critical component of the armamentarium that can be used to treat recurrent bile duct stones. As with most things in modern medicine, a multidisciplinary approach to recurrent CBD stones is important to properly select and sequence the numerous options now available. Gastroenterologists, radiologists, and surgeons should work together closely to assess the most appropriate intervention for an individual patient. In making the choice between open surgery, laparoscopic surgery, percutaneous therapies, and ES, the surgeon must consider not only the published data but institutional expertise and experience. In a patient with a retained stone and a T-tube in place, percutaneous extraction through the T-tube tract or ES should be attempted first. In the absence of a T-tube, ES should be attempted first. If unsuccessful or contraindicated, operative management is a reasonable alternative. Surgical intervention has a high success rate and acceptable rates of mortality and morbidity. Before operation, the surgeon must make an accurate diagnosis of retained stones by using a combination of MRCP, ERCP, and EUS. These findings should be confirmed via intraoperative cholangiography and complete clearance of

the biliary tree documented with completion cholangiography and choledochoscopy. Not all patients require biliary-enteric drainage, but certain patients, particularly those with multiple or incompletely cleared calculi, large ducts (>2 cm), and distal CBD strictures will benefit from drainage procedure.

SURGICAL TECHNIQUES FOR EXPLORATION OF THE COMMON BILE DUCT

The principal techniques for open exploration of the CBD will be detailed in this section. Broadly, the goals of CBDE include complete clearance of calculi from the biliary system and establishment of free flow of bile into the gut. The preferred approach to CBDE is typically through a supraduodenal choledochotomy, with the transduodenal/transampullary route reserved for patients with impacted stones that cannot be removed readily from above. Stones impacted at the ampulla can be broken down and removed through a supraduodenal approach; however, a transduodenal sphincteroplasty is generally less traumatic.

Clearance of the biliary tree should be confirmed by performing postexploratory choledochoscopy and cholangiography. The value of choledochoscopy has been confirmed by many authors.[74,75,100] Postexploratory cholangiography should also be performed before closure of the abdomen, not only because it can locate missed stones, but also because it may reveal unsuspected disruption of the biliary ductal system. If the cholangiography technique is meticulous, issues with false positives from air bubbles and poor opacification of the entire system can be largely eliminated to provide consistent and reliable cholangiograms.

The selective use of biliary-enteric drainage procedures is another method to decrease the incidence of subsequently symptomatic retained stones. Although we do not recommend routine biliary-enteric decompression at initial operation, it should be considered carefully in patients with multiple stones, large stones, dilated duct, distal bile duct stricture, and in selected elderly patients. If these conditions pertain to an elderly or poor-risk patient, choledochoduodenostomy may obviate reexploration. Other indications include (1) the presence of irretrievable intrahepatic stones, (2) proven ampullary stenosis, or (3) an impacted ampullary stone.

Supraduodenal Choledochotomy and Exploration of the Common Bile Duct

Exposure

The liver is retracted superiorly with a broad-bladed, slightly curved retractor, such as a Hartmann ("sweetheart") retractor. This retractor should be deep enough to displace the liver but not so curved as to traumatize it. A pack should be put over the hepatic flexure of the colon down to the hepatorenal pouch and the medial part of the duodenum. This pack is retracted by a similar, broad-bladed retractor to prevent the colon or duodenum from obscuring vision (Fig. 37A.1). The lesser omentum and stomach are retracted to the left after placement of another pack. The gallbladder is usually removed before exploration of the CBD and the cystic duct ligated with a suture that can be left long and used for retraction if necessary. Palpation of the CBD and handling of its lower part during exploration and subsequent choledochoscopy is best facilitated by mobilizing the duodenum and head of pancreas with the performance of a Kocher maneuver (Fig. 37A.2).

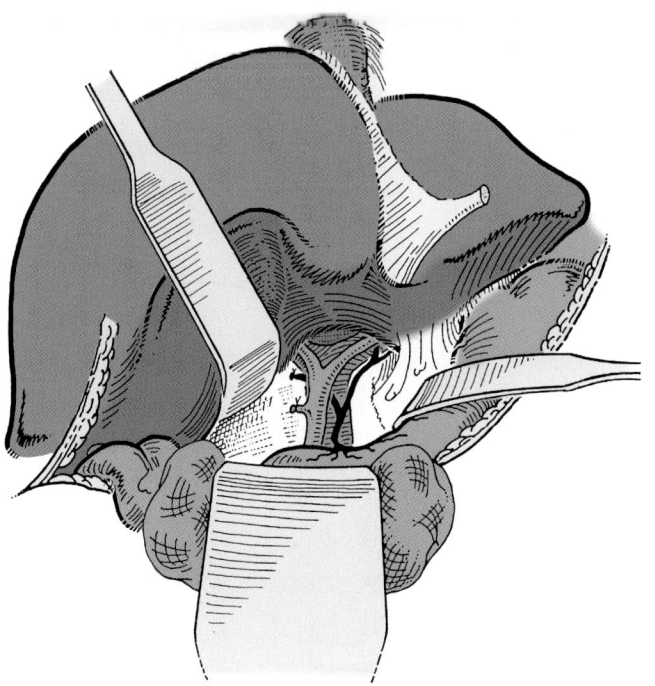

FIGURE 37A.1 Exposure of the common bile duct by packs and retractors.

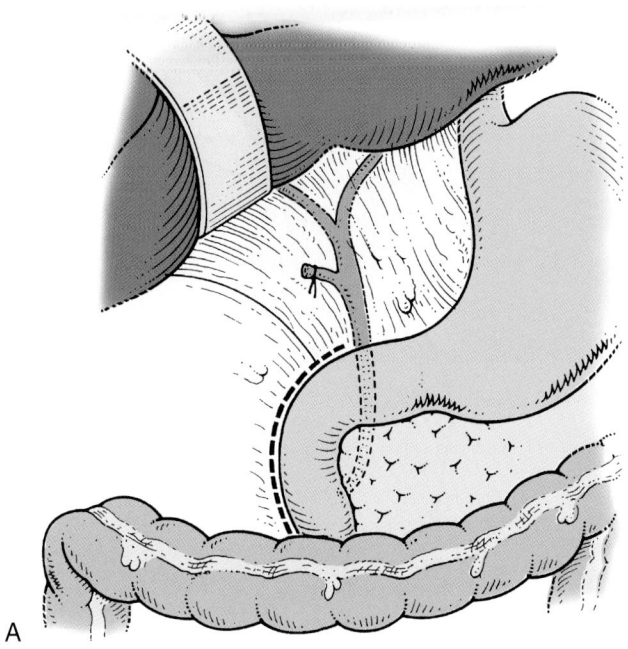

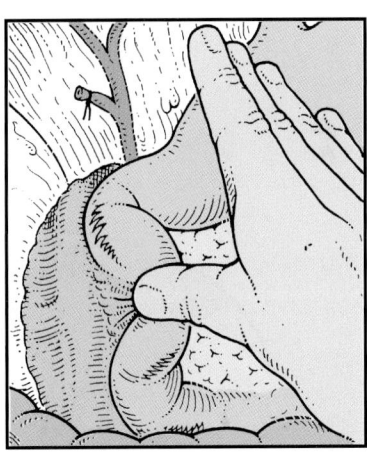

FIGURE 37A.2 **A,** The gallbladder has been removed. The *dotted line* indicates the incision in the retroperitoneum to allow mobilization of the duodenum by the Kocher maneuver **(B)**.

Choledochotomy

A distal vertical supraduodenal choledochotomy is generally preferred for several reasons. First, because a choledochoduodenostomy may be required (see Chapter 31), the opening should be positioned in the lowest part of the supraduodenal CBD such that an anastomosis can be created easily and without tension (Figs. 37A.3 and 37A.4). Second, a distal choledochotomy leaves the maximal amount of bile duct proximally so that it may be used in the future for an additional procedure (e.g., repair of a stricture). Third, the usual distance from this point to the papilla measures 7 cm or more, which is the exact length of the rigid choledochoscope sometimes used for CBDE; this is less of an issue when using a flexible scope, which is typically much longer.

The anatomy of the cystic duct is highly variable, and care must be exercised to open the correct duct (see Chapter 2). A cystic duct lying anterior or closely applied to the CBD can be easily opened in error, particularly if dilated. Bile is aspirated by gentle suction, and a specimen should be sent for culture (Fig. 37A.5).

Exploration of the Duct

All efforts must be made to minimize trauma related to the exploration, and rigid instruments should be avoided if possible, as false passages into the duodenum and pancreas can be created.[101] Grasping forceps of any type can catch the duct wall and result in delayed stricture formation. Use of the Fogarty balloon catheter (5- to 6-Fr) can avoid these issues and has been found to be suitable for CBDE.[102,103]

The Fogarty catheter is held in long forceps with the surgeon's dominant hand, introduced into the CBD (Fig. 37A.6), and passed into the duodenum. The balloon is inflated, and the catheter is withdrawn until it impinges against the papilla (Fig. 37A.7). The balloon is identified in the second part of the

duodenum by palpation, and the location is noted as the site of duodenotomy should a sphincteroplasty become necessary. Stones can usually be felt against the shaft of the catheter within the duct. The balloon is deflated and gently withdrawn through the papilla, and then the balloon is reinflated immediately. Passage back through the ampulla can be detected by a sudden easing of the pull on the catheter. At this point, the syringe is held in the surgeon's nondominant hand, and the degree of balloon inflation is controlled by the thumb and the plunger. With gentle traction superiorly from long forceps held in the surgeon's dominant hand, the catheter is gradually pulled up to the choledochotomy site (Fig. 37A.8), with care being taken to prevent any stone slipping into the proximal biliary tree. If the traction is anterior rather than superior, there is the risk of lacerating the opening into the duct (Fig. 37A.9), and the risk is increased when the opening in the duct is longitudinal. The procedure is repeated until the distal duct is considered to be clear.

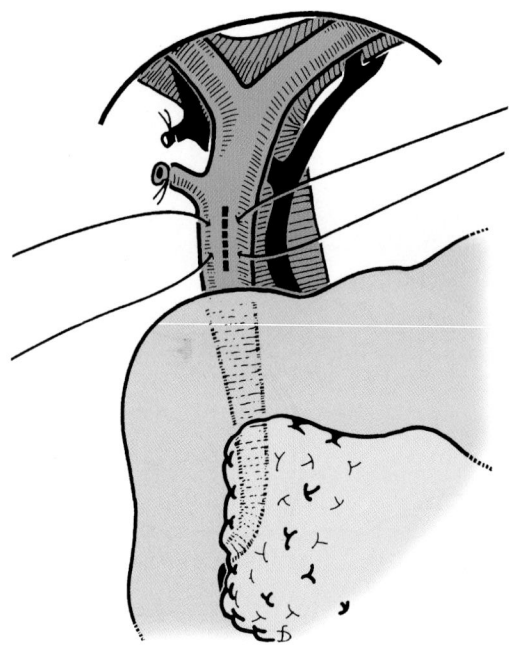

FIGURE 37A.3 The common bile duct is opened just above the duodenum to leave room for a choledochoduodenostomy if necessary.

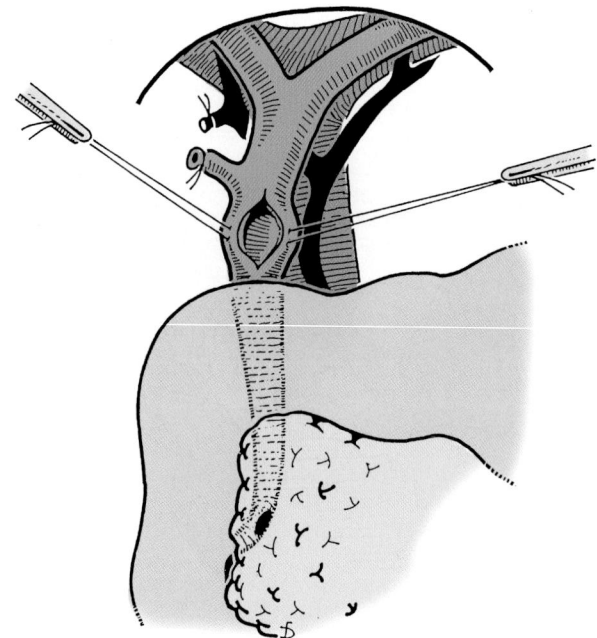

FIGURE 37A.4 Two fine absorbable stay sutures are used to lift and render the common bile duct (CBD) tense for an incision about 1 to 2 cm long, depending on the size of the duct and the size of the stones. If the CBD is not made tense, damage can be done to the posterior wall, or an irregular incision can be made.

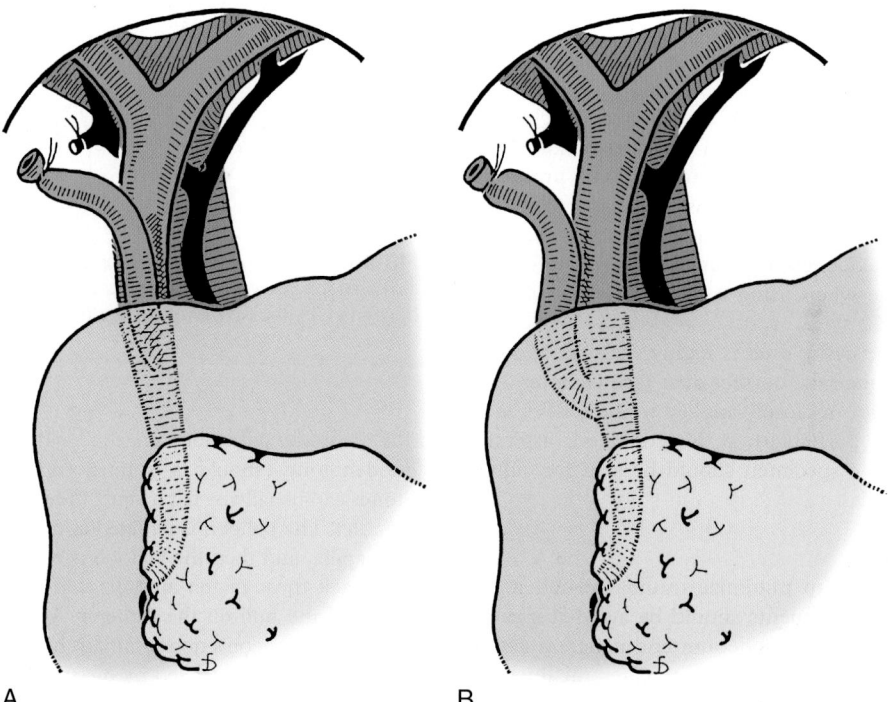

A   B

FIGURE 37A.5 **A,** The cystic duct may lie anterior to the common bile duct (CBD) and may be opened in error. **B,** The cystic duct may run parallel to the CBD with a low entrance, mimicking a dilated duct.

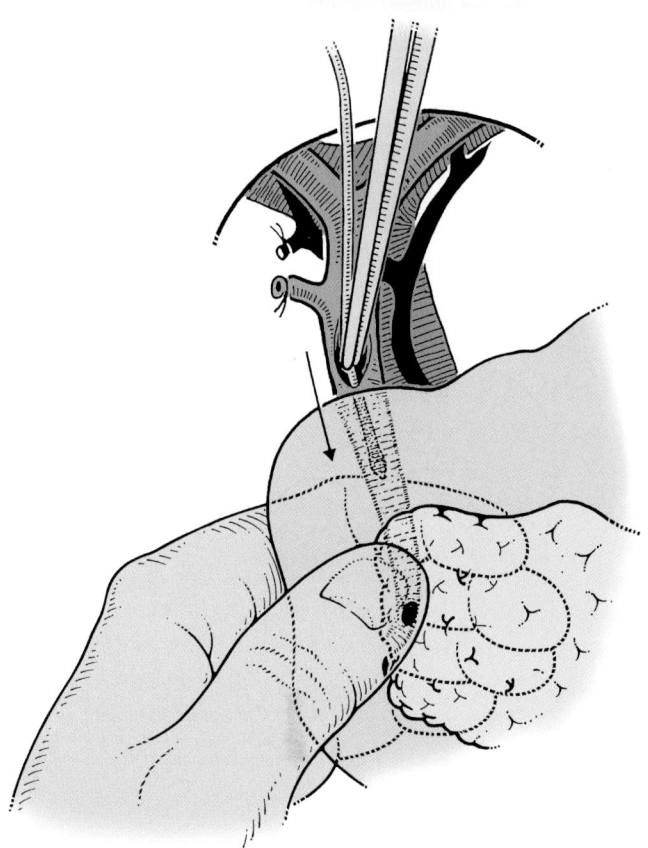

FIGURE 37A.6 A Fogarty catheter is fed into the duct with forceps by using the dominant hand. The operator's nondominant hand is used to grasp the mobilized duodenum, which allows palpation of the passage of the catheter and of any stones within the intrapancreatic portion of the common bile duct.

Next, this procedure is repeated for the proximal ducts by reinserting the catheter upward into each of the main hepatic ducts. The degree of balloon inflation is of great importance here, as overinflation will result in damage to the ducts and underinflation risks missing stones. Correct inflation can be achieved by inflating the balloon until the tension of the syringe plunger can be felt in the fingers. This tension is maintained as the catheter is withdrawn into the gradually widening duct. It is important to remove the stone when it appears at the choledochotomy opening and to avoid letting it fall into another part of the duct.

The next step in CBDE is to irrigate the duct generously with saline. Small stones, sludge, and debris can be flushed into the duodenum or back into the choledochotomy opening by irrigating the ductal system. Finally, the Fogarty catheter is passed again into the duodenum, and the balloon is inflated and retracted against the papilla. Although the catheter is held in the surgeon's dominant hand, the index and middle fingers of the other hand are placed posterior to the duodenum with the thumb anterior; this allows palpation of the duct against the wall of the catheter for any residual stones.

Postexploratory Investigations

Following exploration, the surgeon must make every effort to ensure that the duct system is normal using choledochoscopy or cholangiography (see Chapter 23).

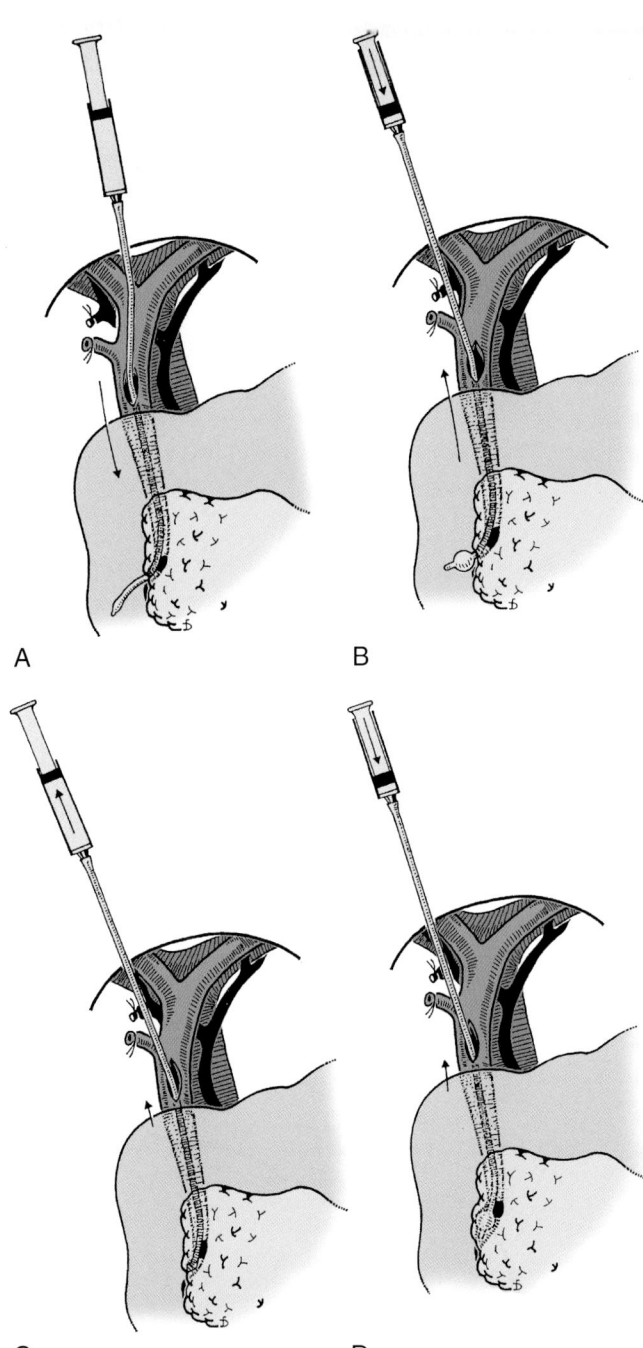

FIGURE 37A.7 **A,** The Fogarty catheter is attached to a syringe, and the balloon is inflated in the duodenum. **B,** The Fogarty catheter is retracted with the balloon against the papilla. **C** and **D,** The balloon is deflated and gently withdrawn until it slips through the papilla; the balloon is then reinflated.

Choledochoscopy

Choledochoscopy is a well-established method to ensure that the duct system is normal. Modern instruments are small enough to allow visualization of the major right and left hepatic ducts and intermediate hepatic ducts and to allow visualization of the orifices of the smaller biliary radicles. Although flexible scopes carry a higher cost and are more difficult to maintain compared with rigid scopes, they allow for less traumatic choledochoscopy and are more versatile because of their increased

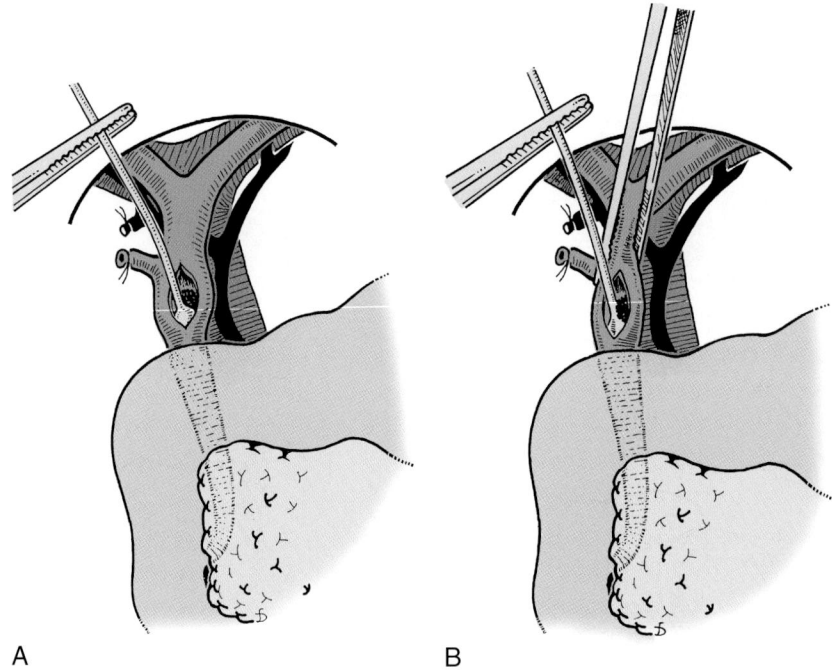

FIGURE 37A.8   A, The balloon is withdrawn gently, revealing the stone. **B,** Long forceps can be used to obstruct the common hepatic duct to prevent the stone from slipping upward.

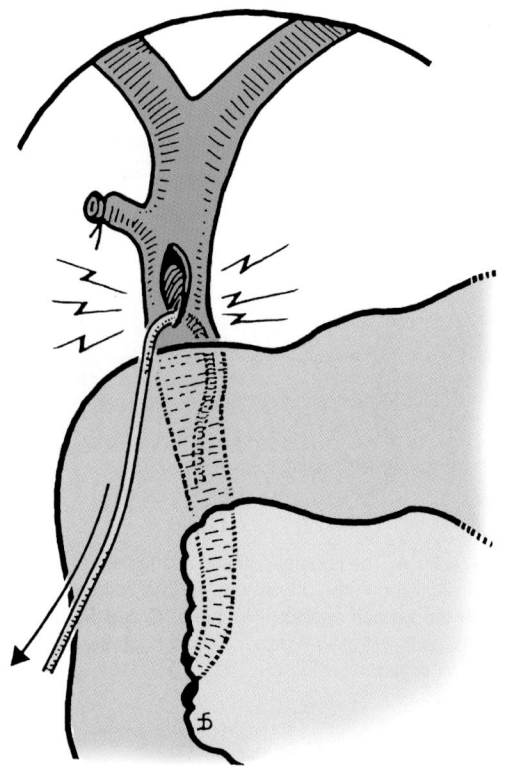

FIGURE 37A.9 Angled traction on the Fogarty catheter can result in tearing of the lower end of the choledochotomy.

length. Flexible scopes also allow the introduction of therapeutic instruments through the working channel. Some surgeons experienced in choledochoscopy recommend exploration of the CBD and removal of stones under direct vision by using the choledochoscope.[99] This can be facilitated by use of a stone basket through the working port of a flexible choledochoscope. The use of grasping or biopsy forceps should be avoided if possible because these instruments can damage the bile duct.

T-Tube Cholangiography

After insertion of a T-tube and closure of the choledochotomy, T-tube cholangiography should be performed to ensure adequate clearance of the biliary system. With proper technique and use of fluoroscopy, T-tube cholangiography is an excellent tool for detecting residual stones after CBDE (Fig. 37A.10). The cystic duct stump, a possible location of residual stones, can be delineated, and incorrect placement of the T-tube can be detected to prevent complications after the operation. In case of residual stones, the T-tube has to be removed, and the duct needs to be explored again; this necessitates a second suture of the CBD, which is a disadvantage of T-tube cholangiography.

T-TUBE DRAINAGE. The standard practice is to use a T-tube to allow spasm or edema of the sphincter to settle after the trauma of the exploration. Failure to drain the duct might theoretically result in a buildup of pressure in the extrahepatic ductal system and cause leakage at the disruption of the closure of the duct, along with biliary peritonitis. As noted earlier in this chapter, several series have not found any decreased risk for bile leak with placement of a T-tube and have in fact noted increased operative times and length of stay.[81] Routine use of a T-tube has, therefore, been questioned. The main role of T-tube placement, therefore, is not to prevent a bile leak but rather to allow an avenue for subsequent treatment of retained stones in high-risk patients. In the event of a retained stone, the T-tube can be useful later for interventional radiologic techniques through the tract created by the tube (Fig. 37A.11) or even direct choledochoscopy. The size of the T-tube should be adapted to the

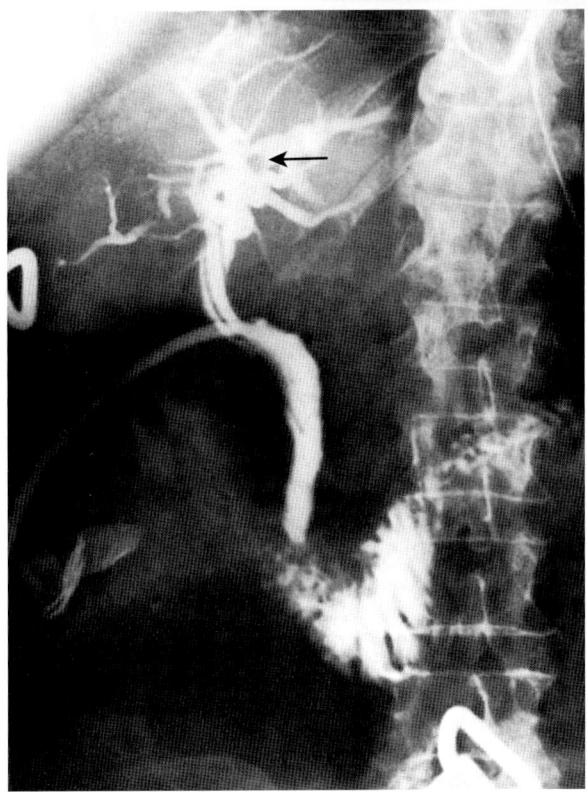

FIGURE 37A.10 A postexploration T-tube cholangiogram identifies a residual stone *(arrow)* in the intrahepatic bile ducts that was missed during operative exploration of the bile duct.

diameter of the CBD, and 14-Fr is the smallest size that should be used. Use of a smaller tube will not result in a satisfactory tract for subsequent interventional radiology procedures.

T-TUBE PLACEMENT. First, the limbs of the T-tube must be shortened (Fig. 37A.12A). T-tubes can become obstructed, particularly if they are tight fitting, and they can be difficult to extract. This situation can be avoided by cutting off a strip of the wall (see Fig. 37A.12B). The practice of dividing the back wall of the T-tube makes subsequent interventional radiology more difficult because the guidewire lodges in the posterior defect. This problem can be avoided by making the length of the T-tube appropriate or by limiting the division of the T-tube. The modified T-tube is held in Desjardin forceps, which conveniently grasps the T-junction of the tube, allowing it to be slipped into the choledochotomy (Fig. 37A.13). The long limb of the tube is placed at the lower end of the opening, and repair is begun just above the upper apex of the incision by using continuous or interrupted absorbable fine sutures. The final stitch should close the opening against the T-tube (Fig. 37A.14).

AVOIDING PROBLEMS IN THE CLOSURE OF THE CHOLEDOCHOTOMY. When closing the choledochotomy over a T-tube, care must be taken to ensure that the wall of the T-tube is not caught in one of the sutures or accidentally affixed to the CBD wall. If this occurs, there is a risk of laceration of the CBD when the T-tube is eventually removed. The proximal limb of the T-tube should be shortened so that it does not enter and obstruct one of the hepatic ducts (Fig. 37A.15). The distal limb should be similarly shortened so that it does not enter the duodenum because, if

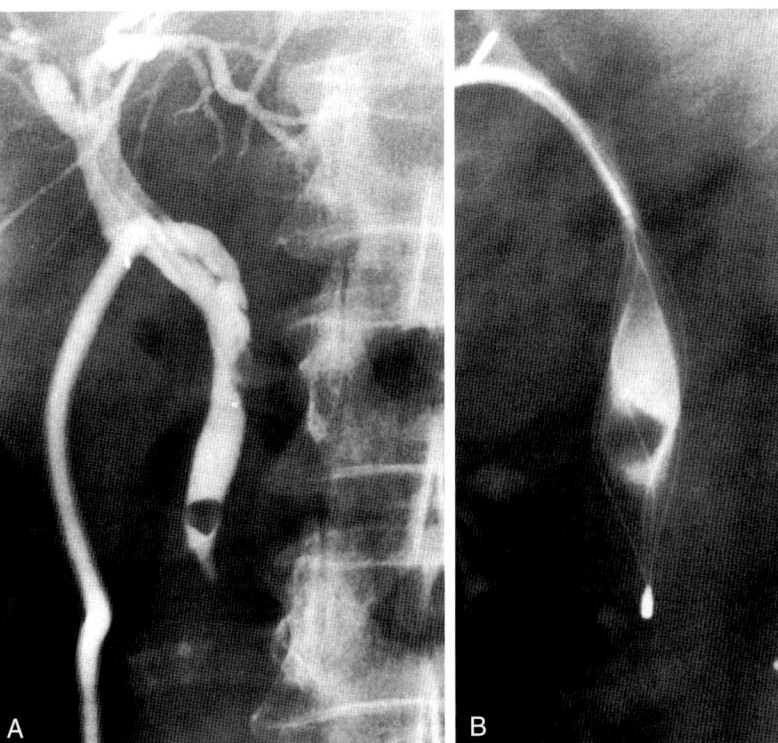

FIGURE 37A.11 **A,** Faceted retained distal common bile duct (CBD) stone on T-tube cholangiography 1 week after operation. The T-tube is inserted in the common hepatic duct above the confluence of the cystic duct. **B,** The retained CBD stone is ensnared in the wire basket before extraction. This stone measured 5 mm in diameter and was extracted intact through the sinus tract of a 14-Fr T-tube.

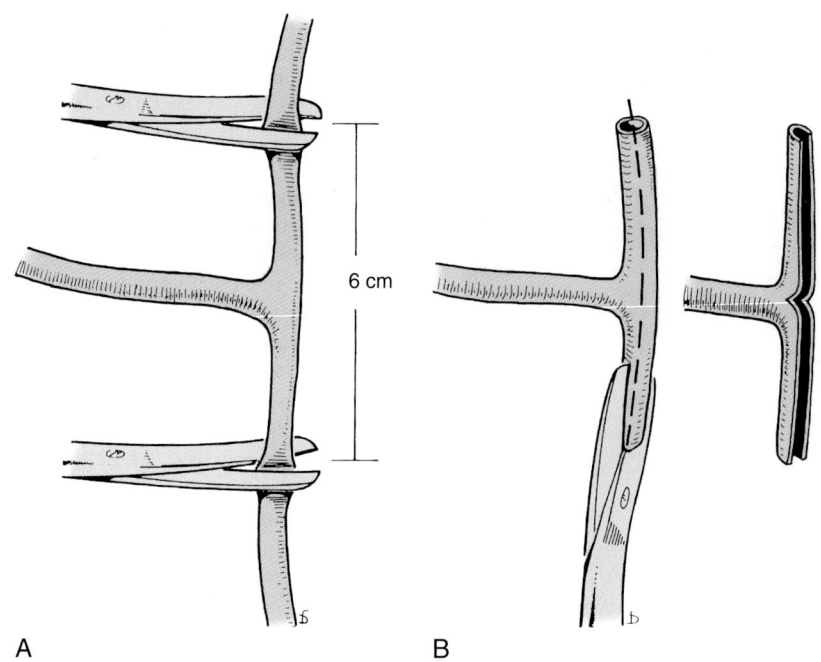

A   B

FIGURE 37A.12 **A,** The T-tube is modified by shortening the limbs to prevent proximal obstruction and distal entry into the duodenum. **B,** A T-tube is modified by removing half the diameter to prevent obstruction and enable easy removal.

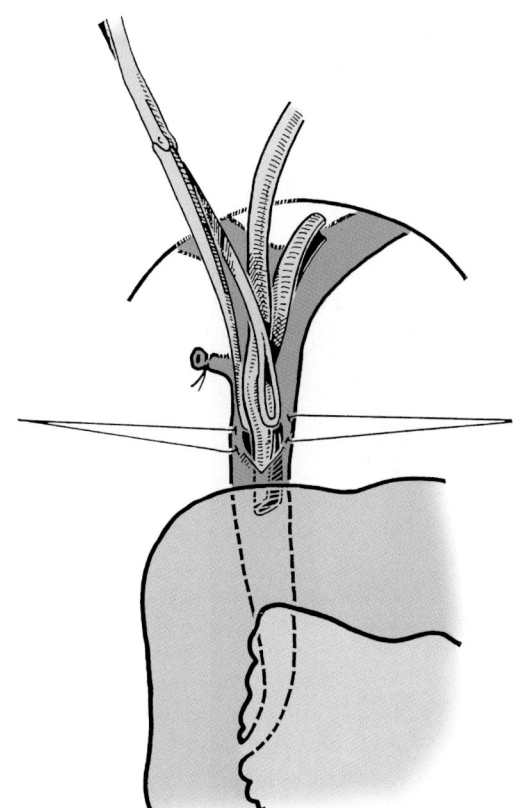

FIGURE 37A.13 The T-tube is introduced by Desjardin forceps.

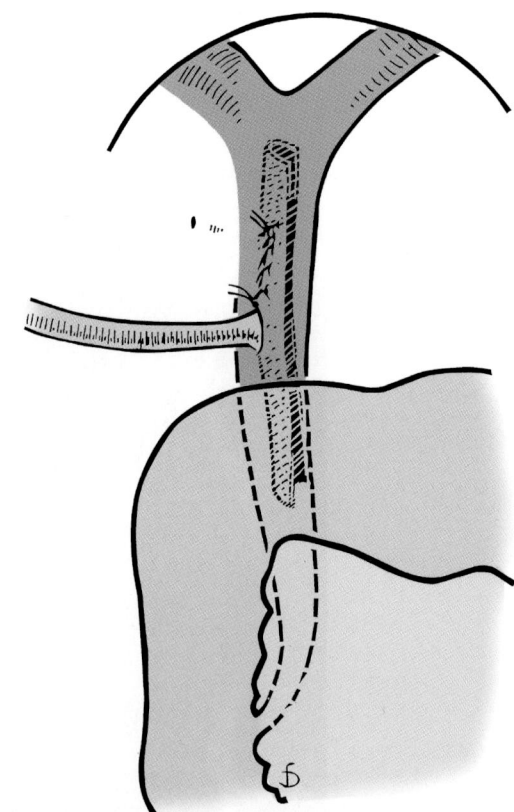

FIGURE 37A.14 The choledochotomy closure is begun above, with the T-tube emerging at the lower end of the repair.

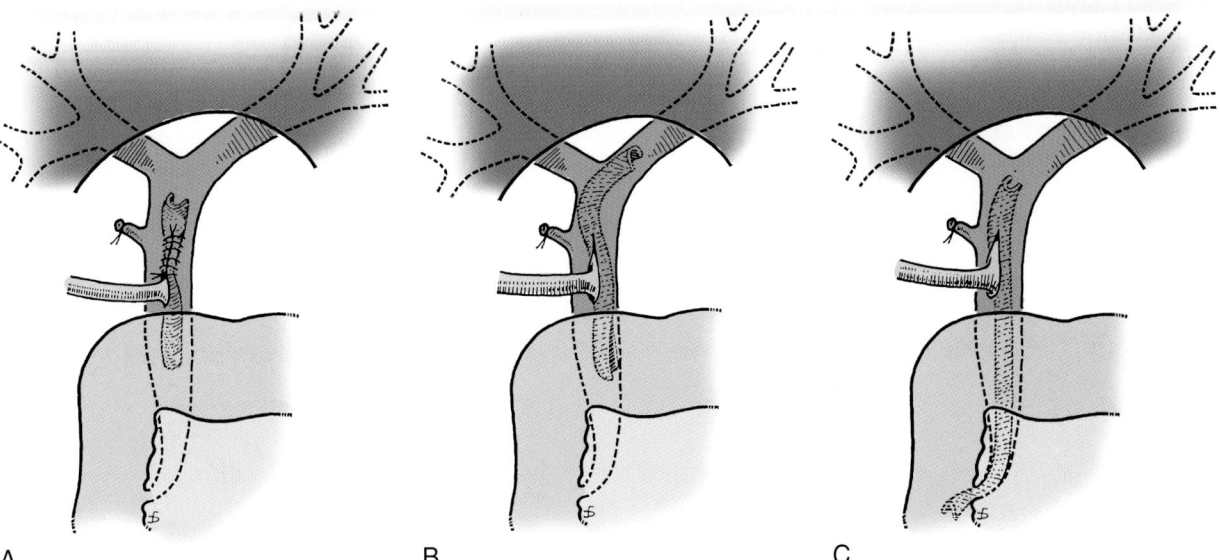

A   B   C

FIGURE 37A.15   A, The suture must not catch the tube as shown here. **B,** The T-tube limb should not enter the hepatic duct, as shown here. **C,** The distal end of the T-tube should not enter the duodenum, as shown here.

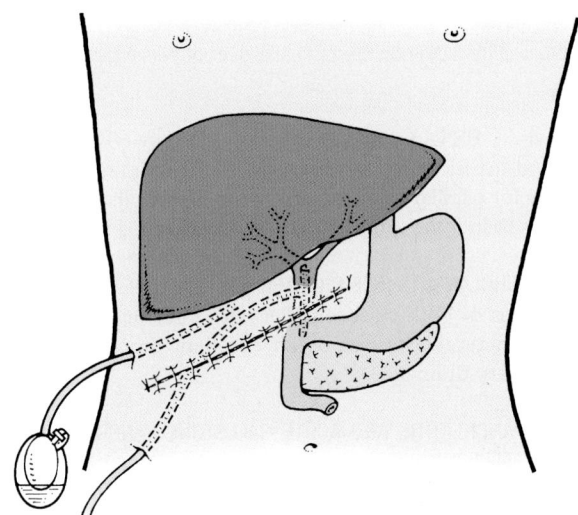

FIGURE 37A.16   The T-tube should be brought out lateral to the wound, and a closed-suction drain should be placed in the hepatorenal space beneath the liver.

the tube does, it can act as a siphon. Furthermore, a tube extending through the papillary orifice may incite pancreatitis. The correct position of the T-tube is with the long limb emerging under the costal margin laterally (Fig. 37A.16). This position facilitates radiologic techniques for later postoperative removal of stones should this be necessary. A suction drain is placed on the right, within the abdomen as high as possible in the hepatorenal pouch.

POSTOPERATIVE MANAGEMENT. Initially, bile is allowed to drain freely into a bile bag to allow any spasm or edema of the sphincter to settle before testing the suture line of the choledochotomy. The volume drained externally should decrease as the bile flow through the ampulla improves. Persistently elevated

volume of externally drained bile should raise concerns for continued distal obstruction or to the distal T-tube limb lying within the duodenum. Similarly, there is a problem if there is no external drainage of the bile or if bile drains around the T-tube, and may indicate that the tube is blocked or dislodged from the duct. Issues with T-tube drainage should be evaluated by T-tube cholangiography. If cholangiography does not reveal any issues, management is aimed at waiting for the bile to flow easily through the papilla into the duodenum. The T-tube should be left to external gravity drainage until this occurs. Once it appears that bile is flowing into the duodenum, a T-tube cholangiogram can be taken about 5 to 7 days postoperatively. If it appears normal, the tube is removed on day 7 or 8 by gentle traction.

If there are residual stones or unclear findings on T-tube cholangiography in the first 1 to 2 weeks after surgery, intervention does not necessarily need to be undertaken unless the patient has signs of cholangitis or rising bilirubin. A repeat cholangiogram several days later will often show spontaneous passage of the stone. If a stone is still seen in an otherwise well patient, the patient can safely be sent home with a sealed drainage system and instructions to open the drain to a bag in the event of any problems. After about 5 weeks, further cholangiography is carried out. If the stone is still present, it is extracted via interventional radiology or endoscopic papillotomy (Fig. 37A.17).

Transduodenal Sphincteroplasty

The role of transduodenal sphincteroplasty in the treatment of choledocholithiasis centers predominantly around management of impacted stones at the ampulla. It also has a role in treating patients with anatomy that prevents ES (e.g., Billroth II gastrectomy), failures of ES, and sometimes in patients with pancreatitis where a drainage procedure of the duct of Wirsung is indicated.[104] Similarly, hydatid cyst remnants and membranes can be readily extracted from the CBD. Exploration may extend to the left and right hepatic ducts, and angled Randall forceps are useful for this purpose.

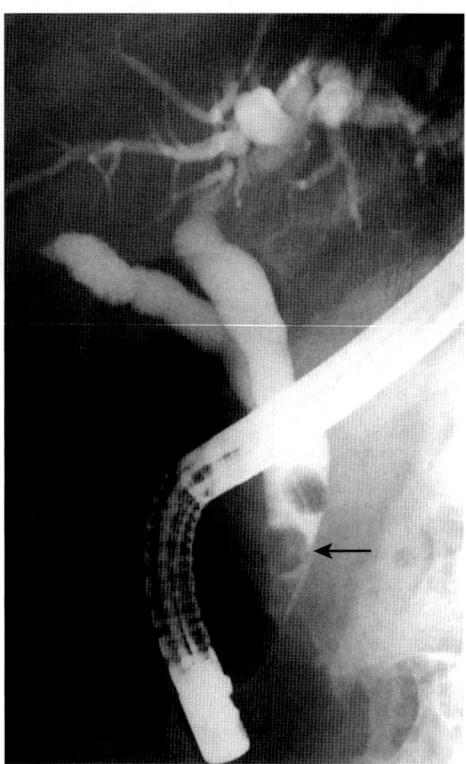

FIGURE 37A.17   Balloon extraction of a single stone *(arrow)*.

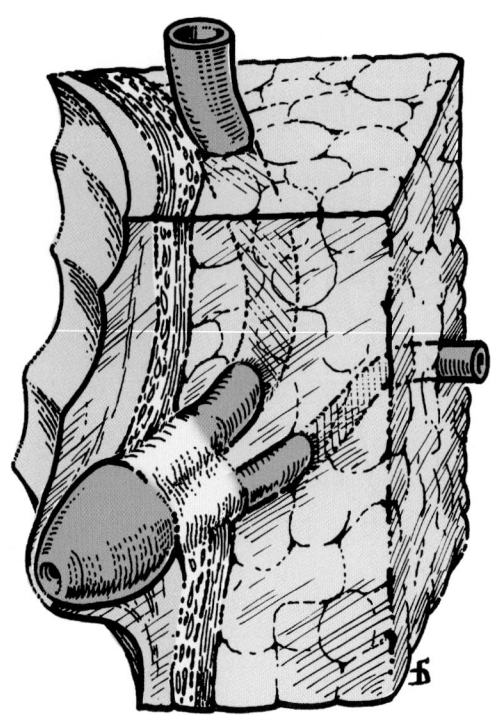

FIGURE 37A.18   A section of the sphincter of Oddi. Note the distinction between the papilla, the common portion of the sphincter, and the sphincters of the common bile duct and duct of Wirsung.

Sphincteroplasty consists of suturing the outer edge or both edges of a surgical sphincterotomy to avoid possible future stenosis of the incision. The stitches achieve hemostasis of the incision margins and help to avoid possible leakage of the duodenal contents should the excision extend beyond the common portion of the sphincter, incurring the risk of retroduodenal perforation. Transduodenal sphincteroplasty is contraindicated in the presence of a large CBD (>2 cm) or where there is a long suprasphincteric stricture. It also should not be attempted in the presence of a duodenal diverticulum or where there is severe periampullary inflammation.

Indications

The most common indications for transduodenal sphincteroplasty relate to bile duct stones and cholangitis (see Chapter 43).

STONES IMPACTED IN THE DISTAL AMPULLARY REGION. An impacted stone is often readily palpable, and the incision may be made safely using the stone as a guide. In such cases, extraction through a supraduodenal choledochotomy is often impossible without undue risk of creating a false passage and without significant risk of postoperative pancreatitis.

MULTIPLE AND RECURRENT COMMON BILE DUCT STONES. In cases of multiple and recurrent CBD stones, sphincteroplasty should provide long-term biliary drainage. When 20 or more stones are removed from the CBD, it is probable that one or more stones are still present.[58] In this situation, choledochoduodenostomy or sphincteroplasty yields excellent results.

PAPILLARY STENOSIS. Papillary stenosis is encountered less frequently than in the past. When it is found at operation, transduodenal sphincteroplasty ensures good biliary drainage and prevents restenosis.[105] ES is technically successful in only 60% to 80% of cases, and the mortality rate exceeds 1%.[106] In addition, sphincterotomy for papillary stenosis is five times more likely to lead to restenosis than if the same procedure is performed for calculi.[107]

PYOGENIC CHOLANGITIS (SEE CHAPTER 43). If papillary stenosis or CBD stones or both exist together with cholangitis, transduodenal sphincteroplasty can be an excellent procedure for definitive biliary drainage.

CHRONIC PANCREATITIS AND ACUTE GALLSTONE PANCREATITIS (SEE CHAPTERS 55–58). In chronic pancreatitis, some authors report good long-term results with transduodenal sphincteroplasty alone[108] or in addition to transpapillary septectomy[109] or with other drainage procedures of the duct of Wirsung.[110] The presence of a stone at the lower end of the CBD or pancreatic duct may cause biliary pancreatitis, and transduodenal sphincteroplasty with clearance of the CBD is a treatment option.

Technique

Sphincteroplasty consists of the incision of the common portion of the sphincter of Oddi (Fig. 37A.18) with partial suture of the incision margin. Using this procedure, the sphincters of the CBD and the duct of Wirsung are not involved, and their functions are not impaired. The procedure also can be called a *subtotal lower sphincteroplasty* (Fig. 37A.19).[111] The approach to the sphincter of Oddi is through a minimal duodenotomy in the second part of the duodenum.

Preparation, Position of the Patient, and Incision

Preoperative preparation is routine. The patient is placed in a supine position on a radiotransparent operating table. A transverse incision below the right costal margin is preferred.[112] This

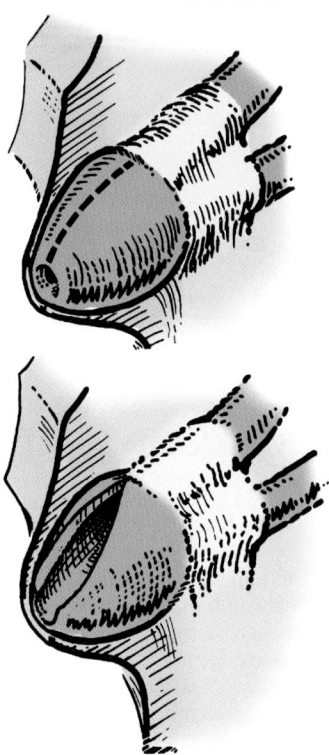

FIGURE 37A.19 Subtotal lower sphincteroplasty involves only the papilla, whereas the common bile duct and the duct of Wirsung are preserved.

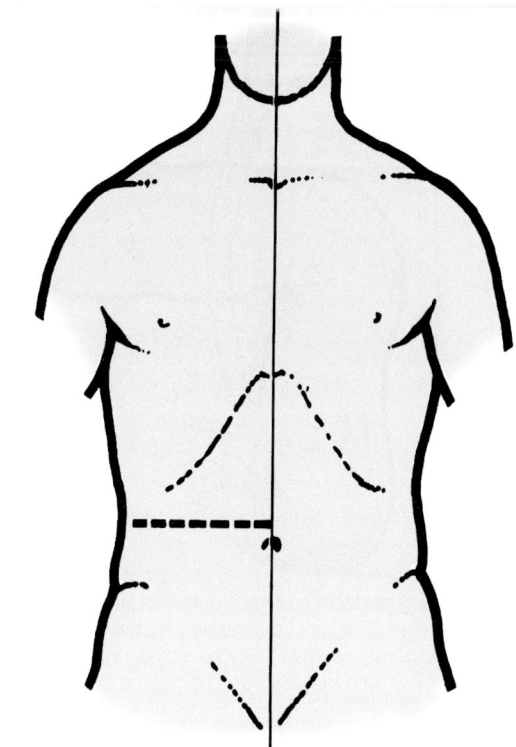

FIGURE 37A.20 Transverse subcostal incision offers excellent exposure with a low incidence of postoperative incisional hernia.

incision allows optimal light and excellent access; it is particularly suitable in obese patients, and the incidence of postoperative incisional hernia is probably lower than with vertical and oblique incisions. The incision of the abdominal wall follows a transverse line, from the midaxillary to the median line at the level of the 11th and 12th ribs (Fig. 37A.20).

Preparation of the Operative Field and Exposure

The abdomen is opened, and a large retractor is positioned at the upper margin of the wound. The hepatic flexure of the colon is displaced inferiorly, and the stomach is displaced to the left by means of two surgical pads. Viscera are maintained in this position with two large, curved retractors. For the performance of the sphincteroplasty, extended mobilization of the duodenum and pancreas (Kocher maneuver) is mandatory.[109] The assistant surgeon displaces the second portion medially and forward, and the peritoneum is incised posteriorly along the curved lateral margin of the duodenum. The mesocolon of the right colic flexure is mobilized and retracted inferiorly. At this point, the assistant surgeon also should displace the duodenum superiorly (Fig. 37A.21). Access is provided to the avascular space between the posterior aspect of the head of the pancreas anteriorly and the perinephric fat and inferior vena cava posteriorly; elevation of the structures should reach the left margin of the inferior vena cava. It is important to expose and mobilize the third portion of the duodenum to allow easy access to the papilla and for closure of the duodenotomy without tension (see Fig. 37A.21).

Duodenotomy

Duodenotomy is performed in the lateral duodenal wall by surgical diathermy. The cut is 10 to 15 mm long immediately above

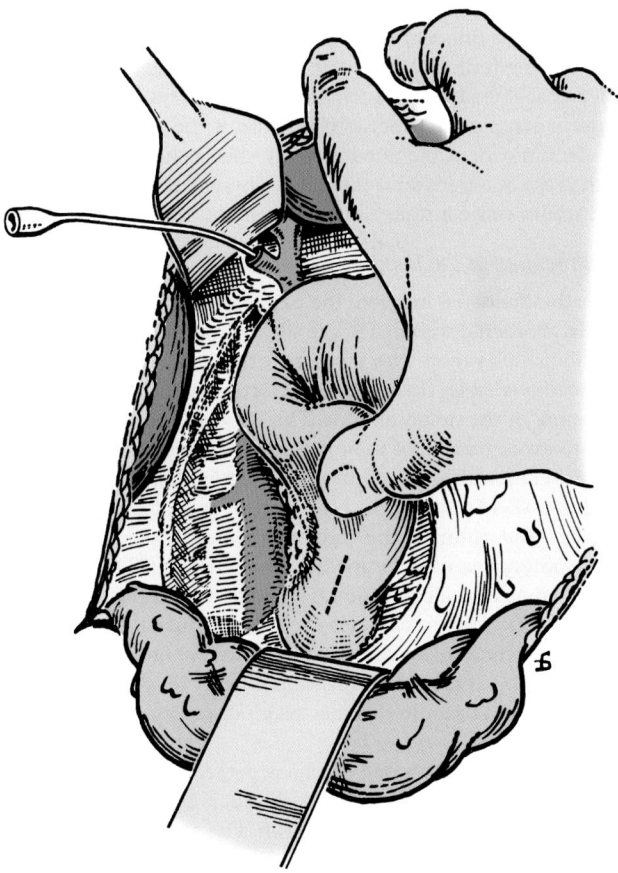

FIGURE 37A.21 It is important to expose and mobilize the third portion of the duodenum to easily identify and operate on the papilla and allow facile closure of the duodenotomy.

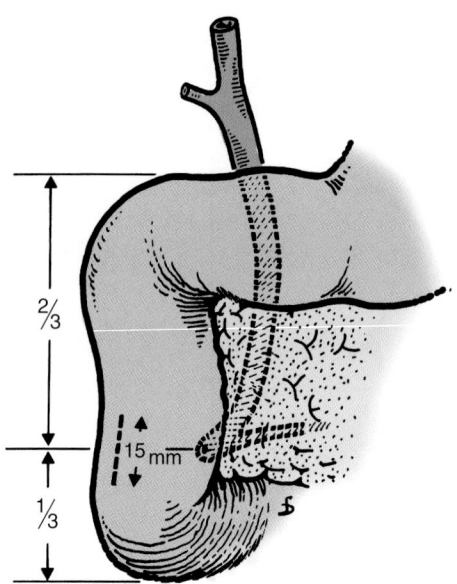

FIGURE 37A.22   The duodenotomy is performed above the junction of the second and third portions of the duodenum; the surgeon takes into account that the papilla usually is located at the junction of the upper two-thirds and lower third of the second part of the duodenum.

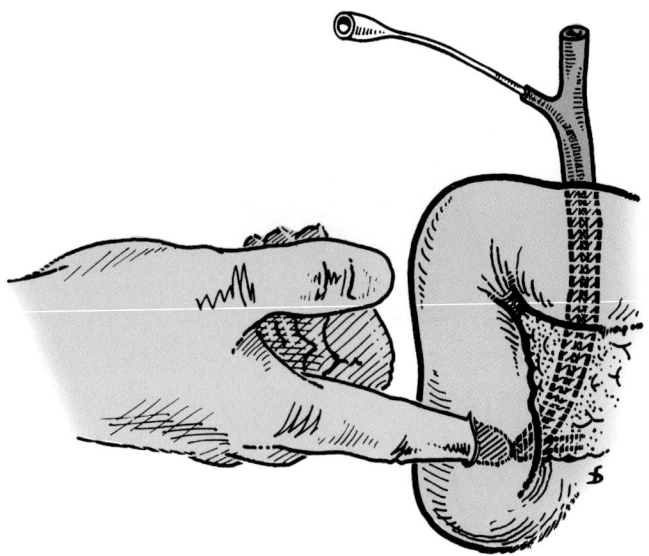

FIGURE 37A.23   If the papilla is not easily seen, it can often be palpated as a small elevation in the medial duodenal wall. If the papilla is still not easily seen, a small Nélaton catheter is introduced through the cystic duct stump until it is seen to protrude from the papillary orifice. The forefinger, introduced through the duodenotomy, detects the papilla as a small, thick elevation.

the inferior knee of the duodenum, with the surgeon taking account of the fact that the papilla usually is located at the junction of the lower third with the upper two-thirds of the second portion of the duodenum (Fig. 37A.22). The duodenal incision may be longitudinal or transverse; both types are suitable, provided that the suture of such incisions is always transverse. We prefer a longitudinal incision, because if the retractor on the duodenum widens the duodenotomy, this occurs longitudinally. In the case of a transverse duodenotomy, any inadvertent extension would cause a transverse enlargement of the wound.

Identification of the Papilla

After the duodenal incision, the papilla is readily shown on the medial duodenal wall in 15% to 20% of patients. It appears as a roundish elevation with a central orifice. When the papilla is not readily visible, it should be detected by displacement and flattening of the mucosal folds. This should be done with great care to avoid tearing of the mucosa, which would hinder good exposure. Identification of the papilla under direct vision is possible in 80% of patients. If this is not the case, digital palpation can be used running the forefinger, introduced through the duodenotomy, across the medial duodenal wall. The papilla is identified as a small elevation. If digital palpation fails, a small (5- to 6-Fr) Nélaton catheter can be introduced via the cystic duct stump and advanced downward to emerge at the papilla (Fig. 37A.23). This maneuver should never be performed with rigid catheters because this may result in the formation of false passages.

Sometimes a very small papilla is detected, and its catheterization is difficult or impossible. In such cases, the orifice is probably that of the duct of Santorini. The major papilla should be searched for in a lower position.

Sphincteroplasty

After the papilla has been identified, it is exposed by gentle extraction with an Allis or similar clamp. This clamp is applied

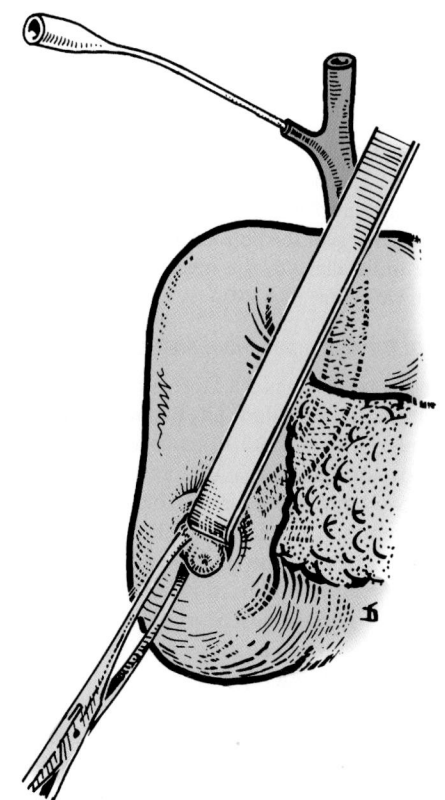

FIGURE 37A.24   The duodenotomy is kept open by a suitable retractor placed in the upper margin of the duodenal incision. The papilla is exposed by gentle traction with an Allis clamp placed laterally, never medially, to avoid trauma to the duct of Wirsung.

laterally, never medially, to avoid trauma to the duct of Wirsung (Fig. 37A.24).[113] A Nélaton catheter (4- to 5-Fr) is introduced from the outside or via the cystic duct. Following the line of the catheter and avoiding plastic catheters, which melt when surgical

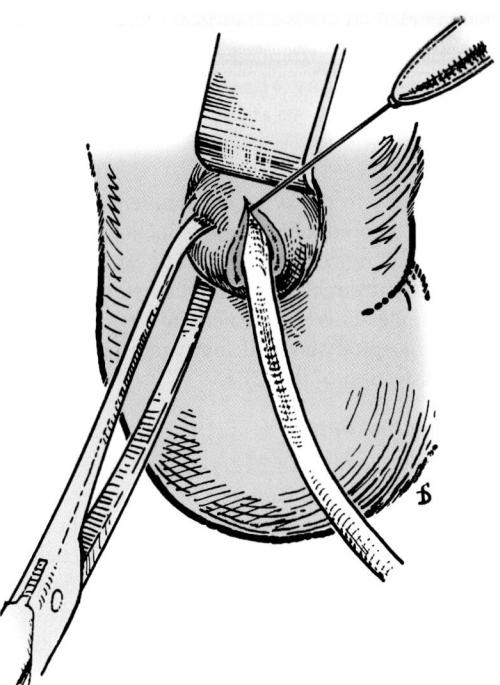

FIGURE 37A.25   With a Nélaton catheter as a guide, a cut is made using surgical diathermy on the medial wall of the duodenum extending superiorly and slightly externally (11 o'clock position). With diathermy, good hemostasis is achieved.

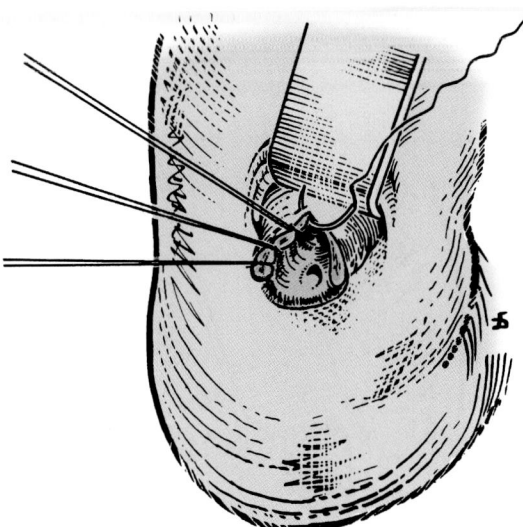

FIGURE 37A.26   After sphincterectomy is performed, several stitches are placed between the duodenal mucosa and the wall of the common bile duct (CBD) by using an atraumatic needle and 3-0 suture. Sutures should be placed only on the outer margin of the sphincterotomy to avoid the risk of damaging the duct of Wirsung, which in its distal portion runs inferiorly and medially along the length of the CBD.

diathermy is applied, the surgeon makes a cut using surgical diathermy. This cut is made superiorly (at the 11 o'clock position) for 4 to 5 mm (Fig. 37A.25). We prefer surgical diathermy because the instrument ensures good hemostasis. When a sample for biopsy is required, it should be obtained with a scalpel and be taken only from the outer margin of the incision. Possible bleeding from the cut, usually modest, can be arrested with a stitch. After sphincterotomy, two or three stitches are placed between the duodenal mucosa and the wall of the CBD on the outer margin by using an atraumatic needle and fine sutures. Traction is applied to these sutures, and incision of the sphincter is extended for another 6 to 7 mm with sutures placed every 2 to 3 mm, all laterally, until the entire common tract of the sphincter of Oddi has been incised (Fig. 37A.26). The incision is complete when it is 10 to 12 mm long and an appropriate forceps can be easily introduced (Fig. 37A.27). Its entry into the CBD allows an abundant flow of bile because of distension of its sphincter. Sutures should be placed only on the outer margin of the sphincterotomy to prevent the risk of damage to the duct of Wirsung. The opening of the duct of Wirsung usually is identified as a small orifice from which clear, colorless pancreatic juice flows.

Instrumental Exploration of the Common Bile Duct

After sphincteroplasty, instrumental exploration of the CBD and extraction of stones is performed.[114] An angled Randall forceps is introduced into the CBD, and the bile duct is carefully explored. The maneuver should be repeated several times to extract all stones. The next step is to rinse with saline solution, introduced under slight pressure with a Nélaton catheter (8- to 9-Fr) and abruptly withdrawn so that small fragments flow downstream with the siphoning (Fig. 37A.28). Other means to extract stones from the CBD are with a Fogarty catheter and Dormia basket. The problem of residual stones is best

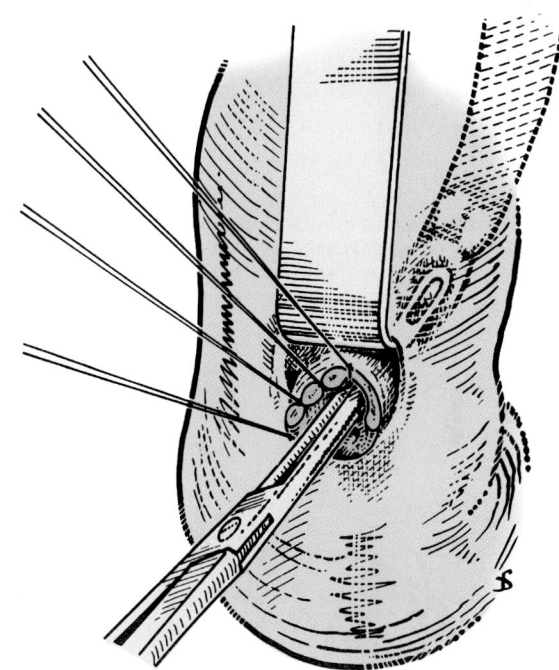

FIGURE 37A.27   Sphincteroplasty is completed when the incision is 10 to 21 mm long, and a Randall forceps can be introduced easily into the common bile duct to extract stones or other foreign bodies.

prevented with choledochoscopy; the endoscope is introduced via the sphincteroplasty.

Duodenal Closure

As already emphasized, initial longitudinal duodenotomy should be closed transversely to avoid stenosis of the duodenum. A number of approaches to the closure exist including linear stapling, a running inverting suture line, and interrupted single

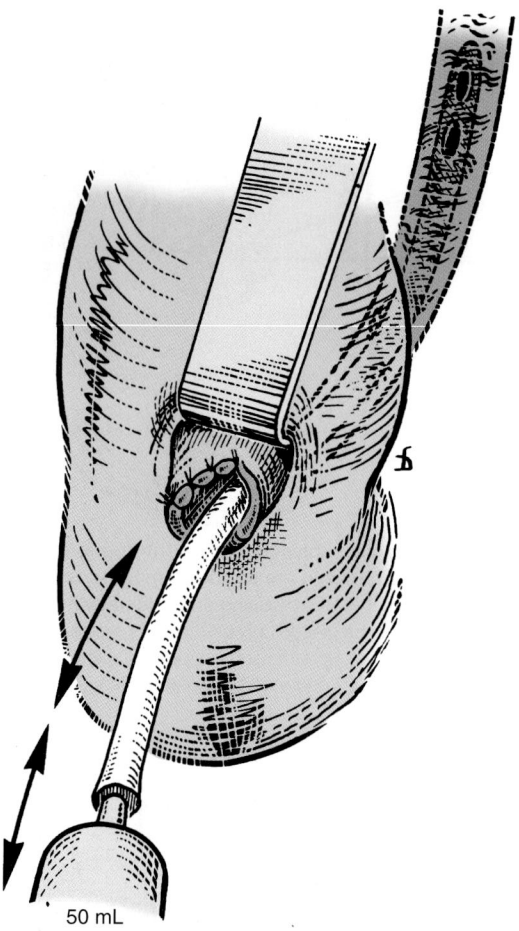

FIGURE 37A.28 After the extraction of stones, the common bile duct is rinsed with saline solution introduced under slight pressure with a Nélaton catheter and with subsequent siphoning so that small fragments can run downstream.

layer closure. The suture should not be under tension, and for this reason, preliminary extended mobilization of the duodenum and pancreas is mandatory. The operation is now complete, and the wound is closed without abdominal drains.

Comment

It is not necessary to perform transduodenal sphincteroplasty combined with supraduodenal choledochotomy, which has a higher associated mortality rate.[115] The cystic duct remnant may be used to introduce a Nélaton catheter to assist recognition of the papilla. There is no need to insert a T-tube, which lengthens the hospital stay and may predispose the patient to stenosis and infection of the CBD.[115,116]

Review of Reported Results

In a retrospective analysis of 25,541 transduodenal sphincteroplasties performed by 130 surgeons in different countries, early transduodenal sphincteroplasty–related complications were bleeding (0.65%), acute pancreatitis (0.60%), dehiscence of the duodenal closure (0.55%), and cholangitis (0.50%), for an overall morbidity rate of 2.3% and a mortality rate of 0.8%.[117] A retrospective study found that the factors affecting mortality in 2.1% of 333 patients (but only in 0.9% for sphincterectomy-related complications) were older than 70 years of age, and had a bilirubin level greater than 85 mmol/L, diabetes, renal failure, and coagulopathy. The mortality rate increased when supraduodenal choledochotomy was combined with transduodenal sphincteroplasty and when a T-tube was used.[118] Transduodenal sphincteroplasty alone[108] or associated with transampullary septectomy[119] has led to good long-term results in patients with chronic and acute recurrent pancreatitis, even in cases with pancreas divisum and in selected patients with abdominal pain of hepatobiliary origin.

The references for this chapter can be found online by accessing the accompanying Expert Consult website.

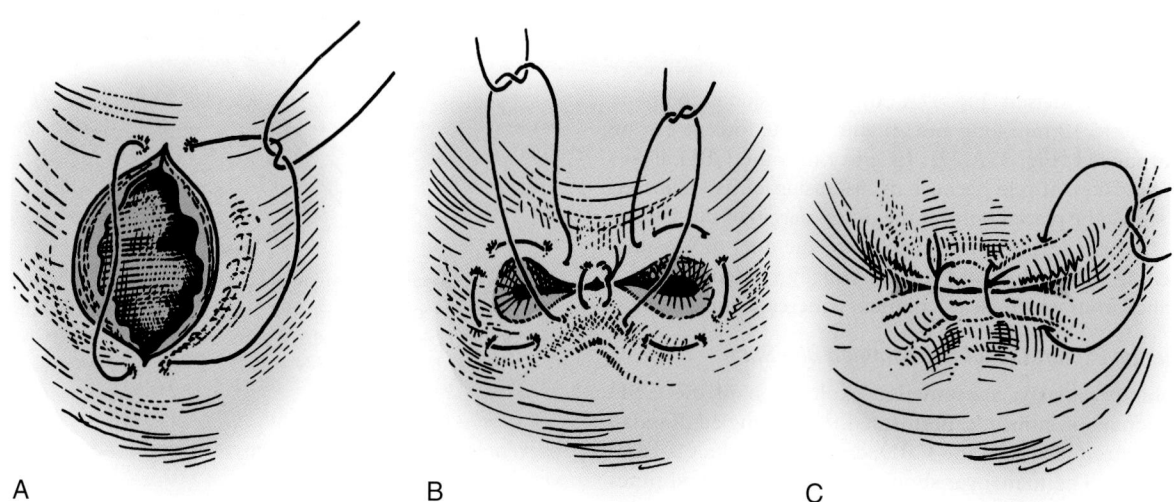

A   B   C

FIGURE 37A.29 The duodenotomy always should be closed transversely to avoid stenosis of the duodenum. **A,** The superior and inferior angles are approximated. **B,** The resulting lateral gaps are sutured with two extramucosal nonabsorbable purse-string sutures. **C,** Three to four nonabsorbable seromuscular stitches are added as a second layer. The sutures should not be under tension.

Stones in the bile duct: Minimally invasive surgical approaches

Michele L. Babicky and Paul D. Hansen

INTRODUCTION

Epidemiology of Choledocholithiasis

The prevalence of cholelithiasis is approximately 15% in the general population, with up to 10% of patients having concomitant choledocholithiasis (CDL; for more information, see Chapter 33). The prevalence of gallstones is increased in the elderly population over 65 years of age, reaching up to 35% in women.[1] Risk factors for gallstones include: obesity, type 2 diabetes and insulin resistance, genetic defects in cholesterol metabolism, female gender, rapid weight gain or loss (as seen with bariatric surgery and pregnancy), systemic inflammatory diseases (such as Crohn disease and rheumatoid arthritis[2]), hemolytic disorders, and conditions leading to biliary stasis (cystic fibrosis, chronic total parenteral nutrition [TPN], estrogen hormonal supplementation).[3] The majority of common bile duct (CBD) stones in Western countries are secondary to gallstone formation within the gallbladder, with an extraordinarily higher prevalence in Native American (73%) and Hispanic (27%) populations.[4] In Eastern countries, the incidence of primary hepatolithiasis and CDL is higher (see Chapter 39), with reported prevalence ranging from 2% to 25%, related to endemic infectious organisms that colonize the liver and biliary tree (e.g., *Clonorchis sinensis*, liver fluke; see Chapter 45) and cause a predisposition to recurrent pyogenic cholangitis[5,6] (see Chapter 44).

CDL is identified in up to 18% of patients undergoing cholecystectomy.[7] Additionally, some patients may be asymptomatic with intra- and extrahepatic biliary dilation and/or CBD stones incidentally identified on cross-sectional imaging performed for other clinical indications. These clinical scenarios can vary significantly in presentation and morbidity, ranging from minimal symptoms to critical illness caused by septic cholangitis. If left untreated, chronic CDL can also cause inflammatory strictures, recurrent infections, or biliary cirrhosis.

Clinical Presentation

The index of suspicion for the presence of CBD stones should be high in patients presenting with gallstone pancreatitis (see Chapters 54 and 55), ascending cholangitis (see Chapter 43), or obstructive jaundice in the setting of acute or chronic cholecystitis with a history of biliary colic (see Chapter 34). Hyperbilirubinemia, defined as elevation of the total bilirubin level greater than 1.3 mg/dL with a predominant unconjugated (direct) component, is most suggestive of biliary obstruction in a patient with otherwise no evidence or history of underlying liver disease (see Chapter 4). Elevation of the alkaline phosphatase (AP) levels (>150 IU/L) out of proportion to changes in the aminotransferase enzyme levels can be seen in the presence of nonobstructing stones or sludge, and an upward trend can be indicative of ongoing cholestasis and/or inflammation of the biliary tree. Elevated gamma-glutamyl transferase levels (>50 IU/L) can confirm a hepatobiliary source of the elevated AP in complex or asymptomatic patients.

Depending on the clinical presentation, first-line imaging modalities include abdominal ultrasound (most sensitive test for identifying gallstones and ductal dilation) and/or single phase abdominal CT scan (most sensitive for identifying acute cholecystitis).[8,9] Intra- or extrahepatic biliary dilation, dilation of the CBD more than 8 mm, or the presence of a filling defect can be informative and guide the treatment algorithm. The caliber, number, and location of the stones combined with the clinical status of the patient will also influence treatment decisions (see Chapter 13).

In patients where the diagnosis of CDL is unclear, either magnetic resonance cholangiopancreatography (MRCP; see Chapter 13) or endoscopic ultrasound (EUS; see Chapter 22) with or without endoscopic retrograde cholangiopancreatography (ERCP; see Chapter 20) can be considered. Recent meta-analyses demonstrate that both EUS and MRCP have high specificity for identifying CDL, with a slightly higher sensitivity for EUS and the added therapeutic benefit of performing ERCP if stones are identified.[10-12] MRCP can be useful when ERCP is not available and may provide anatomic delineation before surgery. Some centers advocate MRCP to avoid the risk of unnecessary ERCP; however, this is associated with an increased cost. The choice of modality may depend on clinical factors of the patient. For example, a patient with a history of Roux-en-Y gastric bypass (RNYGB) surgery complicates the ability to perform routine EUS/ERCP without the use of single or double balloon enteroscopy via the Roux limb. In contrast, a patient with a pacemaker, severe claustrophobia, or inability to hold their breath may preclude MRCP as an option in the diagnostic work-up.

Historical Management of Choledocholithiasis

The management of CDL has evolved dramatically over the last four decades (see Chapter 38). Before the advent of laparoscopy in the 1980s, stones in the CBD were identified and removed at the time of open surgical exploration for cholecystectomy. Even after the introduction of ERCP in the 1970s, laparotomy remained the mainstay for CBD exploration (CBDE; see Chapter 37A).[13] At that time, the tools and techniques used for surgical clearance of the CBD were superior to those available via ERCP, and as long as a laparotomy was used to perform the cholecystectomy, minimally invasive treatment of CDL was unnecessary. It was not until the introduction of the laparoscopic cholecystectomy (LC) in the late 1980s that finding an associated less invasive method of treating CDL became a priority.

During the initial adoption of LC, most general surgeons did not have the skill set, experience, or equipment to facilitate a laparoscopic CBDE. As the skills, experience, and tools have developed, the advantages and disadvantages of laparoscopic CBDE versus ERCP have been a frequent source of debate (see Chapter 37C).

This chapter will discuss laparoscopic techniques for managing CDL, including indications and technical aspects of laparoscopic transcystic, transcholedochal, and transduodenal CBDE, as well as laparoscopic biliary-enteric bypass procedures and laparoscopic-assisted ERCP.

CLINICAL SCENARIOS

Indications for Intervention

The standard of care for the management of most CBD stones is minimally invasive, whether laparoscopic, endoscopic, or percutaneous. The minimally invasive techniques used and the sequence in which they are used depends on the specific clinical scenario. In addition, the capability and experience of the available personnel at each institution will affect the treatment algorithm. The most common clinical scenarios encountered by surgeons include known or suspected stones before cholecystectomy, the diagnosis of stones intraoperatively, and stones identified subsequent to cholecystectomy.

Preoperative Choledocholithiasis

Ascending cholangitis, gallstone pancreatitis, and symptomatic cholelithiasis or acute cholecystitis with evidence of CDL on imaging or liver function tests require evaluation for the presence of CDL (see Chapter 33). For CBD stones confirmed at the time of initial clinical presentation, the decision making is often based on surgeon preference and institutional capabilities. The two primary strategies include ERCP followed by LC or LC with intraoperative cholangiogram (IOC). In the latter case, laparoscopic CBDE can be performed simultaneously or postoperative ERCP is performed if CBD stones are identified on the cholangiogram.

ERCP has become widely available in urban settings within the United States with more than 150,000 procedures performed annually (see Chapters 20, 30, and 37C). In general, ERCP is more accessible than laparoscopic CBDE and is also highly effective with successful clearance of the CBD in more than 95% of cases.[14] In most centers, CBD stones up to 1.5 cm can be extracted and centers that use lithotripsy can treat stones as large as 3 cm in diameter.[15] Therefore, in settings where laparoscopic CBDE is not available, the debate centers on preoperative versus postoperative ERCP. The central argument against an ERCP-first strategy is that 80% of known or suspected CBD stones will have passed before the intervention, making the risks and cost of the intervention unnecessary.[16] The risks of ERCP include acute pancreatitis (3%–7%), bleeding (0.3%–1.4%), ascending cholangitis (1.4%), and perforation (0.6%). The mortality associated with ERCP is 0.2% to 0.9%.[17] Proponents of performing preoperative ERCP argue that if ERCP is unsuccessful a CBDE can be performed at the time of cholecystectomy without requiring a third procedure.

A randomized controlled trial (RCT) of 100 patients undergoing either preoperative ERCP followed by LC or LC with CBDE demonstrated comparable outcomes with similar rates of stone clearance (98% vs. 88%, respectively, not significant),

with slightly shorter hospital length of stay (LOS) and decreased professional fees in the LC+CBDE group.[18] Our preferred strategy in most patients is to proceed straight to LC with selective intraoperative cholangiogram. Laparoscopic CBDE or postoperative ERCP are used when CBD stones are identified (see later). In patients with cholangitis (see Chapters 43, 55, and 56; severe pancreatitis) with hemodynamic instability and persistent hyperbilirubinemia, we recommend preoperative ERCP.[19] This allows for both clearance of the duct and assessment for additional or alternative pathologies such as impacted stones, strictures, or malignancy. In the case of ascending cholangitis, broad-spectrum antibiotics and urgent biliary decompression with ERCP is typically the best option because it is the least invasive and both diagnostic and therapeutic[20] (see Chapters 20, 30, and 43). If ERCP is unavailable or not possible (e.g., history of RNYGB), percutaneous transhepatic biliary decompression (PTC) should be considered (see Chapters 20 and 31). Surgical options, laparoscopic or open, are indicated when less invasive methods are not immediately available, and the patient's condition warrants immediate biliary decompression (see Chapter 37A). In both cholangitis and pancreatitis, once the patient has sufficiently recovered, cholecystectomy should be completed during the same hospitalization because recurrent symptoms are common and can lead to significant morbidity.[21,22]

Intraoperative Choledocholithiasis

When CDL is diagnosed on IOC, and the surgeon experience and diameter of cystic duct are favorable (greater than 8 mm), our preference is to proceed with laparoscopic transcystic CBDE (Fig. 37B.1). If clearance cannot be achieved via the transcystic route, the options are to proceed with transcholedochal CBDE or a postoperative ERCP. Intraoperative ERCP, although uncommon, is also available at some institutions.[23,24] Our preference is to proceed with postoperative ERCP if the stones are less than 2 cm and do not appear to be impacted.

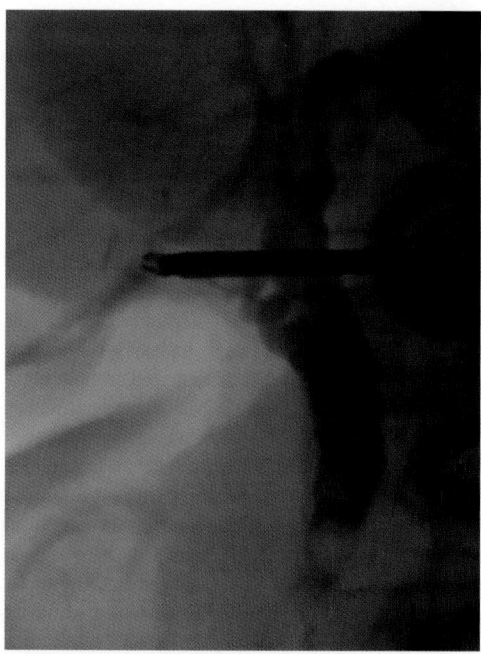

FIGURE 37B.1 Intraoperative cholangiogram demonstrating retained common bile duct stone impacted just above ampulla.

ERCP avoids complications associated with a transcholedochal exploration, including biliary strictures and bile leaks.[25] When the probability of endoscopic clearance is questionable or low, we proceed with a transcholedochal exploration. A number of retrospective studies have shown that LC with CBDE as a single operative procedure is more cost effective and results in shorter hospital LOS than LC and ERCP.[18,26,27] A recent prospective RCT showed that both options were highly effective and equivalent in overall cost, although the hospital LOS was shorter for laparoscopic CBDE.[18]

Postoperative Choledocholithiasis

CDL identified after a cholecystectomy or when there is not a plan to perform a cholecystectomy is typically managed with ERCP; however, occasionally endoscopy is unsuccessful or cannot be performed because of altered anatomy. ERCP fails to cannulate the CBD in 1% to 2% of cases. In this situation we proceed with laparoscopic CBDE. Similarly, if stone extraction fails because of the size of the stones, then laparoscopic exploration is a reasonable next step. In the case of impacted or large stones that cannot be removed endoscopically or surgically, biliary-enteric bypass with either a choledochoduodenostomy (CD) or Roux-en-Y hepaticojejunostomy (RNY-HJ) should be considered (see Chapter 37A).

TECHNIQUES

Laparoscopic Transcystic Common Bile Duct Exploration

The primary method for performing laparoscopic CBDE with minimal morbidity is via the cystic duct. Transcystic exploration is typically performed using standard LC trocar placement, with the cholangiogram catheter placed through the epigastric port into the cystic duct. An additional trocar may be placed in the right midclavicular line to facilitate access to the cystic duct, if necessary (Fig. 37B.2A). The gallbladder is left in situ to provide retraction and counter-traction on the cystic duct, allowing easier passage of wires, catheters, and the choledochoscope.

First, an intraoperative cholangiogram is performed. The cystic duct should be dissected along its length from the insertion into the gallbladder to its origin from the CBD. This allows for adequate exposure and assessment of the caliber of the cystic duct. The cystic duct is clipped distally and partially transected, allowing enough room for final ligation with clips but close enough to the CBD so that a tortuous cystic duct does not need to be navigated for stone extraction. A cholangiogram is performed with 1:1 dilution of saline and contrast to lessen the viscosity of the contrast solution and better visualize filling defects. Care should be taken not to introduce air bubbles into the biliary tree because these can be confused for filling defects on fluoroscopy. This approach works best for stones less than 1 cm and when the cystic duct is short and dilated. If the cystic duct is diminutive, cholangiogram and stone extraction will prove difficult. At times, the cystic duct can be serially dilated with balloon catheters to facilitate access to the CBD.

The first and easiest step in facilitating passage of stones through the ampulla is pharmacologic relaxation of the Sphincter of Oddi using intravenous glucagon (1 mg).[28] Next, the duct is vigorously irrigated with saline or contrast to flush the stones through the ampulla. This technique is most successful for sludge and stones less than 4 mm.[29]

If flushing is unsuccessful, two additional techniques are used: dilation of the ampulla and choledochoscopy. Ampullary dilation is performed by passing a wire through the cystic duct and into the duodenum under fluoroscopic guidance. A 4- to 6-mm diameter, 4-cm long ureteral balloon is advanced over the wire and positioned across the ampulla. After fluoroscopic confirmation of the balloon's position, it is inflated, dilating the ampulla (Fig. 37B.3A). After dilation, the balloon is removed, and the duct is again vigorously irrigated. Finally, a cholangiogram is performed to assess for residual stones.

If ampullary dilation is unsuccessful, choledochoscopy is the next step. Some surgeons prefer to proceed straight to choledochoscopy without attempting ampullary dilation because it allows for direct visualization of the duct and stones. A cholangioscope or ureteroscope is passed transcystically into the common duct. If the cystic duct is too small, the same balloon used for ampullary dilation can be used to gently dilate the cystic duct until it is large enough to allow the cholangioscope to pass. Once the stones are identified, they can be gently

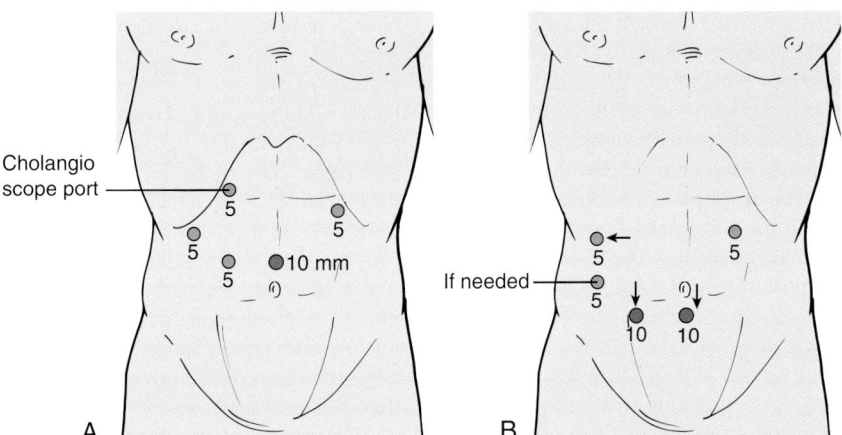

FIGURE 37B.2   A, Illustration demonstrating trocar placement for performing laparoscopic transcystic or transcholedochal common bile duct exploration. An additional trocar may be placed in the right midclavicular line for access to the cystic duct, if necessary. **B,** Illustration demonstrating trocar placement for performing laparoscopic transduodenal common bile duct exploration and sphincterotomy. The trocar position is slightly lower to facilitate mobilization of the duodenum. An additional camera trocar in the right lower quadrant allows for easier visualization of the ampulla.

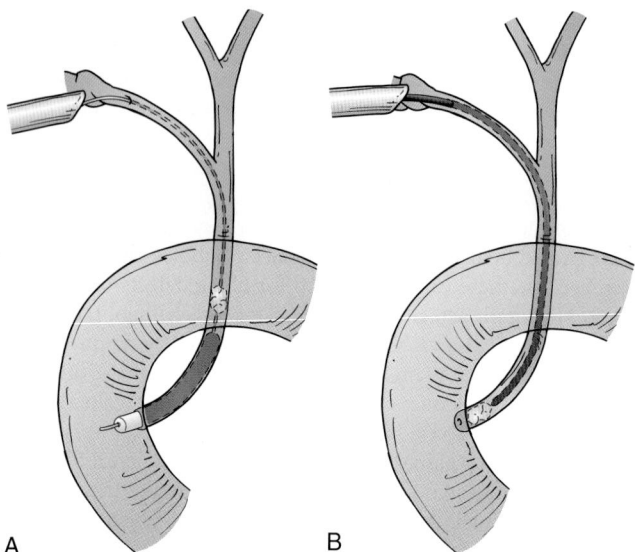

FIGURE 37B.3   A, Illustration demonstrating advancement of a ureteral balloon catheter across the ampulla with dilation. **B,** Illustration demonstrating dislodgement of common bile ducts stones with a cholangioscope. The stones can then be pushed across the ampulla with the scope.

pushed through the ampulla with the tip of the cholangioscope (see Fig. 37B.3B) or they can be snared. To snare the stones, we recommend a helical stone retrieval basket, which is passed through the working channel of the cholangioscope. Under direct visualization the basket is then passed beyond the stone. Once the basket is distal to the stone, it is opened and withdrawn until the stone is captured. The snare is then closed, and the stone is removed through the cystic duct. Care must be taken to avoid causing injury with the snare. It is a stiff instrument and ductal perforation or penetration into the pancreas is possible, particularly with snares that have a blunt tip. Some authors recommend blind or fluoroscopically guided wire basket stone capture and extraction. In our experience, this has proven less successful and the risk for injury is higher. There are two options to deal with large stones that cannot be extracted through the cystic duct. Large stones that are soft can often be crushed by tightening the snare around them. The debris can then be snared individually or pushed through the ampulla and into the duodenum. For large stones that are too hard to crush, a laser or mechanical lithotripsy catheter can be passed through the cholangioscope allowing the stone to be fractured under direct visualization.[30] Finally, in ducts with significant inflammation or strictures, biopsy should be considered. Malignancy may be an inciting event in the development of ductal debris or ductal obstruction. Complications of transcystic CBDE, as observed by Paganini et al., include bile leak (1%), acute pancreatitis (0.5%), and rupture of the cystic duct (6.8%).[31]

The success rate of a laparoscopic transcystic approach to CDL by experienced surgical teams is 80% to 90%.[29] There are a number of reasons a transcystic CBDE can fail. In some cases, the cystic duct is too small, tortuous, or even obliterated and passage of a catheter into the CBD is difficult or impossible. It can be difficult to pull stones retrograde into the cystic duct from the CBD because the tendency is for stones to slip upward into the common hepatic duct. Occasionally the cystic duct inserts into the very distal CBD or at an acute angle. This

can make accessing the proximal CBD challenging. Large stones, impacted stones, and significant inflammation can all increase the difficulty of clearing the duct transcystically. In such cases, the surgeon must decide whether to proceed with a transcholedochal exploration or defer to postoperative ERCP. If the CBD is less than 1 cm in diameter and in the absence of large impacted stones, our preference is to proceed with postoperative ERCP because it has a high rate of success and less potential morbidity.

Laparoscopic Transcholedochal Common Bile Duct Exploration

As discussed, laparoscopic choledochotomy is indicated when the transcystic approach fails or in the presence of multiple, large, or impacted stones (Fig. 37B.4A). Choledochotomy should be avoided if the CBD is less than 1 cm in diameter.[25] The CBD is accessed by exposing the second portion of the duodenum and mobilizing the duodenum down to the level of the pancreas. Excessive mobilization and skeletonization of the CBD should be avoided to preserve blood supply to the proximal duct. Stay sutures may be placed anteriorly on either side of the choledochotomy (preserving the 3 o'clock and 9 o'clock blood supply) to allow for traction on the CBD. A longitudinal choledochotomy is then made on the distal CBD. The choledochotomy should be long enough for removal of the largest stone and passage of the choledochoscope. Typically, a 1 cm incision is sufficient to meet both of these goals (see Fig. 37B.4B–C).

A cholangioscope is passed directly into the duct and a thorough exploration of the proximal and distal duct is performed. Stones may be flushed out of the ductotomy, removed directly with atraumatic graspers (see Fig. 37B.4D–E), or extracted using a snare passed through the cholangioscope as described in the transcystic approach. There is a mechanical advantage to removing impacted stones directly through a choledochotomy, although stones impacted in the head of the pancreas may require a transduodenal approach.

After clearance of the duct and completion of the exploration, the ductotomy is closed primarily or over a T-tube. Historically, T-tubes were used to decompress the biliary tree and were thought to minimize bile leaks (see Chapter 37A). They also allow postoperative percutaneous access to the CBD. T-tubes, however, have potential morbidity including inadvertent displacement, erosion, cholangitis, and nutritional deficiencies from bile loss.[32] In addition, T-tubes can be painful and problematic to manage. Several RCTs have concluded that primary closure of the duct does not result in a higher rate of bile leaks.[33] These studies have uniformly shown a decreased hospital LOS, shorter operative time, lower hospital expenses, and earlier return to normal activity in patients who did not have a T-tube.[34] In addition, because of the high success rates of duct clearance by choledochotomy, the need for T-tubes to provide percutaneous access for retained stones is unlikely.[33] A recent meta-analysis of 16 studies and 1770 patients concluded that primary duct closure is feasible after laparoscopic CBDE and is associated with fewer postoperative complications, decreased operative time, shorter LOS, and lower median hospital expenses.[35]

If clearance of the duct has been achieved with confidence and there are no concerns of distal obstruction, our preference is to primarily close the choledochotomy, without a T-tube, with simple interrupted sutures spaced evenly to avoid duct ischemia. We generally use 5-0 monofilament slowly absorbable

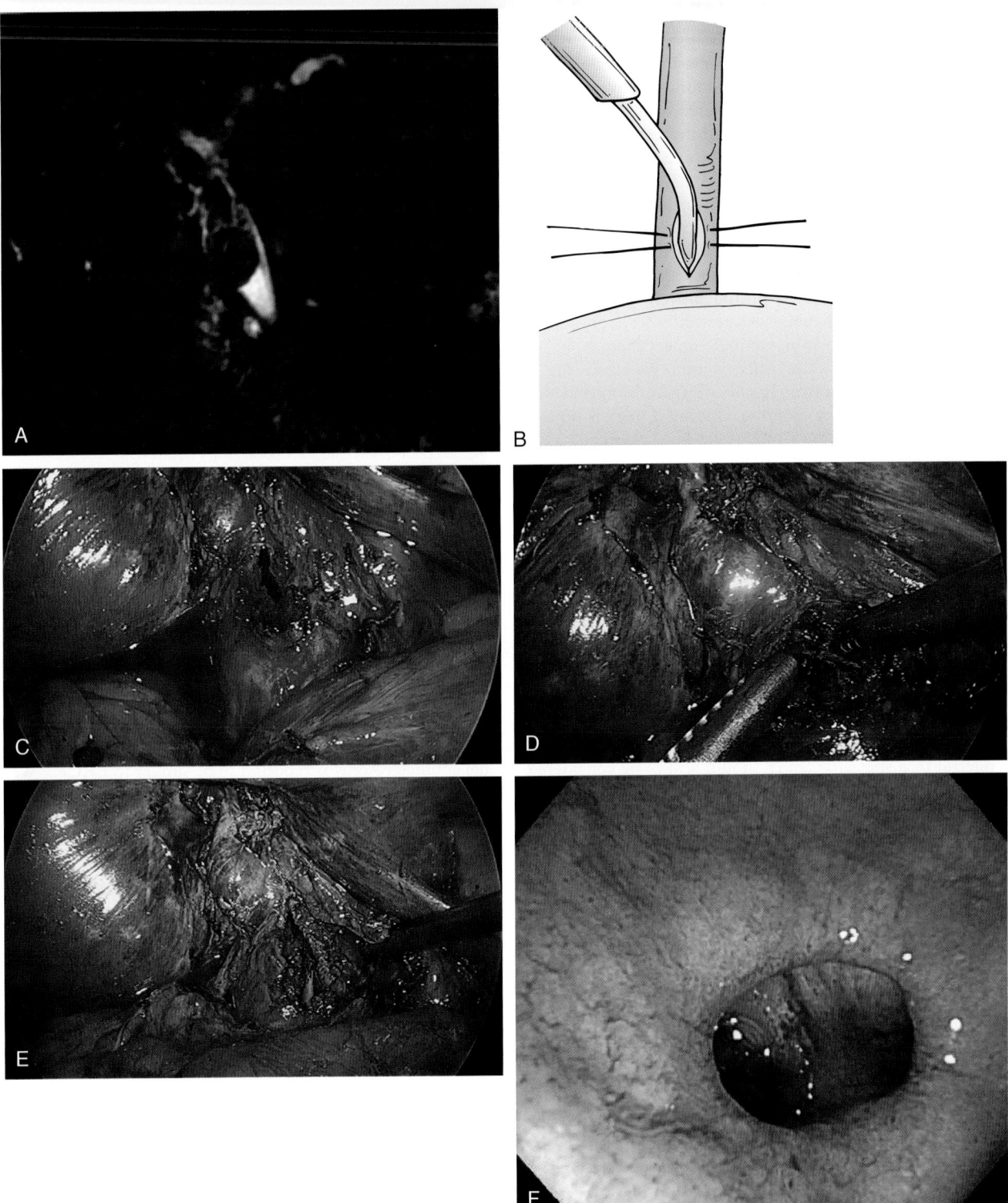

FIGURE 37B.4   A, Preoperative magnetic resonance cholangiopancreatogram (MRCP) demonstrating a significant burden of common bile duct stones refractory to endoscopic lithotripsy. **B,** Illustration demonstrating an anterior choledochotomy made to accommodate the cholangioscope. Two stay stitches are placed at 3 o'clock and 9 o'clock to allow for traction on the common bile duct. **C,** Intraoperative photograph of anterior ductotomy at the time of laparoscopic transcholedochal common bile duct exploration. **D,** Intraoperative photograph demonstrating transcholedochal stone extraction. **E,** Intraoperative photograph demonstrating the residual ductotomy and endoscopically placed stent after stone extraction. This defect was repaired with a choledochoduodenostomy. **F,** Endoscopic image of choledochoduodenal anastomosis 3 months postoperatively.

suture. T-tubes may be used if there is concern for residual stones or if the caliber or quality of the tissue of the CBD is friable and inadequate for primary closure. In these cases, biliary-enteric bypass should be considered for definitive management (see Chapter 37A). If a T-tube is used, once in place, the ductotomy is closed around the base of the tube using a few sutures adjacent to the side of the T-tube and the tube is exteriorized through a lateral trocar site. A final cholangiogram through the T-tube is performed at the conclusion of the case. Tubes are left in place for 3 weeks to promote formation of an inflammatory tract around the tube. The T-tube can then be gently removed, and the tract will collapse and seal spontaneously. If stones are discovered postoperatively, percutaneous stone extraction via the T-tube is successful in 95% of cases.[36] Surgical drains are not placed routinely unless there is an increased risk for bile leak or a T-tube is used. We clamp the T-tube once the patient is tolerating a diet if there is no evidence of obstruction. The surgical drain is removed if there is no evidence of a bile leak after the T-tube is has been clamped.

The overall success rate of laparoscopic choledochotomy is 83% to 96%, with a morbidity rate of 5% to 10% and mortality rate of 1%.[25] As mentioned previously, this procedure is not without complications. Bile leak (reported as high as 14%) and postoperative CBD strictures are the most feared complications.[27] Choledochotomy has similar rates of pancreatitis (7.3% vs. 8.8%), retained stones (2.4% vs. 4.4%), reoperation (7.3% vs. 6.6%), and overall morbidity (17% vs. 13%) as ERCP.[27] Major advantages of the transcholedochal approach include easier access to both upper and lower ductal system and extraction of any size stone. Conversion to an open procedure must always be considered in difficult cases, although challenging laparoscopic cases are frequently also challenging open cases, and referral to a specialty center should always be considered before converting to a laparotomy. In patients with a high risk of recurrent stone disease or formation of a biliary stricture, usually because of inflammation or a small duct, a definitive bypass should be considered (see Fig. 37B.4F).

Laparoscopic Transduodenal Sphincterotomy and Common Bile Duct Exploration

For impacted stones refractory to clearance by endoscopy or CBDE, laparoscopic transduodenal exploration with sphincterotomy is an alternative modality for duct clearance. Nevertheless, this procedure is technically challenging and should be reserved for unique circumstances and only attempted by experienced laparoscopic surgeons. This procedure can typically be performed with a 4 or 5 trocar technique. We have found it useful to place the trocars lower than the typical approach to cholecystectomy. An additional camera trocar in the right lower quadrant will also provide a better angle for visualization of the ampullary reconstruction (see Fig. 37B.2B).

To gain access to the duodenum, the right colon is mobilized and a Kocher maneuver is completed. With the duodenum elevated, it may be useful to place a surgical sponge posterior to the head of the pancreas. This will elevate the duodenum and absorb enteric fluids leaked into the field once the duodenotomy is created. A longitudinal incision is made in the antimesenteric wall of the second portion of the duodenum using electrocautery or ultrasonic shears to expose the major duodenal papilla. If the papilla is not easily located and the cystic and CBD are patent, a cholangiogram catheter or wire can be inserted via the cystic duct and passed through the

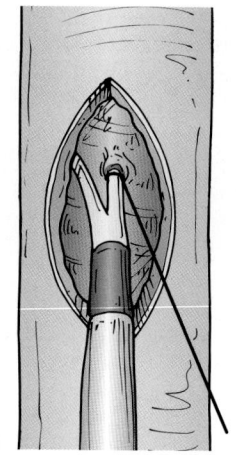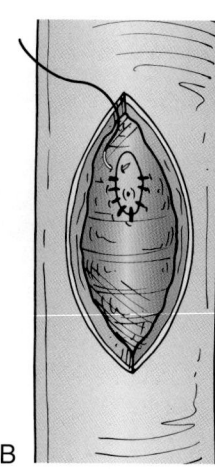

FIGURE 37B.5 A, Illustration of transduodenal sphincterotomy made at the 11 o'clock position of the ampulla with a cautery device. **B,** Illustration of laparoscopic interrupted suture repair of the ampulla re-approximating the bile duct mucosa to the duodenum.

ampulla to aid in identification. Once the papilla is identified, the CBD is intubated using a wire or silicone tube. Electrocautery or ultrasonic shears are then used to create a sphincterotomy at the 11 o'clock position on the papilla (Fig. 37B.5A).[37] This facilitates a transduodenal CBDE using cholangiocatheters, balloons, or a cholangioscope. Once clearance of the CBD is achieved, the mucosa of the bile duct is sutured to the duodenum with interrupted 5-0 monofilament slowly absorbable sutures (see Fig. 37B.5B).[37] The duodenotomy is then closed to complete the case. The risk of complications from transduodenal sphincterotomy is reported to be similar to ERCP.[38] We use surgical drains selectively and, if used, they are removed within a few days of the operation if there is no evidence of bile leak.

Laparoscopic Biliary-Enteric Bypass

In patients at moderate to high risk for recurrent CBD stones, or in patients with distal inflammatory strictures, biliary-enteric bypass may provide the most durable result (see Chapters 37A and 42). The two primary options for bypass are CD or RNY-HJ. Currently there is inadequate comparative data to recommend one technique over another. There are a number of retrospective studies comparing the two anastomoses that show equivalent outcomes and morbidity, and selection of the appropriate technique depends on intraoperative technical factors, clinical findings, and patient anatomy.[39–41] CD has been criticized in the past because of concern for reflux of enteric contents into the CBD leading to chronic inflammation and recurring bouts of cholangitis, referred to as *sump syndrome*.[42,43] Results of analyses by several authors suggest that symptoms associated with sump syndrome may actually be because of a mechanical problem associated with a narrow anastomosis and/or stricture.[44–46]

Our current preference is laparoscopic CD because it is technically easier, leads to a more physiologic reconstruction, and allows direct access to the biliary system should further evaluation or manipulation of the duct prove necessary.[47,48] Nevertheless, CD can be difficult in the setting of significant duodenal inflammation or inadequate duodenal mobility after Kocherization. In these cases, we proceed with laparoscopic RNY-HJ.

To perform a laparoscopic CD, we use a trocar placement similar to that described for the transduodenal sphincterotomy (see Fig. 37B.1B). A Kocher maneuver is performed, and the duodenum is mobilized to perform a tension-free anastomosis to the CBD. The degree of Kocherization ultimately depends on individual anatomy and mobility of the duodenum. Next, approximately 2 cm of the inferior and anterior surface of the distal CBD is exposed. The dissection plane should remain anterior to the duct to avoid injury of the blood supply to the proximal duct. A thorough laparoscopic ultrasound examination should be performed to identity the CBD and verify the location of any stones. A 1.5 cm supraduodenal longitudinal choledochotomy is made in the anterior wall of the duct using electrocautery or ultrasonic shears. A choledochoscope is then inserted through the choledochotomy and a thorough examination both proximal and distally is performed. The appearance of any stricture should raise concern for underlying malignancy, and biopsies should be performed at this point if there are any concerns for a neoplastic process. A 1 cm longitudinal duodenotomy is made in the adjacent post bulbar duodenum. The duodenotomy is made slightly shorter than the ductotomy because of the inevitable stretching of the duodenotomy (Fig. 37B.6A).

With the advent of the absorbable barbed suture,[49] we now perform a single layer running CD with two 3-0 absorbable

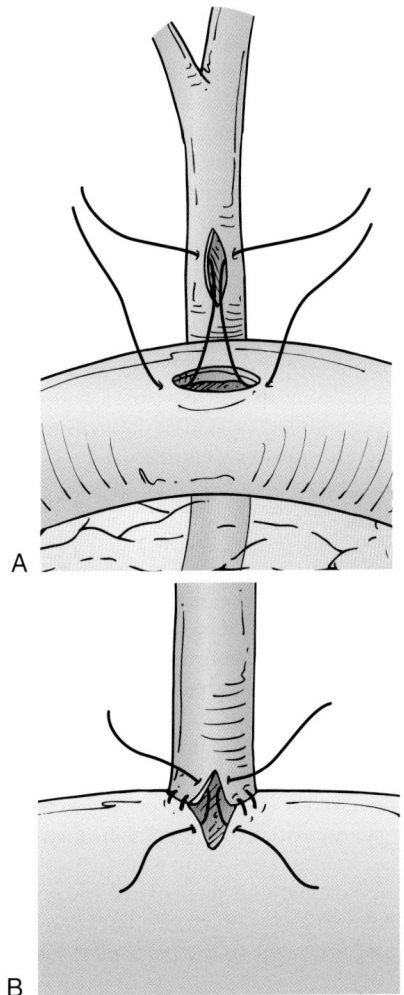

FIGURE 37B.6   A, Illustration demonstrating the setup of a choledochoduodenostomy anastomosis. Stay sutures can be placed to ensure appropriate alignment. **B,** Illustration demonstrating completion of the choledochoduodenostomy with the final sutures placed in the superior apex.

barbed sutures. We place two to three interrupted posterior 3-0 Vicryl sutures to secure the inferior apex of the anastomosis. The posterior sutures are tied internally. The lateral and medial sides are then run sequentially from the inferior apex, rolling the duodenum up to complete the anastomosis (see Fig. 37B.6B). To complete the anastomosis, two to three additional buttressing stitches can be placed in the duodenum to secure it to bile duct, before cutting the suture and removing the needle. No knots are required in the barbed suture. Alternatively, an interrupted anastomosis can be performed with multiple 3-0 Vicryl sutures. Tying the sutures as they are placed can limit access during placement of the subsequent sutures, but leaving too many sutures untied makes it difficult to identify the appropriate sutures and frequently leads to tangling of the sutures. To avoid these problems, we typically place two to three sutures at a time, tying the deeper sutures after the shallower sutures are placed. Alternating dyed and undyed sutures and clipping the suture tails also helps in identification of the sutures and prevents tangling. Final inspection of the anastomosis should confirm that there is no leakage of bile from the anastomosis and no tension on the duodenum or duct. Similar to laparoscopic sphincterotomy, drains are used selectively and removed early. We also use upper gastrointestinal contrast studies selectively before starting a diet in patients who are at high risk of an anastomotic leak.

Trocar placement for laparoscopic RNY-HJ is similar to that used for sphincterotomy and CD, although a slightly lower placement may facilitate access to and division of the jejunum. Access to the common hepatic duct may require mobilization of the right colon and more extensive Kocherization of the duodenum. Laparoscopic ultrasound examination is again used to facilitate identification of the portal structures. We typically prefer an end-to-side hepaticojejunostomy (Fig. 37B.7A), although this requires circumferential dissection and division of the duct distally. In some cases, significant periportal inflammation makes circumferential dissection of the CBD near impossible and fraught with potential iatrogenic injury to the portal vein or right hepatic artery. In these cases, a side-to-side hepaticojejunostomy should be considered (see Fig. 37B.7B).

To create the Roux limb, the jejunum is divided using an endostapler approximately 20 cm distal to the ligament of Trietz. The mesentery is then divided to allow the Roux limb to reach the bile duct without tension. The limb is preferentially passed antecolic; however, if this results in too much tension, it can be passed retrocolic through the transverse mesocolon just to the right of the middle colic vessels. The jejunojejunostomy is created in the infracolic position 30 to 40 cm distal to the future bilioenteric anastomosis.

The hepaticojejunostomy is created in a single layer using 3-0 absorbable barbed suture or 4-0 or 5-0 interrupted absorbable sutures (Vicryl or PDS). Depending on the size of the duct, this anastomosis may be created using interrupted sutures (ducts less than 1 cm), in a fashion similar to that described for the CD, or running sutures (ducts greater than 1 cm). Again, drains are used selectively.

SPECIAL CIRCUMSTANCES

Choledocholithiasis after Roux-en-Y Gastric Bypass

Laparoscopic CBDE or laparoscopic-assisted ERCP may be the only options in patients with a history of gastrointestinal surgery. With the introduction and rapid expansion of RNYGB

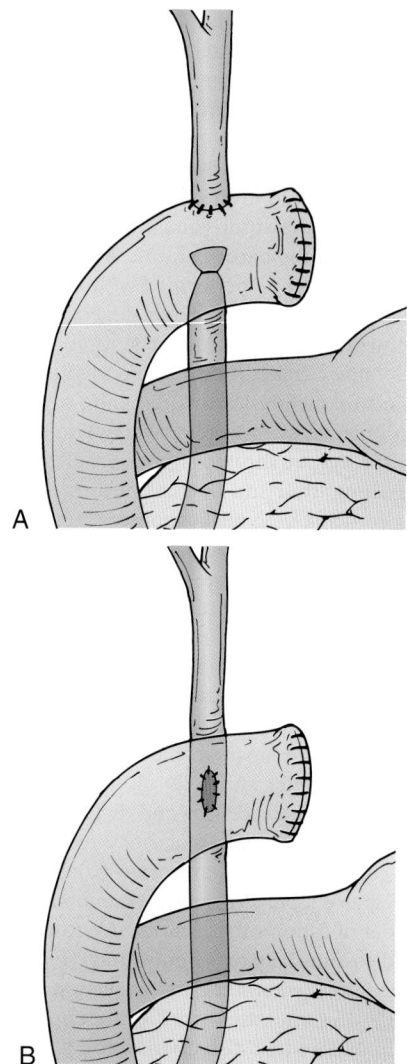

FIGURE 37B.7 **A,** Illustration demonstrating an end-side hepaticojejunostomy. **B,** Illustration demonstrating a side-side hepaticojejunostomy.

single-balloon endoscopes can facilitate successful performance of ERCP in nearly 80% of patients[53] (see Chapter 30). Nevertheless, the majority of centers do not currently have access to these technologies, and the procedures are time consuming and technically difficult to perform.[54] Some studies have suggested that EUS-guided gastrogastrostomy formation to facilitate ERCP may be an alternative to double- or single-balloon endoscopy.[55] In these cases, laparoscopic access to the distal gastric remnant may be a straightforward solution to allow performance of an intraoperative ERCP and/or EUS, minimizing time, cost, and potential postprocedure complications. One study has even shown this technique to be more cost-effective than double-balloon enteroscopy.[23]

Laparoscopic-Assisted Endoscopic Retrograde Cholangiopancreatography

At laparoscopy, the gastric remnant is identified, and the front wall of the stomach is exposed. The gastric remnant may need to be mobilized from surrounding adhesions to adequately reach the anterior abdominal wall, with care being taken to avoid injury to the mesentery of the gastrojejunal limb. We place two 0 sutures through the abdominal wall and through the anterior wall of the stomach adjacent to the future gastrotomy site with a Keith needle or suture passer. These sutures are used to retract and stabilize the stomach to the anterior abdominal wall. Hardy sutures should be used because they can snap from torque on the trocar site during ERCP causing the stomach to fall away from the abdominal wall and subsequent loss of access. A gastrotomy is then made in the location that will allow easy passage of the endoscope through the pylorus. A 15-mm, radially dilating trocar with a balloon tip or a single port device is inserted through the abdominal wall and directly into the gastrotomy. A sterile drape with Ioban is placed around the trocar and used to preserve the sterile field. The endoscope can then be placed through the trocar or single port device into the stomach to perform the ERCP. After the conclusion of the ERCP, the gastrotomy is sutured closed with 3-0 absorbable suture in either a single or double layer. Surgical drains are rarely indicated after this procedure.

CONCLUSION

The first laparoscopic biliary surgery was performed more than 35 years ago. During the last three decades, substantial progress has been made in surgical skill sets, experience, and technology. Our understanding of how and when to apply these minimally invasive tools has greatly reduced the suffering of patients with CDL. We now have the ability to diagnose biliary stone disease, differentiate it from neoplastic processes, and treat it with very high levels of success and decreasing levels of morbidity.

We have reviewed a wide range of approaches to the management of patients with CBD stones. In managing these patients, surgeons must assess their own skill set and the capabilities of their hospital and team. They must understand the tools and talent available within their institutions. Finally, they must apply this knowledge to the particular clinical scenario of their patient.

The references for this chapter can be found online by accessing the accompanying Expert Consult website.

procedures, it is becoming increasingly common to have patients present in whom an ERCP is either not possible or extremely challenging. A recent review of the National Inpatient Sample demonstrated that nearly 2 million bariatric surgeries were performed between 1993 and 2016, with substantial improvements in complication rates.[50] Approximately 160,000 procedures are performed annually, with more than 98% of procedures now performed laparoscopically, 28% of which are RNYGB. Approximately 40% of patients undergoing bariatric procedures will develop gallstones or biliary sludge within six months of surgery, with less than 50% of patients becoming symptomatic.[51] The performance of LC at the time of gastric bypass surgery remains controversial, with some studies demonstrating increased operative times and hospital LOS. Prophylactic ursodiol has been shown in an RCT to reduce the incidence of gallstone formation after gastric bypass surgery.[52] Because of these factors, late presentation of gallstone disease and CDL will continue to be a persistent clinical challenge.

In patients who have undergone a previous RNYGB procedure, access to the ampulla of Vater using double- and

Stones in the bile duct: Endoscopic and percutaneous approaches

Satish Nagula

HISTORICAL OVERVIEW

In the 1970s and 1980s, endoscopic retrograde cholangiopancreatography (ERCP) transformed the diagnostic approach to suspected biliary disease and jaundice (see Chapters 20 and 30). Similarly, in the years since it was first performed in humans,[1,2] endoscopic sphincterotomy (ES) has had a dramatic impact on the management of biliary disease, specifically in the treatment of common bile duct (CBD) stones. The widespread availability of ES has made endoscopic stone extraction the primary modality for the management of choledocholithiasis. Interest in ERCP and endoscopic sphincterotomy as definitive therapy for CBD stones grew in the 1990s after the introduction of laparoscopic cholecystectomy (see Chapter 36). Patient-related factors, clinical judgment, availability of expertise, and current evidence from clinical trials must be combined to decide on an endoscopic, percutaneous, or surgical approach. Although ERCP as a diagnostic modality has been replaced by noninvasive imaging modalities such as magnetic resonance cholangiopancreatography (MRCP) (see Chapter 13), it remains the major nonoperative tool for the management of biliary diseases such as choledocholithiasis and obstructive jaundice.

INDICATIONS FOR ENDOSCOPIC THERAPY

Patients with choledocholithiasis may present with asymptomatic stones on noninvasive imaging or direct cholangiography or with a variety of clinical symptoms (see Chapter 33), such as cholestasis, pain, cholangitis (see Chapter 43), and pancreatitis (see Chapter 55). In the early days of ES—at a time when few endoscopy centers could offer the technique and criticisms by surgical experts were common—it was considered justifiable only in elderly postcholecystectomy patients with recurrent or retained bile duct stones who were at high risk of serious complications from open surgical CBD exploration or reexploration.[3] The impressive success of ES in this group, combined with expanded availability, a low rate of complications, and strong patient preference, has led to ERCP becoming the primary modality for the management of CBD stones.

The endoscopist now must consider several clearly defined conditions for which endoscopic management may be indicated in patients with definite or suspected bile duct stones[4,5]:

1. Acute cholangitis
2. Visualized CBD stone on abdominal ultrasound, endoscopic ultrasound (EUS), computed tomography (CT), MRCP, or intraoperative cholangiogram
3. High suspicion of CBD stones: cholelithiasis, dilated CBD, and abnormal liver biochemical tests
4. Worsening gallstone pancreatitis
5. Recurrent CBD stones or gallstone pancreatitis, nonsurgical candidate for cholecystectomy

ENDOSCOPIC TECHNIQUES

An endoscopy service that treats CBD stones must have access to an appropriate endoscopy facility and high-quality fluoroscopy. The endoscopy team must be fully cognizant of all basic ERCP maneuvers, less frequently used techniques, and potential complications and their management. It is essential to explain the nature of the procedure to the patient and to outline the purpose, benefits, advantages, alternatives, and potential hazards (see Chapters 20 and 30).

On successful deep biliary cannulation with a sphincterotome, a cholangiogram is initially performed, which defines the ductal anatomy and the extent of the stone burden. ES is usually the first therapeutic step in stone extraction. Balloon dilation of the biliary sphincter is an alternative to ES, but this has fallen out of favor due to increased risks of severe post-ERCP pancreatitis.[6–8] Standard pull-type sphincterotomes allow a vertical incision to be made from the papillary orifice in a cephalad direction along the intramural course of the CBD for a variable length (average, 10 to 15 mm), depending on local anatomy, the degree of CBD dilation, and the size of the stone to be removed (Fig. 37C.1). The incision is produced by the controlled application of monopolar electrocautery delivered by a generator specifically designed for endoscopic use. It is fundamental to ES technique that complete control of wire tension and electrocautery be maintained at all times. "Smart" generators incorporate a pulsed generator (Erbe, Tubingen, Germany; ConMed Endoscopic Technologies, Billerica, MA) with feedback-controlled power output, thus avoiding a "zipper effect" and reducing pancreatitis and bleeding.

Occasionally, a *precut sphincterotomy*, also referred to as an *access papillotomy*, is needed to initiate ES when the standard instrument cannot be inserted deeply. This incision is often needed when cannulation has been prevented by an impacted stone. The needle-knife is more useful in this situation because the intramural CBD is usually grossly distended and easily incised, starting from the papilla and extending cephalad. Needle-knife fistulotomy is a variant of this technique; the incision is begun above the papilla to form a choledochoduodenal fistulotomy. This technique is similar in efficacy to precut sphincterotomy, but more often it requires mechanical lithotripsy (ML) and may have a lower rate of pancreatitis.[9] Patients with Billroth II partial gastrectomy (Fig. 37C.2) and Roux-en-Y bypass operations present special problems to the endoscopist, and numerous methods have been described to obtain successful cannulation[10,11] and removal of CBD stones[12] (see Chapter 37B).

It is standard practice to attempt stone extraction from the CBD immediately after ES. The two accessory instruments used most commonly for this are the Dormia-type basket (Fig. 37C.3) and the Fogarty-type balloon (Figs. 37C.4 and 37C.5), which

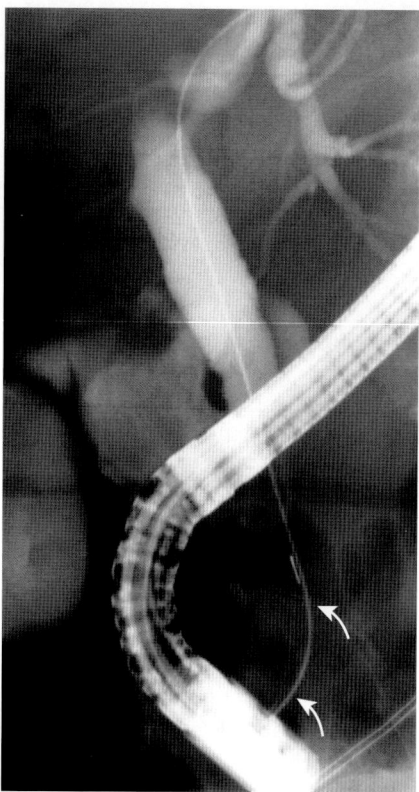

FIGURE 37C.1 Endoscopic retrograde cholangiopancreatography showing a dilated bile duct, a single duct stone just below the endoscope, a guidewire, and a sphincterotome in position during sphincterotomy *(arrows)*.

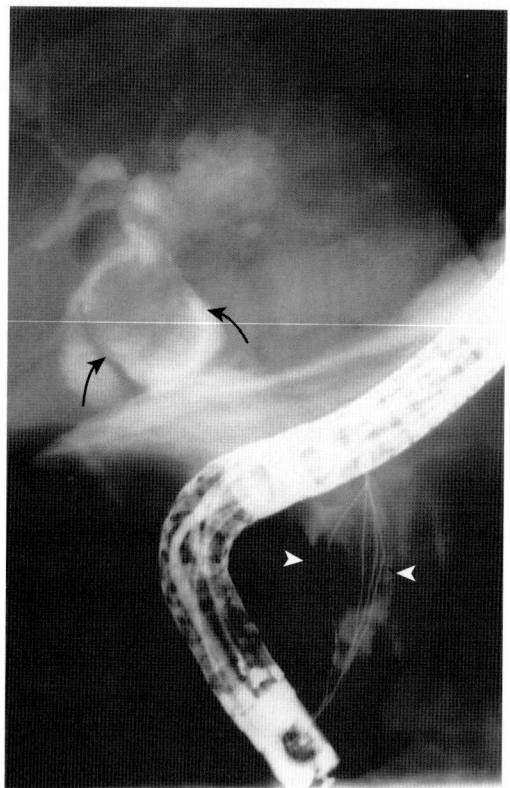

FIGURE 37C.3 Endoscopic retrograde cholangiopancreatography showing large stone in the proximal bile duct *(arrows)* and basket extraction of a distal bile duct stone *(chevrons)* after endoscopic sphincterotomy.

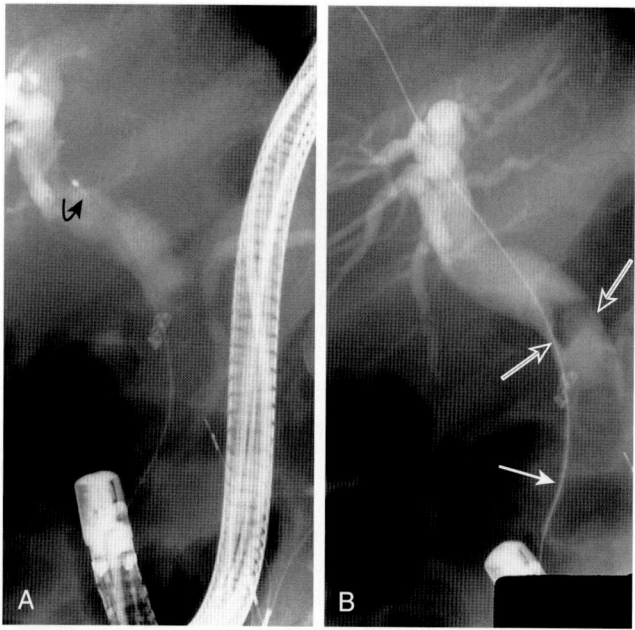

FIGURE 37C.2 Endoscopic retrograde cholangiopancreatography in a patient with Billroth II partial gastrectomy showing insertion of a catheter *(curved arrow)* **(A)** and placement of a guidewire and short biliary endoprosthesis *(solid arrow)* **(B)** immediately before needle-knife sphincterotomy and demonstration of common bile duct stones *(open arrows)*.

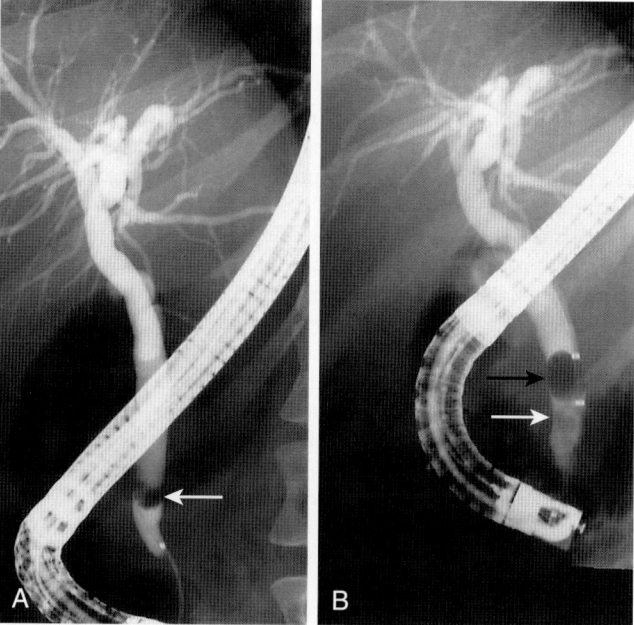

FIGURE 37C.4 Endoscopic retrograde cholangiopancreatography showing a nondilated bile duct containing a single distal stone *(white arrow)* **(A)** and extraction balloon *(black arrow, right)* **(B)** placed above the stone immediately before its removal after endoscopic sphincterotomy.

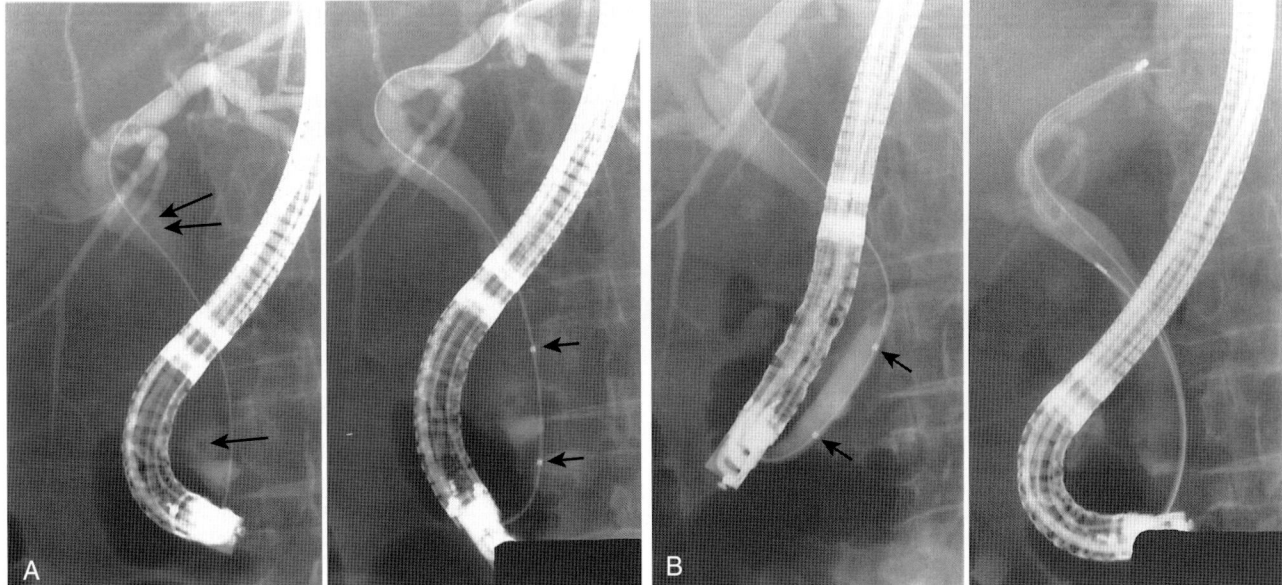

FIGURE 37C.5   Endoscopic retrograde cholangiopancreatography series showing technique of balloon dilation of the papilla for extraction of small stones. **A,** Initial cholangiography with demonstration of three small stones *(long arrows, left)* and placement of a guidewire and insertion of an 8-mm dilating balloon located between two radiopaque markers *(small arrows, right).* **B,** Inflation of the dilating balloon *(left)* followed by insertion of an extraction basket for stone removal *(right).*

are greater than 90% successful in clearing the CBD. Occlusion cholangiography is performed after stone extraction to confirm complete ductal clearance.

Difficult Stones

Difficulties in extraction of CBD stones are either related to anatomic factors affecting the ability to perform an adequate ES or related to complex morphology of the stones themselves (see Chapters 30 and 37B). An inaccessible papilla may be related to aberrant anatomy or unfavorable duodenal or papillary structures, such as a periampullary diverticulum, or prior surgery, such as Billroth II or Roux-en-Y reconstruction. Techniques have been described for the unique challenge of selective bile duct cannulation in a patient with a Billroth II partial gastrectomy.[10] The performance of ES in Billroth II or Roux-en-Y anatomy is also a challenge because the visualized anatomy is inverted. In especially difficult cases, needle-knife sphincterotomy with a stentor guidewire used as a guide may be an option, or specially designed reverse-direction accessories. Roux-en-Y gastric bypass patients pose an extra challenge for the endoscopist due to the long pancreaticobiliary limb. ERCP using overtube-assisted enteroscopy has been performed successfully in patients with Roux-en-Y gastric bypass, with a recent meta-analysis demonstrating a 75% technical success rate and an 8% adverse event rate.[13]

When ES has been successfully performed, extraction may be hindered by a variety of stone factors, including size, number, consistency, shape, and location of stones, as well as ductal factors such as contour and diameter at the level of and distal to the stones, and the presence of coexisting pathology (e.g., stricture or tumor). Stones that are likely to be more difficult to extract and may require adjuvant techniques to remove them are those that appear larger than the endoscope on radiographic imaging (usually >15 mm); stones that are numerous or hard in consistency; stones that are square, piston shaped, or faceted that tightly fit the bile duct or that are packed against each

other; intrahepatic stones; or stones located proximal to a stricture or narrowed distal bile duct or in a sigmoid-shaped duct.

Methods that have been developed to dilate the papillary orifice, reduce stone size, and facilitate endoscopic removal include endoscopic papillary large balloon dilation (EPLBD), ML, intracorporeal lithotripsy with laser or electrohydraulic probes, extracorporeal shockwave lithotripsy (ESWL), and chemical contact dissolution therapy. Treatment options must be discussed jointly by the endoscopist, surgeon, and interventional radiologist when difficulties are encountered (Fig. 37C.6).

Extracorporeal Shockwave Lithotripsy

ESWL with a variety of lithotripsy machines is now an alternative to endoscopic management of difficult bile duct stones. In contrast to intracorporeal techniques, direct contact with the stone is unnecessary. Most centers localize stones with fluoroscopic focusing during contrast perfusion of the bile duct through an endoscopically placed nasobiliary catheter or percutaneous drain.[14,15] Ponchon et al.[16] reported ESWL success with an ultrasound localization system, although it was less effective when multiple stones were present. Several large series indicated success rates for ESWL stone fragmentation of 53% to 91% and duct clearance in 58% to 90%.[17–20] Minor complications are common and include biliary pain, hemobilia, transient liver function test elevations, and cutaneous petechiae. Overall, with the use of endoscopic techniques such as ML, EHL, laser lithotripsy, and ESWL, one report showed successful stone removal in 98% of 217 patients, with only 5 patients requiring surgery.[21] However, given the high efficacy of newer endoscopic techniques, ESWL is currently rarely used for bile duct stones.

Mechanical Lithotripsy

Removal of large CBD stones is a challenge for the most skilled endoscopists (see Chapter 30).[22,23] ML remains an excellent option for stones that cannot be removed by conventional

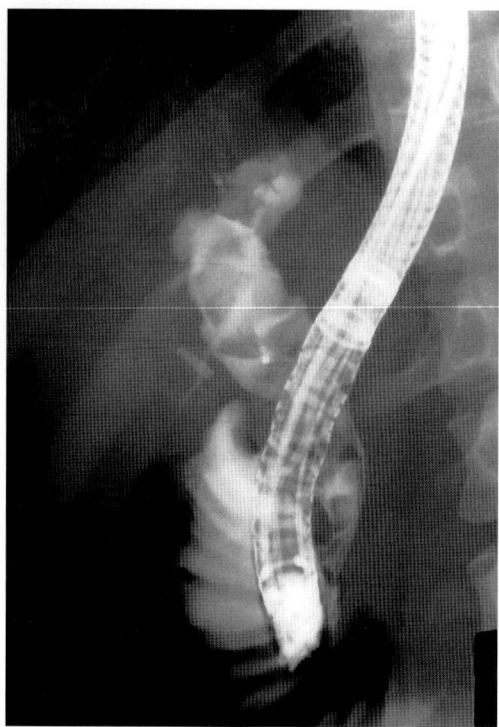

FIGURE 37C.6 Endoscopic retrograde cholangiopancreatography showing a dilated bile duct containing multiple faceted stones in a postcholecystectomy patient positioned such that standard extraction techniques might be difficult.

This procedure can be performed through the endoscope instrumentation channel, or it can be done after the endoscope has been removed from the patient and a metal sheath has been extended over the inner Teflon catheter. The end of the metal sheath is attached to a winding mechanism, which retracts the basket when cranked and impales the stone against the rigid distal end of the metal sheath leading to stone fracturing. The stone fragments can be removed with the same basket or a standard retrieval basket or balloon. In experienced centers, this technique allows removal of more than 90% of difficult bile stones that are refractory to standard extraction techniques, but multiple procedures may be required to achieve complete ductal clearance.[24–27]

Endoscopic Papillary Large Balloon Dilation

EPLBD in conjunction with ES has greatly improved the rates of ductal clearance of difficult stones without the need for advanced ERCP lithotripsy techniques. The first report of EPLBD (12–20 mm) with ES was described in 2003, when a retrospective review demonstrated that 38 out of 40 patients with large stones previously unable to be removed with standard techniques had successful ductal clearance with acceptable complication rates.[28] Further research has shown that endoscopic sphincterotomy with EPLBD can obviate the need for ML. A review of seven studies included 902 patients and compared ES with EPBLD versus ES with standard techniques.[29] The authors found no differences in ductal clearance between the EPLBD and standard-techniques groups (98% vs. 95%, $P = .6$), but patients in the EPLBD group needed less ML. The use of EPLBD had a relative risk reduction of 0.58 (0.32–0.74) in terms of adverse events. For large bile duct stones (>13 mm), EPLBD results in improved ductal clearance (96% vs. 74%, $P < 0.001$) with reduced need for ML (3.9% vs. 35.6%, $P < 0.001$) compared with ES alone.[30]

Although the studies mentioned in the previous sections demonstrate the safety of EPLBD, there has been concern for the rare but serious complications, such as bleeding, perforation,

techniques because it can be used safely and effectively during the initial endoscopic procedure. Mechanical lithotripters are modifications of standard Dormia baskets and possess great tensile strength (Fig. 37C.7). The reinforced basket is opened in the CBD, and the stone is entrapped within the braided wires.

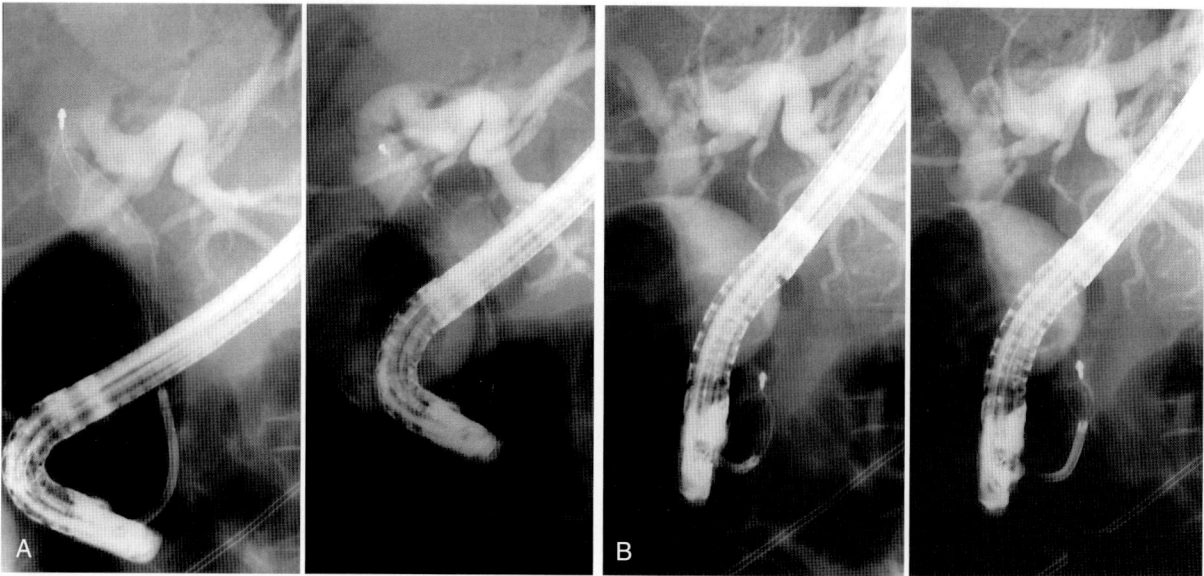

FIGURE 37C.7 Endoscopic retrograde cholangiopancreatography sequence showing use of transendoscopic mechanical lithotripsy. **A,** Positioning of the mechanical lithotripsy basket with its metallic sheath in the proximal bile duct (left) and its slow withdrawal toward the distally placed stone to entrap it (right). **B,** Process of lithotripsy after stone entrapment within the basket (left) as the basket wires cut through the stone (right) to produce stone fragmentation.

and pancreatitis related to stretching the ampullary orifice to such a large size. A review of 33 publications including 2924 total procedures compared the complication rates of EPLBD with a large ES, with limited ES, and without ES.[31] The rate of adverse events was less than 10% in each group and not significantly different. The rates of severe complications such as pancreatitis (all <4%) and perforation (all <0.5%) were acceptable and also not significantly different among the three groups. The rate of bleeding, however, was highest in the large ES group, at 4.1%, which was significantly higher than the limited-ES and no-ES groups (1.3% vs. 1.9%, respectively).

A multicenter retrospective study that included 946 patients who underwent EPBLD for CBD stones greater than 10 mm in size sought to determine the predictive factors of adverse events in EPLBD.[32] Based on their findings, the authors made the following recommendations: (1) Indication should be patients with a dilated CBD without distal CBD strictures. (2) Avoid full-ES immediately before LBD to prevent perforation and bleeding. (3) Inflate the balloon gradually to recognize an occult stricture. (4) Discontinue balloon inflation if resistance is met in the presence of a persistent balloon waist. (5) Do not inflate the balloon beyond the maximal size of the upstream dilated CBD. (6) Do not hesitate to convert into alternative stone removal methods, such as ML or electrohydraulic lithotripsy (EHL), if there is difficulty in removing stones.

If performed correctly (with an incomplete ES and then EPLBD to the size of the CBD), ES with EPLBD is a safe and effective method for removal of multiple or large stones in the CBD, which leads to shorter procedure times with decreased use of lithotripsy techniques.

Electrohydraulic Lithotripsy

Since its development during the 1950s in the former Soviet Union as a method to fragment rocks during mining, EHL has been adapted for medical use in the treatment of nephrolithiasis and biliary tract calculi. The electrohydraulic probe consists of two coaxially isolated electrodes at the tip of a flexible catheter, which is capable of delivering electric sparks in short, rapid pulses leading to sudden expansion of the surrounding liquid environment and generating pressure waves that result in stone fragmentation.[33] Direct cholangioscopy with either mother-daughter cholangioscopes[34] or single-operator cholangioscopy (SOC) systems, such as the SpyGlass DS (Boston Scientific, Natick, MA), are used to directly target stones for fragmentation while avoiding ductal trauma or perforation.[35,36] Continuous saline irrigation is used with the bipolar electrode placed near the surface of the stone to provide a medium for shockwave energy transmission, to flush away debris, and to maintain adequate visualization.[36] Reports document complete stone clearance after multiple sessions in 86% of patients,[34,37–39] and in a prospective nonrandomized trial, EHL was comparable to ESWL in stone clearance.[37]

The largest study of EHL performed to date is a retrospective review of 407 patients with difficult biliary stones who underwent ERCP with SOC, using either EHL (75.2%) or laser lithotripsy (24.8%). On subgroup analysis, 74.5% of patients who underwent EHL achieved complete stone fragmentation and ductal clearance in a single procedure. Adverse events across the entire study population occurred in 15 patients (3.7%), including 6 with cholangitis and 1 with pancreatitis. The adverse events were classified as mild in 10 of 15 patients (66.7%).[40]

Laser Lithotripsy

Reports of the use of a holmium:yttrium-aluminum-garnet (holmium:YAG) laser lithotripsy for choledocholithiasis were first published in 1998.[41,42] During holmium laser therapy, continuous ductal irrigation with normal saline is needed to provide a medium for the transfer of energy and to help clear stone fragments.[43] Despite the fragmentation of stones, standard techniques such as balloon sweep or mechanical lithotripsy may still be required to completely clear the duct of all debris. A study published in 2007 described how the holmium laser can fragment stones regardless of their composition, whether they are cholesterol, pigment, or calcium stones.[44] The holmium laser has a high absorption coefficient in water and therefore has a better safety margin and has more than 100 times the energy absorption than the neodymium laser.[45] Despite the safety profile, to prevent bile duct injury, it is necessary to use direct visual control while performing holmium laser lithotripsy, which also allows real-time assessment of any biliary injuries.[46,47]

Cholangioscopy was classically performed using mother-daughter scopes with two endoscopists, but several recent studies demonstrate the safety and efficacy of the SpyGlass SOC for laser lithotripsy with the holmium:YAG laser. A prospective study in 2011 examined 60 patients with choledocholithiasis who either failed therapy with conventional methods or were referred for management of potentially difficult stone removal.[45] Complete ductal clearance using the Spyglass SOC system with the holmium:YAG laser was achieved in 50 patients (83.3%) in one session, and the remaining patients achieved ductal clearance after one additional session. Complications included fever in 3 patients (although these patients were already admitted with cholangitis), postprocedure pain requiring hospital admission in 4 patients, and a biliary stricture in 1 patient who developed a stricture proximal to the stone, which was successfully treated with dilation using a 10-Fr biliary stent for 3 months. The authors were not sure if the stricture was caused by the laser therapy or the stone itself. A multicenter retrospective study demonstrated even higher rates of complete ductal clearance in a single procedure (97%), with a low adverse event rate (4.1%; 2 with minor bleeding of the bile duct wall, 1 patient with mild pancreatitis).[48]

Endoprosthesis Placement

In the few situations in which stone extraction is incomplete or impossible, a nasobiliary tube or an endoprosthesis (Fig. 37C.8) should be inserted to provide biliary decompression and prevent stone impaction in the distal CBD. This is a temporizing therapy to allow the patient's clinical condition to improve, until complete stone clearance is achieved via additional endoscopic maneuvers or surgery (see Chapters 30 and 37).

Nasobiliary tubes are rarely tolerated beyond a few days. Furthermore, problems with tube placement, such as accidental dislodgment, have led to the alternative therapy of temporary biliary endoprosthesis placement.[49,50] In a poor-risk surgical patient, ES and long-term placement of a plastic biliary endoprosthesis has been proposed as a nonsurgical alternative.[51–54] Of 84 patients intentionally treated with permanent plastic stents for endoscopically irretrievable stones and followed for a mean of 3 years, 49 (58%) developed biliary complications, and 9 died as a result of complications. Most of the patients had a long, symptom-free interval, however, before complications developed, supporting stenting alone as a short-term treatment.[55,56] In a randomized study with a short mean follow-up (1.5 years)

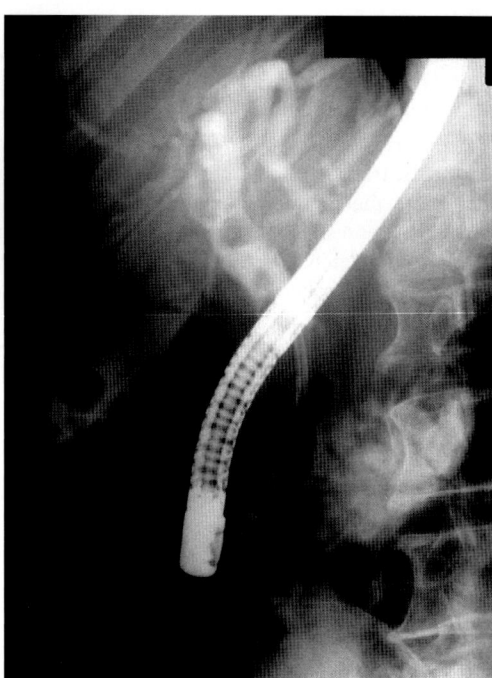

FIGURE 37C.8 Endoscopic retrograde cholangiopancreatography showing placement of a 10-Fr diameter endoprosthesis for the temporary management of cholangitis caused by several bile duct stones.

that compared placement of a plastic biliary stent with ES as definitive therapy with stone clearance by means of the basket, balloon, or mechanical lithotripter, the patients with stents had a significantly greater rate of cholangitis (36%) than the patients managed by a conventional endoscopic duct clearance approach (14%). The high risk of long-term complications does not support the concept of permanent plastic stent therapy except for patients with severe comorbidity and a short life expectancy.

The fully covered self-expanding metal stent (FC-SEMS) was designed to improve patency of traditional self-expanding metal stents by preventing tissue ingrowth in malignant bile duct obstruction. However, the silicone covering on the stent has allowed for delayed stent removal and thus has subsequently been successfully used in an off-label fashion for benign biliary diseases, such as benign biliary strictures and complex bile duct stones.[57,58] It has been postulated that the friction between the stones and the stent reduces the stone size, and that the radial dilating force of the stent across the papilla further assists in the clearance of choledocholithiasis.[59,60] A retrospective review studied 36 patients with complex biliary stones who had incomplete ductal clearance despite the use of advanced extraction techniques.[61] All patients had successful biliary drainage after the initial SEMS was placed. Thirty-three patients (94%) had complete ductal clearance after a mean of 2.2 ERCP sessions. There were no immediate or delayed complications related to FC-SEMS placement or removal, and only 4 patients had spontaneous migration of stents that were deemed clinically insignificant. Another retrospective review evaluated 29 patients with long-term FC-SEMS placement for the management of difficult CBD stones that could not be removed by standard or advanced techniques.[59] All patients had successful procedures in terms of biliary drainage, and the stents were left in place for a median of 200 days. After ERCP, 13 of the patients refused repeat procedures, and therefore only 16 patients returned for successful stent removal. Complete ductal clearance was achieved in 15 of 16 (93.7%) patients after the second ERCP. The 13 patients who refused repeat ERCP were followed for more than 6 months without any complications related to stent placement. In patients in whom complete ductal clearance is not feasible on the index ERCP, FC-SEMS placement can greatly improve the chances of success on the subsequent ERCP while also minimizing the need for advanced lithotripsy techniques.

Dissolution Therapy

Contact chemical dissolution of stones has been attempted by perfusing the CBD with solvents administered via an indwelling nasobiliary tube, percutaneous transhepatic catheter, cholecystostomy tube, or an existing T-tube. The initial results with these agents were disappointing because of incomplete stone dissolution and complications. A semisynthetic vegetable oil, monooctanoin, composed of 70% glycerol-1-monooctanoate and 30% glycerol-1,2-dioctanoate, was used experimentally for the dissolution of CBD stones beginning in 1977. Results collected from 222 clinicians treating 343 patients with CBD stones between 1977 and 1983 reported a success rate for complete stone dissolution of only 25.6% and an additional partial success rate of 28%.[62] Serious adverse events leading to discontinuation of treatment occurred in 5% of patients, including hemorrhage from duodenal ulceration, acute pancreatitis, jaundice, pulmonary edema, acidosis, anaphylaxis, septicemia, and leukopenia, but no deaths were reported. The use of organic solvents, such as the aliphatic ether methyl tert-butyl ether,[63] also has been disappointing, with complete stone dissolution achieved in only 30% to 45% and an unacceptable complication rate related to systemic absorption from spillover of solvent into the duodenum and intrahepatic bile ducts.[64-68] Expectations of developing a solvent-chelating agent (ethylenediaminetetraacetic acid) for pigment stones have not been realized. As a result of its low efficacy and morbidity, contact dissolution therapy has not assumed an important role in patients with refractory CBD stones, and newer agents with better methods for instillation are awaited.

RESULTS OF ENDOSCOPIC THERAPY (SEE CHAPTER 30)

Successful endoscopic treatment of CBD stones requires an adequate ES, which is now achieved in greater than 90% of attempts in most reported series, with noticeable improvement as experience increases.[3,21,69-74] Most experts now would expect to extract stones in at least 90% of successful sphincterotomies. Reported success rates should be interpreted with caution because centers with greater expertise are more likely to be referred difficult cases that may be failures from attempts elsewhere, biasing results. Patient characteristics also vary considerably from unit to unit and country to country, reflecting different referral patterns, patient selection, and attitudes toward endoscopic therapy. Results from centers around the world with individual and collected series of 430 to 9041 patients range from 75% to 96% for duct clearance, with a median value of 91%.[21,69-80]

Complications of Endoscopic Therapy (see Chapter 30)

Despite the disparate indications and selection of patients among centers, the overall incidence of ERCP-related complications seems to be remarkably consistent and ranges between 5% and 10%.[69-75,81-83] A comprehensive review of all major prospective ERCP trials (16,855 patients) revealed the following specific complication rates: acute pancreatitis, 3.5% (range, 1.0%–8.7%); cholecystitis or cholangitis, 1.4% (range, 0%–5%); acute hemorrhage from sphincterotomy site, 1.3% (range, 0.3%–6.2%); perforation, 0.6% (range, 0%–6.2%); and small numbers of other rare complications, such as impacted basket and gallstone ileus. Complication rates must be interpreted with caution because definitions of hemorrhage, acute pancreatitis, cholangitis, and perforation often differ, although many studies use consensus definitions.[84]

Post-ERCP pancreatitis is defined as a rise in serum amylase to at least three times the upper limit of normal with accompanying typical pain of pancreatitis, leading to either a hospital admission or prolongation of current hospitalization (see Chapter 55). It is important to recognize that isolated asymptomatic hyperamylasemia after ERCP is a common and expected finding. Post-ERCP pancreatitis is managed like any typical bout of acute pancreatitis (see Chapter 56), and although most attacks are mild and self-limited, clinicians must remain vigilant in diagnosing severe pancreatitis. Wire-guided cannulation decreases the rate of post-ERCP pancreatitis by approximately 50% compared with conventional contrast-guided approaches.[85] Risk factors for post-ERCP pancreatitis include suspected sphincter of Oddi dysfunction, prior history of post-ERCP pancreatitis, female patients, young age, difficult cannulation, and contrast injections into the pancreatic duct.[75,86–88] Prophylactic pancreatic ductal stent placement and periprocedural administration of rectal nonsteroidal antiinflammatory drugs, such as diclofenac and indomethacin, each reduce the risk of post-ERCP pancreatitis by 50%.[89] The combined protective effect of pancreatic stents and rectal nonsteroidal antiinflammatory drugs is the subject of ongoing study. A new, highly potent protease inhibitor, nafamostat mesylate, has shown significant efficacy in early trials; however, larger clinical studies are needed.[90]

Postsphincterotomy bleeding is often recognized immediately after the sphincterotomy, but some patients may have delayed bleeding. Although there is a paucity of data, use of antiplatelet agents does not appear to increase the risk of bleeding. Controlled sphincterotomy technique with the use of blended current, while avoiding the "zipper" cut, is a recommended method to prevent bleeding. In patients with delayed bleeding, symptoms are similar to any routine upper gastrointestinal bleed, including hemodynamic changes and melena. Mild cholestasis may be evident due occlusion of the biliary orifice with blood clots. Mild to moderate bleeding can often be controlled with endoscopic techniques, including balloon tamponade of the sphincterotomy site, injection of dilute epinephrine (1:10,000), bipolar cautery, and placement of hemostatic clips.[91–93] Temporary placement of FC-SEMS can provide durable hemostasis through long-term tamponade of the bleeding site, with efficacy demonstrated in a small case series.[94] In rare cases of major arterial hemorrhage, the endoscopic view of the papillary area is obscured by blood, precluding any further endoscopic therapies. In these patients, angiography with superselective embolization of the active bleeding site has been shown to be highly effective.[95] Accordingly, surgical management for post-ERCP bleeding has become very uncommon in hospitals with interventional radiology services.

Duodenal perforation is relatively rare and is either a small retroperitoneal perforation related to the sphincterotomy or a large duodenal perforation from the shaft of the scope. The perforation may be asymptomatic and noticed only as retroperitoneal gas (Fig. 37C.9) or extravasation of radiographic contrast material, but even in a symptomatic patient conservative

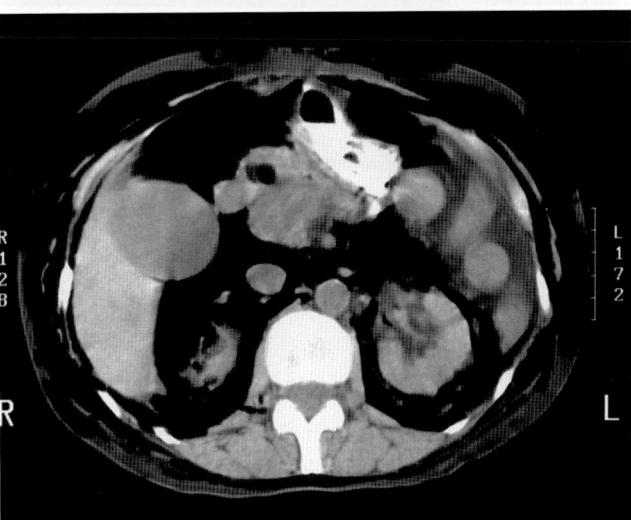

FIGURE 37C.9 Computed tomography scan of the stomach, with oral contrast administration showing extensive retroperitoneal, intraperitoneal, and subcutaneous air caused by a perforation from endoscopic sphincterotomy. The patient made an uneventful recovery on conservative treatment.

treatment is often effective, with spontaneous resolution and avoidance of potentially difficult surgery. Occasionally, this complication presents late after ES with a retroperitoneal collection of bile or pus in the flank or inguinal region[72,96] and requires percutaneous or surgical drainage.

Post-ERCP cholangitis is confined almost completely to patients in whom CBD clearance has not been achieved, and measures should be directed at providing adequate biliary drainage (e.g., by nasobiliary catheter or endoprosthesis) and administering parenteral antibiotics. Gallstone ileus is a rare complication, but its recognition needs to be emphasized because symptoms may be obscure in elderly patients, and they occur many days after ERCP and stone release; treatment is along standard surgical lines (see Chapter 43).

The impaction of an extraction basket within the bile duct during stone extraction occurs rarely in experienced hands because many endoscopic maneuvers have been learned to prevent or salvage this situation. These maneuvers include (1) avoiding basket closure during initial attempts to extract a large stone to prevent impaling the basket wires in the stone surface, (2) converting the standard basket into a crushing type by replacing the handle with a mechanical lithotripter, and (3) extending the ES incision by removing the duodenoscope over the impacted basket catheter and reintroducing it alongside the catheter, introducing a second duodenoscope, or passing a sphincterotome along the same instrument channel as the impacted basket catheter when using large-channel (3.7 mm or 4.2 mm) endoscopes.

Death after ERCP is a rare event, with a mortality rate directly attributable to the procedure ranging between 0% and 0.94%, with an average of 0.3%,[81] with roughly equal distribution of causes between hemorrhage, pancreatitis, cholangitis, and perforation.

Long-Term Morbidity

Reports on long-term follow-up ranging from 1 to 15 years after ERCP with ES in postcholecystectomy patients have demonstrated that more than 90% of patients are well on symptomatic review, and 7% to 11% have significant symptoms secondary to recurrent stones (5%), with or without stenosis of the ES site (1.5%–3%) and cholangitis (2%).[69,73,97–101] Most of these long-term complications are amenable to further endoscopic treatment.

LAPAROSCOPIC AND PERCUTANEOUS APPROACHES TO BILE DUCT STONES

Laparoscopic Common Bile Duct Exploration (see Chapter 37B)

Laparoscopic CBD exploration was first performed in the early 1990s and typically performed at experienced tertiary referral centers.[102–104] Ductal exploration may be accomplished through the cystic duct or directly through a choledochotomy. The transcystic route is the least invasive and generally does not require any direct ductal manipulation or drainage procedure, whereas choledochotomy requires either closure of the duct over a T-tube or primary closure of the choledochotomy with or without a biliary stent placed in an antegrade fashion without need for a T-tube.[104,105] Bile duct clearance rates average 90%, with a median rate of conversion to open operation of 4%.[106] Complication rate is 2.5%, with a median mortality rate of 1%.[107]

Multiple randomized clinical trials have been performed comparing single-stage laparoscopic CBD exploration at the time of cholecystectomy versus a two-stage approach with ERCP preceding or following laparoscopic cholecystectomy.[108–111] The results of these trials have been strikingly similar, demonstrating similar ductal clearance rates for both groups with comparable rates of complications and mortality. Recent meta-analyses have conflicting results, with one meta-analysis favoring the single-stage surgical approach and the other meta-analysis favoring preoperative ERCP followed by cholecystectomy.[112,113] These conflicting conclusions reflect the similarity in outcomes between these two approaches. In studies that examined hospital parameters, the single-stage surgical approach was associated with a shorter length of stay and reduced hospital costs. Length of stay and associated hospital costs can be reduced with improved coordination between the surgeon and the endoscopist. Although the single-stage approach appears at least equivalent to the two-stage approach, implementation of this strategy is restricted to centers with significant expertise in laparoscopic bile duct exploration. Conversely, most facilities have ready access to ERCP services, and thus a two-stage approach is the most common strategy in the United States.

Percutaneous Approach (see Chapters 31 and 35)

In the 5% to 10% of patients for whom the endoscopic approach is unsuccessful at clearing the CBD of stones, two nonsurgical approaches are available: a *rendezvous procedure* and a *complete percutaneous procedure*. If the papillary region can be reached endoscopically and deep biliary cannulation is unable to be achieved, a rendezvous procedure may be used. Although typically used for patients with obstructive jaundice from pancreaticobiliary malignancy, this technique can be used for choledocholithiasis in patients with surgically altered anatomy, such as a Billroth II, or in patients with challenging papillary anatomy, such as a large periampullary diverticulum. This involves a two-stage procedure with the introduction of a percutaneous guidewire through the bile ducts and papilla into the duodenum in the first stage, followed by an ERCP.[114–117] In one report of

rendezvous procedures for choledocholithiasis, 0.9% (15/1753) of ERCPs were unsuccessful at biliary cannulation, usually owing to duodenal diverticula or Billroth II anatomy.[118] Three patients underwent surgery, and 93% of the remaining patients underwent a successful rendezvous procedure. There was one complication with a retroperitoneal perforation that required surgical management, and during follow-up, only one patient developed recurrent choledocholithiasis, requiring a repeat rendezvous procedure. In a multicenter prospective trial of endoscopic biliary sphincterotomy complications,[75] the combined endoscopic-percutaneous approach was a risk factor for the development of complications, with a high rate of complications at 22.6% (6.5% classified as severe). EUS-guided rendezvous procedures have emerged as a viable alternative to percutaneous rendezvous approaches for bile duct access in patients with unsuccessful biliary cannulation[119] (see Chapters 30 and 35).

The complete percutaneous approach has been established as treatment for hepatolithiasis[120] (see Chapters 39 and 44), but it may also be used for choledocholithiasis. Historically, the procedure involves initial establishment of a transhepatic fistula, followed by stone extraction under fluoroscopy or cholangioscopy 7 to 8 days after the fistula forms. In a series of 31 patients with failed endoscopic procedures, percutaneous biliary access was achieved in all patients, and stone clearance was complete in 87% after a mean of 5.6 sessions.[121] All patients underwent balloon dilation of the papilla, and most patients required additional means of stone fragmentation, including ML, EHL, and ESWL. Complications including pancreatitis and bacteremia occurred in 9.7% and did not require surgical intervention. The 4 patients who did not respond to percutaneous management underwent surgery.

Recent advances in the percutaneous approach to bile duct stones have focused on antegrade expulsion of the stones into the duodenum using a Fogarty-type balloon after dilation of the biliary sphincter (sphincteroplasty). This requires a much smaller bore tract as compared with percutaneous extraction of biliary stones. Large series have demonstrated high clinical success with the percutaneous approach (95%) with a 7% major complication rate, including cholangitis, subcapsular hematoma, subcapsular abscess, and arterial injury.[122] In most centers, the percutaneous approach to bile duct stones is limited to patients where ERCP is not feasible due to anatomic considerations.

SPECIFIC CLINICAL SCENARIOS

Pregnancy

Symptomatic choledocholithiasis during pregnancy poses a diagnostic and therapeutic challenge. Biliary tract stone disease occurs in approximately 1.5% of pregnancies.[123] Endoscopic treatment can be performed safely in pregnant patients using techniques to minimize fluoroscopy.[124–127] A recent retrospective study using the Nationwide Inpatient Sample demonstrated a higher risk of post-ERCP pancreatitis in pregnant patients (12%) compared with control patients (5%); multivariable analysis confirmed pregnancy was an independent risk factor for post-ERCP pancreatitis.[128]

Patients With Gallbladder in Situ (see Chapters 37 and 38)

In elderly patients or in patients with significant comorbidity, a deliberate decision often is made to leave the gallbladder in situ after ERCP and CBD stone removal. The short- and long-term results and complications of ERCP with ES in patients with gallbladders do not differ from those in postcholecystectomy patients.[129] The risk of deferring cholecystectomy was examined in a study of 120 patients with known gallstones who underwent successful ERCP with bile duct clearance. The study excluded patients who were not surgical candidates, and patients were randomized to laparoscopic cholecystectomy within 6 weeks after ERCP or a wait-and-see policy with median 2.5-year follow-up. Nearly half the patients in the wait-and-see group developed biliary-related problems, including biliary pain and cholecystitis, which led to cholecystectomy or repeat ERCP or both, whereas none of the patients in the cholecystectomy group experienced biliary-related problems. The wait-and-see group also had a higher rate of conversion to an open procedure at the time of surgery.[130] A meta-analysis of randomized trials comparing the wait-and-see approach with elective cholecystectomy confirmed these findings, with a higher risk of biliary pain (relative risk, 14.6) and cholangitis (relative risk, 2.5) in patients who deferred cholecystectomy.[131] The risk of these future biliary complications needs to be balanced with operative risk in patients with significant underlying comorbidity.

Suspected Choledocholithiasis (see Chapters 33, 34, and 37)

In patients with suspected choledocholithiasis, it is imperative to perform a risk assessment for the presence of CBD stones before cholecystectomy. The following algorithm accounts for the relative efficacy, safety, and cost-effectiveness of each procedure and imaging study.[132] Patients with any very strong predictor of CBD stones (visualized CBD stone on imaging, cholangitis, or bilirubin >4) or two strong predictors of CBD stones (dilated CBD >6 mm, bilirubin between 1.8 and 4) should undergo preoperative ERCP. Moderate predictors are any other abnormal liver function tests, age older than 55 years, and gallstone pancreatitis. Patients without any very strong, strong, or moderate predictors are deemed low risk for CBD stones and should proceed directly to cholecystectomy. All remaining patients are at intermediate risk for CBD stones and should either undergo preoperative MRCP or EUS, followed by ERCP if CBD stones are visualized. Alternatively, depending on local expertise, these intermediate-risk patients can proceed with laparoscopic cholecystectomy with intraoperative cholangiogram; patients can then proceed with laparoscopic bile duct exploration or undergo postoperative ERCP. In patients who undergo preoperative ERCP, it is important to minimize the time between the ERCP and cholecystectomy, to reduce the risk of recurrent CBD stones before surgery. Subsequent studies have found this algorithm to be moderately accurate (60%–70%) for predicting the presence of CBD stones; the remaining patients did not have CBD stones on ERCP despite having criteria suggestive of choledocholithiasis.[133,134]

Acute Cholangitis (see Chapter 43)

Acute cholangitis resulting from CBD stones traditionally was managed by supportive measures and parenteral antibiotics, followed by early surgery if improvement was slow or absent. In early reports, the mortality from emergency surgery ranged from 12% to 16%, with higher rates for elderly patients.[69,135,136] The only randomized trial of emergency endoscopic versus surgical management of severe calculous cholangitis[137] showed a 3-fold difference in mortality rate (10% vs. 32%; $P < .03$) in favor of ERCP. In patients who are hemodynamically stable, it is reasonable

to proceed with ES during ERCP with removal of all calculi. Care must be taken to minimize aggressive contrast injection (particularly during balloon-occluded cholangiography) to reduce the potential risk of bacteremia from the procedure. In patients with hemodynamic compromise, procedure duration can be minimized using a two-stage approach, placing a plastic biliary stent without sphincterotomy to achieve biliary decompression, which leads to resolution of cholangitis.[138] After the patient's clinical status has improved, a second ERCP can be performed with ES, allowing complete ductal clearance of CBD stones.

Gallstone Pancreatitis (see Chapters 55 and 56)

Acute pancreatitis resulting from gallstones in the ampulla of Vater was first reported by Opie in 1901.[139] From his observations in this study, an "obstructive theory" was derived to explain the mechanism responsible for gallstone pancreatitis. Current evidence suggests that transient stone impaction in the common channel of the pancreatic duct and CBD causes increased pancreatic ductal pressure with associated inappropriate activation of pancreatic enzymes.[140] In support of the obstructive theory, gallstones can be recovered from the feces of 85% to 95% of patients,[141–143] and the incidence of CBD stones is 80% in patients undergoing urgent operative or endoscopic intervention compared with a 5% to 30% incidence when the procedure is delayed.[142–146]

The Ranson, Imrie, Glasgow, and Acute Physiology, Age, and Chronic Health Evaluation (APACHE II) assessments provide well-established criteria for assessing the severity of pancreatitis and predicting local adverse events—such as necrosis, hemorrhage, infection, and pseudocyst formation—and systemic complications of acute respiratory distress syndrome, disseminated intravascular coagulation, distant fat necrosis, and renal failure.[147] Stratifying patients by severity based on these criteria has been helpful in directing appropriate management. Most patients experience mild pancreatitis resulting from transient impaction of a stone in the ampulla, followed by spontaneous migration into the duodenum. These patients do well with conservative therapy alone and are unlikely to benefit from urgent intervention. In contrast, it has been proposed that more severe cases of pancreatitis result from persistent stone impaction or choledocholithiasis with infected bile, suggesting the possibility that early stone extraction by surgical or endoscopic techniques would halt progression of the acute event and prevent the development of future attacks in the short term.

Early surgical therapy in cases of acute biliary pancreatitis (ABP) has been challenged owing to the high operative morbidity and mortality. Results and conclusions from numerous series comparing early and late surgical therapy in gallstone pancreatitis are difficult to interpret. The mortality rates range from 2% to 67%, studies are retrospective with frequent comparisons to historical controls, and stratification for severity of illness has not been used.[144,145,148,149] In one study, Kelly and Wagner[150] prospectively randomized 165 patients with gallstone pancreatitis to early or delayed surgery. In the group with severe pancreatitis, mortality was 48% after urgent operative intervention compared with 11% mortality rate in patients in whom surgery for gallstones was delayed for more than 48 hours. In contrast, patients with mild pancreatitis had mortality rates of 3.3% and 0%, respectively. Another study of moderate to severe gallstone pancreatitis with peripancreatic fluid collections confirmed these results, with complications in 44% of patients in the early surgery group compared with 6% in the delayed surgery group.[151]

The results of these aforementioned studies favor avoidance of early operative intervention in the acute phase of biliary pancreatitis, as the previous surgical dictum was that inflammation and edema from pancreatitis can distort biliary anatomy, which would complicate surgery and predispose patients to bile duct injury.[152] However, recent robust clinical data have challenged this thought process, leading to a paradigm shift favoring cholecystectomy during the initial hospitalization for ABP, once the acute inflammatory process has improved (see Chapters 34 and 36).

A UK study retrospectively reviewed admissions to the hospital while awaiting an elective outpatient cholecystectomy after an episode of biliary pancreatitis.[153] Of the 58 patients awaiting laparoscopic cholecystectomy, 21% had unplanned readmissions if waiting for more than 28 days. No patients who had cholecystectomy within 28 days had recurrent admissions. The presence of a sphincterotomy did not affect readmission rates despite the fact that no patients with ES returned with ABP, as they instead returned with cholecystitis or biliary colic. These results were echoed by another European study that retrospectively analyzed 80 patients with ABP who had ERCP with ES.[154] The authors found a 60% rate of recurrent biliary complications (pancreatitis, symptomatic choledocholithiasis, colic) in patients who delayed cholecystectomy versus 2% in the group who underwent early cholecystectomy ($P < .0001$). A multicenter randomized control trial of 266 patients with mild gallstone pancreatitis has been performed. In this study, 129 patients were randomly assigned to same-admission cholecystectomy within 3 days, whereas 137 were randomized to interval cholecystectomy within 25 to 30 days.[152] Readmission for gallstone-related complications (pancreatitis, cholecystitis, cholangitis, jaundice, colic) was significantly more common in the interval group than the same-admission group (17% vs. 5%, $P = .002$). These results remained significant when comparing patients with endoscopic sphincterotomy in a subgroup analysis. As with the previous retrospective studies, there was no difference in length of stay, difficulty of surgery, conversions from laparoscopic to open surgery, or healthcare use between the two groups.

Because of this paradigm shift in the surgical management of biliary pancreatitis, along with the change in guidelines recommending cholecystectomy on the index admission, a retrospective review studied how the implementation of an acute care surgery (ACS) service for biliary disease affected outcomes in biliary pancreatitis.[155,156] The rate of index cholecystectomy increased from 2.4% to 67% ($P < .001$) after the implementation of the ACS service, which correlated with a decrease in readmission rate for biliary-related disease from 16.8% to 7.3% ($P = .04$). Although an ACS service is not a new concept, the study demonstrates the importance of inpatient consultation and prompt evaluation by a surgical service that adheres to the current management guidelines.

The data regarding cholecystectomy in patients with severe ABP with complications such as multiorgan failure or necrosis are not as robust, and a Cochrane Review states that there is currently no evidence to support or refute early laparoscopic cholecystectomy for patients with severe acute pancreatitis.[157] Usually, a delay in surgery in these patients is secondary to critical illness or while awaiting other surgical or endoscopic treatments for complications of pancreatitis such as symptomatic pseudocysts or walled-off pancreatic necrosis. In patients who are too ill or have limiting comorbidities (severe coronary artery disease, cirrhosis) to tolerate any type of surgery, there is a potentially protective effect of an endoscopic sphincterotomy in preventing further biliary complications, although the data for the role of ES in lieu of a cholecystectomy for a high-risk patient in the absence of choledocholithiasis are limited.[158]

In the acute setting, an endoscopic approach to biliary pancreatitis offers the theoretical advantage of immediate relief of biliary obstruction and ductal clearance without the risks of surgery. As animal models and human studies have suggested that the duration of biliary obstruction is a critical factor in determining the severity of pancreatitis, early resolution of obstruction with ERCP would theoretically ameliorate the course of the disease.[159] The timing of ERCP in ABP has been controversial, and until recently, many studies did suggest a role for early ERCP.[160] Three often-quoted studies in previous guidelines and reviews gave the antecedent evidence that early ERCP (within 72 hours) and sphincterotomy reduced complications in ABP.[161–163] These studies included patients with conditions that necessarily required ERCP (cholangitis, jaundice), and therefore the question of a biliary sphincterotomy in all patients with ABP was not adequately addressed.

A randomized multicenter European study avoided these confounding variables by examining the role of early ERCP with sphincterotomy in patients with ABP without cholangitis or jaundice.[164] Two hundred thirty-eight patients were randomly assigned to early ERCP (within 72 hours) or conservative treatment. The overall mortality and complication rates were similar between the two groups regardless of the severity of pancreatitis, but the rate of serious respiratory failure was higher in the invasive group ($P = .03$). A meta-analysis published in 2009 of the seven known well-designed, randomized, controlled trials on this topic confirms these same findings.[165]

According to the published data, the current practice management guidelines state that early ERCP is not needed in patients with ABP who lack the laboratory or clinical evidence of ongoing biliary obstruction or cholangitis. In the absence of jaundice or cholangitis, noninvasive methods such as MRCP and EUS should be used to screen for choledocholithiasis.[156,160]

CONCLUSIONS

Endoscopic management of choledocholithiasis is widely accepted as a highly effective therapy for CBD stones. Endoscopic techniques are well established, and accessories have been developed to enhance success and safety. ERCP with ES is the standard of care in the management of CBD stones in most clinical situations, regardless of the presence or absence of the gallbladder. Improvements in endoscopic techniques allow for the management of complex bile duct stone disease. The endoscopic removal of stones in the perioperative period has been shown to be effective, minimizing the need for surgical CBD exploration. Patients with acute cholangitis should be considered for urgent endoscopic management. ERCP is generally not indicated in the management of gallstone pancreatitis in the absence of associated obstructive jaundice or cholangitis. Integrated, multidisciplinary therapy where surgeons, interventional radiologists, and endoscopists collaborate closely together allows for the development and evaluation of new procedural techniques, as well as the optimal management of patients with both routine and complex biliary stone disease.

References are available at expertconsult.com.

CHAPTER 38

Cholecystolithiasis and stones in the common bile duct: Which approach and when?

Joshua T. Cohen, Rachel E. Beard, Lygia Stewart, and Mark P. Callery

DIAGNOSTIC CONSIDERATIONS

Imaging Modalities: Why and When

Determining the presence of cholecystolithiasis and choledocholithiasis can be challenging and often relies on indirect evidence of obstruction. For choledocholithiasis, clinicians use predictive models based on risk factors that include clinical features, abnormal liver function tests (LFTs), jaundice, and common bile duct (CBD) dilation. These are very sensitive (96%–98%) but not very specific (0%–70%).[1]

The Society of American Gastrointestinal and Endoscopic Surgeons (SAGES) provides a practical strategy for the approach to diagnosis of choledocholithiasis in patients with documented cholelithiasis based on the number of relevant risk factors that are present. These risk factors include visualization of a CBD stone on transabdominal ultrasound (US) or a dilated CBD, clinical evidence of acute cholangitis, and total bilirubin greater than 1.7 mg/dL. Patients with 0, 1, or 2+ risk factors have low (<5%), intermediate (% to <50%), or high (50%–94%) risk for CBD stones, respectively.[2] Low-risk patients require no additional testing to exonerate the duct. High-risk patients should be assumed to have choledocholithiasis and undergo either an endoscopic retrograde cholangiopancreatogram (ERCP) or CBD exploration (CBDE). Intermediate-risk patients require further interrogation of the CBD, either with magnetic resonance cholangiopancreatography (MRCP), endoscopic ultrasound (EUS), or intraoperative cholangiogram (IOC).[2] These imaging modalities are discussed in depth later.

Transabdominal Ultrasound

Transabdominal US is the diagnostic test of choice in evaluating patients with right upper quadrant (RUQ) abdominal pain thought to be related to biliary pathology (see Chapter 16). It can readily identify cholelithiasis and signs of gallbladder inflammation and is an appropriate initial modality in the evaluation of CBD stones.[3–5] US can identify bile duct dilation because of stone obstruction, and it can visualize the actual stone in some cases (sensitivity 0.3, specificity 1.0). If the extrahepatic bile duct diameter is less than 5 mm, CBD stones are exceedingly rare, whereas a diameter greater than 10 mm with signs of jaundice predicts the presence of CBD stones in more than 90% of cases.[6] Axial computed tomography (CT) scans have better sensitivity (84%) for choledocholithiasis than US. Helical CT scans outperform conventional nonhelical CT, with 88% sensitivity and 73% to 97% specificity.[7] In terms of availability, cost, and radiation exposure, US prevails as the first-line diagnostic.

Magnetic Resonance Cholangiopancreatography

MRCP is the most accurate noninvasive modality available (see Chapter 16). It is useful as an adjunct when a definitive diagnosis is not readily apparent on US.[4] MRCP is the standard investigation for CBD stones for patients with intermediate probability or for those who need to be investigated to exclude other differential diagnoses. MRCP is especially helpful when anatomic considerations preclude ERCP (status post–Billroth II gastrectomy, Roux-en-Y biliary bypass, duodenal stenoses). The drawback of MRCP is its high cost, which challenges its routine use as a more front-line diagnostic modality.[8]

Endoscopic Retrograde Cholangiopancreatography

ERCP is still considered the gold standard diagnostic modality, although it is invasive, requires radiation, and has significant complications[9] (see Chapters 20 and 30). Observed complications after ERCP include pancreatitis, hemorrhage, cholangitis, perforation, and a clinically relevant mortality rate.[10] Routine ERCP before all laparoscopic cholecystectomies is impractical and unnecessary and should be reserved for patients with high pretest probability of or known choledocholithiasis.[2] When overused, most cholangiograms are normal, and costs and complication rates are prohibitive. Even in patients at high risk, namely those with jaundice, cholestatic LFTs, CBD dilation, and a history of pancreatitis, half will not have CBD stones at the time of ERCP. The utility of ERCP now lies more with its therapeutic capabilities rather than for diagnostic purposes.[11]

Endoscopic Ultrasound

EUS is very sensitive for choledocholithiasis,[12] and a meta-analysis reveals that EUS can reduce unnecessary diagnostic ERCP[13] (see Chapter 22). A systematic review reveals that patients who undergo EUS can avoid ERCP in 67% of cases, with fewer complications and less pancreatitis compared with those undergoing ERCP initially.[14] The diagnostic efficacy of EUS and MRCP compared with ERCP have revealed the tests to be quite comparable.[15,16]

Intraoperative Cholangiography

IOC during cholecystectomy can accurately diagnose CBD stones and both minimize and maximize the need for ERCP (see Chapter 24). It is best used for intermediate-risk patients.[2] The technique can be performed safely in both open and laparoscopic approaches. Surgeons can respond to such findings, flushing the duct to clear stones or debris. Open and laparoscopic IOC can successfully be completed in about 95% of patients, with sensitivity for detecting CBD stones between

80% and 92% and specificity of 93% to 97%.[17] Regardless, an ongoing debate remains whether IOC should be performed routinely or selectively during cholecystectomy. When used routinely, it has high sensitivity and specificity both for suspected CBD stones and for the 3% to 4% of stones that are not clinically suspected but may become symptomatic postoperatively. Other suggested benefits specifically relate to the prevention of bile duct injuries.[18] The randomized trials that have been performed to address this question are small, and even a systematic review of these trials was not sufficiently powered to demonstrate a significant benefit.[19] Because no large prospective randomized trial has answered the question of whether routine IOC is beneficial, most practicing surgeons perform IOC selectively.

CHOLECYSTOLITHIASIS

Indications for Cholecystectomy

Asymptomatic Gallstones

Gallstones are one of the most common pathologies affecting the general population. From 10% to 20% of the Western population has gallstones, and the majority of patients with gallstones, about 65% to 80%, are asymptomatic.[20] Studies of the natural history of *silent gallstones* have shown that symptoms develop in 1% to 2% of patients per year (see Chapter 33). Among patients with asymptomatic gallstones, about 10% develop symptoms in 5 years, and about 20% develop symptoms by 20 years. Importantly, most patients experience symptoms before the development of a complication.[21–24] Therefore the majority of patients with asymptomatic gallstones can be observed, and surgical intervention (laparoscopic cholecystectomy) should be offered only when symptoms develop.

There are certain groups for which prophylactic cholecystectomy has previously been recommended for asymptomatic gallstones. This is an area of controversy, however, and the recommendations are changing. These populations include solid-organ transplant patients; patients with diabetes; patients with chronic liver disease, sickle cell anemia, or other chronic hemolytic anemias; patients undergoing bariatric or other gastrointestinal (GI) operations; and those with a potentially increased risk of gallbladder carcinoma (Table 38.1).

Prophylactic cholecystectomy for asymptomatic cholelithiasis was previously recommended for patients with diabetes mellitus. Studies in the late 1960s reported a higher mortality after emergency cholecystectomy in patients with diabetes; however, subsequent meta-analysis revealed that diabetes was not an independent variable. Rather, associated risk factors such as cardiovascular, peripheral vascular, cerebrovascular, or prerenal azotemia were associated with more severe acute cholecystitis.[24,25] More recent series have shown similar complication rates for acute cholecystectomy among diabetic and nondiabetic patients. Patients with diabetes with asymptomatic gallstones today are managed expectantly.

The incidence of gallstones is twice as high in patients with chronic liver disease. Most of these patients remain asymptomatic. Operative morbidity and mortality rates for patients with chronic liver disease are also significantly higher (see Chapter 75). Meta-analyses report no increase in mortality in asymptomatic patients with an expectant management approach.[23,24] Although laparoscopic cholecystectomy has been shown to be safe in well-selected Child-Pugh class A and B cirrhotic patients, it is contraindicated

TABLE 38.1	Management of Asymptomatic Gallstones
PATIENT POPULATION	**MANAGEMENT**
Healthy adults	Expectant
Children (without hemoglobinopathy or hemolytic anemia)	Expectant
Diabetes mellitus	Expectant
Chronic liver disease	Expectant
Concomitant cholecystectomy at time of bariatric procedure	Only if symptomatic
Previous bariatric surgery	Expectant
Abdominal aortic aneurysm repair	Expectant
Transplant Kidney or pancreas Cardiac	Expectant Likely cholecystectomy posttransplant, but remains controversial
Undergoing gastrointestinal operation	Incidental cholecystectomy
Hemoglobinopathy/chronic hemolytic anemia (sickle cell disease, spherocytosis, elliptocytosis, β-thalassemia)	Elective cholecystectomy
High-risk group for gallbladder carcinoma (>3 cm gallstones, calcified gallbladder, Native-American race)	Consideration for prophylactic cholecystectomy, although data from randomized controlled trials are lacking

in all but emergent settings in Child-Pugh class C patients because of high complication rates.[26]

Because of the association between morbid obesity and cholelithiasis, a high proportion of patients undergoing bariatric surgery have gallbladder pathology. Patients undergoing bariatric surgery have a higher incidence of cholelithiasis, related both to obesity and rapid weight loss. Studies report a cholelithiasis incidence of 27% to 35% before bariatric operations and a 28% to 71% increase in gallstone formation after bariatric surgery.[27] Some surgeons use bile salt medications during periods of rapid weight change to help prevent cholesterol gallstone formation; however, more recent studies have shown that this approach is not cost-effective.[28] The question of whether or not to perform concomitant cholecystectomy at the time of bariatric surgery is controversial, but an increasing number of studies suggest that prophylactic cholecystectomy in the absence of symptoms is not indicated.[29,30] In the case of gallstone formation after bariatric surgery without concomitant cholecystectomy, management should be expectant because the majority of patients remain asymptomatic.[23] For patients with symptomatic cholelithiasis and concomitant morbid obesity, elective cholecystectomy is indicated. Some favor directed referral for cholecystectomy to bariatric surgical specialists, given their technical experience and enhanced facilities and equipment for the care of such patients.

Several factors must be considered for potential solid-organ transplant patients with asymptomatic cholelithiasis. In these patients, cholelithiasis is common, immunosuppression may increase infectious morbidity, and morbidity and mortality may be increased with emergency surgery. This problem was examined with decision analysis, using probabilities and outcomes derived from a pooled analysis of published studies.[31] For pancreas and kidney transplant patients with asymptomatic cholelithiasis, however, expectant management was recommended, an approach that is widely agreed upon in the literature.[31] Kao and colleagues[32] recommended prophylactic after transplantation cholecystectomy for cardiac transplant recipients with asymptomatic cholelithiasis, an approach advocated by other studies as well because of the increased morbidity and mortality that has been demonstrated with subsequent urgent or emergent cholecystectomy compared with the general populace.[33] This remains an area of debate, however, because other studies have demonstrated that expectant management of asymptomatic gallstones is safe.[34]

Asymptomatic gallstones found at an unrelated open GI operation should prompt a cholecystectomy, if exposure is adequate and if the operation can be done safely. Studies of expectant management for patients with asymptomatic gallstones undergoing laparotomy for other conditions have shown a high (up to 70%) incidence of symptoms and/or complications from the biliary system, and a significant percentage (up to 40%) of patients require a cholecystectomy within 1 year of the initial operation. Further, no increase in morbidity is associated with concomitant cholecystectomy.[24,35]

The management of patients with asymptomatic gallstones undergoing abdominal aortic aneurysm (AAA) repair has evolved, especially with the advent of endovascular aortic procedures. In the past, when AAA repair and cholecystectomy were open operations, concomitant cholecystectomy was recommended to prevent the higher morbidity associated with the development of acute cholecystitis in the postoperative period. Studies reported no increase in graft infection or morbidity when cholecystectomy was performed after closure of the retroperitoneum; however, more recent data show similar mortality rates with or without concomitant cholecystectomy. Current management is typically expectant, and laparoscopic cholecystectomy can be performed after AAA repair without increased morbidity if symptoms develop. Although simultaneous laparoscopic cholecystectomy and endovascular AAA repair has been reported,[36,37] it is not widely practiced and certainly not for asymptomatic gallstones.

Children with asymptomatic gallstones fall into two main etiologic groups: those with hemolytic anemia (sickle cell disease, β-thalassemia, hemoglobinopathies) and those whose cholelithiasis stems from some other cause (total parenteral nutrition, short bowel syndrome, cardiac surgery, leukemia, lymphoma). Expectant management for children with hemolytic anemia is associated with a significant increase in morbidity and postoperative hospital stay, and elective cholecystectomy is therefore recommended.[38] For patients with sickle cell disease and asymptomatic gallstones, elective cholecystectomy is advised because expectant management yields more than a 2-fold increase in morbidity. Further, the diagnosis of acute cholecystitis can be difficult to differentiate from acute vaso-occlusive sickle cell crisis.[38] There is also a high incidence of choledocholithiasis in this population, and studies have demonstrated that ERCP can be safely used in children to perform sphincterotomy and stone extraction.[39] In contrast, children with asymptomatic gallstones caused by other etiologies can be safely managed expectantly, and these gallstones have been shown to regress in 17% to 34% of cases.[38]

Finally, gallstones have a proven association with gallbladder carcinoma[40] (see Chapter 49). In a review of 200 consecutive calculous cholecystitis specimens, Albores-Saavedra and colleagues[41] reported that 83% exhibited epithelial hyperplasia, 13.5% atypical hyperplasia, and 3.5% carcinoma in situ. It is not known whether such data apply today, but chronic cholecystitis changes may equate to hyperplasia and dysplasia if not infrequent. Cholecystectomy alone remains sufficient. In areas endemic for gallbladder cancer, the risk of carcinoma increases with larger gallstones. The relative risk rises from 2.4 for stones 2 to 2.9 cm in diameter to 10 for gallstones larger than 3 cm. Some patients with gallbladder calcification also have a higher incidence of gallbladder cancer. Elective cholecystectomy has been recommended in patients with gallstones greater than 3 cm in diameter, but no proof is available to support that such an approach is warranted from an oncologic standpoint.[40,42,43] Preemptive elective cholecystectomy for asymptomatic gallstones is considered in some parts of the world with unusually high gallbladder cancer rates, including some parts of India, Chile, and Mexico.[44]

Symptomatic Gallstones

Approximately 20% to 30% of patients with gallstones will develop symptoms, and once this occurs, cholecystectomy is usually indicated for both symptomatic improvement and to prevent further complications (see Chapter 33). The spectrum of severity characterizing symptomatic gallstones ranges from episodic pain to life-threatening infection and shock.

BILIARY COLIC. Biliary colic is the most typical clinical presentation of symptomatic gallstones. It usually occurs a few hours after a meal, especially one of high fat or spice content, as a slowly progressive and constant pain that occurs in the epigastrium and RUQ of the abdomen and often radiates posteriorly to the scapula and right shoulder. This visceral pain likely reflects the gallbladder contracting against a cystic duct blocked by an impacted gallstone. If pain persists and escalates, it can herald a worse complication of gallstones, such as cholecystitis, cholangitis, or pancreatitis. Pain often remits after several hours, which can create a false sense of security in some patients. More than 60% of patients will suffer recurrent pain within 2 years of their initial attack, and several studies have indicated that gallstone-associated complications occur more frequently in patients who experience biliary colic. Biliary colic is therefore the most common indication for cholecystectomy.

CHOLECYSTITIS. Acute cholecystitis occurs in about 20% of patients with symptomatic gallstones (see Chapter 34). The pathogenesis is prolonged calculous obstruction of the cystic duct with resulting inflammation. The inflamed gallbladder becomes dilated and edematous, manifested by wall thickening, and an exudate of pericholecystic fluid can develop. If the gallstones are sterile, the inflammation is initially sterile, which can occur in patients with cholesterol gallstones. In other cases, however, gallstone formation occurs as a result of bacterial colonization of the biliary tree, rendering pigmented gallstones containing bacterial microcolonies.[45] In these cases, obstruction of the cystic duct results in a contained infection of the gallbladder. Research on the pathogenesis of gallstone-associated infections has shown that patients with bacteria-laden gallstones have more severe biliary infections. In addition, acute cholecystitis can coexist with choledocholithiasis, cholangitis, or gallstone pancreatitis. In the general population, 5% of patients presenting with cholecystitis have co-existing CBD stones. In the elderly, however, this figure rises to 10% to 20%.[46]

The initial treatment for patients with acute cholecystitis is intravenous (IV) hydration, antibiotics, and bowel rest. Many patients should be offered early cholecystectomy, but others will benefit from delayed intervention, either after conservative therapy or percutaneous gallbladder drainage. Several factors govern the approach to patients with acute cholecystitis. One consideration is patient comorbidity; emergency cholecystectomy in patients with significant comorbidities can be associated with high morbidity (20%–30%) and mortality (6%–30%) rates. Guidelines for the management of acute cholecystitis and acute cholangitis were described at an international consensus meeting held in Tokyo in 2006. Updated guidelines were then published in 2013 and re-adopted without modification in 2018.[4,47,48] The Tokyo Guidelines define three levels of severity for acute cholecystitis and serve as a useful tool in the management of acute cholecystitis (Table 38.2).[4,49]

GRADE I ACUTE CHOLECYSTITIS.

Patients presenting with mild grade I acute cholecystitis should be offered early cholecystectomy, performed laparoscopically if possible. Several studies have documented high success rates for laparoscopic cholecystectomy when the procedure is performed within 72 hours of onset of acute cholecystitis.[50,51] Further, a Cochrane Review of five randomized trials showed a shorter hospital stay for early cholecystectomy patients and no significant difference in complication rates or conversion rates between early laparoscopic cholecystectomy (within 7 days) versus delayed laparoscopic cholecystectomy (6–12 weeks).[52] Conversion rates, however, were 45% among patients randomized to the delayed group, which required a cholecystectomy between 1 and 6 weeks. For patients with significant medical problems, cholecystectomy may need to be delayed to maximize medical therapy. Most of these patients with acute cholecystitis can be safely managed with antibiotics and bowel rest, with resolution of their acute illness; they can then undergo an elective cholecystectomy once their medical problems have been addressed.

GRADE II ACUTE CHOLECYSTITIS.

Patients presenting with grade II acute cholecystitis are a more diverse group. Many will be well managed with early cholecystectomy; this is particularly true for cases with delayed presentation as their only grade II finding. In these cases, laparoscopic cholecystectomy should be performed, if possible, within 7 days of the acute illness. In cases with severe local inflammation, early gallbladder drainage (percutaneous or surgical) is recommended as the initial treatment of choice, followed by elective cholecystectomy once the acute inflammation resolves. The key is to identify which patients have such an inflammatory process. Several studies have correlated such findings as age older than 50 years, male sex, presence of diabetes, elevated bilirubin level (>1.5 mg/dL), and leukocytosis (white blood cell count > 15,000 mm³) with gangrenous cholecystitis.[53] These findings are also frequently associated with a severe inflammatory process. Other factors suggestive of a significant inflammatory process include symptoms of gastric outlet obstruction. Patients with such symptoms should have cross-sectional imaging, with either CT or magnetic resonance imaging (MRI), to determine whether a severe inflammatory process is present (Fig. 38.1), followed by percutaneous cholecystostomy if such is found.[47] In the updated 2013 Tokyo Guidelines, percutaneous transhepatic gallbladder drainage remains the standard drainage method for grade II cholecystitis that does not respond to conservative therapy, although techniques such as percutaneous transhepatic gallbladder aspiration and endoscopic nasobiliary gallbladder drainage were also cited as alternatives.[54]

GRADE III ACUTE CHOLECYSTITIS.

Patients presenting with grade III acute cholecystitis have associated organ dysfunction. Although this occurs rarely, approximately 6% of the time, it is important because these patients require intensive organ support and medical treatment.[55] Because the source of their inflammatory (septic) response and organ dysfunction is the severe cholecystitis, percutaneous cholecystostomy is necessary to treat the

TABLE 38.2	Tokyo Guidelines (TG18/TG13) Severity Grading for Acute Cholecystitis
GRADE	**CRITERIA**
I: Mild	Acute cholecystitis that does not meet the criteria for a more severe grade. Mild gallbladder inflammation, no organ dysfunction
II: Moderate	The presence of one or more of the following: 1. Elevated white blood cell count (>18,000/mm³) 2. Palpable tender mass in the right upper abdominal quadrant 3. Duration of complaints > 72 hr 4. Marked local inflammation (biliary peritonitis, pericholecystic abscess, hepatic abscess, gangrenous cholecystitis, emphysematous cholecystitis)
III: Severe	Associated with dysfunction of any one of the following: 1. Cardiovascular system: hypotension requiring dopamine >5 μg/kg/min or any dose of norepinephrine 2. Nervous system: decreased level of consciousness 3. Respiratory system: Pao₂/Fio₂ ratio < 300 4. Renal system: oliguria, serum creatinine > 2.0 mg/dL 5. Hepatic system: PT-INR > 1.5 6. Hematologic system: platelet count < 100,000/mm³

Fio_2, Forced inspiratory oxygen concentration; Pao_2, partial pressure of oxygen in arterial blood; PT-INR, prothrombin time/international normalized ratio.

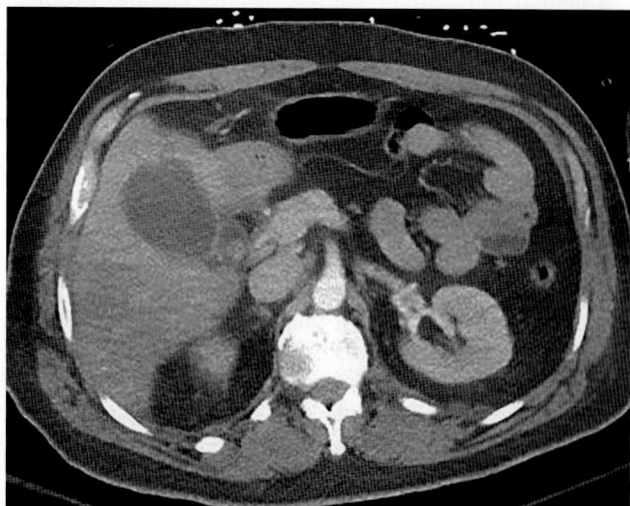

FIGURE 38.1 Computed tomographic scan demonstrating a severe inflammatory process in the setting of acute cholecystitis (see Chapter 16). This patient was treated with percutaneous cholecystostomy (see Chapter 35), followed by elective laparoscopic cholecystectomy once the inflammatory process had resolved.

severe infection as well as the associated organ dysfunction. Numerous studies have documented the success of percutaneous cholecystostomy in achieving control of the underlying infection within 24 to 48 hours.[56] In rare cases, urgent cholecystectomy may be required, such as cases with biliary peritonitis as a result of perforation of the gallbladder; but in general, cholecystectomy in the acute phase of grade III acute cholecystitis should be avoided.[47,57]

DURABILITY OF THE TOKYO GUIDELINES. The Tokyo Guidelines derived for the diagnostic criteria and severity grading of acute cholecystitis and cholangitis originated in 2007.[47] These were embraced and validated worldwide but understandably revisited and modified by consensus experts in 2013 (known as the TG13).[57] The TG13 updates provided better specificity and higher diagnostic accuracy. They have indeed since stood the test of time, and are now offered as TG18/TG13 Guidelines (see Tables 38.2, 38.4, and 38.5). As part of the 2018 interval consensus update, evidence was sought and evaluated from published studies worldwide, which may have prompted additional modifications of the 2013 guideline. Their impact and validity were proven durable.[4]

UNCOMMON PRESENTATIONS OF ACUTE CHOLECYSTITIS. Acalculous cholecystitis arises in the absence of cholecystolithiasis, and associated risk factors include trauma, burns, and GI surgery.[58] Emphysematous cholecystitis is caused by infection with gas-forming anaerobes, such as *Clostridium perfringens*. Patients with diabetes are at risk, and the disease can progress quickly to profound sepsis. Emergent cholecystectomy is indicated. Gallbladder torsion can also occur when the gallbladder is especially mobile because of a connection to the liver by a thin elongated mesentery. Gallbladder perforation can occur as a result of gallbladder wall ischemic and resulting necrosis. A localized perforation can result in formation of a pericholecystic abscess, whereas free perforation can lead to biliary peritonitis. A biliary fistula can also form between the gallbladder and the duodenum as a sequela of cholecystitis, and this can result in a gallstone ileus if a stone passes via this fistula and causes a mechanical obstruction at the ileocecal valve[59] (see Chapter 32).

Cholecystectomy Technique (see Chapter 36)
Choosing Laparoscopic Versus Open Techniques

For typical uncomplicated symptomatic gallstone disease, laparoscopic cholecystectomy is the preferred method of removing the gallbladder.[51,60] Since its origin, cholecystectomy rates have increased worldwide, reflecting general acceptance of the laparoscopic technique. Because the technical aspects of this operation are covered in other chapters, this section will focus on concepts of feasibility and safety that relate to disease severity and the choice between laparoscopic and open cholecystectomy.[61]

Laparoscopic cholecystectomy for severe acute and chronic inflammation is a technically difficult and advanced operation. Less experienced surgeons must recognize this and seek help from a more experienced surgeon, when appropriate, to avoid the potentially disastrous complication of bile duct injury. Furthermore, the surgeon must understand that conversion to open cholecystectomy may be necessary and is more likely in these cases.[62] Biliary injuries are more likely to occur during difficult laparoscopic operations, no different than with open operations, but at a higher incidence. When laparoscopic cholecystectomy is performed for acute cholecystitis, biliary injuries occur three times more often than during elective laparoscopic cases and twice as often compared with open cholecystectomy for acute cholecystitis. Surgeons should therefore not hesitate to convert to an open operation if they experience difficulties with the laparoscopic dissection or are unable to clearly identify the critical view of safety.[63] Surgeons should also be aware of certain patient risk factors, including male gender, advanced cholecystitis, the presence of jaundice, and previous abdominal surgery, which are associated with an increased risk of conversion to open procedure.[51]

The decision to perform open cholecystectomy may be difficult for some. Over the past 20 years, open cholecystectomy has been far less frequently performed. Trainees during this period have less experience with open cases.[64] The experience and training needed to learn the laparoscopic operation likely reduces the level of comfort with the open technique. Finally, there is the pressure related to patient expectation for rapid recovery as well as, perhaps, the hospital expectation for decreased length of stay and cost because conversion is associated with lengthier stays and increased expense.[65] Certain scenarios may thus arise that might subtly account, in part, for static biliary injury rates.[66] Because of inexperience, the surgeon may ignore or resist the sensible default option to convert to the open technique, persists with the laparoscopic approach, and causes injury. In other instances, the surgeon overextends laparoscopic experience when disease severity warrants conversion. To prevent this, patients need to be made fully aware that open cholecystectomy is always a possibility, and the surgeon should not hesitate to seek help if needed, rather than rely on marginal laparoscopic or open cholecystectomy experience. Conversion from laparoscopic to open cholecystectomy is not a defeat but rather is reflective of caution and good judgment.[67,68]

Ideally, a surgeon anticipates the likelihood of conversion on clinical grounds. The anesthesia and operative teams should be so notified and prepared. Open-case instruments need to be readily available, and trocar placement should be along a predrawn right subcostal incision line. Unless there is need to control bleeding, the surgeon enters the RUQ deliberately and is not stressed by the decision to convert. Everyone should be ready for what lies ahead, and it should be clear to all that it will be a difficult operation.

The difficult open cholecystectomy demands adequate exposure, retraction, and identification of anatomy by dissection in the anterior and posterior aspects of the triangle of Calot, followed by dissection of the gallbladder off the liver bed. The surgeon achieves conclusive identification of the cystic structures as the only two structures entering the gallbladder, eliminating the possibility of misidentification.[61] As with the laparoscopic technique, once the critical view is attained, the cystic structures can be ligated and divided. Failure to achieve this critical view should prompt cholangiography to define ductal anatomy. Avoidance of ductal injury in the liver bed depends on a combination of patience and staying in the correct plane of dissection, with meticulous technique and experience. In some cases of acute cholecystitis, the gallbladder "shells out" relatively easily from its edematous hepatic bed. In other cases, and especially in chronic cholecystitis, the dissection of the gallbladder out of the liver bed can be tedious, frustrating, and bloody. Hemostasis can take time and may require an argon beam, cautery, packing, and topical hemostatics. Subtotal cholecystectomy is always a valid option, especially in patients with cirrhosis or in those with severe inflammation that obscures the anatomy within the porta hepatis. Surgeons should indicate in operative notes for open and laparoscopic cholecystectomy precisely how they identified the cystic structures for division. For conversions, they should specify the circumstances, stressing safety and surgical judgment.

Subtotal Cholecystectomy

If subtotal cholecystectomy is determined to be the safest approach to completing the operation, options include whether to proceed with a minimally invasive approach versus converting to an open operation, and whether to fenestrate or reconstitute (see Chapter 36). These terms have recently been clarified and standardized. Subtotal reconstituting cholecystectomy indicates excision of the free, peritonealized portion of the gallbladder, with subsequent closure of the lowest portion with sutures or staples. The risk of a postoperative biliary fistula is reduced, but a remnant gallbladder is created, which could result in recurrence of disease. Subtotal fenestrating cholecystectomy is defined as excision of the gallbladder with the exception of a lip at the lowest portion, with the cystic duct then either being left open or closed from the inside. The risk of postoperative biliary fistula is increased, but there should be no risk of recurrent symptomatic cholecystolithiasis.[69] Advantages and disadvantages of each approach continue to be debated, with some studies suggesting that laparoscopic and reconstituting techniques may reduce the risk of perioperative complications.[70,71] Regardless, as application of these procedure has increased, so have their unique complications, including remnant cholecystitis, recurrent stones, and even remnant gallbladder carcinoma.

Robotic Cholecystectomy

The Da Vinci Surgical System (Intuitive Surgical, Inc., Sunnyvale, CA) was designed to expand on the technical capabilities of minimally invasive surgery (see Chapters 36 and 127). Advantages of robotic-assisted surgery compared with a laparoscopic approach include simulating a surgeon's wrist motion with full articulating movement, an improved three-dimensional camera view of the surgical field, elimination of physiologic tremor, and enhanced instrument dexterity for suturing and dissection. Disadvantages include the equipment expense, a learning curve when the platform is newly adopted, and a perceived loss of tactile feedback for the surgeon, although this last point is somewhat debatable. Several early series demonstrated the safety and feasibility of robotic surgery when employed in abdominal surgery to treat a variety of diseases, including cholecystectomy.[72,73] Most recent studies have redemonstrated low complication rates and equivalent clinical outcomes for robotic-assisted cholecystectomy compared with laparoscopic cholecystectomy, with some studies suggesting lower conversion rates but increased cost with a robotic approach.[74]

Percutaneous Cholecystostomy (see Chapter 35)

The indications for percutaneous cholecystostomy include grade II acute cholecystitis with a severe inflammatory process, grade III acute cholecystitis with associated organ dysfunction, or acute cholecystitis in patients with severe medical morbidity that limits surgical options.[47,51,56,57,75,76] The technical success rate of percutaneous radiologically guided cholecystostomy is 98% to 100%, with few procedure-related complications (mortality and major

complications, 0%–6.5%; minor complications, 0%–20%).[56,77] Potential complications include intrahepatic hematoma, pericholecystic abscess, and biliary peritonitis and pleural effusion caused by puncture of the liver and subsequent migration of the catheter.[51]

Timing of Subsequent Operation for Cholecystitis

Once the inflammatory process has resolved, elective cholecystectomy can be performed early (within 1–7 days) or delayed (6–8 weeks) with excellent success and conversion rates as low as 3%.[78] The optimal timing remains controversial because of a lack of randomized controlled trials; however, early cholecystectomy after percutaneous drainage may be preferable if the procedure is free of complications and the patient's condition improves.[51] Some have reported using percutaneous cholecystostomy as definitive treatment for acute cholecystitis in high-risk, elderly, and debilitated patients. In patients who do not have subsequent cholecystectomy, recurrent biliary symptoms occur in 9% to 33%.[77,79]

CHOLEDOCHOLITHIASIS (SEE CHAPTER 37)

The clinical clues of CBD stones were recognized during the Roman Empire by Soranus of Ephesus, who described jaundice, itching, dark urine, and acholic stools. Not all CBD stones render such a classic clinical scenario, but they still carry risk if left unidentified and untreated. More than 85% of CBD stones originate in the gallbladder and secondarily migrate into the CBD. For patients undergoing cholecystectomy for symptomatic gallstones, the prevalence of choledocholithiasis ranges from 10% to 18%.[80] Primary CBD stones are far less common and are typically associated with conditions of biliary infection and stasis, such as benign biliary strictures, sclerosing cholangitis, and choledochal cysts. Primary CBD stones are more prevalent in Asians and can sometimes be related to parasitic infections.[81]

Silent Common Bile Duct Stones

Published reports using routine intraoperative cholangiography have found that at least 12% of CBD stones are clinically silent,[82] and approximately 6% do not exhibit abnormalities in LFTs or in the diameter of the CBD.[83] When prospectively followed, data suggest that more than one-third of asymptomatic stones will pass spontaneously after the first 6 weeks after cholecystectomy.[84]

Symptomatic Common Bile Duct Stones

The symptoms of CBD stones relate to partial or complete biliary obstruction with and without inflammatory complications, such as cholangitis, hepatic abscesses, or pancreatitis. In chronic scenarios, and depending on the extent and duration of biliary obstruction, choledocholithiasis may also lead to secondary biliary cirrhosis and portal hypertension. Because of the uncertain clinical behavior and potential harmful complications, it is currently accepted that in the great majority of situations, CBD stones should be removed, even if they are asymptomatic.[5]

Definitive Treatment Approaches: Biliary Obstruction
Catheter-Based Approaches

ERCP (SEE CHAPTERS 20, 30, AND 37C). Before the laparoscopic era, ERCP was not commonly used because open surgical bile duct clearance was superior to ERCP in terms of success and morbidity.[85] This changed as laparoscopic cholecystectomy emerged and outpaced the abilities of most surgeons to perform laparoscopic CBD stone removal (see Chapter 37B). Indeed, ERCP captured and has held its role as the first-line approach to CBD stones, being successful in more than 90% of patients.[86] Although well tolerated in most, a 10% rate of complications remains constant for ERCP,[9] with a serious morbidity rate of 1.5% and an overall mortality rate of 0.2% to 0.5%.[87] When surgical and endoscopic teams are inexperienced with CBD stones, the perceived need for preoperative ERCP increases. In this setting, ERCP allows laparoscopic cholecystectomy to be performed quickly and with confidence that CBD stones are already managed. If ERCP fails, the surgical plan will need to consider intraoperative management of choledocholithiasis. Conversely, in centers where successful sphincterotomy and stone extraction is almost assured, the rate of preoperative ERCP will be lower. If the surgeon finds a stone at operation, ERCP becomes a reliable postoperative option. Current consensus accepts the use of ERCP before laparoscopic cholecystectomy for patients with a high probability of choledocholithiasis. It is recommended that patients with a low or intermediate index of suspicion for choledocholithiasis undergo additional imaging techniques (MRCP, EUS, IOC) to avoid unnecessary biliary instrumentation.[5,88,89]

PERCUTANEOUS TRANSHEPATIC CHOLANGIOGRAPHY (SEE CHAPTERS 20, 31, AND 37C).

Compared with ERCP, percutaneous transhepatic cholangiography (PTC) is time-consuming, more involved, and likely more stressful for a patient. It is usually reserved for patients in whom anatomic considerations preclude safe ERCP, such as in the case of an impossible ampullary cannulation. Experienced PTC groups have reported successful stone removal rates in more than 90% of cases, with complication rates around 5%,[90] although these are hardly the norms. PTC stone removal takes time, involving insertions of catheters that are upsized over time, before stones are actually retrieved with stone baskets. Consequently, there are many reports of attempts to make it easier. Gil and colleagues[91] have reported the safety and utility of balloon dilation of the papilla in the clearing of CBD stones using occlusion balloon pushing. This has also gained some popularity for the laparoscopic surgeon during IOC.

Surgical Approaches: Open and Laparoscopic Techniques (see Chapters 37A and 37B)

The same issues discussed in choosing open versus laparoscopic cholecystectomy are accentuated when CBDE is considered. Today, many trainees will graduate residency having never performed an open CBDE. Their ability to succeed with laparoscopic CBDE is quite variable because many train with a default dependence on ERCP.

Approach to Recurrent Common Bile Duct Stones

In some instances, even after successful decompression and stone removal of the common duct with ERCP, patients will continue to present with recurrent choledocholithiasis. Such patients present a management challenge, with varying treatment options. One possible endoscopic approach is balloon dilation of the papilla with concurrent stone removal, which has been shown to decrease subsequent CBD stone recurrences compared with stone extraction alone.[92,93] For patients who fail nonoperative treatments, surgical drainage may be necessary.

Described approaches include choledocholithotomy and T-tube drainage, choledochoduodenostomy, and choledochojejunostomy, and there is evidence indicating that choledochoduodenostomy is the most successful approach for preventing future recurrences.[94-96]

CHOLECYSTECTOMY WITH INTRAOPERATIVE CHOLANGIOGRAPHY (SEE CHAPTERS 24, 37A, AND 37B).

Open and laparoscopic IOC can successfully be completed in the majority of patients by the majority of surgeons.[17] IOC can be performed through the direct insertion of contrast medium into the gallbladder or more often by intubating the cystic duct. Plain radiographs have largely been replaced by digital fluoroscopic imaging. IOC is common, and most surgeons receive sufficient training. Laparoscopic ultrasound cholangiography is also efficacious but not broadly used, and its utility is limited by its longer learning curve.[97] Newer techniques such as hyperspectral cholangiography and near-infrared fluorescence cholangiography hold promise and may become more widely used in the future.[98]

Since the introduction of laparoscopic cholecystectomy, the debate over routine versus selective IOC has been rekindled because of the increased incidence of CBD injuries and the inability to palpate the CBD during laparoscopy. IOC accurately defines the biliary anatomy and may protect against intraoperative bile duct injuries[18] and may reduce their severity.[99] Opponents claim that routine IOC may lead to bile duct injury and unnecessary CBDEs because of false positives and that it may add time and costs unnecessarily.

Selective IOC relies on predicting the probability of choledocholithiasis. In general, patients with a low probability (normal LFTs, normal CBD diameter) may undergo cholecystectomy with no further preoperative investigation and selective IOC. Patients with intermediate risk (isolated abnormal LFTs or CBD dilation) may undergo further preoperative imaging (MRCP) and routine IOC at an absolute minimum. Patients with high risk (jaundice, cholangitis) warrant confirmatory/therapeutic ERCP[88] at most centers. In fact, today many patients are triaged for this purpose, but in years past, many would undergo open CBDE. Ultimately, the choice of modality depends on local availability and expertise in minimally invasive treatments coupled with considerations of cost and convenience.

COMMON BILE DUCT EXPLORATION: TRANSCYSTIC VERSUS CHOLEDOCHOTOMY ACCESS (SEE CHAPTERS 37A AND 37B).

When IOC reveals CBD stones, they can be removed during cholecystectomy. The open choledochotomy to allow cholangioscopy, flushing, forceps and balloon clearance, and T-tube placement is rarely performed or taught today. Instead, laparoscopic CBDE (LCBDE) has evolved as an efficient and more commonly used technique, as described in other chapters. Several studies have shown LCBDE to be at least as efficient as preoperative or postoperative ERCP in terms of stone clearance, morbidity, mortality, and short hospital stay, and thus LCBDE is recommended for surgeons with appropriate skills and facilities.[85] A 2013 Cochrane Review of randomized trials actually demonstrated the superiority of both open and laparoscopic CBDE when compared with ERCP in clearing the CBD, without any associated increased morbidity.[80] For capable surgeons, LCBDE is as safe and efficient as ERCP, thus avoiding the discomfort, costs, and potential complications of an extra procedure.[85,100]

Although LCBDE can be safely performed through either transcystic or choledochotomy approaches, most surgeons prefer the transcystic approach. It is feasible in most cases, saves time, does not violate the CBD, and shows no higher morbidity than standard laparoscopic cholecystectomy alone.[101,102] Techniques available for transcystic CBD stone extraction mirror those used in an open approach. After a cholangiogram, 1 to 2 mg of glucagon can be administered and small stones (<4 mm) can be flushed out of the duct with 30 mL of saline through the cholangiogram catheter.[103] Larger stones can be extracted with a 4 French (F) Fogarty balloon or wire basket under fluoroscopic guidance or direct visualization using a choledochoscope. To accommodate the choledochoscope and allow for extraction of larger stones, the cystic duct often will need to be dilated with a 5 to 8 mm angioplasty balloon.[103,104]

The most consistent risk factor for failing transcystic stone clearance is the size of the stone. Once stones exceed 5 mm, the likelihood of transcystic extraction falls considerably,[105] and laparoscopic choledochotomy becomes necessary. However, many surgeons do not have the laparoscopic dissection and suturing expertise to perform this procedure; they rely instead on ERCP, or they convert to an open operation. Experienced surgeons can remove larger or multiple CBD stones with reported success rates of up to 90%.[106]

The question of how to close the CBD after exploration remains a topic of debate. A 2007 Cochrane Review was not able to conclude significant differences in outcomes for primary closure of the CBD versus the routine use of T-tube drainage after open CBDE.[107] However, two 2013 Cochrane Reviews reported that T-tube drainage results in longer operating times and hospital stays without any apparent benefit over primary closure in both open and laparoscopic CBDE.[108,109] Another 2012 meta-analysis of randomized controlled trials confirmed the superior safety and effectiveness of primary closure over T-tube drainage after laparoscopic CBDE.[110]

Gallstone Pancreatitis (see Chapters 54 and 55)

Acute gallstone pancreatitis is the most frequent form of acute pancreatitis in Western countries. The two most commonly accepted mechanisms for the pathogenesis of gallstone pancreatitis are reflux of bile into the pancreatic duct and transient ampullary obstruction caused by temporary impaction of a stone in the ampulla. The disease is mild in approximately 80% of patients, but 20% experience a more severe clinical course that includes complications such as pancreatic necrosis, multisystem organ failure, and even death.[111–113]

In many patients, the biliary obstruction has spontaneously resolved at the time of presentation, so biliary decompression is not needed. These patients should undergo elective cholecystectomy once the pancreatitis has resolved, with many favoring operation during the index hospitalization. At the other end of the spectrum are patients with gallstone pancreatitis and associated acute cholangitis. Clear evidence shows that endoscopic biliary drainage is beneficial in patients with acute cholangitis; thus these patients should have early biliary decompression.

A secondary question is whether patients with gallstone pancreatitis, without cholangitis, benefit from biliary decompression. Clinical and experimental studies suggest that impacted ampullary stones and persistent biliopancreatic obstruction are associated with a more severe clinical course. In theory, early endoscopic removal of obstructing ampullary gallstones should improve outcomes.[111,112] Between the late 1970s and

mid 1980s, urgent surgery with biliary decompression was studied as a treatment of choice for patients with acute gallstone pancreatitis, but this approach was associated with an increased mortality rate among patients with severe pancreatitis. As such, surgical treatment during the acute phase of the gallstone pancreatitis is not recommended.

The role of nonsurgical intervention, before definitive surgical therapy, has been examined in several prospective randomized studies in which patients with cholangitis were excluded. Integral to any interpretation of treatment approach is the severity of the gallstone pancreatitis. These studies defined *severe pancreatitis* using a number of systems that included the Ranson criteria (>3), Glasgow criteria (>3), or the Acute Physiology and Chronic Health Evaluation (APACHE) II score (>8). The Ranson and Glasgow criteria have the advantage of ease of use and considerable areas of overlap (Table 38.3). A meta-analysis analyzed five prospective randomized studies that examined the use of early biliary decompression in cases of gallstone pancreatitis without cholangitis[114] (see Chapters 54 and 55). This study reported a significant reduction in pancreatitis-related complications in patients with predicted severe pancreatitis (rate difference of 38.5%; 95% confidence interval, –53% to –23.9%; $P < .0001$), but no advantage was seen in cases with mild pancreatitis, and no difference in mortality rate was noted. A 2012 Cochrane Review did not demonstrate any differences between early ERCP and conservative management in pancreatitis of any severity without evidence of cholangitis or biliary obstruction. However, in patients with concurrent cholangitis or biliary obstruction, early ERCP significantly reduced mortality and systemic complications.[115]

TABLE 38.3 Ranson and Glasgow Criteria for Severity of Acute Pancreatitis

CRITERION[a]	ACTION
Ranson	
Age > 55 years	Admission
WBC count > 16,000/mm^3	Admission
Glucose > 200 mg/dL	Admission
AST > 250 IU/L	Admission
LDH > 350 IU/L	Admission
Increased BUN > 8 mg/dL	48 hr
Pao$_2$ < 60 mm Hg	48 hr
Calcium < 8.0 mg/dL	48 hr
Base deficit < 4 mEq/L	48 hr
Fluid sequestration ≥ 6 L	48 hr
Glasgow	
Age > 55 years	Admission
WBC count > 15,000/mm^3	Admission
Glucose > 200 mg/dL	Admission
AST/ALT > 96 IU/L	48 hr
LDH > 219 IU/L	48 hr
BUN > 45 mg/dL	Admission
Pao$_2$ < 76 mm Hg	Admission
Calcium < 8.0 mg/dL	48 hr
Albumin < 3.4 g/dL	48 hr

[a]Mortality rates: 0–2 = 2%, 3–4 = 15%, 5–6 = 40%, >7 = 100%.

ALT, Alanine aminotransferase; *AST*, aspartate aminotransferase; *BUN*, blood urea nitrogen; *LDH*, lactate dehydrogenase; *Pao$_2$*, partial pressure of oxygen in arterial blood; *WBC*, white blood cell count.

The severity of the patient's illness guides the timing of intervention. Patients whose biliary obstruction has spontaneously resolved at the time of presentation and those who have mild predicted pancreatitis should have early elective cholecystectomy once their pancreatitis has resolved. Patients with severe predicted pancreatitis and those with associated cholangitis should undergo early biliary decompression (ERCP or PTC). Among cases of escalating pancreatitis, biliary decompression should be performed within 24 to 72 hours of admission.[114] For cases with associated cholangitis, biliary decompression should occur within 24 hours of presentation. Elective cholecystectomy can then be performed once the severe illness has resolved.

Risk of Recurrence

Historically, recurrence rates of gallstone pancreatitis have been reported as high as 25% to 76% for patients who do not undergo a cholecystectomy at their index presentation.[116] A more contemporary report of 1,119 patients described an overall recurrence rate of 14.6% at a median follow up of 2.3 years. The risk of recurrence was mitigated by ERCP and sphincterotomy with an estimated 5-year recurrence rate of 11.1% compared with 22.7% in patients who underwent no intervention. Median time to recurrence was under 1 year in both groups. Cholecystectomy restores the risk of recurrence of gallstone pancreatitis to that of the general population but does not prevent it entirely.[117]

Cholangitis (see Chapter 43)

Clinical findings associated with acute cholangitis include RUQ abdominal pain, jaundice, fever and chills—also known as *Charcot's triad* (1877). Charcot's triad demonstrates high specificity but low sensitivity because not all patients with cholangitis manifest all findings: 90% develop fever, but only about 50% to 70% of patients develop all three symptoms.[118] *Reynold's pentad* (1959)—Charcot's triad plus shock and altered mental status—represents a form of severe (grade III) cholangitis, which can also manifest with multiorgan dysfunction.

Severe cholangitis is reported in 12% to 30% of patients with acute cholangitis.[118,119]

The 2013 updated Tokyo guidelines, which were subsequently re-affirmed in 2018, provide a more sensitive (91.8%) and specific (77.7%) definition for cholangitis based on signs of systemic inflammation, laboratory evidence of cholestasis, and imaging findings consistent with biliary obstruction (Table 38.4).[120] Patients with systemic inflammation and evidence of either cholestasis or biliary obstruction are said to have a suspected diagnosis, whereas patients with both cholestasis and biliary obstruction are said to have a definitive diagnosis.[120]

Cholangitis is a localized infection of the biliary tree, and an understanding of the pathophysiology of cholangitis guides treatment decisions. Research into this disease has shown that bacteria-laden gallstones are often the source of infection. These bacteria exist in a bacterial microcolony (biofilm) within the pigmented matrix of gallstones (Fig. 38.2).[45] The bacteria must detach from the biofilm to cause a localized infection,

TABLE 38.4 Tokyo Guidelines (TG18/TG13) Diagnostic Criteria for Acute Cholangitis	
CRITERIA	**THRESHOLD**
A. Systemic inflammation	Fever >38°C WBC <4 or >10 CRP ≥ 1
B. Cholestasis	T-Bili ≥ 2 ALP > 1.5 × upper limit of normal GGT > 1.5 × upper limit of normal AST > 1.5 × upper limit of normal ALT > 1.5 × upper limit of normal
C. Imaging	Biliary Dilation Evidence of the etiology on imaging (stricture, stone, stent, etc.)

ALP, Alkaline phosphatase; *ALT,* alanine aminotransferase; *AST,* aspartate aminotransferase; *CRP,* c-reactive protein; *GGT,* r-glutamyltransferase; *T-Bili,* total bilirubin; *WBC,* white blood cell count.

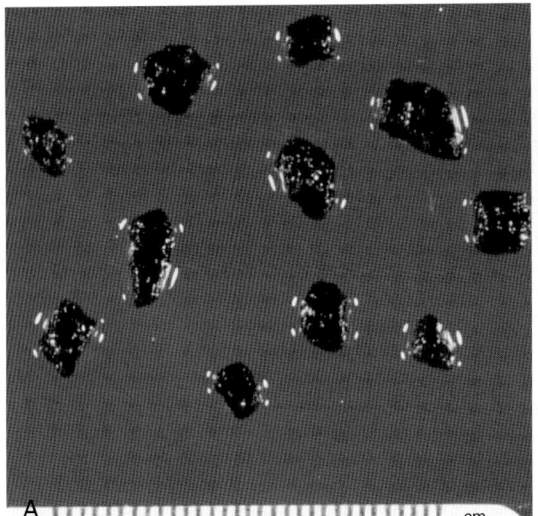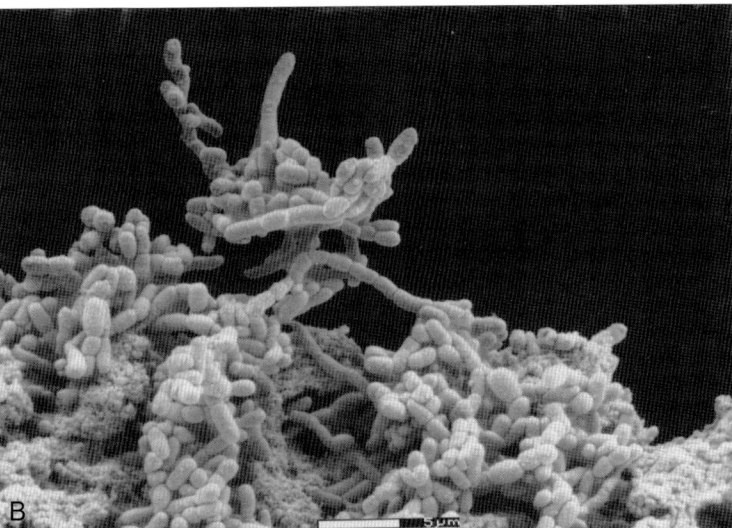

FIGURE 38.2   A, Black-pigment gallstones. **B,** Scanning electron micrograph of the black-pigment stones demonstrating bacterial microcolonies. Note the bacterial bridges and three-dimensional nature of the biofilm. (From Stewart L, Oesterle AL, Erdan I, Griffiss JM, Way LW. The pathogenesis of pigment gallstones in Western societies: The central role of bacteria. *J Gastrointest Surg.* 2002;6:891–904.)

and it must reflux into the cholangiovenous circulation to cause a more severe illness, including bacteremia and organ dysfunction.[121,122] Cholangiovenous reflux occurs with biliary pressures greater than 20 cm H_2O, and even at this pressure, bacterial characteristics (slime production) influence cholangiovenous reflux. In addition, bacterial breakdown by complement releases endotoxin, and this influences the induction of inflammatory cytokines that drive the septic manifestations. It is important to note that although choledocholithiasis is a common cause of biliary obstruction, benign and malignant biliary stenosis and biliary anastomotic strictures are also etiologies.[118]

The 2018/2013 updated Tokyo Guidelines describe three grades of acute cholangitis (Table 38.5): *grade III* is associated with organ failure, *grade II cases* should undergo prompt early biliary drainage, and *grade I* is all others.[120] All patients with suspected cholangitis should be treated with IV hydration and antibiotics that cover the most common biliary organisms: *Escherichia coli, Klebsiella* spp., *Enterococcus, Enterobacter cloacae, Pseudomonas* spp., and anaerobic pathogens. Patients with severe grade III cholangitis also require organ support and stabilization of organ dysfunction.

The critical component of the treatment of cholangitis is biliary decompression. Because elevated biliary pressure drives cholangiovenous reflux, decompression of the biliary tree with ERCP is crucial; PTC may be used if ERCP is not available. Not only does biliary drainage prevent bacterial cholangiovenous reflux, it has also been shown to be associated with a marked decreased in bile and serum endotoxin levels. In the setting of acute cholangitis, biliary drainage via a noninvasive procedure is preferable. Drainage can be achieved using ERCP

or PTC cannulation of the biliary tree. Open surgical drainage may be necessary in medical centers lacking interventional radiology or gastroenterology ERCP capability, or in rare cases where anatomic abnormalities limit noninvasive approaches.[57]

The Tokyo Guidelines provide a useful tool for the management of acute cholangitis (see Table 38.5). Patients with grade I cholangitis who respond to medical therapy can be treated with ERCP (within 24 hours), followed by definitive surgical treatment (laparoscopic cholecystectomy), or the surgeon can proceed to laparoscopic cholecystectomy with intraoperative LCBDE after medical stabilization.[47,123] Factors guiding these choices include the patient's clinical findings and the surgeon's experience with LCBDE. Patients with grade II cholangitis require urgent biliary decompression, whereas patients with severe (grade III) cholangitis require urgent endoscopic or percutaneous transhepatic biliary drainage after stabilization of organ dysfunction. For patients with grade II or III cholangitis, the initial therapy should emphasize biliary decompression rather than definitive removal of all CBD stones. Prolonged procedures with excessive manipulation in an attempt to remove large stones should be avoided in patients with active infectious manifestations. Once the acute illness has resolved, early cholecystectomy can be performed within 6 weeks of biliary decompression with no increase in postoperative complications.[124]

Need for Cholecystectomy After Endoscopic Retrograde Cholangiopancreatography/Sphincterotomy

There has been considerable debate over whether cholecystectomy is required after ERCP/sphincterotomy for patients who initially present with choledocholithiasis. Retrospective studies have reported a low incidence of cholecystectomy among patients with a gallbladder in situ after ERCP/sphincterotomy managed by watchful waiting (10%–15% over 5–14 years).[77,125] Many of these studies involved older patient populations and patients with multiple medical illnesses. A Cochrane Review of prospective randomized studies reported that elective cholecystectomy is recommended to decrease mortality, recurrent biliary symptoms, and the need for repeat interventions such as ERCP and cholangiography.[126] Other contemporary studies also support this recommendation, particularly if there is a history of pancreatitis or if more than 6 months have passed since sphincterotomy was performed.[127] However, when the combined surgical and anesthetic risks are prohibitive, usually because of comorbidities and age, reliance on a sufficient protective sphincterotomy is certainly reasonable.

CHALLENGES IN ADHERING TO THE STANDARD OF CARE

Events have unfolded in the modern era that have forced surgeons to develop new approaches to surgical diseases and modify what is generally considered to be the standard of care. Since 2020, the COVID-19 pandemic profoundly impacted healthcare worldwide and hospitals struggled to cope as their capacities and resources were strained. In March of 2020, as COVID-19 cases in the United States surged, both the American College of Surgeons (ACS) and SAGES issued guidelines encouraging the postponement of elective surgical and endoscopic cases. The care of cholelithiasis/choledocholithiasis was particularly impacted because both endoscopy and laparoscopy

---

TABLE 38.5 Tokyo Guidelines (TG18/TG13) Severity Assessment Criteria for Acute Cholangitis

GRADE	CRITERIA
I: Mild	Does not meet the criteria of grade III (severe) or grade II (moderate) acute cholangitis at initial diagnosis
II: Moderate	Associated with any two of the following conditions: 1. Abnormal WBC count (>12,000/mm³, <4,000/mm³) 2. High fever (≥39°C) 3. Age (≥75 years) 4. Hyperbilirubinemia (total bilirubin ≥ 5 mg/dL) 5. Hypoalbuminemia (<STD × 0.7)
III: Severe	Associated dysfunction in at least one of the following organ systems: 1. Cardiovascular system: hypotension requiring dopamine >5 μg/kg/min or any dose of norepinephrine 2. Nervous system: disturbance of consciousness 3. Respiratory system: Pao₂/Fio₂ ratio < 300 4. Renal system: oliguria, serum creatinine > 2.0 mg/dL 5. Liver: PT-INR > 1.5 6. Hematologic system: platelet count < 100,000/mm³

Fio₂, Forced inspiratory oxygen concentration; *Pao₂,* partial pressure of oxygen in arterial blood; *PT-INR,* prothrombin time/international normalized ratio; *STD,* standard deviation; *WBC,* white blood cell count.

were considered aerosol-generating procedures (AGPs), which increased the risk of healthcare workers. The ACS advised that AGPs should only be performed while wearing full personal protective equipment (PPE) including an N95 mask or power, air-purifying respiratory (PAPR) designed for the operating room. Likewise, SAGES emphasized the enhanced risk of viral exposure to endoscopists and encouraged the use of N95 masks and face shields. Given the profound shortages of PPE in many regions, the challenges in adhering to these guidelines were profound. SAGES additionally advocated for the use of air filtration devices for the evacuation of pneumoperitoneum during laparoscopic or robotic cases to prevent aerosolization, which were not necessarily readily available.[128]

On March 25, 2020, the ACS issued the COVID-19 Guidelines for Triage of Emergency General Surgery Patients, wherein they offered more specific advice for the management of average risk, non–COVID-19 positive patients with surgical diseases during the pandemic. They specifically advised that patients with symptomatic cholelithiasis should have surgery delayed if possible, with consideration of laparoscopic cholecystectomy for those with crescendo symptoms or refractory to medical management. Laparoscopic cholecystectomy was also recommended in healthy patients with cholecystitis to minimize hospital stays, with antibiotics and possible percutaneous cholecystostomy tube advised for high-risk patients or if an operating room was not available. Expectant management was recommended in the setting of choledocholithiasis in the absence of cholangitis, but ERCP and sphincterotomy, with appropriate precautions, were advised if necessary. Another ACS communication by Hughes and Strasberg agreed with postponing surgery in the setting of biliary colic and biliary dyskinesia but proceeding with cholecystectomy in the setting of cholecystitis when resources allowed it.[129]

As the pandemic progressed, additional information was gained, illustrating the significantly increased risk for COVID-19 patients undergoing operations. An international multicenter cohort study analyzed 1,128 patients with SARS-CoV-2 infection who underwent surgery, including 372 who had GI or general surgery[130]; 51.2% of all patients and 53.6% of those undergoing GI/general surgery developed pulmonary complications and an exceedingly high 30-day mortality rate of 23.8% overall and 23.1% after GI/general surgery was demonstrated. Nonoperative management was encouraged whenever possible for COVID-19 patients, particularly male patients and those aged 70 and older who were at increased risk for perioperative mortality.

In 2021, with the improvement of COVID-19 treatments, vaccination strategies and patient safety and distancing guidelines, there has been at least some return to normalcy. COVID-19 testing is providing important reassurance of the safety to proceed more and more often along elective guidelines. Questions remain, and will for some time, especially as case numbers continue to rise worldwide, new COVID variants emerge, and breakthrough infections occur.

SPECIAL POPULATIONS: MANAGEMENT OF CHOLELITHIASIS AND CHOLECYSTITIS IN PREGNANCY

Out of concern for spontaneous abortion and preterm labor, traditional recommendations dictated that operations should be avoided in the first and third trimesters of pregnancy.[131] With the introduction of laparoscopic surgery, further concerns were raised over the risk of trocar injuries to the gravid uterus.[132] Over the past 3 decades as prenatal care and laparoscopic techniques have improved, there has been a concerted effort to delineate better the optimal management of cholelithiasis and cholecystitis in pregnant patients.

Sedaghat et al. performed a meta-analysis of 11 studies and 10,632 patients comparing open and laparoscopic cholecystectomy in pregnancy. They found a significant decrease in the rate of fetal and maternal complications, with a shorter length of hospital stay when laparoscopy was employed. Patients who underwent laparoscopic cholecystectomy had a gestational age 6 weeks younger compared with the open approach in this study (18 vs. 24 weeks). The conversion rate from laparoscopic to open cholecystectomy was reported to be relatively low at 3.8%.[133]

As patients exit the first trimester, there are important technical adaptations that are required to accommodate the gravid uterus. Patients should be placed in partial left lateral decubitus to prevent compression of the inferior vena cava (IVC). Initial access and subsequent port placement should be adjusted for fundal height but can be safely accomplished with a Veress needle or open Hassan technique. Typically, a right subcostal trocar allows for safe access to the peritoneal cavity. Standard insufflation pressures can ordinarily be used but should be adjusted based on the patient's hemodynamics.[134]

Regarding the timing of surgery, there is no difference in the rates of preterm delivery and spontaneous abortion when symptomatic cholelithiasis is managed conservatively or by laparoscopic cholecystectomy regardless of trimester.[135] However, when patients present with complicated biliary disease, the rates of preterm labor and spontaneous abortion increase, with studies reporting rates of fetal loss as high as 60% in severe disease. Patients are at high risk of recurrent disease, with rates as high as 92%, 64%, and 44% in the first, second, and third trimester, respectively.[134] Ultimately, 50% of these patients will require hospitalization, with 23% of those patients developing complicated biliary disease.[134,136] Given the high rates of recurrence and risk of preterm labor and spontaneous abortion, in 2017 SAGES published guidelines for the evaluation and management of cholecystitis in pregnancy, advocating for the use of laparoscopic cholecystectomy in all trimesters for the treatment of cholecystitis.[134]

CONCLUSION

In 1970, who could have predicted that the common ailments of cholecystolithiasis and choledocholithiasis would soon face historical advances in technology? Patients now benefit from improved imaging and minimally invasive endoscopic and laparoscopic techniques, especially when combined. Nevertheless, although our technical strategies only occasionally resemble those of a bygone era in biliary surgery, our treatment strategies should reflect enduring principles. Disease severity grading, diagnostic criteria, drainage, timing and patient selection will always be critical. By combining technical versatility and flexibility upon these principles, we can continue to drive improved outcomes worldwide for these conditions.

References are available at expertconsult.com.

CHAPTER 39

Intrahepatic stone disease

Itaru Endo, Ryusei Matsuyama, Norifumi Kumamoto, and Yuki Homma

OVERVIEW

Hepatolithiasis (intrahepatic stones) is defined as the presence of gallstones in the bile ducts peripheral to the confluence of the right and left hepatic ducts. These intrahepatic stones can simultaneously be present with stones in the common bile duct (CBD) and/or gallbladder. Hepatolithiasis, which is most prevalent in East Asia, is characterized by recurrent bouts of cholangitis and can lead to sepsis, biliary cirrhosis, and even death if not properly treated (see Chapters 43 and 44). Hepatolithiasis is also associated with intrahepatic cholangiocarcinoma (ICC; see Chapter 50). Although the incidence of primary hepatolithiasis has decreased as a result of urbanization in endemic areas, the prevalence of secondary hepatolithiasis associated with past biliary surgery has increased with recent increases in hepatobiliary surgery and increased long-term survival.

Hepatolithiasis can be diagnosed by ultrasonography (US), computed tomography (CT), and magnetic resonance imaging (MRI). Direct cholangiography and three-dimensional CT are useful in deciding treatment strategies (see Chapter 16).

Treatment for hepatolithiasis can be divided broadly into partial hepatectomy and endoscopic treatment. Treatment must be tailored to each patient, depending on performance status, liver function, stone location, and liver atrophy. With liver resection, bile duct strictures can also be eliminated, so stone recurrence rates are generally lower. Although satisfactory stone removal rates can be achieved with endoscopic treatment, rates of clinical failure are higher if bile duct strictures are not completely resolved, which can lead to recurrent cholangitis and subsequent ICC. Hepatectomy can be performed when the disease is limited to the right or left hemiliver with ipsilateral atrophy. In patients with multiple bile duct strictures in both hemilivers, percutaneous transhepatic cholangioscopic lithotomy (PTCSL) with balloon dilation is generally applied to remove stones and treat biliary strictures (see Chapters 20 and 31). Bilateral hepatic resections may offer better stone clearance and a reduced risk of ICC because of effective clearance of the affected liver in selected patients. Hepatolithiasis requires careful management for the possible presence of ICC, even after stone clearance. Long-term follow-up for at least 10 years is recommended.

EPIDEMIOLOGY

Hepatolithiasis is commonly seen in East Asian patients, but the incidence varies, even among Asian countries (Table 39.1).[1–12] In Japan, the Ministry of Health, Labour, and Welfare organized a research group to evaluate the epidemiology of hepatolithiasis and improve outcomes. This research group has conducted nationwide surveys seven times in the past 40 years. Their studies revealed that the incidence of hepatolithiasis among all patients with gallstone disease has decreased from 3% to 1.8%.[13] Although hepatolithiasis has largely been limited to Asia, the incidence has increased in Western countries as a result of more common worldwide travel and increasing Asian immigration.

ETIOLOGY

The etiology of hepatolithiasis is unknown in about 70% to 80% of cases. Intrahepatic stones are classified by composition into calcium bilirubinate or cholesterol stones (see Chapter 8). Calcium bilirubinate stones are predominant, representing about 75% of cases, whereas stones formed within the gallbladder are composed mainly of cholesterol, suggesting differences in the lithogenic mechanism of gallbladder stones.

Hepatolithiasis is thought to be generated by four factors: infection, bile metabolism changes, anatomic abnormalities, and bile stasis.[14,15] The higher incidence of hepatolithiasis in rural compared with urban areas also suggests that poor nutrition and environmental factors play additional roles.[16,17] In Japan, as the urbanization of society has advanced, the chance of bacterial contamination decreased, which may also explain the decreasing incidence of bile pigment stones. In fact, a decrease in the presence of bactibilia, from 92.1% in 1913 to 67.3% in 1961, has been documented.[18] A survey conducted in the town of Kamigoto in Nagasaki Prefecture, an area in Japan with a high incidence of hepatolithiasis (about 30% of all gallstone diseases), reported that the expression of specific human leukocyte antigens—A26, B44, BW54, CW7, and DR6—was higher in patients with than in those without intrahepatic stones.[19] However, the etiologic role of these genetic factors remains undefined.

Infection of the biliary tree has long been regarded as a cause of bile pigment stones. Maki and colleagues found increased β-glucuronidase activity in bile harboring bile pigment stones.[20,21] It has been suggested that the increased activity of β-glucuronidase caused by bacterial contamination may be an important factor in lithogenicity. Glucuronic acid–conjugated bilirubin, the major component of bile bilirubin, is water soluble. However, it converts to unconjugated bilirubin, which is less soluble, when hydrolyzed by β-glucuronidase, which may be derived from bacteria. It is thought that unconjugated bilirubin combines with a calcium ion in bile before being deposited as bilirubin calcium. Despite reports of an association between *Escherichia coli* and CBD stones in Western Europe, the incidence of intrahepatic stones remains very low, and therefore biliary infection alone is an unlikely cause of hepatolithiasis.

The presence of chronic biliary inflammation has been shown to accelerate stone formation via increased secretion of mucin core proteins (MUCs). In addition, in biliary tract infection, pathogen-associated molecular patterns, such as increased

TABLE 39.1 Incidence of Intrahepatic Stones in Studies Involving Patients With Hepatolithiasis				
REFERENCE, YEAR	**COUNTRY**	**TOTAL PATIENTS**	**HEPATOLITHIASIS**	**PERCENTAGE (%)**
Asia				
King[1]	Malaysia	661	120	18.2
Nakayama[2]	Singapore	647	11	1.7
Nakayama[3]	China	394	83	21.1
Su[4]	Taiwan	17,182	3,486	20.3
Han[5]	Korea	1344	145	10.8
Uchiyama[6]	Japan	10,5062	2,353	2.2
North and South America				
Best[7]	United States	456	35	7.6
Glenn[8]	United States	169	22	13.0
Bove[9]	Brazil	2000	20	1.0
Yarmuch[10]	Chile	17,200	251	1.5
Europe				
Lindström[11]	Sweden	804	5	0.6
Simi[12]	Italy	2700	36	1.3

bacterial lipopolysaccharide and lipoteichoic acid, bind to Toll-like receptors on bile duct epithelial cell membranes. The production of inflammatory cytokines from biliary epithelium is also increased. This activates intracellular signal molecules and increases the expression of protein kinase, nuclear factor kappa B (NF-κB), MUC2, and MUC5. Tian et al. reported that neutrophil elastase can stimulate MUC5AC expression in human biliary epithelial cells.[22] The increased secretion of mucin induces gel formation of bile and may accelerate bile stasis, leading to crystallization. Therefore these factors are considered to be associated with stone formation and chronic proliferative cholangitis (CPC).

This disease entity includes recurrent pyogenic cholangitis (see Chapter 44), which is endemic in Southeast Asia, as first reported by Digby and colleagues at Hong Kong University.[23] Clonorchiasis (*Clonorchis sinensis*), ascariasis (*Ascaris lumbricoides*), and fascioliasis (*Fasciola* spp.; see Chapter 45) can lead to inflammation of the biliary epithelium. Patients with clonorchiasis (*C. sinensis*) are usually asymptomatic when the number of flukes is small, but bile duct obstruction, suppurative cholangitis, and intrahepatic stones usually occur when 500 to 1000 flukes (hepatic distomiasis) are present because the parasite's fragments or eggs can act as a nidus for stone formation. Fluke eggs in the feces or bile and peripheral blood eosinophilia are important diagnostic findings for this disease. The presence of hepatolithiasis in regions without endemic parasitic infection supports the concept that biliary parasites may not be regarded as a primary cause of hepatolithiasis.

In regard to bile metabolic changes, a feature of intrahepatic calcium bilirubinate stones is that, compared with calcium bilirubinate stones in the gallbladder and CBD, a relatively high cholesterol content has been reported.[24,25] Cholesterol in hepatic bile may result from relative cholesterol supersaturation because of increased cholesterol secretion from hepatocytes or to relatively decreased bile phospholipids and acids.[26] Specifically, decreased phospholipid secretion leads to reduced cholesterol dissolution and easier formation of lithogenic bile.[27-29]

Transporter proteins in the bile canalicular membrane are involved in secretion and thus may also be a factor leading to changes in bile composition[30] (see Chapter 8). Multidrug resistance-associated protein 3 (MRP3), encoded by the *ABCB4* gene, is involved in phospholipid secretion. MRP2, encoded by the *ABCC2* gene, is involved in bilirubin excretion, and bile salt export pump protein (BSEP), encoded by the *ABCB11* gene, is involved in bile acid secretion.[31-33] Therefore the role these transport proteins play as membrane proteins leading to changes in bile composition and the development of hepatolithiasis has received increasing attention.[33] Recent studies have revealed that a single nucleotide polymorphism of the *ABCB4* and *ABCB11* genes might affect the expression of pertinent transporter proteins.[34,35] Gan et al. (2019) reported that rs497692 and rs118109635 mutations affected translation of the *ABCB11* gene, resulting in the downregulation of BSEP expression.[36] Dysregulation of these transporter proteins may change the composition of bile and lead to cholestasis and cholelithiasis. These genetic changes could explain the different racial and regional distributions of hepatolithiasis.

Whether simple anatomic bile stenosis or bile stasis alone can cause stone formation remains unclear; however, biliary stenosis and bile stasis usually co-exist, and can cause a high rate of stone formation. Indeed, numerous studies have reported that biliary stricture and stasis are strong predictors of stone recurrence and cholangitis after treatment for hepatolithiasis.

SECONDARY HEPATOLITHIASIS

Secondary hepatolithiasis associated with past biliary surgery or congenital biliary malformation is an example of a case in which the etiology can be presumed.[37] With recent increases in hepatobiliary surgery and long-term survival, secondary hepatolithiasis because of bilioenteric stenosis or duct-to-duct biliary anastomoses has increased[38,39] (see Chapters 32 and 42).

Congenital choledochal cysts (CCs), including those in Caroli syndrome, are well known for their anatomic features, which include dilation and strictures of the intrahepatic and extrahepatic biliary tract (see Chapter 46). Congenital CCs are associated with intrahepatic stones (12%–17% of adult patients),[40–42] as well as a high incidence of biliary tract carcinoma (10.6%–20.3%).[42,43] Hepatolithiasis occurs in 3.5% to 23.5% of patients after flow-diversion surgery for congenital CCs.[44–48] Bile contamination and anastomotic strictures resulting from hepaticojejunal (Roux-en-Y) anastomosis may be contributing factors,[49] but much remains unknown about the mechanisms of onset. Type IV-A cysts are most commonly associated with cholangitis and intrahepatic stone formation.[45,46] Aota et al. (2018) reported a higher postoperative incidence of hepatolithiasis in Type IV-A than in Type I cysts (7/20 [35%] vs. 1/20 [5.0%], respectively).[50] Because complete resection of the dilated left and right hepatic ducts is difficult in Type IV-A cysts, part of the dilated ducts often remains, possibly leading to bile stasis. In such instances, creating a wide anastomosis by extending the incision along the lateral wall of both hepatic ducts by common hepatic duct-plasty is often attempted to obtain a wide hepaticoenterostomy at the hepatic hilum.

In addition to the possible carcinogenesis related to long-term stimulation of the biliary mucosa by pancreatic juices, bilioenteric anastomosis itself may accelerate carcinogenesis as a result of irritation from contaminated bile, even in benign conditions (see Chapter 51).[51–53] The risk of subsequent biliary malignancy in patients undergoing cyst excision for congenital CCs has been reported to be 0.7% to 5.4%.[46,54–56] Indeed, the risk of biliary malignancy remains elevated, even more than 15 years after CC excision.[57] Therefore long-term surveillance is important after hepaticojejunostomy for congenital biliary cysts because the risk of cancer is suspected to be doubled.[58]

Bile duct stones, sludge, and casts, which represent bile duct filling defects, occur in approximately 5% of patients after living donor liver transplantation (LDLT),[59] with the majority of such defects caused by stones[60] (see Chapter 111). Because the anastomotic site is more peripheral to that in orthotopic liver transplantation, hepatic ducts at the anastomotic site are usually small and thin walled. Therefore anastomotic stricture is likely to occur more frequently in LDLT than in deceased donor liver transplantation. Persistent cholangitis caused by small stones is sometimes difficult to discriminate from T-cell–mediated rejection and drug-induced liver dysfunction. Because delayed diagnosis and treatments may affect both long-term graft and patient survival, early recognition and prompt treatment of intrahepatic stones after liver transplantation is essential.

CHOLANGIOCARCINOMA

The development of cholangiocarcinoma (CCA) in patients with hepatolithiasis is associated with poor outcomes (see Chapters 50 and 51). The incidence of CCA in patients with hepatolithiasis reported from Asian centers ranges from 2.1% to 15.6% (Table 39.2).[61–78] By contrast, hepatolithiasis is uncommon in Western countries, with a reported incidence of only 2.4%.[11,12,79,80] Vetrone and colleagues (2006) found only one case with intramucosal adenocarcinoma of the extrahepatic bile duct out of 22 patients with hepatolithiasis who underwent surgical therapy.[70] On the other hand, Tabrizian and colleagues

TABLE 39.2 Incidence of Intrahepatic Cholangiocarcinoma in Hepatolithiasis

REFERENCE	HEPATOLITHIASIS	ICC	PERCENTAGE (%)
Koga, 1985[61]	61	3	4.9
Chen, 1989[62]	1105	55	5.0
Sheen-Chen, 1991[63]	101	5	5.0
Kubo, 1995[64]	113	10	8.8
Liu, 1998[65]	96	15	15.6
Huang, 2003[66]	209	5	2.4
Chen, 2004[67]	103	10	9.7
Cheung, 2005[68]	174	10	5.7
Herman, 2005[69]	48	1	2.1
Vetrone, 2006[70]	22	1	4.5
Lee, 2007[71]	123	3	2.4
Al-Sukhni, 2008[72]	42	5	12
Uenishi, 2009[73]	87	10	11.5
Suzuki, 2012[74]	336	23	6.8
Tabrizian, 2012[75]	30	7	23.3
Lin CC, 2013[76]	211	10	4.7
Guglielmi, 2014[77]	161	23	14.3
Zhu QD, 2014[78]	2056	107	5.2

ICC, Intrahepatic cholangiocarcinoma.

(2012) reported a much higher incidence of concomitant CCA (7/30 [23.3%]) during a 14-year follow-up period.[75] In addition, Al-Sukhni and colleagues (2008) reported identifying CCA in 5 (12%) of 42 patients during a 20-year study period.[72] Guglielmi and colleagues (2014) prospectively collected a cohort of 161 patients with hepatolithiasis from five Italian tertiary hepatobiliary centers.[77] From their database, 23 (14.3%) patients with concomitant ICC were identified. From the aforementioned reports, although the overall incidence of hepatolithiasis is low in Western countries, the incidence of CCA arising in conjunction with hepatolithiasis is similar when comparing Eastern and Western countries. Therefore hepatolithiasis needs to be carefully evaluated for the possible presence of ICC, even in Western countries.

Although the association between hepatolithiasis and CCA is well recognized, the exact mechanism of carcinogenesis remains unclear. Persistent inflammation because of cholangitis can cause repeated tissue damage and regeneration; this recurrent inflammatory process may lead to carcinogenesis. Hyperplastic epithelial cells often show a papillomatous or adenomatous pattern, which is frequently associated with the presence of stones.[61] Ohta and colleagues (1991) reported that various degrees of hyperplastic biliary epithelium exist around impacted stones and are associated with CPC.[81] Mucosal dysplasia accompanied by MUC and cytokeratin expression may be a precursor to CCA.[82] Recent studies have suggested that multiple factors, including NF-κB, epidermal growth factor receptor, prostaglandin E_2, c-Met, and p16, are associated with cell proliferation, inflammation, and carcinogenesis.[83]

However, no clear symptoms or clinical presentations have been reported to be associated with the presence of CCA in patients with hepatolithiasis. Therefore the possibility of co-existing CCA should be considered in all cases but especially in unusual presentations, such as weight loss, anemia, and intractable pain.[63]

Some risk factors for ICC concomitant with hepatolithiasis have been reported (Box 39.1).[74,84,85] Atrophic liver segments with persistent cholangitis are well-accepted risk factors. CCA is likely to be found in atrophic liver with obliterated portal flow.[64] Therefore hepatectomy of an atrophic liver with intrahepatic stones and biliary strictures may reduce the risk of CCA.[73]

Concomitant CCA has been reported to be a strong negative predictive factor for overall survival after hepatectomy for hepatolithiasis.[67] Zhu et al. (2014) found that 107 of 2056 patients who had undergone surgical treatment for hepatolithiasis had CCA.[78] Overall, the 5-year survival rate was 20.2%, and a subgroup of patients who had undergone potentially curative resection showed good 5-year survival (50.0%). However, only about 40% (38/97) of patients underwent curative resection; the other 60% underwent either palliative resection, radiofrequency ablation, or were not resected. Zhang et al. (2018) reported that patients with hepatolithiasis-associated CCA had worse long-term outcomes than those with conventional ICC.[86] Five-year overall survival among patients with hepatolithiasis-associated ICC was 18.3% compared with 38.0% for those with conventional ICC.

It should be noted that subsequent ICC may occur even after primary treatment for hepatolithiasis. Chijiiwa and colleagues (1995) reported that among 85 patients with hepatolithiasis, 6 (7%) died of subsequent CCA during a mean follow-up period of 6 years.[87] Cheon et al. (2009) also reported that the rate of late development of CCA in patients with intrahepatic stones during follow-up was 4.8% (11/225).[88] More recently, Kim et al. (2018) analyzed Korean National Health Insurance data.[89] Among the 7419 patients who had undergone liver resection for hepatolithiasis, subsequent ICC developed in 107 (1.98%). Table 39.3 shows the incidence of subsequent ICC (approximately 0.3%–9.1%) among patients with hepatolithiasis.[58,61,66,71,73,76,88–95] The mean interval from initial treatment to the development of CCA was 10.7 years (range, 6.6–19.7 years). Half of those patients developed CCA at a site different from the initial site of hepatolithiasis.

Regarding the risk factors for subsequent ICC, age older than 65 years and stone removal only as the initial treatment were significant risk factors for the subsequent development of CCA.[13] Further, the study revealed that age older than 65 years and the presence of biliary strictures were significant risk factors for the development of CCA in patients with a history of bilioenteric anastomosis. On the other hand, in patients

TABLE 39.3 Rate of Metachronous ICC After Primary Treatment for Intrahepatic Stones

REFERENCE	YEAR	HL	ICC	PERCENTAGE (%)
Koga[61]	1985	61	2	3.3
Chijiiwa[90]	1993	109	8	7.3
Jan[91]	1996	427	12	2.8
Furukawa[92]	1998	122	3	2.5
Huang[66]	2003	209	5	2.4
Lee[71]	2007	123	2	1.6
Uenishi[73]	2009	77	2	2.6
Cheon[88]	2009	227	11	4.8
Li[93]	2012	718	2	0.3
Lin[76]	2013	137	12	6.1
Tsuyuguchi[58]	2014	121	11	9.1
Kim[94]	2015	236	16	6.8
Meng[95]	2017	981	55	5.6
Kim[89]	2018	7419	107	1.98

HL, Hepatolithiasis; *ICC*, intrahepatic cholangiocarcinoma.

without a history of a bilioenteric anastomosis, left lobe location and stone recurrence were significant risk factors for the development of subsequent CCA. Although partial hepatectomy as the initial treatment was associated with a reduced risk of CCA, it did not reach the level of statistical significance ($P = .066$). On the other hand, Kim et al. (2015) reported that subsequent CCA occurred with similar rates in patients treated with and without hepatic resection (6.3% vs. 7.1%, respectively).[83] They emphasized that the presence of residual stones was the most significant risk factor for subsequent CCA regardless of the initial treatment; therefore hepatic resection is considered to have limited value in preventing CCA. Meng et al. (2017) reported that the presence of stone-affected remaining liver segments after initial hepatic resection was also a predictive factor for subsequent CCA.[95]

Long-term outcomes of patients with subsequent CCA after treatment for hepatolithiasis are extremely poor. The mean interval from diagnosis of CCA to disease-related death has been reported to be 4 months, compared with 41 months for patients with concomitant CCA at the time of initial diagnosis.[76] Based on a Korean national database, patients with subsequent CCA had very poor survival outcomes compared with those with concomitant CCA, with a median survival time of 0.9 years.[89] Intensive follow-up is therefore mandatory, especially in patients with risk factors for subsequent CCA, such as residual stones, hepaticojejunostomy, and a remaining stone-affected liver segment.

SYMPTOMS

Charcot's triad of symptoms—abdominal pain, fever, and jaundice—occur in about 60% of patients with hepatolithiasis[65] (see Chapter 43). These pyogenic cholangitis-related symptoms tend to recur over the long term. Severe cholangitis is sometimes concomitant with liver abscess and septic shock. Patients with septic shock often develop disseminated intravascular

BOX 39.1 Predictive Factors for Concomitant Cholangiocarcinoma

Liver atrophy (Suzuki[74])
Smoking (Liu[84])
Family history of cancer (Liu[84])
Duration of symptoms > 10 years (Liu[84])
History of gastrectomy (Jo[85])
History of cholechochoenterostomy (Suzuki[74]; Jo[85])
Elevated serum CA19-9 (Jo[85])

cholangiopathy. On the other hand, some patients with hepatolithiasis present without any symptoms. According to a Japanese survey, 20% of patients with hepatolithiasis showed no symptoms.[96] In another study, 14 (11.5%) of 122 patients with asymptomatic hepatolithiasis developed symptoms during long-term follow-up.[97] In difficult-to-treat cases, when stones cannot be completely removed or bile duct strictures are not eliminated, hepatolithiasis is likely to recur. Symptoms occur in patients with biliary cirrhosis because of chronic recurrent cholangitis; this often progresses to liver failure. Patients in whom CCA develops during follow-up often present with an abdominal mass, bloating because of ascites, and weight loss.

DIAGNOSIS

Acute cholangitis accompanied by hepatolithiasis is diagnosed by findings of systemic inflammation, cholestasis, and imaging showing intrahepatic biliary dilation, strictures, and stone formation.[98] Acute cholangitis can present with a wide range of severity. The diagnosis of acute cholangitis is usually made, or at least suspected, on the basis of a physical examination and the patient's medical history. Charcot's triad—abdominal pain, fever, and jaundice—is the classic presentation of acute cholangitis. However, only 50% to 70% of patients show all three features at acute presentation (see Chapter 43).

Blood test findings commonly show an elevated white blood cell count, elevated levels of hepatobiliary enzymes, and hyperbilirubinemia. Amylase levels are also elevated in about 20% of patients. Blood cultures are often positive, and the most commonly isolated microorganisms are *E. coli*, *Morganella morganii*, *Klebsiella* spp., and *Enterobacter* spp.[69] Bacteria in bile, when tested, are isolated from cultures in about 85% of cases. Biliary cultures usually grow Gram-negative bacteria, such as *E. coli*, *Klebsiella* spp., and *Enterobacter* spp. Cholangitis caused by *Enterococcus* spp. and *Pseudomonas aeruginosa* has become more common.[99,100] In one study, serum carbohydrate antigen 19-9 was elevated in 18 (78.3%) of 23 patients with CCA.[101]

IMAGING DIAGNOSIS

The presence of stones in intrahepatic bile ducts represents an important imaging finding for diagnosing hepatolithiasis, but the location of the bile duct branches in which intrahepatic stones are present is also very important in planning treatment.[102–104]

Concerning the location of stones, the Japan Research Group for the Study of Hepatolithiasis classifies patients with stones only in the intrahepatic bile duct as type I and those with stones both in the intrahepatic and extrahepatic bile ducts as type IE. Furthermore, patients are classified by the location of stones as follows: right side: type R; left side: type L; right and left sides: type LR; and caudate lobe: type C. Several other classifications according to the location of biliary strictures have been proposed. Figure 39.1 summarizes the classification system proposed by Takada and colleagues (1978).[105]

Useful imaging modalities include US, CT, and MRI (see Chapter 13), but direct imaging techniques such as percutaneous transhepatic cholangiography (PTC), endoscopic retrograde cholangiography (ERC), and transpapillary or percutaneous cholangioscopy are available (see Chapters 20, 30, 31, 37, and 52). The radiologic diagnosis of hepatolithiasis can be difficult because of changes and technical constraints associated with

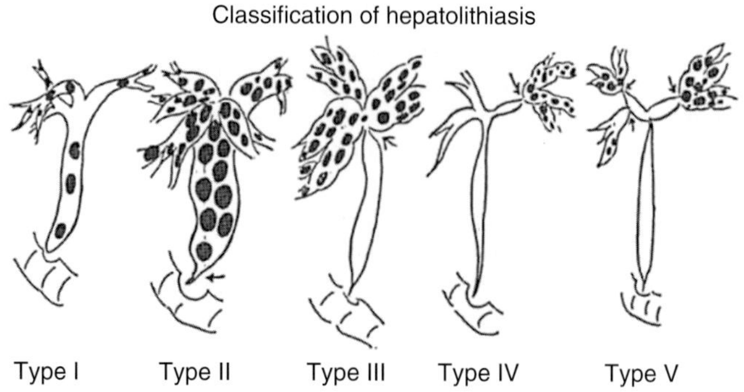

Classification of hepatolithiasis

Type I   Type II   Type III   Type IV   Type V

FIGURE 39.1 Classification of hepatolithiasis proposed by Takada and colleagues (1978). This classification is divided into five types according to the location of the stones and strictures. Type I: no strictures in the intrahepatic and extrahepatic biliary tract, with mild dilation of the biliary system. Type II: biliary stricture in the lower bile duct or ampulla of the duodenum, showing remarkable dilation of the bile ducts. Type III: stricture at the hepatic hilum. Type IV: biliary stricture in the unilateral hepatic lobe. Type V: multiple biliary strictures in the bilateral hepatic lobe or bilateral congenital biliary cysts.

cholangitis, which may also co-exist with cholelithiasis, and previous biliary surgery. Therefore highly technical procedures such as hepatectomy and/or several kinds of endoscopic lithotripsy may be required. As a result, unlike patients with cholecystitis or choledocholithiasis, patients with hepatolithiasis are often treated at high-volume tertiary centers.

The number of new cases of primary hepatolithiasis has recently decreased, whereas the number of cases of secondary hepatolithiasis is increasing in patients with prior biliary reconstructive surgery. In the latter case, the diagnosis may be more difficult because of previous biliary reconstruction such as hepaticojejunostomy.

The diagnosis of co-existing ICC is important (see Chapter 50). CCA may occur at biliary stricture sites; however, differential diagnosis based on imaging alone may be difficult because of the background presence of stones, inflammation, or pneumobilia. As a result, ICC is often incidentally found during surgery.[64,81,106] Preoperative bile cytology and intraoperative frozen-section examination of resection margins are recommended in older patients with severe biliary strictures.

Intrahepatic stones include calcium bilirubinate and cholesterol stones. Calcium bilirubinate stones are often present in the left and right bile ducts near the porta hepatis, and severe morphologic changes, such as strictures and dilation, are common. On the other hand, cholesterol stones, which are smaller and may be multiple, are found in segmental and peripheral biliary branches. Biliary dilation (cholangiectasis) is usually limited to sites where stones are present, and the dilation of upstream bile ducts is uncommon. In addition, a stricture of downstream bile ducts is not usually seen, a finding that differs from calcium bilirubinate stones. In addition, cholesterol stones cannot be visualized on CT.

When a diagnosis of hepatolithiasis is suspected, noninvasive abdominal US should initially be performed. If hepatolithiasis is strongly suspected, performing CT or magnetic resonance cholangiography (MRC) is also important to avoid other unnecessary tests. If the presence of stones is confirmed, further testing to identify the site of stones, such as direct cholangiography, is useful in planning a treatment strategy.

ABDOMINAL ULTRASOUND

Abdominal US is a convenient and noninvasive method that provides excellent depiction of stones and dilated bile ducts; therefore it is the initial imaging modality of choice when hepatolithiasis is suspected (see Chapter 15). Calcium bilirubinate stones, which are common in hepatolithiasis, show the same or slightly higher echogenicity than the liver, and a weaker acoustic shadow (Fig. 39.2A–B). Bile ducts above the stone site are often dilated. Meanwhile, cholesterol stones have higher echogenicity than surrounding liver parenchyma and a stronger acoustic shadow (see Fig. 39.2C). Areas of biliary dilation are often limited to where the stones are located.[107,108]

Other findings that suggest the presence of hepatolithiasis include segmental liver atrophy and decreased segmental blood flow.[109] An important point is that stones may not always have acoustic shadows. Pneumobilia can also appear as a hyperechoic area with acoustic shadows within bile ducts, so careful attention should be paid to the differential diagnosis with intrahepatic stones (see Fig. 39.2C). Another pitfall is that bile ducts may not be depicted if filled with biliary sludge and showing high echogenicity.[65]

ABDOMINAL COMPUTED TOMOGRAPHY

Abdominal CT can depict not only stones but also the location they are located within the intrahepatic ducts, in addition to any bile duct dilation or strictures proximal and distal to the stone sites[110] (see Chapter 13). Calcium bilirubinate stones with high calcium content appear as hyperintensities on CT (Fig. 39.3). However, intrahepatic stones often have a lower calcium content than CBD stones and may not be depicted because of CT density values similar to those of bile. Cholesterol stones show almost the same pixel value as bile, and thus may not be depicted on CT (Fig. 39.4).

Segmental hepatic atrophy in hepatolithiasis is an indication for liver resection and, therefore, atrophy on CT is an important finding. Segmental atrophy on CT may appear as a crowding of

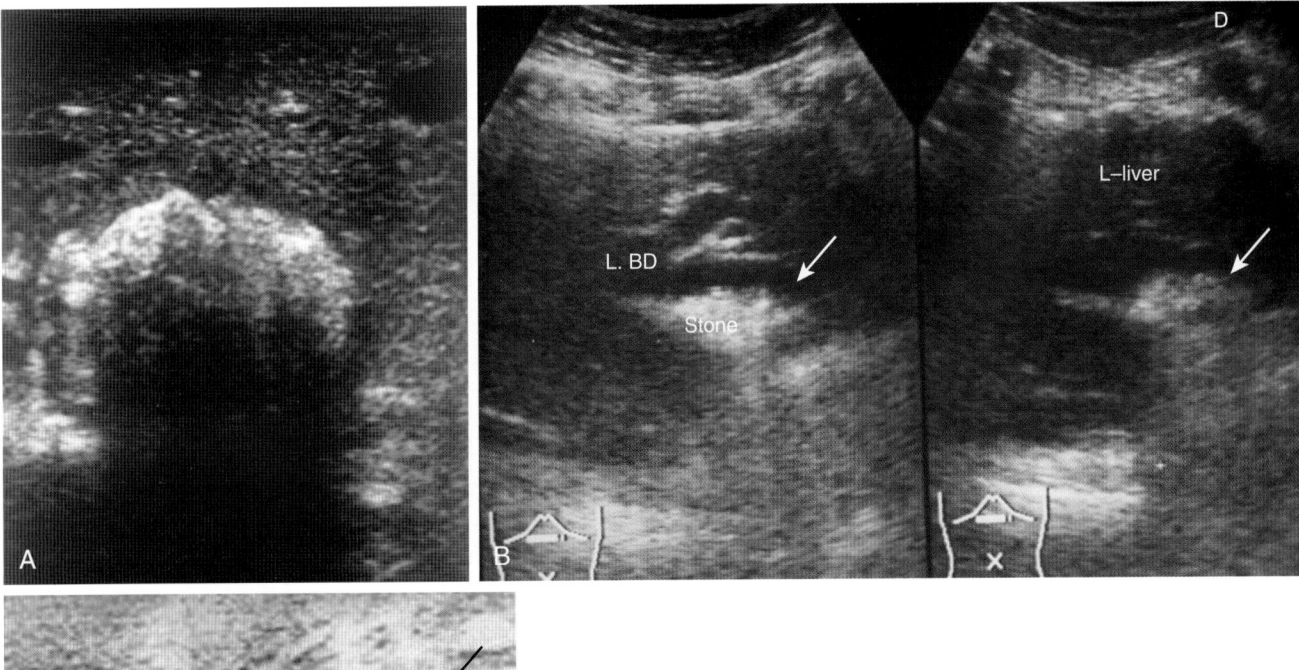

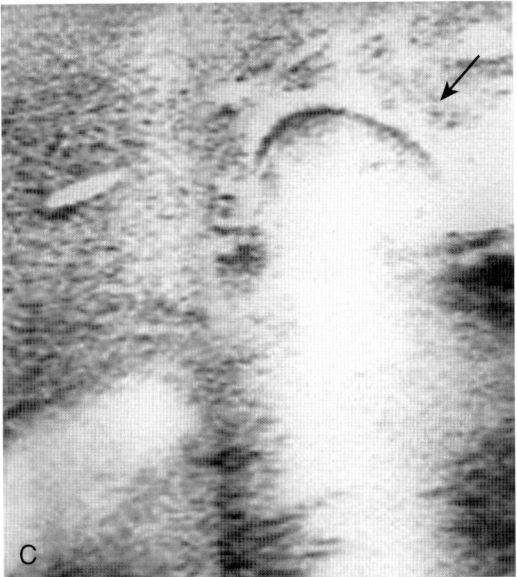

FIGURE 39.2   A, Abdominal ultrasound of the liver shows a shadowing echogenic mass. **B,** A cluster of small echogenic stones without shadowing *(arrows)*. Note the moderate dilation of subsegmental bile ducts with a thick wall. **C,** A strong shadowing stone with linear round-shaped echo *(arrow)*. *L. BD,* left bile duct. (See Chapter 13.)

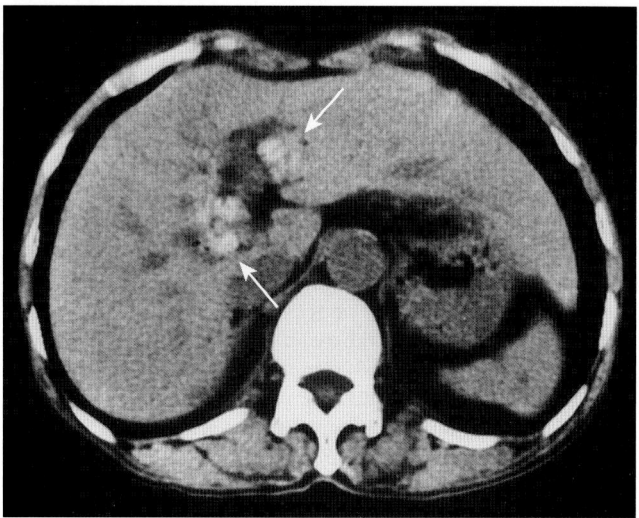

FIGURE 39.3 Noncontrast computed tomography shows high-density shadows in the bilateral hepatic lobe *(arrows)*. (See Chapter 13.)

bile duct branches, diminished portal blood flow, and a loss of portal vein branches (Fig. 39.5). Patients with severe liver damage may also show splenomegaly.[111]

In most cases, intrahepatic calcification, a finding often observed on screening, is not because of intrahepatic stones but rather because of tuberculosis, bleeding, or parasitic infestation. Therefore other findings must also be present for a diagnosis of hepatolithiasis. When clay-like stones fill the biliary branch segments, they may not be easily identifiable in imaging studies.

MAGNETIC RESONANCE IMAGING

MRI carries no radiation exposure risks, can identify intrahepatic stones and bile duct strictures, and is useful in diagnosing hepatolithiasis[112–114] (see Chapter 13). In MRC, stones with little water content have relatively low signal intensity compared with signal-hyperintense bile and appear as filling defects (Fig. 39.6). However, if bile stasis is present, inspissated bile demonstrates low signal intensity. Therefore stones may not be able to be diagnosed, and bile ducts may not be

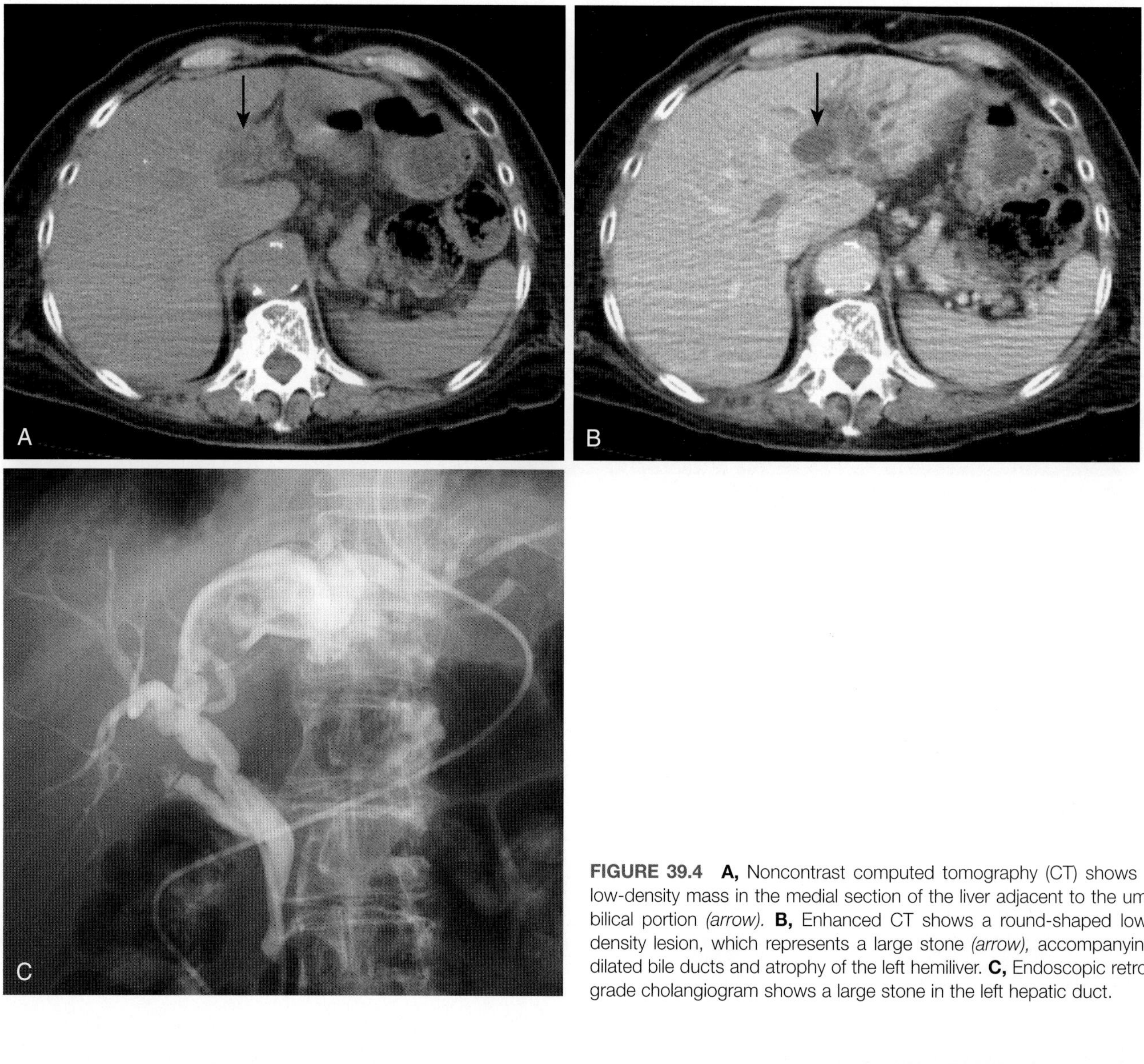

FIGURE 39.4 **A,** Noncontrast computed tomography (CT) shows a low-density mass in the medial section of the liver adjacent to the umbilical portion *(arrow)*. **B,** Enhanced CT shows a round-shaped low-density lesion, which represents a large stone *(arrow)*, accompanying dilated bile ducts and atrophy of the left hemiliver. **C,** Endoscopic retrograde cholangiogram shows a large stone in the left hepatic duct.

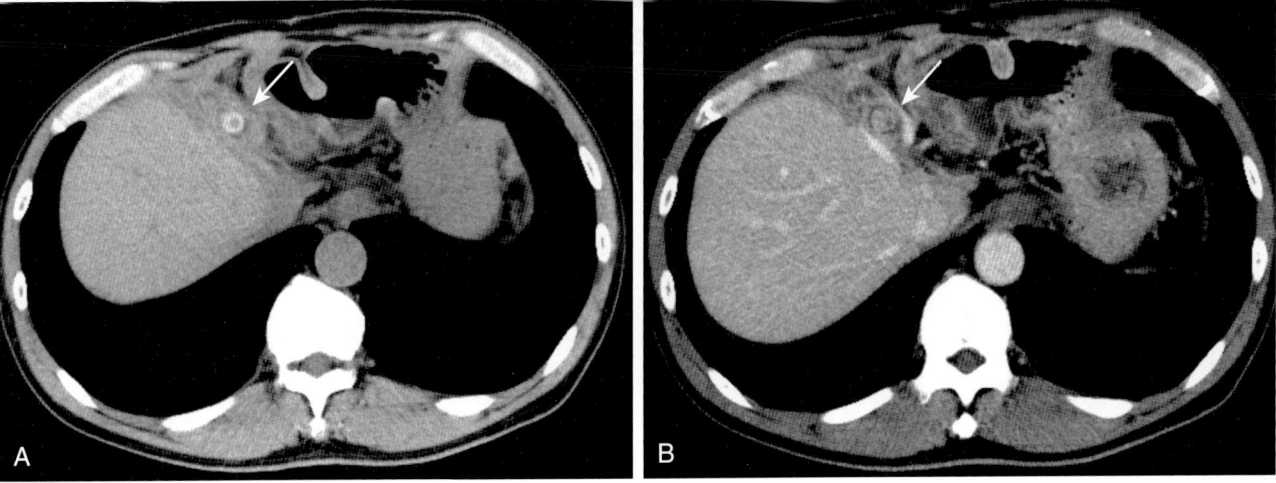

FIGURE 39.5   A, Noncontrast computed tomography (CT) reveals a stone *(arrow)* with ring-like calcification in the left hemiliver, showing marked atrophy. **B,** Enhanced CT shows severe atrophy of the left hemiliver. *Arrow* indicates an intrahepatic stone. (See Chapter 13.)

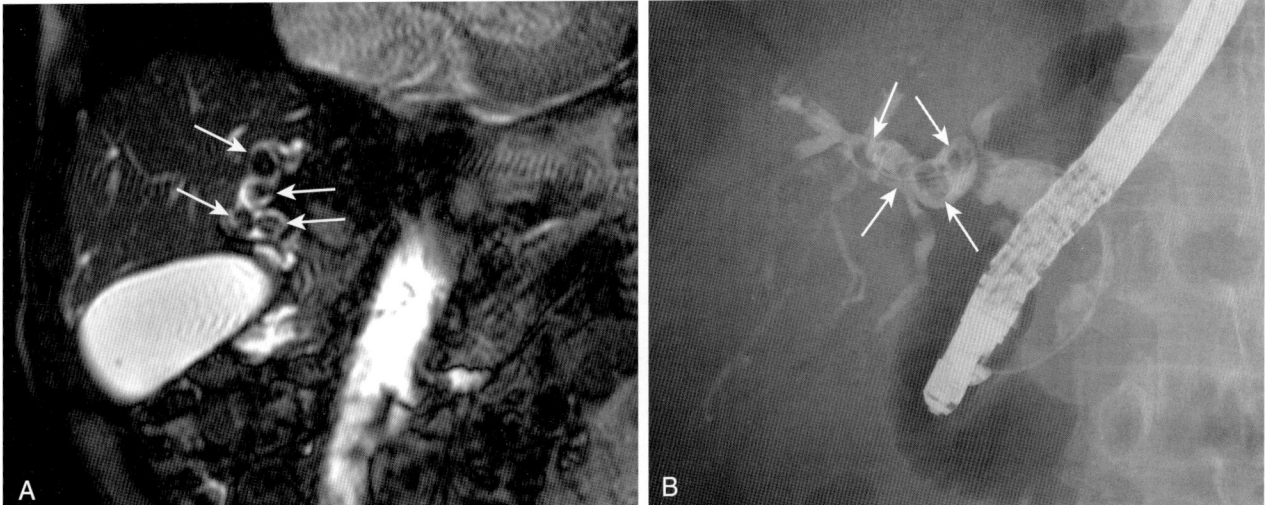

FIGURE 39.6   A, Magnetic resonance cholangiography shows multiple low-intensity nodules *(arrows)* in the anterior sectoral bile duct. (See Chapter 13.) **B,** Endoscopic retrograde cholangiography shows multiple filling defects *(arrows)* in the dilated anterior sectorial branch. (See Chapters 20 and 30.)

depicted. Pneumobilia also shows low signal intensity, and misdiagnosis as a "stone" frequently occurs, so careful attention must be paid to the differential diagnosis. In addition, tumors must be considered in the differential diagnosis when diagnosing intrahepatic duct filling defects and bile duct strictures in MRC.

PERCUTANEOUS TRANSHEPATIC CHOLANGIOGRAPHY AND ENDOSCOPIC RETROGRADE CHOLANGIOGRAPHY

PTC and ERC are invasive and, as such, are now performed less frequently for diagnostic purposes (see Chapters 20, 30, 31, and 52). However, no superior diagnostic modalities for direct cholangiography are available (Fig. 39.7). Bile duct findings may include straightening, rigidity, decreased arborization, and increased branching angles[111] (Fig. 39.8). When intrahepatic stones are present, identifying the bile duct branches in which the stones are located is important for choosing a treatment strategy, which often makes direct cholangiography essential.

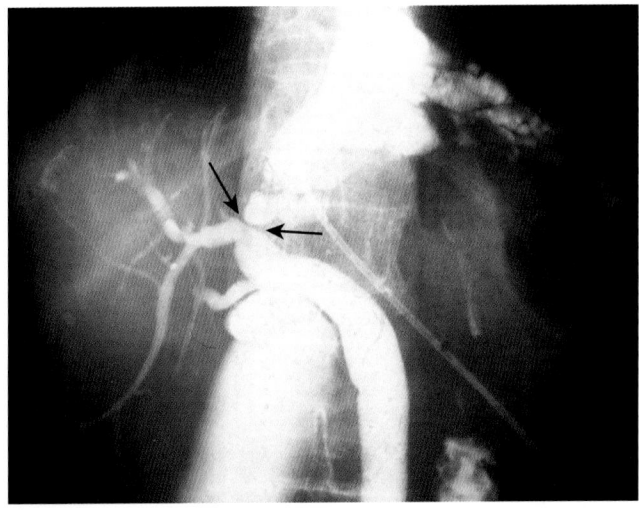

FIGURE 39.7   Cholangiogram through percutaneous transhepatic biliary drainage catheter shows markedly dilated left hepatic duct with proximal stricture *(arrows)*.

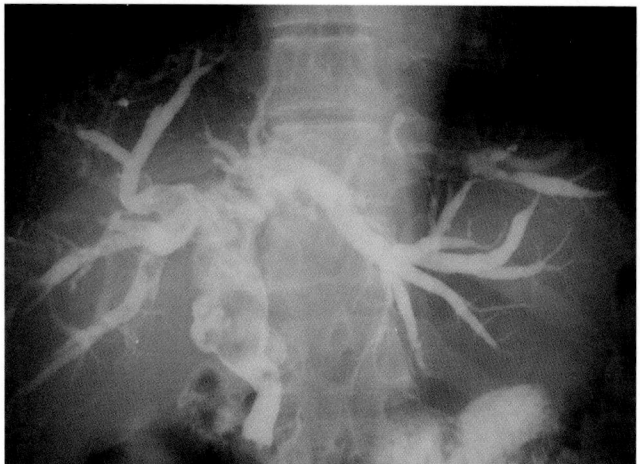

FIGURE 39.8 Endoscopic retrograde cholangiogram shows multiple filling defects in both intra and extrahepatic bile ducts. Intrahepatic ducts show straightening, rigidity, decreased arborization, increased branching angles, and abrupt tapering.

Cholangioscopy can also be a helpful examination; it can be performed after access routes to bile ducts used for imaging are sequentially dilated and a fistula is created (Fig. 39.9). Stones and strictures can be directly visualized by cholangioscopy, and biopsy and treatment such as stone removal (lithotomy) can be performed. In hepatolithiasis that occurs after Roux-en-Y hepaticojejunostomy for congenital CCs, ERC can be technically challenging. Recently, double-balloon enteroscopy has been used for examinations and stone removal in this situation[115] (Fig. 39.10A–B).

TREATMENT FOR HEPATOLITHIASIS

For more information, see Chapter 44.

The initial management of all patients with acute cholangitis should include intravenous fluid resuscitation and antibiotics. Supportive measures may also include invasive monitoring, intensive care, and inotropic and ventilation support in patients with severe cholangitis. Given the wide range of possible infecting organisms and the likelihood of mixed infection, broad-spectrum

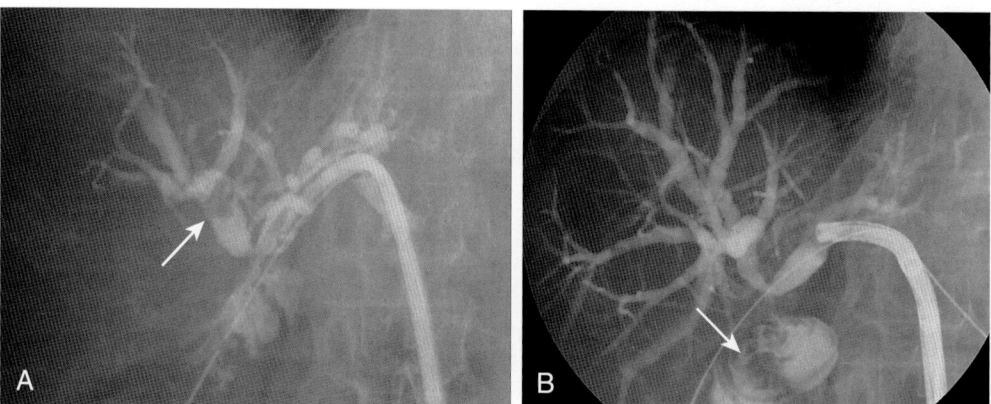

FIGURE 39.9 **A,** A case of secondary hepatolithiasis after excision of congenital choledochal cysts. Cholangiogram through percutaneous cholangioscopy shows a stone in the right hepatic duct *(arrow)*. **B,** The stone was pulled down into the jejunum *(arrow)* using basket forceps.

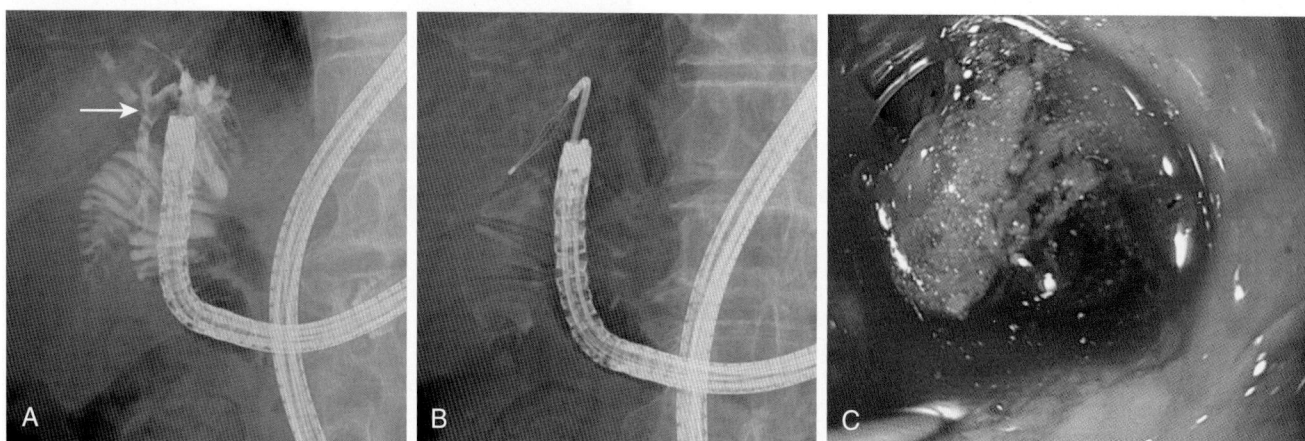

FIGURE 39.10 **A,** A case of secondary hepatolithiasis after left hemihepatectomy and caudate lobectomy for hilar cholangiocarcinoma. Cholangiogram through double-balloon enteroscopy shows multiple stones in the posterior branch. **B,** The stones were removed using basket forceps. **C,** Brownish stones were observed in the posterior duct.

antibiotics are required.[116] The severity of cholangitis must be assessed, and treatment with biliary drainage is necessary.[98] With advances in drainage procedures and appropriate antibiotic therapy, death from acute cholangitis is now less frequent. However, mortality rates of 2.1% to 14.3% are still reported in cases of severe cholangitis[117]; therefore careful management is required in such patients.

On the other hand, some patients show no symptoms. Kusano et al. (2001) reported that 122 (39.2%) of 311 patients with hepatolithiasis were asymptomatic.[97] Approximately 5.3% to 11.5% of these patients may develop some symptoms attributed to hepatolithiasis.[118] In particular, patients with peripheral-type hepatolithiasis have been reported to be less symptomatic than those with main duct-type hepatolithiasis (8/31 [25.8%] vs. 1/39 [2.6%], respectively).[118] Therefore patients with asymptomatic, peripheral-type hepatolithiasis can be observed without the need for invasive treatment; however, long-term observation is required.

Definitive treatment of intrahepatic stones generally includes complete clearance of stones and elimination of bile stasis. Biliary strictures, which are found in 35% to 96% of patients with hepatolithiasis, are a major factor in the recurrence of stones and cholangitis. If strictures are not treated, a high rate of stone recurrence is observed. When complete stone removal and elimination of biliary strictures cannot be achieved, progression to biliary cirrhosis and the subsequent development of CCA is inevitable.[73]

When stone removal (lithotomy) is considered, stricture sites, severity, variations in stone sites, prior biliary surgery, and the possibility of concomitant CCA must be evaluated. Specifically, when one side of the liver is atrophied with severe bile duct strictures and dilation, liver resection should be considered. However, when stones are present in multiple liver segments or in both the left and right lobes, complete stone removal, even with hepatectomy, is sometimes difficult. In such cases, serial cholangioscopic lithotomy in addition to hepatectomy may be effective. In patients with a poor general condition, history of multiple surgeries, or biliary cirrhosis, cholangioscopic lithotomy, in addition to or without hepatectomy, should be the treatment of choice.

A treatment algorithm based on symptoms, liver atrophy, and past history of biliary surgery was proposed by the Guideline Committee for the Japanese Society of Gastroenterology.[119] This algorithm is highly dependent on individual conditions such as the severity of comorbidities, accessibility to the biliary system, and liver functional reserve. Generally, treatment modalities are classified into pharmacologic, percutaneous transhepatic, peroral cholangioscopic, and surgical approaches often combined with an endoscopic approach.[120]

PHARMACOLOGIC THERAPY

Because the etiology of intrahepatic stone formation has not been elucidated, drug therapy for hepatolithiasis has yet to be established, and no pharmacologic agents have been proven to be effective for stone dissolution in large-scale clinical trials. Therefore medical therapy plays only a supplementary role. Ursodeoxycholic acid (UDCA), a hydrophilic bile acid, offers liver cytoprotection and promotes accelerated bile acid/bilirubin metabolizing enzyme activity, ABC transporter protein activity, an increased bile flow rate, and reduced bile mucin viscosity.[121,122] In an observational study conducted between

1981 and 1991, 17 of 20 patients with a diagnosis of Caroli syndrome were found to have intrahepatic stones.[123] Complete dissolution of intrahepatic stones was observed in three patients after treatment with UDCA (pretreatment stone diameters, 6–9 mm) after 12, 18, and 48 months. Nine patients showed partial dissolution, three had no further decrease in stone size or number after treatment for 18 to 36 months, and six had stones that were still dissolving.

Simvastatin reduces plasma and biliary cholesterol levels primarily by inhibiting cholesterol synthesis.[124] The reduction in CBD bile lithogenicity and bile acid hydrophobicity caused by simvastatin suggests that this agent might be useful for patients in the early stages of cholesterol gallstone development, especially when stones have higher levels of cholesterol content. The long-term use of statins in Europe has been reported to be associated with a decreased risk of gallstones requiring cholecystectomy.[125] On the other hand, a study in East Asia did not provide support for a beneficial association between the use of statins and gallstone disease.[126]

Because prostaglandin E receptor (PGE) is thought to be associated with CPC, selective COX-2 inhibitors and PGE antagonists may play a role in improving inflammatory changes in hepatolithiasis.[127]

Japanese/Chinese herbal medicine, *inchin-ko-to*, has long been considered to have choleretic effects in Asia. *Inchin-ko-to* increases bile flow through the upregulation of MRP2, which results in the expectation of reduced stone formation.[128] *Inchin-ko-to* also has a potent cytoprotective effect against ischemia–reperfusion stress to the liver,[129] and thereby a preventive effect against postoperative liver dysfunction.[130] Furthermore, Uji et al. (2018) revealed that the administration of *inchin-ko-to* was associated with a reduction of so-called harmful bacteria in feces.[131] However, these potential beneficial effects in regard to hepatolithiasis should be confirmed in large-scale clinical trials.

PERCUTANEOUS TRANSHEPATIC CHOLANGIOSCOPIC LITHOTOMY

With the technical development of percutaneous transhepatic biliary drainage and dilation procedures, it is now possible to place catheters into the intrahepatic duct without laparotomy[132,133] (Fig. 39.11; see Chapters 31 and 52). Before 2006, PTCSL was the most frequently performed treatment for nonsurgical lithotripsy in Japan, but recently, ERC with stone extraction has been performed more frequently than PTCSL (22.7% vs. 11.7%, respectively).[13] However, PTCSL may be a suitable alternative when endoscopic retrograde cholangioscopic lithotomy cannot be performed. Thus PTCSL may still play a role in stone clearance among patients in whom hepatectomy is not suitable or serial lithotripsy after liver resection with bilioenterostomy is required.

Stones are removed according to size using basket forceps, an electric hydraulic lithotripter, or a laser lithotripter.[132,134,135] When bile duct strictures exist, narrow segments should be dilated using a balloon or dilators.[136–138]

In selected cases, the rate of complete stone removal with PTCSL has been reported to range from 63.9% to 96.4% (Table 39.4). Biliary strictures are a factor that can impede the complete removal of stones. Takada and colleagues (1996) reviewed 86 patients who underwent PTCSL and analyzed data from 27 patients in whom complete stone removal was unsuccessful: 15 patients (56%) had severe strictures, 7 (26%) had

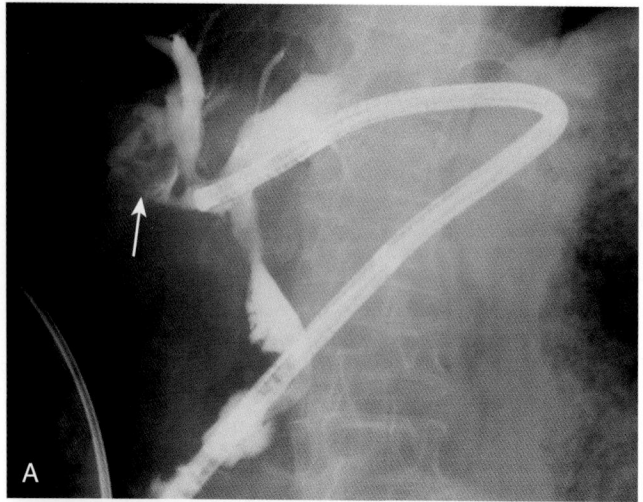

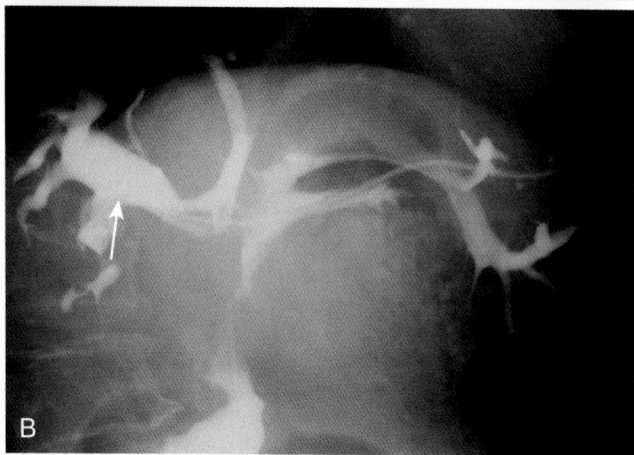

FIGURE 39.11 A, Percutaneous transhepatic cholangioscopic lithotomy from the left hepatic duct. *Arrow* indicates stones in the right anterior branch. **B,** Stones in the right anterior section were removed using an electrohydraulic lithotripter and basket forceps. *Arrow* indicates no filling defects after lithotripsy.

drainage variation in the posterior sectoral duct, and 4 (15%) had drainage variations with severe strictures.[139] According to Otani and colleagues (1999), 18.2% of patients (4/22) who underwent partial hepatectomy had residual strictures, whereas 58.3% of patients (14/24) who underwent PTCSL (despite dilation in all cases) still had residual strictures.[138] The time required for complete stone removal is also an issue. The mean reported number of treatments ranges from 3.9 to 6.

Stone recurrence despite complete removal ranges from 14.5% to 50.8% (see Table 39.4) and tends to be higher than after hepatectomy. Biliary strictures are a common cause of stone recurrence. Although Huang and colleagues (2003) reported no significant difference in stone recurrence rates based on the presence or absence of strictures, they identified a significantly shorter mean time (11 vs. 18 years, respectively) until stone recurrence in patients with bile duct strictures.[66] Lee and colleagues (2001) reported strictures and co-existing biliary cirrhosis as risk factors (Child's type B and C = 89%, Child's type A = 29%).[137] Tsuyuguchi and colleagues (2014) reported that patients with liver atrophy treated with nonsurgical modalities showed a poor long-term prognosis.[58]

An important point to keep in mind is that stone recurrence is associated with the late development of cholangiocarcinoma (see Chapters 50 and 51). Among 209 patients with complete stone removal, 4 (6.6%) of 61 with recurrent intrahepatic stones during follow-up had ICC[66]; on the other hand, only 1 of 148 patients without stone recurrence had ICC. In patients with recurrent hepatolithiasis because of biliary strictures, Jeng and colleagues (1999) compared repeated placement of external–internal stents and expandable metallic stents (EMS) and found significantly lower rates of stone recurrence in the EMS group.[140] Meanwhile, with placement of self-EMS in stricture areas, 2-year patency rates were estimated to be approximately 40%.[141] However, these results are somewhat controversial and include some recommendations that these stents should not be used for dilation.

PERORAL CHOLANGIOSCOPIC LITHOTRIPSY

Since the description of endoscopic sphincterotomy and stone extraction in the early 1970s, endoscopic management has

TABLE 39.4 Treatment Outcomes				
REFERENCE	COMPLETE STONE REMOVAL (%)	RECURRENT STONES (%)	PROCEDURE-RELATED MORBIDITY (%)	IN-HOSPITAL MORTALITY (%)
Peroral Cholangioscopic Lithotripsy				
Tanaka, 1996[142]	36.8	0	—	—
Okugawa, 2002[148]	63.9	21.7	2.8	0
Cheon, 2009[88]	57.1	17.9	—	—
Tsuyuguchi, 2014[58]	57.8	—	—	—
Percutaneous Transhepatic Cholangioscopic Lithotomy				
Yeh, 1995[149]	80.0	32.6	28.5	—
Jan, 1995[150]	83.3	40.0	14.5	—
Otani, 1999[138]	96.4	31.5	21.4	3.6
Lee, 2001[137]	80.4	29.4	10.9	—
Huang, 2003[66]	85.3	49.8	1.6	—
Chen, 2005[136]	82.4	50.8	17.6	0
Cheon, 2009[88]	63.9	14.5	3	—

TABLE 39.4   Treatment Outcomes—cont'd

REFERENCE	COMPLETE STONE REMOVAL (%)	RECURRENT STONES (%)	PROCEDURE-RELATED MORBIDITY (%)	IN-HOSPITAL MORTALITY (%)
Common Bile Duct Exploration + T-Tube Drainage + Postoperative Cholangioscopy				
Hwang, 1980 [151]	83	—	—	0
Yamakawa, 1980[147]	92.1	0	—	—
Choi, 1982[145]	—	23.6	—	5.4
Takada, 1995[133]	68.6	3.4	—	—
Jan, 1996[91]	84.9	28.2	—	—
Li, 2006[152]	66.0	35.7	16.0	
Hepaticojejunostomy (With/Without Subcutaneous Jejunostomy)				
Fan, 1993[153]	92.7	15.8	—	—
Akiyama, 1994[154]	81.3	30.8	—	0
Ker, 1994[155]	—	13.8	—	0
Kusano, 2001[156]	68.6	30.6	—	—
Li, 2006[152]	74.1	27		
Hepatectomy				
Tsunoda, 1985[157]	—	25.7	—	—
Jeng, 1996 (bilat.)[158]	92.5	11.9	—	5.5
Fan, 1993[153]	—	15.9	32	1.6
Chen, 1997 (bilat.)[159]	40-84	12	—	1.7
Kim, 1998[160]	64	11	—	3.9
Liu, 1998[65]	77.0	3.0	29.0	1.0
Otani, 1999[138]	96.2	5.6	38.5	3.8
Chen, 2004[67]	98	7.9	28	2
Cheung, 2005[68]	98	13	44.2	0
Lee, 2007[71]	96	5.7	33.3	1.6
Uchiyama, 2007[161]	100	13.9	23.7	0
Cheon, 2009[88]	83	18	—	0
Uenishi, 2009[73]	95	10	—	3.5
Yang, 2010 (bilat.) [162]	83.1	29.3	46.3	2.2
Shah, 2012 (unilat.)[163]	97.8	5.2	—	0
Li, 2012[93]				
(unilat.)	99.3	6.2	20.4	0.4
(bilat.)	90.2	16.7	38.5	0.4
Li, 2019 (bilat.)[164]	92.9	13.5	26.8	2.9

bilat., Bilateral stones; *unilat.,* unilateral stones.

become the optimal mode of treatment for many patients with various conditions, including acute cholangitis with hepatolithiasis.[13] The aim of ERC with endoscopic sphincterotomy is to decompress the biliary tract quickly to resolve biliary sepsis (see Chapter 30); this choice allows the extraction of stones via the duodenal papilla.

However, the incidence of residual and recurrent stones after ERC with stone removal is higher than after PTCSL and hepatectomy. Suzuki and colleagues (2014) reported that biliary strictures and dilation were predictive factors for stone recurrence after ERC with stone removal.[13] In addition, peripheral stone impaction and ductal angulation can lead to difficulties.

Because endoscopic sphincterotomy induces bile reflux and contamination, the divergent effects of endoscopic sphincterotomy on long-term hepatolithiasis outcomes, especially in patients with remaining stones, have been noted.[142] Therefore the complete clearance of intrahepatic calculi is mandatory if adverse effects are to be avoided.

Endoscopic therapeutic interventions are sometimes difficult in patients with Roux-en-Y anastomosis and hepaticojejunostomy. However, recent advances in double-balloon enteroscopy and cholangioscopy have allowed direct lithotripsy and biliary stricture treatments in some cases[115] (see Fig. 39.10).

Endoscopic US-guided hepaticogastrostomy is another option to access intrahepatic stones.[143,144] This method is useful for patients with a surgically altered anatomy, such as Roux-en-Y hepaticojejunostomy, when it is difficult to approach by double-balloon enteroscopy (Fig. 39.12).

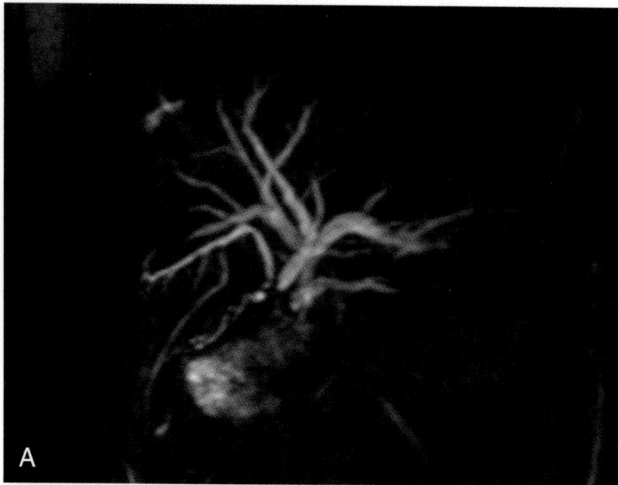

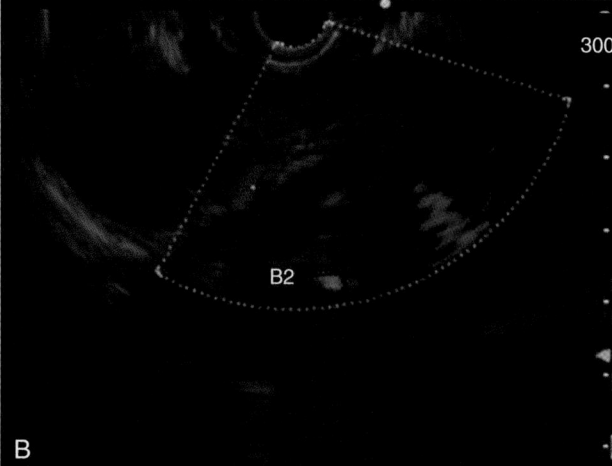

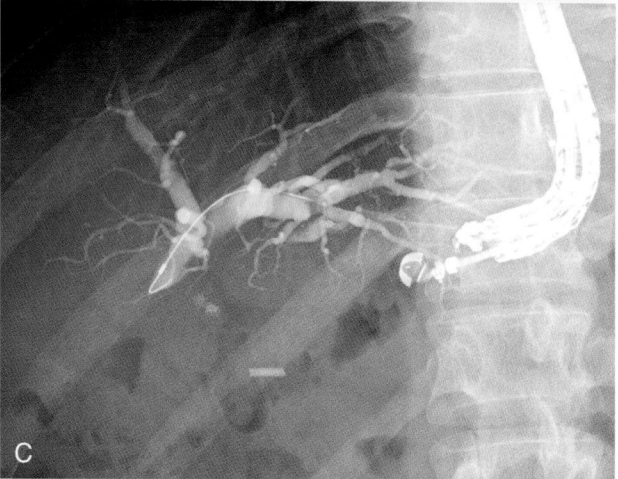

FIGURE 39.12 **A**, A case of Bismuth type IV benign biliary stricture caused by laparoscopic cholecystectomy, which was reconstructed by multiple hepaticojejunostomy in the hospital. The left hepatic duct, anterior sections, and posterior sections were reconstructed separately. **B**, Endoscopic ultrasonography (EUS) from the stomach showed a dilated bile duct of segment 2. **C**, Left hepatic duct was opacified through an EUS-guided hepaticogastrostomy showing complete obstruction of hepaticojejunostomy.

SURGICAL TREATMENT (SEE CHAPTER 44)

In the 1970s, the primary surgical treatment was cholecystectomy with stone removal and insertion of a T-tube to allow removal of remnant stones by postoperative cholangioscopy.[145–147] Using this treatment, stones were successfully removed in repeated postoperative examinations in 66% to 83% of cases (see Table 39.4).[58,65–68,71,73,88,91,93,133,136–138,142,145,147–149,150–164] However, high stone recurrence rates of 23.6% to 35.7% after T-tube removal have been reported.[145,152] Recently, the use of cholecystectomy with stone removal and insertion of a T-tube has decreased remarkably (50.2% in 1985–1988 vs. 1.0% in 2011).[13] Choledochojejunostomy and transduodenal pupilloplasty were also performed in the 1970s but are now seldom performed.

Generally, stones localized in a unilateral hemiliver, severe biliary strictures, atrophy, and the presence of ICC are indications for partial hepatectomy (Fig. 39.13; see Chapter 101). Intrahepatic stones limited to the left lobe, accounting for about half of cases, are a good indication for liver resection alone from the perspectives of cure and treatment time.[163]

The incidence of residual stones after hepatectomy is usually lower than that after endoscopic lithotripsy (see Table 39.4). Stones recur at rates of 0% to 18% in cases without bilateral disease. Moreover, the resection of atrophic liver and stricture areas is expected to reduce the future incidence of ICC.[73,91] Jan and colleagues (1996) reported significantly superior results with hepatectomy versus nonsurgical treatment (stone recurrence: 9.5% vs. 29.6%, secondary biliary cirrhosis: 2.1% vs. 6.8%, and late development of ICC: 0% vs. 2.8%, respectively).[91]

The management of bilateral hepatolithiasis is more complicated than that of unilateral hepatolithiasis. Even in patients with affected liver segments on both hemilivers, resection of the atrophied segments is often applied (Fig. 39.14). In such instances, hepatectomy combined with postoperative stone removal from a T-tube fistula, or with stone removal by PTCSL, is recommended to obtain high complete stone removal rates. Indeed, Chen and colleagues (1997) reported that the rate of complete stone clearance was 84% 1 year after operation, despite 60% of the patients having remnant stones immediately after the operation.[159] In addition, combining hepatectomy and hepaticojejunostomy with anchoring of the jejunal limb to the abdominal wall within subcutaneous tissue for the purpose of postoperative stone removal and treatment of bile duct strictures has long been performed (Fig. 39.15; see Chapter 101B). If stones recur several years after complete stone clearance, this jejunal limb can be used as an access route to the biliary system under local anesthesia. Some consider this to be a useful procedure for the prevention of bacterial reflux into the liver.[165] However, complementary hepaticojejunostomy itself may cause cholangitis.[97] Herman and colleagues (2010) confirmed that all patients undergoing liver resection showed good results, whereas 7 (41.2%) of 17 patients who underwent liver resection associated with hepaticojejunostomy had late complications during the follow-up period.[165] In an attempt to clarify the drawbacks of bilioenteric anastomosis, they compared only patients with unilateral disease with and without hepaticojejunostomy; a significant difference was found between groups, indicating the negative effects of bilioenteric anastomosis on patient outcomes. Likewise, Li et al. (2006) noted that if intrahepatic stone clearance could not be achieved during surgery,

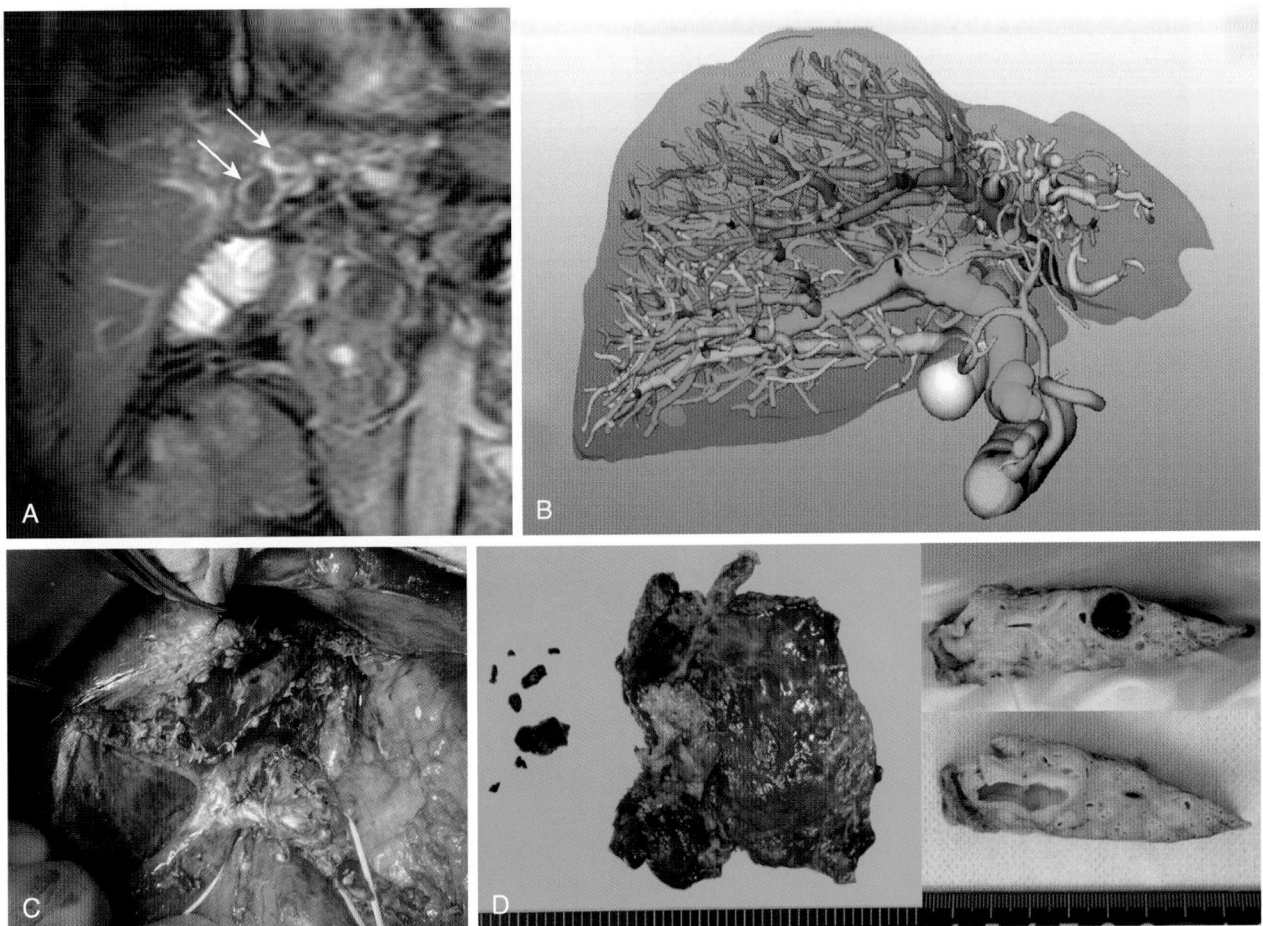

FIGURE 39.13 A, A case of secondary hepatolithiasis after excision of congenital choledochal cysts. Some filling defects *(arrows)* in the left hepatic duct are seen on magnetic resonance cholangiopancreatography. **B,** Three-dimensional computed tomography shows marked atrophy of the left hemiliver with diminished portal flow. **C,** Left hemihepatectomy with caudate lobectomy was carried out. The anastomotic site of the right hepatic duct and the jejunal limb were intact. The jejunal orifice for the left hepatic duct anastomosis was closed. **D,** Resected specimen shows marked atrophy and impacted stones in the left hemiliver.

T-tube placement within the CBD rather than hepaticojejunostomy would facilitate postoperative choledochoscopic lithotripsy.[152]

Bilateral partial resection of the liver may provide good long-term results, even in patients with bilateral intrahepatic stones and stenosis.[162] In that study, the incidences of stone recurrence after bilateral and unilateral hepatectomy for bilateral intrahepatic stones were 11.8% and 34.1%, respectively. It should be noted, however, that three hospital deaths related to postoperative liver failure occurred in 54 patients in the bilateral resection group. Extended parenchymal resections to eliminate the persistence of CPC may reduce stone recurrence. Even in patients with bilateral stones, stone recurrence rates are low and comparable with that of unilateral stones if the extent of liver resection is equal to the stone-affected segments.[93] Recently, a combination of intraoperative lithotomy with hepatectomy achieved satisfactory stone clearance of 92.9% (52/56) in patients with complicated bilateral hepatolithiasis.[164] In addition, resection of liver parenchyma with CPC may also reduce the late development of ICC because CPC is thought to be a possible precursor lesion of ICC.[81]

The safety of hepatectomy has improved, but postoperative complication rates, including those for wound infection, hemobilia, and biliary fistula, still range from 15.7% to 38.5%.[159] Li and colleagues (2012) reported that left lobectomy or hepatectomy within 1 month of the last episode of cholangitis is a risk factor for postoperative bile leakage.[93]

With recent advances in laparoscopic techniques, laparoscopic liver resection is increasingly being performed for hepatolithiasis.[166] Although the number of patients is still limited, operative mortality and residual stone rates are comparable to those of open hepatectomy.[167,168] On the other hand, increased postoperative complications have been reported[169] and thus no consensus has been reached regarding its clinical utility. Further investigation in a larger number of patients is therefore necessary.

Because of its complicated clinical features, such as repeated cholangitis and multiple operations, diffusely distributed hepatolithiasis is untreatable by hepatectomy, cholangiojejunostomy, or choledochoscopy, and thus often leads to portal hypertension and liver failure. Liver transplantation has been performed in patients who have progressed to liver failure[170–173] (see Chapter 105).

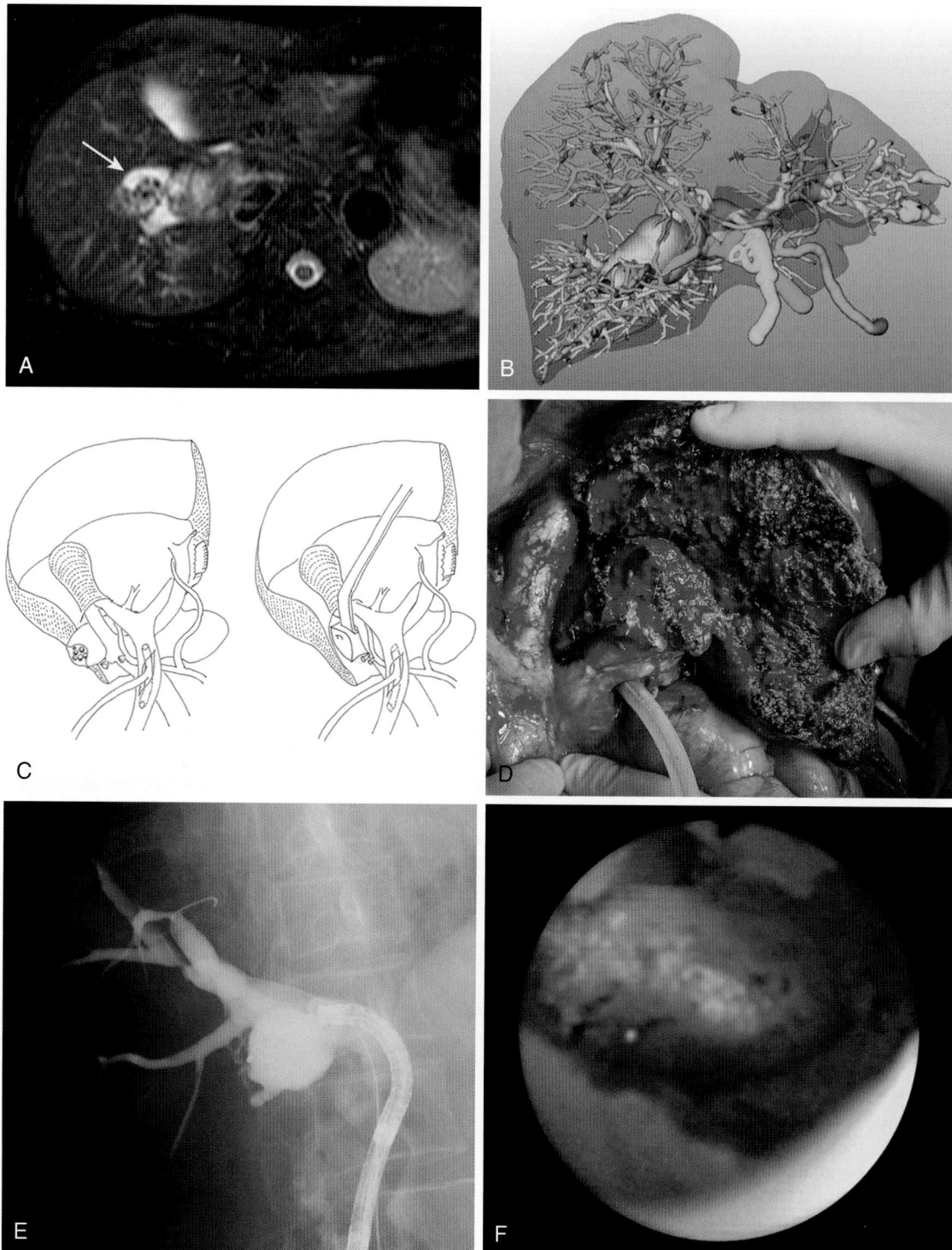

FIGURE 39.14 **A,** A case of primary hepatolithiasis. Magnetic resonance image demonstrating dilated right posterior intrahepatic duct containing multiple stones. *Arrow* indicates filling defects in the dilated right to posterior segment branch. **B,** Three-dimensional computed tomography shows multiple biliary stenosis and dilation in the left lateral section. In addition, remarkable cystic dilation is observed from the right to the posterior hepatic duct. Portal flow is decreased to both the left lateral and right posterior sections. Note the absence of right posterior ductal strictures. **C,** Bilateral hepatectomy, left lateral sectionectomy, and posterior sectionectomy with T-tube insertion were carried out. Stones were extracted from the cut end of the posterior sectional branch. The orifice was then additionally resected and sutured to reduce the size of the remnant dilated posterior duct to be as small as possible. At that time, attention was paid not to tuck the caudate lobe branches. **D,** After closure of the posterior sectional branch stump. **E,** Cholangiography through the cholangioscopy. **F,** Postoperative cholangioscopy reveals a remnant stone that was subsequently removed using basket forceps.

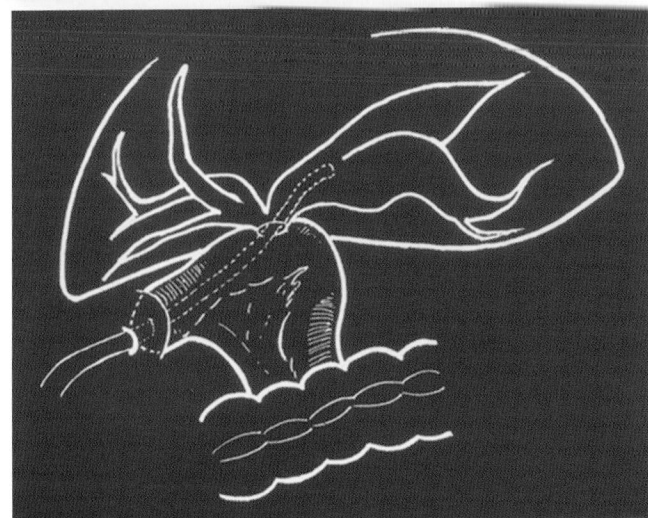

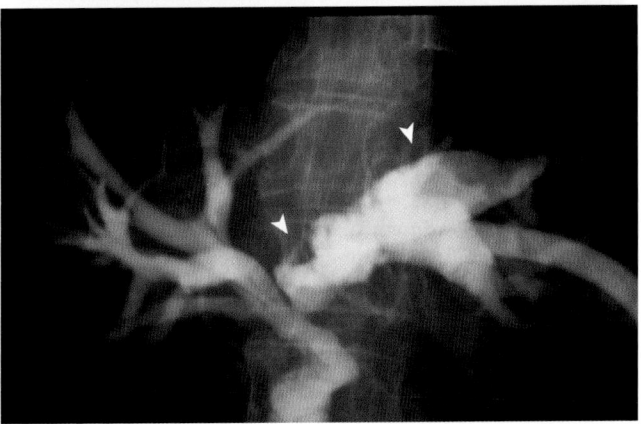

FIGURE 39.15 A drawing of combining hepaticojejunostomy with anchoring of a Roux-en-Y jejunal limb to the abdominal wall for the purpose of postoperative stone extraction *(upper)*. A cholangiogram after lithotomy shows no remnant stones in the dilated left hepatic duct *(arrowheads) (lower)*.

PROGNOSIS

Even when intrahepatic stones are completely removed, stone recurrence rates are high. The major factors that predict the long-term outcome of intrahepatic stones are concomitant CCA, cholangitis, liver abscess, and biliary cirrhosis because of repeated cholangitis. Recurrence rates, depending on the type of treatment and the presence or absence of bile duct strictures, range from 0% to 50.8% (see Table 39.4). Patients with recurrence may have repeated/chronic cholangitis and develop biliary cirrhosis over a period of 10 to 20 years. In addition, the rate of late development of CCA is about 0.3% to 9.1% (see Table 39.3). Long-term outcomes of patients with subsequent CCA are extremely poor. Based on Korean national data, patients with subsequent CCA had very poor survival outcomes compared with concomitant CCA.[89] Therefore patients with risk factors should be observed carefully over the long term because cancer is known to emerge even after 10 to 20 years. The overall 10-year survival rate for patients with hepatolithiasis is about 80% to 90%.[73,91] Nevertheless, a 5-year survival rate of only 9% has been reported in patients with concomitant ICC.[67]

References are available at expertconsult.com.

SECTION I. Inflammatory, Infective, and Congenital

B. Biliary Stricture and Fistula

CHAPTER 40

Extrahepatic biliary atresia

Alex G. Cuenca and Heung Bae Kim

INTRODUCTION

Extrahepatic biliary atresia or biliary atresia (BA) is an obstructive fibroinflammatory disease that presents in infancy. First described in a case series of 49 patients by John Thompson in 1892, this disease is characterized by a destructive inflammatory cholangiopathy that can affect both the intrahepatic and extrahepatic biliary tree. If left untreated, the disease is progressive and leads to death from complications of biliary cirrhosis by age 2 years in most cases (see Chapters 74 and 76). There are two therapies that are currently used and widely accepted for this condition: the Kasai hepatoportoenterostomy (HPE) and liver transplantation (see Chapters 105 and 110). Although there is still some controversy as to whether patients should proceed to transplant as the primary therapy, most centers, including ours, agree with performing the HPE first and as early as possible to allow for the possibility of biliary drainage and delay the need for transplant.

BA affects approximately 1 in every 10,000 live births with higher incidences in Asian/Polynesian and black South African ethnicities. For example, the populations of Taiwan, Japan, and Hawaii have been shown to have 1.5 to 2 times the rate of BA compared with European countries.[1] The reasons for this are unclear, but a study of Asians born in the United States (US) shows a higher prevalence of BA than the general US population, suggesting a strong genetic component to the disease.[2]

Several classification schemes have been proposed to describe the anatomic variants of BA, but the most widely used is the Japanese Association of Pediatric Surgeons classification, which groups BA into three main variants (Fig. 40.1).[3] Type I, or the distal BA present in approximately 5% of cases, affects only the common bile duct (CBD) distal to the cystic duct, with the cystic duct and hepatic ducts remaining patent. In type II BA (approximately 5% of cases), the hepatic duct is obliterated but the proximal intrahepatic ducts are patent and frequently terminate in an extrahepatic cystic structure. Type II is further subdivided into IIa, in which the gallbladder and CBD are patent, and IIb, in which the gallbladder, CBD, and hepatic ducts are scarred and atretic. The most common variant of BA is type III or complete BA, present in greater than 90% of cases, in which the intrahepatic as well as extrahepatic ducts are completely obliterated.

Although most patients have isolated BA, a minority (10%–20%) of patients with BA have a congenital or syndromic association with additional anatomic anomalies affecting the spleen, heart, hepatic anatomy and orientation, and intestinal rotation; this is known as BA splenic malformation syndrome (BASM).[1] In contrast to isolated BA, patients with BASM are more likely to be found in European populations.[1] This is further supported by Japanese BA registry data, which found associated anomalies in only 2% of their patients.[4]

ETIOLOGY

Despite advances in medical and surgical care in the management of BA, its etiology remains a mystery. The association of multiple anatomic anomalies in addition to a significant poorly understood inflammatory component suggest a multifactorial origin to BA. This is further supported by the fact that animal models have failed to isolate a specific gene that leads to the BA phenotype. This section will outline our current progress and understanding of the etiology of the disease.

A Genetic Component

BASM describes a distinct association of anatomic anomalies found in a minority of BA patients, including cardiovascular defects, situs inversus or heterotaxy, intestinal malrotation, polysplenia, preduodenal portal vein, and interrupted inferior vena cava with azygous continuation.[1] Mutations in the developmental genes *CFC1* and *inversin*, which have been associated with heterotaxy/malrotation, have been speculated to be associated with BASM.[5,6] However, CFC1, despite a higher association, was not found in all patients with BASM and although *inversin* mutations cause *situs inversus* as well as hyperbilirubinemia in mice, *inversin* was not found to be associated with these findings in BASM patients.[7,8]

Using a powerful tool that can determine the association of individual common genetic variants to a given disease, known as single nucleotide repeats (SNPs), genome-wide association studies (GWAS) have identified several genes associated with BA. For example, a Chinese study identified an SNP variant in the *ADD3* gene, which led to lower expression levels of *ADD3* and was associated with BA in the Han population of China.[9] Another candidate identified through GWAS in China is *glypican 1* or *GPC1*.[9] This gene, when knocked out in a zebrafish animal model, leads to disorganized biliary tract/ductule formation.[10] *ADD3* SNPs have been examined in Caucasians, and although a different SNP of *ADD3* was found to be correlative of BA in Caucasians, the data suggest that defects in *ADD3* expression may have implications in the development of BA.[11] Other SNPs that have been examined and are thought to be associated are *ARF6* and *EFEMP1*.[12] More definitive analyses

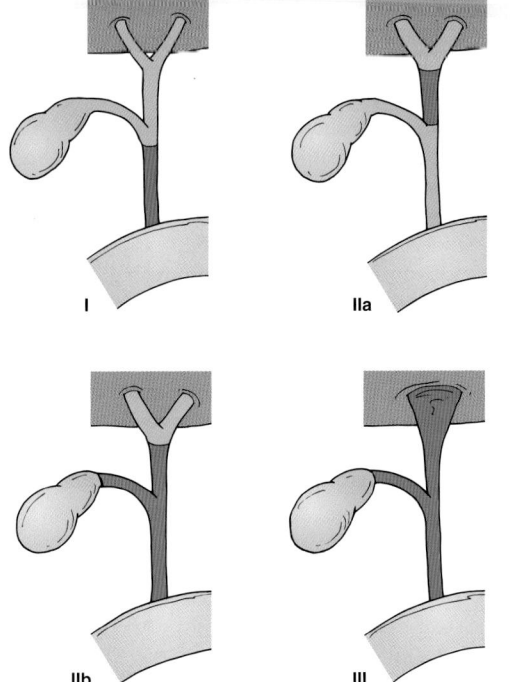

FIGURE 40.1 Classification and anatomy of biliary atresia. Type 1: Obliteration of common bile duct. Type IIa: Atresia of common hepatic duct with cystic dilations of the proximal intrahepatic ducts. Type IIb: Atresia of the gallbladder, cystic duct, and common hepatic ducts. Type III: Obliteration of the entire intrahepatic and extrahepatic biliary trees.

TABLE 40.1 Genes Associated With the Development of Biliary Atresia and Their Cellular Function

GENE	FUNCTION
ADD3 (Aducin)	Regulation of cell-cell contact
GPC1 (Glypican-1)	Signaling/developmental pathways
ARF6 (adenosine diphosphate-ribosylation-6)	Bile duct development (?)
EFEMP1 (extracellular matrix protein 1)	Bile duct development (?)
JAG1 (Jagged 1)	Cell-cell signaling, associated with Allagile's syndrome
CFTR (Cystic fibrosis transmembrane conductance receptor)	Ion transport
ZIC3 (Zic family member 3)	Zinc finger protein
INVS (Inversin)	Left-right axis development
VEGF (Vascular endothelial growth factor)	Growth factor
FXR (Farnesoid X receptor)	Bile acid receptor
CFC1 (Cryptic)	Growth factor, associated with heterotaxy
SOX17	

of these SNP variants in other populations have not been done but are underway.

Other developmental genes that have been investigated and implicated in clinical investigations or preclinical models in the development of BA are listed in Table 40.1. Although the exact mechanism in which they may contribute to the development of BA in patients is unknown, it has been inferred from their function and/or association with BA tissue samples. These are

genes that are important for bile duct/system development, bile acid transport, vasculogenesis, left-right axis/development, and organogenesis. Although still unclear, efforts to elucidate the role of these genes in the biology of BA continues with the goal of targeted therapy for BA patients.

Infection and Inflammation in Biliary Atresia

Because no clear single genetic factor has been found in all BA patients, some investigators have suggested that infection may play a critical role in the etiology of BA, particularly given the well-known seasonal variation in the incidence of BA.[13] It has been proposed that a virally induced bile duct injury could lead to a progressive fibroinflammatory and obliterative process that ultimately leads to the destruction of the biliary tree. Several viruses have been implicated in BA, such as cytomegalovirus (CMV), reovirus, and rotavirus.

With a worldwide seroprevalence that ranges from 70% to 100% depending on the country, infection with CMV in most patients is typically benign, with most infections described as asymptomatic. The association of CMV with the development of BA varies widely depending on the study referenced.[14–17] CMV infection has also been suggested to delay the resolution of jaundice in BA patients.[18] However, results are inconclusive because these studies suffer from low numbers and associative nonmechanistic findings that make interpretation of the data difficult.

Reovirus has also been implicated in BA development. This association is based on murine studies and the identification of reoviral particles in neonates with BA.[17] Unlike CMV or other viruses, however, reoviral infections produce no identifiable symptomology in patients and no study has demonstrated a definite link between the two processes. Another virus that has been associated with the development of BA is rotavirus. Animal models using specific rotaviral strains appear to cause similar cholangiopathy to what is seen in humans and studies examining for the presence of rotavirus suggest an increase in viral titers or rotavirus antibody compared with controls.[19] As with all of the viral studies previously described, however, the numbers of patients included within these studies is small and it is still unclear as to whether or not any of these viral infections lead to or exacerbate BA.

Because inflammatory infiltrates are typically found throughout the liver of explants of patients with BA at the time of transplant, many have speculated that inappropriate innate/adaptive immune responses or even an autoimmune component may be driving the progressive fibro-obliterative process in BA.[20,21] In this setting, the innate immune response is responsible for the production of many inflammatory cytokines and chemokines such as tumor necrosis factor (TNF)-α, interleukin (IL)-1β, and IL-6. This can be through the stimulation of pathogen recognition receptors (PRRs) such as Toll-like receptors (TLRs), which are present not only on innate immune effector cells but also on cholangiocytes. These PRRs are designed to respond to pathogens but can also be stimulated by damage-associated molecular patterns (DAMPs), which are intracellular "self" proteins that are released during cell death. Therefore it is possible that cholangiocyte cell death, through either infection or other processes, could set off an unchecked cyclical inflammatory response that could lead to the pathology we associate with BA. Pang et al. examined the serum of 124 BA patients pre-Kasai and found that 56.5% of these patients were positive for one or multiple autoantibodies compared with less than 5% in healthy controls.[22] In addition, a study of T-cell receptors (TCR) in BA patients demonstrated that the TCR repertoire was more limited and oligoclonal in nature, suggesting that these patients might be mounting an immunologic response to an autoantigen.[23] Also, cholangiocytes from BA patients have also been found to express not only major histocompatibility complex (MHC) Class I but also MHC Class II, which is likely caused by the inflammatory milieu.[24] This is important because this aberrant expression of MHC Class II on cholangiocytes could also be propagating an adaptive immune response in situ as well as systemically.

Although the antigen that may be responsible for or contributing to this inflammatory response is unknown, another possibility is that BA may result from the activation of maternal resident T cells against a variety of paternal antigens resulting from maternofetal microchimerism. This suggestion comes from data in which infants with BA have been shown to have high numbers of maternally derived CD8[+] T cells within their livers.[25] In support of this, longitudinal studies of living related liver transplant recipients with maternal grafts have demonstrated increased graft survival, decreased rejection, and more successful undergoing of intentional withdrawal of immunosuppression.[26]

CLINICAL FEATURES DIAGNOSIS AND WORKUP

The clinical presentation of infants with BA can be variable but usually includes jaundice lasting longer than the first 2 weeks of life, acholic stools, choluria, and hepatomegaly. If left untreated, all patients will progress to cirrhosis with the development of ascites, splenomegaly, and the stigmata of portal hypertension. Coagulopathy may also develop early in the course of disease, not from liver failure, but rather from poor fat-soluble bile acid absorption, malnutrition, and Vitamin K deficiency. This coagulopathy can be severe and lead to mortality from intracranial or gastrointestinal (GI) hemorrhage.

Evaluation of an infant with suspected BA begins with standard laboratory testing including a liver function test (including γ-glutamyl transpeptidase [GGT]), standard chemistries, prothrombin time (PT)/ international normalized ratio (INR), and complete blood counts (CBCs). Infants with BA typically have direct hyperbilirubinemia greater than 2 mg/dL and elevated alkaline phosphatase and GGT. Transaminases are typically mildly elevated, whereas chemistries and CBC are usually within normal limits. PT/INR elevation that cannot be corrected with Vitamin K administration is a late finding of decompensated cirrhosis. Numerous other conditions can cause conjugated hyperbilirubinemia in newborns, including neonatal infection with the TORCH pathogens (toxoplasma, other viruses, rubella, cytomegalovirus, and hepatitis), as well as metabolic disorders, cystic fibrosis, and alpha 1-antitrypsin deficiency, and should be considered during the evaluation as well.

An abdominal ultrasound is typically performed to evaluate the liver parenchyma and vascular flow and the presence of a gallbladder or intra/extrahepatic bile ducts. In infants with BA, the gallbladder is typically shrunken or absent and intrahepatic ducts are typically not visualized. The presence of the "triangular cord sign" on ultrasound is highly suggestive of BA and when combined with some novel ultrasound modalities to identify liver fibrosis has been suggested to increase the diagnostic sensitivity of ultrasound to greater than 90%.[27] However, although these new data are promising, these are small preliminary studies and more rigorous evaluations are required (see Chapter 13).

Additional studies have also been suggested to be important in the evaluation of an infant with hyperbilirubinemia. The hepatobiliary iminodiacetic acid (HIDA) scan is typically performed during the patient evaluation (see Chapter 18). Although the HIDA scan is highly sensitive for detecting excretion of bile from the liver, it is not very specific to the diagnosis of BA. However, a HIDA scan demonstrating excretion rules out BA. Magnetic resonance cholangiopancreatography (MRCP) has also been suggested as a possible tool in the diagnosis of BA because of the increased fidelity and visualization of the intra- and extrahepatic biliary tree. Studies from the late 1990s and early 2000s suggested a reported sensitivity and specificity of greater than 90%.[28,29]

Regardless of the imaging study, the vast majority of infants in whom the suspicion for BA is high will progress to the gold standard for diagnosis of intraoperative cholangiography with biopsy. Although some centers perform a liver biopsy before operative cholangiography, we generally do not because the pathologic findings in the liver of BA patients early in the disease are not pathognomonic and therefore cannot entirely rule out BA.

SURGICAL MANAGEMENT

Preoperative Care and Surgical Technique

The preoperative management of a child with BA includes the correction of coagulopathy if present and the administration of broad-spectrum antibiotics with biliary coverage. Developed by Morio Kasai in 1959, the Roux-en-Y hepatoportoenterostomy (HPE) is the gold standard approach in the surgical management of BA. Although there has been some recent controversy over whether or not liver transplant should be offered as the primary operative treatment, most centers agree that HPE should be performed first to give each child the chance to have improved biliary drainage and to delay the progression to end-stage liver failure requiring liver transplant.

The entire operation may be performed through a small right upper quadrant incision approximately one fingerbreadth below the costal margin. Keeping the incision well below the costal margin will ensure that the same incision can be used in the future should liver transplantation be required. Incisions made too close to the costal margin may ultimately migrate to the lower ribs as the child grows. The gallbladder of BA patients is typically shrunken, contracted, or absent and is often partially intrahepatic below a cleft in the liver edge. Upon entry into the gallbladder for the introduction of a cholangiogram catheter, "white bile" is often encountered, which confirms the lack of continuity between the intrahepatic bile ducts and the gall bladder. Unless this is proven to result from isolated cystic duct obstruction, the presence of "white bile" is confirmatory for BA and some surgeons would not proceed with the cholangiogram. If normal golden bile is encountered, a cholangiogram should be performed via the gall bladder to further delineate the biliary anatomy.

To perform the cholangiogram, a purse string suture is placed in the fundus of the gallbladder and a small catheter (3.5 French [F] feeding tube or angiocatheter) is placed within the lumen for the instillation of contrast. If it appears that contrast flows into the intrahepatic ducts and duodenum, BA is excluded. If the intrahepatic ducts, extrahepatic ducts, and/or the duodenum do not fill with contrast, surgical correction is typically required. The cholangiogram can be performed laparoscopically, but most centers perform an open procedure because of the high likelihood of proceeding to HPE.[30]

Once the decision has been made to proceed with HPE, the biliary tract is carefully dissected to the portal plate, which is typically at the bifurcation of both the portal vein and hepatic artery. The extrahepatic biliary tree is then excised, leaving a thin layer of fibrotic portal plate in place. It is at this interface that any remaining biliary ductules will be found. Care is taken to limit the use of cautery in this area because this may cause destruction of the remaining ductules. We often place dilute epinephrine–soaked gelfoam directly on the portal plate for hemostasis while a retrocolic Roux-en-Y limb of approximately 45 cm is created from the proximal jejunum. We typically anastomose the open end of the Roux-en-Y limb around the remnant portal plate with 6-0 PDS sutures placed into any appropriate surrounding tissue including portal vein adventitia posteriorly and liver capsule anteriorly. It is critical to avoid suturing any areas of the portal plate where bile flow is observed. Postoperative abdominal drainage is not necessary.

Although the open approach is most commonly used to perform HPE, some groups have attempted a minimally invasive approach. Several studies, including larger meta-analyses, have found no difference in the clearance of jaundice between the laparoscopic and open approaches with short-term follow-up. However, longer-term outcomes of laparoscopic HPE have been shown to be inferior to the open procedure with respect to native liver survival in several studies and therefore the majority of centers have abandoned the laparoscopic approach to HPE.[31,32]

We and others have adapted a minimally invasive open approach to HPE to facilitate the future liver transplant that is required in the majority of these patients.[33] This includes a smaller abdominal incision (approximately 3–4 cm), minimal dissection of the porta hepatis structures, and minimal to no dissection of the peritoneal/ diaphragmatic attachments to the liver. These modifications serve to minimize adhesions and preservation of dissection planes, resulting in fewer intraabdominal varices and a less hostile abdomen at the time of future liver transplantation. In addition, because the Roux-en-Y will also be used for biliary drainage at the time of transplant, it is our practice to perform a retrocolic Roux-en-Y and leave a significant amount of Roux limb above the colonic mesentery so that the Roux-en-Y does not have to be mobilized during the liver transplant. In our experience, these small modifications do not compromise the safety of the operation but do significantly reduce some of the technical challenges that may be encountered during a future liver transplant.

Although liver transplant is typically considered the definitive treatment in the algorithm for those with an unsuccessful HPE, some centers have advocated for a redo HPE in certain circumstances. In 2012 the Cincinnati group published their experience with redo HPE in a select group of patients that either had recurrent cholangitis or had sudden cessation of bile drainage.[34] Although the differences were not statistically significant, they found that 39% that underwent HPE revision versus 22% of those that did not were alive with their native livers after 15 years.[34] These findings have also been supported by additional studies suggesting an increase in survival of the native liver with redo HPE versus those with no revision.[35,36] Despite this, the decision to perform a redo HPE is controversial. Given that additional surgery in these patients can increase adhesions, which become vascularized in the setting of portal hypertension and can increase operative times, blood loss, and mortality during liver transplant, most centers do not perform redo HPE.

POSTOPERATIVE OUTCOMES

Although previously uniformly fatal within the first 2 years of life, outcomes in BA have improved substantially since the development of the HPE. After HPE, patients are followed for the production of pigmented stool, which is usually associated with successful biliary drainage and an associated decrease in serum bilirubin. This process can take up to 2 to 3 months after HPE, although improvements are usually noted within the first few weeks. Most centers cite initial success in approximately 60% of patients and a 5-year native liver survival ranging from 20% to 80% depending on the study[4,37,38] (Table 40.2). Recently, several longitudinal studies of 20-year native liver survival have been published and range from approximately 20% to 50% depending on the country (see Table 40.2).

Unfortunately, approximately half of patients in whom the HPE is initially successful will have continued inflammation, cholangitis, fibrosis, and eventual liver failure that may occur over months to years. In those patients in whom HPE was unsuccessful, end-stage liver disease will develop more rapidly and liver transplantation will be required within the first 2 years of life. In either case, liver transplantation is the only option and

TABLE 40.2   National Patient Outcomes and Native Liver Survival

STUDY	YEAR	COUNTRY	ERA	N	TIME TO HPE (DAYS)	CLEARANCE OF JAUNDICE (%) CLEARANCE OF JAUNDICE	NATIVE LIVER SURVIVAL (%) 4 TO 5 YEARS	10 YEARS	20 YR.	30/40 YR.
Nio et al.	2003	Japan	1989	108	>65	NR	62	53	NR	NR
Schneider et al.	2006	US	1997–2000	104	61	40	56	NR	NR	NR
Schreiber	2007	Canada	1985–1995	349	65	NR	36	26	NR	NR
Wildhaber et al.	2008	Switzerland	1994–2004	48	68	40	37	33	NR	NR
Davenport et al.	2011	England and Wales	1999–2009	443	54	55	46	40	NR	NR
Leonhardt et al.	2011	Germany	2001–2005	137	57	NR	20	NR	NR	NR
Nio	2017	Japan	1989–2015	3160	68	60	NR	NR	49	
Chan et al.	2019	China	1993–2007	20	53	45	85	85	NR	
Parolini et al.	2019	Italy	1975–1996	174	60	52	41	32	18	15
Fanna et al.	2019	France	1986–2015	1428	NR	40	41	35	26	22

HPE, Hepatoportoenterostomy; NR, not reported.

Table adapted from prior Blumgart chapter.

referral to a pediatric transplant center for evaluation should be initiated.

We and others have examined outcomes related to success or failure after HPE. In a study of 185 BA patients, Chung et al. found that repeated cholangitis was a significant risk factor for early and late (>3 years) failure after HPE.[39] In our study of 81 BA patients that had undergone HPE, we identified two factors that seemed to be important predictors of failure and need for transplantation. These included total bilirubin greater than 2 mg/dL and albumin less than 3.5 g/dL at 3 months after HPE.[40] This was further supported by a recent study published by Wang et al. in which they found that the high rates of jaundice clearance over the course of 4 weeks was protective and was directly proportional to native liver survival.[37]

POSTOPERATIVE COMPLICATIONS

Although the development of HPE is an important bridge and temporizing measure to transplant, complications associated with the pathophysiology of BA and end-stage liver disease occur. These include cholangitis, portal hypertension, hepatopulmonary syndrome, and malignancy. A brief overview of these complications will be described next.

Cholangitis

Continued inflammation, intermittent obstruction of bile flow, and reflux of intestinal contents likely contribute to cholangitis after HPE. This is the most common complication of HPE and affects approximately 50% of patients, usually within the first 2 years postoperatively.[41] Patients will present with fevers, increasing liver function tests, elevated white blood cell count, and acholic stools. Not surprisingly, gram-negative bacteremia with *Escherichia coli, Klebsiella pneumoniae,* and *Pseudomonas aeruginosa* is also frequent.[42]

Most centers recommend postoperative oral or intravenous (IV) antibiotic prophylaxis, but evidence to support this is not strong. The only randomized control trial (RCT) to date found that postoperative antibiotics were protective (risk ratio [RR] 0.42–0.52), but the study population was very small (n = 34).[43] Some authors have advocated for redo HPE in this setting to ensure proper drainage through the Roux and prolong native liver survival; however, this remains controversial.[34,44]

Portal Hypertension

Because of the persistence of liver injury and the progression of liver fibrosis in most patients after HPE, approximately 70% of BA infants will develop portal hypertension with esophageal varices (see Chapter 76). Although most are asymptomatic, up to 25% of these patients present with a variceal bleed within a year of HPE and half will have at least one variceal bleed over time.[45] Many studies have developed predictive models in an attempt to identify patients that would be most at risk for variceal bleeding. These studies suggested that patients with thrombocytopenia (platelet count < 100 X 10⁹/L), transient elastography, or Fibroscan value greater than 31.5 kPa and/or failure clear jaundice early after HPE were at higher risk.[46–49] Although there is no consensus on the appropriate surveillance or variceal bleeding prophylaxis of children with portal hypertension, a recent survey of centers in France found that 75% of centers used endoscopy as primary prophylaxis and only 20% of centers use nonselective beta-blockers.[50]

The most serious sequela of portal hypertension is variceal bleeding, which can present as melena/hematemesis with or without hemodynamic instability. Treatment for variceal bleeding is fairly standard across centers and involves endoscopy with banding and/or sclerotherapy after resuscitation (see Chapters 80 and 81). Medical adjuncts such as octreotide, vasopressin, antibiotic prophylaxis, and/or proton pump inhibitors are often employed as well. In addition to these therapies, surgical shunts and transjugular intrahepatic portosystemic shunt (TIPS) procedures have been considered and will be discussed in more detail (see Chapter 85).

Pulmonary Vascular Complications

In addition to the abdominal manifestations of portal hypertension previously described, patients with portal hypertension are prone to develop pulmonary complications such as hepatopulmonary syndrome (HPS) and portopulmonary hypertension (PoPHTN; see Chapter 76). Although the pathophysiology of HPS is not completely understood, it is thought that intrapulmonary vessel dilation and increased pressure leads to the stimulation of angiogenesis and the development of intrapulmonary shunting and hypoxemia. This is typically diagnosed using contrast-bubble echocardiography, lung perfusion scans, and/or pulmonary arteriography. It has been estimated that the incidence of HPS in children with BA occurs in 3% to 20% of children with end-stage liver disease.[51] Although cardiac catherization or pulmonary angiography may identify a treatable lesion or shunt, there is no definitive medical or surgical therapy for HPS except for liver transplantation.

Portopulmonary hypertension (PoPHTN) related to cirrhosis occurs in a minority of patients and develops in response to pulmonary arterial vasoconstriction secondary to soluble mediators (e.g., endothelin-1), which are increased in the setting of end-stage liver disease. Although more common in adult patients, PoPHTN does occur in the pediatric population but usually in adolescents secondary to long-standing cirrhosis.[51] Pulmonary vasodilators such as sildenafil and a fairly novel class of drugs designed to target the endothelin receptor antagonists are currently being used in these patients.[51,52]

Malignancy

With significant liver inflammation and the development of fibrosis and cirrhosis in the native liver, there is thought to be a significant risk for malignant transformation. Hadzic et al. reported that 5 of 387 BA patients developed hepatocellular carcinoma (HCC) at a median age of 2.1 years.[53] An earlier study by Esquivel et al., which examined the histology of 72 livers from pediatric patients that underwent liver transplantation, found that 9 had HCC or severe dysplasia.[54] Two of these livers were from patients with BA and were found to have liver cell dysplasia in one and HCC in the other. Case reports of cholangiocarcinoma and hepatoblastoma have also been reported but are more rare than HCC.[55,56]

CONTROVERSIES IN THE MANAGEMENT OF BILIARY ATRESIA

Postoperative Steroids

Because of the persistent inflammatory response that exists after HPE in BA patients, steroids have been used postoperatively after HPE for over 3 decades. In addition to their antiinflammatory

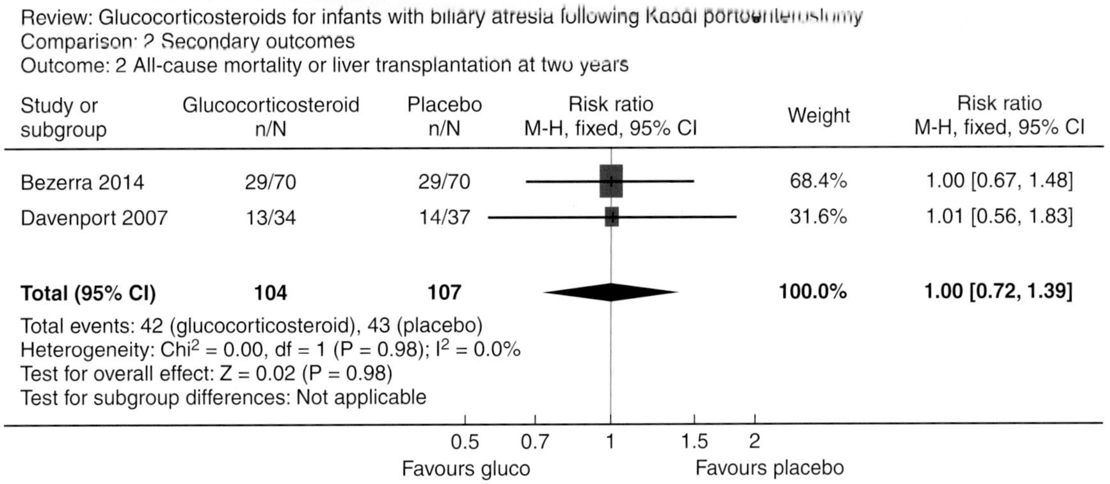

Review: Glucocorticosteroids for infants with biliary atresia following Kasai portoenterostomy
Comparison: 2 Secondary outcomes
Outcome: 2 All-cause mortality or liver transplantation at two years

Study or subgroup	Glucocorticosteroid n/N	Placebo n/N	Risk ratio M-H, fixed, 95% CI	Weight	Risk ratio M-H, fixed, 95% CI
Bezerra 2014	29/70	29/70		68.4%	1.00 [0.67, 1.48]
Davenport 2007	13/34	14/37		31.6%	1.01 [0.56, 1.83]
Total (95% CI)	**104**	**107**		**100.0%**	**1.00 [0.72, 1.39]**

Total events: 42 (glucocorticosteroid), 43 (placebo)
Heterogeneity: Chi^2 = 0.00, df = 1 (P = 0.98); I^2 = 0.0%
Test for overall effect: Z = 0.02 (P = 0.98)
Test for subgroup differences: Not applicable

0.5   0.7   1   1.5   2
Favours gluco   Favours placebo

FIGURE 40.2 Forrest plot depicting efficacy of glucocorticoid on overall native liver survival. (Tyraskis A, Parsons C, Davenport M. Glucocorticosteroids for infants with biliary atresia following Kasai portoenterostomy. *Cochrane Database Syst Rev.* 2018;2018[5]).

response, steroids are thought to have choleretic properties. However, data supporting the use of steroids in the early or late postoperative setting are equivocal. Multiple studies have either demonstrated a trend towards significance or significant increases in the rate of jaundice clearance in those patients treated with steroids. However, the majority of studies fail to show any differences in long-term native liver or patient survival.

A recent Cochrane review of glucocorticoids in BA identified two RCTs in which glucocorticoids were administered to BA patients after HPE.[57] When the glucocorticoid-treated groups were compared with placebo/no intervention, there was no significant difference in all-cause mortality (Fig. 40.2), serious adverse events (defined as events leading to disability or death), clearance of jaundice, or liver transplantation at 2 years.[57] Despite these findings, the majority of centers around the world except the US use high-dose steroids postoperatively.[15]

TIPS or Surgical Shunts

BA patients with severe portal hypertension (portosystemic gradient [PSG] > 12 mm Hg) are at high risk for variceal hemorrhage. Although GI bleeding in children is typically managed through endoscopy, some centers have advocated for the use of TIPS in cases where further endoscopy has been deemed inadequate/futile or in diuretic refractory ascites (see Chapter 85). In one study of 34 pediatric patients with a median age of 12, TIPS was used in patients that had either a GI bleed, ascites, or splenomegaly with sequestration.[58] Of these, BA was the etiology of liver disease in 5 patients. Technical success was defined as the decrease in PSG to less than 12 mm Hg or a decrease of the PSG by half in those with PSG less than 12 mm Hg. Of the BA patients, all had early technical success with good outcomes except one that had ongoing bleeding and was transplanted 3 days later. No details of the transplant were offered in the report. In another retrospective series of 59 patients, of whom 12 (20%) were BA patients, TIPS was successful in 94% of patients that presented with bleeding in preventing subsequent variceal bleeding.[59] Interestingly, three of the four technical failures were in BA patients secondary to their hepatic venous anatomy, which included an interrupted inferior vena cava with azygous extension. In addition, one of the five deaths was as a result of sepsis from puncture of the portal plate during TIPS placement that resulted in bowel perforation. These anatomic differences in the BA population versus other pediatric end-stage liver failure patients must be considered when a TIPS procedure is being considered.

Other groups have challenged the utility of TIPS and have advocated for the creation of surgical shunts to control bleeding or ascites or delay time to transplant (see Chapters 83 and 84). For example, Guerin et al. recently published a series of 38 patients with BA and significant variceal hemorrhage (Grade 2/3 varices with stigmata of bleeding) after HPE who underwent surgical shunt (SS) creation.[60] Also included in the analysis were 7 BA patients that underwent a TIPS procedure for similar reasons. This study demonstrates that a SS may be used in place of TIPS or repeated endoscopy to delay time to transplant and stabilize a bleeding patient. Because of the sample size and short follow-up, it is difficult to draw other conclusions. The TIPS cohort in their study population had poor outcomes with four patients experiencing immediate technical failure, one mortality, and one with hepatic encephalopathy, suggesting that the SS may be better. However, because GI bleeding is a common complication of portal hypertension in BA patients, these interventions should be discussed in the event that endoscopy fails to control ongoing hemorrhage.

Liver Transplantation

Despite our best efforts, most studies demonstrate that only 30% of native livers of BA patients that have undergone an HPE survive after 15 years and BA remains the most common reason for liver transplantation in the pediatric population[4,38] (see Chapter 110). Although the factors that are associated with failure of the native liver and progression to transplant are still somewhat unclear, many studies have found that early clearance of bilirubin after HPE as well as age at HPE are critical for HPE success[40,61] (Fig. 40.3). In support of this, our group has found that total bilirubin greater than 2 and albumin less than 3.5 at 3 months post-HPE were the most significant factors associated with progression to transplant or mortality.[40]

Given this poor long-term native liver survival, some centers have questioned the role of HPE in BA. A recent study by LeeVan et al. examining a California administrative database

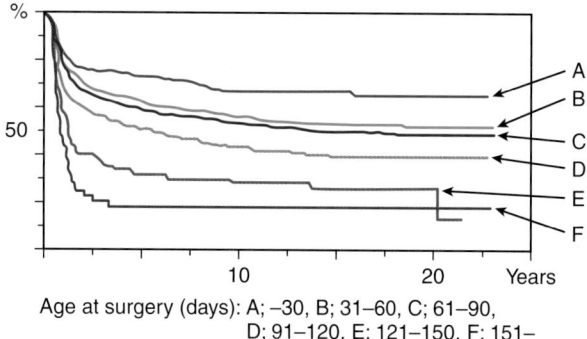

Age at surgery (days): A; –30, B; 31–60, C; 61–90,
D; 91–120, E; 121–150, F; 151–

FIGURE 40.3 Long-term native liver survival by age at hepatoportoenterostomy. (Nio M. Japanese biliary atresia registry. *Pediatr Surg Int.* 2017;33[12]:1319–1325.)

has suggested that BA patients should undergo liver transplant as a primary therapy, completely eliminating HPE as an option.[62] This conclusion was based on their findings that BA patients undergoing primary liver transplant had significantly better outcomes compared with those patients who underwent HPE (after 2002) or those who underwent salvage liver transplant after HPE (hazard ratio [HR] 0.16–0.43). Although these data are thought provoking, there are several major limitations to the study. The majority of centers still recommend HPE as

the initial surgical therapy for most patients suspected to have BA because of the high potential benefit and low morbidity of the procedure as it is currently performed.[63]

CONCLUSIONS

Infants diagnosed today with BA can expect to have an excellent long-term survival rate because of the surgical advances made over the past 50 years (Fig. 40.4). The HPE developed by Morio Kasai remains the gold standard for the initial treatment of these infants when diagnosed before the development of decompensated cirrhosis. Liver transplantation outcomes in children have improved dramatically and with the additional surgical options including living donation and split liver transplantation that have become commonplace, waitlist mortality among infants and children awaiting liver transplantation has become rare. Future advancements in the management of BA patients are likely to result from research to identify and/or modulate the genetic components and/or the inflammatory response, which continues to destroy the biliary system in these patients. Our hope is that these advances will ultimately convert BA from a surgical to a medical disease.

The references for this chapter can be found online by accessing the accompanying Expert Consult website.

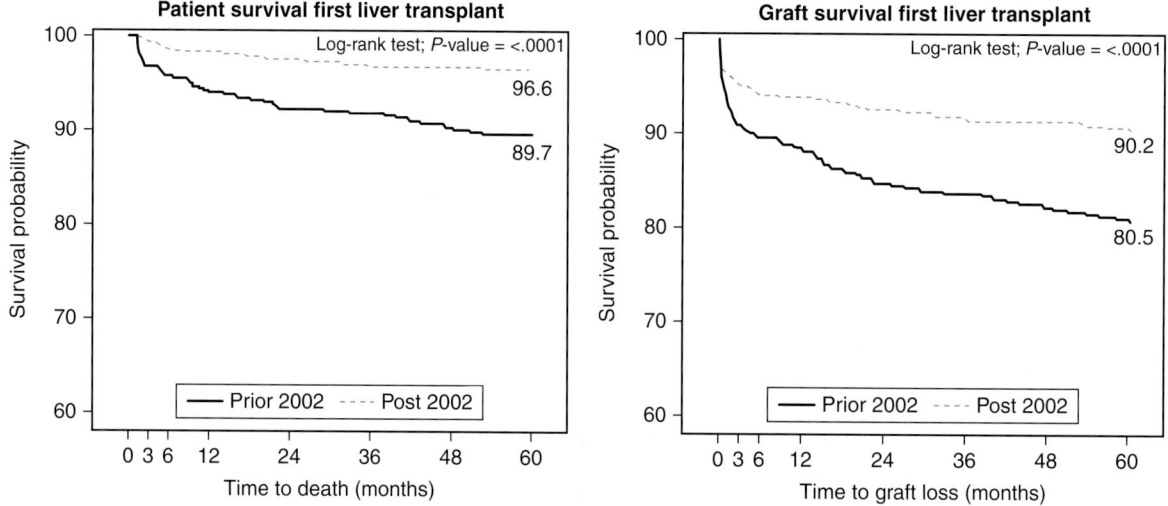

FIGURE 40.4 Survival data of biliary atresia patients post liver transplant by era. (From Taylor SA, Venkat V, Arnon R, et al. Improved outcomes for liver transplantation in patients with biliary atresia since Pediatric end stage liver disease implementation: Analysis of the society of Pediatric Liver Transplantation Registry. *J Pediatr.* 2020;219:89–97.)

CHAPTER 41

Primary sclerosing cholangitis

Navine Nasser-Ghodsi, James H. Tabibian, and Nicholas F. LaRusso

OVERVIEW

Primary sclerosing cholangitis (PSC) is a chronic, idiopathic cholangiopathy characterized histologically by peribiliary inflammation and fibrosis. PSC can progress to cirrhosis and is a risk factor for hepatobiliary and colonic carcinogenesis. The median liver transplant (LT) free survival time is approximately 15 years.[1-3] Despite ongoing research over the past several decades, the etiopathogenesis of PSC remains poorly understood; as a result, effective pharmacologic therapy for PSC has not been established.[4,5] Despite being a relatively rare disorder, PSC is the fifth most common indication for LT in the United States (US) (UNOS) and the leading indication for LT in several other countries[2,6] (see Chapter 105). LT is presently the only proven life-extending therapy for patients with end-stage PSC; although LT is potentially curative, it is offered to only selected patients, and even suitable candidates can experience recurrent PSC or hepatobiliary malignancy post-LT.[7,8]

EPIDEMIOLOGY

PSC more commonly affects men than women (2:1) and has a peak incidence in the fourth decade of life.[9,10] The age-adjusted incidence of PSC in the US is 1.25 per 100,000 for Caucasian men and 0.54 per 100,000 for Caucasian women.[11] Recent data suggest the prevalence of PSC has been rising in both sexes, which may be attributable to an increase in incidence and not decrease in deaths.[10] The calculated prevalence of PSC in the US has been reported as 20.9 and 6.3 per 100,000 people, respectively, corresponding to approximately 30,000 cases nationwide.[11] Similar statistics on PSC prevalence have been reported in Canada,[12] Northern Europe,[10,13] and New Zealand.[14] Limited available data suggest a similar prevalence for African American patients in the US compared with European American patients, but African American patients tend to be younger and have a higher model for end-stage liver disease (MELD) at the time of LT listing.[15] Epidemiologic data regarding the geographic distribution of PSC remains poorly defined in most other countries.[16]

PSC is strongly associated with inflammatory bowel disease (IBD). Approximately 70% of Western (e.g., US, UK) patients with PSC are co-diagnosed with IBD, most commonly ulcerative colitis (UC)[17,18]; conversely, only approximately 3% to 5% of patients with IBD have PSC.[19-21] It is worth noting, though, that in far Eastern cohorts, only approximately one-third of patients with PSC have concomitant IBD, a discrepancy that may be attributable to genetic and/or environmental factors.[22]

CLINICAL PRESENTATION

Up to 40% of patients with PSC are asymptomatic at the time of diagnosis and incidentally found to have elevated serum liver enzymes, most commonly alkaline phosphatase (ALP) and alanine aminotransferase (ALT), which leads to further evaluation and ultimately the diagnosis of PSC.[12,23-25] When present, the most common symptoms at the time of PSC diagnosis include abdominal pain, pruritus, diarrhea, jaundice, fatigue, and fever. The two most frequently encountered physical examination signs are hepatomegaly and splenomegaly, although the physical examination is often unrevealing. On occasion, a patient may present with manifestations of advanced cirrhosis and portal hypertension, including ascites or gastrointestinal bleeding secondary to varices. Children with PSC relatively frequently have liver disease with features of autoimmune hepatitis (AIH) as discussed later (see "Associated Diseases" section).[26,27] Therefore the clinical presentation of PSC varies considerably, depending in part on the disease stage at the time of diagnosis and the age at diagnosis.

DIAGNOSIS

The most common biochemical abnormality in patients with PSC is an elevated ALP, reflecting chronic cholestasis, and may be the only laboratory abnormality identified. Although some patients may have a normal ALP, it is typically about twofold to threefold higher than the upper limit of normal. Unlike other autoimmune liver diseases, such as autoimmune hepatitis or primary biliary cirrhosis, there is no serologic test that aids in diagnosis but often just nonspecific elevated autoantibodies.[28]

Noninvasive imaging, in particular magnetic resonance cholangiopancreatography (MRCP), can be used to diagnose PSC (see Chapter 16). Cholangiographic features of PSC include multifocal intra and/or extrahepatic biliary strictures, proximal segmental ductal dilatation, and a "pruned" biliary tree (Fig. 41.1). Given advances in noninvasive imaging techniques, including MRCP, endoscopic retrograde cholangiopancreatography (ERCP) is generally no longer needed to make a diagnosis of PSC. Instead, ERCP is now typically reserved for evaluation of unexplained hepatobiliary symptoms, biliary obstruction caused by a suspected dominant stricture, or possible/known malignancy, among other indications[29] (Fig. 41.2; see Chapters 20 and 30).

A liver biopsy is not required for the diagnosis of PSC, especially if the patient fits the classical pattern, including a patient with underlying IBD, elevated ALP, and typical findings on MRCP. The major role of liver biopsy in PSC, if performed, is to: (1) exclude other or co-existing causes of liver disease (e.g., autoimmune hepatitis), (2) diagnose small-duct PSC, and (3) determine the disease stage.[30] Pathologic features compatible with PSC include chronic cholangitis, ductular proliferation, and periductal fibrosis (Fig. 41.3) but can vary depending on disease stage.[4,31,32]

It is important to distinguish between PSC and other causes of liver disease, especially secondary sclerosing cholangitis

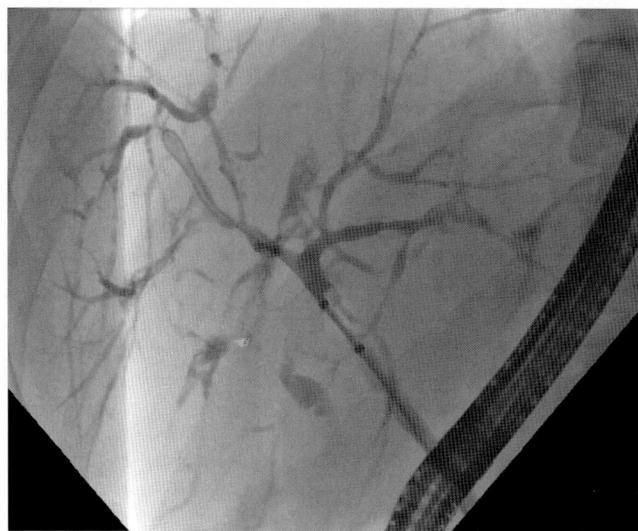

FIGURE 41.1 Endoscopic retrograde cholangiography demonstrating typical cholangiographic findings of primary sclerosing cholangitis, namely diffuse irregularity and multifocal stricturing, with proximal dilation of bile ducts.

(Table 41.1), because secondary sclerosing cholangitis generally originates from known pathologic processes (e.g., biliary trauma, malignancy, infection) and may respond well to pharmacotherapy.[33] An important example of secondary sclerosing cholangitis is IgG4-associated cholangiopathy, which is part of a spectrum of systemic fibroinflammatory disorders (IgG4-related diseases) that can affect multiple organ systems, are characterized by elevated serum and/or tissue IgG4 levels, and generally respond to corticosteroid therapy.[34] Novel qPCR quantifying the IgG4/IgG RNA ratio in blood and next-generation sequencing showing dominant IgG4+ B-cell receptor clones in patients with IgG4-related disease are both new tests that can aid in differentiating patients with IgG4-realted disease from those with PSC[35,36] (see Chapter 43).

OTHER SEROLOGIC ABNORMALITIES

Although the classic serum biochemical pattern in PSC is cholestatic, other or concomitant abnormalities may also be seen.

For instance, serum aminotransferase levels may also be increased in many patients, albeit only modestly (to less than three times the upper limit of normal).[37] Those with markedly elevated aminotransferase levels may show concomitant serologic and histologic features of AIH,[38] thus suggesting PSC-AIH overlap syndrome, as discussed further in a subsequent section (see "Associated Diseases" section). Because patients with PSC may develop an overlap syndrome years after the initial diagnosis of PSC, periodic monitoring of aminotransferases (together with ALP and bilirubin) is advisable.

Serum bilirubin levels are normal in 60% of patients at diagnosis but tend to rise as PSC progresses.[24] An abrupt, sustained increase in conjugated bilirubin may indicate the presence of a dominant biliary stricture, bile duct stone, or the development of cholangiocarcinoma (CCA)[39]; therefore it should prompt additional investigation (e.g., MRCP). Serum copper and ceruloplasmin and hepatic and urinary copper levels are often abnormal. Hepatic copper levels can be increased to the degree seen in Wilson's disease and primary biliary cirrhosis (PBC) and is a reflection of prolonged cholestasis.[40]

Elevated serum IgM, IgE, IgG, and total IgA has been reported in approximately 45%, 40%, 25%, and 10% of patients with PSC, respectively.[16,27,41,42] Patients with an increase in one immunoglobulin isotype will generally have increased levels of other isotypes as well.[27] Although the relevance of hyperglobulinemias in PSC remains uncertain, it is conceivable that they may have as yet unrecognized prognostic and/or pathophysiologic implications (e.g., as with IgG4-related cholangiopathy). Auto-antibody testing in PSC is of limited value.[43]

IMAGING MODALITIES

Cholangiography is necessary for diagnosing large-duct PSC. MRI/MRCP is a noninvasive modality that visualizes the biliary tree and has largely replaced the prior gold standard invasive technique of ERCP (see Chapters 16, 20, and 30). The International PSC Study Group has recommended MRCP as the initial diagnostic imaging technique in patients suspected of having PSC.[44] Classically, both the intrahepatic and extrahepatic biliary tree is involved, but variations of PSC exist (Table 41.2), and involvement may become more extensive over time in those presenting with only intra or only extrahepatic disease. In addition to location, strictures can also vary in length and

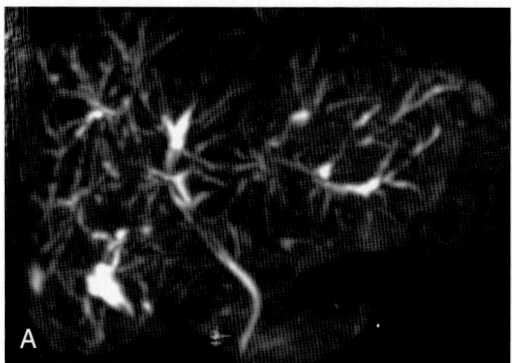
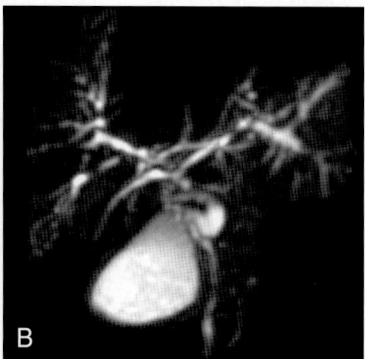
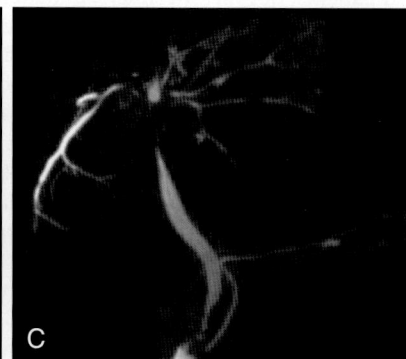

FIGURE 41.2 **Magnetic resonance cholangiopancreatography in primary sclerosing cholangitis *(PSC)*.** Shown are three separate cases demonstrating characteristic yet heterogeneous features of PSC on maximal intensity projection images. **A,** Proximal common bile duct stricture and diffuse intrahepatic stricturing with focal upstream dilation. **B,** Multifocal extrahepatic bile duct stricturing and bilateral intrahepatic duct stricturing with proximal dilation. **C,** Severely pruned intrahepatic biliary tree, right posterior hepatic ductal system dilation proximal to a perihilar stricture, and dominant-appearing common hepatic duct stricture. (See Chapter 16.)

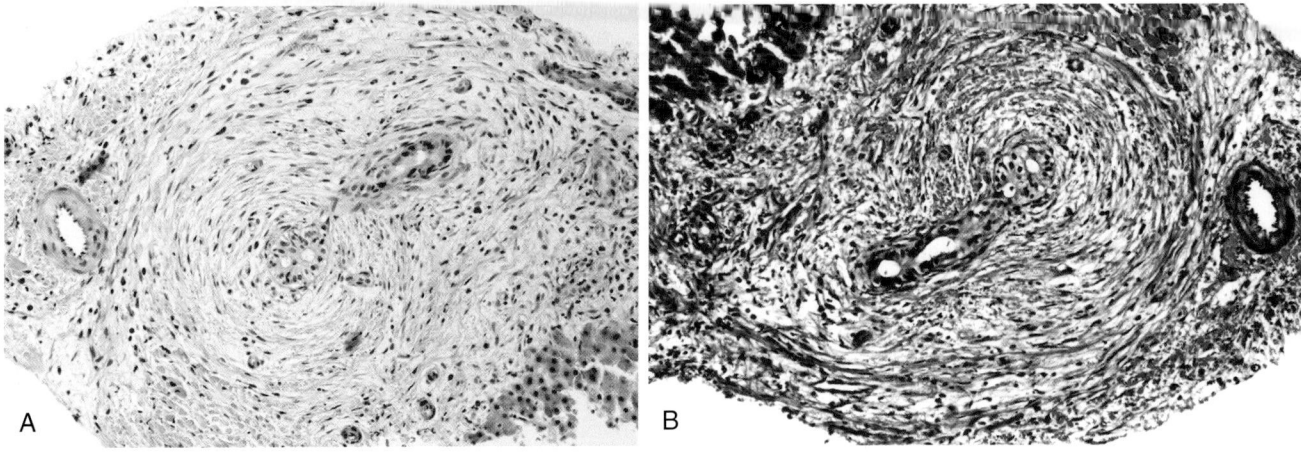

FIGURE 41.3   Histologic features of primary sclerosing cholangitis. A, Typical changes of cholangitis, periportal inflammation, and biliary fibrosis (hematoxylin and eosin stain, ×40). **B,** Classic finding of periductal, that is, "onion-skin," fibrosis (trichrome stain, ×40).

severity (i.e., degree of fibrosis and obstruction). Some strictures may also harbour malignancy, and indeed distinguishing between benign and malignant dominant strictures in PSC represents a major ongoing challenge,[23,45] as discussed later (see "Cholangiocarcinoma" section).

The emergence of MRCP has been partly driven by ERCP being an invasive procedure requiring anaesthesia and carrying a considerable risk of adverse events, such as acute pancreatitis, bleeding, perforation, and acute cholangitis. Patients with PSC, in particular, have a higher incidence of acute cholangitis compared with patients without PSC undergoing ERCP, whereas the risk of other adverse events appears to be similar.[46] Because of the risks of ERCP, MRCP has emerged as a noninvasive substitute for ERCP (see Fig. 41.2). MRCP has diagnostic accuracy comparable with that of ERCP and results in cost savings when used as the initial diagnostic strategy.[28,47–49] MRCP also lends itself well to simultaneous MR elastography of the liver, which is a technique used to quantify hepatic fibrosis (expressed in kilopascals) and distinguish patients with and without cirrhosis.[50]

Abdominal ultrasound and computed tomography (CT) are useful in monitoring patients and evaluating for biliary stones, hepatobiliary malignancy, and other disease complications once a diagnosis of PSC has already been made (see Chapter 16). Percutaneous cholangiography (PTC) allows access to the biliary tree when ERCP is not technically feasible (see Chapters 20 and 31). Positron emission tomography (PET)/CT has a high sensitivity for CCA in a dominant stricture and has a role in combination with brush cytology for monitoring PSC patients who have a dominant stricture.[51]

HISTOPATHOLOGY

Classic histologic findings on liver biopsy include paucicellular, mixed, nonsuppurative portal tract inflammation, cholangitis

TABLE 41.1   Causes of Secondary Sclerosing Cholangitis and Mimics of Primary Sclerosing Cholangitis

Infectious	AIDS cholangiopathy (e.g., *Cryptosporidium parvum*, CMV) Helminth infection (e.g., *Clonorchis, Opisthorchis, Ascaris*) Recurrent pyogenic cholangitis (i.e., Oriental cholangiohepatitis)
Chronic intrinsic or extrinsic compression (benign or malignant)	Choledocholithiasis (e.g., Mirizzi syndrome) Cholangiocarcinoma Diffuse intrahepatic malignancy (e.g., metastatic disease) Compressive lymphadenopathy Portal hypertensive biliopathy Postoperative injury or stricture Chronic or necrotizing pancreatitis
Immunologic	IgG4-associated disease Eosinophilic cholangitis Mast cell cholangiopathy Histiocytosis X Systemic vasculitis Hepatic allograft rejection Primary biliary cirrhosis (small-duct PSC mimic)
Ischemic	Post-transplant nonanastomotic strictures Intra-arterial chemotherapy Radiation therapy
Congenital and/or idiopathic	Choledochal cyst (e.g., Caroli disease) Progressive familial intrahepatic cholestasis (small-duct PSC mimic)

AIDS, Acquired immune deficiency syndrome; *CMV*, cytomegalovirus; *PSC*, primary sclerosing cholangitis.

TABLE 41.2   Classification and Features of PSC

DIAGNOSTIC TERM	CHOLANGIOGRAPHY	LIVER HISTOLOGY
Classic PSC	Multifocal intrahepatic and extrahepatic strictures and resultant proximal ductal dilation	Typical (i.e., biliary inflammation, periductal fibrosis [staged by Ludwig classification], ductular proliferation, and ductopenia)
Intrahepatic PSC	Multifocal *intrahepatic*-only strictures and resultant proximal ductal dilation	Typical
Extrahepatic PSC	*Extrahepatic*-only strictures and resultant proximal ductal dilation	Nondiagnostic, particularly in early disease
Small-duct PSC	Normal	Typical

PSC, Primary sclerosing cholangitis.

(with or without ductopenia), cholestasis, and a periductal cuff of fibrous sheets and edema that acquires a classic "onion skin" appearance (see Fig. 41.3).[52] This classic finding is nearly pathognomonic but is seen in fewer than 10% of PSC liver biopsies (but more frequently in larger surgical specimens).[53]

It is important to recognize and distinguish fibro-obliterative cholangitis of PSC from alternative etiologies including: (1) PBC, (2) mechanical obstruction of larger bile ducts, (3) ductopenic rejection after LT, (4) cholangiopathy of acquired immunodeficiency syndrome (AIDS), and (5) patients having undergone hepatic arterial infusion of floxuridine (FUDR). Distinguishing PSC from PBC, for example, can be based on the involvement of extrahepatic and large intrahepatic bile ducts in the former, as well as the milder, mixed inflammatory infiltrate, but this distinction may be difficult to make in some cases without appropriate clinical correlation.[50] Moreover, granulomata, thought to be a feature of PBC, may be seen in approximately 4% of liver biopsies from patients with PSC[54] (thus further emphasizing the importance of additional clinical data.

There are three main liver histology grading systems relevant to PSC: Nakanuma, Ishak, and Ludwig. The Ludwig system has been the most commonly used[55] and is based on the degree of extension of fibroinflammatory changes in the hepatic parenchyma, ranging from stage 1 (portal inflammation) to stage 4 (biliary cirrhosis; Table 41.3). A head-to-head comparison of the three scoring systems has shown that all are independent predictors of long-term outcomes in patients with PSC but that the Nakanuma has the highest predictive value.[56]

ETIOPATHOGENESIS

Although the pathogenesis of PSC remains unclear, it is generally accepted that environmental exposures and genetic underpinnings drive inflammation and fibrosis in PSC via alterations in the gut microbiota, autoimmunity, bile acid composition, and a proinflammatory cholangiocyte phenotype.[57-60] Cholangiocytes, the epithelial cells lining the bile ducts, are a morphologically, biochemically, and functionally heterogeneous and highly dynamic population of cells that are not only a target of injury in PSC but may also be directly and actively involved in its pathogenesis.[61,62] For example, in response to recognition of pathogen associated molecular patterns (PAMPs) and other stimuli such as infection or ischemia, cholangiocytes are activated to express a number of proinflammatory cytokines (e.g., tumor necrosis factor [TNF]-α, interleukin [IL]-6, IL-8) and other bioactive molecules.[63-65] Biosynthesis and secretion of these signaling mediators makes up part of the biliary innate immune and repair response and mediates recruitment and

activation of T cells, macrophages, neutrophils, natural killer cells, and other resident and recruited cells in the peribiliary environment.[59,66,67]

Several hypotheses regarding the etiopathogenesis of PSC have been proposed,[68,69] of which two are described herein, and both of which are compatible with cholangiocytes (and cholangiocyte senescence) playing a central role in PSC, as previously mentioned: (1) the PSC-microbiota hypothesis[70,71] and (2) the gut lymphocyte homing hypothesis. The PSC-microbiota hypothesis is based, in part, on the association between PSC and IBD and represents an expansion of what has been termed the "leaky gut" hypothesis.[72] It posits that PSC may develop as a result of: (1) increased enterohepatic circulation of microbial molecules (possibly facilitated by compromised intestinal barrier function), (2) alterations in gut microbial diversity and/or the repertoire of metabolites (e.g., because of intestinal microbial dysbiosis), and/or (3) an aberrant or exaggerated cholangiocyte or other hepatic cell response to microbial molecules. This hypothesis is supported by various findings in vitro,[73-75] in animal models,[76-81] and in vivo.[60,8-87] Human studies have evaluated the bacterial diversity of stool in healthy controls, patients with PSC, and patients with UC without liver disease; patients with PSC had a unique microbial composition compared with the other two groups and reduced bacterial diversity, although there was no significant difference among patients with PSC with or without IBD.[88]

The gut lymphocyte homing hypothesis postulates that intestinal T lymphocytes are: (1) activated in gut-associated lymphoid tissue, (2) primed by dendritic cells to express the cell surface receptors integrin α4β7 and CCR9, and (3) recruited to the liver as a result of aberrant hepatic expression of their cognate ligands, namely the addressin protein MAdCAM-1 and the chemotactic protein CCL25, which are usually restricted to the intestine.[67,89] Although the hepatic expression of these ligands on periportal endothelial cells and subsequent homing of α4β7+, CCR9+ lymphocytes to the liver appears to be relatively specific to PSC,[90,91] the pathobiologic relevance of this process has not been well-defined but is believed to represent a means of initiating peribiliary inflammation and cholangiocyte injury.[67] The discovery of α4β7 as a possible therapeutic approach led to the human studies of vedolizumab, which will be discussed later in this chapter.

Genetic factors appear to play a role in the development of PSC or in modifying its phenotype and may well interconnect with the aforementioned hypotheses. Several lines of evidence support a role for genetic factors in PSC: first, the risk of PSC is significantly increased within offspring and siblings of patients with PSC (hazard ratio of approximately 11).[92,93] Second, data from genome-wide association studies suggest that the human leukocyte antigen (HLA) gene family collectively represents the strongest risk locus associated with PSC.[94] Third, various non-HLA susceptibility and modifier genes have been identified, including but not limited to stromelysin-1 (i.e., matrix metalloproteinase 3), intracellular adhesion molecule 1 (ICAM1), and matrix metalloproteinase (MMP) 1 and 3.[95-97]

There have been numerous mouse and rat models developed to study various features of PSC. Given the uncertainties regarding the etiopathogenesis of PSC, it is not surprising that no single animal model has recapitulated all of the biochemical, cholangiographic, histologic, and pre-malignant features of PSC. Indeed, although the Mdr2−/− (ABCB4 gene) knockout mouse[98] has been the most widely studied model and exhibits

TABLE 41.3	Staging of Primary Sclerosing Cholangitis According to Ludwig
Stage I (portal)	Portal edema, inflammation, and ductular proliferation; abnormalities do not extend beyond the limiting plate.
Stage II (periportal)	Periportal fibrosis and inflammation in addition to stage I features; piecemeal necrosis may be present.
Stage III (septal)	Septal fibrosis or bridging necrosis in addition to stage I and II features; ductopenia may be present.
Stage IV (cirrhotic)	Biliary cirrhosis; ductopenia may be present.

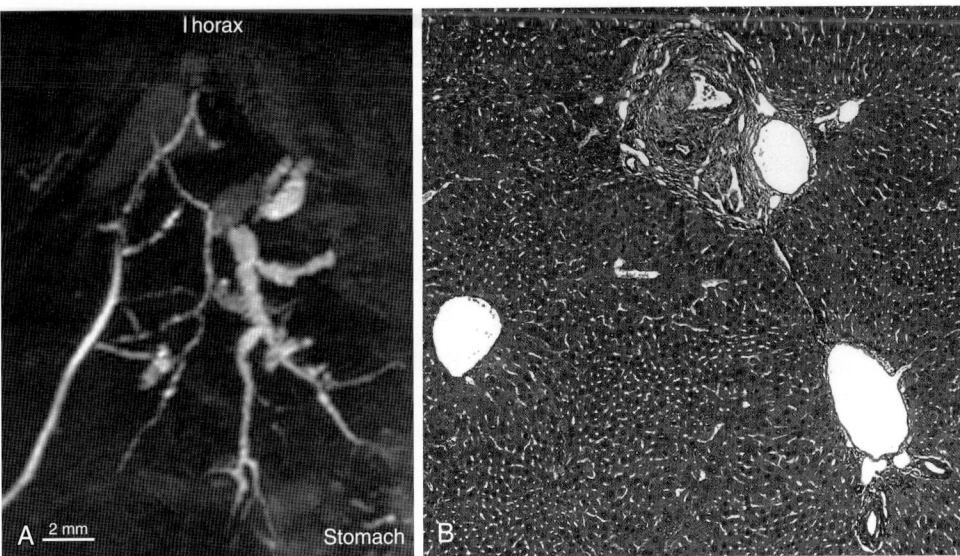

FIGURE 41.4   The multidrug-resistance 2 (*ABCB4* gene) knockout mouse model demonstrates multiple features of primary sclerosing cholangitis. **A,** Maximal intensity projection of a live adult *ABCB4* gene knockout mouse by using a 16.4-tesla small animal magnetic resonance imaging spectrometer exhibiting characteristic biliary ductal irregularity. **B,** Histologic appearance of the liver with features of biliary fibrosis. (**A,** Modified from Tabibian JH, Macura SI, O'Hara SP, et al. Micro-computed tomography and nuclear magnetic resonance imaging for noninvasive, live-mouse cholangiography. *Lab Invest.* 2013;93[6]:733–743.)

biochemical,[99–101] histologic,[98] and cholangiographic[102] features of the human PSC (Fig. 41.4), it is discordant from PSC in several aspects. For instance, disease severity in the Mdr2[-/-] mouse appears to be worse in female mice, and there is no apparent association with IBD or CCA.[98,100] Moreover, the mechanism of injury in the model (decreased biliary phospholipids resulting in hydrophobic bile-mediated epithelial injury and leakage of bile into portal tracts) has not been shown to correspond to human PSC. Thus there is no consensus to date regarding the optimal animal model, and this has hindered development and testing of potential therapies for PSC.[96]

NATURAL HISTORY

PSC is a chronic disorder that generally progresses to end-stage liver disease, even among asymptomatic patients.[103] The median LT-free survival from the time of PSC diagnosis is approximately 20 years.[1–3,10,104] LT-free survival in children with PSC appears to also be within this range.[105,106] It should be noted that data from large academic centers may suggest shorter median survival as a result of referral bias, whereas early diagnosis of PSC may be associated with longer survival because of lead-time bias.[5,107,108]

Prognostic models for PSC have been developed to predict survival and hepatic decompensations and to identify the ideal timing of LT.[103,109–113] A commonly used prognostic model, which does not require liver histologic data, is the revised natural history model for PSC (i.e., the revised Mayo PSC risk score,) which utilizes patient age, serum bilirubin, albumin, aspartate aminotransferase, and history of variceal bleeding).[110] Similarly, the Model for End-Stage Liver Disease (MELD) and MELD-Na are used for LT allocation for PSC and non-PSC patients and are a surrogate marker for mortality risk[114,115] (see Chapter 4). Normalization of ALP has been evaluated in several studies as a biomarker of improved survival and decreased risk of major adverse PSC-related events but continues to be a subject of uncertainty and ongoing investigation.[116–119] The limitations of current prognostic models are several, including, for instance, their inaccuracy in predicting development of CCA and impairment of health-related quality of life; indeed, no consensus exists regarding the optimal model.[120]

Patients with small-duct PSC (5% of all PSC), a term that refers to patients with biochemical and histologic features consistent with PSC but a normal cholangiogram (Table 41.2), appear to have a better long-term prognosis compared with those with non–small-duct PSC.[121] In a multi-institutional and multi-national study, 83 patients with small-duct PSC were matched by age, sex, year of diagnosis, and institution in a 1:2 fashion to patients with large-duct (i.e., classic) PSC.[122] Patients with small-duct PSC did not develop CCA unless their disease progressed to large-duct PSC (which occurred in 23% over a median of 7.4 years) and had significantly longer LT-free survival (13 compared with 10 years).

ASSOCIATED DISEASES

A variety of diseases are associated with PSC. These associations are listed in Box 41.1, of which two are discussed below.

BOX 41.1   Diseases Associated With Primary Sclerosing Cholangitis

Ulcerative colitis
Crohn disease
Autoimmune hepatitis
Hypothyroidism/Riedel thyroiditis
Sicca syndrome
Celiac disease
Autoimmune hemolytic anemia
Sarcoidosis
Glomerulonephritis
Type 1 diabetes mellitus

Inflammatory Bowel Disease and Colorectal Cancer

Of the approximately 70% of (Western) patients with PSC who have IBD, the majority of patients have UC, and the remainder have Crohn disease or indeterminate colitis.[123–125] The diagnosis of IBD may precede that of PSC by years, although there is no clear temporal association, and cases of IBD being diagnosed concurrently with or years after the diagnosis of PSC have been reported.[17,126,127] Compared with patients with IBD alone, patients with PSC-IBD have a unique disease phenotype characterized often by pancolitis with rectal sparing and backwash ileitis.[106,126] Colitis is usually milder (even if more extensive) in patients with PSC-IBD compared with those with IBD alone.[128] Additionally, PSC does not appear to be associated with small bowel-only Crohn disease,[129,130] although ileal pouchitis is more common post-colectomy for patients with PSC-IBD.

The presence of and duration of IBD (irrespective of severity) has been associated with greater PSC-related morbidity and mortality,[14,131,132] and the presence and activity of IBD as well as an intact colon before LT both appear to be predictors of recurrent PSC post-LT.[133,134] Despite its association with milder colitis, PSC-IBD confers nearly a fivefold increased risk of colorectal cancer compared with IBD alone.[135,136] In a study from Sweden, the absolute cumulative risk of developing colorectal dysplasia or carcinoma in patients with PSC-UC was 9%, 31%, and 50% after 10, 20, and 25 years of disease duration, respectively, compared with 2%, 5%, and 10%, respectively, in patients with UC alone.[137] Subsequent studies have demonstrated similar findings in other cohorts of PSC-IBD patients.[135,138–140] Societal guidelines recommend that colonoscopy surveillance (with extensive random mucosal biopsies)[141,142] be performed annually from the time of PSC diagnosis in patients with IBD and approximately every five years in patients with PSC alone.[4,143]

Autoimmune Hepatitis

An overlap syndrome between PSC and AIH has long been recognized but remains an area of etiopathogenic uncertainty[144,145] (see Chapter 68). PSC-AIH overlap syndrome is seen in up to 35% of pediatric patients with PSC[104,105] and approximately 5% of adult patients with PSC.[146,147] Cases of PSC-AIH overlap syndrome typically fulfill criteria for both diseases, including elevated serum ALP and cholangiographic abnormalities, biliary tract lesions and elevated serum aminotransferases, IgG, and antinuclear and/or anti–smooth muscle antibody titers. Liver biopsy generally reveals both nonsuppurative cholangitis and interface hepatitis. A clinical clue to this overlap syndrome may come in one of two forms: (1) a patient with AIH who does not respond completely to immunosuppressive therapy and subsequently develops a cholestatic serum liver profile or (2) a patient who has features of PSC but also aminotransferase level elevations that are beyond what would be expected of PSC alone (i.e., more than three times the upper limit of normal). Patients with suspected PSC-AIH overlap syndrome, particularly those in whom AIH seems to be the "dominant" disease, should be treated with immunosuppressive therapy.[4] Compared with AIH alone or PBC-AIH overlap, patients with PSC-AIH have increased mortality and are more likely to require LT.[148,149]

COMPLICATIONS

Clinical complications of PSC include cholelithiasis, choledocholithiasis, dominant biliary strictures, recurrent acute bacterial cholangitis, and CCA.[4,150,151] Other complications and symptoms in patients with PSC include: (1) those secondary to chronic cholestasis (e.g., fat-soluble vitamin deficiency, hepatic osteodystrophy, and pruritus) and (2) those associated with cirrhosis and portal hypertension (e.g., esophageal varices, ascites, and hepatocellular carcinoma), which are managed similar to patients with non-PSC related cirrhosis (Fig. 41.5), and (3) those seen among patients with PSC who have undergone proctocolectomy and ileostomy for IBD (e.g., peristomal varices and pouchitis).[152–154] These complications are further discussed in the forthcoming sections.

Gallbladder Disorders and Choledocholithiasis

Approximately 30% of patients with PSC will have calculi in the gallbladder or in the biliary tree (see Chapter 33). For example, in a study of 121 patients with PSC, 26% had gallstones, half of which were pigment stones.[155] The spectrum of gallbladder pathology in PSC is not limited to stones; patients with PSC can also develop an unusual form of acalculous cholecystitis characterized by a diffuse lymphoplasmacytic infiltrate.[156] In addition, patients with PSC are at increased risk for gallbladder masses and related malignancy.[157] Studies have found gallbladder masses are present in about 10% to 20% of patients with PSC, with a median size of 4 mm.[158] Given the risk of dysplasia and carcinoma within gallbladder masses in patients with PSC, annual surveillance is recommended (see Fig. 41.5).[159] Management recommendations of gallbladder mass lesions are variable; for example, the European Association for the Study of the Liver and American Association for the Study of Liver Diseases recommend cholecystectomy regardless of gallbladder lesion size, whereas the American College of Gastroenterology recommends cholecystectomy for those with a gallbladder lesion greater than 8 mm.[4,160,161]

Choledocholithiasis is present at any given point in time in approximately 8% of patients with PSC based on a cross-sectional radiologic series[162] (see Chapter 37). Choledocholiths are a nidus for bacterial infection, although clinical acute bacterial cholangitis is uncommonly seen in the absence of a dominant stricture or prior bile duct manipulation (e.g., surgery or ERCP). In patients with choledocholithiasis visualized on noninvasive imaging, ERCP (with or without sphincterotomy and/or plastic stent placement) is indicated for duct clearance and, if present, dilation of associated biliary strictures. Because patients with PSC are believed to be at increased risk for post-endoscopic retrograde cholangiography (ERC) bacterial cholangitis, even with successful choledocholith extraction, prophylactic coverage with antibiotics before (i.e., a single intravenous dose) and after ERC (i.e., oral ciprofloxacin for three to seven days) is advisable,[150] although high-quality evidence for this practice is lacking.[163-165]

Dominant Strictures

Formation of a dominant stricture occurs in approximately 45% of patients with PSC over the course of disease and typically presents with progressive jaundice, pruritus, bacterial cholangitis, and right upper quadrant pain. A "dominant stricture" is loosely defined as a stenosis with a diameter of up to 1.5 mm in the common bile duct or up to 1 mm in the hepatic duct.[150] If diagnosed by noninvasive imaging, cholangiography (preferably ERCP) is necessary to evaluate the biliary tree and perform therapeutic dilation with or without biliary stenting depending on stricture characteristics. ERCP also allows for

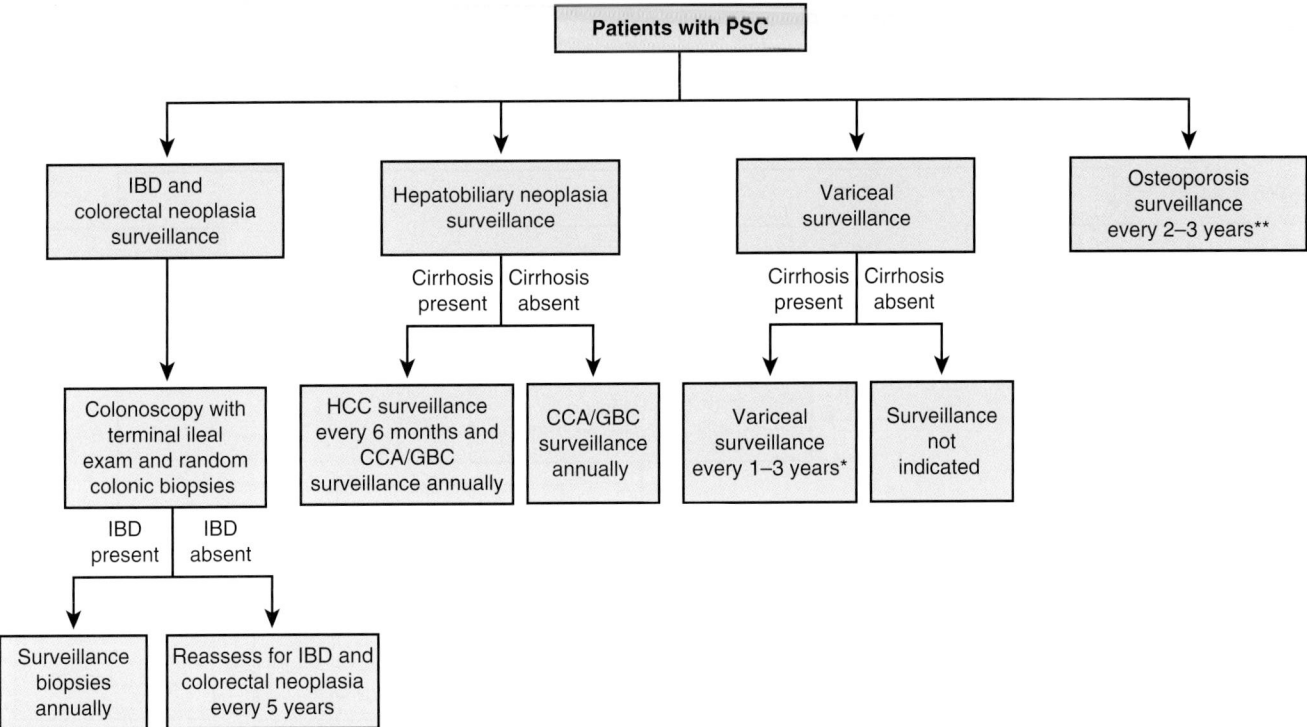

FIGURE 41.5 **Overview of surveillance in patients with primary sclerosing cholangitis beginning at the time of diagnosis.** *Based on American Association for the Study of Liver Disease practice guidelines (generally every one to three years). **May be performed more frequently in patients at higher risk or with known hepatic osteodystrophy/osteoporosis. *CCA,* Cholangiocarcinoma, *GBC,* gallbladder carcinoma, *HCC,* hepatocellular carcinoma; *IBD,* inflammatory bowel disease.

sampling (i.e., brushings, biopsies) of the biliary tree and stricture to evaluate for CCA. Satisfactory dilation of dominant strictures may require multiple ERCP sessions, following which a subset of patients will demonstrate sustained biochemical and symptomatic improvement, as shown in several prior studies.[166–169]

Cholangiocarcinoma

PSC is a premalignant condition, with the most ominous neoplastic complication being the development of CCA, which accounts for approximately 30% of all-cause mortality in this population[10] (see Chapters 50 and 51). CCA is estimated to have an annual incidence of 1% and a lifetime occurrence of 15% among patients with PSC.[18,137,138,170] Studies have demonstrated that screening for CCA in patients with PSC can lead to improved survival and diagnosis of CCA at an earlier stage, thus routine CCA surveillance is recommended (Fig. 41.6; see also Fig. 41.5).[4,44,171] Patients with PSC and CCA have poor survival because of the aggressive nature and late diagnosis (related to the insidious nature) of CCA. For example, in a retrospective study of 30 patients with PSC-related CCA, 63% had metastatic disease at diagnosis, and 47% considered to have localized disease had abdominal metastasis at surgical exploration; median survival in this cohort was five months from the time of CCA diagnosis.

Diagnosis of CCA is challenging because most of the signs and symptoms of CCA are typical of PSC itself. Additionally, there are no clinical or biochemical features that can accurately predict the development of CCA, although several associations have been made, including an elevated enhanced liver fibrosis (ELF) score in patients with PSC, plus CCA compared with

PSC alone, and a clinical history notable for smoking or prior colectomy.[135,172–176] As with carcinogenesis in other parts of the digestive tract, chronic inflammation is believed to play a central role in CCA development, but nevertheless, duration of PSC does not appear to be associated with risk of CCA.[173]

Further hindering early diagnosis of CCA is the low diagnostic performance characteristics (particularly sensitivity) of existing modalities. In addition, perihilar lymphadenopathy is common in PSC but not specific for CCA. ERCP can be a complimentary or superior (albeit invasive) approach to evaluating for CCA,[177] but accurate cholangiographic distinction between benign and malignant lesions is often not possible.[24] Biliary brush cytology specimens and, when technically feasible, biliary epithelial biopsies are thus typically obtained at ERCP and add to the specificity of cholangiographic findings but are at best 30% to 40% sensitive for securing a diagnosis of CCA. A newer method for detection of CCA is fluorescence in situ hybridization (FISH) performed on biliary brush cytology specimens. FISH is a molecular diagnostic technique that employs fluorescently labeled DNA probes that hybridize to selected chromosomal loci (e.g., 9p21) to identify nuclear aneusomy (i.e., numerical gain or loss of chromosomal loci).[178,179] FISH has complementary value to conventional cytology and improves its sensitivity by approximately 20% when the latter is negative.[180–182] In addition, FISH polysomy has been shown to indicate a significantly increased risk for CCA presence or development when serially positive or multi-focally positive.[178,183,184]

With respect to serologic tests to detect CCA in PSC, carbohydrate antigen 19-9 (CA 19-9) is the primary biomarker, although its performance characteristics are suboptimal and

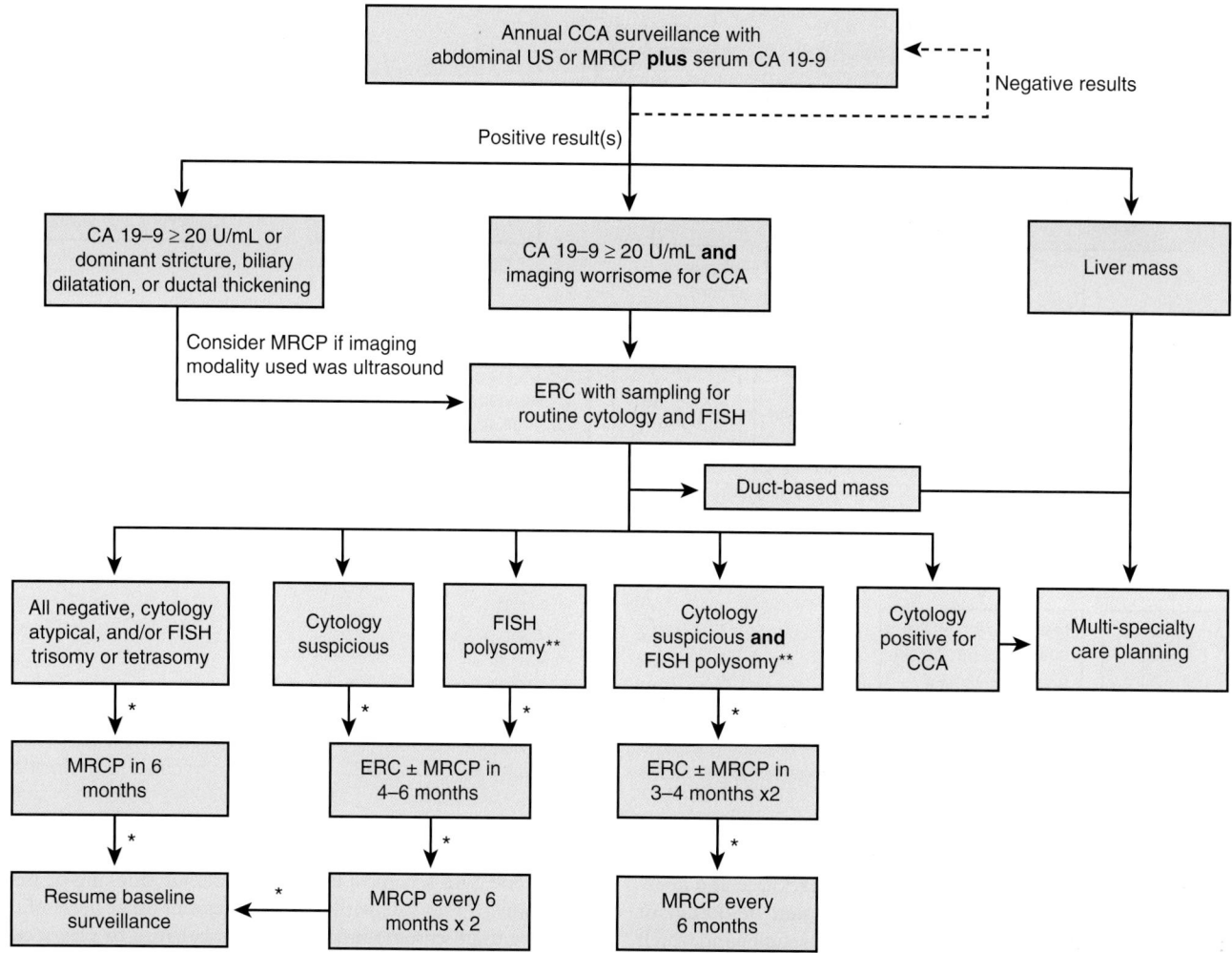

FIGURE 41.6 **Cholangiocarcinoma surveillance in patients with primary sclerosing cholangitis.** *Assumes clinical stability and absence of new signs or symptoms; serum CA 19-9 and liver biochemistries to be checked along with ERC or MRCP, and cytology and FISH to be checked with ERC. **Consider early referral to transplant center if worsening in serum tests or other signs or symptoms. *CA 19-9,* Carbohydrate antigen 19-9; *ERC,* endoscopic retrograde cholangiography; *FISH,* fluorescence in situ hybridization; *MRCP,* magnetic resonance cholangiopancreatography. (Adapted from Tabibian JH, Lindor KD. Challenges of cholangiocarcinoma detection in patients with primary sclerosing cholangitis. *J Anal Oncol.* 2012;1[1]:50–55.)

vary depending on the cutoff used. For example, studies have found a cutoff value of 129 U/mL to provide sensitivity of 13% to 79% and specificity of 99% to 100%, whereas lower cutoffs (e.g., 40 U/mL) provide greater sensitivity at the expense of specificity.[39,185] Specific limitations to serum CA19-9 include that: (1) it can also be elevated in pancreatic malignancies, bacterial cholangitis, nonmalignant pancreaticobiliary obstruction, and active smokers; and (2) it is not synthesized in individuals negative for the Lewis[a] blood antigen, which corresponds to 6% and 22% of Whites and Blacks, respectively, in the US.[4,186] Despite these limitations, annual CA19-9 testing is recommended as part of surveillance for development of CCA in patients with PSC (see Fig. 41.6).

Other methods for early detection and diagnosis of CCA are on the horizon and include serologic and biliary biomarkers (e.g., proteomic profiling, microRNAs, extracellular vesicles, next-generation sequencing)[187–191] and advanced endoscopic imaging techniques. The latter include: (1) intraductal endoscopic ultrasound,[192] (2) probe-based confocal laser endomicroscopy,[193–195] and (3) cholangioscopy with or without narrow band imaging and site-directed biopsy.[196–198] Endoscopic ultrasound

(EUS) is better than CT and magnetic resonance imaging (MRI) for evaluating regional lymph nodes as part of CCA staging and operative planning.

Treatment of CCA is discussed in forthcoming sections.

Cirrhosis and Portal Hypertension (see Chapters 74, 77, and 78)

Patients with PSC who progress to liver cirrhosis may experience complications of portal hypertension similar to patients with other causes of cirrhosis. Such complications include development of esophageal varices, ascites, and hepatocellular carcinoma. The manifestations, surveillance, and treatment of these complications are similar to patients with non-PSC related cirrhosis.[152–154]

Pruritus

At least one third of patients with PSC will experience pruritus at initial presentation or later during their disease course.[109] Pruritus contributes to sleep disturbance, emotional/psychological distress, impaired quality of life, and even suicidal ideation.[199–201] It may be localized or diffuse, is usually worse at night, and can be exacerbated by contact with wool, heat, or during pregnancy. The cause of pruritus in PSC is multifactorial, and there are likely several pruritogens that contribute, including bile salts, endogenous opiates, progesterone derivatives, lysophosphatidic acid, and bilirubin.[202–205]

In patients with new-onset pruritus, development of dominant bile duct strictures should be ruled out with serum biochemical tests and noninvasive imaging. If there is no evidence of a dominant stricture, pruritus in PSC may be treated similar to that of other chronic cholestatic conditions, including with stepwise use of cholestyramine, rifampicin, naltrexone, and/or sertraline.[160,161] Although lacking high-quality evidence to support their use, antihistamines (e.g., hydroxyzine) and ursodeoxycholic acid (UDCA) can provide symptomatic improvement in some patients, but use of the former is limited by sedative effects.[9] One small recent retrospective study found significant improvement in pruritus in patients with PSC treated with fenofibrate or bezafibrate for at least six months in combination with UDCA.[206] In patients who have failed these options and, as a result, are suffering with poor quality of life, antihistamines, gabapentin, ondansetron, antibacterials,[32,71,207] extracorporeal albumin dialysis, plasmapheresis, and other less-established therapies may be considered.[160,161] LT is reserved as a consideration for patients with intractable pruritus who have failed all other available options.

Fatigue

The etiology of fatigue in chronic cholestatic disease, including PSC, is unclear, and, to date, remains without specific therapy. Fatigue is nonspecific and does not correlate with liver disease severity[208] but is associated with depression and can have significant negative impact on quality of life.[209]

Before ascribing fatigue to PSC, however, it is important to rule out other causes that may be amenable to specific intervention. This includes AIH overlap syndrome (which may be amenable to immunosuppressive therapy), clinical depression, sleep disturbance/poor sleep hygiene, hypothyroidism, and autonomic dysfunction.[210] Although there are no specific interventions to treat fatigue related to PSC, supportive and understanding clinical care can improve patients' ability to cope.

Fat-Soluble Vitamin Deficiency and Steatorrhea

As with other chronic cholestatic diseases, patients with PSC can develop fat malabsorption secondary to diminished delivery of bile acids to the small intestine. If prolonged, this can lead to fat-soluble vitamin deficiency and symptomatic steatorrhea. In one study of a cohort of patients with advanced PSC undergoing LT evaluation, deficiencies of vitamins A, D, and E were present in 82%, 57%, and 43%, respectively.[211] Overall, the epidemiology of fat-soluble vitamin deficiency and steatorrhea specifically in PSC has not been well studied.

With respect to management, deficiencies of fat-soluble vitamins should be treated with oral supplementation. In patients who develop steatorrhea, evaluation should be performed to rule out celiac sprue (or other enteropathy) and pancreatic exocrine insufficiency because either entity can coexist with PSC, and both conditions are readily treatable causes of fat malabsorption.[212,213]

Hepatic Osteodystrophy

Hepatic osteodystrophy refers to demineralizing metabolic bone disease occurring in chronic liver disease. The diagnosis is made by bone mineral density measurement, with a T-score between one to 2.5 standard deviations below normal (i.e., the density observed in healthy young individuals) being consistent with osteopenia, and a T-score greater than 2.5 standard deviation below normal being consistent with osteoporosis. Hepatic osteodystrophy is relatively common in and an important complication of PSC; indeed, the incidence of osteoporosis in PSC is between 4% to 10%, and up to half of patients have a bone mineral density below the fracture threshold.[214] Risk factors for hepatic osteodystrophy include lower body mass index, longer duration of PSC and/or IBD, more advanced PSC, and higher age.[215] Hepatic osteodystrophy should thus be looked for in all newly diagnosed patients with PSC.

Unfortunately, there is no well-established therapy for the treatment of hepatic osteodystrophy. It is considered reasonable, however, to screen for hepatic osteodystrophy at approximately two- to three-year intervals and treat with oral calcium and vitamin D if osteopenia or osteoporosis is present. In the case of osteoporosis, a bisphosphonate may also be added, but referral to endocrinology may be advisable before doing so given evolving therapeutic practices. Gentle weight-bearing exercise should also be encouraged.

Peristomal Varices and Pouchitis After Proctocolectomy

The presence of PSC in patients with IBD affects the management of the latter. For example, although colectomy should be performed for indications pertinent to/necessitated by the IBD (e.g., medically-refractory UC, colonic dysplasia), the decision to perform an end ileostomy or an ileal pouch–anal anastomosis (IPAA) is greatly influenced by the presence of PSC. In a retrospective study of patients with PSC and UC treated with either end ileostomy or IPAA, eight of 31 patients (26%) with ileostomy developed peristomal varices and subsequent bleeding, but none of the 40 patients who underwent IPAA developed perianastomotic varices or perianal bleeding[216]; however, the cumulative risk of one or more episodes of acute pouchitis at 10 years post-IPAA was significantly more common in patients with PSC-UC compared with UC alone (60% vs. 15%).[217] The risk of *chronic* pouchitis is also higher in patients with PSC-UC compared with UC alone.[218] Nevertheless, among patients with PSC who are in need of colectomy, IPAA is typically recommended over end ileostomy because bleeding peristomal varices may be more life-threatening and have fewer and more invasive treatment options (e.g., transjugular intrahepatic portosystemic shunt).[4,18,216] Recent advances suggest that microcoils injected under EUS and fluoroscopic guidance at the site of peristomal varices may represent a less invasive approach.[219]

TREATMENT OF PRIMARY SCLEROSING CHOLANGITIS

Pharmacotherapy

To date, a specific medical therapy for PSC has yet to be established or recommended, despite numerous clinical trials of numerous categories of pharmacologic agents, including immunosuppressants, cupruretics, antifibrotics, antiinflammatories, and, most recently, oral antibacterials.[32,71,220] Examples of such agents include prednisone, mycophenolate mofetil, tacrolimus, pentoxifylline, D-penicillamine, pirfenidone, silymarin, oral and transcutaneous nicotine, and oral vancomycin.

The most extensively investigated drug in PSC is UDCA, a hydrophilic, 3,7-dihydroxy bile acid.[221] The mechanisms by which UDCA is thought to exert beneficial effects in cholestatic disorders include cholangiocytoprotection against hydrophobic bile acids, hepatocytoprotection against bile acid-induced apoptosis, stimulation of bile acid excretion, and bicarbonate-rich choleresis.[4,222,223] Prospective clinical studies of UDCA in PSC were first reported in the late 1980s,[224] and albeit uncontrolled, demonstrated both symptomatic and objective improvement.[117] These studies soon led to the first randomized controlled trial (RCT) of UDCA (13–15 mg/kg/day), which demonstrated significant improvements in multiple biochemical and histologic endpoints.[225] Since then, seven other RCTs have been conducted, initially with low- (10–15 mg/kg/day), then intermediate- (17–23 mg/kg/day), and most recently high-dose (28–30 mg/kg/day) UDCA. In brief, whereas low-dose UDCA was associated with significant biochemical improvements but no differences in "hard endpoints" such as CCA, LT, or death, high-dose UDCA was associated with an approximately 2-fold increase in serious adverse events, ostensibly because of toxic metabolites of supratherapeutic UDCA.[226] The most promising data come from intermediate-dose UDCA, with which significant improvements in serum liver tests, hepatic fibrosis stage, and cholangiographic appearance have been reported.[227] Subsequently, the largest trial to date reported a 22% relative reduction in CCA, 34% relative reduction in need for LT, and 31% relative reduction in mortality[228]; however, these results did not reach statistical significance. As a result of the lack of high-quality evidence to support the use of UDCA in patients with PSC, societal guidelines have recommended against or offered no specific recommendation regarding the use of UDCA for PSC.[4,160]

There is extensive ongoing research into novel therapeutics for PSC, although none have been shown to alter the disease course. Vedolizumab treats IBD by blocking integrin $\alpha 4\beta 7$ and was hypothesized to decrease lymphocyte infiltration into the liver in patients with PSC; however, a large multicentered trial found no evidence for a biochemical response, although vedolizumab is considered safe and can be effective for treating IBD in patients with PSC.[229,230] Other ongoing therapeutic trials target different aspects of the pathophysiology of PSC, including bile acid–based therapy (*Nor*UDCA and cilofexor, a farnesoid X receptor [FXR] antagonist), therapy targeting peroxisome proliferator-activated receptor (PPAR), therapy aimed at the gut microbiota, and immune-modulating therapy.[231]

Surgical Therapy

The two main hepatobiliary surgical interventions for PSC or associated CCA are hepatic resection and LT.

Resection of Cholangiocarcinoma

In the absence of PSC, resection is an effective and potentially curative treatment for CCA (see Chapters 50 and 51). In patients with PSC and CCA, however, resection is discouraged for several reasons: (1) CCA is often multifocal, (2) underlying hepatic fibrosis and/or low hepatic reserve may preclude safe resection, and (3) recurrent disease and consequent death occur in more than 90% of patients. These observations are attributable, in part, to the fact that PSC is essentially a premalignant disorder.[232] Nevertheless, if a patient presents with a CCA that is surgically resectable, does not have cirrhotic-stage PSC, and is not a candidate for LT, an attempt at resection should be considered, although estimated five-year survival rates are at best only 25%.[233,234]

Orthotopic Liver Transplantation (see Chapter 105)

PSC is the fifth most common indication for LT in the US and the leading indication in Nordic countries, as mentioned earlier. With one- and five-year rates of survival surpassing 90% and 80%, respectively, patients with PSC have among the most successful outcomes post-LT, and thus LT is the optimal treatment for patients with PSC presenting with end-stage liver disease and/or associated complications that are not amenable to medical treatment.[235]

Potential predictors of post-LT outcomes have been identified in patients with PSC and may include disease severity at LT, previous biliary or shunt surgery, concurrent CCA, and IBD, but study findings have been somewhat inconsistent.[233,234,236]

Recurrent PSC remains a problem post-LT and has been found to occur in up to 34% of deceased donor LTs[237] and 67% of living-related donor LTs.[238,239] These statistics have been somewhat difficult to quantify because of the variable metrics used to make the diagnosis of recurrent PSC, although well-defined criteria have been established and recommended.[235] Proposed risk factors for recurrent PSC include IBD with intact colon (i.e., pre-LT colectomy may play a protective role), prolonged ischemic time, acute cellular rejection episodes, cytomegalovirus infection, and lymphotoxic cross match.[8,240–242] These proposed risk factors were recently explored in a large retrospective study that included 10 German transplant centers and found that donor age, IBD, and international normalized ratio (INR) at the time of transplant were independent risk factors for post-transplant biliary strictures and recurrence of PSC.[243] A recent study comparing recurrent PSC in a deceased donor with living donor LTs did not demonstrate a significant difference between the two groups. The risk of PSC recurrence was associated with a history of biliary complications, CCA, higher MELD score, and donor age.[244] Median survival without redo-LT for these patients has not been well-studied but is estimated to be approximately four years.[245]

Patients with PSC undergoing LT for hilar CCA merit additional discussion. Historically, CCA had been regarded as a contraindication for LT, given the prohibitively high rate of tumor recurrence and lack of superiority in disease-free and overall survival compared with resection alone. However, specialized LT centers have shown promising outcomes for patients with stage I or II hilar CCA (with or without PSC) using a protocol consisting of neoadjuvant radiosensitizing chemotherapy, external beam radiotherapy, and ERC-delivered transluminal brachytherapy, followed by oral capecitabine up until staging laparotomy immediately before LT to re-verify candidacy[246,247] (see Chapters 51 and 108B). Based on a study examining 12 US LT centers, the five-year rate of recurrence-free survival was 65% after excluding the 12% who dropped out pre-LT (e.g., did not tolerate the regimen), and all centers had similar survival rates.[248] An even better prognosis is seen in patients with PSC who undergo LT and are found to have *incidental* CCA (defined as tumors less than 1 cm in diameter discovered only at the time of pathologic sectioning of the explanted liver), with five-year overall survival of approximately 80%.[249] Limited research has shown early promise of neoadjuvant treatment in downstaging unresectable locally advanced hilar or intrahepatic CCA before LT[250] (see Chapters 50 and 51).

CONCLUSION

PSC is a chronic, cholestatic, premalignant cholangiopathy of unknown etiology characterized by fibrous obliteration of the intrahepatic and/or extrahepatic biliary tree and a strong association with IBD. PSC generally progresses to cirrhosis, is a major risk factor for hepatobiliary and colonic neoplasia, and confers a median survival to death or LT of only 15 years. During the course of PSC, patients may develop various disease-specific and nonspecific complications. Management is challenging and often requires a multidisciplinary approach. Effective medical therapy has yet to be established, but LT is an excellent option in carefully selected patients with PSC-associated liver failure or hepatobiliary malignancy. More studies are needed to better understand the etiopathogenesis of this disease and develop more therapeutic options.

The references for this chapter can be found online by accessing the accompanying Expert Consult website.

CHAPTER 42

Benign biliary strictures and biliary fistulae

Carlos U. Corvera and Andrew D. Wisneski

OVERVIEW

In this chapter we cover biliary fistulae and strictures from benign etiologies. There is significant overlap in conditions that lead to benign biliary fistulae and strictures, thus these two topics are combined in one chapter.

By definition, a biliary fistula is an abnormal communication between the biliary tract and another organ or potential space. In contrast, a biliary stricture is defined as an abnormal narrowing of the bile duct that may lead to obstruction and subsequent fistula. Biliary fistulae are grouped into two main types: internal or external. *Internal biliary fistulae* are rare, and usually form spontaneously from an inflammatory condition (e.g., cholecystitis), and bile usually drains into another organ's lumen without forming a substantial collection. *External biliary fistulae* are more commonly encountered, often resulting from iatrogenic injury (e.g., bile duct injury in laparoscopic cholecystectomy) or trauma. Biliary stricture formation may be a long-term sequela of this injury with or without persistent bilious drainage. The terms *benign biliary stricture* and *fistula* are often used interchangeably when referring to external biliary fistula and iatrogenic injuries. This is because both conditions can occur at some point in the course of the patient's condition and treatment. Additionally, in this new edition of the chapter, we mention more newly characterized entities such as ampullary stenosis and immunoglobulin G4 (IgG4)–related disease that have been found to be associated with biliary strictures.

Benign biliary strictures pose difficult management problems. In contrast to malignant biliary obstruction, in which short-term palliation is often the goal of therapy, benign strictures require durable repair because most patients are expected to live for many years. Regardless of the nature of the biliary fistulae and strictures, management of patients with this condition is optimized when treatment is directed by a highly specialized multidisciplinary team of experienced hepatobiliary surgeons, interventional radiologists, diagnostic radiologists, and gastroenterologists.

INTERNAL BILIARY FISTULAE

Incidence and Etiology

Whether occurring as a consequence of calculous biliary tract disease, trauma, neoplasm, or congenital anomalies, internal biliary fistulae are uncommon. Estimates of incidence are crude, gleaned only from many small series, usually with fewer than 50 patients. If all types of internal biliary fistula are included, calculous biliary tract disease accounts for 90%; peptic ulcer disease, 6%; and neoplasm, trauma, parasitic infection, and congenital anomalies make up the remaining 4%.[1]

Overall, 1% to 3% of patients with cholelithiasis in Western countries develop biliary-enteric fistula, with a female-to-male ratio of approximately 3:1.[2–5] The pathogenic sequence of events for calculous biliary tract disease has been well described by Glenn et al.[2] It consists of pressure necrosis and erosion of part of the biliary tract wall into an adjacent structure to which it has become adherent in the course of repeated bouts of inflammation, often with distal biliary tract obstruction. The likelihood of the branches of the hepatobiliary tree to become inflamed and anatomic proximity to adjacent hollow viscera largely determine the relative incidence of the different types of spontaneous biliary-enteric fistulae secondary to calculous disease. Indeed, repeated attacks of cholecystitis may result in progressive fibrosis and shrinking of the gallbladder, which ultimately obliterates the triangle of Calot. The inflammatory process may spread to involve the common hepatic duct, causing inflammatory stenosis or stricture resulting in jaundice and cholangitis. Patients with inflammatory strictures of the extrahepatic bile duct in association with chronic cholelithiasis may have radiologic features that are indistinguishable from cholangiocarcinoma.[6–8]

The various types of biliary-enteric fistulae can best be subclassified from an anatomic point of view, by the names of the principal organs involved (Fig. 42.1).

Fistulae Involving the Gallbladder

In Western countries, where cholesterol cholelithiasis abounds, the gallbladder is most often the site of severe inflammation and obstruction. Cholecystoenteric fistulae, an abnormal connection between the gallbladder and the enteric tract, constitute 70% to 85% of all biliary fistulae reported in the world literature.[9,10] Of these, 55% to 75% are cholecystoduodenal (gallbladder and duodenum), 15% to 30% are cholecystocolic (gallbladder and colon), and 2% to 5% are cholecystogastric (gallbladder and stomach) (see Fig. 42.1). Multiple fistulae (e.g., cholecystoduodenocolic) are very rare.[11]

Gallstone ileus, the historical misnomer for distal ileal obstruction from gallstone impaction, is a dramatic clinical presentation of a cholecystoenteric fistula that is reported in 8% to 20% of large series of patients with biliary-enteric fistulae.[9,10,12–16] Modern series of bowel obstructions report gallstone ileus to be a very uncommon cause (well under 1%).[12,17–21]

Although most fistulae between the gallbladder and intestinal tract are obvious preoperatively or intraoperatively, cholecystocholedochal fistulae are insidious and may not be appreciated even at surgery. These biliobiliary fistulae develop between the gallbladder or cystic duct and the proximal common hepatic or common bile duct (CBD) (see Fig. 42.1D). In either instance, the mechanism of formation is the same: pressure necrosis into the common duct by a large solitary impacted calculus. Recently, cholecystocholedochal fistula has been estimated to

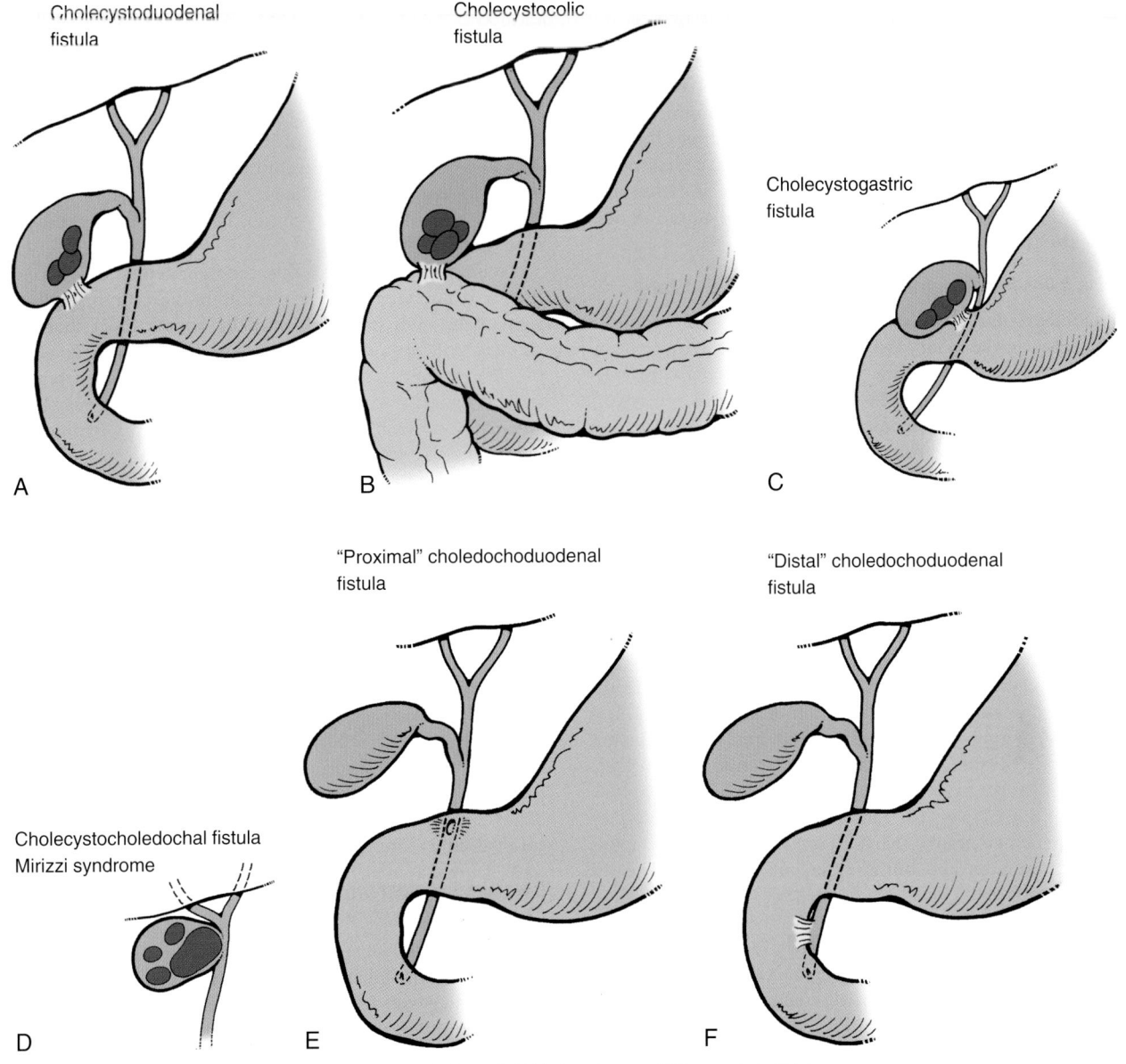

Cholecystoduodenal fistula

Cholecystocolic fistula

Cholecystogastric fistula

A

B

C

"Proximal" choledochoduodenal fistula

"Distal" choledochoduodenal fistula

Cholecystocholedochal fistula
Mirizzi syndrome

D

E

F

FIGURE 42.1   A through **F,** Various types of biliary-enteric fistulae.

be present in 0.7% to 1.4% of biliary operations for calculous disease.[22] Awareness of this condition is important and may help avoid damage to the common duct at operation.

Fistulae Involving the Common Bile Duct, Cystic Duct Remnant, and Other Extrahepatic Ducts

Choledochoduodenal fistulae are classified as either proximal or distal (see Fig. 42.1E and 42.1F). A *proximal choledocho-duodenal fistula* is the most common form of abnormal communication between the CBD and adjacent structures (often the duodenum) and represents 4% to 20% of all biliary-enteric fistulae. In the past, the majority were caused by peptic ulcer erosion from the first portion of the duodenum into the proximal CBD. This cause is now much less common as a result of effective medical therapy for peptic ulcer disease. Other, less common causes of choledochoduodenal fistula include cholelithiasis, operative trauma, duodenal diverticula,

echinococcal infection, and Crohn's disease, as well as neoplasms of the stomach, distal bile duct, ampullary region, and duodenum.[23–30]

Distal choledochoduodenal fistulae connect to the duodenum in the distal 2 cm of the CBD, and the fistula opening can be seen during percutaneous transhepatic cholangiography (PTC) (see Chapters 12 and 31) and endoscopic retrograde cholangiopancreatography (ERCP). The incidence of distal choledochoduodenal fistula secondary to cholelithiasis or operative trauma is variable in different parts of the world. With the development of radiologic studies of biliary anatomy, it is becoming apparent that many patients with biliodigestive complaints and gallstone disease may in fact have a distal choledochoduodenal fistula. A large series from Argentina reported the incidence of distal choledochoduodenal fistula to be 0.7%.[31]

In Japan, where there is a high incidence of primary intrahepatic biliary tract calculous disease, Tanaka et al.[32] reported a

5.3% incidence of parapapillary fistula in ERCP studies of 1500 patients. Ikeda et al.[33] classified these as a *type I fistula*, characterized by a small fistula opening on the longitudinal fold of the duodenum just proximal to the papilla, probably caused by penetration of a small calculus through the intramural portion of the common duct into the duodenum; and *type II fistula*, a larger opening of the duodenum wall adjacent to the longitudinal fold, probably caused by a relatively large stone eroding from the extramural portion of a greatly dilated common duct into the duodenum.

Fistulae Involving the Intrahepatic Ducts, Liver, and Lung

Thoracobiliary and bronchobiliary fistulae refer to communications between the biliary tree and the pleural cavity or bronchial tree, and are rare entities.[34-36] The three major categories of bronchobiliary fistula are those resulting from (1) infection, (2) trauma, and (3) congenital causes.[37-40] Worldwide, the most common cause of bronchobiliary fistula in adults is parasitic disease of the liver, either echinococcal (see Chapter 72) or amoebic disease (see Chapters 45 and 71).[41] In developed countries, iatrogenic injury to the biliary system is the most frequent cause.

The hallmark symptom of a bronchobiliary fistula is bilioptysis, coughing up bile, in conjunction with other pulmonary complaints.[37] Jaundice, cholangitis, and external biliary fistula or subphrenic abscess may also occur. Radiographic confirmation of the diagnosis is possible by a variety of methods. In the presence of an external fistula, injection of contrast solution is the most direct approach. PTC and ERCP are equally effective and have the potential for therapeutic intervention.[37] Bronchobiliary fistulae also have been shown by cholescintigraphy.[42-48] Computed tomography (CT) and magnetic resonance imaging cholangiopancreatography (MRCP) are also useful in assessing the upper abdomen and biliary tract but rarely visualize the fistula tract.[24,49-51]

The treatment of parasitic diseases of the liver is discussed elsewhere in this edition (see Chapters 45, 71, and 72). In large series of surgically treated cases of hepatic echinococcal disease in Greece and Turkey, only 2% were complicated by rupture into the lung or bronchi.[52] Amoebic abscess of the liver has been reported in association with bronchobiliary fistula in 8% of cases.[53] The successful treatment of these fistulae depends on the use of appropriate surgical drainage or resection in conjunction with appropriate pharmacologic therapy.[54]

The incidence of bronchobiliary fistula as a consequence of surgical treatment for hepatobiliary tract neoplasm or calculi has decreased, as patients are operated on earlier in the course of their disease with better-established surgical techniques.[37,55-57] Reports of bronchobiliary fistula caused by liver tumor ablative therapies, such as radiofrequency ablation, have been described.[58-61] These cases resolved with biliary drainage alone; however, there are two reported cases of successful treatment using drainage and pleurocentesis with α-cyanoacrylate glue.[62,63]

Untreated choledocholithiasis complicated by repeated episodes of biliary obstruction and cholangitis is another, albeit infrequent, cause of bronchobiliary fistula. Brem et al.[64] reported the successful treatment of an 87-year-old patient with this clinical situation by endoscopic papillotomy alone. Bronchobiliary fistulae should be treated by transampullary biliary decompression to reduce the fistula tract pressure. Patients with a persistent fistula or infection may require transthoracic debridement and drainage.

Posttraumatic thoracobiliary fistulae are extremely rare (see Chapter 113).[65,66] Historically, successful treatment required pulmonary decortication, repair of the diaphragm, and adequate drainage above and below the diaphragm. More recent publications have described successful treatment through endoscopic decompression of the biliary system and pleural drainage.[37,66] Although the optimal management strategy remains undefined, reports suggest that aggressive surgical intervention should be reserved for cases that fail conservative management.[39,67-69]

Neuhauser et al.[70] first described congenital bronchobiliary fistula in an infant with a tract communicating between the right main stem bronchus and the hepatic duct that passed through the posterior mediastinum. Tommasoni et al.[71] described two newborn infants with this condition treated surgically. It has also been documented that there is a very high incidence (approximately 36%) of co-existing hypoplasia or biliary atresia and congenital diaphragmatic hernia.[44,72,73] There are several options for reestablishing communication with the intestinal tract, including Roux-en-Y choledochojejunostomy, fistula enteric anastomosis, and portoenterostomy in cases of extrahepatobiliary atresia[74] (see Chapter 32). On microscopic examination, the proximal portion of the fistula in most patients resembles the bronchus, and the distal segment resembles the esophagus; the embryologic explanations for this anomaly are conjectural.[38,75] Transthoracic excision of the fistula with surgical correction of associated biliary anomaly is usually curative.[40]

Diagnostic Tests

A variety of imaging modalities can be used to establish the diagnosis of biliary fistula and define the anatomy to guide surgical intervention.

Computed Tomography and Magnetic Resonance Imaging Cholangiopancreatography

CT and MRCP (see Chapter 16) are able to demonstrate gallstones, air in the biliary tree, the presence of additional stones, and a biliary-enteric fistula.[76,77] In the case of gallstone ileus, these studies are useful for estimating the size of an impacted stone and determining the site of intestinal obstruction for planning operative approaches (Fig. 42.2). Newer multidetector CT scanners, which use three-dimensional volume-rendering reconstruction, are better able to estimate stone size as well as the presence of additional stones and may be able to detect an impacted stone before severe clinical symptoms are evident. Modern magnetic resonance imaging (MRI) and MRCP have been shown to accurately detect most small fistulous tracts.[78-80] MRI scanning can also be used to show other important pathologic changes, such as distal common duct stones, other obstructive processes, the presence of a subphrenic abscess, pleural effusion, or parasitic disease of the liver.[81] Scanning can also be used to verify and localize contrast extravasation after invasive cholangiography or after contrast injection of an existing controlled external fistula (Fig. 42.3).

Direct Cholangiography

Direct injection of contrast material is the best way to outline the normal and pathologic anatomy of the biliary tract (see Chapter 20). This imaging can be accomplished by ERCP, PTC, or through a fistulogram. Intraoperative cholangiograms are another method of directly imaging the biliary tree.

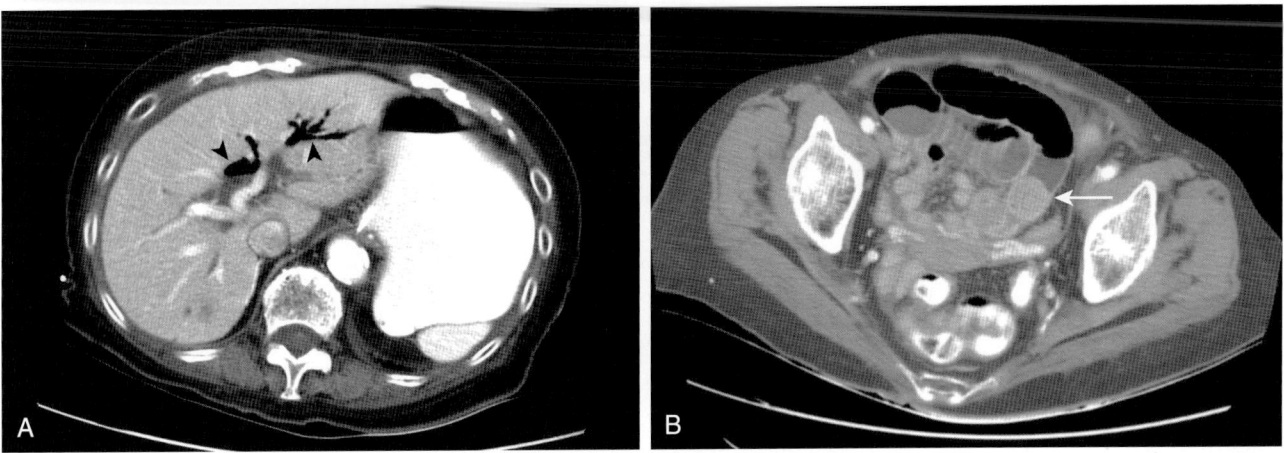

FIGURE 42.2   A 92-year-old woman with recurrent pyogenic cholangitis and increasing abdominal pain, anorexia, constipation, nausea, and vomiting over a 36-hour period. **A,** Computed tomography through the liver showing extensive pneumobilia *(arrowheads)*. **B,** In the pelvis, a soft tissue–attenuated, round, 2.5-cm gallstone *(arrow)* is seen at the transition point between dilated and decompressed bowel. (Courtesy Dr. Fergus V. Coakley.)

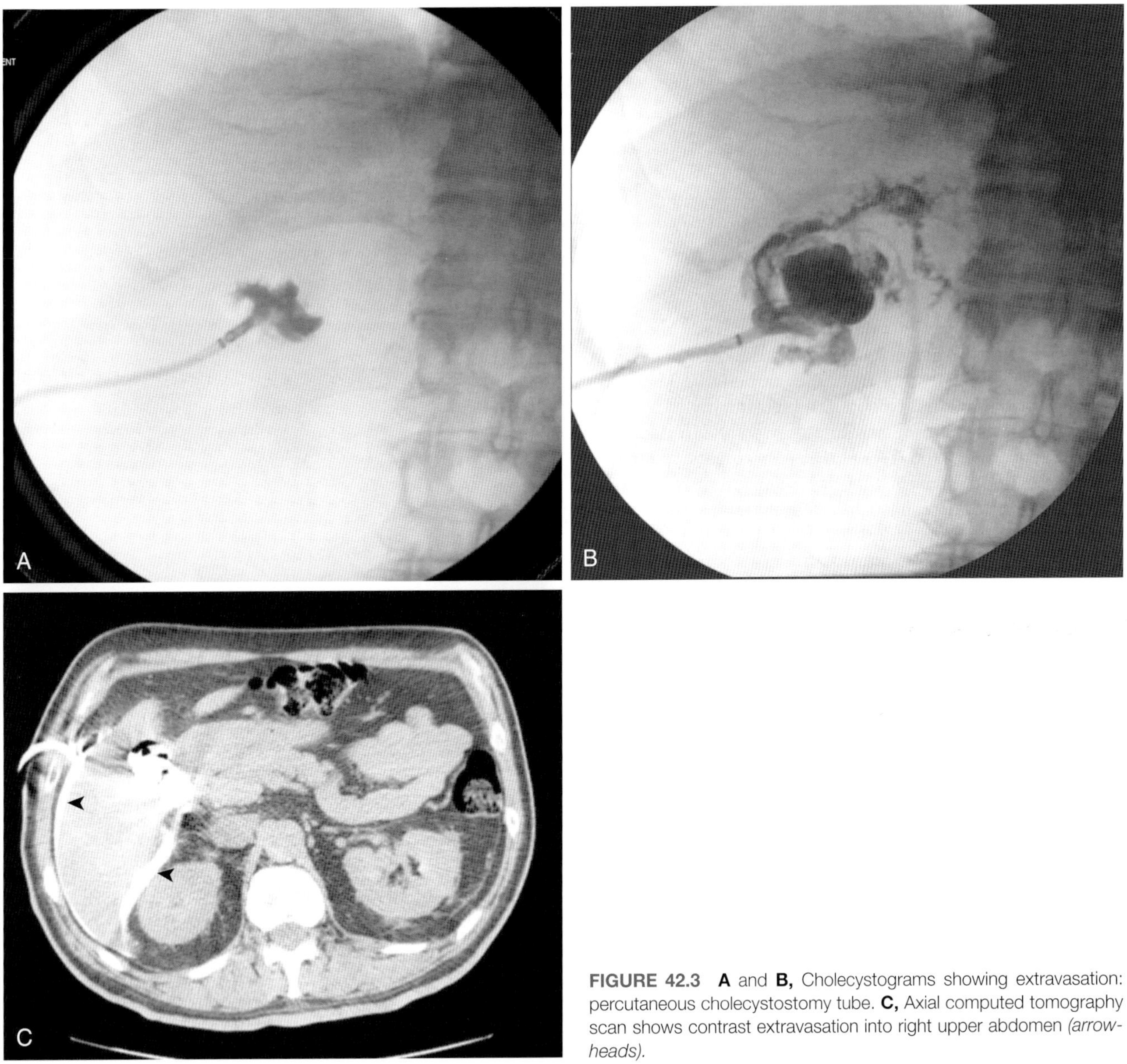

FIGURE 42.3   **A** and **B,** Cholecystograms showing extravasation: percutaneous cholecystostomy tube. **C,** Axial computed tomography scan shows contrast extravasation into right upper abdomen *(arrowheads)*.

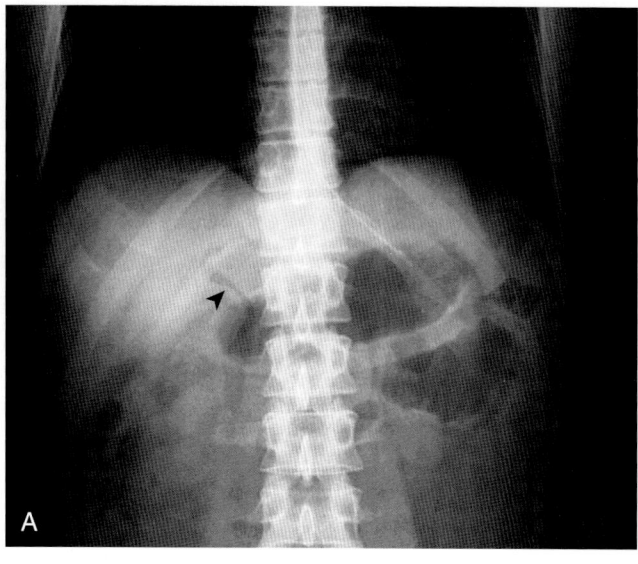
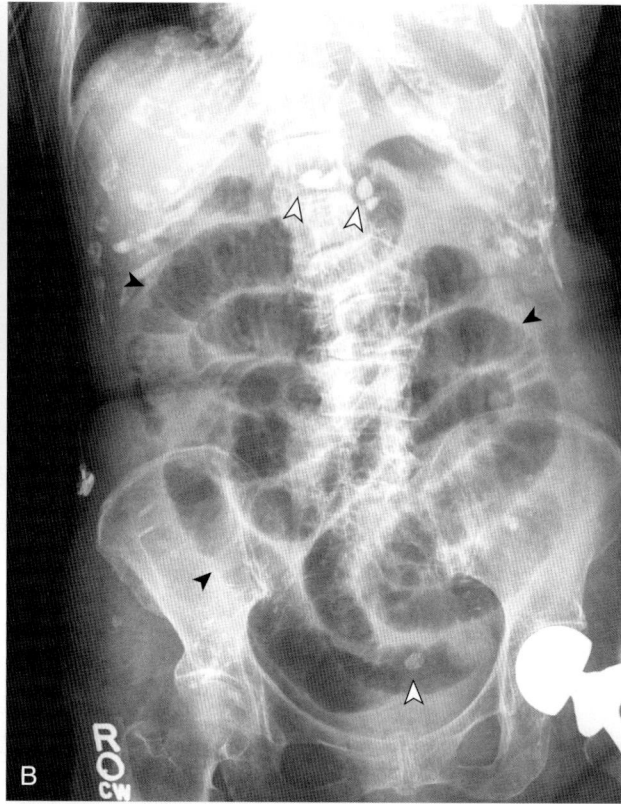

FIGURE 42.4   A, Plain radiograph shows pneumobilia *(arrowhead).* **B,** Plain radiograph shows multiple dilated loops of small bowel *(black arrowheads),* several calcified gallstones *(white arrowheads),* three gallstones located in small bowel in the upper abdomen, and one obstructing gallstone in the pelvis. (**A,** Courtesy Dr. Rizwan Aslam; **B,** courtesy Dr. Fergus V. Coakley.)

Numerous reports have documented the efficacy of ERCP in demonstrating biliary fistulae.[32,82–85] Endoscopically, the alimentary side of a fistula near the ampulla of Vater can sometimes be cannulated to obtain a high-quality radiograph of the communicating biliary anatomy.[78,86,87] In fact, the largely unappreciated and frequently asymptomatic parapapillary choledochoduodenal fistula has been found to be quite common.[24,32,88,89] There have been far fewer reports of the role of PTC in demonstrating biliary fistulae, but PTC can be helpful in the diagnosis and treatment of various types of biliary fistulae associated with dilated intrahepatic ducts.[90–92]

Plain and Contrast Radiographs

Pneumobilia, the presence of air in the biliary tree, may be noted on plain films of 30% to 50% of patients with gallstone ileus (Fig. 42.4A). Other classic radiographic signs of gallstone ileus are visualization of a calcified gallstone in the abdominal cavity at a distance away from the gallbladder (see Fig. 42.4B), serial imaging demonstrating migration of a previously observed calcification, and a change in the level of mechanical intestinal obstruction—the so-called "tumbling obstruction."[16,93] However, only 30% of gallstones are sufficiently calcified to be radiopaque.

A barium meal or upper gastrointestinal (GI) series shows reflux of contrast material into the fistula in 40% of cholecystoduodenal communications and 75% of choledochoduodenal fistulae of peptic ulcer origin.[94,95] If the plain film and barium swallow are used in concert, more than 60% of biliary enteric fistulae are correctly diagnosed preoperatively[96] (Fig. 42.5).

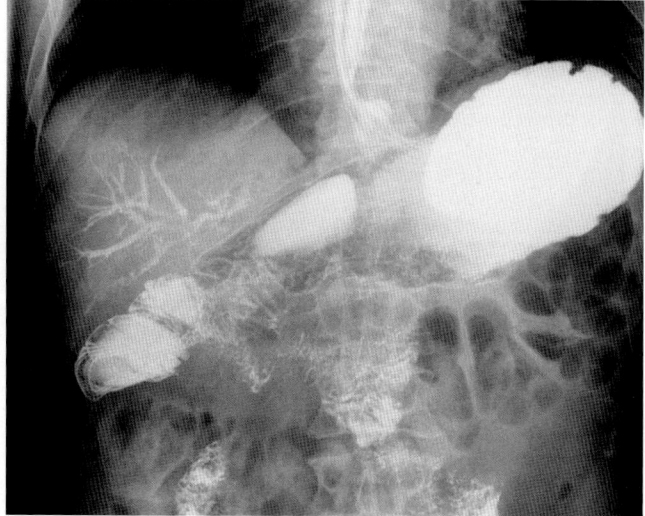

FIGURE 42.5   Upper gastrointestinal series shows a choledochoduodenal fistula with reflux of contrast medium into the biliary tree. (Courtesy Dr. Benjamin M. Yeh.)

Barium enema demonstrates greater than 95% of cholecystocolic fistulae (Fig. 42.6).

Sonography

Sonography is a useful noninvasive diagnostic aid in the preoperative evaluation of a patient with a suspected biliary fistula (see Chapter 16). Although a radionuclide scan may readily

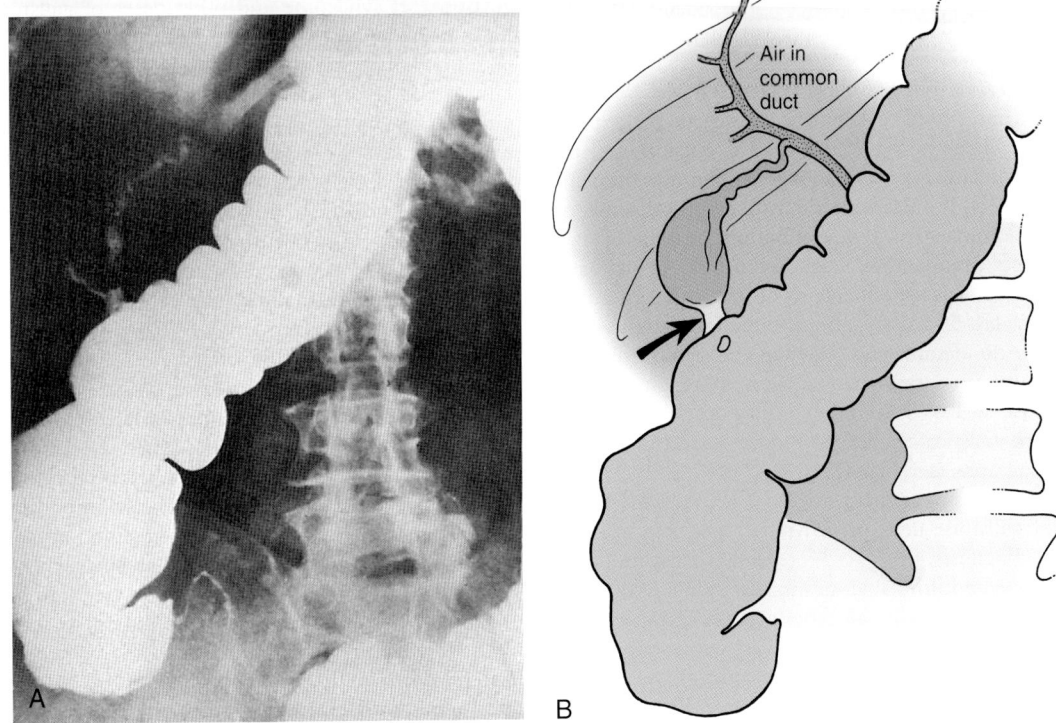

FIGURE 42.6 **A** and **B,** Cholecystocolic fistula seen by barium enema.

show a fistula, a sonogram can assess for the presence of calculi in the gallbladder; common duct stones; and inflammatory, cystic, or infiltrative disease of the liver and pancreas.[97] Sonography can be useful to detect pneumobilia, indicating a high likelihood of a biliary-enteric fistula. In gallstone ileus, sonography can detect an ileal stone not seen on plain films.[98] Ripollés et al.[99] reported that 22 of 23 patients who had undergone surgery for gallstone ileus were found on sonogram to have pneumobilia. In contrast, Lassandro et al.[18] were able to identify pneumobilia in 56% of their 27 patients and often required additional investigation to characterize the obstruction. Sonography is also useful to document the persistence or closure of biliary enteric fistulae after initial emergent surgical or combined endoscopic lithotripter treatment of gallstone ileus, and it has aided the decision for or against further surgery.[12]

Laboratory Testing

Serum liver function tests, electrolytes, and blood counts are useful in the comprehensive evaluation and management of a patient with a symptomatic biliary fistula. Sputum analysis for bilirubin and viable scolices or membranes can be used as laboratory evidence to establish the diagnosis of bronchobiliary fistulae secondary to echinococcosis.[100]

Radionuclide Imaging

Radionuclide scans with imidoacetic acid agents bound to technetium (*p*-isopropylacetanilido iminodiacetic acid [PIPIDA] and hepatobiliary iminodiacetic acid [HIDA]) have become an effective method of assessing normal and pathologic anatomy of the extrahepatic bile passages (see Chapter 18). Prolonged (24 hours) accumulation of radioactivity, measured by scanning or quantitative isotopic counts of body secretions (e.g., sputum), has been used to demonstrate small or intermittent

fistulae from the biliary tract to the respiratory passages and the colon.[43,45,47,101–105]

Specific Clinical Presentations and Treatment

This section elaborates on the clinical presentation, evaluation, and management of specific kinds of internal biliary fistulae.

Gallstone Ileus

Gallstone ileus is the blockage of the intestinal tract by a gallstone large enough to occlude its lumen partially or completely (see Chapter 33). Often, the site of obstruction is the distal ileum. This rare presentation of intestinal obstruction is too indelibly fixed in the medical imagination to permit amendment of the inappropriate term *ileus;* perhaps this derives from the frequent initial clinical impression of an unexplained ileus, in that many patients with gallstone obstruction are initially seen without any clinical history or physical signs to suggest mechanical intestinal obstruction. Similar to other patients in Western Europe and English-speaking countries, where cholesterol cholelithiasis predominates, patients seen with this manifestation of advanced biliary tract disease are usually elderly, female, and beset by multiple other medical conditions that may delay or complicate prompt diagnosis and appropriate treatment.

When an elderly person presents with typical signs and symptoms of intestinal obstruction or, perhaps less dramatically, an unexplained ileus without an obvious cause, gallstone ileus should be considered. Approximately half of patients presenting with gallstone ileus describe a history suggesting prior calculous biliary tract disease. At the time of clinical presentation, however, signs of active gallstone disease, cholangitis, and jaundice may be absent. Laboratory data are consistent with fluid and electrolyte disturbances related to intestinal obstruction. Some abnormalities of liver function tests (LFTs) may suggest chronic disease of the liver and biliary tract in approximately one quarter of patients.

The classic plain abdominal film triad of small bowel obstruction, pneumobilia, and ectopic gallstone is considered pathognomonic of gallstone ileus; however, the triad is encountered in only 30% to 35% of cases.[106] Pneumobilia is often not appreciated even in retrospect. If biliary-enteric fistula is suspected and a barium meal is administered, reflux of barium into the biliary tree yields a correct preoperative diagnosis in 60% of patients (see Fig. 42.5). Calculi large enough to obstruct the intestine usually do so in the last 50 cm of ileum, although sometimes also in the jejunum or duodenum and rarely in the sigmoid colon. Such calculi are usually larger than 2.5 cm, although smaller stones may increase in size via accretion as they descend through the GI tract.[79] If partially calcified, these stones are readily apparent on plain radiographs (see Fig. 42.2B).

Abdominal ultrasound, as mentioned earlier, may establish the diagnosis of gallstone ileus or provides other information relevant to the diagnosis,[12,98,99,107,108] revealing pneumobilia, the site of the fistula, additional stones in the gallbladder or in the common duct, and occasionally the location of an ectopic calculus. The diagnostic superiority of CT over abdominal plain films and sonography for gallstone ileus is now well established.[76,79,109,110] In fact, the clinical significance of Rigler's triad has been revitalized by CT because all three findings are more consistently detected (~78%) by this method.[17,111]

The clinical presentation of gallstone ileus has not changed. In patients with intestinal obstruction, preoperative diagnostic accuracy is approximately 75%.[2] Preoperative diagnostic accuracy has contributed to an improved outcome of therapy.[112] The frequent use of CT in patients with symptoms of intestinal obstruction has led to additional improvement in the diagnostic accuracy of gallstone ileus and has resulted in a decrease in the high mortality rate encountered with this disease.[17,18,110,113]

The overriding consideration in patients presenting with gallstone obstruction of the intestine should be relief of the life-threatening cause of obstruction (i.e., enterolithotomy). This surgical emergency should be approached expeditiously and without a period of waiting in the hope that a suspected stone will pass; it will not. The only reason for delay should be to provide adequate preoperative fluid and electrolyte resuscitation to these critically ill patients and, if possible, to assess the presence of other gallstones in the gallbladder and common duct by means of sonography or MRCP. The use of nasogastric decompression and preoperative antibiotics is recommended to minimize the risks of aspiration and postoperative wound infection.

Unless the obstructed segment is ischemic or has perforated and requires a small bowel resection, the obstructing calculus can be manipulated proximally to a healthy section of bowel, where a safe enterotomy and stone removal may be executed. Jejunal impaction, often by stones larger than 4 cm, occurs approximately 15% of the time, and enterotomy may be made at the site or just proximal to it. Duodenal obstruction, usually in the bulb, is known as *Bouveret syndrome*, which occurs in 10% of patients and may be handled by duodenostomy or pyloroplasty.[114–120] It occasionally may be possible to manipulate the stone back into the stomach and remove it via gastrotomy. Rarely, a gastroenterostomy or duodenal exclusion procedure is necessary to protect a severely traumatized duodenum at the site of impaction.

Bouveret syndrome and other cases of gallstone impaction high in the jejunum have also been managed successfully by a combination of endoscopy and electrohydraulic lithotripsy.[121–126] However, a review of 128 cases by Cappell et al.[127] noted marginal success with endoscopy. We are aware of one case report of a failed endoscopic extraction that led to spontaneous uneventful passage of the stone. In rare instances, the sigmoid colon is the site of obstruction of a calculus that has managed to pass through the terminal ileum or enter the colon via a cholecystocolic fistula.[12,128] Almost invariably, some other pathologic process, such as diverticulitis, has produced an area of colonic narrowing. An early report by Milsom et al.[129] suggested that surgical management should include colostomy to decompress the proximal bowel and Hartmann closure of the distal bowel if the impacted stone cannot be manipulated to a transverse colostomy. However, reports have described successful management with enterolithotomy and resection of the fistulous segment.[130] Colostomy with Hartmann's pouch was reported in a case of sigmoid perforation with purulent-free abdominal fluid due to an impacted gallstone in an elderly patient.[131]

Open exploration and enterolithotomy has been the standard surgical approach for the treatment of classic gallstone ileus. It not only allows removal of the obstructing stone but also permits careful palpation of the entire bowel and gallbladder region, to determine whether other gallstones are in transit more proximally or if any still reside in the diseased gallbladder (see Fig. 42.2B). These calculi may be poised for passage through the fistula, possibly to induce a recurrent episode of gallstone ileus, a phenomenon estimated to occur in 5% of cases.[12,132,133] Several authors have described laparoscopic or laparoscopic-assisted treatment for patients with gallstone ileus.[134–141] Yu et al.[140] reported on 34 cases of gallstone ileus treated laparoscopically with satisfactory results. Although the global experience with laparoscopic management of gallstone ileus is growing, the existing literature is based entirely on small numbers of patients and case reports. Because of these limitations, the efficacy and safety of this approach remain unclear, although the available reports suggest favorable outcomes in selected patients.

There is considerable debate in the surgical literature as to whether cholecystectomy, common duct exploration, and/or dismantling and closure of the cholecystenteric fistula should accompany enterotomy and relief of the obstruction or await a second operation.[111,142,143] Historical data of published reports showed a lower mortality rate of 11.7% in the enterolithotomy-alone group compared with 16.7% for patients who underwent a one-stage operation.[19] Several published reports indicated that operative mortality is lower in these critically ill, elderly patients when only the gallstone obstruction is relieved.[13,14,16,142,144] This has led to the general agreement that enterolithotomy alone should be done for fragile patients with significant comorbidities and that the single-stage procedure should be reserved for young, fit, and low-risk patients. However, data from the American College of Surgeons National Surgical Quality Improvement Program (ACS-NSQIP) database have challenged this conservative approach. Mallipeddi et al.[145] evaluated 127 cases of gallstone ileus and noted a 6% 30-day mortality and 35% morbidity rate; 14 patients underwent cholecystectomy at the time of index operation. Interestingly, there was no significant difference between the two cohorts with regard to age, comorbid conditions, preoperative sepsis, classification as an emergent procedure, or differences in morbidity or mortality rates. Taken together, this report suggests that cholecystectomy and enterolithotomy may be safer than historically reported.[140,145] We recommend maintaining a conservative approach in such patients and would only consider cholecystectomy in the clinically stable patient. Indeed, careful follow-up of patients treated with enterolithotomy alone indicates that one third to one half will have minimal or no symptoms after relief of the gallstone ileus, and no further treatment will be necessary.[12,144,146] It is important to remember that recurrence of gallstone ileus in patients treated with enterolithotomy alone is estimated to be between 5% and 10%.[79,145] Common duct stones are found in 40% of patients with biliary-enteric fistula; thus it is likely that patients who continue to be symptomatic will require endoscopic or open surgical removal of their common duct stones in addition to cholecystectomy and repair of the fistula. As mentioned, operative mortality rates were reported at 15% to 25% in large reported series until the early 1970s. Reductions in operative mortality rates have been possible by limiting treatment to enterotomy and stone removal alone without further surgical therapy in high-risk patients.[2,142,144,145,147]

Cholecystoduodenal Fistulae

Most cholecystoduodenal fistulae do not result in gallstone ileus (see Fig. 42.1A). Rather they are typically asymptomatic or occur in association with common digestive complaints consistent with gastric or biliary tract disease. They may be found during an upper GI barium study or at the time of abdominal surgery for an unrelated problem.

If an asymptomatic or mildly symptomatic cholecystoenteric fistula is diagnosed preoperatively, many of the management decisions regarding gallstone ileus discussed previously may apply. Elective surgery may never be necessary in a completely asymptomatic individual, and surgery may present an unfavorable risk-to-benefit ratio in an elderly, minimally symptomatic patient. Along with dismantling of the fistula and management of common duct stones, other alternatives to cholecystectomy should be considered, such as a period of expectant management with careful observation, endoscopic papillotomy and stone extraction (in the case of common duct stones) with the gallbladder left in situ, or interval cholecystectomy if symptoms of pain or cholangitis persist after endoscopic biliary surgery. In a relatively healthy patient, we believe that cholecystectomy, closure of the fistula, and treatment of any common duct pathology promise the best long-term therapeutic result.[80,148-152]

If an incidental cholecystoduodenal fistula is discovered at the time of surgery, the major intraoperative decision revolves around the patient's need for, and ability to tolerate, additional surgical manipulations. If the patient is judged an unsound risk, or if the biliary tract pathology is not believed to be pertinent to the major indication for operation, observation alone should be considered. One operative consideration is to perform a cholecystostomy and extraction of large calculi, which should add little additional risk. Usually, the gallbladder is shrunken, barely palpable, and stuck to the duodenum. If one is going to proceed with definitive cholecystectomy and closure of the fistula, consideration should be given to performing an operative cholangiogram to rule out common duct stones.

Cholecystocolic Fistulae and Choleric Enteropathy

A cholecystocolic fistula may develop acutely in patients with long-standing mild or moderately symptomatic biliary tract disease and may be heralded by a sudden change in bowel habits with multiple, loose stools and the development of fever, chills, and other signs of cholangitis from colonic bacterial reflux into the biliary tract. There is a female predominance with approximately a 3:1 ratio.[153] Many patients either weather or ignore these symptoms without seeking medical attention, and some develop signs and symptoms that may incriminate the entire GI tract. Increased stool frequency persists, particularly after ingestion of food, and bouts of fever and malaise subside. Other characteristic symptoms then appear, such as eructation, nausea, weight loss, and increasing diarrhea and steatorrhea. These latter symptoms precede the onset of choleric enteropathy, a dramatic complication of cholecystocolonic fistula.[154] This enteropathy also is seen in other major disturbances of bile acid metabolism, such as with major ileal resection or blind loop syndrome.

Choleric enteropathy comprises a wide spectrum of anatomic, physiologic, and biochemical changes produced by a significant alteration of the enterohepatic circulation. The malabsorption syndrome secondary to cholecystocolonic fistula was clinically documented first by Augur and Gracie and has since been studied by others.[9,155] Ordinarily, 95% of bile acids are passed down the jejunum, aiding in fat and cholesterol absorption, before being largely reabsorbed in the terminal ileum as part of an efficient enterohepatic circulation. Two or three cycles of the bile acid pool per meal occur, with further metabolism of bile acids in the colon and very little lost. With a cholecystocolic fistula, however, a large part of all of the primary bile acid pool is lost directly into the colon, resulting in a high luminal concentration of bile acids. In the colon, the primary bile acids undergo deconjugation and dehydroxylation by fecal bacteria, and this increased concentration of bile acids induces a water secretory diarrhea.

Depending on the amount of bile still passing via the common duct into the small bowel, fat absorption is affected, which over time may result in fatty-acid diarrhea. More immediately, however, colonic secretion of water and electrolytes is maximally stimulated by bile acids. At this point, even with a partial shunt to the colon, the bile acid concentration still normally passing down the common duct and through the small intestine may be too small to effect micellar solubilization of dietary fat. Until the fistula is dismantled, massive shunting of bile acids to the intestine persists and promotes continued watery diarrhea, diminished bile salt pool, and a variable degree of fat malabsorption.

Cholangitis (see Chapter 43) seems to be a more prominent feature of cholecystocolic fistula compared with other biliary-enteric fistulae. This may be related to a narrow fistula that is prone to intermittent obstruction.[3,10,103] We are also aware of one case report of a patient with a cholecystocolic fistula who presented with massive lower GI hemorrhage.[156] Given the higher likelihood of cholangitis, serum levels of bilirubin, alanine aminotransferase, and γ-glutamyltransferase may be slightly elevated at presentation.

Because of the unusual initial complaints, a full investigation for malabsorption, which includes upper GI studies, GI sonography, and jejunal biopsy, may be undertaken but usually does not clarify the diagnosis. A pathognomonic triad consisting of pneumobilia, chronic diarrhea, and vitamin K malabsorption was recently suggested by Savvidou et al. to aid in the diagnosis of cholecystocolic fistula. Although the condition of bile acid malabsorption can be diagnosed by the selenium-75-homocholic acid taurine (SeHCAT) test, this study is time consuming and is not widely available.[157] Plain abdominal radiographs have been reported to reveal air in the biliary tree in only 50% of cases. The diagnosis is most readily made by a barium enema (see Fig. 42.6) demonstrating air and contrast in the gallbladder and bile ducts.[158] Failure of a barium enema to show a cholecystocolic fistula has been reported, but this is rare. In such cases, the cholecystocolic fistula can be diagnosed by ERCP.[159]

There is little controversy about the appropriate treatment for cholecystocolic fistulae. Except in the most extenuating circumstances, the fistulae should be dismantled because of the risk of sepsis and previously mentioned metabolic disturbances. Cholecystectomy and, if indicated, common duct exploration should be performed at the same time. Laparoscopic surgical treatment of cholecystocolic fistulae has been reported.[78,80,151,160,161] Preoperative imaging of the CBD and treatment of CBD stones, if present, is mandated in all cases of cholecystocolic fistulae.[162]

Cholecystocholedochal Fistula, Including Mirizzi Syndrome

The pathogenesis of cholecystobiliary fistula is similar to the mechanism of fistula formation between the gallbladder and other adjacent segments of the alimentary tract: The offending calculus remains impacted in the ampulla of the gallbladder or cystic duct, and the resultant inflammation causes adherence and then perforation into the adjacent structure (see Fig. 42.1D). In 1948 Mirizzi[163] described the clinical picture in detail and called it *functional hepatic syndrome*. It is now commonly referred to as *Mirizzi syndrome*. The mechanism of jaundice was postulated by Mirizzi to be due to spasm of the hepatic sphincter secondary to inflammation in the region of the cystic duct junction with the common hepatic duct; however, extensive histologic studies have failed to disclose a "sphincter" in the common hepatic duct. The large size of the stone and the acute cholecystitis with marked pressure necrosis and inflammatory reaction at the site of stone intrusion into the common hepatic duct combine to produce jaundice with variable components of extrinsic compression and intrinsic calculous blockage of bile flow.

The early phase of a cholecystobiliary fistula presumably exists when a large gallstone is impacted in the ampulla of the gallbladder or in the intramural segment of the cystic duct, which often courses parallel to the common duct. The jaundice that occurs as a consequence of this pathologic anatomy is clinically indistinguishable from choledocholithiasis. McSherry et al.[164] suggested that this classic picture (Fig. 42.7) of Mirizzi's "functional hepatic syndrome" be subclassified as type 1. With progression of the disease, extrusion of the stone into the common hepatic duct may occur, and a fistula forms between the gallbladder and the hepatic duct. This is classified as type 2 (see Fig. 42.1D), which is characteristically diagnosed intraoperatively by observing a "gush" of bile on removal of the impacted stone. Csendes et al.[165] further subclassified type 2 patients into three categories based on the percentage of the wall of the common duct that was eroded by the calculus. In this subclassification, type II is a fistula involving less than one third of the circumference of the bile duct, type III involves two thirds, and type IV is a fistula with complete bile duct destruction.[165] This classification scheme was recently updated to include a type V,

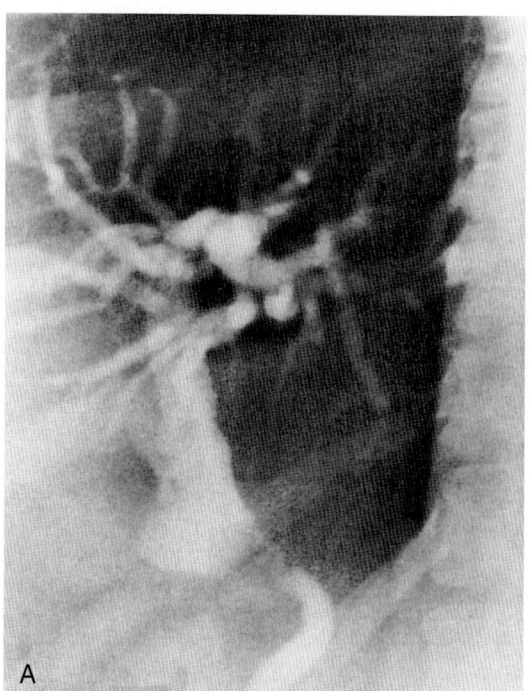
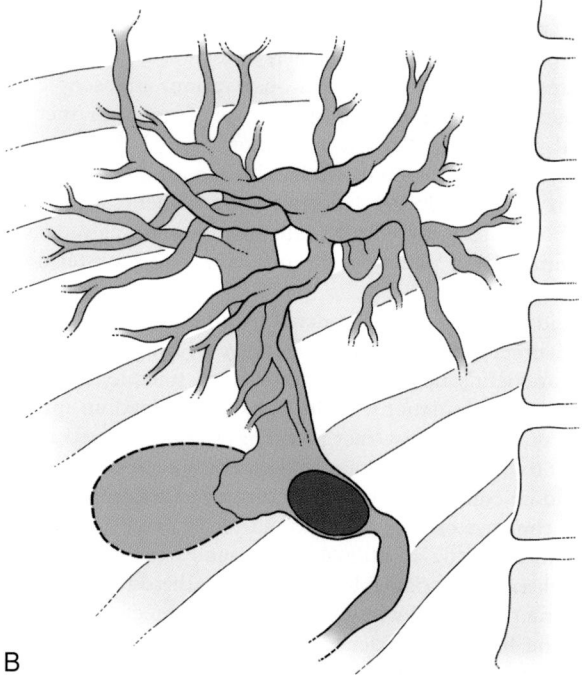

FIGURE 42.7 **A** and **B,** Mirizzi syndrome type 1 (without cholecystocholedochal fistula). Percutaneous cholangiography shows an impacted cystic stone with extrinsic compression of the proximal hepatic ducts (see Chapters 20 and 31).

which describes cholecystoenteric fistula, with or without gallstone ileus, co-existing with any of the other types.[166]

The classic findings on ultrasonography include dilation of the biliary tree proximal to the gallbladder neck, a stone impacted in the gallbladder, and an abrupt change in the caliber of the common duct below the stone.[167] Because most of these patients present with jaundice or abnormal LFTs, a preoperative ERCP or PTC frequently is performed.[168] These imaging studies permit a precise delineation of the condition, assisting with surgical strategy.

Historically, biliobiliary fistulae have been referred to as a "trap" in the surgery of cholelithiasis.[169] This term is appropriate because the presence of such a fistula frequently is not recognized until the time of surgery, often not soon enough to prevent injury to the common duct in an attempt to dissect the ampulla of the gallbladder or the cystic duct. Lygidakis et al.[3] emphasized the technical problems in operating on these patients. Other authors emphasized the importance of preoperative direct cholangiography.[170–172] In patients with jaundice, biliary drainage may be necessary in the preoperative management. The endoluminal biliary stent can be palpated during surgery and used for orientation to the biliary anatomy. In these cases, the acute inflammation is often intense, resulting in severely distorted hilar anatomy. The hepatoduodenal ligament is often "accordioned" or tethered to the base of the liver, making recognition of the CBD difficult. Although some centers are increasingly advocating a minimally invasive approach, we manage these patients by an open technique. For the Mirizzi type 1, our practice is to perform a near-total cholecystectomy leaving the biliary stent in place, if present, throughout the postoperative recovery until the inflammation subsides. For Mirizzi type 2, direct choledochotomy with removal of the stone, followed by direct closure of the gallbladder, may be performed. Alternatively, the opened gallbladder may be anastomosed to the duodenum or a Roux-en-Y loop of jejunum.[6,170,173] It is important to emphasize that stenosis of the biliary tree typically resolves spontaneously in the postoperative period, and choledochotomy is seldom indicated.

A minimally invasive approach to the management of patients with Mirizzi syndrome can be undertaken.[150,152,174–184] To address the utility of laparoscopic treatment of Mirizzi syndrome, Antoniou et al.[185] conducted a systematic review of the literature on this topic. Because of the strict study criteria, the authors identified only 10 of 66 articles for analysis. The total number of patients treated by laparoscopy was 124, of which 73 (59%) were successfully completed. Interestingly, patients from studies reporting a high preoperative diagnosis rate (>80%) had a significantly lower risk for conversion. The main reasons for conversion included technical failure as a result of dense adhesions in the triangle of Calot, unclear anatomy, and unsuccessful stone retrieval. The analysis showed a complication rate of 16%, with residual stones and bile duct injury the most common complications. The authors concluded that laparoscopic treatment of Mirizzi syndrome cannot be recommended as a standard procedure because of the high failure rate and hazard posed by dissection in this area.[150,184,185] However, greater advances with advanced laparoscopy and endoscopy may offer newer treatment paradigms that preserve patient safety and afford acceptable outcomes. A study by Yuan et al.[186] described 49 patients with type II Mirizzi syndrome successfully managed by laparoscopic subtotal cholecystectomy with ERCP, without need for conversion to open approach, with minimal morbidity,

and with reduced postoperative complications compared with a group treated by purely open approach. An approach with combined endoscopic and robotic subtotal cholecystectomy is described by Lee et al.[187,188] Recent reviews on management advocate for careful patient selection, and for combined minimally invasive/endoscopic approaches for type I and II Mirizzi syndrome to be performed with proper surgical and endoscopic expertise.[189,190]

Proximal Choledochoduodenal Fistulae and Chronic Peptic Ulcer Disease

Chronic duodenal ulcer can cause inflammation and fibrosis in the entire periampullary area and result in a distal biliary stricture or proximal choledochoduodenal fistulae. Patients may be asymptomatic, or they may present with jaundice and cholangitis in a patient with a long history of duodenal ulcer (see Fig. 42.1E). Biliary tract symptoms are usually absent, and these patients generally do not have associated cholelithiasis. The diagnosis may be suggested by pneumobilia in 15% to 60% of patients. More often, the diagnosis is made as contrast material from an upper GI study refluxes up the common duct to outline a normal gallbladder. Endoscopy with direct visualization of the ulcer and fistula and ERCP are the best studies to confirm the diagnosis and evaluate the extent of disease.

Given the paucity of reported experience with choledochoduodenal fistula, it is not surprising that, until recently, treatment recommendations have been controversial.[23,25,95,191] Most authors now agree that treatment should be directed at the ulcer diathesis and not at the biliary tract or the fistula itself. Medical management with proton-pump inhibitors and therapy for *Helicobacter pylori* is often sufficient to control the ulcer disease and even result in closure of the fistula.

Modern success rates of medical management for peptic ulcer disease have resulted in a drastic reduction in the number of case reports of patients with proximal choledochoduodenal fistulae.[192–194] Although choledochoduodenal fistula because of peptic ulcer is now rare, clinicians should remain aware of this clinical entity, especially in symptomatic patients with refractory peptic ulcer disease. In such patients, surgery may be indicated to prevent major complications.[195] If indicated, an exclusion type of gastric resection or duodenal bypass procedure, such as a Billroth II gastrectomy or gastroenterostomy, should be performed in addition to a vagotomy. There is no need to close the fistula and doing so may injure the duodenum or bile duct. Cholecystectomy and biliary enteric reconstruction may be done, but these are reserved for cases of biliary stricture. It should be stressed that in modern times these operations are rarely necessary.

Distal Parapapillary Choledochoduodenal Fistula

Whether caused by spontaneous gallstone erosion or by iatrogenic damage to the distal common duct, parapapillary fistulae have a clinical presentation similar to that of other advanced calculous biliary tract diseases. In the series reported by Tanaka in 1983,[32] the following observations were made: a history of biliary symptoms longer than 10 years' duration in 46%; pain and/or jaundice in 88% and 69%, respectively; prior biliary surgery in 54%; air or barium in the biliary tree in 41%; cholelithiasis in 71%; and choledocholithiasis in 38%. Additionally, there are more recent case reports of fistulae in patients who present with biliary tumors and who have no prior history of gallstone disease but a history of endoscopic or

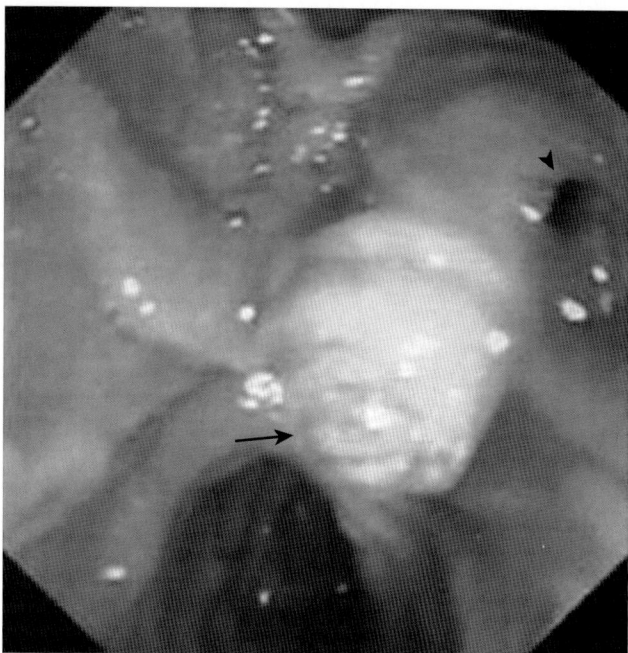

FIGURE 42.8 Duodenoscopy showing the papilla of Vater *(arrow)* and a distal or peripapillary choledochoduodenal fistula *(arrowhead)*. (Courtesy Dr. Melih Karincaglu.)

surgical biliary manipulation. Chronic reflux of bilious material and biliary stasis are thought to precede obstructive biliary tumors that may lead to parapapillary choledochoduodenal fistula.[24,196] The anatomic diagnosis rests on meticulous endoscopic observation and expertise in the technique of ERCP (Fig. 42.8; also see Fig. 42.1F).

The management of these biliary fistulae is still evolving, and a variety of endoscopic techniques have been advocated.[84,197–200] These techniques involve using endoscopic sphincterotomy to widen the choledochal fistula enough to permit free drainage or to create a common channel between the fistula and natural ampullary orifice. When necessary, open surgical procedures, such as hepaticodochojejunostomy, have been used.[88]

Fistula to the Hepatic Veins or Portal Veins

Biliary-venous fistula is a rare occurrence that results in bilhemia (see Chapter 116), a condition associated with high biliary pressures and flow of bile into the systemic circulation via hepatic/portal veins. This can be dangerous, especially if there is related biliary infection, which can result in systemic sepsis. This fistula can also be associated with interventional transhepatic maneuvers. Case reports describe portobiliary fistula after ERCP.[201,202] When a large-caliber intrahepatic bile duct is injured during the creation of a transjugular intrahepatic portosystemic stent-shunt, this may be complicated by a biliary-venous fistula. The resulting biliary leak plays an important role in the subsequent risk of stenosis and occlusion of the portosystemic shunt.[203]

EXTERNAL BILIARY FISTULAE AND STRICTURES

Clinically significant external biliary fistulae are often unintended consequences following surgical procedure or intervention directly on or adjacent to the biliary system. Causes of external biliary fistulae include invasive radiologic procedures, cholecystostomy, cholecystectomy (with or without common duct exploration), liver surgery or injury, intentionally created surgical biliary-enteric anastomosis, and other abdominal operations. In contrast to internal biliary fistulae, discussed in the previous section, external biliary fistulae are characterized by persistent biliary drainage into the peritoneum or transcutaneously. This is often the result of an unrecognized disease affecting the bile ducts or complications from an intervention or surgical procedure. We introduce discussion on biliary strictures in this chapter section, as the nature of certain conditions often can produce both fistulae and strictures. Other times, biliary stricture presentation is one of "malignant mimicry" where challenges lay in ruling out neoplastic entity. However, many principles of evaluation and repair for external fistulae and biliary stricture have much in common.

Etiology and Prevention of External Biliary Fistulae

External biliary fistulae are best considered according to the type of preceding intervention. The following are the more commonly associated surgical antecedents of fistulae.

Fistula After Cholecystostomy Tube or Other Radiologic Procedures

Percutaneous cholecystostomy is the percutaneous placement of a catheter into the lumen of the gallbladder (see Chapter 35). This procedure only requires local anesthesia and can be performed under ultrasound guidance at the bedside of critically ill patients.[204–206] Typically, the catheter is allowed to drain externally to treat underlying infection in an obstructed gallbladder. Persistently elevated cholecystostomy tube drainage or cutaneous drainage of biliary contents after cholecystostomy tube removal may indicate ongoing obstruction in the cystic duct or distally in the common bile duct (Fig. 42.9). A case report by Lofgren et al.[207] describes discovery of an external biliary fistula after cholecystostomy tube removal after a large abdominal wall abscess developed, which was treated by incision and drainage and subsequent cholecystectomy. A retrospective study by Peters et al.[208] found rates of fistula and abscess after percutaneous cholecystostomy tube placement to be 3.6% and 1.8%, respectively.

Biliary fistulae may follow any invasive radiologic procedure involving the hepatobiliary system and are usually the consequence of ongoing distal biliary obstruction. Published rates of clinically significant biliary leak after interventional radiologic procedures vary significantly and depend on patient selection and practitioner experience. Complications result from suboptimal puncture location, incorrect selection of biliary catheter size, and inadequate postprocedural tube care.[209] Burke et al.[210] classified bile leakage, sepsis, and infected biloma as major complications that occur at rates of 2% after PTC and biliary drainage procedures (see Fig. 42.4).

Clinical Presentation

The clinical presentation of a biliary fistula may be excessive, abnormal biliary drainage from a drain site or wound or, alternatively, of a localized or generalized peritonitis resulting from an intraabdominal collection of bile. Cross-sectional imaging such as an abdominal CT scan is often useful in arriving at this diagnosis and characterizing the size and location of the bile collection. Depending on the circumstances, percutaneous external drains placed by international radiologists is an effective

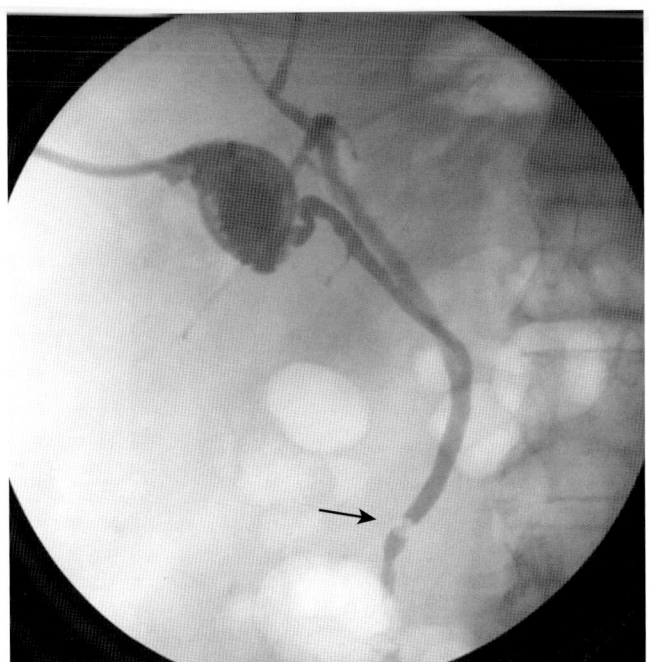

FIGURE 42.9 An 85-year-old man with severe cardiomyopathy (unfit for surgery) was treated by percutaneous cholecystostomy tube drainage. Six weeks after tube insertion, a cholecystogram shows a retained gallstone impacted in the distal common bile duct (*arrow*). The patient was treated definitively by endoscopic retrograde cholangiopancreatography and papillotomy (see Chapter 30).

way to initially drain and control an external biliary fistula. After a diagnosis of biliary fistula has been established, it is most important to assess the adequacy of bile drainage. In well-controlled fistulae, external biliary drainage is adequate, with no signs of localized or generalized infection, and cholestasis is not present.

In an uncontrolled external biliary fistula, biliary drainage is inadequate, resulting in an intraabdominal bilious collection. Because the bile is usually infected, the presentation is mostly of a subphrenic or subhepatic abscess or generalized peritonitis. The situation may be complicated further by cholangitis with or without intrahepatic abscess and septicemia that demands urgent treatment. In patients with sterile bile, large volumes may accumulate within the peritoneal cavity with minimal clinical findings apart from a distended abdomen. The presence of skin excoriation and digestion implies that activated digestive enzymes from the GI tract are present in the fistula effluent because bile alone contains no digestive enzymes.

Pathologic Consequences of External Biliary Fistulae

The pathophysiologic effects of an external biliary fistula depend on the volume of bile drained, the length of time the fistula has been present, and the degree to which bile is diverted from the GI tract. Consequences of biliary fistulae are mainly due to depletion of electrolytes and fluid, to the absence of bile from the gut, and to the possibility of ascending biliary infection. The important practical considerations are that the volume of bile secreted daily by the liver is approximately 1000 mL, and the electrolyte composition of bile is similar to that of blood.

Total biliary loss for short periods (≤3 weeks) may not result in a serious depletion of electrolytes and fluid because the body is able to compensate for this loss. Long-term total external biliary fistula results in fluid and electrolyte disturbances if replacement therapy is not instituted. Sodium loss is usually greater than chloride loss, leading to metabolic acidosis.[211] The serum potassium level is initially lowered, but the accompanying fluid loss may lead to a decrease in plasma volume, low-output renal failure, and hyperkalemia.[212] Absence of bile from the GI tract causes interference with the absorption of fat-soluble vitamins. Vitamin A and D deficiencies are associated with long-term total biliary fistula and are rarely seen today, whereas vitamin K deficiency is evident earlier and can be easily diagnosed by a prolonged prothrombin time. Other adverse effects of total biliary loss are disruption of intestinal barrier function and bacterial translocation.[213] These findings are supported by an observation that bile replacement was able to restore intestinal barrier function in patients with malignant obstruction undergoing external biliary drainage.[214] Even in the short term, patients with an external biliary fistula feel unwell, weak, and lethargic. In advanced and neglected cases, caloric and protein malnutrition results in gradual weight loss, whereas the electrolyte changes may result in stupor and vasomotor collapse.

Diagnostic Procedures and Initial Management

The presence of a biliary fistula may first become apparent at reoperation for peritonitis. More commonly, and particularly after laparoscopic cholecystectomy, the biliary fistula becomes apparent at cholangiography or after percutaneous drainage of a perihepatic collection. Reoperation or percutaneous drainage may be required for peritonitis or for management of an intraabdominal collection. The basic principle of initial management of an uncontrolled biliary injury is conversion of the leak into a controlled fistula, usually by means of tube drainage. No attempt at definitive repair should be made when there is uncontrolled infection because the involved bile ducts are collapsed, friable, and usually embedded within a severe local inflammatory reaction. In this situation, it is virtually impossible to expose healthy bile ducts for any form of long-lasting definitive repair, and any attempt to do so is bound to fail and renders further operation more difficult.

It is important to ensure adequate drainage and to create a well-controlled fistula. Biliary drainage is ideally carried out using a sealed drainage-bag system.[215] Drainage initially should be carried out using a low-pressure, closed-suction system, which is valuable in reducing the cavity of the intraabdominal bile collection and in controlling the abscess. Improvement of the clinical picture and repeated radiologic studies eventually should show proper positioning of the drain and reveal no residual collection or abscess. Cross-sectional imaging and contrast tube studies are helpful in this respect.

After the fistula is controlled, conservative treatment is instituted, the patient is nourished, deficits of electrolytes and vitamins (mostly vitamin K) are corrected, and infection is treated. It is important to know whether the biliary fistula contains bile only or whether it also contains duodenal, pancreatic, or intestinal juice. When the latter is present, appropriate measures to protect the skin should be taken. Parenteral nutrition may be necessary in the management of significant duodenal and pancreatic fistulae. It has been shown that treatment with somatostatin can reduce bile secretion and decrease outputs from pancreatic and small intestine fistulae.[216–219] However, the benefit of somatostatin therapy in promoting closure of

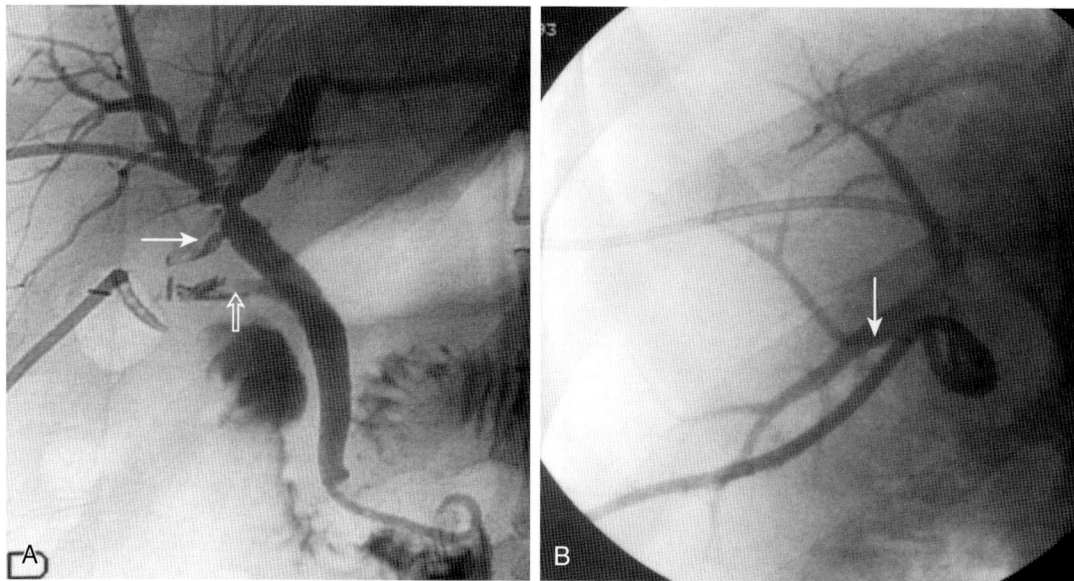

FIGURE 42.10 Injury to a right posterior sectoral hepatic duct at laparoscopic cholecystectomy. **A,** Percutaneous transluminal cholangiography. Note the remnant of the duct draining into the common bile duct (CBD) *(solid arrow)* and cystic stump *(open arrow)*. Note the low entry of this duct into the CBD. **B,** Tube fistulography. The biliary ductal system of the orphaned sectoral duct is outlined *(solid arrow)*.

biliary fistulae arising entirely from the biliary tree remains unproven.[220]

After the establishment of a controlled fistula, various radiologic investigations are performed with the aim of assessing the (1) origin of the fistula, (2) presence and extent of an injury to the extrahepatic biliary system, (3) adequacy of drainage, and (4) presence of biliary-enteric bile flow. The anatomy of the entire intrahepatic and extrahepatic biliary tree should be shown, and this is achieved by a variety of radiologic studies. All contrast examinations that directly assess the biliary tree/fistula should be covered with antibiotic prophylaxis to minimize the risk of a bacteremic episode.

Tube cholangiography should be performed routinely before removal of cholecystostomy or choledochostomy tubes or tube drainage across biliary-enteric anastomoses. Whenever an obstruction to free biliary-enteric bile flow is present, it should be treated. Removal of a tube in the presence of a distal stricture or a retained bile duct stone results in a persistent external biliary fistula.

Fistulography is a simple and effective means of determining whether biliary drainage is adequate and whether a fistulous cavity has converted to a fistulous tract. The site and underlying cause of the biliary fistula often can often be demonstrated by fistulography (Figs. 42.10 and 42.11). Direct cholangiography (PTC or ERCP) can be used when the findings of fistulography are equivocal and unable to demonstrate the pathology (see Chapter 20). ERCP is a useful diagnostic and therapeutic tool where there is a continuity of the extrahepatic biliary system, particularly after laparoscopic cholecystectomy and after liver transplantation.[221–224] CT after fistulography can help verify maturation of a fistula tract and define perihepatic bile collections or isolated liver segments.

HIDA scintigraphy, as mentioned earlier, is a useful noninvasive method of evaluating liver function and bile secretion.[225] Although it may not supply accurate anatomic details, information such as the presence of a fistula, its origin (liver or extrahepatic biliary system), and adequacy of its drainage (Fig. 42.12) can be obtained[226] (see Chapter 18).

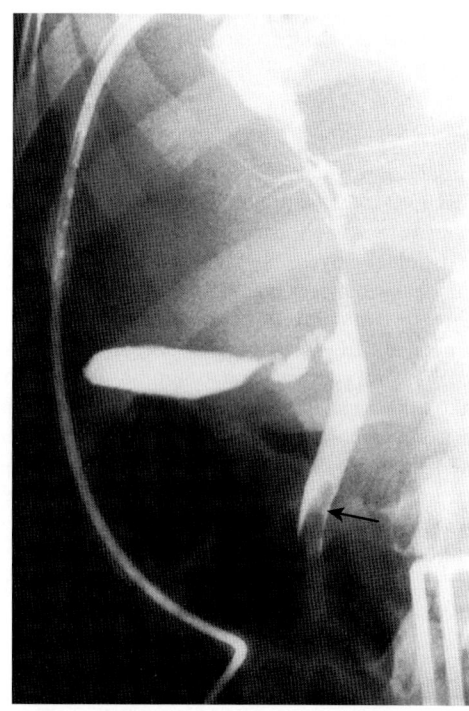

FIGURE 42.11 Fistulography obtained after excision of a right hepatic hydatid cyst. Note the persistent fistula as a consequence of retained hydatid material in the common bile duct (CBD) *(arrow)*. Treatment was by exploration of the CBD and surgical removal of the retained hydatid material. The fistula rapidly closed.

Treatment

The principles of management of postoperative biliary fistulae are essentially the same regardless of the underlying etiology; these principles are summarized in Fig. 42.13. The first critical step is to establish a controlled fistula, preferably with image-guided drainage of the collection. Operation is indicated when

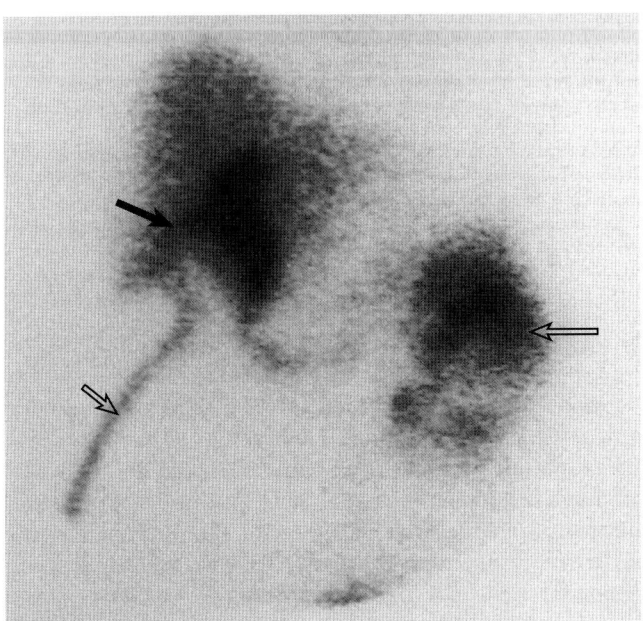

FIGURE 42.12   Hepatobiliary iminodiacetic acid scan (right lateral view) showing a controlled biliary fistula *(small open arrow)* resulting from an incomplete closure of a wide cystic stump *(solid arrow)* at laparoscopic cholecystectomy. Free biliary-enteric bile flow is shown *(large open arrow)*. The fistula closed spontaneously after 2 weeks (see Chapter 18).

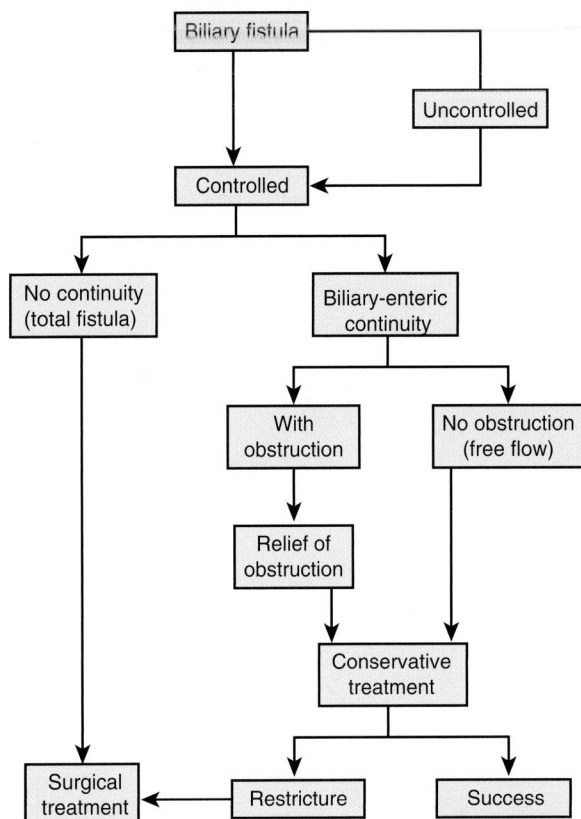

FIGURE 42.13   Proposed management plan for postoperative biliary fistula. The initial treatment is most important and includes the establishment of a controlled fistula. This is achieved radiologically, by percutaneous drainage of a collection, or surgically, at which time no attempt at primary repair is made. The fistula is evaluated for biliary-enteric continuity. When a total fistula has been diagnosed, it is most important to ensure that it is controlled. Definitive surgical repair is attempted after a reasonable period of conservative treatment. When biliary-enteric continuity is present with free biliary-enteric bile flow, conservative treatment is instituted and results in spontaneous closure in most cases. The presence of biliary-enteric continuity with distal obstruction calls for some form of treatment to relieve the obstruction, and this is done endoscopically or, preferably, percutaneously by balloon dilation. After the establishment of free biliary-enteric bile flow, patients are treated conservatively. In suitable cases, nasobiliary intubation is followed up carefully after fistula closure for early signs of stricture. Highly complex hilar fistulae are treated conservatively with prolonged periods of drainage. The fistula is expected to close, and this usually occurs together with the development of stricture. After a stricture develops, it is treated surgically.

percutaneous measures are not feasible or in patients with severe peritonitis or sepsis. During operation for uncontrolled peritonitis or sepsis, the temptation to attempt primary repair at this stage must be resisted; only good drainage should be established. Occasionally, persistent drainage of large amounts of bile with significant fluid and electrolyte loss may necessitate early operation, when the external fistula may be converted to an internal fistulojejunostomy using a mobilized and approximated Roux-en-Y jejunal loop[227] (see Chapter 32). In this procedure, the drainage tube is led from the fistula origin through the jejunal loop to the exterior; this allows control, but it creates an almost certain necessity to reoperate for restenosis at a later stage.

It is important to identify the presence or absence of biliary-enteric bile flow, which differentiates a total biliary fistula from a partial fistula with some residual biliary-enteric continuity. Subsequent management is influenced significantly because operation is usually unavoidable in the former, and a nonoperative approach may be successful in the latter. A total biliary fistula rarely closes spontaneously when an internal fistula develops between the divided upper duct and the gut.[228]

When biliary-enteric continuity is present and bile flow is not obstructed distal to the origin of the fistula, a prolonged period of conservative treatment is indicated because spontaneous closure of the fistula is common. Fistula closure may be facilitated by temporary placement of a stent across the fistulous opening in the bile duct, excluding bile flow through the fistula. This method may be attempted when the bile duct is intact above the fistula origin and the defect in the common duct is not too large. Stenting may be achieved by endoscopic placement of an endoprosthesis or a nasobiliary tube with its tip above the origin of the fistula. When a short period of stenting is anticipated, nasobiliary intubation is preferred because it enables follow-up cholangiography, damage to the papilla is minimal, and a second endoscopic procedure is avoided.[229,230] Using this method, some fistulae close within 2 weeks.[231,232] It

is also useful after liver transplantation in patients who have undergone duct-to-duct biliary reconstruction.

Endoscopic treatment of fistulae with intact biliary-enteric flow by sphincterotomy, stenting, or both is effective in most patients[222,233,234] (see Chapter 30). In most instances, a biliary endoprosthesis is used and is left in place for several weeks, until the fistula closes. Closure is verified by HIDA scan before removal of the stent. If standard endoscopic therapy fails, an alternative endoscopic technique using *n*-butyl-2-cyanoacrylate glue occlusion of the fistula has been shown to be effective and helps avoid the need for surgery.[235]

Some authors recommend endoscopic sphincterotomy alone with the intention of reducing the pressure gradient between the biliary system and the duodenum.[236] This procedure is rarely necessary, because the fistula will close if no distal obstruction is present. Sphincterotomy may also be associated with short- and long-term complications; therefore it should be avoided unless specifically indicated (e.g., in patients with a papillary stricture).[24,237] It also has been shown that stenting is more effective than sphincterotomy alone in the resolution of biliary fistulae.[233,238] As stated earlier, we believe that although endoscopic approaches are useful, they generally should be delayed for weeks to allow spontaneous closure of the fistula, which occurs the majority of the time.

An obstruction distal to the fistula requires specific treatments to allow healing of the fistula. Obstruction is most commonly caused by a retained stone or a stricture. Retained stones are usually removed by endoscopic means, and relief of a benign stricture can be achieved using balloon dilation. The patient is treated conservatively for fistula closure or for recurrent stricture, and fistula closure can be facilitated by temporary stenting (Fig. 42.14) if the location and the size of the defect in the bile duct are suitable.

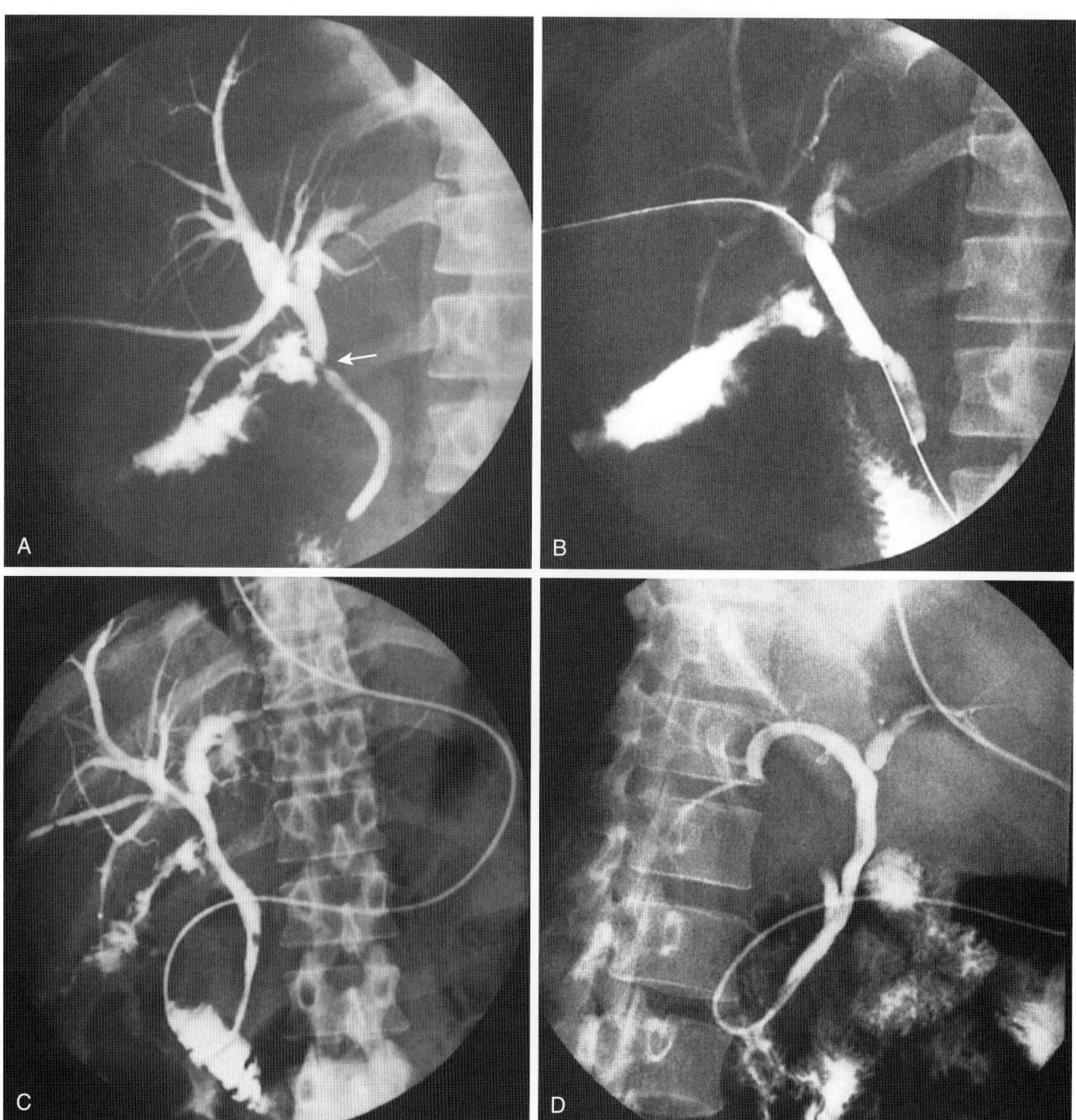

FIGURE 42.14 Combined surgical/endoscopic/radiologic management of a biliary fistula diagnosed 3 weeks after an open cholecystectomy. **A,** Percutaneous transluminal cholangiography shows a biliary fistula with a significant distal stricture *(arrow).* **B,** Percutaneous transhepatic balloon dilation of the stricture. **C,** Percutaneous transhepatic guide is exchanged for a nasobiliary tube, which is placed endoscopically with its tip above the origin of the fistula. Free biliary-enteric bile flow is obtained. The fistula is still present but is smaller. **D,** Check-up cholangiography (lateral view) after 2 weeks of nasobiliary drainage shows fistula closure. The nasobiliary drain was removed.

After closure of the fistula, patients are followed up carefully with regular LFTs and imaging to detect early signs of the development of a biliary stricture, which may take months and sometimes years. Stricture is most likely to occur where a stricture has already been present or where a fistula is associated with an injury to a major bile duct.[239] The proposed plan may involve relatively prolonged management, but it improves the chances of a successful and long-lasting bile duct repair, especially after injury at cholecystectomy. In this situation, early and untimely surgical attempts at definitive repair carry a high risk of biliary leak and anastomotic stricture.

Management of the rare patient with excluded segmental bile ducts that do not connect to the main biliary tree is extremely challenging. This complication most commonly occurs after partial hepatectomy and often results from unrecognized anatomic biliary variations or when normal anatomic planes are violated during hepatic transection. The end result is that a portion of liver tissue remains well perfused but disconnected from the biliary tract. Multiple interventional treatments have been described, the majority consisting of sclerotic agents that are injected directly into the fistula tract. These substances include tetracycline, ethanol, and acetic acid.[240–244] Other agents such as fibrin glue, thrombin, and *n*-butyl cyanoacrylate have been used with variable success.[245,246] We are aware of one successful case report of a patient who was treated by percutaneous intraductal laser ablation after failing other treatments.[247] When these nonoperative treatments fail, repeat liver resection may be required.[248] The authors have successfully used microwave energy ablation of the liver tissue containing the orphaned biliary segment to treat persistent biliary fistulae.

Benign Biliary Strictures

Several causes of benign biliary stricture are listed (Box 42.1). Broadly speaking, benign biliary strictures can be congenital, iatrogenic, a result of inflammatory process, or autoimmune, to list several. The following discussion focuses on several unique

---

BOX 42.1   Causes of Benign Biliary Strictures

I. Congenital Strictures
  A. Biliary atresia (see Chapter 40)
II. Bile Duct Injuries
  A. Postoperative strictures
    1. Cholecystectomy or common bile duct exploration
    2. Biliary-enteric anastomosis
    3. Hepatic resection
    4. Portocaval shunt
    5. Pancreatic surgery
    6. Gastrectomy
    7. Liver transplantation
  B. Strictures after blunt or penetrating trauma
  C. Strictures after endoscopic or percutaneous biliary intubation
III. Inflammatory Strictures
  A. Cholelithiasis or choledocholithiasis
  B. Chronic pancreatitis
  C. Chronic duodenal ulceration
  D. Abscess or inflammation of liver or subhepatic space
  E. Parasitic infection
  F. Recurrent pyogenic cholangitis
IV. Primary Sclerosing Cholangitis
V. Radiation-Induced Stricture
VI. Papillary Stenosis

---

noniatrogenic conditions that are almost entirely associated with bile duct stricture development, in contrast to many other entities in this chapter that have potential to produce both strictures and fistulae. Certain diagnoses present as *malignant masquerades* or *mimics* rendering differentiation from malignancy difficult. Distinguishing these benign conditions from a cancer is difficult and in the majority of cases a cancer operation is necessary. The diversity of the clinical presentation of these conditions varies widely, and therefore comprehensive evaluation of these patients by expert hepatobiliary surgeons, radiologists, and gastroenterologists is important.

Etiology and Incidence

Noniatrogenic benign biliary strictures are rare, and prevalence rates are difficult to estimate. Most literature on the topic are single-center retrospective case series. One of the largest retrospective reviews on benign biliary stricture describes 22 benign biliary strictures out of 275 patients (8%) who were referred for evaluation of proximal biliary obstruction at a tertiary surgical center over an 11-year period.[249] These 22 patients had presumed malignancy and underwent operations that would have been appropriate for an oncologic diagnosis. On postoperative histopathologic analysis, it was determined that these strictures were of fibroinflammatory nature. Five pathologic diagnoses were provided: lymphoplasmacytic sclerosing cholangitis, sclerosing cholangitis, nonspecific inflammatory process, granulomatous process, and choledocholithiasis.

Clinical Manifestations

Patients often present with typical signs and symptoms of biliary obstruction, including jaundice, pruritus, and abdominal pain. Some patients may report decreased appetite and weight loss, as a result of feeling unwell, which lends credible plausibility to an oncologic diagnosis.

Diagnosis

Standard serum laboratory values for liver function tests and cancer markers (CA19-9, CA-125) should be obtained; however, there are significant limitations of the sensitivity and specificity of these markers. Standard cross-sectional abdominal imaging may help reveal periportal lymphadenopathy or telltale signs of locoregional malignancy. Dedicated biliary tract imaging with ERCP, MRCP, or PTC is standard, as the morphology and pattern of biliary stricture(s) often yields clues to the diagnosis. Direct biliary tract imaging (PTC or ERCP) with cytology or biopsy should be interpreted with caution given the limitations of the biopsy/cytology specimen quality, as well as sensitivity and specificity. Sensitivity and specificity of biliary cytology were 45% and 99%, and biliary tract biopsy 48.1% and 99.2%, respectively.[250] Other than a biopsy revealing malignancy, no isolated study or laboratory value should be used to provide a diagnosis and treatment plan for these cases, and multimodal imaging and discussion with a multidisciplinary team are essential.

Obtaining a thorough patient history to establish whether prior biliary tract surgery, trauma, intervention, abdominal radiation therapy, biliary tract parasitic infection, or chronic pancreatitis had occurred will help in determination the nature of a biliary stricture. Nevertheless, a handful of diagnoses are idiopathic conditions of immune-mediated inflammatory conditions whose diagnosis is challenging to obtain even with extensive multimodal evaluation.

Causes

Several specific disease entities and diagnoses are described here. We expand on the entities of IgG4 sclerosing cholangitis and ampullary stenosis as two particular examples of malignant mimics that have recently gained more attention in the literature.

Recurrent Pyogenic Cholangitis

Recurrent pyogenic cholangitis is addressed in detail in Chapters 39 and 44. This condition is seen mainly in Southeast Asia and is associated with intrahepatic calcium bilirubinate stones and intrahepatic strictures.[251–254] Recurrent episodes of cholangitis and sepsis are the major threat to life in these patients, along with a significantly increased risk of cholangiocarcinoma.[255–258] Hepatic resection combined with Roux-en-Y biliary-enteric reconstruction that optimizes drainage may be most effective in relieving symptoms and clearing stones. This is particularly true if the disease is unilateral, but even patients with bilateral disease may benefit from a combination of resection and postoperative balloon dilation and stone extraction.[259,260] Because of the high incidence of recurrent stricture and stone formation, a team approach that includes experienced surgeons, interventional radiologists, and gastroenterologists is required to obtain the best results.[261] Careful operative planning is important, and the operation can be tailored to help provide future access to the biliary tract. For example, we have successfully used a Roux-en-Y biliary-enteric reconstruction that not only includes the long-segment limb anchored to the abdominal wall for interventional radiology access, but a jejunoduodenostomy is also constructed, using the proximal end of the Roux limb, for easy endoscopic access in patients at high risk for recurrent stones. Some authors have reported success using balloon dilation combined with transhepatic choledochoscopic lithotripsy, either as initial therapy or for recurrent stones after surgery.[262,263] Numerous patients have advanced parenchymal disease at presentation and die from related complications, despite aggressive intervention.[255]

Chronic Pancreatitis

Chronic pancreatitis is a well-known cause of distal bile duct stenosis and stricture (see Chapters 57 and 58). The incidence of biliary stricture in these patients is difficult to know with certainty, but it has been reported in 30% of patients.[264] The characteristic lesion is a long, narrow stricture involving the retropancreatic portion of the CBD, but other variants have been described.[264,265] Although more common in association with alcohol-related chronic pancreatitis, it may occur in chronic pancreatitis unrelated to alcohol use. In addition to jaundice, pain is common, which may be intermittent and similar to biliary colic; cholangitis and fever are less frequent.[265–267]

IgG4 Systemic Disease and Sclerosing Cholangitis

IgG4 systemic disease is a rare autoimmune condition that can affect multiple organ systems. IgG4 sclerosing cholangitis is the biliary tract manifestation of this condition that has an estimated prevalence and incidence of 1.8 and 0.5 per 100,000 individuals with strong male predominance based on a 2011 epidemiologic study by Kanno et al.[268,269] IgG4 sclerosing cholangitis is histologically characterized by biliary tract strictures featuring lymphoplasmacytic infiltration, storiform fibrosis, and obliterative phlebitis. The morphology of the biliary stricture(s) can easily masquerade as hilar cholangiocarcinoma (see Chapter 51) or primary sclerosing cholangitis[250,270–273] (see Chapter 41). IgG4 sclerosing cholangitis has an association with autoimmune pancreatitis, which is the pancreatic manifestation of IgG4 disease often termed *type I autoimmune pancreatitis*. Oh et al.[270] describe a series of 16 patients with IgG4 sclerosing cholangitis, of which 10 had prior history of autoimmune pancreatitis. Extrapancreatobiliary manifestations of IgG4 disease include sialadenitis, renal infiltrates, interstitial lung disease, ocular disturbances, and hypopituitarism.

Although an elevated serum IgG4 level greater than 135 mg/dL aids in diagnosis of IgG4 systemic disease, it may not be elevated in up to 10% to 40% of patients who have this condition.[269] Full biliary tract imaging is necessary, and patterns of strictures may lend clues to the diagnosis. A classification scheme of IgG4 sclerosing cholangitis has been proposed by Nakazawa et al.[274] to aid in differentiation from primary sclerosing cholangitis (Fig. 42.15). Biliary tract biopsy is useful, but results may not entirely exclude cholangiocarcinoma as it has been demonstrated that malignancy can induce reactive histopathologic changes that share features of IgG4 sclerosing cholangitis.[250] Steroids are the mainstay of therapy for IgG4 disease, with dramatic improvements to the extent that often no procedural or surgical intervention is required to address the stricture.[270,271,273]

To aid in differentiation of IgG4 sclerosing cholangitis from biliary tract malignancy, a combination of serum IgG4, thorough evaluation for other systemic manifestations of IgG4 disease, interpretation of cholangiogram findings, review of bile duct cytology and biopsy, and careful monitoring of the clinical course should be undertaken. The limited sensitivity and specificity of

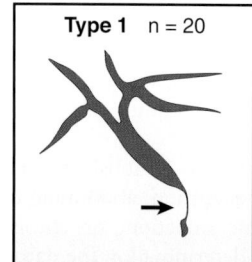
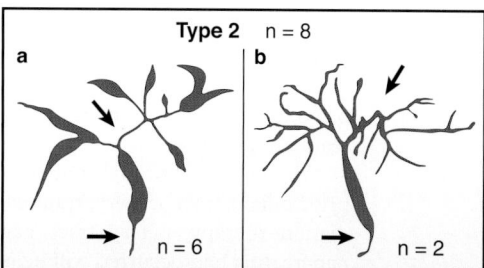
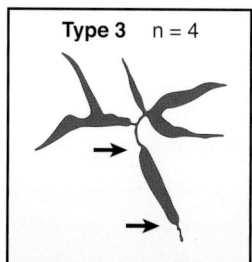
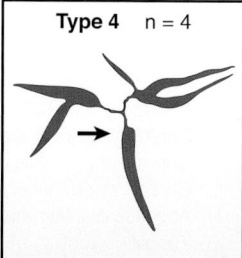

FIGURE 42.15 Cholangiogram classification for IgG4 sclerosing cholangitis proposed by Nakazawa et al, Pancreas 2006. **Type 1:** stenosis in distal portion of common bile duct. **Type 2:** stenosis of intrahepatic bile ducts with prestenotic dilation (2a), and without dilation and reduced number of bile ducts (2b). **Type 3:** stenosis at bilateral hepatic hilar bile ducts and distal common bile duct. **Type 4:** Stenosis only localized to bilateral hepatic hilar ducts.

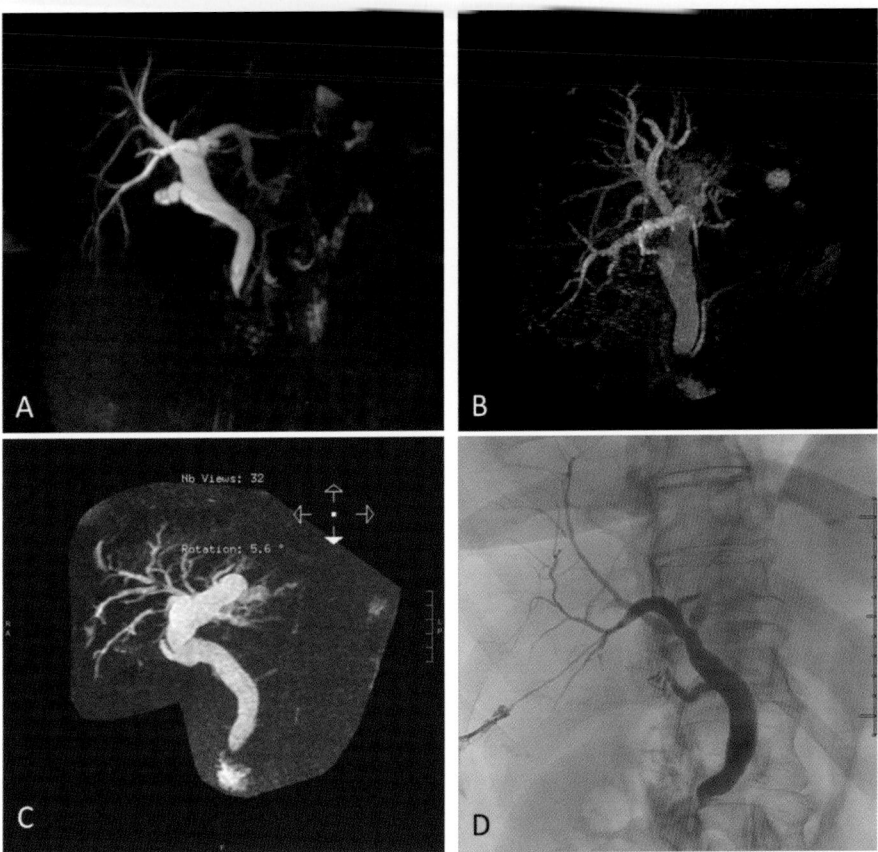

FIGURE 42.16   Imaging of Roux-en-Y gastric bypass patients who developed ampullary stenosis. Images in **A–C** are magnetic resonance cholangiopancreatography and **D** is a percutaneous transhepatic cholangiogram demonstrating biliary duct dilatation. (**A–D,** Courtesy Dr. Carlos Corvera and Dr. Andrew Wisneski.)

each modality or study in isolation mandate a comprehensive evaluation with exercise of clinical judgement.[269,270,273] Ultimately, a short course of steroids with imaging resolution confirms the diagnosis and is recommended if the diagnosis is suspected.

Ampullary Stenosis Associated With Roux-en-Y Gastric Bypass

Several case series have been published describing an association between benign distal common bile duct stricture at the ampulla in patients who had previously underwent Roux-en-Y gastric bypass for morbid obesity.[275–279] The mechanism for this process is not completely understood, but presentation can raise concern for distal cholangiocarcinoma or pancreatic adenocarcinoma. A series by Wisneski et al.[275] detailed 15 cases of this phenomenon, where initial workup was prompted by symptoms from abdominal pain to severe cholangitis. Patients were predominantly female with mean age of 54 years old. All patients underwent biliary imaging with MRCP or PTC (Fig. 42.16). A mean 7.5 years passed from the Roux-en-Y gastric bypass occurred until ampullary stenosis was diagnosed. No cases out of several published studies ever reported malignant pathology. Treatment has evolved from open ampullectomy or biliary bypass to less invasive combined laparoscopic transgastric ERCP with sphincterotomy or advanced endoscopic techniques that enable access to the ampulla with the more difficult Roux-en-Y

anatomy.[278,280,281] More invasive surgical intervention is reserved if sphincterotomy alone fails to provide adequate decompression, restenosis occurs, or malignancy is strongly suspected.

The pathophysiology of ampullary stenosis associated with Roux-en-Y gastric bypass remains to be elucidated, but it has been postulated that association with patient autoimmune conditions, chronic opioid use causing sphincter of Oddi hypertension, or GI regulatory hormonal changes after Roux-en-Y may contribute. Though this particular phenomenon appears benign, surgeons should still maintain appropriate suspicion for malignancy during workup of these patients.

BILE DUCT INJURY AT CHOLECYSTECTOMY

Laparoscopic cholecystectomy is one of the most commonly performed general surgery operations around the world and remains the leading cause of iatrogenic bile injury (see Chapter 36). This can produce biliary leaks or external biliary fistulae, and delayed formation of bile duct strictures. Hepatobiliary surgeons will often be sought to provide evaluation, management, and surgical repair of these injuries and should be familiar with all aspects of this condition and the requirements needed to provide adequate repair of bile duct injuries.

Incidence

Because of the great frequency with which the operation is performed, cholecystectomy remains the greatest source of

---

BOX 42.2   Classification of Causes of Laparoscopic Biliary Injuries

- Misidentification of the bile ducts as the cystic duct
- Misidentification of the common bile duct as the cystic duct
- Misidentification of an aberrant right sectoral hepatic duct as the cystic duct
- Technical causes
- Improper techniques of ductal exploration
- Failure to occlude the cystic duct securely
- Plane of dissection away from gallbladder wall into the liver bed
- Excessive traction on cystic duct with tenting upward of common hepatic duct
- Injudicious use of electrocautery for dissection or bleeding control
- Injudicious use of clips to control bleeding

Modified from Strasberg SM, Hertl M, Soper NJ. An analysis of the problem of biliary injury during laparoscopic cholecystectomy. *J Am Coll Surg.* 1995;180:101–125.

---

iatrogenic biliary injuries (see Chapters 34 and 36), with national incidence rates of 0.2% to 0.6%.[282,283] Laparoscopic cholecystectomy is currently the standard procedure for symptomatic cholelithiasis and for all forms of cholecystitis, including acute cholecystitis.[284–286]

Pathogenesis (Contributing Factors)

Several factors are associated with an increased risk of bile duct injury at cholecystectomy, some of which are general and some unique to the laparoscopic approach. Ultimately, the final common pathway of most injuries is either a technical error or misinterpretation of the anatomy[283,287,288] (Box 42.2). Many authors classify biliary injuries as major, such as transection of the CBD, or minor, such as biliary leak, but the line separating the two is often blurred. In general, major injuries are more serious and usually require reoperation to repair. Minor injuries are not always trivial, however, and they may require operative intervention. The classification of biliary injuries is discussed later.

Anatomic Variations

Any surgeon operating on the biliary tree must be familiar with the wide range of anatomic variations that may be encountered. Anomalies of the cystic duct insertion into the common hepatic duct are most commonly seen (Fig. 42.17). The cystic duct may join the common hepatic duct quite high, almost at the biliary confluence, or it may run parallel to the common hepatic duct for a long distance before joining it very low, occasionally at the level of the ampulla (see Chapter 2). In up to 25% of patients, the right hepatic duct per se is absent, and the right anterior and posterior sectoral hepatic ducts join the left hepatic duct independently. In some cases, one of the right sectoral hepatic ducts, usually the anterior, may follow a prolonged extrahepatic course and enter the common hepatic duct quite low, and it may receive drainage from the cystic duct (see Fig. 42.17D). Such unrecognized, low-entry right sectoral hepatic ducts are at particular risk of injury during laparoscopic cholecystectomy[289] (Fig. 42.18).

Vascular anomalies are also common, occurring in approximately 20% of patients (see Chapter 2). In the most common of these, the right hepatic arterial supply arises in part or in whole from the superior mesenteric artery. Such an aberrant vessel usually courses to the right of the portal vein, lateral and posterior to the CBD. During cholecystectomy, this vessel is

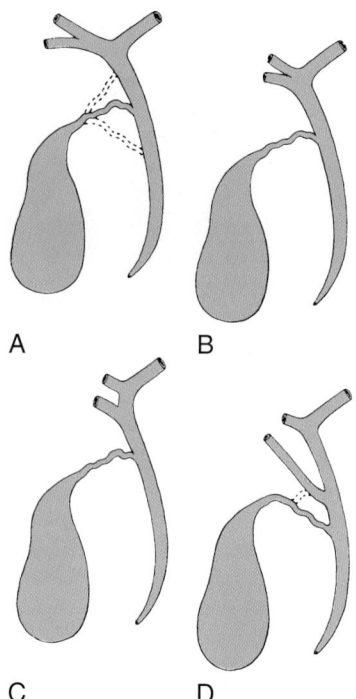

FIGURE 42.17   Schematic representations of various junctions of the cystic duct with the main extrahepatic biliary channel. **A,** The cystic duct may join the main bile duct very high, almost at the confluence of the hepatic ducts, or it may run parallel to the common hepatic duct before entering almost at the level of the ampulla of Vater. In this illustration, the right anterior and posterior sectoral hepatic ducts join to form a main right hepatic duct. **B,** The right anterior and posterior sectoral hepatic ducts may join the left hepatic duct at a common confluence. **C,** The right anterior and posterior sectoral hepatic ducts may join the left hepatic duct independently. **D,** The right anterior or posterior sectoral hepatic duct may join the common hepatic duct at a much lower level. The cystic duct may drain into such a duct. Another variation, not shown and probably not relevant for postcholecystectomy injuries, is entry of the right anterior or posterior sectoral hepatic duct into the left hepatic duct (see Chapter 2).

prone to injury at the junction of the cystic and common hepatic ducts. Vascular injuries are not limited to patients with anatomic anomalies; biliary injury during laparoscopic cholecystectomy, in which the surgeon mistakes the CBD for the cystic duct, is frequently associated with injury to the right hepatic artery.[290] This problem has been documented to occur in as many as 0.6% of patients after laparoscopic cholecystectomy and may not be apparent at the initial operation but may come to attention later as a hepatic artery pseudoaneurysm.[291–293] Rarely, concomitant vascular injury may involve both the right hepatic artery and right portal vein, which can be life threatening (Fig. 42.19).

Biliary Ischemia

In the absence of overt injury, delayed biliary stricture formation may result from extensive periductal dissection and consequent interruption of the major ductal arterial supply. Most of the arterial supply to the extrahepatic bile duct is provided by two small arteries that travel along the lateral duct borders in the 3 and 9 o'clock positions (see Chapter 2). Sixty percent of the blood supply runs upward from the major inferior vessels

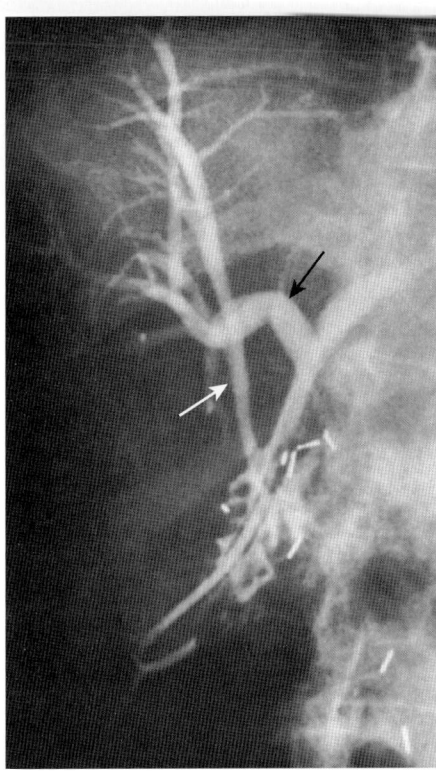

FIGURE 42.18 The right anterior sectoral hepatic duct *(white arrow)* drains into the common hepatic duct, and the right posterior sectoral hepatic duct *(black arrow)* joins a main left hepatic duct. In this patient, cholecystectomy was accompanied by a biliary injury at the point of confluence of the common hepatic duct and the right anterior sectoral hepatic duct (Bismuth type 5). Repair has been carried out by Roux-en-Y hepaticojejunostomy (see Chapter 2).

(retroduodenal, gastroduodenal), and approximately 40% runs downward from the right hepatic artery.[294] Extensive circumferential dissection of the duct may disrupt this axial blood flow and has been proposed as a mechanism of biliary stricture formation. Although there is no direct evidence to support this, it would seem reasonable not to pursue extensive skeletonization of the common duct during cholecystectomy. Also, damage to these vessels is likely to be a contributing factor, if not the central factor, in the formation of strictures attributed to electrocautery use.

Pathologic Factors

Patients with acute cholecystitis may have severe inflammation in the porta hepatis and triangle of Calot, which greatly distorts the anatomy. In addition, the gallbladder is often distended, friable, and difficult to grasp, and persistent oozing of blood often obscures the field. Some or all of these factors may conspire to preclude safe laparoscopic cholecystectomy. When laparoscopic cholecystectomy is performed for acute cholecystitis, studies have also revealed a greater potential for biliary injury[295] (see Chapter 34). Fletcher et al.[296] reported that complex cases that include patients with acute cholecystitis, cholangitis, and gallstone pancreatitis are associated with a dramatically increased incidence of bile duct injuries (1.7%), although acute cholecystitis alone is not an independent risk factor. Other authors have shown that acute cholecystitis increases the incidence of bile duct injuries 2-fold to 3-fold.[297–299] Given this increased risk of

biliary injury in these settings, alternative techniques need to be in the armamentarium of the biliary surgeon.

Fluorescent Cholangiography for Bile Duct Visualization

Intraoperative cholangiography is a technique that helps delineate biliary anatomy and is helpful to verify anatomy during laparoscopic cholecystectomy to prevent common bile duct injury (see Chapter 24). However, it exposes the surgical team to radiation and requires a fluoroscopic C-arm that can be cumbersome to set up. Additionally, direct cannulation of the cystic duct and injection of contrast can be harmful to the bile ducts particularly in cases with severe inflammation. Fluorescent cholangiography with indocyanine green (ICG) is a newly pioneered alternative to fluoroscopic cholangiography and has become more widely available with greater adoption of robotic surgical platforms in general surgery and hepatobiliary surgery.[300–303] It requires intravenous (IV) injection of ICG and on near-infrared imaging, viable tissues are highlighted. Fluorescent cholangiography requires no radiation, no C-arm, and the infrared image can be obtained almost instantly at any point during the operation.

Several studies have reported the benefits of fluorescent cholangiography during laparoscopic cholecystectomy with or without a robotic surgical platform and concluded that it is safe and effective. Success rates in visualizing the cystic duct, common bile duct, and common hepatic duct were reported at 97.8%, 96.1%, and 94%, respectively.[304] Visualization of accessory hepatic ducts, variants of cystic duct insertion to the common bile duct (classic vs. parallel vs. spiral type), have been described.[301,302,305] Operative times were not adversely affected and may even be quicker than when using traditional fluoroscopic cholangiography.[303,304,306] The use of ICG as an IV contrast agent is safe, with an adverse reaction rate of 0.003%.[301,305]

The near-infrared light emitted for fluorescent cholangiography imaging can only penetrate tissue to a depth of 5 to 10 mm, thus its effectiveness could be reduced in excessively fatty tissues in patients with higher body mass index.[306] It is important to emphasize that fluorescent cholangiography cannot detect the presence of common bile duct stones.[304] To date, most studies on fluorescent cholangiography represent single-center series and no randomized controlled trials have been published. There is not yet enough data to draw broad conclusions about its impact on CBD injury rate. Fluorescent cholangiography shows promise as a useful adjunct to perform safe laparoscopic cholecystectomy, especially with greater availability of robotic surgical platforms.

Subtotal Cholecystectomy for Severe Cholecystitis: Fenestration Versus Reconstruction

When confronted with severe acute cholecystitis, the surgeon must consider alternative strategies to safely visualize key structures in the triangle of Calot, obtain the critical view of safety, and avoid injury to vital structures (see Chapters 34 and 36). Historically, open cholecystectomy is considered a standard alternative if the laparoscopic approach is difficult. This notion has recently been challenged because the concern that trainees no longer encounter open cholecystectomy frequently enough to become competent with this procedure.[307] A study from The Netherlands challenged the assertion that open cholecystectomy was a safe approach to the difficult cholecystectomy. A retrospective analysis was performed on

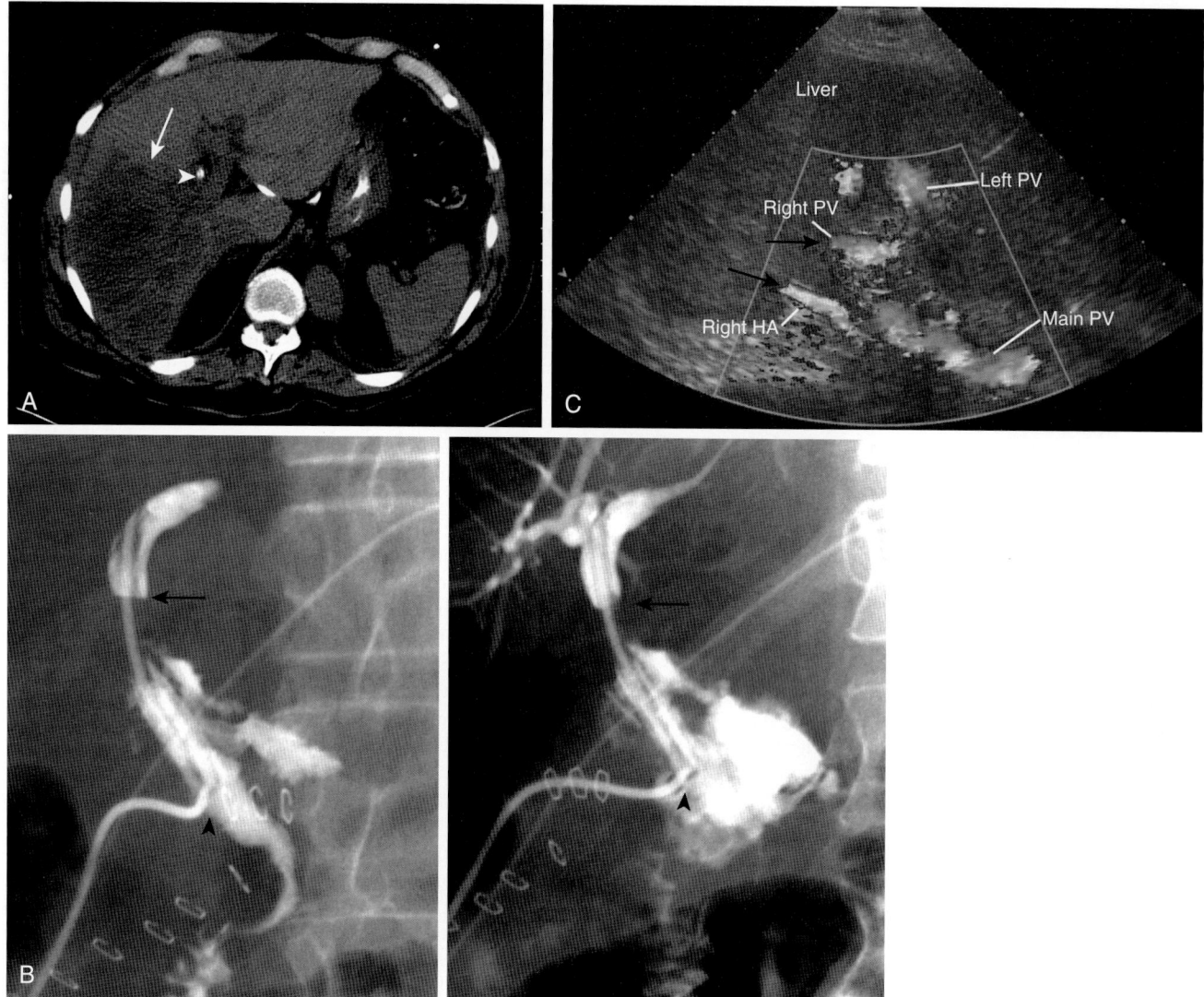

FIGURE 42.19 **A,** Transaxial computed tomography scan without intravenous contrast demonstrating the hypoperfused right lobe *(white arrow)* and an intraoperatively placed biliary tube *(arrowhead)*. In this patient, the surgeon was confronted with significant bleeding during laparoscopic cholecystectomy and converted to open operation. Bleeding involved the right hepatic artery *(HA)* and portal vein *(PV)*; these were suture ligated to control the hemorrhage. **B,** A tube cholangiogram demonstrates the "classic" biliary injury during laparoscopic cholecystectomy: the common bile duct was mistaken for the cystic duct, and a long section of the common duct was excised up to the common hepatic duct *(arrow)*. The *arrowhead* points to the tube insertion site in the distal common duct. **C,** Doppler ultrasonography demonstrates lack of flow in both the right HA and PV *(arrows)*.

bile duct injury patients, and it was found that a greater percentage of more complex bile duct injuries (defined as Bismuth III–V) occurred *after* conversion from laparoscopic to open approach than to when no conversion occurred (65% vs. 34%; $P = .013$). Merely converting from laparoscopic to an open cholecystectomy was fraught with heightened risk for bile duct injury, and in the absence of extensive training with safe open cholecystectomy technique, it was advocated for greater use of subtotal cholecystectomy or drainage.

Subtotal cholecystectomy, by definition, removes the majority of the gallbladder. The anterior free portion of the gallbladder is removed, and the posterior gallbladder wall adherent to the liver aspect is either removed if possible, or if remaining in situ is ablated with cautery. The lower portion of the gallbladder at the infundibulum remains in place. How the remnant gallbladder is addressed differentiates two variants of subtotal

cholecystectomy technique: fenestration versus reconstitution. With the fenestration technique, the remnant is left open; with reconstitution the remnant is sutured or stapled closed.[308] A meta-analysis of 30 articles and 1231 subtotal cholecystectomies determined that this approach was overall a safe alternative to total cholecystectomy.[309] When comparing open versus laparoscopic subtotal cholecystectomy, the laparoscopic approach resulted in fewer subhepatic collections, retained stones, wound infections, and reoperations but lead to a greater rate of bile leakage. Rates of bile leakage comparing fenestration and reconstitution techniques were 42.0% versus 16.5%, but this did not attain statistical significance. There was only one case of CBD injury (0.08%) during subtotal cholecystectomy.

There is little evidence examining direct comparison of the fenestration versus reconstitution techniques. One recently published study by Van Dijk et al.[310] examined 191 patients who underwent subtotal cholecystectomy where both techniques were used. Per operation reports, fenestration was performed more often when fibrosis was noted, whereas reconstitution was done when anatomic visualization was incomplete. As might be predicted, bile leak occurred more frequently after fenestration (18% vs. 7%). However, at a median 6-year follow-up, recurrence of biliary events was lower after fenestration than reconstitution (9% vs. 18%). Overall reintervention rate did not significantly differ between the two groups. Contrary to expectations, completion cholecystectomy was performed more often in the fenestration group with patients having CBD stones, cholecystitis of the remnant, and cholangitis. One case describes findings of an inflammatory mass resected en bloc, with histopathology confirming presence of gallbladder tissue with chronic inflammation. It is difficult to offer a blanket recommendation with such limited and biased data, but surgeons should be aware of the two subtotal cholecystectomy techniques. The decision driving use of fenestration versus reconstitutions may be influenced by intraoperative assessment of the anatomy, degree of inflammation or fibrosis, and surgeon comfort with techniques.

Location and Classification

The ease of management, operative risk, and outcome of biliary injuries vary considerably and depend on the type of injury and its location.[311,312] It has long been recognized that strictures involving the CBD or distal common hepatic duct are easier to repair than are more proximal injuries. The anatomic classification of Bismuth has been widely adopted in recognition of this fact[313] (Fig. 42.20). In this classification scheme, five stricture

types are recognized, reflecting the location with respect to the hepatic duct confluence (types 1–4) or the involvement of an aberrant right sectoral hepatic duct with or without a concomitant hepatic duct stricture (type 5).

The Bismuth classification is useful for localization and for prognosis after repair, but it does not encompass the entire spectrum of injuries that are possible. No provision is made for simple bile leaks or major ductal injuries without stricture. Even within the group of patients with bile leaks, there are varying degrees of severity. In an effort to fill this gap, Strasberg et al.[283] proposed a comprehensive classification system that incorporates Bismuth's scheme but is much broader in scope (Fig. 42.21). Injuries are classified as type A to type E, with the latter representing biliary strictures and further subdivided as E1 to E5 according to the Bismuth classification. *Type A* injuries are bile leaks from minor ducts still in continuity with the

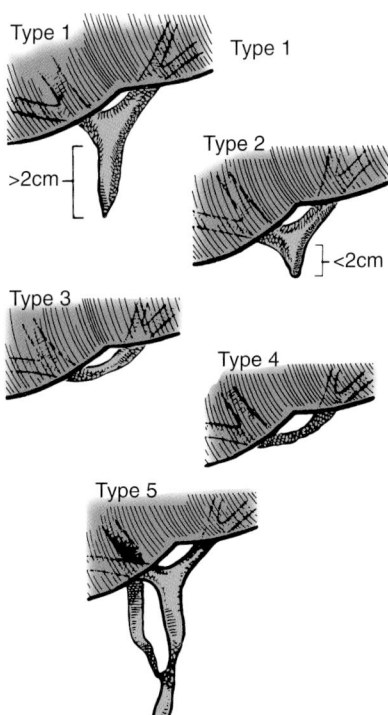

FIGURE 42.20 Classification of bile duct strictures based on location with respect to the hepatic duct confluence (see Table 42.1). (From Bismuth H: Postoperative strictures of the bile duct. In Blumgart LH [ed]: *The biliary tract: Clinical surgery international.* Edinburgh, 1982, Churchill Livingstone, pp 209–218.)

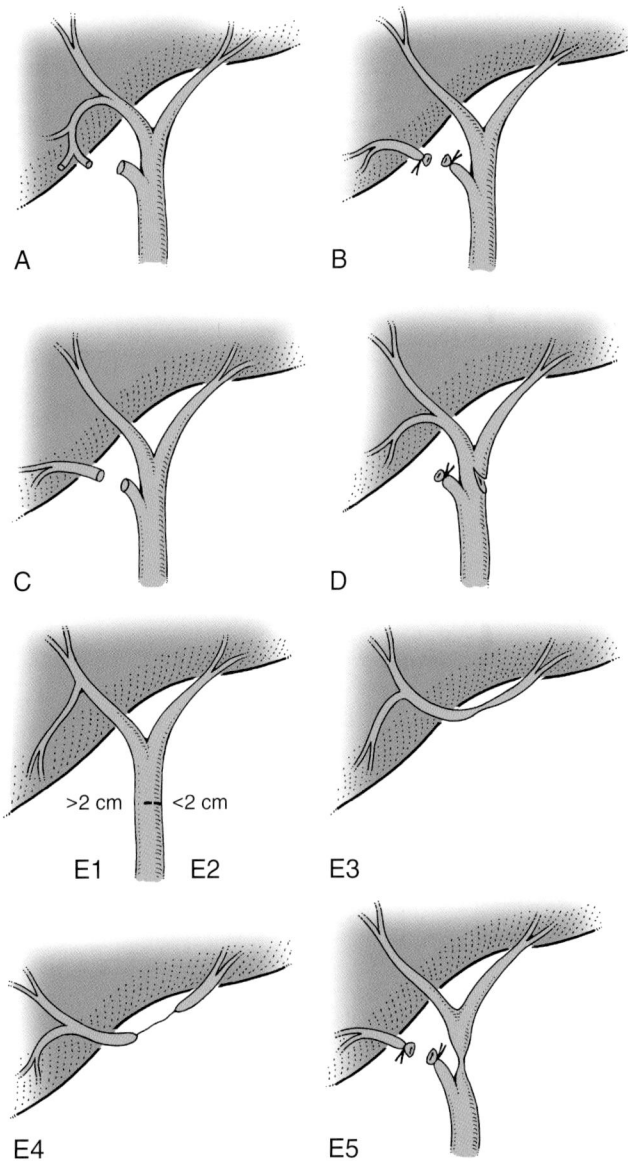

FIGURE 42.21 Classification of laparoscopic biliary injuries according to Strasberg et al. (1995).[283] Injuries are stratified from type A to type E. Type E injuries are subdivided further into E1 to E5 according to the Bismuth classification system.

CBD. This encompasses the most common causes of bile leaks seen after laparoscopic cholecystectomy—leakage from the cystic duct and from a subvesical duct of Luschka. *Type B* injuries involve occlusion of part of the biliary tree, which for practical purposes almost always is an aberrant right sectoral hepatic duct. When this duct is transected without ligation, the injury is termed *type C*, reflecting the differences in presentation and management between the two. A lateral injury to an extrahepatic bile duct is termed *type D*, which is similar to type A injuries in that the extrahepatic biliary tree remains in continuity but is classified separately to underscore the greater severity and potential need for major reconstruction.

The Stewart-Way classification of laparoscopic bile duct injury was published in 2003, after analysis of 252 cases of major bile duct injury that occurred during laparoscopic cholecystectomy (Fig. 42.22).[288] Four classes of injury are described. Class I injury (7%) results from incomplete transection of the CBD with no loss of duct. Class II injury (22%) occurs from lateral damage to the common hepatic duct that produces stricture or fistula, usually from clips or cautery damage to the lateral aspect of the duct. Class III injuries were the most common (61%) and involved full transection of the CBD and a variable portion of the proximal duct. Class IV injuries (10%) entailed transection or damage to the right hepatic duct, and many had concurrent right hepatic artery injury.

The incidence of each type of biliary injury is difficult to ascertain with certainty. Most literature reports are derived from tertiary referral centers and are biased toward more severe injuries. Most surgical series focus on management of Strasberg type E biliary strictures, whereas endoscopic and radiologic reports are concerned mainly with the treatment of bile leaks. Type A injuries may be the most common, but many are managed successfully without referral and are underrepresented in reports from major centers.[283]

Biliary Injury: Clinical Presentation

The range of injury can result in bile leak or external biliary fistulae, which may be recognized or present in the immediate postoperative period. Vascular injuries, thermal injury, or traction injury to the duct not causing frank bile leak may lead to delayed formation of a stricture, which may present weeks to months postoperatively with obstructive liver function tests, jaundice, or ascending cholangitis. Most patients with postcholecystectomy biliary injuries, if not diagnosed at operation, come to medical attention early in the postoperative period.[290,314,315]

The clinical presentation depends on the type of injury; conversely, the type of injury may be inferred based on the clinical picture at presentation. Patients with significant bile leaks (types A, C, and D) generally present within the first week after operation, but some leaks may not become apparent for several weeks, and few are diagnosed intraoperatively.[283] Most patients have abdominal pain coupled with fever or other signs of sepsis or bile leakage from an incision. A few patients have none of these signs and symptoms but rather have nonspecific complaints of weakness, fatigue, or anorexia. Elevated alkaline phosphatase levels are characteristic, as is mild hyperbilirubinemia, but markedly elevated serum bilirubin levels (>3 mg/dL) are uncommon.[316,317]

Major injuries to the common duct (type E injuries) are more likely to be discovered intraoperatively, although most remain unrecognized until after operation. Similar to bile leaks, these injuries are more often diagnosed within the first few postoperative weeks, although patients with a slowly evolving stricture may not come to attention for several months, which is distinctly uncommon for patients with bile leaks.[283] Most patients with these injuries present with jaundice, often coupled with pain and occasionally sepsis. Jaundice is not always present early in the course of the illness. In some patients, the stricture may evolve slowly or cause only partial obstruction. Such patients may have nonspecific complaints, pruritus, or derangements in LFTs, any or all of which should prompt an investigation. In addition, patients with an isolated right sectoral hepatic duct injury (type B) or an internal biliary fistula may be seen initially with a history of unexplained fevers, pain, or general debilitation.

The findings on physical examination are often nonspecific. Jaundice, if present, is usually obvious, and there may be multiple skin excoriations from pruritus. Abdominal distention and pain may be seen in patients with bile peritonitis, whereas focal tenderness suggests a localized collection or abscess. Hepatomegaly may be seen with long-standing biliary obstruction. Splenomegaly or other signs of portal hypertension are uncommon, but if present, should alert the surgeon to the possibility of concomitant portal venous injury or severe underlying hepatocellular damage. The presence of portal hypertension in association with a biliary stricture portends a poor outcome, and its identification is therefore important.

Pathologic Consequences

Fibrosis

Biliary obstruction is associated with the formation of high local concentrations of bile salts at the canalicular membrane, and these initiate pathologic changes in the liver.[318] Bile thrombi form within dilated centrilobular bile canaliculi, and secondary changes develop in adjacent hepatocytes. A complex cascade of molecular and cellular events ensues, collectively termed *fibrogenesis*, which ultimately leads to the deposition of collagen and other extracellular matrix proteins and eventually to fibrosis and scarring around bile ducts and ductules[319–323]

**Stewart-Way Classification
Laparoscopic Bile Duct Injuries**

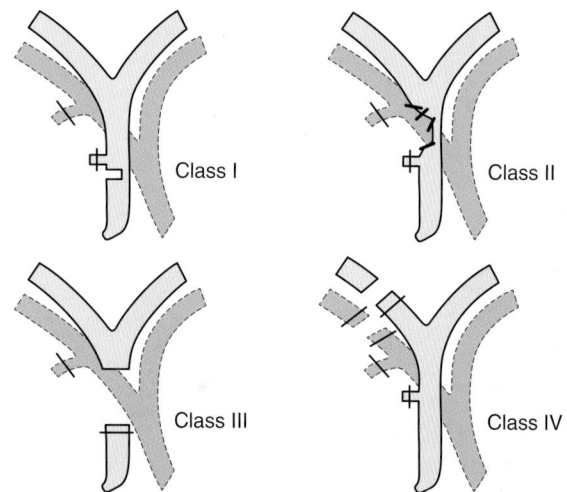

FIGURE 42.22 The Stewart-Way classification of laparoscopic bile duct injury. (Courtesy Dr. Lawrence Way and Dr. Lygia Stewart.)

(see Chapter 7). As this process progresses, mechanical interference with bile flow develops in these intrahepatic biliary radicles and perpetuates cholestasis.

Fibrosis is accompanied by liver cell hyperplasia; this is not true in secondary biliary cirrhosis because the lobular structure of the liver is usually well preserved (Fig. 42.23), and the marked fibrosis that occurs in advanced cases only rarely progresses to true cirrhosis.[324] This knowledge is important in planning therapy because many of these pathologic changes are reversible.[325] A histologic return of normal liver parenchyma is seen after relief of obstruction in both animal and human models, which correlates with the return to near-normal liver function after relief of biliary obstruction.[326–328] Fibrosis also may develop in the extrahepatic ducts proximal to the stricture, which is especially likely after biliary intubation. Upward retraction of the ducts is accompanied by a sequence of mucosal atrophy, squamous metaplasia, inflammatory infiltration, and further fibrosis in the subepithelial layers of the ducts.

Atrophy

The distribution of liver mass is regulated by a poorly understood balance of bile flow, portal venous inflow, and hepatic venous outflow (see Chapter 6). Segmental or lobar atrophy may result from portal venous obstruction or bile duct occlusion in the affected area. Unilobar atrophy is associated with hypertrophy of the contralateral lobe and may present diagnostic and operative difficulties. Liver lobe atrophy and compensatory hypertrophy are frequently found in benign strictures and may be associated with asymmetric involvement of lobar or sectoral hepatic ducts, interference with portal venous blood supply, or decreased portal perfusion owing to secondary fibrosis. In benign strictures, the dilated ducts within the atrophic segments often are filled with infected bile and debris, and even though drainage of an atrophic segment would not be effective in relieving jaundice, cholangitis may continue unabated unless satisfactory drainage of the atrophic and hypertrophic segments is achieved.

The presence of significant atrophy and compensatory hypertrophy greatly influences the approach to repair (see Chapter 32). The most common situation is gross hypertrophy of the left lobe accompanied by right lobe atrophy.[329] Anastomosis in the region of the hilum is made difficult by the rotational deformity and anatomic distortion imposed by this condition. A thoracoabdominal approach to such strictures may be necessary to provide more direct exposure and access for repair by allowing rotation of the liver to the left.[313] Reports verify that atrophy and contralateral hypertrophy are associated with significantly longer reconstructive operations, higher intraoperative blood loss, and greater blood transfusion requirements.[330] Similar problems may occur in bile duct strictures after right hepatic resection.

Portal Hypertension

It is estimated that approximately 15% to 20% of patients with benign biliary stricture have concomitant portal hypertension[311,331] (see Chapter 74). Patients with biliary strictures may develop portal hypertension as a result of secondary hepatic fibrosis or direct damage to the portal vein. Alternatively, portal hypertension may be due to preexisting liver disease. It is important that these patients undergo further workup to exclude underlying chronic parenchymal disease. Iatrogenic biliary injuries are often the subject of medicolegal proceedings, and precise documentation of all injuries is essential to provide an accurate assessment of the cause of symptoms and prognosis. The outcome of patients with biliary strictures and portal hypertension is much worse than for patients without portal hypertension, with an in-hospital mortality rate of 25% to 40%.[311,331] It has been suggested, however, that adequate biliary drainage may be followed by some resolution of fibrosis and perhaps a reduction in portal pressure.[328]

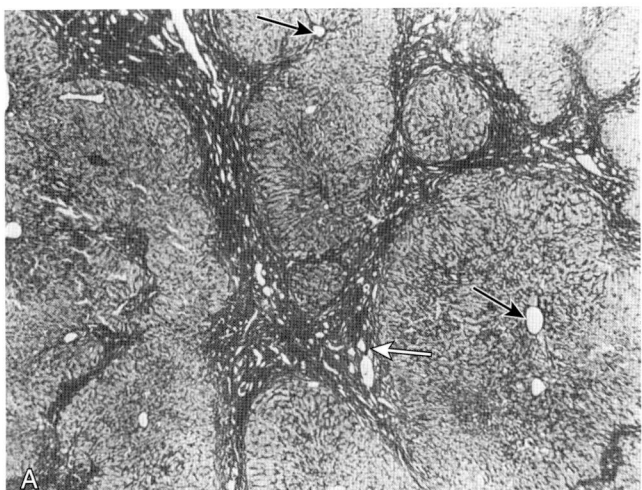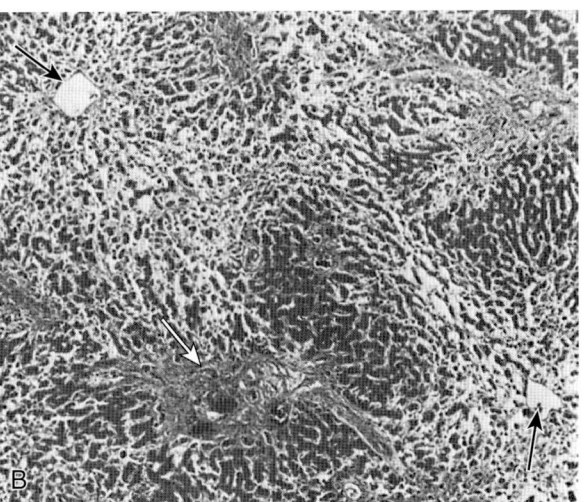

FIGURE 42.23 A, Photomicrograph showing the effect of long-standing biliary obstruction secondary to benign biliary stricture. Hepatic fibrosis is present, but with preservation of the basic hepatic architecture, with the portal tract *(white arrow)* and hepatic venous radicles *(black arrows)* maintaining their normal relationships. The fibrosis extends between the lobules, but the pattern is not one of true cirrhosis, in which there is destruction of the basic hepatic architecture. **B,** Extensive fibrosis with a substantially normal relationship of hepatic venous radicles *(black arrows)* to portal tracts *(white arrow)* in a patient with portal hypertension (see Chapter 7). (From Weinbren K, Hadjis NS, & Blumgart LH. Structural aspects of the liver in patients with biliary disease and portal hypertension. *J Clin Pathol.* 1985;38:1013–1020.)

Management

Successful management of patients with postcholecystectomy bile duct injuries requires careful planning. The importance of thorough investigation and patient preparation cannot be overemphasized. Before any intervention, the surgeon must define the type and extent of injury and treat life-threatening co-existing conditions such as sepsis, cholangitis, ongoing biliary leakage, and abscess. Hasty treatment decisions based on incomplete data are more likely to exacerbate an already difficult situation. Imaging studies play a central role in assessing patients with biliary injuries and should be directed at answering the following questions: Is there a bile collection or abscess? Is there ongoing bile leakage? What is the level and extent of injury in the biliary tree? Are there associated vascular injuries? Is there evidence of lobar atrophy?

Radiologic Investigations

In patients with biliary strictures, complete delineation of the level and extent of injury is necessary. All branches of the right and left intrahepatic biliary tree must be outlined, particularly in cases of high bile duct stricture and recurrent stricture after previous reconstruction. Displaying the hepatic duct confluence (if intact) and the left ductal system and its branches is especially important in selecting the appropriate reconstruction.

CT is often the best initial study, the results of which help direct further investigations. A good-quality CT scan with arterial and portal venous phases shows a dilated biliary tree and helps localize the level of ductal obstruction in patients with strictures and can identify related vascular issues (see Chapter 16). In addition, CT identifies fluid collections or ascites and lobar atrophy. Duplex ultrasonography is an excellent, noninvasive means of showing intrahepatic ductal dilation and may reveal a subhepatic fluid collection or evidence of vascular damage. Although ultrasound may provide valuable information regarding the level of biliary injury, it is of little value in assessing the extent of a stricture and is of no value if the biliary tree is decompressed.

Complete biliary imaging is a necessity in preoperative planning for repair of bile duct injury or stricture. Several modalities have been mentioned previously, and PTC has often been considered a gold standard for this purpose. However, with the advent of MRCP in the 1990s coupled with advances in imaging technology and resolution, MRCP alone can often provide adequate complete biliary tract imaging in a noninvasive manner.[332–334] Multiple studies have confirmed the accuracy and utility of MRCP in biliary tract pathology evaluation, especially for bile duct injury characterization.[333,335–341] Expanding the use of MRI for detection of bile leaks has been made possible with recent advances in IV contrast agents that are hepatocyte specific.

ERCP is invasive, and has a shortcoming of being unable to provide high-quality delineation proximal to the injury site depending on severity of the stricture or injury due to discontinuity of the CBD preventing adequate visualization of the intrahepatic biliary tree.[342] PTC is also invasive and is accompanied with 2% major risk of complications from the procedure itself, including hemorrhage, cholangitis, or bile leak. Additionally, ERCP and PTC may miss isolated bile ducts.[336,337,341,343]

MRCP can offer complete biliary tract imaging proximal and distal to the injury in a noninvasive manner, without the need for contrast agents. At our institution, we do not require all patients to undergo ERCP or PTC before bile duct injury repair if a high-quality MRCP has been obtained. PTC or ERCP do offer therapeutic advantage if a need for biliary decompression or stenting was determined to be necessary as part of the treatment plan.[336,342] We encourage institutions to consider use of noninvasive modalities if imaging is to be obtained solely for diagnosis and preoperative planning purposes.

PTC remains a standard investigation in this setting (see Chapters 31 and 52). Drainage catheters should be left in place following PTC if a complex injury is identified on cholangiogram because palpation of the catheter intraoperatively may help guide identification of ductal structures during definitive repair. The risk of PTC-related cholangitis can be reduced with prophylactic antibiotics. ERCP is seldom of value in the precise diagnosis of complete proximal bile duct strictures because there is often discontinuity of the CBD preventing visualization of the intrahepatic ductal system. ERCP may be more helpful for incomplete strictures (stenoses) and is appropriate for patients with a history of sphincteric damage at previous common duct exploration, or if there is suspicion of papillary stenosis or other periampullary pathology. ERCP also has a role in the diagnosis and treatment of patients with bile leakage from the cystic duct stump or from a laceration of the common duct[316] (see Chapter 30). These patients have evidence of an intraabdominal fluid collection on CT. After percutaneous drainage, biliary scintigraphy (e.g., HIDA scan) can be used to establish the presence of a persistent bile leak (see Chapter 18). ERCP may then be applied to identify the location of the leak, and placement of a stent may reduce or eliminate bile leakage; however, many bile leaks resolve with percutaneous drainage alone, and ERCP is probably unnecessary in the absence of radiographic or clinical evidence of ongoing bile drainage.[316]

Isotopic scanning techniques may be valuable in assessing bile duct strictures, particularly the functional assessment of incomplete strictures, previous biliary reconstructions, and isolated sectoral hepatic duct strictures. HIDA scanning offers a dynamic and quantitative assessment of liver function and of the clearance of bile across anastomoses and stenoses[344] (Fig. 42.24) (see Chapter 18). In patients with hepatocellular disease, HIDA scanning may be valuable in distinguishing the contribution of the biliary obstruction from that of the intrinsic liver disease to the overall biochemical and symptomatic picture. In such cases, the bilirubin level may be normal, but the alkaline phosphatase level is increased. HIDA scanning also is valuable during follow-up of patients after surgical repair. Because it can be repeated and is noninvasive, it is of particular value in showing anastomotic patency and function when no tube has been left across the anastomosis at the time of repair (see Fig. 42.24B). An isolated sectoral hepatic duct stricture is suggested by delayed clearance of isotope from a portion of the liver.

Arteriography and delayed-phase portography can be obtained to assess for vascular injury (see Chapter 21). However, modern CT techniques with appropriate multiphasic radiologic protocols are nearly always sufficient to analyze vascular injuries and patency. The combination of biliary and vascular injuries often leads to segmental or lobar atrophy, but this may also be seen with long-standing biliary obstruction alone. An atrophic lobe may be evident on the initial ultrasound or CT scan and appears as a small, often hypoperfused area with dilated, irregular, and crowded bile ducts (see Chapters 51B and 52). Isotopic scanning may show what appears to be a filling defect in the affected area. It is important to recognize lobar atrophy

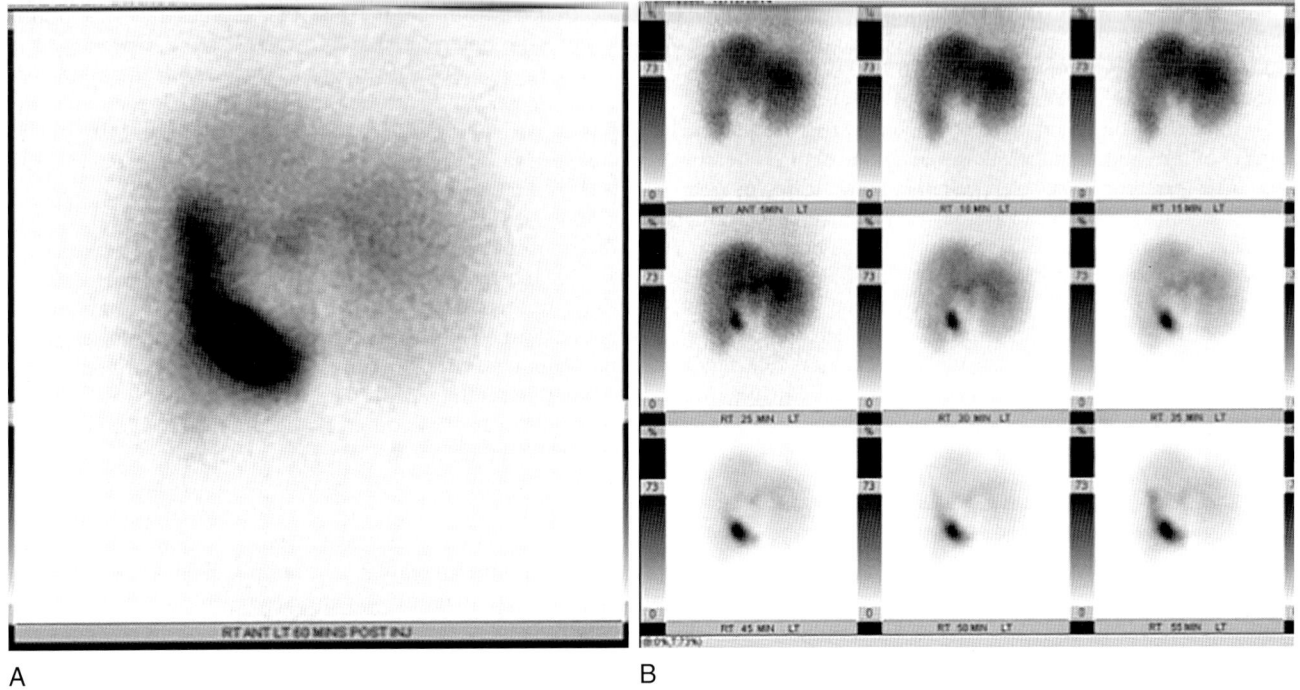

FIGURE 42.24   A hepatobiliary iminodiacetic acid scan was obtained several days after biliary injury. After 60 minutes, there is contrast retention in an isolated sectoral duct, suggestive of stricture causing delayed biliary excretion (see Chapter 18).

on the cross-sectional imaging studies, not only because it is an indicator of a likely concomitant vascular injury, but also because it would change the operative approach during repair.[345] In addition, patients with combined bile duct and hepatic artery injuries seem to be at increased risk for severe complications, such as hepatic necrosis and abscess, after reconstructive surgery. A patient undergoing biliary reconstruction in the setting of hepatic artery occlusion may also be at greater risk of late stricture recurrence.[346]

Occasionally, injection of contrast material into an established biliary fistula or percutaneous drain outlines the ductal system. Such studies may complement information provided by formal PTC, particularly if the fistula or tube tract drains an excluded sectoral duct. Because bacterial colonization or biliary infection is inevitable in such cases, it is wise to administer prophylactic antibiotics before and after these studies.

Preoperative Preparation

In general, operative repair of bile duct injuries need not be rushed, the exceptions being treatment of bile duct injuries recognized at the time of initial cholecystectomy or, rarely, emergency treatment of suppurative cholangitis or peritonitis. For most patients, there is ample time to treat co-existing conditions and to perform a full investigation, both of which increase the likelihood of a successful outcome.[311,347]

Cholangitis is a frequent occurrence in patients with bile duct strictures, especially after ductal intubation (see Chapter 43). Administration of IV antibiotics is important before surgical treatment, and the results from bile cultures obtained at PTC should be used to direct therapy. Patients with severe cholangitis and sepsis are unlikely to respond to antibiotics alone and should be submitted to percutaneous drainage before surgery. Preoperative antibiotics are usually adequate to manage milder

attacks and should be used in patients with no clinical evidence of cholangitis, given the high incidence of bacterial contamination. Antibiotic regimens should consider the frequent presence of anaerobic organisms and enterococci in patients with biliary obstruction.[348,349] We use antibiotics immediately before operation and continue appropriate treatment for 5 to 7 days postoperatively if cholangitis is a preoperative feature. Van Lent et al.[350] reported that nearly 50% of patients in their series who presented with biliary obstruction and underwent endoscopic drainage demonstrated culture-positive bacteremia. Emerging reports suggest that a shorter duration of antibiotics may be reasonable once the patient is afebrile, if the biliary tract can be drained.[351] Although no firm data exist to guide the duration of treatment, the markedly increased incidence of postoperative infectious complications in patients with endoscopic or percutaneous stents suggests that a prolonged course of treatment is justified.[348] These data further suggest that jaundice without evidence of cholangitis is not an indication for biliary intubation.

Anemia should be corrected and coagulation defects, which typically manifest as a prolongation of the prothrombin time, should be treated with vitamin K or fresh frozen plasma. Patients with prolonged illness may be seen with malnutrition. Enteral feedings through a fine-bore nasal catheter may be successful in some cases but may not be tolerated in sufficient amounts, and parenteral nutrition may be necessary. Despite these measures, however, weight gain is sometimes difficult to achieve, and to date no prospective randomized trials have shown a benefit from short-term preoperative nutritional support. A significant external bile fistula predisposes to excessive fluid and electrolyte loss and may lead to hyponatremia and acidosis.[344] It is imperative to correct fluid deficits and electrolyte imbalances before operation.

The preoperative management of complications of biliary injuries, such as biliary peritonitis, subphrenic or subhepatic abscess, hemorrhage from erosive gastritis or esophageal varices, or hepatic failure secondary to fibrosis, must be addressed before biliary reconstruction can be considered. In general, drainage of intraabdominal abscesses and control of GI hemorrhage takes priority; however, if systemic sepsis arises from an obstructed biliary tree, a factor that may contribute to other complications, immediate biliary drainage is essential. In such desperately ill patients, it is preferable to perform rapid percutaneous drainage to allow further resuscitative measures with IV antibiotics and hydration to prevent renal insufficiency. Management of portal hypertension and external bile fistula occurring in association with stricture is addressed subsequently.

Surgical Treatment

This section provides an overview pertaining to surgical management of bile duct injuries, and the reader is advised to review Part 10 for further details on specific operative techniques. The most appropriate management of bile duct injuries depends on the injury type and the timing of injury diagnosis relative to the index operation.

INJURY RECOGNIZED AT INITIAL OPERATION. If injury to the extrahepatic biliary tree is recognized at the time of initial cholecystectomy, the surgeon should consider his or her experience and ability to repair it immediately. The advice of a more experienced surgeon should be sought if possible. The situation is not immediately desperate, and there is always time to wait a short while for another opinion and for additional assistance. Substantial evidence suggests that immediate open conversion and repair by an experienced surgeon is associated with reduced morbidity, shorter duration of illness, and lower cost.[347,352] A multivariate analysis of bile duct injuries by Stewart and Way identified timing of biliary reconstruction as being insignificant when patient preoperative condition, complete cholangiography, surgical technique, and surgeon experience are optimized.[353]

Despite the apparent ability to perform biliary reconstruction electively, several studies have cited the benefits of early referral to a tertiary center, as such institutions have specialized hepatobiliary surgeons and radiologists to diagnose and treat biliary complications in a timely fashion.[354,355] Each failed repair is associated with some loss of bile duct length and greatly exacerbates an already difficult situation.[356] This is particularly true of injuries involving the biliary confluence, in which failure of the initial repair and loss of bile duct length may result in isolation of the right and left hepatic ducts; repair becomes more difficult, and the likelihood of a successful outcome is reduced.[311] If the surgeon cannot perform a reasonable repair and experienced help is unavailable, drains should be placed to control any biliary leak, and the patient should be referred to a specialist center.

INJURY RECOGNIZED IN THE IMMEDIATE POSTOPERATIVE PERIOD. Biliary injuries not appreciated intraoperatively may appear in the first few days after operation. In the setting of an external biliary fistula, the essential consideration in management is to avoid early reoperation. It is wiser to take full stock of the situation, to carry out appropriate investigations as described earlier, and to keep the patient well-nourished and free of

infection. If fistulography or other studies reveal continuity between the biliary system and the GI tract, a prolonged period of drainage is warranted and may result in spontaneous closure, provided that there is no distal obstruction to bile flow. This is particularly true of bile leakage from the cystic duct or a subvesical duct of Luschka (type A) or from a noncircumferential laceration (type D).

More severe lacerations or complete transections of the common duct or an aberrant right sectoral hepatic duct with ongoing bile leakage require careful consideration. Because the biliary tree is decompressed, the proximal ducts are small in caliber. Immediate surgical treatment of these injuries is difficult. Adequate repair requires exposing healthy bile duct mucosa within a sufficiently dilated proximal duct to allow precise anastomosis. In the setting of a decompressed biliary tree and significant inflammation, this exposure can be quite demanding or even impossible. A delayed approach may be the most appropriate course of action. If fluid losses from the biliary fistula remain high over a prolonged period, a useful but rarely used technique is creation of a temporary internal fistulojejunostomy, with definitive repair deferred for a later date.[227] Alternatively, placement of an endoscopic or percutaneous stent across the defect may reduce output from the fistula, hasten closure, and make operative management easier (Fig 42.25). Long-term results of such interventions have shown excellent results, and often, greater than 90% of patients with peripheral leaks or strictures can be treated endoscopically, although this therapy can be associated with complications, including cholangitis, hepatic abscess, and stent occlusion and migration.[357,358] Some authors advocate early endoscopic sphincterotomy to decrease the relative resistance of transpapillary bile drainage to promote closure.[359–362] Although these approaches are occasionally useful, no evidence is available to show that

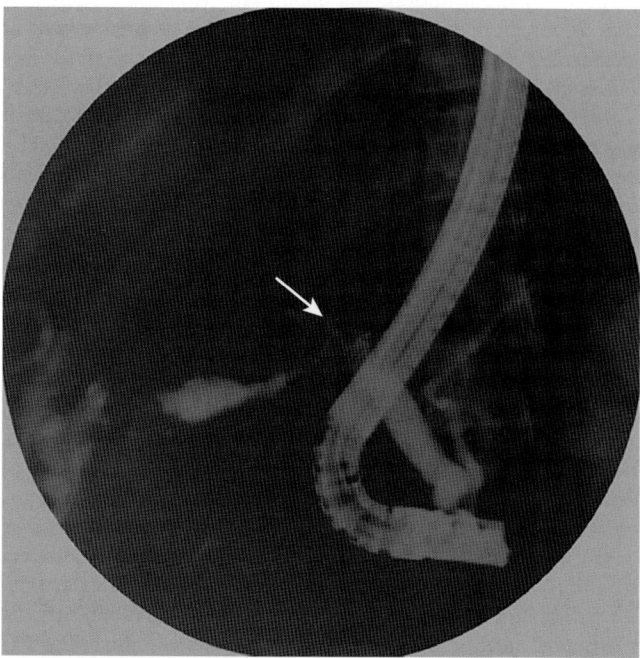

FIGURE 42.25 After transection of the bile duct in this patient, an endoscopic retrograde cholangiopancreatography was undertaken with deployment of biliary stents. Contrast is noted to extravagate from the blind end at the site of transection *(arrow).*

they provide a significant advantage. In our practice, we discourage the use of endoscopic stenting across the defect and prefer early surgical repair of the injury.

Patients with bile peritonitis are often desperately ill, especially if the bile is infected, although some patients with sterile bile may accumulate large volumes without overt signs of sepsis. Drainage of the bile collection and control of ongoing bile leak is the primary objective and often requires percutaneous abscess drains in combination with percutaneous biliary catheters. Definitive repair is seldom possible initially, with the bile ducts collapsed, deeply bile stained, and friable; repair is best delayed until the biliary leak has been controlled completely and the patient has been fully resuscitated.

INJURY PRESENTING AT AN INTERVAL AFTER INITIAL OPERATION. The principles of the surgical management of late bile duct strictures include (1) exposure of healthy proximal bile ducts draining all areas of the liver, (2) preparation of a suitable segment of distal mucosa for anastomosis, and (3) creation of a mucosa-to-mucosa sutured anastomosis of the bile ducts to the distal conduit, which is most commonly a Roux-en-Y loop of jejunum (see Chapter 32).

It may be necessary to consider a staged approach to stricture repair in the presence of intraabdominal infection, portal hypertension, or poor general condition of the patient. Repair attempts in the face of uncontrolled local infection, acute complications of portal hypertension, or general debilitation are doomed to fail. The initial approach in such cases should be limited to establishing external bile drainage, controlling sepsis, and treating other co-existing conditions that are life threatening. In this manner, the clinical condition of the patient may be improved before attempts at definitive repair. In a patient with portal hypertension, initial interventional radiologic management by percutaneously placed biliary drainage catheters is probably safer than operation, given the danger of intraoperative hemorrhage.[363]

Technical Approaches to Biliary Repair (see Chapter 32)

END-TO-END DUCT REPAIR. Excision of the stricture with end-to-end anastomosis was one of the earliest techniques used for reconstruction. This repair reestablishes normal anatomic continuity and drainage via an intact sphincter of Oddi. Such an approach has been tried even for high strictures after extensive mobilization of the duodenum and common duct. End-to-end repair is associated with a 50% to 60% incidence of long-term failure.[347,363,364] These figures reflect the failure rates in the most favorable of cases because patients with more extensive injuries usually were treated to biliary-enteric anastomosis.[365] These data suggest that end-to-end repair has a limited role in the surgical treatment of benign biliary strictures.

BILIARY-ENTERIC REPAIR. For most cases of bile duct transection or stricture, biliary-enteric anastomosis is the procedure of choice. For strictures of the retropancreatic or immediate supraduodenal portion of the CBD, choledochoduodenostomy is an ideal procedure. The anastomosis may be performed either side-to-side or end-to-side. This technique is appropriate only in the setting of a dilated bile duct and almost certainly would result in recurrent stricture if created to a decompressed duct. Most postcholecystectomy strictures are not amenable to choledochoduodenostomy because such low injuries are unusual in

contrast to postgastrectomy strictures, which often involve the distal bile duct. Strictures involving the common hepatic duct are more difficult to manage, especially strictures involving the biliary confluence, and they almost always require Roux-en-Y hepaticojejunostomy for reconstruction.[331,366]

There are a variety of approaches to the proximal hepatic ducts. When the stricture is below the confluence (Bismuth type 1 or 2), a direct anastomosis to the hepatic duct stump is usually straightforward. By contrast, when the stricture encroaches on the confluence of the right and left hepatic ducts (type 3) or extends proximally so as to isolate the ducts (type 4), the problem becomes more complex, and good results are more difficult to achieve. The choice of surgical approach should be tailored to the height and extent of the lesion. The technical descriptions that follow should be read in conjunction with Chapter 32.

Attempts to identify the duct below the stricture are unnecessary because the distal duct generally cannot be used for anastomosis; it is usually encased in dense scar tissue, and extensive dissection to free it risks injury to the hepatic artery and portal vein. The essential point is identification of the bile ducts proximal to the stricture, and a systematic, careful, and patient approach is necessary.

Strictures at or above the level of the biliary confluence are much more challenging. Adequate exposure of the bile ducts is usually achievable by dissecting the left hepatic duct system. This approach is based on the anatomic studies of Couinaud and Hepp and is well described.[331,367–369] For type 2 and type 3 strictures, biliary-enteric anastomosis to the left hepatic duct provides complete drainage of the left and right ductal systems. For type 4 strictures, however, the confluence is obliterated, and it is necessary to provide drainage of the right lobe as well, often by dissection across the stricture and creation of a second anastomosis to the right ductal system. Occasionally, mobilization or even partial excision of segment IV of the liver may be necessary in some type 4 strictures.

It is occasionally difficult to expose the left hepatic duct because of adhesions or fibrosis. Excessive bleeding may be encountered, or a large, overhanging portion of liver may prevent access to the left duct. Occasionally, the extrahepatic length of the left duct, normally much greater than the right, is short, and access to it is difficult. In such instances, repair can be accomplished by dissection of the left duct within the umbilical fissure, known as the *ligamentum teres* or *round ligament approach* (Fig. 42.26). This approach rarely is indicated for benign strictures and should not be used unless the biliary confluence is intact, so that a left-sided anastomosis would drain the entire liver.

LIVER SPLIT AND LIVER RESECTION. To expose the bile ducts for repair, it is sometimes necessary to open the liver tissue as a hepatotomy.[370] The most frequent situations involve opening the umbilical fissure to obtain access to the segment III duct or extending the subhepatic approach to expose the origin of the right hepatic duct. This latter approach involves opening the liver in the line of the gallbladder fossa. Upward mobilization of segment IV by this maneuver combined with opening the umbilical fissure facilitates access for selected type 4 strictures.

ISOLATED SECTORAL HEPATIC DUCT INJURIES. Injuries to aberrant or "low entry" right sectoral hepatic ducts can be particularly

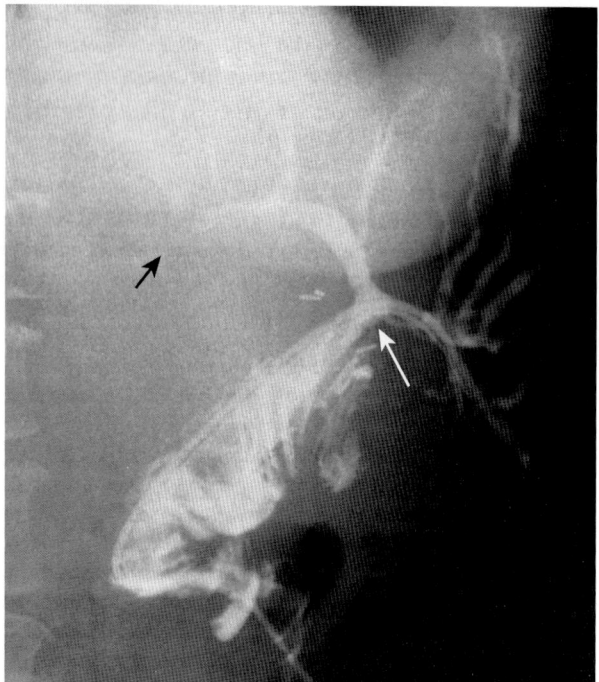

FIGURE 42.26 Roux-en-Y hepaticojejunostomy to the segment III duct after postcholecystectomy stricture initially treated by hepaticojejunostomy, using the mucosal graft technique with a transhepatic tube through the right liver. At referral, the patient had a grossly atrophic right lobe and a high bile duct stricture *(black arrow)*. At operation, the left hepatic duct was exposed using the ligamentum teres approach, and anastomosis was carried out *(white arrow)*. Subsequent repeat stricture occurred 1 year later and was treated by refashioning of the anastomosis and subsequent transtubal balloon dilation with a satisfactory outcome. The patient was well and symptom free 2 years after operation (see Chapter 32).

difficult to diagnose and manage (Figs. 42.27 and 42.28). Patients with a stricture but no bile leak (type B) may remain asymptomatic for months or years after the injury and only then present with pain or evidence of cholangitis. Some patients may remain essentially asymptomatic and come to attention because of abnormal LFTs. These injuries are not associated with jaundice unless concomitant stricture of the common hepatic duct (type E5) is present. Long-standing obstruction may result in atrophy of the corresponding hepatic sector drained by the occluded duct. Biliary drainage to a Roux-en-Y loop of jejunum should be done in symptomatic patients. In patients with symptoms, especially recurrent cholangitis, and evidence of liver atrophy, drainage alone may be insufficient, and resection of the atrophic sector may be required. Asymptomatic patients may not require intervention, especially if the injury was remote, and significant atrophy is already evident; however, patients with a relatively recent injury and no atrophy probably are best served with operative drainage to prevent future problems.[283] However, successful nonoperative management and interventional procedures with sclerotherapy have been described.[371,372]

COMBINED MODALITY APPROACHES. The standard surgical techniques of biliary reconstruction described are suitable for most cases. In the most complex and difficult strictures, and especially in the presence of intrahepatic strictures and stones, even optimal surgical management is met with a disappointingly high incidence of postoperative intrahepatic stone formation, cholangitis, and recurrent stricture. Interventional radiologic and endoscopic techniques, used as primary therapy in this setting, are similarly unsuccessful because of recurrent cholangitis associated with stent occlusion or recurrent stricture after balloon dilation. Often, nonoperative techniques are technically impossible because of limited access.

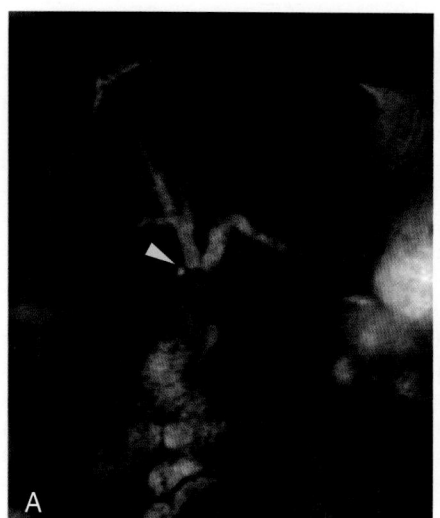
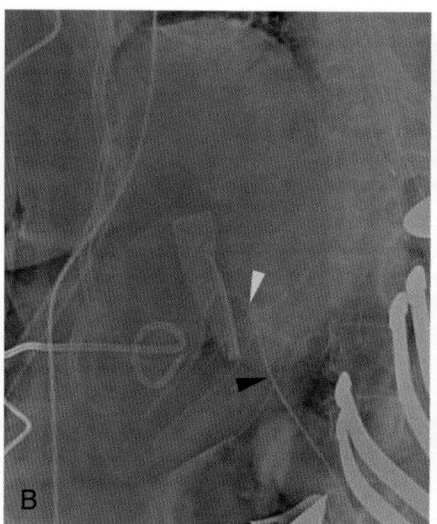
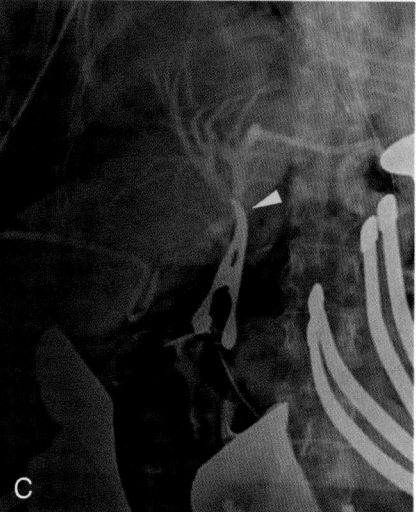

FIGURE 42.27 Common bile duct injury sustained during laparoscopic cholecystectomy with transection of common bile duct at hilum and exclusion of an isolated right posterior sectoral branch. **A,** Magnetic resonance imaging cholangiopancreatography before operative repair of bile duct injury. The excluded right posterior sectoral branch can be seen in discontinuity *(yellow arrow)*. **B,** Intraoperative cholangiogram with direct cannulation of the lumen of the right posterior sectoral branch bile duct. *Black arrow* indicates cholangiogram catheter, and *yellow arrow* indicates right posterior sectoral branch. **C,** Intraoperative cholangiogram with direct cannulation of the hilar confluence *(yellow arrow)* demonstrates opacification of the left and right hepatic ducts. (**A–C,** Courtesy Dr. Carlos Corvera.)

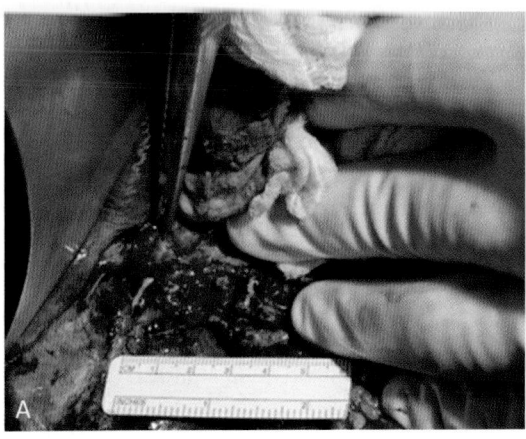
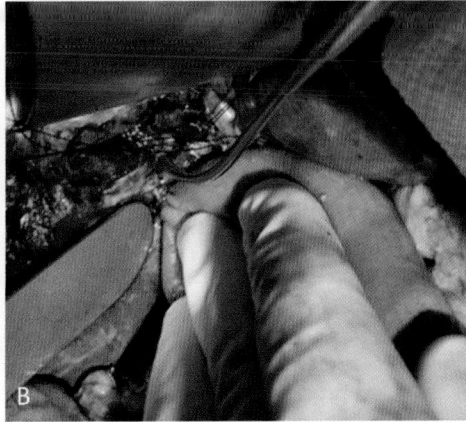

FIGURE 42.28   Intraoperative repair of common bile duct injury with exclusion of isolated right posterior sectoral branch. **A,** The hilar plate. The right hepatic artery supplying the right posterior sector was found to have been transected. **B,** Reconstruction with hepaticojejunostomy to the isolated right posterior sectoral duct, sewn with 6-0 interrupted sutures over a 6-French stent. The same hepaticojejunostomy was used for anastomosis to the hepatic hilum as well. (**A, B,** Courtesy Dr. Carlos Corvera.)

Under such adverse circumstances, when the risk of recurrent stricture or stone formation is believed to be high, hepaticojejunostomy may be performed over a transjejunal tube brought to the exterior across the blind end of the Roux limb. The defunctionalized Roux limb is deliberately left long, and the end is secured subcutaneously or subperitoneally (Fig. 42.29); this allows easy subsequent access for cholangiography, cholangioscopy, dilation, or stone removal. The blind end of the Roux limb may be re-accessed by percutaneous puncture under fluoroscopic guidance or via a small incision made under local anesthetic for late diagnostic or therapeutic procedures long after the transjejunal tube has been removed. In our experience, this approach is rarely necessary but can provide an improved chance of excellent outcome in difficult cases and may spare the patient the need for repeated major surgical intervention months or years later.[373,374] It is generally unnecessary to add the morbidity of a formal stoma, although such an approach has been reported.[375]

HEPATIC RESECTION (SEE CHAPTER 101). Patients who have undergone prior unsuccessful repairs or have concomitant vascular injury or long-standing cholangitis may develop sectional duct strictures or interruptions between the right-sided and left-sided biliary tree, effectively precluding biliary-enteric revision. Such patients may require formal liver resection to eliminate atrophied liver or the biliary duct confluence. The surgical aim in such instances is to create a more functional biliary-enteric anastomosis using the remnant liver. Although mostly described as isolated cases, several groups have reported their experience with formal resections for benign biliary stricture.[312,376,377] At a median follow-up of 8 years, 94% of patients had good or excellent results. Another report described eight patients who underwent either right hepatectomy or left lateral sectionectomy, and it demonstrated similar, excellent results.[378] Hepatic resection remains an important option in the treatment of refractory benign biliary stricture or complex injury with vascular involvement, especially in patients suffering from recurrent bouts of cholangitis or sepsis.[379]

LIVER TRANSPLANTATION (SEE CHAPTER 105). Transplantation for iatrogenic biliary injury can be performed acutely but is usually

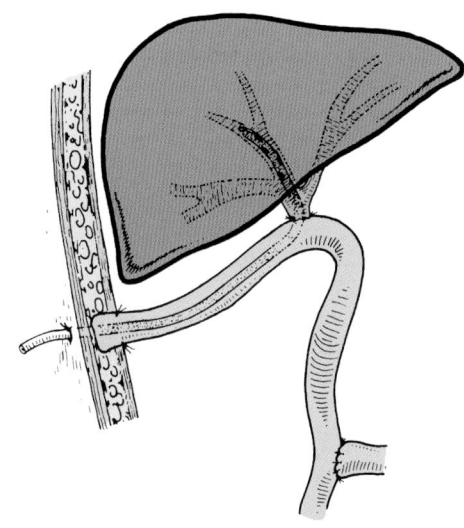

FIGURE 42.29   Hepaticojejunostomy with a long, defunctionalized Roux limb with the end secured subcutaneously or subperitoneally to allow access for future diagnostic or therapeutic studies (see Chapter 32).

done because of a devastating combined vascular and biliary injury.[380,381] Only rarely does secondary biliary fibrosis resulting from long-standing biliary obstruction progress to true cirrhosis. In such cases, orthotopic liver transplantation should be considered as an alternative to biliary reconstruction. Thomson et al.[378] reported their series of 14 patients who either underwent hepatic resection or transplantation for secondary biliary cirrhosis. Of the 5 patients who ultimately required transplant for survival, 2 were deemed unsuitable for the procedure, 1 died awaiting an organ, and 2 underwent the procedure. Even in experienced transplantation centers, surgical reconstruction is preferred for most patients with benign strictures.

PORTAL HYPERTENSION AND BILIARY STRICTURE (SEE CHAPTER 74). Patients with co-existing portal hypertension and biliary stricture are an especially difficult group to manage. This combination has been reported in 10% to 20% of patients at the time of referral.[311,331] Portal hypertension may result from secondary biliary fibrosis or direct injury to the portal vein or from coincident hepatocellular disease. The presence of splenomegaly or a history of GI bleeding in a patient with biliary stricture should prompt further investigation for portal hypertension. Bleeding esophageal varices, particularly if accompanied by hypersplenism or ascites, render the overall prognosis far worse.[311] Collateral venous channels in the subhepatic region and within adhesions make dissection difficult and bloody. Patients with portal hypertension often have a proximal stricture, and some have had multiple previous attempts at repair, further reducing the likelihood of a successful outcome.

In seriously ill patients with jaundice and portal hypertension, it is preferable to attempt nonoperative stenting or balloon dilation than to proceed to immediate definitive repair.[363,382–385] In the face of severe GI bleeding, initial measures must be directed at stopping the hemorrhage and resuscitating the patient (see Chapters 80 and 81). If bleeding continues, consideration should be given to immediate splenorenal (see Chapters 83 and 84) or transjugular intrahepatic portosystemic shunting (see Chapter 85) to achieve control, with bile duct reconstruction deferred until a later date. Occasionally, successful biliary-enteric reconstruction can be performed under these circumstances with no need to create a portosystemic shunt.[386,387]

If hemorrhage is encountered during stricture repair, hepaticostomy drainage may be performed as an initial measure, and a splenorenal shunt may be undertaken at a later date. Bile duct stricture repair done at the time of the shunting procedure can be extremely difficult and in any event is unwise at a time of severely compromised liver function. Occasionally, patients present with variceal hemorrhage after an otherwise successful stricture repair. In these instances, portosystemic shunting may be indicated as an emergency measure or, preferably, after initial conservative management. Injection sclerotherapy or banding may control the variceal bleeding successfully and obviate the need for operative intervention.

RESULTS OF BILIARY RECONSTRUCTION. Given the wide spectrum of injuries that are possible at cholecystectomy, it is difficult to assess the results of operative repair. Most surgical series report results of repair of biliary strictures (type E) and do not address operative intervention for other injury types. In addition, a percentage of patients are subjected to immediate repair at the time of initial injury; the more difficult cases and the failures generally are referred to specialist units, but the long-term outcome of the other cases is often not reported. Studies detailing bile duct injury repairs are listed in the tables, with several providing long-term outcomes[388–396] (Tables 42.1 and 42.2).

OPERATIVE MORBIDITY AND MORTALITY. Several studies have suggested significant morbidity associated with repair of benign strictures.[239] The most common postoperative complications seen were intraabdominal abscess, wound infection, cholangitis, sepsis, biliary fistula, postoperative hemorrhage, and pneumonia (see Table 42.1). These figures generally do not consider patients who die from biliary tract–related sepsis while awaiting definitive treatment. Factors frequently associated with perioperative death include advanced age, significant comorbid medical conditions, and biliary sepsis. Significant underlying liver disease is perhaps the most important predictor of adverse outcome. Chapman et al.[311] reported a perioperative mortality rate of 23% in patients with biliary strictures and portal hypertension subjected to any operative procedure.

A significant proportion of patients in many reports were referred after one or more repair attempts. Failed repairs nearly always render subsequent attempts more difficult and have a negative impact on the ultimate outcome. The reported morbidity and mortality rates reflect this point and underscore the serious nature of these injuries. Nevertheless, in experienced hands, operative repair of biliary strictures is a relatively safe procedure, and this fact must be considered when comparing surgery with nonoperative techniques.

TABLE 42.1 Selected Historic Series Reporting Outcome After Repair of Benign Biliary Strictures From Bile Duct Injury

REFERENCE	NO. PATIENTS	MECHANISM OF INJURY	PREVIOUS REPAIR ATTEMPT	MORBIDITY/ MORTALITY	SUCCESSFUL OUTCOME	FOLLOW-UP
Chapman et al., 1995[311]	122	OC (all)	80 (66%)	NR/1.8%[a]	76%	86 mo
McDonald et al., 1995[396]	45	OC, 26	11 (24%)	36%/0%	95%[b]	55 mo
		LC, 16				
		Other, 3				
Stewart & Way, 1995[347]	45	LC (all)	27 (60%)	4%/0%	94%	NR
Tocchi et al., 1996[356]	84	OC, 60	4 (5%)	21%/2.2%	83%[c]	108 mo
		CBDE, 4				
		Trauma, 4				
		Other, 16				
Lillemoe, 1997[315]	59	LC (all)	15 (25%)	NR/0%	92%[c]	33 mo
Pottakkat et al., 2007[397]	36	LC and OC, 22	36 (100%)	31%/0%	94%	37 mo (median)

[a]Postoperative deaths in two patients subjected to mucosal grafts; no deaths occurred in patients submitted to direct biliary-enteric repair.
[b]Includes some asymptomatic patients with mild elevations of liver function tests.
[c]Includes patients with excellent or good outcomes.
CBDE, Common bile duct exploration; *LC,* laparoscopic cholecystectomy; *NR,* not reported; *OC,* open cholecystectomy.
Most repairs were performed as hepaticojejunostomy or choledochojejunostomy (Roux-en-Y). *Previous repair attempt* refers to the number and percentage of patients referred after at least one attempt at repair. *Successful outcome* refers to the percentage of patients requiring no further intervention after initial, definitive surgical management at the reporting institution; most series reported salvaging some of the initial failures with interventional radiologic or further surgical intervention.

TABLE 42.2 Contemporary Studies on Outcomes of Bile Duct Injury Repair

REFERENCE	NO. PATIENTS	ORIGIN OF STUDY	STUDY TYPE	MECHANISM OF INJURY	CONCOMITANT VASCULOBILIARY INJURY	PREVIOUS REPAIR ATTEMPT	TIME FROM INJURY TO REPAIR	REPAIR TECHNIQUE	POSTOPERATIVE MORBIDITY/ MORTALITY	REPAIR OUTCOMES	LONG-TERM FOLLOW-UP
Iannelli et al., 2013[395]	543	France	National database	Predominantly laparoscopic cholecystectomy	n/a	n/a	36% immediate, 40% early, 25% late	52% primary suture repair, 48% biliodigestive (HJ or CD)	29%/2%	Failure rates[b]: immediate repair, 64%; early repair, 43%; late repair, 8%	n/a
Stilling et al., 2015[388]	139	Denmark	Multicenter	Laparoscopic cholecystectomy	26%	4%	Median 5 days	All HJ	46%/2%	30% HJ stricture median 12 mo; treated with re-HJ or PTC	132 mo
Sulpice et al., 2014[389]	38	France	Single center	Laparoscopic cholecystectomy	26%	68%	<72 hr: 39%; 72 hr-6 wk: 18%; >6 wk: 11%.	66%: HJ, 34%: reconstruction of prior HJ, 24%: HJ with hepatectomy	26%/0%	5% HJ stricture at median 60 mo; treated with re-HJ	93 mo
AbdelRafee et al., 2015[390]	120	Egypt	Single center	>90% open cholecystectomy	4%	0%	Median 1.5 mo	All HJ	36%/0%	12% HJ stricture median 63 mo; treated with re-HJ or PTC	149 mo
Felekouras et al., 2015[391]	92	Greece	Single center	Laparoscopic cholecystectomy	4%	20%	<2 wk: 57%, >12 wk 43%[a]	63% HJ, 12% primary biliary repair, 14% PTC, 11% other	23%/2%	14% HJ stricture	93 mo
Dominguez-Rosado et al., 2016[392]	614	Mexico	Single center	62% open cholecystectomy	4%	44%	<7 days 10%, 26% 8 days-6 wk, 64% >6 wk	94% HJ	30%/1%	22% with anastomotic complication at median 5.8 mo, 13% stenosis	40.5 mo
Ismael et al., 2016[393]	293	USA	National database	Cases identified by bile duct injury, specific mechanism not included	n/a	n/a	<30 days: 42%, >30 days: 58%	All HJ	26%/2%	Morbidity of repair <30 days 24% vs. >30 days 23%; P = 0.88 Mortality 5.0 vs. 0.0%; P = 0.01	n/a
Kirks et al., 2016[394]	61	USA	Single center	70% cholecystectomy; remainder trauma or non-biliary procedure	20%	n/a	<48 hr: 44%, >48 hr: 56%	All HJ	30-day readmission: 13%; 90-day mortality: 7%	No significant difference in outcomes with early vs. delayed repair	n/a

[a]For subset treated by specialized hepatobiliary surgeon.
[b]Failure defined as need for intervention or surgery needed.
CD, choledochoduodenostomy; HJ, hepaticojejunostomy; n/a, not available; PTC, percutaneous transhepatic cholangiography.

LONG-TERM RESULTS AND FOLLOW-UP. Several factors must be considered when analyzing the long-term results of biliary reconstruction. First, there is no consistently used algorithm for postoperative investigation. Likewise, the measures used to assess outcome vary considerably. Approaches to follow-up range from simple observation and measurement of LFTs to performance of cholangiography or HIDA scans. Consistency in analyzing long-term results is important and should include an assessment of symptoms, LFTs, and radiographic studies. Such a triad of criteria is useful for clarifying the results and is the only way to compare accurately the results from various series or interventions[374] (Table 42.3). In addition, long-term follow-up is crucial in analyzing the final results of any series and when comparing different treatment modalities. Pitt et al.[314] reported that two thirds of recurrent strictures were apparent within 2 years, but 20% were diagnosed 5 or more years after the initial repair. Similarly, Tocchi et al.[356] observed that 40% of recurrent strictures were identified more than 5 years after the initial operation, although greater than 90% of restrictures were identified within 1 year of surgical repair in the series by Pottakkat et al.[397] Complete and accurate assessment of the results of surgery or any other intervention may require longer-term follow-up of at least 5 years. More contemporary studies (see Table 42.2) cite a wide range of repair outcomes, with reconstruction "failures" often being defined as need for additional intervention (repeat surgery, endoscopic, or PTC) to address stricture or complications of obstruction (i.e., cholangitis). Hepaticojejunostomy stricture rates range from 5% to 30% over the course of several years of follow-up.[398]

Excellent outcomes can be achieved in many patients reconstructed with Roux-en-Y biliary-enteric anastomosis (see Tables 42.1 and 42.2 and Chapter 32). Many of these studies also identified factors associated with an adverse outcome (Box 42.3). Chapman et al.[311] found that long-term failure and the need for reintervention were significantly greater in patients with injuries involving the biliary confluence and those subjected to three or more repair attempts before referral. Tocchi et al.[356] observed that the best results correlated directly with the degree of biliary ductal dilation, independent of stricture location. Surgeon experience and the type of repair also are important determinants of outcome. In the series reported by Stewart and Way, primary end-to-end repairs over a T-tube were always unsuccessful when the duct had been completely transected.[347]

Some authors have advocated the use of anastomotic stents,[399–401] but the impact of such stents on long-term patency is questionable. Transanastomotic stents seem to have little impact on outcome and are not recommended to be used

routinely.[347,356,369] Although stents may be useful in selected cases, they cannot prevent the inevitable failure of a poorly constructed anastomosis.

The results of surgical reconstruction for injuries other than those involving the main extrahepatic bile duct have not been reported in great numbers and are not known precisely. Lillemoe et al.[402] reported the results of nine cases of reconstruction for isolated sectoral hepatic duct strictures over an 18-year period. All patients in this series incurred injuries to aberrant right sectoral hepatic ducts at laparoscopic or open cholecystectomy, and all had associated bile leaks. After Roux-en-Y hepaticojejunostomy, 6 (66.6%) of the 9 patients had a successful outcome, whereas 3 patients developed late strictures that required reintervention. Colovic[403] likewise analyzed 19 patients with isolated segmental, sectoral, and right hepatic duct injuries over a 26-year period. Twelve patients underwent surgical reconstruction, and the rest were managed expectantly or with percutaneous drainage with good to excellent results.

Patients with recurrent strictures after reconstruction at a specialist unit may be salvaged with further intervention, either anastomotic revision or balloon dilation. Several authors have reported some measure of success with surgical revision in these patients.[311,347,356,400,404] The likelihood of a good outcome is less than with the initial reconstruction, however. Other groups have reported nearly equivalent surgical outcomes for reoperated patients when compared with primary repairs at the same institution.[397] As discussed previously, the loss of bile duct length associated with a failed repair is a major factor that limits the success of subsequent interventions.

Duodenal ulceration has been reported in 10% of patients after Roux-en-Y biliary-enteric reconstruction and constitutes an additional cause of late morbidity.[405,406] Most patients respond to antiulcer medication, but some may develop significant hemorrhage.

NONOPERATIVE APPROACHES. Advances in interventional radiology have resulted in a broader application of nonoperative approaches to bile duct stricture[407–410] (see Chapters 20, 31, and 52). The largest reported experience has been with percutaneous balloon dilation. With this technique, the biliary tree is accessed percutaneously, and a guidewire is passed through the stricture. The stricture is dilated with an angioplasty-type balloon catheter, after which a transhepatic stent is left in place

---

BOX 42.3 Factors Associated With Stricture Recurrence or Poor Outcome After Operative Reconstruction

- Proximal stricture (Bismuth types 3 and 4)
- Multiple prior attempts at repair
- Portal hypertension
- Hepatic parenchymal disease (cirrhosis or hepatic fibrosis)
- End-to-end biliary anastomosis
- Surgeon inexperience
- Intrahepatic or multiple strictures
- Concurrent cholangitis or hepatic abscess
- Intrahepatic stones
- External or internal biliary fistula
- Intraabdominal abscess or bile collection
- Hepatic lobar atrophy
- Advanced age or poor general health

TABLE 42.3 Suggested Criteria for Assessing the Late Results of Biliary Stricture Management

CLASSIFICATION	SYMPTOMS	BIOCHEMISTRY[a]	RADIOLOGY[b]
Excellent	None	Normal	Normal
Good	None	Elevated	Abnormal
Fair	Improved	Elevated	Abnormal
Poor	Persistent/worse	Elevated	Abnormal

[a]Serum bilirubin and alkaline phosphatase.
[b]Hepatobiliary iminodiacetic acid scan or cholangiography or both.

for follow-up cholangiography and repeat dilation. In most cases, multiple dilations and prolonged biliary intubation with increasing stent sizes are required. Results have been encouraging, with several authors reporting good results in 55% to 98% of patients.[315,411-416]

These results must be viewed with considerable caution, however. First, the mean follow-up in most of these studies was less than 3 years, which is insufficient to make a definitive comment regarding long-term efficacy. Second, balloon dilation is limited in its application to patients in whom biliary continuity is intact or has been restored by a previous attempt at repair; it has no role for strictures at or above the confluence and cannot be used if the bile duct has been transected.[315] Third, complications related to balloon dilation or to the percutaneous catheter are frequent and include hemobilia, bile leak, and cholangitis in 20% of patients.

Another nonoperative approach used is endoscopic stenting.[407,409,410] With this technique, multiple plastic or metallic stents are placed across the stricture endoscopically, necessitating removal later. Kassab et al.[417] reported their experience with 88 patients with benign biliary stricture after cholecystectomy and who underwent endoscopic stenting during ERCP. They reported that 69.1% of patients were successfully treated, with a mean of 1.6 stents placed for an average duration of 14 months and no stricture recurrence at a mean follow-up of 28 months after stent removal. Other groups have reported higher success rates, albeit at shorter follow-up intervals.[418,419] As with balloon dilation, the results of stenting are tempered with caveats of short follow-up periods and no randomized studies. Additionally, stents may be prone to migration and plastic stents require exchange every few months to maintain patency. Stent migration rates have been reported at 20% to 66%, and up to one third of patients may experience cholangitis or pancreatitis.[409]

Comparing the results of balloon dilation or endoscopic stenting with operative reconstruction is difficult because of differences in the types of injuries selected for each type of treatment, inconsistencies in defining successful outcomes, and differences in reporting complications and length of follow-up. To date, no randomized studies have compared these techniques. In two retrospective analyses, biliary reconstruction was more likely to result in a successful outcome: 89% versus 52%,[414] 92% versus 64%,[315] and 94% versus 58%.[411] Because balloon dilation requires multiple readmissions and repeat interventions, the overall cost and morbidity seem to be similar to those of operatively treated patients.[414] The data suggest that, in most cases, biliary-enteric anastomosis is more effective and provides more durable relief of symptoms than balloon dilation, although balloon dilation is preferable in patients who otherwise would not tolerate an operation; it may be tried as an initial treatment in patients with biliary anastomotic strictures, for which the success rate seems to be greater than for primary bile duct strictures and may limit the need for an invasive procedure and its associated risks.[420,421]

CONSIDERATIONS OF BILE DUCT INJURY AFTER OTHER OPERATIONS

Robotic Cholecystectomy (see Chapter 127)

Robotic technologies have been gaining more attention in the field of general and hepatobiliary surgery. In theory, the robot provides the ability for more refined movements and superior visualization with three-dimensional views. Groups have reported routine use of robotic surgical platforms for elective cholecystectomy, for acute cholecystitis, and even as a salvage mechanism for completion cholecystectomy.[30,422,423] It is believed that the increased precision allows better visualization and dissection in a hostile abdomen than is provided by traditional open or laparoscopic approaches.[304,424] Several series have reported favorable outcomes with robotic cholecystectomy; however, there is no randomized controlled trial to date comparing laparoscopic versus robotic techniques.[422,425,426] Application of this new technology needs further careful safety evaluation before it can be widely recommended, and best training practices should be established given the learning curve needed for surgeons to achieve proficiency and ensure safe outcomes. Another important consideration is the increased cost associated with this technology that will be a significant barrier for wider acceptance.[423] A review by Angelou et al.[426] pooled 16 studies together, and reported bile duct injury rate of 8 out of 2264 cases analyzed for an incidence of 0.35%. However, with limited numbers of studies or a database on outcomes, it is challenging to obtain accurate national trends in adverse events.

Biliary Reconstructive Operations

Postoperative stricture or fistula can complicate procedures that require biliary-enteric anastomoses, such as reconstruction after pancreaticoduodenectomy (see Chapters 62 and 117A), bile duct resection for mid–bile duct tumors (see Chapter 51A), and excision of choledochal cysts (see Chapter 46). Typically, these procedures involve choledochoenteric or hepaticoenteric anastomosis. Late strictures after such procedures are most likely to occur when enteric anastomosis is performed to a normal-caliber duct, or when the duct itself is diseased, as in cases of choledochal cysts. When biliary-enteric anastomosis has been performed for long-standing biliary obstruction, the duct is dilated and thickened. In these cases, the anastomosis is usually easy to construct, and late stenosis is uncommon.[356] In most cases, stricture of a biliary-enteric anastomosis after resection for malignancy is the result of cancer recurrence. However, in a retrospective study of 1595 patients, no difference was apparent in postoperative stricture rate (2.6%) between benign and malignant indications for resection following pancreaticoduodenectomy.[427] Only 9% of strictures were caused by recurrent malignant disease, and preoperative biliary drainage and postoperative biliary stenting were the only risk factors for stricture. Duconseil et al.[428] noted a postoperative stricture rate of 4.2%, with most strictures resulting from benign perianastomotic fibrosis. Bile duct size of less than 5 mm was noted to be the most significant risk factor in this series.

Late stricture may also occur after side-to-side choledochoduodenostomy performed for choledocholithiasis or as a bypass procedure for chronic pancreatitis. This complication is rare if the anastomosis is performed to a sufficiently dilated duct (at least 1.5 cm) and the final diameter of the anastomosis is at least 2 to 2.5 cm.[429,430] The so-called sump syndrome after choledochoduodenostomy—in which particulate matter, stones, and food debris accumulate and stagnate within the distal, "blind" end of the common duct—is an occasional cause of recurrent cholangitis that can result in anastomotic stricture.[431,432] Endoscopic management, consisting of sphincterotomy with or without balloon dilation of the anastomosis or even placement of an occlusion device, has been reported for this condition.[433-435] This approach may not be adequate, however, to remove the thick, infected, and sometimes large debris that is often densely adherent to the wall of the inflamed distal CBD, and restricture of the anastomosis is common. We prefer reoperation with end-to-side hepaticojejunostomy, Roux-en-Y, to prevent persistent regurgitation of intestinal contents and to remove the "sump" permanently.[431] When dissection in the hilus is rendered hazardous because of dense scarring, an alternative maneuver is to perform a pyloric exclusion and gastrojejunostomy, which accomplishes the same objective of preventing reflux of intestinal contents into the biliary tree.

Open Cholecystectomy (see Chapter 36)

The occurrence of unexpected biliary fistulae after cholecystectomy almost always indicates operative injury to a major bile duct. A 0.21% incidence of bile duct injuries was found in a study by Roslyn et al.[282] of 42,474 patients who underwent an open cholecystectomy and up to 0.7% in a more recent report by Jablonska and Lampe.[436] Bile duct injury is recognized at the time of cholecystectomy in only a few patients; in approximately 25% to 40% of patients with unrecognized bile duct injury, the injury becomes apparent only when the presence of a biliary fistula is recognized.[437,438] In the remaining patients, the injury is recognized only later, when a biliary stricture develops.[239] Inadequately ligated or sloughed ligatures on the cystic duct are rarely responsible for biliary fistulae, and for this reason, transfixion suturing of the cystic stump is recommended. However, the presence of an unrecognized significant distal obstruction may be followed by a blowout of the cystic duct stump, resulting in a biliary fistula or bile peritonitis.

Currently, open cholecystectomy is done under difficult circumstances, as in the presence of a gangrenous gallbladder associated with fibrosis and inflammation in the region of the triangle of Calot. In these instances, proper identification and transfixion of the cystic stump may not be possible, and the patient is left with a temporary biliary fistula. As described previously, type 2 Mirizzi syndrome may pose significant technical difficulties, and specific surgical techniques have been devised to deal with this situation.[170]

If a defect in the bile duct is found during operation, and if immediate repair is impossible, it may be better to end the procedure with adequate drainage, expecting a future controlled fistula. In all these difficult instances in which a biliary fistula is anticipated, it is important to ensure controlled and adequate drainage of bile and to exclude the presence of a distal obstruction to biliary-enteric bile flow. Under these circumstances, most fistulae close spontaneously after conservative treatment.

Common Duct Exploration

The classic open common duct exploration is now less frequently performed, having been replaced by laparoscopic and endoscopic techniques. Whether it occurs after open or laparoscopic exploration of the CBD or persists after removal of a T-tube, a biliary fistula is almost always due to distal obstruction, most commonly a residual common duct gallstone. It is essential to perform cholangiography and rule out the presence of retained stones before removal of a T-tube or biliary stent.

Less commonly, an overlooked malignant distal obstruction is the causative factor. In addition, the passage of metal bougies through the papilla during common duct exploration may result in the creation of a false tract, which may result in a choledochoduodenal fistula and may cause jaundice, ascending cholangitis, and acute or chronic recurrent pancreatitis. Treatment may be by endoscopic papillotomy or sphincterotomy, joining the fistulous orifice with the papillary opening.[31,89,439]

Liver Resection

Biliary injury during liver resection is uncommon in experienced hands (see Chapter 101). The incidence of bile leak after hepatic resection ranges from 1.7% to 12% in large series.[440-446] If there is a suspicion of iatrogenic ductal injury that cannot be readily identified, or if the biliary anatomy is unclear, intraoperative cholangiography should be performed; deliberate choledochotomy with passage of fine bougies into the right and left ducts may assist identification. Injury is most common when resection is done for lesions near the hilus. In such instances, we recommend that the bile duct be freed from the tumor by careful dissection of hilum and clear identification of the right and left main ducts. Special care should be exercised when using the pedicle ligation and stapler technique to prevent inadvertent injury or complete occlusion of the left bile duct in right-sided resections. In most patients, bile leak resolves spontaneously, but sometimes a persistent fistula requires reoperation.[248] Liver resection performed for tumor may be followed by biliary fistula, which may result from inadequate ligation of the bile ducts at the cut liver surface or from failure to secure the bile ducts at the hilus[447] (see Fig. 42.28). This failure is more likely after right hepatectomy, in which the anatomy of the right sectoral ducts is variable in the hilar region (see Chapter 2). Extended left hepatic lobectomy also has been associated with a high incidence of biliary fistula. In Japan, Yamashita et al.[445] reported a biliary fistula rate of 4% (31/781) after hepatic resection. Their analysis identified operative procedures exposing the major Glisson capsule and including the hilum—anterior sectorectomy, central hepatectomy, and caudate resections—to be high-risk operations for development of postoperative bile leakage. Other factors that may contribute to a persistent bile fistula may include underlying cirrhosis or chronic hepatitis that impairs wound healing.[443] The large experience reported by Zimmitti et al.[446] identified that extended right hepatectomy, repeat hepatectomy, and en-bloc diaphragmatic resection were predictive of bile leak.

NONSURGICAL CONDITIONS CAUSING FISTULAE AND STRICTURES

Liver Trauma

Hepatic and biliary injuries from trauma are discussed more fully in Chapter 113. The gallbladder or biliary tree may be damaged by blunt or penetrating abdominal injuries. The CBD is susceptible to disruption from deceleration injuries, usually at the level of the pancreaticoduodenal junction, where it is relatively fixed compared with the more proximal duct. Delayed common duct stricture has been reported after blunt abdominal trauma.[448,449] Late problems also may arise after hepatic trauma, in which prolonged fistulization occurs from a segment of liver isolated by the injury, particularly when bile drains from a large portion of the liver through the fistulous tract. Such fistulae may occur in association with damage to the liver and the bile ducts or may follow sequestration and infection of areas of liver necrosis. Blunt or penetrating grade III or IV liver trauma may be complicated by bile collections and biliary fistulae in 0.5% to 14% of patients.[150–155]

Hydatid Disease

Biliary fistula may develop after operation for hydatid disease in up to 16% of patients in certain situations[456] (see Chapter 72). First, a communication between the cyst cavity and the biliary system is missed at operation and is not directly secured. It is prudent to drain all cyst cavities, particularly those of multiloculated hydatid cysts, to ensure that if a biliary fistula were to develop, it would be controlled. Unless a distal obstruction is present, these fistulae usually close spontaneously. Second, and rarely, the presence of hydatid material within the biliary tract produces biliary ductal obstruction that results in a persistent biliary fistula that is relieved only when the hydatid material passes or is removed. Removal is achieved by exploration of the CBD with or without a bypass procedure or by endoscopic methods.[457–459]

Assessment of the biliary tree, preferably by endoscopic cholangiography, should be performed before surgery in patients with a history of jaundice or cholangitis or in the presence of a large cyst located centrally and abutting the hilar structures. Kayaalp et al.,[460] in a series of 113 patients, showed that the location of the hydatid cyst near the hilum is a risk factor for the development of a cystobiliary communication and cavity-related complications. When a cystobiliary communication is shown, the biliary system should be cleared of all debris and cyst remnants, and endoscopic sphincterotomy should be performed before surgical intervention.[461] Percutaneous treatment of hydatid cysts is associated with a 10% to 11% incidence of biliary fistula.[462,463] Such fistulae may close spontaneously.

References are available at expertconsult.com.

SECTION I. Inflammatory, Infective, and Congenital

C. Biliary Infection and Infestation

CHAPTER 43

Cholangitis

Matthew Iyer and Vinod P. Balachandran

OVERVIEW

Cholangitis, also called acute cholangitis or ascending cholangitis, occurs when obstructed biliary flow leads to cholestasis and infection of the biliary tree. Cholangitis is commonly caused by choledocholithiasis and a variety of pathologies that obstruct the biliary tree. The severity of cholangitis ranges from mild to life-threatening, with mortality rates approaching 10% for the most severe cases.[1] Prompt diagnosis followed by fluid resuscitation, administration of antibiotics, and biliary decompression constitute the fundamental management principles.

The urgency of biliary decompression depends on disease severity; all patients who fail to improve or deteriorate within 12 to 24 hours of instituting medical therapy (i.e., supportive care and antibiotic therapy) should undergo immediate biliary decompression by either endoscopic (see Chapters 20 and 30) or percutaneous (see Chapters 31 and 52) approaches based on the type and suspected location of the obstruction in the biliary tree. A distal biliary tree obstruction is best decompressed endoscopically, whereas obstructions proximal to the hepatic bifurcation or from biliary-enteric anastomoses should be decompressed percutaneously in most situations. Procedures to achieve goals beyond decompression, such as papillotomy, balloon stricture dilation, or biliary tract debris clearance, should be avoided in the setting of recent or present sepsis. Operative biliary decompression should be reserved only for those patients who fail nonoperative decompression, as it is associated with high morbidity and mortality. The extent of operative biliary decompression, should, in most cases, be limited to T-tube type decompression of the common bile duct (CBD) with definitive management of the underlying cause of the biliary obstruction deferral until the patient's condition has improved. Continuation of antibiotic therapy should be guided by the persistence of residual biliary obstruction because of the increased risk of recurrent cholangitis.

An international consensus on evidence-based care for patients with cholangitis was first published in 2007 as the Tokyo Guidelines (TG) and was subsequently updated in 2013 (TG13) and 2018 (TG18).[2] These guidelines are referenced throughout this chapter.

CHOLANGITIS

Cholangitis presents along a spectrum of severity ranging from mild, intermittent, and recurrent episodes of fever, jaundice, and abdominal pain, as described by Charcot in 1877, to rapidly progressive systemic illness that results in shock, mental status changes, and death.[3] The pathogenesis of cholangitis involves (1) obstruction of bile flow, (2) elevation of intraductal biliary pressure, (3) colonization of bile with microorganisms, and (4) translocation of bacteria into the vascular and lymphatic system, with a subsequent systemic inflammatory response that can progress to life-threatening sepsis.[1] Complications include hepatic abscesses, recurrent cholangitis, and secondary biliary cirrhosis.

The most common causes of biliary obstruction are choledocholithiasis (see Chapter 37), neoplasia (see Chapters 49, 51, 62, and 63), and occluded biliary stents.[4] Other notable causes (Box 43.1) include benign biliary strictures (see Chapter 42), conditions that cause extrinsic compression of the bile duct, parasites, and inflammatory/immune-mediated syndromes.

Diagnosis

Biliary infection is suspected in patients who present with any combination of fever, chills (often severe rigors), abdominal pain, jaundice, nausea, vomiting, or altered mental status. A detailed medical history is obtained with specific attention to constitutional symptoms, gallstone or biliary disease, malignancy, autoimmune disease, prior biliary interventions, and prior abdominal surgery. A thorough physical examination is undertaken in which the presence or absence of altered mental status, jaundice, focal or generalized abdominal tenderness, and peritonitis are noted. Vital signs should be measured, and the situation is deemed urgent when significant hemodynamic changes are present. Laboratory testing includes complete blood count (CBC) with platelet count and differential, basic metabolic panel (BMP), and hepatic function panel. When feasible, blood cultures should be drawn in the presence of fever, rigors, or before empiric antimicrobial administration. Arterial blood gas analysis is indicated in patients with hemodynamic instability, respiratory insufficiency, alterations in mental status, or when other laboratory testing suggests the presence of organ dysfunction. In terms of diagnostic imaging, abdominal ultrasound and computed tomography (CT) imaging are useful first-line studies for detecting biliary obstruction.[5]

The diagnosis of cholangitis based on the Charcot's triad (fever, right upper quadrant abdominal pain, and jaundice) or Reynaud's pentad (the Charcot's triad plus lethargy and hypotension) provides high specificity but low sensitivity.[6] More

---

BOX 43.1   Causes of Cholangitis

1. Biliary stones
   a. Choledocholithiasis
   b. Hepatolithiasis
   c. Mirizzi syndrome
2. Benign biliary strictures
   a. Congenital factors
   b. Biliary surgery
      i. Damaged bile duct
      ii. Strictured choledochojejunostomy
   c. Chronic pancreatitis
   d. Primary sclerosing cholangitis
   e. Orthotopic liver transplantation
   f. Cholangiopathy in patients with AIDS
3. Malignant biliary obstruction
   a. Pancreas
   b. Bile duct/gallbladder
   c. Ampulla
   d. Duodenum
4. Nonsurgical biliary interventions
   a. ERCP
   b. PTC
   c. Biliary stents
5. Parasitic infection
6. Miscellaneous

AIDS, Acquired immunodeficiency syndrome; *ERCP,* endoscopic retrograde cholangiopancreatography; *PTC,* percutaneous transhepatic cholangiography.
Adapted from Kimura Y, et al. TG13 current terminology, etiology, and epidemiology of acute cholangitis and cholecystitis. *J Hepatobiliary Pancreat Sci.* 2013 Jan;20(1):8–23.

BOX 43.2   Tokyo Guidelines Criteria for Acute Cholangitis

Diagnostic Criteria
A. Systemic Inflammation
   A-1. Fever (>38°C) and/or shaking chills
   A-2. Laboratory evidence of inflammatory response (WBC <4 or >10, C-reactive protein >1)
B. Cholestasis
   B-1. Jaundice (total bilirubin >2 mg/dL)
   B-2. Abnormal liver function tests
C. Imaging
   C-1. Biliary dilatation
   C-2. Imaging evidence of biliary obstruction
Suspected diagnosis: one item in A + one item in either B or C.
Definite diagnosis: one item in A, one item in B, and one item in C.

Severity Grading
Grade III (severe) acute cholangitis – acute cholangitis associated with the onset of dysfunction in at least one of the following organs/systems:
1. Cardiovascular dysfunction: hypotension requiring dopamine ≥5 Ig/kg per min, or any dose of norepinephrine
2. Neurologic dysfunction: disturbance of consciousness
3. Respiratory dysfunction: PaO_2/FiO_2 ratio <300
4. Renal dysfunction: oliguria, serum creatinine >2.0 mg/dL
5. Hepatic dysfunction: PT-INR >1.5
6. Hematologic dysfunction: platelet count <100,000/mm^3
Grade II (moderate) acute cholangitis - acute cholangitis associated with any two of the following conditions:
1. Abnormal WBC count (>12,000 cells/mm^3, <4000 cells/mm^3)
2. High fever (≥39°C)
3. Age (≥75 years old)
4. Hyperbilirubinemia (total bilirubin ≥5 mg/dL)
5. Hypoalbuminemia
Grade I (mild) acute cholangitis - acute cholangitis that does not meet the criteria of "grade III (severe)" or "grade II (moderate)" acute cholangitis at initial diagnosis. Early diagnosis, early biliary drainage and/or treatment for etiology, and antimicrobial administration are fundamental for all grades of acute cholangitis.

PT-INR, Prothrombin time-international normalized ratio; *WBC,* white blood cell count.
Adapted from Kiriyama S, et al. Tokyo Guidelines 2018: diagnostic criteria and severity grading of acute cholangitis (with videos). *J Hepatobiliary Pancreat Sci.* 2018;25(1):17–30.

---

updated diagnostic criteria are provided by TG, which are based on several multicenter outcomes studies and establish a common definition and diagnostic criteria (Box 43.2) that incorporates clinical, laboratory, and imaging findings.[7] Given the importance of early recognition and treatment, these diagnostic criteria prioritize sensitivity over specificity, providing an overall accuracy of 90% to diagnose cholangitis.[8] Although not included in the criteria, the presence of abdominal pain and history of biliary disease or previous biliary instrumentation are helpful adjunct factors. Acute cholecystitis and acute hepatitis represent common etiologies and must be considered in the differential diagnosis.

In addition to providing a standardized diagnostic approach, TG also established a prognostic severity grading system based on clinical and laboratory parameters (see Box 43.2): a large retrospective study (*n* = 7294) found mortality rates of 2.4%, 4.7%, and 8.4% for TG18 severity grades I (mild), II (moderate), and III (severe), respectively.[4] Furthermore, this study noted a significantly lower 30-day mortality in patients with grade II disease who were treated with biliary decompression within 24 to 48 hours, suggesting that TG18 severity grading may be useful for identifying patients most likely to benefit from early biliary drainage. Nonetheless, biliary decompression/drainage should be performed for any patients regardless of severity grade who do not respond to initial supportive care and antimicrobial therapy.

Imaging Studies

Noninvasive imaging modalities to visualize the biliary tree and gallbladder include transabdominal ultrasound, CT, magnetic resonance cholangiopancreatography (MRCP; see Chapter 16),

and radionuclide imaging (e.g., hepatobiliary iminodiacetic acid [HIDA] scan; see Chapter 17). Nonoperative invasive modalities requiring sedation and/or local or general anesthesia include endoscopic ultrasonography (EUS; see Chapter 22), intraductal ultrasonography (IDUS), endoscopic retrograde cholangiopancreatography (ERCP; see Chapters 20 and 30), and percutaneous transhepatic cholangiopancreatography (PTC; see Chapters 31 and 52). The most widely used initial diagnostic imaging test remains a contrast-enhanced CT scan of the abdomen and pelvis.

Transabdominal Ultrasound

Transabdominal ultrasound is the preferred first-line imaging study when evaluating a patient with suspected cholangitis due to its low cost, wide availability, and lack of ionizing radiation.[9] Ultrasound can reliably detect the presence of intrahepatic and extrahepatic biliary dilation with a sensitivity of 85% to 95%.[10] It is important to note that biliary dilation may be absent in acute obstruction, as this takes time to develop. Transabdominal ultrasound has limited sensitivity, however, for detecting choledocholithiasis, particularly small stones or lesions in the distal CBD that are often obscured by bowel gas.[11] The sensitivity of ultrasound to detect CBD stones varies between 20% and 75%, with increased sensitivity in the case of multiple large stones within a dilated CBD and less sensitivity in the case of stone impaction in the retropancreatic segment of the CBD.[12]

Computed Tomography

CT imaging overcomes the technical limitations of ultrasound and can accurately detect biliary obstruction and characterize the cause of biliary stenosis.[13] In cholangitis, contrast-enhanced CT may reveal bile duct thickening and enhancement (see Chapter 16). The arterial phase may reveal inhomogeneous enhancement of hepatic parenchyma.[14] Findings of biliary ductal dilatation or abrupt termination of the CBD are indirect findings in choledocholithiasis. However, because up to 24% of gallstones have the same density as bile, the sensitivity of CT for detecting CBD stones ranges from 25% to 90%.[15] CT can also detect complications of cholangitis, including hepatic abscess (Fig. 43.1) and pylephlebitis (suppurative thrombosis of the portal vein). Due to its availability and convenience, CT imaging may be completed ahead of transabdominal ultrasound or magnetic resonance imaging (MRI) when other abdominal pathologies are considered in the differential diagnosis. A key drawback of CT is the risk of nephrotoxicity associated with the use of contrast material, particularly in under resuscitated or hemodynamically unstable patients.

Magnetic Resonance Cholangiopancreatography

MRCP provides noninvasive three-dimensional (3D) imaging of the biliary tree using a heavily T2-weighted scheme that emphasizes the intensity of stationary fluids (see Chapter 16). It outperforms both ultrasound and CT in its ability to delineate the bile duct and identify both malignant disease and CBD stones causing obstruction.[16] In a systematic review, the sensitivity and specificity of MRCP for the detection of choledocholithiasis were 93% and 96%, respectively.[17] MRCP cannot differentiate stones from air bubbles, sludge, or blood clots, as all of these lack liquid. Furthermore, MRCP cannot detect stones less than 3 mm in size, nor can it detect impacted stones in the ampulla, which require evaluation of T1 images before and after gadolinium injection. The drawbacks of MRCP are cost, limited accessibility, and specific contraindications, such as morbid obesity and metallic foreign bodies/devices. Therefore MRCP is typically reserved for cases in which diagnosis proves difficult with ultrasound or CT.

Endoscopic Ultrasound

EUS can provide additional diagnostic information and allows therapeutic intervention (see Chapter 22). Once endoscopically passed through the stomach and into the duodenum, the ultrasound probe is in close proximity to the CBD. By using high-frequency ultrasound (7.5–12 MHz), the resolution of EUS is exceptional (<1 mm), and allows accurate detection of small gallstones or other obstructive etiologies. EUS has a sensitivity approaching 100% and a specificity of greater than 90%, with an overall accuracy of 96% to detect bile duct stones.[18] EUS can be combined with fine-needle aspiration to provide tissue diagnosis or ERCP during the same session if clinically warranted. The major limitations of endoscopic techniques are that they cannot be performed in patients with altered anatomy, such as those with a prior distal gastrectomy or gastric bypass, or in the presence of a significantly calcified pancreas or hilar biliary pathology.

Intraductal Ultrasonography

IDUS can be performed endoscopically or percutaneously by introducing a flexible, thin-caliber (2-mm) ultrasound probe into the biliary and/or pancreatic ducts using wire guidance.[19] IDUS utilizes high-frequency ultrasound (12.30 MHz) to provide high resolution (0.07–0.018 mm) at the cost of decreased depth of penetration (2–3 cm).[20] Specialized centers have reported the cannulation rate of the major papilla to approach 100%, obviating the need for sphincterotomy in most cases. In addition, IDUS may identify lesions missed by traditional imaging, making it a useful adjunct to ERCP for the identification and characterization of bile duct lesions.[21] Drawbacks include the need for specialized equipment, cost, and operator expertise.

Direct Cholangiography

Although historically considered the reference radiologic modality, direct cholangiography for purely diagnostic purposes has been replaced by noninvasive cross-sectional imaging techniques that provide additional anatomic detail of adjacent organs and allow a more complete assessment. In addition to inferior image quality, there are various complications associated with the use of direct cholangiography, including biliary infection, pancreatitis, and hemorrhage.[22] Currently, given that cholangitis can be accurately detected based on noninvasive studies endoscopic retrograde or percutaneous cholangiography is largely limited to the first step of a therapeutic procedure.[23]

Management

The management of cholangitis follows three principles: (1) vigorous resuscitation and hemodynamic support, (2) parenteral administration of broad-spectrum antibiotics, and (3) biliary decompression.[5]

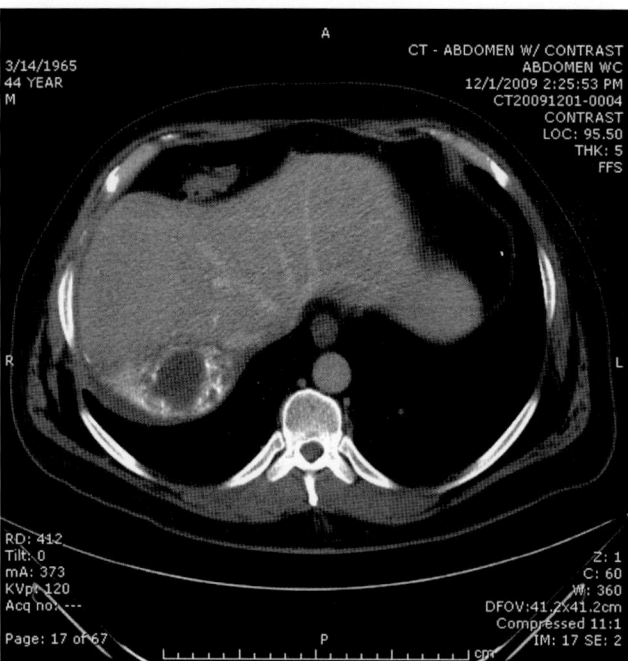

FIGURE 43.1 Abdominal computed tomograghphy (CT) scan demonstrating a hepatic abscess involving the right hepatic lobe with surrounding inflammatory changes.

Initial Management

Figure 43.2 illustrates a suggested management algorithm for patients with cholangitis. Supportive medical care for all patients with cholangitis includes aggressive fluid resuscitation, correction of electrolyte imbalances, appropriate intravenous (IV) antibiotic administration, and analgesia. Heart rate, blood pressure, mental status, and urine output must be closely monitored while awaiting results of diagnostic studies to determine the location and cause of the underlying biliary obstruction. Patients should be fasted in case immediate procedural intervention becomes necessary.

In conjunction with supportive therapy and diagnostic studies, severity should be assessed according to the TG18 severity grading criteria (see Box 43.2) and repeated whenever the clinical status changes or new data become available. The proposed TG18 management bundles tailor subsequent therapy by severity grade.[24] Briefly, grade I patients can defer biliary drainage as long as they improve within 24 hours, whereas all grade II and III patients should receive biliary decompression and drainage.[5] Blood cultures should be obtained before the initiation of antibiotics. If biliary drainage cannot be performed due to lack of facilities or specialized personnel, transferring the patient should be considered.

Antimicrobial Therapy

Empiric antimicrobial therapy serves to temporize the development of life-threatening sepsis in lieu of adequate source control and prevent the spread of infection and the development of complications (e.g., intrahepatic abscess). A variety of culture-identified pathogens and frequently polymicrobial isolates necessitate treatment with broad-spectrum agents.[25] The most common isolates from blood and bile of patients

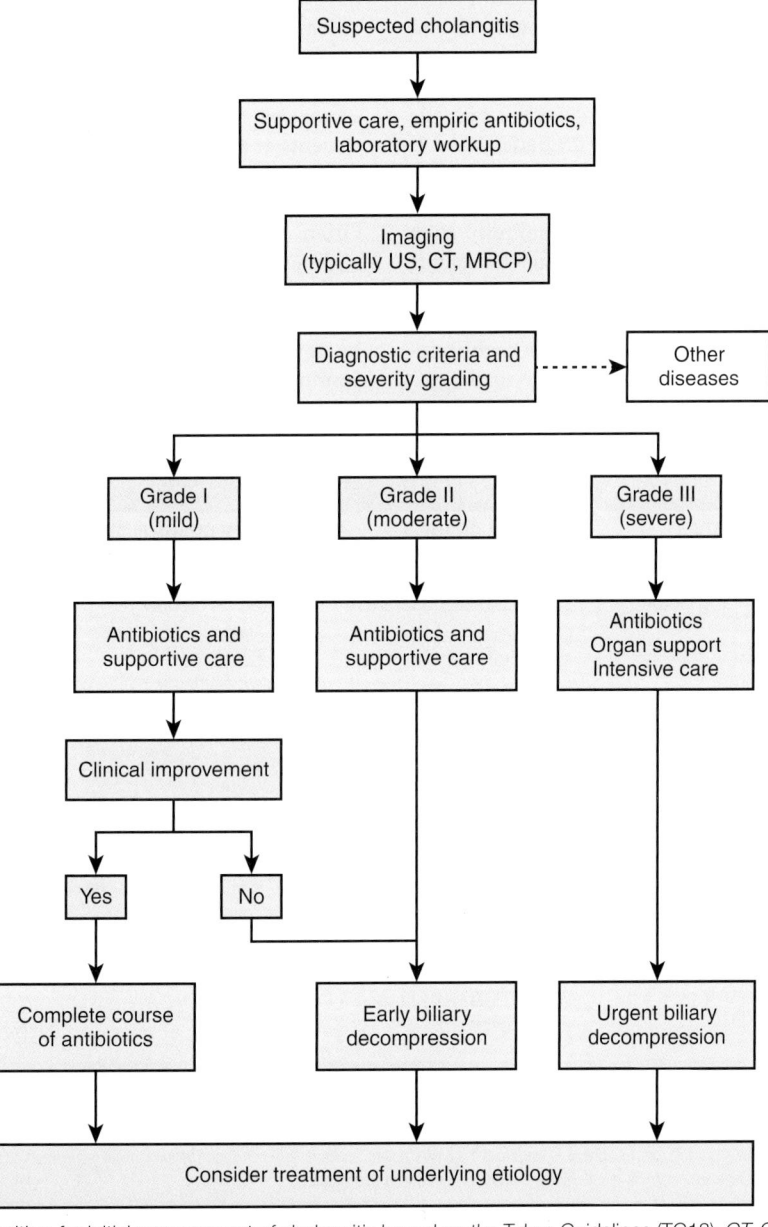

FIGURE 43.2 Suggested algorithm for initial management of cholangitis based on the Tokyo Guidelines (TG18). *CT,* Computed tomography; *MRCP,* magnetic resonance cholangiopancreatography; *US,* ultrasound.

with cholangitis include the gram-negative aerobes *Escherichia coli* and *Klebsiella* spp. and gram-positive *Enterococcus* spp.[26] Anaerobes represent an infrequent isolate but must be considered in the presence of a biliary-enteric anastomosis. Liver transplantation and immunosuppression have been associated with fungal cholangitis due to *Candida* spp.[27]

Over the last several decades, the microbiology of acute cholangitis reflects the emergence of healthcare-associated multidrug-resistant organisms. Extended-spectrum β-lactamase (ESBL), and carbapenemase-producing Enterobacteriaceae, and vancomycin-resistant enterococci pervade healthcare systems and complicate empirical antibiotic selection.[28] The incidence of infections from resistant organisms has been associated with previous biliary procedures, operations, recent antibiotic use, or prolonged hospitalization. Resistance patterns vary widely and reflect local and institution-specific antibiotic use, making it essential to incorporate the local epidemiologic milieu (antibiogram) into therapeutic decision making.

TG18 provides guidelines for the use of empiric antibiotics that takes into account bacterial species commonly found in community-acquired and healthcare-associated infections (Table 43.1).[26] Antibiotic recommendations are stratified by severity grade to balance adequate pathogen coverage with the risk of bolstering antimicrobial resistance.[29] For grades I and II cholangitis, the recommended agents do not cover resistant species, such as ESBL-producing *E. coli*. If the prevalence of these organisms exceeds 10% to 20% in the community, then carbapenems, tigecycline, amikacin, and other newer agents such as ceftazidime/avibactam and ceftolozane/tazobactam may also be used.[26] TG18 recommends adding anti-pseudomonal coverage for grade III community-acquired and healthcare-associated cholangitis. Although an uncommon biliary pathogen,

Pseudomonas aeruginosa may account for excess mortality in critical illness when neglected.

The administration of empiric antibiotics should not be delayed by more than 1 hour for patients with septic shock.[30] For less acutely ill patients, antibiotics should be administered within 6 hours of diagnosis. Blood cultures should be drawn before antibiotic administration, and bile cultures should be obtained at the start of any biliary interrogation or drainage procedure. Antimicrobial agents should be modified based on culture-identified pathogens and susceptibility testing results. This antimicrobial stewardship practice (i.e., de-escalation) promotes evidence-based use of broad-spectrum antibiotics.[30]

The optimal duration of antimicrobial therapy for cholangitis remains unknown, but the TG18 recommendations are based on a number of studies exploring this issue.[31-33] General guidelines are to continue antibiotic therapy until biliary obstruction is relieved, biochemical liver function tests have improved or normalized, and the patient is afebrile for at least 48 hours. Per TG18, a duration of 4 to 7 days is recommended after source control with three notable exceptions. First, the presence of gram-positive bacteremia (e.g., *Enterococcus* spp.) requires at least 2 weeks of treatment. Second, patients at risk for recurrent cholangitis due to residual calculi or persistent partial obstruction warrant continuation of antibiotics until the underlying cause can be completely treated. Often these patients can be transitioned to oral antibiotic regimens, such as trimethoprim/sulfamethoxazole and levofloxacin or ciprofloxacin alone or in combination with metronidazole. Finally, if a liver abscess is present, treatment should be continued until there is adequate drainage and complete resolution (see Chapter 70).

TABLE 43.1	Antimicrobial Recommendations For Cholangitis (TG18)		
	SEVERITY GRADE I	**SEVERITY GRADE II**	**SEVERITY GRADE III AND HEALTHCARE-ASSOCIATED INFECTIONS**
Vancomycin[a]	No	No	Yes
Penicillins	Piperacillin/tazobactam	Piperacillin/tazobactam	Piperacillin/tazobactam
Cephalosporins	Cefazolin[b], or cefotiam[b], or cefuroxime[b], or ceftriaxone, or cefotaxime, ± metronidazole[c] Cefmetazol[b] Cefoxitin[b] Flomoxef[b] Cefoperazone/sulbactam	Ceftriaxone, or cefotaxime, or cefepime, or cefozopran, or ceftazidime ± metronidazole[c] Cefoperazone/sulbactam	Cefepime, or ceftazidime, or cefozopran ± metronidazole[c]
Carbapenems	Ertapenem	Ertapenem	Imipenem/cilastatin, meropenem, doripenem, ertapenem
Monobactams			Aztreonam ± metronidazole[c]
Fluoroquinolones[d]	Ciprofloxacin, or levofloxacin, or pazufloxacin ± metronidazole[c] Moxifloxacin	Ciprofloxacin, or levofloxacin, or pazufloxacin ± metronidazole[c] Moxifloxacin	

[a]Vancomycin is recommended to cover *Enterococcus* spp. for grade III community-acquired and healthcare-associated acute biliary infections. Linezolid or daptomycin is recommended if there is known colonization of vancomycin-resistant *Enterococcus*, if previous treatment included vancomycin, and/or if the organism is common in the community.

[b]Local antimicrobial susceptibility patterns (antibiogram) should guide use.

[c]Antianaerobic therapy, including metronidazole, tinidazole, or clindamycin, is warranted if a biliary-enteric anastomosis is present. The carbapenems piperacillin/tazobactam, ampicillin/sulbactam, cefmetazole, cefoxitin, flomoxef, and cefoperazone/sulbactam have sufficient anti-anaerobic activity for this situation.

[d]Fluoroquinolone use is recommended if the susceptibility of cultured isolates is known or for patients with β-lactam allergies. Many extended-spectrum β-lactamase (ESBL)-producing gram-negative isolates are fluoroquinolone resistant.

Adapted from Gomi H, et al. Tokyo Guidelines 2018: antimicrobial therapy for acute cholangitis and cholecystitis. *J Hepatobiliary Pancreat Sci.* 2018;25(1):3–16.

Definitive Management

When the infectious process has been temporized, care should shift toward addressing the underlying cause of cholangitis. Definitive treatment guidelines vary based on the specific disease and individual patient factors. Figure 43.3 provides a general framework for procedural modalities used in the treatment of affected patients. The remainder of this chapter focuses on specific biliary interventions and their application to specific disease entities.

Procedures for Biliary Decompression

Prompt biliary decompression and drainage are the cornerstones of acute cholangitis treatment. Several techniques can be used to ensure effective biliary drainage, including endoscopic, percutaneous, endoscopic ultrasound–guided, or surgical procedures. The preferred method and route to relieve biliary obstruction, and the ultimate clinical success of biliary drainage, depends on a number of factors including availability of the technique, local expertise, etiology, location and severity of obstruction, and the presence of comorbid medical conditions.

Endoscopic Transpapillary Biliary Drainage (see Chapters 20 and 30)

Endoscopic transpapillary biliary drainage has become the gold standard for cholangitis of benign or malignant etiologies because it is less invasive and associated with a lower risk of adverse events than other biliary drainage procedures.[34] Endoscopic transpapillary biliary drainage should be carried out in a monitored setting (i.e., endoscopy laboratory, intensive care unit, or operating room) under either conscious sedation or general anesthesia. A side-viewing scope is used to visualize and cannulate the ampulla of Vater. Contrast is injected into the bile duct under real-time fluoroscopy only in an amount that allows

the level of the obstruction to be visualized, and a guidewire is passed across the obstruction. If the patient has mild to moderate cholangitis and is stable, an effort can be made to definitively clear the duct of calculi. However, if the patient is septic with hemodynamic instability, or if there is purulence within the duct, biliary decompression should be obtained with the least amount of manipulation and effort, and extended maneuvers to remove calculi should be deferred until the patient is more stable and sepsis has resolved.

The two approaches to endoscopic transpapillary biliary drainage are endoscopic nasobiliary drainage (ENBD) and endoscopic biliary stenting (EBS), which provide external and internal drainage, respectively. ENBD is performed by placing a 5- to 7-Fr drainage tube into the biliary tract over a guidewire. Advantages of ENBD include the ability to monitor and lavage the bile and the ability to collect additional culture specimens. Disadvantages include patient discomfort, which can lead to tube dislodgement and potentially fluid loss and electrolyte imbalances. In contrast, EBS involves inserting a 7- to 10-Fr plastic stent into the bile duct over a guidewire. Internal drainage avoids patient discomfort and minimizes fluid and electrolyte loss; however, reports suggest that stent occlusion may occur more frequently than nasobiliary drain occlusion, especially in patients with hilar cholangiocarcinoma.[35,36] Despite these trade-offs, a TG18 meta-analysis noted no statistically significant differences in success or adverse event rates between patients undergoing ENBD versus EBS. Therefore TG18 recommends that either EBND or EBS can be used based on patient preference, etiology, and bile properties.[33,37–40]

Endoscopic Sphincterotomy and Balloon Dilation

Endoscopic sphincterotomy (EST) involves incising the duodenal papilla to facilitate biliary drainage and stone extraction in a

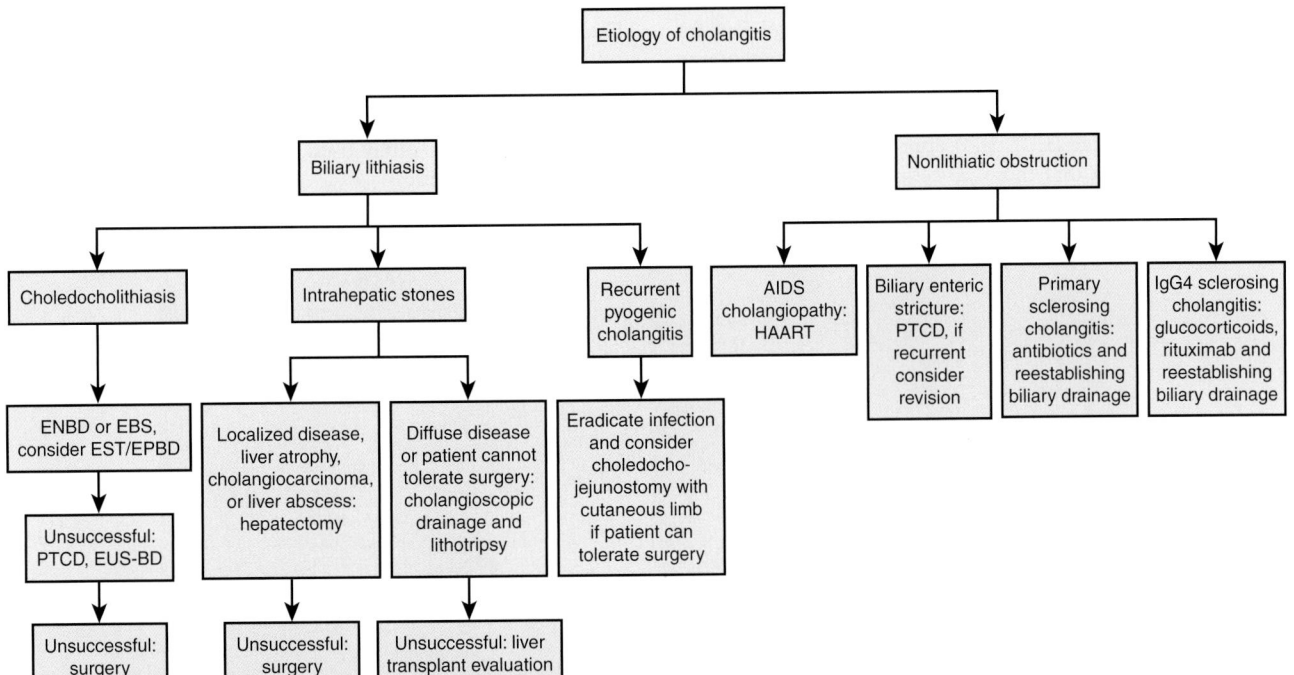

FIGURE 43.3   Indications and procedures for biliary drainage and treatment for nonmalignant causes of cholangitis. *IgG4,* Immunoglobulin G4; *AIDS,* acquired immunodeficiency syndrome; *EBS,* endoscopic biliary stenting; *ENBD,* endoscopic nasobiliary drainage; *EPBD,* endoscopic papillary balloon dilation; *EST,* endoscopic sphincterotomy; *EUS-BD,* endoscopic ultrasound–guided biliary drainage; *HAART,* highly active antiretroviral therapy; *PTCD,* percutaneous transhepatic cholangiography drainage.

single session (see Chapters 20 and 30). Briefly, a high-frequency electrosurgical generator is used to make a controlled incision using various types of sphincterotome devices inserted into the bile duct. The routine use of EST is controversial due to reports of increased risks of hemorrhage, retroduodenal perforation, and pancreatitis.[41,42] A randomized controlled trial comparing ENBD with or without EST in 72 cholangitic patients did not find a statistically significant difference in clinical outcomes or adverse events, suggesting that EST can be cautiously employed to alleviate stone obstruction.[43] Contraindications include coagulopathy, systemic sepsis, and hemodynamic instability. The TG18 states that EST may not be required for biliary drainage and should be deferred until after the resolution of severe sepsis and correction of coagulopathy.[34] For patients with grade I or grade II cholangitis due to stone obstruction who are not coagulopathic, it is acceptable to perform EST and stone removal in a single session.[44]

In contrast to EST, endoscopic papillary balloon dilation (EPBD) preserves the sphincter of Oddi. In this technique, a balloon is passed into the bile duct, inflated, and then withdrawn to dilate the duodenal papilla and facilitate the passage of stones and debris. Comparative studies of EPBD and EST have demonstrated that EPBD is significantly less successful for stone removal and carries a higher risk of pancreatitis; however, there is a significantly lower rate of bleeding with EPBD.[45] Thus EST remains the gold-standard technique to alleviate choledocholithiasis, with EPBD as an alternative when bleeding risk is high.

Single-Balloon and Double-Balloon Endoscopy

Single-balloon and double-balloon enteroscopy (SBE and DBE) are recent innovations that enable access to the duodenal papilla in patients with surgically altered anatomy, such as Roux-en-Y gastric bypass or hepaticojejunostomy[34] (see Chapter 30). There have been many reports of successful SBE- and DBE-guided ERCP in such patients, with high success rates and low frequency of adverse events.[46–50] Disadvantages of balloon enteroscopy include reports of lower success rates and significantly longer procedure times compared with endoscopic ultrasound–guided biliary drainage (EUS-BD) approaches (see the following section).[51] Given that these procedures require specialized training and resources, technical success rates may be institution and practitioner specific.

Percutaneous Transhepatic Cholangial Drainage

Percutaneous transhepatic cholangial drainage (PTCD) is an established and efficacious technique for biliary decompression[52] (see Chapters 20 and 31). In the setting of cholangitis, PTCD is considered a second-line therapy due to the increased risk of adverse events, such as intraperitoneal bleeding (2%), bile peritonitis, tube dislodgement, and superficial site events compared with endoscopic interventions.[53–55] However, when performed at high-volume centers, the complication rates for PTCD versus endoscopic drainage for malignant biliary obstruction were similar.[56] The specific circumstances that warrant PTCD include (1) when the duodenal papilla cannot be accessed due to the presence of gastric outlet obstruction or surgically altered anatomy (e.g., pancreaticoduodenectomy or Roux-en-Y anastomosis), (2) when there is proximal or hilar obstruction that cannot be accessed endoscopically (Fig. 43.4), and (3) in resource-limited settings where advanced endoscopy is not available.

In PTCD, catheterization of a peripheral bile duct with an 18- to 22-gauge needle is performed under ultrasonographic guidance, with care taken to avoid hepatic arterial or portal vessels. Once the biliary system is entered and backflow of bile confirmed, a guidewire is passed and advanced distally under fluoroscopic guidance to traverse the point of biliary obstruction (Fig. 43.5). If the obstructing lesion cannot be traversed, a 7- to 10-Fr locking pigtail catheter is placed to decompress the biliary system proximal to the point of obstruction. Deciding which side of the liver to drain initially depends on the underlying pathology and the location of the obstruction within the biliary tree. Therefore ultrasound and/or CT of the liver should be obtained to assess anatomy, hepatic atrophy, distribution of dilated intrahepatic ducts, and to identify the likely cause and location of the obstruction. When the left hemiliver is punctured, it is preferable to enter into the segment III or IV bile duct through the left lateral segment or the umbilical fissure. When the right hemiliver is punctured, an intercostal approach is often used, preferably aimed toward the main segment VI duct.

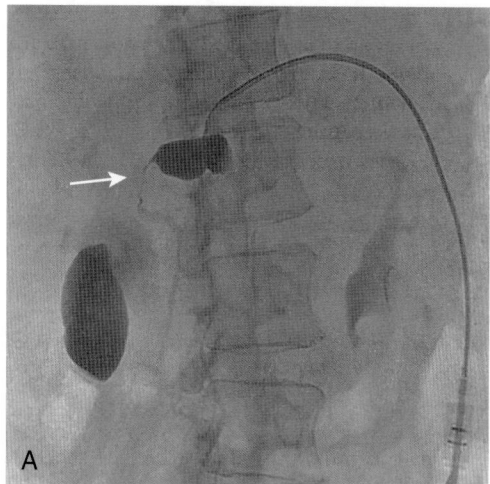
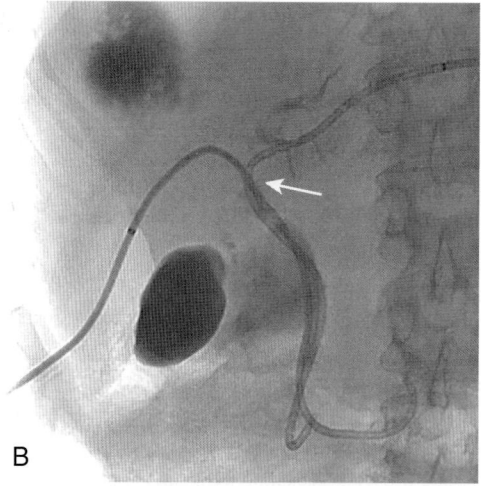

FIGURE 43.4   A, Percutaneous transhepatic cholangiogram (PTC) for cholangitis showing hilar obstruction extending to the left hepatic radical *(arrow)*. **B,** Left and right posterior internal-external biliary drains *(arrow)* placed by PTC to decompress and bypass the obstruction.

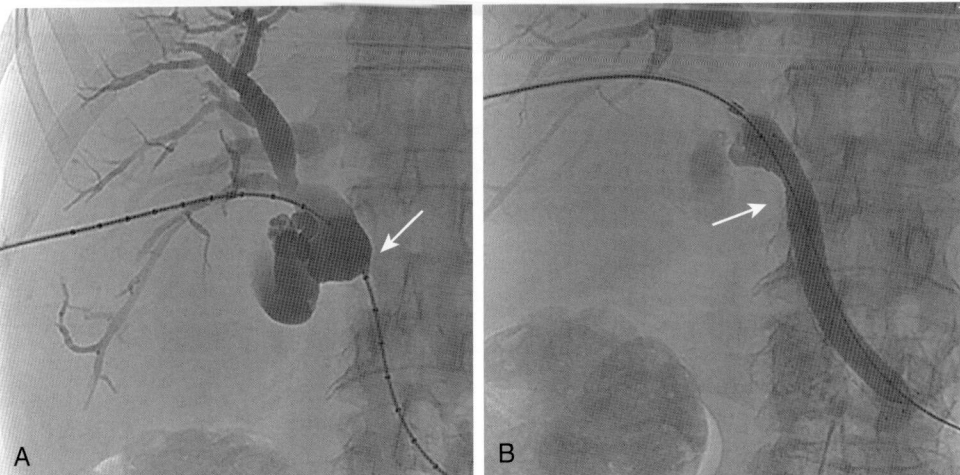

FIGURE 43.5   A, Percutaneous transhepatic cholangiogram (PTC) showing a common bile duct (CBD) obstruction *(arrow)* with dilated bile ducts. **B,** CBD obstruction after balloon plasty *(arrow)* and metallic stent placement through PTC.

In septic or unstable patients, attempting complete clearance of the biliary tree is not recommended, as the goal is decompression. PTCD is contraindicated in patients with significant ascites and should be avoided in anticoagulated or otherwise coagulopathic patients due to the increased risk of bleeding.

Endoscopic Ultrasound–Guided Bile Duct Drainage

EUS-BD has emerged as a viable second-line option after failed endoscopic transpapillary drainage[57,58] (see Chapters 22 and 30). There are three different EUS-BD approaches that can be used: (1) intrahepatic biliary drainage via the transgastric or transjejunal route, (2) extrahepatic biliary drainage by a transduodenal or transgastric approach, or (3) antegrade stenting. The approach is determined by the level of obstruction and whether there is a gastric outlet obstruction.[59] EUS-guided intrahepatic and extrahepatic approaches have a higher technical success rate (95%) compared with EUS-guided antegrade stenting (77%), likely due to difficult technical steps in antegrade stenting, including guidewire passage and stent delivery system insertion.[60] Finally, the "rendezvous" drainage procedure first described in 2004 utilizes combined EUS and PTC-guided transduodenal access to then allow for external access via PTC and internal access via ERCP.[61]

In all EUS-guided techniques, a fine needle is advanced into either an intrahepatic or extrahepatic bile duct under ultrasound visualization. Cholangiography is then performed to confirm successful biliary cannulation, and a guidewire is advanced into the bile duct. The newly created tract is then dilated, and a stent is then placed, which facilitates biliary drainage. Serious adverse events, including peritonitis and stent migration, can result after EUS-BD because artificial tracts create the potential for free extravasation of bile or gastrointestinal contents. As in PTCD, the inadvertent puncture of hepatic vessels can lead to major bleeding complications. The rates of adverse events vary but have been reported to be as high as 20%.[62]

Several studies, including a randomized controlled trial and meta-analyses, have evaluated EUS-BD versus PTCD after failed endoscopic transpapillary biliary drainage and show equivalent success rates of 90% to 100% and lower postprocedure complications after EUS-BD.[63–66] Other notable advantages of EUS-BD include (1) the ability to access the bile duct

in patients with abnormal anatomy and (2) the benefits of internal drainage, including lack of external catheters with the related skin and superficial site events, lack of fluid/electrolyte shifts, and improved nutrition reabsorption and digestion. Key drawbacks of EUS-BD include its dependence on highly skilled pancreaticobiliary endoscopists with access to specialized tools and devices. Thus EUS-BD is a viable second-line intervention at institutions with the requisite resources and expertise; otherwise, either PTCD or transfer to an experienced center should be considered.

Surgical Common Bile Duct Exploration

Surgical CBD drainage carries the highest mortality rate of all biliary drainage options, and due to the significant advances in the aforementioned noninvasive procedures, it is considered a last resort[1] (see Chapters 32 and 37A). At rural or community hospitals that lack interventional radiology or advanced endoscopy, transfer of cholangitic patients to tertiary centers with appropriate technology and specialists is preferred. Surgical intervention may be necessary when failures or complications occur during noninvasive procedures. For example, peritonitis after failed EUS-BD may ultimately warrant laparotomy, washout, and open surgical drainage.

In surgical drainage for cholangitis, the goal is to decompress the biliary system as quickly and effectively as possible. Procedures such as T-tube placement without choledocholithotomy are recommended, as prolonged operations should be avoided. During open CBD exploration, exposure should be obtained along the free border of the lesser omentum, above the duodenum. When dense adhesions are encountered, or the anatomy is unclear, aspiration with a fine needle facilitates localization of the CBD. Once identified, an anterior vertical incision is made parallel to the long axis of the duct on the distal CBD, with stay sutures placed on either side. It is important to emphasize that a vertical, rather than horizontal, incision should be performed; a horizontal incision is limited in extension, yields a stenotic area when closed, and may interrupt the axial arterial blood supply of the CBD, which courses along the 3 o'clock and 9 o'clock positions along the lateral aspects of the bile duct. A T-tube should be placed in the CBD above the level of the obstruction to externally decompress the biliary system and enable bile duct closure. The benefits of T-tube placement and decompression are maintenance of biliary ductal patency in the setting of edema and allowance of subsequent access to the biliary tract. Usually, the T-tube is kept in place for 4 to 6 weeks and is removed after a normal cholangiogram.[67]

OTHER ETIOLOGIES OF CHOLANGITIS

Intrahepatic Biliary Stone Obstruction

Intrahepatic biliary stone disease, or hepatolithiasis, occurs frequently in parts of Asia but is rare in Western countries[68] (see Chapters 39 and 44). Contributing etiologies include genetic defects in bile metabolism, anatomic abnormalities, diet, and bacterial or parasitic colonization.[69] The resulting cholangitis can be difficult to eradicate, and its sequelae include chronic inflammation, biliary fibrosis, ductal strictures, microabscesses, worsening cholestasis, recurrent hepatolithiasis, and liver failure. Hepatolithiasis is also an established risk factor for cholangiocarcinoma, with the overall incidence rate of hepatolithiasis-associated cholangiocarcinoma ranging from 5% to 12%[70] (see Chapter 50). To prevent this cascade of events, treatment of both symptomatic and asymptomatic hepatolithiasis is generally recommended. Treatment options for hepatolithiasis are classified into pharmacologic, endoscopic, and interventional radiology procedures, and surgery. Pharmacologic treatment with ursodeoxycholic acid over long periods (several years) can lead to dissolution of intrahepatic stones but does not effectively treat acute cholangitis.[71]

Lithotripsy

The most common and most well-established nonsurgical approach, percutaneous transhepatic cholangioscopic lithotripsy (PTCSL) utilizes PTCD to create a cutaneobiliary fistula through which cholangioscopy and lithotripsy can be performed. This traditionally requires a long treatment period because serial dilations of the cutaneous tract are performed over days to weeks before cholangioscopy can be performed. Recently, a one-step PTCSL technique was described that uses a protective sheath to enable immediate cholangioscopy without maturation of the sinus tract.[72] Risks of the percutaneous approach are similar to PTCD and include hemobilia, hemoperitoneum, hepatic vascular or ductal injury, and rupture of the sinus tract.[73] An alternative to percutaneous access is peroral cholangioscopic lithotomy (POCSL), which involves ERCP followed by direct intubation of the bile duct with a cholangioscope.[74] This procedure avoids the risks associated with percutaneous biliary access and creation of a cutaneobiliary fistula; however, the ability to access peripheral hepatic ducts may be limited with POCSL.

Once access to the desired segment of the liver is obtained, lithotripsy can be performed using several techniques: (1) mechanical force, (2) electrohydraulic (shockwave), or (3) yttrium-aluminum-garnet (YAG) laser. In mechanical lithotripsy, a lithotripter basket device crushes and removes stones. When stone debris is removed, distal strictures can be traversed with an angioplasty balloon catheter and dilated. Electrohydraulic lithotripsy (EHL) creates short pulses of electric sparks at the tip of a fiber that induce a spherical shock wave that generates sufficient pressure to fragment stones.[75] Holmium:YAG laser lithotripsy ablation of intrahepatic and bile duct stones uses pulses of a laser fiber placed in direct contact with a calculus

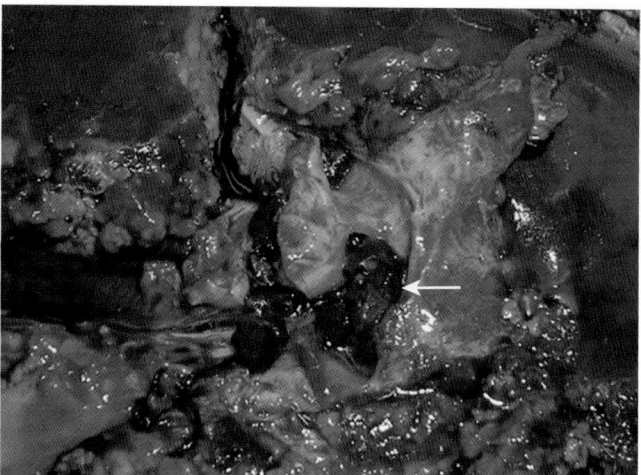

FIGURE 43.6   Intraoperative picture of intrahepatic biliary stones *(arrow)* with strictures and microabscesses.

under direct cholangioscopic visualization.[76] When intraductal techniques fail or access cannot be obtained, extracorporeal shock wave lithotripsy (ESWL) has been described, although this has been reported to be less efficacious.[69]

Stone clearance rates in PTCSL have been reported as high as 85%, with failures mostly due to difficulty manipulating impacted stones proximal to strictures; however, stone recurrence arises in 35% to 50% of hepatolithiasis patients.[69] Stone clearance rates also vary significantly by the modality of lithotripsy used, although there is a paucity of randomized trial data. Two recent randomized controlled trials demonstrated a significantly increased rate of stone clearance in patients treated with laser lithotripsy compared with mechanical lithotripsy without an increase in adverse events.[77,78] The superior efficacy of laser lithotripsy was upheld by a meta-analysis comparing 32 studies with 1969 patients undergoing EHL, laser lithotripsy, or ESWL.[79] Laser lithotripsy had a significantly higher rate of complete ductal clearance (95%) than EHL (88%) and ESWL (84%). The postprocedure complication rate was significantly lower in patients treated with laser lithotripsy (10%) than for patients treated with EHL (14%).

Surgery

Despite advances in noninvasive techniques, surgical management consisting of hepatic resection and/or hepaticojejunostomy remains an effective treatment for patients with complex hepatolithiasis as it simultaneously removes stones and resolves associated pathologic changes, including ductal stricture/fibrosis, and microabscesses (Fig. 43.6), thereby halting the disease process (see Chapters 39 and 44). Indications for hepatectomy include localized disease involving one lobe or a few segments, atrophy or fibrosis of the involved liver, multiple intrahepatic stones causing marked biliary stricture or dilation, presence of a liver abscess, cholangiocarcinoma, and failure of noninvasive treatments.[68] Liver transplantation exists as a salvage option for terminal hepatolithiasis.[80]

Recurrent Pyogenic Cholangitis (see Chapter 43)

Recurrent pyogenic cholangitis (RPC) was first described in 1930[81] and is most common in Southeast Asian populations. It is characterized by recurrent episodes of bacterial cholangitis that occur in association with bile duct strictures, segmental biliary dilation with bile stasis, recurrent episodes of obstructive jaundice and ascending cholangitis, pigmented biliary calculi, and biliary cirrhosis.

The goal of RPC treatment is to eradicate the infection with antimicrobials and eliminate all biliary stones and strictures. As optimal management of stones and strictures will often require multiple treatment sessions, it is usually advised that patients are capable of tolerating a major operation, which may include choledochojejunostomy or hepaticojejunostomy with a biliary access procedure, so that the biliary tree can be readily accessed to clear recurrent stones and to dilate recurrent intrahepatic strictures. Choledochojejunostomy with a cutaneous limb offers a number of distinct advantages over previous approaches in the management of RPC. Following standard cholecystectomy, a portion of the CBD is isolated for choledochoenteric anastomosis. A 60- to 70-cm segment of bowel is used for the Roux-en-Y limb, and a side-to-side choledochojejunostomy is then constructed 10 to 15 cm from the end of the jejunal limb. The blind limb of the jejunal access loop is then brought through the fascia of the abdominal wall in the right upper quadrant at a point that will allow easy access to the biliary tree. Lateral placement of the bowel, just below the skin, will help ensure that the interventional radiologist's hands and instruments are not in the fluoroscopy beam. Although gross stones are removed, no attempt is made at complete clearance of the CBD or hepatic radicles. After closure of the abdomen, the stoma is matured in a "turn-back" fashion. The availability of the cutaneous stoma greatly facilitates subsequent treatment of the residual stones and strictures. After completion of radiologic treatment, the stoma is mobilized, closed, and left buried in the subcutaneous tissues for future access.[82]

The treatment described earlier is far less radical and is associated with lower morbidity and mortality than hepatic resection, with the added benefit of sparing hepatic parenchyma that can potentially recover subsequent to biliary decompression. At the same time, the bypass provides effective initial biliary drainage of the biliary tree and alleviates any immediate biliary sepsis. Clearance of residual stones and dilation of strictures is easily accomplished on an outpatient basis. The treatment of recurrent stones or strictures is greatly simplified by access to the cutaneous jejunal limb, minimizing the need for high-risk reoperative biliary procedures.

Nonlithogenic Biliary Obstruction

Whereas biliary stones are responsible for most cases of cholangitis, other causes include malignancies of the biliary tract and pancreatic head, and nonmalignant etiologies including primary sclerosing cholangitis (PSC), IgG4 cholangitis, acquired immunodeficiency syndrome (AIDS) cholangiopathy, and biliary-enteric anastomotic stricture. As biliary and pancreatic malignancies are discussed in dedicated sections elsewhere, we focus on nonmalignant etiologies here.

Primary Sclerosing Cholangitis

PSC is a chronic cholestatic disease of the liver and bile ducts that frequently progresses to end-stage liver disease[83] (see Chapter 41). The inflammatory process results in patchy areas of fibrosis and obstruction that leads to chronic biliary infection and recurrent episodes of cholangitis. The pathogenesis of PSC involves a combination of autoimmune inflammation of the biliary tree leading to ischemic ductal injury and recurrent bacterial infection. Various diseases are associated with PSC, including inflammatory bowel disease (IBD), celiac sprue, sarcoidosis, chronic pancreatitis, rheumatoid arthritis, retroperitoneal fibrosis, thyroiditis, and vasculitis. Patients with PSC also have a substantial predisposition to develop biliary malignancies.[84]

The diagnosis of PSC is generally made in the setting of chronic cholestatic liver test abnormalities, in particular, elevation of serum alkaline phosphatase, along with cholangiographic (MRCP, ERCP, or PTC) evidence of multifocal strictures of the intrahepatic and extrahepatic bile ducts.[85] Secondary causes of sclerosing cholangitis, including IgG4 disease and AIDS cholangiopathy, must also be excluded. Various autoantibodies have been described in PSC, but the clinical significance of these findings, if any, is unclear. Antineutrophil cytoplasmic antibodies, anticardiolipin antibodies, and antinuclear antibodies have been detected in 84%, 66%, and 53% of patients with PSC, respectively.[84]

The mainstay of treatment for PSC consists of appropriate antibiotic coverage for the bactobilia and reestablishing biliary drainage to the intestinal tract. Long-term antimicrobial prophylaxis is necessary for many patients because of multiple intrahepatic partial biliary strictures; however, no medical therapy is available to halt disease progression or prevent the development of cholangiocarcinoma. The only effective treatment for advanced PSC is orthotopic liver transplantation, which in the absence of cholangiocarcinoma confers a 5-year survival rate of approximately 85%.[86] Patients with cholangiocarcinoma who undergo liver transplantation have a high risk of recurrence and dramatically worsened survival if this occurs. Therefore patients with deteriorating liver function that require liver transplantation should be identified before they develop cholangiocarcinoma.

Immunoglobulin G4–Related Cholangitis

IgG4-related disease (IgG4-RD) is a multiorgan immune-mediated condition that resembles many malignant, infectious, and inflammatory disorders.[87] Originally considered a form of autoimmune pancreatitis (AIP), the concept of IgG4-RD as a unifying diagnosis for its myriad of systemic ramifications did not occur in the literature until 2003.[88] Histopathologic findings of tumefactive lesions, a dense lymphoplasmacytic infiltrate rich in IgG4-positive plasma cells, and storiform fibrosis forms the basis for the diagnosis.[89] Elevated concentrations of IgG4 in tissue and serum are helpful in diagnosing IgG4-RD, but neither one is a specific diagnostic marker.

Biliary tract manifestations of IgG4-RD are termed IgG4-sclerosing cholangitis (IgG4-SC). IgG4-SC frequently occurs in conjunction with IgG4-related AIP.[90] The differential diagnosis of IgG4-SC includes PSC, hilar cholangiocarcinoma, and other causes of secondary sclerosing cholangitis. In particular, distinguishing IgG4-SC from PSC requires careful integration of histology, imaging, serology, pattern of organ involvement, and response to treatment with immunosuppressive therapy (Table 43.2).[91] Accurate diagnosis is of utmost importance to prevent unnecessary surgery and avoid delayed diagnosis of a potentially fatal malignancy. IgG4-RD responds rapidly to immunosuppressive therapy, and the absence of a quick response should prompt reconsideration of the underlying diagnosis. Glucocorticoids and rituximab, a steroid-sparing agent, are the most widely used agents. In the presence of superimposed

TABLE 43.2 Primary Sclerosing Cholangitis versus IgG4-SC

	PSC	IgG4-SC
Age at diagnosis (years)	30–50	50–70
Incidence by sex	Male > Female	Male > Female
Response to steroids	Minimal	Swift
Other organ involvement	Intestinal tract related to inflammatory bowel disease	**Pancreas (organ with primary manifestation)**, salivary glands, kidneys, periorbital tissues, aorta, lymph nodes, lungs, meninges, etc.
Association with cholangiocarcinoma	Yes	No
Serum IgG4 > 140 mg/dL	15%	90%
Cholangiography	Bile duct with short segment strictures and interspersed normal caliber or dilated segments (beads-on-a-string appearance)	Thickened bile duct walls; long strictures with upstream dilatation
Histology	Loss of bile ducts; onion skin-type periductal fibrosis	Dense lymphoplasmacytic infiltrate; storiform fibrosis; obliterative phlebitis; onion skin-type periductal fibrosis (rare)
Immunohistochemistry: >10 IgG4+ cells/HPF or IgG4:IgG ratio >0.4	Occasionally	Usually

HPF, High-power field; *IBD,* Inflammatory bowel disease; *IgG4,* immunoglobulin G4; *PSC,* primary sclerosing cholangitis.
Adapted from Chen JH, et al. IgG4-related disease and the liver. *Gastroenterology Clin North Am.* 2017;46(2):195–216.

cholangitis, urgent interventions to relieve biliary obstruction may be necessary.[92]

AIDS Cholangiopathy

AIDS cholangiopathy occurs when strictures in the biliary tract develop due to opportunistic infections in severely immunocompromised patients (CD4 lymphocyte count <100 cells/mm³).[93] Common pathogens associated with AIDS cholangiopathy include *Cryptosporidium parvum*, cytomegalovirus (CMV), and microsporidia such as *Enterocytozoon bieneusi*. Manifestations of AIDS cholangiopathy resemble PSC and include papillary stenosis, long extrahepatic strictures, acalculous cholecystitis, and intrahepatic and extrahepatic sclerosing lesions.[94]

Highly active antiretroviral therapy (HAART) to restore immune function is the only effective treatment for AIDS cholangiopathy. Treatment of opportunistic infections with antiinfectives has not resulted in significant benefit.[93] ERCP to improve biliary drainage may alleviate symptoms of pain and improve biliary drainage but does not alter the progression of disease nor impact overall survival.[95]

The overall prognosis of patients with AIDS cholangiopathy is poor due to the sequelae of severe immunosuppression. Before the widespread use of HAART, one study reported 1- and 2-year survival rates of 41% and 8%, respectively.[96] In a later study of 94 patients with AIDS cholangiopathy diagnosed between 1983 and 2001,[97] the mean survival was 9 months in those patients with cholangiopathy, and HAART provided a dramatic survival benefit. As in other secondary causes of sclerosing cholangitis, AIDS cholangiopathy may be associated with cholangiocarcinoma.[98] With the increasing availability of HAART, it is hoped that AIDS cholangiopathy might become a disorder of historic interest only.[99]

Biliary-Enteric Anastomosis

Cholangitis is a well-known complication following Roux-en-Y hepaticojejunostomy or choledochojejunostomy for benign or malignant hepatobiliary or pancreatic disease (see Chapters 37A and 42). In a large meta-analysis of 28 studies involving 6904 patients, the pooled incidence of postoperative cholangitis within a median time interval of 10 months was 10%.[100] Postoperative anastomotic strictures and postoperative hepatolithiasis were strongly associated with the occurrence of cholangitis.

Postoperative cholangitis after biliary-enteric anastomosis presents a complex situation for which standardized guidelines do not yet exist. In addition to antibiotic therapy, treatment options to restore biliary drainage include ERCP (facilitated by SBE or DBE), EUS-BD, PTCD, or reoperation. When cholangitis due to anastomotic stricture occurs within the first 30 postoperative days, greater consideration should be given to surgical revision. In contrast, late-onset cholangitis has been reported up to 10 years after the initial surgery, and initial management in this case should be conservative. Patients with recurrent cholangitis and/or failed endoscopic or percutaneous attempts to restore normal bile flow should be evaluated for revision biliary surgery.[100]

Complications of Cholangitis

Inadequately managed cholangitis can be complicated by liver, gallbladder, and subphrenic abscesses, which can be fatal if untreated. When suspected, the diagnosis should be pursued with imaging studies: contrast-enhanced CT will show rim-enhancing fluid collection, and ultrasound findings frequently show a thickened edematous wall with inhomogeneous hypoechoic contents.[101] Treatment follows standard surgical principles of antibiotic administration and drainage of purulent collections. Blood cultures should be sent and empiric antibiotics started as soon as possible. Microbial populations reflect those of the underlying acute cholangitis; therefore the TG18 antimicrobial guidelines serve as an acceptable resource for selecting the empiric antibiotic regimen (see Table 43.1). In general, parenteral antibiotics should be continued until resolution of symptoms and laboratory abnormalities, after which patients should transition to oral antibiotics. The typical duration of antibiotic therapy is 4 to 6 weeks.[101]

Drainage options include percutaneous needle aspiration (PNA) with or without a drainage catheter, endoscopic drainage, and laparoscopic or open surgical drainage. The number of abscesses and their size serve as chief criteria for selecting the optimal drainage strategy. Single abscesses less than 3 cm in size often resolve with antibiotic therapy alone.[102] Abscesses less than 3 cm that fail to resolve with antibiotics or those greater than 3 cm should be percutaneously drained. The outcomes for patients undergoing PNA versus percutaneous catheter drainage (PCD) have been studied in randomized trials. A meta-analysis of 5 randomized controlled trials covering 306 patients showed superior outcomes in patients treated with PCD versus PNA, including success rate, clinical improvement, and time to achieve a 50% reduction in abscess[103]; no significant differences were found in duration of hospitalization or complication rates. Taking into account the variability of the studies, both PNA and PCD appear to be acceptable choices for smaller abscesses (<5 cm).

For large (>5 cm) or multiloculated abscesses, either PCD or surgical drainage should be considered (see Chapter 70). A comparative study of 80 patients with abscesses greater than 5 cm showed that surgical drainage (n = 44) was associated with a significantly lower rate of treatment failure, fewer additional procedures, and shorter hospitalization than percutaneous drainage (n = 36); however, there were no differences in rates of morbidity or mortality.[104] Moreover, retrospective studies of patients undergoing percutaneous drainage for abscesses greater than 10 cm showed acceptable outcomes, suggesting that abscess size alone should not be a contraindication to percutaneous drainage.[105,106] If percutaneous drainage is unsuccessful, either repeat percutaneous drainage or surgical drainage are viable options. Surgical drainage warrants stronger consideration for large or multiloculated abscesses, situations where percutaneous access is infeasible, or for patients with coexisting pathologies thought to be contributing to the perpetuation of infection or hindering abscess resolution.

SUMMARY

Cholangitis occurs due to a wide spectrum of underlying etiologies that lead to cholestasis, obstruction of biliary flow, and infection. It cannot be overemphasized that prompt recognition and treatment are of paramount importance, as inadequately treated cholangitis can rapidly progress to life-threatening sepsis. Standardized diagnostic criteria and severity grading should be applied during patient workup. Intervention should begin with resuscitation and parenteral empirical antibiotics. The timing of and indications for biliary decompression vary from elective to urgent, depending on the severity of disease. An emerging armamentarium of percutaneous and endoscopic biliary drainage interventions has narrowed the indications for surgical drainage to rare and specific situations. The procedural modalities used in the treatment of affected patients require a thorough understanding of the etiology and should be tailored to the specific cause.

The references for this chapter can be found online by accessing the accompanying Expert Consult website.

CHAPTER 44

Recurrent pyogenic cholangitis

Tan To Cheung, Wong Hoi She, Ka Wing Ma, and Simon Tsang

Recurrent pyogenic cholangitis (RPC) is a clinical condition caused by repeated episodes of cholangitis, with biliary sepsis secondary to the accumulation of pigmented stones inside the biliary system (see Chapters 39 and 43), and there may be associated stricture formation of the biliary tree (see Chapter 42). The term RPC was formulated after identification of a series of patients with similar clinical conditions and pathology by Cook in 1954. The condition was also known as Hong Kong disease following an initial description by Professor K. H. Digby in 1930.[1] Other names of this entity include "Oriental cholangiohepatitis,"[2] "intrahepatic stones,"[3] "hepatolithiasis,"[4] and "Oriental infestational cholangitis."[5] Most of these patients originated from Southeast Asia, which raises a postulation that this condition may be associated with lifestyle and dietary habits of the ethnic groups native to this area.

In the past, RPC was associated with patients of a lower socioeconomic background. However, as the standard of living in endemic areas improved in the 1960s and 1990s, this association became less obvious. There is no difference in the incidence among males and females. The median age of the first attack of cholangitis is approximately 60 years old, which means that the condition may require several decades to develop before clinical presentation. Although the number of new cases presented each year in Hong Kong remains similar, the projected incidences are expected to fall as general standards of hygiene, living conditions, and health awareness continue to improve.

ETIOLOGY AND PATHOGENESIS

The etiology of RPC is multifactorial. The essence of stricture formation is the presence of microorganisms in the biliary tract as a result of repeated infections and inflammation (see Chapters 8, 39, and 43). The sequence of events likely begins with contamination of bile with bowel microorganisms. Clinical and experimental studies have shown that organisms isolated from the liver and the biliary tract are nearly identical to the microorganisms found in gut flora, as these organs communicate via venous drainage through the superior mesenteric vein (SMV) and the portal vein (PV). In most healthy individuals, the microorganisms will not breach the portal venous system and cause infection in the liver and biliary tree. However, in individuals with chronic illness, malnutrition, persistent stress, and any condition leading to an immunocompromised state, the microorganism may breach the gut mucosal barrier and migrate to the liver. Liver flukes and worms may also penetrate the gut mucosa and enter the biliary system along the portal venous circulation. Some of these microorganisms will station in the hepatobiliary system and cause infection including micro liver abscess or localized infection of the portal triads. If the infection is serious, hepatocytes may undergo necrosis resulting in cholangiohepatitis. The damage to the biliary system is usually mild if the infection is localized to the cholangioles. Mild infection can be self-limiting; however, if the area of infection is

more extensive, the segmental biliary tree as well as the common bile duct (CBD) may be involved. The presence of repeated infections and inflammation may lead to fibrosis and strictures to the biliary system, causing irreversible morphologic changes to the bile ducts.

The presence of stones is a common finding in patients with RPC. Whether stones or stricture formation develop first remains uncertain. The stones act as a nidus and promote bacterial colonization and infection. Repeated infections are associated with strictures of the biliary system, thereby hindering bile flow, which may further promote stone formation and recurring infection. Endoscopic retrograde cholangiography (ERCP) findings of RPC patients commonly show a ductal stricture followed by clusters of stones. Patients can also develop cholangitis with focal strictures of the biliary system without any obvious stone. Other typical findings at ERCP include multiple stones and dilatation of the bile duct without any obvious stricture. In patients with intrahepatic duct strictures, there can be stone impaction causing a stone cast. The biliary strictures may not be severe, but even a mild narrowing can be sufficient to reduce the normal passage of bile promoting viscous bile and sludge formation as well as early precipitation of bile before discernible stones are formed.

The calculi in RPC are typically pigmented bilirubinate stones, it is postulated that bile turns from a supersaturated solution into an insoluble precipitate inside the affected bile duct (see Chapter 8). It was also postulated that β-glucuronidase, derived from Clostridium perfringens and Escherichia coli, splits the bilirubin diglucuronide into free bilirubin, and ionized unconjugated bilirubin, together with ionic calcium, precipitates to form the insoluble calcium bilirubinate, which eventually form stones inside the biliary system.[4,6,7]

Biliary obstruction combined with bacterial overgrowth will ultimately result in cholangitis. In this vicious cycle the infection leads to intramural inflammation of ducts and results in more frequent infections with structural damage and stenosis in the biliary system.

In the histologic examination of the resected liver, the number of mucus glands in the epithelial lining is increased.[8,9] The increase in mucus formation secondary to focal inflammation together with bacterial colonization triggers a cascade of events culminating in lithogenesis. Lipopolysaccharide may induce overexpression of gel-forming apomucin (MUC2 and MIC5AC) in the biliary epithelial cells through the synthesis of tumor necrosis factor (TNF)-α and activation of protein kinase C.[10] Mucin hypersecretion contributes to further stone formation by slowing the flow of bile and creating a focus for pigment deposit.[11]

The associations between RPC and Clonorchis sinensis or Ascaris lumbricoides have been well established.[12,13] C. sinensis is well known to cause biliary stricture and recurrent cholangitic attacks. The identification of this liver fluke has been documented in approximately 20% of patients with RPC. It can be identified in patients' stool, bile, and resected liver specimens. Transcriptional alterations in bile ducts involved with *C. sinensis* infection have been noted in animal studies.[14] In *C. sinensis*–infected rats, the majority of differentially expressed genes (DEGs) were downregulated, suggesting that potential pathologic changes in the bile ducts start from the early stage of infection. The DEGs are likely to be temporally dysregulated over the time course of the infection.

C. sinensis infiltration of the biliary system produces an easily recognizable cholangiographic picture (see Chapters 45 and 71). The findings consist of characteristic filling defects and changes in the intrahepatic and extrahepatic ducts. The filling defects are usually small, irregular, and uniform in size. The changes in the intrahepatic ducts consist of ductal dilatation typically involving smaller ducts, apparent elongation, tortuosity, and duct wall irregularities. The changes in the extrahepatic ducts consist mainly of duct wall irregularities and a mild degree of dilatation. Recognizing such features is important as the management may have to be modified if cholangitis is the result of clonorchiasis alone.[15] However, biliary infection with other organisms may also give rise to RPC, because RPC is still prevalent in some countries, like the Philippines, where clonorchiasis is not frequently found.

PATHOLOGY

The permanent structural changes caused by RPC are secondary to repeated infections, inflammation, and fibrosis formation leading to strictures of the bile duct and stone formation. The results of repeated infections are progressive epithelial and hepatocellular cell damage, as discussed previously. These changes have been documented by Lam and colleagues.[16] These changes include loss of parallelism of ductal walls, excessive branching, and abrupt termination or "arrowhead" formation of smaller ducts (Fig. 44.1).

The most common site of the ductal strictures is in the larger branches. Main left-sided ducts are more likely to be involved followed by main right ducts and intrahepatic ducts. Proximal dilatation of biliary structures can be observed if the stricture is severe. Long strictures can occur, but these are usually located in the intrahepatic biliary tree and are manifested by tubular narrowing over a length of duct (Fig. 44.2). Main

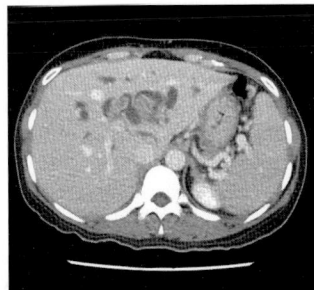

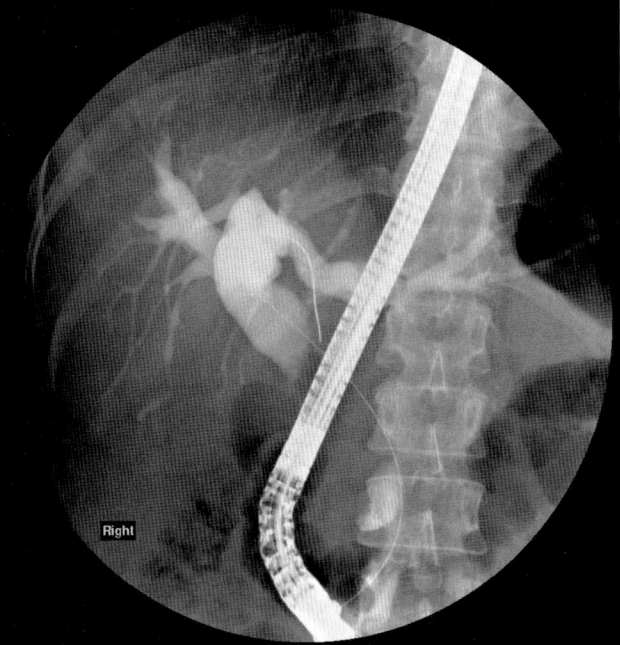

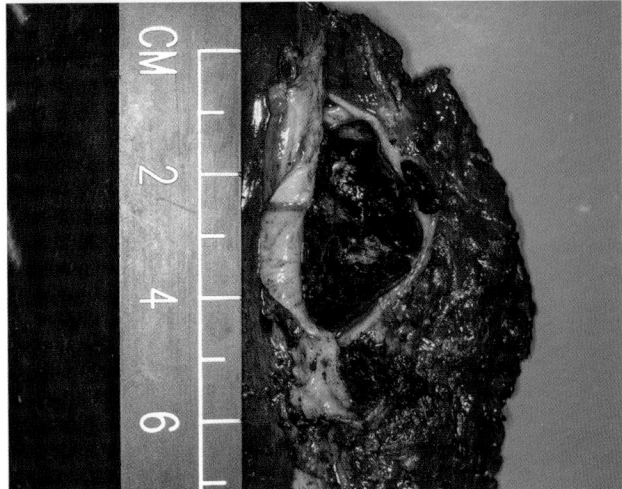

FIGURE 44.2 A, Dilatation of left intrahepatic ducts with multiple stones inside the biliary tree. There is evidence of portal hypertension with splenomegaly and varices formation (see Chapter 16). **B,** Endoscopic retrograde cholangiopancreatography showing stone in common bile duct and absence of S2 duct in the left biliary system, which is suggestive of a stricture or biliary stone impaction in the S2 duct. Liver resection is indicated for infection control and removal of a possibly stenotic biliary segment, which is potentially malignant (see Chapter 30). **C,** Left hepatectomy performed. The left biliary duct was packed with pigmented stones.

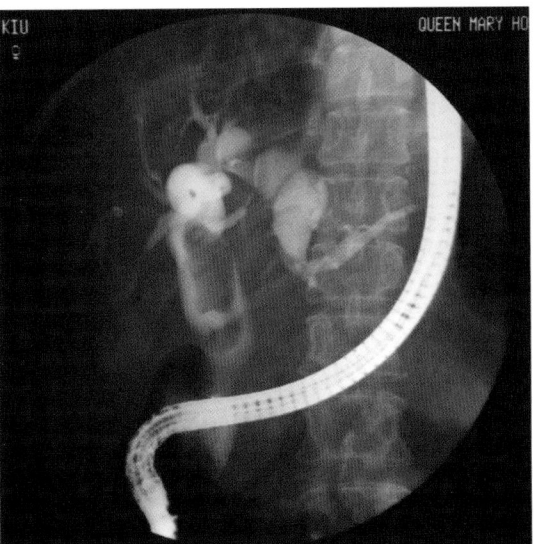

FIGURE 44.1 Endoscopic retrograde cholangiopancreatography showing typical feature of recurrent pyogenic cholangitis with dilated common bile duct (CBD), CBD stone, dilated left intrahepatic duct, and arrowhead stricture of right intrahepatic ducts (see Chapter 30).

left duct structures are found in 40% of patients with RPC. The exact reason for this pattern remains unknown, but it is believed that because the left duct is oriented more horizontally, this may result in a more sluggish flow of bile exacerbating stasis and stone formation. The main right hepatic duct is involved in approximately 20% of patients with RPC. The remaining 40% of patients have bilateral involvement or intrahepatic ductal involvement (Fig. 44.3).[17]

Proximal dilatation of ducts in relation to a stricture are a secondary phenomenon. The dilated portions can be large and are called cisterns.[18] Regression of the hepatocytes in these areas may result in segmental atrophy (see Chapter 16). Stones may or may not be present in these pathologic bile ducts (Fig. 44.4). The walls of these bile ducts are typically thickened and fibrotic, potentially causing difficulties during reconstruction. Attempts to repair them may be complicated by restenosis and cholangitis, eventually requiring resection of the diseased liver segment.

Twenty percent of patients present with isolated extrahepatic CBD dilatation, gallbladder stones, and a diseased gallbladder. In acute cholangitis, where the CBD is obstructed by stone, the gallbladder may be distended. Edema, empyema, gangrenous change, and perforation of the gallbladder can complicate biliary obstruction. With recurrent episodes of cholangitis and gallbladder stones, initial drainage by ERCP, surgical drainage procedures, and cholecystectomy may be required for effective management of extrahepatic manifestations of RPC (Fig. 44.5).

Biliary stones at the distal end of the CBD may cause choledochoduodenal fistulae and acute pancreatitis. Acute pancreatitis is a potentially lethal consequence of RPC. Acute pancreatitis was once associated with RPC in 50% of the patient population and was present in 20% of RPC patients with elevated serum amylase levels.[19] Choledochoduodenal fistula is a chronic sequela of stone erosion, which is usually self-limiting, but it may cause confusion to the clinician during endoscopy.

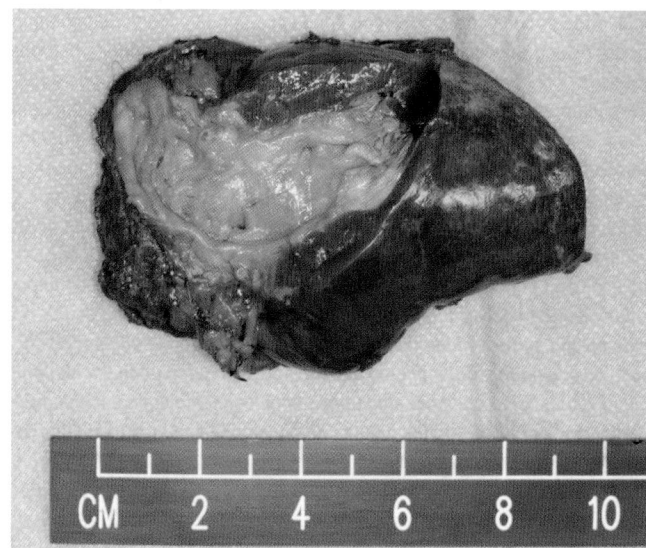

FIGURE 44.4 Resected segment of liver showed gross dilatation of the left duct of the liver without impaction of stone inside the biliary system.

In approximately 10% of cases, no biliary stone can be found in the biliary tree. Muddy debris made up of mucus, pus, parasites, microcalculi, and desquamated epithelium may be found inside a bile duct during ERCP or surgical procedures. Whenever *C. sinensis* is encountered, anthelminthic therapy should be prescribed to eliminate infestation by the liver fluke (see Chapters 45 and 71).

Stones found in RPC patients are bilirubinate stones. These stones are usually characterized by pigmentation and are relatively soft (see Chapter 8). They can accumulate and mold to the configuration of the bile duct in which they reside. When packed together, these stones can have multiple facets. Bilirubinate stone can easily be fragmented during surgery, choledochoscopy, and ERCP.

In the fresh state, the stone surfaces are covered with mucus or a film of viscous bile. In some stones, the outer color may be almost black from prolonged exposure to bile, whereas in others, it is orange or green. Flakes of more recently deposited bile debris are separated from the surface when gently scraped, exposing a light-colored interior, which may appear laminated. Some stones show no organized structure and disintegrate with the slightest compression into irregular, powdery clumps. A nidus may sometimes be identified, and microscopic examination of this area may find dead parasites or clumps of bacteria or cells.[20]

In patients undergoing surgery for RPC during an acute episode of cholangitis, the liver surface is usually found to be "cholangitic" with elements of congestion, bile-stained surfaces, relatively soft consistency, and with a tendency to bleed. In the quiescent phase, avascular adhesions may be found between the surfaces of the liver and the parietal peritoneum. In long-standing patients, the adhesions are dense and vascular. Pus on the liver surface signifies previous abscess formation and rupture with resolution.

Atrophy of a particular liver segment can develop as a consequence of long-standing stone obstruction and stricture of the segmental bile duct. When the left lobe of the liver is atrophic, compensatory hypertrophy of the right lobe is typically found. Conversely, when the right lobe is atrophic, there is

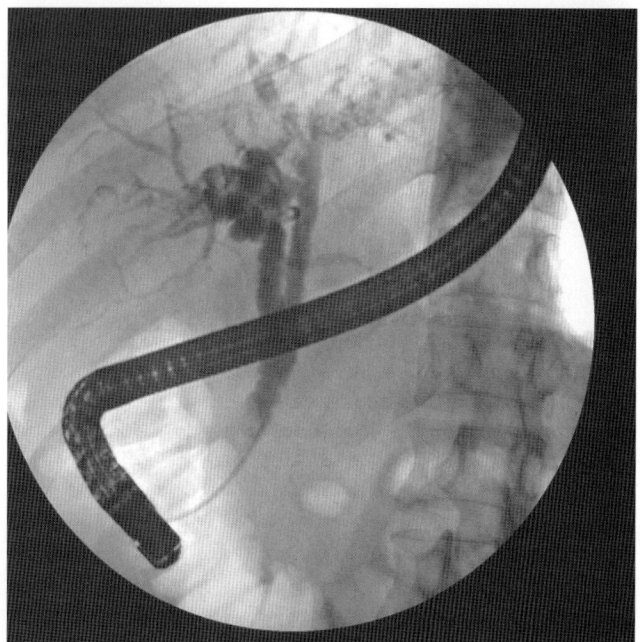

FIGURE 44.3 Endoscopic retrograde cholangiopancreatography showed focal dilatation of intrahepatic ducts with stone accumulation inside the intrahepatic ducts.

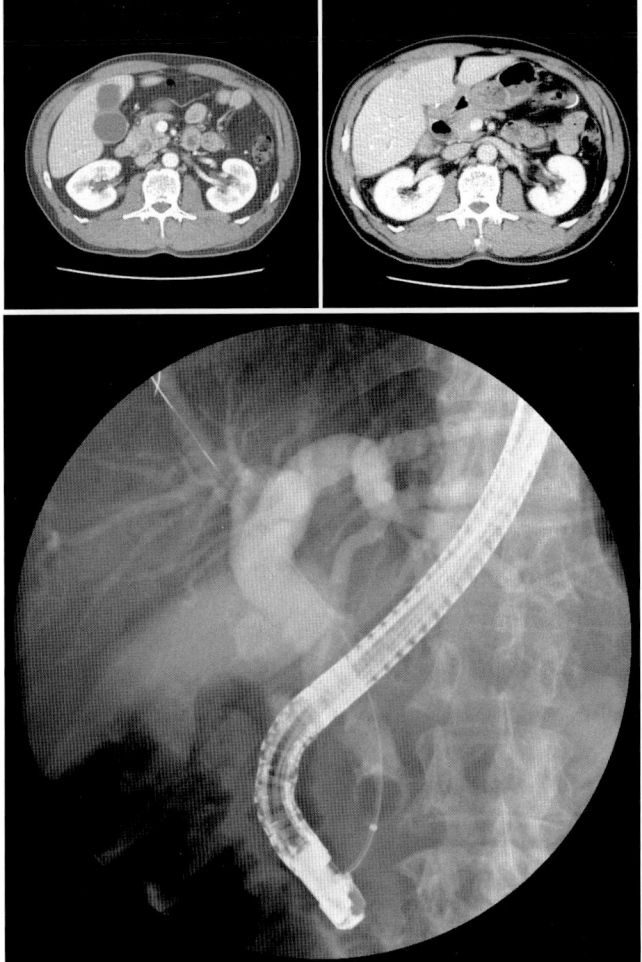

FIGURE 44.5 **A** and **B,** Contrast computed tomography (CT) scan of a patient with extrahepatic recurrent pyogenic cholangitis, which showed dilated common bile duct (CBD) and distended gallbladder. There was a large stone at the lower end of the CBD. This patient had undergone a robotic-assisted cholecystectomy and choledochojejunostomy. The follow-up CT scan showed no more stone and no dilatation of bile ducts (see Chapter 16). **C,** Endoscopic retrograde cholangiopancreatography showing dilated CBD and left intrahepatic duct with no stricture in the intrahepatic ductal system (see Chapter 30).

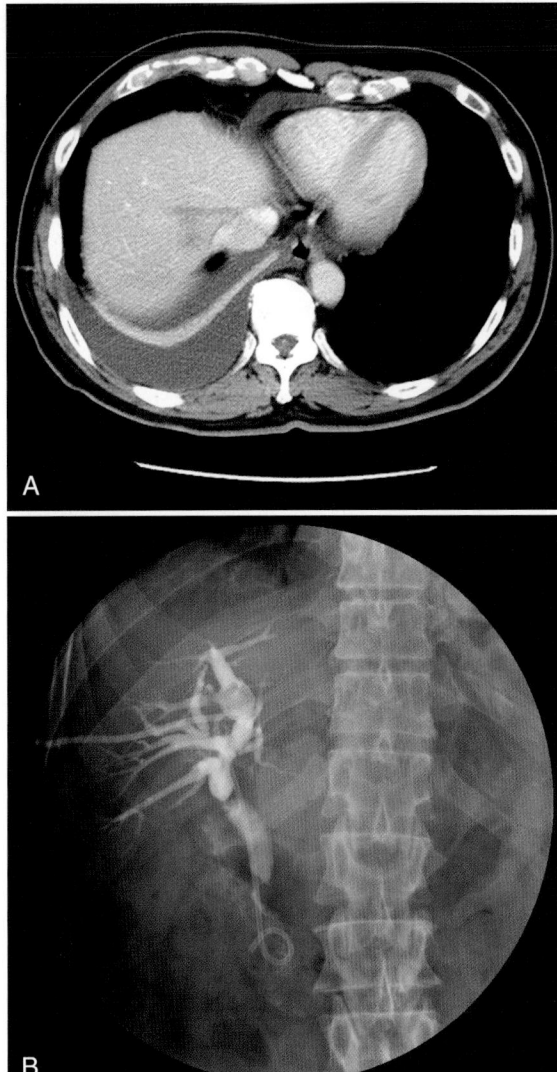

FIGURE 44.6 **A,** Patient who presented with recurrent pyogenic cholangitis (RPC) with recurrent infection and abscess formation in the dome of the liver, resulting in pleural effusion. **B,** Patient presented with RPC, with strictures in the intrahepatic portion of S8 ducts and the left duct was not well shown in endoscopic retrograde cholangiopancreatography due to stone impaction. Right hepatectomy is warranted in view of the focal stricture in the intrahepatic duct. Percutaneous transhepatic biliary drainage was inserted to the S8 duct before liver resection to control the systemic sepsis (see Chapter 30).

usually hypertrophy of the left lobe or caudate lobe leading to rotation of the liver hilum.

When inadequately treated with antibiotics, an infected and obstructed segmental duct may form a liver abscess, resulting in severe localized infection, and potential rupture of the abscess with systemic sepsis. Liver abscesses located in the left lobe of liver may rupture into the pericardial cavity and cause cardiac tamponade,[21] whereas abscesses in the right liver may rupture to form a pleurobiliary or bronchobiliary fistula.[22] These abscesses may bleed into their own cavities or bile ducts, or rupture into the abdominal cavity or into any adjacent hollow viscera with extension into the subphrenic or subhepatic spaces (Fig. 44.6).

Following biliary tract infection, thrombophlebitis of the PV and its branches may occur because of the proximity to the biliary ducts in the portal triad (see Chapter 43). Acute inflammation of the biliary tree can cause edema and compression in the portal venous system, which can result in acute thrombosis

of the PV. Chronic portal venous obstruction leads to segmental liver atrophy.[23] Pulmonary hypertension may follow hepatic venous thrombosis.[24] Microscopically, the portal triads are infiltrated with inflammatory cells and pus, and repeated attacks may result in metaplasia of the ductal mucosal glands. Degeneration and necrosis of hepatocytes will develop when fibrosis extends beyond the thickened duct wall into the adjoining liver parenchyma.

Chronic liver insufficiency, biliary liver cirrhosis, and overt liver failure may develop after a long history of RPC. Patients who have neglected their symptoms or had experienced subclinical symptoms can present with liver failure. Other patients may have undergone multiple operations for RPC, and still develop liver decompensation. Complications of cirrhosis such

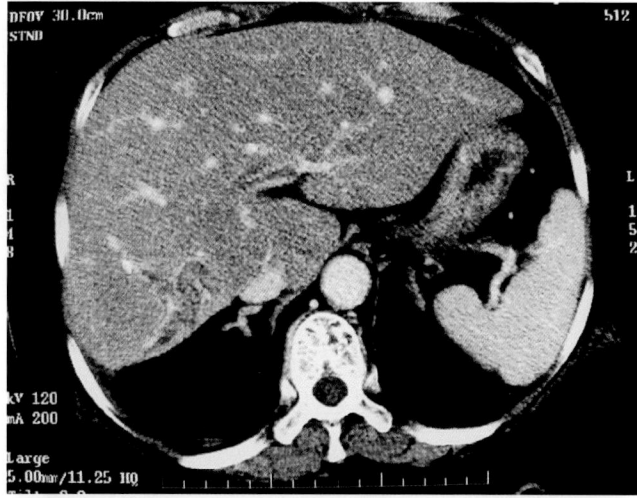

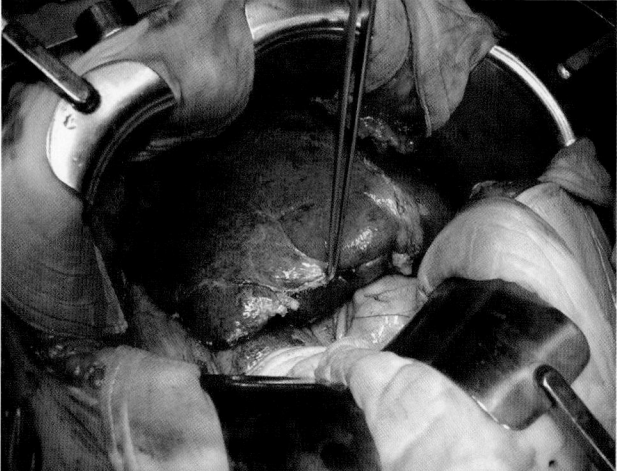

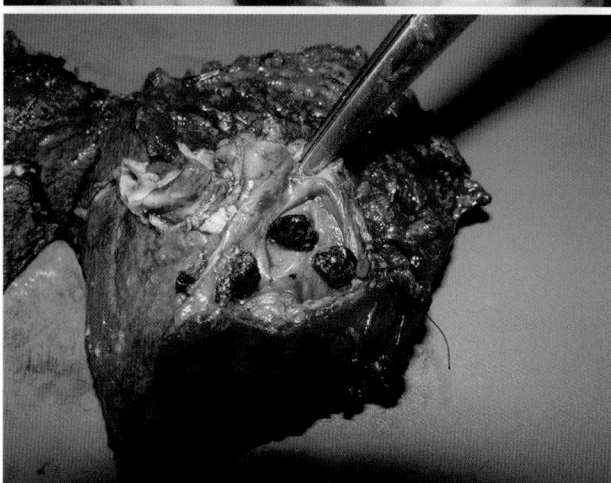

FIGURE 44.7 **A,** Computed tomography scan showed atrophy of the right posterior sector of the liver with stone impaction of the right sectorial duct. Recurrent infection with ductal stricture resulted in the atrophy of the local segment of liver (see Chapter 16). **B,** Operative photo of right posterior sectionectomy for an atrophic liver, secondary to recurrent pyogenic cholangitis. The right anterior section of the liver has undergone hypertrophic changes. **C,** Right posterior section of liver is atrophic, with stricture at the origin of the duct and multiple stones impacted inside the diseased duct.

as portal hypertension and bleeding esophageal varices may ensue. Portosystemic shunting or liver transplant is warranted in cases of recurrent bleeding or liver decompensation.

Chronic cholangitic abscesses may be indistinguishable from cholangiocarcinoma clinically, during surgery, or in contrast imaging studies. The definitive diagnosis can only be confirmed by histology after liver resection. The association between RPC and cholangiocarcinoma is well estrablished.[25,26]

The incidence of cholangiocarcinoma is high in patients with RPC (see Chapters 50 and 51). From the experience of Queen Mary Hospital in Hong Kong, the incidence of cholangiocarcinoma was 7.5% in patients with RPC from 2000 to 2020. The incidence of cholangiocarcinoma, however, has been decreasing. A possible explanation for this trend may be that the strongest risk factors for cancer formation, such as severe clonorchiasis (Fig. 44.7)[27] and intrahepatic stones,[26,28–30] more often lead to liver resection for infection control, potentially preventing the later progression to cancer. Autopsy studies suggest that recurrent cholangitis can induce progressive changes, leading to atypical hyperplasia of the ductal epithelium, followed by dysplasia and carcinoma formation.[26] Evidence has shown that patients with RPC may develop cholangiocarcinoma in a multistep process of transformation including biliary intraepithelial neoplasia and intraductal papillary neoplasia formations (Fig. 44.8).[31] The tumor may take the form of a nodular or papillary growth, and stones may be found within the tumor mass or within the ductal lumen with tumor invasion. A low threshold of suspicion for malignancy should be adopted. When an abnormal lesion is found during imaging studies or an abnormal serum carcinoembryonic antigen (CEA) level is detected in an RPC patient, complete workup for cholangiocarcinoma should be performed.[32]

Cholangiocarcinoma tends to develop in an atrophic segment of liver. In case series, up to 88% of cholangiocarcinoma was located in atrophic hepatic segments.[33] It is postulated that RPC patients who have undergone surgical treatment early with resection of diseased liver can remain free of malignancy. Vigilant surveillance and early intervention are essential in high-risk patients.[34]

Clinical Manifestation of the Recurrent Pyogenic Cholangitis and Nonsurgical Management Option of Recurrent Pyogenic Cholangitis

Clinical Features

In contrast to biliary calculous diseases seen in Western countries (see Chapter 33), RPC affects men and women equally, with a predilection for the lower socioeconomic classes. In Hong Kong, with improved socioeconomic conditions, there is a trend toward fewer new cases and fewer young patients with RPC. In a survey in which the median age of patients with RPC was 59.5 years, 56% had prior biliary surgery for stone disease.[35] The incidence of RPC has been constantly decreasing in recent years, with fewer complications and emergencies.

The symptoms of RPC overlap with acute cholangitis, often presenting with pain, fever, and jaundice (Charcot's triad) (see Chapter 43). The usual symptoms of an acute attack resemble those of acute cholangitis, including pain, fever, and jaundice. The overall presentation can range from subtle complaints of nausea and vomiting with slightly deranged liver function tests, to florid symptoms with the characteristics of Charcot's triad or Reynold's pentad. The pain is typically worst in the right

Incidence of RPC in Queen Mary Hospital Hong Kong

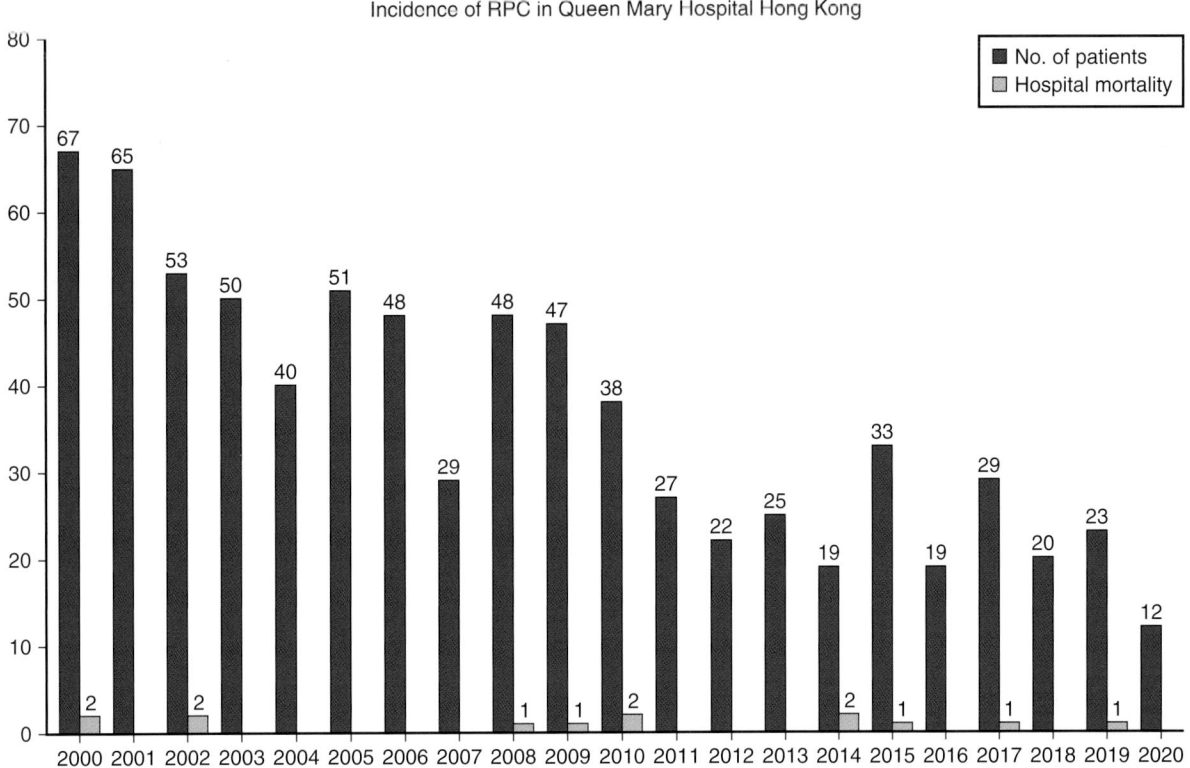

FIGURE 44.8 The incidence of Hong Kong disease in diminishing with improved standards of living, more proactive intervention, and adoption of early definitive surgery. *RPC,* Recurrent pyogenic cholangitis.

hypochondrium or in the epigastrium, and it may be distending, sharp, gnawing, or cutting, with frequent radiation to the back. It is constant, seldom colicky, and may last for hours. In cases with high fever, septicemia or liver abscess formation should be suspected; the temperature chart often shows spikes rather than a continuous fever pattern. Patients may have a tinge of jaundice, which is suggestive of incomplete obstruction. Pruritus and pale stools are rarely noted. Passage of tea-colored urine is a more common symptom.

Physical examination during an acute attack reveals a restless patient, slightly jaundiced, and generally unwell, which may suggest sepsis. Old abdominal scars such as a right subcostal incision with upper midline extension, or bilateral subcostal scars, provide clues to the possibility of previous hepatobiliary surgery. There may also be evidence of a previous stoma in the upper abdomen such as those used for a hepaticocutaneous jejunostomy (HCJ; Fig. 44.9). Tenderness is typically elicited in the epigastrium or the right hypochondrium, and there may be guarding. The liver is enlarged in 60% of patients, but this may be masked by guarding. Similarly, a distended gallbladder may not be palpable. In patients with advanced disease following repeated attacks and complications, cirrhosis may result. Signs of cirrhosis may be present, with stigmata of chronic liver disease, ankle edema secondary to hypoalbuminaemia, and ascites. The spleen is enlarged in 25% of patients.

The therapeutic strategy is typically a step-up approach beginning with endoscopic or radiologic interventions. However, emergency surgery may be necessary if there are signs of clinical deterioration, such as shock, or peritonitis. In the elderly or diabetic, the clinical signs may be subtle and may present late. A high index of suspicion is required to offer timely intervention.

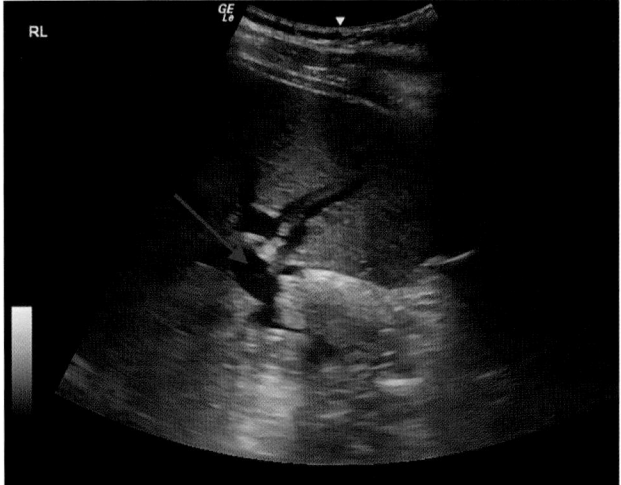

FIGURE 44.9 A patient who had received previous left hepatectomy with hepaticocutaneous jejunostomy.

A transient increase in blood pressure in a patient with acute cholangitis may be a prelude to shock, and must be regarded as a sign of impending deterioration rather than a positive response to treatment. Between attacks, there are few if any significant clinical features. Some patients present with symptoms of cirrhosis caused by RPC. Recent weight loss in elderly patients known to have RPC should raise the suspicion of cholangiocarcinoma, which should also be suspected during follow-up when a patient's serum alkaline phosphatase (ALP) level increases greatly,[36] or when intrahepatic stones involving both

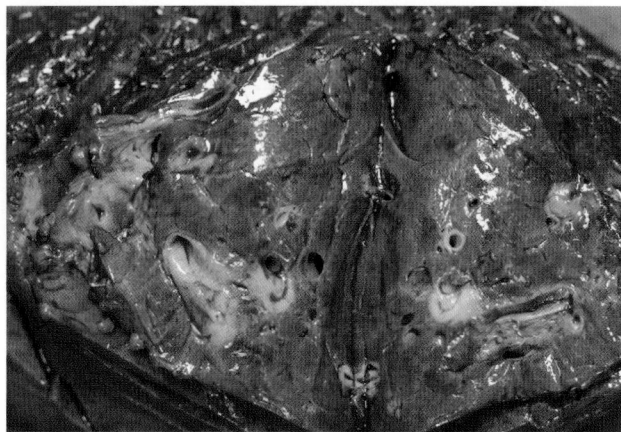

FIGURE 44.10 Resected right lobe of liver with focal stricture of the intrahepatic duct. Histopathology found cholangiocarcinoma changes in the stricture.

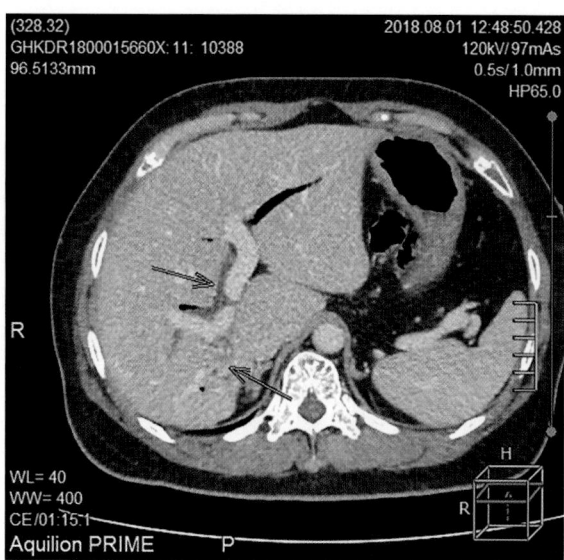

FIGURE 44.11 Contrast computed tomography scan showing right posterior ductal stones in the presence of pneumobilia (arrow) (see Chapter 16).

lobes have not been completely cleared in previous operations.[37] Tumor markers including carbohydrate antigen (CA) 19-9 and CEA should be checked, and they may be elevated with cholangiocarcinoma. With cholangiocarcinoma, higher tumor markers are associated with higher mortality[38] (see Chapters 50 and 51). A computed tomography (CT) scan of the abdomen could reveal the presence of cholangiocarcinoma when the tumor markers are elevated (Fig. 44.10).

Investigations

The results from baseline blood tests can be misleading in some of the cases, as the derangement of the liver function can be minimal and may be undistinguished from other patterns of septicemia. Leukocytosis is often present, and liver function tests often show an obstructive picture with a moderately elevated serum bilirubin level and high serum ALP and γ-glutamyltransferase (GGT) levels. There can be associated acute pancreatitis during which the amylase level will be elevated. Occasionally, patients with RPC have completely normal liver biochemistry even during an acute attack. Imaging studies remain the most important diagnostic tools to establish the diagnosis of an acute attack of RPC, while excluding other sources of sepsis. Also, imaging studies are critical tools to help evaluate the extent of disease, detect complications, and formulate treatment plans to treat the underlying RPC. Ultrasonography (US), CT, direct cholangiography, and magnetic resonance imaging (MRI) are complementary to each other in achieving such goals (see Chapters 16, 30, and 31).

When applied optimally, US can measure the diameter of the common and intrahepatic ducts and confirm the presence and location of stones. It may also diagnose complications, such as liver abscesses, biloma, tumor, or ascites if any of these are present. Color Doppler US is useful in studying PV hemodynamics, where there may be absent portal flow with severe cholangitis, or cholangiocarcinoma with tumor invasion. Intrahepatic stones are readily identified if they cast sonic shadows, but some stones found in RPC are isoechoic with respect to the surrounding tissue.[39] This fact, combined with the propensity of these stones to form biliary casts, may lead to failure of US to identify intrahepatic stones in some patients.[40] Pneumobilia is a common finding in patients with RPC who have undergone ERCP with internal stent placement or biliary-enteric drainage

procedures. In 30% of patients with RPC, prominent periportal echogenicity is found.[40] Unfortunately, highly reflective echoes due to the presence of pneumobilia may mask the acoustic shadowing seen in the presence of stones, limiting the use of US.[39] These changes could also represent pericholangitis and periportal fibrous thickening found in advanced stages of RPC, a finding that should prompt the ultrasonographer to search for other evidence of RPC.

CT is now the investigation of choice (see Chapter 16). In addition to providing the information offered by US, CT can accurately differentiate intrahepatic stones from pneumobilia, which may be confusing on US, and can provide accurate topographic localization for drainage of liver abscesses[41] (Fig. 44.11). Examination of a plain scan is mandatory to establish the baseline liver status, as some stones may become less conspicuous on postcontrast scans against the contrast-enhanced hepatic parenchyma. On CT scan, information regarding the presence of the liver abscess, cholangiocarcinoma, and features of cirrhosis can be detected; volumetric and contour alterations of the liver can also be readily seen. Lobar atrophy, hypertrophy, and rotation of the liver hilum are present in long-standing cases. Other notable findings include parenchymal changes, the anatomy of the PV or hepatic artery, and the presence of varices. During an acute attack, persistent segmental enhancement is observed in 36% of patients,[28] representing parenchymal suppuration analogous to the angiographic finding of diffuse hypervascularity and arteriovenous shunting described in RPC.[42]

Ultrasound and CT are complementary examinations to cholangiography, which provides clear delineation of the ductal anatomy (see Chapters 16, 30, and 31). The patterns of ductal disease can be so diverse in RPC that detailed delineation of the entire biliary tract is essential. ERCP and percutaneous transhepatic cholangiography (PTC) are the direct cholangiographic methods of choice for RPC, which are both diagnostic and therapeutic. Our initial investigation of choice is ERCP for patients without previous hepaticojejunostomy, because the extrahepatic ducts, which are affected in more than 50% of patients with RPC, are better visualized (Fig. 44.12). Additionally,

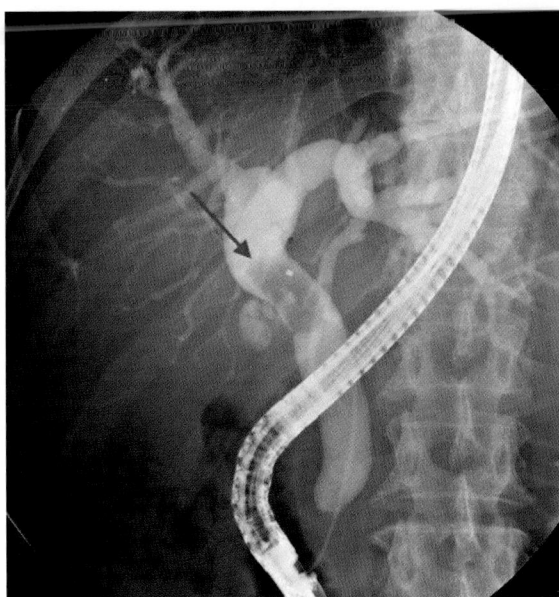

FIGURE 44.12 This patient suffered from acute cholangitis from recurrent pyogenic cholangitis with initial cholangiogram showing a dilated common bile duct and a large obstructing stone *(red arrow)* (see Chapter 30).

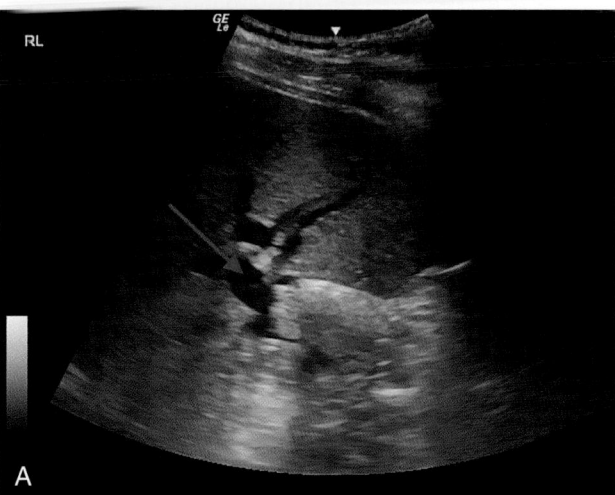

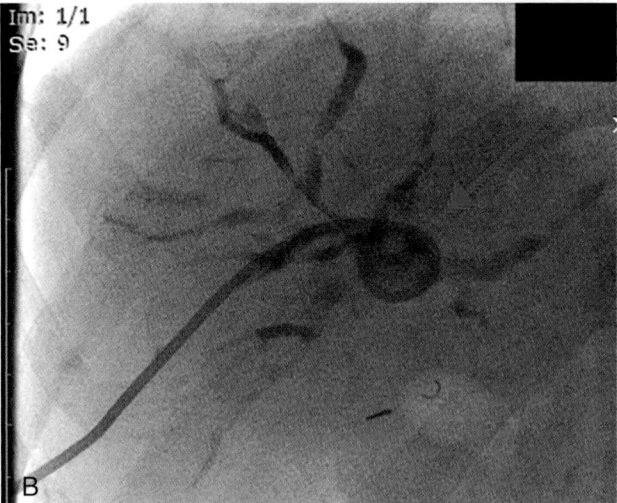

FIGURE 44.13 **A,** Patient who had previous left lateral sectionectomy with hepaticocutaneous jejunostomy had recurrent attacks of recurrent pyogenic cholangitis (RPC). USG found a dilated intrahepatic duct with a hyperechoic filling defect *(red arrow)*. **B,** An acute attack of RPC in the same patient required urgent percutaneous transhepatic biliary drainage. The cholangiogram showed typical features of RPC with intrahepatic ductal stones just proximal to the hepaticojejunostomy *(red arrow)*.

repeated procedures can be performed with ease because blockages of previously placed internal biliary stents can be managed endoscopically. PTC is preferred when there has been a hepaticojejunostomy or choledochojejunostomy and when a stone or stricture located at the biliary confluence prevents filling of the intrahepatic ducts (see Chapter 31). PTC is also preferred when there is a peripheral stricture that ERCP may not be able to diagnose. One advantage of PTC is that it can be targeted to a particular segment. CT or US-guided percutaneous puncture of the targeted bile ducts have been shown to be very safe (Fig. 44.13A,B). When interpreting cholangiograms of patients with RPC, care should be exercised in looking for missing segmental ducts, especially with a paucity of intrahepatic filling; however, in case of sepsis, a complete cholangiogram may be risky because hepaticovenous reflux secondary to excessive contrast filling the entire biliary tree may worsen the septicemia (Fig. 44.14A,B). Correlation of cholangiography with US or CT can yield useful information in defining the cause of repeated attacks of cholangitis in patients who have seemingly cleared all stones.

Similar to CT and US, MRI is a sensitive modality for demonstrating the volume and contour changes in RPC (see Chapter 16). Contrast-enhanced T1-weighted MRI can show the acute suppurative changes by enhancement of the ductal walls and parenchyma. Periportal inflammation is seen on MRI as an intermediate signal between that of the liver and bile on T2-weighted images.[43] T2-weighted images are best for showing ductal dilatation and stones, because bile appears with high signal intensity, whereas stones (without free protons) are signal void and appear as an intraductal filling defect. Compared with US and CT, MRI is slightly better in detecting intrahepatic stones, ductal dilatation, and strictures[44]; however, the presence of pneumobilia, which is also signal void, may adversely affect the stone detection rate. This could be helped with the addition of T1-weighted gradient-echo in-phase images to standard MR cholangiopancreatography

(MRCP) sequences, and which may improve the detection and differentiation between hepatolithiasis and intrahepatic pneumobilia.[45] Three-dimensional display of the biliary system by MR cholangiography is indicated when ERCP cannot be performed, and it may supplant direct cholangiography for diagnostic purposes (Fig. 44.15A,B).[46] MR cholangiography may be more sensitive and effective than ERCP in detecting intrahepatic stones,[47] because intrahepatic strictures inhibit filling of intrahepatic branches by contrast material in ERCP, which is further enhanced by adding the T1-weighted sequence to MRCP.[48,49] It has been suggested that MR cholangiopancreatography may replace ERCP when a therapeutic procedure is not mandatory.[50]

A differential diagnosis should be made to distinguish RPC from other conditions with secondary hepatolithiasis. Unlike Caroli disease, RPC predominantly affects the left side of the liver and has no evidence of ductal plate malformation (see Chapter 46). Bilirubinate stones and chronic proliferative cholangitis are not seen in uncomplicated Caroli disease. However,

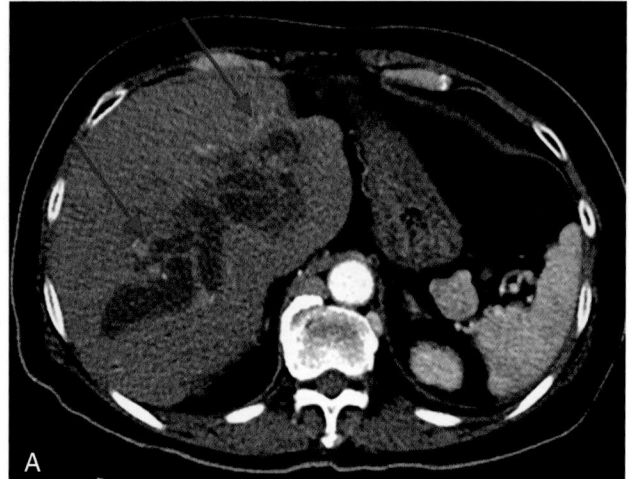

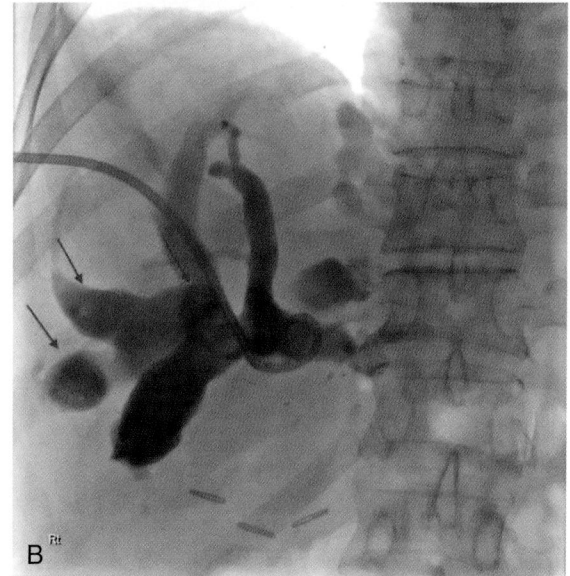

FIGURE 44.14 **A,** This patient had previous left hepatectomy with hepaticocutaneous jejunostomy. She had recurrent attacks of recurrent pyogenic cholangitis. Computed tomography scan showed that the right intrahepatic ducts were dilated and filled with stones (*red arrow: intrahepatic ductal stones*). **B,** Acute attack from the same patient was settled after placing percutaneous transhepatic biliary drainage. The cholangiogram revealed multiple intrahepatic ductal stones in the dilated right ductal system (*arrows: intrahepatic ductal stones*).

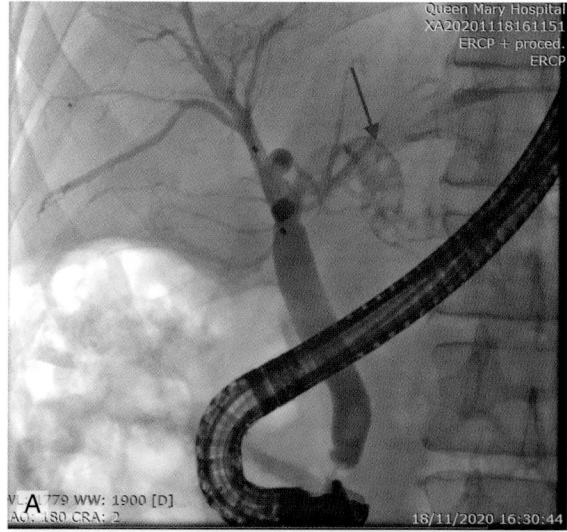

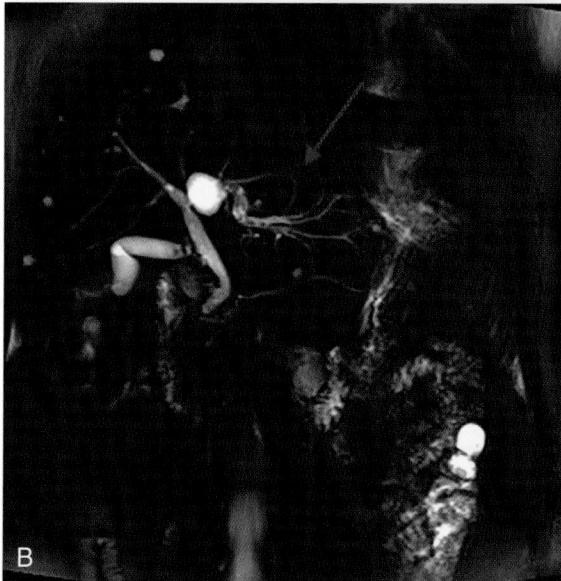

FIGURE 44.15 **A,** Endoscopic retrograde cholangiopancreatography image showing stricture and the dilated segment of the left duct. There were multiple filling defects compatible with stones (*arrow*) (see Chapter 30). **B,** Magnetic resonance cholangiopancreatography image of the same patient showing the stricture and the dilated segment of the left duct. The proximal left duct was filled with stones (*arrow*) (see Chapter 16).

ductal dilatation and even stone formation have been observed in primary sclerosing cholangitis, which may be mistaken for RPC, especially if only the peripheral liver parenchyma is examined. In RPC, ductopenia is not significant. A multimodal imaging approach is sometimes needed to make an accurate and detailed diagnosis.[51]

Management

Most patients present with repeated acute attacks of RPC, and radiologic examinations are required for diagnosis. Acute attacks usually resolve with antibiotics and endoscopic or surgical treatment. After the acute condition has settled, the site of the strictures, location of stones, size of the ducts, volume of the liver parenchyma involved, presence of cholangiocarcinoma, and any associated complications can be ascertained before a decision is made regarding the need for or type of intervention. If the patient's liver function is normal and the volume of the future liver remnant is adequate, definitive treatment by liver resection is often indicated. The few patients for whom liver resection is not recommended generally include frail patients with minimal ductal strictures and no stones, and rarely those whose bile ducts are filled with *C. sinensis* and whose attack of cholangitis is presumably caused by bacterial infection superimposing a heavy infestation of liver flukes. These patients can be treated with antibiotics, antifungals, antihelminthic medications, and endoscopic or radiologic interventions (see Chapter 45).

Acute Attacks

The initial management of an acute attack involves noninvasive, conservative measures. This phase of treatment is regarded as preoperative or preinterventional. Intravenous (IV) fluids, broad-spectrum antibiotics, and analgesics are given, and the gastrointestinal tract is rested. Antibiotics must cover gram-positive and gram-negative organisms, particularly *E. coli*, *Klebsiella* species, and anaerobes, especially in patients with a previous biliary-enteric anastomosis.[52] Drainage procedures should be considered.

Conservative treatment for an acute attack fails in approximately 30% of RPC patients. On the other hand, complications occur in approximately 35% of the patients who require emergent surgical, endoscopic, or radiologic procedures.[53,54] A retrospective analysis suggested that conservative treatment is more likely to fail with obstruction of the entire biliary tract by stones or strictures in the CBD than when the biliary obstruction only involves an isolated segment. In other words, sepsis involving the entire biliary tract seems to be more serious than sepsis with segmental involvement. Factors such as age, incidence of comorbidities, previous surgery, bacteremia, bacterial strains resistant to antibiotics, and multiplicity of bacterial cultures seem to be less important determinants.[54]

Failure of conservative treatment is suggested by persistent fever, mental obtundation, spreading signs of peritonitis, tachycardia, oliguria, and hypotension. Urgent biliary decompression is required before the patient lapses into irreversible shock and death. This is achieved by an endoscopic, radiologic, or surgical approach.

Nonsurgical Treatment of an Acute Attack

Biliary decompression can be achieved by endoscopic or percutaneous means (see Chapters 30 and 31). Endoscopic papillotomy with internal stent insertion is now the first-line approach for acute cholangitis.[55] Endoscopic biliary decompression has the advantage of immediate relief of biliary obstruction if the site of obstruction is within the CBD in an unaltered biliary system, but it is not beneficial if the disease is predominantly intrahepatic. In this situation, percutaneous transhepatic biliary drainage (PTBD) of the obstructed segmental ducts under US guidance may be helpful.[56,57] The drainage tubes used in these procedures are small, and the lumen is even smaller; these can easily be blocked in the presence of thick, infected bile and soft stones,[58] and multiple and repeated drainage may be necessary. As multiple strictures are often present inside and outside the liver, a single drain may be insufficient in affording total decompression; therefore repeated drainage and multiple catheters should be anticipated.

Careful assessment of the patient's clinical condition after endoscopic or radiologic biliary decompression is necessary, and the patients should be monitored in an intensive care or high-dependency unit. If the patient's condition does not improve, further imaging is necessary to identify the location of sepsis and the presence of any complications, and to determine whether operative management is warranted. Possible causes of ongoing sepsis include acute cholecystitis, empyema of the gallbladder with perforation and bile peritonitis, one or more undrained segmental ducts, liver abscess, and blockage of the lumen of a previously placed drainage tube by thick bile, or even pancreatitis. Biliary pancreatitis can potentially be severe and fatal in the presence of the CBD stones. Regardless of the cause of sepsis, prompt surgical intervention is indicated.

In the past, biliary decompression was performed when a patient's condition deteriorated or failed to improve after conservative treatment. The mortality of this approach was about 10% and is unacceptable currently. The latest evidence suggests that mortality could be less than 1% if endoscopic decompression could be performed within 72 hours.[59] With the availability of an emergency endoscopic service, we advocate emergency ERCP and endoscopic decompression within 24 to 48 hours of admission, hoping to avoid surgical intervention in the presence of unfavorable physiologic parameters. ERCP is the best initial step, because the pathology leading to failure of conservative treatment usually resides in the CBD,[54,60] and adequate decompression can be achieved by the use of a large-bore endoprosthesis. With this approach, there is almost no hospital mortality for an acute attack[35]; however, the condition of the patient must be meticulously observed. If signs of immediate improvement are not apparent, surgery must be considered.

Surgical Treatment During an Acute Attack

In an acute attack, surgical treatment is the last resort and is usually considered when nonsurgical interventions have failed. The aim of surgery is to decompress the obstructed bile duct and achieve free biliary drainage. The standard approach is exploration of the CBD through a choledochotomy, and insertion of a large-bore T-tube. The CBD is often a few centimeters in diameter and may be very thick walled. However, in the presence of RPC, the operative field may contain dense adhesions; when the CBD is extremely large and fibrosed, the normal anatomy can be distorted (Fig. 44.16); under such circumstances, recognition of the relevant anatomic structures may not be straightforward, especially with a history of previous surgery. When the duct is opened, thick, infected biliary mud or pus exudes. After this material has been aspirated, stones within the duct are gently removed with forceps; a scoop is useful in retrieving soft stones and thick mud. Balloon catheters, such as a Fogarty catheter or an endoscopic balloon catheter, may be used to trawl out the stones via the choledochotomy.

Intrahepatic strictures and stones may not be dealt with definitively during the emergency operation, but intrahepatic ductal infection must be relieved by dilatation of strictures with graduated biliary sounds. When tight strictures are dilated, a gush of infected bile emerges from the duct. One should be careful when using the sound for dilatation, as a false track may be created. To establish drainage and decompression of the

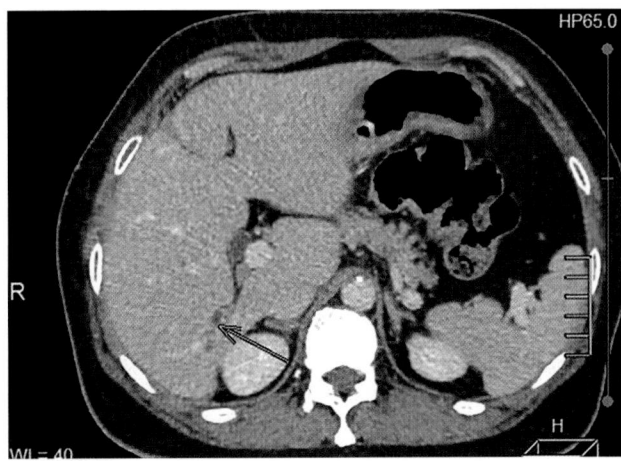

FIGURE 44.16 Computed tomography scan showing an atrophic right posterior segment and distorted liver hilum *(arrow)* (see Chapter 16).

intrahepatic segmental ducts, a transhepatic tube can be inserted on the same principle as a percutaneous transhepatic biliary drain inserted by radiologic means.[61] During exploration of the CBD, irrigation of the bile duct with warm saline solution must be done gently, because syringing at high pressure may induce bacteremia. For this reason, among others, choledochoscopic examination of the intrahepatic duct should not be performed. Choledochoscopy can safely be performed on the distal end of the CBD, provided that the choledochotomy is large and allows free egress of saline. A stone impacted at the lower end of the CBD that cannot be extracted by choledochotomy should be dealt with by fragmentation of the stone using electrohydraulic lithotripsy[62] in the same setting.

After clearing the CBD, patency of its lower end can be established by gently passing a biliary Fogarty catheter or an endoscopic balloon dilator. Inflation of the balloon without choledochoscopic/fluoroscopic guidance is not recommended, because inflation of the balloon at the sphincter of Oddi may damage the sphincter or induce acute pancreatitis. Similarly, blind passage of a biliary sound is not recommended, because it may create a false passage or injure the sphincter. Digital exploration also is helpful to detect stones and strictures in the CBD and the proximal hepatic ducts, but it is not reliable in ascertaining complete clearance of stones.

After bile flow from both lobes of the liver is established, a large-bore T-tube is inserted in the CBD, and the choledochotomy is closed over the tube with absorbable sutures. This T-tube allows debris to pass unimpeded, and because residual stones are found in more than 30% of patients following emergency exploration, it affords a large tract for any future percutaneous manipulation. The T-tube should be kept straight and taut to avoid kinking and angulation, in case any further procedure is necessary.

Cholecystectomy is performed at the same setting, especially where there is acute cholecystitis, empyema, or gangrene of the gallbladder, or the gallbladder is distended, unless the patient's condition is unstable. Cholecystostomy may be considered when operating on a gravely unstable patient. When the patient's condition is unstable, the presence of stones in an otherwise normal gallbladder is not an indication for cholecystectomy during surgery for an acute attack. Palpable liver abscesses can be drained externally, whereas smaller, multiple abscesses should resolve following adequate biliary drainage and antibiotics (see Chapter 70). If the patient's cardiovascular condition is stable, hepatic resection can be performed safely for multiple liver abscesses in a destroyed left lateral segment.[63]

Postoperatively, the patient's improvement is often dramatic. Patients who undergo surgery for septic shock may need a prolonged convalescence in the intensive care unit to recover from hepatic and renal dysfunction; temperature, pulse rate, and blood pressure may take some time to return to normal levels. However, mortality may occur even after definitive surgery, usually because of failure of multiple organs, sepsis, and generalized bleeding secondary to coagulopathy.

Patients with heavy *C. sinensis* infection may pass large volumes of thin bile through the T-tube despite demonstrated patency of the lower end of the CBD. The mechanism for this choleresis is unknown. Praziquantel should be given to eradicate the infection, and adequate fluid and electrolyte replacements must be given to avoid complications (see Chapters 45 and 71).

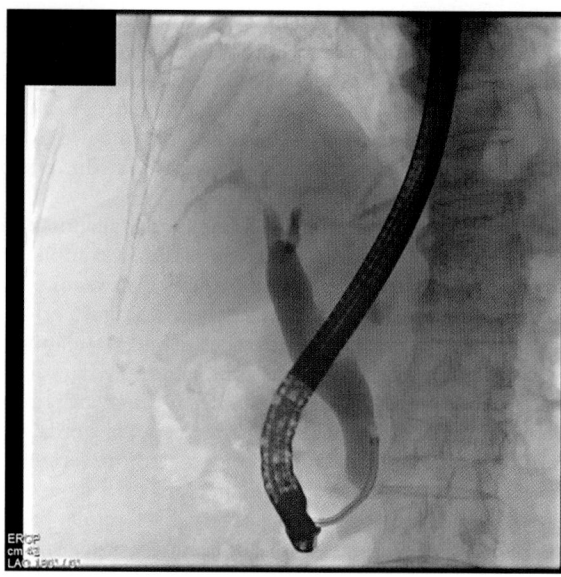

FIGURE 44.17 Cholangioscope can facilitate fragmentation of a large stone inside the biliary system. This allows direct visualization of any pathology, and facilitates biopsy (see Chapter 30).

Definitive Treatment

Endoscopic Management of the Intrahepatic Stones

On some occasions, cholangiography may not elucidate the complete anatomy of the biliary tract. Direct endoscopic visualization of the biliary and pancreatic ducts represents a recent advance in digestive endoscopy. It allows identification of lesions that were previously not visible by cholangiography alone. Directed biopsy can provide a more accurate characterization of biliary lesions. The use of power sources through the cholangiopancreatoscope is now making it possible to fragment and remove refractory lithiasis using traditional endoscopic systems. Large stones in patients with RPC can be fragmented with laser, whereas strictures in the biliary system can be directly visualized. Biopsies of these strictures can be taken under direct visualization (see Chapter 30; Fig. 44.17).

Surgery

RPC is characterized by intrahepatic stone formation, bile duct strictures, repeated bile duct infection, lobar atrophy, and even malignant transformation. Surgical procedures are designed to tackle these problems, which include cholecystectomy, exploration of the CBD (see Chapters 32 and 37), hepatotomy, and hepaticojejunostomy (see Chapters 32 and 42), hepatectomy (see Chapter 101), and even liver transplantation (see Chapter 105).

Cholecystectomy and Approach to Diseased Bile Duct Segment

This is usually the only procedure that is required in patients with milder forms of RPC, in which the disease is mainly extrahepatic. This group of patients can present with symptoms associated with CBD stone or cholangitis. Even when there is no gallstone in the gallbladder and the CBD stone is most likely to have arisen from the bile ducts, cholecystectomy should be performed to prevent future complications of cholecystitis. Exploration of the CBD should be performed as usual (see Chapter 32). When it is difficult to approach the

CBD because of severe periportal adhesions secondary to previous surgery or repeated cholangitis, the CBD can be approached from its posterior aspect. This is performed by medialization of the duodenum and exposing the CBD posteriorly. The posterior approach is particularly useful when there is gross anatomic distortion caused by previous operations, which can be seen after right hepatectomy. In some cases, left lobe hypertrophy combined with postoperative adhesions will alter the position of the CBD to become more lateral and posterior to the main PV. In this situation, the area posterior to the bile duct can have an avascular plan, providing an ideal alternative approach to the difficult CBD. For stone or stricture located higher up in the bile duct, the choledochotomy can be extended to the biliary confluence and the area around the right and left main ducts to facilitate stone removal and stricturoplasty.[61] For stones located in the left lateral section of the liver, distant from the hilar region, they can be approached using the round ligament approach. By tracing along the round ligament to the left side of the umbilical fissure, with the aid of CUSA dissection and intraoperative USG guidance, the segment 3 bile duct can usually be isolated.[64] For stones impacted at the periphery of the liver, a hepatotomy[65] can be performed directly on the diseased section with the aid of palpation and USG. Minimal bleeding can be expected if the hepatotomy is made at superficially located bile ducts instead of the deep-seated ones. A transduodenal approach can be adopted for stones impacted at the distal CBD or ampulla (see Chapter 117D). Following kocherization of the duodenum, a 3-cm longitudinal duodenotomy is made at the antimesenteric aspect of the descending duodenum. After that, the ampulla will be directly in view. A biliary sound is then used to cannulate the CBD, and a biliary sound-guided sphincteroplasty[66] can be performed to provide access to the lower CBD. After stone removal, sphincteroplasty using 4-0 Vicryl should be done to ensure adequate bile outflow to the duodenum, and the duodenotomy is closed horizontally.

Drainage Procedures

Strictures as a result of chronic inflammation are common in patients with RPC. They commonly contribute to infection and stone formation. A drainage procedure is therefore used to achieve unobstructed bile flow from the liver. It is commonly done by a hepaticojejunostomy (see Chapters 32 and 42). There are two approaches: side-to-side anastomosis of a jejunal loop to the anterior wall of the common hepatic ducts or by division of the common hepatic duct to fashion an end-to-side hepaticojejunostomy. There are pros and cons for each option. For the former one, because the CBD is still in continuity, future access to the biliary system with ERCP is possible; however, the blood supply and the size of the anastomosis is considered inferior, which may predispose to an anastomotic stricture. In addition, the bile flow from the common hepatic duct to the jejunum is in a "right-angle" configuration, which is not physiologic and might theoretically compromise drainage. Therefore, in the authors' center, the latter option is preferred. During hepaticojejunostomy, the common hepatic duct is divided as close to the hilar plate as possible to maximize the blood supply and the size of the anastomosis. If the biliary stricture is close to the hilum, an attempt should be made to resect the stricture site for pathologic assessment. To allow easy future access to the biliary system should the need arise, instead

of a hepaticojejunostomy, a IICJ is fashioned.[67,68] There are different ways to perform an HCJ[69]; in our center it is done by leaving a longer jejunal stump, which is just long enough to be tagged under the abdominal wall using suture, preferably at the left upper quadrant (see Chapters 32 and 42). The location of the jejunal stump is radiologically marked with a few large metallic clips[70] for future reference. In the case of recurrence of hepatolithiasis or any need for access to the biliary system, a small incision can be made under x-ray guidance, and a choledochoscope can then be inserted via the new jejunal opening to the skin. Subsequent choledochoscopy via the HCJ can be performed under conscious sedation. When stone clearance is achieved, the fistula can be closed and buried without mobilization of the jejunal stump, which is important for "reopening" of the HCJ when deemed necessary in the future. Alternatively, hepaticolithotomy can be performed via a PTBD tract following serial tract dilatation until the choledochoscope could be accommodated through the tract.[71-74] The merits of either technique are compared and shown in Table 44.1. Generally speaking, the HCJ approach is the preferred option for patients with heavy stone load with multiple sessions of stone clearance procedures anticipated. On the other hand, PTBD avoids general anesthesia and does not have stoma-related complications. Additionally, new stent developments incorporate expandable and biodegradable features, which may theoretically reduce the number of treatment sessions required, albeit convincing data are still eagerly awaited.[75] Therefore the choice of either PTBD or HCJ approaches should be individualized according to each patient's needs.

In cases with severe adhesion and anatomic distortion, such that HCJ at the hilar region is deemed impossible, the Longmire operation can be considered.[76] It is achieved by transecting the edge of the left lateral section with CUSA, and an HCJ can be

TABLE 44.1 Comparison of Hepaticolithotomy Using Percutaneous Transhepatic Biliary Drainage and Jejunal Loop Access

	VIA PTBD ROUTE	VIA JEJUNAL LOOP
Creation of access	Local anaesthesia plus conscious sedation	General anaesthesia
Magnitude of access creation	Minor procedure	Major procedure
Choledochoscopy	Painful at skin entry	Minimal discomfort at stoma site
Size of stone extraction	Stone fragment might not be removed through small PTBD tract	Large stone can be removed via stoma
Access to different segmental duct	Segmental duct adjacent to the PTBD might not be accessible because of sharp angulation	Can reach all segment theoretically
Loss of access	Tract disruption after repeated use	Unlimited access
Wound complication	Granuloma at PTBD exit site	Stoma dermatitis due to bile irritation
Tube blockage and dislodgement	Common	No such concern

PTBC, Percutaneous transhepatic biliary drainage.

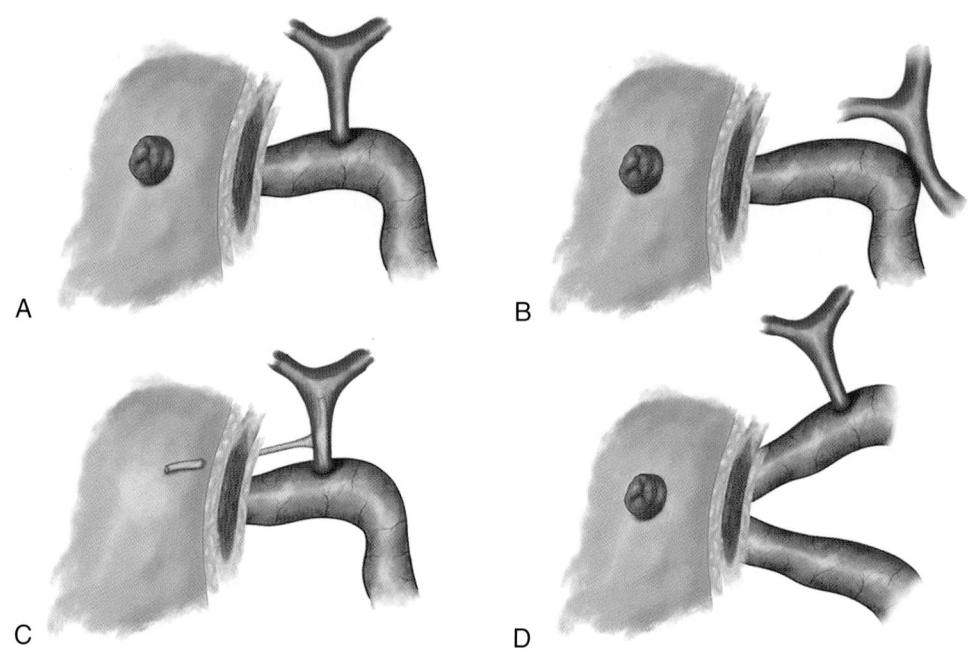

FIGURE 44.18 Diagram showing the operation of hepaticojejunostomy **(A)** and modification in selected conditions **(B, C,** and **D)**. Method B is used when separation of the common bile duct from the portal vein is dangerous. Method C is used when a stoma is not required immediately after the operation. Method D is used on patients with previous choledochojejunostomy (see Chapters 32 and 42).

performed with an exposed segment 3 bile duct. In cases in which the hilum is inaccessible, interventional endoscopy could be considered. With the help of endoscopic ultrasound, endoscopic hepaticogastrostomy can be performed by inserting a fully covered metal stent between the lesser curve of the stomach and the segment 2 or 3 bile duct to provide drainage. Similarly, this technique can be applied to a segregated right biliary system, where a fully covered metal stent can be inserted between the antimesenteric side of the duodenum and segment 5 or 6 bile duct. After removal of the stent at 6 weeks, the hepaticogastrostomy or hepaticoduodenostomy fistula is matured, allowing access to endoscopic lithotripsy.[77] Having said that, use of the endoscopic hepaticoenteric route of biliary access requires cautious case selection and should only be performed in experienced centers (Fig. 44.18).

Removal of Stones During Laparotomy

During laparotomy, stones can be removed by flushing, stone forceps, stone removal balloon, and basket via the choledochotomy, or a hepatotomy (see Chapters 32 and 37). In the case of difficult stones,[59,78,79] (i.e., stone behind a stricture, impacted stones, large and hard stones), choledochoscopic electrohydraulic lithotripsy is an ideal option.[62] The choledochoscope can be advanced to the site where the stone is located, and the lithotripsy probe is then brought in contact with the stone, which is fragmented by the sparks generated by the lithotripter. Care should be taken not to activate the probe while touching the bile duct wall, as it might cause hemobilia, which can obscure the view, forcing one to prematurely abort the procedure. Holmium:yttrium-aluminium-garnet laser[80] and plasma shockwave lithotripters may be viable alternatives, as they do not damage the ductal wall, and they can clear intrahepatic stones in almost all the cases.

Hepatic Resection

Recurring liver abscesses and malignancy are common indications for hepatectomy in patients with RPC[81–83] (see Chapter 101). The principles of liver resection follow that of hepatectomy in other situations, with a few specific precautions. At the preoperative stage, patients should be worked up to ensure that there is adequate functional and volumetric reserve after liver resection. Because RPC mostly affects the left lobe or the left lateral section,[84,85] the liver remnant following left hepatectomy or left lateral section usually provides sufficient volume and physiologic reserve. In cases in which right hepatectomy is contemplated, care should be taken during measurement of the left lobe volume as the principal plane may be skewed as a result of lobar atrophy. Hepatectomy should best be performed in an elective setting because the mortality rate is much higher when performed in patients with active sepsis (Fig. 44.19). Prophylactic antibiotics should be carefully selected, because the biliary tracts of these patients are commonly colonized by resistant bacteria. During hepatic transection, liberal use of ligatures and clips should be adopted because of a higher chance of bile leak resulting from scattered strictures and dilated ductopathy. A drain is recommended and should be placed in proximity to the transection surface, which can be removed early postoperatively in case the output is not bilious. In the case of hepatectomy for malignant indications, frozen sections should be considered of margins that are a concern. Adjuvant treatment should be considered. Long-term surveillance with CT/MRI scan should be scheduled at least yearly for stone and disease recurrence. Regarding surgical approaches, studies[86,87] and meta-analysis[88] have shown that laparoscopic hepatectomy is safe and feasible (see Chapters 127D and E). In experienced hands, the laparoscopic approach may shorten the length of hospital stay and reduce complication rates compared with open hepatectomy. With the use of a robotic-assisted approach, an intracorporeal

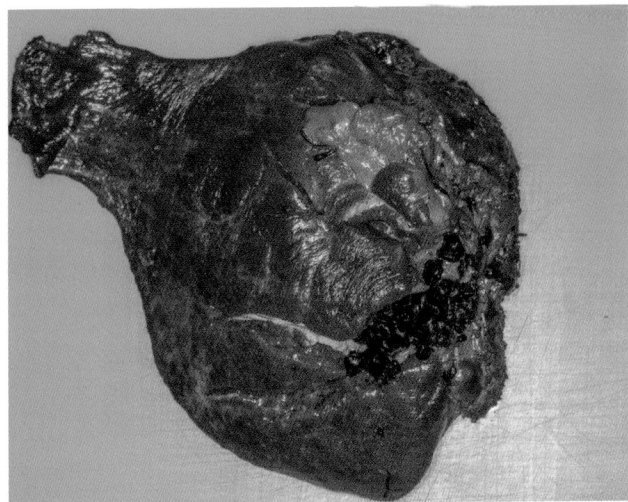

FIGURE 44.19 Resected left lobe of liver showing the biliary system in the specimen full of pigmented stones.

TABLE 44.2 Comparison of Patients Treated During Different Periods at Queen Mary Hospital

	1984-1989 (S. T. FAN ET AL., 1991 1991)	1991-1996 (LIU ET AL., 1998)	2000-2020 (UNPUBLISHED DATA)
Number of patients	137	96	765
Age (median)	56	59.5	70
Intrahepatic strictures	46 (33.6%)	31 (32.3%)	95 (12.4%)
Emergency ERCP	1 (0.7%)	61 (63.5%)	88 (11.5%)
Hepatectomy	45 (32.8%)	60 (62.5%)	159 (20.8%)
Major	1 (0.7%)	5 (5.2%)	87 (11.4%)
Minor	44 (32.1%)	55 (57.3%)	72 (9.4%)
Hepatico-cutaneous jejunostomy	19 (13.9%)	70 (72.9%)	176 (23.0%)
Stone clearance rate	114 (83.2%)	96 (100%)	749 (97.9%)
Hospital mortality	4 (2.9%)	1 (1.0%)	13 (1.7%)

ERCP, Endoscopic retrograde cholangiopancreatography.

anastomosis for hepaticojejunostomy is made possible even in unfavorable locations.[89]

Liver Transplantation

Secondary biliary cirrhosis can result from repeated cholangitis secondary to widespread intrahepatic ductal strictures or long-standing severe hepatolithiasis. Liver transplantation is indicated for patients who have features of end-stage liver cirrhosis or repeated life-threatening cholangitis (see Chapter 105). Model for End-Stage Liver Disease (MELD) score should be calculated as per other cirrhotic patients on the liver transplant waiting list (see Chapter 4). Because concomitant cholangiocarcinoma should be actively ruled out, tumor markers such as CEA and CA 19-9 must be checked. Brush cytology with ERCP or cholangioscopic focused biopsy should be obtained in cases of suspicious biliary strictures in cholangiography (see Chapter 30). Positron-emitted tomography with an 18-fluorodeoxyglucose tracer should be considered in cases with a clinical suspicion of cholangiocarcinoma, although the findings in cancer are not always distinguishable from cholangitis (see Chapter 18). Acute uncontrolled biliary sepsis precludes transplantation because of the obvious risk of overwhelming sepsis in an immunosuppressed patient. The surgeon performing the liver harvest should preserve the vasculobiliary structure for as long a distance as possible, because the inflow vessel at the recipient side will most likely be short and unfavorable. A backup organ recipient should always be prepared for the worst-case scenario of a stuck down liver in the original recipient.[90] In liver transplantation for RPC, bile duct reconstructions with hepaticojejunostomy might have an advantage over duct-to-duct

anastomosis, as this avoids using a native fibrotic CBD, which is prone to biliary anastomotic strictures and may subsequently compromise the graft function.

Result of Treatment

Complication rates vary among different cohorts, and range from 17.5% to 45%.[91-93] Most of the complications following surgery are related to wound infection, which is secondary to contamination by the infected bile.[81,94] Bile leak after liver resection remains the most worrying morbidity, but it can be managed conservatively most of the time if the leakage is well drained and the sepsis is under control (see Chapter 28). Reoperation for management of bile leakage is sometimes required. The mortality rate for surgical treatment for RPC should be around 1% to 2% in experienced centers (Table 44.2). Regarding long-term outcomes, the results are usually favorable.[92] Stone clearance rate should be high, and our center's overall average is approximately 90%. Concerning cholangiocarcinoma in the background RPC,[95] the long-term oncologic outcomes are inferior to cholangiocarcinoma without underlying RPC,[96] such that the thresholds for adjuvant chemotherapy and close postoperative surveillance should be considered. Transplantation for RPC without malignancy is usually associated with very good long-term outcome with 5-year overall survival over 90% (Fig. 44.20).

References are available at expertconsult.com.

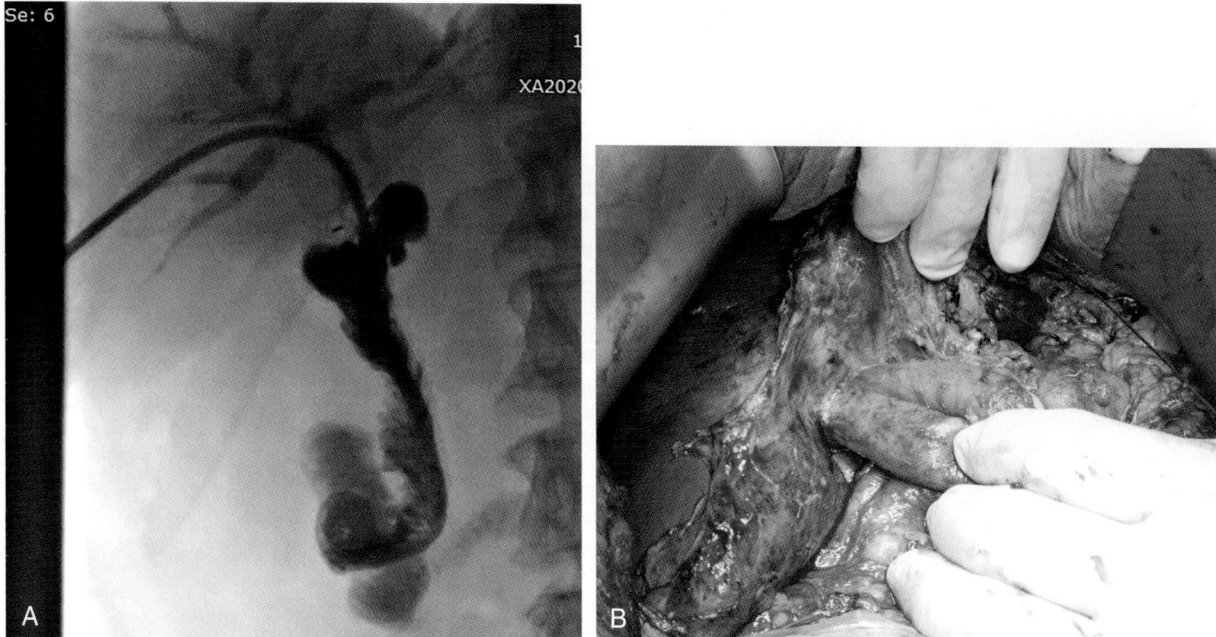

FIGURE 44.20   A, Percutaneous transhepatic biliary drainage cholangiogram showed a stricture at the hepaticojejunostomy 10 years after an operative drainage procedure. Dilatation, stenting, redo anastomosis, and liver transplant are options that need to be considered if stricture develops (see Chapter 31). **B,** Operative photos of a patient who had previous left hepatectomy and hepaticojejunostomy and developed an anastomotic stricture. Redo anastomosis should be performed. Liver transplant is reserved for patients with decompensated liver function.

CHAPTER 45

Biliary parasitic disease

John A. Steinharter and Michael D'Angelica

Parasitic infections of the biliary tract are a common cause of biliary obstruction in tropical developing countries and less frequently, in developed countries. These infections are important because they can lead to serious complications such as cholelithiasis (see Chapters 33 and 39), recurrent pyogenic cholangitis (see Chapter 44), cirrhosis (see Chapter 74), pancreatitis (see Chapters 54, 55, and 57), and cholangiocarcinoma (see Chapters 50 and 51B). The most common parasites of the biliary tract reported in humans are *Fasciola*, *Opisthorchis*, *Clonorchis*, and *Ascaris* spp. Opisthorchiidae (which includes species of *Clonorchis* and *Opisthorchis*) and Fasciolidae (which includes species of *Fasciola*) are two families that make up a category called liver flukes. The number of people affected by liver flukes worldwide is approximately 15.3 million for *Clonorchis*, 8.4 million for *Opisthorchis*, and 2.6 million for *Fasciola*. Although these flukes are unlikely to cause mortality, significant morbidity has been reported and calculated as disability-adjusted life years (DALYs) (*Clonorchis*: 275,380 DALYs; *Opisthorchis*: 74,367 DALYs; *Fasciola*: 35,206 DALYs)[1,2] (see Chapter 71).

FASCIOLIASIS

Fascioliasis, or distomatosis, is a zoonosis (disease that can be transmitted from animals to humans) caused by *Fasciola hepatica* or *Fasciola gigantica* (Trematoda: Fasciolidae). *Fasciola* is globally distributed and present in all continents except Antarctica, especially in sheep- and cattle-raising areas. *F. hepatica* and *F. gigantica* are mostly reported in temperate zones and tropical regions, respectively (Fig. 45.1). In approaching a patient with suspected fascioliasis, epidemiologic, clinical, and imaging features can provide clues for the diagnosis before the physician orders a diagnostic test to confirm the infection. An algorithm for diagnosis and management is recommended (Fig. 45.2).[3]

Epidemiology

The first case of *F. hepatica* infection was documented in the Gallo-Roman period.[4] Despite the recent developments in diagnostic and surveillance techniques, some countries are still lacking in data on human fascioliasis. This may be due to underreporting and underdiagnosis occurring in resource-limited regions of the world. Cases are mostly reported as a complication from the infection, and therefore the current denominator of patients with fascioliasis is unknown and likely underestimated. On the other hand, globalization and migration of populations from rural areas to large cities have led to cases of fascioliasis in areas where this fluke is typically not endemic. In fact, because of most clinicians' lack of familiarity with this parasitic infection in nonendemic areas, the rate of complications may increase because of late diagnosis.[5] Currently, the estimated number of human infections ranges from 35 to 72 million and 180 million are at risk of infection worldwide.[6] In the past, fascioliasis was limited to specific and typical geographic areas, but it is now widespread throughout the world (see Fig. 45.1). According to

the reported cases, *F. hepatica* transmission has increased in Europe, the Americas, and Oceania, as well as in Africa and Asia, where *F. gigantica* and *F. hepatica* overlap. The geographic distribution is determined by the intermediate host (*Lymnaea* spp.) and certain other conditions, such as climate, alimentary behaviors, and poverty (Table 45.1).

Examples of countries with estimates of the infected population include 830,000 in Egypt, 742,000 in Peru, 360,000 in Bolivia, 37,000 in Yemen, 20,000 in Ecuador, and 10,000 in Iran.[7] Furthermore, other countries have reported patients with *Fasciola* infection, including Argentina,[8] Venezuela,[9] Chile,[10] Ecuador,[11] Mexico,[12] Turkey,[13,14] Thailand,[15] Japan,[16] Korea,[17] the United States,[18–20] Tunisia,[21] India,[22] Lebanon,[23] and South Africa,[24] among others.

The Andean region of South America is likely the area most affected by the *Fasciola* fluke in the world, with point prevalence rates ranging from 6% to 68%.[25–27] Although fascioliasis is mainly reported in rural areas, new evidence has shown that proximity of medium- to high-income industrialized cities to rural areas creates a potential source of infection because of the importation of contaminated vegetables to the high-consuming markets in large cities. Thus cases of fascioliasis may be seen in areas where this fluke is not endemic. Another factor that contributes significantly to the dissemination of the infection to new areas is the highly adaptable capacity of both the parasite and the lymnaeid snail host to challenging meteorologic conditions (e.g., 4200 m above sea level, Andean region). Paleoparasitologic studies have shown that the introduction of *F. hepatica* and its snail host from Europe into the Americas has been relatively recent. Given this evidence, fascioliasis is the vector-borne disease with the widest latitudinal, longitudinal, and altitudinal distribution in the world.[28]

To facilitate the classification of fascioliasis cases based on transmission, the following epidemiologic pattern has been proposed[29]: (1) cases imported to areas where neither human nor animal fascioliasis is transmitted; (2) autochthonous, isolated, nonconstant cases of sporadic infection in areas where animal fascioliasis is present; (3) endemic fascioliasis (hypoendemic ≤1%, mesoendemic 1%–10%, hyperendemic ≥10%); and (4) epidemic fascioliasis (a) in animal endemic areas and (b) in human endemic areas. Epidemiology is an important determinant of the initial evaluation of a patient with probable fascioliasis.

Life Cycle

The trematodes *F. hepatica* (also known as the common liver fluke or the sheep liver fluke) and *F. gigantica* are large liver flukes (*F. hepatica*: up to 30 by 15 mm; *F. gigantica*: up to 75 by 15 mm), which are primarily found in domestic and wild ruminants (their main definitive hosts). The adult *F. hepatica* flukes are large, broadly flattened, measuring 30 mm long and 15 mm wide, with a broad anterior portion covered with scale-like spines (Fig. 45.3). The adult fluke lives in the common and

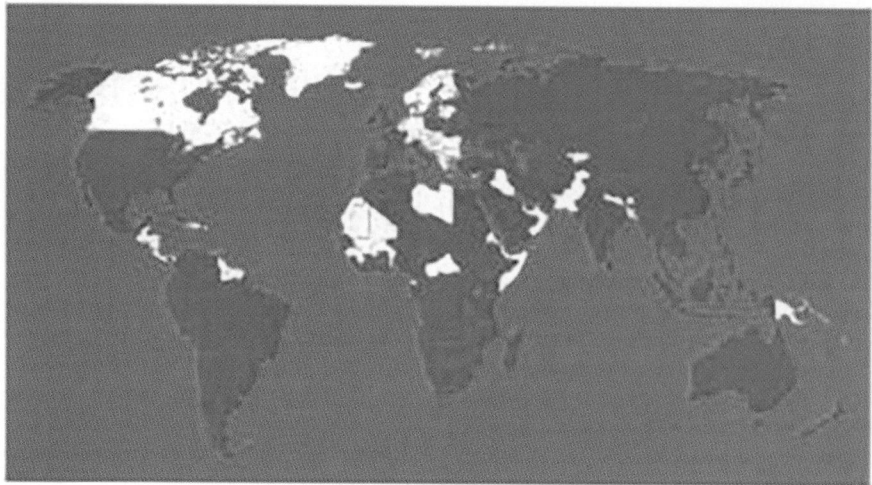

FIGURE 45.1 Global distribution of fascioliasis, 2015. Countries reporting cases of fascioliasis shaded in *blue*. The figure implies that fascioliasis is distributed in over 90% of the world.[84] (From Nyindo M, Lukambagire A-H. Fascioliasis: An ongoing zoonotic trematode infection. *Biomed Res Int.* 2015;786195:1–5.)

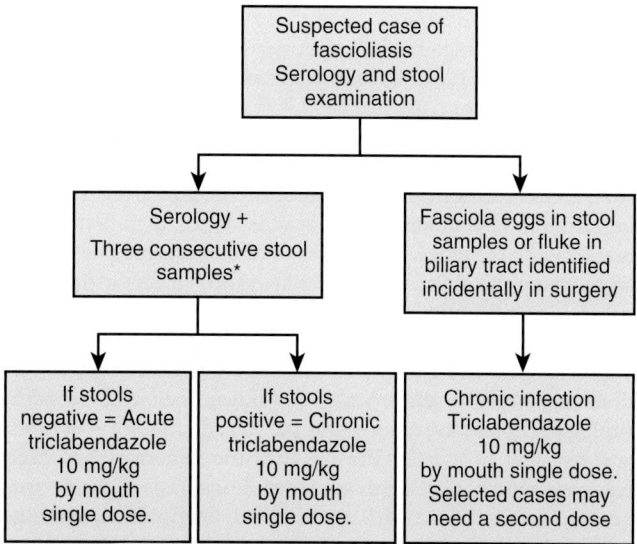

FIGURE 45.2 **Summary of management and treatment of a patient suspected to have fascioliasis.**[*] Three consecutive stool samples must be examined by a sedimentation technique[3] before ruling out the infection. Stool examination is preferred versus serologic studies because of cost effectiveness and availability. In highly suspected cases, a trial of triclabendazole is warranted. Single-dose triclabendazole (10 mg/kg) has a cure rate greater than 90%. A second single dose may be used in select cases (e.g., high intensity of infection in feces, large numbers of parasites in surgery, refractory cases).

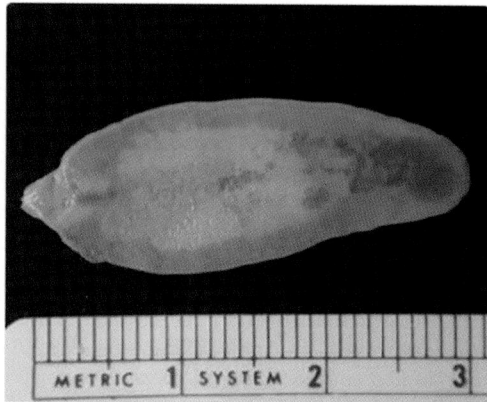

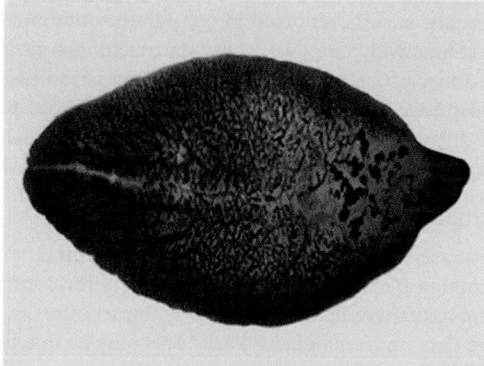

FIGURE 45.3 **A,** Unstained adult of *Fasciola hepatica* fixed in formalin. **B,** Adult of *F. hepatica* stained with carmine. (From Centers for Disease Control and Prevention. Fascioliasis. https://www.cdc.gov/dpdx/fascioliasis/index.html.)

TABLE 45.1	Epidemiology of Human Fascioliasis	
GEOGRAPHIC AREA	**RISK FACTORS**	**POPULATION AT RISK**
Latin America (Andean region)	Watercress	Children in endemic areas
Europe	Drinking alfalfa juice	Travelers
Africa	Green vegetables	Women
Asia	Contaminated water	Vegetarians
Australia	Travel to endemic areas	
	Living close to irrigation canals	
	Eating salads	

hepatic bile ducts of the human or the animal host; the worm can live in the biliary tract for a long time—between 9 and 14 years (Fig. 45.4). Animals susceptible to becoming reservoir hosts for *Fasciola* spp. mainly include cattle, sheep, pigs, buffaloes, and donkeys, although it has been also reported in horses, dogs, goats, llamas, alpacas, dromedaries, and camels. The eggs are oval, yellowish-brown, and measure approximately 130 to 150 by 60 to 90 μm (Fig. 45.5).

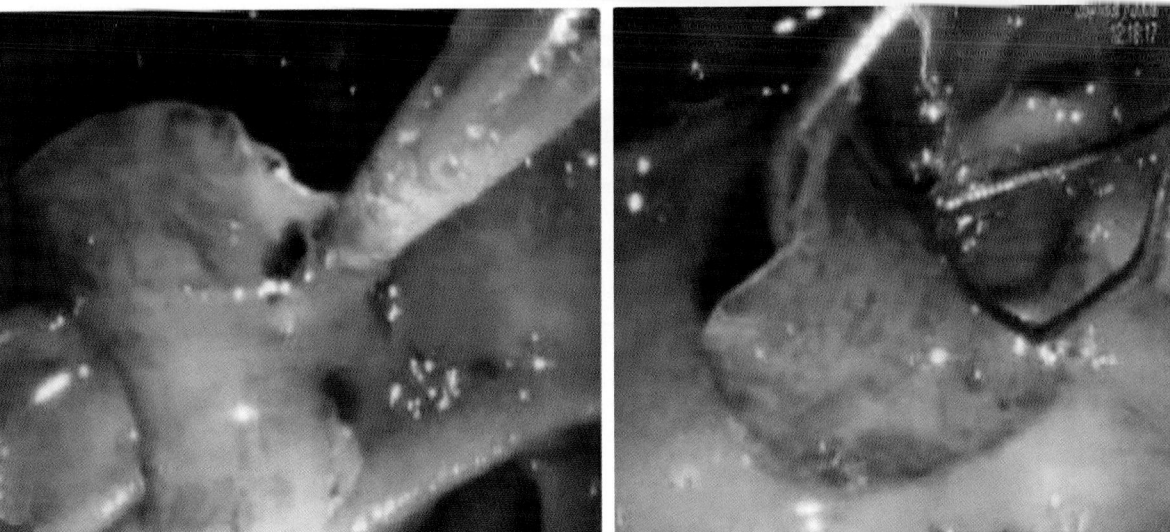

FIGURE 45.4 Adults of *Fasciola hepatica* observed with endoscopic retrograde cholangiopancreatography (ERCP) imaging. (From the Centers for Disease Control and Prevention. Fascioliasis. https://www.cdc.gov/dpdx/fascioliasis/index.html.)

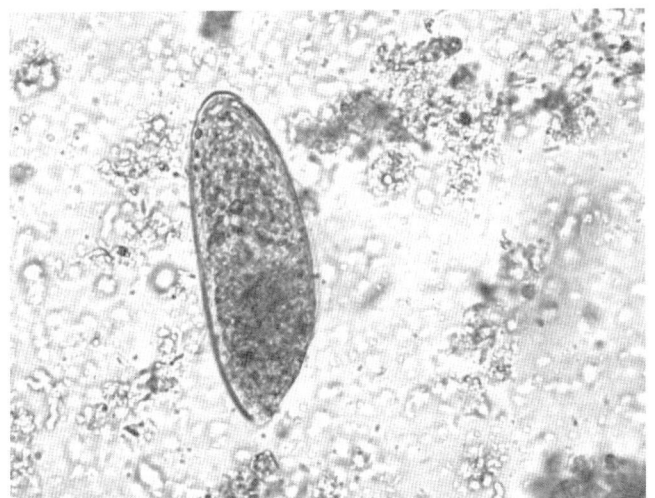

FIGURE 45.5 Adult egg of *Fasciola hepatica* in microscopic examination of stools by the rapid sedimentation technique.

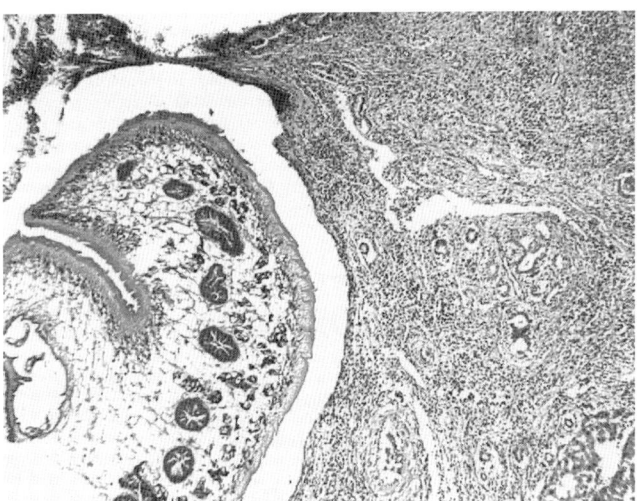

FIGURE 45.6 Liver biopsy of an infected rat with *Fasciola hepatica* shows adult parasite in a bile duct.

The life cycle begins when the parasite eggs in stool are deposited in tepid water (22°–26°C); miracidia appear, develop, and hatch in 9 to 14 days. These miracidia then invade many species of freshwater snails, in which they multiply as sporozoites and redia for 4 to 7 weeks. They leave as free-swimming cercariae that subsequently attach to watercress, water lettuce, alfalfa, mint, parsley, or khat. Free-swimming cercariae may remain suspended in water and encyst over a few hours, and infection of the human host begins after consumption of plants or water contaminated with the metacercariae. In the first week, the larvae excyst in the duodenum and migrate through the bowel wall and peritoneal cavity. After 4 weeks, the juvenile larvae penetrate the liver through the Glisson capsule to initiate the acute larval, hepatic, and invasive stages of human infection.

Sometimes the larvae deviate to other locations; these are called *extrahepatic forms* or *ectopic infections.* Maturation from juvenile larvae into adult flukes takes approximately 3 to 5 months, during which time the larvae mature and migrate through the liver into the large hepatic and common bile ducts (Figs. 45.4 and 45.6). Mature flukes consume hepatocytes and duct epithelium and reside for years in the hepatic and common bile ducts and occasionally in the gallbladder. Adult fluke worms produce eggs within 4 months after infection (range, 3–18 months); these eggs traverse the sphincter of Oddi and intestine and then continue the cycle of infection. Interestingly, acute and chronic stages can overlap; this is often seen in endemic areas, and it is not unusual to find eggs in the stool samples of patients with acute infection.

Life Cycle

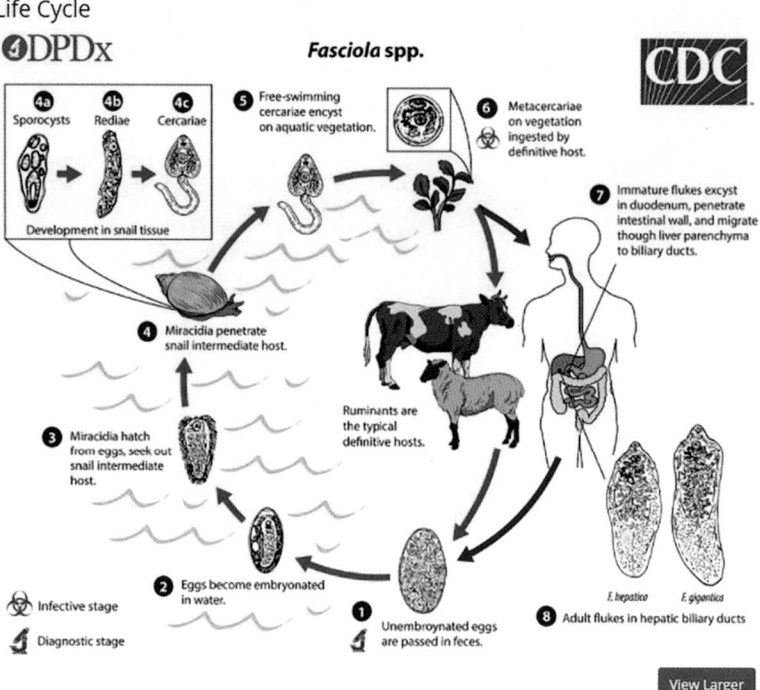

Immature eggs are discharged in the biliary ducts and passed in the stool ❶ . Eggs become embryonated in freshwater over ~2 weeks ❷ ; embryonated eggs release miracidia ❸ , which invade a suitable snail intermediate host ❹ . In the snail, the parasites undergo several developmental stages (sporocysts ④ₐ , rediae ④ᵦ , and cercariae ④c). The cercariae are released from the snail ❺ and encyst as metacercariae on aquatic vegetation or other substrates. Humans and other mammals become infected by ingesting metacercariae-contaminated vegetation (e.g., watercress) ❻ . After ingestion, the metacercariae excyst in the duodenum ❼ and penetrate through the intestinal wall into the peritoneal cavity. The immature flukes then migrate through the liver parenchyma into biliary ducts, where they mature into adult flukes and produce eggs ❽ . In humans, maturation from metacercariae into adult flukes usually takes about 3–4 months; development of *F. gigantica* may take somewhat longer than *F. hepatica*.

Life Cycle

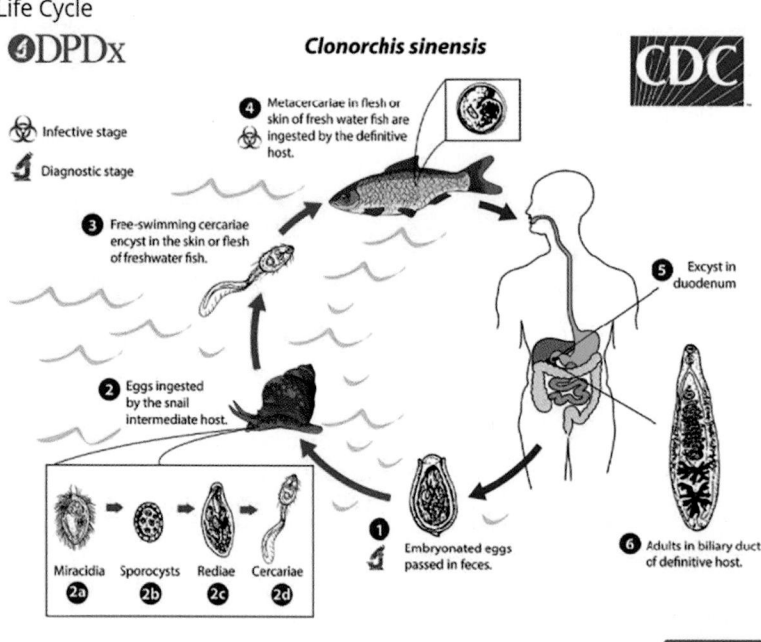

Clonorchis sinensis eggs are discharged in the biliary ducts and in the stool in an embryonated state ❶ . Eggs are ingested by a suitable snail intermediate host ❷ . Eggs release miracidia ②ₐ , which go through several developmental stages (sporocysts ②ᵦ , rediae ②c , and cercariae ②d). The cercariae are released from the snail and, after a short period of free-swimming time in water, they come in contact and penetrate the flesh of freshwater fish, where they encyst as metacercariae ❸ . Infection of humans occurs by ingestion of undercooked, salted, pickled, or smoked freshwater fish ❹ . After ingestion, the metacercariae excyst in the duodenum ❺ and ascend the biliary tract through the ampulla of Vater ❻ . Maturation takes approximately one month. The adult flukes (measuring 10 to 25 mm by 3 to 5 mm) reside in small and medium sized biliary ducts.

Life Cycle:

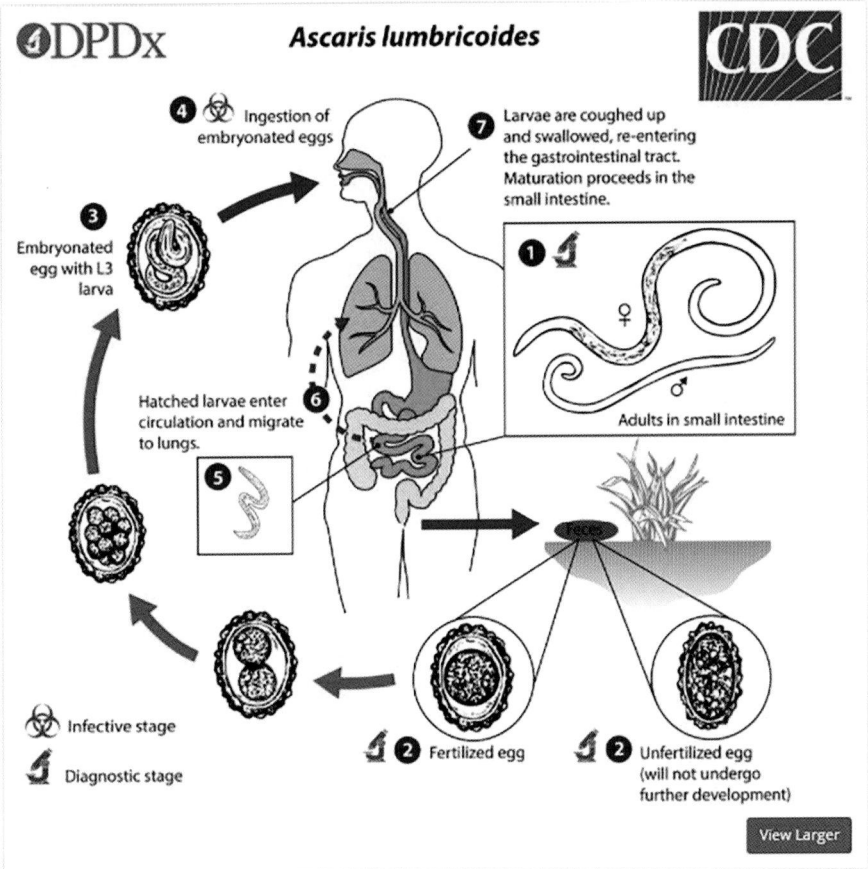

Adult worms ❶ live in the lumen of the small intestine. A female may produce approximately 200,000 eggs per day, which are passed with the feces ❷ . Unfertilized eggs may be ingested but are not infective. Larvae develop to infectivity within fertile eggs after 18 days to several weeks ❸ , depending on the environmental conditions (optimum: moist, warm, shaded soil). After infective eggs are swallowed ❹ , the larvae hatch ❺ , invade the intestinal mucosa, and are carried via the portal, then systemic circulation to the lungs ❻ . The larvae mature further in the lungs (10 to 14 days), penetrate the alveolar walls, ascend the bronchial tree to the throat, and are swallowed ❼ . Upon reaching the small intestine, they develop into adult worms. Between 2 and 3 months are required from ingestion of the infective eggs to oviposition by the adult female. Adult worms can live 1 to 2 years.

Risk Factors

Ingestion of metacercariae in infected raw vegetables (e.g., watercress, lettuce, alfalfa juice, mixed green salads) is a major source of the infection in humans and animals.[30,31] Water contaminated with metacercariae also has been described as a potential source of infection in poor rural areas with inadequate sanitation and water supplies.[32] People living in urban areas may be at risk for acquiring fascioliasis. Contaminated vegetables imported from endemic areas can be consumed by people living in large cities. Fascioliasis has been reported in people (e.g., tourists) who have eaten salads in luxury restaurants or hotels in endemic countries, and watercress has traditionally been the most common known source of infection.[33] The plants that have been described associated with *Fasciola* infection are *Medicago sativa* (alfalfa in juice) in Peru; *Taraxacum dens leonis* (dandelion leaves), *Valerianella olitoria* (lamb's lettuce), and *Mentha viridis* (spearmint) in France; green leafy *Nasturtium* spp. and *Mentha* spp. in Iran; *Juncus andicola* and *Juncus ebracteatus* (Juncaceae), *Mimulus glabratus* (Scrophulariaceae), and *Nostoc* spp. (Cianofitas) in the Bolivian Altiplano.[29,34] Treatment of contaminated plants with high doses of potassium permanganate decreases metacercariae viability and could be used to prevent infection.[35]

Epidemiologic studies have been carried out in endemic areas to measure the impact of alimentary habits on the acquisition of infection. Drinking beverages made from watercress or alfalfa leaves, called *emollients*, and living close to irrigation channels were found to be risk factors in a multivariate analysis in the Andean region.[30] Eating salads is the common factor among infected families, and it carries a 3.3-fold increased risk of acquiring the infection.[25] In a logistic regression analysis, an age- and gender-matched case-control study comparing 60 infected children found that drinking alfalfa juice carries a 4.5-fold increased risk of acquiring fascioliasis and familiarity with aquatic plants a 4.3-fold increased risk.[36] Similar risk factors have been found in other parts of the world. In Mexico, aquatic plants and alfalfa juice have been associated with fascioliasis.[37] Socioeconomic factors and drinking untreated water may represent additional risk factors in poor people from endemic areas.[32] Therefore aquatic plants (e.g., watercress, alfalfa) and the irrigation channels that carry the metacercariae play a key role in the transmission of fascioliasis in Andean endemic areas. Table 45.2 summarizes risk factors with studies reporting odds ratios.

More women are affected with fascioliasis than men. Women have higher prevalence rates, more severe infections, and more

TABLE 45.2   *Fasciola hepatica* Infection in Endemic Areas in Peru[*]

RISK FACTOR	OR (95% CI)	P VALUE	REFERENCE
Multivariate Analysis			
Drinking emollients	5.2 (1.7-15.6)	.05	Marcos et al., 2004[30]
Living close to irrigation channels	17.2 (2.8-106.7)	.05	
Eating salads	3.3 (1.2-9.0)	.05	Marcos et al., 2005[25]
Drinking alfalfa juice	4.5 (1.7-11.1)	.001	Marcos et al., 2006[36]
Familiarity with aquatic plants	4.3 (1.7-10.5)	.001	
Univariate Analysis			
Water supply from channels	2.4 (1.1-5.3)	.03	Marcos et al., 2006[36]
Consumption of aquatic plants	2.5 (1.1-5.6)	.028	
Breeding five or more heads of cattle	2.5 (1.1-5.6)	.028	
Owning dogs	3.2 (1.3-8.1)	.1	
Defecation site in fields	2.6 (1.3-5.6)	.01	
Familiarity with aquatic plants	3.9 (1.8-8.3)	.0001	
Breeding more than five sheep	0.3 (0.1-0.7)	.003	

[*]These studies were performed in the Andean region of South America. Risk factors in other parts of the world may be similar.

CI, Confidence interval; *OR*, Odds ratio.

TABLE 45.3   Clinical Manifestations, Laboratory Data, and Imaging in Fascioliasis

CLINICAL PICTURE	IMAGING AND LABORATORY RESULTS
Acute	
Prolonged fever (weeks or months)	Eosinophilia (any cell count)
Abdominal pain (mostly upper abdomen)	Anemia
	Anicteric hepatitis
	Biliary hemorrhage or hemobilia
Hepatomegaly	Subscapular hematoma or hepatic rupture (seen on CT)
Weight loss	Hepatic abscesses
Urticaria	Track-like lesions on CT
Ectopic lesions[*]	
Chronic	
Abdominal pain in right upper quadrant	Eosinophilia (sometimes)
Biliary colic	Cholestasis
Nausea and vomiting	Hepatic abscesses
Recurrent or intermittent jaundice	Liver fibrosis and ultimately cirrhosis
Urticaria	Necrotic granuloma (increased ALT and AST levels)
	Cystic tumors
	Cholangitis caused by *Klebsiella* spp., *Escherichia coli*, *Enterococcus* spp.
	Choledocholithiasis
	Eosinophilic cholecystitis
	Acalculous cholecystitis

[*]Ectopic migration and other clinical manifestations. *Acute stage:* Migratory nodule under the skin or peritoneal cavity, arthralgias, lymphadenopathies, hemolytic anemia, seizures, and pleural effusion. *Chronic stage:* Subcutaneous nodules and gastric nodules.

ALT, Alanine aminotransferase; *AST*, aspartate aminotransferase; *CT*, computed tomography.

reported liver or biliary complications.[36] Children are affected more than adults in endemic areas,[38] which probably reflects partial acquired immunity, exposure to the metacercaria, genetic susceptibility, and other factors. Reinfection is frequently seen in highly endemic areas, and the intensity of the infection depends on the number of metacercariae ingested (this fluke does not multiply in the host).

Clinical Manifestations

Fascioliasis has two distinct clinical phases: acute and chronic. Signs and symptoms depend on the worm burden, duration, and phase of infection. In general, the *chronic* infection is usually diagnosed in epidemiologic studies in endemic areas as a cause of biliary obstruction or in routine stool tests. On the other hand, the *acute* infection has a more florid clinical picture that brings the patient to the emergency department (Table 45.3). The clinical manifestations are so variable that mild right upper quadrant abdominal pain may call for a step-by-step workup that can lead to the final diagnosis of fascioliasis.[39]

Acute Infection

The first acute or invasive phase lasts from 3 to 5 months and is caused by the migration of the immature larvae from the duodenum to the liver. Finally reaching the bile ducts, parasites migrate through the liver parenchyma and digest hepatic tissue, causing intense inflammation and hemorrhage proportionate to the number of worms. Migration tracks can be observed in histologic sections, and flukes may die, leaving cavities filled with necrotic debris; these are eventually replaced by scar tissue. Symptoms include prolonged fever, hepatomegaly with abdominal pain, and mild eosinophilia (early infection) or hypereosinophilia (mid- or late-acute infection). Multiple hypodense lesions can be seen on computed tomography (CT) scan, similar to metastases.[40] Of note, one of the most frequent manifestations in this acute phase is hypereosinophilia, which is seen in almost all cases. If no eosinophilia is detected at the initial visit, it may be too early in the acute infection; a repeat blood cell count 3 to 5 days later will detect a significant increase in the eosinophil count. Absence of persistent eosinophilia reduces the suspicion for acute infection. In summary, acute fascioliasis is a clinical syndrome similar to acute cholecystitis with significant eosinophilia.

The acute phase manifests with subcapsular hematomas, hepatic cysts, residual hepatic calcifications, and severe anemia. Hyperbilirubinemia is absent in the acute phase,[41] which distinguishes it from other forms of acute hepatitis. Other manifestations are anorexia, weight loss, nausea, vomiting, cough, diarrhea, urticaria, lymphadenopathies, and arthralgias.[42] Occasionally, the juvenile larvae reach other anatomic locations, such as the subcutaneous tissue, pancreas, eye, brain, and stomach wall.[43]

Chronic Infection

The chronic phase begins approximately 3 to 6 months after the consumption of the metacercariae, when the parasite reaches the bile ducts. On macroscopic examination, the liver has large, dilated, thick-walled, and calcareous bile ducts with yellowish-brown bile. On microscopic examination, the bile ducts have a thickened hyperplastic wall with marked fibrosis.[38,44] Symptoms usually reflect biliary obstruction with colicky pain in the right upper quadrant, epigastric area, or upper abdomen.[13,15,16] Fascioliasis also can be a silent, potential threat: the parasites can survive for longer than 10 years, and infection is usually asymptomatic.[30]

Liver function tests during this phase are consistent with an extrahepatic cholestasis syndrome,[47] which can lead to surgery to treat the biliary obstruction.[45] Asymptomatic cholestasis can be frequently found in infected people from endemic areas. In Egypt, it was found that patients with fascioliasis had significant liver enzyme abnormalities, the most common being an increase in the γ-glutamyltransferase and alkaline phosphatase.[48]

Imaging abnormalities can also be found on ultrasound (US), including hepatomegaly, splenomegaly, periportal fibrosis, thickened gallbladder wall, dilated common bile duct, parasites in the gallbladder and common bile duct, stones in the gallbladder, stones in bile duct, cystic lesions in the liver, focal lesions in the liver, and ascites.[49] *Fasciola* may also cause acute eosinophilic cholecystitis,[50] along with pruritus and intermittent jaundice.[51] The parasites appear as small, intrahepatic cystic lesions[15] or as a large, multiloculated cyst that causes abscesses. On imaging, parasites may appear very similar to echinococcosis.[52] Bacterial superinfection of *Fasciola* cysts is a complication of the chronic phase. Recent studies in a rat model have shown a significantly increased risk of bacterobilia in the chronic infection[53] and with concomitant gallstones.[54] Even after successful treatment, abdominal pain and weight loss still may be present in approximately 2% to 4% of patients for several months,[55] which emphasizes the risk for morbidity even after eradication of the infection.

Eosinophilia is not as common a finding in chronic fascioliasis as in the acute stage. On admission to a tertiary health center, 47% of 277 patients with complicated disease had eosinophilia.[56] A similar percentage was found in 101 chronic cases from the Andean region and other endemic areas: 48% had eosinophilia above normal levels, and only 14% had more than 1000 eosinophils/mL.[57] In another study, approximately half of a group of 61 children in the Peruvian Altiplano with chronic fascioliasis had eosinophilia.[51] In Turkey, only 11% of 18 patients with fascioliasis had eosinophilia.[14] Likewise, mild eosinophilia may be present in a minority of fascioliasis patients.[58] Few patients in the chronic phase have high-grade eosinophilia, in contrast with the acute phase, which presents with hypereosinophilia in almost all patients. A wide variety of other infectious agents are associated with eosinophilia, such as *Strongyloides stercoralis*, *Ascaris lumbricoides*, and hookworms or other helminths. Although these are the most common parasitic causes of eosinophilia, they do not typically cause hepatic lesions and do not reach the high levels observed in patients with acute fascioliasis. In summary, chronic fascioliasis may manifest without eosinophilia.

Another presentation of the chronic infection is hemobilia as a result of ulcerative lesions in the biliary tract caused by the adult parasite (see Chapter 116).[59] Severe iron deficiency anemia has been frequently reported in patients with chronic fascioliasis.[32,60,61] A granulomatous chronic inflammation also may be triggered by parasite ova in the liver or other locations.[62,63]

Chronic fascioliasis may suppress the immune system. In an animal model, persistent immune suppression has been demonstrated in advanced chronic infection,[64] suggesting that the infected host may be susceptible during the chronic phase to any T helper cell type 2 (Th2)-suppression–dependent infection. This chronic immunosuppression may predispose to bacterial infection that can be life threatening.

Fasciola and Liver Fibrosis

An association exists between fascioliasis and liver fibrosis. It appears that hepatic fibrosis may evolve in some susceptible hosts, depending on the time and burden of infection. For example, almost 50% of cattle infected chronically by fascioliasis had cirrhosis.[38] Data support that cathepsin L1 and its collagenolytic function are associated with tissue invasion in the pathogenesis of hepatic involvement associated with *F. hepatica* infection.[65] Fascioliasis causes bile duct hyperplasia,[66] increased levels of proline,[67,68] and types I and III collagen in the liver[69]; these anomalies are similar to the progression observed in cirrhosis and other pathologic conditions, including wound healing (see Chapter 7). However, few studies have attempted to identify factors associated with liver fibrosis, which is an important clinical outcome of the infection.[38,70–72] In addition, liver cirrhosis has been reported in both children and adults with fascioliasis.[31,73–75] In an endemic country, preliminary studies have shown that approximately 9% of cirrhotic patients have antibodies against *Fasciola*.[76] In vitro and in vivo studies have shown a significant correlation between fibrogenic gene expression and both intensity and duration of infection, demonstrating that longer and higher burden of infection stimulates fibrogenesis in the infected liver.[77] In conclusion, the chronic infection may lead to liver fibrosis (see Chapter 7)

Imaging Studies

Table 45.4 summarizes the most common imaging findings in fascioliasis.

Abdominal Ultrasound

Findings in the acute phase of fascioliasis include focal areas of increased echogenicity; multiple nodular or irregular lesions of variable echogenicity; or a single, complex mass in the liver that resembles malignancy mimicking malignancy[78,79] (see Chapter 14). In frequent travelers, an abnormal liver US scan showing a complex cystic lesion warrants a workup for fascioliasis or other parasitic disease, such as echinococcal infection. In the chronic phase, US is even less specific, although the adult parasites can be visualized in the gallbladder[80–82] as echogenic nonshadowing particles.[83] Overall, the detection rate is extremely low if used as the sole diagnostic tool. For example,

TABLE 45.4	Imaging Findings in Fascioliasis	
ULTRASONOGRAPHY	**COMPUTED TOMOGRAPHY**	**MAGNETIC RESONANCE IMAGING**
Focal areas	Multiple hepatic metastatic-like lesions	Homogeneous hyperintense T2-weighted turbo spin-echo image
Multiple nodules		
Irregular lesions	Change in position, attenuation, shape in time	
Variable or increased echogenicity		Subscapular multiple hypointense areas
	Abscess-like lesions	
Single complex mass	Low-density serpiginous tortuous tunnel-like branching	Hypointense T1-weighted three-dimensional gradient-echo image
Complex cystic mass		
	Subscapular hematoma	
Parasites moving in gallbladder	Cystic calcifications	
	Glisson capsule contrast enhancement	
	Single non–contrast-enhanced hypodense irregular mass	

of 76 patients with chronic fascioliasis evaluated by abdominal US, only 11 (14%) had visualized parasites and in only 2 (2.6%) the parasites were spontaneously moving into the gallbladder. Therefore the detection rate of *F. hepatica* chronic infection by US is disappointingly low[84] and not specific.[14]

Computed Tomography

The most common CT findings in acute fascioliasis include multiple hepatic metastasis-like lesions that change in position, attenuation, and shape over time[41] (see Chapter 14). Initial lesions may be easily confused with hepatic metastases. Other findings are hepatomegaly, tract-like hypodense lesions with subcapsular location, subcapsular hematoma, and cystic calcifications.[41,85] The hepatic lesions correlate with the time of infection. Early infection is associated with contrast enhancement of the Glisson capsule as a result of inflammation stimulated as the juvenile parasite penetrates the liver capsule. This occurs in the early stage of the acute infection (first month of infection). In the intermediate stage (after the first month), multiple hypodense nodular areas (abscess-like lesions) or low-density serpiginous, tortuous, tunnel-like branching lesions that range from 2 to 10 mm are created by parasite migration through the liver and are typically visualized in the subcapsular region.[40,86] In the late stage of the acute infection (≥3 months), a necrotic granuloma is seen that appears as a single, non–contrast-enhanced hypodense irregular mass in the liver parenchyma, more central than peripheral.[87–89] Part of the differential diagnosis of liver calcification is fascioliasis, which generally means an old infection of at least 6 months' duration. Although the characteristics of these cyst calcifications seem to be unique to fascioliasis, this finding adds a new agent to the list of infectious diseases associated with tissue calcifications, such as echinococcosis, paragonimiasis, histoplasmosis, and toxoplasmosis.

Magnetic Resonance Imaging

Only a few cases visualized on magnetic resonance imaging (MRI) have been reported. T2-weighted turbo spin-echo MRI showed a homogeneous hyperintense area in a subcapsular location containing multiple hypointense areas (see Chapter 14). A T1-weighted three-dimensional gradient-echo image displayed homogeneous contrast enhancement.[90] The hypodense lesions observed in the CT scan are of hypointense signal in T1-weighted and hyperintense in T2-weighted MR images.[91,92]

Diagnosis

The diagnosis of fascioliasis should be considered in patients with abdominal pain and hepatomegaly accompanied by peripheral eosinophilia. A careful dietary history should be obtained, including a history of watercress ingestion or consumption of raw vegetables washed in potentially contaminated water.[93] The diagnosis of the fascioliasis is confirmed mainly by eggs in stool and serologic examination, based on epidemiology, clinical picture, and adjunct imaging results or surgical techniques. In poor endemic areas, the diagnosis can be a challenge and sometimes a trial of antiparasitic drug may be needed. Clinical improvement and reduction in the eosinophil counts after 3 to 5 days of triclabendazole can be used as a diagnostic criterion.[41] Fig. 45.7 shows the results of the serologic examination and stool sampling, the possible stage of the infection, and the clinical significance.

Acute Phase

Enzyme-linked immunosorbent assay (ELISA) against excretory-secretory proteins has the highest sensitivity in the acute form of fascioliasis. The so-called *Fas2-ELISA* (cathepsin L1–based antibody) is more specific than Western blot and Arc II and has a sensitivity of 92.4%, specificity of 83.6%, and negative predictive value of 97.2%.[94,95] A classic presentation of a patient with acute *F. hepatica* infection is eosinophilia, prolonged fever, abdominal pain, multiple hepatic abscesses, or metastasis-like lesions in the peritoneum or liver. Recognizing the clinical scenario early may allow timely and noninvasive identification of this infection.

Chronic Phase

The gold standard for the diagnosis of chronic infection is visualization of the eggs in the stool or bile or duodenal aspirates or recovery of the adult parasites during surgery. A serologic test can be used as a diagnostic test when the stool examination is persistently negative for *Fasciola* eggs. A sedimentation technique should be performed on serial stool specimens (at least three) from different days to increase the likelihood of detecting

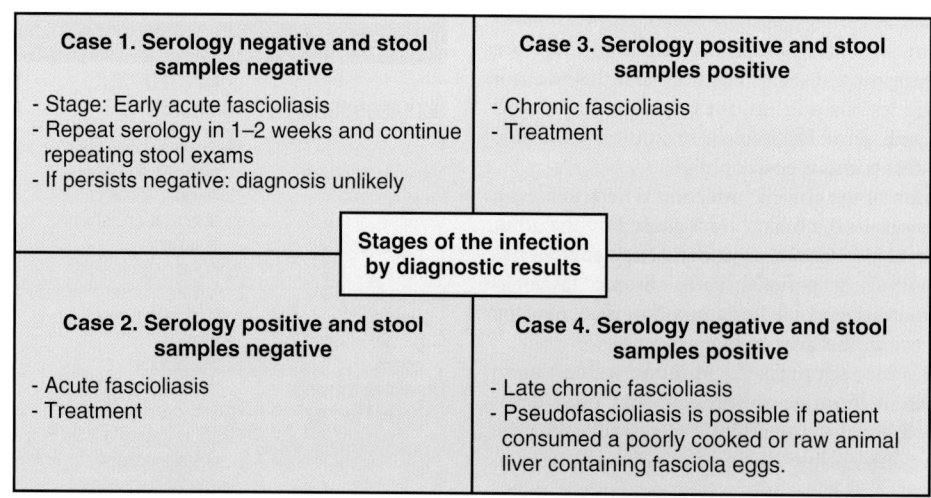

FIGURE 45.7 **Most common possible scenarios of diagnostic results in fascioliasis.** Cases 2 and 3 are the most commonly found in clinical practice. Cases 1 and 4 are uncommon.

the eggs in the stools. The intermittent deposition of parasite ova in the biliary duct can decrease the sensitivity of the sedimentation technique, so frequent stool examinations may be considered. One technique is the rapid sedimentation technique described by Lumbreras et al.[3] in Peru. This test is inexpensive, easy to perform, and sensitive, with a higher sensitivity than the ether-formalin concentration method.[26] Another technique, the Kato-Katz method, can be used to measure the intensity of infection.[96] The FLOTAC technique also can be used to detect *Fasciola* eggs in the stool.[97]

Diagnosis of Fascioliasis by Surgery

In the cases reported in the literature, most patients who underwent a surgical or invasive procedure had chronic *Fasciola* infection and their initial clinical problem was biliary obstruction and choledocholithiasis.[98,99] However, the detection rate of the adult parasite during surgery of the biliary tract is low overall. In a series of 162 patients who had cholecystectomy in an endemic area, only 1.2% had *F. hepatica* in the gallbladder[57]; however, several cases have been diagnosed in the operating room incidentally.

A mild eosinophilia in the clinical setting of biliary obstruction in a traveler or immigrant from endemic areas should suggest fascioliasis. Several cases have been diagnosed and managed by endoscopic retrograde cholangiopancreatography (ERCP), and only a few had mild eosinophilia.[100–102] A single dose of triclabendazole should be given after the procedure to ensure elimination of any parasites missed by endoscopy or remaining in other locations. The adult parasite also can be found incidentally during an elective laparoscopic cholecystectomy.[103] Even in highly endemic areas, the diagnosis can be missed initially, and cases of parasites accidentally obstructing percutaneous biliary drainage catheters have been reported.[46] Biliary obstruction by *Fasciola* associated with cholangitis requires both surgical intervention and antiparasitic agents.

Interestingly, fascioliasis can be misdiagnosed as echinococcal disease (see Chapter 72) because the former may have a strong cross-reactivity with ELISA. Patients may have surgical intervention to remove the pseudocyst of *Echinococcus*, when parasites of *F. hepatica* cause an intrahepatic cyst.[104] In other situations, adult parasites were found when trying to remove a possible malignancy or metastasis-like lesion from the colonic wall,[105] neck,[106] epidural space,[107] eye,[108] and breast.[63]

When fascioliasis affects the pancreatic duct,[109] the management, either surgical or conservative, should be individualized. However, when indicated, drainage can be a reasonable approach, followed by a trial of triclabendazole along with antispasmodics to reduce the severe abdominal pain experienced after the death of the parasite. Complications such as pancreatic duct obstruction and consequent pancreatitis may be life threatening but are rare.[110]

In patients with cholangitis,[111] emergent percutaneous drainage is recommended, because despite the antiparasitic medication, the dead parasites will remain in the biliary duct for a few days before clearing, obstructing drainage through the ampulla of Vater (see Chapters 30, 31, and 43). The most common bacterial organisms causing cholangitis identified in an animal model were *Escherichia coli* (45%), *Enterococcus faecalis* (45%), and *Klebsiella pneumoniae* (10%).[53] No data in humans are available, but the presence of *E. faecalis* in almost half the cases of bacterobilia in the animal model should be taken with special consideration for antibiotic choice. It is recommended that a single antibiotic be given, such as a β-lactam/lactamase inhibitor for mild to moderate infection or a carbapenem for severe infection. A combination therapy of cephalosporin or fluoroquinolone is also acceptable. However, antimicrobial therapy should be adjusted according to the organism identified, with susceptibilities to common antimicrobials.

In summary, in a patient from an endemic area who presents with a clinical picture similar to that of acute cholecystitis, normal US, or abscess-like lesions on imaging, the diagnosis of fascioliasis should be considered. Furthermore, during diagnostic laparoscopy, metastatic-like liver lesions with eosinophilia are strongly suggestive of acute fascioliasis.

Treatment

Triclabendazole is the treatment of choice for both phases of *Fasciola* infection; bithionol and nitazoxanide are alternative choices.[112] The cure rate exceeds 90% for acute stages after a single dose of 10 mg/kg,[41] and similar results have been obtained in the therapy for chronic infection.[113–115] This drug has better absorption in the postprandial setting, preferably with a fatty meal, and the most frequent adverse event is biliary colic caused by obstruction by dead parasites, but it is a generally well-tolerated regimen.[116,117] Triclabendazole was introduced in the early 1980s for the treatment of *F. hepatica* infections in livestock, and it has been placed on the World Health Organization (WHO) List of Essential Medicines (http://www.who.int/medicines/publications/essentialmedicines/en/) because of its efficacy and cost effectiveness.

Treatment of fascioliasis with triclabendazole has been shown to reduce the prevalence significantly, from 5.2% to 1.2% in 7 years.[118] However, the intensive use of triclabendazole in animals has resulted in the development of resistance.[119,120] On the other hand, in places where triclabendazole for humans is not available, the veterinary form can be used and more recently has been shown to have some resistance in humans as well. A study conducted by Terashima et al.[121] showed patients labeled as having "TCBZ resistance" may respond to multiple regimens of TCBZ with a cure rate of 74%. Most cases of human fascioliasis are successfully treated with TCBZ, but some continue excreting eggs in the stools despite one or two standard of care regimens of TCBZ.[122] The US Food and Drug Administration has approved a recommendation of a total dose of 20 mg/kg (two doses of 10 mg/kg given 12 hours apart) for treatment of patients aged 6 years or more.[112,123] The most important adverse effect was abdominal pain or biliary colic during the first week of treatment. Antispasmodic drugs may decrease or completely alleviate the transient episodes of abdominal pain and should be used in most cases at the beginning of therapy. Given the unlikelihood of any new drugs against *F. hepatica* being developed in the foreseeable future, the emergence of animal resistance to triclabendazole represents an important threat,[119] and there is also evidence of resistance in humans according to recent studies.[124]

Many years ago, parenteral dehydroemetine at doses of 1 mg/kg for 10 days was used. Then, bithionol was applied at doses of 30 to 50 mg/kg every third day for a total of 10 to 15 doses, although it is cardiotoxic and very expensive. Other drugs, such as nitazoxanide, have been evaluated for fascioliasis, but cure rates have been disappointingly low. Adult patients who received a 7-day course of nitazoxanide had a cure rate of 60%, but the rate was only 40% in children.[125] New drugs have been evaluated and tested in animals with fascioliasis. Artesunate, artemether, and OZ78 have fasciocidal properties in animals and are promising drugs for the near future, should resistance to triclabendazole become a problem.[126,127] Albendazole, metronidazole, and praziquantel are not recommended for fascioliasis treatment.

Future Directions and Vaccines

Because fascioliasis constitutes a major economic impact, development of effective vaccines would be an important advance. Major advances have been made in identifying potential vaccine molecules for the control of fasciolosis in livestock but we have yet to reach the level of efficacy required for commercialization.[128] Cysteine proteinases released by *F. hepatica* play a key role in parasite feeding and migration through host tissues and in immune system evasion. A recombinant cysteine proteinase (CPFhW) expressed as inclusion bodies in *E. coli* was used for enteral vaccination of rats against fascioliasis. In that study, oral vaccination reduced the parasite burden by 78% to 80% after a challenge with metacercariae.[129] The glutathione transferase superfamily from liver fluke plays Phase II detoxification and housekeeping roles and has been shown to contain protective vaccine candidates.[130] Promising future research will yield meaningful immunologic targets to prevent the infection, especially in the well-recognized endemic areas and particularly in children, but so far the vaccines are targeted only to animals.

CLONORCHIASIS AND OPISTHORCHIASIS

Liver fluke infection caused by trematodes belonging to the family Opisthorchiidae—*Opisthorchis viverrini*, *Opisthorchis felineus*, and *Clonorchis sinensis*—is a major public health problem in many parts of the Far East, Southeast Asia, and Eastern Europe. Clonorchiasis is an infection caused by *C. sinensis*, the Chinese or Oriental liver fluke, whereas opisthorchiasis is caused by *O. viverrini* and *O. felineus* (class Trematoda). Similar to fascioliasis, migration and global tourism are responsible for cases diagnosed in areas where the disease is not endemic (see Chapters 50 and 51).

Epidemiology

C. sinensis and *O. viverrini*, small Asian liver flukes 8 to 15 mm in length, are very similar in adult morphology and genetics but differ in geographic distribution.[131] It is estimated that more than 35 million people are infected worldwide, approximately 15 million of whom are Chinese, with another 600 million people at risk of infection. *C. sinensis* is endemic in northeast China, southern Korea, Japan, Taiwan, northern Vietnam, and the far eastern part of Russia,[132] and *O. viverrini* is endemic in Laos, Thailand, Vietnam, and Cambodia. *O. felineus* infection is the most prevalent foodborne liver fluke infection of humans in Russia, Ukraine, and Kazakhstan (Fig. 45.8). Approximately 10 million people are infected with *O. viverrini*, with four in five infections having occurred in Thailand and the remainder in

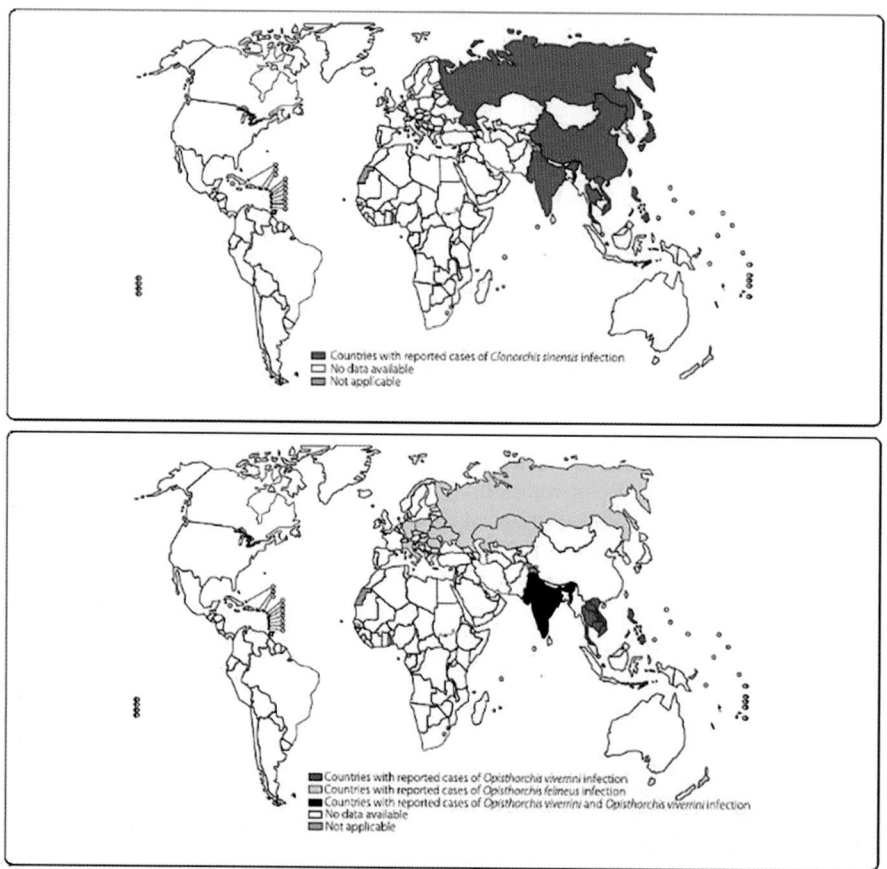

FIGURE 45.8 **A,** Global distribution of clonorchiasis. **B,** Global distribution of opisthorchiasis. (From Lu XT, Gu QY, Limpanont Y, et al. Snail-borne parasitic diseases: An update on global epidemiological distribution, transmission interruption and control methods. *Infect Dis Poverty*. 2018;7(1):28.

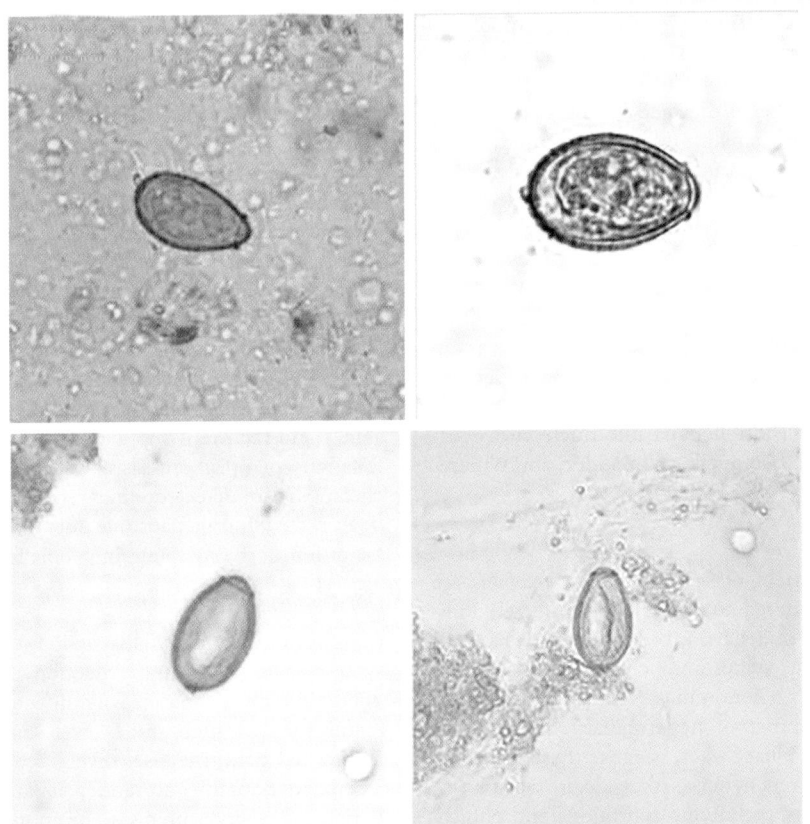

FIGURE 45.9   **A,** *Clonorchis sinensis* egg: the small knob at the abopercular end is visible in this image. **B,** *C. sinensis* egg. Note the operculum resting on the "shoulder"; image taken at 400× magnification. **C,** *C. Sinensis* egg; image taken at 400× magnification. **D,** *C. Sinensis* egg; image taken at 400× magnification. (From Centers for Disease Control and Prevention. Fascioliasis. https://www.cdc.gov/dpdx/clonorchiasis/index.html.)

Laos. It is thought that 1.2 million people are infected with *O. felineus,* which is endemic to the area encompassing the former Soviet Union.[133] In China, *Clonorchis* infections have more than tripled over the last decade, with 15 million people infected in 2004.[134] Similar to fascioliasis, the geographic pattern of these small flukes is not uniform. For instance, in Thailand, the greatest prevalence of opisthorchiasis is in the north (19.3%) and northeast (15.7%) compared with the central (3.8%) and southern regions (0%). In general, the infection is acquired by eating raw or uncooked cyprinoid fish products in rural areas or dishes such as *koi-pla.*[135] Some cases are documented in North America, mainly imported by Asian immigrants.

Life Cycle

The life cycles of *Clonorchis* and *Opisthorchis* flukes are similar. Starting from a human host, the adult worms deposit fully developed eggs (Fig. 45.9); the eggs are then passed to the environment through the feces, and they must get into water to hatch and infect their first intermediate host, a freshwater snail. After being ingested by a suitable snail, the eggs release miracidia, which undergo several developmental stages in the snail: as sporocysts, redia, and cercariae. The snail intermediate hosts for *Opisthorchis* are *Bithynia goniompharus, Bithynia funiculata,* and *Bithynia siamensis. Parafossarulus manchouricus* often serves as a first intermediate host for *C. sinensis,* and snail hosts also include other *Bithynia, Tarebia, Alocinma,* and *Bulimus* spp. (Fig. 45.10). Once inside the snail's body, the miracidium hatches from the egg and parasitically grows inside of the snail, where it develops into a sporocyst that houses the

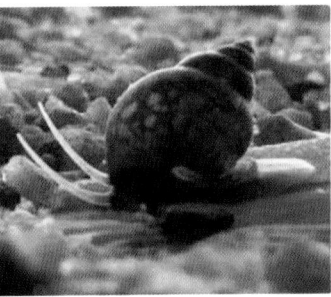

FIGURE 45.10   *Bithynia* sp., another common intermediate host of *C. sinensis.* (Image courtesy of Michal Maňas. From Centers for Disease Control and Prevention. Fascioliasis. https://www.cdc.gov/dpdx/clonorchiasis/index.html.)

asexual reproduction of redia, the next stage. The redia house the asexual reproduction of free-swimming cercariae. This system of asexual reproduction allows for an exponential multiplication of cercaria individuals from one miracidium. Once the redia mature, having grown inside the snail body until this point, they actively bore out of the snail body into the freshwater environment and seek out fish. Cercariae are released from the snail and then penetrate freshwater fish—the second intermediate host (*Cyclocheilichthys* and *Puntius* spp., *Hampala dispar*), encysting as metacercariae in the muscles or under the scales. Once inside the fish muscle, the cercaria creates a protective metacercarial cyst with which to encapsulate its body.

This protective cyst proves useful for when the fish muscle is consumed by a human or other host, such as a cat, dog, pig, or any other fish-eating mammal. The acid-resistant cyst enables the metacercariae to avoid being digested by the gastric acids and allows them to reach the small intestine unharmed.

Reaching the small intestine, the metacercariae navigate toward the human liver—the final habitat. In contrast with the larger *F. hepatica* fluke, metacercariae of *Opisthorchis* and *Clonorchis* migrate through the ampulla of Vater after excysting in the duodenum; they then travel into the bile ducts, where they mature into adult worms within 4 weeks and deposit yellow, operculated eggs. The parasites may live for up to 45 years in the liver of a human host, producing 1000 to 2500 eggs per day. The adult flukes, measuring 10 to 25 mm by 3 to 5 mm, reside in medium-sized and small intrahepatic bile ducts and occasionally in the extrahepatic bile ducts, gallbladder, and pancreatic duct.

Clinical Manifestations

The clinical manifestations of *Opisthorchis* and *Clonorchis* are similar and may be considered together. Most infected individuals are asymptomatic and have a benign course. Even in heavily infected individuals, symptoms occur in only approximately 10% of patients.[136] Clonorchiasis and opisthorchiasis are associated with a number of hepatobiliary diseases but mainly with disease in the biliary tract, because these flukes do not penetrate the liver parenchyma as they do in fascioliasis. The frequency and types of pathologic conditions and clinical disease seem to differ for *C. sinensis* and *O. viverrine* occasionally. For example, cholelithiasis is one of the more serious complications of clonorchiasis (see Chapters 32 and 39) but is a rare complication of opisthorchiasis. In both species the prominent inflammatory process within the biliary tract is the main pathologic characteristic of these infections, which can sometimes lead to cholangiocarcinoma, especially with *O. viverrini*. *C. sinensis* has been classified by the International Agency for Research on Cancer (IARC) as a probable carcinogen (group 2A), and *O. viverrini* has been definitively validated as a carcinogen (class 1).[137]

Flukes can occasionally gain access to the pancreatic duct, where they can cause obstruction and pancreatitis. The pathologic and clinical consequences of opisthorchiasis are related to the intensity and duration of cumulative infections. Because adult flukes are long lived, they can produce eggs and symptoms long after the human host has emigrated from the area. Most people with these Asian fluke infections have no symptoms, and only 5% to 10% of those heavily infected have nonspecific chronic symptoms such as right upper quadrant abdominal pain, flatulence, and fatigue. Cholangiocarcinoma is a known complication.

Clonorchis Sinensis

Acute infection by *C. sinensis* is usually asymptomatic, but some patients may have fever, rash, malaise, and right upper quadrant abdominal discomfort. Chronic infection reflects the worm burden and may appear as recurrent pyogenic liver cholangitis, cholecystitis, obstructive jaundice, hepatomegaly, cholecystitis, multiple hepatic tumors,[138] and cholelithiasis.[139,140] Occasionally, *Clonorchis* can cause acute acalculous cholecystitis[141] and eosinophilic cholecystitis.[142]

An association between clonorchiasis and cholangiocarcinoma has been reported[143] (see Chapters 50 and 51). Severe

C. sinensis infection is a significant risk factor for malignant changes in bile ducts and surrounding liver tissues occurring as a result of direct contact with *C. sinensis* worms and their excretory-secretory products.

Opisthorchis Viverrini

With acute *O. viverrini* infection, most infected individuals have low fluke counts and therefore are asymptomatic. In acute *O. viverrini* infection, only 5% to 10% of heavily infected patients have nonspecific symptoms, such as right upper quadrant abdominal pain, flatulence, fatigue, and a hot sensation over the abdomen. In the chronic phase, mild hepatomegaly occurs, mainly in more heavily infected patients (egg counts >10,000 eggs/g). Jaundice and splenomegaly are not observed, but intrahepatic duct stones and recurrent suppurative cholangitis are common manifestations of opisthorchiasis. Whenever jaundice and ascending cholangitis are detected, fluke-related cholangiocarcinoma should be suspected. Intrahepatic bile duct dilatation is the most common factor for morbidity found in people from endemic areas.[144]

Opisthorchis Felineus

O. felineus infection yields acute symptoms more frequently symptomatic than that infection, usually beginning 10 to 26 days after eating heavily infected undercooked fish and manifesting as high-grade fever, anorexia, nausea, vomiting, abdominal pain, malaise, myalgia, arthralgia, and urticaria.[145] Lymphadenopathy and tender hepatomegaly may be observed. Peripheral eosinophilia is a common finding, especially during the first 2 to 6 weeks of the infection, together with increased liver enzyme levels. In chronic infection, eosinophilia is usually milder, but patients may present with suppurative cholangitis (see Chapter 43) and liver abscess (see Chapter 70) as a result of biliary obstruction.

Consequences of Chronic Infection

Chronic infection with *C. sinensis* and *O. viverrini* may manifest with symptoms similar to those of chronic fascioliasis, or they may manifest with more sinister symptoms in the form of different types of cancer. Similar to fascioliasis, mechanical complications from a chronic infection of clonorchiasis and opisthorchiasis include physical bile duct obstruction, fatigue, abdominal discomfort, anorexia, weight loss, dyspepsia, and diarrhea. An elevated alkaline phosphatase level may be observed, but transaminases are generally normal. The gallbladder is often nonfunctional and enlarged. Dead parasites or ova can serve as a nidus for stone formation. Severe disease can result in obstructive jaundice, pancreatitis, recurrent cholangitis, and pyogenic liver abscesses.[146]

More serious complications of chronic infection include cholangitis, cholangiohepatitis, and cholangiocarcinoma (see Chapters 44, 50, and 51) Carcinogenesis associated with helminth infections is a complex process that may involve several different mechanisms, but chronic inflammation is a key feature. The human liver fluke *O. viverrini* infects millions of people throughout Southeast Asia and is a major cause of cholangiocarcinoma (see Chapters 50 and 51). The mechanisms by which chronic infection with *O. viverrini* results in cholangiocarcinogenesis are likely multifactorial, but one mechanism is the secretion of parasite proteins with mitogenic properties into the bile ducts, driving cell proliferation and creating a tumorigenic environment. A possible pathway for the development of cholangiocarcinoma is the presence of Ov-GRN-1, a major growth factor present in *O. viverrini* excretory-secretory products that induces proliferation of host cells, which supports a role for this fluke protein to establish a tumorigenic environment.

In general, these flukes cause inflammation around the biliary tree that leads to severe hyperplasia of epithelial cells, metaplasia of mucin-producing cells in the mucosa, and progressive periductal fibrosis. Clear associations exist between *O. viverrini* infection and cholangiocarcinoma in the context of the intensity of infection, parasite-specific antibody response, and abnormalities of the biliary tract.

The higher the intensity of anti–*O. viverrini* antibody titers, the higher is the risk for cholangiocarcinoma.[147] In 2009 the International Agency for Research on Cancer recognized *C. sinensis* and *O. viverrini* as group I human carcinogens.[148,149] The lesions that predispose to malignant changes in *O. viverrini* are evident as a dilatation of subcapsular medium-sized and large bile ducts with a prominent fibrotic wall, periductal inflammatory cell infiltration, goblet cell metaplasia, epithelial and adenomatous hyperplasia, and periductal fibrosis. The pathogenesis of *O. viverrini*–mediated hepatobiliary changes may be caused by mechanical irritation or its metabolic products.[150] Several *N*-nitroso compounds and their precursors occur at low levels in fermented food, such as preserved mud fish paste *(pla ra)*, a condiment ubiquitous in the cuisine of northeastern Thailand and Laos.[151] The study of *O. viverrini* genes should expedite molecular studies of cholangiocarcinogenesis and accelerate research focused on developing new interventions, drugs, and vaccines that might help in controlling *O. viverrini* and related flukes.[152] Similarly, studies show a strong association between *C. sinensis* and development of cholangiocarcinoma.[143] An epidemiologic study in Korea correlated the prevalence of *C. sinensis* and the incidence rate of cholangiocarcinoma: *C. sinensis* prevalence was 2.1% in Chuncheon, 7.8% in Chungju, and 31.3% in Haman; cholangiocarcinoma incidence rate was 0.3, 1.8, and 5.5 per 100,000 population, respectively.[153] The mechanism of *C. sinensis* infestation causing cholangiocarcinoma is not completely clear. Recent studies show that this fluke can promote the expression of focal and cell–cell adhesion proteins in cholangiocarcinoma cells and secretion of matrix metalloproteinases, leading to the proliferation and invasion of this cancer.[154]

Hepatocellular carcinoma also has been associated with clonorchiasis, along with hepatitis B virus and alcohol consumption as cofactors[155] (see Chapter 89). Moreover, gallbladder tubulovillous adenoma has been reported with *Clonorchis* infection.[156] It seems plausible that cholangiocarcinogenesis associated with clonorchiasis is the cumulative end result of a multifactorial carcinogenic mechanism, although the mechanisms involved are not completely understood.

Improving diagnosis with new serologic tests may be helpful, but such tests cannot distinguish between recent or past infection. Currently, the Ov-CP-1–based ELISA shows a sensitivity of 95% and specificity of 96% in serum coinfected with hookworm, minute intestinal fluke, *S. stercoralis, Taenia* spp., *Giardia lamblia,* and *E. coli* infection.[157] The sensitivity and specificity are similar to those in other studies using an ELISA based on recombinant trematode cysteine protease such as *C. sinensis* (sensitivity 81.3%–96%, specificity 92.6%–96.2%).[158,159]

Human clonorchiasis and opisthorchiasis are primarily diagnosed by the detection of eggs in feces. The Kato-Katz method is accepted as the best for fecal examination, although sometimes the eggs may not be detected because of biliary obstruction or intermittent egg excretion, similar to that encountered with fascioliasis. Thus multiple Kato-Katz thick smears may increase the detection rate of *Clonorchis* eggs.[160] In light infections, with fewer than 10 adult worms in the biliary tract, a polymerase chain reaction detecting the DNA of the adult parasite in stools may be helpful.[161] In low-resource settings, a serologic test for *O. viverrini* such as loop-mediated isothermal amplification has 100% sensitivity and 61.5% specificity.[162] Early detection of these liver fluke infections is important to prevent the appearance of cholangiocarcinoma in the untreated individuals. Promising diagnostic testing for cholangiocarcinoma from the infection by *O. viverrini*, including the detection of miRNA profiles, is being developed,[163] which may lead to early diagnosis and treatment.

Intrahepatic duct dilatation is the most common finding on US imaging (76% of patients), and increasing periductal echogenicity and gallbladder sludge are seen only in patients with extensive infection.[164] Ruangsittichai et al.[165] reported high sensitivity and specificity using a recombinant eggshell protein, with potential for the serodiagnosis of human opisthorchiasis. However, detection of *O. viverrini* DNA is expensive and requires skilled personnel.

Treatment

Praziquantel, a derivative of pyrazino isoquinoline, is the drug of choice for *O. viverrini, O. felineus,* and *C. sinensis* treatment. For *O. viverrini,* a single dose of 40 mg/kg of praziquantel has a cure rate of 71.4%, whereas a total dose of 75 mg/kg (50 mg/kg plus 25 mg/kg, 4 hours apart) has a cure rate of 96.6%.[166] For clonorchiasis, the recommended dose of praziquantel is 25 mg/kg three times at 5-hour intervals in 1 day (total dose, 75 mg/kg), with a cure rate of 83% to 85%.[132] Side effects of praziquantel include headache, dizziness, insomnia, nausea, and vomiting.

Tribendimidine appears to be at least as efficacious as praziquantel for treatment of opisthorchiasis.[167] In a randomized trial including more than 600 patients with *O. viverrini* infection treated with tribendimidine (single oral dose: 200 mg for children, 400 mg for adolescents and adults) or praziquantel (two doses: 50 mg/kg followed 25 mg/kg, 6 hours apart), the cure rate (defined as no parasite eggs in stool at 3 weeks observation) were 94% and 97%, respectively; adverse events were mild but were more frequent in the praziquantel group.[168]

Albendazole is another potential agent for treatment of *Clonorchis* infection. Albendazole (10 mg/kg orally with fatty meal for 7 days) shows good efficacy for clonorchiasis (>90% cure rate) but modest efficacy for opisthorchiasis (63% cure rate).[169] Occasionally, coinfection with *Fasciola* and *Clonorchis* has been reported in areas where both parasites are endemic, and therapy should include both praziquantel and triclabendazole.[170]

Although successful treatment of infection may take only a handful of days, symptoms of infection may take months to resolve. As more people need liver transplants, it seems that livers infested with *C. sinensis* can be used as donor organs for liver transplantation.[171]

OTHER PARASITOSES OF THE BILIARY TRACT

A. lumbricoides is the largest intestinal nematode parasitizing the human intestine, with females measuring 25 to 35 cm in length (Fig. 45.11). *A. lumbricoides* infections (ascariasis) are endemic in tropical countries, where access to personal hygiene and proper sanitation practices are not available and in places where human feces is used as fertilizer. *A. lumbrocoides* may occasionally migrate from its normal habitat in the small bowel to other locations, such as the biliary tract or pancreatic duct. Because

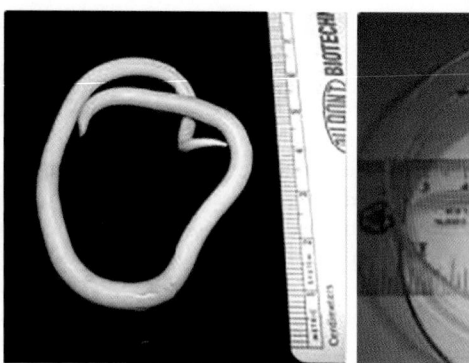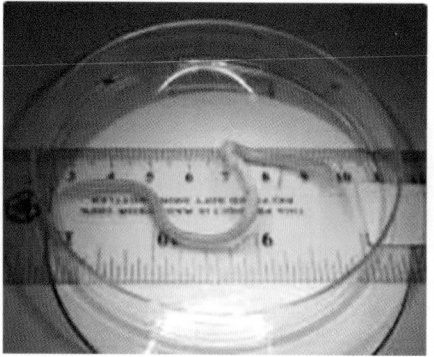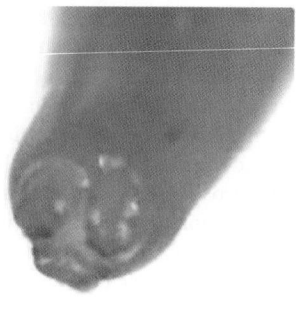

FIGURE 45.11   Adults of *Ascaris lumbricoides* are large roundworms. Females measure 20 to 35 cm long with straight tails; males are smaller at 15 to 31 cm and tend to have curved tails. Adults of both sexes possess three "lips" at the anterior end of the body. (https://www.cdc.gov/dpdx/ascariasis/index.html.)

TABLE 45.5   Distribution, Clinical Complications, and Treatment of Other Biliary Parasites

PARASITE	DISTRIBUTION	COMPLICATIONS	TREATMENT
Opisthorchis and *Clonorchis*	Far East, Southeast Asia, and Eastern Europe	Recurrent pyogenic liver cholangitis Cholelithiasis Cholangiocarcinoma	PZQ ± antibiotics PZQ ± surgery Surgery/chemotherapy/PZQ
Ascaris	Worldwide	Biliary obstruction with cholangitis Pancreatitis Ileal volvulus, perforations, intussusceptions, and impacted multiple worm boluses	ERCP to remove adult parasite + albendazole
Echinococcus granulosus	Worldwide	Hepatic hydatid cyst rupture into biliary tree	Albendazole followed by ERCP ± sphincterotomy

ERCP, Endoscopic retrograde cholangiopancreatography; *PZQ,* praziquantel.

of the high intensity of infection in endemic areas, *A. lumbrocoides* is more often seen as a clinical picture of jaundice, abdominal right upper quadrant pain, and fever, although it can occasionally cause biliary obstruction and result in obstructive jaundice or pancreatitis. Other surgical complications reported are ileal volvulus, perforations, intussusception, and impacted multiple worm boluses.[172]

Occasionally, ERCP may diagnose parasitosis of the biliary tract. For example, of 3548 ERCPs performed for extrahepatic cholestasis, cholangitis, and choledocholithiasis in a moderate endemic area in Eastern Europe, only 24 (0.66%) showed biliary parasitosis, such as hydatid cystic disease (*n* = 16) (see Chapter 74). In addition, 8 showed partial obstruction of the biliary tract, and 8 found ruptured cysts; *F. hepatica* (*n* = 4) and *A. lumbricoides* (*n* = 4) were also found. Endoscopic sphincterotomy was performed, after which the choledochus was examined carefully using a balloon catheter and basket procedure. ERCP is very useful in the therapy of biliary parasitic infections. The treatment for *Ascaris* in the biliary tract is elimination of the adult parasite through the endoscope, followed by a single oral dose of albendazole (400 mg).

Hepatic hydatid cyst (larval cystic stage of adult parasite tapeworm *Echinococcus granulosus*) rupture into the biliary tree occurs in 5% to 25% of patients and constitutes the most common complication of hepatic echinococcal cysts (see Chapter 72). In this setting, ERCP plays a pivotal role in the therapeutic management of the disease, even as a definitive therapy in some cases. However, oral albendazole (400 mg) twice daily can be started before the procedure. Typically, ERCP will show diffuse dilatation of the biliary tree, with several laminated defects occupying the distal common bile duct with multiple white germinative membranes; a sphincterotomy will help eliminate the membranes causing the obstruction. The treatment of choice for hepatic echinococcosis usually involves anthelmintic therapy and surgical resection or percutaneous aspiration. However, when hydatid material, comprising daughter cysts and hydatid membranes, is released into the biliary tree through a fistulous tract, ERCP is mandatory before surgery to ensure the retrieval of hydatid biliary material to treat or prevent biliary obstruction complications, mainly acute cholangitis. Regardless of management, anthelmintic drugs always should be started before endoscopic or surgical therapy to inactivate intracystic material and minimize allergic disorders or postoperative recurrence.

Table 45.5 summarizes the distribution, clinical complications, and treatment of *Opisthochis, Clonorchis, Ascaris,* and *E. granulosus.*

The references for this chapter can be found online by accessing the accompanying Expert Consult website.

SECTION I. Inflamatory, Infective, and Congenital

D. Cystic Disease of the Biliary Tract

CHAPTER 46

Bile duct cysts in adults

Michael R. Driedger, Patrick Starlinger, and David M. Nagorney

First reported by Vater and Ezler in 1723, bile duct cysts represent a rare pathology. They exist most commonly as a pediatric surgical problem.[1] The majority of bile duct cysts are diagnosed in infants and children within the first decade of life, and an estimated 25% are detected by 1 year of age with an additional 35% to 55% by the age of 10 years.[2–5] Presentation occurs in adulthood in approximately 25% of patients.[6,7] Although clinically similar, the presentation and therapeutic strategies for bile duct cysts in adults differ substantially from those of younger patients.[8–10] In contrast to the pediatric experience, adult patients have an increased rate of acute presentation with biliary and/or pancreatic symptoms,[11] are more commonly associated with hepatobiliary pathology,[12–14] and they are often first seen with complications of previous cyst-related procedures.[12,15–18] The surgical management of bile duct cysts in adults is therefore complicated by co-existing hepatobiliary disease and the added technical difficulties of reoperative biliary surgery. Despite the heterogeneity of the disease and the absence of clinical trials, a collective consensus for excision of extrahepatic bile duct cysts has been generally accepted. However, the management of intrahepatic bile duct cysts remains controversial and the method of choice for reestablishing bilioenteric continuity after excision is debatable. This chapter examines the spectrum of hepatobiliary pathology encountered in adults with bile duct cysts and describes the surgical approaches for managing such patients.

DIAGNOSIS

Classification (Fig. 46.1)

Bile duct cysts are classified according to their anatomic distribution within the biliary ductal system as well as the extent and morphology of the cystic anomaly. Although the term *choledochal cyst* is often used, *bile duct or biliary cyst* semantically is more appropriate because cystic dilation can occur anywhere throughout the biliary ductal system, not only within the common bile duct (CBD; choledochus). The first systematic classification of extrahepatic bile duct cysts was proposed by Alonso-Lej and colleagues in 1959 in which cysts were classified into three types. Although this classification did not include intrahepatic bile duct cysts, this simple and practical scheme has provided the basis for all other classification systems. Interestingly, the size of the dilation of bile duct to

qualify as "cystic" dilation has not been defined clearly by either absolute size (diameter in millimeter) or ratio of measured-to-expected duct size at the cyst site in the biliary tree. Lack of specific criteria for defining bile duct cysts can be difficult clinically, particularly in patients after cholecystectomy, in whom the extrahepatic bile duct dilates as a physiologic response to an intact sphincter of Oddi. Whether secondary cystic dilation of bile ducts has the same clinicopathologic consequences and requires similar operative management is unknown. Operative intervention in these patients is avoided, unless symptoms develop.

In 1958 Caroli and colleagues described the entity of "multiple intrahepatic bile duct cysts." The recognition of intrahepatic bile duct cysts led to modification of the original classification system. In 1977 Todani refined the classification system of bile duct cysts by combining the Alonso-Lej classification and the variants of Caroli disease.[19] The classification system was further expanded on in 2003 to incorporate the presence of an anomalous pancreaticobiliary junction (APBJ)[20] (see Chapter 2).

Type I cysts are solitary fusiform or saccular dilations of the CBD and common hepatic duct (CHD). The CHD proximal to the cyst and ductal confluence is normal. Type I cysts are the most common bile duct cyst, comprising 50% to 90% of cysts and are subclassified further according to anatomic extent.[4,21]

- Type IA cysts are the most common subtype and are associated with an APBJ. They involve cystic dilation of the CBD and the CHD and may extend to the extrahepatic right or left hepatic ducts. The cystic duct and gallbladder arise from the cyst.
- Type IB cysts demonstrate focal, segmental dilation of the extrahepatic bile duct, most commonly involving the distal CBD and are not associated with an APBJ.
- Type IC refers to a smooth, fusiform, diffuse, or cylindrical dilatation of the extrahepatic ducts and are associated with an APBJ. Typically, the dilation extends from the pancreatobiliary junction to the CHD or extrahepatic main left and right hepatic ducts.
- Type ID cyst is a recently proposed modification of the Todani classification.[22,23] They are characterized by dilation of the cystic duct as well as CBD and CHD, resulting in a bicornal configuration of the cyst. An association with an APBJ has not been defined.

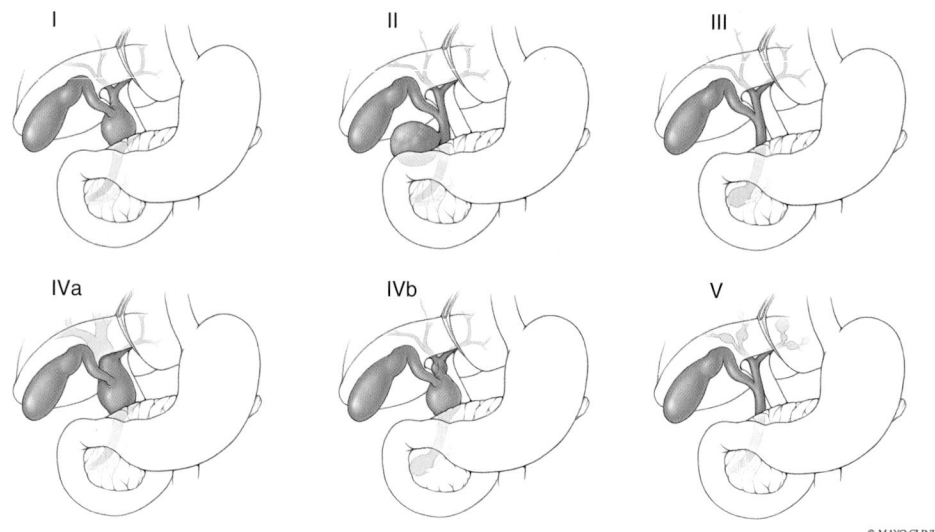

FIGURE 46.1 Classification of bile duct cysts.

© MAYO CLINIC

Type II bile duct cysts occur in approximately 2% to 3% of patients.[24,25] They are a discrete, true diverticulum of the extrahepatic bile duct system. They often project off the right lateral side of the bile duct and can resemble a duplication of the gallbladder. Approximately 60% are located between the CHD and biliary bifurcation, whereas 20% arise from the suprapancreatic CBD and another 20% from the intrapancreatic portion of the CBD.[26]

Type III cysts comprise 1% to 6% of bile ducts cysts and are characterized by cystic dilation of the intraduodenal portion of the distal CBD.[7,27,28] They are also referred to as choledochoceles. Type III cysts may represent a disparate disease entity and can be lined by duodenal or biliary epithelium. Type III cysts are more likely to be encountered incidentally during endoscopic retrograde cholangiopancreatography (ERCP) and are managed primarily with endoscopic therapy. Pancreatitis is often seen with type III cysts, whereas biliary tract symptoms are less common.[29] They are commonly divided into two subtypes based on their anatomic morphology.[30,31] Type A choledochoceles are cystic dilatations of a segment of the intramural bile duct. The bile duct and pancreatic duct enter the cyst and the cyst communicates with the duodenum at a separate orifice. Type B choledochoceles are diverticula of the intraampullary common channel. The bile duct opens normally into the duodenum.

Type IV cysts are the second most common subtype, comprising 15% to 35% of all cysts.[7] They are defined by the presence of multiple cysts and can be stratified by intrahepatic bile duct involvement. Type IVa is the most prevalent and involves multiple cysts in both the intrahepatic and extrahepatic bile ducts (Fig. 46.2). Intrahepatic dilation can affect both lobes, although the left lobe is predominantly involved.[32] Isolated dilation within the right liver is rare.[33] A primary hilar stricture or discrete change in duct caliber at the hilum may be seen. Type IVb, by contrast, consists of multiple dilations of the extrahepatic biliary tree with an uninvolved intrahepatic biliary tree. It is classically described as having a "string-of-beads" configuration.[34]

Last, type V cysts are characterized by one or more saccular or fusiform dilations of the medium- and large-sized intrahepatic ducts with no underlying obstruction or extrahepatic ductal system involvement. This entity is also known as Caroli disease, or communicating cavernous ectasia, and accounts for up to 20% of bile duct cysts. When type V bile duct cysts are associated with congenital hepatic fibrosis, the condition is termed Caroli syndrome or Grumbach disease.[35] Specifically, Caroli syndrome is characterized by the presence of intrahepatic ductal ectasia and periportal fibrosis. Both Caroli disease and syndrome have been described as inheritable in an autosomal recessive pattern and may be associated with autosomal recessive polycystic kidney disease as well as other hepatorenal fibrocystic diseases.[36]

A type VI bile duct cyst has recently been proposed and is characterized by an isolated dilation of the cystic duct in the absence of CBD or CHD involvement. This finding is quite rare and limited to a few case reports.[37,38]

Forme fruste bile duct cyst (an atypical or attenuated manifestation of a disease process) is simply a normal biliary ductal system associated with an APBJ.[39] Patients present with typical symptoms of abdominal pain and obstructive jaundice. A predisposition to recurrent pancreatitis is present. Similar evidence of histologic inflammatory change and malignant potential has been described; thus some authors have posited inclusion of this entity in the spectrum of bile duct cysts.[40–42]

Matsumoto also modified the Alonso-Lej classification system based on adding configuration to the location of the cysts.[43] Clinical management of bile duct cysts is dictated by cyst location, not configuration. Indeed, no data have shown clinical differences in presentation for similar type cysts with varying configurations. Therefore this subtyping has limited clinical utility.[44,45]

There are advantages and disadvantages to the increasingly complex alphanumeric modifications of the widely used Todani classification. Although the principle critique of the original Todani classification is that multiple distinct subtypes have been consolidated, whether the anatomic subtypes differ with respect to pathogenesis, natural history, clinical management, associated hepatobiliary pathology, and complication profile remains unclear. Additionally, mixed or variant types of cysts exist and are unclassifiable by the Todani classification (see Fig. 46.1). Visser and colleague's recent recommendation for descriptive terminology alone in lieu of Todani classification, although more exact, may provide clinical evidence for the value of subtyping.[47]

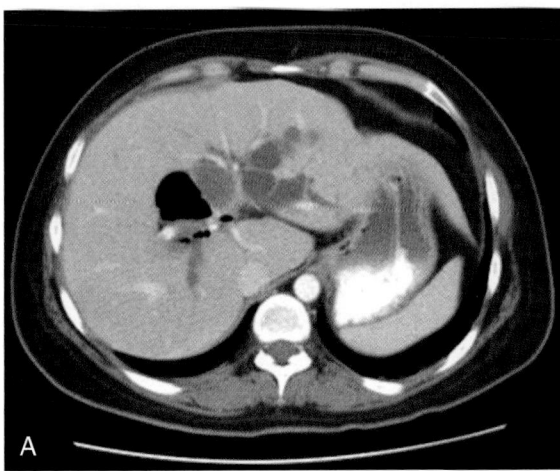

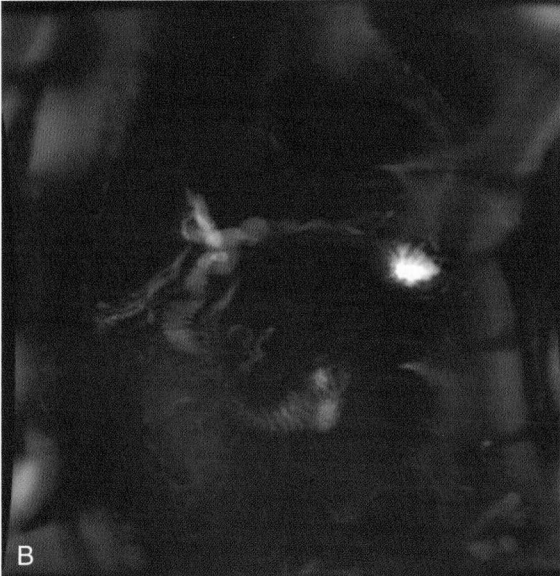

FIGURE 46.2 Computed tomography **(A)** and three-dimensional magnetic resonance imaging (MRI) reconstruction **(B)** of a type IVa cyst with multiple fusiform intrahepatic cysts accompanied by involvement of the common bile duct.

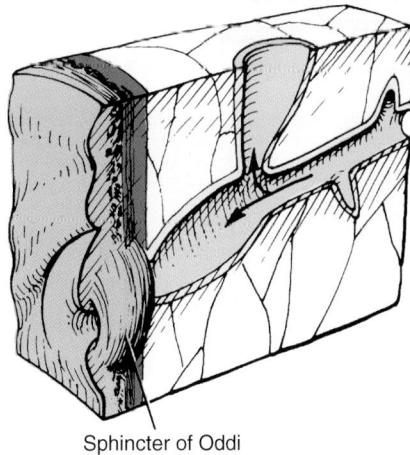

Sphincter of Oddi

FIGURE 46.3 A long common channel in the pancreaticobiliary ductal confluence is the most accepted cause of choledochal cysts.

ETIOLOGY

A single mechanism for the pathogenesis of bile duct cysts is unlikely because bile duct cysts represent a spectrum of distinct anatomic subtypes. Bile duct cysts may be either congenital or acquired. Both environmental and genetic factors have been postulated. Moreover, the increased incidence is predominant in Asian populations with rare reports of familial inheritance.[6,48,49] Bile duct cysts have been associated with numerous developmental anomalies including biliary atresia, duodenal atresia, colonic atresia, imperforate anus, pancreatic arteriovenous malformation, multiseptated gallbladder, OMENS (orbital, mandibular, ear, neural, and soft tissue) plus syndrome, ventricular septal defect, aortic hypoplasia, congenital absence of the portal vein, heterotopic pancreatic tissue, familial adenomatous polyposis, and autosomal recessive and autosomal dominant polycystic kidney disease[50] (see Chapter 1).

Multiple theories have been proposed for the origin of bile duct cysts. The most widely accepted hypothesis is that cystic dilation of the bile ducts is related to an anomalous arrangement of the pancreaticobiliary ductal junction.[45,51–55] Babbitt's theory of the "common channel" describes the APBJ in which the pancreatic and bile duct junction lies outside of the duodenal wall and sphincter of Oddi (Figs. 46.3 and 46.4).[21,27,52] This anatomic anomaly results in reflux of pancreatic juices into the biliary system and resultant activation of pancreatic enzymes. Elevated pancreatic secretory pressure relative to biliary secretory pressure promotes reflux and mixing of secretions within the biliary system. Intraductal activation of proteolytic pancreatic enzymes induces an inflammatory response resulting in deterioration of the ductal wall, dilation, and bile duct cyst formation.[56] Furthermore, epithelial damage may lead to mucosal dysplasia and potential malignant transformation. This hypothesis has been supported by biliary manometric studies[57]; high concentrations of pancreatic enzymes in cyst fluid[58]; and histopathologic studies of ductal epithelial hyperplasia, round cell infiltration, and marked ductal fibrosis.[59] Moreover, experimental canine studies of pancreaticocholecystostomy and pancreaticocholedochostomy have resulted in cystic dilation of the extrahepatic bile duct.[59,60] Indeed, an association among amylase concentration, earlier age of symptom onset and presentation, and grade of dysplasia has been described.[61] Amylase likely represents a surrogate measure; trypsinogen and phospholipase A2 levels have also been demonstrated to be elevated in APBJ.[62–64] Although trypsinogen requires activation by enterokinase, normally absent in the biliary epithelium, it is secreted by dysplastic biliary epithelium.[63,65] Thus, in the setting of a diseased biliary epithelium, enterokinase will activate trypsinogen to trypsin that in turn activates phospholipase A2. Trypsin itself induces damage and inflammatory change, whereas activated phospholipase A2 exacerbates the situation by hydrolyzing epithelial lecithin to lysolecithin, leading to enhanced inflammation and deterioration of the bile duct wall.

APBJ is a rare congenital anomaly that may result from failure of appropriate embryonic duct migration from the duodenum (see Chapter 1). It is present in 50% to 80% of patients with bile duct cysts.[21,27,66] Yamao and colleagues[67] defined the prevalence of APBJ as 0.3% in a Japanese cohort. The length of the common channel is variable; however, a length of greater than 8 mm has been suggested as a diagnostic criterion in addition to an intraductal amylase level exceeding 8000 IU/L.[66]

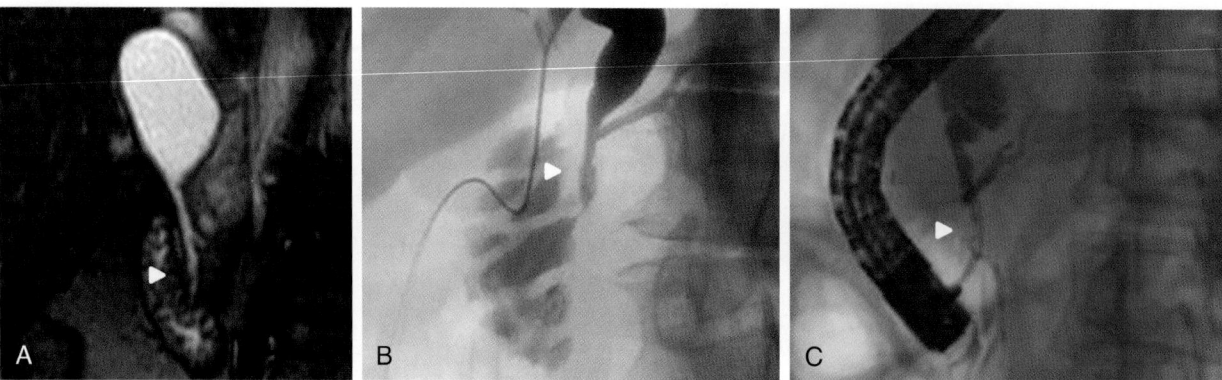

FIGURE 46.4   A long common channel, a characteristic finding in biliary cyst patients, is seen via magnetic resonance imaging (MRI; see Chapter 16) **(A)** and endoscopic retrograde cholangiopancreatography (ERCP; see Chapters 20 and 30) **(B and C)** as marked by the *white arrowhead*.

Sphincter of Oddi pressures may also be elevated in the setting of APBJ, further contributing to the pathogenesis of bile duct cysts.[57,68] APBJ has also been implicated in biliary tract cancer in the absence of a biliary cyst[69,70] (see Chapters 49 and 51).

APBJ has been associated with Type IA, IC, and IV bile duct cysts; therefore a significant proportion of bile duct cyst patients will lack this predisposing congenital anomaly. The absence of APBJ may be a true normal pancreaticobiliary junction, or secondary to inadequate resolution on diagnostic imaging, or exclusion by arbitrarily defined diagnostic criteria of the length of the common channel. A further detraction of the APBJ mechanism is that immature neonatal pancreatic acini are incapable of producing sufficient pancreatic enzymes to explain antenatally diagnosed bile duct cysts.[71,72] These observations make it difficult to invoke pancreatobiliary maljunction as a unifying etiologic factor.

Congenital cysts may develop from embryologic overproliferation of biliary epithelial cells during the cannulation phase of development, resulting in dilation.[10,27,51] Viral infection of the fetus also has been implicated as a possible etiologic agent responsible for inducing the inflammatory changes that result in congenital bile duct cysts.[73] An additional mechanism for congenital bile duct cyst formation is oligoganglionosis in the distal neck of the cyst. The reduction in ganglion cells in the narrow portion of the cyst wall may be the biliary equivalent of Hirschsprung disease of the colon.[74,75] Whether this histologic finding accounts for the presence of bile duct cysts in the absence of an APBJ is unknown.

Acquired bile duct cysts in adults have been attributed to terminal ductal obstruction, including sphincter of Oddi dysfunction or stenosis. Pancreatobiliary reflux in the absence of an APBJ was documented in 81% of adults with bile duct cysts and previous cholecystectomy.[76]

Type III bile duct cysts (choledochoceles) may arise embryologically as duodenal duplications that involve the ampulla.[77] Alternatively, increasing evidence has suggested they are acquired. Mechanisms include inflammation of the papilla leading to obstructive dilation of the intramural CBD as well as sphincter of Oddi dysfunction or stenosis, with the increased sphincter pressure resulting in cystic dilatation.[29,78,79] Given the variety of proposed pathogeneses and wide range of age at presentation, it is plausible that both congenital and acquired forms of choledochocele exist.[30]

Caroli disease and syndrome are unique from the other bile duct cysts. The pathogenesis may be secondary to disruption or cessation of remodeling of the ductal plate during development of the intrahepatic bile ducts. The molecular basis is incompletely understood and has been posited to result from the gene implicated in autosomal recessive polycystic kidney disease.[80]

DEMOGRAPHICS

Bile duct cysts are uncommon, with fewer than 5000 cases reported.[4,81] The incidence ranges from 1 in 100,000 to 1 in 150,000 individuals in Western countries to 1 in 1000 in certain parts of Asia.[11,26,82] The incidence has been reported as great as 1 in 13,500 births in the United States and 1 in 15,000 births in Australia.[15] Estimates of the actual clinical incidence range from 1 in 13,000 to 1 in 2 million patients,[83] and biliary cysts account for approximately 1% of all benign biliary disease.[27,84] An elevated geographic incidence has been appreciated in Japan,[13,85,86] where between one-half and two-thirds of reported cases have occurred.[87,88] Although the number of reported cases has increased recently, this finding probably reflects advances in diagnosis through improvements in hepatobiliary imaging rather than a true increase in incidence.

A female preponderance among patients with bile duct cysts is well known. Regardless of cyst type, the female to male ratio is 3 to 4:1.[10,15,19,87] The current pathogenesis of bile duct cysts has not implicated sex hormones or congenital intrauterine endocrine disturbances as possible factors, and the explanation for this finding is unknown.

CLINICAL FEATURES

Bile duct cysts often remain asymptomatic for years. Indeed, clinical presentation that occurs initially in adulthood occurs in nearly 25% of patients.[7,85,86] Diagnosis may be an incidental finding on imaging studies for unrelated processes. If symptomatic, bile duct cysts usually present with symptoms mimicking calculous biliary tract disease, regardless of cyst type. The classic triad of symptoms includes abdominal pain, jaundice, and a palpable mass, and it is more common in children than adults.[16] The triad of symptoms is observed in approximately 25% of adults; however, approximately 85% of children will have at least two features of the triad.[9,11,82]

Symptoms typically are intermittent, nonspecific, and vague. They include recurrent epigastric or right hypochondrial pain, abdominal tenderness, fever, and mild jaundice. Pain may radiate to the right infrascapular region or to the midback. If present, it generally persists for hours. Patients also may report nausea, vomiting, anorexia, pruritus, and weight loss. Biliuria precedes the onset of clinical jaundice. Abdominal pain or discomfort can be overshadowed by signs of cholangitis, such as fever and rigors. An abdominal mass is rare in adults; however, if a mass is present, cyst-associated malignancy must be strongly suspected (see Chapter 51).

The development of nonmalignant complications of bile duct cysts will contribute to clinical presentation. Complications include stone disease (cystolithiasis, cholelithiasis, cholecystitis, choledocholithiasis, and hepatolithiasis; see Chapters 33 and 39), cholangitis (see Chapter 43), acute and chronic pancreatitis (see Chapters 55 and 57), intraperitoneal rupture of the bile duct cyst, intussusception, gastric outlet obstruction, secondary biliary cirrhosis and hemorrhage from cyst erosion, and portal hypertension following development of cirrhosis, portal vein thrombosis, or mechanical compression of the portal vein by the cyst.[10,27,90] Spontaneous intraperitoneal rupture has been reported in 1% to 12% of patients.[91,92] These patients will present with acute-onset abdominal pain, signs of peritonitis, and sepsis.

Complications that arise from all subtypes of bile duct cysts often result from bile stasis, stone formation, recurrent infection, and inflammation. Dilated cysts as well as distal obstruction in the setting of strictures, stenosis, and sphincter of Oddi dysfunction contribute to proximal bile stasis, resulting in stone and sludge formation and secondary bile infection. Stone and protein plug development in the distal CBD and pancreatic duct results in pancreatitis. Protein plug formation may be secondary to chronic inflammatory changes with the formation of

an albumin-rich exudate or a result of hypersecretion of mucin in the setting of a dysplastic biliary epithelium.[93]

Clinical pancreatitis is present in almost 30% of patients with bile duct cysts.[12] In contrast to patients with cholangitis, patients with pancreatitis have more intense and prolonged epigastric pain and vomiting. Fever and jaundice are less prominent. Weight loss, although unusual, is noteworthy because almost 70% of adults with this finding will harbor an associated bile duct malignancy.

Approximately 15% of adults with type I or type IV bile duct cysts present overtly with secondary biliary cirrhosis or hepatic fibrosis from chronic biliary obstruction (see Chapter 74). Such patients typically have had multiple operations for complications of type I or IVa cysts or Caroli disease. Hepatomegaly and splenomegaly are common in patients with cirrhosis and portal hypertension. Hematemesis, melena, and ascites may accompany portal hypertension. Interestingly, other signs of chronic liver disease (muscle wasting, fatigue, spider angiomas, and pruritus) are uncommon. Liver failure is seen late in Caroli disease.

IMAGING

Accurate preoperative imaging of biliary cysts is key to adequately assess cyst extent, potentially identify malignancy, and define aberrant anatomy relevant for surgical planning (Fig. 46.5)[94] (see Chapter 16). Abdominal ultrasound, endoscopic ultrasonography (EUS), magnetic resonance cholangiopancreatography (MRCP),

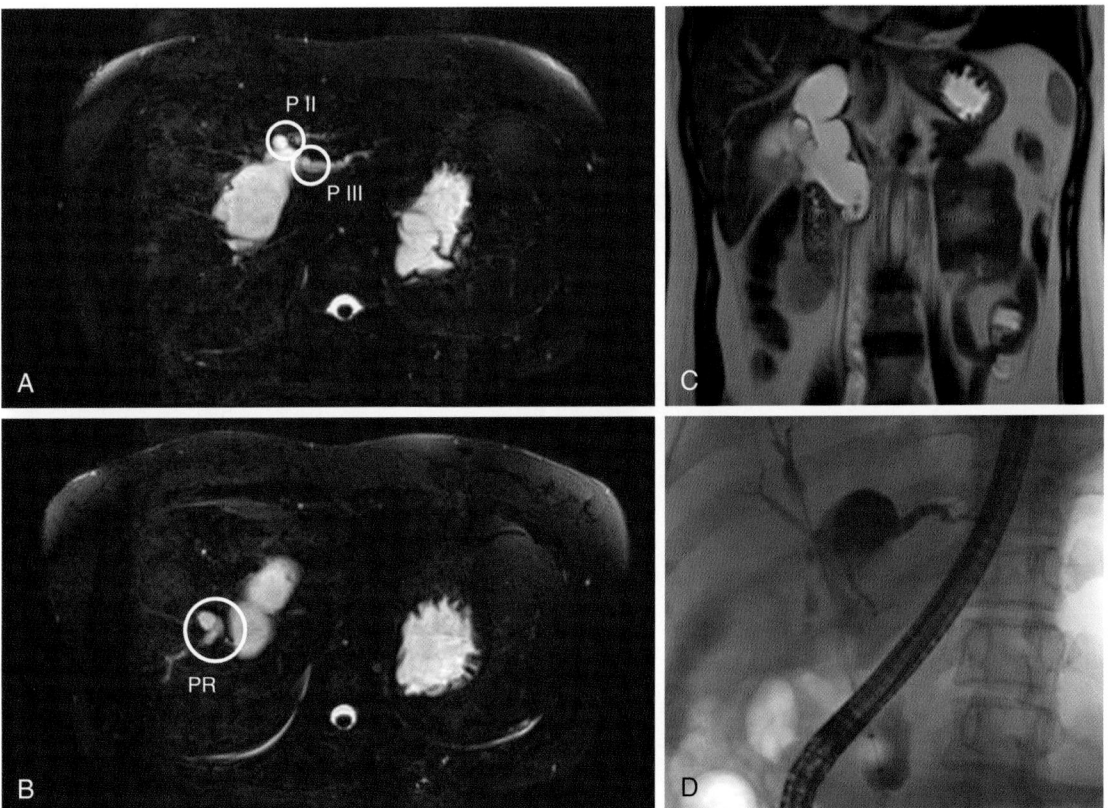

FIGURE 46.5   Detailed preoperative workup of a patient with a type IVa biliary cyst utilizing magnetic resonance imaging (MRI). (A–C) (see Chapter 16) and endoscopic retrograde cholangiopancreatography (ERCP; see Chapters 20 and 30) **(D). A,** Involvement of the main left pedicle up to the pedicle of segment II *(P II)* and III *(P III).* **B,** The right main pedicle *(PR)* is uninvolved by the biliary cyst. **C,** Extrahepatic fusiform dilatation of the bile duct. **D,** The entirety of the cyst is visualized by ERCP. This patient required a left hepatectomy with extrahepatic bile duct resection and Roux-en-Y reconstruction.

computed tomography (CT), direct cholangiography by ERCP (see Chapters 20 and 30), or percutaneous transhepatic cholangiography (PTC; see Chapters 20 and 31) are potential options for preoperative imaging (Fig. 46.6). Current reviews of the diagnostic imaging modalities of bile duct cysts with representative images are referenced.[34,95]

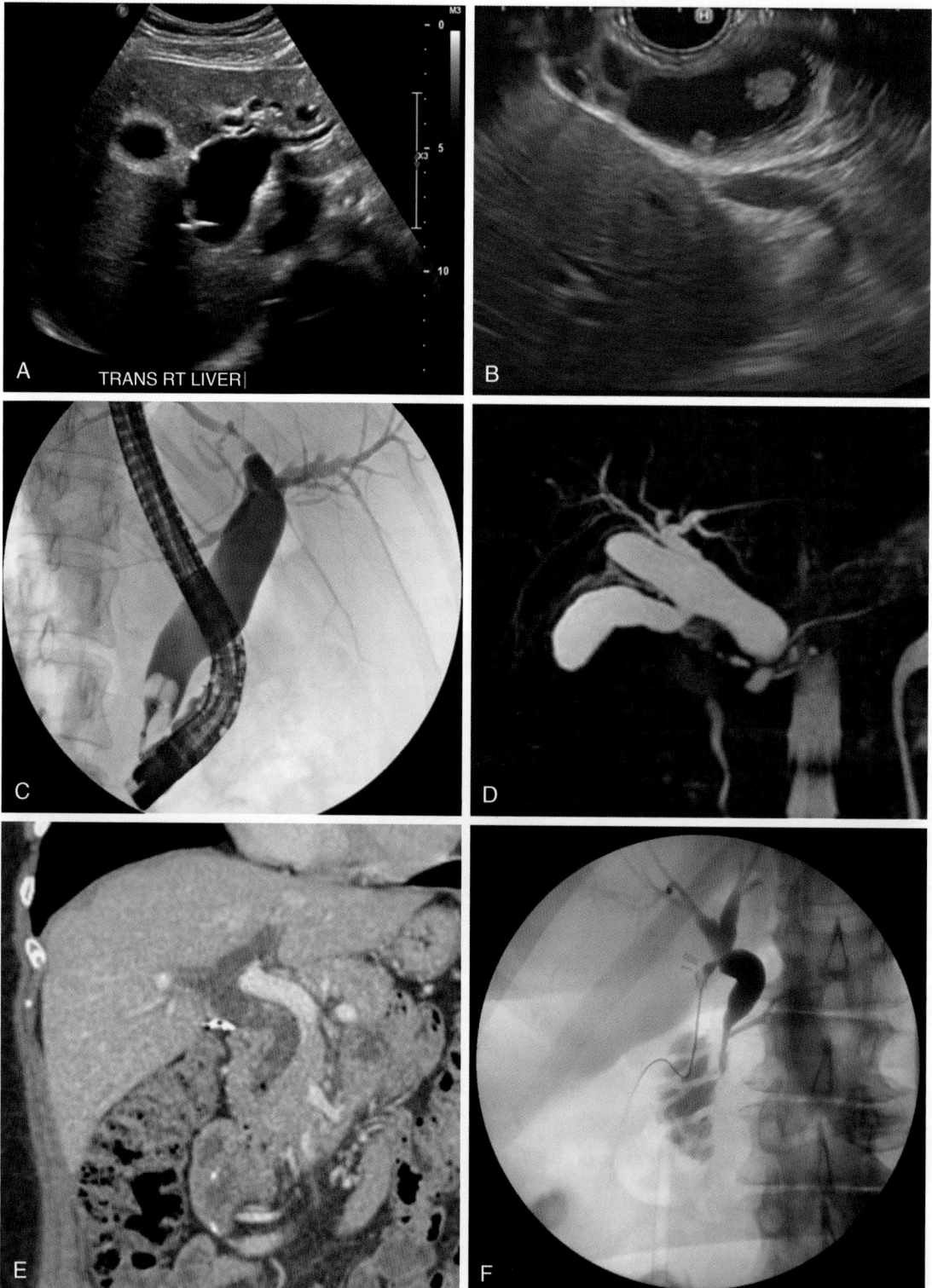

FIGURE 46.6 **Commonly applied imaging modalities for biliary cysts (see Chapters 16, 20, and 30).** **A,** Ultrasound findings of a type IVa cyst with cystic extension to the segment II pedicle. **B,** Endosonographic picture of a type 2 biliary cyst with intracystic polyps. **C,** Endoscopic retrograde cholangiopancreatography (ECRP) using an occlusive balloon to illustrate the entirety of cystic extent. **D,** Three-dimensional magnetic resonance imaging (MRI) reconstruction of a type I biliary cyst. **E,** Computed tomography (CT) image of a type I cyst with intracystic sludge. **F,** Intraoperative cholangiogram via the cystic duct of a type I cyst with visualization of a long common channel.

General Principles

Both cholangiographic and dimensional imaging of the bile duct, liver, and pancreas are essential. Anatomic definition of the pancreatobiliary ductal junction is critical for operative management of bile duct cysts to avoid intraoperative damage to the pancreatic duct during cyst excision, to recognize stones impacted within the common channel or junction, and to exclude distal tumors. The angle of fusion between the distal bile duct and pancreatic duct varies widely and has led to a subclassification of cyst types.[45] Typically, the bile duct cyst joins the pancreatic duct 2 to 4 cm proximal to the duodenum (see Figs. 46.2 and 46.3), resulting in a long common channel (ampulla).[14,17,45,96] Additionally, clear definition of the intrahepatic extent of the cyst is important (see Fig. 46.5). Detailed assessment of the liver including intrahepatic and extrahepatic bile ducts is of critical importance, as previous reports suggest that almost 80% of adults with bile duct cysts have liver-associated pathology.[12,17,97] Although increased incidental detection of cysts certainly has decreased this rate, assessment for concomitant pathology remains indispensable for surgical planning.

Significant advancements in imaging and endoscopic modalities in recent years have resulted in different diagnostic approaches for bile duct cysts. Today, MRCP, CT, and ERCP have become the mainstays of diagnostic workup.

Ultrasound

Ultrasound is frequently used as the initial diagnostic step in the workup of patients with biliary cysts. It remains a relevant noninvasive screening and surveillance modality.[98] The detection rate of biliary cysts ranges from 71% to 97%.[7] The sonographic features of bile duct cysts have been well defined for type I bile duct cysts and the variants of Caroli disease.[3,24,99,100] Ultrasound of type I cysts simply shows an irregular, hypoechoic segmental dilatation of the extrahepatic bile duct (see Fig. 46.6). Focal duct wall thickening or nodularity should arouse suspicion for cancer in an adult and requires further investigations. Ductal stones within the cyst are identified by typical echogenic features and acoustic shadowing. The absence of septations on ultrasound distinguishes bile duct cysts from extrahepatic cystadenomas.[101] Although the sensitivity of ultrasound is excellent for cysts involving the bile duct proximal to the pancreas, it is limited in adults in identifying choledochoceles because of the frequency of bowel gas overlying the terminal CBD and the small size of these cysts.[102] EUS is not limited by bowel gas or body habitus, and it allows biopsy if malignancy is suspected. Overall, EUS represents a useful, selective diagnostic adjunct (see Chapters 16 and 22).

Computed Tomography

CT has led to a significant increase in the incidental detection of biliary cysts. It provides excellent initial assessment of the type and extent of bile duct cysts. Although certainly sufficient for initial assessment, CT has significant limitations for detailed biliary anatomy.[103] Despite frequent use of CT cholangiography in the past,[104] its utility has been replaced by MRCP, which provides similar dimensional information and detailed cholangiography (see Chapter 16).

Magnetic Resonance Cholangiopancreatography

MRCP has now become the gold standard for the assessment of biliary cysts compared with other imaging modalities.[95] It provides an accurate anatomic definition of the intrahepatic and extrahepatic bile duct cysts and relevant hepatic and pancreatic anatomy.[78,105,106] MRCP has the greatest diagnostic accuracy for detection of bile duct cysts, assessment of biliopancreatic junction, choledocholithiasis, and cholangiocarcinoma concurrent with bile duct cysts.[34,107] Continued advances in three-dimensional (3D) cholangiogram results in detailed preoperative illustration of the biliary anatomy. The noninvasive nature of this imaging modality avoids potential complications such as intestinal perforation, hemorrhage, pancreatitis, or cholangitis associated with endoscopic cholangiography. However, limitations include minor ductal anomalies and very small cysts that may be overlooked by MRCP[108] and its lack of therapeutic capability. Selective hepatobiliary contrast agents might better visualize the bile ducts than heavily T2-weighted MRCP sequences because of their elimination through the biliary system. MRCP can be used in difficult cases to evaluate for communication between a cystic lesion and the biliary tree[95] (see Chapter 16).

Endoscopic Retrograde Cholangiopancreatography and Percutaneous Transhepatic Cholangiography

ERCP remains one of the most widely utilized diagnostic tools for assessment of biliary cysts because of its interventional capability[27,30] (see Chapters 20 and 30); however, ERCP also has disadvantages. Large volumes of radiographic contrast may be required for complete visualization of the bile ducts and such volumes may obscure ductal details. ERCP in adults without previous cystenterostomy defines the pancreaticobiliary ductal junction through the papilla well.[45,109] However, in adults with prior cystenterostomy, assessment of the pancreaticobiliary ductal junction might be more challenging as contrast rapidly empties into the bowel. Carcinoma can be confirmed by biopsy or brush cytology. Intracystic stones can be extracted after papillotomy to relieve severe cholangitis before surgery. Cholangitis can be relieved temporarily by endoscopic biliary stenting until definitive operation. Endoscopy also allows visualization of the esophagus and stomach to exclude signs of portal hypertension. The endoscopist should attempt to examine the ductal bifurcation and the lining of the cyst if a prior cystoduodenostomy allows introduction of the endoscope into the biliary tree. Endoscopic directed biopsy of an intracystic mass can be performed to exclude malignancy. Obstructing balloons should be available to ensure that complete radiographic filling of the biliary tree is possible (see Fig. 46.6), especially in patients with prior cystoduodenostomy. Endoscopy of the cyst through a cystenterostomy may also permit diagnosis of intraductal stenoses by membranes or septae at the confluence of the major bile ducts in patients with type IVa cysts.[110] The procedure of choice for a symptomatic type III cyst or choledochocele is ERCP because endoscopic papillotomy is potentially therapeutic.[111,112]

PTC is an efficacious alternative to ERCP in the diagnosis of bile duct cysts, although its use has continued to decline because of the versatility of ERCP (see Chapters 20 and 31). PTC is most advantageous in patients with a prior Roux-en-Y cystojejunostomy or hepaticojejunostomy, because of limited endoscopic access dependent on the length of the Roux limb, and in patients with type IV bile duct cysts in whom ductal strictures or tumor prevent complete visualization of intrahepatic cysts by ERCP.[109] Percutaneous biliary drainage (PBD) may be performed after PTC for control of biliary sepsis or for stenting after surgical reconstruction. PTC is limited, particularly in patients with a widely patent cystenterostomy in whom runoff of the contrast precludes complete evaluation of the cyst or in patients with huge extrahepatic cysts in which intracystic contrast is superimposed over the pancreaticobiliary junction and obscures its radiographic definition.

Scintigraphy

Although hepatobiliary scintigraphy has been useful in the past, its clinical value is limited because of the lack of both cholangiographic and dimensional anatomic detail. Scintigraphy has no current utility (see Chapter 18).

Follow-Up

Regardless of operative intervention, radiologic follow-up of patients with bile duct cysts remains relevant. Even after complete cyst resection, patients remain at an increased risk for cholangiocarcinoma (as outlined later). However, the optimal strategy and algorithm for radiologic follow-up of these patients remains unclear. Routine radiologic follow-up has not been substantiated to date. However, as 53% of patients will present with unresectable disease if they develop cholangiocarcinoma and as this might occur with significant delay from initial operation,[113] routine surveillance of these patients seems warranted.

ASSOCIATED HEPATOBILIARY PATHOLOGY

Concurrent hepatobiliary pathology is frequently associated with bile duct cysts in adults. Cystolithiasis (see Chapter 33), hepatolithiasis (see Chapters 37 and 39), calculous cholecystitis (see Chapter 34), pancreatitis (see Chapters 55 and 57), cholangiocarcinoma (see Chapter 51), intrahepatic abscess (see Chapter 70), and cirrhosis with or without portal hypertension (see Chapter 74) are conditions that may either precipitate or complicate treatment. Studies in adults showed that almost 80% of adults with bile duct cysts have complications from one or more of the previously mentioned conditions.[12,17,97] However, with the more recent increased use of cross-sectional imaging, more cysts are identified incidentally. Moreover, complications in adults may decrease if excision is used routinely in infants and children.[15]

Cystolithiasis is the most frequent accompanying condition in adults with bile duct cysts. In contrast to the low prevalence of cystolithiasis in pediatric patients,[14,43,46,85] the prevalence of intracystic stones ranges from 2% to 72% in adults.[12,114,115] Although their composition has not been analyzed biochemically, most intracystic stones have been described as soft, earthy, and pigmented in appearance, thus supporting bile stasis as a primary etiologic factor[43,46] (see Chapter 8). Intracystic stones typically are associated with thick, viscous bile that may form bile duct or cyst casts. Cystolithiasis may complicate anastomotic strictures after previous cystoenterostomies, which further supports stasis and cholangitis as major factors in the pathogenesis of these stones.

Hepatolithiasis has been recognized increasingly with prolonged follow-up and may occur with or without evidence of anastomotic stricture (Fig. 46.7).[15,116,117] Some patients develop complete or partial strictures of the cystoenteric anastomosis. Hepatolithiasis develops as a consequence of proximal bile stasis or migration of intracystic stones (see Chapters 8 and 39).

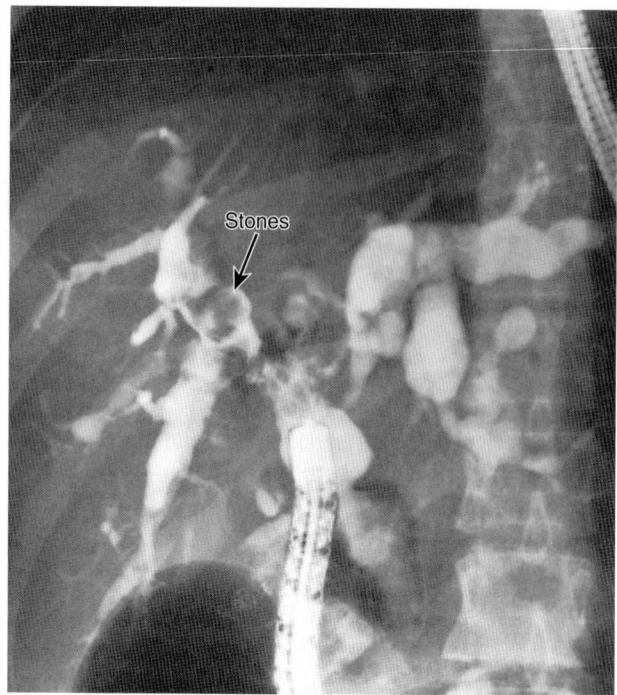

FIGURE 46.7 Endoscopic retrograde cholangiogram of a type IVa bile duct cyst showing multiple intrahepatic stones and a patent choledochoduodenostomy (see Chapters 20 and 30).

Hepatolithiasis usually occurs in type IV bile duct cysts. More than 80% of type IV bile duct cysts are associated with either a membranous or a septal stenosis of the major lobar bile ducts near the confluence.[110] Stenosis of the major ducts should be assessed in all patients with hepatolithiasis. Intrahepatic stones may be sequestered in segmental ducts, leading to further localized intrahepatic ductal dilation, segmental or sectional hepatic atrophy, or intrahepatic abscesses.

Gallbladder disease is a frequent complication in patients with bile duct cysts. Gallbladder disease can occur de novo, leading to the incidental discovery of bile duct cysts, or it can evolve after treatment for bile duct cysts. In particular, a gallbladder left in situ during initial treatment for symptomatic bile duct cysts is frequently a subsequent source of biliary tract disease. Both acute and chronic cholecystitis, with or without stones, has been recognized in these patients. Similar to stones within cysts, stones in in situ gallbladders after cyst operations are typically bilirubinate or stasis stones.

The association of pancreatitis with bile duct cysts is well recognized, particularly in adults. The reported prevalence has ranged from 2% to 70%.[12,14,53,89,118] The clinical pattern of pancreatitis is acute and often relapsing (see Chapter 55). Chronic pancreatitis, or endocrine or exocrine insufficiency associated with bile duct cysts, is rare (see Chapter 57). Obstruction of the pancreatic duct at the pancreaticobiliary junction or distally in the common channel (ampulla) by stones is postulated as the precipitating factor. A few studies[12,14] have shown an association between biliary tract stones in patients with bile duct cysts and pancreatitis, and stone impaction within the pancreaticobiliary junction may cause pancreatitis (see Fig. 46.7). An alternative mechanism for pancreatitis is bile reflux into the pancreatic duct.[118,119] Although the anatomy of the pancreaticobiliary ductal system is conducive to bile reflux, there is little evidence to support this theory. Some patients with bile duct cysts and pancreatitis have normal pancreaticobiliary anatomy.[118] Moreover, some patients with choledochoceles also may have recurrent acute pancreatitis.[102,120] Thus the etiology of pancreatitis associated with bile duct cysts is multifactorial.

Rare hepatobiliary problems arising in adults with common duct cysts include intrahepatic abscess and portal hypertension. Both conditions usually result from recurrent cholangitis and biliary obstruction, often after strictures of prior cystoenterostomies. Large, solitary hepatic abscesses represent the end stage of obstructive cholangitis and are usually completely obstructed, pus-filled intrahepatic cysts. These intrahepatic abscesses occur predominantly in the left intrahepatic ducts[121,122] and may be related partly to angulation of the left main duct. Adjacent liver parenchyma is fibrotic and atrophic and may harbor miliary abscesses within the peripheral bile duct radicles.

Portal hypertension associated with bile duct cysts may be caused by secondary biliary cirrhosis or fibrosis, portal vein thrombosis, or Caroli disease with congenital hepatic fibrosis.[17,123,124] Portal hypertension in adults generally is preceded by numerous operations for cyst drainage.[89,125,126] Portal hypertension in patients with bile duct cysts is manifested clinically by hepatosplenomegaly, hematemesis, melena, or ascites. Portal hypertension causes a hypervascularity of the hepatoduodenal ligament with prominent pericholedochal varices that increase risk of resection. Hepatic functional reserve deteriorates progressively, and hepatic coma and renal failure may be precipitated by recurrent cholangitis.

MALIGNANCY AND BILE DUCT CYSTS

The true incidence of malignancy associated with bile duct cysts is unknown. Most reported malignancies have been detected in excised surgical specimens and thus may underestimate incidence. However, the association of bile duct cysts and hepatobiliary and pancreatic malignancy exists.[127–133] Bile duct cysts are most notably associated with an increased risk of cholangiocarcinoma (see Chapters 50 and 51), and pancreatic (see Chapters 59, 61, and 62) and gallbladder carcinomas (see Chapter 49). The risk of malignancy is greater in elderly patients and in those with type I and IV cysts. The overall incidence of cancer has ranged from 10% to 30%.[134,135] A recent systematic review showed 434 reported cases of malignancy in resected bile duct cysts, demonstrating an incidence of 7.5%.[81] Hepatobiliary malignancies arising within or associated with bile duct cysts have included cholangiocarcinoma, adenoacanthoma, squamous cell carcinoma, anaplastic carcinoma, bile duct sarcoma, hepatocellular carcinoma, pancreatic carcinoma, and gallbladder carcinoma.[17,128,132,133,136] Cholangiocarcinoma is the most common malignancy, representing more than 70% of associated malignancies.[81] The incidence of malignancy in association with bile duct cysts is approximately 20 to 30 times greater than that of bile duct carcinoma in the general population.[85,134] Gallbladder carcinoma (see Chapter 49) is the second most common cyst-associated malignancy, accounting for about 20% of associated malignancies, with the previously mentioned malignancies making up the remainder. The incidence of cyst-associated malignancy is age related, increasing from 0.4% to 0.7% in the first decade of life to more than 14% after age 20.[81,137] The mean age of patients with cancer associated with bile duct

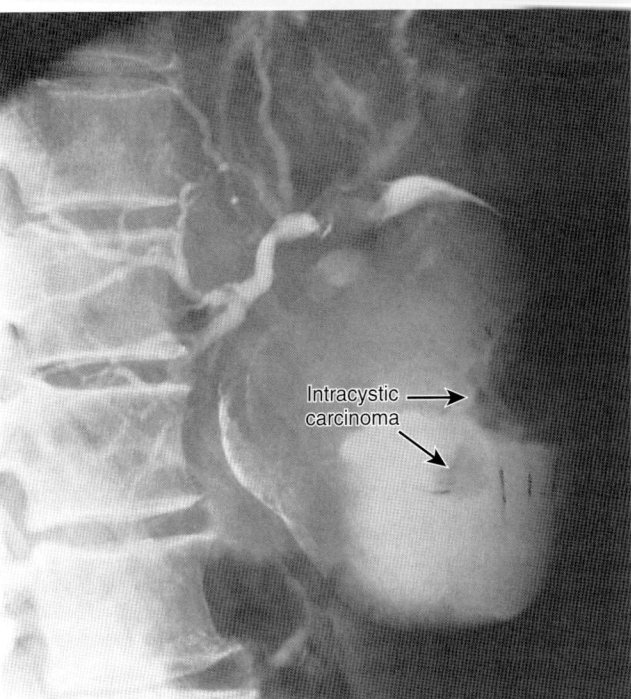

FIGURE 46.8 Percutaneous transhepatic cholangiography of a type I choledochal cyst with a polypoid intracystic cholangiocarcinoma (see Chapters 20 and 31).

cysts is 32.[17] In patients older than 60, malignancy rates may be as high as 38%. Histopathologic examination reveals increasing dysplasia with increasing age.[138,139] These findings underscore the necessity for a high index of suspicion of carcinoma in adults with biliary cystic disease.

Malignancies associated with bile duct cysts may arise within the cyst or elsewhere within the liver or pancreaticobiliary tract. Indeed, it has been reported that only 57% of tumors are intracystic (Fig. 46.8).[129] Moreover, malignancies may occur after cyst excision.[101,140] The risk of malignancy is not reduced in patients with prior cystoenterostomy or incomplete cyst excision.[141] Malignancies may be associated with any type of bile duct cyst, although the prevalence of cancer is significantly greater in type I and IV cysts. Todani and colleagues published a series in which 68% and 21% of malignancies occurred in type I and IV cysts, respectively. The incidence of malignancy has been reported in 7.6% of patients with type I, 4.3% with type II, 4.0% with type III, 9.2% with type IV, and 2.5% with type V.[81] In type III bile duct cysts, the incidence of malignancy has been reported to be as high as 10%.[142] Interestingly, the risk is elevated in choledochoceles with a biliary, rather than a duodenal, epithelium.[143]

The presence of an APBJ increases the risk of malignancy, even in the absence of a bile duct cyst.[144,145] Furthermore, the risk of cyst-related malignancy is greater in patients with an APBJ. In a European, multicenter review, Ragot and colleagues[66] demonstrated that synchronous biliary cancer had an incidence of 8.7% in all patients with bile duct cysts versus 11.1% in those with bile duct cysts and documented APBJ. The etiology of cyst-associated malignancies is unknown. Carcinogenesis is thought to occur through multistep genetic events in which early K-Ras and p53 mutations are seen in more than 60% of related carcinomas[146] (see Chapter 9E).

Intracystic carcinoma

Bile stagnation with the development of intrabiliary carcinogens leading to epithelial malignant degeneration is postulated as the most likely mechanism.[129,132] Unconjugated deoxycholate and lithocholate have been associated with biliary metaplasia and mutagenicity, which may lead to neoplasia. Secondary bile acids have been found in bile duct cysts with cancer,[147] although neither their relative nor their absolute concentration in patients with bile duct cysts has differed in the presence or absence of cancer,[148] suggesting other factors as primary carcinogens. An association between cystolithiasis and malignancy has not been established. Bile stasis and bacterial overgrowth associated with stones may lead to secondary bile acid formation.

Long-term survival of patients with bile duct cysts and malignancy is rare, with a reported overall survival of 6 to 21 months.[149] Delayed diagnosis, advanced stage of disease, intraabdominal seeding from previous surgery, and tumor multicentricity generally preclude curative resection.

TREATMENT

General Principles

The surgical management of adults with bile duct cysts is based on cyst type and the presence of associated hepatobiliary pathology. The aims of preoperative management are complete cholangiographic definition of the extent of the cystic process and associated ductal pathology and control of biliary infections. Careful review of high-quality preoperative imaging is required to plan for aberrant biliovascular anatomy. Any patient with recurrent symptoms after prior cyst-related surgery must be evaluated for anastomotic stricture, ductal stones, biliary tract malignancy, cirrhosis, and portal hypertension. Broad-spectrum antibiotics concentrated in bile and effective against proximal enteric bacteria are preferred for control of biliary infections. When sepsis fails to resolve with intravenous antibiotics, percutaneous or endoscopic drainage of infected bile duct cysts usually controls the infections before definitive surgery. Management of cyst rupture should include laparotomy or laparoscopy and washout of the bile, external drainage, and antibiotics for stabilization before definitive management. However, a definitive, single-stage operation has been revealed to be safe with excellent outcomes in children.[150]

The definitive treatment of bile duct cysts is predominantly surgical.[99] Fig. 46.9 shows the therapeutic options for the treatment of each type of bile duct cyst. Intraoperative examples of type I and type II cysts are given in Fig. 49.10. Type I, II, and IV bile duct cysts mandate resection in an appropriate operative candidate. Type I and IV cysts, specifically, should be completely resected and bile flow established by mucosa-to-mucosa bilioenteric anastomosis (see Chapter 32). External drainage alone has no role in the definitive management of bile duct cysts.

Reduction in risk of malignancy is based on three presumptions: (1) the potential carcinogenic effect of pancreatic secretions is eliminated because of total diversion from the biliary tract, (2) the production of mutagenic secondary bile acids is reduced because bacterial overgrowth in the bile is less frequent, and (3) abnormal cyst epithelium is excised. The clinical results of cyst excision and Roux-en-Y hepaticojejunostomy have been excellent. Moreover, most reports with late follow-up have confirmed that the majority of patients remain asymptomatic after excision.[12,14,15,17,117,148,151,152] The rate of anastomotic stricture following hepaticojejunostomy ranges from 1.5% to 13%.[151,153–155]

Long-term follow-up must be considered in adults because of the age-related risk of malignancy and the frequency of late anastomotic strictures in patients treated without complete cyst resection (cystenterostomy). Although the risk of malignancy is significantly reduced in those who have undergone bile duct cyst resection, these patients remain at increased risk of carcinoma relative to the general population within the remnant

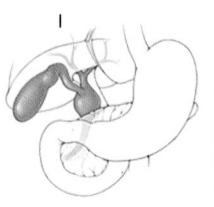

I

EXCISION,
ROUX-EN-Y HEPATICOJEJUNOSTOMY,
HEPATICODUODENOSTOMY
Roux-en-Y choledochocystojejunostomy
Choledochocystoduodenostomy

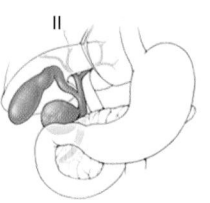

II

EXCISION

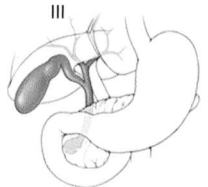

III

TRANSDUODENAL EXCISION,
Transduodenal sphincteroplasty
Endoscopic sphincterotomy

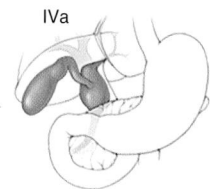

IVa

Extraheptic component:
EXCISION, ROUX-EN-Y HEPATICOJEJUNOSTOMY
EXCISION, HEPATICODUODENOSTOMY
Intrahepatic component:
HEPATIC RESECTION +/– Roux-en-Y Hepaticojejunostomy

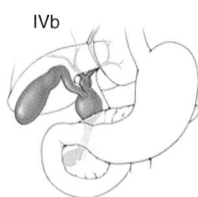

IVb

EXCISION,
ROUX-EN-Y HEPATICOJEJUNOSTOMY,
HEPATICODUODENOSTOMY
+/– transduodenal sphincteroplasty

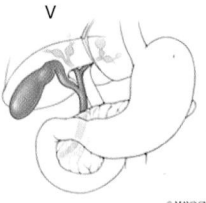

V

HEPATIC RESECTION
Roux-en-Y intrahepatic cholangiojejunostomy
Transhepatic intubation
Orthotopic liver transplantation

© MAYO CLINIC

FIGURE 46.9 **Surgical options for treatment of choledochal cysts.** The preferred treatment appears in capital letters.

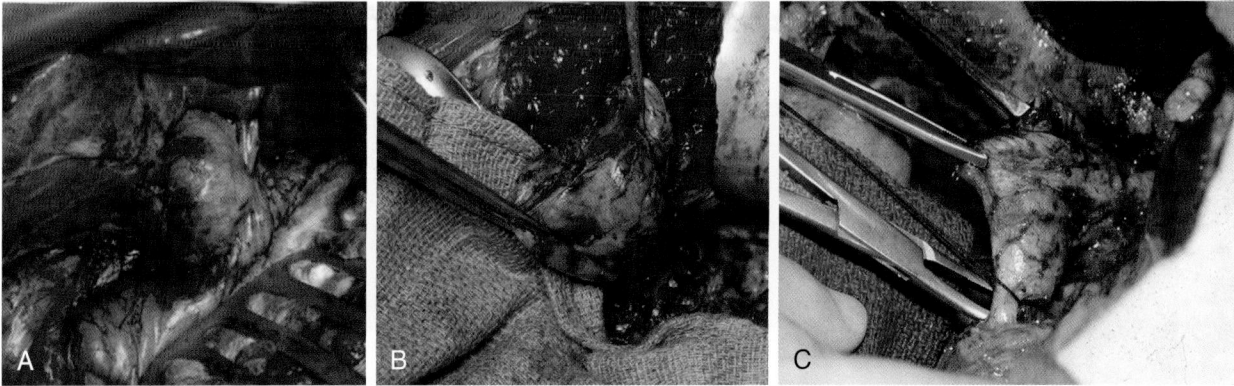

FIGURE 46.10   Type I biliary cyst **(A and C)** and a type II biliary cyst with the typical neck **(B).**

biliary tree and pancreas. Previous publications demonstrate postexcisional malignant disease is experienced in 0.7% to 6% of patients.[156–159] Recently, the overall the risk of subsequent carcinoma during long-term follow-up was estimated at 3.4%.[160] Stratified by operative approach, malignant transformation occurred in 1.9% of those treated with cyst resection and hepaticojejunostomy versus 18.4% in those managed with cystenterostomy.[160] Furthermore, in patients managed with prior cystenterostomy, the rate of malignancy or the development of nonmalignant complications, including cholangitis, hepatolithiasis, and pancreatitis, can be as high as 70%.[161] A review of the current literature reveals that development of cholangiocarcinoma following bile duct cyst resection occurs 10 or more years following operative intervention in two-thirds of patients.[113] Unfortunately, only 47% of these patients were resectable at time of diagnosis, underlining the relevance of systematic follow-up in these patients.

A clearly defined follow-up protocol for patients after treatment of bile duct cysts is lacking. Clearly, those with carcinoma in the resected specimen should follow treatment and surveillance in accordance with appropriate consensus guidelines. In patients who have undergone prior cyst resection with bilioenteric anastomosis, consideration of annual liver biochemistry to screen for anastomotic stricture is warranted. It remains unknown if surveillance with tumor markers or imaging for development of postresection malignancy results in earlier detection or improved patient outcomes.[113]

In patients who have previously undergone internal drainage with cystenterostomy, reoperative intervention with complete cyst resection and bilioenteric reconstruction is recommended. This patient population is predisposed to high rates of long-term complications and malignant transformation.[27] Reflux of enteric contents into the retained cyst and biliary tract results in recurrent cholangitis, inflammation, and anastomotic stricture, whereas the rate of malignancy is as high as 18% to 30%.[160,162,163]

Portal decompression may be required before biliary reconstruction in patients who develop portal hypertension because of secondary biliary cirrhosis, recurrent inflammation with resultant portal vein thrombosis, or mechanical compression by the cyst[12,164] (see Chapter 74). Cirrhosis is the most common etiology of portal hypertension in adult bile duct cyst patients, whereas mechanical compression predominates in the pediatric population.[164] Preoperative assessment of these patients should include CT angiography or MR angiography of abdominal

vessels in addition to evaluation of liver function and candidacy for operative intervention. In general, central or proximal splenorenal shunts are preferred because portal decompression is performed remote from the subhepatic pericystic inflammation (see Chapters 83 and 84) and site of subsequent operation. Resection typically is undertaken 6 to 12 weeks after portosystemic shunting. Although transjugular intrahepatic portosystemic shunting (TIPS) can be used for preoperative portal decompression, it should be avoided. Importantly, the risk of infection of the TIPS endovascular prosthesis leading to recurrent sepsis is increased with any bilioenteric anastomosis because of expected bactibilia and its contamination of the small bile duct traversed by the TIPS prosthesis (see Chapter 85).

Type I Cyst

The treatment of choice for type I bile duct cysts in adults is total cystectomy from the ductal confluence to the pancreatic duct and Roux-en-Y hepaticojejunostomy.[5,98] Resection of the intrapancreatic portion of the bile duct cyst is important as dysplastic changes identified within the cyst likely represent a field defect of the residual biliary mucosa.[11] A surgical specimen of a type I and type II cyst is displayed in Fig. 46.11. If a significant remnant of the bile duct cyst is left in situ, the intrapancreatic portion can predispose to stones or malignancy.[165,166] Careful surgical planning mandates anatomic delineation of the cyst and biliopancreatic junction with preoperative imaging to facilitate identification of the distal resection margin (see Fig. 46.5). The proximal margin of resection is based primarily on cyst morphology and proximal extent. Cyst excision eliminates the primary site of bile stasis and permits a bilioenteric anastomosis of normal jejunum or duodenum and epithelial-lined proximal bile duct. The theoretic advantages of this approach include a reduced incidence of anastomotic stricture, stone formation, cholangitis, and intracystic malignancy. The advantages of a mucosa-to-mucosa anastomosis have been extrapolated from similar biliary reconstructions for other biliary tract problems: benign strictures, CBD stones, and suppurative cholangitis (see Chapter 32). Interestingly, a recent publication has suggested that adequate bile flow, not radical cyst excision, is the most critical factor in reducing long-term complications in type IA and IVa bile duct cysts,[167] which underscores the importance of a technically precise bilioenteric anastomosis.

Hepaticoduodenostomy represents an alternative option for reconstruction in both benign and malignant disease.[168] It has been associated with reduced operative time, ease of

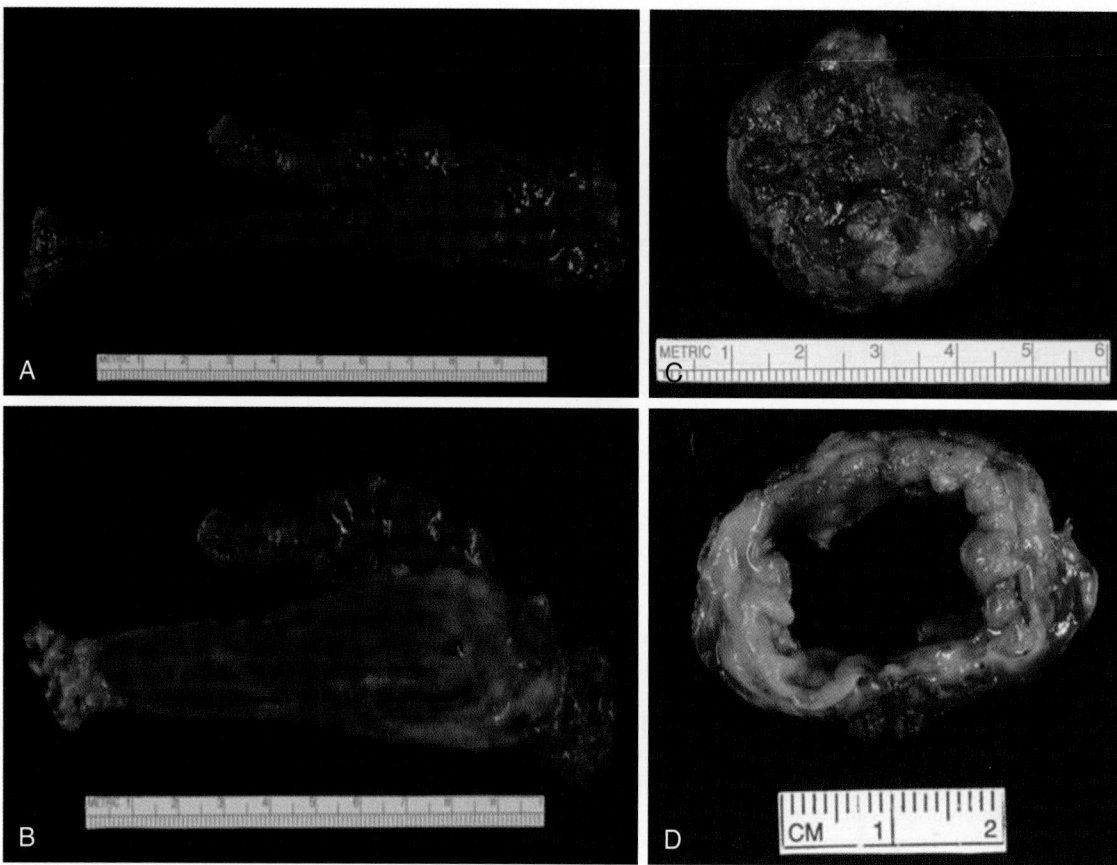

FIGURE 46.11   Surgical specimens of a type I biliary cyst **(A and B)** and a type II biliary cyst **(C and D)**. The fusiform dilatation of the common bile duct in the type I cyst and the characteristic neck of the type II cyst are both appreciable.

laparoscopic approach, a decreased length of hospital stay, and more direct endoscopic access of the biliary tree during follow-up.[151,169] Fig. 46.12 illustrates an endoscopic picture of a hepaticoduodenostomy and demonstrates the easy visualization and access after this type of reconstruction. Bile gastritis and reflux is increased in some reports and equivalent to hepaticojejunostomy in others.[151,170–172] In the pediatric population, hepaticoduodenostomy confers equivalent long-term outcomes with respect to anastomotic stricture, cholangitis, and reoperative intervention.[172] Technical factors influencing choice of hepaticoenterostomy (Roux-en-Y hepaticojejunostomy vs. hepaticoduodenostomy) include aberrant hilar ductal anatomy, ductal strictures, ductal size, and hilar arterial anatomy.[173] Although mobility of the duodenum may limit its use in some patients, generally apposition the duodenum to the hilar ducts for anastomosis is straightforward.

In situations in which dense pericystic fibrosis or varices precludes safe resection with increased risk of vascular injury, resection of the majority of the cyst and mucosa with retention of the most densely adherent portion of the cyst wall on the hepatoduodenal ligament (portal vein and hepatic artery) has been recommended. Alternatively, mucosectomy or ablation of the mucosa with diathermy is then performed to remove the cyst epithelium.[27,174,136] Generally, this technique should not be used unless there are no safe alternatives.

Technically, cyst excision in adults can be accomplished by initially mobilizing the gallbladder from its bed to expose the hilar plate. The proximal cyst is encircled and dissected

from the hilar structures. The portal vein and hepatic arteries are isolated and protected. Proximal control of the hepatic artery before dissection of the posterior cyst wall can be very helpful, especially if hypervascularity and dense adhesions are encountered. Before division of the cyst, the distal cyst is dissected circumferentially from the pancreas to identify the pancreaticobiliary ductal junction.[175] The intrapancreatic portion of the cyst is separated from the pancreas along the areolar plane between these structures. Meticulous fine-suture ligature of collateral vessels will prevent potentially troublesome and postoperative hemorrhage. Knowledge of the anatomy by preoperative cholangiography, which might be significantly distorted in these patients, becomes particularly important to avoid damage to the pancreatic ducts. The cyst is transected distally within the head of the pancreas. The distal bile duct is ligated or stapled several millimeters above the pancreatic duct to prevent subsequent narrowing of the pancreatic duct. The decision to ligate the distal CBD was explored by Diao and colleagues[176] who published a series of 270 laparoscopic radical cyst resections with hepaticojejunostomy reconstruction. Ligation of the distal stump was predicated on preoperative radiographic morphology. In the majority of patients (77%) the distal CBD was stenotic and therefore left unligated. After 3 years of follow-up, no patients experienced a pancreatic fistula in either group. The distal bile duct remnant or cyst should be minimal to avert recurrent symptoms or complications. Dissection of the intrapancreatic portion of the cyst, although tedious, is seldom precluded

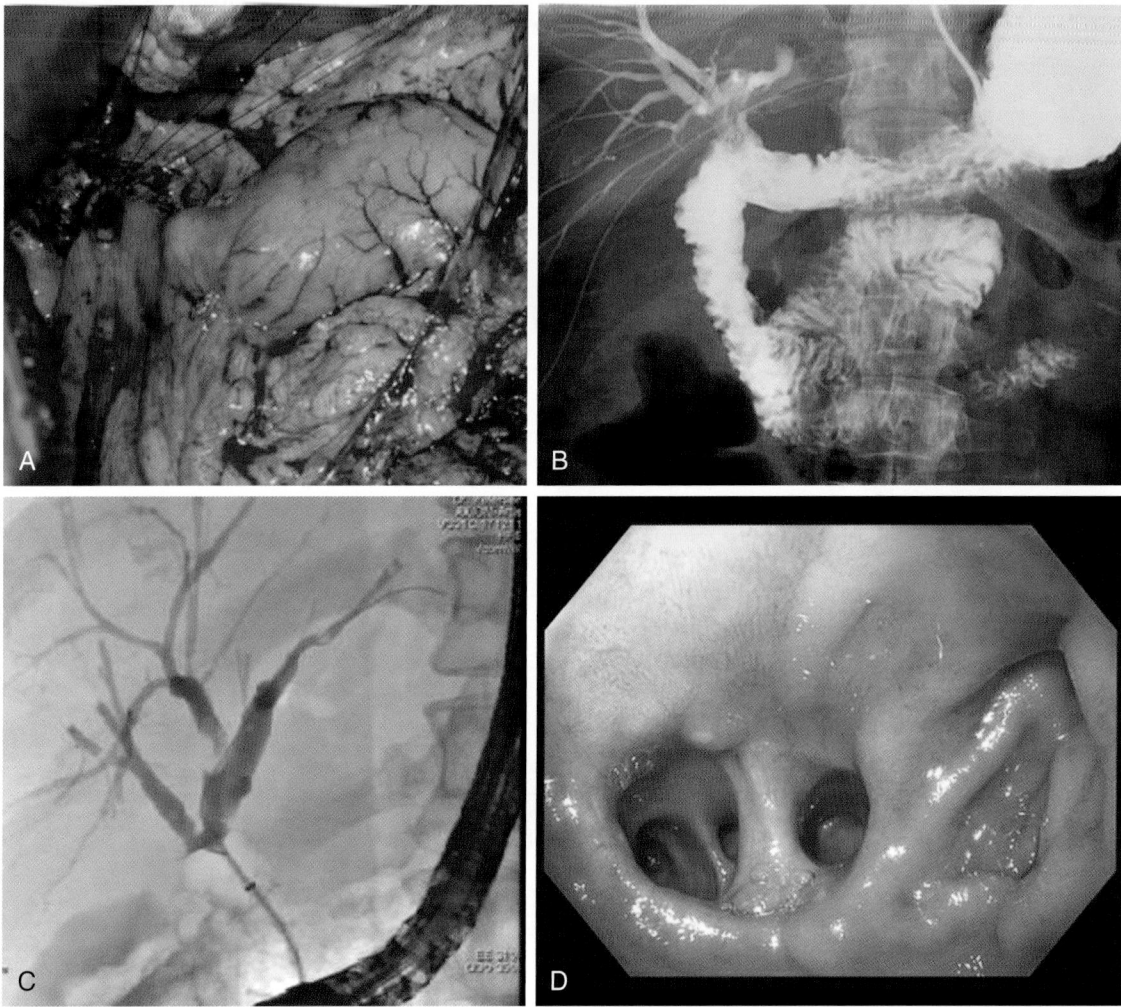

FIGURE 46.12   **A,** Hepaticoduodenostomy after resection of a type I biliary cyst. **B,** Abdominal x-ray after application of oral contrast media illustrating easy accessibility of a hepaticoduodenostomy. **C,** Endoscopic retrograde cholangiopancreatography (ERCP) with cholangiography for recurrent hepaticolithiasis. **D,** Excellent visualization of the hepaticoduodenostomy for surveillance and potential intervention.

technically from inflammation. Indeed, only rarely in the absence of malignancy does inflammation require pancreaticoduodenectomy. The cyst is mobilized proximally to the ductal confluence. After confirmation of the ductal confluence, the proximal cyst is transected and the cyst removed. Bilioenteric flow is reestablished through a wide mucosa-to-mucosa Roux-en-Y hepaticojejunostomy at the level of the hilum or with a hepaticoduodenostomy (Fig. 46.13). If a previous cystenterostomy has been performed, the same technique is used for excision after the cystoenterostomy has been divided. An existing Roux loop can be reused for the new anastomosis. The right hepatic artery should be positioned posterior to the cystoenterostomy to reduce the potential risk of injury in case of reoperation.

Type II Cyst

Excision is the treatment of choice for type II bile duct cysts.[13,85] Despite the low incidence and limited experience, reported results after excision have been excellent.[12,13,26,177,178] Ideally, the bile duct cyst is selectively excised with preservation of the normal extrahepatic bile duct.[26,27,179] Technically, excision of type II bile duct cysts is similar to a cholecystectomy

except the artery runs along the base of the cyst wall rather than entering the cyst separately. Depending on the size of the neck of the cyst at its junction with the common duct, the neck can either be ligated, stapled, or closed primarily. Alternatively, closure can be achieved with T-tube decompression of the CBD. Despite the consideration of selective excision of type II bile duct cysts as standard of care, greater than 50% of reported cases in the literature require resection of the associated extrahepatic bile duct, hemihepatectomy, or pancreaticoduodenectomy.[26] Intimate adhesion between the cyst and adjacent structures challenges the surgeon's ability to dissociate the diverticulum from the bile duct. When cholangitis, pancreatitis, and jaundice are present preoperatively, bile duct resection was always required[26]; therefore planning and preparation for more extensive resection should be made in those with symptomatic type II cysts.

Type III Cyst

Preoperative delineation of distal CBD and pancreatic duct anatomy in relation to the choledochocele is critical in directing treatment. ERCP remains the standard diagnostic modality and provides the option for concurrent definitive manage-

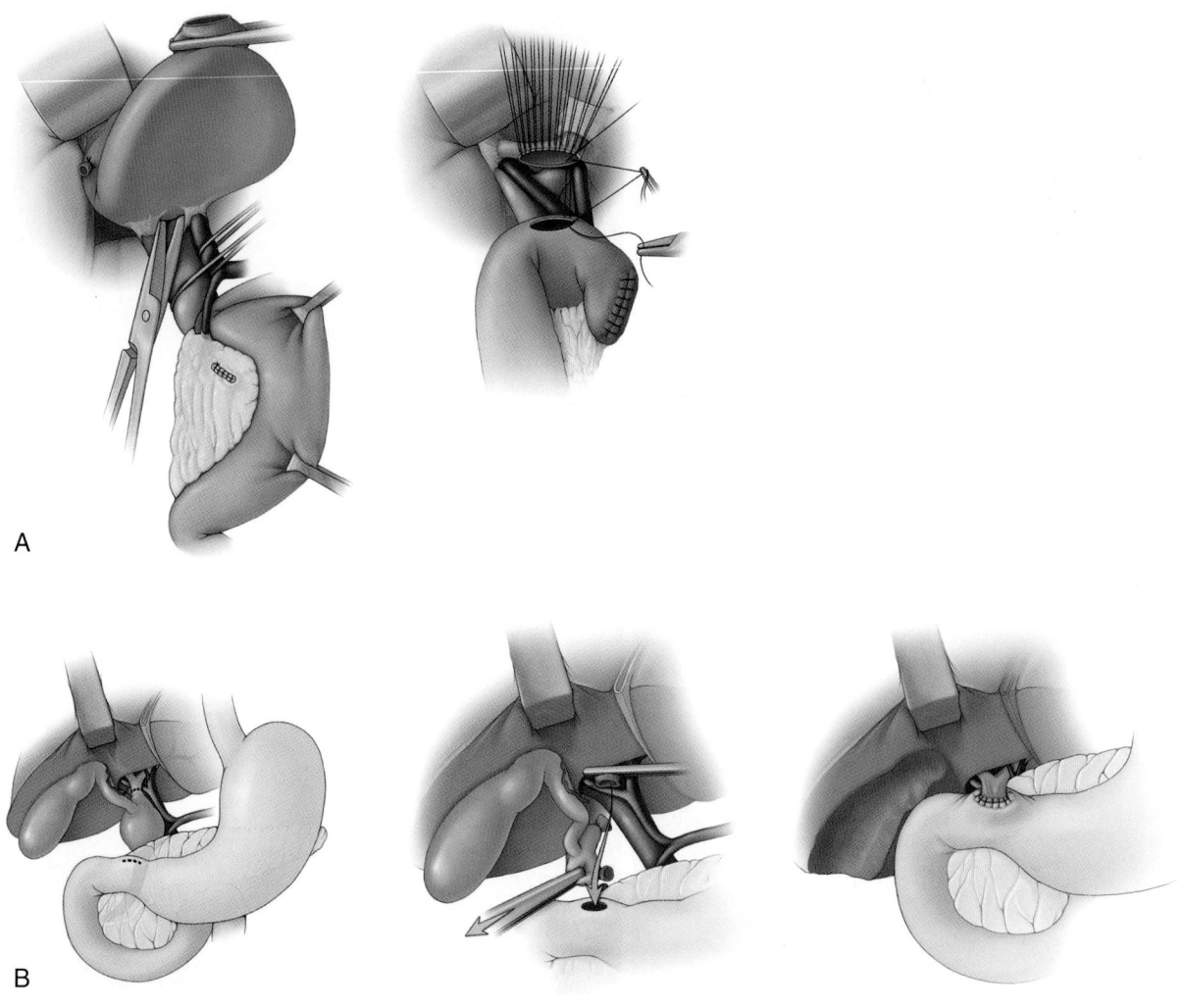

© MAYO CLINIC

FIGURE 46.13   A and B, Isolation of vascular structures, complete excision of the cyst with closure of the distal stump, and bilioenteric reconstruction with hepaticojejunostomy with a Roux-en-Y loop (see Chapter 32).

ment.[142] The reported diagnostic sensitivity of ERCP is 97%.[102] Although the incidence of carcinoma has previously been estimated at 2.5%,[180] a recent systematic review of published case reports demonstrated a 12% incidence of carcinoma in the 25 patients with choledochoceles for which pathology was reported.[142] Choledochoceles may be lined by either duodenal or biliary epithelium. The presence of biliary epithelium represents a risk factor for malignant transformation.[30]

Choledochoceles may be treated with either drainage or resection.[30] The principal goal in the treatment of choledochoceles is maintaining normal outflow of biliary and pancreatic ducts and minimizing future risk of malignancy. The choice of treatment is predicated on age and comorbidity profile, the presence of symptoms, cyst subtype, size of the lesion, and local anatomic relationships. Type A choledochoceles are most commonly treated with endoscopic sphincterotomy given their proximal location to the orifice of the ampulla and continuity with the bile duct. Biopsy of the cyst lining for histologic assessment should be performed, and in the presence of biliary epithelium, snare resection of the cyst.[30] Type B choledochoceles are located distal to the ampullary orifice. These lesions should undergo endoscopic or

surgical resection. Lobeck and colleagues[142] have recently developed a more aggressive treatment algorithm based on cyst size rather than subtype of choledochocele. Lesions less than 3 cm in diameter, composed of intestinal epithelium, should be managed with endoscopic sphincterotomy. Lesions composed of biliary epithelium should undergo local resection (endoscopic or open) and surveillance versus pancreaticoduodenectomy. Cysts greater than 3 cm are also stratified by histologic evaluation. Those with intestinal epithelium should be managed with cyst excision, whereas cyst excision with surveillance versus pancreaticoduodenectomy is recommended for those with biliary epithelium.

The excellent long-term results with endoscopic treatment coupled with the diagnostic advantage of ERCP in defining the terminal pancreaticobiliary anatomy clearly favor the endoscopic approach. Although transduodenal excision eliminates the risk of malignancy, only a few cases of carcinoma in choledochoceles have been documented and the incidence is likely subject to reporting bias.[102,142] Surgical intervention should likely be reserved for cases in which malignancy is present or lesions are not amenable to appropriate endoscopic therapy. The role of surveillance has yet to be defined following management, and consideration of endoscopic re-evaluation at 6 to 12 months has been proposed.[181]

Type IV Cyst

The extrahepatic component of type IVa and IVb cysts is approached as a type I bile duct cyst. The treatment of choice is excision of the extrahepatic cyst, cholecystectomy, and Roux-en-Y hepaticojejunostomy.[12,18,27,121] The challenge of a type IVa cyst is the management of the intrahepatic component. The principle therapeutic objective is optimal biliary drainage. In the absence of hilar or intrahepatic ductal strictures, intrahepatic stones, intrahepatic abscess, or malignancy, type IVa bile ducts cysts may be managed with extrahepatic duct resection and a wide hilar hepaticoenterostomy. However, patients often have symptoms of concomitant intrahepatic disease.[182,183] If the intrahepatic involvement is localized, an anatomic partial hepatectomy of the cystic intrahepatic component should be performed in addition to the standard resection of the extrahepatic cyst.[184] Complications involving the intrahepatic component that prompt such resections include hepatolithiasis, intrahepatic strictures as the source of cholangitis, and focal biliary cirrhosis.[163,184,185] If intrahepatic disease is untreated, the rate of postoperative morbidity is increased regardless of the appropriate treatment of the extrahepatic cyst. The incidence of cholangitis may approach 30% to 40% in the presence of remnant intrahepatic disease.[186] Combined partial hepatectomy is deemed most appropriate for patients with severe cystic dilation of lobar intrahepatic ducts and a demonstrable hilar stenosis. In the setting of bilobar disease and hilar stenoses, extended hepatectomy with resection of the hemiliver comprising the greatest disease burden should be considered.[98,187] Xia and colleagues reported a series of 59 patients with type IVa bile duct cysts who underwent combined extrahepatic cyst excision and partial hepatectomy.[184] Only 6% of patients had incomplete cyst excision, predominantly a consequence of wide disease distribution. Long-term outcomes included excellent or good biliary function in 86% of patients with a cholangitis rate of 12% and anastomotic stricture rate of 6%.

Importantly, recognition of the presence of variant ductal anatomy and stenoses at the hilum is critical to optimal management. If intrahepatic ductal stenosis or aberrant ducts are not recognized and addressed during extrahepatic cyst excision, subsequent operation will often be necessary. Membranous or bridge-like stenoses should be excised circumferentially to their base. The long-term results of the treatment of type IVb cysts in adults are similar to those of type I choledochal cysts. Although patients with type IVa cysts and portal hypertension may be approached by proximal splenorenal shunts before cyst drainage, liver transplantation may provide a more durable solution. Resection of intrahepatic cysts in cirrhotic patients is associated with an increase in morbidity and mortality rates and is generally contraindicated.

Type V Cyst/Caroli Disease

The treatment of Caroli disease is dependent on the distribution of intrahepatic bile duct cysts and the presence of congenital hepatic fibrosis, secondary biliary cirrhosis, or carcinoma. Caroli disease in adults may present in a localized form, limited to one hepatic lobe or segment, or a diffuse form, involving the entire intrahepatic biliary tree.[121,127,188,189] Most adults with Caroli disease have a unilobar fusiform dilation of the intrahepatic ducts.[121,122] The left intrahepatic ductal system is most often involved.[149]

Treatment can be supportive in nature and should be individualized given the considerable heterogeneity in presentation.[190,191] Supportive, nonoperative management includes the medical treatment of recurrent cholangitis and sepsis and stone extraction when possible. Endoscopic management of extrahepatic ductal stones is effective; however, retrieval of intrahepatic stone diseases is more difficult.[192] Additional endoscopic options for intrahepatic stone disease include peroral cholangioscopy, extracorporeal shockwave lithotripsy, and intraductal electrohydraulic lithotripsy.[193-194] Dissolution or litholytic therapy has been previously described. In a small series of patients with Caroli syndrome and intrahepatic stones, ursodeoxycholic acid was employed resulting in sustained clinical remission and partial or complete dissolution of intrahepatic stones on ultrasound.[195]

When medical management fails, operative intervention is indicated. Surgical options include hepatic resection (see Chapter 101) and orthotopic liver transplantation[196] (see Chapter 105). Approximately 80% of patients will have unilobar disease, therefore, partial hepatectomy represents the procedure of choice.[197-200] Good long-term outcomes can be achieved in those with localized disease and preserved hepatic function after complete resection of intrahepatic disease is achieved.[201-203] After hepatic resection, bilioenteric reconstruction is only considered if disease is present at the level of the bifurcation of the CHD. This finding occurs in approximately 10% of patients.[149] In the setting of extensive bilobar disease, or those with portal hypertension and cirrhosis, it is recommended to proceed with evaluation for candidacy of liver transplantation.[199] In a large series of 148 patients undergoing surgical management of type V bile duct cysts, hepatic resection in those with unilobar disease and liver transplant in those with diffuse, bilobar disease complicated by cholangitis and/or portal hypertension resulted in excellent long-term outcomes and survival.[149] Liver transplantation is often precluded in those with preoperatively diagnosed cholangiocarcinoma.[204-206]

The natural history of Caroli disease includes cirrhosis, variceal bleeding, and liver failure. Liver transplantation facilitates complete resection of hepatobiliary pathology and prevention of malignant transformation[149] (see Chapter 105); however, liver transplantation does expose the patient to increased perioperative morbidity, mortality, and immunosuppressive therapy. This indication represents less than 0.2% of all liver transplants and produces equivalent outcomes to those undergoing transplant for end-stage liver disease.[196,207,208] This disease is not associated with an APBJ and the extrahepatic bile duct system is not at increased risk of carcinoma. Routine resection of the extrahepatic biliary tree and bilioenteric anastomosis is not recommended.[149] If the diagnosis of bilobar Caroli disease is made, nonsurgical medical treatment should be used until the patient is considered a transplant candidate. Avoidance of numerous ineffective surgical procedures will reduce the technical risk of transplantation.

ADVANCES IN MINIMALLY INVASIVE SURGICAL MANAGEMENT (SEE CHAPTER 127)

Laparoscopic excision of bile duct cysts and Roux-en-Y hepaticojejunostomy were first reported in a pediatric patient with a type I cyst.[209] Subsequently, large pediatric case series have

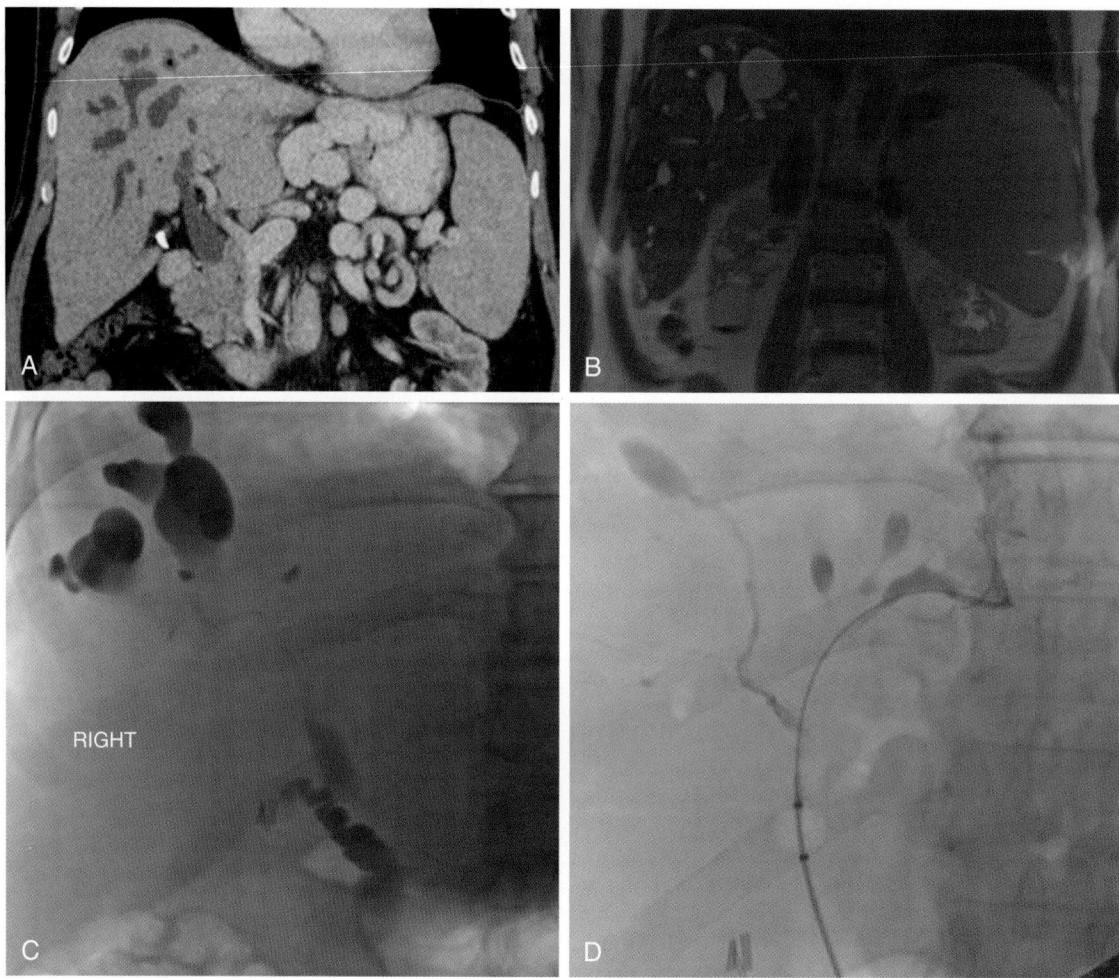

FIGURE 46.14 Caroli disease. Computed tomography **(A)**, magnetic resonance imaging (MRI) **(B),** and endoscopic retrograde cholangiopancrea-tography (ERCP) documenting multiple saccular cysts of only the intrahepatic bile ducts **(C and D).**

been reported from Asia, in which a greater prevalence of bile duct cysts has been observed.[210–221] Minimally invasive approaches are used increasingly in most visceral operations, and outcomes consistently suggest patient advantages over conventional approaches regarding pain, wound complications, length of hospital stay, and recovery time. A major advantage of the laparoscopic approach in bile duct cysts is the reputed superior visualization of the structures around the cyst and at the hepatic hilum. The magnification conferred by the laparoscope helps assess neovascularity around the cyst, separation of the posterior cyst wall from the portal vein, and dissection and anastomosis in the hilar area. It also may aid dissection and identification of the narrow intrapancreatic bile duct close to the APBJ because of the magnified laparoscopic view. However, it must be emphasized that laparoscopic excision of bile duct cysts is technically challenging and requires experience in both complex biliary operations and advanced laparoscopic surgery. Bile leakage rate with laparoscopic cyst excision and hepatico-jejunostomy has been reported from 1.6% to 8.1%. Liem and colleagues[222] described a series of 400 pediatric patients with no perioperative deaths and a leak rate of 2%. Stringer has voiced concern regarding the increased adoption of laparoscopic management of bile duct cysts in the pediatric population.[223] Under closer inspection, the optimal procedure may

not have been utilized for many patients with type I and IVa cysts. The performance of a less-than-radical cyst resection to facilitate completion laparoscopically predisposes the patient to long-term postoperative morbidity. Clearly, whatever operative approach is selected, performance of the operation in accordance with sound surgical principles is paramount.

Although experience is more limited in adults, outcomes have been similar. Duan and colleagues (2015)[224] reported a 5-year experience with totally laparoscopic cyst excision and Roux-en-Y hepaticojejunostomy in adults. In this series of 31 patients, hepatobiliary morbidity was limited to one biliary leak and one biliary stricture, with no perioperative mortality. In another series of 110 patients (55 adults and 55 children), outcomes were largely equivalent between the two populations with low rates of postoperative morbidity (10%) and bile leak (3.6%).[225] All adult patients underwent hepaticojejunostomy, whereas in the pediatric population 53% underwent hepatico-jejunostomy and 47% hepaticoduodenostomy. Three adult patients were converted to an open procedure due to dense adhesions or adherence to the portal vein.

Conversion to an open procedure, intraoperative complications, and postoperative morbidity are elevated in the early stages of laparoscopic series.[211,222] In a review of 104 patients undergoing laparoscopic cyst excision and Roux-en-Y hepaticojejunostomy by

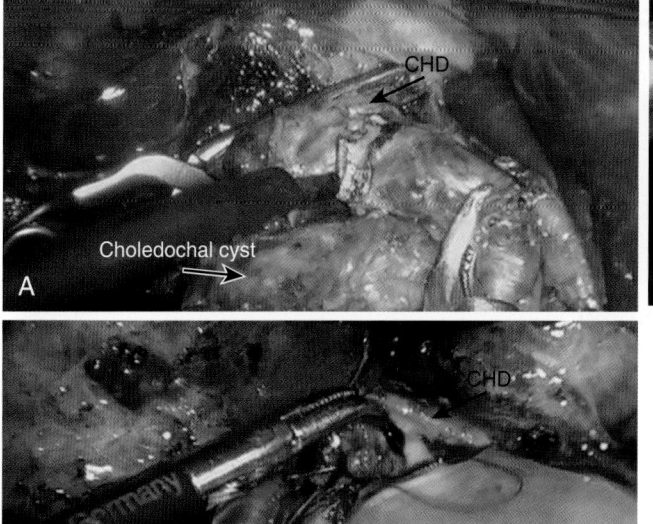

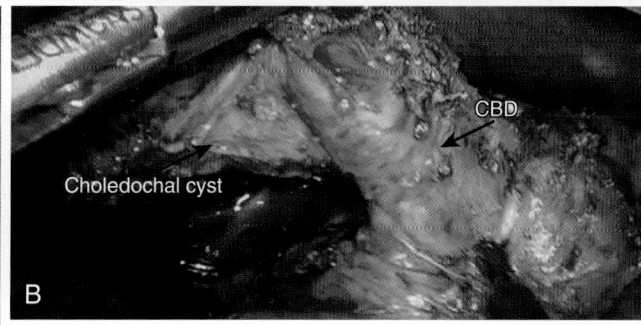

FIGURE 46.15   Laparoscopic resection of type II bile duct cyst. A, Transection of common hepatic duct. **B,** Elevated cyst attached to distal common bile duct *(CBD)*. **C,** Roux-en-Y anastomosis (see Chapter 127).

a single surgeon, the learning curve was calculated to be 37 cases.[226] After completion of the learning curve, surgeon-specific outcomes significantly improved with respect to operative time, overall postoperative complication rate, and the length of hospital stay. An example is given in Fig. 46.15.

Several publications of robotic bile duct cyst resection with reconstruction have been described in the adult population with acceptable outcomes.[227–230] In two recent retrospective reviews of patients undergoing robotic or laparoscopic resection and reconstruction, the robotic approach was associated with equivalent or potentially improved postoperative outcomes.[228,231] Given the current advances in laparoscopic and robotic-assisted resection of complex pancreaticobiliary pathology in adults, further application of such approaches in patients with bile duct cysts is expected in the future.

SUMMARY

Bile duct cysts represent a rare pathology in which single or multiple cysts may be present throughout the biliary ductal system. They are associated with malignancy as well as numerous benign complications. The surgical management of adults with bile duct cysts is based on cyst type and the presence of associated hepatobiliary pathology. Although the risk of malignancy is significantly reduced in those who have undergone bile duct cyst resection, these patients remain at increased risk of carcinoma relative to the general population, within the remnant biliary tree and pancreas.

The references for this chapter can be found online by accessing the accompanying Expert Consult website.

SECTION II. Neoplastic

A. General

CHAPTER 47

Tumors of the bile ducts: Pathologic features

Olca Basturk and David S. Klimstra

The biliary tract is lined by simple columnar epithelial cells of foregut origin (Fig. 47.1).[1] The vast majority of biliary neoplasms arise from this cell type and therefore show major similarities to other foregut tumors, particularly those of pancreatic ductal origin (see Chapter 1). By far the most common neoplasm of the biliary tract is adenocarcinoma, referred to collectively with pancreatic ductal adenocarcinoma as a pancreatobiliary-type adenocarcinoma (Figs. 47.2–47.5), reflecting the similarities between these two neoplasms (see Chapter 59).

Tumors arising from the gallbladder and the different segments of the bile ducts have overlapping histologic characteristics; therefore their pathologic classification is also very similar.[2–4] On the other hand, the risk factors, clinical findings, and biologic behavior may vary (see Chapters 49, 50, 51, and 59). For example, although gallstones are the main risk factor for gallbladder adenocarcinoma, adenocarcinomas of the proximal bile ducts have a much stronger association with primary sclerosing cholangitis (PSC; see Chapter 41) or anomalous pancreatobiliary duct junction.[5] This variability also is partially reflected in the molecular alterations, which, although not specific for the histologic subtype of the tumor, may affect the management and prognosis (see Chapter 9E). The different presentations of biliary adenocarcinoma also influence the mode by which a specimen is obtained for pathologic examination. For example, many gallbladder adenocarcinomas are currently identified in "routine" cholecystectomy specimens from primary care facilities, performed with a preoperative diagnosis of chronic cholecystitis or symptomatic cholelithiasis, whereas extrahepatic bile duct lesions are seldom resected without a strong preoperative suspicion of carcinoma, and this is usually performed in tertiary care facilities.

This chapter discusses the pathologic aspects of biliary tract neoplasia, with special emphasis on adenocarcinomas. The tumor types are discussed by viewing the biliary system as a whole; site-specific characteristics are mentioned only when pertinent to pathologic classification. For the details of clinical findings, risk factors, and site-specific management, the reader is referred to other chapters.

INVASIVE CARCINOMAS OF THE BILIARY TRACT

Most "biliary tract cancers" are conventional adenocarcinomas (pancreatobiliary-type), which are morphologically very similar to pancreatic ductal adenocarcinoma.[2–4] This tumor is referred to as

intrahepatic cholangiocarcinoma in the intrahepatic biliary tract (see Chapter 50) and *adenocarcinoma* in the extrahepatic biliary tract (see Chapters 51 and 59) and in the gallbladder (see Chapter 49).[6] As in adenocarcinomas of other organs, these are usually tumors of elderly persons. The association of biliary adenocarcinomas with preceding chronic inflammation has been well established,[7,8] mostly by epidemiologic data showing the high incidence of gallbladder cancer in areas with a high prevalence of gallstones[9] and by the pathologic observation that many individual carcinomas have associated gallstones or cholecystitis (see Chapter 49). Also, the risk of adenocarcinoma is relatively high in patients with PSC (see Chapter 41) and indirectly in those with ulcerative colitis. The association of biliary cancers with some infectious agents, especially *Salmonella* serovar Typhi[10] and parasites (e.g., *Clonorchis sinensis*),[11,12] as well as with choledochal cysts (see Chapter 46), is also presumably related to the potential for chronic inflammation from constant epithelial injury and repair that can lead to neoplastic alterations.[12] The role of *Helicobacter* spp.,[13] especially *Helicobacter bilis*, has been studied in gallbladder cancers.[14,15]

Growth Patterns and Macroscopic Features

Based on their macroscopic growth pattern, biliary carcinomas have been divided into four types: (1) polypoid, (2) nodular

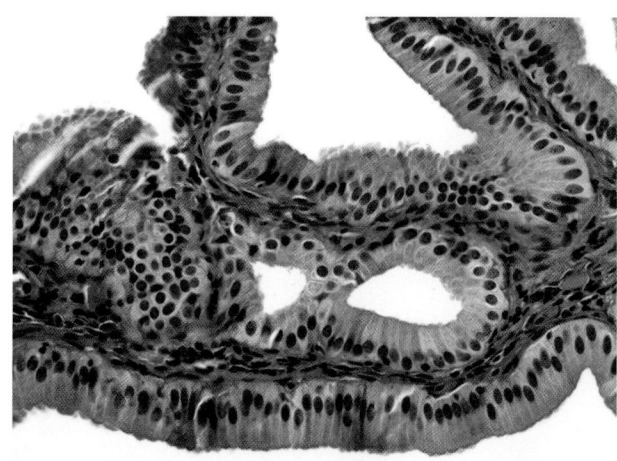

FIGURE 47.1 **Benign epithelium.** The biliary epithelium is composed of a layer of columnar cells with acidophilic cytoplasm.

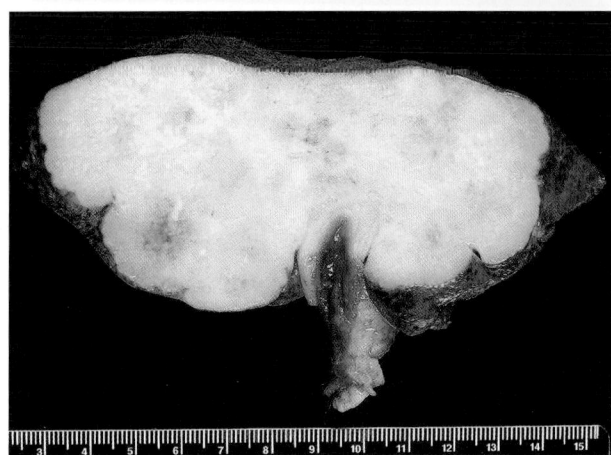

FIGURE 47.2   Macroscopic appearance of an adenocarcinoma. The cut surfaces of adenocarcinomas of the biliary tract (an intrahepatic cholangiocarcinoma is depicted here) typically have a firm, white, sclerotic appearance because of the abundance of desmoplastic stroma.

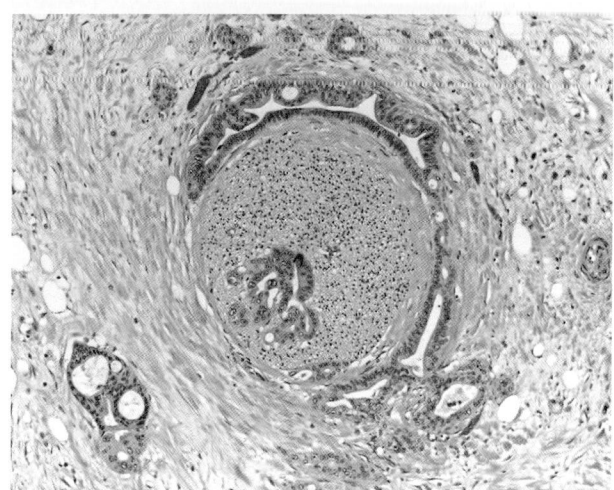

FIGURE 47.4   Adenocarcinoma with perineural invasion. Carcinoma cells wrapping around nerves is a very common finding in biliary adenocarcinomas.

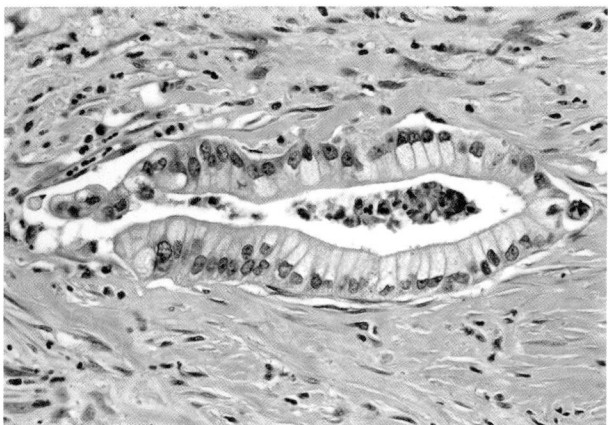

FIGURE 47.3   Well-differentiated adenocarcinoma. Most adenocarcinomas of the biliary tract are of the pancreatobiliary type, characterized by simple tubular units lined by well-polarized, relatively bland-appearing cells.

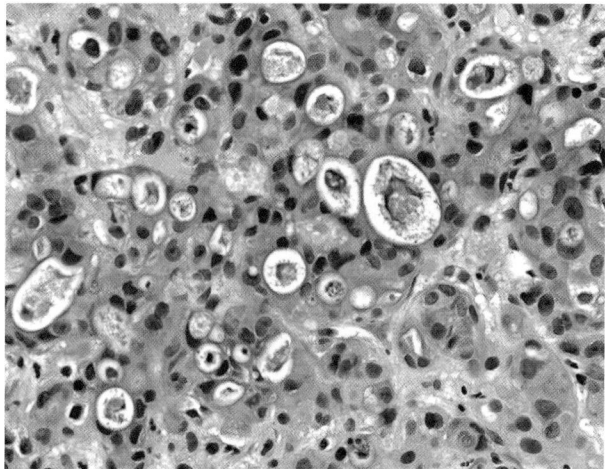

FIGURE 47.5   Adenocarcinoma with mucin. Intracytoplasmic and intraluminal mucin often are present in biliary adenocarcinomas. In this example, the material in the lumina represents mucin admixed with necrotic debris.

(nodular-sclerosing), (3) scirrhous-constricting, and (4) diffusely infiltrative.[4,16] Polypoid growth typically is found in carcinomas, with an associated component of intraductal papillary or tubulopapillary neoplasms, previously designated noninvasive papillary carcinoma, which are associated with a better prognosis.[17–20] The nodular and scirrhous-constricting types have a propensity to infiltrate surrounding tissues and are therefore difficult to resect. The scirrhous-constricting and diffusely infiltrative patterns may be difficult to differentiate from chronic inflammatory conditions, especially PSC and autoimmune cholangitis.[21] The diffusely infiltrating type tends to spread linearly along the ducts. Significant histologic overlaps occur among these different growth patterns, so their utility in pathologic tumor classification is limited.

On cut sections, the intraluminal components of biliary carcinomas, especially those with a polypoid gross appearance, may appear more friable, soft, and tan.[22] This reflects the presence of intraductal neoplastic elements growing into the lumen, and ulceration and necrosis may be evident in larger tumors; so much so that the tumor may appear to represent "debris" in the lumen.[18] The infiltrating components of adenocarcinomas are more scirrhous (scar-like), with a firm, white, gritty appearance because of the abundance of desmoplasia, the fibrotic tissue reaction associated with infiltrating carcinoma (see Fig. 47.2).

When adenocarcinoma invades the adjacent liver, the growth pattern often becomes more expansile, and the liver-carcinoma interface appears deceptively well demarcated. This allows for easier detection of the boundaries of these carcinomas in hepatic resections. In contrast, the boundaries of carcinomas invading the hilar soft tissue are typically poorly defined and difficult to appreciate. In the literature, porcelain gallbladder, which had been defined as extensive calcification in the gallbladder wall, has been reported to have a particularly strong association with carcinoma, but recent studies have shown that a distinctive type of hyalinizing cholecystitis with minimal or no calcifications (incomplete porcelain gallbladder) actually has the higher risk for carcinoma.[23–25]

Microscopic Features

Most adenocarcinomas of the gallbladder and bile ducts show the characteristic features of a pancreatobiliary-type adenocarcinoma (see Figs. 47.3–47.5): both simple and complex, irregularly shaped glands mixed with small clusters of cells, often with associated stromal desmoplasia.[2–4,26,27] The glands often are well formed, lined by cuboidal cells, and show dilated lumina. The nuclear grade may be unexpectedly high for the degree of glandular differentiation, and marked variation in nuclear size, shape, and intracellular location may occur between different cells within the individual glands. The cytoplasm may be acidophilic and granular in some cases and pale or clear in others. Variable amounts of intracytoplasmic and intraluminal mucin are present; in some cases, mucin is readily evident by routine histologic examination; in others, it is only demonstrable by histochemical stains.

Perineural invasion (see Fig. 47.4) and vascular invasion are common, and carcinoma cells, when they invade these structures, may have a deceptively well-differentiated appearance. In fact, the distinction of a well-differentiated adenocarcinoma from a benign reactive process in this region is one of the more challenging differential diagnoses in surgical pathology.

Dysplasia, or biliary intraepithelial neoplasia (BilIN; Fig. 47.6), is often present in the adjacent biliary epithelium.[28] Sometimes the intraepithelial component includes a papillary neoplasm (Fig. 47.7). In such cases, the noninvasive and invasive components of the tumor should be evaluated separately, and the extent of invasion should be quantified because those with "minimal invasion" have been shown to have a relatively favorable outcome.[29–31] In contrast, widely invasive cases typically have an aggressive clinical

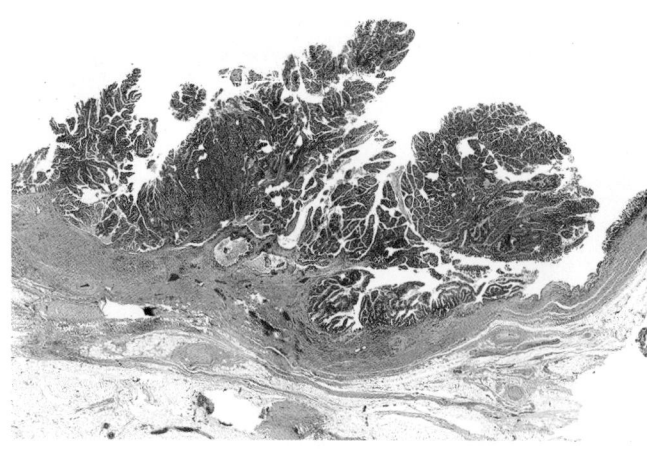

FIGURE 47.7 **Intraductal papillary neoplasm.** This polypoid lesion shows papillary fronds lined by neoplastic cells.

course. Even in the absence of invasive carcinoma, these tumors may recur and metastasize, possibly because of the presence of an undetected focus of invasive carcinoma, or a "field-effect" phenomenon that predisposes the remaining segments of biliary tract to the development of carcinoma.[18]

Tumors that infiltrate the adjacent liver may acquire a more trabecular pattern, presumably by growing along the sinusoidal backbone of the liver parenchyma. Entrapped reactive bile ductules and hepatocytes are often present within the tumor and may create a diagnostic problem in biopsy specimens.[32]

Anatomic Variants

For therapeutic and prognostic purposes, tumors of the extrahepatic biliary tract are traditionally separated by their anatomic distribution into peri-hilar (arising predominantly in the main lobar extrahepatic ducts, distal to segmental bile ducts and proximal to the cystic duct), mid-duct, and distal (located between the confluence of the common hepatic duct and cystic duct and Ampulla of Vater, excluding ampullary carcinoma; see Chapter 2). Mid-duct carcinomas, however, do not include a separate site for staging.[33] The distinctive clinical characteristics of adenocarcinomas that occur in different segments of the biliary tract are discussed in other chapters, and only a few issues pertinent to pathologic aspects are mentioned here. Most extrahepatic biliary tract carcinomas are peri-hilar and tend to be the scirrhous-constricting and diffusely infiltrative types. Studies have shown that many originate within 5 mm of the cystic duct junction or within the cystic duct itself. Hilar carcinoma, located at the confluence of the right and left hepatic ducts, sometimes referred to as a *Klatskin tumor*,[34,35] has distinctive clinical features. Klatskin tumors usually grow into the liver rather than distally toward the duodenum,[36] and the component that invades the liver is often well demarcated. Carcinomas in the middle third tend to be the nodular sclerosing type (thickened along a long segment, with a narrow lumen and inflammatory changes in the surrounding tissues) and thus are difficult to differentiate from extrahepatic sclerosing cholangitis. These have a very high propensity for perineural invasion and involvement of radial surfaces, making curative resection difficult.[37] Carcinomas in the distal common bile duct (CBD) have the best prognosis because of their resectability by pancreatoduodenectomy and because many, especially those close to the ampullary region, are composed predominantly of noninvasive neoplastic elements.[2–4]

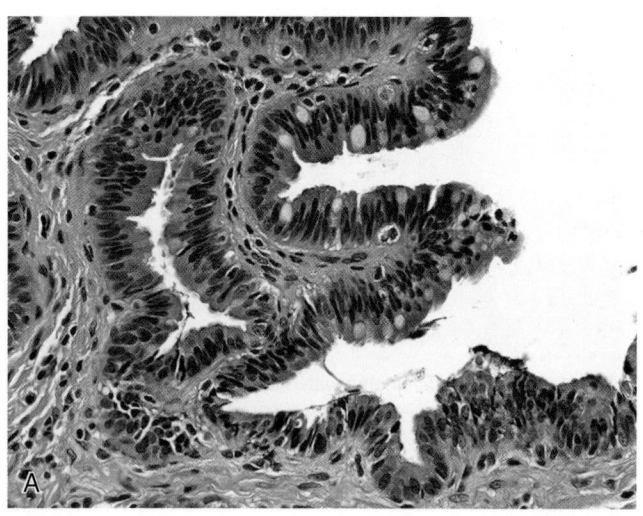

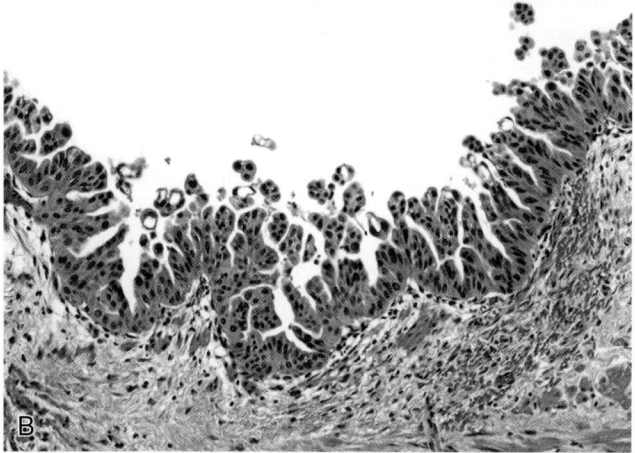

FIGURE 47.6 **Dysplasia (biliary intraepithelial neoplasia).** Loss of polarity of the cells is associated with nuclear atypia, including enlargement, hyperchromatism, and pleomorphism. **A,** Low-grade dysplasia. **B,** High-grade dysplasia.

Pathologic Differential Diagnosis

The difficulty at the clinical level of distinguishing biliary adeno-carcinomas from benign inflammatory conditions, such as scle-rosing cholangitis, is also problematic at the microscopic level.[38] Reactive changes in the accessory biliary ductules in the wall of the bile ducts can mimic adenocarcinomas, although nonneoplas-tic ductules may retain a lobular configuration, and they lack the density of cellularity of a carcinoma. Pancreatobiliary adenocarci-nomas can be deceptively benign appearing, composed of well-formed glandular elements lined by fairly organized, cytologically bland glandular cells (see Fig. 47.3). The distinction of reactive changes in the surface epithelium from dysplasia/BilIN often proves to be even more challenging, especially because any injury to the biliary epithelium, including instrumentation and stent placement, has a tendency to induce marked cytologic atypia that can mimic the appearance of high-grade dysplasia (Fig. 47.8). Marked nuclear enlargement or irregularity, hyperchromasia, loss of polarity, mitotic figures, apoptotic cells, and intraluminal ne-crosis are findings in favor of a neoplastic process (see Fig. 47.6). Overlaps are common, however, and at times this distinction may not be possible on the basis of biopsies or frozen sections.

Biliary carcinomas that grow into the liver must be distin-guished from primary hepatocellular carcinomas (see Chapter 89). The presence of true glandular elements and mucin are common findings in biliary carcinomas and typically are absent in hepatocellular carcinomas. In contrast, hepatocellular carci-nomas may have intracellular bile and generally lack significant stromal fibrosis and desmoplasia. Other distinctive features of hepatocellular carcinomas—the solid and trabecular growth pattern, centrally located nuclei with prominent nucleoli, and abundant eosinophilic cytoplasm—usually are identifiable; im-munohistochemical demonstration of hepatocellular differentia-tion with markers such as hepatocyte-1 or arginase-1 can be used in problematic cases.

Differentiation between ampullary and duodenal neoplasms and CBD tumors can be difficult because carcinomas of these sites often infiltrate neighboring structures (see Chapters 59 and 63). In such cases, the correct classification of the tumor greatly depends on determining where it is centered, which often can be achieved only by close correlation of the radio-graphic and macroscopic findings. In addition, any dysplasia or other preinvasive neoplasm may be an important clue to the site of origin.[39] In this complex region, the origin of the tumor (by site) should be evaluated separately from the type of the carci-noma, such as ampullary carcinomas of the pancreatobiliary-type. Intestinal-type carcinomas in this region are more likely to be of either ampullary or duodenal origin.[40,41]

Biliary carcinomas metastatic to other sites may mimic the primary tumors of those organs. In particular, metastases to the ovary often become cystic and are mistaken for primary ovarian mucinous cystic neoplasms, and lung metastases can resemble mucinous pulmonary adenocarcinomas.

Immunohistochemical and Molecular Characteristics (see Chapter 9E)

By immunohistochemistry, biliary adenocarcinomas typically express CK7, CK19, B72.3, CA19-9, CEA, MUC1 (Fig. 47.9), and MUC5AC.[2–4,26,27,42] On occasion, these markers can be helpful in distinguishing certain other carcinomas that do not express these markers, such as hepatocellular carcinoma (see Chapter 89). None of these markers, however, is specific enough to prove biliary origin for an adenocarcinoma when a metastasis from another organ is under consideration (see Chapters 90–92). Biliary adenocarcinomas generally lack expression of CK20 and CDX2, typically found in intestinal adenocarcinomas; TTF-1 and napsin, found in pulmonary primary tumors; and hormone receptors. In situ hybridization for albumin has recently been shown in intrahepatic (peripheral) cholangiocarcinomas and represents a method to distinguish these from metastatic adeno-carcinoma, but hilar cholangiocarcinomas and extrahepatic bile duct adenocarcinomas are negative for this marker.[43]

In approximately 65% of cases, positive immunoreactivity for the protein product of the *TP53* gene is noted.[44,45] Some studies

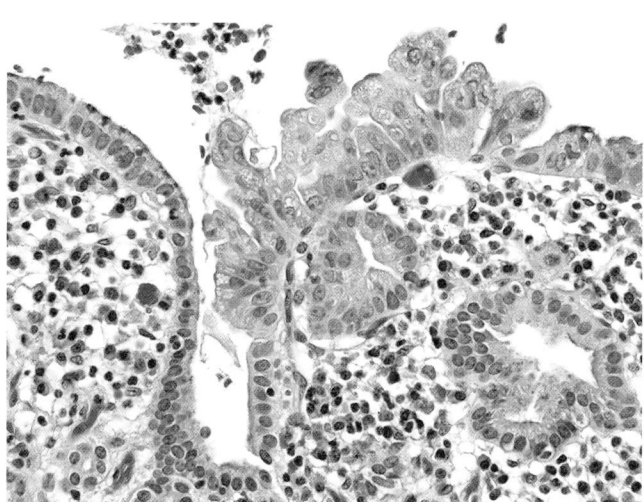

FIGURE 47.8 Reactive atypia. Injury to the bile duct epithelium—whether from a primary inflammatory process, such as sclerosing cholan-gitis, or from instrumentation during endoscopic retrograde cholangiopan-creatography or stent placement—often induces cytologic atypia and complex architectural changes, including cribriforming and micropapillary formations. Although the differential diagnosis in such a case includes high-grade dysplasia, the marked background inflammation and the fact that changes wax and wane throughout the involved epithelium would favor this as reactive atypia.

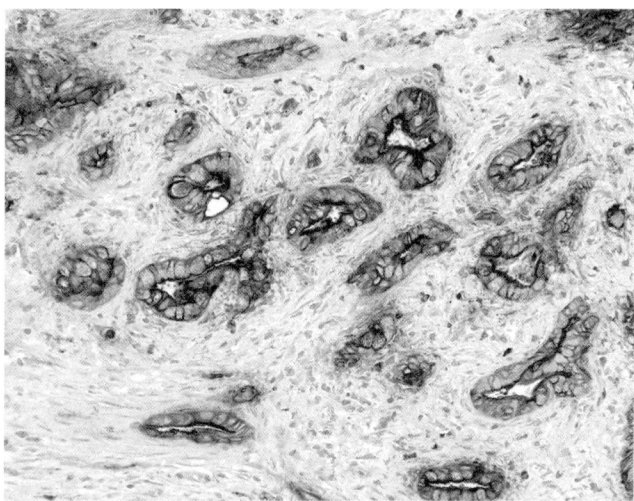

FIGURE 47.9 Mucin 1 (MUC1) in adenocarcinoma. Immunohisto-chemical studies may be useful in the differential diagnosis of biliary neoplasia. In this example, carcinoma cells show expression of MUC1, which often is negative in intestinal-type adenocarcinomas.

have shown this to be fairly specific for carcinoma, as opposed to the nonneoplastic changes associated with PSC.[46] It should be used cautiously, however, because of significant overlap.

Mutations at codon 12 of the *KRAS* oncogene, seen in more than 90% of pancreatic ductal adenocarcinomas (see Chapter 9D), are much less common in biliary adenocarcinomas,[45] and the frequency of *KRAS* mutation appears to decrease from distal to proximal along the biliary tree.[45,47,48] Similarly, loss of *SMAD4*, present in approximately half of pancreatic ductal adenocarcinomas, is almost as common in distal CBD carcinomas. However, *SMAD4* is retained in most proximal extrahepatic bile duct carcinomas.[49] More than half of the cases have loss of heterozygosity at 8p, 9q, and 18q; amplification of *ERBB2* is also reported in more than half.[50] Overexpression of *HER* family receptors, including epidermal growth factor receptor (EGFR) and c-met, has also been reported.[51,52]

In gallbladder carcinomas, other common mutations include alterations in *CDKN2A* or *CDKN2B* (19%), *ARID1A* (13%), *PIK3CA* (10%), and *CTNNB1* (10%).[53,54] Of these, microsatellite instability and *CDKN2A* inactivation by promoter methylation, which have been reported in both preinvasive and invasive lesions,[55] may have therapeutic implications in the future.[56] Also, mechanistic target of rapamycin pathway alterations[57] and cyclooxygenase-2 overexpression have been found to be associated with adverse prognosis.[58,59]

Not surprisingly, the adenoma-carcinoma sequence appears to go through different pathways, with paucity of mutations in *TP53* and *CDKN2A* and a higher frequency of mutations in *CTNNB1* (encoding β-catenin).[60] A higher *KRAS* mutation rate in lesions associated with pancreatobiliary maljunction has also been reported.[61,62]

Other Types of Carcinomas in the Biliary Tract

Other, less common carcinomas of glandular epithelial origin in the gallbladder and biliary tract are classified separately from pancreatobiliary-type adenocarcinomas.[2-4] Intestinal-type adenocarcinomas[63] are morphologically similar to their counterparts in the gastrointestinal (GI) tract. Signet ring cell carcinomas are characterized by a diffusely infiltrative pattern of individual cells, often with signet ring morphology because of intracellular mucin; a cord-like growth pattern may also occur in the biliary tract but is exceedingly uncommon. Mucinous adenocarcinomas may be seen in some cases, with extensive mucin production associated with stromal mucin deposition (Fig. 47.10), usually mixed with conventional adenocarcinomas[64]; this subtype can occur in association with intraductal papillary neoplasms.[18] In the past, it has been suggested that the prognosis of mucinous adenocarcinomas may be more favorable than that of conventional pancreatobiliary-type adenocarcinoma,[35] but a recent study has shown that these are typically large and advanced tumors at diagnosis and thus exhibit more aggressive behavior than conventional adenocarcinomas.[64] Adenosquamous carcinomas[65] are rare tumors in which a mixture of glandular and squamous differentiation is seen in variable amounts. These are also highly aggressive carcinomas, partly attributed to their higher stage at diagnosis.[66] In some recent studies, however, their adverse outcome persisted even in stage-matched cases.[65] Clear-cell carcinomas[67] are described, in which the morphologic features resemble those of renal cell carcinoma.

Some patterns of biliary carcinoma lack gland, mucin, or papilla formation. Undifferentiated carcinomas (Fig. 47.11)

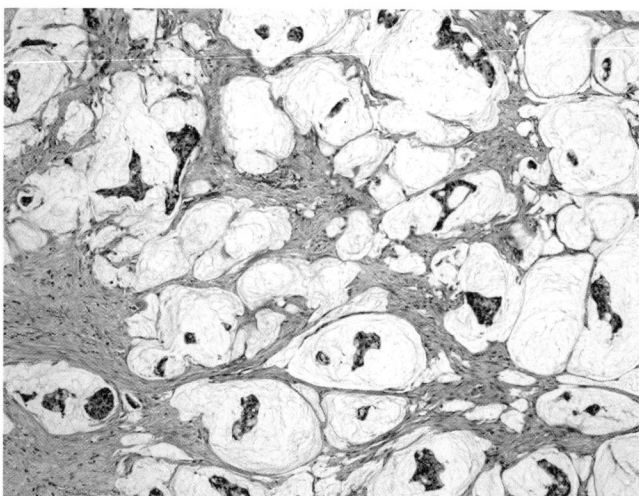

FIGURE 47.10 **Mucinous carcinoma.** Rarely, a biliary adenocarcinoma may be associated with abundant stromal mucin deposition. In this example, scant carcinoma cells are floating within the mucin pools.

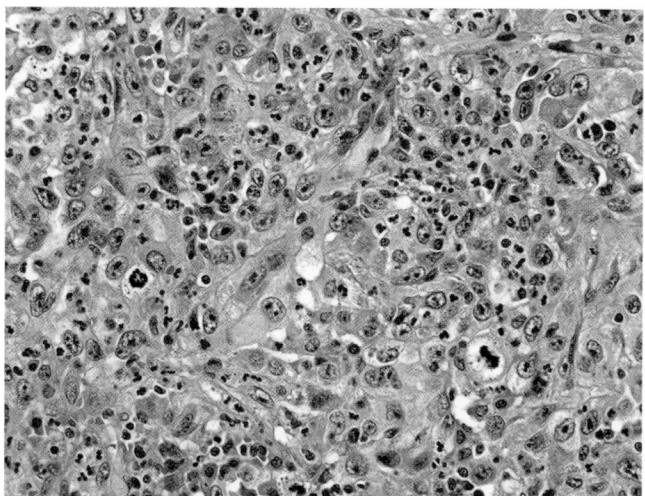

FIGURE 47.11 **Undifferentiated carcinoma.** This carcinoma is characterized by a diffuse, sheet-like growth pattern of large cells with prominent nucleoli. Note frequent mitoses.

and sarcomatoid carcinomas[68] represent the least differentiated end of the spectrum of adenocarcinomas, in which glandular differentiation is no longer detectable. These patterns can coexist with conventional adenocarcinomas, pointing to the close relationship of these tumor types. In sarcomatoid carcinomas, the cells acquire mesenchymal characteristics, including a spindle shape; in some cases, "heterologous" elements, such as bone and cartilage, occur. In the absence of a more epithelioid or glandular component or preinvasive neoplasia within the bile ducts, these tumors may be difficult to distinguish from true sarcomas. Some examples of undifferentiated carcinomas are associated with abundant osteoclast-like giant cells and are referred to as *undifferentiated carcinoma* with *osteoclast-like giant cells*. It has been well documented that these giant cells are of histiocytic origin, and the malignant cells in this tumor are the mononuclear cells in the background.[69-71]

Clinically Relevant Pathologic Parameters in Biliary Carcinomas

TUMOR TYPE. Whether the tumor is a conventional pancreatobiliary-type invasive adenocarcinoma or another type of neoplasm is important. For example, undifferentiated carcinoma has a worse outcome.[68]

INVASIVE VERSUS NONINVASIVE COMPONENTS. For carcinomas with predominantly intraductal/intracholecystic growth (discussed later), the extent of the noninvasive and invasive components should be reported separately.[18,22,72] In fact, cases of biliary adenocarcinomas associated with an unusually protracted clinical course are often predominantly intraductal/intracholecystic papillary neoplasms.[18]

PATHOLOGIC STAGE. The size and depth of the tumor are the most important aspects of pathologic staging of biliary carcinomas.[18,31,33,73,74] There are, however, pitfalls in establishing the depth of the tumor in some parts of the biliary tract, where unlike other sites, such as the GI tract, the layers that constitute the duct walls are not well defined. In particular, in parts of the CBD, the interface of the mucosa with the muscular layer and the interface of the muscle with the perimuscular tissue are highly irregular, which hinders the accurate evaluation of tumor depth.[74] Similarly, in the intrapancreatic segment of the CBD, the demarcation of the CBD from pancreatic lobules is highly variable, and how to evaluate invasion into the pancreas is controversial.[75] More strikingly, because the gallbladder mucosa is highly irregular, there is no clear-cut definition of what constitutes high-grade dysplasia (carcinoma in situ; Tis) versus early invasion of the lamina propria. Furthermore, there is no clear demarcation of the lamina propria (T1a) from the tunica muscularis (T1b) because the muscularis of gallbladder is irregular and lacunar, allowing for frequent mucosal invaginations. These distinctive aspects of the gallbladder render the "T" category of American Joint Committee on Cancer (AJCC) staging less applicable for many cases. Thus it is not surprising that several groups from regions where the incidence of gallbladder cancer is very high have independently adopted the term *early gallbladder carcinoma*[31,76–78] for carcinomas confined by the tunica muscularis, a concept encompassing the spectrum of cases that were meant to be classified as Tis, T1a, or T1b in the AJCC staging system. When penetration of the muscularis has been ruled out by thorough sampling, early gallbladder carcinoma has a very good prognosis.[31] These cases appear to be curable in most instances, reaching survival rates up to 92% at five years and 90% at 10 years with no significant differences between intramucosal and muscular cases.[79] In contrast, extension to Rokitansky-Aschoff sinuses with no definitive perisinusal infiltration has proven to be an independent prognostic factor in an early gallbladder carcinoma series.[31] Moreover, a preliminary study indicates that the amount/depth of perimuscular invasion may also be of importance, and cases that have only very minimal pT2 invasion may have a prognosis closer to that of early gallbladder carcinoma, if total sampling is performed to exclude deeper invasion.[80]

GRADING. The grading scheme, as advocated in the *Atlas of Tumor Pathology* series,[4] is based on the percent of the tumor that shows glandular differentiation (specifically, tubule formation). If more than 95% of the tumor is composed of tubules, it is well differentiated; 40% to 95% is moderately differentiated, and 5% to 39% is poorly differentiated. Tumors without glandular differentiation are regarded as undifferentiated.

PERINEURAL AND VASCULAR INVASION. Although the prognostic significance of perineural and vascular invasion has not been fully established, these findings are nevertheless regarded as components of the pathologic evaluation, especially in resection specimens.

ASSESSMENT OF SURGICAL MARGINS. Proper orientation of the specimen with identification of the margins by the surgical team using sutures or dyes often proves very helpful for accurate evaluation of the surgical margins, especially in complex specimens. The status of the resection margins is an important factor predictive of survival[81] and recurrence[82] (see Chapters 49, 50, and 51). Bile duct margins typically are amputated from the specimen and submitted *en face*, whereas hepatic and soft tissue margins are inked and sections are submitted perpendicular to the margin.

NONINVASIVE EPITHELIAL NEOPLASIA

Dysplasia/Biliary Intraepithelial Neoplasia

For microscopic, incidental forms of biliary preinvasive epithelial lesions, *dysplasia* is still more widely used in daily practice, especially for gallbladder lesions. In the 2019 World Health Organization (WHO) classification, however, the term *biliary intraepithelial neoplasia* (BilIN; see Fig. 47.6) is endorsed,[83] in analogy to pancreatic intraepithelial neoplasia (PanIN) in the pancreas. Recently, it has been reported that *KRAS* mutations are present in approximately 33% of intrahepatic BilIN lesions and, similar to the frequent clonal mutations in the *KRAS* oncogene found in PanIN lesions, these occur as an early molecular event during the progression of BilIN to cholangiocarcinoma, whereas *TP53* overexpression is identified as a later molecular event[84] (see Chapter 9E).

Dysplasia/BilIN can be seen in the mucosa adjacent to invasive biliary carcinomas and, occasionally, as an incidental finding in specimens obtained for other reasons. In general, it is a radiographically and grossly occult process characterized by cytoarchitectural atypia of the biliary epithelium, including nuclear enlargement, irregularities, loss of polarity, and mitotic activity.[28,83] Although various growth patterns and cell lineages have been described in the gallbladder, and certain lineages are reported to progress possibly more than others to invasive carcinoma,[85,86] large series with clinicopathologic correlation are needed to confirm this impression. Based on the degree of atypia, dysplasia/BilIN is graded as *low-* or *high-grade* (the former BilIN-1 and BilIN-2 categories are now classified as low-grade and the former BilIN-3 as high-grade).[83] Of note, in South America (especially Chile) and the Far East where these lesions are much better analyzed, the term *carcinoma in situ (CIS)* is preferred instead of high-grade dysplasia/BilIN.

Among biliary sites, dysplasia is the most common and best studied in the gallbladder, where low-grade dysplasia is reported in as many as 15% and high-grade dysplasia in as many as 3.5% of routine cholecystectomy specimens in geographic regions with a higher prevalence of gallbladder carcinoma[87–90] (see Chapter 49). In contrast, in an analysis of routine cholecystectomy specimens in a North American population, the incidence of low-grade dysplasia was less than 5% and high-grade dysplasia less than 1%.[91] The incidence of dysplasia in surgical specimens in the remainder of the biliary tract appears to be even lower. However, choledochal cysts (see Chapter 46) are associated with a high rate of BilIN (28.5%).[92] Similarly, when hepatic explants for cirrhosis resulting from alcohol abuse or hepatitis C are systematically evaluated, dysplasia—particularly low to intermediate grade—is found in more than half of cases.[93]

It should be kept in mind that the true frequency of dysplasia in the biliary tract is difficult to determine. Because the diagnostic criteria for dysplasia are highly subjective and reactive atypia in the biliary epithelium caused by inflammation or stenting are difficult to distinguish from dysplasia, it can make intraoperative frozen-section evaluation of bile duct margins challenging. Moreover, in patients with invasive carcinoma, dysplasia may be difficult to distinguish from retrograde mucosal involvement by invasive carcinoma, a phenomenon referred to as *colonization* of the surface epithelium.

In the gallbladder, dysplasia associated with invasive carcinomas appears to have no bearing on the prognosis (see Chapter 49). Cases of gallbladder dysplasia detected incidentally in the absence of invasive carcinoma appear to be clinically silent and have no documented clinical consequences, provided that the gallbladder has been thoroughly examined histologically to exclude occult foci of invasive carcinoma. However, data from the Surveillance, Epidemiology, and End Results (SEER) program of the National Cancer Institute indicate a 10-year age-adjusted survival of 80% to 90% for high-grade dysplasia (carcinoma in situ) of the gallbladder, suggesting that either a small invasive carcinoma was missed or that a second malignant neoplasm developed elsewhere in the patients' biliary systems.[94] Extrapolating from these observations, a field-effect phenomenon may occur in some cases, and patients with high-grade gallbladder dysplasia, especially if extensive, probably should have some surveillance to screen for a subsequent invasive biliary carcinoma. High-grade dysplasia (carcinoma in situ) of the gallbladder extending to the cystic duct margin can also be associated with invasive carcinoma more distal within the cystic duct, based on some anecdotal cases.[95] In the bile ducts, high-grade dysplasia (carcinoma in situ) rarely is detected in the absence of invasive carcinoma, so the clinical significance of isolated dysplasia is unclear. Such patients would presumably also have an increased risk for invasive bile duct carcinomas, and careful examination of the biliary tree to exclude a synchronous, discontinuous focus of invasive carcinoma would seem prudent.

Mass-Forming Intraepithelial Neoplasms

Mass-forming preinvasive epithelial neoplasms that project into the lumina of the gallbladder or bile ducts include a family of related entities that have been designated by many different terms depending on the location of the tumor, its architecture, and the cell types that it comprises. In the 2019 WHO classification, these lesions were regrouped as *intraductal papillary neoplasm*[22] in the bile ducts and *pyloric gland adenoma*[96] and *intracholecystic papillary neoplasm*[72] in the gallbladder. There are remarkable overlaps, however, and excessive subjectivity in classifying these lesions into *pyloric gland adenoma* and *intracholecystic papillary neoplasm* categories.[97] Therefore Adsay et al. proposed the unifying term of "intracholecystic papillary

tubular neoplasm" in the gallbladder to embrace lesions that form large (>1 cm) tumors that are distinguishable from the background mucosa and/or lesions that have a convincingly dysplastic epithelium.[18] The 1 cm cutoff point is arbitrary. It was chosen because it is used as a cutoff point for the indication to perform cholecystectomy,[98] and it is used for pancreatic lesions (i.e., intraductal neoplasms).[99] On the basis of the highest degree of cytoarchitectural atypia in the epithelium, intraductal papillary neoplasms and intracholecystic papillary tubular neoplasms are graded as low-grade or high-grade.[22,72] Recently, the biliary counterparts of pancreatic intraductal tubulopapillary neoplasm (ITPN), *intraductal tubular (or tubulopapillary) neoplasm of the bile ducts*[19,60,100,101] and *intracholecystic tubular nonmucinous neoplasms*,[102] have also been described.

In contrast to dysplasia/BilIN, these intraductal/intracholecystic neoplasms can be identified grossly as soft, polypoid tumors within the bile duct lumen.[18,19,60,102] Most are relatively localized, although multicentric or diffuse involvement can occur, as in so-called *papillomatosis*.[103–105] Cystic dilation of the bile ducts may occur[19,106] and, in some cases, may exhibit mucin hypersecretion.[107] The epithelial cell types in intraductal papillary neoplasms and intracholecystic papillary neoplasm include pancreatobiliary, gastric, intestinal, and oncocytic,[4,22,72] similar to the spectrum of intraductal papillary mucinous neoplasms (IPMNs) of the pancreas (see Chapter 60). Therefore some authors have referred to these tumors as *biliary IPMNs*.[107–111] In contrast, intraductal tubular (or tubulopapillary) neoplasms of the bile ducts and intracholecystic tubular nonmucinous neoplasms contain nonmucinous pancreatobiliary-type epithelium. It should be kept in mind that differences in the frequency and types of associated invasive carcinoma, as well as the morphology and immunophenotype, of these intraductal/intracholecystic neoplasms are significant.[18,19,22,60,83,102,112] Although the most associated invasive carcinomas are conventional tubular (pancreatobiliary-type) adenocarcinomas, similar to other bile duct carcinomas,[18,19,60] some cases have a mucinous (colloid) pattern, usually when the intraductal neoplasm is of the intestinal-type. Undifferentiated carcinoma and poorly differentiated neuroendocrine carcinoma have also been reported.[4]

Unlike with pancreatic IPMNs, *GNAS* codon 201 mutations are uncommon in intraductal papillary neoplasms of the bile ducts,[84,113] and the molecular alterations observed in intraductal tubular (or tubulopapillary) neoplasms of the bile ducts include *CDKN2A/p16* and *TP53*, but mutations in *KRAS*, *PIK3CA*, and loss of *SMAD4/DPC4* are rare[60] (see Chapters 9D and 9E). Of note, accumulating data suggest regional geographic differences in the proportion of intraductal papillary neoplasms with the different cell types, perhaps related to varying etiologic factors in different parts of the world.[107] In Asian patients, for example, an association of intraductal papillary neoplasms with *Clonorchis* infection has been reported[114] (see Chapter 45).

Noninvasive intraductal/intracholecystic neoplasms have an excellent prognosis. However, some noninvasive cases still follow an aggressive clinical course, likely because of missed foci of invasion or a field-effect phenomenon with multicentric biliary neoplasia, and therefore long-term follow up is recommended. Interestingly, even those associated with an invasive carcinoma have a better clinical outcome compared with conventional pancreatobiliary-type biliary carcinomas.[18,19,29,60,115]

One lesion to be distinguished from intraductal papillary neoplasms of the bile ducts is biliary mucinous cystic neoplasm, also known as *hepatobiliary cystadenoma.*[116,117] Biliary mucinous cystic neoplasms are analogous to mucinous cystic neoplasms of the pancreas and are also regarded as a type of mass-forming preinvasive neoplasm. They form cystic lesions that occur predominantly in adult women and exhibit pathognomonic hormone receptor-expressing ovarian-type subepithelial stroma.[117,118] The lining epithelium is composed of cuboidal to columnar cells, sometimes with abundant apical mucin. Papillary projections may be identified in the cyst lumen. Although most biliary mucinous cystic neoplasms show benign cytoarchitectural features, some may harbor foci of high-grade dysplasia (carcinoma in situ) or invasive carcinoma. Carcinoma can be focal, so thorough histologic examination is warranted.[117]

NEUROENDOCRINE NEOPLASMS

Well-differentiated neuroendocrine tumors (NETs; 2019 WHO Grade 1, 2 and 3 NETs) are rare but may occur in any part of the biliary tract.[119–123] They are seen predominantly in young or middle-aged adults. Most cases are nonfunctioning, and patients are seen with signs and symptoms of biliary obstruction. Rare examples may be associated with von Hippel-Lindau syndrome.[124] Grossly, well-differentiated NETs form relatively well-demarcated nodules and may be polypoid and mucosa covered. They are fleshy, firm, and homogeneous on cut sections. Microscopically, well-differentiated NETs are characterized by distinct nests separated by a fibrovascular stroma and strands of cells with round uniform nuclei, coarsely granular chromatin, and abundant cytoplasm (Fig. 47.12). Rarely, the cytoplasm may exhibit clear-cell, oncocytic, or signet ring-like changes.[125] The data on prognosis of biliary NETs are highly limited because of the rarity of these tumors, but their prognosis seem to be similar to that of NETs in the GI tract. Metastases can occur.[123] In the SEER database, the 10-year survival rate was 36% for gallbladder NETs and 80% for extrahepatic bile duct NETs, although these data may not be entirely reliable because pathologic confirmation is lacking.[121]

Rarely, paraganglioma,[126,127] a tumor that also displays neuroendocrine differentiation, may occur in the biliary tract.

Poorly-differentiated neuroendocrine carcinomas, namely *small-cell carcinoma* and *large-cell neuroendocrine carcinoma*, also occur in the region of biliary tree, predominantly in the gall bladder or distal CBD. Although these were classified as grade 3 neuroendocrine carcinomas in the previous (2010) WHO classification system, giving the impression that they are part of a continuum with the well-differentiated NETs, there is now evidence that poorly-differentiated neuroendocrine carcinomas actually constitute a genetically and biologically distinct tumor entity.[128,129] Therefore, in the current (2019) WHO classification, well-differentiated NETs and poorly differentiated neuroendocrine carcinomas are classified separately.[123]

Small-cell carcinomas (Fig. 47.13) are defined by the same histologic criteria applied to their counterparts in the lung (high nucleus/cytoplasm ratio, molding of nuclei, diffuse chromatin pattern, absence of nucleoli).[121,130-133] In cases with the typical cytologic features of small-cell carcinoma, it is not necessary to document neuroendocrine differentiation by immunohistochemistry. For large-cell neuroendocrine carcinomas,[134] however, positive immunohistochemical staining for chromogranin or synaptophysin should be obtained to confirm the diagnosis. Half of small-cell carcinomas are pure, but a significant proportion of large-cell neuroendocrine carcinomas are admixed with conventional adenocarcinomas.[131,132] These are classified as mixed neuroendocrine-nonneuroendocrine neoplasm (MiNEN).[123] Additionally, there is often associated dysplasia on the surface mucosa.[132]

These poorly differentiated neuroendocrine carcinomas are highly aggressive tumors with a rapidly fatal course and an overall prognosis that is worse than that of conventional pancreatobiliary-type adenocarcinoma.[121,132] However, these tend to be sensitive to chemotherapy with platinum-based protocols.[123]

OTHER TUMORS

Mesenchymal Tumors

Among the extremely rare mesenchymal tumors of the biliary tree, the one that warrants specific attention is embryonal (botyroid) rhabdomyosarcoma[135] because it is relatively more

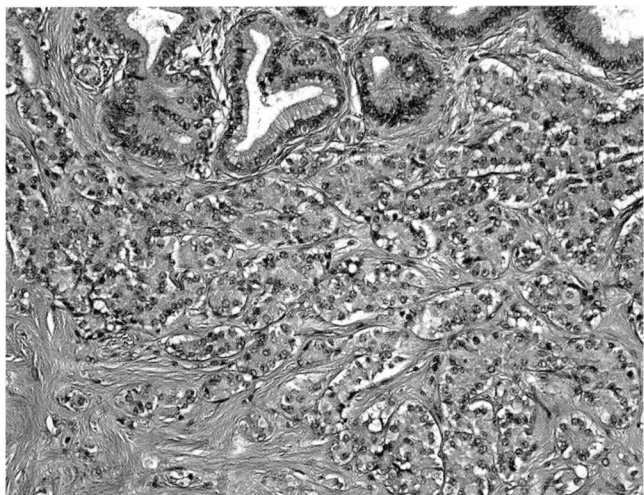

FIGURE 47.12 Well-differentiated neuroendocrine tumor. These tumors are characterized by relatively uniform cells with round nuclei and abundant cytoplasm, usually arranged in nests separated by prominent, delicate vasculature.

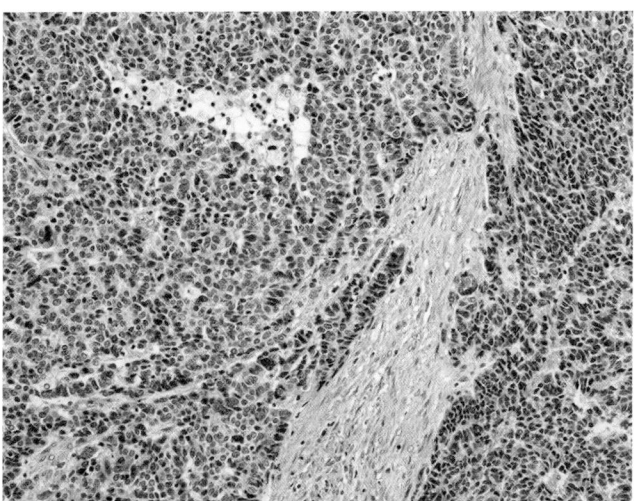

FIGURE 47.13 Small-cell carcinoma. The cells are relatively small, with a high nucleus-to-cytoplasm ratio, hyperchromatic nuclei, and nuclear molding.

common and well characterized in this region. These are predominantly seen in children three to four years old and constitute 1% of all rhabdomyosarcomas (see Chapter 93). The tumor consists of a conglomerate of soft, mucosa-covered polyps filling the lumen. Size ranges from 3 to 14 cm, and the most common site is the CBD. Beneath the surface layer of flattened biliary epithelium is a dense zone of primitive spindle cells, representing the cambium layer. Cytoplasmic cross-striations may be seen, and skeletal muscle differentiation is demonstrable by immunohistochemical staining for actin, desmin, or myoD1. Although the prognosis is poor, multimodal therapy has resulted in long-term survival in some patients. Metastases occur in 40% of patients, but death usually is caused by the local effects of the tumor.

Granular cell tumor is another mesenchymal tumor that occurs in this region, predominantly in the CBD. It is characterized by cells containing abundant acidophilic granular cytoplasm, occasionally with larger globules. This tumor is of uncertain origin, but most evidence, including expression of S-100 protein, indicates a relationship to Schwann cells. Although it has an infiltrative appearance, granular cell tumor is benign with only minimal recurrence potential, even when incompletely excised.[136–138]

A variety of other mesenchymal tumors have been documented in the biliary tree, both benign and malignant. Benign tumors include hemangioma,[139] lymphangioma,[140] neurofibroma,[141] schwannoma,[142] ganglioneuroma (almost always associated with multiple endocrine neoplasia type 2b),[143] leiomyoma,[144] myofibroblastic tumors, lipoma,[144] and osteoma.[145] Malignant mesenchymal tumors include angiosarcoma,[146] Kaposi sarcoma,[147] leiomyosarcoma,[148] chondrosarcoma, peripheral nerve sheath tumor,[149] and malignant fibrous histiocytoma. These tumors are documented mostly as case reports.[2–4,150] Before a case is classified as sarcoma, the possibility of a sarcomatoid carcinoma must be carefully considered.

Secondary Tumors

The biliary tree may be involved by a variety of carcinomas originating in other organs, especially the pancreas, stomach, colon, kidney, and breast, either by metastasis or direct invasion.[2–4,150] Among these, metastatic renal cell carcinoma is notorious for mimicking a primary tumor because it may form a polypoid luminal lesion, and the history of the primary tumor may be remote. Similarly, melanomas may also form polypoid lesions and mimic primary tumors (Fig. 47.14), and often the history of melanoma may not be apparent. Metastases from primary colorectal cancer to the biliary epithelium have also been described[151] and can mimic intraductal papillary neoplasms.

Hematopoietic Malignancies

The biliary tree may be involved by hematopoietic malignancies (lymphoma, myeloma, or leukemia) as a part of systemic disease; rarely, this may be the initial presentation.[2–4,150] Primary lymphomas of the mucosa-associated lymphoid tissue type also have been reported.

TUMOR-LIKE LESIONS

In addition to sclerosing cholangitis (see Chapter 41), a few other nonneoplastic conditions of the biliary tract may present as tumors

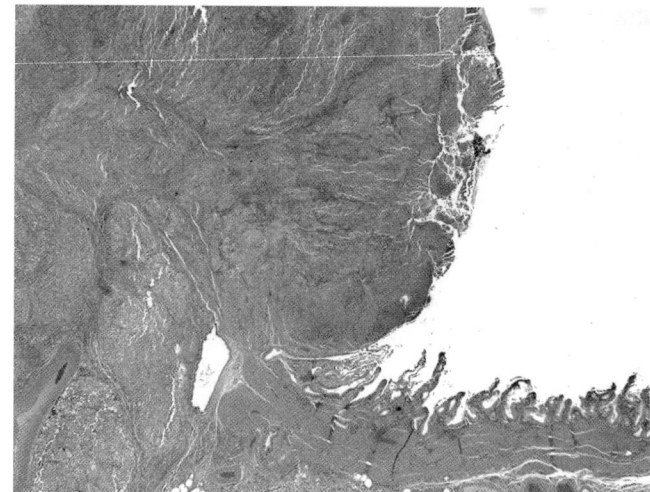

FIGURE 47.14   Melanoma. Metastatic melanomas may mimic primary carcinomas in the gallbladder and biliary tract, sometimes even forming polypoid tumors.

(see Chapter 48). Rarely, heterotopic tissue, especially pancreatic tissue,[152,153] may form a mass. Traumatic, or "amputation," neuroma,[154,155] which is an exuberant regenerative proliferation of transected nerves, may form a tumor-like nodule, typically in the cystic duct stump, that may mimic a carcinoma. These are very rare and may be seen with obstruction-related signs and symptoms, sometimes several years after the intervention.

Certain types of tumor-like lesions occur rather frequently in the gallbladder but not often in the remainder of the biliary tree. Two distinct categories were delineated: (1) injury-related polyps such as fibro(myo)glandular polyps, metaplastic pyloric glands forming polypoid collections, and inflammatory-type polyps associated with acute/subacute injury, and (2) cholesterol polyps.[15] Cystic change in Rokitansky-Aschoff sinuses and adenomyomatous hyperplasia also frequently form pseudotumors in the gallbladder; however, these are not seen in the bile ducts.

Immunoglobulin G4 (IgG4)-related sclerosing disease may affect the bile ducts and gallbladder.[157] As in autoimmune pancreatitis type 1, a prototypical organ manifestation of IgG4-related disease, this is characterized by a dense, subepithelial lymphoplasmacytic inflammatory infiltrate; dense fibrosis, often with a storiform pattern; and obliterative venulitis. There is an association with elevated levels of IgG4 in the serum, and IgG4-expressing plasma cells can be found in large numbers within the lesions by immunohistochemistry.[158] These processes form a tumor-like mass that can be mistaken for carcinoma on imaging studies[21] (see Chapter 42). Some cases are associated with autoimmune pancreatitis type 1,[159] whereas others present with disease limited to the gallbladder or bile ducts. In such cases, a more specific diagnosis of IgG4-related sclerosing cholecystitis may be justifiable.[157,160] However, careful clinical correlation with exclusion of other etiologies is required before such a diagnosis can be rendered. These autoimmune lesions are sensitive to corticosteroid therapy, so their distinction from carcinomas is clinically important.

References are available at expertconsult.com.

CHAPTER 48

Benign tumors and pseudotumors of the biliary tract

Eva Galka and David Linehan

Although uncommon, benign tumors and pseudotumors may arise from the intrahepatic and extrahepatic biliary ducts and gallbladder. These lesions may originate from both the epithelial and nonepithelial structures that comprise the biliary ducts and gallbladder (Box 48.1). Epithelial tumors include adenomas, cystadenomas, and biliary papillomatosis, and nonepithelial tumors consist of granular cell tumors, neurofibromas, and leiomyomas. Finally there are the tumor-like lesions and pseudotumors, including primary sclerosing cholangitis, sclerosing pancreatitis/autoimmune pancreatitis (AIP), and heterotopia. These entities are difficult to diagnose before surgical intervention because of their shared symptoms of obstructive jaundice and lack of specific imaging findings. These are the malignant masqueraders that create the ultimate diagnostic and therapeutic challenges.

Although most are benign, a few also represent premalignant lesions in which surgical intervention would be curative. Tissue biopsy does not often alter therapy in appropriate-risk patients with resectable lesions. The majority of these tumors show nonspecific clinical and radiographic features that make diagnosis difficult, if not impossible, without resection. Intraoperative frozen section will not always reveal an accurate diagnosis but is helpful for ensuring clear margins.

In this chapter, we will first review the embryology and anatomy of the biliary tract and then discuss the clinical presentation and diagnostic evaluation of patients with benign tumors and pseudotumors of the biliary tract. Benign tumors and pseudotumors of the biliary tract can broadly be classified into the following general categories: papilloma and adenoma, granular cell tumor, neurofibroma, leiomyoma, neuroendocrine tumor, and pseudotumor. Pseudotumors of the biliary tract comprise inflammatory entities such as primary sclerosing cholangitis, sclerosing pancreatitis, immunoglobulin G4 (IgG4) cholangitis, and heterotopia.

EMBRYOLOGIC AND ANATOMIC FACTORS
(SEE CHAPTERS 1 AND 2)

Benign tumors comprising a variety of histologic types have been observed in the extrahepatic ducts and gallbladder because of their common embryology. During the fourth week of embryogenesis, the biliary system will arise from the most caudal aspect of the foregut as a ventral bud. This small outpouching is the anlage of the liver, extrahepatic biliary ducts, gallbladder, and the ventral bud of the pancreas.

The diverticulum divides into a superior and inferior bud as it grows into the ventral mesogastrium (Fig. 48.1A) A ventral pancreatic bud develops from the superior surface of the diverticulum, proximal to the enlarging terminal sacculations. The cranial sacculation, the larger of the two, pushes ventrally and cranially into the septum transversum, which separates the thoracic from the celomic cavity. Composed of a solid mass of endodermal cells, the cranial sacculation spreads out into the substance of the septum transversum, eventually forming the right and left lobes of the liver. Cephalad growth and extension of the cranial sacculation results in stretching of the endodermal cell mass from the duodenum to the liver, which will form into the extrahepatic biliary tree. At approximately the seventh week of intrauterine life, vacuolization takes place within the solid mass of cells of the primitive extrahepatic biliary tree leading to a ductal lumen.

Before the 7-mm stage, the common bile duct (CBD) is attached to the ventral surface of the duodenum close to the ventral pancreatic bud. At the 7-mm stage, left-to-right rotation of the ventral pancreas and duodenum takes place so that the CBD ultimately enters the posteromedial surface of the duodenum (see Fig. 48.1B–C). The gallbladder and cystic duct develop concurrently from the caudal portion of the primitive hepatic diverticulum during the same period.[1]

The extrahepatic duct lies in the right border of the hepatoduodenal ligament between serosal surfaces and is composed of mucosa, fibrous tissue, and serosa. The dense connective tissue beneath the mucosa comprises collagen, elastic fibers, and scattered smooth muscle fibers, which are not a prominent component. The muscle layer becomes more prominent at the cystic duct, forming the valves of Heister and near the sphincter of Oddi.[2] The CBD most often will join the pancreatic duct at the terminal portion but may fail to unite and enter separately.[3] The thickness of the duct wall varies from 0.8 to 1.5 mm, with an average of approximately 1.1 mm.[4]

The extrahepatic ducts are lined by a single layer of columnar epithelium which rests on the basement membrane and lamina propria and contains mucous glands (see Chapter 47). Scattered chromogranin-positive cells can be found in glands of the normal gallbladder neck, and rare cells immunoreactive for somatostatin have been found between the lining epithelium of

---

BOX 48.1   Benign Tumors and Pseudotumors That Can Cause Bile Duct Obstruction

Epithelial Tumors
Adenoma
Papilloma
Cystadenoma (intrahepatic)

Nonepithelial Tumors
Leiomyoma
Lipoma
Hemangioma
Lymphangioma
Granular cell tumor
Osteoma

Neural Tumors
Neurofibroma
Schwannoma
Neuroendocrine tumors

Pseudotumors
Idiopathic benign focal stricture
Lymphoplasmacytic sclerosing pancreatitis
Sclerosing cholangitis
Heterotopic tissue

Modified from Levy AD, Murakata LA, Abbott RM, Rohrmann Jr CA. Benign tumors and tumor-like lesions of the gallbladder and extra-hepatic bile ducts: radiologic–pathologic correlation. *Radiographics.* 2002;22:387–413.

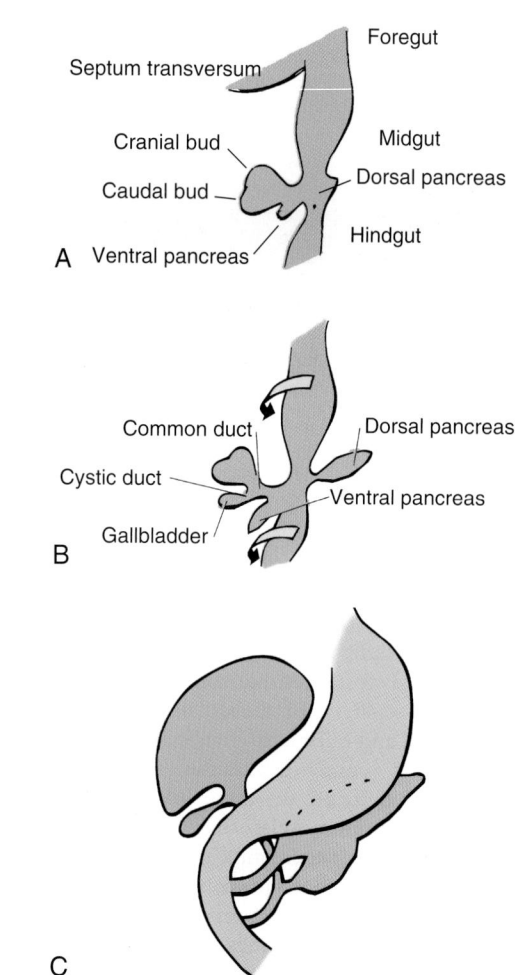

FIGURE 48.1   A, At approximately the fifth week of intrauterine life, a diverticulum evolves near the junction of the midgut and hindgut and grows into the ventral mesogastrium. The ventral pancreatic bud develops from the superior surface as the cranial sacculation and pushes cephalad into the septum transversum. **B,** The gallbladder and extrahepatic ducts develop from the caudal bud, and the liver develops from the cranial bud. The ventral pancreas evolves in close relationship to the developing common bile duct. **C,** At the 7-mm stage, left-to-right rotation occurs, resulting in subsequent fusion of the pancreas, gallbladder, duodenum, and extrahepatic bile ducts into their normal anatomic relationship. (See Chapter 1.)

the hepatic duct in patients with biliary disease.[5] Chronic inflammation of the biliary tract leading to intestinal metaplasia of the mucosa and increase in enterochromaffin (Kulchitsky) cells is a possible basis for development of carcinoid tumors of the biliary tree.[6] The epithelial surface of the duct is generally flat except for tiny pits in the mucosa known as *sacculi of Beale,* which are luminal openings for the intramural mucous glands. As the duct penetrates the wall of the duodenum, the mucosa appears to become thickened and the surface roughened by longitudinal folds of mucosa, or *valvules,* particularly at the terminal end of the duct. The valvules were first described in the *Fabrica* of Vesalius[7] in 1543, followed later by a more detailed description by Santorini[8] in 1724. Brown and Echenberg[9] described a more frequent occurrence of transverse oriented flaps or valvules that face the duodenal lumen and probably function to prevent reflux of duodenal contents into the biliary tree and pancreatic ducts (Fig. 48.2). Baggenstoss[10] also reported that free folds of ductal epithelia in the form of papillary processes may extend 2 to 3 mm beyond the ampullary orifice. Microscopically, a definite transition exists between the mucosa of the duct within the ampulla and the surrounding duodenal mucosa. The ductal mucosa of the ampulla exhibits numerous papillary processes much larger than the adjacent duodenal villi.

The gallbladder wall is composed of a columnar epithelial mucosa with an underlying basement membrane and lamina propria, irregular smooth muscle, perimuscular connective tissue, and serosa. The perimuscular connective tissue is composed of nerves, blood vessels, lymphatics, and paraganglia.[11]

CLINICAL PRESENTATION AND DIAGNOSIS

Patients with benign biliary tract tumors and inflammatory pseudotumors present with symptoms of jaundice as a result of obstruction of the bile duct. The icterus may be insidious and intermittent and may be associated with epigastric pain. Most benign biliary duct tumors are slow in growth and therefore symptoms may be gradually progressive. There are no clinical symptoms that can differentiate benign tumors from malignant counterparts. Likewise, the physical findings are nonspecific but may include hepatic enlargement, palpable gallbladder, tenderness in the right hypochondrium, and jaundice. The lack of characteristic signs and symptoms contributes to the lack of diagnosis before surgical intervention.

Percutaneous transhepatic cholangiography (PTC) and endoscopic retrograde cholangiopancreatography (ERCP) have

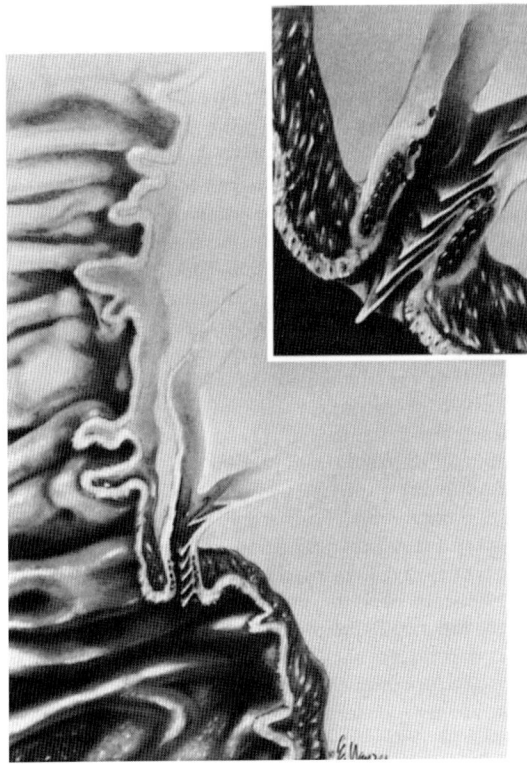

FIGURE 48.2 Artist's representation of the macroscopic anatomy of the choledochoduodenal junction, depicting the transverse valvules described by Brown and Echenberg (1964) that prevents reflux from the duodenum.

historically been the mainstay of preoperative diagnosis of extrahepatic biliary obstruction for several decades. Noninvasive imaging of the biliary tree with magnetic resonance cholangiopancreatography (MRCP) and multiphase computed tomography (CT) play a more dominant role in diagnosis of these lesions currently. Endoscopic ultrasound (EUS) is another useful modality in the assessment of biliary lesions. EUS may visualize lesions not detected by magnetic resonance imaging (MRI) and CT and provides additional assessment of regional lymphadenopathy and vascular involvement.

Unfortunately, none of the described imaging modalities can reliably distinguish benign from malignant obstruction of the biliary ducts but allow visualization and characterization of biliary obstruction with either mass, stricture or ulceration as well as provide tumor location, size, and extent of biliary involvement.

PAPILLOMA AND ADENOMA

Although all benign lesions of the extrahepatic biliary tree are uncommon, the most prevalent are those characterized as papilloma, adenomatous papilloma, or adenoma. Papilloma and adenomas arise from the glandular epithelium of the bile duct. The distinctive quality of papilloma is growth of the superficial epithelium into a frond-like tumor compared with that of the adenoma, which arises from glandular tissue deep within the crypts of Lieberkuhn.[12]

The pathogenesis of bile duct adenomas remains unclear, but mounting evidence suggests reactivity to injury. High MUC6 expression (94%) was found by Hughes et al.,[13] which

was indistinguishable from pyloric gland metaplasia. Based on the similarities to pyloric gland metaplasia it is concluded that adenomas develop as a biliary healing response to injury similar to metaplasia in the foregut.[13] Elevated Ki-67 and p53 staining support malignant potential of these lesions.[14] Several groups have reported atypia, dysplasia, and foci of carcinoma in situ in papilloma and adenoma, supporting the idea that these lesions have a malignant potential.[15,16] Malignancy potential is also supported by clinical findings of recurrence and development of metastasis in incomplete resection.[17]

There is a female predominance (70%), with a mean age at presentation of between 48 and 58.[18,19] Adenomas of the extrahepatic duct can be classified as solid, cystic, or mixed. The least common subtype is cystadenoma, which has a higher female predominance of 90% and was first reported in 1929.[18] Adenomas also may be classified by their architecture as tubular, papillary, and tubulopapillary and by their cytoarchitecture as pyloric gland, intestinal type, and biliary type.[17] The pyloric gland adenoma is more common in the gallbladder, whereas biliary-type adenoma is more common within the extrahepatic biliary tract.[17] Papillomatosis describes papillary lesions that are multifocal within the biliary tract and have a high incidence of high-grade dysplasia.[20] This entity will be described in more detail later.

Anatomic distribution within the biliary tree is shown in Figure 48.3. They are most commonly present within or adjacent to the ampulla and distal CBD. Because of their prevalence in the distal bile duct, adenomas may protrude through

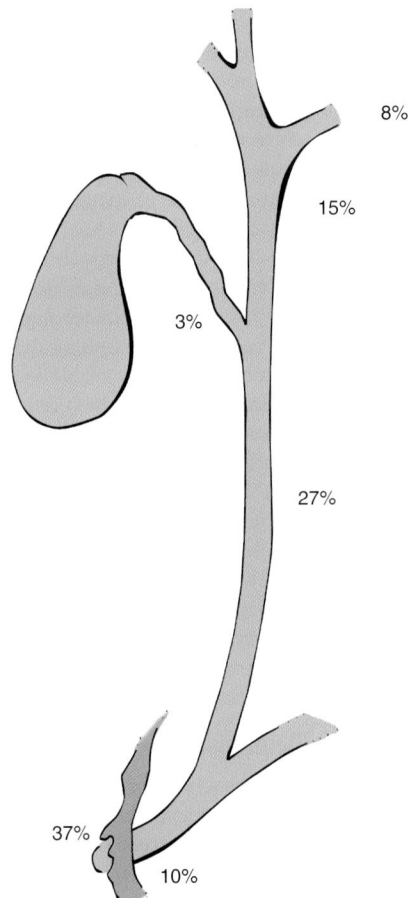

FIGURE 48.3 Location and frequency of papillomas and adenomas reported between the hepatic duct confluence and the ampulla of Vater.

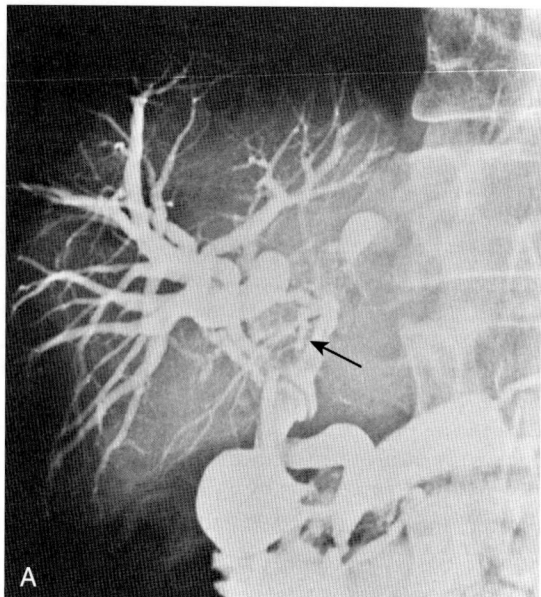
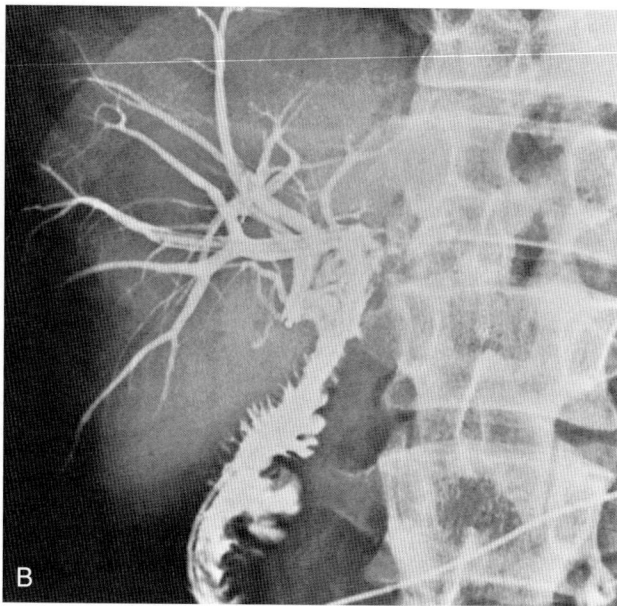

FIGURE 48.4   A, T-tube cholangiogram obtained after initial choledochotomy in a patient who presented with intermittent attacks of jaundice. At surgery, loose tumor particles were found in the common bile duct and proved to be fragments of papilloma. The T-tube enters the main right hepatic duct, and a residual filling defect is seen in the left ducts *(arrow).* **B,** Tube cholangiogram following subsequent left hepatic lobectomy and reconstruction by hepaticojejunostomy Roux-en-Y. The anastomosis is widely patent. The tube was removed, and the patient was alive and well 4 years later. (Reproduced with permission from Gouma DJ, Mutum SS, Benjamin IS, et al, Intrahepatic biliary papillomatosus. *Br J Surg.* 1984:71:72–74.)

the ampulla, leading to intermittent obstruction. These lesions are generally soft and pliable, which may also contribute to intermittent obstruction. Symptoms of right upper quadrant abdominal pain are often intermittent. Jaundice is present in 90% of patients and may be intermittent in 40% of these patients,[21] which may be due to intermittent obstruction. Lesions may remain dormant for many years.[14,22]

There are no distinguishing features radiographically to differentiate from cholangiocarcinoma (Fig. 48.4) (see Chapters 16 and 51A). Ultrasound may show a nonshadowing mass with a pedicle. ERCP will reveal an intraluminal filling defect. Lesions protruding through the ampulla may be visible via endoscopy. This is in contrast to malignant lesions, which tend to infiltrate and have overlying ulceration.

Several studies have indicated high recurrence rates in patients with local tumor excision alone.[3,18,23] Surgical resection is recommended in appropriate candidates and should include complete resection of the lesion with the duct wall to prevent recurrence and malignant transformation. Complex endoscopic resection has been performed in an adenoma of the biliary tree[24] and for papillomas,[25] but longer-term follow-up is lacking to support this treatment. Ongoing surveillance would be recommended in these cases.

Multiple Biliary Papillomatosis

Multiple biliary papillomatosis (MPB) is an entity characterized by multiple mucin-secreting papillary adenomas within the intrahepatic and extrahepatic biliary tree. In 2010 the (WHO) adopted the term *intraductal papillary neoplasm of the bile duct* (IPNB) to describe these biliary epithelial tumors with papillary projections within the biliary tree. This term encompasses previously described MPB. Previously considered a low-grade malignancy, it is now regarded as a precursor for cholangiocarcinoma.

Histologically, the tumors are a papillary or villous neoplasm with a fibrovascular stalk covered by epithelial cells. The epithelium is composed of columnar or cuboidal cells with basal nuclei, which in some cases are mucin secreting. Generally, there is minimal pleomorphism.

Proposed risk factors include hepatolithiasis (see Chapter 39), clonorchiasis infection (see Chapter 45), primary sclerosing cholangitis (see Chapter 41), biliary malformation, and familial adenomatous polyposis or Gardner syndrome.[26] Induction of metaplasia or hyperplasia is incompletely understood but may be due to chronic biliary inflammation by stones, infection, or pancreatic enzyme secretion.

The pathogenesis of IPNB is becoming better understood with a plethora of investigations. Carcinoma within the bile duct occurs through a multistep process via separate precursor pathways. Mimicking the sequence of pancreatic intraepithelial neoplasm progression to pancreatic cancer, biliary intraepithelial neoplasia (BIN) begins as biliary dysplasia and progressively advances from mild dysplasia to moderate dysplasia, to severe dysplasia/carcinoma in situ. In the setting of IPNB, an alternative pathway is thought to exist, with proliferation of the epithelium on fibrovascular stalks within the biliary tract.[27,28]

Three clinicopathologic subtypes have been described: exophytic and papillary proliferation of epithelial cells with fibrovascular stalk within the bile duct lumen; a similar variant with mucin hypersecretion; and lastly, prominent dilatation with multilocular cystic changes with prominent dilatation.[28] Cytologic features of the neoplastic epithelial cells are classified into three phenotypes similar to intraductal papillary neoplasm of the pancreas: pancreaticobiliary, intestinal, gastric, and oncocytic.[27,29] The oncocytic subtype appears to be the least common. Assessment of expression of mucin proteins and molecular analysis of mutations has been increasing in the literature and comparison to the findings in IPMN has been of particular interest. The relative frequency of the subtypes of IPNB has generally shown a greater frequency of the pancreaticobiliary subtype in several studies in America and Europe[29–32]; however, the intestinal subtype was the most frequent in Asian patients.[33] The gastric subtype appears to be less common in IPNB as compared with the pancreas counterpart.

Whereas subtype has well-established prognostic significance in IPMN of the pancreas, this is less clear in IPNB. IPNB Reports of incidence of invasive carcinoma has been found to be as high as 70% to 80% of resected specimens[28,30]; however, subtype analysis has not shown consistency in studies. Two groups were unable to show prognostic differences in subtypes in their large series.[28,30]

Emerging studies support that IPNB have a strong similarity to IPMN of the pancreas (see Chapter 60); however, the profile of IPNB appears more similar to that of main duct pancreatic IPMN, with greater expression of pancreaticobiliary and intestinal subtype, MUC expression, and risk of malignancy.[28]

The median age at presentation for intraductal papillary lesions of the biliary duct is 60 to 66 years, with male predominance (male to female 2:1). There is a higher incidence in Asian countries, accounting for 10% to 30% bile duct tumors in Korea, Japan, and China[34,35] compared with 7% to 11% in Western countries.[30] Most commonly, the disease affects both intrahepatic and extrahepatic bile ducts (42%) whereas 27% may involve the intrahepatic ducts alone and another 27% have only extrahepatic involvement.

Patients usually present with obstructive jaundice that may be intermittent but recurrent and complicated by cholangitis (see Chapter 43). Intermittent obstruction may be due to episodes of intermittent shedding of tumor fragments, mucin obstruction, or bleeding. Rarely, cholelithiasis and choledocholithiasis are encountered.

Sonographic imaging in biliary papillomatosis primarily shows intrahepatic and extrahepatic biliary dilation; however, nonshadowing single or multiple intraluminal masses may be present with medium echotexture.[36,37] CT imaging will demonstrate biliary dilation and may show intraductal soft-tissue masses before contrast. MRI has been less commonly described; however, it shows low signal intensity on T1-weighted images and hyperintense on T2-weighted images.[11] Tumors that produce significant mucin may have a jelly-like consistency.[37] Cholangiography classically shows multiple, polypoid filling defects within dilated bile ducts that do not clear with irrigation[36] (Fig. 48.5). Endoscopic examination of the papilla of Vater may show a wide-open orifice filled with mucin similar to that seen in main duct IPMN. Endoscopic ultrasound may have added benefit in assessing involvement of the bile duct wall and visualization and biopsy of adjacent lymph nodes indicating regional metastasis.[38–40]

Because of the multifocal nature, therapeutic intervention has several challenges. In cases of involvement confined to a lobe of the liver or solitary extrahepatic involvement, surgical resection should be considered. Pancreatectomy, hemihepatectomy, bile duct resection, segmental liver resection, and liver transplant have been performed with success. Radical resection with hepatectomy, extrahepatic biliary duct resection and pancreaticoduodenectomy for diffuse disease is not supported in the literature as beneficial at this time given the elevated recurrence risk. Palliation with choledochoscopic laser ablation, iridium-192 intraluminal therapy, percutaneous cholangioscopic electrocoagulation,

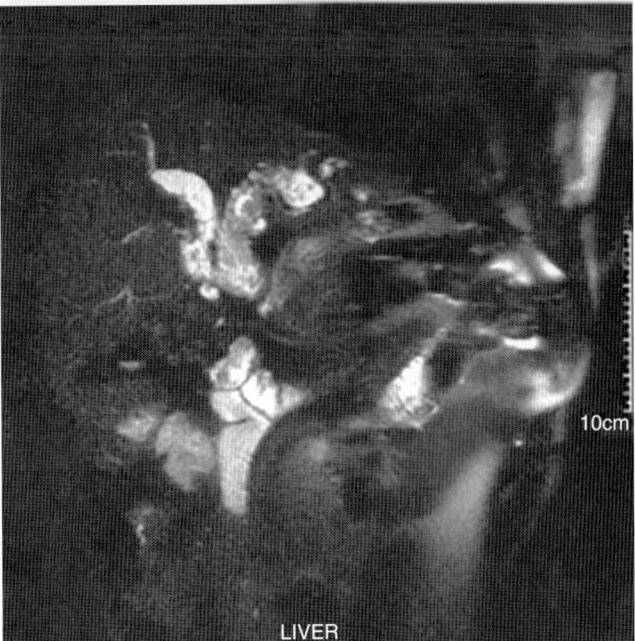

FIGURE 48.5 T2-weighted magnetic resonance imaging demonstrates biliary papillomatosis involving the left hepatic duct system in a 60-year-old patient who presented with intermittent jaundice and pruritus. The patient underwent a left hemihepatectomy with caudate lobe resection and excision of the extrahepatic biliary tree with hepaticojejunostomy. Histopathologic findings were consistent with biliary papillomatosis, with mild to moderate dysplasia involving a majority of the extrahepatic biliary tree and extending into the intrahepatic biliary tree. The patient ultimately developed progressive papillomatosis requiring liver transplantation. (Reproduced from White AD, Young AL, Verbeke C, et al. Biliary papillomatosis in three Caucasian patients in a Western centre. *Eur J Surg Oncol.* 2012;38:181–184.)

and external beam radiotherapy have all been described, with limited benefit.[41]

GRANULAR CELL TUMORS

Granular cell tumors (GCTs) are rare soft tissue tumors usually found in the skin, soft tissues, and oral cavity, although they may arise anywhere in the body. Presence in the extrahepatic bile duct is rare with case reports of fewer than 100 in the literature. First described in the skeletal muscle of the tongue by Abrikossoff[42] in 1926 as granular cell myoblastoma (myoblastic myomata), more recently the myoblast cell origin has been questioned and several groups have suggested Schwann cell origin. The pathogenesis remains poorly understood. There is mounting evidence for Schwann cell origin as suggested by ultrastructural and immunohistochemical patterns, including staining for S-100, polyclonal neuron-specific enolase (NSE), myelin basic protein, laminin, Leu 7, and cathepsin B, as well as lack of staining for neurofilament glial fibrillary acidic protein (GFAP).[43] The classic ultrastructural characteristics include myelin figures and membrane-bound vacuoles with debris and fragments of mitochondria and endoplasmic reticulum.

Generally considered benign, evidence of malignancy has been rarely discovered (<2%) but none have been described in GCTs of the biliary tree.[44–46] They are considered benign because of lack of atypia, necrosis, mitosis, and low Ki-67 proliferation index.[47] Prognosis is excellent when complete surgical excision is performed. Complete excision reduces the risk of recurrence, but recurrence has been noted in at least two studies in 6 in 92 cases[46] and 5 of 118 cases.[48] GCTs located in the bile duct are indistinguishable from those in the skin and soft tissues. Grossly they appear as a firm, round mass or infiltration of the duct wall. Clinically patients develop obstructive jaundice with abdominal pain and pruritus indistinguishable from malignant causes. Imaging notes a bile duct stricture with proximal dilation of the biliary tree. The most frequent sites of occurrence within the extrahepatic biliary tree is the CBD, but they have been noted in the common hepatic duct, cystic duct and gallbladder.[43]

Usually solitary, few cases of multifocal lesions have been reported in GCT or the biliary tree. In some series, upward of 16% of patients had multiple primary lesions.[46] There is a rare familial component with one study indicating a familial occurrence in 3 of 37 patients.[46,49]

The median age of diagnosis in this tumor is 34 years.[50] There is a female predominance with a female-to-male ratio of 4:1 in all GCTs, and this is consistent in tumors involving the biliary tree. There is also a predominance in individuals of African descent, with larger case series noting as high as 66% of patients.[46,48,51] Multiple lesions in the biliary tree have been described but account for only five reported cases.[52,53] Multiple lesions were more frequent in Blacks as was a higher propensity for malignancy.[49]

Although granular cell tumors are uncommon, they should remain in the differential in young Black women with biliary obstruction, stricture, and lack of gallstones.

NEUROFIBROMA

Neurofibroma is another rare tumor of the bile duct. These benign tumors arise from Schwann cells of nerve sheaths. Although they most often occur in the setting of neurofibromatosis, solitary tumors are possible. In the bile duct these arise from the sympathetic and parasympathetic nerve fibers that make up the wall of the CBD.[54]

In the absence of neurofibromatosis, almost all are secondary to operative trauma and have been described after cholecystectomy and hepatic transplantation.[55,56] Traumatic neurofibromas are proposed to be due to traumatic rupture of the epineurium leading to proliferation of the nerve fibers in the connective tissue surrounding the nerve. Primary neurofibroma in the absence of surgical injury has been described and likely occurs as a result of chronic inflammation from inflammatory lesions, infection, or gallstones. In these cases, it is postulated that the chronicity of inflammation leads to primary axonal proliferation within the epineurium.[57]

Grossly, these appear as a distinct mass with thickening of the bile duct wall. Histologically they appear as a mass with nerve bundles or nerve stump with infiltration of the bile duct. Pathologic evaluation shows long spindle cells arranged in a palisading pattern that are positive for S100, a marker for neurofilament protein.[54]

Clinically they create the same symptoms as malignant counterparts with obstructive jaundice and variable abdominal pain, pruritus, and/or fever. Imaging characteristics are nondiagnostic with presence of a homogeneous mass or biliary stricture. These tumors should be considered in the differential in the setting of delayed biliary obstruction after hepatic transplantation specifically when there is failure of percutaneous dilation or stenting[56] (see Chapter 111).

NEUROENDOCRINE TUMORS

Neuroendocrine tumors (NETs) of the extrahepatic bile duct are exceedingly rare (see Chapter 47). They arise from Kulchitsky cells, which are present throughout the gastrointestinal and respiratory tracts. Presence in the biliary tree is sparse, but somatostatin D cells have been demonstrated in the extrahepatic bile duct.[5] A recent report indicated that the incidence of neuroendocrine tumors of the extrahepatic bile duct was 0.67% of all GEP-NETs.[58]

Almost all NETs are nonfunctional hormonally; however, a case of peptic ulcer resulting from CBD carcinoid with gastrin production has been described. In this case, the ulcer resolved without therapy after resection of the tumor indicating the presence of a functional tumor.[59] None of the reported series have reported carcinoid syndrome. Although there are no known predisposing factors, it has been suggested that chronic inflammation of the bile duct may cause intestinal metaplasia, increasing the proliferation of neuroendocrine cells.

According to the World Health Organization (WHO) classification, neuroendocrine tumors of the extrahepatic bile ducts and gallbladder are classified according to differentiation and biologic aggressiveness.[60] Grades 1 and 2 are considered neuroendocrine tumors of less aggressive behavior and Grade 3 is considered neuroendocrine carcinoma. The last classification is that of mixed adenoneuroendocrine carcinoma (MANEC).

NETs may arise from all areas of the extrahepatic biliary tree but appear to be more common in the CBD than common hepatic, cystic duct, or gallbladder. There is a female predominance with female-to-male ratio of 1.05 to 2.2:1 and peak incidence is in the fifth decade.[61]

NETs may be distinguished by shape, involvement of bile duct, and upstream dilation. In one study that evaluated the radiographic findings of extrahepatic biliary NETs, three growth patterns were noted: nodular, intraductal growth, and periductal infiltration. A nodular growth pattern describes a mass with stricture of the bile duct, whereas the intraductal growing pattern was noted to have a mass without bile duct constriction. The periductal infiltrating subtype was defined as presence of bile duct thickening without a definite mass. There was an equal distribution between the nodular and intraductal growing radiographic findings (45% each) and less commonly the periductal infiltrating type.[62] This is in contrast with adenocarcinoma of the extrahepatic biliary duct in which periductal infiltration is more commonly seen.

CT and MRI are both useful for diagnosis and surgical evaluation of NETs (see Chapter 16) Figure 48.6. Signal intensity of NETs vary with each modality but appear to have hyperintensity of tumor and wall thickening in the arterial phase of CT imaging. It has been suggested that positron emission tomography (PET)/CT is of less use in neuroendocrine tumors due to low sensitivity; however, enhancement has been noted in neuroendocrine carcinoma. Functional imaging with PET/CT-68Ga-DOTATATE shows improved sensitivity in well-differentiated NET in comparison to neuroendocrine carcinoma in which PET/CT-FDG[63] (see Chapter 18).

LEIOMYOMAS

Exceedingly rare because of the scant presence of muscle fibers in the bile duct, leiomyomas have been reported in the extrahepatic biliary tree. The first report of this tumor's existence was

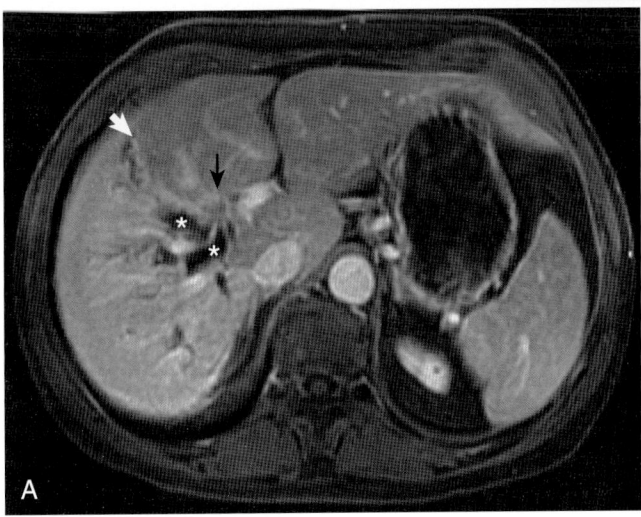 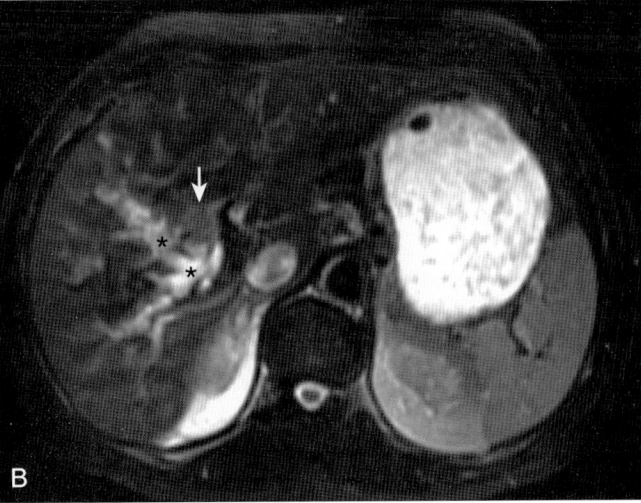

FIGURE 48.6 Magnetic resonance cholangiopancreatogram (MRCP) showing a carcinoid tumor arising from the right hepatic duct. **A,** Contrast-enhanced axial T1-weighted sequence. The tumor *(black arrow)* is located at the confluence of the right anterior and posterior sectoral ducts, which are dilated *(asterisks)*. Despite the absence of vascular inflow involvement by tumor, a notable difference in perfusion was found between the right and left hemilivers *(arrowhead)*, with hypertrophy of the left side, the apparent result of long-standing biliary obstruction. **B,** Axial MRCP image of the same patient. The tumor *(arrow)* at the confluence of the dilated right and left anterior sectoral ducts *(asterisks)*, which appear *white* in this sequence.

in 1952 in a 31-year-old woman. Single case reports have documented leiomyoma of the hepatic bifurcation[64] and distal CBD.[65–68] Symptoms of malignant obstruction with jaundice, abdominal pain, and pruritus lend no diagnostic help. Use of direct cholangioscopy for diagnosis and endoscopic resection was performed in one case series.[68]

PSEUDOTUMORS

Nonneoplastic lesions may cause obstruction of the extrahepatic biliary ductal system and may closely resemble neoplasms by preoperative imaging and at the time of surgery. Pseudotumors occur frequently enough to require consideration of lesions suspected to be biliary tumors. Figure 48.7. The incidence of benign pseudotumors has been reported to range from 3% to 20% in large surgical series. The term is used to describe inflammatory fibrotic or erosive lesions and include primary sclerosing cholangitis, sclerosive pancreatitis (AIP), IgG4-mediated cholangitis, and heterotopia.

Primary Sclerosing Cholangitis

Primary sclerosing cholangitis (PSC) is an inflammatory disorder characterized by chronic inflammatory strictures resulting from fibrosis (see Chapter 41). There is a 70% association with inflammatory bowel disease (IBD), and therefore PSC should be strongly suspected in any patient with biliary strictures in the setting of IBD. Colonic involvement is most commonly ulcerative colitis; however, it also may be interpreted as Crohn disease or indeterminate colitis. Imaging shows characteristic multifocal strictures and dilation of the intrahepatic and extrahepatic ducts on cholangiography. PSC typically manifests in the fourth to fifth decades of life and there is a male preponderance. Impaired bile flow occurs secondary to inflammation, and fibrosis leads to progressive disease of the liver. If left untreated, PSC can lead to cholestasis and ultimately hepatic failure. Additionally, there is an increased risk of cholangiocarcinoma, gallbladder carcinoma, and colon cancer.[69,70] Hepatobiliary

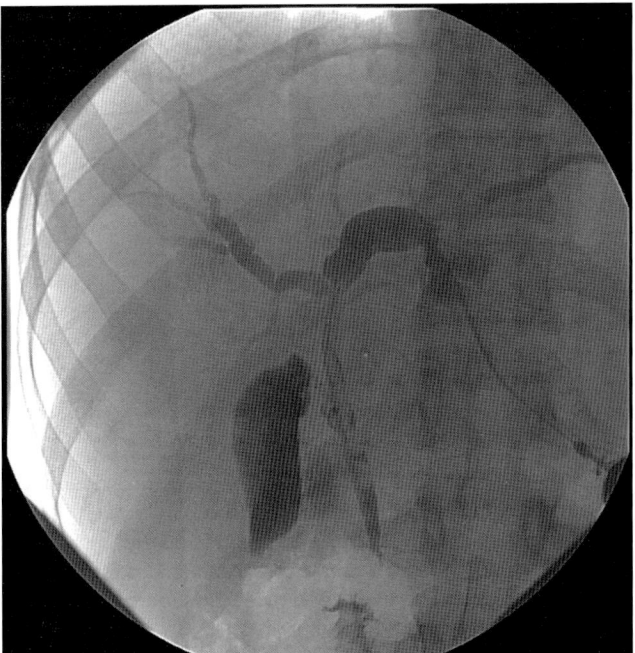

FIGURE 48.7 Percutaneous transhepatic cholangiography reveals obstructing hilar mass in an asymptomatic 25-year-old patient who presented with jaundice. The patient underwent a right hemihepatectomy, caudate resection, bile duct resection, and hepaticojejunostomy. Pathologic examination revealed acute and chronic cholangitis with abscess formation, fibrosis, and capsular serositis; specifically, there was no evidence of malignancy. (Courtesy Dr. Christine Menias.)

malignancy was present in 10.9% of patients with PSC in a multicenter study of 7119 patients.[71]

PSC affects both the intrahepatic and extrahepatic bile ducts and most commonly manifests with involvement of both the small and large bile ducts. Involvement of large bile ducts alone occurs in 10%.[72]

Gallbladder mass lesions were present in 6% of patients with PSC as reported by Said et al.[73] reviewing 286 patients with PSC. Gallbladder adenocarcinoma was present in 56% of the specimens with mass lesions.

Patients may be asymptomatic or have symptoms of jaundice, pruritus, and right upper quadrant pain. Less commonly, symptoms of end-stage liver disease, such as encephalopathy, variceal bleeding, and ascites, can be the first symptoms in occult disease.

Genetic and environmental factors are thought to play a role. A comprehensive study by Liwinski et al.[74] found alterations in the microbiome of the upper alimentary tract and bile between samples from patients with PSC and controls with reduced biodiversity in PSC samples. There also was an increased presence of *Enterococcus faecalis*. A strong correlation was found between concentration of *Enterococcus* and bile acid taurolithocholic acid.[74] This study suggests that the altered microbiome and increase in noxious lithocholic acid may contribute to the pathogenesis of cholangiocarcinoma.

Biliary obstruction is usually due to progressive multifocal cholestasis but may also occur as a result of a dominant stricture within an area of disease. Transplantation is currently the only established curative treatment option[75] (see Chapter 110). Cholecystectomy should be considered in patients with imaging abnormalities and symptoms in the setting of primary sclerosing cholangitis because of the high risk of involvement.

Lymphoplasmocytic Sclerosing Pancreatitis

Lymphoplasmacytic sclerosing pancreatitis (LP) is a rare inflammatory cause of pancreatitis, which may result in biliary obstruction and be indistinguishable from pancreatic cancer (see Chapter 54). This entity is now referred to as AIP and may lead to diffuse or focal abnormality of the pancreas. The concept of AIP was first proposed in 1995 by Yoshida et al.[76] and has since been further elucidated. Histologic features include lymphoplasmacytic infiltration of the pancreas, interstitial fibrosis, periductal inflammation, and phlebitis. Hypergammaglobulinemia (IgG4 subtype) and response to steroids further define the disorder.[77] Further classification of autoimmune pancreatitis as guided by the International Consensus Criteria for Autoimmune Pancreatitis defined subtypes AIP types 1 and 2, in which the latter has duct-centric pancreatitis and is not associated with serum IgG4 elevation.[78] Additionally type 1 AIP exhibits extrapancreatic manifestations such as retroperitoneal fibrosis, sialadenitis, and pulmonary and renal abnormalities.

Clinically patients present with painless jaundice and a pancreatic mass that cannot be distinguished from pancreatic cancer based on imaging characteristics. Elevated IgG4 may assist in avoidance of unnecessary pancreatic resection; however, the proportion of type 2 AIP with normal IgG4 levels is high in European and American series making this less reliable.[80]

Although pancreaticoduodenectomy was initially thought to be effective at treating this disorder, a series reported by Weber et al.[79] found a 28% recurrence of jaundice resulting from biliary stricture. Consensus guidelines now recommend steroids as first-line treatment of AIP with surgical intervention left for refractory symptoms after failure of steroids and alternative therapies.[80]

Immunoglobulin G4–Mediated Cholangitis

A distinct entity of IgG4-mediated cholangitis associated with AIP has been reported that is difficult to distinguish from sclerosing cholangitis or malignancy. Deshpande et al.[81] reported patients with IgG-4 cholangitis were older than those with sclerosing cholangitis and had higher portal and lobular inflammatory scores. Similar to AIP, this disorder shows an increase in IgG4-positive plasma cells and is responsive to steroids compared with primary sclerosing cholangitis, which is typically resistant to steroids.[81] Imaging and clinical findings may mimic those of AIP, primary sclerosing cholangitis, and cholangiocarcinoma; however, steroids and rituximab may induce and maintain remission.[82] This disease appears to be more common in older men, with mean age of onset in eighth decade.[83]

Heterotopic Tissue

Although heterotopic tissue in the gallbladder and extrahepatic biliary tree is exceedingly rare, cases of gastric and pancreatic heterotopia have been reported. Possible causes postulated include displacement of cells during embryologic development and irregular differentiation of multipotential cells. Symptoms related to heterotopia are consistent with the origin of the heterotopic tissue and location of the heterotopia. Hemorrhage and pain resulting from ulceration are common in cases of gastric heterotopia and pancreatitis, and jaundice may occur in the setting of pancreatic heterotopia.[11] Heterotopia is present in the gallbladder more commonly than the extrahepatic biliary tree, and gastric heterotopia has been described more commonly than pancreatic in the literature.[84]

Heterotopia was first observed in a cystic duct with clinical evidence of gallbladder obstruction in 1967 by Whittaker et al.[85] Gastric heterotopia manifesting as a 1-cm papillary tumor of the common hepatic duct,[86] tumor of ampulla of Vater,[87] and stricture of biliary tract[88] have been reported. Heterotopic pancreatic tissue has been reported in the bile duct and gallbladder.[89–92]

In the gallbladder, imaging may show an echogenic polypoid mass in the lumen of the gallbladder, focal wall thickening, or nodularity.[11] CT scan may show a soft tissue mass with mild enhancement after contrast administration.[84] Topic mucosa of the bile duct may be discovered as an intraluminal polyp or stricture. O'Reilly et al.[92] described a case of pancreatic heterotopia discovered in a 12-year-old boy presenting with jaundice. ERCP showed a stricture of the distal biliary tree without mass.

Symptomatic heterotopic tissue arising in the extrahepatic biliary tree is exceedingly rare. Resection is required for symptom control and diagnosis.

The references for this chapter can be found online by accessing the accompanying Expert Consult website.

CHAPTER 49

Tumors of the gallbladder

Rachel M. Lee and Shishir K. Maithel

BENIGN TUMORS OF THE GALLBLADDER

Although gallbladder cancer is a rare and aggressive malignancy that generally carries a dismal prognosis, there are a number of benign conditions of the gallbladder that can radiographically mimic malignancy and deserve consideration in a robust differential diagnosis because preoperative determination of a benign lesion may significantly alter treatment strategy.[1]

Gallbladder Polyps

Gallbladder polyps are found in approximately 3% to 7% of abdominal ultrasound examinations and 2% to 12% of cholecystectomy specimens.[2–5] The majority (50%–80%) of polypoid lesions of the gallbladder are cholesterol polyps, which carry no malignant potential.[1,4,6,7] Cholesterol polyps are most commonly found in women aged 40 to 50 years during evaluation for epigastric or right upper quadrant abdominal pain. They may be single or multiple and generally are less than 10 mm in size.[1,8,9] Pathologically, cholesterol polyps are nonneoplastic collections of lipid laden macrophages covered in normal gallbladder epithelium.[8] They are typically smooth or lobulated and attached to the gallbladder wall by a stalk.[8] Radiographically, cholesterol polyps are brightly echogenic without shadowing on ultrasound (Fig. 49.1). Although larger polyps are less echogenic than smaller ones, they contain characteristic echogenic foci that may differentiate large cholesterol polyps from adenomas or adenocarcinomas.[1,9] These lesions may be safely observed as long as they are less than 10 mm in size.

Adenomatous polyps, or adenomas, are neoplastic lesions derived from the gallbladder epithelium that make up approximately 15% of gallbladder polyps.[1,10] Adenomas are more commonly found in women and are typically asymptomatic but may be associated with chronic right upper quadrant abdominal pain if large or obstructing the cystic duct.[1] Adenomas are commonly associated with cholelithiasis.[1] Histologically, adenomas may be tubular, papillary, or tubulopapillary as well as sessile or pedunculated.[1,8] Radiographically, adenomas are smooth intraluminal masses, although occasionally they may appear lobulated or cauliflower-like (Fig. 49.2). Importantly, the adjacent gallbladder wall maintains a normal thickness of less than 3 mm in the case of a benign adenoma[1,9] (see Chapter 47).

Although the minority of adenomatous polyps transform into adenocarcinoma, malignant transformation does occur, and a high degree of suspicion is warranted given the vastly improved overall survival in patients with early-stage gallbladder cancer compared with advanced disease. Previously cited risk factors for gallbladder cancer include older age, specifically older than 50 years, presence of gallstones, larger polyp size (>10 mm), and isolated gallbladder wall thickening.[11] Classically, guidelines have recommended cholecystectomy for polyps greater than 10 mm in size on preoperative imaging, and several studies have cited polyp size as the most reliable indication of malignant potential. For example, in a study of over 2000 patients who underwent cholecystectomy for polypoid lesions, Li and colleagues found that 90% of patients with gallbladder cancer had lesions greater than 10 mm.[4] Further, Zielinski and colleagues found that 100% of gallbladder cancers occurred in patients with polyps at least 6 mm in size.[12] Additional characteristics independently associated with malignancy in the setting of polypoid lesions included a history of primary sclerosing cholangitis, local gallbladder wall invasion, and polyp vascularity.[12] Based on these data, citing a negative predictive value of 100%, and the absence of randomized controlled trials (RCTs) to guide decision making, the most recent guidelines from the Society of American Gastrointestinal and Endoscopic Surgeons (SAGES) recommend cholecystectomy for larger, especially single, polyps and those causing symptoms, and watchful waiting for asymptomatic polyps less than 5 mm in size.[13] Generally speaking, polyps greater than 10 mm in size should be removed with a cholecystectomy.

Adenomyomatosis

Adenomyomatosis, also known as adenomyomatous hyperplasia, is present in 8% to 10% of cholecystectomy specimens and is associated with chronic inflammation of the gallbladder.[1,14] Adenomyomatosis can present in three variants: (1) localized (30%), presenting as a mass in the gallbladder fundus and accounting for approximately 11% of gallbladder polyps, (2) segmental (>60%), presenting as focal, circumferential gallbladder wall thickening, and (3) diffuse (<5%), presenting with diffuse gallbladder wall thickening and intramural diverticulae.[1] Histologically adenomyomatosis is characterized by epithelial and smooth muscle proliferation, causing epithelial invaginations,

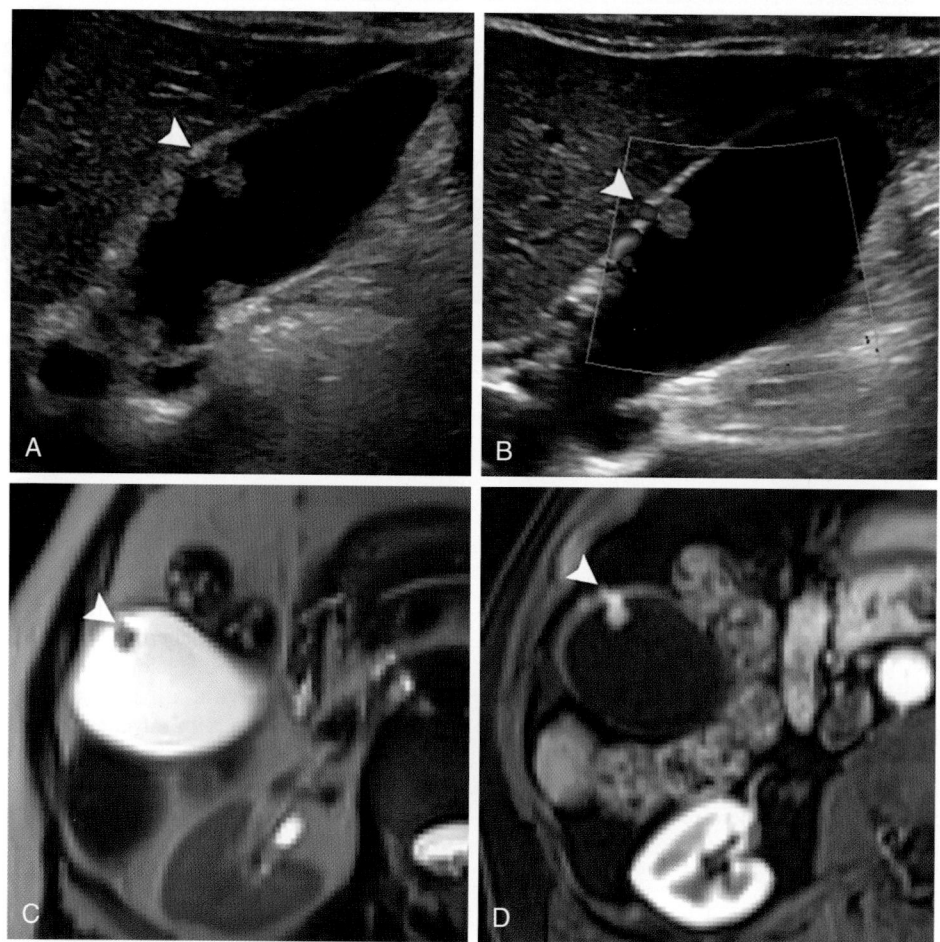

FIGURE 49.1 Radiographic appearance of cholesterol polyp. **A–B,** Ultrasound images. **C,** Magnetic resonance imaging (MRI) T2-weighted sequence. **D,** MRI venous phase (see Chapter 16).

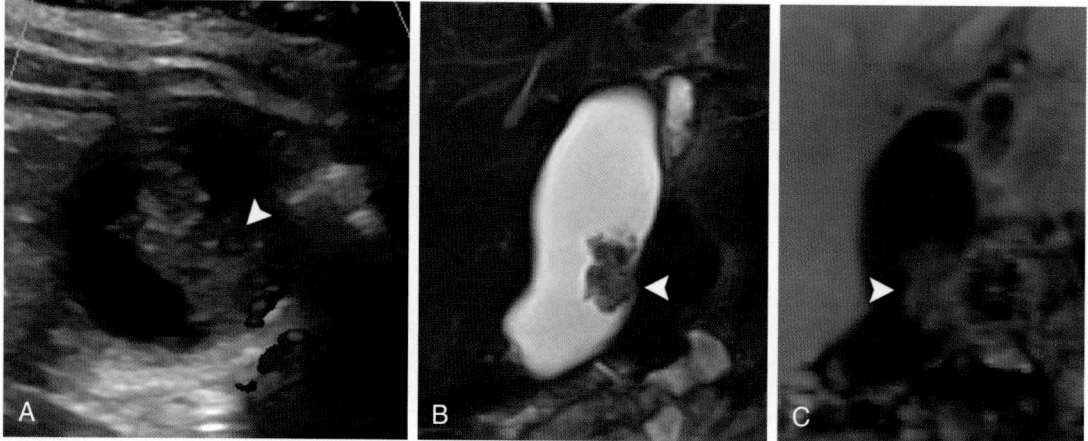

FIGURE 49.2 Radiographic appearance of gallbladder adenoma. **A,** Ultrasound with Doppler. **B,** Magnetic resonance imaging (MRI) T2-weighted sequence. **C,** MRI precontrast phase (see Chapter 16).

or Rokitansky-Aschoff sinuses that form cystic spaces within the gallbladder wall (Fig. 49.3).[1] Adenomyomatosis is responsible for approximately one-quarter of cases of gallbladder wall thickening and is identified on abdominal ultrasound by the characteristic comet-tail artifacts, resulting from acoustic reverberations from calcium deposits trapped in the Rokitansky-Aschoff sinuses.[15] Although dysplasia, carcinoma in situ, and invasive adenocarcinoma can form within the epithelium of adenomyomatous hyperplasia, adenomyomatosis itself is considered a benign lesion and not a malignant precursor.[1,15] Cholecystectomy is indicated in symptomatic cases or when differentiation from neoplastic thickening is a concern.[15]

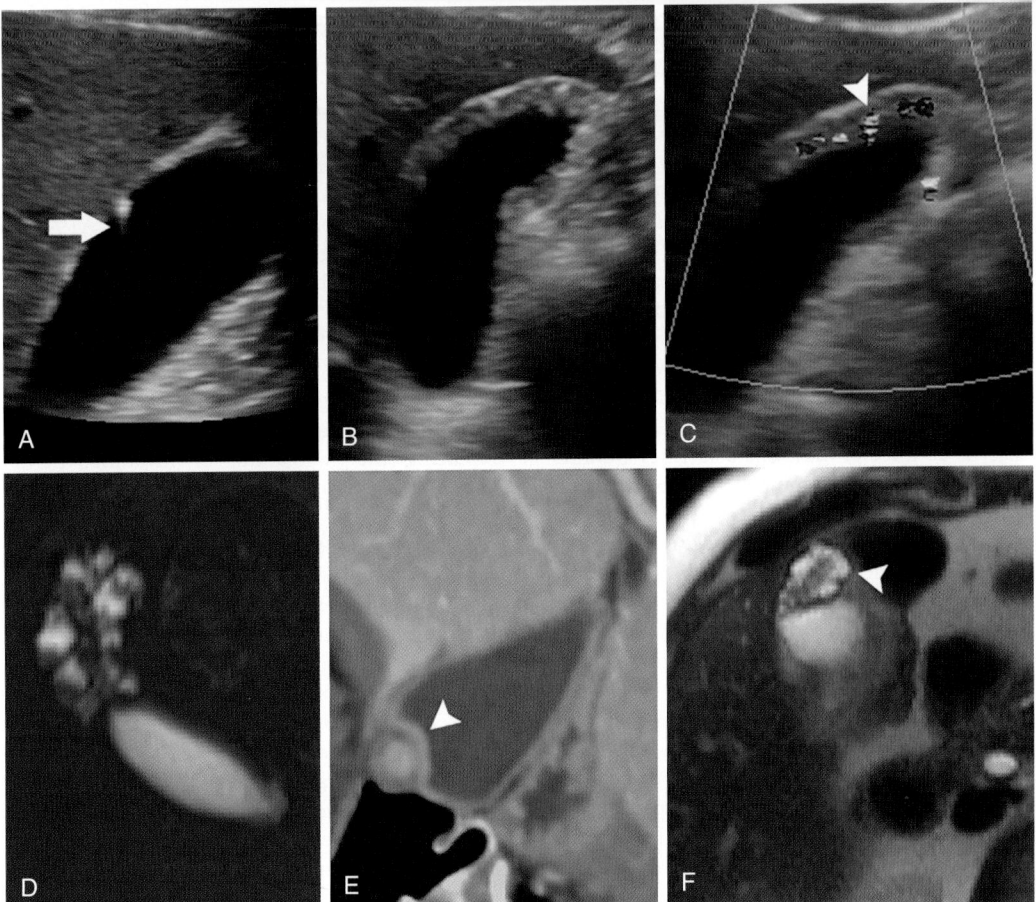

FIGURE 49.3   Radiographic appearance of adenomyomatosis. Characteristic "comet tail" artefact is depicted by the arrow in image **A**. **A–C**, Ultrasound images. **D,** Magnetic resonance imaging (MRI) T2-weighted sequence. **E,** Computed tomography (CT) scan venous phase. **F,** MRI T2-weighted sequence (see Chapter 16).

Granular Cell Tumors

Granular cell tumors are nonepithelial tumors that occur throughout the body. One percent of granular cell tumors occur in the biliary tract, and 4% of these biliary granular cell tumors occur in the gallbladder, thus making them very rare tumors.[1,16] The vast majority (90%) of patients with granular cell tumors are women and the average age of presentation is 34 years. Granular cell tumors occur predominantly in African Americans and often present with symptoms of biliary colic or acute cholecystitis.[1,16] Histologically granular cell tumors are thought to be of Schwann cell origin and are S-100 positive on immunohistochemical staining. Radiographically, granular cell tumors appear as heterogeneous, mildly hyperechoic, poorly defined masses on ultrasound, and as nonspecific soft tissue masses on computed tomography (CT).[1] Cholecystectomy is indicated for symptomatic lesions or when there is difficulty distinguishing it from a neoplastic polyp.[1]

A comprehensive list of benign tumors of the gallbladder is presented in Table 49.1.

GALLBLADDER CANCER

Epidemiology

Incidence of gallbladder cancer varies greatly worldwide and is highest in India (10–22 cases per 100,000), Asia (5–8 per 100,000), Eastern Europe (2–4 per 100,000), and South America (9–14 per 100,000).[17–19] Incidence in the United States is

TABLE 49.1	Benign Tumors of the Gallbladder		
EPITHELIAL LESIONS	**NONEPITHELIAL LESIONS**	**NEUROGENIC LESIONS**	**TUMOR-LIKE LESIONS**
• Adenoma • Papilloma • Cystadenoma	• Leiomyoma • Lipoma • Hemangioma • Lymphangioma • Granular cell tumor	• Neurofibroma • Paraganglioma	• Cholesterol polyp • Inflammatory polyp • Fibrous polyp • Xanthogranulomatous cholecystitis • Adenomyomatosis

Adapted from Levy AD, Murakata LA, Abbott RM, Rohrmann CA, Jr. From the archives of the AFIP. Benign tumors and tumorlike lesions of the gallbladder and extrahepatic bile ducts: Radiologic-pathologic correlation. Armed Forces Institute of Pathology. *Radiographics*. 2002;22(2):387–413.

comparatively low, with 1 to 2 cases per 100,000 persons; however, gallbladder cancer is the sixth most common gastrointestinal (GI) malignancy and the most common biliary tract malignancy in the United States.[20] Geographic differences in risk factor prevalence likely explain some of this variation. For example, gallstone disease is a well-cited risk factor for gallbladder cancer because of mechanical injury, promotion of bacterial colonization, and chronic inflammation.[21] Gallstone disease is highly prevalent in Chile (where 36% of women and 16% of men are affected); similarly, cholelithiasis is common in Hispanic and Native American populations in the United States, who also are at higher risk for gallbladder cancer compared with the general population.[17,22] Higher risk of gallbladder cancer with obesity, multiparity, and an approximately 3-fold increased risk in women compared with men is also presumably linked to higher incidence of gallstone disease, as all three of these characteristics are independent risk factors for stone development.[22] Interestingly, although gallstones are present in 80% of cases of gallbladder cancer in India, the incidence of gallbladder cancer is higher than expected based on the prevalence of cholelithiasis in this country, indicating other risk factors may be playing a larger role[21] (see Chapter 33). Additional risk factors, including low socioeconomic status, as a surrogate for decreased access to healthcare and specifically cholecystectomy, chronic *Salmonella typhi* infection, *Helicobacter pylori* infection, exposure to various pollutants and chemicals, and smoking, have also been implicated in higher rates of gallbladder cancer in specific populations.[21] In contrast, the majority of gallbladder cancers diagnosed in Japan are not associated with gallstone disease, and furthermore, incidence is equal between men and women.[23] However, presence of a *K-ras* mutation, anomalous pancreaticobiliary junction, and deregulatory mutations in the *TP53* gene are more common in Japan and these molecular differences may result in the high incidence in that country.[17,24,25]

Despite these etiologic or pathogenic differences, from a prognostic standpoint, disease extent at diagnosis is the most important predictor of survival as demonstrated by Butte and colleagues. In examining cases of gallbladder cancer from three academic centers in the United States, Chile, and Japan, the authors found no differences in disease-specific survival (DSS) between countries after curative intent resection but instead cited higher T-stage and lymph node involvement as being associated with decreased overall survival on multivariable analysis.[17]

Clinical Presentation

Patients with gallbladder cancer present in one of three ways: (1) malignancy is diagnosed on final pathology after cholecystectomy for presumed benign disease, (2) malignancy is discovered *during* cholecystectomy for presumed benign disease, and (3) malignancy is suspected preoperatively.[26] Malignancy diagnosed during or after cholecystectomy for benign disease will further be referred to as "incidental" gallbladder cancer. Clinical presentation of incidental gallbladder cancer most commonly involves abdominal pain or symptoms consistent with biliary colic and/or acute or chronic cholecystitis. More advanced disease may present with jaundice, malaise, weight loss, and a palpable mass.[26]

Generally, there is no set pattern of laboratory values that raises specific suspicion for gallbladder cancer. However, Pitt and colleagues found that along with age over 65 years, female sex, and Asian or African American race, elevated alkaline phosphatase was associated with an increased risk of incidental gallbladder cancer diagnosis.[27] Laboratory values consistent with chronic disease, including anemia, hypoalbuminemia, and leukocytosis, can be seen in the context of advanced disease, as well as hyperbilirubinemia and an elevated alkaline phosphatase.[28]

Tumor markers are generally not helpful in diagnosing gallbladder cancer. However, both carcinoembryonic antigen (CEA) and carbonic anhydrase 19-9 (CA19-9) may be elevated in patients with gallbladder cancer and can be used to monitor for recurrence after treatment.[29]

Radiologic Evaluation

Ultrasonography is typically the initial imaging modality employed to investigate the gallbladder (see Chapter 16). On ultrasound examination, gallbladder cancer may appear as a mass replacing the gallbladder or invading the gallbladder bed (45%–60% of cases), irregular wall thickening (20%–30% of cases) or as an intraluminal polyp or mass (15%–25% of cases).[26,30,31] In cases of advanced disease, standard ultrasonography has a sensitivity of 85%; however, gallbladder cancer can also mimic intramural changes of complicated cholecystitis (see Chapter 34). Early-stage disease, especially when associated with sessile polyps or gallstones, is difficult to identify.[26,32,33] The use of color Doppler ultrasonography can identify increased blood flow to a lesion, which has been associated with malignancy; however, this is of controversial diagnostic value.[26,34,35] Intravenous (IV) contrast enhanced ultrasound (CEUS) was developed over the past two decades and historically used for liver tumor pathology. In 2012 guidelines for examination of extrahepatic biliary structures were introduced, but these guidelines differentiated benign and malignant lesions by polyp size greater than 10 mm and clinical characteristics.[34,36] However, CEUS has been studied by several groups to identify characteristics of gallbladder malignancy.

Liu and colleagues, in a multicenter study of 9 hospitals in China, evaluated 192 patients with histologically confirmed gallbladder pathology, including 51 cases of adenocarcinoma.[37] The authors found that while both benign and malignant lesions enhanced during the arterial phase of CEUS, malignant lesions were more likely to enhance heterogeneously and had a faster washout time of 41.4 seconds compared with 58.2 seconds in benign lesions. Malignant lesions were also more likely to have branched or linear intralesional vessels during the arterial phase, whereas benign lesions were more likely to present with dotted intralesional vessels.[37] On multivariable analysis, the authors found branched or linear intralesional vessels (sensitivity 74.8%, specificity 98%) and gallbladder wall destruction adjacent to the lesion (sensitivity 78.4%, specificity 92.9%) as the best predictors of gallbladder cancer using CEUS (Fig. 49.4).[37]

Zhang and colleagues performed a similar study comparing CEUS with conventional ultrasound on 105 gallbladder lesions, including 18 cases of gallbladder cancer.[38] Lesions were evaluated by both conventional ultrasound and CEUS and rated as benign, probably benign, probably malignant, and malignant using both modalities. CEUS was found to have higher sensitivity (94.1% vs. 82.4%), specificity (95.5% vs. 89.8%), positive predictive value (80.0% vs. 60.9%), negative predictive value (98.8% vs. 96.3%), and accuracy (95.2% vs. 88.6%) compared with conventional ultrasound, and although these differences were not statistically significant, the authors concluded that CEUS may provide value in the differential diagnosis of gallbladder lesions.[38] The most recent guidelines written in 2017 by

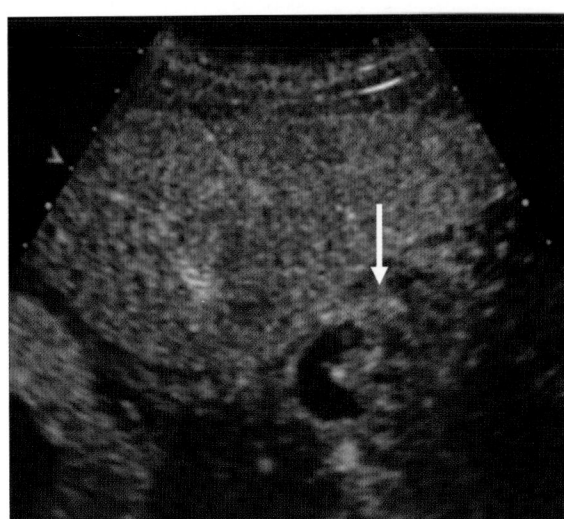

FIGURE 49.4 Contrast-enhanced ultrasound of gallbladder carcinoma. *Arrow* indicates heterogeneously enhancing mass on arterial phase with intra-tumoral vessel (see Chapter 16).

the European Federation of Societies for Ultrasound in Medicine and Biology state that CEUS "improves the diagnosis of malignant gallbladder polyps and wall thickening over [conventional] ultrasound. In gallbladder malignancy (protruding lesions as well as circumferential wall thickening), a heterogeneous enhancement pattern, the presence of perfusion defects, and an irregular vessel pattern were found to be typical features with [CEUS]."[39] Although the microbubble contrast agent used in CEUS has been approved by the Food and Drug Administration (FDA) in the United States, as of this writing, its use is mostly limited to research activities, rather than standard clinical practice. However, CEUS is widely used in Europe and Asia.[40]

If gallbladder cancer is suspected preoperatively, a multiphase CT scan or contrasted magnetic resonance imaging (MRI) of the abdomen and pelvis and a CT of the chest is indicated[41] (see Chapter 16). The purpose of cross-sectional imaging is 3-fold: to define local extent of disease, to evaluate for nodal metastases, and to evaluate for distant metastatic disease.[26] Because complete resection is the only possibility for cure in gallbladder cancer, accurate determination of tumor resectability is paramount, especially given that only 20% to 30% of patients present with tumors amenable to resection.[42] Choi and colleagues investigated the association between CT findings and final resection margin and found that liver invasion, bile duct invasion, and hepatic artery involvement were associated with a positive margin on final pathology with a specificity of 93.3% when combining two or three of the aforementioned criteria.[43] Tumor size, tumor morphology, hepatic versus peritoneal side involvement, and portal vein involvement were not independent predictors of positive resection margin on multivariable regression.[43] Adequate radiographic evaluation of distant lymph nodes is likewise critically important because prognosis after resection is drastically reduced when lymph node metastases outside of the hepatoduodenal ligament are present.[44] There is debate as to the ideal imaging modality for lymph node evaluation; de Savornin Lohman and colleagues performed a systematic review investigating the diagnostic accuracy of CT and MRI in identification of lymph node

metastases.[44] The sensitivity of both CT and MRI in the included studies varied widely, from 25% to 93% in CT and 59% to 92% in MRI exams. The modalities were not directly compared.[44] In current clinical practice, the majority of patients are evaluated with a CT scan of the abdomen and pelvis, likely because of ease of examination performance in conjunction with a CT of the chest, less time required to complete the examination, and patient comfort. Of note, all false-negative lymph nodes identified in the included studies were less than 10 mm in size, and there is potential that newer technology, including thinner slices, higher resolution, and diffusion-weighted MRI may improve diagnostic accuracy, although this has not yet been proven for gallbladder cancer.[44]

Finally, ^{18}F-fluorodeoxyglucose positron emission tomography (FDG-PET) may provide additional information in the staging and work-up of patients with gallbladder cancer (see Chapter 18). Most biliary tract cancers are FDG-PET avid, and this has been used to detect occult metastatic disease before resection of known cancers and to detect residual disease after cholecystectomy in incidentally diagnosed cases. Corvera and colleagues evaluated preoperative staging FDG-PET scans on 31 patients with gallbladder cancer.[45] The results of these FDG-PET scans changed the stage and treatment of 23% of patients (the majority of whom had previously undergone multiple additional imaging studies) by identifying occult metastatic disease, rendering operative exploration unnecessary. The sensitivity and specificity of FDG-PET in these patients were 86% and 50%, respectively, for detecting the primary tumor, and 87% and 89%, respectively, for detecting metastatic disease, both local and distant.[45]

In patients with incidental gallbladder cancer, FDG-PET has been shown to have a high specificity and accuracy in diagnosing residual disease in the gallbladder fossa (specificity 89.4%, accuracy 85.7%), regional disease (specificity 80.9%, accuracy 70.8%), liver metastases (specificity 100%, accuracy 100%), and lymph node metastases (specificity 95.2%–100%, accuracy 90.4%–100%) after cholecystectomy.[46] These data were published by Shukla and colleagues who evaluated 24 patients referred for consideration for radical resection after cholecystectomy and incidentally diagnosed gallbladder cancer. Patients received both FDG-PET-CT and multidetector CT (MDCT) scans. The authors concluded that the imaging modalities have complimentary uses in patients with incidental gallbladder cancer, with the specific strength of FDG-PET-CT cited as detection of occult metastatic disease in the body outside the fields captured by MDCT.[46] Of note, residual inflammation in the gallbladder fossa from the index cholecystectomy must be considered when interpreting a positive finding on FDG-PET done before performing re-resection of an incidentally discovered gallbladder cancer.

Butte and colleagues likewise examined patients with incidental gallbladder cancer with FDG-PET-CT for evaluation of residual disease before radical re-resection.[47] Of 32 patients studied, 13 had a FDG-PET-CT that indicated no residual disease (negative), and 19 had evidence of residual disease (positive). Nine of these patients had evidence of locoregional and potentially resectable disease, and 10 had evidence of distant metastases. Of patients with negative FDG-PET-CT scans, 4 underwent reoperation; 3 had no residual disease on final pathology, and 1 patient was found to have peritoneal dissemination intraoperatively. Of patients with positive scans indicating potentially resectable disease, 4 underwent reoperation;

2 received a resection confirming locoregional disease, and 2 were found to have peritoneal dissemination.[47] The authors concluded that use of FDG-PET in patients with incidental gallbladder cancer may reduce the number of patients undergoing nontherapeutic re-exploration after cholecystectomy; however, it is important to note the poor sensitivity of FDG-PET in detecting peritoneal disease, quantified as 28.5% by Shukla and colleagues in the previously discussed study.[46,47] Ultimately, identifying the optimal imaging modality or modalities for staging and determining resectability in occult gallbladder cancer and for identifying residual disease, restaging, and determining resectability in incidental gallbladder cancer requires further investigation. Overall, it appears that a multimodal approach may provide the most accurate and detailed information for treatment planning.

Preoperative Pathologic Diagnosis

Because gallbladder cancer has the tendency and ability to seed the peritoneum, biopsy tracts, and surgical wounds, preoperative tissue diagnosis via fine-needle aspiration or core biopsy is generally not recommended.[48–50] Cholecystectomy, in the case of known gallbladder cancer to provide a preoperative pathologic diagnosis, is also not advised because disruption of the gallbladder integrity and iatrogenic tumor dissemination leading to peritoneal implants may preclude curative resection, as has been described by Fong and colleagues.[48] Risks of dissemination aside, Akosa and colleagues determined that fine-needle aspiration had an acceptable sensitivity for preoperative diagnosis of gallbladder cancer of 88%. Exfoliative cytology of bile was found to have a sensitivity of 50%; however two cases of endoscopic brushings evaluated yielded false-negative results.[51]

Current clinical guidelines recommend biopsy only in the case of unresectable disease. Patients with resectable disease should proceed to definitive resection and the surgeon and patient should be prepared for the possibility of a resection being performed for benign disease, which, given the dismal prognosis of gallbladder cancer, is an acceptable risk when a high degree of suspicion for malignancy is present based on preoperative imaging.[41,50]

Histology

The vast majority of gallbladder cancers are adenocarcinomas and the association of adenomatous polyps with increased risk of cancer suggests that the adenoma to adenocarcinoma sequence occurs in some patients (see Chapter 47). Approximately 60% of tumors originate in the fundus, 30% in the body, and 10% in the neck of the gallbladder. Tumors of the neck, infundibulum, or cystic duct may infiltrate the porta hepatis, in a presentation that mimics hilar cholangiocarcinoma, resulting in major vascular invasion and obstructive jaundice.[52–54] Grossly, gallbladder cancers may be categorized as (1) infiltrative, causing diffuse thickening and induration of the gallbladder wall, (2) nodular, presenting as a well-circumscribed mass, (3) combined nodular-infiltrative, (4) papillary, with a frondlike, cauliflower appearance and the best prognosis because of limited invasion into the gallbladder wall, and (5) combined papillary-infiltrative forms.[52–54]

Although adenocarcinoma makes up 90% of malignant gallbladder tumors, there are several rare histologies that deserve mention (Box 49.1). Squamous differentiation is not uncommon in gallbladder cancer, often mixed with adenocarcinoma; pure squamous cell carcinoma (SCC) accounts for 2% to 3%

> **BOX 49.1**   Malignant Tumors of the Gallbladder
>
> - Adenocarcinoma (90%)
> - Squamous/adenosquamous (2%–3%)
> - Neuroendocrine (2%–3%)
> - Clear cell
> - Sarcoma
> - Melanoma
> - Lymphoma
> - Metastases

---

of all malignant gallbladder tumors. The available data regarding this histology are limited to case reports, although from these cases, SCC appears to proliferate at a faster rate than adenocarcinoma and tends to involve locally advanced/infiltrative tumors, often invading the entire gallbladder wall. Interestingly, SCC tumors appear to have less of a tendency to metastasize to regional lymph nodes than adenocarcinoma, and the poor 5-year overall survival of approximately 1% has been attributed to early direct invasion into the liver and other adjacent organs.[55–58] Adenosquamous carcinoma of the gallbladder is similarly rare and often grouped with SCC in the literature. Chan and colleagues compared 12 patients with adenosquamous carcinoma of the gallbladder and 2 patients with SCC with 140 patients with adenocarcinoma. The authors found similar clinical characteristics in the two groups, but more advanced T stage and higher rates of liver involvement in the predominantly adenosquamous group and similarly poor outcomes for all histologies.[59]

Primary neuroendocrine tumors (NET) of the gallbladder account for approximately 2% to 3% of malignant gallbladder tumors. Ayabe and colleagues conducted an analysis of 754 patients with primary neuroendocrine tumors of the gallbladder in the National Cancer Database from 2004 to 2015. The authors found a longer median overall survival in patients with neuroendocrine gallbladder tumors compared with patients with gallbladder adenocarcinoma (25 months vs. 17 months, $P = .001$). However, overall survival (OS) in resected gallbladder neuroendocrine tumors was significantly worse than in neuroendocrine tumors of other sites (Median OS: gallbladder NET: 25 months; small bowel NET: 130 months; colon NET: 65 months; pancreas, appendix, stomach, rectum NET: median not reached, $P < .001$).[60] Reports of both primary and metastatic melanoma of the gallbladder, gallbladder sarcoma, lymphoma, and clear cell carcinoma of the gallbladder have been published, but these tumors are exceedingly rare.[61–65]

Staging

Historically, multiple staging systems were used for gallbladder cancer, but the American Joint Committee on Cancer (AJCC) staging system is now most commonly used and considered the standard.[66,67] The 8th edition of the AJCC staging system was published in December 2016 and employs the standard tumor (T), nodal (N), and metastatic (M) nomenclature.[66,68,69] Tumor stage is determined by depth of invasion: T1a tumors are limited to the lamina propria, whereas T1b tumors invade the muscular layer. An important change from the 7th to the 8th edition was the division of T2 tumors into two categories. Previously, T2 tumors were classified as invading the perimuscular connective tissue of any location; however, in the

8th edition, these tumors were divided into T2a, invading the perimuscular connective tissue on the peritoneal side, and T2b, invading the perimuscular connective tissue on the hepatic side.[66,68,69] More advanced T-stage designations remained the same: T3 tumors either perforate the serosa in any location or directly invade the liver or other adjacent organs, including the stomach, duodenum, colon, pancreas, omentum, or extrahepatic bile ducts, and T4 tumors invade the main portal vein, hepatic artery, or two or more adjacent structures.[66,68,69]

Changes to the T-stage designation were largely driven by an international, multicenter study performed by Shindoh and colleagues.[68] The authors found that patients who had T2 tumors located on the hepatic side of the gallbladder had higher rates of vascular invasion, neural invasion, and nodal metastases compared with patients with T2 tumors located on the peritoneal side of the gallbladder. These patients also had worse overall survival at 3 and 5 years; 3-year survival was 73.7% for peritoneal sided tumors compared with 52.1% for hepatic sided tumors, and 5-year survival after a median follow-up of 58.9 months was 64.7% versus 42.6%, respectively.[68] Further, tumor location was independently associated with OS on multivariable analysis, including potential confounders such as age, sex, institution, year of treatment, nodal involvement, liver metastasis, resection type (radical vs. simple, bile duct resection), margin status, tumor grade, and receipt of neoadjuvant and/or adjuvant chemotherapy.[68] Anatomically, these differences may be explained by differences in lymphatic and venous drainage. A classic injection study performed in 1932 by Karlmark and colleagues identified between 2 and 20 cholecystic veins on the hepatic side of the gallbladder that drain directly into segment IV of the liver after a very short course.[70,71] In contrast, on the peritoneal side of the liver, one to two cholecystic veins exist, and although they may terminate directly into the liver, they also often take a longer course and join the venous plexus surrounding the common bile duct and then enter the liver at the quadrate lobe.[70,71] Similarly, through detailed cadaver dissections, Ito and colleagues demonstrated that lymphatic drainage on the hepatic side of the gallbladder tends to have a more direct course to regional lymph nodes, whereas lymphatics from the peritoneal side must descend spirally and posteriorly before nodal drainage.[72] There is therefore an anatomic rationale that may explain why hepatic and peritoneal sided tumors would have differing rates of spread and prognosis, supporting the change in staging paradigm.

External validation of the 8th edition T-stage designations has yielded conflicting results. Sung and colleagues evaluated 348 resected gallbladder cancers and found no difference in OS in a pairwise comparison of patients with T2a and T2b tumors (5-year OS: 52.4% vs. 47.3%, P = .223).[69] Owiera and colleagues used the Surveillance, Epidemiology, and End Results (SEER) database to evaluate 3892 patients with gallbladder cancer. They determined that the 7th and 8th edition staging systems had comparable prognostic value, with the outcome of OS; however, they were unable to directly compare stage IIa and IIb cancers.[67] Finally, Wang and colleagues evaluated 327 patients with gallbladder cancer from the Fudan University Zhongshan Hospital database and in a supplementary analysis found a significant difference in OS on univariate analysis between patients with T2a and T2b tumors (P = .040).[73]

The second notable difference in the 8th edition staging system was the change in nodal status from location of positive nodes to number of positive nodes. Nodal categories are defined as N0 (no positive nodes), N1 (1–3 positive regional lymph nodes), and N2 (≥4 positive regional lymph nodes).[66] Importantly, distant lymph node involvement outside the porta hepatis, such as celiac, para-aortic, and aorto-caval lymph nodes, are still considered metastatic and are given an M1 designation. In addition, the updated edition recommended examination of at least six lymph nodes for accurate staging.[66] Sung and colleagues also sought to externally validate changes to the nodal stage and evaluated patients who had less than six and at least six lymph nodes retrieved separately. In patients with adequate lymph node retrieval according to the 8th edition guidelines, there was a significant difference in 5-year OS by nodal stage in both overall and pairwise comparisons (5-year OS: N0: 72.2%; N1: 28.8%; N2: 7.1%, P < .001 overall, P = .001 N0–N1; P = .039 N1–N2).[69] Recurrence-free survival (RFS) was likewise significantly different between groups (5-year RFS: N0: 64.6%; N1: 9.1%; N2: 0%, P < .001).[69] However, when the authors examined patients with one to five lymph nodes evaluated, although 5-year OS was significantly different between the groups overall, it was not different in the pairwise comparison of patients with N1 and N2 disease (5-year OS: N0: 73.0%; N1: 29.2%; N2: 50.0%, P < .001 overall, P < .001 N0–N1, P = .624 N1–N2). Analysis of 5-year RFS yielded similar results (5-year RFS: N0: 63.3%; N1: 17.3%; N2: 50.0%, P < .001 overall, P < .001 N0–N1, P = .430 N1–N2).[69] Although these data must be taken in the context of relatively small sample sizes from a single institution, they support both the new nodal staging guidelines and guidelines for appropriate lymph node yield.

Current T, N, and M stage definitions and the resultant stage groupings according to the 8th edition AJCC guidelines are presented in Table 49.2.

EXTENT OF PRIMARY RESECTION BY T STAGE

Complete resection is the only potential for cure for gallbladder cancer, and an R0 resection yields the best prognosis. In patients with incidental gallbladder cancer submitted to reoperation and definitive resection (see later), the presence of gross residual disease portends a similar prognosis to stage IV gallbladder cancer.[50,74] The extent of primary resection varies based on T stage. For T1a tumors, which invade no further than the lamina propria, simple cholecystectomy is appropriate and curative in approximately 90% of cases.[75] These tumors are rare and generally found only on pathologic review of cholecystectomy specimens performed for benign disease, but for these patients re-resection is not necessary.[75] For T1b tumors, or tumors invading the muscular layers of the gallbladder, however, simple cholecystectomy has been demonstrated to be insufficient in a significant fraction of cases. Principe and colleagues found a 1-year OS of 50% after simple cholecystectomy for patients with T1b tumors, compared with 100% for patients with T1a tumors.[50,76] Additionally, approximately 10% of patients have been reported to have residual disease after simple cholecystectomy for T1b tumors, and these tumors have been associated with a 10% to 20% rate of lymph node metastases on re-exploration, supporting a more extensive surgical approach.[18,77,78] Current National Comprehensive Cancer Network (NCCN) guidelines recommend a definitive oncologic resection consisting of a cholecystectomy and en-bloc resection adjacent liver parenchyma in segments IVb and V and portal lymphadenectomy for T1b, as well as T2 tumors after appropriate cross-sectional imaging to evaluate for metastatic disease.[41]

TABLE 49.2 American Joint Committee on Cancer 8th Edition Staging for Gallbladder Cancer

Tumor Stage

Tis	Carcinoma in situ
T1a	Invading lamina propria
T1b	Invading muscular layers
T2a	Invading perimuscular connective tissue on *peritoneal* side
T2b	Invading perimuscular connective tissue on *hepatic* side
T3	Invading or perforating serosa and/or directly invades the liver and/or *one* adjacent organ
T4	Invading main portal vein or hepatic artery and/or invading *two or more* adjacent organs

Nodal Stage

N0	No regional lymph node involvement
N1	Metastasis to 1–3 regional lymph nodes
N2	Metastasis to ≥4 regional lymph nodes

Metastasis Stage

M0	No distant metastasis
M1	Distant metastasis, including to the peritoneum, liver (beyond direct extension), lungs, pleura, and periaortic, pericaval, superior mesenteric artery, and/or celiac artery lymph nodes

Combined Stage

0	TisN0M0
I	T1(a-b)N0M0
IIa	T2aN0M0
IIb	T2bN0M0
IIIa	T3N0M0
IIIb	T1(a-b)N1M0 *or* T2(a-b)N1M0 *or* T3N1M0
IVa	T4N0M0 *or* T4N1M0
IVb	T(any)N2M0 *or* T(any)N(any)M1

Adapted from Amin M, Edge S. *AJCC Cancer Staging Manual.* 8th ed. Springer; 2017.

Finally, for T3 and T4 tumors, the extent of appropriate resection is debatable. The NCCN guidelines make a blanket statement regarding principles for resection, which include "radical cholecystectomy including segments IVb and V and lymphadenectomy and extended hepatic or biliary resection as necessary to obtain a negative margin."[41] Because T3 and T4 tumors invade adjacent organs, en bloc resection becomes more complicated. D'Angelica and colleagues retrospectively examined 109 patients who underwent resection for gallbladder cancer at a single institution over a 12-year period, 21 of whom underwent adjacent organ resection.[75] The authors found that adjacent organ resection was not associated with DSS and concluded that disease biology and stage, rather than extent of resection, drove outcomes. However, half of patients who underwent adjacent organ resection for adhesions to the involved organ (most commonly the colon and duodenum) that could not be differentiated from malignant involvement had malignant involvement of the resected organ, emphasizing the importance of resecting adherent adjacent organs to achieve an R0 resection because the same group demonstrated severely decreased disease-free survival (DFS) and DSS in patients with residual disease at any site (11.2 vs. 93.4 months, $P < .001$ and 25.2 months vs. median not reached, $P < .001$, respectively).[74] Additionally, the authors found no association between adjacent

organ involvement and increased postoperative morbidity.[75] However, major hepatic resections with bile duct resection and/or vascular resection and reconstruction for T4 tumors have been shown to have increased postoperative morbidity and mortality and the expert consensus from the Americas Hepatobiliary Association recommends careful assessment of performance status and lymph node metastases, with patients with T3 or T4 N1 disease encouraged to seek clinical trials with neoadjuvant therapy rather than aggressive upfront resection.[79]

TREATMENT

Incidental Gallbladder Cancer (see Chapter 119)

Incidental gallbladder cancer, or gallbladder cancer diagnosed during or after cholecystectomy for presumed benign disease, is discovered in 0.2% to 3% of all cholecystectomy specimens[80] (see Chapter 33). Estimates of the proportion of incidental gallbladder cancer to all gallbladder cancer vary, from 27% up to 70% of all gallbladder cancers discovered during cholecystectomy or on pathologic review.[81-83] The majority of these cases are early-stage gallbladder cancer, or pathologic T stage 1 or 2, and thus the potential for cure exists, making appropriate and timely management decisions paramount to achieving long-term survival.[84] Rathanaswamy and colleagues published an algorithmic approach to the management of incidental gallbladder cancer, which is closely mirrored by the most recent NCCN guidelines.[41,81] This general algorithm is depicted in Figure 49.5 and centers around re-resection for incidentally discovered gallbladder cancers.

The rationale for re-resection is centered on data showing improved OS for patients who undergo re-resection compared with those who do not; Fuks and colleagues found an increase in 5-year OS from 0% to 62% in patients with T2 tumors who underwent re-resection ($P = .001$) and from 0% to 19% in patients with T3 tumors ($P = .04$).[85] This survival advantage with re-resection is associated with removing residual disease in the liver and locoregional lymph node metastasis. Pawlik and colleagues showed that the incidence of residual disease in the liver bed and lymph node metastasis increases with higher T stage: in an analysis of 225 patients, 0% of patients with T1 tumors had residual disease in the liver at the time of re-resection, compared with 10.4% of patients with T2 and 36.4% of patients with T3 tumors ($P = .006$). Similarly, the authors found that 12.5% of patients with T1 tumors had locoregional lymph node metastases, compared with 31.2% of patients with T2 tumors and 45.5% of patients with T3 tumors ($P = .04$).[78] Ethun and colleagues developed a risk score to predict the presence of locoregional residual and distant disease at re-resection and to predict OS. The authors found that T stage, tumor differentiation, lymphovascular invasion, and perineural invasion were associated with increased odds of locoregional residual and distant disease, as well as OS.[86]

Although pathologic variations within T stage can further risk-stratify patients, aid in patient selection and in counseling patients regarding prognostic expectations, management decisions continue to center around T stage in incidental gallbladder cancer. Consensus has long existed regarding performance of re-resection for gallbladder cancer; however, several aspects of re-resection have provided some controversy regarding appropriate management and will be discussed in detail.

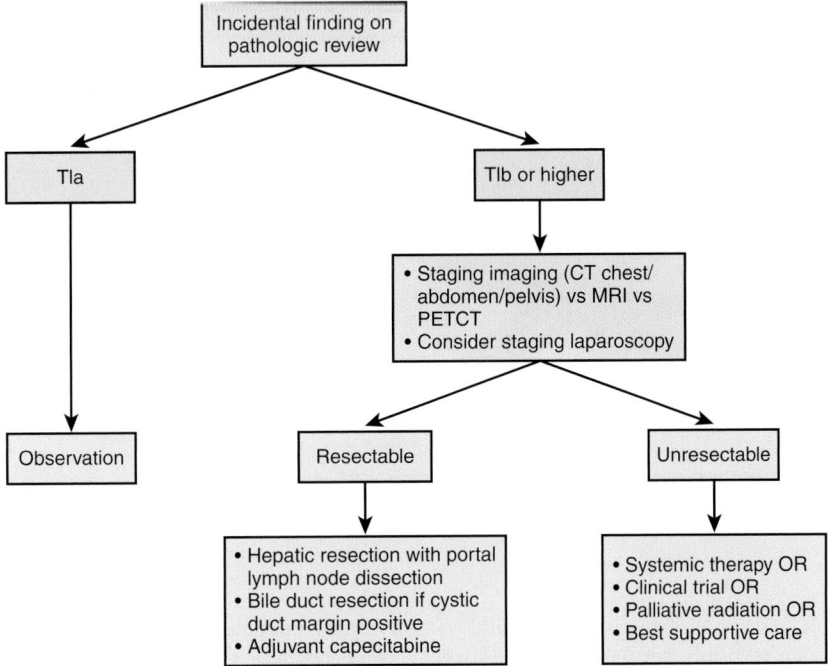

FIGURE 49.5   **Treatment algorithm for incidental gallbladder cancer.** Adapted from National Comprehensive Cancer Network (NCCN) Guidelines 3.2020

Staging Laparoscopy

After diagnosis of incidental gallbladder cancer on pathologic review, cross-sectional imaging is indicated for disease staging and evaluation for metastatic disease. However, despite no evidence of metastatic disease on high-quality cross-sectional imaging, 10% to 57% of patients will have radiographically occult metastatic disease at re-exploration.[18] Staging laparoscopy allows for the identification of occult metastatic disease before subjecting the patient to the morbidity, hospital cost, and length of stay associated with a laparotomy for re-resection.[87] Peritoneal dissemination is common in gallbladder cancer, occurring in 30% to 75% of patients, with the risk of peritoneal metastasis increasing with increasing tumor stage.[18] Weber and colleagues evaluated 44 patients with potentially resectable gallbladder cancer who underwent staging laparoscopy after thorough preoperative imaging evaluation between October 1997 and May 2001, followed by laparotomy and resection if appropriate.[88] Twenty-one patients were identified as having unresectable disease on staging laparoscopy, resulting in an overall yield of 48%. Of the 23 patients who underwent laparotomy, 15 were found to be unresectable, resulting in an overall accuracy of detecting unresectable disease via staging laparoscopy of 58%.[88] In subgroup analysis examining patients with incidentally diagnosed gallbladder cancer after simple cholecystectomy, however, the yield of staging laparoscopy was only 20%, compared with 56% in patients undergoing staging laparoscopy as an initial step for known gallbladder cancer, indicating that staging laparoscopy may not be *mandatory* for patients with incidental gallbladder cancer before re-resection.[88] The current NCCN guidelines recommend *consideration* of staging laparoscopy for patients with incidental gallbladder cancer of T stage 1b and greater.[41]

It is also important to consider improvements in imaging studies, increasing use of PET-CT as previously discussed, and

their ability to detect peritoneal dissemination and accurately stage gallbladder cancer when deciding whether staging laparoscopy is warranted. A more recent series reported by Butte and colleagues examined 136 patients with incidental gallbladder cancer who were referred for consideration for re-resection between 1998 and 2009.[17] Of these patients, 44 underwent staging laparoscopy before laparotomy. The yield of staging laparoscopy was 4.8% in this cohort, with an overall accuracy of 20%.[17] The authors also redemonstrated the association between disseminated disease and more advanced T stage: 0% of patients with T1b tumors had disseminated disease, compared with 7% of T2 tumors, and 26% of T3 tumors.[17]

The results of these two studies indicate that the yield of staging laparoscopy is relatively low in cases of incidental gallbladder cancer. Consideration of staging laparoscopy is most appropriate in patients with incidental gallbladder cancer with disruption of the gallbladder wall during cholecystectomy, T3 tumors, a positive resection margin, poorly differentiated tumors, and lymphovascular or perineural invasion, because these factors have been associated with increased risk of disseminated disease.[17] Ultimately, staging laparoscopy is not necessary in every patient with incidental gallbladder cancer before re-resection, but a careful analysis of the risks and benefits of the procedure must be performed and considered.

Indications for Major Hepatectomy

Although consensus exists that radical, or extended, cholecystectomy is warranted for T1b and more advanced tumors, the extent of hepatic resection is a subject of some controversy. Rationale for hepatic resection is 3-fold: (1) to achieve an R0 resection margin by removing direct neoplastic invasion into the gallbladder bed, (2) to prevent local recurrence in the gallbladder bed by removing micrometastatic disease, and (3) to prevent potential invasion of the hepatoduodenal ligament.[89–92] Surgical options

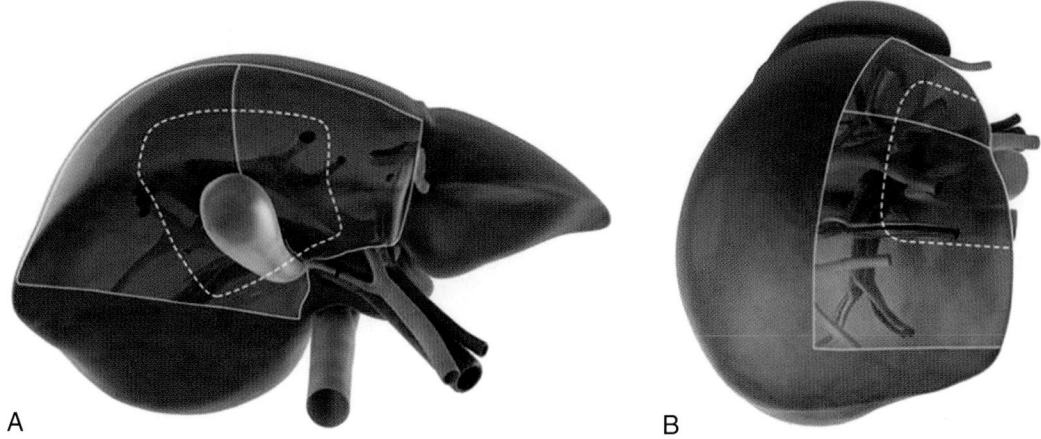

A   B

FIGURE 49.6   Anatomic IVb/V segmentectomy *(solid white line)* compared with nonanatomic wedge resection *(dotted white line)* of the liver for radical resection of gallbladder cancer in two views (see Chapter 119).

include a formal anatomic resection of segments IVb and V, nonanatomic wedge resection of visibly normal liver tissue with a 2 to 3 cm margin around the gallbladder fossa, and major hepatectomy.[93] Although there is no level I evidence to guide this decision, retrospective studies have concluded that parenchymal sparing wedge resection, contingent on achieving an R0 resection, has equivalent oncologic efficacy to anatomic segmental resection (Fig. 49.6). Araida and colleagues conducted a survey of 112 institutions in the Japanese Association of Biliary Surgery and reviewed outcomes of 485 cases of T2 and T3 gallbladder cancer who underwent re-resection consisting of either wedge resection or formal segmentectomy of IVb and V over a 10-year period.[89] The authors found no difference in 5-year OS between patients who received a formal segmentectomy and those who underwent a wedge resection (72% vs. 74%, respectively, $P = .7713$) and, further, found that there was no difference in liver metastasis (3.4% vs. 7.8%, $P = .2696$).[89] In a nationwide study using the Japanese Biliary Tract Registry, Horiguchi and colleagues likewise found no difference in hepatic metastasis or OS in patients with T2 tumors who underwent wedge resection versus IVb/V segmentectomy.[94] They cited the most common mode of hepatic recurrence in patients who underwent wedge resection as distant bilobar disease, rather than in the remaining portions of segments IVb/V, indicating that wedge resection was oncologically effective for locoregional control.[94] Similarly, Tewari and colleagues evaluated 30 patients with T1b, T2, or T3 gallbladder cancer who underwent radical cholecystectomy with wedge resection of the gallbladder fossa including at least 2 cm nonneoplastic liver parenchyma between October 2012 and June 2015. All patients had an R0 resection, and no hepatic recurrences were observed in a follow-up period of 43 months.[93] In aggregate, these studies support wedge resection to address hepatic invasion in T1b, T2, and T3 tumors, as long as an R0 resection is achieved.

There is some evidence that location of the neoplasm within the gallbladder may affect the needed resection. Lee and colleagues examined 192 patients with T2 gallbladder cancer at six institutions in Korea.[95] The authors found that in patients with peritoneal sided tumors, there was no difference in 5-year OS between patients who underwent simple cholecystectomy with lymph node dissection and patients who underwent cholecystectomy,

lymph node dissection, and hepatic resection (54.8% vs. 70.5%, respectively, $P = .111$). In contrast, in patients with hepatic-sided tumors, there was a significant difference in OS between these two groups (hepatic resection: 5-year OS 80.3%; no hepatic resection: 5-year OS 30.0%, $P = .032$).[95] However, extent of hepatic resection did not affect outcomes. It is important to note that in this series patients who did not receive a liver resection did not because of older age or worse general preoperative condition, introducing an obvious bias into this retrospective survival analysis.[95] Cho and colleagues conducted a similar analysis in 81 patients with T2 tumors and found that although patients with hepatic sided tumors had decreased 3-year OS compared with those with peritoneal sided tumors (96.6% vs. 76%, $P = .041$), hepatic resection did not confer improved 3-year OS in any group over cholecystectomy with lymph node dissection (T2a: hepatic resection 94.1%; no hepatic resection 100%, $P = .552$, T2b: hepatic resection 70.9%, no hepatic resection 100%, $P = .365$).[90] Particularly in light of changes to the staging guidelines regarding peritoneal versus hepatic tumor location, this is an interesting question to be explored further, although current guidelines recommend hepatic resection for all tumors T1b and above that are considered resectable, regardless of T2a or T2b designation.[41]

Because achieving an R0 resection is paramount to improving prognosis in patients with gallbladder cancer, major hepatectomy, in the form of a right or extended right hepatectomy, is only warranted if necessary, to achieve negative margins. This was demonstrated by Pawlik and colleagues in an analysis of 225 patients with incidental gallbladder cancer who underwent re-resection at six major hepatobiliary centers in the United States.[78] On multivariable analysis, the authors found that major hepatic resection was not associated with decreased OS (hazard ratio [HR] 1.25, 95% confidence interval [CI] 0.54–2.92, $P = .60$). Rather, independent predictors of decreased OS included increasing stage and residual carcinoma in the liver bed.[78] Invasion into the hepatoduodenal ligament or Glisson's capsule or vascular inflow involvement, however, necessitates right hepatectomy for complete oncologic tumor clearance.[75,92] In the early 2000s, extended operations such as the hepatopancreaticoduodenectomy (HPD) were performed for tumors with hepatoduodenal ligament invasion to retrieve all peripancreatic lymph nodes. Prophylactic pancreaticoduodenectomy (PD) for lymphatic resection, however, has been shown to not improve survival, with Araida and colleagues demonstrating a 5-year OS after curative HPD of 4%, and is associated with significant postoperative complications.[96] PD is currently only indicated for direct pancreatic invasion, and guidelines for these locally advanced cancers include consideration for clinical trials and neoadjuvant therapy.[41]

Finally, regardless of resection extent, the timing of re-resection after discovery of incidental gallbladder cancer has been shown to impact long-term outcomes. Using a large, multi-institutional database, Ethun and colleagues examined 207 patients who underwent re-resection for gallbladder cancer after simple cholecystectomy and found that definitive operation at an interval of 4 to 8 weeks after the index operation was associated with the best prognosis (median OS: < 4 weeks: 17.4 months, 4–8 weeks: 40.4 months, > 8 weeks: 22.3 months, $P = .03$).[97] Further, time interval to re-resection was independently associated with OS on multivariable analysis, including presence of residual disease, final resection margin, T stage, and lymph node involvement.[97]

Bile Duct Resection

The utility and benefit of common bile duct resection has likewise been debated and consensus is likewise guided by retrospective analyses rather than level I evidence. Current NCCN guidelines recommend hepatic resection and lymphadenectomy *with or without bile duct excision for malignant involvement*.[41] Routine common bile duct excision has not been reliably shown to be associated with improved survival. D'Angelica and colleagues examined 32 patients who underwent empiric common bile duct excision during resection.[75] The authors found no difference in DSS between those who did and did not undergo a common bile duct excision, nor did bile duct excision increase lymph node yield.[75] Fuks and colleagues similarly found no significant difference in survival between patients who did and did not undergo common bile duct resection, but both studies reported trends toward worse survival in the resected group.[75,85] Further, Fuks et al. demonstrated increased postoperative complication rates in the common bile duct resection group (60% vs. 23%, $P = .0001$) and no difference in R0 resection rates.[85]

However, a positive cystic stump margin, if not able to be cleared with a more proximal cystic duct dissection and transection, mandates common bile duct resection to ensure negative margins and an R0 resection.[50] Pawlik and colleagues, in a review of 225 patients, found residual disease in the common bile ducts of 21.4% of patients who underwent bile duct resection, and microscopic cystic stump margin predicted residual common bile duct disease; 42% of patients with a positive cystic stump margin had residual ductal disease compared with 4% of patients with negative cystic stump margins ($P = .01$).

The presence of jaundice because of malignant infiltration of the bile duct portends advanced disease, a dismal prognosis, and low likelihood of an R0 resection.[33]

Portal Lymph Node Dissection

Lymphatic spread is an important mechanism of gallbladder metastasis; approximately 12% of T1b tumors, 31% of T2, and 45% of T3 tumors have associated lymph node involvement.[78] In 1992 Shirai and colleagues performed a dye injection study to identify the route of lymphatic drainage from the gallbladder. The authors found that lymphatic drainage flows initially to the cystic and pericholedochal node groups, then to the posterosuperior pancreaticoduodenal, celiac, and retroportal nodes.[98] Lymph node dissection as part of resection for gallbladder cancer was described and practiced much earlier, however. In 1954 Glenn and Hays first described the "radical cholecystectomy" for gallbladder cancer, in which at least a 1-cm margin of liver parenchyma and the lymph nodes of the hepatoduodenal ligament were excised during cholecystectomy, which quickly became standard of care.[99] Studies performed since that time have supported this practice.

Lymph node metastases have been repeatedly shown to be independently associated with worse prognosis in gallbladder cancer. For example, in a review of 149 patients who underwent resection for gallbladder cancer, Bartlett and colleagues found nodal stage to be the only independent predictor of decreased OS in a multivariable analysis including T stage, M stage, level of hepatic involvement, and level of bile duct involvement.[100] Liu and colleagues, in an analysis of 78 patients who underwent radical resection for gallbladder cancer, similarly found significantly better DSS in patients with no lymph node metastases (median DSS 40 months vs. 7 months, $P < .001$).[101] Benoist and colleagues, in an analysis of 86 patients from 25 centers in France, likewise found a significant difference in postoperative OS in patients who had lymph node metastases (5-year OS 0%) and those without (5-year OS 44%, $P < .05$).[102]

Although lymph node metastases confer a poor prognosis, lymph node resection is associated with improved survival. Jensen and colleagues conducted a study of 4614 patients who received surgical treatment for T1b, T2, or T3 gallbladder cancer in the SEER database between 1988 and 2004.[103] The authors found that 56% of patients who underwent radical resection and 28% of patients who underwent cholecystectomy had lymph nodes evaluated, and 49.5% of patients who had lymph nodes evaluated had nodal metastases on pathologic evaluation. Patients who were more likely to have nodes evaluated were younger than 70 years and those with higher T stage and higher grade tumors. Lymph node evaluation was associated with improved median OS in tumors of all T stages; patients with T1b and T2 tumors who underwent radical resection with evaluation of at least one lymph node had a median OS of 123 months, compared with 22 months for patients who did not have lymph nodes resected ($P < .001$), and patients with T3 tumors who had evaluation of at least one lymph node had a median OS of 10 months, compared with 6 months for patients who did not have lymph nodes resected ($P = .014$).[103] Further, lymph node evaluation remained associated with improved DSS and OS on multivariable analysis accounting for age, sex, race, tumor grade, receipt of radiation, and year of treatment (DSS: T1b/T2: HR 0.759, 95% CI 0.635–0.907, $P = .024$; T3: HR 0.74, 95% CI 0.647–0.848, $P < .001$; OS: T1b/T2: HR 0.752, 95% CI 0.649–0.872, $P = .002$; T3: HR 0.717, 95% CI 0.635–0.808, $P < .001$).[103] Importantly, without lymphadenectomy, radical resection and simple cholecystectomy conferred similar OS (7 months vs. 6 months, respectively). The authors concluded that lymph node evaluation was an important component of surgical therapy for gallbladder cancer and portal lymphadenectomy remains the standard of care.[41,103]

Although consensus exists regarding the importance of a lymph node dissection, optimal lymph node yield has been a subject of some debate. In the previously discussed study, Jensen and colleagues found no difference in mortality when multiple lymph nodes were retrieved rather than a single node.[103] Birnbaum and colleagues, in an analysis of 112 patients, similarly found that the number of lymph nodes retrieved during radical resection (1–6 vs. >6) was not associated with OS.[104] In contrast, multiple studies have identified an "optimal" cutoff for lymph node yield. Negi and colleagues, in an analysis of 98 patients, found a total lymph node count of 6 or greater to be associated with improved DFS compared with a lymph node yield of fewer than 6 nodes in patients without lymph node metastases (median DFS: not reached vs. 32 months, $P = .012$).[105] Lymph node yield was not prognostic of recurrence in patients with lymph node metastases.[105] However, Liu and colleagues found prolonged DSS in patients with positive lymph nodes who had six or more nodes resected (median DSS: 33 months vs. 15 months, $P < .001$).[101] In both studies, location of positive lymph nodes was not associated with study outcomes. These results support the changes to the AJCC staging guidelines to defining nodal stage by number of lymph nodes rather than location and the resection of at least six lymph nodes, which appears to accurately stage patients. Although debatable, some studies suggest that nodal dissection in and of itself is associated with improved outcomes by decreasing recurrence via eliminating a common method of metastatic spread, and by removing lymph node–positive disease.[66,101,105]

Port Site Resection

The incidence of port site metastases after laparoscopic cholecystectomy in incidental gallbladder cancer is approximately 10%.[106] Incidence of port site recurrence or metastasis has been shown to increase with gallbladder perforation during cholecystectomy and to be highest at the extraction port.[106,107] Because port site recurrence not surprisingly correlates with peritoneal dissemination and advanced disease, the utility of port site resection as part of definitive resection for incidental gallbladder cancer has been questioned.[107]

Maker and colleagues conducted a retrospective analysis of 113 patients seen at a single center. Patients with port site metastases on final pathology did have decreased OS compared with patients without port site involvement; however, port site resection was not associated with improved OS or RFS, and the authors concluded that port site resection was not mandatory to improve outcomes during re-resection.[107] Fuks and colleagues conducted a similar study using a French multicenter database and found similar 1, 3, and 5-year OS in patients who underwent port site resection compared with those who did not (1-year OS: 77% vs. 78%; 3-year OS: 58% vs. 55%, 5-year OS 21% vs. 33%, $P = .37$).[108] Notably, 8% of patients who underwent port site resection developed incisional hernias at the resection site; thus, although port site resection does not appear to be associated with improved survival, it may confer additional morbidity.[108] Finally, Ethun and colleagues evaluated 193 patients from the United States Extrahepatic Biliary Malignancy Consortium database with incidentally discovered gallbladder cancer who underwent re-resection.[109] The authors found no difference in 3-year OS between patients whose re-resection included resection of previous port sites and those who did not undergo port site resection (65% vs. 43%, respectively, $P = .07$). Distant disease recurrence rates were likewise similar between groups (80% vs. 81%, $P = 1.0$).[110]

Based on the results of these studies, port site resection in incidental gallbladder cancer is not considered standard of care

for all patients undergoing re-resection, which is reflected in the current NCCN guidelines.[41]

Nonincidental Gallbladder Cancer (see Chapter 119)

Nonincidental or per primum gallbladder cancer represents the minority of gallbladder cancer diagnoses in the United States and other Western countries. Commonly, patients present with symptoms of advanced disease, including jaundice and weight loss.[110] Although nonincidental gallbladder cancer has been uniformly cited as portending worse outcomes compared with incidentally diagnosed cancers, two groups have investigated specific clinicopathologic differences between incidental and nonincidental gallbladder cancers.[110,111] Mazer and colleagues found patients with nonincidentally diagnosed gallbladder cancer to be more likely to present with higher T-stage tumors and nodal metastases, vascular, perineural, and lymphatic invasion to be less likely to have well-differentiated tumors, compared with patients with incidentally diagnosed tumors. Consequently, patients with nonincidental gallbladder cancer were less likely to undergo resection. Patients with incidentally diagnosed tumors were more likely to have only been evaluated with ultrasonography preoperatively, consistent with suspicion of benign disease.[111] The findings of Ethun and colleagues confirm and expand on those of Mazer et al. These authors found that patients with nonincidental gallbladder cancer often had lower body mass index (BMI), were less likely to be of non-Hispanic White race, and were more likely to present with jaundice. Nonincidental gallbladder cancer was also associated with increased rates of distant disease at surgical exploration leading to aborted procedures, higher incidence of R1 or R2 resections, higher T stage, poor tumor differentiation, and higher rates of lymphovascular invasion and lymph node positivity.[110]

The surgical principles concerning incidental and nonincidental, or suspected, gallbladder cancer are largely similar. For suspected gallbladder cancers without preoperative tissue diagnosis, however, one expert consensus report recommends intraoperative core needle biopsy with immediate frozen-section analysis to confirm the diagnosis before committing to radical resection.[79] Additionally, because of the increased risk of both disseminated disease and locally advanced unresectable disease at presentation in nonincidental cancers, staging laparoscopy is recommended before laparotomy for all cases of suspected gallbladder cancer.[110] The general treatment algorithm for nonincidental gallbladder cancer is depicted in Figure 49.7.

ADJUVANT THERAPY

Despite appropriate resection, recurrence rates in gallbladder cancers are high and almost 70% of patients will develop a recurrence postoperatively.[112] The majority of recurrences occur distantly; Jarnagin and colleagues studied the recurrence patterns in patients with gallbladder cancer who had appropriate surgical resection and found that 72% of recurrences were distant, most commonly to the peritoneum, followed by the liver, lung or mediastinum, and abdominal wall/incision, whereas 17% of recurrences were local, and 11% were regional, defined as metastasis to the retroperitoneal lymph nodes.[112] These recurrence patterns emphasize the need for effective systemic therapies for gallbladder cancer in the adjuvant setting. However, because of the rarity of this malignancy, until recently there have been a paucity of data to guide treatment recommendations.

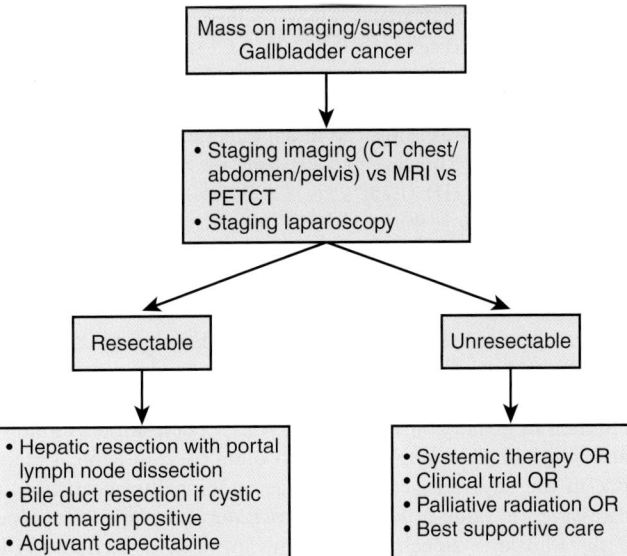

FIGURE 49.7 Treatment algorithm for nonincidental gallbladder cancer. Adapted from National Comprehensive Cancer Network (NCCN) Guidelines 3.2020

Multiple retrospective studies have been published, which are nicely summarized in a systematic review and meta-analysis by Horgan and colleagues who reviewed studies published between 1960 and 2010 that investigated adjuvant chemotherapy, radiotherapy, or chemoradiotherapy for resected biliary tract cancers.[113] In the overall population on pooled analysis, there was no difference in OS in patients who received any adjuvant therapy or those who did not; however, when the two large studies from the SEER database were removed, leaving 17 institutional studies to be analyzed, patients who received adjuvant therapy had an improved OS (HR 0.53, 95% CI 0.39–0.72, $P < .001$). Additionally, patients who received adjuvant

chemotherapy or chemoradiotherapy had significantly improved survival compared with patients who did not receive adjuvant therapy (chemotherapy: HR 0.39, 95% CI 0.23–0.66, $P < .001$; chemoradiotherapy: HR 0.61, 95% CI 0.38–0.99, $P = .049$), whereas survival was similar among patients who received adjuvant radiotherapy alone compared with no adjuvant therapy (HR 0.98, 95% CI 0.67–1.43, $P = .90$).[113] An association between adjuvant therapy including chemotherapy or chemoradiotherapy and improved OS was also seen on subgroup analysis in patients with node-positive disease and those who underwent R1 resections.[113] Although this analysis supported the use of adjuvant therapy in general, it does not specify the relative utility of chemotherapy or chemoradiotherapy in biliary tract cancers, nor does it specify the optimal agent or combination and dosing schedule. The study analyzes biliary tract cancers as a whole and provides no targeted information on gallbladder cancer. The lone phase III trial performed in this time period by Takada and colleagues included patients with resected pancreatic, gallbladder, bile duct, or ampullary cancers. Patients were randomized to receive adjuvant therapy with mitomycin C and 5-fluorouracil (5-FU) or surgery alone. When analyzing the subset of patients with gallbladder cancer, patients who received adjuvant chemotherapy had a 5-year OS of 26.0% compared with 14.4% in patients receiving surgery alone ($P = .0367$). Patients with gallbladder cancer who received adjuvant chemotherapy also had an improved DFS at 5 years (20.3% vs. 11.6%, $P = .0210$).[114]

Since 2010, five major RCTs, four investigating chemotherapy alone and one investigating chemoradiotherapy, have been reported to guide adjuvant therapy using more modern chemotherapeutic regimens. These trials are summarized in Table 49.3.

ABC-02

The Cisplatin plus Gemcitabine versus Gemcitabine for Advanced Biliary Tract Cancer (ABC-02) trial conducted by Valle

TABLE 49.3   Modern Published Randomized Controlled Trials of Adjuvant Therapy for Gallbladder Cancer

	ABC-02	PRODIGE-12/ ACCORD-18	BILCAP	BCAT	SWOG0809
Study design	Randomized phase III	Randomized phase III	Randomized phase III	Randomized phase III	Single-arm phase II
Study arms	Gemcitabine/cisplatin vs. gemcitabine alone	Surgery plus GEMOX vs. surgery alone	Surgery plus Capecitabine vs. surgery alone	Surgery plus Gemcitabine vs. surgery alone	Gemcitabine/ Capecitabine then capecitabine + radiotherapy
Recruitment period	Feb 2002 – Oct 2008	Jul 2009 – Feb 2014	Mar 2006 – Dec 2017	Sept 2007 – Jan 2011	Dec 2008 – Oct 2012
Country	United Kingdom	France	United Kingdom	Japan	United States
Number of sites	37	33	44	48	10
Primary endpoint	Overall survival (OS)	Recurrence-free survival (RFS)	OS	OS	OS
Result	OS: Gem/Cis: 11.7 months Gem alone: 8.1 months $P < .001$	RFS: GEMOX: 30.4 months Surgery alone: 18.5 months $P = .48$	OS: Cap: 51.1 months Surgery alone: 36.4 months $P = .09$	OS: Gem: 62.3 months Surgery alone: 63.8 months $P = .96$	2-year OS: R0: 67% R1: 60%

ABC-02, Cisplatin plus Gemcitabine versus Gemcitabine for Advanced Biliary Tract Cancer trial; *BCAT*, Bile Duct Cancer Adjuvant trial; *BILCAP*, Capecitabine or Observation after Surgery in Treating Patients with Biliary Treat Cancer trial; *Cap*, Capecitabine; *Cis*, cisplatin; *Gem*, gemcitabine; *GEMOX*, adjuvant gemcitabine and oxaliplatin; *PRODIGE-12/ACCORD-18*, Gemcitabine Hydrochloride and Oxaliplatin or Observation in Treating Patients with Biliary Tract Cancer that Has Been Removed by Surgery trial; *SWOG0809*, Adjuvant Capecitabine Tund Gemcitabine Followed by radiotherapy and Concurrent Capecitabine in Extrahepatic Cholangiocarcinoma and Gallbladder Carcinoma trial.

and colleagues compared gemcitabine and cisplatin doublet therapy in locally advanced or metastatic cholangiocarcinoma and gallbladder cancer.[115] Between February 2002 and October 2008, 410 patients were randomized, and the authors found improved OS and progression-free survival (PFS) in patients who received the combination therapy compared with gemcitabine alone (OS: 11.7 vs. 8.1 months, $P < .001$, PFS: 8 vs. 5 months, $P < .001$) without an increase in adverse events. Although this study focused on patients with advanced biliary malignancy, these results have been extrapolated to the adjuvant setting and the use of gemcitabine-based chemotherapy regimens formed the basis of future trials.[115]

PRODIGE-12/ACCORD-18

The Gemcitabine Hydrochloride and Oxaliplatin or Observation in Treating Patients with Biliary Tract Cancer that Has Been Removed by Surgery (PRODIGE-12/ACCORD-18) trial conducted by Edeline and colleagues compared adjuvant gemcitabine and oxaliplatin (GEMOX) to best supportive care in patients with cholangiocarcinoma of all sites and gallbladder cancer who underwent an R0 or R1 resection.[116] Patients with gallbladder cancer made up 20% of the study population. Between July 2009 and February 2014, 196 patients were randomized. The authors found no difference in relapse-free survival (HR 0.88, 95% CI 0.62–1.25, $P = .48$), OS (HR 1.08, 95% CI 0.70–1.66, $P = .74$) and quality of life score at 12 months (adjuvant GEMOX: 70.8 vs. best supportive care: 83.3, $P = .18$). This statistically negative trial has drawn criticism because of its design to detect a 40% reduction in relapse-free survival, suggesting that it was underpowered to detect smaller, yet clinically relevant differences between the groups. Additionally, the population enrolled in the trial was composed primarily of patients who underwent R0 resections and those without lymph node metastases, patients who are generally considered lower risk, whereas analysis of higher risk patients might demonstrate a benefit to adjuvant therapy.[116]

BCAT

The Bile Duct Cancer Adjuvant (BCAT) trial by Ebata and colleagues also compared adjuvant gemcitabine with best supportive care in patients with extrahepatic cholangiocarcinoma. Between September 2007 and January 2011, 226 patients were randomized. A minority of patients, 11%, had microscopically positive resection margins, whereas 54% of patients in the gemcitabine group and 35% in the best supportive care group had lymph node metastases. The authors found no significant differences in OS or RFS (OS: HR 1.01, 95% CI 0.70–1.45, $P = .964$; RFS: HR 0.93, 95% CI 0.66–1.32, $P = .693$).[117]

BILCAP

The Capecitabine or Observation after Surgery in Treating Patients with Biliary Treat Cancer (BILCAP) trial by Primrose and colleagues compared adjuvant capecitabine with best supportive care in patients with cholangiocarcinoma of all sites and muscle-invasive gallbladder cancer after complete macroscopic resection.[118] Patients with gallbladder cancer made up 18% of the study population. In contrast to PRODIGE-12/ACCORD-18, 54% of patients had microscopically positive margins after resection, and 38% of patients had lymph node–positive disease. Between March 2006 and December 2014, 447 patients were randomized. The authors found significantly improved OS in patients randomized to receive adjuvant therapy

in intention to treat analysis when adjusting for nodal status, disease grade, and sex (HR 0.71, 95% CI 0.55–0.92, $P = .01$), although no statistical difference was demonstrated in unadjusted intention to treat analysis (HR 0.81, 95% CI 0.63–1.04, $P = .097$). RFS was improved in patients randomized to receive adjuvant therapy; however, it was only for the first 24 months after resection (HR 0.75, 95% CI 0.58–0.98, $P = .033$).[118] Importantly, this is the only RCT to date to demonstrate improved outcomes with receipt of adjuvant chemotherapy in biliary tract malignancies. Because of the results of this trial, adjuvant capecitabine for a duration of 6 months is currently one recommended strategy for patients who undergo resection of gallbladder cancer.[119] Despite the results of the BILCAP trial, given its negative intention to treat analysis, a doublet regimen of gemcitabine combined with a platinum chemotherapy (cisplatin or oxaliplatin) is still often used in clinical practice in the adjuvant setting. A large ongoing European trial is assessing the value of adjuvant gemcitabine/cisplatin compared with adjuvant capecitabine (Adjuvant Chemotherapy With Gemcitabine and Cisplatin Compared to Standard of Care After Curative Intent Resection of Biliary Tract Cancer [ACTICCA-1]).

SWOG0809

The Adjuvant Capecitabine and Gemcitabine Followed by radiotherapy and Concurrent Capecitabine in Extrahepatic Cholangiocarcinoma and Gallbladder Carcinoma (SWOG0809) trial by Ben-Josef and colleagues analyzed a single-arm trial of 105 patients with hilar or distal cholangiocarcinoma or gallbladder cancer between December 2008 and October 2012 to receive adjuvant gemcitabine and capecitabine followed by concurrent capecitabine and radiotherapy to the tumor bed and regional lymph nodes if no tumor progression was noted after adjuvant chemotherapy alone.[120] Patients with gallbladder cancer made up 32% of the study population. Analysis was stratified by final margin status. OS was 67% in the R0 group and 60% in the R1 group. Local recurrence at 2 years was 9% in the R0 group and 16% in the R1 group. The authors' predetermined goal was to demonstrate OS of at least 65% for patients with R0 resections and of at least 45% for patients with R1 resections, both of which were met; however, the lack of a control arm limits the applicability of these data to clinical practice. Despite this, the American Society of Clinical Oncology Clinical Practice Guidelines state that patients with microscopically positive surgical resection margins may be considered for adjuvant chemoradiotherapy after a course of adjuvant chemotherapy.[119,120]

NEOADJUVANT THERAPY

The role of neoadjuvant therapy in gallbladder cancer is not well defined. The rationale for neoadjuvant therapy includes downstaging of the primary tumor, providing an in vivo test of chemosensitivity, immediate treatment of micrometastatic disease, and to optimize patient selection for re-resection, possibly sparing patients the morbidity of a radical resection if disease biology declares itself to be particularly aggressive.[121] However, the risk of progression during therapy and decreased functional status because of toxicity affecting surgical candidacy must also be considered. There is currently no level I evidence guiding neoadjuvant treatment decisions. The NCCN guidelines advise consideration of neoadjuvant therapy after an incidental finding of gallbladder cancer "if there is evidence of locoregional advanced disease (big mass invading liver and/or nodal disease, including cystic duct node positive)...largely to rule out rapid progression and avoid futile surgery" while acknowledging "there are limited data to define a standard regimen or definitive benefit."[41]

Hakeem and colleagues performed a systematic review of the literature through May 10, 2018 and included six retrospective and two prospective cohort studies investigating the role of neoadjuvant therapy in gallbladder cancer.[122] Patients in the evaluated studies who were selected to receive neoadjuvant therapy were diagnosed with stage IIIa disease or greater. Approximately one-third of patients (30.6%) had progressive disease despite receipt of neoadjuvant therapy, and two-thirds (66.6%) demonstrated clinical benefit. One-half of patients (50.4%) were considered suitable for surgical resection after neoadjuvant therapy; however, the resectability rate upon exploration in included studies ranged from 13.5% to 66.7%. The overall R0 resection rate for included patients was 35.4%.[122] The authors concluded that there was insufficient evidence to support routine use of neoadjuvant therapy; however, the inclusion, because of natural selection bias inherent to retrospective studies, of only patients with locally advanced disease limits the applicability of these results to patients with earlier-stage, incidentally diagnosed gallbladder cancers.

Goetze and colleagues are currently recruiting patients for a multicenter phase III trial, "Neoadjuvant Chemotherapy With Gemcitabine Plus Cisplatin Followed by Radical Liver Resection Versus Immediate Radical Liver Resection Alone With or Without Adjuvant Chemotherapy in Incidentally Detected Gallbladder Carcinoma After Simple Cholecystectomy or in Front of Radical Resection of BTC," which will randomize patients with incidentally diagnosed T2 or T3 node negative or T1, 2, or 3 node positive tumors to receive neoadjuvant gemcitabine and cisplatin followed by radical resection or radical resection alone, followed by adjuvant chemotherapy at the investigators' discretion. The primary endpoint for this study will be OS, with the secondary endpoints of quality of life, PFS, toxicity, and perioperative morbidity and mortality.[123] Additionally, a recently approved phase II/III trial by Maithel and colleagues, "EA2197: Perioperative Chemotherapy Prior to and After Re-Resection for Incidental Gallbladder Cancer – A Randomized Phase II/III Trial" through the National Cancer Trials Network will evaluate the role of perioperative gemcitabine/cisplatin in patients with T2 or T3 gallbladder cancer compared with only adjuvant gemcitabine/cisplatin. The results of these and future RCTs are eagerly awaited.

TARGETED THERAPY

Multiple genetic alterations have been identified in gallbladder cancer, many of which are potential targets for novel therapies (see Chapter 9E). As previously mentioned, these alterations or mutations vary in prevalence by region. Overall, the most common mutation is in the Tp53 gene, occurring in approximately 55% of gallbladder cancers, followed by CDKN2A in 26%, HER2/neu in 15%, and ERBB2 in 12%.[124,125] Other genes affected include Kras, ARID1A, PBRM1, PIK3CA, BAP1, and SMAD4.[124] Although targeted therapy in gallbladder cancer is not currently used as a part of standard practice, its efficacy has been demonstrated in smaller studies and targeted therapy is included in multiple current RCTs.

For example, Javle and colleagues retrospectively reviewed patients with advanced gallbladder cancer and cholangiocarcinoma with HER2/neu genetic mutations or overexpression who received HER2/neu-directed therapy (trastuzumab, lapatinib, or pertuzumab) over a 7-year period.[125] Of eight patients with gallbladder cancer studied, three demonstrated disease stability, four a partial response, and one a complete response with HER2/neu-directed therapy.[125]

Li and colleagues performed whole genome sequencing on 157 patients with gallbladder cancer and performed functional experiments on gallbladder cancer cell lines.[126] Because activating ERBB2 mutations have been shown to be sensitive to ERBB inhibitors in multiple other cancer types, the authors exposed gallbladder cancer cells expressing mutant ERBB2/ERBB3 to the ERBB3 tyrosine kinase inhibitor sapitinib and found significant inhibition of phosphorylation levels and tumor growth, although cells with wild type ERBB2/ERBB3 were unaffected.[126–129] Additionally, the authors found that PD-1 was upregulated in cancers with ERBB2/ERBB3 mutations and that combination therapy with anti-PDL1 and anti-ERBB therapy decreased cellular viability in a gallbladder cancer cell line with mutant ERBB2/ERBB3 by 70%, compared with 30% with anti-PDL1, and 45% with anti-ERBB alone.

Iyer and colleagues performed co-immunoprecipitation of EGFR and ERBB2 in gallbladder cancer cell lines, the results of which suggested that ERBB2 requires EGFR for activation and that downregulation of EGFR may suppress the functionality of ERBB2 and provide an effective target for therapy in gallbladder cancer.[130] However, the authors found that a Kras mutation, specifically on codon 12, may render gallbladder cancers resistant to anti-epidermal growth factor receptor (EGFR) therapy, a differential response that has also been seen in colon cancers.[130] These preclinical studies suggest that targeted therapy will be the next frontier in treatment of gallbladder cancer, and several RCTs are underway to investigate the role of these therapies. The integration of this personalized approach in the neoadjuvant and adjuvant setting is the next horizon.

SURVEILLANCE

There are no data to support a specific surveillance schedule after radical resection for gallbladder cancer. However, given the high rates of recurrence, particularly distant recurrence, most surgeons agree that some manner of surveillance is advisable. Current NCCN guidelines recommend the schedule presented by Primrose and colleagues in the BILCAP trial: imaging of the chest, abdomen, and pelvis every 3 to 6 months for the first 2 years, then every 6 to 12 months for up to 5 years, or as clinically indicated.[41]

SUMMARY

Gallbladder cancer remains a highly lethal malignancy, but significant improvements in our understanding of this rare disease and in effective treatments, both surgical and systemic, have been made in recent decades. Surgical management, specifically with an R0 resection, remains the cornerstone of treatment for localized gallbladder cancer; however, advances in adjuvant and neoadjuvant therapy, chemotherapeutic regimens for locally advanced and metastatic disease, and in targeted therapies will continue to improve outcomes for patients. Ultimately, clinical trials investigating these novel therapies, advancements in imaging enabling earlier stage at diagnosis, and the maintaining of a high index of suspicion are needed. Multidisciplinary management of patients with gallbladder cancer is paramount to optimize outcomes and leverage available treatment options. Finally, given the rarity of this disease, national and international cooperation/ collaboration is necessary to conduct relevant and meaningful clinical trials that will improve the outcome of patients with this disease.

The references for this chapter can be found online by accessing the accompanying Expert Consult website.

CHAPTER 50

Intrahepatic cholangiocarcinoma

Jonathan B. Koea

INTRODUCTION

Intrahepatic cholangiocarcinoma (IHCC) is a primary adenocarcinoma of the liver. Like other primary adenocarcinomas of the upper gastrointestinal tract, IHCC often presents with symptoms due to advanced local disease or metastatic disease. IHCC is a biologically aggressive disease; complete resection, where possible, is the only known potentially curative therapy. In addition, there are few effective systemic therapies.

IHCC is also known as peripheral cholangiocarcinoma, cholangiolar carcinoma, or cholangiolocellular carcinoma, and these terms have previously been used interchangeably. The term *cholangiolocellular carcinoma* was first used in 1959 by Steiner and Higginson[1] to describe a subtype of cholangiocarcinoma in which the glands are small and regular with inconspicuous lumens and resemble proliferating cholangioles. Recent evidence suggests that these tumors represent a distinct subtype of intrahepatic cholangiocarcinoma and develop from hepatic stem cells.[2] Current nomenclature uses the term *intrahepatic cholangiocarcinoma* to define tumors arising from biliary epithelium in intrahepatic bile ducts above the level of the left main and right main ducts.[3,4] These tumors constitute 10% of primary hepatic malignancies and 20% of all cholangiocarcinomas.[2] Although much is known about extrahepatic cholangiocarcinoma, IHCC is less well understood.

Hepatic resection for IHCC was infrequently described until recently. Foster and Berman[5] reported only 13 cases in their summary of hepatic surgery in the United States, whereas they presented 112 resections for hepatocellular carcinoma and 47 cases of hepatoblastoma. This low number of resections likely represented the frequency with which advanced disease was diagnosed at presentation. In addition, the recognition of IHCC as a discrete primary liver tumor was slow to occur and many were historically diagnosed as metastatic lesions from unknown primary sites. However, with increased recognition of IHCC significant clinical effort has been directed at developing comprehensive treatment strategies incorporating surgery, systemic therapies, and regional therapies for patients with this malignancy.

EPIDEMIOLOGY AND DEMOGRAPHICS

IHCC is the second most common primary liver cancer after hepatocellular carcinoma and represents 3% of all gastrointestinal cancers.[6] The geographic incidence of cholangiocarcinoma is highly variable (Fig. 50.1), reflecting the influence of locally prevalent risk factors. The highest incidence rates are observed in Chile, Bolivia, South Korea, and Northern Thailand,[6] where IHCC constitutes 89% of all primary liver cancers.[7] Overall, the worldwide incidence of IHCC has been increasing both in areas of high and low incidence,[6] while the worldwide incidence of extrahepatic cholangiocarcinoma has decreased.[6,9] IHCC is more commonly diagnosed in males and usually presents in the 7th or 8th decades of life.[10] However, for individuals with specific risk factors (primary sclerosing cholangitis or untreated choledochal cysts), the average age of primary presentation falls to between 30 and 50 years of age.[11]

The incidence of IHCC also shows marked ethnic variation. In the United States approximately 5000 patients present annually with a diagnosis of cholangiocarcinoma.[12] The age-adjusted incidence of IHCC is highest in Hispanic Americans, is lowest in African Americans, and shows an annual rate of increase of 5% per year for the last two decades that is most marked in males and in Hispanic Americans.[13] In addition, Hispanics and African Americans have a poorer survival compared with Caucasians. There are significant variations in treatment related to patient socioeconomic status, demographics, and geographic region.[12,14]

ETIOLOGY AND RISK FACTORS

In Western countries over 90% of patients presenting with IHCC do not have a recognized risk factor.[8,15] However, a number of factors are understood to increase the risk of developing cholangiocarcinoma via sometimes overlapping effects of sustained, chronic inflammation of biliary epithelia, the presence of specific at-risk precursor lesions, and more general conditions that may intensify the effects of known carcinogens.[16] Many of these risk factors contribute to the development of both intrahepatic and extrahepatic cholangiocarcinoma.

Primary Sclerosing Cholangitis

Primary sclerosing cholangitis (PSC) is the most common risk factor for cholangiocarcinoma in Western countries[17,18] (see Chapter 41). The cumulative annual risk of cholangiocarcinoma in patients with PSC is 1.5% per year,[18] and the prevalence of cholangiocarcinoma in these patients is between 8% and 40%.[19–21] The risk for PSC patients developing cholangiocarcinoma is increased in those with associated inflammatory bowel disease where the 10 and 20 year rates for cholangiocarcinoma is 14% and 31% respectively versus 2% and 2% in patients without inflammatory bowel disease.[19] Cholangiocarcinoma often develops two to three decades earlier in patients with PSC than in those with sporadic tumors (30–50 years versus 60–70 years of age),[11,18] and PSC-associated tumors often present with advanced stage disease because of difficulties in detecting malignant change in inflammatory strictures. Surgical treatment can be difficult because of the presence of chronic liver disease. Patients are also often ineligible for orthotropic liver transplantation at presentation, because of the cancer diagnosis, and they consequently have a poor prognosis[22] (see Chapter 105). Factors predictive of cholangiocarcinoma in patients with PSC

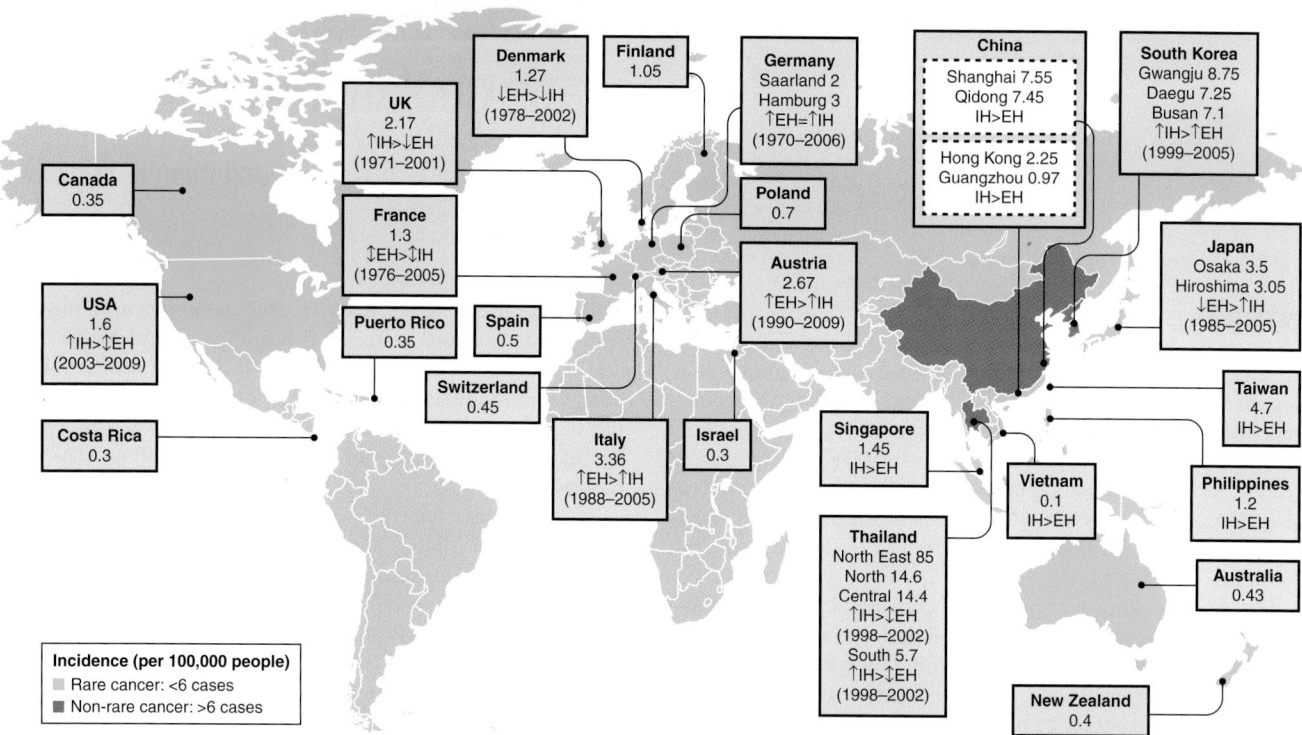

FIGURE 50.1 Graphic summarizing the worldwide incidence (cases per 100,000 population) of cholangiocarcinoma for the period 1971–2009. The green color identifies countries with lower incidence (<6 cases per 100,000 population, rare cancer) and the pink color identifies countries with higher incidence (>6 cases per 100,000 population). When available, incidence data from intrahepatic cholangiocarcinoma (IH) and extrahepatic cholangiocarcinoma (EH) and the temporal trend of incidence (↑ increasing trend; ↕ stable trend; ↓ decreasing trend) is presented. (With permission under the Creative Commons Attribution 4.0 International License, http://creativecommons.org/licenses/by/4.0/.)

are sudden development of jaundice, weight loss, marked biliary dilation proximal to a dominant stricture, a sudden rise in carbohydrate antigen 19-9 (CA 19-9), the presence of a hypovascular mass with late contrast enhancement on radiologic imaging, and cytologic evidence of dysplasia or malignancy obtained on brushings.[23]

Parasitic Infections

Chronic infection with the liver flukes (*Opisthorchis viverrini* and *Clinorchis sinensis*) is the most common risk factor for developing cholangiocarcinoma in Southeast Asia[24–26] (see Chapter 45). The mechanism of carcinogenesis is unclear. However, mechanical irritation, excreted metabolic products, and the actions of proinflammatory cytokines, particularly those that stimulate the release of nitric oxide from activated white cells, are all important.[16,17,27]

A further parasitic hepatic infestation is caused by the Trematodes *Fasciola hepatica* or *Fasciola gigantica* (see Chapters 45 and 71). These parasites are widely spread throughout Asia, Africa, the Americas, and Oceania. *Fasciola* species migrate into the liver from the duodenum and cause hepatic fibrosis.[28] There is no evidence that fascioliasis increases the risk of cholangiocarcinoma per se, although the radiologic and fibrotic pathologic changes accompanying an infection can be difficult to distinguish from carcinoma.[29,30]

Hepatolithiasis

Recurrent pyogenic cholangiohepatitis (previously known as oriental cholangiohepatitis) is characterized by recurrent episodes of ascending cholangitis, hepatolithiasis, biliary strictures, and biliary dilation (see Chapters 39 and 44). The syndrome is present in one fifth of the population of Southeast Asia and up to 10% of these patients develop IHCC,[31–34] possibly because of chronic bile stasis leading to chronic infection and inflammation with malignant transformation.[16] Patients present with recurrent episodes of cholangitis and, on investigation, have significant hepatolithiasis and associated inflammatory biliary strictures.[35] The mean interval between the treatment of hepatolithiasis and the development of cholangiocarcinoma is between 3 and 8 years,[36] and patients remain at risk of developing IHCC following hepatectomy if affected parts of the liver remain.[37] Infection with liver flukes may also occur concurrently in many patients, but recurrent pyogenic cholangitis is a separate condition and can develop in the absence of parasitic infection.[38]

Congenital Biliary Cystic Disease

Untreated choledochal cysts and Caroli disease carry an increased risk of developing cholangiocarcinoma (see Chapter 46). The incidence of cholangiocarcinoma is estimated at between 10% and 20% if the cyst is not resected by a patient age of 20 years.[39,40] Correspondingly, patients who have had their cysts resected have a very low incidence of cholangiocarcinoma,[41] although subsequent development of cholangiocarcinoma has been recorded following cyst excision.[42] The mechanism of malignant transformation is not understood but many patients with choledochal cysts have an abnormally high union of the pancreatic and bile ducts, suggesting that biliary stasis and chronic reflux of pancreatic secretions may contribute to the development of chronic inflammation of biliary epithelium. In patients with pancreaticobiliary maljunction alone there is a 7% risk of cholangiocarcinoma.[43]

Hepatic Cirrhosis and Viral Infections

The risk of developing IHCC is increased in patients with cirrhosis (10.7% versus 0.7% in the general population),[44,45] and 1% of explanted cirrhotic livers will harbor a previously unsuspected IHCC[46] (see Chapters 9B, 9C, 68, 74, and 89). An association between hepatitis C infection and IHCC was postulated in 1991.[47] A case control study from Japan demonstrated that the risk of developing IHCC is 3.5% at 10 years in patients with hepatitis C–related cirrhosis.[48] A separate large cohort study found a significant association between IHCC and hepatitis C after adjusting for potential confounders, including the presence of cirrhosis with a relative risk of 2.55 (95% confidence intervals 1.3–4.95).[49] In these patients carcinogenesis may be due to a direct viral effect since biliary dysplasia is more commonly observed in explanted livers of patients transplanted for hepatitis C–related cirrhosis than in other conditions.[50] IHCC is also more frequent in patients with chronic hepatitis B viral infection (11.5% versus 5.5% in the general population),[51] although the relative risk (RR) is less than for hepatitis C infection (RR 1.8, 95% confidence interval 1.4–2.4).[52] IHCC developing in the setting of hepatitis B infection is more likely to present with a mass-forming growth pattern, which carries a more favorable prognosis following resection.[53] It has been suggested the increasing incidence of IHCC in the West is related to the increasing prevalence of chronic liver disease and chronic viral infection.[8,54] Co-infection with both hepatitis B and *Opisthorchis viverrini* or *Clinorchis sinensis* is an important factor in the high incidence of IHCC observed in Asia.[54] In addition there is evidence that nonalcoholic steatohepatitis is present in up to 20% of patients with IHCC, although this may reflect lifestyle rather than representing an etiologic factor.[55] Diabetes and obesity have been associated with an increased risk of cholangiocarcinoma,[56–58] although this association may be stronger for carcinoma of the gallbladder.[17]

Human immunodeficiency virus (HIV) does not cause cirrhosis, but cholangiocarcinomas have been found in up to 0.5% of patients infected with the virus compared with 0.1% in controls, suggesting that it too is associated with an increased risk of biliary carcinogenesis.[59]

Benign Biliary Tumors

The development of biliary cystadenocarcinomas from biliary cystadenomas is rare and, in general, occurs if a cystadenocarcinoma is untreated for many years. Biliary cystadenomas without ovarian stromal tissue appear to be at higher risk of malignant change and patients present with cystadenocarcinomas in the 6th or 7th decades of life, whereas cystadenomas present at an earlier age.[60] IHCCs have also been reported developing in patients with biliary papillomata,[61,62] and three related pathologic precursor lesions are now recognized for IHCC—flat intraepithelial neoplasia (BilIN), intraductal papillary mucinous neoplasm of the bile duct (IPNB; previously recognized as biliary papillomatosis), and intraductal tubulo-papillary neoplasm (ITNB).[63] All three lesions are often seen in the context chronic biliary inflammation.[63] Progression of bile duct adenoma to IHCC has been reported, and Von Meyenberg complex has also been suggested as a possible premalignant lesion for IHCC due to the occasional association of Von Meyenberg complexes and IHCC.[64]

Chemical Agents

Thorotrast (thorium dioxide) was used as a radiologic contrast agent between 1928 and 1950. It is an alpha emitter with a biologic half-life of 400 years. Thorotrast accumulates in reticuloendothelial cells in the liver and spleen, and increases the risk of cholangiocarcinoma by 300 times in comparison to the general population.[65] It is now no longer in use, although the latency period of 16 to 45 years means that patients will occasionally still present having received this agent during childhood radiologic examinations.[66]

A number of other agents have been implicated in the development of cholangiocarcinoma. Associations have been shown for asbestos,[67] vinyl chloride,[68] nitrosamines,[69] the antituberculosis agent isoniazid,[70] and first-generation oral contraceptives.[71]

General Risk Factors

Surgical biliary-enteric bypass and surgical sphincteroplasty increase the risk of developing cholangiocarcinoma.[72] Tobacco smoking is a significant risk factor for the development of cholangiocarcinoma in patients with PSC,[73] although the relationship is less marked in the general population.[59] Finally, congenital hepatic fibrosis has also been associated with an increased risk of developing cholangiocarcinoma in later life.[8]

PATHOGENESIS

IHCC develops within the hepatic biliary system in second-order and more proximal bile ducts (septal, interlobular bile ducts, and ductules).[63] Hepatic bile ducts are lined with specialized cholangiocytes whose function centers around the modification of bile at the canalicular surface and detoxification of xenobiotics.[74]

Cell of Origin

Within the liver the segmental and septal bile ducts are lined with cylindrical mucin-producing cholangiocytes. IHCC that develop from these cells form adenocarcinomas with significant mucus secretion.[75] These tumors may invade along the biliary tree and morphologically form periductal infiltrating or large nodular mass-forming tumors. However, the interlobular bile ducts and ductules are lined with cuboidal cholangiocytes that do not secrete mucus. IHCCs developing from these cells are non–mucin-secreting adenocarcinomas and usually form mass lesions at the periphery of the liver.[75] The ductules also contain hepatic progenitor stem cells, which can display varying degrees of hepatocyte or cholangiocytic differentiation. Cholangiolocellular carcinoma is considered to develop from these progenitor cells and also forms mass lesions at the periphery of the liver.[75,76]

Chromosomal Aberrations

Recent investigations have defined chromosomal aberrations in patients with IHCC (see Chapter 9E). Deleted genomic areas were defined in 1p, 3p, and 4q, and the main areas of amplification were present in 1q, 7p, 7q, and 8q.[77,78] Interestingly, these investigations suggest that hepatocellular carcinoma and IHCC may be closely related at a molecular level as they share chromosomal gains at 1q, 8q, and 17q, as well as chromosomal losses at 4q, 8p, and 17p (Fig. 50.2).[79]

Genomic and Epigenetic Alterations

Two distinct genomic classes have been characterized in IHCC (see Chapter 9E): an inflammatory class with predominant

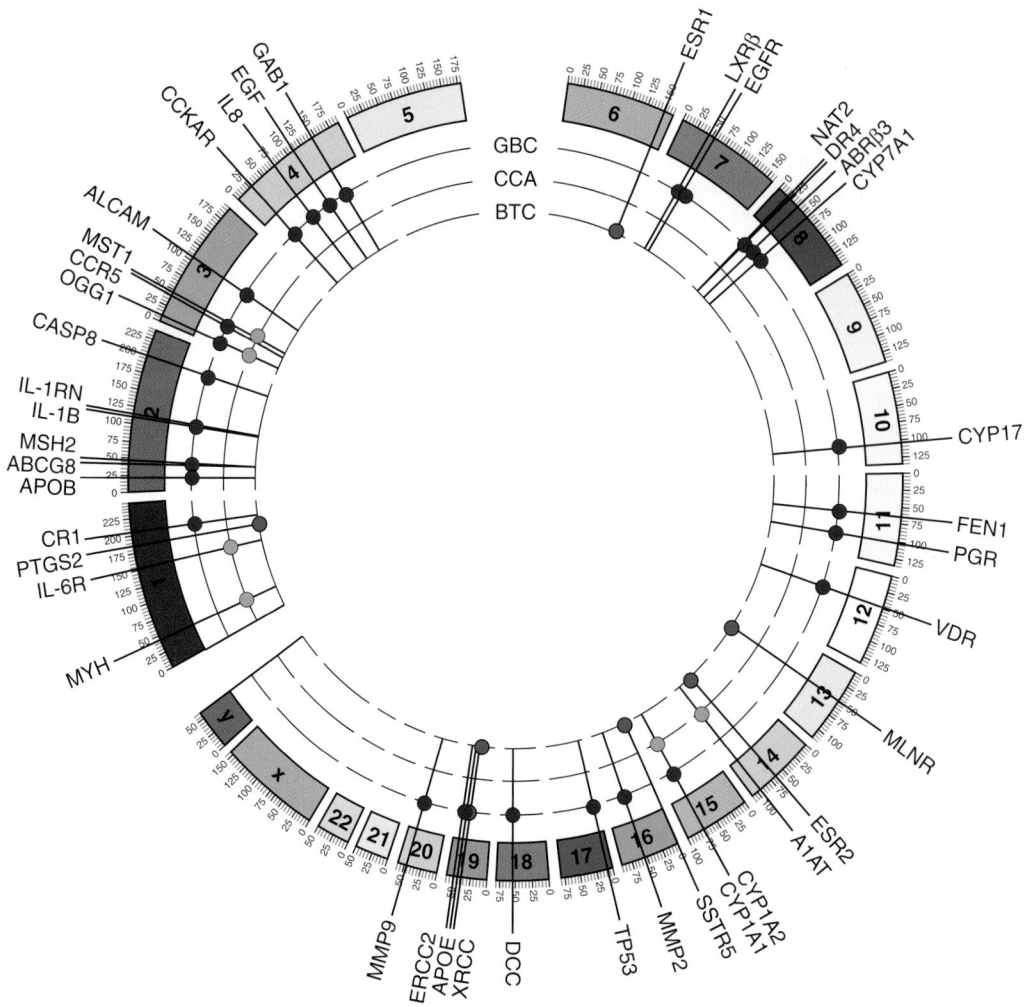

FIGURE 50.2 Circa plot of the gene variants and chromosomal locations associated with cholangiocarcinoma (CCA), as well as gallbladder cancer (GBC) and biliary tract cancer (BTC). (Reproduced from Marcano-Bonilla L, Mohamed EA, Mounajjed T, Roberts LR. Biliary tract cancers: Epidemiology, molecular pathogenesis and genetic risk associations. *Chin Clin Oncol.* 2016;5[5]:11. With permission.)

activation of inflammatory pathways (38% of IHCCs) and a proliferation class (62% IHCCs) with predominant activation of oncogenic signaling pathways, the latter correlating with a worse prognosis (Fig. 50.3).[80] Within the inflammatory group of tumors STAT3 activation and overexpression of interleukin-6 (IL-6) is common. IL-6 stimulates cholangiocyte growth via activation of the MAPK pathway and epigenetic control of gene expression and apopotosis.[81] In addition, inflammatory cytokines induce the expression of nitric oxide synthetase, which in turn enhances the expression of COX-2, a proliferative stimulus for cholangiocytes. Nitric oxide synthetase also increases tissue levels of nitric oxide, which promotes DNA damage and inhibits DNA repair mechanisms.[82,83]

Within the proliferative class of tumors there are widespread alterations in pathways related to DNA repair (TP53),[84] the WNT-CTNNB1 pathway,[85] tyrosine kinase signaling (KRAS, BRAF, SMAD4, and FGFR2),[86,87] protein tyrosine phosphatase (PTPN3),[88] epigenetic remodeling factors (IDH1, IDH2),[86,87] chromatin-remodeling factors (histone-lysine N-methyltransferase 2C),[89] the SW1/SNF complex, and deregulated Notch signaling.[90,91] Variations have also been found in the genetic signaling for human telomerase reverse transcriptase (TERT) in IHCC associated with chronic hepatitis.[81]

Growth and Tissue Factors

The presence of numerous hormones (estrogens, secretin, gastric, cholecystokinin), bile acids, and growth factors (serotonin, dopamine, leptin, histamine, endothelin-1, opioids, and endocannabinoids)[8] promote or retard proliferation and apoptosis in cholangiocytes, indicating that the development of a malignant phenotype is a complex, multistep process and confirming the clinical observation of significant biologic heterogeneity with IHCC. In addition, it has been suggested that specific cancer-associated fibroblasts, derived from activated hepatic stellate cells that form the characteristic desmoplastic stroma of IHCC, contribute to cholangiocyte proliferation, migration, and invasion.[92,93] The extent of neovascularization has also emerged as an important determinant of IHCC prognosis, with patients having a high tumor microvessel density having a poorer outcome following resection than those with low microvessel density.[94]

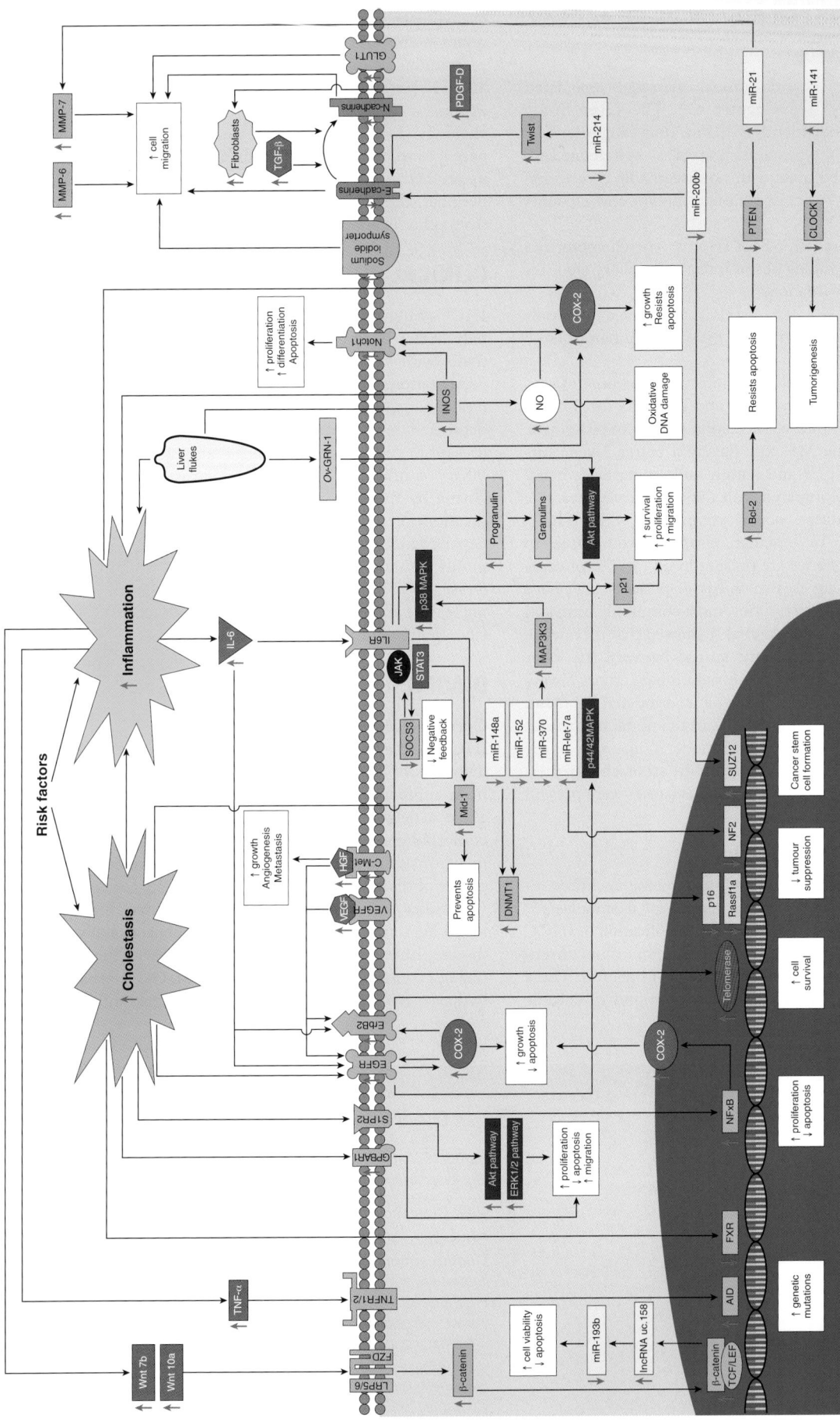

FIGURE 50.3   The molecular pathogenesis of cholangiocarcinoma. The majority of the risk factors cause chronic inflammation or cholestasis. Inflammatory mediators (IL-6 and TNF-α) activate a number of pathways, such as JK-STAT, p38 MAPK, and Akt, resulting in increased cell growth, survival, and proliferation. Macrophages secrete ligands that activate the Wnt/β-catenin pathway, leading to TCF/LEF-mediated gene transcription. Prolonged exposure to bile acids leads to up-regulation of COX-2 and Mcl-1 resulting in resistance to apoptosis. Liver flukes can also cause activation of the Akt pathway and upregulation of iNOS, increasing cell survival and proliferation. A number of microRNAs are up- or down-regulated in cholangiocarcinoma. (Reproduced from Labib PL, Goodchild G, Pereira S. Molecular pathogenesis of cholangiocarcinoma. *BMC Cancer.* 2019;19:7. With permission under the Creative Commons Attribution 4.0 International License, http://creativecommons.crg/licenses/by/4.0/.)

PATHOLOGIC SUBTYPES AND MODE OF SPREAD

Macroscopic Appearance

IHCCs are firm, white sclerotic tumors often with associated satellite lesions nearby (see Chapter 47). The Liver Study Group of Japan has subdivided IHCC into four categories[95,96]:

1. Mass-forming (MF) type consisting of a well-delineated, firm, nonencapsulated mass with no discernable connection to a bile duct. This is the most common subtype and accounts for 65% of all IHCCs.
2. Periductal infiltrating (PI; 6% of IHCC) type characterized by growth spreading along portal tracts with biliary stenoses and proximal biliary dilation.
3. Intraductal growth (IG; 4% of IHCC) type, usually a polypoid or papillary lesion growing within the lumen of large bile duct.
4. Mixed growth pattern which demonstrates features of several of the other growth patterns and accounts for 25% of IHCC. This morphologic classification does have prognostic implications with the MF type having a better 5-year survival than the PI type[53] and lymph node metastases being rare in the IG type compared with the other histotypes.[63]

Intrahepatic metastases occur commonly with IHCC, usually on the basis of vascular invasion. Metastases to intraabdominal lymph nodes are present in up to 75% of cases at presentation,[97] and up to two thirds of patients may have evidence of remote organ metastases, most commonly lung and bone, at presentation.[9,97] Nozaki et al.[98] showed that there were significant differences in lymphatic spread between left lobar and right lobar tumors. Patients with right lobar tumors always had lymph node metastases in the hepaticoduodenal ligament; in patients with left lobar tumors, 50% of the nodal metastases were found distant from the hepaticoduodenal ligament in the cardia and around the lesser curvature of the stomach. Furthermore, in these patients, no lymph node metastases were present in the hepatoduodenal ligament.

Microscopic Appearance

Histologically, IHCCs are usually well-to-moderately differentiated adenocarcinomas with varying degrees of desmoplasia.[63] Sempoux et al.[100] proposed a detailed subclassification of IHCC (Box 50.1). Of these, the pathologic classification of unconventional IHCC is the subject of significant investigation. These tumors most commonly develop on a background of chronic liver disease and cirrhosis and may mimic hepatocellular carcinoma in appearance[63] (see Chapter 47).

Immunohistochemistry examination demonstrates CK 7 and CK 19 (biliary subtype cytokeratin) expression. N-cadherin expression is increased in IHCC compared with extrahepatic cholangiocarcinomas. Hepatocyte markers (HepPar1 and arginase 1) are occasionally seen in IHCCs, and albumin mRNA in-situ hydridization is also useful in distinguishing IHCC from perihilar cholangiocarcinoma and metastatic adenocarcinoma from other primary malignancies.[63]

CLINICAL PRESENTATION

IHCCs often present as asymptomatic hepatic masses incidentally detected on cross-sectional imaging examinations. In patients with symptoms, abdominal pain is the most common presentation.[101,102] A significant proportion of patients may also report nonspecific constitutional symptoms such as weight loss, decreased energy, and diminished appetite.[103] Jaundice may be present in centrally placed tumors that compress or invade the biliary confluence. Extensive replacement of hepatic parenchyma by tumor, portal vein compromise, intrabiliary tumor invasion, or mucobilia can also present with jaundice due to hepatic failure. An increase in serum liver enzymes, most commonly alkaline phosphatase (ALP) or gamma glutamyl transferase (GGT), without symptoms may also be the only presenting feature and prompt further investigations, including physical examination and cross-sectional imaging.

DIAGNOSIS AND EVALUATION

Currently, resection is the only potentially curative therapy for IHCC, and evaluation of patients is focused on establishing the diagnosis of IHCC and ruling out metastatic adenocarcinoma from another primary tumor. Thorough evaluation should include a detailed history, physical examination, assessment of comorbid conditions, assessment of hepatic function, measurement of tumor markers, and radiologic imaging to assess the extent of disease.

History and examination may reveal presenting symptoms and a liver mass, signs of jaundice, and occasionally metastatic disease. Liver function should be assessed with measurement of platelet count, serum levels of bilirubin, GGT, aspartate transaminase (AST), ALP, albumin, total protein, and prothrombin

---

BOX 50.1 Pathologic Classifications of IHCC

World Health Organization Classification[4]

Adenocarcinoma
Well differentiated
Moderately differentiated
Poorly differentiated

Rare Variants
Adenosquamous
Squamous
Mucinous
Signet-ring cell
Clear cell
Lymphoepithelial
Sarcomatoid
Others

New Classification by Komuta et al.[99]
Mucin-IHCC (large bile duct type)
Mixed-IHCC (small bile duct type)
Cholangiocellular carcinoma

New Classification by Sempoux et al.[100]

Conventional IHCC
Unconventional IHCC
Trabecular subtype
Hilar subtype
Intraductal neoplasia of intrahepatic bile ducts
    Intraductal papillary neoplasm of the bile duct
    Intraductal tubulopapillary neoplasm of the bile duct
IHCC with ductal plate malformation
Cholangiocellular carcinoma

time or international normalized ratio (INR). Any abnormality in hepatic function, particularly signs of underlying chronic liver disease, should be investigated in more detail.

The diagnosis of IHCC is established with the typical finding of a hypovascular mass present on cross-sectional imaging[104] (see Chapter 16). Gastrointestinal metastases are excluded by performing upper and lower gastrointestinal endoscopies without the finding of a primary tumor. The absence of other primary malignancies (e.g., pancreas, kidney, lung, breast) on cross-sectional imaging of the chest, abdomen, and pelvis is mandated. Routine tumor biopsy is not recommended in patients with resectable tumors because of the small risk of tumor dissemination associated with biopsy.[105] Biopsy is indicated only to establish the diagnosis in the presence of irresectable disease, which is present in over half of patients at their initial presentation.[9] Irresectability is determined by local tumor factors such as involvement of the vascular supply or biliary drainage of the future liver remnant or the presence of metastatic disease. Staging laparoscopy is also useful in the evaluation of IHCC to exclude peritoneal disease, nodal disease, or abdominal wall invasion, particularly when these are suspected on preoperative imaging.[106]

SCREENING

The Cholangiocarcinoma Screening and Care Program (CASCAP) was developed in Thailand and is functioning in Northern Thailand where there is a high incidence of cholangiocarcinoma. Patients 40 years of age or older with a history of liver fluke infection or having eaten uncooked freshwater fish are screened with hepatic ultrasound every 12 months, increasing to every 6 months for patients with periductal fibrosis, steatosis, or cirrhosis. Referral for computed tomography (CT) or magnetic resonance imaging (MRI) is made if a liver mass or biliary dilation is detected[107] (see Chapter 16). This screened cohort includes 150,000 individuals living in high-risk areas. In addition, a further 25,000 surveillance patients will be added following treatment for cholangiocarcinoma.[107]

BIOMARKERS FOR CHOLANGIOCARCINOMA

Serum Tumor Markers

CA 19-9 and carcinoembryonic antigen (CEA) are the most widely used serum markers used in the diagnosis and monitoring of IHCC. For CA 19-9, a recent meta-analysis confirmed a sensitivity of 72% and specificity of 84% in distinguishing patients with cholangiocarcinoma and benign biliary disease.[108] Similarly, the sensitivity and specificity of CEA for cholangiocarcinoma ranges between 42% to 85% and 70% to 89%, respectively.[109,110] Consequently both these markers are a useful part of the workup and monitoring of patients with cholangiocarcinoma, but normal results are not necessarily diagnostic. Elevations in both serum CEA and CA 19-9 have been shown to be independent prognostic markers, but the cutoff values vary significantly between investigations.[111]

Other biomarkers investigated, but not yet in clinical practice, have included osteopontin,[111] IL-6,[111] matrix metalloproteinase 7,[111–113] S110A6,[101] DKK1,[101,112] SSP411,[107] KL-6 mucin,[111,112] MUC5AC,[112,113] hTERTmRNA,[112,113] RCAS1,[112] cytokeratin fragment 19,[113] and C-reactive protein.[113] Using multiple tumor markers, Lumachi et al.[114] have used CEA, CA

19-9, cytokeratin-19 fragment, and matrix metalloproteinase-7, which collectively achieved a sensitivity of 92% and a specificity of 96% in diagnosing cholangiocarcinoma. Yoh et al.[115] have also shown that elevations in CA 19-9, C-reactive protein, and the neutrophil-to-lymphocyte ratio are predictive of poor survival following treatment. Collectively this indicates that multiple diagnostic markers may be required to diagnose and monitor treatment outcomes in cholangiocarcinoma.

Bile Markers for Cholangiocarcinoma

Bile markers of cholangiocarcinoma have been investigated for their use in the diagnosis of biliary obstruction and may have a significant role in the evaluation of extrahepatic biliary obstruction because they can be easily measured if bile is collected during endoscopic retrograde cholangiopancreatography (ERCP). These have included a variety of specific proteins, including WFA-L1Cam, SSP411, and Mac-2BP,[112] as well as micro-RNAs.[116] It is uncommon for IHCC to present with biliary obstruction and their use in this tumor is, therefore, limited.

IMAGING

IHCCs often present with vague and nonspecific symptoms.[117] Accurate cross-sectional imaging is required to diagnose and stage the tumors as well as plan resection or other possible treatments. Most patients will be imaged with a number of modalities.

Transabdominal Ultrasound

Ultrasound is often used as a screening examination by primary healthcare practitioners investigating patients with right upper quadrant pain, a palpable mass, or unexplained jaundice. IHCC has a nonspecific appearance with the mass-forming subtype appearing as a hypoechoic hepatic mass, whereas the periductal infiltrating type presents as a small mass-like lesion with diffuse periductal thickening and distal dilation[118,119] (see Chapter 16).

The intraductal subtype usually presents as diffuse segmental or lobar biliary dilation, and an intrabiliary polypoid mass may be visible.[118] Satellite lesions may be seen as well as capsular retraction. The tumors are hypovascular and usually have minimal Doppler evidence of internal blood flow. Ultrasound is useful for defining associated biliary dilatation, portal venous invasion, hepatic venous invasion, and, rarely, portal lymphadenopathy.[120] Contrast-enhanced ultrasound is useful in distinguishing between IHCC and hepatocellular carcinoma based on the presence of peripheral arterial enhancement commonly observed in IHCC.[121]

Computed Tomography

Triple-phase CT scan is widely available and is the single most effective investigation in diagnosing and staging IHCC. Mass-forming tumors present as hypodense lesions with irregular, infiltrative margins and a variable degree of delayed enhancement in the portal venous phase (see Chapter 16). Progressive enhancement may be observed on delayed images (3–6 minutes following contrast injection) and is related to the amount of fibrous stroma present.[122] In periductal infiltrating and intraductal IHCC, CT will detect biliary dilation and in the intraductal type may demonstrate an expanded bile duct containing a mass lesion.[119] In all tumor subtypes CT scan will also demonstrate portal or hepatic venous involvement,[123] and lobar atrophy due to longstanding biliary obstruction or portal venous involvement.[124] CT scan is also useful in detecting metastatic disease affecting regional lymph nodes, peritoneum, or lung fields.[122] Data from newer multiphase, fast acquisition scanners can also be used to construct three-dimensional models of hepatic and tumor anatomy to facilitate resection,[125] as well as accurate assessment of hepatic volumetry, particularly in relation to remnant volume and the risk of postoperative liver failure.[126]

Magnetic Resonance Imaging

Mass-forming IHCCs appear as hypointense lesions on T1-weighted images and mild to moderately hyperintensity on T2-weighted images, depending on the content of desmoplastic stroma and mucin. There is also typically pooling of contrast within the lesions on delayed images (6–8 minutes after contrast injection).[122] Periductal infiltrating tumors demonstrate diffuse periductal thickening with enhancement with biliary stricturing and proximal biliary dilation.[119,122] However, differentiation of benign intrahepatic fibrous strictures from periductal tumors is challenging and relies on the presence of contrast enhancement within the stricture, and an irregular stricture margin, asymmetry, or the presence of an associated soft tissue mass.[118,122] Most commonly the intraductal subtype is seen as dilated bile duct with a polypoid mass.[118] MRI is also useful in defining venous and arterial involvement by tumor, and magnetic resonance cholangiography is useful in defining biliary anatomy to facilitate resection and reconstruction, if required (see Chapter 16).

Positron Emission Tomography

Positron emission tomography (PET) scanning is now a commonly used modality for staging gastrointestinal malignancy, and the integration of PET and CT scans now provides the opportunity to obtain anatomic and functional information in a single scan[122] (see Chapter 18). IHCCs are present as glucose avid lesions within the liver; however, PET is most effective in detecting mass-forming tumors ≥ 1 cm in diameter but is less effective in assessing infiltrating periductal tumors.[122,127] PET/CT is also useful in tumor staging detecting intraabdominal lymph node metastases (sensitivity 42%, specificity 80%) and distant metastases (sensitivity 56%, specificity 88%).[128] However, PET is limited by the finding of false-positive results in patients with biliary inflammation,[129] and patients with mucinous tumors can present with false-negative scans.[130]

STAGING

IHCCs are classified as primary cancers of the liver by the American Joint Committee on Cancer (AJCC), and Western hepatobiliary centers commonly use the AJCC systems to stage tumors. Before the 7th edition of the AJCC staging manual, a single staging system was applied to both hepatocellular carcinomas and IHCCs. The 8th edition of the AJCC staging manual[131] presents a revised version (Table 50.1) of the dedicated IHCC staging system first presented in the 7th edition.[132] This new staging incorporates tumor size of 5 cm to separate the T_1 category into T_{1A} and T_{1B} because tumor size has been shown to be an independent prognostic factor and increasing size is associated with increasing tumor grade and the presence of microscopic vascular invasion.[133,134] For T_4 tumors the presence of periductal invasion has been removed because of a paucity of data on its prognostic significance.[130] Three investigations[135–137] have confirmed that the 8th edition staging system is effective in stratifying patients' overall survival.

Two other staging systems have been described (see Table 50.1) from the Liver Cancer Study Group of Japan[138] and the National

---

TABLE 50.1 Staging Systems for IHCC

AMERICAN JOINT COMMISSION ON CANCER, 8TH EDITION[131]	LIVER CANCER STUDY GROUP OF JAPAN[138]	NATIONAL CANCER CENTRE HOSPITAL OF JAPAN[139]
	Criteria • Tumor size ≤ 2 cm • Tumor number = 1 • No portal vein, hepatic vein, or serosal invasion	

T_1
  T_{1A}: Solitary tumor ≤ 5 cm without vascular invasion
  T_{1B}: Solitary tumor >5 cm without vascular invasion
	T_1 All three criteria present	T_1 Solitary tumor without vascular invasion

T_2 Solitary tumor with vascular invasion or multiple tumors with or without vascular invasion	T_2 two of three criteria present	T_2 Solitary tumor with vascular invasion
T_3 Tumor perforating the visceral peritoneum	T_3 One of three criteria present	T_3 Multiple tumors with or without vascular invasion
T_4 Tumor involving extrahepatic structures by direct invasion	T_4 None of three criteria present	
N_0 No regional lymph node metastases	N_0 No regional lymph node metastases	N_0 No regional lymph node metastases
N_1 Regional lymph node metastases	N_1 Regional lymph node metastases	N_1 Regional lymph node metastases
M_1 Distant metastases	M_1 Distant metastases	M_1 Distant metastases
STAGE GROUPING	**STAGE GROUPING**	**STAGE GROUPING**
I_A $T1_A N_0 M_0$ I_B $T1_B N_0 M_0$ II $T_2 N_0 M_0$ III_A $T_3 N_0 M_0$ III_B T_4 and/or $N_1 M_0$ IV Any T, any N, M_1	I $T_1 N_0 M_0$ II $T_2 N_0 M_0$ III $T_3 N_0 M_0$ IV_A $T_4 N_0 M_0$, Any T N_1, M_0 IV_B Any T, Any N, M_1	I $T_1 N_0 M_0$ II $T_2 N_0 M_0$ III_A $T_3 N_0 M_0$ III_B Any T, N_1, M_0 IV Any T, Any N, M_1

Cancer Centre of Japan.[139] Although these systems are not in common usage in Western hepatobiliary centers, the AJCC staging manual does recommend collection of tumor growth patterns (mass-forming, periductal infiltrating, or mixed) based on the Liver Cancer Study Group of Japan classification.[138]

TREATMENT

Patients with untreated IHCC have a median survival of less than 12 months.[140,141] Resection of IHCC has been the only treatment associated with a significant disease-free survival and it remains the only potentially curative treatment modality. Orthotopic liver transplantation has now been studied in some detail, and the roles of neoadjuvant and adjuvant systemic and regional chemotherapy, immunotherapy, conformal radiation, intraarterial radiation therapy, and ablative therapies are under intense investigation and have led to the early development of multimodality treatment pathways for IHCC.[142]

Surgical

Hepatic Resection

Complete resection of IHCC is based on the surgical principles applied to resections for hepatocellular carcinoma and metastatic tumors (see Chapter 101). Staging laparoscopy can be used before resection to investigate areas of potential extrahepatic disease[106] (see Chapter 24). Criteria for irresectability of IHCC are locally advanced solitary tumors involving either inflow or outflow bilaterally, multiple intrahepatic tumors, and distant metastatic disease.[9] An R_0 resection is the goal of surgical

therapy.[133] Ideally, hepatic resection is undertaken with the aim of obtaining a clear margin of 1 cm or greater, while leaving a well-vascularized remnant with adequate venous and biliary drainage. However, tumor size and proximity to vascular structures often mandate a close margin. Resection of up to 80% of hepatic volume can be contemplated in patients with good liver function and 60% in patients with compromised liver function.[143] However, often resections of this magnitude will need to be proceeded by portal vein embolization,[126] or other interventions to optimize remnant volume.[144]

The results of contemporary series of IHCC treated with hepatic resection are summarized in Table 50.2.[145-165] Although there is a role for minimally invasive surgical approaches (see Chapters 127D and 127E),[166] all reported series emphasize the use of aggressive, open hepatic resection to achieve R_0 margins including associating liver partition and portal vein ligation for staged hepatectomy (ALPP)[144] and the use of re-resections in patients with localized recurrences.[159] Recent experience confirms single-figure perioperative mortality, except when ALPP is employed (see Chapter 102D),[164] and 5-year survival of approximately 40% (see Table 50.2). There is also a steady increase in utilization of adjuvant therapy following resection, particularly in patients with nodal metastases, multiple tumors, and vascular invasion.[147,148,153,157,158] For patients undergoing resection survival is reduced in those with multiple tumor foci (median survival 15 months versus 38 months with solitary lesions).[164] Raoof et al.[161] have shown that multifocality, extrahepatic tumor extension, high tumor grade, lymph node positivity, and age greater than 60 years were independently associated with worse survival following resection. Using these factors,

TABLE 50.2 Summary of Contemporary Results for Surgical Resection of Intrahepatic Cholangiocarcinoma

AUTHOR	YEAR	COUNTRY	NUMBER OF PATIENTS	PERIOPERATIVE MORTALITY	ADJUVANT THERAPY	SURVIVAL (%) 1 YR	3 YR	5 YR
Lanthaler et al.[145]	2010	Austria	25	4%	No	84	57	45
Saxena et al.[146]	2010	Australia	40	2%	No	79	48	29
Cho et al.[147]	2010	Korea	63	2%	Yes	68	50	32
De Jong et al.[148]	2011	USA/Europe	449	NR	Yes	78	44	31
Ellis et al.[149]	2011	USA	31	6%	NR		40	
Farges et al.[150]	2011	France	212	NR	NR	77	44	28*
Saiura et al.[151]	2011	Japan	44	0	No	87	56	39
Sulpice et al.[152]	2012	France	87	5%	NR	79	47	31
Dhanasekaran et al.[153]	2013	USA	53	NR	Yes	82	33	19
Sriputtha et al.[154]	2013	Thailand	73	NR	NR	52	23	11
Luo et al.[155]	2014	China	1333	0.6%	NR	58	25	17
Murakami et al.[156]	2014	Japan	45	2%	Yes			42
Schiffman et al.[157]	2014	USA	34	6%	Yes	68	40	30
Ali et al.[158]	2015	USA	150	NR	NR	84		43
Bergeat et al.[159]	2015	France	107	9.2%	Yes	80	49	35
Tabrizian et al.[160]	2015	USA	82	1%	NR	60	24	16
Raoof et al.[161]	2017	USA	275	4.4%	NR	80	46	36
Reames et al.[162]	2017	USA/Europe	1087	4.8%	NR	80	51	40
Le Roy et al.[163]	2018	France	82	10%	Yes		45	24
Buettner et al.[164]	2019	Multinational	1013	4.4%	NR	80	55	40
Schnitzbauer et al.[165]	2020	Germany	511	3%	NR	70-95	40-70	28-70
Li et al.[144]	2020	Multinational	102	21.2%	NR	64	52	39

NR, Not reported; *USA*, United States of America.

and assigning each a score of 1, these investigators developed the MEGNA prognostic score (minimum score: zero, no factors present; maximum score 5, five factors present), which Schnitzbauer et al.[165] have confirmed correctly stratifies patient survival at 1, 3, and 5 years (see Table 50.2). A more recent study showed that genomic alterations in TP53, KRAS and/or CDKN2 predicted much worse outcome after resection or treatment with systemic chemotherapy.

The Status of Lymphadenectomy

Lymph node metastases are present in between 30% and 40% of patients presenting with IHCC and are an important prognostic factor,[132] although the role of routine lymph node dissection in the surgical treatment of patients with IHCC continues to be debated. Amini et al.[167] have reported that over 75% of patients now undergo lymph node dissection in addition to resection. However, the current 8th edition of the AJCC staging system[131] recommends resecting at least six lymph nodes for adequate staging, and a recent review demonstrates that only 25% of patients undergoing lymphadenectomy for IHCC have at least six lymph nodes present in the operative specimen.[168] On the other hand, two recent publications showed that patients with N0 disease based on lymph node sampling/lymphadenectomy had a median survival that was no different than patients deemed N0 based on imaging and intraoperative assessment.

The composition of lymph node dissection is also debated. There is agreement that portal nodes should be included, and Nozaki et al.[98] have recommended routine dissection of cardia and lesser curvature nodes for left-sided tumors and dissection of the hepatoduodenal ligament for right-sided tumors. Because preoperative imaging is insensitive at detecting nodal metastases, routine lymphadenectomy has been advocated for all IHCCs[168,169] to provide accurate staging information, to assist in selecting patients for adjuvant therapies, and to potentially decrease locoregional recurrence. Currently the European Society for Medical Oncology (ESMO) recommends routine lymphadenectomy within the hepatoduodenal ligament,[170] the National Comprehensive Cancer Network (NCCN) considers lymphadenectomy reasonable,[171] and the European Association for the Study of the Liver (EASL) states that lymphadenectomy should be strongly considered at the time of resection.[172] This uncertainty has encouraged the development of preoperative tools to predict the presence of nodal metastases assisting in the application of therapeutic nodal dissection. Yoh et al.[173] have shown that elevated CA 19-9 levels, IHCC with hilar invasion, and the presence of lymph nodes larger than 10 mm in short-axis diameter accurately predicted the presence of nodal metastases with a false-negative rate of 2.3%.

Liver Transplantation

Currently IHCC is a contraindication for liver transplant in most centers worldwide[172,173] (see Chapter 105). Historically, outcomes for transplantation for IHCC were poor with the first report[174] noting a median survival of 5 months and a 1-year survival of 14% in 18 patients treated with liver transplantation. Several studies confirmed these findings,[175,176] although Cherqui et al.[177] reported two long-term survivors and concluded that an intrahepatic tumor with no extrahepatic spread that cannot be resected for anatomic reasons may be a candidate for liver transplantation. Subsequently, Robles et al.[178] reported a

5-year survival of 42% in 23 patients undergoing liver transplant, although in 10 patients the IHCC was discovered incidentally after transplant. Similarly, Sapisochin et al.[179] reported a 47% 5-year survival in patients who underwent transplant for presumed hepatocellular carcinoma (HCC) but were found to have IHCC on explant pathology. Facciuto et al.[180] compared patients with IHCC with matched patients with HCC. When patients were stratified by the Milan criteria,[180] overall survival was equivalent for tumors within the criteria (78% IHCC versus 79% for HCC) and also for patients outside the criteria (48% IHCC versus 53% HCC). A multicenter study reviewed 48 patients with IHCC on explant pathology and found that 15 patients with tumors ≤2 cm in diameter ("very early" IHCC) had a 5-year actuarial survival of 65% compared with 45% in patients with "advanced" disease (single tumor >2 cm in diameter or multifocal disease).[181] These findings indicate that patients with "very early" IHCC could be considered for transplantation.[182] However, transplantation was undertaken either for a presumed diagnosis of HCC or hepatic decompensation in all of the reported patients found to have an IHCC in the explant. The outcomes of patients with known IHCC before transplant are yet to be fully investigated, and the role, if any, of pretransplant neoadjuvant chemotherapy or radiotherapy in IHCC is unknown.[183]

Tumor Ablation

Tumor ablation refers to the destruction of tumors using thermal energy. Historically cryotherapy has been employed, but radiofrequency and microwave ablation are currently most commonly used. Ablation is performed under ultrasound guidance with the aim to ablate the index lesion and a 5- to 10-mm margin of uninvolved tissue. Usually, a single electrode is placed for small tumors (≤3 cm in diameter) and larger lesions require the use of multiple or clustered applicators with multiple overlapping ablation zones. Multivariate analysis confirms that tumor diameter is a significant factor in determining the effectiveness of ablation and patient survival.[184] In a meta-analysis of radiofrequency ablation for IHCC the rate of incomplete ablation following one treatment was 21% and the rate of major complication was 8%.[185] The 1-, 3-, and 5-year survival rates were 82%, 47%, and 24%, respectively,[185] although only 5% of patients with IHCC are treated with ablation therapy alone,[186] due to the size and multiplicity of tumors at presentation. Consequently, in patients who cannot be considered for resection due to significant comorbidity but who have small, solitary IHCC, ablation therapy is a useful primary treatment. Similarly, Zhang et al.[187] have shown that, in patients with solitary liver only recurrence, percutaneous ablation has an efficacy similar to repeat resection but is associated with a complication rate of 4% compared with a complication rate of 47% in patients undergoing repeat resection.

Chemotherapy

IHCC has proven to be difficult to treat with chemotherapy. Much of the information on the effectiveness of chemotherapy for this tumor has been derived from phase 2 trials rather than phase 3 trials, and many of these trials have been carried out in groups of patients with all tumors arising from biliary epithelia and include patients with intrahepatic and extrahepatic cholangiocarcinoma, gallbladder cancer, and even pancreatic cancer. However, the publication of Valle et al.[188] established systemic gemcitabine and cisplatin as the standard of care for treatment of biliary cancers. In addition, regional delivery of chemotherapy has been explored and recent investigations evaluating biologic agents have been driven by better understanding of the potential genetic and regulatory targets in IHCC.[189]

Regional Chemotherapy

TRANSARTERIAL CHEMOEMBOLIZATION OR TRANSARTERIAL DRUG-ELUTING BEADS. Patients with unresectable liver disease without extrahepatic disease have been considered for treatment with transarterial chemoembolization (TACE; commonly with cisplatin, doxorubicin, and mitomycin C) or transarterial treatment with drug-eluting beads (DEB-TACE; doxorubicin, oxaliplatin, or irinotecan).[190] A large multi-institutional study[191] evaluated both treatments and found similar overall survivals in patients treated with TACE (13.4 months) and DEB-TACE (10.5 months). In a prospective study, Kiefer et al.[192] have reported 62 patients treated with intraarterial doxorubicin, cisplatin, and mitomycin C with a median overall survival of 20 months. Survival was improved in those patients receiving concomitant systemic chemotherapy (overall survival 28 months). Combination therapy appears to be more effective than single-agent therapy,[193] with large tumor size, tumor hypovascularity, and Child-Pugh class B being adverse prognostic factors.[194] A survival benefit of up to 7 months over best supportive care can be expected.[190]

TACE (5-fluorouracil, epirubicin, and hydroxycamptothecin) has also been used as an adjuvant therapy following resection of IHCC. One investigation gave mixed results where adjuvant TACE was associated with an improved survival but a greater risk of intrahepatic recurrence.[195] In a second study, 5-year recurrence rates were reduced in patients treated with TACE following an R_0 resection and an improved overall 5-year survival noted (38% versus 30% in patients treated without TACE).[196]

Hepatic Artery Infusion

Using an implanted, subcutaneous pump, patients with IHCC have been treated with continuous hepatic artery infusions of floxuridine (FUDR),[197] 5-fluorouracil and oxaliplatin,[198] gemcitabine,[199] epirubicin, and cisplatin.[200] A number of investigations have also administered concurrent systemic chemotherapy.[193,200,201] In an early report, Jarnagin et al.[197] demonstrated an objective response rate of 47% and converted one initially unresectable patient to resection with intraarterial FUDR treatment. A recent investigation using FUDR combined with systemic gemcitabine and oxaliplatin confirmed a response rate of 46% with a 2-year overall survival of 53%,[201] although 10% of patients developed significant complications (portal hypertension, gastroduodenal artery aneurysm, catheter displacement, and jaundice). Consequently, hepatic artery infusion chemotherapy remains an attractive concept to potentially downstage large, localized IHCC for subsequent resection, or to prevent intrahepatic tumor progression, and appears to be more effective than TACE or intraarterial radioembolization.[202] Importantly, thorough pre-treatment staging must be undertaken to exclude extrahepatic disease, and patients with underlying cirrhosis cannot be treated because of the risk of liver-related complications.[197]

Systemic Chemotherapy

NEOADJUVANT CHEMOTHERAPY. There are several case reports of the use of neoadjuvant systemic therapy, most commonly with gemcitabine and platinum-based chemotherapy, in the literature.[203] However, Le Roy et al.[163] have published a comprehensive series using neoadjuvant systemic therapy in a group of patients with initially unresectable IHCC. Seventy-four patients were treated with neoadjuvant therapy, most commonly with gemcitabine and oxaliplatin, of whom 24% responded, 45% stabilized tumor growth, and 31% progressed. Overall, 53% (39 patients) of this cohort underwent resection (R_0 resection in 31%) with 3- and 5-year overall survival rates of 45% and 24%, respectively. Only the presence of lymph node metastases was a significant adverse prognostic factor on multivariate analysis. Importantly, this investigation confirmed that neoadjuvant therapy is feasible for IHCC and outcomes can be achieved that are comparable to patients who are treated with upfront resection. However, the rate of major hepatectomy is higher and the R_1 resection rates are twice those observed in patients able to undergo resection without neoadjuvant treatment.

ADJUVANT CHEMOTHERAPY. Two retrospective investigations have evaluated adjuvant therapy (most commonly with gemcitabine and platinum) following resection of IHCC. Sur et al.[204] reported that patients receiving adjuvant therapy were more likely to have lymph node metastases and positive resection margins, and in these patient groups administration of adjuvant therapy, both alone and in combination with radiation therapy, was associated with a significant improvement in survival. Miura et al.[205] also demonstrated in a matched cohort study that administration of adjuvant chemotherapy was associated with improved survival in patients resected with positive margins and those with lymph node metastases. The phase III BILCAP trial, published in 2019,[206] compared capecitabine with observation in patients with resected biliary tract cancer (of whom one fifth had a diagnosis of IHCC) and demonstrated a significant trend toward improved survival in a per-protocol analysis (median survival 51 months versus 36 months in the observation group). In contrast, the PRODIGE-12 study[207] demonstrated no significant survival benefit for adjuvant gemcitabine and oxaliplatin. The results of the ACTICCA-1 trial comparing gemcitabine and cisplatin with capecitabine in patients with resected biliary cancers are awaited.[208] Of the current guidelines the NCCN suggests that adjuvant chemotherapy may be an option for patients with either negative or positive surgical margins and lymph node metastases,[171] whereas ESMO guidelines suggest that adjuvant therapy should be considered in all patients because of the high rate of recurrence following resection.[170] In 2019 the American Society for Clinical Oncology suggested, in a clinical practice guideline, that patients with resected biliary tract cancer should be offered adjuvant capecitabine for 6 months on the basis of the BILCAP study,[209] and this is supported by a recent meta-analyisis.[210]

Chemotherapy for Advanced Disease

In 1996 Glimelius et al.[211] reported that patients with advanced biliopancreatic tumors treated with chemotherapy had an improved quality of life and survival over those treated with best supportive care. Subsequently, eight further randomized trials of systemic therapy in advanced cholangiocarcinoma have been published (Table 50.3).[212-219] The publications of Valle et al.[188,214] established gemcitabine and cisplatin as the standard of care first-line treatment for advanced cholangiocarcinoma, and a further trial carried out in Japan confirmed this

TABLE 50.3 Summary of Randomized Clinical Trials of Chemotherapy in Advanced Cholangiocarcinoma

AUTHOR	YEAR	INTERVENTION	PATIENT NUMBER	ORR/DCR (%)	MEDIAN OS (MONTHS)
Morizone[212]	2018	Gem vs Cis/Gem	354	29.8 vs 32.4 / NA	15.1 vs 13.4
Kang[213]	2012	Gem vs Cis/Gem	96	23.8 vs 19.6 / 85.7 vs 71.7	10.1 vs 9.9
Valle[214]	2010	Cis/Gem vs Gem	86	27.8 vs 22.7 vs 58	11.7 vs 8.1
Okusaka[215]	2010	Cis/Gem vs Gem	84	19.5 vs 11.9 / 68.3 vs 50	11.2 vs 7.7
Valle[188]	2009	Cis/Gem vs Gem	86	27.8 vs 22.7 vs 58	NA
Ducreux[216]	2005	5FU/FA/Cis vs HD5FU	58	18.5 vs 7.1 / 62.5 vs 53.1	8 vs 5
Rao[217]	2005	ECF vs FELV	54	19.2 vs 15 / 65.4 vs 60	9 vs 12
Kornek[218]	2004	MMC/CAPE vs MM/Gem	51	65 vs 56 / 31 vs 20	9.2 vs 6.7
Glimelius[211]	1996	5FU ± etoposide vs BSC	90	8/46	6 vs 2.5

C, CAPE, Capecitabine; *Cis,* cisplatin; *ECF,* epirubicin/cisplatin/5-fluorouracil; *FA,* folinic acid; *FELV,* 5-fluorouracil, etoposide, folinic acid; *Gem,* gemcitabine; *HD5FU,* high-dose 5-fluorouracil; *MMC,* mitomycin; *NA,* not available; *ORR/DCR,* overall response rate/disease control rate; *OS,* overall survival.
Redrawn from Adeva et al.[219]

finding.[215] Treatment with both agents is associated with neutropenia in up to 25% of patients as well as fatigue in up to 20% of patients; however, up one quarter of patients demonstrate a response, and median survival in treated patients now approaches 12 months.[188,215,216]

Other agents have been assessed in nonrandomized trials. Three investigations have evaluated the use of oxaliplatin in addition to gemcitabine (GEMOX) and have confirmed response rates of between 22% and 50% and median overall survivals between 11 and 15 months, which are comparable to gemcitabine and cisplatin.[220–223] Similarly, combination oxaliplatin with capecitabine has shown similar response rates to cisplatin and gemcitabine but a median survival of less than 12 months.[224] FOLFOX (5-fluorouracil, folinic acid, and oxaliplatin) has also shown similar results to gemcitabine and cisplatin,[225,226] and combination gemcitabine/capecitabine has shown a similar response rate of 25% to gemcitabine/cisplatin and has become established as a reasonable alternative first-line therapy in patients in whom cisplatin or oxaliplatin are not recommended.[227,228]

There are currently no randomized phase III trials of second-line chemotherapy in advanced biliary cancer and therefore no established second-line therapy.[228] A retrospective analysis of patients receiving second-line therapy, most commonly fluoropyrimidine doublet therapy, following first-line gemcitabine and cisplatin demonstrated a 3.4% response rate and an overall survival of 7 months.[229,230] Consistent predictors of a response to second-line therapy are good performance status, low CA 19-9 levels, and absence of distant metastatic disease.[229,231]

Targeted Biologic Treatments

Contemporary genomic analysis of IHCC has highlighted the presence of common genetic mutations, specifically isocitrate dehydrogenase (IDH), KRAS, and TP53,[189] demonstrating that increasing understanding of the genetic and metabolic aberrations observed in IHCC will facilitate targeted biologic therapy.[232] In vitro, RNA synthesis inhibitors, microtubule-targeting agents, topoisomerase and pololike kinase 1 inhibitors, and mTOR pathway modulators exhibited the greatest efficacy.[189] Early clinical use of the IDH inhibitor ivosidenib in IDH-mutated patients resulted in a 12-month progression-free

survival of 21%.[233] A recent phase 2 study of pemigatinib showed promising results in patients with FGFR2 fusions or rearrangements, with objective response rate of 35.5%. Treatment with the BRAF inhibitors dabrafenib and trametinib was associated with a 42% response rate and median overall survival of 12 months in a cohort of cholangiocarcinoma patients pre-treated with at least two lines of chemotherapy.[234] Other agents now under active investigation are MET inhibitors (tivantinib), AKT selective inhibitors (everolimus), TRK inhibitors (iarotrectinib), PD-1 inhibitors (pembrolizumab and nivolumab),[219,232] and the fibroblast growth factor inhibitor (pemigatinib).[235]

Radiation Therapy

Cholangiocarcinomas are radiosensitive tumors, although careful targeting and dosimetry are required to minimize radiation-related damage to non–tumor-bearing liver and adjacent visceral structures.

HEPATIC ARTERY RADIOEMBOLIZATION. Radioembolization using Yttrium-90 (^{90}Y)–loaded microspheres administered via the hepatic artery has been used to treat unresectable IHCC,[146,236,237] with acceptable adverse effects and median survival following the procedure of 15 to 22 months.[237] In early series of patients treated with advanced unresectable disease up to 5% of patients also downstaged sufficiently to be considered for resection.[236-238] Rayer et al.[239] have reported on the neoadjuvant use of ^{90}Y infusion when used in association with gemcitabine/cisplatin chemotherapy. Of 45 patients in their series with unresectable IHCC, 8 patients with single IHCC in noncirrhotic livers were resected following downsizing in tumor volume of between one third and one half. The median disease-free survival was 19 months following resection, although there was a 25% perioperative mortality rate.

EXTERNAL BEAM RADIATION THERAPY. Three investigations have assessed the efficacy of external beam radiation therapy in achieving local control of large, irresectable IHCC. Tao et al.[240] achieved a local control rate of 78% with a treatment dose of 85 Gy, and Hong et al.[241] demonstrated a local control rate of 94% for patients treated with a median dose of 58Gy. Smart et al.[242] reported a 2-year local control rate of 84% for all patients (93% for patients with liver only disease). Overall, 11% of patients reported grade 3 or 4 toxicity—significantly less than reported for gemcitabine-cisplatin chemotherapy.[188,214] In addition, radiation treatment was well tolerated in patients with reduced performance status who are not always able to manage systemic chemotherapy.[229] External beam radiation therapy can be considered as a viable treatment modality in patients with large, unresectable IHCC with the aim of achieving local disease control.[243]

BEST SUPPORTIVE CARE

Over half of patients presenting with IHCC may not be candidates for resection because of patient comorbidity or extent of disease and will be managed with best supportive care alone or in conjunction with other treatments.[244] Important priorities for these patients are management of capsular-related pain, ascites, maintenance of adequate nutritional intake, and psychological support for patients and their family members.

SUMMARY

IHCCs develop in intrahepatic biliary epithelium and constitute 10% of primary hepatic tumors. Although many are sporadic, conditions leading to chronic inflammation of biliary epithelium constitute significant risk factors for their development. For patients with liver only disease, R_0 resection offers the chance of cure, which occurs in 30% to 40% of patients. The last 5 years has seen significant advances in the effectiveness of systemic and regional chemotherapy, as well as radiation and liver-directed therapies such as TACE and radioembolization. Combination gemcitabine/cisplatin is now standard of care for the neoadjuvant treatment and the treatment of advanced disease, and capecitabine is the preferred adjuvant agent. Trials of targeted biologic agents, driven by improved understanding of the molecular pathogenesis of IHCC, are ongoing.

The references for this chapter can be found online by accessing the accompanying Expert Consult website.

CHAPTER 51A

Extrahepatic biliary tumors

Kevin C. Soares, Michael I. D'Angelica, and William R. Jarnagin

OVERVIEW

Extrahepatic biliary tumors are rare. Patients classically present with painless jaundice secondary to biliary obstruction. Management of bile duct tumors is challenging and best approached with input from an experienced multidisciplinary team. This chapter focuses on the cause of most common of these tumors, cholangiocarcinoma. We describe its epidemiology, preoperative evaluation, management, surgical technique, and long-term outcomes.

EPIDEMIOLOGY AND RISK FACTORS

Cholangiocarcinoma accounts for 3% of all digestive cancers and is classically divided into three subtypes: intrahepatic cholangiocarcinoma (ICC) (20% of all cholangiocarcinoma in the United States) (see Chapter 50) and extrahepatic cholangiocarcinoma (EHC), which includes both perihilar cholangiocarcinoma (HC) (50%–60%) and distal cholangiocarcinoma (DC) (20%–30%).[1] Although derived from biliary epithelial cells, the subtypes of cholangiocarcinoma differ in epidemiology, prognosis, and treatment paradigms.[2] The incidence of both ICC and EHC are increasing over time. The incidence of EHC increased 20% from 1973 to 2012, from 1.6 per 100,000 individuals in 1973 to 1975 to 2.3 per 100,000 in 2011 to 2012 (Fig. 51A.1).[3] In the United States, there are approximately 2500 new cases of EHC annually. The incidence of EHC is evenly distributed between sexes.[4] Rates among blacks and whites appear to be increasing in contrast to those of Hispanics and people of non-Hispanic ethnicity.[3,4] Although most cases of EHC occur in older patients, approximately 20% of EHCs are diagnosed before the age of 60, with the largest rise in incidence seen in 18- to 44-year-olds.[4]

Several risk factors are associated with an increased incidence of cholangiocarcinoma; however, it must be noted that most cholangiocarcinoma cases in Western countries are sporadic, with no obvious risk factors. Conditions associated with cholangiocarcinoma include primary sclerosing cholangitis (PSC) (see Chapter 41), choledochal cysts (see Chapter 46), recurrent pyogenic cholangiohepatitis (see Chapter 44), hepatolithiasis (see Chapter 39), and biliary parasites (see Chapters 45 and 71). Commonalities across these risk factors include the likelihood of these conditions to cause cholestasis and chronic inflammation.

Cholestatic liver diseases such as PSC, congenital hepatic fibrosis, Caroli disease, and choledochal cysts are well-recognized risk factors. Genetic disorders with an increased risk of EHC are rare and include Lynch syndrome and bile salt transporter protein gene defects[5] (see Chapter 9E).

More recently, metabolic conditions such as type 2 diabetes have been found to be associated with an increased risk of EHC. For example, in a meta-analysis, individuals with type 2 diabetes had an increased risk of cholangiocarcinoma (relative risk [RR], 1.60; 95% CI 1.38–1.87), EHC (RR, 1.63; 95% CI, 1.29–2.05) and ICC (RR, 1.97; 95% CI, 2.57–2.46).[5] Nonalcoholic fatty liver disease, obesity, dyslipidemia, and hypertension are also associated with an increased risk of EHC.[7,8] These conditions are increasing worldwide and, in part, may explain the rising incidence of EHC.

TUMOR LOCATION AND HISTOPATHOLOGY

Extrahepatic cholangiocarcinoma can arise anywhere from first-order bile ducts within the liver down to the ampulla of Vater. Perihilar cholangiocarcinoma (HC or Klatskin tumors) was first described in 1965 by Klatskin and comprises 50% of all cholangiocarcinomas.[9] HC arises in the right or left hepatic duct or at the confluence of the right and left ducts, whereas DC arises in the common bile duct distal to the takeoff of the cystic duct (Fig. 51A.2). Any extrahepatic biliary strictures are highly suggestive of malignancy; however, histopathologic assessment with brushing or biopsy has limited sensitivity although are highly specific.[1] Thus, in the absence of histologic findings indicating malignancy, preoperative differentiation between cholangiocarcinoma and benign strictures (also known as malignant masquerade) is difficult.[10,11] Benign strictures may arise from autoimmune cholangiopathy, autoimmune pancreatitis, stone-related disease, or primary sclerosing cholangiopathy and should be treated accordingly when recognized (see Chapter 42).

Adenocarcinoma is the dominant histologic group, comprising more than 75% of extrahepatic biliary tumors. Precancerous lesions include biliary intraepithelial neoplasia, intraductal papillary neoplasm of the biliary tract, intraductal tubular papillary neoplasm, and mucinous cystic neoplasm. Common immunohistochemical markers of EHC include mucin, MUC5AC, MUC6, S100P, SMAD4 loss, and BAP1.[9] Adenocarcinomas are subdivided into three subtypes: sclerosing, nodular, and papillary (Figs. 51A.3 and 51A.4). Papillary tumors are seen in up to 25% of EHCs and are associated with improved survival compared with nodular sclerosing lesions (see Fig. 51A.4).[12,13]

Molecular profiling of cholangiocarcinoma is distinct, depending on the subtype. KRAS (55%) and TP53 (40%) mutations in HC are common.[14,15] *IDH*, *EPHA2*, and *BAP1* mutations and *FGFR2* fusions are more common in ICC, whereas EHCs contain *PRKACA* and *PRKACB* fusions and mutations in *ELF3*, *ERBB2*, and *ARID1B*.[9,16,17] In contrast to ICC, targetable mutations in extrahepatic cholangiocarcinoma are rare.

CLINICAL PRESENTATION

Clinical presentation depends on tumor size and location. HC presents with jaundice in 90% of patients.[18] Nonspecific symptoms such as abdominal pain, weight loss, nausea, and pruritus

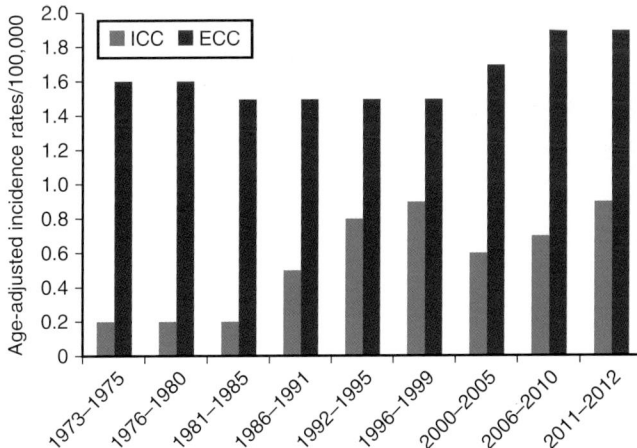

FIGURE 51A.1 Temporal trends in age-adjusted incidence rates of cholangiocarcinoma by anatomic location. *ECC,* Extrahepatic cholangiocarcinoma; *ICC,* intrahepatic cholangiocarcinoma (From Mukkamalla SKR, Naseri HM, Kim BY, et al. Trends in incidence and factors affecting survival of patients with cholangiocarcinoma in the United States. *J Natl Compr Canc Netw.* 2018;16[4]:370–376.)

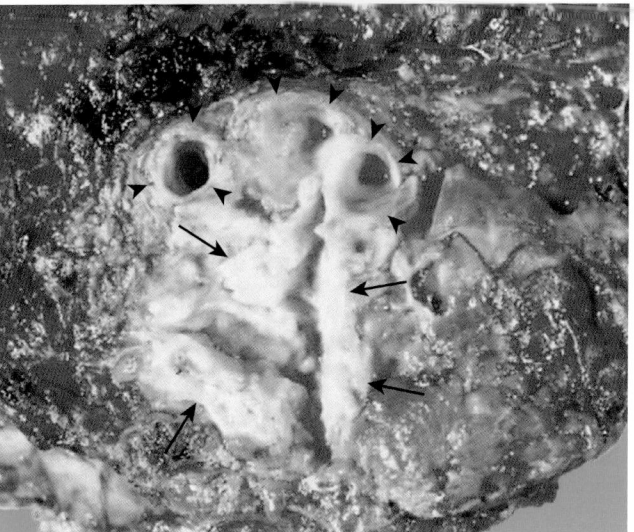

FIGURE 51A.3 Gross appearance of sclerosing cholangiocarcinoma with thickening of the bile duct walls *(arrows)* and dilation of intrahepatic bile ducts *(arrowheads).* (From Lee WJ, Lim HK, Jang KM, et al. Radiologic spectrum of cholangiocarcinoma: emphasis on unusual manifestations and differential diagnoses. *Radiographics.* 2001;21[Spec No]:S97–S116, 2001.)

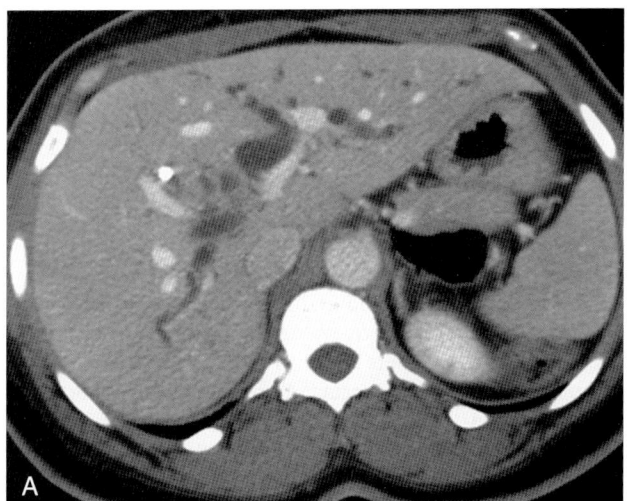

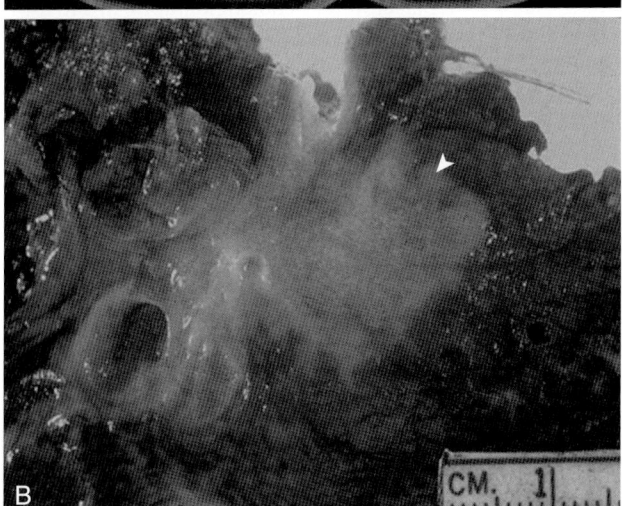

FIGURE 51A.2 A, Contrast-enhanced computed tomography scan showing hilar bile duct tumor involving the right and left hepatic ducts (see Chapter 16). **B,** Gross appearance of a nodular-sclerosing tumor invading the hepatic parenchyma *(arrowhead).*

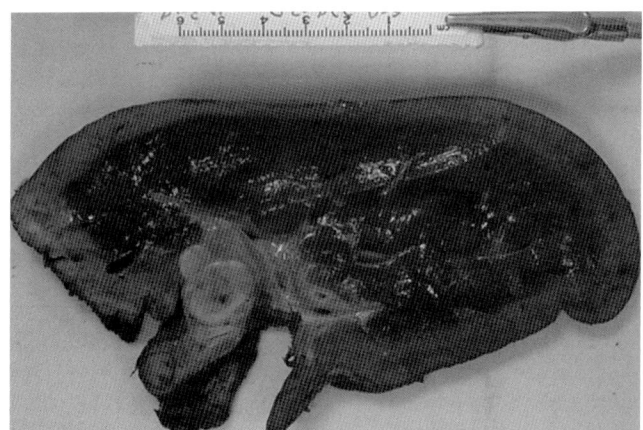

FIGURE 51A.4 Gross appearance of a papillary-type cholangiocarcinoma within the right hepatic duct. Note the expansion of the duct lumen.

are also common.[19] In general, tumors become clinically apparent as a result of jaundice and jaundice-related symptoms such as pruritus, acholic stools, choluria, or abnormal liver function tests. Cholangitis is rare at the time of initial presentation because of a lack of bactibilia in an uninstrumented biliary tree. Laboratory evaluations are consistent with biliary obstruction and includes elevated total bilirubin, direct bilirubin, alkaline phosphatase and gamma-glutamyl transferase. Tumor markers such as carbonic anhydrase 19-9 (CA19-9) and carcinoembryonic antigen (CEA) are elevated; however, the former is often markedly elevated in the setting of jaundice.

The presentation of DC is similar to those of other periampullary tumors in which painless jaundice is classically described. HC presenting with jaundice can be indicative of a late finding in the disease course because early on, incomplete obstruction of the biliary tree or unilateral obstruction does not cause jaundice and may manifest with nearly normal liver function tests. A common finding in these scenarios is an isolated elevation in alkaline phosphatase (even minimal changes) which ultimately leads to the diagnosis. Additionally, papillary hilar tumors may manifest with intermittent jaundice as a result of small fragments of tumor detaching from a friable papillary tumor of the right or left hepatic duct or a mobile main tumor causing a ball valve effect at the hepatic duct confluence.

The level of bilirubin elevation may help determine the cause of obstruction. Significantly elevated bilirubin levels (>10 mg/dL) suggests malignant obstruction, whereas obstruction from choledocholithiasis is often associated with lower bilirubin levels typically ranging from 2 to 4 mg/dL, although there is significant overlap.[20] Cholangitis at presentation in patients without a history of biliary manipulation is rare; however, the incidence of bactibilia is 100% after biliary instrumentation that compromises the sphincter of Oddi. Although common bile duct stones or gallstones may coexist with bile duct cancer, it is rare for choledocholithiasis to cause obstruction at the hepatic confluence in the absence of predisposing conditions such as PSC, choledochal cyst, or hepatolithiasis. A thorough and complete evaluation outlining the level of obstruction and nature of obstructing lesion is critical to avoid missing a diagnosis of carcinoma.

The physical examination, other than the presence of jaundice, is generally unremarkable. Evidence of liver dysfunction, enlarged liver, and portal hypertension may be noted in cases of long-standing biliary obstruction and portal vein involvement. An enlarged gallbladder on examination prompts consideration of biliary obstruction distal to or involving the cystic duct. With proximal biliary obstruction the gallbladder is typically collapsed.

DIAGNOSTIC STUDIES (SEE CHAPTER 16)

Patients are usually referred after undergoing initial evaluation. Imaging for staging and assessing resectability should be performed before biliary decompression. Abdominal ultrasound is commonly performed as a first method of evaluation. Although noninvasive and cost effective, ultrasound findings are typically nonspecific and consist of biliary dilatation. The level of biliary obstruction is sometimes noted; however, ultrasound has low sensitivity in this regard.[21] Duplex ultrasonography in experienced hands can accurately predict vascular involvement (Fig. 51A.5). Duplex ultrasound can be particularly useful for assessing portal venous invasion. In a series of 63 consecutive patients from Memorial Sloan Kettering Cancer Center (MSKCC), duplex US predicted portal vein involvement in 93% of cases, with a specificity of 99% and a positive predictive value of 97%.[22] With the now more widespread availability of liver-specific multiphasic contrast enhanced imaging with CT and MRI/MRCP, ultrasound is less used in preoperative assessment; however, it can be a valuable adjunct when there is questionable vascular involvement.

Preoperative imaging should be performed with multidetector multiphasic CT or MRI of the abdomen and pelvis. Contrast-enhanced cross-sectional imaging such as liver angiogram CT with chest and pelvis is a highly sensitive diagnostic modality to delineate the level of biliary obstruction, vascular involvement, relevant anatomy, hepatic lobar atrophy as well as assess for evidence of metastatic disease. Appropriate CT protocols consist of thin (1 mm) cuts in the arterial and portal venous phases of intravenous contrast. These can then be used to create

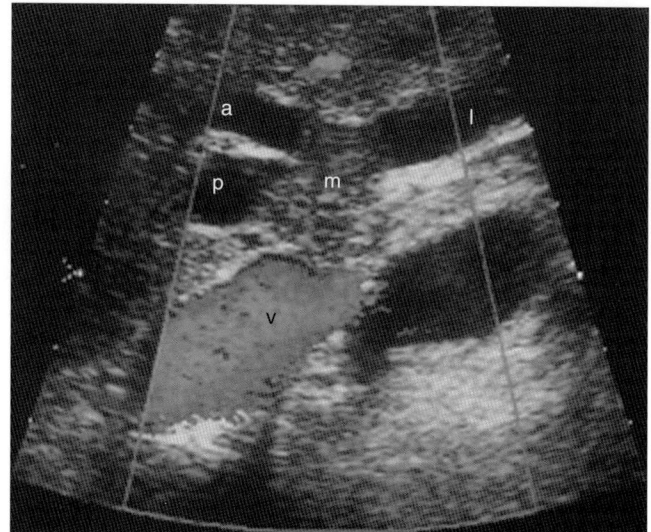

FIGURE 51A.5 Transverse color Doppler ultrasound of the biliary confluence shows a papillary cholangiocarcinoma *(m)* extending into the right anterior *(a)* and posterior *(p)* sectoral ducts and the origin of the left duct *(l)*. The adjacent portal vein *(v)* is not involved and has normal flow. (See Chapter 16.) (From Hann LE, Fong Y, Shriver CD, et al. Malignant hepatic hilar tumors: can ultrasonography be used as an alternative to angiography with CT arterial portography for determination of resectability? *J Ultrasound Med.* 15:37–45, 1996.)

high-quality three-dimensional images such as CT arteriography in a single session. The anatomy of the biliary tree, portal vein, and hepatic arteries, along with their relationship to the tumor, are specifically assessed (Fig. 51A.6).

MRI with MRCP, including biliary tree reconstruction, has been increasingly utilized to evaluate biliary tree abnormalities. MRCP accurately depicts the level of biliary obstruction, biliary anatomy as well as obstructed or isolated ducts not always appreciated on percutaneous or endoscopic evaluations[23] (Fig. 51A.7) Vascular involvement, lobar atrophy, and regional nodal and distant metastases are also assessed (Fig. 51A.8). MRCP has now replaced direct cholangiography in the initial assessment of biliary malignancy. Direct cholangiography with ERCP (see Chapters 20 and 30) and/or PTC (see Chapters 20, 31, 51B, and 52) should be used for therapeutic intervention. Specifically protocoled MRI with MRCP and contrast-enhanced CT have comparable outcomes in assessing tumor resectability.[24]

The role of PET/CT in EHC is limited (see Chapter 18). In a systematic review and meta-analysis of 2125 patients from 47 eligible studies exploring the diagnostic test accuracy of [18F] fluoro-2-deoxy-D-glucose (18FDG-PET) as a diagnostic tool for diagnosis of primary tumor, lymph node invasion, distant metastases, and relapsed disease, the sensitivity and specificity of 18FDG-PET for the diagnosis of primary tumor were 91.7% (95% CI, 89.8–93.2) and 51.3% (95% CI, 46.4-56.2), respectively. For lymph node involvement, sensitivity was 88.4% (95% CI, 82.6–92.8) and specificity was 69.1% (95% CI, 63.8–74.1). For distant metastases, sensitivity was 85.4% (95% CI, 79.5–90.2) and specificity was 89.7% (95% CI, 86.0–92.7). In identifying relapse after resection, sensitivity was 90.1% (95% CI, 84.4–94.3) and specificity was 83.5% (95% CI, 74.4–90.4).[25] Routine use of PET/CT in the preoperative setting remains unproven although unstudied in prospective trials.

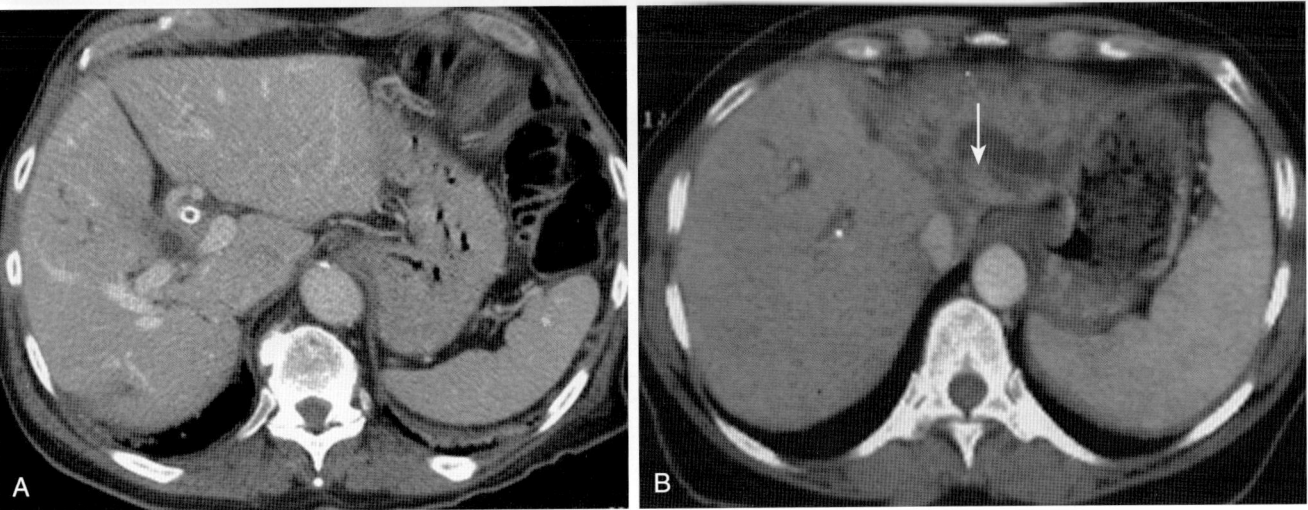

FIGURE 51A.6   A, Computed tomography images from a patient with hilar cholangiocarcinoma and jaundice. The right portal vein is invaded by tumor, and there is right-sided lobar atrophy with compensatory left hemiliver hypertrophy. **B,** Left portal vein is occluded, causing left lobar atrophy with crowding of dilated ducts *(arrow)*. Note that there is no defined mass in either image. (See Chapter 16.)

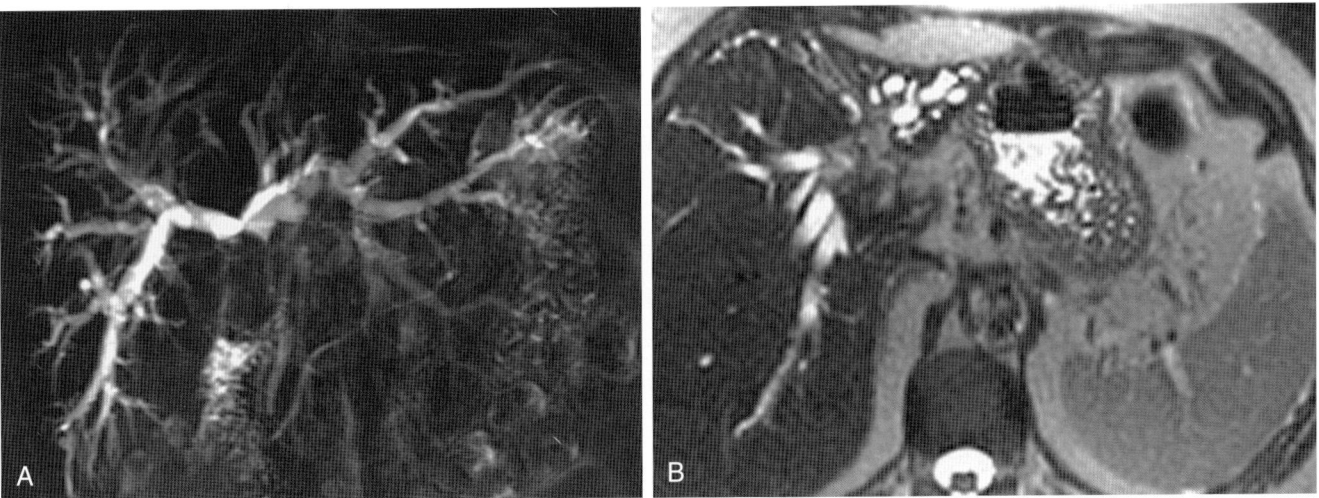

FIGURE 51A.7   Coronal **(A)** and axial **(B)** magnetic resonance cholangiopancreatographic images of a patient with hilar cholangiocarcinoma. The tumor involves the right and the left hepatic ducts. The bile ducts in this study appear *white*. (See Chapter 16.)

PET/CT is best used as a problem-solving tool when there is an equivocal finding on cross-sectional imaging.

Direct cholangiography via ERCP or PTC encompasses highly sensitive, invasive techniques which delineate the biliary tree, tumor or stricture location and extent of biliary disease. Moreover, these studies allow for biopsy to establish a diagnosis and biliary drainage can be performed when necessary (Fig. 51A.9). Both ERCP and PTC have a sensitivity and specificity of approximately 70% to 75% for obtaining a tissue diagnosis.[26,27] However, a tissue diagnosis is not mandatory before proceeding with attempted resection for cholangiocarcinoma, and a negative biopsy sample in the setting of a high clinical suspicion for malignancy does not provide helpful data. Noninvasive imaging has replaced direct cholangiography for the staging of EHC, and direct cholangiography is limited to biliary decompression and tissue sampling.

Although most patients with hilar strictures and jaundice have cholangiocarcinoma, alternative diagnoses are possible in 10% to 15% of patients. The most common of these are gallbladder carcinoma, Mirizzi syndrome, and benign focal strictures, such as autoimmune cholangitis, lymphoplasmacytic sclerosing pancreatitis/cholangitis, granulomatous disease, and PSC. A thickened, irregular gallbladder wall with infiltration into segments IV and V of the liver, selective involvement of the right portal pedicle, and obstruction of the mid–bile duct with occlusion of the cystic duct on endoscopic cholangiography all suggest gallbladder carcinoma (Figs. 51A.10 and 51A.11).

Distal bile duct tumors frequently are mistaken for adenocarcinoma of the pancreatic head, the most common periampullary malignancy (see Chapter 17). Cross-sectional imaging and direct cholangiography can provide valuable information regarding the level of obstruction and may show clearly that

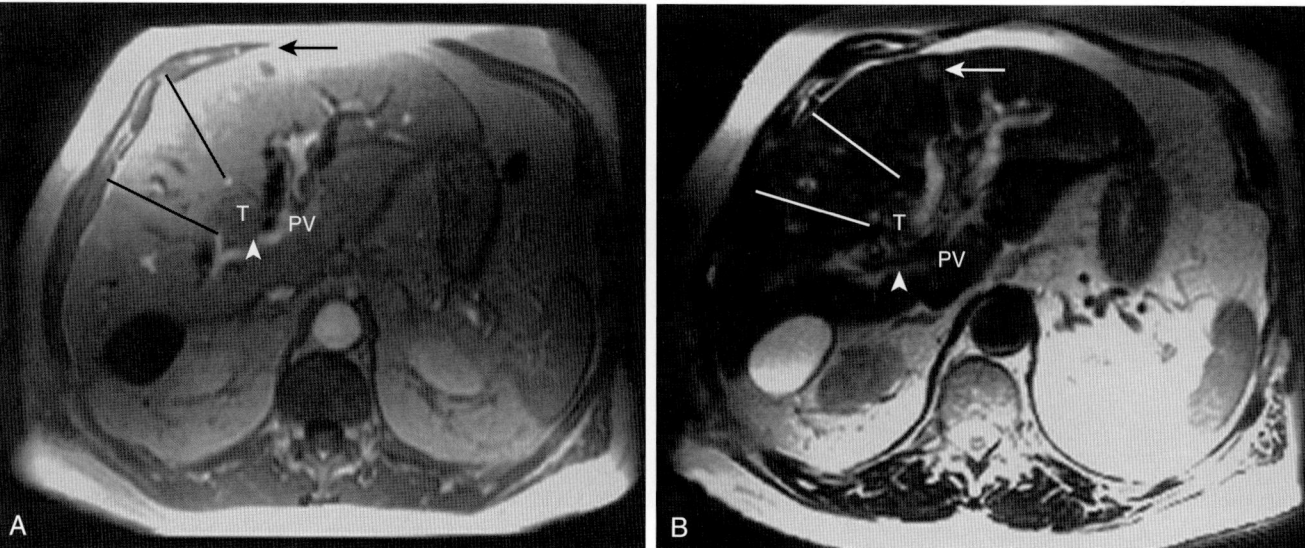

FIGURE 51A.8 **A,** T1-weighted, gadolinium-enhanced magnetic resonance image of a patient with hilar cholangiocarcinoma. The bile ducts appear *black*. A hilar tumor is seen *(T)*, apparently adherent to or encasing the right portal vein branch *(PV; arrowhead)*. The tumor has occluded the right anterior sectoral branch of the portal vein, and the anterior sector appears atrophic *(black lines)* with crowded, dilated ducts. The *arrow* points to intrahepatic metastases. **B,** Magnetic resonance cholangiopancreatography cut through the same area of the liver. Similar findings are indicated in this image, in which the bile ducts appear *white*. (See Chapter 16.)

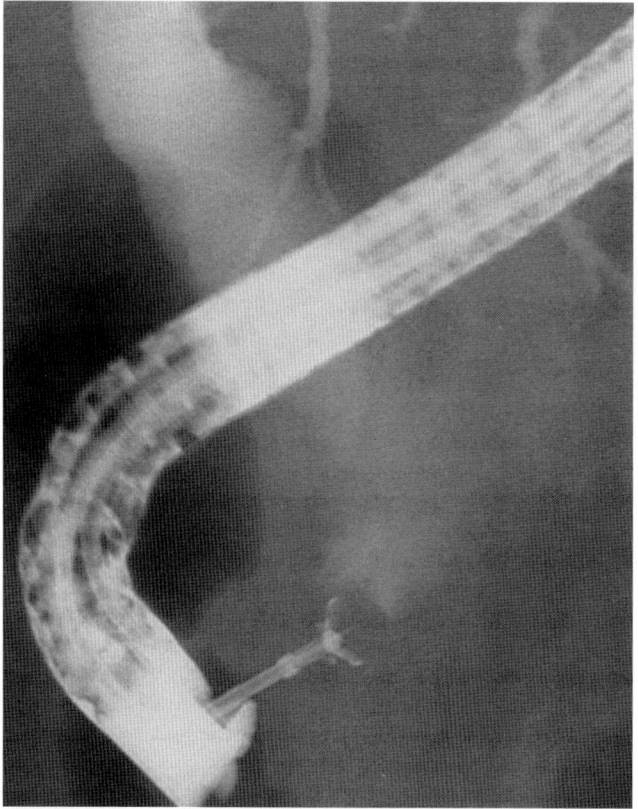

FIGURE 51A.9 Endoscopic retrograde cholangiopancreatography–guided grasp biopsy of a distal bile duct tumor in a patient presenting with obstructive jaundice and requiring biliary drainage. Cross-sectional imaging had previously staged the patient with metastatic disease, and a tissue diagnosis was sought. (See Chapters 20 and 30.)

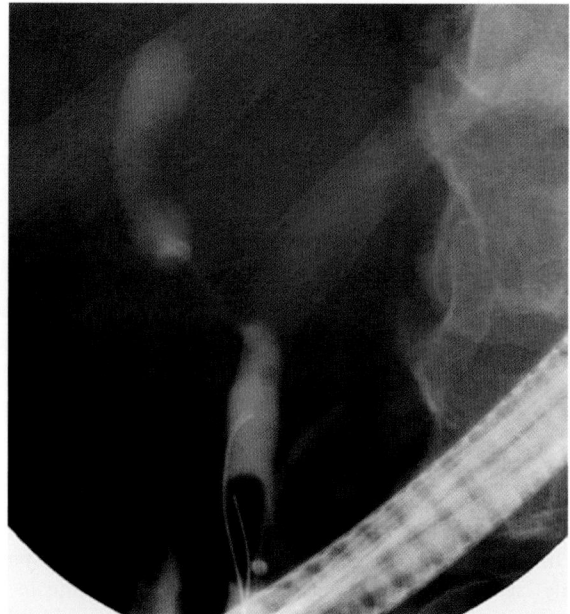

FIGURE 51A.10 Endoscopic retrograde cholangiopancreatography findings of a mid–common bile duct stricture are typically associated with carcinoma of the gallbladder or cystic duct. (See Chapters 20 and 30.)

the obstruction is arising from the bile duct and does not involve the pancreatic duct. MRCP is noninvasive and evaluates for choledocholithiasis as well as visualizes the distal bile duct. ERCP is therapeutic for patients with choledocholithiasis and can clearly show the level of obstruction of the distal bile duct. A dilated extrahepatic bile duct terminating abruptly at its

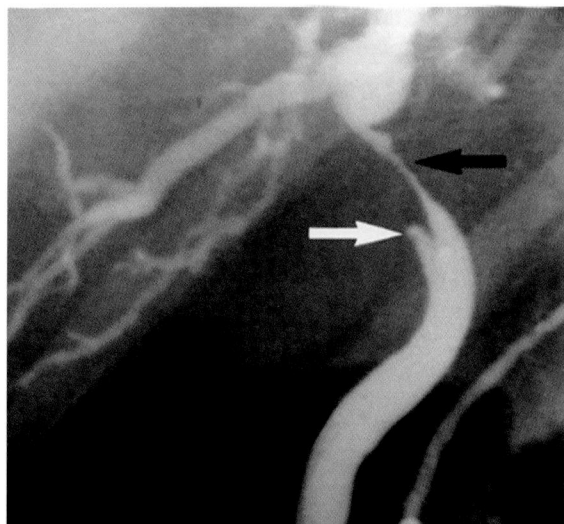

FIGURE 51A.11 Endoscopic retrograde cholangiopancreatography from a patient with a benign stricture of the proximal bile duct. The smooth, tapered appearance *(black arrow)* is in contrast to the irregular stricture typical of a sclerosing tumor. Nonfilling of the cystic duct *(white arrow)* is an important finding, and in the appropriate setting, it should raise the suspicion of gallbladder carcinoma. In this patient, the chronic inflammatory process had involved the hepatic duct and cystic ducts. Most cases of benign strictures of the proximal bile duct spare the cystic duct. (See Chapters 20 and 30.)

distal aspect without a concomitantly dilated pancreatic duct suggests a distal bile duct carcinoma.

Benign strictures such as inflammatory strictures, sclerosing cholangitis or immunoglobulin G4 (IgG4)-related cholangiopathy account for 10% to 15% of resected strictures[10,28] (see Chapter 42). These can be difficult to differentiate from malignant strictures without resection. Biopsy approaches such as endoscopic brushings of the bile duct, endoscopic ultrasound–fine needle aspiration (EUS-FNA) and PTC endobiliary forceps biopsy have a high false-negative rate, and repeat attempts at biopsy can delay resection and increase procedure-related complications.[29,30] In patients with a stricture of the bile duct and a clinical presentation consistent with cholangiocarcinoma, histologic confirmation of malignancy is generally unnecessary, unless nonoperative therapy is planned.[31,32] Serum IgG4 levels can be helpful in diagnosing benign autoimmune strictures treatable with steroids.

PREOPERATIVE EVALUATION AND MANAGEMENT

When extrahepatic cholangiocarcinoma is suspected, evaluation should focus on determining resectability, hepatic reserve

and overall performance status (see Chapters 51B and 52). Significant baseline comorbidities such as portal hypertension, cirrhosis, and poor performance status can preclude surgical resection. Patients with metastatic disease do not benefit from resection and should be offered palliative systemic chemotherapy. In unresectable or metastatic cases, biliary decompression in jaundiced patients and confirmation of the diagnosis with tissue sampling are warranted to move forward with palliative systemic chemotherapy.

Resectability is determined by assessing four criteria: (1) extent of biliary tree involvement, (2) lobar atrophy, (3) vascular involvement, and (4) the presence of metastatic disease[12,33] (Table 51A.1). High-quality cross-sectional imaging, ideally performed before biliary decompression, provides an assessment of potential portal vein and hepatic artery involvement and the extent of biliary involvement. Obstructed bile ducts appear dilated up to the level of the tumor. A dilated gallbladder on examination or cross-sectional imaging should alert the physician to the possibility of distal cholangiocarcinoma, pancreatic cancer, or gallbladder cancer rather than hilar cholangiocarcinoma. Portal vein involvement is suggested by a change in contour of the vein or occlusion.

Assessment of hepatic atrophy is a critical component of assessing resectability because this may indicate extent of tumor involvement, which has implications in treatment decisions. Long-standing biliary obstruction may cause moderate atrophy, whereas concomitant ipsilateral portal venous compromise induces rapid and severe atrophy of the involved segments. Atrophy is noted on cross sectional imaging by a shrunken, hypoperfused liver with crowding of dilated bile ducts along with concomitant hypertrophy of the contralateral lobe (Fig. 51A.12).

The right hepatic artery generally courses posterior to the common hepatic duct. Involvement of the right hepatic artery in left-sided biliary tumors requiring a left-sided liver resection precludes resection or requires arterial reconstruction in highly selected cases. Lymph node–positive disease has an adverse effect on long-term survival and significantly decreases the likelihood of cure; however, lymphadenopathy on cross-sectional imaging is neither sensitive nor specific for metastatic disease. Enlarged regional nodes on preoperative imaging are often reactive and nonneoplastic, particularly after biliary instrumentation; therefore surgical exploration can still be considered in these instances.

Pretreatment Biliary Drainage

Identification of the level of biliary obstruction followed by selective and appropriately planned biliary drainage is a critical decision. Biliary decompression is necessary to start systemic therapies and address symptoms such as anorexia, weight loss, and pruritus. Patients with resectable tumors often require major

TABLE 51A.1 Criteria for Nonresectability in Hilar Cholangiocarcinoma		
PATIENT FACTORS	**LOCAL TUMOR EXTENT**	**DISTANT TUMOR SPREAD**
Patient medically unfit for major operation	Bilateral hepatic duct involvement up to secondary biliary radicals	Positive lymph nodes outside the hepatoduodenal ligament
Cirrhosis with portal hypertension	Encasement/occlusion of the main portal vein	Metastases to liver, lung, peritoneum, or other distant organs
	Encasement of portal vein branch with atrophy of contralateral hepatic lobe	
	Hepatic duct involvement up to secondary biliary radicles with atrophy of contralateral hepatic lobe	

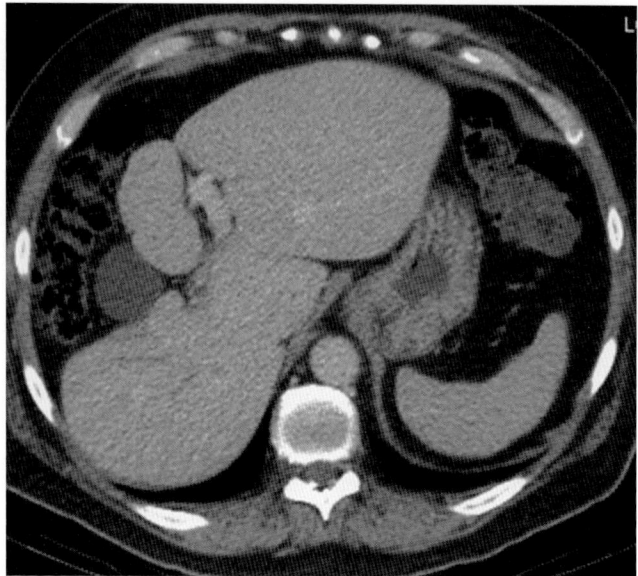

FIGURE 51A.12 Axial computed tomography demonstrates severe atrophy of the right anterior sector in a patient with a hilar cholangiocarcinoma that had invaded the respective sectoral portal vein selectively. (See Chapter 16.)

hepatectomy; therefore adequate drainage of a jaundiced future liver remnant (FLR) is often necessary to optimize postoperative liver regeneration and decrease postoperative morbidity and mortality. Cholangitis and infectious complications in resectable patients are common after biliary instrumentation and are an important source of perioperative morbidity (see Chapter 43) Appropriate resuscitation and treatment of these infections is imperative before resection. Inappropriate or misplaced biliary drains can lead to significant infectious complications which can

preclude resection. Early input from a hepatopancreatobiliary surgeon is highly recommended.

Obstructive jaundice associated with HC differs from that associated with middle or distal bile duct cancer. In distal bile duct cancer, a single catheter or stent is sufficient for complete biliary drainage, whereas in HC, multiple biliary drainage catheters of the FLR may be necessary. Percutaneous and endoscopic approaches to biliary drainage are both acceptable. Internal drainage is preferred to limit bile loss, malabsorption, and dehydration. Cholangitic patients, jaundiced patients requiring systemic chemotherapy, patients with hyperbilirubinemia-induced malnutrition, those with hepatic insufficiency, and jaundiced patients undergoing portal vein embolization (PVE) require immediate biliary decompression.[33]

The indications for biliary drainage in resectable HC are highly debated. Routine biliary drainage before resection to reach a baseline bilirubin below 3 mg/dL has been proposed with the rationale that routine drainage improves the regenerative capacity of the FLR and thus reduces morbidity and mortality.[35] Contrarily, multiple series have demonstrated an association with improved outcomes with selective biliary drainage.[36–38] Kennedy et al.[38] analyzed the impact of FLR volume and preoperative biliary drainage on postoperative hepatic insufficiency and mortality rates. They identified 60 patients who underwent hepatic resection for HC. Preoperative biliary drainage of the FLR appears to improve outcome if the predicted volume is less than 30% in contrast to patients with FLR greater than 30% where no patients experienced hepatic insufficiency and preoperative biliary drainage did not appear to improve outcomes (Fig. 51A.13). A subsequent multi-institutional study combined the experiences of MSKCC and the Academic Medical Center in Amsterdam. In this study, biliary drainage appeared to reduce risk of postoperative liver failure in patients with a small FLR (defined as ≤50%) compared with undrained patients.[39] Conversely, patients with a large FLR

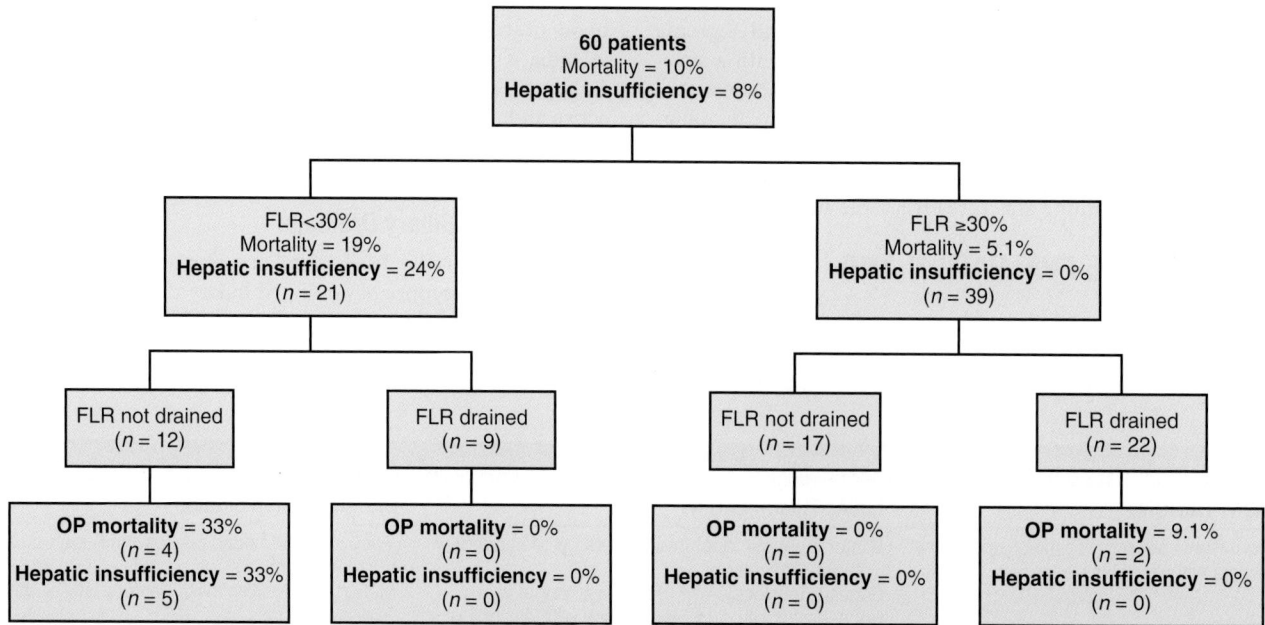

FIGURE 51A.13 Outcomes in patients stratified by future liver remnant volume and adequacy of biliary decompression. *FLR,* Future liver remnant; *OP,* operative. (From Kennedy TJ, Yopp A, Qin Y, et al. Role of preoperative biliary drainage of liver remnant prior to extended liver resection for hilar cholangiocarcinoma. *HPB (Oxford).* 2009;11[5]:445–451.)

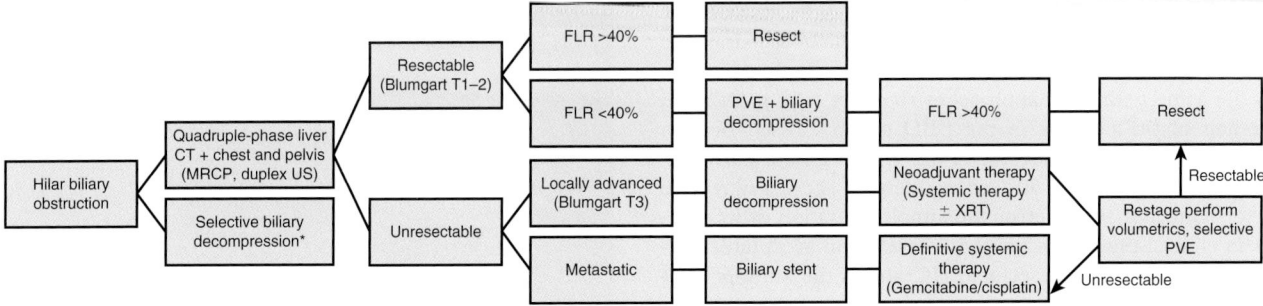

FIGURE 51A.14 **Algorithm illustrating general approach to patients with hilar cholangiocarcinoma.** *Patients presenting with obstructive cholangitis must undergo biliary decompression. *CT,* Computed tomography; *FLR,* future liver remnant; *MRCP,* magnetic resonance cholangiopancreatography; *PVE,* portal vein embolization; *US,* ultrasound. (From Lidsky ME, Jarnagin WR. Surgical management of hilar cholangiocarcinoma at Memorial Sloan Kettering Cancer Center. *Ann Gastroenterol Surg.* 2018;2[4]:304–312.)

(>50%) had increased mortality after biliary drainage compared with patients without percutaneous biliary drainage (PBD) (12% vs. 0% mortality). Taken together, these studies indicate that patients with a large FLR are able to undergo major resection without preoperative biliary drainage and that biliary drainage in these patients likely introduces morbidity and mortality without any added benefit. Small FLR, on the other hand, requires preoperative biliary drainage to improve postoperative liver regeneration and likely reduces morbidity and mortality[34] (Fig. 51A.14). When indicated in resectable HC, biliary drainage should be limited to the FLR. If segmental cholangitis develops after biliary drainage, urgent decompression of the affected ducts should be performed. It should be stressed that predrainage imaging to determine resectability and a multidisciplinary decision regarding the method and target of the drainage procedures are critically important.

Biliary drainage can be accomplished via endoscopic biliary drainage (EBD) (see Chapters 30 and 51B), percutaneous transhepatic biliary drainage (PTBD) (see Chapters 31 and 51B), or endoscopic nasobiliary drainage (END) (see Chapters 51B and 119B). In most centers, either EBD or PTBD is performed, with END occurring mainly in Asian centers (see Chapter 119B). The advantage of EBD versus PTBD is the ability to avoid external drains; however, stent misplacement is not uncommon, with up to half of patients requiring PTBD after inadequate or inappropriate drainage via EBD (Fig. 51A.15).[40] Moreover, there is a high incidence of cholangitis, particularly when multiple obstructed ducts are instrumented but not drained.[40] PTBD allows for precise placement of drainage catheters in the FLR, as well as delineation of the extent of tumor involvement in the biliary tree, which are both critical for operative planning. Additionally, PTBD allows for internal drainage of proximal bile duct strictures with termination of the stent or catheter above the ampulla. This improves catheter patency and decreases the risk of contamination of the biliary tree and infectious related complications.[42] In a Surveillance, Epidemiology, and End Results (SEER)-Medicare analysis of patients with supra-ampullary cholangiocarcinoma who did not undergo resection, biliary drainage procedures that violated the sphincter of Oddi were associated with increased rates of cholangitis.[43] Drawbacks to PTBD include catheter-associated discomfort and concerns with tract seeding. Tract seeding, however, is associated with distant metastatic disease and is rare.[44]

A multicenter, randomized controlled trial (RCT) in the Netherlands evaluated PTBD versus EBD in patients with

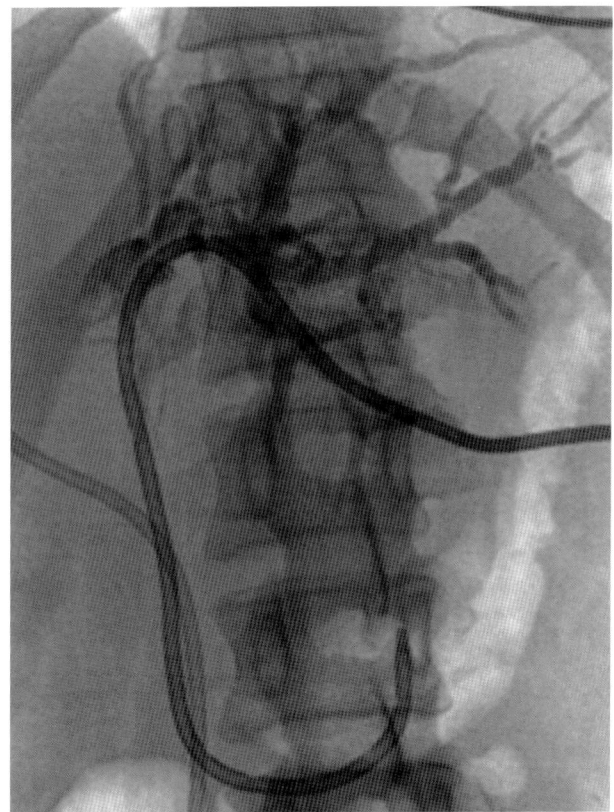

FIGURE 51A.15 Percutaneous transhepatic cholangiogram (PTC) shows a left hepatic duct stricture with no apparent isolation of the segment IV and left lateral ducts. PTC guides safe placement of a percutaneous biliary drain, which can permit internalization of bile flow. (See Chapter 31.)

potentially resectable HC requiring major liver resection and PBD.[40] The primary end point was the rate of severe complications with a planned accrual of 106 patients; however, the study was stopped after accruing 54 patients due to increased mortality in the PTBD group versus EBD (41% vs. 11%; RR, 3.67; 95% CI, 1.15–11.7; $P = .03$). Of the 11 deaths in the PTBD cohort, 3 patients died preoperatively, and there was no difference in the preoperative mortality rate in patients who had PTBD alone ($n = 3/26$), EBD alone ($n = 0/11$), or crossed over to PTBD from EBD ($n = 0/16$) ($P = 0.2$). Patients died from liver failure, bile leak complications, cholangitis, and disease progression, and there was no direct link to the biliary drainage procedure as the cause of death. The overall complication rate was the same with both approaches (63% vs. 67%). Of note, over half of the patients in the EBD group crossed over to PTBD compared with just 4% of the PTBD group. Early termination of the study at 50% of its intended accrual may have led to significant type I error thus implementation of its findings in clinical practice is limited. PTBD is an acceptable modality in patients with resectable HC and is the authors' preferred approach.

Advocates for ENBD over EBD cite decreased complication rates and more durable biliary drainage. Kawakubo et al.[45] evaluated the complications associated with temporary ENBD in patients with HC being assessed for resection compared with EBD and PTBD. ENBD was associated with a lower risk of biliary reintervention (odds ratio [OR], 0.26; 95% CI, 0.08–0.76, P = .012). The E-POD hilar study was a multicenter retrospective review of 374 malignant hilar biliary obstruction cases undergoing either ENBD or EBD for HC and showed no advantage of ENBD over EBD as the initial approach in resectable HC.[46] Moreover, there is significant patient discomfort because of the nasal drainage, which cannot be ignored.

Internal biliary drainage is preferred to external drainage, when possible, because of impaired intestinal barrier function from decreased intestinal cell regeneration and disruption of tight junctions between the cells in patients with prolonged external biliary drainage.[47] Animal models showed that bile replacement after bile duct ligation is essential to maintain intestinal barrier function.[48] Bile replacement can restore the intestinal barrier function primarily because of repair of physical damage to the intestinal mucosa. Bile replacement during external biliary drainage has been recommended for planned hepatectomy for hilar cholangiocarcinoma because of the substantial infectious morbidity associated with these resections.

Portal Vein Embolization

PVE was first described by Makuuchi et al.[49] in cases in which volumetric analysis predicts an inadequate FLR portending a high risk of postoperative liver dysfunction (see Chapter 102C). Originally this procedure required a transileocolic approach; however, a percutaneous transhepatic approach is more commonly performed, which obviates the need for general anesthesia and laparotomy (Fig. 51A.16). General indications for PVE consist of a FLR less than 25% in normal healthy liver, less than 30% in a setting of chemotherapy-induced liver toxicity, or less than 40% in patients with cirrhosis and underlying liver dysfunction. PVE allows for assessment in gross change in liver volume as well as a dynamic assessment of liver hypertrophy by measuring the kinetic growth rate (KGR). KGR is calculated by the degree of hypertrophy over the number of weeks since PVE and is highly predictive of postoperative liver failure. In a series of 153 patients undergoing major hepatectomy after PVE, no patients with a KGR greater than 2.66% per week experienced postoperative liver insufficiency.[50] PVE is safe with a low morbidity (2%–2.5%) and mortality (0.1%) rate and increases FLR by an absolute value of 8% to 37.9%.[51,52] Given that most patients present with cholestatic liver failure and commonly have advanced tumors requiring neoadjuvant chemotherapy, we typically prefer PVE in cases in which FLR is expected to be less than 40%.

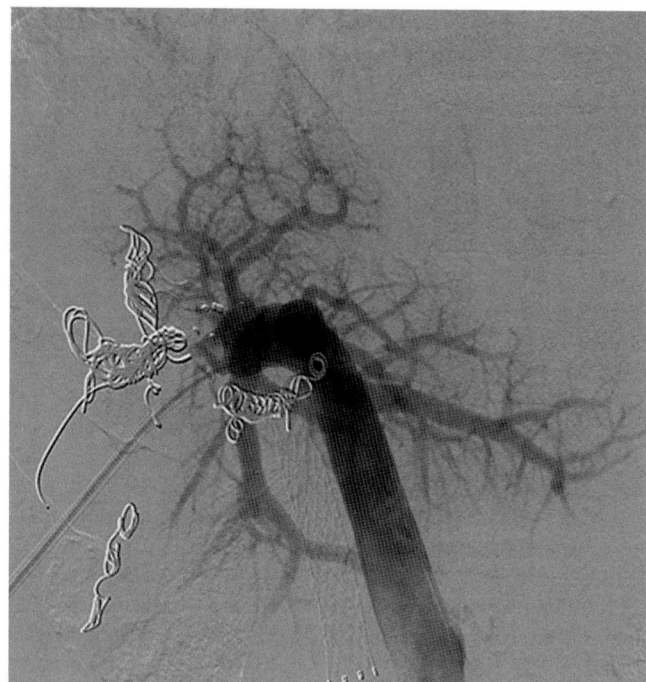

FIGURE 51A.16 Portal vein embolization can be used to induce hypertrophy of the planned functional liver remnant *(FLR)* after major hepatectomy for hilar bile duct cancer. Percutaneous transhepatic embolization is the most widely used technique. In this patient, right portal vein branches were coil embolized 4 weeks before a planned right hepatectomy. Three-dimensional volumetric calculations of the planned FLR were analyzed before and after embolization. (See Chapter 102C.)

Preoperative Staging

Various staging systems exist for HC that can help determine prognosis and resectability. The modified Bismuth-Corlette classification stratifies patients based on extent of biliary involvement (Fig. 51A.17).[53] Type I tumors are distal to the biliary confluence, type II tumors involve the confluence, type IIIA tumors extend past the confluence to the right hepatic duct, and type IIIB tumors involve the confluence and left hepatic duct. Type IV tumors involve the confluence and bilateral hepatic ducts. A limitation of the Bismuth classification is that it does not describe involvement of vascular structures, resectability, or prognosis.

The American Joint Commission for Cancer (AJCC) tumor-node-metastasis staging system (Table 51A.2) predicts survival after resection; however, it is based on pathologic findings and therefore has no utility in preoperative management. The eighth edition of the *Cancer Staging Manual* has a separate staging system for HC. Its utility is limited to the postoperative setting in patients with resectable disease and assessing prognosis in the metastatic setting.

Given the limitations of both the Bismuth classification and AJCC staging, Jarnagin et al.[54] proposed a staging system that aimed to address prognosis, resectability, and the need for hepatic resection. The MSKCC staging system describes the T stage of the tumor by describing the extent of tumor within the biliary tree, vascular involvement, and lobar atrophy (Table 51A.3) and predicts resectability as well as the likelihood of achieving an R0 resection.[54] Despite the fact that this system does not account for N stage or M stage, it is significantly associated with overall survival.[55]

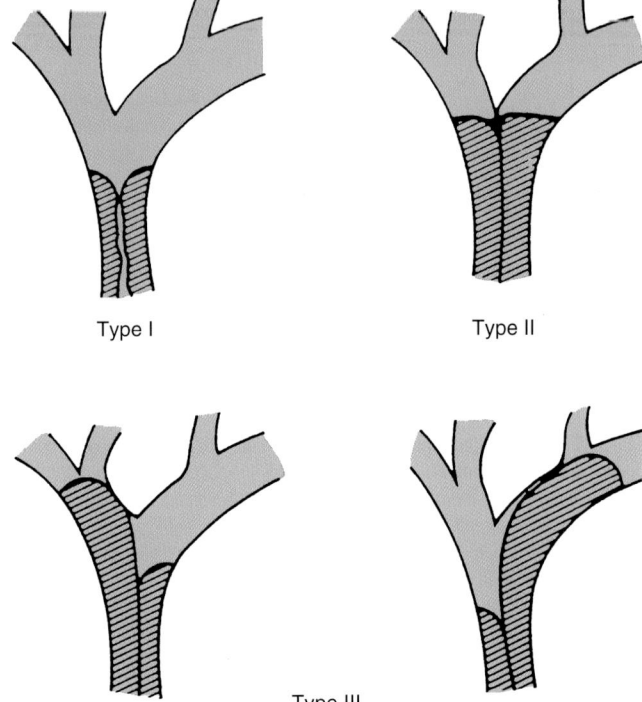

FIGURE 51A.17 **Bismuth-Corlette classification scheme of biliary strictures.** (See Chapter 42.)

Type I

Type II

Type III

Diagnostic Laparoscopy

Despite significant improvement in imaging sensitivity and techniques, up to 50% of patients will have unresectable disease at exploration.[12] Diagnostic laparoscopy can avoid a nontherapeutic laparotomy in approximately 25% of patients undergoing resection for HC.[56,57] In a retrospective review of patients diagnosed with potentially resectable HC between January 2010 and April 2015 in the United Kingdom, 27.2% of patients were spared a nontherapeutic laparotomy.[56]

Another retrospective review out of MSKCC analyzed 56 patients with radiographically resectable HC, in which 14 (25%) of patients were found to have metastatic disease.[57] The yield of diagnostic laparoscopy increased to 36% in patients with T2/T3 tumors. Overall, the data suggest a significant yield in staging laparoscopy for HC, particularly in patients with locally advanced, potentially resectable HC (see Chapter 24).

TREATMENT

Most patients with unresectable bile duct cancer die within 1 year of diagnosis. The most common causes of death are liver failure and infectious complications related to biliary obstruction and biliary instrumentation. Although some have suggested a worse prognosis for unresectable tumors involving the hilum compared with distal bile duct tumors, the associated worse outcome is likely secondary to a higher incidence of infectious complications and later presentation in hilar tumors. Patients with resected proximal and distal cholangiocarcinoma experience similar disease-specific survival.[58,59]

Resection of Hilar Cholangiocarcinoma

The main objective in HC resection is complete tumor extirpation and reconstitution of biliary enteric continuity (see

TABLE 51A.2 American Joint Committee on Cancer Staging System for Perihilar Bile Duct Tumors (Eighth Edition)

CLASSIFICATION	CRITERIA
Primary Tumor (T)	
TX	Primary tumor cannot be assessed
T0	No evidence of primary tumor
Tis	Carcinoma in situ
T1	Tumor confined to the bile duct, with extension up to the muscle layer or fibrous tissue
T2a	Tumor invades beyond the wall of the bile duct to surrounding adipose tissue
T2b	Tumor invades adjacent hepatic parenchyma
T3	Tumor invades unilateral branches of the portal vein or hepatic artery
T4	Tumor invades main portal vein or its branches bilaterally, or the common hepatic artery, or unilateral second-order biliary radicles with contralateral portal vein or hepatic artery involvement
Regional Lymph Nodes (N)	
NX	Regional lymph nodes cannot be assessed
N0	No regional lymph node metastasis
N1	One to three positive lymph nodes typically involving the hilar, cystic duct, common bile duct, hepatic artery, posterior pancreatoduodenal and portal vein lymph nodes
N2	Four or more positive lymph nodes from the sites described for N1
Distant Metastasis (M)	
M0	No distant metastasis
M1	Distant metastasis (includes lymph node metastasis distant to hepatoduodenal ligament)

Anatomic Stage/Prognostic Groups

Stage 0	Tis	N0	M0
Stage I	T1	N0	M0
Stage II	T2a, T2b	N0	M0
Stage IIIA	T3	N0	M0
Stage IIIB	T4	N0	M0
Stage IIIC	Any T	N1	M0
Stage IVA	Any T	N2	M0
Stage IVB	Any T	Any N	M1

From Amin MB, Edge SB, Green FL et al., eds. *AJCC Cancer Staging Manual.* 8th ed. New York, NY: Springer; 2017.

TABLE 51A.3 Memorial Sloan Kettering Preoperative T-Stage Criteria for Hilar Cholangiocarcinoma

STAGE	CRITERIA
T1	Tumor involving biliary confluence ± unilateral extension to second-order biliary radicles
T2	Tumor involving biliary confluence ± unilateral extension to second-order biliary radicles **and** *ipsilateral* portal vein involvement ± *ipsilateral* hepatic lobar atrophy
T3	Tumor involving biliary confluence ± unilateral extension to second-order biliary radicles; **or** Unilateral extension to second-order biliary radicles with *contralateral* portal vein involvement; **or** Unilateral extension to second-order biliary radicles with *contralateral* hepatic lobar atrophy; **or** Main or bilateral portal venous involvement

Chapters 101B and 119B). Preoperative assessment of resectability with contrast-enhanced cross-sectional imaging should be performed before biliary interventions because biliary stents and catheters can induce inflammation, thus making assessment and exploration more difficult. Criteria for irresectability include patient factors such as performance status and baseline liver disease, local factors such as involvement of secondary biliary radicles bilaterally, and distant disease (see Table 50A.1). If deemed unresectable, biliary stents combined with nonoperative therapies can achieve reasonable palliation and control local tumor growth.

In patients with potentially resectable tumors, the primary goal should be complete resection with negative margins and intent to cure. The operative approach depends on biliary tumor location. Tumors involving the distal bile duct are typically removed with pancreaticoduodenectomy. To achieve an R0 resection, hilar tumors generally require a major hepatectomy with en bloc bile duct excision and often with en bloc caudate lobectomy, particularly with centrally located tumors.[54]

The importance of achieving negative margins has important implications for long-term survival. We routinely use hepatic resection but perform caudate resection selectively in cases with suggested tumor extension into the ducts of the caudate lobe. The main caudate lobe ducts drain into the left hepatic duct; therefore tumors extending into the left hepatic duct often involve the caudate duct requiring caudate resection.[60] A dilated caudate duct suggestive of tumor involvement can usually be seen on imaging performed before biliary drainage.

The improvement in long survival after complete resection of HC over time likely reflects increased implementation of en bloc partial hepatectomy and improved R0 resection rates.[61] The association between disease-specific survival (DSS) and pathologic margin status after resection of HC was evaluated in retrospective series of 101 patients. The median DSS for patients with wide margins was 56 months compared with 38 months for patients with narrow margins and 32 months for margin-positive patients ($P = .01$).[62] Survival after an R1 resection (histologically involved resection margins) appears to be similar to survival in patients with unresectable, locally advanced tumors identified at exploration (Fig. 51A.18). Moreover, nearly 10% of patients had a misleading interpretation of proximal bile duct margin on frozen section. Whether the ability to obtain adequate margins truly improves survival or if this is simply a surrogate for underlying tumor biological processes remains undetermined. Transection of the proximal bile duct should be performed as high as technically feasible with appropriate consideration of additional operative morbidity.

Determining resectability requires a thorough evaluation of preoperative and intraoperative findings. Bilateral second-order biliary radicle involvement precludes resection. Although portal vein resection can be performed in well-selected patients, unreconstructible main portal vein encasement or occlusion is a contraindication to resection. Ipsilateral lobar atrophy and ipsilateral involvement of the bile duct and portal vein are amenable to resection, whereas contralateral involvement typically precludes this (see Chapter 122).

Invasion of the main portal vein or its branches by tumor is a major determinant of resectability. The preoperative assessment of vascular involvement and ductal extension of tumor is an essential part of operative planning and gives valuable information to the surgeon with respect to the extent of operation and operative strategy. Limited tumor involvement of the portal

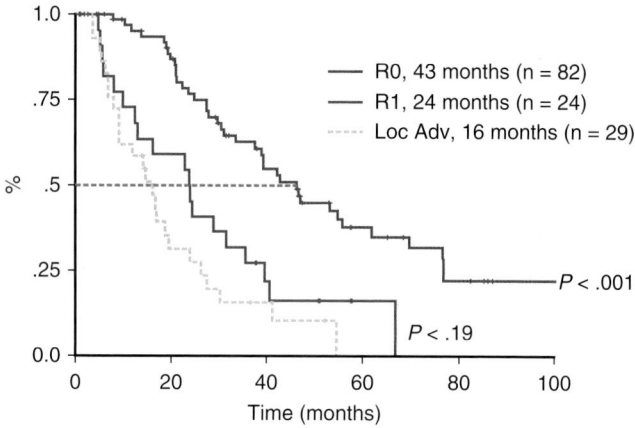

FIGURE 51A.18 Actuarial survival curves after resection of hilar cholangiocarcinoma. *R0* indicates complete resection with histologically negative resection margins (median survival, 43 months). *R1* indicates histologically involved resection margins (median survival, 24 months; $P < .001$ R0 vs. R1). *Loc Adv* indicates a patient explored but found to have unresectable tumors because of local invasion (no metastatic disease; median survival, 16 months; $P < .19$ R1 vs. Loc Adv).

venous confluence or the main portal vein may be amenable to resection and portal vein reconstruction.

Several technical steps during the exploration and resection of hilar cholangiocarcinoma are crucial to the success of the operation. After assessing for the presence of metastatic disease, one of the next steps in assessing resectability is assessing vascular involvement. This is particularly pertinent for planned left-sided resections in which involvement of the right hepatic artery coursing along the tumor is commonly seen. Bile duct resection alone without concomitant partial hepatectomy is sometimes possible. In this situation, resection must include removal of the entire supraduodenal bile duct, gallbladder, cystic duct, and extrahepatic hepatic ducts with clearance of the supraduodenal tissues and portal lymphadenectomy. However, local resections are associated with worse overall survival even after resection with clear margins. In 106 resections at MSKCC, 19 were local resections, and 9 of these were R0; however, no patient submitted to an R0 bile duct resection was among the 5-year survivors.[12]

In most patients, the option of a local resection does not exist because of intrahepatic extension of the tumor, right or left portal vein involvement, or both. In these cases, en bloc liver resection, often with caudate lobectomy, is necessary to achieve tumor clearance. Portal vein involvement by the tumor can be managed by segmental portal vein resection and reconstruction.[63–65] This procedure can be done only if intraoperative assessment shows that a tumor-free remnant with intact biliary drainage and blood supply can be left in situ. Some centrally located tumors may be amenable to a more limited hepatic resection. Such resections, which include segments IV and V or IV and I, are limited in their application and are inappropriate in the face of lobar atrophy and involvement of a main portal vein branch, both of which are common findings.

Operative exploration is carried out through a right subcostal incision with proximal extension to the xiphoid, a so-called "hockey stick" incision or midline incision. The exploration should begin with a thorough inspection of the peritoneal cavity and distant nodal sites because metastatic disease is common in patients with hilar cholangiocarcinoma. In our experience, 73 (50%) of 145 unresectable patients had metastases to regional lymph nodes or distant sites.[54] Careful bimanual palpation of the liver and intraoperative ultrasound is performed to rule out unsuspected masses in the liver. Palpation of the caudate lobe is performed after incision of the lesser omentum, allowing access to the lesser sac. A Kocher maneuver is performed to allow access to the retroduodenal lymph nodes, and the ligamentum teres is elevated, exposing the undersurface of the liver and allowing thorough examination of the subhilar and retroduodenal area. Precise assessment of tumor extension and biopsy of any suspicious lesions or distant lymph nodes with frozen section analysis should be performed. Evidence of intrahepatic metastases or spread to distant sites precludes resection. With any of these findings, the patient should be considered for palliative biliary drainage.

In all cases, the surgeon must be prepared to perform a liver resection. The general principles of intraoperative management are discussed in detail in other chapters (see Chapters 101B and 119B). Preparation for surgery includes suitable intraoperative monitoring and the possibility for rapid transfusion. The patient's central venous pressure is kept at less than 5 mm Hg during the operation to keep blood loss from hepatic veins at a minimum during retrohepatic dissection, dissection of the hepatic veins, and parenchymal transection.

The following description summarizes the initial steps of dissection, exposure of the hilar structures, dissection and resection of the hilar structures, and subsequent biliary-enteric reconstruction as performed for a segmental bile duct resection. The specifics of en bloc liver resection, including caudate lobectomy, are discussed in other chapters (see Chapters 101B and 118B).

To reach the confluence of the bile ducts and assess its relationship to the portal vein, the common bile duct first must be transected above the duodenum and turned upward. The liver hilus is fully exposed anteriorly by taking down the gallbladder and lowering the hilar plate by incising the Glisson capsule along the base of segment IV. Exposure of the left hepatic duct is improved by dividing the bridge of liver tissue that often connects the base of segment IV and the left lateral segment; this may be quite substantial in some patients. The entire extrahepatic biliary apparatus and adjacent lymphatic tissues are turned upward to expose the portal vein. A plane can be developed between the posterior aspect of the bile duct tumor and the portal vein, provided no tumor has invaded into the vessels (Fig. 51A.19). The dissection is continued upward toward the hilus, skeletonizing the portal vein and hepatic artery.

At this point, the surgeon should assess the proximal extent of tumor by palpation and, if necessary, by biopsy. Segmental bile duct resection is possible only if an adequate length of the hepatic ducts can be achieved beyond the tumor, and if no vascular involvement is evident. This is rarely possible. If the tumor extends to the second-order biliary radicles unilaterally such that clearance cannot be achieved, or if the ipsilateral portal vein branch is involved, partial hepatectomy must be performed. Tumors extending well into the left hepatic duct may involve the caudate ducts as well and require en bloc caudate lobectomy. If partial hepatectomy is required, inflow control is obtained by ligation and transection of the ipsilateral branch of the portal vein and hepatic artery. Extrahepatic control and division of the ipsilateral hepatic vein are performed before parenchymal transection.

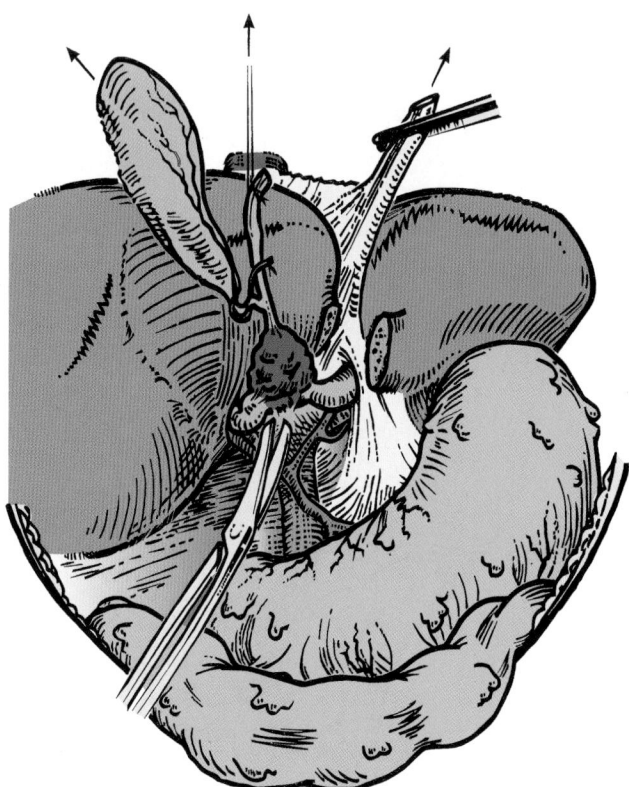

FIGURE 51A.19 Entire extrahepatic biliary apparatus is elevated together with associated portal connective tissue and nodes to allow dissection anterior to the bifurcation of the portal vein and elevation of the tumor, which is now completely mobilized. The hepatic artery and portal vein are skeletonized. (See Chapter 119B.)

When it has been established that segmental bile duct excision is feasible and will result in an R0 resection, the left and right hepatic ducts are divided above the tumor. Occasionally, irresectability as a result of main portal vein invasion or extensive bilateral intrahepatic duct involvement will not be determined until the extrahepatic biliary tree has been divided and mobilized. In both situations, biliary enteric continuity is restored by hepaticojejunostomy to a Roux-en-Y loop of jejunum. (see Chapter 32) When residual disease remains at the final level of the transected duct, appropriate consideration should be made for placement of retrograde transhepatic biliary stents (Fig. 51A.20). After removal of the tumor, the surgeon may be faced with multiple exposed duct orifices, all of which require suitable drainage. Frequently, removal of the tumor results in discontinuity of the right anterior and posterior sectoral ducts, separation of one or more caudate ducts from the left hepatic duct, or both. The sidewalls of adjacent ducts can be brought into apposition with sutures and regarded as a single duct for purposes of anastomosis. In cases of multiple exposed ducts, it is often possible to make it so that no more than two or three separate ducts need to be anastomosed. A Roux-en-Y loop of jejunum is prepared and brought up, usually in a retrocolic fashion, and anastomosis is carried out in an end-to-side fashion between the exposed ducts and the side of the jejunal loop using a single layer of interrupted absorbable sutures.

High biliary anastomoses to multiple ducts can be difficult and require careful planning. Multiple disconnected ducts that

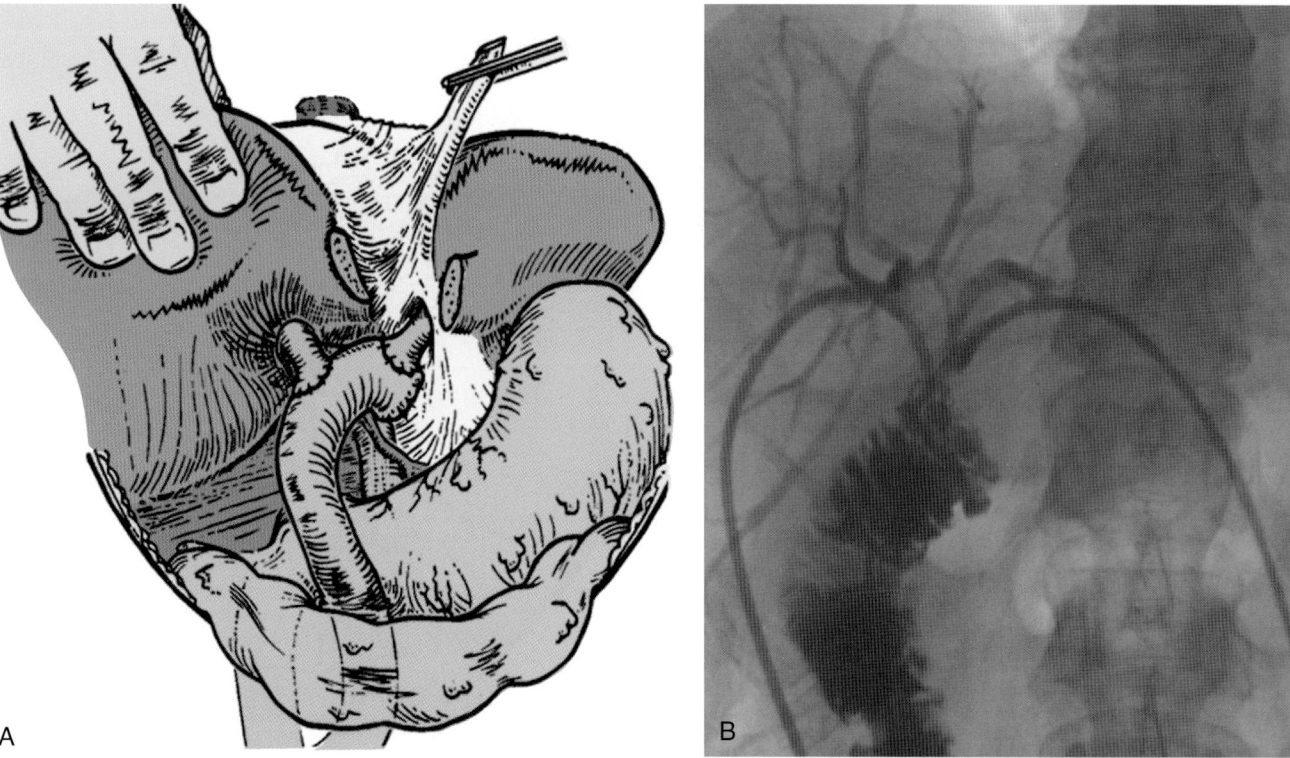

FIGURE 51A.20   **A,** In rare circumstances, the extrahepatic biliary tree can be excised alone with curative intent without the need for partial hepatectomy. In other situations, tumor unresectability may not be determined until the extrahepatic bile ducts are divided. The exposed right and left hepatic ducts are anastomosed individually to a retrocolic Roux-en-Y loop of jejunum. **B,** Retrograde transhepatic biliary stents can be passed at surgery to provide long-term palliation of obstructive jaundice and facilitate photodynamic therapy. (See Chapter 119B.)

cannot be approximated should be similarly viewed as a single duct for purposes of the anastomosis. It is usually impossible to perform sequential anastomoses in this location. The safest and most reliable method is to place the entire anterior row of sutures to all exposed ducts and separately place the entire posterior row of sutures to the duct and jejunum. The jejunum is railroaded up on the posterior sutures so that the back wall of the duct is flush with the back wall of the jejunum. The posterior layer of sutures to all exposed ducts is tied first, and the previously placed anterior sutures are passed sequentially through the anterior jejunal wall to complete the anastomosis. We routinely employ dependent drainage near the anastomosis.

Associating Liver Partition and Portal Vein Embolization for Staged Hepatectomy (see Chapter 108D)

Associating liver partition and portal vein embolization for staged hepatectomy (ALPPS) is a two-stage hepatectomy combined with in situ splitting of the liver and concomitant portal ligation during the first stage. This approach leads to rapid hypertrophy of the FLR with the cost of high perioperative morbidity and mortality rates (80% and 12%, respectively) (Fig. 51A.21).[66-68] Although the first ALPPS procedure was performed for HC, ALPPS for this disease is now rare largely because of the high complication rates associated with perihilar resections, which can be compounded in the setting of an ALPPS resection.[68] For example, most HC patients have bactibilia, which increases the likelihood to infectious complications. Additionally, intraabdominal collections and abscesses

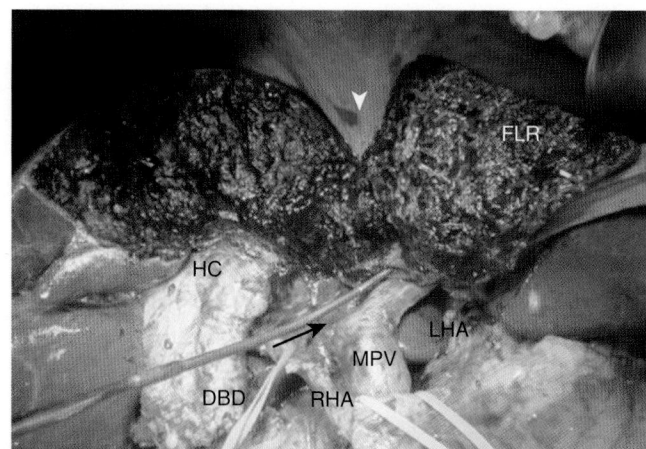

FIGURE 51A.21   Intraoperative photograph demonstrating the first stage of an associating liver partition and portal vein embolization for staged hepatectomy (ALPPS) procedure. The right portal vein has been ligated *(arrow)*, and the liver has undergone in situ splitting *(arrowhead)*. A probe has been inserted into the left hepatic duct. *DBD,* Cut distal common bile duct; *FLR,* future liver remnant; *HC,* hilar cholangiocarcinoma with en bloc dissection of the extrahepatic bile duct and lymph nodes; *LHA,* left hepatic artery; *MPV,* main portal vein; *RHA,* right hepatic artery. (From de Santibañes E, Alvarez FA, Ardiles V. How to avoid postoperative liver failure: a novel method. *World J Surg.* 2012;36[1]:125–128, 2012. (See Chapter 102D.)

are common, resulting in significant morbidity and mortality with the ALPPS procedure. The international ALPPS registry reported a 90 day-mortality rate of 27% in patients with HC who underwent ALPPS.[66] A multicenter study comprising six Italian centers (ALPPS Italian registry group) reported a 40% 90-day mortality rate for ALPPS performed for biliary tumors prompting the authors to recommend against ALPPS in patients with biliary tumors.[69] Finally, a matched case–control study compared outcomes of 29 ALPPS patients from the international ALPPS registry with 29 standard resection patients based on similar future liver remnant volume. The mortality rate in the ALPPS group was twice as high as that among patients who did not undergo ALPPS (48% vs. 24%).[70] The median survival was 6 months in the ALPPS group versus 29 months in the matched control group.[70] Modified ALPPS approaches, including partial parenchymal transection with PVE in the first stage (rather than portal vein ligation/transection), have been suggested.[67] The hilum is not dissected in the first stage; thus this approach could potentially decrease the morbidity, this has not been convincingly demonstrated in HC.

Liver Transplantation in Hilar Cholangiocarcinoma (see Chapter 108B)

Initial reports of orthotopic liver transplantation for unresectable HC demonstrated dismal results.[71–74] Meyer et al. reviewed 207 patients who underwent orthotopic liver transplantation OLT for unresectable cholangiocarcinoma. Half of the patients recurred in their series and 84% of these recurrences occurred within 2 years of transplantation. The 2-year overall survival was 48%.[73] Additional studies reported similar findings, and liver transplantation for HC was initially thought not appropriate.[71,72]

More recently, however, the implementation of intense pretransplant protocols for unresectable hilar cholangiocarcinoma, which includes neoadjuvant chemotherapy, radiation, and strict diagnostic protocols, including diagnostic laparoscopies and biopsy techniques, has resulted in improved patient selection and more encouraging long-term data.[75,76] Transplant is now a well-recognized and accepted treatment modality in highly selected HC patients.

The Mayo HC transplant protocol consists of neoadjuvant chemotherapy, radiation, and operative assessment of regional lymph nodes and distant metastases before transplant.[77] Patients are deemed eligible for transplant by meeting one of the following criteria: a mass lesion at the biliary stricture, tissue diagnosis obtained via endoluminal biopsy, or CA19-9 greater than 100. Contraindication to transplant include tumors larger than 3 cm, positive nodal or metastatic disease, previous resection attempt or transperitoneal biopsy, history of prior malignancy, and previous therapy that precludes completing neoadjuvant therapy.[34,78] Approximately one third of patients will drop out pretransplant because of disease progression or death.[79–81] Long-term results for this treatment approach are encouraging. Rosen et al.[81] from the Mayo clinic reported on 148 patients enrolled in their HC liver transplant protocol since 1993. Of these, 90 patients went on to receive a liver transplant with a 75% 5-year overall survival.

The encouraging long-term outcomes with HC transplant protocols spurred interest in broader applicability of this liver transplant for HC patients. The US Extrahepatic Biliary Malignancy Consortium performed a retrospective review of 304 patients with suspected HC who underwent resections

($n = 234$) or transplant $n = 70$).[80] Transplant was associated with a significant improvement in 5-year overall survival compared with resection (64% vs. 18%, $P < .001$). Transplant remained associated with improved survival on intention-to-treat analysis, even after accounting for tumor size, lymph node status, and PSC ($P = .049$) By contrast, the Mayo group evaluated patients with de novo HC treated by their liver transplant protocol ($n = 90$) versus standard resection ($n = 124$) and saw no difference in overall survival after adjusting for age, lymph node status, and tumor size.[79] The TRANSPHIL study (NCT02232932) is a prospective, randomized multicenter study comparing liver transplantation with liver and bile duct resection in potentially resectable HC without evidence of PSC. This study is ongoing, with a primary outcome of overall survival and a planned enrollment of 60 patients.

Although the data are compelling, liver transplant is applicable to only a small fraction of patients because of the highly specific selection criteria and the high incidence of lymph node metastases and distant occult metastases in this disease. There are no level 1 data to evaluate resection versus transplant in resectable HC, and organ availability for transplant remains limited. Given this, resectable tumors should continue to be treated with resection when an R0 resection is feasible. Unresectable locally advanced HC or HC in the setting of PSC should be referred for liver transplantation.[32,33]

Resection of Distal Cholangiocarcinoma

Resection of most distal bile duct cancers requires pancreatoduodenectomy (see Chapters 62 and 117A). Compared with patients with pancreatic cancer, those with distal bile duct cancer are more often amenable to resection, less often have microscopic disease at the resection margin, and less frequently have spread of tumor to adjacent lymph nodes.[82] In addition to completeness of resection, lymph node status is an important prognostic factor. Ethun et al.[82] found that lymph node involvement was the only independent predictor of long-term survival in resected patients, with positive nodes conferring a 1.63 times greater likelihood of death.

OUTCOMES AFTER RESECTION

After resection of hilar cholangiocarcinoma, 5-year survival rates range from 11% to 44%.[12,34,64,83] Postoperative mortality ranges from 4% to 17%.[39,84,85] One of the strongest associations with survival is margin status, and patients with positive bile duct margins have significantly decreased survival compared with patients with negative margins.[62] Recurrences are seen in up to 75% of patients.[86–88] Along with the status of the resection margin, other factors that are associated with outcome are involvement of resected regional lymph nodes, grade of the tumor, and tumor histology (nodular sclerosing vs. papillary).[19,89] Table 51A.4 reviews outcomes of selected series of hilar cholangiocarcinoma resection.[90–95]

ADJUVANT THERAPY

Resection remains the only modality to achieve long-term survival; however, recurrence is common even after R0 resection. Common sites of recurrence after resection of HC are locoregional recurrences and in the peritoneum and liver.[88] In a single institution retrospective review of 404 patients who

TABLE 51A.4	Selected Reports of Outcomes After Hilar Cholangiocarcinoma Resection			
STUDY	RESECTIONS	MORBIDITY (%)	MORTALITY (%)	SURVIVAL (5-YR)
Nakeeb et al. (1996)[84]	109	47	4	11
Klempnauer et al. (1997)[72]	151	NR	10	28
Neuhaus et al. (1999)[64]	80	55	8	22
Launois et al. (2000)[85]	131	NR	17	NR
Lee et al. (2000)[90]	128	64	10	35
Gerhards. et al (2000)[91]	112	65	17	NR
Nishio et al. (2005)[92]	301	NR	7.6	22
Jarnagin et al. (2005)[12]	106	50	7.5	40
Igami et al. (2010)[93]	298	43	2	42
Unno et al. (2010)[94]	125	49	8	35
Matsuo et al. (2012)[95]	157	59	7	32
Nagino et al. (2013)[61]	574	57	4.7	33
Wiggers et al. (2016)[39]	287	NR	14	NR
Komaya et al. (2018)[83]	402	NR	NR	43.7

NR, Not reported.

From Soares KC, Jarnagin WR. The Landmark Series: hilar cholangiocarcinoma. *Ann Surg Oncol.* 2021;28(8):4158–4170.

underwent R0 resection of HC with long-term follow-up, 60% of patients developed a recurrence and recurrence reached nearly 50% at 10 years after resection.[88] Similarly, in a multi-institutional analysis of 306 consecutive patients with resected HC, 76% of patients recurred after resection.[86] Over 25% of patients recurred after 5 years of recurrence-free survival. Moreover, node-positive disease precluded recurrence-free survival beyond 7 years.

Distant metastases are more common than locoregional recurrence after R0 resection of HC.[88,96] Therefore a role for systemic adjuvant therapies has been considered as a means of decreasing recurrence. Until recently, analysis of adjuvant strategies in HC and DC consisted of single-arm retrospective reviews with mixed findings. However, multiple randomized prospective studies evaluating adjuvant therapies after resection of HC and DC have now been reported, albeit also with mixed results. Takada et al. reported a phase III trial in 2002 where 508 patients with resected bile duct cancer, pancreatic, gallbladder and ampullary cancer were randomized to surgery alone versus adjuvant mitomycin C and 5-fluorouracil.[97] The primary end point was overall survival, and the study showed no significant differences in overall or disease-free survival in resected bile duct tumors.

The BILCAP trial was a phase III multi-institutional clinical trial in the United Kingdom investigating adjuvant capecitabine versus observation after R0/R1 resection of HC (29%), gallbladder cancer (18%), distal cholangiocarcinoma (35%), and ICC (19%).[98] The primary end point of the study was overall survival designed to detect an effect size of HR 0.71.

Of the 447 randomized patients between 2006 and 2014, 430 were evaluable for the primary end point by intention-to-treat analysis. Approximately 50% of patients had node-positive disease, and 38% of patients had an R1 resection. By intention-to-treat analysis, there was no significant difference in overall survival (hazard ratio [HR], 0.81; 95% CI, 0.63–1.04; P = .097). However, a per-protocol analysis was performed after excluding 17 patients who could not receive at least one cycle of chemotherapy or could not be randomized. This analysis showed a statistically significant improvement in both overall (HR, 0.75;

95% CI, 0.58–0.97; P = .03) and recurrence free survival (HR 0.70; 95% CI, 0.54–0.92; P = .009) in the capecitabine arm and prompted the routine use of 6 months of adjuvant capecitabine after bile duct cancer resection.[34,99]

The Advanced Biliary Tract Cancer (ABC)-02 trial established gemcitabine and cisplatin as the standard of care for unresectable locally advanced and metastatic biliary tract cancers.[100] Subsequently, a multicenter study in France, the PRODIGE 12-Accord 18 trial, randomized 196 patients with R0/R1 resected biliary tract cancers to gemcitabine plus oxaliplatin (GEMOX) versus surveillance.[101] This study included gallbladder cancer (n = 38), ICC (n = 86), HC (n = 15), and DC (n = 55) patients. Ultimately, 155 patients were evaluable for the primary end point of relapse-free survival, which showed no difference between the groups (HR, 0.88; 95% CI, 0.62–1.25; P = .48). The planned subgroup analyses failed to suggest any subgroup with a benefit with adjuvant GEMOX. However, it should be noted that only 37% of patients in this study had lymph node–positive disease, which could theoretically derive more benefit from adjuvant strategies. Thus further studies are necessary to determine adjuvant therapy utility in high-risk tumors.

The Bile Duct Cancer Adjuvant Trial (BCAT) was a phase III RCT in Japan evaluating adjuvant gemcitabine versus observation in 225 resected patients with DC or HC.[102] The primary end point was overall survival, and secondary end points included relapse-free survival and toxicity. Similarly to the PRODIGE study, there was no significant difference in overall survival (HR, 1.01; 95% CI, 0.7–1.45) or relapse-free survival.

Although distant recurrence in HC is most common, isolated locoregional recurrence can be seen in up to 27% of patients.[86,88] Thus adjuvant strategies targeting locoregional disease in HC patients have been suggested.

Analyses of such adjuvant strategies in HC have consisted of small, single-center reports. Two separate reports from Johns Hopkins suggest no benefit for adjuvant external beam or intraluminal radiation therapy.[103,104] In contrast, other series have suggested that radiation may improve overall survival, particularly in patients with histologically positive hepatic duct margins.[105–108] More recently, the single arm phase II SWOG S0809 trial reported on adjuvant gemcitabine and capecitabine followed by concurrent capecitabine and radiotherapy in resected R0/R1 stage pT2-4 or node-positive extrahepatic cholangiocarcinoma and gallbladder cancer.[109] The radiation protocol called for 45 Gy to regional lymphatics and 54 to 59.4 Gy to the tumor bed.[109] The 2-year overall survival for the entire 79 patient cohort was 65% (95% CI, 53%–74%; 67% and 60% in R0 and R1 patients, respectively). This met the primary end point of a 95% CI for the 2-year overall survival estimate greater than 45%, and R0 and R1 2-year overall survival estimates 65% or greater and 45%, respectively. Although this trial met its prespecified end point, the lack of a comparison arm limits its interpretation and widespread applicability. We do not routinely use adjuvant radiation therapy after R0 resection of HC or DC; however, this approach may benefit patients with positive resection margins.[34]

Further studies are needed to address the question of optimal adjuvant strategies in EHC. The ACTICCA-1 trial is a multicenter, prospective, randomized, controlled phase III trial comparing adjuvant gemcitabine and cisplatin to standard of care after curative resection of biliary tract cancer (NCT02548195).[110] Of note, this trial was ongoing when BILCAP results were reported therefore the standard of care arm was switched to capecitabine rather than observation alone. Similarly, a phase II study in Asia (NCT03079427) randomizes resected EHC patients with positive lymph node to either adjuvant capecitabine or adjuvant doublet gemcitabine plus cisplatin. The primary end point is 2-year disease-free survival. The Adjuvant S-1 for Cholangiocarcinoma Trial (ASCOT) is a multicenter trial in Japan randomizing patients with resected biliary tract cancer to adjuvant S-1 versus observation (UMIN000011688) with a planned sample size of 440 patients.[111]

The widespread implementation of genetic analyses has led to novel approaches using immunotherapy and targeted. Emerging evidence indicates the utility of these approaches in extrahepatic cholangiocarcinoma.[1] KRAS, TP53, and SMAD4 mutations in HC are common.[14] HER2 gene amplification can be seen in nearly 20% of extrahepatic cholangiocarcinoma.[112] Additionally, ALK and TP53 mutations are associated with a worse prognosis in extrahepatic cholangiocarcinoma.[113] Mismatch repair deficiency is seen in up to 5% of HC suggesting a potential role for immunotherapy approaches in this subset of patients.[9,114,115] Molecular testing of extrahepatic cholangiocarcinoma is recommended. A better understanding of the genomic drivers and epigenetic, immunologic, and molecular heterogeneity of this disease holds promise for successful combinations of targeted therapy and immunotherapy (see Chapter 9E).

PALLIATIVE THERAPY

Most patients with HC are not suitable for resection. In this setting, management options include some form of biliary decompression or supportive care. Jaundice alone, without pruritus or cholangitis, is not necessarily an indication for biliary decompression, especially in a patient whose only goal is palliation. For biliary decompression in inoperable patients, our current indications are to relieve intractable pruritus, treat cholangitis, lower bilirubin, and allow recovery of hepatic parenchymal function in patients who are potential candidates for chemotherapy. Supportive care is strongly considered for

elderly patients with significant comorbid conditions, provided that pruritus is not a major feature. Patients who are found to be unresectable at operation represent a different group, and operative biliary decompression is usually performed successfully. In patients with unresectable HC, segment III bypass provides excellent palliation with relatively few late complications and can be performed with minimal morbidity and mortality[116] (see Chapters 29, 30, 31, and 52).

Assessment of palliative biliary drainage procedures is difficult, because the spectrum of patients ranges from those critically ill and unresectable to those in relatively good health with potentially resectable tumors. All patients should be assessed properly by experienced personnel with a view toward possible resection. If the patient is deemed unresectable, the diagnosis should be confirmed with a biopsy. Biliary decompression can be achieved by percutaneous transhepatic puncture or by endoscopic stent placement. Hilar tumors are more difficult to traverse with the endoscopic technique, which should be approached only by skilled endoscopists with extensive ERCP experience. The failure rates and incidence of subsequent cholangitis after endoscopic drainage can be high (see earlier discussion of pretreatment biliary drainage). Initial endobiliary drainage, even in the palliative setting, should use plastic stents.[117] Exchange for metallic stents can be considered after close monitoring for adequate palliative biliary drainage with plastic stents in the short and intermediate term.

Percutaneous transhepatic biliary drainage and subsequent placement of a self-expandable metallic endoprosthesis (SEM) can be performed successfully in most patients with hilar obstruction (see Chapters 31 and 52). Satisfactory drainage of only 25% to 30% of functional hepatic parenchyma is required for resolution of jaundice.[118] Still, hilar tumors frequently isolate all three major hilar ducts—left hepatic, right anterior sectoral hepatic, and right posterior sectoral hepatic—and two or more uncovered stents must be placed for adequate drainage (Fig. 51A.22). In the setting of cholangitis, all infected ductal systems need to be drained. Bile duct(s) unintentionally opacified upstream from a malignant hilar stricture should be drained during the same procedure.[117] Otherwise, bilateral drainage is not better or more effective than unilateral drainage, provided that an adequate volume of liver parenchyma can be decompressed. It also must be considered that jaundice may result from hepatic dysfunction secondary to portal vein occlusion. Jaundice in this setting, without intrahepatic biliary dilation, is not correctable with biliary stents. In addition, lobar atrophy is an important factor when considering palliative biliary procedures. Percutaneous drainage through an atrophic lobe does not relieve jaundice and should be avoided. The presence of multiple intrahepatic metastases or ascites also may add to the technical difficulty of the procedure.

The median patency of plastic stents is only 1.4 to 3 months. SEMs are wider diameter, resulting in a median patency of approximately 6 months. Raju et al.[119] reviewed 100 patients with inoperable HC at a tertiary cancer hospital. Of these, 48 patients had SEMs placed and 52 patients had plastic stents placed. The median patency times were 1.86 months in the plastic stent group and 5.56 months in the SEM group ($P < .0001$). A mean of 1.53 and 4.60 reinterventions were performed in the SEM and plastic groups, respectively and the complication rates between both groups were similar (8.3% SEMS and 7.7% plastic stent). Similarly, Liberato and

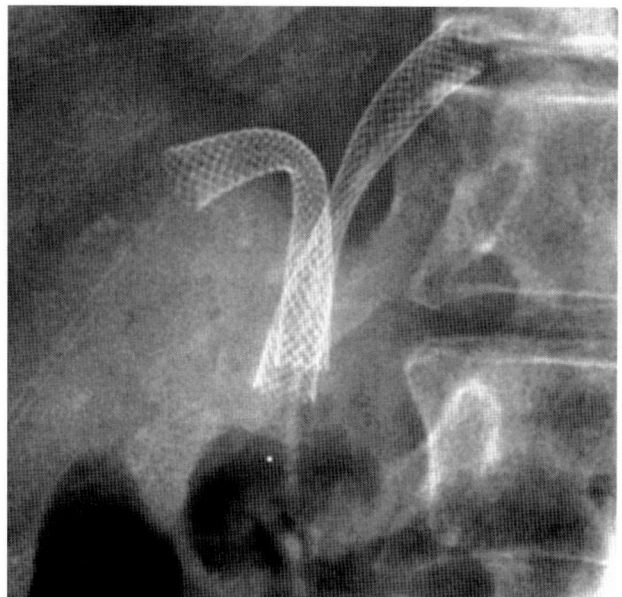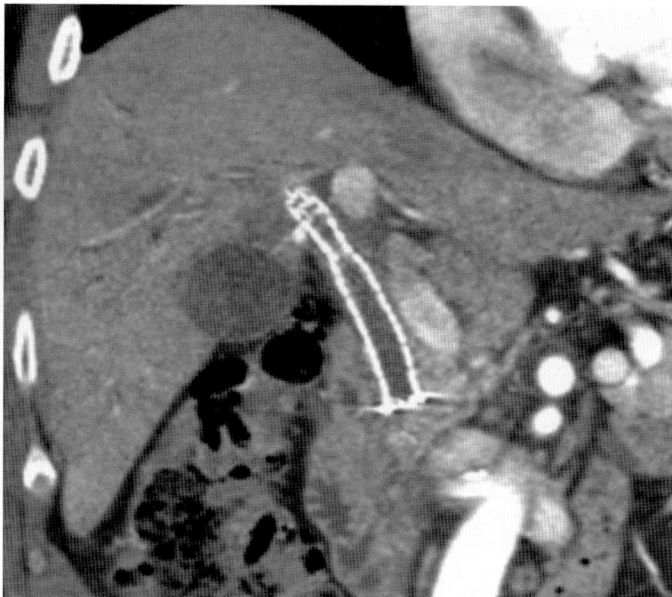

FIGURE 51A.22 Unresectable hilar cholangiocarcinoma tends to isolate all major hilar bile ducts from one another. In this patient, two expandable metallic stents were required for adequate biliary drainage. Self-expanding metal stents are shown here on plain radiography and coronal computed tomographic imaging. (See Chapter 16.)

Canena[120] evaluated 480 patients undergoing endoscopic biliary drainage for HC. Technical success was more common with SEM versus plastic stents (98.8% vs. 88.3%, $P < .001$). Additionally, in an intention-to-treat analysis, functional success in patients treated with SEMs was significantly higher than in patients treated with PS (97.9% vs. 84.8%, respectively, $P < .001$). Finally, in a prospective trial, patients presenting for percutaneous biliary drainage for malignant biliary obstruction had a dismal survival and experienced no improvement in quality of life with drainage. The exception in this trial was an improvement in pruritus-related quality of life, which was significantly better.[121]

Palliating distal biliary obstruction in unresectable patients can be achieved with an operative bypass (hepaticojejunostomy or choledochojejunostomy) (see Chapter 32) or with placement of a biliary stent (see Chapters 30, 31, and 52). Endoprostheses for distal biliary obstruction are typically easy to place and have a greater long-term patency than endoprostheses placed for hilar obstruction. Operative biliary-enteric bypass, either open or laparoscopic, will provide excellent relief of jaundice and can be done with an acceptably low morbidity and mortality. Patients who are found to have unresectable disease at the time of operative exploration should be considered for biliary-enteric bypass, particularly in instances in which endoscopic or percutaneous techniques have failed. Planned palliative operative bypass should be reserved for patients expected to survive longer than 6 months,[122] and SEMs should be used in patients with clear-cut metastatic disease on cross-sectional imaging or discovered with staging laparoscopy. Multiple studies evaluating surgical and nonsurgical palliative biliary drainage have failed to show a significant difference between surgical and nonsurgical approaches.[122–125]

Patients with hilar tumors found to be unresectable at operation may be candidates for hepaticojejunostomy or intrahepatic biliary-enteric bypass. (see Chapter 32) The segment III duct usually is the most accessible and is our preferred approach, but the right anterior or posterior sectoral hepatic ducts also can be used.[116] Typically, a segment III bypass is used to restore biliary-enteric continuity after the bile duct has been divided and a locally invasive, unresectable tumor has been discovered. Segment III bypass provides excellent biliary drainage, resolves jaundice in approximately two thirds of HC patients and is less prone to occlusion by tumor than a SEMs[126,127] because the anastomosis can be placed some distance from the tumor (Fig. 51A.23). Relief of jaundice is achieved in 70% of patients if the functioning hepatic parenchyma is adequately drained.[122] Communication between the right and left hepatic ducts is unnecessary, provided the undrained lobe has not been percutaneously drained or otherwise contaminated. In this circumstance, there is a high risk of persistent biliary fistula and cholangitis. Bypass to an atrophic lobe or a lobe heavily involved with tumor is ineffective. In a report of 55 consecutive bypasses in patients with malignant hilar obstruction, segment III bypass in patients with hilar cholangiocarcinoma ($n = 20$) yielded the best results. The 1-year bypass patency in this group was 80%, with no perioperative deaths.[116]

Patients with unresectable, locally advanced tumors but without evidence of widespread disease may be candidates for palliative radiation therapy. External beam radiation and stereotactic body radiation therapy (SBRT) can be delivered percutaneously. Although there is little evidence to support this, this approach appears safe in well-selected patients.[128,129] Moureau-Zabotto et al.[127] performed a retrospective review of 30 patients with locally advanced extrahepatic cholangiocarcinoma treated with external beam radiotherapy: 24 with a primary tumor and 6 with a local relapse. Toxicity was acceptable, and median overall survival the cohort was 12 months. The 1-year and 3-year progression-free survivals were respectively 38% and 16%. Radiation therapy is inappropriate in patients with widespread disease. Systemic chemotherapy is the only option for these patients, but response rates are low.

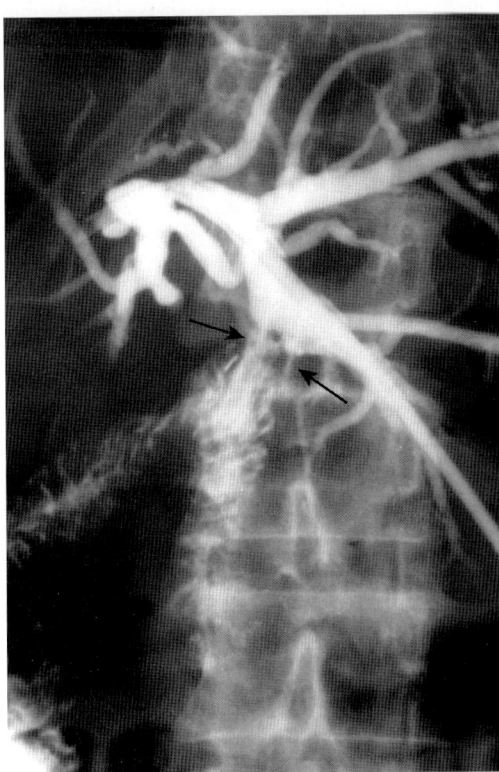

FIGURE 51A.23 Transhepatic cholangiography obtained through a temporary percutaneous drainage tube shows a widely patent anastomosis from the segment III duct to a Roux-en-Y loop of jejunum *(arrows)*. (See Chapter 31.)

Palliative systemic chemotherapy has been investigated. The Advanced Biliary Cancer (ABC) 02 trial randomized 410 patients with locally advanced or metastatic cholangiocarcinoma, gallbladder cancer, or ampullary cancer to receive either cisplatin followed by gemcitabine or gemcitabine alone for up to 6 months.[100] This study showed an improvement in median survival from 8.2 to 11.7 months for patients receiving cisplatin plus gemcitabine without the addition of substantial toxicity. This regimen remains the first-line recommendation for patients with unresectable or metastatic biliary tract cancers.

A systematic review of 761 patients with advanced biliary tract cancer evaluated the efficacy of second-line chemotherapy.[130] Eligible studies reported survival and/or response data for patients with advanced biliary cancer. The authors concluded that there is insufficient evidence to recommend a second-line chemotherapy schedule in advanced biliary cancer. Further prospective randomized trials are needed.

Photodynamic therapy is an ablative therapy used in unresectable hilar cholangiocarcinoma. This method has been used in the treatment of tumors of the esophagus, colon, stomach, bronchus, bladder, and brain. It is a two-step procedure. First, a photosensitizing drug is injected, followed by direct illumination with a light of a specific wavelength via cholangioscopy, which activates the compound, causing tumor cell death. Two randomized studies in patients with unresectable cholangiocarcinoma suggested improved survival with biliary stenting combined with photodynamic therapy compared with biliary stenting alone.[131,132] The improved survival observed with photodynamic therapy is likely related to better biliary decompression and avoidance of early segmental duct isolation and subsequent cholangitis, rather than any significant reduction in tumor burden.[133]

SUMMARY

Improvements in high-resolution cross-sectional imaging have permitted better patient selection and enhanced preoperative planning and preparation before the safe performance of operations for hilar cholangiocarcinoma. Long-term disease-free survival is the primary goal of operative resection. Judicious use of adjunctive preoperative interventions that include biliary drainage and PVE may help improve outcomes, especially when major perioperative and postoperative complications are anticipated. Selection of appropriate nonoperative therapies for palliation of unresectable tumors arising from the proximal and distal bile ducts should be tailored, according to the patient's expected longevity and technical expertise of the multidisciplinary team charged with treating bile duct cancer. Future studies in extrahepatic cholangiocarcinoma should focus on adjuvant strategies along with implementation of genomics, epigenetics, targeted therapies, and immunotherapy.

References are available at expertconsult.com.

CHAPTER 51B

Perihilar cholangiocarcinoma: Presurgical management

Roeland F. de Wilde and Bas Groot Koerkamp

The perihilar region is among the most common site of origin of cholangiocarcinoma (perihilar cholangiocarcinoma [pCCA]).[1–3] However, considering the incidence of 1 to 2 per 100,000 in Western countries, which is significantly lower than in Asia, the disease remains rare.[2,4] By the American Joint Cancer Committee (AJCC) definition, pCCA originates distal to the second-order intrahepatic bile ducts and proximal to the insertion of the cystic duct into the extrahepatic bile duct.[5] It may be difficult to discriminate pCCA from intrahepatic cholangiocarcinoma extending into the hepatic hilum.[6]

Complete resection is associated with 5-year overall survival (OS) rates of up to 35%.[7] However, only approximately one-third of patients are considered resectable. A resection generally requires a hemihepatectomy or greater, en bloc caudate resection with extrahepatic bile duct resection and lymphadenectomy. Reconstruction often entails complex biliary and sometimes vascular reconstruction to obtain negative surgical margins and an adequate future liver remnant (FLR).[8–10] Nonetheless, positive surgical margins are observed in about one-third of patients, adversely affecting outcome[11,12] (see Chapter 119B).

Surgery for pCCA is associated with considerable 90-day postoperative mortality rates of 5% to 18% in Western centers. However, much lower mortality rates of 1% to 3% have been reported in recent Eastern series.[12–16] Multidisciplinary treatment of pCCA is complex and should take place in tertiary referral centers. Upon suspicion of pCCA, before any intervention, referral or consultation of an expert center should take place. Failure to do so may result in a lost opportunity to obtain adequate imaging before biliary drainage, unnecessary or inadequate drainage increasing surgical risk, and lost opportunity for resection or liver transplantation. In this chapter, we will cover management of patients with pCCA before surgery.

DIAGNOSING pCCA

Patients with pCCA typically present with painless jaundice (90%). Concomitant cholangitis is uncommon and occurs in 10% of patients.[17,18] pCCA rarely arises in the left or right hepatic duct without jaundice. Anorexia, fatigue, weight loss, and sarcopenia are each observed in about 50% of patients.[18,19] Physical examination of the abdomen may reveal a palpable mass in the upper abdomen indicative of unilateral hepatic lobe hypertrophy because of the concomitant contralateral lobar atrophy (Fig. 51B.1).[20,21]

Blood analysis generally reflects cholestasis and sometimes cholangitis. Serum carbohydrate antigen (CA) 19-9 level is high in most patients, but elevated CA 19-9 may be partially attributable to biliary obstruction. Moreover, about 10% of patients do not produce CA 19-9 because of the lack of the Lewis antigen.[22,23] Determination of immunoglobulin G4 (IgG4) serum level can help in diagnosing eosinophilic cholangiopathy (i.e.,

lymphoplasmatic cholangiopathy, more commonly referred to as auto-immune cholangitis), which is one of the benign diagnoses that may present as a hilar biliary obstruction[24] (see Chapters 47 and 48). However, IgG4 can be normal in patients with auto-immune cholangitis and IgG4 can be elevated in patients with pCCA. A 4-fold increase in IgG4 nearly excludes pCCA. The HISORt criteria predict the presence of IgG4-associated disease based on histology, imaging (typically smooth concentric biliary wall thickening with a visible lumen, absence of a mass, skip lesions, and involvement of the extrahepatic bile duct), serology, other organ manifestation, and response to steroid treatment.[25,26] Finally, liver fluke infestation (*Clonorchis sinensis* and *Opisthorchis viverrini*) can be ruled out with serology if in an endemic area[27] (see Chapter 45).

High-quality presenting imaging is a crucial step in the preoperative work-up of pCCA, enabling diagnosis, staging, liver volumetry, and determination of the extent of resection[22] (see Chapters 16 and 102). High-resolution thin-slice computed tomography (CT) with multiphase scanning using intravenous (IV) contrast (i.e., arterial and portovenous phases) enables a diagnostic accuracy to detect arterial involvement up to 93% and portal vein involvement as high as 87%. However, sensitivity of detecting lymph node metastases is poor (54%) and the proximal biliary extent of the tumor is often underestimated.[28] Magnetic resonance imaging (MRI) with magnetic resonance cholangiopancreatography (MRCP) is superior to CT in assessing the intrahepatic biliary extent of pCCA and to help discriminate benign etiologies from pCCA (e.g., Mirizzi syndrome, intrahepatic lithiasis, and primary sclerosing cholangitis [PSC]; Fig. 51B.2).[29] The role of positron emission tomography (PET) scanning is limited because of false-positive results related to inflammation and is reflected by a specificity of 67%[30,31] (see Chapter 18). It is of utmost importance to realize that the diagnosis and staging after biliary stenting are considerably impaired because of decompression of the biliary system and imaging artefacts induced by stenting-related inflammation. Patients with a perihilar obstruction should be referred to an expert center before biliary drainage because high-quality imaging is essential before biliary drainage, not all patients with pCCA require biliary drainage, and drainage of the FLR is only possible after an expert team has determined the resection plan (see later).

Tissue diagnosis is challenging because of the low sensitivity (typically less than 40%) of an endoscopic or percutaneous brush.[20,32] A tissue diagnosis is not mandatory for surgical exploration. The application of fluorescent in situ hybridization (FISH) to determine polysomy in addition to conventional cytology typically doubles the sensitivity to detect a malignancy.[33] In a study on PSC patients with a dominant stricture without visible mass and equivocal cytology undergoing routine endoscopic brushing, multivariable analysis revealed FISH to be the only significant predictor of malignancy (see Chapter 43). Once

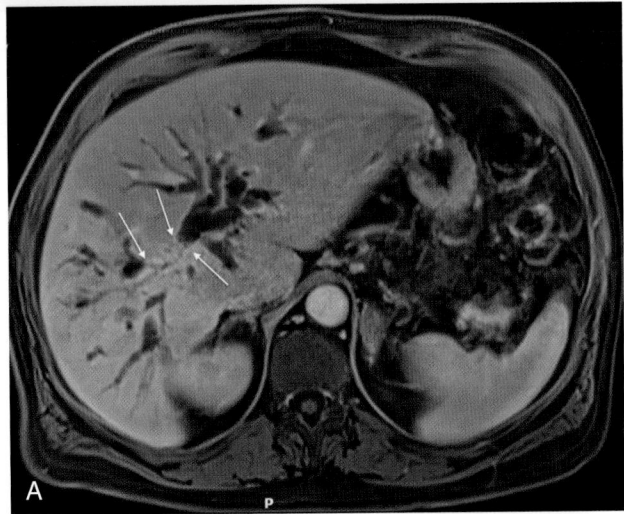

FIGURE 51B.1 Diagnostic computed tomography (CT) scan of a patient with Bismuth type 3B perihilar cholangiocarcinoma (pCCA). This image features lobar atrophy of the left liver lobe. The demarcation line is indicated with an *arrow* (see Chapter 16).

CA 19-9 was at least 129, a hazard ratio (HR) of 11 was found when combined with polysomy on FISH.[34] Percutaneous biopsy of pCCA should be avoided in patients that may be eligible for a liver transplant (LT; see later).[35] Biopsy may cause needle track metastases and LT is therefore contraindicated in many centers after any transperitoneal biopsy. Suspicious lymphadenopathy may be subjected to fine needle aspiration (FNA) through endoscopic ultrasound (EUS) or resection at staging laparoscopy.[22]

The current expert consensus statements of the American Hepato-Pancreato-Biliary Association (AHPBA), the National Comprehensive Cancer Network (NCCN), and the European Network for the Study of Cholangiocarcinoma (ENS-CCA) on the initial evaluation of pCCA dictate[22,36–38]:

- The minimum diagnostic and staging work-up in suspected pCCA includes liver function, CA 19-9 level, and high-quality cross-sectional imaging (preferably before biliary stenting) of the chest, abdomen and pelvis, besides cholangiography.
- Early consultation of a multidisciplinary team includes a surgeon with expertise in pCCA.
- Pathologic confirmation is not required before surgical exploration for resection or initiation of an LT protocol, provided that benign etiologies have been excluded and a complete staging evaluation has been completed.
- Percutaneous or laparoscopic biopsy of the primary tumor is not recommended in patients who may be candidates for transplantation because of the risk of biopsy tract metastases.
- Imaging by fluorodeoxyglucose-PET lacks the sensitivity and specificity required to be a routine staging tool for patients with pCCA.

The diagnostic work-up for pCCA is imperfect because, after surgery for anticipated pCCA, approximately 10% of patients are diagnosed with benign disease at pathologic examination of the resected specimen.[10,12,39,40]

CLASSIFICATION AND STAGING

Clinical staging of pCCA should first rule out metastatic disease by means of chest and abdominal/pelvic CT. Patients with

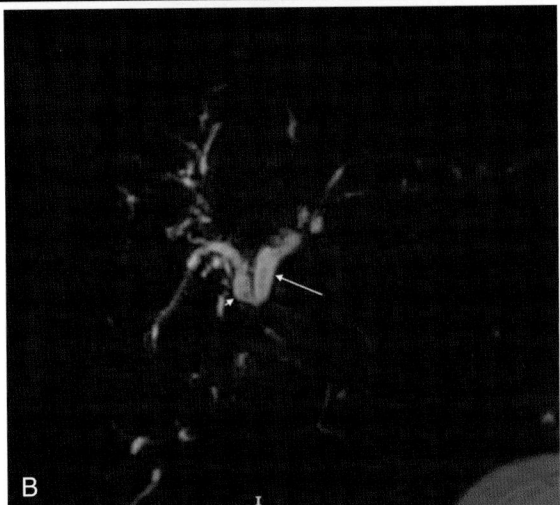

FIGURE 51B.2 Diagnostic magnetic resonance imaging (MRI) of two patients with perihilar cholangiocarcinoma (pCCA). The left panel depicts an axial view of a Bismuth type 3A pCCA. The tumor is often iso-intense with the surrounding liver parenchyma but can be located at the abrupt cut-off *(arrows)* of the intrahepatic bile ducts. The right panel depicts a coronal view of a magnetic resonance cholangiopancreatography (MRCP) of a Bismuth type 2 pCCA with secondary biliary dilatation of the right *(short arrow)* and left *(long arrow)* intrahepatic bile ducts (see Chapter 16).

distant metastases (e.g., in lung and peritoneum) and lymph node involvement beyond the hepatoduodenal ligament (e.g., aortocaval) have Stage IV disease and should rarely be considered for upfront resection.[9,41]

Several tumor-staging systems aim to determine local disease extent, guide treatment decisions (i.e., determine resectability), and inform prognosis.[42] Unfortunately, current staging of pCCA remains challenging and imperfect and most systems are based on surgical pathology and therefore not applicable to the majority of patients that do not undergo resection.[43–46]

The Bismuth-Corlette system was the first tumor-staging system to classify pCCA based solely on the extent of involvement of the biliary tree (Fig. 51B.3).[47] However, this classification does not take into account the radial extent of pCCA into surrounding structures such as the liver, hilar soft tissue, and vasculature. Bismuth stage is insufficient to determine resectability; for example, a large study found excellent outcomes of

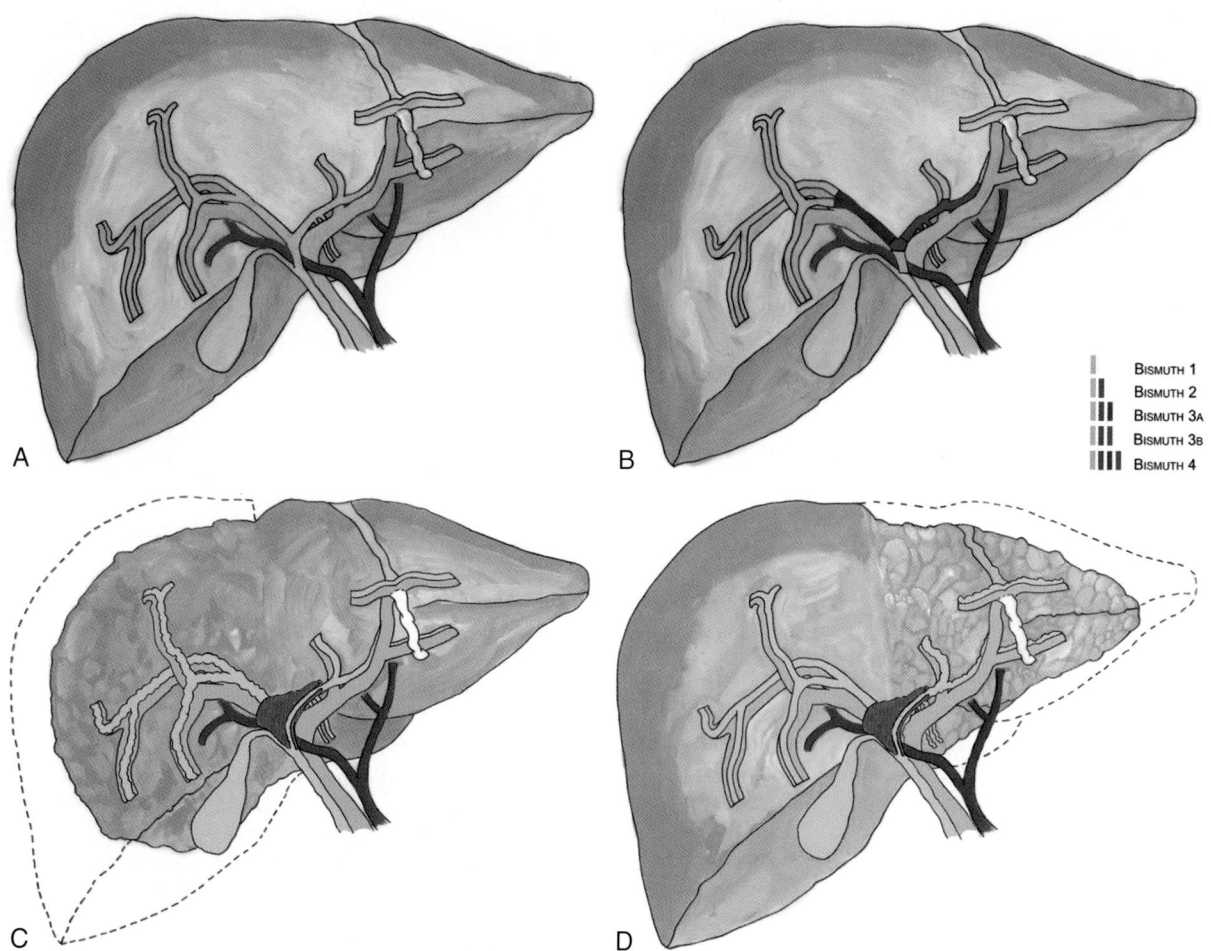

FIGURE 51B.3 Summary of different classification systems of perihilar cholangiocarcinoma (pCCA). **A,** Key anatomic structures (portal vein, hepatic artery, and bile ducts) considered in staging pCCA. **B,** Bismuth-Corlette staging system. Blumgart/ Memorial Sloan-Kettering Cancer Center (MSKCC) stage T1: tumor involving the bile duct bifurcation and/or unilateral extension into second-order bile ducts. **C,** Blumgart/MSKCC stage T2: unilateral vascular involvement and/or unilateral lobar atrophy. **D,** Blumgart/MSKCC stage T3: bilateral/contralateral involvement of second-order bile ducts, vascular involvement, and/or lobar atrophy. (Adapted from Hartog H, Ijzermans JN, van Gulik TM, et al. Resection of perihilar cholangiocarcinoma. *Surg Clin North Am.* 2016;96[2]:247–267.Original artwork by Mrs. Elsbeth Leeffers.)

resection for Bismuth IV pCCA.[41] In addition to the biliary extent of the tumor, the Memorial Sloan-Kettering Cancer Center (MSKCC) staging system involves portal venous involvement and lobar atrophy (Fig. 51B.3).[10] However, both classification systems perform poorly in predicting resectability because in most series about 50% of patients undergoing surgical exploration with curative intent undergo a resection.[48,49]

The third staging-system is the AJCC/International Union Against Cancer (UICC) tumor-node-metastasis (TNM) system, which is currently in its eighth edition.[5] The T-stage of pCCA relies heavily on vascular invasion (unilateral or bilateral of portal vein or hepatic artery) but does not describe how pathologic vascular invasion can be determined on imaging or what extent of vascular invasion is still potentially resectable. Evaluation of the current eighth edition compared with the seventh edition showed slightly improved prognostic accuracy for patients after resection but remained poor in patients with unresectable disease.[50,51] To inform prognosis after resection of pCCA, staging systems have been developed that perform better than the TNM staging.[7]

PREOPERATIVE CONSIDERATIONS TO SURGERY FOR pCCA

The median OS of patients with pCCA without surgery is around 8 months compared with up to 40 months after resection with curative intent.[7] Actual cure (i.e., 10-year OS) is rarely seen outside of patients with papillary or well-differentiated pCCA.[52] The expected benefit of surgery should outweigh the substantial postoperative morbidity and mortality.

Resectability

The aim of resection for pCCA is a margin negative resection and an adequate FLR[11] (see Chapters 101B, 118A, and 119B). Because of the anatomic location and propensity for infiltration into the central liver, a hemihepatectomy or greater with enbloc caudate resection is typically required for complete resection of pCCA.[53] Whether a right-sided or left-sided resection is necessary is determined by unilateral lobar atrophy, unilateral second-order bile duct involvement, unilateral portal vein, or unilateral hepatic artery involvement.[9] In patients with a

Bismuth I or II tumor without unilateral atrophy or vascular involvement, both right- and left sided resections could result in an R0 resection. The disadvantage of a right-sided resection is that the right liver is larger than the left liver, resulting in a higher risk of postoperative morbidity and liver failure. In 80% of patients, the volume of the left lateral sector is below 20% and in 10% of patients the volume of the left hemiliver is below 20%.[54] In general, when possible, a left-sided resection leaves a much larger FLR, minimizes the risk of postoperative liver failure, and is the preferred approach.

An adequate FLR must include at least two contiguous liver segments with sufficient functional capacity and intact arterial venous inflow, portal venous inflow, and portal venous outflow.[9] The FLR volume is measured by image-guided volumetry where the FLR should constitute at least 25% of the total liver volume before resection in the absence of underlying liver disease, hepatotoxic preoperative chemotherapy, or biliary obstruction. Most patients with pCCA require a larger FLR volume (>30%–40%) because of biliary obstruction to avoid postoperative liver failure.[55] Obtaining an R0 resection may require portal vein reconstruction and a complex biliary reconstruction with often more than one hepaticojejunostomy. In Western countries, arterial reconstructions are rarely performed to obtain an R0 resection of pCCA: postoperative mortality rate is increased, and survival is generally poor in patients, which makes it difficult to justify.[56]

Patient-Related Variables

Several patient-related variables should be taken into consideration to compare the benefit and risk of resection for patients with pCCA. A risk score model was developed to predict postoperative mortality after resection of pCCA.[16] Independent prognostic factors for postoperative mortality included age, preoperative cholangitis, FLR volume of less than 30%, incomplete biliary drainage of the FLR in patients with an FLR volume of less than 50%, and portal vein reconstruction (Table 51B.1). Age was the most important poor prognostic factor with the risk of both postoperative liver failure and death increasing rapidly with advanced age. The predicted 90-day postoperative mortality risks were 2% (low risk: 0–2 points), 11% (intermediate risk: 3 or 4 points), or 37% (high risk: 5–9 points). Another study identified similar factors to

predict postoperative liver failure, including albumin level below 3.5 mg/dL, preoperative cholangitis, preoperative total bilirubin level above 3 mg/dL (51 mmol/L), and FLR volume of less than 30% (see Table 51B.1).[57]

In summary, several patient-related factors contribute significantly to the risk of postoperative liver failure, such as age, low serum albumin level, cholangitis, hyperbilirubinemia/jaundice and incomplete drainage of the FLR, low FLR volume, and portal vein reconstruction. These factors should be taken into account and optimized when considering a resection in patients with pCCA.

OPTIMIZING THE FUTURE LIVER REMNANT

Biliary Drainage (see Chapters 30, 31, 52)

Biliary drainage aims to restore the regenerative capacity of the FLR. Preoperative biliary drainage is necessary in patients with:
- cholangitis,
- jaundice and the need to undergo neoadjuvant therapy,
- liver or renal insufficiency possibly related to hyperbilirubinemia, and
- small FLR volume (<50%), especially before PVE.[22]

There are several approaches to biliary drainage. The two most commonly used techniques worldwide are endoscopic biliary drainage (EBD) and percutaneous transhepatic biliary drainage (PTBD; Fig. 51B.4).[58,59] There is currently no universal consensus on the preferred method of preoperative biliary drainage in patients with pCCA. Several small retrospective studies have reported higher technical success and fewer

TABLE 51B.1 Risk Factors (Multivariate Analysis) for Postoperative Mortality After Resection of pCCA from Two Studies

RISK FACTOR	OR	95% CI	P VALUE
Age (per 10 years)[a]	2.1	1.4–3.3	.001
Preoperative cholangitis	4.1*	1.8–9.4	.001
	7.5†	1.5–29.0	.016
Incomplete biliary drainage + FLR <50%[a]	2.8	1.1–7.5	.04
FLR <30%	2.9[a]	1.2–6.9	.02
	7.2[b]	1.4–37.0	.019
Portal vein reconstruction[a]	2.3	0.9–5.8	.09

CI, Confidence interval; *FLR*, future liver remnant; *OR*, odds ratio; *pCCA*, perihilar cholangiocarcinoma.

[a]Data from Wiggers JK, Groot Koerkamp B, Cieslak KP, et al. Postoperative mortality after liver resection for perihilar cholangiocarcinoma: Development of a risk score and importance of biliary drainage of the future liver remnant. *J Am Coll Surg.* 2016;223(2):321–331.e1.

[b]Data from Ribero D, Zimmitti G, Aloia TA, et al. Preoperative cholangitis and future liver remnant volume determine the risk of liver failure in patients undergoing resection for hilar cholangiocarcinoma. *J Am Coll Surg.* 2016;223(1):87–97.

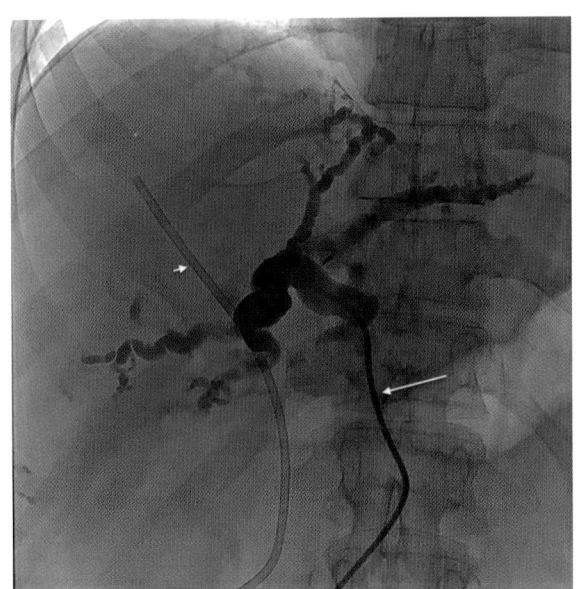

FIGURE 51B.4 Diagnostic fluoroscopic image of a patient with Bismuth type 3A/B perihilar cholangiocarcinoma (pCCA) in whom a right extended hemihepatectomy was intended. Upon the initial attempt to biliary drainage through endoscopic retrograde cholangiopancreatography (ERCP), the left biliary system could not be reached to drain the future liver remnant (FLR). Thus a plastic endoprosthesis *(short arrow)* was placed in the right biliary system. Drainage of the FLR (i.e., the left biliary system) was accomplished through additional percutaneous transhepatic biliary drainage (PTBD) in this case *(long arrow;* see Chapters 31 and 52)

complications after PTBD.[58,60] A multicenter randomized controlled trial (RCT) in four expert centers investigated the incidence of severe drainage-related complications of EBD or PTBD in patients with potentially resectable pCCA.[61] Interim analysis after randomization of 54 patients (50% accrual) revealed a statistically significant difference in mortality at 90-day follow-up after surgery between the PTBD group (41%) and the EBD group (11%, relative risk [RR] 3.67, 1.15–11.69, $P = .03$), which led to the decision to stop the trial. This RCT included all patients who had resectable pCCA on imaging, compared with retrospective studies that only included the subgroup (typically 50%–65%) who underwent a resection.[61] Mortality was higher than in retrospective studies because it also included substantial mortality in the preoperative period, as well as mortality from patients who were explored but did not undergo a resection. Technical success of biliary drainage was higher in the PTBD group than the EBD group (93% vs. 74%; $P = .07$), whereas therapeutic success one week after drainage was equal in both groups (78% vs. 63%; $P = .21$, respectively for PTBD and EBD). Crossover treatment was significantly higher in the EBD group (56%) versus the PTBD group ($n = 1$, 4%, $P < .0001$), and 76% of patients underwent more than one drainage procedure before surgery. One or more severe drainage-related complications were observed in 67% of EBD patients and 63% of PTBN patients (RR 0.94, 0.64–1.40, absolute risk difference [ARD] 3.7%), of which cholangitis was most frequently observed (59% vs. 37%, $P = .1$, respectively amongst PTBD and EBD). Severe complications within 90-days after surgery were observed in 65% of PTBD patients and 55% (RR 1.19, 0.73–1.96, ARD 10.4%) of EBD patients. The percentage of cholangitis that occurred in the PTBD group was relatively high compared with the historical series where the prevalence of cholangitis was reported below 20%.[62-64] The INTERCPT trial also compared PTBD and EBD as the initial approach when managing a patient with suspected hilar malignant obstruction.[65] Unfortunately, the trial was terminated in the beginning of 2020 because of slow accrual.[66]

A third technique to biliary drainage, as recommended by The Japanese Clinical Practice Guidelines for Biliary Tract Cancer, is the use of endoscopic nasobiliary drainage (ENBD) because of less frequently observed cholangitis in ENBD versus EBD.[67] Subgroup analysis of two studies (comprising a total of 198 patients) in a meta-analysis confirmed a higher incidence of preoperative cholangitis in pCCA patients drained with EBD (47.1%, 25/53) compared with ENBD (25.5%, 37/145, odds ratio [OR] 0.40, 0.21–0.75, $P = .005$). In addition, the stent dysfunction rate was higher in EBD (62.3%, 33/53) compared with ENBD (29.7%, 43/145, OR 0.26, 0.13–0.50, $P < .0001$).[58,68,69] A recent study by Nagino and colleagues reported a cholangitis rate of 37% in a cohort of 191 patients who underwent ENBD, and 27% of patients required a reintervention.[59] We conclude that ENBD appears superior in the Japanese centers and that EBD is at least noninferior compared with PTBD for patients with resectable pCCA who require preoperative biliary drainage.

Incomplete or no biliary drainage in patients with an FLR volume above 50% has not been identified as a risk factor for mortality.[16] In fact, postoperative mortality at 90 days was higher with biliary drainage in patients with an FLR volume above 50%, implying that biliary drainage should be avoided in these patients.[16] Farges et al. also found that mortality after left hemihepatectomy (typically with an FLR above 50%) for

pCCA was lower without preoperative biliary drainage.[70] In jaundiced patients with an FLR volume below 50%, the risk of an undrained small FLR appears more important than the risk of post-drainage cholangitis and other subsequent infectious complications.[16,57,71] Experts advocate to postpone surgery until the serum bilirubin level is below 2 mg/dL (i.e., 34 mmol/L).[14] A bilirubin above 3 mg/dL has been associated with a 4-fold increased risk of postoperative liver failure.[57] Preoperative biliary drainage should decompress the FLR. Therefore it is important that patients be referred to an expert center before biliary drainage to determine the FLR and therefore the drainage strategy. However, the contralateral liver must also be drained if it is the focus of cholangitis (e.g., after previous endoscopic contamination without drainage).[9]

Portal Vein Embolization (see Chapter 102C)

The substantial morbidity and mortality associated with (extended) liver resection for pCCA is primarily mediated by postoperative liver failure.[72] An FLR volume below 40% to 50% is the most important modifiable risk factor for postoperative mortality.[57,73] PVE has been demonstrated to induce an increase in FLR volume in both healthy and compromised liver parenchyma by means of hypertrophy of the FLR.[74,75]

In 1990 Makuuchi presented the initial result of PVE in 14 pCCA patients without major side effects, and only temporary moderate increases of serum transaminase or bilirubin were observed after preoperative PVE.[76] Postoperatively, the authors observed mortality in a patient with jaundice and suppurative cholangitis after 30 days and after 3 months in a patient with untreated hepatitis. In a meta-analysis, Jiao and colleagues examined the impact of PVE on liver resection (regardless of diagnosis) in 1,088 patients.[77] The authors demonstrated that PVE is a safe and effective procedure with a morbidity rate of 2.2% and no mortality. It was demonstrated that the increase in remnant liver volume was slightly larger after percutaneous transhepatic portal embolization versus transileocolic portal embolization (11.9% vs. 9.7%, $P = .00001$). In an international study including 1,484 patients who underwent liver resection for pCCA, PVE was less frequently performed in Western centers (7%) compared with Eastern centers (55%, $P < .001$).[12,78] Overall liver failure rate was 17% and the 90-day mortality rate was 13%. Most PVE procedures (93%) were right-sided. PVE was more frequently performed before right-sided resections (38% vs. 3%, $P < .001$) and most frequently in extended right hemihepatectomy (45%). Propensity score matching was possible in a cohort of 98 patients, which revealed a relative increase of liver volume after PVE of 42% (18–59) in a median of 22 (19–29 days). The use of PVE was associated with a 4.4-fold reduction in liver failure (from 36% to 8%), a reduction in postoperative bile leakage by 3.5-fold (from 35% to 10%) and a decrease in 90-day postoperative mortality from 18% to 7% (2.6-fold reduction). A drawback of PVE is that the multidisciplinary team has to decide preoperatively whether a left- or right-sided resection is best. In some patients, imaging may allow for both a left- or right-sided resection. In this regard, a left hemihepatectomy is preferable; however, involvement of the right hepatic artery may be found at surgical exploration because of the proximity of this artery to the central biliary tree.

Additional ipsilateral hepatic vein embolization may be performed to induce liver regeneration even further if the desired gain of volume by PVE is not accomplished.[79] The international prospective multicenter DRAGON trial 1 (NCT04272931) is aimed to assess enrolment capacity and safety of PVE combined with hepatic vein embolization in patients with colorectal liver metastases planned for liver resection.[80] The results of this trial will form the basis for the anticipated RCT DRAGON 2 to compare outcomes of PVE with PVE and hepatic vein embolization.

In conclusion, PVE can be performed safely and is recommended in patients with pCCA and an FLR below 40%.[81] Future studies should investigate whether patient selection for PVE can be improved by functional FLR tests such as indocyanine green-clearance testing or ^{99m}Tc-mebrofenin hepatobiliary scintigraphy.[82–84]

Associating Liver Partition and Portal Vein Ligation for Staged Hepatectomy for pCCA (see Chapters 102D and 123)

Associating liver partition and portal vein ligation for staged hepatectomy (ALPPS) has been performed in a patient with pCCA and found to rapidly induce hypertrophy of the FLR.[85] The procedure is based on the concept of a complete or partial portal venous devascularization of the tumor-carrying liver with preservation of arterial blood flow and division of the liver substance, triggering tremendous hypertrophy of the contralateral liver lobe.[86] After 2007, ALPPS gained some popularity over PVE in select cases with insufficient FLR volumes. Currently, the technique is selectively used for extended liver resections, mainly to resect colorectal liver metastases otherwise deemed unresectable.[86] The application of ALPPS for pCCA has been criticized because of a reported high postoperative mortality of 27% in the initial 11 patients.[87–90] More recently, van Gulik and colleagues analyzed data on 37 patients who underwent ALPPS for pCCA in 23 centers. Only 29 patients had available data for analysis, with a 90-day mortality of 48% (14/29).[91] Matching the 29 ALPPS patients to patients with the same FLR without ALPPS from an international cohort revealed postoperative mortality to be twice as high in the ALPSS cohort (14/29 patients vs. 7/29 patients, $P = .100$). Median OS was 6 months in the ALPPS group and 29 months for the matched controls ($P = .048$). Survival was comparable between the two groups once perioperative mortality was excluded. Based on these studies, ALPPS is not recommended for pCCA.

Liver Transplantation for pCCA (see Chapter 108B)

For patients with pCCA confined to the liver that is considered unresectable, LT is a treatment option.[22,92] Technically, LT avoids the risk of positive surgical margins observed in around one-third of patients undergoing resection, solves the risk of an inadequate FLR, and treats the underlying liver disease in patients with PSC.[12,93] In order for patients to qualify for LT, strict criteria apply (e.g., the Mayo Clinic transplantation protocol): pCCA must be unresectable and confined to the liver and the tumor should be located proximally to the cystic duct with a maximum radial tumor diameter of 3 cm without evidence of metastases. Patients must be pretreated with induction chemoradiation therapy to qualify for LT. Once patients are eligible, staging surgery with lymph node biopsy is performed to rule out metastatic disease. Recommendations from the Working Group from the International Liver Transplantation

Society (ILTS) Transplant Oncology Consensus Conference further include:[92]

- Diagnostic criteria for pCCA in the setting of LT include a dominant stricture of the perihilar bile duct and one or more of the following: positive cytology by endoscopic brushing or biopsy demonstrating pCCA, fluorescence in situ hybridization polysomy, or elevated CA 19-9 greater than 100 U/mL in the absence of cholangitis (moderate level of evidence, conditional recommendation).
- LT for pCCA can be considered in patients with unresectable disease after neoadjuvant chemoradiation therapy in centers with a specific protocol (moderate level of evidence, conditional recommendation).
- Transplant teams should prepare for arterial and venous jump grafts in the setting of LT for pCCA (moderate level of evidence, strong recommendation).

Initial results of LT for pCCA were unacceptable considering 3-year survival rates of 30% to 38% and a 5-year survival rate of 23% with high recurrence rates.[94–96] Since these results fell short compared with outcomes after resection for pCCA, induction therapy was introduced before LT. Several studies have reported 5-year survival rates after LT of 64% (up to 80% in patients with underlying PSC) and intention-to-treat survival rates (i.e., including all patients who started the preoperative neoadjuvant regimen) of 53% to 56% at 5 years.[97,98] These results compare favorably with resection of pCCA. However, in LT series, typically about two-thirds of patients have underlying PSC (see Chapter 41) compared with about 5% in resection series. Many of these series also include substantial proportions of patients who have never had a histologically proven cholangiocarcinoma on preoperative biopsies or on final pathology.

A retrospective study comparing patients after resection for pCCA with those after LT and neoadjuvant therapy revealed overall 5-year survival rates of 18% and 64%, respectively.[99] Subset analysis of patients with R0 resection without PSC who fulfilled the Mayo Clinic transplant criteria still showed lower 5-year survival (29%) versus transplanted patients (54%, $P = .049$). The randomized multicenter TRANSPHIL study compares overall survival at 5 years and 3-year recurrence free survival of neoadjuvant chemoradiation with LT versus liver resection.[100] The rationale for the latter trial was a retrospective study that assessed the role of neoadjuvant therapy before LT for pCCA.[101] Five-year OS was 59% in 28 patients with pCCA who met LT criteria but did not undergo neoadjuvant treatment before LT. The authors concluded that selection, rather than induction therapy, is key.

Neoadjuvant Therapy for Liver Resection in pCCA

Induction chemoradiation therapy in the setting of LT found excellent results in patients judged unresectable by conventional hepatectomy.[97] Naturally, this raises the question of whether neoadjuvant therapy would be beneficial in patients deemed upfront resectable. In a systematic review assessing neoadjuvant chemo(radio)therapy before resection of pCCA, only 7 studies were included.[102] These studies included a total number of 87 pCCA patients treated in a median period of 14 years (range 4–31). In only two studies, patients ($n = 28$ and $n = 9$) were upfront resectable.[103,104] Chemoradiation protocols differed and the reported survival in one of the studies with the most pCCA patients also included patients with other diagnoses. In summary, to date there are insufficient data available on the effect of neoadjuvant (chemo)radiation therapy for patients with resectable pCCA.

Prehabilitation to Surgery for pCCA

Enhanced Recovery After Surgery (ERAS; see Chapter 27) is aimed to improve recovery after major surgery by means of a multimodal perioperative pathway that has been validated for many surgical procedures.[105] ERAS guidelines that have yet to be validated specific to liver surgery were published in 2016.[106] The preoperative part of ERAS (i.e., prehabilitation) aims to improve the physical, nutritional, and psychological aspects of a patient's health to reduce the risk of postoperative complications and facilitate a swift recovery of physical performance status.[107]

Patient-related factors that are significantly associated with postoperative mortality in pCCA include age, albumin level of less than 3.5 mg/dL, and sarcopenia.[16,19] The albumin level and sarcopenia reflect nutritional and physical health and can be modified in a prehabilitation program.

Exercise prehabilitation had a positive effect on physical fitness after hepatopancreatobiliary (HPB) surgery, although the effect on postoperative outcomes remains inconclusive.[108,109] A prospective cohort study in patients with HPB malignancies evaluated protein supplementation combined with unsupervised home-based aerobic and resistance exercises on postoperative outcome.[110] Results from this study showed a significantly shorter hospital stay for patients after prehabilitation versus those who enrolled the standard preoperative course (23 vs. 30 days, $P = .045$), without a significant difference in postoperative complications. The latter studies seem to justify prehabilitation of patients before resection of pCCA, especially in patients with modifiable risk factors such as low albumin level and sarcopenia.

The references for this chapter can be found online by accessing the accompanying Expert Consult website.

CHAPTER 52

Interventional techniques in hilar and intrahepatic biliary strictures

Karen T. Brown

Malignant disease resulting in proximal or high bile duct obstruction (Fig. 52.1)—that is, in close proximity to or involving the biliary confluence—may arise from a variety of cancer types and is a common clinical problem. Historically, the proximal biliary tree was defined as above the level of the cystic duct insertion into the common hepatic duct (CHD). Given the wide anatomic variability of the cystic duct/CHD confluence (see Chapter 2), this definition is not accurate, and high bile duct obstruction is best thought of as obstruction involving the hepatic confluence and the 2 to 4 cm of CHD distal to the confluence.

Although frequently seen with hilar cholangiocarcinoma and intraductal tumor (see Chapters 50 and 51), hilar obstruction can result from other common malignancies, such as colorectal, breast, and pancreatic cancers (see Chapters 62 and 90–92). Significant technical progress has occurred in both endoscopic (see Chapter 30) and percutaneous approaches to biliary drainage (see Chapter 31), allowing for safer palliative treatment of patients with such obstructions. Because these patients may be asymptomatic at presentation, the goals of treatment should be clearly defined before the physician commits the patient to any biliary drainage procedure. The most important question concerns resectability. With the exception of clearly palliative situations, these patients are ideally discussed in a multidisciplinary group with hepatobiliary surgeons, interventional radiologists, oncologists, and gastroenterologists to outline a plan of treatment. A thorough understanding of this plan (specifically involving details of the potential surgical approaches), and of the patient's prognosis, facilitates concomitant development of a strategy for drainage, when indicated. Accepted indications for palliative biliary drainage include intractable pruritus, cholangitis, the need to restore liver function to allow for administration of chemotherapeutic agents with biliary metabolism/excretion, access for intraluminal brachytherapy, and diversion for bile leak. Given the availability of high-quality magnetic resonance cholangiopancreatography (MRCP; see Chapter 16), direct cholangiography as a diagnostic tool is rarely warranted (see Chapter 20).[1,2]

INDICATIONS FOR BILIARY DRAINAGE

Neither isolated hyperbilirubinemia nor imaging findings of bile duct dilation are an indication for biliary drainage. Pruritus, cholangitis, and the need to lower the bilirubin to administer certain chemotherapeutic agents, on the other hand, are all accepted indications for biliary drainage. Postoperative bile leaks that require drainage for diversion may develop in patients who have undergone biliary-enteric bypass as part of curative resection for a benign or malignant lesion (see Chapter 28). In some cases, access to the biliary tree may be undertaken as a method of delivering local treatment for primary bile duct

cancer, such as brachytherapy or photodynamic therapy. Many physicians have the impression that patients feel better and have improved performance status after relief of jaundice, but this has never been definitively demonstrated in clinical studies. Indeed, in a prospective trial, Robson and colleagues[3] showed that percutaneous drainage of high biliary obstruction does not significantly improve the quality of life (QOL) of patients with malignant biliary obstruction, except for the minority with associated pruritus. Controversy remains with regard to the role of biliary drainage before surgery.[4-6] Preoperative drainage of the future remnant liver is often performed for jaundiced patients that require major hepatectomy[7,8] or before preoperative portal vein embolization (see Chapters 51B, 102C, and 119B). When preoperative drainage is necessary for relief of symptoms (pruritus, cholangitis), if neoadjuvant therapy is planned, or when surgery will be delayed, endoscopic methods are preferred for low bile duct obstruction because of the lower complication rate, whereas high obstruction is treated with carefully targeted percutaneous methods to reduce the risk of cholangitis in

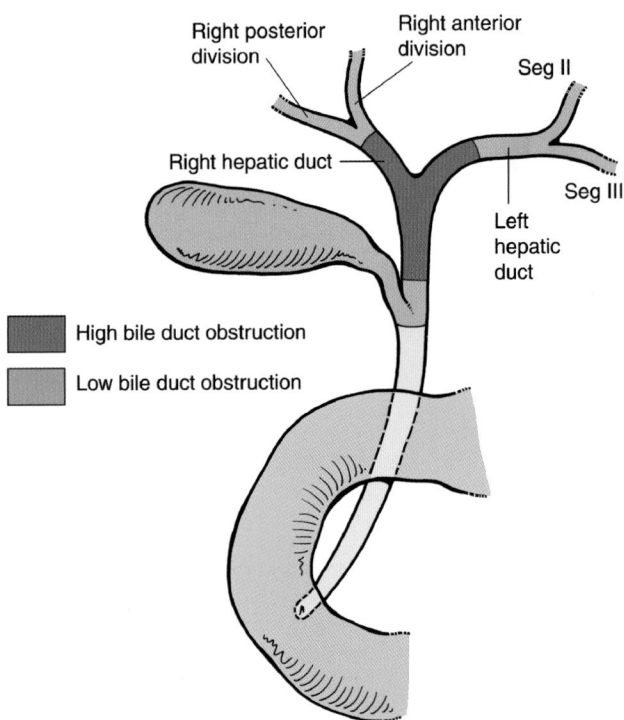

FIGURE 52.1 High bile duct obstruction refers to obstruction at or above confluence; low bile duct obstruction occurs below the common hepatic duct. *Seg,* Segment. (Courtesy Memorial Sloan Kettering Cancer Center Medical Graphics.)

undrained segments.[9] Patients with Bismuth type II and higher levels of obstruction are at high risk for requiring multiple drainage procedures[10] (see Chapter 42).

ENDOSCOPIC VERSUS PERCUTANEOUS DRAINAGE (SEE CHAPTERS 20, 30, AND 31)

Patients with low bile duct obstruction are typically treated endoscopically. Patients with high bile duct obstruction, particularly when the obstruction extends above the hilus, have traditionally been treated percutaneously. The success rate of percutaneous drainage is higher, and the complication rate lower, when compared with endoscopic methods.[11,12] This perspective is evolving while technologic advances in endoscope design occur and endoscopists become better trained and more experienced in wire-guided procedures, with access to better drainage devices and accessories. Currently, however, high bile duct obstruction, with rare exception, should be approached percutaneously. This has been called into question with a randomized trial

of percutaneous versus endoscopic preoperative drainage in patients with hilar cholangiocarcinoma that was stopped prematurely because of high overall mortality in the percutaneous group. The reported 11% mortality in the percutaneous group is vastly higher than any recent report on percutaneous biliary drainage. It is also well outside the 1.7% mortality threshold established by the Society of Interventional Radiology in 2010,[13] calling into question the experience and expertise of those involved in performing the trial.

Two major drawbacks to endoscopic drainage for high bile duct obstruction are the lack of ability to reliably target a specific area of the liver for drainage and the risk of enteric contamination, by retrograde injection of contrast, of parts of the biliary tree that will not be drained. In a patient thought to have undergone successful endoscopic stenting of the right and left liver, repeat imaging may reveal that this is not the case at all (Fig. 52.2). Despite improvements in endoscopic techniques, a paper from Wiggers et al.[14] in 2015 reported a high risk of inadequate preoperative endoscopic drainage, with 108 of 288

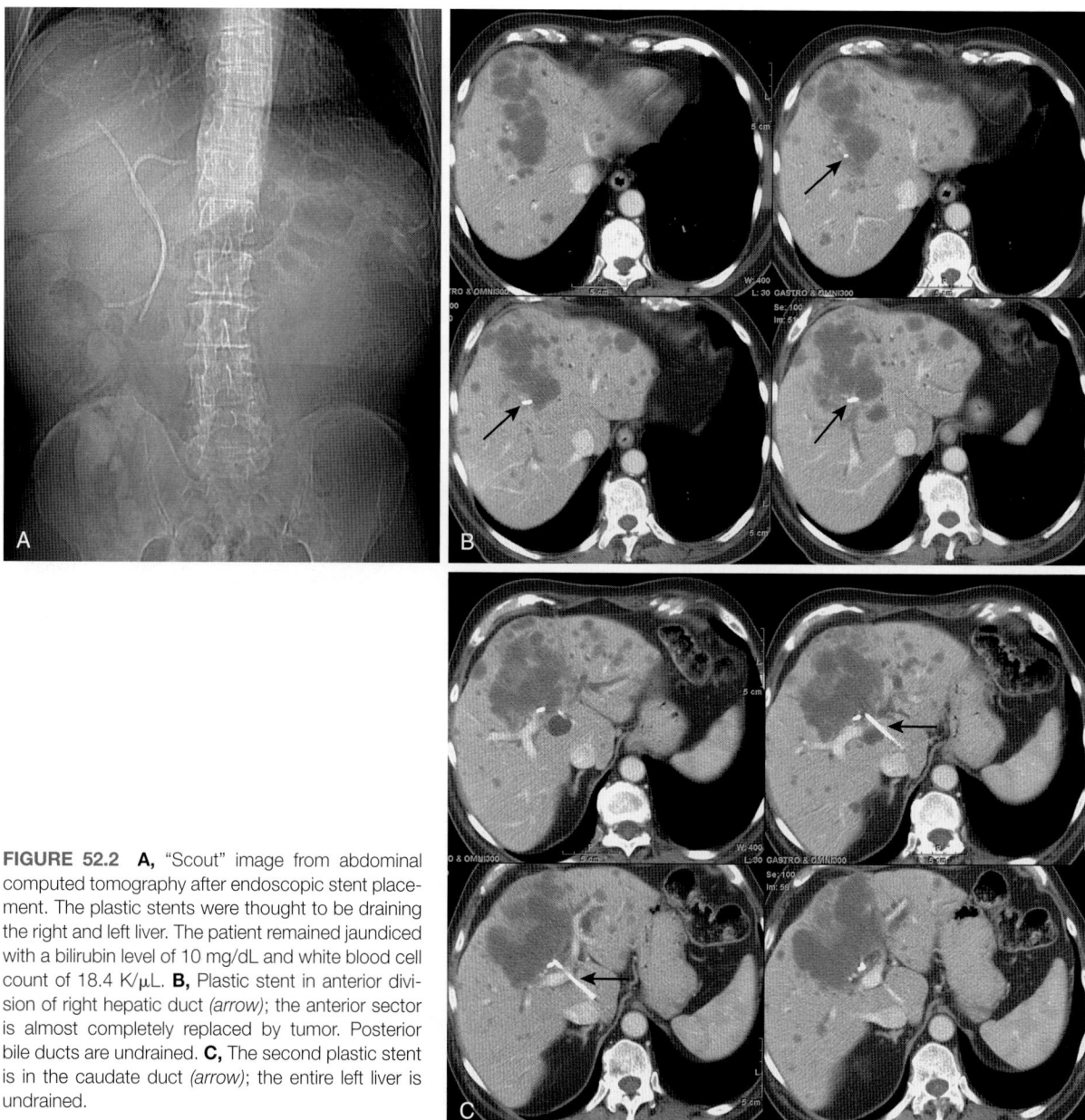

FIGURE 52.2 A, "Scout" image from abdominal computed tomography after endoscopic stent placement. The plastic stents were thought to be draining the right and left liver. The patient remained jaundiced with a bilirubin level of 10 mg/dL and white blood cell count of 18.4 K/μL. **B,** Plastic stent in anterior division of right hepatic duct *(arrow)*; the anterior sector is almost completely replaced by tumor. Posterior bile ducts are undrained. **C,** The second plastic stent is in the caudate duct *(arrow)*; the entire left liver is undrained.

(38%) patients with perihilar cholangiocarcinoma requiring additional percutaneous procedures subsequent to endoscopic retrograde cholangiopancreatography (ERCP).[14]

Development of the linear-array echoendoscope has allowed for the expansion of endoscopic ultrasound–guided biliary drainage procedures, including choledochoduodenostomy and hepaticogastrostomy.[15] Hepaticogastrostomy may be considered when a patient is best treated by draining the left lateral segment,

anatomy is favorable, and the percutaneous approach is technically difficult, or when the risk of contaminating the right-sided bile ducts is thought to be prohibitive. This is particularly the case when draining the right liver would be of no clinical benefit, either because of replacement of the liver by tumor or occlusion of the right portal vein (Fig. 52.3). High technical success rates with few complications are reported by some authors,[15,16] whereas others report high technical success with less favorable

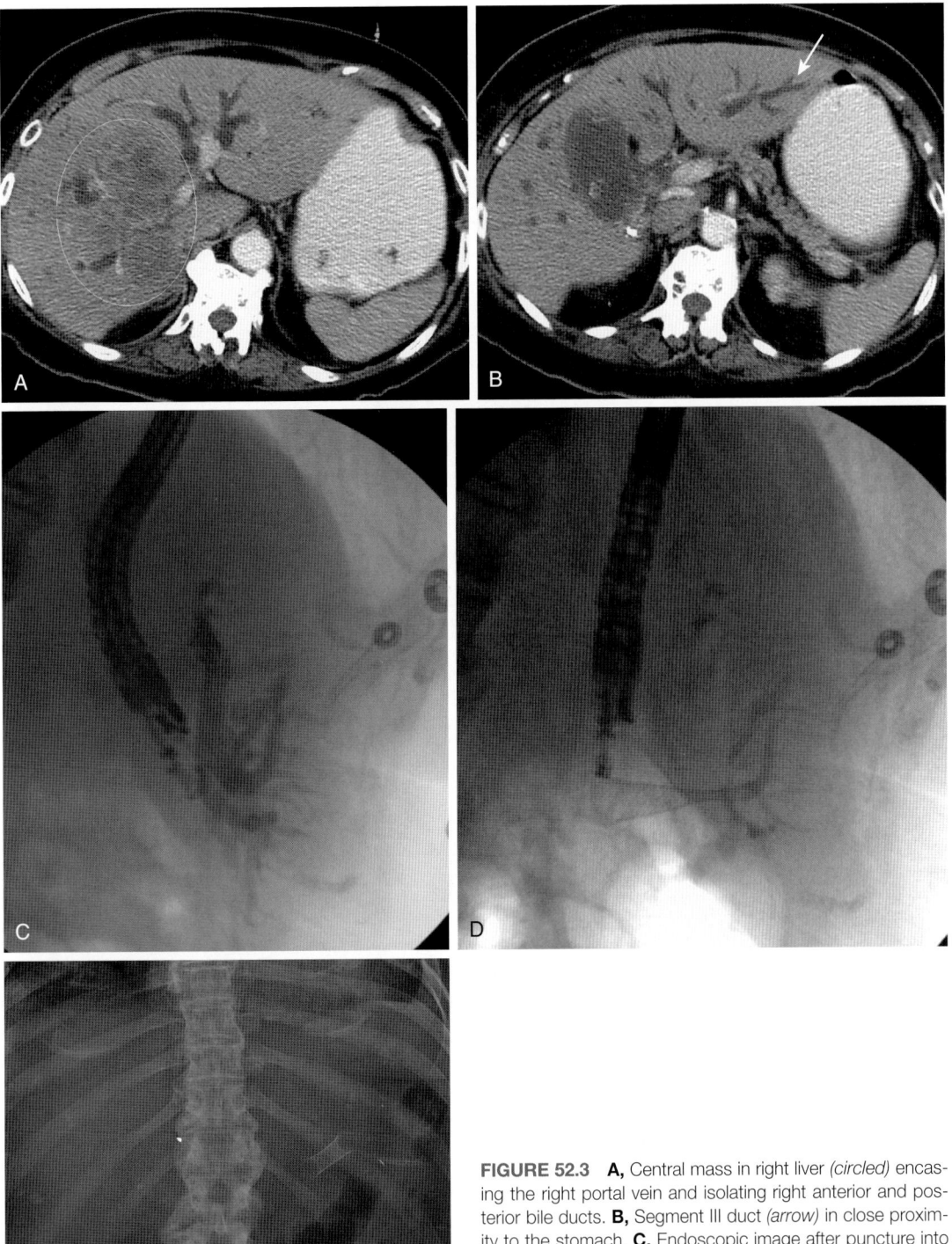

FIGURE 52.3 A, Central mass in right liver *(circled)* encasing the right portal vein and isolating right anterior and posterior bile ducts. **B,** Segment III duct *(arrow)* in close proximity to the stomach. **C,** Endoscopic image after puncture into segment III duct and injection of contrast. **D,** Image after placement of transgastric segment III stent. **E,** Image of the abdomen the next day demonstrates a well-expanded stent between the lesser curvature of the stomach and the segment III bile duct.

complication and stent patency rates.[17] Most operators are early on the learning curve at present. When technically feasible, and in the hands of highly trained endoscopists, this procedure can be gratifying for the patient, with relief of pruritus and lowering of bilirubin without the added burden of a percutaneous catheter.

Endoscopic drainage is rarely indicated in patients with papillary intraductal tumor because of inevitable tumor ingrowth into the metallic stent with early stent occlusion. Intraductal tumor can arise from cancers other than papillary cholangiocarcinoma, including colorectal metastases, gallbladder cancer, and hepatocellular carcinoma. When intraductal tumor occurs in the setting of metastatic colorectal cancer or hepatocellular cancer, it is usually the direct extension of a parenchymal metastasis into the duct (Fig. 52.4A). Patients with intraductal tumor often require permanent indwelling catheter drainage, with an indwelling, multi-sidehole catheter allowing bile to drain around the intraductal tumor, but they may be stented when the intraductal tumor can be effectively excluded (see Fig. 52.4B–D).

A realistic idea of what is feasible endoscopically and percutaneously is important when the initial decision is made regarding who will treat the patient. This depends on a thorough understanding of the goal of treatment as well as knowledge of the skill level of the interventional radiologists and endoscopists available to care for the patient.

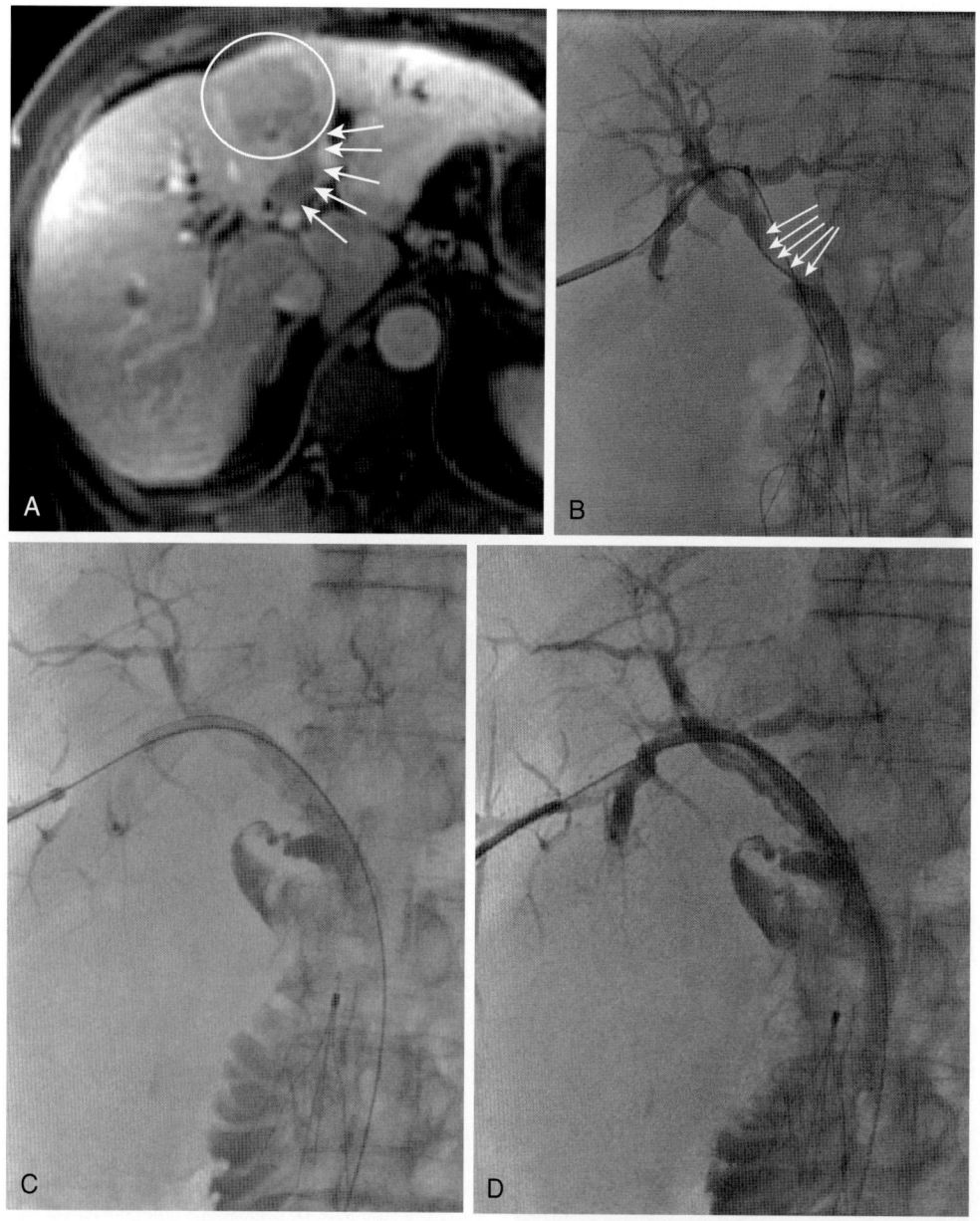

FIGURE 52.4   A, Patient with hilar cholangiocarcinoma arising in segment IV *(circle)* with tumor extension into left hepatic duct *(arrows).* **B,** Cholangiogram at time of drainage demonstrates tumor in left hepatic duct (LHD) compressing hilus and extending into the common hepatic duct (CHD) *(arrows).* **C,** Image at time of stent placement. Stent extends from right side to CHD, essentially excluding tumor in LHD. **D,** Cholangiogram after stent placement.

PREPROCEDURE PREPARATION

Imaging

The importance of excellent preprocedure imaging in patients with bile duct obstruction cannot be overemphasized. This imaging should include, at a minimum, a contrast-enhanced computed tomography (CT) scan of the abdomen (see Chapter 16). Ultrasound is often used to establish the presence of dilated bile ducts, identify the level of obstruction, evaluate portal vein patency, and demonstrate intraductal tumor, but ultrasound is not adequate for drainage planning. Although MRCP provides a detailed three-dimensional (3D) rendering of the obstructed

bile ducts and is effective at delineating intraductal abnormalities and depicting isolated bile ducts (Fig. 52.5), it excludes certain details that can serve as targeting aides for percutaneous drainage. These shortcomings of MRCP include poor visualization of surgical clips, dystrophic calcifications, and bony landmarks (see Chapter 16). In addition, if the patient is unable to breath-hold during image acquisition, MRCP will be suboptimal. CT scans performed on multi-slice scanners in a picture-archiving and communication system (PACS) environment allow a 3D rendering of the anatomy, while identifying relevant landmarks that can be used for targeting and demonstration of other structures that should be avoided, such as liver tumors and bowel. Also, as with magnetic resonance imaging (MRI), one may identify ancillary

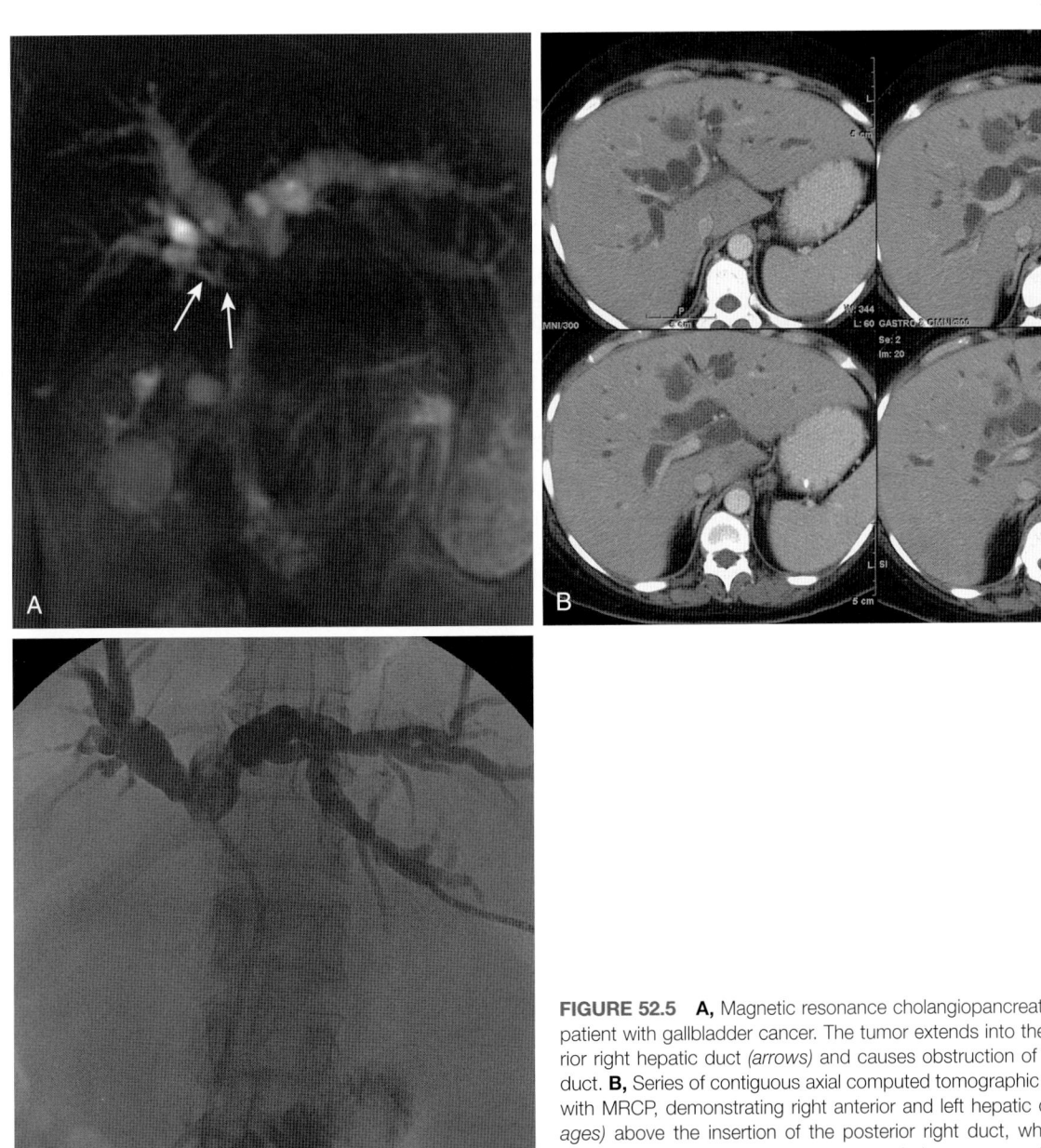

FIGURE 52.5 A, Magnetic resonance cholangiopancreatography (MRCP) in a patient with gallbladder cancer. The tumor extends into the low-inserting posterior right hepatic duct *(arrows)* and causes obstruction of the common hepatic duct. **B,** Series of contiguous axial computed tomographic images correlate well with MRCP, demonstrating right anterior and left hepatic ducts joining *(top images)* above the insertion of the posterior right duct, which contains material of soft tissue density (tumor) that extends into common hepatic duct *(bottom images)*. **C,** Image taken at biliary drainage demonstrates the left hepatic duct joining the anterior division; a low-inserting posterior duct is isolated and thus is not opacified. The filling defect in left hepatic duct is a blood clot related to the placement of percutaneous catheter, not a tumor.

important findings, such as ascites, hepatic lobar atrophy, and portal vein occlusion or encasement. All this information is critical to make prognostic assessments and determine the best approach for drainage.

The amount of functional parenchyma that can be drained should be estimated. Functional parenchyma is that part of the liver that is not replaced by tumor and that has an intact portal venous supply and hepatic venous drainage. If 75% of the hepatic parenchyma is replaced by tumor, even if it were possible to drain the entire biliary tree, it is unlikely that normal hepatic function or normalization of serum bilirubin level would result. The portal vein provides the trophic blood supply to the liver, and occlusion results in atrophy of the affected segment(s), particularly when the ipsilateral bile duct is also occluded (see Chapter 5).[18] Atrophy may be recognized by the diminutive size of the involved part of the liver, accompanied by crowding of the bile ducts (Fig. 52.6; see Chapters 16 and 51A). When portal vein occlusion causes atrophy, drainage of the atrophied liver does not improve liver function. In addition, it is frequently difficult to manipulate catheters through the obstructed/atrophied portion of the liver into the central biliary tree. The end result is an external drainage catheter that provides no clinical benefit to the patient and only serves to risk complications and degrade QOL.

Central tumors frequently obstruct the right and the left biliary tree, isolating them from one another. Obstruction may extend even higher, isolating the ductal system at the sectoral, segmental, or subsegmental level. When drainage is undertaken for relief of pruritus, draining even a segment of the liver may result in relief of symptoms.[19,20] When isolation is present, and drainage is undertaken to lower the serum bilirubin, as mentioned previously, it is important to estimate how much functional parenchyma can be drained with one catheter. Drainage of at least 75% of the liver is associated with a significantly increased probability of returning the serum bilirubin to normal or near-normal levels.[21] In some cases, this goal may be impossible to achieve, unless more than one drainage catheter or stent is placed. Recognition of this allows for informing both the patient and the referring physician about the potential need for more than one catheter or stent.

Cholangitis is rarely the primary indication for drainage in patients with malignant bile duct obstruction, except in patients who have undergone prior biliary instrumentation and in those who have a contaminated biliary tree related to previous biliary-enteric bypass, cross-ampullary stenting, or sphincterotomy.[22] Drainage of an isolated region of the liver, either percutaneously or endoscopically, may contaminate other functionally "isolated" parts of the biliary tree. In this case, subsequent cholangitis may drive the placement of additional catheters to relieve infection. Widespread contamination of a severely isolated biliary tree with drainage of only part of the obstructed system can result in chronic recurrent cholangitis. Whether induced by endoscopic or percutaneous means, this situation can be difficult to manage and should be anticipated and avoided if possible.

Laboratory Studies

Preoperative labs for biliary drainage include a complete blood count, hepatic function panel, and coagulation studies. The serum bilirubin can change rapidly when patients become obstructed. Because decisions regarding the need for further drainage in high obstruction with isolated bile ducts depend, in part, on the serum bilirubin, it is important to draw this reference laboratory value within 24 hours of drainage. The bilirubin is typically rising at the time of drainage and the serum bilirubin may be higher the morning after the drainage procedure than the morning of the procedure. Serum bilirubin values drawn 48 hours after drainage more accurately predict effectiveness of drainage. The lack of bile salts in the intestine impairs vitamin K absorption and may result in elevation of the prothrombin time (PT), international normalized ratio (INR), and the partial thromboplastin time (PTT); therefore these values should also be checked within a few days of the procedure. Coagulation abnormalities may be exacerbated if there is

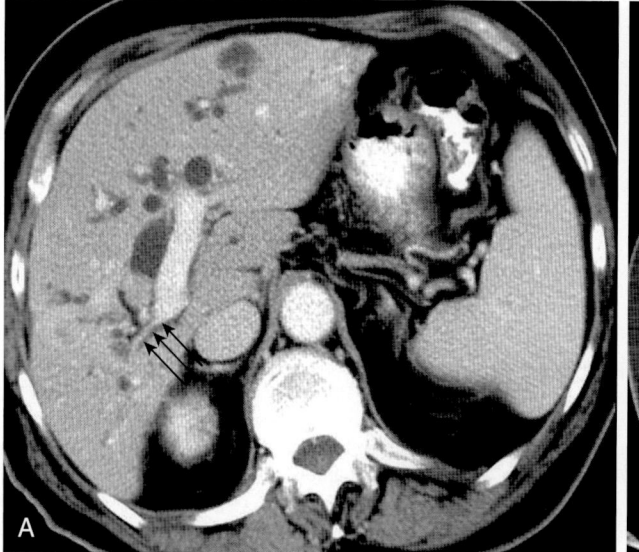
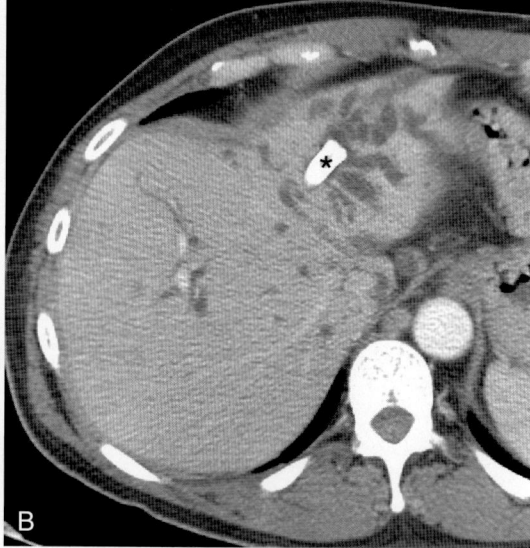

FIGURE 52.6 **A,** Right hepatic atrophy. Volume of the right hemiliver is greatly diminished, with severe attenuation of the right portal vein *(arrows)*. **B,** Left hepatic atrophy. Note the small size of the left hemiliver and crowding of dilated bile ducts secondary to portal vein occlusion. Endoscopic stent *(asterisk)* had been placed at another hospital, and subsequently the patient returned with jaundice and cholangitis.

also poor hepatic synthetic function. This can be corrected by the administration of vitamin K or fresh frozen plasma, depending on the urgency of drainage.

Antibiotics

Preprocedure antibiotic prophylaxis is given to all patients undergoing biliary drainage. Both a history of previous instrumentation and fever have been shown to be highly predictive of bactibilia, but up to 5% of patients without these signs may have positive bile cultures[23] (see Chapter 11). Many patients become bacteremic during or after the procedure, even in the absence of preexisting signs or symptoms of infection, particularly when they are known to have a colonized biliary tree. Generally, patients receive broad coverage with an agent such as ticarcillin-clavulanate or ceftriaxone, but the prophylactic antibiotic chosen should reflect common biliary organisms at the individual institution and is best chosen in consultation with institutional infectious disease stewards. When cholangitis is not present, administration of intravenous (IV) antibiotics beyond the prophylactic dose is not warranted. Patients with a history of cholangitis or sepsis or those presumed to have a contaminated biliary tree associated with transampullary stenting, biliary-enteric bypass, sphincterotomy, or recent instrumentation may be best covered with an agent such as piperacillin-tazobactam (Zosyn), which is excreted into the bile. Appropriate postprocedure coverage is determined based on bile cultures obtained at drainage.

Psychological Preparation

Managing patient expectations is a major part of the process. A thorough discussion of possible outcomes is particularly important before biliary drainage in patients with high bile duct obstruction. Patients should understand that, although every effort will be made to establish internal drainage with stents, this may not be achieved. Although it is usually possible to cross an obstructing lesion into the common bile duct, internalization might be precluded by extensive isolation of the biliary tree, intraductal tumor, concomitant duodenal obstruction, or other factors. Two or more catheters or self-expanding stents may be required when the tumor extends beyond the secondary confluence on one side or the other, depending on the clinical objective. Such a discussion is not intended to distress the patient but rather to promote an understanding of the complexity of the situation to mitigate sentiments of surprise or anger if stent placement is not possible at the initial encounter and subsequent procedures are necessary.

Even in the presence of segmental isolation, pruritus often resolves after biliary drainage. Unfortunately, it is not always possible to lower the serum bilirubin, particularly to levels that would allow for the administration of certain chemotherapeutic agents. In certain situations, two or more biliary drainage catheters may be placed without a significant decrease in bilirubin; sometimes, the bilirubin may even increase. It is possible that a single biliary drainage catheter may drain one portion of the liver well while converting near-complete obstructions in other areas to complete obstructions (Fig. 52.7). It also is conceivable that intervening cholangitis or progression of disease may play a role. Patients who have realistic expectations and some understanding of these issues before the initial biliary drainage procedure are less likely to become distressed if multiple procedures are required or if the ultimate outcome is less than satisfactory (see Chapter 29).

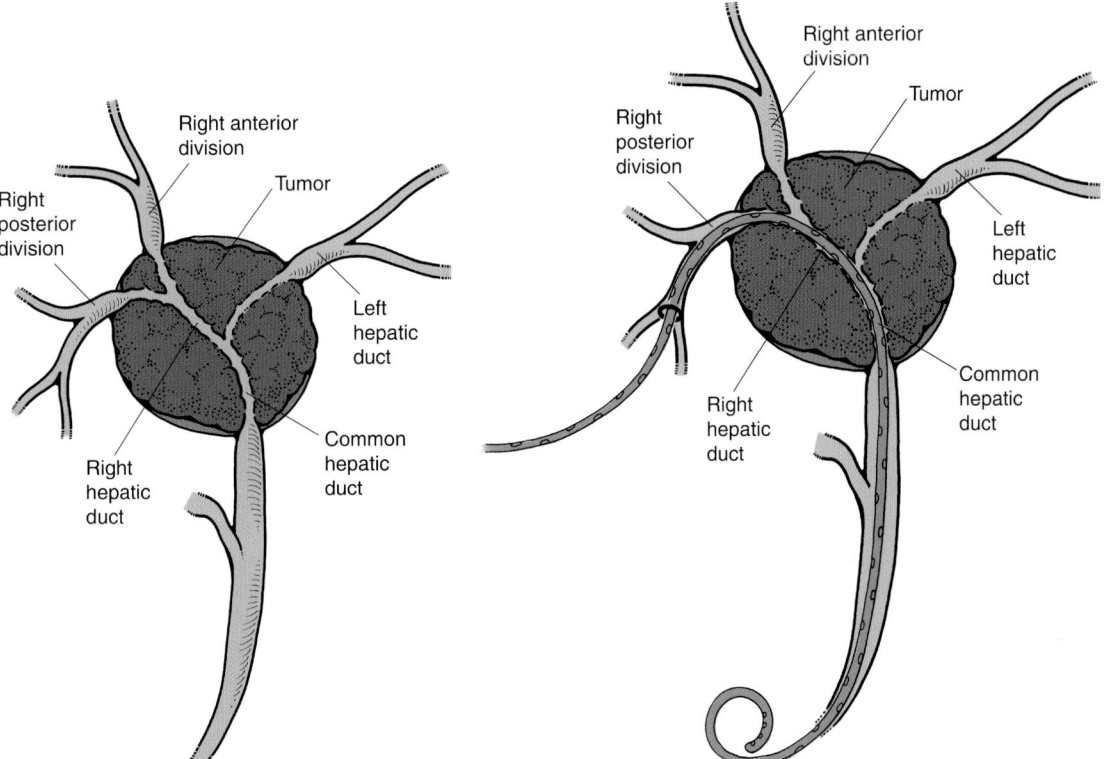

FIGURE 52.7 **A,** Obstruction caused by tumor severely narrows the biliary tree up to the secondary confluence on right. **B,** After placement of a multiple sidehole catheter, the right posterior sector is well drained by the catheter, which compromises near-complete obstruction of the right anterior division duct and left hepatic duct. (Courtesy Memorial Sloan Kettering Cancer Center Medical Graphics.)

INTRAPROCEDURAL ISSUES

Approach

Many interventional radiologists prefer a right-sided approach to the biliary tree. The right side of the liver is larger and more accessible than the left. Approach from the right side more easily avoids direct x-ray exposure to the hands of the operator and allows a direct approach to the hepatic hilus and common bile duct, making catheter and guidewire manipulations easier and often more successful. In addition, approach from the right side is thought to be safer because there are fewer structures between the skin and right liver that may be injured and, some believe, a lower risk of bleeding. To date, a higher risk of bleeding with a left-sided approach has not been conclusively demonstrated.[24,25] Patients with low bile duct obstruction that cannot be drained endoscopically may be approached from either side.

The direct approach from the right is sometimes complicated when the site of puncture is the right posterior duct and this duct enters the left hepatic duct. This anatomic variant is often evident on preprocedure imaging studies (see Chapter 2) and should be specifically evaluated; it occurs in 20% of patients and may add a 180-degree turn to the approach to the hepatic hilum, making it more difficult to traverse the obstruction. On the other hand, when the obstruction extends to involve the left-right confluence but no higher, approach from the posterior right duct will drain the right posterior sector and the entire left liver when the posterior duct joins the left. The main disadvantages to a right-sided approach are the discomfort associated with intercostal catheters and leaking of ascites around a more gravity-dependent right-sided catheter. Both of these issues can be mitigated with primary stent placement at the time of initial biliary drainage.

A left-sided approach to the biliary tree is preferred in several situations. When an obstructing tumor extends above the biliary confluence, it may isolate the right and left bile ducts and may involve a secondary confluence or higher. The right hepatic duct is typically shorter than the left (see Chapter 2); as a result, tumor is more likely to extend to and isolate the right anterior and posterior sectoral ducts, while the left medial and lateral sectors continue to communicate. In such cases, it may be possible to drain more functional hepatic parenchyma by placing a single catheter or stent on the left depending on the size of the left liver. Patients with ascites are less likely to have leakage around a left anterior catheter, so a left approach is preferred when possible. When atrophy or compromise of the portal vein is present, the patient will always derive more benefit from drainage of the contralateral functional liver, as previously discussed.

Image Guidance

In most cases, biliary drainage is performed with fluoroscopic guidance (see Chapter 31). Ultrasound is often used for duct puncture from a left-sided approach; but less often from the right because bile duct orientation and the need to image through an intercostal space make the use of ultrasound more challenging. Careful review of a high-quality CT scan is helpful for identifying radiopaque landmarks that may be used to target a specific region of the biliary tree or even a specific bile duct. This review is particularly important when isolation is suspected, and the objective is to target a specific duct. If the right anterior duct is the target, it would be unfortunate to enter a segment IV duct by being too anterior or medial. Previously placed stents, surgical clips, or other radiopaque landmarks can frequently be used to facilitate targeting.

Sedation

Although general anesthesia is not necessary, and biliary drainage can be performed with conscious sedation, general anesthesia can be quite helpful when available. This is particularly true when the bile ducts are not dilated, or only minimally dilated, and in patients with sleep apnea in whom variable respirations can make targeting and entering a bile duct difficult. To allow for either general anesthesia or conscious sedation, patients take nothing by mouth for 8 hours before the procedure. They are well hydrated and have functional venous access, particularly if cholangitis has been present. These patients can become septic and hypotensive, requiring rapid volume expansion.

Technical Aids

The most significant technical development to facilitate biliary drainage and other fluoroscopically guided procedures in recent years has been the advent of multidetector CT (MDCT), particularly when used within a PACS environment. The ability to scan the liver in a single breath hold and then cine through the images facilitates identification of the level of obstruction and the likelihood of isolation (see Chapter 16). It also enables the formulation of a 3D mental image of the biliary tree. Understanding the biliary anatomy in this way facilitates a successful, uncomplicated procedure. It is frequently possible to anticipate normal variants of bile duct anatomy, which can have a significant impact on preprocedure planning (see Chapter 2). In addition, most PACS workstations allow cross-reference of the axial images (Fig. 52.8A) with the "scout" image (see Fig. 52.8B), which is a simulated frontal radiograph used for programming the extent of the scan. In this way, targeting of a specific region, or even a specific duct, is made much easier—and the final catheter resides within the planned segment of the liver (see Fig. 52.8C). Although this degree of sophistication may be unnecessary for obstruction below the hepatic hilum, MDCT facilitates drainage in patients with complex high bile duct obstruction such that it is always worth performing MDCT if a recent scan does not exist.

Drainage Catheter Versus Primary Stent Placement

The suitability of a patient for primary stent placement is determined at the time of biliary drainage based on the indication for the drainage, evidence of infected bile, presence of blood or tumor within the biliary tree, and cholangiographic findings. The goal of biliary drainage is to solve the patient's clinical problem by placing as few catheters or stents as possible, intending that the bile should drain internally when the intervention is complete. In patients with a presumed sterile biliary tree, ideally an attempt should be made to accomplish this without ever placing a drainage catheter into the duodenum. There is evidence that when stent occlusion occurs, the patient is less likely to present with cholangitis if the sphincter of Oddi has not been compromised.[26] Patients with high bile duct obstruction without cholangitis may be stented primarily at the initial drainage procedure, provided significant blood is not present within the biliary tree. Blood clot within the intrahepatic bile ducts impairs drainage and may compromise flow of bile through the stent, which may result in bile leaking into the peritoneal cavity from the site of duct puncture. When clots are visible within the biliary tree, the best course might be to place a drainage catheter

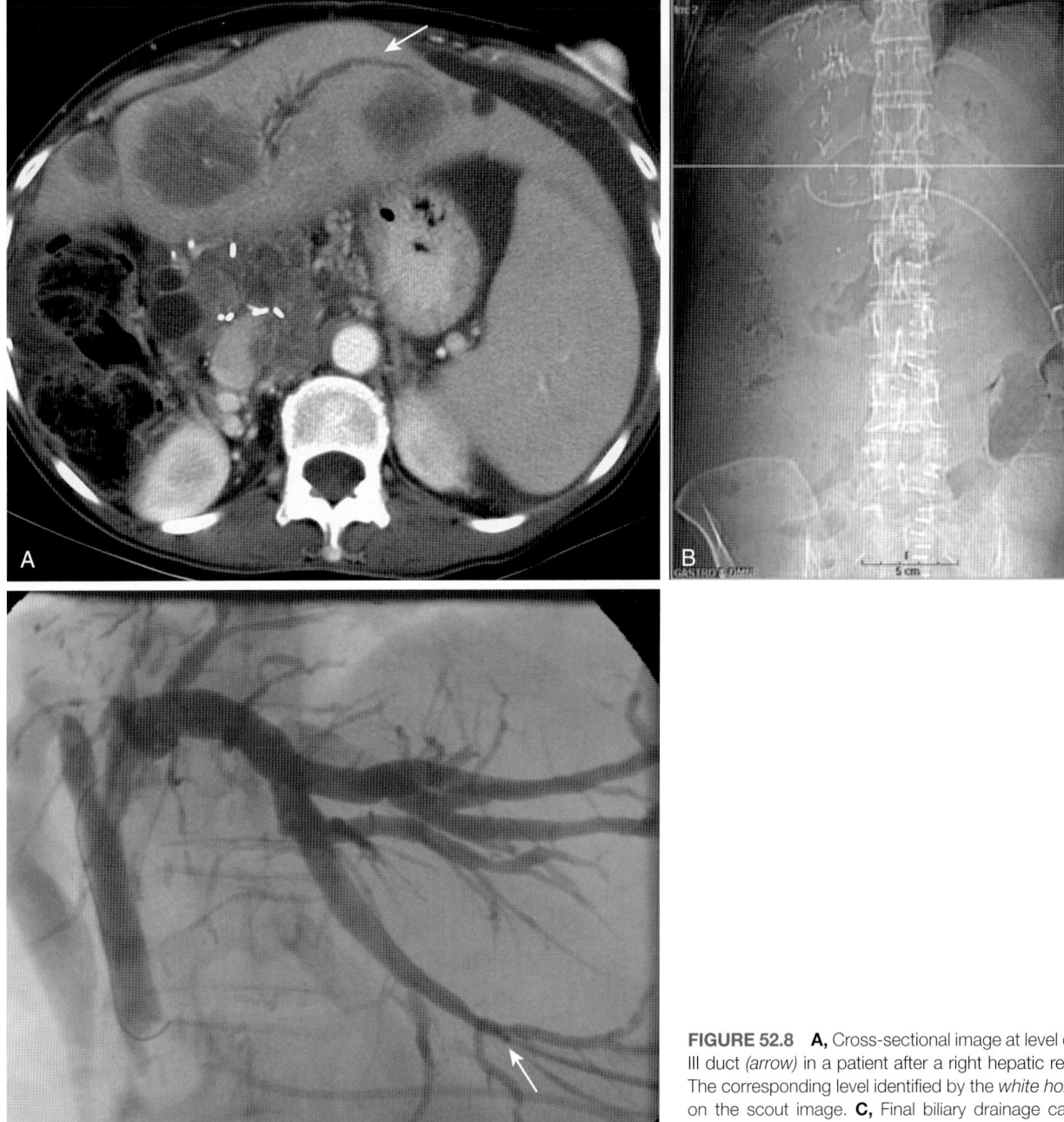

FIGURE 52.8 A, Cross-sectional image at level of segment III duct *(arrow)* in a patient after a right hepatic resection. **B,** The corresponding level identified by the *white horizontal line* on the scout image. **C,** Final biliary drainage catheter that clearly enters segment III duct at planned peripheral puncture site *(arrow)*.

until the bile clears, at which time the patient is stented. Patients undergoing drainage for cholangitis should not be stented primarily in most cases. Catheter manipulation in this group of patients is kept to a minimum to diminish the risk of procedure-related sepsis. Once the biliary tree is drained and cholangitis resolves, a stent can be placed.

Having addressed the decisions regarding patients who clearly can or cannot be stented, the more difficult situations that occur in patients with high bile duct obstruction must be addressed. In 1975 Bismuth and Corlette[27] classified obstruction of the hepatic confluence as types I through IV (Fig. 52.9; see Chapter 42). Predictions about the level of obstruction and degree of isolation of the biliary tree can be made based on the

preprocedure imaging studies. These predictions are not always accurate, however, and it is sometimes necessary to modify the stenting approach based on cholangiographic findings; in rare cases, it may be necessary to abandon the procedure altogether. Patients with Bismuth type I obstruction can have the entire liver drained with one catheter or stent because right and left ducts communicate freely. Barring one of the previously mentioned contraindications, these patients have a primary stent placed.

Patients with Bismuth type II obstruction cannot be completely drained with one catheter, although it is sometimes possible to opacify ducts in both sides of the liver. Some suggest that survival is better when both sides of the liver are drained.[28]

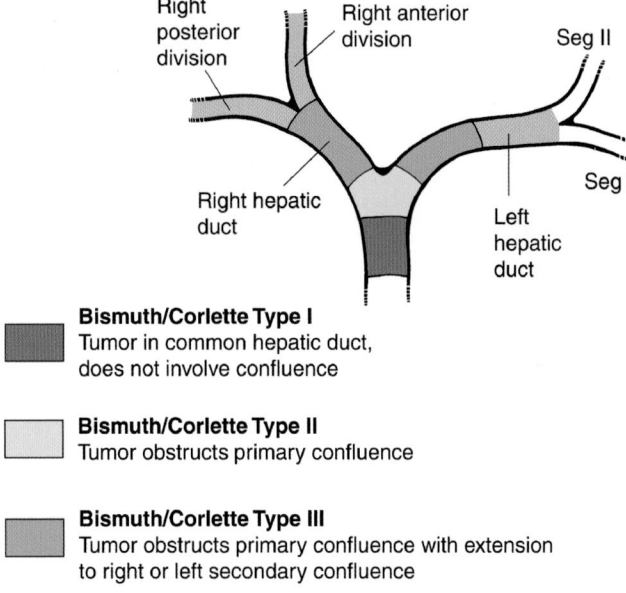

Bismuth/Corlette Type I
Tumor in common hepatic duct, does not involve confluence

Bismuth/Corlette Type II
Tumor obstructs primary confluence

Bismuth/Corlette Type III
Tumor obstructs primary confluence with extension to right or left secondary confluence

FIGURE 52.9 Bismuth-Corlette classification for malignant high bile duct obstruction. Type IV involves both right and left ducts to secondary confluence. *Seg,* Segment. (Courtesy Memorial Sloan Kettering Cancer Center Medical Graphics.)

Even in Bismuth type II and III hilar obstructions, however, Inal and colleagues[29] saw no significant difference in clinical response to treatment or stent patency rate with unilobar versus bilobar drainage.

When contrast material enters the obstructed side opposite the puncture, it usually does not drain effectively, and in the presence of risk factors for infection, that side may be contaminated. These patients can be stented from the ipsilateral approach by inserting one stent from the ipsilateral side to the contralateral side and a second stent from the ipsilateral side into the common bile duct or duodenum (Fig. 52.10) in a T-shaped configuration. The other option is to puncture the contralateral side and place side-by-side stents (Fig. 52.11) in a Y-shaped configuration. In either case, stenting into the common bile duct is preferred rather than into the duodenum if possible so as to preserve function of the sphincter of Oddi. Barring any contraindication, this could be done primarily at initial drainage, as advocated by Inal and colleagues,[30] who found that whether stents were placed primarily or at a second sitting, cholangitis did not subsequently develop in patients without cholangitis at the time of stenting. In the Inal et al.[29] study, all patients with a Bismuth type I or II obstruction achieved a serum bilirubin of 2 mg/dL or less. One advantage of the more anatomic Y-shaped configuration stent placement is

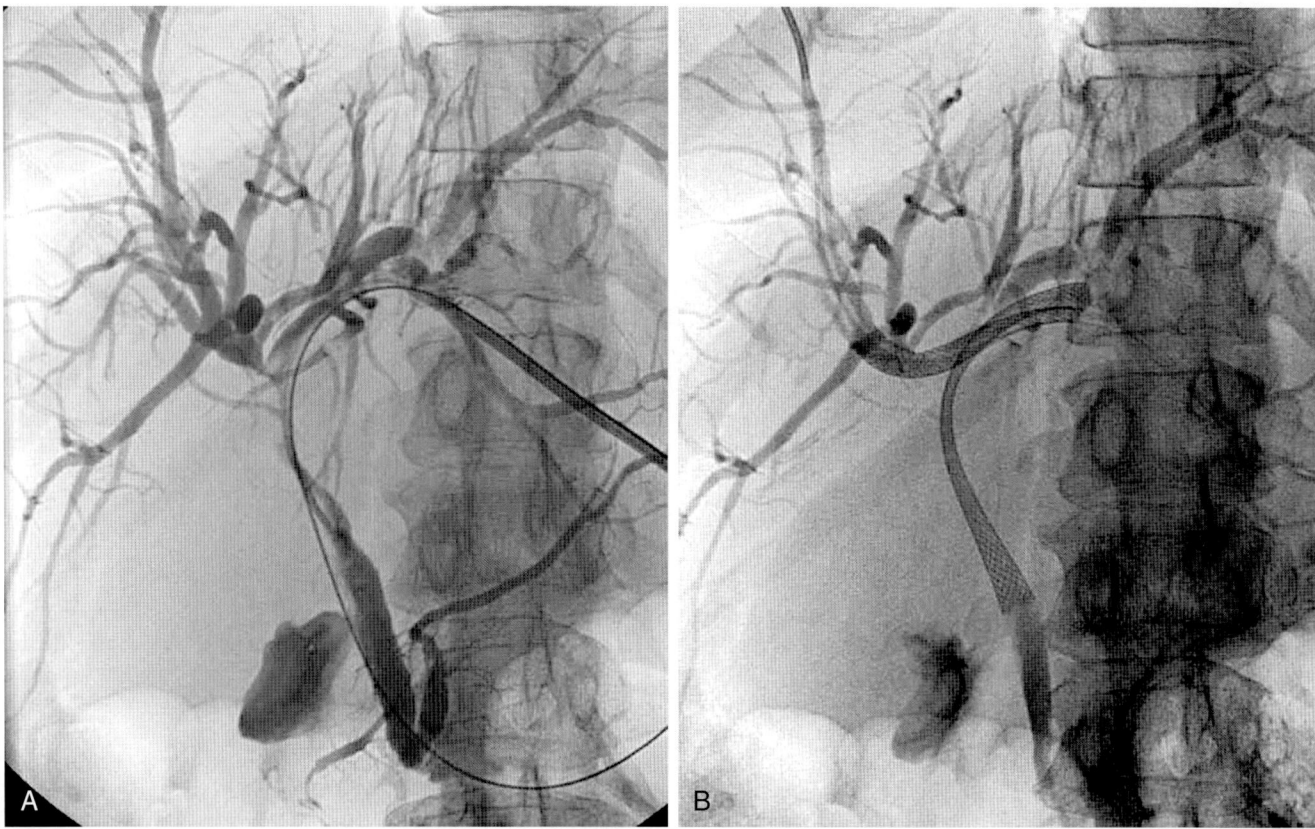

FIGURE 52.10 **A,** Patient with cholangiocarcinoma that resulted in Bismuth-Corlette type II obstruction, with near-complete isolation of right and left hepatic ducts. **B,** Same patient treated with side-by-side T-shaped configuration. Wall stents were placed simultaneously, with one stent placed from the left hepatic duct (LHD) to the right hepatic duct and the other from the LHD into the common bile duct (CBD). The stent from the LHD to CBD ends well short of the duodenum but extends several centimeters on either side of the obstructed segment.

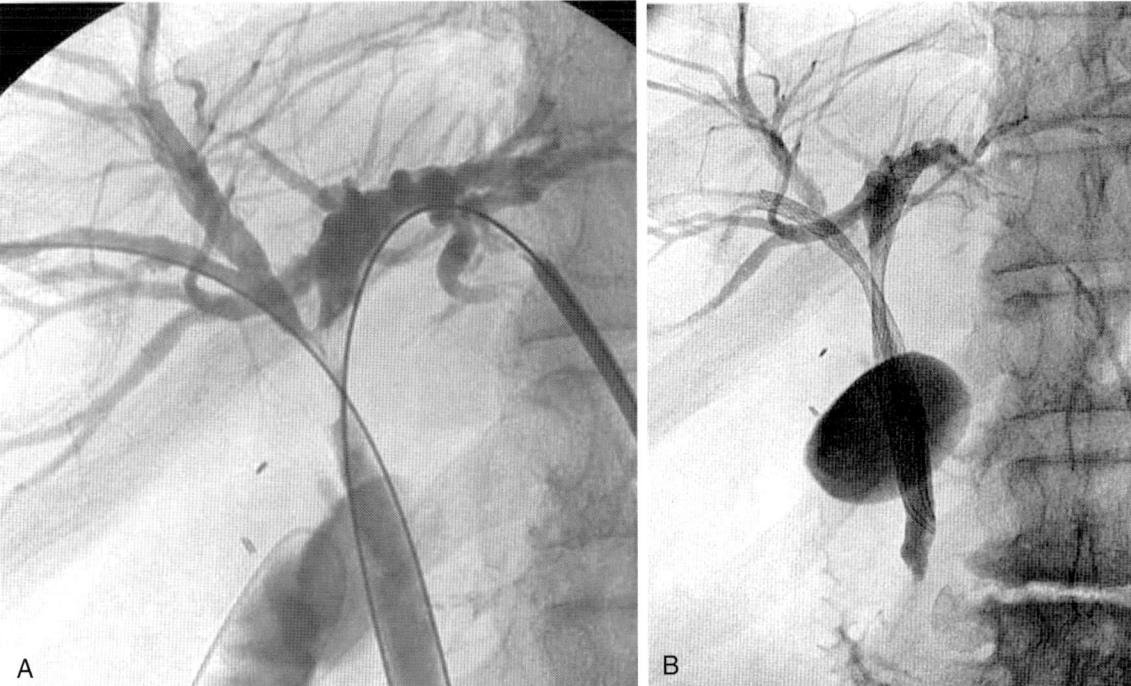

FIGURE 52.11   A, Patient with history of pancreatic cancer after a Whipple procedure with recurrence at the biliary-enteric anastomosis and type II obstruction. **B,** Same patient after simultaneous placement of side-by-side Y-shaped configuration stents.

that if stent occlusion occurs, both stents are approachable either percutaneously or endoscopically and the patient can be restented. In addition, the patency rate of the Y-shaped configuration may be better in patients with type IV obstruction.[29] Specially constructed stents have been developed that allow placement of one stent through an opening in the midbody of the other,[31] but these are not in widespread use. In the absence of risk factors for bactibilia, a single ipsilateral stent can be placed. If the goal of drainage is not achieved, the patient can return after a period of observation for contralateral stenting.

When the contralateral biliary tree is not opacified, precluding knowledge of the type of obstruction, or the ipsilateral obstruction is a Bismuth type III obstruction, or worse, in the absence of some other contraindication, patients being drained for pruritus alone should have a primary stent placed. If the patient is being drained in an attempt to lower the bilirubin level for chemotherapy, a stent should be considered when it is thought that 30% or more of the liver will be drained. We use this as a rule of thumb despite the fact that, in a series of 149 patients drained at Memorial Sloan Kettering Cancer Center, there was only a marginally significant difference in the number of patients attaining a bilirubin less than 2 mg/dL, based on the estimated volume of liver drained. In this analysis, 6 (29%) of 21 patients with less than one third of the liver drained attained a bilirubin level below 2 mg/dL, whereas this was achieved in 65 (51%) of 128 patients with more than one third of the liver drained ($P = .06$).[32] After stent placement, if the bilirubin fails to fall to the desired level, a second drainage procedure can be performed. Given the QOL issues for the patient, as well as the risk of contaminating an undrained part of the liver by having an externalized catheter in place, the slight inconvenience of working alongside a previously placed stent is warranted.

Alternatively, a drainage catheter can be placed and when the serum bilirubin normalizes, the patient can return for secondary stent placement. If an internal/external catheter has been placed, and the bilirubin does not fall to a level that allows treatment, or cholangitis develops, it may be necessary to drain more of the isolated undrained liver.

If the initial drainage is on the right side, and the tumor has extended up the right hepatic duct so as to isolate the anterior and posterior divisions from each other and from the left hepatic duct, stenting either the anterior or posterior division is often adequate. Alternatively, side-by-side self-expanding metallic stents can be placed on the right to drain both the anterior and posterior ducts. In challenging cases, one has to devise creative drainage solutions with placement of multiple stents into isolated parts of the liver when clinically indicated. Although a significant difference in patency is reported when more than one stent is placed in a noncoaxial manner,[33] the mean patency of multiple stents is almost 6 months, justifying stent placement. Even when one part of the liver is not functional, drainage may be necessary to eliminate a source of ongoing cholangitis (Fig. 52.12).

The concepts of biliary drainage are simple, but when high bile duct obstruction is present, the planning is complex, and execution can be difficult. The patient must have enough of the liver drained to be free of cholangitis and pruritus to reduce the serum bilirubin sufficiently to receive chemotherapy, if indicated. Given that no difference in stent patency is reported if the stent is inserted for proximal or distal obstruction, that a significant difference in patency is seen when more than one stent is placed, and that lower complication rates are reported when stents are placed primarily, primary stent placement should be considered whenever possible.[29,33,34] Additional

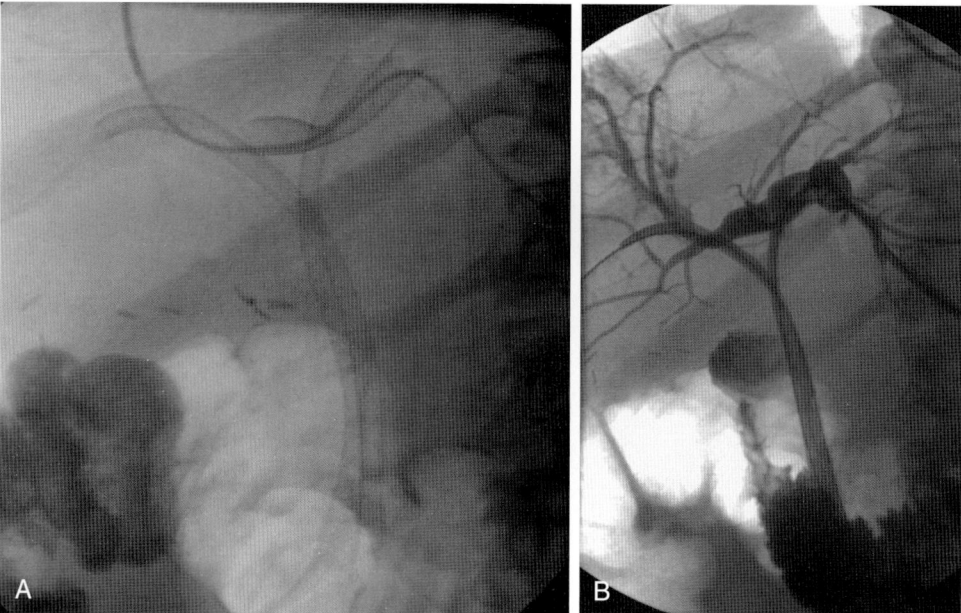

FIGURE 52.12 Stents placed from right anterior hepatic duct to the common bile duct, from the left hepatic duct to the common bile duct, and from the left hepatic duct to the residual undrained posterior right duct. **A,** Without contrast. **B,** After injection of contrast.

stents can be placed later if necessary. Patients with Bismuth type I or II obstructions may be treated with a single stent, whereas patients with type III or IV obstructions may require placement of additional stents.[29]

POSTPROCEDURE CARE

Patients are monitored carefully for the first 24 hours after drainage for signs of bleeding or sepsis. With proper technique, including peripheral bile duct puncture, serious bleeding complications are uncommon. Because the hepatic artery, portal vein, and bile duct travel side by side within portal triads, at the time of drainage blood may enter the bile duct during catheter exchanges, resulting in hemobilia in the immediate postprocedure period (see Chapter 116). Hemobilia usually clears within 24 hours, and new or recurrent hemobilia within the first few days of drainage typically is related to catheter malposition. If the catheter has pulled out from its original position, a catheter sidehole may become positioned outside the biliary tree adjacent to a portal vein branch; this problem can be corrected by simply repositioning the catheter, and we often upsize the catheter as well. Significant arterial bleeding during this period is rare. No matter where the initial puncture is performed to opacify the biliary tree, attempts are always made to puncture a peripheral bile duct for catheter placement, preferably a fourth-order or fifth-order branch. The more peripheral the bile duct punctured, the smaller the accompanying hepatic artery branch, mitigating the risk of arterial injury and postprocedure bleeding.[24]

When bleeding occurs 1 week or more after biliary drainage—especially when the event is sudden in onset, and there is not only hemobilia but also bleeding around the catheter entry site—arterial injury should be suspected, and the patient should be studied angiographically. Although a pseudoaneurysm or extravasation of contrast is sometimes seen, as in other cases of vascular trauma, any abnormality of a hepatic arterial branch adjacent to the biliary drainage catheter should be taken as presumptive evidence of injury to the branch, and the vessel should be selectively coil embolized (Fig. 52.13; see Chapter 116). If the operator is determined to demonstrate extravasation of contrast material angiographically, it is sometimes necessary to remove the biliary drainage catheter over a guidewire during the angiogram. In the correct clinical setting, empiric superselective embolization of the arterial branch corresponding to the bile duct punctured is acceptable. There is little downside to this approach, and the patient's bleeding is stopped; the biliary catheter is exchanged at this point because it is usually at least partially occluded by thrombus.

Despite prophylactic antibiotic coverage, sepsis may occur immediately after or within several hours of drainage and should be treated appropriately.[35] This is most frequently manifested by the development of rigors with normal or low body temperature, but hypotension and fever may also occur. Sepsis is managed with typical measures: continued administration of appropriate antibiotics, expansion of intravascular volume, and pressor support if necessary. Blood cultures should be drawn to identify organisms responsible for the bacteremia. Cultures of bile obtained at drainage are routinely sent for all patients. This is particularly important for those with preprocedure fever, biliary-enteric anastomosis or sphincterotomy, previous ERCP, or an indwelling stent or catheter. Although positive bile cultures are more common in patients with benign bile duct obstruction, cultures are positive in many patients with malignant obstruction, particularly in the setting of fever and known contamination of the biliary tree. As mentioned earlier, 5% of patients without fever, previous biliary surgery, or endoscopic or percutaneous intervention can have positive bile cultures.[23]

Bile may leak around a biliary drainage catheter. Leaking is most often related to the catheter becoming malpositioned so that one or more sideholes are no longer within the biliary tree but are in the catheter tract or even outside the patient. This problem is managed by repositioning the catheter. Leakage may also be seen with lack of adequate sideholes above the

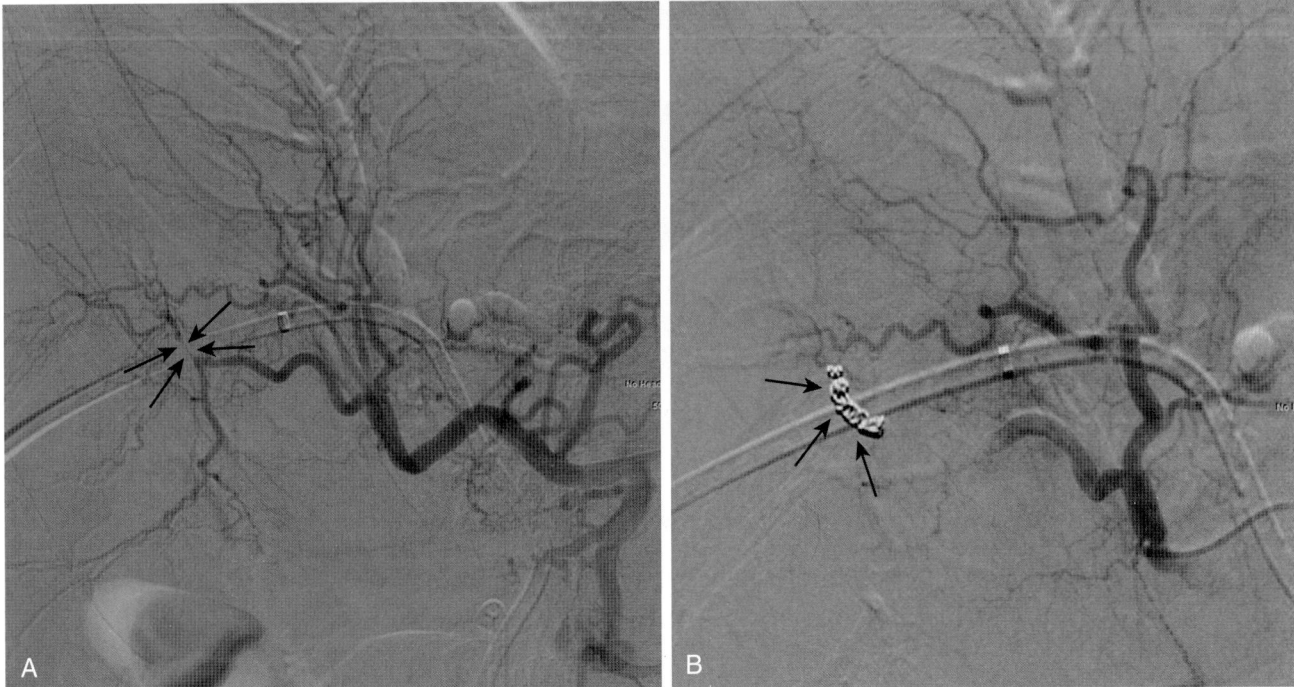

FIGURE 52.13   A, Proper hepatic angiogram in patient with hemobilia and bleeding around biliary drainage catheter 1 week after drainage. Note spasm of right hepatic artery branch *(arrows)* adjacent to catheter at site of duct puncture. **B,** Right hepatic angiogram after coil embolization *(arrows)* of right hepatic artery branch.

level of obstruction. Anything that impedes the flow of bile from above the obstruction, either through the catheter to below the obstruction or into a drainage bag, will result in bile leaking back along an established tract. For a properly positioned catheter with an appropriate number of sideholes, the problem is typically related to catheter occlusion and is remedied by catheter exchange. Patients with capped internal-external catheters may have bile leak back along the catheter tract when egress of bile is obstructed internally. Distal sidehole occlusion is the most common cause, and this problem is easily remedied initially by opening the catheter to gravity drainage and then definitively by catheter exchange. Patients with duodenal obstruction or impaired small bowel motility may be relegated to obligate external drainage.

Ascites may leak around the catheter and may be mistaken for bile. This happens in patients with jaundice, when the ascitic fluid is bile colored. Leaking of ascites can be difficult to manage. The best treatment is to establish internal biliary drainage with stent placement as expeditiously as possible. If the patient cannot be stented, the catheter may be upsized to tamponade the site more effectively, but eventually the leak will recur. Ascites can be tapped frequently or drained by a Tenckhoff catheter in an attempt to allow time for tract maturation. These

strategies often fail eventually, and as a last resort, a stoma device is placed around the entry site to contain the ascites.

SUMMARY

Treatment of malignant high bile duct obstruction presents unique challenges to the interventional radiologist. The outcome depends on the condition of the underlying hepatic parenchyma, the degree of isolation of the biliary tree, and the technical skills of the operator. A thorough understanding of functional biliary anatomy and the availability of high-quality imaging are necessary to optimize outcome. Although pruritus may be palliated by draining even one segment of the liver, lowering the serum bilirubin to normal or near normal is best achieved by draining at least 30% of the liver, assuming the underlying parenchyma is relatively normal. Contamination of undrained parts of the biliary tree may result from drainage catheter placement, with ongoing or recurrent cholangitis becoming a problem. For this reason, primary stent placement should be considered when 30% or more of the liver can be drained at the initial procedure.

References are available at expertconsult.com.

PART 6

Pancreatic Disease

SECTION I. Inflammatory, Infective, and Congenital

A. Congenital Disorders

CHAPTER 53

Congenital disorders of the pancreas: Surgical considerations

Ewen M. Harrison and Rowan W. Parks

The pancreas is a glandular organ that lies on the posterior abdominal wall in the retroperitoneum (see Chapter 2) It is an exocrine gland that secretes enzymes of digestion into the duodenum; it also performs endocrine functions, producing insulin, glucagon, somatostatin, pancreatic polypeptide, and ghrelin (see Chapter 3) Congenital abnormalities of the pancreas may be so severe that they are diagnosed in utero or in the neonatal period, such as pancreatic agenesis. However, many congenital conditions go undetected until adulthood, when the patient comes to medical attention with nonspecific symptoms or an abnormality is discovered incidentally. This chapter describes the diagnosis, investigation, and treatment of the various congenital pancreatic abnormalities.

EMBRYOLOGIC DEVELOPMENT OF THE PANCREAS

The basis for the understanding of congenital abnormalities of the pancreas is the embryologic development of the organ (see Chapter 1). The pancreas develops from two buds originating from the endodermal lining of the duodenum. The dorsal bud forms posteriorly within the mesentery, whereas the ventral bud is associated with the hepaticopancreatic duct (Fig. 53.1). During the second month of development, the stomach rotates and the duodenum becomes C-shaped. As part of this process, the ventral pancreatic bud migrates dorsally, coming to lie postero-inferiorly to the dorsal bud, forming what will become the inferior head/uncinate process of the pancreas. In the majority of individuals, the main pancreatic duct (of Wirsung) is formed by the entire ventral duct and the distal dorsal duct and enters the duodenum at the major papilla. Persistence of the proximal part of the dorsal duct occurs in approximately 25% and results in an accessory duct (of Santorini), which enters the duodenum by the minor papilla (see Fig. 53.1).[1] There is no known pathologic consequence of this normal variation. Failure of fusion of the ductal system occurs in roughly 10% of the normal population,[2,3] resulting in the entire dorsal pancreas—superior head, body, and tail—draining through the minor papilla, and ventral pancreas—the inferior head and uncinate process—draining through the major papilla (Fig. 53.2). This abnormality is termed *pancreas divisum* (PD) and is described in more detail later (see Chapter 1).

Annular pancreas is a rare congenital abnormality, the embryologic basis of which is poorly understood. A complete or incomplete ring of pancreatic tissue is found around the second part of the duodenum, and it may cause symptoms (also discussed later). A number of published studies have identified mechanisms by which the pancreas is specified from the early endoderm.[4] Retinoic acid and bone morphogenic peptide both appear to have important roles in defining early endodermal compartments in the embryo.[5,6] The origins of the signaling mechanisms involved in the specification of the dorsal and ventral pancreas are different.[7] In the dorsal pancreas, signals arising from the notochord[8] and dorsal aorta[9] are required; in the ventral pancreas, the lateral plate mesoderm is important.[10] The specific identity of these signals has not yet been established, although the Hedgehog family of signaling molecules appears to be significant.[11]

PANCREAS DIVISUM

PD results from incomplete fusion of the dorsal and ventral pancreatic ducts toward the end of the second month of embryogenesis. The distal dorsal pancreatic duct typically fuses with the ventral pancreatic duct to drain the entire pancreas into the duodenum by the major papilla (see Chapter 1). The proximal dorsal duct can persist as an accessory pancreatic duct and may drain by the minor papilla. Complete PD exists when there is no communication between the dorsal and ventral systems and the majority of the pancreas drains by the dorsal duct through the minor papilla (see Fig. 53.2). Variations exist in which a small branch may connect the two ducts, termed *incomplete pancreas divisum*. The prevalence of this variant is about 15%.[12–14]

Investigations have suggested that PD may be explained by distinct patterns of incomplete fusion of branches of the dorsal and ventral pancreatic ducts,[12] confirming theories first proposed in early anatomic studies.[2] The first description of PD is from 1865, attributed to Josef Hyrtl[15] (1810–1894), Professor of Anatomy at the Universities of Prague and Vienna. However, as discussed by Stern (1986),[16] a number of anatomists were aware of it much earlier than this, including Regnier de Graaf, who described the finding in 1664.

In postmortem studies performed throughout the 20th century, the prevalence of PD is reported to be approximately 8%

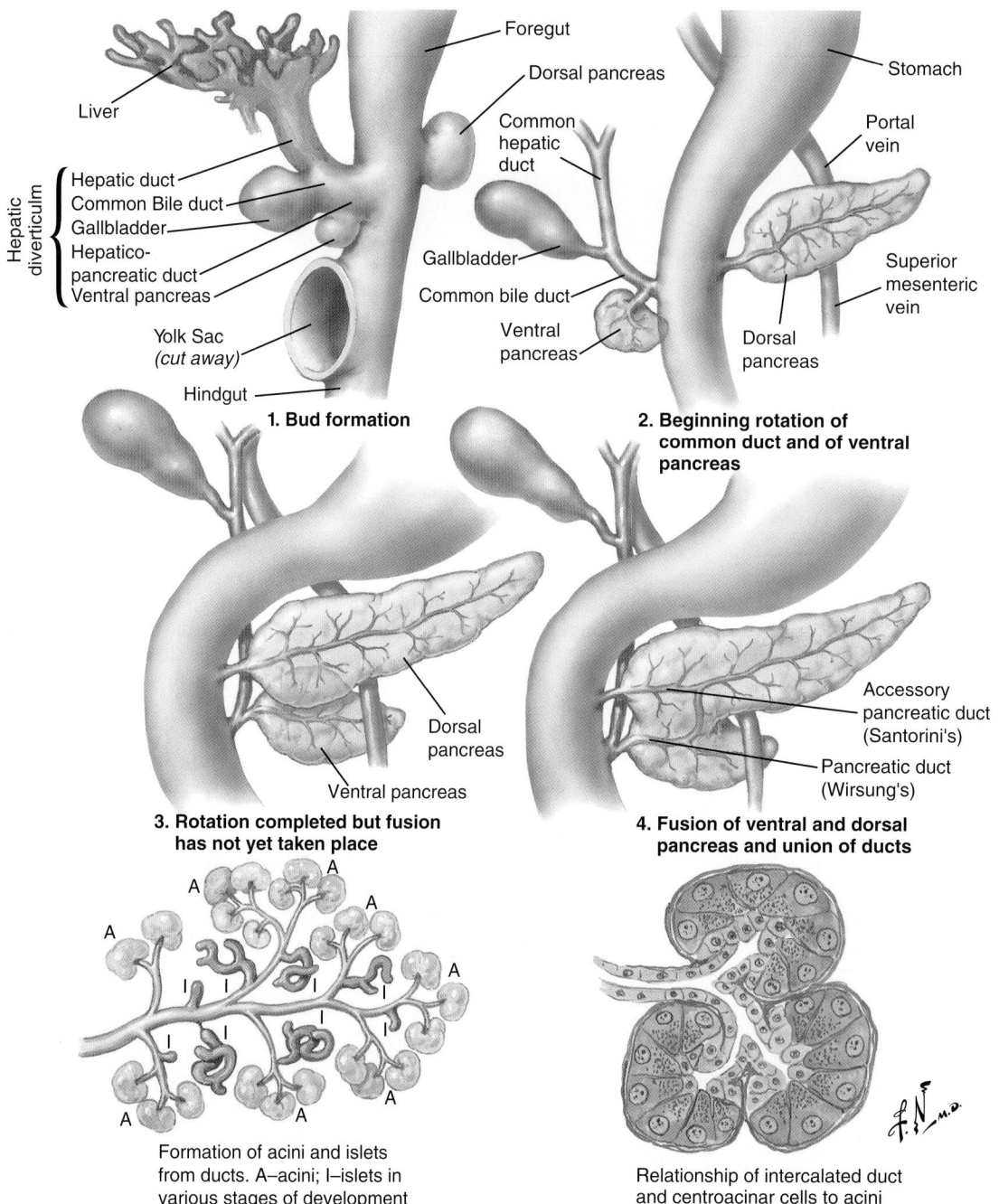

Liver

Foregut

Dorsal pancreas

Stomach

Hepatic duct

Common
hepatic
duct

Portal
vein

Common Bile duct

Gallbladder

Hepatico-
pancreatic duct

Ventral pancreas

Gallbladder

Superior
mesenteric
vein

Hepatic diverticulum

Common bile duct

Yolk Sac
(cut away)

Ventral
pancreas

Dorsal
pancreas

Hindgut

1. Bud formation

**2. Beginning rotation of
common duct and of ventral
pancreas**

Accessory
pancreatic duct
(Santorini's)

Dorsal
pancreas

Pancreatic duct
(Wirsung's)

Ventral pancreas

**3. Rotation completed but fusion
has not yet taken place**

**4. Fusion of ventral and dorsal
pancreas and union of ducts**

Formation of acini and islets
from ducts. A–acini; I–islets in
various stages of development

Relationship of intercalated duct
and centroacinar cells to acini

FIGURE 53.1 Embryologic development of the pancreas. (See Chapter 1.) (Netter illustration from http://www.netterimages.com. Copyright Elsevier, Inc. All rights reserved.)

(range, 4%–14.5%).[17–37] With the development of endoscopic retrograde cholangiopancreatography (ERCP, see Chapters 20 and 30) in the late 1960s, however, the considerable congenital variation in the ductal system of the pancreas became more widely appreciated.[38–41] The prevalence of PD is lower in published ERCP series than in anatomic series for reasons that are not clear, although it may be due to referral bias, difficulty in the interpretation of pancreatograms, or inability to cannulate the minor papilla. The reported prevalence is particularly low in Asian series (0.3%–0.6%) compared with Western populations (~5%).[41–43]

PD is clinically relevant for three reasons.[22] First, the small ventral duct seen in PD must be differentiated from a similar appearance seen in some cases of pancreatic cancer. It is important for those performing ERCP to be aware of the anomaly to become proficient in interpreting pancreatograms (Fig. 53.3). Other forms of imaging, such as computed tomography (CT) or magnetic resonance imaging, must be used if there is uncertainty whether a mass lesion is present and causing a ductal abnormality (see Chapter 17). Second, on cannulating the major papilla at ERCP, only the ventral portion of the pancreas may be visualized in PD, which risks missing important pathologic conditions if a pancreatogram is not performed via the minor papilla (see Chapters 20 and 30). It is important to become proficient at cannulation of the minor papilla, which is considerably more challenging than cannulating the major papilla. The minor papilla commonly sits in a superior, more ventral position. Cannulation may be facilitated by having the duodenoscope in the "long position" and by administration of intravenous secretin.[44] Third, PD may be associated with pancreatitis or other pathologic condition (see Chapters 54 and 55), and this will be discussed in detail in this chapter.

Possible Association Between Pancreas Divisum and Pancreatitis

The question of whether PD causes recurrent acute pancreatitis, chronic pancreatitis, or pancreas-related pain has been debated for many years (Table 53.1). An up-to-date systematic review concluded that "current research fails to define a clear association between PD and pancreatic disease."[45] Those proposing the theory suggest that obstruction occurs at the level of the minor papilla, the caliber of which is too narrow to provide adequate drainage of the pancreatic secretions. This is supported by an early study reporting an elevated pressure in the dorsal duct (23.7 ± 1.3 mm Hg) compared with the ventral duct (10.8 ± 1.9 mm Hg) in six patients with PD, whereas pressures were similar when two ducts existed in patients without PD.[46] This

was contradicted in a subsequent study in which no difference in duct pressures was observed between the major and minor papillae in four patients with recurrent acute pancreatitis and PD.[47] Another early report demonstrated chronic pancreatitis confined to the dorsal pancreas in two pancreatoduodenectomy specimens from patients with PD who had resections for symptom control[48] (see Chapters 54 and 55).

Difficulty exists in demonstrating an epidemiologic relationship between PD and pancreatitis because early anatomic studies were small and confounded by differing definitions, and ERCP series have been skewed by selection bias.[48] In the largest early series of 1850 successful major ampulla cannulations, Rösch et al.[1] identified PD in 63 cases (3.4%). The indications for pancreatography were not given, but pathologic findings were seen in 13 of 63 patients with PD; changes were consistent with pancreatitis in 12 patients and tumor in 1 patient. In another large series by Gregg,[50] 33 patients with PD were identified among 1100 patients (3%) referred primarily for investigation of pancreatic-type pain or pancreatitis. Documented pancreatitis was present in 15 patients, and another 11 had recurrent episodes of pain typical of pancreatitis.

These and similar studies have been used as evidence of a link between PD and pancreatitis, but the absence of a suitable control group makes the assertion weak. Mitchell et al.[52] identified this problem and performed a retrospective analysis of patients who had undergone ERCP and observed that 21 (4.7%) of 449 patients had PD, whereas 4 (3.3%) of 120 patients with pancreatitis defined by clinical and/or ERCP criteria had PD. Thus, in this series, the prevalence of PD in patients with pancreatitis was the same as the prevalence of PD in the series as a whole. This has been supported by the largest published ERCP series of 304 patients, in which the dorsal duct was visualized in 97 patients.[58] The frequency of PD was similar in patients with acute or chronic pancreatitis (6.9%) as in all patients in the series undergoing ERCP (5.7%).

Contrary to these findings, Cotton[42] reported that in patients with primary biliary disease who had an incidental pancreatogram at the time of endoscopic retrograde cholangiogram, the prevalence of PD was 3.6%. This was compared with a prevalence of 16.4% in those with chronic or recurrent acute

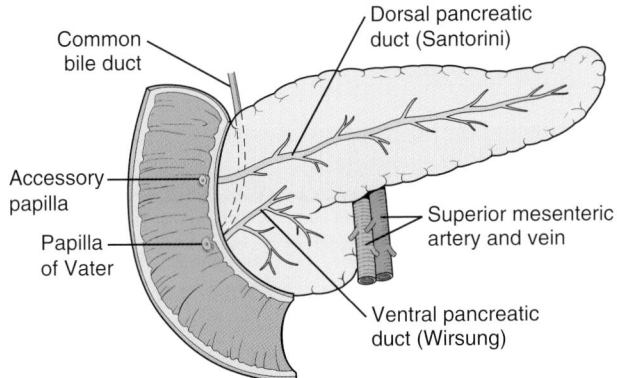

FIGURE 53.2 Pancreas divisum describes the incomplete fusion of the dorsal and ventral pancreatic ducts.

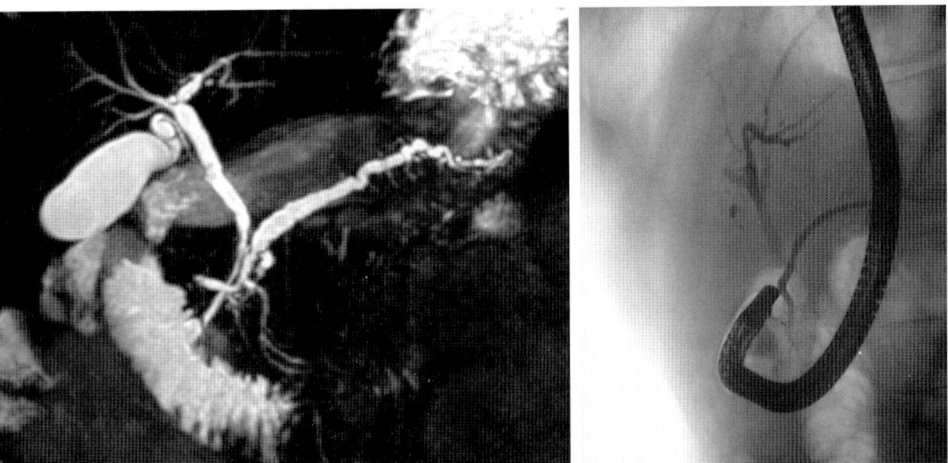

FIGURE 53.3 **Imaging in pancreas divisum (PD).** A magnetic resonance cholangiopancreatography image shows PD with the dorsal pancreatic duct draining through the minor papilla *(left)*. Endoscopic retrograde cholangiopancreatography in PD performed through the minor papilla *(right)*. Contrast can still be seen in the common bile duct after cannulation of the major papilla. (See Chapters 17 and 20.) (Courtesy Dr. K. Palmer, Edinburgh.)

TABLE 53.1 Early Series Reporting Pancreas Divisum

STUDY	PANCREATITIS RELATIONSHIP SUPPORTED	STUDY TYPE	N (%)	INTERVENTION
Phillip J et al., 1974[49]	—	ERCP series	18/911 (2.0)	—
Rösch et al., 1976[1]	—	ERCP series	63/1850 (3.4)	—
Gregg, 1977[50]	—	ERCP series	33/1100 (3.0)	—
Heiss & Shea, 1978[51]	Yes	ERCP series	4	—
Mitchell et al., 1979[52]	No	ERCP series	21/449 (4.7)	—
Cotton, 1980[42]	Yes	ERCP series	47/810 (5.8)	—
Tulassay & Papp, 1980[53]	Yes	ERCP series	33/2410 (1.4)	Unspecified surgery in 11; no outcomes described
Richter et al., 1981[54]	Yes	ERCP series	519	Open sphincteroplasty to minor ampulla in 9; decreased pain: 5/6 with acute pancreatitis, 0/3 with chronic
Thompson et al., 1981[55]	Yes	ERCP series	11/850 (1.3)	—
Cooperman et al., 1982[56]		Case series	21/314 (6.7)	Open sphincteroplasty to minor ampulla in 5; 4 of 6 "have done well" at 28 months
Sahel et al., 1982[57]	Yes	ERCP series	41/812 (5.0)	—
Blair et al., 1984[48]	Yes	Case series	14	15 operative resections in 14 patients with RAP; 7/14 had no pain after surgery
Delhaye et al., 1985[58]	No	ERCP series	304 total; 6.9% AP/CP, 5.7% no pancreatitis	—
Sugawa et al., 1987[59]	No	ERCP series	55/1529 (3.6)	Open sphincteroplasty to minor ampulla in 3; no improvement in symptoms
Bernard et al., 1990[40]	Yes	ERCP series	137/1825 (7.5)	—

AP, Acute pancreatitis; *CP,* chronic pancreatitis; *ERCP,* endoscopic retrograde cholangiopancreatography; *RAP,* recurrent acute pancreatitis.

pancreatitis. In 83 patients with idiopathic pancreatitis, recurrent pancreatitis with no clear cause, such as gallstones, alcohol, or trauma, the prevalence of PD was 25.6%.

This controversy is a good example of the difficulty in determining a causal relationship between two factors that appear to have a clinical association. The traditional criteria used in evaluating such a relationship can be applied: (1) strength of association, (2) consistency across studies, (3) dose-response relationship, and (4) biologic plausibility. The relationship is not a strong one, and many of those in the general population who have PD (~10%) never have any related symptoms, and many with pancreatitis do not have PD; less than 5% of individuals with PD are estimated to ever develop pancreatic symptoms. Furthermore, those with a more pronounced form of the anomaly (i.e., complete PD) do not seem to be more likely to develop pancreatitis than those with incomplete PD.

Imaging in Pancreas Divisum

One of the difficulties in relating PD to pancreatitis is the inconsistency in making the diagnosis. ERCP studies of patients without pancreatitis consistently report a lower prevalence of PD when compared with magnetic resonance cholangiopancreatography (MRCP) or postmortem studies (Table 53.2) (see Chapters 17, 20, and 30). The use of secretin during MRCP (S-MRCP) improves the detection rate of PD,[60] yet it is still reported to be missed on S-MRCP, possibly because of suboptimal magnetic resonance techniques or inexperience of those reporting the MRCP (see Chapter 19).[61] A more recent study reported the use of portal venous phase 64–multidetector-row CT (MDCT). Of 93 patients, 5 had PD diagnosed on MRCP or ERCP. Of these, one observer detected three cases, and a second observer found four cases by reviewing the MDCT images.[62] ERCP features of the minor papilla that suggest the

TABLE 53.2 Prevalence of Pancreas Divisum in Patients Without Pancreatitis by Method of Investigation or Imaging Modality

INVESTIGATION TYPE	N	% PREVALENCE OF PD (95% CI)
Postmortem	2895	7.8 (6.8-8.8)
MRCP	505	9.3 (6.8-11.8)
S-MRCP	156	17.9 (11.9-24.0)
ERCP	16,078	4.1 (3.8-4.4)

CI, Confidence interval; *ERCP,* endoscopic retrograde cholangiopancreatography; *MRCP,* magnetic resonance cholangiopancreatography; *PD,* pancreas divisum; *S-MRCP,* secretin-enhanced MRCP; cholangiopancreatography.

From Fogel EL, et al: Does endoscopic therapy favorably affect the outcome of patients who have recurrent acute pancreatitis and pancreas divisum? *Pancreas.* 2007;34:21–45.

presence of PD include an enlarged papilla or open orifice and are thought to moderately predict the presence of PD; however, a significant number of patients with PD do not have these features.[63,64] Endoscopic ultrasound (EUS) as an alternative imaging modality has gained in popularity and is reported to be useful in the investigation of patients with acute recurrent pancreatitis of unknown cause (see Chapter 22).[65] The sensitivity of EUS for PD has been shown to be 85% to 95%,[65–67] which was superior to the sensitivity of CT (50%–60%)[69,70] or MRCP (50%–70%),[61,71–73] but similar to that with secretin-enhanced MRCP (83%–86%).[74,75]

Therapy to the Minor Papilla in Those With Pancreas Divisum and Pancreatitis

If PD is associated with obstruction at the minor papilla, which in turn contributes to the occurrence of pancreatitis and pancreatic pain, it follows that surgical intervention to relieve this obstruction would be beneficial. As has been discussed, significant controversy exists as to whether this assumption is correct. A number of studies have been performed examining whether therapy to the minor papilla is beneficial in patients with acute recurrent pancreatitis, chronic pancreatitis, or pancreas-related pain; however, little in the way of randomized controlled data has been generated (Table 53.3) (see Chapters 54 to 58). Interventions examined include endoscopic dilation; papillotomy; sphincterotomy of the minor papilla, with or without stent placement; and surgical sphincteroplasty.

The first minor papilla endoscopic sphincterotomy was described by Cotton in 1978,[91] and the majority of publications since have been small case series with short follow-up times. Lehman et al.[80] described the effects of minor papilla sphincterotomy in 52 PD patients with chronic pancreatic pain ($n = 24$), recurrent acute pancreatitis ($n = 17$), or chronic pancreatitis ($n = 11$) with long-standing symptoms refractory to conservative management. Minor papilla sphincterotomy was performed with a needle knife over a previously placed dorsal pancreatic duct stent, with a mean follow-up of 1.7 years. When compared with the chronic pain and chronic pancreatitis groups, patients with recurrent acute pancreatitis had a significant reduction in mean symptom score (recurrent acute pancreatitis, 76.5%; chronic pancreatitis, 27.3%; chronic pain, 26.1%) and inpatient hospital stay. This reflects other published results that consistently show less benefit after minor papilla therapy in those with chronic pancreatitis or chronic pain compared with those with recurrent acute pancreatitis. Complications were seen in 15%, and one patient died of a pancreatic abscess after a failed cannulation. Of concern, 50% of patients evaluated at the time of stent removal had stent-induced dorsal duct changes.

In a prospective, randomized, controlled trial published by Lans et al.,[79] 19 patients with PD and recurrent acute pancreatitis—two or more episodes of abdominal pain associated with a rise in amylase greater than twice the upper limit of normal—and no other identified cause were recruited. Of these, 10 patients were randomized to stent placement, and 9 were randomized to no treatment, with observation for 1 year. In the stent group, no patients subsequently came to the hospital with pain, but 5 patients in the control group were admitted, and 2 more came in with pain. Furthermore, 9 patients in the stent group rated their pain improved by 50% or more, but only 1 patient in the control group reported a similar improvement.

It has been pointed out that a significant period of time can exist between attacks of pancreatitis in this patient group, and this study has since been criticized on the basis of the short duration of observation. Sherman et al.[82] have also published randomized data in abstract form in which patients with chronic abdominal pain thought to be pancreatic in origin and PDs were randomized to minor papilla sphincterotomy ($n = 16$) or no intervention ($n = 17$). Mean observation time in the treated and untreated groups was 2.1 and 1.2 years, respectively. Although an improvement in pain was seen in 43.8% of treated patients compared with 23.5% in the control group, this trend did not reach statistical significance.

Borak et al[90] published the long-term outcomes after endoscopic minor papilla therapy in 145 patients with PD over a 6-year period. Follow-up data were available for 113 patients (78%), and the median observation time was 43 months. The majority of patients had a needle-knife sphincterotomy (82%) and temporary stent placement (90%). Primary success, defined as the patient being better or cured after a single ERCP session, was seen in 53.2% of patients with recurrent acute pancreatitis, 18.2% of those with chronic pancreatitis, and 41.4% of those with chronic/recurrent epigastric pain. Two or more ERCP sessions were required in 41.6%, with success in

TABLE 53.3	Endoscopic Therapy to the Minor Papilla in Pancreas Divisum							
		MEAN FOLLOW-UP	**RAP**		**PAIN ONLY**		**CP**	
STUDY	**THERAPY**	**(mo)**	**N**	**% IMPROVED**	**N**	**% IMPROVED**	**N**	**% IMPROVED**
Soehendra et al., 1986[76]	MiES	3	2	100	0	—	4	75
Liguory et al., 1986[77]	MiES	24	8	63	0	—	0	—
McCarthy et al., 1988[78]	Stent	21	19	89	0	—	0	—
Lans et al., 1992[79]	Stent	30	10	90	0	—	0	—
Lehman et al., 1993[80]	MiES	22	17	76	23	26	11	27
Coleman et al., 1994[81]	MiES/stent	23	9	78	5	0	20	60
Sherman et al., 1994[82] (RCT)	MiES	28	0	—	16	44	0	—
Kozarek et al., 1995[83]	MiES/stent	20	15	73	5	20	19	32
Ertan, 2000[84]	Stent	24	25	76	0	—	0	—
Heyries et al., 2002[85]	MiES/stent	39	24	92	0	—	0	—
Linder et al., 2003a[86]	Stent	NG (range, 3-36)	83	66	48	23	38	38
Bierig et al., 2006[87]	MiES	19	16	94	7	43	16	38
Linder et al., 2003b[88]	MiES	NG (range, 1-120)	38	58	12	0	4	25
Vitale et al., 2007[89]	Stent	59.6	—	—	—	—	24*	58
Borak et al., 2009[90]	MiES/stent	43	62	71	29	62	22	46
Total		**25**	**328**	**77**	**145**	**33**	**135**	**41**

*11 patients required open surgery.

CP, Chronic pancreatitis; *MiES*, minor papilla sphincterotomy; *NG*, not given; *RAP*, recurrent acute pancreatitis; *RCT*, randomized, controlled trial.

From Fogel EL, et al. Does endoscopic therapy favorably affect the outcome of patients who have recurrent acute pancreatitis and pancreas divisum? *Pancreas* 34:21–45, 2007.

71% of patients with recurrent acute pancreatitis, 46% of those with chronic pancreatitis, and 55% of those with chronic, recurrent epigastric pain. In a multivariate analysis that corrected for age, sex, symptom frequency/duration, and length of observation, chronic pancreatitis and younger age both independently predicted failure of improvement after treatment. Complications occurred in 13% after ERCP, including mild and moderate pancreatitis, mild bleeding, and anesthetic complications.

Surgical sphincteroplasty to the minor papilla, usually combined with cholecystectomy and major papilla sphincteroplasty, has been used in the treatment of recurrent acute pancreatitis, chronic pancreatitis, and chronic pancreatic-type pain associated with PD (see Chapter 117D) (Table 53.4). In the largest published series by Warshaw et al.,[92] 88 patients with recurrent acute pancreatitis (49%) or "pancreatic pain" (51%) had minor papilla sphincteroplasty with a mean observation of 53 months; 70% of patients were reported to show improvement, 85% if the minor papilla was stenotic at surgery, compared with 27% if it was not ($P < .01$). Of those with recurrent acute pancreatitis, 82% were reported to have improved compared with 56% in the chronic pain group ($P < .01$). Preoperative ultrasonography (US) with secretin stimulation was compared with examination of the minor papilla and had a sensitivity of 78% and a specificity of 97%. Thus preoperative US with secretin stimulation was judged to be a good predictor of surgical success (92% success if positive, 40% success if negative). Seven patients were documented to have developed a restenosis at the minor papilla, six of whom had further surgery. The study concluded that a demonstrable stenosis at the minor papilla was a necessary cofactor in the development of recurrent acute pancreatitis or pancreatic pain in patients with PD.

Surgical sphincteroplasty is not without risk, however. In a recent large series of 446 patients, complications were reported in 34.8% of patients; pancreatitis (8.8%), asymptomatic hyperamylasemia (6.0%), and wound/abdominal infection (7.1%) were the most common morbidities. One death occurred after a duodenal leak.[101]

A recent study evaluated the question of whether children with acute recurrent pancreatitis or chronic pancreatitis should be treated differently? In this report, 38 pediatric patients were presented in whom 74 ERCPs were performed.[102] The frequency of pancreatitis episodes decreased significantly (from 2.31 to 0.45) during a median 41-month observations period. The authors concluded that therapeutic ERCP may be useful in this population.

Resection in Those With Pancreas Divisum and Pancreatitis

The place of duodenum-preserving pancreatic head resection and longitudinal pancreaticojejunostomy (Frey procedure) for painful chronic pancreatitis associated with PD has been presented elsewhere[103] (see Chapter 58). In this study, 14 patients (6 PD, 5 alcohol, and 3 idiopathic) who underwent a Frey procedure for chronic pancreatitis and disease-related intractable pain were compared. The series is clearly small, but outcomes for those with PD treated with the Frey procedure were equivalent to those with other etiologies. The authors commented on the potential advantage of this approach over minor duct sphincteroplasty as lateral pancreaticojejunostomy is associated with removal of the fibrotic tissue of the head of the pancreas,

the potential origin of the pain. It was pointed out in the accompanying editorial that PD patients with abdominal pain but no evidence of chronic pancreatitis were unlikely to benefit from this approach.[104]

The Case Against an Association Between Pancreas Divisum and Pancreatitis

Those making the case against an association between PD and pancreatitis begin by highlighting problems with the epidemiologic studies. It is argued that in ERCP series, the true incidence of PD is underdiagnosed. This is supported by autopsy studies that demonstrate the prevalence of PD to be approximately 10%, whereas ERCP series show it to be less than 5%. It is argued that if ERCP were able to accurately diagnose PD, then its prevalence in control and pancreatitis groups would be the same. Patients in groups used as controls often only have cholangiography and do not undergo intentional pancreatography. Pancreatitis patients, on the other hand, have the pancreatic ducts imaged intentionally; therefore PD may be diagnosed more accurately. Furthermore, the ERCP prevalence of PD in pancreatitis patients is the same as the prevalence of PD in the general population in autopsy studies (7.6% vs. 7.8%). The argument therefore follows that if ERCP accurately diagnosed PD in the general population, no difference would exist.

An argument is also made against the theory of minor papilla obstruction. It is argued that patients with pancreatitis secondary to PD should have a dilated ductal system, but this has not been shown to be the case in the majority of studies.[22] Similarly, if pancreatitis were associated with PD, only the dorsal pancreas should be affected, yet ventral duct pancreatitis is present in up to 11.8% of patients with PD and is the only duct involved in 4.2% of patients.

Cystic Fibrosis and Recurrent Pancreatitis

Cohn et al.[105] and Sharer et al.[106] first described the link between cystic fibrosis gene mutations and idiopathic pancreatitis (see Chapters 3 and 54 to 57). More recently, Choudari[107] demonstrated that mutations of the cystic fibrosis transmembrane conductance regulator (CFTR) gene were present in 8 (22%) of 37 patients with PD and pancreatitis compared with 0 of 20 patients with PD and no history of pancreatitis (odds ratio, 11.8; confidence interval [CI], 8.9 to 14.7; $P = .02$). The authors concluded that in patients with PD, CFTR mutations increased the risk for pancreatitis. Furthermore, Gelrud et al.[108] directly measured CFTR gene function in nasal epithelium in response to isoproterenol and demonstrated that those with PD and recurrent acute pancreatitis had results somewhere between those observed for healthy controls and those for classic cystic fibrosis patients. Thus CFTR dysfunction may explain why some PD patients have recurrent acute pancreatitis but others with PD do not. Moreover, of 12 patients with PD and recurrent acute pancreatitis, 10 had undergone therapy to the minor papilla, and only 2 had resolution of their symptoms. Finally, Bertin et al.[109] evaluated the presence of PD with MRCP in 40 patients with idiopathic pancreatitis. The frequency of PD was 7% in those without pancreatic disease, 7% in those with alcohol-induced pancreatitis, and 5% in those with idiopathic pancreatitis. However, PD was seen in 47% of those with CFTR-associated pancreatitis, and further associations between other functional genetic anomalies were demonstrated (SPINK1, PRSS1). The authors propose that although

TABLE 53.4 Surgical Therapy in Pancreas Divisum

STUDY	TOTAL (N)	PATIENTS IMPROVED (%)*	RAP		PAIN ALONE†		CP‡		RESTENOSIS	MAJOR COMPLICATIONS	DEATHS	MEAN FOLLOW-UP (mo)
			N	PATIENTS IMPROVED (%)	N	PATIENTS IMPROVED (%)	N	PATIENTS IMPROVED (%)				
Warshaw et al., 1990[92]	88	77	43	82	45	56	0	0	7/88	1/88	0	53
Brenner et al., 1990[93]	13	54	10	70	3	0	0	0	0/13	0/13	0	18
Cooperman et al., 1982[56]	4	75	4	75	0	0	0	0	1/4	NG	0	14
Bragg et al., 1988[94]	4	100	3	100	1	100	0	0	0/4	NG	0	21
Rusnak et al., 1988[95]	4	75	NG	—	NG	—	NG	—	1/4	0/4	0	≈48
Madura, 1986[96]	32	75	11	82	19	68	2	0	NG	3/32	0	31
Britt et al., 1983[97]	5§	60	4	75	0	0	1	0	1/5	NG	0	21
Russell et al., 1984[98]	7	71	NG	—	NG	—	NG	—	1/7	NG	0	8
Gregg et al., 1983[99]	19	53	NG	—	NG	—	NG	—	1/19	1/19	1	NG
Keith et al., 1989[100]	22§	86	13	100	8	75	1	0	1/22	2/22	0	53

All series used sphincteroplasty, except that by Keith et al.,[100] which performed sphincterotomy alone.

*Includes patients graded excellent, good, and fair (if more than 50% improved and off opioids).

†Pain suggestive of pancreatic origin (generally epigastric with back radiation) without serologic, ultrasound, computed tomographic scan, or ductographic evidence of pancreatitis.

‡Some patients had a history of heavy alcohol ingestion.

§Plus one patient who did not respond to minor papilla identification at laparotomy.

CP, Chronic pancreatitis; RAP, recurrent acute pancreatitis; NG, not given.

From Fogel EL, et al: Does endoscopic therapy favorably affect the outcome of patients who have recurrent acute pancreatitis and pancreas divisum? Pancreas. 2007;34:21–45.

the frequency of PD was not different in patients with idiopathic pancreatitis compared with control patients, the frequency of PD was higher in those with genetic pancreatitis, suggesting a cumulative effect of these two factors.

Summary

Despite the association of pancreatitis and PD being described in the 1970s, significant controversy continues regarding whether a causal relationship exists. Although many case series report the benefit of therapy to the minor papilla in patients with PD and pancreatitis, a lack of randomized, controlled data means interpretation of these studies must be guarded. At best, careful case selection is paramount before embarking on any such therapy. Patients most likely to benefit are older, have documented recurrent acute pancreatitis, and have been thoroughly investigated for a recognized cause of pancreatitis. Those with chronic pancreatitis or pancreas-type pain are much less likely to benefit. Recurrence of symptoms is common, and repeat therapy involving the minor ampulla may be required. More recent data showing an association between functional genetic anomalies and PD may begin to explain why few patients with PD experience pancreatitis. Genetic testing in those with symptomatic PD is likely to become more commonplace.

ANNULAR PANCREAS

Annular pancreas is a rare congenital abnormality in which the head of the pancreas completely encircles the second part of the duodenum (Fig. 53.4) (see Chapter 1). It was first described in 1862 by Ecker,[110] who reported a "ring derived from the head of the pancreas which surrounded the descending portion of the duodenum and was formed by uninterrupted glandular tissue."[110,111] The prevalence in autopsy studies is approximately 3 in 20,000[111] but is higher in patients undergoing

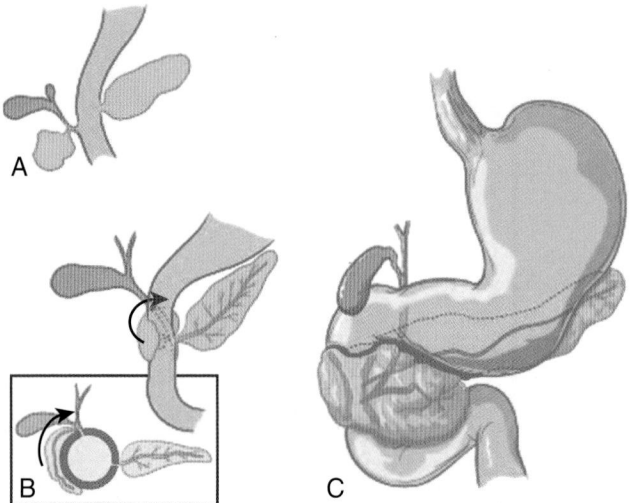

FIGURE 53.4 Embryologic development of annular pancreas. **A,** Dorsal and ventral buds of the gut tube at about 4 weeks of development. **B,** Tethering of the ventral bud tip to the duodenum and rotation lead to a ring of pancreatic tissue encircling the duodenum. **C,** Annular pancreas depicting pancreas divisum, which was present in 29% of adults in this series. (See Chapter 1.) (Modified from Zyromski, et al: Annular pancreas: dramatic differences between children and adults. *J Am Coll Surg.* 2008;206:1019–1025.)

ERCP, at approximately 3 in 1000.[112] Given the difficulty in making the diagnosis during autopsy and the highly selected patient population undergoing ERCP, the true prevalence likely lies somewhere in between.

Pathogenesis

In early development, the ventral pancreas is formed by two buds (see Chapter 1). In mammals, the left ventral pancreatic bud is thought to regress,[9,113] and the larger right ventral pancreatic bud migrates to take up the position seen in the adult. A number of hypotheses have been proposed to explain the occurrence of annular pancreas. The most persistent is that of Lecco,[114] who suggested that adherence of the right ventral pancreatic bud to the duodenum before gut rotation resulted in a partial or complete ring of pancreatic tissue around the duodenum. A competing hypothesis offered by Baldwin[115] postulates that the left ventral bud persists to form the annulus. Although in most annular pancreas specimens, only one ventral lobe is apparent, reports of a bilobar ventral pancreas have surfaced that support Baldwin's theory.[116] Neither of these theories explains the variation in the position of the annular duct seen in various specimens, and Kamisawa et al.[117] proposed a new theory that the tip of the left ventral bud adheres to the duodenum and stretches to form a ring. The exact location of this attachment in relation to the bile duct determines the final arrangement of the annular duct.

Reports of familial annular pancreas support a genetic basis for the disease. Annular pancreas has been described in siblings,[118–120] a mother and three of her children,[121] a mother and son,[122] a mother and daughter,[123,124] and a father and son,[125] and a recent report describes the anomaly in monozygotic twins.[126]

Clues as to the genetic basis of the disease are beginning to emerge. Only recently has it been shown that the cells that form the annulus are derived entirely from the ventral pancreas.[127] In the same report, it was demonstrated that in *Xenopus* embryos, inactivation of transmembrane 4 superfamily member 3 *(TM4SF3),* a member of the tetraspanin family, inhibited fusion of the dorsal and ventral pancreatic buds. Overexpression of the same gene promoted development of annular pancreas. This would suggest that the product of this gene directly regulates the migration of ventral pancreatic bud cells, although whether it plays a role in the formation of annular pancreas in humans remains unknown.

Another recent study has demonstrated a link between the Hedgehog signaling pathway and the development of annular pancreas. Members of the Hedgehog family of genes promote growth and differentiation of organs, and defects are associated with congenital malformations of the foregut.[128] In 42% of mice embryos with a targeted inactivation of the Indian Hedgehog *(IHH)* gene, a member of the mammalian Hedgehog family, changes in the morphology of the ventral pancreatic bud similar to annular pancreas were seen.[129] In most, the annulus was complete, although pancreas cells were not seen within the muscularis of the duodenum, as has been described in humans. Annular pancreas is also frequently seen after inactivation of Sonic Hedgehog *(SHH),* although the incidence of the anomaly is closely related to the background strain of the transgenic mouse, suggesting interaction with other genetic modifiers.[130] *SHH* is not expressed in pancreatic tissue; therefore it has been suggested that a defect in duodenal Hedgehog signaling may lead to the anomaly because both *SHH* and *IHH* are expressed in the developing gut.[129,131] *SHH* knockout mice embryos also demonstrate a number of other abnormalities, including gut malrotation (100%), intestinal transformation of the stomach (100%), duodenal stenosis (67%), and imperforate anus (100%), strikingly similar to congenital malformations seen in humans with annular pancreas (see later).

Clinical Presentation and Diagnosis in Adults

An estimated half to two thirds of cases of annular pancreas in adults remain asymptomatic.[132] Annular pancreas presents with equal frequency in adults and children. In a recent series of 103 patients with annular pancreas, 55 (53.4%) were diagnosed as adults (median age, 47 years), and 48 (46.6%) were diagnosed as children (median age, 1 day).[133] Of those diagnosed as adults, 41 (75%) presented with pain, and 12 (22%) had pancreatitis; only 13 (24%) had gastrointestinal (GI) symptoms that included vomiting, and six (11%) had obstructive jaundice and/or abnormal liver function test results. In addition, 16 patients (29%) were also found to have PD, a higher prevalence than is seen in the general population (see previous section), which may suggest that similar genetic abnormalities link the two conditions. The diagnosis of annular pancreas was made by ERCP in 26 patients (47%), by abdominal CT in 10 patients (18%), by MRCP in 9 patients (16%), and at operation in 7 patients (13%) (Fig. 53.5).[133]

In a recent ERCP series, 39 (85%) of 46 patients with annular pancreas without previous bypass were noted to have duodenal narrowing but retained gastric contents was seen only in 2 of these patients.[134] ERCP was technically successful in 42 of 46 (91%) patients, and PD was found in 21 patients (45.7%), 18 of whom had complete divisum.

Improvements in imaging have led to the identification of incomplete annular pancreas, in which the annulus does not fully encircle the duodenum.[132] The presence of pancreatic tissue on cross-sectional imaging posterolateral to the second part

of the duodenum has a high sensitivity (92%) and specificity (100%) for this condition. Three of nine patients (33%) found to have incomplete annular pancreas on imaging had gastric outlet obstruction.[132]

A number of case reports describe annular pancreatitis in association with neoplasm, most commonly periampullary or pancreatic malignancy, raising the question as to whether annular pancreas predisposes to neoplasia[135-140] (see Chapter 61). In a recent series, a pancreatobiliary neoplasia was the indication for ERCP in 7 of 42 patients (15.2%) found to have annular pancreas.[134]

The adult population in whom annular pancreas is diagnosed is a highly select group with a variety of symptoms. The incidence of annular pancreas is too small to be certain, but it is likely that the association is a result of study bias rather than pathogenesis. What should be remembered is that the symptoms of a patient diagnosed with annular pancreas are not necessarily secondary to the annular pancreas; a second condition may be present. For instance, annular pancreas rarely manifests with obstructive jaundice; therefore, when a patient with obstructive jaundice is found to have annular pancreas, a high index of suspicion for an underlying malignancy must be maintained.

Clinical Presentation and Diagnosis in Children

A significant difference between the adult and pediatric populations with annular pancreas is the prevalence of associated congenital abnormalities in children. The majority of children with annular pancreas show evidence of the condition in the first days after birth. In a recent series of 16 patients, 12 (75%) came to medical attention during the first week of life, one during the first month, and the remainder within the first year (Table 53.5).[141] If complete duodenal obstruction is present, polyhydramnios will usually be a feature; primary biliary obstruction and jaundice are not typical.[142]

Preampullary obstruction resulting in nonbilious vomiting has been reported to be more common in annular pancreas than in other causes of duodenal obstruction (94% vs. 10%).[141,144] In the series by Zyromski et al.[133] 27 (56%) of 48 children with annular pancreas were suspected to have the condition based on prenatal US, and the remainder were seen with GI obstruction, 37 (77%) of whom were diagnosed within the first two days of life; 34 (71%) children with annular pancreas were reported to have at least one other congenital abnormality, the most common being trisomy 21 (Down syndrome), seen in 10 (21%) children. GI abnormalities included intestinal malrotation in 10 of the 48 children (21%), tracheoesophageal fistula in four (8.3%), and 1 each of mobile right colon, omphalocele, nonrotation, duodenal atresia, and situs inversus. In addition, 10 children (21%) had significant cardiac anomalies, and genitourinary abnormalities were seen in 5 children (10%).

Diagnosis was made in a similar way in both the Jimenez and Zyromski series; plain abdominal radiographs showed the "double-bubble" sign or air in the stomach and first part of the duodenum, in 14 (88%) of 16 and 30 (63%) of 48 patients, respectively. Upper GI contrast was used in 9 (56%) of 16 and 9 (19%) of 48 patients, respectively, and neonatal ultrasonography was used in 3 infants (6%) of 48 in the Zyromski series only.

Therapy for Annular Pancreas

A review of the existing literature published in 1980 concluded that "while there is no single operative procedure of choice,

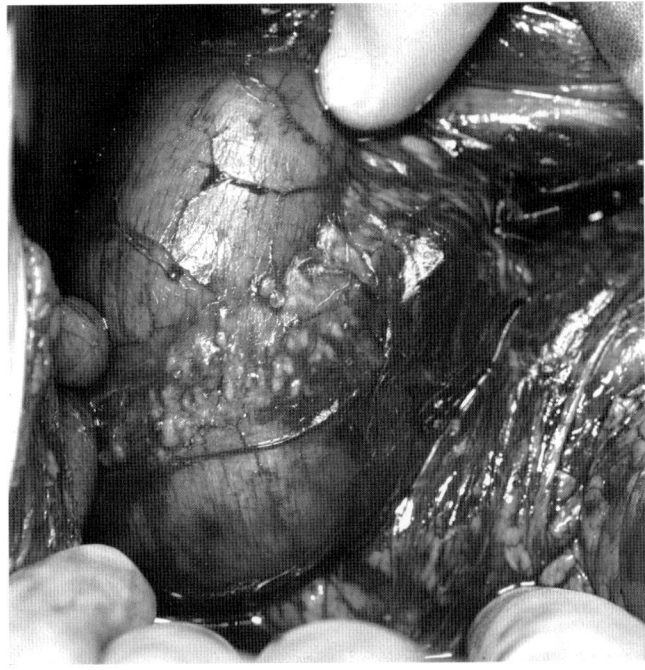

FIGURE 53.5 Annular pancreas.

TABLE 53.5 Annular Pancreas Case Series

STUDY	NO.	SEX (% MALE)	NEONATAL PRESENTATION (%)	PREMATURITY (%)	CHROMOSOMAL ABNORMALITIES (%)	MAJOR CONGENITAL ABNORMALITIES (%)	PREAMPULLARY OBSTRUCTION (%)	COMPLETE OBSTRUCTION (%)	SURVIVAL (%)
Kiesewetter & Koop, 1954[143]	6	67	83	NR	17	33	NR	3	17
Hays et al., 1961[144]	7	NR	100	29	29	43	100	NR	57
Merrill & Raffensperger, 1976[142]	24	38	96	NR	29	54	NR	54	75
Kiernan et al., 1980[145]	6	67	100	NR	17	NR	NR	NR	67
Sencan et al., 2002[146]	7	29	100	14	14	14	0	43	100
Current series	16	69	81	23	31	38	94	33	100

NR, Not reported.

From Jimenez JC, et al: Annular pancreas in children: a recent decade's experience. *J Pediatr Surg.* 2004;39:1654–1657.

experience dictates against any direct attack on the offending annulus."[145] This conclusion stands, and any attempt to divide the annulus itself risks the formation of a pancreatic fistula. Early pediatric series established duodenal bypass as the treatment of choice, although mortality rates remained high, likely related to the presence of other congenital malformations and the lack of supportive care.[142–144] Duodenoduodenostomy has replaced duodenojejunostomy as the treatment of choice because it has a lower incidence of postoperative complications, particularly obstruction and blind-loop syndromes.[141] Before the procedure, care should be given to ensure adequate fluid replacement and correction of electrolyte abnormalities. A right upper quadrant incision gives excellent access, and a full examination should be performed to exclude other congenital abnormalities. An end-to-end or side-to-side duodenoduodenostomy should be performed, ensuring adequate mobilization of proximal and distal ends. Where the first part of the duodenum is distended, a tapering duodenoplasty or plication can be performed, although this may not always be required. Consideration should be given to the placement of a gastrostomy tube; however, this should be reserved for those patients who are likely to have long-term problems, such as those with complex GI malformations or chromosomal abnormalities. An enteral feeding tube is often useful and allows early feeding to be commenced.

A recent series of 11 neonates described laparoscopic diagnosis and treatment of annular pancreas.[147] All of the patients presented with bilious vomiting and had the double-bubble sign on plain radiograph. A laparoscopic duodenal "diamond" anastomosis was performed in all patients, some of whom had additional procedures for other congenital abnormalities. One patient with the complication of anal atresia died of pneumonia 6 months after the procedure, but the other patients continue to do well. The laparoscopic approach for annular pancreas is clearly a highly technical procedure, but the early results suggest it can be performed successfully in the neonatal period.

More generally, outcomes after surgery have improved markedly, with early mortality rates decreasing from 83% in the 1950s[143] to less than 10% in most recent series.[133,141] These improvements are largely secondary to improved surgical decision making, advances in operative technique, and advances in neonatal intensive care and anesthesia. Deaths in contemporary series are usually attributed to severe associated congenital anomalies.

In the series from Zyromski, 35 of 55 (63%) adults were reported to have had surgical therapy for symptoms related to annular pancreas. Duodenal bypass was performed in 13 adult patients (24%) compared with 100% of the children. Adults also underwent a number of other surgical procedures, including cholecystectomy, pancreatoduodenectomy, pancreatic sphincteroplasty, lateral pancreatojejunostomy, hepaticojejunostomy, and biliary sphincteroplasty. Therapeutic ERCP with sphincterotomy/stenting was performed in 37 (67%) of 55 adults.

Summary

Annular pancreas is a rare condition that is being increasingly diagnosed as a consequence of improvements in modern imaging. Children are seen at birth with GI obstruction and often have other congenital abnormalities. Adults come to medical attention with pain or vague upper abdominal symptoms, and diagnosis can be confirmed using CT, MRCP, or ERCP. In children, duodenoduodenostomy is the treatment of choice,

and laparoscopic approaches are now being used; in adults, an array of interventions may be required, often in the treatment of a coexisting pathology.

PANCREATOBILIARY MALJUNCTION

Pancreatobiliary maljunction was first described by Babbitt in 1969,[148] and it since has been defined as "a congenital anomaly in which a junction of the pancreatic duct and biliary ducts is detected radiologically and/or anatomically outside the duodenal wall" (see Chapter 1).[149] It is often associated with congenital bile duct dilation (choledochal cyst) (see Chapter 46), which is significant because it results in regurgitation of pancreatic juice into the biliary tree (pancreatobiliary reflux) and of bile into the pancreatic duct (biliopancreatic reflux). It has been associated with a number of pathologic conditions, most notably carcinoma of the biliary tree (see Chapters 49, 51, and 59).

Pathogenesis

The anatomic relationship between the junction of the duodenum and the pancreatobiliary ducts is subject to significant variation.[150,151] The pancreatic and bile duct may open into the duodenum in one of three configurations: (1) separately, (2) through a single opening with no common channel, or (3) through a single opening with a common channel (Fig. 53.6). Within the wall of the duodenum, the pancreatic and bile ducts are under the control of the sphincter of Oddi; proximal to this extend the sphincter choledochus (of Boyden) and the sphincter pancreaticus. A single opening with a short common channel is usual, but when the common channel extends beyond the duodenal wall, the pancreatobiliary ductal junction is not controlled by these sphincter mechanisms, allowing regurgitation to occur between the two ducts. This is termed *pancreatobiliary maljunction*, which was reported to have a prevalence of 3.1% in a recent ERCP series.[152] A further 3.7% of patients were shown to have a high confluence of the pancreatobiliary ducts, and although sphincter function existed at the junction, the group was still susceptible to the same pathologic consequences as those with maljunction. The incidence of maljunction is higher in Asian compared with Western populations, although the reasons for this remain unclear.

The embryologic origins of pancreatobiliary maljunction have not been fully elucidated. Small pancreatic radicals arising from the long common channel have led to the suggestion that it originates from the ventral pancreatic duct.[153–155] In one such hypothesis, it is suggested that the persistence of the left ventral duct, usually seen to regress in normal development, associated with regression of the distal bile duct results in a long common

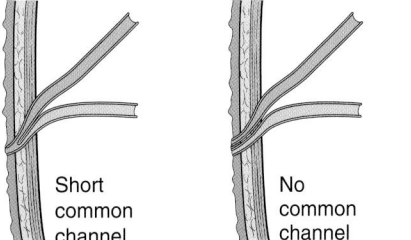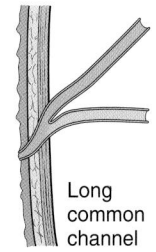

Short common channel   No common channel   Long common channel

FIGURE 53.6 Normal variations in the configuration of the pancreatic and bile ducts. (See Chapter 2.) (Modified from Rizzo RJ, et al: Congenital abnormalities of the pancreas and biliary tree in adults. *Radiographics.* 1995;15:49–68.)

channel.[156] An alternative hypothesis suggests that maljunction results from a disturbance in embryologic connections of the terminal bile duct and the ductal system of the ventral pancreas.[153] A case report of pancreatobiliary maljunction in monozygotic twins provides strong support for a genetic basis for the disease.[157]

Diagnosis and Investigation

Maljunction is closely associated with choledochal cyst and in one series was described in all patients with type I choledochal cysts (see Chapter 46).[158] Clinical presentation in this context can be at any age and may feature a right upper quadrant mass, hepatomegaly, jaundice, abdominal pain, cholangitis, or pancreatitis. In maljunction without bile duct dilation, patients may be asymptomatic (30%), or they may be seen with abdominal pain (24%), recurrent acute pancreatitis (18%), obstructive jaundice (18%), or acute cholangitis (9%).[159] When pancreatic maljunction is suspected, the lack of effect of the sphincter muscle on the pancreatobiliary ductal junction can be confirmed radiologically, and regurgitation can be demonstrated by MRCP, ERCP, EUS, operative cholangiography, or percutaneous transhepatic cholangiography. Biliary amylase levels have been shown to be high in this group.[160] On hepatobiliary scintigraphy, the passage time from the bile duct to the second part of the duodenum was significantly longer in maljunction patients than in control patients (49 ± 13 vs. 3 ± 14 minutes, respectively).[161] The diagnostic criteria for pancreaticobiliary maljunction have been formalized by the Japanese Study Group on Pancreaticobiliary Maljunction, taking into account advanced diagnostic imaging techniques[162] (Box 53.1).

Carcinogenesis in Pancreatobiliary Maljunction

The association of bile duct cancer and choledochal cyst is well established,[163] and resection of the extrahepatic bile duct and gallbladder with biliary reconstruction is now standard treatment[164] (see Chapters 9E and 46). A number of published series have described a high incidence of gallbladder cancer in patients with pancreatobiliary maljunction in the absence of a dilated bile duct (see Chapters 46 and 49).[152,165–172] The hydrostatic pressure in the pancreatic duct is greater than that of the bile duct,[173,174] so it follows that when free communication exists between the two ducts, pancreatic juice flows from the pancreatic duct into the bile duct. The pathogenesis of malignant change is not fully characterized but is likely due to the effect of activated pancreatic enzymes on the biliary epithelium, together with biliary stasis. *KRAS* and *p53* mutations have been reported in noncancerous biliary epithelium of patients with maljunction, which may be important given the apparent higher incidence of carcinoma in this group.[175–179] The Japanese Study Group on Pancreaticobiliary Maljunction has published comprehensive clinical practice guidelines for pancreaticobiliary maljunction.[180] These highlight the lack of good evidence in this area and rely on expert opinion. However, the guidelines cover definitions, pathogenesis, diagnosis, and treatment and are a useful addition for clinicians managing this condition (see Chapter 9E).

Takeshita et al.[181] have recently published a 40-year series describing the management of patients with pancreaticobiliary maljunction with biliary dilation. In a retrospective review of 144 patients who underwent flow diversion surgery with no

---

BOX 53.1   Diagnostic Criteria for Pancreaticobiliary Maljunction

I. Definition
Pancreaticobiliary maljunction is a congenital malformation in which the pancreatic and bile ducts join anatomically outside the duodenal wall.

II. Pathophysiology
In pancreaticobiliary maljunction, the duodenal papillary sphincter (sphincter of Oddi) fails to exert any influence on the pancreaticobiliary junction due to the abnormally long common channel. Therefore reciprocal reflux between pancreatic juice and bile occurs, resulting in various pathologic conditions, such as inhibiting the excretion of bile and pancreatic juice, and biliary cancer, in the biliary tract and pancreas.

III. Diagnostic Criteria
Pancreaticobiliary maljunction is diagnosed by either imaging test or anatomic examination.

Imaging Diagnosis
a. An abnormally long common channel and/or an abnormal union between the pancreatic and bile ducts must be evident on direct cholangiography, such as endoscopic retrograde cholangiopancreatography, percutaneous transpehatic cholangiography, or intraoperative cholangiography; magnetic resonance cholangiopancreatography, or three-dimensional drip infusion cholangiography computed tomography. However, in cases with a relatively short common channel, it is necessary to confirm that the effect of the papillary sphincter does not extend to the junction by direct cholangiography.
b. Pancreaticobiliary maljunction can be diagnosed if the pancreaticobiliary junction outside the wall can be depicted by endoscopic ultrasonography or multiplanar reconstruction images provided by multidetector-row computed tomography.

Anatomic Diagnosis
It should be confirmed by surgery or autopsy that the pancreaticobiliary junction lies outside the duodenal wall, or pancreatic and bile ducts unite abnormally.

IV. Supplementary Diagnosis
The following findings strongly suggest the existence of pancreaticobiliary maljunction.

Elevated Amylase Levels in Bile
Pancreatic enzymes, especially amylase, in the bile within the bile duct and gallbladder obtained immediately after laparotomy (endoscopically or percutaneously), are generally at extremely high levels. However, levels close to or below the normal serum value are occasionally observed in patients with pancreaticobiliary maljunction.

Clinical features similar to those of pancreaticobiliary maljunction, including elevation of pancreatic enzymes in bile, are observed in some cases with a relatively long common channel, showing the effect of the sphincter on the pancreaticobiliary junction.

Extrahepatic Bile Duct Dilation
Pancreaticobiliary maljunction includes one type that is associated with bile duct dilation (congenital biliary dilation), and another that is not (pancreaticobiliary dilation without biliary dilation). When cystic, fusiform, or cylindrical dilation is detected in the extrahepatic bile duct, careful investigations are needed to determine whether pancreaticobiliary maljunction is present.

Standard values for the maximum diameter of the common bile duct at each age are useful for diagnosing pancreaticobiliasry maljunction with or without biliary dilation.

From Kamisawa T, et al. Diagnostic criteria for pancreaticobiliary maljunction 2013. *J Hepatobiliary Pancreat Sci.* 2014;21(3):159–161.

known existing malignancy, 137 had complete cyst excision, with 7 undergoing head of pancreas resection. During a mean observation of approximately 8 years, 14 patients (10%) had long-term postoperative complications, including cholangitis, pancreatitis, intrahepatic calculi, and pancreatic calculus. One patient developed an intrahepatic cholangiocarcinoma. In comparison to outcomes from case series of untreated patients, these results are excellent and support an aggressive surgical approach to prevent the development of malignancy.

Therapy for Pancreatobiliary Maljunction Without Bile Duct Dilation

Given the risk of malignant transformation in patients with pancreatobiliary maljunction without biliary dilation, resectional surgery is generally advocated. However, significant controversy exists as to whether a complete excision of the extrahepatic biliary tree is required or just a prophylactic cholecystectomy. Those arguing the former cite case reports of choledochal cyst patients developing cancer in the hepatic duct above the reconstruction after bile duct resection.[182,183] This, together with the *p53/KRAS* mutation, suggests the biliary epithelium is in a "premalignant state."[184-188] Other investigators argue that cholecystectomy alone is sufficient and base this on reasonable follow-up data, albeit small cohorts, showing no patients developed bile duct malignancy in this group.[189-192] It is currently impossible to confirm which strategy is correct, and any decision must be made on an individual basis.[193]

CONGENITAL CYSTS OF THE PANCREAS

Of the cystic diseases of the pancreas (see Chapters 1 and 60), true congenital cysts are uncommon and comprise less than 1% of the total.[194] Cysts may be solitary, but this is rare—fewer than 30 have been described in the world literature. They are usually multiple, and some are associated with a systemic disorder, such as von Hippel-Lindau syndrome or polycystic kidney disease.[195] Enteric duplication cysts of the GI tract are also rare (2 in 9000 fetal/neonatal autopsies)[196] and can lie in the pancreatic head in isolation or in communication with the pancreatic duct.[197] They are lined with GI mucosa and take a layer of smooth muscle from their associated viscus. Several hypotheses on their embryologic origins exist, but no consensus has been reached.[198-201]

Congenital pancreatic cysts are most commonly seen in neonates or infants as an asymptomatic epigastric mass. It is very rare for them to manifest in adulthood, although case reports do exist.[202] In the case of duplication cysts, presentation with acute pancreatitis is not uncommon. This is likely to be due to the secretions of the GI mucosa within the cyst activating pancreatic enzymes. Other modes of presentation relate to compression of other structures by the cyst and include abdominal pain, obstructive jaundice, and splenic vein thrombosis.[195]

Diagnosis can be difficult, and most of the published cases describe extensive investigation of patients with recurrent abdominal pain or pancreatitis before the diagnosis is established. In patients with solitary congenital pancreatic cysts, US, CT, and ERCP have all been used in making the diagnosis[202] (see Chapter 17) Enteric duplication cysts involving the head of the pancreas can be differentiated from pseudocysts on US by the identification of hyperechoic mucosa and hypoechoic smooth muscle.[203] Peristalsis also has been seen in these lesions.[204] CT

helps further characterize the lesion and MRCP and ERCP can determine ductal relationships.[205]

Complete resection of solitary pancreatic cysts has been advocated, given that cystic neoplasms represent a possible differential diagnosis.[195] Drainage procedures have been performed successfully, but multiple biopsies of the cyst wall should be taken to exclude malignancy. Drainage procedures have been performed for enteric duplication cysts but are not usually definitive because patients often return with further pain or pancreatitis. When possible, local or mucosal resection is preferable to major resection, such as pancreatoduodenectomy, which should be reserved for when malignancy cannot be excluded. The spleen should be preserved whenever possible, particularly in the pediatric population.

HETEROTOPIC PANCREAS

Heterotopic pancreas is defined as pancreatic tissue outside the boundaries of the pancreas that lacks anatomic or vascular continuity with the organ (Fig. 53.7). The first description is credited to Jean Schultz in 1729, and sporadic cases have been described since.[206] Heterotopic pancreas is a congenital anomaly that is usually asymptomatic but can become clinically apparent when the inflamed or enlarged pancreas compresses adjacent viscera. The prevalence in the general population is difficult to determine; estimates range from 0.6% to 13.7%.[206,207]

The pathogenesis of heterotopic pancreas is unclear. It has been hypothesized that during embryologic development, pancreatic tissue may become attached to the duodenum and be carried proximally or distally as the bowel elongates[208] (see Chapter 1). This, however, does not explain the rare instances of heterotopic pancreas at sites distant from the GI tract (e.g., in the uterine tube).[209] As has been described, the pancreas is endodermal in origin, and contemporary studies are beginning to uncover the mechanisms by which cells destined to become pancreas are specified from surrounding tissues.[4] The observation that heterotopic pancreas tissue usually drains into the GI tract by a primitive duct[210] suggests in situ differentiation rather than migration from elsewhere.[211] Thus it is possible that heterotopic pancreas is the result of a process in which cells

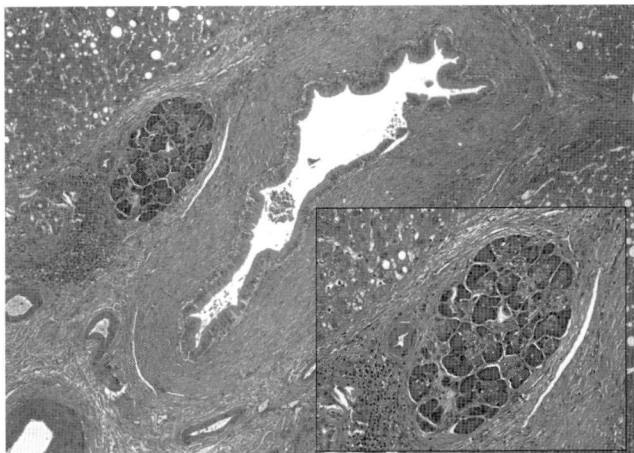

FIGURE 53.7 Heterotopic pancreas *(inset)* in a large portal tract in the liver found incidentally. The liver resection was for metastatic colorectal cancer. (Courtesy Dr. Barbara Langdale-Brown, Edinburgh.)

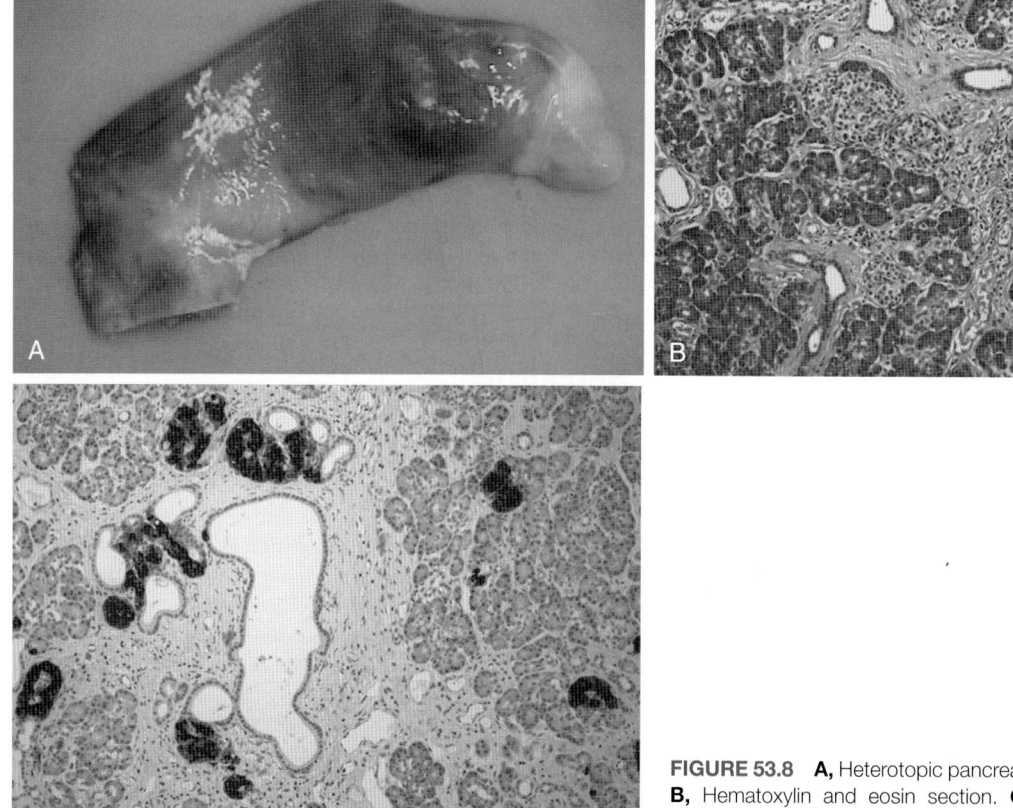

FIGURE 53.8 **A,** Heterotopic pancreas found in Meckel diverticulum. **B,** Hematoxylin and eosin section. **C,** Immunohistochemistry with primary antibody specific for human insulin. (Courtesy Dr. Kathryn McKenzie, Edinburgh.)

destined for other endodermal structures are anomalously diverted to a pancreatic fate.

Clinical presentation depends entirely on anatomic site. An early series of 34 patients by Armstrong et al.[212] is representative: Heterotopic tissue was found in the stomach (24%), duodenum (32%), jejunum (29%), Meckel diverticulum (15%) (Fig. 53.8), and gallbladder (3%). Occurrences have also been documented in the esophagus, bile duct, spleen, mesentery, and fallopian tubes. In the same series, heterotopic pancreas was thought to be clinically significant in 13 patients (38%) and possibly significant in 4 patients (12%). All gastric lesions, and 4 of 11 duodenal lesions, manifested with epigastric pain. Two of the duodenal lesions manifested with ulcer bleeding and one with chronic anemia.

Investigation and diagnosis again depend on the mode of presentation. In a contemporary series, diagnosis was made at gastroduodenoscopy in 36% and at surgery in 64%.[213] It was noted that definitive diagnosis was obtained only with histologic assessment. Heterotopic pancreas was the indication for surgery in 36% of cases, and in 45%, it was diagnosed incidentally during surgery. In 18% it was diagnosed on gastroduodenoscopy and definitive surgical management was not required.

In the majority of cases found at open surgery, the lesion was resected even when thought to be asymptomatic. This is advised because the diagnosis cannot be made clinically, and the main differential is malignancy. A frozen histologic section is an alternative approach but is rarely worthwhile unless an extensive resection is required. When identified at endoscopy, initial biopsies are often negative because the overlying mucosa may be normal. Recently, endoscopic US-guided core biopsies have been ideal. If the lesion is thought to be symptomatic, a resection can be planned, but many can be treated conservatively with no negative long-term consequences.

The references for this chapter can be found online by accessing the accompanying Expert Consult website.

SECTION I. Inflamatory, Infective, Congenital

B. Pancreatitis

CHAPTER 54

Definition and classification of pancreatitis

Giovanni Marchegiani, Giuseppe Malleo, Roberto Salvia, and Claudio Bassi

OVERVIEW

Despite five international consensus meetings over the last 40 years, the definition and classification of pancreatitis (see Chapters 55–58) continues to evolve. The main reason is the actual difficulty, in contrast to other common inflammatory diseases of the gastrointestinal (GI) tract, of obtaining pancreatic tissue specimens to define the diagnosis during the inflammatory process. As a consequence, classifications of pancreatitis are necessarily based on clinical, morphologic, and laboratory features.

The main historical landmark in defining and classifying pancreatitis was the development of the distinction between acute pancreatitis (AP) and chronic pancreatitis (CP; see Chapters 55 and 57), as first stated by Lagerlof in 1942.[1] In more recent years, with an improved understanding of the clinical presentation of pancreatitis, an increase in the number of experimental trials, and improved accuracy of imaging studies—particularly magnetic resonance imaging (MRI) of the bile ducts and the duct of Wirsung (see Chapters 2 and 17)—the classic distinction between AP and CP has undergone extensive revision.

The process leading to fibrotic changes in the glandular tissue usually begins with typical acute abdominal pain, with increased serum amylase and lipase and subsequent resolution. AP leads to CP because of episodes of obstruction secondary to edema or inflammation of the sphincter of Oddi. As in other inflammatory diseases, timing seems to play the main role in determining whether glandular inflammation leads to a chronic condition or self-limits with no further sequelae.

The most typical natural history regarding the correlation between AP and CP is what is known as *recurrent pancreatitis*. It is not possible to define this condition as acute or chronic, per se, and it represents the best example of the new understanding of the pathologic process. Nevertheless, distinguishing between AP and CP still represents a milestone in helping to develop further diagnostic and therapeutic algorithms.

HISTORY OF THE DEFINITION AND CLASSIFICATION OF PANCREATITIS

Pancreatitis is an inflammation of glandular parenchyma, leading to injury or possibly irreversible destruction of acinar components. This inflammatory pathologic process could acutely result in either a self-limited disease with no sequelae or in catastrophic autodigestion with systemic cytotoxic effects and life-threatening complications. In the case of chronic inflammation, permanent fibrosis and calcification are the characteristic features of the disease.

The history of the definition and classification of pancreatitis is summarized in Table 54.1. The first effort to classify and define pancreatitis by a worldwide group of experts led to the Marseille Consensus Meeting in 1963.[2] In this initial effort at consensus, it was agreed that AP and CP were different diseases mainly because of their different morphologic patterns. Relapsing pancreatitis was defined as the presence of multiple episodes in a morphologic pattern of AP or CP. The distinctive features of the two diseases were the pathologic benign course of acute inflammation, with biologic restitution in the acute condition, and the progressively worsening parenchymal lesions in the chronic condition (Table 54.2). This histology-based classification did not provide clinically useful definitions, making it impossible to compare different clinical experiences. From a clinical point of view, AP and CP show a similar pattern, at least in the early phases.

After the Cambridge meeting,[3] the distinction between AP and CP was maintained, and the term *relapsing pancreatitis* was abandoned. The importance of the clinical impact of the different severity of systemic responses was emphasized (Table 54.3), and the importance of defining a morphologic characterization of the inflammatory process was recognized, particularly for the AP group. The Cambridge group pointed out the relevant problem of etiology, and the role of imaging in CP was addressed.

Endoscopic retrograde cholangiopancreatography (ERCP) classification (Box 54.1) is still in use in some centers. Several studies in the literature showed that ERCP findings are not pathognomonic of CP but could coexist with many clinical conditions. In particular, cholelithiasis and its complications (see Chapters 33 and 37) lead to demonstrable alterations in the morphology of the duct of Wirsung, as stated in the Cambridge classification,[4,5] and these morphologic changes could persist for many months. In biliary cirrhosis, Sjögren's syndrome, and sclerosing cholangitis (see Chapter 41), pancreatic duct changes are commonly observed at ERCP.[6–8] For all these reasons, the ERCP morphology of the duct of Wirsung is not a specific finding that allows for a diagnosis of CP. In addition, increasing use of MRI of the bile ducts and duct of Wirsung can

TABLE 54.1 A Synopsis of Pancreatitis Classification From 1965–2015

CLASSIFICATION	DEFINITION
Marseille, 1965	Description of morphologic characteristics and etiologic factors of the disease; no categorization according to disease severity; no imaging findings
Cambridge, 1984	Classification of disease severity based on pancreatic imaging criteria (US, CT, ERCP); discussion of etiologic factors and pancreatic function
Revised Marseille, 1985	Description and further subclassification of morphologic changes; definition of "obstructive chronic pancreatitis" as a distinct form; no discussion of the correlation between anatomic and functional changes; no inclusion of pancreatic imaging findings
Marseille-Rome, 1988	Further description of "chronic calcifying" and "chronic inflammatory" pancreatitis as distinct forms; description of etiologic factors; no further elaboration of clinical, functional, or imaging criteria
Atlanta, 1992	Description of clinical and morphologic features of pancreatitis; dynamic classification system able to characterize the individual patient and predict severity
Zurich, 1997	Description of clinical presentation and classification of the disease into "definite" and "probable" chronic pancreatitis categories according to imaging findings, functional testing, and histologic examination
Japan Pancreas Society, 1997	Description of clinical presentation and classification of the disease into "definite" and "probable" chronic pancreatitis categories according to imaging findings, functional testing, and histologic examination; definition of radiologic and laboratory features in patients lacking etiologic and pathogenetic features
TIGAR-O, 2001	Detailed categorization of etiologic risk factors and correlation between acute and chronic pancreatitis
ABC, 2002	Disease grading according to clinical criteria; limited separation of different disease severities; not all clinical presentations categorized
Manchester, 2006	Disease grading according to clinical criteria; limited separation of different disease severities
M-ANNHEIM, 2007	Categorization of patients according to etiology, clinical stage, and severity of disease; severity of pancreatic inflammation assessed using a specific scoring system
Revised Atlanta, 2012	Comprehensive classification of acute pancreatitis: severity and peripancreatic collections; differentiation of acute peripancreatic fluid, pancreatic pseudocyst, acute necrotic collection, and walled-off necrosis
Determinant based, 2012	Classification based on the actual local (peripancreatic necrosis) and systemic determinants (organ failure) of severity

CT, Computed tomography; *ERCP,* endoscopic retrograde cholangiopancreatography; *US,* ultrasound.

TABLE 54.2 Marseille Classification of Pancreatitis

FEATURE	ACUTE PANCREATITIS/ACUTE RELAPSING PANCREATITIS	CHRONIC RELAPSING PANCREATITIS/CHRONIC PANCREATITIS
Clinical characteristics	Single/multiple episodes	Multiple episodes/no acute exacerbations is common
Morphologic characteristics	Not defined	Irregular sclerosis with destruction and focal segmental or diffuse loss of parenchyma, with varying dilation of ductal system; strictures, intracanalicular stones (calcifications), cysts, pseudocysts; islets of Langerhans involved much later in the course of the disease; morphologic picture is similar, independent of cause
Course	Clinical and biologic restitution if the cause is removed	Functional and morphologic lesions persist or progress after the cause is removed

Modified from Sarles H. Proposal adopted unanimously by the participants of the symposium of acute pancreatitis in Marseille, 1963. *Bibl Gastroenterol.* 1965;7:7–8.

TABLE 54.3 Cambridge Classification of Pancreatitis

FEATURE	ACUTE PANCREATITIS	CHRONIC PANCREATITIS
Clinical characteristics	Clinically defined as an acute illness because of inflammatory pancreatic disease that typically presents with abdominal pain and usually is associated with an increase in pancreatic enzymes in blood or urine Mild pancreatitis: if no multisystem failure occurs and no complications in recovery are seen Severe pancreatitis: if multisystem failure occurs, or early or late local or systemic complications occur	Defined as a continuing inflammatory disease of the pancreas; typically presents with abdominal pain or features of pancreatic insufficiency; also can remain painless; only sign of an inflammatory process may be fibrosis, indicating earlier pancreatic inflammation
Morphologic characteristics	Early: subcellular changes Later: fat necrosis or pancreatic tissue necrosis, which may be associated with hemorrhage **Complications** Phlegmon: an inflammatory mass in or around the pancreas Pseudocyst: a localized collection of fluid containing high concentrations of pancreatic enzymes within, adjacent to, or remote from the pancreas Abscess: pus in or around the pancreas	Not clearly defined; characterized by "irreversible morphologic changes"; classification is based on results of imaging studies
Course	Acute pancreatitis may recur	Many patients may have acute exacerbations of pain

Modified from Sarner M, Cotton PB. Classification of pancreatitis. *Gut.* 1984;25:756–759.

BOX 54.1	Grading of Chronic Pancreatitis by Endoscopic Retrograde Cholangiopancreatography

Normal	Visualization of the Gland Without Abnormal Signs
Equivocal	1.1 <3 abnormal branches
Mild	1.2 >3 abnormal branches
1.3 Moderate	1.4 Above + abnormal main duct
1.5 Marked	1.6 Above + one or more of:
	1.7 Cavity >10 mm
	Intraductal filling defects
	Calculi/pancreatic calcification
	Duct obstruction (stricture)
	Severe duct dilation or irregularity
	Contiguous organ invasion on ultrasound or CT

CT, Computed tomography.
Modified from Sarner M, Cotton PB. Classification of pancreatitis. *Gut.* 1984;25:756–759.

provide excellent morphologic imaging of the main- and side-branch ducts so that many centers currently have completely replaced the routine use of ERCP with MRI cholangiopancreatography (see Chapter 17).

The increasing attention to duct morphology resulted in new terminology at the second Marseille meeting held in 1984.[9] In addition to the classic distinction between AP and CP, a new entity was identified: *obstructive chronic pancreatitis* (Table 54.4). The role of duct obstruction in the chronic inflammatory process was recognized as a distinctive pathway to developing pancreatitis. This new concept has gained importance over the years in distinguishing chronic calcifying pancreatitis in alcoholics from obstructive CP initially presenting as relapsing acute attacks because of strictures from different conditions, such as solid tumors, mucinous plugs typical of intraductal papillary mucinous neoplasms (IPMN; see Chapter 60), severe pancreatitis with duct disruption (see Chapters 55 and 56), and scar and inflammation of the sphincter of Oddi of biliary origin. Regarding AP, another hallmark was recognized by the second Marseille meeting: the absence of necrosis in mild pancreatitis. The recognition of the pivotal role of necrosis in severe pancreatitis opened the doors to studies on severity assessment and prevention of complications.[10]

A new classification system was established after the Rome 1988 consensus (Table 54.5). The main feature of the new classification[11] concerned the reversibility of lesions observed in the course of AP; even the severe forms showed complete clinical response in almost half of severe pancreatitis patients. In contrast, in CP, some pathologic features were defined as permanent, and the condition was described as *chronic inflammatory pancreatitis*, morphologically characterized by loss of exocrine parenchyma and fibrosis with mononuclear cell

TABLE 54.4	Revised Marseille Classification of Pancreatitis		
FEATURE	ACUTE PANCREATITIS	CHRONIC PANCREATITIS	SPECIAL FORM: OBSTRUCTIVE CHRONIC PANCREATITIS
Clinical characteristics	Acute-onset abdominal pain and increase in pancreatic enzymes	Relapsing or persistent abdominal pain; occasionally painless; evidence of pancreatic insufficiency; steatorrhea or diabetes may be present	
Morphologic characteristics	Mild form: interstitial edema, pancreatic necrosis absent; possible peripancreatic fat necrosis	Irregular sclerosis with focal, segmental, or diffuse destruction and permanent loss of exocrine parenchyma; varying degrees of dilation of segments of the ductal system; protein plugs, intraductal calculi, edema, focal necrosis, inflammatory cells, cysts, and pseudocysts; islets of Langerhans are relatively well preserved The following descriptive terms can be used: chronic pancreatitis with focal necrosis, chronic pancreatitis with segmental or diffuse fibrosis, chronic pancreatitis with or without calculi	Dilation of the ductal system proximal to occlusion of one of the main ducts (e.g., by tumor or scar)
	Severe form: extensive peripancreatic and extrapancreatic fat necrosis, parenchymal necrosis, and hemorrhage; lesions may be either localized or diffuse		
Course	Usually benign but severe forms may be fatal; seen as a single episode or recurrent disease; exocrine and endocrine functions impaired to a variable degree for a variable duration Restitution to normal occurs if primary cause and complications are removed; rarely, acute pancreatitis may lead to chronic pancreatitis	Progressive and permanent loss of pancreatic exocrine and endocrine function Further investigation needed about the possibility to regress after removal of primary cause	Structural and functional changes tend to improve when the obstruction is removed

From Singer MV, Gyr K, Sarles H. Revised classification of pancreatitis. Report of the Second International Symposium on the Classification of Pancreatitis in Marseille, France, March 28-30, 1984. *Gastroenterology.* 1985;89(3):683–685.

TABLE 54.5 Marseille-Rome Classification of Pancreatitis

FEATURE	ACUTE PANCREATITIS	CHRONIC PANCREATITIS	CHRONIC INFLAMMATORY PANCREATITIS
Clinical characteristics	Not defined	First stages: attacks of acute pancreatitis responsible for recurrent pain, which may be the only clinical symptom Generally, after some years, exocrine and endocrine insufficiency develop; acute attacks decrease and disappear	
Morphologic characteristics	Edema, necrosis, hemorrhagic necrosis, fatty necrosis	*Chronic calcifying pancreatitis:* Irregular fibrosis, lobular spotty distribution of lesions of different density in between neighboring lobules; intraductal protein precipitates or plugs are always found and, at least in late stages, calcified precipitates (calculi) Atrophy and stenosis of duct frequent, more often than in the obstructive form; structural and functional changes may progress, even if primary cause is removed *Chronic obstructive pancreatitis:* As defined by the revised Marseille meeting (1984)	Loss of exocrine parenchyma, replaced by a dense fibrosis infiltrated by mononuclear cells —
Etiology	Extrapancreatic: gallstones, trauma, drugs, surgery, ERCP, hyperlipoproteinemia	Chronic alcohol consumption, high-protein diet, abnormally low- or high-lipid diets frequently associated with disease and probably represent etiologic factors, as does hypercalcemia	—
	Intrapancreatic: tumors, chronic pancreatitis, pancreas divisum (?), alcohol (?)	Other clinical forms: *nonalcoholic, tropical, hereditary*	—
Course	Generally considered reversible; necrosis may be infected; fluid collection filled with pancreatic juice, blood, and necrotic fragments may follow; pseudocysts may form If necrosis involves a segment of the main pancreatic duct, stenosis may result, leading to obstructive chronic pancreatitis distal to necrosis	Generally progresses from painful to painless disease; may progress despite removal of cause. Intrapancreatic retention cysts form when these cysts expand into peripancreatic tissues; necrotic pseudocysts form after an acute exacerbation; infected cysts or pseudocysts, called *abscesses,* form	—

ERCP, Endoscopic retrograde cholangiopancreatography.

Modified from Sarles H, Adler G, Dani R, et al. Classifications of pancreatitis and definition of pancreatic diseases. *Digestion.* 1989;43(4):234–236.

TABLE 54.6 Atlanta Classification

TERMINOLOGY	DEFINITION	CLINICAL MANIFESTATION	PATHOLOGY
Acute pancreatitis	Acute inflammatory process with involvement of other organs	Mild with minimal organ involvement; severe disease characterized by organ failure	Interstitial edema, intrapancreatic or extrapancreatic necrosis
Acute fluid collections	Occur early, lack a wall	30% to 50% in severe pancreatitis	Absence of well-defined wall
Pancreatic necrosis	Devitalized pancreatic parenchyma	Multiorgan failure	Extensive vessel, acinar cell, islet cell, and pancreatic duct damage
Postacute pseudocysts	Nonepithelialized collection of pancreatic juice	Main symptom pain; rarely palpable	Well-defined wall with clear, often sterile contents
Pancreatic abscess	Circumscribed intraabdominal collection of pus	If present, infection	Pus confined within a wall of granulation tissue

Modified from Bradley EL, 3rd. A clinically based classification system for acute pancreatitis. *Arch Surg.* 1993;128:586–590.

infiltration. For the first time, etiology specifically was addressed, with pancreas divisum and alcohol as possible causes of AP (see Chapters 53 and 55).

The need for further effort to better define AP resulted from the observation that the terminology of the Rome meeting was conflicting and not widely applied worldwide.[12] In 1992 40 pancreatologists met in Atlanta and developed a new classification system of AP (Table 54.6).[13] The clinical and morphologic features of pancreatitis were considered, resulting in a dynamic ongoing classification system better able to characterize the individual patient and predict disease severity.

The Zurich classification for alcoholic CP (Table 54.7)[14] specifically addresses the most common cause of the disease and gives less importance to other causes, which are sometimes difficult to diagnose, resulting in a quite complex classification system not widely adopted (see Chapter 57). In 1997 a new definition of CP was published, dividing *definite* from *probable* CP (Table 54.8).[15] This definition provided a list of radiologic

TABLE 54.7   Zurich Classification for Alcoholic Chronic Pancreatitis

DEFINITE ALCOHOLIC CHRONIC PANCREATITIS	PROBABLE ALCOHOLIC CHRONIC PANCREATITIS
In addition to a typical history or a history of excessive alcohol intake (≥80 g/day), one or more of the following criteria establish the diagnosis: Calcification in the pancreas Moderate to marked ductal lesions (Cambridge criteria) Marked exocrine insufficiency defined as steatorrhea (>7 g fat/24 hr) normalized or markedly reduced by enzyme supplementation Typical histology of an adequate surgical specimen	In addition to a typical history or a history of excessive alcohol intake (≥80 g/day), the diagnosis of probable chronic pancreatitis is likely if any of the following criteria are present: Mild ductal alterations (Cambridge criteria) Recurrent or persistent pseudocysts Pathologic secretin test Endocrine insufficiency

Etiologic Factors[a]

Alcoholic chronic pancreatitis

Nonalcoholic chronic pancreatitis

Tropical (nutritional) chronic pancreatitis

Hereditary chronic pancreatitis

Metabolic (hypercalcemic, hypertriglyceridemic) chronic pancreatitis

Idiopathic (early and late onset) chronic pancreatitis

Autoimmune chronic pancreatitis

Chronic pancreatitis resulting from miscellaneous causes (e.g., radiation injury, phenacetin abuse)

Chronic pancreatitis associated with anatomic abnormalities (anatomic chronic pancreatitis—periampullary duodenal wall cysts, pancreas divisum, obstructive pancreatitis, posttraumatic pancreatic duct scars)

Clinical Staging

Early stage: Recurrent attacks of clinical alcoholic acute pancreatitis (with or without local complications) without evidence of chronic pancreatitis abnormalities

Late stage: Any evidence of probable or definite chronic pancreatitis

[a]These diagnostic definitions also may be used for nonalcoholic chronic pancreatitis.

From Amman RW. A clinically based classification system for alcoholic chronic pancreatitis: Summary of an international workshop on chronic pancreatitis. *Pancreas*. 1997;14:215–221.

TABLE 54.8   Diagnostic Criteria for Chronic Pancreatitis From the Japan Pancreas Society

DEFINITE CHRONIC PANCREATITIS	PROBABLE CHRONIC PANCREATITIS
Ultrasound: Pancreatic stones evidenced by intrapancreatic hyperreflective echoes with acoustic shadows behind CT: Pancreatic stones evidenced by intrapancreatic calcifications	Ultrasound: Intrapancreatic coarse hyperreflective echoes, irregular dilation of pancreatic ducts, or pancreatic deformity with irregular contour CT: Pancreatic deformity with irregular contour
ERCP: Irregular dilation of pancreatic duct branches of variable intensity, with scattered distribution throughout the entire pancreas or irregular dilation of the main pancreatic duct and branches proximal to complete or incomplete obstruction of the main pancreatic duct (with pancreatic stones or protein plugs)	ERCP: Irregular dilation of the main pancreatic duct alone; intraductal filling defects suggest noncalcified pancreatic stones or protein plugs
Secretin test: Abnormally low bicarbonate concentration combined with either decreased enzyme outputs or decreased secretory volume Histologic examination: Irregular fibrosis with destruction and loss of exocrine parenchyma in tissue specimens obtained by biopsy, surgery, or autopsy; fibrosis with an irregular and patchy distribution in the interlobular spaces; intralobular fibrosis alone not specific for chronic pancreatitis	Secretin test: Abnormally low bicarbonate concentration alone or decreased enzyme output plus decreased secretory volume Tubeless tests: Simultaneous abnormalities in benzoyl-tyrosyl-*p*-amino benzoic acid and fecal chymotrypsin tests observed at two points several months apart Histologic examination: Intralobular fibrosis with one of the following findings: loss of exocrine parenchyma, isolated islets of Langerhans, or pseudocysts
Protein plugs, pancreatic stones, dilation of the pancreatic ducts, hyperplasia and metaplasia of the ductal epithelium, and cyst formation	

CT, Computed tomography; *ERCP*, endoscopic retrograde cholangiopancreatography.

Modified from Homma T, Harada H, Koizumi M. Diagnostic criteria for chronic pancreatitis by the Japan Pancreas Society. *Pancreas*. 1997;15(1):14–15.

and/or laboratory features in CP patients lacking etiologic and pathogenetic features. The TIGAR-O risk factor classification system (*t*oxic-metabolic, *i*diopathic, *g*enetic, *a*utoimmune, *r*ecurrent severe, *o*bstructive; Table 54.9) provides a complete overview of the risk factors for CP development, with special attention to the relationship between acute and chronic disease.[16] In recent years, two separate categorization systems have been proposed: the ABC system[17] and the Manchester classification

(Box 54.2).[18] The aim of these systems is to provide an accurate description of CP while underlining various therapeutic approaches and prognoses depending on disease stage. The ABC system divides patients into grades depending on the presence or absence of abdominal pain, complications, and deficiency in pancreatic function. The Manchester classification uses the terms *mild, moderate,* and *end stage* to represent disease progression, allowing comparison between patient groups.

TABLE 54.9 TIGAR-O Classification System for Chronic Pancreatitis

TOXIC-METABOLIC	IDIOPATHIC	GENETIC	AUTOIMMUNE	RECURRENT AND SEVERE ACUTE	OBSTRUCTIVE

Alcoholic
Tobacco smoking
Hypercalcemia
Hyperlipidemia
Chronic renal
  failure
Medications
  (phenacetin abuse)
Toxins (organotin
  compounds)
	Early onset
	Late onset
	Tropical (tropical
	  calcific and
	  fibrocalculous
	  pancreatic
	  diabetes)
	Other
		Autosomal dominant:
		  cationic trypsinogen
		  gene (codon 29 and
		  122 mutations)
		Autosomal recessive/
		  modifier genes:
		  CFTR mutations,
		  SPINK1 mutations,
		  cationic trypsinogen
		  (codon 16, 22,
		  and 23 mutations),
		  α_1-antitrypsin
		  deficiency possible
			Isolated autoimmune
			  chronic pancreatitis
			Syndromic autoimmune
			  chronic pancreatitis
			  (Sjögren's syndrome–
			  associated,
			  inflammatory
			  disease–associated,
			  primary biliary
			  cirrhosis–associated)
				Postnecrotic (severe
				  acute pancreatitis)
				Recurrent acute
				  pancreatitis
				Vascular disease/
				  ischemic
				Radiation injury
					Pancreas divisum
					Sphincter of Oddi
					  disorders
					  (controversial)
					Duct obstruction
					  (e.g., tumor)
					Periampullary
					  duodenal
					  wall cysts
					Posttraumatic
					  pancreatic
					  duct scars

CFTR, Cystic fibrosis transmembrane conductance regulator; *SPINK1,* serine protease inhibitor, Kazal type 1

Modified from Etemad B, Whitcomb DC. Chronic pancreatitis: Diagnosis, classification, and new genetic developments. *Gastroenterology.* 2001;120:682–707.

BOX 54.2 Manchester Classification System for Chronic Pancreatitis

Mild: Five Essential Criteria
1. ERP/MRP/CT evidence of chronic pancreatitis
2. Abdominal pain
3. No regular analgesia
4. Preserved endocrine and exocrine function
5. No peripancreatic complications

Moderate: Five Essential Criteria
1. ERP/MRP/CT evidence of chronic pancreatitis
2. Abdominal pain
3. Regular (weekly) opiates
4. Evidence of impaired endocrine/exocrine function
5. No peripancreatic complications

End Stage
1. ERP/MRP/CT evidence of chronic pancreatitis
2. One or more of the following "extrapancreatic features":
    i. Biliary stricture
    ii. Segmental portal hypertension
    iii. Duodenal stenosis
3. Plus one or more of the following:
    i. Diabetes
    ii. Steatorrhea
    Note that abdominal pain may or may not be present.

CT, Computed tomography; *ERP,* endoscopic retrograde pancreatography; *MRP,* magnetic resonance pancreatography.
Modified from Bagul A, Siriwardena AK. Evaluation of the Manchester classification system for chronic pancreatitis. *JOP* 2006;7(4):390–396.

A different classification attempt is represented by the M-ANNHEIM multiple risk factor system (Table 54.10), which was developed to provide a standardized method for the clinical diagnosis of CP according to etiology, clinical stage, and severity of disease and, finally, to direct clinical practice.[19]

DEFINITION AND CLASSIFICATION OF PANCREATITIS IN THE MODERN ERA

The different classifications of the last 30 years have provided crucial advances in the definition of the inflammatory processes of pancreatitis and oriented clinical strategies. Nevertheless,

---

TABLE 54.10 M-ANNHEIM Multiple Risk Factor Classification System

MULTIPLE RISK FACTOR CLASSIFICATION	CLINICAL STAGING OF CHRONIC PANCREATITIS
Alcohol consumption	*Asymptomatic chronic pancreatitis*
Nicotine consumption	0. Stage of subclinical chronic pancreatitis
Nutritional factors	*Symptomatic chronic pancreatitis*
Hereditary factors	I. Stage without pancreatic insufficiency
Efferent duct factors	II. Stage of partial pancreatic insufficiency
Immunologic factors	III. Stage of painful complete pancreatic insufficiency
Miscellaneous and rare metabolic factors	IV. Stage of secondary painless disease (burnout)

Diagnostic Criteria of Chronic Pancreatitis
The diagnosis requires a typical clinical history of chronic pancreatitis, such as recurrent pancreatitis or abdominal pain, except for primary painless pancreatitis. Based on these features, the three forms of chronic pancreatitis are (1) definite chronic pancreatitis, (2) probable chronic pancreatitis, and (3) borderline chronic pancreatitis.

Scoring System for the Grading of Clinical Features of Chronic Pancreatitis Points

Patient report of pain	0–4
Pain control	0–2
Surgical intervention	0 or 4
Exocrine insufficiency	0–2
Endocrine insufficiency	0 or 4
Morphologic status on pancreatic imaging	0–4
Severe organ complications	0, 2, or 4

Severity Index of Chronic Pancreatitis

Severity Level	Point Range
M-Annheim A: minor	0–5
M-Annheim B: increased	6–10
M-Annheim C: advanced	11–15
M-Annheim D: marked	16–20
M-Annheim E: exacerbated	>20

Modified from Schneider A, Löhr JM, Singer MV. The M-ANNHEIM classification of chronic pancreatitis: Introduction of a unifying classification system based on a review of previous classifications of the disease. *J Gastroenterol.* 2007;42(2):101–119.

TABLE 54.11	Revised Atlanta Classification
Mild acute pancreatitis	No organ failure
	No local or systemic complications
Moderately severe acute pancreatitis	Organ failure that resolves within 48 hours
	Local or systemic complications without persistent organ failure
Severe acute pancreatitis	Persistent organ failure >48 hours

The Revised Atlanta Classification includes definitions of acute peripancreatic fluid collection, pancreatic pseudocyst, acute necrotic collection, walled-off necrosis, and infectious necrosis.

Modified from Banks PA, Bollen TL, Dervenis C, et al. Classification of acute pancreatitis—2012: Revision of the Atlanta classification and definitions by international consensus. *Gut.* 2013;62(1):102–111.

there is still the need for a definite clinical assessment of its severity and more objective terms to describe its local complications. In 2012 two major contributions were published in an attempt to address the remaining clinical questions.

First, the Atlanta Classification of 1992 was updated through an international consensus.[20] In this revised Atlanta Classification, a new severity classification was proposed, together with a clear definition for diagnosing AP. Both interstitial and necrotizing pancreatitis were defined, as well as the individual local complications. In particular, the Revised Atlanta Classification outlined the early and late phases of the disease, with the late phase typically limited to patients with moderate or severe disease. Finally, severe AP was defined solely by the presence of persistent organ failure, which is acknowledged as the main determinant of mortality. Table 54.11 highlights the main novelties of this classification and, in particular, the standardization of terminology that was introduced.

In the same year as the publication of the Revised Atlanta Classification, the determinant-based classification of AP severity was published by a multidisciplinary panel of experts.[21] This classification used persistent organ failure and infectious peripancreatic necrosis as determinants of mortality in AP to classify patients into four categories (Table 54.12). The main rationale for this classification was that either event could occur at any stage of disease so two specific phases (early and late) are not recognized.

Very recently, several studies have independently validated the two newer classifications and compared their performances with the original Atlanta Classification of 1992.[22] Both newer classifications were found to perform better than the previous one in all outcome measures; however, the Revised Atlanta Classification appears more relevant in the day-to-day clinical care of patients.

AUTOIMMUNE PANCREATITIS

After isolated reports of pancreatitis associated with increased serum immunoglobulin levels, Kawaguchi et al. described a variant of primary sclerosing cholangitis extensively involving the pancreas, called lymphoplasmacytic sclerosing pancreatitis (LPSP; see Chapters 48 and 55).[23] The association of CP with autoimmune diseases was described by Chari et al., who proposed that this be classified separately as "chronic autoimmune pancreatitis."[24] The concept of autoimmune pancreatitis (AIP) was finally established by Yoshida et al. by demonstrating a sharp response to steroids in a case of CP with elevated immunoglobulin levels.[25] Later, it was shown that IgG4 antibodies were elevated in patients with AIP and that histologic changes, including tissue infiltration with IgG4-positive plasma cells along with storiform fibrosis and obliterative phlebitis, occurred in multiple sites.[26] This form of AIP characterized by multiple organ involvement is now known as Type 1 AIP and is associated with elevated IgG4 levels and the presence of LPSP histologically. Meanwhile, investigators from Europe described a subset of patients with non-alcoholic duct destructive CP. Although some of the described features overlapped with LPSP, the presence of a duct-centric neutrophilic infiltrate and duct destruction were characteristically different. This form of inflammation was termed idiopathic duct-centric pancreatitis (IDCP), and the neutrophilic lesion was termed granulocyte epithelial lesion (GEL) and is now well described as the histologic hallmark of IDCP.[27] IDCP was eventually defined as a distinct type of AIP (Type 2 AIP), characterized mainly by a younger age at presentation, the absence of extrapancreatic involvement, lack of association with elevated IgG4 elevation, and an association with inflammatory bowel disease.[28] International consensus diagnostic criteria for AIP were established in 2011 and formally defined criteria for the diagnosis of type 1 and type 2 AIP[29] is summarized in Table 54.13. Despite the increasing knowledge of AIP, the precise antigen responsible for triggering the inflammation remains unknown. Also, it is not known why AIP is painless despite intense inflammation, as compared with AP and CP, which are associated with intense pain.[30]

THE FUTURE OF PANCREATITIS DEFINITION AND CLASSIFICATION

The thorough analysis of the history of pancreatitis classification shows how all these more recent advances in the "definition dilemma" abandoned the mere clinical purpose of a classification to better investigate different specific features of this complex disease. The classification systems will likely come full circle with the recognition of the deep but still controversial correlation between acute and chronic inflammation.

As a take-home message for clinical practice, the history of every patient must be carefully considered to identify risk factors that may include alcohol abuse, obstruction, genetics, and autoimmune disease. The clinical evidence of pancreas-related abdominal pain associated with alterations of serum amylase

TABLE 54.12	Determinant-Based Classification of Acute Pancreatitis Severity			
	MILD AP	**MODERATE AP**	**SEVERE AP**	**CRITICAL AP**
(Peri)pancreatic necrosis	No	Sterile	Infected	Infected
	And	And/or	Or	And
Organ Failure	No	Transient	Persistent	Persistent

AP, Acute pancreatitis.

Modified from Dellinger EP, Forsmark CE, Layer P, et al. Determinant-based classification of acute pancreatitis severity: An international multidisciplinary consultation. *Ann Surg.* 2012;256(6):875–880.

TABLE 54.13 Clinical and Histologic Features of Type 1 and Type 2 Autoimmune Pancreatitis

FEATURE	TYPE 1 AIP (LPSP)	TYPE 2 AIP (IDCP)
Clinical		
Age	7th decade	5th decade
Gender (M:F)	3:1	1:1
Increased serum IgG (>2×)	~2/3rd	~1/4th
Extrapancreatic involvement/ association with IgG4 RD	Yes	No
Association with IBD	Weak	Strong (10%-20%)
Imaging	Similar imaging features in LPSP and IDCP	
Histology		
Lymphoplasmacytic infiltration	Yes	Yes
Periductal inflammation	Yes	Yes
Storiform fibrosis	More prominent	Less prominent
Obliterative phlebitis	Characteristic	Rare
GEL	Absent	Characteristic
IgG4 staining	Abundant; >10/hpf	Rare; <10/hpf
Treatment		
Response to steroids	~100%	~100%
Relapse	Up to 60%	<10%

AIP, Autoimmune pancreatitis; *GEL,* granulocyte epithelial lesion; *IDCP,* idiopathic duct-centric pancreatitis; *LPSP,* lymphoplasmacytic sclerosing pancreatitis.

Adapted from Nagpal SJS, Sharma A, Chari ST. Autoimmune pancreatitis. *Am J Gastroenterol.* 2018;113(9):1301.

and lipase led to the term *pancreatitis*. The ongoing clinical observations obtained with imaging studies that include ultrasound, computed tomography (CT), and especially MRI of the bile ducts and duct of Wirsung should address the required treatment patient by patient. The early stage is the most difficult to diagnose, but it is also important to give the right medical or surgical option. Only the dynamic observation of patients with controlled follow-up enables us to classify pancreatitis and to better define the disease, assigning the definitive labels supported by the biochemical and radiologic sources well characterized by the different classification systems available. The clinician should recognize pancreatitis at an early stage but avoid assigning a "definitive" classification immediately, instead investigating all the factors available to determine whether a first acute attack could lead to chronic changes with fibrosis, permanent disruptions, and exocrine endocrine insufficiency.

POSTOPERATIVE ACUTE PANCREATITIS: A NEW KID ON THE BLOCK

AP in a medical context is an inflammatory process of the pancreatic parenchyma that presents with features that have been deeply investigated over the years and led to a universally shared definition of AP and common terminologies on its complications (see Chapter 117).

Recently the presence of a pancreatic process that partially shares with the medical AP some typical pathologic findings in a continuum between inflammation and necrosis of the pancreatic parenchyma[31] has been described in the postpancreatic surgery setting. This phenomenon, called postoperative acute pancreatitis (POAP), seems, however, to have specific characteristics. The ischemia/inflammation process of POAP may be limited to the area of the pancreatic stump without involving the entire pancreatic remnant.

POAP appears from the recent literature as an extremely early event that occurs in the first postoperative days. POAP is characterized by postoperative serum hyperamylasemia (POH) and the ability to trigger additional morbidity.[32,33] The immediate consequences of POAP manifested mainly in impaired healing of the pancreatic stump, whether or not a pancreatic anastomosis is made. Therefore the main clinical manifestations of POAP may be both local, with the development of postoperative pancreatic fistula (POPF), abdominal abscess and bleeding from the pancreatic stump area,[3] and systemic, characterized by a systemic inflammatory response syndrome (SIRS).[34] Risk factors related to the development of POAP were crucially linked to the presence of a healthy pancreatic parenchyma, such as a soft pancreatic texture and a preserved functionality.[35]

The pathologic mechanism underling POAP still remains unclear because of the limited possibility of investigating specific changes in the pancreatic parenchyma occurring in the early postoperative period, the clinical and radiologic criteria commonly used in the diagnosis of AP may not be adequate for the assessment of POAP because the clinical picture is hidden by postoperative analgesia, and CT imaging criteria overlaps with early common postsurgical findings.

The designation of POAP and its presence is currently very controversial among pancreatic surgeons. Whether this condition is separate from, or simply related to, POPF is unclear. However, its recognition and interpretation as a stand-alone postoperative complication will allow for promising early therapeutic interventions aimed at the prevention or mitigation of other morbidities, especially POPF. Its actual definition and grading is currently ongoing and will be likely available in the very near future.

References are available at expertconsult.com.

CHAPTER 55

Etiology, pathogenesis, and diagnostic assessment of acute pancreatitis

Ser Yee Lee, Adrian Kah Heng Chiow, Brian Kim Poh Goh, and Chung Yip Chan

Acute pancreatitis (AP) is an inflammatory condition of the pancreas that can lead to injury or destruction of acinar components and is clinically characterized by abdominal pain and elevated blood levels of pancreatic enzymes.[1–3] The clinical spectrum is as diverse as its causes and pathogenesis, ranging from a relatively mild set of symptoms to a severe illness with potentially life-threatening complications. In the recent Atlanta classification revision, AP is differentiated into two types: interstitial edematous pancreatitis and necrotizing pancreatitis.[1] AP is the most common diagnosis for hospitalization among the gastrointestinal (GI) conditions in the United States, accounting for as many as 300,000 hospitalizations per year.[4,5] The incidence is on an increasing trend during the past decades and has ranged from approximately 5 to 100 per 100,000 population per year.[6–13] AP with its associated complications is a major cause of morbidity and mortality worldwide; mortality ranges from approximately 1% in mild cases to almost 30% in severe cases with persistent organ failure.[11,14–16] As a result, AP poses a huge financial healthcare burden as well.[12,17] In a recent study by Brindise et al., the incidence of AP was observed to increase from 9.48 to 12.19 per 1000 hospitalizations with cost of hospitalization increasing from \$27,827 to \$49,772 from 2002 compared with 2013 and an aggregate cost of over \$2.6 billion per year in the US alone.[2,12,18] In-hospital mortality and mean length of stay (LOS) has decreased from 2.99 to 2.04 per 100 cases and 6.99 to 5.74 days, respectively, in the same period.[18]

ETIOLOGY AND PATHOGENESIS OF ACUTE PANCREATITIS

Gallstones and alcohol abuse together account for as many as 60% to 80% of all AP cases.[11,19] The relative frequency of each of these etiologies depends largely on the population being evaluated. In both the East and the West, biliary pancreatitis is more common in women, whereas alcoholic pancreatitis is more common in middle-aged men.[6,15] Approximately 10% of cases are caused by diverse causes, such as malignancy, hyperlipidemia, hypercalcemia, viral infection, drugs, and iatrogenic causes. As many as 30% of cases are idiopathic.[7,20]

Acute Biliary Pancreatitis

Between 4% and 8% of patients with gallstones eventually experience biliary pancreatitis secondary to migratory gallstones (Fig. 55.1A; see Chapters 33 and 37).[21,22] The incidence of acute biliary pancreatitis is higher in women than in men (69% vs. 31%) and increases with age.[23] The natural history of acute biliary pancreatitis is different from that of alcohol-induced disease. There is a spectrum of severity similar to alcoholic pancreatitis, but if the patient recovers, endocrine and exocrine deficiencies are much less likely than in alcoholic patients, and in most cases the gland is histologically normal after clinical recovery.[24]

Opie first observed an impacted gallstone at the papilla of Vater in two patients with severe pancreatitis in 1901. Since then, investigations have shown that the pathogenesis of biliary pancreatitis is multifaceted, with ampullary obstruction, biliopancreatic reflux, gallstone-related factors, and genetics each playing a role.

Experimental and clinical studies have shown that ampullary obstruction by gallstones not only initiates but also sustains and aggravates biliary pancreatitis.[25,26] On the other hand, Acosta et al. found small gallstones in the stool of 94% of patients with biliary pancreatitis compared with 8% of control subjects with gallstones who did not have pancreatitis, demonstrating that the crucial event is probably not the impaction of a stone in the common bile duct (CBD) but rather the passage of a gallstone of a suitable size through the ampulla of Vater.[27] In the absence of an obstructing stone at the ampulla, based on findings of inflamed ampulla in patients operated on early (<36 hours after admission) for biliary pancreatitis versus those operated on late (>3 months after admission), it is hypothesized that local edema or spasm of the ampulla can also lead to obstruction of the pancreatic duct.[28] Either way, transient obstruction increases pressures in the pancreatic duct, which then leads to extravasation of pancreatic juice in the interstitium and subsequent injury of the gland. Pancreatic hypersecretion after a meal may then enhance the increasing pressure in an already-obstructed duct from the migrating gallstone and intensify the injury.[29] The causative role of transient obstruction by gallstones in pancreatitis is further supported by the observation that recurrent attacks of biliary pancreatitis can be prevented or reduced by endoscopic sphincterotomy.[30] In patients with separate orifices of the CBD and pancreatic duct, biliary pancreatitis can still occur, likely because of the stone in the distal bile duct compressing the adjacent pancreatic duct directly or from the resulting edema.[31]

Opie proposed in 1901 that bile reflux into the pancreatic duct caused by stone obstruction of the common biliary pancreatic channel initiates the inflammation. Since then, however, the evidence suggests that the common channel focus is invalid.[32] Under physiologic circumstances, the pressure in the pancreatic duct is 3-fold higher than in the CBD, thereby preventing reflux of bile into the pancreatic duct.[33] During ampullary obstruction, the pressure gradient between the biliary tree and the pancreatic duct may reverse.[34] Nonetheless, although sterile refluxate can cause an increase in the permeability of the pancreatic ductal system through activation of pancreatic enzymes, it does not lead to pancreatitis and would remain a harmless event.[35,36] However, when there is temporary biliary and pancreatic obstruction, followed by decompression and

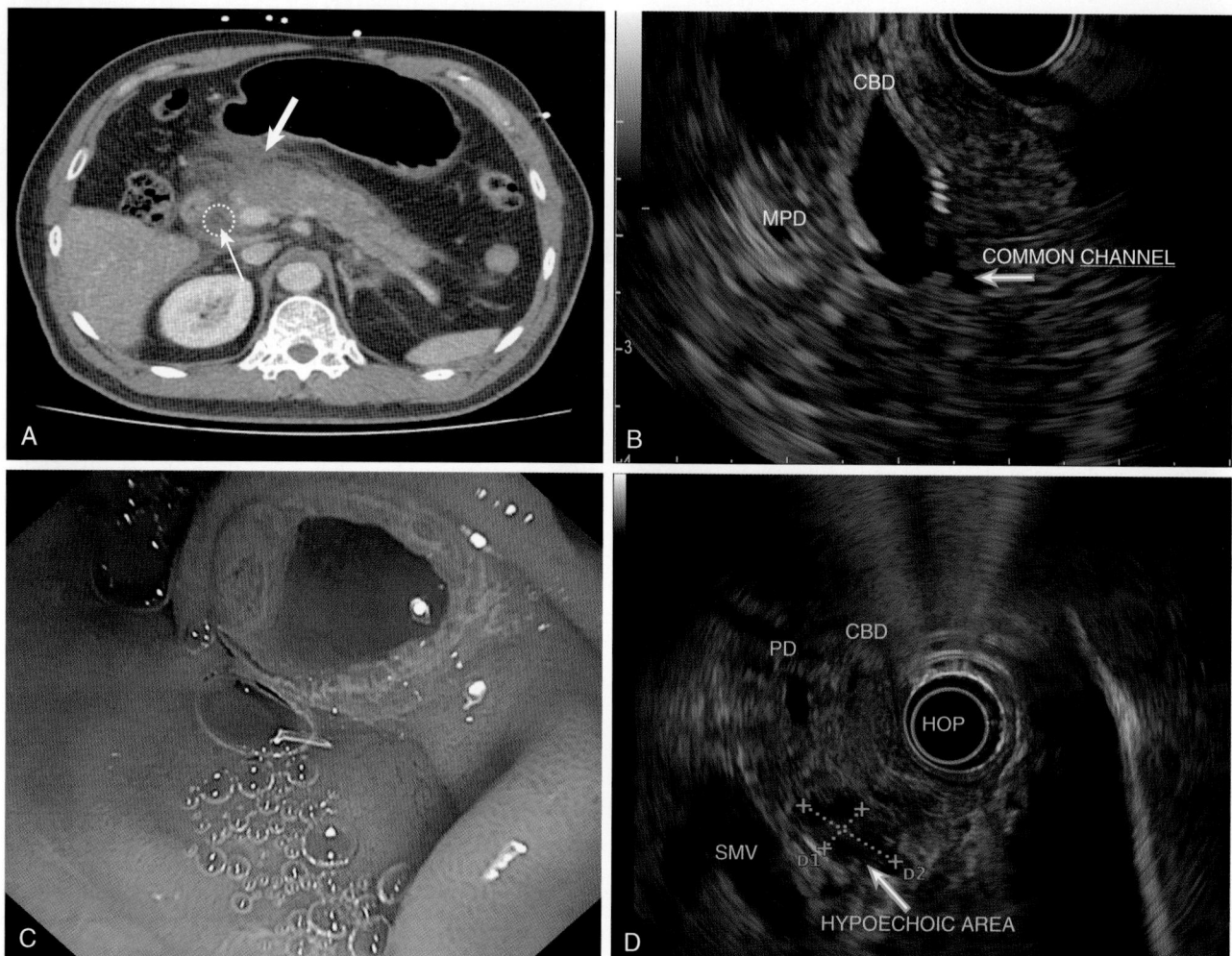

FIGURE 55.1 **Causes of acute pancreatitis. A,** Cross-sectional computed tomography (CT) image of acute biliary pancreatitis. *Thin arrow,* Small gallstones within common bile duct (*circle*); *thick arrow,* edematous head and neck of pancreas with peripancreatic fluid (see Chapters 33 and 37). **B,** Anomalous pancreaticobiliary duct junction (ABPJ) on endoscopic ultrasound (EUS). *Arrow,* Common channel. (see Chapter 46). **C,** Endoscopy picture of fish-mouth papilla with mucus coming out, main duct. Intraductal papillary mucinous neoplasm causing pancreatitis (see Chapters 54 and 60). **D,** Initially diagnosed idiopathic pancreatitis, cross-sectional imaging (e.g., CT) did not detect a cause, but further workup with EUS reveals the lesion as a hypoechoic area (*arrow*), which proved to be a pancreatic adenocarcinoma (see Chapter 62). *CBD,* Common bile duct; *HOP,* head of pancreas; *MPD,* main pancreatic duct; *PD,* pancreatic duct; *SMV,* superior mesenteric vein. (Images courtesy Dr. Damien Tan and Dr. Ser Yee Lee.)

flow of infected bile at high pressure into the pancreatic duct, AP is induced.[34]

Contributing to the pathogenesis of biliary pancreatitis are factors that facilitate the passage of gallstones from the gallbladder into CBD and then through the ampulla. A recent study showed that small gallstone diameter (<5 mm), wide cystic duct (>5 mm) and high stone load (>20 gallstones) were significant risk factors for biliary pancreatitis.[37] Other gallstone-associated features that increase the risk for development of biliary pancreatitis include mulberry shape and irregular surfaces.[38,39] Excess cholesterol crystals in the gallbladder and good emptying of the gallbladder are also associated with an increased risk of pancreatitis.[40]

In recent years, variations or mutations in the genes that encode pancreatic enzymes or their inhibitors have been suggested as potential risk factors for development of AP. *SPINK1* encodes a potent inhibitor of trypsin activity within the pancreas, and it has been found that mutations in *SPINK1* are significantly higher in patients with AP (all causes) compared

with a healthy control group.[41] A case of recurrent biliary pancreatitis has reportedly been associated with a mutation in *ABCB4* gene, which encodes a multidrug resistance protein involved in the transport of phosphatidylcholine across the canalicular membrane of hepatocytes.

Acute Alcoholic Pancreatitis

Alcoholic pancreatitis is more common in men, which may be secondary to greater alcohol intake in men rather than a gender-based difference in susceptibility.[42] The peak age for presentation of alcoholic pancreatitis is uniformly 40 to 60 years. Incidence and prevalence also differ in terms of race and geographic distribution.[6] The average daily alcohol consumption among patients with alcoholic pancreatitis averages 100 to 150 g/day. Although the risk for pancreatitis increases with greater doses of alcohol, epidemiologic studies shows that clinically evident pancreatitis develops in only a minority of heavy drinkers.[19,43] On the other hand, findings consistent with pancreatitis have been reported in as many as 75% of autopsies performed on alcohol abusers.[44] These observations suggest that alcohol alone may not cause pancreatitis unless accompanied by additional genetic and/or environmental factors. As such, it is probable that alcohol sensitizes the pancreas, with these additional genetic and environmental factors then initiating pancreatitis. Interestingly, binge drinking in the absence of long-term, heavy alcohol use does not appear to precipitate AP and the type of alcohol intake (e.g., wine vs. beer) does not change risk.[45]

The direct effect of alcohol on the pancreatic duct and the acinar cells has been studied. Alcohol increases secretion of two nondigestive proteins, lithostathine and glycoprotein GP2, in the pancreas, which precipitate within the ducts and form aggregates that eventually enlarge and calcify to form intraductal calculi.[46,47] Whether these protein plugs and ductal calculi play a role in the initiation of alcoholic pancreatitis is yet to be determined, although it is accepted that these events have the potential to facilitate disease progression. In animal studies, chronic administration of alcohol has been found to increase the pancreatic content of the digestive enzymes trypsinogen, chymotrypsinogen, and lipase, as well as the lysosomal enzyme cathepsin B.[48] Trypsinogen can be activated by cathepsin B within acinar cells, leading to a cascade of autodigestion characteristic of pancreatitis.[49] The pancreas can metabolize alcohol via both oxidative and nonoxidative pathways, yielding the toxic metabolites acetaldehyde and fatty acid ethyl esters (FAEEs), respectively.[50,51] Oxidative alcohol metabolism results in the generation of reactive oxygen species (ROS) as a byproduct and, at the same time, depletion of the ROS scavenger glutathione. The products of alcohol oxidation (acetaldehyde and ROS) and those of nonoxidative metabolism of alcohol (FAEEs) have all been reported to cause acinar cell injury.[52–54] Clinical and experimental studies have demonstrated that oxidant stress from the metabolism of alcohol induces destabilization of zymogen granules and lysosomes, resulting in pancreatic injury. Similarly, FAEEs from nonoxidative metabolism of alcohol destabilize lysosomes in acinar cells, thus increasing the potential for contact between lysosomal and digestive enzymes, leading to their intracellular activation and autodigestion of the gland. This is mediated by the sustained increases in intracellular calcium levels, leading to trypsinogen activation, alterations in endoplasmic reticulum (ER) luminal environment, activation of mitochondrial permeability transition pore (MPTP), and depletion of ATP leading to cellular necrosis. Ethanol itself can affect cellular autophagy, an important cellular process by which unneeded or damaged cellular components are sequestered in autophagic vacuoles and targeted to the lysosome for degradation. This is postulated to result in the accumulation of large vacuoles within acinar cells, one histologic characteristic seen in pancreatitis. Furthermore, it has been shown that the induction of pancreatic stellate cells by ethanol or acetaldehyde leads to their transformation to highly proliferative myofibroblast-like cells. This leads to accumulation of extracellular matrix proteins, which can lead to fibrosis. Furthermore, stellate cells can induce the synthesis of cytokines and growth factors involved in their activation, resulting in an autocrine loop that may explain the inability of the pancreas to fully recover from injury in the presence of continued alcohol ingestion, leading to chronic pancreatitis (CP).[55]

Despite the many pathways of direct toxic injury of alcohol to the pancreas, the low numbers of patients with alcoholism in whom pancreatitis develops suggests that a susceptibility factor, environmental or genetic, is at play to provide a second hit for triggering clinical pancreatitis. Among the environmental factors studied, smoking has garnered the most interest. A recent cohort study showed that smoking was a dose-dependent risk factor for alcoholic pancreatitis after controlling for age, gender, body mass index (BMI), and alcohol consumption.[56] As for genetic factors, to date, studies on hereditary factors as well as mutations in genes related to digestive enzymes and their inhibitors have shown no conclusive association with alcoholic pancreatitis. A potential cofactor that does have relevance to the clinical situation is bacterial endotoxemia. A recent study has demonstrated a key role for lipopolysaccharide, an endotoxin found in the cell wall of gram-negative bacteria, in the initiation and progression of alcoholic pancreatitis.[57]

Nonbiliary and Nonalcoholic Acute Pancreatitis

Although less frequent, there are a variety of other etiologic factors that have been found to cause AP, accounting for as many as one-quarter of the cases. Improved understanding of AP, coupled with advances in genetics, molecular biology, and pathology, has shed new light on its pathogenesis; AP is often the result of a complex interaction between host and environmental factors. This section examines some of these nonbiliary and nonalcoholic causes of AP.

Metabolic Causes

HYPERTRIGLYCERIDEMIA. Hypertriglyceridemia is well documented and accounts for 1% to 10 % of all AP cases.[7,58,59] AP secondary to hypertriglyceridemia seldom occurs unless it is severe (defined as >10 mmol/L fasting), although the exact pathophysiologic mechanism is unclear.[60,61] The prevalence of AP development among dyslipidemia patients is approximately 5% and 20% of patients, with serum triglycerides levels higher than 1000 and 2000 mg/dL, respectively.[61] The clinical course of AP from hypertriglyceridemia is often similar to other causes of AP; however, the morbidity and mortality are reported to be significantly higher in these patients.[61]

This is confounded by the frequent presence of other factors coexisting in some of these patients, such as poorly controlled diabetes mellitus, obesity, alcohol abuse, pregnancy, and hypothyroidism. Triglyceride-induced AP is associated with types I, IV, and V hyperlipidemia.[19] A common theory is that excess triglycerides are hydrolyzed by pancreatic lipase and released in the pancreatic microvasculature, resulting in high concentrations of free fatty acids (FFAs), which overwhelm the binding capacity of albumin and self-aggregate to micellar structures with detergent properties. This promotes acinar cell and pancreatic capillary injury, which results in ischemia and forms an acidic milieu that starts the vicious cycle of triggering more FFA toxicity. At the same time, the ischemia is exacerbated by the increased viscosity of blood from the elevated levels of chylomicrons. The damage to the acinar cells and microvasculature leads to amplification of inflammatory mediators and free radicals, ultimately leading to necrosis, edema, and inflammation of the pancreas.[58,62,63]

Mild to moderate hypertriglyceridemia (<5 mmol/L) occurs in almost half of patients in the early phase of AP from any etiology, but some speculate that this is an epiphenomenon rather than a true precipitant because of the high prevalence of hypertriglyceridemia in the general population.[64,65] Some studies have proposed a genetic predisposition to hypertriglyceridemic AP. Lipoprotein lipase deficiency associated with chylomicronemia is a rare autosomal recessive disorder caused by multiple/different lipoprotein lipase gene mutations, characterized by high fasting plasma triglyceride levels.[66] The frequency of mutations in cationic trypsinogen *(PRSS1)*, serine protease inhibitor Kazal type 1 *(SPINK1)*, cystic fibrosis transmembrane conductance regulator *(CFTR)*, and tumor necrosis factor superfamily member 2 *(TNF2)* genes were studied in 128 patients with hypertriglyceridemia with or without AP. The prevalence of polymorphisms in *CFTR* and *TNF* genes was found to be significantly higher in those with hypertriglyceridemia.[67]

HYPERCALCEMIA. Hypercalcemia is a rare cause of AP, with a reported prevalence of 1% to 4%.[68] There is no clear pathophysiologic mechanism, but elevated parathyroid hormone (parathormone, PTH) and hypercalcemia could be responsible for calcium deposit in the pancreatic ducts. Hypercalcemia-induced cellular injury occurs through activation of pancreatic enzymes by a trypsin-mediated mechanism, resulting in acinar cell damage, pancreatic autodigestion, and subsequent pancreatitis. Another mechanism is the formation of pancreatic calculi, which, by modifying pancreatic secretion, may lead to protein plug formation, resulting in ductal obstruction. Acute hypercalcemia also increases the permeability of the pancreatic ductal membrane, allowing enzymes to leak and injure the pancreatic parenchyma. Parathormone may have direct toxic effects on the pancreas as well.[69] Coexistence of primary hyperparathyroidism and AP has widely been reported, with a prevalence of 1.5% to 13%, but a causal relationship remains unclear.[70,71] Hypercalcemia results from calcium infusion during total parenteral nutrition and occurs in patients with myeloma, leukemia, vitamin D poisoning, disseminated cancer, or severe hyperthyroidism, all of which have been associated with pancreatitis.[19,72,73] Reciprocally, treatment of the hypercalcemia, regardless of the cause, has been reported to resolve the AP.[70]

INBORN ERRORS OF METABOLISM. AP has been associated with a variety of inborn errors of metabolism; these entities are rare but more common in neonatal and pediatric patients. These familial disorders cause hyperlipidemias, disorders of branched-chain amino acid degradation, homocystinuria, hemolytic disorders, acute intermittent porphyria, and several amino acid transporter defects.[74] AP also has been reported in patients with type I glycogen storage disease (von Gierke). The mechanism is not clear, but the common physiobiochemical processes are hyperlipidemia, lactic acidosis, hypoglycemia, and hyperuricemia, any of which could initiate pancreatitis.[75] Other metabolic conditions associated with AP are maple syrup urine disease, cystathionine β-synthase deficiency, 3-hydroxy-3-methylglutaryl-CoA lyase deficiency, pyruvate kinase deficiency, cystinuria, lysinuric protein intolerance, and other cationic aminoacidurias.[76] In the majority of these diseases, pancreatitis is not common, and its pathogenesis is poorly understood.[74]

Chronic Renal Failure and Dialysis-Related Causes

AP can be caused by and associated with end-stage renal disease, including chronic renal failure and dialysis-related complications. Although rare, AP contributes to significant morbidity and mortality in patients whose health is already compromised. The diagnosis of AP is also confounded by renal dysfunction caused by altered levels of pancreatic enzyme estimation and the contribution of pancreatic damage from dialysis and uremia.[77] Multiple studies attempting to determine the incidence of AP in dialysis patients have demonstrated mixed

results. However, the incidence of pancreatitis is generally accepted to be significantly higher in patients undergoing peritoneal dialysis (PD) versus those receiving hemodialysis (HD).[78,79] In a recent large prospective cohort study of 2603 HD patients who were followed for 4 consecutive years after initial diagnosis of chronic HD, it was shown that the incidence of AP was more than three times higher in patients receiving HD compared with the general population. These results conflicted with older small retrospective studies reporting similar rates of AP between HD and the general population.[80,81] Based on postmortem studies, pancreatic abnormalities are reported in as many as 60% of patients undergoing long-term dialysis.[80] Toxic substances in PD dialysate, alterations in serum calcium and PTH levels, and coexisting bacterial and viral infections are postulated factors that can initiate AP.[82] The increase in various GI hormones in patients with end-stage renal disease, such as cholecystokinin, glucagon, and gastric inhibitory polypeptide, can stimulate hypersecretion of pancreatic enzymes such as trypsin, which can also initiate AP.[83] Local accumulation of calcium in the pancreas from calcium in the PD solution has also been postulated. Another mechanism is peritoneal infusion of a large amount of nonphysiologic fluid under high intraabdominal pressure, which renders the pancreas more susceptible to parenchymal injury and hypoxemia, inducing premature activation of proteolytic enzymes, with higher risk of AP. These and other factors are cited to explain why the incidence of AP is higher in patients with PD than in patients with HD.[80]

In conventional HD, there is a risk of hypotension, which is referred to as intradialytic hypotension. It is defined as a decrease of systolic blood pressure greater than or equal to 20 mm Hg or a mean arterial pressure by 10 mm Hg. This can lead to mesenteric ischemia via ischemic-reperfusion injury, a well-established cause of AP. Furthermore, excess GI hormones are not cleared in HD, increasing the risk of AP as mentioned above.[84]

Drug-Induced and Toxin-Induced Pancreatitis

Drug-induced pancreatitis (DIP) is a rare entity with a reported incidence of 0.1% to 2% of AP cases.[85,86] In a World Health Organization (WHO) database, 525 different drugs were listed to cause AP as an adverse effect. Epidemiologic studies report that at-risk populations for DIP include the elderly and pediatric age-groups, females, and patients with inflammatory bowel disease or human immunodeficiency virus (HIV).[85–87] Management and prevention of DIP requires an updated, evidence-based database of drugs associated with pancreatitis because prompt withdrawal of the offending agent is necessary along with supportive care. Little is clear, especially in patients on multidrug therapy; much controversy exists about the precise causes of DIP, and most theories center around a few mechanisms. Accumulation of a toxic metabolite/intermediary and hypersensitivity reactions cause immune-mediated injuries and pancreatic duct constriction, localized angioedema effect in the pancreas, and arteriolar thrombosis.[88,89] Adverse effects of drugs causing hypercalcemia or hypertriglyceridemia are also mechanisms for DIP.[90] The family of drugs often reported to cause AP are the angiotensin-converting enzyme (ACE) inhibitors, antidiabetic agents, statins, 5-ASA and derivatives, antibiotics (e.g., metronidazole, tetracycline), and valproic acid. Table 55.1 summarizes the various classifications and drugs.[86,89–95] A recent publication developed a data-driven classification system, based loosely on the system

TABLE 55.1 Classifications of Drug-Induced Acute Pancreatitis (AP) and Common Drugs and Toxins Reported in the Literature[a]

ASSOCIATIONS	DEFINITE		PROBABLE	POSSIBLE
Definitions Karch & Lasagna, 1975	1. Drug reaction that follows a reasonable temporal sequence from administration of the drug that follows a known response pattern 2. That is confirmed by cessation of the drug (dechallenge) 3. That is confirmed by reappearance of the symptoms on repeated exposure to the drug (rechallenge)		3. That could not be explained by the known characteristics of patient's clinical state	2. That could have been produced by patient's clinical state or other modes of therapy administered to patient
Definitions Mallory & Kern, 1980	*Criteria* 1. Pancreatitis develops during the treatment with a suspected drug. 2. There is no evidence of any other etiologic factors. 3. Symptoms disappear after withdrawal of the drug. 4. Recurrence of pancreatitis on reintroduction of the pharmacologic agent.		Criteria fulfilled without proof of recurrent pancreatitis after rechallenge of the pharmacologic agent	Single case reports on pancreatitis

DEFINITION/ CLASS	CLASS 1A	CLASS 1B		CLASS II	CLASS III	CLASS IV
Badalov et al., 2007	At least 1 case report, evidence of positive rechallenge Exclusion of other causes of AP.	At least 1 case report with positive rechallenge Other causes such as alcohol, gallstones, hypertriglyceridemia, and other drugs were not excluded.		At least 4 case reports with a consistent latency period for 75% or more of cases	At least 2 cases in the literature No consistent latency among cases No rechallenge	Not fitting into cases described earlier Single case report in published literature, without rechallenge
Wolfe et al., 2020	At least 1 case report in humans, with positive rechallenge; All other causes ruled out[b]	At least 1 case report in humans, with positive rechallenge; All other causes not ruled out[b]	At least 1 case report in humans, without positive rechallenge; All other causes not ruled out[b]	At least 2 cases in humans reported in literature, without positive rechallenge; All other causes not ruled out, Consistent latency[c]	At least 2 cases in humans, reported in literature without positive rechallenge; All other causes not ruled out; Inconsistent latency[c]	At least 1 case in humans reported in literature, drugs not fitting into earlier described classes

DRUGS						
Wolfe et al., 2020; Badalov et al., 2007 Jones MR, 2015 Kaurich, 2008 Hung, 2014 Nitsche et al., 2010 Trivedi & Pitchumoni, 2005 Mallory & Kern, 1980	5-acetylsalicylic acid (mesalamine 6-mercaptopurine (6-MP) Acetaminophen All-trans retinoic acid Azathioprine Azodisalicylate/olsalazine Bezafibrate Captopril Carbimazole Cimetidine Codeine Dapsone Erythromycin Fluvastatin Furosemide Interferon-alpha Isoniazid Lisinopril L-asparaginase Metformin Methimazole Methylprednisolone[a] Metronidazole Nitrofurantoin Orlistat[a] Piroxicam[a]	Amiodarone Ampicillin Antilymphocyte Globulin[a] Carbamazepine Ciprofloxacin[a] Clomiphene Clothiapine[a] Clozapine Cytarabine[a] Dexamethasone Didanosine Diphenoxylate + atropine Eluxadoline[a] Enalapril Everolimus[a] Growth Hormone[a] Hydrochlorothiazide Lamivudine Hydrocortisone Ifosfamide Indalpine[a] Losartan Mefenamic acid[a] Meglumine antimoniate Methyldopa Mirtazapine	Adefovir dipivoxil[a] Amoxicillin + clavulanic acid[a] Artesunate[a] Atorvastatin Axitinib[a] Boceprevir[a] Bortezomib[a] Canagliflozin[a] Candesartan[a] Celecoxib[a] Clarithromycin Danazol Dexfenfluramine[a] Diclofenac Diethylstilbestrol[a] Dilantin[a] Dimethyl fumarate[a] Doxycycline[a] Ezetimibe[a] Finasteride Flurbiprofen[a] Gadolinium[a] Glicazide[a] Glimepiride[a] Ibuprofen[a] Indomethacin	Ceftriaxone Clofibrate[a] Exenatide[a] Isotretinoin Levetiracetam[a] Sitagliptin[a]	Acetylsalicylic acid[a] Gold Nivolumab[a] Ondanseton[a] Tacrolimus[a]	Ado-trastuzumab Emtansine[a] Albiglutide[a] Alendronate Amineptine[a] Benazepril Brentuximab vedotin[a] Calcium carbonate[a] Capecitabine Chlorthalidone Ciprofibrate[a] Cisplatin Clomipramine[a] Clonidine[a] Demeclocycline[a] Doxylamine succinate[a] Ertapenem[a] Estramustine Phosphate[a] Famcyclovir Gatifloxacin[a] Gemfibrozil Granisetron[a] Interleukin-2 Lacosamide[a] Lamotrigine Linagliptin[a] Linezolid[a]

Continued

TABLE 55.1   Classifications of Drug-Induced Acute Pancreatitis (AP) and Common Drugs and Toxins Reported in the Literature—cont'd

DRUGS

Pravastatin	Nelfinavir	Interferon beta	Lixisenatide[a]
Prednisone	Octreotide	Irbesartan	Loperamide[a]
Premarin	Omeprazole	Itraconazole[a]	Lovastatin
Procainamide	Oral contracep-	Ixazomib[a]	Maprotiline[a]
Pyritinol	tive	Ketoprofen	Methandrostenolone[a]
Ramipril	Oxyphenbuta-	Ketorolac	Micafungin[a]
Ranitidine	zone	Lanreotide[a]	Miltefosine[a]
Rosuvastatin	Paclitaxel	Lenvatinib[a]	Mizoribine[a]
Simvastatin	Paromomycin[a]	Liraglutide[a]	Montelukast[a]
Sorafenib[a]	Pentamidine	Meprobamate[a]	Mycophenolate
Sulindac	Perindopril[a]	Metolazone	mofetil[a]
Tamoxifen	Prednisolone	Minocycline	Nifuroxazide[a]
Telaprevir[a]	Propofol	Naltrexone[a]	Norfloxacin[a]
Tetracycline	Quetiapine[a]	Naproxen	Pazopanib[a]
Tigecycline[a]	Rifampicin[a]	Nilotinib	Phenformin[a]
Thalidomide[a]	Risperidone	Olanzapine[a]	Phenolpthalien
Trimethoprim-	Salazopyrine[a]	Pantoprazole[a]	Polyethylene
sulfamethox-	Saxagliptin[a]	Propylthiouracil[a]	glycol bowel
azole	Stibogluconate	Riluzole[a]	Preparation[a]
Vemurafenib^	Sulfasalazine	Rofecoxib[a]	Pregabalin[a]
Valproic acid	Valsartan[a]	Secnidazole[a]	Procetofene[a]
	Voriconazole[a]	Sirolimus[a]	Rasburicase[a]
		Theophylline[a]	Rifampin
		Tiaprofenic acid[a]	Ritonavir
		Tinidazole[a]	Roxithromycin
		Vedolizumab[a]	Stavudine[a]
		Vildagliptin[a]	Sunitinib[a]
			Tacalcitol[a]
			Telmisartan[a]
			Tocilizumab[a]
			Ursodeoxycholic
			acid[a]
			Venlafaxine[a]
			Zidovudine[a]
			Ziprasidone[a]

ASSOCIATIONS	DEFINITE	PROBABLE	POSSIBLE/SHOWN IN ANIMAL STUDIES
Toxins (sources) Khurana & Barkin, 2001	Ethyl alcohol (antifreeze, organic solvent) Methanol (solvent, nail vanish, gasoline additive) Organophosphate insecticides (pesticide, agricultural sprays, household insecticides, herbicides) Scorpion's venom	Alpha toxin (*Clostridium perfringens*, *Staphylococcus aureus*) Diesel exhaust fumes (diesel engines) Pentachlorophenol (paper, leather, wood preservatives, fungicide) Tricholorethylene (degreaser for metals, veterinary anesthetic)	Aflatoxin (contaminated food, peanuts, grains) Carbon tetrachloride (organic solvent, dry cleaning, fire extinguishers, refrigerants) Cobalt (metal alloys) Neutral red (coloring agent, tropical viricide)

Drug list adapted from Wolfe et al (2020).
[a]The associations for new drugs are not reported in Badalov et al. (2007)
[b]Causes such as alcohol, hypertriglyceridemia, gallstones, and other drugs.
[c]Consistent latency defined as greater than 75% of cases falling into the same latency category (category 1: < 24 hours, category 2: 1–30 days, category 3: >30 days)

developed by Badalov et al., that reclassified drugs into six classes based on: (1) evidence of a positive rechallenge, (2) a simplified measure of the rigor of causality assessment conducted, and (3) the consistency of the latency for drugs for cases in which a positive rechallenge or rigorous causality measurement was not reported.[91,96]

Toxins are reported causes of AP, but this is rare. Many cases may, in fact, be erroneously labeled "idiopathic pancreatitis." Mechanisms may be similar to how certain drugs can initiate AP. The commonly reported toxins include scorpion's venom,[97] organophosphate anticholinesterase insecticides,[98] organic solvents, pentachlorophenol,[99] and diethyl glycol (see Table 55.1).[100,101] Data on AP associated with herbal or alternative medicines are limited.[92] Reports documenting saw palmetto–induced AP postulate that saw palmetto (*Serenoa repens*, extract of American dwarf palm tree fruit) stimulates estrogen receptors, which may result in hypertriglyceridemia or induce a hypercoagulable state that leads to pancreatic necrosis. Saw palmetto also inhibits cyclooxygenase, which is associated with the development of AP.[102,103]

The challenge with DIP lies in the lack of a standardized definition for the diagnosis of DIP. Although AP diagnostic criteria have been generally accepted, a recent review of DIP noted a substantial difference in criteria used by researchers to determine causality for DIP and an inconsistent application of the standard criteria for AP diagnosis. This potentially leads to challenges in classifying drugs with respect to their association with DIP. Furthermore, this can lead to information bias from misdiagnosis of other GI disease as AP and incorrect attribution of cause to a drug when it is not.[96,104]

Infectious Causes

A variety of bacterial, viral, and parasitic infections have been established to cause AP, but the true incidence is not known, although it has been postulated to up to 10% of AP may be attributed to an infectious etiology.[105] The value of treating the infectious agent to reverse pancreatitis is also not well established. Diagnostic criteria have been defined to evaluate the relationship between the microorganism and AP, based on histologic and imaging evidence of pancreatitis and combined with laboratory data on the infectious agent, after exclusion of the common causes (Table 55.2).[106] AP may manifest as a mild interstitial form, which constitutes 80% of patients and has a low morbidity and mortality rate (<1%). In 20% of patients, however, they may develop a more severe form characterized by an early vasoactive and toxic phase, and a late, more septic phase. Each organism works in a peculiar way to cause AP.[105]

BACTERIAL CAUSES. Pancreatitis caused by bacteria has been reported with hematogenous, lymphatic seeding or ascending infection of the pancreatic duct from the biliary tree or the GI tract. *Mycoplasma pneumoniae* has been implicated as a cause of pancreatitis from antibody detection.[107,108] Studies in the 1970s have reported high *Mycoplasma* antibody titer in patients with AP.[105,109,110] Nevertheless, the exact mechanism and relationship between AP and *Mycoplasma* infection remains unclear; postulated factors include ascending infection of *Mycoplasma* organisms, seeding via the hematogenous or lymphatic routes, autoimmune-mediated response to *Mycoplasma* infection, and an organ-specific toxin.[111] Other pathogenic bacteria, such as *Leptospira interrogans, Campylobacter jejuni, Salmonella typhi, Salmonella paratyphi Brucella, Yersinia enterocolitica, Y. pseudotuberculosis, Legionella, Nocardia, Mycobacterium tuberculosis,* and *M. avium,* have been reported as causes of sporadic cases of AP.[105,112–114]

VIRAL CAUSES. Viruses are the first and largest group of infectious agents found associated with AP. Diagnosis is based on detection of antiviral antibodies coupled with the clinical diagnosis of pancreatitis after exclusion of the common causes. Mumps (single-stranded DNA paramyxovirus) was implicated as a cause of AP in 1905, when Lemoine and Lapasset described the first case of AP associated with mumps virus infection on autopsy.[115] Since the mass vaccination of the general population with the measles, mumps, rubella (MMR) vaccine, the associated AP rarely has been reported.[111,116] In 1944 Linsey first described the association between AP and viral hepatitis, which now is well recognized. In most cases, AP is a complication in the course of fulminant liver failure, and AP in nonfulminant viral hepatitis is uncommon, with only isolated case reports.[117] Hepatitis B is the hepatitis virus most implicated in AP (see Chapter 68).[118–120] This is typically observed after liver transplantation where immunosuppression therapy may play a role.[120,121] In one study, 4 out of 27 HBsAg carriers who underwent liver transplantation had AP post-transplantation; the diagnosis was based on presence of HBsAg in pancreatic juice and acinar cells.[120,121] There have been recent studies reporting hepatitis A and E virus causing AP as well.[105,122,123] Studies have reported pathologic changes in the pancreas of HIV patients. Coexisting conditions such as alcohol use, biliary disease, and malignancy associated with acquired immunodeficiency syndrome (AIDS; e.g., Kaposi sarcoma, lymphoma) in HIV/AIDS patients; the use of antiretroviral and other medications in their treatment (e.g., corticosteroids, ketoconazole, sulfonamides, pentamidine, metronidazole, isoniazid); and opportunistic infections (e.g., mycobacteria, cytomegalovirus, herpes simplex, cryptosporidiosis) all can contribute to the pathogenesis of AP.[124] Other viruses reported to cause AP include coxsackievirus type B, cytomegalovirus, varicella-zoster, and herpes simplex.[105,111,125–127]

FUNGAL AND PARASITIC CAUSES. Fungal and parasitic infestation is a rare cause of AP. The fungi *Aspergillus* and *Candida* have been reported to cause AP.[106,128] *Ascaris lumbricoides* (nematode) is the most common parasite involved. It is a common infection in developing countries and endemic in certain tropical countries (20%–82% of the population).[129,130] AP is likely triggered by the obstruction of the pancreatic duct, especially in pediatric patients, in whom the duct is much narrower relative to the

TABLE 55.2	Diagnostic Criteria for Infectious Causes of Acute Pancreatitis		
CRITERIA	DEFINITE	PROBABLE	POSSIBLE
Pancreatitis	Evidence of pancreatitis at surgery, autopsy, *or* Radiologic evidence	Threefold increase in amylase and/or lipase *and* Characteristic symptoms (e.g., abdominal pain, tenderness)	Threefold increase in amylase and/or lipase without characteristic symptoms
Infection	Organism identified in pancreas or pancreatic duct by stain or culture	Culture of organism from blood or pancreatic juice *or* Serologic diagnosis (Fourfold or greater rise in titer) *with* Characteristic clinical or epidemiologic setting	Culture of organism from other body sites *or* Serologic diagnosis (Fourfold or greater rise in titer)

Modified from Parenti DM, Steinberg W, Kang P. Infectious causes of acute pancreatitis. *Pancreas.* 1996;13(4):356–371.

parasite. Other parasites implicated in AP by similar mechanisms include *Clonorchis senensis, Opisthorchis* spp., *Dicrocoelium dendriticum, Fasciola hepatica, Schistosoma haematobium, S. mansoni, Toxoplasma, Cryptosporidium, Plasmodium falciparum, Echinococcus granulous, Opisthorchis species,* and *Paragonimus westermani* (see Chapter 45).[92,105,106,130,131]

Iatrogenic or Traumatic Pancreatitis

Post–endoscopic retrograde cholangiopancreatography (ERCP) pancreatitis (PEP) is the most common and feared iatrogenic cause of AP, occurring in approximately 1% to 3% of patients undergoing diagnostic ERCP, 2% to 5% receiving therapeutic ERCP, and as many as 25% having sphincter of Oddi studies (see Chapters 20 and 30). PEP accounts for substantial morbidity and mortality, with mortality reported at 0.7%[132,133]; and healthcare expenditures in excess of $200 million annually in the United States.[134] PEP is defined as new or increased abdominal pain that is clinically consistent with AP and associated pancreatic enzyme elevation, at least three times the upper normal limit within 24 hours after the procedure and resulting in hospitalization of 2 nights or more.[132,133,135] Based on a recent meta-analysis and several large studies, patient-related factors, such as female gender, sphincter of Oddi dysfunction, intraductal papillary mucinous neoplasm (IPMN), previous or recurrent pancreatitis, and procedure-related factors such as previous PEP, precut/endoscopic sphincterotomy, difficult cannulation, and main pancreatic duct injection are all independent risk factors for PEP.[136–140]

Patients with pancreatic trauma are seen usually with a triad of abdominal pain, leukocytosis, and elevated serum amylase levels. Both blunt and penetrating trauma can injure the pancreas, although these injuries are uncommon because of its retroperitoneal location (see Chapter 114). Traumatic AP occurs in less than 2% of blunt trauma cases and is mainly in connection with multiple injuries after bicycle or vehicle accidents but in as many as 12% to 30% of penetrating trauma caused by gunshot or stab wounds.[141,142] Pancreatic injury is challenging to recognize because of coexisting abdominal injuries and thus requires a high index of suspicion. The damage can be mild to very severe, from a contusion to a severe crush injury or transection of the gland, particularly where the pancreas crosses over the spine, resulting in pancreatic ascites and acute duct rupture. Healing of pancreatic ductal injuries can lead to scarring and stricture of the main pancreatic duct, with resultant obstructive pancreatitis proximally.

Autoimmune Pancreatitis

Autoimmune pancreatitis (AIP) is a rare but distinct disorder with a reported prevalence up to 4.6 per 100,000.[7,143–145] AIP often has a dramatic response to corticosteroid treatment (see Chapters 54 and 57).[143,146,147] The incidence seems to be increasing, probably because of increased recognition of this distinct entity. Radiologically, AIP is characterized by segmental, diffuse, or irregular narrowing of the main pancreatic duct and diffuse enlargement of the pancreas, elevated levels of serum immunoglobulin G (more than twice the upper limit of IgG, particularly of the IgG4 subtype), and the presence of autoantibodies. Histopathologically it is characterized by lymphoplasmacytic infiltration and fibrosis. An international consensus on diagnosis based on histopathologic characteristics has been proposed and subdivided AIP into type 1 (lymphoplasmacytic sclerosing pancreatitis [LPSP]) and type 2

(idiopathic duct-centric pancreatitis [IDCP]). Cardinal features include imaging of pancreatic parenchyma and duct, serology, extrapancreatic involvement, histology, and an optional criterion of response to corticosteroid therapy. Each feature was categorized as level 1 or 2 depending on the reliability of the diagnosis.[148] Types 1 and 2 AIP have similarities but also different clinical features and associations (Table 55.3).[143,147,149,150] Other autoimmune-related disease such as vasculitic conditions (e.g., glomerulonephritis, Wegener's granulomatosis) and rheumatic diseases such as rheumatoid arthritis and systemic lupus erythematosus have been reported to be associated with AP, but the pathogenesis is still unclear.[147,151–155] Some typical features of AIP on CT and MRI are shown in Fig. 55.2 (see Chapter 17).

Anatomic or Congenital Causes

Anatomic variants or congenital anomalies can lead to AP. Based on autopsy and ERCP studies, *pancreas divisum* (PD) is the most common congenital variation of pancreatic ductal anatomy, occurring in as many as 5% to 12% of individuals (see Chapters 1, 2, and 53).[138,156,157] The failure of the derived ventral and dorsal pancreas to fuse embryologically in approximately the seventh week of intrauterine life can result in separate ductal systems.[146,147] Partial fusion results in the incomplete PD, and the dorsal duct drains through the major papillae via the ventral duct.[158] This communication is generally narrow and may be inadequate for drainage. The inability of minor papillae to accommodate the flow when the pancreas is stimulated over time leads to relative obstruction and ductal hypertension, causing injury and leading to pancreatitis.[159] There is considerable debate as to the causative role of PD in pancreatitis.[7,157,158] Some observational studies of patients with idiopathic recurrent acute pancreatitis (I-RAP) and CP have shown similar frequency of pancreatitis in patients with PD compared with normal ductal variants. The prevalence of I-RAP and CP is as high as 50% in patients with PD when associated with certain genetic mutations such as serine protease inhibitor Kazal type 1 (SPINK1), cystic fibrosis transmembrane conductance regulator gene (CFTR), and chymotrypsin C gene (CTRC), suggesting that it may be a co-factor rather than causative for pancreatitis (see Chapter 53). Furthermore, it has been postulated that the presence of PD reduces the threshold for AP from other known primary factors such as alcohol and trauma.[160]

Annular pancreas is another rare anatomic condition, affecting about 1 in 20,000 newborns,[161] resulting in the entrapment of both the CBD and duodenum by the annular growth of the pancreas[138] (see Chapter 53). Approximately one third of patients with annular pancreas have PD, but it is not clear whether pancreatitis depends on the annular variant or the PD.[7] The sphincter of Oddi (SO) is a complex of smooth muscle surrounding the terminal CBD, main pancreatic duct, and common channel. Its main functions are regulating pancreatic and bile flow and preventing reflux of duodenal contents into the ducts. *Sphincter of Oddi dysfunction* (SOD) refers to the abnormality of SO contractility that can manifest clinically as pain, pancreatitis, or deranged liver function tests. *Anomalous pancreaticobiliary duct junction* (APBJ) results in pancreatic reflux in the biliary tree. Reflux of bile into the pancreas seldom occurs because of the higher pressure in the pancreatic duct compared with the bile duct (see Fig. 55.1B). Other anatomic lesions that can cause AP include anomalies in the biliary tree

TABLE 55.3 Features of Types 1 and 2 Autoimmune Pancreatitis (AIP)

CLINICAL FEATURES	TYPE 1 AIP	TYPE 2 AIP
Synonyms	Lymphoplasmacytic sclerosing Pancreatitis; AIP without GEL	Idiopathic duct-centric chronic pancreatitis; AIP with GEL
Epidemiology	Asia > USA, Europe	Europe > USA > Asia
Age at diagnosis, mean	Old, 7th decade	Young, 5th decade
Gender	Male predominance, 75% in males	Equal, 50% in males
Clinical presentation	Painless obstructive jaundice	Painless obstructive jaundice; abdominal pain, acute pancreatitis
Serum IgG4 level	Often elevated; ~66%	Normal, occasionally elevated; ~25%
Extrapancreatic involvement	Proximal bile duct, salivary gland, kidney, retroperitoneum; ~50%	No
Inflammatory bowel disease, association with ulcerative colitis	Occasionally	Common; ~10%–20%
Response to corticosteroids	Excellent; ~100%	Excellent; ~100%
Recurrence	High (20%–60%)	Low (<10%)
Associated with IgG4-related disease	Yes	No

HISTOLOGIC FEATURES	TYPE 1 AIP	TYPE 2 AIP
IgG4 tissue staining	Abundant (>10 cells/hpf)	Scant (<10 cells/hpf)
GEL	—	+ + +
Lymphoplasmacytic infiltration	+ +	+ +
Periductal inflammation	+ +	+ +
Obliterative phlebitis	+ +	+
Storiform fibrosis	+ +	+

GEL, Granulocytic epithelial lesion; *hpf*, high-power field; *IgG4*, immunoglobulin G4.
From Hart PA, Zen Y, Chari ST. Recent advances in autoimmune pancreatitis. *Gastroenterology.* 2015;149(1):39–51; and Kamisawa T, Chari ST, Lerch MM, Kim MH, Gress TM, Shimosegawa T. Recent advances in autoimmune pancreatitis: Type 1 and type 2. *Gut.* 2013;62(9):1373–1380.

such as choledochal cyst, choledochocele (type III choledochal cyst), and duodenal duplication cyst.[162]

Tumors

Pancreatitis can be the first presentation of pancreaticobiliary and periampullary tumors (see Chapter 62). This should be considered in patients with the index pancreatitis episode who are older than 40 years, especially if they have constitutional symptoms such as loss of weight and appetite or new onset of diabetes. The most common neoplasms associated with pancreatitis are IPMN (see Fig. 55.1C), mucinous cystic neoplasms, ampullary tumors, islet cell tumors, and pancreatic adenocarcinoma (see Fig. 55.1D).[7,163] Benign or premalignant tumors that arise at the major papillae have the same potential to cause pancreatitis by causing ductal obstruction (e.g., adenoma, lipoma, fibroma, lymphangioma, leiomyoma, harmatoma).[164]

Genetic Causes

There is increasing evidence for a genetic basis for pancreatitis.[165–167] Hereditary pancreatitis (HP) was first described in 1952, in six family members across three generations. Since then, more than 100 families with HP have been reported. Studies from Europe reported a prevalence ranging from 0.125 to 0.57 per 100,000 people.[7,166,168] This was led by the discovery that gain-of-function mutations in trypsinogen lead to HP. Molecular, epidemiologic, and genetic studies have identified several pancreas-targeting factors associated with the susceptibility for AP and CP. These include *SPINK1, CFTR, PRSS1,* anionic trypsinogen (*PRSS2*), MCP-1-2518 G allele, calcium-sensing receptor (*CASR*), chymotrypsinogen C (*CTRC*),

CTRB1/CTRB2 locus, *CPA1* gene, *CEL/ CEL-HYB* allele and *CLDN2* variants (Fig. 55.3).[165,166,169,170] Patients with these mutations are at increased risk for pancreatitis caused by a variety of mechanisms involving hypercalcemia and hyperlipidemia. Other mechanisms exist, but most are not well elucidated. Mitochondrial disorders may very occasionally suffer from AP, but the pathogenesis is unclear as well.[171] Recent studies have also shown that patients with idiopathic AP and idiopathic CP may have different genetic backgrounds[169] (see Chapter 54).

Idiopathic Acute Pancreatitis

The cause for AP is unidentifiable in as many as 30% of patients, despite a comprehensive history (drug, alcohol, metabolic disorder), physical examination, laboratory investigations, and radiologic evaluation (of at least two second-level imaging techniques including endoscopic ultrasound [EUS] and magnetic resonance cholangiopancreatography [MRCP]).[7,20] These patients are conventionally classified as having idiopathic AP (IAP).[172] Idiopathic acute recurrent pancreatitis (IARP) is defined when patients have more than one episode of IAP. This accounts for 3% to 59% of all cases of recurrent AP.[7,173,174] Evaluation of IAP/IARP is prudent because most untreated patients with IARP experience recurrent episodes that may result in chronic pancreatitis.[175] Many of these IAP/IARP cases may, in fact, be caused by previously unrecognized causes, such as genetic mutations or drugs/toxins.[7] For example, it has been shown that chronic cigarette smoking impairs CFTR ion channel conductance in pancreatic ductal cells, one possible mechanism predisposing to IAP, particularly in persons carrying a

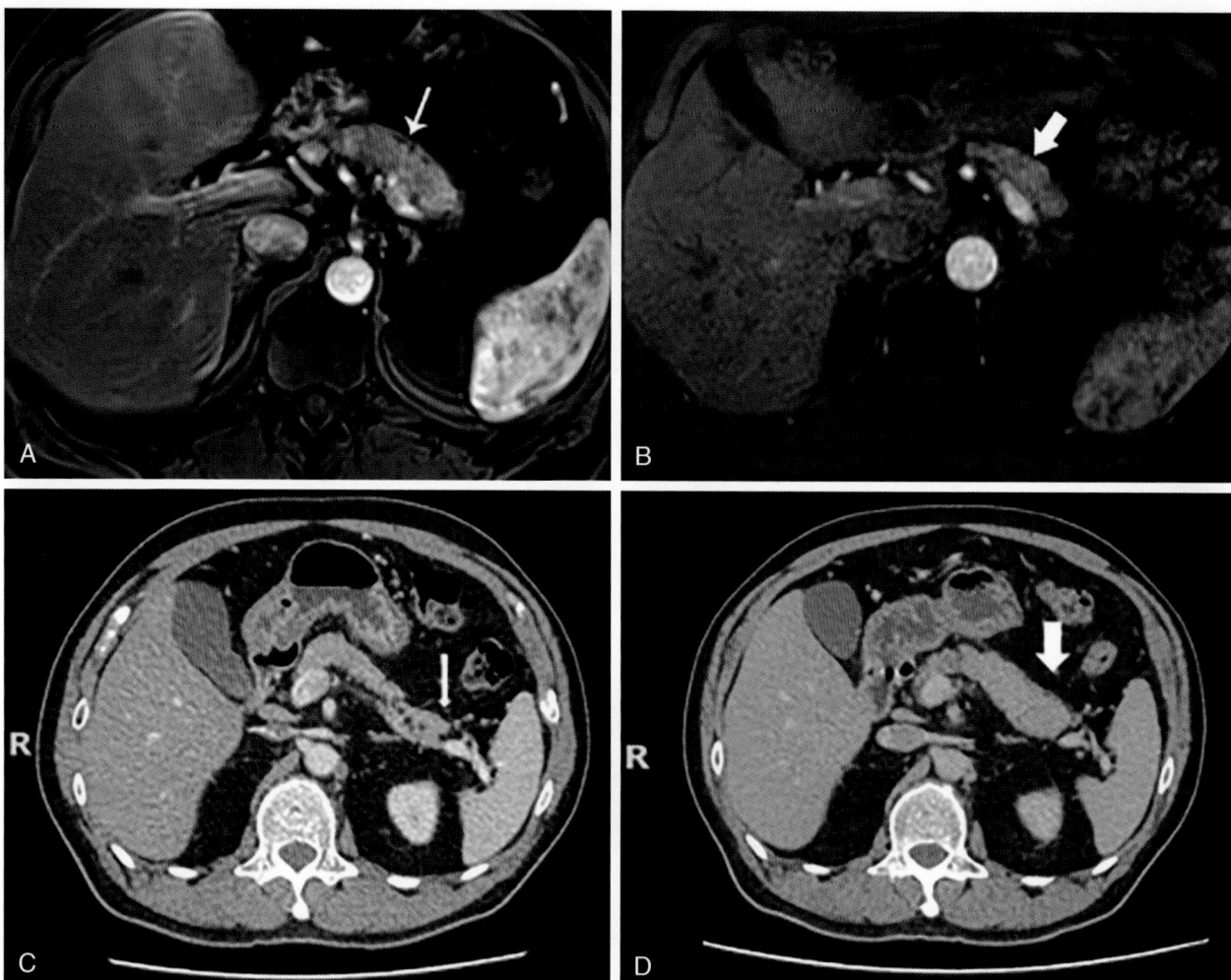

FIGURE 55.2   Diagnostic magnetic resonance imaging (MRI) **(A–B)** and computed tomography (CT) **(C–D)** of the pancreas in type 1 autoimmune pancreatitis (AIP; see Chapters 54). **A,** MRI T1-weighted arterial-phase postcontrast image of a 60-year-old man showing enlargement of the pancreatic gland with a peripheral enhancing rim *(thin arrow)*. **B,** MRI imaging in the same patient obtained 6 months after treatment with oral corticosteroids showing normalization of the pancreatic parenchyma and resolution of the peripancreatic halo *(thick arrow)*. **C,** Normal lobular architecture and contour of the pancreas in another patient before AIP *(thin arrow)*. **D,** The pancreas is featureless with effacement of the normal lobular contour resulting in the commonly known "sausage shaped pancreas" classic of AIP in the same patient during AIP *(thick arrow)*. (Images A and B used with permission from Hafezi-Nejad N, Singh VK, Fung C, Takahashi N, Zaheer A. MR imaging of autoimmune pancreatitis. Magn Reson Imaging Clin N Am. 2018;26(3):463–478; Images C and D courtesy of Dr. Adrian Chiow/Dr. Andrew Kwek.)

CFTR mutation.[157] It is hoped that this AP patient group will decrease while our understanding of the disease process improves with time and future studies.

ASSESSMENT OF ACUTE PANCREATITIS

Diagnostic Assessment

The diagnosis of AP is based on the clinical presentation of the patient supported by serum levels of amylase and lipase and imaging findings. The diagnosis of AP requires at least 2 of the following features: (1) characteristic abdominal pain; (2) biochemical evidence of pancreatitis (i.e., amylase or lipase elevated >3 times the upper limit of normal); and/or (3) evidence of pancreatitis on cross-sectional imaging[1] (see Chapter 54 and 56). History should also focus on possible causes, such as gallstones and heavy alcohol intake.[2,9] AP is characterized by acute and constant pain localized in the epigastrium or right upper quadrant that usually radiates to the back.[176] The pain typically lasts for several days and can be associated with nausea and vomiting. In metabolic causes or those associated with alcohol abuse, however, the pain may be poorly localized and less acute in onset.[177] AP presents along a clinical spectrum and can be categorized as mild, moderately severe, or severe, based on the revised Atlanta classification. Physical signs depend on the severity of pancreatitis.[176] In mild pancreatitis, abdominal examination usually reveals upper abdominal tenderness without features of peritonitis, such as rigidity or rebound tenderness. In severe cases, however, pancreatitis may mimic other causes of acute abdominal emergencies. Severe pancreatitis with necrosis may also result in exudates tracking along the falciform ligament and retroperitoneum, resulting in Cullen and Grey Turner signs. There are two overlapping phases of AP: early and late. The early phase of AP generally takes place in the first 2 weeks after onset and the late phase can last weeks to months after initial symptoms develop.

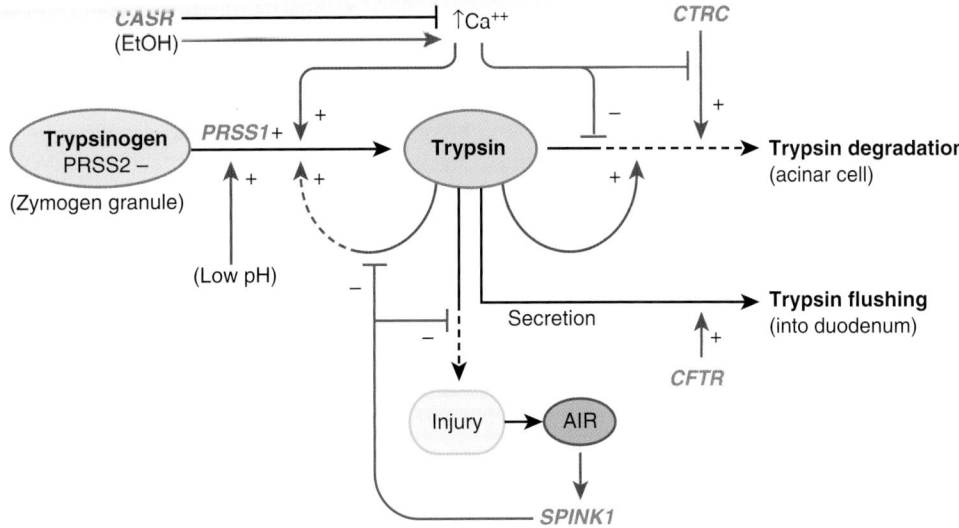

FIGURE 55.3   Genetic basis of acute pancreatitis. Activation of trypsinogen to trypsin within the pancreas is crucial in the pathogenesis of pancreatitis. Trypsinogen activation is promoted by cationic trypsinogen mutations *(PRSS1+)*, high calcium (Ca^{2+}), active trypsin, and low pH. Ca^{2+} levels are regulated by calcium-sensing receptor *(CASR)* and dysregulated by alcohol *(EtOH)*. Active trypsin degradation is facilitated by cystic fibrosis transmembrane conductance regulator *(CFTR)* and by other active trypsin molecules but is blocked by high Ca^{2+}. Active trypsin leads to pancreatic injury, which leads to an acute inflammatory response *(AIR)*. This upregulates expression of serine protease inhibitor Kazal 1 *(SPINK1)*, which blocks active trypsin and therefore prevents further activation of trypsinogen and limits further tissue injury. CFTR is an extra–acinar cell mechanism to eliminate trypsin by flushing it out of the pancreatic duct. Mutations in *CFTR* reduce fluid secretion and trypsinogen/trypsin washout. Genes in *blue italic* type indicate that genetic variants are associated with pancreatitis. (From Whitcomb DC. Genetic aspects of pancreatitis. *Annu Rev Med.* 2010;61:413–424.)

Serum levels of amylase and lipase are frequently obtained for the diagnosis of AP. An elevation exceeding three times the normal upper limit of serum amylase or lipase supports the diagnosis of pancreatitis. There is no standardized reference range for serum amylase or lipase levels because of different laboratory techniques, with the upper limit of normal ranges being between 100–300 U/l for amylase and 50–160 U/l for lipase.[178] Serum amylase concentrations generally rise within a few hours after symptom onset and return to normal within approximately 5 days.[176] It is important to note that amylase levels may not be elevated in as many as 19% of AP patients on admission. Furthermore, amylase levels may also be elevated in the absence of pancreatitis in patients with renal impairment, salivary gland diseases, and other extrapancreatic abdominal conditions (e.g., acute appendicitis, perforated viscus, intestinal obstruction, mesenteric ischemia). Serum lipase levels have the added advantage of remaining elevated for a longer period and have a higher specificity versus amylase. Other laboratory tests, such as trypsinogen activation peptide and trypsinogen-2 levels, have been shown to be more specific than serum amylase or lipase levels, but these tests are not readily available.[177,179]

Occasionally, diagnosis of AP based on the clinical presentation and biochemical investigations alone may be difficult. In these patients, cross-sectional imaging such as ultrasound, contrast-enhanced computed tomography (CT), or magnetic resonance imaging (MRI) should be performed on admission to confirm the diagnosis and exclude other abdominal conditions.[177] CT scan has a reported sensitivity of 87% to 90% and specificity of 90% to 92% for detecting pancreatitis.[176] Imaging may also identify the cause of pancreatitis and its associated complications (see Chapter 17).

Definition and Classification of Severity of Acute Pancreatitis

Most cases (around 80%) are mild and have a self-limiting course with only interstitial changes of the pancreas without local and/or systemic complications[9,180] (see Chapter 56). Nevertheless, approximately 20% of cases may progress to severe pancreatitis, resulting in major local and systemic complications with a significant risk of mortality. The definition and stratification of the severity of pancreatitis are of utmost importance both in clinical practice and for consistency in research.[1,181] In the clinical setting, early identification of patients on admission allows for timely intervention and treatment. In the secondary care setting, patients needing transfer to a tertiary care center may be identified. Physicians treating severe pancreatitis may triage these patients to optimize and tailor their management accordingly. Targeted therapy such as enteral feeding, endoscopic sphincterotomy, or antibiotics may be initiated at the appropriate time in select patients.[182] For research purposes, accurate stratification of patients is important for recruitment in clinical trials and for valid comparison between studies.[9,181]

The first classification system for pancreatitis was established in Marseille in 1965[183] (see Chapter 54). Since then, the standard tool for defining severe pancreatitis has been the Atlanta classification, which was proposed in 1992.[184] This was based on clinical, radiologic, and pathologic findings and categorized pancreatitis into mild interstitial and severe necrotizing pancreatitis. Despite its value, however, it has several limitations. The main drawback is that no distinction was made between predicted (based on Ranson and APACHE II criteria) and actual (based on organ failure) severity for severe AP. The initial Atlanta classification also failed to recognize that the number of organs failing and the duration of organ failure were important prognosticators for AP.[185]

Because of a better understanding of the pathophysiology and outcomes of necrotizing pancreatitis and organ failure, the Atlanta classification was revised in 2012 based on an international Internet-based consensus (Table 55.4).[1] The updated classification defined three degrees of severity for AP instead of two and recognized that pancreatitis is an evolving, dynamic condition in which disease severity may change during the course of disease. Another important revision included the

definitions for pancreatic and peripancreatic collections and the distinction between collections composed of fluid versus those arising from necrosis, containing solid components.

Parallel to the development of the revised Atlanta classification, the determinant-based classification (DBC) was developed based on a large international survey.[181] In this system, pancreatitis was stratified into four degrees of severity: mild, moderate, severe, and critical (see Table 55.4). The DBC was based on two main principles to overcome the limitations of the original Atlanta criteria. First, it was based on actual factors of

TABLE 55.4   Atlanta and Determinant-Based Classification Systems for Severity of Acute Pancreatitis

CLASSIFICATION	MILD	MODERATE	SEVERE
Atlanta 2012[1]	No organ failure	Presence of transient organ failure (usually resolves within 48 hr) *and/or*	Persistent organ failure: may be single or multiple
	No local or systemic complications	Local or systemic complications without persistent organ failure	Usually have at least 1 local complications
	Mortality is very rare.	Mortality is much lower than that of severe acute pancreatitis.	Infected necrosis with persistent organ failure is associated with extremely high mortality, reported as high as 36%–50%.
Atlanta 1992[184]	Minimal organ dysfunction and an uneventful recovery Responds to appropriate fluid administration with prompt normalization of physical signs and laboratory values Lacks the described features of severe acute pancreatitis	Not defined	Associated with organ failure and/or local complications, such as necrosis, abscess, or pseudocyst Further characterized by ≥3 on Ranson criteria or ≥8 on APACHE II
Determinant-based classification[181,186]	No peripancreatic necrosis No organ failure Mortality 0%	Presence of sterile peripancreatic necrosis *and/or* Transient organ failure Mortality 3.6%	*Severe:* Presence of *either* infected peripancreatic necrosis *or* persistent organ failure Mortality 33.8% *Critical:* Presence of infected peripancreatic necrosis *and* persistent organ failure Mortality 87.5%

		LOCAL COMPLICATIONS	
DEFINITIONS	**ORGAN FAILURE**	**EARLY (WITHIN 4 wk)**	**LATE (>4 wk)**
Atlanta 2012[1]	Score of ≥2 for one of three organ systems—respiratory, cardiovascular, or renal—using modified Marshall scoring system[187] Score: 0–4 *Respiratory* Pao_2/Fio_2: 400; 301–400; 201–300; 101–200; ≤101 *Renal* Serum creatinine (μmol/L): ≤134; 134–169; 170–310; 311–439; >439 *Cardiovascular* Systolic blood pressure (mm Hg): >90; <90, fluid responsive; <90, not fluid responsive; <90, pH <7.3; <90, pH <7.2	Acute peripancreatic fluid collection: fluid seen usually develops in early phase, associated with interstitial edematous pancreatitis CECT: no well-defined wall, homogeneous, confined by normal fascial planes in retroperitoneum; may be multiple Acute necrotic collection (ANC): containing variable amounts of fluid and necrotic tissue Infected necrosis: diagnosis of infection of ANC or WON suspected by patient's clinical course or by presence of gas within collection on CECT	Pancreatic pseudocyst: fluid collection in peripancreatic tissues, surrounded by well-defined wall with minimal or no necrosis; after onset of interstitial edematous pancreatitis Walled-off necrosis (WON): mature, encapsulated collection of pancreatic and/or peripancreatic necrosis with well-defined inflammatory wall; after onset of necrotizing pancreatitis Infected necrosis: infection of ANC or WON, suspected by patient's clinical course or by presence of gas within collection on CECT
Determinant-based classification[181]	Persistent organ failure: ≥48 hr Transient organ failure: ≤48 hr Cardiovascular: need for inotropic agent Renal: creatinine: ≥171 μmol/L Respiratory: Pao_2/Fio_2 ≤300 mm Hg Persistent organ failure: organ failure in same organ system for ≥48 hr Transient organ failure: ≤48 hr	Peripancreatic necrosis: nonviable tissue located in pancreas alone and/or in peripancreatic tissues; can be solid or semisolid, without radiologically defined wall Sterile peripancreatic necrosis: absence of proven infection in necrosis Infected peripancreatic necrosis (when at least one of following is present): gas bubbles within peripancreatic necrosis on CT; positive culture of peripancreatic necrosis obtained by image-guided fine-needle aspiration or during first drainage and/or necrosectomy	

APACHE, Acute Physiology and Chronic Health Evaluation points; *CECT,* contrast-enhanced computed tomography.

severity, such as necrosis and organ failure, rather than predictive factors of severity, such as the APACHE II and Ranson criteria. Second, the factors of severity used in this system had a direct causal association with severity. The DBC was recently validated prospectively, and it accurately stratified the patients according to mortality. Patients classified as mild, moderate, severe, and critical had mortality rates of 0%, 3.6%, 33.8%, and 87.5%, respectively.[186]

At present, it remains uncertain whether the revised Atlanta classification or the DBC will become the dominant classification system in the future.[188,189] Both systems have recently been validated in a prospective study and have been shown to represent an improvement to the original 1992 Atlanta classification.[190]

Clinical Assessment (see Chapter 56)

Prediction of the likely course and outcome of AP is of utmost importance when the patient with pancreatitis is admitted to the hospital. However, this can be challenging, even for experienced clinicians. In the vast majority (75%–80%) of patients, AP is a mild disease with a benign course and without associated mortality. The main challenge, however, is to identify patients who are most likely to progress to severe pancreatitis and experience major complications. These patients could potentially benefit from early intensive care monitoring and treatment. In addition to the initial clinical assessment, several prognostic criteria have been developed to aid the clinician in predicting the clinical course of pancreatitis. These prognostic criteria include severity scoring systems based on clinical parameters and laboratory results (e.g., Ranson criteria), radiology-based criteria (e.g., Balthazar score), and single biomarkers (e.g., C-reactive protein [CRP]).[176,177]

Mortality from AP follows a biphasic distribution. Early death is usually from the development of severe and irreversible multiorgan dysfunction, whereas late death occurs in the latter phase of the illness, with organ failure as the end result of sepsis and its sequelae. Several authors have reported the important prognostic significance of distinguishing between transient and persistent organ failure for predicting mortality from severe AP.[1,181] It has been shown that persistent or deteriorating multiorgan dysfunction in the first 7 days after admission is the most significant predictor of death.[180,191,192]

Scoring Systems for Assessing Severity of Pancreatitis

Since the 1970s, several scoring systems have been devised to predict the clinical course of AP[180] with some combining clinical and laboratory findings to determine the likelihood of a severe disease (e.g., the Acute Physiology and Chronic Health Evaluation II [APACHE-II], Ranson score, modified Glasgow/Imrie score, SIRS criteria, Bedside Index for the Severity in Acute Pancreatitis and Harmless Acute Pancreatitis Score) and some using a single laboratory parameter, such as CRP.[9] Before severity scoring systems were introduced, patients were assessed solely on clinical progression, which was clearly inadequate. Early prediction of severe disease is important to identify patients who are at greater risk for subsequent severe morbidity and mortality. The first, most widely used scoring system was the Ranson criteria.[193] The Ranson criteria were formulated based on the identification of 11 significant prognostic factors from 43 clinical and laboratory variables assessed in 100 acute episodes of pancreatitis (Table 55.5). The main limitations associated with the Ranson criteria are that prognostication is only complete after 48 hours and that it only functions accurately at

the extremes of the scale (less than three criteria predicted survival, and more than three predicted death) and less well at intermediate scores.[180] Subsequently, several modifications of this system have been proposed, such as the Glasgow (Imrie) severity scoring system. This system was simplified down to nine variables and has been shown to have prognostic accuracy similar to the Ranson criteria.[194,195] In Japan, the Japanese Severity Score (JSS) is used to predict severity and mortality from AP.[179,196]

Currently, the APACHE II system together with the Ranson criteria remain two of the most commonly used systems for the risk assessment of AP (see Table 55.5). The APACHE system was not developed specifically for pancreatitis but was devised for patients in the intensive care unit.[197] It is a complex, physiologically based classification system based on the most abnormal values of 34 variables, taking into account the patient's baseline health status. The APACHE system was simplified to the APACHE II scoring system, based on 12 physiologic variables, age, and five organ-based chronic health points.[198] The APACHE II system has the added utility of not only allowing determination of disease severity on admission but also allowing daily recalculation and thus assessment of disease progression.[180] Because obesity has been shown to be an important prognostic factor of mortality from pancreatitis, the APACHE-O scale has been proposed as an improvement to APACHE II and has been shown to improve its prognostic value.[185,199] Other organ-failure–related scores (e.g., MOF/Goris, Marshall, SOFA) have also been applied to AP but have only been used in a limited number of studies for pancreatitis (see Table 55.5).[183] Because these scores were not developed specifically for pancreatitis, these systems have several shortcomings and perform variably in ICU versus non-ICU patients.[200]

Most recently, a new scoring system termed the Bedside Index for Severity in Acute Pancreatitis (BISAP) was proposed as a simple and accurate method for the early (<24 hours of admission) identification of patients at risk of mortality (see Table 55.5).[201,202] The BISAP was proposed as a model that clinicians could use at the bedside with routinely available data. It was developed based on retrospective data on 17,992 patients and validated in another 18,256 patients.[203,204] Subsequent validation studies[201,205,206] have demonstrated that although the BISAP is comparable to other scoring systems, its major advantage is its simplicity, not its accuracy.[203] Also, calculation of the BISAP score may not be as simple as it seems because systemic inflammatory response syndrome (SIRS) calculation requires multiple variables.[201]

More recently, a new scoring system was developed by a panel of international experts as a tool for dynamic measurement of disease activity in AP. The Pancreatitis Activity Scoring System (PASS) incorporated five weighted parameters of organ failure, systemic inflammatory response syndrome, abdominal pain, requirement for opiates, and ability to tolerate oral intake.[207] This scoring system showed distinct patterns of disease activity related to duration of illness with an early and persistent elevation of disease activity amongst patients with severe AP defined as persistent organ failure. This was subsequently validated in a large cohort of 439 patients where an admission score of greater than 140 was associated with moderately severe and severe pancreatitis, ICU admission, local complications, and prolonged LOS.[208] Further validation in large international cohorts are required to determine the role of this novel score.

TABLE 55.5   Acute Pancreatitis (AP) Prognostic Scoring Systems

SCORING SYSTEMS	YEAR	PARAMETERS[a]
Ranson[192]	1974	At admission: age (>55 yr), WBC (>16,000/mL), glucose (>200 mg/dL), LDH (>350 IU/mL), AST (>250 IU/mL) At 48 hours: hematocrit (decrease >10%), BUN (increase >5 mg/dL), calcium (>8 mg/dL), Pao$_2$ (>60 mm Hg), base deficit (>4 mEq/L), fluid sequestration (>6 L)
Glasgow	1984	Age (>55 yr), WBC (>15,000/mL), glucose (>180 mg/dL), BUN (>45 mg/dL), Pao$_2$ (<60 mm Hg), calcium (<8 g/dL), albumin (<3.2 g/dL), LDH (>600 IU/L)
APACHE II Acute Physiology and Chronic Health Evaluation	1989	Temperature, MAP, heart rate, respiratory rate, Pao$_2$, arterial pH, bicarbonate, sodium, potassium, creatinine, hematocrit, WBC, GCS score, age, chronic health points
SOFA Sepsis-related Organ Failure Assessment	1996	MAP, Pao$_2$/Fio$_2$, creatinine, GCS, platelet count, bilirubin Score: 1–5, based on severity of each parameter
SIRS Systemic inflammatory response syndrome	2006	Temperature (<36°C or >38°C), heart rate (>90/min), respiratory rate (>20/min) or Paco2 (<32 mm Hg), WBC (<4000/mm^3, >12,000/mm^3, or >10% bands)
POP Pancreatitis Outcome Prediction score	2007	Age, MAP, Pao$_2$/Fio$_2$, arterial pH, BUN, calcium (these scores use normal ranges)
PANC 3	2007	Hematocrit (>44 mg/dL), body mass index (>30 kg/m^2), pleural effusion
BISAP Bedside Index for Severity in Acute Pancreatitis	2008	BUN (>25 mg/dL), impaired mental status (GCS score <15), SIRS (>2), age (>60 yr), pleural effusion
Haps Harmless Acute Pancreatitis Score	2009	Abdominal tenderness, hematocrit (>43 mg/dL for men or >39.6 mg/dL for women), creatinine (>2 mg/dL)
JSS Japanese Severity Score	2009	Base excess (≤3 mEq/L), Pao$_2$ (≤60 mm Hg or respiratory failure), BUN (≥40 mg/dL) or creatinine (≥2 mg/dL), LDH (≥2× upper limit of normal), platelet (≤100,000/mm^3), calcium (≤7.5 mg/dL), C-reactive protein (≥15 mg/dL), SIRS (≥3), age (≥70 yr)
Pancreatitis Activity Scoring System (PASS)	2018	Organ failure x100 (for each system),[b] SIRS x 35 for each criteria, Abdominal pain (0–10) x5, Morphine equivalent dose (mg) x5, Tolerating solid diet (yes = 0, no = 1) ×40

[a]At admission and at 48 hours, unless otherwise stated.

[b]Organ failure definition: Modified Marshall or SOFA score ≥ 2 points any category

AST, Aspartate transaminase; *BUN*, blood urea nitrogen; *GCS*, Glasgow Coma Scale; *LDH*, lactate dehydrogenase; *MAP*, mean arterial pressure; *SIRS*, systemic inflammatory response syndrome; *WBC*, white blood cell count.

Adapted from Mounzer R, Langmead CJ, Wu BU, et al. Comparison of existing clinical scoring systems to predict persistent organ failure in patients with acute pancreatitis. *Gastroenterology.* 2012;142(7):1476–1482; quiz e1415–1476.

There is still no single system that is completely reliable for prognostication in patients with AP.[209] A recent study evaluated and compared seven CT scoring systems (CT severity index [CTSI], modified CT severity index [MCTSI], pancreatic size index [PSI], extrapancreatic score [EP], extrapancreatic inflammation on CT score [EPIC], mesenteric edema and peritoneal fluid score [MOP], and Balthazar grade]) and two clinical scoring systems: APACHE-II and BISAP. The authors found on admission (within 24 hours) that the predictive accuracy of CT scoring systems for severity of AP is similar to clinical scoring systems.[182,210] Existing scoring systems have moderate accuracy (about 80%) and seem to have reached their maximal efficacy in predicting outcomes in AP.[211,212]

New approaches and biomarkers are needed to improve prognostication.[213] Regular clinical review and timely intervention remains the mainstay of treatment in AP. It is interesting to note that only the 2015 Japanese guidelines[179] recommend the use of scoring systems in the assessment of pancreatitis (i.e., JSS). Neither the International Association of Pancreatology (IAP) nor the American Pancreas Association (APA) guidelines,[214] the American College of Gastroenterology (ACG) guidelines,[60] or American Gastroenterological Association (AGA)[2] presently recommend or mention the use of scoring systems.

Laboratory Assessment

Single-Parameter Biochemical Markers

Because of the lack of accuracy and the cumbersome nature of the complex prognostic models to date, simple single predictors have some advantages.[178]

C-REACTIVE PROTEIN. CRP is an acute-phase protein predominantly synthesized in the liver in response to various infective and noninfectious stimuli, resulting in elevated serum levels.[183] Because of its easy availability in clinical practice, CRP has been used widely to distinguish mild from severe AP and, at a cutoff level of 150 mg/L, has been shown to have a diagnostic accuracy of 70% to 80% when measured within the first 48 hours of disease onset.[183,185,215] Presently, CRP is frequently considered the "gold standard" single biochemical marker for the risk stratification of AP and is used as the comparison when assessing new potential biomarkers.[183] A major limitation of CRP is the relatively long delay in achieving peak systematic values at 72 to 96 hours after onset of disease, making very early assessment of severity impossible.

HEMATOCRIT. The hematocrit value has been shown to be a prognostic marker for the severity of AP, and its prognostic significance emphasizes the pathophysiologic role of fluid loss in the severity of pancreatitis and the role of vigorous fluid replacement in the course of disease. A hematocrit of more than 44% on admission or the absence of a fall in hematocrit during the first 24 hours after admission was found to be a clear risk factor for pancreatic necrosis, organ failure, or pancreatic infection.[216] Hematocrit greater than 50% has also been shown to predict severe pancreatitis.[217] A study reported that hemoconcentration is best used as a measure of increased fluid sequestration to guide the aggressiveness of fluid resuscitation in AP patients.[218] However, the value of hematocrit remains controversial, because several large studies failed to demonstrate its prognostic value on admission.[183,210] Nonetheless, other investigators have reported that hematocrit less than 40% to 44% had a high predictive value of approximately 90% in excluding severe pancreatitis.[219,220]

PROCALCITONIN. Procalcitonin (PCT) has been widely used as a biomarker of bacterial infection or sepsis.[183] At a cutoff level of 1.8 ng/mL, PCT was able to predict the development of infected necrosis in patients with pancreatitis with a sensitivity and specificity of more than 90%.[221] The utility of PCT as a prognostic marker in AP was subsequently confirmed by several other studies. Notably, a prospective international multicenter study in 104 patients with severe pancreatitis reported that PCT was able to predict serious complications such as pancreatic infections and death with a sensitivity of 79% and specificity of 93% at a cutoff level greater than 3.8 ng/mL within 48 to 96 hours from symptom onset.[222] A meta-analysis of 24 studies demonstrated that the sensitivity and specificity of PCT for the development of severe AP was 72% and 86%, respectively, but with a significant degree of heterogeneity. The sensitivity and specificity of PCT for prediction of infected pancreatic necrosis were 80% and 91%, respectively, with no significant heterogeneity.[223] Based on currently available data, PCT is a promising parameter for the early risk stratification of patients at risk for severe complications from pancreatitis.

Blood Urea Nitrogen. Blood urea nitrogen (BUN) at admission and its trend during the first 24 hours of admission has been used as a marker of severity. In a prospectively validated study of more than 1000 AP cases at three institutions, it showed that an increased BUN at admission and an increase of BUN during the first 24 hours correlated with increased mortality in AP.[224,225]

Other Biomarkers

Other biomarkers, such as the proinflammatory cytokines, have also been proposed as prognostic of disease severity in pancreatitis. A meta-analysis concluded that interleukin-6 (IL-6) and IL-8 may potentially be used as prognostic biomarkers for pancreatitis.[226] Trypsinogen and trypsinogen activation peptide (TAP) have also been evaluated as prognostic markers for pancreatitis.[227,228] Urinary TAP concentrations have been reported to correlate well with the severity of AP at admission. Presently, however, measurements of IL-6, IL-8, or TAP are not routinely available outside the laboratory setting, which severely limits their use in clinical practice.

Imaging Assessment (see Chapter 17)
Computed Tomography

There are two main indications of cross-sectional imaging in AP: confirmation of the diagnosis in cases of diagnostic uncertainty and prognostication and detection of complications in the latter course of disease. Dynamic contrast-enhanced CT (CECT) scan is the imaging modality of choice for staging AP and for detecting complications. CT has been reported to detect pancreatic necrosis with a sensitivity of 87%.[229,230] Pancreatic necrosis might not develop until 72 hours after symptoms onset; therefore a CT scan before 72 hours is discouraged in some guidelines (e.g., ACG and AGA). The morphologic abnormalities and changes associated with pancreatitis are now well recognized, well documented, and defined in the revised 2012 Atlanta classification.[1] In early-phase inflammation, interstitial edema and fluid collections are recognized on CT. Subsequently, with progression of disease, pseudocysts, acute necrotic collections, and walled-off pancreatic necrosis may develop. These morphologic developments form the basis for current radiologic scoring systems. Presently, CT scoring systems can be stratified into two groups. Unenhanced CT scoring systems evaluate the extent of pancreatic and peripancreatic inflammatory changes, which include the Balthazar grade and pancreatic size index (PSI), or both peripancreatic inflammatory changes and extrapancreatic complications, such as the "mesenteric edema and peritoneal fluid" (MOP) score, extrapancreatic score (EP), and extrapancreatic inflammation on CT (EPIC) score.[182] CECT scores determine the presence and extent of necrosis, including the CTSI and the MCTSI (Table 55.6).

The first radiologic scoring system was based on morphologic criteria detected on noncontrast CT.[231] With the absence of contrast, however, important features such as necrosis could not be assessed, and this system was revised by the same group in 1990 and termed the "CT severity index" (CTSI).[232] Based on the CTSI, the severity of AP is classified into five grades (0–4) on unenhanced CT, whereas the degree of necrosis is

TABLE 55.6   Modified Computed Tomography (CT) Severity Index

POINTS, GRADE	CRITERIA
Evaluation of Pancreatic Morphology	
0, A	Normal pancreas consistent with mild pancreatitis
2, B/C	Focal or diffuse enlargement of the gland, including contour irregularities and inhomogeneous attenuation with or without peripancreatic inflammation
4, D/E	Pancreatic or peripancreatic fluid collection or peripancreatic fat necrosis
Additional 2 points	Extrapancreatic complications, one or more of the following: pleural effusion, ascites, vascular complications, parenchymal complications, or gastrointestinal tract involvement
Scoring Pancreatic Necrosis	
0	No pancreatic necrosis
2	≤30% pancreatic necrosis
4	>30% pancreatic necrosis

PREDICTING MORBIDITY AND MORTALITY WITH THE CT SEVERITY INDEX COMBINING SCORES

INDEX	MORBIDITY	MORTALITY
0–3	8%	3%
4–6	35%	6%
7–10	92%	17%

From Mortele KJ, Wiesner W, Intriere L, et al. A modified CT severity index for evaluating acute pancreatitis: improved correlation with patient outcome. *AJR Am J Roentgenol.* 2004;183(5): 1261–1265.

measured and given a score of 0 to 6. The sum of these two scores is used to calculate the CTSI, and a score of 7 or greater has been shown to be predictive of high morbidity and mortality.[232] CTSI of 3 or less correlated with a mortality of 3% versus 92% with CTSI greater than 7.[183] A modified CTSI was subsequently proposed, which took into account extrapancreatic complications such as pleural effusion and vascular complications (see Table 55.6).[233] However, it has not proved to be superior in accuracy to the original CTSI.[183] In 2007 De Waele and colleagues[234] proposed a CT score based on factors in extrapancreatic inflammation, such as ascites, pleural effusion, retroperitoneal inflammation, or mesenteric inflammation, termed the "extrapancreatic inflammation on CT score" (EPIC). The authors demonstrated that with a score of 4 or greater within the first 24 hours, EPIC could predict severe AP and mortality with 100% sensitivity and 71% specificity.[183] This system also has the added advantage of not requiring the use of CECT, unlike previous CT-based systems.

A study analyzing 159 episodes of AP in 150 patients compared the accuracy of seven CT scoring systems (CTSI, MCTSI, PSI, EP, EPIC, MOP, and Balthazar) with two clinical scoring systems (APACHE II and BISAP) in predicting severity of AP within the first 24 hours of hospitalization.[182] It demonstrated that the predictive accuracy of CT scoring systems are similar to the more easily obtainable clinical scoring systems. Therefore based on these findings, the authors concluded that CT scan should not be routinely performed on admission for the assessment of disease severity.[182] This finding was concordant with earlier studies that report the utility of CT scan is low early in the course of pancreatitis.[235] Presently, CT is recommended in

patients with persistent organ failure, for those who have the SIRS or sepsis, for those who do not improve within 6 to 10 days into the disease course, and for those with probable infected pancreatic necrosis (evidence-based medicine recommendation grade B).[236]

Magnetic Resonance Imaging

Although dynamic CECT remains the gold standard in imaging for AP, it may be contraindicated in select patients with significant renal impairment on contrast allergies. The utility of MRI in pancreatitis has been investigated in several studies and has been shown to be a useful alternative and complementary role to CT.[237] In certain situations (e.g., AIP), MRI/MRCP and its various sequences, such as diffusion-weighted imaging (DWI), can be used to assess the pancreatic parenchymal changes and pancreaticobiliary ductal involvement (see Fig. 55.2).[238]

SUMMARY

AP is a challenging disease to manage with a myriad of etiologies; however, gallstones and alcohol-related causes remain the two most common etiologies. In recent years, significant improvement has been achieved in understanding the underlying etiopathogenesis and factors involved in the occurrence of disease because of advanced diagnostic tools ranging from cross-sectional imaging and endoscopic procedures to genetic testing.

The references for this chapter can be found online by accessing the accompanying Expert Consult website.

CHAPTER 56

Management of acute pancreatitis and pancreatitis-related complications

Euan J. Dickson, Maria Coats, and C. Ross Carter

ACUTE PANCREATITIS

Acute pancreatitis (AP) is common with an incidence of 15 to 45 per 100,000 population per year.[1] This has increased over the last two decades largely because of a rising prevalence of obesity and gallstone disease. Recurrent AP represents a subgroup of patients who have had at least two distinct episodes of pancreatitis with complete resolution in between and no evidence of chronic pancreatitis (CP). This may occur in up to 20% of patients, 35% of whom develop recurrent AP and will go on to develop features of CP.[2]

AP is a potentially life-threatening illness. It may result in a prolonged hospital admission associated with significant morbidity and mortality; however, for the majority, it is a self-limiting disease. Successful management of pancreatitis relies on the early recognition of the high-risk subgroup and a multidisciplinary approach to manage complications of pancreatitis under the supervision of a pancreatic specialist. For the majority of patients who have mild uncomplicated attacks of pancreatitis, management is centered around early supportive care until resolution followed by appropriate measures to alleviate the precipitating cause and minimize further attacks, including lifestyle modification.

AP as defined by the revised Atlanta Classification 2012 requires two or more of the following: (1) abdominal pain characteristic of pancreatitis, (2) serum levels of amylase/lipase more than three times the upper limit of normal, and/or (3) imaging characteristics of pancreatitis[3] (see Chapters 54 and 55). There are several causes of a solitary hyperamylasemia, especially in critical care patients. These include chronic renal failure, severe burns, liver failure, diabetic ketoacidosis, or after transplant or neurosurgery, and therefore results must be interpreted in context with clinical findings.[4] Gallstones and alcohol are the two most common etiologic factors responsible for AP and their relative importance differs between populations across the world. There is an overall lifetime risk of AP in asymptomatic gallstones and heavy drinkers of 2% to 3%.[5,6]

Historically, pancreatitis was categorized into mild and severe groups with the emphasis being placed on clinical scoring systems and "predictive" indicators that would allow early triage into one category or another.[7,8] This overly simplistic classification, however, has been recognized and reflected in the revised Atlanta criteria where an additional category of "moderately severe" pancreatitis is defined[9] to accommodate those patients who experience transient organ failure (Table 56.1A and B; Atlanta Classification). The importance of early systemic organ dysfunction and multiple organ failure is key to determining disease severity and outcome, and the management of local complications is heavily influenced by the degree of systemic disturbance.

Pancreatitis is a dynamic illness, and its severity may change during the course of the disease. Two distinct phases are seen in AP that correlate with two recognized peaks in mortality. Early death (defined as within two weeks of onset) occurs as a consequence of progressive multiple organ failure driven by cytokine cascades and systemic inflammatory response syndrome (SIRS).[10,11] Later mortality is often a consequence of local pancreatic complications because of pancreatic necrosis and therefore only manifests in those with moderate to severe pancreatitis.

Although intervention during the early phase of illness is usually counterproductive, timely and appropriate intervention for local complications in the late phase can be lifesaving and significantly alter the course of the illness. The incidence of AP has been rising but the overall mortality has been falling for several decades, and despite mortality rates in patients with severe AP being disproportionately high, we have seen a downward trend in recent years. This decrease in mortality can be attributed to widespread improvements in intensive care management, the use of minimally invasive approaches to treat complications, advances in interventional and vascular radiologic methods, better and more aggressive nutritional support, and, most importantly, the adoption of a multidisciplinary approach to this systemic disease through the development of specialist centers. The main impact of these improvements is that patients are given more optimal support, earlier and for longer periods during the early phase of the illness, allowing interventions for local complications to be carried out later and by less invasive methods.

Despite multiple randomized control trials (RCTs), there are no effective drug therapies that have shown any significant benefit in preventing organ failure through the use of agents such as glucagon, gabexate, somatostatin, or lexipafant.[12] Although it is recognized that acinar cellular injury underpins the pathophysiology of the disease process, there have been very few trials targeting this and a distinct lack of translational studies.

INITIAL MANAGEMENT

Management of AP requires a multimodal approach that is addressed in a number of national and international guidelines, with the most cited being the American Pancreatic Association (APA)/International Association of Pancreatology (IAP) guidelines of 2013.[13]

Analgesia

Pain is a cardinal feature of AP and should be managed along similar lines to pain caused by other intraabdominal emergencies to improve the patient's immediate quality of life. Most

TABLE 56.1A Local Complications in Acute Pancreatitis[9]

TIME SCALE	NECROSIS ABSENT	NECROSIS PRESENT
<4 weeks	Acute peripancreatic fluid collection (peripancreatic fluid associated with interstitial edematous pancreatitis with no associated peripancreatic necrosis)	Acute necrotic collection (a collection containing variable amounts of both fluid and necrosis; the necrosis can involve the pancreatic parenchyma or the extrapancreatic tissues)
>4 weeks	Pancreatic pseudocyst (an encapsulated collection of fluid with a well-defined inflammatory wall usually outside the pancreas with minimal or no necrosis)	Walled-off necrosis (a mature, encapsulated collection of pancreatic or extrapancreatic necrosis that has developed a well-defined inflammatory wall)
Infection	Each collection type may be sterile or infected	

TABLE 56.1B Grades of Severity (2012 Revised Atlanta Classification)[9]

Mild acute pancreatitis	No organ failure No local or systemic complications
Moderately severe acute pancreatitis	Organ failure that resolves within 48 hours (transient organ failure) and/or Local or systemic complications without persistent organ failure
Severe acute pancreatitis	Persistent organ failure (>48 hours) • Single organ failure • Multiple organ failure

patients will require parenteral opiate analgesia after hospital admission, but the duration and severity of pain is variable. The choice of analgesic is largely dependent on local protocols, physician preference, and patient's prior drug histories because no single approach has been shown to be beneficial. Historically, opiates, and morphine in particular, were thought to induce sphincter of Oddi spasm, thereby potentially exacerbating the severity or duration of AP. These were once contraindicated, but there is little evidence to support this.[14] A Cochrane review in 2013[15] of five RCTs comparing different analgesics in AP found no evidence of increased complications relating to opioid use.

Several RCTs have been conducted comparing different analgesic modalities in AP. Collectively these have shown no contraindications to opiate-based drugs, no benefit from parenteral local anaesthetic agents, and although transdermal and rectal analgesia may be effective, no trials have compared them directly with conventional routes.[16] Administration of opioids by patient-controlled analgesia (PCA) is recommended for patients with protracted and severe pain.

There has been growing interest in the potential role of epidural analgesia, particularly in patients with severe AP, because of their known effects on splanchnic perfusion and tissue oxygenation in experimental models[17] as well as potential improvements in respiratory complications and shock.[18] One RCT has shown that epidural analgesia has better analgesic coverage than parenteral intravenous (IV) opioids, improves pancreatic perfusion, and trends toward a reduced rate of necrosectomy, but the latter failed to reach statistical significance.[19] Further

larger trials are ongoing. However, epidural analgesia carries a risk of infective complications and systemic physiologic disturbances such as hypotension, which may be counterproductive in those who experience large fluid shifts, and thus this approach to analgesia is not often used.[20]

Fluid Therapy and Resuscitation

Current guidelines for managing AP strongly recommend early and appropriate fluid therapy within the first 12 to 24 hours of admission to reduce the incidence of persistent SIRS and subsequent organ failure.[13] Rapid and effective restoration of circulating volume is the single intervention most likely to improve outcome and reduce mortality and morbidity. There is limited evidence to support the fluid type, volume, rate of delivery, and markers to confirm adequate restoration of perfusion. Volume resuscitation as a fundamental principle remains the Holy Grail of critical care.

The choice of initial resuscitation fluid is becoming less contentious, although the lack of high-quality evidence leads to wide variations in practice worldwide. The colloid versus crystalloid debate is moving in favor of crystalloids after the SAFE trial.[21] The American Gastroenterological Association (AGA) makes no specific recommendation over whether normal saline or Ringer's lactate is better and instead recommends goal-directed therapy. RCTs have been conducted comparing Ringer's lactate and normal saline in relation to local complications (necrosis, infection), systemic complications (renal failure, shock, respiratory failure, and persistent organ dysfunction) and mortality. Two of these trials demonstrated a clinical benefit with Ringer's lactate in reducing SIRS in the first 24 hours, but it made no difference to SIRS or mortality at 48 hours.[22,23] These outcomes are consistent with the known proinflammatory effect of normal saline, which should be used cautiously because it can also cause hyperchloraemic metabolic acidosis when used in large volumes during resuscitation.[24] Evidence, however, remains low quality and there is a lack of any well-designed RCTs.

The addition of hydroxyl ethyl starch (HES) has demonstrated theoretical benefits when used in the resuscitation of patients with AP by reducing intraabdominal hypertension (IAH) and the subsequent need for mechanical ventilation.[25,26] However, the use of HES in severe sepsis in intensive care has been shown, in several large multicenter studies, to increase the need for renal replacement therapy and overall mortality.[27–29] Interestingly, a meta-analysis of nonseptic critical care patients has shown that HES does not increase mortality and morbidity in the same way[30]; however, the studies included were small and there is sufficient concern to recommend against the use of HES in resuscitation of AP.

The volume and rate of fluid resuscitation are similarly not well defined, but several liters may be required in the first 24 hours and there is a move away from rapid fluid infusions toward a more controlled approach with goal-directed therapy.[31] Studies have demonstrated an adverse effect with large volumes of resuscitation fluids (>4 L) in the first 24 hours associated with more respiratory complications, acute collections, persistent organ failure, and a higher mortality.[31–33]

Current evidence supports a rate of 5 to 10 mL/kg/h, demonstrating a decreased requirement for mechanic ventilation, abdominal compartment syndrome, sepsis, and mortality with this fluid regimen compared with patients assigned to lower infusion rates.[33,34] An initial fluid bolus of 20 mL/kg before commencing fluid infusions to deliver 3 L to 4 L over the first

24 hours has been recommended in a few studies and closely correlates with fluid resuscitation guidelines in septic shock.[23]

There are no recommended national or international algorithms for the recommended fluid resuscitation in AP. It is crucial that patients have tailored fluid regimens delivered in a closely monitored environment, with frequent reviews by specialists with the aim of maintaining end organ perfusion and restoring physiologic homeostasis. Early identification and treatment of organ failure is key. This can be achieved using adjuncts such as a urinary catheter, arterial line and central venous line to allow monitoring of these variables. More advanced and invasive techniques to determine stroke volume variation or intrathoracic blood volume are only suitable for critically ill patients who are in an intensive care unit.

CRITICAL CARE AND THE MANAGEMENT OF SYSTEMIC COMPLICATIONS

Patients with uncomplicated mild AP can be safely managed in a ward environment with close monitoring and regular clinical reviews to ensure high-risk patients, who may deteriorate, are identified early. Those with persistent or worsening organ dysfunction should be managed in a critical care environment, either in a high-dependency unit (HDU) or an intensive care unit (ICU). In general, an HDU will provide enhanced monitoring and single organ support, whereas an ICU provides multiorgan support and the ability to invasively ventilate (see Chapter 26). Critical care is not a treatment per se, but it provides organ support until the pathologic process driving organ failure improves. This may be achieved either with time or by using an additional treatment modality (e.g., surgery) or managing sepsis with source control and antibiotics. It should be noted that critical care requires significant physiologic reserve from the patient and should be used appropriately; not all patients have the reserve to survive critical illness, particularly if they have severe comorbid disease or increased frailty.

The need for critical care may manifest early in the disease course reflecting acute physiologic changes occurring as a result of the inflammatory process from the pancreatitis triggering organ failure. Admission to critical care later in the disease process is usually because of superimposed infective complications and sepsis. Systemic complications, including organ failure, are not binary processes but rather a dynamic continuum with the potential for rapid deterioration; hence early discussion with the critical care team is recommended. This is driven by the patient's pathophysiology and not the anatomy of the disease process, and therefore close monitoring in all pancreatitis patients is recommended. The management of severe pancreatitis requiring critical care should involve a multidisciplinary team including surgeons, ICU clinicians, radiologists, microbiologists, physiotherapists, and dieticians.

Organ Failure

Respiratory, cardiovascular, renal, and gastrointestinal (GI) dysfunction are the most common systemic complications encountered in AP and careful monitoring of each of these systems is key to determining medium- and long-term outcomes for these patients. Respiratory failure usually mandates transfer to the critical care unit, either for maximizing noninvasive support such as continuous positive airway pressure (CPAP) or high-flow nasal cannula or intubation and mechanical ventilation with lung protective strategies.

Cardiovascular collapse is managed primarily by volume resuscitation and vasoactive agents if necessary. This should be guided by invasive monitoring and goal-directed therapy as previously described. Renal failure usually occurs in the context of severe AP as a result of prolonged renal hypoperfusion causing renal tubular necrosis, IAH or nephrotoxic drugs, or computed tomography (CT) contrast. Management involves restoration of circulating volume, ensuring there is adequate blood pressure to provide renal perfusion. Despite this, renal failure may still occur and renal replacement therapy may be required. Recovering renal function is a useful marker of global physiologic improvement.

GI failure also occurs as a result of reduced perfusion, and the use of vasopressors for cardiovascular support can exacerbate the splanchnic vasoconstriction that occurs in these critically ill patients. It manifests as nausea, vomiting, and abdominal distension. The two most clinically relevant consequences of this phenomenon are failure to tolerate enteral nutrition (EN), and the breakdown of the intestinal barrier function with subsequent bacterial translocation, bacteremia, and ultimately infected pancreatic necrosis. Adequate nutrition is extremely important for patients with pancreatitis because a nutritional debt will rapidly develop with muscle wasting and an increased risk of additional complications, particularly respiratory ones.

Intraabdominal Hypertension and Abdominal Compartment Syndrome

Raised intraabdominal pressure (IAP) contributes to organ dysfunction and represents a growing area of interest in the management of patients with severe AP. IAH is defined as a persistently raised IAP of 12 mm Hg or higher (Grade I: 12–15 mm Hg; Grade II: 16–20 mm Hg; Grade III: 21–25 mm Hg; Grade IV: >25 mm Hg). Abdominal compartment syndrome (ACS) occurs when IAP is sustained at greater than 20 mm Hg and is associated with failure of at least one organ.[35] The majority of the literature on ACS refers to trauma patients, but it is a recognized complication of severe AP and has been reported to occur in approximately 15%[36] of these patients. When present, there is an associated 49% mortality.[37]

IAH is an indicator of disease severity, organ failure, and mortality, but raised IAP may simply be a surrogate marker indicating a poor outcome and there are no data to suggest that this risk of mortality is improved by surgical decompression. Although controversial, international consensus guidelines advocate the following approach: First, measurement of IAP should be considered in mechanically ventilated patients with severe AP, especially in the context of clinical deterioration. Second, the mainstay of treatment is medical intervention to target the most important contributors to IAH (hollow viscera volume, careful attention to intravascular and extravascular volume status and abdominal wall compliance). Finally, and most controversially given the lack of evidence, invasive treatment for ACS in AP should only be considered after a multidisciplinary discussion for patients with a sustained IAP greater than 25 mm Hg and new-onset organ failure refractory to medical therapy and nasogastric/rectal tube decompression. Invasive treatment options include percutaneous catheter drainage of ascites, laparostomy, or subcutaneous linea alba fasciotomy.[13] The major challenges of the surgical approach include the risk of infecting previously sterile pancreatic necrosis and the difficulty of managing the significant fluid losses that may ensue with an open abdomen. It cannot be overemphasized that these recommendations lack a solid evidence base and high-quality RCTs are required to determine the benefit, if any, of this approach.

Referral to a Specialist Unit

It is strongly recommended that patients with severe AP should be discussed with, but not necessarily transferred to, a specialist pancreatic unit at an early stage. Increasingly, these patients are managed "remotely" by the base hospital in conjunction with the specialist unit. This is particularly relevant during the early phase of the illness, where specialist intervention is rarely required, to avoid overwhelming the resources of the regional unit. Current guidelines advocate transfer to a specialist unit when patients with severe AP require radiologic, endoscopic, or surgical intervention.

Nutrition

AP is associated with a hypercatabolic state and despite the historic practice of dietary restriction, recent evidence supports that early oral nutrition or EN is beneficial and should be commenced within 24 to 72 hours of admission[38,39] (see Chapter 26). Those with clinically mild AP do not usually require additional nutritional support and may be maintained on a normal diet. Patients with severe AP, however, commonly require additional nutritional support.

The enteral route is preferred over parenteral nutrition (PN) in these patients for several reasons. Enteral feeding maintains normal gut integrity, stimulates intestinal motility, reduces bacterial translocation, and increases splanchnic blood flow, which all potentially reduce the incidence of infected pancreatic necrosis and organ failure. Gastric colonization by pathogenic bacteria, which may also increase the risk for septic complications, is reduced with EN support. PN is associated with more complications (e.g., line sepsis, trace element deficiencies, and liver dysfunction). EN is also significantly cheaper.

There are several RCTs and meta-analyses that support the use of EN over PN in AP. EN is associated with a reduction in systemic infections (including infected pancreatic necrosis), multiorgan failure, need for surgical intervention, and mortality.[40,41] Some studies have also shown a trend towards shorter length of stay (LOS) in patients who are enterally fed, although this fails to reach statistical significance.[42,43] A meta-analysis of 20 RCTs also supports the use of any EN formula and did not find any benefit with immuno-nutrition.[44]

The benefits of EN over PN are well recognized, but there has been a long-standing debate regarding the best mode of delivery of EN. Nasogastric (NG) feeding is tolerated in up to 85% of patients and should be tried preferentially to nasojejunal (NJ) feeding. NG tubes are easier to place and are also more convenient and cheaper. Patients who do not tolerate NG feeding usually suffer with delayed gastric emptying, and NJ feeding can work well for these patients.[45]

Contraindications for EN include prolonged paralytic ileus, ACS, and mesenteric ischemia, and a relative contraindication may include enteric fistulae. PN should be reserved for patients in whom the enteral route is not tolerated or inappropriate and although it may be used on its own, it is often used in conjunction with EN to allow patients to adequately meet their nutritional requirements. Glutamine supplementation has been found to be beneficial and is advised where PN is needed; two recent meta-analyses demonstrated elevated serum albumin, reduced C-reactive protein (CRP), less infective complications, shorter LOS, and lower mortality when used.[46,47]

There is no evidence to support the use of probiotics in the management of AP.[48] Pancreatic enzyme replacement therapy (PERT) is not currently recommended for routine use in AP unless there is evidence of pancreatic exocrine insufficiency (PEI) by testing fecal elastase or demonstrated as malabsorption with steatorrhea. This has been evaluated in two small RCTs: one showed a slightly better outcome with PERT in patients with obvious PEI only and the other showed no difference.[49,50]

Antibiotics

In patients who survive the early systemic complications of AP, secondary infection of pancreatic necrosis leads to a second peak in mortality between 2 to 4 weeks after disease onset. It can be difficult to differentiate infection from inflammation, although markers such as procalcitonin have shown promise.[51] However, the outcomes of a large RCT, PROCAP, which may help guide antibiotic use in AP, are still awaited.[52] In the absence of a sufficiently specific and sensitive test, the decision to commence antibiotics is based on a variety of factors, including patient trajectory.

Infection occurs in some 40% of patients with pancreatic necrosis and the potential prevention of this by prophylactic antibiotic therapy has been the subject of much research interest. Mortality in this subgroup of patients with co-existing organ failure have a 2-fold increase in their overall mortality.[53] However, there is no evidence to suggest that the routine use of prophylactic antibiotics alters the incidence of infected pancreatic necrosis or overall mortality.[13,54,55] A Cochrane review of 7 RCTs[56] and a meta-analysis of 14 studies[57] have found no benefit from routine antibiotic prophylaxis either in mortality or in the incidence of infected pancreatic necrosis, and current international guidelines are clear in advising against routine antibiotic use.[13]

Antibiotic treatment (as opposed to prophylaxis) is indicated in those with proven sepsis. This may occasionally occur at presentation because of co-existing cholangitis, and these patients require urgent relief of biliary obstruction, as discussed later in the next section. In the absence of cholangitis, antibiotics should be reserved for those patients with proven or strongly suspected sepsis because many patients may exhibit signs of SIRS in the absence of infection. In the event that antibiotics are commenced, they should ideally be targeted by culture and sensitivity results, and the duration should be limited to avoid antibiotic resistance.

Endoscopic Retrograde Cholangiopancreatography

An urgent endoscopic retrograde cholangiopancreatography (ERCP; <24 hrs after presentation) is indicated in gallstone pancreatitis in the presence of cholangitis (see Chapters 30 and 43). True cholangitis (jaundice, rigors, and pyrexia) is extremely rare, and a more common scenario is abnormal liver function tests in the context of pancreatitis, and these patients do not benefit from early intervention.

The first RCT of ERCP in pancreatitis was published in 1988[58] and reported fewer complications and shorter hospital LOS in patients randomized to early ERCP with sphincterotomy and stone extraction if stones were present. A second trial from Hong Kong[59] suggested early ERCP was mainly effective in reducing the incidence of biliary sepsis rather than the severity of AP, and subsequent trials, meta-analyses, and reviews have drawn conflicting conclusions. The most recent Cochrane review of the five RCTs suggested that ERCP done within 72 hours may be associated with a nonsignificant trend toward a reduction in local and systemic complications.[60] A retrospective study compared the outcomes in 73 patients with AP and no cholangitis who underwent urgent ERCP (<24 hours) or early ERCP (24–72 hours) and found that there was no difference in LOS or development of complications from pancreatitis or directly because of the ERCP.[61] Being a small and retrospective study, however, its application is limited and highlights the need for an adequately powered RCT.

In the absence of cholangitis, for patients in whom bilirubin levels persist or rise, magnetic resonance cholangiopancreatography (MRCP) or endoscopic ultrasound (EUS) may be an alternative to ERCP to determine the presence of ductal stones. Given that in the majority of cases, most stones will pass spontaneously, identification of stones before performing ERCP is warranted.

Nontherapeutic ERCP in this group of patients should be avoided and, in a RCT of ERCP, was associated with a higher complication rate than EUS.[62] The APEC trial, undertaken by the Dutch Pancreatitis Study Group, was a multicenter RCT whose aim was to determine if early nontherapeutic ERCP and sphincterotomy was better than conservative management in patients with severe acute biliary pancreatitis without cholangitis.[63] They concluded that early ERCP was not associated with better outcomes with regard to developing organ failure, pancreatic necrosis, pancreatic endocrine, exocrine insufficiency, or pneumonia/bacteremia. In the group who underwent ERCP,[64] however, they observed a reduction in what they described as cholangitis, although this was not defined by conventional cholangitic criteria.

IMAGING (SEE CHAPTER 17)

At initial presentation, the primary focus is on resuscitation, and early imaging rarely influences management. An urgent CT is indicated only in cases of diagnostic uncertainty. The role of CT thereafter is in the assessment and follow-up of local complications. Although upper abdominal ultrasound (US) is indicated to determine the presence of gallstones, this does not influence early management and should be performed after the patient has been adequately resuscitated. If the initial US is negative, this should be repeated before discharge because there are many factors that may contribute to false negative results (i.e., operator experience, stones <3 mm, patient body habitus).

In patients with proven gallstones, MRCP, EUS, or intraoperative cholangiography (IOC) may be indicated to evaluate the extrahepatic biliary tree as clinically appropriate. In patients with negative biliary imaging, no alcohol history, or alternative etiology, EUS may be helpful to exclude microlithiasis (Fig. 56.1; see Chapter 22) or neoplastic pancreatic pathology. If the latter is expected, cross-sectional imaging should be performed, particularly in the older patient or in a patient with other symptoms suggestive of pancreatic malignancy such as significant pre-incident weight loss.

MANAGEMENT OF NECROSIS

As previously discussed, there is consensus advocating a principle of early targeted organ support, with nutritional optimization, ideally by the enteral route where possible.[65] In previous

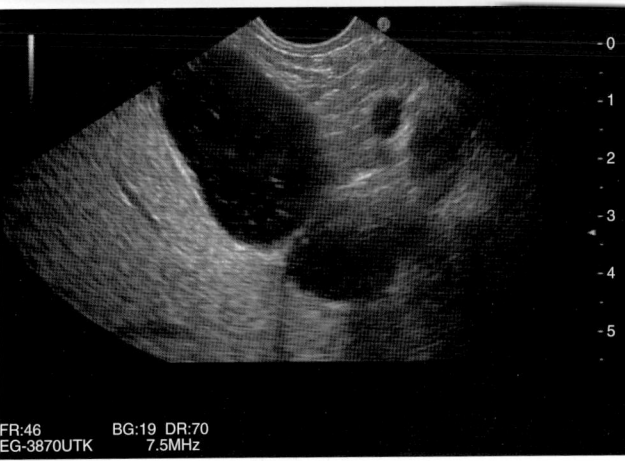

FIGURE 56.1 Endoscopic ultrasound (EUS) confirming gallbladder microlithiasis as a cause for acute pancreatitis.

editions of this chapter, the focus has been on the timing of open necrosectomy, the role of bacterial fine-needle aspiration to facilitate early intervention, and the management of the post-debridement cavity as described by Bradley,[66] Warshaw,[67] and Beger.[68] This approach has since been largely superseded by the concept of minimally invasive intervention within a "step-up" framework.[69]

The 2012 revision of the Atlanta Classification[9] has taken account of these changes and provides guidelines on how to structure the management of what are invariably complex and individual management algorithms (see Chapter 54). This classification divides AP into three categories: mild, moderately severe, and severe disease. A subsequent paper suggested an additional category of "critical pancreatitis" to recognize those patients with sepsis and organ failure, which was associated with the highest mortality.[70]

These categories are based on the absence or presence of local and/or systemic complications. In addition to disease severity, early mortality is strongly associated with age and comorbidity.[71] The classification further categorizes local complications on the basis of time from presentation (< or > 4 weeks) and on the presence of necrosis (Table 56.1). The vast majority of acute fluid collections (AFC) without necrosis (Fig. 56.2) will resolve within 4 weeks and a persistent fluid collection with minimal or no necrotic component ("acute pancreatic pseudocyst") is very rare, with the majority having at least a small amount of necrosis. In addition, collections may be sterile or infected.

The majority of peripancreatic complications are therefore related to either acute necrotic collections (<4 weeks) or walled-off pancreatic necrosis (WOPN; >4 weeks; Fig. 56.3A–B). This temporal separation is somewhat arbitrary because the clinical management and surgical approach is determined by multifactorial individual patient factors. Where possible, it is recommended that any planned intervention for necrosis be delayed until at least 4 weeks after presentation.

The systemic clinical course does not always correlate with the presence or severity of the local complications. One in five cases, however, will develop organ failure with or without local complications, a setting that defines severe AP. Half of the deaths attributable to AP occur within the first 7 days of admission,[72] with the majority in the first 3 days. Patients with severe

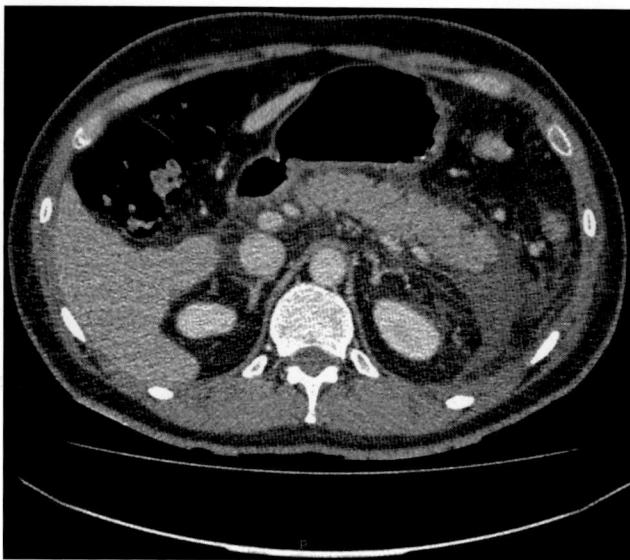

FIGURE 56.2 Acute fluid collection with normal pancreatic attenuation of contrast-enhanced computed tomography (CECT).

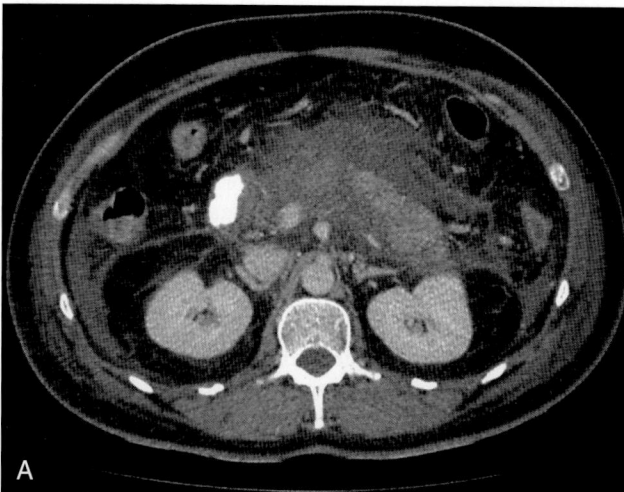

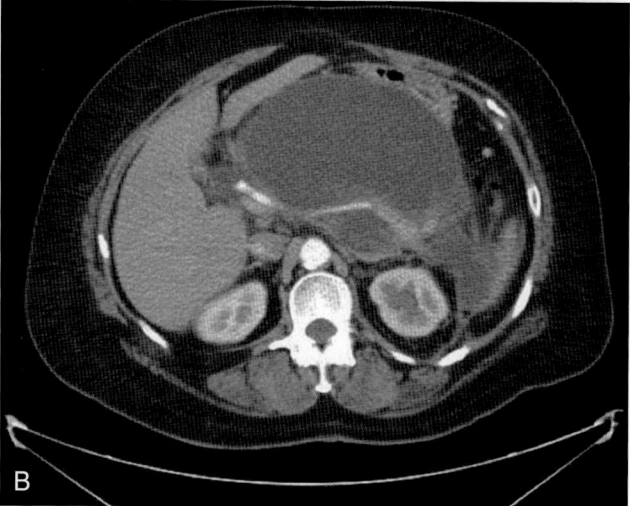

FIGURE 56.3 A, Acute necrotic collection (ANC). **B,** Walled-off pancreatic necrosis (WOPN).

AP who survive this first phase of illness, particularly those with persistent SIRS or organ failure,[10,71,73] are particularly at risk for developing secondary infection of pancreatic necrosis. Mortality in patients with infected necrosis and organ failure may reach 20% to 30%.

Acute Fluid Collections

These are common within the first few days and are identified radiologically as poorly demarcated fluid in the vicinity of the pancreas. Patients with this finding may be monitored with serial imaging but do not usually require intervention. These immature collections tend to resolve spontaneously in the majority of patients. They reflect local peripancreatic edema, and failure of resolution is probably related to the presence of parenchymal necrosis and duct disruption.

Intervention for Acute Necrotic Collections or Walled-Off Pancreatic Necrosis

There is clearly some degree of overlap between the early and late patient populations, and most studies in the literature include heterogeneous groups. There have been repeated attempts to compare different approaches to the management of pancreatic necrosis, either within cohort series or RCTs. The Holy Grail of identifying a single superior technique is, however, a flawed approach because the heterogeneity of presentation, anatomy, and physiology has a much greater influence on outcome than any differences in the technique of intervention. The choice of intervention is guided by the clinical picture, anatomic position of the collection, and local expertise. All of the described approaches can have their role, but increasingly the choice lies between endoscopic or minimally invasive surgical drainage.[73]

Indications include:
1. Infection/sepsis, either suspected radiologically or as a part of the clinical picture
2. Nutritional failure
3. Persistent abdominal pain
4. Management of complications

Indications for intervention vary with time from onset, initially being limited to the management of early complications, a middle phase focusing on sepsis control, and lastly addressing failure to thrive or late-onset complications. Surgical intervention for necrosis in the first 2 weeks carries a high risk for morbidity and mortality and is therefore to be avoided[74] in the absence of specific complications, such as bleeding or ischemia. Although intervention may be eventually required for a persistent symptomatic walled-off necrotic (WON) collection, intervention for an acute necrotic collection before it has matured sufficiently to become encapsulated is usually only indicated in the presence of secondary infection. This may be evidenced by a secondary clinical and biochemical deterioration, coupled with CT evidence of infection such as a small pockets of gas.[75] The identification of gas within a collection is not in itself an indication for intervention because spontaneous enteric discharge of a collection may be associated with clinical improvement. In this situation, there is often a gas/fluid level (Fig. 56.4), and therefore any imaging result needs to be interpreted within the overall clinical context.

Once a decision is made that intervention is required, these pancreatic (and peripancreatic) collections can be managed by a variety of approaches. Freeny and colleagues[76] showed in the 1990s that aggressive percutaneous sepsis control would

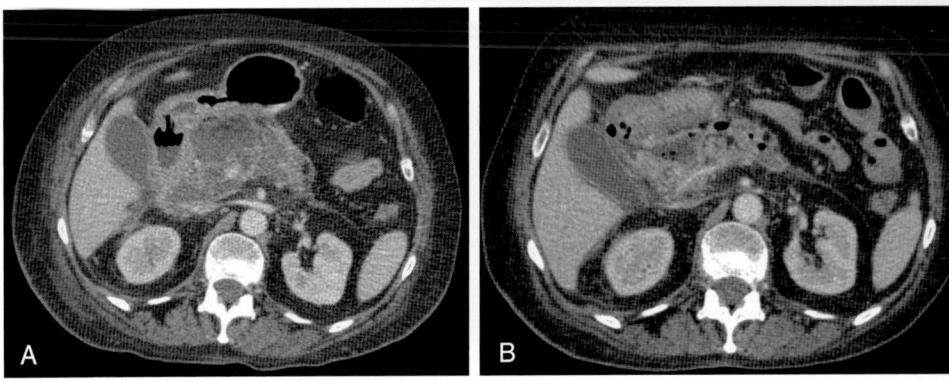

FIGURE 56.4 Spontaneous duodenal discharge of a walled-off necrosis (WON) collection resulting in clinical improvement.

promote recovery in the absence of formal necrosectomy, although 50% required subsequent surgical intervention. A number of minimally invasive approaches have been described, including percutaneous necrosectomy (MIRP),[77] video-assisted retroperitoneal debridement (VARD),[78] endoscopic cystgastrostomy,[79] and laparoscopic cystgastrostomy.[80] Laparoscopic direct necrosectomy was described in the 1990s but failed to gain popularity because of its technical difficulty.[81] Dual-modality drainages are commonly employed during a disease episode.[82] There is evidence that minimal access techniques may pose less of a challenge to the patient's systemic inflammatory response and, in our own experience, patients have reduced requirements for the intensive care management.[83] Connor and colleagues[84] reported half as many deaths in patients treated with a minimal access approach when compared with those having laparotomy.

Although a number of differing minimally invasive techniques had been described in cohort series showing benefit of historical controls, the PANTER trial[85] from the Dutch Pancreatitis Study Group provided randomized data regarding the management of infected pancreatic necrosis (IPN). Patients with IPN were randomized to either open necrosectomy or a "step-up" approach based on endoscopic or percutaneous drainage as the initial intervention, with progression to retroperitoneal debridement with lavage if no improvement was observed. The composite endpoint of death or major complication demonstrated a significant benefit with the step-up approach. Indeed, 35% were successfully managed with percutaneous drainage alone and did not require subsequent debridement. There is now a consensus advocating a principle of early organ support and nutritional optimization, followed ideally by delayed minimally invasive intervention within a "step-up" framework where possible.

The choice of one approach over another is determined by the clinical condition of the patient, local experience and expertise, anatomic position/content of the collection, and the time from presentation/maturation of the wall of the collection. There is an acceptance that because of the complexity of presentation, no single technique is applicable in all circumstances. The optimal approach is developing through an evolution of the management concepts introduced over the last decade and has been informed by the publication of two RCTs comparing percutaneous and endoscopic intervention. The TENSION trial,[86] again by the Dutch Pancreatitis Study Group, compared a step-up endoscopic drainage with a VARD-based surgical approach and is discussed in more detail later in this chapter. The MISER trial[87] compared an endoscopic step-up approach with a primary laparoscopic cystgastrostomy intervention, although 19% were managed by VARD, and the trial design failed to recognize that laparoscopic cystgastrostomy is more suited to management of organized WON, with only 20% of interventions occurring more than 6 weeks from presentation.

The choice of initial percutaneous or endoscopic drainage is now largely based on the position of the collection relative to the stomach, colon, liver, spleen, and kidney. Although both the aforementioned trials can be critiqued as having biased intervention protocols, the results favored endoscopic intervention and, where available, this has become the primary intervention of choice. Furthermore, the ability to perform EUS-guided puncture within an ICU setting, without moving the patient to the radiology department for CT-guided drainage, may influence the management decision where a patient is in extremis.

In general, our practice has been to approach lateral collections and those extending behind the colon from the left or right flank percutaneously and to prefer endoscopic drainage for those medial collections where a percutaneous route may be compromised by overlying bowel, spleen, or liver. The route of percutaneous drainage should ideally take into account the probability of subsequent "step-up" escalation, siting the drain as lateral and inferior as possible and avoiding the costal margin, but the initial priority must be sepsis control. If the initial drain placement is suboptimal, secondary alternative access can be obtained, sometimes involving a combination of percutaneous and endoscopic techniques.

Retroperitoneal "Step-Up" Management Techniques

Both MIRP and VARD retroperitoneal techniques are modifications of the open lateral approach initially described in the 1980s by Fagniez,[88] which used a loin/subcostal and retrocolic approach to allow debridement of pancreatic and peripancreatic necrosis. This open approach was associated with major morbidity (enteric fistula 45%, hemorrhage 40%, and colonic necrosis 15%) and failed to gain popularity. For both minimally invasive techniques, a left-sided small diameter percutaneous drain is ideally placed into the acute necrotic collection between the spleen, kidney, and colon under CT guidance. The key to successful upsizing is choosing a drainage route that facilitates subsequent step-up management. Right-sided or transperitoneal drainage are also possible. In those who fail to respond adequately to simple drainage, this access drain is then used as a guide to gain enhanced drainage of the collection.

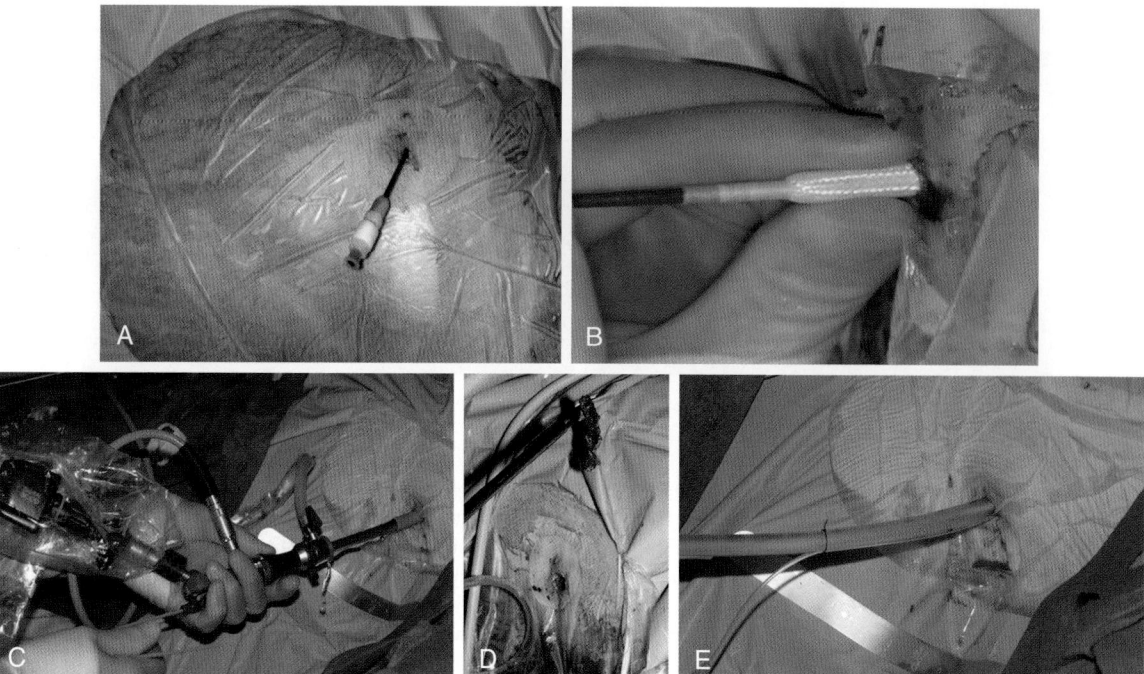

FIGURE 56.5   A–E, Technique of minimally invasive percutaneous necrosectomy (MIPN).

Minimally Invasive Pancreatic Necrosectomy

For percutaneous necrosectomy (Fig. 56.5A–E), the catheter is exchanged for a radiologic guidewire, then a low-compliance balloon dilator is inserted into the collection and dilated to 30 FG. Access to the cavity is then maintained by an Amplatz sheath through which is passed an operating nephroscope to allow debridement under direct vision. The nephroscope has an operating channel that permits standard (5 mm) laparoscopic graspers and an irrigation/suction channel. The directed high-flow lavage promotes rapid evacuation of pus and liquefied necrotic material, revealing black or grey devascularized pancreatic tissue and peripancreatic fat, which, if loose, is extracted in a piecemeal fashion until, after several procedures, a cavity lined by viable tissue or granulating pancreas is created. At the end of the procedure, an 8 FG catheter sutured to a 24 FG drain is passed into the cavity to allow continuous postoperative lavage of warmed 0.9% normal saline initially at 250 mL an hour. Subsequent conversion of the lavage system to simple drainage may be all that is required before recovery or the procedure may be repeated until sepsis control is achieved and interval CT confirms resolution.

Video-Assisted Retroperitoneal Debridement

A VARD procedure is performed with the patient placed in a supine position with the left side 30 to 40 degrees elevated. A subcostal incision of 5 cm is placed in the left flank at the mid-axillary line, close to the exit point of the percutaneous drain. Using the in situ percutaneous drain as a guide, the retroperitoneal collection is entered. The cavity is cleared of purulent material using a standard suction device. Visible necrosis is carefully removed with the use of long grasping forceps. Deeper access is then facilitated using a 0-degree laparoscope, and further debridement performed with laparoscopic forceps under videoscopic assistance. As with a percutaneous necrosectomy, complete necrosectomy is not

the aim of this procedure and only loosely adherent pieces of necrosis are removed, minimizing the risk for hemorrhage. Two large-bore single lumen drains are positioned in the cavity, and the fascia is closed to facilitate a closed continuous postoperative lavage system.

Open Surgical Necrosectomy

Three general variations of open necrosectomy are currently practiced and remain widespread while experience of minimally invasive approaches increases. These can also be used within a step-up framework with preoperative percutaneous drainage, allowing control of sepsis before intervention. Although the procedures are broadly similar in terms of the necrosectomy, they differ in terms of how they prevent recurrence of an infected collection within the debridement cavity:

1. Open necrosectomy with open or closed packing
2. Open necrosectomy with continuous closed postoperative lavage
3. Programmed open necrosectomy

In all approaches, the abdomen is entered though a midline or preferably a bilateral subcostal incision because this minimizes contamination of the lower abdomen and allows lateral access. The pancreas is exposed by dividing the gastrocolic omentum or gastrohepatic omentum to access the pancreas through the lesser sac.

Open Necrosectomy with Open Packing

Bradley described this technique in 1987 where sepsis control is achieved by leaving the abdomen open after debridement, packing the cavity as a laparostomy.[66] Planned reintervention with sequential pack changes allows for resolution with healing by secondary intention. Drains may be placed in addition to the packing. Open packing techniques have been reported to have higher incidences of fistulae, bleeding, and incisional hernias and a slightly higher mortality rate.[89]

Open Necrosectomy with Closed Packing

The goal of necrosectomy with closed packing is to achieve sepsis control by performing a thorough debridement and removal of necrotic and infected tissue to minimize the need for reoperation or subsequent drainage.[90] Primary closure of the abdomen is the intention over gauze-stuffed Penrose drains with the intention to fill the cavity and provide some compression.[67] Additional silicone drains (Jackson-Pratt) may be placed in the pancreatic bed and lesser sac for fluid drainage. The drains are removed sequentially, starting 5 to 7 days postoperatively, allowing a gradual involution of the cavity.

Open Necrosectomy with Continuous Closed Postoperative Lavage

After debridement, where possible, a closed peripancreatic compartment is reconstituted by suturing the gastrocolic and duodenocolic ligaments over large-bore drains to allow for side to side continuous lavage.[68] Postoperative continuous lavage is instituted at 1 to 10 L per day and continued until the effluent is clear and the patient shows improvement in clinical and laboratory parameters.[91] No evidence is available to suggest the best irrigation fluid, the optimal number or caliber of drains, or the duration of irrigation.

Programmed Open Necrosectomy

In response to the bleeding and fistulation that can arise after aggressive necrosectomy, this approach attempts to initially perform a more conservative debridement, with the intention of performing repeat procedures every 48 hours until debridement is no longer required. This mimics concepts associated with the step-up approaches. The pancreatic bed is drained or packed, and the abdomen is closed by suturing mesh or a zipper to the fascial edges of the wound.[92] The addition of intraabdominal vacuum dressings may encourage granulation of the pancreatic bed, and it has been suggested that they may reduce the number of operations and mortality, but there are little data to support this and they have been associated with enteric fistulation.[93]

Open or Laparoscopic Cystogastrostomy

Open transgastric debridement has been proposed to minimize postoperative peritoneal contamination.[94] The procedure can equally be performed laparoscopically and may be the intervention of choice for mature WOPN presenting with failure to thrive because resolution may be achieved safely with a single intervention.[95] The risk of inadequate initial drainage, and requirement for repeated tract dilatation with the EUS-guided transgastric approach, coupled with parallel improvements in laparoscopic equipment and operative technique, have refocused interest on the potential of a single laparoscopic intervention for patients with WOPN. Our current technique for laparoscopic cystgastrostomy is described.

First, an open subumbilical cut down is employed. Blunt trocars are then inserted on the patient's left and right side with the specific port site placement being determined by the position of the retrogastric collection on cross-sectional imaging, thus optimizing triangulation over the cystgastrostomy site. Adhesions from recent inflammation are common and are divided to expose the anterior gastric wall. An anterior gastrotomy (5–10 cm long) is then performed using the harmonic scalpel (Ethicon Endo-Surgery, Inc, Cincinnati, Ohio, USA). The superior leaf of the opened stomach is lifted toward the anterior abdominal wall to maximize access and delineate the area of adherence between the cyst and the posterior aspect of the stomach. This is achieved by passing a straight needle 2/0 suture through the abdominal wall, then the anterior stomach wall, and back out of the abdomen.

The key advance has been the use of a "STEP" dilatation port system (Covidien plc, Dublin, Ireland) to achieve initial cyst puncture, allow tract dilatation, and maintain access until insertion of the initial staple device. The puncture trocar is inserted through the abdominal wall and, having chosen an appropriate epigastric/stomach puncture site under guidance of laparoscopic ultrasound, the sharp trocar enters the collection via the exposed posterior gastric wall. The port is dilated, allowing 12-mm access to the cyst cavity, apposition of the posterior stomach wall and cyst being maintained by the radial resistance of the dilatation sleeve. After aspiration of the collection to relative dryness, the port is withdrawn, leaving the suction instrument within the collection to maintain access, and a stapled cystgastrostomy is performed using 4 to 5 firings of the angulating Universal Endo GIA stapler (Covidien plc, Dublin, Ireland; image 2). Necrotic debris within the cavity is removed and placed in the fundus of the stomach (image 3). Once adequate debridement and hemostasis have been assured, the anterior gastrotomy is closed using a running 3/0 monofilament suture (Biosyn, Covidien plc, Dublin, Ireland), with the integrity of the closure then tested by insufflating the stomach through an orogastric tube, while the anastomosis is held under lavage fluid. Postoperative fluid and diet is allowed as tolerated. In this complex cohort of patients, suitability for hospital discharge is often multifactorial but may be within 36 hours of surgery when dietary intake is adequate. Where gallstones are present, a simultaneous laparoscopic cholecystectomy is performed.

Transmural Drainage

EUS-guided drainage was initially reported as a management strategy for an established pancreatic abscess in the context of minimal necrosis. The procedure has, however, evolved in the last 15 years and is now best considered a NOTES (natural orifice transluminal endoscopic surgery) procedure. Advances in both technique and equipment now facilitate endoscopic transmural exploration and debridement of the retroperitoneum. The presence of significant WOPN is no longer considered a contraindication to this approach, but concerns do remain regarding the adequacy of endoscopic drainage, particularly in solid predominant or larger collections. It is important to establish dependent drainage, and this is not always possible via the EUS route in these settings.

The principles remain the same regardless of the approach: initial simple drainage of a collection under pressure, followed by subsequent "step up" tract dilatation and even necrosectomy apply to the endoscopic approach as they do to the surgical techniques. Initial experience was promising (Seifert et al., 2009), and an early pilot study exploring the outcome of endoscopic transmural drainage versus minimally invasive intervention (VARD; the PENGUIN trial)[96] suggested at least equivalence, if not benefit, from endoscopic drainage. This study has been criticized because of very small numbers and an excessive mortality, compared with historical results, within the VARD arm.

The TENSION trial provided further insights on the relative merits of the endoscopic and surgical approaches for infected pancreatic necrosis.[86] This multicenter RCT in 98 patients did not demonstrate superiority of the endoscopic over the surgical step-up approach in reducing major complications or death. Unsurprisingly, the rate of pancreatic fistulae and the hospital LOS were lower in the patients managed endoscopically. By definition, external (surgical) drainage will create a pancreatic fistula which, if controlled, is not a significant clinical issue. The hospital LOS reflects both the magnitude of intervention and the challenge of managing an external versus internal pancreatic fistula. The authors concluded that this trial will probably influence current management in favor of endoscopy. Although this is one interpretation of the data, the decision making regarding this complex patient cohort is often more nuanced.

Endoscopic Ultrasound–Guided Cystgastrostomy/ Necrosectomy

Transgastric drainage of pancreatic necrosis was first described by Baron and colleagues in a series of 11 patients with WOPN.[97] Since then the procedure has evolved and with the introduction of EUS, guidance has been widely adopted in the management of pseudocysts and WOPN. As discussed earlier, true pancreatic pseudocysts are rare after AP because some degree of necrosis is usually present in persistent pancreatic collections and the great majority of collections requiring intervention are best considered WOPN, with varying degrees of fluid content. Infection with or without organ failure may be present. There are now many cohort series and one RCT attesting to the utility and safety of this procedure, at least in selected patients, and several different modifications to the technique have been described.

WOPN may be drained by either a transgastric or less commonly a transduodenal route. The procedure is best carried out under EUS guidance as two RCTs have shown an increased success rate compared with conventional transmural drainage.[98–100] EUS allows for identification of the collection where there is no obvious bulge seen within the stomach and helps identify a safe route for puncture. Early reports used EUS to identify and mark a puncture site followed by drainage using conventional endoscopic techniques, but a one-step EUS-guided procedure is now the norm.[101]

There are several methods described, but all involve an initial puncture of the collection with a needle or cystotome. Our previously preferred method was to puncture the collection using a cystotome (Cook Medical, Bloomington USA) under EUS guidance, the outer sheath of the cystotome is then advanced into the collection, again under EUS guidance, although radiologic screening may also be employed. The inner sheath and guidewire of the cystotome are then removed and the collection aspirated, a sample being taken for bacteriology. Two guidewires are then inserted into the collection through the outer (10 French [F]) sheath of the cystotome and the sheath then removed, leaving the wires coiled inside the collection. The puncture site is then dilated using an over-the-wire dilatation balloon (CRE) to 12 mm and two 7F pigtail stents then inserted into the cavity using a combination of endoscopic and fluoroscopic control. A nasocystic catheter can then be inserted alongside the two pigtail stents for lavage where there is extensive necrotic debris. Where the collection is mainly fluid, this procedure is associated with high success rates, but problems may arise in the presence of extensive necrosis or in very large and complex collections with retroperitoneal extension.[102] In these patients, repeated procedures with progressive dilatation of the cystgastrostomy site and cavity lavage may be required.

Modifications to the technique that may be considered in complex necrotic collections include the multiple gateway technique and formal endoscopic necrosectomy. In the multiple gateway technique,[98] two or three transmural stents are placed under EUS guidance, one of which is used for nasocystic cavity lavage and the others to facilitate drainage of necrotic debris. Endoscopic necrosectomy was described by Seifert and colleagues[100] in the same year as we described our own experience with percutaneous necrosectomy.

A recent systematic review[103] of 14 studies including 455 patients found an overall success rate of 81% and mortality of 6%, although all but one study was retrospective. One small RCT[96] has compared endoscopic with minimally invasive surgical drainage and found a reduction in significant complications with the endoscopic approach. Endoscopic necrosectomy is, however, a challenging procedure and not without risk. Major complications including fatal air embolism, bleeding, and perforation occurred in 26% of patients in the multicenter GEPARD[104] study. Removal of necrotic debris with existing endoscopic baskets and snares is time consuming and often ineffective. Endoscopic access to the cavity is not always straightforward and may require repeated dilatations before an adequately sized cystgastrostomy is achieved.

The introduction of self-expanding metal stents (SEMS) to facilitate endoscopic access to the necrotic collection (Fig. 56.6A–B) is now our preferred method of transmural

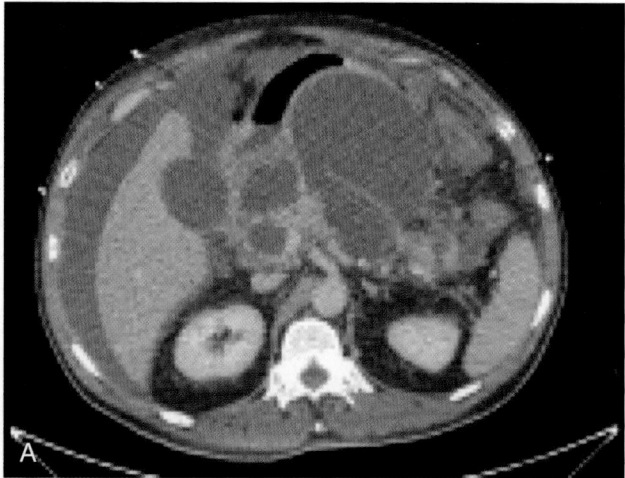

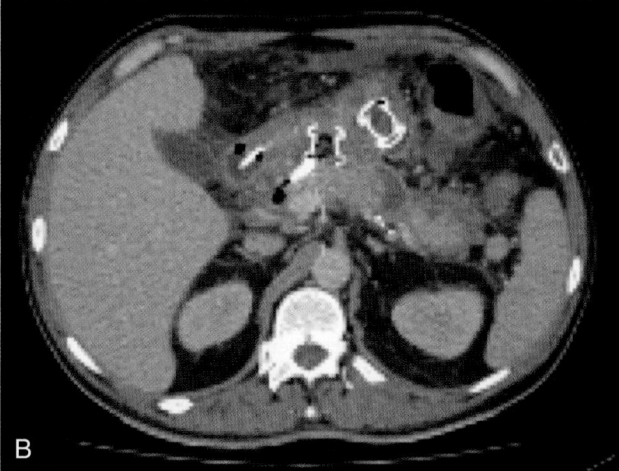

FIGURE 56.6 A, Centrally placed walled-off necrosis (WON) collection. **B,** Computed tomography (CT) after successful LAMS(Axios) cystgastrostomy drainage.

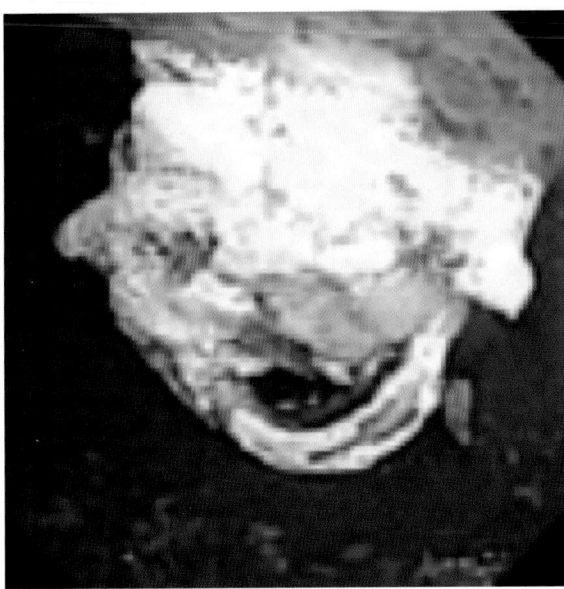

FIGURE 56.7 Solid necrotic debris after an endoscopic transmural cystgastrostomy preventing drainage.

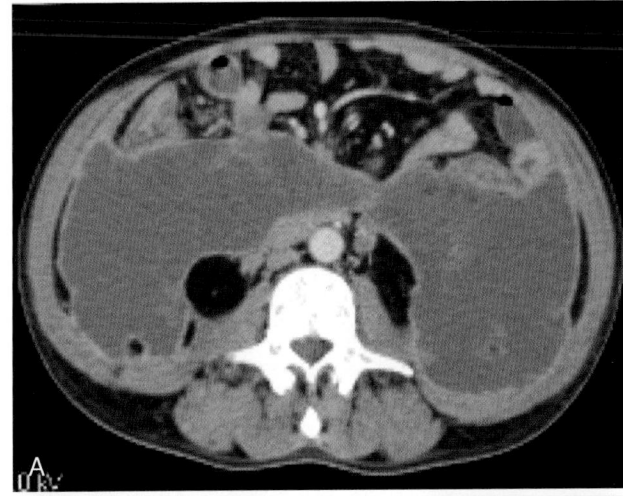

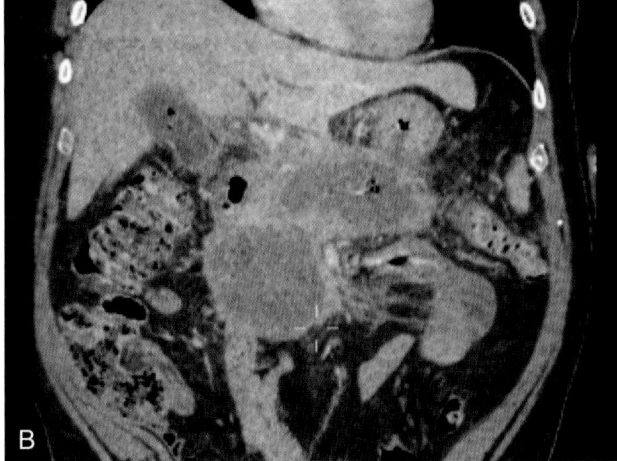

FIGURE 56.8 **Problematic collections. A,** Retro-colic extension. **B,** mesenteric extension.

drainage. The NAGI stent was one of the first technical developments in this field, but initially there was little evidence that it increased resolution rates over conventional pigtail stents.[105] More recently, the Hot AXIOS stent was introduced and our results with this are more favorable. Unlike previous stents for this purpose, this is the first lumen-apposing metal stent (LAMS), which confers significant advantages, particularly when draining collections that are poorly opposed to the gastric or duodenal wall. The deployment mechanism makes the procedure technically less demanding and losing access to the cavity during placement of the stent is less frequent. Our approach has evolved further to perform over-the-wire CRE balloon dilatation of the AXIOS to 12 to 15 mm once deployed. A premarked 7F 4-cm double pigtail stent is then deployed across the AXIOS in an effort to avoid "ball-valving" of necrotic debris within the lumen (Fig. 56.7). The AXIOS is usually removed 1 to 2 weeks after the index procedure. The cystgastrostomy is dilated further, and drainage is then maintained with one or two double pigtail stents.

A further modification is the use of intracavity hydrogen peroxide to facilitate necrosectomy, although further experience is required before this can be recommended for routine practice.[106] Regardless of the technique employed, all patients require a tailored approach to follow-up depending on the extent of necrosis and degree of systemic organ dysfunction. Patients with retroperitoneal extension of necrosis (Fig. 56.8A) may need further percutaneous procedures, and large necrotic collections may need many repeated procedures to achieve resolution. Small bowel mesenteric extension creates specific challenges because achieving drainage endoscopically or percutaneously can be troublesome, particularly in the obese patient (see Fig. 56.8B)

COMPLICATIONS

SIRS/Bacteremia Requiring Critical Care Support

After any intervention on an infected collection, it is common for patients to develop significant SIRS as a result of postprocedural

bacteremia. This usually occurs in the first 12 to 24 hours after intervention, regardless of route or technique, and may require critical care admission for organ support, most often vasopressor therapy. With minimally invasive intervention, this is usually of moderate severity and frequently resolves within 24 to 48 hours. More significant deterioration may follow open necrosectomy and has underpinned the improvements in mortality that have been seen with a minimally invasive step-up protocol. If possible, it is often beneficial for these patients to be observed in a critical care environment after intervention, particularly if they were not receiving level two care preprocedure.

Acute or Delayed Hemorrhage

Intraoperative hemorrhage may complicate early or overenthusiastic necrosectomy. Venous bleeding is more common in this situation and usually settles with correction of any coagulopathy and with local pressure (by simple drain occlusion, a modified Sengstaken-Blakemore tube having amputated the gastric balloon [MIRP; Fig. 56.9], or gauze packing if there is sufficient cutaneous access [VARD]).

Secondary hemorrhage is occasionally sudden and massive, but there is usually a prelude with a self-terminating "herald bleed," presenting clinically with hemorrhage into a retroperitoneal drain or occasionally a GI bleed. In contrast to intraoperative

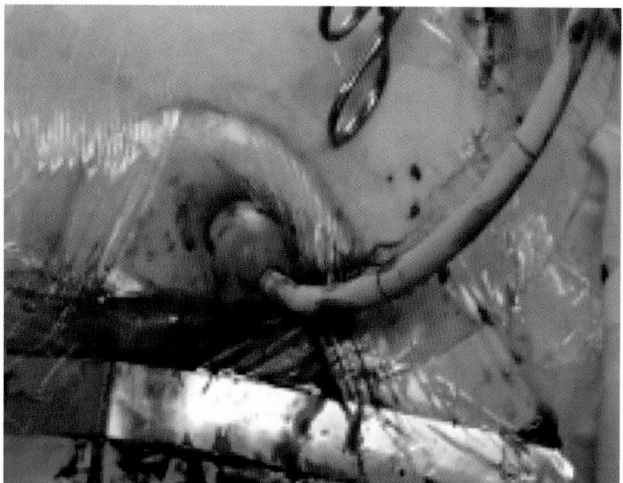

FIGURE 56.9 Modified Sengstaken–Blakemore tube used to control venous hemorrhage after percutaneous necrosectomy.

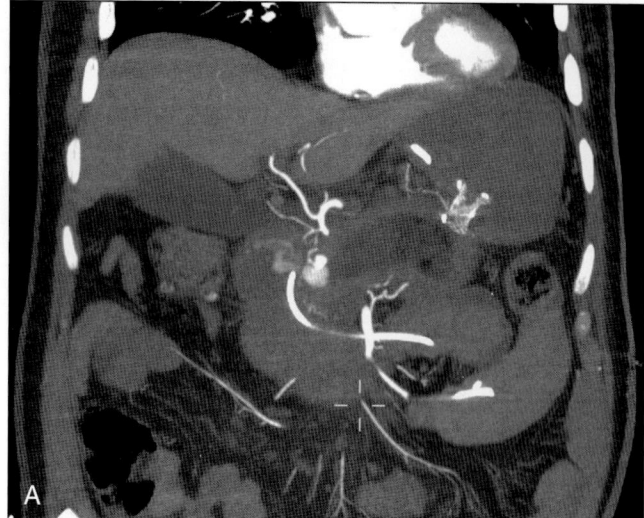

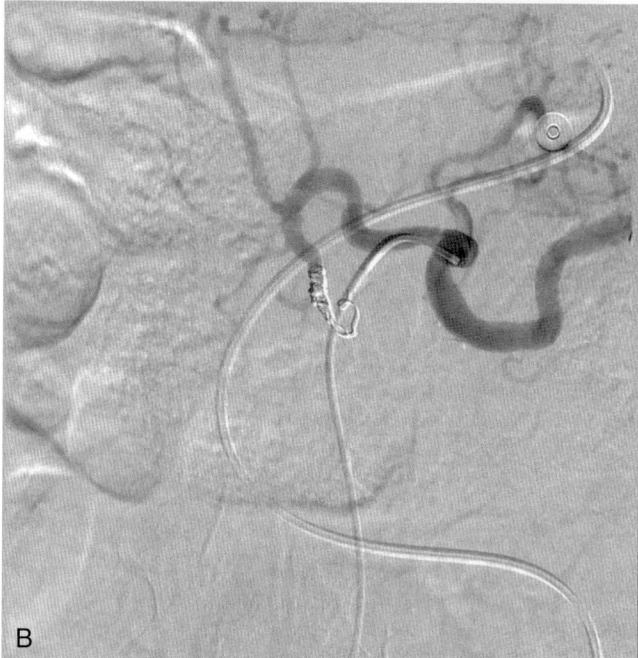

FIGURE 56.10 **Management of hemorrhage. A,** Identification of source of hemorrhage by computed tomography angiography (CTA). **B,** Control of hemorrhage by angiographic embolization.

bleeding, an arterial origin is more common because this usually results from uncontrolled sepsis around a major vessel. Overall, the mortality exceeds 30% to 40% and a high index of suspicion is to intervene before major bleeding with controlled volume support of the circulation and a simultaneous emergency CT angiogram followed by angiography and embolization (Fig. 56.10A–B), if appropriate. Upper GI endoscopy in this setting is usually nondiagnostic and so should not delay radiologic assessment, which allows definitive management. The increased intracavity pressure, associated with hemorrhage into an infected cavity, may also often be followed by escalating organ dysfunction through bacteremia and sepsis; therefore early introduction of targeted antimicrobials is essential. Further early intervention may be required to evacuate infected hematoma and re-establish adequate drainage.

Occasionally massive delayed venous bleeding may occur. This is significantly more challenging to control. There are rarely interventional radiology options and surgery in this group of patients, who are often already physiologically compromised with sepsis, carries a high mortality. The patient in extremis may require bedside laparotomy as a damage control maneuver, and although this is rare, we have used this to good effect, particularly in the younger patient with reasonable reserve. The goal in this scenario is control of hemorrhage, concurrent with resuscitation, using the most rapid and simplest technique, usually packing. The site of bleeding is usually either difficult to identify or multifocal, and it is critical to perform an abbreviated procedure at the bedside rather than pursue definitive control. Further procedures may be performed in the operating room in a controlled environment.

Enteric Fistulation

Spontaneous discharge of a post-acute collection into the adjacent GI tract is a recognized complication, often later in the patients' hospital course. Broadly, we divide these into foregut and hindgut fistulae. The former may decompress the collection and result in clinical improvement without intervention, particularly where the fistulous communication involved is the stomach or duodenum (Fig. 56.11A). This essentially replicates the outcome after endoscopic cystgastrostomy. Although spontaneous resolution is possible, fistulation into the colon—hindgut (see Fig. 56.11B)—will

often result in persistent sepsis and poorly controlled collections. There is often a marked clinical deterioration and, in this situation, a defunctioning colostomy/ileostomy or resection may be required. The decision will be determined by the condition of the patient, CT evidence of the site of fistulation, and any evidence of persistent undrained sepsis.

Pancreatic Fistula

An acute necrotic collection with significant parenchymal loss is commonly associated with disruption of the main pancreatic duct, frequently at the neck of the gland. After resolution of associated sepsis, leakage of amylase rich fluid is common, leading to a pancreatic fistula. Early endoscopic transpapillary intervention should be discouraged while collections remain because this may introduce infection and usually proves detrimental. After resolution of sepsis and any significant collection, pancreatic duct

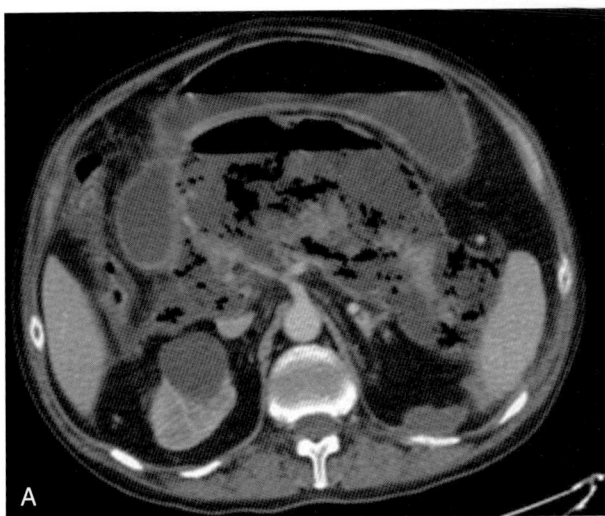

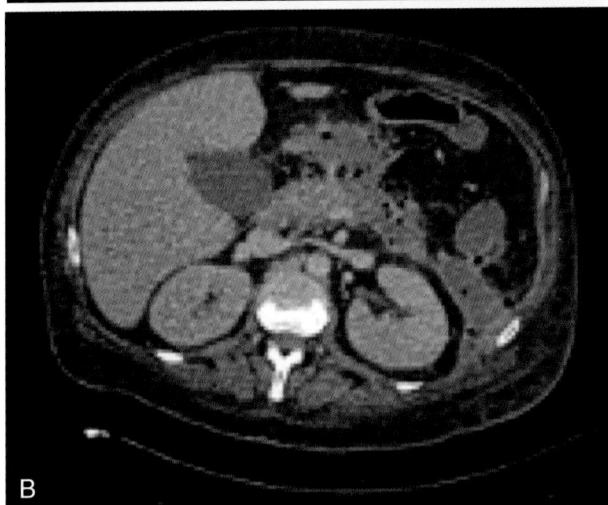

FIGURE 56.11   Computed tomography (CT) of enteric fistulation. A, Foregut fistulation. **B,** Hindgut fistulation.

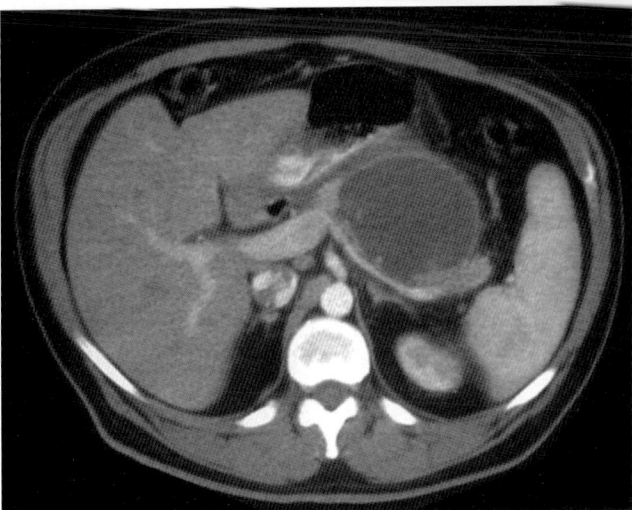

FIGURE 56.12   Disconnected tail with recurrent pseudocyst as late complication after resolution of necrotizing pancreatitis.

EXTREME PANCREATITIS

Pancreatitis occurs on a spectrum of severity, complexity, and chronology. Although the vast majority of patients do not progress to significant systemic or local complications, a subset will develop potentially devastating complications. We have termed this entity extreme pancreatitis (EP). It encompasses a wide range of profound physiologic disturbance and complex anatomic derangement, posing significant management challenges.

Here, we describe our current approach to EP, including management strategies and a novel classification. This is offered as a practical guide to deconstruct the process and facilitate care.

Dilemmas

Decision making in the patient with EP is the most challenging aspect of pancreatology. This is best appreciated if we contrast this with the patient with pancreatic cancer. The latter revolves around the two Ps of surgical oncology decision making: is the *patient* suitable for surgery and is the *pathology* appropriate for surgical management. This is a relatively straightforward, non-time-critical, multidisciplinary endeavor, which may occur over days to weeks.

In comparison, the patient with EP often has a significant, complex, and time-critical illness. There is a large volume of physiologic and anatomic data to interpret and synthesize in a relatively short time frame of perhaps hours or days. Successful management therefore requires a deep understanding of the pathophysiology to allow the careful construct of an appropriate strategy.

General Principles of Management

There are broadly two aspects to managing EP: decision making and the requisite practical skill set if intervention is necessary. Of these, the greatest challenge is the decision making in determining the need for a practical skill (or intervention) rather than in the skill itself.

EP occurs along a spectrum of disease punctuated by critical decision nodes. A reductionist approach is therefore required and is key to decision making. There are only two questions to consider:

1. Do I need to intervene?
2. If yes, how?

stent insertion at ERCP may result in resolution of a persistent fistula. Persistent drainage is often associated with more extensive parenchymal loss or with loss of continuity of the main pancreatic duct. Prolonged catheter drainage will lead to maturation of the fistula tract and planned interval drain removal may result in spontaneous resolution or development of a late pseudocyst.

Disconnected Pancreatic Duct

Necrosis extending across most of the transverse diameter of the body or tail results in complete separation of the gland and the main pancreatic duct on either side. This may lead to a persistent fistula and "disconnected duct syndrome" (Fig. 56.12). Ductal occlusion occurs at the level of parenchymal loss, usually at the pancreatic neck, and often precludes transpapillary access. If this is not the case, transpapillary stenting may result in resolution. If transpapillary access is not possible, the options are transmural EUS-guided drainage or to perform a "salvage" distal pancreatectomy to resect the residual disconnected pancreatic parenchyma, often in combination with a splenectomy. This operative intervention may be technically challenging as a result of dense postinflammatory fibrosis with obliteration of surgical planes. Further, occlusion of the splenic vein by this process can result in large venous collaterals adding a further layer of complexity to the surgery.

This decision making can be simplified and is largely governed by three factors:

1. Timing: Early versus late in disease course
2. Physiology: Organ failure/sepsis
3. Anatomy: What's achievable and is there a route

Synthesis of these three factors in the context of institutional capabilities ultimately governs the systematic approach to management. In addition, the key to success includes meticulous attention to detail within a multidisciplinary team; a dynamic and flexible mind set; individualized multimodal therapy; nutrition; targeted antimicrobials; and critical care support.

Extreme Pancreatitis Classification

The following novel classification of EP facilitates early pattern recognition, diagnosis, and management. Essentially a pancreatic fistula may be free, contained, or intraorgan. It may occur in the abdomen or the thorax or both. Pancreatic juice can track to a variety of extra-pancreatic anatomic regions and a high index of suspicion is required (Table 56.2).

Presentation and Clinical Scenarios (see Table 56.2)

Pancreatic Ascites

Pancreatic ascites usually presents with abdominal pain and acute physiologic deterioration. Previous imaging may demonstrate a contained pancreatic collection, which has now at least partially decompressed into the peritoneal cavity. These patients may be profoundly unwell.

Pseudocyst

A pseudocyst may present with local symptoms, such as pain or early satiety, or systemic issues such as sepsis or bleeding. These may be treated by drainage into an adjacent hollow viscus—usually the stomach—as an EUS, laparoscopic cystgastrostomy, or open cystgastrostomy.

Intraorgan Abdomen

Intraorgan abdomen presents with abdominal pain and often with superimposed sepsis. Liver and spleen are the most commonly affected end organs. The pathophysiology in this group of patients introduces the concept of "hilar tracking" (i.e., pancreatic juice tracking along the hilum of the liver or spleen to collect in the parenchyma or subcapsular space).

Pancreatico-Pleural Fistula

Patients often present with respiratory compromise. Imaging may demonstrate a pancreatic duct disruption, which then tracks behind the diaphragm or via the hiatus to the chest. Frequently, however, it is not possible to delineate the track on

imaging and the diagnosis is based on amylase-rich pleural aspirate. The resultant pleural effusion may be unilateral or bilateral (Fig. 56.13A).

Mediastinal Pseudocyst

A mediastinal pseudocyst may present with respiratory compromise and occasionally dysphagia. It may be completely contained or associated with a pancreatico-pleural effusion. Per abdominal pseudocyst, these are drained into an adjacent hollow viscus, usually the esophagus.

Intraorgan Chest

Pancreatico-bronchial fistula will present with respiratory compromise and sepsis. The patient may be in extremis and require urgent intubation and critical care support. There is often gas in the collection on imaging as a consequence of communication

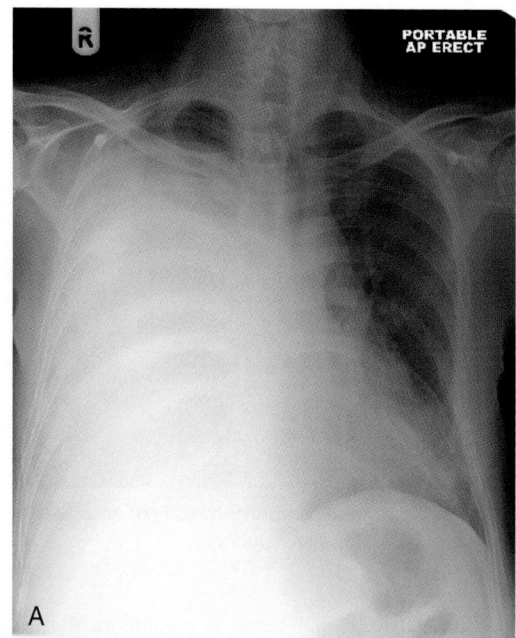

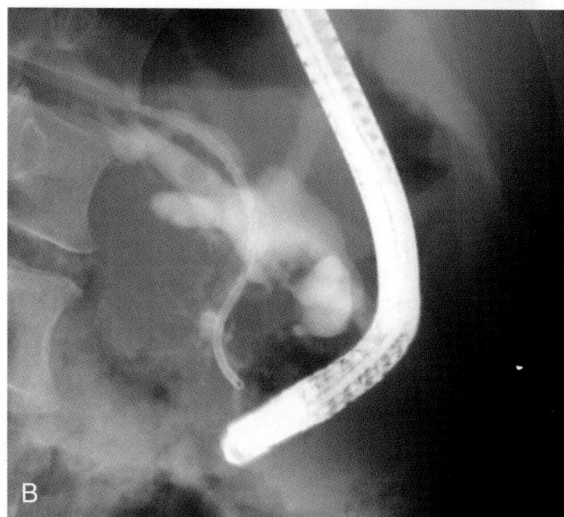

FIGURE 56.13 Tension pancreatico-pleural fistula. A, Chest X-ray with mediastinal shift. **B,** Endoscopic retrograde cholangiopancreatography (ERCP) confirming neck duct disruption and showing insertion of pancreatic duct stent.

TABLE 56.2 The Glasgow Clinical Classification of Post-Acute Pancreatic Collections		
	ABDOMEN	**INTER-THORACIC**
Free	1A pancreatic ascites	1C pancreatico-pleural fistula
Contained	2A AFC/pseudocyst	2C mediastinal pseudocyst
Intraorgan	3A intrahepatic/splenic collection	3C pancreatico-bronchial fistula

A, Abdomen; *AFC,* acute fluid collection; *C,* chest.

with the airways. The diagnosis is made on sputum amylase, frequently as an endotracheal tube aspirate.

Specific Management Principles

Regardless of the ultimate location of pancreatic juice, the management principles are always the same. They may be best deconstructed to three phases to simplify and guide care:

1. External control with percutaneous drainage
2. Internal control (initial) achieved endoscopically (ERCP or EUS; see Fig. 56.13B)
3. Internal control (definitive): Surgery for the rare patient who fails phase 2

In addition, nutritional support and critical care may be required at any or all of the above phases. In our experience, the Glasgow Porcupine Approach is often required, which involves multiple percutaneous drains as part of phase 1 until control is achieved. These principles serve as a reminder that there are only three safe locations for pancreatic juice: the pancreas, the hollow GI viscera, and a drain bag.

DISCUSSION

There is general agreement that intervention in the first two weeks of severe AP should be avoided if at all possible.[74] During this period, many patients may require intensive care management, with escalating organ failure associated with a significant mortality.[72] Intervention for the pancreatic or peripancreatic inflammatory mass has not been shown to enhance recovery and may be detrimental. Several observational studies have shown improved outcome for operation beyond 28 days from onset,[107] although in the absence of randomized evidence this may reflect the requirement to intervene earlier in the sickest patients. Some authors[108,109] have expressed concern that to delay beyond this point confers unnecessary risk, with resultant impaired nutritional and immune status. However, where slow improvement continues, delay until there is an established walled-off collection simplifies intervention.

Indications for intervention include strong suspicion or documented infection of necrosis. In the absence of infection, persistent organ failure for several weeks, with a drainable walled-off collection and persistence of symptoms such as pain and ileus, may also require intervention. Timing of intervention requires judgment by an experienced and specialist pancreatic team, involving a multifactorial algorithm based on radiologic, clinical, and nutritional progress. Once the decision for intervention has been made, there are often several possible options and no single approach is ideal for use in all patients. There is growing consensus that intervention where required should involve a minimally invasive technique within a step-up framework. In practice, a range of options may be required, often in combination,[109] based on the position of the acute necrotic or walled-off collection taken in context with the patient's overall clinical condition.

Minimally invasive approaches have been criticized because they often require repeated intervention before resolution, with increased inpatient stay. In a clinically well patient with established

WON, whose principal symptom is failure to thrive, a laparoscopic transgastric cystgastrostomy offers the potential of a single intervention with the possibility of simultaneous definitive management of cholelithiasis.[80]

Complications after enhanced drainage are common and may be either disease or procedure related. Enteric fistulation is relatively common, and the requirement for secondary control is dependent on whether the fistula arises from the proximal or distal gut, colonic fistulae often requiring surgical enteric diversion to control persistent sepsis. Bleeding may occur intraoperatively and may be controlled by balloon tamponade, conversion to a VARD procedure with gauze packing, or occasionally angiography. Venous bleeding is more common intraoperatively. Secondary hemorrhage may arise on the background of poorly controlled sepsis and in the presence of an enteric fistula may result in GI bleeding or direct bleeding within a surgical drain. Angiographic control or again local pressure via the drain tract or VARD wound is preferred to open surgery, which historically was often an agonal intervention.

Operator experience is a key determinant to the choice of which minimally invasive approach to adopt. There is no evidence supporting the use of one approach over another. Many units may have experience in only one method, and this will influence the decision process. The differences between a VARD and MIRP are small, and in practice these procedures are interchangeable, whereas the addition of either an endoscopic or laparoscopic cystgastrostomy can increase management options, particularly where collections are centrally placed and percutaneous access is difficult.

A "gold standard" minimally invasive management algorithm would take into account the clinical condition of the patient, the anatomic location of the collection, and, in an ideal world, expertise in all four techniques. This allows for adaptability and flexibility in the interventional approaches to what is often an extremely challenging clinical problem. An important point to note is that many patients may benefit from the use of a multimodal approach with the use of more than one technique during the course of their illness. For example, a patient with escalating multiorgan failure can be stabilized within the ICU setting with EUS-guided transgastric drainage and after a period of stabilization, more definitive intervention employed by either MIRP, VARD, or even laparoscopic cystgastrostomy.

Ultimately, there are principles and preferences. The principles should be universal, such as drainage of pus under pressure to control sepsis. Interventional preference will be determined by patient physiology and trajectory and by institutional capabilities with regards to the experience and techniques available. It is possible to become "procedure-focused" rather than "patient-focused" if a unit or individual can only offer a limited range of interventions. It is for this reason that these patients are best managed in a specialist center, with expertise in the full range of techniques, to match the intervention to each point on the patient journey and provide individualized care.

The references for this chapter can be found online by accessing the accompanying Expert Consult website.

CHAPTER 57

Etiology, pathogenesis, and diagnosis of chronic pancreatitis

Kevin N. Shah and Theodore Pappas

Pancreatitis, marked by inflammation of the pancreatic parenchyma and injury to the acinar cells, has been traditionally divided into categories of acute or chronic (see Chapters 54–56 and 58). Initial attempts to distinguish acute from chronic pancreatitis centered on the resolution of symptoms and inflammation in acute pancreatitis, contrasted with the permanent changes observed in chronic pancreatitis.[1] Chronic pancreatitis, while broadly and classically defined by progressive and irreversible fibrosis of the pancreas, is marked by complexity, heterogeneity, and an evolution in understanding of cause, course, and treatment[2–5] (see Chapter 54).

The primary challenge of using the traditional clinicopathologic framework is that relying on the "irreversible" component of the definition requires years of delay between symptom onset and diagnosis, poor prediction of the entire clinical course, and a deemphasis on addressing the underlying etiology.[6] In 2016 a new mechanistic definition was proposed to define chronic pancreatitis as "a pathologic fibroinflammatory syndrome of the pancreas in individuals with genetic, environmental and/or other risk factors who develop persistent pathologic responses to parenchymal injury or stress." Common features of chronic pancreatitis include "pancreatic atrophy, fibrosis, pain syndromes, duct distortion and strictures, calcifications, pancreatic exocrine dysfunction, pancreatic endocrine dysfunction, and dysplasia," but may not be seen in all patients.[7] The definition is linked to a progressive model to organize risk factors, clinical scenarios, disease biomarkers, sequential and progressive features, and individual variables within a lifetime. It was also designed to assess the differential diagnosis of disorders with pathologic features that overlap with early chronic pancreatitis, such as fibrosis, atrophy, maldigestion, and diabetes[6] (see Chapter 54).

CLASSIFICATION SYSTEMS

To better understand the heterogenous etiologic and clinical considerations of chronic pancreatitis, a number of classification systems have been proposed. The basis for classification of chronic pancreatitis comes from four major consensus conferences and one study: Marseille in 1963, Marseille-Rome in 1986, Cambridge in 1984,[1,8–10] the Zurich symposium, and the Manchester classification[11] (see Chapter 54).

The Cambridge and Rosemont classification systems established discrete categories based on morphologic changes (adapted for computed tomography [CT] and endoscopic ultrasonography [EUS]); however, the correlation between morphologic changes and clinical symptoms is imperfect at best and etiology is not incorporated.[12,13] The TIGAR-O (Table 57.1) system considers major etiologic sources, but it does not offer clinical severity staging.[4,5,14,15] Others, like the Manchester and Heidelberg systems, classify patients based on discrete clinical features into three severity stages and were conceived as practical clinical tools. The Heidelberg classification in particular offers guidance on which clinical stages are most likely to require surgical intervention.[16]

Although each of these systems offers some clinical utility, each has its own shortcomings, and none facilitate complete classification of chronic pancreatitis heterogeneity. A combination of the previously mentioned clinical and etiologic classification systems may be necessary to facilitate clinical care and allow for use of common language when referring to chronic pancreatitis. In contrast to the previously mentioned classification/scoring systems, the M-ANNHEIM system (**M**ultiple risk factors: **A**lcohol, **N**icotine, **N**utrition, **H**ereditary, **E**fferent duct factors, **I**mmunological, **M**iscellaneous) is the most comprehensive classification at present, and includes severity scoring and diagnostic criteria in addition to a multifactorial risk factor classification. Although the detailed nature may not lend to easy clinical usage in some situations, it remains the most complete classification and clinical grading tool. As such, it will be used here as the basis of exploring the etiology of chronic pancreatitis.

ETIOLOGY OF CHRONIC PANCREATITIS (SEE CHAPTER 54)

It is likely that multiple genetic and environmental cofactors, as well as risk modifiers, interact to produce expression of the disease in a given individual, but fundamentally the development of pancreatitis depends on two main factors: host and environment (e.g., toxin).[17–22] Chronic pancreatitis will develop depending on the type, duration, and amount of toxin or infectious agent exposure and the patient's individual susceptibility and genetic makeup. This general concept explains why individuals respond differently to the same amounts of a toxin, such as alcohol, or why less amounts of the same toxin produce disease in a susceptible individual. Furthermore, the low prevalence of chronic pancreatitis among patients with alcoholism would seem to suggest other cofactors are important in many with diagnosed alcoholic pancreatitis. One of these cofactors is smoking.[5] In fact, the presence of multiple risk factors may be required for progression to fibrosis. The various etiologies of chronic pancreatitis based on the TIGAR-O and M-ANNHEIM systems provide a further advancement in the etiologic and mechanistic classification of chronic pancreatitis.[22–28] We present the etiology of chronic pancreatitis based on the TIGAR-O classification and include the M-ANNHEIM counterpart (in parentheses).

TABLE 57.1 TIGAR-O Classification System (Version 2) of Chronic Pancreatitis Etiologic Groups	
Toxic-metabolic	Alcohol
	Cigarette smoking
	Hypertriglyceridemia
	Hypercalcemia (Total calcium >12.0 mg/dL)
	Medications
	Metabolic (Diabetes mellitus or other)
	Chronic renal failure
Idiopathic	Early onset <35 years of age
	Later onset >35 years of age
Genetic	Suspected (genotypic not available)
	Autosomal dominant (PRSS1)
	Autosomal recessive (CFTR, SPINK1)
	Complex genetics
Autoimmune	IgG related (type I)
	IgG4 negative (type II)
Recurrent/severe acute pancreatitis	
Obstructive	Pancreas divisum
	Main pancreatic duct strictures
	Pancreatic duct scar
	Main duct pancreatic stones
	Widespread pancreatic calcifications
	Localized mass causing duct obstruction
	Ampullary stenosis

CFTR, Cystic fibrosis transmembrane regulator.

From Whitcomb DC. North American Pancreatitis Study Group. Pancreatitis: TIGAR-O Version 2 Risk/Etiology Checklist With Topic Reviews, Updates, and Use Primers. *Clin Transl Gastroenterol.* 2019;10(6):e00027.

Toxic and Metabolic (A, N = Alcohol and Nicotine in MANNHEIM)

Alcohol is the most common cause of chronic pancreatitis in most developed countries, and this association was first described by Comfort and colleagues (1946).[29] Notably, clinically apparent chronic pancreatitis develops in only 5% to 10% of patients with alcoholism, pointing to the multifactorial pathophysiology.[30–35] Although the cumulative toxin dose required for alcohol to cause chronic pancreatitis varies, 60% to 90% of patients will have 10 to 15 years of heavy alcohol consumption before development of clinical disease. The critical threshold of daily alcohol intake has been estimated to be approximately 40 g daily for women and 80 g daily for men (four to five drinks a day). The type of alcoholic beverage does not appear to be a modifying factor, but early age of alcoholism may result in shorter duration before onset of symptoms.[5,34,36,37] In the past it was believed that at the time of the initial attack, most patients with alcohol-induced chronic pancreatitis already had underlying fibrosis and calcifications of the pancreas, but the Zurich group has demonstrated that acute attacks preceded the development of chronic disease.[31,38] Of patients with chronic pancreatitis, those with alcohol-induced disease may be more likely to develop necrosis and pseudocysts (Fig. 57.1; see Chapter 58).

As only a minority of alcoholic individuals develop symptoms, cofactors in the evolution of clinical chronic pancreatitis have been investigated.[3] Several lines of evidence have shown that in addition to the direct effects of alcohol, various predisposing factors, such as genetics, smoking, intestinal infection, high-fat diet, compromised immune function, gallstones, gender, hormonal factors, and drinking patterns, may render the pancreas more susceptible to alcohol-induced tissue injury.[33,39–44] Many patients thought to have chronic pancreatitis as a result of alcohol abuse may indeed have a higher inherited susceptibility to alcohol-induced pancreatic damage, or genetic defects that cause pancreatitis independent of alcohol exposure.[25,45]

Tobacco smoke is a common cofactor in the development of alcoholic pancreatitis, and there is convincing evidence that smoking is independently associated with an increased risk for chronic pancreatitis, with an odds ratio (OR) as high as 17.3.[5,46] Smoking increases the risk of chronic pancreatitis in a dose-dependent manner, and the risk for chronic pancreatitis in individuals smoking less than 1 pack of cigarettes per day is 2.4, increasing to 3.3 in individuals who smoke more than 1 pack per day.[5] In smokers with alcoholic chronic pancreatitis, the course was accelerated and a major threshold effect is seen at 20 pack-years.[47] Just as abstinence from alcohol after an

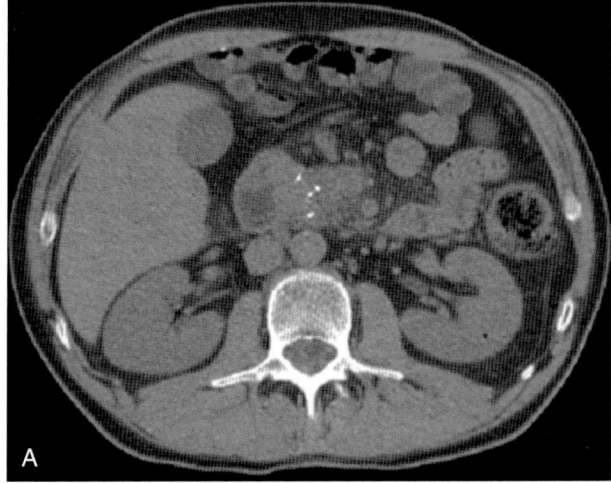
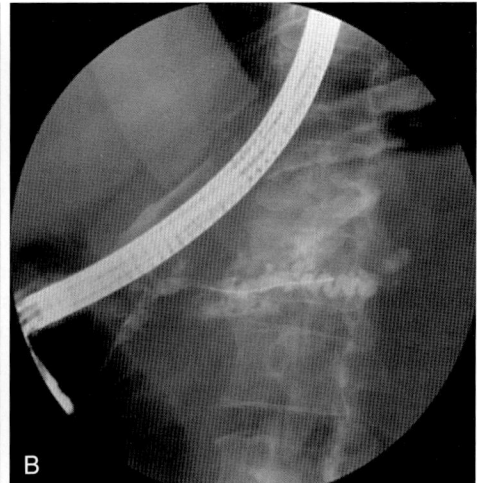

FIGURE 57.1 In patients with alcohol-induced pancreatitis, necrosis and pseudocyst formation are more common. **A,** Computed tomographic image shows a pseudocyst in the head of the pancreas and multiple calcifications. **B,** Endoscopic retrograde cholangiopancreatogram shows a tortuously dilated pancreatic duct with multiple irregular side branches (see Chapter 17).

episode of acute pancreatitis can significantly decrease the risk of progression to chronic pancreatitis, smoking cessation reduces the risk ratio estimate for chronic pancreatitis.[48,49] In a large cohort of US Veterans Administration (VA) patients, including almost one-half million individuals, Munigala and colleagues also found that smoking is an independent risk factor for acute pancreatitis and augmented the effect of alcohol on the risk, age of onset, and recurrence of pancreatitis.[42]

Tobacco induces oxidative stress and alters the secretion and composition of pancreatic juice, resulting in decreased juice and bicarbonate secretion and inflammation.[18,25,49,50] In a large study involving 146 patients with chronic pancreatitis, 52 patients with pancreatic cancer, and 235 healthy controls, the genomic DNA for expression of uridine 5′-diphosphate (UDP) glucuronosyltransferase (UGT1A7) genes was analyzed by Ockenga and colleagues (2003).[43] These proteins are vital biochemical factors for detoxification and cell defense. The incidence of this mutation was much more common in patients with chronic pancreatitis and tobacco abuse, but not in patients with nonalcoholic chronic pancreatitis. This study established the possible connection between genetic predisposition and external triggering factors. It is possible that smoking is the main factor of chronic pancreatitis in some patients, whereas in others smoking may increase the damage induced by alcohol, and in another group it might potentiate another yet unidentified factor or pathogen (see Chapter 9D).[50]

Calcium plays a central role in trypsinogen secretion and trypsin stabilization. Hypercalcemia as a result of primary or secondary hyperparathyroidism results in recurrent acute pancreatitis, which progresses to chronic pancreatitis, likely from trypsinogen activation, which in turn results in necrosis and fibrosis of the parenchyma.[51-53] Increased serum calcium concentration is also believed to induce direct damage to acinar cells, and increased secretion of calcium results in intraductal stone formation. It also appears that hypercalcemia modifies pancreatic secretion and leads to protein plug formation, in turn resulting in varying degrees of pancreatic fibrosis with calcifications.[52]

Nutritional Factors (N = Nutritional in M-ANNHEIM)

Evidence for the role of diets rich in fat and protein in the development of chronic pancreatitis come predominantly from animal studies, in which it has been found to induce pancreatic injury and alcohol induced damage.[54,55] There are limited data in humans that high-fat diets may result in more pain symptoms and earlier age of onset.[40,56] As will be discussed later in this chapter, the availability of excess substrate in the form of lipid and protein is thought to be an important catalyst for cytochrome P-450 activation and subsequent induction of oxidative stress. Additional support comes from the association between hyperlipidemia and recurrent acute pancreatitis, and in some cases, chronic pancreatitis.[15] In sum, however, the evidence for the causative effect of nutritional factors in the pathogenesis of chronic pancreatitis is limited mostly because of the challenges of retrospectively collecting accurate dietary data.[57]

Idiopathic (I = Idiopathic in M-ANNHEIM)

Based on the bimodal age of onset of the clinical symptoms, idiopathic pancreatitis is traditionally separated into two distinct entities. Early idiopathic chronic pancreatitis is seen during the first 2 decades of life, with abdominal pain the predominant clinical feature, whereas pancreatic calcifications and exocrine and endocrine pancreatic insufficiency are rare at the first diagnosis.[58] In contrast, the clinical presentation of late-onset idiopathic chronic pancreatitis typically occurs in patients during their fifth decade of life, and is marked by greater incidence of exocrine and endocrine pancreatic insufficiency and pancreatic calcifications rather than pain.[36,58] A more modern prospective study performed by Lewis and colleagues demonstrated that the median age for early-onset idiopathic pancreatitis was 20, whereas late-onset symptoms started at a median age of 58.[59] Both groups were predominantly women (62% and 81%, respectively, for early and late onset). As in earlier studies, pain was a more prominent feature in early-onset disease (96% vs. 69%), and exocrine insufficiency was more typical in the late-onset group (85%). Histologically, many cases of idiopathic chronic pancreatitis have T-lymphocyte infiltration, ductal obstruction, acinar atrophy, and fibrosis, raising the possibility of autoimmune etiology.

As the understanding of chronic pancreatitis matures and diagnostic tools become more sophisticated, the category of idiopathic pancreatitis will likely continue to shrink. Approximately 30% of patients with chronic pancreatitis have been labeled as having an idiopathic cause in the past, but in many cases risk factors ranging from underreported alcohol and tobacco abuse, undiscovered underlying genetic or hereditary abnormalities, or currently undiscovered factors are the actual stimulants of disease.[27,60] Mutations of the serine protease inhibitor Kazal type 1 (SPINK1 gene) have been described in up to 25% of patients with "idiopathic" chronic pancreatitis.[27,61] Other genetic alterations have been described in patients with idiopathic chronic pancreatitis. In a series published by Jalaly and colleagues, 47.8% of patients with acute recurrent or chronic idiopathic pancreatitis had variants in PRSS1, CFTR, SPINK1, or CTRC.[62] Similarly, nearly 50% of patients with early-onset idiopathic pancreatitis were found to have a mutation in cystic fibrosis transmembrane regulator (CFTR), chymotrypsin C (CTRC), or SPINK1 by Lewis and colleagues.[59] A strong association between CFTR mutations and idiopathic chronic pancreatitis has also been demonstrated.[20,63,64] In patients without evidence of cystic fibrosis, the frequency of CFTR mutations was six times that of patients without mutations. Subsequently, Cavestro and colleagues reported that one-third of all patients with idiopathic chronic pancreatitis have CFTR mutations.[19] Mutations in the SPINK1 gene are associated with familial patterns of idiopathic pancreatitis.

Until recently, tropical pancreatitis or nutritional pancreatitis was considered a form of idiopathic chronic pancreatitis and up to 60% to 70% of chronic pancreatitis in India and China have been labeled idiopathic.[65-67] Initial attempts to understand the disease implicated malnutrition and excess consumption of cyanogenic glycosides in cassava.[68] This conception of tropical pancreatitis has been the subject of significant debate, however, and several studies have confirmed that many of these patients have gene mutations that are associated with acute and chronic pancreatitis. Several studies have shown that variants in SPINK1, cathepsin B, CTRC, CFTR, and carboxypeptidase A1 predict the risk for tropical calcific pancreatitis.[67,69] Therefore many of these patients, once labeled as having idiopathic pancreatitis, would be more accurately categorized as genetic.

Genetic (H = Hereditary in M-ANNHEIM)

Several genetic variations have been associated with pancreatitis, including cationic trypsinogen (PRSS1), anionic trypsinogen

(PRSS2), *SPINK1*, *CTRC*, calcium-sensing receptor (*CASR*), and *CFTR*, all of which are closely linked with the trypsin pathway, either through early activation or failure to inhibit the activated enzyme.[5] Until recently, data on the genetic basis of chronic pancreatitis were scarce. Cystic fibrosis is the classic example of chronic pancreatic insufficiency and probably the best studied.[20,64] Many cases of chronic pancreatitis represent a variable part of the cystic fibrosis syndrome, which is caused by mutations in the gene coding for the CFTR. Several groups have reported an increased prevalence of *CFTR* mutations in patients with chronic pancreatitis of different etiologies. Later studies demonstrated that the mutations associated with cystic fibrosis (*CFTR* mutations) were also found with increased frequency in patients with chronic pancreatitis.[70] Interestingly, this mutation was also found to be more frequent in patients with chronic pancreatitis thought to be secondary to pancreas divisum.[71]

Other genetic variants predispose for chronic pancreatitis. Research has focused on the *SPINK1-N34S* gene mutation, which is also closely associated with tropical (50%), alcoholic (6%), or idiopathic (20%) chronic pancreatitis.[65,72] Dysregulated calcium homeostasis has been associated with development of pancreatitis, and mutations in the calcium ion channel gene TRPV6 have been associated with development of chronic pancreatitis.[73] As noted previously, emerging evidence supports an important role for genetic risk factors in tropical pancreatitis.[67] Therefore "classic" tropical pancreatitis may indeed be a form of hereditary pancreatitis related to SPINK1 mutations, similar to forms of chronic pancreatitis seen in Western countries.[67,69] The *SPINK1* pancreatic secretory trypsin inhibitory (*PSTI*) gene is responsible for the encoding of *SPINK1*.[65,69] *PSTI* has the main function of inhibiting activated trypsin. *SPINK1* is the major intrapancreatic "deactivator" of activated trypsinogen.[74] Trypsin has a central role in the digestion of dietary proteins and activation of other digestive enzymes. If the trypsin inhibitory protein malfunctions or cannot bind itself to trypsin, then trypsin is not properly deactivated or destroyed, and it remains active for a longer time. This is called a *gain of function* of trypsin.[25,61,74-77]

One of the major discoveries in chronic pancreatitis was the description of the point mutation in patients with autosomal dominant hereditary pancreatitis.[75] Several variants of *PRSS1* exist, all of which lead to a malfunction of trypsinogen.[71,74,76-80] Consequently, premature intracellular activation of trypsinogen within the pancreatic acinar cell leads to activation of other enzymes, which may ultimately result in autodigestion.[74] Genetic abnormalities have been described more frequently in hereditary pancreatitis, which typically present in a bimodal pattern of childhood and adulthood.[79] Associated with trypsinogen gene mutations, hereditary chronic pancreatitis is an autosomal dominant disease that carries an 80% penetrance.[81-83] It is characterized by recurrent episodes of acute pancreatitis or familial aggregation of chronic pancreatitis, but most patients with this genetic mutation are asymptomatic. The progression of chronic pancreatitis is faster in patients with *SPINK-N34S* mutation than in patients with *PRSS1* mutations.[82,84] Patients with hereditary pancreatitis have a more than 50-fold increased risk of pancreatic ductal cancer compared with the general population[82,85] (see Chapter 9D).

Autoimmune (I = Immunologic in M-ANNHEIM)

Autoimmune pancreatitis (AIP) is a rare but distinct form of chronic pancreatitis characterized by specific histopathologic, immunologic, and imaging features (Fig. 57.2)[86-89] (see Chapters 10, 54, 55, and 59). Its morphologic hallmarks are periductal infiltration by lymphocytes and plasma cells and granulocytic epithelial lesions, with consequent destruction of the duct epithelium and venulitis.[90] Based on etiology, serum markers, histology, and systemic involvement, AIP is classified into two distinct subtypes: type 1, related to immunoglobulin G4 (IgG4) (lymphoplasmacytic sclerosing pancreatitis), and type 2, related to a granulocytic epithelial lesion (idiopathic duct-centric chronic pancreatitis).[88]

The pathogenesis of AIP involves both a cellular (CD4$^+$ and CD8$^+$ T cells) and a humoral immune-mediated attack on the ductal cells that results in cytokine-mediated inflammation and

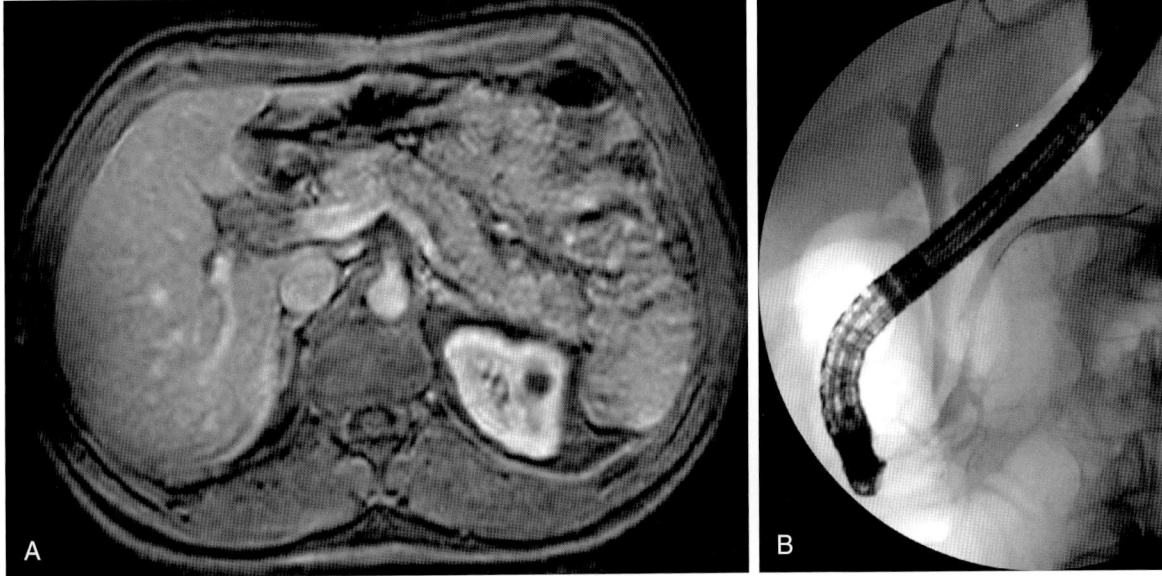

FIGURE 57.2 **Autoimmune pancreatitis is a rare but distinct form of chronic pancreatitis. A,** Magnetic resonance imaging may show a sausage-like and edematous pancreas that may mimic pancreatic cancer. **B,** The pancreatic duct may be dilated or may have stenosis and sacculations (see Chapters 17 and 54).

periductular fibrosis, with subsequent obstruction of the pancreatic ducts (see *primary duct hypothesis*).[91] Unlike type 2 AIP, type 1 AIP is characteristically associated with increasing levels of serum IgG4 and positive serum autoantibodies, abundant infiltration of IgG4-positive plasmacytes, frequent extrapancreatic lesions, and clinical recurrence.[88,92] AIP, especially type 1, is often associated with other autoimmune diseases, such as Sjögren's syndrome, primary sclerosing cholangitis (PSC), and inflammatory bowel disease.[87,89] Nevertheless, more than one-third of patients with AIP do not have other extrapancreatic autoimmune disorders. AIP is clinically characterized by minimal abdominal pain and diffuse enlargement of the pancreas without calcifications or pseudocysts, and it most frequently involves the head of the pancreas and the distal bile duct. On occasion, masses have been described as *inflammatory myofibroblastic tumors*.[86] The presentation and imaging findings of AIP sometimes resemble those of pancreatic malignancy, but the therapeutic approach differs significantly.[88]

On laboratory examination, patients may have hypergammaglobulinemia and autoantibodies, such as antinuclear and anti–smooth muscle antibodies.[93,94] Histopathologic examination of the pancreas reveals inflammatory infiltration of lymphocytes and plasma cells around the pancreatic duct, as well as fibrosis, in a pattern similar to PSC.[89,94] In 2002 the Japan Pancreas Society was the first in the world to propose diagnostic criteria for AIP, and a number of diagnostic criteria have been proposed since that time. The Unifying-Autoimmune-Pancreatitis-Criteria for diagnosis are listed in in Box 57.1.[95,96]

Obstructive (E = Efferent Duct Factors in M-ANNHEIM)

Pancreatic fusion or migration anomalies may result in anatomic variants that predispose patients to specific pancreatic or peripancreatic diseases, such as recurrent acute or chronic pancreatitis, cystic dystrophy of the duodenum, duodenal obstruction, cholangiocarcinoma, and gallbladder carcinoma[97] (see Chapters 46, 53, and 62). Obstruction of the main pancreatic duct is well known to result in chronic pancreatitis. The most common causes of pancreatic duct obstruction resulting in chronic pancreatitis include scars of the pancreatic duct, tumors of the ampulla of

Vater, mucinous duct ectasia, tumors of head of the pancreas, and trauma (Fig. 57.3). Other disorders, such as sphincter of Oddi dysfunction and pancreas divisum, have a more tenuous connection with recurrent acute and chronic pancreatitis (Fig. 57.4).

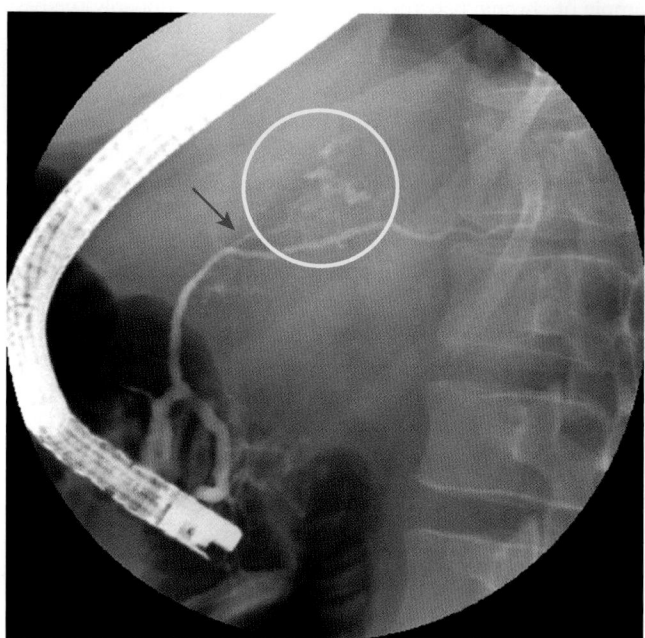

FIGURE 57.3 Tumors such as pancreatic head cancer causing pancreatic ductal obstruction of mucin-secreting tumors, such as main- or side-branch mucinous duct ectasia (MDE), can mimic chronic pancreatitis. Endoscopic retrograde cholangiopancreatogram shows a side-branch MDE. *Red arrow* points to the side branch; *yellow circle* shows the diseased tumorous segment.

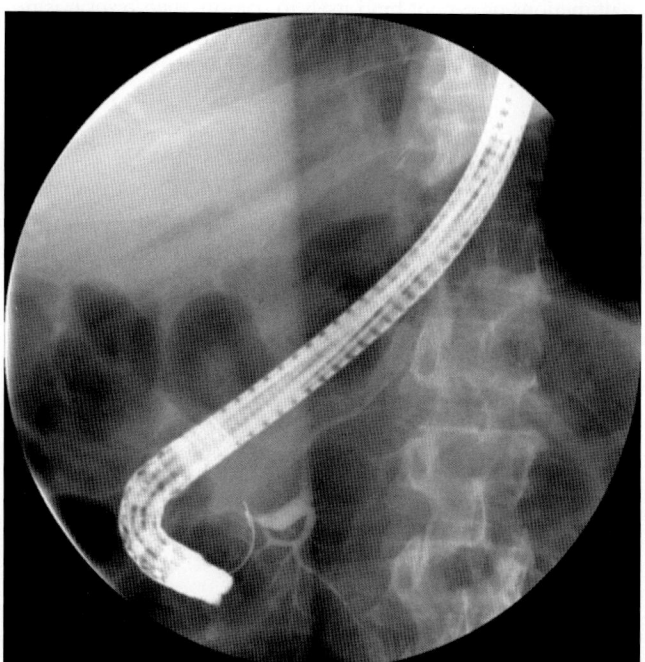

FIGURE 57.4 **Typical pancreatographic appearance of pancreas divisum.** Only the ventral duct can be filled with contrast. The entire dorsal duct empties into the minor papilla (not shown). A separate cannulation of the minor papilla is thus necessary to fill the dorsal duct with contrast (see Chapters 20 and 53).

BOX 57.1 Unifying-Autoimmune-Pancreatitis-Criteria

Diagnos is requires A in combination with B I, B II, or B III.
A. Negative workup for pancreatic cancer
B. Disease features:
  I. Typical histologic features
  II. Typical imaging findings **AND** elevated IgG4 **OR** ANA
  III. Response to steroids
  - With typical imaging
    OR
  - Idiopathic pancreatic disease with features of autoimmune disease
    AND at least one of the following:
  - Elevated IgG4
  - Other organ involvement
  - Elevated autoantibodies
  - Other autoimmune disease
  - Inflammatory bowel disease
  - IgG4 positive biopsy

ANA, Antinuclear antibodies; *IgG4*, immunoglobulin G4.
Adapted from Schneider A, Michaely H, Rückert F, et al. Diagnosing autoimmune pancreatitis with the Unifying-Autoimmune-Pancreatitis-Criteria. *Pancreatology*. 2017;17(3):381–394.

Obstruction of the main pancreatic duct produces changes of chronic pancreatitis within weeks in several animal models.[98,99] Main pancreatic duct obstruction leads to stagnation and stone formation of pancreatic juice (stone and duct obstruction theory) or acute recurrent pancreatitis and periductular fibrosis (necrosis-fibrosis theory). Histopathologic characteristics of human chronic pancreatitis as a result of obstruction include uniform distribution of interlobular and intralobular fibrosis and marked destruction of the exocrine parenchyma in the territory of obstruction, without significant protein plugs or calcifications.[100]

Miscellaneous (M = Miscellaneous in MANNHEIM)

The TIGAR-O system does not contain a letter for miscellaneous forms of chronic pancreatitis, such as primary hypercalcemia, hyperlipidemia, or hyperthyroidism. These etiologic factors are summarized under the second M of MANNHEIM.[4] In addition, tropical calcific pancreatitis is included here in the MANNHEIM classification, whereas it is considered "idiopathic" in the TIGAR-O classification. As previously mentioned, tropical pancreatitis is likely a genetic (hereditary) form of pancreatitis likely triggered by lack of micronutrients or toxins, including alcohol and tobacco.[69]

PATHOGENESIS

As discussed previously, it is well established that chronic pancreatitis is characterized by progressive, irreversible pancreatic inflammation and fibrosis, which can lead to exocrine and endocrine dysfunction.[5,101] The precise mechanism by which this progressive fibrosis develops, however, has been the subject of

some debate. A number of mechanisms have been postulated, and while they provide insight into the pathophysiology of certain etiologies, none in isolation gives a complete picture. Rather than viewing each of these hypotheses as competing models, it is more likely that varying etiologies of chronic pancreatitis progress through differing pathophysiologic mechanisms. Many causes of chronic pancreatitis may result from multiple pathways because of the complex interaction of the inciting trigger, underlying genetic predisposition, the immunologic process, oxidative and toxic-metabolic stress, changes in the consistency and flow of pancreatic juice, and fibrosis and ductal obstruction (Fig. 57.5). The principal theories are summarized in Box 57.2 and will be explored in more detail later.

Necrosis-Fibrosis Hypothesis

Originally proposed by Comfort and colleagues in 1946,[29] the necrosis-fibrosis hypothesis proposes that chronic pancreatitis results from recurrent acute pancreatitis, ultimately leading to necrosis and fibrosis.[102–104] More modern studies have found that acute pancreatitis can lead to development of chronic pancreatitis in up to 24% of cases, and that recurrent acute pancreatitis is the strongest predictor of future chronic pancreatitis.[105,106] Furthermore, a prospective study of subjects following an initial episode of pancreatitis revealed that higher frequency and severity of recurrent acute pancreatitis was associated with a more rapid progression to chronic pancreatitis.[107] Additional support for this model comes from hereditary pancreatitis, where mutation of cationic trypsinogen results in pancreatitis secondary to autodigestion. The majority of these patients go on to develop chronic pancreatitis, providing more support for the role of recurrent acute pancreatitis in the development in

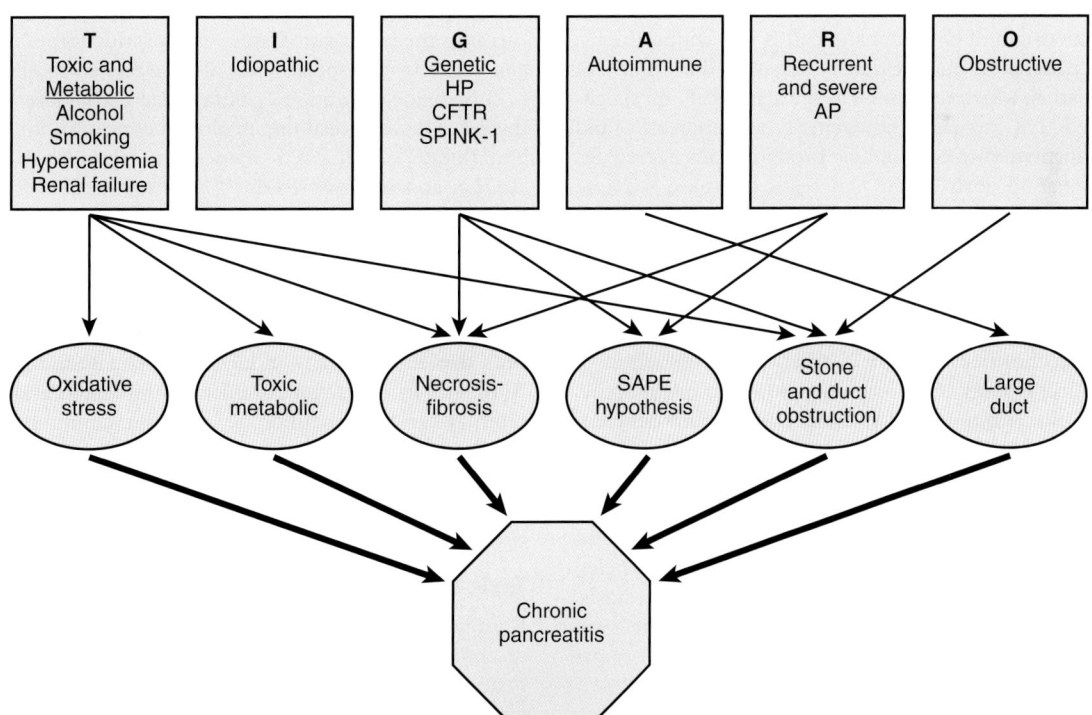

FIGURE 57.5 **Pathophysiologic mechanisms in the development of chronic pancreatitis may vary according to etiology.** Multiple overlapping pathophysiologic pathways may be involved with the development of chronic pancreatitis as seen here, organized by TIGAR-O classification.[25] (Reproduced from Stevens T, Conwell DL, Zuccaro G. Pathogenesis of chronic pancreatitis: an evidence-based review of past theories and recent developments. *Am J Gastroenterol.* 2004;99[11]:2256–2270.)

BOX 57.2 Proposed Mechanisms of Chronic Pancreatitis

Proposed pathophysiologic mechanisms of chronic pancreatitis
Necrosis-fibrosis hypothesis
Protein-plug (stone/ductal obstruction) hypothesis
Oxidative stress theory
Toxic-metabolic theory
Primary duct hypothesis
Sentinel acute pancreatitis event hypothesis
Sustained intraacinar NF-κB activation

---

chronic pancreatitis.[77,108] Acute pancreatitis results in ongoing inflammatory tissue that is ultimately replaced by periductal and parenchymal fibrosis. This fibrosis then impairs flow of pancreatic juice, and calcifications form as a result of precipitated proteins.[109] A cycle of further stasis, plugging, and stone formation leads to progression of fibrosis and, ultimately, atrophy of the gland.[104] Although clinical recurrent acute pancreatitis leading to chronic pancreatitis is the classic scenario in the necrosis-fibrosis pathway, some patients will present with pancreatic calcifications without a history of acute pancreatitis. In this setting, subclinical acinar injury and fibrosis may lead to the development of chronic pancreatitis. In the necrosis-fibrosis hypothesis, chronic pancreatitis is felt to originate from parenchymal and periductal fibrosis.[110,111]

Protein-Plug (Stone/Ductal Obstruction) Hypothesis

Whereas the necrosis-fibrosis hypothesis suggests chronic pancreatitis results from recurrent acute pancreatitis, Henri Sarles proposed alternate mechanisms for acute and chronic pancreatitis: acute pancreatitis results from parenchymal autodigestion and fibrosis, whereas chronic pancreatitis results from plugging of the pancreatic duct.[9,112] These investigators proposed that the origin of chronic pancreatitis was within the lumen of the pancreatic ductules, in contrast to the origins of acute pancreatitis, which tend to be in the acinar cell. Investigators proposed that increased lithogenicity of pancreatic fluid leads to the formation of eosinophilic proteinaceous aggregates that precipitate and obstruct the pancreatic ductules.[113] These plugs then become rich in calcium and precipitate in the ductules because of deficiency of lithostatin ("lithostathine") or pancreatic stone protein (PSP); this protein is synthesized in the acinar cell and is an important factor in avoiding calcification within the ductules.[9,113–116] Indeed, several studies have proved that alcohol decreases the formation and secretion of pancreatic juice, making it more viscous; lower in bicarbonate; richer in protein, enzymes, and calcium crystals; and deficient in PSP or lithostatin.[35,100] Alcohol has also been shown to mediate the release of gastrointestinal hormones by increasing cholecystokinin (CCK)-releasing factor, which in turn affects pancreatic juice formation and flow. The pancreatic stones and plugs are believed to produce ulceration of the ductal epithelial cells, which results in inflammation, fibrosis, obstruction, stasis, and further stone formation. Parenchymal damage in the form of inflammation and fibrosis then follows and is usually worst proximal to the obstruction.[98]

Another protein believed to induce pancreatic plug formation is glycoprotein 2 (GP-2), a major component of the zymogen granule cell membranes.[117] The chain of events of decreased flow, decreased lithostatin production, plug formation, calcification, stone precipitation, ductal ulceration, parenchymal and

periductular inflammation, stenosis, and stasis repeats itself in a constant vicious cycle.[113,118] Although pancreatic stones and plugs are found in late stages of pancreatitis, it has not known whether their formation represents a primary or initiating event in chronic pancreatitis.

A two-hit hypothesis has been postulated as a means to reconcile the necrosis-fibrosis and protein plug hypotheses: (1) early formation of protein plugs and (2) postnecrotic fibrosis from acute pancreatitis resulting in ductal obstruction.[25]

Oxidative Stress Theory

Oxidative stress leading to the generation of free radicals and ultimately ending in parenchymal fibrosis was initially postulated by Braganza.[119] He proposed that by-products of overactive hepatic mixed-function oxidases lead to oxidative damage, and that this was the lead event in the development of chronic pancreatitis. This oxidase overactivity may be triggered by high levels of dietary lipids or proteins that act as a substrate for cytochrome P-450, or triggers like alcohol, cigarette smoke, or other xenobiotics that increase stimulation of cytochrome P-450.[120–122] The hepatic mixed-function oxidases are part of the hepatic detoxification system, and as a consequence of the metabolization process, several by-products such as toxic epoxides, free radicals, and lipid peroxidation products are produced.[123] These are then released into the systemic circulation and reach the pancreatic parenchyma, or they are secreted into the bile and end up refluxing into the pancreatic duct, where they induce inflammatory damage of the acinar and ductular cell. As in the necrosis-fibrosis pathway, the acinar cell is the central area of initial injury in the oxidative stress theory, with "pancreastasis" leading to lysosomal fragility and exocytosis of pancreatic enzymes. Pancreatitis is triggered through interference of the methionine-glutathione transulfuration pathway, resulting in depletion of glutathione, and diversion of free radicals into the pancreatic tissue. Overproduction of reactive oxygen and nitrogen species may also be related to altered activity in superoxide dismutase 1, glutathione peroxidase 1, and glutathione reductase, resulting in altered concentrations of reduced glutathione, conjugated dienes in low-density lipoprotein (LDL), and oxidized LDL.[124] This subsequently leads to inflammation and fibrosis of the ductules and resultant low flow of pancreatic juice, inhibition of lithostatin, and precipitation of proteins and calcium.[120,123,125] Furthermore, alcohol may also contribute to oxidative stress as a result of the depletion of scavengers such as selenium, vitamins E and C, and riboflavin; such depletion helps to induce or propagate the damage.[126–128] With this in mind, micronutrient supplementation with selenium, β-carotene, methionine, and other compounds have been suggested as a method to buttress tissue methyl and thiol groups. There is some data that suggest this may decrease recurrent attacks and control baseline pain in patients with chronic pancreatitis, irrespective of etiology.[120,129–131]

Toxic-Metabolic Theory

Bordalo and colleagues proposed the toxic-metabolic hypothesis of chronic pancreatitis.[132] They described how alcohol and its toxic metabolites cause accumulation of intracellular lipids and fatty acid ethyl esters, which damage the acinar cell. The alterations of intracellular lipid metabolism then lead to fatty degeneration, apoptosis, and scarring of the pancreatic parenchyma with impairment of the pancreatic microcirculation. In a landmark study, biopsies from 42 patients with chronic alcoholism with and without established chronic pancreatitis were evaluated by histology and electron microscopy.[132] Even though many of these patients did not have chronic pancreatitis, many changes were found to be caused by cellular damage, such as cytoplasmic fat droplets of the acinar cells, decreased zymogen granules, and increased mitochondrial size.

Several studies in animals and human pancreatic tissue have demonstrated that the toxic or metabolic insult to pancreatic pericytes plays an important role in the pathogenesis of pancreatic fibrosis similar to Ito cells in the liver.[133–136] These fat cells exist in the human pancreas and can migrate into the periacinar spaces, and they are activated by alcohol and acetaldehyde, transforming into scar-producing cells.[137–139] As demonstrated in immunohistochemical analysis of pancreatic tissue, a clear correlation exists between the expression of activated Kupffer cells and the degree of fibrosis. These cells have been shown to deposit collagen very early in the process of chronic pancreatitis.[140] Therefore an analogy to cirrhosis of the liver can be made regarding macronodular and micronodular fibrosis in chronic pancreatitis.

Primary Duct Hypothesis

Cavallini from Italy proposed that chronic pancreatitis represents a primary autoimmune or inflammatory condition beginning in the pancreatic duct.[141] The primary pathogenic factor leading to chronic pancreatitis is an outflow obstruction, likely the result of duct inflammation, destruction, and fibrosis, probably caused by an immunologic attack to a specific genetic, structural, or acquired antigen of the periductular epithelium. The target of this attack may be some specific genetic or acquired antigen on the duct epithelium. Cavallini proposed that the immune-type mechanism may occur through two channels: one results from aberrant expression of major histocompatibility antigens by the ductal epithelium, and the other results from infiltration of activated lymphocytes that produce a periductular cytotoxic response. Several reports have shown a defect of ductal epithelial aberrant expression, which leads to periductular lymphocyte infiltration.[93,133,142] Therefore it appears that chronic pancreatitis is an autoimmune or "duct-destroying" disease, analogous to PSC. This is supported by several observations: the radiologic and histologic similarity of chronic pancreatitis and PSC, the activation of cytotoxic T lymphocytes in the periductular areas of the pancreas in patients with alcoholic chronic pancreatitis, and the occasional association of chronic pancreatitis with PSC.[87,89,143]

Sentinel Acute Pancreatitis Event Hypothesis

Introduced by Whitcomb, the sentinel acute pancreatitis event (SAPE) hypothesis is fascinating because it incorporates much of the knowledge about the molecular and cellular mechanisms of chronic pancreatitis pathogenesis.[144] SAPE is an effort to link previous hypotheses and provide a "final common pathway" for the many etiologies of pancreatitis. According to Whitcomb, a SAPE is essential to initiate the inflammatory and immunologic process of chronic pancreatitis. In addition, it is necessary for multiple risk factors or insults, such as agents, toxins, and infections, to propagate chronic pancreatitis through membrane and mitochondrial injury as well as through the release of inflammatory cytokines. Susceptibility is essential, either genetic or through some other mechanism, such as ongoing injury (i.e., alcohol toxicity). The critical sentinel event then appears, triggers

the process, and causes acute pancreatitis and chronic pancreatitis. Further activation of the immunologic system and the stellate cells propagates chronic pancreatitis, and the end result is fibrosis and calcification.[144] Most studies demonstrate that an acute attack of pancreatitis tends to be self-limited; other studies have also shown that the continued oxidative stress cannot cause pancreatitis under normal conditions. The disease does not develop spontaneously even in patients with genetic mutations (susceptibility) known to be associated with chronic pancreatitis. Nevertheless, this hypothesis has the merits of placing several of the previous theories under one umbrella.

Sustained Intraacinar Nuclear Factor-κB Activation

Common denominators to most theories are the inflammatory response and activation of intracellular trypsinogen. However, recent advances have challenged the trypsin-centered understanding of pancreatitis etiology, as demonstrated by genetic models lacking trypsinogen activation. These models have shown that nuclear factor (NF)-κB activation occurs very early in the process of pancreatitis, independent of trypsinogen activation. Sustained activation of inflammatory pathways in pancreatic acinar cells may result in chronic pancreatitis. Persistence of the stimulus, which may be any of the recognized etiologic factors (e.g., alcohol, nicotine, hereditary, efferent duct effect) may drive the sustained intraacinar activation of the inflammation pathways in chronic pancreatitis. This novel paradigm does not require the activation of trypsinogen, a necrosis-fibrosis sequence, acute-to-chronic pancreatitis progression, or SAPE.[145–147]

DIAGNOSIS OF CHRONIC PANCREATITIS

As noted previously, a new mechanistic definition was proposed to define chronic pancreatitis as "a pathologic fibro-inflammatory syndrome of the pancreas in individuals with genetic, environmental and/or other risk factors who develop persistent pathologic responses to parenchymal injury or stress," and is marked by features such as "pancreatic atrophy, fibrosis, pain syndromes, duct distortion and strictures, calcifications, pancreatic exocrine dysfunction, pancreatic endocrine dysfunction, and dysplasia"[7] (see Chapter 54). Part of the impetus behind the development of this new diagnosis was to shift emphasis away from end-stage changes and facilitate earlier diagnosis. This definition includes histologic, mechanistic, gross morphologic, and physiologic elements. As such, securing the diagnosis of chronic pancreatitis may involve multiple interventional, imaging, and clinical tools. Using a multimodal approach is particularly important early in the disease, when diagnosis can prove elusive.[7,148]

Chronic pancreatitis is a dynamic disease, and morphologic and functional changes to the pancreas vary depending on which stage it is in. The disease has previously been classified in three distinct stages (Table 57.2).[31,107,149,150] The M-ANNHEIM clinical staging expands on previous staging systems and broadly divides chronic pancreatitis into symptomatic and asymptomatic phases (Box 57.3).[57] The symptomatic phase is further categorized into stages I–IV. Stage I is characterized by abdominal pain without pancreatic insufficiency. Stage II is determined by the presence of partial pancreatic insufficiency, either exocrine or endocrine insufficiency, but not both. This stage may be marked by pain or may be independent of abdominal pain. Stage III is characterized by pain in the presence

TABLE 57.2 Stages of Chronic Pancreatitis: Typical Clinical and Morphologic Pictures, Pancreatic Function, and Recommended Diagnostic Procedures

STAGE	CLINICAL PICTURE PAIN	CLINICAL PICTURE COMPLICATIONS	MORPHOLOGY	PANCREATIC FUNCTION	DIAGNOSTICS
A: Early	Recurrent acute attacks	No complications	Morphologic changes detectable with imaging procedures directed to pancreatic parenchyma and ductal system	Normal pancreatic endocrine and exocrine function	EUS, ERP/MRP, CT, secretin
B: Moderate	Increasing number of attacks and increased intensity	Pseudocysts, cholestasis, segmental portal hypertension	Progredient morphologic changes detectable in several imaging procedures	Impairment of pancreatic function in several degrees, but rarely steatorrhea	Transabdominal ultrasound, ERP/MRP, EUS, CT, fasting blood glucose, oral glucose tolerance test
C: Advanced	Decreasing pain ("burnout" of the pancreas)	Pseudocysts, cholestasis, segmental portal hypertension	Calculi	Marked impairment of pancreatic function, more often steatorrhea than in other stages; diabetes mellitus	Transabdominal ultrasound, ERP/MRP, CT, FE-1, fasting blood glucose, oral glucose tolerance test

CT, Computed tomography; *ERP,* endoscopic retrograde pancreatography; *EUS,* endoscopic ultrasound; *FE-1,* fecal elastase 1; *MRP,* magnetic resonance pancreatography.

BOX 57.3 M-ANNHEIM Clinical Staging of Chronic Pancreatitis

Asymptomatic Chronic Pancreatitis
Stage 0: Subclinical chronic pancreatitis
A. Period without symptoms (determination by chance, e.g., autopsy)
B. Acute pancreatitis: single episode (possible onset of chronic pancreatitis)
C. Acute pancreatitis with severe complications

Symptomatic Chronic Pancreatitis
Stage I: Chronic pancreatitis without pancreatic insufficiency
A. (Recurrent) acute pancreatitis (no pain between episodes of acute pancreatitis)
B. Recurrent or chronic abdominal pain (including pain between episodes of acute pancreatitis)
C. A/B with severe complications[a]

Stage II: Partial pancreatic insufficiency
A. Isolated exocrine (or endocrine) pancreatic insufficiency (without pain)
B. Isolated exocrine (or endocrine) pancreatic insufficiency (with pain)
C. II A/B with severe complications[a]
Stage III: Pain plus complete pancreatic insufficiency
A. Exocrine and endocrine insufficiency (with pain, e.g., requiring pain medication)
B. IIIA with severe complications[a]
Stage IV: Painless disease (burnout phase)
A. Exocrine and endocrine insufficiency without pain and without severe complications[a]
B. Exocrine and endocrine insufficiency without pain and with severe complications[a]

[a]Severe complications are defined as severe organ complications not included in the Cambridge classification. Reversible severe complications include development of ascites, bleeding, pseudoaneurysm, obstruction or stricture of the ductus choledochus, pancreatic fistula, and duodenal stenosis. Irreversible severe complications are portal or splenic vein thrombosis with or without portal hypertension and pancreatic cancer.
Adapted from Schneider A, Löhr JM, Singer MV. The M-ANNHEIM classification of chronic pancreatitis: introduction of a unifying classification system based on a review of previous classifications of the disease. *J Gastroenterol.* 2007;42(2):101–119.

of both exocrine and endocrine insufficiency. Finally, stage IV corresponds with the "burnout" stage, as abdominal pain subsides. Although permanent and complete dissolution of pain can occur after a period of at least 10 years, this does not reliably occur or may be marked by intermittent/incomplete decrease in pain.[57,151,152]

Any evaluation for chronic pancreatitis begins, of course, with a detailed history and physical. In the history, attention should be paid to risk factors, particularly alcohol, as it is the most common etiology of chronic pancreatitis. Abdominal pain is the most common initial symptom, but it may be absent in as many as 15% of patients with alcohol-related chronic pancreatitis and in as many as 23% of patients with nonalcoholic chronic pancreatitis.[148] Abdominal pain is usually located in the epigastrium and radiates to the back. Although abdominal pain may correlate closely with morphologic changes, development of pain does not rely solely on pancreatic ductal hypertension and is best understood as a multimodal event including parenchymal

inflammation leading to neuronal plasticity and increased nociceptor expression (Box 57.4).[153–156] Steatorrhea typically occurs later in the disease course because 90% of exocrine function must be lost before steatorrhea develops. Symptoms of exocrine insufficiency including bloating, abdominal pain, or a change in bowel habits may occur when 60% to 90% of pancreatic function is lost and can precede steatorrhea (Box 57.5). Early in the course, no correlation is seen between morphologic changes and pancreatic function.[31,107] Weight loss is caused by two factors: at first, patients fear eating because of the accompanying pain, whereas later in the disease process, weight loss results from malabsorption related to pancreatic insufficiency.[24,148]

A systematic approach to identifying the etiologic origin of nonalcoholic pancreatitis is required, and forgoing a meticulous history and laboratory workup may lead to patients incorrectly being labeled as idiopathic. In all patients without any obvious identifiable cause, attention on imaging to the characteristic "sausage-like appearance" and testing of IgG4 levels should be

---

BOX 57.4   Causes of Pain in Chronic Pancreatitis

Primary pancreatic pain:
- Duct obstruction and tissue hypertension
- Active inflammation
- Tissue ischemia
- Altered nociception

Secondary pancreatic pain:
- Local complications: pseudocysts, inflammatory mass, biliary and bowel strictures
- Remote complications: peptic ulcer due to changes in blood flow, bacterial overgrowth, diabetes mellitus type 3c-related visceral neuropathy

Treatment related pain:
- Procedural complications
- Adverse medication reaction (e.g., hyperalgesia or bowel dysfunction from opioid use)

Adapted from Kleeff J, Whitcomb DC, Shimosegawa T, et al. Chronic pancreatitis. *Nat Rev Dis Primers*. 2017;3:17060.

BOX 57.5   M-ANNHEIM Diagnostic Criteria for Chronic Pancreatitis

Probable chronic pancreatitis (one or more of the following):
- Mild ductal alterations (as per Cambridge classification (see Table 57.4)
- Recurrent/persistent pseudocyst
- Exocrine insufficiency as diagnosed by testing (e.g., fecal elastase-1 test, secretin test)
- Endocrine insufficiency

Borderline chronic pancreatitis:
- Typical history of chronic pancreatitis but without additional criteria in probable or definite categories *or*
- First episode of acute pancreatitis in the presence of family history of pancreatitis *or* presence of M-ANNHEIM risk factors.

Chronic pancreatitis associated with alcohol consumption (requires the above mentioned criteria plus one of the following):
- History of excessive alcohol consumption (>80 g/day for multiple years)
- History of increased alcohol consumption (20-80 g/day for multiple years)
- History of moderate alcohol consumption (<20 g/day for multiple years)

Note: Diagnosis requires a typical history for chronic pancreatitis and certainty of diagnosis is defined by the above criteria.
Modified from Schneider A, Löhr JM, Singer MV. The M-ANNHEIM classification of chronic pancreatitis: introduction of a unifying classification system based on a review of previous classifications of the disease. *J Gastroenterol*. 2007;42(2):101–119.

---

performed to rule out AIP (see Chapters 54 and 55). In younger patients, particularly pediatric populations and adults under the age of 20, hereditary pancreatitis should be considered even in the absence of family history, and evaluation for PRSS1, CFTR, SPINK1, or other mutations may be informative.[152,157]

Histologic diagnosis, with typical findings of fibrosis and atrophy of the acinar tissue, is the most accurate method of confirming chronic pancreatitis. Because endoscopic ultrasound–guided fine-needle aspiration does not give significant architectural detail and surgical biopsy of the gland is needlessly invasive, histology is rarely used as an initial tool in diagnosing chronic pancreatitis. Therefore imaging modalities are the primary tools of chronic pancreatitis diagnosis, with functional testing of the pancreas playing a more limited role reserved for cases in which standard imaging techniques are not informative; evaluation should generally progress from least invasive to more invasive approaches. The M-ANNHEIM imaging criteria are summarized in Table 57.3.

Imaging Methods

Noninvasive imaging methods are preferred for diagnosing chronic pancreatitis in most patients.[5,148,158] Sensitivity and specificity of different imaging methods vary significantly, depending on the imaging modality used, the stage of the disease, and the experience of the investigator. In general, EUS, magnetic resonance imaging (MRI), and CT are the best imaging methods for establishing a diagnosis of chronic pancreatitis, whereas abdominal ultrasound is the least accurate imaging technique for chronic pancreatitis[157] (see Chapters 17 and 22). Endoscopic retrograde cholangiopancreatography (ERCP) was previously viewed as the standard for pancreatic duct imaging, but because of its invasiveness it has been largely replaced by EUS and magnetic resonance cholangiopancreatography (MRCP; see Chapters 20, 22, and 30). The role of ERCP is now predominantly reserved for therapeutic interventions in chronic pancreatitis.

Transabdominal Ultrasonography (see Chapter 17)

Because it is an inexpensive, noninvasive, and readily available imaging tool, transabdominal ultrasonography is frequently the first imaging method utilized in patients with abdominal complaints. It can be useful in detecting gallstones and investigating biliary origins of pain that may be in the differential diagnosis. With respect to evaluation of the pancreas, a major disadvantage of ultrasound is the difficult examination based on poor

---

TABLE 57.3   M-ANNHEIM Imaging Criteria for Ultrasound, Computed Tomography, Magnetic Resonance Imaging, and Endoscopic Ultrasonography Based on Imaging Features Defined in the Cambridge Criteria

CAMBRIDGE GRADING	CT/MRI/ULTRASOUND[a]	EUS[b]
Normal	Evaluates entire gland without abnormal findings (0 points)	
Equivocal	One abnormal feature (1 point)	Four or fewer abnormal features
Mild	Two or more abnormal features, but normal MPD (2 points)	
Moderate	Two or more abnormal features, including enlargement of MPD between 2 and 4 mm or increased duct wall echogenicity (3 points)	Five or more abnormal features (3 points)
Marked	As above with one or more marked changes (4 points)	

[a]See Table 57.4 for abnormal features.
[b]See Table 57.4 and Box 57.6 for EUS abnormal features.
CT, Computed tomography; *EUS,* endoscopic ultrasonography; *MPD,* main pancreatic duct; *MRI,* magnetic resonance imaging.

Adapted from Schneider A, Löhr JM, Singer MV. The M-ANNHEIM classification of chronic pancreatitis: introduction of a unifying classification system based on a review of previous classifications of the disease. *J Gastroenterol*. 2007;42(2):101–119.

TABLE 57.4 Cambridge Criteria of Chronic Pancreatitis

STAGE	TYPICAL CHANGES
Normal	Normal appearance of side branches and main pancreatic duct
Equivocal	Dilation or obstruction of less than three side branches; normal main pancreatic duct
Mild	Dilation or obstruction of more than three side branches; normal main pancreatic duct
Moderate	Additional stenosis and dilation of main pancreatic duct
Severe	Additional obstructions, cysts, and stenosis of main pancreatic duct; calculi

From Axon AT, et al. Pancreatography in chronic pancreatitis: international definitions. *Gut.* 1984; 25:1107–1112.

BOX 57.6 Endoscopic Ultrasound Criteria for the Diagnosis of Chronic Pancreatitis

Parenchymal features:
- Gland size
- Cysts
- Echo-poor lesions
- Echo-ich lesions (>3 mm)
- Accentuation of lobular patterns (e.g., echo-poor areas surrounded by hyperechoic strands)

Ductal features:
- Increased duct wall echogenicity
- Irregularity of main pancreatic duct
- Dilation of the main pancreatic duct
- Dilated side branches
- Calcification

Adapted from Schneider A, Löhr JM, Singer MV. The M-ANNHEIM classification of chronic pancreatitis: introduction of a unifying classification system based on a review of previous classifications of the disease. *J Gastroenterol.* 2007;42(2):101–119.

TABLE 57.5 Sensitivity and Specificity of Imaging Methods for Chronic Pancreatitis

IMAGING METHOD	SENSITIVITY (%)	SPECIFICITY (%)
Transabdominal ultrasound	48–96	75–90
Computed tomography	56–95	85–100
Endoscopic retrograde pancreatography	68–100	89–100
Endoscopic ultrasound	85–100	85–100

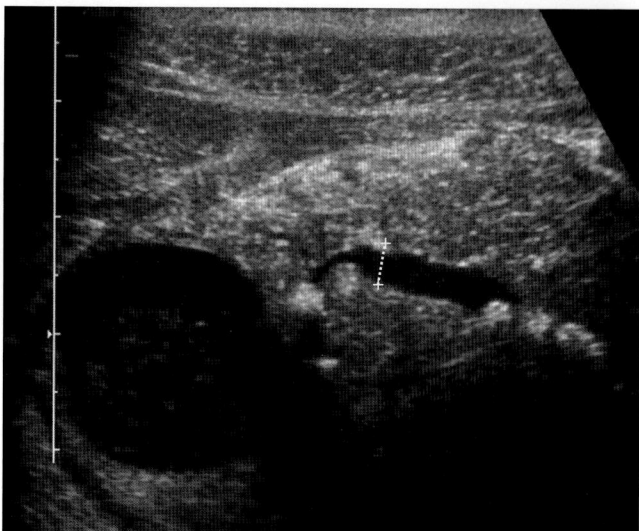

FIGURE 57.6 **Transabdominal ultrasound showing typical changes of chronic pancreatitis.** Note the multiple intrapancreatic calcifications and the dilated pancreatic duct. A large pseudocyst is also present in the region of the head of the pancreas.

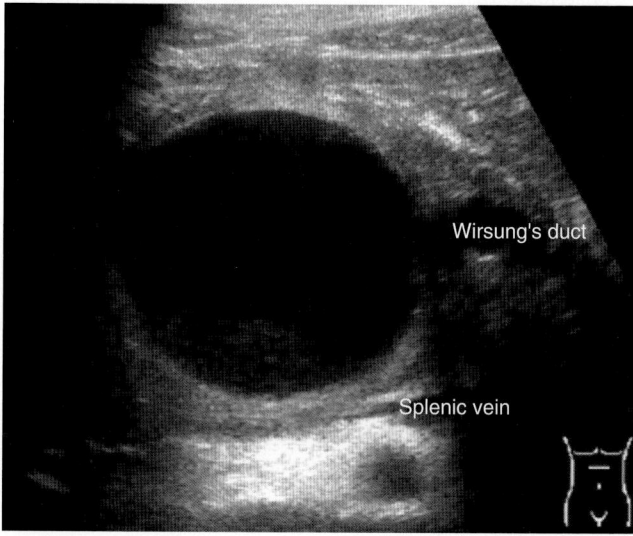

Wirsung's duct

Splenic vein

FIGURE 57.7 Ultrasound image showing a large, solitary pancreatic pseudocyst complicating chronic pancreatitis.

visualization of the pancreas, mainly because of overlying gas-filled bowel loops, obesity, and technical and operator-dependent factors. Given this, the sensitivity of ultrasound to detect chronic pancreatitis is as low as 48%, but with advancing stages of chronic pancreatitis this can increase to 96% and the specificity is described between 75% and 90% (Table 57.5 and Fig. 57.6). It is useful for the detection of calcifications and pseudocysts (see Fig. 57.6; Figs. 57.7 and 57.8).[5] If ultrasound detects changes of chronic pancreatitis, diagnosis is certain (high specificity), but if the pancreas is not completely visualized or appears normal, further examinations are necessary (low sensitivity). Diagnostic criteria for chronic pancreatitis by transabdominal ultrasound are (1) irregular contour (lobulation), (2) pancreatic duct dilation and irregularity of the main pancreatic duct, (3) loss or reduction of pancreatic parenchyma echogenicity (echo-poor or echo-rich areas), (4) cysts or cavities, and (5) pancreatic calcifications.[159,160]

Computed Tomography (see Chapter 17)

International consensus guidelines for cross-sectional diagnosis in chronic pancreatitis were published in 2018 and recommended that

CT is the best initial imaging modality for the evaluation of patients with suspected chronic pancreatitis, because it is widely available and can depict most changes in pancreatic morphology (parenchymal atrophy, parenchymal or ductal calcifications, ductal changes and complications). CT is also useful to detect incidental lesions and pathology of the pancreas, e.g. malignancy or autoimmune etiology.[161]

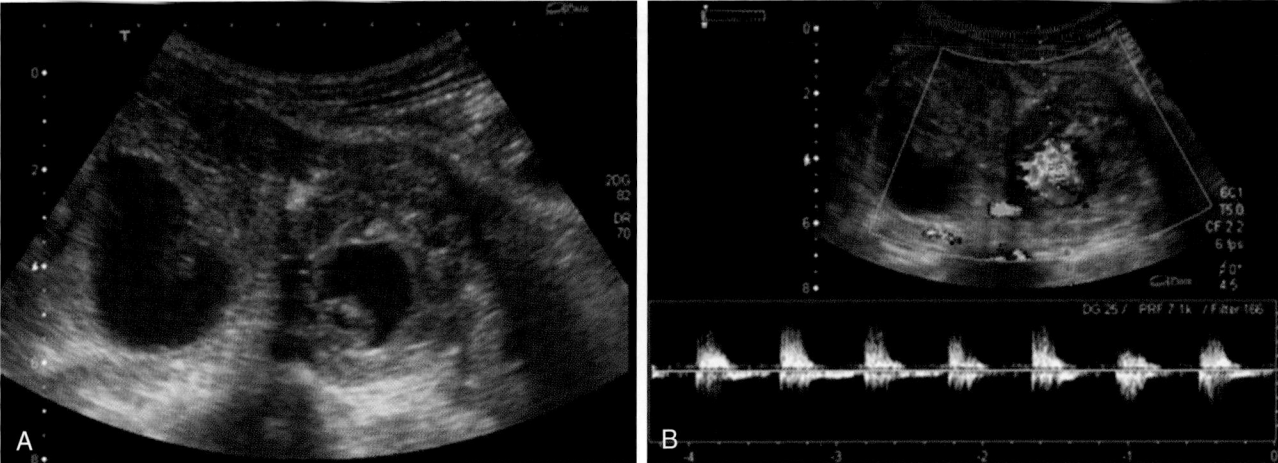

FIGURE 57.8 **A,** Ultrasound image of a cyst-like structure in the pancreas in a 56-year-old woman with chronic pancreatitis and sudden anemia without evidence of overt gastrointestinal blood loss. **B,** Doppler flow studies demonstrating blood flow inside a pseudocyst-like structure. This study confirmed the presence of a pseudoaneurysm with bleeding. Patient underwent percutaneous angiographic therapy with release of an endocoil, which completely obliterated blood flow to the aneurysm, therefore preventing its catastrophic rupture. This pseudoaneurysm is one of the most dreaded and potentially fatal complications of chronic pancreatitis (see Chapters 21, 115 and 116).

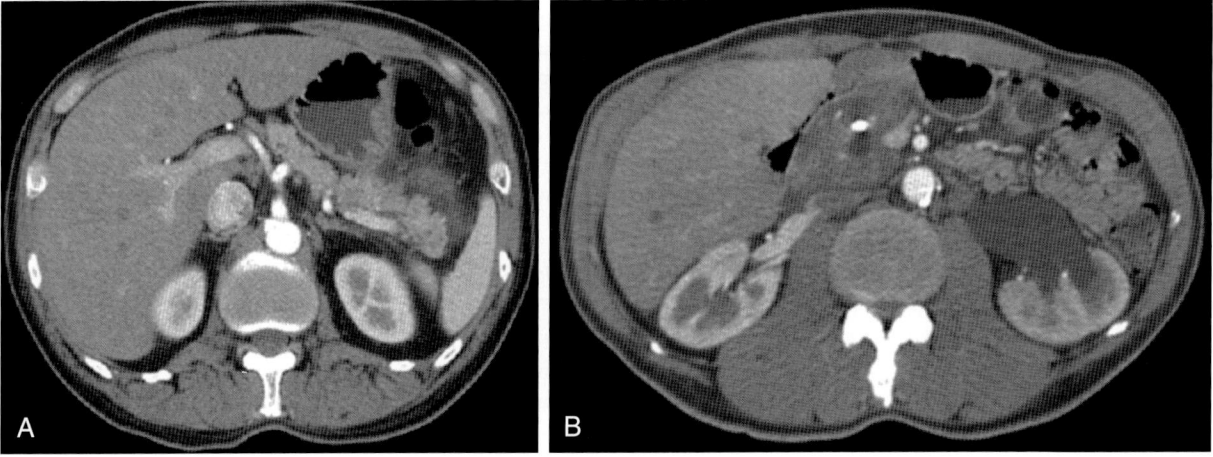

FIGURE 57.9 **Computed tomography of the abdomen. A,** Pancreatic atrophy. **B,** Calcifications. The patient with calcifications **(B)** also had partial outlet gastric obstruction caused by inflammatory enlargement of the head of the pancreas (see Chapter 17).

CT has become one of the most widely employed imaging modalities in the evaluation of chronic pancreatitis. The CT findings of chronic pancreatitis include main pancreatic duct and secondary duct dilation, intraductal calcifications, gland atrophy, and cystic lesions (Figs. 57.9 and 57.10).[5,162] Other significant findings include heterogeneous density of the pancreatic gland with atrophy or enlargement. The inability of CT to detect early parenchymal changes or changes in small pancreatic ducts limits its utility in very early disease, but advanced stages and complications of the disease can be evaluated with high reliability. CT is the most sensitive method to detect calculi, and although it may be technically best evaluated during the noncontrast phase, CT with contrast still allows for adequate detection of parenchymal calcifications.

On imaging, it can sometimes be a challenge to differentiate chronic pancreatitis from pancreatic cancer. Features that favor chronic pancreatitis are intraductal or parenchymal calcifications, lack of obstructing mass, irregular dilation of the pancreatic duct, and relatively limited atrophy of the gland. Findings that favor neoplasia include pancreatic duct dilation with associated mass at the site of obstruction, with associated atrophy of the pancreas, vascular invasion, and metastases.[5,163]

CT has been shown to have a sensitivity of 56% to 95% with a specificity of 85% to 100% for the diagnosis of chronic pancreatitis (see Table 57.5).[162,164] In addition, CT is useful to evaluate the extrapancreatic and peripancreatic organs and tissues and to exclude complications of chronic pancreatitis such as pseudoaneurysms, pseudocysts, and thrombosis of the portosplenic circulation (e.g., splenic vein thrombosis/occlusion).[5,163] In summary, CT is useful as an initial radiologic test and is helpful to visualize calcifications and duct abnormalities and to exclude complications and other etiologies for pain or weight loss.

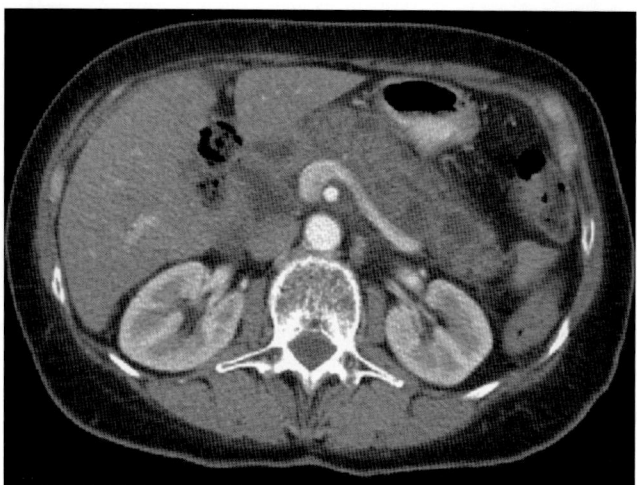

FIGURE 57.10 Computed tomographic image of a 52-year-old female patient with chronic nicotine- and alcohol-induced pancreatitis showing dilated pancreatic duct and multiple pseudocysts.

Magnetic Resonance Imaging and Cholangiopancreatography (see Chapter 17)

Use of MRI/MRCP is more sensitive for the diagnosis of chronic pancreatitis than either CT or ultrasound, and MRI/MRCP is particularly useful in detecting early parenchymal and ductal changes that are typically missed by CT and ultrasound.[5,161,165–167] The international consensus guidelines recommend MRI/MRCP in patients where no specific pathologic changes are seen on CT, but where the clinical suspicion of a diagnosis remains high.[161] The use of secretin-stimulated MRI/MRCP provides a dynamic test to characterize the pancreatic duct and pancreatic parenchyma, and can more accurately detect subtle duct changes. It is particularly useful in patients in which the clinical suspicion is high, but standard MRI/MRCP was not diagnostic.[161] Specifically, intravenous (IV) secretin should lead to an increase in the pancreatic duct diameter of more than 1 mm, with recovery of its size after 10 minutes ("pancreatic duct compliance").[5] MRI/MRCP with IV secretin can also be used to evaluate the exocrine function of the pancreas. By using a multislice, fast T2-weighted sequence, it is possible to estimate the amount of fluid secreted by the pancreas before and after stimulation.

Trikudanathan and colleagues assessed the correlation of MRI and secretin-induced MRCP (sMRCP) findings with surgical histopathology in a cohort of patients with noncalcific chronic pancreatitis who had undergone total pancreatectomy with islet autotransplantation. A total of 57 patients had sMRCP within 1 year of surgery. Using receiver operating characteristic (ROC) curve analysis, the authors found that two or more MRI/sMRCP features provided the best balance of sensitivity (65%), specificity (89%), and accuracy (68%) to differentiate abnormal from normal pancreatic tissue. A linear regression analysis taking age, smoking, and body mass index (BMI) into consideration showed that main pancreatic duct irregularity, T1-weighted signal intensity ratio between pancreas and paraspinal muscle, and duodenal filling after secretin injection were significant independent predictors of fibrosis. This study showed a strong correlation between MRI/sMRCP findings and histopathology of noncalcific chronic pancreatitis.[167]

In summary, MRI/MRCP is useful to evaluate for periductal fibrosis, ductal dilation with ectasia and side-branch abnormalities, intraparenchymal cyst formation, and pancreatic duct strictures and stones leading to obstructed outflow.[5,165] MRI is especially useful to detect early parenchymal changes suggestive of chronic pancreatitis, such as abnormal decreased signal intensity on fat-suppressed T1-weighted images and delayed or limited enhancement after gadolinium administration.[5] Dilation of side branches rather than the main pancreatic duct can also be indicative of early chronic pancreatitis.[168] The primary disadvantage of MRCP is that changes in side branches are not visualized with the same accuracy as in ERCP.

Endoscopic Retrograde Pancreatography (see Chapters 20 and 30)

Endoscopic retrograde pancreatography (ERP) has previously been held as the gold standard among all imaging methods for diagnosis and staging of chronic pancreatitis because it has 90% sensitivity and approaches 100% specificity in diagnosis (see Fig. 57.1B; Fig. 57.11).[8,169] However, in the era of high-quality

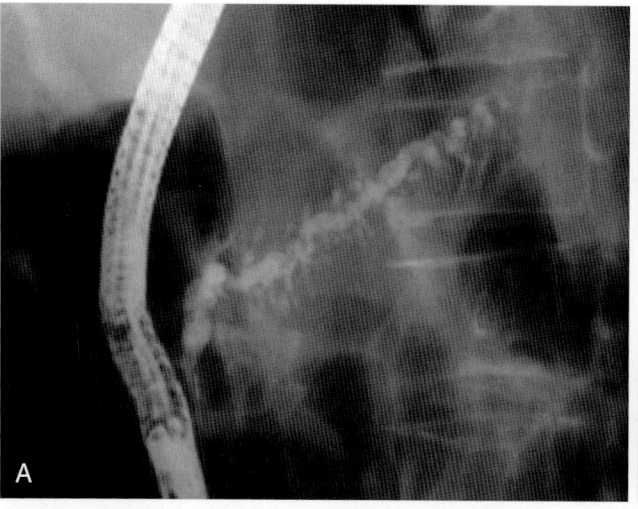
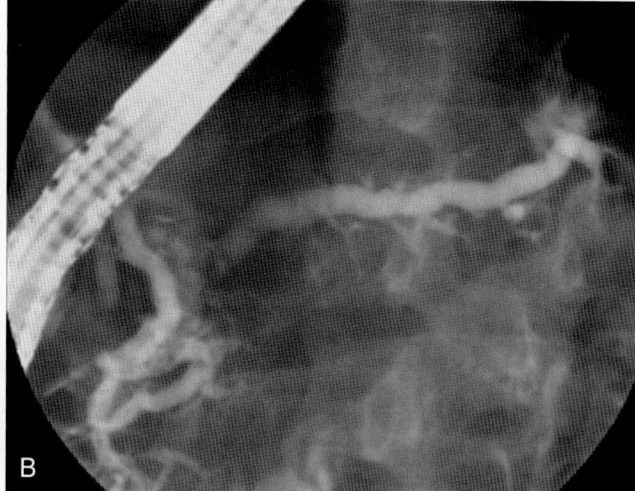

FIGURE 57.11 Pancreatograms **(A and B)** show a dilated and tortuous pancreatic duct with multiple side branches.

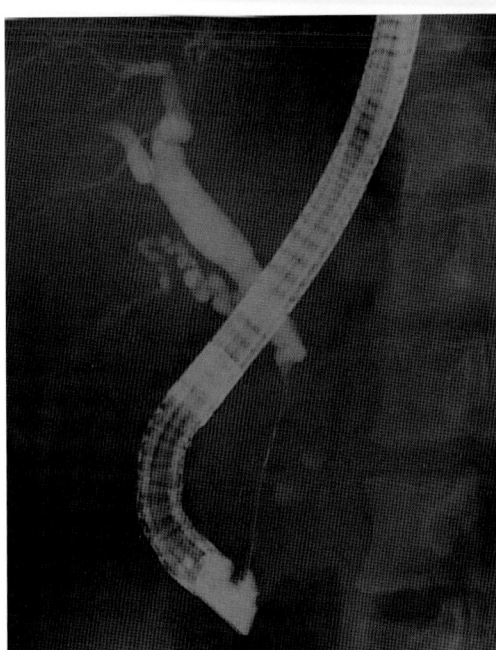

FIGURE 57.12 Endoscopic retrograde cholangiopancreatography in a patient with chronic pancreatitis demonstrates calcification in the region of the pancreatic head and concomitant distal common bile duct stenosis.

imaging tests such as CT and MRI/MRCP, the role of ERP for the diagnosis of chronic pancreatitis has greatly decreased. It must be kept in mind that ERP is an invasive method with a low but important rate of post-ERP pancreatitis in 3% to 10% of patients.[170] Currently, ERP is mainly used as a therapeutic tool in patients with chronic pancreatitis (see Fig. 57.11; see Chapters 30 and 56). An ERP staging system based on pancreatic ductal changes has been developed for the diagnosis of chronic pancreatitis, and international definitions are based on ERP findings published in 1984 as the Cambridge criteria (Table 57.4).[8] Nevertheless, it is important to mention that changes of early chronic pancreatitis may not be seen on ERP, which may assess ductal changes that occur in advanced disease, such as irregularity, dilation, tortuosity, stenosis, cysts, calculi, and bile duct stenosis (see Fig. 57.11; Fig. 57.12). These findings may culminate in a "chain of lakes" appearance of the main pancreatic duct with intermittent points of obstruction in a dilated pancreatic duct. In large multicenter trials, the sensitivity of ERP was described to be 68% to 100%, with a specificity of 89% to 100%.[158,171,172]

The advantage of using ERP for the diagnosis of chronic pancreatitis is its high diagnostic accuracy. However, its invasiveness, costs, and complications preclude its use as an initial diagnostic test.

Endoscopic Ultrasonography (see Chapter 22)

EUS is considered to be the most appropriate and sensitive imaging technique to diagnose parenchymal and ductal changes, mainly during the early stage of the disease. In contrast to other imaging methods, which detect chronic pancreatitis only in its advanced stages, EUS has the ability to detect chronic pancreatitis in patients with early stages of the disease as well as in those with advanced chronic pancreatitis.[173,174] Hence EUS is indicated when CT (and MRI) are negative in patients with clinical suspicion of chronic pancreatitis.[161] EUS

is a common diagnostic tool for evaluating chronic pancreatitis because of its ability to visualize subtle alterations in pancreatic structure before these can be detected using other imaging modalities or pancreatic function tests.[174–177] EUS has a high sensitivity but poor specificity for diagnosing chronic pancreatitis, and care must be taken before basing the diagnosis only on EUS criteria. Indeed, many EUS features of chronic pancreatitis are not necessarily pathologic and may occur as normal aging, smoking, obesity, as a normal variant, or from nonpathologic asymptomatic fibrosis in the absence of endocrine or exocrine dysfunction.[5,161,178]

Wiersema and colleagues described diagnostic criteria of chronic pancreatitis detectable by EUS, and these Milwaukee criteria were further refined with the Rosemont classification[12,174] (see Chapter 54). Parenchymal and ductal changes were divided into major and minor criteria, based on their importance, and subdivided into major A, major B, and minor. The two parenchymal major A criteria are hyperechoic foci with shadowing and well-circumscribed lobularity, and the only ductal major A criterion is calculi in the main pancreatic duct. The only parenchymal major B criterion is lobularity with honeycombing. Minor parenchymal criteria are cysts, stranding, nonshadowing hyperechoic foci, and lobularity with noncontiguous lobules. Minor ductal criteria are dilated ducts (body ≥3.5 mm and tail ≥1.5 mm), irregular main pancreatic duct contour, dilated side branches (≥1 mm), and hyperechoic duct margin.[12] The diagnosis based on the Rosemont classification is consistent if one of the following is present: (1) one major A feature and three or more minor features, (2) one major A feature and one major B feature, and (3) two major A features. All other combinations of features are categorized as suggestive, indeterminate, or normal. The advantage of this classification system compared with others is the use of weighted criteria. However, it should be noted that there is often relatively poor interobserver agreement for EUS, even among expert endosonographers, which limits the diagnostic accuracy and overall utility of EUS for diagnosing chronic pancreatitis.[5]

In early stages of chronic pancreatitis, EUS has a number of potential advantages compared with other imaging modalities. In a series of patients with a history of chronic alcohol abuse and recurrent abdominal pain with normal ERP, typical changes of chronic pancreatitis were detected by EUS. After a median follow-up of 18 months, typical changes of chronic pancreatitis by repeat ERP were seen in 68.8% of patients who initially presented with normal ERP but who showed typical changes of chronic pancreatitis on EUS. This study showed that EUS has a higher sensitivity to detect chronic pancreatitis compared with ERP in a typical clinical and patient history setting.[179]

The disadvantage of this method is the need for expert EUS endoscopists and a dedicated EUS unit. The advantages of EUS are the reliable visualization of the pancreatic parenchyma and ductal system without risk for pancreatitis.

Tests of Exocrine Pancreatic Function (see Chapter 4)

Presently, function tests play only a relatively minor, complementary role in the diagnosis of chronic pancreatitis. There are four main reasons for this: (1) noninvasive tests of exocrine pancreatic function show high sensitivity only in advanced stages of chronic pancreatitis, (2) there is low clinical availability of most direct tests, (3) utility of function tests is limited to the diagnosis of more advanced disease, and (4) these tests have low specificity (70%).[180–183] Indeed, direct pancreatic function tests may be limited by, among other factors, false-positive results for at least several months after a bout of acute pancreatitis and false-negative results in some patients who have early chronic pancreatitis.[5] The problem with chronic pancreatitis is that any clinical manifestation of exocrine pancreatic insufficiency occurs late in the course of disease, after approximately 90% of the exocrine parenchyma has been destroyed.[184] The majority of these pancreatic function tests are only able to diagnose chronic pancreatitis when approximately 70% to 80% of the pancreatic function has been lost.

Invasive (Direct) Pancreatic Function Tests (see Chapter 4)

One of the most sensitive tests to detect exocrine insufficiency is invasive and requires duodenal intubation and aspiration of duodenal juice after pancreatic stimulation.[158] The secretin stimulation test can be used for the detection of functional impairment in all stages of chronic pancreatitis and has a reported sensitivity and specificity between 75% and 95%.[185,186] The secretin stimulation test, with or without concomitant CCK-8 or cerulein administration, measures the volume of secretion and the concentration of output of bicarbonate and pancreatic enzymes (by 60-minute continuous duodenal fluid aspiration) in response to IV secretin. Bicarbonate levels less than 50 mEq/L are consistent with chronic pancreatitis; levels of 50 to 75 mEq/L are normal. False-positive results may be seen in the setting of diabetes mellitus, Billroth II gastrectomy, celiac sprue, and cirrhosis. Invasive tests like the secretin stimulation test have several obvious disadvantages including cost, invasiveness, and risk. Although these tests have shown a good correlation with the fibrosis scores detected by EUS, their clinical use is mostly of historical interest and are limited predominantly to answer scientific questions related to chronic pancreatitis.[187–189]

Noninvasive (Indirect) Pancreatic Function Tests (see Chapter 4)

Indirect tests of pancreatic function noninvasively assess pancreatic function by measuring the absorption of some compound (e.g., fat), which first requires digestion by pancreatic enzymes, and measuring the level of enzymes or zymogens secreted by the pancreas (serum trypsinogen or fecal elastase [FE-1]). A low serum amylase or lipase is a potentially useful indirect test of pancreatic function, but these noninvasive tests have the disadvantage of low sensitivity in early stages of chronic pancreatitis. The diagnostic accuracy increases slightly when moderate or severe disease is present. Importantly, these tests should always be accompanied by CT or MRI/MRCP when assessing chronic pancreatitis.[5]

Previously, 3-day tests of stool quantity and weight were proposed for the diagnosis of malabsorptive chronic pancreatitis,

but this never gained clinical popularity.[24] The evaluation of gross stool fat no longer plays a significant role in the diagnosis of chronic pancreatitis, because fat malabsorption occurs only in later stages, after more than 90% of the exocrine pancreatic parenchyma has been destroyed.[184] Therefore only a minority of patients will have significant steatorrhea even with marked exocrine insufficiency.

Stool tests for the quantification of fat (with subsequent correction after pancreatic enzyme replacement), chymotrypsin, and FE-1 have been well studied. Measurement of fecal chymotrypsin is still popular in Europe today, but the diagnostic accuracy of this test is not acceptable. Fecal chymotrypsin may be useful in detecting compliance with exogenous pancreatic enzyme supplementation. The best accuracy of all stool tests is obtained by measurement of FE-1. Along with high stability of pancreatic elastase during passage throughout the intestine, the commercial test measures only human elastase. This is an advantage in patients receiving therapeutic oral enzyme supplementation, because this lipase is of porcine origin. Even if FE-1 measurement is superior to other stool tests, its diagnostic value should not be overrated; sensitivity and specificity are low in the early stages of chronic pancreatitis, with only mild to moderate exocrine insufficiency.[181,183]

SUMMARY

Chronic pancreatitis is classically defined as progressive pancreatic inflammation and fibrosis that irreversibly damages the pancreas and results in loss of exocrine and endocrine function. The most common etiologies of chronic pancreatitis in adults in Western societies are long-term alcohol abuse and smoking. Multiple underlying environmental, genetic, epigenetic, cellular, and molecular aspects contribute to the development of chronic pancreatitis. There is no unifying theory for the pathogenesis of chronic pancreatitis; instead, multiple overlapping hypotheses have varying roles depending on the etiology of disease. These hypotheses include necrosis-fibrosis theory, toxic-metabolic causes, oxidative stress, plug and stone formation with duct obstruction, primary duct obstruction, and SAPE. Currently, the two-hit hypothesis seems to explain the process best: (1) a patient with underlying susceptibility (e.g., hereditary, efferent duct, immunologic) has a first attack of acute pancreatitis from an insulting factor (alcohol, nicotine, gallstones), and an inflammatory immunologic process ensues, and (2) the pancreas recovers, or more hits occur, promoting disease progression. Regardless of etiology or underlying mechanism, chronic pancreatitis remains a debilitating condition with limited therapeutic interventions.

References are available at expertconsult.com.

CHAPTER 58

Management of chronic pancreatitis: Conservative, endoscopic, surgical

Thilo Hackert, John P. Neoptolemos, and Markus W. Büchler

BACKGROUND

Chronic pancreatitis (CP) is characterized by a progressive inflammatory process, the etiologies of which vary depending on geographic and sociocultural circumstances.[1] Therefore incidence and prevalence of CP differs between the respective regions, which has been shown in studies that include Western and Asian countries as well as India. The reported rates show an incidence of approximately 5 to 15 per 100,000 and prevalence of 40 to 120 per 100,000 inhabitants calculated on the basis of an estimated median survival time of 20 years. Especially in Asian countries, these numbers have increased in recent decades.[1–3] Etiology of CP includes chronic alcohol consumption as the most common cause with an increasing impact accounting for 70% of all CP cases.[1,2] A persistent alcohol intake of 70 g/day for a duration of more than 12 months is the threshold for developing CP, and tobacco smoking is a co-risk factor and also an independent factor of CP.[3]

Hereditary CP was recognized as a distinct entity in the 1990s and the underlying genetic mutations were defined in the following years, including mainly mutations in gene loci of cationic trypsinogen (PRSS1), serine protease inhibitor Kazal-type 1 (SPINK1), carboxypeptidase A1 (CPA1), as well as cystic fibrosis transmembrane conductance regulator (CFTR), chymotrypsinogen C (CTRC), and carboxyesterlipase (CEL).[1,4,5] Today, the proportion of hereditary CP is estimated at 20% to 30% of all CP patients. Especially in previously reported "idiopathic" CP, there may be a considerable number of patients with an unrecognized genetic background, reducing the actual incidence of "idiopathic" CP, which is only accepted as a terminology after exclusion of all other risk factors and may account for approximately 10% of all cases today.[5] Moreover, the term "tropical CP" is now falling into disuse as it has become evident that an aggressive form of idiopathic CP reported from India and other tropical countries in which this term was at first applied is actually strongly associated with genetic mutations/polymorphisms in multiple genes, including SPINK1, CFTR, CTRC, Cathepsin B, and CLDN2/MORC4, with clinical characteristics similar to CP in more temperate countries.[6]

A gallstone etiology of CP remains controversial because this type of CP was exclusively described in Chinese patient cohorts. Besides the fact that no other region in the world observed this type of CP, the pathophysiology of gallstones themselves leading to CP is not explained and it has been assumed that recurrent episodes of gallstone-induced acute pancreatitis (AP) not definitely treated after the first episode finally lead to the picture of CP, rather than this pathophysiology representing a separate etiology of CP itself[2] (see Chapter 33).

Autoimmune pancreatitis (AIP) was first described in 1995[7] and has gained increasing attention since the early 2000s as an important and distinctly different entity of CP in terms of diagnostic measures and therapy. It is found in approximately 5% to 6% of all CP patients. As a presumed systemic IgG4-related sclerosing disease, AIP is addressed in different guidelines and recommendations than CP by most national and international societies today[8] (see Chapters 54 and 60)

From a pathophysiologic point of view, CP leads to a fibrosclerotic transformation of the pancreatic tissue often associated with calcifications. Local fibro-inflammatory and neuroimmunologic changes lead to a chronic progressive destruction of functional pancreatic tissue. These changes primarily affect exocrine function by acinar cell destruction followed by late symptoms of endocrine failure in most patients when the endocrine cells are affected. The clinical symptoms of exocrine failure include steatorrhea, weight loss, and maldigestion with intolerance of fatty food and malabsorption with vitamin deficiency; endocrine failure leads to symptoms of and eventually complications of diabetes mellitus (DM)[9,10] (see Chapter 54).

In addition, pain is a key feature of CP and clinically the most important symptom in nearly all patients. Pain in CP has been characterized by immunologic and neural modulations, which lead to a reactive change in peripheral nerve diameter, density, and function correlating with pain intensity in the long-term course of CP.[11,12] After pain generation on a peripheral level, an increasing and stimulus-independent pain sensation develops with characteristics of an autonomous pain caused by neural plasticity and memory function of the peripheral and central nervous system. This neural plasticity finally induces an irreversible change of pain sensation because of cerebral cortical reorganization.[11] Clinically, this cascade is represented by the fact that many CP patients who typically present in a later stage of the disease are already opioid-dependent and highly disabled.[11,12]

The morphologic macroscopic correlate of CP is characterized by an inflammatory tumorous mass, which is often focused on the head of the gland, pseudocysts, calcifications, and a dilation of the main pancreatic duct with obvious diameter irregularities and stenotic segments. In addition, the bile duct can be obstructed by these changes with a consequent cholestasis.[13] Depending on the enlargement of the inflammatory mass, signs of local compression can be found with a stenosis or occlusion of the portal, superior mesenteric, or splenic vein. This may result in a—mostly left-sided—portal hypertension with collateral circulation via the short gastric veins and can cause a cavernous transformation of the proximal portal vein. Furthermore, the enlarged pancreatic head may result in duodenal and gastric outlet obstruction with subsequent reduction of oral intake, which can further aggravate malnutrition and weight loss.[13–15]

The major aims of therapy in CP are prevention of acute pain attacks, long-lasting pain relief, prevention of disease progression, correction of metabolic consequences, and restoration of a good quality of life combined with a preservation of endocrine and exocrine function of the pancreas. Furthermore, psychosocial problems should be addressed and managed.[16] Because of the complex pathophysiology of CP, this requires an interdisciplinary management team that includes gastroenterologic, radiologic, pathologic, psychological and surgical expertise.

CONSERVATIVE THERAPY

Exposition to Nutritional and Toxic Risk Factors

In alcoholic CP, stopping alcohol intake and nicotine use with sustained abstinence are principal steps in management. These steps require a high level of patient compliance, and the cessation of both risk factors that usually coincide may be challenging and require accompanying psychological therapy.[17–19] If not achieved synchronously, the preferable sequence may be smoking cessation before alcohol abstinence which, however, should also be achieved to improve pain frequency, intensity, and therapy response and to maintain the remaining pancreatic function.[20,21] Abstaining from the mentioned toxic risk factors may not only reduce symptoms and deterioration of pancreatic function but also contribute to a reduction of disease-associated mortality.[22,23]

Psychological Symptoms

Social re-integration and professional rehabilitation are important therapy aims in the typically young (35–60 years old) cohort of CP patients. A psychological therapy approach in CP should address the complex mechanisms of pain-associated disability in social and professional function, dependency on alcohol and smoking, self-blaming, and the patient's personal economic deterioration. Interventions to address these issues should start as early as possible in the disease course to prevent or reverse the vicious cycle of one factor enhancing the other and can be performed by educational programs and continuous psychological support, as well as self-conducted supportive measures.[17,24] Despite such approaches, CP patients seem to be at a higher risk of attempted and completed suicide, which underlines the importance of accompanying CP therapy with psychological support.[25]

Exocrine Dysfunction

Exocrine dysfunction, characterized by steatorrhea, malabsorption, maldigestion, lack of fat-soluble vitamins and weight loss, must be addressed by adequate oral substitution of pancreatic enzyme preparations (PEPs). PEPs containing high lipase activity must be resistant to gastric acid provided by enteric coating and should homogenously mix with the nutritional components. This provides coordinated gastric emptying with nutrients and an early activation in the duodenum. Different compositions and galenic forms, including capsules and powders, have been developed and tested with variable results. Especially after pancreatic resections for CP, gastric acid blockade is important to facilitate PEP activity and prevent ulcer development. A fat restricting diet to treat steatorrhea is no longer recommended. CP patients often suffer from a reduced body mass index (BMI) because of maldigestion and reduced food intake to avoid abdominal pain. Therefore a sufficient calorie intake is required and must be adjusted to individual patient needs. The dose of PEPs follows fat intake, with approximately 2000 international units (IU) of lipase per gram of fat ingested[26] resulting in dose ranges from 25,000 to 75,000 units of lipase, depending on the fat content of the meal, that must be provided during the meal to achieve an optimal treatment effect.[27,28] In case of therapy failure, the first step in treatment recommendations is to increase PEP dosage.[26] Even in countries with high-standard healthcare, many patients with CP-related exocrine pancreatic failure are insufficiently treated.[29] The supportive prescription of proton pump inhibitors in addition to an enteric-coated PEP is often necessary in surgical CP patients if PEP alone is not effective and a dose augmentation of PEP does not lead to a satisfying improvement of symptoms.[30,31] The success of PEP therapy should primarily be judged by the improvement of clinical symptoms (weight gain, improvement of abdominal symptoms). Besides the improvement of digestive and absorptive function, PEPs themselves may lead to pain reduction and—more importantly—contribute to a normalization of intestinal motility and reduction of dyspepsia.[32,33]

Deficiency in fat-soluble vitamins, especially vitamin A, D and E, is observed in up to 75% of all CP patients,[34] which may lead to clinically manifest osteoporosis, as observed in approximately 25% of CP patients.[35] Fat-soluble vitamin monitoring and replacement should be performed according to current guidelines and supplemented by vitamin B_1, B_2, and B_6 therapy in case of persistent alcohol abuse.

Endocrine Dysfunction

CP-related endocrine pancreatic insufficiency is defined as DM type 3c, which is characterized by deficiency of insulin and glucagon as well as pancreatic polypeptide. The treatment primarily follows the recommendations of DM type 1 with absolute insulin deficiency.[36,37] Three main criteria for the diagnosis of DM type 3c are mandatory: exocrine pancreatic insufficiency (tested by monoclonal fecal elastase-1 testing or direct function tests), consistent morphologic pancreatic abnormalities on imaging (endoscopic ultrasound, magnetic resonance imaging [MRI], or computed tomography [CT] scan), and absence of related autoimmune markers of DM type 1.[38] In addition, minor criteria include impaired β-cell function (i.e., measured by C-peptide or glucose concentrations), absence of insulin resistance (defined by homoeostatic model assessment for insulin resistance), impaired incretin secretion (glucagon-like peptide-1 [GLP-1] or pancreatic polypeptide, or both), and low serum concentrations of fat-soluble vitamins (A, D, E, and K). In addition to CP, DM type 3c is found in pancreatic cancer patients, patients after pancreatic surgery, and genetic and metabolic disorders affecting the pancreas (i.e., hemochromatosis or cystic fibrosis) and accounts for 5% to 10% off all DM patients worldwide.[36]

Metformin is recommended as first-line therapy of DM type 3c for CP patients but in most patients an additional therapy with insulin is unavoidable. CP patients show a high risk of hypoglycemia, which can be explained by a lack of compliance, persisting alcohol consumption, and a co-existing autonomous neuropathy.[5] Especially in alcoholic CP, this is associated with a high risk of mortality. Consequently, the avoidance of hypoglycemia must be a major goal that can often be achieved by simple insulin regimens that increase compliance and reduce therapy-associated severe complications.[39]

Pain Management

As previously mentioned, abstinence from alcohol and smoking as well as PEP contribute to conservative pain management in CP to a certain extent. Despite this fact, nearly all CP patients require pain medication, although a significant variability between individual patients is observed. Therefore pain sensation needs to be characterized diligently concerning character, intensity, frequency, and possible causes. The backbone of pain medication in CP is the current World Health Organization (WHO) recommendation for analgesic therapy after a stepwise use of analgesic drugs.[40-42] The first step is represented by nonopioid peripheral analgesics (i.e., acetaminophen, nonsteroidal antiinflammatory drugs [NSAIDs]) supported by adjuvant medication (i.e., antidepressants, anticonvulsants) and the prescription of these drugs "around the clock" instead of as "on-demand" use. The next step of the WHO ladder includes mild opioids (i.e., tramadol) in addition to the ongoing basic medication. This is followed by an escalation to strong opioid drugs, if needed, as the third step of the WHO scheme. In all of the steps, oral application of drugs should be preferred to increase compliance and reduce injection-associated complications and potential accidental overdosage. Despite the fact that high-potent opioids may provide complete pain relief, one must consider that narcotic addiction will most likely occur after long-term use. Because of this, alternative therapy approaches should be considered early in the course of CP to provide a causal solution of the associated pain because CP patients—in contrast to palliative cancer patients—should not reach a state of chronic opioid dependency as long as other solutions can be achieved.

A currently added "fourth" step of the WHO ladder includes interventional approaches of pain management. These approaches include treatments such as endoscopic ultrasound (EUS)–guided plexus block, splanchnic nerve, block, spinal cord stimulation, transcranial magnetic stimulation, and acupuncture. According to current guidelines of the United European Gastroenterology (UEG), such interventions may be effective in selected cases of CP; however, only a small number of patient will ultimately qualify for these approaches after failure of all other therapeutic measures.[2,41] Nerve destruction may lead to an increase in pain because of neuropathic mechanisms that develop later, and there are potential severe side effects, such as hypotension, hemorrhage, infections, and neurologic complications.[11,42] Any beneficial effect lasts for less than 3 months and after the neurolysis any neuropathic pain will worsen. Taken together with the potential severe side effects, the use of neurolysis in CP is not supported by the International (International Association of Pancreatology [IAP]/American Pancreatic Association [APA]/Japan Pancreas Society [JPS]/European Pancreatic Club [EPC]) Consensus Guidelines.[11,42]

Autoimmune Pancreatitis

AIP as a special type of CP related to IgG4 autoimmune diseases is distinctly different than other forms of sclerosing or calcifying CP with relevant consequences in clinical management and is primarily managed conservatively (see Chapters 54 and 55). Two different subtypes of AIP have to be differentiated. AIP type 1 with histologic features of dense periductal lymphoplasmacytic immune cell infiltrates, so-called "storiform fibrosis," and obliterative venulitis is mostly associated with increased serum levels of IgG4, which underlines the theory that the pancreas is only one target organ of a systemic autoimmune disease in these patients.[43] In line with this consideration, other affected organs include bile duct, kidneys, salivary glands, and the retroperitoneum. AIP type 2 shows a typical duct-destructive pathology, infiltrating neutrophil and plasma cells as well as lymphocytes. Furthermore, serum markers found in AIP type 1 are often not elevated.[44] As a consequence, AIP type 2 is difficult to differentiate from pancreatic masses of other etiologies, especially pancreatic ductal adenocarcinoma (PDAC).[45]

AIP imaging morphology shows typical features of a diffusely swollen pancreas ("sausage") in only 50% of patients (see Chapter 17), whereas localized mass formation (pronounced in the tail or head of the pancreas) is also often observed and can lead to PDAC misdiagnosis.[45] The most reliable imaging feature is found in late-phase contrast-enhanced MRI ("late enhancement") and—if conservative treatment is started—is a rapid regression of the characteristic swelling and mass formation.[46] No feature, however, is pathognomonic, and the differential diagnosis of PDAC has always to be considered. Also, EUS-guided core biopsies may not result in a definite diagnosis in all patients because typical (i.e., IgG4 positivity) findings are present in only 20% of biopsies and—vice versa—false-positive IgG4 staining has been reported in PDAC.[47]

The conservative management of AIP starts with high-dosage corticosteroid therapy (0.6–0.8 mg/kg body weight/day orally prednisone equivalent) for 4 weeks to induce remission and then be tapered within 2 additional months. Response to initial treatment should be assessed at week 2 to 4 with clinical, biochemical, and morphologic markers (i.e., MRI). In patients with multiorgan disease or relapse, glucocorticoids should be considered as maintenance treatment. If the disease relapses during the 3 months of treatment, immunosuppressive drugs should be added.[7] Importantly, if there is no change in disease activity and symptoms within 3 months, the diagnosis of AIP should be critically re-evaluated and—in doubtful cases and the potential differential diagnosis of PDAC—surgery must be strongly considered.[48]

ENDOSCOPIC THERAPY

Bile Duct/Pancreatic Duct Stenosis

Since the early 2000s, there has been an ongoing debate about the superiority of endoscopic versus surgical treatment of bile and pancreatic duct stenosis in CP, especially with regard to indications and duration of endoscopic treatment and the question of whether endoscopic therapy can serve as a definitive treatment option and prevent surgery (see Chapters 20, 30, 31, and 52). A number of studies, including randomized controlled trials (RCTs), have addressed these topics in the meantime.[48-52] An early trial with 61 patients with CP-associated bile duct stenosis and 1 year of endoscopic treatment, including three to four stenting procedures, showed a success rate of 60% for patients without calcifications of the pancreas but only 8% when calcifications were present, with an overall operation rate of 50% after one year.[47] Another multicenter trial with more than 1000 patients resulted in endoscopic success rates of 46% to 76%, reinterventions in 5% to 19% and a secondary operation rate of 24% to 48% depending on CP morphology (strictures alone, stones alone, a combination of both, or miscellaneous).[49] No improvements in pancreatic function were observed in this study after completed endoscopic therapy. Two RCTs addressed the outcome of endoscopic versus surgical therapy for pancreatic duct obstruction in the pancreatic head with regard to primary success, pain relief, and quality of life in the short-term and long-term follow-up.[50,51] In the first study of 72 patients, endoscopic therapy included sphincterotomy with stenting and/or stone removal (52% and 23% of the patients, respectively; see Chapters 20 and 30), whereas surgery consisted of resection (80%) and drainage (20%) procedures (see Chapters 37A and 42). After initially similar success rates for both groups, long-term observation after 5 years revealed that complete absence of pain was more frequent after surgery (37% vs. 14% endoscopy) with a similar rate of partial pain relief (49% vs. 51%). In addition, a 20% to 25% greater increase in body weight was observed in surgical patients, but postinterventional new-onset diabetes rates were comparable in both groups (34%–43%).[50] Perhaps the most prominent RCT was published by the Dutch study group and included 19 patients receiving endoscopic drainage for pancreatic duct obstruction versus 20 patients with surgical drainage.[51] This study demonstrated the superiority of surgical drainage in terms of less interventions, more complete pain relief (75% surgery vs. 32% endoscopy), and a higher proportion of exocrine and endocrine function preservation after 2 and 5 years of follow-up. Furthermore, half of the patients initially treated by endoscopy ultimately underwent surgery.[52] Based on these studies, today endoscopic treatment can be considered as a first-line management for bile and pancreatic duct stenosis for a limited time in CP. It should be generally performed using plastic stents, which need to be exchanged in most patients after 3 to 4 months. If endoscopic therapy is not successful after a maximum treatment of 12 months, surgery should be strongly considered as the definitive treatment for a good long-term outcome. These recommendations have been adopted by most international and interdisciplinary guidelines[42,53]; however, daily practice shows that the acceptance is limited and many CP patients are still referred to a surgical center very late in their CP disease course. A current Dutch RCT on the timing of surgery compared 44 patients with early surgery for pancreatic drainage with 44 patients receiving an endoscopy-first approach.[54] After a median of 18 months follow-up, patients undergoing early surgery showed lower pain scores and higher rates of complete or partial pain relief (58% early surgery group vs. 39% endoscopy-first group). In addition, early surgery patients underwent fewer interventions, whereas treatment complications (27% vs. 25%), mortality (0% vs. 0%), hospital admissions, pancreatic function, and quality of life were not significantly different between both groups.

Pseudocyst Management

Pancreatic pseudocysts occur as a late complication of CP in 20% to 40% of all patients and are classified according to the Atlanta classification as acute or chronic pseudocysts, potentially superinfected, leading to pancreatic abscesses[55,56] (see Chapters 54 and 56). In contrast to pseudocysts in AP, which show a spontaneous regression rate of approximately 50%, in CP patients, only 10% of pseudocysts regress spontaneously.[57] Treatment indications for pseudocysts in CP include local complications such as vascular compression; gastric, duodenal, or bile duct stenosis; infection; hemorrhage; and pancreatopleural fistula development.[58] In addition, abdominal distension, nausea, vomiting, or pain may be indications for pseudocyst treatment as well as large cysts (>5 cm) without regression over 3 to 6 months, solid wall (>5 mm), and suspected cystic

tumors. Endoscopic pseudocyst management can be achieved by transgastric, transduodenal, or transpapillary access to the pseudocyst, depending on the location and a potential connection to the main pancreatic duct. A duct connection can be found in up to 50% of all patients, allowing a transpapillary stent insertion as the simplest approach to decompress the pseudocyst. The transpapillary drainage may be hampered by duct stenosis or calculi, which do not allow access and guide wire and consecutive stent insertion. In such cases, or if a clear duct connection is not demonstrated by endoscopic retrograde cholangiopancreatography, a transmural approach (stomach or duodenum) under EUS guidance is a feasible alternative (see Chapter 30). A temporary stent placement after initial evacuation of the cyst allows for a prolonged drainage and decreases recurrence rates.[59] A number of studies have shown technical success rates of endoscopic pseudocyst drainage of 80%, recurrence rates of approximately 8%, and procedure-related complications in 10% to 15% with very low mortality rates.[57] Endoscopic treatment should therefore be regarded as the first-line therapy for pseudocyst in CP, and surgery should be considered if endoscopic treatment fails or if a cystic tumor is suspected.[2]

Lithotripsy

Extracorporeal shock wave lithotripsy (ESWL; see Chapters 30 and 39) for pancreatic duct stones in CP is usually combined with ERCP and endoscopic stone extraction (i.e., using a Dormia basket). However, a recent RCT comparing both procedures did not show a benefit in adding ERCP and stone extraction.[60] The indication for ESWL can occur in calcified radiopaque stones of the main pancreatic duct measuring more than 5 mm in diameter, although smaller stones can also be treated with ESWL. To ensure technical success, preferably single stones within the pancreatic head should be targeted because they allow an endoscopic extraction more easily than stones located in the pancreatic neck or even further to the left side of the pancreas. Because the combined procedure requires a high level of expertise and the number of suitable patients is rather low, ESWL is infrequently performed in CP. Data from a meta-analysis pooling 27 mainly retrospective studies with nearly 3200 patients showed ductal clearance in 70%, complete pain control by ESWL in 53%, and mild to moderate persistent pain in 34% of the patients.[61] This resulted in reduced use of narcotics in 80%, stable or increasing body weight in 81%, and an improvement in quality of life in 88% of the reported patients. Morbidity includes ESWL-associated pancreatitis in 4% to 5% and secondary surgery because of therapeutic failure in 4% to 5%. According to these results, ESWL can be chosen as a therapy option for selected patients who fulfill the aforementioned criteria when centers have adequate experience with this approach. Table 58.1 summarizes endoscopic therapy options and indications.

SURGICAL THERAPY

Pain is the most frequent indication for surgery in CP; besides this, recurrent episodes of pancreatitis, cholestasis, compression of the surrounding structures (including duodenum, stomach, and portal vein), and suspicion of malignancy represent common reasons for CP operations.[62–68] Table 58.2 gives an overview on the relative proportions of the different indications. Acute complications such as pseudocyst rupture, bleeding, or organ perforation (duodenum, stomach, or colon) are

TABLE 58.1 Endoscopic Therapy Options, Indications, and Limitations	
Therapy Options	Indications
Internal Drainage	
Cysto-gastrostomy / Cystoduodenostomy	Treatment of pseudocysts, no RCs with comparison to surgery, if anatomically possible less invasive than surgery, recurrence/stent dislocation possible
Endoscopic Ductal Drainage	
Papillotomy	Pancreas divisum, sphincter of Oddi dysfunction
Papillotomy + dilation/stenting of pancreatic duct	Proximal short segment stenosis of pancreatic duct
Papillotomy + lithotripsy and stone extraction	Pancreatolithiasis in the proximal duct segment
Papillotomy + bile duct stenting	Bile duct stenosis
Indicators of Poor Outcome:	
Distal/long segment stenosis of pancreatic duct Calcifying chronic pancreatitis (CP) Unsuccessful therapy >12 months	

TABLE 58.2 Indications for Surgery in Chronic Pancreatitis and Estimated Proportions of the Different Indications	
INDICATION	**RELATIVE PROPORTION**
Intractable pain	80%
Bile duct stenosis	15%
Other local compression symptoms (portal vein stenosis, gastric outlet/duodenal stenosis)	10%
Suspicion of malignancy	5%
Pseudocysts	5%
Emergency indications (bleeding, organ perforation)	<5%

uncommon indications for surgery in CP; however, if present, they may require emergency surgery, which can result in advanced operative procedures, including unplanned pancreatic resections.[66]

The major aims of surgical therapy in CP are long-lasting pain relief and restoration of a good quality of life combined with a preservation of endocrine and exocrine function of the pancreas. Furthermore, professional and social rehabilitation of the mostly young CP patients should be achieved. The prevention of malignancy is another indication for surgery in CP because the risk for pancreatic cancer is elevated; however, this risk may have been overestimated in the past for CP patients who do not have a hereditary background of the disease[65] (see Chapter 61). In sporadic CP, an up to 16 times elevated risk of developing malignancy has been assumed in older studies, whereas in more recent investigations, this is currently assumed to be about only a 4-fold to 5-fold increase.[64,65] In contrast, cancer risk in hereditary CP is approximately 40 to 50 times higher than the normal risk of the average population, with a lifetime probability of 40% to suffer from pancreatic cancer, which justifies a more aggressive surgical approach in these patients.[67,68]

Timing of Surgery

Timing of surgery should be carefully considered so as not to miss the phase in CP patient history when reversible pain becomes autonomous and neuronal plasticity generates stimulus-independent pain generation. Consequently, the aspect of pain medication is of high importance and chronic intake of strong opioids with imminent dependency must be avoided. Because the second step of the WHO pain medication concept already includes regular medication with opioid drugs, definitive management of CP-associated symptoms and morphologic changes should be considered. Therefore endoscopic management and the number of interventions should be restricted, and after 1 year of endoscopic therapy without persisting success, a surgical consultation and decision about a potential operative therapy should be achieved (Fig. 58.1). This time frame is reasonable because it is long enough to evaluate the efficacy of endoscopic therapy and yet short enough not to induce chronic opioid dependency.[69]

The major technical aim of CP surgery is the decompression of the obstructed pancreatic and, if necessary, the bile duct, which can be combined with a removal of the fibrotic and calcified tissue that caused the obstruction. Consequently, there are two major groups of surgical procedures that have to be differentiated: drainage procedures alone and resection procedures (Table 58.3).

Drainage Procedures

Drainage procedures in CP address either the obstructed main pancreatic duct or pseudocysts. In the 1950s, two procedures approaching the dilated pancreatic duct from the left side were described by Duval[70] and Puestow and Gillesby.[71] In both operations, a small part of the pancreatic tail was resected and the duct opened to allow free drainage into a jejunal loop defunctioned by a Roux-en-Y reconstruction. The Puestow modification included a longer opening of the pancreatic duct toward the body of the pancreas based on the consideration that many patients demonstrated not only one stricture but also sequential stenotic segments ("chain-of-lakes"), and this could effectively be decompressed by a longer and larger opening. In 1960 this approach was modified by Partington and Rochelle,[72] who abandoned the tail resection and opened the pancreatic duct throughout the entire aspect of the gland. Reconstruction is

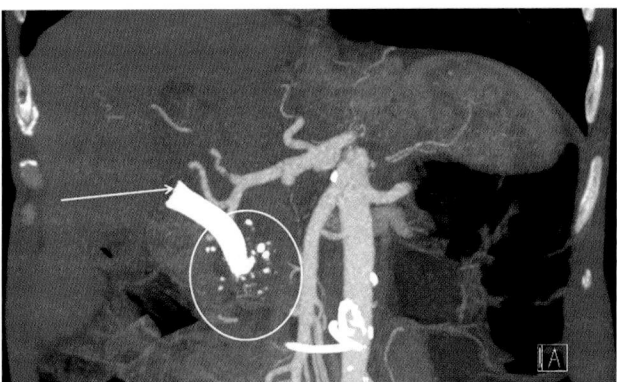

FIGURE 58.1 Typical computed tomography (CT) morphology after long-lasting endoscopic interventions, arterial phase coronary reformatting. Covered metal stent bridging bile duct strictures *(white arrow)* surrounded by multiple calcifications *(white circle)*.

TABLE 58.3   Surgical Procedures and Specific Indications in Chronic Pancreatitis

Drainage Procedures

Cystojejunostomy	Pseudocysts after failure of endoscopic therapy
Caudal drainage (Puestow operation)	Rare indication, replaced by other procedures
Latero-lateral pancreatojejunostomy (Partington-Rochelle operation)	Duct dilation > 7 mm without inflammatory mass

Resection Procedures

Partial pancreaticoduodenectomy	Suspected malignancy, irreversible duodenal stenosis, procedure of choice when technically possible, limited by perivascular inflammation or portal vein thrombosis/portal hypertension
Duodenum-preserving pancreatic head resection (DPPHR) Beger	Inflammatory head mass, no suspected malignancy, portal vein axis technically accessible
DPPHR Berne	Inflammatory head mass, technically easier that DPPHR Beger, also possible in portal vein thrombosis/collateralization
DPPHR Frey	Long segment obstruction of the pancreatic duct, no prominent inflammatory head mass
Distal / segmental pancreatectomy	Rare indication for isolated left-sided inflammation (i.e., post-traumatic)
Total pancreatectomy	Rare indication in patients with severe chronic pancreatitis changes in the entire gland, preexisting IDDM
Total pancreatectomy with islet cell autotransplantation	Indication for selected patients (i.e., pediatric patients)

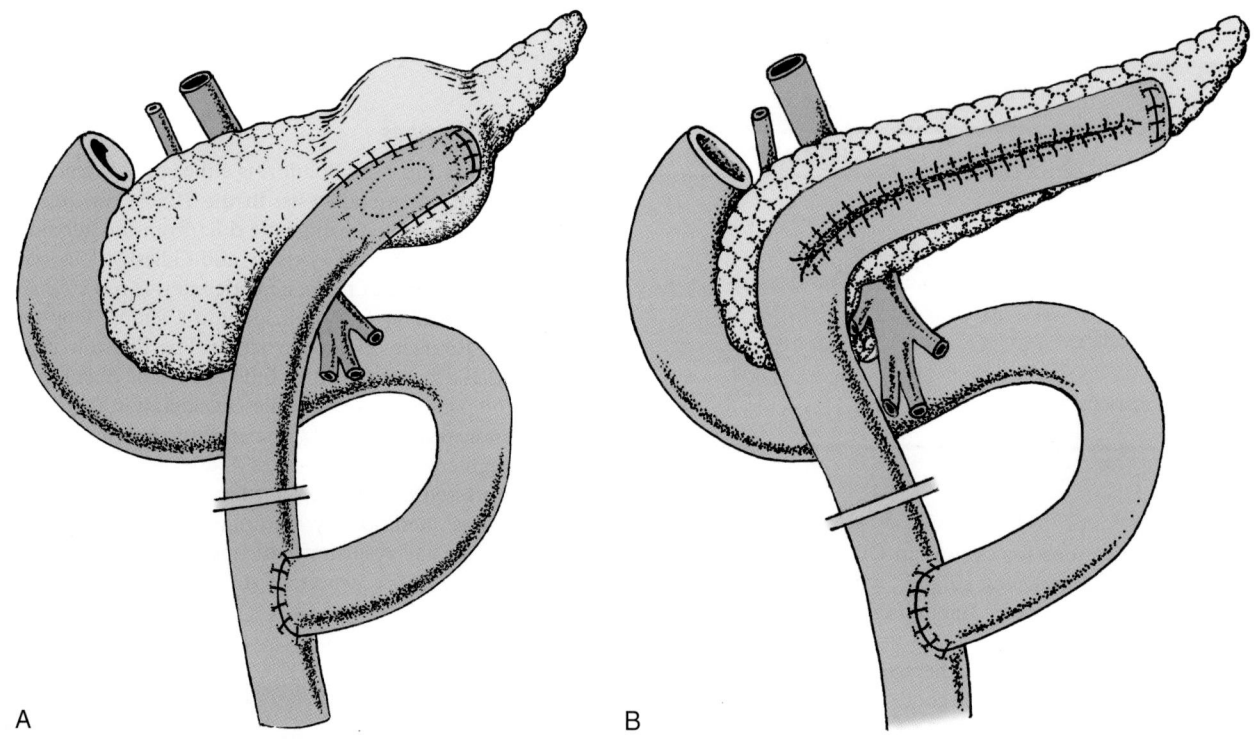

A   B

FIGURE 58.2   Drainage procedures in chronic pancreatitis. **A,** In rare patients with dilation of the pancreatic duct and no inflammatory mass, a latero-lateral pancreaticojejunostomy—Partington-Rochelle procedure—may be performed. **B,** If the cyst wall is thick enough, a pancreatic pseudocyst can be safely and effectively treated by drainage with a cystojejunostomy and Roux-en-Y reconstruction.

performed as a latero-lateral pancreatojejunostomy (Fig. 58.2A). This procedure shows very low surgical morbidity (<10%) and mortality (<1%) and preserves nearly all pancreatic tissue.[73,74] Today, these procedures are not performed very frequently because of often poor long-term outcome in terms of persisting pain relief and only a few patients showing the morphologic features required (diffuse enlargement of the pancreatic duct > 7 mm, no accompanying mass-forming fibrosis); however, in pediatric CP patients, they still have a certain impact.[76,77]

Surgical pseudocyst drainage after failure of endoscopic treatment is feasible and a cystojejunostomy can be performed with a high success rate (see Chapter 56). This procedure, however, is required only infrequently because the majority of pseudocysts either resolve spontaneously or can be treated endoscopically (i.e., by transgastric drainage).[57] Only in symptomatic and complicated pseudocysts (pain or gastrointestinal discomfort caused by compression of the stomach, duodenum, or the proximal small bowel), which are not suitable or already treated with endoscopic approaches, is surgery indicated. Surgical pseudocyst-jejunostomy can be performed with an open, laparoscopic, or robotic approach. The draining site should be located at the most caudal point of the cyst to ensure optimal drainage. Regarding this goal, the lesser sac is opened, and the anterior aspect of the cyst is exposed after releasing inflammatory adhesions of the posterior wall of the stomach. Many pseudocysts extend toward the transverse mesocolon and should consecutively be drained using a transmesocolic approach. To confirm cyst location, an intraoperative puncture of the cyst can be performed with an injection needle and the most caudally located point of the cysts can be defined. The wall of the cyst is afterwards incised liberally, and fluid and solid material is evacuated. A side-to-side cystojejunostomy is performed after transection of the jejunum approximately 40 cm distal to the ligament of Treitz, and continuity of the bowel is afterwards restored by a Roux-Y reconstruction (see Fig. 58.2B). Results after surgical pseudocyst-jejunostomy show a long-term success rate of approximately 90%, and surgical morbidity and mortality are very low.[57,58]

Resection Procedures

In contrast to drainage alone, resection offers the advantage that a large portion of the fibrosclerotic and calcified tissue can be removed in combination with the restoration of free drainage of the pancreatic and, when required, bile duct. If patients undergo a resection procedure early in their disease history, this provides a causal and symptomatic therapy as the obstructive tissue is removed and the otherwise ongoing process of neuroimmunologic changes previously described is broken.[11,12] In most patients, CP-associated morphologic changes, such as inflammatory tumor, fibrosis, and calcification, are pronounced on the region of the pancreatic head, causing an obstruction of the pancreatic and possibly bile duct. Different types of pancreatic head resections are suitable for these patients that are superior to drainage procedures alone.

Historical approaches in CP surgery included total pancreatoduodenectomy for pain relief as described by Allan Whipple

in the 1940s.[78] Later, pancreaticoduodenectomy (PD) has been the most common procedure for CP patients,[79] with the typical finding of an inflammatory pancreatic head mass (Fig. 58.3A). The potential advantage of PD is the removal of the entire head of the gland, which implies that the pancreatic and bile ducts are opened and drainage is restored while the body and tail of the pancreas are not resected, implying some functional preservation. The potential disadvantages of PD in CP are the relatively great loss of tissue by removal of the entire head and the possible difficulties to perform this resection with regard to the inflammatory changes in the surrounding tissue of the pancreatic head. Especially dissection along the portal vein and tunneling the pancreas before transection of the pancreatic neck is often challenging, and accidental injuries of the mesenteric-portal vein can be associated with a considerable blood loss and may even prohibit performance of PD.

Based on these experiences, and the fact that CP resections do not have to follow principles of oncologic surgery, other techniques of pancreatic head resection have been developed in CP surgery since the 1970s.[80] All of them are summarized under the terminology of duodenum-preserving pancreatic head resection (DPPHR) although variations in the extent of resection characterize the different modifications of DPPHR. The common features of all DPPHR modifications are the partial resection of the pancreatic head and the preservation of the physiologic gastroduodenal passage. The original method introduced by Beger in 1972 consists of a transection of the pancreas on the portomesenteric axis to open the pancreatic duct toward the body and tail of the gland and an excavation of the fibrotic tissue in the pancreatic head under preservation of the duodenum and a dorsal tissue layer in the area of the head.[80,81] During the operation, the bile duct can be opened longitudinally on its ventral aspect, especially in the case of preoperative cholestasis, to ensure free bile drainage into the excavation cavity. Continuity is restored with a two-step anastomosis of a transected jejunal loop: terminal-lateral pancreatojejunostomy towards the pancreatic body—similar to reconstruction in PD—and an additional side-to-side pancreatojejunostomy using the same jejunal

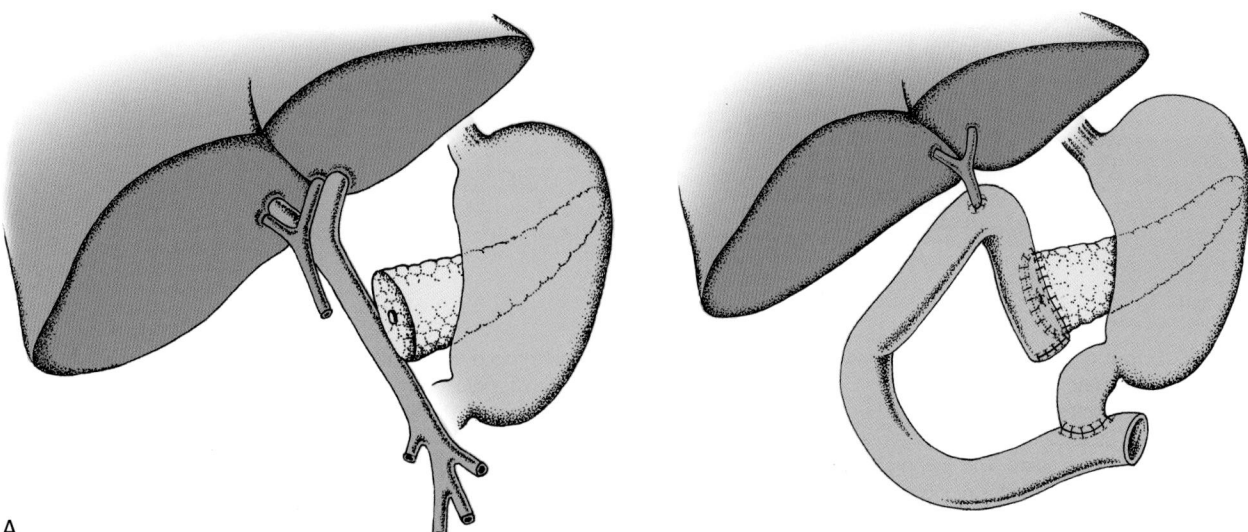

A

FIGURE 58.3 **Techniques of pancreatic head resection for chronic pancreatitis.** Resections are shown on the left, reconstructions on the right side. **A,** Partial pancreatoduodenectomy (here shown as a pylorus-preserving procedure). The pancreatic head and duodenum are removed. The reconstruction is performed by a pancreaticojejunostomy, hepaticojejunostomy, and a duodenojejunostomy (if pylorus preserving).

Continued

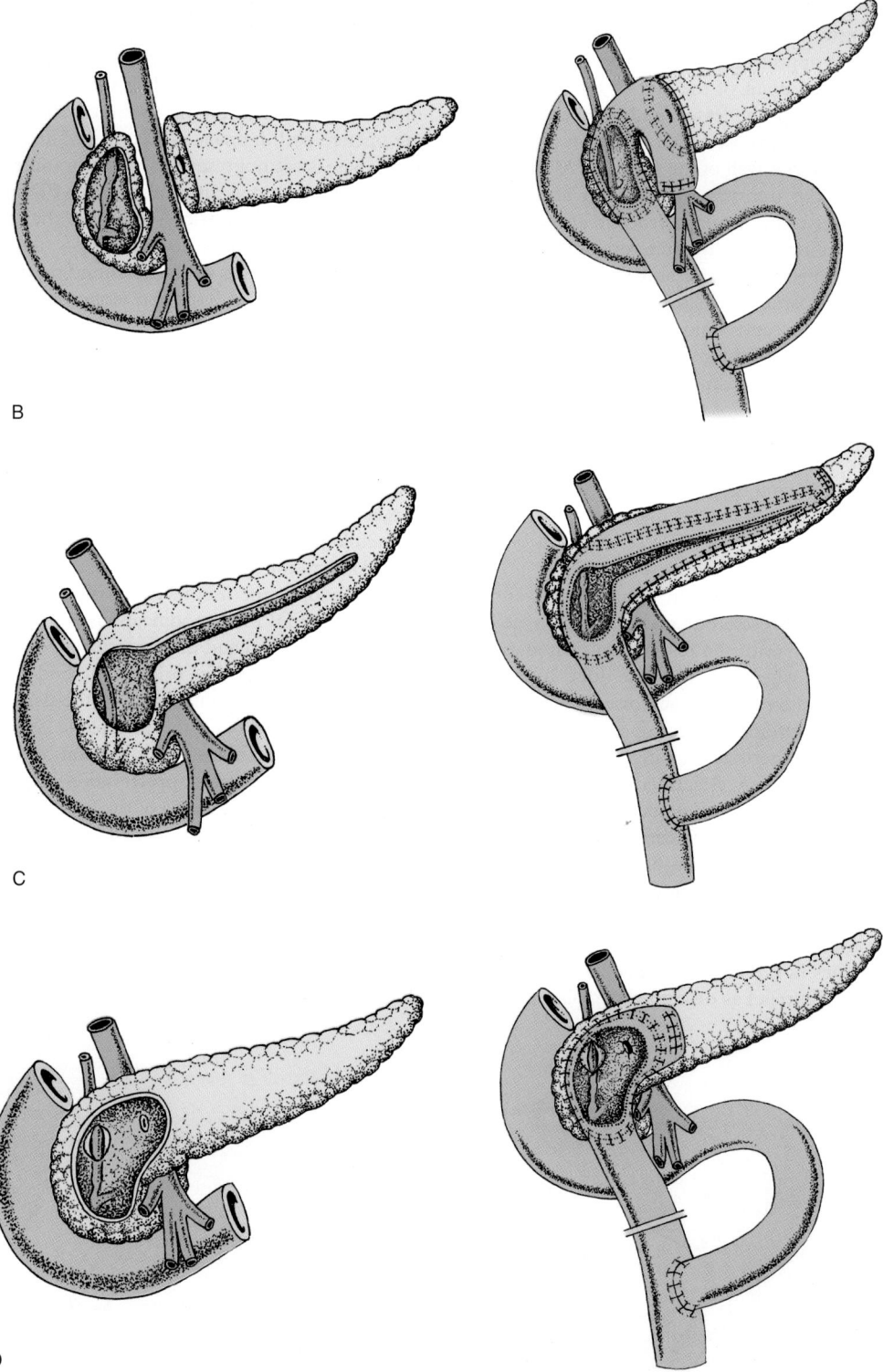

FIGURE 58.3, cont'd   B, Duodenum-preserving pancreatic head resection: Beger procedure. The pancreas is dissected on the level of the portal vein. The pancreatic head is excavated, and the duodenum is preserved with a thin layer of pancreatic tissue. If the bile duct is obstructed, it can be opened, and an internal anastomosis with the excavated pancreatic head can be performed (not shown). The reconstruction is performed with a Roux-en-Y jejunal loop including two anastomoses, one to the pancreatic tail remnant and one to the excavated pancreatic head. **C,** Duodenum-preserving pancreatic head resection: Frey procedure. The Frey procedure combines a circumscript excision in the pancreatic head with longitudinal dissection of the pancreatic duct toward the tail. Reconstruction is performed with an anastomosis to a Roux-en-Y jejunal loop. Compared with the Beger procedure, the extent of pancreatic head resection is less; however, reconstruction is easier because it only requires one anastomosis to the pancreas. **D,** Duodenum-preserving pancreatic head resection: Bern modification. The Bern modification is a technical simplification of the Beger procedure. The extent of resection of the pancreatic head is comparable to the Beger procedure. Nevertheless, the pancreas is not dissected on the level of the portal vein. Thus reconstruction can be performed with one single anastomosis of the pancreas to a Roux-en-Y jejunal loop. The bile duct may be opened if necessary, with an internal anastomosis to the loop (as demonstrated). The pancreatic duct toward the tail has to be probed to rule out distal stenosis.

loop to cover the excavation cavity in the pancreatic head. Intestinal passage is restored by a Roux-en-Y reconstruction of the transected efferent loop and the corresponding afferent loop (see Fig. 58.3B). Low morbidity and mortality rates have been shown for the Beger modification of DPPHR in experienced centers; however, the transection of the pancreatic neck on the portal-mesenteric venous axis, which is required, is occasionally very difficult because of the inflammatory changes around the vessel. Despite this, the efficacy of the Beger procedure with regard to long-term pain relief and good quality of life has been demonstrated in large collectives.[81,82]

The clinical observation that morphologic changes of CP patients in the United States seem to differ compared with European patient collectives led to a modification of the Beger procedure in the 1980s, although the distinct reasons for these differences remain unclear. In the United States, many CP patients present with a less pronounced pancreatic head mass but more extended fibrosclerotic tissue changes toward the tail of the pancreas.[83] Consequently, the Frey modification of DPPHR has been introduced to address these specific findings. It describes a smaller excavation of the pancreatic head and a longitudinal opening of the main pancreatic duct toward the tail of the gland without transecting the pancreatic neck above the portal vein, comparable with a Partington-Rochelle drainage operation. Reconstruction is performed by a single side-to-side anastomosis of a transected jejunal loop and Roux-en-Y reconstruction as previously described (see Fig. 58.3C).[84]

The third type of DPPHR is the Berne modification, which was introduced in the late 1990s.[85] This procedure combines aspects of both techniques previously described. The pancreatic head is resected without transection of the pancreas above the portal vein under preservation of the dorsal parenchyma layer and the duodenum. The main pancreatic duct and, if necessary, bile duct are widely opened during the resection but the pancreatic duct does not necessarily need to be opened too far to the left side of the portal vein axis as soon as free drainage is achieved. This procedure offers the advantage of a tissue-sparing resection and is often technically easier to perform than PD or the Beger procedure because the preparation of the portal vein and tunneling of the pancreas is not required (see Fig. 58.3D). Especially in case of severe chronic peripancreatic inflammation and portal hypertension or venous collaterals, uncontrolled vessel injury and severe bleeding can be prevented by this procedure.

An extensive DPPHR procedure with an excavation of the entire pancreatic head, body, and tail has been developed by the Liverpool group for patients with end-stage fibrosclerotic morphologic changes affecting the entire pancreas, including a duodenum-and spleen-preserving near-total pancreatectomy.[86] A large number of studies have investigated the efficacy of the different modifications of DPPHR and compared these approaches with PD in mainly observational studies or smaller single-center RCTs.[87–96]

Basically, all DPPHR and PD procedures are comparable with respect to surgical morbidity and mortality, which is low (10%–15% and 0%–2%, respectively), mainly because of the low risk for postoperative pancreatic fistula in CP. Regarding long-term outcomes, a high level of pain control is achieved, with a 70% to 90% proportion of patients who are pain-free and a major improvement in quality of life in up to 80%, which is associated with occupational rehabilitation in 70% to 80% of patients. These results underline the general superiority of resectional procedures for CP therapy, regardless of whether DPPHR or PD is the chosen approach.

Important differences between DPPHR modifications and PD have been reported for operative outcome parameters. DPPHR as the less invasive procedure was considered to be superior in terms of blood loss, need for transfusion, and operation time and therefore was regarded as the procedure of choice in any CP patient undergoing surgery for symptoms caused by the typical findings of an inflammatory head mass with fibrosis and calcifications.[87–96]

To evaluate this hypothesis with a high level of evidence, DPPHR and PD were compared in the multicenter CHROPAC RCT.[97,98] Including a total number of 226 patients (DPPHR $n = 115$, PD $n = 111$), quality of life after 24 months was analyzed as the primary endpoint, as well as other perioperative outcome parameters. Operation time was the only surgical parameter that was significantly different (DPPHR < PD), whereas all short-term outcomes were similar in both groups. After 24 months, DPPHR and PD resulted in a similar quality of life; however, DPPHR patients underwent rehospitalization for CP-associated problems significantly more often (27% vs. 11%). These results show that the presumed superiority of DPPHR as seen in many single-center series could not be reproduced in a multicenter setting and that consequently PD should be the standard procedure because it offers the more definitive surgical treatment (Fig. 58.4).[98] Despite this, DPPHR represents an alternative procedure that is especially important in CP patients who show portal venous hypertension and collateralization that may make performance of a standard PD technically impossible (Fig. 58.5), which was observed in 12% of all patients included in the CHROPAC trial.

Less frequently, CP shows its main morphologic manifestation in the body or tail of the pancreas alone. In this situation, fibrosis, calcifications, and pseudocysts are the most important findings predominantly located on the left side of the portal vein axis. Besides alcoholic or idiopathic CP, this situation can be caused by blunt abdominal trauma and subclinical pancreatic contusion in the area of the pancreatic neck and body by compression or stretching because of the inflexible position in

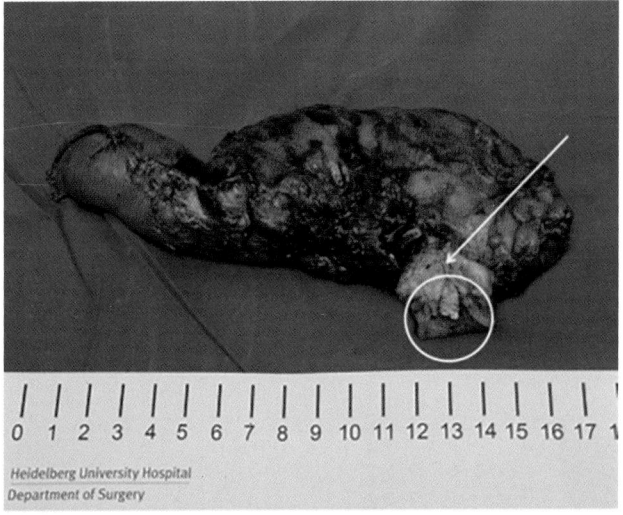

FIGURE 58.4 Resection specimen after pancreaticoduodenectomy *(PD)* showing the duodenum and pancreatic head with fibroic stenosis in the pancreatic neck area *(white arrow)* and consecutive dilation with intraductal concrements *(white circle)*.

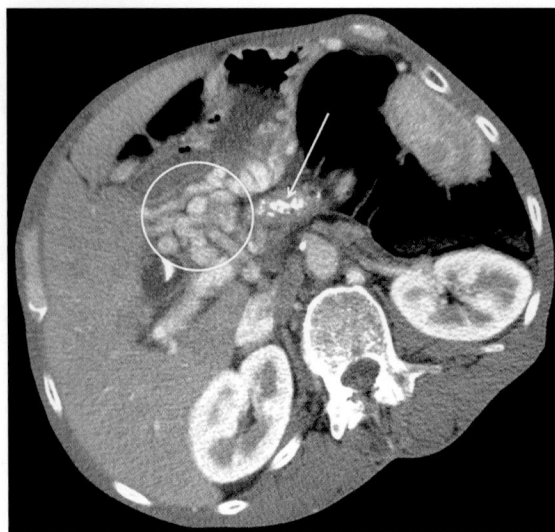

FIGURE 58.5 Computed tomography *(CT)* scan (axial reformatting, porto-venous phase) showing chronic pancreatitis *(CP)* with massive intraductal calcifications *(white arrow)* and complete cavernous transformation of the portal vein *(white circle)* making pancreaticoduodenectomy *(PD)* technically impossible.

front of the spinal column. Depending on the localization of the pathology, distal pancreatectomy can be performed. The pancreas is divided above the mesenteric-portal vein axis, most commonly by stapler or scalpel with sutures, and the pancreatic body tail is removed toward the left side. Principally, this procedure can be performed without splenectomy either under preservation of the splenic vessels or, in the case of strong inflammatory adhesion, with resection of the splenic artery and vein, even if the spleen is not removed (Warshaw procedure).[99]

In many CP patients, however, the spleen is removed during distal pancreatectomy because of inflammatory adhesions around the splenic vessels, the pancreatic tail, and the splenic hilum or for bleeding control in case of venous collaterals if the splenic vein is obstructed because of chronic inflammatory alterations (Fig. 58.6). If the spleen is preserved, the development of left-sided portal hypertension is a postoperative complication in the long-term follow-up because the splenic vein

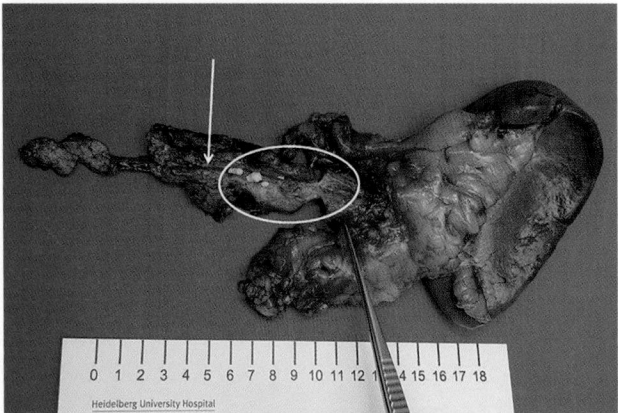

FIGURE 58.6 Resection specimen after distal pancreatectomy and splenectomy for chronic pancreatitis (CP). Fibrotic stenosis in the body of the pancreas *(white arrow)* with consecutive dilation of the pancreatic duct and multiple intraductal concrements *(white circle)*.

may show thrombosis, resulting in the development of gastric varices and upper gastrointestinal bleeding.[100]

The most important postoperative complication after distal pancreatectomy is the occurrence of a pancreatic fistula, which is observed in approximately 30% of all patients, regardless of synchronous splenectomy. This clinical problem remains unsolved, and no technical modifications regarding parenchyma transection of the pancreas or stump closure have shown any superiority for fistula prevention. The most common techniques of stapler transection and closure or scalpel transection with suture closure remain equivalent, which has been confirmed by RCTs and meta-analyses.[101,102] Adding any type of autologous patch covering of the pancreatic stump may be beneficial; however, fistula rates are still unsatisfying.[103] A history of CP has been controversially described as a patient-related risk factor for postoperative fistula development but could not be confirmed in a recent meta-analysis.[104] The risk of new-onset insulin-dependent DM after distal pancreatectomy correlates with the amount of removed tissue and the preoperative endocrine function. Although in distal pancreatectomy for other indications, this risk is approximately 15%, it increases to 40% in CP patients.[105] Therefore the amount of resected tissue should, whenever possible, not exceed 40% to 50% of the gland.

Total Pancreatectomy with Islet Cell Autotransplantation

Total pancreatectomy with islet autotransplantation (TPIAT) was reported in 1978, driven by the concept that complete removal of the pancreas leads to complete relief of intractable pain in CP and islet cell autotransplantation can avoid brittle DM in the respective patients.[106] After initial experiences in adult patients, the indication for TPIAT was extended to pediatric CP patients and favorable outcomes in terms of reduced opioid medication and improved quality of life have been observed.[107-110] TPIAT requires a high level of surgical expertise as well as the facilities and multidisciplinary knowledge for islet cell preparation and autotransplantation. Today, TPIAT is performed in centers in the United States, Europe, and Australia, with reasonable results showing that the risk of TPIAT has to be carefully weighed against other treatment options in CP, especially as other surgical procedures, exocrine and endocrine medical management, and pain therapy have considerably improved over the decades.

The procedure of TPIAT consists of total (potentially spleen-preserving) pancreatectomy, harvesting and purification of the islet cells, and reinfusion of the resulting suspension into the liver, either unselectively via the splenic vein stump or selectively to the left liver lobe via a more centrally placed catheter in the left portal vein.[107,108] The islet cells can take up function immediately after the operation.

Outcomes of TPIAT show an overall improvement in quality of life in 90% of patients after 2 years and 85% after 5 years, respectively. Especially in children, complete pain relief is reported in 95% to 100% of cases, making TPIAT in pediatric patients an extremely beneficial procedure. In adult patients, pain relief with opioid independency is achieved in approximately 50% in the long-term course, depending on the underlying etiology of CP, with alcoholic CP resulting in worse outcomes than CP of other causes.[111,112]

After TPIAT, complete insulin independency is achieved in only one third of patients because the function of the isolated and transplanted islet cells is often compromised in the long-term course. Even if insulin independency is not reached in the remaining patients, TPIAT can still lead to reduced dosages of insulin and improved glycemic control compared with brittle DM with absolute insulin deficiency.[111] The timing and patient selection for TPIAT remains challenging and no high-level evidence is available comparing TPIAT with other surgical procedures in CP in terms of pain relief and endocrine function. Based on expert consensus statements, outcomes of TPIAT seem to be favorable, especially in younger CP patients without morphologic end-stage features of pancreatic parenchyma destruction or endocrine insufficiency. To achieve complete pain relief—the only indication for TPIAT—patients should be chosen for this procedure before reaching a stage of long-standing opioid intake to avoid autonomous pain remodeling processes with stimulus-independent neuropathic pain generation.[112] The International (IAP/APA/JPS/EPC) Consensus Guidelines have emphasized that patient selection for TPIAT remains a major challenge and that adults with CP who have end-stage disease with exocrine and complete endocrine failure are not suitable for it if there are few or no functioning islets present.[112]

Minimally Invasive and Robotic Surgery

Surgery for CP can be performed using a minimally invasive approach that includes both laparoscopic and robotic techniques. For standard resections (i.e., partial pancreatoduodenectomy, distal pancreatectomy), these procedures are carried out similarly to those for other indications; however, the inflammatory changes, especially within the retroperitoneal margins or around the portal vein, can be challenging Also, portal hypertension with collateral circulation may limit successful minimally invasive resection and require conversion to open surgery.[113–115] Patients who need drainage procedures (pseudocyst-jejunostomy or lateral pancreatojejunostomy) may also be considered for minimally invasive approaches.[116–117] CP-specific resections, such as DPPHR, have been reported by robotic approaches.[118,119] These results show the principal feasibility of minimally invasive surgery in CP in experienced centers; however, no RCTs have addressed this topic to date

and potential advantages compared with standard open surgery remain speculative.

CONCLUSIONS

The adequate and tailored therapy for CP is adjusted to the symptoms of the patient, the stage of disease, and the morphology of pathologic changes of the pancreas. Conservative therapy is the basis of treatment for all patients and includes pain medication, abstinence from alcohol and smoking, and enzyme supplementation. These basic steps must also be a part of endoscopic and surgical therapies. Endoscopy seems to be effective as an initial approach, showing good results in pseudocyst drainage or ductal stenosis without calcifications. Endoscopic treatment often requires frequent re-interventions and should be limited to a maximum time frame of 1 year. Especially in calcifying CP, surgery should be considered early to achieve good long-term results. Surgical procedures in CP patients can be carried out with low postoperative morbidity and very low mortality rates. The procedure-specific features should be defined and reported according to a recent ISGPS consensus on reporting standards in CP.[120] Long-term outcome shows that pain control and even complete absence of pain as the major aim of CP therapy is achieved in 4 out of 5 patients and scales of physiologic, emotional, and social functioning show rates that are nearly comparable with those of the normal population. The progression of exocrine and endocrine failure during the natural course of CP can be prolonged or even stopped, especially if surgery is performed in an early disease stage as soon as morphologic changes are visible. Persistent chronic risk factor exposition (especially ongoing alcohol consumption) is associated with progression of the disease and consequently represents the major determinant of long-term mortality in CP patients.

The references for this chapter can be found online by accessing the accompanying Expert Consult website.

SECTION II. Neoplastic

A. General

CHAPTER 59

Tumors of the Pancreas and Ampulla

Laura H. Tang, MD, PhD, and Christine E. Orr, MD, FRCPC

TUMORS OF THE PANCREATIC DUCT OR DUCTAL-RELATED ORIGIN

Pancreatic Intraepithelial Neoplasia

Pancreatic intraepithelial neoplasia (PanIN) is a noninvasive lesion confined to the pancreatic ducts and observed only microscopically (<0.5 cm). The mucin-containing duct epithelium exhibits a spectrum of architectural and cytologic atypia, which is designated as low-grade (PanIN-1 and PanIN-2) or high-grade dysplasia (PanIN-3). Low-grade PanIN may be associated with age, obesity, and diabetes mellitus (DM); it can be found in more than 50% of people older than 50 years of age. Molecular and genomic studies have indicated that high-grade PanIN is the key precursor of pancreatic ductal (PD) adenocarcinoma[1-3]; thus it is staged carcinoma in situ.

Pathologic Features

Low-grade PanIN lesions have flat or mildly papillated and polarized mucinous epithelium, which reveal mild to moderate nuclear atypia (Fig. 59.1A–B). High-grade PanIN lesions exhibit increased architectural complexity with prominent epithelial papillation, cribriforming, budding micropapillae, loss of cellular polarity, marked cytologic atypia with nuclear pleomorphism, and frequent mitosis (see Fig. 59.1C). The biomarker expression in high-grade PanIN usually mirrors that of ductal adenocarcinoma with positive immunoreactivity to mucin 1 (MUC1) and abnormal expression of carcinoembryonic antigen (CEA).

The presence of high-grade PanIN is virtually indicative of invasive adenocarcinoma in the pancreas. When PanIN-3 is identified in the absence of established invasive adenocarcinoma, it is prudent to re-examine the specimen thoroughly to exclude any occult or overlooked early-stage adenocarcinoma. When high-grade PanIN is present at the resection margin, it is considered to be a microscopically positive margin (R1).

Molecular Biology and Genetics

Most PanINs, including both high- and low-grade lesions, harbor *KRAS* mutations, with significantly increased clonality in high-grade PanINs.[2] High-grade PanIN shares some genetic abnormalities with invasive ductal adenocarcinoma, including biallelic inactivation of *CDKN2A* (p16) and a wide spectrum of clonal copy number changes but lacks *TP53* and *SMAD4*

mutations, which are commonly seen in invasive ductal adenocarcinoma[1,4] (see Chapter 9D).

Ductal Adenocarcinoma and the Variants

Pancreatic ductal adenocarcinoma (PDAC) is an aggressive malignant epithelial neoplasm derived from the pancreatic duct and has predominant glandular/tubular differentiation with or without mucin production. The less common variants include adenosquamous carcinoma, neuroendocrine carcinoma (NEC; small-cell or large-cell type), colloid carcinoma, anaplastic undifferentiated carcinoma, sarcomatoid undifferentiated carcinoma, undifferentiated carcinoma with osteoclastic giant cells, medullary carcinoma, hepatoid carcinoma, signet ring cell carcinoma, and mixed ductal and nonductal carcinoma.[5,6]

Epidemiology and Clinical Features

PDAC is the most common neoplasm of the pancreas (>90%). Most cases of PDAC are sporadic, but about 10% of cases have a documented familial history of the disease,[5] in which a deleterious germline mutation has been identified in 10% to 20% of patients. Adenocarcinoma is more commonly located in the head of the pancreas (two thirds) than in the distal portion of the gland. Although extremely rare, it can also occur in pancreatic heterotopia present in the upper gastrointestinal (GI) tract.[7] The median age at diagnosis for PDAC is approximately 70 years. The most common clinical presentation is unexplained weight loss, back pain, jaundice, decreased appetite, and new-onset DM. Rare symptoms include migratory thrombophlebitis and acute pancreatitis (AP).

PDAC is usually diagnosed when an infiltrative solid mass is detected by computed tomography (CT) scans with multiphase-dynamic contrast or by magnetic resonance imaging (MRI). Endoscopic ultrasound (EUS) can facilitate sampling of the mass or lymph node for definitive diagnosis. Serum biomarker CEA and CA 19-9 may be elevated (see Chapter 17).

The prognosis of PDAC remains poor for most patients with an overall 5-year survival of less than 10%.[5] The most effective treatment is complete surgical resection of the tumor and adjuvant systemic therapy with a corresponding 5-year survival of about 12% to 20%, but, unfortunately, this modality is only possible in approximately 20% of patients at the time of diagnosis (see Chapter 62). Neoadjuvant therapy may improve

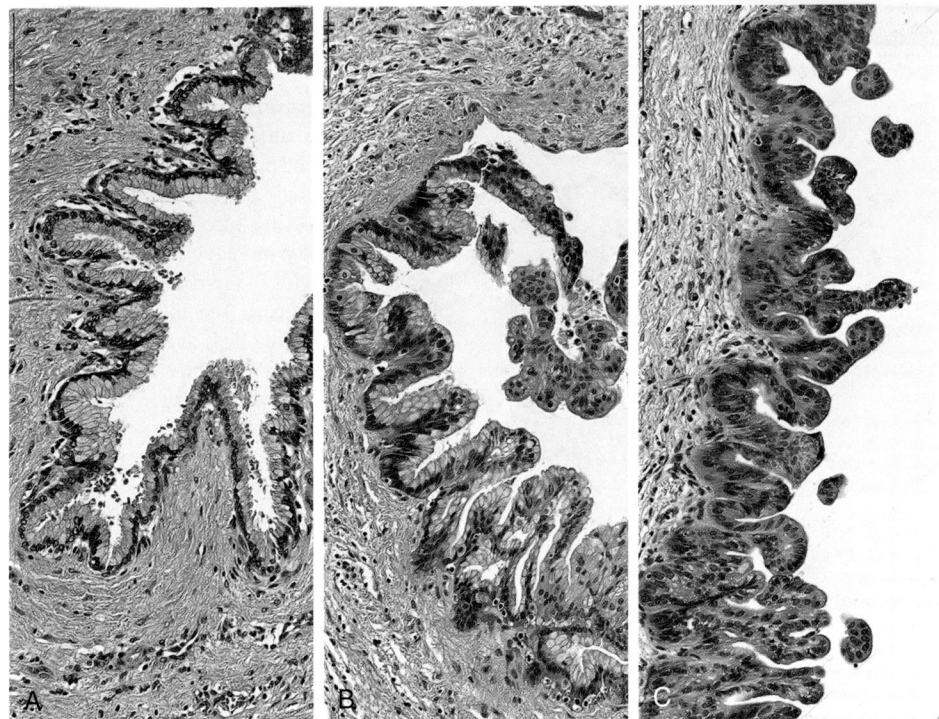

FIGURE 59.1   Pancreatic intraepithelial neoplasia (PanIN).   A, Low-grade PanIN-1 with small and basally oriented nuclei and flat to minimally papillated mucinous epithelium. **B,** Low-grade PanIN-2 with mildly enlarged and basally oriented nuclei and increased papillary architecture. **C,** High-grade PanIN-3 with marked cytologic atypia, loss of nuclear polarity, and increased architectural complexity.

surgical resectability and survival of PDAC patients in some cases.[8] Patients with untreated PDAC, or with metastatic disease, have a mean survival of less than 6 months.

Pathologic Features

The macroscopic appearance of PDAC is a solid firm mass with an irregular contour. The mean size of lesions amenable to resection is roughly 3.5 cm, although tumors located in the distal pancreas are usually larger. Focal cystic changes may be observed distal to the tumor secondary to obstruction of pancreatic ducts. Obstruction of the common bile duct (CBD) and the main pancreatic duct is common when the tumor is located in the head of the pancreas (Fig. 59.2). The tumor may grossly infiltrate the ampulla, duodenal wall, superior mesenteric vein, or uncinate process and retroperitoneum.

CONVENTIONAL DUCTAL ADENOCARCINOMA. Microscopically, most PDAC has gland formation but exhibits significant heterogeneity in an histologic pattern with distorted glands/tubules of varying sizes and shapes. Large glands may have a cribriform and papillary pattern, and the small units may reveal incomplete gland/tubular structure or single cell–infiltrating pattern (Fig. 59.3A). Both intracellular and extracellular mucin are common within the tumor. A desmoplastic reaction surrounding the malignant epithelium is typical in PDAC, although, in some cases, the tumor stroma may appear hypocellular with dense and pink collagen. The epithelium in PDAC can be either columnar or cuboidal with considerable nuclear pleomorphism. The nuclear membrane of the neoplastic cells is irregular and has a smudged appearance. Better differentiated PDAC with well-formed glands usually shows vesicular/foamy intracellular mucin with a condensed and thickened apical border of the

cytoplasmic membrane (see Fig. 59.3B). PDAC metastases to the lung and omentum may present paradoxically with better differentiation and may be diagnostically challenging during the pathologic workup to exclude lung or other potential primary sites (see Fig. 59.3C). Immunohistochemical and molecular studies can facilitate a more definitive diagnosis.

The immunoprofile of conventional PDAC is that of typical pancreatobiliary phenotype, which is not entirely specific, and the workup is usually for a diagnosis of exclusion of adenocarcinoma from other primary sites. The tumor cells of typical PDAC are positive for CK7 and negative for CK20 and CDX2; they express carcinoma biomarkers MUC1, CEA, CA125, and B72.3. PDAC with *DPC4* and *CDKN2A* gene mutations has loss of nuclear SMAD4 and p16 expression, respectively (see Chapter 9D).

ADENOSQUAMOUS CARCINOMA. Although homogenous squamous cell carcinoma of the pancreas is uncommon, varying extents of squamous differentiation can occur in association with conventional ductal adenocarcinoma (Fig. 59.4A). The classification of an adenosquamous carcinoma requires the presence of greater than or equal to 30% squamous component.[5] The pitfall associated with this subtype is that exclusively squamous carcinoma may be present in small biopsies or at the site of metastasis, which would raise the differential diagnosis of a primary squamous cell carcinoma from other sites including the lung—which is a common metastatic site for PDAC.

NEUROENDOCRINE CARCINOMA. Neuroendocrine carcinoma (NEC) of the pancreas is rare and accounts for less than 1% of pancreatic neoplasms. This subtype includes small-cell and large-cell variants (see Fig. 59.4B). It is crucial to recognize that NEC is

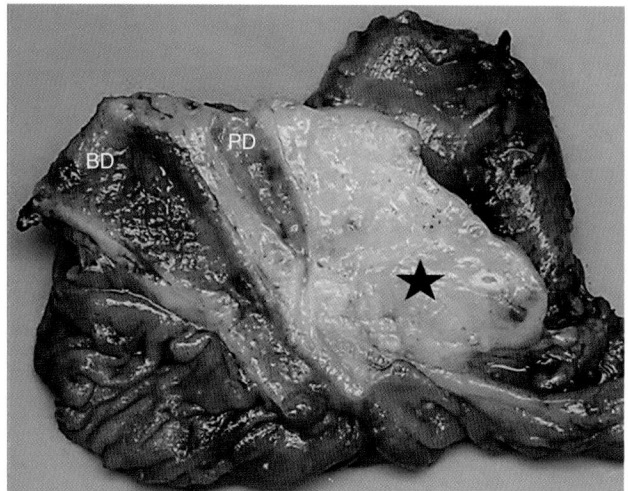

FIGURE 59.2 Macroscopic appearance of pancreatic ductal adenocarcinoma. An example of ductal adenocarcinoma (*) in the head of the pancreas near the uncinate process, which obstructs the pancreatic duct *(PD)* and impinging common bile duct *(CBD)*, causing distal dilatation of both ducts.

clinically, pathologically, and genetically distinct from well-differentiated neuroendocrine tumor (NET) of the pancreas (see Chapter 65). NEC is more akin to PDAC in its pathogenesis, including its commonly observed association with an adenocarcinoma component, and has frequent *TP53* and *RB1* mutations or inactivation of the *RB1/P16* pathway.[9,10] Diagnosis requires the morphologic characteristics of NEC and immunoreactivity for neuroendocrine markers (chromogranin and synaptophysin). The small-cell subtype of NEC has distinctive morphologic features, including nuclear hyperchromasia and molding with minimal

cytoplasm and loss of Rb protein expression in most cases, as evaluated by immunohistochemistry. Carcinoma with partial immunoreactivity for neuroendocrine markers and without typical morphologic features may be considered adenocarcinoma with neuroendocrine differentiation. The diagnosis of large-cell variant NEC can be challenging, particularly in small biopsies, which can reveal morphologic features overlapping with high-grade pancreatic neuroendocrine tumors (PanNET), acinar cell carcinoma, and other solid pancreatic neoplasms. Combining clinicopathologic features with biomarkers and results of genetic tests can facilitate the diagnosis (see the section on PanNET). Pancreatic NECs are inevitably high grade with a proliferative index (Ki67) of greater than 80% for the small-cell subtype and more than 20% for the large-cell subtype.

COLLOID CARCINOMA. This variant of PDAC is usually derived from intestinal type intraductal papillary mucinous neoplasia (IPMN). The defining feature of colloid carcinoma is that at least 80% of the neoplastic epithelium of the tumor is suspended in mucin. The tumor cells can have focal poorly differentiated signet ring cell morphology, although the majority of them are arranged as strips, clusters, or glands that are well to moderately differentiated. The tumor is immunoreactive for CK20, CDX2, and MUC2. Patients with colloid carcinoma have more favorable outcomes than those with conventional PDAC, with a 5-year survival of greater than 55%.[11]

UNDIFFERENTIATED CARCINOMA. Undifferentiated carcinoma of the pancreas lacks a recognizable cell line of differentiation with hypercellularity and a confluent growth pattern. The tumor cells may have partial or complete loss of immunoreactivity for cytokeratin and are usually positive for vimentin. Sarcomatoid carcinoma and carcinosarcoma have a significant component of malignant spindle cells with or without heterologous elements.

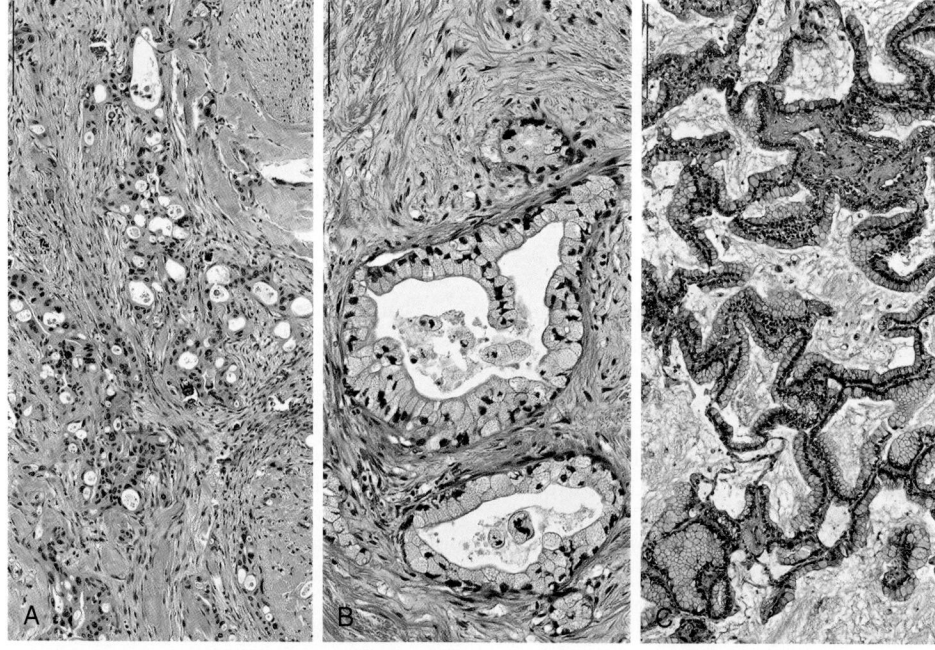

FIGURE 59.3 Microscopic appearance of pancreatic ductal adenocarcinoma (PDAC). **A,** Primary PDAC with histologic and cytologic heterogeneity. **B,** Primary PDAC with foamy intracellular mucin and thickened atypical cytoplasmic membrane. **C,** Metastatic PDAC to lung showing paradoxical better differentiation.

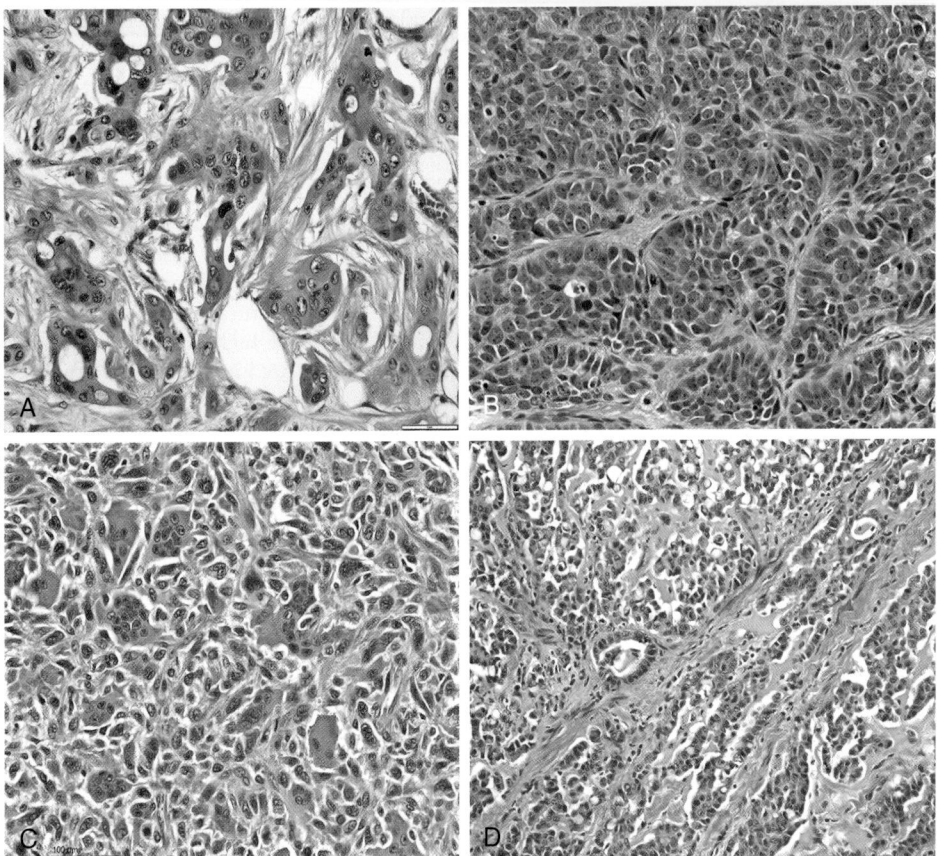

FIGURE 59.4 Variants of pancreatic ductal adenocarcinoma. **A**, Adenosquamous carcinoma. **B**, Neuroendocrine carcinoma, non-small cell type. **C**, Undifferentiated carcinoma with osteoclastic giant cells. **D**, Mixed ductal *(upper left)* and acinar carcinoma *(lower right)*.

Tumors with rhabdoid morphology may be associated with SWI/SNF pathway abnormalities and corresponding loss of nuclear expression of SMARCA2 or SMARCA4 proteins, which are designated as SMARC-deficiency malignancies.[12] Undifferentiated carcinoma with osteoclastic giant cells has loss of epithelial differentiation and is composed of both neoplastic and non-neoplastic mononuclear cells, including osteoclast-like multinucleated giant cells (see Fig. 59.4C), which are immunoreactive to the histiocytic makers CD68 and CD163.

MIXED DUCTAL AND NONDUCTAL CARCINOMA. This entity includes ductal-NEC, ductal-acinar cell carcinoma (see Fig. 59.4D), and the ductal-neuroendocrine-acinar carcinoma combination, which have been discussed in the corresponding sections of acinar cell carcinoma and NEC.

Molecular Biology and Genetics

Somatic genetic drivers of PDAC include oncogenic mutations of *KRAS* (>90%) and mutation or deletion of *TP53* (75%), *SMAD4* (55%), or *CDKN2A* (80%).[13–16] Other less common somatic mutations are found in genes involved in DNA repair and epigenetics, including *PALB2, ATM, CHEK2,* and *RAD51.*[17–19]

Hereditary cases of PDAC are associated with several, well-established susceptibility genes, including *BRCA2, ATM, BRCA1, PALB2, CDKN2A, STK11, PRSS1,* and *SPINK1,* as well as DNA mismatch repair genes.[5] However, the majority of familial aggregations of PDAC have uncertain underlying genetic abnormalities.

Tumors Associated With Cystic Intraductal Neoplasm

This entity includes a group of neoplasms that have a prominent intraductal papillary growth pattern with grossly visible cystic lesions in most cases (>5 mm), which may involve the main pancreatic duct or its accessory branch ducts. Depending on the phenotype of the epithelium, the subtypes of intraductal neoplasm include IPMN, intraductal oncocytic papillary neoplasm (IOPN), and intraductal tubulopapillary neoplasm (ITPN). The neoplastic epithelium can exhibit a spectrum of histologic and cytologic atypia, which is further designated as low-grade or high-grade neoplasm, or invasive carcinoma when stroma invasion is present.

Epidemiology and Clinical Features

Pancreatic intraductal neoplasms can occur in a wide range of age groups but are more common in older adults in their 50s and 60s. Location in the head of the pancreas is more common than in the distal portion of the pancreas and lesions can be multifocal. The most common and better evaluated intraductal neoplasm is IPMN, which can involve (1) the main pancreatic duct with prominent dilation, (2) branch ducts with an isolated cystic lesion but no apparent communication with the main duct, or (3) mixed main-branch duct type. Clinical symptoms associated with intraductal neoplasms are relatively nonspecific and include pain, chronic pancreatitis (CP), DM, and jaundice. In the absence of invasive carcinoma, markers such as CEA and CA19-9 may not be elevated in serum but only in the cyst fluid from aspiration samples.[20–22]

The prognosis of IPMN without invasive carcinoma is favorable, particularly in those cases with branch-duct subtype (5-year survival of >85%). The main-duct subtype is often associated with multifocal lesions, greater risk of high-grade dysplasia and carcinoma, and higher risk of recurrence.[23-25] The prognosis of IPMN with invasive carcinoma depends on the tumor stage and subtype; the 5-year survival ranges from 35% to 90%. Patients with IPMN and associated colloid carcinoma have a significantly better outcome than those with conventual PDAC.[26,27] The subtypes of IOPN and ITPN with invasive carcinoma also appear to have better prognoses, although this observation may not be conclusive given the recent establishment of these pathologic entities and the rarity of the disease.[28,29]

Pathologic Features

INTRADUCTAL PAPILLARY MUCINOUS NEOPLASM (SEE CHAPTER 60). Main-duct IPMN may involve a portion of the duct or the entire duct, including the ampulla where mucin extrusion may be visualized by upper GI endoscopy or endoscopic retrograde cholangiopancreatography (ERCP). The dilated duct is usually filled with mucin and soft papillary projections (Fig. 59.5A). Branch-duct IPMN may lack a visible connection to the main duct and is usually present as multilocular cysts filled with mucin (see Fig. 59.5B). Larger IPMNs (>3 cm) and those with mural nodules or intracystic masses are more likely to harbor high-grade dysplasia or invasive carcinoma.

Microscopically, IPMNs show intraductal proliferation of columnar epithelium with abundant intracellular and extracellular mucin. The neoplasm is categorized as either low- or high-grade dysplasia based on the histologic complexity and cytologic atypia.

Intestinal-type IPMN is commonly associated with main-duct IPMN (Fig. 59.6A). The neoplastic epithelium forms villous papillary architecture and contains tall columnar intestinal-type cells with elongated nuclei and apical intracellular mucin. High-grade dysplasia is commonly observed in this subtype.[30] The neoplastic cells are immunoreactive to CK20, CDX2, and MUC2; they are negative for CK7 and MUC1.

Gastric-type IPMN is often found in branch ducts (see Fig. 59.6B). The lining epithelium has a gastric foveolar phenotype, often with low-grade dysplasia, although high-grade dysplasia and invasive carcinoma can occur as well.[31,32] The neoplastic cells are immunoreactive to CK7 and MUC5AC, and they are negative for CK20, CDX2, MUC2, and MUC1.

Pancreatobiliary-type IPMN usually involves the main pancreatic duct. The neoplastic epithelium has a more complex architecture with anastomosing papillae composed of cuboidal cells with eosinophilic or amphophilic cytoplasm that may or may not contain intracellular mucin. Most pancreatobiliary-type IPMNs have high-grade dysplasia within the lesion. The neoplastic cells are immunoreactive to CK7, MUC1, and MUC5AC; they are negative for CK20, CDX2, and MUC2.

Adenocarcinoma arising in IPMN can be either of the colloid type (see Fig. 59.6A) or conventional PDAC type. The former is associated with intestinal-type IPMN, and the latter is commonly associated with pancreatobiliary-type or gastric-type IPMN. It is important to emphasize that thorough examination and adequate sampling are crucial to identify occult carcinoma within IPMNs, particularly in large lesions or cysts with complex architecture.

INTRADUCTAL ONCOCYTIC PAPILLARY NEOPLASM. IOPN is considered a variant of intraductal cystic papillary neoplasm but IOPN has some unique pathologic and molecular characteristics. IOPN has an exophytic growth pattern with friable papillary projections into the dilated pancreatic ducts. Histologically, the neoplastic epithelium forms back-to-back papillary or cribriform complexes, which are lined by multilayered columnar cells with characteristic eosinophilic (oncocytic) and granular cytoplasm (see Fig. 59.6C). Focal mucin containing neoplastic epithelium can also be observed in IOPN. The oncocytic neoplastic cells are positive for MUC1, MUC6, and hepatocyte antigen (Heppar-1), and the mucin-containing goblet cells are positive for MUC2 and MUC5AC.

INTRADUCTAL TUBULOPAPILLARY NEOPLASM. ITPN is the least common pancreatic intraductal neoplasm and exhibits a predominant tubule-forming neoplasia with PD epithelial phenotype but a lack of mucin production. Macroscopically, the tumor has a more solid, less cystic appearance, and intraductal growth may be difficult to recognize. Microscopically, the tubules are tightly packed and form cribriform-appearing nests of varying sizes (see Fig. 59.6D). The tumor cells are cuboidal in shape and have scant eosinophilic or amphophilic cytoplasm. Foci of necrosis and high-grade dysplasia are common in ITPN. Invasive carcinoma has been identified in 70% of reported cases.[28,29] The neoplastic cells are immunoreactive to CK7, MUC1, and MUC6; they are negative for MUC2 and MUC5AC.

Molecular Biology and Genetics

Somatic mutations of *KRAS* and *GNAS* are identified in 60% to 80% and 50% to 70% of IPMN cases, respectively, particularly the intestinal phenotype.[33,34] *RNF43* mutations have been found in approximately 50% of IPMN cases.[33,35] Although *KRAS* mutation is also common in PDAC, *GNAS* mutation appears to be unique to IPMN (see Chapter 9D).

There are no defining genomic alterations in most IOPN and ITPN cases, which may be because of the rarity of these entities. Recurrent mutations of *ERBB4*, *ARHGAP26*, *ASXL1*, and

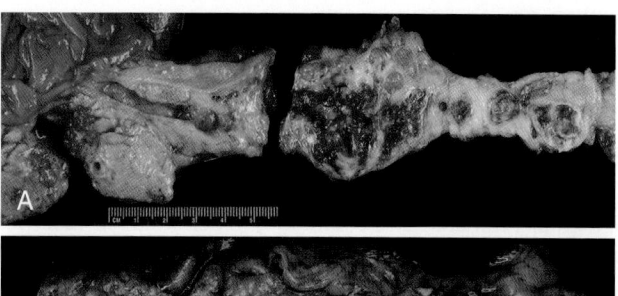
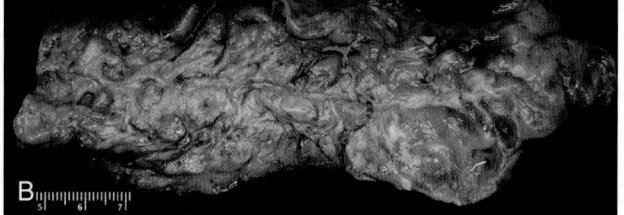

FIGURE 59.5 Macroscopic appearance of intraductal papillary mucinous neoplasm (IPMN). **A,** Total pancreatectomy *(head left, tail right)* with multifocal IMPN involving the entire main duct. **B,** Distal pancreatectomy with mixed main-duct and branch-duct IPMN.

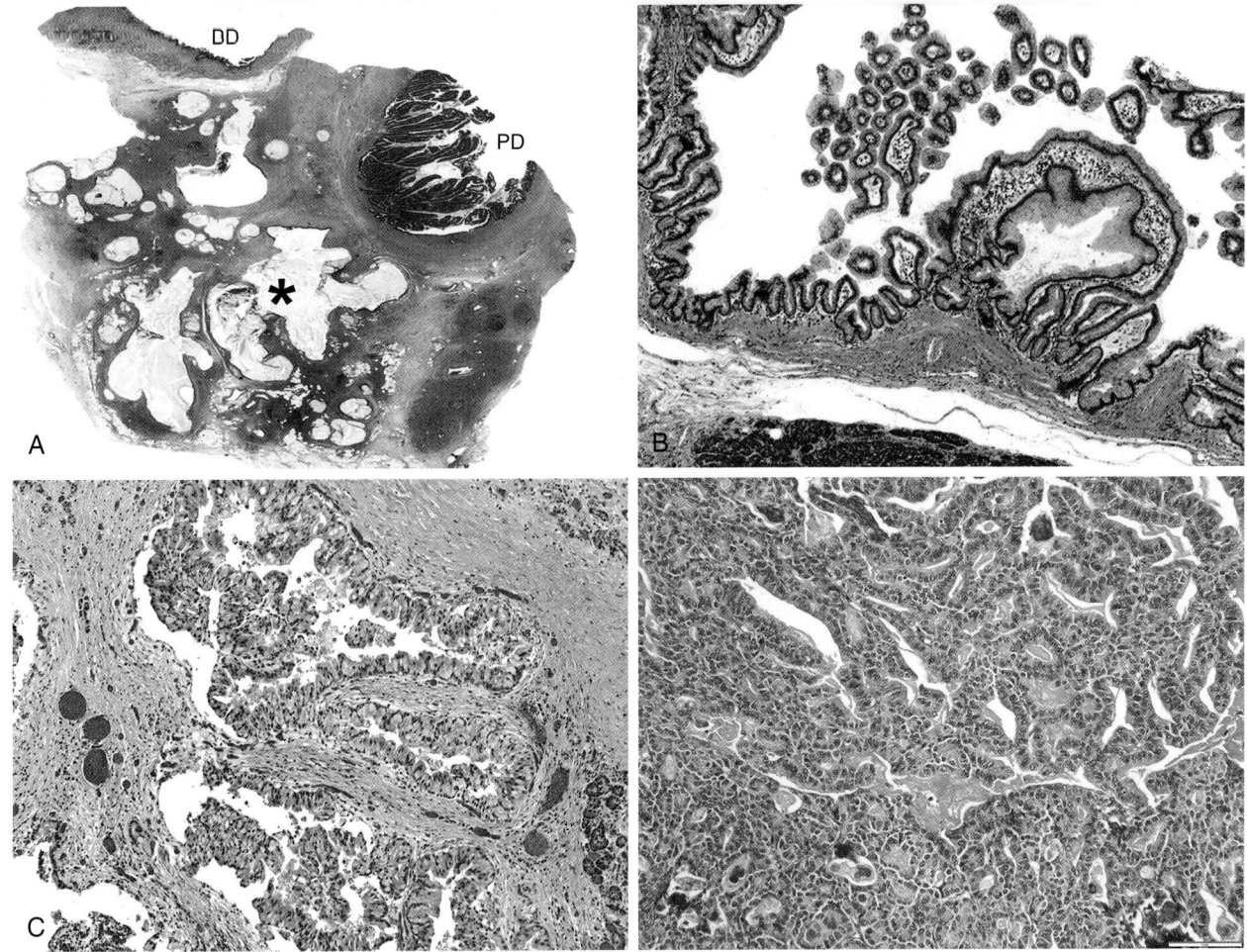

FIGURE 59.6 Histopathology of intraductal papillary mucinous neoplasm (IPMN) and variants. **A**, Intestinal-type IPMN present in main pancreatic duct *(PD)* with associated invasive colloid carcinoma (*); common bile duct *(CBD)* is not involved by tumor. **B**, Gastric-type IPMN with foveolar-type epithelium. **C**, Intraductal oncocytic papillary neoplasm *(IOPN)* with a papillary growth pattern and eosinophilic/oncocytic cytoplasm. **D**, Intraductal tubulopapillary neoplasm *(ITPN)* with complex tubular and cribriform pattern and lack of intracellular mucin.

EPHA8 have been identified in some IOPN cases.[36] ITPN has been reported to have alterations in certain chromatin remodeling genes, such as *MLL1-3, BAP1,* and PI3K pathway genes.[37]

Mucinous Cystic Neoplasm

Mucinous cystic neoplasms (MCN) are cystic lesions of the pancreas lined by mucin-producing neoplastic epithelium, which can exhibit low-grade to high-grade dysplasia (see Chapter 60). Noninvasive MCN is synonymous with mucinous cystadenoma, whereas in the presence of invasion, it is designated as mucinous cystadenocarcinoma.

Epidemiology and Clinical Features

MCN occurs almost exclusively in women (>98%) and the mean onset age is 48 years. Patients with mucinous cystadenocarcinoma are 5 to 10 years older on average than those with mucinous cystadenoma at the time of diagnosis, suggesting a potential malignant progression from mucinous cystadenoma carcinoma.[38] The majority of the tumors are located in the body and tail of the pancreas (>98%). Radiographically, MCNs present as thick-walled cystic lesions without communication with the pancreatic ducts. Cystic fluid from preoperative aspiration shows elevated CEA levels, which can help to distinguish MCNs from nonmucinous cystic lesions, such as serous cystadenoma, cystic neuroendocrine tumor, and solid pseudopapillary neoplasm.[22]

The prognosis for noninvasive MCN is favorable with a 5-year survival of 100%. The outcome for patients with invasive mucinous cystadenocarcinoma depends on the pathologic stage (i.e., tumor size and metastatic status), with an estimated 5-year survival of 26%.[39]

Pathologic Features

The median diameter of MCN is approximately 6 cm. The cyst wall is fibrotic and may have peripheral calcifications that have been termed "egg-shell calcifications." MCNs with invasive carcinoma are reportedly larger.[39] The cyst lining is relatively smooth in low-grade MCNs (Fig. 59.7A), whereas irregularities, such as papillary projections and nodules of various sizes, may be present in high-grade MCNs or mucinous cystadenocarcinoma. The cyst can be unilocular or multilocular and contains thick mucin or necrotic debris.

Microscopically, typical MCN is lined by tall columnar cells with abundant apical intracellular mucin (see Fig. 59.7B). In many cases, however, the cyst wall may be denuded and lack epithelial lining; in other cases, the epithelium is cuboidal in

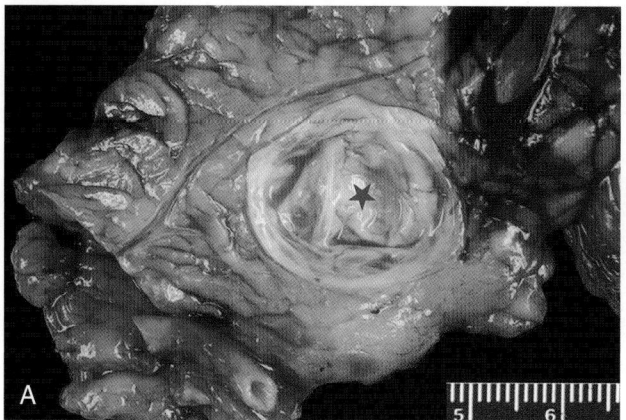

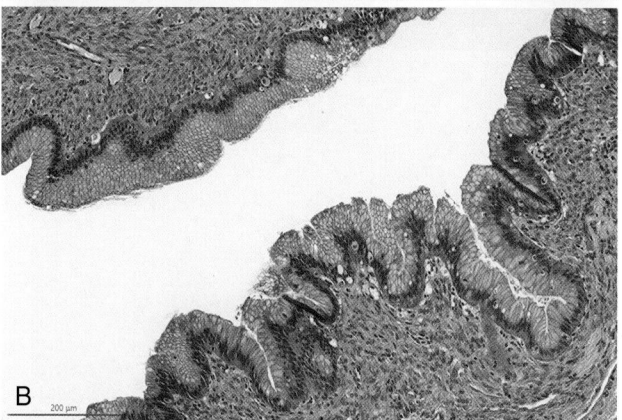

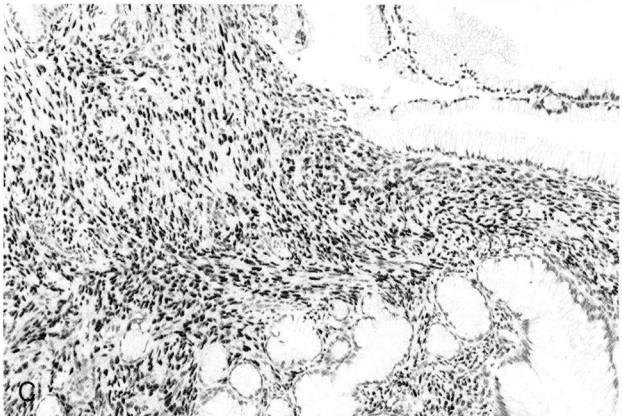

FIGURE 59.7 Macroscopic and microscopic appearance of mucinous cystic neoplasm (MCN). **A**, Gross photo of MCN with a unilocular cyst in the tail of pancreas without involvement of pancreatic duct. **B**, Low-grade MCN is lined by a single layer of tall columnar mucinous epithelium overlying dense ovarian-like stroma. **C**, Ovarian-like stroma is immunoreactive to the estrogen receptor.

appearance and devoid of intracellular mucin. The defining features of MCN are the presence of subepithelial spindle cell–rich and ovarian-like stroma (see Fig. 59.6B). Within this stroma, nests of epithelioid cells resembling luteinized cells can be identified. The density of the ovarian-like stroma varies depending on the age of the patient (more cellular in younger patients and less so in postmenopausal patients) and on the size of the tumor (larger tumors tend to have less dense stroma).[39]

The grading of mucinous cystic adenoma is based on the degree of epithelial atypia as either low- or high-grade dysplasia. Low-grade MCN maintains cellular polarity with minimal nuclear stratification and mild to moderate cytologic atypia. High-grade MCN exhibits increased architectural complexity with cribriform and branching epithelium and budding papillae; there is loss of cellular polarity with significant cytologic atypia and frequent mitotic activity.

When invasive carcinoma is present in MCN, it recapitulates the phenotype of PDAC, including conventional tubular type adenocarcinoma, adenosquamous carcinoma, or undifferentiated carcinoma with osteoclast-like giant cells.[5]

Because the neoplastic epithelium lining MCNs is predominately of the pancreatobiliary type, MCNs also exhibit the pancreatobiliary immunophenotype with reactivity to CK7 and CEA. Mucinous cystadenocarcinoma expresses MUC1 and may lose nuclear SMAD4 expression. The ovarian-like stromal cells are positive for estrogen and progestogen receptors (see Fig. 59.7C), and luteinized cells are immunoreactive to α-inhibin and calretinin.

Molecular Biology and Genetics

The malignant epithelium of MCNs harbor activating *KRAS* mutations in codon 12 and *RNF43* gene alterations in 50% to 66% of cases[40] (see Chapter 9D).

Serous Cystic Tumors

The exact pathogenesis of the serous cystic tumor is not known. Abnormal VHL/HIF pathway regulation in cells of centroacinar origin has been postulated as the potential tumor cytogenesis[41–44] (see Chapter 60).

The vast majority of serous cystic tumors are benign; thus they have a synonymous terminology with serous cystadenoma. They can be further classified as microcystic serous adenoma (most common type), oligocystic serous adenoma, solid serous adenoma, von Hippel-Lindau (VHL) syndrome–associated serous cystic adenoma, or mixed serous-neuroendocrine neoplasm.[5] Rare cases of serous cystadenocarcinoma (1%–3%) have been reported. There are currently no specific morphologic criteria or molecular alterations characterizing the malignant transformation; the strict criteria for the diagnosis of serous cystadenocarcinoma require the presence of distant metastasis, which occurs in fewer than 0.2% of cases.[45]

Epidemiology and Clinical Features

Serous cystadenoma accounts for 1% to 2% of all pancreatic neoplasms and 10% to 16% of operation for pancreatic cystic lesion. Most serous cystadenomas are discovered incidentally by abdominal imaging. They are typically identified in the age group of 50 to 60 years old (mean age of 58) with a female predominance of 7 to 3.[5] Patients may have nonspecific symptoms secondary to local mass effect, but more than 50% are asymptomatic.

On CT scans, the tumor is a well-circumscribed and multinodular cystic or microcystic mass. A characteristic central scar with a sunburst calcification pattern is observed in approximately 30% of cases. The tumor does not have communication with the PD system.[46,47]

Considering its indolent clinical behavior, the prognosis for patients with serous cystadenoma is generally excellent and surgical resection is almost always curative.[48] Because of its benign nature, radiographic observation is considered appropriate for patients with asymptomatic tumors after establishment of the diagnosis.

Pathologic Features

Serous cystadenomas are most commonly located in the body or the tail of the pancreas (>50%) as a solitary tumor. When they are associated with germline *VHL* gene alterations, however, they can present as multifocal lesions throughout the entire pancreas.[49,50] The size of serous cystadenomas varies and can be relatively large (up to 25 cm). The microcystic variant of serous cystadenoma is usually well demarcated and typically composed of numerous minute cysts (1 to 2 mm in diameter), which gives rise to the macroscopic appearance of a sponge-like texture (Fig. 59.8A). Calcifications may be observed in the central scar. The macrocystic (oligocystic) type lacks the central scar and can present with larger cysts (1–3 cm in diameter) that are either unilocular or multilocular. No cystic formation is apparent in the rare solid-type serous cystadenoma. Serous cystadenomas do not usually communicate with the PD system.

Microscopically, the cysts of serous tumors are lined by a single layer of nonmucinous and cuboidal epithelium with sharp cell borders, glycogen-containing clear cytoplasm, and homogeneously hyperchromatic, round nuclei. A distinctive capillary-rich network underlies the tumor epithelium (see Fig. 59.8B). Nuclear atypia and mitotic activity are uncommon in serous cystadenomas. The cytoplasm of the tumor cells and the cyst contents are devoid of the mucin and mucin-related glycoproteins and oncoproteins (e.g., monoclonal CEA, CA125, CA19.9, MUC1) that are typically found in ductal adenocarcinomas of the pancreas. This feature may help to establish the preoperative diagnosis by analyzing biomarkers in either the cystic fluid or biopsy tissues by immunohistochemistry. The cytologic features of microcystic-serous tumors, macrocystic-serous tumors, and solid serous tumors are identical. The solid variant lacks cystic dilation and is composed of back-to-back acinar architecture with or without appreciable small lumens.

When associated with VHL disease (50%–90% of cases), serous cystadenoma usually presents as multifocal lesions throughout the entire pancreas (diffuse serous cystadenoma) and can occur in either the microcystic or macrocystic form. There is no significant morphologic distinction between sporadic and familial VHL-associated serous cystadenoma.

In addition to serous cystadenoma, neuroendocrine neoplasms, including neuroendocrine microadenomatosis, can also develop in VHL disease (10%–17% of PanNET and 70% of neuroendocrine microadenomas, respectively).[5] Serous and neuroendocrine tumors can exist independently or intermingle with each other to give rise to the mixed serous-neuroendocrine phenotype (see Fig. 59.8C).

Unequivocal examples of malignant serous tumors (serous cystadenocarcinomas or carcinomas ex serouscysticadenoma) are exceedingly rare (<0.2%) and require evidence of distant metastasis, which is often to the liver.[51] Large tumors may exhibit locally aggressive features, such as direct extension or adhesion to the adjacent organs or structures, including the liver, but they do not fulfill the typical definition of malignancy.

Serous neoplasms appear to recapitulate centroacinar cells in terms of both histopathology and immunophenotype.[52] They express low molecular weight, as well as broad-spectrum cytokeratins, EMA, MUC6, and inhibin.

Molecular Biology and Genetics

VHL gene alterations account for both familial and sporadic serous cystic tumors. Somatic *VHL* mutations at 3p25.3 and loss of heterozygosity of 3p are observed in 50% and 90% of

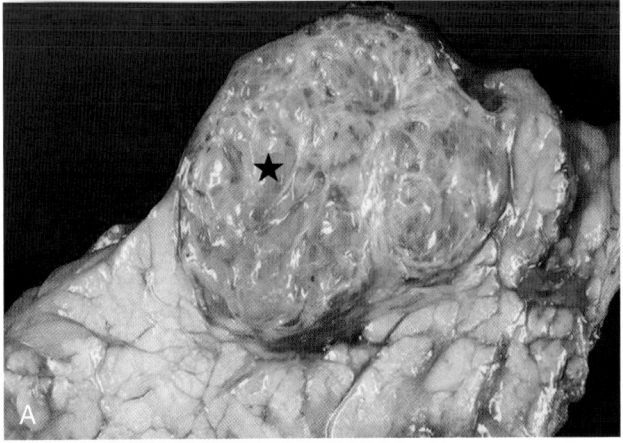
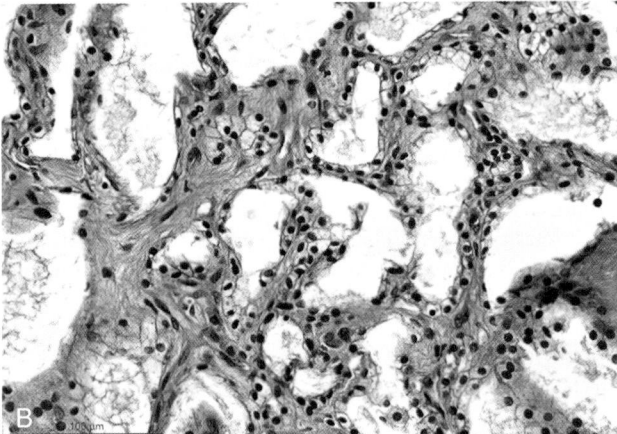
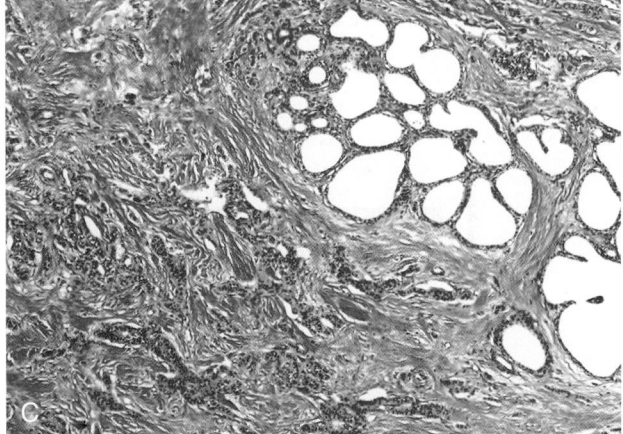

FIGURE 59.8 **Macroscopic and microscopic appearance of serous cystadenoma.** **A,** Gross photo of serous cystadenoma (*) with numerous minute cysts. **B,** Microscopically the cysts are lined by a single layer of cuboidal epithelium with clear cytoplasm and homogeneously hyperchromatic nuclei. **C,** Co-existing serous cystadenoma (*upper right*) and neuroendocrine tumors (*lower left*) in a case of von Hippel-Lindau (*VHL*) syndrome.

cases, respectively.[40,43] In addition, allelic loss of chromosome 10p has been reported in 50% of serous cystadenomas.[53]

Lymphoepithelial Cyst

Lymphoepithelial cysts (LECs) are benign unilocular or multilocular lesions lined by squamous epithelium and a surrounding cuff of lymphocytes in the cyst wall.[54] LECs are rare and account for less than 1% of all pancreatic cystic lesions.[55]

The pathogenesis of LECs is unknown and hypothetical etiologies include development from squamous metaplasia of the pancreatic ducts, derivation from epithelial remnants in lymph nodes, displacement of branchial cysts and fusion with the pancreas during embryogenesis, or the possibility that LECs are a form of teratoma.[56]

LEC has a strong male preponderance with a male to female ratio of 3 to 4:1 and a mean age of 56 years old. About half of the patients present with the lesion incidentally and the remaining are associated with nonspecific symptoms. Because of its relatively nonspecific clinical and radiographic presentations, the preoperative differential diagnosis includes other cystic lesions of the pancreas, such as serous cystadenoma, MCN, IPMN, and pseudocyst.

The mean size of LEC at presentation is 4.7 cm.[6] The lesion is well circumscribed without communication with pancreatic ducts and is sharply demarcated from the adjacent normal pancreas. The cyst is filled with chalky keratin debris and the inner cyst wall is smooth to granular (Fig. 59.9A). Most LECs are lined by keratinized squamous epithelium, although nonkeratinizing squamous epithelium, transitional epithelium, and flat cuboidal epithelium can be present as well. The lining epithelium may exhibit reactive atypia secondary to inflammation, but dysplasia is absent. The layer of lymphoid stroma with varying thickness is immediately beneath the squamous epithelium and may have germinal center formation.

NEUROENDOCRINE TUMORS OF THE PANCREAS (SEE CHAPTER 65)

Islet cell tumor was first recognized in an autopsy specimen by Nicholls in 1902.[57] After the discovery of the glucose regulatory function of insulin by Banting and Best et al. in 1921,[58] insulinoma derived from β-cell of the islet was reported in 1924.[59,60] Virginia K. Franzt at Columbia University in New York described a case of glucagonoma in great detail in the first one-stage pancreatoduodenectomy specimen obtained by Allan Whipple in 1940.[61] The production of glucagon by the tumor could not be confirmed until radioimmunoassay became available in 1966. Subsequently, other functional islet tumors of the pancreas were documented, including gastrinoma associated with multiple endocrine neoplasia type 1 (MEN-1) syndrome and vasoactive intestinal peptide tumors (VIPoma) associated with Verner-Morrison syndrome. In addition, nonfunctional PanNET were initially designated as "endocrine-inactive islet cell tumors." Despite evolving concepts and ongoing efforts to update classifications, misperceptions still exist regarding terminology, tumor grade, and differentiation of pancreatic neuroendocrine neoplasms (PanNEN).

The current World Health Organization (WHO; 2019) classifies PanNENs as follows[5]: (1) pancreatic neuroendocrine microadenoma (<5 mm); (2) well-differentiated PanNET, including nonfunctional and functional PanNET (with clinical evidence of hormone release, such as insulinoma, glucagonoma, gastrinoma, and VIPoma); and (3) poorly differentiated pancreatic NEC (PanNEC), including small cell and large cell PanNEC. The last entity is considered a variant carcinoma and discussed in the section on PDAC.

Pancreatic Neuroendocrine Microadenoma

Although arbitrarily designated by its size, smaller than 5 mm, pancreatic neuroendocrine microadenoma is considered a precursor neoplasm of well-differentiated PanNET, particularly in the setting of hereditary conditions and functional PanNETs, in which numerous microadenomas of varying sizes can be seen in the background before they are large enough (>5 mm) to be designated as PanNETs. One common issue is how to distinguish an enlarged islet, or an aggregate of islets, from a microadenoma. Normal pancreatic islets are made up of two predominant endocrine cell populations: glucagon-producing α-cells and insulin-producing β-cells. The α-cell and β-cell distribution can be delineated by immunohistochemical stains

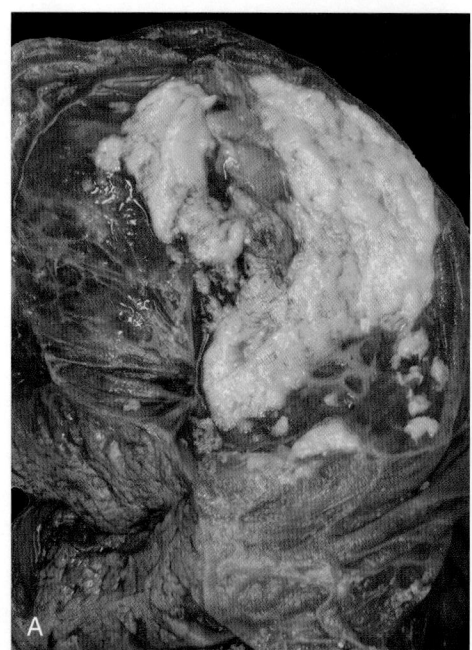
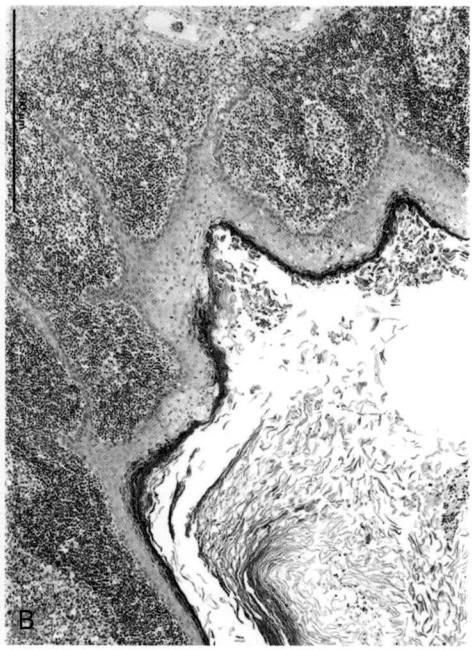

FIGURE 59.9 Macroscopic and histopathology of lymphoepithelial cyst (LEC). **A,** Gross photo of LEC filled with chalky keratin debris. **B,** LEC is lined by keratinized squamous epithelium overlying lymphoid tissue, and keratin debris is present in the cyst content.

for glucagon and insulin. Regardless of the size of the islet, if the glucagon and insulin distributions reveal a normal pattern, it is not a neoplasm (Fig. 59.10A–C). Because a microadenoma represents a neoplastic process, hormone production is either clonal with abnormal distribution or derives from the random expression of multiple pancreatic or nonpancreatic peptide hormones (see Fig. 59.10D–F).

Aggregation of islets is a phenomenon commonly seen in the atrophic pancreas, secondary to either duct obstruction by tumor or diffuse CP. Islet aggregates are sometimes considered synonymous to "nesidioblastosis," but this is a misconception. George F. Laidlaw coined the term *nesidioblastosis* in 1938 by combining the Greek words for islet *(nesidion)* and builder *(blastos)* to emphasize that cells differentiate and bud from the PD epithelium to form new islet tissue[62]; this was believed to be the pathogenic mechanism of congenital hyperinsulinemia. Thus in the 1970s and 1980s, nesidioblastosis was synonymous with congenital hyperinsulinemia. In 1995 the genetic basis for

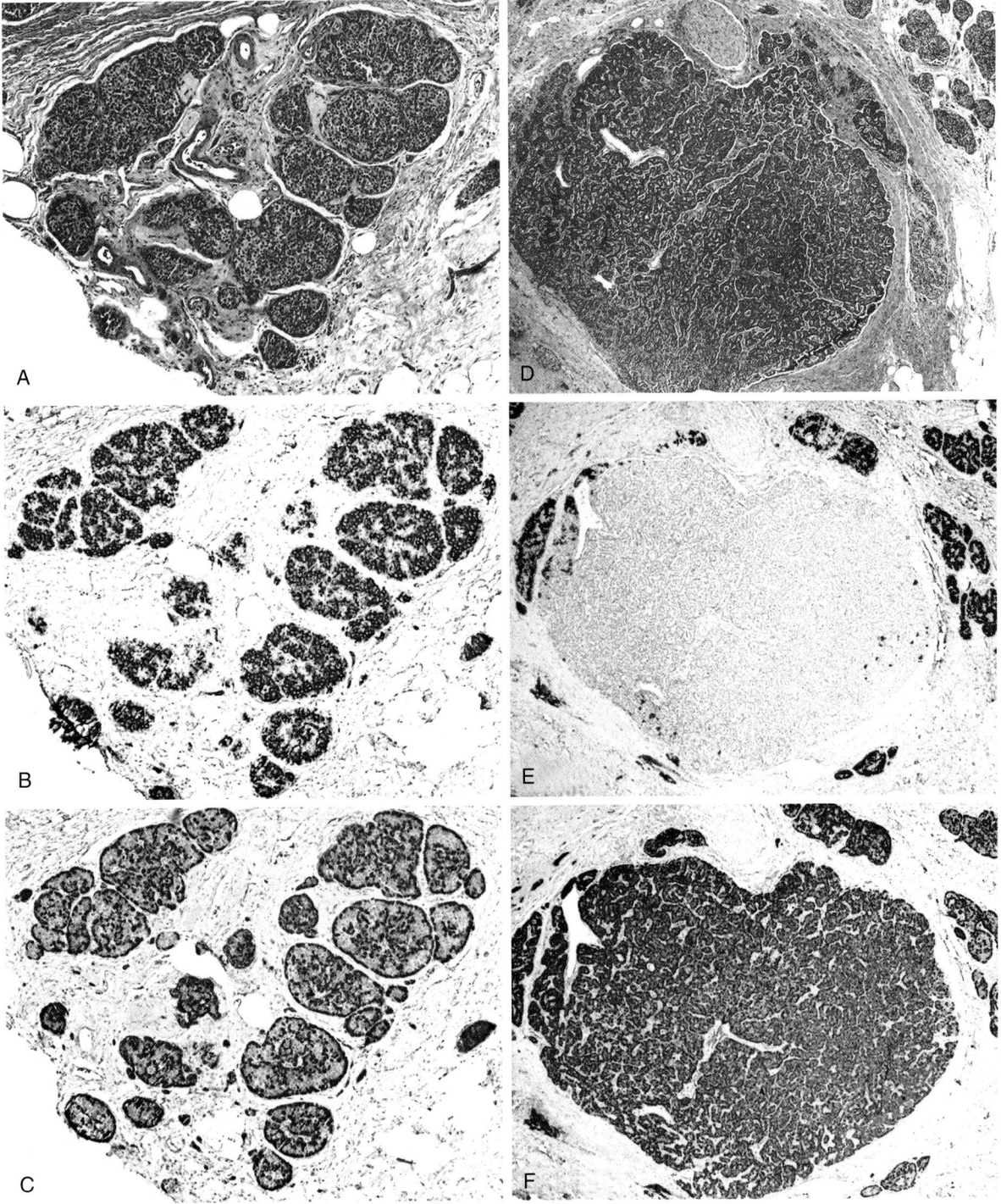

FIGURE 59.10 Pancreatic neuroendocrine microadenoma versus islet cell hyperplasia. Nonneoplastic islet aggregate **(A)** with a normal central insulin **(B)** and peripheral glucagon **(C)** distribution on immunostains. A pancreatic neuroendocrine microadenoma **(D)** lacks insulin expression **(E)** and has clonal production of glucagon **(F).**

congenital hyperinsulinemia was identified as an inactivating mutation in the subunit that forms the β-cell plasma membrane ATP-dependent potassium channel.[63] Therefore it is the malfunction, and not the proliferation, of β-cells that is accountable for the condition of hyperinsulinemia. The preferred terminology now is *idiopathic hyperinsulinism of infant or adult*. To avoid confusion, the term *nesidioblastosis* is not recommended for hyperinsulinism or islet aggregates in atrophic pancreas.

Pancreatic Neuroendocrine Tumors

PanNETs are historically classified as either: (1) functional NETs with clinical evidence of hormone release and associated symptoms or (2) nonfunctional NETs. They are further stratified by tumor differentiation and tumor grade, and the two categories have sometimes been used interchangeably or mixed, which has generated considerable confusion. In view of the pathogenesis of PanNENs, and the impact on clinical management, PanNENs are best classified as either well-differentiated PanNET or poorly differentiated PanNEC (discussed in the section on PDAC).[5,64,65]

Well-differentiated PanNETs vary in size and have a solid and fleshy appearance. They exhibit the characteristic pathologic features of neuroendocrine lineage and morphologically resemble their nonneoplastic counterpart, neuroendocrine cells of the islet, in most cases.[6,66] The tumor cells contain neuroendocrine secretory granules in the cytoplasm, which is reflected in the diffuse and strong immunoreactivity to neuroendocrine markers, such as chromogranin-A and synaptophysin. Most PanNETs are low- to intermediate-grade (WHO G1 and G2) with clinically stable disease but can, albeit rarely, progress to high-grade (WHO G3) with mitotic activity greater than 20 per 10 high-power fields and Ki67 proliferative index above 20%. The high-grade component in a PanNET is usually not homogenous and a lower-grade counterpart can often be observed in resection specimens or in specimens from different sites, namely primary versus metastasis.[65] G3 PanNET is rarely seen at initial presentation without obvious progression. Distinguishing between a high-grade PanNET (WHO G3) and PanNEC in small biopsy specimens can be challenging (see later). Poorly differentiated PanNECs do not resemble neuroendocrine cells of the islet; they rarely resemble any nonneoplastic epithelial cell counterparts and have high-grade cytologic features with only partial expression of neuroendocrine markers as revealed by immunohistochemistry.[64] PanNEC does not represent genetic progression from a lower-grade PanNET.[65]

It should be emphasized that high-grade PanNENs include both G3 PanNET and PanNEC because of their considerable clinical significance.[64,65] Both neoplasms are relatively rare, and mitotic activity and Ki67 proliferative index are for grading but not for classification between PanNET and PanNEC in isolation. The distinction between these two high-grade neuroendocrine neoplasms can be challenging in small biopsy specimens, particularly when the NEC is non–small cell type and requires clinicopathologic correlation and ancillary immunohistochemistry and molecular tests.[65]

Pathologic Features

Most PanNETs are sharply demarcated from the adjacent pancreatic parenchyma or are encapsulated. Small tumors are usually homogeneous and fleshy in consistency (Fig. 59.11A). Partially cystic tumors are not uncommon and are secondary to degenerative changes. Large PanNETs are often bosselated or

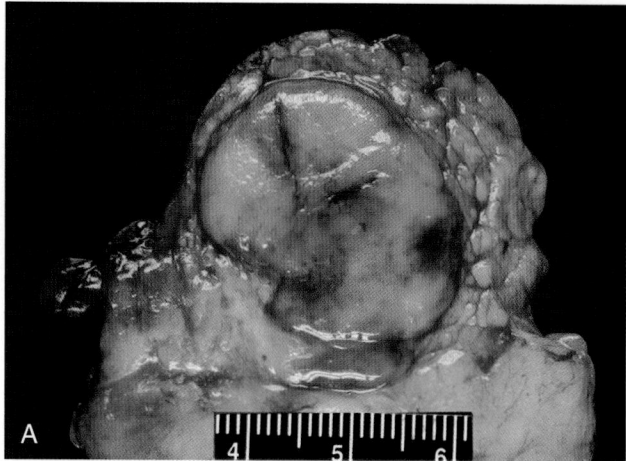
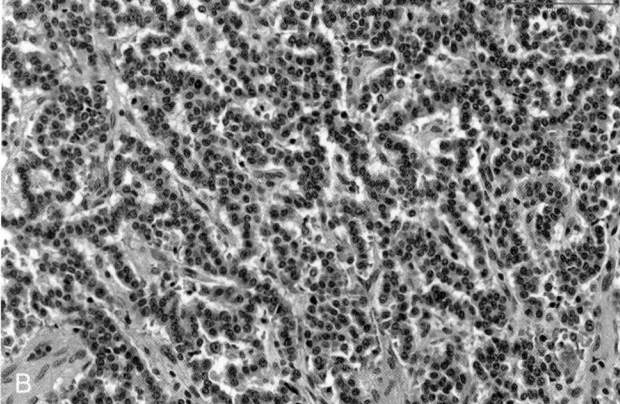

FIGURE 59.11 Macroscopic and histopathology of well-differentiated pancreatic neuroendocrine tumor (PanNET). **A,** Gross photo of PanNET with a well-circumscribed and flashy appearing lesion. **B,** PanNET showing a trabecular pattern with low-grade cytologic features.

multinodular lesions and can exhibit gross invasion into peripancreatic tissues, mesentery, or adjacent organs (stomach, duodenum, colon, and spleen). Vascular invasion may be grossly evident, particularly into the splenic vein. Most PanNETs do not involve the pancreatic duct; however, a variant of serotonin-producing PanNET has been described that arises from the pancreatic duct with associated fibrosis similar to the mesenteric fibrosis seen in NETs of the small intestine. These tumors may generate a clinical impression of ductal adenocarcinoma because of the presentation of duct obstruction and jaundice.[67]

Microscopically, most PanNETs are easily recognized by a few characteristic histologic patterns: loosely cohesive, nested, trabecular/gyriform, hyaline vascular architecture, clear cell change, or pleomorphic type (see Fig. 59.11B). Groups of neoplastic cells are separated by enriched and delicate vessels.[66] Most PanNETs are hypercellular and stroma poor. The tumor cells have copious and granular eosinophilic or amphophilic cytoplasm and are usually polygonal without distinct cell borders. The nucleus is centrally or peripherally located, the latter resulting in a plasmacytoid appearance. The nuclei are usually uniform in size and shape and characteristically have a finely stippled appearance, which is better appreciated in well-fixed tissue. PanNET with high-grade transformation may be morphologically subtle on routine histopathology evaluation (Fig. 59.12A) and an immunostain of Ki67 can be helpful (see Fig. 59.12B).

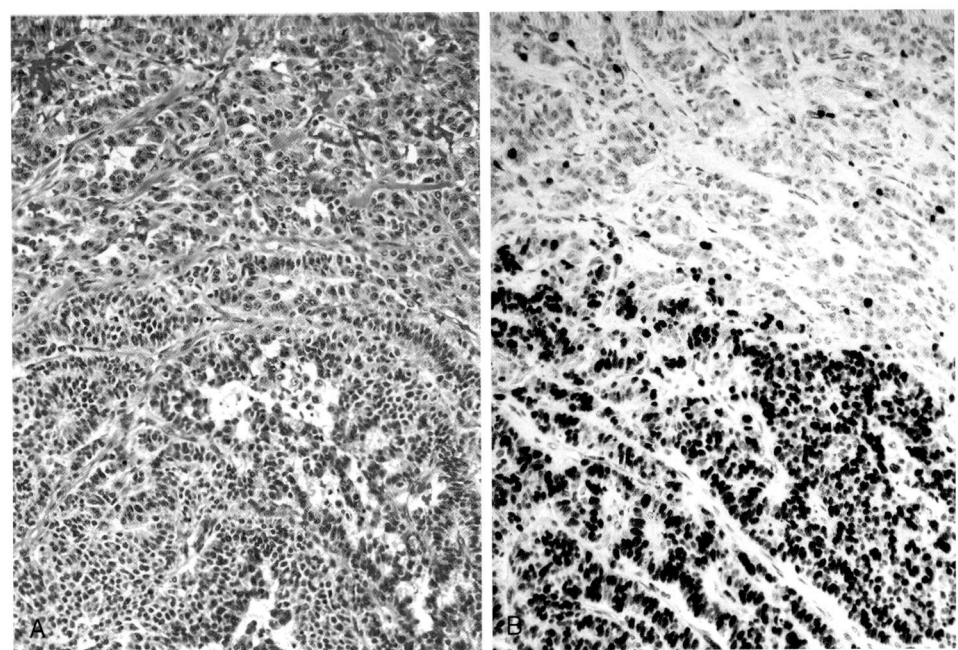

FIGURE 59.12 Pancreatic neuroendocrine tumor (PanNET) with high-grade transformation. **A**, Hematoxylin- and eosin-stained PanNET with subtle morphologic alteration from low-grade *(upper)* to high-grade transformation *(lower)*. **B**, The grade transformation is better delineated on Ki67 immunostain.

Uncommon morphologic variants of PanNET, including oncocytic phenotype or clear cell change, should be distinguished from renal cell carcinoma, which is the most common metastatic malignancy in the pancreas. PanNETs with marked nuclear atypia have been designated as pleomorphic PanNETs. Tumors with such features can be confused with poorly differentiated or undifferentiated ductal adenocarcinomas.[68] Despite their bizarre cytologic features, most pleomorphic PanNETs do not demonstrate an increased proliferative activity or correlate with an unfavorable outcome.

Hereditary Pancreatic Neuroendocrine Tumor Syndromes

Four hereditary associations with PanNET have been previously established and include: (1) MEN-1/4; (2) VHL disease; (3) neurofibromatosis type 1 (NF1); and (4) tuberous sclerosis (TSC). All four conditions are inherited as autosomal dominant disorders. The frequencies of PanNET are high in MEN1 (30%–80%) and VHL (17%)[69,70]; they are extremely rare in NF1 and TSC.[71] NF1-associated duodenal and ampullary somatostatinoma, however, is more common (see section on ampullary neuroendocrine tumors).[72] Recently, a fifth hereditary PanNET has been described in a few isolated cases and is currently given the name of *Mahvash disease*, which is an autosomal recessive hereditary condition with homozygous or biallelic heterozygous mutation of the gene-encoding glucagon receptor.[73] The patients present with asymptomatic hyperglucagonemia and develop multiple glucagonomas. Based on limited case reports, the penetrance is 100% by 60 years of age.[74] Insulinomatosis, which is not associated with MEN-1/4, has been described and its molecular and genetic mechanisms remain to be further delineated.[75,76]

The pathologic relevance in examining pancreatic specimens with these hereditary conditions is that precursor microadenomas are present in MEN-1 (predominantly insulin- and glucagon-producing in the pancreas and gastrin-producing in the duodenum) and in Mahvash disease (glucagon-producing). The microscopic finding of a spectrum of abnormal islets with varying sizes in the background should raise the possibility of one of these two hereditary conditions (Fig. 59.13A). Multiple PanNETs are often observed in MEN-1, VHL, and Mahvash disease. This can be a challenge in management when the patient is symptomatic and the source of hormone production can be from one of several tumors. Patients with VHL can also develop serous cystadenomas that can coexist with PanNETs (see Fig. 59.13B).[66]

Molecular Biology and Genetics

In addition to hereditary syndromes, which account for less than 10% of PanNETs, germline mutations in DNA damage repair genes such as *CHEK2* and *MUTYH* have been identified in 17% of sporadic cases without apparent familial association.[77] In early cytogenetic and molecular genetic studies, many chromosomal alterations were identified in sporadic PanNETs, which appear to be the result of progressive accumulation associated with clinical tumor stage and disease progression. Deletions are more frequently detected in primary PanNET, whereas increased copy numbers are seen in metastatic tumors.[70] Activation of oncogenes does not appear to play a major role in PanNET development. Advances in next-generation sequencing (NGS) technology have enabled genome-wide analyses of PanNETs, which have highlighted the molecular heterogeneity of the disease.[77–79] Many of the genes implicated in the development of PDAC (including PanNEC and mixed ductal-NEC) are not affected in PanNETs. In particular, *KRAS2*, *TP53*, *p16/cdkn2A*, and *SMAD4* are usually not mutated in PanNETs.[10,80] Nevertheless, even in the absence of *TP53* mutation, an impaired p53 pathway in PanNETs is evident by amplifications of the negative regulators of p53: MDM2, MDM4, and WIP1.[81] In contrast, *MEN1* (44%) and *DAXX/ATRX* (43%) genes involved in histone modification/remodeling and telomere maintenance are frequently mutated in sporadic PanNETs.[78] Although *DAXX* and

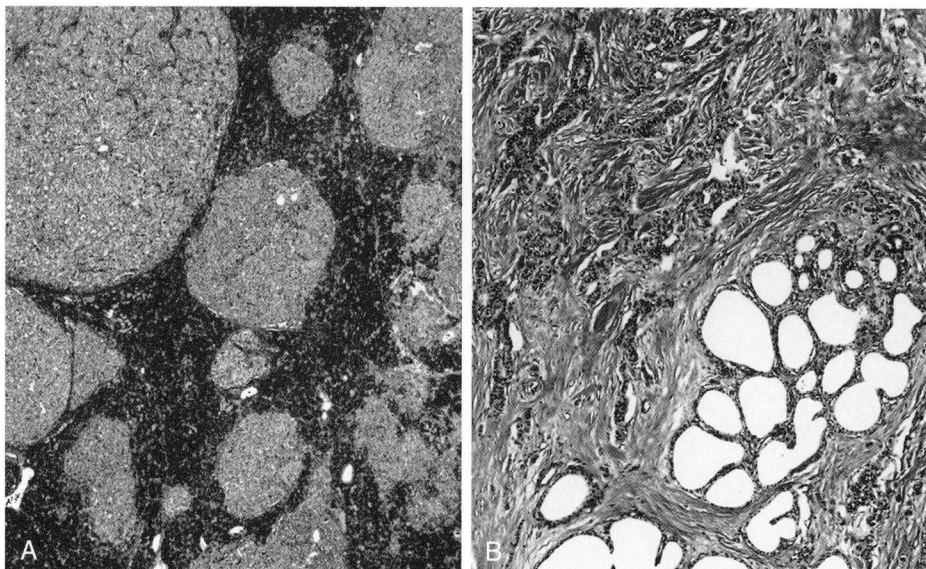

FIGURE 59.13 Hereditary pancreatic neuroendocrine tumor (PanNET). **A**, Hereditary PanNET with abnormal islets of varying sizes and neuroendocrine microadenoma and PanNET. **B**, von Hippel-Lindau (VHL) with serous cystadenoma *(lower right)* and co-existing well-differentiated neuroendocrine neoplasm *(upper left)*.

ATRX mutations are mutually exclusive, more than 20% of tumors can harbor either *DAXX* or *ATRX* and *MEN1* mutations. Thus, collectively, about 60% of PanNETs carry *MEN1/DAXX/ATRX* mutations.[70,79] Because these genes affect the epigenetic landscape, the epigenome, including DNA methylation, histone modification, posttranscriptional regulation, and ultimately gene expression, likely plays a critical role in the pathogenesis of PanNET.[70] Although the precise molecular mechanisms associated with these gene mutations remain to be further delineated, PanNETs with *MEN1/DAXX/ATRX* mutant genotype as a group correlate with a worse clinical prognosis than tumors carrying the wild-type alleles of *MEN1/DAXX/ATRX*.[79] From their differential gene expression profiles, *MEN1/DAXX/ATRX*-mutant PanNETs exhibit gene signatures of islet α-cell lineage of the pancreas, whereas *MEN1/DAXX/ATRX* wild-type PanNETs are more heterogenous in gene expressions.[79] These findings suggest that although PanNETs may seemingly present as a single clinical disease, they can be further characterized into different subtypes on the basis of their cell lineage and the associated molecular genotype. Understanding the epigenetic and transcriptional dysregulation of PanNETs will require comparison to their proper cells of origin, which may explain the unpredictable outcome of the disease and facilitate the development of unique and targeted therapeutic strategies (see Chapter 9D).

Mutations in the *PI3K/AKT*/mTOR pathway occur in 14.7% of PanNETs.[78] This pathway involves vital cellular processes of cell cycle progression, angiogenesis, DNA repair, epigenetic regulation, and gene expression. Most importantly, treatment with the mTOR inhibitor everolimus has shown improved survival in a subset of patients with advanced PanNETs.[82]

TUMORS WITH ACINAR DIFFERENTIATION

Acinar Cell Cystadenoma (Acinar Cyst Transformation)

Acinar cell cystadenoma is considered a non-neoplastic cystic lesion lined by mixed acinar and ductal epithelium. The proposed etiology includes obstruction or a metaplastic process.[6]

Epidemiology and Clinical Features

The exact incidence of acinar cell cystadenoma is unknown because less than 50 cases have been reported in the literature.[83,84] This may suggest that the pathologic entity is underrecognized or misdiagnosed. Acinar cell cystadenoma can occur at any age with a female predominance (3:1). Because these lesions vary significantly in size (from less than 1 cm to 20 cm), some are clinically evident, whereas others are incidental microscopic findings in pancreatic specimens removed for other indications. Patients with a large acinar cell cystadenoma can experience mass-related clinical symptoms. All reported cases have been clinically benign without evidence of recurrence or malignant transformation. There is no pathologic association between acinar cell cystadenoma and acinar cell carcinoma or pancreatoblastoma (see later).

Pathologic Features

Radiographically identified acinar cell cystadenomas range from 1.5 cm to 17.9 cm (mean size of 5.8 cm) in greatest dimension, and multicentricity is common. The lesions can form unilocular or multilocular cysts and have a smooth, thin inner wall with clear fluid; they do not communicate with pancreatic ducts.

Microscopically, there are many cysts of varying sizes that are separated by either atrophic pancreatic parenchyma or incomplete fibrotic septa. Some cysts are filled with eosinophilic proteinaceous material. Acinar cell cystadenoma is lined by one or two layers of simple cuboidal epithelium with pale eosinophilic or granulated cytoplasm. Acinar differentiation can be appreciated when the granular and intense eosinophilic cytoplasm is apically located, and nuclei are basally oriented (Fig. 59.14A). The presence of intervening columnar epithelium with ductal differentiation (with or without mucin) can create a diagnostic challenge and the differential diagnosis would include serous cystadenoma, squamoid cysts of pancreatic ducts, retention cyst, low-grade pancreatic intraepithelial neoplasia, and variants of intraductal papillary neoplasm.

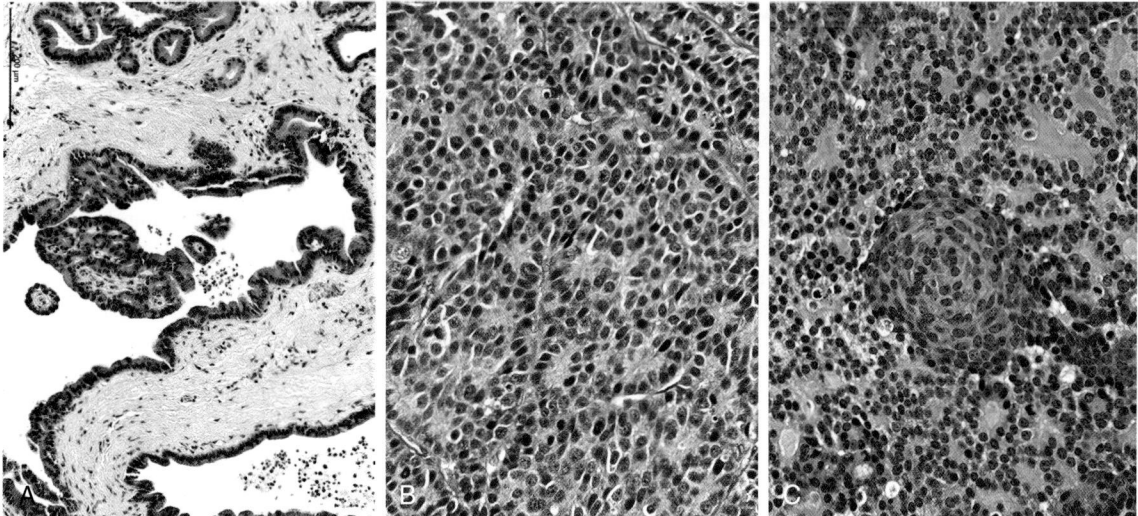

FIGURE 59.14 **Histopathology of tumors with acinar differentiation.** **A**, Acinar cystadenoma is lined by mixed acinar and ductal type epithelium. **B**, Acinar cell carcinoma with acinar architecture and polarized apical eosinophilic and granular cytoplasm. **C**, Pancreatoblastoma with a squamoid nest.

Immunostains for cytokeratin, including CK7, are positive in acinar cell cystadenoma and reveal the ductal differentiation of the cyst-lining cells.[6] Cells with apparent acinar differentiation are positive for periodic acid-Schiff (PAS) stain with resistance to diastase and also stain positive for pancreatic enzymes, including trypsin and chymotrypsin by immunohistochemistry.

Rare cases of malignant transformation of acinar cell cystadenoma to cystadenocarcinoma have been reported,[85] and the diagnosis is based on the combination of morphologic features and distant metastasis. The microscopic findings of acinar cell cystadenocarcinoma include the recognizable acinar cell cystadenoma with increased architectural complexity resembling acinar cell carcinoma (see the following section). Most of these reported cases had liver or peritoneal metastasis with a mean survival of 14.3 months.[85]

Molecular Biology and Genetics

No pathogenic gene alterations have been identified in acinar cell cystadenoma, although some studies have reported random X-chromosome inactivation.[86]

Acinar Cell Carcinoma

Acinar cell carcinoma is a malignant epithelial neoplasm derived from acinar cells of the pancreas. The subtypes of this entity include acinar cell cystadenocarcinoma, mixed acinar-NEC, mix acinar-neuroendocrine-ductal carcinoma, and mixed acinar-ductal combination.[5] These subtypes appear to share the same cytogenetic background.[87]

Epidemiology and Clinical Features

Acinar cell carcinoma has a male sex predominance (2:1) and accounts for less than 2% of pancreatic neoplasms in adults and 15% in children.[5] The age of onset is 60 to 70 years of age (age range 2–88 years). Although uncommon, up to 6% of acinar cell carcinomas can occur in children. The majority of cases are sporadic, but rare cases have been diagnosed in association with familial adenomatous polyposis (FAP), Lynch syndrome, and Carney's complex.[88–90]

Clinical symptoms are usually related to mass effect because acinar cell carcinoma is commonly large. When associated with disseminated metastasis, patients may present with subcutaneous fat necrosis and polyarthralgia because of hypersecretion of pancreatic enzymes (particularly lipase) from the tumor cells.[6] Alpha-fetal protein may be present at increased levels in young patients.[91,92] Acinar cell carcinoma usually appears as a well-demarcated, large enhancing mass on radiographic studies. The median survival for patients with this tumor is 19 months and the 5-year survival is approximately 25%.

Pathologic Features

The average size of an acinar cell carcinoma at the time of presentation is approximately 9 cm. It has a fleshy and homogenous appearance but friable consistency because of its hypercellular nature. Focal necrosis and cystic change may occur because of the large-size-associated degeneration.

Microscopically, acinar cell carcinoma is characteristically hypercellular with minimal thin fibrous septa and lacks stromal desmoplasia. Viewed at low magnification, the tumor cells are arranged in sheets and large nests with a lobulated growth pattern. The acinar pattern of the small units is most characteristic of this neoplasm, which can be recognized by its resemblance to normal pancreatic acini with either minute luminal spaces or solid central eosinophilic rosettes (see Fig. 59.14B). Other histologic patterns include solid, glandular, and trabecular, which can bear a resemblance to a well-differentiated pancreatic neuroendocrine tumor. Less common histology subtypes include the oncocytic, clear, spindle, and pleomorphic variants.[93,94]

The tumor cells of acinar carcinoma are usually monotonous with mild to moderate nuclear atypia and prominent nucleoli, although the latter is not always present. Tumor mitotic activity is variable but usually increased. The apically located abundant eosinophilic zymogen granules in the cytoplasm are highly suggestive of the diagnosis of acinar cell carcinoma, although they are not always histologically appreciated.

The definitive diagnosis requires documentation of pancreatic enzyme production in the tumor cells. Zymogen granules stain positively with PAS with resistance to diastase.

Immunohistochemical staining of trypsin and/or chymotrypsin has the highest degree of sensitivity. In addition, the C-terminal portion of BCL10 is also specific in identifying acinar differentiation by recognizing pancreatic lipase.[93,95] β-catenin nuclear reactivity is observed in about 10% of cases of acinar cell carcinoma.

Mixed acinar cell carcinoma is defined as having greater than 30% of each line of cell differentiation.[5] The most encountered type is mixed acinar-NEC, and, in most cases, the two cell types are intermingled without morphologically distinct acinar and neuroendocrine components. Thus the diagnosis is usually established based on co-expression of acinar and neuroendocrine markers by immunohistochemistry. Mixed acinar-NEC should be regarded as a subtype of acinar cell carcinoma because it shares both clinical and genomic characteristic with pure acinar cell carcinoma.

The subtype of mixed acinar-ductal carcinoma usually has a distinct component of gland-forming ductal adenocarcinoma. This entity is uncommon and is associated with poor clinical outcome.[96] The combined line of cell differentiation may also include acinar-neuroendocrine-ductal carcinoma.

Molecular and Genetics

There are no consistent genetic alterations in most cases of acinar cell carcinoma. A small subset of the tumors carry *SMAD4*, *CDKN2A*, and *CDKN2B* mutations. Although abnormalities in the APC/β-catenin pathway have been documented, mutations in the *APC* and *CTNNB1* genes each occur in less than 10% of cases. *APC* gene loss (48% of cases) or promoter hypermethylation (56% of cases) may be more frequent in acinar cell carcinoma.[97] *BRAF* and *RAF1* gene rearrangements are found in 23% of cases of acinar cell carcinoma.[87,98]

Pancreatoblastoma

Pancreatoblastoma is a malignant acinar cell neoplasm with distinct squamoid nests. Endocrine, ductal, and mesenchymal differentiation can also be uncommonly observed within the tumor.

The prognosis of pancreatoblastoma is more favorable in children than adults. The 5-year survival is 65% for those with resectable tumors, 18% of whom develop locoregional recurrence.[99] Distant metastasis, mostly to the liver, is associated with poor outcome.

Epidemiology and Clinical Features

Pancreatoblastoma is a rare neoplasm in adults but accounts for 25% of pancreatic neoplasms in early childhood with a median age of 4 to 5 years. Although most cases of pancreatoblastoma are sporadic, its association with Beckwith-Wiedemann syndrome and familial adenomatous polyposis has also been reported.[100,101]

The most common clinical presentation is a palpable mass and its associated symptoms. Inappropriate adrenocorticotropic hormone (ACTH) secretion from the tumor can cause Cushing syndrome in rare cases.[102] Markedly elevated serum alpha-fetoprotein (AFP) is common in two-thirds of cases, particularly in children.

Pathologic Features

Pancreatoblastoma is usually a large solitary mass with a mean diameter of 10 cm. Focal necrosis and cystic change can occur secondary to degeneration. Beckwith-Wiedemann syndrome-associated pancreatoblastoma may be predominantly cystic.[5]

Pancreatoblastoma is a hypercellular neoplasm with a lobulated growth pattern that is separated by fibrous septa. Similar to acinar cell carcinoma, tumor cells with acinar differentiation in pancreatoblastoma form small units of acini with either polarized eosinophilic and granular cytoplasm or tiny lumina in the center. The presence of squamoid nests is the essential feature for the diagnosis of pancreatoblastoma. These nests are composed of epithelial cells with varying degree of squamous differentiation with or without keratinization (see Fig. 59.14C). Heterologous stromal elements, including bone and cartilage, may also be present in the tumor.

Immunostaining for β-catenin should reveal a nuclear pattern of reactivity in most cases and the acinar component of the tumor is positive for PAS with resistance to diastase, pancreatic enzymes, and BCL10.

Molecular Biology and Genetics

The loss of chromosome 11p occurs in more than 80% of both sporadic pancreatoblastomas and cases of children with Beckwith-Wiedemann syndrome.[103] In addition, APC pathway alterations, which involve *CTNNB1* mutations (resulting in abnormal β-catenin nuclear labeling), are present in 50% to 80% of pancreatoblastomas.[104]

TUMOR OF UNCERTAIN CELL LINEAGE

Solid Pseudopapillary Neoplasm

The cell lineage of solid pseudopapillary neoplasm (SPN) is unknown. The striking predominance among females and the young age distribution suggest a potential hormonal effect, although no apparent association with endocrine imbalances has been reported. SPNs have been described in the ovary and testis.[105–107] It has been suggested that the cells giving rise to SPN occur in the genital ridges and migrate to the pancreas during embryogenesis.[108]

Epidemiology and Clinical Features

SPN accounts for 0.9% to 2.7% of all exocrine pancreatic neoplasms in adults and represents about 5% of all cystic pancreatic neoplasms.[5] This neoplasm is seen predominantly in young women (mean age 28 years; >85% female) with no apparent ethnic predilection. When SPN does occur in men, the age of onset is usually 5 to 10 years older than that of women.[6]

SPN is a low-grade malignant neoplasm for which complete surgical resection is curative in most cases. Metastasis occurs in less than 15% of patients and is usually to the liver or peritoneum. Even in the presence of metastasis, patients usually have a protracted clinical course with a reported 10-year disease-specific survival rate of 96%.[109] . However, rare cases of highly aggressive SPNs that exhibit transformation from a conventional SPN to either a high-grade malignancy or carcinoma phenotype have been reported.[110]

Pathologic Features

Grossly, SPNs are well demarcated and at the time of presentation may be as large as 8 to 10 cm in diameter. The tumor has a solid appearance when small, but cystic degeneration transformation and intratumor hemorrhage are common when the tumor is large (Fig. 59.15A). Calcifications may be present in the septa or the wall of the tumor.

Microscopically, SPNs have a heterogeneous histologic pattern with various proportions of solid, cystic, and pseudopapillary

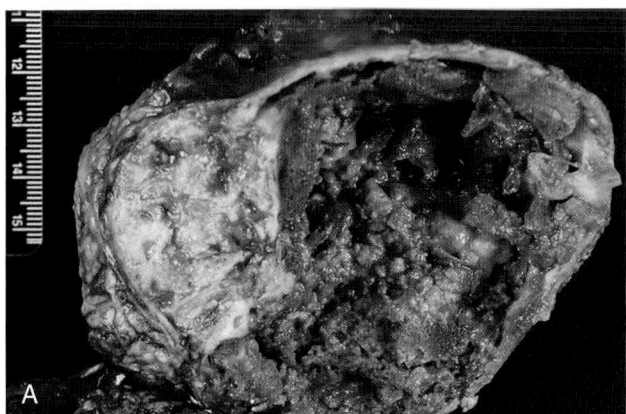

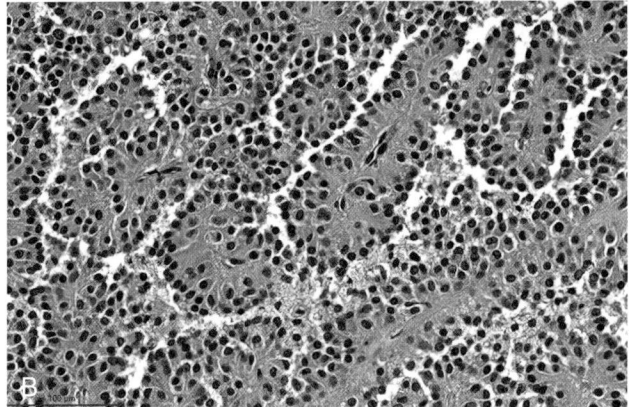

FIGURE 59.15 Macroscopic and microscopic appearance of solid pseudopapillary neoplasm (SPN). **A**, Gross photo of a large SPN with degenerative changes. **B**, Microscopic photo of SPN with prominent papillary structure.

structures (see Fig. 59.15B). The periphery of the tumor may interweave with the adjacent pancreatic parenchyma, creating a poorly defined margin. Neoplastic cells are round to oval with eosinophilic or vacuolated cytoplasm often containing diastase-resistant PAS–positive hyaline globules. The solid component, which may resemble a well-differentiated PanNET or acinar cell carcinoma, is composed of uniform cells arranged in a poorly or loosely cohesive pattern with intertwined capillary vessels. The pseudopapillary morphology is secondary to the detachment of neoplastic cells distant from the vessels, leaving some tumor cells clinging to hyalinized or myxoid fibrovascular cords. Nuclei of tumor cells are round to oval and often grooved or indented with finely dispersed chromatin. Tumor mitotic activity is nil. Lymphovascular and perineural invasion are uncommon. In the area of the tumor with hemorrhage and cystic degeneration, foamy macrophages and deposits of cholesterol crystals can be observed.

The immunophenotype of SPN is distinctive, which is helpful in the differential diagnosis, with its morphologic mimics including well-differentiated PanNET and pancreatic acinar cell carcinoma. However, this immunoprofile fails to delineate the line of specific cellular differentiation. Tumor cells of SPN characteristically reveal nuclear or cytoplasmic immunoreactivity for β-catenin and typically express vimentin, progesterone receptors, CD10, and some of the less specific neuroendocrine markers, such as CD56 and synaptophysin.[111] Chromogranin, the most specific neuroendocrine marker, is negative in SPN and this is important for the differential diagnosis with PanNETs. Pancreatic enzymes (e.g., trypsin and chymotrypsin) are not expressed, which distinguishes SPN from pancreatic acinar cell carcinoma. CD99 shows a dot-like paranuclear expression pattern. Tumor cells in SPN may show patchy reactivity to pan-cytokeratin or low-molecular-weight cytokeratin but are often negative for cytokeratin and never reveal a diffusely positive pattern.

Molecular Biology and Genetics

SPN is known to have somatic activating mutations in exon 3 of the *CTNNB1* gene, which is involved in the Wnt/β-catenin signaling pathway. These mutations prevent the phosphorylation of β-catenin in the cytoplasm, resulting in loss of membranous expression as β-catenin is translocated to the nucleus.[112]

MESENCHYMAL AND OTHER NON-EPITHELIAL TUMORS

Primary mesenchymal or nonepithelial neoplasms of the pancreas are rare and account for 1% to 2% of pancreatic tumors. The pathologic classification of these tumors of the pancreas is similar to that of the same neoplasms arising outside of the pancreas. These neoplasms can be either solid or cystic and distinguishing them from a spectrum of the more common epithelial neoplasms can be diagnostically challenging both clinically and radiographically.

Mesenchymal Tumors

Benign Mesenchymal Tumors

MATURE CYSTIC TERATOMA. Mature cystic teratomas are of germ cell origin and are commonly found in the ovaries and testes, but they may arise anywhere along the path of germ cell migration during embryogenesis, usually along the midline of the body. The pancreas is the least common site of this lesion.[113] The majority of mature cystic teratomas are composed of ectodermal elements (hair follicles, sebaceous glands, skin) and are also referred to as dermoid cysts. Mature cystic teratomas are usually diagnosed in younger patients with a mean age of 36 years (ranging from 4 months to 74 years).

When possible, it is important to differentiate mature cystic teratoma from mucinous neoplasms, including MCN and IPMN, particularly given their potential for malignant transformation. Difficulty in definitive preoperative diagnosis, particularly for larger lesions (>3 cm), often leads to surgical resection.

Slow-growing mature cystic teratomas can be large at presentation with a mean size of 7 to 8 cm (ranging from 2–20 cm). Macroscopically, they are heterogeneous with both solid and cystic areas. The cystic contents may appear pasty, containing hair, keratinous debris, and sebaceous material. Microscopically, the cyst wall is lined by epithelium that may be squamous, respiratory, or glandular. All reported cases of pancreatic teratomas have been classified as mature and thus benign.[114] Complete sampling of the resected specimen is still recommended, however, to exclude the presence of any immature elements.

The prognosis of cystic teratoma is excellent with complete resection. Neither recurrence nor malignant transformation has been reported.[115]

LYMPHANGIOMA. Lymphangiomas are benign tumors arising from the lymphatic system, with 95% of cases occurring in the neck/axilla and less than 5% occurring in the mesentery/retroperitoneum. Pancreatic lymphangiomas account for less than

1% of all abdominal lymphangiomas, which may arise from the pancreatic parenchyma or adjacent tissue.[116] A possible etiology could be that congenital lymphatic malformations lead to lymphatic obstruction and development of lymphangiectasia.

Symptoms vary, are nonspecific, and are typically based on locoregional effects of the tumor. Pancreatic lymphangiomas have been reported in all age groups but are more commonly seen in women.[117]

Macroscopically, lymphangiomas appear as cystic masses, which are usually multilocular. The cysts may be interconnected, representing dilated lymphatic channels. The cysts contain chylous, serous, or serosanguineous fluid. Microscopically, pancreatic lymphangiomas present as either the cystic or cavernous subtype. The cyst walls are lined with endothelial cells and are composed of varying amounts of collagenous connective tissue, smooth muscle, focal adipose tissue, and lymphocytes. The lining endothelial cells are immunoreactive to CD31 and D2-40 but are usually negative for CD34; they are negative for epithelial markers.

Differential diagnosis includes pancreatic mucinous cystic neoplasm, IPMN of the branch-duct type, serous cystadenoma, retention cysts, pseudocysts, and other solid tumors with cystic degeneration. The diagnosis of lymphangioma can be made when the cystic fluid, obtained by EUS aspiration, is found to have an elevated triglyceride level (above 5000 mg/dL; 56.5 mmol/L).[118] The cyst fluid should be tested for CEA to rule out epithelial lesions. Although lymphangiomas are generally benign, they may be locally invasive. Surgical excision is curative, but incomplete resection may result in recurrence.[119]

SCHWANNOMA.

Schwannomas are predominantly benign peripheral nerve sheath tumors that are composed of Schwann cells. Most schwannomas are solitary; multiple schwannomas are associated with neurofibromatosis type 2.

Pancreatic schwannoma is extremely rare, with only 37 reported cases in the English literature.[120] It typically occurs in adults, affecting men and women equally. Schwannomas of the pancreas arise from the autonomic sympathetic or parasympathetic nerves within the pancreas and have been identified more often in the head, body, and uncinate process, but less frequently in the tail of the pancreas.

Schwannomas are slow-growing but the tumor may be large at the time of diagnosis with an average size of 9 cm (range from 2–20 cm). The most common symptom is vague abdominal pain.

Macroscopically, schwannomas are well-circumscribed, round, firm, and encapsulated masses. Large tumors may have secondary degenerative alterations including cyst formation, hemorrhage, calcification, and yellowish xanthomatous change. Histologically, schwannomas present as an intertwined hypercellular (Antoni-A) and hypocellular (Antoni-B) spindle cell neoplasm. Lymphocytes may be present at the periphery of the tumor, and the hypocellular area of the tumor can have myxoid changes. Schwannomas are diffusely positive for S100 on immunohistochemistry.

The treatment is surgical resection. The prognosis should mirror its counterpart of nonpancreatic primaries and the presence of underlying neurofibromatosis adversely affects the prognosis.[120]

GANGLIONEUROMA.

Ganglioneuromas are benign mesenchymal tumors that arise from sympathetic ganglion cells and consist of mature gangliocytes and stroma. Pancreatic ganglioneuromas are exceedingly rare[121] and may arise from the peripancreatic sympathetic nerve fibers. When present, symptoms are related to mass effect on adjacent structures, but most ganglioneuromas are detected incidentally.

The average size of ganglioneuromas at the time of presentation is approximately 8 cm. The tumors are firm and well-circumscribed, although not usually encapsulated. Microscopically, ganglioneuromas consist of Schwann cells and variable amounts of mature ganglion cells. The tumor cells are immunoreactive to neuron-specific enolase, neurofilament protein, and synaptophysin.

The treatment for ganglioneuroma is complete surgical resection, and recurrence is rare.

GRANULAR CELL TUMOR.

Granular cell tumors are of benign nerve sheath origin. Only rare cases in the pancreas have been reported. Clinical diagnosis of this tumor type may be challenging because it may mimic ductal adenocarcinoma.[6] Microscopically, granular cell tumors have characteristic eosinophilic granular cytoplasm with small and inconspicuous nuclei. Definitive diagnosis can be established by the tumor cells' positive immunoreactivity to S100.

DESMOID TUMOR.

Desmoid tumors are locally aggressive mesenchymal tumors. They are typically associated with FAP and Gardner syndrome but may occur sporadically or as a result of trauma or surgery.

Ten cases of desmoid tumors of the pancreas have been described over the past several decades.[122,123] These tumors have no metastatic potential but exhibit locally aggressive growth and invade adjacent structures with an estimated morbidity of 10%. Patients may be asymptomatic or have symptoms related to mass effect and complications associated with encasement of adjacent structures.

Macroscopically, desmoid tumors are homogeneous, firm, white masses and usually have infiltrative borders. The tumor can occasionally be cystic.[123] Desmoid tumors are composed of bland proliferative fibroblasts within a collagen matrix. The tumors are low-grade and lack pleomorphism, atypia, and significant mitotic activities. Positive nuclear β-catenin immunoreactivity is effective in distinguishing desmoid tumors from other spindle-cell neoplasms with fibroblastic and myoblastic differentiation.

The differential diagnosis includes solitary fibrous tumor, GI stromal tumor (GIST), or a low-grade sarcoma, all of which have a characteristic immunophenotype that does not overlap with that of desmoid tumors.

Although surgery is the mainstay treatment of desmoid tumors, achievement of clear resection margins may be challenging because of their infiltrative growth pattern. The risk of recurrence ranges from 20% to 75%, with a higher rate in patients with FAP or Gardner syndrome.[122]

LEIOMYOMA.

Leiomyomas are benign smooth muscle tumors that usually arise in organs composed primarily of smooth muscle. Primary leiomyoma of the pancreas is exceedingly rare and likely arises from the smooth muscle wall of the blood vessels.[124]

Microscopically, the tumors are composed of spindle cells with characteristic blunt-ended and cigar-shaped nuclei and eosinophilic cytoplasm. Leiomyomas are diffusely positive for smooth muscle actin and desmin by immunohistochemistry.

The differential diagnosis includes other mesenchymal tumors of the pancreas, such as leiomyosarcoma.

LIPOMA. Lipomas are benign mesenchymal tumors composed of mature adipose tissue. They are uncommon in the pancreas.[6] Pancreatic lipomatosis or diffuse fatty change of the pancreas can be seen in patients with cystic fibrosis, Shwachman-Diamond syndrome, CP, obesity, or DM and may be age-related.[125] The differential diagnosis includes other fat-containing neoplasms, such as cystic teratoma, liposarcoma, fibrolipoma, and lipoblastoma.

Grossly, pancreatic lipomas are well-circumscribed and fatty lesions. Given the classic imaging findings of lipomas, histologic confirmation may not be necessary. Microscopically, lipomas are composed of mature adipocytes with delicate fibrous septa and a thin collagen capsule.

Lipomatosis and lipomas of the pancreas can be observed and managed conservatively. The presence of solid nodules, thick septa, calcification, or rapid growth observed by radiographic imaging raise the concern for malignant transformation to liposarcoma or other malignancies.

PERIVASCULAR EPITHELIOID CELL TUMOR. Perivascular epithelioid cell tumor (PEComa), also known as angiomyolipoma, is a mesenchymal tumor arising from perivascular epithelioid smooth muscle cells with clear cytoplasm. PEComa of the pancreas is very rare and only a few cases have been described in the literature, but there is a strong female predominance.[126] Some cases are related to a genetic alteration in the tuberous sclerosis gene complex.[127] Tumors are usually located in the head and body of the pancreas.

Grossly, PEComas are well-circumscribed tumors with an average size of 2.5 cm, which may demonstrate hemorrhage or cystic degeneration. Microscopically, they are composed of nests of large low-grade epithelioid cells with eosinophilic or clear (glycogen-rich) cytoplasm. Although uncommon, macrovesicular fat may be present in pancreatic PEComas.[6] The glycogen-rich clear cells are positive for PAS and diastase sensitive. PEComas co-express smooth muscle actin (SMA) and melanocytic markers (HMB-45 and Melan-A) but are negative for cytokeratin by immunohistochemistry.

The differential diagnosis includes other cellular epithelial tumors of the pancreas, such as pancreatic neuroendocrine tumor and uncommon variants of adenocarcinoma that express cytokeratin and other lineage-specific markers.

PARAGANGLIOMA. Paragangliomas are tumors that arise from the extra-adrenal paraganglia, which are nests of specialized neural crest cells dispersed along the sympathetic ganglia and plexuses throughout the body. Retroperitoneal paragangliomas that arise in a peripancreatic location can manifest as primary pancreatic neoplasms.

The incidence of paraganglioma is the same for both men and women, and the tumor is most often detected in patients between the ages of 42 and 85 years. Most retroperitoneal/pancreatic paragangliomas are nonfunctional and are discovered either incidentally or in patients with either abdominal pain or a palpable abdominal mass.[128]

Functioning paragangliomas can cause symptoms of catecholamine excess, including palpitations, headache, sweating, and hypertension. These tumors are associated with elevated urine and plasma metanephrine and normetanephrine levels.

All paragangliomas share similar pathologic features regardless of their site of origin. Grossly, they appear as a well-marginated fleshy and tan-brown mass. Microscopically, they are characterized by the typical *zellballen* arrangement of variably sized nests of tumor cells with an entwined reticular vascular network. The tumor cells contain abundant granular amphophilic cytoplasm and eccentric nuclei. The tumor nests are surrounded by delicate sustentacular cells. Immunohistochemistry shows that the tumor cells express chromogranin and synaptophysin; and the sustentacular cells are positive for S100. Immunostains for cytokeratin should be negative in tumor cells, which distinguishes paraganglioma from an epithelial neuroendocrine neoplasm. Although metastasis of paraganglioma rarely occurs, there are no morphologic criteria that can unequivocally define the malignancy.

Preoperative diagnosis of paraganglioma can be challenging. The differential diagnosis includes other hyper-enhancing tumors of the pancreas on CT scans, such as well-differentiated pancreatic neuroendocrine tumors. When dealing with a neuroendocrine neoplasm in small biopsies, an immunostain of cytokeratin should be performed in addition to neuroendocrine markers because a diagnosis of paraganglioma (negative for cytokeratin) requires preoperative preparation to prevent intraoperative hypertensive crisis.

Malignant Mesenchymal and Nonepithelial Tumors

This group of malignant neoplasms in the pancreas consists primarily of sarcomas resembling their soft-tissue counterparts. Ten percent of sarcomas arise in the retroperitoneum and, when they occur in the peripancreatic retroperitoneal space, malignant sarcomas can infiltrate the pancreas and simulate a primary pancreatic neoplasm. Less commonly, they can occur primarily within the pancreas. Sarcomas represent 0.1% of all pancreatic malignancies. The classification and clinical behavior of sarcomas in the pancreas are similar to those of the same neoplasms arising outside of the pancreas.

LEIOMYOSARCOMA. Although very rare, leiomyosarcoma is the most common primary sarcoma of the pancreas, which affects women more often than men with a mean age in the mid-50s. The tumor can be large, some as big as 30 cm. Large tumors are usually associated with cystic degeneration, hemorrhage, and necrosis. Microscopically, the spindled tumor cells are arranged in long and storiform fascicles with marked nuclear pleomorphism and eosinophilic cytoplasm. The neoplastic cells are immunoreactive to the muscle markers SMA and desmin. The differential diagnosis includes primary undifferentiated/sarcomatous carcinoma of the pancreas, which, by immunohistochemistry, may show partial expression of muscle markers and should have some expression for cytokeratin (although the reactivity can be focal).

LIPOSARCOMA. Liposarcoma, which affects middle-aged or older patients, is the most common sarcoma of the retroperitoneum. The tumor can be as large as 20 cm. This malignant neoplasm exhibits a wide spectrum of differentiation and phenotypes with distinct clinical, radiologic, and cytogenetic features.[129] Well-differentiated liposarcomas have areas that follow fat attenuation or signal intensity by CT and MRI.[130]

Microscopically, high-grade liposarcoma usually contains pleomorphic adipocytes and lipoblasts. Well-differentiated liposarcomas may have minimal cytologic atypia of the neoplastic adipocytes and often require ancillary studies. Dedifferentiated tumors reveal hypercellularity and significant pleomorphisms and are indistinguishable from other high-grade sarcomas. The diagnosis can be confirmed if amplification of the *MDM2* and *CDK4* genes is revealed by in situ hybridization or Mdm2 and Cdk4 protein overexpression is detected by immunohistochemistry.

PRIMITIVE NEUROECTODERMAL TUMOR AND EXTRAOSSEOUS EWING SARCOMA. Primitive neuroectodermal tumor (PNET) and extraosseous Ewing sarcoma (EES) are rare tumors arising from ectopic neural and neuroectodermal tissue that can occur anywhere in the body. These tumors are grouped together in the Ewing sarcoma family because of their similar morphology, immunophenotype, and cytogenetic alterations (t[11;22]). EES and PNET are aggressive malignancies that occur almost exclusively in children and young adults with equal sex distribution. Like other types of sarcoma, they manifest as large solid masses (mean size of 8.2 cm). Clinical presentations of pancreatic PNET and EES include abdominal pain and jaundice.[131]

Grossly, PNET and EES are fleshy and lobulated masses that frequently invade into peripancreatic soft tissue and adjacent structures. Microscopically, the tumors are composed of sheets or nodules of small round blue cells with open and coarse chromatin, frequent mitoses, and scant cytoplasm. The tumor cells show strong and membranous immunoreactivity to CD99. Cytokeratin may also be positive in PNET and EES; the results should be interpreted with caution in the differential diagnosis of an undifferentiated and sarcomatous carcinoma (although the latter usually occurs only in much older adults). The t(11:22) chromosomal translocation is characteristic and can be confirmed by in situ hybridization or other genetic testing platforms.

EXTRAGASTROINTESTINAL STROMAL TUMOR. GISTs, spindle cell neoplasms originating from the interstitial cells of Cajal, are primarily located in the GI tract, although they have been identified in the pancreas as well.[132] Extra-GISTs (E-GISTs) represent less than 10% of all GISTs[6] and are exceedingly rare in the pancreas.[133] E-GISTs of pancreatic origin affect middle-aged adults and represents less than 1% of all GISTs.

Primary pancreatic E-GISTs can be large, reaching up to 13 cm. Microscopically, the tumor cells are arranged in fascicles or nests and can exhibit either spindled or epithelioid morphology with perinuclear vacuoles. The epithelioid morphology can simulate other primary pancreatic epithelial tumors. E-GIST cells are immunoreactive to CD117, DOG-1, and CD34 and exhibit variable expression of SMA.

The differential diagnosis includes leiomyosarcoma, which can be confirmed by immunohistochemistry with expression of muscle markers (desmin and SMA). Primary desmoid tumor, schwannoma, solitary fibrous tumor, and inflammatory myofibroblast tumor should all be considered as well during the diagnostic workup.

The prognosis of primary pancreatic E-GIST is similar to that of small bowel GIST, which is relatively aggressive compared with GIST from other sites of the GI tract.

SOLITARY FIBROUS TUMOR. An extrapleural solitary fibrous tumor (SFT) is a rare fibroblastic mesenchymal tumor with a hemangiopericytoma-like branching vascular pattern that develops in soft-tissue sites such as the thorax, extremities, orbit, and retroperitoneum. Pancreatic SFT has been reported in middle-aged

to elderly women (age range 41–78 years).[134,135] Most SFTs manifest as slow-growing and painless masses. Patients with large tumors can present with compressive symptoms or, rarely, hypoglycemia (Doege-Potter syndrome). Most SFTs are indolent but should not be considered benign; they may display aggressive local invasion or recur after treatment. Rare cases of metastases from pancreatic SFTs have also been reported.[136]

Grossly, SFTs are well circumscribed and may be exophytic with a thin fibrous capsule. Microscopically, they are composed of short spindle cells with indistinct cell borders that are arranged around a branching vasculature of variable caliber, frequently with a staghorn-like appearance. Aggressive SFTs tend to be hypercellular with an increased mitotic count and tumor necrosis. Immunohistochemical staining demonstrates reactivity to CD34, CD99, and STAT6. Epithelial membrane antigen (EMA) and SMA are immunoreactive only in a small portion of cases.

The differential diagnosis includes other primary spindle cell tumors of the pancreas, as discussed in this section.

INFLAMMATORY MYOFIBROBLASTIC TUMOR. Inflammatory myofibroblastic tumors (IMTs) are low-grade and uncommon mesenchymal neoplasms of unknown etiology with variable myofibroblastic proliferation and inflammatory infiltrate. These tumors most commonly occur in the mesentery, omentum, retroperitoneum, pelvis, and abdominal soft tissues. In the most recent WHO classification of tumors of soft tissue, IMTs are classified as tumors of intermediate biologic potential because of a tendency for local recurrence and rare metastasis.[129]

Primary pancreatic IMT is uncommon[137] but is slightly more prevalent in women with a wide age distribution (0.5–70 years). Symptoms are vague and may include abdominal pain, weight loss, or a palpable mass. When IMT involves the pancreatic head, obstructive jaundice may occur. Although prognosis of IMT is considered favorable after surgical resection, rare cases of malignant transformation have been described.[138]

Grossly, these tumors are nodular, lobulated masses. Microscopically, IMTs consist of spindled and stellate-shaped cells of variable cellularity with myxoid to collagenous stroma in a background of mixed inflammatory infiltrate containing lymphocytes, plasma cells, and, frequently, eosinophils. The spindle cells of IMT can be pleomorphic. Lymphoid follicles with germinal centers may be present within the tumor. Malignant transformation may be associated with local invasion, vascular invasion, and marked nuclear polymorphism. The tumor cells are immunoreactive with SMA and about one-third may be positive for cytokeratin. Many IMTs harbor clonal *ALK* rearrangements; therefore immunoreactivity with anaplastic lymphoma kinase 1 (ALK-1) is a diagnostic hallmark of this tumor. Differential diagnosis includes other primary spindle cell tumors of the pancreas, as discussed in this section, and undifferentiated and sarcomatous carcinoma of the pancreas, which is a much more common primary neoplasm.

Lymphomas

Most cases of lymphoma found in the pancreas are associated with the systemic disease. When the disease is localized to the pancreas, even in the presence of contiguous nodal involvement or distant spread, it is considered to be a primary pancreatic lymphoma (PPL).[139] Non-Hodgkin lymphoma is the most common subtype of PPL, and the histologic subtype is diffuse large B-cell lymphoma (DLBCL), followed by follicular lymphoma.

PPL accounts for 0.5% of all pancreatic tumors and 0.6% of extranodal lymphomas.[139] Most PPLs occur in middle-aged patients with a mean age of 63 years (range 15–85 years). It is more common in immunocompromised patients, including those with associated organ transplantation or human immunodeficiency virus (HIV)/acquired immunodeficiency syndrome (AIDS).[140] Common symptoms for patients with PPL include abdominal pain and weight loss. Jaundice is not common despite the frequent location of PPL in the head of the pancreas.[140]

Since the treatment and prognosis of PPL are considerably different from those of PDAC, accurate diagnosis is crucial. PPL has a high complete response rate to chemotherapy and a long disease-specific survival, similar to those of nodal non-Hodgkin lymphoma.

Grossly, lymphomas are characterized as soft masses of variable size with a white and fleshy appearance on cut surface. Higher-grade PPL such as DLBCL can show areas of necrosis.

Pathologically, lymphomas are monoclonal and can be characterized by means of histopathology, flow cytometry, immunohistochemistry, cytogenetics, and molecular genetic testing.

The infiltrative and sclerosing form of lymphoma can mimic PDAC or pancreatitis and distinguishing these entities can be extremely challenging preoperatively. Given the drastic difference in management, biopsy diagnoses may be prudent when radiographic and clinical presentations are not typical for a conventional ductal carcinoma.

PSEUDOTUMORS OF THE PANCREAS

Pseudocyst

Pancreatic pseudocysts are circumscribed collections of fluid rich in pancreatic enzymes with hemorrhage and necrosis (see Chapters 54 and 56). They usually form as a complication of pancreatitis, although in children they frequently occur after abdominal trauma. Pancreatic pseudocysts have an inflamed fibrous capsule with no epithelial lining. They develop after acute injury resulting in the release and activation of pancreatic enzymes, leading to tissue necrosis. The dissolved tissue is confined within surrounding granulation tissue and ultimately forms an encapsulated cyst.[6]

Most patients with pseudocysts have a clinical history of repeated attacks of AP, which can be secondary to alcohol abuse, duct obstruction by a non-neoplastic ideology such as stones, or trauma.

Macroscopically, most pseudocysts are unilocular and of varying sizes, with some as large as 20 cm. The cyst contents are hemorrhagic, oily, or necrotic and the cyst wall is thick and fibrotic. Microscopically, the cyst wall lacks any epithelial lining and is composed of organized granulation tissue with varying degrees of inflammatory infiltrate and fibroblastic proliferation. Aggregates of foamy histocytes and fat necrosis can be observed in the inner cyst wall.

The differential diagnosis includes neoplastic cystic lesions of the pancreas, such as mucinous cystic neoplasm, solid pseudopapillary tumor, and serous cystadenoma. Although radiographic diagnosis can be challenging, an established clinical history of repetitive episodes of AP or trauma can facilitate the establishment of a diagnosis. In addition, cyst fluid aspirations accompanying the cytology specimen can be used for measurement of amylase and CEA levels and other molecular tests.

Markedly elevated amylase along with the clinical history could bolster the diagnosis of pseudocysts. In contrast, elevated CEA levels and other molecular profiles would suggest potential mucinous neoplasms.[141]

Retention Cyst

Pancreatic retention cysts are usually unilocular and developed by the dilatation of an obstructed pancreatic main or branch duct because of either stones, inflammation, or tumors (Fig. 59.16). Although isolated retention cysts are benign, they can be observed distal to pancreatic adenocarcinoma, which impedes the duct proximally. Multiple retention cysts with viscose content can be seen in patients with cystic fibrosis.[6]

Retention cysts are thin walled and vary in size from incidental microscopic findings (a few millimeters) to grossly detectable cysts. Careful examination of the pancreatic duct proximal to the cyst is prudent to exclude a potential occult adenocarcinoma. The inner cyst wall has a smooth and shiny appearance. The cyst is lined by a single layer of cuboidal epithelium mirroring normal PD epithelium. The epithelium can exhibit low-grade PanIN, which raises the differential diagnosis of true neoplastic lesions such as MCN and branch-duct IPMN. MCNs usually occur in women and have characteristic cellular ovarian-like stroma. Distinguishing between a retention cyst with PanIN and a branch-duct IPMN can be challenging; the latter usually has at least focal papillae formation and may be associated with multiple, microscopically dilated ducts in the vicinity.

Chronic Pancreatitis

Benign chronic inflammatory and fibrosing conditions of the pancreas may be difficult to distinguish from carcinomas, both clinically and pathologically (see Chapters 57 and 58). CP associated with alcohol abuse, ductal obstruction, or other inflammatory conditions may lead to localized fibrosis and mass-forming lesions. Certain subtypes of CP are especially inclined to form pseudotumors and simulate malignant carcinomas.

Groove Pancreatitis

Groove pancreatitis (GP) is a localized form of CP that occurs in the pancreaticoduodenal space between the medial wall of the first and second portions of the duodenum and the superior-posterior aspect of the head of the pancreas. GP is also

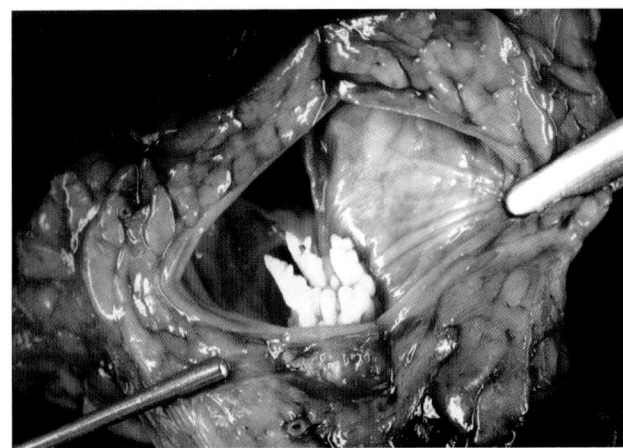

FIGURE 59.16 Macroscopic appearance of pancreatic retention cyst. Gross photo of a retention cyst formed secondary to obstruction by stones.

known as paraduodenal pancreatitis, cystic dystrophy of heterotopic pancreas, myoadenomatosis, periampullary duodenal wall cyst, and pancreatic hamartoma of the duodenum.[142] The etiology of GP is multifactorial, involving structural and anatomic factors as well as stasis of pancreatic secretions, which lead to PD obstruction with extravasation of activated proteolytic enzymes triggering pancreatitis and a cascade of chronic inflammation, cyst formation, and fibrosis. Primary or secondary obstruction of the accessory duct of Santorini and its outlet minor papilla appears to be a leading cause of GP; this is supported by the frequent finding of cystic dilatation of the accessory duct on pathologic examination.[143] Heterotopic pancreatic tissue and Brunner's gland hyperplasia that infiltrate the wall of the second portion of duodenum can lead to partial obstruction of the minor papilla. Because the minor papilla lacks a well-developed sphincter, it is more susceptible to partial obstruction.

Patients with GP are typically males in their fifth or sixth decade. Most patients have a history of chronic alcohol and/or nicotine abuse and up to 50% of patients may have a history of prior episodes of AP.[144] The clinical presentation may mimic AP, including severe abdominal pain, nausea, and vomiting. Nevertheless, the clinical presentation of GP often has a more chronic and relapsing course with repeated episodes of abdominal pain and weight. Jaundice may be present in patients with involvement of the CBD and postinflammatory strictures. These symptoms of GP can simulate those of PDAC.

The variability of GP on imaging analysis can render a definitive preoperative diagnosis challenging, particularly with the differential diagnosis of pancreatic or ampullary carcinomas.

Macroscopic findings include thickening of the medial aspect of the duodenal wall with mucosal nodularity in the vicinity of the minor papilla. The ampulla of Vater is usually unremarkable. A fibrotic mass is present in the pancreaticoduodenal space, which reveals some degree of microcystic change. Foci of pancreatic parenchyma can be found within the fibrotic mass.

Microscopically, the pseudotumor of GP is composed of varying amounts of dense fibrosis, lymphoplasmacytic or histiocytic type inflammation, granulation tissue, microabscesses, Brunner's gland hyperplasia, smooth muscle hyperplasia, and myoadenomatosis of the duodenal wall. Fibrosis may lead to duodenal encasement and stenosis with resultant gastric outlet obstruction. Biliary obstruction may occur when the lesion extends to the CBD.

Autoimmune Pancreatitis

Autoimmune pancreatitis (AIP), also known as lymphoplasmacytic sclerosing pancreatitis (LPSP) or nonalcoholic destructive pancreatitis, is a chronic inflammatory condition increasingly being recognized as an uncommon but important cause of recurrent AP or painless jaundice and can be radiographically and endoscopically mistaken for PDAC (see Chapters 54–57 and 60). It is reported to account for up to 2% of all cases of CP.[145] The etiology of AIP is considered to be autoimmune, as demonstrated by the presence of lymphoplasmacytic infiltration on histology. AIP has been classified into two clinical subtypes: Type 1 (IgG4-related pancreatitis, associated with high serum IgG4 concentration and IgG4-bearing plasma cell infiltration of the pancreas with a background of lymphoplasmacytic sclerosing pancreatitis) and Type 2 (idiopathic duct-centric pancreatitis, granulocytic epithelial lesions in pancreatic duct without IgG4-positive cells or systemic involvement).

Patients with AIP can present with recurrent episodes of abdominal pain, with or without attacks of pancreatitis. Obstructive jaundice is a common presentation that can be accompanied by nonspecific symptoms such as nausea, vomiting, loss of appetite, or weight loss.[146] AIP responds generally well to treatment with corticosteroids and has a favorable prognosis.

The diagnostic criteria for AIP include imaging of the pancreas and pancreatic duct, serologic studies of IgG4 levels, and histopathology, as well as the presence of other associated conditions such as multifocal fibrosclerosis syndrome, retroperitoneal and mediastinal fibrosis, Riedel thyroiditis, inflammatory pseudotumor of the orbit, and sclerosing cholangitis.[147]

If resected, pancreatic parenchyma may or may not have discrete lesions and usually have a rigid appearance (Fig. 59.17). Microscopically, dense periductal and perivenular lymphoplasmacytic infiltrates, obliterative phlebitis, and the presence of both interlobular and intralobular fibrosis along with acinar atrophy are characteristic features of AIP (Fig. 59.18).[148] Immunohistochemistry for IgG4 reveals numerous positive plasma cells diffusely distributed in the periductal infiltrates in Type 1 AIP.[149]

Heterotopic Spleen

Nodules of heterotopic spleen tissue (splenules) can be present within pancreatic parenchyma, and most of them are located in the distal pancreas. Radiographically, splenules may appear as a solid primary pancreatic neoplasm.

Macroscopically, splenules are well-circumscribed, red-tan soft lesions usually less than 3 cm in diameter. Microscopically, they are made up of unremarkable spleen tissue.

Hamartoma

Pancreatic hamartomas are benign tumor-like nodules composed of an overgrowth of mature parenchymal elements, usually acini and/or ducts with distorted architecture and lacking discrete islets of Langerhans.

Macroscopically, hamartomas form sharply demarcated nodulus with an average diameter of 3.3 cm. The cut surface may be solid or focally cystic. Microscopically, tumors include epithelial elements and fibrous stroma. The epithelial elements (acini or ducts) tend to distribute in the periphery of the tumor, whereas fibrotic stroma is situated more centrally.[150]

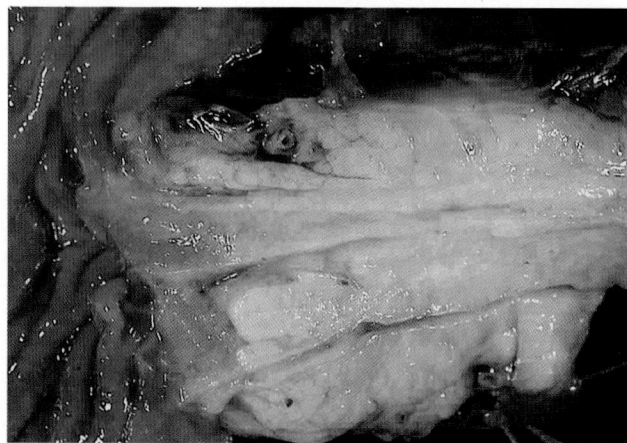

FIGURE 59.17 Macroscopic appearance of lymphoplasmacytic sclerosing pancreatitis (LPSP). Gross photo of a pancreatoduodenectomy with rigid pancreatic parenchyma without discrete lesion/mass. Both pancreatic duct and common bile duct are not obstructed.

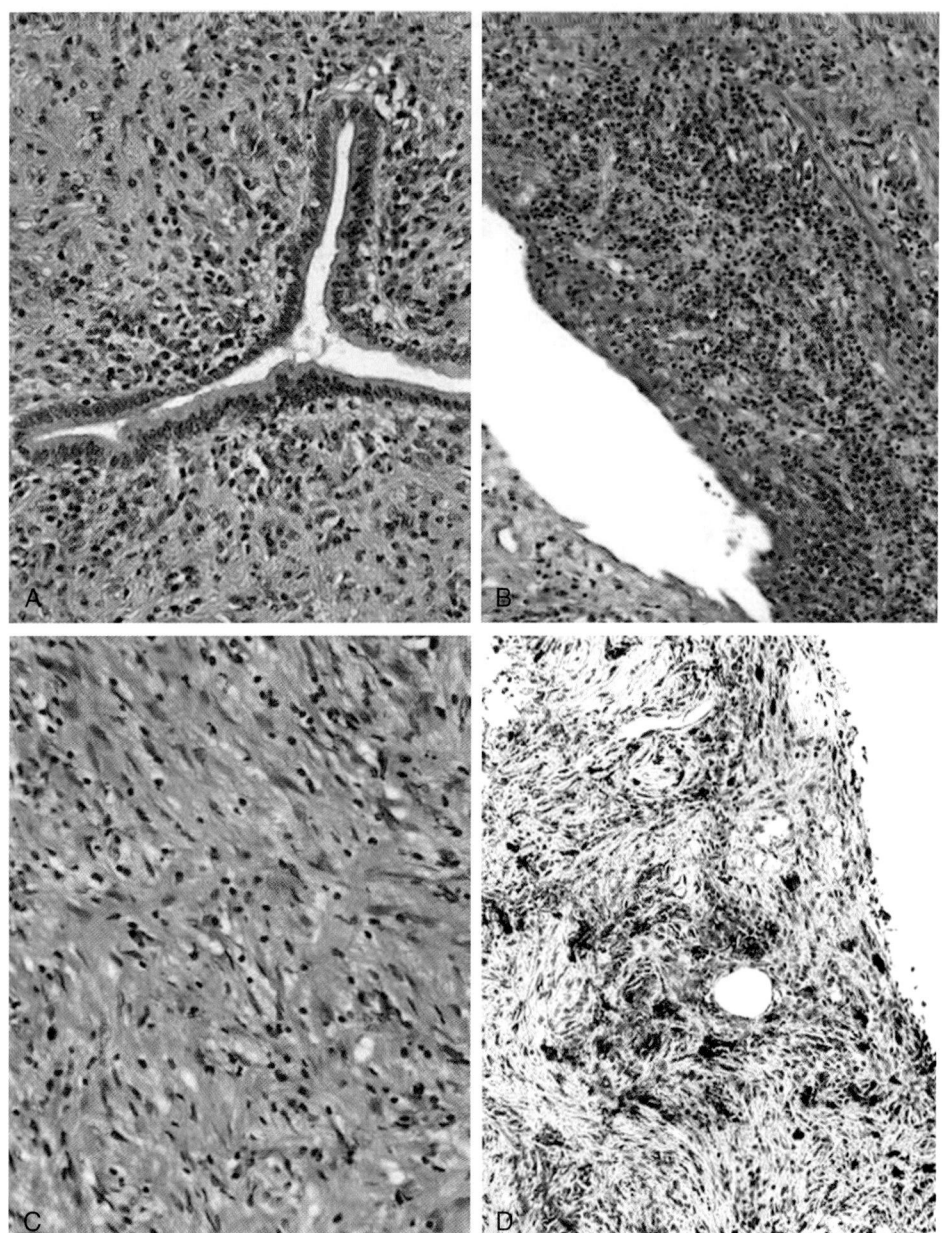

FIGURE 59.18 **Histopathology of lymphoplasmacytic sclerosing pancreatitis (LPSP). A,** Dense periductal lymphoplasmacytic infiltrate. **B,** Dense perivenular lymphoplasmacytic infiltrate (venulitis). **C,** Interstitial and periductal fibrosis. **D,** Diffuse and intense staining for IgG4 by immuno-histochemistry.

METASTATIC TUMORS (SEE CHAPTER 64)

The most common metastatic tumors that involve the pancreas are carcinomas of the lung and of GI origin followed by lymphomas and renal cell carcinoma. Secondary tumors account for almost half of the pancreatic masses detected at autopsy.[151] The common metastatic tumors present in surgical resection specimens are lymphomas, renal cell carcinomas, and melanomas, which are resected either as a result of occult primary tumors, unrecognized clinical history of the primary tumors, or as therapeutic modality, either because of complications caused by these secondary tumors or for curative attempts. In these situations, the tumors are usually solitary with no other detectable masses. Lymphomas (discussed in section V-B) and renal

cell carcinomas are particularly prone to involve the pancreas in the absence of other metastatic foci, thus mimicking a primary carcinoma of the pancreas.

Metastatic Renal Cell Carcinoma

Renal cell carcinomas often involve the pancreas as a solitary mass in the absence of other metastatic foci; it is thus amenable to surgical resection and is associated with long-term survival.[152] Clear cell carcinoma is the most common subtype to metastasize to the pancreas. This can manifest more than a decade after initial presentation and diagnosis of the primary kidney tumor. Macroscopically, they are well-circumscribed, fleshy, and bright yellow-tan lesions. Microscopically, the tumor cells are arranged in nests, sheets, or cords with a rich sinusoid-pattern of a vascular network and prominent clear cytoplasm. The differential diagnosis includes primary pancreatic, well-differentiated, neuroendocrine tumor of clear cell subtype and other solid tumors with clear cytoplasm such as ductal adenocarcinoma with a clear cell appearance, solid serous adenoma, the clear cell variant of solid pseudopapillary tumor, and PEComa.[153]

Metastatic Melanoma

Metastatic melanoma in the pancreas of unknown primary site is rare. According to reviews from the literature, the major primary sites of melanoma metastasizing to the pancreas are cutaneous and ocular; however, in up to 13% of cases, the primary site may not be identified,[154] which suggests the possibility of a misdiagnosis of a primary pancreatic malignancy.

Some have proposed that patients with isolated pancreatic melanoma may benefit from surgery when complete resection is possible.[155] Patients with unknown primary melanoma appear to have equivalent or better outcomes than patients with known primaries of a similar stage.[156]

The gross appearance of metastatic melanoma in the pancreas may be black if the tumor is intensely pigmented. On microscopic examination, melanoma can have a wide spectrum of morphologic features. In general, the tumor cells are not arranged in a particular pattern but display diffuse and noncohesive infiltration. Although malignant melanocytes are described as having large round nuclei with macronucleoli, they can notoriously mimic many types of malignancies including carcinoma, sarcoma, and lymphoma, particularly when the tumor is not pigmented. Immunoreactivity for melanocytic markers (S100, SOX10, Melan-A, HMB45) and negative labeling for cytokeratin can confirm the diagnosis.

TUMOR OF AMPULLA AND PERIAMPULLA

A variety of neoplasms can arise at the ampulla of Vater, minor papillae, and the surrounding periampullary duodenum at the confluence of the pancreatic and biliary ducts. The ampulla is comprised of several types of epithelia: the intestinal-type duodenal mucosa covering the papilla, the PD epithelium, biliary epithelium of the distal CBD, and the epithelium lining the common channel uniting the PD and CBD within the duodenal wall. The lining epithelia of the PD, CBD, and their common channel are histologically similar, pancreatobiliary-type epithelium. Neoplasms arising in the ampulla may have predominantly intestinal, pancreatobiliary, or mixed phenotype. Most ampullary neoplasms are adenocarcinomas or their precursor lesions, but rare specific types of neuroendocrine tumors also involve this region. Tumors that develop in this region often extend to involve not only the ampulla but also the pancreas, distal bile duct, and duodenum.

Adenoma and Noninvasive Intraampullary Papillary-Tubular Neoplasm

This entity has two subtypes based on the location and histologic phenotype of the neoplasm: (1) Those arising from the duodenal surface mucosa overlying the ampulla are intestinal-type adenomas (Fig. 59.19A), which are similar to colorectal adenomas and can occur in association with FAP or Lynch syndromes; and (2) those arising within the intraampullary channel (distal CBD and PD) are usually pancreatobiliary-type and designated as intraampullary papillary-tubular neoplasm (IAPN; see Fig. 59.19B; see also Chapter 63).[5]

Most patients with ampullary adenomas and IAPNs are asymptomatic when the tumors are small. Larger tumors can cause jaundice, cholangitis, and pancreatitis secondary to obstruction of CBD or PD.

Microscopically, intestinal-type ampullary adenomas resemble their colorectal counterparts and may have a tubular, villous, or tubulovillous configuration. The intestinal-type epithelium reveals nuclear pseudostratification of tall-columnar cells with elongated nuclei, and the degree of dysplasia is assessed based on cytologic atypia and architectural complexity.

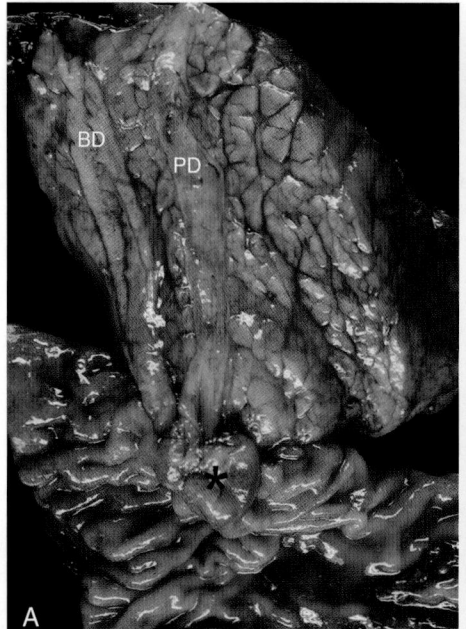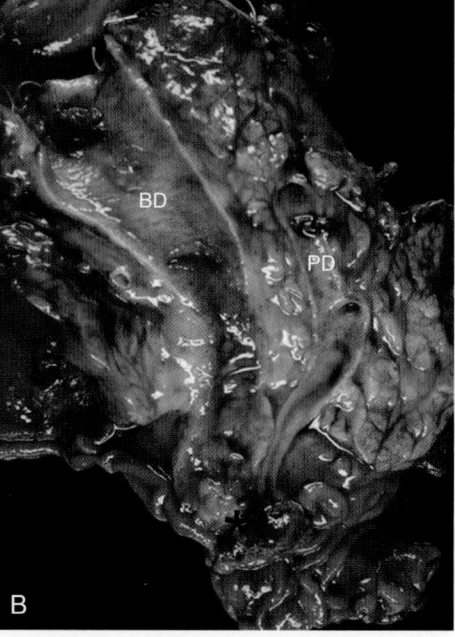

FIGURE 59.19 Ampullary adenoma. A, An adenoma (*) arising from the duodenal surface mucosa overlying the ampulla at the converge of distal common bile duct *(CBD)* and pancreatic duct *(PD)*. **B,** An intraampullary papillary-tubular neoplasm (*) arising within the intraampullary channel (distal CBD and PD).

High-grade dysplasia is characterized by complex, cribriform glands with significant nuclear atypia and loss of epithelial polarity. Immunohistochemistry reveals expression of intestinal markers, such as CK20, MUC2, and CDX2, and generally a lack of expression of CK7 and MUC1.

IAPNs are defined as predominantly pancreatobiliary type, although nearly half of the cases have mixed pancreatobiliary and intestinal phenotype. They form exophytic polypoid masses in the ampulla and grow within the ampullary channel with minimal or no involvement of PD, CBD, or duodenal papilla. This leads to a protuberant ampulla with a widened orifice seen by endoscopic examination. Microscopically, most cases of IAPN exhibit a markedly complex villous and papillary architecture, with branching papillae lined by cuboidal cells that have round and atypical nuclei lacking the nuclear pseudostratification of intestinal-type adenomas. Most IAPNs (>80%) have both low-grade and high-grade-dysplasia.[5] The degree of dysplasia is assessed by the architecture complexity and nuclear atypia.

Ampullary adenomas and IAPNs may be treated effectively by endoscopic resection or transduodenal papillectomy rather than pancreatoduodenectomy. Specimens from these procedures should be carefully examined to determine the complete excision of the lesion and to search for occult foci of carcinoma. Patients with noninvasive carcinomas have a very good prognosis but may occasionally develop recurrence in long-term follow-up.[157] The presence of carcinoma can give rise to recurrence after local therapy and a more radical operative approach is commonly preferred.[158]

Adenocarcinoma and the Variants
Epidemiology and Clinical Features

The ampulla is the most common site for small intestinal adenocarcinoma, which accounts for 15% of all pancreatoduodenectomies performed.[5] Because of the complex anatomy at the papillae and biliary/pancreatic effluents, many carcinomas arising in the duodenum, pancreas, or CBD can secondarily extend into the ampulla and may be incorrectly designated as an ampullary primary tumor. Establishment of the tumor's ampullary origin may be challenging preoperatively and may ultimately require the examination of the pancreatoduodenectomy specimen. The median age for ampullary adenocarcinoma (Fig. 59.20) is approximately mid-60s. The typical presentation is biliary obstruction and associated symptoms, such as cholestasis and jaundice, which lead to a relatively early diagnosis. Periampullary duodenal subtype carcinomas can cause GI bleeding because of mucosal ulceration.

Patients with ampullary carcinomas have a relatively favorable survival prognosis compared with those with pancreatic ductal carcinomas. The 5-year survival rate is 50% with localized disease and 28% with lymph node metastases, respectively.[159]

Ampullary adenocarcinomas can arise from: (1) periampullary duodenal mucosa, usually with an associated adenoma and prevalent in patients with FAP; or (2) the intraampullary channel, either with an associated IAPN or flat dysplasia of ampullary ducts.

Pathologic Features

The macroscopic appearance of ampullary adenocarcinomas depends on the specific subtype. When the tumor involves surface duodenal mucosa, it can form a polypoid or ulcerated mass evident at the endoscopic evaluation, whereas intraampullary carcinomas are relatively small and covered by intact duodenal mucosa, which may only present as a subtle and raised module elevated from the duodenal mucosa.

Microscopically, most ampullary carcinomas have gland formation and either an intestinal or pancreatobiliary phenotype, although about 30% to 40% of cases have mixed phenotype.[160]

INTESTINAL-TYPE ADENOCARCINOMA. This subtype of carcinoma usually arises in association with an ampullary adenoma and

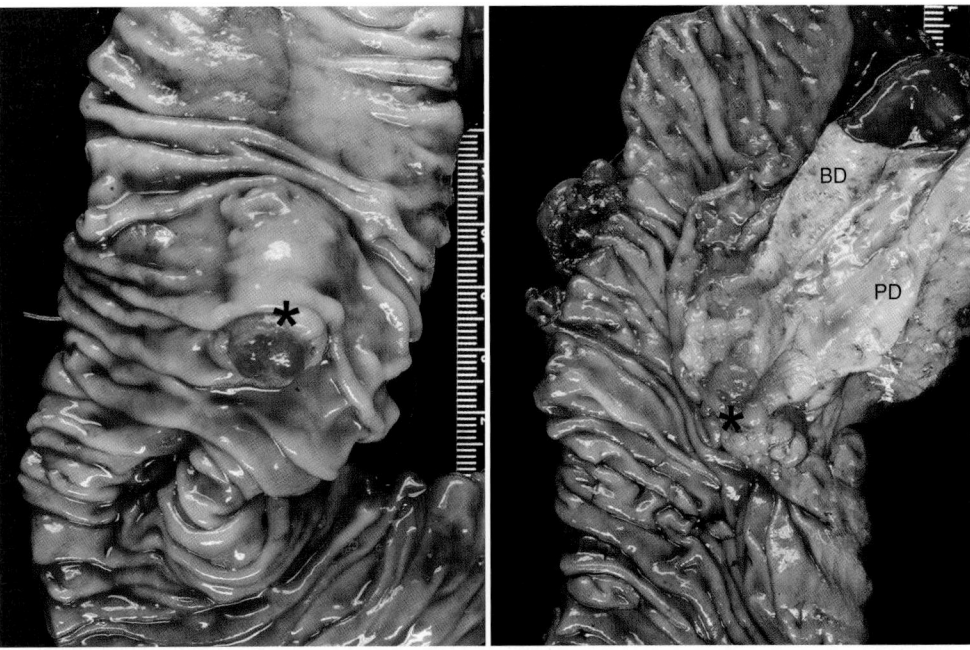

FIGURE 59.20   Ampullary adenocarcinoma in a Whipple specimen.   A, An adenocarcinoma (*) protruding from the ampulla. **B,** Bi-valved pancreas head showing the tumor (*) at the ampulla involving distal bile duct *(BD)* and pancreatic duct *(PD)* causing proximal ductal dilatation.

resembles its large intestinal adenocarcinoma counterpart. The tumors are composed of cribriform glands with tall columnar cells that have elongated nuclei. The intestinal phenotype can be confirmed by immunohistochemistry with positive reactivity for CDX2 and MUC2.

PANCREATOBILIARY-TYPE ADENOCARCINOMA. This subtype of carcinoma shares morphologic features and immunophenotype with PDAC. The tumors are composed of simple or branching glands lined by a single layer of cuboidal cells with round or pleomorphic nuclei and prominent stromal desmoplasia. The tumor cells are immunoreactive to CK7 and MUC1.

NEUROENDOCRINE CARCINOMA. Poorly differentiated NECs represent a rare phenotype of ampullary carcinoma. Many NECs arise in association with an adenoma and may have mixed components of glandular or squamous differentiation. The NEC subtype of small-cell carcinoma has fusiform cells with minimal cytoplasm, hyperchromatic chromatin, and nuclear molding. The large-cell variant NECs have moderate amounts of cytoplasm and round nuclei with prominent nucleoli. Poorly differentiated NECs are high-grade, aggressive malignancies and geographic necrosis is commonly observed. Neuroendocrine differentiation is required for the diagnosis and is generally assessed by checking the expression of chromogranin or synaptophysin.

OTHER HISTOLOGY VARIANTS. Many other, but less common, histologic variants of ampullary carcinoma have been described, including adenosquamous carcinoma, mucinous adenocarcinoma, signet ring cell carcinoma, medullary carcinoma, and undifferentiated carcinoma. Although the morphologic features of each of these subtypes are distinctive, they do not have specific clinical or genetic differences when compared with the more common histologic subtypes.[5]

Neuroendocrine Tumors

Epidemiology and Clinical Features

Duodenal NETs are rare among intestinal NETs (2%–3%) and represent the most diverse group of neoplasms (see Chapter 63). They often present with unusual clinical features and unique pathologic characteristics, involve several subtypes of neuroendocrine cells, and are associated with multiple hereditary associations.[161] Ampullary NETs predominantly involve the submucosa and muscularis of the duodenum and ampulla, although extension into the mucosa with subsequent bleeding can occur. The diagnosis can be established via endoscopic mucosal biopsy.

Ampullary duodenum is the primary location of somatostatin-producing D-cell NET (somatostatinoma) and gangliocyticparaganglioma, which constitute about 30% of all duodenal NETs. Both entities have known associations with the hereditary conditions of NF1 and MEN1, although the hereditary association is much less common in gangliocyticparaganglioma.[72] In contrast to its extremely rare pancreatic counterpart somatostatinoma, which presents with somatostatin hypersecretion–related symptoms of diarrhea, cholelithiasis, dyspepsia, and diabetes, somatostatinoma of the duodenum is almost never functional. Given its exclusive location at or around the major or minor ampulla, somatostatinomas frequently cause obstructive symptoms such as AP, jaundice, and intestinal bleeding.

Pathologic Features

Somatostatin-producing D-cell NETs commonly exhibit a glandular growth pattern with psammomatous calcifications present in the lumen of the glands; they are also known as glandular carcinoid and psammomatous somatostatinoma (Fig. 59.21). They are usually less than 1 to 3 cm in size and typically located in either the major or minor ampulla or periampullary region.[162] The presence of calcification phenomena is associated with 100% of NF1-associated tumors and 60% of sporadic somatostatinomas.[72] When present in the submucosa, they may have an appearance mimicking benign Brunner's glands of the duodenum. The tumor does not form a well-circumscribed border and infiltrates deeply into the smooth muscle of the Sphincter of Oddi; abutting or invading the pancreas is common without eliciting a desmoplastic reaction. As a result, negative deep resection margins can be difficult to achieve from local excisions via either endoscopic intervention or papillectomy. Given the combined clinical presentation of jaundice and the glandular-forming histology, it is not uncommon for somatostatinomas to be misinterpreted as adenocarcinoma of the ampulla in biopsy specimens.[163]

Somatostatinomas exhibit relatively homogenous and round to ovoid nuclei with stippled chromatin and a moderate amount of granular cytoplasm at the cytologic level (see Fig. 59.21). Tumor necrosis is almost never seen in small tumors and mitotic activity is in the range of 0 to 2 mitoses/10 high power fields (WHO G1 grade), although Ki67 proliferative index of greater than 2% may place them in the WHO G2 grade.

Gangliocyticparaganglioma may present as a polypoid or pedunculated ampullary or periampullary lesion and usually measure 1 to 3 cm (Fig. 59.22A). It is a unique type of neuroendocrine tumor with trilineage differentiation, including neuroendocrine epithelium, schwannian/nerve sheath, and ganglion components (see Fig. 59.22B). Immunohistochemically, the tumor cells are generally reactive for chromogranin and synaptophysin. The epithelial component may not be immunoreactive to cytokeratin in up to 50% cases, but the tumor cells are usually positive for pancreatic polypeptide, somatostatin, or vasoactive intestinal peptide (VIP). The schwannian competent of the tumor is immunoreactive for S100.

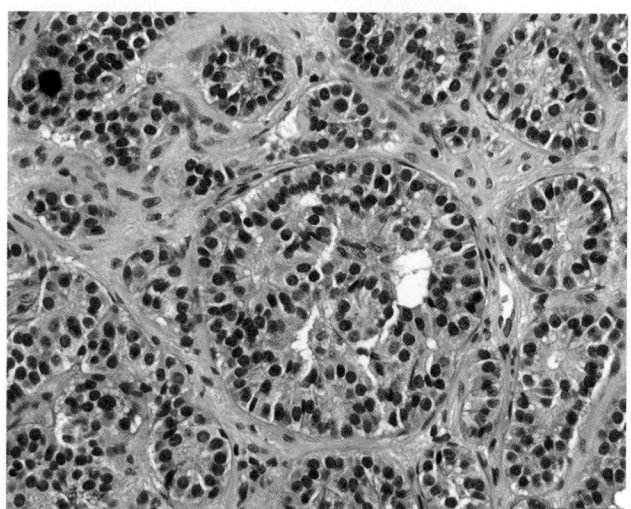

FIGURE 59.21 Ampullary somatostatinoma. A, Somatostatinoma with prominent glandular formation, bland cytologic features, and a psammoma body *(upper left).*

Although lymph node metastasis (~30%) and liver metastasis (~5%) occur in somatostatinoma and gangliocyticparaganglioma, most patients have favorable outcomes after complete removal of the disease but may require pancreatoduodenectomy because of the ampullary location of the tumor, with a 10-year survival of over 70%.[163]

References are available at expertconsult.com.

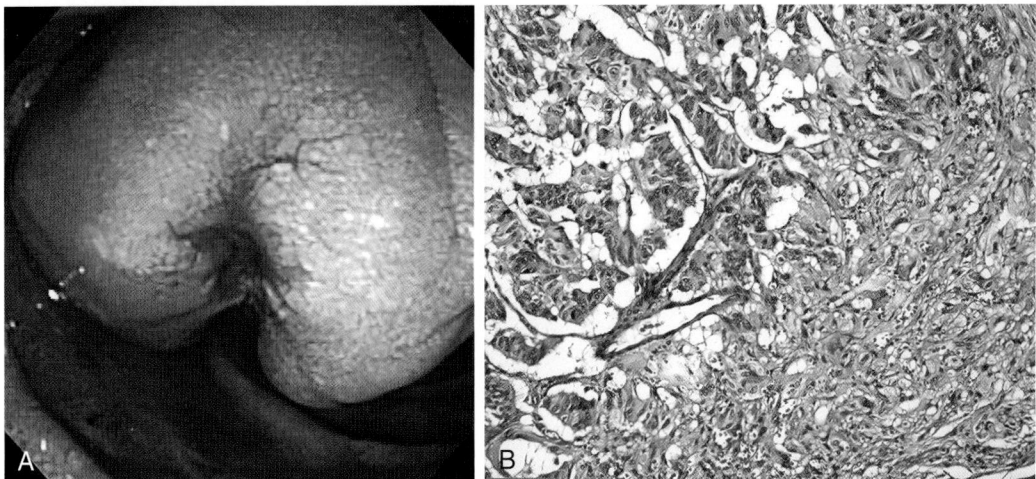

FIGURE 59.22 Ampullary gangliocyticparagonglioma (GCP). A, Endoscopic appearance of a polypoid mass. **B**, GCP with trilineage differentiation including neuroendocrine epithelium *(upper left)*, spindled schwannian/nerve sheath, and ganglion components *(lower right)*.

SECTION II. Neoplastic

B. Benign and Premalignant Tumors

CHAPTER 60

Cystic neoplasms of the pancreas: Epidemiology, clinical features, assessment, and management

Neda Amini and Christopher L. Wolfgang

INTRODUCTION

Cystic neoplasms of the pancreas have become a well-defined radiographic entity during the last decade. With the increasing use of cross-sectional imaging, the better quality of imaging modalities, and the aging population, the diagnosis rate has increased to an estimated 2.6 cystic lesions per 100 individuals per year.[1,2] Abdominal ultrasonography only detects pancreas cysts in 0.21% of tested individuals,[3] whereas computed tomography (CT) can detect pancreas cysts in 2.6%[4] and magnetic resonance imaging (MRI)/magnetic resonance cholangiopancreatography (MRCP) reveal pancreas cysts in 2.4% to 49.1% of tested individuals[1] (see Chapter 17). In autopsy studies, pancreas cysts were detected in up to 50% of patients.[5] Cystic lesions of the pancreas can be categorized as neoplastic (intraductal papillary mucinous neoplasms [IPMNs], mucinous cystic neoplasms [MCNs], serous cystadenomas [SCAs], solid pseudopapillary neoplasm [SPTs]) or nonneoplastic (i.e., pseudocysts) based on World Health Organization (WHO) classification (see Chapter 59).[6] The neoplastic cysts can be further categorized as mucin-producing (IPMNs, MCNs) versus nonmucin producing (SCAs, SPTs). The mucinous cysts are considered malignant precursor lesions and are covered with endoderm-derived columnar epithelium (see Chapters 61 and 62), whereas the nonmucinous cysts are lined by a simple cuboidal epithelium. The ability to differentiate among neoplastic pancreatic cystic neoplasms without the need for resection continues to evolve. Serous cysts can often be differentiated from mucinous cysts by using cross-sectional imaging and endoscopic ultrasound (EUS) with cyst fluid analysis.[7,8] The recent development of next-generation sequencing of the pancreas cyst fluid is also a useful marker to distinguish cyst types and predict the risk of invasive carcinoma.[9]

Cystic lesions of the pancreas remain a diagnostic challenge. Although the incidence of these lesions increases, so does the differential diagnosis. With increasing knowledge of the clinicopathologic variables predictive of invasive carcinoma or high-grade dysplasia, and an improved understanding of the natural history of many of the common cystic lesions, management has changed to one of selective resection.

Herein we summarize the current literature on the diagnosis and management of patients with cystic neoplasms of the pancreas.

CLINICOPATHOLOGIC VARIABLES

The majority of patients with pancreatic cysts will have non-neoplastic inflammatory pseudocysts that develop as a complication of acute pancreatitis (AP; see Chapters 54–57).[10,11] A pseudocyst is a fluid collection that is devoid of an epithelial lining. Pseudocysts have been reported to develop in as many as 50% of patients who experience AP.[11] Of note, up to 20% of unexplained pancreatitis occurs because of the presence of cystic neoplasms.[12] Hence, a cystic neoplasm of the pancreas should be considered as a differential diagnosis of an incidental cyst associated with pancreatitis. Pseudocysts can be managed with observation, endoscopic drainage, or operative drainage. The particulars of the management of patients with pancreatic pseudocysts are beyond the scope of this chapter.

Cystic neoplasms are a heterogeneous group of lesions. They make up approximately 10% to 15% of cystic lesions of the pancreas and are a heterogeneous group of lesions that range from benign to malignant. Cystic lesions that harbor the risk of invasive carcinoma include IPMNs and MCNs. SPTs and SCAs have a very low risk for invasive carcinoma. The other end of the spectrum includes benign cystic lesions such as lymphoepithelial cysts, simple cysts, and mucinous nonneoplastic cysts. Even though there are numerous neoplasms that can present as a cystic lesion, the most common cystic neoplasms encountered by surgeons include IPMNs, MCNs, and SCAs. In a study by the Massachusetts General Hospital (MGH) of 851 resected pancreatic cystic neoplasms, these three lesions made up 77% of all lesions.[13] The clinicopathologic factors associated with the more common cystic neoplasms are shown in Table 60.1.

Serous Cystadenomas

SCAs were first characterized by Compagno and Oertel in 1978 as microcystic and glycogen rich. Their paper in 1978 was a seminal article that clearly distinguished SCAs from mucinous cysts (MCNs and IPMNs; see Chapter 59).[14,15] Around half of patients with SCAs are found incidentally. In symptomatic patients, abdominal pain, palpable mass, and weight loss are the most common manifestations. These symptoms are usually related to the mass effect of the cyst. Jaundice, because of bile duct compression, is infrequent. Of note, SCAs can be associated

TABLE 60.1   Characteristics of Common Cystic Neoplasms of Pancreas

	AGE OF PRESENTATION (DECADE)	GENDER DISTRIBUTION	IMAGING CHARACTERISTICS	MACROSCOPIC FEATURES	CONNECTION WITH MPD	INVASIVE OR HGD POTENTIAL	CYST FLUID ANALYSIS
IPMN-BD	5th to 7th	Equal	Macrocytic, grape-like cystic lesion, Unilocular or multilocular	Mucine producing epithelium with papillae	Yes	12%–30%	mucin, high CEA, GNAS frequently mutated, RNF43 mutated
IPMN-MD	5th to 7th	Equal	Segmental or diffuse dilation of main pancreatic duct	Mucine producing epithelium with papillae	Yes	36%–100%	mucin, high CEA, GNAS frequently mutated, RNF43 mutated
MCN	4th to 5th	Female > male	Macrocytic, unilocular body/tail location, peripheral calcification	Tall columnar mucin-producing epithelium Ovarian-type stroma	No	10%–50%	mucin, high CEA, GNAS wild, RNF43 mutated
SCA	5th to 7th	Female > male	Microcystic characteristic honeycomb pattern Stellate scar	Clear cytoplasm, well defined borders, uniform nuclei, glycogen-rich cells	No	Negligible	serous, very low CEA, VHL gene mutated, RNF43 wild
SPT	2nd to 3rd	Female > male	Macrocytic, Solid, and cystic, area of hemorrhage	Solid sheets of variable cells	No	10%–15%	Bloody, necrotic debris
Pseudocyst	4th to 5th	Equal	Unilocular associated with pancreatitis	No epithelial lining	common	0%	nonmucinous, high amylase, low viscosity, Dark, low CEA

BD, Branch duct; *CEA*, carcinoembryonic antigen; *HGD*, high-grade dysplasia; *IPMN*, intraductal papillary mucinous neoplasm; *MCN*, mucinous cystic neoplasm; *MD*, main duct; *MPD*, main pancreatic duct; *SCA*, serous cystadenoma; *SPT*, solid pseudopapillary tumor.

with von Hippel-Lindau (VHL) disease. SCAs were reported between 2.7% and 9.5% of patients with VHL disease. In these patients, SCAs are generally diagnosed at a younger age (25 years) compared with the general population and have a benign course.[16]

SCAs presents with morphologic varieties including microcystic, macrocystic (or oligocystic), mixed microcystic and macrocystic, and solid SCA. Grossly, these cysts are characterized by septations and thick fibrous walls and have what appear to be innumerable small cysts containing clear thin fluid. Microcystic SCAs often have a classic honeycomb appearance and a calcified central scar with or without hemorrhage. The septa may centrally coalesce into a characteristic "stellate scar" with or without calcification itself, which is pathognomonic for SCAs. These lesions may also be oligocystic (single large cyst) in appearance on imaging and, if so, are very difficult to distinguish from mucinous lesions. Because of the fibrous nature of this lesion, a solid component is often visualized and, if noted in the presence of the other characteristic findings of SCA, should not be considered as concerning for invasive carcinoma.

SCAs are generally considered benign lesions. Serous cystadenocarcinoma is extremely uncommon and usually reported as case reports. Currently, about 30 cases of serous cystadenocarcinoma have been reported in the literature.[8] Many of these case reports describe the "malignant" SCA as locally invasive, whereas only 14 of 30 cases (46.6%) had evidence of metastasis. Despite the presence of metastasis, long-term prognosis was excellent in these patients.[17,18] It appears that the true incidence of invasive carcinoma within SCAs is much less than 1%. In a multinational study from 23 countries including 2622 patients with SCAs, 61% underwent surgical resection with only 0.1% of patients diagnosed with serous cystadenocarcinoma.[19]

The more common problem caused by these lesions is local invasion resulting in symptoms such as early satiety, obstructive jaundice, and pain. Intuitively, large lesions are more likely to produce symptoms; several factors such as female gender, older age of patients when first detected, and larger cyst size (>10 cm) were associated with the risk of invasive carcinoma.[20,21]

Mucinous Cystic Neoplasms

MCNs are mucin-producing cystic tumors that lack communication with the pancreatic duct and contain mucin-producing columnar epithelium. An ovarian-like stroma surrounding the columnar epithelium is considered a pathognomonic finding and is the presumed reason that MCNs are almost exclusively found in females (see Chapter 59). The ovarian stroma is a characteristic that pancreatic MCNs share with mucinous cysts found in the ovary and the liver. MCNs have been classified separately from IPMNs by WHO since 1996.[22] Pancreatic MCNs are most commonly found in the body and tail and can range in size from small (2 cm) to large (25 cm). Many MCNs are discovered incidentally, but patients may have symptoms such as abdominal pain, nausea or vomiting, back pain, recurrent pancreatitis, or rarely jaundice.[23,24]

Any macrocystic lesion in the distal pancreas of a female patient should be considered highly suspicious for MCN. These lesions are often unilocular but may contain septa within the primary lesion. When these lesions are multilocular, they are typically macrocystic, in contrast to SCAs (microcystic). These lesions may also have peripheral "eggshell" calcifications that are best demonstrated on the noncontrast phase of CT imaging. Any evidence of mural nodularity in these lesions is considered concerning for invasion. Upon gross inspection, these tumors are round with a smooth surface and fibrous pseudocapsule.

These tumors, in contrast to SCAs, have a risk for harboring invasive carcinoma. Rates of invasive disease range from 10% to 50%, which may be an underestimate because both benign and malignant epithelium may coexist within the same cyst. Only an extensive pathologic evaluation may detect both entities and is critical for an accurate diagnosis. Clinical factors that increase the risk of invasive carcinoma in MCNs are not well characterized. In a multicenter analysis of data from eight academic centers in the United States, the overall rate of invasive carcinoma in MCN lesions reported up to 15%. Factors associated with the risk of invasive carcinoma were male gender, pancreatic head and neck location, larger MCN, mural nodules, and duct dilation.[25] Because of the rarity of these lesions, the natural history is not well defined. The 5-year disease-specific survival for patients with invasive carcinoma was estimated between 57% and 64%.[23,25]

Intraductal Papillary Mucinous Neoplasms

IPMNs are epithelial tumors that arise from the main pancreatic duct or the branch ducts, causing ductal dilation from mucin production. It is a recently described entity and was first classified into a unified diagnosis by WHO in 1996.[26] Because of the increasing use of high-quality cross-sectional imaging, the identification of asymptomatic cystic lesions of the pancreas has increased, and a significant percentage of patients with incidentally discovered cysts will have IPMNs.[27] In contrast to MCNs, IPMNs occur equally in men and women and are more often found in older individuals, with the peak incidence between 50 and 70 years.[28] Among cystic neoplasms diagnosed in large series, IPMNs represent approximately 15% to 30% of all lesions.[7,13,29] Because of the recent evolution in the understanding of IPMN, many early reports likely included a mixture of patients with IPMN and MCN and should be interpreted with caution.

IPMN is believed to be a process that involves the entire pancreas; however, radiographically detectable disease may present as involving the main duct alone, branch ducts alone, or both (mixed variant). The main-duct IPMN (MD-IPMN) is characterized by diffuse or segmental dilatation of the main pancreatic duct (>5 mm) without other reasons for obstruction. Cysts that have communication with the main pancreatic duct without significant dilation of the main pancreatic duct are defined as branch-duct IPMN (BD-IPMN). They may be unilocular, multilocular, and have septations or mural nodularity. In the absence of septations, mural nodules, or a solid component, BD-IPMNs may be radiographically and endoscopically indistinguishable from pancreatic retention cysts, MCNs, small cystic endocrine tumors, or even pancreatic pseudocysts. IPMN is classified as mixed-IPMN when branch-duct dilation is associated with main-duct dilation (main pancreatic duct > 5 mm).

This radiographic classification of IPMN into MD-IPMN, BD-IPMN, or the mixed variant has formed the backbone of the management paradigm of IPMN because the radiographic subtype is one of the strongest predictors of high-grade dysplasia or invasive cancer (see Chapter 17). As many as 60% of MD-IPMNs are malignant (high-grade dysplasia and invasive cancer), and as many as 45% have invasive adenocarcinoma, thus forming the basis of the recommendation that, in general, patients with MD-IPMN should undergo resection.[30,31] Invasive carcinoma or high-grade dysplasia is reported in 12% to 30% of patients who undergo resection for BD-IPMN.[30,32–34] Series of patients who have undergone resection for mixed IPMN have generally reported rates of invasive carcinoma or

high-grade dysplasia in between those of BD-IPMN and MD-IPMN (see Chapter 59).

IPMN can also be classified based on cellular morphology as gastric, intestinal, pancreatobiliary, or oncocytic. This classification is based on histologic appearance, mucin (MUC) gene expression, and tissue architecture. Each subtype exhibits a particular risk of invasive carcinoma. The gastric-type papillae are often mingled with tubular glands resembling pyloric glands. Intestinal-type IPMNs have villous papillae consisting of tall columnar cells with pseudostratified cigar-shaped nuclei and basophilic cytoplasm with variable amounts of apical mucin. Pancreatobiliary-type IPMNs have complex branching papillae consisting of columnar cells with marked atypical nuclei and neutral or basophilic cytoplasm. Finally, the oncocytic-type has arborizing papillae consisting of cells with enlarged round nuclei and eosinophilic cytoplasm secondary to an abundance of mitochondria.[35,36]

Histologically, the mucosa of IPMN can express a range of dysplasia. IPMNs were graded based on the revised classification system and recommendations from the Baltimore consensus into low-grade dysplasia, high-grade dysplasia, or invasive carcinoma.[37] Multiple degrees of dysplasia can coexist in a resected specimen of IPMN, and generally pathologists will report this as the highest grade of dysplasia in the resected lesion (see Chapter 59).

Intraductal Papillary Mucinous Neoplasm–Associated Cancer

Invasive carcinoma arising from IPMN is well documented, and several large series have been reported in the literature.[34,38–40] Invasive cancer is found in 20% to 50% of resected IPMN specimens, which is why these lesions are typically resected. In a recent Japanese series of 1404 patients with BD-IPMN, the overall incidence rate of invasive carcinoma was 3.3%, 6.6%, and 15.0% at 5, 10, and 15 years, respectively.[41] In another study from MGH, the rate of high-grade or invasive cancer was 5.5% and invasive cancer was developed in 4.4%.[42] Factors shown to be associated with the presence of invasive cancer in large series include symptoms at presentation such as jaundice, pancreatitis, and new-onset diabetes; larger lesions (cyst size ≥ 3 cm); an abrupt change in caliber of the pancreatic duct with distal pancreatic atrophy; mural nodules; main-duct dilation; cyst growth over time; and elevated serum cancer antigen (CA) 19-9 levels. In addition, patients with IPMN are at an increased risk for developing conventional pancreatic ductal adenocarcinoma (between 1% and 8%) elsewhere in the pancreas.[43–45]

The reported outcome associated with invasive cancer in patients with IPMN (43%–60% 5-year survival) has been thought to be improved when compared with patients with ductal adenocarcinoma (15% 5-year survival) after resection. Poultsides et al. reported the Johns Hopkins experience of IPMN-associated invasive cancers and found that compared with patients with ductal adenocarcinoma, IPMN patients had lower rates of advanced T stage and lymph node metastasis. Patients with ductal adenocarcinoma more often had high-grade lesions and evidence of perineural invasion, vascular invasion, and positive margins. Despite patients with IPMN-associated cancers having an overall better outcome, if any of the adverse tumor-related factors were present, the outcome was similar to patients with ductal adenocarcinoma.[33] One may infer from this study that the improved outcome of IPMN-associated cancer is a factor of the earlier stage of disease at resection. These findings were confirmed in a meta-analysis of

12 comparative studies between conventional pancreas adeno-carcinoma and IPMN-associated cancer.[46]

Variants of IPMN-associated cancers have different progno-ses. Patients with colloid-subtype invasive IPMN had significantly better survival than both matched patients with conventional pancreatic carcinoma and patients with invasive tubular IPMN.[47] Among IPMN-associated cancers, tubular-variant and lymph node involvement were negative prognostic factors associated with outcome. Patients with conventional adenocarcinoma more often were seen with obstructive jaundice and had more speci-mens with evidence of perineural/vascular invasion and regional lymph node metastasis. In a pooled analysis of literature, tubular adenocarcinoma had a poor overall survival (HR 1.90) compared with colloid carcinoma and similar to the survival of pancreatic ductal adenocarcinoma.[48]

Genetics of Intraductal Papillary Mucinous Neoplasm

Although IPMN shares many molecular alterations with pancre-atic cancer, there are some significant differences with respect to both the prevalence of these mutations and the presence of novel mutations. Like the genetic landscape of pancreatic cancer, *KRAS* mutations, loss of *p16*, and *TP53* mutations are fre-quently observed in IPMN. Besides the similarities, the genetic makeup of pancreatic cancer and IPMN has some contrasting differences. SMAD4/DPC4 expression, which is inactivated in more than half of patients with pancreatic adenocarcinoma, is preserved in virtually all noninvasive IPMNs[49] and is lost only in 10% of colloid cancers arising in the background of intestinal-type IPMN.[50] Another prominent difference is the mutations of the *GNAS* gene in IPMN. *GNAS* mutations have been de-scribed in as many as 66% of IPMN cases. *GNAS* mutations were not found in other types of cystic neoplasms of the pan-creas or in invasive adenocarcinomas not associated with IPMNs.[51] *GNAS* mutations are the predominant mutation in patients with colloid carcinoma (*KRAS* uncommon), and *KRAS* mutations are much more common in tubular carcinoma (*GNAS* uncommon). It also seems concomitant pancreas ade-nocarcinoma tends to develop in the pancreas with IPMNs with wild-type *GNAS*, irrespective of the BD- or MD-IPMN sub-type.[52] The whole-exome sequencing of pancreatic cysts showed IPMNs had alterations of RNF43, *GNAS*, or *KRAS* and never had VHL or CTNNB1 mutations.[51] These findings emphasize the role of molecular genetic analysis in combination with clini-cal and radiologic data to have a more accurate diagnosis. Un-derstanding the mutation type may also be helpful to predict progression to invasive cancer (see Chapters 9D and 59).

DIAGNOSTIC EVALUATION OF PANCREATIC CYSTIC NEOPLASMS

High-quality cross-sectional imaging is the key to the diagnos-tic evaluation of any cystic lesion of the pancreas. Multidetector CT allows thin-section imaging of the pancreas and is the most common method for the evaluation of pancreatic cysts. A pan-creatic protocol CT scan can carefully delineate and character-ize the pancreatic parenchyma near a cystic lesion, which is critical in assessing for a radiographically occult invasive cancer–causing adjacent dilation of a pancreatic duct. In addition, care-ful visualization of the cystic lesion allows evaluation of septa-tions, mural nodules, and calcifications. MRCP can also be used to define cyst morphology and may actually be better than CT for determining a connection with the pancreatic duct,

presence of an enhancing mural nodule, or internal septa-tions.[53] Secretin-enhanced MRCP also has been introduced to improve the visualization of a connection between a pancreatic cyst and the main pancreatic duct[54] (see Chapter 17).

An improvement in endoscopic techniques has significantly improved the clinician's ability to evaluate pancreatic cystic neoplasms. The indication for EUS is implied as an adjunct to other imaging modalities if the pancreas cyst has either con-cerning or radiologic features or to obtain cyst fluid for cytol-ogy and biochemical analysis for a more precise diagnosis (Box 60.1). Because this procedure is operator dependent, a gastroenterologist with expertise in performing EUS is highly valuable.[55,56] Distinction between mucin clots or debris and mural nodules is clinically important. Contrast-enhanced EUS is one of the most accurate diagnostic modalities for the dis-crimination between mural nodules and mucin clots. Contrast-enhanced EUS can characterize vascularity by detecting signals from microbubbles in vessels produced by intravenously (IV) administered contrast agents[57] (see Chapter 22).

Confocal laser endomicroscopy (CLE) is a new promising technique to differentiate between the different pancreatic cyst types. CLE shows real-time visualization of the pancreatic cyst with microscopic detail using an endoscopic probe introduced through a 19-gauge needle.[58] Each pancreatic cyst type has a specific imaging pattern; for example, superficial vascular net-work or "fern pattern" is highly specific for SCAs.[59] MCN characteristic findings are single or multiple layers of epithelium without a papillary configuration (epithelial bands), whereas IPMN finger-like papillae is a characteristic feature.[60,61]

Cyst fluid analysis has been extensively studied as a diagnos-tic tool in the assessment of cystic lesions of the pancreas.[62,63] EUS–fine-needle aspiration (FNA) is considered a low-risk pro-cedure with a complication rate of 2% to 3%. Numerous mark-ers have been evaluated, including CA19-9, cancer embryonic antigen (CEA), CA15-3, mucin proteins, KRAS, and amylase. In a landmark study by Brugge and colleagues,[64] cyst fluid CEA greater than 192 ng/mL was the best predictor of a mucinous lesion, which accurately defined these lesions in 79% of cases. An elevation of cyst fluid CEA in combination with the presence of extracellular mucin has been shown to have a positive predic-tive value as high as 85% in some series. SCAs and pancreatic

---

BOX 60.1 Indications for Evaluation of Pancreatic Cyst With EUS

European 2018
- If the EUS changes clinical management
- Cyst clinical or radiologic features of concern identified during the initial investigation or surveillance

IAP 2017
- Growth rate ≥ 5 mm over 2 years
- Increased levels of serum CA19-9
- MPD dilatation between 5 and 9 mm
- Cyst diameter ≥ 3 cm
- Acute pancreatitis (caused by IPMN)
- Enhancing mural nodule (< 5 mm)
- Abrupt change in caliber of MPD with distal pancreatic atrophy
- Lymphadenopathy
- Thickened/enhancing cyst walls

CA19-9, Cancer antigen 19-9; *EUS,* endoscopic ultrasound; *European,* European Study Group on Cystic Tumors of the Pancreas; *IAP,* International Association of Pancreatology; *IPMN,* intraductal papillary mucinous neoplasm; *MPD,* main pancreatic duct.

retention cysts uniformly have undetectable levels of CEA.[65] The ability to predict the presence of invasive disease, however, has not been demonstrated by the measurement of cyst fluid CEA.[64,66] Pancreatic cyst fluid glucose levels have also been described as a potential biomarker for mucinous pancreatic cyst, with similar diagnostic accuracy to the standard CEA, amylase, and cytology tests but with improved efficiency.[67,68] Cyst fluid amylase is another cyst fluid protein marker; low amylase levels are useful to exclude a pseudocyst,[65] but a high cyst fluid amylase level is not helpful because it may be found in multiple types of pancreatic cysts including SCAs, IPMNs, and MCNs.[69]

The limitations of cyst fluid cytology stem from the very small volume of evaluable fluid and the low cellular content of aspirates. Furthermore, the samples are often contaminated with mucin and mucin-producing cells from the stomach or duodenum, through which the EUS needle is passed to reach the cyst. A through-the-needle forceps device has been recently introduced as a novel approach for EUS-guided tissue acquisition. These microforceps can be passed through a 19-gauge EUS needle to obtain samples of the cyst wall and/or mural nodule. This technique might improve diagnostic accuracy. However, experience with this sampling technique is limited to case reports and small pilot studies, and therefore this technique remains investigational.[70]

Limitations of cyst fluid CEA measurements and cytology coupled with increasing understanding of the molecular events leading to cyst formation (KRAS mutation, p53 mutation, and loss of p16 and SMAD4)[9,71] has led investigators to search for markers of dysplasia in patients with IPMN. Mutations or deletions in SMAD4, CDKN2A, TP53, PIK3CA and/or PTEN are associated with advanced neoplasia.[72]

Furthermore, KRAS mutation followed by allelic loss was initially felt to be strongly predictive of a malignant cyst.[73] An attempt has been made to validate these results in other studies, and the results have been mixed,[74] with KRAS mutation alone having high specificity but very low sensitivity at only 11%. This study also demonstrated that molecular analysis alone had lower sensitivity (76.5%) when compared with CEA measurement alone (detected 82.4% of all mucinous lesions). Recently, a novel murine monoclonal antibody (mAb) Das-1 has been developed and multiple studies showed high sensitivity and specificity of this biomarker for the detection of high-risk and invasive carcinoma.[75,76]

A machine-learning method, CompCyst, is a new technique that integrates high-dimensional clinical (symptoms), imaging (solid component), and genetic mutations based on cyst fluid analysis (KRAS, GNAS, RNF43, CDKN2A, CTNNB1, TP53, BRAF, VHL, PIK3CA) to diagnose and determine the likely best course of action for patients with pancreatic cysts. A previous study from the Johns Hopkins group showed this method is more accurate than the management dictated by conventional clinical and imaging criteria alone.[77] Therefore CompCyst has the potential to reduce the patient morbidity and economic costs associated with the current standard of the care.

TREATMENT OF PANCREATIC CYSTIC NEOPLASMS

If the histopathology of a cystic neoplasm can be diagnosed by clinical and imaging criteria, then treatment recommendations should be made based on the known behavior of that specific histologic entity. In some instances, most often in patients with small cysts, the exact histopathologic diagnosis cannot be determined without formal pancreatectomy. It is under these circumstances that treatment recommendations are based on the radiographic and *inferred* histopathology once a comprehensive diagnostic evaluation is complete.

Serous Cystadenoma

When radiographic and/or endoscopic findings are characteristic of SCA (microcystic, central scar, low cyst fluid CEA), resection should be reserved for young patients with lesions that have experienced significant growth or when the lesion is clearly symptomatic or to prevent complications related to occlusion of the splenic and/or portal veins. As discussed earlier in this chapter, asymptomatic patients have a risk of invasive carcinoma of less than 1%. For these lesions, the risk associated with pancreatectomy is much greater than the risk of cancer. It is well documented that the risk of cancer in SCA is exceedingly rare, and therefore resection should not be based on the risk of invasive carcinoma.

Tseng and colleagues[78] radiographically followed 24 patients with SCA for a median time of 23 months. The authors reported a 0.6 cm per year median growth rate for these lesions and noted that larger lesions (≥4 cm) had a higher growth rate (1.98 cm/yr) compared with lesions smaller than 4 cm (0.12 cm/yr). The authors recommended that all patients with SCAs larger than 4 cm should be resected, regardless of symptoms. However, in a study from Memorial Sloan Kettering, no association was found between larger size and faster growth.[79] In another multicenter study of 2622 patients with a diagnosis of SCA, the risk of invasive carcinoma was estimated very low. Surgical treatment was recommended only to a minority of patients with uncertain diagnosis remaining after complete workup, patients with significant and related symptoms, or exceptionally when concern with invasive carcinoma exists.[19]

Management of SCAs should mainly follow a conservative approach, following asymptomatic patients and monitoring if any progression in size and appearance or onset of symptoms happen. Surgical resection should be considered only for symptomatic patients, potentially malignant tumor, or a diagnostic dilemma. Decisions in large SCAs should be made on a case-by-case basis, considering the patient's age, tumor location, and patients' comorbidities. A young patient without comorbidity with a potentially growing lesion in the body/tail of the pancreas could be a candidate for function-preserving minimally invasive surgical resection. Apart from that, large SCAs can be strictly followed and resection considered only in cases of symptoms or rapid increase in cyst size.

Mucinous Cystic Neoplasms

The 2012 International Association of Pancreatology (IAP) guidelines recommend resection for all MCNs regardless of size, whereas the European guidelines (2018) recommend resection for MCNs with cyst dimension 4 cm or larger, enhancing mural nodules, or symptoms related to the cyst (jaundice, acute pancreatitis, new-onset diabetes). This latter group suggests that patients with MCN less than 4 cm and otherwise asymptomatic can be safely followed every 6 months for 1 year and then yearly.[80,81] Multiple studies showed that small indeterminate MCNs without symptoms or high-risk features can safely be observed.[25,82] MCNs are more often located in the distal pancreas and therefore may be amenable to splenic preservation and laparoscopic resection, which has been demonstrated to be safe and feasible.

A systematic review including 13 studies with 773 patients found no risk of progression after resection of MCN without invasive cancer.[24] Therefore patients with surgically resected MCN with low-grade or high-grade dysplasia do not require surveillance. This is an additional argument for resection, particularly in young patients, because unlike for patients with IPMN, there is no long-term, lifelong follow-up required. Patients with features that are concerning for invasive carcinoma should have formal pancreatectomy, and if a patient has a mucinous cystadenocarcinoma, they should undergo postoperative surveillance, as for patients with pancreatic cancer.

Main-Duct IPMN and Combined-Type IPMN: Indication and Extent of Resection

When MD-IPMN is identified based on cross-sectional imaging, operative resection is generally recommended because these lesions have a high risk of harboring high-grade dysplasia or invasive disease. Even when invasive carcinoma or high-grade dysplasia does not exist at the time of presentation, it is believed that most, if not all, MD-IPMNs will progress to invasive carcinoma.[83] Because of the frequency of invasive disease within MD-IPMN, a careful assessment of local resectability should be performed before operative intervention.

Historically, mixed-type IPMNs have been treated like MD-IPMN, assuming a similar risk of invasive carcinoma because of the involvement of the main pancreatic duct. The MGH group demonstrated that a minimal involvement of the main pancreatic duct does not carry the same malignant potential as a true MD-IPMN.[84] On the other hand, during the international consensus for main-duct/mixed-type IPMNs with pancreatic duct dilation (≥ 5 mm), 41% of experts advised nonoperative surveillance every 3 to 6 months, whereas 59% of experts advised operative intervention.[85] The European guidelines in 2018 defined main pancreatic duct dilation of 10 mm or greater as an absolute indication for surgical resection and 5 to 9 mm diameter as a relative indication for surgical resection.[80] Similarly, IAP 2017 recommended surgical resection for all MD-IPMNs with a main pancreatic duct of at least 10 mm. The main pancreatic duct 5 to 9 mm is considered as "worrisome features" with no recommendation for immediate surgical resection, but EUS evaluation is recommended.[83]

The extent of pancreatic resection for patients with MD-IPMN is controversial. The goal of surgery in MD-IPMN is the resection of invasive carcinoma and high-grade dysplasia and, if possible, removal of all high-risk disease. When the presence of invasive cancer can be ascertained preoperatively, a standard resection with lymphadenectomy should be considered (see Chapters 117A and 117B). The prognosis of patients with invasive IPMN is dominated by the biology and outcome of the invasive component, and the development of additional invasive or noninvasive disease in the remnant MD-IPMN is of less concern. Thus total pancreatectomy is generally avoided when preoperative testing suggests an invasive cancer in the setting of IPMN (see Chapter 117C).

In patients with MD-IPMN in which the disease is limited to a part of the pancreas and there is no overt radiographic evidence of invasive cancer, resection of the IPMN-containing pancreas, with pancreaticoduodenectomy for the head of the pancreas and distal pancreatectomy for the body and tail of the pancreas, should be performed. When performing partial pancreatectomy for IPMN, intraoperative frozen-section evaluation focused on the identification of high-grade dysplasia or an occult invasive cancer at the margin should be performed because data suggest that high-risk disease at the margin is a significant predictor of future remnant progression.[86,87] The 2017 IAP guidelines recommend that when low-grade dysplasia is present at the margin, no further resection is required because of the risk of progression to cancer, and local progression are minimal.[83] Conversely, high-grade dysplasia, as well as invasive carcinoma at the margin, should prompt additional resection, with some advocating that total pancreatectomy is a negative margin that cannot be achieved. In addition, it should be noted that frozen section is not able to capture discontinuous lesions ("skipped lesions") of the main pancreatic duct.

Patients with MD-IPMN diffusely involving the whole gland pose a difficult management dilemma. Ductal dilation throughout the pancreas could be because of MD-IPMN extending throughout the pancreatic duct or because of outflow obstruction caused by invasive carcinoma or IPMN in the head of the pancreas. Furthermore, dilation may also occur proximal or distal to the high-risk lesion because of the overproduction of mucus. Thus, in the absence of clear signs of invasive carcinoma (mass effect, intraductal mass, or nodules), ductal dilation does not help in the localization of invasive cancer. Because IPMN is considered to represent a field defect within the entire ductal system, there is concern that in cases with ductal dilation throughout the pancreas, removal of just part of the pancreas leaves the patient with a remnant pancreas with significant risk for developing pancreatic adenocarcinoma. This is even more of a concern in young patients, in whom the pancreatic remnant has a longer time for development of invasive carcinoma. However, this risk needs to be balanced with the morbidity, mortality, and reduced quality of life (QoL) with total pancreatectomy (see Chapter 117C). In a study of 329 patients who underwent total pancreatectomy in two high-volume centers (Johns Hopkins and University of Verona) between 2000 and 2014, the operative morbidity was 59.3% and 30-day operative mortality rate was 2.1%. QoL assessment was performed in a subset of patients using Short Form (SF) 36, European Organization for Research and Treatment of Cancer QLQ-PAN26, and Audit of Diabetes Dependent questionnaires, as well as an original survey. Young age, abdominal pain, and worse perception of body image were negatively associated with the physical component of SF-36, whereas diabetes, sexual satisfaction, and perception of body image affected the mental component of SF-36.[88] In another study of 93 patients who underwent total pancreatectomy from a multicentric French database between 2004 and 2013, postoperative mortality and morbidity were reported at 4.3% and 47.3%, respectively.[89] These results suggest that total pancreatectomy is a viable option for patients with main-duct IPMN with diffuse involvement of pancreas and should be discussed with patients who have a gland at very high risk for developing invasive carcinoma.

When less than a total pancreatectomy is performed, postoperative surveillance is warranted in all patients. Patients with noninvasive IPMN should be followed for the development of additional lesions within the remnant gland, and patients with invasive disease should be followed for both distant recurrence and gland recurrence. There is no consensus for the best follow-up strategy after pancreatectomy for patients with noninvasive IPMN. IAP 2017 guidelines recommend follow-up at least twice a year in patients with a family history of pancreatic cancer or a surgical resection margin with high-grade dysplasia or a resected IPMN of the nonintestinal subtype, and follow-up every 6 to 12 months in all other patients with resected

IPMNs.[83] On the contrary, the 2018 European guidelines recommend follow-up every 6 months for the first 2 years, followed by yearly surveillance, for IPMNs with high-grade dysplasia or main duct involvement after pancreatectomy. IPMN with low-grade dysplasia should be followed up in the same way as nonresected IPMN.[80] Completion pancreatectomy is indicated for the treatment of any detected progression thought to be representative of high-grade dysplasia or invasive disease.

Branch-Duct Intraductal Papillary Mucinous Neoplasm: Indication for Resection

Resection is reserved for selected patients with BD-IPMN. The 2017 IAP guidelines have classified the concerning radiographic features into "worrisome features" and "high-risk stigmata."[83] Based on these recommendations, patients with "high-risk stigmata" (obstructive jaundice in a patient with a cystic lesion of the pancreatic head, enhancing mural nodule ≥ 5mm, and main pancreatic duct ≥ 10 mm) should undergo resection without further testing. Cysts with worrisome features (pancreatitis, cyst ≥ 3 cm, enhancing mural nodule < 5 mm, thickened/enhancing cyst walls, main duct size 5–9 mm, an abrupt change in caliber of the pancreatic duct with distal pancreatic atrophy, lymphadenopathy, increased serum level of CA19-9, and cyst growth rate > 5 mm/2 years) should undergo further evaluation with EUS. These guidelines also recommend EUS evaluation of cysts greater than 3 cm without any worrisome features to verify the absence of thickened walls or mural nodules. A multicentric study has analyzed the outcomes and predictors of survival in nonoperative patients with presumed IPMNs. The authors found that patients with IPMNs who had "worrisome features" had a 5-year disease-specific survival of 96%, suggesting that conservative management is appropriate in these patients. On the other hand, the presence of "high-risk stigma" was associated with a 40% risk of IPMN-related death, indicating the policy of surgical resection in patients with "high-risk stigma."[43]

The 2018 European guidelines also have similar recommendations to the 2017 IAP for resection of BD-IPMN; absolute indications for surgery are jaundice, cytology positive for high-grade dysplasia or cancer, the presence of a contrast-enhancing mural nodule (≥5 mm) or solid mass. Patients with relative indications for surgery (growth rate ≥5 mm/year, increased serum CA 19.9 level >37 U/mL in the absence of jaundice, main pancreatic duct diameter between 5 and 9.9 mm, cyst size ≥4 cm, new-onset of diabetes mellitus or AP, and contrast-enhancing mural nodules < 5 mm) should undergo closer follow-up or resection based on their comorbidities.

Branch-duct lesions in the head of the pancreas should be resected with pancreatoduodenectomy and in the tail with distal pancreatectomy with or without splenectomy (see Chapters 117A and 117B). Recently, pancreas-sparing procedures, such as enucleation and central pancreatectomy, have been reported in an effort to maintain the exocrine and endocrine pancreatic function (see Chapter 117B). A single institutional study demonstrated that pancreas-sparing pancreatectomy is feasible in the treatment of IPMN and can be performed with acceptable mortality.[90] In this study, pancreas-sparing pancreatectomy was attempted in 91 patients and was feasible in 81 patients (89%). Enucleation was the most common pancreas-sparing pancreatectomy procedure. Other procedures included central pancreatectomy and resection of the uncinate process. Although these procedures were performed with acceptable mortality, there was higher-than-expected morbidity when compared with standard pancreatic resections, mainly in the form of pancreatic fistula. Whether or not pancreas-sparing pancreatectomy allows for preservation of pancreatic exocrine and endocrine function will require further investigation.

Solid Pseudopapillary Tumor and Other Cystic Pancreatic Neoplasms

SPTs are also known as Frantz or Hamoudi tumors after the pathologists who first described this unique entity in the 1950s.[91,92] SPTs are rare tumors that account for as many as 2.5% of resected pancreatic neoplasms. They are predominately in young women and are often discovered when patients experience symptoms. A review of SPTs[93] described the clinicopathologic factors of 2744 patients collected from the English literature. The female to male ratio was 9:1, and the mean age was 29 years. Only 38% of the patients in the review were asymptomatic at presentation, with 64% of patients having pain and 33% having a mass. Tumors were often large, and the mean tumor size was 8.6 cm. The most common location for SPTs was the tail and body pancreas (59.3%). SPT tumors may also present acutely with rupture of the capsule and resulting hemoperitoneum, although this is uncommon. Mao et al. reviewed 292 reported cases in the literature and found 8 cases with acute rupture.[94]

Cross-sectional imaging characteristically reveals encapsulated lesions with irregular areas of hypodensity secondary to necrosis or hemorrhage (see Chapter 17). The wall may reveal calcifications. Because of the cystic degeneration exhibited by these lesions, they are often difficult to differentiate from pseudocyst or other pancreatic cystic neoplasms. However, when a well-encapsulated pancreatic mass with cystic and solid components is encountered in a young female patient, SPT should be at the top of the differential diagnosis. What differentiates these lesions from other cystic tumors is a combination of solid and cystic components, with gradual degenerative changes resulting in pseudopapillae formation.[95,96] SPTs are distinct from the normal pancreatic parenchyma and, like other cystic neoplasms, rarely cause ductal dilation because of the lack of invasion. On MRI, SPTs can present as areas of high signal intensity on T1-weighted images correspond to areas of hemorrhagic necrosis or hemorrhagic debris.

Grossly, these tumors appear tan or yellow and are well circumscribed and smooth on palpation. When opened, the tumors show irregular cystic cavities with some areas of necrosis or hemorrhage. Most SPTs can be diagnosed with routine histologic evaluation by the presence of polygonal epithelial cells arranged in a discohesive pattern. The boundaries resemble a mass effect as opposed to being invasive. Immunohistochemical staining for vimentin, keratin, neuron-specific enolase, CD10, and progesterone is common.[97,98] These lesions rarely will express chromogranin or estrogen. In contrast to ductal adenocarcinoma, abnormal β-catenin expression has been shown to be present in SPTs, whereas KRAS, p53, and DPC4 appear to be unaltered[98,99] (see Chapters 9D and 59). Aggressive phenotypes of SPT have been demonstrated and histologically exhibit a high mitotic rate, nuclear atypia, spindling of tumor cells, and anaplastic giant tumor cells consistent with sarcomatoid carcinoma.[95] Park et al. demonstrated the existence of new molecular alterations involved in SPT. The results of a 1686 gene analysis revealed that the Wnt/β-catenin, Hedgehog, and androgen receptor signaling pathways, as well as genes involved in epithelial mesenchymal transition, are activated in SPTs.[100] The role of genetic testing in the diagnosis of SPTs has not been extensively investigated, and further studies are needed to characterize specific, clinically related mutations for this entity.

Clinically, SPTs are generally indolent and typically cured with complete surgical extirpation. Many series have demonstrated long-term survival after resection.[101,102] Significant vascular invasion is the most common reason for the inability to resect these lesions. Metastatic disease has been noted to be present in as many as 15% of patients. Criteria for defining SPTs as "malignant" may be a locally advanced disease with vascular invasion precluding resection, or lymph node or hepatic metastasis. Long-term survival is often possible despite the presence of malignant factors such as metastatic disease and should not preclude resection in selected cases.[97,101] In a meta-analysis of literature between 2002 and 2017, the progression rate after initial surgery in patients with nonmetastatic SPTs was estimated around 2.6%. Male gender, positive lymph nodes, positive margin at the time of resection, and lymph vascular invasion were associated with a risk of progression.[103]

CONCLUSIONS

The diagnosis of cystic lesions of the pancreas is increasing, and the most common lesions are IPMNs, MCNs, and SCAs. Despite multiple clinical guidelines, there is no definitive strategy to differentiate between various cyst types. Therefore patients with pancreas cysts should be discussed by a multidisciplinary team in centers with expertise in diagnosis (imaging, endoscopy, pathology) and surgical treatment of pancreatic cysts. SCAs should be considered benign, and in the asymptomatic patient, they can be followed radiographically. Most patients with mucinous lesions should undergo resection, especially in the setting of concerning features such as size greater than 3 cm, solid component, and ductal dilation. The initial evaluation of a small, benign-appearing cyst should include one early interval image to ensure no occult invasive carcinoma or high-grade dysplasia is present that has resulted in a retention cyst.

Although more clinicians are adopting a selective approach, improvements have been made in the ability to determine histopathologic subtypes without resection. High-quality cross-sectional imaging and EUS with cyst fluid analysis can help subtype many pancreatic cystic neoplasms. Advancements are also being made in the development of biomarkers from cyst fluid. Continued improvements in all these modalities should lead to better identification of mucinous subtypes, obviating the need for resection.

The references for this chapter can be found online by accessing the accompanying Expert Consult website.

SECTION II. Neoplastic

C. Malignant Tumors

CHAPTER 61

Pancreatic cancer: Epidemiology

Theresa Pluth Yeo, Geoffrey W. Krampitz, and Charles J. Yeo

OVERVIEW

The pancreas, an organ located in the retroperitoneum, has both exocrine and endocrine functions. The exocrine pancreas is composed of duct cells and acinar cells that produce enzymes needed to break down carbohydrates, proteins, and lipids, thus promoting digestion. The majority of malignant pancreatic neoplasms are presumed to arise from the exocrine component.[1]

Pancreatic ductal adenocarcinoma (PDAC) is the most common type of pancreatic cancer (PC), representing greater than 90% of the exocrine pancreas cases (see Chapter 59). The other 10% of exocrine tumors are mucinous tumors, mixed adenosquamous tumors, or acinar cell tumors.[1] Endocrine neoplasms (pancreatic neuroendocrine tumors) contribute approximately 5% of the total pancreatic cancer cases.[1] In this chapter, the abbreviations PDAC and PC may be used interchangeably, depending on how the term was defined in different investigations.

Of the 2,820,034 deaths recorded in the United States (US) in 2017, 21% were from cancer.[2] Overall, the cancer death rate has declined 29% from its peak in 1991 (215.1 per 100,000 population) to 2017 (152.4 per 100,000 population).[2] The lower cancer death rate is largely driven by declining cigarette smoking and improvements in early detection and treatment and fewer annual deaths from lung cancer in particular.

PDAC is responsible for 3.0% of all new cancers, but 8% of all cancer deaths in the US.[2] PDAC is the fourth leading cause of cancer death in men, after lung, prostate, and colorectal cancer, and as of 2014, it is also the fourth leading cause of cancer death in women, after lung, breast, and colorectal cancer.[2] The incidence of PC continues to increase with more than 57,600 new cases of PC predicted for the US and approximately 47,050 deaths in 2020.[2] The diagnosis of PDAC continues to confer an unfavorable prognosis, with an increase in the death rate for PDAC cases of 0.4% between 1998 and 2017.[2] In the past 10 years, however, the 5-year survival rate has tripled to 9.3%, as a result of the persistent efforts by oncologists, research scientists, and surgeons alike. PDAC is predicted to become the second leading cause of cancer death by 2030.[2,3] This is mainly because of greatly improved survival for the other leading cancers (lung, breast, colorectal, and prostate cancer) and limited success in improving the chemotherapeutic and radiotherapeutic treatment options for PDAC because of multilayered therapeutic resistance. These layers include but

are not limited to a dense, desmoplastic tumor stroma that creates a hypoxic environment, reduced vascular density, immune suppression, and early, undetected microscopic metastases.[4] Current research targeting each of these challenges offers hope for progress in the laboratory and in clinical practice.

PC is the seventh leading cause of cancer-related deaths worldwide with 432,242 deaths in 2018, representing 2.5% of all cancers.[5,6] Globally, 458,918 new cases of pancreatic cancer were reported in 2018. The annual incidence rate worldwide for all histologic types of pancreatic cancer is approximately 4.9 new cases per 100,000 persons, ranking 12th among all cancers globally (Figs. 61.1 and 61.2).[7] On a worldwide basis, PC is also more common in men (5.5 cases per 100,000 men) than in women (4.0 cases per 100,000 women).[6] The risk of developing PDAC is highest in Hungary (10.8 cases per 100,000 persons), Uruguay (10.7 cases per 100,000 persons), the Republic of Moldova (10.5 cases per 100,000 persons), and Latvia (10.3 cases per 100,000 persons).[8] The lowest rates are in Guinea (0.35 cases per 100,000 persons) and Malawi (0.40 cases per 100,000 persons).[8] There are few to no cases in certain African regions, such as Comoros and Sao Tome and Principe.[8] Tables 61.1 and 61.2 show the global incidence and mortality of PC by country.

NONMODIFIABLE RISK FACTORS

Gender and Age

The US National Center for Health Statistics estimates the number of new cases of PC in 2020 will be 30,400 in men and 27,200 in women, accounting for 3% of all cancers in the US.[2] The US population risk for PC is 14.0 per 100,000 for men and 10.7 per 100,000 for women. Women in high development index countries have 5 times greater risk of PC than women in lower development index countries.[7] A systematic review of 15 studies found no reproductive factors associated with the risk of developing PC in women.[22]

In the US, the peak incidence of PDAC occurs in the seventh and eighth decades of life.[23,24] The main risk factor for PC is advancing age. Between 2007 and 2011, the median age at diagnosis for cancer of the pancreas was 71 years, and the median age at death was 73 years according to Surveillance, Epidemiology, and End Results (SEER) data.[23] More than 60% of new PDAC cases occur between the ages of 65 and 84 years. The peak age of incidence varies between countries; for example, in

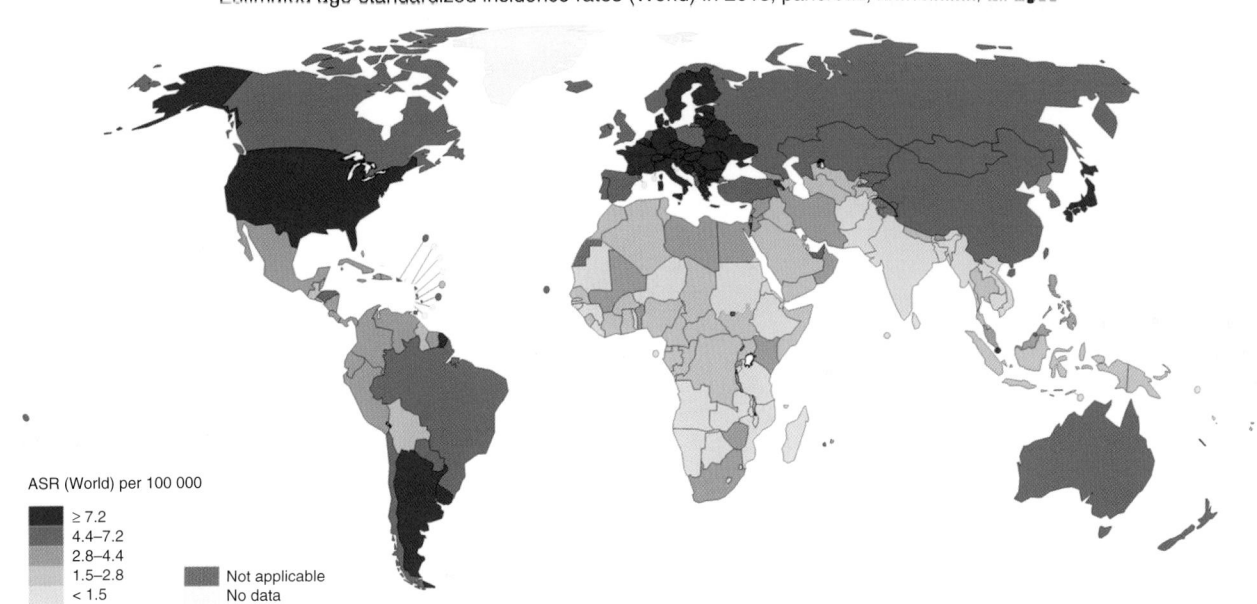

FIGURE 61.1   Heatmap of the global incidence of pancreatic cancer. (From Ferlay J EM, Lam F, Colombet M, Mery L, Piñeros M, Znaor A, Soerjomataram I, Bray F. Global cancer observatory: Cancer today. *International Agency for Research on Cancer.* https://gco.iarc.fr/today. 2018. Accessed June 6, 2020.)

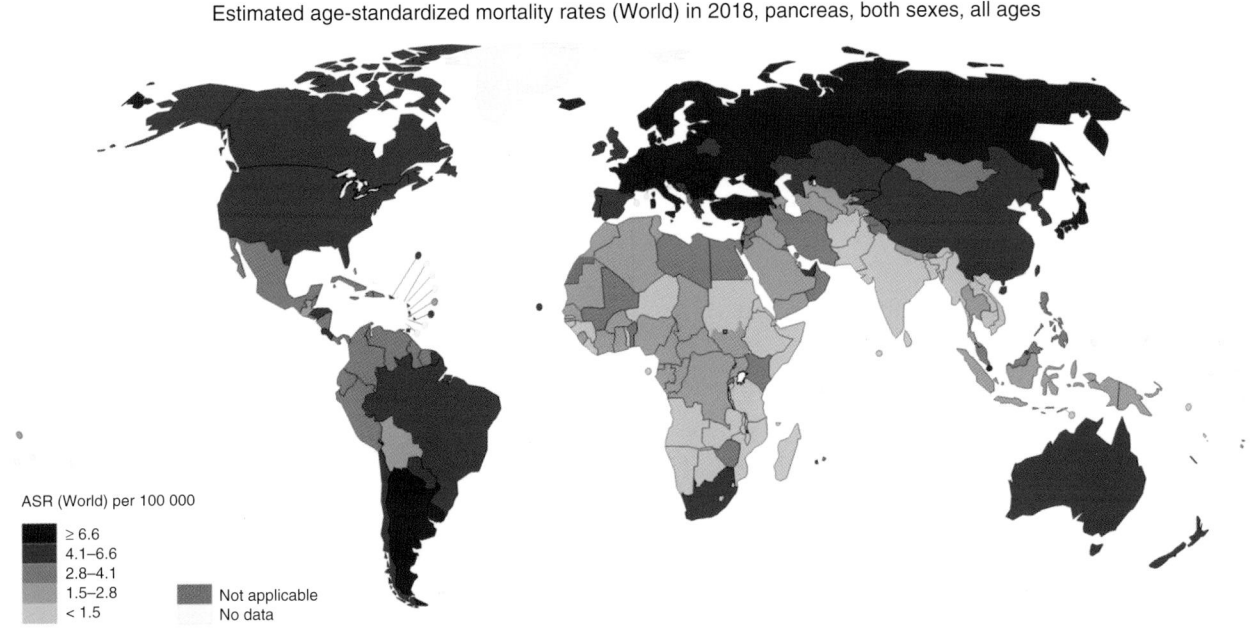

FIGURE 61.2   Heatmap of the global mortality of pancreatic cancer. (From Ferlay J EM, Lam F, Colombet M, Mery L, Piñeros M, Znaor A, Soerjomataram I, Bray F. Global cancer observatory: Cancer today. *International Agency for Research on Cancer.* https://gco.iarc.fr/today. 2018. Accessed June 6, 2020.)

India, the peak age is the sixth decade.[25] An emerging age-specific trend has been identified in individuals 20 to 29 years old and in those persons over the age of 80 years in the US.[26]

Race and Ethnicity

The incidence of PDAC remains highest for black Americans, with rates of 17.2 per 100,000 in men and 14.2 per 100,000 in women.[2] The lowest risk of pancreatic cancer is among Asian/Pacific Islander men and women (10.7 and 8.9 per 100,000,

respectively). African Americans have the highest death rates from cancer and the shortest survival period of all racial groups.[27,28] African American males specifically have higher incidence rates for all cancers combined and also for the most common cancers (prostate, lung, colorectal, and pancreas). Death rates, per 100,000 population, from PDAC are 15.5 for African American men and 12.6 for African American women, compared with 12.4 for white men and 9.3 for white women. African Americans of lower socioeconomic status are more

TABLE 61.1   Estimated Global Incidence and Mortality of Pancreatic Cancer[8]

ISO CODE	POPULATION	INCIDENCE	MORTALITY	ISO CODE	POPULATION	INCIDENCE	MORTALITY
HUN	Hungary	10.8	9.4	TUR	Turkey	6.7	6.6
URY	Uruguay	10.7	9.9	NOR	Norway	6.7	7.4
MDA	Republic of Moldova	10.5	8.5	ESP	Spain	6.6	5.9
LVA	Latvia	10.3	7.8	BRB	Barbados	6.4	6.4
JPN	Japan	9.7	7.8	CAN	Canada	6.4	5.9
SVK	Slovakia	9.6	7.9	GLP	France, Guadeloupe	6.1	6.3
EST	Estonia	9.2	7.9	IRL	Ireland	5.9	5.5
CZE	Czechia	9	8.3	CYP	Cyprus	5.9	6.2
FRA	France	8.9	7.7	REU	France, La Réunion	5.9	4.8
ARM	Armenia	8.9	8.5	KAZ	Kazakhstan	5.8	5.7
SRB	Serbia	8.8	7.9	ISL	Iceland	5.7	8.4
AUT	Austria	8.7	8.1	PRT	Portugal	5.6	5.4
BEL	Belgium	8.7	6.6	MNE	Montenegro	5.6	5.2
NCL	France, New Caledonia	8.6	6.1	CHL	Chile	5.6	5.4
BGR	Bulgaria	8.4	7.6	BRN	Brunei	5.4	4.8
MLT	Malta	8.3	8.7	CPV	Cabo Verde	5.4	5.3
DEU	Germany	8.3	7.8	TTO	Trinidad and Tobago	5.3	5.3
SVN	Slovenia	8.2	7.6	GUA	Guam	5.3	4.8
BIH	Bosnia and Herzegovina	8	6.3	CHN	China	5.2	4.9
HRV	Croatia	8	7.1	PRY	Paraguay	5.1	4.8
GUF	French Guiana	8	5.4	HND	Honduras	4.9	4.6
FIN	Finland	7.9	8.1	PYF	French Polynesia	4.8	4.8
DNK	Denmark	7.8	7.7	BRA	Brazil	4.7	4.4
MKD	The former Yugoslav Republic of Macedonia	7.8	6.9	MNG	Mongolia	4.6	3.9
LUX	Luxembourg	7.8	6.8	KGZ	Kyrgyzstan	4.5	4.4
SWE	Sweden	7.7	7.7	PRI	Puerto Rico	4.5	4.4
USA	United States of America	7.7	6.6	ALB	Albania	4.5	4.1
ISR	Israel	7.6	7.8	SUR	Suriname	4.4	4
LTU	Lithuania	7.6	7.2	ARE	United Arab Emirates	4.4	4.4
SGP	Singapore	7.6	6.7	PER	Peru	4.4	4.1
ITA	Italy	7.5	6.6	DOM	Dominican Republic	4.3	4.1
ROU	Romania	7.4	6.9	ZAF	South Africa	4.3	4.3
ARG	Argentina	7.3	6.9	LBY	Libya	4.3	4.1
GRC	Greece	7.3	6.5	VEN	Venezuela, Bolivarian Republic of	4.2	4
UKR	Ukraine	7.3	6.9	CUB	Cuba	4.1	3.8
KOR	Korea, Republic of	7.2	6.1	PRK	Korea, Democratic Republic of	4.1	4.2
BLR	Belarus	7.2	6.5	CRI	Costa Rica	4	4.1
CHE	Switzerland	7.2	6.6	COL	Colombia	4	3.7
RUS	Russian Federation	7.2	7.4	PSE	Gaza Strip and West Bank	3.8	3.8
POL	Poland	7.1	6.9	KWT	Kuwait	3.8	3.7
GBR	United Kingdom	7.1	6	PHL	Philippines	3.8	3.8
WSM	Samoa	7	2.1	EGY	Egypt	3.7	3.6
NLD	The Netherlands	7	7	LBN	Lebanon	3.7	3.7
MTQ	France, Martinique	7	6.3	JOR	Jordan	3.7	3.7
AUS	Australia	6.9	5.9	MUS	Mauritius	3.7	3.6
NZL	New Zealand	6.8	6	HTI	Haiti	3.6	3.1

TABLE 61.1 Estimated Global Incidence and Mortality of Pancreatic Cancer—cont'd

ISO CODE	POPULATION	INCIDENCE	MORTALITY	ISO CODE	POPULATION	INCIDENCE	MORTALITY
BHR	Bahrain	3.6	3.5	TJK	Tajikistan	1.9	1.8
MEX	Mexico	3.6	3.3	SSD	South Sudan	1.9	1.9
NIC	Nicaragua	3.6	3.5	CAF	Central African Republic	1.8	1.8
SYR	Syrian Arab Republic	3.3	3.3	TCD	Chad	1.8	1.8
RWA	Rwanda	3.3	3.3	BFA	Burkina Faso	1.8	1.8
MLI	Mali	3.3	3.3	COG	Congo, Republic of	1.7	1.6
BTN	Bhutan	3.2	3.2	GAB	Gabon	1.6	1.6
KEN	Kenya	3.2	3.2	SOM	Somalia	1.6	1.5
SLV	El Salvador	3.2	3.2	MMR	Myanmar	1.5	1.4
MYS	Malaysia	3.2	3	TLS	Timor-Leste	1.5	1.5
ECU	Ecuador	3.2	3	MRT	Mauritania	1.5	1.5
PAN	Panama	3.2	3	SLE	Sierra Leone	1.5	1.5
ZWE	Zimbabwe	3.2	3.2	LBR	Liberia	1.4	1.3
JAM	Jamaica	3.2	3.1	AFG	Afghanistan	1.4	1.4
IRN	Iran, Islamic Republic of	3.1	2.9	NER	Niger	1.4	1.4
BEN	Benin	3.1	2.9	GNB	Guinea-Bissau	1.4	1.4
GEO	Georgia	3.1	3	BDI	Burundi	1.4	1.5
OMN	Oman	3	3	NAM	Namibia	1.3	1.2
BLZ	Belize	2.9	2.9	AGO	Angola	1.2	1.1
LCA	Saint Lucia	2.8	2.8	LAO	Lao People's Democratic Republic	1.2	1.2
GUY	Guyana	2.8	2.9				
QAT	Qatar	2.7	2.7	MDV	Maldives	1.1	1.1
CMR	Cameroon	2.7	2.7	KHM	Cambodia	1.1	1.1
UZB	Uzbekistan	2.7	2.5	TGO	Togo	0.99	0.97
AZE	Azerbaijan	2.7	2.6	SDN	Sudan	1	1
BOL	Bolivia, Plurinational State of	2.7	2.7	BWA	Botswana	1	1
FJI	Fiji	2.6	2.6	BGD	Bangladesh	1	0.99
TUN	Tunisia	2.6	2.5	ETH	Ethiopia	0.92	0.72
TKM	Turkmenistan	2.6	2.6	VNM	Vietnam	0.88	0.82
IRQ	Iraq	2.5	2.5	ERI	Eritrea	0.94	0.92
CIV	Côte d'Ivoire	2.5	2.5	IND	India	0.85	0.82
COD	Congo, Democratic Republic of	2.5	2.5	LSO	Lesotho	0.72	0.72
DZA	Algeria	2.4	2.3	PAK	Pakistan	0.74	0.71
UGA	Uganda	2.4	2.4	SWZ	Eswatini	0.7	0.77
NGA	Nigeria	2.3	2.3	ZMB	Zambia	0.67	0.66
SAU	Saudi Arabia	2.2	2.1	TZA	Tanzania, United Republic of	0.55	0.55
GTM	Guatemala	2.2	2.2	MOZ	Mozambique	0.56	0.58
MAR	Morocco	2.2	1.9	SLB	Solomon Islands	0.64	1.3
YEM	Yemen	2.1	2.1	LKA	Sri Lanka	0.62	0.56
GHA	Ghana	2.1	2.1	VUT	Vanuatu	0.57	0.57
BHS	Bahamas	2.1	2.2	DJI	Djibouti	0.64	0.64
GNQ	Equatorial Guinea	2.1	2.1	MDG	Madagascar	0.52	0.53
IDN	Indonesia	2.1	2	GMB	The Republic of the Gambia	0.52	0.52
NPL	Nepal	2	1.8	MWI	Malawi	0.4	0.42
PNG	Papua New Guinea	2	1.9	GIN	Guinea	0.35	0.32
THA	Thailand	2	2	COM	Comoros	0	0
SEN	Senegal	2	2	STP	Sao Tome and Principe	0	0

TABLE 61.2 Risk Factors Associated With Cancer of the Pancreas: Summary of Previous Reports[9–21]

Lifestyle and Environmental Factors

Cigarette smoking (dose-response relationship)
Environmental tobacco smoke exposure, particularly early in life
Alcohol
Residential radon
Physical inactivity

Race/Ethnic Factors

African American men and women
Native female Hawaiians
Ashkenazi Jews

Inherited Predisposition

Hereditary pancreatitis
Hereditary nonpolyposis colorectal cancer
Hereditary breast and ovarian cancer
Familial atypical multiple mole melanoma syndrome
Peutz-Jeghers syndrome
Ataxia-telangiectasia
Fanconi anemia
Cystic fibrosis

Medical Conditions

Chronic pancreatitis
Cirrhosis
Diabetes (and pre-diabetes)
Helicobacter pylori infection
Periodontal disease

Dietary Factors

High fat/cholesterol
Overweight and obesity
Nitrosamines in food

Occupational Exposure to Carcinogens

Asbestos, 2-naphthylamine, benzidine, gasoline products, PAHs, dry-cleaning agents, DDT, radon

Selected High-Risk Occupations

Dry cleaning or chemical plant work, sawmill work, electrical equipment manufacturing work, mining, and metal-working occupations

Height

RR, 1.81 (CI, 1.31 to 2.52) when comparing tallest- and shortest-height categories for men and women

Previous Surgery

Cholecystectomy
Gastrectomy

Not all listed factors have been definitively proven to cause pancreatic cancer.
CI, Confidence interval; *DDT,* dichlorodiphenyl-trichloroethane; *PAHs,* polyaromatic hydrocarbons; *RR,* relative risk.

likely to be diagnosed with advanced stage pancreatic cancer and are less likely to undergo surgery or to receive chemotherapy.[27–29] Other known risk factors for PDAC (such as obesity, diabetes, and pancreatitis) are more common in African Americans.

It has been reported that, among smokers, serum cotinine levels, the primary metabolite of nicotine, are consistently higher in African Americans than in Whites and Mexican Americans, even after adjustment for the number of cigarettes smoked per day, the number of smokers in the home, the number of hours of environmental tobacco smoke (ETS) exposure at work, the number of rooms in the home, and the region of the country where the subject lived.[30] This suggests that genetic differences in cigarette product metabolism may influence rates of PDAC.

Ashkenazi Jews

PC occurs more commonly in the Jewish population, particularly those of Ashkenazi heritage.[9] The age-standardized rates for PDAC are significantly different for Jewish versus non-Jewish patients in Israel (7.2 per 100,000 for all Jewish men and 5.7 per 100,000 for Jewish women vs. 4.0 per 100,000 for non-Jewish men and 2.9 per 100,000 for non-Jewish women). Approximately 5% to 10% of this discrepancy is attributed to the *BRCA2* mutation, 6174delT, which is also associated with breast, gastric, ovarian, and bile duct cancers. The 6174delT

mutation is present in approximately 1% of Ashkenazi Jews and in approximately 4% of all patients with PDAC.[31,32] A *BRCA1* (185delAG, 5382insC) founder mutation occurs less commonly than the *BRCA2* mutation. In a study of 187 Jewish patients with PC, a *BRCA1* founder mutation was identified in 1.3% of the patients as compared with the *BRCA2* mutation, which was present in 4.1% of the patients[31] (see Chapter 9D).

Asians

Asian patients with PDAC have been reported to have less aggressive tumors than non-Asians (either Black or White patients) and higher survival rates when assessed on a stage-adjusted basis.[33] A recent population-based study using three SEER geographic areas with large Asian populations, namely Hawaii, San Francisco, and Seattle, examined whether Asians develop a histologically different type of PDAC than Western populations.[34] They compared PC cases in Japanese, Chinese, Filipino, Hawaiian, Black, and White patients in these areas. The study revealed that Japanese patients had the highest fraction of localized tumors with the lowest grade, and that Chinese, Filipino, and Japanese women had longer survival times than did Whites, although survival time was significantly different for Japanese women only. The reason for these differences is unknown, but race-related genetic and environmental exposure factors may be the cause of these survival discrepancies.

RISK FACTORS FOR PANCREATIC DUCTAL ADENOCARCINOMA AND PANCREATIC CANCERS

The risk factors for developing PC have been extensively studied, and new information continues to be uncovered. The etiology of PC is multifactorial and involves several common underlying pathways: insulin resistance, inflammation, hemostasis, and infection.[10] PC is also characterized by multiple germline and somatic genetic mutations.[11] (This topic is covered extensively in Chapter 9D.) Most PCs (>80%) are because of sporadically occurring mutations. It is estimated that less than 3% of PCs are truly hereditary and because of inherited germline mutations and their respective syndromes.[35] A 2015 investigation of the prevalence of germline mutations in PC patients found 11 pathogenic mutations of the genes: *ATM, BRCA1, BRCa2, MLH1, MSH6, TP53,* for a mutation carrier rate of 3.8%.[36] None of the mutations correlated with known family history of PC, age at diagnosis, or stage of disease.[36] There were also no carriers of *PALB2, CDK2NA, PRSS1,* or *STK11.*

Personal risk factors for PC include tobacco exposure, including cigarette, cigar, and pipe smoking; ETS exposure, also known as *secondhand smoke* or *passive smoke exposure;* exposure to occupational and environmental carcinogens; African-American race; Ashkenazi Jewish heritage; high-fat and high-cholesterol diets; obesity; alcohol abuse; pancreatitis; diabetes; blood group subtype; and infectious agents (see Table 61.2).[10,12,37–39] A recent extensive meta-analysis of 117 studies on putative causative factors for PC calculated the population attributable risk for many of the known risk factors.[10]

Familial Pancreatic Cancer and Inherited Genetic Disorders (see Chapter 9D)

PC is generally considered to be familial if two or more first-degree relatives (mother, father, sister, brother) have a confirmed diagnosis of pancreatic cancer. A more stringent definition used at some institutions requires three first-degree relatives to have PC to be considered familial cases.[13] A family history is found in about 5% to 10% of PC cases. Just having a family history of PC confers a 9-fold greater risk for PC than not having a family history.[40]

Findings from the 2017 Australian Pancreatic Cancer Genome Initiative found that 10% to 20% of PCs likely have an inherited component.[41] This is a higher percentage than previously estimated and relates to deleterious mutations in *BRCA1, BRCA2, MLH1, ATM, PALB2,* and *CDK2NA,* as well as mismatch repair gene mutations found in families with Lynch syndrome (see Chapter 9D). Germline mutations have also been detected in 7% of patients unselected for a family history of PDAC. In the classic prospective studies of family members of PC kindreds from the National Familial Pancreas Tumor Registry at Johns Hopkins Hospital, a 2-fold increased risk of PC was found in the first-degree relatives of persons with sporadic PC and a 9-fold increased risk in first-degree relatives of those with familial PC.[35,42] Germline mutations of *BRCA2* are found in 6% to 19% of familial pancreatic cancer patients.[43] When a more stringent definition of familial PC is used, a 57-fold increased risk of PC was reported in kindreds with three or more family members affected with PC.[44] This corresponds to a notably high incidence rate of 301 cases per 100,000 per year, compared with the SEER age-adjusted rate for the entire US population of only 8.8 cases per 100,000 per year. A recent report identified a germline truncating mutation of the *PALB2* gene in 3% of familial pancreatic cancer patients.[45,46] Despite these many advances in the understanding of the mutations involved in the pathogenesis of PC, no single "pancreatic cancer gene" has been identified.

Two recent studies have documented an increased risk of PC in persons with A, B, and AB blood types.[46,47] This risk has been attributed to an *ABO* single nucleotide polymorphism, rs505922. Overall, 56% of the population has a non-O blood group and the proportion of PDAC because of non-O blood group is 13% to 19%.[10]

Six Genetic Syndromes Associated with Pancreatic Ductal Adenocarcinoma (see Chapter 9D)

Six genetic familial syndromes and their respective predisposing genes have been identified and linked to the development of PC; these are described briefly later (Table 61.3). Although individuals with these syndromes have an increased risk of developing PC, collectively these syndromes account for less than 5% of the familial aggregation of PC. The mean age of onset of familial PC is similar to that of nonfamilial cases: 65.8 years versus 65.2 years.[11] Familial cases have also been noted to have a somewhat increased incidence of secondary primary cancers (23.8%) when compared with their nonfamilial counterparts (18.9%).

Hereditary Pancreatitis

Hereditary pancreatitis (HP) is an autosomal dominant inherited disease that begins in childhood or adolescence. Children and adolescents with HP develop severe pancreatitis at a young age, with a resultant 50-fold to 80-fold increased risk of PC developing over their lifetime. HP results from germline or new somatic mutations in the *PRSS1* cationic trypsinogen gene.[14] A *PRSS1* (7q35) mutation has been identified, and the cumulative risk of PC is 50% to 80% in these individuals. Approximately 40% of those with HP will develop PC when the additional risk factor of cigarette smoking is added. Cigarette

TABLE 61.3 High-Risk Genetic Disorders Associated With Familial Pancreatic Cancer

GENETIC SYNDROME	GENE/CHROMOSOMAL MUTATION REGION	ESTIMATED INCREASED RISK OF PDA
Hereditary pancreatitis	*PRSS1* (7q35)	50–80 times
Hereditary nonpolyposis colorectal cancer (Lynch II variant)	*hMSH2, hMSH1, hPMS2, hMSH3, hPMS1, hMSH6/GTBP*	Undefined
Hereditary breast and ovarian cancer	*BRCA2* (13q12-q13)	3.5–10 times
FAMMM syndrome	*p16* (9p21)	20–34 times
Peutz-Jeghers syndrome	*STK11/LKB1* (19p13)	75–132 times
Ataxia-telangiectasia	*ATM* (11q22-23)	Undefined

FAMMM, Familial atypical multiple mole melanoma; *PDA,* pancreatic ductal carcinoma.

smoking in combination with HP may lower the age at diagnosis. The risk of cancer seems to be limited to the pancreas and not tumors in other organs.[14]

Hereditary Nonpolyposis Colorectal Cancer (Lynch Syndrome)

Hereditary nonpolyposis colorectal cancer is an autosomal dominant inherited disease that predisposes affected persons to colorectal cancer and PC.[48] It is usually caused by germline mutations in a number of DNA mismatch repair genes, such as *MLH1, MSH2, MSH6,* and *PNMS2.*[36] Those with mismatch repair gene mutations are estimated to develop PC at eight times the rate of the general population.[49] Of the inherited syndromes associated with an increased risk of PDAC, hereditary nonpolyposis colorectal cancer is the least strongly linked to pancreatic cancer.

Hereditary Breast and Ovarian Cancer

Patients with germline *BRCA2* mutations have up to a 10-fold increased risk (range, 3.5- to 10-fold) of PC, even in patients without a strong family history of breast cancer. Germline *BRCA2* mutations have been identified in 7% of sporadic (nonfamilial) PC patients screened, none of whom had a family history of breast cancer or PC.[50] *BRCA1* mutation carriers followed in a breast and ovarian cancer evaluation center, had a 3-fold increased risk of PC, a twofold increased risk for colon cancer, a 4-fold increased risk for gastric cancer, and a 120-fold increased risk for fallopian tube cancer compared with SEER population–based estimated risk.[51]

Familial Atypical Multiple Mole and Melanoma Syndrome

Familial atypical multiple mole and melanoma (FAMMM) syndrome is a rare condition associated with *p16* germline mutations, a tumor suppressor gene that may be mutated or may have its expression altered by post-transcriptional methylation. The syndrome predisposes affected individuals to melanomas, multiple nevi, atypical nevi, and PC.[52] Those with FAMMM have a 20- to 34-fold increased risk of PC over their lifetime.

Peutz-Jeghers Syndrome

Peutz-Jeghers syndrome is a rare autosomal dominant disease associated with alterations in the *STK11* gene, in which affected individuals develop hamartomatous polyps of the gastrointestinal tract and lip freckles referred to as *mucocutaneous melanocytic macules.*[48] Individuals with this syndrome have a roughly 100-fold increased risk of developing PC, and they also appear to have a tendency to form intraductal papillary mucinous neoplasms.[53]

Ataxia-Telangiectasia

Ataxia-telangiectasia is an autosomal recessive inherited disorder associated with *ATM* gene mutations, in which affected persons present with cerebellar ataxia, conjunctival telangiectasias, a hypofunctioning thymus gland, and oculomotor abnormalities. An association between ataxia- telangiectasia and the subsequent development of PC has been reported, but it is less well established than with the other five familial syndromes.[9]

Cigarette Smoking

Cigarette smoking has been definitively identified as a causative agent in 25% to 35% of the cases of PDAC and is the most consistently reported risk factor.[54-56] Smoking is associated with increased risk of PC in at least 29 epidemiologic studies, and smokers have a 70% increased risk of PC compared with nonsmokers.[38] The International Agency for Research on Cancer has confirmed that smoking is casually related to PDAC.[57,58] Cigarette smoking also contributes to death in PDAC patients. In a meta-analysis of 20 studies including 2,517,623 PDAC patients, there were 15,341 PC deaths were identified.[59] Compared with never-smokers, the hazard ratio for death for current smokers with PDAC was 1.56 (confidence interval [CI] 1.34–1.83) and 1.15 (CI 1.06–1.26) for former smokers.[59] This effect was independent of alcohol use, body mass index, and diabetes.[59]

It is reported that 15% or 40 million Americans continue to smoke cigarettes.[60] The gender difference in cigarette smoking rates narrowed in the mid-1980s. Currently, cigarette smoking in the US varies by race, with 15.1% of white men identifying as smokers, compared with 13% of white women, 21% of African American men and 13% of African American women, 15% of Hispanic men and 8% of Hispanic women, and 12.6% of Asian men and 3.5% of Asian women.[2,60] Persons of American Indian and Alaskan Native descent have the highest rates of smoking. Rural areas and southern states have a higher prevalence of smoking than northern states.[60]

Smoking habits in the 13 years preceding the diagnosis of PC appear to be more relevant to increased risk, whereas former smokers who have quit for more than 13 years decrease their PC risk to that of lifetime nonsmokers.[52,61] A meta-analysis of 83 epidemiologic studies found that the overall relative risk of PC in current and former smokers was 1.74, a 74% increased risk of PC in these groups.[54] A retrospective analysis comparing smoking in cases of familial PC and sporadic PC found that 57% and 60%, respectively, of patients reported prolonged cigarette smoking, with an overall mean of 35 packs/year history.[13]

A dose-response relationship between PDAC and the number of cigarettes consumed has been documented in several investigations.[15,61] For current smokers who also have a family history of PC, the relative risk of PC was found to be as high as 8.23.[62] Individuals with familial PC tend to smoke more than those with sporadic PC.[14] A younger age at diagnosis was found in those with familial PC compared with those with sporadically occurring PC.[13] These observations raise the possibility that smoking is interactive, perhaps multiplicatively, with genetic mutations known to be present in persons with familial PC. Postmortem examinations of the pancreatic ducts of smokers have found widespread ductal hyperplasia, that is, lesions termed *pancreatic intraepithelial neoplasia*, which are considered to be premalignant lesions. There is also a relationship between cigarette smoking and the development of PC as a second malignancy in patients with a smoking-related first malignancy, such as lung, head and neck, or bladder cancer.[63] This relationship is likely because of overlapping smoking-related genetic mutations among these different malignancies.

Eighteen percent of adults and 14% of high school students in the US report current smoking.[60] A 2003 study of adults aged 30 to 39 years that included parental occupation, adult educational attainment, and household income as indicators of socioeconomic status (SES) found that those of lower SES were more likely to start smoking and to become regular smokers and were less likely to quit smoking than their higher SES counterparts.[60,64] Smoking prevalence has decreased in all education groups over recent decades, but the largest decrease has been in college-educated persons.[60]

The carcinogenic components of cigarette smoke are usually cleared from the bloodstream and excreted into bile and reach the pancreas from the bile duct through biliary-pancreatic reflux or may be carried into the pancreatic parenchyma directly by the bloodstream. Cigarette smoke contains more than 60 known carcinogens, including polycyclic aromatic hydrocarbons (PAHs), nitrosamines, benzo[a]pyrene, β-naphthylamine, methylfluoranthenes, and arylamines.[65]

The numerous chemical carcinogens identified in cigarette smoke led to the development of PC via a variety of mechanisms. Some of the carcinogenic components of cigarette smoke may bind to DNA and form adducts, which increase the risk of somatic mutations and cancer if unrepaired. Nitrosamines are known to be organ specific, causing pancreatic carcinomas in hamsters; such tumors are histologically like the type found in humans.[35] Another possible mechanism by which cigarette smoke leads to PC is unrelated to the carcinogens in the smoke. Rather, higher cholesterol (lipid) levels are measured in smokers than in nonsmokers. The pathophysiologic mechanism of hypercholesterolemia may be partially because of nicotinic stimulation of circulating catecholamines, which increase serum cholesterol levels. Elevated lipid levels may also be causative in the induction of PC.[66] Cigarette smoking also induces a state of chronic inflammation, which may also contribute to its carcinogenic effects.[60,67-69] Cigarette smoke and inflammation may not only contribute to the development of PC but may also be integral to reactivation of metastatic disease.[70,71]

Environmental Tobacco Smoke and Second-Hand Smoke

Environmental tobacco smoke (ETS) is related to the development of PC, with a likely dose-response relationship.[15,72] A mildly elevated odds ratio (OR, 1.21; CI, 0.60–2.44) has been reported, suggesting a weak association between PDAC and ETS exposure in nonsmokers who reported ETS exposure both as an adult and in childhood. The effect was more pronounced in smokers who reported ETS exposure. Findings from a 2009 retrospective case-only analysis of familial and sporadic PDAC indicated that nonsmokers with PC who were exposed to ETS early in life (<21 years of age) were diagnosed with PC at a significantly younger mean age (64.0 years) when compared with nonsmoker, non–ETS-exposed cases (66.5 years).[13] Moreover, both cigarette smoking and ETS exposure in nonsmokers younger than 21 years are associated with a younger mean age of diagnosis in familial, sporadic, and Ashkenazi Jewish cases of PC.

In 2006 the US Surgeon General determined that second-hand smoke contains at least 69 human carcinogens for which there is no safe exposure level.[73] There are more than 45,000 annual deaths in the US from lung cancer and heart disease in persons who have no personal smoking history but did report exposure to secondhand smoke.[74]

Cigar, Waterpipe Smoking, E-Cigarettes, and Smokeless Tobacco

Cigars contain the same carcinogens as cigarettes. Regular cigar smokers, including users of large cigars, cigarillos, and small cigars, have an increased risk for lung, oropharyngeal, larynx, and esophageal cancers and 4 to 10 times the risk of dying from these cancers compared with never-cigar smokers.[2] Waterpipe smoking, reported by 4% of high school students on a regular basis, is less well studied and is considered more socially acceptable than cigars and cigarettes. The smoke moves through water as a filter before being inhaled, implying less harm; however, it delivers the same toxins as other forms of smoking. The adverse effects are under investigation. E-cigarettes, an aerosolized delivery system of nicotine, emerged in the early 2000s. The aerosolized liquid contains nicotine, propylene glycol, vegetable glycerin, and flavorings (ACS 2020). Between 2017 and 2018, use of e-cigarettes increased 78% among high school students and 3% of adults report current use.[75] More than 200 possible cases of severe pulmonary disease among e-cigarette users have been reported.[76] The long-term association with PC remains to be determined.

Smokeless Tobacco

Smokeless tobacco includes dry snuff, chewing tobacco, snus (moist smokeless tobacco), and dissolvable nicotine products. Sales of these products are increasing at a faster rate than cigarettes. The use of smokeless tobacco is being promoted as safer than cigarette smoking and as a method to quit smoking. There is no evidence that smokeless tobacco is an effective method of smoking cessation. These products do, however, cause oral cancer, esophageal cancer, and PC, as well as bone loss around teeth and nicotine addiction.[77]

High-Risk Occupations

The evidence linking occupational exposures to PC is inconsistent, reflecting the difficulty of quantifying workplace exposure to carcinogens and of differentiating these exposures from other risk factors. A number of epidemiologic investigations have suggested excess risk of PC in certain occupations (Table 61.4). Definitively establishing certain occupations as high risk for the development of PC is difficult because of the problems with self-reported exposures, lack of objective quantitative monitoring data, personal comorbidities, and the presence of other confounding and modifying risk factors.

Occupational Exposures

Studies examining specific occupational exposures that increase a worker's risk of developing PC have been conducted both in the US and in Europe, particularly in the Scandinavian countries. Occupational exposures linked to PC are summarized in Table 61.5. Overall, the occupational etiologic fraction for PC was estimated at 12% in a meta-analysis of 20 occupational studies conducted between 1969 and 1998.[5,22] A retrospective analysis of more than 22 occupational and environmental studies reporting on people with PC found that exposure to asbestos, pesticides and herbicides, residential radon, coal products, welding products, and radiation were the most commonly reported exposures.[13]

TABLE 61.4   **Occupations Associated With Excess Risk of Pancreatic Cancer**

OCCUPATION	RISK ESTIMATE	95% CI
Chemical processor[78]	1.22 OR	NR
Chemical fertilizer[78]	1.20 OR	NR
Chemist[79]	10.2 MH	NR
Auto mechanic (gasoline exposure)[66,78]	5.1 RR if >10 years exposure	NR
Service station worker[78]	1.6 SMR	NR
Machine repairer[78]	2.45 OR	NR
Dry cleaner[66]	2.1 RR	NR
Leather tanner[80]	3.1 MH	(1.1-9.2)
Oil refinery worker[81]	2.11 OR	(0.86-5.20)
Aluminum mill worker[82]	125.2 SMR	NR
Floor polisher[83]	1.3 SMR	NR
Electrical assembler/installer/repairer[78]	2.20 OR	NR
Metalworker[84]	2.0 SMR	(0.9-3.8)
Manufacturing plant worker[85]	3.0 SMR	(1.2-6.24)
Assembly worker[86]	3.0 SMR	(1.0-7.5)
Foundry and engine plant workers[87]	3.0 SMR	(121-624)
Plant/system operator[88]	6.1 OR	(1.1-33.9)
Pharmacist, dietician, therapist[88]	7.1 OR	(1.8-27.5)

CI, Confidence interval; *MH*, Mantel-Haenszel estimate; *NR*, not reported; *OR*, odds ratio; *RR*, relative risk; *SMR*, standardized mortality ratio.

TABLE 61.5   **Occupational Exposures Linked to Pancreatic Cancer (PC)**

CHEMICAL	EXPOSURE ROUTE	PC RISK ESTIMATES
Methylene chloride (chlorinated hydrocarbons)	Spray paints	1.61 OR
	Paint strippers	1.40 OR
	Aerosol propellant	1.6 RR
	Metal degreasing agent	
	Paint/paint thinners	
	Varnish	
	Solvents	
Pesticides/herbicides	Corn wet milling	1.4 OR
DDT	Farming	4.8 RR
DDD	Flight attendants	4.3 RR
Ethylan		5.0 RR
Asbestos	Industrial	3.0 OR
Fertilizer	Farming	1.2 OR
Cotton dust	Farming	4.37 OR
Cement	Construction work (manufacturing of cement)	1.28 OR
Lead	Various	1.28 OR
Metalworking fluids	Machinist	2.0 OR

DDD, Dichlorodiphenyl-dichloroethane; *DDT*, dichlorodiphenyl-trichloroethane; *OR*, odds ratio; *RR*, relative risk.

Data from references cited in Table 61.4.

A review supported by the National Institute for Occupational Safety and Health (NIOSH) of five cohort studies reported an association between the use of metalworking fluids (MWFs) used in industrial machining and grinding operations and the development of all types of cancer, including

PDAC.[22,84,89-91] More than 1 million workers are exposed to MWFs according to NIOSH estimates.[92] Substantial evidence was found for an increased risk of cancer at several sites, including the pancreas, larynx, rectum, skin, scrotum, and bladder. MWFs contain a number of compounds suspected to be cancer initiators or promoters, including long-chain aliphatics, PAHs, nitrosamines, sulfur-containing compounds, formaldehyde-releasing biocides, and heavy metals.[84]

Diabetes

Diabetes and prediabetes are risk factors for PC and may also be a consequence of PC.[93] The majority of PDAC patients (50%–80%) have either subclinical impaired glucose tolerance or type 2 diabetes at the time of diagnosis.[94,95] PC causes alteration of islet cell function—specifically, the loss of β-cell mass from tumor growth—or a result of disruptions in acinar–islet cell interactions. The chronic hyperinsulinemia and hyperglycemia associated with type 2 diabetes has been proposed as the underlying mechanism of PC. Experimental evidence suggests that insulin promotes proliferation and reduces apoptosis in pancreatic cancer cells, both directly and indirectly through increased bioavailability of insulin-like growth factor.[96-98] Hyperglycemia can also enhance proliferation and the invasion capability of PC cells. A 2015 meta-analysis of nine prospective studies involving 2408 patients examined the association between elevated blood glucose and PC and found that every 0.56 mmol/L increase in fasting blood glucose was associated with a 14% increase in the rate of PC.[93]

In a population-based case-control study of 484 PDAC cases and 2099 control subjects in three geographic areas of the US, those diagnosed with diabetes at least 10 years before the development of PDAC had a 50% increased risk of PDAC compared with the control group.[16] Insulin treatment did not appear to alter the risk of development of PDAC (OR, 1.6 with insulin and 1.5 without). Two other recent investigations found a self-reported history of new-onset diabetes before PC diagnosis in 26% and 31% of the study populations.[13,99]

During an 18-year follow-up study of 88,802 women in the Nurses' Health Study (NHS), 180 incident cases of PC were reported.[17] A positive association was observed between fructose intake and impaired glucose metabolism and increased PC risk. The risk was most apparent in women with an elevated body mass index (BMI) above 30 kg/m^2 and low physical activity. A diet high in glycemic load (defined as the glucose response to each unit of carbohydrate-containing foods) may increase the risk of PC in women with underlying insulin resistance because of obesity. Increased PC risk has been associated with chronically elevated plasma glucose levels, further suggesting that impaired glucose tolerance, insulin resistance, and hyperinsulinemia are involved in the etiology of PC.[100]

Pancreatitis

Pancreatitis has been widely studied as a risk factor for PC (see Chapters 54–57). The population-attributable fraction of pancreatitis to the development of PC was 1.34% (i.e., a 34% excess risk) in an analysis of 10 pooled studies.[101] When the pancreatitis occurred more than 3 years before the diagnosis of PC, the association was stronger (OR, 4.0; CI, 2.5–6.0). Acute pancreatitis (AP) may be the initial clinical presentation of PDAC, preceding the malignant diagnosis by weeks or months (see Chapter 55). A 2014 Veterans Health Administration retrospective study found that 10.7% of veterans diagnosed with PC had a history of AP within 2 years of the cancer diagnosis.[102] The risk was greatest in the first year after the episode of AP and further elevated in persons 70 years of age or older.

Chronic pancreatitis (CP) has been linked to the development of PC (see Chapter 57). The standardized incidence ratio of PDAC in individuals with a diagnosis of CP was 16.5 compared with the 1.76 expected number of cases.[103] A review of the records of patients with AP, CP, or unspecified pancreatitis was conducted on all inpatient medical institutions in Sweden from 1965 to 1983. In 7956 patients with pancreatitis, 46 PCs were diagnosed compared with 21 expected cases, a standardized incidence ratio of 2.2 (CI, 1.6–2.9).[18] Pooled results from seven studies investigating CP found a significant 13-fold higher risk of PC (risk ratio [RR] 13.3, 95% CI: 6.1–28.9) in CP patients compared with the general population or controls.[104] Although it seems reasonable to conclude that the cellular destruction and glandular dysfunction caused by pancreatitis may yield an environment favoring the initiation of tumor growth, it remains problematic that some premalignant lesions such as intraductal papillary mucinous neoplasms (IPMNs) may be initially incorrectly diagnosed as CP, clouding the arguments concerning chronic pancreatitis as a risk factor.

Pancreatic Cysts

Pancreatic cysts are fairly common, and most are incidentally found when individuals undergo MRI or CT imaging for another indication. Incidentally identified pancreatic cysts are present in the general population at rates that vary from 2.6% to 15% or higher, and some of these represent premalignant lesions such as IPMN and mucinous cystic neoplasm (MCN).[104] Seventy-five percent of PDACs arise from solid lesions and about 25% from cystic lesions.[104] The risk of PDAC increases with the size of the cystic lesion; beyond 3 cm, the risk of cancer is estimated at 18% to 25%.[104] Removing premalignant pancreatic cysts at the appropriate time can reduce the incidence of PDAC (see Chapter 60).

Lifestyle Factors and Height and Weight

The Health Professional Follow-up Study (HPFS) and the NHS are two large, prospective cohort studies that first reported on the relationship between BMI, height, weight, physical activity, and smoking and the risk of PC.[17] The HPFS, initiated in 1986, includes 51,529 men aged 40 to 75 years who responded to a mailed questionnaire; the NHS began in 1976 and includes 121,700 registered nurses. Activity levels and body weight were ascertained prospectively. A higher risk of PDAC was found among obese men and women: 10% higher for overweight persons and 20% higher in obese persons as compared with normal-weight persons. A 5-unit increase in BMI corresponded to a 10% excess risk of PC.[105] The proportion of PC attributable to obesity ranges from 3% to 16%.[10]

A direct association between above-average height and risk of PC was also observed, such that an additional 2.54 cm of height above average height increased the risk of PC by 6% in the HPFS and by 10% in the NHS. Although the association between height and general cancer risk has been identified in other studies, a pooled meta-analytical study found no association between height and PC.[10,106,107] Height may serve as a proxy for calorie intake or exposure to growth factors, such as insulin or insulin-like growth factor-1, in childhood.

The proportion of all cancers attributable to physical inactivity is estimated at 3%.[108] An inverse relationship between moderate physical activity and PC has been reported.[17] Walking or hiking 1.5 hours or more per week in an overweight cohort was associated with a 50% reduction in PC risk. BMI had no effect on risk if the participant was a moderate exerciser. Those individuals with a BMI of at least 30 kg/m² had an elevated risk of PC (RR, 1.72; CI, 1.19–2.52) compared with those with a BMI of less than 23 kg/m².

Diet

It is estimated that 30% to 50% of PCs may be attributable to dietary factors. Both butter consumption and saturated fat intake were positively associated with PDAC risk (hazard ratio [HR], 1.40; CI, 0.87–2.25; and HR, 1.60; CI, 0.96–2.64, respectively) in the Finnish Cancer Registry.[109] Higher consumption of saturated fat and calorie-rich foods may influence mortality trends in PC.[110] Fat entering the duodenum stimulates cholecystokinin secretion, and it is possible that chronic hypercholecystokininemia may be associated with an increased susceptibility of the pancreas to carcinogens. Other possible explanations include that the increased intake of saturated fat may lead to insulin resistance and the development of diabetes or that foods with a high soluble fat content may be contaminated with carcinogenic organochloride compounds from the environment.

Processed meats have been linked to the development of PC. In a prospective study of more than 200,000 people, 482 individuals developed PC during 7 years of follow-up.[111] Those who had consumed the greatest number of processed meats had a 67% increased risk of PC. Diets laden with pork and red meat intake were associated with a 50% increase in PC risk, but poultry, fish, dairy products, and egg consumption conferred no additional risk. Heterocyclic amines and polycyclic aromatic hydrocarbons that form during high-temperature cooking are known to be carcinogenic and may be responsible for the increased risk of PC observed with processed and barbecued meats.

Several recent investigations have focused on the relationship between *glycemic load* and *glycemic index*. Consumption of fruit juices and soda has been evaluated in six studies to date with conflicting results.[109,111–114] Two studies found no relationship between PDAC and glycemic load; carbohydrate intake; or sugar, sucrose, or fructose intake.[114,115] Three studies reported mixed findings.[109,111,112] In the Multiethnic Cohort Study, BMI modified the effect of high sucrose intake and the occurrence of PDAC, with elevated BMI increasing the risk and normal BMI decreasing the risk.[111] A positive association with PDAC was also observed with a high fructose intake, but no association was observed with consumption of soft drinks (diet or regular).

Coffee and Alcohol Consumption

Cohort studies from the 1970s and 1980s indicating that heavy coffee and alcohol consumption led to an excess risk of PDAC were often confounded by excessive smoking among the heavy coffee and alcohol drinkers.[17]

A 2002 study hypothesized that because heavy alcohol intake often causes CP, which may be a risk factor for PDAC, the ideal group to examine would be those with a diagnosis of alcoholism, alcoholic CP, and alcoholic liver cirrhosis. Using the Swedish National Board of Health and Welfare, data were collected on 178,688 patients over a 30-year period. A total of 305 incident cases of PDA were identified in the group, representing a 40% excess risk in observed compared with expected cases.

Alcoholics with CP or cirrhosis had a 2-fold increased risk of PDAC. A major limitation of the study was the lack of information on smoking. The authors estimated that the observed excess risk of PDAC in the alcoholic group "may be almost totally attributable to the confounding effect of smoking."[116]

The NHS and the HPFS examined data on coffee and alcohol consumption and other dietary factors obtained at baseline in two large national cohort studies.[17] Follow-up information was gathered via a mailed questionnaire from both cohorts (NHS & HPFS) on age, marital status, weight, height, medical history, medication use, smoking status, physical activity, and intake of coffee and alcohol. The results regarding coffee and alcohol are compelling: During 1,907,222 person-years of follow-up, 288 incident cases of PDAC were diagnosed. Data were analyzed separately for each of the cohorts and then pooled to compute overall RR estimates. The results revealed that neither coffee consumption nor alcohol consumption conferred an excess risk of PDAC; a pooled RR of 0.62 was reported (95% CI, 0.27–1.43) for more than three cups of coffee per day versus no coffee, and a pooled RR of 1.00 (95% CI, 0.57–1.76) for more than 30 g alcohol per day versus no alcohol.

Based on 37 case-control studies and 17 cohort studies (total 10,594 cases) of PC and coffee consumption, after adjusting for smoking, Turati et al. (2011) found the RR was 1.10 (CI 0.92–1.29) for the case-control studies, 1.04 (0.8–1.36) for the cohort studies and 1.8 (0.94–1.25) for all cases. They concluded that coffee consumption is not appreciably related to PC, even at high doses.

Two recent meta-analyses found that heavy alcohol consumption is associated with an increased risk of PC.[117,118] A pooled meta-analysis of 19 studies including 4,211,129 persons examined the effect of alcohol intake on PC occurrence.[117] Low to moderate intake had little to no influence, but high alcohol and hard liquor intake were associated with a RR 1.15 to 1.43 increase in PC incidence. Alcohol intake was defined as light if less than 12 g alcohol/day, moderate was 12 to 24 g/day, and heavy was more than 24 g/day, where 1 drink equaled 12 g. Lucentefore and colleagues from the International Pancreatic Cancer Case–Control Consortium (PanC4) pooled data from case-control studies to assess the relationship between alcohol and PC risk. Compared with nondrinkers and occasional drinkers (<1 drink/ day), there was no association between light to moderate alcohol consumption (~4 drinks per day) and PC risk. There was a positive association between PC and high consumption levels (9 drinks/day) with an OR of 1.6, (95% CI, 1.2–2.2). The results persisted after adjustment for smoking and excluding those with a history of pancreatitis.

Infectious Agents

Helicobacter pylori has emerged as a moderate risk factor for PDAC in an analysis of seven studies.[119] The global prevalence of *H. pylori* infection ranges from 25% to 50% in Westernized countries. It is thus estimated that 25% to 45% of PC cases in these countries may involve *H. pylori*.[10] Chronic infection with the hepatitis B virus (HBV) increases the risk of PDAC (OR, 1.42) in blood group A individuals. HBV can infect the pancreas and the liver. A recent report demonstrated a 40% to 60% excess risk of PC in HBV-positive persons.[120]

A 2017 systematic review found that lower levels of *Neisseria elongate* and *Streptococcus mitis* and high levels of *Porphyromonas gingivalis* and *Granulicatella adiacens* in the gut were associated with an increased risk of PC.[121]

SUMMARY

PDAC is a complex biologic process, the etiology of which is multifactorial, although certain risk factors are amenable to modification. There are a number of strategies for persons to reduce their risk of PC.

One strategy is avoiding the use and proximity to tobacco products. Do not start smoking, and if one does smoke cigarettes or cigars, quit. Do not use smokeless tobacco products. Avoid persons who are actively smoking. Ask smokers to not smoke in the home. Discourage the use of cigars, water pipe smoking, e-cigarettes, and smokeless tobacco. Refer smokers to smoking cessation programs.

Another strategy is to make healthy dietary and exercise modifications. If one is overweight or obese, reduce weight through menu-based and calorie restriction programs. One should consider surgical obesity intervention, if appropriate. One should also increase daily intake of fruits and vegetables, reduce intake of simple carbohydrates and saturated fats, avoid processed meats, limit red meat intake, increase fish and poultry portions, and increase physical activity to 20 minutes of moderate exercise three to five times a week.

Yet another strategy is to consider occupational and environmental exposures and protections. For individuals engaged in high-risk occupations or environmental exposure, regular use of the Occupational Safety and Health Administration–recommended personal protective equipment will minimize the risk.

Still another strategy is to screen high-risk individuals to detect precursor lesions and early-stage tumors. High-risk individuals include older smokers with new-onset diabetes, persons experiencing unintentional weight loss, individuals with suspicious pancreatic or biliary tree lesions that are incidentally found and may be asymptomatic, and people with a family history of pancreatic or related cancers.

A considerable amount of epidemiologic data point to PC causes that are largely avoidable. Nearly two-thirds of the major, noninherited genetic risk factors are modifiable through increased public awareness, screening of high-risk individuals to detect advanced precursor lesions, and promotion of healthier lifestyles. This knowledge offers an opportunity for prevention and perhaps bending the curve on the predicted rise of PC.

The references for this chapter can be found online by accessing the accompanying Expert Consult website.

CHAPTER 62

Pancreatic cancer: Clinical aspects, assessment, and management

Jeffrey A. Debrin

CLINICAL PRESENTATION

Pancreatic adenocarcinoma, or pancreas cancer, is one of the most lethal malignancies. While a relatively uncommon cancer, ranking 8th among cancer types in women and 10th in men, it is among the most common causes of cancer death in the United States.[1] Pancreas cancer currently ranks third behind lung and colorectal cancer as a cause of cancer death, and is expected to become the second most common cause of cancer death in the coming decade. The increasing frequency of pancreas cancer in recent decades reflects both a true increase in its age-adjusted incidence, and the fact that pancreas cancer risk approximately doubles for each decade of life between age 50 and 90[2]; thus the increasing average age of our population results in a larger number of patients with a new diagnosis of pancreas cancer (see Chapter 61).

The lethality of pancreas cancer reflects both its intrinsic biologic aggressiveness and that most patients are diagnosed when their tumor is relatively advanced. Surgical resection is the only treatment modality associated with long-term survival of pancreas cancer patients, but unfortunately only a small minority of pancreas cancer patients are candidates for surgery at the time of their diagnosis.[3] Over half of pancreas cancer patients have systemic metastases identified at the time of diagnosis, and another third have locally advanced disease precluding immediate surgery, although some may become resectable with preoperative (neoadjuvant) chemotherapy, as will be discussed in the following sections. Only 15% to 20% of patients initially present with surgically operable pancreas cancer and, despite improvements in perioperative chemotherapy, cancer will recur in many of these patients. For unresectable patients, and those who recur after surgery, survival with current chemotherapy and radiation therapy approaches generally ranges from several months to several years. Recent therapeutic advances that have contributed to improved outcomes in other cancer types, in areas like targeted cancer therapy and immunotherapy, have thus far been of relatively limited benefit in pancreas cancer.

Pancreas cancer is rarely diagnosed "early" because it is often relatively asymptomatic in its initial stages. Tumors in the head of the pancreas can obstruct the bile duct, causing jaundice, and the phrase "painless jaundice" has been used to define a classic presentation of pancreas cancer. Most operable tumors occur in the pancreatic head and are identified in patients by the occurrence of jaundice. However, it is important to recognize that many tumors occur in areas of the pancreas that do not obstruct the bile duct, and that most pancreas cancers are not in fact painless by the time they are diagnosed. Many patients have a nonlocalized upper abdominal discomfort related to tumor growth and infiltration that is present for weeks or months before diagnosis. Pain radiating to the back is a particularly ominous symptom reflecting tumor involvement of retroperitoneal nerves. This pain is often worse at night when supine, and relieved with sitting. Other signs and symptoms of pancreas cancer include weight loss, nausea and vomiting reflecting gastric outlet obstruction, a palpable mass, gallbladder distension (Courvoisier's sign), peripheral venous thrombosis (Trousseau's sign), pancreatitis in the absence of other potential precipitants such as gallstones or regular alcohol use, and pancreatic insufficiency (either exocrine and/or endocrine). In fact, new-onset insulin-dependent diabetes after the age of 60 is associated with a 1% to 2% incidence of a previously undiagnosed pancreas cancer.[4] Unfortunately, most of these signs and symptoms are nonspecific and, with the exception of jaundice, are generally subacute, contributing to the relative rarity of diagnosing pancreas cancer at an early stage.

DIAGNOSIS

Laboratory Tests

Patients in whom a suspicion of pancreas cancer is raised are often initially evaluated with serum blood tests. These laboratory studies may show a marked elevated bilirubin and alkaline phosphatase, confirming the clinical impression of obstructive jaundice, often with some elevation of liver alanine aminotransferase and aspartate aminotransferase. The serum tumor marker CA19-9 is often elevated in pancreas cancer, but it may also be markedly elevated in patients with biliary obstruction because of benign causes. Furthermore, CA19-9 is a carbohydrate antigen linked to the Lewis blood group antigens and approximately 15% to 20% of patients are incapable of synthesizing CA19-9.[5] Thus the use of CA19-9 in making the diagnosis of pancreas cancer, particularly in patients with jaundice, is of limited value. Its primary utility is in following treatment response when it is elevated in nonjaundiced patients with a known pancreatic malignancy, whereas a reduction in CA19-9 levels is associated with improved survival.[6-8] It is also a negative prognostic factor if markedly elevated in nonjaundiced patients and those who have undergone successful biliary decompression.[9]

Other serum markers, such as carcinoembryonic antigen (CEA), are similarly too insensitive or nonspecific to be of use in the initial diagnosis of pancreas cancer. An evolving approach is the evaluation of circulating cancer cells[10] or circulating tumor DNA[11] in the diagnosis of pancreas cancer. The combination of such approaches with evaluation of CA19-9 and other blood markers may offer a relatively sensitive and specific approach to the early diagnosis of pancreas cancer,[12] although this is still experimental.

Imaging Studies

The identification of a pancreatic tumor is generally made by cross-sectional imaging (see Chapter 17). High-resolution triple-phase contrast-enhanced computed tomographic (CT) scanning of the abdomen is the primary tool used to identify a pancreatic mass.[13,14] Pancreatic carcinomas are generally hypoenhancing on the arterial phase and hypointense or isointense on the venous phase. CT scanning can also define regional adenopathy and potential extrapancreatic extension with involvement of adjacent vascular structures and is useful in detecting evidence of metastatic disease to the liver or peritoneum. Magnetic resonance imaging (MRI) scanning is of similar utility in assessing a pancreatic mass and may be more useful for defining small liver metastases.[15] MRI may be preferentially used over CT in patients with limited renal function or allergy to the intravenous contrast used in CT. Patients rarely require both modalities except that MRI is more useful for characterizing small or indeterminate lesions (see Chapter 17). MRI is of particular utility in assessing cystic lesions of the pancreas and in their long-term follow-up, as MRI provides excellent resolution of high-risk features such as mural nodules, and the absence of radiation exposure is a benefit in long-term surveillance imaging (see Chapter 60).

Positron emission tomographic (PET) scanning using the 18-fluoro-2-deoxyglucose (FDG) tracer to assess tumor metabolic activity is of more limited utility because 10% to 30% of pancreas cancers fail to take up this tracer, and thus are PET negative.[16] Furthermore, benign sites of inflammation may take up FDG and thus be erroneously PET positive. FDG-PET scanning is of greatest utility in helping to define small indeterminate lesions that cannot be well characterized by CT or MRI scanning, when the suspicion for a benign inflammatory process is low. Advances in the use of alternative tracers, such as 68-gallium dotatate for neuroendocrine malignancies,[17] while useful in the diagnosis and staging of certain tumors, is outside the scope of this chapter (see Chapter 18).

Diagnostic Biopsy

The definitive diagnosis of pancreatic adenocarcinoma requires evaluation of histopathology. However, not all operable pancreatic masses require a preoperative biopsy.[18] A lesion that has radiographic characteristics of a pancreatic carcinoma and which is amenable to surgical resection after radiologic staging may, in some cases, be best managed by proceeding directly to surgery. For patients with a pancreas mass that has a high likelihood of being malignant based on radiologic findings alone and in whom surgery can be performed with low morbidity and mortality, performing preoperative biopsy may be of no benefit. In contrast, for patients who are at higher risk for surgery because of their age or underlying medical conditions and/or who wish to have a diagnosis made before consenting to surgery, obtaining a preoperative biopsy may be quite useful. Such biopsy-proven confirmation of the presence of pancreas cancer is also generally required for patients who will receive neoadjuvant chemotherapy.

For patients requiring a biopsy of a pancreas mass, endoscopic ultrasound (EUS)–guided fine-needle aspiration (FNA) has become the most common nonoperative or preoperative approach to identifying the presence of pancreas cancer[19,20] (see Chapter 22). Although occasionally limited by intervening vascular structures, in experienced hands the vast majority of pancreas lesions can be sampled with EUS-FNA. However, it is important to recognize that pancreas cancers are often highly fibrotic with relatively small areas of cancer cellularity. In some patients less than 10% of the area containing the cancer on histopathologic analysis will harbor nests of cancer cells, with the remainder composed of fibrous stroma. Sampling error in FNA of such lesions may fail to obtain material sufficient to make the diagnosis of cancer on cytology, accounting for the approximately 10% to 20% false-negative rate for EUS-FNA-guided biopsy of pancreas cancer. Although highly operator dependent, EUS may be more sensitive than axial imaging in identifying vascular involvement and suspicious peripancreatic lymph nodes,[19] and thus may contribute to more accurate tumor staging as described next.

Alternative nonoperative approaches to obtaining a tissue diagnosis include endoscopic retrograde cholangiopancreatography (ERCP) with brushings for lesions causing biliary obstruction (see Chapter 20) and percutaneous biopsy under radiologic (ultrasound or CT) guidance (see Chapter 23). ERCP for diagnosis alone is rarely performed in the presence of a radiologically evident pancreatic mass. The sensitivity of ERCP with brushings is inferior to EUS-FNA[21] and the complications of ERCP, particularly pancreatitis, which can be severe in a small fraction of patients, can be responsible for significant morbidity and rare mortality, and may complicate subsequent treatment decisions.

ERCP may be useful in placing a stent and decompressing the biliary tree to relieve the symptoms of jaundice, particularly pruritus, if patients are not able to have surgical resection with biliary reconstruction because of inoperable disease or planned neoadjuvant chemotherapy (see Chapters 20 and 30). Because plastic stents require replacement every 2 to 3 months, candidates for neoadjuvant treatment should generally have a metallic wall stent placed, as such stents provide a superior duration of biliary drainage that will generally not require another intervention during the period of neoadjuvant treatment. Data from randomized studies do not support the routine placement of biliary stents in jaundiced patients with resectable tumors who are anticipated to have surgery and biliary reconstruction within a relatively short time period.[22] There is no evidence that endoscopic biliary decompression improves postsurgical outcomes. In addition to the small risk of severe pancreatitis mentioned earlier, there is growing literature demonstrating that preoperative biliary intervention is associated with a higher postoperative surgical infection rate, presumably caused by seeding of the biliary tree with enteric microorganisms.[23]

In the relatively rare patient who requires a nonoperative biopsy and in whom EUS-FNA is unsuccessful because anatomic factors, percutaneous needle biopsy under radiologic guidance remains an option.[24] Such biopsies may target the primary tumor mass, or suspected metastases in the liver or elsewhere. Seeding of tumor cells intraperitoneally as a result of percutaneous needle biopsy is a theoretical concern but is quite rare; in the largest series reported it occurred in 0.1% of cases.[25] Given the relative difficulty in accessing the pancreas percutaneously, it is often easiest and most definitive to biopsy a suspected site of metastasis if such sites exist.

Diagnostic Laparoscopy

The critical impact of metastatic disease in guiding both prognosis and treatment decisions (as discussed later), and the limitations of imaging technology in determining the presence of metastatic disease, has led to the use of staging laparoscopy to rigorously define or exclude metastatic disease before proceeding with surgical resection. Early studies suggested that 20% to 30% of patients thought to have localized resectable disease would in fact have metastatic disease at laparoscopy.[26–28] However, with improvements in radiologic technique, CT scanning has become more accurate in defining the presence or absence of metastases, and the yield of staging laparoscopy to the workup in identification of radiographically occult metastatic disease in recent series is less than 10%.[29] Thus a selective approach to employing staging laparoscopy seems warranted. When there is a large tumor (T3 or T4) present, or there are indeterminate liver lesions seen on imaging, or the CA19-9 is markedly elevated, staging laparoscopy may be of particular use[30,31] (see Chapter 24).

Cancer Staging

The current staging system for pancreas cancer is described in the eighth edition (2016) of the American Joint Committee on Cancer (AJCC) *Cancer Staging Manual*,[32] and demonstrated in Table 62.1. Like most staging systems, this one combines tumor (T) factors, nodal (N) involvement, and the absence or presence of distant metastases (M) to define prognostically important stages from I to IV. The current staging system is different than prior AJCC staging schemes that included principally tumor size less than or greater than 2 cm (previously T1 vs. T2), the presence or absence of any nodal metastases (previously N0 vs. N1), and extrapancreatic extension of tumor not involving the superior mesenteric artery or celiac artery (previously T3).[33]

In the new system, the size of the tumor is divided into less than 2 cm (T1), 2 to 4 cm (T2), and over 4 cm (T3). Tumor involvement of the superior mesenteric artery or celiac artery is defined as T4 in both the old and new systems, although in the new system this is not classified as necessarily "unresectable" (discussed further in the following sections). Similarly, the nodal status is now stratified as node negative (N0), having one to three involved nodes (N1), or more than three involved nodes (N2), recognizing that an abundance of involved nodes is a negative prognostic factor. The presence of metastatic disease is defined as M1 in both old and new systems. The important differences in the new staging system are that stage IIA

disease is more objectively characterized as tumor greater than 4 cm than by the less definitive criterion of extrapancreatic extension. Similarly, stage IIB is defined as T1-3 with N1 nodal involvement but not N2 nodal involvement; patients with N2 nodal involvement and any T stage are now included with patients having T4 tumor stage in stage III. This staging system has been validated using multiple data sets from the United States, Europe, and Asia.[34–37] Five-year actuarial survivals by stage, obtained by averaging these validation sets, are approximately IA, 40%; IB, 30%; IIA, 25%; IIB, 13%; and III, 10%.

TREATMENT

Surgical resection is the only treatment associated with long-term survival, thus assessment for resectability is an important initial step in patient management (see Chapters 117A and B). An experienced pancreatic surgeon working in a medical center that does a high volume of pancreatic surgery is most likely to achieve a good surgical outcome,[38,39] and the evaluation by such an experienced surgeon, ideally as part of a multidisciplinary tumor board, should be part of a potentially resectable patient's treatment planning. Based on preoperative imaging, patients may be categorized as resectable, borderline resectable/locally advanced, or metastatic. Resectable patients have no evidence of metastatic disease, no evidence of superior mesenteric artery or celiac artery involvement or abutment by tumor, and generally have either no involvement of the portal/superior mesenteric vein, or venous involvement that can be readily resected en bloc to achieve a margin negative (R0) resection (Fig. 62.1).

Borderline resectable disease has been defined independently by multiple groups.[40,41] Although the definitions differ slightly, in general borderline resectable disease refers to tumor proximity to, or direct involvement of, venous or arterial structures, with venous involvement that is potentially resectable with reconstruction and/or arterial involvement including less than 180 degrees of the circumference of the superior mesenteric or celiac artery. Such tumors may be grossly resectable in experienced hands but are likely to have at least a positive microscopic (R1) or macroscopic (R2) resection margin. Not surprisingly, patients having microscopically positive resection margins (R1) or grossly positive resection margins (R2) have

TABLE 62.1	American Joint Commission on Cancer Staging of Pancreatic Cancer			
STAGE	**PRIMARY TUMOR (T)**	**REGIONAL LYMPH NODES (N)**	**DISTANT METASTASES (M)**	**DESCRIPTION**
0	Tis	N0	M0	Carcinoma in situ, includes PanIN3
IA	T1	N0	M0	Tumor limited to the pancreas, ≤2 cm in greatest dimension
IB	T2	N0	M0	Tumor limited to the pancreas, >2 cm and <4 cm in greatest dimension
IIA	T3	N0	M0	Tumor >4 cm in greatest dimension without involvement of the celiac axis or the superior mesenteric artery
IIB	T1, T2, T3	N1	M0	1-3 regional lymph node metastasis
III	T4	N2	M0	Tumor involves the celiac axis or the superior mesenteric artery and/or four or more lymph node metastases
IV	Any T	Any N	M1	Distant metastasis

PanIN3, pancreatic intraepithelial neoplasia.

From Kakar S, Pawlik TM, Allen PJ, et al. Exocrine pancreas. Pancreatic adenocarcinoma. In: Amin MB, ed. *AJCC Cancer Staging Manual.* 8th ed. New York: Springer-Verlag; 2017: 337–347.

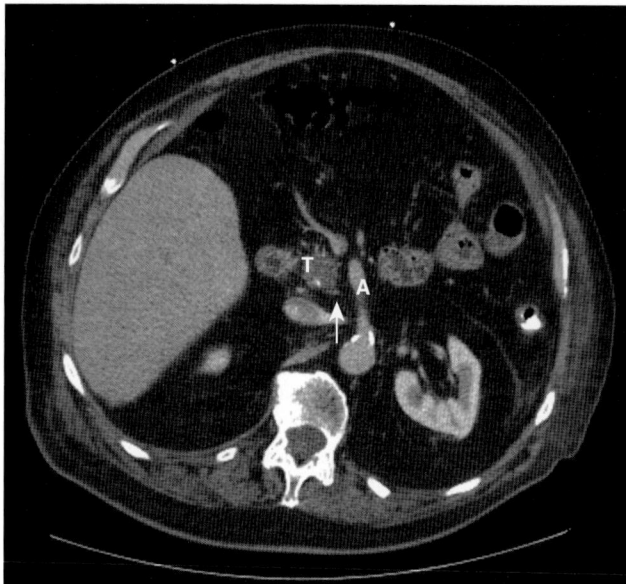

FIGURE 62.1 Resectable pancreatic adenocarcinoma in the head and uncinate process, showing well-preserved fat plane *(arrow)* between tumor *(T)* and superior mesenteric artery *(A)*.

markedly diminished survival.[42,43] Thus the phrase borderline resectable might be better termed "borderline unresectable," and such patients should be treated initially with chemotherapy and in some cases radiation to attempt to downstage their tumors and permit an R0 resection (see Chapter 66).

Patients with locally unresectable disease generally have more extensive vascular involvement, such as complete encasement of the portal or superior mesenteric vein that is not reconstructible and/or more extensive arterial involvement (Fig. 62.2). Such tumors would only be potentially resectable with a grossly positive (R2) resection. Locally advanced tumors in general have a low, but still some, potential to respond to treatment with tumor

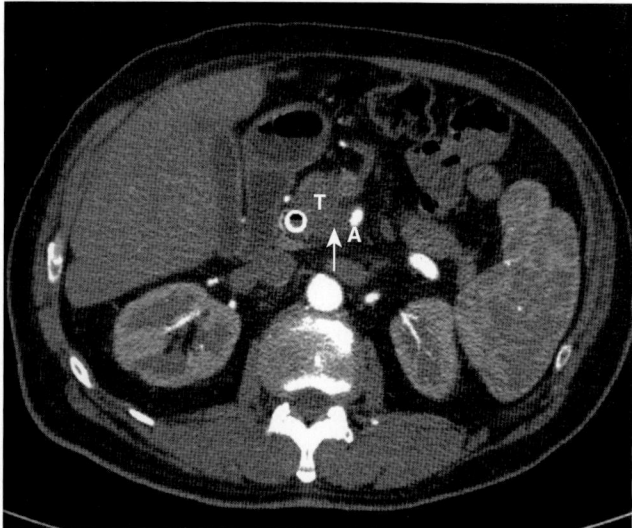

FIGURE 62.2 Unresectable pancreatic adenocarcinoma in the head and uncinate process, showing loss of fat plane *(arrow)* between tumor *(T)* and superior mesenteric artery *(A)*. A metallic endoprosthesis is seen as a circular structure in the distal common bile duct.

downstaging permitting surgical resection (see Chapter 66). At a minimum such treatment slows tumor growth and is associated with improved survival.[44-46]

Patients with metastatic disease, unfortunately the largest subset of pancreas cancer patients,[32] are generally managed with systemic chemotherapy (see Chapter 66) as opposed to surgery or radiation, except in the context of palliation of specific symptoms (see Chapter 67).Systemic therapy for metastatic pancreas cancer has improved in recent years, and those improvements are translated into improved outcomes in the adjuvant setting for resectable tumors, and improved response to neoadjuvant treatment to permit resection of borderline resectable/locally unresectable tumors in some cases.

Advances in Chemotherapy for Metastatic Disease

Until the last decade, chemotherapy for metastatic pancreas cancer had made very little progress (see Chapter 66). Before 1997 single-agent 5-fluorouracil (5-FU) was the standard of care, but it was unclear whether such treatment had any impact on survival or quality of life. In 1997 it was demonstrated in a prospective randomized trial by Burris and colleagues[47] that single-agent gemcitabine was superior to 5-FU in terms of a significant though modest survival benefit (5.6 vs. 4.4 months, $P < .003$), and in improvement of a composite quality of life measure termed clinical benefit response that evaluated pain, Karnofsky performance scale, and maintenance of weight. This study led to the approval of gemcitabine for advanced pancreas cancer specifically based on improving the quantity and quality of patient survival. Over the ensuing 16 years multiple clinical trials combining gemcitabine with other agents failed to show evidence of incremental benefit compared with single-agent gemcitabine.[48]

In 2011 a randomized trial of three agents (5-FU, irinotecan, and oxaliplatin, known as FOLFIRINOX) demonstrated significantly longer survival compared with gemcitabine monotherapy in patients with advanced pancreas cancer.[49] Not only was median survival nearly doubled, from 6 months to 11 months, but quality of life was improved, tumor shrinkage consistent with a radiologic partial response was much more common (31% vs. 9%), and a significant number of patients receiving FOLFIRINOX survived beyond 12 months. Two years later, Von Hoff and colleagues published the results of a different prospective randomized trial, demonstrating that the combination of gemcitabine plus nab-paclitaxel (GA) was superior to single-agent gemcitabine, with improvement in survival from 7 to 9 months and significant tumor shrinkage in 23% of patients treated with the combination versus 7% of those treated with single-agent gemcitabine.[50] Although not directly comparable, it has been concluded from these studies that both combinations are superior to single-agent gemcitabine and that FOLFIRINOX, although more toxic, may be superior to GA. These studies have led to the evaluation of these agents in combination with other drugs and biologics for metastatic disease that is ongoing, and to their use in the adjuvant setting and in the treatment of locally unresectable disease, as will be discussed in the following section.

Surgical Treatment for Resectable Patients

Resectable pancreatic cancers may arise from the pancreatic head, which are generally treated with a pancreaticoduodenectomy (see Chapter 117A) or the pancreatic body and tail, which are generally treated with a left-sided or distal pancreatectomy plus or minus splenectomy (see Chapter 117B). Very rarely extensive intrapancreatic cancer spread without the presence of metastatic disease may warrant a total pancreatectomy (see Chapter 117C). Recent decades have seen marked improvements in short-term outcomes from these procedures in terms of morbidity and mortality[51,52] and in parallel, although not directly related, the advent of minimally invasive surgical approaches using laparoscopy or the DaVinci robot.[53] Thus far, in individual institutional series, comparable short-term results are being obtained with open and minimally invasive approaches. There is a paucity of data on the impact of specific surgical approaches on long-term oncologic outcomes, although most studies to date have not demonstrated significant differences. Unfortunately, despite extensive efforts to operatively improve cancer-specific survival after pancreatectomy, beyond reinforcing the importance of achieving an R0 resection, modifications of technical factors in surgery have not resulted in improved long-term outcomes.

Adjuvant Therapy

There has been an improvement in long-term survival following surgical resection of pancreas cancer associated with the use of more effective adjuvant chemotherapy (see Chapter 66). The field is changing rapidly and today's solutions are unlikely to be the state-of-the-art tomorrow; for this reason enrollment in clinical trials should be encouraged. Despite recent improvements, long-term survivors after resection of pancreatic cancer are still in the minority. With better staging/patient selection and more effective adjuvant therapies, median survivals beyond 2 years and 5-year survivals of over 30% are being achieved in select patients.

There has been stepwise progress in the adjuvant therapy of resected pancreas cancer, based on information gleaned from prospective clinical trials. Although underpowered with just 43 enrolled patients, and largely of historic interest, the GI Tumor Study Group (GITSG) trial was the first prospective randomized study to demonstrate a benefit for postoperative adjuvant therapy, in this case adjuvant 5-FU plus radiation therapy.[54] Median survival in the treatment group, at 20 months, was almost double the survival of 11 months in untreated patients. Two-year survival was more than doubled by treatment (to 43%), but an impact on longer-term survival was not provided. The French Conko-001 trial randomizing between adjuvant single-agent gemcitabine and no treatment showed a near doubling of 5-year survival at 21% versus 9% ($P < .005$).[55] The European ESPAC-3 trial showed similar median and 5-year survival rates for resected patients randomized to gemcitabine or 5-FU plus leucovorin. Notably, the 5-year survivals in the high teens in both arms were essentially identical to that seen in the gemcitabine treatment arm of the Conko-001 trial.[56]

The ESPAC-4 trial compared the combination of gemcitabine plus capecitabine with single-agent gemcitabine, and demonstrated a 29% 5-year survival for the combination versus a 17% 5-year survival for single-agent gemcitabine.[57] Of note, for patients undergoing a margin negative (R0) resection who received the combination therapy, the median survival was 39 months and the 5-year survival exceeded 40%. The promising results of FOLFIRINOX in advanced disease have subsequently been translated to the adjuvant setting. French and Canadian researchers conducted the Prodige-24 trial, comparing resected patients who were randomized to receive adjuvant FOLFIRINOX with patients receiving single-agent gemcitabine.[58] This study demonstrated a median survival of 54 months in patients receiving FOLFIRINOX versus 35 months in the gemcitabine arm, although with increased toxicity in the FOLFIRINOX arm. Thus the application of increasingly effective chemotherapy combinations has resulted in long-term survival benefits in resected patients.

Neoadjuvant versus Adjuvant Chemotherapy for Resectable Disease

The evidence of increasing potency for adjuvant chemotherapy combinations has led to enthusiasm among some surgical and medical oncologists for the use of such combinations preoperatively[59,60] (see Chapter 66). Advantages of such neoadjuvant chemotherapy include the ability to ensure that all patients receive at least some chemotherapy (because those having surgical complications may not receive adjuvant therapy), a biologic test of the tumor's aggressiveness and responsiveness to chemotherapy (because some patients will have early demonstration of metastatic disease despite chemotherapy and such patients can avoid surgery), and potential tumor shrinkage with an increase in the fraction of R0 resections. The counter arguments for up-front surgery and postoperative adjuvant chemotherapy include the possibility of tumor progression despite neoadjuvant chemotherapy administration with loss of the window to perform a potentially curative resection, the relatively low rate of tumor shrinkage in metastatic disease (31%), and the possibility that chemotherapy side effects may be lethal or so substantial that surgical resection is delayed or abandoned because of toxicity.

The only prospective randomized trial of neoadjuvant versus adjuvant therapy for resected pancreas cancer that has been published to date is the Dutch PREOPANC trial.[61] This study randomized both borderline resectable and resectable patients to chemoradiation with single-agent gemcitabine, followed by surgery and then additional gemcitabine in the neoadjuvant arm versus initial surgery followed by adjuvant single-agent gemcitabine alone. This trial is open to a number of criticisms, including different oncologic treatments given to the neoadjuvant and adjuvant groups, the inclusion of both resectable and borderline resectable/locally unresectable patients, and relatively small numbers that made the study underpowered, particularly for subgroup analysis. Based on an intention to treat analysis, there was no difference in survival in the neoadjuvant group, and a more substantial benefit in patients with borderline/locally unresectable disease than with resectable disease. Several multi-institutional prospective randomized trials, using FOLFIRINOX or GA and randomizing to neoadjuvant versus adjuvant treatment for resectable tumors are in progress and should help address the relative merit of neoadjuvant versus adjuvant therapy in the coming years.

Borderline Resectable and Locally Unresectable Disease

A substantial fraction of pancreas cancer patients present with borderline resectable or locally unresectable disease. Neoadjuvant chemotherapy may result in sufficient tumor response to render the lesion resectable with a negative margin in 30% to 60% of borderline resectable and a smaller fraction of locally unresectable patients.[40,41] Such patients who undergo surgical resection appear to have survival equal to patients presenting with initially resectable disease that undergo resection. Data from some centers support the view that patients responding to neoadjuvant chemotherapy for borderline resectable or locally advanced pancreas cancer benefit from the addition of subsequent radiation therapy to their treatment, before surgical exploration, although this is controversial,[62,63] and the recently completed Alliance trial closed the radiation arm early due to lack of efficacy.[64] In addition, the LAP07 trial, which randomized locally advanced pancreas cancer patients to chemotherapy, or chemotherapy followed by chemoradiation, also did not find an advantage to chemoradiation.[65] Recent work by Crane and colleagues suggests that delivery of a higher tumor radiation dose using stereotactic ablative radiation therapy may improve local control and survival more than conventional dosing.[66]

Regardless of which specific neoadjuvant treatment is carried out, it has been suggested in recent years that post-treatment radiologic assessment for borderline resectable and locally advanced tumors does not accurately predict resectability.[40,62,67] These studies have found that preoperative imaging is unable to accurately discriminate residual pancreas cancer adjacent to or involving major blood vessels from residual scar tissue in sites rendered free of tumor by treatment. Thus surgeons caring for such patients need to have a low threshold for proceeding to surgical exploration, and the skill to mobilize and, when possible, to safely remove tumors along with tissue abutting major arterial structures.

Formal Arterial Resection and Reconstruction

In an effort to achieve an R0 resection for patients with T4 tumors involving the celiac and/or superior mesenteric arteries, trials were carried out in the 1970s and 1980s at Memorial Sloan Kettering Cancer Center by Fortner (1984)[68] and at the National Cancer Institute by Sindelar (1989).[69] Although technical aspects varied depending on the specifics of a given patient's tumor, these centers pioneered what was called "regional pancreatectomy," in which arterial and venous resections were performed en bloc with extensive pancreatectomy and regional lymphadenectomy, followed by vascular reconstruction. These were technically demanding procedures that had an extraordinarily high morbidity and mortality. Most significantly, despite undergoing these extensive surgical procedures, there were few long-term survivors. These experiences led to the view among most pancreatic surgeons that arterial involvement by tumor requiring an arterial resection to achieve an R0 tumor resection margin was, in general, not appropriate for surgery (see Chapter 122).

An exception to the principal that arterial resection is of uncertain benefit in pancreatic resection applies to patients with locally advanced pancreatic body tumors involving the upper portion of the celiac artery. If the celiac origin from the aorta is free of tumor and the patient has an intact gastroduodenal artery and proper hepatic artery that are uninvolved by tumor (and even better if the patient has an aberrant right hepatic artery arising from the superior mesenteric artery that is also uninvolved by tumor) it is possible in such patients to resect the celiac and common hepatic artery en bloc with the tumor, most commonly with a left-sided pancreatectomy.[70,71] This is actually a modification of the original Appleby procedure described for gastric cancer[72] and depends on retrograde flow in the gastroduodenal artery to provide the liver with an arterial blood supply. Not surprisingly, liver failure is one of the major sources of morbidity and mortality in patients undergoing an Appleby procedure. The use of an arterial bypass graft to "supercharge" the gastroduodenal blood flow and reduce the risk of liver failure has been recently described.[73] Select patients undergoing an Appleby procedure

appear to have cancer-specific survival similar to that of patients presenting with a resectable tumor[70]; thus it may represent a useful treatment option in carefully selected patients (see Chapters 117A and B).

Because certain patients with tumor abutting major arteries can be successfully resected with R0 margins following neoadjuvant treatment has led some experienced surgeons to selectively perform arterial resection and reconstruction of the celiac and/or superior mesenteric arteries following neoadjuvant treatment.[67,74] This is done to attempt to achieve an R0 margin when the arterial wall is still extensively involved by viable cancer despite neoadjuvant treatment. Such arterial resections are clearly higher risk in terms of morbidity and mortality,[75] and it is not yet clear that patients surviving such procedures have a meaningful chance of long-term survival. The majority of pancreas cancer patients regardless of their initial stage at presentation and the successful performance R0 resection eventually succumb to metastatic disease, and more extensive surgery for stage III disease may not influence prognosis. Furthermore, the impressive locoregional control achieved with ablative radiation therapy described earlier[66] may render arterial resection and reconstruction even less necessary for local control. Thus arterial resection and reconstruction should be considered outside the range of standard therapy and should only be employed on a highly selective basis by surgeons with the individual and institutional skill to manage these complex procedures and their complications.

Surgical Palliation

Many unresectable or recurrent pancreas cancers cause obstruction of the biliary tree, the duodenum, or the intestine. Surgical management of these problems with the historic but now rarely performed "double bypass" procedure (gastrojejunostomy and choledochojejunostomy) has significant morbidity and mortality[76] and has been largely supplanted by nonoperative approaches. Most biliary obstructions can be managed with endoscopic or percutaneous transhepatic wall stents.[77] Duodenal obstruction can similarly be often managed with endoscopically placed endoluminal stents.[78] Although there is still an occasional need for surgical palliation, generally in the form of a gastrojejunostomy for unstentable duodenal obstruction, at most large medical centers this has become infrequent (see Chapter 67).

Advances in Cancer Biology: Impact on Pancreas Cancer Diagnosis and Treatment

Although occasional pancreatic cancer patients may benefit from the most radical surgical treatments, further improvements in outcome for most patients will require earlier diagnosis and/or more effective systemic treatment, rather than even more aggressive surgery. Advances in cancer biology are beginning to make an impact (see Chapters 9A and D). Circulating tumor DNA has been demonstrated to predict recurrence months ahead of axial imaging in resected pancreatic patients,[11] and in combination with other blood markers may be useful in the early identification of pancreas cancer in high-risk populations.[12] Radiomic analysis of primary pancreas tumors has the potential to define tumor prognosis.[79] Genomic characterization has defined distinct subsets of pancreas cancer with markedly different prognoses[80,81]; some genomic subtypes may be more likely to benefit from specific chemotherapy agents.[82] Such stratification may define which patients are more likely to benefit from FOLFIRINOX and which will likely benefit from GA.[83,84]

Newer therapeutic agents are on the horizon, and the recent demonstration of drug targeting of a mutant K-ras oncogene[85] may lead to the ability to target this common molecular driver of pancreas cancer. The finding that pancreas cancers arising in patients with DNA mismatch repair deficiency (Lynch syndrome) may have a marked response to checkpoint inhibitor-based immunotherapy,[86] which offers immediate hope for the small fraction of patients with Lynch syndrome. Of greater significance, it suggests the possibility that additional stimulation of a patient's immune system might generate antitumor responses against more standard forms of pancreatic cancer. Surgical tumor resection is likely to remain a critical factor in permitting long-term survival of pancreas cancer patients; in combination with advances on the horizon in diagnosis and treatment it can be hoped that more patients will be able to benefit from such surgery.

CHAPTER 63

Duodenal adenocarcinoma

Sophia K. McKinley and Cristina R. Ferrone

OVERVIEW

Duodenal adenocarcinoma (DA) is a rare malignancy that accounts for less than 1% of all gastrointestinal (GI) cancers and occurs at a rate of less than 6 cases per million person years.[1-4] In 2018 it was estimated that within the United States there were 10,470 cases of small bowel cancer with 1450 deaths.[5] Even though the duodenum comprises a relatively small portion of the small intestine, DA represents the majority of small bowel adenocarcinomas (SBAs), with reported rates ranging between 55% and 82% of cases.[3] With regard to histology, adenocarcinoma accounts for approximately 40% of all small bowel cancers, and it is the most common histologic subtype of malignancy of the duodenum compared with lymphoma, carcinoid, and GI stromal tumors.[4,6] Interestingly, epidemiologic studies suggest there may be an increasing incidence of DA.[6,7]

Unfortunately, prognosis for DA remains poor, with 5-year overall survival less than 50%, even with attempted curative surgical resection, and with 5-year survival rates between 15% and 33% when patients at all stages at diagnosis are considered.[3,8,9] One persistent challenge to advancing treatment for DA is its rarity, which is why many studies include DA alongside analysis of all small bowel cancers or periampullary tumors. In fact, clinical practice guidelines for SBA were only recently published, first by a French intergroup in 2018 and then by the National Comprehensive Cancer Network in 2019.[10,11]

PRESENTATION

DA demonstrates a slight male predominance with the most common presentation during the 6th or 7th decade of life.[12-14] The clinical presentation of DA may be delayed until the tumor has grown large enough to cause symptoms. The most common symptoms are bleeding or those related to gastric outlet obstruction, such as nausea, vomiting, anorexia, early satiety, and weight loss. Nonspecific or vague abdominal pain is also commonly reported. Additionally, patients may be seen with jaundice if the cancer is in the second portion of the duodenum. A retrospective Japanese study of 205 patients with SBA found that 64 patients (43.0%) with DA were asymptomatic at the time of diagnosis, because 85.9% of asymptomatic cases were found by esophagogastroduodenoscopy (EGD) completed for unrelated reasons.[13] In contrast, 47 patients (83.8%) with jejunoileal adenocarcinoma were symptomatic at the time of diagnosis. This asymptomatic progression of DA leads to high rates of late stage or unresectability at the time of diagnosis, with 24.2% of new DA cases found to be stage 3, and 20.8% found at stage 4 disease in the Japanese cohort study.[13] In Western countries where EGD for gastric cancer surveillance is not routine, the risk for late presentation of DA may be even higher. As a consequence, a significant proportion of DA patients do not proceed to curative intent surgical resection, with a recent

systematic review indicating 29% of patients with DA receiving palliative treatment only.[8] Similarly, a recent prospective cohort study from France demonstrated that less than 60% of SBAs were resectable at the time of diagnosis.[15] Periampullary tumors often present earlier than extra ampullary tumors, and perhaps for this reason, a slightly greater percentage of these lesions are resectable at presentation.[14]

Grossly, DAs appear as circumferential "napkin-ring" type masses or as polypoidal fungating masses (Fig. 63.1). Median tumor size at presentation is approximately 4.0 to 4.6 cm.[12,16,17] However, it is important to note that size may not be a factor in resectability of DA.[14]

Pathogenesis and Risk Factors

The pathogenesis of DA is incompletely understood, but the available data suggest a multistep process of malignant transformation from adenomatous polyp to carcinoma.[18] Acquired mutations in key oncogenes and tumor suppressor genes, including SMAD4, KRAS, TP53, ERBB2, and TGFBRII, have been reported to be drivers in the malignant transformation of preexisting polyps (see Chapters 9A, 9D). As with colon cancer, villous adenomas harbor the most malignant potential. Importantly, the genetic profile of SBA appears to be distinct from both gastric cancer and colorectal cancer.[19] The specific etiology of most cases remains unknown, but a number of predisposing risk factors and conditions have been described. As with other types of malignancy, a role for chronic inflammation, perhaps secondary to exposure to intestinal carcinogens, has been suggested as a factor leading to the accumulation of somatic mutations, with eventual malignant transformation. Lifestyle factors including body mass index (BMI), alcohol intake, and smoking have all been suggested to be associated with increased risk for DA.[20-22]

The most important hereditary syndrome contributing to the development of DA is familial adenomatous polyposis (FAP). These patients harbor a germline mutation in the adenomatous polyposis coli (APC) gene that promotes polyposis and tumor formation within the colon and duodenum. DAs will develop in nearly all patients with FAP, with the periampullary segment of the duodenum most commonly affected. DA and desmoid tumors are the leading causes of death in patients with FAP who have undergone colectomy.[23] FAP patients with duodenal polyps are staged from 0 to IV according to histologic and macroscopic findings based on the Spigelman classification.[24] Progression to stage 4 is often slow, with one group finding a 22.4-year median time to progression to stage 4 disease from first EGD.[25] Patients with advanced stage Spigelman polyps are offered duodenal resection in an attempt to precede progression to carcinoma.

Unfortunately, screening to prevent development of DA in patients with FAP has been found to be variably effective. In a study of 304 patients with FAP, a Danish group found significantly improved survival after screening-diagnosed DA versus

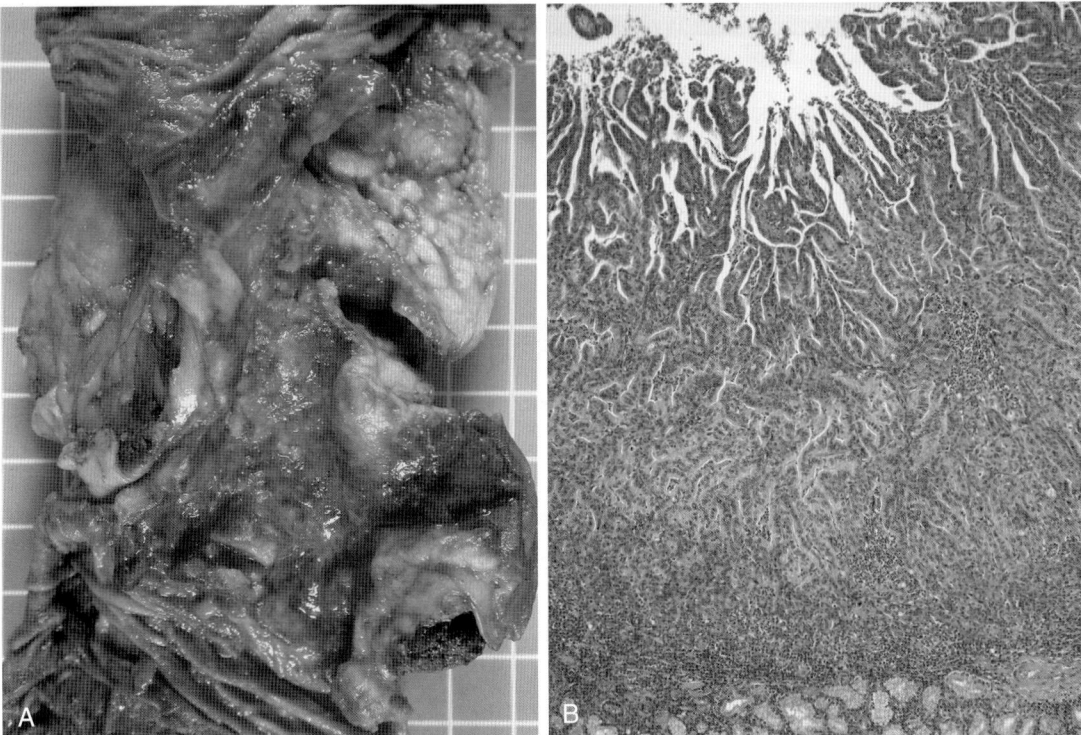

FIGURE 63.1   A, Macroscopic photograph of a resected duodenal adenocarcinoma. **B,** Microscopic image of a duodenal adenocarcinoma.

DA diagnosed on workup of symptoms (8 years vs. 0.8 years, $p < .0001$).[26] Although the Danish group found a benefit to screening, others identified patients who undergo screening and may still develop late-stage DA.[27] Importantly, not all patients who develop duodenal cancer in FAP have preceding Spigelman stage IV polyposis, and even patients who undergo resection for Spigelman stage III and IV polyposis are frequently upstaged to duodenal carcinoma on final pathologic analysis.[28,29] A large French series of 437 patients undergoing over 1900 endoscopies also demonstrated that surveillance is not fool-proof in preventing a DA diagnosis in patients with FAP, with over 20% of the patients undergoing surgical resection for advanced duodenal polyposis upstaged to adenocarcinoma.[30] Although the extent of surgical resection for duodenal polyposis depends on the number and distribution of polyps that cannot be removed endoscopically, patients undergoing more limited resection may require a second, more radical resection for recurrent late stage polyposis.[28]

Lynch syndrome and Peutz-Jeghers syndrome also confer a risk of DA, although the risk is lower compared with FAP.[10] Still, aggressive endoscopic surveillance is also required in these patients. In Lynch syndrome, the relative risk (RR) of DA is estimated to be 100-fold the general population, with a lifetime risk of approximately 4%.[31] Risk of DA in patients with Peutz-Jeghers syndrome has been estimated to be between 1.7% and 13%, significantly higher than the general population.[32–35] Inflammatory bowel disease (IBD) and celiac disease are also thought to be associated with increased risk for DA. In a retrospective study of over 9000 patients with IBD, there was significantly increased risk of small bowel cancer relative to the background population (RR = 3.70; 95% confidence interval [CI] = 1.23–11.1).[36] Case reports and epidemiologic studies suggest celiac disease may also have an increased association with SBA.[10,37]

Diagnostic Workup and Staging

The initial study that identifies a patient's DA will vary depending on the patient's symptoms and individual risk factors. The evaluation of any duodenal mass will include the need to obtain a tissue diagnosis, and then once adenocarcinoma is confirmed, complete staging to determine (1) resectability of the lesion and (2) evidence of distant metastases. Staging of DA is based on the tumor, node, metastasis (TNM) staging system.[38] Tissue diagnosis and location of the lesion relative to the ampulla can be obtained during upper GI endoscopy. Computed tomography or magnetic resonance imaging can be used to assess resectability and rule out metastatic disease. Radiologic findings concerning a duodenal malignancy include an intraluminal exophytic mass or an intramural mass with ulceration (Fig. 63.2). Central necrosis can also be present. Potentially resectable primary tumors demonstrate no evidence of major vascular encasement, distant lymphadenopathy, or distant metastases. If a segmental resection is planned, the patient should undergo endoscopy to confirm the relationship of the tumor to the ampulla. National Comprehensive Cancer Network (NCCN) guidelines indicate that laboratory studies should include CA19-9 and carcinoembryonic antigen (CEA), and that patients should be evaluated for celiac disease and/or IBD depending on their overall clinical picture.[10] DNA mismatch repair (MMR) or microsatellite instability (MSI) testing on tumor tissue is also recommended by NCCN to identify patients who should be tested for Lynch syndrome. The French intergroup guidelines include colonoscopy to assess for synchronous lesions in all patients with DA.[11]

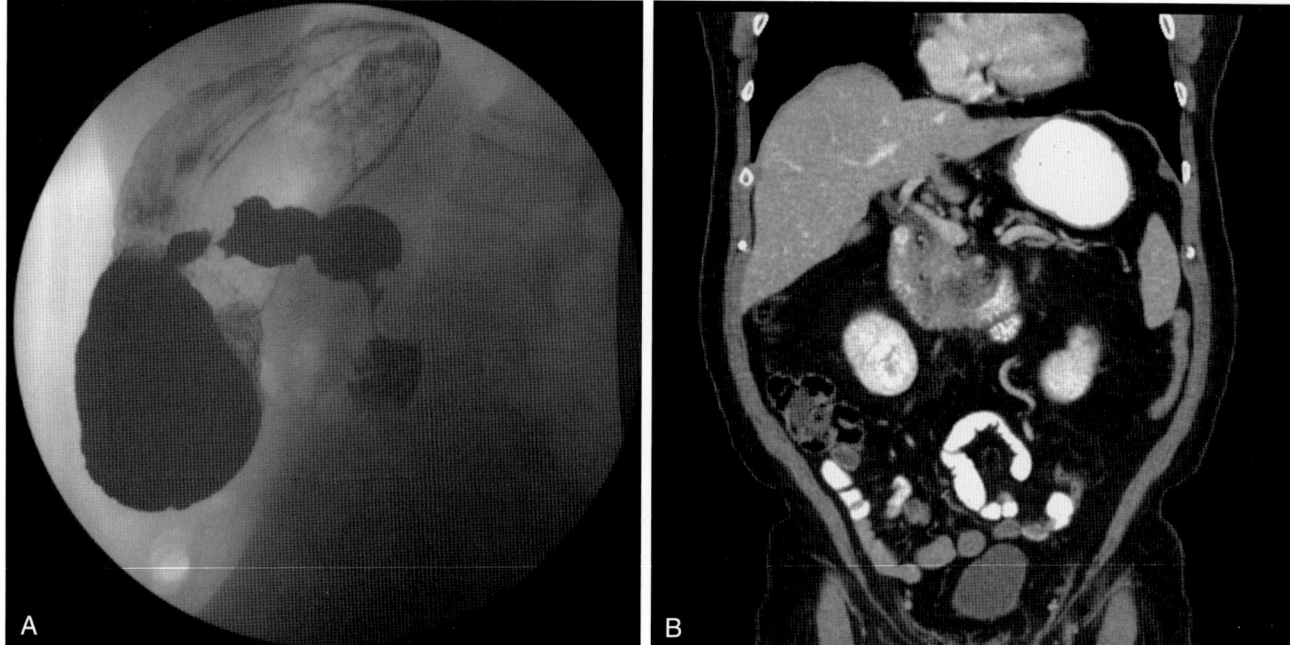

FIGURE 63.2 A, Barium swallow demonstrating narrowing of the duodenum secondary to duodenal adenocarcinoma. **B,** Abdominal computed tomographic image demonstrating mass in the second portion of the duodenum.

Treatment

Surgical Therapy

Surgical resection is the strongest predictor of long-term survival in DA. For patients with invasive adenocarcinoma, most series report a 5-year overall survival of approximately 40%. A 2018 meta-analysis pooling outcomes of 26 observational studies, including 6438 patients with DA, demonstrated a 5-year overall survival of 36% and median survival of 31 months.[8] Two different meta-analyses demonstrated that patients undergoing curative intent surgery had an increased 5-year overall survival to 46% compared with less than 1% for patients receiving palliative treatment only.[8,9] As such, only patients with dysplasia or carcinoma in situ may be candidates for endoscopic submucosal excision (see Chapters 22 and 30). Any patient with invasive adenocarcinoma requires a more extensive operation such as a segmental resection or pancreaticoduodenectomy. The technical details of these procedures are discussed in Chapter 117A.

The optimal extent of resection continues to be a subject of debate, and given the rarity of these cancers, relatively few studies have examined the association of the type of resection on long-term outcomes. There is uniformity in agreement regarding the necessity of pancreaticoduodenectomy in the treatment of periampullary tumors. A number of retrospective series and a review of the Surveillance, Epidemiology, and End Results (SEER) database from 1998 to 2010 (1611 patients) have demonstrated no survival difference between pancreaticoduodenectomy and segmental resection for extra-ampullary tumors that do not invade the pancreas.[8,12,39] This appears to be true even after controlling for confounding factors, including the extent of disease.

When considering type of surgical resection, it should be recalled that the typical lymphatic drainage patterns for tumors in the third and fourth portions of the duodenum are into the small bowel mesentery and not via the pancreaticoduodenal lymphatic basins. Lymphatic drainage from tumors in the first portion of the duodenum is often to the pyloric nodes. These anatomic considerations are critical given that lymph node metastases are an important prognostic factor for DA. Series from the Massachusetts General Hospital (MGH) and Mayo Clinic demonstrated a decrease in 5-year overall survival from 65% to 25% and 68% to 22%, respectively, in the presence of lymph node metastases.[12,40] Meta-analysis of 11 studies including 654 patients undergoing resection for DA demonstrated significantly improved 5-year survival in patients with node-negative disease (65% vs. 21%), with most studies demonstrating prognostic importance even after correction for other factors including tumor size, grade, differentiation, and overall disease stage.[8] NCCN guidelines recommend at least eight lymph nodes be evaluated for adequate staging of small bowel and duodenal cancer.[41–43] Thus the extent of resection should be based on the tumor's location with respect to the ampulla, and the ability to obtain an R0 resection with adequate lymph node sampling.

In addition to lymph node metastases, other histopathologic factors may affect prognosis. The MGH series was the first to identify perineural invasion as the most powerful independent predictor of survival.[12] The 5-year overall survival was 56% versus 19% for patients with and without perineural invasion, respectively. A recent report examined morphologic and immunophenotypic characteristics of extra-ampullary DAs and characterized them as either gastric type (50%), intestinal type (37%), or pancreaticobiliary subtype (5%), with intestinal-type tumors having the most favorable prognosis. Intestinal-type tumors generally express CDX2, MUC2, and CD10, whereas gastric-type tumors express MUC5AC and MUC6.[44]

Neoadjuvant and Adjuvant Therapy

Several small retrospective series of patients with DA undergoing neoadjuvant therapy have demonstrated occasions of pathologic complete response and conversion of unresectable to resectable lesions.[45-48] A Mayo Clinic series of 10 patients with unresectable DA demonstrated conversion to resectability for nine patients with three patients demonstrating either complete or near complete pathologic response.[45] For this reason, NCCN guidelines recommend neoadjuvant therapy for locally unresectable or medically inoperable DA, with monitoring for conversion to resectable disease.[10]

Currently, many patients with DA have been offered postoperative adjuvant therapy on the grounds that it may share features with colorectal cancer, in which the benefit of adjuvant therapy is well established.[15] NCCN guidelines recommend adjuvant therapy for patients with DA with positive lymph nodes (stage III disease), and consideration of adjuvant therapy for patients with stage II disease and high-risk tumor features such as T4 tumors, poorly differentiated histology, lymphovascular or perineural invasion, or tumor perforation.[10] Adjuvant chemoradiation was noted as a treatment possibility for patients with stage II or stage III disease and positive or close surgical margins. With regard to particular treatment regimens, the NCCN guidelines acknowledge that their recommendations are extrapolated from the colorectal cancer literature without proven efficacy in the context of SBA. The preferred treatment regimen, therefore, is enrollment in a clinical trial. French guidelines are similarly adopted from the treatment of colon cancer, with a recommendation for adjuvant chemotherapy in the setting of stage III disease and then consideration or adjuvant chemotherapy in patients with stage II disease and T4 tumors.[11]

Retrospective data supporting these treatment practices and guidelines are mixed. A systematic review of surgical outcomes of DA did not demonstrate a benefit of adjuvant therapy when pooling results of 6 studies and comparing 5-year overall survival for 148 patients who did receive any regimen of adjuvant therapy to 263 patients who did not (48% vs. 46%, odds ratio [OR] 1.14, 95% CI 0.60–2.15).[8] The study was unable to compare adjuvant chemotherapy regimens. Another systematic review pooling outcomes for 607 patients with DA also did not demonstrate an overall survival benefit for adjuvant therapy (hazard risk [HR] = 0.96, 95% CI 0.75–1.23).[49] However, a retrospective study of the National Cancer Database (NCDB) did show increased median overall survival of adjuvant chemotherapy for patients with stage III SBA, 42.4 versus 26.1 months.[50] Comparison of patients with SBA undergoing adjuvant chemotherapy alone versus chemoradiation did not demonstrate any benefit for the addition of radiotherapy, even in patients with positive surgical margins.[51] For both of these latter studies, analyses aggregated patients who received any adjuvant therapy and were not stratified by chemotherapy regimen.

To address the paucity of high-quality data, there is currently an ongoing international prospective, randomized study intended to clarify the benefit of adjuvant therapy for stage I–III DA called the Benefit of Adjuvant Chemotherapy for Small Bowel Adenocarcinoma (BALLAD) trial.[52,53] The objective of the BALLAD trial is 2-fold: (1) compare disease-free survival in patients undergoing adjuvant therapy versus observation and (2) compare disease-free survival between patients undergoing fluoropyrimidine-based adjuvant therapy with or without oxaliplatin. In the BALLAD trial, patients in whom the value of chemotherapy is uncertain will be randomized to observation versus adjuvant chemotherapy using leucovorin and 5-fluorouracil (LV5FU2). Patients in whom the benefit of chemotherapy is certain will be randomized to either LV5FU2 versus leucovorin, fluorouracil, and oxaliplatin (FOLFOX). Primary outcomes will be 3-year disease-free survival and overall survival. Until the BALLAD trial results are available, there appears to be a standard for neoadjuvant therapy in select unresectable patients, and adjuvant therapy in patients with surgically resected disease and evidence for aggressive tumor biology, positive margins, and/or lymph node metastases.

Patterns of Disease Recurrence

Different patterns of recurrence have been reported by different case series. In a series of 83 patients with DA from MGH treated between 1982 and 2010, recurrence was documented in 37 patients (44.6%) at a median follow-up time of 14.5 months.[12] An approximately equal proportion of recurrences were first noted locoregionally (16 of 37, 43.2%) or distantly (17 or 37, 47.2%), with a small number of patients found to have both locoregional and distant recurrence (4 of 37, 10.8%). In a more recent Norwegian series of 69 patients with DA treated from 2000 to 2015, over 80% of first disease recurrence was distant (29 of 36, 80.6%).[54] For both series, the liver was the most common site of distant recurrence. The high rate of disease recurrence and associated poor prognosis underscores the importance of ongoing, collaborative research to improve systemic therapy in hopes of obtaining more durable disease control after curative intent surgical resection of DA.[55]

The references for this chapter can be found online by accessing the accompanying Expert Consult website.

CHAPTER 64

Pancreas as a site of metastatic cancer

Patryk Kambakamba and Kevin C. Conlon

INTRODUCTION

The pancreas is a rare site of distant metastasis. In 1950 in an autopsy study, Abrams et al. were one of the first to highlight the pancreas as a potential site for metastatic spread.[1] Overall, these metastatic lesions constitute only a minor portion (approximately 2%–5%) of all pancreatic neoplasms.[2,3] The most common sites of primary carcinoma for metastatic spread to the pancreas are renal cell carcinoma (~50%) followed by colorectal cancer (~10%). Still, a variety of different cancer sites have been described as a source of spread, such as melanoma, lung cancer, and gastric cancer.[4] The majority of patients metastatic disease to the pancreas also have widespread systemic disease at the time of diagnosis and are not candidates for surgical resection.

Given the rarity of solitary pancreatic metastasis, surgical experience is mainly restricted to case series of limited size. Whereas pancreatectomy remains essential in the curative treatment of primary pancreatic cancer (see Chapter 62), the role of resection is less well understood for metastasis into the pancreas. Historically, resected pancreatic metastases were often misdiagnosed as primary cancers and were identified as metastatic disease by post-operative histologic assessment of the specimen. In 1972 Guttmann et al. presented one of the first cases of a renal cell metastases to the pancreas treated by total pancreatectomy.[5] Similar to a later case series by Zgraggen et al., it was assumed that the disease was a primary pancreatic tumor before resection.[5,6] Still, over time a number of encouraging reports suggested potential oncologic benefits from pancreatic metastasectomy in selected patients.[3,4,7–14]

CLINICAL PRESENTATION AND THE CHALLENGE OF DIAGNOSIS

Clinical Presentation

Pancreatic metastasis are not necessarily associated with symptoms. The literature suggests that approximately 50% of patients are asymptomatic at the time of diagnosis.[4,10,15] In symptomatic patients, the spectrum of symptoms is similar to clinical manifestations of primary pancreatic neoplasia. Abdominal pain, obstructive jaundice and gastric outlet obstruction or hemorrhage are commonly described.[4,16,17] However, many patients present with incidental findings during the extent of disease work-up for the primary cancer or during disease surveillance after treatment of the primary disease.

Diagnosis

The major challenges for the diagnosis are, firstly, to distinguish metastasis from primary pancreatic cancer and then to exclude the presence of disseminated disease. Often a suspicious lesion detected on computed tomography (CT) is the first indication of a pancreatic metastasis[18] (see Chapter 17). From a morphologic standpoint, metastases to the pancreas may display similar characteristics to a primary tumor. In that context, intravenous (IV) contrast protocols for axial imaging are essential to enable a description of vascularization patterns and already may hint to the primary source. Metastasis originating from hypovascular primaries (i.e., colon, gastric, or lung cancer) mostly occur as hypoattenuated lesions, metastasis from hypervascular cancers (i.e., renal cell, hepatocellular, or thyroid cancer) display increased vascularity on CT.[18] This is of particular importance for metastases from renal cell carcinomas that display strong early enhancement at CT and MRI, a pattern that mirrors the hypervascularity of the primary tumor tissue (Fig. 64.1A–B).

Routine use of magnetic resonance imaging (MRI) is not mandatory but may help identify duct infiltration, indicating a primary originating from the pancreatic duct itself[18] (see Chapter 17). Endoscopic ultrasound (EUS) with fine needle aspiration (FNA) is also a valuable diagnostic tool[19] (see Chapter 22). Histologic analysis may be extended by specific immunohistochemistry for certain entities: that is, neuroendocrine tumor (Synaptophysin, Somatostatin), breast cancer (ER, PR, Her2/neu) or lung and thyroid cancer (TTF-1).[20] Tumor markers such as carbohydrate antigen 19-9 (CA 19-9) or carcinoembryonic antigen (CEA) may be helpful laboratory parameters to discriminate a primary from a metastatic pancreatic lesion.

Some authors have recommended preoperative fluorodeoxyglucose–positron-emission tomography (FDG-PET),[21] excluding the presence of extra pancreatic disease (see Fig. 64.1C–D) (see Chapter 18). We believe that this is useful particularly if the patient has a colonic, renal, or melanoma primary. Metastasis from renal cell carcinoma may express somatostatin receptors and can show a similar uptake pattern as neuroendocrine tumors on OctreoScan scintigraphy.[22]

The pattern of metastasis is of no less importance for surgical planning. Whereas the solitary lesion is reported to be the most common manifestation of metastasis to the pancreas (50%–75%), diffuse infiltration or multinodular disease may prevent a pancreas preserving surgical strategy and result in total pancreatectomy.[23,24]

PATIENT SELECTION

In general, the patient needs to be "fit" for surgery, and a proper detailed preoperative assessment by the surgeon and anesthetist is mandatory (see Chapter 117).

Given the variety of entities and constantly evolving therapeutic options, a decision for surgery should be made after multidisciplinary discussion. The indication to resect a pancreatic metastasis should be very carefully weighed against the natural history of the primary disease and the availability of other effective antineoplastic therapies. The clinician should

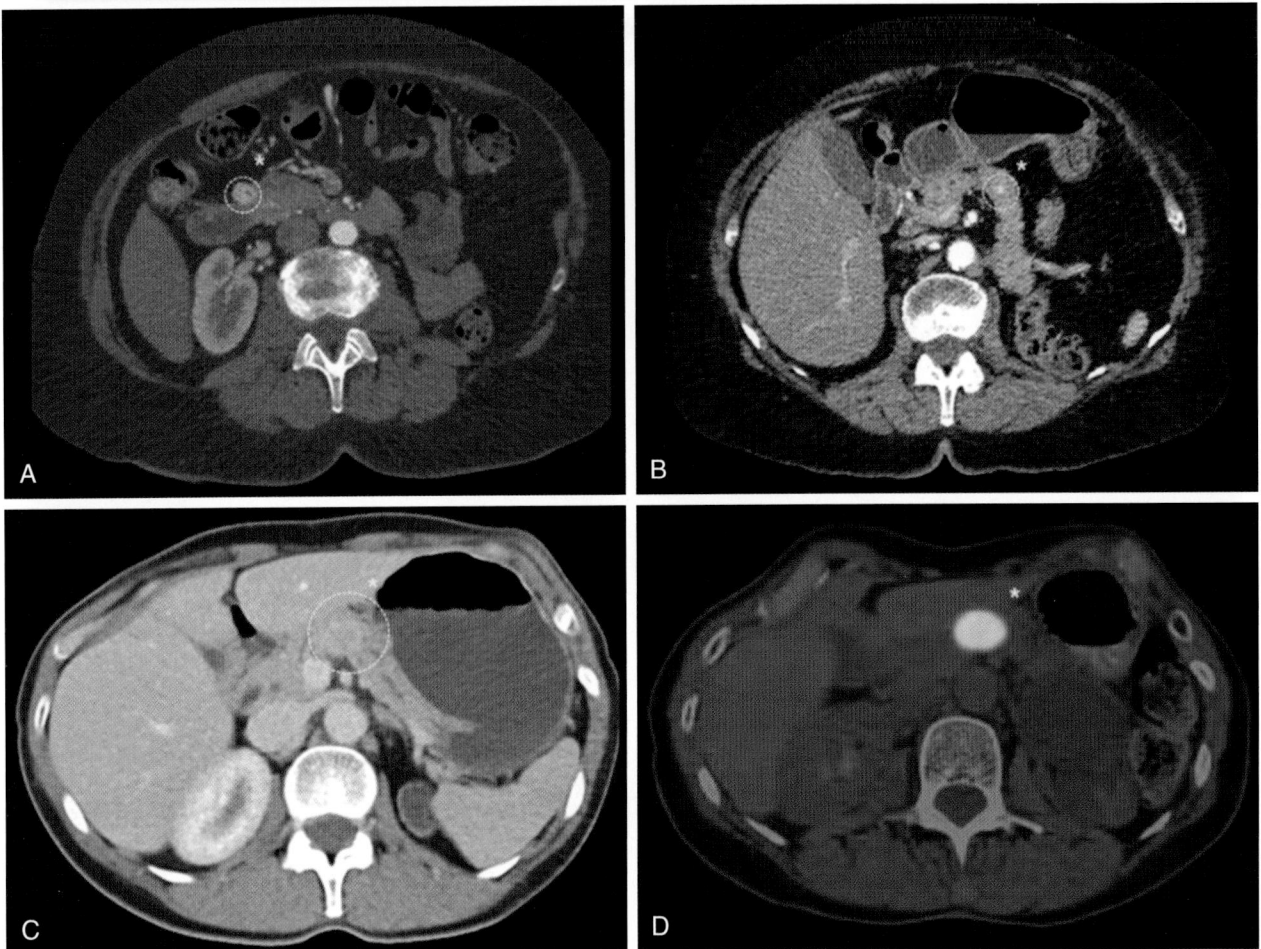

FIIGURE 64.1   Imaging of Pancreatic Metastases. A and B, Patient: 71-year-old female patient with renal cell carcinoma metastases pancreas, with a 6 years disease free interval from after nephrectomy. **A,** Computed tomography shows characteristic arterial enhancement in the lesion in the head of the pancreas and **(B)** multifocality with additional smaller lesions in the body of the pancreas. Patient underwent total pancreatectomy. **C and D,** Patient: 61-year-old female patient with an isolated metastases to the pancreas, originating from a papillary thyroid cancer. Disease free interval after thyroidectomy was 5 years. **C,** Computed tomography demonstrate the tumor in the body of the pancreas, **(D)** which showed strong metabolic activity in positron emission tomography. Patient underwent distal pancreatectomy and splenectomy. Legend: * and *yellow circle* demonstrate the lesion.

always consider the prognosis, time from treatment of the primary disease and the disease natural history of the primary tumor. In general, the presence of synchronous metastatic disease to the pancreas is a poor prognostic sign often signaling subclinical disseminated disease.

SURGICAL STRATEGY

In principle, the whole armamentarium of pancreatic surgery can be considered. Caution should be exercised with pancreas parenchyma preserving strategies, such as duodenum preserving pancreatic head resections, middle pancreatectomies, and enucleations, which although allowing for preservation of pancreatic tissue have been associated with increased operative morbidity, and even associated with inferior oncologic outcomes.[25] Therefore the typical approach to resection used for primary pancreatic adenocarcinoma should be considered for metastases.[25] In this regard, we believe that an R0 resection with a regional lymphadenectomy are the key elements of the surgical approach. Nonetheless, the role of lymph node re-

trieval for pancreatic metastases is controversial. Metastasis originating from renal cell carcinoma rarely show lymph node involvement, but other entities are associated with lymph node infiltration in >60%.[4,8]

Extensive vascular involvement is a relative contraindication for surgical resection. There are only a few reports that exist on concomitant portal vein resection.[4] If limited portal vein attachment to the metastasis is encountered intraoperatively, a limited vascular resection may be performed if the surgeon believes it can be done safely and the risk:benefit ratio is in the patient's favor (see Chapter 62).

Perioperative Morbidity

All pancreatic resections are associated with a 5% to 25% risk for major morbidity. For resections of pancreatic metastases, a recent review described mortality rates of <2% and morbidity rate <50%.[4] This data is similar to that reported after resection for pancreatic ductal adenocarcinoma (PDAC) (see Chapter 117). The most common complication is postoperative pancreatic fistula (POPF), which was described in approximately 10% of patients for a variety of pancreatic resections. In patients with metastatic disease to the pancreas, the pancreatic duct is often normal in caliber. Therefore the surgeon will often face the challenge of a soft pancreas and a small pancreatic duct. Strategies to monitor or reduce the risk for POPF such as placement of drains, application of octreotide, pasireotide, or stenting may be considered for patients undergoing pancreaticoduodenectomy.[26]

Overall, resection of metastatic lesions to the pancreas can be achieved with acceptable risk for adverse events, not exceeding complication rates in the treatment of primary tumors.

The following paragraphs will summarize the most common sources of metastasis to the pancreas.

RENAL CELL CARCINOMA

Metastasis deriving from renal cell carcinoma are the most common and therefore the most thoroughly investigated entity. As mentioned above, metastasis from renal cell carcinoma constitute approximately 50% of all reported resected pancreatic metastases.[4,11] Despite being the predominant entity to be reported in literature, single center reports on resection of renal cell carcinoma metastases to the pancreas rarely include more than 20 patients.[7,9,10,14] The reason for this high prevalence of reports of resected renal cell carcinoma metastases remains unclear but is likely associated with the relatively indolent biology of this particular entity and the reportedly good prognosis after resection.[14,27,28]

In addition, there are few reports of obstruction of the bile duct or gastric outlet, or presentation with gastrointestinal or intraperitoneal hemorrhage, as a consequence of the hypervascularization of the mass.

Little data is available to compare the outcome after resection of synchronous and metachronous disease. It would appear that metastasectomy for synchronous disease is associated with poorer prognosis, possibly because of undetected extrapancreatic metastatic sites.[29] In that context Masetti et al. described improved survival after pancreatic metastasectomy for patients without symptoms and a disease free interval from the primary of over 2 years.[29]

Although a solitary metastasis to the pancreatic tail can be resected at the time of the primary resection, a metastatic lesion in the head of the gland requiring a pancreaticoduodenectomy

should be dealt with at a separate setting. Our preference is to give treatment with a tyrosine kinase inhibitor for 3 to 6 months before proceeding with a resection.[30] This may help control tumor growth during the recovery from the primary tumor resection and also allow the detection of other metastatic sites in case of rapidly disseminating disease. It has been suggested that this leads better selection of candidates for resection and improves outcome.[21]

Enucleation or partial pancreatic resection may be pursued for selected cases.[16] In that context, Yazbek et al. described reduced occurrence of postoperative diabetes for atypical resections, whereas survival was comparable to standard resections such as pancreaticoduodenectomy or distal pancreatcetomy.[16]

However, some authors prefer to perform standard pancreatic resection, even in cases of small pancreatic metastases, because data from Bassi et al. indicate that atypical resections may be associated with an increased risk for recurrence (50% vs. 18%).[13,25] A possible reason is that multifocality is common (60%–70%), and atypical resections bear a risk for missing radiographically occult lesions. In an effort to decrease this latter challenge, intraoperative gland palpation and ultrasound examination should be routinely performed.[10]

In the reported series of resected RCC metastasis to the pancreas, only 7% to 30% of patients had positive lymph nodes in their resected specimens.[4] There are no data to support that an extended lymphadenectomy improves survival. However, we believe that a lymphadenectomy as performed for primary pancreatic cancers is advised for staging purposes whenever technically feasible.

The literature provides encouraging results with a 5 years survival of over 70% after resection of RCC metastasis to the pancreas (Table 64.1).[4,31] leading to some authors recommending an aggressive approach.[25,31] A recent report by Di Franco et al. postulates encouraging results for pancreatic metastasectomy in combination with resection of other gastrointestinal organs, such as the stomach or colon, for synchronous extrapancreatic disease.[14] Nevertheless, radical approaches cannot be recommended in general and are only justified in highly selected cases. Besides surgical resection the tumor biology itself seems to be a prognostic key factor. A prolonged disease free interval from the initial primary treatment appears to be associated with improved outcome.[29]

TABLE 64.1	Surgical Treatment of Renal Cell Carcinoma Metastases to the Pancreas					
AUTHOR	YEAR	PATIENTS [$n =$]	MONTHS FROM PRIMARY	2 YEAR SURVIVAL	5 YEAR SURVIVAL	MEDIAN SURVIVAL [MONTHS]
Hiotis et al.	2002	10	90	75%	—	57.6
Law et al.	2003	14	83	78%	—	—
Moussa et al.	2004	10	108	—	—	61
Schauer et al.	2008	10	110	80%	80%	74
Zerbi et al.	2008	23	144	95%	88%	—
Konstanidis	2010	20	104.4	—	61%	104.4
Yazbek et al.	2012	11	136.8	—	63.7%	78
Niess et al.	2013	16	73.5	88%	68.8%	—
Untsch et al.	2014	27	—	—	—	96
Lee et al.	2017	57	109.2	—	—	57.6
Di Franco et al.	2019	21	107.5	—	71.6%	—
TOTAL		**219**	**108**	**80%**	**63.7%**	**67.5**

Only studies with n ≥10 cases of renal cell carcinoma.

In the context of multimodal treatment, a retrospective study found a median survival 103 months for patients undergoing resection versus 86 months for patients treated with tyrosine kinase inhibitors (TKIs) alone.[25] Although there was a trend favoring resection, the difference was not significant. A multimodal approach combining surgery with TKI may show an advantageous impact on outcome, however this field warrants more exploration.

COLORECTAL CANCER

In recent years, a number of studies have suggest a benefit for hepatic and pulmonary resection for metastatic colorectal carcinoma.[32–34] Limited data exist to evaluate the outcome of pancreatectomy for metastatic colon cancer. Most reported series are single-institutional reviews of pancreatic resection for metastatic disease and contain only a small number of cases[3,4,11,14]

In 2014 Adler and coworkers identified 399 patients who had a pancreatic metastasectomy,[13] 25 (6.2%) of which had a colorectal primary. Sperti et al. reviewed 24 studies and identified 37 out of 418 patients (8.8%) who underwent pancreatic resection for a colorectal primary.[21] In patients who recurred after resection, the median disease-free interval was 21 months (range 5–105 months). In an earlier study, this group detailed 9 patients who underwent resection for colon ($n = 7$) and rectal ($n = 2$) cancers. The median disease-free interval between initial therapy and recurrence was 32.5 months and they achieved an overall median survival of 17 months (range 5–30 months).[17] Others have reported a 5-year survival of 42% after resection.[29] In a more recent study, Huang and colleagues reported that a 5-year survival of 50% can be achieved in selected patients undergoing resection for colorectal cancer metastases to the pancreas.[4] Lymph node involvement was reported in 25% of cases, leading them to recommend a regional lymphadenectomy in all operative cases.

It appears that, in common with other primary sites, the median survival after resection of colorectal pancreatic metastases is significantly shorter as compared with renal cell carcinoma metastases and can be estimated to be approximately 2 years (Table 64.2). Of note, multifocality was observed in up to half of reported cases and this finding should be considered before proceeding with operative resection.

These data, as with other nonrenal cell primary sites, are highly selected and rarely take into account the potential impact of nonsurgical therapies such as chemotherapy or biological approaches. Nonetheless, it would appear than in selected patients who present incidentally, with a prolonged disease-free interval, and have an absence of other disease, that pancreatic resection may be associated with extended survival. However, resection of pancreatic metastases from colorectal cancer should be made on a case by case basis and after a detailed extent of disease work-up and multidisciplinary discussion.

LUNG CANCER

Solitary pancreatic metastases deriving from the lung are extremely rare, and pancreatic disease usually represents metachronous lesions.[35] Small cell lung cancer (SCLC) represents the most typical histologic subtype based on the few reports available in the literature.[21]

Overall, isolated metastases to the pancreas are uncommon, and despite single reports of median survival of almost 40 months, the majority of reports suggest a poor outcome after resection.[8,15] Therefore treatment strategies for metastatic lung cancer lesions to the pancreas should be considered palliative and surgical resection confined to very highly selected patients.

MELANOMA

Gastrointestinal metastases of malignant melanoma are common. However, isolated disease of the pancreas is rare, and surgical experience is limited to small case series.[8,21,36–40] Reports of pancreatic metastasectomy for melanoma metastases rarely include more than five patients.[38,40] Metastases to the pancreas have been described to originate disproportionately from primary ocular melanoma.[36,41]

Besides limitation of disease to the pancreas the tumor biology seems to play an essential role for the prognosis of this disease. A prolonged disease-free interval after the treatment of the primary appears to be associated with improved survival after resection.[8,37] Small series suggest a 5-year survival of 50% for R0 resected isolated melanoma metastases, as compared with 9% for patient who were treated with non-operative management.[38] These data however are retrospective and highly selective; thus a clear benefit of resection cannot be assessed.

There are not sufficient data in the literature to compare surgical treatment with evolving forms of chemotherapy and/or immunotherapy. Therefore surgical resection for pancreatic metastases from melanoma should be considered a palliative

TABLE 64.2	Surgical Treatment of Colorectal Cancer Metastases to the Pancreas			
AUTHOR	**YEAR**	**PATIENTS [$n = $]**	**MONTHS FROM PRIMARY**	**MEDIAN SURVIVAL [MONTHS]**
Moussa et al.	2004	4	61	33
Varker et al.	2007	9	—	—
Sperti et al.	2009	9	32.5	17
Konstanidis et al.	2010	3	—	14.4
You et al.	2011	2	—	30
Alzharani et al.	2012	2	11	—
Niess et al.	2013	2	7	21
Lee et al.	2017	2	22.8	24
TOTAL		**33**	**22.8**	**22.5**

Only studies with n ≥2 cases of colorectal cancer metastases.

treatment, and generally, should be performed in patients with long disease-free intervals, a negative extent-of-disease workup, and after a multidisciplinary discussion.

OTHER SITES

Theoretically, every cancer has the potential to reach the pancreas through a hematogenous or lymphatic pathway. To name a few, pancreatic metastases originating from breast cancer, gastric cancer, Merkel cell carcinoma, and sarcoma have been reported in literature.[4] Most reports are anecdotal small case series and studies often report pooled outcome data of nonrenal cell carcinoma metastases.[4,8,14] As such, it is difficult to draw conclusions for specific entities.

A review by Sperti et al. identified 19 patients in literature who underwent pancreatic resection for metastatic breast cancer, and describes a successful relief of obstructive symptoms in all patients.[21] The 5-year survival was estimated over 30%.[29]

Metastatic sarcoma generally is associated with a poor outcome and isolated sarcoma to the pancreas are extremely rare. Data for these variants are too limited to define proper biology and natural history. Overall, despite some promising results for metastasis from sarcoma,[3,42,43] the outcome for resections of pancreatic metastasis of these entities show poor 5-year survival and should rather be part of palliative concepts. A comprehensive review by Reddy et al. identified only 9 cases and reported a 5-year survival of 14% for resected metastases of this entity.[12]

CONCLUSION

The identification of solitary metastatic disease to the pancreas is often found in asymptomatic patients during routine follow-up. In general, synchronous disease at presentation, a disease free interval less than 1 year after resection of the primary tumor, a nonrenal cell primary, and the presence of significant co-morbidities are associated with poorer outcomes. A "multi-factorial" algorithm should guide the management with younger patients without comorbidities, a prolonged disease-free interval and metachronous solitary metastases to the pancreas considered for resection, whereas patients with significant medical comorbidities should be considered for a non-surgical therapies. Going forward, ablative techniques may be additionally explored to expand the multimodal options.[44] For all patients with metastatic pancreatic disease, a multidisciplinary approach is advocated to "tailor" the appropriate therapy for each individual patient.

The references for this chapter can be found online by accessing the accompanying Expert Consult website.

SECTION II. Neoplastic

D. Endocrine Tumors

CHAPTER 65

Pancreatic neuroendocrine tumors: Classification, clinical picture, diagnosis, and therapy

Haley Hauser, Diane Reidy-Lagunes, and Nitya Raj

INTRODUCTION

Neuroendocrine tumors (NETs) represent a group of heterogenous neoplasms that originate from the diffuse neuroendocrine cell system, most commonly arising in the lung or gastrointestinal (GI) tract.[1] Although NETs represent a rarer group of neoplasms, NET incidence and prevalence continues to increase and NETs are now the second most prevalent GI cancer.[2] Well-differentiated NETs can be subdivided largely based on their tissue of origin, with pancreatic neuroendocrine tumors (PNETs) representing those NETs that originate from endocrine tissue of the pancreas (i.e., islets of Langerhans).[3]

PNETs are the second most common tumor arising from the pancreas.[4,5] A comprehensive PNET diagnosis relies on the evaluation of clinical symptoms, imaging, and histopathology. The management and treatment of PNETs can be challenging because of the heterogeneity in tumor behavior, as well as clinical presentation, with approximately 30% of PNETs presenting as functional tumors, producing clinical symptoms from hormone hypersecretion.[5] Although many advanced PNETs can be monitored initially because of indolent growth patterns, with time the disease will require treatment; the decision to start a therapy occurs because of increasing clinical symptoms (from hormone secretion and/or tumor bulk), high tumor burden, and/or progressive disease while on observation. Treatment options for PNETs are multidisciplinary and include surgical resection, liver-directed therapies, and systemic treatments. For metastatic PNETs, treatment is almost always noncurative, and although survival for patients can often be measured on the order of years, most patients will die of the disease.[6,7] This chapter reviews the classification, clinical features, diagnosis, and treatment of PNETs.

EPIDEMIOLOGY

PNETs account for approximately 7% of all NETs and 1% to 2% of pancreatic tumors[8-10] (see Chapters 59 and 61). The incidence of PNETs has risen over the past 30 years from 0.17 to 0.43 cases per 100,000 people.[11] Males and females are affected equally. Most patients are diagnosed between the ages of 60 to 80 years.[12] Approximately 5% of patients will have an underlying familial syndrome predisposing to PNET development, such as multiple endocrine neoplasia type 1 (MEN1), von Hippel-Lindau (VHL), tuberous sclerosis (TS), or neurofibromatosis type I (NF1), and these patients tend to be diagnosed at a younger age.[10] A family history significant for NET is the only well-established risk factor for PNET development[13]; risk factors for pancreatic adenocarcinoma, such as cigarette smoking, diabetes mellitus, chronic pancreatitis, and obesity, have not been found to be associated with the development of PNET.[14]

MOLECULAR BIOLOGY AND SOMATIC ALTERATIONS

Apart from the germline syndromes previously described, in recent years, understanding of the genetic basis of sporadic PNETs has advanced (see Chapter 9D).

In one of the earliest studies, whole-exome sequencing was performed in 10 nonfamilial PNETs, and the most commonly mutated genes were screened in an additional 58 PNET specimens.[15] In the tested tumors, an increased number of mutations were identified in chromatin remodeling genes (MEN1, DAXX, ATRX), and in genes of the mammalian target of rapamycin (mTOR) pathway (notably in PTEN, TSC2, and PIK3CA).

Whole-genome sequencing was subsequently performed.[16] In this analysis of 102 PNETs, somatic point and gene fusion mutations were observed in genes along four pathways (chromatin remodeling, DNA damage repair, mTOR, telomere maintenance). In addition, a larger than anticipated germline contribution was identified, with previously unreported germline mutations seen in DNA repair genes (MUTYH, CHEK2, and BRCA2).

Building on the findings from whole-exome and whole-genome sequencing, additional efforts have evaluated a role for genetic testing in the routine clinic setting. The benefit of next-generation sequencing (NGS) was assessed in 96 tumor samples from 80 patients with metastatic PNETs.[17] In this study, somatic alterations were identified in 95% of the tested tumor samples, with the most commonly altered genes being MEN1, DAXX, ATRX, and TSC2. In this study, sequencing of pre- and post-treatment samples was also conducted, revealing progression in tumor grade as well as clonal evolution in the tumors. Germline analysis was also performed, with alterations identified in high-penetrance autosomal dominant cancer susceptibility genes (*MEN1*, *TSC2*, and *VHL*).

Of note, poorly differentiated pancreatic neuroendocrine carcinomas (PNECs) are clinically and genetically distinct from PNETs. The most commonly mutated genes in PNECs are the tumor suppressors *p53* (95%) and *Rb* (74%).[18,19]

PATHOLOGY AND STAGING

PNETs are generally well-circumscribed, solitary masses that can occur anywhere in the pancreas.[10] The majority of PNETs are well differentiated.[20] All PNETs have the potential to grow and eventually metastasize, and because of this, these tumors are considered malignant. Because the likelihood of metastatic spread is very low in subsets of patients with PNETs, the term "benign" has been used as a classification variable. Most classification schemes have considered PNET to be malignant if it invades locoregionally; has metastasized distantly or to regional lymph nodes; is greater than 2 cm in size; displays vascular, lymphatic, or perineural invasion; or has a proliferative index greater than 2%[21,22] (see Chapter 59).

PNETs are classified according to the 2017 World Health Organization (WHO) classification of pancreatic neuroendocrine neoplasms (PNENs).[23] The pathologic classification by WHO 2017 criteria remains the most significant prognostic tool for the clinician because it offers information to predict tumor behavior and guide the selection of treatment.

The 2017 WHO classification stratifies PNENs by differentiation (well or poorly differentiated) and grade (grade 1, low; grade 2, intermediate; grade 3, high), with grade classified by proliferative index measured by Ki-67 and/or mitotic count.[24] The mitotic index is expressed as the number of mitotic figures per 10 high-powered microscopic fields (HPFs), and it is recommended that 40 to 50 HPFs be examined.[25] Ki-67 labeling tags neoplastic cells with an antibody and then reports the percentage of cells that stain positively[26] (Table 65.1). Well-differentiated NENs are defined as tumors (NETs), whereas poorly differentiated NENs are defined as carcinomas (NECs). The 2017 classification recognizes the heterogeneity of grade 3 pancreatic NENs, differentiating well-differentiated NETs and poorly differentiated NECs within the grade 3 category as distinct subtypes.[24] Changes in the WHO classification for pancreatic NENs from 2010 to 2017 evolved through an understanding of distinct treatment responses and clinical outcomes for grade 3 PNETs in comparison to PNECs[27–31] (see Chapter 58).

The staging system most commonly used in the United States for classifying PNETs is the 2017 American Joint Committee on Cancer tumor-node-metastasis system.[32] Stage I indicates localized tumors, stages II and III more advanced local or regional disease, and stage IV distant metastases. The 5-year overall survival (OS) rates (nonfunctional and functional tumors combined) derived from analysis of the Surveillance Epidemiology and End Results (SEER) database are 62% for patients with localized tumors, 54% for those with regionally advanced disease, and 20% for patients with distant metastases.[7]

PROGNOSIS

Despite being classified as well differentiated, the majority of PNETs have pathologic features that increase the likelihood of future recurrence or have metastatic disease at the time of diagnosis.[10] Low- and intermediate-grade (G1 and G2, respectively) PNETs have significantly better 5-year OS (75% and 63%, respectively) than do G3 tumors (7%),[33] and functional tumors are associated with better survival than nonfunctional PNETs because they are more often identified at an earlier stage (68% vs. 60% 5-year OS).[34] Approximately 60% of PNET cases have distant metastases at presentation, which is associated with decreased survival compared with those with local or locoregional disease.[35] In addition to grade and the presence of distant metastases, age at diagnosis can also help stratify patients into prognostic categories because an older age at diagnosis correlates with impaired survival (<55 years, 67.8% 5-year OS vs. >75 years, 40.8% 5-year OS).[34]

FAMILIAL SYNDROMES

PNETs are associated with four familial diseases: MEN1, VHL, NF1, and TS. MEN1 is the most common of these syndromes, and approximately 5% to 7% of patients with PNETs will have MEN1.[34] MEN1 is inherited in an autosomal dominant fashion and characterized by the development of parathyroid adenomas that will cause hyperparathyroidism in 90% of patients, multiple functional or nonfunctional PNETs in 75%, and pituitary adenomas in 40%.[36] Adrenocortical tumors (both functional and nonfunctional), thymic tumors, and bronchial NETs are also seen in some patients.[10] Genetic testing for MEN1 should be performed in all first-degree relatives (including children younger than 5 years) of affected patients and those who have had a germline mutation identified in the *MEN1* gene.[37] Approximately 30% to 50% of patients will present with

TABLE 65.1	Grading System for Pancreatic Neuroendocrine Tumors[a]			
TERMINOLOGY	DIFFERENTIATION	GRADE	MITOTIC RATE (mitoses/2 mm^2)	Ki-67 INDEX (PERCENT)
NET, G1	Well differentiated	Low	<2	<3
NET, G2	Well differentiated	Intermediate	2 to 20	3 to 20
NET, G3	Well differentiated	High	>20	>20
NEC (small cell or non-small cell)	Poorly differentiated	High	>20	>20

[a]Poorly differentiated NECs are not formally graded but are considered high grade by definition. This system is recommended by European Neuroendocrine Tumor Society (ENETS) and World Health Organization. It is the most widely used grading system and the method used by most surgical pathology laboratories.
NEC, Neuroendocrine carcinoma; *NET*, neuroendocrine tumor.

From Lloyd RV, Osamura RY, Klöppel G, et al. *WHO Classification of Tumours of Endocrine Organs*. International Agency for Research on Cancer; 2017.

metastases, complications of which are the most common cause of death from MEN1.[38,39] The surgical management of these tumors is complex and discussed in greater detail later (see Chapters 66 and 67).

VHL is an autosomal dominant syndrome caused by inactivation of the *VHL* gene, which is thought to play a role in angiogenesis.[40] VHL predisposes patients to several cancers: renal cell carcinoma, pheochromocytoma, cerebellar and spinal hemangioblastoma, retinal angioma, endolymphatic sac neoplasms, epididymal cystadenoma, and cystic and solid pancreatic neoplasms.[41] Between 10% and 15% of VHL patients will develop PNETs, although the most common pancreatic manifestation of this syndrome is serous cystadenoma.[10,42]

PNETs may also develop in TS and NF1. The tuberous sclerosis complex 1/2 (TSC1/2) inhibits mTOR, and a defect in the *TSC2* gene leads to development of TS. *NF1*, the gene responsible for NF1, regulates the activity of *TSC2*. Loss of *NF1* leads to constitutive mTOR activation. In TS, hamartomas may develop in the brain, eyes, heart, lungs, skin, kidneys, and pancreas. In NF1, the primary manifestation is the development of benign neurofibromas in multiple locations of the peripheral nervous system. Patients are also at risk for pheochromocytomas and sarcomas. In both TS and NF1, multiple PNETs may develop in the pancreas and duodenum.[40,43]

FUNCTIONAL TUMORS: CLINICAL FEATURES

PNETs are clinically classified into two categories: functional and nonfunctional. Functional PNETs produce clinical syndromes because of the hypersecretion of biologically active peptides. Functional PNETs tend to have better 5-year OS compared with nonfunctional PNETs.[34] This is likely because they are detected earlier than nonfunctional PNETs because of the presence of symptoms.

Insulinoma

Insulinomas secrete insulin and/or proinsulin, causing hypoglycemia. They represent 1% to 2% of all pancreatic tumors and are typically small (<2 cm), solitary (except in MEN1), and intrapancreatic. In the rare cases where these tumors are malignant, 5-year OS is 56%,[20] and 10-year OS declines to 29%.[44] A critical part of the history includes establishment of the presence of Whipple's triad: plasma glucose less than 40 mg/dL, symptoms of hypoglycemia, and resolution of symptoms with a meal. The diagnosis can be confirmed by drawing plasma glucose, insulin, C-peptide, and proinsulin levels during a 72-hour fast. This panel will detect 90% of insulinomas.[45] Malignant insulinomas tend to produce higher levels of insulin and proinsulin and thus more severe symptoms because their metastases also secrete these hormones. Although most insulinomas are identified with computed tomography (CT) or ultrasound (US), when they are very small these methods may not localize the tumor, and arterial stimulation venous sampling may then be helpful. To perform this test, the right and left hepatic veins are catheterized via a femoral puncture. Calcium is injected successively into the gastroduodenal, proximal splenic, superior mesenteric, and proper hepatic arteries. After each injection, venous blood is sampled from the hepatic veins at 30, 60, and 120 seconds, and a positive localization corresponds to a 2-fold increase in hepatic vein insulin levels.[46] The accuracy of this method to localize the tumor to a region of the pancreas (i.e., head, body, tail) is 94% to 100%.[44]

Gastrinoma

Gastrinomas secrete gastrin, causing Zollinger-Ellison syndrome. This syndrome is named for Zollinger and his colleagues[47] who, in 1955, published a case series detailing the clinical courses of two patients with gastric acid hypersecretion, severe peptic ulceration, and pancreatic tumors. The extraordinarily high levels of gastrin secreted by these tumors are the cause of the recurrent peptic ulcers, diarrhea, and reflux esophagitis experienced by most patients and cause the thickened mucosal folds in the stomach that are a hallmark of the disease.[48,49] These functional PNETs may be sporadic (67%) or familial (33%)[48] and tend to be solitary tumors unless seen in the context of MEN1, in which case they are small, multiple, and most likely found in the duodenum (>85%).[49] Regardless of their etiology, they are generally found within the gastrinoma triangle (Fig. 65.1), which was described in 1984 to aid surgeons in finding these frequently diminutive tumors.[50] The majority of gastrinomas are considered malignant (60%) and have spread to regional lymph nodes by the time they are diagnosed. Liver metastases are often associated with gastrinomas that arise in the pancreas.[48] Laboratory diagnosis of the disease requires demonstration of hypergastrinemia and abnormal gastric acid secretion. This can be done by obtaining a fasting serum gastrin and a gastric pH. If the gastrin level is 10 times normal and the gastric pH is less than 2, the diagnosis is confirmed.[45] If results are equivocal, a secretin or glucagon stimulation test can be performed because gastrinomas frequently express both receptors and respond by secreting abnormally large amounts of gastrin to the injected reagent.[49,51]

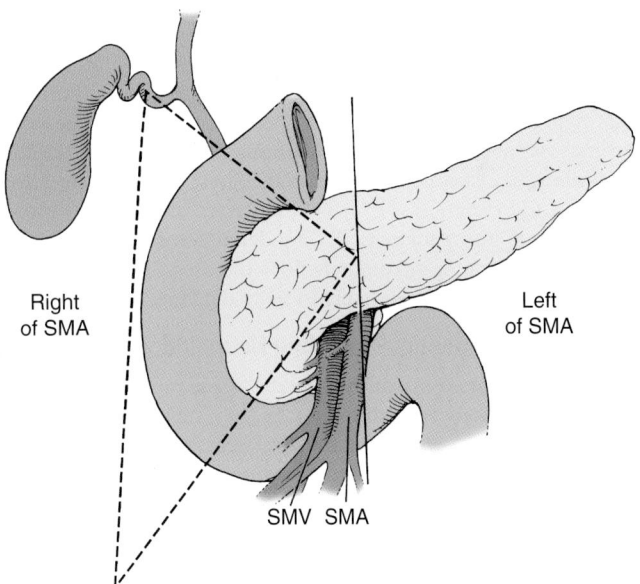

Right of SMA

Left of SMA

SMV SMA

FIGURE 65.1 Gastrinoma triangle. Approximately 90% of gastrinomas are thought to arise in this anatomic location. The apex is at the junction of the cystic duct and common bile duct, the inferior aspect lies at the junction of the second and third parts of the duodenum, and the medial extent lies at the junction of the head and body of the pancreas. *SMA,* Superior mesenteric artery; *SMV,* superior mesenteric vein. (From Howard TJ, Stabile BE, Zinner MJ, Chang S, Bhagavan BS, Passaro Jr E. Anatomic distribution of pancreatic endocrine tumors. *Am J Surg.* 1990;159:258–264.)

Glucagonoma

Glucagonomas secrete glucagon, causing hyperglycemia. These tumors are extremely rare, and only about 400 cases of glucagonomas have been reported in the literature.[52] These tend to be large (>6 cm) and solitary pancreatic tumors. The most common symptoms of the disease are glucose intolerance, migratory necrolytic erythema, and weight loss.[49] The migratory rash is often the first manifestation.[53] It tends to start in the perineum and then spreads to the trunk and extremities. The diagnosis is achieved when an elevated plasma glucagon level is found in the context of an enhancing pancreatic mass on CT. Approximately 60% will have liver metastases at diagnosis.[49] In a case report of 23 glucagonomas, the 5-year OS (regardless of treatment) was nearly 75%.[54]

Vasoactive Intestinal Peptide-Secreting Neuroendocrine Tumor

Vasoactive intestinal peptide (VIP)-secreting neuroendocrine tumors (VIPomas) secrete VIP, causing severe secretory diarrhea. These tumors tend to be solitary, intrapancreatic tumors, greater than 50% of which are metastatic at presentation.[49] The hypersecretion of VIP, a neurotransmitter and intestinal secretagogue, leads to the development of "pancreatic cholera,"[55] also known as Verner-Morrison syndrome,[56] which is characterized by large-volume (average, 4.5 L) watery diarrhea that leads to metabolic acidosis, achlorhydria, and hypokalemia. If not properly identified and treated, patients will eventually succumb to renal failure secondary to hypovolemia.[57] As with the other functional PNETs, the diagnosis is made by radiographic evidence of a pancreatic tumor and a history consistent with the syndrome associated with hypersecretion of VIP. Further confirmation is made by demonstration of an elevated plasma VIP level.

Somatostatinoma

Somatostatinomas (SSomas) have a less-defined clinical syndrome than do the other functional PNETs, and not all tumors that hypersecrete somatostatin will cause symptoms. The syndrome may include glucose intolerance, cholelithiasis, weight loss, diarrhea, steatorrhea, or anemia. These tumors may arise either in the pancreas (56%) or duodenum and may be more aggressive if intrapancreatic.[58] Duodenal SSomas are associated with NF1 in approximately 50% of cases. If discovered in this context, they are less likely to be malignant.[59]

Pancreatic Polypeptide-Secreting Neuroendocrine Tumors

PNETs that predominantly secrete pancreatic polypeptide (PP) are extremely rare and whether they should be classified as functional is a matter of debate because no specific syndrome has been defined. Patients may present with intermittent abdominal pain, pancreatitis,[60] and some patients may develop glucose intolerance.[61] If these tumors occur in the context of MEN1, they tend to be multifocal and malignant.[60] PP can be used as a marker for PNETs in MEN1 patients, as fasting PP levels greater than three times normal have been shown to correlate with the presence of a PNET that will likely be large enough to detect by standard imaging.[62]

NONFUNCTIONAL TUMORS: CLINICAL FEATURES

Nonfunctional PNETs are characterized by their lack of hormone production and hormone-associated syndromes. They have the potential to produce peptides (pancreatic polypeptide, chromogranin A, ghrelin, neurotensin, subunits of chorionic gonadotropin, neuro-specific enolase), but these peptides do not cause hormone producing symptoms.[63] Patients that present with tumors classified as nonfunctional can develop symptoms of hormone secretion further into their disease course.[64]

It is difficult to know what proportion of PNETs are truly nonfunctional because reports vary widely, ranging from 10% to 91%.[7,8,65-67] This wide range is because of two main factors. Rates calculated from single institutions may be lower because of a referral bias for functional tumors at academic medical centers. If rates are calculated using large, public databases such as SEER or the National Cancer Database (NCDB), they often will identify higher numbers of nonfunctional tumors because these repositories do not collect data on specific symptoms or hormone levels. Thus the default in these databases is categorization of a PNET as nonfunctional unless a specific functional histology code is recorded, such as insulinoma, glucagonoma, VIPoma, or gastrinoma. Therefore a reasonable estimate of the proportion of nonfunctional PNETs is approximately 75%.[68]

In one report, 39% of these tumors were discovered because of symptoms related to the tumor's mass effect—abdominal pain, jaundice, weight loss, abdominal mass, nausea, vomiting, back pain, or pancreatitis.[69] Nonfunctional PNETs causing symptoms tend to be larger than those PNETs found incidentally (2.5 vs. 1.8 cm) and are more likely to have involved nodes at diagnosis.[69]

Approximately 35% of PNETs are discovered incidentally, and this is occurring with greater frequency as the use of high-quality axial imaging is increasing[70] (see Chapter 17). In one series of incidentally discovered PNET, 19% were classified as having benign histopathologic findings, 52% had uncertain histology, and 28% were considered to have malignant pathologic features. The benign tumors and those with uncertain histology were associated with a 5-year OS of 89% and 93%, respectively, whereas malignant tumors had 50% 5-year OS.[71]

Whether discovered incidentally or because of symptoms, it is important to note that although some blood biomarkers can be elevated in the presence of a PNET (chromogranin A, pancreastatin, pancreatic polypeptide, neuron specific enolase, tachykinins), there is a lack of laboratory standards, as well as varying sensitivity and specificity in measuring these biomarkers; serum chromogranin A, which is often checked, can be elevated in many conditions, including kidney and/or heart disease, proton-pump inhibitor usage, and other non-NEN tumors.[72,73] Currently there are no data justifying the use of these biomarkers in isolation for diagnosis or treatment decision making.

IMAGING

Imaging and endoscopy are used for primary tumor detection, staging, surgical planning, and evaluation of somatostatin receptor (SSTR) expression. The modalities used most often are CT, magnetic resonance imaging (MRI; see Chapter 17), endoscopic US (EUS; see Chapter 22), standard US (see Chapter 17), somatostatin receptor scintigraphy (SRS), and positron-emission tomography (PET; see Chapter 18).

CT is often the first modality used to image PNETs because it is valuable for detection of the primary, regional, and

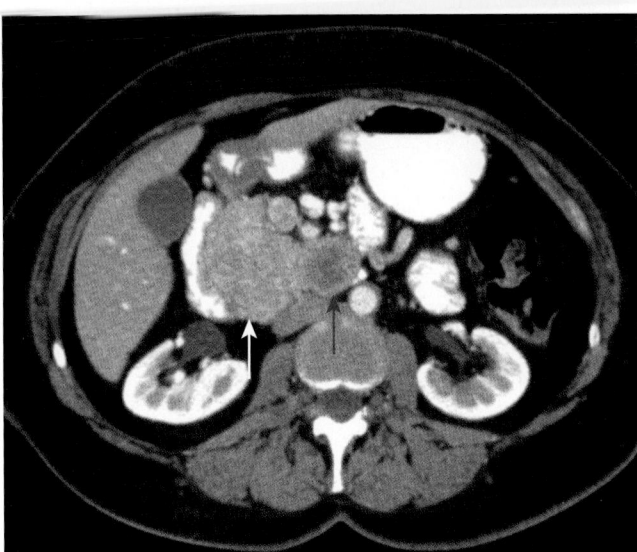

FIGURE 65.2 Arterial phase of a contrast-enhanced computed tomography of the abdomen showing an early enhancing pancreatic neuroendocrine tumor in the head and uncinate process of the pancreas *(white arrow),* with a necrotic node medially *(red arrow).*

metastatic disease (Fig. 65.2; see Chapter 17). Its sensitivity for tumors greater than 2 cm is 80% to 100%,[9] although it is more sensitive for hepatic metastases than it is for primary tumors.[74,75] This modality can detect some PNETs smaller than 0.5 cm,[76] although it is more likely to miss these small lesions when compared with EUS.[77] CT imaging should be obtained with oral and intravenous (IV) contrast. IV contrast is important for the detection of the primary tumor and metastases because PNETs and their metastases tend to be hypervascular and best seen in the arterial phase. These lesions will wash out in the venous and delayed phases.[78] Oral contrast is helpful for visualizing the duodenum.[9]

MRI should be considered a second-line test for detection of primary PNETs and used when superior delineation of hepatic metastases is required,[79] when patients have an iodinated contrast allergy, or in cases of renal failure.[80] This study should also be obtained with IV contrast. The tumors will be hypointense on T1 and hyperintense on T2 images. As with CT, lesions less than 1 cm may be missed, regardless of contrast administration[9] (see Chapter 17).

US is most commonly combined with endoscopy or used intraoperatively in the localization of PNETs (see Chapter 22). EUS may be used to identify the primary tumor and local nodal involvement and, when combined with fine needle biopsy, to obtain tissue diagnosis with a diagnostic accuracy of 90%.[81,82] It has a sensitivity of 79% to 82%[83] and can detect tumors as small as 2 to 3 mm.[9] US is commonly used intraoperatively to localize small tumors such as insulinomas. In this role, it has a sensitivity of 80% to 100%,[44] although like EUS, it is highly operator dependent.

Imaging is critical to clarify the SSTR status of the disease, and scintigraphy with radiolabeled SST analogs has proven to be a useful tool in diagnosis and treatment determination.[84] There are five types of somatostatin receptors (SSTR1 to SSTR5), and SSTR2 is frequently expressed on well-differentiated NETs and serves as the primary receptor for both somatostatin analogue imaging and treatment[85] (see Chapter 18).

The original somatostatin analogue–based imaging modality is the OctreoScan, which uses the radiotracer indium-111–DPTA-octreotide.[86] In its most basic form, this study produces a whole-body planar image with dark spots indicating where radiotracer has bound to SSTR2 (and to a lesser extent, SSTR5 and SSTR3).[87] In most centers, these planar images are enhanced by combining the OctreoScan with single-photon emission computed tomography (SPECT), which adds axial three-dimensional imaging to the functional scintigraphic image, greatly improving the diagnostic accuracy.[88] In one study, the addition of SPECT to OctreoScan improved lesion detection by 52%.[89]

The most modern iteration of SSTR–based imaging combines PET with CT and uses the positron emitter gallium-68 to label various somatostatin analogues—most commonly ^{68}Ga-DOTA-Tyr(3)-octreotide (DOTATOC), ^{68}Ga-DOTA-1-Nal(3)-octreotide (DOTANOC), and ^{68}Ga-DOTA-Tyr(3)-octreotate (DOTATATE)—which then bind to their respective SSTR subtypes.[90] ^{68}Ga-PET/CT is the preferred functional imaging of choice over OctreoScan. Each ligand varies in its affinity for the various SSTR subtypes, but these differences are not clinically significant.[80] ^{68}Ga-PET/CT will detect both functional and nonfunctional PNETs.[52,91,92] Studies comparing ^{68}Ga-PET/CT and conventional imaging modalities (CT, MRI, OctreoScan) consistently demonstrate the superiority of ^{68}Ga-PET/CT in the detection of NET primary tumors and metastases.[93–95] However, care must be taken to differentiate NETs from physiologic uptake of ^{68}Ga, as is seen in the uncinate process of the pancreas,[96] pituitary, spleen (or accessory spleen), and kidneys.[97] Given its demonstrated utility in NET imaging, ^{68}Ga-PET/CT was approved for general use in the United States in 2016.

18-Fluoro-deoxy-glucose PET ([18]FDG PET) is most often used in PNETs when the tumor is high grade.[98] Patients found to have PNETs with uptake on [18]FDG PET are more likely to have early disease progression than those who are [18]FDG PET negative.[99] (see Chapter 18)

SURGICAL MANAGEMENT

Resection of the Primary Tumor: Surgical Considerations

Surgical excision of the primary PNET, regional nodal disease, and distant metastases are required to achieve cure of the disease, although cure is unlikely in the setting of distant metastases. Despite this, patients may derive benefit from surgical resection in the setting of metastatic disease and should therefore be evaluated and treated by a surgeon familiar with the nuances of NET-directed operations (see Chapter 117). In general, resection is indicated for (1) functional, symptomatic PNETs; (2) isolated G1 or G2 PNETs greater than 2 cm; and (3) patients with metastatic disease in which all visible metastases can be resected.[9] Palliative resection of the primary PNET and hepatic debulking may be considered for those patients with symptomatic, advanced disease where the liver is the only focus of distant metastases, however, whether this affects overall survival is unknown.[100,101]

It is generally accepted that nonfunctional PNETs greater than 2 cm should be resected, given their metastatic potential. However, much debate exists around what to do about smaller PNETs. In many centers, these small tumors are observed with serial imaging and resected if they show signs of progression. Evidence for this approach is conflicting. Lee and colleagues (2012)[102] compared patients with nonfunctional PNETs less than 4 cm who were managed nonoperatively ($n = 77$; median tumor size, 1 cm) with patients who underwent resection ($n = 56$; median tumor size, 1.8 cm). Nine percent of the operative group had positive nodes and a median tumor size of 2.4 cm. The study had a mean follow-up of 3.75 years (maximum, 12.75 years). The median primary tumor size in the nonoperative group did not change during follow-up, nor was there disease progression or disease-specific mortality in this group, suggesting that small PNETs can be safely managed nonoperatively. Sadot et al. also reviewed 464 incidentally discovered sporadic small (<3 cm) stage I to II PNETs of which 104 were recommended observation.[103] In the observation group, at the time of last follow-up, median tumor size had not changed (1.2 cm, $P = .7$), and no patient developed evidence of metastases. Within the resection group, low-grade pathology was recorded in 72 (95%) tumors and 5 (6%) developed a recurrence, which occurred after a median of 5.1 (range 2.9–8.1) years. No patient in either group died from disease. Death from other causes occurred in 11 of 181 (6 %) patients. The authors concluded that observation for stable, small, incidentally discovered PNETs is reasonable in selected patients.

In contrast, a study examining the survival of patients in the NCDB with localized, nonfunctioning PNETs less than 2 cm ($n = 380$) showed that OS was significantly improved in those patients who underwent resection of their primary (median survival > 5 years, compared with 2.3 years in observation group).[104] However, because inclusion in NCDB requires a tissue diagnosis, this study would not have included many patients with incidentally found tumors that were being followed by imaging. Therefore the optimal management of nonfunctional tumors less than 2 cm is unclear. In patients with significant comorbidities, it seems reasonable to observe these tumors. Furthermore, pancreas-directed operations are not without risk. In the series from Lee and colleagues (2012),[102] 46% of the surgically treated patients had some sort of perioperative complication, the most common of which was development of a pancreatic fistula.

Lesions in the body and tail are generally treated with distal pancreatectomy (Fig. 65.3). As larger tumors commonly invade the splenic vein, splenectomy is often performed, although in cases where the tumors are small and do not invade the vein, splenic preservation should be considered. Tumors in the head, especially if large, will require pancreaticoduodenectomy (PD). Small tumors in the head can be considered for enucleation (see Chapter 117).

More limited procedures, such as enucleation, are acceptable for the resection of small, isolated PNETs and in well-selected patients are associated with relatively low rates of complications (Fig. 65.4). Three recent studies reported on the safety and efficacy of enucleation to treat small (1–3 cm) PNETs. Compared with patients who underwent PD or distal pancreatectomy for their tumors, patients having enucleation experienced less blood loss, shorter operative times, fewer postoperative complications, and less pancreatic insufficiency.[105–107] Enucleation can be approached safely either via laparotomy or laparoscopy[108,109] but should be reserved for those PNETs most likely to be benign. This procedure is generally performed on insulinomas and small, isolated gastrinomas or nonfunctional PNETs.[49] From a technical standpoint, enucleation

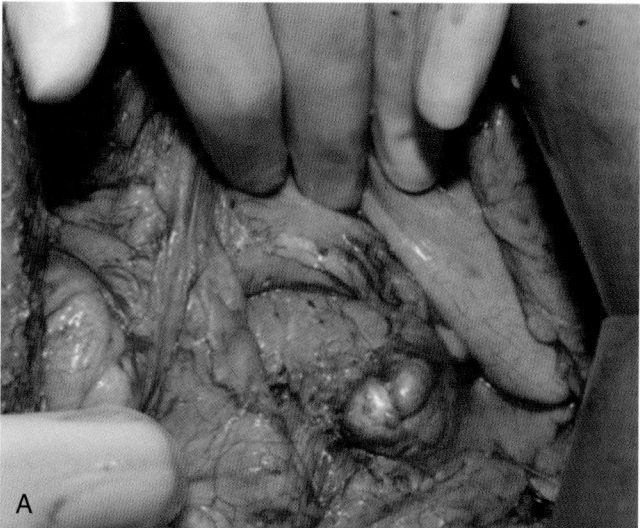

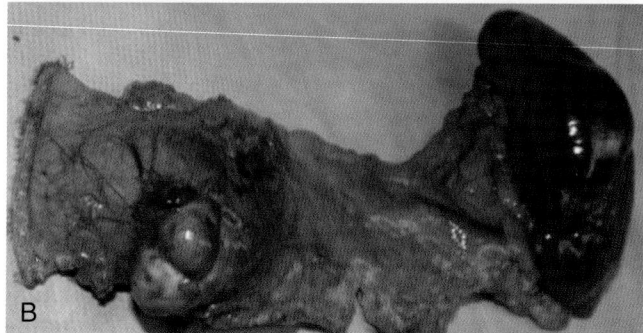

FIGURE 65.3 **A,** Intraoperative view of a pancreatic neuroendocrine tumor located in the body of the pancreas. **B,** Specimen resulting from distal pancreatectomy and splenectomy.

should only be considered for PNETs that are 2 to 3 mm away from the main pancreatic duct, less than 2 cm in size, and located relatively near the surface of the pancreatic parenchyma. In addition, intraoperative US should be used to help visualize the location of the pancreatic duct during the procedure.[105–107]

To improve patient recovery, distal pancreatectomy may be performed laparoscopically or robotically.[110] A meta-analysis examined 18 studies that included 1814 patients with pancreatic tumors amenable to resection via distal pancreatectomy. Forty-three percent of patients underwent laparoscopic resection, and the rest were approached with laparotomy. The laparoscopic group had a shorter length of stay, less blood loss, and fewer postoperative complications. Encouragingly, there was no difference in margin positivity, postoperative pancreatic fistula development, or mortality, although there did seem to be a trend toward fewer lymph nodes being sampled with the laparoscopic approach[111] (see Chapter 127).

A common debate in the management of NETs is whether to resect the primary tumor in the presence of advanced disease. One argument against resection is that the patient is unlikely to obtain a curative (R0) resection and thus bears the risk of a large operation without the potential benefit of improved survival. Hill and colleagues (2009)[65] compared patients with all stages of disease who underwent surgical resection with those who did not. They found that those who had surgery had significantly better OS (median, 114 months) compared with

inhibitors (PPIs), and the dose should be titrated to effect. If patients are not candidates for surgery, they can be sustained on PPI over the long term because studies show patients treated for more than 10 years do not develop tachyphylaxis, although they may develop achlorhydria, which can lead to nutritional deficiencies.[49]

SYSTEMIC THERAPY

Given the heterogeneity of PNETs, systemic therapy strategy depends on several factors: tumor functional status, pathologic grade of the tumor, SSTR avidity on functional imaging, disease bulk, and disease behavior.

Somatostatin Analogs

Most well-differentiated NETs express SSTRs on their surface, most commonly subtype 2, and are avid on functional imaging (OctreoScan or gallium-68 Dotatate PET/CT). Somatostatin analogs (SSAs; octreotide and lanreotide) are typically considered for first-line treatment of advanced and progressive SSTR-avid PNETs and can also be used to moderate symptoms in a number of functional PNETs.[20,54,132–134] SSAs mediate antiproliferative activity by binding primarily to SSTR2, SSTR5, and SSTR3, which eventually stimulate cell-cycle arrest and inhibition of mitosis.[135] This class of drugs is well tolerated, with the most common side effects being flatulence, diarrhea or steatorrhea, nausea, cholelithiasis, and glucose intolerance.[49,136]

A role for SSAs in cytostatic control was demonstrated in the PROMID and CLARINET studies. In the PROMID study, 85 patients with well-differentiated, functioning and nonfunctioning, metastatic midgut NETs were randomly assigned, 42 to receive octreotide long-acting-release (LAR) and 43 to receive placebo intramuscularly monthly with a primary endpoint of progression-free survival (PFS).[137] At 6 months, 66.7% of octreotide recipients and 37.2% of placebo recipients had stable disease with a significant difference in median time to tumor progression (14.3 and 6 months respectively, $P < .001$). In the CLARINET study, a similar benefit of prolonged PFS was demonstrated with use of the SSA lanreotide.[138] In CLARINET, 204 patients with advanced, well- or moderately differentiated, nonfunctioning, low- or intermediate-grade NETs were randomly assigned, 101 receiving lanreotide and 103 receiving placebo monthly. At 24 months, 65.1% of lanreotide recipients and 33% of placebo recipients were estimated to be progression free (median PFS not reached vs. 18 months, $P < .001$).

The findings from PROMID and CLARINET illustrated the clinically relevant antiproliferative effects of SSAs in patients with NETs. The National Comprehensive Cancer Network (NCCN) guidelines recommend use of either octreotide LAR or lanreotide in the first-line for relief of symptoms (in the setting of hormone release) as well as for tumor control in patients with SSTR avid NETs.[139,140]

Targeted Therapies

The targeted therapies sunitinib and everolimus have both demonstrated activity and are approved for the treatment of advanced PNETs. Because of the highly vascular nature of PNETs, inhibition of angiogenesis is a favorable target. Everolimus is an mTOR inhibitor, and sunitinib is a multitargeted receptor tyrosine kinase inhibitor that blocks vascular endothelial growth factor (VEGF), platelet-derived growth factor (PDGFR), and c-KIT.

Everolimus

The mTOR pathway regulates cell survival, proliferation, and metabolism; several genes in the pathway are important in the development of familial syndromes (NF1, TS).[141] The efficacy of everolimus and its Food and Drug Administration (FDA) approval for use in treating PNETs was established through RADIANT-3.[142] In RADIANT-3, 410 patients with advanced and progressive PNETs were randomly assigned, with 207 patients receiving everolimus and 203 patients receiving placebo daily in conjunction with best supportive care. In this study, treatment with everolimus was associated with an improved median PFS by 6.4 months (11 months vs. 4.6 months) and increased response rate (5% vs. 2%) when compared with placebo. Everolimus was well tolerated, and most adverse events were grade 1 or 2 (stomatitis, rash, diarrhea, fatigue, upper respiratory infections). In a later survival analysis, patients who were randomly assigned to receive everolimus had a median OS of 44 months, the longest OS reported in a phase III study for this population.[143] Crossover from placebo to open-label everolimus was allowed at disease progression and 172 patients (85%) initially randomized to receive placebo did crossover to receive everolimus, with a 37.7 month OS reported for the placebo cohort.

It is also important to note that everolimus can be effective in treating insulinomas because one of the drug's known side effects is induction of glucose intolerance, which may eliminate the symptoms of hypoglycemia in some patients.[20,144] A phase II study investigated the synergistic effects of everolimus and octreotide in a group of 50 NET patients, 14 of whom had PNETs. Of the PNETs, 14% had a partial response, and none had a complete response. Although the response rates were relatively poor, the clinical benefit rate for this regimen was 92%, which is better than many other drug combinations.[145]

Sunitinib

Sunitinib is an effective therapy for PNETs. The efficacy of sunitinib for advanced PNETs was demonstrated in a randomized, multinational, phase III study, where 171 patients with advanced and well-differentiated PNETs were randomized to receive best supportive care with the addition of daily sunitinib or placebo.[146] The study was stopped early because serious adverse events and deaths were observed in the placebo group and the PFS favored sunitinib (median PFS 11.4 months in the sunitinib arm vs. 5.5 months in the placebo arm). A notable difference in objective overall response was also seen (9.3% in the sunitinib arm and 0% in the placebo arm). The findings from this study led to the FDA approval of sunitinib in PNETs. In a later survival analysis, a five-year overall survival (OS) difference of 9.5 months was confirmed for the sunitinib arm versus the placebo arm.[147]

Cytotoxic Chemotherapy

Chemotherapy is typically reserved for treatment in PNET patients who have high-grade disease, heavy tumor burden, and/or an aggressive clinical course. The role for chemotherapy in PNET treatment has been examined in several single and combination-drug studies, and while evidence for a survival benefit is conflicting, the results demonstrate symptomatic and cytostatic benefits. Previously investigated and commonly used chemotherapy agents include alkylating agents and platinum drugs.

Alkylating Agents

Alkylating agents that have been investigated for PNET treatment include streptozocin, dacarbazine, and temozolomide. The earliest evidence for use of alkylating drugs in PNETs comes from a case series describing patients with insulinoma who were treated with streptozocin and saw relief in hormonal symptoms and cytostatic control.[148] A randomized study from the Eastern Cooperative Oncology Group (ECOG) later demonstrated activity with streptozocin; however, in the ECOG study, streptozocin therapy was associated with symptoms (nausea and vomiting) compromising quality of life and treatment compliance.[149] Follow-up retrospective efforts demonstrated mixed findings with regards to a role for treatment with streptozocin.[150,151]

Dacarbazine was first studied in carcinoid tumors, where tumor shrinkage and improvement in quality of life were noted.[152,153] A role for the use of dacarbazine in the treatment of PNETs came from the phase II ECOG study (E6282), which included 50 patients with advanced PNETs. The observed response rate was 34%, with the majority of responses occurring in chemonaïve patients; median OS was 19.3 months. Notable lethal toxicities were observed, including septic shock and myocardial infractions, as well as multiple grade 4 hematologic adverse events. Given the potential adverse events, widespread use of dacarbazine has been limited.[154]

Temozolomide was investigated as a therapy for PNETs in an effort to identify a less toxic alternative to dacarbazine.[155] Notable phase II data demonstrated a role for both single-agent temozolomide, as well as temozolomide in combination with capecitabine (CAPETEM), for advanced PNET treatment.[156–160] The most notable toxicity with temozolomide is myelosuppression, and blood counts must be carefully monitored during treatment with this drug.

The question regarding the benefit of single versus combination temozolomide therapy was addressed in the prospective ECOG E2211 study.[161] In ECOG E2211, 144 PNET patients with advanced low or intermediate grade progressive disease were enrolled onto a two-arm, phase II trial, and were randomized to receive temozolomide alone or CAPETEM. The median PFS in the temozolomide and CAPETEM arms were 14.4 and 22.7 months, respectively. The median OS in the temozolomide arm was 38 months. Although data review is ongoing and the OS for the CAPETEM arm has not been reached, there was an association noted between CAPETEM and an improved PFS and OS compared with temozolomide alone.

Platinum Agents

Chemotherapy regimens incorporating cisplatin and carboplatin have been investigated as a treatment options for PNETs; however, the benefit may be limited largely to those patients with higher grade tumors.[162,163] In the largest retrospective study, 305 patients with advanced GI NENs were included. The study concluded that tumors with Ki-67 less than 55% were less responsive to platinum-based chemotherapy; however, importantly, patients with tumors of Ki-67 less than 55% did still experience longer survival, highlighting the varying biology within the high-grade cohort of NENs.[27]

Oxaliplatin-based regimens have also been investigated. Two prospective phase II studies suggested antitumor activity in previously progressing NETs based on radiographic responses and prolonged disease stability.[164] The first study evaluated treatment with oxaliplatin, leucovorin, and 5-flurouracil (FOLFOX) plus bevacizumab in progressing and advanced carcinoid, PNETs, and poorly differentiated NECs; after 12 treatment cycles, in the 12 PNET patients eligible for response assessment, response rate was 41.7% (5/12) and median PFS was 21 months. The second study evaluated 40 advanced NET patients treated with oxaliplatin and capecitabine plus bevacizumab for four cycles with the option to continue bevacizumab plus or minus capecitabine thereafter; response rate was 18% and median PFS was 16.7 months.

PNECs are most commonly treated with a platinum drug (cisplatin or carboplatin) and etoposide because these tumors are histologically like small-cell lung cancers. Response rates vary from 42% to 67%, and median survival hovers just at more than 1 year.[165,166] Newer drug combinations have been suggested, but response rates do not exceed those obtained with platinum and etoposide.[145]

Peptide Receptor Radionuclide Therapy

Peptide receptor radionuclide therapy (PRRT) targets and treats NETs with radiolabeled SSAs. In PRRT, a SSA is linked to a therapeutic beta-emitting radioisotope via a chelator allowing for the systemic delivery of targeted radiation to tumors.[167] When the radiolabeled SSA binds to the surface of the tumor, targeted radiation is emitted, killing the tumor cells as well as neighboring cells.[168] Given the mechanism of action, it is well recognized that SSTR expression on functional imaging is an important predictor of response to PRRT.[169,170]

The first-generation radionuclide investigated for use in PRRT was a gamma-emitting ^{111}Indium, which had short particle ranges and weak therapeutic (cytotoxic) effects.[171] The next-generation radionuclides investigated were beta-emitting ^{90}Yttrium (^{90}Y) and ^{177}Lutetium (^{177}Lu), which increased the particle ranges, killing neighboring tumor cells and improving cytotoxicity.[172]

A role for PRRT in the treatment of advanced PNETs has been demonstrated in several studies, and the most notable toxicities of PRRT include myelosuppression and nephrotoxicity.[173] Most efforts have used ^{177}Lu-based radiolabeled SSAs, with results showing a benefit in reduction of tumor size, survival, and quality of life.[172,174] In a large study, 504 advanced NETs treated with four cycles of ^{177}Lu-DOTATATE at 6- to 10-week intervals, showed a median OS of 46 months (128 months from diagnosis) from the start of treatment, with an increased survival benefit of 40 to 72 months from time of diagnosis when compared with historical controls.[175] In the largest retrospective effort, the outcomes of more than 1200 patients treated at Erasmus Medical Center who received ^{177}Lu-DOTATATE infusion for four treatments at 8-week intervals were reviewed.[176] In this cohort, an objective response rate of 39% was observed with 43% of patients achieving stable disease and PFS and OS were 29 months and 63 months, respectively. Long-term toxicities were primarily hematologic and included acute leukemia in 4 patients (0.7%) and myelodysplastic syndrome in 9 patients (1.5%).

The NETTER-1 trial was the first prospective, randomized trial of PRRT.[177] In NETTER-1, 229 patients with progressive, well-differentiated metastatic midgut NETs were randomized to receive either ^{177}Lu-DOTATATE plus octreotide LAR or octreotide LAR alone. At analysis, the PFS at 20 months were 65.2% in the ^{177}Lu-DOTATATE group versus 10.8% in the control group, and the observed overall response rate was 18% in the ^{177}Lu-DOTATATE group versus 3% in the control group. Fourteen deaths were observed in the ^{177}Lu-DOTATATE group versus 26 deaths in the control group. The grade 3/4 toxicities observed in the ^{177}Lu-DOTATATE group included neutropenia (1%), thrombocytopenia (2%), and lymphopenia (9%). ^{177}Lu-DOTATATE was FDA approved for the treatment of advanced gastroenteropancreatic NETs in 2018 because of the data reported from Erasmus Medical Center study and the NETTER-1 trial.[176,177]

SURVEILLANCE AND FOLLOW-UP

The National Comprehensive Cancer Network has guidelines outlining the surveillance and follow-up of PNETs. If a patient has been resected, biochemical markers and a contrast-enhanced CT or MRI can be obtained at least once in the 3 to 12 months after surgery, as clinically indicated. Thereafter, if the patient does not recur, they should be followed every 6 to 12 months for 10 years with an examination, as well as biochemical markers and cross-sectional imaging as clinically indicated. The exception to this would be in the case of a benign insulinoma, which may only need to be followed for 1 to 2 years unless the patient had multiple lesions or has MEN1.

If the patient experiences a recurrence, has G3 disease, or has locoregional or distant unresectable disease, follow-up will be determined by the patient's clinical condition and the behavior of the tumor. An asymptomatic patient with a low tumor burden can be followed every 3 to 12 months with clinical examination and imaging. Onset of new symptoms or evidence of disease progression should prompt more frequent follow-up.

The references for this chapter can be found online by accessing the accompanying Expert Consult website.

CHAPTER 66

Chemotherapy and radiotherapy for pancreatic cancer: Adjuvant, neoadjuvant, and palliative

Fiyinfolu Balogun, Naveen Premnath, and Eileen M. O'Reilly

ADJUVANT CHEMORADIOTHERAPY

Early studies examining the role of external beam radiotherapy (EBRT) combined with 5-fluorouracil (5-FU) as a radio-sensitizing agent in advanced, unresectable, pancreatic adenocarcinoma identified increased median survival over radiotherapy alone.[1,2] One study published in 1979 by the Gastrointestinal Tumour Study Group (GITSG) demonstrated a survival benefit with radiotherapy and concurrent chemotherapy. In this trial, 43 patients were randomized, following potentially curative pancreatic resection, to either chemoradiotherapy (40 Gy EBRT, concurrent with 5-FU and subsequent 5-FU for up to 2 years) or no adjuvant treatment. Median, 2-year, and 5-year survival rates were all increased in the treatment group (Table 66.1). However, recruitment was slow, and the trial enrolled only 43 patients after 8 years instead of the intended 150.[3] Furthermore, this trial suffered from poor compliance and quality assurance because only 9% of patients completed the intended 2 years of therapy, and 32% had violations of the intended radiation therapy. An additional 30 patients were entered into a treatment group, without randomization (see Table 66.1).[4] Several subsequent studies showed similar advantages,[5,6] although they were nonrandomized studies and included small numbers of patients.

Later, Klinkenbijl and colleagues,[7] on behalf of the European Organization for Research and Treatment of Cancer (EORTC), randomized 218 patients after curative resection for pancreatic cancer to chemoradiotherapy (40 Gy EBRT with concurrent 5-FU) or no adjuvant treatment.[8] This phase III trial enrolled 114 patients with pancreatic cancer and 92 with periampullary cancer. Patients with pancreatic cancer experienced a nonstatistically significant trend towards survival benefit in the treatment group; with median survival of 1 year (95% confidence interval [CI], 0.8–1.4) and 1.3 years (95% CI, 1.1–1.8) in the observation and treatment groups respectively ($P =$ .099). A similar trend had also been noted in the overall study population (see Table 66.1). About 20% of patients randomized to the chemoradiotherapy arm did not receive the intended treatment, raising the question of whether the benefit would have been significant if the study was adequately powered.

These early studies set the stage for the European Study Group for Pancreatic Cancer (ESPAC) to conduct a randomized controlled trial (RCT) of adjuvant chemotherapy and chemoradiotherapy for patients who had undergone resection of pancreatic cancer. In the ESPAC-1 trial, about half of the patients were randomized to chemotherapy (bolus 5-FU for 6 months) versus no chemotherapy and chemoradiotherapy (20 Gy concurrent with 5-FU) versus no chemoradiotherapy. A novel two-by-two (2 × 2) factorial design was utilized for the other half of patients, whereby they were randomized to chemoradiotherapy, chemotherapy, both, and observation. A total of 541 patients were enrolled from 61 centers in 11 countries, making it the largest adjuvant therapy trial in pancreatic cancer at the time. A total of 289 patients were randomized into the 2 × 2 factorial design, whereas 256 patients were randomized to either chemotherapy or chemoradiation versus observation outside the original design (ESPAC-1 plus). Results from the overall study failed to demonstrate a survival benefit for chemoradiotherapy over observation but revealed a statistically significant survival benefit for chemotherapy.[9] These findings were maintained when data from only the 2 × 2 factorial design study was evaluated.[10]

ESPAC-1 has been criticized for the 2 × 2 trial design. Variation in the amount of radiotherapy received and lack of adjuvant chemotherapy in the radiation arm raised doubts about the observed lack of benefit to radiotherapy. Nonetheless, data from both patient sets are relevant[10] and indicate the benefit of chemotherapy (Table 66.2), evident in both resection margin–positive (R1) and resection margin–negative (R0) patients. The 2 × 2 factorial design was used to answer the two most important questions for intervention: (1) Is there a benefit for adjuvant chemoradiotherapy? and (2) Is there a benefit for adjuvant chemotherapy? Meta-analyses have confirmed this survival advantage of adjuvant chemotherapy, with a reduced risk of death in pancreatic cancer patients after resection of 25% (95% CI, 0.64–0.90; $P =$ .001; see Chapter 62).[11] This benefit is more pronounced in patients with an R0 margin compared with those with an R1 margin.[12] In addition, the reported survival advantage for adjuvant chemotherapy was maintained when adjusted for quality of life during the 24 months after resection.[13] Overall, these studies suggested that chemotherapy, as opposed to radiotherapy, in the adjuvant treatment of resected pancreatic cancer provides significant survival impact.

To evaluate the potential role of gemcitabine in conjunction with adjuvant chemoradiotherapy, the Radiation Therapy Oncology Group (RTOG) 9704 trial compared gemcitabine versus 5-FU administered before and after 5-FU–based chemoradiotherapy.[14] Chemotherapy was given for 3 weeks before and 10 to 12 weeks after chemoradiotherapy (50.4 Gy EBRT concurrent with infusional 5-FU). Four hundred and fifty-one patients were stratified by tumor size, nodal involvement, and resection margin status. Median survival was not improved in the gemcitabine arm (20.5 months) compared with the 5-FU arm (16.9 months; hazard ratio [HR] = 0.84; 95% CI, 0.67–1.05; $P =$ .12; Table 66.3). Analysis of the 5-year data of RTOG 9704 demonstrated no changes to the original inferences drawn.[15]

ESPAC-1 reported a survival benefit for adjuvant chemotherapy, without exploring the question of whether chemoradiotherapy could improve on that benefit. The EORTC 40013/ FFCD/GERCOR Phase II trial randomized 90 patients to

TABLE 66.1 Early Studies Examining Adjuvant Chemoradiotherapy in Pancreatic Cancer

STUDY		NO. OF PATIENTS	REGIMEN	SURVIVAL			
				MEDIAN (mo)	2 YEAR (%)	3 YEAR (%)	5 YEAR (%)
GITSG-9173 (1985)[3]		21	60 Gy EBRT 5-FU Follow-on 5-FU	20	42	—	18[a]
		22	Surgery, observation	11	15	—	0[a]
GITSG (1987)[4]		30	60 Gy EBRT 5-FU Follow-on 5-FU	18	46	—	—
EORTC[7,8]	PDAC RR 0.7 (0.5–1.1) P = .099	60	40 Gy EBRT 5-FU	17.1	37	—	20
		54	Surgery, observation	12.6	23	—	10
	Periampullary RR 0.9 (0.5–1.6) P = .737	44	40 Gy EBRT 5-FU	39.5	70	—-	38
		49	Surgery, observation	40.1	64	—	36

[a]Estimated.

EBRT, External beam radiotherapy; *EORTC*, European Organization for Research and Treatment of Cancer; *5-FU*, 5-fluorouracil; *GITSG*, Gastrointestinal Tumour Study Group; *PDAC*, pancreatic ductal adenocarcinoma; *RR*, relative risk.

TABLE 66.2 European Study Group for Pancreatic Cancer (ESPAC-1) Data[10]

STUDY	MODALITY	MEDIAN SURVIVAL (mo)	2-YEAR SURVIVAL (%)	5-YEAR SURVIVAL (%)
ESPAC-1 2 × 2 chemoradiotherapy analysis	Chemoradiotherapy	15.9	28.5	10
	No chemoradiotherapy	17.9	41.4	19.6 (P = .053)
ESPAC-1 2 × 2 chemotherapy analysis	Chemotherapy	20.1	39.7	21.1
	No chemotherapy	15.5	30	8.4 (P = .009)
ESPAC-1 2 x 2 factorial design	Observation	16.9	38.7	10.7
	Chemoradiotherapy	13.9	21.7	7.3
	Chemotherapy	21.6	44	29 (P = .0005)
	Chemoradiotherapy + follow-on chemotherapy	19.9	35	13.2

TABLE 66.3 Key Studies Examining Effect of Gemcitabine-Based Chemoradiation in Pancreatic Cancer

STUDY	PATIENT NO.	REGIMEN	MEDIAN SURVIVAL (mo)	2-YEAR SURVIVAL (%)	3-YEAR SURVIVAL (%)
EORTC-40013[16]	45	4 cycles of Gem	24.4	50.2	—
	45	2 cycles of Gem + Gem and 50.5 Gy EBRT	24.3	50.6	—
RTOG-9704[14] (Head of pancreas only, eligible = 388)	187	Gem pre-CRT, 50.4 Gy EBRT + 5-FU, Gem post-CRT	20.5[a]	—	31
	(201)	5-FU pre-CRT, 50.4 Gy EBRT + 5-FU, 5-FU post-CRT	16.9	—	22

[a]Hazard ratio, 0.82; confidence interval, 0.65–1.03; P = .09.

CRT, Chemoradiotherapy; *EBRT*, external beam radiotherapy; *EORTC*, European Organization for Research and Treatment of Cancer; *5-FU*, 5-fluorouracil; *Gem*, gemcitabine; *RTOG*, Radiation Therapy Oncology Group.

receive chemotherapy alone with four cycles of gemcitabine, or chemoradiotherapy with two courses of gemcitabine followed by 50.4 Gy EBRT concurrent with weekly gemcitabine for 5 to 6 weeks.[16] This trial included only R0 resection patients, who received gemcitabine-based chemoradiotherapy after systemic chemotherapy. Toxicity was the primary endpoint and was comparable in both arms. There were no differences between the two groups for the secondary endpoints of overall survival (24 months in both arms; see Table 66.3) and disease-free survival (12 months in chemoradiotherapy arm and 11 months in chemotherapy-alone arm). Local relapse rates were lower in the chemoradiotherapy arm (11% vs. 24%), although there was no difference in distant metastases rates (42% vs. 40%). This study suggested that chemoradiotherapy added to chemotherapy can reduce the incidence of local recurrence even though it does not demonstrate an overall survival benefit. Use of a more intense chemotherapy regimen before chemoradiotherapy did not increase survival as observed in a Phase II RCT that compared 3 months of induction chemotherapy using cisplatin, epirubicin, 5-FU, and gemcitabine (PEFG) versus gemcitabine. Chemotherapy was followed by chemoradiotherapy (54–60 Gy RT, concurrent with infusional 5-FU).[17]

A systematic review and network meta-analysis identified nine high-quality studies with 3033 total patients who had been randomized to one of six treatment arms including chemotherapy and/or chemoradiotherapy.[18] The analysis demonstrated that adjuvant chemotherapy with either 5-FU or gemcitabine reduces mortality by at least one-third in patients with resected pancreatic adenocarcinoma. It was unclear whether chemoradiation plus chemotherapy is more effective than chemotherapy alone in prolonging survival; however, the addition of radiotherapy added toxicity. Nonetheless, in many parts of North America, the use of adjuvant chemoradiation continues, in contrast to Europe and Asia, where adjuvant chemotherapy is considered the standard of care.[19] Guidelines in North America favor adjuvant chemotherapy, while making allowance for the addition of chemoradiotherapy, particularly for settings with high risk of recurrence (such as positive resection margins). Interferon-based adjuvant protocols have evaluated and demonstrated no improvement in survival and with significant toxicity.[20–23]

Ongoing Trials Evaluating Perioperative Chemoradiotherapy

The joint NRG (National Radiation Group)/RTOG-0848 Phase III trial (NCT01013649) commenced recruitment in 2009 aiming to randomize 950 patients with resected pancreatic head cancer to adjuvant gemcitabine or gemcitabine and erlotinib. After five cycles of gemcitabine, patients with no disease progression were then randomized to concurrent fluoropyrimidine and radiotherapy or to continue with adjuvant gemcitabine-based chemotherapy. Results of the erlotinib randomization have been reported.[24] Specifically, 163 were randomized to gemcitabine and 159 to gemcitabine and erlotinib. At a median follow-up of 42.5 months for surviving patients, the median OS was 29.9 months (95% CI, 21.7–33.4) for gemcitabine and 28.1 months (95% CI, 20.7–30.9; HR 1.04, $P = .062$) for gemcitabine and erlotinib. The overall study design was modified to include gemcitabine-based combinations (stratifying for single agent vs. combination) and aiming to address the radiation question and has completed recruitment with final results for the randomization of radiation anticipated in 2022.

ADJUVANT CHEMOTHERAPY

The ESPAC-1 trial provided the first evidence that survival benefit can be derived from adjuvant chemotherapy (see Table 66.2), when based on regimens of biomodulated 5-FU. The benefit of chemotherapy was evident in both R1 and R0 resections. As noted previously, two meta-analyses confirmed a reduced mortality risk of 25% (95% CI, 0.64–0.90; $P = .001$)[11] and an advantage of adjuvant chemotherapy in R0 margin versus R1 margin patients.[12] The reported survival advantage for adjuvant chemotherapy was maintained when adjusted for quality of life during the 24-month period after resection.[13] The advance made by ESPAC-1 has driven the next generation of adjuvant chemotherapy trials,[25] notably ESPAC-3 (version 2) and ESPAC-4, as well as translational runoffs.

Emerging evidence in the 1990s demonstrated the value of gemcitabine for treatment of pancreas cancer, initially in the setting of advanced disease.[20,26] The CONKO-001 multicenter Phase III RCT demonstrated improved median disease-free survival (DFS) with adjuvant gemcitabine (13.4 months; 95% CI, 11.4–15.3) compared with observation (6.9 months; 95% CI, 6.1–7.8; $P < .001$; Table 66.4).[27] The estimated DFS at 3 years and 5 years was 23.5% and 16.5%, respectively, in the gemcitabine group versus 7.5% and 5.5% in the observation group. There was, however, no significant improvement in median overall survival (OS) with gemcitabine (22.1 months; 95% CI, 18.4–25.8), compared with observation alone (20.2 months; 95% CI, 17–23.4; $P = .06$). Estimated OS at 3 years and

TABLE 66.4 Key Gemcitabine-Based Single-Agent Adjuvant Chemotherapy for Pancreatic Cancer

STUDY	PATIENT NO.	REGIMEN	SURVIVAL OVERALL MEDIAN (mo)	1 YEAR (%)	2 YEAR (%)	3 YEAR (%)	5 YEAR (%)
CONKO-001[27]	179	Gemcitabine	22.1	72.5	47.5	34	22.5
	175	Surgery, observation	20.2	72.5	42	20.5	11.5
Yoshitomi et al[29]	50	Gemcitabine	29.8	85.7	—	46.9	—
	50	Gemcitabine + uracil/tegafur	21.2 ($P = .28$)	80	—	30.4	—
JSAP-02[30]	58	Gemcitabine	22.3	77.6	48.5	—	23.9
	60	Surgery alone	18.4[a]	75	40	—	10.6
ESPAC-3[31]	537	Gemcitabine	23.6 ($P = .39$)	80.1	49.1	—	—
	551	5-FU/FA	23	78.5	48.1	—	—
JASPAC-01[33]	190	Gemcitabine	25.5	—	—	38.8	24.2
	187	S-1	46.5 (HR 0.57[†])	—	—	59.7[b]	44.1[b]

[a]Hazard ratio, 0.77; confidence interval, 0.51–1.14; $P = .19$
[b]$P < .0001$ vs. gemcitabine. Per protocol.
5-FU, 5-Fluorouracil; *FA*, folinic acid.

5 years was 34% and 22.5%, respectively, for gemcitabine patients versus 20.5% and 11.5% for observation patients. Subsequent analyses of the 5- and 10-year data[28] continued to demonstrate significantly improved median OS: 20.7% and 12.2%, respectively, in the gemcitabine arm versus 10.4% and 7.7% in the observation arm. Two smaller studies provided similar survival estimates for gemcitabine, with a survival benefit over observation that was not further improved by the addition of fluoropyrimidines (see Table 66.4).[29,30]

As previously illustrated, CONKO-001 showed that gemcitabine improved survival compared with observation in resected pancreatic cancer patients, and Yoshitomi et al. found that the addition of fluoropyrimidine to gemcitabine did not improve on survival. It remained unclear, however, whether gemcitabine was superior to 5-FU for adjuvant treatment of patients with resected pancreatic cancer. The ESPAC-3 trial set out to answer this question. This study recruited 1088 patients with pancreatic ductal adenocarcinoma and reported no difference in OS between 5-FU/leucovorin (LV; also known as folinic acid [FA]) and gemcitabine by treatment ($P = .39$), treatment effect by resection status ($P = .56$), or by progression-free survival ($P = .44$). There were, however, key advantages to the use of gemcitabine, such as its significantly reduced side effect and toxicity profile[31] (see Table 66.4). Evaluating ESPAC-3 to determine the optimal duration and time to initiate chemotherapy, Valle and colleagues[32] concluded that completion of all six cycles of adjuvant chemotherapy was an independent prognostic factor after resection for pancreatic adenocarcinoma. No survival disadvantage was seen by delaying chemotherapy initiation for up to 12 weeks after resection. Interestingly, within the sub-group that completed less than 6 months of chemotherapy, those that started chemotherapy after 8 weeks fared better than those that started before 8 weeks after resection. These sub-analyses suggest a benefit to delaying chemotherapy for up to 12 weeks to allow for adequate postoperative recovery. Caution should be taken, however, in the interpretation of data obtained from subgroup analyses that were not pre-specified, as in this case.

The JASPAC-01 phase III multi-institutional trial randomized 385 patients in Japan to receive either gemcitabine or S-1, an orally active fluoropyrimidine. S-1 contains a prodrug of 5-FU (tegafur) along with two other agents designed to minimize gastrointestinal and systemic toxicity (gimeracil and oteracil), effectively increasing the tolerable tumor dose of 5-FU.[33] In advanced pancreatic cancer, S-1 has been shown to be noninferior to gemcitabine,[34,35] so this study set out to evaluate noninferiority in the adjuvant setting. After the interim analysis for efficacy, the study was stopped early in accordance with the prespecified criteria for discontinuation. At the time of stoppage, all protocol treatments had been completed and the data analysis reported 5-year OS of 44.1% and 24.4% in the S-1 and gemcitabine groups, respectively. Median OS was observed to be 46.5 and 25.5 months, respectively, in the per protocol analysis (see Table 66.4). From these results, S-1 was determined to be noninferior to gemcitabine in Japanese patients. Because S-1 is not approved in the West, it is uncertain how generalizable these findings are outside of Japan.

Several studies have attempted to explore the potential benefit of multi-agent fluoropyrimidine-based chemotherapy in the adjuvant setting. Bakkevold and colleagues[36] randomized patients who had undergone pancreatic resection (61 with radical pancreatic resection, including 14 patients with periampullary cancers) to 5-FU, doxorubicin (Adriamycin), and mitomycin C (FAM) or observation. Although there was a significant increase in median survival of 23 months versus 11 months ($P = .02$) favoring the FAM-treated group, there was no improvement in 3-year or 5-year survival. Increased toxicity was also noted, and only 56% of the FAM treatment group was able to complete the six courses of chemotherapy (Table 66.5). In another study, Takada, and colleagues[37] enrolled 508 patients with mixed pancreaticobiliary cancers ($n = 158$ pancreatic cancer) who were randomized to surgery alone or surgery with combined mitomycin C and 5-FU. The 5-year survival rates were not significantly different, at 18% versus 11.5%, respectively. Of note, this study used oral 5-FU, which has lower bioavailability compared with intravenous administration because of the phenomenon of

TABLE 66.5	Comparison of Main Studies Using Combination Chemotherapy for Resected Pancreatic Cancer						
STUDY	PATIENT NO.	REGIMEN	MEDIAN SURVIVAL (mo)	2-YEAR SURVIVAL (%)	3-YEAR SURVIVAL (%)	5-YEAR SURVIVAL (%)
Bakkevold et al.[36]	30	5-FU Doxorubicin Mitomycin C	23 ($P = .02$)	70	27	4
	31	Observation	11	45	30	8
Takada et al.[37]	81	5-FU Mitomycin C	—	—	—	11.5
	77	Observation	—	—	—	18
Kosuge et al.[38]	45	5-FU Cisplatin	12.5	—	—	26.4
	44	Observation	15.8	—	—	14.9 ($P = .94$)
PRODIGE-24[45]	247	mFOLFIRINOX	54.4	—	63.4	—
	246	Gemcitabine	35.0	—	48.6	—
APACT[46]		Gemcitabine nab-paclitaxel	19.4[a]			
		Gemcitabine	18.8[a]			

[a]Disease-free survival.
5-FU, 5-Fluorouracil; *nab*, albumin-bound.

first-pass hepatic metabolism. Kosuge and colleagues[38] undertook a multicenter RCT of surgery versus surgery and combination cisplatin and 5-FU, with 60% of patients also receiving 30 Gy of intraoperative radiotherapy. They concluded that although cisplatin with 5-FU was safe and well tolerated, it conferred no survival benefit (see Table 66.5).

Gemcitabine combined with the orally active 5-FU prodrug capecitabine (GemCap) has produced a small improvement in survival compared with gemcitabine alone in the advanced disease setting.[39–42] Subsequently, GemCap was evaluated in the adjuvant setting in the ESPAC-4 trial. This study enrolled 732 patients who had undergone curative resection for pancreatic ductal adenocarcinoma and randomized them to gemcitabine ($n = 366$) or GemCap ($n = 364$).[43] The median OS was 28 months (95% CI, 23.5–31.5) in the GemCap group and 25.5 months (95% CI, 22.7–27.9) in the gemcitabine group, with an HR of 0.82 (95% CI, 0.68–0.98; $P = .032$). In an updated analysis, this benefit was maintained with a median OS of 30.2 months (95% CI, 25.8–33.5) and 27.9 months (95% CI, 24.8–29.9), respectively.[44] This study established GemCap as an option for adjuvant therapy, and it is now typically used for older patients and/or for patients with an ECOG performance status greater than 1.

More recently, the value of adjuvant-modified FOLFIRINOX (mFOLFIRINOX; 5-FU, oxaliplatin, leucovorin, irinotecan) has been established as the standard adjuvant recommendation for fit patients who have undergone curative surgery for pancreatic cancer based on the results of the PRODIGE (Parternariat de Recherche en Oncologie Digestive)/ACCORD (Action Concertées dans les Cancers Colorectaux et Digestifs) 24/CCTG (Canadian Clinical Trials Group) PA.6 trial.[45] In total, 493 patients were randomized to either adjuvant mFOLFIRINOX or adjuvant gemcitabine for 6 months. Specific eligibility included World Health Organization (WHO) performance status 0 to 1, CA19-9 less than 180 U/mL, and either an R0 or R1 resection. At a median follow-up of 33.6 months for surviving patients, the median DFS was 21.6 months in the mFOLFIRINOX group and 12.8 months in the gemcitabine group (HR 0.58; 95% CI, 0.46–0.73; $P < .001$). The median OS was notable at 54.4 months in the mFOLFIRINOX and 35.0 months in the gemcitabine group, respectively (HR 0.64; 95% CI 0.48–0.86; $P = .03$). There was a higher rate of grade 3 to 4 adverse events in the mFOLFIRINOX arm of 75.9%, and 52.9% in the gemcitabine group. These data immediately changed practice and support the recommendation for adjuvant mFOLFIRINOX for good performance status patients.

The APACT (Adjuvant PAnCreas Trial) results have been preliminarily reported and provide insight into the role of gemcitabine and nab-paclitaxel in the adjuvant setting.[46] This large adjuvant study randomized 866 patients to either gemcitabine and nab-paclitaxel or gemcitabine alone for six cycles. Eligibility criteria were like the adjuvant PRODIGE trial. The primary endpoint was DFS adjudicated by blinded independent central review. At a median follow-up of 38.5 months, the DFS for gemcitabine and nab-paclitaxel was 19.5 months versus 18.8 months for the gemcitabine group (HR 0.88; 95% CI 0.729–1.063; $P = .18$). The interim median OS was 40.5 months for the doublet and 36.2 months for the gemcitabine group (HR 0.82; 95% CI 0.68–0.99; $P = .045$). Mature OS data are awaited because the interim analysis did not show significant benefit with the doublet regimen. Currently, the use of gemcitabine and nab-paclitaxel in the adjuvant setting remains investigational.

Overall key factors that are moving the benchmark for adjuvant therapy for pancreatic cancer include improved patient selection (such as limiting by CA19-9 level), integration of optimal supportive therapy measures, and improvements in therapy.

Ongoing Trials Evaluating and Emerging Directions in Adjuvant Therapy

A preponderance of ongoing trials evaluating adjuvant systemic therapy in pancreatic cancer are attempting to recruit the immune system in the management of this disease. These are primarily in the form of vaccines and checkpoint blockade given after completion of standard adjuvant regimens with some examples described herein. A pilot nonrandomized study from Memorial Sloan Kettering Cancer Center (NCT04161755) combines a personalized RNA-based cancer vaccine, R07198457, with atezolizumab (PD-L1 antibody) and chemotherapy for the treatment of resected pancreatic cancer. The vaccine uses tumor antigens obtained from surgical resection of the tumor, thus making it unique to each individual patient's cancer. Other studies use vaccines derived from KRAS (Kirsten RAt Sarcoma) mutant peptides: a study from Johns Hopkins (NCT04117087) combines a KRAS-vaccine with dual checkpoint blockade (nivolumab, anti-PD-1; and ipilimumab, anti-CTLA4); another study from University of Pennsylvania (NCT03592888) administers a KRAS-vaccine after depletion of the patients' regulatory T-cells with cyclophosphamide. Another emerging direction in pancreatic cancer treatment is the incorporation of minimal residual disease (MRD) status in the decision to treat. One study that is currently underway is the AMPLIFY trial, where patients with KRAS mutated disease are treated with KRAS targeted immunotherapy if they have MRD detected via circulating tumor DNA testing. In addition to these studies that target the immune system, the APOLLO study (NCT04858334) is underway in resected pancreatic cancer. This is a Phase II RCT that investigates the benefit of a targeted drug in pancreatic cancer patients with a mutation in BRCA1, BRCA2, or PALB2. Additional details of this study are described later, in the section on targeted therapy. Other studies in resected pancreatic cancer focus on treatment in the neoadjuvant setting, the concepts of which will be discussed (Table 66.6).

NEOADJUVANT TREATMENT OF PANCREATIC CANCER

Neoadjuvant treatment is increasingly being incorporated into the management of localized pancreatic cancer. Even in patients that are deemed to have resectable disease, a large number have microscopically incomplete resections (R1) after surgery.[47] A mathematical and computational analysis of primary pancreatic tumors and associated metastases described pancreatic tumors growing in an exponential manner, and the authors predicted that patients are likely to have metastases at diagnosis.[48] The computational modeling suggested that targeting tumor cells while they are rapidly growing is crucial and that any delay in treatment may be detrimental. This provides a strong rationale for neoadjuvant therapy, which aims to increase the number of patients with resectable disease and to treat micrometastases not evident at staging.

Although neoadjuvant treatment for pancreatic cancer was proposed more than 30 years ago,[49,50] and despite the benefit demonstrated in some other tumor types, limited data from

TABLE 66.6 Summary Ongoing Trials for Systemic Therapy in Adjuvant and Neoadjuvant Pancreatic cancer

STUDY ID	TREATMENT	COMPARATOR	START DATE (PLANNED ACCRUAL)	ADJUVANT/ NEOADJUVANT
NCT04858334 (APOLLO)	• Olaparib (PARPi) • Chemotherapy	• Placebo • Chemotherapy	2021 (152 patients)	Adjuvant
NCT04161755	• RO7198457 (personalized neoantigen vaccine) • Atezolizumab • mFOLFIRINOX	N/A (Phase I)	2019 (20)	Adjuvant
NCT04117087	• KRAS vaccine • Nivolumab • Ipilimumab	N/A (Phase I)	2020 (30)	Adjuvant
NCT03592888	• mDC3/8-KRAS vaccine • Cyclophosphamide	N/A (Phase I)	2018 (12)	Adjuvant
NCT01088789	• Allogeneic pancreatic tumor cell vaccine • Cyclophosphamide	N/A (Phase II)	2010 (72)	Adjuvant
Netherlands Trial Register: NL7094 (PREOPANC-2)	• FOLFIRINOX (neoadjuvant)	• Gemcitabine/RT (neoadjuvant) • Gemcitabine (adjuvant)	2018 (368)	Neoadjuvant
NCT04340141 (A021806)	• FOLFIRINOX x 8c (neoadjuvant) • FOLFIRINOX x 4 (adjuvant)	• FOLFIRINOX x 12 (adjuvant)	2020 (344)	Neoadjuvant
NCT04536077	• CDX 1140 (ANTI-CD40) (Neoadjuvant)	• CDX 1140 • CDX 301 (RFLT3 ligand) (Neoadjuvant)	2021 (24)	Neoadjuvant
NCT04853017 (AMPLIFY)	• ELI-002 (mutant KRAS peptides + immune-stimulant) in MRD-positive	• N/A in Phase 1A/B • Observation in Phase 2	2021 (159)	Adjuvant

N/A, Not available.

phase III RCTs are available in this disease. Many prior neoadjuvant trials have suffered from poor recruitment, subsequently closing early,[51,52] and have grouped locally advanced with borderline resectable cancers.[53-55] In addition, debate is ongoing regarding the most appropriate patient groups to treat, the optimal regimen, and the definition of borderline disease.[56]

A phase II RCT attempted to investigate the role of neoadjuvant chemoradiation therapy with gemcitabine and cisplatin followed by surgery versus immediate surgery in resectable pancreatic cancer.[57] This study required 254 patients but was terminated early because of slow recruitment, with only 33 eligible patients in each arm. Tumor resection was performed in 23 versus 19 patients, respectively; the R0 resection rate was 48% versus 52%; the pN0 rate was 30% versus 39%; postoperative complications were comparable; and the median OS was 14.4 versus 17.4 months, respectively.

A large meta-analysis of neoadjuvant therapy has provided further insight. Gillen and colleagues[58] reviewed 111 studies (56 phase I/II), with a median patient number per study of 31 (interquartile range, 19–46), comparing treatment of resectable tumors (group 1) and nonresectable (borderline resectable/ unresectable) tumors (group 2). In patients that received neoadjuvant chemotherapy, 96.4% were treated with gemcitabine, fluoropyrimidines, mitomycin C, and platinum compounds. In the group that were treated with neoadjuvant radiotherapy, 93.7% of them received doses ranging from 24 to 63 Gy. In group 1, resectability was estimated at 73.6%, compared with 33.2% in group 2, who also had higher resection-associated morbidity and mortality rates. Combination chemotherapy resulted in higher estimated response and resection probabilities for patients initially staged as unresectable compared with monotherapy regimens. Overall, the median survival after resection was 23.3 months (range, 12–54) for group 1 and

20.5 months (range, 9–62) for group 2 patients. Therefore these data argue that there is no advantage to using neoadjuvant treatment in patients with resectable disease versus the current practice of resection and adjuvant therapy. Although it is recognized that apparent early-stage pancreatic cancer can metastasize frequently, current guidance indicates that neoadjuvant therapy in the setting of resectable disease is optimally evaluated in clinical trials or when poor prognostic factors are evident (elevated CA19-9, large primary tumors, large regional lymph nodes, equivocal extrapancreatic imaging lesions, excessive weight loss, extreme pain).[56,59,60]

However, in patients initially staged as locally advanced or unresectable, approximately 20% to 30% may be able to undergo resection after neoadjuvant treatment, with comparable survival rates relative to resectable cases. This meta-analysis highlighted the difference between the historical concepts of neoadjuvant treatment—to avoid surgery in patients who are poor responders because of aggressive tumor biology—and the modern thinking that neoadjuvant treatment may improve the survival of patients that respond.[58,61-64] The findings suggest a need for trials to focus on investigating the use of neoadjuvant therapy in patients that are initially staged as borderline/unresectable disease.

A crucial point in the evaluation of neoadjuvant therapy is the criteria for defining resectability (see Chapters 61 and 62). To arrive at a universally accepted terminology, a multi-institutional and multidisciplinary team of experts, including radiologists, gastroenterologists, and hepatobiliary surgeons, came together to formulate a consensus statement.[66] The definition of a resectable pancreatic cancer, according to preoperative reporting template, includes (1) no evidence of superior mesenteric vein (SMV) or portal vein (PV) distortion and (2) clear fat planes around the celiac axis (CA), hepatic artery (HA), and superior mesenteric artery (SMA).[65] Borderline resectable pancreatic cancer, according to this criteria, includes (1) venous involvement of SMV or PV with distortion or narrowing of the vein or occlusion of the vein, yet allowing for safe resection and replacement; (2) gastro-duodenal artery encasement up to the HA with either short-segment encasement or direct abutment of the HA, without extension to the CA; and (3) tumor abutment of the SMA with no greater than 180 degrees of the circumference of the vessel wall.[65] The definition of unresectable pancreatic cancer involved (1) unreconstructable SMV or PV vein occlusion, but the arterial involvement depends on tumor location: for pancreatic head tumor (2) more than 180 degree SMA encasement, any CA abutment, or IVC; and for pancreatic body/tail tumor (3), SMA or CA encasement greater than 180 degrees.[65]

Although most definitions overlap, there exist a few differences between the two main classifications originating from North America: the MD Anderson Classification[54] and the American Hepato-Pancreato-Biliary Association/Society of Surgical Oncology/Society for Surgery of the Alimentary Tract (AHPBA/SSO/SSAT) consensus guidelines,[66] which define potentially resectable, borderline resectable, and locally unresectable pancreatic cancer (Table 66.7). These classifications, combined with the radiology reporting template as reported by Al-Hawary et al., form the most recent National Comprehensive Cancer Network[67] guidelines (Table 66.8) and are also largely endorsed by the International Study Group for Pancreatic Surgery.[68]

A review of 129 patients with borderline disease from MD Anderson Cancer Center identified considerable discrepancies in the classification of potentially resectable, borderline resectable, and locally unresectable disease between the MD Anderson and AHPBA/SSO/SSAT systems.[69] Of 122 patients who had restaging after receipt of neoadjuvant therapy, 84 (69%) had stable disease, 15 (12%) had a partial response, and 23 (19%) had progressive disease using Response Evaluation Criteria in Solid Tumors (RECIST, version 1.1).[70] Although only one patient (0.8%) had radiographic downstaging, 85 patients (66%) underwent a pancreatectomy. The median survival for all 129 patients was 22 months and 33 months for the patients who underwent resection. The current consensus is that the RECIST criteria cannot be used to accurately determine tumor response and the efficacy of neoadjuvant therapy.

PREOPANC represents an important landmark study in that it was one of the first phase III RCTs of neoadjuvant versus adjuvant therapy to be reported in pancreatic cancer,[71] with an updated analysis presented after a median follow-up of 56 months.[72] This trial randomized 246 patients with both resectable and borderline resectable pancreatic cancer to either initial surgery and adjuvant gemcitabine ($n = 127$) or neoadjuvant gemcitabine, gemcitabine concurrent with radiation, and subsequent surgery followed by adjuvant gemcitabine ($n = 119$). The R0 resection rate was 72% versus 43% ($P < .001$) favoring the neoadjuvant group. The primary endpoint of median OS by intent to treat was 15.7 months for the neoadjuvant group and 14.3 months for the initial surgery group (HR 0.73; 95% CI 0.56–0.96; $P = .025$). In addition, neoadjuvant chemoradiotherapy was associated with improved disease-free survival, lower lymph node involvement at resection, and less neurovascular disease invasion. For the subset of patients who were able to undergo resection, the neoadjuvant group had improved survival compared with the initial surgery group at 33.7 months and 17.3 months, respectively (HR, 0.47; 95% CI, 0.32–0.67; $P = .029$). This study demonstrated that neoadjuvant chemoradiotherapy with gemcitabine and radiotherapy had several benefits over adjuvant gemcitabine alone, including improvement of long-term survival. As expected, this benefit was particularly pronounced in patients who were able to successfully undergo resection after neoadjuvant therapy.

Another RCT that investigated the benefit of neoadjuvant therapy is the Preop-02/JSAP-05 trial, which was conducted in Japan. This was a phase II/III study where patients with resectable or borderline resectable disease were randomized to 6 weeks of neoadjuvant chemotherapy (gemcitabine and S-1) or initial surgery. All patients who underwent resection went on to receive adjuvant S-1 chemotherapy for 24 weeks.[73] The median OS for the neoadjuvant group was 36.7 months, and it was 26.7 months for the surgery first group (HR 0.72; 95% CI, 0.55–0.94; $P = .015$). This study provides phase III evidence to support the role of neoadjuvant therapy in an Asian population.

A small single-institution study performed by the Massachusetts General Group investigated a total neoadjuvant treatment (TNT) strategy[74]. Forty-eight patients with borderline resectable pancreatic cancer received 8 cycles of FOLFIRINOX, after which those with no vascular involvement were

TABLE 66.7 AHPBA/SSO/SSAT and MD Anderson Definition of Resectability[a] in Pancreatic Cancer

	AHPBA/SSO/SSAT CLASSIFICATION			MD ANDERSON CLASSIFICATION		
LOCALIZATION	**POTENTIALLY RESECTABLE**	**BORDERLINE RESECTABLE**	**LOCALLY ADVANCED**	**POTENTIALLY RESECTABLE**	**BORDERLINE RESECTABLE**	**LOCALLY ADVANCED**
SMV/PV	No abutment or encasement	Abutment, encasement, or occlusion	Not constructible	Abutment or encasement without occlusion	Short-segment occlusion	Not constructible
SMA	No abutment or encasement	Abutment	Encasement	No abutment or encasement	Abutment	Encasement
CHA	No abutment or encasement	Abutment or short-segment encasement	Long-segment encasement	No abutment or encasement	Abutment or short-segment encasement	Long-segment encasement
Celiac trunk	No abutment or encasement	No abutment or encasement	Abutment	No abutment or encasement	Abutment	Encasement

[a]Abutment, <180 degrees of vascular circumference; encasement, ≥180 degrees of vascular circumference.
AHPBA/SSO/SSAT, American Hepato-Pancreato-Biliary Association/Society of Surgical Oncology/Society for Surgery of the Alimentary Tract; *CHA,* common hepatic artery; *PV,* portal vein; *SMA,* superior mesenteric artery; *SMV,* superior mesenteric vein.

TABLE 66.8	NCCN Pancreatic Adenocarcinoma Guidelines Version 2.2021, Criteria Defining Resectability Status at Diagnosis		
	RESECTABLE	**BORDERLINE RESECTABLE**	**LOCALLY ADVANCED**
Venous	No radiographic evidence of tumor contact with SMV or PV or ≤ 180 degree contact without vein distortion	Solid tumor contact with SMV or PV > 180 degrees, contact ≤ 180 degrees with distortion or thrombosis of the vein but with suitable vessel proximal and distal to allow for complete resection with vein reconstruction. Solid tumor contact with IVC	Unreconstructable SMV of PV because of tumor involvement or occlusion
Arterial, *Pancreatic head/uncinate process*	No arterial tumor contact involving CA, SMA, or CHA.	Solid tumor contact with CHA without extension to CA or hepatic artery bifurcation, allowing for complete resection and reconstruction. Solid tumor contact with SMA ≤ 180 degrees Solid tumor contact with variant arterial anatomy	Solid tumor contact with SMA > 180 degrees Solid tumor contact with CA > 180 degrees
Arterial, *Pancreatic body/tail*		Solid tumor contact with CA ≤ 180 degrees	Solid tumor contact > 180 degrees with SMA or CA
		Solid tumor contact with CA > 180 degrees without involvement of aorta and with intact and uninvolved GDA that permits modified Appleby procedure	Solid tumor contact with CA and aortic involvement

CA, Celiac axis; *CHA,* common hepatic artery; *GDA,* gastroduodenal artery; *IVC,* inferior vena cava; *PV,* portal vein; *SMA,* superior mesenteric artery; *SMV,* superior mesenteric vein.

treated with short course radiation while those with residual vascular involvement received standard 5.5 weeklong-course radiation. Radiotherapy was administered concurrently with capecitabine. The median progression-free survival (PFS) for the entire cohort was 14.7 months and the median OS was 37.7 months; 65% (32) of the patients were able to undergo surgery, with 97% undergoing an R0 resection. The median PFS in this group was 48.6 months and the median OS was not reached at the time of reporting. The survival rates in this study compare favorably to those seen in the adjuvant setting, particularly PRODIGE-24. This gives promise to the benefit of neoadjuvant therapy and calls for a large RCT to investigate further the role of neoadjuvant chemotherapy with or without radiotherapy.

In 2021 preliminary results of the A021501 study were reported.[75] This phase II trial RCT conducted in patients with borderline resectable pancreatic cancer evaluated two parallel arms of mFOLFIRINOX followed by hypofractionated radiation or mFOLFIRINOX alone; both followed by surgery. Both arms were compared with historical control and the trial was not designed to compare the arms directly. The primary endpoint was 18-month median OS. The radiation arm closed early because of lack of efficacy at a preplanned interim analysis. For the radiation arm, the 18-month median OS was 47.3% (95% CI 33.7–59.7) and for the chemotherapy-alone arm, it was 67.9% (95% CI, 54.6–78.0). The chemotherapy arm compared favorably to historical controls and met the predefined benchmark of relative efficacy (>50%). The conclusion from the study supports the use of neoadjuvant systemic therapy in borderline resectable pancreatic cancer.

The Southwest Oncology Group (SWOG) S1515 phase II RCT provided important insights into the perioperative use of mFOLFIRINOX and gemcitabine and nab-paclitaxel in resectable pancreatic cancer.[76] This study concluded that both regimens performed with similar efficacy. For the primary endpoint of 2-year OS, 47% (95% CI, 31%–61%) was observed in the mFOLFIRINOX arm and 48% (95% CI, 31%–63%) in the gemcitabine and nab-paclitaxel arm. The median OS was 23.2 months (95% CI, 17.6–45.9) and 23.6 months (95% CI, 17.8–31.7); median DFS after resection was 10.9 months for

mFOLFIRINOX and 14.2 months for gemcitabine and nab-paclitaxel, respectively. Although the design of this study did not allow for direct comparison between the FOLFIRINOX and gemcitabine and nab-paclitaxel arms, the latter arm performed better than expected, thus suggesting a larger than previously expected role for the gemcitabine and nab-paclitaxel regimen in a perioperative setting.

The ESPAC-5F phase II RCT is a small 4 arm study that compared three neoadjuvant regimens to upfront surgery followed by adjuvant GemCap in borderline resectable pancreatic cancer.[77] The three neoadjuvant arms included GemCap, FOLFIRINOX, or chemoradiation with capecitabine as a radiosensitizer. Ninety patients were enrolled with a resection rate of 62% for the upfront surgery group and 55% for the combined neoadjuvant arms (P = .668). The 1-year survival rate was 40% (95% CI 26%–62%) for the upfront surgery group and 77% (95% CI 66%–89%) for the neoadjuvant therapy, HR 0.27 (95% CI, 0.13–0.55; P < .001). The investigators concluded from this small RCT that there was a survival advantage to neoadjuvant therapy over upfront surgery.

Ongoing Trials Evaluating Neoadjuvant Therapy

The Dutch Pancreatic Cancer Group recently completed enrollment of the PREOPANC-2 trial (EudraCT Number: 2017-002036-17; Netherlands Trial Register: NL7094). This trial evaluates an all-neoadjuvant approach and randomized patients with either resectable or borderline resectable pancreatic cancer to neoadjuvant mFOLFIRINOX for 8 cycles followed by surgery or the successful regimen from the PREOPANC study of neoadjuvant gemcitabine followed by gemcitabine/radiation, subsequent surgery, and adjuvant gemcitabine. The Alliance cooperative group trial, A021806 (NCT04340141), is a phase III RCT that is planned to enroll 344 patients with resectable pancreatic cancer to either initial surgery and adjuvant mFOLFIRINOX or neoadjuvant mFOLFIRINOX for 8 cycles, followed by surgery and 4 additional cycles of adjuvant mFOLFIRINOX. This trial was activated in 2020 and is of relevance because it is currently the only North American RCT to address specifically the question of neoadjuvant versus adjuvant chemotherapy. Other smaller studies include the randomized phase II/III NEPAFOX study comparing neoadjuvant/adjuvant FOLFIRINOX with surgery and adjuvant gemcitabine.[78] This study was planned for 310 patients but stopped early due to slow accrual—40 patients after 3 years. The findings suggested an advantage for adjuvant gemcitabine over perioperative FOLFIRINOX; however, it was too underpowered to serve as more than descriptive.[79]

TREATMENT FOR UNRESECTABLE PANCREATIC CANCER

Unresectable pancreatic cancer encompasses locally advanced disease that is not amenable to surgical resection and disease with de novo metastases. RCTs have demonstrated that 5-FU and 5-FU–based regimens improve survival and quality of life when compared with best supportive care for patients with advanced disease.[42] Gemcitabine replaced 5-FU as a gold standard for palliative therapy in the late 1990s when a pivotal phase III trial demonstrated an improvement in several quality of life parameters (Clinical Benefit Response) and a modest improvement in median OS (Table 66.9).[26]

Over time, several studies have shown that multiagent chemotherapy can improve survival in pancreatic cancer patients. The GemCap trial compared gemcitabine with capecitabine to gemcitabine monotherapy in 553 patients with advanced pancreatic cancer. There was a significantly better objective response rate for the combination compared with gemcitabine alone at 19.1% versus 12.4%, respectively ($P = 0.034$) and improved progression-free survival (HR, 0.78; 95% CI, 0.66–0.93; $P = .004$).[39] There was also a trend toward improved OS favoring the GemCap group (HR, 0.86; 95% CI, 0.72–1.02; $P = .08$, see Table 66.9). This survival benefit was confirmed in meta-analysis (HR, 0.86; 95% CI, 0.75–0.98; $P = .020$),[39–42] thus making GemCap an accepted regimen in the treatment of advanced pancreatic cancer.[56] This benefit applied to both locally advanced and metastatic disease as was seen in the GemCap trial, 155 patients with locally advanced disease and 377 with metastatic disease had similar OS benefit by stage (see Table 66.9). A National Cancer Institute of Canada Clinical Trials Group-3 (CCTG3) study that compared gemcitabine-erlotinib to gemcitabine alone reported a survival benefit in the whole population, which included both locally advanced and metastatic disease[80] (reviewed in Table 66.9). This benefit was less pronounced in the locally advanced group, which was 138 of 569 the patients studied, likely because of being underpowered for subset analysis.

Additional studies have built on the benefit of multiagent therapy, leading to the current gold standard regimens for advanced pancreatic cancer. Both FOLFIRINOX from the PRODIGE-4/ACCORD-11 trial[81] and nab-paclitaxel with gemcitabine from the MPACT trial,[82] summarized in Table 66.9, are recommended in patients with metastatic disease with good performance and normal liver function tests. In the phase III PRODIGE-4 study, median OS in the FOLFIRINOX arm was 11.1 months compared with 6.8 months in the gemcitabine arm.[81] In MPACT, median OS in the gemcitabine/nab-paclitaxel arm was 8.5 months and 6.7 months in the gemcitabine monotherapy arm.[82] FOLFIRINOX has not been thoroughly compared head-to-head with gemcitabine and nab-paclitaxel in this setting, except in retrospective analyses. Of note, MPACT allowed for patients older than 75 years old and ECOG performance status 2, both of which were excluded from the PRODIGE study. European guidelines specifically recommend that FOLFIRINOX should be used in patients up to 75 years of age, with an ECOG performance status 0-1 and a level of bilirubin up to 1.5 upper limit of normal.[59] The JCOG1407 study was a phase II RCT that compared mFOLFIRINOX with gemcitabine and nab-paclitaxel in patients with locally advanced pancreatic cancer.[83] One hundred and twenty-six patients were enrolled from Japanese institutions with 62 randomized to FOLFIRINOX and 64 patients to gemcitabine and nab-paclitaxel. One-year OS was 77.4% (95% CI, 64.9–86.0) and 82.5% (95% CI, 70.7–89.9) initially favoring gemcitabine and nab-paclitaxel. The 2-year OS was in a different direction and was 48.2% (95% CI, 33.3–61.7) for FOLFIRINOX and 39.7% (95% CI, 28.6–52.5) for gemcitabine and nab-paclitaxel. Median OS was 2 years (95% CI, 1.6–2.7) and 1.8 years (95% CI, 1.5–2.0), respectively. With the significant confidence interval overlap in the 2-year and median OS, we await further maturity of the data. This is one of the first trials to compare FOLFIRINOX with gemcitabine and nab-paclitaxel in a prospective and randomized manner.

TABLE 66.9   Summary of Pivotal Randomized Phase III Trials in Locally Advanced and Metastatic Pancreatic Cancer

STUDY	REGIMEN	NO. OF PATIENTS	LOCALLY ADVANCED DISEASE NO. (%)	RESPONSE RATE (%)	OVERALL SURVIVAL (mo)	P VALUE
Burris et al.[26]	Gemcitabine	63	NA	5.4	5.65	.0025
	Bolus 5-FU	63	NA	0	4.41	
Moore et al.[80]	Gemcitabine	284	67 (25)	8.0	5.91	.038
	Gemcitabine + erlotinib	285	71 (24)	8.6	6.24	
Cunningham et al.[39]	Gemcitabine	266	76 (29)	12.4	6.2	.08 (meta-analysis = .02)
	Gemcitabine + capecitabine	267	80 (30)	19.1	7.1	
Conroy et al.[81]	Gemcitabine	171	0	9.4	6.8	<.001
	Folinic acid + 5-FU + irinotecan + oxaliplatin	171	0	31.6	11.1	
Von Hoff et al.[82]	Gemcitabine	430	0	7	6.7	<.001
	Gemcitabine + nab-paclitaxel	431	0	23	8.5	

NA, Not available

Moving beyond the front-line, the NAPOLI-1 trial reported a significant survival advantage for the combination of nanoliposomal irinotecan (formulation of irinotecan encapsulated in a liposome), fluorouracil (5-FU), and leucovorin (LV) compared with 5-FU/LV in 417 patients with pancreatic cancer whose disease had progressed after gemcitabine-based first-line chemotherapy.[84] The median OS for the liposomal-irinotecan combination arm was 6.1 months (95% CI 4.8–8.9) compared with 4.1 months (95% CI 3.3–5.3) in the 5FU/LV group (HR 0.67; 95% CI 0.49–0.92; $P = .012$). These results led to the Food and Drug Administration (FDA) approval of the triplet regimen in 2015. RCTs are currently underway to investigate a role for liposomal irinotecan-based regimens in the front-line treatment of metastatic pancreatic cancer. Liposomal-irinotecan combined with 5-FU/LV is being compared with gemcitabine/nab-paclitaxel in older patients (EA2186; NCT04233866). Another trial is comparing liposomal-irinotecan/5-FU/LV and oxaliplatin (NALIRIFOX) to gemcitabine/nab-paclitaxel in all ages (NAPOLI-3; NCT04083235).

Although multiagent treatment regimens have been demonstrated to improve survival over monotherapy, they do so at the risk of increased toxicity.[42,81,82,84–86,56] Gemcitabine and capecitabine or single-agent therapies are recommended for patients unable to tolerate regimens associated with greater toxicity.[56]

Regarding a role for radiation in advanced pancreatic cancer, chemoradiotherapy is superior to radiotherapy alone for locally unresectable disease; however, there is no evidence that radiation prolongs life over chemotherapy alone.[87,88] The French 2000–2001 FFCD/SFRO trial was halted after 119 patients who were randomized as survival were significantly worse in the chemoradiotherapy arm compared with the chemotherapy arm.[89] The median OS was 8.6 months (99% CI, 7.1–11.4) with chemoradiotherapy compared with 13 months (99% CI, 8.7–18.1) with gemcitabine monotherapy ($P = .03$). Although these results have been explained by significantly higher toxicity in the chemoradiation arm, the median OS in the ECOG 4201 trial—as described later—with chemoradiotherapy of 9.2 months (95% CI, 7.9–11.4) was no different than that seen in the chemoradiotherapy arm of the FFCD/SFRO trial. Only 42% of the patients received 75% or more of planned radiotherapy or chemotherapy. High-grade (3/4) side effects were increased with chemoradiotherapy (66%) compared with gemcitabine (40%; $P = .008$).

In the ECOG 4201 trial, the median survival for a gemcitabine-based chemoradiotherapy arm was 11.1 months (95% CI, 7.6–5.5) and 9.2 months (95% CI, 7.9–11.4) for the gemcitabine-alone arm.[90] The study was notable for more grade 4/5 toxicity in the chemoradiotherapy arm at 41%, compared with 9% in the gemcitabine only arm. Only 74 of the planned 316 patients were recruited and the study was terminated early in view of accrual concerns. The authors reported significance, using a one-sided analysis. Criticism of this study includes the overlapping confidence intervals for survival that indicates no significant difference between the two groups, thus it should be considered a failed trial. An accompanying editorial in the *Journal of Clinical Oncology* concluded that the findings were not convincing.[91] Similarly, no survival benefit was seen for the addition of radiotherapy in the French LAP 07 trial. Here, 449 patients with locally advanced pancreatic cancer were randomized to gemcitabine or gemcitabine combined with erlotinib, with a second randomization after 4 months of therapy to continue chemotherapy for 2 more months or chemoradiotherapy.[92] The median OS in the

chemotherapy arm was 16.5 months (95% CI, 14.5–18.5) and 15.2 months (95% CI, 13.9–17.3) in the chemoradiotherapy arm with HR 1.03 (95% CI, 0.79–1.34; $P = .083$).

The SCALOP trial set out to evaluate concurrent gemcitabine or capecitabine, added to radiation. This was a Phase II RCT whereby patients with locally unresectable pancreatic cancer received 12 weeks of induction therapy with gemcitabine/capecitabine, after which those with stable or responding disease were randomized to receive gemcitabine-based or capecitabine-based chemoradiotherapy.[93] The primary end point of 9-month progression-free survival identified 22 (62.9%) of 35 assessable patients (80% CI, 50.6–73.9) in the capecitabine group, and 18 (51.4%) of 35 assessable patients (80% CI, 39.4–63.4) in the gemcitabine group had not experienced disease progression. Although a trend towards favorability of the capecitabine-based regimen was seen, there was no significant difference in the primary endpoint.

Several other techniques are under exploration to better control locally advanced pancreatic cancer; to date, however, there have been no RCTs. There is little evidence that stereotactic body radiotherapy is superior to conventional treatment.[94,95] Radiofrequency ablation (RFA) is a technique performed during laparotomy with general anesthesia, with a single or multiple hook needle placed into the tumor with ultrasound guidance. A median survival of 34 months was observed in a highly selected group of 32 patients that received a combination of RFA, chemoradiotherapy, intra-arterial chemotherapy, and then systemic chemotherapy.[96] Irreversible electroporation uses electrical pulses to increase cell membrane permeability by changing the transmembrane potential, leading to tumor cell death while preserving the surrounding stroma. It appears to be relatively safe and can be used either alone or in conjunction with pancreatectomy in select patients.[97,98] More recently, highly innovative radiotherapy approaches using "ablative" dosing of radiation (98 Gy biologically effective dose) has been reported in a single institution cohort of 119 selected patients with locally advanced inoperable pancreatic cancer and a median OS from diagnosis of 26.8 months was observed with a two year local-regional failure of 32.8% (95% CI, 21.6%–44.1%).[99] Further evaluation of this approach is required.

TARGETED THERAPY FOR PANCREATIC CANCER

The genomic profile and pathobiology of pancreatic cancer is increasingly understood (see Chapter 9D). Over 90% of pancreatic cancer patients have somatic mutations in one or more driver oncogenes, including *KRAS*, *p53*, *SMAD4* and *CDKN2A*, which are not therapeutically targetable.[100] Olaparib, a poly-ADP ribose polymerase inhibitor (PARPi), is the first targeted therapy that has received a pancreatic cancer-specific FDA approval in the US; approved for use in metastatic pancreatic cancer with germline mutation in *BRCA1/2* as a maintenance therapy. Approximately 5% to 7% of patients with pancreatic cancer have a germline *BRCA1/2* mutation. Results from the Pancreas OLaparib Ongoing (POLO) trial support the use of olaparib in a maintenance setting after at least 4 months of platinum-based therapy.[101] In the POLO trial, 154 patients with a germline *BRCA1/2* mutation were randomized to either olaparib ($n = 92$) or placebo ($n = 62$) in a 3:2 ratio. PFS, the primary endpoint, was significantly longer in the olaparib group compared with the placebo group (7.4 vs 3.8 months; HR 0.53, 95% CI 0.35–08.82; $P = 0.004$). An interim analysis of OS with 46% data maturity showed no difference in outcome between the two groups, with median OS of 18.9 months for the olaparib group and 18.1 months for the placebo group (HR 0.91, 95% CI 0.56–1.46; $P = .68$). These data, although not without controversy given the absence of an active comparator arm, support the use of a targeted therapy in a subset of genomically defined pancreatic cancer patients. A more recent phase II non-RCT confirms the value of maintenance PARPi therapy with rucaparib in a similar maintenance setting and extends the evidence for use of such drugs beyond germline *BRCA1/2*, to somatic *BRCA* and *PALB2* variants.[102] These findings, combined with evidence of PARPi benefit in the adjuvant setting,[103] have led to the investigation of maintenance olaparib in pancreatic cancer patients with resected disease. In the APOLLO trial (EA2192; NCT04858334), patients with germline or somatic mutations in *BRCA1/2* or *PALB2* who have undergone successful resection are randomized to 1 year of maintenance olaparib or placebo upon completion of perioperative therapy. Endpoints include relapse free survival and OS.

The *KRAS* wild-type subset makes up about 6% to 8% of all pancreatic cancer patients and up to 16% to 18% in patients younger than 50 at diagnosis.[104] In *KRAS* wild-type disease, there are other rare oncogenic drivers that may be targetable in small subsets of patients, including those with *NRG-1, NTRK1-3, Alk, ROS1, RET*, and other uncommon fusions. The importance of targeting a genomic alteration with a related matched therapy was reported in an analysis from the "Know Your Tumor Program," a community and academic-based next-generation sequencing program for pancreatic cancer. In a retrospective analysis of 189 patients who possessed an actionable alteration, 24% received a targeted therapy as the "matched" group, whereas 76% (the "unmatched" group) did not.[105] The median OS was significantly longer in the matched group compared with the unmatched group (2.58 vs. 1.51 years; HR 0.42; 95% CI: 0.26–0.68; $P = .0004$). These data collectively underscore the importance of comprehensive germline and somatic profiling in pancreatic cancer.[56,106,107]

Approximately 15% to 20% of pancreatic cancers are deficient in homologous recombination repair (HRD) related to defects in germline and somatic genes, including *BRCA1/2, PALB2, ATM*, and *FANCA*, amongst other genes.[108] For these individuals with HRD, platinum-based therapy is preferred as an initial treatment approach. A phase II RCT evaluated cisplatin and gemcitabine with or without the PARPi, veliparib, in 50 patients with untreated locally advanced or metastatic pancreatic cancer who harbored a germline *BRCA1/2* or *PALB2* mutation.[109] Response rates in both treatment arms were very high at 74% for the triplet and 65.2% for the doublet ($P = .55$) with median OS of 15.5 months (95% CI 12.2–24.3 months and 16.4 months, respectively; 95% CI 11.7–23.4 months; $P = .06$). Notably, 2-year and 3-year OS for the entire cohort was prolonged compared with historical data, at 30.6% (95% CI 17.8%–44.4%) and 17.8% (95% CI 8.1%–30.7%), respectively. These data support the use of a cisplatin-based doublet as initial treatment for advanced pancreatic cancer in patients with a germline *BRCA1/2* or *PALB2* mutation.

Pancreatic cancer is characterized by an immunosuppressive hypoxic microenvironment with a dearth of effector T cells, an abundance of regulatory T cells, macrophages of the M2 category, hyaluronan, and other cellular components that mitigate against generating an effective immune response.[110] Immunotherapy has had a major impact in multiple malignancies; however, single or double agent checkpoint inhibitors have demonstrated no significant benefit in pancreatic cancer[111] (see Chapter 10). Nonetheless, there are multiple strategies in development attempting to overcome inherent resistance by combining multiple immune agents together, combining chemotherapy with immunotherapy,[112] and targeting the tumor microenvironment. Currently, the role of immunotherapy in the treatment of pancreatic cancer is limited to pembrolizumab, which is FDA approved for a disease agnostic indication in the setting of mismatch repair deficiency.[113,114] However, mismatch repair deficiency is identified in less than 1% of patients with pancreatic cancer.[115] Many ongoing trials will report out over the next few years and are likely to provide important insights into targeting the immune system in pancreatic cancer.

SUMMARY

The understanding of pancreatic cancer pathobiology has significantly evolved over the last decade, providing enhanced opportunities for improving survival. The current data strongly support adjuvant systemic chemotherapy with modified FOLFIRINOX for individuals with a good performance status and gemcitabine/capecitabine or gemcitabine alone for less fit individuals. To date, no studies provide sufficient evidence to support routine use of adjuvant chemoradiation, and its use in the adjuvant setting remains controversial. Results from the adjuvant NRG/RTOG 0848 trial are awaited and will specifically inform this use. Neoadjuvant therapy is increasingly being used in the treatment of localized pancreatic cancer, and current guidelines (expert consensus) endorse its use for borderline resectable disease and for resectable disease with high-risk features, although definitive phase III data are lacking. A key national US study underway, A028106, is evaluating perioperative FOLFIRINOX versus a paradigm of initial surgery followed by adjuvant FOLFIRINOX. In the advanced disease setting, current standards include (m)FOLFIRINOX or gemcitabine and nab-paclitaxel in the first-line setting and nanoliposomal irinotecan/5-FU in a beyond front-line setting. For the subset of patients with a germline *BRCA1/2* mutation maintenance therapy, olaparib is an option. With the expanding role of targeted/personalized disease management, it is now standard of care to conduct germline and somatic testing in all patients with pancreatic cancer to identify rare subsets that have other targetable alterations. A major investigational strategy includes incorporating immune therapeutics into the treatment of all stages of pancreatic cancer, although value remains to be definitively established.

References are available at expertconsult.com.

CHAPTER 67

Palliative treatment of pancreatic and periampullary tumors

Motaz Qadan and Roi Anteby

INTRODUCTION

Pancreatic and periampullary tumors are a common cause of cancer death, with rising incidence in the Western world. In 2018 the incidence of pancreatic cancer in the United States (US) was 13.7 per 100,000 persons, compared with 11.6 per 100,000 persons in 2000.[1] Pancreatic cancer is the fourth most common cause of cancer death in men and women in the US[2] (see Chapters 61 and 62). Periampullary tumors, in particular pancreatic adenocarcinoma, confer an extremely poor prognosis. Unfortunately, the vast majority of patients with pancreatic or periampullary cancer (approximately 75%–85%) are not candidates for curative-intent surgery at diagnosis because of extensive local disease or metastases.[3,4] According to the National Cancer Institute 2009 to 2018 records, only about 12% of patients with pancreas cancer present with localized disease confined to the pancreas, 30% present with regional locally advanced disease (including resectable and unresectable disease), and half have distant metastases at diagnosis.[1] Furthermore, even patients undergoing curative-intent resections have a relatively poor prognosis secondary to rapid disease progression or recurrence. The corresponding estimated 5-year survival rates by stage of diagnosis are 37%, 12%, and 3% for localized, regional, and metastatic disease.[2] These data clearly demonstrate that noncurative intent care represents a substantial portion of care for patients with pancreatic and periampullary tumors because the vast majority of patients will most likely require palliation at some point. Therefore surgeons should be knowledgeable in various aspects of palliative options, including both surgical and nonsurgical strategies that have evolved over the years.

Palliation is performed with the intent to improve the patient's quality of life through prevention and relief of suffering.[5,6] The goal of treatment transitions from an attempt to cure or prolong survival to that of offering durable solutions for debilitating symptom relief.[7] Considering operative intervention for palliation is complex; possible benefits of intervention must be weighed against the inherent risks of the intervention, while accounting for longevity associated with advanced disease. In pancreatic and periampullary cancer, surgical palliation should be considered specifically for three commonly debilitating entities: biliary obstruction, gastric outlet obstruction, and tumor-related pain.

In the last decade, several advances in care have resulted in moderate improvements in survival for patients with pancreatic cancer. Most importantly, treatment with combinations of modern systemic agents (such as gemcitabine plus a taxane agent or oxaliplatin, irinotecan, fluorouracil, and leucovorin [FOLFIRINOX]) have demonstrated superior survival benefit compared with conventional gemcitabine mono-chemotherapy,[8,9] with reported median survival of up to 54 months for patients in resected pancreatic cancer (see Chapter 62).[10] Other advances in care include use of neoadjuvant therapy for borderline/locally advanced disease,[11] introduction of targeted therapy (biological agents and immunotherapy),[12] improved multidisciplinary management of chemotherapy-associated toxicities, and optimization of surgical technique, including use of minimal invasive surgery and enhanced postoperative care and recovery pathways.[13] As patients live longer with incurable disease, the need of palliative treatment becomes increasingly pertinent. This is especially true in locally advanced disease given the potentially locally obstructive and destructive nature of periampullary or pancreatic head tumors. In general, surgical palliation is mostly used to relieve the effects of advanced locoregional disease.[14] Patients with distant metastases may be candidates for palliative surgical intervention. Metastatic spread, however, is associated with more aggressive disease, fewer local signs and symptoms, and generally a shorter overall life expectancy. In a National Cancer Database (NCDB) analysis of patients with metastatic pancreatic adenocarcinoma diagnosed between 2003 to 2011, only 19% of the patients underwent operative palliation, with the majority receiving nonoperative palliation (chemotherapy, radiation, or pain management alone; see Chapter 66).[15]

This chapter focuses on palliative surgical treatment of biliary obstruction, gastric outlet obstruction, and tumor-related pain. We also discuss local ablative therapies, palliative pancreatectomy, and strategies for end-of-life care for terminally ill patients. The role of chemotherapy and radiotherapy is discussed in Chapter 66. It is critical that readers recognize that palliative treatment in pancreatic and periampullary tumors should be tailored to the individual patient with multidisciplinary support. Ideally, the patient's clinical presentation, functional status, comorbidities, tumor stage, tumor biology, and patient and tumor genetics should all be accounted for.[16] Finally, any care should be consistent with the patient's goals of care, which should be thoroughly and expertly evaluated with shared decision making to determine the role of any interventions.

BILIARY OBSTRUCTION

Jaundice secondary to extrinsic mechanical obstruction of the biliary tree is the presenting symptom in 50% to 70% of patients with pancreatic head adenocarcinoma and develops in as many as 80% during the course of the disease[17,18] (see Chapters 61 and 62). Obstructive jaundice can manifest clinically with jaundiced skin and sclera, pruritis, nausea, vomiting, cachexia, dark colored urine, and clay-colored stool. Bile stasis secondary to obstruction can eventually lead to recurrent ascending cholangitis, fat malabsorption, progressive malnutrition, hepatic dysfunction and failure, and eventually death. In patients with reasonable life expectancy, relieving the obstruction is of paramount importance because successful biliary drainage has been shown to improve quality of life (see Chapters 29–31). Decompression of the biliary obstruction relieves the patient from the often-debilitating symptoms previously described and prevents rapid clinical deterioration that can accompany cholangitis in previously instrumented settings. Treating biliary obstruction is associated with improved liver function and nutritional status, and, on a cellular level, has been shown to reverse proinflammatory immune responses in both animal and human models.[19,20] Finally, in patients who are candidates for chemotherapy, unobstructed bile flow and resolution of jaundice are a prerequisite for successful and safe administration of systemic chemotherapy to avoid toxicity secondary to inadequate biliary excretion of metabolites (see Chapter 66).

Importantly, patients report improved quality of life after biliary decompression. In a prospective study of 50 patients with malignant biliary obstruction and unresectable disease, 1 month after successful endoscopic biliary drainage, patients with reduction in plasma bilirubin levels reported substantial improvement in social function (relative risk [RR]: 0.11; 95% confidence interval [CI]: 0.03–0.19) and mental health (RR: 0.04; 95% CI: 0.01–0.08) compared with pre-decompression.[21] Another small single institution study found that patients with locally advanced or metastatic disease ($n = 64$) who underwent biliary or enteral stent placement reported an increase in quality of life at 6 months compared with baseline.[22]

Interventions for biliary drainage in obstructive jaundice include operative biliary bypass, endoscopic stent placement, percutaneous external drainage, and endoscopic ultrasound (EUS)-guided biliary drainage (the most novel technique).

These various tools in the armamentarium of the multidisciplinary treatment team have ensured the cases of biliary obstruction that are completely unreachable for drainage are minimized. In the last several years, the pendulum has shifted away from operative palliation of the biliary tree, largely because of enhanced durability of decompressive endoscopic metal stents (see Chapters 30 and 31). In a large case series from Johns Hopkins Hospital of patients with unresectable pancreatic adenocarcinoma, between the years 1996 to 2010 there was a consistent temporal decrease in the use of palliative surgical bypass (Fig. 67.1); in 1996 to 2001, 10% of the patients received hepaticojejunostomy bypass, whereas since 2002 under 4% of patients underwent this procedure.[18]

Biliary Stenting

The current standard of care is biliary drainage via endoscopic self-expandable metallic stents (see Chapter 30).[23] Endobiliary stent placement has been shown to be associated with lower complication rates and faster recovery compared with operative palliative biliary drainage and results in durable relief with similar success rates (80%–100%) and an even higher postintervention quality of life.[24,25] The effectiveness of endoscopic biliary stenting has improved thanks to the usage of self-expanding metal stents introduced in the 1990s that are far superior to previously relied-on Teflon/polyethylene plastic stents.[26] Interestingly, covered metal stents have been shown to possess longer patency compared with uncovered stents in three randomized controlled trials (RCTs).[27] Importantly, while easier than major surgical interventions, endoscopic retrograde cholangiopancreatography (ERCP) and biliary stent placement carry a risk for complications, such as perforation, cholecystitis,

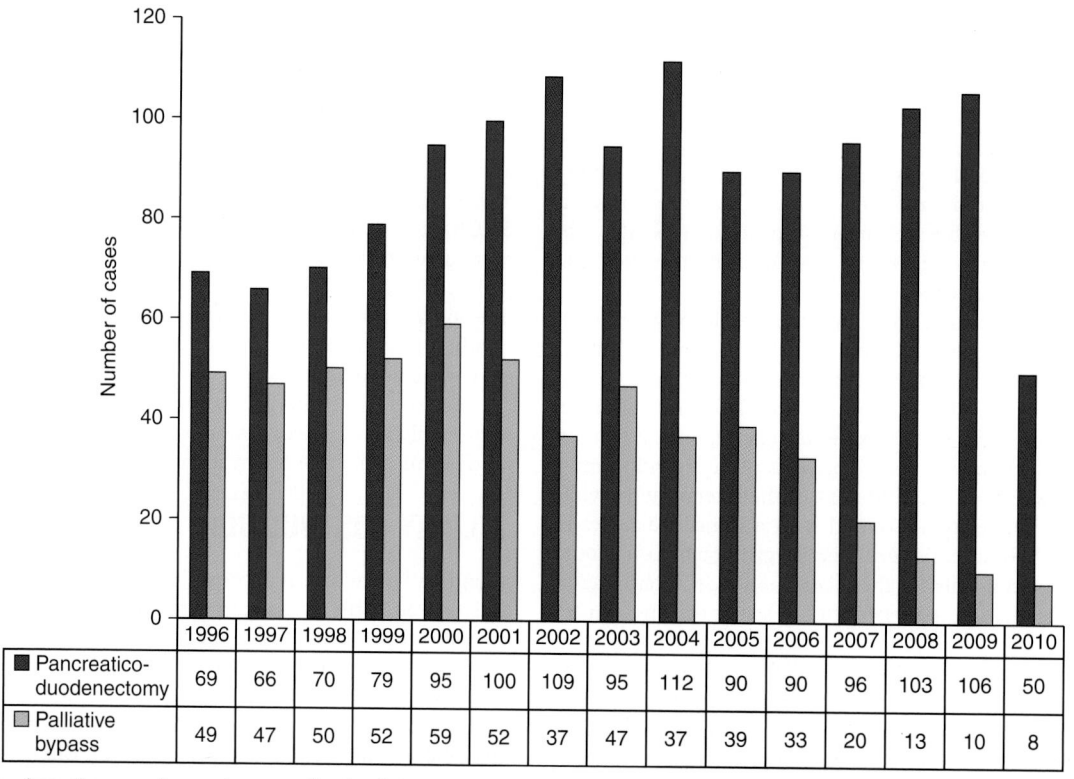

FIGURE 67.1 Annual case volume of pancreaticoduodenectomy versus bypass for pancreatic adenocarcinoma at the Johns Hopkins Hospital. (Modified from Kneuertz PJ, Cunningham SC, Cameron JL, et al. Palliative surgical management of patients with unresectable pancreatic adenocarcinoma: trends and lessons learned from a large, single institution experience. *J Gastrointest Surg.* 2011;15:1917.)

	1996	1997	1998	1999	2000	2001	2002	2003	2004	2005	2006	2007	2008	2009	2010
■ Pancreaticoduodenectomy	69	66	70	79	95	100	109	95	112	90	90	96	103	106	50
□ Palliative bypass	49	47	50	52	59	52	37	47	37	39	33	20	13	10	8

TABLE 67.1 Prospective Randomized Controlled Trials Comparing Surgical Biliary Drainage With Percutaneous Drainage or Endoscopic Drainage

	BORNMANN ET AL., 1986[32]		SHEPERD ET AL., 1988[33]		ANDERSEN ET AL., 1989[34]		SMITH ET AL., 1994[35]		NIEVEEN VAN DIJ-KUM ET AL., 2003[31]		ARTIFON ET AL., 2006[28]	
	BYPASS	STENT[a]	BYPASS	STENT	BYPASS	STENT	BYPASS	STENT	BYPASS	STENT	BYPASS	STENT
No. patients	25	25	25	23	25	25	101	100	13	14	15	15
Success (%)	76	84	92	80	88	96	93	95	100	100	100	100
Morbidity (%)	32	28	56	30	20	36	58	29	8	7	47	33
30-day mortality (%)	20	8	20	9	24	20	14	3	0	0	0	0
Hospital stay (days)	24	18	13	5	27	26	26	19	12	3	19	5
Readmission(s) (%)	-	-	12	43	-	-	-	-	11	14	40	26
Recurrent jaundice or cholangitis (%)	16	38	0	30	0	0	2	36	-	-	0	27
GOO (%)	0	14	4	9	0	0	11	19	-	-	7	0
Survival (weeks)	15	19	18	22	14	12	26	21	27	17	29	23

[a]Percutaneous transhepatic biliary drainage
GOO, Gastric outlet obstruction; *No.*, number.

cholangitis, hemorrhage, and acute pancreatitis. Furthermore, endobiliary stents can fail because of obstruction or migration, necessitating complex reinterventions and readmissions, which, in turn, increase the risk of complications. Five RCTs have compared surgical biliary drainage (see Chapter 32) to endoscopic drainage (Table 67.1). The majority of these studies were conducted before 1994, with the most recent one published in 2006.[28] The studies enrolled small patient cohorts and included a variety of stent types (in size and material). In a 2007 meta-analysis, the pooled plastic stent treatment arm showed fewer complications (RR 0.6; 95% CI 0.45–0.81) but a higher risk of recurrent biliary obstruction compared with surgery (RR 18.59; 95% CI 5.33–64.86).[24] An updated meta-analysis from 2014 reported similar technical success rates (RR 0.99; 95% CI 0.93–1.05), complications, and mortality (RR 1.54; 95% CI 0.87–2.71) between surgical biliary bypass and endoscopic biliary stent placement but with consistently lower rates of recurrent jaundice after surgical bypass (RR 0.14; 95% CI 0.03–0.63; Fig. 67.2). Furthermore, patients with prolonged survival in the stent group had more hospital days (a 2-fold increase for stent patients in the total number of hospital days from the index procedure until death).[29] A 2015 meta-analysis comparing the same 5 studies concluded that stenting has lower procedure-associated complications (risk difference of –0.19 to –0.24 favoring stenting).[30] These pooled estimates should be interpreted with caution. In the two most recent meta-analyses, 4 of the 5 studies included were conducted before 1994 and used plastic stents. In addition, the meta-analyses did not include a more recent small RCT from 2003, with similar procedure-related morbidity (7% in the stent group [n = 14] and 8% in the surgical bypass group [n = 13]).[31] Although contemporary high-quality evidence is lacking, these data allow for some general conclusions to be drawn (i.e., that endoscopic stent placement is associated with slightly lower morbidity). However, surgical bypass offers a more durable long-term solution.

Surgical Bypass (see Chapter 32)

There is no agreed on consensus regarding the exact indications for surgical palliation in biliary obstruction because of periampullary tumors. About 20% of patients with pancreatic head adenocarcinoma have unresectable disease at the time of surgical exploration for curative-intent.[36] Interestingly, these numbers have persisted throughout the years, with a similar proportion reported in more recent cohort studies, despite advancements in preoperative imaging.[37–39] These cases lead to intraoperative dilemmas on whether to perform palliative surgery "while there." In these cases, surgical biliary bypass may be indicated in patients who presented with recurrent cholangitis. On the other hand, proceeding with a bypass procedure for prophylactic symptom control is largely not indicated because of associated high postoperative morbidity[36] and relatively short survival in patients who may never develop biliary obstruction.[37] Studies on biliary bypass procedures, with or without gastroenterostomy for advanced pancreatic cancer, have reported high mortality (up to 6.5%–8%) and morbidity (up to 55%; Table 67.2). For jaundiced patients with disease that is determined as unresectable outside of the setting of operative exploration, endoscopic biliary bypass is preferred over surgery. There is less controversy when endoscopic biliary stent is technically impossible, as is the case in patients with duodenal obstruction or a history of prior gastric bypass or gastrectomy. In these patients, surgical palliation may be superior to percutaneous transhepatic biliary drainage that involves initial external drainage and is associated with high complication rates and unsatisfactory improvement in quality of life.[40] There have also been improvements in this approach, however, and in many cases internalization of the external catheter(s) by interventional radiology or combined with advanced gastroenterology technique ("rendezvous") is possible. Another possibility that has evolved in this setting is EUS-guided biliary drainage, which involves the creation of a duodenal to bile duct conduit proximal to the site of ampullary obstruction. Although the data remain limited, this modality has been shown to have similar success rates compared with percutaneous transhepatic drainage, but with lower need for reintervention and potentially fewer complications.[41]

Technical Considerations

Surgical bypass of the biliary tree can be performed in various techniques and approaches (open surgery or minimally-invasive). Roux-en-Y hepaticojejunostomy or choledochojejunostomy are

A

Study or subgroup	Surgery Events	Total	Stent Events	Total	Weight	Risk ratio M–H, Random, 95% CI	Risk ratio M–H, Random, 95% CI
Andersen 1989	22	25	24	25	13.2%	0.92 [0.78, 1.08]	
Artifon 2006	15	15	15	15	23.4%	1.00 [0.88, 1.13]	
Bornman 1986	19	25	21	25	4.7%	0.90 [0.68, 1.20]	
Shepherd 1988	23	25	19	23	7.5%	1.11 [0.89, 1.39]	
Smith 1994	92	101	92	100	51.3%	0.99 [0.91, 1.08]	
Total (95% CI)		**191**		**188**	**100.0%**	**0.99 [0.93, 1.05]**	
Total events	171		171				

Heterogeneity: Tau^2 = 0.00; Chi^2 = 2.35, df = 4 (P = 0.67); I^2 = 0%
Test for overall effect: Z = 0.43 (P = 0.67)

0.5 0.7 1 1.5 2
Stent successful Surgery successful

B

Study or subgroup	Surgery Events	Total	Stent Events	Total	Weight	Risk ratio M–H, Random, 95% CI	Risk ratio M–H, Random, 95% CI
Andersen 1989	5	25	9	25	17.3%	0.56 [0.22, 1.43]	
Artifon 2006	9	15	6	15	21.1%	1.50 [0.71, 3.16]	
Bornman 1986	8	25	6	25	18.0%	1.33 [0.54, 3.29]	
Shepherd 1988	10	25	5	23	17.9%	1.84 [0.74, 4.58]	
Smith 1994	43	101	14	100	25.6%	3.04 [1.78, 5.20]	
Total (95% CI)		**191**		**188**	**100.0%**	**1.54 [0.87, 2.71]**	
Total events	75		40				

Heterogeneity: Tau^2 = 0.25; Chi^2 = 10.37, df = 4 (P = 0.03); I^2 = 61%
Test for overall effect: Z = 1.49 (P = 0.14)

0.02 0.1 1 10 50
Stent complications Surgery complications

C

Study or subgroup	Surgery Events	Total	Stent Events	Total	Weight	Risk ratio M–H, Random, 95% CI	Risk ratio M–H, Random, 95% CI
Andersen 1989	0	25	0	25		Not estimable	
Artifon 2006	0	15	3	15	16.5%	0.14 [0.01, 2.55]	
Bornman 1986	4	25	8	25	35.3%	0.50 [0.17, 1.45]	
Shepherd 1988	0	25	7	23	17.0%	0.06 [0.00, 1.02]	
Smith 1994	2	101	36	100	31.2%	0.06 [0.01, 0.22]	
Total (95% CI)		**191**		**188**	**100.0%**	**0.14 [0.03, 0.63]**	
Total events	6		54				

Heterogeneity: Tau^2 = 1.33; Chi^2 = 8.07, df = 3 (P = 0.04); I^2 = 63%
Test for overall effect: Z = 2.56 (P = 0.01)

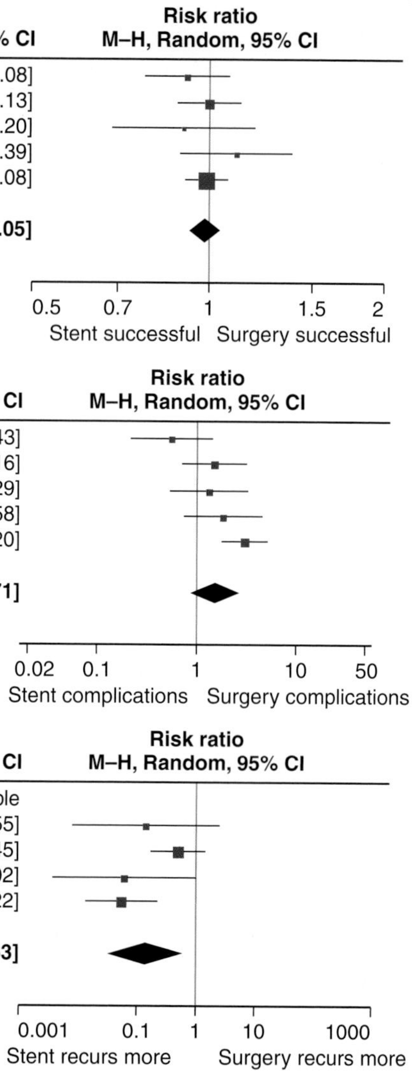

0.001 0.1 1 10 1000
Stent recurs more Surgery recurs more

FIGURE 67.2 Meta-analysis of prospective randomized controlled trials comparing technical success **(A)**, complications and mortality **(B)** and recurrent obstructions **(C)** between biliary stents and surgical bypass in malignant biliary obstruction. (From Glazer ES, Hornbrook MC, Krouse RS. A meta-analysis of randomized trials: Immediate stent placement vs. surgical bypass in the palliative management of malignant biliary obstruction. *J Pain Symptom Manage.* 2014;47[2]:307–314.)

usually the procedures of choice for biliary drainage because pancreatic surgeons are most experienced with using the common bile duct or common hepatic duct as biliary conduits to the small bowel. Other possible techniques include gallbladder bypass (cholecystogastrostomy, duodenostomy, or jejunostomy) or, alternatively, common bile duct or hepatic duct bypass options (choledochoduodenostomy or hepaticoduodenostomy; see Chapter 32).

Cholecystenteric Bypass

The gallbladder can serve as a conduit for biliary-digestive bypass, with minimal alteration to the normal anatomy. In the setting of biliary obstruction, the gallbladder is often distended (Courvoisier's sign), further strengthening the technical appeal of this approach as the anastomosis becomes simpler. The bypass can be done to the stomach, duodenum, or jejunum. With cholecystojejunostomy, the procedure is more extensive as a jejunal loop needs to be approximated to the gallbladder in an anticolic or retrocolic configuration, and an additional Roux

limb or Braun enteroenterostomy created to avoid reflux. The anastomosis can be safely performed handsewn or using a staple device (Fig. 67.3). Cholecystogastrostomy and cholecystoduodenostomy are procedures that are largely of historic interest. Tumors involving the proximal gastroduodenal tract at the time of surgery preclude these procedures. If pursued, they require mobilization of the gallbladder fundus from the cystic plate. With gallbladder bypass, the surgeon must rule out tumor involvement in the cystic duct/common hepatic duct juncture to ensure effective drainage of the biliary tree. An intraoperative cholecystogram is recommended to ensure free-flowing bile into the gallbladder (see Chapter 24).

Direct Choledochoenteric and Hepatoenteric Bypass

The common bile duct or common hepatic duct are commonly used conduits for bypassing biliary obstructions. These are advantageous to the gallbladder because involvement of the proximal biliary tree is less likely with periampullary or pancreatic cancer, even with large tumors. Anastomosis to the duodenum

TABLE 67.2 Outcomes of Biliary Bypass Procedures With or Without Gastric Bypass for Advanced Pancreatic Cancer

STUDY	NO. PATIENTS	BILIARY BYPASS	GASTRIC BYPASS	MORTALITY	MORBIDITY	HOSPITAL STAY (DAYS)	RECURRENT JAUNDICE	SURVIVAL (MONTHS)
Lillemoe et al. 1993a[42]	118	89	107	3%	37%	14	2%	7.7
Park et al. 1997[43]	61	61	0	8%	21%	10	8%	7
van Wagensveld et al. 1997[44]	126	124	120	2%	17%	17	NA	6
Lesurtel et al. 2006[45]	83	83	83	5%	27%	16	2%	9.2
Singh et al. 2008[46]	204	195	167	1%	27%	9	1%	8
Mann et al. 2009[47]	102	102	102	6%	26%	12	2%	9.5
Kneuertz et al. 2011[18]	553	397	513	2%	14%	10	5%	6
Wellner et al. 2012[48]	117	87	109	3%	23%	12	2%	6
Spanheimer et al. 2014[36]	34	21	18	0%	55%	7.5	14%	6.6
Ueda et al. 2014[49]	69	69	NA	0%	15%	NA	NA	NA
Bartlett et al. 2014[50]	1126	407	720	7%	29%	8	NA	6
Bliss et al. 2016[51]	312	312	197	5%	4.5%[a]	11	NA	NA
Pencovich et al. 2020[52]	42	11	31	17%	36%	18	NA	14.4
Azari et al. 2020[53]	79	49	30	7%-19%	14%-17%	8-9	NA	11.9

[a]Cholangitis, evidence of biliary obstruction, or acute pancreatitis on first revisit.

NA, Not available; *No.*, number.

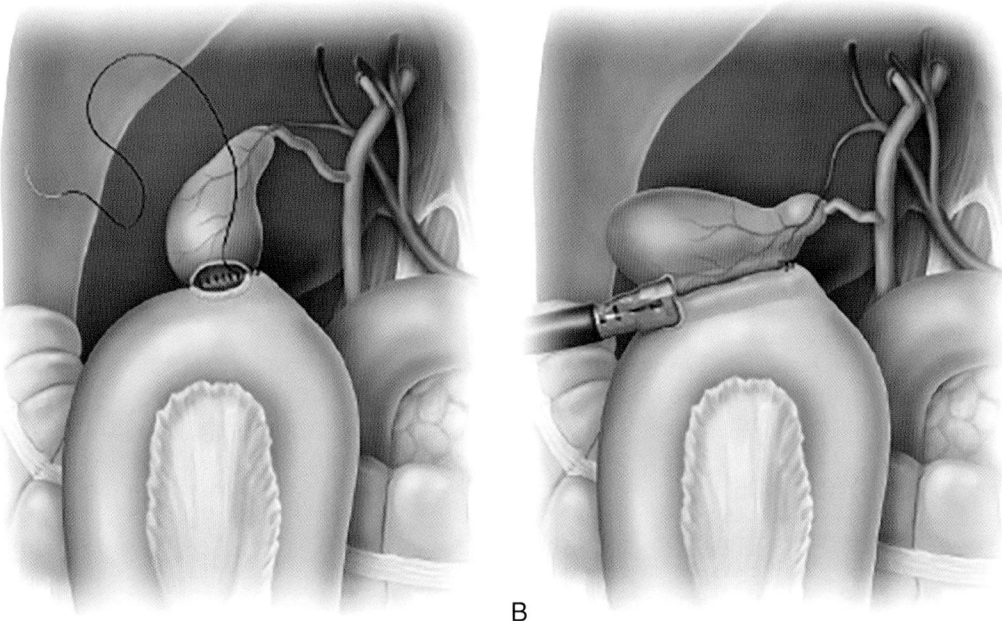

FIGURE 67.3 Cholecystojejunostomy for biliary enteric bypass performed using hand-sewn **(A)** or stapled **(B)** techniques. (From Lillemoe K, Jarnagin W [eds]. *Master Techniques in Surgery – Hepatobiliary and Pancreatic Surgery.* Wolters Kluwer; 2013.)

(choledochoduodenostomy or hepaticoduodenostomy) is a possibility, necessitating a Kocher maneuver to bring the duodenum toward the biliary duct. Both side-to-side or end-to-side anastomosis are possible, with concurrent cholecystectomy (Fig. 67.4). Complications include cholangitis, gastritis caused by bile reflux, and sump syndrome. In sump syndrome, the defunctionalized distal common bile duct reservoir accumulates bile debris and sludge, potentially causing cholangitis and hepatic abscess.[54] Sump syndrome is usually a long-term complication, often occurring 5 to 6 years after the biliary-enteric bypass.[55] Treatment of sump syndrome may necessitate revision of the bypass with Roux-en-Y hepaticojejunostomy and

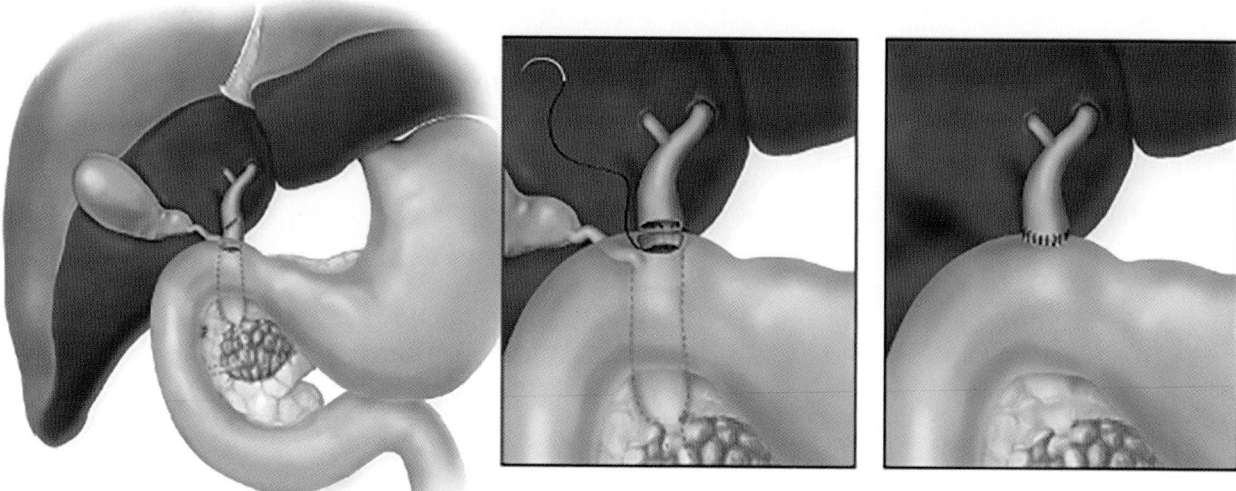

FIGURE 67.4 Choledochoduodenostomy or hepaticoduodenostomy for biliary enteric bypass performed as an end-to-end anastomosis. (From Lillemoe K, Jarnagin W [eds]. *Master Techniques in Surgery – Hepatobiliary and Pancreatic Surgery.* Wolters Kluwer; 2013.)

occurs after older operations used to treat biliary stone disease. Endoscopic resolution of the sump is frequently technically not possible in patients with malignant obstruction who were initially treated with a surgical bypass. As with cholecystoduodenostomy, tumor involvement in the proximal gastrointestinal (GI) tract is a contraindication for choledochoduodenostomy or hepaticoduodenostomy (see Chapter 32).

The jejunum is usually the preferred GI anastomosis site for the common bile duct or common hepatic duct, being distant from the tumor location in the proximal GI tract and because of surgeon's familiarity with the procedure as part of every Whipple procedure. Roux-en-Y hepaticojejunostomy is a durable technical solution used by pancreatic surgeons to drain the biliary tree and one that minimizes the risk of cholangitis secondary to enteric reflux in the defunctionalized limb of small bowel. Hepaticojejunostomy and its various techniques are reviewed in Chapter 32. One recommended option, depicted in Fig. 67.5, is to perform a single layer interrupted anterior and posterior row with 4-0 absorbable sutures (preferable polydioxanone [PDS]). Possible reasons that preclude hepaticojejunostomy include previous history of small bowel resections and extensive peritoneal adhesions in the setting of peritoneal carcinomatosis (frozen abdomen).

GASTRIC OUTLET OBSTRUCTION

Gastric outlet obstruction in pancreatic cancer was historically estimated to occur in 10% to 20% of cases, based on studies from the 1980s and 90s.[56-58] Because of recent advancements in systemic therapies, however, the incidence may be higher because of the prolonged longevity of patients. In a 2014 retrospective single-center study of patients with unresectable pancreatic adenocarcinoma who underwent palliative biliary stent placement for obstructive jaundice, 40% of these patients eventually developed gastric outlet obstruction within almost a year of diagnosis (mean 11.4 ± 4.9 months).[59] Symptoms of gastric outlet obstruction include nausea, vomiting, abdominal pain, early satiety, and subsequent dehydration and malnutrition.[60] Mechanical gastric outlet obstruction is defined as complete or near complete obstruction of the distal stomach or proximal

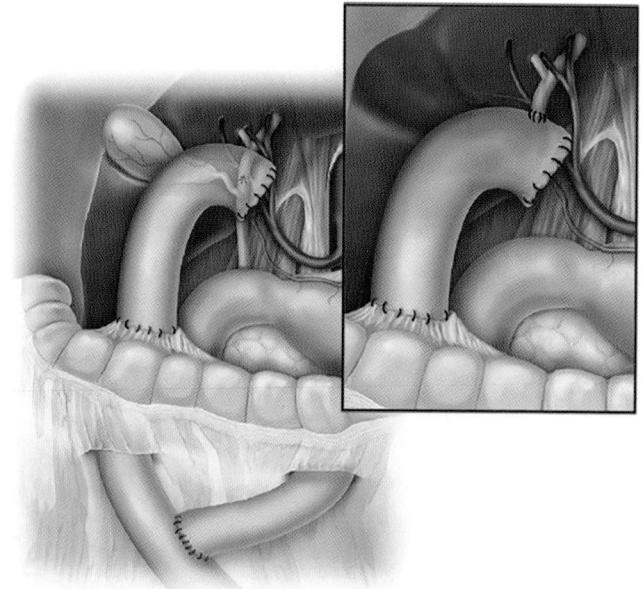

FIGURE 67.5 Roux-en-Y hepaticojejunostomy for biliary enteric bypass performed using a single layer of interrupted anterior and posterior row 4-0 polydioxanone (PDS) sutures placed radially from the jejunum to the hepatic duct following transection of the duct and oversewing of the distal portion (From Lillemoe K, Jarnagin W [eds]. *Master Techniques in Surgery – Hepatobiliary and Pancreatic Surgery.* Wolters Kluwer; 2013.)

duodenum. Malignant obstruction can be the result of direct tumor in-growth in the bowel lumen or indirect compression of the bowel by adjacent tumor. Diagnosis of mechanical gastric outlet obstruction should be confirmed via imaging and/or endoscopy.[60] Importantly, pancreatic cancer can also cause gastric outlet obstruction symptoms secondary to motility dysfunction of the stomach and duodenum caused by tumor infiltration to the celiac nerve plexus.[61]

Management modalities for mechanical gastric outlet obstruction include surgical bypass, enteric stent placement, EUS-guided gastroenterostomy, and percutaneous endoscopic gastrostomy (PEG) with or without jejunostomy. In enteric obstruction because of locally advanced disease, the preferred intervention for treatment of obstruction or impending obstruction has not been demonstrated, although surgical decompression tends to be favored. Unlike biliary stenting, endoscopic enteric stenting is less reliable and requires more frequent reinterventions because of stent migration and obstruction.[62] Some reports have also shown enteric stenting to be associated with a slightly lower success rate (96% vs. 99%) with ongoing dietary restrictions.[63] In addition, surgical palliation, including minimally invasive decompression, is simpler for gastric outlet obstruction than biliary bypass. Surgical bypass offers long-term efficacy and recovery to full oral dietary intake of solids and liquids alike.

Surgical Bypass

Indications for palliative gastrojejunostomy include patients with unresectable pancreatic or periampullary cancer who present with symptomatic gastric outlet obstruction, as long as they have reasonable life expectancy and acceptable performance status. For patients without signs of gastric outlet obstruction, in the setting of intraoperative discovery of unresectable disease, a prophylactic gastrojejunostomy may be performed, although the need for prophylactic interventions are again debatable. Prophylactic surgical bypass of the stomach is relatively easier than the biliary tree and so is considered, and it may even be considered among patients not expected to undergo attempt at surgical resection of the tumor. Interestingly, data from two prospective RCTs in 1999 and 2003 showed that prophylactic gastrojejunostomy resulted in reduced incidence of subsequent obstruction, without adversely affecting short-term outcomes (Table 67.3).[57,64] A 2013 Cochrane review that included the aforementioned trials compared gastrojejunostomy with no-gastrojejunostomy and reported no evidence of difference in the overall survival (hazard ratio [HR] 1.02; 95% CI 0.84–1.25), perioperative morbidity or mortality, or hospital stay (mean difference [MD] 0.97 days; 95% CI –0.18 to 2.12) between the two groups. In the prophylactic gastrojejunostomy group, 2.5% of the patients developed long‚Äìterm gastric outlet obstruction compared with 27.8% in the no-gastrojejunostomy group (RR 0.10; 95% CI 0.03–0.37). The authors concluded that routine prophylactic gastrojejunostomy is indicated in patients with unresectable periampullary cancer, at least among patients already undergoing exploratory laparotomy (with or without biliary bypass).[65]

Technical Considerations

Historically, patients with gastric outlet obstruction were treated with open gastrojejunostomy, the first described in 1881 by the Polish surgeon Ludwik Rydygier, who operated on a person with benign gastric outlet obstruction (duodenal ulcer) and separately in the same year by the Austrian surgeon Anton Wolfler, who operated on a patient with malignant gastric outlet obstruction (gastric cancer).[67,68] Today, the most prevalent technique for surgical gastric bypass remains gastrojejunostomy with a simple loop side-to-side procedure in an open or minimally invasive approach. A Roux-en-Y gastrojejunostomy can also be employed, although it is rarely used because of an additional, largely unnecessary anastomosis and associated complications (Roux stasis syndrome and functional nonemptying of the stomach) and limited additional benefit. Technical variations in simple gastrojejunostomy include retrocolic versus antecolic routing and isoperistaltic and antiperistalsic loop anastomoses. Different types of anastomoses are possible: Two-layer or one-layer hand-sewn anastomosis (with running versus interrupted sutures) or stapled anastomosis. These techniques are all relatively equivalent in efficacy. However, older data suggest that a retrocolic isoperistaltic configuration is associated with a lower incidence of delayed gastric emptying.[69] Delayed gastric emptying despite a patent gastrojejunostomy is a possible complication of surgical bypass. Vagotomy for prevention of this complication is not routinely done at time of surgery. However, postoperative administration of acid-reducing drugs, such as proton pump inhibitors and histamine type-2 blockers, is recommended.

Double Bypass

Combined biliary and gastric surgical bypass is a more complex procedure with various reconstruction options. One preferred option would be to use a Roux-en-Y biliary anastomosis (see section on biliary obstruction) and a loop gastrojejunostomy using the pancreaticobiliary limb. To allow for the formation of the loop gastrojejunostomy anastomosis before the jejunojejunostomy, the pancreaticobiliary limb should be longer at the point of the jejunal transection (20-40 cm compared with 10–15 cm).

Enteric Stenting

Duodenal stents are longer and of larger caliber compared with those employed for biliary decompression. The commonly used self-expanding metal stents can be covered or uncovered. Covered stents may prevent tumor ingrowth but have a higher rate

TABLE 67.3 Two Prospective Randomized Controlled Trials of Prophylactic Gastrojejunostomy in Patients With Unresectable Periampullary Cancer and Biliary Bypass and One Trial of Gastrojejunostomy Versus Stent for Symptomatic GOO

| | LILLEMOE ET AL., 1999[57] | | VAN HEEK ET AL., 2003[64] | | JEURNINK ET AL., 2010[66] | |
	GASTRO-JEJUNOSTOMY	NO GASTRO-JEJUNOSTOMY	DOUBLE BYPASS	SINGLE BYPASS	GASTRO-JEJUNOSTOMY	ENDOSCOPIC STENT
No. patients	44	43	36	29	18	21
Morbidity (%)	32	33	31	28	0	19
Mortality (%)	0	0	3	0	0	0
Hospital stay (days)	8.5	8	11	9	15	7
Late GOO (%)	0	19	6	41	6	24
Survival (months)	8.3	8.3	7.2	8.4	2.6	1.9

GOO, Gastric outlet obstruction; No., number.

of stent migration, although there is no evidence indicating that either type have superior results.[62,70] Complications of duodenal stent placement include mechanical irritation with subsequent bleeding and perforation, stent migration, and stent obstruction. Three RCTs comparing endoscopic with surgical bypass for malignant gastric outlet obstruction were published in 2006, 2010, and 2013, all relatively small and of variable quality.[66,71,72] A Cochrane meta-analysis of these studies showed that stenting for malignant GOO has higher early clinical success (shorter time to oral intake and length of stay) but increased symptom recurrence and need for further intervention.[62] These results were reaffirmed in meta-analyses that also included non-RCT trials and compared gastrojejunostomy with endoscopic stents for all types of malignant gastric outlet obstruction.[73,74] To summarize, patients with anticipated long-term survival should be considered for surgical gastric bypass at the time of surgery because of the relatively low risk of the procedure and more durable results.

Other Palliative Interventions

An emerging alternative for palliation of gastric outlet obstruction is EUS-guided gastroenterostomy with or without placement of a lumen-apposing metal stent. This technique has shown comparable results to enteric stenting, with the advantage of fewer reinterventions.[75,76] EUS-guided gastroenterostomy has not been shown to offer superior outcomes compared with surgical gastrojejunostomy in early small cohort studies, despite the rapid recovery (patients can eat the following day).[77] High-quality evidence is needed to further evaluate the efficacy and safety of this novel technique, which is currently available in specialized centers. PEG, with or without jejunostomy, is also a possible treatment modality, especially for patients who are not surgical candidates for venting (and feeding) purposes.

TUMOR-RELATED PAIN

Abdominal pain in the tumor site is a disturbing and potentially incapacitating symptom in pancreatic and periampullary cancers. It is reported in about 60% to 80% of patients at presentation and becomes a feature in almost all patients with advanced disease (see Chapters 61 and 62).[78] The classic clinical presentation is central epigastric pain radiating to the back. It is often most noticeable during sleep at night when patients are supine. Pain is believed to stem from neural invasion of infiltrating tumor and stimulation of visceral afferent neural fibers traveling from the celiac plexus through the splanchnic.[79] In pancreatic cancer, abdominal pain is often a sign of advanced disease. In early-stage disease, there is decreased facilitation of pain development in various pathways, including via noxious stimulation that gradually suppresses transmission of nociceptive information from the pancreas to the central nervous system (CNS).[80] Constant severe pain has a detrimental effect on quality of life; thus alleviating pain is a key component of care. Initial pain management with pharmacologic medication is often inadequate. Furthermore, the side effects of systemic analgesics (i.e., narcotics) are also a troublesome to patients in the current era of heightened awareness against narcotic use.

Invasive procedures for severe tumor-related pain include celiac axis blockade and thoracoscopic splanchnicectomy. These may be considered to control, delay, or prevent pain when oral or transdermal pain medication fail. Of the two,

celiac axis blockade is used more frequently, whereas splanchnicectomy is usually indicated for chronic pancreatitis and should be considered if celiac axis blockade fails. Celiac axis blockade prevents painful stimuli from reaching the CNS. It can be achieved surgically or via endoscopic or percutaneous techniques.[81] The latter are limited by access to the celiac plexus and often poor visualization. Furthermore, nonsurgical interventions are highly operator dependent and should be considered only in centers that are experienced in such techniques. To achieve neurolysis, 20 milliliters of 50% alcohol injections are used, aiming at the plexus or ganglia propria, which are located behind the hepatic and splenic arteries. Chemical splanchnicectomy, aiming for the splanchnic nerves, can be achieved by injecting on each side of the aorta at the level of the celiac trunk.

Level 1 evidence supporting surgical chemical splanchnicectomy dates back to the late 1980s, from a prospective double-blind RCT conducted at Johns Hopkins Hospital.[82] Patients with unresectable pancreatic cancer were either injected with alcohol ($n = 65$) or received a sham injection ($n = 72$) during surgical exploration. The trial demonstrated significant differences in pain between the groups. Compared with placebo, alcohol injections significantly reduced the mean pain score at 2, 4, and 6 months. In a subgroup analysis of patients without preexisting pain, alcohol injection resulted in a longer pain-free interval (mean number of months without significant pain of 7.2 months vs. 3 months). No differences were observed in hospital stay or procedure-related complications. The results of this trial suggested that prophylactic surgical splanchnicectomy or celiac plexus block was advantageous in delaying pain with minimal side effects and should be routinely employed.

Neurolytic celiac plexus block has also been reported via laparoscopy. In a 2010 prospective study at Memorial Sloan Kettering Cancer Center, celiac plexus block was performed in 20 patients with elevated pain scores scheduled for staging laparoscopy.[83] Injection was made possible with a 23-gauge needle passed through the abdominal wall under direct visualization. The injections were made into the fat pad on both sides of the celiac vasculature, at the base of the left gastric artery. Median total operative time was 57 minutes (range 29–92 minutes) and all patients except for one were discharged on the day of surgery. No major complications were reported. The mean score for worst pain at 24 hours and 1 month after the procedure decreased in the study population. However, pain was not fully controlled and the use of narcotic pain medication was similar before operation and 1 month after.

An alternative invasive procedure to palliate pain is unilateral or bilateral thoracoscopic splanchnicectomy. There is variability in the techniques for trocar placement to achieve optimal pleural visualization. The greater splanchnic nerve should be identified inferior and medial to the sympathetic trunk. After pleural incision, all roots of the greater and lesser splanchnic nerves are transected.[84] There are few reports focused on thoracoscopic splanchnicectomy for pancreatic cancer-related pain. Although some report a significant decrease in pain and use of narcotics after the procedure,[84,85] there is also a risk for operative complications, including pneumothorax.

High-quality evidence comparing different techniques for pain control are lacking. A small randomized study ($n = 65$) in the UK, comparing opioid analgesia, celiac plexus block, and thoracoscopic splanchnicectomy did not find any differences between the groups in pain scores or opioid consumption.[86]

PALLIATIVE PANCREATECTOMY

Palliative pancreatectomy includes resection of less than all gross disease (R2 resection). There is no high-quality evidence to justify planned palliative pancreatectomy. Thus it is not recommended in the setting of locally advanced disease or metastatic spread. Studies on tumor debulking versus palliative bypass in patients with pancreatic cancer without metastasis showed that palliative resection had higher morbidity and mortality, with marginal improvement in survival (Table 67.4). In a 2012 meta-analysis of four cohort studies comparing 138 patients who underwent R2 resections with 261 who underwent surgical bypass procedures, the pooled median survival was 8.2 months compared with 6.7, respectively. The pooled risk ratio for surgical morbidity and mortality were 1.75 (95% CI 1.35–2.26) and 2.98 (95% CI: 1.31–6.75) for the R2 group compared with bypass alone.[87] Furthermore, quality of life scores in patients who underwent palliative pancreatectomy have been reported to be lower compared with bypass.[88]

Recently, the role of pancreatectomy in the setting of (treated) metastatic disease has been revisited by many, given the substantial improvements in efficacy of systemic therapies. With anecdotal data on palliative pancreatectomy for patients with low volume disease that is stable with modern systemic therapy,[89,90] early reports suggest that palliative pancreatectomy may be beneficial in highly selected patients with exceptionally favorable tumor biology. Currently the evidence to justify such intervention is largely limited to case series at most, and it remains questionable whether the additive morbidity of complex pancreatic surgery justifies possible improvement in survival, which remains to be definitively established.

LOCAL ABLATIVE THERAPY

There are experimental data on treatment of locally advanced unresectable pancreatic cancer with local ablation. Approaches include needle ablation or noninvasive ablation. Ablation can be performed using alcohol, cryoablation, radiofrequency ablation, irreversible electroporation, high-intensity focused ultrasound, microwave ablation, and intraoperative radiation therapy (IORT).[94] Surgical use of these modalities is not considered standard of care. However, some reports have shown association with survival in small-scale studies. These modalities may be recommended in specialized centers if locally advanced unresectable disease is encountered intraoperatively (see Chapter 66).

At Massachusetts General Hospital, IORT has been successfully used to treat locally advanced pancreas cancer, showing promising results in its ability to arrest tumor progression.[95,96] In a recent retrospective analysis of 46 patients with locally advanced unresectable disease, IORT alone after FOLFIRINOX-based neoadjuvant therapy was associated with a median survival of 23 months and with reports of long-term survival (72 and 93 months) in a few patients. In this cohort, mean radiation dose given was 15 Gy (± 1.6 Gy) through a median cone size of 5 cm (range 2–8 cm). Postoperative morbidity from the radiation per se is limited. Interestingly, IORT has also been shown to improve local control for patients who undergo curative-intent resection with close/positive margin accentuation with intraoperative radiation (see Chapter 66).[97]

END-OF-LIFE CARE

Physicians involved in the management of patients with pancreatic and periampullary cancer should have adequate training in end-of-life care. Beyond procedural interventions, other palliative care process measures should be discussed among surgeons, patients, and their families. These include goals-of-care discussions, code status clarification, specialist palliative-care referral, and hospice assessment. Data from two large tertiary care centers in the US demonstrated that patients with advanced pancreatic cancer treated by surgeons were less likely to have these processes performed.[98] Only 25% of patients hospitalized for palliative procedures had all four performed, but 68% had at least one. Performance of these processes was associated with subsequent reduced use of healthcare (fewer emergency department visits and hospital and intensive care unit [ICU] readmissions), even after adjusting for differences in survival. There is growing evidence on the significant benefits of these basic processes of care, such as conversations about goals, including improved quality of life for patients and better closure for bereaved family members[99] (see Chapter 29).

Medical orders for life-sustaining treatment (i.e., code status clarification) include do not resuscitate (DNR), do not intubate (DNI), and, ideally, do not operate (DNO).[100] Clarifying the patient's wishes for invasive interventions at the end of life can reduce suffering from nonbeneficial procedures because palliative surgery is associated with significant 30-day perioperative morbidity, longer hospitalizations, and high rates of recurrent or additional symptoms.[101] Identifying patients for whom surgical intervention is not desired can be optimally achieved via patient-centered discussions. An important component of palliative care communication is discussing overall goals and values in the context of meaningful outcomes. As such, there is a need to explore the patient goals and values to outline principles of care: prioritizing time at home with family, ability to eat and drink, alleviation of pain, prolonging longevity as much as possible, and dying peacefully. Patients' wishes may be dynamic and require iterative exploration by physicians. Recommended questions that help decipher patients' goals include: *What are you most worried about?; What are you hoping for?; What is most important to you?* and *What makes your life meaningful?*[102] Decisions on palliative interventions in pancreatic cancer can be challenging to patients and families because risk and exact prognosis are uncertain. A possible strategy to promote shared decision making and clarify outcomes is the best case/worst case framework.[103] This includes presenting a range of plausible

---

TABLE 67.4 Outcomes of Nonradical Resection (R2) versus Bypass Procedure in Patients With Nonmetastatic Unresectable Pancreas Cancer

	KONINGER ET AL., 2008[91]		BOCKHORN ET AL., 2009[92]		TOL ET AL., 2015[93]	
	R2	BYPASS	R2	BYPASS	R2	BYPASS
No. patients	38	45	40	39	11	203
Morbidity (%)	47	22	43	18	73	34
Mortality (%)	8	2	5	5	0	2
Survival (weeks)	10.7	10.7	11.5	7.5	8.5	9

No., number.

scenarios within the boundaries of a best and worst outcome, so that patients maintain hope for the best and prepare for the worst. As opposed to focusing on enumerating the chances for risks and benefits, use language of informed consent.

SUMMARY

Most patients with pancreatic and periampullary cancer will eventually arrive at a common endpoint where palliative care is at the forefront of decision making. The role for surgical palliative care has evolved over the past several decades, with advances in other invasive and noninvasive techniques. However, surgical intervention is still an important tool when managing uncurable pancreatic cancer. Compared with other treatment modalities, surgery is usually the most durable intervention and may confer the greatest benefit; however, it is also associated with greater risk. Given the progressive improvement in life expectancy for patients with advanced pancreas cancer, the benefit of durable relief of symptoms via surgery may be enhanced. This is especially true in locally advanced disease given the better prognosis

and tendency for biliary and/or enteric obstruction. For biliary obstruction, in patients with symptomatic jaundice that undergo exploration and are found to have unresectable disease, palliative surgical biliary bypass in the form of a Roux-en-Y hepaticojejunostomy should be considered. In most other cases, biliary decompression can be achieved via endoscopic stenting using self-expandable metallic stents. For gastric outlet obstruction, loop gastrojejunostomy (open or minimally invasive) is indicated at time of exploration for most patients with unresectable disease, with or without symptoms of gastric outlet obstructions. Endoscopically placed duodenal stents are less reliable and often require reinterventions. For tumor-related pain, prophylactic celiac axis blockade has shown to control, delay, and even prevent severe pain and should be considered at times of exploration because it is associated with minimal risk or morbidity. Holistic palliative care should incorporate noninvasive processes, including code clarifications, goals-of-care discussions, and hospice assessment. Surgeons should be acquainted with communication strategies to facilitate shared goal-centered decision making for patients with terminal disease.